Contents

Order of Assigned Readings

Wk. ch. Lecture   Seminar/lab   Clinical

1/22 ch 28 breast feeding

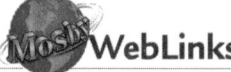
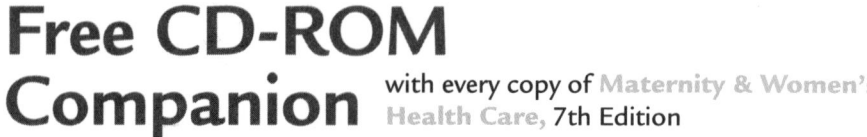
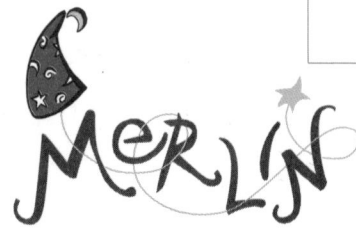

Maternity & Women's Health Care

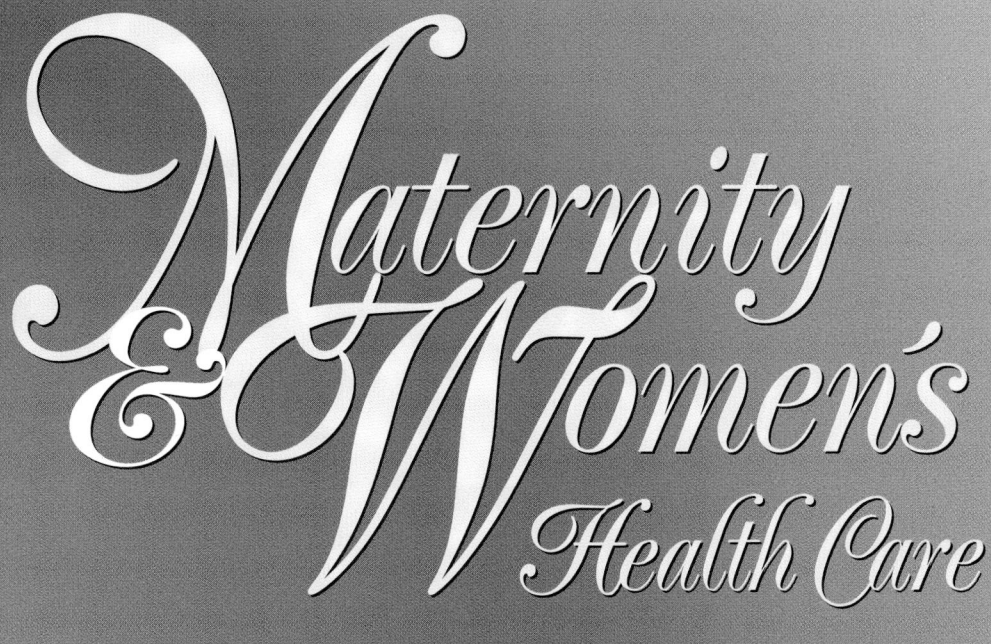

Maternity & Women's Health Care

SEVENTH EDITION

DEITRA LEONARD LOWDERMILK, RNC, PHD, FAAN

Clinical Professor, School of Nursing
University of North Carolina at Chapel Hill
Chapel Hill, North Carolina

SHANNON E. PERRY, RN, CNS, PHD, FAAN

Professor, School of Nursing
San Francisco State University
San Francisco, California

IRENE M. BOBAK, RN, PHD, FAAN

Professor Emerita
San Francisco State University
San Francisco, California

www.mosby.com

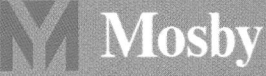 **Mosby**

A Harcourt Health Sciences Company

St. Louis   London   Philadelphia   Sydney   Toronto

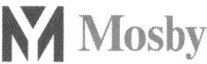

A Harcourt Health Sciences Company

Vice President, Nursing Editorial Director: Sally Schrefer
Senior Editor: Michael S. Ledbetter
Senior Developmental Editor: Laurie K. Muench
Project Manager: Catherine Jackson
Designer: Amy Buxton

SEVENTH EDITION

Mosby, Inc.
A Harcourt Health Sciences Company
11830 Westline Industrial Drive
St. Louis, Missouri 63146

Printed in the United States of America

ISBN: 0-323-00961-1

00 01 02 03 04 / GW/KPT 9 8 7 6 5 4 3 2 1

Contributors

KATHRYN RHODES ALDEN, MSN, RN, IBCLC
Clinical Assistant Professor, School of Nursing
University of North Carolina at Chapel Hill
Chapel Hill, North Carolina;
Lactation Consultant, Rex Healthcare
Raleigh, North Carolina

KARI ANDERSON, RN, MSN, EdD
Assistant Professor, School of Nursing
University of North Carolina at Wilmington
Wilmington, North Carolina

DEBBIE FRASER ASKIN, MN, RNC
Assistant Professor, Faculty of Nursing
University of Manitoba
Winnipeg, Manitoba, Canada

JEAN A. BACHMAN, DSN
MSN Program Director and Associate Professor
Barnes College of Nursing
University of Missouri
St. Louis, Missouri

KITTY CASHION, RN, C, MSN
Clinical Nurse Specialist
University of Tennessee College of Medicine
Department of Obstetrics & Gynecology
Division of Maternal–Fetal Medicine
Memphis, Tennessee

JANE G. CONNER, MSN, WHCNP, RNC
Assistant Professor, Department of Nursing
California State University
Los Angeles, California

GAYLE TART DAVIS, BSN, MSN, EdD, CPNP
Associate Professor, School of Nursing
University of North Carolina at Chapel Hill
Chapel Hill, North Carolina

LIENNE D. EDWARDS, RN, PhD
Assistant Professor and Director, Office
  of Continuing Education
College of Nursing and Health Professions, University
  of North Carolina at Charlotte
Charlotte, North Carolina

ANNE H. FISHEL, PHD, RN, CS
Professor, School of Nursing
University of North Carolina at Chapel Hill
Chapel Hill, North Carolina

CATHERINE INGRAM FOGEL, RNC (WHNP), PHD, FAAN
Professor, School of Nursing
University of North Carolina at Chapel Hill
Chapel Hill, North Carolina

MARGARET COMERFORD FREDA, RN, EdD, CHES, FAAN
Associate Professor, Obstetrics & Gynecology
  and Women's Health
Montefiore Medical Center
Albert Einstein College of Medicine
Bronx, New York

CYNTHIA GARRETT, RNC, BSN, MSN
Women's Health Clinical Nurse Specialist
University of North Carolina Hospitals
Chapel Hill, North Carolina

S. KIM GENOVESE, RNC, MSN, CARN, MSA
Associate Professor of Nursing
Purdue University
Westville, Indiana

BETTE B. HAMMOND, RN, BSN, MSN
Assistant Professor Emerita
St. Charles County Community College
St. Peters, Missouri

BETTY G. HARRIS, RN, PHD
Dean, Health Sciences Division
Wake Technical Community College
Raleigh, North Carolina

MILDRED G. HARVEY, BSN, MSN, RNC
Obstetrical Clinical Nurse Specialist
Obstetrical Nursing Consultant
Lakeland, Tennessee

SHARON E. LOCK, PhD, RN, FNP
Assistant Professor, College of Nursing
University of Kentucky
Lexington, Kentucky

JANE McATEER, RN, BSN, MN
Professor of Nursing
San Mateo Community College District
San Mateo, California

ESTHER MEGERMAN, MA, PhD
Psychologist
Kansas City, Missouri

MARGARET SHANDOR MILES, RN, MSN, PhD, FAAN
Professor, School of Nursing
University of North Carolina at Chapel Hill
Chapel Hill, North Carolina

MARY COURTNEY MOORE, RN, RD, PhD
Research Assistant Professor
Vanderbilt University
Nashville, Tennessee

AMY A. NICHOLS, RN, PCNS, EdD
Associate Professor, School of Nursing
San Francisco State University
San Francisco, California

KAREN PIOTROWSKI, RNC, MSN
Assistant Professor of Nursing
D'Youville College
Buffalo, New York

JUDITH H. POOLE, PhD, RNC, FACCE
Perinatal Outreach Education Coordinator
Carolinas Medical Center
Charlotte, North Carolina

BARBARA C. RYNERSON, RN, MS, CS
Associate Professor Emerita, School of Nursing
University of North Carolina at Chapel Hill
Chapel Hill, North Carolina

REBECCA BURDETTE SAUNDERS, RNC, PhD
Associate Professor, School of Nursing
University of North Carolina at Greensboro
Greensboro, North Carolina

BARBARA PETERSON SINCLAIR, MN, RNC, OGNP, FAAN
Interim Dean, School of Health
California State University, Dominguez Hills
Carson, California

LINDA H. SNELL, DNS
Associate Professor of Nursing
D'Youville College
Buffalo, New York

SUSAN M. TUCKER, MSN, RN, PHN, CNAA
Healthcare Consultant
Quality Management and Perinatal Systems
Roseville, California

WENDY WETZEL, RN, MSN, FNP, HNC
Nurse Practitioner
A Woman's Place
Flagstaff, Arizona

RHEA P. WILLIAMS, RN, MN, PHD
Professor, Department of Nursing
California State University at Los Angeles
Los Angeles, California

JAN LAMARCHE ZDANUK, RNC, MSN, CNS, CFNP
Certified Family Nurse Practitioner
Private Practice
Bedford, Texas

Consultants

VICKIE CARTER, ASN, BSN, MSN, FNP
BSN Faculty
University of Indianapolis School of Nursing
Indianapolis, Indiana

BUNNY FORGIONE, RN, MSN, CNS
Assistant Professor of Nursing
Texas A&M University
Corpus Christi, Texas

KATHY GOODWIN, RN, BSN, MSN, CNM
SDBD
St. Louis, Missouri

IRENE GONZALES, RN, PhD, CNNP, CLNC
Assistant Professor of Pediatrics
San Francisco State University
San Francisco, California

JUDITH JOHNSON HILTON, BSN, MSN, RNC
Assistant Professor of Nursing
Lenoir-Rhyne College
Hickory, North Carolina

JUDITH M. KACHEL, RN, EdD
Nurse Educator
Joliet Junior College
Joliet, Illinois

JANE KIRKPATRICK, BSN, MSN
Associate Professor
Purdue University
West Lafayette, Indiana

MAUREEN LANGE, RNC, CNOR, MS
Professor
Elgin Community College
Elgin, Illinois

MARTHA LEBRON, RN
Clinical Nurse II
UNC Women's Hospital
Chapel Hill, North Carolina

EDWARD L. LOWDERMILK, BS, RPH
Lowdermilk Associates
Chapel Hill, North Carolina

MARTHA SLEUTEL, BSN, ADN, MSN
Assistant Professor
Angelo State University
San Angelo, Texas

CHERYL SMITH, RNC, MSN
DeKalb County Board of Health
Decatur, Georgia

SUE G. THACKER, RNC, AS, BSN, MS, PhD
Professor
Wytheville Community College
Wytheville, Virginia

ANN TUMBLIN, BA, LCCE, FACCE, CD (DONA)
Perinatal Educator
Wake Medical Center
Raleigh, North Carolina

Preface

Women's health care is more than reproductive health care even though reproductive health concerns and problems are a primary focus. Women's health care encompasses the unique physical, psychologic, and social needs of women throughout their life span. The specialty of maternity and women's health nursing offers both challenges and opportunities. Nurses are challenged to assimilate knowledge and to develop technical and critical thinking skills needed to apply that knowledge to practice. Each woman, with her individual needs that must be identified and met, presents a new challenge. However, the opportunities are sufficiently extraordinary to make this one of the most fulfilling specialties of nursing practice.

The goal of nursing education is to prepare today's students to meet the challenges of tomorrow. This preparation must extend beyond mastery of facts and skills. Nurses must be able to combine competence with caring and critical thinking. They must address both the physiologic and psychosocial needs of their clients. They must look beyond the condition and see the woman as an individual with distinctive needs. Above all, they must strive to improve nursing practice on the basis of sound research information. In a time of shrinking financial and personnel resources for health care, nurses can use evidence-based practice to produce measurable outcomes that can validate their unique role in the health care delivery system.

Maternity & Women's Health Care was developed to provide students with the knowledge and skills they need to become competent, think critically, and attain the necessary sensitivity to become caring nurses. This seventh edition would not have been possible if the sixth edition had not been so successful. *Maternity & Women's Health Care* is one of the leading maternity nursing texts, and we are proud of the continued support this text has received.

This seventh edition has been revised and refined in response to comments and suggestions from educators, clinicians, and students. It includes the most accurate, current, and clinically relevant information available. Many exciting changes will be noted throughout the book; they demonstrate the different dimensions of women's health care. However, we have retained the underlying philosophy that has been the strength of previous editions: our belief that pregnancy and childbirth and developmental changes in a woman's life are natural processes. We have also retained a strong integrated focus on the family and research-based practice.

APPROACH

Professional nursing practice continues to evolve and adapt to society's changing health priorities. The ever-changing health care delivery system offers new opportunities for nurses to alter the practice of maternity and women's health nursing and to improve the way care is given. Consumers of maternity and women's health care vary in age, ethnicity, culture, language, social status, marital status, and sexual preference. They seek care with obstetricians, gynecologists, family practice physicians, nurse-midwives, nurse-practitioners, and other health care providers in a variety of health care settings, including the home. Increasingly, many are self-treating, using a variety of alternative and complementary therapies.

Nursing education must reflect these changes. Clinical education must be planned to offer students a variety of maternity and women's health care experiences in settings that include hospitals and birth centers, home health, clinics and private physician offices, shelters for the homeless or women in need of protection, prisons, and other community-based settings. The changing needs of nursing students also must be addressed. Today's nursing students are challenged to learn more than ever before and often in less time than their predecessors. Students are diverse. They may be new high school graduates, college students, or older adults with families. They may be male or female. They may have college degrees in other fields and be interested in changing careers. They may represent various cultures; English may not be their primary language.

As we move into the twenty-first century, this seventh edition of *Maternity & Women's Health Care* is designed to meet the needs of women during their reproductive years and beyond, as well as the needs of students in all types of nursing programs. This edition presents tighter, more focused content in a clearly written and easily read manner while retaining the comprehensiveness of previous editions.

To ensure a logical and consistent presentation of material, *Care Management* has been used as an organizing framework for discussion in the nursing care chapters. This approach incorporates the nursing process and collaborative care strategies to demonstrate how nursing care is combined with care from other health care providers to give the most comprehensive care to women and newborns. Assessments, nursing diagnoses, expected outcomes, nursing and collaborative interventions, and evaluations of care are highlighted throughout the chapters for emphasis. Nursing plans of care reinforce the problem-solving approach to client care. In chapters that focus on complications of childbearing and reproductive conditions, medical care is often the priority for client care. Therefore, in these discussions, the specific condition and medical therapy are discussed first, followed by the nursing care management.

Health care today emphasizes *wellness*. This focus is an integral part of our philosophy. Likewise, the developmental changes a woman experiences throughout her life are considered natural and normal. In women's health care, the goal is promotion of wellness for the woman through knowledge of her body and its normal functioning throughout her life span, while developing an awareness of conditions that require professional intervention. The unit on women's health care has been expanded to emphasize the wellness aspect of care. This unit has been placed before the units on pregnancy because many of the aspects of assessment and care can be applied to later chapters. Pregnancy and childbirth are also part of a natural developmental process. We believe that students need to thoroughly understand and recognize the normal processes before they can identify complications and comprehend their implications for care. Therefore we present the entire normal childbearing cycle before discussing potential complications.

Teaching for self-care is an essential component of nursing care of women and newborns. In recognition of integrative health care models that provide both traditional and nontraditional health care and in seeking to provide options for women that encourage them to take more responsibility for their health, we have added a **NEW** chapter on Alternative and Complementary Therapies. The chapter on women's health promotion and screening emphasizes teaching for self-care to promote wellness and to encourage preventive care. A **NEW** chapter on Transition to Parenthood focuses on caring for new mothers and infants at home. Special boxed features highlight teaching guidelines, client self-care, and home care throughout the text. To implement *preventive care*, perinatal and women's health nurses must be able to recognize signs and symptoms of emergent problems. Throughout the discussion of assessment and care, we alert the nurse to signs of potential problems and provide boxed information highlighting warning signs and emergency situations.

Today's perinatal and women's health nurses will encounter women from diverse backgrounds. The family chapter includes a discussion of cultural implications and focuses on specific customs related to childbearing and women's health. This chapter also stresses the importance of assessing both the nurse's and the client's cultural beliefs. Cultural implications are integrated throughout the text to emphasize the wide range of ethnic diversity and its effects on maternity and women's health. **NEW** English-Spanish Guidelines/Guías boxes have been added to provide students with common terms to make assessments and provide teaching. Boxes throughout the text highlight cultural aspects of care. A **NEW** chapter on Community and Home Care has been added to prepare the student to provide maternity and women's health care in a variety of settings. Community aspects of care are also integrated throughout nursing care chapters to emphasize that care can take place wherever the woman and her family may be.

To truly meet the specific needs of each woman, the nurse must include family members and significant others in the plan of care. *Family dynamics* are rarely more prominent than in pregnancy and childbirth. The nurse is often the family's primary advocate. A separate chapter on the family as well as integrated family considerations throughout the chapters on pregnancy, labor and birth, postpartum, and newborn care demonstrate the importance of the entire family. Issues concerning grandparents, siblings, and different family constellations are also addressed.

Nursing research is an integral part of nursing education and practice. Nursing research has been incorporated throughout the text to demonstrate the effect of research utilization on the practice of maternity and women's health nursing. Conclusions from research studies on care practices are described and highlighted. Students and practicing nurses will be challenged to think critically and improve nursing practice by questioning traditional nursing practices that have no scientific basis. In addition, boxed research highlights describe selected studies and discuss clinical implications.

Maternity and women's health nurses confront ethical and legal challenges daily. Nurses need to develop a reflective stance that assesses new reproductive and women's health technologies and policies in light of their potential to influence human well-being. Although we have chosen not to include separate chapters on legal or ethical issues, highlighted information on ethical considerations and legal tips throughout the text emphasize these issues as they relate to maternal and women's health nursing.

FEATURES

The seventh edition features a contemporary design and spacious presentation. Students will find that the logical, easy-to-follow headings and attractive full-color design highlight important content and increase visual appeal. More than 600 color photographs and drawings throughout the text illustrate important concepts and techniques to further enhance comprehension. Each chapter begins with a list of *Key Terms* that alerts students to new vocabulary; these terms are then boldfaced and defined within the chapter. *Learning Objectives* focus students' attention on the important content to be mastered.

The organizing framework, *Care Management,* is used consistently to discuss collaborative care and specifically nursing care. The five steps of the *Nursing Process* are incorporated into this framework. *Plans of Care* are included to help students apply the nursing process in the clinical setting. The Plans of Care use only NANDA-approved nursing diagnoses, describe expected outcomes for client care, provide rationales for interventions, and include evaluation of care. *Care Paths, Protocols,* and *Procedures* for care are included to provide students with examples of various approaches to implementation of care.

Special boxed features are highlighted and visually identifiable. *Teaching Guidelines* supplement the narrative and emphasize the information needed by the nurse in teaching the client. **NEW** for the seventh edition are English-Spanish *Guidelines/Guías* boxes that provide common English-to-Spanish phrases for client assessments and teaching. *Client Self-Care* boxes and *Home Care* boxes emphasize guidelines for the client to practice self-care and provide information to help students transfer learning from the hospital to the home setting. *Emergency* boxes alert the students to the signs and symptoms of various emergency situations and provide interventions for immediate implementation. **NEW** *Nurse-Alerts* highlight critical information for the student. *Research* boxes include a brief summary of the study and a discussion of application to practice. Also **NEW,** research findings summarized in the Cochrane Pregnancy and Childbirth Database that confirm effective practices or identify practices that have unknown, ineffective, or harmful effects are integrated throughout the text and identified by the ▮▮ icon in the margin.

Although childbearing is a normal process, complications may occur. When making assessments, the nurse must be alert for *Signs of Potential Complications;* therefore we have included these signs in chapters that cover uncomplicated pregnancy and childbirth. Other features include *Cultural Considerations* boxes, which describe beliefs and practices about pregnancy, childbirth, parenting, and women's health concerns. *Legal Tips* and *Ethical Considerations* are integrated throughout to provide students with relevant information to deal with these important areas in the context of maternity and women's health nursing. **NEW** *Medication Guide* boxes include key information about medications used in maternity and women's health care, including their indications, adverse effects, and nursing considerations. Alternative and complementary therapies are discussed for many women's health and pregnancy-related problems.

At the end of each chapter, *Key Points* summarize important content. *Critical Thinking Exercises* guide the students in applying their knowledge and in increasing their ability to think critically about maternity and women's health care issues. References have been updated significantly, with most citations being less than 5 years old and all chapters having citations within 1 year of publication.

ORGANIZATION

The seventh edition of *Maternity & Women's Heath Care* comprises eight units organized to enhance understanding and learning and to facilitate easy retrieval of information.

Unit One, *Introduction to Maternity and Women's Health Nursing,* begins with an overview of contemporary issues in maternity and women's health nursing practice. It then addresses the family as a unit of care, incorporating cultural aspects of care. The unit concludes with two **NEW** chapters. One is on Community and Home Care that provides understanding of these practice settings in relation to maternity and women's health nursing. The other describes Alternative and Complementary Therapies, providing an overview of the important therapies that can be used instead of or in addition to traditional techniques used in maternity and women's health care.

Unit Two, *Reproductive Years,* is a revised and expanded unit on women's health that has been moved earlier in the book. Nine chapters discuss health promotion, screening, and physical assessment, and then present common reproductive concerns. The chapter on Health Assessment is **NEW** and incorporates normal anatomy and physiology of the female reproductive system. There are separate chapters on menstrual problems, sexually transmitted infections and other infections **(NEW),** contraception and abortion, infertility, violence, problems of the breast, and structural disorders and neoplasms of the female reproductive system.

Unit Three, *Pregnancy,* describes nursing care of the woman and her family from conception through preparation for childbirth. Nursing care during pregnancy has been streamlined into one chapter that now includes both physiologic and psychologic aspects of care. A separate chapter on maternal and fetal nutrition emphasizes the important aspects of care, highlights cultural variations on diet, and stresses the importance of early recognition and management of nutritional problems. The preparation for childbirth chapter has been updated and revised to include information on incorporating doula care during pregnancy and labor and birth.

Unit Four, *Childbirth,* focuses on collaborative care among physicians, nurse-midwives, nurses, and women and their families during the processes of labor and birth. Separate chapters deal with the nurse's role in management of discomfort during labor and childbirth and fetal monitoring. These chapters familiarize students with current childbirth practices and focus on interventions to support and educate the woman and her family.

Unit Five, *Postpartum,* deals with a time of significant change for the entire family. The mother requires both physical and emotional support as she adjusts to her new role. A **NEW** chapter on Transition to Parenthood discusses family dynamics in response to the birth of a child and describes ways nurses can facilitate parent-infant adjustment, including anticipatory guidance for the first few days at home and home follow-up care.

Unit Six, *The Newborn,* has been extensively revised and addresses physiologic adaptations of the newborn and assessment and care of the newborn. Information on the nutritional needs of the newborn and nursing care associated with breastfeeding and formula feeding are highlighted in a separate chapter.

Unit Seven, *Complications of Childbearing,* discusses the conditions that place the woman, fetus, infant, and family at risk. This unit has been extensively reorganized and includes a chapter on high risk assessment of pregnancy complications and three **NEW** chapters—Antepartal Hemorrhagic Disorders, Preterm Labor and Birth, and Postpartum Complications. Chapters on hypertensive disorders, endocrine and metabolic problems, medical-surgical problems, obstetric critical care, mental health problems and substance abuse, and labor and birth complications have been updated. Care management focuses on achieving the best possible outcomes, as well as supporting the woman and family when expectations are not met.

Unit Eight, *Newborn Complications,* addresses the most common acquired conditions of the neonate and hematologic disorders and congenital anomalies. It then describes the nursing care for high risk newborns, emphasizing the care of the preterm infant. All chapters have been greatly revised and updated. This unit addresses the continuing trend of providing care to moderately compromised newborns in the newborn nursery. A separate chapter on loss and grief discusses care management of the family experiencing a fetal, neonatal, or maternal loss.

The text concludes with appendixes that provide valuable resource information, including websites; a glossary of important terms; and a detailed, cross-referenced index.

TEACHING AND LEARNING PACKAGE

A number of ancillaries to this text have been developed to assist instructors and students in the teaching and learning process. For the instructor, these include an *Instructor's Resource Manual and Test Bank,* a **NEW** CD-ROM version of the test bank, and a **NEW** CD-ROM product, *Mosby's Electronic Image Collection.* For the student, the seventh edition includes a *Study Guide* and a **NEW** interactive CD-ROM product, *Mosby's Maternity & Women's Health Care CD-ROM.* Also **NEW** for the instructor and student is *Mosby's Electronic Resource Links and Information Network (MERLIN).*

The Instructor's Resource Manual and Test Bank is keyed chapter by chapter to the text to help coordinate course objectives to chapter content. Each chapter includes an outline of content with course guidelines, suggested learning activities, and a summary of key concepts. A sample syllabus that includes a proposed class schedule and reading assignments for 6- to 7-week courses as well as 14- to 16-week courses is provided. This provides educators with suggestions for using the text in the most essential manner or in a more comprehensive way. New editions to the manual are the case study presentations and additional critical thinking activities (many with community-based applications) that can be used by educators to foster critical thinking skills. The Test Bank includes approximately 900 questions that parallel the NCLEX format. The answer key provides page references and coding of questions according to the NCLEX test plan categories of nursing process and client needs. The Test Bank is also available in a **NEW** CD-ROM version with the optional use on either Windows or Mac formats.

NEW to the seventh edition is *Mosby's Electronic Image Collection CD-ROM.* This valuable tool for instructors provides easy access to electronic images from the main textbook. Each image can be imported to a slide presentation (e.g., Power Point) to enhance lecture materials.

A separate *Study Guide* includes *Chapter Review Activities* and *Critical Thinking Exercises* to reinforce learning and evaluate comprehension. The *Study Guide* can be used for homework assignments or for remedial practice. The exercises in the guide were developed to assist students in synthesizing knowledge of maternity and women's health care and to foster critical thinking.

NEW to the seventh edition is *Mosby's Maternity & Women's Health Care CD-ROM.* This exciting, interactive program provides students with a resource to solve critical thinking case studies, review questions, and review vocabulary. The vocabulary review includes a sound card so that students can easily hear and practice the correct pronunciations.

Also **NEW** for both the instructor and student is *Mosby's Electronic Resource Links and Information Network* (MERLIN). This exciting new resource is provided through Mosby's website at www.mosby.com/MERLIN/Lowdermilk/MatWmnHlth and allows access to information and resources based on topics covered in *Maternity & Women's Health Care,* seventh edition.

Acknowledgments

Maternity & Women's Health Care would not have been possible without the contributions of many people. First, we want to thank the many nurse educators, clinicians, and nursing students in the United States, Canada, Australia, and Taiwan whose comments and suggestions about the manuscript led to this collaborative effort by an outstanding group of contributors. A special thanks goes to these contributors, many of whom are new to this edition, whose names are listed in the Contributor list. Their expertise and knowledge of current clinical practice and research have added to the relevancy and accuracy of the materials presented. Karen Piotrowski deserves special recognition for her extra efforts. We acknowledge the contributions to the chapter on Alternative and Complementary Therapies from The American Holistic Nurses' Association, and Phillip Fenske, LAc. We thank Lisa B. Fikac for her contributions to the chapter on Nursing Care of the High Risk Newborn. We also thank Kari Anderson for contributing to the Research boxes, Jane McAteer for developing Plans of Care, Martha Lebron for assisting with Spanish translations, and Ed Lowdermilk for his assistance with Medication Guides.

We are also appreciative of the critiques given by the reviewers, especially their attention to validating the accuracy of content and their challenge to present content differently and to include new ideas. These combined efforts have resulted in a revision that incorporates the most recent research and current information about the practice of maternity and women's health care.

We offer thanks for shared expertise and photographs to the staffs of University of North Carolina Hospitals; University of North Carolina School of Nursing; the staff of Spa Health Club of Chapel Hill, NC; Nurses Certificate program in Interactive Imagery; Jane Stansbury (SRS Medical Systems, Inc.); Phil Wilson, (Momentum, Inc.); Leonard Nihan (Sea-Band International); Gayle Kipnis, RNC, CHTP, HNC; Tina Whitehorn; Polly Perez, Cutting Edge Press; and Barbara Harper, Global Maternal/Child Health Association.

We would also like to thank the following photographers: Marjorie Pyle, RNC, Lifecircle, Costa Mesa, CA; Kim Molloy, Knoxville, IA; Jonas N. McCoy, Raleigh, NC; Michael S. Clement, MD, Mesa, AZ; Leslie Canerday, Phoenix, AZ; Ed Lowdermilk, Chapel Hill, NC; and Amy and Ken Turner, Cary, NC.

This edition also contains artwork by George Wassilchenko, Broken Arrow, OK, and Julie Perry, Phoenix, AZ. Their talent is evident in the precise detailed illustrations throughout the text.

Special words of gratitude are extended to Michael Ledbetter, our editor; Laurie Muench, our developmental editor; Catherine Jackson, our production editor; and Amy Buxton, our designer, for their encouragement, inspiration, and assistance in preparation and production of this text. These talented and hardworking people helped change our manuscript into a beautiful book by editing the manuscript, designing an attractive format for our special features, and overseeing the production of the book from start to finish. We are especially thankful to Laurie Muench who always had time to answer our questions, kept track of innumerable details, found just the right photo or resource, obtained that elusive permission, and always reassured us that we were doing a great job. We also thank Sally Schrefer, our publisher, for support and encouragement throughout the project.

Finally, we thank Irene Bobak for her continued support and encouragement as we have taken on the responsibility for this seventh edition. We hope that we have continued her tradition of excellence.

Deitra Leonard Lowdermilk
Shannon E. Perry

Contents

33 Medical-Surgical Problems in Pregnancy, 887

34 Obstetric Critical Care, 912

35 Mental Health Disorders and Substance Abuse, 940

36 Preterm Labor and Birth, 964

42 Loss and Grief, 1134

Maternity & Women's
Health Care

1

Contemporary Issues in Maternity and Women's Health Care

Shannon E. Perry

LEARNING OBJECTIVES

- Define the key terms.
- Describe the scope of maternity and women's health nursing.
- Evaluate contemporary issues and trends in maternity and women's health nursing.
- Describe sociopolitical issues affecting the care of women and infants.
- Compare selected biostatistical data among races.

- Examine social concerns in maternity and women's health care.
- Explain quality management and standards of practice in the delivery of nursing care.
- Debate ethical issues in perinatal nursing.
- Identify topics for nursing research related to maternity and women's health nursing.

KEY TERMS

Association of Women's Health, Obstetric, and Neonatal Nurses (AWHONN)
best practice
birthrate
clinical benchmarking
Cochrane Pregnancy and Childbirth Database

evidence-based practice
fertility rate
infant mortality rate
integrative health care
low-birth-weight (LBW) infants
managed care
maternal mortality rate
maternity nursing

outcomes-oriented care
preterm infants
risk management
self-care
standard of care
telemedicine
women's health nursing

Maternity nursing focuses on the care of childbearing women and their families through all stages of pregnancy and childbirth, as well as the first 4 weeks after birth. Throughout the prenatal period, nurses, nurse-practitioners, and nurse-midwives provide care for women in clinics and physician's offices and teach classes to help families prepare for childbirth. They also care for childbearing families during labor and birth in hospitals, in birthing centers, and less frequently in the home. Nurses with special training may provide intensive care for high risk neonates in special care units and for high risk mothers in antepar-

tum units, in critical care obstetric units, or at home. Maternity nurses teach about pregnancy, the process of labor, birth and recovery, and parenting skills. Investment in health promotion during childbearing can make a significant difference in the health of women and their infants and also in society.

Women's health nursing focuses on the physical, psychologic, and social needs of women throughout their lives. The term *women's health* emphasizes the overall experience of women: diseases, childbearing functions, and general physical and psychologic well-being. Women's health nurses specialize in and investigate conditions unique to women (such as reproductive malignancies and menopause) and sociocultural and occupational factors that may be related to women's health problems (such as poverty, lower wages, rape, incest, sexual harassment, and family violence).

Nurses caring for women have helped make the health care system more responsive to women's needs. The changing health care delivery system offers opportunities for nurses to alter nursing practice and improve the way care is delivered through **managed care,** integrated delivery systems (IDSs), and redefined roles (Barter et al., 1995). Nurses have been critically important in developing strategies to improve the well-being of women and their infants. Nurses have led the efforts to implement clinical practice guidelines developed through the Agency for Health Care Policy and Research (AHCPR) (Kaegi, 1995).

In the United States, serious problems related to the health and health care of mothers and infants exist. Access to prepregnancy and pregnancy-related care for all women and the lack of reproductive health services for adolescents are major concerns. Nurses can influence health policy by actively participating in the education of the public and state and federal legislators (Hastings, 1995).

Racial and ethnic diversity are increasing within North America. It is estimated that within 40 years, 50% of the population will be European-American, 22% will be African-American, 18% will be Hispanic, and 10% will be Asian-American (Gary, Sigsby, & Campbell, 1998). People who are ethnically diverse have preferences in their lifestyles, health needs, and health care. They may have dietary preferences and health practices that are not understood by caregivers. To meet the health care needs of a culturally diverse society, it is essential that the nursing workforce reflect the diversity of its clients.

This chapter presents a general overview of issues and trends related to the health and health care of women and infants.

CONTEMPORARY ISSUES AND TRENDS

Changing Health Care Delivery Structure

Changes in the health care market are influencing the way health care providers can care for their clients (Box 1-1). Health care consumed 13.6% of the gross domestic product in 1995. To control costs, managed care links providers and insurers; health maintenance organizations were the prototype for this system (Barter et al., 1995). Hospital consolidation, merger, and integration provided services throughout the continuum of care (Barter et al., 1995). The number of professional nurses in hospitals has declined, and unlicensed assistive personnel and multiskilled workers have been substituted. The role of the nurse is evolving from primary caregiver to leader of the interdisciplinary care team. Documentation of client outcomes has become essential (Barter et al., 1995). Advanced practice roles will increase as nurses assume more responsibility for client care.

BOX 1-1 Trends in the Health Care Market

1. Growth of the health care labor force
2. Economics as a driving force
3. Continued movement of health care away from acute care hospitals
4. Growth of managed care
5. Changing demographics—the aging populace
6. Changing demographics—increasing multiculturalism
7. Profound growth of information and technology
8. Nursing's lack of involvement in political change
9. Replacement of registered nurses with unlicensed assistive personnel
10. Increasing complexity

Data from Huston, C., & Fox, S. (1998). The changing health care market: Implications for nursing education in the coming decade. *Nurs Outlook* 46, 109-114.

Integrative Health Care

Integrative health care encompasses complementary and alternative therapies in combination with conventional Western modalities of treatment. Eisenberg and colleagues (1993) reported that approximately 60 million Americans used an alternative medical therapy in 1990, that the number of visits to providers of alternative medicine exceeded the number of visits to U.S. primary care physicians, and that over 70% of users of alternative therapy did not tell their physician. Eisenberg (1997) suggested that providers use a step-by-step approach with clients who seek alternative therapies:

1. Ask the client to identify the principal symptom.
2. Have the client maintain a symptom diary.
3. Discuss the client's preferences and expectations.
4. Review issues of safety and efficacy.
5. Identify a licensed provider.
6. Provide key questions for the alternative therapy provider during the initial consultation.
7. Schedule a follow-up visit (or telephone call) to review the treatment plan.
8. Follow up to review the response to treatment after a reasonable period (usually 4 to 8 weeks).
9. Provide documentation in the medical record.

Changing Childbirth Practices

Maternity care has changed dramatically. Women can choose physicians or nurse-midwives as primary care providers. In 1996 physicians attended 93% of all births and nurse-midwives attended less than 1% of all births. Approximately 1% of births occurred out of the hospital (Ventura et al., 1998); home births made up 0.6% of all births, and births in freestanding birthing centers were 0.26% of all births (Ventura et al., 1998). Women can give birth in a hospital labor room (rather than a delivery room), in a birthing room, in a freestanding birthing center, or at home (Ernst, 1994).

Certified nurse-midwives provide safe, quality care (Fischler & Harvey, 1995). Women who choose nurse-midwives as their primary providers participate actively in childbirth decisions and receive fewer interventions such as epidural analgesia for labor (Callister, 1995).

The method of analgesia and positions for labor and birth also vary, depending on the condition and choice of the mother and preferences of the providers. Mothers typically are awake and aware during labor and birth. Contrasting philosophies exist regarding analgesia during labor. Some women prefer to experience the sensations of birth with little or no analgesia; others opt for epidural analgesia to provide comfort and control over their behavior during the experience.

No longer are laboring mothers and their support people separated. With family-centered care, fathers, partners, grandparents, siblings, and friends may be present for labor and birth. Fathers or partners may be present for cesarean births. Newborns remain with the mother and may breastfeed immediately after birth. Parents participate in the care of their infants in nurseries and neonatal intensive care units.

Childbirth education and parenting classes encourage the participation of a support person; teach breathing and relaxation techniques; and give general information about birth, infant development, and parenting. Other classes or parent support groups may be organized for the weeks and months after birth.

In some cases a woman labors, gives birth, and recovers in the same room (labor-delivery-recovery). In some settings, the mother stays in the same room for the entire birth experience (labor-delivery-recovery-postpartum). Instead of having one nurse care for the baby and another nurse care for the mother, some hospitals have one nurse care for both the mother and baby (couplet or mother-baby care). In some hospitals, central nurseries have been eliminated, and babies "room-in" with their mothers. Many hospitals employ lactation consultants to assist mothers with breastfeeding.

Discharge of a mother and baby within 24 hours of birth has resulted in a growing need for follow-up or home care. In some settings, discharge may occur as early as 6 hours after birth. Legislation has been passed to ensure that mothers and babies are permitted to stay in the hospital for at least 48 hours after vaginal birth and 96 hours after cesarean birth. There is a need for focused and efficient teaching to enable the parents and infant to safely make the transition from the hospital to the home. Nurses may use follow-up telephone calls or home visits to assist families needing information and reassurance.

Neonatal security in the hospital setting is receiving increasing attention. A number of cases of "baby-napping" and sending home the wrong baby have been reported. Parents have expressed concerns for their infant's safety.

Security systems are being placed in nurseries, and nurses are being required to wear a photo identification or some other security badge.

Changing Women's Health Practices

To understand women's health, practitioners must view women holistically and in the context in which they live. Physical, mental, and social factors must be considered because these interdependent components influence women's health and illness (Breslin, 1995). Even the language used to describe women and their problems must be examined (Freda, 1995). For example, practitioners describe women who have an "incompetent cervix," who "fail to progress," and who have an "arrest" of labor or describe a fetus with intrauterine growth "retardation." They also "allow" women a "trial" of labor. Practitioners should use the phrases "women who have recurrent premature dilation of the cervix" or "fetuses whose intrauterine growth has been restricted" (Freda, 1995). There is a movement to refer to spontaneous pregnancy loss as a miscarriage instead of the more politically charged "abortion," especially when talking to clients (Freda, 1999). Practitioners must avoid punitive terms associated with confinement and prison (Peterson & Cefalo, 1990).

The social context of health care changed in the United States during the 1990s, and women's health received increasing attention. The Society for the Advancement of Women's Health Research was founded in 1991 (Wood & Ransom, 1994) to address the prevention of disease and violence toward women, women's wellness, and women's access to health care (Bass & Howes, 1992). In 1992 the Office of Research on Women's Health was authorized by Congress (Wood & Ransom, 1994). As a result of these actions, women must be included in studies, and funding was increased for studies of osteoporosis and heart disease in women.

A variety of factors and conditions affect the health of women. Race is a major factor: Caucasian females have a life expectancy at birth of 79.8 years in contrast with 74.7 years for African-American females (Guyer et al., 1998). There are 110 cases of breast cancer per 100,000 women (American Cancer Society, 1999). Early detection of breast cancer through breast self-examination and mammography can reduce the mortality rate resulting from this type of cancer. However, through lack of information or lack of insurance and access, many women never have mammograms. There is wide disparity between Caucasian women and women of other races and between older and younger women in their rates of mammography, detection and treatment of breast cancer, and survival rates (McCool, 1994).

The population has grown older; approximately 50 million women are older than age 50, the median age for menopause. Hormone replacement therapy for menopausal women has been used for many years and has benefits and risks (see Chapter 7).

Violence is a major factor affecting women. Violence includes battery, rape or other sexual assaults, and attacks

Statistics 1

with various weapons. The incidence of violence has increased, possibly because of better assessment and reporting mechanisms. The incidence of battering may increase during pregnancy; an estimated 8.3% of pregnant women are battered (Loring & Smith, 1994). Alcoholism in and substance abuse by the woman and her abuser are associated with violence and homelessness, which affect a growing number of women and children, placing them at risk for a variety of health problems.

The rates of pregnancy and abortion among adolescents have declined but are still higher in the United States than in any other industrialized country (Burnhill, 1994). Single mothers gave birth to almost one third of the babies born in the United States in 1997; among women younger than 20 years of age, 25.8% of the births were to single Caucasian mothers, 69.1% were to single African-American mothers, and 40.9% were to Hispanic women (Guyer et al., 1998).

The human immunodeficiency virus (HIV) and acquired immunodeficiency syndrome (AIDS) increasingly affect women and children. Approximately 30% of neonates of pregnant HIV-infected women will be infected with the virus before or during birth (Kass, 1994). By the year 2000, AIDS will be one of the top five causes of death in women of childbearing age (Covington & Collins, 1994). Policy makers and scientists are discussing whether HIV-infected women should be permitted to become pregnant or carry a fetus to term (Kass, 1994), and practitioners now engage in mass screening of infants and mothers (Grady, 1994).

Society has begun to address the following significant problems associated with women's health:

- New specialties within nursing and medicine are devoted to women's health.
- Encouraging progress is being made in treating breast cancer.
- Increased attention is being devoted to violence, abuse, and homelessness.
- More research dollars are being spent to study the problems of women.

Through care for women throughout their lives and research dedicated to women's problems, nurses and other women's health practitioners can significantly improve the quality of life for women and children.

Trends in Fertility and Birthrate

Fertility trends and birthrates reflect women's needs for health care. (See Box 1-2 for an explanation of biostatistical terminology useful in analyzing maternity and women's health care.) In 1997 the **fertility rate** was 65.3 (Guyer et al., 1998). The highest birthrates occurred among women between the ages of 20 and 29 (Table 1-1). The **birthrate** was 14.6 in 1997 (Guyer et al., 1998). In 1997 the birthrate for unmarried women varied widely among racial groups in the United States: African-American, 69.1 per 1000; Hispanic, 40.9 per 1000; Caucasian, 25.8 per 1000 (Guyer et al., 1998). Births to unmarried women are frequently related to less favorable out-

---

BOX 1-2 Maternal-Infant Biostatistical Terminology

Abortus—Embryo or fetus that is removed or expelled from the uterus at 20 weeks of gestation or less, that weighs 500 g or less, or that measures 25 cm or less.

Birthrate—Number of live births in 1 year per 1000 population.

Fertility rate—Number of births per 1000 women between the ages of 15 and 44 (inclusive), calculated on a yearly basis.

Infant mortality rate—Number of deaths of infants under 1 year of age per 1000 live births.

Maternal mortality rate—Number of maternal deaths from births and complications of pregnancy, childbirth, and puerperium (first 42 days after termination of the pregnancy) per 100,000 live births.

Neonatal mortality rate—Number of deaths of infants under 28 days of age per 1000 live births.

Perinatal mortality rate—Number of stillbirths and neonatal deaths per 1000 live births.

Stillbirth—Neonate who demonstrates no signs of life, such as breathing, heartbeat, or voluntary muscle movement.

TABLE 1-1 Birthrate According to Age—1996

AGE	RATE PER 1000 WOMEN
15-17	33.8
18-19	86
20-24	110.4
25-29	113.1
30-34	83.9
35-39	35.3
40-44	6.8

Data from Guyer, B. et al. (1998). Annual summary of vital statistics. *Pediatrics* 102, 1333-1349.

---

comes, such as low birth weight or preterm birth, because a large number of these women are teenagers.

Incidence of Low Birth Weight

The risks of morbidity and mortality increase for newborns weighing less than 2500 g (5 lb, 8 oz)—**low-birth-weight (LBW) infants.** In 1997 the incidence of LBW rose to 7.5%, the highest rate since 1973 (Guyer et al., 1998). For African-American births, the incidence of LBW was 13.0%, whereas the rate was 6.5% for Caucasian births (Guyer et al., 1998). African-American infants are more than twice as likely as Caucasian infants to be LBW and to die in the first year of life.

The percentage of **preterm infants** (those infants born before 38 weeks of gestation) was 17.4% for African-American births. The rate of Caucasian preterm births was 9.8%. Multiple births contribute to the incidence of preterm births. The number of multiple births is increasing; in 1996 the rate was 27.4 per 1000. The rise in multiple births is attributed to the use of fertility-enhancing drugs (Guyer et al., 1998).

Infant Mortality in the United States

A common indicator of the adequacy of prenatal care and the health of a nation as a whole is the **infant mortality rate.** The U.S. infant mortality rate for 1997 was 7.1, the lowest ever recorded (Guyer et al., 1998). The infant mortality rate continues to be higher for African-American infants than for Caucasian infants by a ratio of 2:3 (Guyer et al., 1998). Limited maternal education, young maternal age, unmarried status, poverty, lack of prenatal care, and smoking appear to be associated with higher infant mortality rates. The current emphasis on high-technology medical interventions must shift to the improvement of access to preventive care for low-income families. Infant mortality rates and pregnancy outcomes must improve as a result of better access to care that prevents health problems and recognizes the changing socioeconomic and behavioral factors that place infants at risk.

International Infant Mortality Trends

The infant mortality rate of Canada ranks fourteenth and that of the United States ranks twenty-third when compared with other industrialized nations (Guyer et al., 1998). Even though the infant mortality rate has decreased in the United States, it did not keep pace with the rates of other industrialized countries. One reason for this is the high rate of LBW infants in the United States in contrast with the rate in other countries.

Maternal Mortality Trends

Although life expectancy in 1997 was 79.8 years for Caucasian females and 74.7 years for African-American females (Guyer et al., 1998), pregnancy poses some risk to childbearing women. The annual **maternal mortality rate** (number of maternal deaths per 100,000 live births) in the United States remained the same between 1982 and 1996 at approximately 7.5. There are significant racial differences in the rates: African-American women have a maternal mortality rate three times higher than do Caucasian women. Maternal mortality ranges from 10 to 22 per 100,000 for African-American women in contrast with 5 to 6 per 100,000 for Caucasian women. The predominant causes of death are hemorrhage, infection, pregnancy-induced hypertension, and ectopic pregnancy. *Healthy People 2000* proposed a goal of 3.3 maternal deaths per 100,000. To achieve this goal, early diagnosis and appropriate intervention must occur (CDC, 1998).

Trends of Consumer Involvement, Self-Care, and Focus on Health Care

In the 1960s clients began to demand information about medical technology and their medical care. A movement toward self-help and assumption of responsibility for wellness has also occurred. No longer do clients passively accept and adhere to the advice of health care providers. Clients demand information and take active roles in their health care. Women make changes in health behaviors to improve pregnancy outcome (Higgins, Frank, & Brown, 1994). Consumers are demanding a choice of health plans and providers that is based on knowledge of their options. In efforts to influence choice, increasing numbers of agencies, health plans, and employers are issuing report cards, that is, reports that contain ratings or scores that indicate quality or measure performance (Grimaldi, 1997). Consumers can use these ratings to judge quality or safety and make selections of providers or care delivery systems based on this information.

Self-care has been appealing to both clients and the health care system because of its potential to reduce health care costs. Maternity care is especially suited to self-care because childbearing is essentially health focused, women are usually well when they enter the system, and visits to health care providers can present the opportunity for health and illness interventions. Measures to improve health and reduce risks associated with poor pregnancy outcomes and illness can be addressed. Visits to health care providers provide opportunities to address topics such as nutrition education, stress management, smoking cessation, alcohol and drug treatment, improvement of social supports, and parenting education.

Trend Toward Earlier Prenatal Care

First trimester care has increased among Caucasian (from 84.0% to 84.7%), Hispanic (from 72.2% to 73.7%), and African-American (from 71.4% to 72.3%) mothers. Only 3.3% of Caucasian, 7.3% of African-American, and 6.2% of Hispanic mothers had late (beginning in the third trimester) or no care (Guyer et al., 1998). Comprehensive and timely care can enable health care providers to detect and manage conditions that preexisted the pregnancy or develop during pregnancy. In addition, education about health-promoting behaviors can occur (Guyer et al., 1998).

Trend Toward High-Technology Care

Advances in scientific knowledge and the large number of high risk pregnancies have contributed to a health care system that emphasizes high-technology care. Obstetrics has branched out to preconception counseling, more and better scientific techniques to monitor the mother and fetus, more definitive tests for hypoxia and acidosis, and neonatal intensive care units. Robotic aids may become common (Eckberg, 1998). Strides are being made in identifying genetic codes; genetic engineering is occurring in laboratories. Women's health has expanded to emphasize care of older women, new cancer screening techniques, advances in the diagnosis and treatment of breast cancer, and work on an AIDS vaccine. In general, high-technology care has flourished, whereas "health" care has become relatively neglected. These technologic advances have also contributed to higher health care costs.

Home Health Care Flourishes

A shift in settings from acute care institutions to the home has been occurring. Even high risk childbearing women are increasingly cared for in the home. Technology previously available only in the hospital is now found in the home. This has affected the organizational structure of care, the skills required in providing such care, and the costs to consumers. Home health care also has a community focus. Nurses are involved in providing care for women and infants in homeless shelters; school-based care for adolescents; and health promotion and prevention activities in community sites, such as schools, churches, and shopping malls. Nursing education curricula are increasingly community based.

High Risk Pregnancies Escalate

High risk pregnancies have increased, which means that a greater number of pregnant women are at risk for poor pregnancy outcomes. Escalating drug use (11% to 27% of pregnant women, depending on the geographic location) has contributed to higher incidences of prematurity, LBW, congenital defects, learning disabilities, and withdrawal symptoms in infants. Alcohol use in pregnancy has been associated with miscarriages (spontaneous abortions), mental retardation, LBW, and fetal alcohol syndrome.

The two most frequently reported maternal medical risk factors are hypertension associated with pregnancy and diabetes (Guyer et al., 1998). The multiple birthrate is increasing, with the higher-order multiple (triplet, quadruplet, and greater) birthrate climbing 20% in 1996 for a rate of 152.6 per 100,000 live births (Guyer et al., 1998). The cesarean birthrate increased to 20.8% for 1997, making it unlikely that the *Healthy People 2000* goal of 15% can be accomplished (Guyer et al., 1998).

Managed Care Expands

Managed care continues to expand. Stahl (1997) predicted that enrollment in health maintenance organizations would increase to 100 million people by the year 2000. Managed care focuses on meeting the clients' needs while promoting efficiency and cost-effectiveness. The drive to contain costs may compromise quality of services. Access to services and quality outcomes are hallmarks of success in managed care. The concept of care management is applied to maternity and women's health nursing in this text. Approaches such as protocols and critical paths are used where applicable. Care paths for public health nurses working with high risk maternal-child clients are available (Lowry et al., 1998).

Trends and Issues of High Cost

Health care is one of the fastest-growing sectors of the U.S. economy. National health expenditures constitute one seventh of the U.S. economy (Vincenzino, 1994). Perinatal care cost $27.8 billion in 1989, representing $6,850 for each mother-infant pair (Long, Marquis, & Harrison, 1994). A shift in demographics, an increased emphasis on high-cost technology, and the liability costs of a litigious society contribute to the high cost of care. Most researchers agree that the costs of caring for the increased number of LBW infants in neonatal intensive care units contributed significantly to the overall health care costs, especially since 19% of all uninsured women gave birth to an LBW infant (National Commission to Prevent Infant Mortality, 1990).

Insurance coverage varies markedly by age, marital status, race, and ethnicity (Horton, 1995). Caucasians of all ages are more likely than African-Americans and other racial or ethnic groups to have private insurance. Caucasians possess insurance 2.5 times more often than Hispanics and 1.8 times more often than African-Americans. Single, separated, or divorced individuals are less likely to have insurance.

In 1991 Medicaid funded 32% of all births in states reporting such data (Singh, Gold, & Frost, 1994). Midwifery care has helped contain some health care costs, but not all insurance carriers reimburse nurse-practitioners and clinical nurse-specialists as direct care providers, a situation that continues to be a problem (Ernst, 1994).

Although total health care spending does not necessarily generate positive health outcomes, public funding of health care for women increases the life expectancy for women (Babazono & Hillman, 1994), probably because of the effectiveness of screening programs for breast and cervical cancer.

Early postpartum discharge programs are also used to reduce costs (Brooten et al., 1994). Practitioners must demonstrate the safety of shorter hospital stays and not just fail to show that they are unsafe (Department of Health and Human Services, 1995). The American Academy of Pediatrics has published minimum criteria for early discharge of a newborn (American Academy of Pediatrics Committee on Fetus and Newborn, 1995).

Nursing data must be identified and placed in a database to be included in public policy decisions; nursing variables such as education and support care must become part of the national data-gathering system. Nurses should also deal with the politics involved in cost-containment health care policies, because they, as knowledgeable experts, can provide solutions to many of the health care problems at a relatively low cost (Hastings, 1995).

Access to Care Problems

Access to prenatal care continues to be an issue. The percentage of women who began prenatal care in the first trimester reached 82.5% in 1997, the highest level ever reported; only 4% delayed care until the third trimester or had no care (Guyer et al., 1998). Many women with access to prenatal care enter the health care system late or come only sporadically. Minority women are less likely than Caucasian women to receive early prenatal care (Guyer et al., 1998). Homelessness inhibits access to care.

Barriers to access must be removed so pregnancy outcomes can be improved. The most significant barrier to access is the inability to pay. Lack of transportation and dependent child care are other barriers. When barriers are removed, low-income women seek care earlier and more often (Piper, Mitchel, & Ray, 1994). Simple incentives to increase participation in prenatal care do not work (Laken & Ager, 1995). In addition to a lack of insurance and high costs, there is a shortage of providers for low-income women because many physicians either refuse to take Medicaid clients or take only a few such clients. This presents a significant problem because one in six births is to a mother who receives Medicaid.

TRENDS IN NURSING PRACTICE

The increasing complexity of care for maternity clients has contributed to specialization of nurses working with these clients. This specialized knowledge is being gained through experience, advanced degrees, and certification programs. Nurses in advanced practice—nurse-practitioners and nurse-midwives—may provide primary care throughout a woman's life, including during the pregnancy cycle. In some settings, the clinical nurse specialist and nurse practitioner roles are blended and nurses deliver high-quality, comprehensive, and cost-effective care in a variety of settings (Sperhac & Strodtbeck, 1997). Lactation consultants provide services in the postpartum unit or on an outpatient basis.

Nursing Interventions Classification

When the National Institutes of Medicine proposed that all client records be computerized by the year 2000, a need for a common language to describe the contributions of nurses to client care became evident (Eganhouse, McCloskey, & Bulachek, 1996). Nurses from the University of Iowa developed a comprehensive standardized language that describes interventions that are performed by generalist or specialist nurses. This language is included in the Nursing Interventions Classification (NIC). Interventions commonly used by maternal-child nurses include those in Box 1-3.

BOX 1-3   Childbearing Care Interventions

LEVEL 1 DOMAIN: FAMILY
Care that supports the family unit

LEVEL 2 CLASS: CHILDBEARING CARE
Interventions to assist in understanding and coping with the psychologic and physiologic changes during the childbearing period

LEVEL 3: INTERVENTIONS
Amnioinfusion
Anticipatory guidance
Attachment promotion
Birthing
Bleeding reduction: antepartum uterus
Bleeding reduction: postpartum uterus
Bottle feeding
Breastfeeding assistance
Cesarean-section care
Childbirth preparation
Electronic fetal monitoring: antepartum
Electronic fetal monitoring: intrapartum
Environmental management: attachment process
Family integrity promotion: childbearing family
Family planning: contraception
Family planning: infertility
Family planning: unplanned pregnancy
Genetic counseling

Grief work facilitation: perinatal death
High risk pregnancy care
Infant care
Intrapartal care
Kangaroo care
Labor induction
Labor suppression
Lactation counseling
Lactation suppression
Newborn care
Newborn monitoring
Nonnutritive sucking
Parent education: childbearing family
Phototherapy: neonate
Postpartal care
Preconception counseling
Pregnancy termination care
Prenatal care
Reproductive technology management
Resuscitation: fetus
Resuscitation: neonate
Risk identification: childbearing family
Surveillance: late pregnancy
Teaching: infant care
Tube care: umbilical line
Ultrasonography: limited obstetric

From Iowa Intervention Project. (1996). *Nursing interventions classification (NIC)* (2nd ed.). St. Louis: Mosby.

Evidence-Based Practice

There is increasing emphasis on providing **evidence-based practice** gained through research and clinical trials. As much as possible, nursing practice should be based on such evidence. Although not all practice can be based on evidence, practitioners must use the best available information on which to base their interventions. Health care providers may write practice guidelines based on findings of research. The American College of Obstetricians and Gynecologists (ACOG) issues *Practice Patterns* based on evidence that has been evaluated and graded (Zinberg, 1997). The first consensus initiative of the Coalition for Improving Maternity Services, the *Mother-Friendly Childbirth Initiative,* is an evidence-based model that focuses on prevention and wellness as alternatives to costly programs of screening, diagnosis, and treatment (*The Mother-Friendly Childbirth Initiative,* 1997). *Standards and Guidelines for Professional Nursing Practice in the Care of Women and Newborns* (Association of Women's Health, Obstetric, and Neonatal Nurses [AWHONN], 1998) includes an evidence-based approach to practice.

Outcomes Orientation

Outcomes of care, that is, the effectiveness of interventions and quality of care, are receiving increased emphasis (Table 1-2). **Outcomes-oriented care** measures effectiveness of care against benchmarks or standards based on results achieved by others. Quality indicators include cost, length of stay, and client satisfaction. This focus requires nurses to take more responsibility for their actions and monitor the effects of their interventions.

Best Practices as Goal of Care

A program or service that has been recognized for excellence is considered to be a **best practice.** A best practice must provide a better or a new way to achieve goals (Lewis, 1998) and be sound from operational, clinical, and financial perspectives (Fitzgerald, 1998). To determine best practices, information is collected from similar institutions. Staff members then identify solutions that have been suc-

cessful in addressing specific needs and select one that incorporates the best resolutions of the problem that fit the agency's unique population and mission characteristics. The agency continually compares its performance against the best in the industry and the best of a specific function.

Clinical Benchmarking

Clinical benchmarking is a process used to compare one's own performance against the performance of the best in an area of service (Fitzgerald, 1998). Benchmarking is used for identification and evaluation to improve performance and strengthen the organization. Benchmarking supports and promotes continuous quality improvement, assisting the organization to remain competitive within the health care market.

Perinatal nursing has an advantage in the process of benchmarking because a number of standards already exist. The standards have been set by such organizations as the **Association of Women's Health, Obstetric, and Neonatal Nurses (AWHONN),** ACOG, and the American Academy of Pediatrics. Figure 1-1 provides an example of a template for areas of practice that are routinely monitored in perinatal nursing.

Telemedicine

Telemedicine is an umbrella term for the use of communication technologies and electronic information to provide or support health care when the participants are separated by distance (Thrall & Boland, 1998). Nurses can interact with clients and physicians using live, real-time, two-way audiovisual interaction. It is estimated that this technology will save billions of dollars annually for health care (Fishman, 1997). There are two types of telenursing: teletriage nursing and home health nursing (see also Chapter 3). Teletriage nursing is conducted over the telephone and involves timely referral of clients to appropriate health care resources. Nurses use protocols or guidelines to assess needs and symptoms and prioritize the urgency of the needs of the client. In home health nursing, nurses use interactive video-based applications in the home. Clients can be monitored and reminded to take

▌TABLE 1-2 **Most Commonly Employed Outcome Indicators**		
COST PERFORMANCE	**SERVICE QUALITY**	**CLINICAL**
Expenditures per unit of service	Overall client satisfaction with care	Morbidity and mortality rates
Staffing levels	Customer service measures	Appropriateness indicators (e.g.,
Staffing ratios	(friendliness, expertise of staff, etc.)	hysterectomies, cesarean births, neonatal intubations)
Staff mix	Physician satisfaction	Readmission rates
Productivity measures	Employee satisfaction	Infection rates
Capital expenditures	Community perceptions	Functional status
Supply costs	Access indicators	

From Arnold, L., Angelini, D., & Possinger, T. (1997). The state of perinatal nursing: Current and future profiles as described by perinatal nursing service directors. *J Perinat Neonatal Nurs* 10(4), 27-35.

medications or vital signs. When telephone outreach crosses state lines, regulatory issues such as license to practice in more than one state cause concern. The National Council of State Boards of Nursing is addressing the issue of multistate regulation and licensing (Stuckey, 1998).

A Global Perspective

Advances in medicine and nursing have resulted in increased knowledge and understanding in the care of mothers and infants and reduced perinatal morbidity and mortality. However, these advances have affected predominantly the industrialized nations. As the world becomes smaller because of travel and communication technologies, nurses and other health care providers are gaining a global perspective and participating in activities to improve the health and health care of people worldwide. Nurses participate in medical outreach, providing obstetric, surgical, ophthalmologic, orthopedic, or other services; attend international meetings; conduct research; and provide international consultation. International student and faculty exchanges occur. More articles about health care in various countries are appearing in nursing journals. Several schools of nursing in the United States are World Health Organization Collaborating Centers.

STANDARDS OF PRACTICE AND LEGAL ISSUES IN DELIVERY OF CARE

Nursing standards of practice in perinatal and women's health nursing have been described by several organizations, including the American Nurses' Association (ANA), which publishes standards for maternal-child health nursing; AWHONN, which publishes standards of practice and education; and the National Association of Neonatal Nurses (NANN), which publishes standards of practice for neonatal nurses. These standards reflect current knowledge and represent levels of practice agreed on by leaders in the specialty (AWHONN, 1998) (Box 1-4). Because nursing practice, society, and the health care system are dynamic rather than static, standards change over time.

In addition to these more formalized standards, agencies often have their own policy and procedure books that outline standards to be followed in that setting. In determining legal negligence, the care given is compared with the standards of care. If the standard was not met and harm resulted, negligence occurred. The number of legal suits in the perinatal area has typically been high. As a consequence, malpractice insurance costs are high for physicians, nurse-midwives, and nurses in labor and delivery.

Areas for improvement	Agency target	AWHONN	ACOG	AAP	HCFA	Hospital 1	Hospital 2
Hospital length of stay							
Maternal mortality*							
Infant mortality**							
Cesarean delivery rate							
Hysterectomy rate							
Epidural rate							
Episiotomy rate							

*Deaths per 100,000 live births
**Deaths per 1,000 live births

Key:
AWHONN, Association of Women's Health, Obstetric, and Neonatal Nurses
ACOG, American College of Obstetricians and Gynecologists
AAP, American Academy of Pediatrics
HCFA, Health Care Financing Administration

Fig. 1-1 Example of a template for a worksheet for benchmarking. *(Adapted from Fitzgerald, K. [1998]. Clinical benchmarking: Implications for perinatal nursing. J Perinat Neonatal Nurs 12[1], 23-40.)*

BOX 1-4   Standards of Care for Women and Newborns

STANDARDS THAT DEFINE THE NURSE'S RESPONSIBILITY TO THE CLIENT

Assessment

Collection of health data of the woman or newborn

Diagnosis

Analysis of data to determine nursing diagnosis

Outcome Identification

Identification of expected outcomes that are individualized

Planning

Development of a plan of care

Implementation

Performance of interventions for the plan of care

Evaluation

Evaluation of the effectiveness of interventions in relation to expected outcomes.

STANDARDS OF PROFESSIONAL PERFORMANCE THAT DELINEATE ROLES AND BEHAVIORS FOR WHICH THE PROFESSIONAL NURSE IS ACCOUNTABLE

Quality of Care

Systemic evaluation of nursing practice

Performance Appraisal

Self-evaluation in relation to professional practice standards and other regulations

Education

Participation in ongoing educational activities to maintain knowledge for practice

Collegiality

Contribution to the development of peers, students, and others

Ethics

Use of Code for Nurses to guide practice

Collaboration

Involvement of client, significant others, and other health care providers in the provision of client care

Research

Use of research findings in practice

Resource Utilization

Consideration of factors related to safety, effectiveness, and costs in planning and delivering client care

Practice Environment

Contribution to the environment of care delivery

Accountability

Legal and professional responsibility for practice

Source: Association of Women's Health, Obstetric, and Neonatal Nurses (AWHONN). (1998). *Standards and guidelines for professional nursing practice in the case of women and newborns* (5th ed.). Washington, D.C.: AWHONN.

LEGAL TIP **Standard of Care**

When you are uncertain about how to perform a procedure, consult the agency procedure book and follow the guidelines printed therein. These guidelines are the standard of care for that agency.

Risk Management

Risk management is an evolving process that identifies risks, establishes preventive practices, develops reporting mechanisms, and delineates procedures for managing lawsuits. Nurses should be familiar with concepts of risk management and their implications for nursing practice. Effective risk management minimizes the risk of injury to clients and the number of lawsuits against nurses. Nurses should view the concepts as systems of checks and balances that ensure high-quality client care from preconception care until after delivery (Foust, 1997). Each facility or site develops site-specific risk management procedures based on accepted standards and guidelines.

ETHICAL ISSUES IN PERINATAL NURSING

Ethical concerns and debates have multiplied with the increased use of technology and scientific advances. For example, with reproductive technology, pregnancy is now possible in women who thought they would never bear children, including some who are menopausal or postmenopausal. Should practitioners devote scarce resources to achieving pregnancies in older women? Is giving birth to a child at an older age worth the risk? Should older parents be encouraged to conceive a baby when they may not live to see the child reach adulthood? Should third-party payers assume the costs of reproductive technology? Potential clients, nurses, physicians, ethicists, and lawmakers must discuss and debate these questions. With induced ovulation and in vitro fertilization, multiple pregnancies occur and multifetal pregnancy reduction (selectively terminating one or more fetuses) may be considered (Lipitz, Mashiach, & Seidman, 1994). Innovations such as intrauterine fetal surgery, fetoscopy, therapeutic insemination, genetic engineering, surrogate childbearing, surgery for infertility, "test tube" babies, fetal research, and treatment of very low-birth-weight (VLBW) babies have resulted in questions about informed consent and allocation of resources. The introduction of long-acting contraceptives has created moral choices and policy dilemmas for health care providers and legislators; that is, should some women (substance abusers, women with low incomes, or women who are HIV positive) be required to take the contraceptives (Moskowitz, Jennings, & Callahan, 1995)? With the potential for great good that can come from fetal tissue transplantation, what research is ethical? What are the rights of the embryo (Sams, 1997)? Discussion and debate about these issues will continue for many years; nurses and clients, as well as scientists, physicians, attorneys, and clergy, must be involved in the discussions.

RESEARCH IN MATERNITY AND WOMEN'S HEALTH

Research plays a vital role in the establishment of a maternity and women's health science. Nurses should promote research funding and conduct research on maternity and women's health, especially concerning the effectiveness of nursing strategies for these clients. Research can validate that nursing care makes a difference. For example, although prenatal care is clearly associated with healthier infants, no one knows exactly which nursing interventions produce this particular outcome. The research into women's health must increase. In the past, medical researchers rarely included women in their studies, so more research in this area is crucial. Many possible areas of research in maternity and women's health care exist. The clinician can identify problems in the health and health care of women and infants. Through research, nurses can make a difference for these clients. Research boxes throughout this text provide examples of the clinical application of research in perinatal and women's health nursing.

RESEARCH INTO PRACTICE

The incorporation of research findings into practice is essential in developing a science-based practice. Practicing nurses can identify problems and read research literature to identify studies that address their clinical concerns.

AWHONN has conducted four research-based practice projects: Transition of an Infant from an Incubator to an Open Crib, Management of Second-Stage Labor, Urinary Continence in Women, and Neonatal Skin Care. These projects were multistate, and staff nurses were involved in implementation of and data collection in the projects. The next

projects planned by AWHONN are on pelvic pain and comfort management and the nursing management of preterm labor. AWHONN is also creating new practice guidelines to incorporate evidence-based practices for second-stage labor management, continence for women, breastfeeding support, assessment of midlife women, and intrapartum-perioperative-perianesthesia care. Using such guidelines and published reports, nurses can develop evidence-based protocols and procedures. Maternity and women's health nurses are encouraged to participate in research endeavors identified by AWHONN as priorities through 2001. These priorities include the above topics as well as family violence, fetal surveillance, genetics, infertility, and early parenting.

Cochrane Pregnancy and Childbirth Database

The **Cochrane Pregnancy and Childbirth Database** was first planned in 1976 with a small grant from the World Health Organization to Dr. Iain Chalmers and colleagues at Oxford. In 1993 the Cochrane Collaboration was formed, and the Oxford Database of Perinatal Trials became known as the Cochrane Pregnancy and Childbirth Database. The Cochrane Collaboration oversees up-to-date, systematic reviews and dissemination of reviews of randomized controlled trials of health care. The underlying premise of the project is that the most reliable evidence about the effects of care is provided by these types of studies.

The evidence from these studies should encourage practitioners to implement useful measures and to abandon those that are useless or harmless. Studies are ranked in six categories:
1. Beneficial forms of care
2. Forms of care that are likely to be beneficial
3. Forms of care with a trade-off between beneficial and adverse effects
4. Forms of care with unknown effectiveness
5. Forms of care that are unlikely to be beneficial
6. Forms of care that are likely to be ineffective or harmful

Practices that have been reviewed by the collaboration will be identified with a ▉▉ throughout this text.

BIAS IN HEALTH RESEARCH

Bias against women exists in health research. This research bias has recently been recognized and publicized. The bias encompasses the following areas: exclusion of women from clinical trials, lack of analysis of the results of studies by gender, inadequate funding of research on diseases of women, and inadequate numbers of female researchers.

To remedy the underrepresentation of women in research and the underfunding of research on diseases of women, the Women's Health Equity Act (WHEA) of 1991 was introduced into the U.S. Congress. This act, a comprehensive package of 22 bills, requires inclusion of women and minorities in studies, authorizes $25 million for research on breast cancer, and provides funding for AIDS research on women and the study of ovarian cancer and osteoporosis (NAACOG: Women's Health Equity Act introduced, 1991).

Ethical Guidelines for Nursing Research

Nurses must protect the rights of human subjects (that is, clients) in all of their research. For example, nurses may collect data on or care for clients who are participating in clinical trials. The nurse ensures that the subjects are fully informed and aware of their rights as subjects.

In 1995 the ANA published "Ethical Guidelines in the Conduct, Dissemination, and Implementation of Nursing Research" (Box 1-5). The guidelines contain nine ethical principles and a commentary on the principles. These guidelines help nurses ensure ethically conducted research.

Research with perinatal clients may create ethical dilemmas for the nurse. For example, participating in research may cause additional stress to a woman concerned about outcomes of genetic testing or one who is waiting for an invasive procedure. Obtaining amniotic fluid samples or performing cordocentesis poses risks to the fetus; the nurse may be involved in determining whether the benefits of research outweigh the risks to the mother and the fetus. Perinatal nurses must protect the rights of their clients by understanding ethical principles and the rights of clients and must use this knowledge to advocate for pregnant women and their fetuses.

BOX 1-5 Ethical Principles in the Conduct, Dissemination, and Implementation of Nursing Research

1. The investigator respects autonomous research participants' capacity to consent to participate in research and to determine the degree and duration of that participation without negative consequences.
2. The investigator prevents harm, minimizes harm, and/or promotes good to all research participants, including vulnerable groups and others affected by the research.
3. The investigator respects the personhood of research participants, their families, and significant others, valuing their diversity.
4. The investigator ensures that the benefits and burdens of research are equitably distributed in the selection of research participants.
5. The investigator protects the privacy of research participants to the maximum degree possible.
6. The investigator ensures the ethical integrity of the research process by use of appropriate checks and balances throughout the conduct, dissemination, and implementation of the research.
7. The investigator reports suspected, alleged, or known incidents of scientific misconduct in research to appropriate institutional officials for investigation.
8. The investigator maintains competency in the subject matter and methodologies of his or her research, as well as in other professional and societal issues that affect nursing research and the public good.
9. The investigator involved in animal research maximizes the benefits of the research with the least possible harm or suffering to the animals.

From Silva, M. (1995). *Ethical guidelines in the conduct, dissemination, and implementation of nursing research.* Washington, D.C.: American Nurses' Association.

KEY POINTS

- Maternity nursing focuses on women and their infants and families during the childbearing cycle.
- Women's health nursing focuses on the special physical, psychologic, and social needs of women throughout their life spans.
- Nurses caring for women can actively shape health care systems to be responsive to the needs of contemporary women.
- Childbirth practices have changed to become more focused on the family and allow alternatives in care.
- Home care is cost-effective and has become an alternative health care setting.
- A variety of factors, including race, aging, and violence, affect women's health.
- The United States ranks twenty-third and Canada ranks fourteenth among industrialized nations in infant mortality rates.
- Evidence-based practice, outcomes orientation, best practices, and clinical benchmarking are emphasized in current practice.
- Ethical concerns have multiplied with the gradual increase in the use of technology and scientific advances.
- Research plays a vital role in establishing a maternity and women's health science.

CRITICAL THINKING EXERCISES

1 *Consult the yellow pages of the telephone directory. What kind of and how many pregnancy-related services are you able to identify? Select one of the services and call to inquire if there is a bus stop close to the service and who can use the services. What does this information say about access to services?*

2 *Select five issues of a newspaper at random. Are there any articles that have relevance for mothers, infants, and families? Is there a theme to the articles? What "slant" do you perceive in the articles (e.g., welfare mothers need to work; teenage pregnancy is a problem). As a regular reader of that newspaper, would your view of women, infants, and families be influenced?*

References

American Academy of Pediatrics Committee on Fetus and Newborn (1995). Hospital stay for healthy term newborns. *Pediatrics* 96(4 pt. 1), 788-790.

American Cancer Society. (1999). *1999 Cancer facts and figures.* New York: American Cancer Society.

Arnold, L., Angelini, D., & Possinger, T. (1997). The state of perinatal nursing: Current and future profiles as described by perinatal nursing service directors. *J Perinat Neonatal Nurs* 10(4), 27-35.

Association of Women's Health, Obstetric, and Neonatal Nurses (AWHONN) (1998). *Standards and guidelines for professional nursing practice in the care of women and newborns* (5th ed.). Washington, D.C.: AWHONN.

Babazono, A., & Hillman, A. (1994). A comparison of international health outcomes and health care spending. *Int J Technol Assess Health Care* 10(3), 376-381.

Barter, M. et al. (1995). The changing health care delivery structure: Opportunities for nursing practice and administration. *Nurs Admin Q* 19(3), 74-80.

Bass, M., & Howes, J. (1992). Women's health: The making of a powerful new public issue. *Women's Health Issues* 2(1), 3-5.

Breslin, E. (1995). Integrating women's health concepts in a nursing course. *Nurs Educ* 20(1), 30-33.

Brooten, D. et al. (1994). A randomized trial of early hospital discharge and home follow-up of women having a cesarean birth. *Obstet Gynecol* 84(5), 832-838.

Burnhill, M. (1994). Adolescent pregnancy rates in the US. *Contemp Obstet Gynecol* 39(2), 26-28.

Callister, L. (1995). Beliefs and perceptions of childbearing women choosing different primary health care providers. *Clin Nurse Res* 4(2), 168-180.

Centers for Disease Control and Prevention (1998). Maternal mortality—United States, 1982-1996. *MMWR* 47(34), 705-707.

Covington, C., & Collins, J. (1994). Back to the future of women's health and perinatal nursing in the 21st century. *J Obstet Gynecol Neonatal Nurs* 23(2), 183-194.

Department of Health and Human Services (1995). *Maternal and newborn length of hospitalization: summary status report.* Washington, D.C.: The Department.

Eckberg, E. (1998). Opinion. The future of robotics can be ours. *AORN J* 67(5), 1018, 1020-1023.

Eganhouse, D., McCloskey, J., & Bulachek, G. (1996). How NIC describes MCH nursing. *MCN Am J Matern Child Nurs* 21(5), 247-252.

Eisenberg, D. (1997). Advising patients who seek alternative medical therapies. *Ann Intern Med* 127(1), 61-69.

Eisenberg, D. et al. (1993). Unconventional medicine in the United States. *N Engl J Med* 328(4), 246-252.

Ernst, E. (1994). Health care reform as an ongoing process. *J Obstet Gynecol Neonatal Nurs* 23(2), 129-138.

Fischler, N., & Harvey, S. (1995). Setting and provider of prenatal care: Association with pregnancy outcomes among low-income women. *Health Care Women Int* 16(4), 309-321.

Fishman, D. (1997). Telemedicine: Bringing the specialist to the patient. *Nurs Manage* 28(7), 30-32.

Fitzgerald, K. (1998). Clinical benchmarking: Implications for perinatal nursing. *J Perinat Neonatal Nurs* 12(1), 23-30.

Foust, R. (1997). Maternity risk management: From preconception to after delivery. *J Care Management* 3(1), 22-28, 33-35, 39-42.

Freda, M. (1995). Arrest, trial, and failure. *J Obstet Gynecol Neonatal Nurs* 24(5), 393-394.

Freda, M. (1999). MCN Editorial. The power of words. *MCN Am J Matern Child Nurs* 24, 63.

Gary, F., Sigsby, L., & Campbell, D. (1998). Preparing for the 21st century: Diversity in nursing education, research, and practice. *J Prof Nurs* 14(5), 272-279.

Grady, G. (1994). HIV mass screening of infants and mothers: Historical, technical, and practical issues. *Acta Paediatr Suppl* 400, 39-42.

Grimaldi, P. (1997). Report cards can improve choice. *Nurs Manage* 28(5), 26.

Guyer, B. et al. (1998). Annual summary of vital statistics–1997. *Pediatrics* 102(6), 1333-1347.

Hastings, K. (1995). Health care reform: We need it, but do we have the national will to shape our future? *Nurse Pract* 20(1), 52-54, 56-57.

Higgins, P., Frank, B., & Brown, M. (1994). Changes in health behaviors made by pregnant women. *Health Care Women Int* 15(2), 149-156.

Horton, J. (1995). *The women's health data book* (2nd ed.). New York: Elsevier.

Huston, C., & Fox, S. (1998). The changing health care market: Implications for nursing education in the coming decade. *Nurs Outlook* 46, 109-114.

Iowa Intervention Project. (1996). *Nursing interventions classification (NIC)* (2nd ed.). St. Louis: Mosby.

Kaegi, L. (1995). Nurses leading the charge to take national AHCPR guidelines into local settings: The Joint Commission. *Jt Comm J Qual Improv* 21(1), 45-49.

Kass, N. (1994). Policy, ethics, and reproductive choice: Pregnancy and childbearing among HIV-infected women. *Acta Paediatr Suppl* 400, 95-98.

Laken, M., & Ager, J. (1995). Using incentives to increase participation in prenatal care. *Obstet Gynecol* 85(3), 326-329.

Lewis, J. (1998). Best practices–ideas that work. *AORN J* 68(3), 444-446.

Lipitz, S., Mashiach, S., & Seidman, D. (1994). Multifetal pregnancy reduction: The case for nondirective patient counseling. *Hum Reprod* 9(11), 1978-1979.

Long, S., Marquis, M., & Harrison, E. (1994). The costs and financing of perinatal care in the United States. *Am J Public Health* 84(9), 1473-1478.

Loring, M., & Smith, R. (1994). Health care barriers and interventions for battered women, US Department of Health and Human Services. *Public Health Rep* 109(3), 328-338.

Lowry, L., Hays, B., Lopez, P., & Hernandez, G. (1998). Care paths. A new approach to high-risk maternal-child home visitation. *MCN Am J Matern Child Nurs* 23, 322-328.

McCool, W. (1994). Barriers to breast cancer screening in older women: A review. *J Nurse Midwifery* 39(5), 283-289.

Moskowitz, E., Jennings, B., & Callahan, D. (1995). Long-acting contraceptives: Ethical guidance for policymakers and health care providers. *Hastings Cent Rep* 25(1), S1-S8.

The Mother-Friendly Childbirth Initiative. (1997). The first consensus initiative of the coalition for improving maternity services. *J Nurse Midwifery* 42(1), 59-63.

NAACOG: Women's Health Equity Act introduced. (1991). *NAACOG Newsletter* 18(9), 15.

National Commission to Prevent Infant Mortality. (1990). *Troubling trends: The health of America's next generation.* Washington, DC: The Commission.

Peterson, R., & Cefalo, R. (1990). Terms of confinement. *Obstet Gynecol* 76(2), 308-309.

Piper, J., Mitchel, B., & Ray, W. (1994). Presumptive eligibility for pregnant Medicaid enrollees: Its effects on prenatal care and perinatal outcome. *Am J Public Health* 84(10), 1626-1630.

Robertson, J. (1995). Symbolic issues in embryo research. *Hastings Cent Rep* 25(1), 37.

Sams, L. (1997). Ethical dilemmas in maternal-fetal research. *MCN Am J Matern Child Nurs* 22, 67-71.

Silva, M. (1995). *Ethical guidelines in the conduct, dissemination, and implementation of nursing research.* Washington, D.C.: American Nurses' Association.

Singh, S., Gold, R., & Frost, J. (1994). Impact of the Medicaid eligibility expansions on coverage of deliveries. *Fam Plann Perspect* 26(1), 31-33.

Sperhac, A., & Strodtbeck, F. (1997). Advanced practice nursing: New opportunities for blended roles. *MCN Am J Matern Child Nurs* 22, 287-293.

Stahl, D. (1997). Managed care trends: The effect on subacute care. *Nurs Manage* 28(3), 17-19.

Stuckey, C. (1998). Nursing practice across fiber optics. *Nurs Manage* 29(7), 24-25.

Thrall, J., & Boland, G. (1998). Telemedicine in practice. *Semin Nucl Med* 28(2), 145-147.

Ventura, S., Martin, J., Curtin, S., & Mathews, T. (1998). Report of final natality statistics, 1996. *Monthly Vital Statistics Report* 46(11 suppl), 1-99.

Vincenzino, J. (1994). Development in health care costs—An update. *Stat Bull* 75(1), 30-35.

Wood, S., & Ransom, V. (1994). The 1990s: A decade for change in women's health care policy. *J Obstet Gynecol Neonatal Nurs* 23(2), 139-143.

Zinberg, S. (1997). A guest editorial: Evidence-based practice guidelines: a current perspective. *Obstet Gynecol Surv* 52(5), 265-266.

2

The Family and Culture

Rhea P. Williams

LEARNING OBJECTIVES

- Define the key terms.
- Identify key factors in determining the quality of family health.
- Identify and describe the key characteristics of various family forms.
- Explain the functions carried out by a family for the well-being of its members and society.
- Explain components of family dynamics and how these contribute to accomplishing family functions.

- Explain three theoretic approaches (family systems theory, family developmental theory, and family stress theory) for working with childbearing families. Describe the nursing implications of each theory.
- Relate the role and impact of culture on childbearing families.
- Identify topics for nursing research related to the family and culture.

KEY TERMS

binuclear family
cultural competence
cultural context
extended family
family

family developmental theory
family dynamics
family functions
family stress theory
family systems theory

homosexual (lesbian and gay) family
nuclear family
reconstituted family
single-parent family

aternity nurses have a unique privilege and opportunity to affect the future through their work with families. In traditional or nontraditional settings, whether in hospitals, homes, or communities, they are among the first health care practitioners to touch the lives of families. Thus the nurse acknowledges the family unit as the focus of care.

The **family,** one of society's most important institutions, represents a primary social group that influences and is influenced by other people and institutions. The family is recognized as the fundamental social unit because most people have more continuous contact with this social group than with any other. The family assumes most of the responsibility for the introduction and socialization of people. A family transmits its fundamental cultural background to its members. Despite modern stresses and strains, the family forms a social network that acts as a potent support system for its members.

To deliver safe, comprehensive, and holistic care, nurses working with childbearing families in hospitals and in the community need a clear understanding of the family as an institution in our society.

DEFINING THE FAMILY

Families are defined in many ways. Definitions of the family usually involve explaining family *structure, functions, composition,* and *affectional ties.*

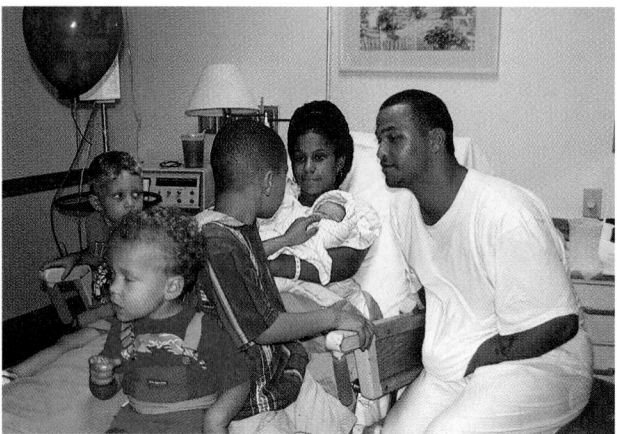

Fig. 2-1 Nuclear family. *(Courtesy Marjorie Pyle, RNC, Lifecircle, Costa Mesa, CA.)*

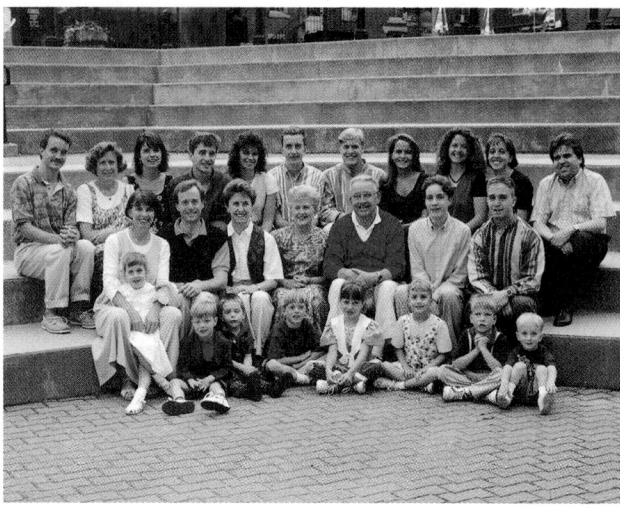

Fig. 2-2 Extended family. *(Courtesy Elizabeth Shaughnessy, San Francisco, CA.)*

Friedman (1998) offers a broad definition of family, emphasizing the importance of emotional involvement as a necessary characteristic. She states that the family is "two or more persons who are joined together by bonds of sharing and emotional closeness and who identify themselves as part of the family." Wright and Leahey (1994) offer an even broader interpretation: "The family is who they say they are." These definitions include a variety of family forms such as the nuclear family, the extended family, the binuclear family, and the reconstituted family.

Nuclear Family

The **nuclear family** consists of parents and their dependent children (Fig. 2-1). The family lives apart from either the husband's or wife's family of origin and is usually economically independent.

The nuclear family has long represented the "traditional" American family. In this family group, parents of different genders once played complementary roles of husband-wife and father-mother in giving emotional and physical support to each other and their children. Recent trends in contemporary society, however, have caused many variations in the "ideal" family structure. The "idealized" two-parent, two-child nuclear family, in which the father is the sole provider and the mother is the homemaker, represents a small number of modern American families; this type of family constitutes fewer than 8% of all households (Walsh, 1993).

Extended Family

The **extended family** includes the nuclear family and other people related by blood. Called *kin,* these people include grandparents, aunts, uncles, and cousins (Fig. 2-2) (Friedman, 1998). Through its kinship network, the extended family provides role models and support to all members.

Alternative Family Forms

Variations of the traditional nuclear and extended families have always existed. Until recently, most of these alternative family forms have been considered deviations from the norm. Today, society recognizes and generally accepts these forms.

Single-Parent Family

The **single-parent family** is becoming an increasingly recognized structure in our society. The single-parent family may result from the loss of a spouse by death, divorce, separation, or desertion; from the out-of-wedlock birth of a child; or from the adoption of a child. Today almost 4 out of every 10 children in the United States are either currently living with a single parent or have lived with one in the past (Bianchi, 1994). Of all children 17 years old or younger, approximately 26% live in a family with a single parent, another relative, or a nonrelative. Fewer than 4% live with fathers in a single-parent household (Evolving American Family, 1993).

The single-parent family tends to be vulnerable economically and socially. Many single-mother households are poor, with the most disadvantaged being children living with mothers who were never married (Bianchi, 1994). Unless buttressed by a concerned society, single-parent families may create an unstable and deprived environment for the growth potential of children.

For other adults, the single-parent family is a chosen lifestyle that provides a free and open system for development of parents and children. In these families decision making and communication are seen as joint commitments between parent and child, and the parent-child relationship is considered a major source of life fulfillment.

Binuclear Family

Binuclear family refers to the family after divorce, in which the child is a member of both the maternal and paternal nuclear households (Ahron & Perlmuller, 1982, as cited in Friedman, 1998). In these families, the degree of cooperation between the parents varies.

Ideally the family uses its resources to provide a safe, intimate environment for the biopsychosocial development of the family members. The family nurtures the newborn and teaches gradual *socialization* of the growing child. Children form their earliest and closest relationships with their parents or guardians; these affiliations continue throughout their lifetime. For better or worse, parent-child relationships influence self-worth and the ability to form later relationships. The family also influences the child's perceptions of the outside world. The family provides the growing child with an identity that possesses both a past and a sense of the future. Cultural values and rituals are passed from one generation to the next through the family (Friedman, 1998).

Through everyday interactions, the family develops and uses its own patterns of verbal and nonverbal *communication*. These patterns give insight into the emotional exchange within a family and act as reliable indicators of interpersonal functioning. Family members not only react to the communication or actions of other family members, but also interpret and define them.

Over time the family develops protocols for *problem solving*, particularly regarding important decisions such as having a baby, buying a house, or sending children to college. The criteria used in making decisions are based on *family values* and *attitudes* concerning the appropriateness of the behavior and the moral, social, political, and economic events of society. The *power* to make critical decisions is given to a family member through tradition or negotiation. This power is not always stated. Power reflects the family's concepts of male or female dominance and the cultural practices, social customs, and community norms. As a result, family members attain certain *statuses* or *hierarchies*. They play out these statuses by assuming various *roles*. Most families have a member who "takes charge" or "is supportive" or "can't be expected to do anything."

FAMILY THEORIES

Many academic disciplines study the family and have developed theories that provide differing perspectives for assessment and interventions. By knowing these theories, nurses can understand family functioning and dynamics. The theories provide a basis for planning and intervening in the day-to-day care of families and help predict events that may necessitate a modification of care.

Family Systems Theory

Wright and Leahey (1994) define *system* as a complex of elements in mutual interaction. When applied to families, the systems theory allows nurses to "view the family as a unit and thus focus on observing the interaction among family members rather than studying family members individually" (Wright & Leahey, 1994). The individual maintains uniqueness and importance as an individual system. However, as a family member, the individual remains a part of a larger system (the family) and also a subsystem.

Wright and Leahey outline the key characteristics of the **family systems theory**:

- A family system is part of a larger suprasystem and comprises many subsystems. The target or focal system (the family) must relate to a suprasystem (e.g., community, cultural group, church, or health care system) and its subsystem (e.g., spousal or parent-child subsystem). As with all systems, the family has boundaries that identify its members. These boundaries have various degrees of permeability, which determine the extent of influence by those outside the system.
- The family as a whole is greater than the sum of its individual members. Viewing the interaction of the whole family helps nurses more fully understand the functioning of individual family members.
- A change in one family member affects all family members.
- The family is able to create a balance between change and stability. This balance allows the family to remain flexible and adapt to changes.
- Family members' behaviors are best understood from a view of circular rather than linear causality (With circular causality, an individual's behavior affects and is affected by the behavior of others) with the linear view, one behavior simply causes another.

Implications for Maternity Nursing and Women's Health Care

The family systems theory encourages nurses to view individual family members as part of a larger family system influenced by and influencing others. Application of these concepts can guide assessment and interventions for the family. For example, the childbearing family as a system interacts with many elements in the environmental suprasystem, including the health care community (The extent to which this suprasystem influences the family in matters such as prenatal care, childbirth education, and infant care depends on the family's boundary permeability.) A relatively closed family may want instructions only from others within the family, whereas a relatively open family may be more receptive to instruction from health care providers.

Family Developmental Theory

The **family developmental theory** focuses on the family as it moves in time. Family members pass through phases of growth, from dependence through active independence to interdependence. The family's structure and function also vary over time. Together, these stages constitute the family life cycle. Carter and McGoldrick (1988) outline the tasks of the family life cycle in Table 2-1.

Mercer (1989) summarizes the essence of the developmental approach in family nursing:

Developmental concepts include movement to a higher level of functioning. This implies continuous, unidirectional progression. However, during transitional periods from one stage or phase to the next, disequilibrium occurs, during which time the individual may revert to an earlier level of developmental responses. Families face normative and unexpected transitions that also create a period of disorganization, during which the family functions at a lower level than usual. Resolution of the disequilibrium or crisis has potential to lead to a higher level of family functioning.

Implications for Maternity Nursing and Women's Health Care

The developmental perspective provides many useful insights into family functioning. Knowing about the phases of the life cycle can assist nurses in providing anticipatory guidance for families. For example, helping childbearing families prepare for the birth of a newborn may minimize the development of crises.

The family as a group and as individuals simultaneously engages in developmental tasks (Duvall, 1977; Erikson, 1968). If the developmental task of the family does not correspond with that of the person, disharmony occurs. Examples include the adolescent father who is grappling with the need to break from his own family ties but is also expected to establish monetary and other support for his new family, and a toddler learning socially acceptable behaviors who may revert to infantile behavior when introduced to a new sibling. Using this knowledge, the nurse helps the family develop appropriate coping mechanisms.

The developmental approach presents a realistic, constantly evolving concept of family. The phases of the life cycle are easier to plot in the nuclear family than in an extended family because the extended family may involve many generations (Fig. 2-3). Sometimes it may be difficult to document the life cycle of a family because it often changes or disintegrates before the nurse can grasp its significance.

Family Stress Theory

Hill originally developed the **family stress theory** in 1949. Known as the *ABCX theory*, it describes how families adapt differently to the same stressor. Researchers use three factors to explain the outcome (X): the stressor itself (A), the family's existing resources (B), and the family's perception of the stressor (C). Other researchers, including Boss (1996), modified and expanded Hill's theory. Boss views this linear approach to understanding family stress as no longer valid. She believes that family stress must be studied within the internal and external contexts in which the family is living. The internal context involves elements that a family can change or control, such as family structure (i.e., boundaries and roles), psychologic defenses (i.e., perception of the event), and philosophic values and beliefs. On the other hand, the external context consists of the time and place in which a particular family finds itself. A family has no control over these elements, which include the culture of the larger society, time in history in which the events happen to the family, economic state of society, maturity of the individuals involved, success of the family in coping with stressors, and genetic inheritance. According to Boss,

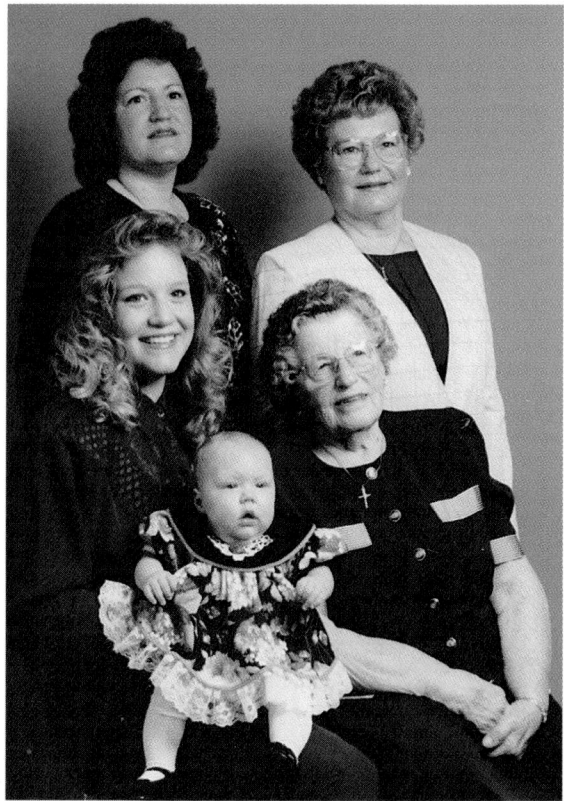

Fig. 2-3 Five generations of a family.

the nurse should ascertain a family's internal context before helping its members manage stress.

Implications for Maternity Nursing

Nurses working with childbearing families may find the family stress theory particularly useful because of its realistic and practical approach. As expressed by Boss (1996), because today's families experience a great deal of pressure, they must develop stress-management strategies. Maternity nurses usually care for healthy but highly stressed families. Nurses who understand the components of the family stress theory and stress management can intervene to reduce the stress level.

Boss considers birth one of the expected developmental (maturational) stressor events. Although a birth is expected and normal, its occurrence causes family dynamics to shift, thus having the potential to change the family's stress level. Boss says that families "experience increased levels of stress at each transition point, at least until the process of reorganization is accomplished after each addition or loss of a family member."

Maternity nurses work with families experiencing nonnormative (unexpected or situational) stressor events such as complicated pregnancies. These highly stressful events require the interventions of nurses who understand family stress management.

Nurses can assist families in changing their stress levels by helping families control internal context factors. For example, if a family's perception of a stressful event is based on incorrect or incomplete information, the nurse intervenes through educational strategies. Nurses can also explain various dimensions of the external context. For example, explaining normal infant growth and development (maturation) may reduce the stress of parenting.

KEY FACTORS IN FAMILY HEALTH

Family dynamics, family socioeconomics, and family response to stress and culture are important in determining the quality of family health. For example, family dynamics (see previous discussion) encompass the coordination of intrafamilial roles, distribution of power within the family, and decision-making process. Family dynamics also affect the use of health services.

Family socioeconomic characteristics influence the family's ability to access and use health care services. Socioeconomic factors govern expectations, obligations, and rewards, all of which influence the use of health services. In addition, the family acts as the primary economic unit in which incomes may be pooled, expenditure decisions made jointly, and services rendered internally.

Friedman (1998) considers a family's social class as the prime molder of its lifestyle. She says that socioeconomic factors and cultural background "exert the greatest overall influence on family life, influencing family values and practices, family behavior patterns, socialization, and world experiences families have." The interplay among stress, perception, and resources affects the level of support given to family members. The family's response to stress influences its members' physiologic and psychologic well-being. Cultural responses to childbearing and women's health concerns and the use of related health care services also play central roles in family health.

CULTURAL FACTORS

Cultural Context of the Family

The **cultural context** of the family should concern nurses, especially when they provide care to the childbearing family. A critical life experience, such as childbearing, often involves traditional beliefs and practices. A culture's economic, religious, kinship, and political structures pervade its beliefs and practices regarding childbearing (Research box). All cultures maintain behavioral norms and expectations for each stage of the perinatal cycle. These norms and expectations evolve from a culture's view of how people stay healthy and prevent illness. To practice with **cultural competence,** nurses must focus on the way people of different cultures perceive life events and the health care system. Clients have a right to expect that their physiologic and psychologic health care needs will be met and that their cultural beliefs will be respected.

Culture has many definitions. Helman (1990) views culture as a set of guidelines, which individuals inherit as members of a particular society, that tell people how to view the

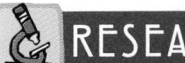 **RESEARCH**

Giving Birth: Guatemalan Women's Voices

Collaborative multicultural research studies have been undertaken with a myriad of ethnically and culturally diverse groups. However, most previous research focused on rites and rituals rather than the subjective meaning of the experience to women.

This ethnographically designed study focused on the birth stories of Guatemalan women and their perceptions of the sociocultural context of childbearing. Thirty Guatemalan women (15 primiparas and 15 multiparas) of mixed Mayan and Latino heritage who had given birth to healthy full-term infants were interviewed during the early postpartum weeks. Open-ended, culturally sensitive interview questions were used to promote spontaneity and to provide insight into what was perceived as important for the participants to share with the researchers about their childbirth experiences.

The sociocultural context of giving birth in Guatemala was described, including common beliefs about pregnancy and childbirth and the meaning and significance of having children. The predominant themes were the sacred nature of childbirth; the need for reliance on God during pregnancy, childbirth, and childrearing; and the bittersweet paradox of giving birth. The researchers concluded that nurses need knowledge of cultural values, needs, and health care practices to provide culturally sensitive care. Further research was recommended with populations of Hispanic women to establish baselines for appropriate health interventions, including educational programs, and to evaluate current provisions for health care for vulnerable populations.

CLINICAL APPLICATION

It is imperative that nurses deliver culturally and spiritually sensitive nursing care to childbearing women and their families. With the increasing number of refugees and immigrants of childbearing age entering the United States, it is important for nurses to recognize, acknowledge, and respect specific cultural practices related to childbearing.

Source: Callister, L., & Vega, R. (1998). Giving birth: Guatemalan women's voices. *J Obstet Gynecol Neonatal Nurs* 27(3), 289-295.

world and how to relate to other people, supernatural forces, and the natural environment. Cultural knowledge includes beliefs and values about each facet of life. These guidelines have been tested over time. They relate to food, language, religion, art, health and healing practices, kinship relationships, and all other systems of behavior.

Many subcultures may be found within each culture. *Subculture* refers to a group existing within a larger cultural system that retains its own characteristics. A subculture may be an ethnic group or a group organized in other ways. For example, in the United States, many ethnic subcultures such as African-Americans, Asian-Americans, and Mexican-Americans exist, as do subcultures within these groups. Nurses should also remember that the Caucasian population in America has diverse and multiple subcultures. Although the recent literature in the area of ethnicity and health has focused on people of color, little has been written about Caucasian ethnic communities (e.g., Italian-, Polish-, and German-Americans) (Spector, 1996). In issues of health, illness, and major life transitions, there may be greater differences among Caucasian groups than has generally been acknowledged.

Each subculture holds rich and complex traditions, including health practices. These traditions vary from group to group. In a multicultural society, many groups can influence these traditions and practices. As cultural groups come in contact with each other, acculturation and assimilation may occur.

Acculturation refers to changes that take place in one or both groups when people from different cultures come in contact with one another. People may retain some of their own culture while adopting some of the cultural practices of the dominant society. This familiarization among cultural groups results in much overt behavioral similarity, especially in mannerisms, styles, and practices. Dress, language patterns, food choices, and health practices especially reveal differences among cultural groups within a society. In the United States, acculturation is generally thought to take three generations. The adult grandchild of the immigrant is usually fully Americanized (Spector, 1996). An example of acculturation would be the adoption of ethnic food practices in the United States. It is important to note that even when individuals have become acculturated, during times of childbearing, child rearing, crisis, and illness, a person may rely on old cultural patterns (Ramer, 1992).

Assimilation, on the other hand, refers to when a cultural group loses its identity and becomes a part of the dominant culture. According to Friedman (1998), "assimilation denotes the more complete and one-way process of one culture being absorbed into the other." Assimilation is the process by which groups "melt" into the mainstream, thus accounting for the notion of a "melting pot," a phenomenon that has been said to occur in the United States. In contrast, Spector (1996) asserts that in the United States, the melting pot, with its dream of a common culture, "has proved to be a myth and faded; it is now time to identify the mosaic phenomenon and both accept and appreciate the differences among people."

A wide range of cultural diversity exists within society. The health care provider striving to provide culturally appropriate health care must assess the beliefs and practices of the client. Nurses must also be aware of factors that may prevent some health care practitioners from providing op-

timal care. Understanding the concepts of ethnocentrism and cultural relativism may help nurses care for families in a multicultural society.

Ethnocentrism refers to "the view that one's culture's way of doing things is the right and natural way" (Galanti, 1997). Essentially, ethnocentrism supports the notion "my group is best." Although the United States is a culturally diverse nation, the prevailing practice of health care is based on the beliefs and practices held by members of the dominant culture, primarily Caucasians of European descent. This practice is based on the biomedical model that represents pregnancy and childbirth as phenomena with inherent risk most appropriately managed through specific knowledge and technology. When encountering behavior in women unfamiliar with this model, the nurse may become frustrated and impatient. The nurse may label the women's behavior inappropriate and believe that it conflicts with "good" health practices. If this system, the Western health care system, provides the nurse's only standard for judgment, the behavior of the nurse is called *ethnocentric.*

Cultural relativism, the opposite of ethnocentrism, refers to learning about and applying the standards of another person's culture to activities within that culture. To be culturally relativistic, the nurse recognizes that people from different cultural backgrounds comprehend the same objects and situations differently. In other words, culture determines a person's viewpoints.

Cultural relativism does not require nurses to *accept* the beliefs and values of another culture; rather nurses recognize that others' behavior may be based on a system of logic different from their own. Cultural relativism affirms the uniqueness and value of every culture. Spector (1996) states that "because health care providers learn from their culture the way and the how of being healthy or ill, it be-

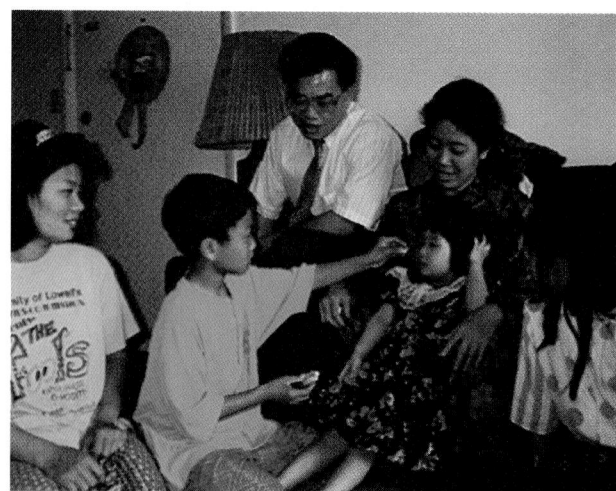

Fig. 2-4 Southeast Asian families may be large and closely spaced. They are often a closely knit group. *(From Dickason, E., Silverman, B., & Kaplan, J. [1998]. Maternal-infant nursing care [3rd ed.]. St. Louis: Mosby.)*

hooves them to treat each patient with deference to his own cultural background."

Childbearing Beliefs and Practices

Nurses working with childbearing families in the United States and Canada care for families from different cultures and ethnic groups (Fig. 2-4). To provide culturally competent care, the nurse should be aware of the cultural beliefs and practices important to individual families. Countless beliefs and practices stem from a religious or an ethnic origin and may be observed by families with differing cultural backgrounds. Spector (1995) observed that people who have maintained a strong sense of their heritage may hold onto traditional health beliefs.

A nurse should consider the products of culture, including communication, space, time, and family roles, when working with childbearing families (Giger & Davidhizar, 1995). Communication often creates the most difficult problem for nurses working with clients from diverse cultural groups. Communication includes understanding not only the individual's language, varied dialect, and style, but also volume of speech and meaning of touch and gestures. Whenever the client, family, or both do not speak the same language as the nurse, the nurse can use an interpreter to address the family's health care needs in a culturally competent manner. When using an interpreter, the nurse respects the family by addressing questions to them and not the interpreter (Box 2-1).

BOX 2-1 Working with a Translator

STEP 1: BEFORE THE INTERVIEW

A. Outline your statements and questions. List the key pieces of information you want/need to know.
B. Learn something about the culture so that you can converse informally with the translator.

STEP 2: MEETING WITH THE TRANSLATOR

A. Introduce yourself to the translator and converse informally. This is the time to find out how well he or she speaks English. No matter how proficient or what age the translator is, be respectful. Some ways to show respect are to ask a cultural question to acknowledge that you can learn from the translator, or you could learn one word or phrase from the translator.
B. Emphasize that you do want the client to ask questions because some cultures consider this inappropriate behavior.
C. Make sure the translator is comfortable with the technical terms you need to use. If not, take some time to explain them.

STEP 3: DURING THE INTERVIEW

A. Ask your questions and explain your statements (see Step 1).
B. Make sure that the translator understands which parts of the interview are most important. You usually have limited time with the translator, and you want to have adequate time at the end for client questions.
C. Try to get a "feel" for how much is "getting through." No matter what the language is, if in relating information to the client the translator uses far fewer or far more words than you do, "something else" is going on.
D. Stop every now and then and ask the translator, "How is it going?" You may not get a totally accu-

rate answer, but you will have emphasized to the translator your strong desire to focus on the task at hand. If there are language problems: (1) speak *slowly;* (2) use gestures (e.g., fingers to count or point to body parts); and (3) use pictures.
E. Ask the translator to elicit questions. This may be difficult, but it is worth the effort.
F. Identify cultural issues that may conflict with your requests or instructions.
G. Use the translator to help problem solve, or at least give insight into possibilities for solutions.

STEP 4: AFTER THE INTERVIEW

A. Speak to the translator and try to get an idea of what went well and what could be improved. This will help you to be more effective with this or another translator.
B. Make notes on what you learned for your future reference or to help a colleague.

Remember:
Your interview is a *collaboration* between you and the translator. *Listen* as well as speak.

Notes:
1. The translator may be a child, grandchild, or sibling of the client. Be sensitive to the fact that the child is playing an adult role.
2. Be sensitive to cultural and situational differences (e.g., an interview with someone from urban Germany will likely be different from an interview with someone from a transitional refugee camp).
3. Younger females telling older males what to do may be a problem for both a female nurse and a female translator. This is not the time to pioneer new gender relations. Be aware that in some cultures it is difficult for a woman to talk about some topics with a husband or a father present.

Courtesy Elizabeth Whalley, PhD, San Francisco State University.

Personal space needs and feelings of territoriality develop in a cultural setting. Although personal space varies from person to person and with the situation, the dimensions of comfort zones differ from culture to culture. Actions such as touching, placing the client in proximity to others, taking away personal possessions, and making decisions for the client can decrease personal security and heighten anxiety. On the other hand, if nurses respect the need for distance, they allow the client to maintain control over personal space and support the client's autonomy, thereby increasing the client's sense of security. For example, since Chinese-Americans have traditionally been a noncontact group, some may consider closeness, increased eye contact, and touch offensive or impolite. Nurses can avoid misunderstandings by providing explanations whenever performing tasks that require close contact (Chang, 1995). Nurses often use touch, especially in areas such as labor and delivery. The acceptance and effectiveness of these approaches must be considered in a cultural context.

Nurses must also understand time as it pertains to culture. People in cultural groups may be oriented to the past, present, or future. People who focus on the past strive to maintain tradition and have little motivation for formulating future goals. Some individuals who focus on the present neither save for the future nor appreciate the past; these individuals do not necessarily adhere to strict schedules. Individuals oriented to the future use the present to achieve future goals.

The time orientation of the childbearing family may affect nursing care. For example, talking to a family about bringing the infant to the clinic for follow-up examinations (events in the future) may be difficult for the family that focuses on the present. On the other hand, a family with a future-oriented sense of time, in which events are planned, may be more likely to return as scheduled for follow-up visits. Despite the differences in time orientation, each family may be equally concerned for the well-being of its newborn.

Family roles involve the expectations and behaviors associated with a member's position in the family (e.g., mother, father, or grandparent). Social class and cultural norms also affect these roles; distinct roles for men and women may be stressed. For example, culture may influence whether a man actively participates in the pregnancy and childbirth. The way that health care practitioners manage this family's care in turn molds its experience in and perception of the Western health care system. Maternity care practitioners expect fathers to be involved, but this role expectation may conflict with that of Mexican-Americans and Arab-Americans, who usually view the birthing experience as a female affair (see Cultural Considerations box).

The nurse must be familiar with each woman as an individual and validate her cultural beliefs. The nurse supports and nurtures the beliefs that promote physical or emotional adaptation to childbearing. However, if certain beliefs might be harmful, the nurse should carefully explore them with the woman and use them in the reeducation and modification process.

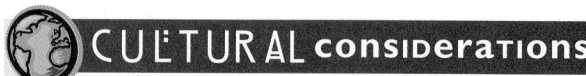

CULTURAL consiDerations

Questions to Obtain Cultural Explanations About Childbearing

1. What do you and your family think you should do to remain healthy during pregnancy?
2. What are the things you can do or not do to improve your health and the health of your infant?
3. Who do you want with you during your labor?
4. What things or actions are important to you and your family after the infant's birth?
5. What do you and your family expect from the nurse or nurses caring for you?
6. How will family members participate in your pregnancy, childbirth, and parenting?

Table 2-2 provides examples of some cultural beliefs and practices regarding childbearing among European-Americans (Caucasians), Hispanics, Asian-Americans, African-Americans, and Native Americans. Most of these cultural beliefs and customs reflect the traditional culture and are not universally practiced by all members of the cultural group in every part of the country. Callister (1995) states that "stereotypical assumptions should not be made based on identified sociocultural-spiritual affiliations; rather, there is a need for sensitivity to the individual family, who may uniquely apply cultural background to their lives." Variables such as an individual subculture within the primary group, degree of acculturation, educational and income levels, and amount of contact with the older generations influence the extent to which people practice these customs. Women from these cultural and ethnic groups may adhere to some, all, or none of the practices listed.

In planning the care of a family or an individual family member, the nurse may find it useful to view the family at a developmental phase in the life cycle, facing stressful life events, and operating as a system. A family assessment tool such as the one outlined by Friedman (1998) (Fig. 2-5, p. 28) can be used as a guide for assessing aspects of the family discussed in this chapter, including family development, family structure, family functions, and family stress and coping. Specific data within each area can provide valuable information for planning care.

No one family member has a problem; if a problem exists, the whole family has a problem. The best solutions evolve through family participation when the nurse uses knowledge of family dynamics and culture and works with the family as a unit.

TABLE 2-2 Traditional* Cultural Beliefs and Practices

PREGNANCY	CHILDBIRTH	PARENTING

HISPANIC

(Members of the Hispanic community have their origins in Spain, Cuba, Central and South America, Mexico, Puerto Rico, and other Spanish-speaking countries. These beliefs are based primarily on knowledge of Mexican-Americans.)

PREGNANCY	**Labor** / **Postpartum period**	**Newborn**
Pregnancy is desired soon after marriage. Prenatal care is sought late. Expectant mother is influenced strongly by mother or mother-in-law. Cool air in motion is considered dangerous during pregnancy. Unsatisfied food cravings cause birthmarks. Some pica is observed in eating ashes or dirt (not common). Milk is avoided because it causes large infants and difficult births. Many predictions are made about sex of the infant. It may be unacceptable and frightening to have pelvic examination by a male health care provider. Women use herbs to treat common complaints of pregnancy. Drinking chamomile tea is thought to ensure effective labor.	**Labor** Use of "partera" or lay midwife is preferred in some places; expectant mother may prefer presence of mother rather than husband. After birth of infant, mother's legs are brought together to prevent air from entering the uterus. Loud behavior occurs during labor. **Postpartum period** Diet may be restricted after birth; for first 2 days, only boiled milk and toasted tortillas are permitted. (These are special foods to restore warmth to the body.) Mother has bed rest for 3 days after birth. Mother is to keep warm and delay bathing. Mother's head and feet are protected from cold air; bathing is permitted after 14 days. Mother is often cared for by her own mother. There is 40-day restriction on sexual intercourse.	**Newborn** Breastfeeding begins after third day; colostrum may be considered "filthy" or "spoiled"; belief that there is no milk. Olive or castor oil is given to stimulate passage of meconium. Male infant is not circumcised. Female infant's ears are pierced. Belly band is used to prevent umbilical hernia. Religious medal worn by mother during pregnancy is placed around the infant's neck. Infant is protected from "evil eye." Various remedies are used to treat "mal ojo" and fallen fontanel (depressed fontanel).

AFRICAN-AMERICAN

(Members of the African-American culture have their origins in Africa, many of whom are descendants of slaves. Today a number of blacks have immigrated from Africa, the West Indian Islands, the Dominican Republic, Haiti, and Jamaica. The following beliefs are based primarily on knowledge of southern, rural African-Americans.)

PREGNANCY	**Labor**	**Newborn**
Acceptance of pregnancy depends on economic status. Pregnancy is thought to be state of "wellness," which is often reason for delay in seeking prenatal care, especially by lower-income African-Americans.	Use of "Granny midwife" occurs in certain parts of the United States. Varied emotional responses occur: some cry out, whereas some display stoic behavior to avoid calling attention to themselves.	Feeding is very important: "Good" infant eats well. Early introduction of solid foods occurs. Mother may breastfeed or bottle feed; breastfeeding may be considered embarrassing. Parents fear spoiling infant.

Data compiled from Amaro (1994), Bar-Yam (1994), Galanti (1997), Geissler (1994), Mattson (1995), Spector (1996), Williams (1989). See also Lipson, Dibble, and Minarik (1996).

*Variations exist in some beliefs and practices within subcultures. Most of these cultural beliefs and customs reflect the traditional culture and are not universally practiced. These lists are not intended to stereotype clients; rather they serve as guidelines while discussing meaningful cultural beliefs with a client and her family. Examples of other cultural beliefs and practices are found throughout this text.

Continued

TABLE 2-2 Traditional* Cultural Beliefs and Practices—cont'd

PREGNANCY	CHILDBIRTH	PARENTING
Old wives' tales include the following: having picture taken during pregnancy will cause stillbirth and reaching up will cause cord to strangle baby.	Emotional support is often provided by other women, especially own mother.	Client may arrive at hospital in far-advanced labor.
Mother may crave certain foods, including chicken, greens, clay, starch, and dirt.	**Postpartum period**	Parents commonly call infant by nicknames.
Pregnancy may be viewed by men as sign of virility.	Vaginal bleeding may be seen as sign of sickness; tub baths and shampooing of hair are prohibited.	Parents may use excessive clothing to keep infant warm.
Self-treatment occurs for various discomforts of pregnancy, including constipation, nausea, vomiting, headache, and heartburn.	Sassafras tea is thought to have healing power.	Belly band is used to prevent umbilical hernia.
	Eating liver is thought to cause heavier vaginal bleeding because of its high "blood" content.	Large amounts of oil are used on infant's scalp and skin.
		Strong feeling of family, community, and religion exists.

ASIAN

(The term *Asian* commonly refers to groups from China; Korea; the Philippines; Japan; and Southeast Asia, particularly Thailand, Indochina, and Vietnam.)

Pregnancy is considered time when mother "has happiness in her body."	**Labor**	**Newborn**
Pregnancy is seen as natural process.	Mother is attended by other women, especially her own mother.	Birth of boy is preferred.
Strong preference for female health care provider exists.	Father does not actively participate.	Parents may delay naming child.
Mother believes in theory of hot and cold.	Labor occurs in silence.	Some groups (e.g., Vietnamese) believe colostrum is dirty; therefore they may delay breastfeeding until milk comes in; belief that there is no milk.
Mother may omit soy sauce from diet to prevent dark-skinned baby.	Cesarean birth is not welcome.	
Mother prefers soup made with ginseng root as general strength tonic.	**Postpartum period**	
Milk is usually excluded from diet; is thought to cause stomach distress.	Mother must protect herself from yin (cold forces) for 30 days.	
Inactivity or sleeping late is thought to cause difficult birth.	Ambulation is limited.	
	Shower and bathing are prohibited.	
	Warm environment to restore warmth to body.	
	Diet:	
	Warm fluids.	
	Some clients are vegetarians.	
	Korean mother is served seaweed soup with rice.	
	Chinese diet is high in hot foods.	
	Chinese mother avoids fruits and vegetables.	
	Concept of family is important and valued.	
	Father is head of household; wife plays subordinate role.	

TABLE 2-2   Traditional* Cultural Beliefs and Practices—cont'd

PREGNANCY	CHILDBIRTH	PARENTING

CAUCASIAN/EUROPEAN-AMERICANS

(These beliefs are based primarily on knowledge of European-Americans.)

Pregnancy is viewed as condition that requires medical attention to ensure health.
Emphasis is placed on early prenatal care.
Variety of childbirth education programs are available, and participation is encouraged.
Technology driven.
Emphasis is placed on nutritional science.
Involvement of the father is valued.
Written information is valued.

Labor
Birth is public concern.
Technology dominated.
Birthing process in institutional setting is valued.
Varied emotional response; stoic or cry out.
Involvement of the father is expected.
Physician is seen as head of team.

Postpartum period
Emphasis or focus on early bonding occurs.
Medical interventions for dealing with discomfort are valued.
Early ambulation and activity are emphasized.
Self-care is valued.

Newborn
Breastfeeding has increased in popularity.
Breastfeeding begins as soon as possible after childbirth.

Parenting
Motherhood and transition to parenting are seen as stressful times.
Nuclear family is valued, although single parenting and other forms of parenting are more acceptable than in past.
Women often deal with multiple roles.
Early return to prepregnancy activities occurs.

NATIVE AMERICAN

(There are many different tribes within the Native American culture; viewpoints vary according to tribal customs and beliefs.)

Pregnancy is considered as normal, natural process.
Prenatal care is late.
Mother avoids heavy lifting.
Herb teas are encouraged.

Labor
Mother prefers female attendant, although husband, mother, or father may assist with birth.
Birth may be attended by whole family.
Herbs may be used to promote uterine activity.
Birth may occur in squatting position.

Postpartum period
Herb teas are used to stop bleeding.

Newborn
Infant is not fed colostrum.
Use of herbs increases flow of milk.
Cradle boards are used for infant.
Babies are not handled often.

The Friedman Family Assessment Model (Short Form)

Identifying Data

1. Family name
2. Address and phone
3. Family composition
4. Type of family form
5. Cultural (ethnic) background
6. Religious identification
7. Social class status
8. Family's recreational or leisure-time activities

Developmental Stage and History of Family

9. Family's present developmental stage
10. Extent of family developmental tasks fulfillment
11. Nuclear family history
12. History of family of origin of both parents

Environmental Data

13. Characteristics of home
14. Characteristics of neighborhood and larger community
15. Family's geographical mobility
16. Family's associations and transactions with community
17. Family's social support system or network (See Fig. 2-6.)

Family Structure

18. Communication patterns
    Extent of functional and dysfunctional communication (types of recurring patterns)
    Extent of emotional (affective) messages and how expressed
    Characteristics of communication within family subsystems
    Extent of congruent and incongruent messages
    Types of dysfunctional communication processes seen in family
    Areas of open and closed communication
    Familial and contextual variables affecting communication
19. Power structure
    Power outcomes
    Decision-making process
    Power bases
    Variables affecting family power
    Overall family system and subsystem power
    (Family power continuum placement)
20. Role structure
    Formal role structure
    Informal role structure
    Analysis of role models (optional)
    Variables affecting role structure
21. Family values
    Compare the family to American or family's reference group values and/or identify important family values and their importance (priority) in family.
    Congruence between the family's values and the family's reference group or wider community

Congruence between the family's values and family member's values
Variables influencing family values
Values consciously or unconsciously held
Presence of value conflicts in family
Effect of the above values and value conflicts on health status of family

Family Functions

22. Affective function
    Family's need–response patterns
    Mutual nurturance, closeness, and identification
    Separateness and connectedness
23. Socialization function
    Family child-rearing practices
    Adaptability of child-rearing practices for family form and family's situation
    Who is (are) socializing agent(s) for child(ren)?
    Value of children in family
    Cultural beliefs that influence family's child-rearing patterns
    Social class influence on child-rearing patterns
    Estimation about whether family is at risk for child-rearing problems and if so, indication of high risk factors
    Adequacy of home environment for children's need to play
24. Health care function
    Family's health beliefs, values, and behavior
    Family's definitions of health–illness and their level of knowledge
    Family's perceived health status and illness susceptibility
    Family's dietary practices
    Adequacy of family diet (recommended 3-day food history record).
    Function of mealtimes and attitudes toward food and mealtimes.
    Shopping (and its planning) practices.
    Person(s) responsible for planning, shopping, and preparation of meals.
    Sleep and rest habits
    Physical activity and recreation practices (not covered earlier)
    Family's drug habits
    Family's role in self-care practices
    Medically based preventive measures (physicals, eye and hearing tests, and immunizations)
    Dental health practices
    Family health history (both general and specific diseases—environmentally and genetically related)
    Health care services received
    Feelings and perceptions regarding health services
    Emergency health services
    Source of payments for health and other services
    Logistics of receiving care

Family Stress and Coping

25. Short- and long-term familial stressors and strengths
26. Extent of family's ability to respond, based on objective appraisal of stress-producing situations
27. Coping strategies utilized (present/past)
    Differences in family members' ways of coping
    Family's inner coping strategies
    Family's external coping strategies
28. Dysfunctional adaptive strategies utilized (present/past; extent of usage)

Family Composition Form

Name (last, first)	Gender	Relationship	Date/place of birth	Occupation	Education
1. (Father)					
2. (Mother)					
3. (Oldest child)					
4.					
5.					
6.					
7.					
8.					

Fig. 2-5 The Friedman Family Assessment Model (Short Form). *(From Friedman, M. [1998]. Family nursing theory and assessment [4th ed.]. New York: Appleton & Lange.)*

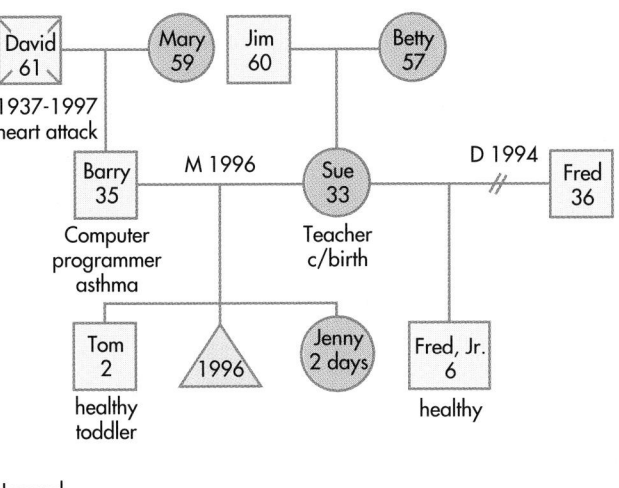

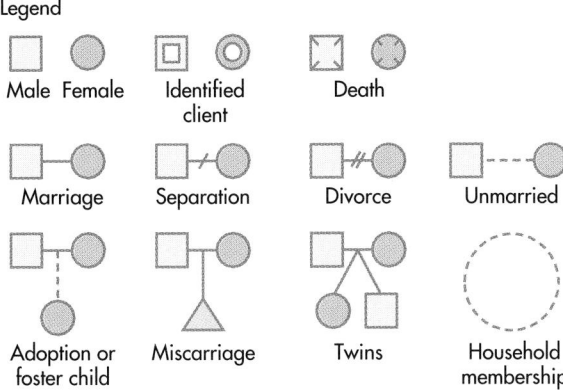

Fig. 2-6 Example of a family genogram.

CRITICAL THINKING EXERCISES

1 *Using one of the family theories discussed in this chapter (family systems theory, developmental theory, family stress theory), explain how you would assess family function and dynamics for families representing various family forms.*

2 *In a prenatal clinic, interview families from various cultural backgrounds. Determine their expectations of the childbearing experience. Discuss strategies and possible interventions for providing culturally competent care to these families during the childbearing cycle.*

KEY POINTS

- Contemporary American society recognizes and accepts a variety of family forms.

- The family is a social network that acts as an important support system for its members.

- Ideally, the family provides a safe, intimate environment for the biopsychosocial development of its children and adult members.

- The family systems, developmental, and stress theories provide nurses with useful guidelines for understanding family function.

- Family socioeconomics, response to stress, and culture are key factors influencing family health.

- The reproductive beliefs and practices of a culture are embedded in its economic, religious, kinship, and political structures.

- The expression of parental roles and the way that children are viewed reflect cultural differences.

- To provide quality care to women in their childbearing years and beyond, nurses should be aware of the cultural beliefs and practices important to individual families.

References

Amaro, H. (1994). Women in the Mexican-American community: Religion, culture, and reproductive attitudes and experiences. *J Comp Psychol* 16(1), 6-19.

Bar-Yam, N. (1994). Learning about culture: A guide for birth practitioners. *Int J Childbirth Educ* 9(2), 8-10.

Bianchi, S. (1994). The changing demographics and socioeconomic characteristics of single-parent families. In S. Hanson & S. Boyd (Eds.). *Family health care nursing: Theory, practice and research*. Philadelphia: F.A. Davis.

Boss, P. (1996). *Family stress management* (2nd ed.). Newbury Park, CA: Sage.

Callister, L. (1995). Cultural meanings of childbirth. *J Obstet Gynecol Neonatal Nurs* 24(4), 327-331.

Carter, B., & McGoldrick, M. (1988). *The changing family life cycle: A framework for family therapy* (2nd ed.). Needham Heights, MA: Allyn & Bacon.

Chang, K. (1995). Chinese Americans. In J. Giger & R. Davidhizar (Eds.). *Transcultural nursing: Assessment and interventions* (2nd ed.). St. Louis: Mosby.

Cox, R. (1997). Family health care delivery for the 21st century. *J Obstet Gynecol Neonatal Nurs* 26(1), 109-118.

Dickason, E., Silverman, B., & Kaplan, J. (1998). *Maternal-infant nursing care* (3rd ed.). St. Louis: Mosby.

Duvall, E. (1977). *Marriage and family development* (5th ed.). Philadelphia: J.B. Lippincott.

Erikson, E. (1968). *Identity: Youth and crisis*. New York: W.W. Norton.

Evolving American family. (1993). *Stat Bull* 74, 2.

Friedman, M. (1998). *Family nursing theory and assessment* (4th ed.). New York: Appleton & Lange.

Galanti, G. (1997). *Caring for patients from different cultures: Case studies from American hospitals*. Philadelphia: University of Pennsylvania.

Geissler, E. (1994). *Pocket guide to cultural assessment*. St. Louis: Mosby.

Giger, J., & Davidhizar, R. (1995). *Transcultural nursing: Assessment and interventions* (2nd ed.). St. Louis: Mosby.

Hanson, S., & Boyd, S. (Eds.). (1996). *Family health care nursing: Theory, practice and research*. Philadelphia: F.A. Davis.

Helman, C. (1990). *Culture, health and illness*. London: Wright.

Hill, R. (1949). *Families under stress*. New York: Harper & Row.

Laird, J. (1993). Lesbian and gay families. In F. Walsh (Ed.). *Normal family processes* (2nd ed.). New York: Guilford.

Lipson, J., Dibble, S., & Minarik, P. (1996). *Culture and nursing care: A pocket guide*. San Francisco: UCSF Nursing Press.

Mattson, S. (1995). Culturally sensitive prenatal care for Southeastern Asians. *J Obstet Gynecol Neonatal Nurs* 24(4), 335-341.

Mercer, R. (1989). Theoretical perspective on the family. In C. Gillis et al. (Eds.). *Toward a science of family nursing*. California: Addison-Wesley.

Quimby, S. (1994). Women and the family of the future. *J Obstet Gynecol Neonatal Nurs* 23(2), 113-123.

Ramer, L. (1992). *Culturally sensitive caregiving and childbearing families*. New York: March of Dimes Birth Defects Foundation.

Spector, R. (1995). Cultural concepts of women's health and health promoting behaviors. *J Obstet Gynecol Neonatal Nurs* 24(3), 241-245.

Spector, R. (1996). *Cultural diversity in health and illness* (4th ed.). New York: Appleton & Lange.

Visher, E., & Visher, J. (1993). Remarried families and stepparenting. In F. Walsh (Ed.). *Normal family processes* (2nd ed.). New York: Guilford.

Walsh, F. (1993). Conceptualization of normal family processes. In F. Walsh (Ed.). *Normal family processes* (2nd ed.). New York: Guilford.

Williams, R. (1989). Issues in women's health care. In B. Johnson (Ed.). *Psychiatric mental health nursing: Adaptation and growth*. Philadelphia: J.B. Lippincott.

Wright, L., & Leahey, M. (1994). *Nurses and families* (2nd ed.). Philadelphia: F.A. Davis.

3

Community and Home Care

Jane G. Conner

LEARNING OBJECTIVES

- Define the key terms.
- Compare community-based health care and community health (population or aggregate focused) care.
- Select appropriate methods of community assessment for specific situations.
- List health indicators of community health status and their relevance to perinatal health care.
- Explain how age, gender, socioeconomic status, health status, and life experiences can predispose people to vulnerability.
- Discuss perinatal concerns and related nursing interventions for selected vulnerable populations: homeless, migrant laborers, and refugees.
- Define *service learning* and describe opportunities across the perinatal health continuum.

- List the potential advantages and disadvantages of home visits.
- Explore telephonic nursing care options in perinatal nursing.
- Describe the way home care fits into the maternity continuum of care.
- Discuss types of agencies providing home care.
- Identify and define common perinatal conditions amenable to home care.
- Discuss safety and infection control principles as they apply to the care of clients in their homes.
- Describe the nurse's role in perinatal home care.
- Identify topics for nursing research related to perinatal home care.

KEY TERMS

aggregates
census data
clinical integration
community
community-as-partner
home health care
homeless

key informants
levels of prevention
Medicaid
migrant laborers
participant observation
proprietary agencies
refugees

surveys
service learning
telephonic nursing
third-party payers
vulnerable populations
windshield (or walking) survey

In the past, nurses have been employed primarily in hospitals, and the content of nursing textbooks has reflected that. However, most health care actually occurs outside of secondary and tertiary institutions, in primary care facilities or clients' homes. In the future hospitals will assume a smaller role, limiting their services to technologically complex care for the acutely ill.

The movement to reduce health care costs has shortened hospitalization time and led to exploration of home- and community-based options for the provision of care

(Henry, 1997). Attention to the role of health care providers in community-oriented health promotion and disease prevention activities is increasing (Expert Panel on Women's Health, 1997; Zyzanski, Williams, & Flocke, 1996). Managed care organizations have a vested interest in maintaining the health of all of their members, not just those who present themselves for care. Publication of the U.S. national health objectives in *Healthy People 2000* and *Healthy Communities 2000* focused attention on the unequal distribution of disease and disability and the need to reach out to vulnerable populations not being adequately served by the current health system. *Healthy People 2010* will continue the focus on health goals. Hospital-based nurses are increasingly involved in follow-up of clients and families after discharge (Fowler et al., 1997). Professional organizations cite the need for all nurses to be prepared to function in community settings and hospitals (Zotti, Brown, & Stotts, 1996). Chapter 2 provided an overview of

family and cultural theory and assessment. In this chapter we discuss the larger system of which the family is a part— the community. Methods of community assessment and the special perinatal health needs of vulnerable aggregates in the population are identified. Guidelines and issues related to the provision of home care for clients across the perinatal continuum are included.

ASSESSING LEVELS OF COMMUNITY WELLNESS

Definitions of Community

There are many definitions of **community,** but most share three characteristics: people, place, and interaction or function. We are all simultaneously part of several communities, such as an ethnic or religious group or a professional organization, but this discussion is limited to geographically based communities. The people are the

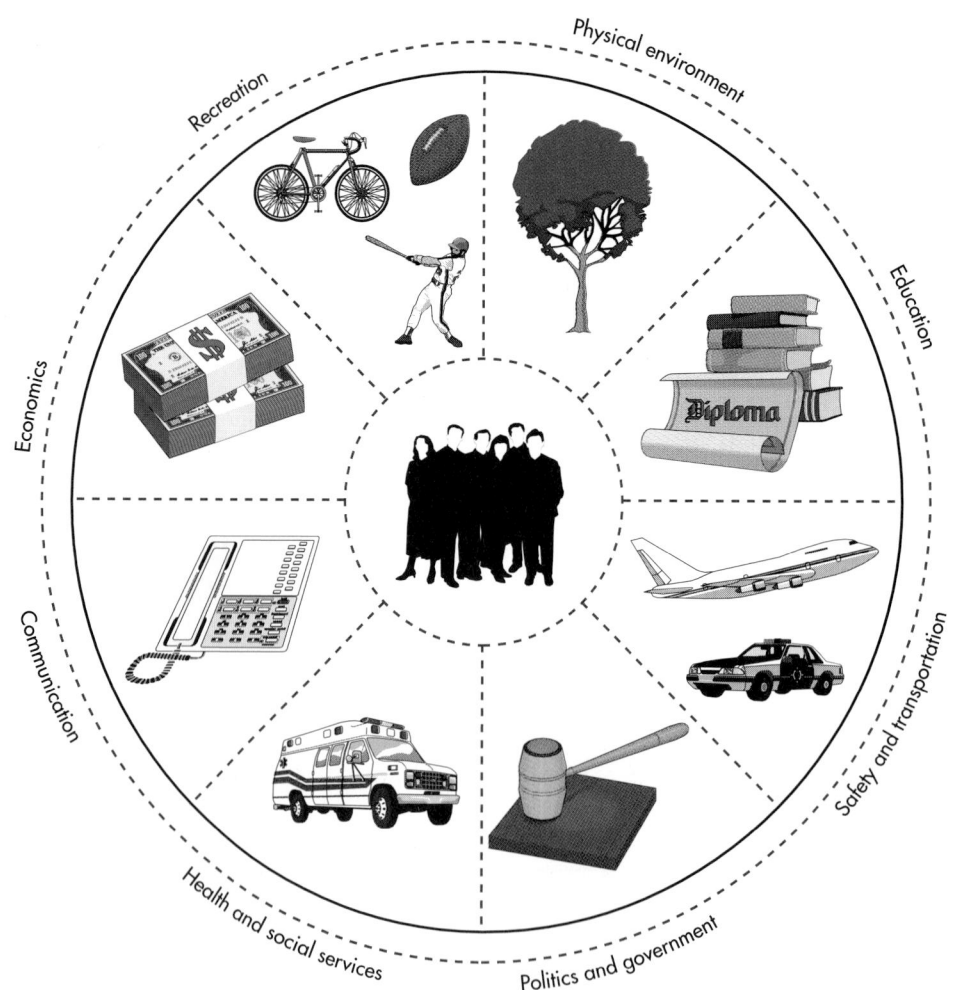

Fig. 3-1 The community assessment wheel, the assessment segment of the community-as-partner model. *(From Anderson, E., & McFarlane, J. [1996]. Community-as-partner: Theory and practice in nursing [2nd ed.]. Philadelphia: J.B. Lippincott.)*

residents of the community; place refers to geographic dimensions; function refers to the activities of the community that meet the needs of the residents (Schuster & Goeppinger, 1996). Figure 3-1 shows the core of the community surrounded by the multiple systems that serve to meet their collective needs. The people who reside there make up the core of the community. Significant characteristics include the demographics of the population and their values, beliefs, and culture. As residents of the community, the people affect, and are influenced by, the subsystems of the community. Economics, education, public safety, environmental factors, and availability of health and social services all have significant impact on community health and well-being. The broken lines between the segments emphasize the interaction and interdependence among the subsystems of the community (Anderson & McFarlane, 1996).

Methods of Community Assessment

Perinatal Health Strategies for the 21st Century (Maternal Child Health Bureau, 1992), a plan produced by a federally funded expert panel, has as one of its basic principles that the organization and focus of perinatal care at the community level must be responsive to the unique characteristics of the populations and their special needs.

Multiple sources of data about communities are available. The extent and nature of the assessment to be performed depends on the time and resources available and the way the information is to be used. A nurse who is providing family-focused home care may be primarily interested in becoming familiar with the neighborhoods and resources with which his or her clients interact. A community health agency must conduct a comprehensive needs assessment in order to plan and evaluate health services for the community as a whole. A variety of methods may be used to obtain both the community's perceptions of its strengths and problems and quantitative analyses of health and well-being, which can be compared with state and national statistics. Methods of data collection include windshield survey, participant observation, interviews, focus groups, analysis of existing data, and surveys.

Using one's senses while traveling through a community is the essence of the **windshield (or walking) survey** (Table 3-1). By focusing skills of observation during a trip through a community, a nurse can obtain significant information about its sociocultural characteristics and the environment, housing, transportation, and local community agencies. Using **participant observation,** in which nurses are part of the situation they wish to learn about, it is possible to more fully understand the people and processes involved and to validate perceptions and inferences. **Service learning** is one type of participant observation (Box 3-1).

Every 10 years the U.S. government conducts a national census. **Census data** offer a broad range of information that is extremely helpful to nurses and other health care providers who wish to become familiar with a community. Data include population size, age, sex and ethnic distribution, socioeconomic status, educational level, employment, and housing characteristics. Reports are available in libraries, in print, on CD-ROM, and through the Internet. Summaries are prepared for municipalities; large metropolitan areas; zip codes; and the smallest unit, a census tract. A census tract is a portion of a larger urban area, usually consisting of 3000 to 6000 persons and often corresponding to a neighborhood. Depending on the density of the population, this can be a few square blocks or several square miles. Looking at individual census tracts helps to identify subpopulations, or **aggregates,** with differing needs that would be obscured by the statistics gathered on the entire community. Census tract–level data on socioeconomic status and environmental stressors have been used to identify women at risk for delivery of a low-birth-weight (LBW) infant. Based on this information, outreach activities can be appropriately targeted (O'Campo et al., 1997).

Vital Statistics and Other Sources of Health Data

Official records of births and deaths are reported annually for the preceding year by city, county, and state health departments. In addition to the number of births and deaths, certificates include the type of birth and any complications, as well as causes of death. Local health departments compile extensive statistics about the incidence of communicable and other diseases within their jurisdictions. The National Center for Health Statistics publishes annual National Health Survey data, which describe health trends on a national sample. Many state and local government reports from health and planning agencies provide data that assist the nurse in assessing the community. Hospitals and voluntary agencies may conduct detailed assessments focused on a particular health area. The March of Dimes Birth Defects Foundation, for example, has supported perinatal needs assessments in many communities across the United States. Other local sources of information include the Chamber of Commerce, newspapers, community center newsletters, libraries, public safety agencies, school districts, and the American Red Cross.

Interviews with selected individuals in positions of leadership, **key informants,** allow input from many different perspectives. Persons such as health care providers or administrators, religious leaders, government officials, representatives of voluntary health organizations, service clubs, and cultural groups can provide an "insider's" viewpoint not available in published documents. Similarly, focus groups can be conducted with potential clients or collaborators to discuss needs and services important to the community. Using structured open-ended questions, exploration of community strengths and needs can be

TABLE 3-1 Windshield Survey Components

ELEMENT	DESCRIPTION
Housing and zoning	What is the age of the houses, their architecture, of what materials are they constructed? Are all the neighborhood houses similar in age, architecture? How would you characterize the differences? Are they detached from or connected to others? Do they have space in front and behind? What is their general condition? Are there signs of disrepair—broken doors, windows, leaks, locks missing? Is there central heating, modern plumbing, air conditioning?
Open space	How much open space is there? What is the quality of the space—green parks or rubble-filled lots? What is the lot size of the houses? Lawns? Flower boxes? Do you see trees on the pavements, a green island in the center of the streets? Is the open space public or private? Used by whom?
Boundaries	What signs are there of where this neighborhood begins and ends? Are the boundaries natural—a river, a different terrain? Physical—a highway, railroad? Economic—difference, in real estate or presence of industrial, commercial units along with residential? The neighborhood has an identity, a name? Do you see it displayed? Are there unofficial names?
"Commons"	What are the neighborhood hangouts? For what groups, at what hours (e.g., schoolyard, candy store, bar, restaurant, park, 24-hour drugstore)? Does the "commons" have a sense of "territoriality" or is it open to the stranger?
Transportation	How do people get in and out of the neighborhood? Car, bus, bike, walk, etc.? Are the streets and roads conducive to good transportation and also to community life? Is there a major highway near the neighborhood? Whom does it serve? How frequent is public transportation available?
Service centers	Do you see social agencies, clients, recreation centers, signs of activity at the schools? Are there offices of doctors, dentists? Palmists, spiritualists, etc.? Parks? Are they in use?
Stores	Where do residents shop? Shopping centers, neighborhood stores? How do they travel to shop?
Street people	If you are traveling during the day, who do you see on the street? An occasional housewife, a mother with a baby? Do you see anyone you would not expect? Teenagers, unemployed males? Can you spot a welfare worker, an insurance collector, a door-to-door salesman? Is the dress of those you see representative or unexpected? Along with people, what animals do you see? Stray cats, dogs, pedigreed pets, "watchdogs"?
Signs of decay	Is this neighborhood on the way up or down? Is it "alive"? How would you decide? Trash, abandoned cars, political posters, neighborhood meeting posters, real estate signs, abandoned houses, mixed-zoning usage?
Race	Are the residents white, black, Asian,* or is the area integrated?
Ethnicity	Are there indices of ethnicity—food stores, churches, private schools, information in a language other than English?
Religion	Of what religion are the residents? Do you see evidence of heterogeneity or homogeneity? What denomination are the churches? Do you see evidence of their use other than on Sunday mornings?
Health and morbidity	Do you see evidence of acute or of chronic diseases or conditions? Of accidents, communicable diseases, alcoholism, drug addiction, mental illness, etc.? How far is it to the nearest hospital? Clinic?
Politics	Do you see any political campaign posters? Is there a headquarters present? Do you see any evidence of a predominant party affiliation?
Media	Do you see outdoor TV antennas? What magazines, newspapers do residents read? Do you see Forward Times, Hampton Post, Enquirer, Readers' Digest in the stores? What media seem most important to the residents? Radio? TV?

Source: Anderson, E., & McFarlane, J. (1996). *Community as partner: Theory and practice in nursing* (2nd ed.). Philadelphia: J.B. Lippincott.
*Added by author.

facilitated. Formal **surveys,** either by mail, telephone, or face-to-face, are expensive and time consuming but can be sources of information not available from secondary sources. Knowledge of support groups, educational programs, and social service agencies allows the nurse to make appropriate referrals for perinatal clients. Information about community resources may be obtained from many of the sources listed previously, as well as the local United Way organization, telephone directory, or community services directory.

BOX 3-1 Service Learning

In 1990 Congress established the Federal Corporation for National and Community Service. Students from elementary through higher education are encouraged to participate in meaningful volunteer efforts that help them to develop knowledge, "character, skills and self-confidence while making their own unique contributions to the life of their communities" (Clinton, 1998).

Service learning goes beyond the traditional clinical experiences that are part of every nursing curriculum. It has broad goals: increasing community empowerment and well-being and challenging students to reflect, think critically, and learn from less-structured, real-life experiences (Ciaccio & Walker, 1998).

BENEFITS OF SERVICE LEARNING

- Provides real-life meaningful experience
- Increases understanding of the lives of people from other cultural and socioeconomic groups
- Develops problem-solving skills
- Develops skills in collaboration and negotiation
- Increases knowledge of community needs and resources

Many nursing programs now include service learning activities as required or elective elements in the curriculum. San Jose State University in California (Yoder, Cohen, & Gorenberg, 1998) has developed a "nursing center without walls" that facilitates student participation in various community agencies, including a postpartum home visiting program.

There is also much interest in interdisciplinary education and practice models involving nursing, medicine, and other health-related professions (Sternas et al., 1999). Several schools have reported on successful community-based service learning projects ranging from health fairs to academic health centers that provide ongoing health care services to underserved communities (Dillon & Sternas, 1997; Hales, 1997; Henley et al., 1998; Simoni & McKinney, 1998).

BOX 3-2 Consensus Set of Indicators* for Assessing Community Health Status

INDICATORS OF HEALTH STATUS OUTCOME

1. Race/ethnicity-specific infant mortality, as measured by the rate (per 1000 live births) of deaths among infants younger than 1 year of age

Death rates (per 100,000 population)† for
2. Motor vehicle crashes
3. Work-related injury
4. Suicide
5. Lung cancer
6. Breast cancer
7. Cardiovascular disease
8. Homicide
9. All causes

Reported incidence (per 100,000 population) of
10. Acquired immunodeficiency syndrome
11. Measles
12. Tuberculosis
13. Primary and secondary syphilis

INDICATORS OF RISK FACTORS

14. Incidence of LBW, as measured by percentage of total number of liveborn infants weighing less than 2500 g at birth
15. Births to adolescents (females age 10 to 17 years) as a percentage of total live births
16. Prenatal care, as measured by percentage of mothers delivering live infants who did not receive prenatal care during first trimester
17. Childhood poverty, as measured by the proportion of children younger than 15 years of age living in families at or below the poverty level
18. Proportion of persons living in counties exceeding U.S. Environmental Protection Agency standards for air quality during previous year

Source: U.S. Department of Health and Human Services. (1991). Consensus set of indicators for assessing community health status. *MMWR* 40(27), 449.
*Position or number of the indicator does not imply priority.
†Age-adjusted to the 1940 standard population

HEALTH AND WELLNESS IN THE COMMUNITY

Community Health Status Indicators

Just as norms have been developed for individual health assessment, the data collected about communities can be compared with state or national standards to assess the well-being of the population as a whole. What percentage of the population has income below the poverty level? What is the unemployment rate? Do most women begin prenatal care in the first trimester? What are the fetal and infant mortality rates?

Box 3-2 displays a set of community health status indicators developed by a committee of experts from many community health-related organizations. Infant mortality, because it is affected by the preconceptional health, prenatal, and intrapartal care of the mother, as well as living conditions for the infant after birth, is a statistic widely used to compare the health status of different populations. Three of the five indicators of risk—incidence of low birth rate, adolescent pregnancy, and early prenatal care—refer to maternal-infant health. Poverty and a high percentage of young children in a community are strongly associated with significant community health needs (Zyzanski, Williams, &

Flocke, 1996). *Healthy People 2000* has set national goals for maternal-child health. One of the overall goals is to reduce disparities in health between groups within the population. Infant mortality in the African-American population remains twice that of the nation as a whole in spite of efforts to address this concern. The rate of pregnancy in young adolescents is still higher than the targeted goal. Reported child abuse and neglect continue to increase. These and many other health problems require intervention at the community level in addition to assisting individuals to improve their personal health behaviors.

Population- or Aggregate-Focused Care

Levels of Prevention

Population-focused health care uses a framework of **levels of prevention.**

- Primary prevention includes efforts made before the development of illness to promote general health and well-being. It also includes the use of specific protection, such as immunizations or approved infant car seats.
- Secondary prevention involves early detection of health problems so that treatment can begin before significant disability occurs. This includes various methods of health screening.
- Tertiary prevention is the treatment and rehabilitation of persons who have developed disease. Because most women are healthy during pregnancy, maternal-newborn nursing emphasizes primary and secondary prevention activities regardless of where care is provided. However, in general, the ill, hospitalized client is the focus of tertiary prevention.

Health Promotion in Group Settings

The use of established groups for health promotion activities has many advantages. Members are used to meeting on a regular basis and are comfortable with each other. Their shared experience may help them focus on a new goal and provide support to each other in initiating new health behaviors. Settings for community health promotion may include day care centers and schools; work sites; religious, service, or social organizations; community nursing centers; and the community at large (Pender, 1996). School-based programs can address many of the needs of adolescents regarding sexual and reproductive health. Employers are concerned about rising health insurance costs and absenteeism and are increasingly willing to sponsor prevention and health promotion programs for employees (Lassiter, 1996; Meurer, Meurer, & Holloway, 1997; Pender, 1996). The March of Dimes Birth Defects Foundation (1991) developed and supports "Babies + You," a campaign using volunteers to bring prenatal health education to women at work. In the growing parish nursing movement, coalitions of religious groups sponsor community health nursing activities for the areas they serve (Bergquist & King, 1994; Dixon, 1996). With **community-as-partner,** nurses can function as members, leaders, advisors, or consultants. Community nursing centers have been established in many areas to provide primary care, health promotion, and home care (Clear, Starbecker, & Kelly, 1999). Two such centers, based in low-income housing projects and cosponsored by the University of Pennsylvania School of Nursing, in collaboration with other health care organizations, were able to reduce the incidence of LBW infants born to residents from 13.6% to only 2% in just 3 years. They offer a comprehensive range of services, staffed by nurse practitioners who provide primary care, prenatal care, home visits, group health education, parenting and grandparenting support and education, mental health services, violence prevention education, and drug and alcohol treatment (U.S. Department of Health and Human Services, 1997).

High Risk Aggregates or Vulnerable Populations

Definition of Vulnerability

The health care system is moving toward managed care rather than fee-for-service. Providers recognize the need to target health education and outreach programs toward vulnerable populations. **Vulnerable populations** are groups who are at higher risk of developing physical, mental, or social health problems or who are more likely to have worse outcomes from these health problems than the population as a whole (Aday, 1997; Sebastian, 1996). People often have problems along more than one of these dimensions. Increasingly the need for multidisciplinary approaches to the needs of vulnerable populations has been recognized (Pew Health Professions Commission, 1995).

Many special population groups are more vulnerable to reproductive health risks, including pregnant adolescents, substance abusers, violence-prone families, the mentally ill, those with sexually transmitted or other communicable diseases, and those with malnutrition. These groups are often served by community health nurses who participate in community outreach (i.e., seeking underserved individuals, families, and groups and facilitating their entry into the health care system) and family and community-based health promotion interventions. In the following section, selected vulnerable populations who may have some or all of these problems are discussed: homeless families, immigrants and refugees, and migrant laborers. These groups, living in poverty and marginalized by mainstream society, have many common characteristics and needs.

Homeless

The term **homeless** as defined by the U.S. Department of Housing and Urban Development includes those who are homeless (i.e., living on the streets or in shelters) and those who are at risk of being homeless, such as those sharing housing and transients. Each year an estimated 2.5 to 3 million people lack access to a conventional dwelling; families are the fastest growing segment of that population. Families with children account for 33% to 43% of the homeless. Young, single women head 53% of homeless families. Many of these women have a history of physical or sexual abuse as children and have also abused alcohol or drugs (American Academy of Pediatrics, 1996; Stanhope & Lancaster, 1996). It is estimated that as many as 2 million homeless adolescents may be living on the streets of major cities. Many engage in "survival sex," exchanging sexual favors for food, clothing, and shelter, making them vulnerable to sexually transmitted diseases and unintended pregnancies. They seldom appear at agencies serving the adult homeless population (Rew, 1996).

Homeless people have fewer resources than other poor families. Preexisting health problems are complicated by homelessness, and other health problems are caused by homelessness. Living conditions contribute to higher levels of infectious disease, including respiratory infections, especially antibiotic-resistant tuberculosis and enteric infections. Anemia and other nutritional deficits are common. Obesity is often present because of lack of storage and cooking facilities and reliance on fast foods and convenience stores. Family members are at higher risk for injury because of accidents, violence, or environmental exposure. Access to health care, especially preventive care, is limited because of the energy required for the daily struggle to meet needs for food and shelter and by frequent moves and reliance on emergency rooms for the most acute needs (American Academy of Pediatrics, 1996; Burg, 1994).

Killion (1995) followed 15 homeless pregnant women living in several different shelters in southern California for periods of several weeks to more than 1 year. Conception among this group of women was rarely planned and usually occurred during the period of homelessness as a result of factors such as victimization, economic survival, lack of access to contraceptives, need for closeness and intimacy, and doubt of fertility. None had consistent prenatal care. Some did not admit to being homeless when seen in clinics or emergency departments for fear of having children removed by protective services. They reported difficulty in dealing with the normal discomforts of pregnancy such as fatigue and nausea and vomiting. Some addicted women found that the stress of pregnancy increased their reliance on drugs, whereas for others the pregnancy was an impetus to help them work toward reestablished stability in their lives.

Although most research has focused on urban homeless families, Wagner, Menke, and Ciccone (1995) studied the needs of rural homeless families. These families were similar to those in cities, but as a group had been homeless for longer periods because fewer resources were available in their communities. Often, because rural populations are sparse and composed largely of elderly families, there may be few or no services for childbearing women and their children (Henly et al., 1998).

Many homeless women are covered by **Medicaid** and may go to private offices and hospitals for care. Because of distrust of the system, they may try to hide their status. Nurses working with homeless women and families agree that treating clients with dignity and respect is basic to establishing a therapeutic relationship. Case management is recommended to coordinate the various agencies and disciplines that may be involved in meeting the multiple needs of these families. Time for appointments must be flexible, and clients should not be penalized if they fail to appear when scheduled. Health is of lower priority than food and shelter, except in emergencies. Whenever possible, the service must be provided when the woman seeks treatment. Each interaction should be purposeful and offered with the awareness that this may be the only encounter possible with the woman. Health information and strategies that are feasible within the context of her living situation are offered. The health care provider builds on existing coping strategies and strengths. The woman is allowed to do as much as possible for herself to reduce her feelings of powerlessness. The woman (and her family) is helped to reconnect with her social support system. At the local, state, and federal levels, health care providers can advocate for adequate funding for homeless prevention programs and comprehensive health care for all homeless people, with a focus on continuity of preventive care (Acquaviva & Lancaster, 1996; American Academy of Pediatrics, 1996; Burg, 1994; Killion, 1995).

Migrants

An estimated 3 to 5 million people are classified as migrant farm workers, 16% of whom are women (Maternal Child Health Bureau, 1997). **Migrant laborers** are those who must establish temporary residence in various areas on a seasonal basis in order to obtain employment. Most live in temporary housing for at least 6 months out of the year; others move continuously throughout the year. They may be thought of as episodically homeless because their shelter is often dependent on employment, and as the seasons change, they become homeless until the next job is obtained. Ethnic groups among migrants include African-Americans, European-Americans, Hispanics, Haitians, and some Southeast Asians. Those in the western and central states are predominantly Mexican; the population in the east, traveling north from Florida, is more varied (Lambert, 1995; Rodriguez, 1996).

Migrant laborers and their families face many problems, including financial instability, child labor, poor housing, lack of education, language and cultural barriers, and limited access to health and social services (Clemen-Stone, Eigsti, & McGuire, 1998). Migrant farm work is one of the most hazardous occupations in the United States because of heavy physical demands, fatigue, operation of potentially dangerous machinery, exposure to pesticides and naturally occurring irritants, and limited enforcement of Occupational Safety and Health Administration (OSHA) standards. Housing is often substandard and overcrowded because of lack of availability or cost (Jones & Schenk,

1996). Although comprehensive studies of migrant health have not been reported, analyses of records of clients seen at Migrant Health Centers indicate that there are high rates of poor dental health, diabetes, hypertension, malnutrition, tuberculosis, substance abuse, and parasitic infections. The average life expectancy for migrant laborers is 49 years as compared with 75 years for the population as a whole. Substance abuse and domestic violence are significant problems. Most farm workers do not view illness as a problem unless the condition prevents working. Health promotion and disease prevention are not values to those with orientation to the present, limited education, and lack of access to health care (Jones & Schenk, 1996).

A typical day for the mother of a migrant family may begin at 4 or 5 AM when she arises to prepare food for the family. She works in the fields until 5 or 6 PM and then continues her workday with housework and child care (Rodriguez, 1996). Higher rates of miscarriage, inadequate prenatal care, and infant mortality are reported. There is concern about the reproductive effects of exposure to toxic chemicals. Less consistent use of contraception and increased rates of sexually transmitted diseases, including human immunodeficiency virus (HIV), and inflammatory conditions of the cervix, vagina, and vulva are reported (Lambert, 1995). Compared with other poor women attending public nutrition clinics, migrants are more likely to have late initiation of prenatal care and inadequate pregnancy weight gain. The incidence of preterm birth and the birth of an LBW infant was similar for both groups and higher than the *Healthy People 2000* objective targets (Maternal Child Health Bureau, 1997). The infant mortality rate is 2.5 times the national average (Sandhaus, 1998).

Although a system of 100 federally funded Migrant Health Centers has been established in the United States and Puerto Rico, they see less than 15% of the 3 to 5 million farm workers, and the gap is not closed by the various voluntary agencies that also serve this community. Many migrants seek help at local community hospitals and clinics in the areas in which they are working. Lack of time is a major barrier to obtaining health care. Even if services are free, the loss of wages incurred in leaving the fields is a deterrent to preventive care. To ensure access, offices should be open after the migrants' usual working hours. Lack of trust (i.e., reluctance to share personal problems with a stranger or fear of being reported to the Immigration and Naturalization Services if they are undocumented) prevents many from obtaining care. Domestic violence is a significant problem, and men's control over women's activities limits women's ability to seek help (Rodriguez, 1996).

Providing culturally competent care to a multiethnic population is a challenge for health care workers (Jones & Schenk, 1996; Lambert, 1995). (See Chapter 2 for discussion of cultural competence.) One approach that has been successful is the use of lay camp aides to assist in outreach and health education. Among Hispanic women the use of camp volunteers, known as "romotoras," who assist families in obtaining prenatal, postpartum, and infant care and meeting other health needs, has been effective. This partnership with the community provides a link between the formal health care system and traditional practices (Rodriguez, 1996). Guidance and information about other resources are available to health care providers through the National Migrant Resource Program and the Migrant Clinicians Network (Lambert, 1995).

Refugees and Immigrants

From 1975 through 1993, 1.85 million **refugees** were admitted to the United States, with 1 of every 140 persons of the U.S. population being of refugee origin (U.S. Committee on Refugees, 1995). The surge in refugee immigration began with Southeast Asians after the Vietnam War and continued with those from Ethiopia, Cuba, Bosnia and Eastern Europe, and the Kurds from Iraq. Other countries whose emigrants are not always officially recognized as refugees include Haiti, China, and uncounted numbers from Central America. Governmental agencies make a distinction between those who voluntarily immigrate for economic reasons and refugees, who are forced to flee for political reasons. Refugees are automatically eligible for permanent resident status and additional services and support. However, the differences are not always clear, and many voluntary immigrants come from countries in political turmoil (Bollini & Siem, 1995). Although most immigrants find adaptation to a new language and culture stressful, refugees share common characteristics that significantly increase the difficulties families experience. These include the following:

- Leaving their homeland without hope of return
- Surviving the trauma of war or refugee camps—women are commonly raped while in transit or in refugee camps
- Grief related to deaths of family members and loss of home
- Multiple health problems, including malnutrition, infectious disease, and stress-related mental health disorders (e.g., posttraumatic stress disorder)
- Lack of previous experience with the Western health care system, in particular no previous experience with prenatal care and family planning
- Unique cultural beliefs that are unfamiliar to most U.S. health workers (Kemp, 1996).

In addressing the needs of refugee women, the World Health Organization recommends that reproductive health programs include a minimum package of care related to issues of family planning; maternal mortality; unwanted pregnancy; sexually transmitted diseases, including HIV and acquired immunodeficiency syndrome (AIDS); and physical and sexual violence. If they have lost children during the exodus from their country, women may want to rebuild their families soon after resettlement. A participatory approach is needed to bring together the many agencies and groups working with refugees and to allow for input into decision making by the refugees themselves (Djeddah, 1995). Foss (1996) explored the difficulty of experiencing the overlapping transitions of adjustment to a new country and parenthood while grieving for the many losses experienced as refugees. Health workers with immigrant and refugee groups have found that most are receptive to new health education but prefer to receive it in their own language from someone who is part of their culture. Bicultural professionals and trained community workers from the refugee group have successfully reached women and families who were reluctant to interact with the health system of the new country (Lipson & Omidian, 1997). When refugee and other immigrant women are hospitalized, a cultural liaison who can interpret not only language but also differing cultural expectations is invaluable. Understanding reproductive health needs through the eyes of refugee communities is an essential step toward providing appropriate and culturally sensitive services and information (Djeddah, 1995; Gany & Bocanegra, 1996). Many immigrants who have strong ties to traditional medical practices from their homeland also respect Western or scientific practices. This pluralistic view allows them to combine both modalities without conflict (Kang, Kahler, & Tesar, 1998; Rodriguez, 1996).

HOME CARE ACROSS THE PERINATAL CONTINUUM OF CARE

A continuum of care is defined as a range of clinical services provided for an individual or group that reflects care given during a single hospitalization or care for multiple conditions over a lifetime. Home care is one delivery component available along the perinatal continuum of care (Fig. 3-2). This continuum begins with family planning and continues with preconception care, prenatal care, intrapartum care, postpartum care, newborn care, interconceptional care, and infant care until the infant is 1 year old. Independent self-care, ambulatory care, home care, low risk hospitalization, or specialized intensive care may be appropriate at different points along this continuum.

Current Trends and Historical Perspectives

A priority for future decades will be the development of innovative, cost-effective methods of health care delivery. Large health care organizations are developing clinically integrated health care delivery networks. The goals of **clinical integration** are improved coordination of care and care outcomes; better communication among health care providers; increased client, payer, and provider satisfaction; and reduced cost. With clinical integration the focus changes from illness to health, from the individual to the population, and from care provided in one setting to care across the continuum (Kastens, 1998). The following several factors make home care a growth area in perinatal services:

- Increased interest in family birthing alternatives
- Shortened hospital stays
- Availability of new technologies that allow sophisticated assessments and treatments to be performed in the home setting
- Increasing reimbursement by third-party payers.

In 1877 the Women's Branch of the New York City Mission provided the first training program for **home health care** nursing. These home care nurses focused on caring for the sick within their homes. In 1893 Lillian Wald established the Henry Street Settlement House and expanded this visitation to include some preventive care. Modern home care nursing has its foundation in public health nursing, which provided comprehensive care to sick and well clients within their own homes.

Specialized maternity home care nursing services began in the 1980s when public health maternity nursing services were limited and services had not kept pace with the changing practices of high risk obstetrics and emerging technology. Lengthy antepartal hospitalizations for such conditions as preterm labor and pregnancy-induced hypertension created nursing care challenges for staff members on inpatient units. Many women expressed their concern for the negative effect of antepartal hospitalizations on the family. Although clinical indications showed that a new nursing care approach was needed, home health care did not become a viable alternative until **third-party payers** (i.e., public or private organizations or employer groups that pay for health care expenses) pushed for cost containment in maternity services.

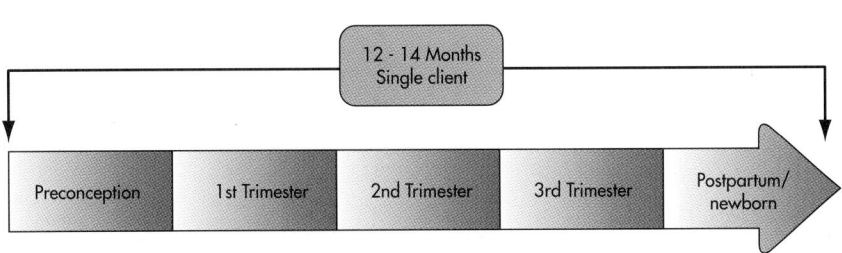

Fig. 3-2 Perinatal continuum of care.

Antepartal home care that prolongs gestation and reduces neonatal intensive care hospitalization is cost effective. Even home infusion services at a cost of $225 to $325 per day provides a substantial saving over an average ($1500 per day) hospitalization (Monical, 1998).

Communication to Bridge the Continuum

As maternity care continues to consist of frequent and brief contacts with health care providers throughout the prenatal and postpartum periods, nurses must develop innovative nursing delivery methods, as well as innovative ways to communicate that care is provided. Bakewell-Sachs and Persily (1995) and Brooten (1995) discussed the need for the development of services that link maternity clients throughout the perinatal continuum of care, including critical pathways, telephonic nursing assessments, discharge planning, specialized education programs, parent support groups, home visiting programs, nurse advice lines, and perinatal home care. Some hospitals have provided cross-training for hospital-based nurses to make postpartum home visits (Fowler et al., 1997; Pignatello et al., 1998). Another approach is the development of outpatient centers for postpartum follow-up, staffed by nurses from the maternity unit (Blystad-Keppler, 1995).

Telephonic Nursing Care

Telephonic nursing care through services such as warm lines, nurse advice lines, and telephonic nursing assessments are emerging as valuable services to manage health care problems and bridge the gaps among acute, outpatient, and home care services. This type of nursing care occurs by telephone and is very interactive and responsive to the immediate health care questions consumers have about particular health care needs. Warm lines are telephone lines that are offered as a community service to provide new parents with support, encouragement, and basic parenting education. Nurse advice lines, or toll-free nurse consultation services, provide answers to medical questions, guide callers through urgent health care situations, suggest treatment options, and provide health education (Bleich, 1998). Telephonic nursing assessments, or nurse consultation, assessment, and health education that take place during a telephone conversation, can be added to the plan of care in conjunction with skilled nursing visits or may be a separate nursing contact for the woman. Telephonic nursing assessments are commonly used after a postpartum home care visit to reassess a woman's knowledge about the signs and symptoms of adequate hydration in breastfeeding, or, after initiating home phototherapy, to assess the caregiver's knowledge regarding problems with equipment. In the new health care environment with limited resources, warm lines, nurse advice lines, and telephonic nursing assessments can influence clients' health care decisions by empowering them with knowledge to make wiser and more cost-efficient health care decisions.

Some hypothesize that most future health care will be provided in clients' homes using two-way telecommunication systems (Kinsella, 1998).

Guidelines for Nursing Practice

Although the home care industry continues to grow rapidly, perinatal home care nursing practice is still emerging. Clarifying the role of the perinatal home care nurse and the ways this role differs from other health care providers is still being molded by clinical practice and regulatory and accreditation organizations.

The Association of Women's Health, Obstetric, and Neonatal Nurses (AWHONN) (1998) defines *home care* as

> the provision of technical, psychological, and other therapeutic support in the patient's home rather than in an institution. The scope of nursing care delivered in the home setting is necessarily limited to practices deemed safe and appropriate to be carried out in an environment that is physically separated from a health care institution and its resources. . . . Nursing practice at home is consistent with federal and state regulations . . . that direct home care practice. The nurse demonstrates practice competence through formalized orientation and ongoing clinical education and performance evaluation in the respective home care agency. Standards for practice from key specialty organizations such as AWHONN, the American College of Obstetricians and Gynecologists (ACOG), the American Academy of Pediatrics, and the Intravenous Nursing Society (INS) provide the basis for clinical protocols and pathways and organizational programs in home care practice. The Joint Commission on Accreditation of Health Care Organizations (JCAHO) provides criteria for home care operations.

AWHONN (1994) developed standards of practice and identified essential knowledge and skills to provide safe perinatal home care. Health care agencies and individuals can use these to assess the nurse's skills and learning needs.

According to the Health Care Financing Administration (HCFA), a client who meets the following criteria may receive home health care services: homebound status, need for intermittent skilled care, medically reasonable and necessary need for treatment, and has a plan of care authorized by the health care provider (Health Care Financing Administration, 1990).

A wide range of professional health care services and health products can be delivered or used in the home. The primary difference between health care in a hospital and home care is the absence of the continuous presence of professional health care providers in a client's home. Most home health care is given as intermittent care with the professional staff visiting in the client's home or providing care on site for fewer than 4 hours at a time. The home health care agency maintains on-call professional staff to assist home care clients who have questions about their care and for emergencies, such as equipment failure.

Perinatal Services

Home care perinatal services may be provided by hospital-based programs, independent **proprietary** (for profit) **agencies** or nonprofit home care agencies, and official or tax-supported agencies (Table 3-2). Innovative programs may be supported by research grants for a period of years, but ultimately they must be sponsored by an agency with long-term funding. Home visits have both advantages and disadvantages. The mother is able to maintain bed rest if indicated, and vulnerable neonates are not exposed to the weather or external sources of infection. The nurse can observe and interact with family members in their most natural and secure environment. Adequacy of resources and safety factors can be assessed. Teaching can be tailored to the actual home conditions and other family members included. A home visit is less expensive than a day's hospitalization, but a 60- to 90-minute visit requires 2.5 to 3 hours of nursing time, including travel and documentation. It is more cost effective to see clients in an office setting where professional time is not spent in travel. Availability of nurses with expertise in maternity care may be limited, and concerns about the nurse's physical safety in some communities may limit visits.

Visits for outreach and health promotion are an integral part of community (or public) health nursing. In countries with national health systems, a nurse may see all women during pregnancy and after birth. In the United States visits of this sort have been provided mainly to low-income families without health insurance who use the clinics provided by local health departments (Koniak-Griffin et al., 1999; Olds et al., 1997). Until recently, private insurers did not reimburse for health promotion visits. Managed care organizations now recognize that anticipatory guidance is cost effective, but home visit programs are still targeted to specific high risk populations, such as young adolescents or women at risk for preterm labor.

Home care agencies are subject to regulation by governmental and professional organizations and provide interdisciplinary services including social work, nutrition, and occupational and physical therapy. Increasingly their caseloads are made up of clients who require high-technologic care, such as infusions or home monitoring. Although the home health nurse develops the care plan, all care must be ordered by a physician. Interventions must meet the insurer's criteria for reimbursement, and services are limited to the registered clients. Preconception care and low risk

TABLE 3-2	**Types of Home Health Care Agencies in the United States**
TYPE OF AGENCY	**DESCRIPTION OF AGENCY**
Official	A governmental or public agency, usually a local health department, which is supported by state and local taxes. Official agencies are mandated by law to provide certain specific services, such as communicable disease follow-up. They provide health promotion and disease prevention services as well as home health care.
Voluntary	A private, nonprofit agency whose operating funds come largely from individual contributions, fees-for-service, united community funds, contracts for service, grants, and other nonofficial sources of funding. Voluntary agencies are governed by a board of directors. These agencies are not required by law to provide specific types of services; they primarily, but not exclusively, provide home health care services. The visiting nurse associations traditionally have been the major voluntary organizations which provide home health care services in a local community.
Combination	A combined governmental (a local health department) and voluntary agency (a VNA), whose operating funds came from both official and nonofficial sources. This organizational structure was promoted for the purposes of preventing duplication of services, decreasing continuity of care difficulties, and reducing the cost of delivering local health care services. A combination agency provides both health promotion/disease prevention and home health care services.
Private, nonprofit	A privately owned agency which is tax exempt because of its nonprofit status. Unlike voluntary agencies, these agencies are governed by the owner(s) of the organization. Their major source of revenue is fee-for-service. Private, nonprofit agencies are usually established to provide home health care services only.
Proprietary	A private agency established to make a profit. These agencies are not eligible for tax exemption. They are governed by their owner(s), who are increasingly large corporations. Their major source of revenue is a fee-for-service. Like the private, nonprofit agencies, proprietary agencies are usually established to provide home health care services only.
Hospital-based	A home health care agency run and governed by a hospital. Sources of revenue and tax status vary depending on the type of hospital (governmental, voluntary, private, nonprofit, or proprietary) which has established the home health care agency.

Source: Health Care Financing Administration. (1989). *Medicare program: Home health agencies—Conditions of participation and reductions in record-keeping requirements.* Washington, D.C.: U.S. Department of Health and Human Services.

antepartum care can usually be provided more efficiently in office settings and are not currently reimbursable. High risk antepartum care is often provided by home care agencies. Women with hyperemesis gravidarum who require parenteral nutrition may be treated at home. Conditions requiring bed rest, such as preterm labor and hypertension, are common indications for home care. Other conditions may include cardiac disease and substance abuse (Kemp & Hatmaker, 1996) and diabetes in pregnancy (Persily, Brown, & York, 1996).

Postpartum home care is a growing area of perinatal services. Some insurers reimburse for at least one visit to families after early discharge or in the presence of high risk factors. Home phototherapy is used for treatment of neonatal hyperbilirubinemia and to avoid separation of mother and infant. Many other neonates who require long-term high-technology care are also managed with home care. The American Academy of Pediatrics (1998) recommends home visits as an effective early-intervention strategy to improve child health in families at risk. Consumer demand and education of insurers by case managers is increasing the availability of home care options (Malnory, 1997; Women's Health Center Management, 1997).

Client Selection and Referral

The office- or hospital-based nurse is often the key person in making effective referrals to home care. When considering a referral to home care, the following factors must be evaluated:
- Health status of mother and fetus or infant: Is condition serious enough to warrant home care, and is it stable enough for intermittent observation to be sufficient?
- Availability of professionals to provide the needed services within the client's community.
- Family resources, including psychosocial, social, and economic resources: Will the family be able to provide care between nursing visits? Are relationships supportive? Is third-party reimbursement available or can it be negotiated with the insurer? Is there a voluntary or tax-supported community agency that could provide needed care without payment?
- Cost-effectiveness: Is it more reasonable for the client to receive these services at home or to go to a local outpatient facility to receive them?

Community referrals should not be limited to women with physiologic complications of pregnancy that require medical treatment. Clients at risk (e.g., young adolescents, families with history of abuse, members of vulnerable population groups, developmentally disabled individuals) may need follow-up care at home. In consultation with the social worker, the hospital-based nurse should become familiar with local agencies that accept such referrals.

Standardized referral forms simplify the referral process and ensure that all needed information will be forwarded to the home health agency. The nursing assessment should include the woman's physical and psychologic status, her level of knowledge about self-care activities, her willingness to learn, the availability of caregivers and social support in the home, and her level of comfort with home care. If the referral is for a mother and infant home care visit, the nursing assessment should include newborn data.

High-technology home care requires additional information to be collected from the chart and consultation with the referring physician and other members of the health care team before making a home care referral. These additional data include the medical diagnosis, medical prognosis, prescribed therapies, medication history, drug dosing information, potential ancillary supplies, and type of infusion access device. The nursing assessment and therapies data provide baseline information for the home care nurse and pharmacist.

Whenever a referral is called into a home health care agency, a member of the nursing or admission staff determines the agency's ability to accept the client for service. The use of fax machines to transmit information has eliminated delays in initiating home care services.

Admission to Home Care

Once the client is admitted to the agency, the determination of staffing is addressed by nursing management. Client assignments are generally determined according to diagnosis, geographic location, potential length of service, and skill level of the home care nurse. An agency may have a number of nurses with various clinical backgrounds and certifications. Clinical nurse specialists are assuming leadership roles in many perinatal home care agencies (Broussard, 1996; Christian, 1996).

Preparing for the Home Visit

The home care nurse reviews the available clinical data, demographic information, and completed plan of care form and consults with the home care pharmacist or other health care team members who have previously contacted the woman to determine the goals of the visit. At this point the nurse uses the medical diagnosis and stage on the perinatal continuum as a starting point to organize the woman's care. The nurse reviews agency policies and procedures, professional literature about diagnosis, and community resources as part of the previsit preparation work (Box 3-3).

Before going on a home visit, the nurse contacts the woman to make necessary arrangements. Contact by telephone has several goals besides establishing a convenient visit date and time and obtaining directions to the woman's home. Setting the stage for the first home care visit is essential.

The nurse identifies himself or herself by name, title, and agency. He or she then explains who referred the woman to the agency for home care and the purpose of the home care visits. The nurse briefly explains what will occur during the visit and approximately how long the visit will last. The woman should be asked to restrain any pets during the visit. Last, the nurse asks about health supplies that may be needed for the woman's care.

BOX 3-3 Protocol for Perinatal Home Visits

PREVISIT INTERVENTIONS

1. Contact family to arrange details for home visit.
   a. Identify self, credentials, and agency role.
   b. Review purpose of home visit follow-up.
   c. Schedule convenient time for visit.
   d. Confirm address and route to family home.
2. Review and clarify appropriate data.
   a. All available assessment data for mother and fetus or infant (i.e., referral forms, hospital discharge summaries, family identified learning needs).
   b. Review records of any previous nursing contacts.
   c. Contact other professional caregivers as necessary to clarify data (i.e., obstetrician, nurse-midwife, pediatrician, referring nurse).
3. Identify community resources and teaching materials appropriate to meet needs already identified.
4. Plan the visit, and prepare bag with equipment, supplies, and materials necessary for assessments of mother and fetus or infant, actual care anticipated, and teaching.

IN-HOME INTERVENTIONS: ESTABLISHING A RELATIONSHIP

1. Reintroduce self and establish purpose of visit for mother, infant, and family; offer family opportunity to clarify their expectations of contact.
2. Spend brief time socially interacting with family to become acquainted and establish trusting relationship.

IN-HOME INTERVENTIONS: WORKING WITH FAMILY

1. Conduct systematic assessment of mother and fetus or newborn to determine physiologic adjustment and any existing complications.
2. Throughout visit, collect data to assess the emotional adjustment of individual family members to pregnancy or birth and lifestyle changes. Note evidence of family-newborn bonding and sibling rivalry; note relationships among mother, father, children, and grandparents.
3. Determine adequacy of support system.
   a. To what extent does someone help with cooking, cleaning, and other home management tasks?
   b. To what extent is help being provided in caring for the newborn and any other children?
   c. Are support persons encouraging the new mother to care for herself and get adequate rest?
   d. Who is providing helpful information? Emotional support?
4. Throughout the visit, observe home environment for adequacy of resources:
   a. Space: privacy, safe play of children, sleeping.
   b. Overall cleanliness and state of repair.
   c. Number of steps pregnant woman/new mother must climb.

d. Adequacy of cooking arrangements.
e. Adequacy of refrigeration and other food storage areas.
f. Adequacy of bathing, toilet, and laundry facilities.
g. Arrangements in home for newborn: sleeping, bathing, formula preparation (if needed), layette items, and diapers.

5. Throughout the visit, observe home environment for overall state of repair and existence of safety hazards:
   a. Storage of medications, household cleaners, and other substances hazardous to children.
   b. Presence of peeling paint on furniture, walls, or pipes.
   c. Factors that contribute to falls, such as dim lighting, broken steps, scatter rugs.
   d. Presence of vermin.
   e. Use of crib or playpen that fails to meet safety guidelines.
   f. Existence of emergency plan in case of fire; fire alarm or extinguisher.
6. Provide care to mother, newborn, or both as prescribed by their respective primary care provider or in accord with agency protocol.
7. Provide teaching on basis of previously identified needs.
8. Refer family to appropriate community agencies or resources, such as warm lines and support groups.
9. Ascertain that woman knows potential problems to watch for and whom to call if they occur.
10. Ensure that used disposable items have been handled appropriately and that reusable items are cleaned and repacked appropriately in the nurse's bag.

IN-HOME INTERVENTIONS: ENDING THE VISIT

1. Summarize the activities and main points of the visit.
2. Clarify future expectations, including schedule of next visit.
3. Review teaching plan and provide major points in writing.
4. Provide information about reaching the nurse or agency if needed before the next scheduled visit.

POSTVISIT INTERVENTIONS

1. Document the visit thoroughly, using the necessary agency forms to serve as a legal record of the visit and to allow third-party reimbursement, as possible.
2. Initiate the plan of care on which the next encounter with the woman/family will be based.
3. Communicate appropriately (by telephone, letter, progress notes, or referral form) with primary care provider, other health professionals, or referral agencies on behalf of woman/family.

Before going out on the first visit, the home care nurse collects the woman's clinical record, client education materials, medical supplies, and equipment necessary for the visit. Medications and specialized equipment should be ordered before the visit and delivered at the time of the scheduled visit.

CARE MANAGEMENT

First Home Care Visit

Making the first home care visit can be stressful for the nurse and the woman. The home care nurse is faced with an unknown environment controlled by the woman and her family. The woman and her family also experience feelings of the unknown, such as anxiety about the way the nurse will treat them or what the nurse will do during the visit. The challenge for the home care nurse is to establish a nurse-client relationship and provide the prescribed home care services within the time provided for the initial home visit.

Introductions generally begin the visit; the nurse identifies self and home care agency (Fig. 3-3). The woman introduces herself and the other family members who are present. Sometimes, the woman may feel uncertain of her role or be uncomfortable in taking the lead in introductions, so other people in the home may not be introduced to the nurse. In these situations the nurse can politely ask about other people in the home and their relationship to the woman.

Before performing any services, the home care nurse must obtain written agreement and consent for the home health care services. This consent-for-care serves two major purposes: agreement for care and authorization to release medical information. Many third-party payers require written documentation of the services provided; therefore the agency obtains authorization from the woman to give information to her physician and any individual or company involved in payment for the services. Agencies that bill third-party payers for the rendered services will include agreement language for assignment of benefits and financial remuneration. By agreeing to assign insurance benefits to the agency, the woman allows her insurance company to pay the home health care agency directly.

All clients have the right to actively participate in their home care plan of care. These client rights and responsibilities should begin the discussion about the nurse-client roles during this initial visit.

Assessment and Nursing Diagnoses

The primary goals of the assessment phase are to develop a trusting relationship and collect data by various methods to obtain a comprehensive client profile. It may not be feasible or appropriate to collect in-depth information about all areas of assessment during the first visit (Clemen-Stone, Eigsti, & McGuire, 1998). However, in many instances the nurse may be limited to one visit and must obtain information pertinent to the current situation in that hour.

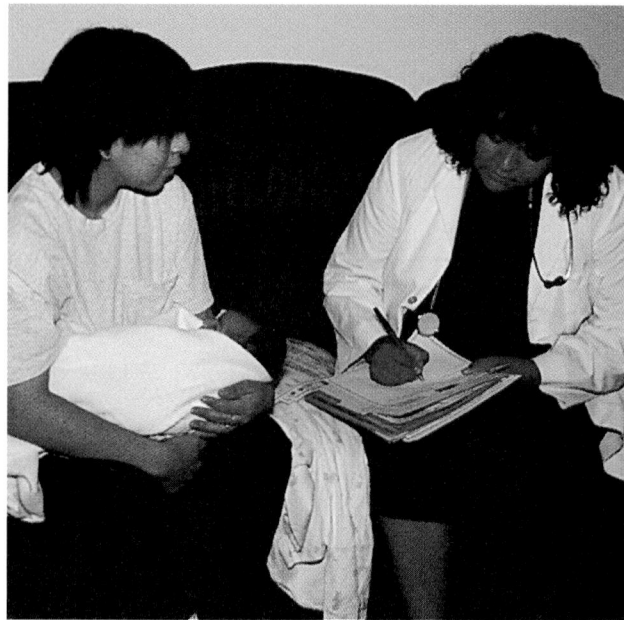

Fig. 3-3 Home care nurse visiting with woman and her infant. *(Courtesy Michael S. Clement, MD, Mesa, AZ.)*

The establishment of a trusting relationship began with the previsit telephone call. An interview style that reflects sensitivity; a nonjudgmental, accepting attitude; and respect for the woman's rights facilitates the development of that trusting relationship. A skillful interviewer avoids barriers to communication such as false reassurance, advice giving, excessive talking, and the showing of approval or disapproval (Clemen-Stone, Eigsti, & McGuire, 1998). This nurse-client relationship continues to develop over the course of home visits.

The nurse is a guest in the woman's home and should show respect for her and her belongings. Some adaptation of the home visit schedule may need to occur if there are numerous distractions during a visit, such as caring for the needs of small children. The nurse may need to ask to have the volume of the television lowered or to suggest moving to another room where it is more quiet and private.

The major areas of the assessment are demographics, medical history, general health history, medication history, sociocultural assessment, home and community environment, and physical assessment. Some of this information can be obtained from client records sent to the home care agency at the time of referral or from the previsit interview. These data will be used to develop the nursing care plan and complete the plan of care, which is required for many licensed home health care agencies. Two areas requiring further discussion are the social assessment and the home environment assessment.

Social assessment includes information regarding the number and roles of each household member, which family members or individuals have taken on the role of caregiver, and the woman's social support network. Identifying

BOX 3-4 Psychosocial Assessment

LANGUAGE

Identify the primary language spoken in the home

Assess whether there are any language barriers to receiving support

COMMUNITY RESOURCES/ACCESS TO CARE

Identify primary and secondary means of transportation

Identify community agencies family currently uses for health care and support

Assess cultural and psychosocial barriers to receiving care

SOCIAL SUPPORT

Determine the people living with the pregnant woman

Identify who assists with household chores

Identify who assists with child care/parenting activities

Identify who the pregnant woman turns to for problems or during a crisis

INTERPERSONAL RELATIONSHIP

Identify the way decisions are made in the family

Identify the family's perception of the need for home care

Identify roles of adults in caring for family members

CAREGIVER

Identify the primary caregiver for home care treatments

Identify other caregivers and their roles

Assess the caregiver's knowledge of treatments and care process

Identify potential strain from the caregiver role

Identify the level of satisfaction with the caregiver role

STRESS AND COPING

Identify what the woman perceives as lifestyle changes and their impact on her and her family

Identify the changes she and her family have made to adjust to her health condition and home health care treatments

---

the roles of each member is helpful for developing the nursing care plan (Box 3-4).

Physical assessment of the home environment is an essential element of the home care assessment. The major areas of the home environment assessment include physical features of the home, access to the home, sanitary conditions, the presence of utilities (for example, telephone, electricity), safety features, and access to transportation and emergency support. Although some of this information can be collected during an interview, physically inspecting many areas of the home essential to care is a critical part of developing an accurate nursing care plan. Before any physical inspection, the home care nurse should ask the client or caregiver for permission and assistance in identifying areas in the home that will be involved in the caregiving activities. During the physical inspection, careful consideration should be taken to avoid moving personal belongings that are not affected by the care.

Each specific plan of care has a different emphasis in the home environment. For example, women on infusion therapy for hyperemesis gravidarum need a safe place to store medications and infusion supplies that are out of reach of small children living in the home. The home care nurse should incorporate the agency policies and procedures for the storage and handling of infusion supplies into her walk-through inspection. During the walk through, the home care nurse looks at the potential storage areas for supplies that are dry, that are clean, and where the temperature can be maintained. The home care nurse should include an inspection of the work areas, such as countertops, tabletops, sinks, and trash areas, that the

woman or caregiver may use for mixing medications, changing infusion tubing, handling supplies, or disposing of used equipment and supplies.

Clients using electronic home health care equipment, such as phototherapy equipment or infusion pumps, require physical inspection of electrical outlets, electrical cords, and extension cords that will be used. Homes with faulty electrical wiring may place the client at risk for being involved in an electrical fire; faulty wiring may require inspection and repair by a professional electrician before electronic devices are used. Findings from the assessment are incorporated into the plan of care.

Nursing diagnoses are derived from the data collected at the first home visit. Nursing diagnoses for perinatal home health care clients include the following:

Nursing Diagnoses

- Knowledge deficit related to
  —management of therapeutic regimen (e.g., nausea and vomiting, preterm labor, gestational diabetes)
- Knowledge deficit related to
  —newborn care and feeding
- Ineffective family coping: compromised, related to
  —lack of child care while mother is on bed rest
- Care of newborn on oxygen therapy
- Risk for parenting, altered, related to
  —maternal immaturity and lack of family support
- Diversional activity deficit related to
  —prolonged bed rest

Expected Outcomes of Care

The home care nurse formulates client-centered expected outcomes. Many of the interventions will be carried out by the woman or the designated caregiver; therefore their participation in the planning process is critical to achieving positive outcomes. Examples of expected outcomes for perinatal clients include the following:

- The woman will verbalize understanding of treatments.
- The woman will report decreased anxiety about performing procedures (e.g., blood glucose monitoring).
- The woman will use support systems to cope effectively with problems (e.g., pregnancy complications, newborn complications/treatments).
- The woman, caregiver, or both will return demonstrate procedures.
- The caregiver will verbalize decreased role strain.

Plan of Care and Interventions

The nursing care plan is developed based on the individual health care needs of the woman. The care plan describes the nursing diagnoses and interventions needed to meet the woman's health care needs.

Home care nurses working in HCFA-regulated home health care agencies use a plan of care that includes client demographics, the health care provider's orders, home care goals, and the level of functioning as a basis for nursing care plans. This document is initiated at the time of referral to the home care agency and must be updated every 60 days or as specified by state regulations.

The frequency of the skilled nursing visit may vary with the individual plan of care, nursing care plan, and reimbursement criteria established by the third-party payers.

Nurse safety and infection control are two important aspects specific to home care.

Safety Issues for the Home Care Nurse

The nurse should be fully aware of the home environment and neighborhood in which the home care is being provided. Unlike hospitals, in which the environment is more predictable and controlled, the client's neighborhood and home have the potential for uncertainty. Home care nurses should take necessary safety precautions and avoid dangerous areas.

Agencies that serve clients in high-crime areas may conduct a violence-potential assessment by telephone before the visit and enlist the client's cooperation in minimizing risk (Hunter, 1997). Others have hired full-time security personnel to accompany nurses on their visits. Personal strategies recommended for nurses visiting families with a history of violence or substance abuse include (1) self-awareness; (2) environmental assessment; (3) using listening and observation skills with clients to be aware of behavioral changes indicating aggression or lack of impulse control; (4) planning for dealing with aggressive behavior (i.e., allowing personal space and taking a nonag-

gressive stance) (Whitley, Jacobson, & Gawrys, 1996); (5) making visits in pairs; and (6) having access to a cellular phone at all times.

Personal safety. The home care nurse must be aware of personal safety behaviors before going on a home visit. Dress should be casual but professional in appearance with a name-identification tag. Limited jewelry should be worn. Valuable personal items, such as an expensive purse or coat, should not be worn on a visit. Carrying an extra set of car keys in the nursing home care bag saves time and frustration if the nurse becomes locked out of the automobile. Automobile keys spread between the fingers with sharp ends outward can be used as a weapon if necessary. The same commonsense behaviors and precautions that guide a person's behavior when alone in any setting should be followed by home care nurses.

The agency should have a copy of the nurse's home care itinerary, including contact telephone numbers if a client does not have a telephone, and information on the nurse's car (make, model, color, and license plate number). Many home care nurses carry agency-provided pagers or cellular telephones that allow the agency to contact the nurse throughout the day to give information about client updates, changes in orders or services, schedule changes, and new clients who require an initial visit. The telephone is also useful to notify clients when the nurse is delayed.

The automobile used for the home care visits, whether a personal or an agency-owned vehicle, should have regular preventive maintenance checks, an adequate fuel level, and road safety items stored in the trunk. Items to carry in the vehicle include change for telephone calls and tolls, maps, emergency telephone numbers, a flashlight, a first aid kit, flares, a blanket, and equipment for inclement weather conditions.

Home care nurses should park and lock their cars in a safe place that is visible from the street and the client's home and away from hidden alleys. While driving to the client's home, the nurse should assess the neighborhood for safety, especially if the neighborhood is unfamiliar. All valuable items should be stored out of sight before leaving the office. While walking to the client's home, nurses should not walk near groups of strangers hanging out in doorways or alleys, enter into vacant buildings, or enter a yard that has an unrestrained dog. The home or building should not be entered if the nurse has any safety concerns. All home care agencies should have policies to follow for such situations (Occupational Safety and Health Administration, 1996).

Client's home. Once inside the woman's home, the nurse may encounter unsafe situations such as the presence of weapons, abusive behavior, or health hazards. Each potentially hazardous situation must be dealt with according to agency policies and procedures. If abuse or neglect is reasonably suspected, the home care nurse should follow home care agency and state and federal regulations for reporting and documenting the situation.

Nurses should maintain their own safety first and act accordingly throughout the visit.

Infection control. The nurse carries the necessary supplies and equipment to provide nursing care to the woman. Home care bags should contain infection control supplies, such as personal protection equipment; disposable nonsterile, sterile, and utility gloves; disinfectants; disposable cardiopulmonary resuscitation (CPR) masks; gowns; shoe covers; caps; leakproof and puncture-resistant specimen containers; sharps container; dry hand disinfectants; and leakproof barriers. Proper infection control techniques should be used in stocking, storing, handling, and transporting this bag. When a procedure is to be performed, the nurse should set up a clean area for necessary supplies. A dirty area is designated with a trash bag for the collection of soiled equipment and supplies. Hands are washed before all supplies and equipment for the visit are removed from the bag and placed in a clean area.

The importance of infection control does not diminish because nursing care is provided in the client's home rather than in a hospital. Clients are not likely to become infected because of their home environment, but the nurse may become exposed to a communicable disease.

The Centers for Disease Control and Prevention (CDC) has recommended standard precaution guidelines for the protection of health care workers from blood-borne pathogens. These guidelines recommend that Standard Precautions should be used whenever a treatment is performed because it is difficult to determine which clients have a communicable disease.

Handwashing remains the single most important infection control procedure. Hands should be washed before and after each client contact. Wearing gloves does not eliminate the necessity for handwashing. If running water or clean facilities are unavailable, the hands can be cleaned with a self-drying antiseptic solution.

Using gloves reduces the incidence of exposure to blood-borne pathogens. Gloves should be selected according to the nursing activity to be performed. Nonsterile latex or vinyl gloves should be worn with each procedure that has the potential for contact with bodily substances (e.g., performing venipunctures, heel sticks on the newborn, and perineal care). Sterile gloves should be worn with clinical procedures requiring sterile technique, such as insertion of peripherally inserted central lines and certain dressing changes. General-purpose utility gloves should be used for housekeeping activities, such as cleaning equipment or spills. Nonsterile and sterile gloves should be discarded after each use in a leak-resistant waste receptacle. Utility gloves may be disinfected and reused.

Disposable personal protection equipment should be removed after each use and discarded in a plastic trash container. Safety glasses or goggles can be cleaned with soap and water after each use.

Whenever specimens are collected, Standard Precautions should be used. Any specimen of bodily fluids should be placed in a leakproof bag and secured in a puncture-proof container. The outside of the container is washed off, if it was soiled, before transporting it. Specimens should be labeled with the woman's name and additional identifying information according to the home health care agency or laboratory policies. If specimens are being transported, they should be placed in a container on a flat surface in the vehicle. An insulated container may be used to keep specimens cool in transit.

Sharps containers are puncture-proof and leakproof containers that are labeled with a biohazard sign on the outside and should be used to collect needles and sharp objects. Clients are instructed to fill containers between two thirds and three fourths full to prevent spillage of their contents. As part of the client teaching process, information about storage and handling is covered by the home care nurse. When the container reaches its maximum capacity, it should be returned to the home health care agency and replaced. Medical waste, such as urine and secretions, can be discarded through the sewer or septic system.

Contaminated dressings and disposable supplies should be placed in a leakproof plastic bag and securely fastened for disposal at the client's home. The client should be instructed regarding the proper disposal of medical waste in the home. Agency policies and procedures and local waste-management ordinances should be consulted before the client is instructed.

Nursing Considerations

In home care the woman or family members are responsible for administration of medications in the absence of the nurse. A careful medication history should be obtained to see if the client is taking her medications correctly and understands the desired action and potential side effects. Sometimes, when orders are changed, women continue to take both the old and new prescriptions, which can lead to dangerous overdoses or medication interactions. The nurse ensures that there is an adequate supply and a safe place for proper storage of medications to prevent deterioration or accidental ingestion by children or pets. The nurse inquires about any other medications that the woman might be taking concurrently. Over-the-counter drugs or herbal supplements may not be considered medications by the women and not mentioned unless such information is specifically asked for.

High-technology home care involves many diagnostic and therapeutic procedures. A focused physical assessment is always part of the visit. Nurses involved in perinatal home care must be skilled in prenatal, postpartal, and newborn assessment (Heaman, 1998). Many women require additional diagnostic tests. The nurse may need to collect blood or other specimens. Portable fetal monitoring equipment or even ultrasound can be used in the home for fetal assessment. Home infusion for women with hyperemesis gravidarum often replaces hospitalization. Women with preterm labor may receive parenteral tocolytic therapy. Phototherapy or apnea monitors can be provided in the home for newborns. The power supply and wiring must be reliable. Family members may need to be taught to monitor equipment between nurse visits and to prevent accidental damage.

Medical emergencies may occur during or between the nurse's visits to the home. Prior planning and education can reduce the risk of problems. All parents of newborns should know infant CPR. There should be immediate telephone access to call for emergency medical assistance. Women and their families should be taught to recognize danger signs related to their condition. For example, women at risk for preterm labor should learn to palpate the uterus and recognize contractions in the absence of pain; women with diabetes must learn the signs of hypoglycemia and what to do if it occurs; women with preeclampsia must know the danger signs that indicate worsening of their condition and notify the health care provider immediately.

Client and family education in home care includes information about the specific high risk condition(s) involved, implications for pregnancy outcome, and measures for self-monitoring. Verbal explanations should be supplemented with clearly written instructions. General information to promote well-being such as nutrition and common discomforts of pregnancy should also be included. The need for preparation for childbirth can be addressed using books or videos and supplemented by individual teaching at home. Coping with bed rest or other limitation of activity is a problem for many women with high risk pregnancies. The nurse may share strategies that others have used, help with time management, and provide information about support services. Teaching about infant care or the special needs of the preterm infant may be appropriate during the prenatal period.

Clear documentation of assessments, problems identified, treatments and interventions performed, and the client's responses is essential. Third-party payers base reimbursement on the nurse's written record of providing skilled nursing care and assessments that support the woman's continuing need for those services. The nurse must promptly inform the health care provider by telephone or facsimile of any significant changes. When new orders are transmitted by telephone, a written copy must be sent for the physician's signature.

The home care nurse continually reassesses the client's condition and response to the interventions during every home visit and revises the nursing diagnoses and care plan. Nursing documentation should reflect an objective description of the nursing assessment data collected at each visit. Statements such as "no change" or "same as last visit" do not accurately reflect the monitoring of the client condition that occurred during the skilled nursing visit. Once the home care outcomes are achieved and the client is discharged from the home care agency, documentation should include information about the client's status at the time of discharge, progress toward attaining health care goals, and plans for follow-up care.

The role of the clinical record in home care has been affected by social, economic, and legal health care changes. Appropriate care should be taken to complete the necessary home health care records accurately and in a timely manner. Documentation guidelines include writing or dictating notes or using a laptop computer at the client's home or shortly after the visit.

Evaluation

Evaluation is based on the expected outcomes of care. The plan is revised as necessary.

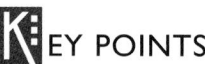

KEY POINTS

- A community is defined as a locality-based entity composed of systems of societal institutions, informal groups, and aggregates that are interdependent and whose function is to meet a wide variety of collective needs.

- Community-oriented practice is targeted to the community, the population group in which healthful change is sought.

- Of necessity, most changes aimed at improving community health involve partnerships among community residents and health workers.

- Assessing community health requires gathering and interpreting data.

- Methods of collecting data useful to the nurse working in the community include windshield surveys, analysis of existing data, informant interviews, participant observation, and service learning.

- The health care system is giving increasing attention to health promotion and disease prevention for populations and aggregates.

- Knowledge of the community in which clients live helps in the planning and organization of care that is responsive to their unique characteristics and needs.

- Vulnerable populations are groups who are at higher risk for developing physical, mental, or social health problems.

- Perinatal home care is a unique nursing practice that incorporates knowledge from community health nursing, acute care nursing, family therapy, health promotion, and client education.

- Social and economic factors affect the scope of perinatal nursing practice.

KEY POINTS—cont'd

- External organizations, such as federal and state government, professional organizations, and health care accrediting agencies, influence the standards of perinatal home health care practice.

- Perinatal home care can be provided for women and infants throughout the perinatal period, beginning before conception and ending in the postpartum period.

- Perinatal home care nurses should incorporate personal safety and infection control practices into the nursing care plan.

- Telephonic nurse advice lines, telephonic nursing assessments, and warm lines are low-cost health care services that facilitate continuous client education, support, and health care decision making even though health care is delivered in multiple sites.

- Communication protocols among members of the home health care team are critical to diminish fragmentation and duplication of health care services.

- Service learning, focusing on meeting community-identified health care needs, allows students to deepen their understanding of communities and themselves.

CRITICAL THINKING EXERCISES

1 *Read your local newspaper and identify articles illustrating community partnerships to meet health needs of vulnerable populations. Were these needs identified by providers or consumers? What needs are unmet?*

2 *Prepare education materials that could be used for teaching clients self-care for preterm labor. Describe the difference between hospital teaching and home care teaching. What follow-up is necessary?*

3 *The home care nurse receives a referral for home visits to a 14-year-old mother with a wound infection following cesarean birth. The new mother and her healthy preterm infant are living with the maternal grandmother in a one-bedroom apartment.*

   a. *What additional information is needed to develop the care plan?*

   b. *How might wound care in the home differ from hospital practice?*

   c. *What health teaching should be provided in addition to wound care?*

   d. *Assuming that the wound heals promptly and the skilled nursing visits are discontinued, what other resources could be used by this family?*

References

Acquaviva, T., & Lancaster, J. (1996). Poverty and homelessness. In M. Stanhope & J. Lancaster (Eds.). *Community health nursing: Promoting the health of aggregates, families and individuals* (4th ed.). St. Louis: Mosby.

Aday, L. (1997). Vulnerable populations: A community-oriented perspective, part 1. *Fam Comm Health* 19(4), 1-16.

American Academy of Pediatrics Committee on Community Health Services. (1996). Health needs of homeless children and families. *Pediatrics,* 98(4 pt 1), 789-781.

American Academy of Pediatrics Council on Child and Adolescent Health. (1998). The role of home-visitation programs in improving health outcomes for children and families. *Pediatrics* 101, 486-489.

Anderson, E., & McFarlane, J. (1996). *Community as partner: Theory and practice in nursing* (2nd ed.). Philadelphia: J.B. Lippincott.

Association of Women's Health, Obstetric, and Neonatal Nurses (AWHONN). (1994). *Didactic content and clinical skills verification for professional nurse providers of perinatal home care.* Washington, D.C.: AWHONN.

Association of Women's Health, Obstetric, and Neonatal Nurses (AWHONN). (1998). *Standards and guidelines for professional nursing practice in the care of women and newborns* (5th ed.). Washington, D.C.: AWHONN.

Bakewell-Sachs, S., & Persily, C. (1995). Perinatal partnerships in practice: A conceptual framework for giving care across the childbearing continuum. *J Perinat Neonatal Nurs* 9(1), 31-37.

Bergquist, S., & King, J. (1994). Parish nursing—a conceptual framework. *J Holist Nurs* 12(2), 155-170.

Bleich, M. (1998). Growth strategies to optimize the functions of telephonic nursing call centers. *Nurs Econ* 4(6), 215-218.

Blystad-Keppler, A. (1995). Postpartum care center: Follow-up care in a hospital-based clinic. *J Obstet Gynecol Neonatal Nurs* 24(1), 17-21.

Bollini, P., & Siem, H. (1995). Health needs of migrants. *World Health* 48(6), 20-21.

Brooten, D. (1995). Perinatal care across the continuum: Early discharge and nursing home follow-up. *J Perinat Neonatal Nurs* 9(1), 38-44.

Broussard, B. (1996). The role of the perinatal home care clinical specialist. *Home Healthc Nurse* 14(11), 855-860.

Burg, M. (1994). Health problems of sheltered homeless women and their dependent children. *Health Soc Work* 19(2), 125-131.

Christian, A. (1996). Clinical nurse specialists: Creating new programs for neonatal home care. *J Perinat Neonatal Nurs* 10(1), 54-63.

Ciaccio, J., & Walker, G. (1998). Nursing and service learning: The kobyashi maru. *Nurs Healthc Perspect* 19, 175-177.

Clear, J., Starbecker, M., & Kelly, D. (1999). Nursing centers and health promotion: A federal vantage point. *Fam Community Health* 21, 1-15.

Clemen-Stone, S., Eigsti, D., & McGuire, S. (1998). *Comprehensive community health nursing: Family, aggregate, and community practice* (4th ed.). St. Louis: Mosby.

Clinton, W. (1998). Proclamation 7141–National Character Counts Week. *34 Weekly Comp Pres,* Doc 2073.

Dillon, D., & Sternas, K. (1997). Designing a successful health fair to promote individual, family and community health. *J Community Health Nurs* 14, 1-14.

Dixon, S. (1996). Parish nurse ministry improves health outcomes of low-income community. *Aspens Advis Nurse Exec* 11(11), 7-8.

Djeddah, C. (1995). Refugee families. *World Health* 48(6), 10-11.

Expert Panel on Women's Health. (1997). Women's health and women's health care: Recommendations of the 1996 AAN expert panel on women's health. *Nurs Outlook* 45, 7-15.

Foss, G. (1996). A conceptual model for studying parenting behaviors in immigrant populations. *Adv Nurs Sci* 19(2), 74-87.

Fowler, B. et al. (1997). Cross-training to develop a home visit program: A rural experience. *Mother Baby Journal* 2(2), 30-38.

Gany, F., & Bocanegra, H. (1996). Maternal-child immigrant health training: Changing knowledge and attitudes to improve health care delivery. *Patient Educ Couns* 27, 23-31.

Hales, A. (1997). Service learning within the nursing curriculum. *Nurs Educ* 22, 15-18.

Health Care Financing Administration. (1989). *Medicare program: Home health agencies—conditions of participation and reductions in record-keeping requirements.* Washington, D.C.: U.S. Department of Health and Human Services.

Health Care Financing Administration. (1990). *Home health insurance manual.* Pub. no. 11-Rev 229. Washington, D.C.: USDHHS.

Heaman, M. (1998). Antepartum home care for high-risk pregnant women. *AACN Clinical Issues: Advance Practice in Acute and Critical Care* 9, 362-376.

Henly, S. et al. (1998). Innovative perspectives on health services for vulnerable rural populations: Community interventions. *Fam Community Health* 1, 22-31.

Henry, J. (1997). Community nursing centers: Models of nurse managed care. *J Obstet Gynecol Neonatal Nurs* 26(2), 224-228.

Hirsh, L., Klein, M., & Marlowe, G. (1967). *Combining public health nursing agencies: A case study in Philadelphia.* New York: NLN.

Hunter, E. (1997). Violence prevention in the home health setting. *Home Healthc Nurse* 15(6), 403-409.

Jones, K., & Schenk, C. (1996). Migrant health issues. In M. Stanhope & J. Lancaster (Eds.). *Community health nursing: Promoting the health of aggregates, families, and individuals* (4th ed.). St. Louis: Mosby.

Kang, D., Kahler, L., & Tesar, C. (1998). Cultural aspects of caring for refugees. *Am Fam Physician* 57, 1245-1246, 1249-1250, 1253-1254.

Kastens, J. (1998). Integrated care management: Aligning medical call centers and nurse triage services. *Nurs Econ* 16, 320-322, 329.

Kemp, C. (1996). Refugee health and community nursing—Dallas, Texas. In E. Anderson & J. Mc Farlane (Eds.). *Community as partner.* Philadelphia: Lippincott-Raven.

Kemp, V., & Hatmaker, D. (1996). Perinatal home care: Issues in family and community health. *Fam Community Health* 18(4), 40.

Killion, C. (1995). Special health care needs of homeless pregnant women. *Adv Nurs Sci* 18(2), 44-56.

Kinsella, A. (1998). Trends for telehealthcare equipment development and disease management. *Remington Report* 6(4), 20-23.

Koniak-Griffin, D. et al. (1999). An early intervention program for adolescent mothers: A nursing demonstration project. *J Obstet Gynecol Neonatal Nurs* 28, 51-59.

Lambert, M. (1995). Migrant and seasonal farm worker women. *J Obstet Gynecol Neonatal Nurs* 24(3), 65-68.

Lassiter, P. (1996). Group approaches in community health. In M. Stanhope & J. Lancaster (Eds.). *Community health nursing: Promoting the health of aggregates, families and individuals* (4th ed.). St. Louis: Mosby.

Lipson, J., & Omidian, P. (1997). Afghan refugee issues in the U.S. social environment. *West J Nurs Res* 19(1), 110-126.

Malnory, M. (1997). Mother-infant home care drives quality in a managed care environment: The quality challenge in managed care. *J Nurs Care Qual* 4(11), 3-26.

March of Dimes Birth Defects Foundation. (1991). *Babies + you: A prenatal health promotion program.* White Plains, NY: March of Dimes Birth Defect Foundation.

Maternal Child Health Bureau. (1992). *Perinatal health strategies for the 21st century.* Washington, D.C.: Maternal Child Health Bureau.

Maternal Child Health Bureau. (1997). Pregnancy-related behaviors among migrant farm workers—four states, 1989-1993. *MMWR* 46(13), 283.

Meurer, L., Meurer, J., & Holloway, R. (1997). New models of health care in the home and in the worksite. *Am Fam Physician* 2(56), 384-386, 389.

Monical, W. (1998). Managing high risk pregnancies at home. *Home Health Cons* 5, 28-31.

O'Campo, P. et al. (1997). Neighborhood risk factors for low birth-weight in Baltimore: A multilevel analysis. *Am J Public Health* 87(7), 1113-1118.

Occupational Safety and Health Administration. (1996). *Guidelines for preventing workplace violence for health care and social service workers—OSHA 3148-1996.* Washington, D.C.: United States Department of Labor (Internet: http://www.osha.gov/oshapubs/workplace/).

Olds, D. et al. (1997). Long term effects of home visitation on maternal life-course and child abuse and neglect. *JAMA* 278(8), 637-643.

Pender, N. (1996). *Health promotion in nursing practice* (3rd ed.). Stamford, CT: Appleton & Lange.

Persily, C., Brown, L., & York, R. (1996). A model of home care for high-risk childbearing families: Women with diabetes in pregnancy. *Nurs Clin North Am* 31, 327-332.

Pew Health Professions Commission. (1995). *Critical challenges: Revitalizing the health professions for the 21st century.* San Francisco: Pew Charitable Trust.

Pignatello, C. et al. (1998). Expanding the role of the pediatric nurse from inpatient to community health. *Nurs Adm Q* 4, 48-53.

Rew, L. (1996). Health risks of homeless adolescents: Implications for holistic nursing. *J Holist Nurs* 14(4), 348-359.

Rodriguez, R. (1996). Promoting healthy partnerships with migrant farm workers—Colorado. In E. Anderson & J. McFarlane (Eds.). *Community as partner.* Philadelphia: Lippincott-Raven.

Sandhaus, S. (1998). Migrant health: A harvest of poverty. *Am J Nurs* 98, 52, 54.

Sebastian, J. (1996). Vulnerability and vulnerable populations: An introduction. In M. Stanhope & J. Lancaster. (Eds.). *Community health nursing: Promoting the health of aggregates, families and individuals* (4th ed.). St. Louis: Mosby.

Shuster, G., & Goeppinger, J. (1996). Community as client: Using the nursing process to promote health. In M. Stanhope & J. Lancaster (Eds.). *Community health nursing: Promoting the health of aggregates, families, and individuals* (4th ed.). St. Louis: Mosby.

Simoni, P., & McKinney, J. (1998). Evaluation of service learning in a school of nursing: Primary care in a community setting. *J Nurs Educ* 37, 122-128.

Stanhope, M., & Lancaster, J. (1996). *Community health nursing: Promoting the health of aggregates, families, and individuals* (4th ed.). St. Louis: Mosby.

Sternas, K. et al. (1999). Nursing and medical student teaming for service learning in partnership with the community: An emerging holistic model for interdisciplinary education and practice. *Holistic Nurs Pract* 2, 66-70.

U.S. Committee on Refugees. (1995). *World refugee survey.* Washington, D.C.: Immigration and Refugee Services of America.

U.S. Department of Health and Human Services. (1991). Consensus set of indicators for assessing community health status. *MMWR* 40(27), 449.

U.S. Department of Health and Human Services. (1997). CHCs staffed by nurses win "models that work" award. *Public Health Rep* 112, 94.

Wagner, J., Menke, E., & Ciccone, J. (1995). What is known about the health of rural homeless families? *Public Health Nurs* 12, 400-408.

Whitley, G., Jacobson, G., & Gawrys, M. (1996). The impact of violence in the health care setting upon nursing education. *J Nurs Educ* 35(5), 211-217.

Women's Health Center Management. (1997). Making insurers want to pay for home care. *Women's Health Care Management* 5(1), 2.

Yoder, M., Cohen, J., & Gorenberg, B. (1998). Transforming the curriculum while serving the community: Strategies for developing community-based sites. *J Nurs Educ* 37, 118-121.

Zotti, M., Brown, P., & Stotts, R. (1996). Community-based nursing versus community health nursing: What does it all mean? *Nurs Outlook* 44, 211-217.

Zyzanski, S., Williams, R., & Flocke, S. (1996). Selection of key community descriptors for community-oriented primary care. *Family Practice* 13(3), 280-288.

4

Alternative and Complementary Therapies

Wendy Wetzel

LEARNING OBJECTIVES

- Define the key terms.
- Describe the differences between standard (allopathic or Western) and holistic health care.
- Define the biopsychosocial and spiritual implications of holistic health care.
- Outline the advantages of a holistic philosophy.
- Compare and contrast touch, energetic, mind-body, and alternative pharmacologic healing modalities.

- Discuss the limitations of research in holistic healing.
- Identify the appropriate modalities for integrative women's health care.
- Propose appropriate topics for holistic nursing research.

KEY TERMS

acupressure
acupuncture
alternative and complementary therapies
biofeedback
energy healing
guided imagery
healing

Healing Touch (HT)
holism
holistic medicine
holistic nursing
homeopathy
massage
meditation
prayer

reflection
relaxation
spirituality
standard (Western or allopathic) medicine
therapeutic touch (TT)
traditional Chinese medicine

INTRODUCTION

It began as a quiet revolution. Consumers, feeling dismayed with the depersonalization of health care and the increasing reliance on high technology and specialization, began investigating alternatives to **standard (Western or allopathic) medicine.** Voicing dissatisfaction with hurried providers, decisions made by insurance companies, and increasing health care costs, some consumers turned to folk healers, spiritual healers, massage therapists, or herbalists.

It has long been argued that the current health care system is disease focused. For example, insurance companies may offer reimbursement for the treatment of various illnesses but not for health maintenance activities; new drugs for chronic illnesses appear in large numbers, but little attention is paid to the role of diet in disease and in health. Stress has been identified as a major health problem, but the treatment of choice has often been pharmaceutical agents rather than lifestyle change and stress-management techniques at a fraction of the cost.

An emerging paradigm now exists in which health is valued and a new appreciation for the connection of body, mind, and spirit is honored and nurtured. Human values, including **spirituality,** ethics, and partnership within health care, are blending with the finest in technology and research. In her classic work, Ferguson (1980) suggested that holistic healing, including **alternative and complementary therapies,** focuses on the correction of underlying disharmony in the interaction of body, mind, and spirit and demonstrates concern and compassion for the whole client, not just the client's symptoms (Box 4-1). **Holism** encompasses attitude, acceptance, perception, and purpose.

Many of the popular alternative **healing** modalities offer human-centered care, with philosophies that recognize the value of the client's input and honor the individual's beliefs, values, and desires. The focus of these modalities is on the whole person, not just a disease complex. Clients often find that alternative modalities are more consistent with their own belief system and allow for more client autonomy in health care decisions (Astin, 1998).

Although standard medical practice excels in many areas, alternative methods are often cited as being more beneficial for the treatment of chronic illness, as well as being more cost-effective because of the emphasis on preventive care and health maintenance (Strohecker, 1994; Weil, 1998a).

As consumer demand grew, the medical community began to investigate. Current researchers suggest that increasing numbers of American adults are seeking alternative and complementary health care and estimate that over 629 million visits were made in 1997 alone, an increase of 47% over previous use. This volume exceeds visits paid to primary health care providers. Expenditures related to alternative therapies are estimated at $27 billion, approximately half of which is out-of-pocket expense and not covered by insurance (Eisenberg et al., 1998; Eisenberg, Kessler, & Forster, 1993).

Although skeptical at first, physicians, nurses, and other providers began to see the value in integrating some of these alternative methods into health care. The research and knowledge base for alternative and complementary therapies has grown and will continue to expand as the interest in and quest for healing continues.

This chapter presents an overview of alternative and complementary therapies, their place in current health care practices, current research endeavors, the role of the nurse in holistic health care, and possibilities for use in women's health care.

OVERVIEW OF ALTERNATIVE AND COMPLEMENTARY MODALITIES

Alternative health care options are many and diverse. Some modalities focus on the body structure and balance, some on the biochemical environment. There are various treatment forms that address the emotional and psychologic health and others that work with the human energy field. It is beyond the scope of this chapter to address all the philosophic and procedural specifics of current alternative and complementary therapies; many texts and reference volumes provide detailed information (Cassileth, 1998; Strohecker, 1994).

Regardless of modality, several concepts are shared by many of these systems. First, there is an emphasis on the client as a whole being, capable of decision making, and as an integral part of the health care team. Clients are encouraged to take responsibility for their health and healing. Equal consideration is provided for all the biopsychosocial and spiritual needs of the client. Each client is seen as a unique individual, and treatment is tailored to that specific person (Dossey, 1997; Dossey, Keegan, Guzzetta, & Kolkmeier, 1995).

Second, proper nutrition, adequate rest, relaxation, exercise, and emotional health are cornerstones of good health and are thought to promote healing. Although various philosophies advocate a variety of dietary regimens, there is agreement that nutrition is often overlooked by mainstream medicine and must be emphasized for healing to occur (Strohecker, 1994).

Third, signs and symptoms of disease states are seen as reflective of deeper processes, including those on the emotional and spiritual levels. Alternative healing modalities attempt to treat those deeper levels and the underlying causes, rather than just the symptoms. Physical symptoms are seen as signals from the mind and the spirit that change is in order (Gerber & Garber, 1996; Starn, 1998; Strohecker, 1994).

The road to healing therefore becomes an individual journey, encompassing the client's entire being, while addressing specific physical, mental, emotional, spiritual, and social needs.

Integrative Health Care

The health care community exists as a fluid and dynamic environment. With a variety of clinicians, from physicians and nurses, physical therapists and mental health counselors, to acupuncturists and massage therapists, energy healers and herbalists, a variety of philosophies and treatment options exist.

Western medicine excels in the treatment of acute diseases, bacterial diseases, surgical emergencies, and trauma. It has also, by necessity, become highly specialized and systematic. With the vast amount of information and research available, it seems impossible for one practitioner to know and absorb all of the current data. With increasing specialization in health care, providers often specialize in one body system or disease, and other symptoms may be overlooked or not evaluated. Clients who seek alternative health care often do so in an attempt to find a practitioner who will address the client as a whole person and who

‖ BOX 4-1   Definitions

An understanding of the following terms used to describe alternative therapies is essential:

- **Acupressure** Massage techniques applied to specific points along certain energy pathways of the body called meridians. A form of treatment based in the theories of traditional Chinese medicine.
- **Acupuncture** A form of treatment using slender needles to stimulate points along energy pathways to correct, enhance, and rebalance the flow of body energy.
- **Alternative and complementary therapies** Nontraditional approaches to health care and healing, often philosophically different from Western medicine. Often involve interventions that are said to induce healing from within the client or improve the internal environment so that the body, mind, or spirit can heal. Often referred to as "natural healing." Can be used in place of or in conjunction with standard health care practices. Also defined as therapeutic modalities not commonly taught by U.S. medical schools or available in U.S. hospitals. Alternative healing often refers to those modalities used *in place of* conventional (or other) health care. Complementary healing refers to those modalities used *in conjunction with* conventional (or other) health care. Many therapies can be either alternative or complementary.
- **Biofeedback** Techniques that teach the client to consciously control certain body functions usually thought of as unconscious (breathing, heart rate, etc.). Often involves electronic instrumentation that provides immediate visual and auditory feedback to assist the learning process.
- **Energy healing** A variety of techniques and disciplines that are said to augment, modulate, stimulate, or remedy certain deficiencies or blocks in the human energy system.
- **Guided imagery** The use of imagination and thought processes in a purposeful way to change certain physiologic and emotional conditions.
- **Healing** The integrating and balancing of the body, mind, and spirit. May or may not effect physical healing from illness. Often perceived as improved sense of well-being, acceptance, and inner peace and harmony.
- **Healing Touch** A combination of energetic healing techniques used by nurses and other health care professionals.
- **Holism** Philosophy that states that the whole is greater than the sum of its parts. In healing, refers to

consideration and treatment of the whole client as a unified being. May include alternative and complementary modalities but is more a philosophic base than a modality in and of itself.
- **Holistic medicine** Health care treatment with techniques not commonly taught in U.S. medical schools or widely available in U.S. hospitals. May include a variety of disciplines involving diet, exercise, vitamin and nutritional supplements, body work, or alternative pharmacologic agents. Philosophy of medicine that encompasses holism.
- **Holistic nursing** Nursing practice that stems from the philosophy of holism, one that views the client as an integrated whole and is influenced by a variety of internal and external factors, including the biopsychosocial and spiritual dimensions of the person, an integrated whole.
- **Meditation** Any activity that focuses the attention in the present moment and, in the process, quiets and relaxes the mind and body.
- **Reflection** Looking within for solutions and answers to certain dilemmas, using intuition and inner wisdom as guides for attainment of healing.
- **Relaxation** The absence or alleviation of mental, physical, and emotional tension through purposeful activities that quiet the mind and body.
- **Spirituality** The individual's connection to one's own values, purpose, and meaning of life. May encompass organized religion or belief in higher power or authority. Recognition of wisdom, imagination, spirit, and intuition. A perception of the unity of nature and the interconnectedness of all beings; inner strength.
- **Standard (Western or allopathic) medicine** Interchangeable terms used to describe the current American health care system. With foundations in germ theory and reductionism, standard medical practice often focuses on one body system or disease complex. Treatments are often pharmaceutical or surgical and produce effects that are different from those of the disease complex.
- **Therapeutic touch** A modern interpretation of the laying on of hands for healing, as interpreted by Dolores Krieger, PhD, RN, and Dora Kunz, a noted healer. Originally taught within nursing programs.
- **Traditional Chinese medicine** Ancient methods of healing that combine herbs, energy healing, and movement as a pathway to health. Seeks to heal on deeper levels rather than just deal with symptoms.

Sources: Cassileth, B. (1998). *The alternative medicine handbook: The complete reference guide to alternative and complementary therapies.* New York: W.W. Norton; Chilton, B. (1998). Recognizing spirituality. *Image J Nurs Sch* 30(4), 400-401; Dossey, B. (Ed.). (1997). *Core curriculum for holistic nursing.* Gaithersburg, MD: Aspen; Dossey, B., Keegan, L., Guzzetta, C., & Kolkmeier, L. (1995). *Holistic nursing: A handbook for practice* (2nd ed.). Gaithersburg, MD: Aspen; Eisenberg, D. et al. (1998). Trends in alternative medicine use in the United States, 1990-1997. *JAMA* 280, 1569-1575; Eisenberg, D., Kessler, R., & Forster, C. (1993). Unconventional medicine in the United States. *N Engl J Med* 329, 246-252; Ferguson, M. (1980). *The Aquarian conspiracy.* Los Angeles: J.P. Tarcher; and Strohecker, J. (Ed.). (1994). *Alternative medicine: The definitive guide.* Puyallup, WA: Future Medicine.

shares the client's own philosophy, convictions, and values (Astin, 1998; Weil, 1998a).

Western medicine has been less successful in the treatment of chronic disease states, such as diabetes, heart disease, immune disorders, and environmental illnesses. Over time, the role of the mind in the health of the body has been forgotten or neglected. Chronic disease states have been treated with an increasing number of pharmaceutical agents or invasive surgery, but the root causes of such ailments have not been considered. The avenues to continued and improved health have not been fully explored (Weil, 1998b; Wetzel, Eisenberg, & Kaptchuk, 1998).

It is imperative that health care become an integrative and cooperative venture, one in which both mainstream and alternative medicine can be accessed and used. Fortunately, that environment is being created, where healing forms are used for what they do best and work side by side in harmony. Medical schools, hospitals, and health care institutions are instituting integrative health care models, and these programs are expected to proliferate as the health care system responds to increased consumer demand (Wetzel et al., 1998). Barriers still exist to complete integration, including a lack of research; opposing or competing philosophies and paradigms; health care cost concerns; lack of consistency in state licensing laws; and lasting biases, attitudes, and prejudices (Phalen, 1998).

Research Efforts

In 1992 the National Institutes of Health (NIH) developed the Office of Alternative Medicine (OAM). Mandated by Congress, the OAM was designed to support research and evaluation of various alternative and complementary modalities and to provide information to health care consumers about such modalities. With a beginning budget of $2 million in 1992, the OAM was awarded a $20 million budget in 1998 to provide research grants; develop and maintain a research database; disseminate information to both health care providers and consumers; support, evaluate, and coordinate domestic and worldwide research; and train researchers. In 1998 Congress instituted the National Center for Complementary and Alternative Medicine (NCCAM), which incorporates the work of the OAM in its mission and function. With additional funding, NCCAM will expand its research focus (Departments of Labor, Health and Human Services, and Education, and Related Agencies Appropriations Act, 1999; Dossey, 1998; National Center for Complementary and Alternative Medicine [NCCAM]/Office of Alternative Medicine [OAM], 1999).

To facilitate definitions and research, NIH established seven categories of alternative and complementary healing (Table 4-1). Although many therapies fall into more than one category, this system provides a starting point for research and data collection.

The creation of OAM and later NCCAM made a substantial statement regarding the willingness of legislators and health care officials to consider integration of these

TABLE 4-1 National Institutes of Health Categories of Alternative Healing Modalities

CATEGORY	EXAMPLES
Alternative systems of medical practice	Acupuncture
	Ayurveda
	Environmental medicine
	Homeopathy
	Native American healing
	Naturopathic medicine
	Shamanism
	Traditional Chinese medicine
Bioelectromagnetic applications	Electroacupuncture
	Neuromagnetic stimulation devices
Diet, nutrition, lifestyle changes	Changes in lifestyle
	Diet
	Macrobiotics
	Megavitamins and other nutritional supplements
Herbal medicine	Herbal approaches from a variety of cultures including the Americas, Europe, and the Far East
Manual healing	Acupressure
	Chiropractic
	Massage therapy
	Osteopathy
	Reflexology
	Therapeutic touch/healing touch
	Trager method
Mind-body control	Art therapy
	Biofeedback
	Counseling
	Dance therapy
	Guided imagery and hypnosis
	Humor therapy
	Meditation
	Music therapy
	Prayer
	Psychotherapy
	Relaxation
	Support and self-help groups
	Yoga
Pharmacologic and biologic treatments	Antioxidizing agents
	Chelation therapy
	Oxidizing agents
	Vaccines (not currently accepted by mainstream medicine)

Sources: Dossey, B. (1998). Holistic modalities and healing moments. *Am J Nurs* 98(6), 44-47; and National Center for Complementary and Alternative Medicine (NCCAM)/Office of Alternative Medicine (OAM). (1999). Internet document: http://altmed.od.nih.gov/nccam/.

modalities into mainstream health care. To date, funding has been granted to researchers investigating guided imagery, biofeedback, prayer, movement (dance, yoga, qi gong, and tai chi), music, acupuncture, chiropractic, massage, homeopathy, herbs, and other therapies for a variety of disease processes and health concerns (NCCAM/OAM, 1999).

THE NURSE'S ROLE: HOLISTIC NURSING

Nursing is coming full circle. As consumers seek medical treatment that is more caring and personal, nurses are playing a key role in the rehumanization of health care. Although it was originally grounded in the holistic theories of Nightingale, nursing has moved into highly technical areas, often losing some of the human-centered caring that was once its hallmark. Many nurses now are rediscovering the value of client-centered care that addresses the whole person, not just a diagnosis or condition. And with that realization, these nurses often self-identify as holistic nurses.

Holistic nurses can be found in every area of nursing practice. Being holistic refers more to one's underlying philosophy than to the tasks assigned to a specific nurse. Holistic nurses provide care that is relationship centered rather than disease or task oriented. By seeing the client as a whole individual, nurses can then provide care that encompasses all of the needs of the individual, be they physical, emotional, spiritual, or social. Seeking to blend technology with healing, holistic nurses are striving to create models of health care that embrace the whole person while enhancing

healing and the interconnectedness of all beings (Dossey et al., 1995). Holistic nurses recognize the need for health care to be based on the interrelated relationships between client and provider, provider and provider, and community and provider. By acknowledging the importance of these levels of relationship, nurses can develop strategies for professional and personal growth (Keegan & Dossey, 1998).

Although many holistic nurses incorporate and integrate alternative and complementary healing modalities into their practices, it must be stated that these techniques are not prerequisites for **holistic nursing** practice. Holistic nursing practice, rather, reflects the attitudes and philosophy brought to the nursing situation, rather than the techniques or modalities employed during the course of nursing care. Holistic nurses also involve themselves in self-care activities, striving to attain their own individual levels of wellness and integration (Box 4-2) (Keegan, 1994; Keegan & Dossey, 1998).

LEGAL TIP

Although a vast array of alternative healing modalities are available, it must be acknowledged that not all of them fall within the scope of nursing practice (Box 4-3). Nurses are advised to consult with their own state's nurse practice act for details.

As the body of knowledge grows, more methods will be integrated into nursing practice.

Many modalities require intensive training, additional certification, or both. As with basic nursing practice, certain competencies must be established before using the skill with clients. With the introduction of dozens of various modalities into health care, nurses are cautioned to carefully examine the reputation, research, and educational criteria of any given program of study.

▪ BOX 4-2 **Description of Holistic Nursing**

Holistic nursing embraces all nursing practice that has healing the whole person as its goal. Holistic nursing recognizes that there are two views regarding holism: that holism involves studying and understanding the interrelationships of the biopsychosocial and spiritual dimensions of the person, recognizing that the whole is greater than the sum of its parts; and that holism involves understanding the individual as an integrated whole interacting with and being acted on by both internal and external environments. Holistic nursing accepts both views, believing that the goals of nursing can be achieved within either framework.

Holistic practice draws on nursing knowledge, theories, expertise, and intuition to guide nurses in becoming therapeutic partners with clients in strengthening the client's responses to facilitate the healing process and achieve wholeness.

Practicing holistic nursing requires nurses to integrate self-care in their own lives. Self-responsibility leads the nurse to a greater awareness of the interconnectedness of all individuals and their relationships to the human and global community, and it permits nurses to use this awareness to facilitate healing. ▪

Source: American Holistic Nurses' Association. (1997). *Leadership council handbook.* Flagstaff, AZ: AHNA.

▪ BOX 4-3 **Holistic Therapies and Modalities Most Commonly Used in Nursing**

- *Body therapies,* including acupressure, healing touch, massage, therapeutic touch, reflexology
- *Mind-body healing,* including art therapy, biofeedback, cognitive therapy, counseling (in cases of addiction, grief, environmental concerns, relationships, spiritual crisis, violence and sexual abuse, and wellness issues), exercise and movement, goal setting and contracts, holistic self-assessment, journaling and self-reflection, meditation, prayer, humor and laughter, imagery, music and sound therapy, play therapy, rituals of healing (combining several modalities)
- *Lifestyle modifications,* including smoking cessation, weight management

▪

Source: Dossey, B. (1998). Holistic modalities and healing moments. *Am J Nurs* 98(6), 4-47; Dossey, B., Frisch, N., Forker, J., & Lavin, J. (1998). Evolving a blueprint for certification: Inventory of professional activities and knowledge of a holistic nurse. *J Holistic Nurs* 16(1), 33-56.

The North American Nursing Diagnosis Association has also acknowledged the emergence of holism with several nursing diagnoses. These include altered/risk for/potential for/enhanced spiritual well-being, spiritual distress, and energy field disturbance. The Nursing Interventions Classification Code lists several alternative modalities as nursing interventions. These include but are not limited to therapeutic touch (TT), simple massage, touch, relaxation, meditation, imagery, and hypnosis (Dossey, 1997).

Support and Education for Holistic Nursing

In 1980 a group of nurses and supporters formed the American Holistic Nurses' Association (AHNA) to assist and support nurses in their own journeys to holism. A vital force in nursing today, AHNA has established certification in holistic nursing and published a core curriculum of holistic nursing practice (Dossey, 1997). It is the mission of AHNA to "develop, implement, and evaluate the standards, education and research for holistic nursing," "to promote the practice of holistic nursing," and "to unite nurses in healing" (American Holistic Nurses' Association

[AHNA], 1997, 1999). This mission is accomplished via various educational offerings, certification, and support of holistic nursing research. AHNA also supports the individual journey toward wholeness and healing by encouraging self-care and personal growth for nurses.

AHNA has also established criteria to guide holistic nursing practice. Although similar to standard nursing principles, the Core Values for Holistic Nursing Practice (AHNA, 1998) reflect the interconnectedness and partnerships that clearly herald a new era of nursing.

Within holistic nursing, other organizations have been established to promote the use of various modalities and healing techniques. Of these, Nurse Healers–Professional Associates International, Inc. (NH-PAI) is one of the largest speciality groups. Focusing on TT with the Krieger-Kunz method, NH-PAI supports TT research and education and sets standards for the practice and scope of the method. They have also been instrumental in creating guidelines and procedures for using TT in health care settings and for practitioner and instructor competency (Box 4-4).

BOX 4-4 | **Resources**

NURSING RESOURCES

American Holistic Nurses' Association
P.O. Box 2130
Flagstaff, AZ 86003-2130
1-800-278-AHNA
http://ahna.org

Healing Touch International, Inc.
12477 W. Cedar Drive, Suite #202
Lakewood, CO 80228
1-303-989-7982
http://www.healingtouch.net

Nurses Certificate Program in Interactive Imagery
Beyond Ordinary Nursing
P.O. Box 8177
Foster City, CA 94404
1-650-570-6157
http://members.aol.com/NCPII/NCPII.html

Nurse Healers–Professional Associates International, Inc.
1211 Locust Street
Philadelphia, PA 19107
1-215-545-8079
http://www.therapeutictouch.org

OTHER RESOURCES

The Academy for Guided Imagery
P.O. Box 2070
Mill Valley, CA 94942
1-800-726-2070
http://www.healthy.net/agi/

Lamaze International
1200 19th Street, NW, Suite 300
Washington, DC 20036-2422
1-800-368-4404 or 202-857-1128
http://www.lamazechildbirth.com/

Momentum98
3509 N. High Street
Columbus, OH 43214
1-800-533-4372
http://momentum98.com

National Center for Complementary and Alternative Medicine (NCCAM)
P.O. Box 8218
Silver Spring, MD 20907-8218
1-888-644-6226
http://altmed.od.nih.gov/nccam/

Sea Band International
580 Thames Street, Suite 440
Newport, RI 02840
1-401-841-5900

Healing Touch International, Inc. (HTI) is another specialty organization that promotes education and research with various forms of **energy healing.** Healing Touch is not restricted to nurses and has grown rapidly in its use and knowledge base. National certification is available to practitioners and instructors. HTI is now recognized in the United States, Canada, and many European countries.

Although these three organizations are representative of nursing involvement in holistic care, many others exist to promote their own specialty or modality. Many welcome nurses as members and supporters. As nurses continue to integrate alternative healing into their practices, additional doors will open for education and support.

ALTERNATIVE AND COMPLEMENTARY THERAPIES IN WOMEN'S HEALTH CARE

Overview

Women's health care is an emerging specialty. There is increased realization that the female human body is biochemically different from that of a male. The long-standing gender biases of Western medicine are giving way to a broader view of women's health care. In the realm of **holistic medicine,** too, an increasing number of modalities are seen as appropriate and are being integrated into care. Thousands of articles and books exist on these topics; this section will address only an overview of a representative sample of those most often used in women's health care and specific to nursing practice (Box 4-5).

Again, nurses are cautioned to be informed regarding the statutes of their state nurse practice act and to seek the additional training required to integrate complementary healing into their nursing practice.

> **BOX 4-5** **Representative Alternative Therapies Commonly Used by Nurses in Women's Health Care**
>
> **TOUCH AND ENERGETIC THERAPIES**
> Massage
> Acupressure
> Therapeutic touch
> Healing touch
>
> **MIND-BODY HEALING**
> Imagery
> Meditation, prayer, reflection
> Biofeedback
> Other modalities that may fall outside of nurse practice guidelines unless the nurse has completed additional training or certification:
> Herbs
> Homeopathy
> Traditional Chinese medicine

Touch and Energetic Healing

One of the most primitive yet effective healing gestures is that of touch. First recorded over 5000 years ago in the records of ancient Asian healers, touch has been a key element of healing throughout the ages. It is a natural instinct to touch that which hurts or needs comfort. The touch of a mother's hand to her child's feverish head and the touch of one friend to another in a time of crisis are clear images of this intuitive healing method.

Archeologic data from ancient cultures, including East Indian, Asian, Native American, and other civilizations, show evidence of touch being integral to the health care systems of these eras. Healing by the laying on of hands was a key element in many spiritual traditions, including those of the ancient Egyptians, Greeks, and Celts. As medicine became an entity unto its own, the realm of hands-on healing declined. Early medical scientists viewed it as a superstition and characteristic of more primitive healing. It was not until the twentieth century that touch became a research topic within modern medicine (Gerber & Garber, 1996).

Early studies showed that touch was vital to human development and had a positive impact on immune function. Other preliminary work documented reduction in heart rate, diastolic blood pressure, and anxiety through touch. Over time, nurses have embraced touch as a therapeutic tool and have studied its effects in client care. Several forms of touch therapy have arisen from this work (Dossey, 1997; Gerber & Garber, 1996; Harlow, 1958).

Using touch for healing has many forms. Most people are familiar with **massage** therapy and its various methods. Massage involves rubbing, stroking, and manipulating the muscle groups and other connective tissue to relieve tension and pain and increase blood flow to the area, thus promoting healing. Various claims are made for the different modes of massage therapy, including increasing circulation, promoting lymphatic drainage, relieving muscle tension, aiding in recovery from certain musculoskeletal injuries, decreasing edema, and improving the functioning of certain body systems. Although simple massage is listed in the nursing intervention categories, therapeutic massage requires additional formal training and has a national certification available (Strohecker, 1994). Massage therapists are subject to individual state laws and regulations.

Other forms of touch within healing combine physical touch and energetic theory. A variety of alternative and complementary therapies use an energy-based philosophy that essentially states that the human body has an energy field around and in it. That energy field is not only detectable, but also can be modulated and changed. Energy-based healing seeks to improve the health of the energy field, balance it, and restore it, so that the body then can heal. Any physical, emotional, or spiritual illness is said to be detectable in the field, as well as healed with the field. In many respects, this is congruent with the nursing theory of Martha Rogers, who spoke of the person as a four-dimensional being (Rogers, 1970).

Energy healing has its roots in the writings of the ancient Hindus (who spoke of *prana*), Asians (who referred to it as *chi* or *qi*), and Greeks and early Christians. The healing ability of Christ is interpreted by some as an energetic healing form. Healing as part of a spiritual path was routinely practiced by clergy and lay people alike within the context of their religious practices until Pope Alexander mandated a halt to the healing mission of the church in the twelfth century. Although this took healing out of the hands of the church, history records many talented healers who continued to employ energetic techniques (Hover-Kramer, Mentgen, & Scandrett-Hibdon, 1996; Starn, 1998).

Acupressure is a variation on massage and touch that has its origins in **traditional Chinese medicine (TCM)**. TCM states that *qi*, or *chi*, is the vital force of life, the energy of the body. If the energy is blocked or stagnated in any way, illness, pain, or other dysfunction can result. Energy travels on defined pathways throughout the body, called meridians, and on each meridian there is a series of points that correspond to body function and various organs. Practitioners of TCM believe that by massaging or compressing a given point, the body energy to that corresponding organ or system can be restored or changed. When the energy flow is restored, healing can occur (Dossey, 1997; Gerber & Garber, 1996; Strohecker, 1994). Although nurses can learn a few select points to use with their clients, a comprehensive education program is desirable for the treatment of more complex health problems.

Within nursing circles, one of the best-known methods of touch healing is **therapeutic touch (TT)**. TT was designed by Dolores Krieger, PhD, RN, a professor of nursing at New York University. She documented a reproducible manner of touch, one in which the practitioner begins in a calm and centered state (called "centering") and holds thoughts of desiring to help or heal (called "intention"). TT has several steps in which the practitioner perceives the client's energy field and notes any areas of uneven activity, deficit, or increase. After observing and feeling the client's energy field, the practitioner can use techniques to modulate the energy and correct the deficiencies or abnormal areas. Krieger's seminal work in the field of human energy is well described in her many publications (Krieger, 1979, 1987, 1993). TT has been widely researched in the nursing field. Early studies documented pain relief, anxiety reduction, and wound healing; later work has focused more on physiologic data (Easter, 1997; Krieger, 1990; Quinn, 1994; Snyder & Lindquist, 1998).

Healing Touch (HT) is another energy-based touch healing modality. Whereas Krieger's work emphasizes a single sequence of energy modulation, HT combines a variety of techniques from a series of disciplines. This gives the practitioner an array of "tools" to use with clients. Practitioners are taught energetic diagnosis and treatment forms and the means for documenting the client's response and progress. These techniques are said to align and balance the human energy field, thereby enhancing the body's ability to heal itself. Proponents assert that HT can be useful for a variety of physical, mental, emotional, and spiritual disorders (Hover-Kramer et al., 1996).

Nursing research on HT is expanding rapidly. Studies focusing on its use by nurses with clients experiencing chronic and acute pain, wound infections, cancer, human immunodeficiency virus infection, depression, fatigue, anxiety, and other health problems are being conducted or have been completed. Nurses are also investigating the phenomenologic implications of this modality, both from the client's and the provider's perspective. Of special note to nurses involved in women's health care are studies on HT with breast cancer clients and those recovering from abdominal hysterectomies (Hutchinson, 1998; Moreland, 1997; Shames & Hover-Kramer, 1997; Silva, 1996; Wetzel, 1993).

TT and HT have been integrated in many health care facilities and institutions, and policies have been written and accepted to make these modalities part of inpatient care. As an independent nursing intervention, they do not require a physician's order for the nurse to provide this service.

Mind-Body Healing

Using the mind as a healing tool is also rooted in ancient teachings. The use of imagination, prayer, and meditation is found in numerous spiritual traditions dating back to the beginning of recorded history.

Guided imagery is used for relaxation, stress management, and enhancing immune function. It is the purposeful development of mental images while in a deep state of relaxation (Giedt, 1997). Imagery allows or guides the normal flow of thoughts within the imagination. It can be likened to the sense of being worried, when mental pictures and thoughts of a dreaded event occur. Although there may not be a direct threat to the person at the time, the mind can induce feelings of fear with associated body symptoms such as tightening the chest or stomach or the onset of sweating. These symptoms are in response to a perception, a thought, but not always to a concurrent event. Imagery uses the power of the mind to induce positive images of healing, improve performance, and reduce anxiety. The mind will then influence the body to meet the image (Dossey et al., 1995).

Proponents also state that using a relaxed body and focused mind can bring about changes in perception and solutions to problems and heal emotional trauma. Imagery has also been used with clients suffering from allergies, musculoskeletal pain, and acute injuries and in preoperative and postoperative situations. Cancer patients have used imagery to decrease the side effects of treatment. Nurses are using guided imagery in private practice as well as within health care settings (Fig. 4-1). Imagery can assist relaxation, reduce anxiety, minimize the need for pain medications, and increase the client's ability to focus while

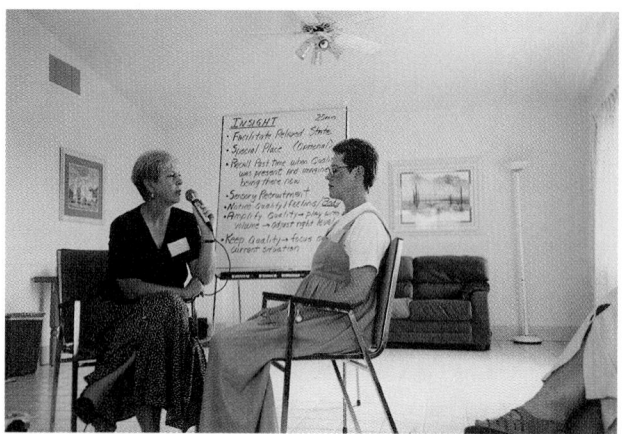

Fig. 4-1 Nurse and client during guided imagery session. *(Courtesy Nurses Certificate Program in Interactive Imagery, Foster City, CA.)*

enhancing creativity. Using recall to enhance change, imagery also may alter emotional and biochemical processes (Dossey et al., 1995; Giedt, 1997; Hoffart & Pross-Keene, 1998).

One of the pioneers of imagery, O. Carl Simonton, MD, used imagery with his cancer patients to enhance their healing. For example, clients are asked to imagine the beams of radiation therapy hitting the cells but leaving the healthy ones intact, or to envision a tumor mass shrinking. Simonton uses these methods in conjunction with other medical treatments, and his success has been well documented (Dossey, 1997; Strohecker, 1994).

Meditation, prayer, reflection, and **relaxation** are similar modalities, all creating an environment of inner quiet. These are ways of looking inside the self and connecting with inner wisdom and intuition. Although some religious traditions define prayer as a communication with God, others simply define it in terms of connecting with a divine or absolute power found within all beings. Prayer is said to be a speaking out, whereas meditation is a quiet listening. Reflection, then, is the evaluation and synthesis of the experience (Dossey, B, 1997; Dossey, L, 1993).

These techniques can aid in the relaxation response and decrease heart rate and blood pressure, thereby reducing stress, decreasing pain perception, and increasing self-understanding. This is thought to allow for insight, cognitive awareness of body functioning, and an intuitive comprehension of what is needed for the individual healing process (Cassileth, 1998; Dossey, B, 1997; Dossey, L, 1993; Snyder & Lindquist, 1998; Strohecker, 1994). Benson's (1984) classic work on the relaxation response indicated that physiologic function was enhanced when meditative and relaxing techniques were integrated into the subject's life. Stress-related illnesses decreased in severity, and the effects of chronic illness were reduced.

Biofeedback combines relaxation with consciously learning to regulate those body functions normally seen as automatic to improve health and decrease pain, blood pressure, and pulse rate. Using specially designed equipment that can monitor heart rate; skin temperature, moisture, and electrical conductivity; and muscle tension, clients are taught the means to reduce tension, induce relaxation, and isolate and exercise certain muscle groups. Biofeedback instruments provide immediate information to the client and show the progress made, thus enabling the client to reinforce the behaviors that brought about the desired change. For example, if a certain breathing technique induces a significant and desired change in heart rate and blood pressure, the client can immediately see the effects on the biofeedback instrumentation and feel the change within her or his body (Cassileth, 1998; Snyder & Lindquist, 1998).

Biofeedback has been used in a variety of settings for stress-related illness, as well as for systemic illnesses such as asthma. Treatment of disorders linked to muscle tension (headaches, temporomandibular joint disorders, hypertension) is especially effective and has been studied extensively (Bray, 1998; Cassileth, 1998; DePalma & Weisse, 1997; Gerber & Garber, 1996).

Biofeedback can also assist with muscle training. By enabling the client to focus on specific muscle groups, correct exercises can be learned with the help of biofeedback. After several sessions, the client is usually able to isolate and exercise the same muscle groups even without the biofeedback equipment.

Alternative Pharmacologic Modalities

Some of the most frequently used alternative therapies employed by American consumers today are those involving alternatives to drug therapy. These modalities involve the use of herbs or other remedies outside the usual scope of pharmaceutical agents. Proper use of these therapies mandates additional education.

The use of herbs and other botanical substances for healing dates back to many ancient civilizations. Although it is often considered a folk remedy, herbal medicine plays a significant role even today. Many of our current pharmacologic agents are derived from or originated in a plant-based model. Digitalis, for example, is a derivative of the foxglove family, and atropine was first derived from the deadly nightshade. Recently, herbal preparations have gained popularity and several have been investigated for their medicinal qualities. St. John's wort has been identified as an antidepressant, and feverfew has been researched in its role in preventing migraines.

By definition, one is practicing herbal medicine if one uses a cup of mint tea to soothe an upset stomach. However, the science of herbal medicine is complex and precise. Herbs can vary in potency from day to day and season to season, and while a small dose may be beneficial, a larger one can be hazardous. Herbal preparations are readily available to the public in a variety of settings, including health food stores and supermarkets. However, they can vary in concentration, and consumers should be advised to carefully read all labels for information about the actual herbal component of the selected preparation.

Herbs are classified according to their properties and effects. Most herbal medicine texts list the desired effect and the properties of the herb itself. Herbs can be delivered in whole form (dried and powdered), as a tea (steeped in water), as extracts and tinctures (small amounts dissolved in an alcohol base), in capsules or tablets, as concentrated "essential" oil, and in creams and salves.

Homeopathy is a system of healing founded by Samuel Hahnemann, a German physician, in the late 1700s. Hahnemann, also known for his work in pharmacology and toxicology, sought to find a more sensible and compassionate alternative to the medical practices of his day (for example, bloodletting with leeches and toxic laxatives). By experimenting with certain botanical agents, he confirmed Hippocrates' observation that small doses of the same agent that caused a disease would cure it. This is also the basis for modern immunologic medicine, wherein a small amount of a toxin, allergen, or virus stimulates the body to create immunity (Jonas, Jacobs, & Dossey, 1998; Weiner & Goss, 1996).

Homeopathic practitioners also believe that each client is a unique individual, and care is directed to create and prescribe a remedy specific to that person. Although many standard remedies exist, practitioners often blend individual remedies based on the client's specific needs. Homeopathy also dictates that illness, as perceived on the physical level, is evidence of disturbances on other, deeper, levels, and the remedies seek to work through those other levels, from the most recent through the oldest, until full healing is achieved (Cassileth, 1998; Jonas et al., 1998; Strohecker, 1994; Weiner & Goss, 1996).

Combining herbal and energy medicine, traditional Chinese medicine (TCM) is experiencing a resurgence of popularity. It has been practiced for over 3000 years and was one of the first methods of healing to be documented. TCM incorporates theories of energetic healing, often describing the energy flow as an excess or a deficiency. The goal of TCM is to restore total harmony on all levels, emotional, spiritual, and physical. Although acupressure is a discipline within TCM, traditional methods include acupuncture (the stimulation of specific points on the body with needles, herbs, or heat) and herbal treatments. Various movement forms such as *tai chi* and *qi gong* may be integrated into a program of TCM (Cassileth, 1998; Elias & Ketcham, 1998; Phalen, 1998; Strohecker, 1994).

Acupuncture is recognized as being widely practiced in the United States for a variety of conditions and is showing promise in the areas of pain management (postoperative states, dental procedures, fibromyalgia, and myofascial pain) and nausea caused by pregnancy or chemotherapy. Research is continuing to determine its efficacy in other areas (Acupuncture: NIH Consensus Development Panel, 1998; Acupuncture: NIH Consensus Statement, 1997).

Applications in Women's Health Care

Many women have sought "natural" alternatives to invasive health care practices. Whether seeking natural childbirth or alternatives for menopause, women have been more open to complementary modalities and have more actively sought care from holistic practitioners. Research is ongoing, and significant strides are being made to open the doors to health care that encompasses the whole patient while providing comprehensive health care (Colbath, 1997).

Pregnancy and Obstetric Care

Pregnancy is usually seen as a naturally occurring event, but highly technical medical practices have shifted the emphasis from a condition of health to one of potential disease. Although there is no disputing the advances in high risk obstetric care, most normal pregnancies will proceed safely with little or no intervention. Several commonly used alternative therapies can assist the expectant mother through her gestation.

Nausea and vomiting of pregnancy can be a difficult problem. Although women with hyperemesis must receive prompt and comprehensive care, the lesser nausea of the first trimester can be effectively treated with herbal teas. Herbs such as peppermint, spearmint, chamomile, and ginger can be used as teas and have been cited as possible remedies for "morning sickness." Other herbs, including fennel, hops, and wild yam, have also been named but are less accessible. Women may need to try several different herbal teas or alternate their use to achieve efficacy (Beal, 1998).

Certain homeopathic remedies are also noted to be effective for nausea. Many are available as over-the-counter products, or a skilled homeopath can construct an appropriate mixture based on the severity of the client's symptoms (Beal, 1998; Weiner & Goss, 1996).

TCM also offers some alternatives in its herbal pharmacy, under the direction of a skilled practitioner. Certain acupressure or acupuncture points assist with the relief of nausea. One of these, pericardium 6 (P6), is a point that women can use for self-treatment. P6 is located two to three finger widths below the flexion crease of the wrist on the dorsal side and between the flexor tendons (Fig. 4-2). By stimulating this point (with a fingertip or other blunt object), nausea can be relieved. Certain elasticized wrist bands (Sea Bands, for example) have been marketed that use a bead or other firm object to stimulate the P6 point and can be worn continuously (Fig. 4-3). Several studies have shown that clients report a decrease in nausea when using the wrist bands on the appropriate point. This acupressure technique has also been studied in cases of nausea occurring with chemotherapy and after anesthesia (Beal, 1992; de Aloysio & Penacchioni, 1992; Elias & Ketcham, 1998; O'Brien, Relyea, & Taerum, 1997).

When appropriate acupressure alone does not relieve nausea or vomiting, acupuncture treatments may be more

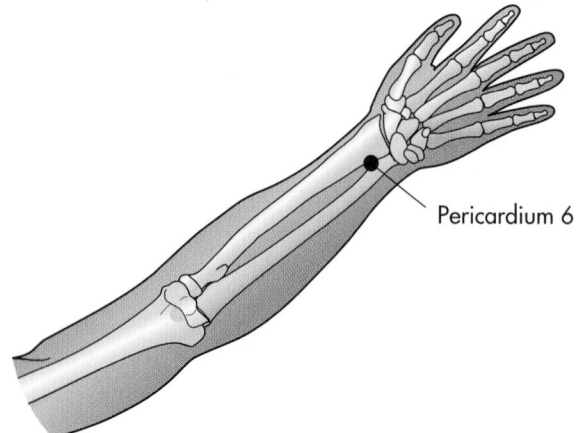

Fig. 4-2 Pericardium 6 (P6) acupressure/acupuncture point for nausea.

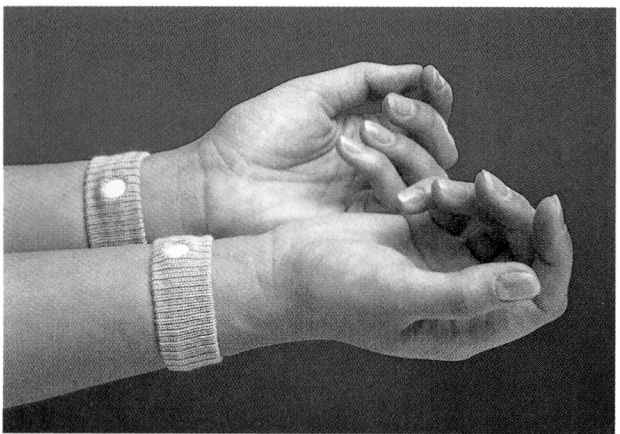

Fig. 4-3 Sea Bands used for stimulation of acupressure point p6. *(Courtesy Sea Band International, Newport, RI.)*

effective. Using slender needles gently inserted into the specific points, licensed acupuncturists can treat not only the P6 point, but also various other points that govern the digestive process. Daily treatments are often required until the nausea subsides (Elias & Ketcham, 1998; P. Fensky, LAc, personal communication, February 3, 1999).

The management of labor pain has long been a nursing function. Prepared childbirth methods that employ learned relaxation and imagery have been practiced since the 1950s. The Lamaze method has been a standard by which other methods are measured. First described by Ferdinand Lamaze, a French obstetrician, the Lamaze method was imported to the United States by Marjorie Karmel, an American woman who gave birth under his care in Paris. She became a staunch believer in his method of pain control and began teaching it to other expectant mothers. Lamaze now encompasses more than labor management and includes a philosophic profile of holistic care. The Lamaze method encourages parents to take an active role in their pregnancy and obstetric care, to make

informed choices, and to be guided by their inner wisdom. Within classes, techniques for stress reduction and pain management are taught as life skills. Modalities such as imagery and progressive relaxation are emphasized along with communication skills and comfort measures (heat and cold, pressure points). The Lamaze method encourages realistic decision making and active participation on the part of the expectant parents (Lamaze International, 1998). Other methods, including the Bradley and Read method, are also taught nationwide, although Lamaze still enjoys the greatest popularity and widest appeal (see also Chapter 18). Energetic healing modalities are also coming into the arena of labor management. Nurses practicing HT and TT have brought these modalities into the hospital setting. Krieger (1987) outlined a study conducted with pregnant couples and the use of TT in labor as an adjunct to the Lamaze method. Although pain control was not measured, couples using TT in addition to the Lamaze method reported a greater marital (relationship) satisfaction for their childbirth experience than the control group. This small study points to the need for further research into pain management in laboring mothers. Healing touch (Fig. 4-4) is also being used for labor care, but to date, no studies have been published (Hover-Kramer et al., 1996; Hutchinson, 1998; G. Kipnis, personal communication, January 18, 1998; Starn, 1998).

Massage techniques are being integrated into labor care. Studies have shown that therapeutic massage decreased labor time, hospital stay, and postpartum depression. Mothers receiving massage during pregnancy and labor had an increased positive outlook, reported less discomfort, and were less agitated than those who did not receive massage (Field, Grizzle, Scafidi, & Schanberg, 1996; Field et al., 1997; Stevenson, 1995).

Gynecology

Gynecologic complaints generate a large number of visits to health care practitioners. Menstrual cramps, irregular periods, pelvic pain, fibroids, and menopausal concerns make up the majority of episodic visits. Women, in increasing numbers, are seeking alternatives to standard surgical and pharmacologic treatments.

Menstrual cramping, or dysmenorrhea, affects a large number of women in all age groups. Various drug therapies, including nonsteroidal antiinflammatory agents, have been proposed over time with a measure of success. However, a vast number of alternatives can provide relief. Dietary changes, such as eliminating milk and dairy products and reducing the intake of complex carbohydrates and red meat, have been shown to decrease the incidence and severity of cramping. Dietary supplements, especially vitamin B_6 (100 mg per day), vitamin E (400 IU per day), and magnesium (up to 600 mg per day), are recommended. Certain herbal preparations, especially those containing cramp bark, white willow, red raspberry, and black cohosh, may also provide relief. Moderate aerobic exercise

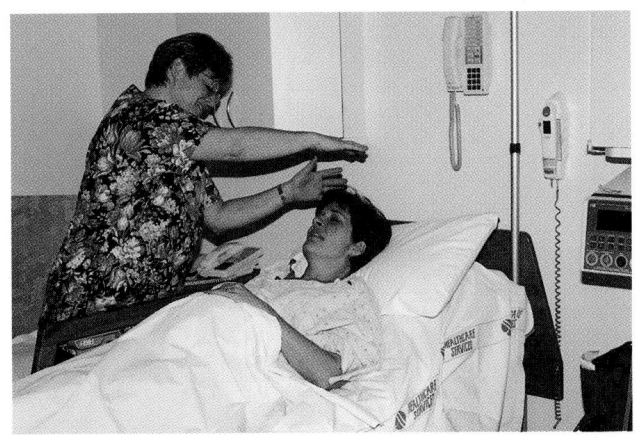
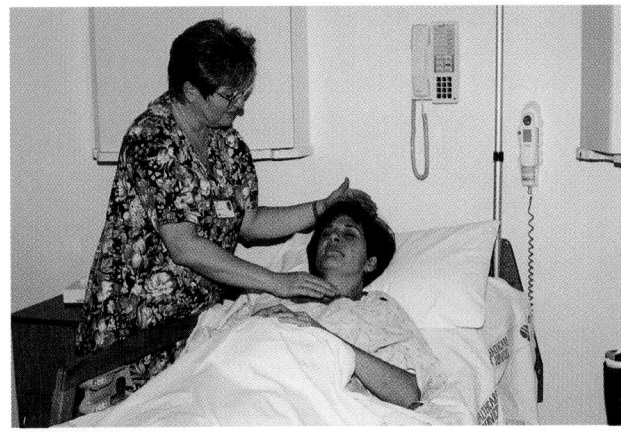
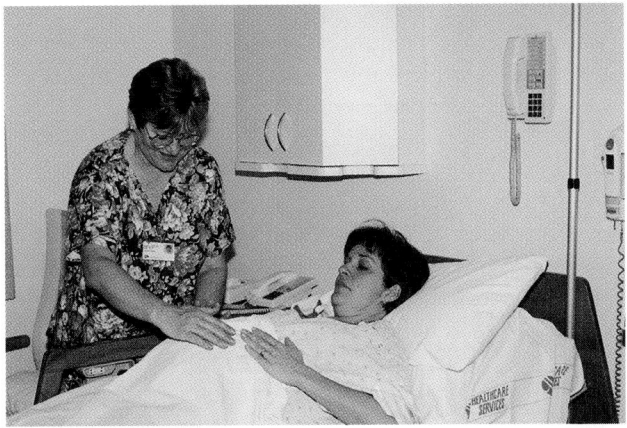
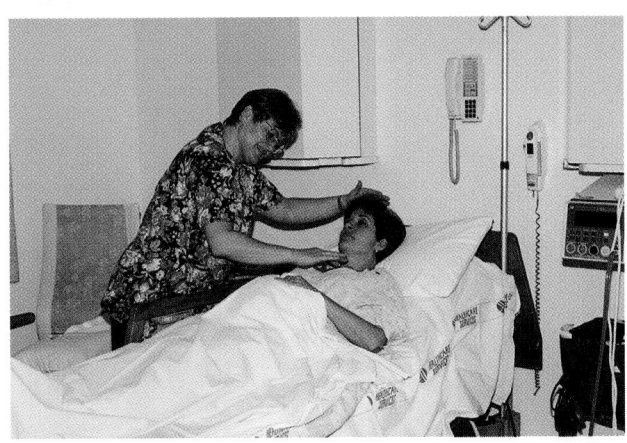
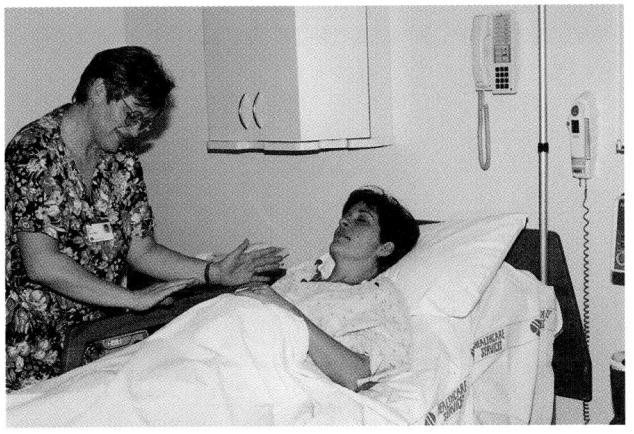
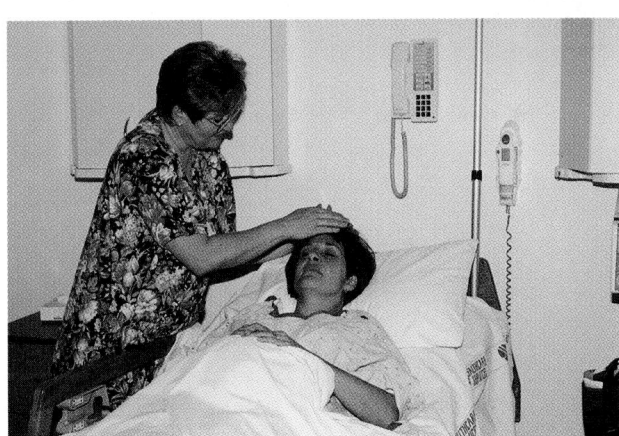
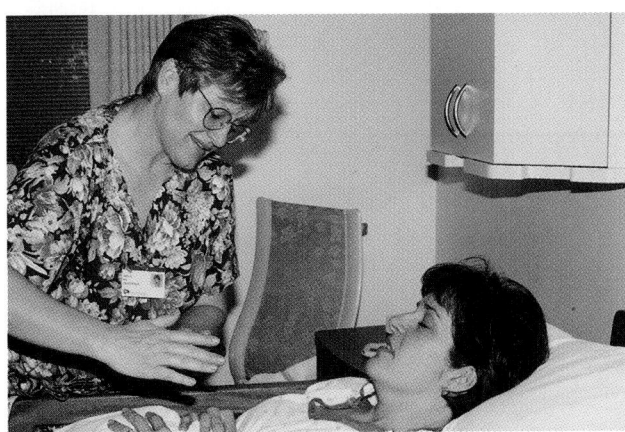

Fig. 4-4 Healing Touch session with pregnant client. *(Courtesy Wendy Wetzel, Flagstaff, AZ.)*

will stimulate blood flow and prevent congestion in the pelvic region. Visualization of healthy pelvic organs with guided imagery can also reduce pain and discomfort. Acupuncture has also been shown to be useful as a complementary modality (Acupuncture: NIH Consensus Development Panel, 1998; Acupuncture: NIH Consensus Statement, 1997; Cassileth, 1998; Northrup, 1998; Strohecker, 1994; Weed, 1989).

Irregular menstrual cycles and heavy menstrual flow are common problems for women. Often a result of hormonal imbalances, dysfunctional uterine bleeding will often respond to synthetic hormone treatment. However, a significant number of women experience adverse effects that cause them to stop therapy. After other physiologic problems (thyroid dysfunction, bleeding disorders, diabetes, and other metabolic diseases) have been ruled out, treatment with human-identical hormones, especially progesterone, may be useful. Herbal therapy with black cohosh, red raspberry, and yarrow are also recommended. Increasing soy in the diet may also provide some additional support (Northrup, 1998; Sauer, 1997; Soffa, 1996; Taylor, 1997; Weed, 1993; Wetzel, 1998).

Premenstrual syndrome (PMS), or premenstrual dysphoria, is a common complaint. Some women experience a variety of disturbing symptoms for the postovulatory period. These symptoms often are alleviated with the onset of menses but cause significant disability and discomfort while they exist. Various theories, including hormonal, emotional, and behavioral, have been proposed. Northrup (1998) suggests that PMS is a social condition brought about by years of shame regarding menstrual functioning; other authors propose that environmental stressors and dietary habits are contributing factors. Suggested remedies include dietary changes; herbal treatments with evening of primrose oil, dandelion, cramp bark, and valerian root; homeopathic remedies to treat the underlying imbalances; body work such as massage and energy healing; and acupuncture (Lee, 1995; Sauer, 1997; Soffa, 1996; Strohecker, 1994).

Increasing attention has been paid to the role of hormones in PMS. Supplementation with "natural" or human-identical progesterone has been reported to provide some relief. Commercially prepared human-identical progesterone appeared on the pharmaceutical market in 1998. Supplementation with this hormone is believed to provide the normal levels of progesterone in the luteal phase and minimize, if not eliminate, the discomforts of PMS (Lee, 1995; Lee & Hopkins, 1996; Wetzel, 1999; Wright & Morgenthaler, 1997).

As the number of menopausal women increases, so do the requests for "natural" hormone therapy. For almost 50 years, women have been offered only estrogens derived from the urine of pregnant horses (conjugated equine estrogens) and synthetic progestins. With the introduction of other botanically based formulas, there are more op-

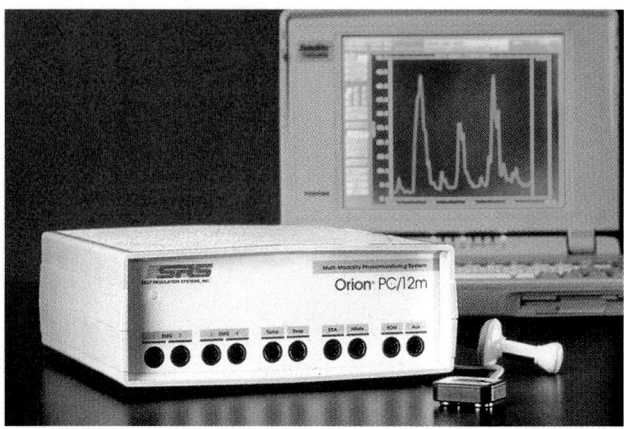

Fig. 4-5 Biofeedback equipment used for pelvic floor training, showing typical display seen with pelvic floor contractions. Vaginal sensor is shown at lower right. *(Courtesy SRS Medical Systems, Inc., Redmond, WA.)*

tions than ever before. Although truly natural hormones may be difficult to obtain, certain plants (soy and yam, for example) have been found to have molecular components that are identical in structure and function to human hormones and can be used in these preparations. These offer a new horizon of menopausal treatment, often without the side effects of standard agents, while offering similar benefits and actions (Lee, 1995; Lee & Hopkins, 1996; Northrup, 1998; Sauer, 1997; Taylor, 1997; Wetzel, 1998; Wright & Morgenthaler, 1997).

For women who cannot take hormonal treatment for menopausal complaints, herbs and homeopathy offer some alternatives. With the increasing awareness and diagnosis of breast cancer, there is consensus that women with a history of breast cancer should not take hormone replacement until they are in remission for several years. However, these women often need some support and treatment for their symptoms. Herbs such as black cohosh, chasteberry, motherwort, burdock, yam, valerian, and St. John's wort can provide symptomatic relief of hot flashes, night sweats, irritability, depression, and insomnia. A skilled herbalist can combine the ingredients into a mixture suited to the individual client. Vitamin E oil can soothe atrophic vaginal tissues, and certain homeopathic remedies can also ease this time of transition. Chinese herbs such as dong quai and ginseng can also provide some essential relief (Jonas et al., 1998; Northrup, 1998; Taylor, 1997; Weed, 1993; Weiner & Goss, 1996).

Women should inform their health care providers that they are using herbal remedies; health care providers should inquire if women are using herbal remedies as part of their history taking.

Biofeedback is being integrated into women's health care as a noninvasive treatment for various forms of urinary incontinence (Fig. 4-5). Incontinence can be a disturbing problem, often compelling women to become homebound because of their loss of urine or embarrassment. Depending on the cause, biofeedback training can enhance the client's ability to exercise the various muscles of the pelvic floor, thereby strengthening them and preventing urinary leakage. Biofeedback can also be used to strengthen pelvic floor muscles, weakened by childbirth, surgery, illness, or aging. These techniques can also be used for clients with pelvic pain related to muscular weakness. Physical therapists and nurses are being trained in this technique, which provides a nonsurgical alternative for incontinence problems. Bladder training also offers a cost-effective means to solve an embarrassing dilemma. Clients should be appropriately screened to determine the cause of incontinence and then referred to a trained therapist for the proper exercises and monitoring (Berghmans et al., 1996; Gallo & Staskin, 1997; Stein et al., 1995).

Implications for Nursing Practice

With increased client awareness of health care models that are different from standard medical practice, the nurse is often the first consulted for her professional opinion and advice. By maintaining an open and compassionate atmosphere, the nurse can determine the client's level of knowledge about a given healing modality, as well as serve as a resource for concise and factual information.

At the intake interview, clients should be asked if they are using any alternative or complementary modalities in their health plan. This also includes asking about the use of vitamins and over-the-counter remedies. Beliefs and values can be explored by the nurse and the client to determine the client's desires and value system. A congruent plan of care can then be formulated that integrates the client's biopsychosocial and spiritual needs. By approaching the client with a nonjudgmental attitude, the nurse can gain the client's trust and assist the client in incorporating the client's desires for alternative and complementary healing into the overall care plan.

Holistic nurses are often called on to guide clients through the healing process and may themselves be the care provider with certain modalities. In ever increasing numbers, nurses are gaining the skills and knowledge to maintain independent practices in various modalities. In this role, they can provide nursing support and guidance along with their chosen modality, thus creating a more comprehensive program of wellness and healing.

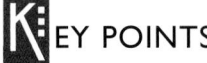EY POINTS

- Integrative medicine combines modern technology with ancient healing practices and encompasses the whole of body, mind, and spirit.
- Alternative and complementary modalities address the whole client and seek to treat on a variety of levels.
- Although holistic research has been limited in the past, increasing efforts and governmental support are paving the way for more inquiries.
- Holistic nursing refers to a philosophic understanding and may integrate alternative and complementary therapies into nursing care.
- Holistic nurses recognize the importance of relationships within healing, as well as the necessity of self-care.
- A variety of alternative and complementary therapies are currently integrated into women's health care.
- Nurses are continuing to identify research opportunities to document the efficacy of integrative women's health care.

RITICAL THINKING EXERCISES

1 *Do an on-line search for resources for holistic health care, holistic medicine, and holistic nursing. What modalities did you find represented? What commonalities did you find in the websites? Did any sites list research studies or other means to verify the efficacy of a given modality? What organizations were listed? After reading the material you found, what impressions did you have? Were there any modalities or specialities you would like more information about? How can you obtain that information?*

2 *Visit a local health food store and observe the various types of vitamins, herbs, and supplements available. Pay particular attention to those products marketed for menopausal women. What claims are made? What are the main ingredients? If possible, interview the store owner or the person in charge of the supplement department. What are their perceptions about women who use "natural" hormones and other nonpharmaceutical remedies for menopause?*

3 *Mrs. Jackson is a new client in your clinic. She is 42 years old, still has regular periods, but is complaining of profound PMS symptoms. She is adamant about wanting only "natural treatment."*

   a. *In taking her history, what symptoms will you be alert for?*

   b. *What recommendations can you provide that are congruent with her needs and desires?*

   c. *What social and spiritual factors might play a role in her PMS?*

   d. *What are your reactions to her history and requests?*

References

Acupuncture: NIH Consensus Statement Online. (1997). Nov 3-5; in press. [1999, February 2]; 15(5):1-34. Internet document: http://odp.od.nih.gov/consensus/cons/107/107_statement.html

Acupuncture: NIH Consensus Development Panel on Acupuncture. (1998). *JAMA* 280:1518-1524 [Abstract].

American Holistic Nurses' Association (AHNA). (1999). *Mission statement*. Flagstaff, AZ.

American Holistic Nurses' Association (AHNA). (1997). *Leadership council handbook*. Raleigh, NC: AHNA.

American Holistic Nurses' Association (AHNA). (1998). *The standards of holistic nursing practice*. Flagstaff, AZ: AHNA.

Astin, J. (1998). Why patients use alternative medicine. *JAMA* 278, 1548-1553.

Beal, M. (1992). Acupuncture and related treatment modalities. Part II: Applications to antepartal and intrapartal care. *J Nurse Midwifery* 37(4), 260-268.

Beal, M. (1998). Women's use of complementary and alternative therapies in reproductive health care. *J Nurse Midwifery* 43(3), 224-234.

Benson, H., & Procter, W. (1984). *Beyond the relaxation response*. New York: Putman/Berkley.

Berghmans, L. et al. (1996). Efficacy of biofeedback, when included with pelvic floor muscle exercise treatment, for genuine stress incontinence. *Neurourol Urodyn* 15(1), 37-52.

Bray D. (1998). Biofeedback. *Complementary Therapies in Nursing and Midwifery* 4(1), 22-24.

Cassileth, B. (1998). *The alternative medicine handbook: The complete reference guide to alternative and complementary therapies*. New York: W.W. Norton.

Chilton, B. (1998). Recognizing spirituality. *Image J Nurs Sch* 30(4), 400-401.

Colbath, J (1997). Holistic health options for women. *Crit Care Nurs Clin North Am* 9(4), 589-599.

de Aloysio, D., & Penacchioni, P. (1992). Morning sickness control in early pregnancy by Neiguan point acupressure. *Obstet Gynecol* 80(5), 852-854.

DePalma, M., & Weisse, C. (1997). Psychological influences on pain perception and nonpharmacologic approaches to the treatment of pain. *J Hand Ther* 10(2), 183-191.

Departments of Labor, Health and Human Services, and Education, and Related Agencies Appropriations Act. (1999). Bill No. S.2440. Sec. 601. Establishment of National Center for Complementary and Alternative Medicine. Internet document: http://altmed.od. nih.gov/nccam/about/history/nccam.shtml

Dossey, B. (1998). Holistic modalities and healing moments. *Am J Nurs* 98(6), 44-47.

Dossey, B. (Ed.). (1997). *Core curriculum for holistic nursing*. Gaithersburg, MD: Aspen.

Dossey, B., Frisch, N., Forker, J., & Lavin, J. (1998). Evolving a blueprint for certification: Inventory of professional activities and knowledge of a holistic nurse. *J Holistic Nurs* 16(1), 33-56.

Dossey, B., Keegan, L., Guzzetta, C., & Kolkmeier, L. (1995). *Holistic nursing: A handbook for practice* (2nd ed.). Gaithersburg, MD: Aspen.

Dossey, L. (1993). *Healing words*. New York: HarperCollins.

Easter, A. (1997). The state of research on the effects of therapeutic touch. *J Holistic Nurs* 15(2), 158-175.

Elias, J., & Ketcham, K. (1998). *The five elements of self-healing: Using Chinese medicine for maximum immunity, wellness, and health*. New York: Random House.

Eisenberg, D., Kessler, R., & Forster C. (1993). Unconventional medicine in the United States. *N Engl J Med* 329, 246-252.

Eisenberg, D. et al. (1998). Trends in alternative medicine use in the United States, 1990-1997. *JAMA* 280, 1569-1575.

Ferguson, M. (1980). *The Aquarian conspiracy*. Los Angeles: J.P. Tarcher.

Field, T., Grizzle, N., Scafidi, F., & Schanberg, S. (1996). Massage and relaxation therapies' effects on depressed adolescent mothers. *Adolescence* 31(124), 903-911.

Field, T., Hernandez-Reif, M., Taylor, S., Quintino, O., & Burman, I. (1997). Labor pain is reduced by massage therapy. *J Psychosom Obstet Gynecol* 18(4), 286-291.

Gallo, M., & Staskin, D. (1997). Cues to action: Pelvic floor muscle exercise compliance in women with stress urinary incontinence. *Neurourol Urodyn* 16(3), 167-177.

Gerber, R., & Garber, R. (1996). *Vibrational medicine: New choices for healing ourselves*. Santa Fe, NM: Bear.

Giedt, J. (1997). Guided imagery: A psychoneuroimmunological intervention in holistic nursing practice. *J Holistic Nurs* 15(2), 112-127.

Harlow, H. (1958). Love in infant monkeys. *Scientific American* 200, 68-74.

Hoffart, M., & Pross-Keene, E. (1998). The benefits of visualization. *Am J Nurs* 98(12), 44-47.

Hover-Kramer, D., Mentgen, J., & Scandrett-Hibdon, S. (1996). *Healing touch: A resource for health care professionals*. Albany, NY: Delmar.

Hutchinson, C. (1998). *The healing touch research survey*. Lakewood, CO: Healing Touch International.

Jonas, W., Jacobs, J., & Dossey, L. (1998). *Healing with homeopathy: The doctor's guide*. New York: Warner Books.

Keegan, L. (1994). *Nurse as healer*. Albany, NY: Delmar.

Keegan, L., & Dossey, B.M. (1998). *Profiles of nurse healers*. Albany, NY: Delmar.

Krieger, D (1979). *The therapeutic touch: How to use your hands to help or to heal*. Englewood Cliffs, NJ: Prentice-Hall.

Krieger, D. (1987). *Living the therapeutic touch: Healing as a lifestyle*. New York: Dodd, Mead.

Krieger, D. (1990). Therapeutic touch: Two decades of research, teaching and clinical practice. *Imprint* 37, 83, 86-88.

Krieger, D. (1993). *Accepting your power to heal: The personal practice of therapeutic touch*. Santa Fe, NM: Bear.

Lamaze International. (1998). Frequently asked questions about the Lamaze method. Internet document: http://www.lamazechildbirth.com.

Lee, J. (1995). *Natural progesterone: The multiple roles of a remarkable hormone*. Sebastopol, CA: BLL.

Lee, J. & Hopkins, V. (1996). *What your doctor may not tell you about menopause*. New York: Warner Books.

Moreland, K. (1997). *The lived experience of receiving healing touch therapy of women with breast cancer who are receiving chemotherapy: A phenomenological study*. Master's Thesis, University of Windsor, Canada.

National Center for Complementary and Alternative Medicine (NCCAM)/Office of Alternative Medicine (OAM). (1999). Internet document: http://altmed.od.nih.gov/nccam/.

Northrup, C. (1998). *Women's bodies, women's wisdom*. New York: Bantam.

O'Brien, B., Relyea, M.J., & Taerum, T. (1997). Efficacy of P6 acupressure in the treatment of nausea and vomiting during pregnancy. *Am J Obstet Gynecol* 176(6), 1395-1397.

Phalen, K. (1998). *Integrative medicine: Achieving wellness through the best of Eastern and Western medical practices*. Boston: Charles Tuttle.

Quinn, J. (1994). *Therapeutic touch: Healing through human energy fields: Theory and research* [videotapes and study guide]. New York: National League for Nursing.

Rogers, M. (1970). *The theoretical basis of nursing*. Philadelphia: F.A. Davis.

Sauer, M. (1997). Progesterone use in reproductive and gynecologic endocrinology: Current and future perspectives. *Contemp Ob Gyn* 42, s4-s11.

Shames, K., & Hover-Kramer, D. (1997). *Energetic approaches to emotional healing. Expanding the art of counseling beyond words.* Albany, NY: Delmar.

Silva, C. (1996). The effects of relaxation touch on the recovery level of postanesthesia abdominal hysterectomy patients [Abstract]. *Alternative Therapies in Health and Medicine* 2(4), 94.

Snyder, M., & Lindquist, R. (Eds.). (1998). *Complementary/alternative therapies in nursing.* New York: Springer.

Soffa, V. (1996). Alternatives to hormone replacement for menopause. *Alternative Therapies* (2)2, 34-39.

Starn, J. (1998). Energy healing with women and children. *J Obstet Gynecol Neonatal Nurs* 27(5), 576-584.

Stein, M., Discippio, W., Davia, M., & Taub, H. (1995). Biofeedback for the treatment of stress and urge incontinence. *J Urol* 153(3, pt 1), 641-643.

Stevensen, C. (1995). Nonpharmacological aspects of acute pain management. *Complementary Therapies in Nurse Midwifery* 1(3), 77-84.

Strohecker, J. (Ed.). (1994). *Alternative medicine: The definitive guide.* Puyallup, WA: Future Medicine.

Taylor, M. (1997). Alternatives to conventional hormone replacement therapy. *Compr Ther* 23, 514-532.

Weed, S. (1989). *Healing wise.* Woodstock, NY: Ash Tree.

Weed, S. (1993). *Menopausal years: The wise woman way.* Woodstock, NY: Ash Tree.

Weil, A. (1998a). *Health and healing.* Boston: Houghton Mifflin.

Weil, A. (1998b). *Natural health, natural medicine: A comprehensive manual for wellness and self-care.* Boston: Houghton Mifflin.

Weiner, M., & Goss, K. (1996). *The complete book of homeopathy.* Garden City Park, NY: Avery.

Wetzel, M., Eisenberg, D., & Kaptchuk, T. (1998). Courses involving complementary and alternative medicine at US medical schools. *JAMA* 280, 784-787.

Wetzel, W. (1993). Healing touch as a nursing intervention: Wound infection following cesarean birth—an anecdotal case study. *J Holistic Nurs* 11(3), 277-285.

Wetzel, W. (1998). Human identical hormones: Real people, real problems, real solutions. *Nurse Pract Forum* 9(4), 227-234.

Wetzel, W. (1999). Micronized progesterone: A new perspective for women's health care, a case study review. *The Nurse Practitioner* 24(5), 62-76.

Wright, J., & Morgenthaler, J. (1997). *Natural hormone replacement.* Petaluma, CA: Smart.

5

Health Promotion and Prevention

Barbara Peterson Sinclair

LEARNING OBJECTIVES

- Define the key terms.
- Describe factors influencing a woman's contact with the health care system.
- Identify reasons for women to enter the health care delivery system.
- Discuss financial, cultural, and gender barriers to seeking health care.
- Explain conditions and characteristics that increase health risks for women during their childbearing years.

- Analyze programs of anticipatory guidance that promote health and prevention.
- Outline health screening schedules for women in the childbearing years.
- Identify topics for nursing research related to health promotion in women.

KEY TERMS

health promotion
infertility
Kegel exercises

menopause
perimenopause

prevention
safer sex

REASONS FOR ENTERING THE HEALTH CARE SYSTEM

In addition to regular human health care needs, women have unique and special health circumstances related to their reproductive capacity. As a result, many women initially enter the health care system because of some reproductive system–related situation such as pregnancy; irregular menses; desire for contraception; or episodic illness, such as vaginal infection. Once in the system, however, it is incumbent on health care providers to recognize the need for health promotion and preventive health maintenance and to provide these services as part of lifelong care for women. It has been demonstrated repeatedly that

lifestyle and health habits influence the development of illness, both chronic and acute. In fact, the leading five causes of death in women are to some degree preventable, or at least modifiable, if individuals eat well, are not exposed to tobacco or environmental hazards, engage in physical activity, are immunized, and maintain appropriate health screening and follow-up (U.S. Preventive Services Task Force, 1996).

One cannot generalize among all women, but rather must view the individual woman within the context of her particular age, family, culture, religion, society, and physical being. Also, women cannot be viewed in the same way as men because women may respond differently physiologically, emotionally, and cognitively. Women's roles in society have changed dramatically during recent decades, and as a result, women's attitudes in regard to health care have changed. In addition to quality health services for themselves and their families, women want information and the opportunity to be involved in decision making and self-care. Nurses have the responsibility to provide health education and health promotion and to show compassion for and understanding of the woman's circumstances while doing so (Sinclair, 1997).

Preconception Counseling

Preconception health promotion provides women and their partners with information that is needed to make decisions about their reproductive future. Preconception counseling guides couples on how to avoid unintended pregnancies, stresses risk management, and identifies healthy behaviors that promote the well-being of the woman and her potential fetus. Some couples simply want information pertaining to normal physiology or the timing of coitus to achieve pregnancy or to have myths or beliefs confirmed or denied.

The initiation of activities that promote healthy mothers and babies must occur before the period of critical fetal organ development, which is between 17 and 56 days following fertilization. By the end of the eighth week after conception and certainly by the end of the first trimester, any major structural anomalies in the fetus are already present. Because many women do not realize that they are pregnant and do not seek prenatal care until well into the first trimester, the rapidly growing fetus may be exposed to many types of intrauterine environmental hazards during this most vulnerable developmental phase. Thus preconception health care should occur well in advance of an actual pregnancy.

Every woman of childbearing age should be viewed as a potential mother. Therefore identifying and treating risk factors and providing anticipatory guidance with emphasis on healthy lifestyles may be the keys to improving the health of the next generation. The components of preconception care, such as health promotion, risk assessment, and interventions, are outlined in Box 18-1.

Preconception care is especially important for women who have had a problem with a previous pregnancy (e.g., miscarriage or preterm birth). Although causes are not always identifiable, in many cases problems can be identified and treated and may not recur in subsequent pregnancies. Preconception care is also important to minimize fetal malformations. For example, research has consistently shown that offspring of women who have type 1 diabetes mellitus have significantly more congenital anomalies than do children of mothers without diabetes. Furthermore, it has been shown that the rate of malformation is greatly reduced when the insulin-dependent diabetic woman has excellent blood glucose control when she becomes pregnant and maintains euglycemia (normal

blood sugar) throughout the period of organ development in the fetus. Therefore education and glucose control must begin before conception for the woman and her fetus to benefit from this knowledge (Casele & Laifer, 1998).

The same concept is true for folic acid as a means to prevent neural tube defects such as spina bifida and anencephaly in the offspring. All women of reproductive age are urged to take a daily vitamin or eat fortified cereal daily to obtain the necessary 400 μg of supplemental folic acid as a means to protect an actual or potential baby (Burke, 1999).

Many examples illustrate effects of maternal age or illnesses; conditions that produce anomalies in the fetus (teratogenic agents), such as drugs, viruses, chemicals, genetically inherited diseases; or conditions that might be harmful to the woman should a pregnancy occur. In many instances, counseling can allow for behavior modification before damage is done or a woman can make an informed decision about her willingness to accept potential hazards. There is no doubt that the concept of counseling bears out the adage that risk reduction before conception may offer greater benefits than risk reduction during a pregnancy.

Pregnancy

A woman's entry into health care is often associated with pregnancy, either for diagnosis or for actual care. Suspicion of pregnancy occurs most commonly when a woman is late with her menses. However, other presumptive symptoms such as breast tenderness, nausea, or urinary frequency may also encourage her to seek confirmation. Pregnancy testing is often the first diagnostic tool to be used and can be performed at home or in the health care provider's clinic, office, or laboratory. Human chorionic gonadotropin (hCG) is the biologic marker on which both serum and urine pregnancy tests are based. Earlier and more accurate results occur from testing the blood, but a first-voided morning urine sample can yield valid findings approximately 1 week after the missed period.

Pregnancy is divided into three 3-month segments called trimesters. It is highly desirous for a woman to enter prenatal care within the first 12 weeks, the first trimester. This allows for early pregnancy counseling, especially for the woman who has had no preconception care. Subjective information is obtained by history taking, and objective findings are gathered by physical examination, laboratory tests, and diagnostic analysis. Major goals of prenatal care are found in Box 5-1 and should be initiated at the first visit.

Gestational age of the fetus and estimated date of birth (EDB) are often predicated on menstrual history. If there is a question about gestational age, ultrasonography during early pregnancy is helpful in accurate dating.

Education and counseling for women in the first trimester include discussion and self-care concepts in the areas of nutrition, exercise, sexual relations, employment, travel, rest, social habits (tobacco, alcohol, drugs), genetic

BOX 5-1 Major Goals of Prenatal Care

- Define health status of mother and fetus.
- Determine the gestational age of the fetus and monitor fetal development.
- Identify the woman at risk for complications and minimize the risk whenever possible.
- Anticipate and try to prevent problems before they occur.
- Provide appropriate education and counseling.

counseling, avoidance of environmental insult to the fetus, physical changes, management of common complaints, prenatal classes, other resources, and what to expect for follow-up (Fahey & Sinclair, 1996). Women should be encouraged to ask questions and to express concerns or fears. It is preferable that the woman's husband or partner is invited to attend prenatal visits and is provided the opportunity to ask questions and express concerns. Extensive discussion of pregnancy is found in Unit Three.

Well-Woman Care

Current trends in the health care of women have expanded beyond a reproductive focus. A holistic approach to women's health care includes a woman's health needs throughout her lifetime. This view goes beyond simply her reproductive needs. This restructuring places women's health within the primary health care delivery system. Women's health assessment and screening focus on a multisystem evaluation emphasizing the maintenance and enhancement of wellness (Allen & Phillips, 1997). Support and reassurance begin with the woman's first contact with the health care team. It is often the nurse's responsibility in health promotion to coordinate the woman's care. A nurse often takes the history, orders diagnostic tests, interprets test results, makes referrals, and directs attention to the problems that require medical intervention and referral. Nurses who function in the expanded role as advanced practice nurses can also perform complete physical assessments, including the gynecologic examination.

Many women first enter the health care delivery system for a Papanicolaou (Pap) smear or contraception. Visits to the nurse may be their only contact with the system unless they become ill. Some women postpone examination until a specific need arises, such as pregnancy, pain, abnormal bleeding, or vaginal discharge. Embarrassing signs and symptoms, such as urinary incontinence, dyspareunia (painful intercourse), and annoying vaginal discharge, are often elicited only by sensitive interviewing and careful examination. Some women report a minor symptom as a way of entering the health care system when stronger motives for seeking care, either conscious or unconscious, underlie their primary complaint. It is not uncommon that

serious concerns, such as fear of pregnancy, sexually transmitted disease, cancer, or sexual dysfunctioning, begin to surface during the interview.

Health care needs vary with culture, religion, age, and personal differences. The changing responsibilities and roles of women, their socioeconomic status, and their personal lifestyles also contribute to differences in the health and behavior of women. Employment outside of the home, physical disability, inadequate or lack of health insurance, divorce, single parenthood, and sexual orientation also can affect women's ability to seek and receive health care in clinical settings (Bartman, 1996). As women age, many continue to address their primary health care needs within their established gynecologic care setting. Therefore well-women's health care should include a complete history, physical examination, and age-appropriate screening (see Chapter 6). In addition, health promotion must be included because it increases the levels of health and well-being and actualizes or maximizes the health potential of all women.

Fertility Control and Infertility

As women become more informed about themselves and their health care, they are more willing to seek counseling and techniques of contraception appropriate to their varied and specific needs. Some women first enter the health care system to obtain such advice. Over half of the pregnancies in the United States each year are unintended, and the majority of these occur in the 10% of women who do not use birth control. Education is the key to encouraging women to make family planning choices based on preference and actual benefit-to-risk ratios. Providers can influence the user's motivation and ability to use the method correctly (Hatcher et al., 1998).

Many types of birth control or contraceptives have a high degree of safety and effectiveness. Included are (1) hormonal methods such as combined oral contraceptives (OCs), pills that contain both estrogen and progestin, and progestin-only systems delivered via injectables, subdermals, or orals; (2) barrier methods with physical deterrents such as latex in diaphragms or condoms and chemical deterrents such as nonoxynol-9, a spermicide found in foams and creams; and (3) natural family planning, which involves a combination of calendar, basal body temperature, and cervical mucus/ovulation record keeping as a basis for periodic abstinence. Information on the specifics of these methods plus intrauterine devices, sterilization, and postcoital options can be found in Chapter 9.

The concept of health promotion applies to contraception as can be seen in Box 5-2. The nurse is in a prime situation to influence women positively regarding the need for child spacing, methods of family planning that are consistent with religious and personal preferences, noncontraceptive benefits of certain methods, the appropriate use of methods selected, and the protection of future fertility when so desired.

BOX 5-2 Contraceptive Health Promotion

- Child spacing and quality maternity care improve perinatal outcomes and health in general of mother and children.
- Achieving desired family size enables a better sharing of all resources with attendant increases in education, health care, and other positive societal parameters.
- Contraceptives themselves may positively affect future health. For example, use of condoms may prevent acquisition of HIV infection; combined OCs may provide some protection against later development of cancer of ovary and endometrium; barrier methods decrease transmission of STDs, which can develop into pelvic inflammatory disease with resultant infertility or sterility and thus affect future childbearing capacity.

Women also enter the health care system because of their desire to achieve a pregnancy. Approximately 15% of couples in the United States have some degree of **infertility** as defined by not becoming pregnant after 1 year of unprotected intercourse or not being able to carry a pregnancy to viability. Infertility can cause emotional pain for many couples, and the inability to produce an offspring sometimes results in feelings of failure and inordinate stress on the relationship. Significant amounts of time, money, and emotional investment can be spent on testing and treatment in efforts to build a family (Epps & Stewart, 1995).

Infertility appears to be an ever-increasing problem. Not only is it addressed more often in the media, but also we may be seeing more couples trying to have babies because America's largest population group, the baby boomers, are well into their reproductive years. Many couples have delayed starting their families until they are in their thirties or forties, which allows for more time to be exposed to situations negatively affecting fertility (including age-related infertility for the woman). In addition, sexually transmitted diseases (STDs), which can predispose to decreased fertility, are on the rise, and many women and men are in workplaces and home settings where they may be exposed to reproductive environmental hazards.

Approximately 30% to 40% of all couples treated for infertility conceive at some point. However, steps toward prevention of infertility should be undertaken as part of ongoing routine health care, and such information is especially appropriate in preconception counseling (Lemcke et al., 1995). Primary care providers can undertake initial evaluation and counseling before couples are referred to specialists. For additional information about infertility, see Chapter 10.

Menstrual Problems

Under the influence of hormones, the initiation of menstruation, called the menarche, heralds the beginning of the ability to reproduce and occurs at a mean age of 13 years. Reproductive capacity extends until menstruation ceases at **menopause** at a mean age of 51 years. Irregularities or problems with the menstrual period are among the most common concerns of women and often cause them to seek help within the health care system. Common menstrual disorders include the following:

- Amenorrhea (absence of menses), which is most often but not always caused by pregnancy
- Dysmenorrhea (cramps or painful menstruation), which is perhaps the most common of all gynecologic problems
- Premenstrual syndrome, which represents a constellation of recurrent physical and psychologic discomforts that occur only during the time period preceding menstruation
- Endometriosis (endometrial tissue outside of the uterus that responds to monthly hormonal changes that cause it to thicken and bleed), which possibly causes discomfort or decreased fertility
- Menorrhagia (excessive bleeding) or metrorrhagia (irregular bleeding), which can be due to a variety of causes and should be investigated to allow for appropriate management

Simple explanation and counseling may handle the concern; however, history and examination must be completed, as well as laboratory or diagnostic tests, if indicated. Questions should never be considered inconsequential and age-specific reading materials are recommended, especially for teenagers. The reader is referred to Chapter 7 for an in-depth discussion of menstrual problems.

Perimenopause

Although menopause or the last menstrual period occurs at an average age of 51 years, it is preceded by a period known as the **perimenopause,** or climacteric, during which ovarian function declines. Ova slowly degenerate, and menstrual cycles are anovulatory, resulting in irregular bleeding; the ovary stops producing estrogen, and eventually menses no longer occurs. The body responds to this natural transition in a number of ways, most of which are due to the decrease in estrogen (Box 5-3). Although fertility is greatly reduced during the climacteric, women are urged to maintain some method of birth control because pregnancies still can occur. Most women seeking health care at this time do so because of irregular bleeding that may accompany the perimenopause. Others are concerned about vasomotor symptoms (hot flashes and flushes). All women need to have factual information, the dispelling of myths, a thorough examination, and periodic health screenings thereafter.

Not all women have the same symptoms, nor do symptoms have the same intensity or duration. Hormone therapy (HT), a combination of estrogen and progestin, relieves many symptoms and also reduces the risk of osteoporosis and heart disease. However, the risk of breast cancer may be increased. Perimenopausal and postmenopausal women

BOX 5-3 Effects of Decreased Estrogen in Perimenopausal Women

- Hot flashes and flushes may occur. These are periodic feelings of warmth that spread over the body and occasionally interfere with sleep.
- Urogenital tissues become dry and less flexible, possibly resulting in painful intercourse, atrophic vaginitis, and urinary problems.
- Accelerated bone loss occurs (osteoporosis), eventually causing bones to be brittle and at risk for fracture.
- Cardiovascular risk increases and continues to rise with aging.
- Mood swings and irritability are occasionally reported but are probably due to poor sleep patterns caused by hot flashes at night.

are encouraged to maintain a well-balanced diet, physical activity, and adequate calcium and vitamin D intake (supplementation is recommended) and to have regular mammograms, pelvic examinations, Papanicolaou tests, and diagnostic tests to evaluate bone density, cholesterol levels, and presence of occult blood in stools. (See Chapter 7 for discussion of perimenopause.)

BARRIERS TO SEEKING HEALTH CARE

Financial Issues

The United States spends almost 15% of its gross domestic product on health, far more than any other industrialized nation in the world, yet major problems still exist (Failure of Health Care Reform, 1995). Employment-based financing of health insurance has resulted in a system in which one's health insurance is linked to a job, and the system is working well for fewer and fewer people, especially women. Fourteen million young women have no health insurance, and 5 million more have coverage so inadequate that it does not even include maternity care (Rosenfeld, 1997).

In the United States disparity occurs among races and socioeconomic classes affecting many facets of life, including health. With limited money and awareness, there is a lack of access to care, delay in seeking care, few prevention activities, and little accurate information about health and the health care system. Women use health services more often than men but are more likely than men to have difficulty in financing them; they are twice as often underinsured (i.e., have limited coverage with high cost copayments or deductibles). Women make up the majority of Medicaid recipients; however, only 42% of poor women are eligible. Medicaid has been expanded to include special benefits for pregnant women, but they are limited to treatment of pregnancy-related conditions and terminate 60 days after birth (Lemcke et al., 1995). Current

questions abound regarding possible changes in the Medicaid coverage related to care for mother and child during the maternity cycle. More and more states are requiring their Medicaid recipients to enroll in managed care programs; whether this improves access and outcomes is yet to be determined.

Insurance coverage varies significantly by age, marital status, race, and ethnicity. Caucasians of all ages are more likely than African-Americans and other racial or ethnic groups to have private insurance. Caucasians possess insurance 2.5 times more often than Hispanics and 1.8 times more often than African-Americans. Single, separated, or divorced individuals are less likely to have insurance. Often unmarried teenagers who are usually covered by their parent's medical insurance do not have maternity coverage because policies have inclusion statements for only the employee or spouse.

Midwifery care has helped contain some health care costs, but not all insurance carriers reimburse nurse-practitioners and clinical nurse-specialists as direct care providers, a situation that continues to be a problem. Nursing data must be identified and placed in a database to be included in public policy decisions; nursing variables such as education and supportive care must become part of the national data-gathering system. Nurses should deal with the politics involved in cost-containment health care policies, because they, as knowledgeable experts, can provide solutions to many of the health care problems at a relatively low cost (Hastings, 1995).

Parts of the health care delivery system remain in a state of flux. Great variation occurs depending on type and size of the system, source of payment for services, private versus public programs, availability of and accessibility to providers, individual preferences, and insurance coverage or ability to pay. The impact of these components can be minimal or great, but in many instances it is not known (Wainess, 1999). The ongoing problems of access, cost, and quality have not been solved. Many providers and consumers are concerned about decreasing safety and quality in relation to the effort to decrease cost and capacity. The existing system continues to be oriented to treatment of acute or episodic conditions rather than the promotion of health and comprehensive care (Heinrich, 1998).

Cultural Issues

Although they are most significant, financial considerations are not the only barriers to obtaining quality health care. As our nation becomes more racially, ethnically, and culturally diverse, the health of minority groups becomes a major issue. The National Center for Health Statistics reports 1997 data that reflect racial differences in health. For example, life expectancy for Caucasian women was 79.8 years, whereas for African-American women it was 74.7 years. The proportion of mothers who began receiving prenatal care during the first trimester of pregnancy was 84.7% for Caucasians, 72.3% for African-Americans, and

73.7% for Latinas (Guyer et al., 1998). According to the 1990 census, one of every four persons in the United States is a person of color; however, it is expected that this ratio will become even greater after the census in 2000. The United States is truly a multicultural, pluralistic society. Cox (1997) suggests that differences for all racial and ethnic groups will be more significant than their aggregate numbers indicate and health care workers will need to deal with even more distinct racially and ethnically diverse populations—obviously presenting another health care challenge.

A variety of reasons converge to explain some of the differences in accessing care when financial barriers are adjusted. Insufficient numbers of providers willing to see low-income women was a powerful disincentive; however, with more of the Medicaid population being admitted into managed care programs, this barrier may be modified. Transportation problems and availability of clinic hours prohibit many women from seeking care. A lack of cross-cultural communication also presents problems. Desired health outcomes are best achieved when the health care provider has knowledge and understanding about the culture, language, values, priorities, and health beliefs of those in minority groups. Conversely, members of the group should understand the health goals to be achieved and the methods proposed to do so. Language differences can produce profound barriers between women clients and those in the health care system. Even when using a translator, information may be skewed in either direction. It is particularly difficult to use a family member to translate when personal information is being requested because cultural mores and personal biases may interfere with accurate interpretations (see Chapter 2).

Providers must consider culturally based differences that could affect the treatment of diverse groups of women, and the women themselves must share practices and beliefs that could influence their management responses or willingness to comply. For example, women in some cultures value privacy to such an extent that they are reluctant to disrobe and as a result avoid physical examination unless absolutely necessary. Other women rely on their husbands to make major decisions, including those affecting the woman's health. Religious beliefs may dictate a plan of care as with birth control measures or blood transfusions. Some cultural groups prefer folk medicine, homeopathy, or prayer to traditional Western medicine, and others attempt combinations of some or all practices. Even the perceived effectiveness of medications may be tempered by route of administration or color of the pill. In any event, it is incumbent on health care providers to value and appreciate their own and their client's various sources of information and beliefs about sickness and health.

Gender Issues

Gender influences provider client communication and may influence access to health care in general. The most obvious gender consideration is that between men and women. Researchers have reported significant male-female differences in receipt of major diagnostic and therapeutic interventions, especially with cardiac and kidney problems. Women tend to use primary care services more often than men—and, some believe, more effectively. The sex of the provider plays a role because studies have shown that female clients have Pap smears and mammograms more consistently if they are seen by female providers. Also, women providers generally engage in greater positive, partnership-building communication that is vital to facilitating clients' lifestyle changes (Lemcke et al., 1995).

Sexual orientation may produce another barrier. Lesbian women have primary erotic attractions and relations with other women. Some lesbians may not disclose their orientation to health care providers because they may be at risk for hostility, inadequate health care, or breach of confidentiality. To offset stereotypes, it is necessary for providers to develop an approach that does not assume that all patients are heterosexual (Roberts & Sorensen, 1995). Primary care of lesbians is not different from caring for any other group of women, and lesbian couples have basic physical and psychologic needs similar to those of any couple. Finding supportive providers to provide quality care may be difficult, and as a result lesbians may have poor access to care.

CONDITIONS AND CHARACTERISTICS THAT INCREASE HEALTH RISKS IN THE CHILDBEARING YEARS

Maintaining optimum health is a goal for all women. Essential components of health maintenance are identification of unrecognized problems and potential risks and the education and health promotion needed to reduce them. This is especially important for women in their childbearing years because conditions that increase a woman's health risks are of concern not only to her well-being but also are potentially associated with negative outcomes for both mother and baby in the event of a pregnancy. Prenatal care is the prime example of prevention that is practiced after conception. However, prevention and health maintenance are needed before pregnancy because many of the mother's risks can be identified and then eliminated or at least modified. An overview of conditions and circumstances that increase health risks in the childbearing years follows.

DEMOGRAPHICS

Age

Adolescents

As a female progresses through development ages and stages, she is faced with conditions that are age related. All teens undergo progressive growth of sexual characteristics and also undertake developmental tasks of adolescence, such as establishing identity, developing sexual preference, emancipating from family, and establishing career goals. Some of these situations can produce great stress for the adolescent, and the health care provider should treat her very carefully. Female teenagers who enter the health care system usually do so for screening (Pap smears start at age 18 or when sexually active) or because of a problem such as episodic illness or accidents. Gynecologic problems are often associated with menses (either bleeding irregularities or dysmenorrhea), vaginitis or leukorrhea, STDs, contraception, or pregnancy.

Most young women begin having sex in their mid to late teens; for those who do not, the likelihood of having intercourse increases steadily with age. A sexually active teen who does not use contraception has a 90% chance of pregnancy within 1 year (Alan Guttmacher Institute, 1998).

Teenage pregnancy. Pregnancy in the teenager who is 16 years of age or younger often introduces additional stress on an already stressful developmental period. The emotional level of such teens is commonly characterized by impulsiveness and self-centered behavior, and they often place primary importance on the beliefs and actions of their peers. In attempts to establish a personal and independent identity, many teens do not realize the consequences of their behavior, and planning for the future is not part of their thinking processes (Muscari, 1998).

Unless very young, teens are sufficiently mature to physically support the pregnancy, but they may not adhere to many areas of prenatal instruction, especially nutrition and continuing care. Children of teen mothers may be at risk for abuse or neglect because of the teen's inadequate knowledge of growth, development, and parenting. Implementation of specialized adolescent programs in schools, communities, and health care systems is demonstrating continued success in lowering the birth rate in teens as evidenced by an overall 15% decline in teenage pregnancy between 1991 and 1997 (National Center for Health Statistics, 1998).

Young and Middle Adulthood

Because women ages 20 to 40 have need for contraception, pelvic and breast screening, and pregnancy care, they may prefer to use their gynecologic or obstetric provider as their primary care provider also. During these years, the woman may be "juggling" family, home, and career responsibilities with resulting increases in stress-related conditions. Health maintenance includes not only pelvic and breast screening, but also promotion of a healthy lifestyle, that is, good nutrition, regular exercise, no smoking, moderate or no alcohol consumption, sufficient rest, stress reduction, and referral for medical conditions and other specific problems. Common conditions in well-woman care include vaginitis, urinary tract infections, menstrual variations, obesity, sexual and relationship issues, and pregnancy.

Parenthood after age 35. The woman over 35 does not have a different physical response to a pregnancy, per se, but rather has had health status changes as a result of time and the aging process. These changes may be responsible for age-related pregnancy conditions. For example, a woman with type 2 diabetes may not have had expression of her diabetes at age 22 but may have full-blown disease at age 38. Other chronic or debilitating diseases or conditions increase in severity with time and these, in turn, may predispose to increased risks during pregnancy. Of significance to women in this age group is the risk for certain genetic anomalies (e.g., Down syndrome), and the opportunity for genetic counseling should be available to all (see Chapter 14).

Late Reproductive Age

Women of later reproductive age are often experiencing change and reordering personal priorities. Generally, the goals of education, career, marriage, and family have been achieved, and now the woman has increased time and opportunity for new interests and activities. Conversely, divorce rates are high at this age, and children leaving home may produce an "empty nest syndrome," resulting in levels of depression. Chronic diseases also become more apparent. Most problems for the well woman are associated with perimenopause (e.g., bleeding irregularities and vasomotor symptoms). Health maintenance screening continues to be of importance because some conditions such as breast disease or ovarian cancer occur more often during this stage.

Social/Cultural

Differences exist among people from different socioeconomic levels and ethnic groups with respect to risk for illness and distribution of disease and death. Some diseases are more common among people of selected ethnicity, for example, sickle cell anemia in African-Americans, Tay-Sachs disease in Ashkenazi Jews, adult lactase deficiency in Chinese, beta thalassemia in Mediterranean peoples, and cystic fibrosis in northern Europeans. Cultural and religious influences also increase health risks because the woman and her family may have life and societal values and a view of health and illness that dictate practices different from those expected in the Judeo-Christian Western model. These may include food taboos or frequencies, methods of hygiene, effects of climate, care-seeking behaviors, willingness to undergo screening and diagnostic procedures, and value conflicts. Culturally induced belief in magic can cause illness and death (Murray & Zentner, 1997).

Socioeconomic contrasts result in major health differences as exemplified in birth outcomes. The rates of perinatal and maternal deaths, preterm births, and low-birth-weight babies are considerably higher in disadvantaged populations (National Center for Health Statistics, 1998). Social consequences for poor women as single parents are great because many mothers with few skills are caught in the bind of insufficient income to afford child care. These families generate fewer and fewer resources and increase their risks for health problems. Multiple roles for women in general produce overload, conflict, and stress, resulting in higher risks for psychosocial health care (Cox, 1997).

Health Behaviors

Smoking

Cigarette smoking is a major preventable cause of death and illness. Smoking is linked to cardiovascular heart disease, various types of cancers (especially lung and cervical), chronic lung disease, and negative pregnancy outcomes. Tobacco contains nicotine, which is an addictive substance that creates a physical and a psychologic dependence. Tobacco smoke contains known carcinogens. An average cigarette smoker shortens life by 6 to 8 years.

The incidence of smoking among persons 18 years of age and over remains stable at 25.5%. However, the age of smoking initiation has been dropping over the last 10 years, and girls as young as age 12 or 13 are currently starting to smoke (Pohl & Caplan, 1998). Among adolescents and young adults, more women than men smoke, with non-Hispanic white women significantly more likely to be frequent smokers than either Hispanic or African-American women (Grimes, 1998). Smoking in persons over age 25 ranges from 12% for college graduates to 38% for those with less than a high school education.

Cigarette smoking impairs fertility in both women and men, may reduce the age for menopause, and increases the risk for osteoporosis after menopause. Passive, or second-hand, smoke (environmental tobacco smoke [ETS]) contains similar hazards and presents additional problems for the smoker, as well as harm for the nonsmoker. The American College of Obstetricians and Gynecologists (ACOG) (1997b) reports widespread exposure to ETS, with 9 of 10 nonsmoking Americans showing blood levels of a chemical metabolized from nicotine.

Approximately one third of women who become pregnant are smokers at the time of conception (ACOG, 1997b). Smoking in pregnancy is known to cause a decrease in placental perfusion and is one cause of low birth weight in infants (ACOG, 1997b). The harmful effects of smoking are numerous because the oxygen-carrying capacity of hemoglobin is decreased when carbon monoxide passes through the placenta. Furthermore, nicotine causes vasoconstriction, and smokers generally have a nutrient-poor diet. Finally, smoking interferes with the body's ability to process essential vitamins and minerals, resulting in calcium loss from the bones, a decreased intestinal synthesis of vitamin B_{12}, and increased usage of vitamin C. The woman who smokes during pregnancy is at risk for a variety of complications (Box 5-4).

Substance Use and Abuse

Use of illicit drugs and inappropriate use of prescription drugs continue to increase and are found in all ages, races,

---

BOX 5-4 Maternal Complications of Pregnancy Associated with Smoking

Ectopic pregnancy
Miscarriage (especially after in vitro fertilization)
Premature rupture of membranes
Preterm birth
Placenta previa
Abruptio placentae
Chorioamnionitis

Source: American College of Obstetricians and Gynecologists. (1997b). *Smoking and women's health. ACOG Technical Bulletin no. 240.* Washington, DC: ACOG.

---

ethnic groups, and socioeconomic strata. When abused, psychoactive (mind-altering) drugs can disturb relationships, cause psychologic and physical dependency, and create serious health problems. Such substances interfere with the brain's neurotransmitters and normal chemistry, which in turn affect an individual's mood. They particularly affect the part of the brain that produces euphoria, pleasure, or pain release and, as a result, lead easily to abuse.

Addiction to substances is seen as a biopsychosocial disease with several factors leading to risk. These include biogenetic predisposition, lack of resilience to stressful life experiences, and poor social support (Jessup, 1997). Women are less likely than men to abuse drugs, but the rate in women is increasing significantly. Substance-abusing pregnant women create severe problems for themselves and their offspring, including interference with optimal growth and development and addiction. In many instances, the use of substances is identified through screening programs in prenatal clinics and obstetric units (Li et al., 1999).

Women ages 35 to 49 have the highest rates of chronic alcoholism, but women ages 21 to 34 have the highest rates of specific alcohol-related problems (Jessup, 1997). About one third of alcoholics are women, and many relate onset of their drinking problem to stressful events. Women who are problem drinkers are often depressed, have more motor vehicle injuries, and have a higher incidence of attempted suicide than women in the general population. Also, they are at particular risk for alcohol-related liver damage. Early case finding and early treatment are important in alcoholism for both the ill individual and for family members. See Chapter 35 for further discussion about alcohol and illicit drug use in women.

Prescription medications

Psychotherapeutic medications. Stimulants, sleeping pills, tranquilizers, and pain relievers are used by an estimated 2% of American women (Epps & Stewart, 1995). Such medications can bring relief from undesirable conditions such as insomnia, anxiety, and pain, but because the medications have mind-altering capacity, misuse can produce psychologic and physical dependency in the same manner as illicit drugs. Risk-to-benefit ratios should be considered when such medications are used for more than very short periods of time. All of these categories of drugs have some effect on the fetus when taken during pregnancy and must be very carefully monitored.

Stimulants. These medications increase energy and reduce appetite. In the past they were occasionally used for weight loss, but because of their tendency to create dependence they are no longer sanctioned for this purpose. They may be prescribed for narcolepsy or attention deficit disorder.

Sleeping pills. Barbiturates and hypnotics are used to relieve insomnia, but with long-term use tolerance develops and larger amounts are needed for the same effect. Larger amounts of the medications can result in poor concentration, mood swings, anxiety, and depression. Again, dependency occurs. Withdrawal symptoms can include emotional distress, anxiety, headache, gastrointestinal disturbances, and restlessness.

Narcotics. The use of opiate narcotics is of great benefit in many circumstances because they act on the brain and nervous system to decrease sensitivity to pain and produce a sense of well-being. However, they are highly addictive over time and can produce severe physical and mental symptoms when withdrawn.

Tranquilizers. Tranquilizers provide short-term relief from anxiety and stress caused by unexpected emotional conflict or trauma. Their effect is similar to that of alcohol; low doses produce relaxation and buoyancy, and higher doses produce intoxication. Tranquilizers are not appropriate for long-term therapy. Withdrawal effects are similar to those of sleeping pills but less severe.

Psychotropic Medications. Depression is the most common mental health problem in women. Everyone has a case of the "blues" periodically, but true depression impairs the ability to live a normal life and involves symptoms of pervasive sadness, isolation, fatigue, changes in eating and sleeping patterns, and general negativity. Severely depressed people are at risk for suicide. Typical medications used to treat depression are tricyclic antidepressants (e.g., imipramine [Tofranil] and amitriptyline [Elavil]), monoamine oxidase (MAO) inhibitors (e.g., phenelzine [Nardil]), selective serotonin reuptake inhibitors (SSRIs) (e.g., fluoxetine [Prozac] or sertraline [Zoloft]), and lithium. Tricyclic antidepressants relieve symptoms of depression without artificial mood enhancement seen with stimulants (see Chapter 35).

Caffeine. Caffeine is found in society's most popular drinks: coffee, tea, and soft drinks. It is a stimulant that can affect mood and interrupt body functions by producing anxiety and sleep interruptions. Heart arrhythmias may be made worse by caffeine, and there can be interactions with certain medications such as lithium. Birth defects have not been related to caffeine consumption; however, high intake has been related to a slight decrease in birth weight. The U.S. Food and Drug Administration recommends that pregnant women eliminate or limit their consumption of caffeine to less than 300 mg per day (3 cups of coffee or cola).

Nutrition

Good nutrition is essential to good health. A well-balanced diet helps prevent illness and also is used to treat certain health problems. Conversely, poor eating habits, eating disorders, and obesity are linked to disease and discomfort.

Nutritional deficiencies. Overt disease caused by lack of certain nutrients is rarely seen in the United States. However, insufficient amounts or imbalances of nutrients do pose problems for individuals and families. Overweight or underweight status, listlessness, fatigue, frequent colds and other minor infections, constipation, dull hair and nails, and dental caries are examples of problems that could be nutritionally related and indicate the need for further nutritional assessment. Poor nutrition, especially related to obesity and high fat and cholesterol intake, may lead to more serious conditions and is said to contribute to 6 of the 10 leading causes of death in the United States: heart disease, cancer, stroke and hypertension, arteriosclerosis, cirrhosis of the liver, and diabetes (Lean et al., 1999).

Obesity. Obesity is the accumulation of excess poundage caused by extra body fat. In addition to the risks previously mentioned, obesity is also a factor in other disorders such as gallbladder disease, gout, breathing problems, varicose veins, and osteoarthritis. Extreme obesity contributes to a shortened life span. Obesity is occurring at earlier ages and is disproportionately high among women (Rosenfeld, 1997). Because it is a chronic condition, short-term approaches to weight loss rarely succeed. Management of obesity requires a lifelong commitment to changes in lifestyle, behaviors, and attitudes toward food and eating. Pregnant women who are morbidly obese are at increased risk for hypertension, diabetes, gallbladder disease, postterm pregnancy, and musculoskeletal problems (de Groot, 1999).

Other considerations. Other dietary extremes can also produce risk. For example, insufficient amounts of calcium can lead to osteoporosis, too much sodium contributes to hypertension, and megadoses of vitamins can create adverse effects in several body systems. Fad weight loss programs and yo-yo dieting (repeated weight gain and weight loss) result in nutritional inequality and, in some instances, medical problems. Such diets and programs are not appropriate for weight maintenance. Adolescent pregnancy produces a special nutritional circumstance because the metabolic needs of pregnancy are superimposed on the teen's own needs for growth and maturation and eating habits, which are often less than nutritious.

Eating disorders

Anorexia nervosa. Some women have a distorted view of their bodies and, no matter what their weight, perceive themselves to be much too heavy. As a result, they undertake strict and severe diets and rigorous extreme exercise.

This chronic and rarest of eating disorders is known as anorexia nervosa. A coexisting depression usually accompanies anorexia. Women can carry this condition to the point of starvation, with resulting endocrine and metabolic abnormalities. If not corrected, significant complications of arrhythmias, cardiomyopathy, and congestive heart failure occur and, in the extreme, can lead to death. The condition commonly begins during adolescence in young women who have some degree of personality disorder. They gradually lose weight over several months, have amenorrhea, and are abnormally concerned with body image. The condition requires both psychiatric and medical interventions.

Bulimia nervosa. Bulimia refers to secret, uncontrolled binge eating alternating with methods to prevent weight gain: self-induced vomiting, laxatives or diuretics, strict diets, fasting, and rigorous exercise. During a binge episode, large numbers of calories are consumed, usually consisting of sweets and "junk foods." Binges occur at least two times per week. Bulimia usually begins in early adulthood (age 18 to 25) and is found primarily in females. Complications can include dehydration and electrolyte imbalance, gastrointestinal abnormalities, and cardiac arrhythmias. Bulimia is somewhat similar to anorexia in that it is an eating disorder and usually involves some degree of depression. Unlike anorexia, individuals may feel shame or disgust about their disorder and tend to seek help earlier.

Physical fitness and exercise. Exercise contributes to good health by lowering risks for a variety of conditions that are influenced by obesity and a sedentary lifestyle. It is effective in the prevention of cardiovascular disease and in the management of chronic conditions such as hypertension, arthritis, diabetes, respiratory disorders, and osteoporosis. Exercise also contributes to stress reduction and weight maintenance. Women report that engaging in regular exercise improves their body image and self-esteem and acts as a mood enhancer. Aerobic exercise produces cardiovascular involvement because increasing amounts of oxygen are delivered to working muscles. Anaerobic exercise, such as weight training, improves individual muscle mass without stress on the cardiovascular system. Because women are concerned about both cardiovascular and bone health, weight-bearing aerobic exercises such as walking, running, racket sports, and dancing are preferred. However, excessive or strenuous exercise can lead to hormonal imbalances, resulting in amenorrhea and its consequences. Physical injury is also a potential risk.

Stress

The modern woman faces increasing levels of stress and as a result is prone to a variety of stress-induced complaints and illness. Stress often occurs because of multiple roles in which coping with job and financial responsibilities conflict with parenting and home. To add to this burden, women are socialized to be caretakers, which is emotionally draining by itself. Also, they may find themselves

BOX 5-5 Physical Symptoms of Stress

Headache
Dizziness or feeling faint
Muscle tension
Backache
Grinding of teeth
Skin rash or hives
Sweaty palms
Indigestion
Nausea, vomiting
Diarrhea
Constipation
Loss of appetite
Shortness of breath
Pounding heart
Nonradiating chest pain
Frequent colds

Source: Modified from Epps, R., & Stewart, S. (1995). *The women's complete healthbook.* New York: The Philip Lief Group, Inc.

in positions of minimal power that do not allow them to have control over their everyday environments (Epps & Stewart, 1995). Some stress is normal and, in fact, contributes to positive outcomes. Many women thrive in busy surroundings. However, excessive or high levels of ongoing stress trigger physical reactions in the body, such as rapid heart rate, elevated blood pressure, slowed digestion, release of additional neurotransmitters and hormones, muscle tenseness, and weakened immune system. Consequently, constant stress can contribute to clinical illnesses such as flare-ups of arthritis or asthma, frequent colds or infections, gastrointestinal upsets, cardiovascular problems, and infertility. Box 5-5 lists physical symptoms that may be related to chronic or extreme stress. Psychologic signs such as anxiety, irritability, eating disorders, depression, insomnia, and substance abuse also have been associated with stress.

Sexual Practices

Potential risks related to sexual activity are undesired pregnancy and STDs. The risks are particularly high for adolescents and young adults who engage in sexual intercourse at earlier and earlier ages. Adolescents report many reasons for wanting to be sexually active, among which are peer pressure, to love and be loved, experimentation, to enhance self-esteem, and to have fun (Murray & Zentner, 1997). However, many teens do not have the decision-making or values-clarification skills needed to take this important step at a young age and are also lacking the knowledge base regarding contraception and STDs. They also do not believe that becoming pregnant or getting an STD will happen to them. Pregnancy raises further issues of continuing the pregnancy versus abortion, adoption versus childrearing, continuing with education and career goals versus quitting school, and accepting jobs that require little skill.

Although some STDs can be cured with antibiotics, many can cause significant problems. Possible sequelae include infertility, ectopic pregnancy, neonatal morbidity and mortality, genital cancers, acquired immunodeficiency syndrome, and even death (Hatcher et al., 1998). Sexually transmitted diseases are increasing rapidly and are in epidemic proportion. Choice of contraception has an impact on the risk of contracting an STD. Natural family planning, hormones, and intrauterine devices offer no protection. Diaphragms offer some cervical protection. Condoms combined with nonoxynol-9 (a spermicide) offer the most protection. No method of contraception offers complete protection. (See Chapter 7 for discussion of STDs and Chapter 9 for contraception.)

Medical Conditions

Most women of reproductive age are relatively healthy. However, certain medical conditions present during pregnancy can have deleterious effects on both mother and fetus. Of particular concern are risks from all forms of diabetes, urinary tract disorders, thyroid disease, hypertensive disorders of pregnancy, cardiac disease, and seizure disorders. Effects on the fetus vary and include intrauterine growth restriction, macrosomia, anemia, prematurity, immaturity, and stillbirth. Effects on the mother can also be severe. Refer to Unit Seven for information on specific conditions.

Gynecologic Conditions Affecting Pregnancy

Gynecologic conditions that may contribute negatively to pregnancy include the following:
- *Pelvic inflammatory disease (PID)* can cause stricture or occlusion of uterine (fallopian) tubes, resulting in infertility or ectopic pregnancy (see Chapter 7).
- *Endometriosis* occurs when endometrial tissue grows outside of the uterus; it responds to hormonal influences and causes scarring and adhesions in the tubes (see Chapter 8).
- Some *STDs* can be vertically transmitted to the fetus (e.g., human immunodeficiency virus [HIV], syphilis) or cause damage during the birth process (e.g., *Chlamydia, Neisseria gonorrhoeae,* herpes simplex virus [HSV], or group B streptococci) (see Chapter 7).
- *Fibroids,* benign fibrous growths from the uterine muscle that are under the influence of estrogen, can press on the lining of the uterus, causing infertility; occasionally, they impinge on the space needed by the growing fetus or require a cesarean birth for a pregnancy occurring after surgical removal of the growth (see Chapter 13).
- *Uterine deformities* (bicornuate uterus) can cause spontaneous abortion, preterm labor, and fetal growth problems.
- *Vaginal infection* caused by *Trichomonas* or *Candida* or

bacterial vaginosis can result in uncomfortable vaginal discharge and be confused with normal leukorrhea. *Candida* has a propensity for the glycogen-laden vaginal epithelium found during pregnancy, and reinfections can occur (see Chapter 7).
- *Reproductive or breast cancer treatments* (radiation, surgery, and chemotherapy) can cause fetal anomalies, miscarriage, and preterm labor (see Chapters 12 and 13).

Risks for Cancer

Women are at risk for cancer. Risk factors differ, depending on the type of cancer.

Cervical cancer. Risks for cervical cancer include the following:
- *Early age of first sexual intercourse:* This introduces foreign bodies to the young teen's rapidly changing cells at the junction of columnar tissue from the endometrium and squamous tissue from the vagina.
- *Cigarette smoking:* Organic residues from tobacco are preferentially deposited in the cervix.
- *Human papillomavirus (HPV) infection:* A few particular strains of HPV, such as types 16, 18, 45, and 56, are associated with cervical cancer.
- *Multiple sexual partners:* This exposes the cervix to many microorganisms.

In the United States, African-American women have the highest rate of cervical cancer, followed by Hispanic women. Abnormal spotting or vaginal bleeding is the primary symptom (American Cancer Society, 1999).

Endometrial cancer. The most common malignancy of the reproductive system is endometrial cancer. Estrogen-related exposures such as nulliparity, unopposed estrogen therapy, infertility, and early or late menopause are the most significant risk factors. Other risk factors include obesity, hypertension, diabetes, gallbladder disease, and family history of breast or ovarian cancer (DiSaia & Creasman, 1997). Use of birth control pills and pregnancy appear to provide some protection against endometrial cancer. It occurs most frequently in Caucasian women and after menopause. Abnormal uterine bleeding is the cardinal sign (American Cancer Society, 1999).

Ovarian cancer. Ovarian cancer is the most malignant of all gynecologic cancers, accounting for the most deaths from these cancers. Risk factors include family history of ovarian or breast cancer and having no children or having them late in life. Native American women have the highest rates of ovarian cancer in the United States. There are usually no early warning symptoms (American Cancer Society, 1999).

Other gynecologic cancers. Cancer of the vulva, vagina, and uterine tubes accounts for less than 6% of all female reproductive cancers. Cancers of the vulva and vagina have been linked to HPV and HSV. The cause of uterine tube cancer is unknown. These cancers occur most often in postmenopausal women. Lesions are often the first sign of vulvar cancer. Women with vaginal or uterine tube cancer may be asymptomatic or have vaginal bleeding (DiSaia & Creasman, 1997).

Other cancers

Lung cancer. Lung cancer is the leading cause of cancer deaths in women. Cigarette smoking is the most important risk factor. Other risks include exposure to certain industrial substances, organic chemicals (e.g., radon, asbestos), and radiation exposure. Symptoms include a persistent cough, blood-tinged sputum, chest pain, and recurring pneumonia or bronchitis (American Cancer Society, 1999). Survival rates are low because most cancers are not detected while they are still localized.

Breast cancer. Cancer of the breast is the second leading cause of cancer deaths in women. Mortality rates since 1991 have declined, probably as a result of earlier detection and improved treatment (American Cancer Society, 1999). Risk factors include family history, early menarche, late menopause, nulliparity or having children later in life, and possibly postmenopausal use of estrogen. The incidence is highest in Caucasian and lowest among American Indian women. The earliest sign is having an abnormality that shows up on a mammogram before it can be detected by the woman or a clinician (American Cancer Society, 1999).

Colon cancer. Colon cancer is the third most common cancer in women. Risk factors include a personal or family history of colorectal cancer or polyps; inflammatory bowel disease; and a high-fat, low-fiber diet. The incidence is highest in African-American women. Signs include rectal bleeding, blood in the stool, and a change in bowel habits (American Cancer Society, 1999).

Environmental and Workplace Hazards

Environmental hazards in the home, workplace, and community can contribute to poor health at all ages. Categories and examples of health-damaging hazards include the following: (1) pathogenic agents (viruses, bacteria, fungi, parasites); (2) natural and synthetic chemicals (natural toxins from animals, insects, and plants; consumer and industrial products such as pesticides and hydrocarbon gases; medical and diagnostic devices; tobacco; fuels; and drug and alcohol abuse); (3) radiation (radon, heat waves, sound waves); (4) food substances (added components that are not necessary for nutrition); and (5) physical objects (moving vehicles, machinery, weapons, water, building materials) (Pender, 1996).

Environmental hazards can affect fertility, fetal development, live birth, and the child's future mental and physical development. Children are at special risk for poisoning from lead found in paint and soil. Everyone is at risk from air pollutants, such as tobacco smoke, carbon monoxide, smog, suspended particles (dust, ash, and asbestos), and cleaning solvents; noise pollution; pesticides; chemical additives; and poor preparation of food. Workers also face safety and health risks caused by ergonomically poor workstations and stress. The lists could go on and on.

It is important that risk assessments continue to be in effect to identify and understand environmental public health problems.

Violence Against Women

Violence against women is a major health care problem in the United States, affecting 2 to 4 million women each year and costing millions of dollars in annual medical costs. Women of all races and of all ethnic, educational, religious, and socioeconomic backgrounds are affected. Pregnancy is often a time when violence begins or escalates. The magnitude of the problem is far greater than the statistics indicate, because violent crimes against women are the most underreported data as a result of fear, lack of understanding, and stigma surrounding violent situations (Stringham, 1999).

Maternity and women's health nurses, by the very nature of their practice, are in a unique position to conduct case finding, provide sensitive care to women experiencing abusive situations, engage in prevention activities, and influence health care and public policy toward decreasing the violence. (For further discussion of violence against women, see Chapter 11.)

ANTICIPATORY GUIDANCE FOR HEALTH PROMOTION AND PREVENTION

Over the last several decades, women have made tremendous strides in education, careers, policy making, and overall participation in today's complex society. There have been costs for these advances, and although women are living longer, they may not be living better. As a result, the health care system needs to pay greater attention to the health consequences for women. In addition, women must be active participants in their own health promotion and illness prevention. Pender (1996) describes **health promotion** as the motivation to increase well-being and actualize health potential. **Prevention** is the desire to avoid illness, detect it early, or maintain optimal functioning when illness is present.

Nurses have a major opportunity and responsibility to help women understand risk factors and to motivate them to adopt healthy lifestyles that prevent disease. Lifestyle factors that affect health over which the woman has some control include diet; tobacco, alcohol, and substance use; exercise; sunlight exposure; stress management; and sexual practices. Other influences, such as genetic and environmental factors, may be beyond the woman's control, although some opportunities for prevention exist (e.g., through environmental legislation activism or genetic counseling services).

Knowledge alone is not enough to bring about healthy behaviors. The woman must be convinced that she has some control over her life and that healthy life habits, including periodic health examinations, are a sound investment. She must believe in the efficacy of prevention, early

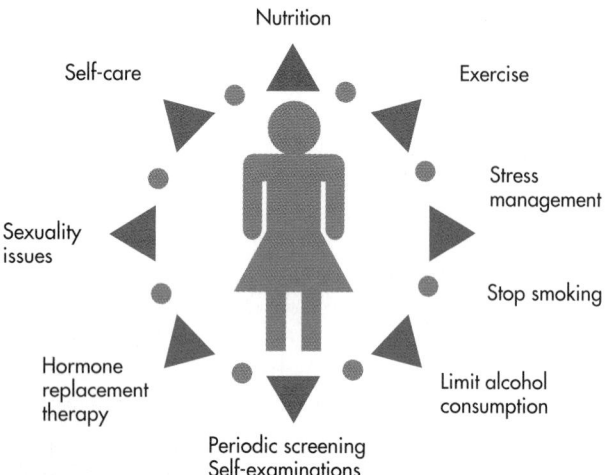

Fig. 5-1 Nursing care model for counseling women about self-care. *(Courtesy University of North Carolina at Chapel Hill School of Nursing, Chapel Hill, NC.)*

detection, and therapy and in her ability to perform self-care practices, such as breast self-examination. Many people believe that they have little control over their health, or they become immobilized by fear and anxiety in the face of life-threatening illnesses, such as cancer, so that they delay seeking treatment. The nurse must explore the reality of each woman's perceptions about health behaviors and individualize teaching if it is to be effective. The model illustrated in Fig. 5-1 incorporates the major aspects to be included when counseling women.

Nutrition

To maintain good nutrition, women should be counseled to include recommended servings from the major food categories of the Food Guide Pyramid (see Fig. 16-5). Complex carbohydrates should make up 45% to 60% of daily intake, including grains, breads, fruits, and vegetables. Moderate amounts of proteins, sugars, and salt should be ingested, and diets should be low in total fat (no more than 30% of total calories), saturated fat (no more than 10%), and cholesterol (up to 300 mg per day). Recommended servings from the food groups also provide for adequate vitamins, minerals, iron, and fiber. Fluid intake is not included in the Food Guide Pyramid, but individuals should be encouraged to drink at least four to six glasses of water every day in addition to other fluids such as juices. Coffee, tea, soft drinks, and alcoholic beverages should be used in moderation.

The technique of basic nutrition counseling does not differ significantly between pregnant and nonpregnant women. The diet can be assessed using a standard assessment form—a 24-hour recall is adequate and quick—and then food likes and dislikes, including cultural variations and typical food portions and dietary habits, should be discussed and incorporated into counseling. The woman should be actively involved in evaluating her intake with the nurse, using a standard food group guide, and should suggest modifications in the diet where needed. Many women have a fair knowledge of food groups and their importance for various nutrients; with guidance they can critique their own intake and suggest changes to improve nutrition. Cultural background and age have a major influence on eating behaviors. A nonjudgmental approach is important, because many women, especially if they are obese or know they are not eating as they should, are sensitive about diet. Unless the motivation to change food habits is intrinsic, efforts to change the diet will fail. If the nurse is supportive, this approach can increase the woman's self-esteem and reinforce good practices while motivating change where needed.

The nurse can provide information about the risks associated with high fat intake and ways to reduce dietary fat intake. Although many people are aware of the association between high fat and cholesterol and disease, they may be ignorant of the major sources of saturated fat and need help in changing eating patterns established during childhood. Because there are more than twice as many calories in fat as there are in protein and carbohydrate, gram for gram, weight control can be facilitated by encouraging women to choose foods relatively low in fat and calories. Fiber-rich foods can be substituted for foods high in fat; they delay digestion and absorption and increase the feeling of satiety.

Most women do not recognize the importance of calcium to health, and their diets are insufficient in calcium. If an adequate bone mass is not achieved at skeletal maturity (usually by about age 20), the woman is at increased risk of developing osteoporosis later in life. Osteoporosis is a disabling, life-threatening disease of epidemic proportions in the United States. The ideal daily calcium intake is unknown, but it is agreed that most women, especially adolescents, should increase their intake. Women under age 50 need 1000 mg of calcium per day, and postmenopausal women over age 50 need 1500 mg. Pregnant and lactating women also need 1500 mg.

Women who are unlikely to get enough calcium in the diet may need calcium supplements in the form of calcium carbonate, which contains more elemental calcium than other preparations.

Long-standing dietary habits are difficult to modify, but given the potential health benefits and positive influence a woman can have on the nutrition of other family members, she may respond to the nurse's encouragement and reinforcement of her good intentions. Chances of success may be enhanced if she becomes involved in a support group or enlists significant others in goal setting.

Exercise

Physical activity and exercise counseling for persons of all ages should be undertaken at schools, worksites, and primary care settings. It is characterized as integrating short bouts of exercise into daily living (Pender, 1996). Specific recommendations include 20 to 30 minutes of moderate activity at least three times per week. Unfortunately, few Americans exercise this often, and physical inactivity increases with age, especially during adolescence and early adulthood.

Nurses are respected care providers who can influence patients to become more active and help them to develop an exercise program geared to their age and personal fitness and goals. Even small increases in activity can be beneficial. The nurse should stress the importance of daily exercise throughout life for weight management and health promotion, suggesting exercises that are enjoyable to the individual (Fig. 5-2). (See Research box.)

Walking, as part of the daily routine, if more vigorous activities cannot be performed, is feasible for most women. Swimming is good for cardiorespiratory fitness but will not prevent osteoporosis, because it is not a weight-bearing exercise (Fig. 5-3). Many women who are sedentary during leisure time can profit from gradually increasing their physical activity. They may be encouraged to exercise with their children or in groups. Worksite fitness programs or community-based programs are increasing. Young women can be involved in physical education activities, games and group sports, and more active pursuits. Home maintenance, yard work, and gardening are other activities that promote health and a sense of well-being, especially for older adults. Attention

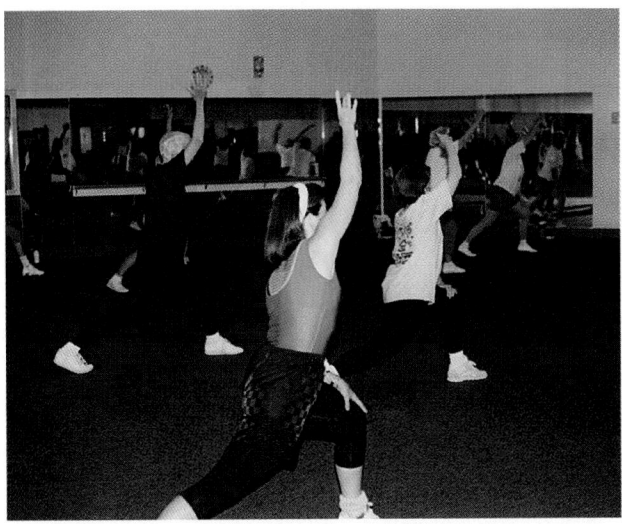

Fig. 5-2 Weight-bearing exercise may delay bone loss and increase bone mass. *(Courtesy Jonas McCoy, Raleigh, NC.)*

to safety factors and wearing clothing and shoes appropriate to each activity are advised. Care should be taken not to aggravate existing conditions or create muscle and joint discomfort by an overly aggressive approach to exercise.

 RESEARCH

Women's Physical Activity Patterns: Nursing Implications

Cardiovascular disease and osteoporosis are two significant health problems facing women as they age. Identifying women's patterns of occupational, household, and leisure activities may provide knowledge from previously unrecognized or untapped sources of activity that can be used in developing intervention strategies for cardiovascular and musculoskeletal health. Previous research studies using physical activity questionnaires have been equivocal and have shown that moderate cardiorespiratory fitness is associated with an improved coronary risk profile in women. The purpose of this study was to develop a method of categorizing patterns of physical activity by describing the frequency, intensity, and duration of women's activities.

This study was designed as a 24-cell quota sample of 200 women stratified by four occupations (academic faculty, telephone personnel, registered nurse, and nursing assistant), two racial groups (Caucasian and African-American), and three age groups (35-43, 44-52, and >53). The main outcome measures consisted of an interview and a self-administered, retrospective occupational, household, and leisure physical questionnaire covering the previous 12 months and lifelong activity.

Results of this study identified five patterns of household and leisure activity: vigorous, continuous, cumulative, occasional, and inactive. Participation in the vigorous pattern was low, but 34% followed a continuous pattern of leisure activity and 75% followed a continuous pattern of household activity. The number of weekly work hours did not affect the household or leisure pattern. It was concluded that women may be able to obtain the recommended levels of physical activity from a combination of occupational, household, and leisure activities.

CLINICAL APPLICATION

Activity patterns begun in early adolescence and young adulthood may be used as predictors in forecasting patterns of activity in later life. Nurses practicing in primary care settings are in a position to help young girls and women identify opportunities to increase their physical activity. Nurses should guide women to increase their regular leisure physical activity or accumulate sessions of moderate-intensity activity by aerobically enhancing daily activities in which they already participate.

Source: Wilbur, J., Miller, A., Montgomery, A., & Chandler, P. (1998). Women's physical activity patterns: Nursing implications. *J Obstet Gynecol Neonatal Nurs* 27(4), 383-392.

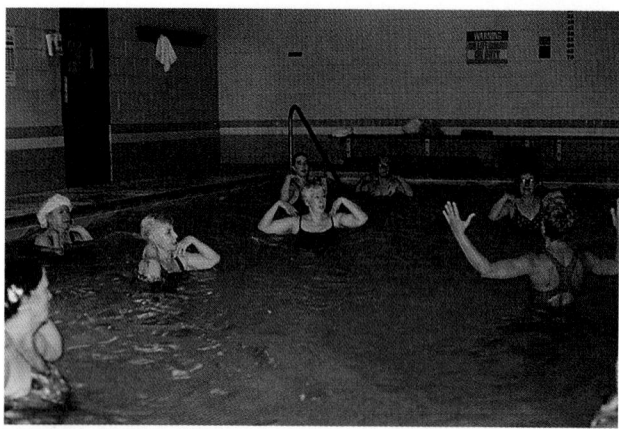

Fig. 5-3 Water aerobics improves cardiovascular function. *(Courtesy Jonas McCoy, Raleigh, NC.)*

During pregnancy, an ongoing exercise regimen can be continued but should be decreased in intensity and duration. Sedentary women should obtain medical clearance to initiate exercise during pregnancy and should begin with low-intensity and low-impact workouts.

Kegel Exercises

Kegel exercises, or pelvic muscle exercises, were developed to strengthen the supportive pelvic floor muscles to control or reduce incontinent urine loss. These exercises are also beneficial during pregnancy and postpartum. They strengthen the muscles of the pelvic floor, providing support for the pelvic organs and control of the muscles surrounding the vagina and urethra.

The Association of Women's Health, Obstetric, and Neonatal Nurses conducted a research utilization project

TEACHING guidelines

Kegel Exercises

DESCRIPTION AND RATIONALE

Kegel exercise, or pelvic muscle exercise, is a technique used to strengthen the muscles that support the pelvic floor. This exercise involves regularly tightening (contracting) and relaxing the muscles that support the bladder and urethra. By strengthening these pelvic muscles, a woman can prevent or reduce accidental urine loss.

TECHNIQUE

The woman needs to learn how to target the muscles for training and how to contract them correctly. One suggestion for teaching is to have the woman pretend she is trying to prevent the passage of intestinal gas. Have her use this tightening motion on the muscles around her vagina and the upper pelvis. She should feel these muscles drawing inward and upward. Other suggested techniques are to have the woman pretend she is trying to stop the flow of urine in midstream or to have her think about how her vagina is able to contract around and move up the length of the penis during intercourse.

The woman should avoid straining or bearing-down motions while performing the exercise. She should be taught how bearing down feels by having her take a breath, hold it, and push down with her abdominal muscles as though she were trying to have a bowel movement. Then the woman can be taught how to avoid straining down by exhaling gently and keeping her mouth open each time she contracts her pelvic muscles.

SPECIFIC INSTRUCTIONS

1. Each contraction should be as intense as possible without contracting the abdomen, thighs, or buttocks.
2. Contractions should be held for at least 10 seconds. The woman may have to start with as little as 2 seconds per contraction until her muscles get stronger.
3. The woman should rest for 10 seconds or more between contractions so that the muscles have time to recover and each contraction can be as strong as the woman can make it.
4. The woman should feel the pulling up and over the three muscle layers so that the contraction reaches the highest level of her pelvis.

OTHER SUGGESTIONS FOR IMPLEMENTATION

1. At first the woman should set aside about 15 minutes a day to do the Kegel exercises.
2. The woman may want to put up reminders, such as notes on her bathroom mirror, her refrigerator, her TV, or a calendar, to do the exercises.
3. Guidelines for practicing Kegel exercises suggest performing between 30 and 80 contractions a day; however, positive results can be achieved with only 30 a day.
4. The best position for learning how to do Kegel exercises is to lie supine with the knees bent. Another position to use is on the hands and knees. Once the woman learns the proper technique, she can perform the exercises in other positions such as standing or sitting. ∎

Sources: Breeding, D. (1996). You don't have to live with incontinence. *Female Patient* 53, 29; Sampselle, C., & Miller, J. (1996). Pelvic muscle exercise: Effective patient teaching. *Female Patient* 21, 29; and Sampselle, C. et al. (1997). Continence for women: Evidence-based practice. *J Obstet Gynecol Neonatal Nurs* 26(4), 375-385.

focused on continence for women (Sampselle et al., 1997). Educational strategies for teaching women how to perform Kegel exercises that were compiled by nurse researchers involved in the project are described in the Teaching Guidelines box.

Stress Management

Because it is neither possible nor desirable to avoid all stress, women must learn how to manage stress. The nurse should assess each women for signs of stress, using therapeutic communication skills to determine risk factors and the woman's ability to function.

Some women must be referred for counseling or other mental health therapy. Women are twice as likely as men to suffer from depression, anxiety, or panic attacks (Japenga, 1998). Nurses must be alert to the symptoms of serious mental disorders, such as depression and anxiety, and make referrals to mental health practitioners when necessary. Women experiencing major life changes, such as divorce and separation, bereavement, serious illness, and unemployment, also need special attention.

For many women the nurse is able to provide comfort, reassurance, and advice concerning helping resources, such as support groups. Many centers offer support groups to help women prevent or manage stress. The nurse can help women become more aware of the relationship between good nutrition, rest, relaxation, and exercise and diversion and their ability to deal with stress. In the case of role overload, determining what needs immediate attention and what can wait is important. Practical advice includes regular breaks, taking time for friends, developing interests outside of work or the home, setting realistic goals, and learning self-acceptance. Discussing how women can maintain meaningful relationships is important. Social support and good coping skills can improve a woman's self-esteem and give her a sense of mastery. Anticipatory guidance for developmental or expected situational crises can help her plan strategies for dealing with potentially stressful events.

There is a great deal of literature on stress management interventions. Role-playing, relaxation techniques, biofeedback, meditation, desensitization, imagery, assertiveness training, yoga, diet, exercise, and weight control are techniques nurses can include in their repertoire of helping skills. Insufficient time prevents one-on-one assistance in many situations, but the more nurses know about these resources, the better able they are to intervene, counsel, and direct women to appropriate resources. Careful follow-up of all women experiencing difficulty in dealing with stress is important.

Substance Use Cessation

All women at all ages will receive substantial and immediate benefits from smoking cessation. However, this is not easy, and most people stop several times before they accomplish their goal. Many are never able to do so.

BOX 5-6   Interventions for Smoking Cessation: The Four A's

ASK

- What was her age when she started smoking? How many cigarettes does she smoke a day? When was her last cigarette? Has she tried to quit? Does she want to quit?

ASSESS

- What are her reasons for not being able to quit before, or what made her start again? Does she have anyone who can help her? Does anyone else smoke at home? Does she have friends or family who have quit successfully?

ADVISE

- Give her information about the effects of smoking on pregnancy and her fetus, on her own future health, and on the members of her household.

ASSIST

- Provide support; give self-help materials. Encourage her to set a quit date. Refer to a smoking cessation program or provide information about nicotine replacement products (not recommended during pregnancy) if she is interested. Teach and encourage use of stress reduction activities. Provide for follow-up with a phone call, letter, or clinic visit.

Source: American College of Obstetricians and Gynecologists. (1997b). *Smoking and women's health. ACOG Technical Bulletin no. 240.* Washington, D.C.: ACOG.

New approaches to increase cessation among smokers and to discourage smoking among young women–especially in adolescence and during pregnancy–are needed. Health care providers can have an impact on smoking behavior and should attempt to motivate smokers to stop (Box 5-6). Raising questions about social consequences–stained teeth, foul-smelling breath and clothes–is sometimes effective with young people.

Those who wish to stop smoking can be referred to a smoking cessation program in which individualized methods can be implemented. At the very least, individuals should be guided to self-help materials available from The March of Dimes Birth Defects Foundation, American Lung Association, and the American Cancer Society. During pregnancy, women seem to be highly motivated to stop or at least to limit smoking to 10 or fewer cigarettes a day. Insult to the fetus can be reduced or even avoided if this is done by the end of the first trimester.

Alcohol and other drugs exact a staggering toll on society, not only in terms of personal health, but also in their

---

BOX 5-7 National Groups Providing Information or Support for Chemical Dependency

Alcoholics Anonymous (for individuals who are alcohol dependent) 1-212-686-1100*
 Al-Anon (for families of alcoholics)
 Al-Ateen (for teenage children of alcoholics)
COCAINE Hotline 1-800-COCAINE
National Alcohol and Drug Abuse Hotline 1-800-252-6465
Narcotics Anonymous (for drug abusers) 1-888-336-4066*

*Also check your telephone book for local listing.

BOX 5-8 "Safer" Sex

"Safer" sex is possible only if there is no oral, genital, or rectal exchange of body fluids.
Correct use of condoms, although greatly reducing risk, is not exclusively protective.
Use of spermicides containing nonoxynol-9 may offer additional protection.
Select sexual partners with extreme care.
Ask partner about history of STDs.

---

association with poverty and homelessness, family disorganization, violence, crime, motor vehicle injuries, reduced productivity, and economic costs. The abuse of alcohol and other drugs increases the risk of victimization and date rape and of acquiring HIV through shared needles or sexual contact. Alcohol use and drug use are the leading preventable causes of birth defects.

A national awareness of the seriousness of problems associated with substance abuse has led to raising the legal drinking age to 21 in all states and tighter controls on advertising. Stronger regulation of advertising and tougher laws and law enforcement for alcohol- and drug-related offenses are being implemented. There is still much that must be done to increase the accessibility to care for low-income people, minorities, and young people. Women have special needs that must be addressed, especially mothers of young children and pregnant women.

All primary care providers should screen for alcohol and other drug use problems, with an understanding of the obvious problems in relying on self-reporting of these behaviors. The use of over-the-counter drugs by women should also be explored. Counseling women who appear to be drinking excessively or using drugs may include strategies to increase self-esteem and teaching new coping skills to resist and maintain resistance to alcohol abuse and drug use. Appropriate referrals should be made, with the health care provider arranging the contact and then following up to be sure that appointments are kept. General referral to sources of support should also be provided. National groups that provide information and support for those who are chemically dependent are listed in Box 5-7. Many of these organizations have local branches or contacts that are listed in the telephone book.

Anticipatory guidance includes teaching about the health and safety risks of alcohol and mind-altering substances and discouraging drug experimentation among preteen and high school students, because the use of drugs at an early age tends to predict greater involvement later.

Safer Sexual Practices

Prevention of STDs is predicated on the reduction of high risk behaviors by educating toward a behavioral change. Behaviors of concern include multiple and casual sexual partners and unsafe sexual practices. Specific self-care measures for **safer sex** are listed in Box 5-8. The abuse of alcohol and drugs is also a high risk behavior resulting in impaired judgment and thoughtless acts.

Behavioral changes must come from within, and therefore the nurse must provide sufficient information for the individual or group to "buy into" the need for change. Education for STDs includes the following: (1) verbal desensitizing (e.g., talking about sex and sexual practices); (2) offering specific information (e.g., the signs and symptoms of diseases and their complications and specifically how to prevent disease); (3) endorsing use of condoms (although not 100% effective, condoms are our best form of protection and should be used each and every time unless abstinence or mutual monogamy is ensured); (4) providing behavioral scripts (e.g., suggest ways to discuss sexual situations before they actually occur); and (5) providing referrals for screening (even in the absence of symptoms), additional information, or treatment (see Chapter 8).

In addition to the prevention of STDs, women of childbearing years need information and behavioral considerations regarding contraception and family planning (see Chapter 9). Education is a powerful tool in health promotion and prevention of sexually associated diseases or pregnancy. However, it works best when delivered in the language or parlance of the intended listener and takes into account the culture and lifestyle of the individual or group to whom it is intended.

Health Screening Schedule

Periodic health screening includes history, physical examination, education, counseling, and selected diagnostic and laboratory tests. This regimen provides the basis for overall health promotion, prevention of illness, early diagnosis of problems, and referral for appropriate management. Such screening should be customized according to a woman's age and risk factors. In most instances, it is completed in health care offices, clinics, or hospitals; however, portions of the screening are now being carried out at events such as Community Health Fairs. An overview of

TABLE 5-1 Health Screening Recommendations for Women 18+ Years of Age

INTERVENTION	RECOMMENDATION*
PHYSICAL EXAMINATION	
Blood pressure	Every visit, but at least every 2 years
Height and weight	
Pelvic examination	
Breast examination	
Self-examination	Initiated/taught at time of first pelvic examination; done monthly at end of menses.
Clinical breast examination†	Every 1 to 3 years starting at age 30; annually over age 40
High risk	Annually over 18 with history of premenopausal breast cancer in first-degree relative
Risk groups	At least annually:
Skin examination	Family history of skin cancer or increased exposure to sunlight
Oral cavity examination	Mouth lesion or exposure to tobacco or excessive alcohol
LABORATORY/DIAGNOSTIC TESTS	
Blood cholesterol†	Every 5 years
High risk	More often per clinical judgment with potential for cardiac or lipid abnormalities
Papanicolaou smear†	Initially at age 18 or when sexually active; after three normal consecutive annual examinations, Pap can be per risk, based on discussion with health care provider‖
Mammography‡	Annually over age 50† Annually over age 40§,‖
Fecal occult blood test	Annually over age 50‖
Sigmoidoscopy	Every 5 years after age 50‖
Colonoscopy	Every 10 years over age 50‖
Risk groups	
Fasting blood sugar	Annually with family history of diabetes, gestational diabetes, or woman who is significantly obese
Hearing	Annually with exposure to excessive noise
STD screen	As needed with multiple sexual partners
Tuberculin skin test	Annually with exposure to persons with tuberculosis or in risk categories for close contact with the disease
Endometrial biopsy	At menopause for women at risk for endometrial cancer‖
IMMUNIZATIONS	
Tetanus-diphtheria	Booster is given every 10 years after primary series
Measles, mumps, rubella	Once if born after 1956 and no evidence of immunity
Hepatitis B	Primary series of three for all who are in risk categories
Influenza	Annually after age 65 or in risk categories, such as chronic diseases, immunosuppression, renal dysfunction

Source: United States Preventive Services Task Force. (1996). *Guide to clinical preventive services* (2nd ed.). Baltimore: Williams & Wilkins.
*Unless otherwise noted, the recommended intervention should be performed routinely every 1 to 3 years.
†United States Preventive Services Task Force (1996).
‡Note: There is no consensus regarding mammograms for women between ages 40 and 49, thus various recommendations are listed. Women are urged to discuss circumstances with their health care provider.
§American College of Obstetricians and Gynecologists (1997a).
‖American Cancer Society (1999).

health screening recommendations for women over 18 years of age is provided in Table 5-1. Consistent with information provided earlier in this chapter, it is important for the nurse to continually educate and counsel on diet, exercise, cessation of smoking, alcohol moderation, help for drug abuse, and stress management.

Health Risk Prevention

Often, simple safety factors are forgotten or perceived not to be important; yet injuries continue to have a major impact on the health status of all age groups. Being aware of hazards and implementing safety guidelines will reduce risks. The nurse should frequently reinforce the following commonsense concepts that will protect the individual:

- Wear seat belts at all times in a moving vehicle.
- Wear safety helmets when riding a motorcycle or bicycle.
- Follow driving "rules of the road."
- Place smoke alarms throughout the home and workplace.
- Avoid secondhand smoke.
- Reduce noise pollution or safeguard against hearing loss.
- Protect skin from ultraviolet light via sunscreen and clothing.
- Handle and store firearms appropriately.
- Practice water safety.

Taking necessary precautions and avoiding dangerous situations are imperative.

KEY POINTS

- Culture, religion, socioeconomic status, personal circumstances, the uniqueness of the individual, and stage of development are among the factors that influence a person's recognition of need for care and response to the health care system and therapy.

- The changing status and roles of women affect their health, needs, and ability to cope with problems.

- Assessment is more comprehensive and learning is best in a safe environment in which the atmosphere is nonjudgmental and sensitive and the interaction is strictly confidential.

- Every woman is entitled to be respected and fully involved in the assessment and educational processes.

- Preconception counseling allows identification and possible remediation of potentially harmful personal and social conditions, medical and psychologic conditions, environmental conditions, and barriers to care before the advent of pregnancy.

- Conditions that increase a woman's health risks also increase risks for her offspring.

- Periodic health screening, including history, physical examination, and diagnostic and laboratory tests, provides the basis for overall health promotion, prevention of illness, early diagnosis of problems, and referral for management.

- Health promotion and prevention assist women to actualize health potential by increasing motivation, providing information, and suggesting how to access specific resources.

Health Protection

Nurses can make a difference in stopping violence against women and preventing further injury. Educating women that abuse is a violation of their rights and facilitating their access to protective and legal services constitute a first step. Also, encouraging health care institutions to implement appropriate domestic violence screening programs is of great value (Gantt & Bickford, 1999). Other helpful measures for women to discourage their fall into abusive relationships are promoting assertiveness and self-defense courses; suggesting support and self-help groups that encourage positive self-regard, confidence, and empowerment; and recommending educational and skills development classes that will enhance independence or at least the ability to take care of oneself.

Numerous national and local organizations provide information and assistance for women experiencing abusive situations. Nurses and victims may find these resources helpful. Box 11-7 lists national resources and hotlines. All nurses who work in women's health care should become familiar with local services and legal options.

CRITICAL THINKING EXERCISES

1 Interview at least two women of different cultures.
   a. Ask them about their beliefs in relation to seeking health care.
   b. Identify reasons for differences and how these would influence planning to teach about preventive health care and health promotion.

2 Identify and visit resources in your community appropriate for referring the following women. Then evaluate the resource in terms of access, costs, and follow-up service.
   a. A woman who wants to stop smoking.
   b. A woman who is battered by her husband.
   c. A woman whose mother is an alcoholic.

3 Interview a 45- to 50-year-old woman.
   a. Identify any risk factors for chronic diseases, cancer, or STDs.
   b. Assess for perimenopausal symptoms and any interventions she may be using.
   c. Evaluate her physical activities and lifestyle to determine what health promotion or prevention activities she engages in.
   d. Based on your findings, develop a plan to meet her specific health needs for the next 10 years.

References

Alan Guttmacher Institute. (1998). *Risks and realities of early child-bearing.* New York: The Institute.

Allen, K. & Phillips, J. (1997). *Women's health across the lifespan: A contemporary perspective.* Philadelphia: J.B. Lippincott.

American Cancer Society. (1999). *Cancer facts and figures 1999.* New York: American Cancer Society.

American College of Obstetricians and Gynecologists. (1997a). *Committee opinion: Routine cancer screening.* Washington, D.C.: ACOG.

American College of Obstetricians and Gynecologists. (1997b). *Smoking and women's health. ACOG Technical Bulletin no. 240.* Washington, D.C.: ACOG.

Bartman, B. (1996). Women's access to appropriate providers within managed care: Implications for the quality of primary care. *Women's Health Issues* 6(1), 45-50.

Breeding, D. (1996). You don't have to live with incontinence. *Female Patient* 53, 29.

Burke, B. (1999). *Preventing neural tube birth defects: A prevention model and resource guide.* Atlanta: Centers for Disease Control and Prevention.

Casele, H., & Laifer, S. (1998). Factors influencing preconception control of glycemia in diabetic women. *Arch Intern Med* 158(12), 1321-1324.

Cox, R. (1997). Family health care delivery for 21st century. *J Obstet Gynecol Neonatal Nurs* 26(1), 109.

deGroot, L. (1999). High maternal body weight and pregnancy outcome. *Nutr Rev* 57(2), 62.

DiSaia, P., & Creasman, W. (1997). *Clinical gynecologic oncology* (5th ed.). St. Louis: Mosby.

Epps, R., & Stewart, S. (1995). *The women's complete healthbook.* New York: The Philip Lief Group, Inc.

Fahey, L., & Sinclair, B. (1996). *Nurse practitioner, certified nurse midwife, physician assistant protocols* (2nd ed). Pasadena, CA: Kaiser Permanente.

Failure of health care reform (special section). (1995). *J Health Polit Policy Law* 20(2), 271.

Gantt, L., & Bickford, A. (1999). Screening for domestic violence. *AWHONN Lifelines* 3(2), 36-42.

Grimes, D. (Ed.). (1998). Helping patients stop smoking: A new treatment option. *Contraceptive Report* 9(3), 12.

Guyer, B. et al. (1998). Annual summary of vital statistics–1997. *Pediatrics* 102(6), 1333-1347.

Hastings, K. (1995). Health care reform: We need it, but do we have the national will to shape our future? *Nurse Pract* 20(1), 52-54, 56-57.

Hatcher, R. et al. (1998). *Contraceptive technology* (17th ed.). New York: Irvington.

Heinrich, J. (1998). Incremental approaches to necessary health care reform lead to more chaos. *Nurs Outlook* 46(3), 137-139.

Japenga, A. (1998, Jan. 2). Depression: Are men hiding? *USA Weekend*, p. 20.

Jessup, M. (1997). Addiction in women: Prevalence, profiles, and meaning. *J Obstet Gynecol Neonatal Nurs* 26(4), 449-458.

Lean, M. et al. (1999). Impairment of health and quality of life using new U.S. federal guidelines for identification of obesity. *Arch Intern Med* 159(8), 837-843.

Lemcke, D. et al. (1995). *Primary care of women.* East Norwalk, CT: Appleton & Lange.

Li, C., Olsen, Y., Kuigne, V., & Weltz, T. (1999). Implementation of substance use screening in prenatal clinics. *S D J Med* 52(2), 59-64.

Murray, R., & Zentner, J. (1997). *Health assessment promotion strategies through the life span* (6th ed.). Stamford, CT: Appleton & Lange.

Muscari, M. (1998). Rebels with a cause. *Am J Nurs* 98(12), 26-30.

National Center for Health Statistics. (1998). *Health, United States, 1998.* Atlanta: Centers for Disease Control and Prevention.

Pender, N. (1996). *Health promotion in nursing practice* (3rd ed.). Stamford, CT: Appleton & Lange.

Pohl, J., & Caplan, D. (1998). Smoking cessation: Using group intervention methods to treat low-income women. *Nurs Pract* 23(12), 13, 17-18, 20.

Roberts, S., & Sorensen, L. (1995). Lesbian health care: A review and recommendations for health promotion in primary care settings. *J Obstet Gynecol Neonatal Nurs* 20(6), 42-47.

Rosenfeld, J. (Ed.). (1997). *Women's health in primary care.* Baltimore: Williams & Wilkins.

Sampselle, C., & Miller, J. (1996). Pelvic muscle exercise: Effective patient teaching. *Female Patient* 21, 29.

Sampselle, C. et al. (1997). Continence for women: Evidence-based practice. *J Obstet Gynecol Neonatal Nurs* 26(4), 375-385.

Sinclair, B. (1997). Advanced practice nurses in integrated health care systems. *J Obstet Gynecol Neonatal Nurs* 26(2), 217-223.

Stringham, P. (1999). Domestic violence. *Prim Care* 26(2), 373-384.

United States Preventive Services Task Force. (1996). *Guide to clinical preventive services* (2nd ed.). Baltimore: Williams & Wilkins.

Wainess, F. (1999). The ways and means of national health care reform. *J Health Polit Policy Law* 24(2), 305.

6

Assessment of Women

Jan Lamarche Zdanuk

LEARNING OBJECTIVES

- Define the key terms.
- Identify the structures and functions of the female reproductive system.
- Summarize the menstrual cycle in relation to hormonal, ovarian, and endometrial response.
- Identify the four phases of the sexual response.
- Compare natural and acquired immunity.
- Discuss the effects of age, lifestyle, environment, and nutrition on the immune system.
- Identify cultural and communication variations that may affect a woman's decision to seek and follow through with health care.
- Discuss how the history and physical examination can be adapted for women with special needs.

- List strategies for teaching safety and injury prevention during routine health examinations.
- Identify indications of abuse, appropriate screening, and referral to community agencies.
- Define components of taking a woman's history and performing a physical examination.
- Identify the correct procedure for assisting with and collecting Papanicolaou smear specimens.
- Review client teaching of breast self-examination.
- Identify risk factors for osteoporosis.
- Identify topics for nursing research related to health assessment of women.

KEY TERMS

acquired immunity	menarche	perineum
active immunity	menopause	prostaglandins (PGs)
breast self-examination (BSE)	menstruation	puberty
climacteric	natural immunity	sexual response cycle
endometrial cycle	ovarian cycle	vaccination
hypothalamic-pituitary cycle	ovulation	vulvar self-examination (VSE)
immunocompetent	Papanicolaou (Pap) smear	
immunology	passive immunity	

The purpose of this chapter is to review female anatomy and physiology, the menstrual cycle, immunology, and gynecologic health assessment. Knowledge of the anatomy and physiology of female structures involved in reproduction is necessary to assess, plan, implement, and evaluate nursing care of women. Each structure has a vital role in expression of human sexuality, generating and maintaining secondary sexual characteristics, and reproduction. The breasts, genitals, and pelvis develop the unique adaptations necessary for childbearing through hormonal influences and organ maturation. The female reproductive system consists of the following four principal components:

1. External genitals
2. Primary sex glands
3. Ducts leading from the gonads to the body's exterior
4. Secondary sex glands

FEMALE REPRODUCTIVE SYSTEM

The female reproductive system consists of external structures visible from the pubis to the perineum and internal structures located in the pelvic cavity. The external and internal female reproductive structures develop and mature in response to estrogen and progesterone starting in fetal life and continuing through puberty and the childbearing years. Reproductive structures atrophy with age or in response to a decrease in ovarian hormone production. A complex nerve and blood supply supports the functions of these structures. The appearance of the external genitals varies greatly among women. Heredity, age, race, and the number of children a woman has borne determine the size, shape, and color of her external organs.

External Structures

The external genital organs, or *vulva*, include all structures visible externally from the pubis to the perineum: the mons pubis, labia majora, labia minora, clitoris, vestibular glands, vaginal vestibule, vaginal orifice, and urethral opening. The external genital organs are illustrated in Fig. 6-1. The *mons pubis* is a fatty pad that lies over the anterior surface of the symphysis pubis. In the postpubertal female, the mons is covered with coarse curly hair. The *labia majora* are two rounded folds of fatty tissue covered with skin that extend downward and backward from the mons pubis. The labia are highly vascular structures that develop hair on the outer surfaces after puberty. They protect the inner vulvar structures. The *labia minora* are two flat, reddish folds of tissue visible when the labia majora are separated. No hair follicles are in the labia minora, but many sebaceous follicles and a few sweat glands are present. The interior of the labia minora is composed of connective tissue and smooth muscle, which are supplied with extremely sensitive nerve endings. Anteriorly, the labia minora fuse to form the *prepuce* (hoodlike covering of the clitoris) and the *frenulum* (fold of tissue under the clitoris). The labia minora join to form a thin flat tissue called the *fourchette* underneath the vaginal opening at midline. The *clitoris* is located underneath the prepuce. It is a small structure composed of erectile tissue with numerous sensory nerve endings. During sexual arousal the clitoris increases in size.

The vaginal *vestibule* is an almond-shaped area enclosed by the labia minora that contains openings to the urethra, Skene's glands, vagina, and Bartholin's glands. The urethra is not a reproductive organ but is considered here because of its location. It usually is found about 2.5 cm below the clitoris. Skene's glands are located on each side of the urethra and produce mucus, which aids in lubrication of the vagina. The vaginal opening is in the lower portion of the vestibule and varies in shape and size. The hymen, a connective tissue membrane, surrounds the vaginal opening. It can be perforated during strenuous exercise, insertion of tampons, masturbation, and vaginal intercourse. Bartholin glands (see Fig. 6-1) lie under the constrictor muscles of the vagina and are located posteriorly on the sides of the vaginal opening, although the ductal openings are usually not visible. During sexual arousal the glands secrete a clear mucus to lubricate the vaginal introitus.

The area between the fourchette and the anus is the **perineum,** a skin-covered muscular area that covers the pelvic structures. The perineum forms the base of the perineal

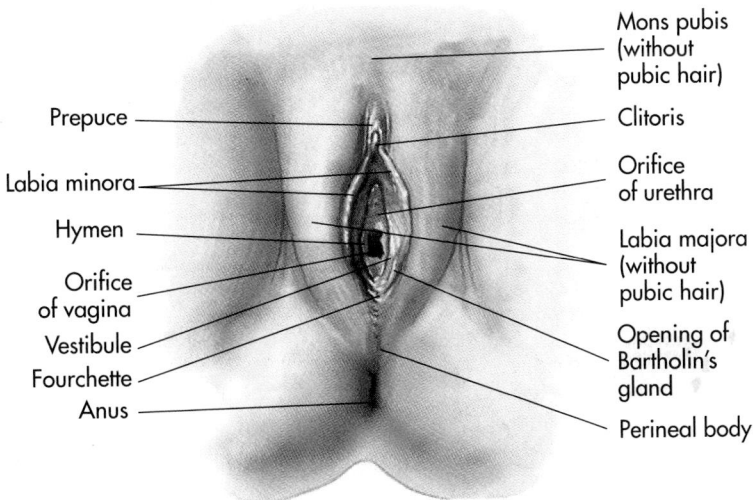

Fig. 6-1 External female genitalia.

Mons pubis (without pubic hair)
Clitoris
Orifice of urethra
Labia majora (without pubic hair)
Opening of Bartholin's gland
Perineal body

Prepuce
Labia minora
Hymen
Orifice of vagina
Vestibule
Fourchette
Anus

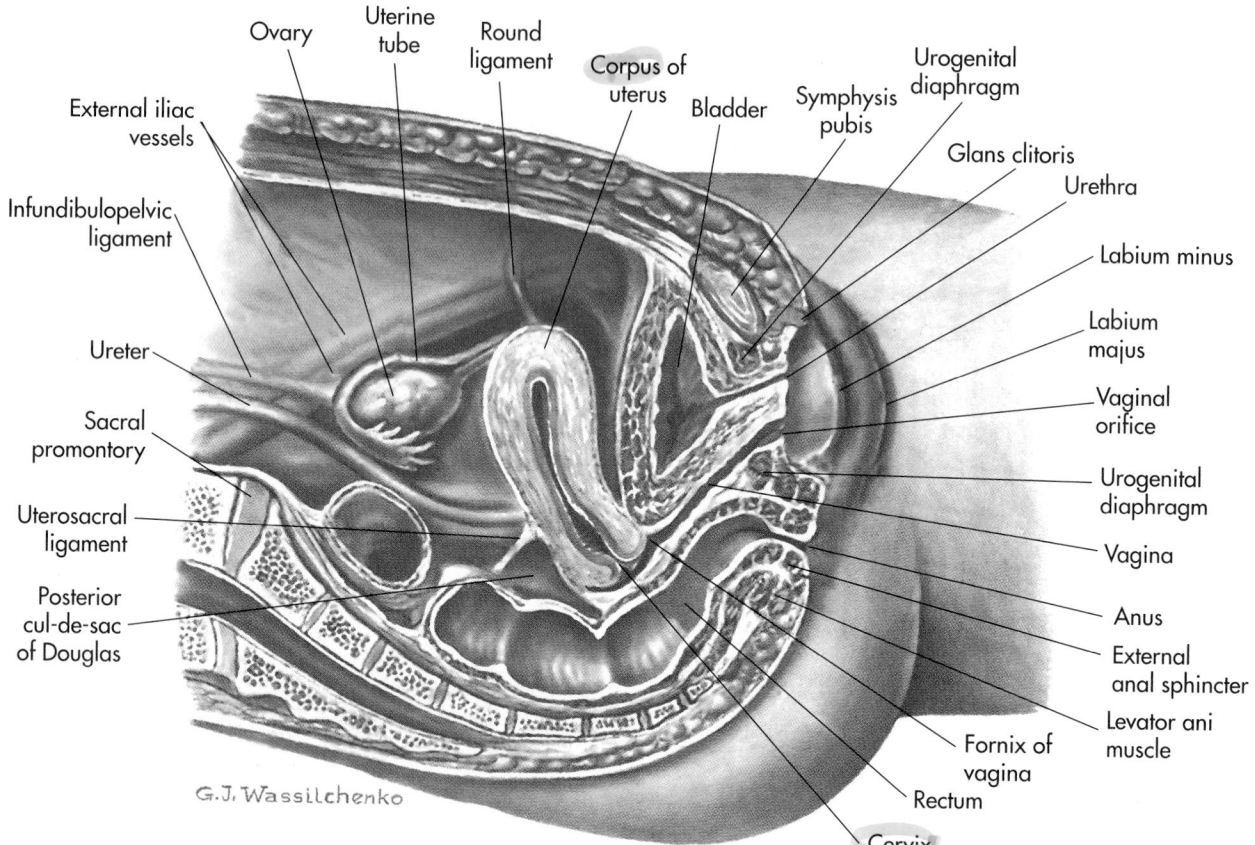

Fig. 6-2 Midsagittal view of female pelvic organs with woman lying supine.

body, a wedge-shaped mass that serves as an anchor for the muscles, fascia, and ligaments of the pelvis. The pelvic organs are supported by muscles and ligaments that form a sling.

Internal Structures

The internal structures include the vagina, uterus, uterine tubes, and ovaries.

The *vagina* is a fibromuscular, collapsible tubular structure that extends from the vulva to the uterus and lies between the bladder and rectum. During the reproductive years the mucosal lining is arranged in transverse folds called *rugae*. These rugae allow the vagina to expand during childbirth. Estrogen deprivation that occurs after childbirth, during lactation, and at menopause causes dryness and thinness of the vaginal walls and the rugae to become smooth. The vagina, particularly the lower segment, has few sensory nerve endings. Vaginal secretions are slightly acidic (pH 4 to 5) so that the vagina's susceptibility to infections is reduced. The vagina serves as a passageway for menstrual flow, a female organ of copulation, and as a part of the birth canal for vaginal childbirth. The uterine cervix projects into a blind vault at the upper end of the vagina. There are anterior, posterior, and lateral pockets called *fornices* that surround the cervix. The internal pelvic organs can be palpated through the thin walls of these fornices.

The *uterus* is a muscular organ shaped like an upside-down pear that sits midline in the pelvic cavity between the bladder and rectum above the vagina. Four pairs of ligaments support the uterus: the cardinal, uterosacral, round, and broad. Single anterior and posterior ligaments also support the uterus. The cul-de-sac of Douglas is a deep pouch, or recess, posterior to the cervix formed by the posterior ligament.

The uterus is divided into two major parts, an upper triangular portion called the corpus and a lower cylindric portion called the cervix (Fig. 6-2). The fundus is the dome-shaped top of the uterus and is the site at which the uterine tubes enter the uterus. The isthmus (lower uterine segment) is a short, constricted portion that separates the corpus from the cervix.

The uterus serves for reception, implantation, retention, and nutrition of the fertilized ovum and later the fetus during pregnancy and expulsion of the fetus during childbirth. It also is responsible for cyclic menstruation.

The uterine wall comprises three layers: the endometrium, the myometrium, and part of the peritoneum. The *endometrium* is a highly vascular lining made up of three layers, the outer two of which are shed during menstruation. The *myometrium* is made up of layers of smooth muscles that extend in three different directions (longitudinal, transverse, and oblique) (Fig. 6-3). Longitudinal fibers of

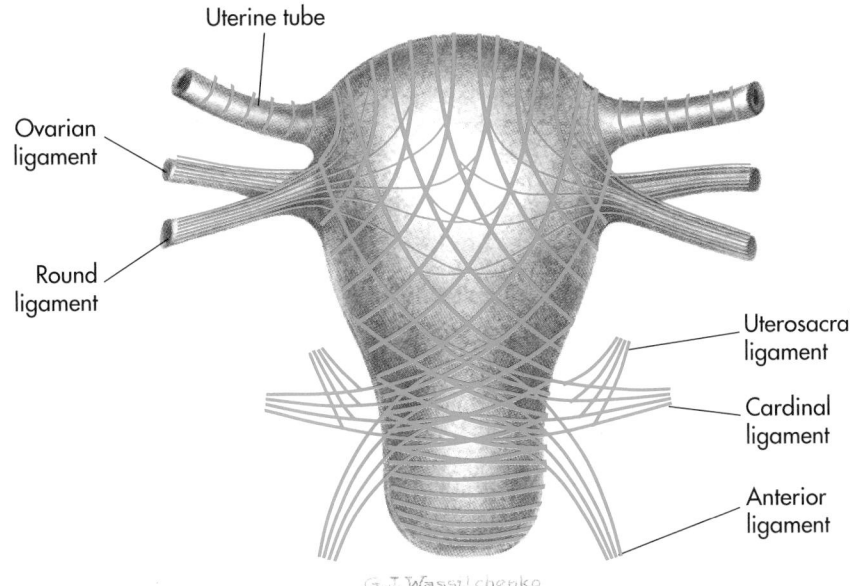

Ovarian ligament

Round ligament

Uterine tube

Uterosacral ligament

Cardinal ligament

Anterior ligament

G. J. Wassilchenko

Fig. 6-3 Schematic arrangement of directions of muscle fibers. Note that uterine muscle fibers are continuous with supportive ligaments of uterus.

the outer myometrial layer are found mostly in the fundus, and this arrangement assists in expelling the fetus during the birth process. The middle layer contains fibers from all three directions, which form a figure-eight pattern encircling large blood vessels. This arrangement assists in ligating blood vessels after childbirth and controls blood loss. Most of the circular fibers of the inner myometrial layer are around the site where the uterine tubes enter the uterus and around the internal cervical os (opening). These fibers help keep the cervix closed during pregnancy and prevent menstrual blood from flowing back into the uterine tubes during menstruation.

The *cervix* is made up of mostly fibrous connective tissues and elastic tissue, making it possible for the cervix to stretch during vaginal childbirth. The opening between the uterine cavity and the canal that connects the uterine cavity to the vagina (endocervical canal) is the internal os. The narrowed opening between the endocervix and the vagina is the external os, a small circular opening in women who have never been pregnant. The cervix feels firm (like the end of a nose) with a dimple in the center, which marks the external os.

The outer cervix is covered with a layer of squamous epithelium. The mucosa of the cervical canal is covered with columnar epithelium and contains numerous glands that secrete mucus in response to ovarian hormones. The *squamocolumnar junction,* where the two types of cells meet, is usually located just inside the cervical os. This junction is the most common site for neoplastic changes, and cells from this site are scraped for the Papanicolaou test (see p. 111).

The *uterine tubes* (fallopian tubes) attach to the uterine fundus. The tubes are supported by the broad ligaments and range from 8 to 14 cm in length. The tubes are divided into four sections: the interstitial portion is closest to the uterus; the isthmus and the ampulla are the middle portions; and the infundibulum is closest to the ovary. The uterine tubes provide a passage between the ovaries and the uterus for the passage of the ovum. The infundibulum has fimbriated ends, which pull the ovum into the tube. The ovum is pulled along the tubes to the uterus by rhythmic contractions of the muscles of the tubes and by the current that is produced by the movement of the cilia that line the tubes. The ovum is usually fertilized by the sperm in the ampulla portion of one of the tubes.

The *ovaries* are almond-shaped organs located on each side of the uterus below and behind the uterine tubes. During the reproductive years, they are approximately 3 cm long, 2 cm wide, and 1 cm thick; they diminish in size after menopause. Before menarche, each ovary has a smooth surface; after menarche they become nodular because of repeated ruptures of follicles at ovulation. The two functions of the ovaries are ovulation and hormone production. **Ovulation** is the release of a mature ovum from the ovary at intervals (usually monthly). Estrogen, progesterone, and androgen are the hormones produced by the ovaries.

The Bony Pelvis

The bony pelvis serves three primary purposes: protection of the pelvic structures, accommodation of the growing fetus during pregnancy, and anchorage of the pelvic support structures. Two innominate (hip) bones (consisting of ilium, ischium, and pubis), the sacrum, and the coccyx make up the four bones of the pelvis (Fig. 6-4). Cartilage and ligaments form the symphysis pubis, sacrococcygeal,

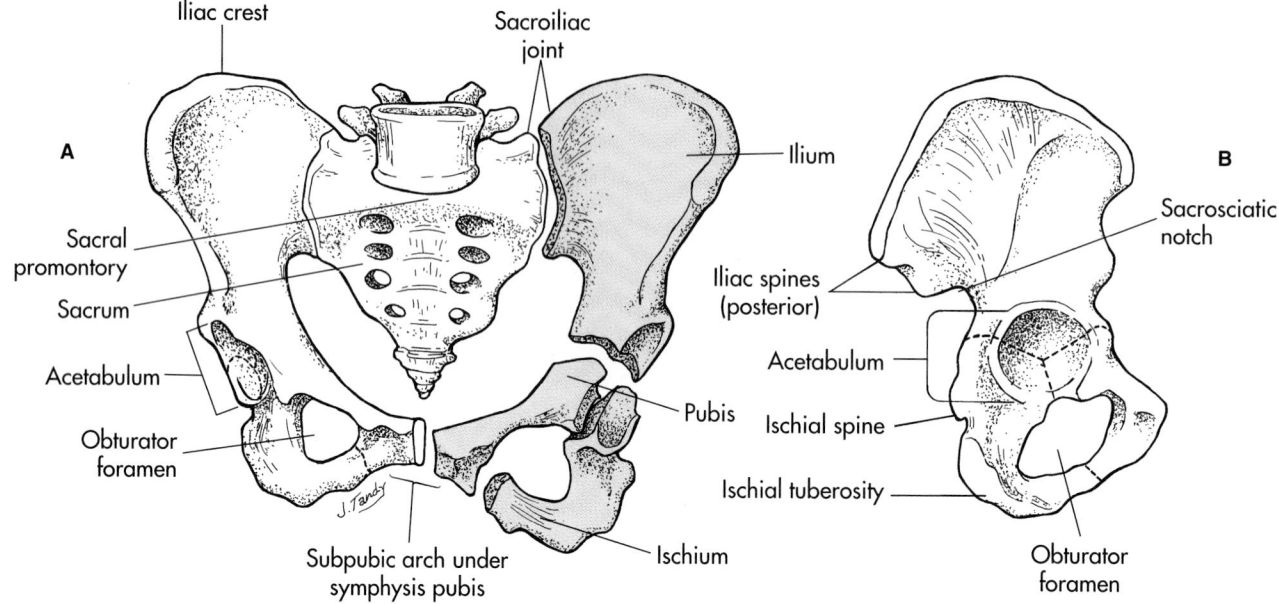

Fig. 6-4 Adult female pelvis. **A,** Anterior view. **B,** External view of innominate bone (fused).

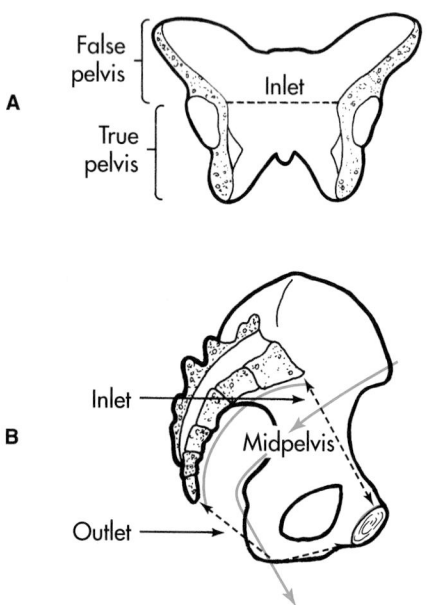

Fig. 6-5 Female pelvis. **A,** Cavity of false pelvis is shallow. **B,** Cavity of true pelvis is an irregularly curved canal *(arrows).*

and two sacroiliac joints that separate the pelvic bones. The pelvis is divided into two parts: the false pelvis and the true pelvis (Fig. 6-5). The false pelvis is the upper portion above the pelvic brim or inlet. The true pelvis is the lower curved bony canal, which includes the inlet, the cavity, and the outlet through which the fetus passes during vaginal birth. The upper portion of the outlet is at the level of the ischial spines, and the lower portion is at the level of the ischial tuberosities and the pubic arch (see

Fig. 6-4). Variations that occur in the size and shape of the pelvis are usually due to age and race. Pelvic ossification is complete at about 20 years of age.

Breasts

The breasts are paired mammary glands located between the second and sixth ribs (Fig. 6-6). About two thirds of the breast overlies the pectoralis major muscle, between the sternum and midaxillary line, with an extension to the axilla referred to as the tail of Spence. The lower one third of the breast overlies the serratus anterior muscle. The breasts are attached to the muscles by connective tissue or fascia.

The breasts of healthy mature women are approximately equal in size and shape, but often are not absolutely symmetric. The size and shape vary depending on the woman's age, heredity, and nutrition. However, the contour should be smooth with no retractions, dimpling, or masses. Estrogen stimulates growth of the breast by inducing fat deposition in the breasts, development of stromal tissue (i.e., increase in its amount and elasticity), and growth of the extensive ductile system. Estrogen also increases the vascularity of breast tissue.

Once ovulation begins in puberty, progesterone levels increase. The increase in progesterone causes maturation of mammary gland tissue, specifically the lobules and acinar structures. During adolescence, fat deposition and growth of fibrous tissue contribute to the increase in the gland's size. Full development of the breasts is not achieved until after the end of the first pregnancy or in the early period of lactation.

Each mammary gland is made of 15 to 20 lobes, which are divided into lobules. Lobules are clusters of acini. An

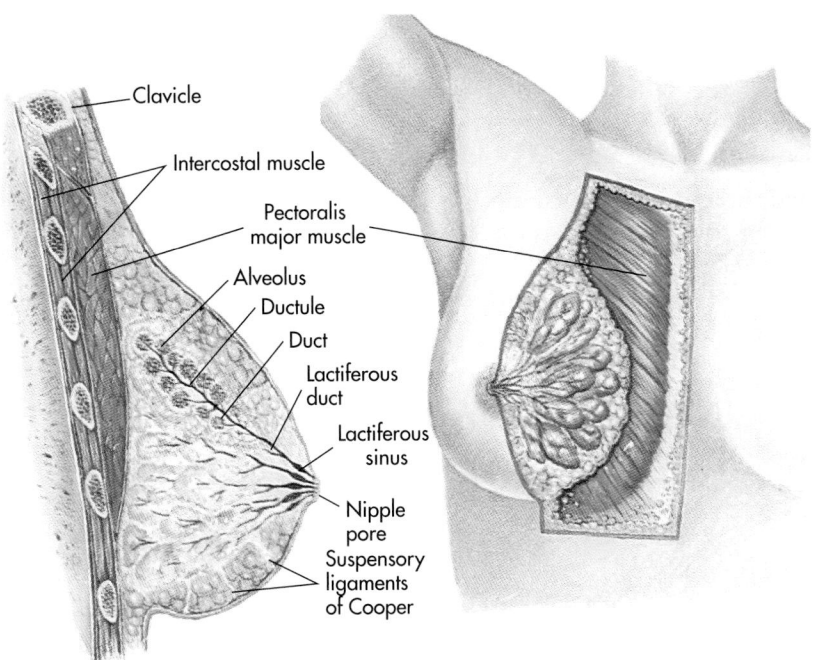

Fig. 6-6 Anatomy of the breast, showing position and major structures. *(From Seidel, H., Ball, J., Dains, J., & Benedict, G. [1999]. Mosby's guide to physical examination [4th ed.]. St. Louis: Mosby.)*

acinus is a saclike terminal part of a compound gland emptying through a narrow lumen or duct. In discussions of mammary glands, the correct anatomic term *(acinus)* is often used interchangeably with the term *alveolus*. The acini are lined with epithelial cells that secrete colostrum and milk. Just below the epithelium is the myoepithelium *(myo,* or muscle), which contracts to expel milk from the acini.

The ducts from the clusters of acini that form the lobules merge to form larger ducts draining the lobes. Ducts from the lobes converge in a single nipple (mammary papilla) surrounded by an areola. Just as the ducts converge, they dilate to form common lactiferous sinuses, which are also called ampullae. The lactiferous sinuses serve as milk reservoirs. Many tiny lactiferous ducts drain the ampullae and exit in the nipple.

The glandular structures and ducts are surrounded by protective fatty tissue and are separated and supported by fibrous suspensory *Cooper's ligaments.* Cooper's ligaments provide support to the mammary glands while permitting their mobility on the chest wall (see Fig. 6-6). The round nipple is usually slightly elevated above the breast. On each breast the nipple projects slightly upward and laterally. It contains 15 to 20 openings from lactiferous ducts. The nipple is surrounded by fibromuscular tissue and covered by wrinkled skin. Except during pregnancy and lactation, there is usually no discharge from the nipple.

The nipple and surrounding areola are usually more deeply pigmented than the skin of the breast. The rough appearance of the areola is caused by sebaceous glands, *Montgomery tubercles,* directly beneath the skin. These glands secrete a fatty substance, thought to lubricate the nipple. Smooth muscle fibers in the areola contract to stiffen the nipple to make it easier for the breastfeeding infant to grasp.

The vascular supply to the mammary gland is abundant. In the nonpregnant state the skin does not have an obvious vascular pattern. The normal skin is smooth without tightness or shininess. The skin covering the breasts contains an extensive superficial lymphatic network that serves the entire chest wall and is continuous with the superficial lymphatics of the neck and abdomen. In the deeper portions of the breasts, the lymphatics form a rich network as well. The primary deep lymphatic pathway drains laterally toward the axillae.

Besides their function of lactation, breasts function as organs for sexual arousal in the mature adult.

The breasts change in size and nodularity in response to cyclic ovarian changes throughout reproductive life. Increasing levels of both estrogen and progesterone in the 3 to 4 days before menstruation increase vascularity of the breasts, induce growth of the ducts and acini, and promote water retention. The epithelial cells lining the ducts proliferate in number, the ducts dilate, and the lobules distend. The acini become enlarged and secretory, and lipid (fat) is deposited within their epithelial cell lining. As a result, breast swelling, tenderness, and discomfort are common symptoms just before the onset of menstruation. After menstruation, cellular proliferation begins to regress, acini begin to decrease in size, and retained water is lost. After

CLIENT SELF-CARE

Breast Self-Examination

1. The best time to do breast self-examination is after your period, when breasts are not tender or swollen. If you do not have regular periods or sometimes skip a month, do it on the same day every month.

2. Lie down and put a pillow under your right shoulder. Place your right arm behind your head (Fig. 1).

3. Use the finger pads of your three middle fingers on your left hand to feel for lumps or thickening. Your finger pads are the top third of each finger.

4. Press firmly enough to know how your breast feels. If you're not sure how hard to press, ask your health care provider, or try to copy the way your health care provider uses the finger pads during a breast examination. Learn what your breast feels like most of the time. A firm ridge in the lower curve of each breast is normal.

5. Move around the breast in a set way. You can choose either circles (Fig. 2, A), vertical lines (Fig. 2, B), or wedges (Fig. 2, C). Do it the same way every time. It will help you to make sure that you've gone over the entire breast area and to remember how your breast feels.

6. Gently compress the nipple between your thumb and forefinger and look for discharge.

7. Now examine your left breast using the finger pads of your right hand.

8. If you find any changes, see your health care provider right away.

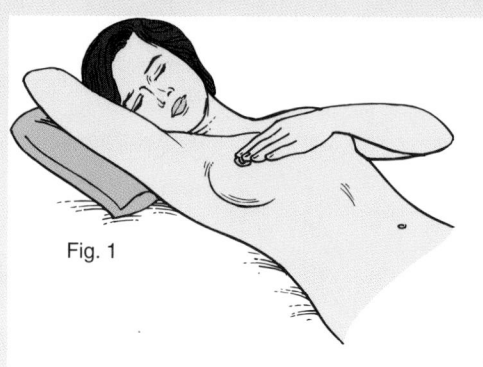

Fig. 1

9. You may want to check your breasts while standing in front of a mirror right after you do your breast self-examination each month. See if there are any changes in the way your breasts look: dimpling of the skin, changes in the nipple, or redness or swelling.

10. You may also want to do an extra breast self-examination while you're in the shower (Fig. 3). Your soapy hands will glide over the wet skin, making it easy to check how your breasts feel.

11. It is important to check the area between the breast and the underarm and the underarm itself. Also examine the area above the breast to the collarbone and to the shoulder.

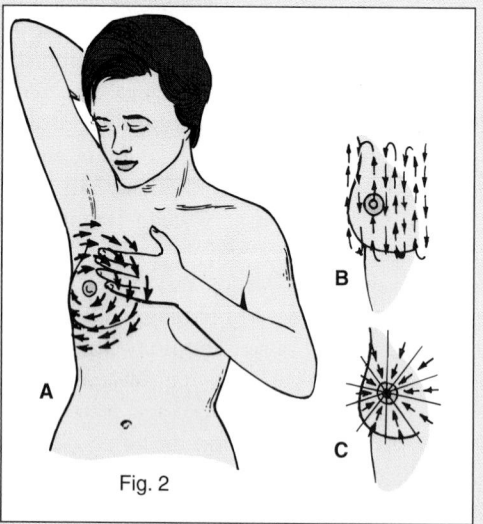

Fig. 2

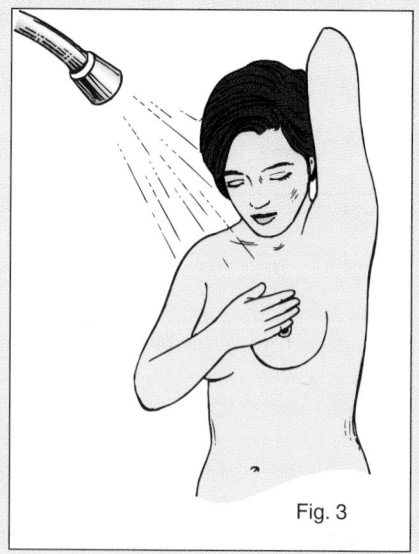

Fig. 3

breasts have undergone changes numerous times in response to the ovarian cycle, the proliferation and involution (regression) are not uniform throughout the breast. In time, after repeated hormonal stimulation, small persistent areas of nodulations may develop. This normal physiologic change must be remembered when breast tissue is examined. Nodules may develop just before and during menstruation, when the breast is most active. The physiologic alterations in breast size and activity reach their minimum level about 5 to 7 days after menstruation stops.

TABLE 6-1 Female Reproductive Physical Assessment Across the Life Cycle

	ADOLESCENT	ADULT	POSTMENOPAUSAL
Breasts	Tender when developing; buds appear; small, firm, one side may grow faster; areola diameter increases; nipples more erect	Grow to full shape in early adulthood; nipples and areolae become pinker and darker	Become stringy, irregular, pendulous, and nodular; borders less well delineated; may shrink, become flatter, elongated, and less elastic; ligaments weaken; nipples are positioned lower
Vagina	Vagina lengthens; epithelial layers thicken; secretions become acidic	Growth complete by age 20	Introitus constricts; vagina narrows, shortens, loses rugation; mucosa is pale, thin, and dry; walls may lose structural integrity
Uterus	Musculature and vasculature increase; lining thickens	Growth complete by age 20	Size decreases; endometrial lining thins
Ovaries	Increase in size and weight; menarche occurs between 8 and 16 years of age; ovulation occurs monthly	Growth complete by age 20	Size decreases to 1 to 2 cm; follicles disappear; surface convolutes; ovarian function ceases between 40 and 55 years of age
Labia majora	Become more prominent; hair develops	Growth complete by age 20	Labia become smaller and flatter; pubic hair sparse and gray
Labia minora	Become more vascular	Growth complete by age 20	Become shinier and dryer
Uterine tubes	Increase in size	Growth complete by age 20	Decrease in size

Therefore **breast self-examination (BSE)** (systematic palpation of breasts to detect signs of breast cancer or other changes) is best carried out during this phase of the menstrual cycle (see Client Self-Care box). Table 6-1 compares the variations in physical assessment related to age differences in women.

MENSTRUATION AND MENOPAUSE

Knowledge of menstruation is important for nurses providing care to women across the life span. Nurses should be knowledgeable about menarche, the endometrial cycle, the hypothalamic-pituitary cycle, the ovarian cycle, other cyclic changes, and the climacteric.

Menarche and Puberty

Although young girls secrete small, rather constant amounts of estrogen, a marked increase occurs between 8 and 11 years of age. The term **menarche** denotes first menstruation. **Puberty** is a broader term that denotes the entire transitional stage between childhood and sexual maturity. Increasing amounts and variations in gonadotropin and estrogen secretion develop into a cyclic pattern at least a year before menarche. In North America this occurs in most girls at about 13 years of age.

Initially, periods are irregular, unpredictable, painless, and anovulatory. After 1 or more years, a hypothalamic-pituitary rhythm develops, and the ovary produces adequate cyclic estrogen to make a mature ovum. Ovulatory periods tend to be regular, monitored by progesterone.

Although pregnancy can occur in exceptional cases of true precocious puberty, most pregnancies in young girls occur after the normally timed menarche. *All girls would benefit from knowing that pregnancy can occur at any time after the onset of menses.*

Menstrual Cycle

Menstruation is the periodic uterine bleeding that begins approximately 14 days after ovulation. It is controlled by a feedback system of three cycles: endometrial, hypothalamic-pituitary, and ovarian. The average length of a menstrual cycle is 28 days, but variations are normal. The first day of bleeding is designated as day 1 of the menstrual cycle, or *menses* (Fig. 6-7). The average duration of menstrual flow is 5 days (range of 3 to 6 days), and the average blood loss is 50 ml (range of 20 to 80 ml), but these vary greatly.

For about 50% of women, menstrual blood does not appear to clot. The menstrual blood clots within the uterus, but the clot usually liquefies before being discharged from the uterus. Uterine discharge includes mucus and epithelial cells in addition to blood.

The menstrual cycle is a complex interplay of events that occur simultaneously in the endometrium, hypothalamus

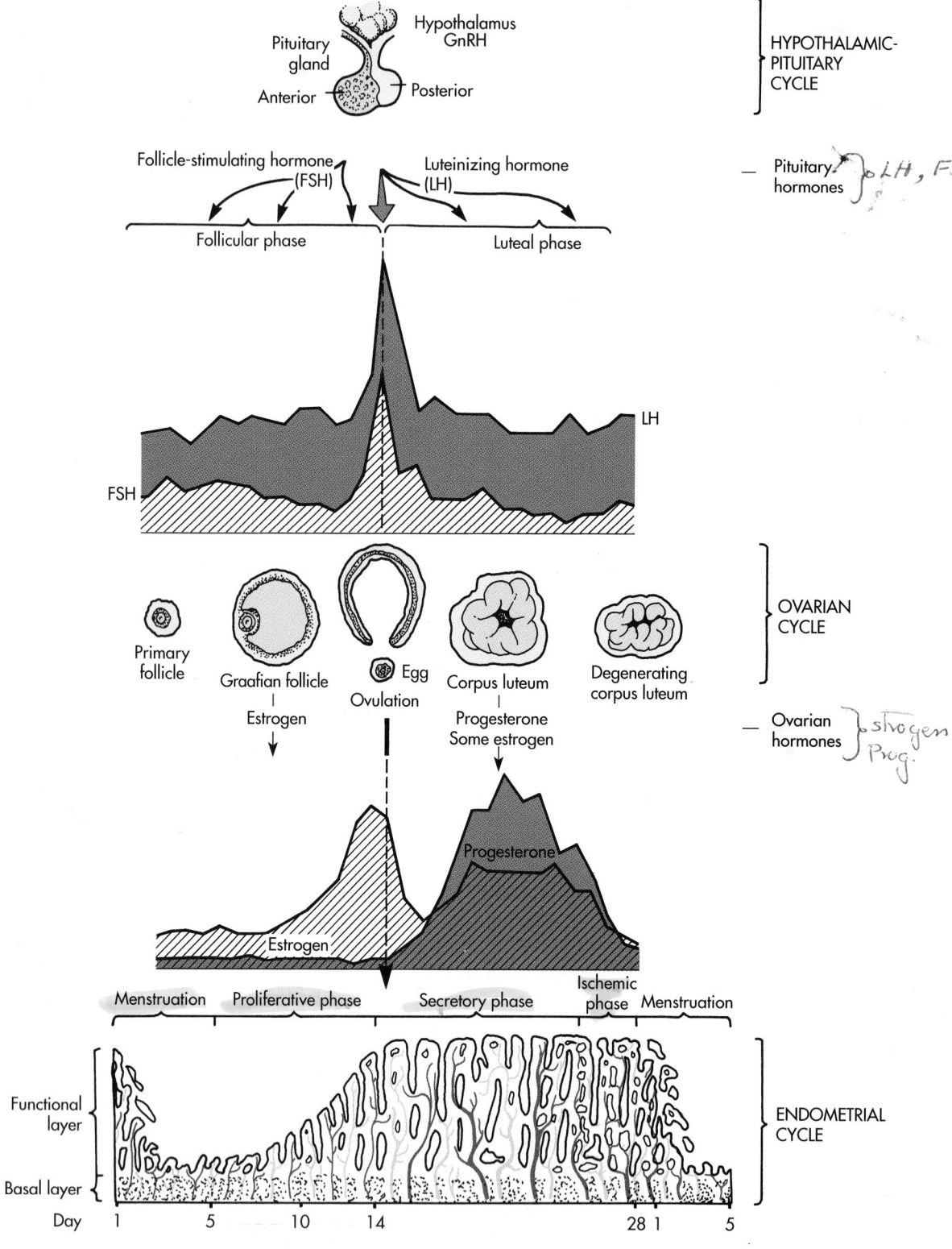

Fig. 6-7 Menstrual cycle: hypothalamic-pituitary, ovarian, and endometrial.

and pituitary glands, and ovaries. The menstrual cycle prepares the uterus for pregnancy. When pregnancy does not occur, menstruation follows. The woman's age, physical and emotional status, and environment influence the regularity of her menstrual cycles.

Endometrial Cycle

The four phases of the **endometrial cycle** are (1) the menstrual phase, (2) the proliferative phase, (3) the secretory phase, and (4) the ischemic phase (see Fig. 6-7). During the *menstrual phase,* shedding of the functional two

(handwritten margin note: is the phase that causes variation in womens cycle length time)

thirds of the endometrium (the compact and spongy layers) is initiated by periodic vasoconstriction in the upper layers of the endometrium. The basal layer is always retained, and regeneration begins near the end of the cycle from cells derived from the remaining glandular remnants or stromal cells in the basalis.

The *proliferative phase* is a period of rapid growth lasting from about the fifth day to the time of ovulation. The endometrial surface is completely restored in approximately 4 days, or slightly before bleeding ceases. From this point on an eightfold to tenfold thickening occurs with a leveling off of growth at ovulation. The proliferative phase depends on estrogen stimulation derived from ovarian follicles.

The *secretory phase* extends from the day of ovulation to about 3 days before the next menstrual period. After ovulation, larger amounts of progesterone are produced. An edematous, vascular, functional endometrium is now apparent.

At the end of the secretory phase the fully matured secretory endometrium reaches the thickness of heavy, soft velvet. It becomes luxuriant with blood and glandular secretions, a suitable protective and nutritive bed for a fertilized ovum.

Implantation of the fertilized ovum generally occurs about 7 to 10 days after ovulation. If fertilization and implantation do not occur, the corpus luteum, which secretes estrogen and progesterone, regresses. With the rapid fall in progesterone and estrogen levels, the spiral arteries go into a spasm. During the *ischemic phase,* the blood supply to the functional endometrium is blocked and necrosis develops. The functional layer separates from the basal layer, and menstrual bleeding begins, marking day 1 of the next cycle (see Fig. 6-7).

Hypothalamic-Pituitary Cycle

Toward the end of the normal menstrual cycle, blood levels of estrogen and progesterone fall. Low blood levels of these ovarian hormones stimulate the hypothalamus to secrete gonadotropin-releasing hormone (GnRH). In turn, GnRH stimulates anterior pituitary secretion of follicle-stimulating hormone (FSH). FSH stimulates development of ovarian graafian follicles and their production of estrogen. Estrogen levels begin to fall, and hypothalamic GnRH triggers the anterior pituitary release of luteinizing hormone (LH). A marked surge of LH and a smaller peak of estrogen (day 12; see Fig. 6-7) precede the expulsion of the ovum from the graafian follicle by about 24 to 36 hours. LH peaks about the thirteenth or fourteenth day of a 28-day cycle. If fertilization and implantation of the ovum have not occurred by this time, regression of the corpus luteum follows. Levels of progesterone and estrogen decline, menstruation occurs, and the hypothalamus is once again stimulated to secrete GnRH. This process is called the **hypothalamic-pituitary cycle**.

Ovarian Cycle

The primitive graafian follicles contain immature oocytes (primordial ova). Before ovulation, from 1 to 30 follicles begin to mature in each ovary under the influence of FSH and estrogen. The preovulatory surge of LH affects a selected follicle. The oocyte matures, ovulation occurs, and the empty follicle begins its transformation into the corpus luteum. This *follicular phase* (preovulatory phase) (see Fig. 6-7) of the **ovarian cycle** varies in length from woman to woman. Almost all variations in ovarian cycle length are the result of variations in the length of the follicular phase. On rare occasions (i.e., 1 in 100 menstrual cycles), more than one follicle is selected, and more than one oocyte matures and undergoes ovulation.

After ovulation, estrogen levels drop. For 90% of women, only a small amount of *withdrawal bleeding* occurs so that it goes unnoticed. In 10% of women, there is sufficient bleeding for it to be visible, resulting in what is termed *midcycle bleeding.*

The *luteal phase* begins immediately after ovulation and ends with the start of menstruation. This postovulatory phase of the ovarian cycle usually requires 14 days (range of 13 to 15 days). The corpus luteum reaches its peak of functional activity 8 days after ovulation, secreting the steroids estrogen and progesterone. Coincident with this time of peak luteal functioning, the fertilized ovum is implanted in the endometrium. If no implantation occurs, the corpus luteum regresses, and steroid levels drop. Two weeks after ovulation, if fertilization and implantation do not occur, the functional layer of the uterine endometrium is shed through menstruation.

Other Cyclic Changes

When the hypothalamic-pituitary-ovarian axis functions properly, other tissues undergo predictable responses. Before ovulation the woman's basal body temperature (BBT) is often below 37° C; after ovulation, with rising progesterone levels, her BBT rises. Changes in the cervix and cervical mucus follow a generally predictable pattern. Preovulatory and postovulatory mucus is viscous (thick) so that sperm penetration is discouraged. At the time of ovulation, cervical mucus is thin and clear. It looks, feels, and stretches like egg white. This stretchable quality is termed *spinnbarkheit.* Some women experience localized lower abdominal pain called *mittelschmerz* that coincides with ovulation.

Prostaglandins

Prostaglandins (PGs) are oxygenated fatty acids classified as hormones. The different kinds of PGs are distinguished by letters (PGE, PGF), numbers (PGE$_2$), and letters of the Greek alphabet (PGF$_{2\alpha}$).

PGs are produced in most organs of the body, including the uterus. Menstrual blood is a potent prostaglandin source. PGs are metabolized quickly by most tissues. They are biologically active in minute amounts in the cardiovascular, gastrointestinal, respiratory, urogenital, and nervous systems. They also exert a marked effect on metabolism, particularly on glycolysis. Prostaglandins play an important role in many physiologic, pathologic, and pharmacologic

TABLE 6-2 Four Phases of Sexual Response

REACTIONS COMMON TO BOTH SEXES	FEMALE REACTIONS	MALE REACTIONS
EXCITEMENT PHASE Heart rate and blood pressure increase. Nipples become erect. Myotonia begins.	Clitoris increases in diameter and swells. External genitals become congested and darken. Vaginal lubrication occurs; upper two thirds of vagina lengthen and extend. Cervix and uterus pull upward. Breast size increases.	Erection of the penis begins; penis increases in length and diameter. Scrotal skin becomes congested and thickens. Testes begin to increase in size and elevate toward the body.
PLATEAU PHASE Heart rate and blood pressure continue to increase. Respirations increase. Myotonia becomes pronounced; grimacing occurs.	Clitoral head retracts under the clitoral hood. Lower one third of vagina becomes engorged. Skin color changes occur—red flush may be observed across breasts, abdomen, or other surfaces.	Head of penis may enlarge slightly. Scrotum continues to grow tense and thicken. Testes continue to elevate and enlarge. Preorgasmic emission of 2 or 3 drops of fluid appears on the head of the penis.
ORGASMIC PHASE Heart rate, blood pressure, and respirations increase to maximum levels. Involuntary muscle spasms occur. External rectal sphincter contracts.	Strong rhythmic contractions are felt in the clitoris, vagina, and uterus. Sensations of warmth spread through the pelvic area.	Testes elevate to maximum level. Point of "inevitability" occurs just before ejaculation and an awareness of fluid in the urethra. Rhythmic contractions occur in the penis. Ejaculation of semen occurs.
RESOLUTION PHASE Heart rate, blood pressure, and respirations return to normal. Nipple erection subsides. Myotonia subsides.	Engorgement in external genitalia and vagina resolves. Uterus descends to normal position. Cervix dips into seminal pool. Breast size decreases. Skin flush disappears.	Fifty percent of erection is lost immediately with ejaculation; penis gradually returns to normal size. Testes and scrotum return to normal size. Refractory period (time needed for erection to occur again) varies according to age and general physical condition.

reactions. $PGF_{2\alpha}$, PGE_4, and PGE_2 are most commonly used in reproductive medicine.

Prostaglandins affect smooth muscle contractility and modulation of hormonal activity. Indirect evidence supports PGs' effects on ovulation, fertility, changes in the cervix and cervical mucus that affect receptivity to sperm, tubal and uterine motility, sloughing of endometrium (menstruation), onset of abortion (spontaneous and induced), and onset of labor (term and preterm).

After exerting their biologic actions, newly synthesized PGs are rapidly metabolized by tissues in such organs as the lungs, kidneys, and liver.

PGs may play a key role in ovulation. If PG levels do not rise along with the surge of LH, the ovum remains trapped within the graafian follicle. After ovulation, PGs may influence production of estrogen and progesterone by the corpus luteum.

The introduction of PGs into the vagina or into the uterine cavity (from ejaculated semen) increases the motility of uterine musculature, which may assist the transport of sperm through the uterus and into the oviduct.

PGs produced by the woman cause regression of the corpus luteum; regression of the endometrium; and sloughing of the endometrium, resulting in menstruation. PGs increase myometrial response to oxytocic stimulation, enhance uterine contractions, and cause cervical dilation. They may be a factor in the initiation of labor, the maintenance of labor, or both. They may also be involved in the following pathologic states: dysmenorrhea, hypertensive states, preeclampsia-eclampsia, and anaphylactic shock.

Climacteric and Menopause

The **climacteric** is a transitional phase during which ovarian function and hormone production decline. This phase spans the years from the onset of premenopausal ovarian decline to the postmenopausal time when symptoms stop. **Menopause** (from the Latin *mensis,* month, and Greek *pausis,* to cease) refers only to the last menstrual period. Unlike menarche, however, menopause can be dated only with certainty 1 year after menstruation ceases. The average age at natural menopause is 51.4 years, with an age range of 35 to 60 years. Perimenopause is the 10 years before menopause, usually from about age 40 on.

SEXUAL RESPONSE

The hypothalamus and anterior pituitary gland in females regulate the production of FSH and LH. The target tissue for these hormones is the ovary, which produces ova and secretes estrogen and progesterone. A *feedback mechanism* between hormone secretion from the ovaries, hypothalamus, and anterior pituitary aids in the control of the production of sex cells and steroid sex hormone secretion.

Physiologic Response to Sexual Stimulation

Although the first outward appearance of maturing sexual development occurs at an earlier age in females, both females and males achieve physical maturity at approximately 17 years of age. However, individual development varies greatly. Anatomic and reproductive differences notwithstanding, women and men are more alike than different in their physiologic response to sexual excitement and orgasm. For example, the glans clitoris and the glans penis are embryonic homologues. Not only is there little difference between female and male sexual response, but the physical response is essentially the same whether stimulated by coitus, fantasy, or masturbation. Physiologically, according to Masters (1992), sexual response can be analyzed in terms of two processes: vasocongestion and myotonia.

Sexual stimulation results in circumvaginal blood vessels (lubrication in the female), causing engorgement and distention of the genitals. Venous congestion is localized primarily in the genitals, but it also occurs to a lesser degree in the breasts and other parts of the body. Arousal is characterized by *myotonia* (increased muscular tension), resulting in voluntary and involuntary rhythmic contractions. Examples of sexually stimulated myotonia are pelvic thrusting, facial grimacing, and spasms of the hands and feet (carpopedal spasms).

The **sexual response cycle** is divided into four phases: excitement phase, plateau phase, orgasmic phase, and resolution phase. The four phases occur progressively with no sharp dividing line between any two phases. Specific body changes take place in sequence. The time, intensity, and duration for cyclic completion also vary for individuals and situations. Table 6-2 compares male and female body changes during each of the four phases of the sexual response cycle.

IMMUNOLOGY

Immunology is the study of the molecules, cells, organs, and systems responsible for the recognition and disposal of foreign material and how the human body defends itself against this material. The human immune system is necessary for survival. Foreign substances can be as diverse as life-threatening infectious microorganisms or a lifesaving organ transplant. The desirable consequences of immunity include natural resistance, recovery, and acquired resistance to infectious diseases.

Body Defenses

The first barrier to infection is unbroken skin and mucous membranes. These surfaces form a physical barrier against many microorganisms. Secretions, such as mucus or those produced in the process of eliminating liquid and solid wastes (i.e., the urinary and gastrointestinal processes), are also important as nonspecific mechanisms for removing potential pathogens from the body. The acidity and alkalinity of the fluids of the stomach and intestinal tract, and the acidity of the vagina, can destroy many potentially infectious microorganisms. These fluids can also have chemical properties that defend the body. For example, lysozyme is an enzyme found in tears and saliva that attacks the cell wall of susceptible bacteria.

The body has a wide variety of barrier-assisting defenses that initially protect the body against disease. Although these barriers vary among individuals, they do assist in the general resistance to infectious organisms. When barrier-assisting defenses break down, the potential for disease increases. For instance, when the new mother's skin integrity is impaired (e.g., through episiotomy or lacerations) or when she has cracking of the nipples, she is at increased risk for infection. In older women, the pH and amount of vaginal fluid is altered, resulting in increased risk of yeast infection (*Candida albicans*).

Types of Immunity
Natural Immunity

Natural (innate or inborn) resistance is one of two ways the body resists infection after microorganisms have penetrated the first line of resistance. The second form, acquired or adaptive resistance, specifically recognizes and selectively eliminates exogenous (or endogenous) agents.

Natural immunity is characterized as a nonspecific mechanism. If a microorganism penetrates the skin or mucous membranes, cellular and humoral defense mechanisms become operational. The elements of natural resistance are phagocytic cells, complement, and the acute inflammatory reaction. Despite their relative lack of specificity, these components are essential, because they are largely responsible for natural immunity to many environmental microorganisms.

Acquired Immunity

If a microorganism overwhelms the body's natural resistance, another form of defensive resistance, **acquired immunity,** allows the body to recognize, remember, and respond to a specific stimulus—an antigen.

Acquired immunity can eliminate microorganisms and commonly leaves the host with antigen-specific immunologic memory. This condition of memory or recall, *acquired resistance,* allows the host to respond more effectively if reinfection with the same microorganism occurs. Acquired immunity, like natural immunity, is composed of cellular and humoral components.

The major cellular component of this mechanism is the lymphocyte; the major humoral component is the antibody. Lymphocytes selectively respond to foreign materials, antigens, which leads to immune memory and a permanently altered pattern of response or adaptation to the environment. The two categories of the adaptive response are antibody-mediated and cell-mediated immunity. Antibody-mediated immunity is the primary defense against bacterial infection. Cell-mediated immunity is the primary defense against viral and fungal infections, intracellular organisms, tumor antigens, and graft rejections.

Antibody-Mediated Immunity

If specific antibodies have been formed to antigen stimulation, they are available to protect the body against foreign substances. The recognition of foreign substances and subsequent production of antibodies to these substances is the specific meaning of immunity. Antibody-mediated immunity to infection occurs when the antibodies are formed by the host or received from another source. These two types of immunity are called *active* and *passive* immunity.

Active immunity can be acquired by natural exposure in response to an infection or acquired by injection of an antigen. This injection of antigen, called **vaccination,** effectively stimulates antibody production and memory (acquired resistance) without suffering from the disease. The selected antigenic agent should produce the antibodies without the clinical signs and symptoms of the disease in an **immunocompetent** host (a person whose immune system is able to recognize a foreign antigen and build specific antigen-directed antibodies) and produce permanent antigenic memory. Booster vaccinations may be needed to expand the pool of memory cells.

Artificial **passive immunity** is achieved by infusion of serum or plasma containing high concentrations of antibody. This provides immediate antibody protection against microorganisms such as hepatitis A or antigens such as Rh-positive (fetal) red blood cells. The antibodies have been produced by another person or animal that has been actively immunized, not by the ultimate recipient. As long as the antibodies persist in the circulation, recipients will benefit from passive immunity. Passive immunity can

also be acquired naturally by the fetus through the transfer of antibodies through maternal circulation in utero. Maternal antibodies are also transferred to the newborn after birth in the prelactation fluid called *colostrum.* For the newborn to have lasting protection, active immunity must occur.

Cell-Mediated Immunity

Cell-mediated immunity consists of immune activities that differ from those of antibody-mediated immunity. Cell-mediated immunity is moderated by the link between T-lymphocytes and phagocytic cells (i.e., monocyte-macrophage cells). Lymphocytes (T-cells) do not directly recognize the antigens of microorganisms or other living cells, such as an *allograft* (a graft of tissue from a genetically different member of the same species [e.g., a human kidney]), but do so when the antigen is present on the surface of an antigen-presenting cell—the macrophage. Lymphocytes are immunologically active through various types of direct cell-to-cell contact and by the production of soluble factors, such as *lymphokines,* for specific immunologic functions. These include the recruitment of phagocytic cells to the site of inflammation. The term *delayed hypersensitivity* is often used synonymously with the term *cell-mediated immunity.* Delayed hypersensitivity refers to the slow appearance of a secondary response in the skin. The term dates back to when antibody responses were detected by immediate hypersensitivity and reflected the difference in the length of time that it took for a delayed response to occur (e.g., tuberculin skin test).

Under some conditions, the activities of cell-mediated immunity may not be beneficial. Suppression of the normal adaptive immune response *(immunosuppression)* by drugs or other means is necessary in conditions such as organ transplantation, hypersensitivity, and autoimmune disorders.

Factors Associated with Immunologic Disease

Factors such as general health and the age of an individual are important considerations in the functioning of the immune system in defense against infectious disease. In the case of noninfectious diseases or disorders, however, additional factors may be important. In caring for women and their families, nurses must consider the effects of the environment, nutritional status, and lifestyle on the developing immune system. Standard precautions should be practiced at all times whether caring for women in the hospital, community, or home.

HEALTH ASSESSMENT

Profound changes in society and the family and in roles and expectations of women make maternity nursing and women's health care a challenging field. Current women's health trends have expanded beyond a reproductive focus to include a holistic approach to health care across the life span. This restructuring deemphasizes tertiary care and places women's health within the scope of primary care. Women's health assessment and screening focus on a systems evaluation beginning with a careful history and physical examination. During the assessment and evaluation, the responsibility for self-care, health promotion, and enhancement of wellness is emphasized. Nursing is an interactive process that begins with establishing trust and a caring relationship with the broader goal of enhancing and maintaining wellness. The nurse provides care that includes assessment, planning, education, counseling, and referral as needed, as well as commendations of good self-care that the woman has practiced. This enables women to make informed decisions about their own health care.

It is the nurse's responsibility to coordinate the woman's care in accordance with established guidelines and protocols (U.S. Department of Health and Human Services, 1997).

In a market-driven system such as managed care, there may be specific guidelines provided for health screening by the insurer or managed care organization. A nurse often takes the history, orders diagnostic tests, interprets test results, makes referrals, coordinates care, and directs attention to problems requiring medical intervention. Advanced practice nurses who have specialized in women's health, such as nurse practitioners, clinical nurse specialists, and nurse midwives, perform complete physical examinations, including gynecologic examinations.

Culturally competent nursing care should be delivered with an awareness of cultural diversity while respecting the unique qualities of each woman. Such care cannot be provided in the absence of self-awareness. Nurses must acknowledge their own values, beliefs, and communication styles in order to understand what they contribute to cross-cultural communication (Lipson et al., 1996).

Interview

The interview should be conducted in a private, comfortable, and relaxed setting (Fig. 6-8). The nurse is seated and makes sure the woman is comfortable. The woman is addressed by her title and name (e.g., Mrs. Gonzalez), and the nurse introduces herself or himself using name and title. It is important to phrase questions in a sensitive and nonjudgmental manner. Body language should match verbal communication. The nurse is cognizant of a woman's vulnerability and assures her of strict confidentiality. For many women, fear, anxiety, and modesty make the examination a dreaded and stressful experience. Many women are uninformed, misguided by myths, or afraid they will appear ignorant by asking questions about sexual or reproductive functioning. The woman is assured that no question is irrelevant. The history begins with an open-ended question such as, "What brings you in to the office/clinic/hospital today? Anything else? Tell me about it." Additional ways to get women to share information include the following:

- **Facilitation:** Using a word or posture that communicates interest; leaning forward; making eye contact; or saying "Mm-hmmm" or "Go on."

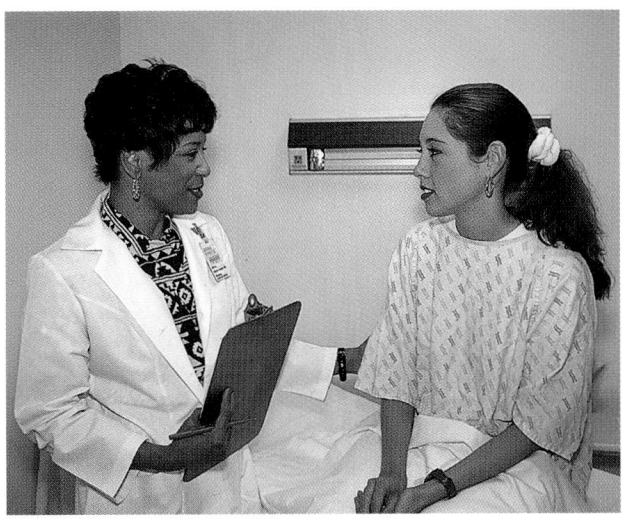

Fig. 6-8 Nurse interviews client as part of annual physical examination. *(From Potter, P., & Perry, A. [1997]. Fundamentals of nursing: Concepts, process, and practice [4th ed.]. St. Louis: Mosby.)*

- **Reflection:** Repeating a word or phrase that a woman has used.
- **Clarification:** Asking the woman what is meant by a word or phrase.
- **Empathic responses:** Acknowledging the feelings of a woman by statements such as, "That must have been frightening."
- **Confrontation:** Identifying something about the woman's behavior or feelings not expressed verbally or apparently inconsistent with her history.
- **Interpretation:** Putting into words what you infer about the woman's feelings or about the meaning of her symptoms, events, or other matters.

Direct questions may be necessary to get specific details. This should be worded in language that is understandable to the woman and expressed neutrally so that the woman will not be led into a specific response. The nurse asks about one item at a time and proceeds from the general to the specific (Seidel et al., 1999).

Biographic Information

At a woman's first visit, she is often expected to fill out a form with biographic and historical data before meeting with the examiner. The nurse is usually responsible for ensuring that the woman's name, age, marital status, race, ethnicity, address, phone numbers, occupation, and date of visit are recorded. The name should be recorded on all pages of the record. Common client names should also have additional identifying client information such as date of birth or Social Security number on each page.

Old records are considered a reliable source of client information. The nurse records a subjective judgment about the reliability of the person giving the history—the woman, parent, spouse, or other historian.

History

A medical history usually includes the following:

1. **Identifying data:** Name, age, race, living household preference, occupation, religion, culture, and ethnicity are obtained.

2. **Chief complaint(s):** A verbatim response to the question, "What problem or symptom brought you here today?" If a lengthy list is recited it may be necessary to tell the woman that her two complaints with the highest priority will be addressed today. Then in order to give all of her problems the full attention they deserve, a follow-up appointment in 1 to 2 weeks will be scheduled. Women are usually appreciative that the nurse is taking extra time and are agreeable to this.

3. **History of present illness:** A chronologic narrative that includes onset of the problem, the setting in which it developed, its manifestations, and any treatments received are noted. The woman's state of health before the onset of the present problem is determined. If the problem is long standing, the reason for seeking attention at this time is elicited. The principal symptoms should be described as to the following:
   - Location
   - Quality
   - Quantity or severity
   - Timing (onset, duration, frequency)
   - Setting
   - Factors that aggravate or relieve
   - Associated manifestations

4. **Past medical history:** Determine general state of health and strength:
   - Infectious diseases: measles, mumps, rubella, whooping cough, chickenpox, rheumatic fever, scarlet fever, diphtheria, polio, tuberculosis (TB), hepatitis
   - Chronic disease and system disorders: arthritis, cancer, diabetes, heart, lung, kidney, seizures, thyroid, stroke, ulcers
   - Adult injuries, accidents, illnesses, disabilities, hospitalizations, blood transfusions; note if the injury occurred on the job (workers' compensation) or if potential litigation is being considered

5. **Present health status:**
   - Allergies: medications, previous transfusion reactions, environmental allergies
   - Immunizations: diphtheria; pertussis; tetanus; polio; measles, mumps, rubella (MMR); hepatitis B; varicella; influenza; pneumococcal vaccine; last TB skin test
   - Screening tests: Pap smear, mammogram, stool for occult blood, sigmoidoscopy/colonoscopy, chest x-ray, hematocrit, hemoglobin, rubella titer, urinalysis, cholesterol test; blood type/Rh; last eye examination; last dental examination
   - Environmental/chemical hazards: home, school, work, and leisure setting; exposure to extreme heat/cold, noise, industrial toxins such as asbestos or lead, pesticides, diethylstilbestrol (DES), radiation exposure, cat feces, cigarette smoke
   - Use of safety measures: seat belts, bicycle helmets, athletic protective devices, designated driver
   - Exercise and leisure activities
   - Sleep patterns: length and quality
   - Sexuality: Is she sexually active? With men, women, or both? Does she use condoms?
   - Diet, including beverages: 24-hour dietary recall; brushes three times daily; flosses daily
   - Medications: name, dose, frequency, duration, reason for taking, and compliance with prescription medications; home remedies, over-the-counter drugs, vitamin and mineral or herbal supplements used over a 24-hour period
   - Nicotine, alcohol, or recreational drugs: type, amount, frequency, duration, and reactions
   - Caffeine: coffee, tea, cola, or chocolate intake

6. **Past surgical history:** Type, date, reason, outcome, and any complications should be noted.

7. **Family history:** Information about age and health of family members may be presented in narrative or genogram (see Fig. 2-6): age, health/death of parents, siblings, spouse, children. Check for history of diabetes, heart disease, hypertension, stroke, respiratory, renal, thyroid, cancer, bleeding disorders, hepatitis, allergies, asthma, arthritis, TB, epilepsy, mental illness, human immunodeficiency virus (HIV), or other disorders.

8. **Social history:** Note birthplace, education, employment, marital status, living accommodations, children, persons at home, and hobbies. Does she enjoy what she is doing?
   - Screen for abuse: Has she ever been hit, kicked, slapped, or forced to have sex against her wishes? Verbally or emotionally abused? History of childhood sexual abuse? If yes, has she received counseling or does she need referral (Seng & Petersen, 1995)?

9. **Review of systems:** It is probable that all questions in each system will not be included every time a history is taken. Some questions regarding each system should be included in every history. The essential areas to be explored are listed in the following head-to-toe sequence. If a woman gives a positive response to a question about an essential area, more detailed questions should be asked.
   - **General:** weight change, fatigue, weakness, fever, chills, or night sweats
   - **Skin:** skin, hair and nail changes, itching, bruising, bleeding, rashes, sores, lumps, or moles
   - **Lymph nodes:** enlargement, inflammation, pain, suppuration (pus), or drainage
   - **Head, eyes, ears, nose, and throat:**
     - **Head:** trauma, vertigo (dizziness), convulsive disorder, syncope (fainting), headache location, frequency, pain type, nausea/vomiting, or visual symptoms

- **Eyes:** glasses, contact lenses, blurriness, tearing, itching, photophobia, diplopia, inflammation, trauma, cataracts, glaucoma, or acute visual loss
- **Ears:** hearing loss, tinnitus (ringing), vertigo, discharge, pain, fullness, recurrent infections, or mastoiditis
- **Nose/sinuses:** trauma, rhinitis, nasal discharge, epistaxis, obstruction, sneezing, itching, allergy, or smelling impairment
- **Mouth/throat/neck:** hoarseness, voice changes, soreness, ulcers, bleeding gums, goiter, swelling, or enlarged nodes
- **Breasts:** masses, pain, lumps, dimpling, nipple discharge, fibrocystic changes or implants; BSE
- **Respiratory:** shortness of breath, wheezing, cough, sputum, hemoptysis, pneumonia, pleurisy, asthma, bronchitis, emphysema, or TB; last chest x-ray
- **Cardiac:** hypertension, rheumatic fever, murmurs, angina, palpitations, dyspnea, tachycardia, orthopnea, edema, chest pain, cough, cyanosis, cold extremities, ascites, intermittent claudication (leg pain), phlebitis, or skin color changes
- **Gastrointestinal:** appetite, nausea, vomiting, indigestion, dysphagia, abdominal pain, ulcers, hematochezia (bleeding with stools), melena (black, tarry stools), bowel habit changes, diarrhea, constipation, bowel movement frequency, food intolerance, hemorrhoids, jaundice, or hepatitis; sigmoidoscopy, colonoscopy, barium enema, ultrasound
- **Genitourinary:** frequency, hesitancy, urgency, polyuria, dysuria, hematuria, nocturia, incontinence, stones, infection, or urethral discharge; dysmenorrhea, intermenstrual bleeding, dyspareunia, discharge, sores, itching, sexually transmitted diseases, gravidity (G), parity (P), problems in pregnancy, contraception, menopause, hot flashes, or sweats (may be included here or as part of endocrine)
- **Vascular:** leg edema, claudication, varicose veins, thromboses, or emboli
- **Endocrine:** heat/cold intolerance, dry skin, excessive sweating, polyuria, polydipsia, polyphagia, thyroid problems, diabetes, or secondary sex characteristic changes; age at menarche, length/flow of menses, last menstrual period (LMP), age at menopause, libido, or sexual concerns
- **Hematologic:** anemia, easy bruising, bleeding, petechiae, purpura, or transfusions
- **Musculoskeletal:** muscle weakness, pain, joint stiffness, scoliosis, lordosis, kyphosis, range-of-motion instability, redness, swelling, arthritis, or gout
- **Neurologic:** loss of sensation, numbness, tingling, tremors, weakness, vertigo, paralysis, fainting, twitching, blackouts, seizures, convulsions, loss of consciousness or memory
- **Psychiatric:** moodiness, depression, anxiety, obsessions, delusions, illusions, or hallucinations

- **Functional assessment:** should be done on women with disabilities and age 70 and over (see later in this chapter)

Cultural Considerations and Communication Variations

Recognition of signs and symptoms of disease and deciding when to seek treatment are influenced by cultural perceptions. Culture evolves over time and is a system of symbols that are learned, shared, and passed on through generations of a social group. Cultural competence in nursing is a complex combination of knowledge, attitudes, and skills mixed with personal attributes of flexibility, empathy, and language facility. It is more than simply acquiring knowledge about another ethnic group. It is essential that a nurse have respect for the rich and unique qualities that cultural diversity brings to individuals. In recognizing the value of these differences, the nurse can modify the plan of care to meet the needs of each woman. Trust that the woman is the expert on her life, culture, and experiences. If the nurse asks with respect and a genuine desire to learn, the client will tell the nurse how to care for her (Lipson et al., 1996). The nurse communicates in an even-toned and nonjudgmental manner, keeps a calm facial expression, and recognizes that modifications may be necessary for the physical examination. In some cultures, it may be considered inappropriate for the woman to completely disrobe for the physical examination. In many cultures, a woman examiner is preferred.

Communication may be hindered by different beliefs even when the nurse and client speak the same language. Communication variations include the following (modified from Lipson et al., 1996):

- **Conversational style and pacing:** Silence may show respect or acknowledgment that the listener has heard. In cultures in which a direct "no" is considered rude, silence may mean no. Repetition or loudness may mean emphasis or anger.
- **Personal space:** Cultural conceptions of personal space differ, based on one's culture. Someone may be perceived as distant for backing off when approached or aggressive for standing too close.
- **Eye contact:** Eye contact varies among cultures from intense to fleeting. In an effort to refrain from invading personal space, avoiding direct eye contact may be a sign of respect.
- **Touch:** The norms about how people should touch each other vary among cultures. In some cultures physical contact with the same sex (embracing, walking hand in hand) is more appropriate than with an unrelated person of the opposite sex.
- **Time orientation:** In some cultures involvement with people is more valued than being "on time." In other cultures, life is scheduled and paced according to clock time, which is valued over personal time.

Women with Special Needs

Women with emotional or physical disorders have special needs. Women who have vision, hearing, emotional, or physical disabilities should be respected and involved in the assessment and physical examination to the full extent of their abilities. The nurse should communicate openly and directly with sensitivity. It is often helpful to learn about the disability directly from the woman while maintaining eye contact. Family and significant others should be relied on only when absolutely necessary. The assessment and physical examination can be adapted to each woman's individual needs.

Communication with a woman who is hearing impaired can be accomplished without difficulty. Most of these women read lips, write, or both; thus an interviewer who speaks and enunciates each word slowly and in full view may be easily understood. If a woman is not comfortable with lip reading, she may use an interpreter. In this case, it is important to continue to address the woman directly, avoiding the temptation to speak directly with the interpreter. The visually impaired woman needs to be oriented to the examination room and may have her guide dog with her. As with all clients, the visually impaired woman needs a full explanation of what the examination entails before proceeding. Before touching her, the nurse explains, "Now I am going to take your blood pressure. I am going to place the cuff on your right arm." The woman can be asked if she would like to touch each of the items that will be used in the examination to reduce her anxiety.

Many physically disabled women cannot comfortably lie in the lithotomy position for the pelvic examination. Several alternative positions may be used, including a lateral (side-lying) position, a V-shaped position, a diamond-shaped position, and an M-shaped position (Fig. 6-9). The woman can be asked what has worked best for her previously. If she has never had a pelvic examination, or has never had a comfortable pelvic examination, the nurse proceeds slowly by showing her a picture of various positions and asking her which one she prefers. The nurse's support and reassurance can help the woman to relax, which will make the examination go more smoothly. The woman is informed that she is in charge, and if the examination must stop for whatever reason, it can be scheduled again at a later date.

Abused Women

Nurses should screen all women entering the health care system for potential abuse (see Chapter 11). It is important to keep in mind the possibility that violence against this woman may have occurred. Abuse is a life-threatening

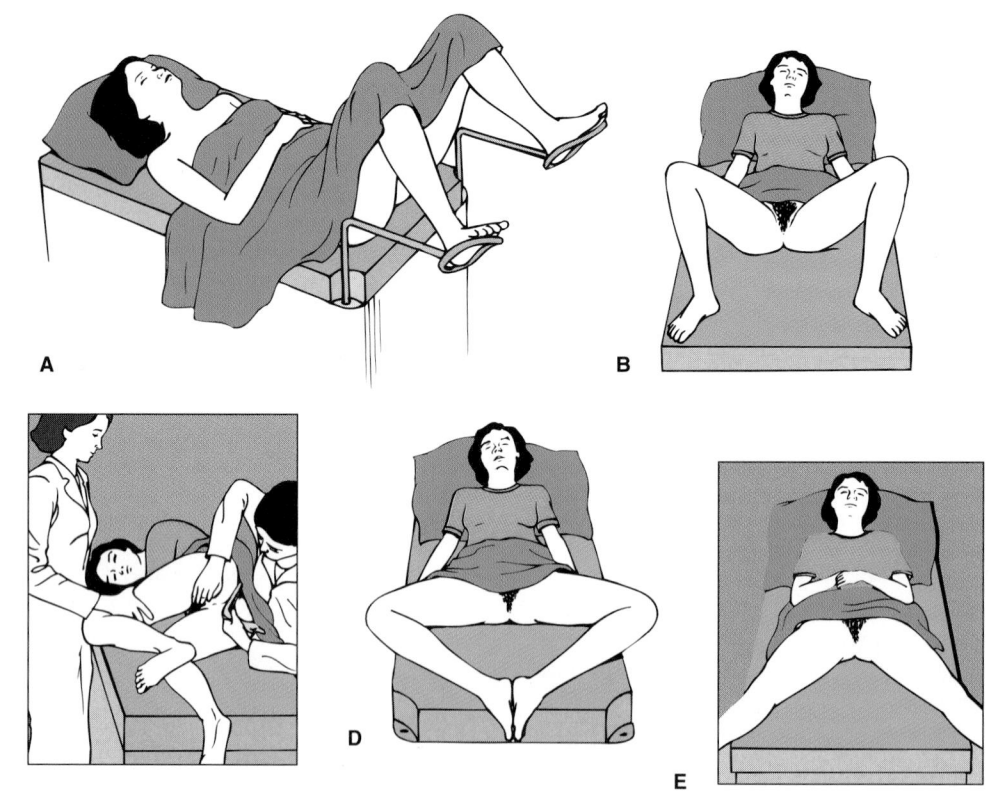

Fig. 6-9 Lithotomy and variable positions for women who have a disability. **A,** Lithotomy position. **B,** M-shaped position. **C,** Side-lying position. **D,** Diamond-shaped position. **E,** V-shaped position.

public health problem that affects millions of women and their children. Abuse of women knows no socioeconomic, racial, ethnic, religious, or age barriers. The risk for domestic violence increases during pregnancy and after separation or divorce. Many health care providers avoid questions about family violence because they are unaware of the extent of the problem, they find it difficult to ask about violence, or they feel helpless to assist the woman. Help for the woman may depend on the sensitivity with which the nurse screens for abuse, the discovery of abuse, and subsequent intervention. The nurse must be familiar with the laws governing abuse in the state in which she or he practices and inform the woman of these laws before eliciting this information. Awareness of the law can ensure the woman's confidentiality and trust.

Pocket cards listing emergency numbers (abuse counseling, legal protection, and emergency shelter) may be available by calling the local police department or women's shelter or going to an emergency department. It is helpful to have these on hand in the setting where screening is done. An abuse assessment screen (Fig. 6-10) can be used as part of the interview or written history (Poirier, 1997). Reports show an increase in identification of victims of domestic violence when screening takes place at each visit. If a male partner is present, he should be asked to leave the room because the woman may not disclose experiences of abuse in his presence, or he may try to answer questions for her to protect himself. The same procedure would apply for partners of lesbians or adult children of older women.

Fear, guilt, and embarrassment may keep many women from giving information about family violence. Clues in the history and evidence of injuries on physical examination should give a high index of suspicion (Box 6-1).

The areas most commonly injured in women are the head, neck, chest, abdomen, breasts, and upper extremities. Burns and bruises in patterns resembling hands, belts, cords, or other weapons and multiple traumatic injuries may be seen. Attention should be given to women who repeatedly seek treatment for somatic complaints such as headaches; insomnia; choking sensation; hyperventilation; gastrointestinal symptoms; and pain in the chest, back, and pelvis. During pregnancy, the nurse should assess for injuries to the breasts, abdomen, and genitals. Assessment requires a detailed history of the woman's abuse and her living arrangements.

If a woman discloses battering as a problem, this disclosure is acknowledged and affirmed that it is unacceptable. The woman is told that she is at risk for recurrence. She also needs to know that battering is a common

---

ABUSE ASSESSMENT SCREEN

1. Have you ever been emotionally or physically abused by your partner or someone important to you?

YES ☐   NO ☐

2. Within the last year, have you been hit, slapped, kicked, or otherwise physically hurt by someone?

YES ☐   NO ☐

If YES, by whom _____

Number of times _____

Mark the area of injury on body map.

3. Within the last year, has anyone forced you to have sexual activities?

YES ☐   NO ☐

If YES, by whom _____

Number of times _____

4. Are you afraid of your partner or anyone you listed above?

YES ☐   NO ☐

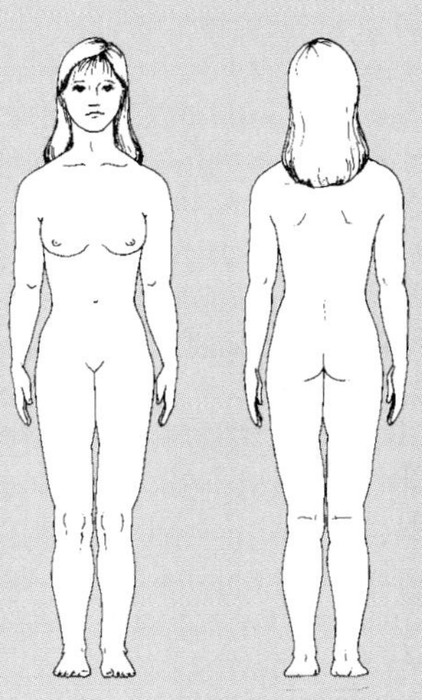

Fig. 6-10   Abuse assessment screen. (Modified from the Nursing Research Consortium on Violence and Abuse. [1991].)

BOX 6-1 Indicators of Possible Abuse

1. Change in appointment pattern, either increased appointments with somatic, vague complaints or frequently missed appointments
2. Self-directed abuse, depression, attempted suicide
3. Severe anxiety, insomnia, or violent nightmares
4. Alcohol or drug abuse; overuse or abuse of prescription medications
5. Bruises

Data from Edge, V., & Miller M. (1994). *Women's health care.* St. Louis: Mosby.

problem, because she may think that she is alone in experiencing violence perpetrated by a family member or loved one. She must be told that help is available and that she does not deserve to be abused. The nurse's goal is to empower the woman. She needs to gain a feeling of control over her life, set her own goals, and make her own decisions. It is vital for the nurse to communicate two messages: (1) the nurse is deeply concerned for her welfare, and (2) the woman does not deserve to be abused (U.S. Department of Health and Human Services, 1997).

The nurse can help the woman formulate a plan: What referrals (shelters, agencies, and legal aid) can help her? Where can she go if she needs to leave immediately? What necessary documents and personal items should be packed that can be easily accessed?

Age-Related Considerations
Adolescents (Age 13 to 19 Years)

As a young woman matures, she should be asked the same questions that are included in any history. Particular attention should be paid to hints about risky behaviors, eating disorders, and depression. Do not assume that a teenager is not sexually active. After rapport has been established it is best to talk to a teen with the parent (partner or friend) out of the room. Questions should be asked with sensitivity and in a gentle and nonjudgmental manner (Seidel et al., 1999).

A teen's first speculum examination is the most important because she will develop perceptions that will remain with her for future examinations. What the examination entails should be discussed with the teen while she is dressed. Models or illustrations can be used to show exactly what will happen. All of the necessary equipment should be assembled so that there are no interruptions. Pediatric specula that are 1 to 1.5 cm wide can be inserted with minimal discomfort. If the teen is sexually active, a small adult speculum may be used.

Injury prevention should be a part of the counseling at routine health examinations with special attention to seat belts, helmets, firearms, recreational hazards, and sports involvement. The use of drugs and alcohol and the nonuse of

seat belts contribute to motor vehicle injuries, accounting for the greatest proportion of accidental deaths in women (Fogel & Woods, 1995). Contraceptive options, including use of condoms, should be addressed during visits.

To provide developmentally appropriate care, it is important to review the major tasks for women in this stage of life. Major tasks for teens include values assessment; education and work goal setting; formation of peer relationships that focus on love and commitment and becoming comfortable with sexuality; and separation from parents. Individuality may be reflected in areas such as sexuality, politics, and career choices. Conflict exists between making and keeping commitments in order to keep options open. The teen is egocentric as she progresses rapidly through emotional and physical change. Her feelings of invulnerability may lead to misconceptions, such as unprotected sexual intercourse will not lead to pregnancy (Youngkin & Davis, 1994).

Midlife and Older Women (Age 50 Years and Older)

The assessment of women age 50 and over presents unique challenges. Women may be experiencing major lifestyle changes such as children leaving home, caretaking for their aging parents, job retirement, divorce or death of a partner, and aging changes and health problems. The nurse has an opportunity to use reflection and empathy while listening and ensuring open and caring communication. It may be necessary to schedule a longer appointment time because older women have longer histories or have a need to talk. Some women may fail to report symptoms because they fear their complaints will be attributed to old age or they feel that they have lived with a chronic condition (e.g., incontinence, dyspareunia, decreased libido) for so long that nothing can be done. Women may choose to ignore a problem if they have symptoms that are life threatening (e.g., chest pain or a breast lump) because they traditionally put the needs of others first. As a result, the nurse should encourage the woman to express her concerns and fears and reassure her that her problems are important and will be addressed. (Hormone therapy, diet, vitamin and calcium supplementation, daily aspirin, breast self-examination, mammogram, sigmoidoscopy, colonoscopy, updating immunizations, and need for exercise and sun protection should be discussed.)

Sexual assessment is important in women age 50 and over. Unless directly asked, women may omit mention of sexual concerns. Questions asked with sensitivity may invite responses regarding changes in sexual desire or response or physical issues that challenge her sexual enjoyment. Open and reflective questions also affirm a woman's right to sexual enjoyment throughout the life span.

Women over age 50 commonly experience menopause (cessation of menses) and have physical changes associated with decreased estrogen. A decrease in estrogen causes thinning of the mucosal tissue layers, resulting in a narrowing and a decrease in lubrication of the vagina. Estrogen also plays a role in the formation of bone matrix, and a decrease may lead to osteoporosis. Decreases in estrogen cause a relaxation of the ligaments and connective tissue, which affects the support of the bladder and uterus. Decreases in estrogen also affect the hypothalamus, causing hot flashes, which are disturbing to most women (Edge & Miller, 1994).

Physical changes can result in increased discomfort during the pelvic examination. It is important to be both gentle and thorough during the examination. A small adult speculum may be used to view the cervix. The uterus in a menopausal woman is small and firm and the ovaries are nonpalpable. In postmenopausal women the specimen from the vaginal pool may be useful to detect endometrial cells (Johnson et al., 1996). A woman with palpable adnexal masses or vaginal bleeding after menopause needs immediate gynecologic referral.

A respectful and reassuring approach toward caring for women age 50 and older will ensure their continued participation in seeking health care. Because the risk of breast, ovarian, uterine, cervical, and colon cancer increases with age, the nurse has the opportunity to educate women about the importance of preventive screening. It is the nurse's responsibility to ensure a positive health care experience that encourages future visits for preventive health, chronic, and acute care.

Advance Directives can be introduced on any entry into a health care system. It is a good idea to have a formal statement in the medical record regarding a woman's wishes in the event of accident or illness regarding life maintenance measures or organ donation. Most states have laws formalizing such statements in writing. The Durable Power of Attorney for Health Care can be used by a client to delegate decision-making authority to a trusted relative or friend.

Functional assessment is included as part of the history in women over age 70 and those with disabilities. In the review of systems, the nurse should ask about self-care activities such as walking, getting to the bathroom, bathing, hair combing, dressing, and eating. Questions about driving, using public transportation or the telephone, hanging up clothes, buying groceries, taking medications, and meal preparation should be included.

Physical Examination

In preparation for the physical examination, the woman is instructed on undressing and given a gown to wear during the examination. She is usually given the opportunity to undress privately. Some guidelines for assisting the Spanish-speaking woman during a physical examination are listed in the accompanying box.

Objective data are recorded by system or location. A general statement of overall health status is a good way to start. Findings are described in detail.

- **General appearance:** age, race, sex, state of health, posture, height, weight, development, dress, hygiene, affect, alertness, orientation, cooperativeness, and communication skills
- **Vital signs:** temperature, pulse, respiration, blood pressure

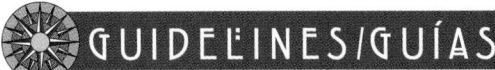

GUIDELINES/GUÍAS

Physical Examination

Take off all your clothes, please.
Quítese toda la ropa, por favor.

Put on the gown, please.
Póngase la bata, por favor.

I'm going to examine you.
Le voy a hacer un examen.

You will feel less discomfort if you relax.
Se sentirá mejor si relaja su cuerpo.

Lie down, please.
Acuéstese, por favor.

Put your feet in the stirrups.
Ponga sus pies en los estribos.

Open your legs, please.
Separa las piernas, por favor.

I'm going to take a sample from the lining of the cervix (Pap smear).
Voy a tomarle una muestra del cuello de la matriz para una prueba del cáncer; se llama la prueba "el pap."

We will test this sample for cancer.
Se le hara la prueba de cáncer.

It won't hurt.
Esto no le va a doler.

Everything looks fine.
Todo está bien.

You may get dressed.
Puede vestirse.

- **Skin:** color; integrity; texture; hydration; temperature; edema; excessive perspiration; unusual odor; presence and description of lesions; hair texture and distribution; nail configuration; color, texture, condition, or presence of nail clubbing
- **Head:** size, shape, trauma, masses, scars, rashes or scaling; facial symmetry; presence of edema or puffiness
- **Eyes:** pupil size, shape, reactivity, conjunctival injection, scleral icterus, fundal papilledema, hemorrhage, lids, extraocular movements, visual fields and acuity
- **Ears:** shape and symmetry, tenderness, discharge, external canal, and tympanic membranes; hearing—Weber should be midline (loudness of sound equal in both ears) and Rinne negative (no conductive or sensorineural hearing loss); should be able to hear whisper at 3 feet
- **Nose:** symmetry, tenderness, discharge, mucosa, turbinate inflammation, frontal or maxillary sinus tenderness; discrimination of odors

- **Mouth and throat:** hygiene, condition of teeth, dentures, appearance of lips, tongue, buccal and oral mucosa, erythema, edema, exudate, tonsillar enlargement, palate, uvula, gag reflex, ulcers
- **Neck:** mobility, masses, range of motion, trachea deviation, thyroid size, carotid bruits
- **Lymphatic:** cervical, intraclavicular, axillary, trochlear, or inguinal adenopathy; size, shape, tenderness, and consistency
- **Breasts:** skin changes, dimpling, symmetry, scars, tenderness, discharge or masses; characteristics of nipples and areolae
- **Heart:** rate, rhythm, murmurs, rubs, gallops, clicks, heaves, or precordial movements
- **Peripheral vascular:** jugular vein distention, bruits, edema, swelling, vein distention, Homans' sign, or tenderness of extremities
- **Lungs:** chest symmetry with respirations, wheezes, crackles, rhonchi, vocal fremitus, whispered pectoriloquy, percussion, and diaphragmatic excursion; breath sounds equal and clear bilaterally
- **Abdomen:** shape, scars, bowel sounds, consistency, tenderness, rebound, masses, guarding, organomegaly, liver span, percussion (tympany, shifting, dullness), costovertebral angle tenderness
- **Extremities:** edema, ulceration, tenderness, varicosities, erythema, tremor, or deformity
- **Genitourinary:** external genitalia, perineum, vaginal mucosa, cervix, inflammation, tenderness, discharge, bleeding, ulcers, nodules, masses, internal vaginal support, bimanual, and rectovaginal; palpation of cervix, uterus, and adnexae
- **Rectal:** sphincter tone, masses, hemorrhoids, rectal wall contour, tenderness, and stool for occult blood
- **Musculoskeletal:** posture, symmetry of muscle mass, muscle atrophy, weakness, appearance of joints, tenderness or crepitus, joint range of motion, instability, redness, swelling, or spine deviation
- **Neurologic:** mental status, orientation, memory, mood, speech clarity and comprehension, cranial nerves II to XII, sensation, strength, deep tendon and superficial reflexes, gait, balance, and coordination with rapid alternating motions.

Pelvic Examination

Many women are intimidated by the gynecologic portion of the physical examination. The nurse in this instance can take an advocacy approach that supports a partnership relationship between the woman and the care provider.

The woman is assisted into the lithotomy position (see Fig. 6-9, *A*) for the pelvic examination. When she is in the lithotomy position, the woman's hips and knees are flexed with the buttocks at the edge of the table, and her feet are supported by heel or knee stirrups.

Some women prefer to keep their shoes or socks on, especially if the stirrups are not padded. Many women express feelings of vulnerability and strangeness when in the lithotomy position. During the procedure the nurse assists the woman with relaxation techniques.

One method of helping the woman relax is to have her place her hands on her chest at about the level of the diaphragm, breathe deeply and slowly (in through her nose and out through her O-shaped mouth), concentrate on the rhythm of breathing, and relax all body muscles with each exhalation (Barkauskas et al., 1998). This breathing technique is particularly helpful for the adolescent or the woman whose introitus may be especially tight or for whom the experience may be new or may provoke tension. Some women relax when they are encouraged to become involved with the examination with a mirror placed so that they can view the area being examined. This type of participation helps with health teaching as well. Distraction is another technique that can be used effectively (e.g., placement of interesting pictures on the ceiling over the head of the table).

Many women find it distressing to attempt to converse in the lithotomy position. Most women appreciate an explanation of the procedure as it unfolds, as well as coaching for the type of sensations they may expect. Generally, however, women prefer not to have to respond to questions until they are again upright and at eye level with the examiner. Questioning during the procedure, especially if they cannot see their questioner's eyes, may make women tense.

External inspection. The examiner sits at the foot of the table for the inspection of the external genitals and for the speculum examination. To facilitate open communication and to help the woman relax, the woman's head is raised on a pillow and the drape is arranged so that eye-to-eye contact can be maintained. In good lighting, external genitals are inspected for sexual maturity, clitoris, labia, and perineum. After childbirth or other trauma there may be healed scars.

External palpation. The examiner proceeds with the examination using palpation and inspection. The examiner wears gloves for this portion of the assessment. Before touching the woman, the examiner explains what is going to be done and what the woman should expect to feel (e.g., pressure). The examiner may touch the woman in a less sensitive area such as the inner thigh to alert her that the genital examination is beginning. This gesture may put the woman more at ease. The labia are spread apart to expose the structures in the vestibule: urinary meatus, Skene's glands, vaginal orifice, and Bartholin's glands (Fig. 6-11). To assess the Skene's glands, the examiner inserts one finger into the vagina and "milks" the area of the urethra. Any exudate from the urethra or the Skene's glands is cultured. Masses and erythema of either structure are assessed further. Ordinarily the openings to the Skene's glands are not visible; prominent openings may be seen if the glands are infected (e.g., with gonorrhea). During the examination, the examiner keeps in mind the data from the review of systems, such as history of burning on urination.

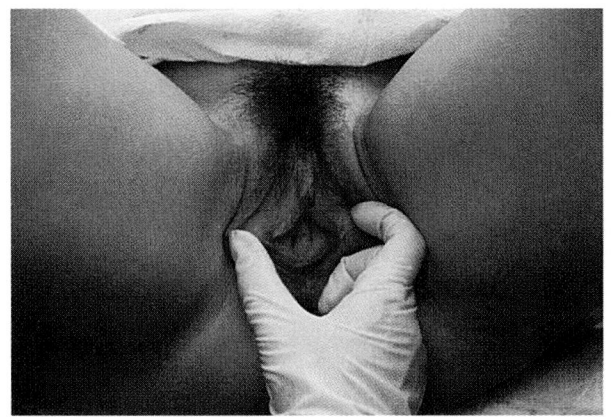

Fig. 6-11 External examination. Separation of the labia. *(From Edge, V., & Miller, M. [1994]. Women's health care. St. Louis: Mosby.)*

Assisting with Pelvic Examination (Fig. 6-12)

Wash hands. Assemble equipment (Fig. 6-13).

Ask woman to empty her bladder before the examination (obtain clean-catch urine specimen as needed).

Assist with relaxation techniques. Have the woman place her hands on her chest at about the level of the diaphragm, breathe deeply and slowly (in through her nose and out through her O-shaped mouth), concentrate on the rhythm of breathing, and relax all body muscles with each exhalation (Barkauskas et al., 1998).

Encourage the woman to become involved with the examination if she shows interest. For example, a mirror can be placed so that she can see the area being examined.

Assess for and treat signs of problems such as supine hypotension.

Warm the speculum in warm water if a prewarmed one is not available.

Instruct the woman to bear down when the speculum is being inserted.

Apply gloves and assist the examiner with collection of specimens for cytologic examination, such as a Pap test. After handling specimens, remove gloves and wash hands.

Lubricate the examiner's fingers with water or water-soluble lubricant before bimanual examination.

Assist the woman at completion of the examination to a sitting position.

Provide tissues to wipe lubricant from perineum.

Provide privacy for the woman while she is dressing.

The vaginal orifice is examined. Hymenal tags are normal findings. With one finger still in the vagina, the examiner repositions the index finger near the posterior part of the orifice. With the thumb outside the posterior part of the labia majora, the examiner compresses the area of Bartholin's glands located at the 8 o'clock and 4 o'clock positions and looks for swelling, discharge, and pain.

The support of the anterior and posterior vaginal wall is assessed. The examiner spreads the labia with the index and middle finger and asks the woman to strain down. Any bulge from the anterior wall (urethrocele or cystocele) or posterior wall (rectocele) is noted and compared with the history, such as difficulty to start the stream of urine or constipation.

The perineum (area between the vagina and anus) is assessed for scars from old lacerations or episiotomies, thinning, fistulas, masses, lesions, and inflammation. The anus is assessed for hemorrhoids, hemorrhoidal tags, and integrity of the anal sphincter. The anal area is also assessed for lesions, masses, abscesses, and tumors. If there is a history of sexually transmitted disease, the examiner may want to obtain a culture specimen from the anal canal at this time. Throughout the genital examination, the examiner notes the odor. Odor may indicate infection or poor hygiene.

Vulvar self-examination. The pelvic examination provides a good opportunity for the practitioner to emphasize the need for regular **vulvar self-examination (VSE)** and to teach this procedure. Because there has been a dramatic increase in cancerous and precancerous conditions of the vulva in recent years, a VSE should be performed as an integral part of preventive health care by all women who are sexually active or 18 years of age or older, monthly between menses or more frequently if there are symptoms or a history of serious vulvar disease. Most lesions, including malignancy, condyloma acuminatum (wartlike growth), and Bartholin's cysts, can be seen or palpated and are easily treated if diagnosed early.

The examination can be performed by the practitioner and woman together, using a mirror. A simple diagram of the anatomy of the vulva can be given to the woman, with instructions to perform the examination herself that evening to reinforce what she has learned. She does the examination in a sitting position with adequate lighting, holding a mirror in one hand and using the other hand to expose the tissues surrounding the vaginal introitus. She then systematically examines the mons pubis, clitoris, urethra, labia majora, perineum, and perianal area and palpates the vulva, noting any changes in appearance or abnormalities, such as ulcers, lumps, warts, and changes in pigmentation.

Internal examination. A vaginal speculum consists of two blades and a handle. Speculums come in a variety of types and styles. A vaginal speculum is used to view the vaginal vault and cervix (see Procedure box). The speculum is gently placed into the vagina and inserted to the back of the vaginal vault. The blades are opened to reveal the cervix and are locked into the open position. The

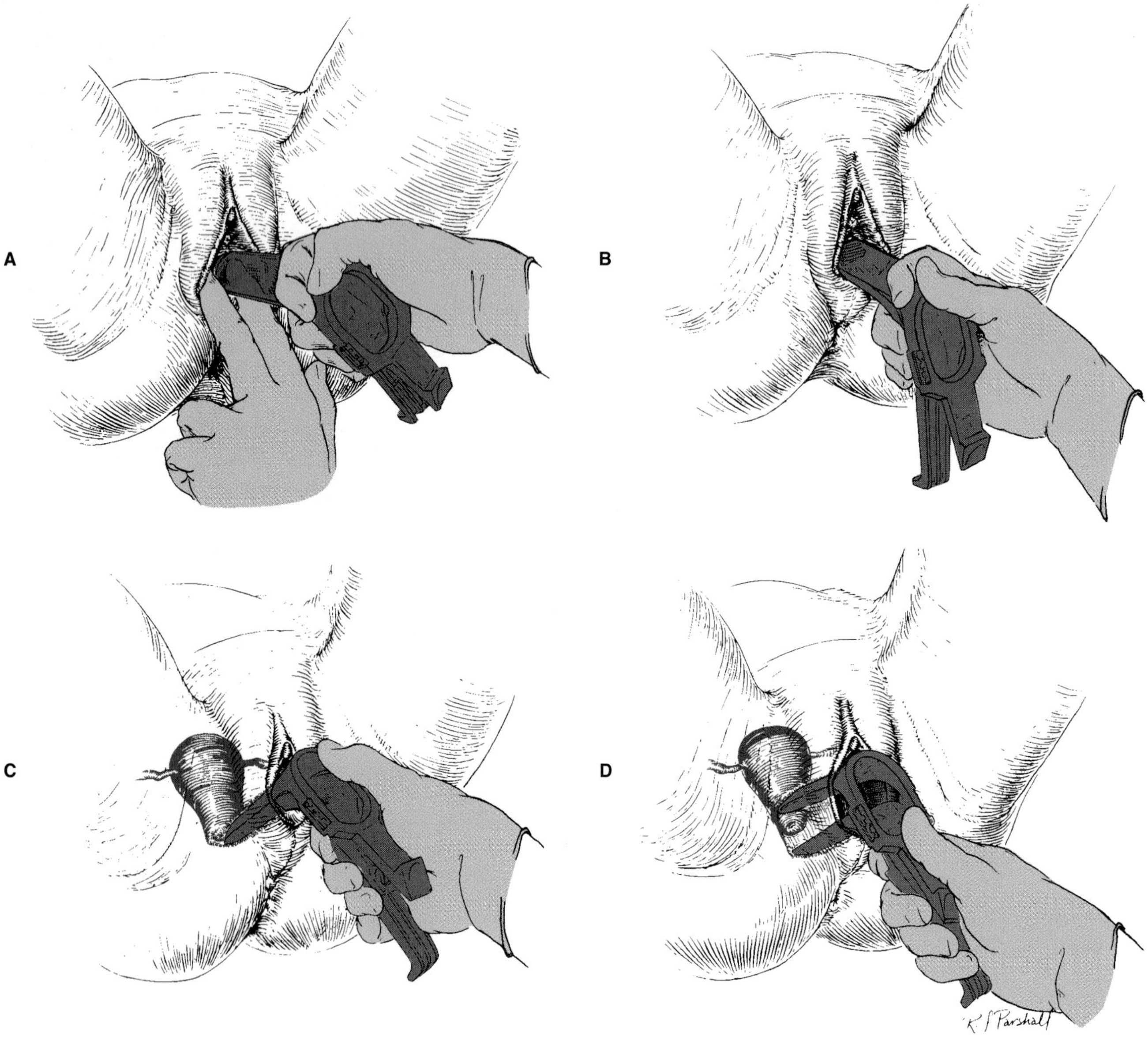

Fig. 6-12 Insertion of speculum for vaginal examination. **A,** Opening of the introitus. **B,** Oblique insertion of the speculum. **C,** Final insertion of the speculum. **D,** Opening of the speculum blades. *(From Barkauskas, V., Stoltenberg-Allen, K., Baumann, L., & Darling-Fisher, C. [1998]. Health and physical assessment [2nd ed.]. St. Louis: Mosby.)*

cervix is inspected for position and appearance of the os: color, lesions, bleeding, and discharge (Fig. 6-12). Cervical findings that are not within normal limits include ulcerations, masses, inflammation, and excessive protrusion into the vaginal vault. Anomalies, such as a cockscomb (a protrusion over the cervix that looks like a rooster's comb), a hooded or collared cervix (seen in DES daughters), or polyps, are noted.

Collection of specimens. The collection of specimens for cytologic examination is an important part of the gynecologic examination. Infection can be diagnosed through examination of specimens collected during the pelvic examination. These infections include *Candida albicans, Trichomonas vaginalis,* bacterial vaginosis, β-hemolytic strep-

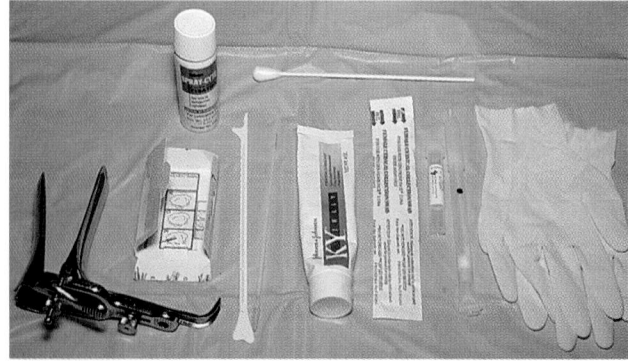

Fig. 6-13 Equipment used for pelvic examination. *(Courtesy Michael S. Clement, MD, Mesa, AZ.)*

Pap Smear

PROCEDURE

Papanicolaou Smear

In preparation, make sure the woman has not douched, used vaginal medications, or had sexual intercourse for at least 24 hours before the procedure. Reschedule the test if the woman is menstruating.

The woman is assisted into a lithotomy position. A speculum is inserted into the vagina.

Explain to the woman the purpose of the test and what sensations she will feel as the specimen is obtained (e.g., pressure but not pain).

The cytologic specimen is obtained before any digital examination of the vagina is made or endocervical bacteriologic specimens are taken with cotton swabbing of the cervix.

The Pap smear is obtained by using an endocervical sampling device (Cytobrush, Cervex-Brush, papette, or broom) (see Fig. 6-14). If the two-sample method of obtaining cells is used, the cytobrush is inserted into the canal and rotated 90 to 180 degrees, followed by a gentle smear of the entire transformation zone using a spatula. Broom devices are inserted and rotated 360 degrees five times. They obtain endocervical and ectocervical samples at the same time. If the client has had a hysterectomy, the vaginal cuff is sampled. Areas that appear abnormal on visualization will require colposcopy and biopsy. If using a one-slide technique, the spatula sample is smeared first. This is followed by applying the cytobrush sample (rolling the brush in the opposite direction from which it was obtained), which is less subject to drying artifact, and then the slide is sprayed with preservative within 5 seconds.

The ThinPrep Pap Test is an improved method of preserving cells that reduces blood, mucus, and inflammation. The Pap specimen is obtained in the manner described above, and the collection device (brush, spatula, or broom) is simply rinsed in a vial of preserving solution that is provided by the lab. The sealed vial with solution is sent off to the appropriate lab. A special processing device filters the contents, and a thin layer of cervical cells is deposited on a slide, which is then examined microscopically. Initial reports state that specimen adequacy is improved by 50% and detection of low-grade and more severe lesions is improved by 65%.

Label the slides with the woman's name and site. Include on the form to accompany the slides the woman's name, age, LMP, parity, and chief complaint or reason for taking the cytologic specimens.

Send specimens to the pathology laboratory promptly for staining, evaluation, and a written report, with special reference to abnormal elements, including cancer cells.

Advise the woman that repeat smears may be necessary if the specimen is not adequate.

Instruct the woman concerning routine checkups for cervical and vaginal cancer. The American Cancer Society advises that women over 18 years of age and those under 18 who are sexually active have the test yearly. After three or more consecutive normal menses, less frequent screening may be performed based on risk.

Record the examination date on the woman's record.

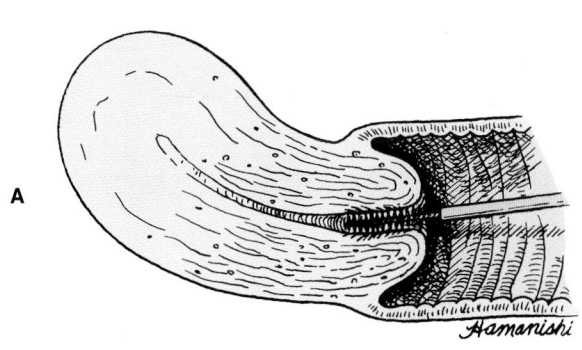
A

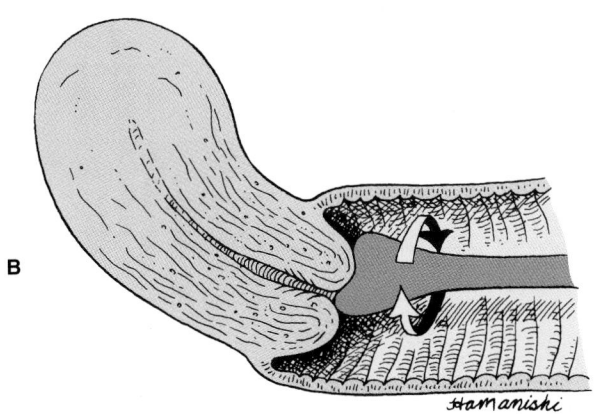
B

Fig. 6-14 Pap smear. **A,** Collecting cells from the endocervix using a cytobrush. **B,** Obtaining cells from the transformation zone using a wooden spatula. *(From Mishell, D., Stenchever, M., Droegemueller, W., & Herbst, A. [1997]. Comprehensive gynecology [3rd ed.]. St. Louis: Mosby.)*

tococci, *Neisseria gonorrhoeae*, *Chlamydia trachomatis*, and herpes simplex virus. Once the diagnoses have been made, treatment can be instituted.

Papanicolaou (Pap) smear. Carcinogenic conditions, potential or actual, can be determined by examination of

cells from the cervix collected during the pelvic examination (see Procedure box) (Fig. 6-14). This is termed a **Papanicolaou (Pap) smear.**

Vaginal examination. After the specimens are obtained, the vagina is viewed when the speculum is rotated.

The speculum blades are unlocked and partially closed. As the speculum is withdrawn, it is rotated and the vaginal walls are inspected for color, lesions, rugae, fistulas, and bulging.

Bimanual palpation. The examiner stands for this part of the examination. A small amount of lubricant is placed on the first and second fingers of the gloved hand for the internal examination. To avoid tissue trauma and contamination, the thumb is abducted and the ring and little fingers are flexed into the palm (Fig. 6-15).

The vagina is palpated for distensibility, lesions, and tenderness. The cervix is examined for position, shape, consistency, motility, and lesions. The fornix around the cervix is palpated.

The other hand is placed on the abdomen halfway between the umbilicus and symphysis pubis and exerts pressure downward toward the pelvic hand. Upward pressure from the pelvic hand traps reproductive structures for assessment by palpation. The uterus is assessed for position, size, shape, consistency, regularity, motility, masses, and tenderness.

With the abdominal hand moving to the right lower quadrant and the fingers of the pelvic hand in the right lateral fornix, the adnexa is assessed for position, size, tenderness, and masses. The examination is repeated on the woman's left side.

Just before the intravaginal fingers are withdrawn, the woman is asked to tighten her vagina around the fingers as much as she can. If the muscle response is weak, the woman is assessed for her knowledge about Kegel exercises.

Rectovaginal palpation. To prevent contamination of the rectum from organisms in the vagina (such as *Neisseria gonorrhoeae*), it is necessary to change gloves, add

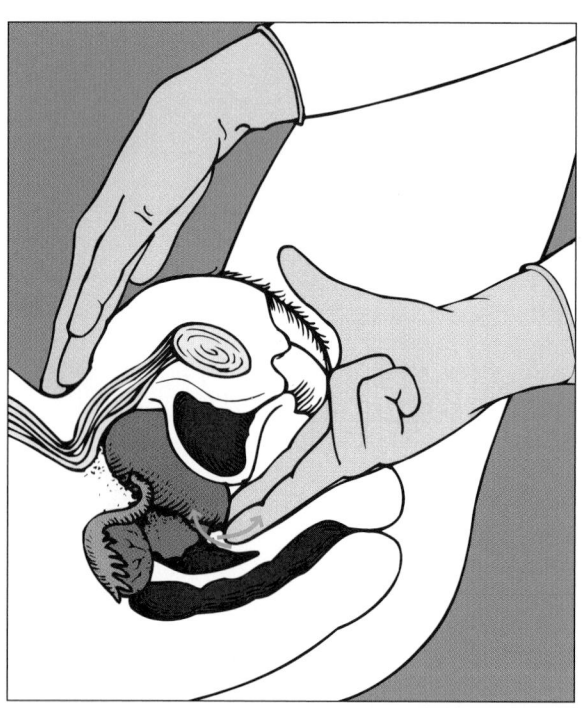

Fig. 6-15   Bimanual palpation of the uterus.

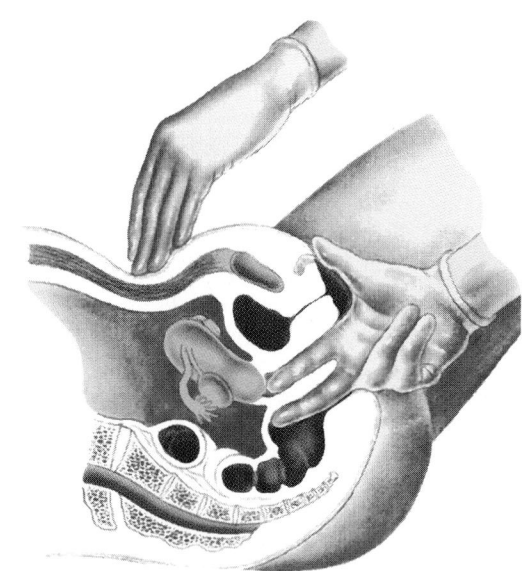

Fig. 6-16   Rectovaginal examination. *(From Seidel, H., Ball, J., Dains, J., & Benedict, G. [1999]. Mosby's guide to physical examination [4th ed.]. St. Louis: Mosby.)*

TABLE 6-3 Pap Smear Screening After Hysterectomy

CLIENT GROUP	SUGGESTED FREQUENCY
After hysterectomy (for benign disease)	Every 2 to 3 years if low cancer risk
After hysterectomy (reason unknown, premalignant or malignant disease)	Annually
Age 65 and older	Screening may be discontinued if three consecutive smears have been normal, if the woman is at low risk for human papillomavirus, and if the woman does not have a partner with human papillomavirus

Source: Johnson, C. (1996). Papanicolaou smear. In C. Johnson, B. Johnson, J. Murray, & B. Apgar (Eds.). *Women's health care handbook.* Philadelphia: Hanley & Belfus.

fresh lubricant, and then reinsert the index finger into the vagina and the middle finger into the rectum (Fig. 6-16). Insertion is facilitated if the woman strains down. The maneuvers of the abdominovaginal examination are repeated. The rectovaginal examination permits assessment of the rectovaginal septum, the posterior surface of the uterus, and the region behind the cervix and the adnexa. The vaginal finger is removed and folded into the palm, leaving the middle finger free to rotate 360 degrees. The rectum is palpated for rectal tenderness and masses.

After the rectal examination, the woman is assisted into a sitting position, given tissues or wipes to cleanse herself, and privacy to dress. The examiner returns after the woman is dressed to discuss findings and the plan of care.

Pelvic Examination During Pregnancy

The pelvic examination is done in the same way as it is during a routine examination on a nonpregnant woman. Pelvic measurements are completed and uterine size is estimated. A Pap smear may be done initially, as well as collection of cytologic specimens to test for infection (gonorrhea, chlamydia, human papillomavirus, herpes simplex virus, group B streptococci). As the pregnancy progresses the nurse will inspect the woman's abdomen, palpate fetal size and position, auscultate fetal heart tones, and measure fundal height at each visit.

While the pregnant woman is in lithotomy position, the nurse must watch for supine hypotension, caused by the weight of the abdomen pressing on the vena cava and aorta, causing a drop in blood pressure. Symptoms of supine hypotension include pallor, dizziness, faintness, breathlessness, tachycardia, nausea, clammy skin, and sweating. The woman should be positioned on her side until symptoms resolve and vital signs stabilize. The vaginal examination can be done with the woman in left lateral position.

Pelvic Examination After Hysterectomy

The pelvic examination is done in a similar manner as it is done on a woman with a uterus, but only a plastic spatula is used for cell sampling during the Pap smear. The Pap smear may be done less frequently at the discretion of the clinician. Because of the epidemic of human papillomavirus, which causes vaginal intraepithelial neoplasia, sampling of the vaginal cuff and vaginal walls after hysterectomy is still recommended. Refer to Table 6-3 for suggested frequency of Pap smear screening after hysterectomy.

Laboratory and Diagnostic Procedures

The following laboratory and diagnostic procedures are ordered at the discretion of the clinician, considering the client and family history: hemoglobin, fasting glucose, total cholesterol, lipid profile, urinalysis, syphilis serology (VDRL or RPR), screening tests for sexually transmitted diseases, Pap smear, mammogram, tuberculosis screening, hearing, visual acuity, electrocardiogram, chest x-ray, pul-

monary function, fecal occult blood, flexible sigmoidoscopy, and bone mineral density (DEXA scan). Tests for human immunodeficiency virus, hepatitis B, and drug screening may be offered with informed consent in high risk populations (see Table 5-1).

KEY POINTS

- Normal feedback regulation of the menstrual cycle depends on an intact hypothalamic-pituitary-gonadal mechanism.
- The female's reproductive tract structures and breasts respond predictably to changing levels of sex steroids across her life span.
- The myometrium of the uterus is uniquely designed to expel the fetus and promote hemostasis after birth.
- Prostaglandins play an important role in reproductive functions by their effect on smooth muscle contractility and modulation of hormones.
- Nurses must be aware of their own feelings and values regarding sexuality before they can competently help clients meet their information needs or refer them for further counseling.
- The desirable consequences of immunity include natural resistance, recovery, and acquired resistance to infectious diseases.
- Vaccination is an effective method of stimulating antibody production and memory.
- Culture, religion, socioeconomic status, personal circumstances, the uniqueness of the individual, and stage of development are among the factors that influence a person's recognition of need for care and responses to the health care system and therapy.
- Profound changes in society and in roles and expectations of women have affected their health needs, and ability to cope with problems.
- Assessment is more comprehensive and learning is best in a safe environment in which the atmosphere is nonjudgmental and sensitive and the interaction is strictly confidential.
- Every woman is entitled to be respected and fully involved in the assessment process to the fullness of her capacity.
- Nurses in all specialties must respond with sensitivity and caring toward women who experience abuse and victimization.
- Well-women's health care includes a complete history, physical examination, and age-appropriate screening.
- Monthly breast self-examination, routine screening mammography, and yearly breast examinations by practitioners are recommended for early detection of breast cancer.

CRITICAL THINKING EXERCISES

1 A young woman who is hearing impaired comes to the clinic for her initial well-woman examination. She is accompanied by her sister, who is skilled in sign language.

   a. What adaptations in the interview, history, and physical examination should be considered?

   b. Are there any barriers at your clinical site that would prevent women with disabilities from receiving care?

   c. What must be changed at your clinical site, and how would you implement these changes?

2 You are assigned to teach breast self-examination (BSE) at a health department clinic for non-English-speaking women from Mexico. The clinic provides you with access to a Hispanic bilingual aide.

   a. Compare the women's perceptions and beliefs about health and BSE with your own.

   b. Analyze how their perceptions may affect their health-seeking behaviors.

   c. How would you incorporate this knowledge into your plan of care?

   d. Using clinic and community resources, draft a sample lesson plan to teach BSE in Spanish.

References

Barkauskas, V., Stoltenberg-Allen, K., Baumann, L., & Darling-Fisher, C. (1998). *Health and physical assessment* (2nd ed.). St. Louis: Mosby.

Edge, V., & Miller, M. (1994). *Women's health care.* St. Louis: Mosby.

Fogel, C., & Woods, N. (1995). *Women's health care. A comprehensive handbook.* Thousand Oaks, CA: Sage.

Johnson, C. (1996). Papanicolaou smear. In C. Johnson, B. Johnson, J. Murray, & B. Apgar (Eds.). *Women's health care handbook.* Philadelphia: Hanley & Belfus.

Lipson, J., Dibble, S., & Minarik, P. (1996). *Culture and nursing care: A pocket guide.* San Francisco: UCSF Nursing Press.

Masters, W. (1992). *Human sexuality* (4th ed.). New York: HarperCollins.

Mishell, D., Stenchever, M., Droegemueller, W., & Herbst, A. (1997). *Comprehensive gynecology* (3rd ed.). St. Louis: Mosby.

Poirier, L. (1997). The importance of screening for domestic violence in all women. *Nurse Pract* 22(5), 105-122.

Potter, P., & Perry, A. (1997). *Fundamentals of nursing: Concepts, process, and practice* (4th ed.). St. Louis: Mosby.

Seidel, H., Ball, J., Dains, J., & Benedict, G. (1999). *Mosby's guide to physical examination* (4th ed.). St. Louis: Mosby.

Seng, J., & Petersen, B. (1995). Incorporating routine screening for history of childhood sexual abuse in well-women and maternity care. *J Nurse Midwifery* 40(1), 26-30.

U.S. Department of Health and Human Services, Public Health Service (1997). *Clinician's handbook of preventive services.* Washington, DC: U.S. Government Printing Office.

Youngkin, E., & Davis, M. (1994). *Women's health. A primary care clinical guide.* Norwalk, CT: Appleton & Lange.

7

Common Reproductive Concerns

Catherine Ingram Fogel

LEARNING OBJECTIVES

- Define the key terms.
- Develop a nursing care plan for the woman with primary dysmenorrhea.
- Outline client teaching about premenstrual syndrome.
- Relate the pathophysiology of endometriosis to associated symptoms.
- Develop an assessment guide for perimenopausal women.
- Develop a nursing care plan for the post-menopausal woman.

- Outline client teaching about menopausal hormone therapy.
- Outline client teaching about prevention of osteoporosis.
- Evaluate the use of alternative therapies for menstrual disorders and menopausal symptoms.
- Identify topics for nursing research related to menstrual disorders and menopause.

KEY TERMS

amenorrhea	hot flush	oligomenorrhea
climacteric	hypogonadotropic amenorrhea	osteoporosis
dysfunctional uterine bleeding	hypomenorrhea	perimenopause
dysmenorrhea	leiomyoma	phytoestrogens
endometriosis	menopause	premenstrual syndrome (PMS)
estrogen replacement therapy	menopausal hormonal therapy	primary dysmenorrhea
hormonal replacement therapy	menorrhagia (hypermenorrhea)	secondary dysmenorrhea
hot flash	metrorrhagia	

 nowledge of the normal parameters of menstruation is essential to the assessment of menstrual cycle experiences and disorders. The menstrual cycle is a result of a complex interplay between the reproductive and endocrine systems. The hypothalamus produces gonadotropin-releasing hormone (GnRH), which stimulates the pituitary gland to produce follicle-stimulating hormone (FSH) and luteinizing hormone (LH). In turn, FSH and LH stimulate the ovaries to produce first estrogen and then progesterone. In response to the hormones, the endometrium, or lining of the uterus, proliferates and then sheds. Chapter 6 provides additional information on the menstrual cycle and endocrine physiology.

Normal menstrual patterns are averages based on observations and reports from large groups of healthy women. When counseling an individual woman, it is important to remember that these values are averages only. As the Federation of Feminist Women's Health Centers (1981) so aptly stated, the 28-day cycle is a medical myth. Although the majority of women do have monthly cycles of approximately 1 month, other healthy and fertile women can have cycles more or less frequently. Although no woman's cycle is exactly the same length every month, the typical month-to-month variation in an individual's cycle is usually plus or minus 2 days. However, greater but still normal variations are noted frequently.

During her reproductive years, a woman may experience more than one physiologic variation in her menstrual cycle. An understanding of the physiologic variations that occur in several age groups is essential knowledge for nurses providing care to women. Menstrual cycle length is most irregular in the 2 years after menarche and the 3 to 5 years before menopause, when anovulatory cycles are most common. Irregular bleeding, both in length of cycle and amount, is the rule, rather than the exception, in early adolescence. It takes approximately 15 months for completion of the first 10 cycles and an average of 20 cycles before ovulation occurs regularly. Cycle lengths of 22 to 40 days are not unusual, and during the first 2 years after menarche, intervals of 3 to 6 months between menses can be normal.

Women typically have menstrual cycles for about 40 years. Once the irregular nature of menses in the first 2 to 3 years following menarche subsides and a cyclic, predictable pattern of monthly bleeding is established, women may worry about any deviation from that pattern, or from what they have been told is normal for all menstruating women. A woman may be concerned about her ability to conceive and bear children or believe that she is not really a woman without monthly evidence. A symptom such as amenorrhea or excess menstrual bleeding can be a source of severe distress and concern for women as they wonder what is wrong with them. Sexual issues often are expressed and must be examined.

Problems may occur at any point in the menstrual cycle. In addition, many factors, including anatomic abnormalities, physiologic imbalances, and lifestyle, can affect the menstrual cycle. Many women seek out nurses as advisors, counselors, and health care providers for information about menstrual cycle experiences, concerns, or disorders. If they are to meet their clients' needs, nurses must have accurate, up-to-date information. This chapter provides information on menstrual cycle experiences, including menarche and menopause, common menstrual disorders, and problems associated with menopause.

COMMON MENSTRUAL DISORDERS

Amenorrhea

Amenorrhea, the absence or cessation of menstrual flow, is a clinical symptom of a variety of disorders. Although the criteria used to determine when a clinical problem of amenorrhea exists are not universal, the following circum-

stances should generally be evaluated: (1) the absence of both menarche and secondary sexual characteristics by age 14; (2) absence of menses by age 16, regardless of presence of normal growth and development (primary amenorrhea); or (3) a 6-month cessation of menses after a period of menstruation (secondary amenorrhea) (Fogel, 1997).

Although amenorrhea is not a disease, it is often the sign of one. Amenorrhea is most commonly a result of pregnancy. It may occur from any defect or interruption in the hypothalamic-pituitary-ovarian-uterine axis. It may also result from anatomic abnormalities, other endocrine disorders such as hypothyroidism or hyperthyroidism, chronic diseases such as type 1 diabetes, medications such as phenytoin (Dilantin), eating disorders, strenuous exercise, emotional stress, and oral contraceptive use.

Assessment of amenorrhea begins with a thorough history and physical examination. An important initial step, often overlooked, is to be sure that the woman is not pregnant. Specific components of the assessment process depend on a client's age—adolescent, young adult, or perimenopausal—and whether she has previously menstruated.

Hypogonadotropic Amenorrhea

Hypogonadotropic amenorrhea reflects a problem in the central hypothalamic-pituitary axis. In rare instances, a pituitary lesion or genetic inability to produce FSH and LH is at fault. Once pregnancy has been ruled out, a diagnostic workup including thyroid-stimulating hormone (TSH) and prolactin levels, x-rays or computed tomography scan of the sella tursica, and a progestational challenge is done to determine the cause of amenorrhea (Kiningham, Apgar, & Schwenk, 1996).

Hypogonadotropic amenorrhea often results from hypothalamic suppression as a result of two principal influences: stress (in the home, school, or workplace) or a body fat–to–lean ratio that is inappropriate for an individual woman, especially during a normal growth period. Research on the interaction between nervous system or neurotransmitter functions and hormonal regulation throughout the body has demonstrated a biologic basis for the relation of stress to physiologic processes. Women who are more than 20% underweight for height or who have experienced rapid weight loss may report amenorrhea, as may women with eating disorders such as anorexia nervosa or bulimia. Amenorrhea is one of the classic signs of anorexia nervosa, and the interrelatedness of disordered eating, amenorrhea, and premature osteoporosis has been described as the female athlete triad (Golden & Shenker, 1994; West, 1998). A loss of calcium from the bone, comparable to that seen in postmenopausal women, may occur with this type of amenorrhea.

Exercise-associated amenorrhea can occur in women undergoing vigorous physical and athletic training (Castiglia, 1996) and is thought to be associated with many factors, including body composition (height, weight, and percentage of body fat); type, intensity, and frequency of exercise; nutritional status; and presence of emotional or physical stressors (McGee, 1997). Women who participate in sports emphasizing low body weight are at greatest risk, including the following (West, 1998):

- Sports in which performance is subjectively scored (e.g., dance, gymnastics)
- Endurance sports favoring participants with low body weight (e.g., distance running, cycling)
- Sports in which body contour–revealing clothing is worn for competition (e.g., swimming, diving, volleyball)
- Sports using weight categories for participation (e.g., rowing, martial arts)
- Sports in which prepubertal body shape favors success (e.g., gymnastics, figure skating).

Management

When amenorrhea is due to hypothalamic disturbances, the nurse is an ideal health professional to assist women because many of the causes are potentially reversible (e.g., stress, weight loss for nonorganic reasons). Counseling and education are primary interventions and appropriate nursing roles. When a stressor known to predispose a client to hypothalamic amenorrhea is identified, initial management involves addressing the stressor. Together the woman and nurse plan how the woman can decrease or discontinue medications known to affect menstruation, correct weight loss, deal more effectively with psychologic stress, and eliminate substance abuse.

The nurse works with the woman to help her identify, cope with, and possibly resolve sources of stress in her life. Deep-breathing exercises and relaxation techniques are simple yet effective stress-reduction measures. Referral for biofeedback or massage therapy also may be useful. In some instances, referrals for psychotherapy may be indicated.

If a woman's exercise program is thought to contribute to her amenorrhea, several options exist for management. She may decide to decrease the intensity or duration of her training if possible or to gain 2% to 3% in body weight. Coming to accept this alternative may be difficult for one who is committed to a strenuous exercise regimen, and the nurse and client may have several sessions before the woman elects to try exercise reduction. Many young female athletes may not understand the consequences of low bone density or osteoporosis; nurses can point out the connection between low bone density and stress fractures. The nurse and woman also should investigate other factors that may be contributing to the amenorrhea and develop plans for altering lifestyle and decreasing stress.

If amenorrhea continues after a woman has decreased her exercise level or gained weight and altered her lifestyle, hormonal therapy may be indicated to prevent additional problems. Because estrogen therapy in postmenopausal women has been shown to protect from bone loss that normally occurs, estrogen therapy also is used in exercise-associated amenorrhea (Castiglia, 1996). Oral contraceptive pills (OCPs) and calcium are frequently used to treat extremely low levels of estrogen seen in exercise-associated amenorrhea to prevent osteoporosis. A daily calcium intake of 1200 to 1500 mg per day, accomplished by drinking 3 glasses of skim milk or taking a calcium supplement, is recommended for women experiencing amenorrhea associated with the female athletic triad (West, 1998). OCPs have the additional advantage of providing pregnancy protection in sexually active women. Furthermore, the few side effects of OCPs often yield higher compliance rates than other forms of hormonal supplementation.

Dysmenorrhea

Dysmenorrhea, painful menstruation, is one of the most common gynecologic problems in women of all ages. Most adolescents experience dysmenorrhea in the first 3 years after menarche. Dysmenorrhea improves in most women after a full-term pregnancy (Speroff, Glass, & Kase, 1999). Between 50% and 80% of women report some level of discomfort associated with menses, and 10% to 18% report severe dysmenorrhea (Fankenauser, 1996; Fogel, 1995); however, the amount of disruption in women's lives is difficult to determine. It has been estimated that up to 10% of women who experience dysmenorrhea have severe enough pain to interfere with their functioning for 1 to 3 days a month (Fankenauser, 1996). Menstrual problems, including dysmenorrhea, are more common in women who smoke (Parazzini et al., 1994). Traditionally dysmenorrhea is differentiated as primary or secondary. Symptoms usually begin with menstruation, although some women experience discomfort several hours before onset of flow. The range and severity of symptoms are different from woman to woman and from cycle to cycle in the same woman. Symptoms of dysmenorrhea may last several hours or several days.

Pain is usually located in the suprapubic area or lower abdomen. Women describe the pain as either sharp, cramping, or gripping or as a steady dull ache; pain may radiate to the lower back or upper thighs.

Primary Dysmenorrhea

Primary dysmenorrhea, a condition associated with ovulatory cycles, is due to myometrium contractions induced by prostaglandins in the second half of the menstrual cycle. During the luteal phase and subsequent menstrual flow, prostaglandin $F_{2\alpha}$ ($PGF_{2\alpha}$) is secreted. The uterine muscle of both normal and dysmenorrheic women is sensitive to prostaglandins; however, the amount of prostaglandin produced is the major differentiating factor (Speroff, Glass, & Kase, 1999). Excessive release of $PGF_{2\alpha}$ increases the amplitude and frequency of uterine contractions and causes vasospasm of the uterine arterioles, resulting in ischemia and cyclic lower abdominal cramps. Systemic responses to $PGF_{2\alpha}$ include backache, weakness, sweating, gastrointestinal symptoms (anorexia, nausea, vomiting, and diarrhea), and central nervous system symptoms (dizziness, syncope, headache, and poor concentration). Pain begins at the onset of menstrual flow and lasts from 8 to 48 hours. Most prostaglandins released during menstruation occur in the first 48 hours, which coincides with the greatest intensity of symptoms (Charlton & White, 1996).

Although primary dysmenorrhea is not a normal condition, it is not caused by underlying pathology; rather it is the occurrence of a physiologic alteration in some women. Primary dysmenorrhea usually appears within 6 to 12 months after menarche when ovulation is established. Anovulatory bleeding, common in the few months or years after menarche, is painless. Because both estrogen and progesterone are necessary for primary dysmenorrhea to occur, it is experienced only with ovulatory cycles. This problem is most commonly experienced by women in their late teens and early twenties; the incidence declines with age. Psychogenic factors may influence symptoms, but symptoms are definitely related to ovulation and do not occur when ovulation is suppressed.

Management. Management of primary dysmenorrhea depends on the severity of the problem and an individual women's response to various treatments. Important components of nursing care are information and support. Because menstruation is so closely linked to reproduction and sexuality, menstrual problems such as dysmenorrhea can have a negative influence on sexuality and self-worth. Nurses can do a lot to correct myths and misinformation about menstruation and dysmenorrhea by providing facts about what is normal. Nurses must support their clients' feelings of positive sexuality and self-worth.

Often more than one alternative for alleviating menstrual discomfort and dysmenorrhea can be offered. Women can then try options and decide which ones work best for them. Heat (heating pad or hot bath) minimizes cramping by increasing vasodilation and muscle relaxation and minimizing uterine ischemia. Massaging the lower back can reduce pain by relaxing paravertebral muscles and increasing pelvic blood supply. Soft rhythmic rubbing of the abdomen (effleurage) may be useful because it provides distraction and an alternative focal point. Biofeed-back, progressive relaxation, hatha yoga, and meditation also have been used successfully to decrease menstrual discomfort.

Exercise has been found to help in relieving menstrual discomfort through increased vasodilation and subsequent decreased ischemia; release of endogenous opiates, specifically beta-endorphins; suppression of prostaglandins; and shunting of blood flow away from the viscera, resulting in less pelvic congestion. Specific exercises that nurses can suggest to their clients include pelvic rock and heels-over-the-head yoga position.

In addition to maintaining good nutrition at all times, specific dietary changes may be helpful in decreasing some of the systemic symptoms associated with dysmenorrhea. Decreased salt and refined sugar intake 7 to 10 days before expected menses may reduce fluid retention. Natural diuretics, such as asparagus, cranberry juice, peaches, parsley, and watermelon, may help reduce edema and related discomforts. Decreasing red meat intake may also help mini-

mize dysmenorrheal symptoms. Some women with primary dysmenorrhea have reported a decrease in symptoms when they switched from a high-fat to a low-fat diet.

Medications used to treat primary dysmenorrhea include prostaglandin synthesis inhibitors, primarily nonsteroidal antiinflammatory drugs (NSAIDs) (Apgar, 1997) (Table 7-1). NSAIDS are effective if begun 2 to 3 days before menses or with the sign of first bleeding; this regimen decreases the possibility of a woman taking these drugs early in pregnancy (Speroff, Glass, & Kase, 1999). All NSAIDs have potential gastrointestinal side effects, including nausea, vomiting, and indigestion. All women taking NSAIDs should be warned to report dark-colored stools because this may be an indication of gastrointestinal bleeding. Women with a history of aspirin sensitivity or allergy should avoid all NSAIDs. Approximately 80% of dysmenorrheic women obtain relief with prostaglandin inhibitors. Often if one NSAID is ineffective, a different one will be effective. If the second drug is unsuccessful after a 6-month trial, OCPs may be used. *oral Contraceptive*

The benefits of OCP use are attributed to decreased prostaglandin synthesis associated with an atrophic decidualized endometrium (Speroff, Glass, & Kase, 1999). No single OCP has been shown to be superior to another for the relief of primary dysmenorrhea. Although generally prescribed on a 21-day cycle of hormones followed by 7 hormone-free days, OCPs can be used continuously in an attempt to produce amenorrhea if women have severe dysmenorrhea during withdrawal bleeding (Lipscomb & Ling, 1997). OCPs are a particularly good choice for therapy because they combine contraception with a positive impact on dysmenorrhea, menstrual flow, and menstrual irregularities. It should be remembered that OCPs have side effects and that women not needing or not wanting them may not wish to use them for dysmenorrhea. OCPs also may be contraindicated for some women. (See Chapter 9 for a complete discussion of oral contraceptives.)

Over-the-counter (OTC) preparations that are indicated for primary dysmenorrhea include the same active ingredients (e.g., ibuprofen, naproxen sodium) as prescription preparations. However, the labeled recommended dose may be subtherapeutic. Preparations containing acetaminophen are even less effective because acetaminophen does not have the antiprostaglandin properties of NSAIDs.

If dysmenorrhea is not relieved by one of the NSAIDs, further investigation into the cause of the symptoms is necessary. Conditions associated with dysmenorrhea include müllerian duct anomalies, endometriosis, and pelvic inflammatory disease.

Secondary Dysmenorrhea

Secondary dysmenorrhea is acquired menstrual pain that developed later in life than primary dysmenorrhea, typically after age 25. This condition is associated with pelvic pathology, such as adenomyosis, endometriosis, pelvic inflammatory disease, endometrial polyps, submucous

TABLE 7-1 Medications Used to Treat Dysmenorrhea (NSAIDs)

DRUG	DOSAGE*	SIDE EFFECTS†	COMMENTS	CONTRAINDICATIONS
Aspirin‡	650-975 mg qid	Gastrointestinal irritation; tinnitus with excess dose	Not as potent a prostaglandin synthesis inhibitor as NSAIDs Do not take with NSAIDs	Hemophilia, hemorrhagic states, bleeding ulcers
Fenoprofen (Nalfon)‡	300-600 mg qid to 2400 mg/day	Diarrhea, abdominal distention, nausea and vomiting, dyspepsia, constipation	For mild-to-moderate pain Take with meals Avoid alcohol	See aspirin
Ibuprofen (Motrin, Advil, Nuprin)	400-800 mg qid to 3200 mg/day	Nausea, dyspepsia, rash, pruritus	Most commonly used Take with meals Do not take with aspirin Avoid alcohol Side effects more likely	See aspirin
Mefenamic acid (Ponstel)	500 mg initially, then 250 mg qid	Diarrhea, nausea, abdominal distention	Very potent and effective prostaglandin synthesis inhibitor Antagonizes already formed prostaglandins Increased incidence of adverse GI side effects	See aspirin
Naproxen sodium (Anaprox, Aleve)	275-550 mg bid	Nausea, abdominal distress, dyspepsia, rash, pruritus	See ibuprofen	See aspirin

Adapted from Fogel, C. (1995). Common symptoms. In C. Fogel & N. Woods (Eds.). *Women's health care.* Thousand Oaks, CA: Sage; Facts and Comparisons. (1995). *Loose-leaf drug information service,* St. Louis: Facts and Comparisons.
qid, Four times a day; *tid,* three times a day; *GI,* gastrointestinal; *bid,* two times a day.
*Dosages are current recommendations and should be verified before use. Recommended dosage for over-the-counter preparations are generally less than recommendations for therapeutic dosage.
†Risk with all NSAIDs is gastrointestinal ulceration, possible bleeding, and prolonged bleeding time. Incidence of side effects is dose related. Reported incidence 3% to 9%.
‡Unlabeled indications for use in treating dysmenorrhea.

or interstitial myomas (fibroids), or use of an intrauterine device (IUD). Women with secondary dysmenorrhea often have other symptoms that may suggest an underlying cause. For example, heavy menstrual flow with dysmenorrhea suggests a diagnosis of leiomyomata, adenomyosis, or endometrial polyps. Pain often begins a few days before menses, but it can be present at ovulation and continue through the first days of menses or start after menstrual flow has begun. In contrast to primary dysmenorrhea, the pain of secondary dysmenorrhea is often characterized by dull, lower abdominal aching radiating to the back or thighs. Often women experience feelings of bloating or pelvic fullness. In addition to a physical examination with a careful pelvic examination, diagnosis may be assisted by ultrasound, dilation and curettage, endometrial biopsy, or laparoscopy. Treatment is directed toward removal of the underlying pathology. Many of the measures described for pain relief of primary dysmenorrhea are also helpful for women with secondary dysmenorrhea.

Premenstrual Syndrome

Approximately 40% of women report problems related to their menstrual cycle, and about 2% to 10% report a degree of impact on work or lifestyle (Speroff, Glass, & Kase, 1999). All age groups are affected, with women in their twenties and thirties most frequently reporting symptoms. These experiences have been categorized as **premenstrual syndrome (PMS).** There is much controversy regarding PMS. The existence, diagnosis, and etiology of PMS are hotly and widely debated. Readers are encouraged to explore current feminist, medical, and social science literature for more information on these topics.

PMS is an appearance of one or more of a large number (more than 100) of physical and psychologic symptoms beginning in the luteal phase of the menstrual cycle, occurring to such a degree that lifestyle or work is affected, and followed by a symptom-free period. Symptoms include fluid retention (abdominal bloating, pelvic fullness, edema of the lower extremities, breast tenderness, and

BOX 7-1 | **Possible Causes of Premenstrual Syndrome**

Low progesterone levels
High estrogen levels
Falling estrogen levels
Changes in estrogen-progesterone levels
Increased aldosterone activity
Increased renin-angiotensin activity
Increased adrenal activity
Endogenous endorphin withdrawal
Subclinical hypoglycemia
Central changes in catecholamines
Response to prostaglandins
Vitamin deficiencies (vitamin B_6)
Excess prolactin secretion

weight gain); behavioral or emotional changes (depression, crying spells, irritability, panic attacks, and impaired ability to concentrate); premenstrual cravings (sweets, salt, increased appetite, and food binges); and headache, fatigue, and backache. In contrast, some women experience a heightened sense of creativity and increased mental and physical energy. A diagnosis of PMS is made only if the following criteria are met:

- Symptoms occur in the luteal phase and resolve within a few days of menses onset.
- Symptom-free period occurs in the follicular phase.
- Symptoms are recurrent.

The cause of PMS is unknown (Box 7-1). It has also been theorized that PMS has a significant psychologic component or may be due to cultural beliefs that lead to the menstrual cycle being associated with a variety of negative reactions. In reality PMS is most likely not a single disorder but rather a collection of different problems. Speroff and associates (1999) suggest that PMS has a basic psychophysiologic origin tied to the menstrual cycle, primarily biologic but with a psychologic overlay. Furthermore, it can be a learned response or a response in vulnerable individuals triggered by normal neuroendocrine and hormonal changes.

Management

There is little agreement on management. A careful, detailed history and daily log of symptoms and mood fluctuations spanning several cycles may give direction to a plan of management. Any changes that assist a woman with PMS to exert control over her life have a positive impact (see Research box). For this reason, lifestyle changes are often effective in the treatment of PMS.

Diet and exercise changes are a useful way to begin and provide symptom relief for some women. Nurses can suggest that clients not smoke and limit their consumption of refined sugar (less than 5 tbsp/day), salt (less than 3 g/day),

 RESEARCH

Positively Reframing Perceptions of the Menstrual Cycle Among Women with Premenstrual Syndrome

Despite more than 60 years of research, investigators have failed to agree on the cause, definition, significance, or management of the cyclic recurrence of a variety of somatic and affective changes manifested during the perimenstrual period. Popularly called *premenstrual syndrome* or *PMS*, symptoms associated with the perimenstrual period have been blamed for a variety of negative behaviors varying from eating disorders to suicide. Although positive changes have been known to exist, researchers have primarily focused on negative changes. This study sought to positively reframe perceptions of menstrual cycle experiences to diminish reports of negative perimenstrual symptoms among women with PMS.

The intervention used in this study was a health promotion program that provided social support and a psychoeducational intervention with a positive reframing psychotherapeutic maneuver. The goal of this intervention was to diminish perimenstrual impairment among women with PMS across four menstrual cycles. Results indicated that negative perimenstrual symptom reports decreased for women in the experimental group. In addition, the participants' personal resources increased significantly. It was concluded that participation in a peer support group provides women with information on positive perceptions of the menstrual cycle that can benefit women with PMS.

CLINICAL APPLICATION

Studies such as this one contribute to the growing awareness of diverse experiences and challenge the belief that menstruation is aberrant. Nurses can effectively work with clients to positively reframe the menstrual cycle events and alter the women's experiences throughout their reproductive life cycle.

Source: Morse, G. (1999). Positively reframing perceptions of the menstrual cycle among women with premenstrual syndrome. *J Obstet Gynecol Neonatal Nurs* 28(2), 165-174.

red meat (up to 3 oz/day), alcohol (less than 1 oz/day), and caffeinated beverages. Clients can be encouraged to include whole grains, legumes, seeds, nuts, vegetables, fruits, and vegetable oils in their diet. Use of natural diuretics (see section on dysmenorrhea management earlier in this chapter) may help reduce fluid retention as well. Nutritional supplements may assist in symptom relief. Calcium (1200 mg), magnesium, and vitamin E have been

PLAN ᵒᶠ CARE | Premenstrual Syndrome

NURSING DIAGNOSIS Pain related to cyclic breast changes as evidenced by client report

Expected outcome *Client will report a decrease in the intensity of pain or discomfort following interventions.*

Nursing Interventions/*Rationales*

Assess timing and intensity of pain or discomfort *to validate relationship to cyclic changes.*

Administer hormonal medications or diuretics if prescribed *to minimize breast tenderness.*

Suggest that client wear a supportive bra *to minimize breast tenderness.*

NURSING DIAGNOSIS Situational low self-esteem related to cyclic hormonal changes as evidenced by client verbal report

Expected outcome: *Client will report increased number of feelings of self-worth.*

Nursing Interventions/*Rationales*

Provide therapeutic communication *to validate client feelings of depression and mood swings.*

Encourage client to limit caffeine and eat small, frequent meals *to lessen irritability aggravated by caffeine and hypoglycemia.*

Refer client to support groups *to encourage the sharing of experiences, feelings, and self-help tips.*

NURSING DIAGNOSIS Fluid volume excess related to cyclic hormonal influences as evidenced by weight gain before start of menstrual period

Expected outcome *Client will report no significant changes in body weight before start of menstrual period.*

Nursing Interventions/*Rationales*

Encourage client to limit intake of salt- and sodium-containing foods *to decrease fluid retention.*

Administer diuretics as prescribed *to facilitate fluid excretion.*

---

shown to be moderately effective in relieving symptoms, to have few side effects, and to be safe. However, vitamin B_6, once widely recommended, is not an effective form of PMS treatment (Carter & Verhoef, 1994). Daily supplements of evening primrose oil are thought to be useful in relieving breast symptoms with minimal side effects. Exercise has been recommended widely for relief of PMS symptoms. Women who exercise regularly seem to have less premenstrual anxiety than nonathletic women. It is thought that aerobic exercise increases beta-endorphin levels to offset symptoms of depression and elevate mood. Clients should exercise for at least 30 minutes, four times per week. A monthly program that varies in intensity and type of exercise according to PMS symptoms is best.

Counseling, in the form of support groups or individual or couple counseling, may be helpful. Stress-reduction techniques may also assist with symptoms management (Baker, 1998).

If these strategies do not provide significant symptom relief in 1 to 2 months, medication is often begun. Many medications have been used in treatment of PMS. At present no single medication alleviates all PMS symptoms. Medications often used in the treatment of PMS include diuretics, prostaglandin inhibitors (NSAIDs), progesterone, and OCPs. Selective serotonin reuptake inhibitors (SSRIs) (e.g., fluoxetine [Prozac] and clomipramine [Anafranil]) are often used for PMS with a resultant decrease in emotional symptoms, especially depression (Baker, 1998; Chandraiah, 1996). Melfenamic acid (250 mg daily during the luteal phase of the menstrual cycle) may relieve or resolve many symptoms—specifically fatigue, headaches, general aches and pains, and mood swings (Chuong, Pearsall-Otey, & Rosenfeld, 1995). Bromocriptine (5 mg daily at night from days 10 to 26 of the cycle) helps reduce breast tenderness and swelling.

Endometriosis

Endometriosis is characterized by the presence and growth of endometrial tissue outside of the uterus. The tissue may be implanted on the ovaries, cul-de-sac, uterine ligaments, rectovaginal septum, sigmoid colon, pelvic peritoneum, cervix, and inguinal area (Fig. 7-1). Endometrial lesions have been found in the vagina and surgical scars, as well as on the vulva, perineum, and bladder and sites far from the pelvic area such as the thoracic cavity, gallbladder, and heart. A chocolate cyst is a cystic area of endometriosis in the ovary. The dark coloring of the contents of the cyst is caused by old blood.

Endometrial tissue contains glands and stoma and responds to cyclic hormonal stimulation in the same way that the uterine endometrium does but often out of phase with it. During the proliferative and secretory phases of the cycle, the endometrial tissue grows. During or immediately after menstruation, the tissue bleeds, resulting in an

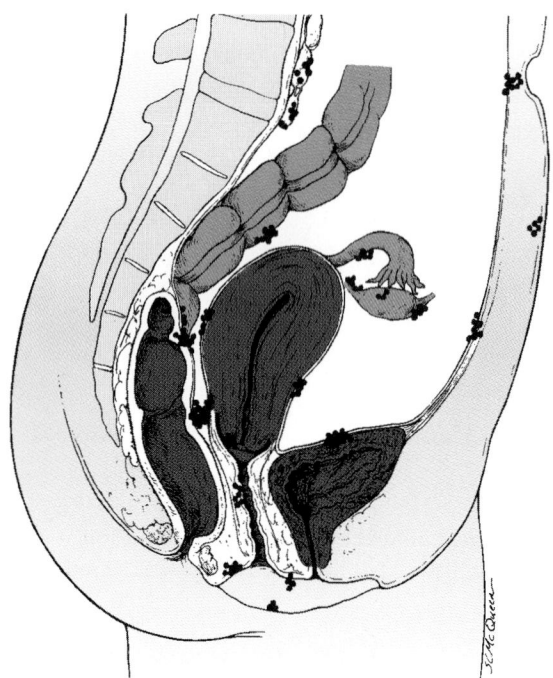

Fig. 7-1 Common sites of endometriosis. *(Source: Mishell, D. et al. [1997]. Comprehensive gynecology. [3rd ed.]. St. Louis: Mosby.)*

inflammatory response with subsequent fibrosis and adhesions to adjacent organs.

The overall incidence of endometriosis is about 10% in reproductive-age women, 25% to 35% in infertile women, and 28% in women with chronic pelvic pain (Corwin, 1997; Speroff, Glass, & Kase, 1999). Endometriosis affects between 1.7 and 5.6 million American women and accounts for about 49,000 hysterectomies each year (Ryan & Taylor, 1997). Although the condition usually develops in the third or fourth decade of life, endometriosis has been found in adolescents with disabling pelvic pain or abnormal vaginal bleeding. Additionally, endometriosis has been reported to occur in about 5% of postmenopausal women on menopausal hormone therapy (Brough & O'Flynn, 1996). At one time endometriosis was believed to be more prevalent in white middle-class women; however, the condition appears equally in Caucasian and African-American women and slightly more in Asian women. Furthermore, endometriosis occurs across all socioeconomic levels (Sangi-Haghpeykar & Poindexter, 1995). There appears to be a familial tendency to develop endometriosis; the incidence of severe endometriosis is higher (61.1%) in family groups than in nonfamily groups (23.8%) (Hadfield et al., 1997). Endometriosis may worsen with repeated cycles, or it may remain asymptomatic and undiagnosed, eventually disappearing after menopause. Endometriosis can occur in women who have been pregnant and may be a cause of secondary infertility (Speroff, Glass, & Kase, 1999).

Several theories to account for the cause of endometriosis have been suggested, yet the etiology and pathology of this condition continue to be poorly understood. One of the most widely accepted, long-debated theories is transtubal migration, or retrograde menstruation. According to this theory, endometrial tissue is regurgitated or mechanically transported from the uterus during menstruation to the uterine (fallopian) tubes and into the peritoneal cavity, where it implants on the ovaries and other organs. Retrograde menstruation has been documented in a number of surgical studies and is estimated to occur in 96% of menstruating women (Corwin, 1997). For most women, endometrial tissue outside the uterus is destroyed before it can implant or seed in the peritoneal cavity or elsewhere. An explanation for why only 10% to 15% of women develop endometriosis may lie in differences in the functioning of an individual's immune system. It may also reflect differences in genetic makeup or environmental challenges (Speroff, Glass, & Kase, 1999).

Symptoms vary among women, from nonexistent to incapacitating. Severity of symptoms can change over time and may be disconnected from the extent of the disease. The major symptoms of endometriosis are dysmenorrhea and deep pelvic dyspareunia (painful intercourse). Women also experience chronic noncyclic pelvic pain, pelvic heaviness, or pain radiating into the thighs. Many women report bowel symptoms such as diarrhea, pain with defecation, and constipation secondary to avoiding defecation because of the pain. Less common symptoms include abnormal bleeding (hypermenorrhea, menorrhagia, or premenstrual staining) and pain during exercise as a result of adhesions.

Impaired fertility may result from adhesions around the uterus that pull the uterus into a fixed, retroverted position. Adhesions around the uterine tubes may block the fimbriated ends or prevent the spontaneous movement that carries the ovum to the uterus or blocks the fimbriated ends.

Management

Treatment is based on the severity of symptoms and the goals of the woman or couple. Women without pain who do not want to become pregnant need no treatment. In women with mild pain who may desire a future pregnancy, treatment may be limited to use of NSAIDs during menstruation (see earlier discussion of these medications).

Suppression of endogenous estrogen production and subsequent endometrial lesion growth is the cornerstone of management of the disease. Two main classes of drugs are currently used to suppress endogenous estrogen levels: gonadotropin-releasing hormone (GnRH) agonists and androgen derivatives. GnRH agonist therapy (leuprolide [Lupron], nafarelin [Synarel]) acts by suppressing pituitary gonadotropin secretion. FSH and LH stimulation to the ovary declines markedly, and ovarian function decreases significantly. A medically induced menopause develops, resulting in anovulation and amenorrhea. Shrinkage of already established endometrial tissue, significant pain relief, and an interruption in further lesion development follow.

The hypoestrogenism results in hot flashes in almost all women. Trabecular bone loss is common, although most loss is reversible within 12 to 18 months after the medication is stopped. Leuprolide (3.75 mg intramuscular injection given once a month) or nafarelin (200 mg administered twice daily by nasal spray) are both effective and well tolerated. Both medications reduce endometrial lesions and pelvic pain associated with endometriosis and have posttreatment pregnancy rates similar to that of danazol therapy (Speroff, Glass, & Kase, 1999). Common side effects of these drugs are those of natural menopause—hot flashes and vaginal dryness. Occasionally women report headaches and muscle aches. Treatment is usually limited to 6 months to minimize bone loss. Although unlikely, it is possible for a woman to become pregnant on a GnRH agonist. Because the potential teratogenicity of this drug is unclear, women should use a barrier contraceptive during treatment.

Danazol (Danocrine), a mildly androgenic synthetic steroid, suppresses FSH and LH secretion, thus producing anovulation and hypogonadotropinism with resulting decreased secretion of estrogen and progesterone and regression of endometrial tissue. This medication was widely used to treat endometriosis in the 1970s and 1980s. Danazol can produce side effects that can cause a woman to discontinue the drug. Side effects include masculinizing traits in the woman—weight gain, edema, decreased breast size, oily skin, hirsutism, and deepening of the voice—all of which often disappear when treatment is discontinued. Other side effects are amenorrhea, hot flashes, vaginal dryness, insomnia, and decreased libido. Migraine headaches, dizziness, fatigue, and depression are also reported. Danazol treatment has been reported to adversely affect lipids, with a decrease in high-density lipoprotein (HDL) levels and an increase in low-density lipoprotein (LDL) levels. Danazol should never be prescribed when pregnancy is suspected, and contraception should be used with it because ovulation may not be suppressed. Danazol can produce pseudohermaphroditism in female fetuses. The medication is contraindicated in women with liver disease and should be used with caution in women with cardiac and renal disease. Because it is an expensive medication, danazol may not be available to all women. The recommended dosage is 200 to 400 mg per day for 3 to 6 months; the average cost for 1 month of treatment is $210.

Women who have severe pain and can postpone pregnancy may be treated with oral contraceptives that have a low estrogen-to-progestin ratio to shrink endometrial tissue. Often the daily dosage has to be increased to two to three pills to maintain amenorrhea. Side effects such as nausea, edema, and breakthrough bleeding often lead to women discontinuing this therapy. When therapy is stopped, clients often experience high rates of recurrence of pain and other symptoms. Most recently, mifepristone (RU-486) has been used to treat endometriosis successfully (Kettel et al., 1998).

Surgical intervention is often needed for severe, acute, or incapacitating symptoms. Decisions regarding the extent and type of surgery are influenced by a woman's age, desire for children, and location of the disease. For women who do not want to preserve their ability to have children, the only definite cure is total abdominal hysterectomy with bilateral salpingo-oophorectomy (TAH with BSO). In women who are in their childbearing years and want children and in whom the disease does not prevent it, reproductive capacity should be retained through careful removal by surgery or laser therapy of all endometrial tissue possible with retention of ovarian function (Garner, 1995).

Regardless of the type of treatment, short of TAH with BSO, endometriosis reoccurs in approximately 40% of women. Thus for many women endometriosis is a chronic disease with conditions such as chronic pain or infertility. Counseling and education are critical components of nursing care for women with endometriosis. Women need an honest discussion of treatment options, with potential risks and benefits of each option reviewed. Because pelvic pain is a subjective, personal experience that can be frightening, support is important. Sexual dysfunction resulting from painful intercourse (dyspareunia) is common and may necessitate referral for counseling if the nurse does not have the necessary skills. Support groups for women with endometriosis may be found in some locations; Resolve, an organization for infertile couples, may also be helpful (see Appendix D). The nursing care discussed in the section on dysmenorrhea is appropriate for managing chronic pelvic pain and dysmenorrhea experienced by the woman with endometriosis.

Alterations in Cyclic Bleeding

Women often experience changes in amount, duration, interval, or regularity of menstrual cycle bleeding. Often women worry about menstruation that is short, that is small in amount, or that occurs too frequently.

Oligomenorrhea/Hypomenorrhea

The term **oligomenorrhea** often is used to describe decreased menstruation, either in amount, time, or both. However, oligomenorrhea more correctly refers to infrequent menstrual periods characterized by intervals of 40 to 45 days or longer and **hypomenorrhea** to scanty bleeding at normal intervals. The causes of oligomenorrhea are often abnormalities of hypothalamic, pituitary, or ovarian function. Oligomenorrhea also can be physiologic, or part of a woman's normal pattern for the first few years after menarche or for several years before menopause.

Treatment is aimed at reversing the underlying cause, if possible. Hormonal therapy using progestins, with or without estrogens, may also be used to prevent complications of unopposed estrogen production (endometrial hyperplasia or carcinoma) or of absent estrogen (vaginal dryness, hot flashes or flushes, osteoporosis).

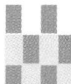

PLAN ᵒᶠ CARE   Endometriosis

NURSING DIAGNOSIS Pain related to menstruation secondary to endometriosis

Expected Outcome *Client will verbalize a decrease in intensity and frequency of pain during each menstrual cycle.*

Nursing Interventions/*Rationales*

Assess location, type, and duration of pain and history of discomfort *to determine severity of dysmenorrhea.*

Administer analgesics *to assist with pain relief.*

Administer hormonal-altering medications if ordered *to suppress ovulation.*

Provide nonpharmacologic methods such as heat *to increase blood flow to the pelvic region.*

NURSING DIAGNOSIS Knowledge deficit related to unfamiliarity with treatment as evidenced by client statements

Expected outcome *Client will verbalize correct understanding of the use of self-care methods and prescribed therapies.*

Nursing Interventions/*Rationales*

Assess client's current understanding of the disorder and related therapies *to validate the accuracy of knowledge base.*

Give information to client regarding the disorder and treatment regimen *to empower the client to become a partner in her own care.*

NURSING DIAGNOSIS Situational low self-esteem related to infertility as evidenced by client's statements of decreased self-worth

Expected outcome *Client will verbalize positive feelings of self-worth.*

Nursing Interventions/*Rationales*

Provide therapeutic communication *to validate feelings and provide support.*

Refer to support group *to enhance feelings of self-worth through group communication.*

NURSING DIAGNOSIS Anxiety related to possible invasive surgical procedure as evidenced by client's verbal report

Expected outcome *Client will report a decreased number of anxious feelings.*

Nursing Interventions/*Rationales*

Provide opportunity to discuss feelings *to identify source of anxiety.*

Reinforce information provided *to keep expectations realistic and dispel myths or inaccuracies.*

Provide emotional support *to encourage verbalization of feelings.*

Women experiencing menstruation characterized by prolonged intervals between cycles need education and counseling. The cause of the condition and the rationale for a specific treatment should be discussed, as should advantages and disadvantages of hormonal therapy. If a woman chooses medical intervention, she should be provided with written instructions, taught how to take the medications, and made aware of side effects of any medications. Teaching and counseling should emphasize the importance of the woman keeping careful records of her vaginal bleeding.

One of the most common causes of scanty menstrual flow is OCPs. If a woman is considering OCPs for contraception, it is important that the nurse explain in advance that the use of OCPs can decrease menstrual flow by as much as two thirds. This effect is caused by the continuous action of the progestin component, which produces a decidualized endometrium with atrophic glands.

Hypomenorrhea also may be caused by structural abnormalities of the endometrium or uterus that result in partial destruction of the endometrium. These conditions include Asherman syndrome, in which adhesions resulting from curettage or infection obliterate the endometrial cavity, and congenital partial obstruction of the vagina.

Metrorrhagia

Metrorrhagia, or intermenstrual bleeding, refers to any episode of bleeding, whether spotting, menses, or hemorrhage, that occurs at a time other than the normal menses. *Mittlestaining*, a small amount of bleeding or spotting that occurs at the time of ovulation (14 days before onset of next menses), is considered normal. The cause of mittlestaining is not known; however, it is a common occurrence that can be documented by its repetition in the menstrual cycle.

Women taking OCPs may experience midcycle bleeding or spotting. (See Chapter 9 for a discussion of the side

TABLE 7-2   Causes of Intermenstrual Bleeding

DISORDER	ABNORMALITY	INFECTIONS
Pregnancy-implantation	Miscarriage	Endometritis
Functional ovarian cyst	Ectopic pregnancy	Sexually transmitted disease
Cervical erosion	Molar pregnancy	disease
Leiomyoma	Retained placenta, abortion	
Polyps, uterine or endocervix	Retained placenta, delivery	
Trauma	Malignancy of reproductive tract	
Foreign body		

effects of OCPs.) If the contraceptive pill does not sufficiently maintain a hypoplastic endometrium, the endometrium will begin to shed, usually in small amounts at a time, a process termed *breakthrough bleeding*. Breakthrough bleeding is most common in the first three cycles of OCPs. The lowered potency of OCPs (resulting in increasing their safety) has decreased the amount of available hormones, making it more important that blood levels be kept constant. Suggesting that women take their pill at exactly the same time each day may alleviate the problem. If the spotting continues, a different formulation of OCP that increases either the estrogen or progestin component of the pill can be tried.

Contraceptive implants, such as Norplant, which are filled with synthetic progestin also may cause midcycle bleeding, especially in the first several cycles after implantation. Women should be advised of this and counseled to report continuation of breakthrough bleeding after the first three to six cycles to their health care provider. Women with an IUD may experience spotting between their periods and heavier menstrual flow.

The causes of intermenstrual bleeding are varied (Table 7-2). It is important that the nurse always consider the possibility that a woman who seeks care for intermenstrual bleeding is or recently has been pregnant.

Treatment of intermenstrual bleeding depends on the cause and may include reassurance and education concerning mittlestaining, observation of three menstrual cycles for presumed functional ovarian cyst, adjustment of an oral contraceptive, removal of foreign bodies, and treatment for vaginal infections. More complex treatment may consist of removal of polyps; evaluation and treatment of an abnormal Pap smear, including colposcopy, biopsy, cautery, cryosurgery, or conization; and surgery, chemotherapy, or radiation treatment for malignancy. Important nursing roles include reassurance, counseling, education, and support.

Menorrhagia

Menorrhagia (hypermenorrhea) is defined as excessive menstrual bleeding, in either duration or amount. The causes of heavy menstrual bleeding are many, including hormonal disturbances, systemic disease, benign and malignant neoplasms, infection, and contraception (IUDs). A single episode of heavy bleeding may occur, or a woman may experience regular flooding as a pattern in which she changes tampons or pads every few hours for several days.

NURSE ALERT

If the woman herself considers the amount or duration of bleeding to be excessive, the problem should be investigated.

Hemoglobin and hematocrit provide objective indicators to actual blood loss and should always be assessed.

A single episode of heavy bleeding may signal an early pregnancy loss. This type of bleeding is often thought to be a period that is heavier than usual, perhaps delayed, and is associated with abdominal pain or pelvic discomfort. When early pregnancy loss is suspected, a hematocrit and serum beta human chorionic gonadotropin (β-hCG) pregnancy test should be done.

Infectious and inflammatory processes such as acute or chronic endometritis and salpingitis may cause heavy menstrual bleeding. Although rare, systemic diseases of nonreproductive origin such as blood dyscrasias, cirrhosis of the liver, and renal disease also can cause hypermenorrhea. In obese women, anovulation caused by increased peripheral conversion of androstenedione to estrogen may develop and manifest as menorrhagia. Medications also may cause abnormal bleeding. Chemotherapy, anticoagulants, neuroleptics, major tranquilizers, and steroid hormone therapy all have been associated with excessive flow.

Uterine **leiomyoma** (fibroids or myomas) are a common cause of menorrhagia. Fibroids are benign tumors of the smooth muscle of the uterus whose etiology is unknown. Fibroids occur in one quarter of women of reproductive age; the incidence of fibroids is 2 to 3 times higher in African-American women than in white or Hispanic women (Speroff, Glass, & Kase, 1999). Fibroids are estrogen sensitive and commonly develop during the reproductive years and shrink after menopause. Fibroids are seen in 1% to 2% of pregnant women and can cause considerable discomfort as the uterus enlarges; furthermore, fetal palpation may be more difficult. The major symptoms associated with fibroids are menorrhagia and the physical effects produced by large myomas. Other uterine growths ranging from endometrial polyps to adenocarcinoma and endometrial cancer are common causes of heavy menstrual bleeding, as well as intermenstrual bleeding.

Treatment for menorrhagia depends on the cause of the bleeding. If the bleeding is related to contraceptive method, the nurse provides factual information and reassurance and discusses other contraceptive options. If bleeding is related to presence of fibroids, the degree of disability and discomfort associated with the fibroids and the woman's plans for childbearing will influence treatment decisions. Treatment options include medical and surgical management. Most fibroids can be followed by frequent examinations to judge growth, if any, and correction of anemia, if present. Women with metrorrhagia should be warned not to use aspirin because of its tendency to increase bleeding. Medical treatment is directed toward temporarily reducing symptoms, shrinking the myoma, and reducing its blood supply (Grabo et al., 1999). This reduction is often accomplished with the use of a GnRH agonist. If the woman wishes to retain childbearing potential, a myomectomy may be done. Myomectomy, or removal of the tumors only, is particularly difficult if multiple myomas must be removed. If the woman does not want to preserve her childbearing function, or if she has severe symptoms (severe anemia, severe pain, considerable disruption of lifestyle), hysterectomy or endometrial ablation may be done (see Chapter 13).

Dysfunctional Uterine Bleeding

Dysfunctional uterine bleeding (DUB) is associated with a wide variety of menstrual irregularities, but most often it is associated with excessive bleeding of some type: flow that is too frequent, too heavy, too prolonged, or irregular. Box 7-2 lists possible causes of dysfunctional uterine bleeding. DUB is most frequently caused by anovulation. Other common causes of DUB are pregnancy-related problems such as miscarriage or ectopic pregnancy. When there is no luteinizing hormonal surge, or if there is not sufficient progesterone produced by the corpus luteum to support the endometrium, it will begin to involute and

shed. This most often occurs at the extremes of a woman's reproductive years—when the menstrual cycle is just becoming established at menarche or when it draws to a close at menopause (Mehring, 1997). DUB can also be found with any condition that gives rise to chronic anovulation associated with continuous estrogen production. Such conditions include obesity, hyperthyroidism and hypothyroidism, polycystic ovarian syndrome, and any of the endocrine conditions discussed in the sections on amenorrhea and oligomenorrhea. Women may also be unknowingly using medications with an impact on the endometrium; for example, ginseng, an herbal root, has been associated with estrogen activity and abnormal bleeding. A diagnosis of DUB is made only after all other causes of abnormal menstrual bleeding have been ruled out (Rosenfeld, 1996).

When uterine bleeding is severe and a woman's hemoglobin level is less than 8 g/100 ml (hematocrit of 23% or 24%), the woman may be hospitalized and given conjugated estrogens (Premarin) 25 to 40 mg intravenously every 4 to 6 hours or 2.5 mg orally every 6 hours (Hillard, 1999) until bleeding stops or slows significantly (up to 3 doses). If the bleeding has not stopped in 12 to 24 hours, dilation and curettage (D&C) may be done to control severe bleeding and hemorrhage. An endometrial biopsy may be collected at the same time to evaluate endometrial tissue or rule out endometrial cancer. Following this treatment, oral conjugated estrogen 2.5 mg to 3.75 mg is given for 21 days. During the last 7 to 10 days of this estrogen regimen, pro-gesterone (e.g., medroxyprogesterone [Provera] 10 mg PO) is added. Alternatively, a combined OCP is given for 21 days after intravenous therapy

---

BOX 7-2   Possible Causes of Dysfunctional Uterine Bleeding

ANOVULATION
- Hypothalamic dysfunction
- Polycystic ovary syndrome

PREGNANCY-RELATED CONDITIONS
- Threatened or spontaneous abortion
- Retained products of conception after elective abortion
- Ectopic pregnancy

LOWER REPRODUCTIVE TRACT INFECTIONS
- Chlamydial cervicitis
- Pelvic inflammatory disease

NEOPLASMS
- Endometrial hyperplasia
- Cancer of cervix and endometrium
- Endometrial polyps
- Hormonally active tumors (rare)

- Leiomyomata (fibroids)
- Vaginal tumors (rare)

TRAUMA
- Genital injury (accidental, coital trauma, sexual abuse)
- Foreign body
- Primary coagulation disorders

SYSTEMIC DISEASES
- Diabetes mellitus
- Thyroid dysfunction (hypothyroidism, hyperthyroidism)
- Severe organ disease (renal or liver failure)

IATROGENIC CAUSES
- Exogenous hormone use (oral contraceptives, menopausal hormone therapy)
- Medications with estrogenic activity
- Herbal preparation (ginseng)

Sources: Hillard, P. (1999). Diagnosing and controlling abnormal uterine bleeding. *Contemporary Adolescent Gynecology* 4(1), 4-11; Speroff, L., Glass, R., & Kase, N. (1999). *Clinical gynecologic endocrinology and infertility* (6th ed.). Baltimore: Lippincott/Williams & Wilkins.

(Starr, Lommel, & Shanon, 1995). Once the acute phase has passed, the woman is maintained on cyclic, low-dose oral contraceptives for 3 to 6 months. Such long-term treatment will help prevent recurrence of the pattern of dysfunctional uterine bleeding and hemorrhage. If she wants contraception, she should continue to take OCPs. If the woman has no need for contraception, the treatment may be stopped in order to assess her bleeding pattern. If her menses does not resume, a pro-gestin regimen (e.g., Provera, 10 mg per day for 10 days before the expected date of her menstrual period) may be prescribed after ruling out pregnancy. This is done to prevent persistent anovulation (Mehring, 1997) with chronic unopposed endogenous estrogen hyperstimulation of the endometrium, which can result in eventual atypical tissue changes.

If the recurrent, heavy bleeding is not controlled by hormonal therapy or D&C, ablation of the endometrium through laser treatment may be performed. Nursing roles include informing clients of their options, counseling and education as indicated, and referring to the appropriate specialists and health care services.

CARE MANAGEMENT

Assessment and Nursing Diagnoses

In addition to taking a careful menstrual, obstetric, sexual, and contraceptive history, the nurse should explore the woman's perceptions of her condition, cultural or ethnic influences, experiences with other caregivers, lifestyle, and patterns of coping. The amount of pain or bleeding experienced and its effect on daily activities should be evaluated (see Guidelines/Guías). Home remedies and prescriptions to relieve discomfort are noted. A symptom diary, in which the woman records emotions, behaviors, physical symptoms, diet, and exercise and rest patterns, is a useful diagnostic tool.

GUIDELINES/GUÍAS

Menstruation

At what age did you begin to menstruate?
¿A qué edad comenzó a menstruar?

When was your last menstrual cycle?
¿Cuándo fue su última menstruación?

Was it normal?
¿Fue normal?

Do you have pains with your period?
¿Tiene dolores con la menstruación?

How many days does your period last?
¿Por cuántos días sangra?

Is the flow light or heavy?
¿Sangra mucho o poco?

Nursing diagnoses for women with menstrual disorders include the following:

Nursing Diagnoses

- Risk for ineffective individual or family coping related to
  - insufficient knowledge of the cause of the disorder
  - emotional and physiologic effects of the disorder
- Knowledge deficit related to
  - self-care
  - available therapy for the disorder
- Risk for body image disturbance related to
  - menstrual disorder
  - sexual dysfunction
- Risk for low self-esteem related to
  - others' perception of her discomfort
  - inability to conceive
- Pain related to menstrual disorder

Expected Outcomes of Care

After data collection and review, mutual expected outcomes are established and a plan of care is developed. The expected outcomes for the woman are that she will do the following:

- Verbalize her understanding of reproductive anatomy, etiology of her disorder, medication regimen, and diary use.
- Verbalize her understanding and acceptance of her emotional and physical responses to her menstrual cycle.
- Develop personal goals that benefit her emotionally and physically.
- Choose appropriate therapeutic measures for her menstrual problems.
- Adapt successfully to the condition if cure is not possible.

Plan of Care and Interventions

During the history and diagnostic workup, the clinician's concern and acceptance of the woman's symptoms as valid are in themselves therapeutic. Data from the daily diary of emotional status, subjective feelings, and physical state are correlated with physiologic changes. If the woman has a partner, both the woman and her partner should keep separate diaries that include how each perceives the other's responses day by day. Through the diaries, feelings are vented, problems are identified and clarified, insights occur, and possible solutions begin to develop. The clinician facilitates insights and suggests therapeutic options. The woman (couple) makes choices considered best for her (them).

Nurses should discuss the options available to women with menstrual disorders. Women must understand basic information about the anatomy and physiology, pathophysiology, psychologic impact, and treatment for the condition, including alternative therapies.

Support groups are an important resource. Nurses can use a local women's center or clinic to bring together women who want to learn more about their condition and support each other.

Evaluation

The nurse can be assured that care has been effective when the woman reports improvement in the quality of her life, skill in self-care, and a positive self-concept and body image.

MENOPAUSE

With the increasing life span of American women, most women can expect to live one third of their life after their reproductive years. As women age, many experience transitions that present challenges such as changing health, work, or marital status that require adaptation. Nowhere is this more true than with the changes associated with menopause. In the United States most women experience menopause during their late forties and early fifties, with the median age being approximately 51 years (McAllister, 1998). The average age for the onset of the perimenopausal transition is 46 years; 95% of women experience the onset between ages 39 and 51. The average duration of the perimenopause is 5 years, with a range of 2 to 8 years for 95% of women (Speroff, Glass, & Kase, 1999). The popular belief that an early menarche predisposes to a late menopause is not substantiated. Unlike menarche, the average age of menopause has remained about the same since the Middle Ages.

Perimenopause is that period of time for a woman that encompasses the transition from normal ovulatory cycles to cessation of menses and is marked by irregular menstrual cycles. Another term used to signal the period of time when a woman moves from the reproductive stage of life through the perimenopausal transition and menopause to the postmenopausal years is the **climacteric**. **Menopause** refers to the complete cessation of menses and is a single physiologic event said to occur when women have not experienced menstrual flow or spotting for 1 year and can be identified only in retrospect. Surgical menopause occurs with hysterectomy and bilateral oophorectomy. Postmenopause is the time after menopause.

Although all women experience similar hormonal changes with menopause, the experience of each woman is influenced by her age, cultural background, health, type of menopause (spontaneous or surgical), childbearing desires, and relationships. Women may view menopause as a major change in their lives—either positive, such as freedom from troublesome dysmenorrhea or the need for contraception, or negative, such as feeling "old" or loss of childbearing possibilities.

Physiology

Knowledge of the normal changes that occur during the perimenopause is essential to the assessment of meno-

pausal experiences and problems. Natural menopause is a gradual process with progressive increases in anovulatory cycles and eventual cessation of menses. In the 2 to 8 years preceding menopause, subtle hormonal changes occur that eventually lead to altered menstrual function and later to amenorrhea. When women are in their forties, anovulation occurs more often, menstrual cycles increase in length, and ovarian follicles become less sensitive to hormonal stimulation from FSH and LH. Because of these changes, a follicle is stimulated to the point that an ovum grows to maturity and is released in some months and in other months no ovulation takes place. Without ovulation and release of an ovum, progesterone is not produced by the corpus luteum. The lining continues to grow until it lacks a sufficient blood supply, at which point it will bleed. During this time, a woman's cycle will become more irregular. She may skip or miss periods; have shorter or lighter periods or longer, heavier periods; and experience clotting. FSH levels become elevated, reflecting an attempt to stimulate a follicle to produce estrogen.

> **NURSE ALERT**
>
> *FSH levels greater than 40 IU/L indicate that menopause is approaching, although women may still be bleeding.*

Physical Changes During the Perimenopausal Period
Bleeding

During the perimenopausal years, women may experience longer menstrual periods that differ in the type of bleeding. They may experience 2 to 3 days of spotting followed by 1 to 2 days of heavy bleeding, or they may have regular menses followed by 2 to 3 days of spotting. Such symptoms are characteristic of degenerating corpus luteum function. After menopause, women continue to have small amounts of circulating estrogen. Although the ovaries do not produce estrogen, androgens (androstenedione and testosterone) are produced for some time after menopause. Androgens produced by the adrenal glands are converted to estrone, a form of estrogen, in the liver and fat cells (Kendig & Sanford, 1998). With advanced age, the ovaries stop producing androstenedione, which further limits the amount of estrone in the body (Woods, 1995). Obese women are more likely to experience dysfunctional uterine bleeding and endometrial hyperplasia because women with more body fat have higher estrone levels.

Genital Changes

The vagina and urethra are estrogen-sensitive tissues, and low levels of estrogen can cause atrophy of both. Age-related vaginal changes not affected by estrogen also occur. Through both processes, the vaginal membranes thin, hold less moisture, and lubricate more slowly. However, not all women experience symptoms of genital atrophy.

GUIDELINES/GUÍAS

Menopause—Vaginal Dryness

Lack of hormone production in menopause can make the vagina dry.
Falta de producción de hormonas durante la menopausia puede causar que se seque la vagina.

Do you have decreased vaginal lubrication?
¿Tiene disminución en la lubricación vaginal?

Is intercourse painful for you?
¿Le da dolor al tener relaciones sexuales?

You may need to use a lubricant with intercourse.
Puede que necesite usar un lubricante en sus relaciones sexuales.

Women who are sexually active have less vaginal atrophy and fewer problems related to intercourse (Avioli et al., 1997). Thin women are more likely to experience more symptoms related to lowered estrogen levels such as vaginal dryness because of lack of adipose tissue and thus stored estrogen. Additionally, vaginal pH increases, lactobacilli growth can be depressed, and other bacteria tend to multiply. This combination of factors can lead to vaginitis.

Dyspareunia (painful intercourse) can occur because the vagina becomes smaller, the vaginal walls become thinner and dryer, and lubrication during sexual stimulation takes longer (Levine, 1998) (see Guidelines/Guías). Intercourse becomes painful and may result in postcoital bleeding. Some women may decide to forego intercourse altogether.

In some women, the shrinking of the uterus, vulva, and distal portion of the urethra associated with aging leads to disturbing symptoms, including urinary frequency, dysuria, uterine prolapse, and stress incontinence. Vaginal relaxation with cystocele, rectocele, and uterine prolapse is not caused by lowered estrogen levels. Urinary frequency sometimes occurs after menopause because the distal portion of the urethra, which has the same embryologic origin as the reproductive organs, shortens and shrinks. Irritants have easier access to the urinary tract with its shorter urethra and may cause frequency and urinary tract infections.

Urinary incontinence and uterine displacement are two other common findings in the postmenopausal period that are age related rather than menopause related. These conditions are discussed in Chapter 13.

Vasomotor Instability

During the past three decades investigators have devoted significant attention to identifying ovarian, hypothalamic, and pituitary hormonal mechanisms that produce symptoms related to menopause. Nonetheless, only two symptoms appear to increase in incidence as women progress through menopause: hot flashes and night sweats (Fogel & Woods, 1995). Many of the other changes commonly associated with menopause, such as decrease in size of genital structures, skin changes, and changes in breast size, are more correctly attributed to aging.

Vasomotor instability in the form of hot flashes or flushes is a result of fluctuating estrogen levels and is the most common disturbance of the perimenopausal years, occurring in up to 75% of menopausal women. Vasomotor instability occurs most frequently in the first 2 postmenopausal years; the number of episodes decreases over time. However, some women experience hot flashes before menopause and continue to have them for 10 to 20 years afterward. During this time, women experience changeable vasodilation and vasoconstriction as a **hot flush** (visible red flush of skin and perspiration) or **hot flash** (sudden warm sensation in neck, head, and chest) and night sweats (Fogel & Woods, 1995). These disturbances vary widely in severity, and only a minority of women seek health care for them (Lemcke, Marshal, & Pattison, 1995). Hot flushes and flashes can occur often throughout the day and may continue for several months or years. For some women, hot flashes may be an infrequent, possibly pleasant, sensation of warmth; for others, they may be an intensely unpleasant sensation of heat or warmth that may occur 20 to 50 times a day, create intense anxiety, and significantly decrease quality of life (Shaw, 1997). Surveys of midlife women have found that, in the absence of menopausal hormonal therapy, most affected women will have disturbances for 1 to 2 years and 25% up to 5 years (Speroff, Glass, & Kase, 1999). Several factors can precipitate or aggravate an episode, including crowded or warm rooms, alcohol, hot drinks, spicy foods, proximity to a heat source, and stress.

Night sweats, characterized by profuse perspiration and heat radiating from the body during the night, are another form of vasomotor instability experienced by many women. Sleep may be interrupted nightly because night clothes and bed linens may be soaked. Women may find that they are not able to go back to sleep. Other problems that may be associated with perimenopausal fluctuations of vasoconstriction or vascular spasms include dizziness, numbness and tingling in fingers and toes, and headaches.

Mood and Behavioral Responses

The tendency to associate hormonal changes with psychologic symptoms in midlife that has been prevalent in medical literature for decades and continues today was fueled by a belief that postmenopausal women suffer from "estrogen deficiency." Contrary to this common belief, there is no concrete evidence that menopause has a deleterious effect on mental health of midlife women. Findings from the Massachusettes Women's Health Study documented that menopause is not associated with an increased risk for mental health problems. Furthermore, a review of epidemiologic studies on menopause and depression concluded that there is no causal relationship between menopause and women's experiences with depression

(Nicol-Smith, 1996). Women who experience hot flashes and night sweats do sometimes report insomnia, fatigue from loss of sleep, and depressed mood. Women complain of feeling more emotionally labile, nervous, or agitated, with less control of their emotions. However, the interaction of psychologic, biologic, and sociocultural factors is so complex that it is difficult to determine whether a woman's reported mood shifts are the result of hormonal changes, normal aging, or cultural conditioning. Most likely a woman's psychologic makeup, cultural background, intercurrent stresses, and changing life roles and circumstances are more important than estrogen levels. Dealing with teenage children; having teenagers leave home; helping aging parents; becoming widowed or divorced; the onset of a major illness or disability (even death) in a spouse, relative, or friend; grieving for friends and family who are ill or dying; retirement; and financial insecurity are among the many stresses that women in their forties and fifties experience.

Cultural messages also influence individual women's perception of menopause. Women's experiences with menopause are not universal and vary among cultural groups. Most American women do not believe that menopause interferes with their quality of life (McAllister, 1998). Women do not find symptoms to be troublesome; however, they do report that symptoms are bothersome. Many women have accepted childbearing and child rearing as their major role in life, and the inability to bear children is a significant loss. Others see menopause as the first step to old age and associate it with a loss of attractiveness, physical ability, and energy. Western culture values youth and physical attractiveness; the wisdom gained from life experience is not valued, and the elderly suffer a loss of status, function, and role. There are no rituals to give older women a special place and function. In cultures where postmenopausal women gain status, such as India, the Far East, and the South Pacific Islands, depression among menopausal women is not observed. Western women, however, may have little to compensate for the losses they experience.

For other women, menopause is not a loss or a symbol of losses, but a relief. For some, menopause is a relief from the fear of pregnancy, the hassle of menstruation, and the inconveniences of contraception.

The ability to cope with any stress involves three factors: the person's perception or understanding of the event, support system, and coping mechanisms. Nurses counseling women in their perimenopausal years must therefore assess their understanding of perimenopausal changes, their perceptions of stressful experiences, their support systems, and their repertoire of coping skills.

Health Risks of Perimenopausal Women
Osteoporosis

Aging is associated with a progressive decrease in bone density in both men and women. **Osteoporosis** is a gener-

alized, metabolic disease characterized by decreased bone mass and increased incidence of bone fractures (Kessenich, 1996). Normally there is a dynamic balance between bone formation (osteoblastic activity) and bone resorption (osteoclastic activity). Because one of the functions of estrogen is to stimulate the osteoblasts, the postmenopausal drop in estrogen levels causes an imbalance between bone formation and resorption. Old bone deteriorates faster than new bone is formed, resulting in a slow thinning of the bones. Estrogen is also required for the conversion of vitamin D into calcitonin, which is essential in the absorption of calcium by the intestine. Reduced calcium absorption from the gut, in addition to the thinning of the bones, places postmenopausal women at risk for problems associated with osteoporosis.

Osteoporosis is a major health problem in the United States, affecting more than 25 million women older than age 45 (Garcini & Strong, 1999). Approximately 50% of American women have some degree of osteoporosis. One in four will have changes severe enough to predispose them to fractures. In the United States, the incidence of osteoporosis-related fractures has increased in the past 20 years. Among those who have a hip fracture, 12% to 20% die within 1 year after the fracture and more than half are unable to return to independent living (Kendig & Sanford, 1998). Of these, the overwhelming majority are older women. During the first 5 to 6 years after menopause, women lose bone six times more rapidly than men. By age 65, one third of women have had a vertebral fracture; by age 81, one third have had a hip fracture. By the time women reach age 80, they have lost 47% of their trabecular bone, concentrated in the vertebrae, pelvis and other flat bones, and the epiphyses. The most well-defined risk factor for osteoporosis is the loss of the protective effect of estrogen associated with cessation of ovarian function, particularly at menopause (Notelovitz, 1997). Women at risk are likely to be Caucasian or Asian, small boned, and thin. Obese women have higher estrogen levels resulting from the conversion of androgens in adipose tissue; mechanical stress from extra weight also helps preserve bone mass. A family history of the disease is common. The influences of heredity, race, and sex may be a result of differences in peak bone mass.

Inadequate calcium intake is a risk factor, particularly during adolescence and into the third and fourth decade, when peak bone mass is attained (Speroff, Glass, & Kase, 1999). An excessive caffeine intake increases calcium excretion, causing a systemic acidosis that stimulates bone resorption. Smoking is associated with earlier and greater bone loss and decreases estrogen production. Excessive alcohol intake interferes with calcium absorption and depresses bone formation. A greater phosphorus than calcium intake, which occurs with soft drink consumption, may be a risk factor. Other risk factors include steroid therapy and disorders such as hypogonadism and hyperthyroidism.

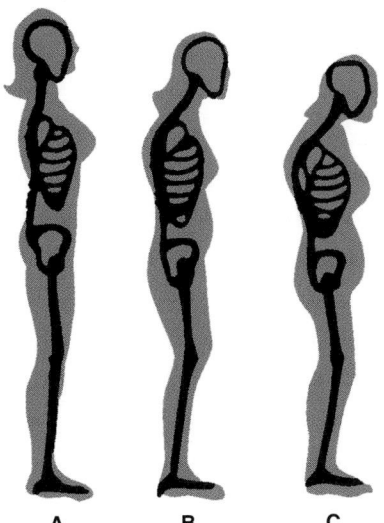

Fig. 7-2 Skeletal changes secondary to osteoporosis assessed by height and body shape at **A**, age 55; **B**, age 65; and **C**, age 75.

The first sign of osteoporosis is often loss of height resulting from vertebral fracture and collapse (Fig. 7-2). Back pain, especially in the lower back, may or may not be present. Later signs include "dowager's hump," in which the vertebrae can no longer support the upper body in an upright position, and fractured hip, in which the fracture often precedes a fall. Damage to the vertebrae usually precedes bone loss in the hip by an average of 10 years. Radiographic techniques to identify women at risk are imprecise, are expensive, and have not been approved for screening by third-party payers. Osteoporosis cannot be detected by x-ray examination until 30% to 50% of the bone mass has been lost, and routine screening is not warranted.

Coronary Heart Disease

During midlife, a woman's risk of developing and dying from cardiovascular disease increases after menopause. Diseases of the heart are the leading cause of death for women in the United States. Known risk factors for coronary heart disease include obesity, cigarette smoking, elevated cholesterol and blood pressure levels, diabetes mellitus, family history of cardiac disease, alcohol abuse, and the effects of aging on the cardiovascular system (Keller, Fullerton, & Fleury, 1998; Speroff, Glass, & Kase, 1999). Postmenopausal women are at risk for coronary artery disease because of changes in lipid metabolism; there is a decline in serum levels of HDL cholesterol and an increase in LDL levels.

These changes can be favorably reduced by diet and exercise (Halm & Penque, 1999). Furthermore, lipid changes at menopause (whether natural or surgical) can be reversed by estrogen treatment (Speroff, Glass, & Kase, 1999; Udoff, Langenberg, & Adashi, 1995). Estrogen has a favorable effect on circulating lipids, decreasing LDL and total cholesterol and increasing HDL, and has a direct antiatherosclerotic effect on arteries.

Menopausal Hormonal Therapy

Menopausal hormonal therapy (MHT)—more commonly known as **estrogen replacement therapy** (ERT), in which a woman takes only estrogen, or **hormonal replacement therapy** (HRT), in which she takes both estrogen and progestins—is the most commonly prescribed therapy for discomforts associated with the perimenopausal years, including hot flashes and vaginal and urinary tract atrophy. The terms *estrogen therapy* (ET) and *menopausal hormonal therapy* are used in this text rather than the more commonly used terms *estrogen replacement therapy* and *hormonal replacement therapy* for several reasons. The serum levels of estrogen and progesterone achieved with oral use are not true replacement levels; there is growing evidence that the benefits and risks of these therapies are due to pharmacologic as well as physiologic effects; and the term *replacement* implies deficiency rather than a natural lessening, which perpetuates the myth that menopause is a deficiency disorder rather than a natural physiologic event in women's lives.

MHT is used for either therapeutic or preventive management. Its use remains a highly controversial issue in women's health. Some authorities recommend MHT or ET for all women; these proponents view the perimenopause as a disease or deficiency state. Others insist that the use of hormones is never indicated for menopausal symptoms. The middle-ground approach advocates the use of hormonal therapy for women who have specific discomforts (therapeutic management) and for women in certain high risk groups (preventive management).

Hormonal Therapy: Therapeutic Management

Numerous studies have demonstrated the usefulness of MHT, including estrogen, progestin, or both, in alleviating vasomotor symptoms and genital changes associated with changing estrogen levels in women with both natural and surgically induced menopause. Although a variety of other hormonal and nonhormonal medical treatments, including phenobarbital, medroxyprogesterone (Depo-Provera), clonidine, and propanolol, have been found effective in relieving hot flashes, none were as effective as ET or MHT, and most had considerable side effects as well.

Whether MHT is indicated for hot flashes depends on the extent to which the individual woman is disturbed by them. The frequency and severity of the flashes and the extent to which they interrupt her sleep and activities of daily life will influence the woman's decision. Short-term therapy of up to 5 years is usually effective for relief of hot flashes or flushes and night sweats. When a woman decides to stop MHT, gradual withdrawal to prevent return of symptoms by rapid withdrawal of estrogen is advised (Moore & Noonan, 1996; Warren & Kulak, 1999). Once symptoms no longer recur, treatment can be stopped.

Although the urogenital changes seen in postmenopausal women are a normal part of aging, they may be quite uncomfortable for individual women and interfere with sexual activity and pleasure. Vaginal symptoms such as dryness, irritation, pruritus, bleeding, and infection have been shown to respond to both vaginal and systemic estrogen therapy (Moore & Noonan, 1996; Warren & Kulak, 1999). However, it may take up to 12 to 18 months after beginning systemic therapy for benefits to be seen. Urinary symptoms respond to oral estrogen use. If estrogen withdrawal occurs, vaginal and urinary symptoms may recur; thus relief may require long-term or even lifelong therapy. Research findings do not support the use of estrogen therapy or menopausal hormonal therapy as a treatment modality for changes or symptoms associated with menopause or aging, except for the relief of hot flashes and urovaginal changes.

Hormonal Therapy: Preventive Management

Estrogen either through ET or MHT may be used as a preventive agent for women at high risk for osteoporosis or cardiovascular disease (Box 7-3).

The protective effects of estrogen on the bone have been well documented. A number of well-designed, tightly controlled studies have shown that estrogen therapy for postmenopausal women significantly slows bone loss for at least as long as the woman continues therapy (Speroff, Glass, & Kase, 1999). ET increases serum levels of calcitonin, which prevents bone resorption, maintains bone density, and decreases the risk of fracture (Notelovitz, 1997).

Estrogen is more beneficial than calcium in preventing osteoporosis, although calcium may increase the effectiveness of estrogen. Estrogen therapy is most effective when begun early in menopause, although delayed therapy may also have beneficial effects. Currently there is no definite answer as to how long ET should be continued for osteoporosis prevention; however, 10 years is considered to be the minimum time needed to account for the years of accelerated bone loss following menopause; thus lifetime therapy must be considered. The minimum effective dose is thought to be 0.625 mg of conjugated estrogens or its equivalent daily (Speroff, Glass, & Kase, 1999). However, any amount of estrogen can have an impact, although it is likely that some degree of protection is lost when the dose is less than the equivalent of 0.625 mg of conjugated estrogen. When ET is stopped, bone mass decreases at a rate similar to that in the immediate postmenopausal period.

Epidemiologic evidence for benefit of estrogen therapy is especially strong for secondary prevention in women with prior cardiovascular heart disease (Keller, Fullerton, & Fleury, 1998). The Postmenopausal Estrogen and Progestin Intervention (PEPI) trials (PEPI, 1995) reviewed evidence that endogenous or exogenous estrogen plays a role in heart disease risk in women and concluded that the evidence suggesting that unopposed oral estrogen re-

BOX 7-3 Menopausal Hormone Therapy

- To relieve discomforts associated with vasomotor instability and genitourinary changes, short-term MHT or ET can be prescribed for women who have no contraindication to estrogen.
- MHT or ET may be prescribed indefinitely (lifelong) for women who are at risk for osteoporosis.
- ET decreases the risk of cardiovascular disease in older women but increases the risk of endometrial cancer in women with a uterus. Adding a progestin to therapy (MHT) decreases this risk.
- It is not known whether ET increases the risk for breast cancer; ET is contraindicated in women at high risk for breast cancer.

duces the risk of cardiovascular heart disease is "strong, reasonably consistent, and biologically plausible." They found that ET is especially beneficial in women who have had an oophorectomy and that its effect is most likely attributable to its favorable influence on lipid and lipoprotein profiles. In contrast to the increased risk of myocardial infarction in women over age 35 taking oral contraceptives, numerous studies indicate that postmenopausal ET is associated with reduced cardiovascular morbidity and mortality. ET has a protective effect, even in women who smoke.

Natural estrogens used in ET or MHT increase HDL levels and decrease LDL levels, thus promoting favorable lipid profiles (Lindsay et al., 1996). Borsage (1995) recommends that the prescription of estrogen solely or primarily to prevent heart disease should be considered for women at high risk—particularly those women who have high LDL cholesterol or low HDL cholesterol. The National Cholesterol Education Program (NCEP) expert panel has recommended estrogen therapy for postmenopausal women with high serum cholesterol (NCEP, 1993). Because combination (estrogen and progesterone) therapy (MHT) is recommended for women with a uterus, the effect of progesterone on lipids and lipoproteins is a critical issue. Epidemiologic evidence suggests that a progesteronal dose that protects the endometrium does not significantly decrease estrogen's cardiovascular benefits (Speroff, Glass, & Kase, 1999). Data from the PEPI trials suggest that estrogen alone and in various combinations with progestin changes blood lipids in a manner that protects women against atherosclerotic disease (PEPI, 1995).

Studies have also shown that estrogen-androgen therapy contributes to prevention of osteoporosis and to decreased levels of cholesterol. This therapy has also been reported to contribute to increased energy levels and libido and an overall feeling of well-being in postmenopausal women, especially those who have had surgical menopause (Bachmann, 1999).

Risks of Hormone Therapy

Currently one in eight American women will experience breast cancer in her lifetime. Studies have shown an increased risk of breast cancer associated with estrogen or estrogen-progestin use (Colditz et al., 1995) and a lack of increased risk with estrogen-progestin use (Stanford et al., 1995). Thus study findings are inconclusive and uncertainty persists. Potential health benefits of MHT (osteoporosis, heart disease, and colon cancer protection) are significant, but two important caveats must be considered. First, no randomized control trial has confirmed protection against heart disease, and selection bias (e.g., lower-risk women electing to take estrogen) may account for the benefits reported. Second, because the use of progestin concurrently is recent in U.S. health care practice, more years are required before the effect of progestin can be adequately studied (Grimes, 1995). At the same time, Col and associates (1997) demonstrated that the benefits of ET in reducing the likelihood of developing coronary heart disease (CHD) appear to outweigh the risk of breast cancer for nearly all women; the only exception appears to be women with two first-degree relatives with breast cancer and no risk factors for CHD. These women should not receive ET.

NURSE ALERT

Nurses are urged to consult the most recent literature available before counseling clients about the risks of MHT and breast cancer.

The risk of endometrial cancer is increased with unopposed estrogen therapy; the risk appears to be negated when a progestin is added at an adequate dose and duration for each cycle of use. Women who are unwilling to have annual endometrial biopsy or endometrial assessment by vaginal ultrasound should not receive unopposed estrogen. The risk of ovarian or cervical cancer does not appear to be increased with estrogen therapy.

Contraindications to Hormonal Therapy

Contraindications to the use of estrogen therapy include presence or suspicion of certain cancers, such as breast cancer or endometrial cancer; current problems with blood clots in the arteries or veins; unexplained vaginal bleeding; and pregnancy (Moore & Noonan, 1996). The breast and endometrium are target tissues of estrogen, and estrogen is contraindicated in women with a history of breast or endometrial malignancies. Carcinoma of the breast may exist for as long as 8 years before it is palpable. Because a small percentage of noncancerous breast lumps contain precancerous lesions, the condition should be evaluated before MHT is begun. Therefore a mammogram must be obtained for all women before ET or MHT is initiated. The importance of regular breast self-examination and follow-up should be empha-

sized. In addition, ET or MHT is not recommended for any woman with a blood relative who has had breast cancer.

MHT may worsen myomas of the uterus and porphyria. Conjugated estrogens are associated with an increased incidence of gallbladder disease, and women with a known history of gallbladder disease should not use ET or MHT. If thrombi develop or if surgery is anticipated, ET or MHT may be discontinued. Smoking decreases the effectiveness of estrogen.

Side Effects

Side effects associated with estrogen include headaches, nausea and vomiting, bloating, ankle and feet swelling, weight gain, breast soreness, brown spots on the skin, eye irritation with contact lenses, and depression. The type of estrogen used for postmenopausal ET is much less potent than ethinyl estradiol used in oral contraceptives and has fewer serious side effects. Side effects that do occur with MHT or ET may disappear with a change in estrogen preparation or a decrease in the dose prescribed.

Decision to Use Hormone Therapy

All women considering ET or MHT must understand that studies on MHT are ongoing and there is still much to be learned. Nurses counseling women considering hormonal therapy must provide information on the benefits and risks of MHT so that their clients can make an informed decision about its use. MHT and ET are currently used for vasomotor symptoms and relief of the discomforts associated with urogenital changes associated with lowered estrogen levels. MHT is approved and recommended for prevention of osteoporosis and cardiovascular disease, especially in women with risk factors for either condition. The long-term effects of MHT on urinary incontinence and cognition are thought to be beneficial but remain to be documented. The decision to use hormone therapy is complex because it involves weighing gains and losses related to physical risk and must be made by the individual woman. There are no clear-cut answers that nurses can give perimenopausal women.

Despite an increasing number of reasons for using MHT, and despite the fact that 70% of women have MHT prescribed at menopause or postmenopause, 20% to 30% never fill their prescription and 10% take the medication sporadically if at all (Moore & Noonan, 1996). Women often do not take or stop taking MHT because of fear of cancer (most often breast) or troublesome side effects such as withdrawal bleeding, irregular bleeding, breast tenderness, fluid retention, nausea, and headache.

Treatment Guidelines

Many different estrogen preparations, natural and synthetic, and ways of administering them—oral tablets, topical creams, transdermal preparations, injectables, suppositories,

TABLE 7-3 Oral and Transdermal Estrogen Equivalences, Vaginal Estrogen Creams, and Progestin Equivalences

TRADE NAME	GENERIC NAME	DOSAGES	METHOD
ESTROGEN EQUIVALENCES			
Premarin	Conjugated estrogens	0.3 mg 0.625 mg 0.9 mg 1.25 mg 2.5 mg	Oral
Estrace	Micronized estradiol	0.5 mg 1.0 mg 2.0 mg	Oral
Estratab Menest	Esterified estrogens	0.3 mg 0.625 mg 1.25 mg 2.5 mg	Oral
Estratest	Esterified estrogens with methyltestosterone	0.635 mg esterified estrogen + 1.25 mg methyltestosterone 1.25 mg esterified estrogens + 2.5 mg methyltestosterone	Oral
Ortho-Est Ogen	Estropipate	0.625 mg 1.25 mg 2.5 mg	Oral
Estraderm Climera FemPatch Esclim Vivelle Alora	Transdermal estradiol	0.05 mg; 0.1 mg 0.05 mg; 0.1 mg 0.025 mg 0.025 mg; 0.0375 mg; 0.075 mg; 0.1 mg 0.0375 mg; 0.05 mg; 0.075 mg; 0.1 mg 0.05 mg; 0.075 mg; 0.1 mg	Transdermal patch Release rates mg/24 hr
VAGINAL ESTROGEN CREAMS/RINGS			
Premarin	Conjugated estrogens	0.625 mg/g	Vaginal
Estrace	Estadiol	0.1 mg/g	Vaginal
Ogen	Estropipate	1.5 mg/g	Vaginal
Dienestrol	Dienestrol	0.01%	Vaginal
Estring	Estradiol	2 mg	Vaginal
PROGESTIN EQUIVALENCIES			
Provera	Medroxyprogesterone acetate	2.5 mg 5.0 mg 10 mg	Oral
Curretabs	Medroxyprogesterone	10 mg	Oral
Aygestin	Norethindrone acetate	5 mg	Oral
Micronor	Norethindrone	0.35 mg	Oral
COMBINATION ESTROGEN-PROGESTIN			
Prempro	Conjugated estrogens Medroxyprogesterone acetate	0.625 mg 2.5 mg or 5 mg	Oral (1 combination tablet/day for 28 days)
Premphase	Conjugated estrogens Medroxyprogesterone acetate	0.625 mg 5 mg	Oral (14 days of estrogen only, then 14 days of both)
COMBINED ESTROGEN/PROGESTIN			
CombiPatch	Estradiol/norethindone acetate (NETA)	0.05 mg estradiol/0.14 mg NETA or 0.05 mg estradiol/0.25 mg NETA	Transdermal (Release rates mg/24 hr)

Source: Facts and Comparisons. (1999). *Loose-leaf drug information service.* St. Louis: Facts and Comparisons; Garner, C. (1994). The climacterium, menopause, and the process of aging. In E. Youngkin & M. Davis (Eds.). *Women's health: A primary care clinical guide.* East Norwalk, CT: Appleton & Lange; CombiPatch package insert. Collegeville, PA., Rhone-Poulenc Rorer Pharmaceuticals, Inc.

and vaginal implants–exist (Table 7-3). However, most women today use either tablets or the transdermal patch.

Previous regimens of sequential MHT prescribed estrogen in combination with progesterone to simulate the normal menstrual cycle. The usual recommended dosage was 0.625 mg of conjugated estrogen or its equivalent for 25 days. This dosage is effective in osteoporosis prevention; higher dosages (0.9 or 1.25 mg) may be necessary to relieve menopausal symptoms. In addition, 5 mg of norethindrone or 5 to 10 mg of medroxyprogesterone acetate was given for 7 to 12 days. Estrogen is taken on calendar days 1 to 25 and progestin on days 16 to 25 of the cycle. This created a 5- to 6-day period at the end of the month when no hormones were taken and breakthrough bleeding occurred. This regimen was cumbersome to explain and difficult for women to follow. Therefore a more convenient regimen of a continuous dose of estrogen (0.625 mg) and intermittent progestins (2.5 mg medroxyprogesterone) has been recommended. It is thought that this dose of progestins will have fewer adverse effects on lipid profiles than do the higher doses. Women usually do not experience cyclical bleeding with this regimen and are less likely to have progestin side effects. An alternative regimen currently used is continuous combined MHT with estrogen and progestin taken daily. The dose of progestin is 2.5 to 5 mg of Provera or its equivalent and is particularly effective in older postmenopausal women.

The transdermal patch is applied one or two times a week to a hairless area of skin. Each patch is designed to last 3.5 to 7 days. Any site on the trunk or upper arms provides adequate absorption. The patches should not be placed on the breasts because of their sensitivity. Some women report minor skin irritation and reddening at the patch site. Generally transdermal estrogen offers the same relief of menopausal symptoms as the oral preparation. The transdermal method of delivery of estrogen does not have the same side effects such as breast tenderness and fluid retention. Oral progestin therapy can be used with transdermal ET. Combined estrogen-progestin transdermal patches are also available.

Alternative Therapies

Women who are unable or do not choose to use MHT or ET may find other modalities useful for relieving some of the changes associated with altered estrogen levels. Homeopathy, acupuncture, and herbs have been used successfully for menopausal problems such as heavy bleeding, hot flashes, irritability, and headaches (Box 7-4).

Homeopathy views menopausal symptoms as the body's efforts to heal itself from the hormonal changes it is experiencing. Examples of remedies commonly prescribed during menopause by homeopaths are sepia, made from the inky juice of the cuttlefish, to relieve symptoms such as dry mouth, eyes, and vagina; nux vomica, derived from the poison nut, to relieve backaches, constipation, and frequent awakenings; and pulsatilla, made from the windflower, to relieve severe menstrual symptoms and hot flashes (Barbach, 1993). Homeopathic remedies are subject to regulation by the U.S. Food and Drug Administration (FDA), although the FDA does not require proof of effectiveness (Beal, 1998).

Acupuncturists also treat hot flashes, but it is important that women evaluate their acupuncturists carefully. The American Association of Acupuncturists and Oriental Medicine will supply a list of acupuncturists in a given state (AAAOR Referrals, 4101 Lake Boone Trail, Suite 201, Raleigh, NC 27607-6518; phone: 919-787-5181). Questions to ask are, Is the acupuncturist certified by the National Commission for the Certification of Acupuncture? Is the acupuncturist certified in the state in which he or she practices? Does the acupuncturist carry malpractice insurance?

Herbal therapy also has been used to treat menopausal discomforts (Box 7-5). Herbs can be ingested as teas or tinctures. Many herbal preparations are also available in capsule form. It is important that women understand mechanisms of action, contraindications, and potential side effects of each herb. Women should always consult with their health care provider before beginning herbal therapy. In addition to resolving physical symptoms, herbs are also used to combat mood swings and depression. Ginseng has been claimed to be helpful in alleviating hot flashes, although research studies have not supported this assertion. Women should be advised against prolonged use of ginseng in high doses because it can increase blood pressure. Oriental herbal teas composed of licorice, ginseng, coptis, and Chinese rhubarb may be of some help in relieving hot flashes. Red raspberry leaf tea may ease hot flashes.

Dong quai and black cohosh have been used to treat menopausal discomforts; both have been investigated for effectiveness, with varying results (Hirata, 1997; Liberman, 1998). Black cohosh has been used by Native Americans for a variety of problems, including gynecologic, and it was a major ingredient in Lydia Pinkham's Vegetable Compound, a well-known nineteenth-century patent medicine (Beal, 1998).

Some plant foods contain **phytoestrogens** (isoflavones) and are capable of interacting with estrogen receptors in the body. These foods include wild yams, dandelion greens, cherries, alfalfa sprouts, black beans, and soybeans (Beal, 1998). Use of soy-rich foods as an alternative to traditional hormonal therapy for menopause has been studied, and beneficial effects on menopausal symptoms and on lowering cholesterol have been documented (Ramsay, Ross, & Fischer, 1999). However, more research is needed to better understand the potential effects of soy intake on prevention of osteoporosis and lowering risks of coronary heart disease (Lindsay & Claywell, 1998). For women who want to add soy to their diets, tofu, roasted soy nuts, and soy milk are good sources. Foods should be added gradually because some women experience gastrointestinal discomfort from the high fiber content of these foods (National Women's Health Report, 1999).

BOX 7-4　Alternatives to Hormonal Therapy for Menopausal Symptoms

HOT FLASH/FLUSH

Vitamin E: 100-600 IU daily (no more than 100 IU in the presence of high blood pressure, diabetes, or rheumatic heart disease). Start with a low dose and increase over 6-8 weeks to 600 IU or less if symptoms improve.

Bioflavonoids (500 mg-1 g) combined with vitamin C. Dietary sources include wheat germ, whole grains, vegetable oils, soybeans, peanuts, spinach and other dark green leafy vegetables, and cold pressed oils.

Herbal therapy:

Dong quai

Ginseng tea—Take on an empty stomach before or between meals. Do not take with vitamin C. Avoid if diabetic or in the presence of cardiac problems. May be associated with postmenopausal bleeding.

Black cohosh (natural estrogen) 40 gtts/day/6 mo

Soy—40 to 100 mg isoflavones or approx. 30 to 50 g soy protein

Vitamin B complex: 1 to 2 daily. Dietary sources include whole grains, wheat germ, yogurt, brewer's yeast, and milk.

Vitamin C

Acupuncture

Medications other than hormone replacement:
　Bellergal (can increase high blood pressure)
　Belladonna (side effects—dry mouth, rapid pulse, constipation)
　Clonidine (side effects—sleepiness, dry mouth, decreased blood pressure)

INSOMNIA

Herbal therapy:
　Valerian (natural tranquilizer)
　Peppermint, catnip, hops, passion flower

HEADACHES

Herbal therapy:
　Natural diuretics (parsley)
　Chasteberry, peppermint oil, feverfew, royal jelly products

UROGENITAL SYMPTOMS

For vaginal dryness and itching:
　Vitamin E—400-600 IU daily or vitamin E oil on the skin
　Evening primrose oil, aloe vera, slippery elm paste
　Witch hazel and glycerin (dip pads in mixture and apply to skin for itching)

NERVOUSNESS/IRRITABILITY

Vitamin B_6: 5 to 25 mg daily. Dietary sources include brewer's yeast, bran, wheat germ, organ meats, molasses, walnuts, peanuts, and brown rice.

Sources: Lowdermilk, D., & Fogel, C. (1996). *Health care issues of midlife women.* Edwardsville, KS: Educational Software; Blumenthal, M. (Ed.). (1998). *The complete German Commission E monographs: Therapeutic guide to herbal medicines.* Austin, TX: The American Botanical Council; Israel, D., & Youngkin, E. (1997). Herbal therapies for perimenopausal and menopausal complaints. *Pharmacotherapy* 17(5), 970-984; Ramsey, L., Ross, B., & Fischer, R. (1999). Phytoestrogens and the management of menopause. *Adv Nurse Pract* 7(1), 27-30.

BOX 7-5　Herbs Commonly Used to Treat Menopausal Symptoms

Dong quai	Estrogen precursor
Black cohosh	Progesterone precursor
Chasteberry	Revitalize vaginal tissue
Nettles	Dysfunctional uterine bleeding
Evening primrose oil	Hot flashes, PMS
Wild yam	Hot flashes
Horsetail	Bone health
St. John's wort	Depression
Oatstraw	Bone health
Raspberry leaf	Hot flashes
Peppermint	Nausea, upset stomach

Source: Kendig, S., & Sanford, D. (1998). *Midlife and menopause: Celebrating women's health.* Washington, DC: AWHONN; Taylor, M. (1997). Alternatives to conventional hormone replacement therapy. *Comprehensive Therapy* 23(8), 514-532.

Vitamin E is a popular alternative among women who do not take MHT. Women who take vitamin E regularly report relief from hot flushes, leg cramps, and loss of energy. Vitamin E is found in a variety of foods, including spinach, peanuts, wheat germ, vegetable oils, and soybeans, or may be taken as a supplement. Dosage varies widely, from 400 to 800 IU per day.

Layered clothing, ice packs, iced water, and fans may offer symptomatic relief from hot flashes (see Client Self-Care box). Women can be counseled to avoid hot curries and other spicy foods. Reassurance that hot flushes will not last forever may be of comfort even if duration of the problem cannot be predicted accurately. Most women find that hot flashes disappear within 4 to 6 years after menopause.

Nurses should be aware of the availability of natural remedies for menopausal symptoms and be knowledgeable about the indications for complementary and alternative therapies so that clients can be counseled appropriately.

CLIENT SELF-CARE

Comfort Measures

HOT FLASHES/FLUSHES

During the day
  Wear layered clothing so you can take things off if you get warm.
  Avoid "triggers" that bring on a flash/flush; these include vigorous exercise on hot days, eating spicy foods, caffeine, hot beverages, and alcohol.
  Splash your face with cool water, drink iced water, or take a cool shower if you get warm.
  Try slow, deep breathing.
Night
  Sleep in cotton clothes, use cotton sheets, and keep room cool.
  Avoid heavy blankets that make you too warm at night.
  Keep a thermos of water by the bed.

INSOMNIA

Avoid caffeine, alcohol, or tobacco in the evening.
Avoid liquids after dinner.
Exercise regularly but limit exercise to the daytime and early evening.
Develop a bedtime routine.
  Identify a regular time to go to bed.
  Try drinking warm milk or having a hot bath.
  Use your bed only for sleeping or sexual activity; don't watch TV, read, etc.

Encourage your body's circadian rhythm.
If you can't sleep, get up and do something until you feel tired.
Avoid naps during the day.
Sprinkle lavender oil on the pillow.
  Drink chamomile tea (do not use if allergic to ragweed or chrysanthemums).

HEADACHES

Try to avoid stress and get plenty of rest.
Eat or drink foods that contain natural diuretics (parsley).

UROGENITAL SYMPTOMS

Drink lots of water and empty bladder frequently.
Practice Kegal exercises daily.
Wear cotton underwear and avoid wet bathing suits for a prolonged time.
Use water-soluble lubricants for vaginal dryness.

NERVOUSNESS, IRRITABILITY

Practice yoga or other meditation.
Do relaxation or deep breathing exercises.
Practice guided imagery.

Source: Lowdermilk, D., & Fogel, C. (1996). *Health care issues of midlife women.* Edwardsville, KS: Educational Software.

: CARE MANAGEMENT

Assessment and Nursing Diagnoses

A thorough health history, physical examination, and laboratory tests are essential to distinguish pathologic conditions from the normal perimenopausal experiences. Personal or family history of breast or uterine cancer, hypertension, thrombophlebitis, liver or gallbladder disease, undiagnosed uterine bleeding, and other acute or chronic diseases are noted, as are hysterectomy and bilateral oophorectomy. Recent changes in menstrual history help identify the phase of the perimenopausal period the woman is experiencing, and risk factors for osteoporosis are identified. The woman's perception of this stage of life, ethnic and cultural factors, and knowledge and concerns about sexuality and care available are all recorded. The practices and remedies the woman has used for menopausal symptoms are assessed, including pharmacologic and alternative therapies.

Nursing diagnoses for perimenopausal women may include the following:

: Nursing Diagnoses

- Knowledge deficit related to
  - menopause and its management
- Family coping, potential for growth related to
  - receiving information about the condition, its management, and prognosis
  - emotional support
- Risk for altered growth and development related to
  - insufficient knowledge of menopause
- Risk for pain related to
  - changing ovarian function
- Risk for injury related to
  - osteoporosis
  - heart disease
- Risk for sexual dysfunction related to
  - changes associated with changing estrogen levels
- Risk for low self-esteem related to
  - physical and emotional changes during the perimenopausal period

Expected Outcomes of Care

Planning requires knowledge of the perimenopausal period and great sensitivity. Informed consent regarding MHT, weight-bearing exercise, and calcium supplements is a major concern because treatment may involve expense, inconvenience, and side effects. Expected outcomes are stated in terms of client behaviors. The woman will do the following:

- Explain the physical changes associated with menopause.
- View the perimenopausal period as a normal developmental phase instead of a deficiency disease.
- Have no discomforts that interfere with daily activities.
- Develop no symptoms or signs of osteoporosis or experience only minimal effect.
- Experience a healthy perimenopausal transition.
- Report concerns about changes associated with menopause and treatment.

Plan of Care and Interventions

Most women know little about menopause, and old wives' tales and misinformation can cause anxiety. They need to know what to expect, why it happens, and what measures will help make them more comfortable. Women appreciate the opportunity to discuss what they are experiencing. They need to know that their discomforts have a normal physiologic basis and that other women experience similar discomforts.

Treatment must be individualized for the specific woman. Menopause clinics are needed where research on the effects of various treatments can be developed and evaluated and where care by the various specialty groups involved, such as endocrinology, radiology, psychosocial resources, exercise physiology, and nutrition, can be effectively coordinated. Women's support groups are also needed. Areas that need further discussion include sexuality, nutrition, exercise, and support.

Sexual Counseling

Sexuality is a lifelong behavior, and contrary to common stereotypes, sex does not end with menopause. Many women remain sexually active throughout their entire lives. However, women and their partners may change their expression of sexuality during and after menopause, depending on physical changes, changes in the partner, and cultural myths and messages. Some women report decreases in interest and desire. These decreases in sexuality with aging are influenced more by culture and attitudes than by nature and physiology (hormones). Although some women report that it takes longer to reach orgasm and that the orgasm is not as intense, the capacity for orgasm is not decreased. There is no way to prevent the inevitable aging process that the body undergoes. For people who see aging as loss, sexuality may become difficult to incorporate into what they perceive to be a less attractive identity. The fear of rejection may be present.

Changes in a male partner may influence whether he continues to want to engage in sexual activity. As men age, they, too, take longer to reach orgasm; erections take longer to occur and are less firm. Men may believe they are becoming impotent or ill and give up sexual activity, viewing it as too frustrating. Women may believe their partners are losing interest in them. Couples may need counseling to understand these changes.

The two most important influences on older women's sexual activity are the strength of a relationship and the physical condition of each partner. The lack of available male partners can have a negative effect on sexual expression for many midlife and older women. Women outlive men, and older widowed and divorced women frequently have fewer opportunities to develop relationships because they are less sought after. In counseling older women who do engage in intercourse, the nurse cannot assume that new or nonmonogamous partners are free of sexually transmitted diseases and should inform clients of their risk for human immunodeficiency virus infection and other sexually transmitted diseases and the need to use condoms.

Older lesbian women largely have been a silent group whose sexual needs and special social circumstances have not been acknowledged or recognized. Although lesbian women in midlife and older do not face the problem of a lack of available male partners, they are faced with negative attitudes accompanying being old, female, and lesbian—all of which can adversely affect sexuality and sexual expression.

As long as women are able to bear children, some accept intercourse as part of their responsibility as wives. When menopause frees them from this duty they may choose to forego intercourse. For other women, libido may increase without the fuss of contraception, fear of pregnancy, or interruption from menses.

Nurses must give accurate information on matters such as appropriate contraception, sexuality, and the physiology of menopause and should offer support and nonjudgmental guidance. Women need advice about contraception, because ovulation may not cease for a year after the last menstrual cycle and menopausal women can still become pregnant. The nurse's attitude toward sex and the older adult is important. Negative attitudes can reinforce the client's misgivings about maintaining an active and satisfying sex life. The nurse can reassure the woman grieving over lost youth and attractiveness that the desire for sex into old age is a natural one and that the body has the capacity for sexual satisfaction. Only minor adjustments may be required.

Muscle tone around the reproductive organs decreases after menopause. Kegel exercises strengthen these muscles, improve tone, and, if practiced regularly, help prevent prolapsed uterus and stress incontinence. This is a low-cost, effective, noninvasive intervention to control symptoms. However, symptoms return if exercises are discontinued.

K-Y lubricating jelly, Replens, and Astroglyde are examples of water-soluble lubricants that provide relief from painful intercourse. They may be applied directly to the vulva and the penis. Oil-based lubricants such as petroleum jelly (Vaseline) should not be used because they clog vaginal glands, which can then be sites for bacterial infection.

The nurse can refer couples to a counselor or physician for problems beyond the scope of nursing practice.

Prolonged hospitalization of an elderly partner may have a significant impact on the couple's sexual relationship. They may have difficulty renewing sexual activity when the separation is over and may need counseling or referral. In the event that a couple is admitted to a nursing home, the nurse should encourage placement of the couple together. With the aging of the American population and changing attitudes about the appropriateness of lifelong sexual expression, long-term care, extended care, and full-term care facilities are more receptive to providing opportunities for sexual activity between marital partners.

Nutrition

Obesity and osteoporosis are common health problems of midlife and older women. As women move out of their childbearing years they may need to change their diets. Because metabolic rates decrease with age and many women exercise less, fewer calories are needed for weight maintenance as women age. In general, foods chosen should be high in nutrients, fiber, and calcium but moderate in calories and low in fat to allow for adequate nutritional intake while maintaining body weight. Nurses can suggest that women substitute skim for whole milk or chicken without skin for steak. Foods high in calcium and low in phosphorus are recommended. Excessive protein should be avoided. Fat-free milk and yogurt are good sources of calcium and vitamin D. It is difficult to eat other foods that contain calcium (sesame seeds, spinach, greens, broccoli, and seaweed) in quantities sufficient to meet daily requirements. Women should avoid excessive intake of alcohol, soft drinks, and caffeinated coffee.

Calcium is an essential part of any therapeutic regimen for women with osteoporosis and those who want to prevent osteoporosis. The best source of calcium is food; however, calcium supplements are recommended when a woman's diet does not supply recommended amounts of calcium. Although calcium cannot reverse loss of bone mass or prevent fractures, calcium supplementation may retard the development of osteoporosis after menopause. Women without contraindications to calcium supplementation (history of kidney stones, kidney failure, hypercalcemia) should be encouraged to consume a diet that has 1200 to 1500 mg of calcium a day or to add an amount of calcium supplementation that will increase their daily intake to this level. Calcium supplements are best taken in divided doses and with meals because of the increase in acid secretions and extended time in the stomach. At least 8 ounces of water to increase solubility is recommended. Calcium is most commonly available as calcium carbonate, calcium lactate, and calcium phosphate. Many of the calcium preparations on the market are useless because they do not dissolve; Tums are most soluble. A combination of vitamin D and calcium (1200 mg) may be recommended as a supplement because vitamin D aids in calcium absorption. Mineral supplements are not classified as drugs by the FDA and are therefore not regulated, making it difficult for consumers to know which product is best.

Exercise

All too often midlife women are sedentary—the demands of family and work constraints increase and energy levels decrease. Unfortunately little or no exercise predisposes women to weight gain and does not help prevent cardiac disease or osteoporosis. Exercise alone cannot prevent or reverse osteoporosis, but data indicate that weight-bearing exercise, such as walking and stair climbing 30 to 60 minutes a day, may delay bone loss and increase bone mass at any age (Fig. 7-3).

Water aerobics is excellent for cardiovascular fitness and is a good choice for older women who may be unable to engage in weight-bearing exercises. The nurse can help women plan an exercise program. Examples of exercises are available from the National Osteoporosis Foundation (Fig. 7-4).

In addition to calcium and exercise, calcitonin, alendronate sodium (Fosamax), or raloxifene (Evista) can be offered to women with postmenopausal osteoporosis. Calcitonin reduces the rate of bone turnover and stabilizes bone mass in women with osteoporosis and may have some analgesic effects. Although it can reduce the incidence of spinal fractures, no data about the use of calcitonin to protect against hip fractures is available (McClung, 1999). Calcitonin may be used with women in whom estrogen is contraindicated or not tolerated. The medication is very safe; however, side effects of nausea, vomiting, and anorexia have been reported. The drug is expensive and must be administered parenterally, thus limiting its use (Box 7-6).

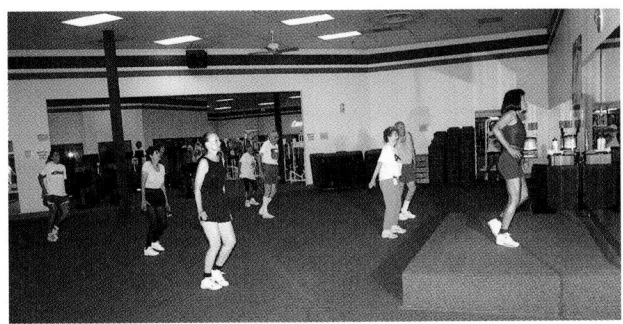

Fig. 7-3 Weight-bearing exercise is beneficial for the midlife woman. *(Courtesy Jonas McCoy, Raleigh, NC.)*

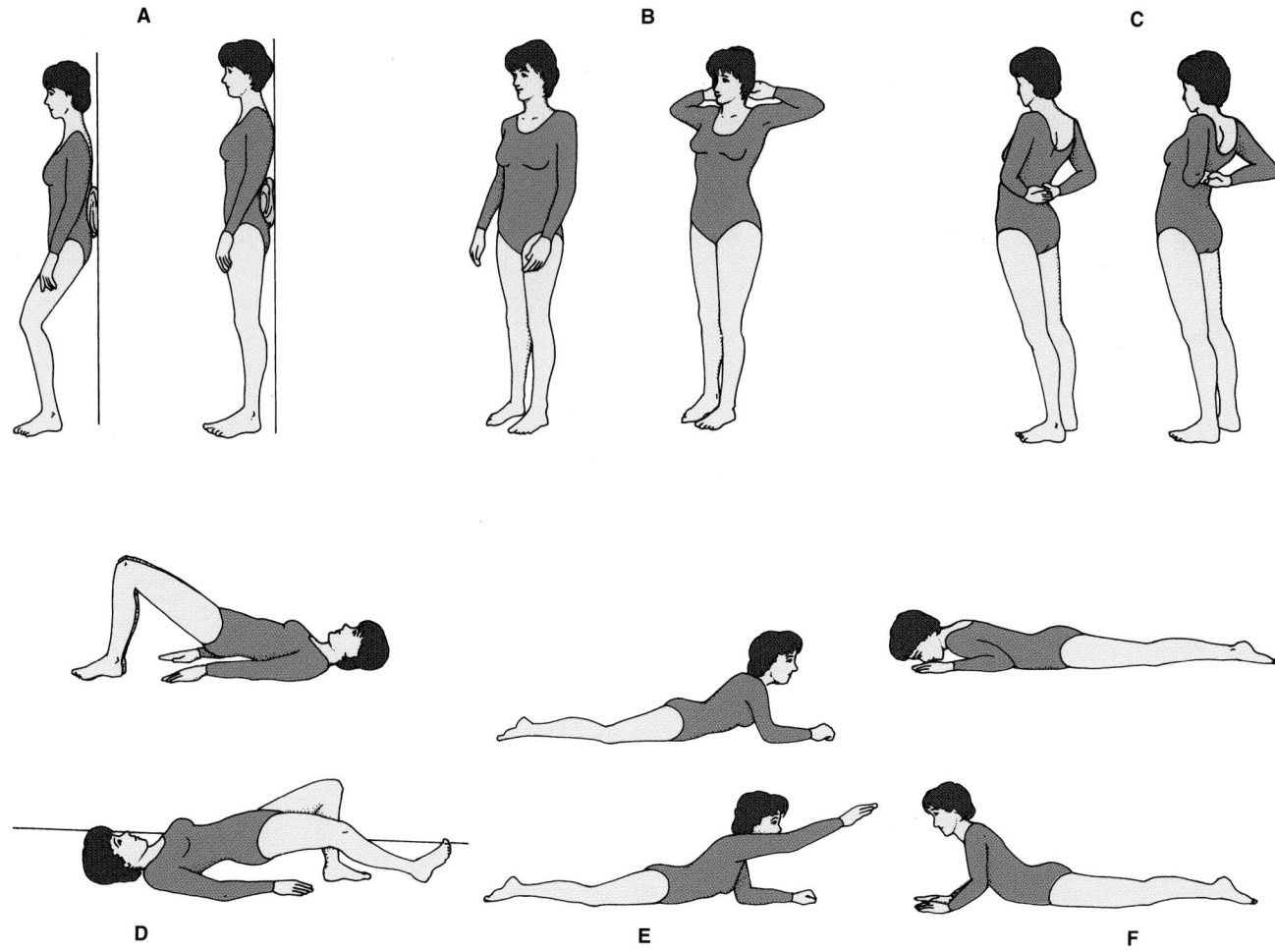

Fig. 7-4 *A,* Wall standing and pelvic tilt. *B,* Isometric posture correction. *C,* Standing back bend. *D,* The bridge. *E,* The elbow prop. *F,* Prone press-ups with deep breathing. *(From "Boning Up on Osteoporosis" courtesy of the National Osteoporosis Foundation.)*

▪ BOX 7-6 Prevention of Osteoporosis

- ET can be prescribed to prevent fractures from osteoporosis. The risks and benefits of ET must be weighed on an individual basis with the health care provider.
- Significant bone loss can be prevented by a well-balanced diet, including 200 to 400 IU of vitamin D and 1000 to 1200 mg of calcium a day, and regular weight-bearing exercise. Good sources of calcium are dairy products, fish, oysters, tofu, dark-green leafy vegetables, and whole-wheat bread.
- Supplements of vitamin D and calcium can be taken but the body cannot use them without the right balance of other vitamins and minerals.

- Eliminating environmental hazards in the home can decrease the risk of falls.
- Weight-bearing exercise 30 to 60 minutes per day may delay bone loss and increase bone mass.
- Raloxifene may be prescribed for prevention of osteoporosis in postmenopausal women.
- Alendronate sodium may be prescribed for women who already have osteoporosis to delay bone loss and increase bone mass.

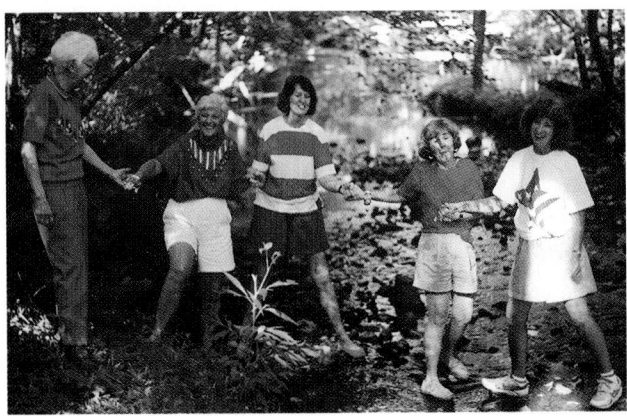

Fig. 7-5 Midlife women can develop a supportive network. *(Courtesy Ed Lowdermilk, Chapel Hill, NC.)*

Alendronate sodium is approved by the FDA for the treatment of osteoporosis in postmenopausal women. The medication assists in delaying bone loss, increasing bone mass, and preventing fractures.

NURSE ALERT

Clients must take alendronate sodium on an empty stomach with 6 to 8 ounces of plain water only at least 30 minutes before eating or drinking to improve absorption (McClung, 1999).

Raloxifene is approved by the FDA for osteoporosis prevention in postmenopausal women only. This medication preserves the beneficial effects of estrogen, including protection against cardiovascular diseases and osteoporosis, without stimulating breast and uterine tissues. It is not effective in reducing hot flashes or flushes. The medication modestly increases bone density (McClung, 1999). Calcium supplements should be taken if dietary intake is inadequate.

Midlife support groups. Nurses should be familiar with local resources and direct women to classes that supply appropriate information and support. They can encourage women to develop a supportive network with other women with whom they can share their concerns (Fig. 7-5).

Women's centers and clinics may have support groups and classes for women who want to discuss menopause and other midlife events (see Appendix D). If no group or class is available in the community, nurses should consider starting one.

Evaluation

The nurse can be reasonably assured that care was effective to the degree that the expected outcomes of care have been met.

KEY POINTS

- Menstrual disorders diminish the quality of life for affected women and their families.
- Premenstrual syndrome (PMS), no longer considered a purely psychologic problem, is a disorder that begins in the luteal phase of the menstrual cycle and ends with the onset of menses.
- Endometriosis is characterized by secondary amenorrhea, dyspareunia, abnormal uterine bleeding, and infertility.
- The perimenopause is a normal developmental phase during which a woman passes from the reproductive to the nonreproductive stage.
- During the perimenopause, women seek care for symptoms that arise from bleeding irregularities, vasomotor instability, fatigue, genital changes, and changes related to sexuality.
- Alternative therapies are beneficial in relieving some discomforts associated with menstrual disorders and menopause.
- MHT and ET are the most commonly used treatments for relieving menopausal discomforts.
- MHT or ET may be used to decrease risk in women at risk for osteoporosis or cardiovascular disease.
- Osteoporosis, a progressive loss of bone mass that results from decreasing levels of estrogen after menopause, can be prevented or minimized with estrogen therapy.
- Estrogen increases calcitonin levels to prevent bone resorption and maintain bone density.
- Sexuality and the ability for sexual expression continue after menopause.

CRITICAL THINKING EXERCISES

1 Interview a woman with primary dysmenorrhea to determine her responses to the condition.
  a. What are her perceptions about how others view her condition?
  b. Examine how her responses compare with theoretic responses, as well as your own perceptions.
  c. Analyze the woman's responses to identify positive and negative aspects of PMS.
  d. Formulate a plan of care using the data from the interview.

Continued

CRITICAL THINKING EXERCISES—cont'd

2 You are assigned to a clinic where women are assessed and treated for menopausal symptoms.

  a. What are some generalizations about women and menopause?

  b. What are your perceptions about women who have numerous complaints or symptoms that they attribute to menopause?

  c. What impact could these perceptions have on providing care to menopausal women?

  d. How can nurses effect a positive change in the care of midlife and older women?

3 Review the literature for studies determining effectiveness of alternative therapies for menstrual problems and menopause. In a clinical conference, discuss therapies that have been shown to be beneficial, are likely to be beneficial, have unknown effects, or have effects that are likely not to be beneficial or may be harmful. Discuss how nurses can use this information in their clinical practices.

References

Apgar, B. (1997). Dysmenorrhea and dysfunctional bleeding. *Prim Care* 24(1), 161-178.

Avioli, V. et al. (1997). *The postmenopausal health curriculum 101*. Chicago: Pramaton.

Bachmann, G. (1999). Androgen cotherapy in menopause. Evolving benefits and challenges. *Am J Obstet Gynecol* 180(3), S308-S311.

Baker, S. (1998). Menstruation and related problems and concerns. In E. Youngkin & M. Davis (Eds.). *Women's health*. Stamford, CT: Appleton & Lange.

Barbach, L. (1993). *The pause*. New York: Dutton.

Barrett-Connor, E. (1998). Efficacy and safety of estrogen/androgen therapy. Menopausal symptoms, bone and cardiovascular parameters. *J Reprod Med* 43(8 suppl), 746-752.

Beal, M. (1998). Women's use of complementary and alternative therapies in reproductive health. *J Nurse Midwifery* 43(3), 224-234.

Blumenthal, M. (Ed.). (1998). *The complete German commission E monograph: Therapeutic guide to herbal medicines*. Austin, TX: The American Botanical Council.

Borsage, P. (1995). Hormone therapy: The woman's decision. *Contemporary Nurse Practitioner* July/August (suppl), 3-10.

Brough, R., & O'Flynn, K. (1996). Recurrent pelvic endometriosis and bilateral uterine obstruction associated with hormone replacement therapy (HRT). *BMJ* 312, 1221-1222.

Carter, J., & Verhoef, M. (1994). Efficacy of self-help and alternative treaments of premenstrual syndrome. *Women's Health Issues* 4(3), 130-137.

Castiglia, P. (1996). Amenorrhea. *J Pediatr Health Care* 10(5), 226-227.

Chandraiah, S. (1996). Premenstrual syndrome. In R. Blackwell (Ed.). *Women's medicine*. Cambridge, MA: Blackwell Science.

Charlton, A., & White, D. (1996). Smoking and menstrual problems in 16-year-olds. *J Royal Soc Med* 89, 193.

Chuong, C., Pearsall-Otey, L, & Rosenfeld, B. (1995). A practical guide to relieving PMS. *Contemp Nurse Pract* 1(3), 31-34, 36-37.

Col, N. et al. (1997). Patient-specific decisions about hormone replacement therapy in postmenopausal women. *JAMA* 277(14), 1140-1147.

Colditz, G. et al. (1995). The use of estrogens and progestins and the risk of breast cancer in postmenopausal women, *N Engl J Med* 332, 1589-1593.

Corwin, E. (1997). Endometriosis: Pathology, diagnosis and treatment. *Nurs Pract* 22(10), 35-36, 38, 40-42, 45, 48, 50-51.

Facts and Comparisons. (1995). *Loose-leaf drug information service*. St. Louis: Facts and Comparisons.

Facts and Comparisons. (1999). *Loose-leaf drug information service*. St. Louis: Facts and Comparisons.

Fankenauser, M. (1996). Treatment of dysmenorrhea and premenstrual syndrome. *Journal of the American Pharmaceutical Association* NS36(8), 503-513.

Federation of Feminist Women's Health Centers. (1981). *A new view of a woman's body*. New York: Simon & Schuster/Touchstone Book.

Fogel, C. (1995). Common symptoms. In C. Fogel & N. Woods (Eds.). *Women's health care*. Thousand Oaks, CA: Sage.

Fogel, C. (1997). Endocrine causes of amenorrhea. *Primary Care Practice* 1(5), 507-518.

Fogel, C., & Woods, N. (1995). Midlife women. In C. Fogel & N. Woods (Eds.). *Women's health care*. Thousand Oaks, CA: Sage.

Garcini, F., & Strong, S. (1999). Care of the perimenopausal and postmenopausal woman. In M.G. Curtis & M.P. Hopkins (Eds.). *Glass's office gynecology* (5th ed.). Baltimore: Williams & Wilkins.

Garner, C. (1995). Infertility. In C. Fogel & N. Woods (Eds.). *Women's health care*. Thousand Oaks, CA: Sage.

Golden, N., & Shenker, I. (1994). Amenorrhea in anorexia nervosa: Neuroendocrine control of hypothalamic dysfuction. *Int J Eat Disord* 16, 53-50.

Grabo, T. et al. (1999). Uterine myomas: Treatment options. *J Obstet Gynecol Neonatal Nurs* 28(1), 23-31.

Grimes, D. (1995). Weighing the benefits and risks of hormone replacement therapy after menopause. *Contraceptive Report* 6(4), 4-14.

Hadfield, R. et al. (1997). Endometriosis in monozygotic twins. *Fertil Steril* 68, 941-942.

Halm, M., & Penque, S. (1999). Heart disease in women. *Am J Nurs* 99(4), 26-32.

Hillard, P. (1999). Diagnosing and controlling abnormal uterine bleeding. *Contemporary Adolescent Gynecology* 4(1), 4-11.

Hirata, J. (1997). Does dong quai have estrogenic effects on postmenopausal women? A double-blind, placebo-controlled trial. *Fertil Steril* 68(6), 981-986.

Isreal, D., & Youngkin, E. (1997). Herbal therapies for perimenopausal and menopausal complaints. *Pharmacotherapy* 17(5), 970-984.

Keller, C., Fullerton, J., & Fleury, J. (1998). Primary and secondary strategies among older postmenopausal women. *J Nurse Midwifery* 43(4), 262-272.

Kendig, S., & Sanford, D. (1998). *Midlife and menopause: Celebrating women's health*. Washington, DC: AWHONN.

Kessenich, C. (1996). Update on pharmacologic therapies for osteoporosis. *Nurs Pract* 21(8), 19-24.

Kettel, L. et al. (1998). Preliminary report on the treatment of endometriosis with low-dose mifepristone (RU 486). *Am J Obstet Gynecol* 178, 1151-1156.

Kiningham, R., Apgar, B., & Schwenk, T. (1996). Evaluation of amenorrhea. *Am Fam Physician* 53(4), 1185-1194.

Lemcke, D., Marshal, L., & Pattison, J. (1995). Menopause and hormone replacement therapy. In D. Lemcke et al. (Eds.). *Primary care of women*. East Norwalk, CT: Appleton & Lange.

Levine, S. (1998). The sexual consequences of perimenopause and menopause. *Women's Health in Primary Care* 1(6), 509-513.

Liberman, S. (1998). A review of effectiveness of cimicufuga nacemosa (black cohosh) for the symptoms of menopause. *J Womens Health* 7(5), 525-529.

Lindsay, R. et al. (1996). Therapeutic controversy. *J Clin Endocrinol Metab* 81, 3829-3838.

Lindsay, S., & Claywell, L. (1998). Considering soy: Its estrogenic effects may protect women. *Lifelines* 2(1), 41-44.

Lipscomb, G., & Ling, F. (1997). Chronic pelvic pain and dysmenorrhea. In S. Scott & S. McNeeley (Eds.). *Gynecology for the primary care provider.* Philadelphia: W.B. Saunders.

Lowdermilk, D., & Fogel, C. (1996). *Health care issues of midlife women.* Edwardsville, KS: Educational Software.

McAllister, M. (1998). Menopause: Providing comprehensive care for women in transition. *Primary Care Practice* 2(3), 256-274.

McClung, B. (1999). Using osteoporosis management to reduce fractures in elderly women. *Nurs Pract* 24(3), 26-42.

McGee, G. (1997). Secondary amenorrhea leading to osteoporosis: Incidence and prevention. *Nurs Pract* 22(5), 38, 41-45.

Mehring, P. (1997). Dysfunctional uterine bleeding. *Adv Nurse Pract* 5(1), 26.

Mishell, D. et al. (1997). *Comprehensive gynecology* (3rd ed.). St. Louis: Mosby.

Moore, A., & Noonan, M. (1996). A nurse's guide to hormone replacement therapy. *J Obstet Gynecol Neonatal Nurs* 25(1), 24-31.

National Women's Health Report. (1999). Fitness and nutrition after menopause. *National Women's Health Report* 21(1), 7.

NCEP. (1993). Summary of the second report of the National Cholesterol Education Program (NCEP) expert panel on detection, evaluation, and treatment of high blood cholesterol in adults (Adult Treatment Panel II). *JAMA* 269, 3015-3025.

Nicol-Smith, L. (1996). Causality, menopause, and depression: A critical review of the literature. *BMJ* 313(7067), 1229-1232.

Notelovitz, M. (1997). Osteoporosis: Alternatives for keeping bones strong. *Cont Nurse Pract* Spring, 7-19.

Parazzini, F. et al. (1994). Cigarette smoking, alcohol consumption, and risk of primary dysmenorrhea. *Epidemiology* 5(4), 469-472.

PEPI. (1995). Effects of estrogen or estrogen/progestin regimens on heart disease risk factors in postmenopausal women. *JAMA* 273(3), 199-208.

Ramsay, L., Ross, B., & Fischer, R. (1999). Phytoestrogens and the management of menopause. *Adv Nurse Pract* 7(5), 26-30.

Rosenfeld, R. (1996). Treatment of menorrhagia due to dysfunctional uterine bleeding. *Am Fam Physician* 53(1), 166-172.

Ryan, I., & Taylor, R. (1997). Endometriosis and infertility: New concepts. *Obstet Gynecol Surv* 52(6), 365-371.

Sangi-Haghpeykar, H., & Poindexter, A. (1995). Epidemiology of endometriosis among parous women. *Obstet Gynecol* 85(6), 983-992.

Shaw, C. (1997). Perimenopausal hot flash: Epidemiology, physiology, and treatment. *Nurs Pract* 22(3), 55-66.

Speroff, L., Glass, R., & Kase, N. (1999). *Clinical gynecologic endocrinology and infertility* (6th ed.). Baltimore: Lippincott/Williams & Wilkins.

Stanford, J. et al. (1995). Combined estrogen and progestin hormone replacement therapy in relation to risk of breast cancer in middle-aged women. *JAMA* 274:137-142.

Starr, W., Lommel, L., & Shanon, M. (1995). *Women's primary health care, protocols for practice.* Washington, DC: American Nurses Publishing.

Taylor, M. (1997). Alternative to conventional hormone replacement therapy. *Compr Ther* 23(8), 514-532.

Udoff, L., Langenberg, P., & Adashi, E. (1995). Combined continuous hormone replacement therapy: A critical review. *Obstet Gynecol* 85, 306-316.

Warren, M., & Kulak, J. (1999). Benefits and drawbacks of hormone replacement therapy. *Women's Health in Primary Care* 2(3), 21-33.

West, R. (1998). The female athlete. The triad of disordered eating, amenorrhea, and osteoporosis. *Sports Med* 26(2), 63-71.

Woods, N. (1995). Women's bodies. In C. Fogel & N. Woods (Eds.). *Women's health care.* Thousand Oaks, CA: Sage.

8

Sexually Transmitted Diseases and Other Infections

Catherine Ingram Fogel

LEARNING OBJECTIVES

- Define the key terms.
- Describe prevention of sexually transmitted infections in women.
- Differentiate signs, symptoms, diagnosis, and management of women with sexually transmitted infections.
- Identify differences in management for pregnant women with sexually transmitted infections.
- Summarize the care of women with selected viral infections (human immunodeficiency virus; hepatitis A, B, C).

- Discuss the effect of group B streptococcus (GBS) on pregnancy and management of pregnant clients with GBS.
- Compare and contrast signs, symptoms, and management of selected vaginal infections.
- Review principles of infection control.
- Identify topics for nursing research related to sexually transmitted infections.

KEY TERMS

bacterial vaginosis
human immunodeficiency virus (HIV)
human papillomavirus (HPV)

pelvic inflammatory disease (PID)
sexually transmitted diseases (STDs)
sexually transmitted infections (STIs)

Standard Precautions
veneral disease
vulvovaginitis

exually transmitted diseases (STDs), or **sexually transmitted infections (STIs),** are infections or infectious disease syndromes primarily transmitted by close, intimate contact (Box 8-1). These terms, used interchangeably in this text, have replaced the older designation, **venereal disease,** which primarily described gonorrhea and syphilis. Caused by a wide spectrum of bacteria, viruses, protozoa, and ectoparasites (organisms that live on the outside of the body such as a louse), STDs are a direct cause of tremendous human suffering, place heavy demands on health care services, and cost hundreds of millions of dollars to treat (Fogel, 1995). The term *sexually transmitted disease* is not specific for any one disease; rather the term includes more

than 25 infectious organisms that are transmitted through sexual activity and the dozens of clinical syndromes that they cause (Institute of Medicine, Committee on Prevention and Control of Sexually Transmitted Diseases, 1997). Despite the U.S. Surgeon General targeting STDs as a priority for prevention and control efforts, STDs are among the most common health problems in the United States (Institute of Medicine, Committee on Prevention and Control of Sexually Transmitted Diseases, 1997). The Centers for Disease Control and Prevention (CDC) estimates that more than 12 million Americans are infected with STDs every year (Centers for Disease Control and Prevention, Division of STD/HIV Prevention, 1995). The

144

BOX 8-1 Sexually Transmitted Diseases

BACTERIA
Chlamydia
Gonorrhea
Syphilis
Chancroid
Lymphogranuloma venereum
Genital mycoplasmas
Group B streptococci

VIRUSES
Human immunodeficiency virus *HIV*
Herpes simplex virus, types 1 and 2
Cytomegalovirus
Viral hepatitis A and B
Human papillomavirus

PROTOZOA
Trichomoniasis

PARASITES
Pediculosis (may or may not be sexually transmitted)
Scabies (may or may not be sexually transmitted)

BOX 8-2 Assessing STD/HIV Risk Behaviors

Answer these questions for all the times in your life from 1977* to now.

SEXUAL RISK
Are you sexually active now?
If no, have you had sex in the past?
Ever had an oral, vaginal, or anal sexual experience with another person?
With how many different people? 1? 2 or 3? 4 to 10? More than 10?
Have your partners been men, women, both?
Ever thought that a sex partner put you at risk for AIDS/STD (IV drug user, bisexual)?
Ever had an STD (herpes, gonorrhea, genital warts, chlamydia)?
Ever had sex against your will?
What do you do to protect yourself from AIDS/STDs?
Do you use male condoms? Female condoms? Other barriers?

DRUG USE–RELATED RISK
Ever injected drugs using shared equipment, including street drugs, steroids?
Ever had sex with a person who uses and shares?
Ever had sex while stoned, high, or drunk, so that you can't remember the details?
Ever exchanged sex for drugs, money, shelter?

BLOOD-RELATED RISKS
Ever had a blood transfusion?
Ever had sex with a person who had a blood transfusion?
Ever had sex with a person with hemophilia?
Ever received donor semen, egg, transplanted organ or tissue?
Ever shared equipment for tattoo, body piercing?

OTHER
Ever had a test for HIV?
Ever worried about AIDS and would like to talk with someone about it?

Adapted from Hatcher, R. et al. (1998). *Contraceptive Technology* (17th ed.). New York: Ardent Media Inc.
*Relates to risk of HIV–infection not known to exist in humans until this time.

most common STDs or STIs in women are chlamydia, human papillomavirus, gonorrhea, herpes simplex virus type 2, syphilis, and human immunodeficiency virus infection and are discussed in this chapter. Neonatal effects are discussed in Chapter 39.

PREVENTION

Preventing infection (primary prevention) is the most effective way of reducing the adverse consequences of STDs for women and for society. With the advent of serious and potentially lethal STDs that are not readily cured or are incurable, primary prevention becomes critical. Prompt diagnosis and treatment of current infections (secondary prevention) also can prevent personal complications and transmission to others.

Preventing the spread of STDs requires that women at risk for transmitting or acquiring infections change their behavior. A critical first step is for the nurse to include questions about a woman's sexual history, sexual risk behaviors, and drug-related risky behaviors as a part of her assessment (Box 8-2). When risk factors or risky behaviors are identified, the nurse has an opportunity to provide prevention counseling. Techniques that are effective in providing prevention counseling include using open-ended questions, using understandable language, and reassuring the woman that treatment will be provided regardless of consideration such as ability to pay, language spoken, or lifestyle (Centers for Disease Control and Prevention, 1998a). Prevention

messages should include descriptions of specific actions to be taken to avoid acquiring or transmitting STDs (e.g., refrain from sexual activity if you have STD-related symptoms) and should be tailored to the individual woman with attention given to her specific risk factors.

To be motivated to take preventive actions, a woman must believe that catching a disease will be serious for her

RESEARCH

Individual, Family, and Relationship Predictors of Young Women's Sexual Risk Perceptions

Unlike past decades, when the primary sexual risk was unintended pregnancy, the risks of the 1990s include a multitude of sexually transmitted diseases (STDs), including human immunodeficiency virus (HIV) infection. Of the millions of new STD cases reported annually, most occur in adolescents and adults in their early twenties. In addition, women now constitute the fastest-growing group of newly acquired immunodeficiency syndrome (AIDS) cases. Given the current rates of STD and HIV infection among young women, and accepting that the perception of self-risk is necessary for risk-reducing behavior change, it is important to identify those factors that promote or impede women's perceptions of their risk for acquiring an STD.

The purpose of this study was to identify the individual, dyad, and family factors that influence the STD risk perceptions of young heterosexual women. A cross-sectional telephone survey using forced choice questioning was the design method used. A convenience sample of 93 young (17 to 26 years old), sexually active, unmarried, heterosexual women was studied. Respondents were asked to estimate their own level of risk for STDs, including HIV. The study results revealed that communication with parents about sexual risk, consistent condom use, relationship satisfaction, and perceiving the partner as no risk were significant predictors of women's perceptions of "no risk" at the $p < .05$ level.

CLINICAL APPLICATION

Nurses can incorporate these and other study findings into the design of sexual risk reduction programs. Programs that enhance parent-teen communication about sexual risks and assist young women to examine their perceptions of their partners may be more effective than programs that provide information only. Nurses should dispel myths equating risk with certain types of people and assist women to personalize and recognize their risk. In addition to recognizing and personalizing the risk for STDs and HIV, nurses should encourage women to practice safer sex behaviors until both partners are clinically documented as free of HIV and STDs.

Source: Hutchinson, M. (1999). Individual, family, and relationship predictors of young women's sexual risk perceptions. *J Obstet Gynecol Neonatal Nurs* 28(1), 60-67.

and that she is at risk for infection. Unfortunately most individuals tend to underestimate their personal risk of infection in a given situation. Thus many women may not perceive themselves as being at risk for contracting an STD, and telling them that they need to carry condoms may not be well received. Though levels of awareness of STDs are generally high, widespread misconceptions or specific gaps in knowledge also exist. Therefore nurses have a responsibility to ensure that their clients have accurate, complete knowledge about transmission and symptoms of STDs and risky behaviors that place them at risk for contracting an infection (see Research box).

Primary preventive measures are individual activities aimed at deterring infection. Risk-free options include complete abstinence from sexual activities that transmit semen, blood, or other body fluids or that allow for skin-to-skin contact (Hatcher et al., 1998). Alternatively, involvement in a mutually monogamous relationship with an uninfected partner also eliminates risk of contracting STDs. When neither of these options is realistic for a woman, however, the nurse must focus on other, more feasible measures.

Safer Sex Practices

An essential component of primary prevention is counseling women regarding safer sex practices, including knowledge of her partner, reduction of number of partners, low risk sex, and avoiding the exchange of body fluids.

No aspect of prevention is more important than knowing one's partner. Reducing the number of partners and avoiding partners who have had many previous sexual partners decreases a woman's chance of contracting an STD. Deciding not to have sexual contact with casual acquaintances also may be helpful. Discussing each new partner's previous sexual history and exposure to STDs will augment other efforts to reduce risk. Cochran and Mays (1990) reported that sizable percentages of men (39%) and women (10%) report lying in order to have sex. Thus women must be cautioned that safer sex measures are always advisable, even when partners insist otherwise. Critically important is whether male partners resist or accept wearing condoms. This is crucial when women are not sure about their partner's history. Women should be cautioned against making decisions about a partner's sexual and other behaviors based on appearances and unfounded assumptions such as the following (Hatcher et al., 1998):

- Single people have many partners and risky practices.
- Older people have few partners and infrequent sexual encounters.
- Sexually experienced people know how to practice safer sex.
- Married people are heterosexual, low risk, and monogamous.
- People who look healthy are healthy.
- People with good jobs do not use drugs.

TABLE 8-1 Safer Sex Guidelines

SAFEST	LOW RISK	POSSIBLY RISKY (POSSIBLE EXPOSURE)	HIGH RISK (UNSAFE)
Behavior:	*Behavior:*	*Behavior:*	*Behavior:*
Abstinence	Wet kissing*	Cunnilingus†	Unprotected anal intercourse
Self-masturbation	Vaginal intercourse with condom	Fellatio‡	Unprotected vaginal intercourse
Monogamous (both partners and no high risk activities)	Anal intercourse with condom	Mutual masturbation with skin breaks	Oral-anal contact
Hugging,* massage,* touching*	Urine contact with intact skin	Vaginal intercourse after anal contact without new condom	Any sex (fisting, rough vaginal or anal intercourse, rape) that causes tissue damage or bleeding
Dry kissing			Multiple sexual partners
Mutual masturbation§			Sharing sex toys, douche equipment
Drug abstinence			Sharing needles
Sexual fantasy			Blood contact, including menstrual blood
Erotic conversation, books, movies, video			
Erotic bathing, showering			
Eroticizing feet, fingers, buttocks, abdomen, ears			
Prevention	*Prevention:*	*Prevention:*	*Prevention:*
Avoid high risk behaviors	Avoid exposure to potentially infected body fluids	Use dental dam or female condom with cunnilingus	Avoid exposure to potentially infected body fluids
	Consistent use of condom and spermicide	Use condom with fellatio	Use condom and spermicide consistently
	Avoid anal intercourse	Use latex gloves	Avoid anal penetration
			If anal penetration occurs, use condom with intercourse, latex glove with hand penetration
			Avoid oral-anal contact
			Do not share sex toys, needles, douching equipment
			If sharing needles, clean with bleach before and after use.

Adapted from Centers for Disease Control and Prevention. (1998a). 1998 guidelines for treatment of sexually transmitted diseases. *MMWR* 47(RR-1), 1-117; Fogel, C. (1995). Sexually transmitted disease. In C. Fogel & N. Woods (Eds.). *Women's healthcare.* Thousand Oaks, CA: Sage; Starr, W., Lommel, L., & Shanon, M. (1995). *Women's primary health care. Protocols for practice.* Washington, DC: American Nurses Publishing.
*Assumes no breaks in skin.
†Cunnilingus: oral stimulation of the female genitalia.
‡Fellatio: oral stimulation of the male genitalia.
§Assumes no contact with semen or vaginal secretions.

Sexually active persons also may benefit from carefully examining a partner for lesions, sores, ulcerations, rashes, redness, discharge, swelling, and odor before initiating sexual activity.

Women should be taught low risk sexual practices and which sexual practices to avoid (Table 8-1). Sexual fantasizing is safe, as are caressing, hugging, body rubbing, and massage. Mutual masturbation is low risk as long as there is no contact with a partner's semen or vaginal secretions. All sexual activities when both partners are monogamous, trustworthy, and known to be free of disease (by testing) are safe.

The physical barrier promoted for the prevention of sexual transmission of human immunodeficiency virus and other STIs is the male condom. Nurses can help motivate clients to use condoms by first discussing the subject with them. This gives women permission to discuss any concerns, misconceptions, or hesitations they may have about using condoms. The nurse may initiate a discussion of how to purchase and use a condom. Information to be discussed includes the importance of using latex or plastic condoms rather than natural skin condoms for STI protection. The nurse should remind women to use a condom with every sexual encounter, to use each one only once, to use a condom with a current expiration date, and to handle it carefully to avoid damaging it with fingernails, teeth, or other sharp objects. Condoms should be stored away from high heat. Though not ideal, women may choose to safely carry condoms in wallets, shoes, or inside a bra. Women can be taught the differences between condoms, price ranges, sizes, and where they can be purchased. Explicit instructions for how to apply a male condom are included in Box 9-3.

The female condom—a lubricated polyurethane sheath with a ring on each end that is inserted into the vagina—is also an effective mechanical barrier to virus, including human immunodeficiency virus (Centers for Disease Control and Prevention, 1998a). Furthermore, clinical studies have documented its effectiveness in providing protection from recurrent trichomoniasis. If used consistently and correctly, the female condom should reduce the risk of contracting or transmitting an STI. Whether condoms lubricated with spermicide are more effective than other lubricated condoms in protecting against STIs (including human immunodeficiency virus) has not been established, nor has it been determined that condoms used with vaginal spermicides are more effective in preventing STI (including human immunodeficiency virus) transmission than when used without spermicide (Centers for Disease Control and Prevention, 1998a). What is important and should be stressed by nurses is the consistent use of condoms for every act of sexual intimacy where there is the possibility of transmission of disease.

With most of the condoms now available to American women, active male cooperation is essential. A key issue in condom usage as a preventive strategy is to stress to women that in sexual encounters, men must comply with a woman's suggestion or request that they use a condom. Moreover, condom usage must be renegotiated with every sexual contact, and women must address the issue of control of sexual decision making every time they request a male partner to use a condom. Women may fear that their partner would be offended if a condom were introduced. Some women may fear rejection and abandonment, conflict, potential violence, or loss of economic support if they suggest the use of condoms to prevent STI transmission (Hatcher et al., 1998). For many individuals condoms are symbols of extrarelationship activity. Introduction of a condom into a long-term relationship where they have not been used previously threatens the trust assumed in most long-term relationships.

Many women do not anticipate or prepare for sexual activity in advance; embarrassment or discomfort in purchasing condoms may prevent some women from using them. Cultural barriers also may impede the use of condoms; for example, Latino gender roles make it difficult for Latina women to suggest using condoms to a partner. Suggesting condom use implies that a woman is sexually active, that she is "available" for sex, and that she is "seeking" sex; these are messages that many women are un-

comfortable conveying given the prevailing mores of our country. In a society that commonly views a woman who carries a condom as overprepared, possibly oversexed, and willing to have sex with any man, expecting her to insist on the use of condoms in a sexual encounter is unrealistic.

Finally, women should be counseled to watch out for situations that make it hard to talk about and practice safer sex. These include romantic times when condoms are not available and when alcohol or drugs make it impossible to make wise decisions about safer sex.

Certain sexual practices should be avoided in order to reduce one's risk of infection. Abstinence from any sexual activities that could result in exchange of infective body fluids will help decrease risk. Anal-genital intercourse, anal-oral contact, and anal-digital activity are high risk sexual behaviors and should be avoided (Hatcher et al., 1998). Sexual transmission occurs through direct skin or mucous membrane contact with infectious lesions or body fluids. Because mucosal linings are delicate and subject to considerable mechanical trauma during intercourse, small abrasions often may occur, facilitating entry of infectious agents into the bloodstream. The rectal epithelium is especially easy to traumatize with penetration. Sexual practices that increase the likelihood of tissue damage or bleeding, such as fisting (inserting a fist into the rectum), should be avoided. Deep kissing when lips, gums, or other tissues are raw or broken also should be avoided (Hatcher et al., 1998). Because enteric infections are transmitted by oral-fecal contact, avoiding oral-anal activities, "rimming" (licking the anal area), and digital-anal activities should reduce the likelihood of infection. Vaginal intercourse should never follow anal contact unless a condom has been used and then removed and replaced with a new condom.

Nurses must suggest strategies to enhance a woman's condom negotiation and communication skills. Suggesting that she talk with her partner about condom use at a time removed from sexual activity may make it easier to bring up the subject. Role playing possible partner reactions with a woman and her alternative responses can be helpful. Asking a woman who appears particularly uncomfortable to rehearse how she might approach the topic is useful, particularly when a woman fears her partner may be resistant. The nurse might suggest her client begin by saying, "I need to talk with you about something that is important to both of us. It's hard for me, and I feel embarrassed, but I think we need to talk about safe sex." If women are able to sort out their feelings and fears before talking with their partners, they may feel more comfortable and in control of the situation. Women can be reassured that it is natural to be uncomfortable and that the hardest part is getting started. Nurses should help their clients clarify what they will and will not do sexually because it is easier to discuss it if they are clear. Women can be reminded that their partner may need time to think about what they have said and that they must pay attention to their partner's response. If the partner seems to be having difficulty with the discussion, a woman may slow down and wait a while. She can be reminded that if her partner resists safer sex, she may wish to reconsider the relationship.

Women may delay seeking care for STDs because they fear social stigma, they have little accessibility to health care services, they are asymptomatic, or they are unaware that they have an infection.

BACTERIAL SEXUALLY TRANSMITTED DISEASES

Chlamydia

Chlamydia trachomatis is the most common and fastest spreading STD in American women, with an estimated 2.6 million new cases each year (Institute of Medicine, Committee on Prevention and Control of Sexually Transmitted Diseases, 1997). These infections are often silent and highly destructive; their sequelae and complications can be very serious. In women, chlamydial infections are difficult to diagnose; the symptoms, if present, are nonspecific, and the organism is expensive to culture.

Early identification of *C. trachomatis* is important because untreated infection often leads to acute salpingitis or pelvic inflammatory disease. Pelvic inflammatory disease is the most serious complication of chlamydial infections, and past chlamydial infections are associated with an increased risk of ectopic pregnancy and tubal factor infertility. Furthermore, chlamydial infection of the cervix causes inflammation resulting in microscopic cervical ulcerations and thus may increase the risk of acquiring human immunodeficiency virus infection. Two thirds of infants born to mothers with chlamydia will develop conjunctivitis or pneumonia following perinatal exposure to the mother's infected cervix (Youngkin, 1995). Chlamydia is the most common infectious cause of ophthalmia neonatorum. Neonatal ocular prophylaxis with silver nitrate solution or antibiotic ointment does not prevent perinatal transmission from mother to infant, nor does it adequately treat chlamydial infection. Systemic treatment with erythromycin is recommended (Centers for Disease Control and Prevention, 1998a).

Sexually active women younger than age 20 years are two to three times as likely to become infected with chlamydia as women between 20 and 29 years. Women over age 30 have the lowest rate of infection. Risky behaviors, including multiple partners and nonuse of barrier methods of birth control, increase a woman's risk of chlamydial infection. Lower socioeconomic status may be a risk factor, especially with respect to treatment-seeking behaviors.

Screening and Diagnosis

In addition to obtaining information regarding the presence of risk factors, the nurse should inquire about the presence of any symptoms. The CDC (Centers for Disease Control and Prevention, 1998a) strongly urges screening of asymptomatic, high risk women in whom infection would otherwise go undetected. CDC guidelines recommend screening of sexually active adolescents, women between ages 20 and 34 years, women who do not use barrier contraceptives, and women with new or multiple partners. In addition, whenever possible, all women with two or more of the risk factors for chlamydia should be cultured. All pregnant women should have cervical cultures for chlamydia at the first prenatal visit. Reculturing late in the third trimester (36 weeks) should be carried out if the woman was positive previously or if she is less than age 25 years or has a new sex partner or multiple sex partners.

Although usually asymptomatic, some women may experience spotting or postcoital bleeding, mucoid or purulent cervical discharge, or dysuria. Bleeding results from inflammation and erosion of the cervical columnar epithelium. Women on oral contraceptives may also experience breakthrough bleeding.

Diagnosis of chlamydia is by culture; these are expensive, require special transport and storage, and take up to 10 days for results. The test procedure requires collection of a sample that contains many epithelial cells. Endocervical (columnar) cells are required; cell scrapings provide better specimens, so the cervix should be swabbed with cotton or rayon swabs before collecting the specimen to remove mucus and discharge from the cervical os. Special culture media and proper handling of specimens are important, so the nurse should always know what is required in her individual practice site. Chlamydial culture testing is not always available, primarily because of expense.

Management

CDC recommendations for treatment of urethral, cervical, and rectal chlamydial infections are doxycycline (100 mg orally twice a day for 7 days) or azithromycin (1 g orally in a single dose) (Table 8-2) (Centers for Disease Control and Prevention, 1998a). Azithromycin is often prescribed when compliance may be a problem because only one dose is needed; however, expense is a concern with this medication. If the woman is pregnant, erythromycin (500 mg orally four times a day for 7 days) or amoxicillin (500 mg orally three times a day for 7 days) is used. Women who have a chlamydial infection and are also infected with human immunodeficiency virus should be treated with the same regimen as those who are not infected with human immunodeficiency virus.

Because chlamydia is often asymptomatic, the woman should be cautioned to take all medication prescribed. All exposed sexual partners should be treated. Woman treated with doxycycline or azithromycin do not need to be retested unless symptoms continue. Women treated with erythromycin may be retested 3 weeks after completing the medication, although the validity of this practice has not been established (Centers for Disease Control and Prevention, 1998a).

TABLE 8-2 Sexually Transmitted Diseases and Drug Therapies for Women

DISEASE	NONPREGNANT WOMEN 13-17 YEARS	NONPREGNANT WOMEN > 18 YEARS	PREGNANT WOMEN	LACTATING WOMEN
Chlamydia	*Recommended:* Azithromycin 1 g orally once or Doxycycline 100 mg orally bid for 7 days *Alternatives:* Erythromycin or sulfisoxazole regimens	*Recommended:* Azithromycin 1 g orally once or Doxycycline 100 mg orally bid for 7 days *Alternatives:* Erythromycin base 500 mg orally qid for 7 days or Erythromycin ethylsuccinate 800 mg orally qid for 7 days or Ofloxacin 300 mg orally bid for 7 days	*Recommended:* Erythromycin base 500 mg orally qid for 7 days or Amoxicillin 500 mg orally tid for 14 days *Alternatives:* Erythromycin base 250 mg orally qid for 14 days or Erythromycin ethylsuccinate 800 mg orally qid for 7 days or Erythromycin ethylsuccinate 400 mg orally qid for 14 days or Azithromycin 1 g orally once (safety not established)	*Recommended:* Erythromycin base 500 mg orally qid for 7 days *Alternatives:* Erythomycin 250 mg orally qid for 14 days or Erythromycin ethylsuccinate 800 mg orally qid for 7 days or Erythromycin ethylsuccinate 400 mg orally qid for 14 days
Gonorrhea	*Recommended:* Ceftriaxone 125 mg IM once PLUS Doxycycline 100 mg orally bid for 7 days (Quinolones are not recommended for women under 18)	*Recommended:* Cefixime 400 mg orally once or Ceftriaxone 125 mg IM once or Ciprofloxacin 500 mg orally once or Ofloxacin 400 mg orally once PLUS Azithromycin 1 g orally once or Doxycycline 100 mg orally bid for 7 days	*Recommended:* Ceftriaxone 125 mg IM once If cephalosporin allergic: Spectinomycin 2 g IM once PLUS Erythromycin base 500 mg orally qid for 7 days or Amoxicillin 500 mg orally tid for 14 days	*Recommended:* Ceftriaxone 125 mg IM once PLUS Erythromycin base 500 mg orally qid for 7 days If cephlosporin allergic: Spectinomycin 2 g IM once PLUS Erythromycin base 500 mg orally qid for 7 days
Syphilis	Primary, secondary, early latent disease *Recommended:* Benzathine penicillin G 2.4 million units IM once	Primary, secondary, early latent disease *Recommended:* Benzathine penicillin G 2.4 million units IM once	Primary, secondary, early latent disease *Recommended:* Benzathine penicillin G 2.4 million units IM once	Primary, secondary, early latent disease *Recommended:* Benzathine penicillin G 2.4 million units IM once

TABLE 8-2 Sexually Transmitted Diseases and Drug Therapies for Women—cont'd

DISEASE	NONPREGNANT WOMEN 13-17 YEARS	NONPREGNANT WOMEN > 18 YEARS	PREGNANT WOMEN	LACTATING WOMEN
Syphilis—cont'd	Late latent or unknown duration disease *Recommended:* Benzathine penicillin G 7.2 million units total, administered as three doses 2.4 million units each at 1-wk intervals Penicillin allergy: Doxyclycine 100 mg orally bid for 14 days or Tetracycline 500 mg orally qid for 14 days	Late latent or unknown duration disease *Recommended:* Benzathine penicillin G 7.2 million units total, administered as three doses 2.4 million units each at 1-wk intervals Penicillin allergy: Doxyclycine 100 mg orally bid for 14 days or Tetracycline 500 mg orally qid for 14 days	Primary, secondary, early latent disease *Recommended:* Benzathine penicillin G 2.4 million units IM once (some experts recommend second dose of benzathine penicillin 2.4 million units 1 wk later) Late latent or unknown duration disease *Recommended:* Benzathine penicillin G 7.2 million units total, administered as three doses 2.4 million units each at 1-wk intervals No proven alternatives to penicillin in pregnancy; pregnant women with history of allergy to penicillin should be desensitized and treated with penicillin	Primary, secondary, early latent disease *Recommended:* Benzathine penicillin G 2.4 million units IM once (some experts recommend second dose of benzathine penicillin 2.4 million units 1 wk later)
Human papillomavirus	Recommended for external genital warts *Client applied:* Podofilox 0.5% solution or gel to wart bid for 3 days followed by 4-day rest for up to four cycles or Imiquimod 5% cream at bedtime 3 times a week for up to 16 weeks *Provider applied:* Cryotherapy with liquid nitrogen or cryoprobe or	Recommended for external genital warts *Client applied:* Podofilox 0.5% solution or gel to wart bid for 3 days followed by 4-day rest for up to four cycles or Imiquimod 5% cream at bedtime 3 times a week for up to 16 weeks *Provider applied:* Cryotherapy with liquid nitrogen or cryoprobe or	Recommended for external genital warts *Provider applied:* Cryotherapy with liquid nitrogen or cryoprobe or TCA or BCA 80%-90% applied weekly Imiquimod, podophyllin, and podofilox should not be used in pregnancy	Recommended for external genital warts *Provider applied:* Cryotherapy with liquid nitrogen or cryoprobe or TCA or BCA 80%-90% applied weekly Imiquimod, podophyllin, and podofilox should not be used during lactation

Continued

TABLE 8-2 Sexually Transmitted Diseases and Drug Therapies for Women—cont'd

DISEASE	NONPREGNANT WOMEN 13-17 YEARS	NONPREGNANT WOMEN > 18 YEARS	PREGNANT WOMEN	LACTATING WOMEN
Human papillomavirus—cont'd	Podophyllin resin 10%-25% in tincture of benzoin compound weekly (wash off in 1-4 hr); repeat weekly as necessary or Trichoacetic acid (TCA) or bichoacetic acid (BCA) 80%-90% applied weekly	Podophyllin resin 10%-25% in tincture of benzoin compound weekly (wash off in 1-4 hr); repeat weekly as necessary or TCA or BCA 80%-90% applied weekly		
Genital herpes simplex virus (HSV type 1 or 2)	Primary infection: Acyclovir 400 mg orally tid for 7-10 days or Acyclovir 200 mg orally 5 times a day for 7-10 days or Famciclovir 250 mg orally tid for 7-10 days or Valacyclovir 1 g orally bid for 7-10 days Recurrent infection: Acyclovir 400 mg orally tid for 5 days or Acyclovir 200 mg orally 5 times a day for 5 days or Acyclovir 800 mg orally bid for 5 days or Famciclovir 125 mg orally bid for 5 days or Valacyclovir 500 mg orally bid for 5 days Suppression therapy: Acyclovir 400 mg orally bid or Famciclovir 250 mg orally bid or	Primary infection: Acyclovir 400 mg orally tid for 7-10 days or Acyclovir 200 mg orally 5 times a day for 7-10 days or Famciclovir 250 mg orally tid for 7-10 days or Valacyclovir 1 g orally bid for 7-10 days Recurrent infection: Acyclovir 400 mg orally tid for 5 days or Acyclovir 200 mg orally 5 times a day for 5 days or Acyclovir 800 mg orally bid for 5 days or Famciclovir 125 mg orally bid for 5 days or Valacyclovir 500 mg orally bid for 5 days Suppression therapy: Acyclovir 400 mg orally bid or Famciclovir 250 mg orally bid or	Safety of acyclovir, valacyclovir, and famciclovir not established in pregnancy	Safety of acyclovir, valacyclovir, and famciclovir not established in pregnancy

TABLE 8-2 Sexually Transmitted Diseases and Drug Therapies for Women—cont'd

DISEASE	NONPREGNANT WOMEN 13-17 YEARS	NONPREGNANT WOMEN > 18 YEARS	PREGNANT WOMEN	LACTATING WOMEN
Genital herpes simplex virus (HSV type 1 or 2)—cont'd	Valacyclovir 250 mg orally bid or Valacyclovir 500 mg orally qd or Valacyclovir 1000 mg orally qd	Valacyclovir 250 mg orally bid or Valacyclovir 500 mg orally qd or Valacyclovir 1000 mg orally qd		

Sources: Centers for Disease Control and Prevention. (1998a). 1998 guidelines for treatment of sexually transmitted diseases. *MMWR* 47(RR-1), 1-117; Youngkin, E. (1995). Sexually transmitted diseases: Current and emerging concerns. *J Obstet Gynecol Neonatal Nurs* 24(8), 743-758.

Gonorrhea

Gonorrhea is probably the oldest communicable disease in the United States. An estimated 800,000 American men and women contract gonorrhea each year. The incidence of drug-resistant cases of gonorrhea, in particular penicillinase-producing *Neisseria gonorrhoeae* (PPNG), is rising dramatically in the United States.

Gonorrhea is caused by the aerobic, gram-negative diplococci *Neisseria gonorrhoeae*. Gonorrhea is almost exclusively transmitted by the contact of sexual activity. The principal means of communication is genital-to-genital contact; however, it is also spread by oral-to-genital and anal-to-genital contact. There is also evidence that infection may spread in females from vagina to rectum. Gonorrhea also can be transmitted to the newborn in the form of ophthalmia neonatorum during birth by direct contact with gonococcal organisms in the cervix. Although the organism has been recovered from inanimate objects artificially inoculated with the bacteria, there is no evidence that natural transmission occurs this way (Schaffer, 1998).

Age is probably the most important risk factor associated with gonorrhea. The majority of those contracting gonorrhea are under 20 years of age. Traditionally the reported incidence of gonococcal disease has been higher in minority groups. Many of the apparent differences in infection rates can be explained by the disproportionate representation of African-Americans among the nation's poor and among inner city dwellers. Rates of gonorrhea are higher in urban areas than in rural areas, with even higher rates in the inner city. Adolescent females have the highest rates of infection, and the incidence is higher in African-American adolescents than in Hispanic or Caucasian teens (Bonny & Biro, 1998). Sex workers and their partners, intravenous drug users, and crack cocaine users are considered high risk groups. Other risk factors include early onset of sexual activity and multiple sexual partners.

Women are often asymptomatic, with one third of infections in adolescent women going unnoticed; when symptoms are present, they are often less specific than the symptoms in men. They may have a purulent endocervical discharge, but discharge is usually minimal or absent. Menstrual irregularities may be the presenting symptom, or women may complain of pain—chronic or acute severe pelvic or lower abdominal pain or longer, more painful menses. Infrequently, dysuria, vague abdominal pain, or low backache prompt woman to seek care. Gonococcal rectal infection may occur in women following anal intercourse, with 10% to 30% of urogenital infections accompanied by rectal infection. Individuals with rectal gonorrhea may be completely asymptomatic or, conversely, experience severe symptoms with profuse purulent anal discharge, rectal pain, and blood in the stool. Rectal itching, fullness, pressure, and pain are also common symptoms, as is diarrhea. A diffuse vaginitis with vulvitis is the most common form of gonococcal infection in prepubertal girls. There may be few signs of infection, or vaginal discharge, dysuria, and swollen, reddened labia may be present.

Gonococcal infections in pregnancy potentially affect both mother and infant. Women with cervical gonorrhea may develop salpingitis in the first trimester. Perinatal complications of gonococcal infection include premature rupture of membranes, preterm birth, chorioamnionitis, neonatal sepsis, intrauterine growth restriction, and maternal postpartum sepsis. Amniotic infection syndrome manifested by placental, fetal, and umbilical cord inflammation following premature rupture of the membranes may result from gonorrheal infections during pregnancy. Ophthalmia neonatorum, the most common manifestation of neonatal gonococcal infections, is highly contagious and if untreated may lead to blindness of the newborn.

Screening and Diagnosis

Because gonococcal infections in women often are asymptomatic, the CDC recommends screening all women at risk for gonorrhea (Centers for Disease Control and Prevention, 1998a). All pregnant women should be screened at the first prenatal visit and infected women and those identified with risky behaviors re-screened at 36 weeks of gestation. Gonococcal infection cannot be diagnosed reliably by clinical signs and symptoms alone. Individuals may have "classic" symptoms, vague symptoms that may be attributed to a number of conditions, or no symptoms at all. Cultures with selective media are considered the gold standard for diagnosis of gonorrhea. Cultures should be obtained from the endocervix, rectum, and when indicated the pharynx. Thayer-Martin cultures are recommended to diagnose gonorrhea in women. Any woman suspected of having gonorrhea should have a chlamydial culture and serologic test for syphilis if one has not been done in the past 2 months because coinfection is common.

Management

Management of gonorrhea is straightforward, and the cure is usually rapid with appropriate antibiotic therapy (see Table 8-2). Single-dose efficacy is a major consideration in selecting an antibiotic regimen for women with gonorrhea. Another important consideration is the high percentage (45%) of women with coexisting chlamydial infections. The treatment of choice for uncomplicated urethral, endocervical, and rectal infections in pregnant and nonpregnant women is ceftriaxone (125 mg IM once). The CDC suggests concomitant treatment for chlamydia because coinfection is common (Centers for Disease Control and Prevention, 1998a). All women with both gonorrhea and syphilis should also be treated for syphilis according to CDC guidelines (see discussion of syphilis in this chapter).

Gonorrhea is a highly communicable disease. Recent (past 30 days) sexual partners should be examined, cultured, and treated with appropriate regimens. Most treatment failures result from reinfection. The client needs to be informed of this, as well as of the consequences of reinfection in terms of chronicity, complications, and potential infertility. Women are counseled to use condoms. All clients with gonorrhea should be offered confidential counseling and testing for human immunodeficiency virus infection.

Gonorrhea is a reportable communicable disease. Health care providers are legally responsible for reporting all cases to the health authorities, usually the local health department in the client's county of residence. Women should be informed that the case will be reported, told why, and informed of the possibility of being contacted by a health department epidemiologist.

Treatment failure following combined ceftriaxone/doxycycline therapy is rare; therefore follow-up culture (test of cure) is not essential. A more cost-effective approach is reexamination with a culture 1 to 2 months after treatment. This approach will detect both treatment failures and reinfections. Clients also should be counseled to return if symptoms persist after treatment.

Syphilis

Syphilis, one of the earliest described sexually transmitted diseases, is caused by *Treponema pallidum*, a motile spiro-

chete. Transmission is thought to be by entry in the subcutaneous tissue through microscopic abrasions that can occur during sexual intercourse. The disease can also be transmitted through kissing, biting, or oral-genital sex. Transplacental transmission may occur at any time during pregnancy; the degree of risk is related to the quantity of spirochetes in the maternal bloodstream.

There are an estimated 120,000 new cases of syphilis in the United States each year. Rates are highest among young adult African-Americans in urban areas and in southern states (Centers for Disease Control and Prevention, 1998b). Much of the rise in cases seen since 1990 is directly attributable to illicit drug use—particularly crack cocaine—and the exchange of sex for drugs and money.

Syphilis is a complex disease that can lead to serious systemic disease and even death when untreated. Infection manifests itself in distinct stages with different symptoms and clinical manifestations. *Primary* syphilis is characterized by a primary lesion, the chancre, that appears 5 to 90 days after infection; this lesion often begins as a painless papule at the site of inoculation and then erodes to form a nontender, shallow, indurated, clean ulcer several millimeters to centimeters in size (Fig. 8-1). *Secondary* syphilis occurs 6 weeks to 6 months after the appearance

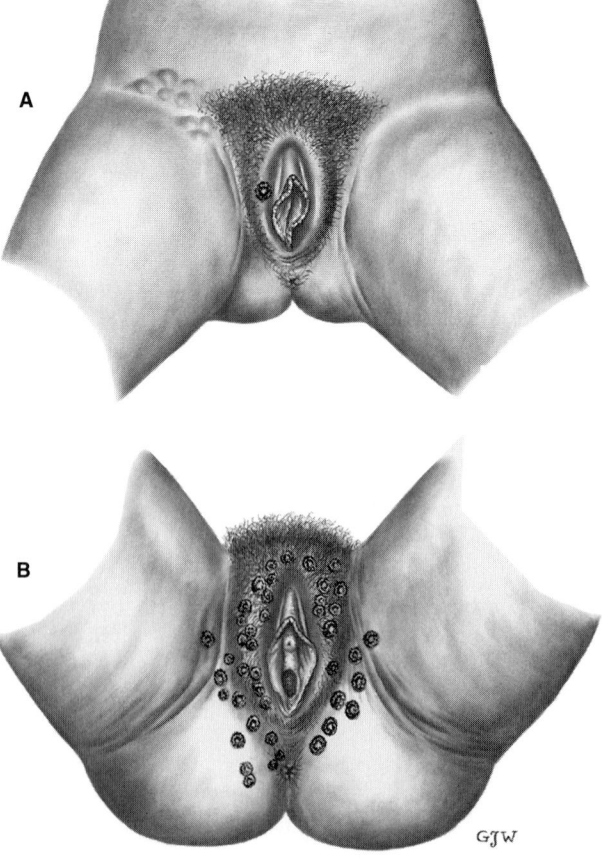

Fig. 8-1   Syphilis. **A,** Primary stage: chancre with inguinal adenopathy. **B,** Secondary stage: condylomata lata.

of the chancre and is characterized by a widespread, symmetric maculopapular rash on the palms and soles and generalized lymphadenopathy. The infected individual also may experience fever, headache, and malaise. Condylomata lata (broad, painless, pink-gray, wartlike infectious lesions) may develop on the vulva, perineum, or anus. If the woman is untreated, she enters a latent phase that is asymptomatic for the majority of individuals. If left untreated, about one third of these women will develop tertiary syphilis. Neurologic, cardiovascular, musculoskeletal, or multiorgan system complications can develop in the third stage.

Screening and Diagnosis

All women who are diagnosed with another STI or with human immunodeficiency virus should be screened for syphilis. All pregnant women should be screened for syphilis at the first prenatal visit and again in the late third trimester. Diagnosis is dependent on microscopic examination of primary and secondary lesion tissue and serology during latency and late infection. Any test for antibodies may not be reactive in the presence of active infection because it takes time for the body's immune system to develop antibodies to any antigens. Two types of serologic tests are used: nontreponemal and treponemal. Nontreponemal antibody tests such as the Venereal Disease Research Laboratories (VDRL) or rapid plasma reagin (RPR) are used as screening tests, and false-positive results are not unusual, particularly when conditions such as acute infection, autoimmune disorders, malignancy, pregnancy, and drug addiction exist and after immunization or vaccination. The treponemal tests, fluorescent treponemal antibody absorbed (FTA-ABS) and microhemagglutination assays for antibody to *T. pallidum* (MHA-TP), are used to confirm positive results. Test results in clients with early primary or incubating syphilis may be negative. Seroconversion usually takes place 6 to 8 weeks after exposure, so testing should be repeated in 1 to 2 months when a suspicious genital lesion exists. Positive treponemal antibody tests stay positive for life regardless of treatment or disease activity (Centers for Disease Control and Prevention, 1998a).

Tests for concomitant STIs should be done, for example wet preps and cultures, and human immunodeficiency virus testing offered if indicated.

Management

Penicillin is the preferred drug for treating clients with syphilis (see Table 8-2). It is the only proven therapy that has been widely used for clients with neurosyphilis, congenital syphilis, or syphilis during pregnancy. Intramuscular benzathine penicillin G (2.4 million units IM once) is used to treat primary, secondary, and early latent syphilis. Women with syphilis of greater than 1 year's duration (late latent or tertiary stages) require weekly treatment of 2.4 million units of benzathine penicillen G for 3 weeks.

Although doxycycline, tetracycline, and erythromycin are alternative treatments for penicillin-allergic clients, both tetracycline and doxycycline are contraindicated in pregnancy, and erythromycin is unlikely to cure a fetal infection. Therefore pregnant women should, if necessary, receive skin testing and be treated with penicillin, or be desensitized (Centers for Disease Control and Prevention, 1998a). Specific protocols are recommended by the CDC.

NURSE ALERT

Clients treated for syphilis may experience a Jarisch-Herxheimer reaction. This is an acute febrile reaction often accompanied by headache, myalgias, and arthralgias that develop within the first 24 hours of treatment. Women treated in the second half of pregnancy are at risk for preterm labor and birth if treatment precipitates this reaction. They should be advised to contact their health care provider if they notice any change in fetal movement or have any contractions.

Monthly follow-up is mandatory so that retreatment may be given if needed. The nurse should emphasize the necessity of long-term serologic testing even in the absence of symptoms. The woman should be advised to practice sexual abstinence until treatment is completed, all evidence of primary and secondary syphilis is gone, and serologic evidence of a cure is demonstrated. Women should be told to notify all partners who may have been exposed. They should be informed that the disease is reportable. Preventive measures should be discussed.

Pelvic Inflammatory Disease

Pelvic inflammatory disease (PID) is an infectious process that most commonly involves the uterine (fallopian) tubes (salpingitis), uterus (endometritis), and, more rarely, the ovaries and peritoneal surfaces. Multiple organisms have been found to cause PID, and most cases are associated with more than one organism. In the past the most common causative agent was thought to be *N. gonorrhoeae;* however, *C. trachomatis* is now estimated to cause one half of all cases of PID. In addition to gonorrhea and chlamydia, a wide variety of anaerobic and aerobic bacteria are recognized to cause PID. Because PID may be caused by a wide variety of infectious agents and encompasses a wide variety of pathologic processes, the infection can either be acute, subacute, or chronic and can have a wide range of symptoms.

Most PID results from ascending spread of microorganisms from the vagina and endocervix to the upper genital tract. This spread most frequently happens at the end of or just after menses following reception of an infectious agent. During the menstrual period, several factors facilitate the development of an infection: the cervical os is slightly open, the cervical mucus barrier is absent, and menstrual blood is an excellent medium for growth. PID also may develop following an abortion, pelvic surgery, or childbirth.

Each year more than 1 million women in the United States have an episode of symptomatic PID (Institute of Medicine, Committee on Prevention and Control of Sexually Transmitted Diseases, 1997). Risk factors for acquiring PID are those associated with the risk of contracting an STD, including young age, multiple partners, high rate of new partners, and a history of STDs. Women who use intrauterine devices (IUDs) may be at increased risk for PID if they have more than one sexual partner or if the partner has other sexual partners because they are at higher risk for acquiring an STD (Hatcher et al., 1998). Most of this risk occurs in the first months after IUD insertion. PID tends to recur, with nearly one in five clients experiencing recurrent PID (Bonny & Biro, 1998).

Women who have had PID are at increased risk for ectopic pregnancy, infertility, and chronic pelvic pain. After a single episode of PID, a woman's risk for ectopic pregnancy increases sevenfold compared with the risk for women who have never had PID. Other problems associated with PID include dyspareunia (painful intercourse), pyosalpinx (pus in the fallopian tubes), tubo-ovarian abscess, and pelvic adhesions.

The symptoms of PID vary depending on whether the infection is acute, subacute, or chronic; however, pain is common to all clinical presentations. It may be dull, cramping, and intermittent (subacute) or severe, persistent, and incapacitating (acute). The woman with acute PID also may complain of intermenstrual bleeding. Physical examination reveals adnexal tenderness, with or without rebound, and exquisite tenderness with cervical movement (Chandelier's sign). Pelvic tenderness is usually bilateral. There may or may not be a palpable adnexal swelling or thickening. A urethral or cervical discharge, often purulent in nature, may be present. A fever of 39° C or above is characteristic. Significant laboratory data include an elevated white blood cell count and markedly elevated erythrocyte sedimentation rate. Fever and peritonitis are more characteristic of gonococcal PID than of PID caused by other organisms that are more likely to be "silent." Because PID caused by chlamydia is more commonly asymptomatic, it more often results in tubal obstruction from delayed diagnosis or inadequate treatment.

Subacute PID is far less dramatic, with a great variety in the severity and extent of symptoms. At times they are so mild and vague that the woman ignores them. Symptoms that suggest subacute PID are chronic lower abdominal pain, dyspareunia, menstrual irregularities, urinary discomfort, low-grade fever, low backache, and constipation. Abdominal examination usually reveals no rebound tenderness; there is slight adnexal tenderness with cervical movement, and cervical or urethral discharge may be present.

Screening and Diagnosis

A careful history is necessary to distinguish between PID and other conditions that cause abdominal pain, such as an ectopic pregnancy or appendicitis. A menstrual history is useful in establishing the relationship of onset of pain to menses and in identifying any variations from normal in the cycle. Other relevant history includes recent pelvic surgery, birth, abortion, or dilation of the cervix; purulent vaginal discharge; irregular bleeding; and a longer, heavier menstrual period. A sexual history will assist in identifying possible increased risk for STD exposure. Symptoms of an STD in a woman's partner(s) also should be noted.

Vital signs are obtained and a complete physical examination performed. CDC routine criteria for diagnosing PID include oral temperature greater than 38.3° C, abnormal cervical or vaginal discharge, elevated erythrocyte sedimentation rate, and laboratory documentation of cervical infection with *N. gonorrhoeae* or *C. trachomatis*. Physical findings of lower abdominal tenderness, bilateral adnexal tenderness, and cervical motion tenderness are important in making a clinical diagnosis of PID. Essential laboratory data are a complete blood count with differential and cervical cultures for gonorrhea and chlamydia.

Management

Perhaps the most important nursing intervention is prevention. Primary prevention would be education in avoiding acquisition of sexually transmitted diseases, whereas secondary prevention involves preventing a lower genital tract infection from ascending to the upper genital tract. Instructing women in self-protective behaviors such as practicing safer sex and using barrier methods is critical. Women using hormonal contraception or the IUD and those who have chosen tubal ligation must be reminded to use a condom with intercourse when indicated. Also important is the detection of asymptomatic gonorrheal and chlamydial infections through routine screening of women who practice risky behaviors or have specific risk factors such as age. Partner notification when an STD is diagnosed is essential to prevent reinfection.

When and if women with PID are hospitalized varies. The CDC recommends hospitalization in the following situations (Centers for Disease Control and Prevention, 1998a):
- Surgical emergencies such as appendicitis cannot be excluded.
- A pelvic abscess is suspected.
- The woman is pregnant.
- Severe illness precludes outpatient management.
- The woman is unable to tolerate or follow an outpatient oral regimen.
- The woman has failed to respond to oral outpatient therapy.
- The woman is immunodeficient.

Many experts recommend that all women with PID be hospitalized so that parenteral antibiotic treatment can be done. It may be particularly important to hospitalize adolescent clients because their adherence to therapy may be unpredictable and the long-term sequelae of PID can be particularly devastating for this group.

TABLE 8-3 Treatment of Pelvic Inflammatory Disease

	TREATMENT OF CHOICE	ALTERNATIVES
Parenteral regimen	Cefotetan 2 g IV every 12 hr or Cefoxitin 2 g IV every 6 hr PLUS Doxycycline 100 mg IV or orally every 12 hr	Clindamycin 900 mg IV every 8 hr PLUS Gentamycin loading dose IV or IM (2 mg/kg of body weight), followed by maintenance dose (1.5 mg/kg) every 8 hr
Oral regimen	Ofloxacin 400 mg orally twice a day for 14 days PLUS Metronidazole 500 mg orally twice a day for 14 days	Cefoxitin 2 g IM PLUS Probenecid 1 g orally in a single dose concurrently or Other parenteral third-generation cephalosporin PLUS Doxycline 100 mg orally twice a day for 14 days

Although treatment regimens vary with the infecting organism, a broad-spectrum antibiotic generally is used. Several antimicrobial regimens have proved to be effective, and no single therapeutic regimen of choice exists (Table 8-3). The woman with acute PID should be on bed rest in a semi-Fowler's position. Comfort measures include analgesics for pain and all other nursing measures applicable to a client confined to bed. Few pelvic examinations should be done during the acute phase of the disease. During the recovery phase, the woman should restrict her activity and make every effort to get adequate rest and a nutritionally sound diet. Follow-up laboratory work after treatment should include endocervical cultures for a test of cure.

Health education is central to effective management of PID. Nurses should explain the nature of their disease to women and should encourage them to comply with all therapy and prevention recommendations, emphasizing the necessity of taking all medication, even if symptoms disappear. Any potential problems, such as lack of money for prescriptions or lack of transportation to return to the clinic for follow-up appointments, that would prevent a woman from completing a course of treatment should be identified and the importance of follow-up visits stressed. Women should be counseled to refrain from sexual intercourse until their treatment is completed. Contraceptive counseling should be provided, including barrier methods such as condoms, contraceptive sponge, or diaphragm. A woman with a history of PID should not choose an IUD as her contraceptive method.

The woman who suffers from PID may be acutely ill or experience long-term discomfort. Either or both take an emotional toll. Pain in itself is debilitating and is compounded by the infectious process. The potential or actual loss of reproductive capabilities can be devastating and can adversely affect the woman's self-concept. Part of the nurse's role is to help the woman adjust her self-concept to fit reality and to accept alterations in a way that promotes health. Because PID is so closely tied to sexuality, body image, and self-concept, the woman diagnosed with it will need supportive care. Her feelings should be discussed and her partner(s) included when appropriate.

VIRAL SEXUALLY TRANSMITTED INFECTIONS

Human Papillomavirus

Human papillomavirus (HPV) infection, previously named genital or venereal warts, is a sexually transmitted infection that was first described in 25 AD and is now one of the most common STIs seen in ambulatory health care settings. HPV, a double-stranded DNA virus, has over 40 known serotypes; more than 20 types can infect the genital tract. Most HPV infections are asymptomatic, subclinical, or unrecognized. The visible genital lesions are usually caused by HPV types 6 and 11. Other types (e.g., 16, 18, 31, 33, and 35) have been strongly associated with cervical dysplasia (Centers for Disease Control and Prevention, 1998a).

Because health care providers are not required to report HPV infections, the true incidence of these infections is not known. An estimated 24 million Americans are infected with HPV, and as many as 1 million new infections occur yearly (Centers for Disease Control and Prevention, 1998a). In addition to the general risk factors for STIs noted earlier, cigarette smoking and use of oral contraceptives for more than 5 years have been found to be risk factors for HPV.

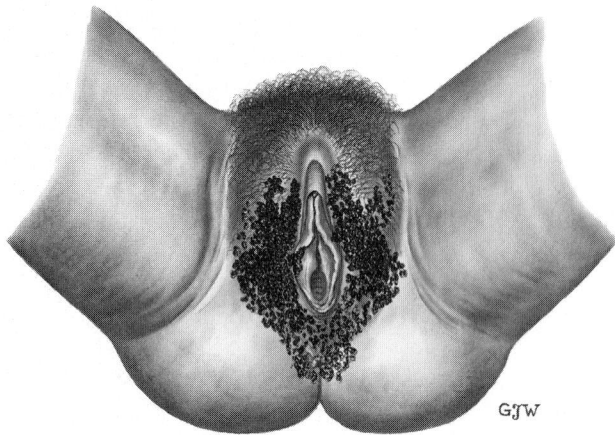

Fig. 8-2 Human papillomavirus infection. Genital warts or condylomata acuminata.

In women, HPV lesions (also called condylomata acuminata) are most frequently seen in the posterior part of the introitus; however, lesions also are found on the buttocks, vulva, vagina, anus, and cervix (Fig. 8-2). Typically the lesions are small, 2 to 3 mm in diameter and 10 to 15 mm in height, soft, papillary swellings occurring singly or in clusters on the genital and anal-rectal region. Infections of long duration may appear as a cauliflower-like mass. In moist areas such as the vaginal introitus, the lesions may appear to have multiple, fine, finger-like projections. Vaginal lesions are often multiple. Flat-topped papules, 1 to 4 mm in diameter, are seen most often on the cervix. Often these lesions are visualized only under magnification. Warts are usually flesh colored or slightly darker on Caucasian women, black on African-American women, and brownish on Asian women. Usually painless, the lesions may also be uncomfortable, particularly when very large, inflamed, or ulcerated. Chronic vaginal discharge, pruritis, or dyspareunia can occur.

HPV infections are thought to be more frequent in pregnant than in nonpregnant women with an increase in incidence from the first trimester to the third. Furthermore, a significant proportion of preexisting HPV lesions enlarge greatly during pregnancy, a proliferation presumably resulting from the relative state of immunosuppression present during pregnancy. Lesions may become so large during pregnancy that they affect urination, defecation, mobility, and fetal descent, although birth by cesarean is rarely necessary (American College of Obstetricians and Gynecologists, 1994). Cesarean birth may be performed when extensive growths are present. However, initial observation of large growths can be misleading, suggesting that the entire vagina is involved; however, all of the growth may derive from one stalk, and in such cases it may be possible to push the large mass to the side, allowing the baby to pass through. HPV infection may be acquired by the neonate during birth; the frequency of such transmission is unknown. Juvenile laryngeal papillomata (JLP) can

occur in children exposed to HPV during birth. JLP can cause death or significant morbidity requiring multiple surgical or laser treatments in affected children. The exact incidence of JLP is not known but is thought to be rare. The preventive value of cesarean birth is unknown and is not recommended solely to prevent transmission of HPV infection to newborns.

Screening and Diagnosis

A woman with HPV lesions may complain of symptoms such as a profuse, irritating vaginal discharge, itching, dyspareunia, or postcoital bleeding. She also may report "bumps" on her vulva or labia. History of a known exposure is important; however, because of the potentially long latency period and the possibility of subclinical infections in men, the lack of a history of known exposure cannot be used to exclude a diagnosis of HPV infection.

Physical inspection of the vulva, perineum, anus, vagina, and cervix is essential whenever HPV lesions are suspected or seen in one area. Because speculum examination of the vagina may block some lesions, it is important to rotate the speculum blades until all areas are visualized. When lesions are visible, the characteristic appearance previously described is considered diagnostic. However, in many instances, cervical lesions are not visible, and some vaginal or vulvar lesions also may be unobservable to the naked eye. Because of the potential spread of vulvar or vaginal lesions to the anus, gloves should be changed between vaginal and rectal examinations.

Diagnosis is made by colposcopy and direct visualization of the growths or by biopsy. It is imperative that women with vulvar HPV or partners with HPV have a cervical examination with a Papanicolaou (Pap) smear. Pap smears of the cervical transformation zone are used as a screening technique; however, because of false-negative results, a negative Pap smear does not indicate absence of disease. The severity of any cervical lesion reported on a Pap smear is best determined by colposcopy and biopsy. Vinegar solution may be used to highlight early or flat cervical lesions; however, it is important to note that a positive reaction may also be obtained with any inflammatory reaction, after sexual intercourse, and with vaginal trauma.

HPV lesions must be differentiated from molluscum contagiosum and condylomata lata. Molluscum contagiosum lesions are half-domed, smooth, flesh-colored to pearly white papules with depressed centers. Condylomata lata are a form of secondary syphilis and generally are flatter and wider than genital warts. A serologic test for syphilis would confirm the diagnosis of secondary syphilis.

Management

Treatment of genital warts is often difficult. No therapy has been shown to eradicate HPV. The goal of treatment therefore is removal of warts and relief of signs and symptoms, not the eradication of HPV (Centers for Disease Control and Prevention, 1998a). The client often must make multiple office visits; frequently, many different treatment modalities will be used. Eradication of the virus is not considered conclusive even after there is no visible evidence of wart tissue because of the high incidence of recurrence.

Treatment of genital warts should be guided by preference of the woman, available resources, and experience of the health care provider. None of the treatments is superior to all other treatments, and no one treatment is ideal for all warts (Centers for Disease Control and Prevention, 1998a). Available treatments are outlined in Table 8-2. Imiquimod, podophyllin, and podofilox, should not be used during pregnancy. Because the lesions can proliferate and become friable during pregnany, many experts recommend their removal using cryotherapy or various surgical techniques during pregnancy (Centers for Disease Control and Prevention, 1998a).

Women who are experiencing discomfort associated with genital warts may find that bathing with an oatmeal solution and drying the area with a cool hair dryer will provide some relief. Keeping the area clean and dry will also decrease growth of the warts. Cotton underwear and loose-fitting clothes that decrease friction and irritation also may decrease discomfort. Women should be advised to maintain a healthy lifestyle to aid the immune system; women can be counseled regarding diet, rest, stress reduction, and exercise.

Client counseling is essential. Women must understand how the virus is transmitted, that no immunity is conferred with infection, and that reacquistion of the infection is likely with repeated contact. Women need to know that their partners should be checked even if they are asymptomatic. Because HPV is highly contagious, the majority of women's partners will be infected and should be treated. All sexually active women with multiple partners or a history of HPV should be encouraged to use latex condoms and a vaginal spermicide for intercourse to decrease acquisition or transmission of condylomata.

Instructions for all medications and treatments must be detailed. Women should be informed before treatment of the possibility of posttreatment pain associated with specific therapies. The importance of thorough treatment of concurrent vaginitis or STD should be emphasized. The link between cervical cancer and HPV infections and the need for close follow-up should be discussed. Annual health examinations are recommended to assess disease recurrence and screening for cervical cancer. Biannual Pap smears should be done for the first 2 years after treatment and annually thereafter on women who have been treated for HPV infections (National Institutes of Health, 1996). When the cervix is treated, a Pap smear should be done in 4 to 6 months; after two negative Pap smears at 6-month intervals, an annual Pap smear can be performed (Centers for Disease Control and Prevention, 1998a). Women should understand the advisability of treatment before becoming pregnant.

Women with HPV infection may radically alter their sexual practices both from fear of transmission to and from a partner and from genital discomfort associated with treatment, which may have a negative impact on their sexual relationships. Unless the partner accepts and understands the necessary precautions, it may be difficult for the woman to follow the treatment regimen. The nurse can offer to discuss feelings that the woman may have. When indicated, joint counseling can be suggested.

Herpes Simplex Virus

Unknown until the middle of the twentieth century, herpes simplex virus (HSV) infection is now widespread in the United States, especially in women. HSV infection results in painful recurrent genital ulcers and is caused by two different antigen subtypes of herpes simplex virus: herpes simplex virus I (HSV-1) and herpes simplex virus II (HSV-2). HSV-2 is usually transmitted sexually and HSV-1 nonsexually. Although HSV-1 is more commonly associated with gingivostomatitis and oral labial ulcers (fever blisters) and HSV-2 with genital lesions, both types are not exclusively associated with the respective sites.

Although HSV infection is not a reportable disease, it is estimated that at least 45 million Americans are infected with genital herpes (Centers for Disease Control and Prevention, 1998a) and that 200,000 to 500,000 persons contract an initial (or primary) infection each year; recurrent HSV infections are much more common (Hatcher et al., 1998). Estimates suggest that at least one in every four women will become infected in her lifetime (Institute of Medicine, Committee on Prevention and Control of Sexually Transmitted Diseases, 1997).

An initial HSV genital infection is characterized by multiple painful lesions, fever, chills, malaise, and severe dysuria and may last 2 to 3 weeks. Women generally have a more severe clinical course than do men. Women with primary genital herpes have many lesions that progress from macules to papules, then forming vesicles, pustules, and ulcers that crust and heal without scarring (Fig. 8-3). These ulcers are extremely tender, and primary infections may be bilateral. Women also may have itching, inguinal tenderness, and lymphadenopathy. Severe vulvar edema may develop, and women may have difficulty sitting. HSV cervicitis also is common with initial HSV-2 infections. The cervix may appear normal or be friable, reddened, ulcerated, or necrotic. A heavy, watery to purulent vaginal discharge is common. Extragenital lesions may be present because of autoinnoculation. Urinary retention and dysuria may occur secondary to autonomic involvement of the sacral nerve root.

Women experiencing recurrent episodes of HSV infections commonly have only local symptoms that are usually less severe than those associated with the initial infection. Systemic symptoms are usually absent, although the characteristic prodromal genital tingling is common. Recurrent lesions are unilateral, are less severe, and usually last 5 to 7 days. Lesions begin as vesicles and progress rapidly to ulcers. Few women with recurrent disease have cervicitis.

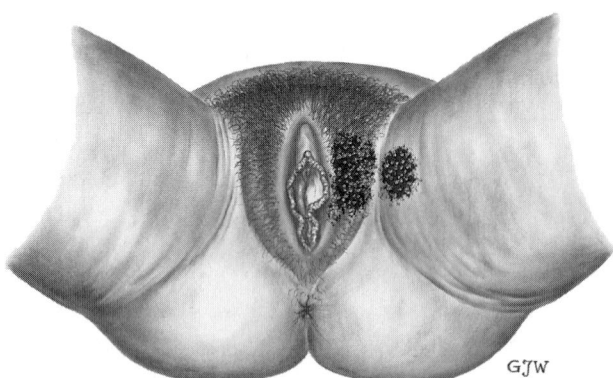

Fig. 8-3 Herpes genitalis.

During pregnancy, maternal infection with HSV-2 can have adverse effects on both the mother and fetus. Viremia occurs during the primary infection, and congenital infection is possible, though rare. Primary infections during the first trimester have been associated with increased miscarriage rates. The most severe complication of HSV infection is neonatal herpes, a potentially fatal or severely disabling disease occurring in 1 in 2000 to 1 in 10,000 live births. Most mothers of infants who contract neonatal herpes lack histories of clinically evident genital herpes. Risk of neonatal infection is highest among women with primary herpes infection who are near term and is low among women with recurrent herpes (Centers for Disease Control and Prevention, 1998a). There is a 60% infant mortality rate associated with infants who contract HSV infection, and about 50% of those who survive suffer serious neurologic damage (Corder-Mabe, 1998).

An association between cervical cancer and HSV-2 has been observed. It is theorized that genital herpes is a marker for high risk sexual behaviors that could transmit other STIs, including HPV (DiSaia & Creasman, 1997).

Screening and Diagnosis

A careful history provides much information when making a diagnosis of herpes. A history of exposure to an infected person is important, although infection from an asymptomatic individual is possible. A history of having viral symptoms such as malaise, headache, fever, or myalgia is suggestive. Local symptoms such as vulvar pain, dysuria, itching or burning at the site of infection, and painful genital lesions that heal spontaneously also are highly suggestive of HSV infections. The nurse should ask about prior history of a primary infection, prodromal symptoms, vaginal discharge, and dyspareunia. Pregnant women should be asked whether they or their partner(s) have had genital lesions.

During the physical examination, the nurse should assess for inguinal and generalized lymphadenopathy and elevated temperature. The entire vulvar, perineal, vaginal, and cervical areas should be carefully inspected for vesicles or ulcerated or crusted areas. A speculum examination may be very difficult for the woman because of the extreme tenderness often associated with herpes infections. Any suspicious or recurrent lesions found during pregnancy should be cultured to document HSV. Although a diagnosis of herpes infection may be suspected from the history and physical, it is confirmed by laboratory studies. A viral culture is obtained by swabbing exudate during the vesicular stage of the disease. Preliminary results are available in 48 hours, final results in 1 to 2 weeks (Youngkin, 1995). In primary HSV infection, viral shedding is prolonged and HSV is more easily isolated.

Management

Genital herpes is a chronic and recurring disease for which there is no known cure. Management is directed toward specific treatment during primary and recurrent infections, prevention, self-help measures, and psychologic support.

Systemic antiviral medications partially control the symptoms and signs of HSV infections when used for the primary or recurrent episodes or when used as daily suppressive therapy. However, these medications do not eradicate the infection, nor do they alter subsequent risk, frequency, or recurrences after the medication is stopped. Three antiviral medications provide clinical benefit: acyclovir, valacyclovir, and famciclovir. Treatment recommendations are given in Table 8-2. Safety and efficacy have been shown clearly in persons taking acyclovir daily for up to 3 years. The safety of acyclovir, valacyclovir, and famciclovir therapy during pregnancy has not been established; however, the first clinical episode of genital herpes during pregnancy may be treated with oral acyclovir. In the presence of life-threatening maternal HSV infection, acyclovir IV is indicated (Centers for Disease Control and Prevention, 1998a). Continued investigation of HSV therapy with these medications in pregnancy is needed.

Cleaning lesions twice a day with saline will help prevent secondary infection. Bacterial infection must be treated with appropriate antibiotics. Measures that may increase comfort for women when lesions are active include warm sitz baths with baking soda; keeping lesions dry by blowing the area dry using a hair dryer set on cool or patting dry with a soft towel; wearing cotton underwear and loose clothing; using drying aids such as hydrogen peroxide, Burow's solution, or oatmeal baths; applying cool, wet, black tea bags to lesions; and applying compresses with an infusion of cloves or peppermint oil and clove oil to lesions.

Oral analgesics such as aspirin or ibuprofen may be used to relieve pain and systemic symptoms associated with initial infections. Because the mucous membranes affected by herpes are extremely sensitive, any topical agents should be used with caution. Nonantiviral ointments, especially those containing cortisone, should be avoided. A thin layer of lidocaine ointment or an antiseptic spray may be applied to decrease discomfort, especially if walking is difficult.

A diet rich in vitamin C, B-complex vitamins, zinc, and calcium is thought to help prevent recurrences. Daily use of kelp powder (2 capsules) and sunflower seed oil (1 tbsp) also have been recommended to decrease recurrences (Ammer, 1989). The amino acid L-lysine has been used in doses of 750 to 1000 mg daily while lesions are active and 500 mg during asymptomatic periods. It is thought that L-lysine has an inhibitory effect on the multiplication of the herpes simplex virus.

Counseling and education are critical components of the nursing care of women with herpes infections. Information regarding the etiology, signs and symptoms, transmission, and treatment should be provided. The nurse should explain that each woman is unique in her response to herpes and emphasize the variability of symptoms. Women should be helped to understand when viral shedding and thus transmission to a partner is most likely, and that they should refrain from sexual contact from the onset of prodrome until complete healing of lesions. Some authorities recommend consistent use of condoms for all persons with genital herpes. Condoms may not prevent transmission, particularly male-to-female transmission; however, this does not mean that the partners should avoid all intimacy. Women can be encouraged to maintain close contact with their partners while avoiding contact with lesions. Women should be taught how to look for herpetic lesions using a mirror and good light source to look and a wet cloth or finger covered with a finger cot to rub lightly over the labia. The nurse should ensure that women understand that when lesions are active, sharing intimate articles (e.g., washcloths, wet towel) that come into contact with the lesions should be avoided. Plain soap and water is all that is needed to clean hands that have come in contact with herpetic lesions; isolation is not necessary or appropriate.

The nurse should explain the role of precipitating factors in the reactivation of the latent virus and recurrent episodes. Stress, menstruation, trauma, febrile illnesses, chronic illness, and ultraviolet light have all been found to trigger genital herpes. Women may wish to keep a diary to identify stressors that seem to be associated with recurrent herpes attacks so that they can then avoid these stressors when possible. The role of exercise in reducing stress can be discussed. Referral for stress reduction therapy, yoga, or meditation classes may be indicated. Avoiding excessive heat and sun and hot baths and using a lubricant during sexual intercourse to reduce friction also may be helpful. Women in their childbearing years should be counseled regarding the risk of herpes infection during pregnancy. They should be instructed to use condoms if there is any risk of contracting any STI from a sexual partner. If they are using acyclovir therapy, they should be counseled to use contraception because of the potential teratogenicity of acyclovir. Women who are breastfeeding should not use acyclovir.

Because neonatal HSV infection is such a devastating disease, prevention is critical. Current recommendations include carefully examining and questioning all women about symptoms at onset of labor (Eisenstat, 1995). Diagnosis of genital herpes in any pregnant women with active, visible lesions should be confirmed with culture. If visible lesions are not present at onset of labor, vaginal birth is acceptable. Cesarean birth within 4 hours after labor begins or membranes rupture is recommended if visible lesions are present. Infants who are delivered through an infected vagina should be carefully observed and cultured. Some experts recommend presumptive treatment of infants who were exposed to HSV during birth. Weekly surveillance cultures from pregnant women with a history of HSV but who do not have visible lesions is not necessary or recommended. Because HSV infection may be associated with cervical dysplasia, women must be encouraged to have yearly Pap smears and gynecologic examinations.

The emotional impact of contracting herpes is considerable. Media publicity regarding this disease has made receiving a diagnosis of genital herpes a devastating experience. No cure is available, and most women will experience recurrences. At diagnosis many emotions may surface—helplessness, anger, denial, guilt, anxiety, shame, or inadequacy. Women need the opportunity to discuss their feelings and help in learning to live with the disease. A woman can be encouraged to think of herself as a person who is not diseased but rather healthy and inconvenienced from time to time. Herpes can affect a woman's sexuality, her sexual practices, and her current and future relationships. She may need help in raising the issue with her partner or with future partners.

Viral Hepatitis

Five different viruses (hepatitis viruses A, B, C, D, and E) account for almost all cases of viral hepatitis in humans. Hepatitis viruses A, B, and C are discussed. Hepatitis D and E viruses, common among users of intravenous drugs and recipients of multiple blood transfusions, are not included in this discussion.

Hepatitis A

Hepatitis A virus (HAV) infection is acquired primarily through a fecal-oral route by ingestion of contaminated food, particularly milk, shellfish, or polluted water, or person-to-person contact. Women living in the western United States, Native Americans, Alaskan Natives, and children and employees in day care centers are at high risk (Centers for Disease Control and Prevention, 1996a).

HAV infection is characterized by flulike symptoms with malaise, fatigue, anorexia, nausea, pruritis, fever, and upper right quadrant pain. Serologic testing to detect the IgM antibody is done to confirm acute infections. The IgM antibody is detectable 5 to 10 days after exposure and can remain positive for up to 6 months. Because HAV infection is self-limited and does not result in chronic infection or chronic liver disease, treatment is usually supportive.

Women who become dehydrated from nausea and vomiting or who have fulminating hepatitis A may need to be hospitalized. Medications that might cause liver damage or that are metabolized in the liver should be used with caution. No specific diet or activity restrictions are necessary. Immune globulin (gamma globulin) or immune-specific globulin is indicated for any pregnant woman exposed to HAV to provide passive immunity through injected antibodies. All household contacts of the woman should also receive gamma globulin.

Hepatitis B

Hepatitis B virus (HBV) infection is a sexually transmitted disease and is the virus most threatening to the fetus and neonate. It is caused by a large DNA virus and is associated with three antigens and their antibodies: hepatitis B surface antigen (HBsAG), HBV antigen (HBeAG), HBV core antigen (HBcAG), antibody to HBsAG (anti-HBs), antibody to HBeAG (anti-HBe), and antibody to HBcAG (anti-HBc). Screening for active or chronic disease or disease immunity is based on testing for these antigens and their antibodies.

Factors considered to place a woman at risk for HBV are those associated with STD risk in general: history of multiple sexual partners, multiple STDs, and intravenous drug use; and behaviors that are associated with blood contact (e.g., work or treatment in a dialysis unit, history of multiple blood transfusions, public safety workers exposed to blood in the workplace, health care workers). Although HBV can be transmitted via blood transfusion, the incidence of such infections has decreased significantly since testing of blood for HBsAG became a routine procedure. Drug abusers who share needles are at risk, as are health care workers who are exposed to blood and needle sticks. In addition, women of Asian, Pacific Islander (Polynesian, Micronesian, and Melanesian), or Alaskan Eskimo descent and of Haitian or sub-Saharan Africa birth are considered to be at risk.

HBV infection is transmitted parenterally and through intimate contact. It is 50 to 100 times more contagious than human immunodeficiency virus. The hepatitis B carrier state affects 5% of the world's population, with higher percentages found in tropical areas and Southeast Asia. Hepatitis B surface antigen has been found in blood, saliva, sweat, tears, vaginal secretions, and semen. Perinatal transmission does occur; however, the fetus is not at risk until it comes in contact with contaminated blood during birth. Infants born to mothers who are highly infectious (positive for both HBsAG and HBeAG) have a 70% to 90% chance of acquiring perinatal hepatitis B infection. Approximately 85% to 90% of infected infants will become chronic carriers. HBV has also been transmitted by artificial insemination.

HBV infection is a disease of the liver and is often a silent infection. In the adult, the course of the infection can be fulminating and the outcome fatal. Symptoms of HBV infection are similar to those of hepatitis A: arthralgias, arthritis, lassitude, anorexia, nausea, vomiting, headache, fever, and mild abdominal pain. Later the woman may have clay-colored stools, dark urine, increased abdominal pain, and jaundice. Between 5% and 10% of individuals with HBV have persistence of HBsAg and become chronic hepatitis B carriers. Twenty-five percent of chronic carriers die from primary hepatocellular carcinoma or cirrhosis of the liver.

Screening and Diagnosis

All women at high risk for contracting HBV should be screened on a regular basis. Screening only individuals at high risk may not identify up to 50% of HBsAg-positive women; therefore current CDC guidelines recommend screening for the presence of HBsAg on all women at the first prenatal visit and repeated later in pregnancy for women with high risk behaviors (Centers for Disease Control and Prevention, 1998a).

Testing for HBV is complex. Clients with acute hepatitis B generally have detectable serum HBsAG levels in the late incubation phase of the disease, 2 to 5 weeks before symptoms appear. Anti-HBs with a negative HBsAG test signals immunity. Anti-HBs with a positive antigen denotes a chronic carrier state; during this time, the disease can be transmitted. During the recovery phase, the client may continue to be infectious even though HBsAG cannot be detected. This is called the "window phase" and is identified by anti-HBc in the absence of anti-HBs. Women should be prepared for repeat testing because HBV screening tests may also be used to monitor the progression of the disease.

Components of the history to be obtained when hepatitis B is suspected include the inquiry about the symptoms of the disease and risk factors outlined earlier. Physical examination includes inspection of the skin for rashes, inspection of the skin and conjunctiva for jaundice, and palpation of the liver for enlargement and tenderness. Weight loss, fever, and general debilitation should be noted. If the HBsAG is positive, further laboratory studies may be ordered (anti-HBe, anti-HBc, serum glutamic-oxaloacetic transaminase [SGOT], alkaline phosphatase, and liver panel). If the HBsAG is negative in early pregnancy and the woman could be in the window phase or if high risk behaviors continue during pregnancy, a repeat HBsAG should be ordered in the third trimester.

Management

There is no specific treatment for hepatitis B. Recovery is usually spontaneous in 3 to 16 weeks. Usually pregnancies complicated by acute viral hepatitis are managed on an outpatient basis. Women should be advised to increase bed rest; eat a high-protein, low-fat diet; and increase their fluid intake. They should avoid medications metabolized in the liver, drugs, and alcohol. Women with a definite exposure to HBV should be given hepatitis B immune globulin and should begin the hepatitis B vaccine series within 14 days of the most recent contact to prevent infection (Centers for Disease Control and Prevention, 1998a). Vaccination during pregnancy is not thought to pose risks to the fetus.

All nonimmune women at high or moderate risk of hepatitis should be informed of the existence of hepatitis B vaccine. Vaccination is recommended for all individuals who have had multiple sex partners within the past 6 months (Centers for Disease Control and Prevention, 1998a). In addition, intravenous drug users, residents of correctional or long-term care facilities, persons seeking care for an STD, prostitutes, women whose partners are intravenous drug users or bisexual, and women whose occupation exposed them to high risk should be vaccinated. The vaccine is given in a series of three (some authorities recommend four) doses over a 6-month period with the first two doses given at least 1 month apart. The vaccine is given in the deltoid muscle (Centers for Disease Control and Prevention, 1998a).

Client education includes explaining the meaning of hepatitis B infection, including transmission, state of infectivity, and sequelae. The nurse should also explain the need for immunoprophylaxis for household members and sexual contacts. To decrease transmission of the virus, women with hepatitis B or who test positive for HBV should be advised to maintain a high level of personal hygiene (e.g., wash hands after using the toilet; carefully dispose of tampons, pads, bandages in plastic bags; do not share razor blades, toothbrushes, needles, manicure implements; have male partner use a condom if unvaccinated and without hepatitis; avoid sharing saliva through kissing, or sharing of silverware or dishes; wipe up blood spills immediately with soap and water). They should inform all health care providers of their carrier state. Postpartum women should be reassured that breastfeeding is not contraindicated if their infants received prophylaxis at birth and are currently on the immunization schedule.

Hepatitis C

Hepatitis C virus (HCV) infection has become an important health problem as increasing numbers of persons acquire the disease. Fourteen percent of the U.S. population is infected with HCV (Hunt, Carson, & Sharara, 1997). Because up to 70% of clients with HCV infection progress to chronic hepatitis, hepatitis C represents nearly 50% of chronic viral hepatitis. Risk factors for pregnant women include women with STDs such as hepatitis B and human immunodeficiency virus, multiple sexual partners, history of blood transmissions, and history of intravenous drug use. Hepatitis C is readily transmitted through exposure to blood and much less efficiently via semen, saliva, or urine.

Most clients with hepatitis C are asymptomatic or have general flulike symptoms similar to hepatitis A. About 10% have fatigue, nausea, and anorexia (Hunt, Carson, & Sharara, 1997). HCV infection is confirmed by the pres-

ence of anti-C antibody during laboratory testing. Testing for hepatitis C is not widely done (Freitag-Koontz, 1996); however, screening of high risk clients is recommended (Hunt, Carson, & Sharara, 1997).

Interferon alfa-2b is the main therapy for HCV infection, although effectiveness of this treatment varies. Currently there is no vaccine for use with hepatitis C. Transmission of HCV through breastfeeding has not been reported.

Human Immunodeficiency Virus

Although **human immunodeficiency virus (HIV)** has traditionally been thought to be a homosexual or gay disease, heterosexual transmission is now the most common means of transmission in women. Furthermore, women are now the fastest-growing population of individuals with HIV infection and acquired immunodeficiency syndrome (AIDS) (Wortley & Flemming, 1997). In 1993 AIDS became the fourth leading cause of death in the United States in women ages 25 to 44 years, and in many of the larger cities on the East Coast it is the leading cause of death (Cotton & Watts, 1997).

Transmission of HIV, a retrovirus, occurs primarily through exchange of body fluids (semen, blood, or vaginal secretions). Severe depression of the cellular immune system associated with HIV infection characterizes AIDS. Although behaviors that place women at risk have been well documented, all women should be assessed for the possibility of HIV exposure. Until recently HIV infection has commonly been reported at a later disease stage in women; however, this is changing with revised CDC definitions of AIDS. For both men and women, the most frequently reported opportunistic diseases are *Pneumocystis carinii* pneumonia (PCP), candida esophagitis, and wasting syndrome. Other viral infections such as HSV and cytomegalovirus infections seem to be more prevalent in women than men (Wildschut, Weiner, & Peters, 1996). PID may be more severe in HIV-infected women, and rates of HPV and cervical dysplasia may be higher. The clinical course of HPV infection in women with HIV infection is accelerated, and recurrence is more frequent.

Once HIV enters the body, seroconversion to HIV positivity usually occurs within 6 to 12 weeks. Although HIV seroconversion may be totally asymptomatic, it usually is accompanied by a viremic, influenza-like response. Symptoms include fever, headache, night sweats, malaise, generalized lymphadenopathy, myalgias, nausea, diarrhea, weight loss, sore throat, and rash.

Laboratory studies may reveal leukopenia, thrombocytopenia, anemia, and an elevated erythrocyte sedimentation rate. HIV has a strong affinity for surface-marker proteins on T lymphocytes. This affinity leads to significant T-cell destruction. Both clinical and epidemiologic studies have shown that declining CD4 levels are strongly associated with increased incidence of AIDS-related diseases and death in many different groups of HIV-infected persons (Cotton & Watts, 1997).

Screening and Diagnosis

Screening, teaching, and counseling regarding HIV risk factors, indications for being tested, and testing are major roles for nurses caring for women today. A number of behaviors that place women at risk for HIV infection have been identified, including intravenous drug use, high risk sexual partners, multiple sex partners, and a previous history of multiple STDs. HIV infection is usually diagnosed by using HIV-1 antibody tests. Antibody testing is first done with a sensitive screening test such as the enzyme immunoassay. Reactive screening tests must be confirmed by an additional test, such as the Western blot or an immunofluorescence assay. If a positive antibody test is confirmed by a supplemental test, it means that a woman is infected with HIV and is capable of infecting others. HIV antibodies are detectable in at least 95% of clients within 6 months after infection. Although a negative antibody test usually indicates that a person is not infected, antibody tests cannot exclude infection that occurred less than 6 months before the test. Because HIV antibody crosses the placenta, its presence in children less than 18 months of age is not diagnostic of HIV infection (Centers for Disease Control and Prevention, 1998a).

CDC guidelines recommend offering HIV testing to all women whose behavior places them at risk for HIV infection (Centers for Disease Control and Prevention, 1998a). It may be useful to allow women to self-select for HIV testing. On entry to the health care system a woman can be handed written information about the risk factors for the AIDS virus and asked to inform the nurse if she believes she is at risk. She should be told that she does not have to say why she may be at risk, only that she thinks she might be.

Counseling for HIV Testing

Counseling before and after HIV testing is standard nursing practice today. It is a nursing responsibility to assess a woman's understanding of the information such a test would provide and to be sure the client thoroughly understands the emotional, legal, and medical implications of a positive or negative test before she is ready to take an HIV test. One's life is profoundly altered by knowledge of HIV seropositivity. A unique stigma is associated with HIV infection that can have a profound impact on the quality of life of those infected. This stigma extends to those who are asymptomatic but seropositive.

Pregnancy is not encouraged for women who are HIV positive, and preconception counseling is recommended. Pregnant women should be counseled about their options and contraceptive counseling offered to HIV-positive women who do not desire pregnancy. HIV-infected women should be informed specifically about the risks for perinatal infection. Current evidence indicates that 15% to 25% of infants born to untreated HIV-infected women are infected with HIV; the virus also can be transmitted through breastfeeding (Centers for Disease Control and Prevention, 1998a).

All pregnant women should be offered HIV testing as early in pregnancy as possible (Centers for Disease Control and Prevention, 1995). This recommendation is essential because of the available treatments that can reduce the likelihood of perinatal transmission and maintain the health of the woman. HIV-infected women should be specifically informed about the risks for perinatal transmission. Insufficient information is available regarding the safety of zidovudine or any other antiretroviral drugs during early pregnancy; however, zidovudine is indicated for the prevention of maternal-fetal HIV transmission. Zidovudine reduces transmission risk to 8% if given in late pregnancy, during labor, and to infants for the first 6 weeks of life (Centers for Disease Control and Prevention, 1994). Therefore zidovudine treatment should be offered to all HIV-positive pregnant women. Current protocol includes oral zidovudine at 14 to 34 weeks of gestation, intravenous zidovudine during labor, and zidovudine syrup to the neonate after birth (Centers for Disease Control and Prevention, 1998a). HIV-infected women should be advised not to breastfeed their infants.

Given the strong social stigma attached to HIV infection, nurses must consider the issue of confidentiality and documentation before providing counseling and offering HIV testing to clients.

LEGAL TIP **HIV Testing**

- *If test results are placed in the woman's chart—the appropriate place for all health information—they are available to all who have access to the chart. The woman must be informed of this before testing. Informed consent must be obtained before an HIV test is performed. In some states written consent is mandated.*
- *Counseling associated with HIV testing has two components: pretest and posttest counseling. During pretest counseling, nurses conduct a personalized risk assessment, explain the meaning of positive and negative test results, obtain informed consent for HIV testing, and help women develop a realistic plan for reducing risk and preventing infection. Posttest counseling includes informing the woman of the test results, reviewing the meaning of the results, and reinforcing infection prevention messages. All pretest and posttest counseling should be documented.*

There is generally a 1- to 3-week waiting period after testing for HIV, which can be a very anxious time for the woman. It is helpful if the nurse informs her that this time period between blood drawing and test results is routine. Test results, whatever they are, always must be communicated in person and women informed in advance that such is the procedure. Whenever possible the person who provided the pretest counseling should also tell the woman her test results. Some women, when informed of negative results, may escalate their risk behaviors because of an equating of negativity with immunity. Others may believe that negative means "bad" and positive means "good." Women's reactions to a negative test should be explored, asking, "How do you feel?" HIV-negative result counseling sessions are another opportunity to provide education. Emphasis can be placed on ways in which a woman can remain HIV free. She should be reminded that if she has been exposed to HIV in the past 6 months she should be retested, and that if she continues high risk behaviors, she should have ongoing testing.

When providing posttest counseling to an HIV-positive woman, privacy with no interruptions is essential. Adequate time for the counseling sessions should also be provided. The nurse should make sure that the woman understands what a positive test means and review the reliability of the test results. Safer sex guidelines should be reemphasized. Referral for appropriate medical evaluation and follow-up should be made, and the need or desire for psychosocial or psychiatric referrals should be assessed.

The importance of early medical evaluation so that a baseline assessment can be made and prophylactic medication begun should be stressed. If possible, the nurse should make a referral or appointment for the woman at the posttest counseling session.

As the number of HIV-infected women escalates, prevention, education, and counseling activities must be directed toward all women. It is very difficult to keep abreast of the ever-changing picture of AIDS. Important sources of information are the National AIDS Hotline (1-800-342-2437 [English], 1-800-344-7432 [Spanish], 1-800-243-7889 [hearing-impaired]) and the National AIDS Information Clearing House, P.O. Box 6003, Rockville, MD 20850 (1-800-458-5231).

Management

During the initial contact with an HIV-infected woman, the nurse should establish what the woman knows about HIV infection. The nurse should ensure that the woman is being cared for by a medical practitioner or facility with expertise in caring for persons with HIV infections, including AIDS. Psychologic referral also may be indicated. Resources such as counseling for death and dying, suicide prevention, financial assistance, and legal advocacy may be appropriate. All women who are drug users should be referred to a substance abuse program. A major focus of counseling is prevention of transmission of HIV to partners.

Nurses counseling seropositive women wishing contraceptive information may recommend oral contraceptives and latex condoms, Norplant implants and latex condoms, or tubal sterilization or vasectomy and latex condoms. The IUD is not an ideal choice for the HIV-infected woman, but it is not totally contraindicated (Johnstone, 1997). Insertion in a woman who is immunocompromised should be avoided. Spermicides, female condoms, or abstinence can be offered to women whose partners refuse to use condoms.

No cure is available for HIV infection at this time. Rare and unusual diseases are characteristic of HIV infection. Opportunistic infections and concurrent diseases should be managed vigorously with treatment specific to the infection or disease. Discussion of the medical care of HIV-positive women and women with AIDS is beyond the scope of this chapter. The reader is referred to the Centers for Disease Control and Prevention AIDS hotlines and Internet websites for the current information and recommendations (see Appendix D).

Routine gynecologic care for HIV-positive women should include a pelvic examination every 6 months. Careful Pap screening is essential because of the greatly increased incidence of abnormal findings. In addition, HIV-positive women should be screened for syphilis, gonorrhea, chlamydia, and other vaginal infections.

Coinfection with syphilis is common in HIV-infected women, and unusual serologic responses have been documented among HIV-infected persons who have syphilis (Centers for Disease Control and Prevention, 1998a). Because treatment failures with benzathine penicillin are common, follow-up and evaluation must be done at 3, 6, 9, 12, and 24 months after therapy. Furthermore, HIV infection increases susceptibility to neurosyphilis, which is difficult to differentiate clinically from HIV dementia.

Group B Streptococcus

Group B streptococcus (GBS) may be considered a normal vaginal flora in a woman who is not pregnant and is present in 10% to 30% of healthy pregnant women. GBS infection has been suggested as a factor in preterm labor, chorioamnionitis, urinary tract infections during pregnancy, and postpartum infections (Clay, 1996; Katz, 1993). Furthermore, GBS infections are an important factor in perinatal and neonatal morbidity and mortality, usually resulting from vertical transmission from the birth canal of the infected mother to the infant during birth (Lieu et al., 1998).

Risk factors for neonatal GBS infection include positive prenatal culture for GBS in the current pregnancy; previous preterm birth of less than 37 weeks of gestation; premature rupture of membranes for longer than 18 hours; intrapartum maternal fever higher than 38° C; and a positive history for early-onset neonatal GBS.

Identification of GBS status during pregnancy is difficult because duration of carrier status is variable. Prenatal screening before the last few weeks of pregnancy may not identify a woman who is a carrier at onset of labor. Current recommendations are to screen all pregnant women for GBS infection at 36 to 37 weeks of gestation. Cultures should be obtained from the anorectal and vaginal areas and not the cervix.

To decrease the risk of neonatal GBS infection, it is recommended that all women who develop risk factors for

GBS during the antepartum and intrapartum period should be treated during labor (Centers for Disease Control and Prevention, 1996b). In addition, all women who test positive for GBS during the 36- to 37-week screening or who go into labor before 37 weeks should be treated. The recommended treatment is penicillin G 5 million units IV loading dose and then 2.5 million units IV every 4 hours during labor. Ampicillin 2 g loading dose IV followed by 1 g IV every 4 hours is an alternative therapy.

VAGINAL INFECTIONS

Vaginal discharge and itching of the vulva and vagina are among the most frequent reasons a woman seeks help from a health care provider. Indeed, more women complain of vaginal discharge than any other gynecologic symptom. Vaginal discharge resulting from infection must be distinguished from normal secretions. Normal vaginal secretions, or leukorrhea, are clear to cloudy in appearance and may turn yellow after drying; the discharge is slightly slimy, is nonirritating, and has a mild, inoffensive odor. Normal vaginal secretions are acidic, with a pH range of 3.8 to 4.2. The amount of leukorrhea present differs with phases of the menstrual cycle, with greater amounts occurring at ovulation and just before menses. Leukorrhea is also increased during pregnancy. Normal vaginal secretions contain lactobacilli and epithelial cells. Women who have adequate endogenous or exogenous estrogen will have vaginal secretions.

Vaginitis, or abnormal vaginal discharge, is related to infection by a microorganism. The most common vaginal infections are bacterial vaginosis, candidiasis, and trichomoniasis. **Vulvovaginitis,** or inflammation of the vulva and vagina, may be caused by vaginal infection; copious amounts of leukorrhea, which can cause maceration of tissues; and chemical irritants, allergens, and foreign bodies, which may produce inflammatory reactions.

Bacterial Vaginosis

Bacterial vaginosis (BV), formerly called nonspecific vaginitis, *Haemophilus* vaginitis, or *Gardnerella*, is the most common type of vaginitis today (Plourd, 1997). BV is associated with preterm labor and birth. The exact etiology of BV is unknown. It is a syndrome in which normal H_2O_2 producing lactobacilli are replaced with high concentrations of anaerobic bacteria (*Gardnerella* and *Mobiluncus*). With the proliferation of anaerobes, the level of vaginal amines is raised and the normal acidic pH of the vagina is altered. Epithelial cells slough and numerous bacteria attach to their surfaces (clue cells). When the amines are volatilized, the characteristic odor of BV occurs.

Most women with BV complain of a characteristic "fishy odor"; however, not all note it. The odor may be noticed by the woman or her partner after heterosexual intercourse because semen releases the vaginal amines. When present, the BV discharge is usually profuse; thin; and white, gray, or milky in appearance. Some women also may experience mild irritation or pruritis.

Screening and Diagnosis

A careful history may help distinguish BV from other vaginal infections if the woman is symptomatic. Reports of fishy odor and increased thin vaginal discharge are most significant, and report of increased odor after intercourse is also suggestive of BV. Women with previous occurrence of similar symptoms, diagnosis, and treatment should be queried, because women with BV often have been treated incorrectly because of misdiagnosis.

Microscopic examination of vaginal secretions is always done (Table 8-4). Both normal saline and 10% potassium hydroxide smears should be made. The presence of clue cells (vaginal epithelial cells coated with bacteria) by wet smear is highly diagnostic because the phenomenon is specific to BV. Vaginal secretions should be tested for pH and amine odor. Nitrazine paper is sensitive enough to detect a pH of 4.5 or greater. The fishy odor of BV will be released when KOH is added to vaginal secretions on the lip of the withdrawn speculum.

Management

Treatment of bacterial vaginosis with oral metronidazole (Flagyl) is most effective (Centers for Disease Control and Prevention, 1998a). Table 8-5 outlines treatment guidelines.

Metronidazole (Flagyl) is an antiprotozoal and antibacterial agent. In the past metronidazole was contraindicated in the first trimester of pregnancy; however, because of the

---

TABLE 8-4 Wet Smear Tests for Vaginal Infections

INFECTION	TEST	POSITIVE FINDINGS
Trichomoniasis	Saline wet smear (vaginal secretions mixed with normal saline on a glass slide)	Presence of many white blood cell protozoa
Candidiasis	Potassium hydroxide (KOH) prep (vaginal secretions mixed with KOH on a glass slide)	Presence of hyphae and pseudohyphae (buds and branches of yeast cells)
Bacterial vaginosis	Normal saline smear	Presence of clue cells (vaginal epithelial cells coated with bacteria)
	Whiff test (vaginal secretions mixed with KOH)	Release of fishy odor

TABLE 8-5 Vaginal Infections and Drug Therapies for Women

DISEASE	NONPREGNANT WOMEN 13-17 YEARS OF AGE	NONPREGNANT WOMEN >18 YEARS OF AGE	PREGNANT WOMEN	LACTATING WOMEN
Bacterial vaginosis	*Recommended:* Metronidazole 500 mg bid for 7 days (no alcohol) or Clindamycin cream 2%, 5 g per vagina for 7 days or Metronidazole gel 0.75%, 5 g per vagina bid for 7 days *Alternatives:* Metronidazole 2 g orally once or Clindamycin 300 mg orally bid for 7 days	*Recommended:* Metronidazole 500 mg bid for 7 days (no alcohol) or Clindamycin cream 2%, 5 g per vagina for 7 days or Metronidazole gel 0.75%, 5 g per vagina bid for 7 days *Alternatives:* Metronidazole 2 g orally once or Clindamycin 300 mg orally bid for 7 days	High Risk asymptomatic or symptomatic women *Recommended:* Metronidazole 250 mg orally tid for 7 days *Alternatives:* Metronidazole 2 g orally once or Clindamycin 300 mg orally bid for 7 days Low Risk symptomatic women *Recommended:* Metronidazole 250 mg orally tid for 7 days *Alternatives:* Metronidazole 2 g orally once or Clindamycin 300 mg orally bid for 7 days or Metronidazole gel 0.75%, 5 g per vagina bid for 5 days	*Recommended:* Clindamycin cream
Trichomoniasis	*Recommended:* Metronidazole 2 g orally once *Alternative:* Metronidazole 500 mg bid for 7 days	*Recommended:* Metronidazole 2 g orally once *Alternative:* Metronidazole 500 mg bid for 7 days	*Recommended:* Metronidazole 2 g orally once	Not recommended during lactation; stop lactation, treat, resume in 48 hours after drug completed
Candidiasis	Numerous over-the-counter topical intravaginal agents: butoconazole, clotrimazole, miconazole, tioconazole, terconazole; treatment with azole drugs more effective than nystatin *Oral agent:* Fluconazole 150 mg oral tablet once	Numerous over-the-counter topical intravaginal agents: butoconazole, clotrimazole, miconazole, tioconazole, terconazole; treatment with azole drugs more effective than nystatin *Oral agent:* Fluconazole 150 mg oral tablet once	Over-the-counter topical azole intravaginal agents: butoconazole, clotrimazole, miconazole, terconazole Use for 7 days	Over-the-counter topical azole intravaginal agents: butoconazole, clotrimazole, miconazole, terconazole Use for 7 days

Source: Centers for Disease Control and Prevention. (1998a). 1998 guidelines for treatment of sexually transmitted diseases. *MMWR* 47(RR-1), 1-117; Youngkin, E. (1995). Sexually transmitted diseases: Current and emerging trends. *J Obstet Gynecol Neonatal Nurs* 24(8), 743-758.

increased risk of preterm birth, current CDC guidelines recommend treatment of all high risk asymptomatic pregnant women, as well as all symptomatic pregnant women (Centers for Disease Control and Prevention, 1998a). The medication is contraindicated if the woman is breastfeeding because high concentrations have been found in infants. If it is necessary to prescribe metronidazole for the lactating woman, she can suspend breastfeeding temporarily and resume it 48 to 72 hours after taking the last dose. Metronidazole is contraindicated in clients with blood dyscrasia or central nervous system disease because in rare cases Flagyl may affect the hematopoietic or central nervous system.

Side effects of metronidazole are numerous, including sharp, unpleasant metallic taste in the mouth; furry tongue; central nervous system reactions; and urinary tract disturbances. When oral metronidazole is taken, the client is advised not to drink alcoholic beverages, or she will experience the severe side effects of abdominal distress, nausea, vomiting, and headache. Gastrointestinal symptoms are common whether alcohol is consumed or not. Treatment of sexual partners is not recommended because sexual transmission of BV has not been proven (Centers for Disease Control and Prevention, 1998a).

Candidiasis

Vulvovaginal candidiasis, or yeast infection, is the second most common type of vaginal infection in the United States. Although vaginal candidiasis infections are common in healthy women, those seen in women with HIV infection are often more severe and persistent. Genital candidiasis lesions may be painful, coalescing ulcerations necessitating continuous, prophylactic therapy.

The most common organism is *Candida albicans;* it is estimated that 80% to 95% of the yeast infections in women are caused by this organism. However, in the past 10 years, the incidence of non–*C. albicans* infections has risen steadily. Women with chronic or recurrent infections often are infected with a higher percentage of non–*C. albicans* species than are women who are experiencing their first infection or who have few recurrences.

Numerous factors have been identified as predisposing a woman to yeast infections, including antibiotic therapy, particularly broad-spectrum antibiotics such as ampicillin, tetracycline, cephalosporins, and metronidazole; diabetes, especially when uncontrolled; pregnancy; obesity; diets high in refined sugars or artificial sweeteners; use of corticosteroids and exogenous hormones; and immunosuppressed states. Clinical observations and research have suggested that tight-fitting clothing and underwear or pantyhose made of nonabsorbent materials create an environment in which a vaginal fungus can grow.

The most common symptom of yeast infections is vulvar and possibly vaginal pruritis. The itching may be mild or intense, interfere with rest and activities, and occur during or after intercourse. Some women report a feeling of dryness. Other may experience painful urination as the urine flows over the vulva; this usually occurs in women who have excoriations resulting from scratching. Most often the discharge is thick, white, lumpy, and cottage cheese–like. The discharge may be found in patches on the vaginal walls, cervix, and labia. Commonly the vulva is red and swollen, as are the labial folds, vagina, and cervix. Although there is not a characteristic odor with yeast infections, sometimes a yeasty or musty smell occurs.

Screening and Diagnosis

In addition to a careful history of the woman's symptoms, their onset, and course, the history is a valuable screening tool for identifying predisposing risk factors. Physical examination should include a thorough inspection of the vulva and vagina. A speculum examination is always done. Commonly saline and KOH wet smear and vaginal pH are obtained. Vaginal pH is normal with a yeast infection; if the pH is greater than 4.5, trichomoniasis or BV should be suspected. The characteristic pseudohyphae (bud or branching of a fungus) may be seen on a wet smear done with normal saline; however, they may be confused with other cells and artifacts.

Management

A number of antifungal preparations are available for the treatment of *C. albicans* (see Table 8-5). In 1990 many of these medications (e.g., Monostat and Gyne-Lotrimin) were made avaliable as over-the-counter (OTC) agents. The first time a woman suspects that she may have a yeast infection, she should see a health care provider for confirmation of the diagnosis and treatment recommendation. If she experiences another infection she may wish to purchase an OTC preparation and self-treat. If she elects to do this, she should always be counseled regarding seeking care for numerous recurrent or chronic yeast infections. If vaginal discharge is extremely thick and copious, vaginal debridement with a cotton swab followed by application of vaginal medication may be useful.

Women who have extensive irritation, swelling, and discomfort of the labia and vulva may find sitz baths helpful in decreasing inflammation and increasing comfort. Adding Aveeno powder to the bath may also increase the woman's comfort. Not wearing underpants to bed may help decrease symptoms and prevent recurrences. Completing the full course of treatment prescribed is essential to removing the pathogen, and women are instructed to continue medication even during menstruation. They should be counseled not to use tampons during menses because the medication will be absorbed by the tampon. If possible, intercourse is avoided during treatment; if this is not feasible, the woman's partner should use a condom to prevent introduction of more organisms. Suggested measures to prevent genital tract infections are outlined in the Client Self-Care box.

Prevention of Genital Tract Infections

- Practice genital hygiene.
- Choose underwear or hosiery with a cotton crotch.
- Avoid tight-fitting clothing (especially tight jeans).
- Select cloth car seat covers instead of vinyl.
- Limit time spent in damp exercise clothes (especially swimsuits, leotards, and tights).
- Limit exposure to bath salts or bubble bath.
- Avoid colored or scented toilet tissue.
- If sensitive, discontinue use of feminine hygiene deodorant sprays.
- Use condoms.
- Void before and after intercourse.
- Decrease dietary sugar.
- Drink yeast-active milk and eat yogurt (with lactobacilli).
- Do not douche.

Trichomoniasis

Trichomonas vaginalis is almost always a sexually transmitted infection. It is also a common cause of vaginal infection (up to 25% of all vaginitis) and discharge and thus is discussed in this section.

Trichomoniasis is caused by *Trichomonas vaginalis*, an anaerobic one-celled protozoan with characteristic flagellae. Although trichomoniasis may be asymptomatic, commonly women experience characteristically yellowish to greenish, frothy, mucopurulent, copious, malodorous discharge. Inflammation of the vulva, vagina, or both may be present, and the woman may complain of irritation and pruritis. Dysuria and dyspareunia are often present. Typically, the discharge worsens during and after menstruation. Often the cervix and vaginal walls will demonstrate the characteristic "strawberry spots" or tiny petechiae, and the cervix may bleed on contact. In severe infections, the vaginal walls, cervix, and occasionally the vulva may be acutely inflamed.

Screening and Diagnosis

In addition to obtaining a history of current symptoms, a careful sexual history should be obtained. Any history of similar symptoms in the past and treatment used should be noted. The nurse should determine whether the client's partner(s) were treated and if she has had subsequent relations with new partners.

A speculum examination is always done, even though it may be very uncomfortable for the woman; relaxation techniques and breathing exercises may help the woman with the procedure. Any of the classic signs may or may not be present on physical examination. The typical one-celled flagellate trichomonads are easily distinguished on a normal saline wet prep. Trichomoniasis also may be iden-

tified on Pap smears. Because trichomonasis is an STI, once diagnosis is confirmed, appropriate laboratory studies for other STDs should be carried out.

Management

The recommended treatment is metronidazole, 2 g orally in a single dose (Centers for Disease Control and Prevention, 1998a) (see Table 8-5). Although the male partner is usually asymptomatic, it is recommended that he receive treatment also, because he often harbors the trichomonads in the urethra or prostate. It is important that nurses discuss the importance of partner treatment with their clients because if they are not treated, it is likely that the infection will recur.

Women with trichomoniasis need to understand the sexual transmission of this disease. The client must know that the organism may be present without symptoms being present, perhaps for several months, and that it is not possible to determine when she became infected. Women should be informed of the necessity for treating all sexual partners and helped with ways to raise the issue with their partner(s).

EFFECTS OF SEXUALLY TRANSMITTED INFECTIONS ON PREGNANCY AND THE FETUS

Sexually transmitted infections in pregnancy are responsible for significant morbidity and mortality. Some consequences of maternal infection, such as infertility and sterility, last a lifetime. Congenitally acquired infection may affect a child's length and quality of life. Table 8-6 describes the effects of several common STIs on pregnancy and the fetus. It is difficult to predict these effects with certainty. Factors such as coinfection with other STIs and when in pregnancy the infection was treated can affect outcomes.

TORCH Infections

One group of infections that can affect a pregnant woman and her fetus is TORCH infections. *T*oxoplasmosis, *o*ther infections (e.g., hepatitis), *r*ubella virus, *c*ytomegalovirus (CMV), and *h*erpes simplex virus, known collectively as TORCH infections, comprise a group of organisms capable of crossing the placenta and adversely affecting the development of the fetus. Generally, all TORCH infections produce influenza-like symptoms in the mother, but fetal and neonatal effects are more serious. TORCH infections and their maternal, fetal, and neonatal effects are shown in Table 8-7.

Toxoplasmosis

Toxoplasmosis is a protozoan infection associated with the consumption of infested raw or undercooked meat and with poor handwashing after handling infected cat litter. Pregnant women with HIV antibodies are at higher risk

TABLE 8-6 Pregnancy and Fetal Effects of Common Sexually Transmitted Infections

INFECTION	PREGNANCY EFFECTS	FETAL EFFECTS
Chlamydia	Premature rupture of membranes Preterm labor	Preterm birth* Conjunctivitis Pneumonia
Gonorrhea	Intraamniotic infection Preterm labor Premature rupture of membranes Postpartum endometritis Miscarriage	Preterm birth Sepsis Conjunctivitis
Group B streptococcus	Preterm labor Premature rupture of membranes Chorioamnionitis Postpartum sepsis Urinary tract infections	Preterm birth* Early-onset sepsis
Herpes simplex	Rare—infection	Systemic infection
Human papillomavirus (HPV)	Dystocia from large lesions Excessive bleeding from lesions following birth trauma	Respiratory papillomatosis (rare)
Syphilis	Preterm labor Miscarriage	Preterm birth Stillbirth Congenital infection

Data from Cunningham, F. et al. (1997). *Williams obstetrics* (20th ed.). Stamford, CT: Appleton & Lange; Gilbert, E., & Harmon, J. (1998). *Manual of high risk pregnancy and delivery* (2nd ed.). St. Louis: Mosby; Walker, C., & Sweet, R. (1992). HIV and other sexually transmitted diseases in pregnancy. In E. Reece et al. (Eds.). *Medicine of the fetus and mother.* Philadelphia: J.B. Lippincott.

because toxoplasmosis is a common accompanying opportunistic infection. The presence of toxoplasmosis can be determined through blood studies, although laboratory diagnosis is difficult. Women at risk for infection should have toxoplasmosis titers evaluated. Acute infection in pregnancy produces influenza-like symptoms and lymphadenopathy in some women but no symptoms in others. Miscarriage may occur.

The pharmaceutic treatment of choice for toxoplasmosis is a combination of pyrimethamine and sulfadiazine. Although pyrimethamine may be potentially harmful to the fetus, treatment of the parasitemia is essential (Fanaroff & Martin, 1997).

Other Infections

The primary infection included in the category of other infections is hepatitis. Hepatitis A, or infectious hepatitis, a virus spread by droplets or hands, is associated with poor handwashing after defecation. Hepatitis A is an uncommon complication of pregnancy, and perinatal transmission is rare but can occur. Pregnancy effects include miscarriage and influenza-like symptoms of fever, malaise, and nausea. Possible effects of untreated exposure to the fetus in the first trimester include fetal anomalies, preterm birth, fetal or neonatal hepatitis, and intrauterine fetal death. Gamma-globulin is given to infected mothers and exposed neonates for prophylaxis (Fanaroff & Martin, 1997).

Hepatitis B virus (HBV) is a major concern in pregnancy. Acute HBV infection occurs in 1 to 2 per 10,0000 pregnancies, and chronic infections occur in 5 to 15 per 1000 pregnancies. The rate of transmission to the fetus varies. The infection is rarely transmitted to the fetus in the second trimester. Women in the third trimester have up to a 60% chance of transmitting the infection to the fetus (Fanaroff & Martin, 1997). Most infections are transmitted during vaginal birth when the newborn infant is exposed to contaminated blood and genital secretions.

During pregnancy, common symptoms include fever, rash, anorexia, malaise, and myalgias and, if the liver is acutely affected, jaundice, right upper quadrant pain, and nausea and vomiting. Fetal and neonatal effects include maternal-fetal transmission (approximately 90% transmission rate), sequelae of prematurity, and fetal or neonatal hepatitis (see previous discussion for treatment guidelines).

Infections other than hepatitis may also be identified as "other" TORCH infections. These include group B streptococci, varicella, and HIV.

Rubella

Rubella, also called German measles or 3-day measles, is a viral infection transmitted by droplets (such as from an infected person's sneeze). Fever, rash, and mild lymphedema are usually seen in the infected mother. Consequences for the fetus are much more serious and include

TABLE 8-7 Maternal Infection: TORCH

INFECTION	MATERNAL EFFECTS	FETAL EFFECTS	COUNSELING: PREVENTION, IDENTIFICATION, AND MANAGEMENT
Toxoplasmosis (protozoa)	Acute infection similar to influenza, lymphadenopathy Woman immune after first episode (except in immunocompromised patients)	With maternal acute infection, parasitemia Less likely to occur with maternal chronic infection Miscarriage likely with acute infection early in pregnancy	Use good handwashing technique Avoid eating raw meat and exposure to litter used by infected cats; if cats in house, have toxoplasma titer checked If titer is rising during early pregnancy, abortion may be considered an option
Other Hepatitis A (infectious hepatitis) (virus)	Miscarriage, cause of liver failure during pregnancy Fever, malaise, nausea, and abdominal discomfort	Exposure during first trimester, fetal anomalies, fetal or neonatal hepatitis, preterm birth, intrauterine fetal death	Usually spread by droplet or hand contact especially by culinary workers; gammaglobulin can be given as prophylaxis for hepatitis A
Hepatitis B (serum hepatitis) (virus)	May be transmitted sexually, symptoms variable—fever, rash, arthralgia, depressed appetite, dyspepsia, abdominal pain, generalized aching, malaise, weakness, jaundice, tender and enlarged liver	Infection occurs during birth Maternal vaccination during pregnancy should present no risk for fetus (however, data are not available)	Generally passed by contaminated needles, syringes, or blood transfusions; also can be transmitted orally or by coitus (but incubation period is longer); hepatitis B immune globulin can be given prophylactically after exposure Hepatitis B vaccine recommended for populations at risk Populations at risk are women from Asia, Pacific Islands, Indochina, Haiti, South Africa, Alaska (women of Eskimo descent); other women at risk include health care providers, users of intravenous drugs, those sexually active with multiple partners or single partner with multiple risks

Continued

TABLE 8-7 Maternal Infection: TORCH—cont'd

INFECTION	MATERNAL EFFECTS	FETAL EFFECTS	COUNSELING: PREVENTION, IDENTIFICATION, AND MANAGEMENT
Rubella (3-day German measles) (virus)	Rash, fever, mild symptoms; suboccipital lymph nodes may be swollen; some photophobia Occasionally arthritis or encephalitis Miscarriage	Incidence of congenital anomalies—first month 50%, second month 25%, third month 10%, fourth month 4% Exposure during first 2 months—malformations of heart, eyes, ears, or brain; abnormal dermatoglyphics Exposure after fourth month—systemic infection, hepatosplenomegaly, intrauterine growth restriction, rash	Vaccination of pregnant women contraindicated; pregnancy should be prevented for 3 months after vaccination; pregnant women nonreactive to hemagglutinin-inhibition antigen can be safely vaccinated after birth.
Cytomegalovirus (CMV) (a herpes virus)	Respiratory or sexually transmitted asymptomatic illness or mononucleosis-like syndrome, may have cervical discharge No immunity develops	Fetal death or severe, generalized disease—hemolytic anemia and jaundice, hydrocephaly or microcephaly, pneumonitis, hepatosplenomegaly, deafness	Virus may be reactivated and cause disease in utero or during birth in subsequent pregnancies; fetal infection may occur during passage through infected birth canal; disease is commonly progressive through infancy and childhood
Herpes genitalis (herpes simplex virus, type 2 [HSV-2])	Primary blisters, rash, fever, malaise, nausea, headache; pregnancy risks include miscarriage, preterm labor, stillbirths	Transplacental infection is rare; congenital effects include skin lesions and scarring, IUGR, mental retardation, microcephaly	Risk of transmission is greatest during vaginal birth if woman has active lesions Acyclovir not recommended in pregnancy; treat symptomatically (see Table 8-2)

miscarriage, congenital anomalies (referred to as congenital rubella syndrome), and death. Vaccination of pregnant women is contraindicated because a rubella infection may develop after the vaccine is administered. Rubella vaccine is given to women who are not immune as part of preconception counseling, with instructions to use contraception for at least 3 months after vaccination.

Cytomegalovirus

Maternal infection with cytomegalovirus (CMV) may begin as a mononucleosis-like syndrome. In most adults the onset of CMV infection is uncertain and asymptomatic; however, the disease may remain subclinical for years. This virus is primarily transmitted by respiratory droplets but has also been isolated from semen, cervical and vaginal secretions, breast milk, placental tissue, urine, feces, and banked blood. Maternal CMV infection may be diagnosed serologically because many women have evidence of CMV infection. Women who show CMV infection in pregnancy (by positive viral titers) usually have chronic or recurrent infections (Fanaroff & Martin, 1997).

Women at risk for infection include those who work in or have children in day care centers, institutions for the mentally retarded, or certain health settings (such as nursery, dialysis, laboratory, and oncology).

In the United States, 1% to 2% of infants have congenital CMV infection. Fetal infection can cause microcephaly; eye, ear, and dental defects; and mental retardation. No treatment is available during pregnancy.

Herpes Simplex Virus

The potential pregnancy effects of primary genital herpes infection include miscarriage, preterm labor, and intrauterine growth restriction. The main route of HSV transmission from mother to neonate is through an infected birth canal. The risk of maternal-infant transmission is greater during a primary HSV-2 infection than during a recurrent episode (Fanaroff & Martin, 1997). Cesarean birth is not recommended for all mothers with HSV. Only mothers with clinical evidence of active lesions during labor should have cesarean birth. Prenatal HSV cultures do not predict the presence of a live virus at time of birth. Cultures in women with HSV lesions at or near term may be done to ensure the absence of the virus at time of birth and increase the likelihood of a vaginal birth (see Table 8-2 for treatment guidelines).

CARE MANAGEMENT

Women may delay seeking care for STIs and other infections because they fear social stigma, have little accessibility to health care services, are asymptomatic, or are unaware that they have an infection.

Assessment and Nursing Diagnoses

A comprehensive assessment focuses on lifestyle issues that are often personal or sensitive. A culturally sensitive, nonjudgmental approach is essential to facilitate accurate data collection. Specific areas to address are listed in Box 8-3. A history that is accurate, comprehensive, and specific is crucial to sound diagnosis.

History

Because many women are embarrassed or anxious, the history should be taken first, with the woman dressed. Information should be collected in a nonjudgmental manner, using open-ended questions and avoiding assumptions of sexual preference. All partners should be referred to as partners and not by gender. A complete history is essential in identifying possible STIs. Factors that may influence the development and management of STIs in women include previous history of STI or PID, number of past or current sexual partners, and types of sexual activity. Lifestyle behaviors that place women at risk for STIs should be specifically queried. Among these are intravenous drug use or partner intravenous drug use, smoking, alcohol use, inadequate or poor nutrition, and high levels of stress or fatigue.

Physical Examination

Before the actual physical examination is performed, the nurse should discuss the examination with the woman

---

> **BOX 8-3** **Essential Areas of Assessment for a Woman at Risk for or Who Has a Sexually Transmitted Infection**
>
> **CURRENT PROBLEM**
> What symptoms are present?
>   Vaginal discharge
>   Lesions
>   Rash
>   Dysuria
>   Fever
>   Itching, burning
>   Dyspareunia
>   Malaise
>
> **PAST MEDICAL HISTORY**
> History of STDs
> Allergies, especially to medications
>
> **MENSTRUAL HISTORY**
> Last menstrual period (possibility of pregnancy)
>
> **PERSONAL AND SOCIAL HISTORY**
> **Sexual History**
> Sexual preference
> Number of partners (past, present)
> Types of sexual activity
> Frequency of sexual activity
>
> **LIFESTYLE BEHAVIORS**
> Intravenous drug use (or partner)
> Smoking
> Alcohol use
> Inadequate/poor nutrition
> High levels of stress, fatigue

---

so she is prepared for it. A thorough assessment of symptoms including a comprehensive physical examination is essential to diagnosing STIs. Because the speculum usually is not lubricated before insertion into the vagina (cultures of vaginal secretions may have to be obtained), insertion may be more uncomfortable than usual. Women should be informed of this and reassured that every effort will be made to make the speculum examination as comfortable as possible.

Laboratory Tests

Appropriate laboratory studies will be suggested, in part, by the history and physical examination results. Bacterial STIs are easily determined from genital tract, urine, and blood studies. Viral agents can also be cultured, but less successfully. Because women often are infected with more than one STI simultaneously and many are asymptomatic, additional laboratory studies may be done, including Pap smear, wet mounts, gonococcal culture, and Venereal Disease

Research Laboratories (VDRL) or rapid plasma reagin (RPR) test for syphilis. Cultures for HSV are obtained when indicated by history or physical examination. The woman should be offered the HIV-antibody test. When indicated, a complete blood count, sedimentation rate, urinalysis, or urine culture and sensitivity should be obtained.

Nursing diagnoses are derived after carefully analyzing assessment findings, medical management, and health care provider directives. The following nursing diagnoses are representative of those used in a plan of care for women with sexually transmitted infections and other vaginal infections:

Nursing Diagnoses

- Anxiety/situational low self-esteem/body image disturbance related to
  - perceived effects on sexual relationships and family processes
  - possible effects on pregnancy/fetus
  - long-term sequelae of infection
- Knowledge deficit related to
  - transmission/prevention of infection/reinfection
  - safer sex behaviors
  - management of infection
- Pain/impaired tissue integrity related to
  - effects of infection process
  - scratching (excoriation) of pruritic areas
  - hygiene practices
- Sexual dysfunction and altered sexuality pattern related to
  - effects of infection process
- Social isolation and impaired social interaction related to
  - perceived effects on relationships with others if STI status is unknown

Expected Outcomes of Care

Care of the woman with an STI focuses on physical and psychologic needs. Avoidance of reinfection and harmful sequelae is critical. Measurable expected outcomes are mutually derived with the woman's input. Outcomes for the woman include that she will do the following:
- Be free of infection, or in the case of viral infection, have remission or stabilization of the infection.
- Identify and be able to discuss the etiology, management, and expected course of the infection and its prevention.
- Be able to identify her risky behaviors and discuss plans for decreasing her risk for infection.

Plan of Care and Interventions

The woman with an STI will need encouragement to seek care at the earliest stage of symptoms. Counseling women about STIs is essential for (1) preventing new infections or reinfection; (2) increasing compliance with treatment and follow-up; (3) providing support during treatment; and (4) assisting women in discussions with their partner(s). Women must be made aware of the serious potential consequences of STIs and the behaviors that increase the likelihood of infection.

The nurse must make sure that the woman understands what infection she has, how it is transmitted, and why it must be treated (see Home Care box). Women should be given a brief description of the infection in language that they can understand. This description should include modes of transmission, incubation period, symptoms, infectious period, and potential complications. Effective treatment of STIs necessitates careful, thorough explanation of the treatment regimen and follow-up procedures. Thorough, careful instructions about medications must be provided, both verbally and in writing. Side effects, benefits, and risks of the medication should be discussed. Unpleasant side effects or early relief of symptoms may discourage women from completing their medication course. Clients should be strongly urged to take all the medication and not stop even if their symptoms diminish or disappear in a few days. Comfort measures to decrease symptoms such as pain, itching, or nausea should be suggested. Providing written information is a useful strategy because this is a time of high anxiety for many women and they may not be able to hear or remember what they were told. A number of booklets on sexually transmitted infections are available, or the nurse may wish to develop literature that is specific to the practice setting and clients.

In general, women will be advised to refrain from intercourse until all treatment is finished and a reculture, if appropriate, is done. After the infection is cured, women

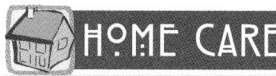

HOME CARE

Sexually Transmitted Infections

Take your medication as directed.

Use comfort measures for symptom relief as suggested by your health care provider.

Keep your appointment for repeat cultures or checkups after your treatment to make sure your infection is cured.

Inform your sexual partner(s) to be tested and treated, if necessary.

Abstain from sexual intercourse until your treatment is completed or for as long as you are advised by your health care provider.

Use safer sex practices when sexual intercourse is resumed.

Call your health care provider immediately if you notice bumps, sores, rashes, or discharges.

Keep all future appointments with your health care provider, even if things appear normal.

should be urged to continue using condoms to prevent repeated infections, especially if they have had one episode of pelvic inflammatory disease or continue to have intercourse with new partners. Women may wish to avoid having sex with partners who have many other sexual partners. All women who have contracted an STI should be taught safer sex practices, if this has not been done already. Follow-up appointments should be made as needed.

Addressing the psychosocial component of STIs is essential. A woman may be afraid or embarrassed to tell her partner or to ask her partner to seek treatment. She may be embarrassed to admit her sexual practices, or she may be concerned about confidentiality. The nurse may need to help the woman deal with the impact of a diagnosis of an STI on a committed relationship, for the woman is now faced with the necessity of dealing with "uncertain monogamy."

In many instances sexual partners should be treated; thus the infected woman is asked to identify and notify all partners who might have been exposed. Often she will find this difficult to do. Empathizing with the client's feelings and suggesting specific ways of talking with partners will help decrease anxiety and assist in efforts to control infection. For example, the nurse might suggest that the woman say, "I care about you and I'm concerned about you. That's why I'm calling to tell you that I have a sexually transmitted disease. My clinician is _____ and she will be happy to talk with you if you would like." Offering literature and role playing situations with the client also may be of assistance. It is often helpful to remind the woman that

---

PLAN ᵒᶠ CARE | Sexually Transmitted Infections

NURSING DIAGNOSIS Altered health maintenance related to prevention of sexually transmitted infections evidenced by client positive diagnosis of sexually transmitted infection

Expected Outcome *Client will verbalize which health practices directly led to positive diagnosis of a sexually transmitted infection.*

Nursing Interventions/*Rationales*

Inquire about client's sexual history and sexual health practices *to provide database for current problem.*

Use therapeutic communication for private, nonjudgmental discussion *to facilitate learning and promote self-esteem.*

Provide emotional support *to indicate awareness of client's feelings about this sensitive topic.*

Provide information about transmission of disease, including cause, symptoms, and treatment for both partners *to enhance client's knowledge base and correct any misinformation.*

Discuss the use and importance of safe sexual practices *to raise client's awareness and motivation to avoid future risk-taking behaviors.*

Instruct client and sexual partner to complete medication regimen *to completely eradicate transmitted organism.*

NURSING DIAGNOSIS: Impaired social interaction related to diagnosis of sexually transmitted disease as evidenced by client verbal report

Expected Outcome *Client will report increased incidences of social interaction.*

Nursing Interventions/*Rationales*

Provide nonjudgmental, confidential therapeutic communication *to increase client's feelings of self-worth.*

Refer to support groups *to provide group interaction, discussion, and information.*

NURSING DIAGNOSIS Impaired tissue integrity related to effects of disease process as evidenced by client report of itching and vaginal discharge

Expected Outcome *Client's tissue integrity will be restored.*

Nursing Interventions/*Rationales*

Assess, monitor, and document characteristics of the damaged skin area, including color, lesions, drainage, and edema *to provide database.*

Instruct client in correct genital hygiene practices *to prevent further infection of damaged tissues with other organisms.*

Provide warm soaks or sitz baths *to promote comfort, circulation, and healing.*

Administer prescribed medications *to promote comfort and eradication of organism.*

Provide written self-help materials and pamphlets *to prevent further skin integrity loss.*

BOX 8-4 Standard Precautions

Medical history and examination cannot reliably identify all persons infected with HIV or other blood-borne pathogens. Standard Precautions should therefore be used consistently in the care of all persons. These precautions apply to blood, body fluids, and all secretions and excretions, except sweat, nonintact skin, and mucous membranes. Standard Precautions are recommended to reduce the risk of transmission of microorganisms from known and unknown sources of infection (Centers for Disease Control and Hospital Infection Control Practices Advisory Committee, 1996).

1. Handwashing is recommended promptly and thoroughly between client contacts. Hands and other skin surfaces should be washed immediately and thoroughly if contaminated with blood or other body fluids. Hands should be washed immediately after gloves are removed.

2. In addition to handwashing, all health care workers should routinely use appropriate barrier precautions to prevent skin and mucous membrane exposure when contact with blood or other body fluids of any person is anticipated. *Latex gloves* should be worn for touching blood and body fluids, mucous membranes, or nonintact skin of all persons; for handling items or surfaces soiled with blood or body fluids; and for performing venipuncture and other vascular access procedures. Gloves should be changed after contact with each client. *Masks and protective eyewear* or face shields should be worn during procedures that are likely to generate droplets of blood or other body fluids to prevent exposure of mucous membranes of the mouth, nose, and eyes. *Gowns or aprons* should be worn during procedures that are likely to generate splashes of blood or other body fluids.

   Leg coverings, boots, or shoe covers also can be worn to provide protection against splashes and may be recommended for certain procedures such as surgery.

3. All health care workers should take precautions to prevent injuries caused by needles, scalpels, and other sharp instruments or devices during procedures; when cleaning used instruments; during disposal of used needles; and when handling sharp instruments after procedures. *To prevent needle-stick injuries,* needles should not be recapped, purposely bent or broken by hand, removed from disposable syringes, or otherwise manipulated by hand. After they are used, disposable syringes and needles, scalpel blades, and other sharp items should be immediately placed in a puncture-resistant container for disposal; puncture-resistant containers should be located as close as is practical to the use area.

4. Although saliva has not been implicated in HIV transmission, to minimize the need for emergency mouth-to-mouth resuscitation, mouthpieces, resuscitation bags, or other ventilation devices should be available for use in areas in which the need for resuscitation is predictable.

5. Health care workers who have exudative lesions or weeping dermatitis should refrain from all direct client care and from handling client care equipment until the condition resolves.

PRECAUTIONS FOR INVASIVE PROCEDURES

An invasive procedure is surgical entry into tissues, cavities, or organs; or repair of major traumatic injuries (1) in an operating or birthing room, emergency department, or out-of-hospital setting, including both physicians' and dentists' offices; and (2) a vaginal or cesarean birth or other invasive obstetric procedure during which bleeding may occur. Standard Precautions, combined with the following precautions, should serve as minimum precautions for all such invasive procedures:

1. All health care workers who participate in invasive procedures must routinely use appropriate barrier precautions to prevent skin and mucous membrane contact with blood and other body fluids of all clients. Gloves and surgical masks must be worn for all invasive procedures. Protective eyewear or face shields should be worn for procedures that commonly result in the generation of droplets, splashing of blood or other body fluids, or the generation of bone chips. Gowns or aprons made of materials that provide an effective barrier should be worn during invasive procedures that are likely to result in the splashing of blood or other body fluids. All health care workers who perform or assist in vaginal or cesarean births should wear gloves and gowns when handling the placenta or the infant until blood and amniotic fluid have been removed from the infant's skin. Gloves should be worn during infant eye prophylaxis, care of the umbilical cord, circumcision site, parenteral procedures, diaper changes, contact with colostrum, and postpartum assessments.

2. If a glove is torn or a needle stick or other injury occurs, the glove should be removed and a new glove used as promptly as patient safety permits; the needle or instrument involved in the incident also should be removed from the sterile field.

3. Any needle stick or other injury should be reported and appropriate treatment obtained as specified by the health care facility.

although this is an embarrassing situation, most persons would rather know than not know that they have been exposed. Health professionals who take time to counsel their clients on how to talk with their partner(s) can improve compliance and case finding.

Interrupting the transmission of infection is crucial to STI control. For treatable and vaccine-preventable STIs, further transmission and reinfection can be prevented with referral of sex partners. Many STIs are reportable; all states require that the five traditional venereal diseases–gonorrhea, syphilis, chancroid, lymphogranuloma venereum, and granuloma inguinale–be reported to public health officials. Many other states require that other STIs such as chlamydial infections, genital herpes, and genital warts be reported. In addition, all states require that AIDS cases be reported; 35 states require that HIV infection be reported. The nurse is legally responsible for reporting all cases of those diseases identified as reportable and should know what the requirements are in the state in which she or he practices. The woman must be informed when a case will be reported and told why. Failure to inform the woman that the case will be reported is a serious breech of professional ethics. Confidentiality is a crucial issue for many clients. When an STI is reportable, women must be told that they may be contacted by a health department epidemiologist. They should be assured that the information reported to and collected by health authorities is not available to anyone without their permission. Every effort, within the limits of one's public health responsibilities, should be made to reassure clients (see Plan of Care).

Management During Pregnancy

Treatment of specific STIs may be different for the pregnant woman and may even be different at different stages of pregnancy. Tables 8-2 and 8-4 describe treatment of common STIs and vaginal infections during pregnancy.

Infection Control

Infection control measures are essential to protect care providers and to prevent nosocomial infection of clients, regardless of the infectious agent. The risk for occupational transmission varies with the disease. Even when the risk is low, as with HIV, the existence of any risk warrants reasonable precautions. Precautions against airborne disease transmission are available in all health care agencies. **Standard Precautions** (precautions to use in care of all persons for infection control) and additional precautions for labor and birth settings are listed in Box 8-4.

Evaluation

Evaluation is a continuous process. To be effective, evaluation is based on client-centered outcomes identified during the planning stage of nursing care. The nurse can be reasonably assured that care was effective to the extent that expected outcomes have been met.

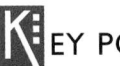 **EY POINTS**

- Safer sex practices are key STI prevention strategies.
- HIV is transmitted through body fluids, primarily blood, semen, and vaginal secretions.
- HPV is the most common viral STI.
- Syphilis has reemerged as a common STI.
- Chlamydia is the most common STI in American women and the most common cause of PID.
- Viral hepatitis has several forms of transmission; hepatitis B virus infections carry the greatest risk.
- Young, sexually active women who do not practice safer sex behaviors and have multiple partners are at greatest risk for STIs and HIV.
- STIs are responsible for substantial mortality and morbidity, great personal suffering, and heavy economic burden in the United States.
- STIs and vaginitis are biologic events for which all individuals have a right to expect objective, compassionate, and effective health care.
- Substance abuse can alter the body's immune system and possibly increase the risk for acquiring AIDS and associated conditions.
- Pregnancy confers no immunity against infection, and both mother and fetus must be considered when the pregnant woman contracts an infection.
- Because history and examination cannot reliably identify all persons with HIV or other blood-borne pathogens, blood and body fluid precautions should be consistently used for everyone all the time.

 RITICAL THINKING EXERCISES

1 You are asked to teach safer sex practices to a group of girls ages 13 through 16.
   a. Examine your personal feelings regarding sexual activity in this age group.
   b. Analyze the significance of your reactions in terms of providing this care.
   c. Formulate a teaching plan for this group.
   d. Determine how you will evaluate the effects of your care.

2 You are assigned to the health department STD clinic.
   a. What resources are available for counseling women who come to the clinic for testing or treatment?

Continued

CRITICAL THINKING EXERCISES—cont'd

b. Develop information sources that would be helpful in the clinic to inform clients about risk factors and safer sex practices.

c. Consider how informational sources should be different for clients of different ages and cultures.

3 You are assigned to a 17-year-old mother who tested positive for syphilis on admission for labor. The baby has a positive urine toxicology screen result for cocaine and also has a positive syphilis test result. The mother is being discharged, but the baby has to remain in the nursery for another week for antibiotic therapy. Social Services has been consulted to evaluate the home situation to determine whether the baby should be discharged to the mother or to foster care.

a. What factors must be considered in evaluating the home situation? What are the pros and cons of the baby going home versus going to foster care?

b. Develop a discharge plan for the mother, including follow-up for drug use and STD counseling.

c. Develop a plan of care for follow-up of the infant if he is allowed to go home to the mother.

References

American College of Obstetricians and Gynecologists. (1994). Genital human papillomavirus infections. *ACOG Technical Bulletin* 194, 1-7.

Ammer, C. (1989). *The new A-to-Z of woman's health: A concise encyclopedia.* New York: Facts on File, Inc.

Bonny, A., & Biro, F. (1998, Spring). Recognizing and treating STDs in the adolescent. *Contemp Nurse Pract* 15-18, 20-24.

Centers for Disease Control and Prevention. (1994). Recommendations of the U.S. Public Health Service Task Force on the use of zidovudine to reduce perinatal transmission of human immunodeficiency virus. *MMWR* 43(RR-11), on-line issue.

Centers for Disease Control and Prevention. (1995). Recommendations of the U.S. Public Health Service Task Force for human immunodeficiency virus counseling and voluntary testing for pregnant women. *MMWR* 44(RR-7), 1-12

Centers for Disease Control and Prevention. (1996a). Prevention of hepatitis A through active or passive immunization: Recommendations of the advisory committee on immunization practice. *MMWR* 45(RR-15), 1-30.

Centers for Disease Control and Prevention. (1996b). Prevention of perinatal group B streptococcal disease: A public health perspective. *MMWR* 45(RR-7), 1-24.

Centers for Disease Control and Prevention. (1998a). 1998 guidelines for treatment of sexually transmitted diseases. *MMWR* 47(RR-1), 1-117.

Centers for Disease Control and Prevention. (1998b). Primary and secondary syphilis–United States, 1997. *MMWR* 47(24), 493-497.

Centers for Disease Control and Prevention, Division of STD/HIV Prevention. (1995). *Annual report 1994. U.S. Department of Health and Human Services.* Atlanta: Centers for Disease Control and Prevention.

Centers for Disease Control and Prevention and Hospital Infection Control Practices Advisory Committee. (1996). Special recommendations: Guidelines for isolation precautions in hospitals. Part II. Recommendations for isolation precautions in hospitals. *Am J Infect Control* 24(1), 24-52.

Clay, L. (1996). Group B streptococcus in the perinatal period: A review. *J Nurse Midwifery* 41(5), 355-363.

Cochran, S., & Mays, V. (1990). Sex, lies, and HIV. *N Engl J Med* 322(11), 774-775.

Corder-Mabe, J. (1998).Complications of pregnancy. In E. Youngkin & M. Davis (Eds.). *Women's health care. A clinical guide* (2nd ed.). Stamford, CT: Appleton & Lange.

Cotton, D., & Watts, D. (1997). *The medical management of AIDS in women.* New York: Willey-Liss.

Cunningham, F. et al. (1997). *Williams obstetrics* (20th ed.). Stamford, CT: Appleton & Lange.

DiSaia, P., & Creasman, W. (1997). *Clinical gynecologic oncology* (5th ed.). St. Louis: Mosby.

Eisenstat, S. (1995). Infectious exposure and immunization during pregnancy. In K. Carlson et al. (Eds.). *Primary care of women.* St. Louis: Mosby.

Fanaroff, A., & Martin, R. (1997). *Neonatal-perinatal medicine: Diseases of the fetus and infant* (6th ed.). St Louis: Mosby.

Fogel, C. (1995). Sexually transmitted disease. In C. Fogel & N. Woods (Eds.). *Women's health care.* Thousand Oaks, CA: Sage.

Freitag-Koontz, M. (1996). Prevention of hepatitis B and C transmission during pregnancy and the first year of life. *J Perinat Neonatal Nurs* 10, 40-55.

Gilbert, E., & Harmon, J. (1998). *Manual of high risk pregnancy and delivery* (2nd ed.). St. Louis: Mosby.

Hatcher, R. et al. (1998). *Contraceptive technology* (17th ed.). New York: Ardent Media, Inc.

Hunt, C., Carson, K., & Sharara, A. (1997). Hepatitis C in pregnancy. *Obstet Gynecol* 89(5, pt 2), 883-890.

Institute of Medicine, Committee on Prevention and Control of Sexually Transmitted Diseases. (1997). *The hidden epidemic: Confronting sexually transmitted diseases.* Washington, DC: National Academy of Sciences.

Johnstone, F. (1997, October). Contraception for the HIV-infected woman. *J Int Assoc Phys AIDS Care* 10-15.

Katz, V. (1993). Management of streptococcal disease in pregnancy. *Clin Obstet Gynecol* 36, 832-842.

Lieu, T. et al. (1998). Neonatal group B streptococcal infection in a managed care population. *Obstet Gynecol* 92(1), 21-27.

National Institutes of Health. (1996). *Consensus development conference statement on cervical cancer.* April 1-3. Bethesda, MD: National Institutes of Health.

Plourd, D. (1997). Practical guide to diagnosing and treating vaginitis. *Medscape Women's Health* 2(1), 1-13.

Schaffer, S. (1998). Vaginitis and sexually transmitted diseases. In E. Youngkin & M. Davis (Eds.). *Women's health. A primary care clinical guide.* Stamford, CT: Appleton & Lange.

Starr, W., Lommel, L., & Shanon, M. (1995). *Women's primary health care. Protocols for practice.* Washington, DC: American Nurses Publishing.

Walker, C., & Sweet, R. (1992). HIV and other sexually transmitted diseases in pregnancy. In E. Reece et al. (Eds.). *Medicine of the fetus and mother.* Philadelphia: J.B. Lippincott.

Wildschut, H., Weiner, C., & Peters, T. (1996). *When to screen in obstetrics and gynecology.* Philadelphia: W.B. Saunders.

Wortley, P., & Flemming, P. (1997). AIDS in women in the United States: Recent trends. *JAMA* 278(11), 911-916.

Youngkin, E. (1995). Sexually transmitted diseases: Current and emerging trends. *J Obstet Gynecol Neonatal Nurs* 24(8), 743-758.

9

Contraception and Abortion

Sharon E. Lock

EARNING OBJECTIVES_____

- Define the key terms.
- Compare the different methods of contraception.
- State the advantages and disadvantages of frequently used methods of contraception.
- Explain the common nursing interventions that facilitate contraceptive use.
- Recognize the various ethical, legal, cultural, and religious considerations of fertility management.

- Describe the techniques used for medical and surgical interruption of pregnancy.
- Examine the various ethical and legal considerations of elective abortion.
- Identify topics in nursing research related to contraception and abortion.

KEY TERMS_____

basal body temperature (BBT)	fertile period	sterilization
calendar rhythm method	fertility awareness methods	symptothermal method
cervical cap	induced abortion	therapeutic abortion
cervical mucus method	intrauterine device (IUD)	toxic shock syndrome (TSS)
condom	laminaria tent	vacuum aspiration
contraception	periodic abstinence	withdrawal bleeding
diaphragm	predictor test for ovulation	
elective abortion	spermicide	

CONTRACEPTION

Contraception is the voluntary prevention of pregnancy. In 1995 more than 90% of U.S. women at risk of pregnancy used a method of contraception. Despite the large numbers of men and women who use contraception, almost half of the 6.3 million pregnancies in the United States every year are unintended (Henshaw, 1998). Those who use contraception may still be at risk for pregnancy simply because their choice of contraceptive method is not perfect or is used incorrectly. Providing adequate instruction in how to use a contraceptive method, when to use a backup method, and information about emergency contraception could decrease the risk of unintended pregnancy (Kowal, 1998). Nurses are instrumental in providing information that contributes to the client's decision making about contraception. To provide accurate information to clients, the nurse must be knowledgeable about the various contraceptive methods.

: CARE MANAGEMENT

A multidisciplinary approach may assist a woman in choosing and correctly using an appropriate contraceptive method. Nurses, nurse-midwives, nurse-practitioners, and other advanced practice nurses and physicians have the knowledge and expertise to assist a woman in making decisions about contraception that will satisfy the woman's personal, social, cultural, and interpersonal needs.

Assessment and Nursing Diagnoses

The woman's knowledge about contraception and her sexual partner's commitment to any particular method are determined. Data are required about the frequency of coitus, number of sexual partners, level of contraceptive involvement, and her or her partner's objections to any methods (see Guidelines/Guías). The woman's level of comfort and willingness to touch her genitals and cervical mucus are assessed. Myths are identified, and religious and cultural factors are determined. The woman's verbal and nonverbal responses to hearing about the various available methods are carefully noted. An individual's reproductive life plan must be considered. A history (including menstrual, contraceptive, and obstetric), physical examination (including pelvic examination), and laboratory tests are usually completed.

Informed consent is a vital component in the education of the client concerning contraception or sterilization. The nurse has the responsibility of documenting information provided and the understanding of that information by the client. Using the acronym BRAIDED may be useful (see Legal Tip).

LEGAL TIP **Informed Consent**

B—Benefits: information about advantages and success rates
R—Risks: information about disadvantages and failure rates
A—Alternatives: information on other methods available
I —Inquiries: opportunity to ask questions
D—Decisions: opportunity to decide or change mind
E—Explanations: information about method and how it is used
D—Documentation: information given and client's understanding

---

Nursing diagnoses reflect analysis of the assessment findings. Examples of nursing diagnoses that may emerge regarding contraception include those listed below.

: Nursing Diagnoses

- Risk for decisional conflict related to
  - contraceptive alternatives
  - partner's willingness to agree on contraceptive method
- Fear related to
  - contraceptive method side effects

: Nursing Diagnoses—cont'd

- Risk for infection related to
  - being sexually active
  - use of contraceptive method
  - broken skin or mucous membrane secondary to surgery, IUD insertion, hormonal implant
- Risk for altered sexuality patterns related to
  - fear of pregnancy
- Pain related to
  - postoperative recovery after sterilization
- Spiritual distress related to
  - discrepancy between religious or cultural beliefs and choice of contraception

Expected Outcomes of Care

Planning is a collaborative effort among the woman, her sexual partner (when appropriate), the primary health care provider, and the nurse. The expected outcomes are determined and stated in client-centered terms and may include that the woman or couple will do the following:
- Verbalize understanding about contraceptive methods.
- Verbalize understanding of all information necessary to give informed consent.
- State comfort and satisfaction with the chosen method.
- Use the contraceptive method correctly and consistently.
- Achieve pregnancy when planned, if childbearing is desired.
- Experience no adverse sequelae as a result of the chosen method of contraception.

Interventions

Unbiased client teaching is fundamental to initiating and maintaining any form of contraception. A care provider relationship based on trust is an important facet in compliance of the client. The nurse counters myths with facts, clarifies misinformation, and fills in gaps of knowledge. Various contraceptive techniques are used in North America. The ideal contraceptive should be safe, easily available, economical, acceptable, simple to use, and promptly reversible. Although no method may ever achieve all these objectives, impressive progress has been made.

Contraceptive failure rate refers to the percentage of contraceptive users expected to experience an accidental pregnancy during the first year, even when they use a method consistently and correctly. Contraceptive effectiveness varies from couple to couple (Box 9-1) and depends on both the properties of the method and the characteristics of the user (Guest, 1998). Failure rates decrease over time either because a user will gain experience and use a method more appropriately or because the less effective users will stop using the method.

Safety of a method depends on the woman's medical history, tobacco use, and age. Barrier methods offer some protection from sexually transmitted infections (STIs), and

BOX 9-1 | **Factors Affecting Method Effectiveness**

Frequency of intercourse
Motivation to prevent pregnancy
Understanding of how to use the method
Compliance with method
Provision of short-term or long-term protection
Likelihood of pregnancy for the individual woman

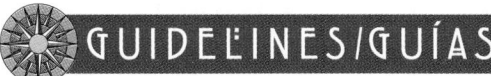

Contraception

Do you plan to have more children?
¿Piensa tener más hijos?

Are you sexually active?
¿Está usted sexualmente activa?

Do you have many partners?
¿Tiene muchos compañeros?

Have you had many partners in the past?
¿He tenido muchos compañeros en el pasado?

Do you presently use contraception/birth control?
¿Usa actualmente anticonceptivos/contol de nacimiento?

The Pill? Condoms? The diaphragm? The I.U.D.?
¿La Píldora? ¿Los condones? ¿El diafragma? ¿El Dispositivo Intrauterino (D.I.U.)?

Spermicides? The rhythm method? Implant (Depo Provera) or injection?
¿Espermaticidas? ¿El método de ritmo? ¿El Implante o inyección?

How long have you used this method?
¿Por cuánto tiempo ha usado este método?

Do you like this method?
¿Le gusta este método?

Why did you stop using it?
¿Por qué dejó de usarlo?

Do you want to change to a different method?
¿Quiere cambiar a otro método?

Have you had a tubal ligation?
¿Le ataron los tubos?

Has he had a vasectomy?
¿Le hicieron a él vasectomía?

oral contraceptives may lower the incidence of ovarian and endometrial cancer but increase the risk of thromboembolic problems.

Methods of Contraception

The following discussion of contraceptive methods provides the nurse with information needed for client teaching. After implementing the appropriate teaching for contraceptive use, the nurse supervises return demonstrations and practice to assess client understanding. The woman is given written instructions and phone numbers for questions. If the woman has difficulty understanding written instructions, she (and her partner, if available) is offered graphic material and a phone number to call as necessary or is offered an opportunity to return for further instruction (see Guidelines/Guías for contraceptive teaching).

Coitus interruptus (withdrawal). Coitus interruptus involves the male partner withdrawing the penis from the woman's vagina before he ejaculates. Although coitus interruptus has been criticized as being an ineffective method of contraception, it is a good choice for couples who do not have another contraceptive available (Kowal, 1998). Effectiveness is similar to barrier methods and depends on the man's ability to withdraw his penis before ejaculation. The percentage of women who will experience an unintended pregnancy within the first year of typical use (failure rate) of withdrawal is about 19% (Kowal, 1998). Coitus interruptus does not protect against STIs or human immunodeficiency virus (HIV) infection.

Periodic abstinence. **Periodic abstinence,** or natural family planning (NFP), provides contraception by using methods that rely on avoidance of intercourse during fertile periods. It is the only method of contraception acceptable to the Roman Catholic Church. **Fertility awareness** is the combination of charting signs and symptoms of the menstrual cycle with the use of abstinence or other contraceptive methods during fertile periods. Signs and symptoms most commonly used are menstrual bleeding, cervical mucus, and basal body temperature (Jennings, Lamprecht, & Kowal, 1998).

Knowledge of the menstrual cycle is basic to the practice of NFP. To review, the human ovum can be fertilized no later than 16 to 24 hours after ovulation. Motile sperm have been recovered from the uterus and the oviducts as long as 60 hours after coitus. However, their ability to fertilize the ovum probably lasts no longer than 24 to 48 hours. Pregnancy is unlikely to occur if a couple abstains from intercourse for 4 days before and for 3 or 4 days after ovulation **(fertile period).** Unprotected intercourse on the other days of the cycle (safe period) should not result in pregnancy. However, there are two principal problems with this method: the exact time of ovulation cannot be predicted accurately, and couples may find it difficult to abstain from sexual intercourse for several days before and after ovulation. Women with irregular menstrual periods have the greatest risk of failure with this form of contraception. Therefore natural family planning methods are not recommended until regular menses has resumed postpartum (Jennings et al., 1998). The typical failure rate for all **fertility**

awareness methods is 25% during the first year of use (Jennings et al., 1998).

Ovulation usually occurs about 14 days before the on-set of menstruation. Therefore variations in the length of menstrual cycles are usually a result of differences in the length of the preovulatory phase. The fertile period can be anticipated by the following:

- Calculating the time at which ovulation is likely to oc-cur based on the lengths of previous menstrual cycles (calendar method)
- Recording the rise in basal body temperature, a result of the thermogenic effect of progesterone (temperature method)
- Recognizing the changes in cervical mucus at different phases of the menstrual cycle (ovulation or Billings method)
- Using a combination of several methods (symptother-mal method)
- Using a predictor test for ovulation

Calendar rhythm method. Practice of the **calendar rhythm method** (also known as the rhythm method or menstrual cycle charting), is based on the number of days in each cycle counting from the first day of menses (Jennings et al., 1998). With the calendar method the fertile period is determined after accurately recording the lengths of menstrual cycles for 6 months. The beginning of the fer-tile period is estimated by subtracting 18 days from the length of the shortest cycle. The end of the fertile period is determined by subtracting 11 days from the length of the longest cycle. If the shortest cycle is 24 days and the longest cycle is 30 days, application of the formula is as follows:

Shortest cycle
24
−18
6th day

Longest cycle
30
−11
19th day

To avoid conception, the couple would abstain during the fertile period–days 6 through 19.

If the woman has regular cycles of 28 days each, the for-mula indicates the fertile days to be as follows:

Shortest cycle
28
−18
10th day

Longest cycle
28
−11
17th day

To avoid pregnancy, the couple abstains from day 10 through 17 because ovulation occurs on day 14 ± 2 days.

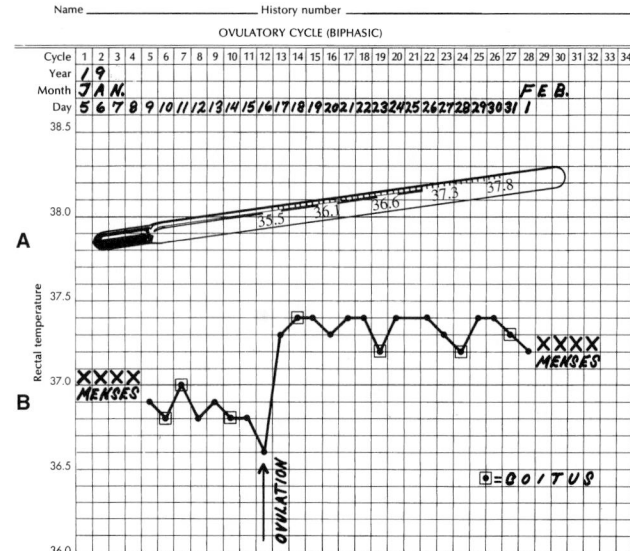

Fig. 9-1 A, Special thermometer for recording BBT, marked in tenths to enable person to read more easily. **B,** Basal temperature record shows drop and sharp rise at time of ovulation. Biphasic curve indicates ovulatory cycle.

A major drawback of the calendar method is that one is trying to predict future events with past data. The unpre-dictability of the menstrual cycle is also not taken into consideration. The calendar rhythm method is most useful as an adjunct to the basal body temperature or cervical mucus method.

Basal body temperature method. The **basal body tem-perature (BBT)** is the lowest body temperature of a healthy person, taken immediately after waking and before getting out of bed. The BBT usually varies from 36.2° to 36.3° C during menses and for about 5 to 7 days afterward (Fig. 9-1).

If ovulation fails to occur, this pattern of lower body temperature continues throughout the cycle. Infection, fa-tigue, less than 3 hours sleep per night, awakening late, and anxiety may cause temperature fluctuations, altering the expected pattern. If a new BBT thermometer is pur-chased, this fact is noted on the chart because the readings may vary slightly. Jet lag, alcohol taken the evening before, or sleeping in a heated waterbed must also be noted on the chart because each affects the BBT.

At about the time of ovulation a slight drop in tempera-ture (approximately 0.05° C) may be seen by some women, but others may see no drop at all. After ovulation, in con-cert with the increasing progesterone levels of the early luteal phase of the cycle, the BBT rises slightly (approxi-mately 0.2° to 0.4° C) (Speroff & Darney, 1996). The tem-perature remains on an elevated plateau until 2 to 4 days be-fore menstruation. Then it drops to the low levels recorded during the previous cycle unless pregnancy has occurred and the temperature remains elevated.

TEACHING guidelines

Basal Body Temperature

Discuss BBT with the woman.

Show the woman a diagram depicting the phases of the menstrual cycle.

Discuss the different hormones in the woman's body that are responsible for her menstrual cycle and ovulation. Leave time for questions.

Show the woman a sample BBT graph (see Fig. 9-1) and the biphasic line seen in ovulatory cycles.

Show the woman the BBT thermometer and how it is calibrated.

Have the woman demonstrate taking the temperature and reading the thermometer and graphing the temperature while the nurse watches.

Instruct the woman to write down on the chart any other activity that might affect her true BBT.

The drop and subsequent rise in temperature are referred to as the thermal shift. When the entire month's temperatures are recorded on a graph, the pattern described is more apparent. It is more difficult to perceive day-to-day variations without the entire picture. Therefore the BBT alone is not a reliable method to predict ovulation (Jennings et al., 1998; Speroff & Darney, 1996). To determine if a rise in temperature is indeed the thermal shift, the woman must be aware of other signs approaching ovulation while she continues to assess the BBT (see later discussion of symptothermal method for other indicators of ovulation).

Most counselors advise couples who wish to prevent conception to avoid unprotected intercourse from the last day of the menses until after 3 days of elevated temperature (Jennings et al., 1998) (see Teaching Guidelines).

Cervical mucus method. The **cervical mucus method** (also called the Billings method and the Creighton model ovulation method) requires that the woman recognize and interpret the characteristic cyclic changes in the amount and consistency of cervical mucus (see Teaching Guidelines). Each woman has her own unique pattern of mucus changes. The cervical mucus that accompanies ovulation is necessary for viability and motility of sperm. Without adequate cervical mucus, coitus does not result in conception. To ensure an accurate assessment of changes, the cervical mucus should be free from semen, contraceptive gels or foams, and blood or discharge from vaginal infections for at least one full cycle. Other factors that create difficulty in identifying mucus changes include douches and vaginal deodorants, being in the sexually aroused state (which thins the mucus), and taking medications such as antihistamines, which dry up the mucus.

Some women may find this method unacceptable if they are uncomfortable touching their genitals. Whether or not the individual wants to use this method for contraception, it is to the woman's advantage to learn to recognize mucus characteristics at ovulation. Self-evaluation of cervical mucus can be highly accurate and can be useful diagnostically for any of the following purposes:

- To alert the couple to the reestablishment of ovulation while breastfeeding and after discontinuation of oral contraception
- To note anovulatory cycles at any time and at the commencement of menopause
- To assist couples in planning a pregnancy

Symptothermal method. The **symptothermal method** combines the BBT and cervical mucus methods with awareness of secondary, cycle phase–related symptoms. The woman gains fertility awareness as she learns the psychologic and physiologic symptoms that mark the phases of her cycle. Secondary symptoms include increased libido, midcycle spotting, mittelschmerz, pelvic fullness or tenderness, and vulvar fullness. The woman is taught to palpate the cervix to assess for changes indicating ovulation: the cervical os dilates slightly, the cervix softens and rises in the vagina, and cervical mucus is copious and slippery (Trent & Clark, 1997). The woman notes days on which coitus, changes in routine, illness, and so on have occurred (Fig. 9-2). Calendar calculations and cervical mucus changes are used to estimate the onset of the fertile period; changes in cervical mucus or the BBT are used to estimate its end.

Predictor test for ovulation. All of the preceding methods discussed are indicative of but do not prove the occurrence and exact timing of ovulation. The predictor test for ovulation is a major addition to the periodic abstinence methods to help women who want to plan the time of their pregnancies and those who are trying to conceive. The **predictor test for ovulation** detects the sudden surge of luteinizing hormone (LH) that occurs approximately 12 to 24 hours before ovulation. Unlike BBT, the test is not affected by illness, emotional upset, or physical activity. Available for home use, a test kit contains sufficient material for several days' testing during each cycle. A positive response indicative of an LH surge is noted by color change that is easy to read. Directions for use of this home test kit vary with the manufacturer.

Barrier methods. Barrier contraceptives have gained in popularity not only as a contraceptive method but also as a protective measure against the spread of STIs. Chemical barriers such as nonoxynol-9 have been shown to slightly reduce the risk of infection with gonorrhea and chlamydia (Cates & Raymond, 1998; Heath & Sulik, 1997). Male and female condoms provide a mechanical barrier to STIs (Stewart, F., 1998).

Spermicides. A vaginal **spermicide** is a physical barrier to sperm penetration that also has a chemical action on sperm. Nonoxynol-9, the most commonly used spermicidal

TEACHING guidelines

Cervical Mucus Characteristics

SETTING THE STAGE

Show charts of menstrual cycle along with changes in the cervical mucus.

Have woman practice with raw egg white.

Supply her with a BBT log and graph if she does not already have one.

Explain that assessment of cervical mucus characteristics is best when mucus is not mixed with semen, contraceptive jellies or foams, or discharge from infections. Douching should not be done before assessment.

CONTENT RELATED TO CERVICAL MUCUS

Explain to woman (couple) how cervical mucus changes throughout the menstrual cycle.

Right before ovulation, the watery, thin, clear mucus becomes more abundant and thick (Fig. A). It feels like a lu-bricant and can be stretched 5+ cm between the thumb and forefinger; this is called spinnbarkheit (Fig. B). This indicates the period of maximum fertility. Sperm deposited in this type of mucus can survive until ovulation occurs.

ASSESSMENT TECHNIQUE

Stress that good handwashing is imperative to begin and end all self-assessment.

Start observation from last day of menstrual flow.

Assess cervical mucus several times a day for several cycles. Mucus can be obtained from vaginal introitus; no need to reach into vagina to cervix.

Record findings on the same record on which BBT is entered.

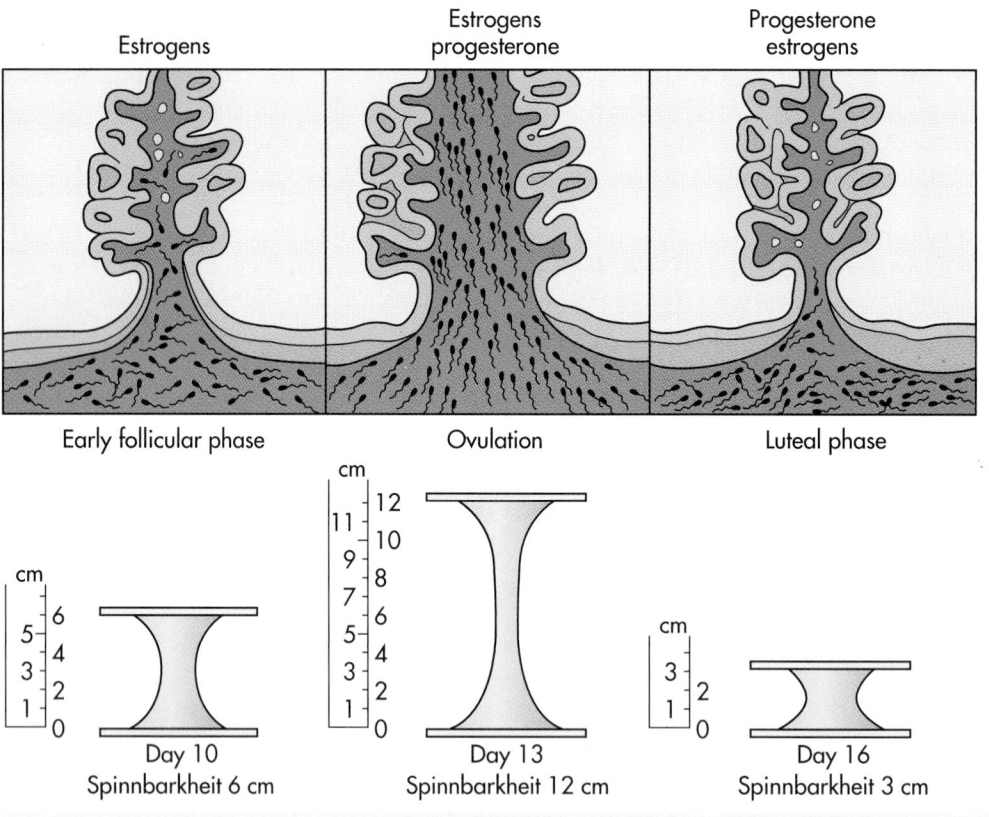

chemical in the United States, is a surfactant that destroys the sperm cell membrane (Cates & Raymond, 1998). Intravaginal spermicides are marketed as aerosol foams, foaming tablets, suppositories, creams, films, and gels (Fig. 9-3). Preloaded, single-dose applicators small enough to be carried in a small purse are available. Effectiveness of spermicides depends on consistent and accurate use. The spermicide should be inserted into the vagina so that it makes contact with the cervix. Spermicide should be inserted no longer than 1 hour before sexual intercourse. Typical fail-

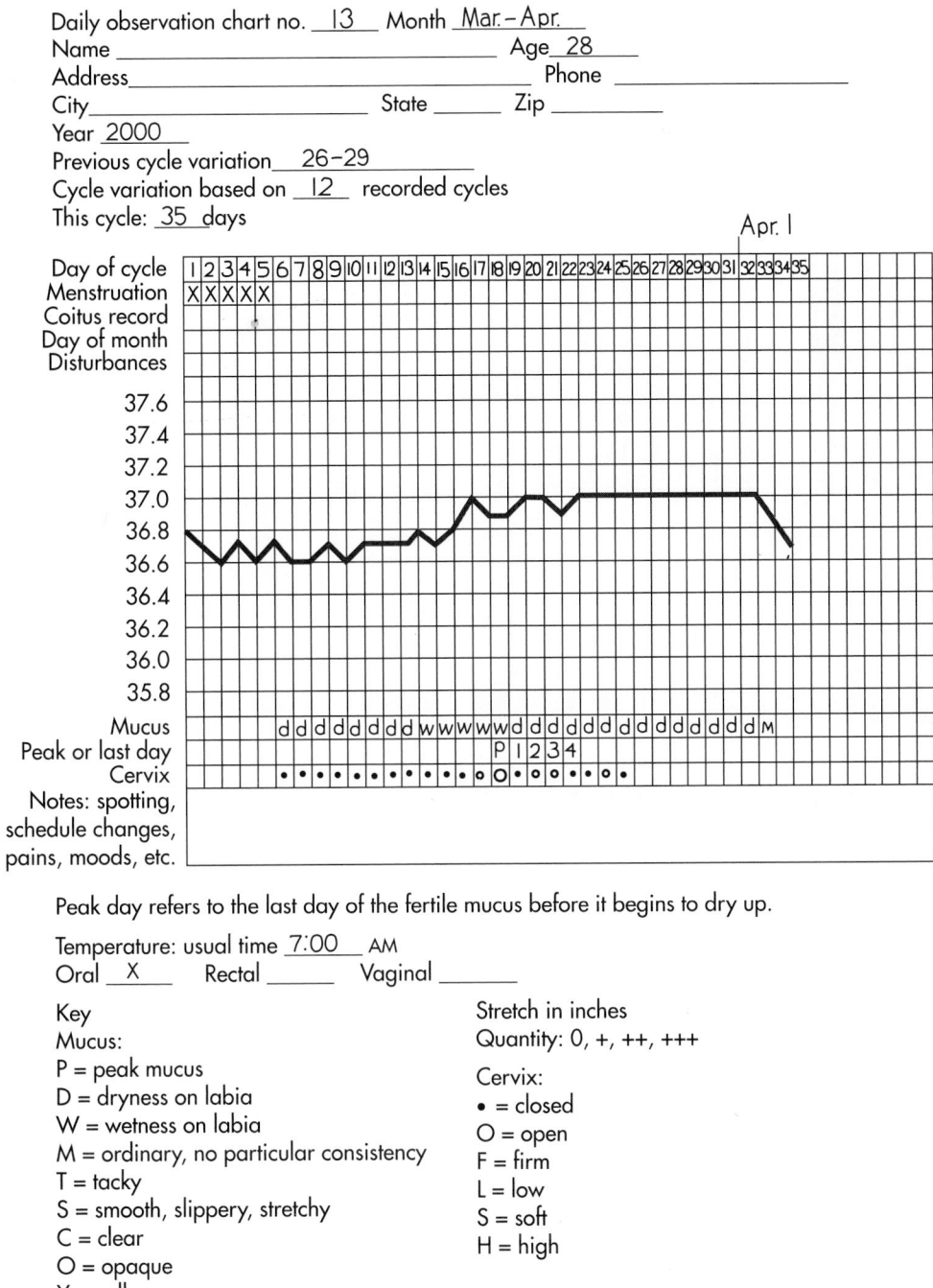

Daily observation chart no. __13__ Month __Mar.–Apr.__
Name _____ Age __28__
Address_____ Phone _____
City_____ State _____ Zip _____
Year __2000__
Previous cycle variation __26–29__
Cycle variation based on __12__ recorded cycles
This cycle: __35__ days

Fig. 9-2 Example of a completed symptothermal chart.

Peak day refers to the last day of the fertile mucus before it begins to dry up.

Temperature: usual time __7:00__ AM
Oral __X__ Rectal _____ Vaginal _____

Key
Mucus:
P = peak mucus
D = dryness on labia
W = wetness on labia
M = ordinary, no particular consistency
T = tacky
S = smooth, slippery, stretchy
C = clear
O = opaque
Y = yellow

Stretch in inches
Quantity: 0, +, ++, +++

Cervix:
• = closed
O = open
F = firm
L = low
S = soft
H = high

ure rate in the first year of spermicidal use alone is 26% (Trussell, 1998). Box 9-2 provides client teaching information about spermicide use.

Condoms. The male **condom** is a thin, stretchable sheath that covers the penis (Fig. 9-4). Most condoms are made of latex rubber. In addition to providing a barrier for sperm, latex condoms also provide a barrier for STIs and HIV. Latex condoms will break down with oil-based lubri-

cants and should be used only with water-based lubricants. A small percentage of condoms are made from the intestinal caecum of lambs (natural skin). Natural skin condoms do not provide the same protection against STIs and HIV infection. Unlike latex condoms, natural skin condoms contain small pores that could allow passage of viruses such as hepatitis B, herpes simplex, and HIV. More recently, condom manufacturers have begun using polyurethane,

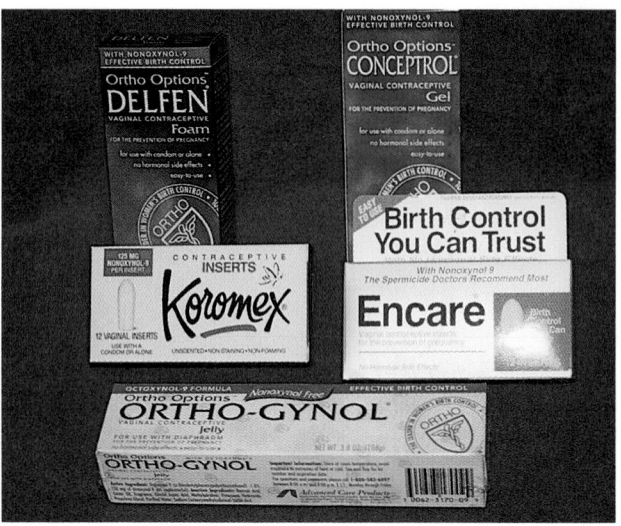

Fig. 9-3 Spermicides. *(Courtesy Marjorie Pyle, RNC, Lifecircle, Costa Mesa, CA.)*

which is thinner and stronger than latex. Unlike latex condoms, polyurethane condoms can be used with oil-based lubricants (e.g., petroleum jelly, suntan oil) (Warner & Hatcher, 1998). Research is being conducted to determine the effectiveness of polyurethane condoms to protect against STIs and HIV.

NURSE ALERT

All clients should be questioned about the potential for latex allergy. Latex condom use is contraindicated for clients with latex sensitivity. Plastic or natural membrane condoms can be used for contraception; however, only plastic condoms should be recommended for prevention of STIs.

A functional difference in condom shape is the presence or absence of a sperm reservoir tip. To enhance vaginal stimulation, some condoms are contoured and rippled or

---

BOX 9-2 Spermicides

MODE OF ACTION

Spermicides provide a physical and chemical barrier that prevents viable sperm from entering the cervix. The effect is local, within the vagina. The spermicide is placed deeply into the vagina in contact with the cervix before each incidence of coitus.

FAILURE RATE

Typical failure: 5% to 50%

ADVANTAGES

- Easy to apply
- Safe
- Low cost
- Available without a prescription or previous medical examination
- Delicate vaginal mucosa is not harmed unless the woman is allergic to a particular preparation
- Aid in lubrication of the vagina
- Alternative for nursing mothers (does not interfere with lactation)
- Alternative for the premenopausal woman (to prevent masking symptoms of onset of the climacteric)
- Backup when the woman forgets her oral contraceptive
- Increases the effectiveness of condoms and other forms of contraception

STI PROTECTION

Spermicides containing nonoxynol-9 provide some protection against STIs through bacteriostatic action. Need

to be used with condoms if protection from STIs is needed.

DISADVANTAGES

- Maximum spermicidal effectiveness lasts usually no longer than 1 hour.
- If intercourse is to be repeated, reapplication of additional spermicide must precede it.
- Some users complain that it is messy and has an unpleasant fizz and taste.
- Allergic response or irritation of vaginal or penile tissue may occur.
- Possible decreased tactile sensation.

NURSING CONSIDERATIONS/CLIENT TEACHING

Can must be shaken to distribute foam spermicide before use.

Tablets and suppositories take from 10 to 30 minutes to dissolve.

Douching must be avoided for at least 6 hours after coitus.

Encourage open communication between sexual partners to discuss intravaginal contraception.

Provide opportunity to see and handle a variety of samples.

Provide anatomic model to practice insertion into the vagina.

have ribbed or roughened surfaces. Thinner construction increases heat transmission and sensitivity; a variety of colors increases their acceptability and attractiveness (Warner & Hatcher, 1998). A wet jelly or dry powder lubricates some condoms. Since 1982 spermicide (0.5 g of nonoxynol-9) has been added to the interior or exterior surfaces of some condoms. Typical failure rate for first year of use of the male condom is 14% (Warner & Hatcher, 1998).

For years, health care providers assumed that everyone knew how to use condoms, so proper instruction was not provided. To prevent unintended pregnancy and the spread of STIs, it is essential that condoms be used correctly. Instructions, such as those listed in Box 9-3, can be used for client teaching.

The vaginal sheath (female condom) is made of polyurethane and has flexible rings at both ends (Speroff & Darney, 1996) (see Fig. 9-4). The closed end of the pouch is inserted into the vagina and is anchored around the cervix, and the open ring covers the labia. The female condom can be inserted up to 8 hours before intercourse and is intended for one-time use. Both women and men report

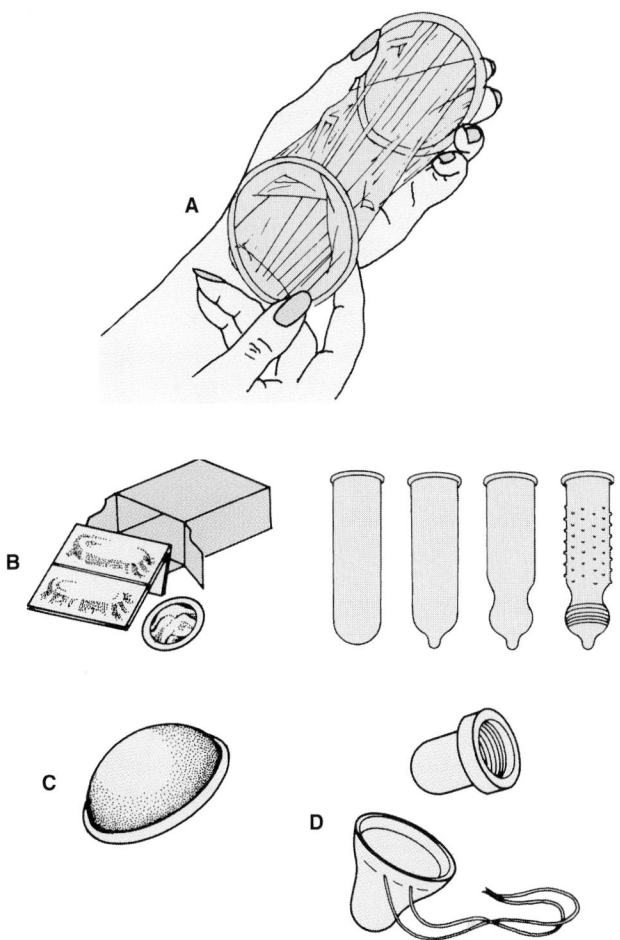

Fig. 9-4 Mechanical barriers. **A,** Female condom. **B,** Types of male condoms. **C,** Diaphragm. **D,** Cervical cap.

that intercourse with the sheath is generally as satisfying as intercourse without the sheath. It comes in one size and is available over the counter. Typical failure rate is 21% in the first year of use (Stewart, F., 1998).

Diaphragm. The vaginal **diaphragm** is a shallow, dome-shaped rubber device with a flexible rim that covers the cervix (see Fig. 9-4). Diaphragms are available in a wide range of diameters (50 to 95 mm) and differ in the inner construction of the circular rim. The types of rims are flat spring, coil spring, arcing spring, and wide seal rim. The diaphragm is a mechanical barrier preventing the meeting of the sperm with the ovum. The diaphragm holds the spermicide in place against the cervix for the 6 hours it takes to destroy the sperm.

The diaphragm should feel comfortable. It should be the largest size the woman can wear without being aware of its presence. Use of a contraceptive gel or cream with the diaphragm offers both mechanical and chemical barriers to pregnancy.

Typical failure rate of the diaphragm alone is 20% in the first year of use. Effectiveness of the diaphragm can be increased when combined with a spermicide (Stewart, F., 1998).

Nursing considerations. The woman is informed that she needs an annual gynecologic examination. The fit of the diaphragm should be assessed every year. The device may need to be refitted after weight loss or weight gain (more than 22 kg), term birth, or second trimester abortion (Stewart, F., 1998). Because there are various types of diaphragms on the market, the nurse uses the package insert for teaching the woman how to use and care for the diaphragm (see Home Care box).

Except for occasional allergic responses to the diaphragm or spermicide, there are no side effects from a well-fitted device. The diaphragm can be inserted as long as 6 hours before intercourse, but spermicide must be inserted into the vagina each time intercourse is repeated (Stewart, F, 1998). The diaphragm must be left in place for at least 6 hours after the last intercourse. The woman who engages in intercourse infrequently may choose this barrier method. The spermicide offers additional lubrication if it is needed. A decreased incidence of vaginitis, cervicitis (including cervicitis caused by *Chlamydia trachomatis* and *Neisseria gonorrhoeae*), and pelvic inflammatory disease has been reported among women who use contraceptive creams, foams, and gels with the diaphragm. A reduced risk of cervical cancer also has been reported among women who use a diaphragm.

Disadvantages of diaphragm use include the reluctance of some women to insert and remove the diaphragm. A cold diaphragm and a cold gel temporarily reduce vaginal response to sexual stimulation if insertion of the diaphragm occurs immediately before intercourse. Some women or couples object to the messiness of the spermicide. These annoyances of diaphragm use, along with failure

BOX 9-3 Male Condoms

MECHANISM OF ACTION

Sheath is applied over the erect penis before insertion or loss of preejaculatory drops of semen. Used correctly, condoms prevent sperm from entering the cervix. Spermicide-coated condoms cause ejaculated sperm to be immobilized rapidly, thus increasing contraceptive effectiveness.

FAILURE RATE

Typical users, 14%
Correct and consistent users, 3%

ADVANTAGES

Safe
No side effects
Readily available
Premalignant changes in cervix can be prevented or ameliorated in women whose partners use condoms
Method of male nonsurgical contraception

DISADVANTAGES

Must interrupt lovemaking to apply sheath.
Sensation may be altered.
If used improperly, spillage of sperm can result in pregnancy.
Occasionally, condoms may tear during intercourse.

STI PROTECTION

If a condom is used throughout the act of intercourse and there is no unprotected contact with female genitals, a latex rubber condom, which is impermeable to viruses, can act as a protective measure against STIs. The addition of nonoxynol-9 increases protection against transmission of STIs, including HIV.

NURSING CONSIDERATIONS

Teach man to do the following:
- Use a new condom (check expiration date) for each act of sexual intercourse or other acts between partners that involve contact with the penis.

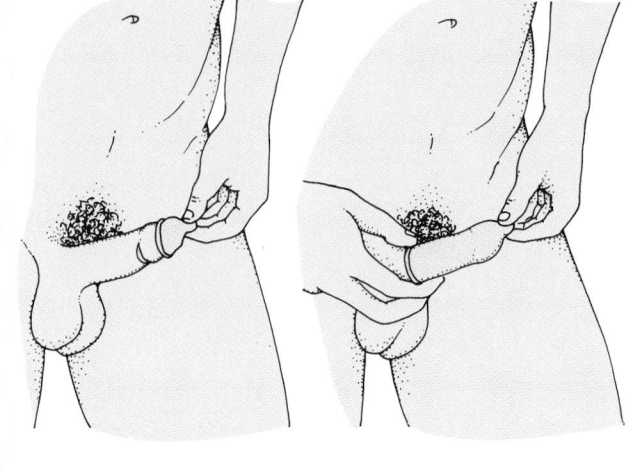

Fig. A   Fig. B

- Place condom after penis is erect and before intimate contact.
- Place condom on head of penis (Fig. A) and unroll it all the way to the base (Fig. B).
- Leave an empty space at the tip (Fig. A); remove any air remaining in the tip by gently pressing air out toward the base of the penis.
- If a lubricant is desired, use water-based products such as K-Y lubricating jelly. Do not use petroleum-based products because they can cause the condom to break.
- After ejaculation, carefully withdraw the still-erect penis from the vagina, holding onto condom rim; remove and discard the condom.
- Store unused condoms in cool, dry place.
- Do not use condoms that are sticky, brittle, or obviously damaged.

to insert the device once foreplay has begun, are the most common reasons for failures of this method. Side effects may include irritation of tissues related to contact with spermicides. Urethritis and recurrent cystitis caused by upward pressure of the diaphragm rim against the urethra may be increased by the use of the contraceptive diaphragm (Stewart, F., 1998). Diaphragms are contraindicated for women with pelvic relaxation (uterine prolapse) or a large cystocele. Women with a latex allergy should not use latex diaphragms.

Toxic shock syndrome (TSS), although reported in very small numbers, can occur in association with the use of the contraceptive diaphragm (Stewart, F., 1998). The nurse should instruct the woman about ways to reduce her risk for TSS. These measures include prompt removal 6 to 8 hours after intercourse, not using the diaphragm during menses, and learning and watching for danger signs of TSS.

NURSE ALERT

The nurse should be alert for signs of TSS in women who use a diaphragm or cervical cap as a contraceptive method. The most common signs include fever of sudden onset greater than 38.4° C, hypotension (systolic less than 90 mm Hg or orthostatic dizziness), and a rash.

HOME CARE

Use and Care of the Diaphragm

POSITIONS FOR INSERTION OF DIAPHRAGM

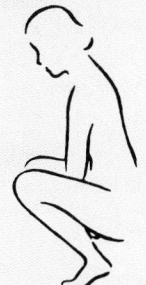

Squatting

Squatting is the most commonly used position, and most women find it satisfactory.

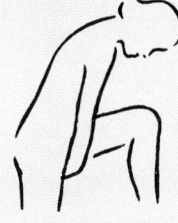

Leg-up Method

Another position is to raise the left foot (if right hand is used for insertion) on a low stool and in a bending position insert the diaphragm.

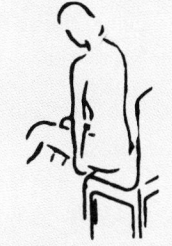

Chair Method

Another practical method for diaphragm insertion is to sit far forward on the edge of a chair.

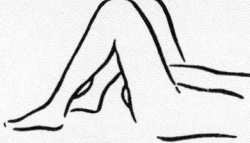

Reclining

You may prefer to insert the diaphragm while in a semi-reclining position in bed.

INSPECTION OF DIAPHRAGM

Your diaphragm must be inspected carefully before each use. The best way to do this is as follows:

Hold the diaphragm up to a light source. Carefully stretch the diaphragm at the area of the rim, on all sides, to make sure there are no holes. Remember, it is possible to puncture the diaphragm with sharp fingernails.

Another way to check for pinholes is to carefully fill the diaphragm with water. If there is any problem, it will be seen immediately.

If your diaphragm is puckered, especially near the rim, this could mean thin spots.

The diaphragm should not be used if you see any of the above; consult your health care provider.

PREPARATION OF DIAPHRAGM

Rinse off cornstarch. Your diaphragm must always be used with a spermicidal lubricant to be effective. Pregnancy cannot be prevented effectively by the diaphragm alone.

Always empty your bladder before inserting the diaphragm. Place about 2 teaspoonfuls of contraceptive jelly or contraceptive cream on the side of the diaphragm that will rest against the cervix (or whichever way you have been instructed). Spread it around to coat the surface and the rim. This aids in insertion and offers a more complete seal. Many women also spread some jelly or cream on the other side of the diaphragm (Fig. A).

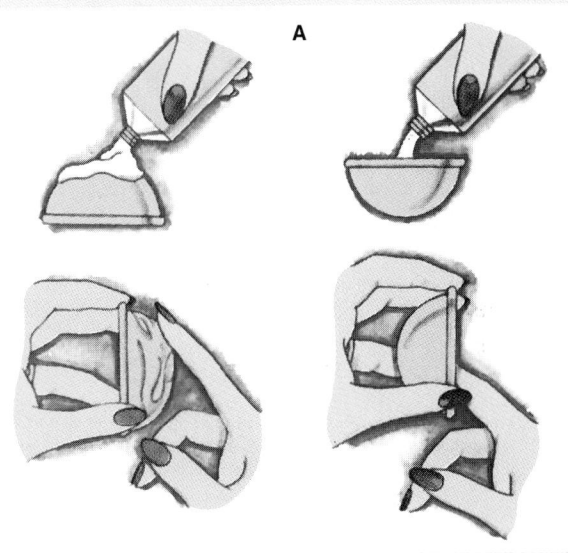

INSERTION OF DIAPHRAGM

The diaphragm can be inserted as long as 6 hours before intercourse. Hold the diaphragm between your thumb and fingers. The dome can either be up or down, as directed by your health care provider. Place your index finger on the outer rim of the compressed diaphragm (Fig. B). Use the fingers of the other hand to spread the labia (lips of the vagina). This will assist in guiding the diaphragm into place.

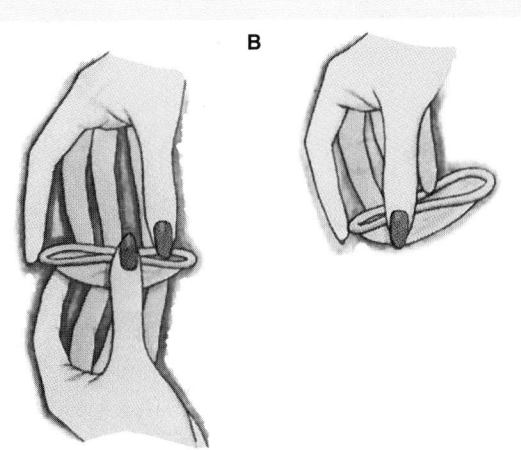

Continued

HOME CARE

Use and Care of the Diaphragm—cont'd

Insert the diaphragm into the vagina. Direct it inward and downward as far as it will go to space behind and below the cervix (Fig. C).

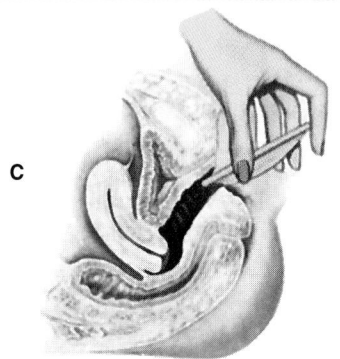

Tuck the front of the rim of the diaphragm behind the pubic bone so that the rubber hugs the front wall of the vagina (Fig. D).

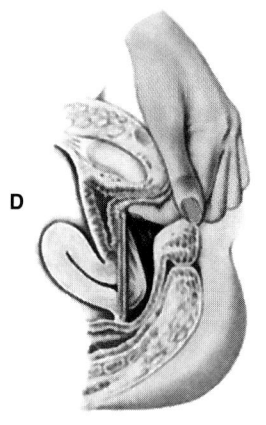

Feel for your cervix through the diaphragm to be certain it is properly placed and securely covered by the rubber dome (Fig. E).

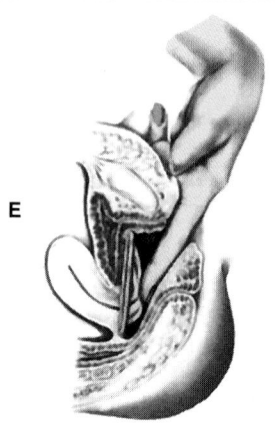

GENERAL INFORMATION

Regardless of the time of the month, you must use your diaphragm each and every time intercourse takes place. Your diaphragm must be left in place for at least 6 hours after the last intercourse. If you remove your diaphragm before the 6-hour period, your chance of becoming pregnant could be greatly increased. If you have repeated acts of intercourse, you need to add more spermicide for each act of intercourse.

REMOVAL OF DIAPHRAGM

The only proper way to remove the diaphragm is to insert your forefinger up and over the top side of the diaphragm and slightly to the side.

Next, turn the palm of your hand downward and backward hooking the forefinger firmly on top of the inside of the upper rim of the diaphragm, breaking the suction.

Pull the diaphragm down and out. This avoids the possibility of tearing the diaphragm with the fingernails. You should not remove the diaphragm by trying to catch the rim from below the dome (Fig. F).

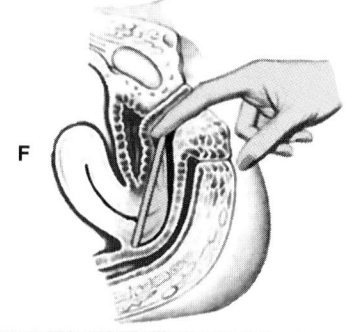

CARE OF DIAPHRAGM

When using a vaginal diaphragm, avoid using oil-based products, such as certain body lubricants, mineral oil, baby oil, vaginal lubricants, or vaginitis preparations. These products can weaken the rubber.

A little care means longer wear for your diaphragm. After each use the diaphragm should be washed in warm water and mild soap. Do not use detergent soaps, cold cream soaps, deodorant soaps, and soaps containing oil products, because they can weaken the rubber.

After washing, the diaphragm should be dried thoroughly. All water and moisture should be removed with a towel. The diaphragm should then be dusted with *cornstarch*. Scented talc, body powder, baby powder, and the like should not be used because they can weaken the rubber.

To clean the introducer (if one is used), wash with mild soap and warm water, rinse, and dry thoroughly.

The diaphragm should be placed back in the plastic case for storage. It should not be stored near a radiator or heat source or exposed to light for an extended period.

Cervical cap. The **cervical cap** has a 22 to 31 mm soft natural rubber dome with a firm but pliable rim (see Fig. 9-4). It fits snugly around the base of the cervix close to the junction of the cervix and vaginal fornices (Stewart, F., 1998). The device is available in four sizes. It is recommended that the cap remain in place no less than 8 hours and not more than 48 hours at a time. It is left in place at least 6 hours after the last act of intercourse. The seal provides a physical barrier to sperm; spermicide inside the cap adds a chemical barrier.

The extended period of wear is an added convenience for women who previously used the diaphragm. Instructions for the actual insertion and use of the cervical cap closely resemble the instructions for the use of the contraceptive diaphragm. Some of the differences are that the cervical cap can be inserted hours before sexual intercourse without a need for additional spermicide later, no additional spermicide is required for repeated acts of intercourse when the cap is used, and the cervical cap requires less spermicide than the diaphragm when initially inserted.

Some women are not good candidates for wearing the cervical cap. They include women with abnormal Papanicolaou (Pap) test results, women who cannot be fitted properly with the existing cap sizes, women who find the insertion and removal of the device too difficult, women with a history of TSS, women with vaginal or cervical infections (Stewart, F., 1998), and women who experience allergic responses to the latex cap or spermicide.

Nursing considerations. The angle of the uterus, the vaginal muscle tone, and the shape of the cervix may interfere with the cervical cap's ease of fitting and use. Correct fitting requires time, effort, and skill from both the woman and the clinician. The woman must check the cap's position before and after each act of intercourse. Current research has not found an association between cervical cap use and Pap smear abnormalities.

Although no link has been discovered between TSS and the use of the cervical cap, such an association is possible. The package insert recommends that another form of birth control be used during menstrual bleeding and for at least 6 weeks postpartum. The cap should be checked for proper fit after any gynecologic surgery or birth and after major weight losses or gains. Otherwise, the size should be checked at least once a year.

Strong client motivation is the most important criterion for successful cap use. Failure rate with typical use for parous women is 40% and for nulliparous women is 20% (Stewart, F., 1998).

The woman must be given the information available for this product as presented previously. The nurse should assess the woman's understanding and skill in the use of the cervical cap (see Home Care box).

Contraceptive sponge. The vaginal sponge was taken off the market in the United States in 1995 because of production problems by the manufacturer. It continued to be available in other countries, and in 1999 the contraceptive

HOME CARE

Use of the Cervical Cap
Push cap up into vagina until it covers cervix.

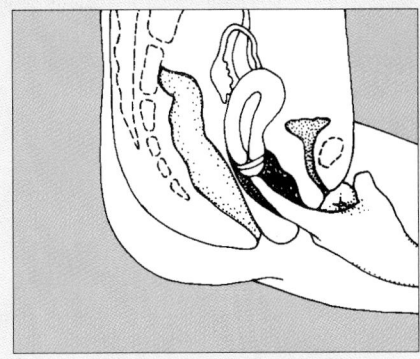

Press rim against cervix to create a seal.

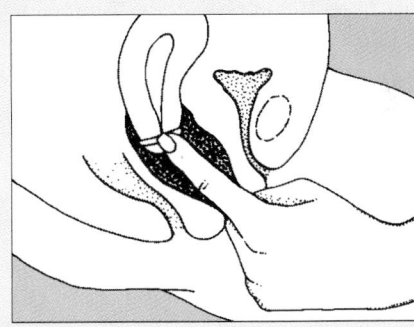

To remove, push rim toward right or left hip to loosen from cervix and then withdraw.

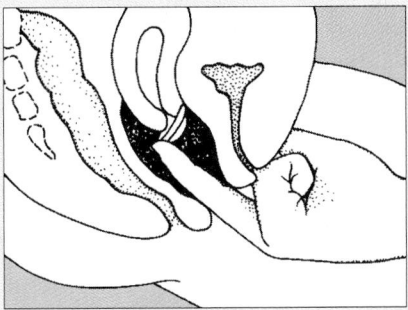

The woman can assume several positions to insert the cervical cap. See the four positions shown for inserting the diaphragm.

sponge again became available as an over-the-counter contraceptive in the United States (Springen, 1999).

The device is a small round polyurethane sponge that contains nonoxynol-9 spermicide. It is designed to fit over the cervix (one size fits all). The side that is placed next to the cervix is concave for better fit. The opposite side has a woven polyester loop to be used in removing the sponge.

TABLE 9-1　Hormonal Contraception

COMPOSITION	ROUTE OF ADMINISTRATION	DURATION OF EFFECT
Combination estrogen and progestin (synthetic estrogens and progestins in varying doses and formulations)	Oral	24 hours
Progestin only		
Norethindrone, norgestrel	Oral	24 hours
Medroxyprogesterone acetate	Intramuscular injection	3 months
Levonorgestrel	Subdermal implant	Up to 5 years
Progesterone	Intrauterine device	1 year

The sponge should be moistened with water before it is inserted into the vagina to cover the cervix. It provides up to 24 hours of protection and for numerous instances of sexual intercourse. The sponge should be left in place for at least 6 hours before its removal. Longer wearing time (greater than 24 to 30 hours) is not recommended because the woman may be at risk for TSS (Stewart, F., 1998).

Hormonal methods. Over 30 different oral contraceptive formulations are available in the United States today. General classes are described in Table 9-1. Because of the wide variety of preparations available, the woman and nurse must read the package insert for information about specific products prescribed. Formulations include combined estrogen-progestin medications and progestational agents. The formulations are administered orally, subdermally, or by implantation. Combined estrogen-progestin medications are discussed first.

Combined estrogen-progestin oral contraceptives

Mode of action. The normal menstrual cycle is maintained by a feedback mechanism. Follicle-stimulating hormone (FSH) and LH are secreted in response to fluctuating levels of ovarian estrogen and progesterone. Regular ingestion of combined oral contraceptive pills (OCPs) suppresses the action of the hypothalamus and anterior pituitary, leading to inappropriate secretion of FSH and LH. Therefore follicles do not mature, and ovulation is inhibited.

Other contraceptive effects are induced by the combined steroids. Maturation of the endometrium is altered, making it a less favorable site for implantation should ovulation and conception occur. It also has a direct effect on the endometrium, so that from 1 to 4 days after the last combined OCP is taken, the endometrium sloughs and bleeds as a result of hormone withdrawal. The **withdrawal bleeding** usually is less profuse than that of normal menstruation and may last only 2 to 3 days. Some women have no bleeding at all.

The cervical mucus remains thick from the effect of the progestin. Cervical mucus under the effect of progesterone does not provide as suitable an environment for sperm penetration as does the thin, watery mucus at ovulation (Hatcher & Guillebaud, 1998).

The possible effect, if any, of altered tubal and uterine motility induced by the combined OCPs is not clear.

Nevertheless, combined OCPs, if taken daily for 3 weeks of every 4, provide virtually absolute protection against conception (Cunningham et al., 1997).

Monophasic pills provide fixed dosages of estrogen and progestin. Phasic pills (e.g., biphasic, triphasic, and multiphasic oral contraceptives) alter the amount of progestin and sometimes the amount of estrogen within each cycle. These preparations reduce the total dosage of hormones in a single cycle without sacrificing contraceptive efficacy or cycle control (Cunningham et al., 1997). To maintain adequate hormonal levels for contraception and enhance compliance, combined OCPs should be taken at the same time each day.

Advantages. Taking the pill does not relate directly to the sexual act; this fact increases its acceptability by some women. Commonly, there is an improvement in sexual response once the possibility of pregnancy is not an issue. For some women, it is convenient to know when to expect the next menstrual flow.

The noncontraceptive health benefits of oral contraceptives include decreased menstrual blood loss and decreased iron-deficiency anemia, regulation of menorrhagia and irregular cycles, and lowered incidence of dysmenorrhea and premenstrual syndrome (PMS). Oral contraceptives also offer protection against endometrial adenocarcinoma and ovarian cancer, reduce the incidence of benign breast disease, improve acne, protect against the development of functional ovarian cysts and some types of pelvic inflammatory disease, and decrease the risk of ectopic pregnancy (Contraception Report, 1997; Hatcher & Guillebaud, 1998; Speroff & Darney, 1996).

Oral contraceptives are considered to be a safe option for older, nonsmoking women until menopause. Perimenopausal women can benefit from regular bleeding cycles, a regular hormonal pattern, and the noncontraceptive health benefits of oral contraceptives (Burkman & Shulman, 1998; Hatcher & Guillebaud, 1998).

Women taking combined oral contraceptives are examined before the medication is prescribed and yearly thereafter. The examination includes medical and family history, weight, blood pressure, general physical and pelvic examination, and screening cervical cytologic analysis (Pap smear). Consistent monitoring by the health care provider is valuable in the detection of noncontraception-related disorders as well, so that timely treatment can be initiated. Most health care providers assess the woman 3 months after beginning combined OCPs in order to detect any complications.

Use of oral hormonal contraceptives is initiated on one of the first 7 days of the menstrual cycle (day 1 of the cycle is the first day of menses). Other women start their use after childbirth or abortion. With a "Sunday start," clients begin taking pills on the first Sunday after the start of their menstrual period. If contraceptives are to be started at any time other than during normal menses, or within 3 weeks after birth or abortion, another method of contraception should be used throughout the first week to avoid the risk of pregnancy (Hatcher & Guillebaud, 1998). The combined estrogen-progestin pill taken daily 3 weeks out of every 4 is the most effective reversible form of contraception available (Cunningham et al., 1997). Taken exactly as directed, oral contraceptives prevent ovulation and pregnancy cannot occur; the overall effectiveness rate is almost 100%. Almost all failures (i.e., pregnancy occurs) are caused by omission of one or more pills during the regimen. The typical failure rate of OCPs due to omission is 5% (Trussell & Kowal, 1998).

Disadvantages and side effects. Since hormonal contraceptives have come into use, the amount of estrogen and progestational agent contained in each tablet has been reduced considerably (Cunningham et al., 1997). This is important because adverse effects are, to a degree, dose related.

Women must be screened for conditions that present absolute or relative contraindications to oral contraceptive use. The World Health Organization (WHO) recommends not providing combined OCPs to women with a history of thromboembolic disorders, cerebrovascular or coronary artery disease, breast cancer, estrogenic-dependent tumors, pregnancy, impaired liver function, liver tumor, lactation less than 6 weeks postpartum, smoking if over 35 years old (more than 20 cigarettes per day), headaches with focal neurologic symptoms, surgery with prolonged immobilization or any surgery on the legs, hypertension (160+/100+), and diabetes mellitus (20 years' duration) with vascular disease (Hatcher & Guillebaud, 1998; Speroff & Darney, 1996).

Certain side effects of OCPs are attributable to estrogen, progestin, or both. Side effects of estrogen excess include nausea and vomiting, dizziness, edema, leg cramps, increase in breast size, chloasma (mask of pregnancy), visual changes, hypertension, and vascular headache. Side effects of estrogen deficiency include early spotting (days 1 to 14), hypomenorrhea, nervousness, and atrophic vaginitis leading to painful intercourse (dyspareunia). Side effects of progestin excess include increased appetite, tiredness, depression, breast tenderness, vaginal yeast infection, oily skin and scalp, hirsutism, and postpill amenorrhea. Side effects of progestin deficiency include late spotting and breakthrough bleeding (days 15 to 21), heavy flow with clots, and decreased breast size. One of the most common side effects of combined OCPs is bleeding irregularities (Contraception Report, 1997; Hatcher & Guillebaud, 1998).

In the presence of side effects, especially those that are bothersome to the woman, a different product, a different drug content, or another method of contraception may be required. The "right" product for a woman contains the lowest dose of hormones that prevents ovulation and that has the fewest and least harmful side effects. There is no way to predict the right dosage for any particular woman; trial and error is the main method for prescribing oral contraceptives, starting with the lowest possible estrogen dose.

The changes in glucose tolerance that occur in some women taking oral contraceptives are similar to those changes that occur during pregnancy. The dosage, type, and potency of progestin (not estrogen) produce some deterioration of glucose tolerance in normal women, as well as in those with a history of gestational diabetes (Hatcher & Guillebaud, 1998; Speroff & Darney, 1996). Women who are insulin dependent may need a small increase in dose if OCPs are taken.

The effectiveness of oral contraceptives is decreased when the following medications are taken simultaneously because these drugs affect liver enzymes and OCPs are metabolized by the liver (Hatcher & Guillebaud, 1998):
- Anticonvulsants (phenytoin sodium, carbamazepine, primidone, topirimate)
- Antifungals (griseofulvin)
- Antibiotics (rifampin)

No strong pharmacokinetic evidence exists that shows a relationship between antibiotic use and altered hormonal levels among OCP users. However, the International Planned Parenthood Federation recommends that women taking broad-spectrum antibiotics use a backup method of contraception for the duration of antibiotic use plus 7 days. The use of oral contraceptives can decrease the effectiveness of several medications (e.g., insulin and oral anticoagulants) (Hatcher & Guillebaud, 1998).

Research on use of oral contraceptives and risk of breast cancer has been inconsistent (Speroff & Darney, 1996); investigation continues on this important concern. Currently the consensus is that the risk of breast cancer is small (Hatcher & Guillebaud, 1998).

After discontinuing oral contraception there is usually a delay before ovulation and menstrual cycles recur, similar to that experienced by a new mother. However, postpill amenorrhea exceeding 6 months should be investigated. Women who discontinue oral contraception for a planned pregnancy commonly ask whether they should wait before attempting to conceive. Studies indicate that these infants have no greater chance of being born with any type of birth defect than do infants born to women in the general population, even if conception occurred in the first month after the medication was discontinued (Hatcher & Guillebaud, 1998; Speroff & Darney, 1996).

Flowchart for Missed *Active* Oral Contraceptive Pills

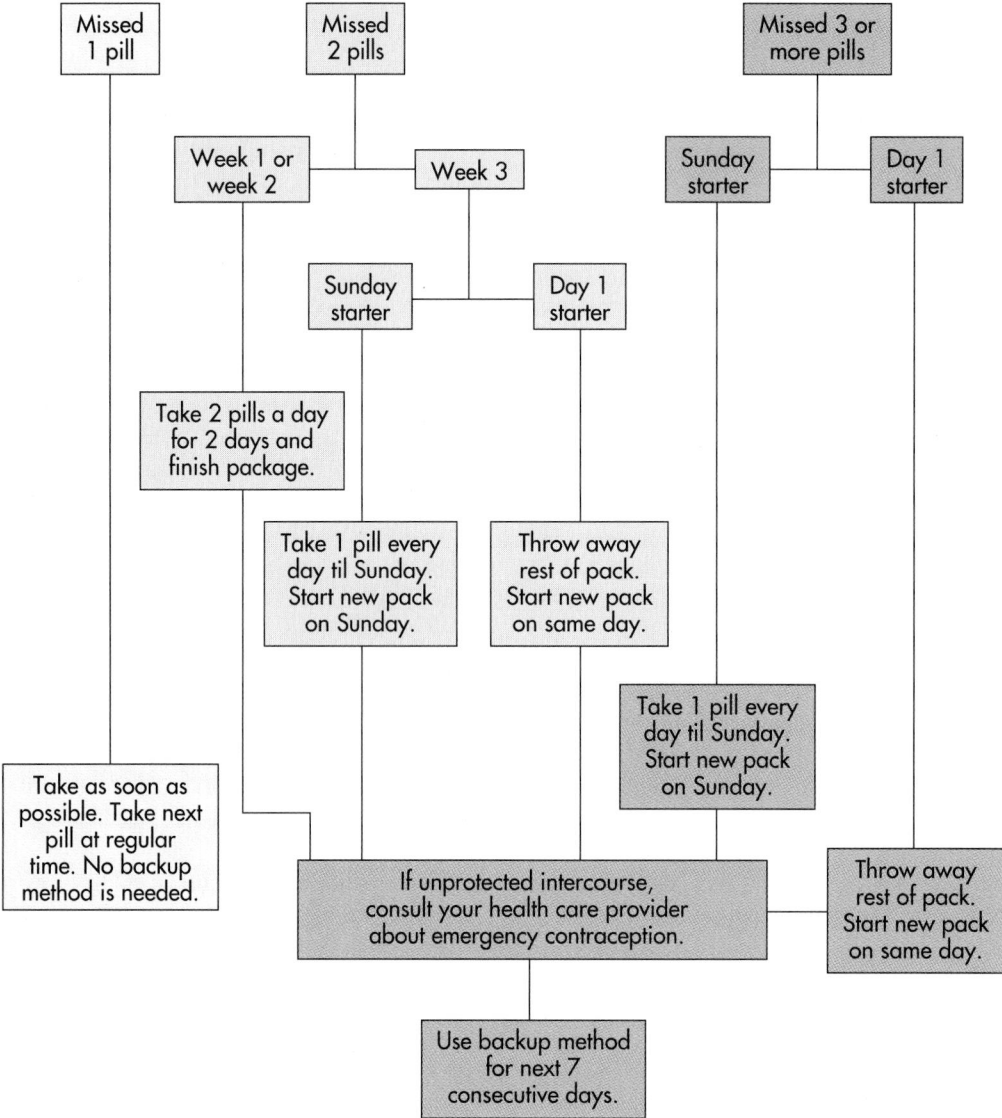

Fig. 9-5 Flowchart for missed contraceptive pills. *(Courtesy Patsy Huff, PharmD., Chapel Hill, NC.)*

Nursing considerations. There are many different preparations of oral hormonal contraceptives. The nurse reviews the prescribing information in the package insert with the woman. Because of the wide variations, each woman must be clear about the unique dosage regimen for the preparation prescribed for her. Directions for care after missing one or two tablets also vary (Fig. 9-5).

Withdrawal bleeding tends to be short and scanty when some combination pills are taken. A woman may see no fresh blood at all. A drop of blood or a brown smudge on a tampon or the underwear counts as a period. This fact may explain why some women have difficulty remembering the first day of their last period.

About 71% of women who start taking oral contraceptives are still taking them after 1 year (Trussell & Kowal, 1998). It is therefore important that nurses recommend that all women choosing to use oral contraceptives be provided with a second method of birth control and that women be instructed and comfortable with this backup method. Most women stop taking oral contraceptives for nonmedical reasons.

The nurse also reviews the signs of potential complications associated with the use of oral contraceptives (see Signs of Potential Complications).

Oral contraceptives do not protect a woman against STIs. A barrier method such as condoms and spermicide

SIGNS of POTENTIAL COMPLICATIONS

Oral Contraceptives (OCs)

Before OCs are prescribed and periodically throughout hormone therapy, the woman is alerted to stop taking the pill and to report any of the following symptoms to the health care provider immediately. The word *aches* helps in retention of this list:

A—Abdominal pain: may indicate a problem with the liver or gallbladder

C—Chest pain or shortness of breath: may indicate possible clot problem within lungs or heart

H—Headaches (sudden or persistent): may be caused by cardiovascular accident or hypertension

E—Eye problems: may indicate vascular accident or hypertension

S—Severe leg pain: may indicate a thromboembolic process

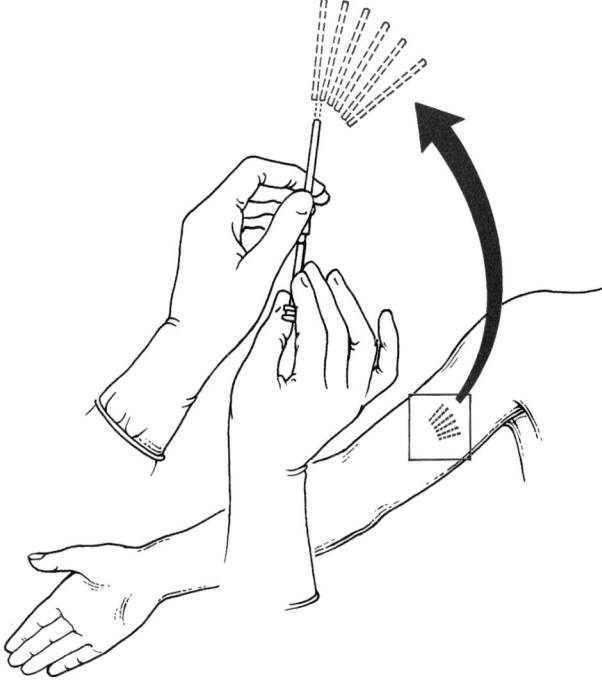

Fig. 9-6 Norplant contraceptive system.

should be used as well if protection is desired (O'Connell, 1996).

Progestin-only contraception. Progestin-only methods impair fertility by inhibiting ovulation, thickening and decreasing the amount of cervical mucus, and thinning the endometrium (Hatcher, 1998).

Oral progestins (minipill). Progestin-only pills are less effective than combined OCPs. Failure rate for typical users is 5% in the first year of use (Hatcher, 1998). Effectiveness is increased if minipills are taken correctly. Because minipills contain such a low dose of progestin, the minipill must be taken at the same time every day (Speroff & Darney, 1996). Users often complain of irregular vaginal bleeding.

Injectable progestins. Medroxyprogesterone (DMPA, Depo-Provera) 150 mg is given intramuscularly in the deltoid or gluteus maximus muscle. A 21- to 23-gauge needle 2.5 to 4 cm long should be used. The injection site should not be massaged because it could lower the effectiveness of the Depo-Provera. Injections should be administered every 12 weeks (Hatcher, 1998) (see Nurse Alert).

NURSE ALERT

When administering an intramuscular injection of progestin (e.g., Depo-Provera), the site should not be massaged after the injection because this action can hasten the absorption and shorten the period of effectiveness.

Advantages of Depo-Provera include a contraceptive effectiveness comparable to combined oral contraceptives, long-lasting effects, the requirement of injections only four times a year, and lactation not likely to be impaired (Cunningham et al., 1997; Hatcher, 1998). Disadvantages

are prolonged amenorrhea or uterine bleeding, increased risk of venous thrombosis and thromboembolism, and no protection against STIs (including HIV).

Implantable progestins (Norplant). The Norplant System consists of six flexible, nonbiodegradable Silastic capsules. The Silastic capsules contain progestin providing up to 5 years of contraception. Insertion and removal of the capsules are minor surgical procedures involving a local anesthetic, a small incision, and no sutures. The capsules are placed subdermally in the inner aspect of the upper arm (Fig. 9-6). The progestin prevents some, but not all, ovulatory cycles and thickens cervical mucus. The effectiveness is greater than 99% over 5 years. Other advantages include reversibility and long-term continuous contraception that is not coitus related.

Irregular menstrual bleeding is the most common side effect (Hatcher, 1998). Less common side effects include headaches, nervousness, nausea, skin changes, and vertigo. No STI protection is provided with the Norplant method, so condoms should be used if protection is desired. The Food and Drug Administration (FDA) has approved Norplant 2, which uses two Silastic capsules (Hatcher, 1998).

ETHICAL CONSIDERATIONS

The nurse may be confronted with an ethical dilemma concerning enforced contraception for a client. There have been some judicial rulings for women convicted of child abuse to either obtain a Norplant device or face a jail term. Other women receiving public assistance for children may be told to receive the implant or be faced with decreased or no payments. Some nurses may consider this punitive approach to be effective in preventing the birth of more children to unsuitable mothers; however, others strongly believe that forcing women to have such procedures is interfering with their constitutional rights.

Emergency contraception. Emergency contraception is used within 72 hours of unprotected intercourse to prevent pregnancy. High doses of combined OCPs are used to prevent ovulation or implantation. Recommended medication regimens for emergency contraception (combined estrogen-progestin) are presented in Table 9-2. The FDA recently approved an emergency contraception kit (Preven) with the exact dosage and instructions for use. There are no medical contraindications for emergency contraception except pregnancy (Van Look & Stewart, 1998). Emergency contraception is ineffective if the woman is pregnant. Effectiveness of emergency contraception is about 75% (Trussell, Rodriguez, & Ellertson, 1998).

Oral contraception for emergency contraception can be offered to a woman who has had unprotected sexual intercourse and requests treatment within 72 hours of that event. To minimize the side effect of nausea that occurs with high doses of estrogen and progestin, the woman can be advised to take an over-the-counter antiemetic 1 hour before each dose. If the woman does not begin menstruation within 21 days after taking the pills, she should be

evaluated for pregnancy (Chez & Chapin, 1997; Lindberg, 1997). Abortion should be offered if the method fails (Lindberg, 1997; Speroff & Darney, 1996; Van Look & Stewart, 1998).

Intrauterine devices containing copper provide another emergency contraception option. The intrauterine device should be inserted within 7 days of unprotected intercourse (Van Look & Stewart, 1998). This method is suggested only for women who wish to have the benefit of long-term contraception.

Contraceptive counseling should be provided to all women requesting emergency contraception, including a discussion of modification of risky sexual behaviors to prevent STIs and unwanted pregnancy.

Mifepristone (RU 486). Progesterone is essential for maintaining pregnancy. Mifepristone (RU 486) is a progesterone antagonist that prevents implantation of a fertilized egg. It is most effective in early gestation, during the luteal phase, within 10 days of the expected onset of what would be the first missed period after conception. A dose of 600 mg of mifepristone within 24 hours of unprotected intercourse is usually effective in preventing pregnancy (Reifsnider, 1997).

Intrauterine devices. An **intrauterine device (IUD)** is a small, T-shaped device inserted into the uterine cavity. Medicated IUDs are loaded with either copper or a progestational agent (Fig. 9-7). These chemically active substances are released continuously, for example, copper-bearing devices for up to 10 years and progesterone devices for 1 year (Speroff & Darney, 1996; Stewart, G., 1998). IUDs are impregnated with barium sulfate for radiopacity. Evidence strongly supports a true contraceptive effect in preventing fertilization (Mishell, 1998). The copper-bearing IUD damages sperm in transit to the uterine tubes and few sperm reach the ovum, thus preventing fertilization (Speroff & Darney, 1996).

The progesterone-bearing IUD causes progestin-related effects on cervical mucus and endometrial maturation (see Fig. 9-7). Because the effect is local, there is no disruption

TABLE 9-2	Dosages for Emergency Contraception	
DRUG	**FIRST DOSE (WITHIN 72 HOURS)**	**SECOND DOSE (12 HOURS LATER)**
Ovral	2 white tablets	2 white tablets
Lo/Ovral	4 white tablets	4 white tablets
Nordette	4 light orange tablets	4 light orange tablets
Levlen	4 light orange tablets	4 light orange tablets
Triphasil	4 yellow tablets	4 yellow tablets
Tri-Levlen	4 yellow tablets	4 yellow tablets
Alesse	5 pink tablets	5 pink tablets
Ovrette*	20 yellow tablets†	20 yellow tablets

Source: Chez, R., & Chapin, J. (1997). Emergency contraception: The pill's little known secret goes public. *Lifelines* 1(5), 28-31; Lindberg, C. (1997). Emergency contraception: The nurse's role in providing postcoital options. *J Obstet Gynecol Neonatal Nurs* 26(2), 145-152.

*Contains only progestin.
†Take within 48 hours.

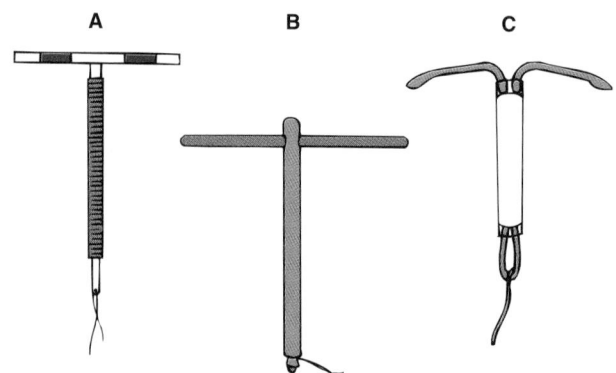

Fig. 9-7 Intrauterine devices. **A,** Copper T380A. **B,** Progesterone T. **C,** Levonorgestrel-releasing IUD.

of the woman's ovulatory pattern. Copper-bearing IUDs have a lower failure rate than the progesterone-releasing IUDs. The typical failure rate of the IUD ranges from 0.1% to 2.0% (Stewart, G., 1998).

The IUD offers constant contraception without the need to remember to take pills each day or engage in other manipulation before or between coital acts. If pregnancy can be excluded, an IUD may be placed at any time during the menstrual cycle. An IUD may be inserted immediately after childbirth or abortion (Speroff & Darney, 1996; Stewart, G., 1998).

The absence of interference with hormonal regulation of menstrual cycles makes the IUD more appropriate than hormonal contraception for heavy smokers, women over 35, women who have hypertension, or those with a history of vascular disease or familial diabetes. Contraceptive effects of the IUD are reversible. When pregnancy is desired, the IUD may be removed by the health care provider.

The progesterone IUD offers two important noncontraceptive progesterone-related advantages: less blood loss during menstruation and decreased primary dysmenorrhea. The average blood loss is increased with the copper IUD. This blood loss may be clinically significant in undernourished populations.

IUD use is contraindicated in women with a history of pelvic inflammatory disease, known or suspected pregnancy, undiagnosed genital bleeding, suspected genital malignancy, or a distorted intrauterine cavity.

Disadvantages of IUD use include risk of pelvic inflammatory disease, especially within 3 months of insertion, and risk of bacterial vaginosis, uterine perforation, and infection at time of insertion. The IUD offers no protection against STIs. The IUD is not recommended for teenagers, but primarily for women who have had at least one child and who are involved in stable monogamous relationships (Stewart, G., 1998).

Nursing considerations. The woman should be taught to check for the presence of the IUD thread after menstruation and at the time of ovulation, as well as before coitus, to rule out expulsion of the device. If pregnancy oc-

curs with the IUD in place, the IUD should be removed immediately, if possible. Retention of the IUD during pregnancy increases the risk of septic spontaneous abortion and ectopic pregnancy (Stewart, G., 1998). Some women who are allergic to copper develop a rash, necessitating the removal of the copper-bearing IUD. Signs of potential complications to be taught to the woman are listed in the accompanying box.

Sterilization. **Sterilization** refers to surgical procedures intended to render the person infertile. Most procedures involve the occlusion of the passageways for the ova and sperm (Fig. 9-8). For the female the oviducts (uterine tubes) are occluded; for the male the sperm ducts (vas deferens) are occluded. Only surgical removal of the ovaries (oophorectomy) or uterus (hysterectomy) or both will result in absolute sterility for the woman. All other sterilization procedures have a small but definite failure rate; that is, pregnancy may result.

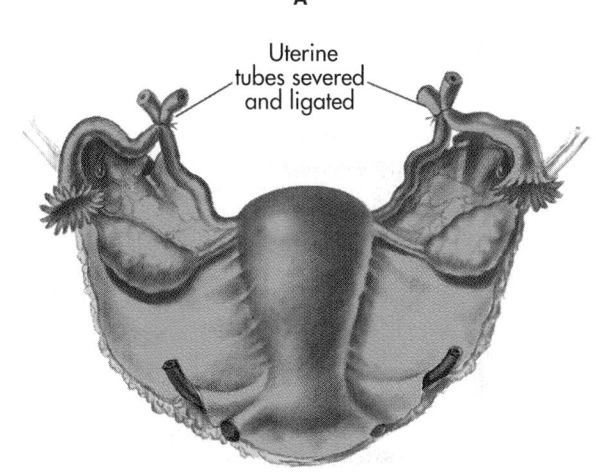

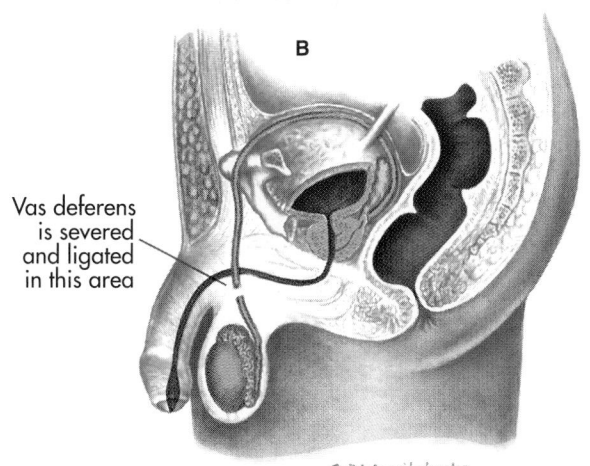

Fig. 9-8 Sterilization. **A,** Uterine tubes severed and ligated (tubal ligation). **B,** Sperm duct severed and ligated (vasectomy).

SIGNS of POTENTIAL COMPLICATIONS

Intrauterine Devices (IUDs)

Signs of potential complications related to IUDs can be remembered in the following manner (Stewart, G., 1998):

P—Period late, abnormal spotting or bleeding
A—Abdominal pain, pain with intercourse
I—Infection exposure, abnormal vaginal discharge
N—Not feeling well, fever, or chills
S—String missing; shorter or longer

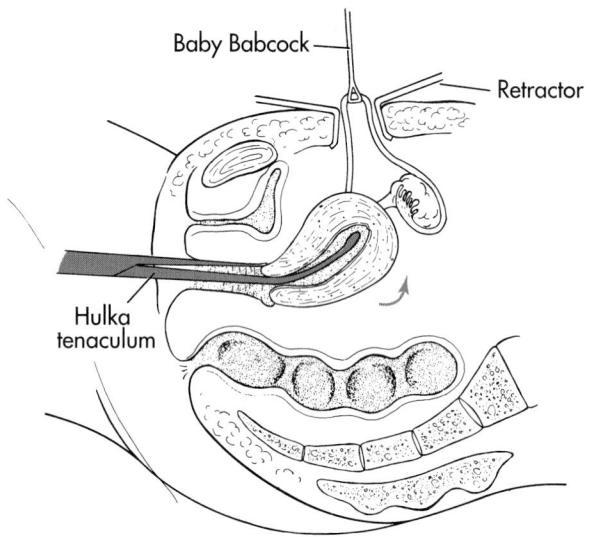

Fig. 9-9 Use of minilaparotomy to gain access to uterine tubes for occlusion procedures. Tenaculum is used to lift uterus upward *(arrow)* toward incision.

Female sterilization. Female sterilization may be done immediately after childbirth (within 24 to 48 hours), concomitantly with abortion, or as an interval procedure (during any phase of the menstrual cycle). If sterilization is performed as an interval procedure, the health care provider must be certain that the woman is not pregnant. Most sterilization procedures are performed immediately after a pregnancy, probably because of heightened motivation or increased practicality. However, there is evidence that sterilization performed after childbirth or abortion is associated with increased feeling of regret. Sterilization procedures can be safely done on an outpatient basis. Failure rate for female sterilization is 0.5% (Stewart & Carignan, 1998).

Tubal occlusion. A minilaparotomy may be used for tubal ligation (Fig. 9-9), tubal electrocoagulation, or the application of bands or clips (e.g., Hulka, Filshe, Wolf). Electrocoagulation and ligation are considered to be permanent methods. Use of the bands or clips has the theoretic advantage of possible removal and return of tubal patency. Transcervical approaches to inject occlusive material into the tubes are being investigated (Reifsnider, 1997).

For the minilaparotomy the woman is admitted the morning of surgery, having received nothing by mouth since midnight. Preoperative sedation is given. The procedure may be carried out with a local anesthetic, but a regional or general anesthetic may also be used. A small incision is made in the abdominal wall below the umbilicus. The woman may experience sensations of tugging, but no pain, and the operation is completed within 20 minutes. She may be discharged several hours later if she has recovered from anesthesia. Any abdominal discomfort usually can be controlled with a mild analgesic (e.g., acetaminophen). Within days the scar is almost invisible (see Client

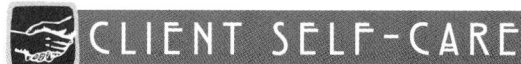

CLIENT SELF-CARE

What to Expect After Tubal Ligation

You should expect no change in hormones and their influence.

Your menstrual period will be about the same as before the sterilization.

You may feel pain at ovulation.

The ovum disintegrates within the abdominal cavity.

It is highly unlikely that you will become pregnant.

You should not experience a change in sexual functioning; in fact, you may enjoy sexual relations more because you will not be concerned about becoming pregnant.

Sterilization offers no protection against STIs; therefore you may need to use condoms.

Self-Care box). As with any surgery, there is always a possibility of complications of anesthesia, infection, hemorrhage, and trauma to other organs.

Tubal reconstruction. Restoration of tubal continuity (reanastomosis) and function is technically feasible except after laparoscopic tubal electrocoagulation. Sterilization reversal, however, is costly, difficult (requiring microsurgery), and uncertain (Cunningham et al., 1997). The success rate varies with the extent of tubal destruction and removal. The incidence of successful pregnancy after reanastomosis ranges from 43% to 88%, depending on the occlusion method. The loss of a segment of tube necessary for sperm capacitation and fertilization is probably the reason for low pregnancy rates.

Male sterilization. Vasectomy is the easiest and most commonly employed operation for male sterilization. In the United States 500,000 men undergo vasectomy each year (Cunningham et al., 1997). Vasectomy can be carried out with local anesthesia on an outpatient basis.

Small incisions are made into the anterior aspect of the scrotum above and lateral to each testis over the spermatic cord (see Fig. 9-8, *B*). Each vas deferens is identified and doubly ligated with fine, absorbable or nonabsorbable sutures. Then each vas deferens is severed between the ligatures. Occasionally the surgeon cauterizes the cut stumps of the sperm ducts. Many surgeons bury the cut ends into scrotal fascia to lessen the chance of reunion. Then the skin incisions are closed. Usually one suture is used for closure of each skin incision and a dressing is applied.

The man is instructed in self-care to promote a safe return to routine activities. To reduce swelling and relieve discomfort, ice packs are applied to the scrotum intermittently for a few hours postoperatively. A scrotal support may be applied to decrease discomfort. Moderate inactivity for about 2 days is advisable because of local scrotal tenderness. The skin suture can be removed 5 to 7 days postoperatively. Sexual intercourse may be resumed as desired; however, sterility is not immediate. Some sperm will remain in the proximal portions of the sperm ducts after vasectomy. One week to several months are required to clear the ducts of sperm (i.e., after approximately 20 ejaculations). Therefore some form of contraception is needed until the sperm count in the ejaculate on two consecutive tests is down to zero (Cunningham et al., 1997).

Vasectomy has no effect on potency (ability to achieve and maintain erection) or volume of ejaculate. Endocrine production of testosterone continues so that secondary sex characteristics are not affected. Sperm production continues, but sperm are unable to leave the epididymis and are lysed by the immune system. Men occasionally may develop a hematoma, infection, or epididymitis (Stewart & Carignan, 1998). Less common are painful granulomas from accumulation of sperm.

Complications after bilateral vasectomy are uncommon and usually not serious. They include bleeding (usually external), suture reaction, and reaction to anesthetic agent. Failure rate for male sterilization is 15% (Stewart & Carignan, 1998).

Tubal reconstruction. Microsurgery to reanastomose (restoration of tubal continuity) the sperm ducts can be accomplished successfully in up to 98% of cases (i.e., sperm in the ejaculate); however, the fertility rate is much lower (16% to 79%) (Stewart & Carignan, 1998). The rate of success decreases as the time since the procedure increases. The vasectomy may result in permanent changes in the testes that leave men unable to father children. The changes are those ordinarily seen only in the elderly (e.g., interstitial fibrosis [scar tissue between the seminiferous tubules]). Some men develop antibodies against their own sperm (autoimmunization). The role of antisperm antibodies in fertility after vasectomy reversal has not been completely determined. Additional research is needed to explore a possible link between vasectomy and prostate cancer.

Laws and regulations. All states have strict regulations for informed consent. Many states permit voluntary sterilization of any mature, rational woman without reference to her marital or pregnancy status. Although the partner's consent is not required by law, the client is encouraged to discuss the situation with the partner, and health care providers may request the partner's consent. Sterilization of minors or mentally incompetent individuals is restricted by most states and often requires the approval of a board of eugenicists or other court-appointed individuals (see Legal Tip).

LEGAL TIP **Sterilization**

- *If federal funds are used for sterilization, the person must be at least 21 years of age.*
- *Informed consent must include an explanation of the risks, benefits, and alternatives; a statement that describes sterilization as a permanent, irreversible method of birth control; and a statement that mandates a 30-day waiting period between giving consent and the sterilization.*
- *Informed consent must be in the person's native language, or an interpreter must be provided.*

Nursing considerations. The nurse plays an important role in assisting people with decision making so that all requirements for informed consent are met. The nurse also provides information about alternatives to sterilization, such as contraception.

The nurse acts as a "sounding board" for people who are exploring the possibility of choosing sterilization and their feelings about and motivation for this choice. The nurse records this information, which may be the basis for referral to a family planning clinic, a psychiatric social worker, or another professional health care provider.

Information must be given about what is entailed in various procedures, how much discomfort or pain can be expected, and what type of care is needed. Many individuals fear sterilization procedures because of the imagined effect on their sex life. They need reassurance concerning the hormonal and psychologic basis for sexual function and that uterine tube occlusion or vasectomy has no biologic sequelae in terms of sexual adequacy (Stewart & Carignan, 1998).

Preoperative care includes health assessment, which includes a psychologic assessment, physical examination, and laboratory tests. The nurse assists with the health assessment, answers questions, and confirms the client's understanding of printed instructions (e.g., nothing by mouth after midnight). Ambivalence and extreme fear of the procedure are reported to the physician.

Postoperative care depends on the procedure performed, for example, laparoscopy, laparotomy for tubal occlusion, or vasectomy. General care includes recovery after anesthesia, vital signs, fluid and electrolyte balance (intake and output, laboratory values), prevention of or early identification and treatment for infection or hemorrhage, control of discomfort, and assessment of emotional response to the procedure and recovery.

Discharge planning depends on the type of procedure performed. In general, the client is given written instructions about observing for and reporting symptoms and signs of complications, the type of recovery to be expected, and the date and time for a follow-up appointment.

Future trends. Contraceptive options are more limited in the United States and Canada than some other industrialized countries. Lack of funding for research, governmental regulations, conflicting values about contraception, and high costs of liability coverage for contraception have been cited as blocks to new and improved methods. However, existing methods of contraception are being improved, and a variety of new ones are being developed.

PLAN ᵒᶠ CARE | Sexual Activity and Contraception

NURSING DIAGNOSIS Decisional conflict related to contraceptive alternatives

Expected Outcome *Client and partner will verbalize understanding of different methods of contraception and will choose the method best suited for their needs.*

Nursing Interventions/Rationales

Provide information regarding reliability, use, indications, contraindications, and side effects of different methods of contraception *to facilitate the decision-making process.*

Utilize privacy and therapeutic communication during discussion of sexual activity and methods of contraception *to provide clarification of information and client trust of caregiver.*

NURSING DIAGNOSIS Risk for infection related to ongoing sexual activity as evidenced by client history

Expected Outcome *Client and her partner will remain free of sexually transmitted infections.*

Nursing Interventions/Rationales

Provide information regarding safer sex practices, use of spermicides and barrier methods *to raise client awareness of methods to prevent infection.*

New formulations of progestin oral contraceptives that have low androgenic and low antiestrogenic effects are in clinical trials, as are gonadotropin-releasing hormone methods. A one-size-fits-all diaphragm or shield that is placed in the posterior fornix of the vagina is being tested, as is a disposable diaphragm that releases nonoxynol-9. Mifepristone (RU 486) has been tested as a contraceptive; it is administered as a single large dose in the follicular phase of the menstrual cycle to inhibit ovulation (Reifsnider, 1997).

Biodegradable hormonal implants and pellets are being tested. Transdermal progestins and vaginal rings that contain estrogen and progestin or progestin only are being investigated. Once-a-month progestin injections and new IUDs containing copper or levonorgestrel are already available outside the United States. Newer versions of the vaginal sponge that contain antiviral spermicides are being tested. Chemical forms of male and female sterilization are being studied. Male contraceptives are also being investigated, including hormonal injections (testosterone), gonadotropin-releasing hormone antagonists, calcium channel blockers, and contraceptive vaccines (Gabelnick, 1998; Reifsnider, 1997).

Evaluation

The nurse can be reasonably assured that care was effective when the client-centered expected outcomes have been achieved: the woman and her partner learn about the various methods of contraception; the couple achieve pregnancy only when it has been planned; and they experience no adverse sequelae as a result of the chosen method of contraception (see Plan of Care).

ABORTION

Induced abortion is the purposeful interruption of a pregnancy before 20 weeks gestation. (Spontaneous abortion [miscarriage] is discussed in Chapter 31.) If the abortion is performed at the woman's request, the term **elective abortion** is used; if performed for reasons of maternal or fetal health or disease, the term **therapeutic abortion** applies. Many factors contribute to a woman's decision to have an abortion. Indications include (1) preservation of the life or health of the mother, (2) genetic disorders of the fetus, (3) rape or incest, and (4) the pregnant woman's request. The control of birth, dealing as it does with human sexuality and the question of life and death, is one of the most emotional components of health care and has been the most controversial social issue in the last half of the twentieth century (Soriano, 1998). Abortion as a surgical alternative to contraception is regulated in most countries (World Health Organization, 1995). Regulations exist to protect the mother from the complications of abortion.

Most women having abortions are Caucasian, younger than 24 years old, and unmarried (Centers for Disease Control and Prevention, 1996). Only one fourth of abortions are obtained by married women (Wallach & Zacur, 1995). Sixty percent of women having abortions say they used a contraceptive, but it failed. The U.S. Supreme Court set aside previous antiabortion laws in January 1973, holding that first trimester abortion is permissible inasmuch as the mortality rate from interruption of early gestation is less than the mortality rate after normal term delivery; 90% of abortions are performed at this point in pregnancy (Wallach & Zacur, 1995). Second trimester abortion was left to the discretion of the individual states (Cates & Ellertson, 1998). Hospitals maintained by Catholics and some of those maintained by strict fundamentalists forbid abortion (and often sterilization) despite legal challenge (see Legal Tip).

LEGAL TIP **Induced Abortion**

It is important for nurses to know the laws regarding abortion in their state of practice before they offer abortion counseling or nursing care to a woman choosing an abortion. Many states enforce a mandatory delay or state-directed counseling before a woman may legally obtain an abortion.

Before the legalization of abortion, many illegal abortions took place, with little documented sequelae other than death from infection, hemorrhage, or both. Although studies indicate that biologic sequelae do occur after abortion (e.g., ectopic pregnancy), rates of biologic complications tend to be low, especially if the woman aborts during the first trimester (Speroff & Darney, 1996). Major psychologic sequelae of induced abortion are rare (Stotland, 1997). Sequelae may be related to circumstances and support systems surrounding the pregnant woman, such as the attitudes reflected by friends, family, and health care workers. Some researchers suggest that emotional distress exhibited by some women after an abortion may be a continuation of symptoms exhibited before the abortion (Grimes, 1995). It must be remembered that the woman facing an abortion is pregnant and will exhibit the emotional responses shared by all pregnant women, including the possibility of postbirth depression.

Nurses often struggle with the same values and moral convictions as those of the pregnant woman. The conflicts and doubts of the nurse can be nonverbally communicated to women who are already anxious and overly sensitive. Health care professionals need assistance to identify and come to terms with their own feelings. It is not uncommon for confusion to arise as beliefs are challenged by the reality of care. Nurses whose religious or moral beliefs do not support abortion have the right to refuse such an assignment. Reassignment is usually an option so that the abortion client receives needed care.

CARE MANAGEMENT

Assessment and Nursing Diagnoses

A thorough assessment is conducted through history, physical examination, and laboratory tests. The length of pregnancy and the condition of the woman must be determined to select the appropriate type of abortion procedure. An ultrasound should be performed before a second trimester abortion is done. If the woman is Rh negative and the pregnancy is greater than 8 weeks of gestation, she is a candidate for prophylaxis against Rh isoimmunization. She will receive $Rh_0(D)$ immune globulin within 72 hours after the abortion if she is D negative and if Coombs' test results are negative (if the woman is unsensitized or isoimmunization has not developed) (Cunningham et al., 1997).

The woman's understanding of alternatives, the types of abortions, and expected recovery is assessed. Misinformation and gaps in knowledge are identified and corrected. The record is reviewed for the signed informed consent, and the client's understanding is verified. General preoperative, operative, and postoperative assessments are performed.

Analysis of data leads to identification of the appropriate nursing diagnoses for the woman undergoing elective abortion. Potential nursing diagnoses are listed below.

Nursing Diagnoses

- Decisional conflict related to
  - perceived conflict related to value system
- Fear related to
  - abortion procedure
  - potential complications
  - implications for future pregnancies
  - what others might think
- Anticipatory grieving related to
  - distress at loss or feelings of guilt
- Risk for infection related to
  - effects of the procedure
  - lack of understanding of preoperative and postoperative self-care
- Pain related to
  - effects of the procedure or postoperative events

Expected Outcomes of Care

Planning is a collaborative effort among the woman, her sexual partner (as appropriate), the physician, and the nurse. Expected outcomes are established collaboratively, should be stated in client-centered terms, and may include that the woman will do the following:
- Verbalize understanding of the information necessary to give informed consent.
- Undergo a successful procedure and uneventful recovery.
- Continue to be satisfied with the decision for induced abortion, the procedure, and her experience with the health care team.

Plan of Care and Interventions

Counseling about abortion includes help for the woman in identifying how she perceives the pregnancy, information about the choices available (i.e., having an abortion or carrying the pregnancy to term and then either keeping the infant or placing the baby for adoption), and information about the types of abortion procedures.

First Trimester Abortion

Methods for performing early elective abortion include vacuum aspiration and medical methods (mifepristone with prostaglandin and methotrexate with misoprostol).

Vacuum aspiration abortion is the most common procedure, with about 97% of all procedures being performed by suction curretage. Very early abortions (menstrual extraction, endometrial aspiration) can be done with a small flexible plastic cannula without cervical dilation or anesthesia. The insertion of a small **laminaria tent** (cone of dried seaweed that swells as it absorbs moisture and dilates the cervix) retained by a vaginal tampon for 4 to 24 hours will usually facilitate the purposeful interruption of a first trimester pregnancy greater than 8 weeks of gestation by dilating the cervix atraumatically (Wallach & Zacur, 1995). On removal of the moist, expanded laminaria tent the cervix will have dilated two or three times its original diameter. Rarely will further mechanical dilation of the cervix be required. The insertion of an adequate-sized aspiration cannula (8.5 to 10.5 mm) is almost always possible. Cervical laceration and bleeding are reduced by the use of laminaria. A disadvantage is the delay necessary and the need for an additional visit to the physician's office or clinic. Prostaglandin gel may also be used to soften the cervix (Cunningham et al., 1997).

Aspiration abortion may be performed in the physician's office, the clinic, or the hospital. For the procedure, the vaginal area is cleansed (shaving is not necessary). The suction procedure for performing an early elective abortion (ideal time is 8 to 12 weeks after the last menstrual period) usually requires less than 5 minutes. During the procedure the nurse or physician keeps the woman informed about what to expect next (e.g., menstrual-like cramping and sounds of the suction machine). The nurse assesses the woman's vital signs. The aspirated uterine contents must be carefully inspected to ascertain whether all fetal parts and adequate placental tissue have been evacuated. After the abortion the woman rests on the table until she is ready to stand. Then she remains in the recovery area or waiting room for 1 to 3 hours for detection of excessive cramping or bleeding; then she is discharged. She may be discharged alone or in the company of a relative or friend, depending on the anesthetic used. If the procedure is done in the physician's office, preoperative sedation is usually not given, and local anesthesia is usually used.

Bleeding after the operation is normally about the equivalent of a heavy menstrual period, and cramps are rarely severe. Excessive vaginal bleeding and infection, such as endometritis or salpingitis, are the most common complications of induced abortion. Retained products of conception are the primary cause of vaginal bleeding. Evacuation of the uterus, uterine massage, and administration of oxytocin or methylergonovine (Methergine) may be necessary (Cates & Ellertson, 1998; World Health Organization, 1995). Prophylactic antibiotics have been shown to decrease the risk of infection and should be considered (Grimes, 1995).

Postabortal instructions differ among health care providers (e.g., tampons should not be used for at least 3 days or should be avoided for up to 3 weeks, and resumption of sexual intercourse may be permitted within 1 week or discouraged for 3 weeks). The woman may shower daily. Instruction is given to watch for excessive bleeding (that is, more than one large pad per hour for 4 hours), cramps, or fever and to avoid douches of any type. The woman may expect her menstrual period to resume 4 to 6 weeks after the day of the procedure. The nurse offers information about the birth control method the woman prefers, if this has not been done previously during the counseling interview that usually precedes the decision to have an abortion. The woman must be strongly encouraged to return for her follow-up visit so that complications can be detected and an acceptable contraceptive method prescribed. A pregnancy test may also be performed to determine if the pregnancy has been successfully terminated.

Other First Trimester Abortions

Mifepristone. Mifepristone (RU 486) can be taken up to 5 weeks after conception. The effectiveness of mifepristone is inversely related to gestational age as determined by β-human chorionic gonadotropin levels and the duration of amenorrhea (Creinin et al., 1996). However, it is considered to be an effective and safe method for termination of early pregnancy.

Uterine bleeding begins within 4 days of administration of the first dose. Usually a period of painless heavy bleeding is reported. Termination of pregnancy occurs for most women. When mifepristone is combined with administration of a prostaglandin agent 36 to 48 hours later, the rate of abortion increases.

Supporters of this method believe that even with known disadvantages, mifepristone offers a reasonable alternative to surgical abortion, which carries the risk of anesthesia and surgical complications, and infertility (Cates & Ellertson, 1998). Others have taken a strong stand against the use of mifepristone. In the United States it is still not readily available for terminating pregnancy.

Methotrexate. Methotrexate can be given intramuscularly followed by vaginal placement of misoprostol (prostglandin analog). Oral methotrexate followed by vaginal misoprostol also has been shown to be effective with few side effects (Carbonell et al., 1998). If abortion does not occur by the next day, misoprostol is repeated (Creinin et al., 1996).

Second Trimester Abortion

Second trimester abortion is associated with an increase of complications and costs (Toppozada, 1995). Dilation and evacuation, induction of uterine contractions, and major operations are methods used.

Dilation and Evacuation

Dilation and evacuation (D & E) can be performed at up to 20 weeks of gestation (Cates & Ellertson, 1998). It is the predominant method of abortion used beyond the first trimester (Wallach & Zacur, 1995). The cervix requires more dilation because the products of conception are larger. Often laminaria are inserted several hours or several days before the procedure. Nursing care includes monitoring vital signs, providing emotional support, administering analgesics, and postoperative monitoring. Disadvantages of D & E may be long-term harmful effects on the cervix.

Prostaglandins

The most common technique for medical termination in the second trimester is the administration of prostaglandins. Prostaglandins can be administered in suppository form, as a gel, or by intrauterine injection. Unpleasant side effects (e.g., nausea, vomiting, and diarrhea) usually occur. Repeated doses may be needed for expulsion of the products of conception.

Other Second Trimester Methods

Other techniques used infrequently are instillation of hypertonic sodium chloride, hypertonic glucose, and urea into the uterine cavity. Uterine contractions usually begin within 12 to 24 hours, and abortion occurs a few hours later. Use of laminaria or oxytocin may facilitate the process. Complications of hypertonic solution injection for second trimester abortion may occur. Complications include infection, need for dilation and curettage to remove retained tissue, failure to abort, and excessive bleeding necessitating transfusion. Hysterotomy and hysterectomy are infrequently used methods of abortion because of increased morbidity and mortality.

Complications After Abortion

The most common complications after abortion include infection, retained products of conception or intrauterine blood clots, continuing pregnancy, cervical or uterine trauma, and excessive bleeding (Cates & Ellertson, 1998; Wallach & Zacur, 1995). Preoperative antibiotic prophylaxis has been effective in reducing the risk of infection. Women are advised to report fever, pelvic pain, and excessive bleeding. Prophylactic chlamydia and gonorrhea treatment and the use of an oral ergonovine postoperatively may reduce the incidence of infection and retained products of conception.

Nursing Considerations

The woman will need help to explore the meaning of the various alternatives and consequences to herself and her significant others. It is often difficult for a woman to express her true feelings (e.g., what abortion means to her now and in the future and what support or regret her friends and peers may demonstrate). A calm, matter-of-fact approach on the part of the nurse can be helpful (e.g., "Yes, I know you are pregnant. I am here to help. Let's talk about alternatives"). Listening to what the woman has to say and encouraging her to speak are essential. Neutral responses such as "Oh," "Uh-huh," and "Umm" and nonverbal encouragement such as nodding, maintaining eye contact, and use of touch are helpful in setting an open, accepting environment. Clarifying, restating, and reflecting statements; open-ended questions; and feedback are

communication techniques that can be used to maintain a realistic focus on the situation and bring the woman's problems into the open. Once a decision has been made, the woman must be assured of continued support. Information about what is entailed in various procedures, how much discomfort or pain can be expected, and what type of care is needed must be given. If family or friends cannot be involved, scheduling time for nursing personnel to give the necessary support is an essential component of the care plan.

Evaluation

The nurse can be reasonably sure that care was effective when the expected outcomes have been met: the client understands all information necessary to give informed consent; the procedure is successful; recovery is uneventful; and the client continues to be satisfied with the decision for elective abortion, the procedure, and the experience with the health care team.

 EY POINTS

- A variety of contraceptive methods are available with various effectiveness rates, advantages, and disadvantages.
- Women and their partners should choose the contraceptive method or methods best suited to them.
- Effective contraceptives are available through both prescription and nonprescription sources.
- A variety of techniques are available to enhance the effectiveness of periodic abstinence in motivated couples who prefer this natural method.
- Hormonal contraception includes both precoital and postcoital prevention through various modalities and requires thorough client education.
- The barrier methods of diaphragm and cervical cap provide safe and effective contraception for women or couples motivated to use them consistently and correctly.
- Proper concurrent use of spermicides and latex condoms provides protection against STIs.
- Tubal ligations and vasectomies are permanent sterilization methods used by increasing numbers of women and men.
- Induced abortion performed in the first trimester is safer than an abortion performed in the second trimester.
- The most common complications of induced abortion include infection, retained products of conception, and excessive vaginal bleeding.
- Major psychologic sequelae of induced abortion are rare.

CRITICAL THINKING EXERCISES

1 You are interviewing a 45-year-old woman in the local health department family planning clinic. She is seeking information about her risks of pregnancy at this time in her life.

a. What information will you need from her to respond?

b. How might you answer her question based on the answers you may receive in part a?

c. Assuming that contraceptive measures are necessary, what methods are appropriate for this client?

d. What further information may you need from this client to make a contraceptive recommendation?

e. What alterations would you make in a teaching plan for her based on her age and previous experiences with contraception?

2 You are working in a health department clinic. A 16-year-old unmarried woman comes in requesting information about options for an unwanted pregnancy.

a. Examine your beliefs about teenage pregnancy. Explore your beliefs about options for an unwanted pregnancy. How might these beliefs affect your ability to provide information about options in a nonjudgmental manner?

b. What client information do you need to know before counseling a client about her options?

c. What information is needed by the pregnant woman in making a decision about her unwanted pregnancy?

d. What are the laws in your state related to abortion, informed consent, and treatment of minors?

e. Select one option for this hypothetic client and justify your choice.

f. Write a care plan addressing the physical and psychosocial needs of a client undergoing abortion.

3 Visit a clinic that provides family planning services in your area.

a. Are there differences in fee schedules for women with and without insurance? Are local, state, or federal funds available?

b. Are the hours of service sufficient to meet the needs of clients? How long are typical waits to be seen during a scheduled appointment?

c. What is the nurse's role in the clinic? What other health care professionals are present and what are their roles? Is there any collaboration among these care providers?

d. Make suggestions for changes in the way care is provided that increase efficacy and client satisfaction.

References

Burkman, R., & Shulman, L. (1998). Oral contraceptive practice guidelines. *Contraception* 58 (suppl 3), 35S-43S.

Carbonell, J. et al. (1998). Oral methotrexate and vaginal misoprostol for early abortion. *Contraception* 57(2), 83-88.

Cates, W., & Ellertson, C. (1998). Abortion. In R. Hatcher et al. (Eds.). *Contraceptive technology* (17 rev. ed.). New York: Ardent Media, Inc.

Cates, W., & Raymond, E. (1998). Vaginal spermicides. In R. Hatcher et al. (Eds.). *Contraceptive technology* (17 rev. ed.). New York: Ardent Media, Inc.

Centers for Disease Control and Prevention. (1996). CDC Surveillance Summaries (Abortion Surveillance–United States, 1991). *MMWR Morb Mortal Wkly Rep* 45(SS-3), 1-43.

Chez, R., & Chapin, J. (1997). Emergency contraception: The pill's little known secret goes public. *Lifelines* 1(5), 28-31.

Contraception Report. (1997). Trends in oral contraceptive development and utilization. *Contraception Report* 7(5), 4-16.

Creinin, M. et al. (1996). Methotrexate and misoprostol for early abortion: A multicenter trial. I. Safety and efficacy. *Contraception* 53(6), 321-327.

Cunningham, F. et al. (1997). *Williams obstetrics* (20th ed.). Stamford, CT: Appleton & Lange.

Gabelnick, H. (1998). Future methods. In R. Hatcher et al. (Eds.). *Contraceptive technology* (17 rev. ed.). New York: Ardent Media, Inc.

Grimes, D. (1995). Sequelae of abortion. In D. Baird, D. Grimes, & P. Van Look (Eds.). *Modern methods of inducing abortion.* London: Blackwell Scientific.

Guest, F. (1998). Education and counseling. In R. Hatcher et al. (Eds.). *Contraceptive technology* (17 rev. ed.). New York: Ardent Media, Inc.

Hatcher, R. (1998). Depo-Provera, Norplant, and progestin-only pills (minipills). In R. Hatcher et al. (Eds.). *Contraceptive technology* (17 rev. ed.). New York: Ardent Media, Inc.

Hatcher, R., & Guillebaud, J. (1998). The pill: Combined oral contraceptives. In R. Hatcher et al. (Eds.). *Contraceptive technology* (17 rev. ed.). New York: Ardent Media, Inc.

Heath, C., & Sulik, S. (1997). Contraception and preconception counseling. *Women's Health* 24(10), 123-133.

Henshaw, S. (1998). Unintended pregnancy in the United States. *Fam Plann Perspect* 30, 24-29, 46.

Jennings, V., Lamprecht, V., & Kowal, D. (1998). Fertility awareness methods. In R. Hatcher et al. (Eds.). *Contraceptive technology* (17 rev. ed.). New York: Ardent Media, Inc.

Kowal, D. (1998). Coitus interruptus (withdrawal). In R. Hatcher et al. (Eds.). *Contraceptive technology* (17 rev. ed.). New York: Ardent Media, Inc.

Lindberg, C. (1997). Emergency contraception: The nurse's role in providing postcoital options. *J Obstet Gynecol Neonatal Nurs* 26(2), 145-152.

Mishell, D. (1998). Intrauterine devices: Mechanisms of action, safety, and efficacy. *Contraception* 58(suppl 3), 45S-53S.

O'Connell, M. (1996). The effect of birth control methods on sexually transmitted disease/HIV risk. *J Obstet Gynecol Neonatal Nurs* 25(6), 476-480.

Reifsnider, E. (1997). On the horizon: New options for contraception. *J Obstet Gynecol Neonatal Nurs* 26(1), 91-100.

Soriano, C. (1998, January 9-11). Abortion: New common ground. *USA Weekend.*

Speroff, L., & Darney, P. (1996). *A clinical guide for contraception* (2nd ed.). Baltimore: Williams & Wilkins.

Springen, K. (1999, April 12). Comeback of a contraceptive: The sponge returns. *Newsweek*, p. 69.

Stewart, F. (1998). Vaginal barriers. In R. Hatcher et al. (Eds.). *Contraceptive technology* (17 rev. ed.). New York: Ardent Media, Inc.

Stewart, G. (1998). Intrauterine devices (IUDs). In R. Hatcher et al. (Eds.). *Contraceptive technology* (17 rev. ed.). New York: Ardent Media, Inc.

Stewart, G., & Carignan, C. (1998). Female and male sterilization. In R. Hatcher et al. (Eds.). *Contraceptive technology* (17 rev. ed.). New York: Ardent Media, Inc.

Stotland, N. (1977). Psychosocial aspects of induced abortion. *Clin Obstet Gynecol* 40(3), 673-686.

Toppozada, M. (1995). Termination of pregnancy after 14 weeks. In D. Baird, D. Grimes, & P. Van Look (Eds.). *Modern methods of inducing abortion.* London: Blackwell Scientific.

Trent, A., & Clark, E. (1997). What nurses should know about natural family planning. *J Obstet Gynecol Neonatal Nurs* 26(6), 643-648.

Trussell, J. (1998). Contraceptive efficacy. In R. Hatcher et al. (Eds.). *Contraceptive technology* (17 rev. ed.). New York: Ardent Media, Inc.

Trussell, J., & Kowal, D. (1998). The essentials of contraception. In R. Hatcher et al. (Eds.). *Contraceptive technology* (17 rev. ed.). New York: Ardent Media, Inc.

Trussell, J., Rodriguez, G., & Ellertson, C. (1998). New estimates of the effectiveness of the Yuzpe regimen of emergency contraception. *Contraception* 57(6), 363-369.

Van Look, P., & Stewart, F. (1998). Emergency contraception. In R. Hatcher et al. (Eds.). *Contraceptive technology* (17 rev. ed.). New York: Ardent Media, Inc.

Wallach, E., & Zacur, H. (1995). *Reproductive medicine and surgery.* St. Louis: Mosby.

Warner, D., & Hatcher, R. (1998). Male condoms. In R. Hatcher et al. (Eds.). *Contraceptive technology* (17 rev. ed.). New York: Ardent Media, Inc.

World Health Organization. (1995). *Complications of abortion.* Geneva: World Health Organization.

10

Infertility

Amy N. Nichols, and Deitra Leonard Lowdermilk

LEARNING OBJECTIVES

- Define the key terms.
- List common causes of infertility.
- Discuss the psychologic impact of infertility.
- List common diagnoses and treatments for infertility.
- Identify reproductive alternatives for couples experiencing infertility.

- Recognize the various ethical and legal considerations of infertility.
- Identify topics for nursing research related to infertility.

KEY TERMS

assisted reproductive therapies (ARTs)
autoimmunization
gamete intrafallopian transfer (GIFT)
infertility
intracytoplasmic sperm injection

in vitro fertilization-embryo transfer (IVF-ET)
isoimmunization
postcoital test (PCT)
referred shoulder pain
semen analysis

therapeutic donor insemination (TDI)
varicocele
zygote intrafallopian transfer (ZIFT)

his chapter addresses infertility, associated tests, and common therapies. The available alternatives and the psychosocial implications of infertility are discussed.

INCIDENCE

Infertility is a serious medical concern that affects quality of life and is a problem for 10% to 15% of reproductive-age couples (ASRM, 1999; Hatcher et al., 1998) Infertility implies subfertility, a prolonged time to conceive, as opposed to sterility, which means inability to conceive. Normally, a fertile couple has approximately a 25% chance of conception in each ovulatory cycle. Primary infertility applies to a woman who has never been pregnant; sec-

ondary infertility applies to a woman who has been pregnant in the past.

The prevalence of infertility is relatively stable among the overall population but increases with the age of the woman. Infertility among all childless women older than 35 years is thought to be 21%. An estimated 1 of every 12 women in the United States is involuntarily childless (Seibel, 1997). Probable causes include the trend toward delaying pregnancy until later in life, when fertility decreases naturally and the prevalence of diseases such as endometriosis and ovulatory dysfunction increases.

There is some controversy regarding whether there has been an increase in male infertility, or whether male infertility is being more readily identified because of improvements in diagnosis. Diagnosis and treatment of infertility require considerable physical, emotional, and financial investment over an extended period. Men and women often perceive infertility differently, with women having more stress from tests and treatments, placing greater importance on having children, being more accepting of indicated treatments, and wanting children more than men (Stephen & Chandra, 1998).

The attitude, sensitivity, and caring nature of those who are involved in the assessment of infertility lay the foundation for the clients' ability to cope with the subsequent therapy and management. Team members must also respect affected individuals' and couples' desires in choosing to stop treatment and to select other alternatives, such as adoption.

INFERTILITY MISCONCEPTIONS

Within the United States, feelings connected with infertility are many and complex. The origins of some of these feelings are myths, superstitions, misinformation, or magical thinking about the causes of infertility. Other feelings arise from the need to undergo many tests and examinations and from a perception of being "different" from others.

It is important that nurses debunk some common myths. These myths include the following (Fogel & Woods, 1995):

1. *If you just relax, you'll get pregnant.* In 90% of all cases of infertility, there is a discernible physiologic explanation.
2. *Adoption improves a couple's chance of conceiving.* No significant increase in conception has been found among couples with infertility who had adopted compared with couples who had not.
3. *Pillows under the hips during and after intercourse enhance fertility.* Sperm are already in the uterine tubes as intercourse is completed. The position of the hips does not really matter.
4. *Jockey shorts cause infertility in men.* Tight underwear alone is insufficient to increase scrotal temperatures. However, daily hot tubs or saunas may increase scrotal temperatures enough to damage spermatogenesis.

FACTORS ASSOCIATED WITH INFERTILITY

The couple is a biologic unit of reproduction. Many factors, both male and female, contribute to normal fertility. A normally developed reproductive tract in both the male and female partner is essential. Normal functioning of an intact hypothalamic-pituitary-gonadal axis supports gametogenesis—the formation of sperm and ova. The life span of the sperm and ovum is short. Although sperm remain viable in the female's reproductive tract for 48 hours or more, probably only a few retain fertilization potential for more than 24 hours. Ova remain viable for about 24

hours, but the optimum time for fertilization may be no more than 1 to 2 hours (Cunningham et al., 1997). Thus timing of intercourse becomes critical.

The male must produce sperm that are normal, adequate in number, and motile. Accessory glands must provide secretions supportive to the sperm to form semen. The tube system to the urethra must be patent. Ejaculation must deposit semen around the cervix at the appropriate time of the female's menstrual cycle. After being deposited, sperm must undergo capacitation to prepare for fertilization. Then they migrate through the uterus to the ampulla of the uterine tube to fertilize a receptive normal ovum.

In the female, a graafian follicle must mature and release a healthy ovum able to be fertilized. The ovum must be drawn by the fimbria into a healthy, patent uterine tube and be fertilized within a few hours. The conceptus must migrate down the tube into a well-developed normal uterus. Implantation of the blastocyst must occur within 7 to 10 days in a hormone-prepared endometrium. The conceptus must develop normally, reach viability, and be born in good condition for extrauterine life.

An alteration in one or more of these structures, functions, or processes results in some degree of impaired fertility. Causes of impaired fertility are sometimes difficult to assign to either the male or female. In general a female factor is responsible for infertility in 50% of infertile couples. Ovulatory dysfunction accounts for 40% of those causes, while pelvic factors also account for 40% (ASRM, 1999). The incidence of infertility increases with increasing age of the woman, so that the probability of conception is greatly reduced as a result of delayed childbearing until later in life. A male factor (sperm and semen abnormalities) is responsible for infertility in about 35% of couples. Unexplained factors and unusual problems account for 10% and 5% of infertility, respectively (Mishell et al., 1997; Session et al., 1998). However, unexplained infertility and recurrent (habitual) miscarriage may be the result of aberrations of the immune system (e.g., antisperm antibodies, failure of implantation and growth of a blastocyst) (Carcio, 1998; Timbers & Feinberg, 1996).

Infertility may also be caused by something as simple as poor timing or inadequate frequency of intercourse. The couple should be taught about the menstrual cycle and the way to detect ovulation (see Chapters 6 and 9).

Female Infertility

Congenital or Developmental Factors

Congenital factors rarely cause impaired fertility. If the woman has abnormal external genitals, surgical reconstruction of abnormal tissue and construction of a functional vagina may permit normal intercourse. However, if internal reproductive tract structures are absent, there is no hope for fertility. Vaginal and uterine anomalies and their surgical repair vary from individual to individual. If a functional uterus can be reconstructed, pregnancy may be possible.

Ovarian Factors

Anovulation may be primary or secondary. Primary anovulation may be caused by a pituitary or hypothalamic hormone disorder or an adrenal gland disorder such as congenital adrenal hyperplasia. It is usually seen in adolescents. Secondary anovulation, usually seen in young to midlife age women, is relatively common and is caused by the disruption of the hypothalamic-pituitary-ovarian-axis. In amenorrheic states and instances of anovulatory cycles, hormone studies usually reveal the problem.

Although it is a relatively rare occurrence, amenorrhea after the discontinuation of oral contraceptives is seen more frequently in women with histories of menstrual dysfunction before initiation of contraceptive use. Because most clients resume menstruating within 6 months, the workup should be delayed until that time in the absence of other symptoms.

Occasionally, women experience menopause before they are 40 years old. In a vast majority of cases of early menopause, the ovaries do not respond to ovulation-inducing drugs.

Increased prolactin levels may cause anovulation and amenorrhea. Many drugs affect the secretion of prolactin, including phenothiazine, opiates, diazepam, reserpine, methyldopa, and tricyclic antidepressants. In general, these agents are thought to inhibit the release of prolactin-inhibiting factor from the hypothalamus. Stress can also inhibit the release of prolactin-inhibiting factor, thereby causing the release of excess prolactin. Physical stressors such as surgery, cranial lesions, or injury may also initiate this response. Another common cause of hyperprolactinemia is benign pituitary adenoma, which is diagnosed through sophisticated radiographic techniques or computed tomographic (CT) scan.

Tubal/Peritoneal Factors

The motility of the tube and its fimbriated end may be reduced or absent as a result of infections, adhesions, scarring, or tumors. Chlamydial infection negatively influences tubal function and impedes fertility (Seibel, 1997). In rare instances there may be congenital absence of one tube. It is also possible to find one tube relatively shorter than the other. This condition is often associated with an abnormally developed uterus.

Inflammation within the tube or involving the exterior of the tube or the fimbriated ends represents a major cause of impaired fertility. Tubal adhesions resulting from pelvic infections (e.g., ruptured appendix, sexually transmitted diseases [STIs]) may impair fertility. When infection with purulent discharge heals, scar tissue adhesions form. In the process the tube may be blocked anywhere along its length. It can be closed off at the fimbriated end, or it can be distorted and kinked by adhesions. Adhesions may permit the tiny sperm to pass through the tube but may prevent a fertilized egg from completing the journey into the intrauterine cavity. This results in an ectopic pregnancy that may completely destroy the tube. In other cases, adhesions of the tubes to the ovary or bowel may follow endometriosis (see Chapter 7). Endometriosis is more commonly seen in women who delay childbearing until they are more than 30 years of age. Women who have a first-degree relative with a history of endometriosis also have a slightly higher risk.

Uterine Factors

Abnormalities of the uterus are more common than might be expected. Minor developmental anomalies of the uterus are fairly common; major anomalies occur rarely. Hysterosalpingography may reveal double uteri or other anomalous congenital variations (Fig. 10-1). Endometrial and myometrial tumors (e.g., polyps or myomas) may also be revealed by x-ray studies of infertile women. These anomalies can affect implantation and maintenance of a pregnancy.

Asherman's syndrome (uterine adhesions or scar tissue) is characterized by hypomenorrhea. The adhesions, which may partially or totally obliterate the uterine cavity, are sequelae to surgical interventions such as too vigorous curettage (scraping) after an abortion (elective or spontaneous). The hysteroscope is useful in the verification of intrauterine anomalies.

Endometritis (inflammation of the endometrium) may result from any of the causes of infection of the cervix or uterine tubes (e.g., *Chlamydia*). Women who have numer-

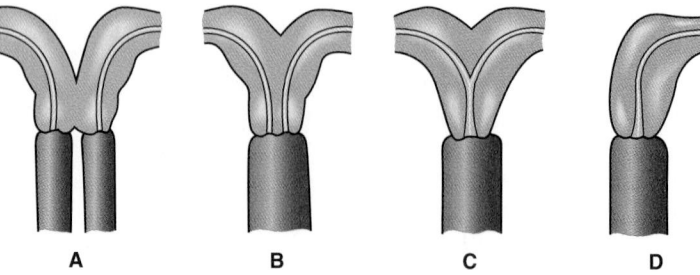

A   **B**   **C**   **D**

Fig. 10-1   Abnormal uterus. **A,** Complete bicornuate uterus with vagina divided by a septum. **B,** Complete bicornuate uterus with normal vagina. **C,** Partial bicornuate uterus with normal vagina. **D,** Unicornuate uterus.

ous sexual partners are more susceptible to endometrial infection than are women in monogamous relationships.

Vaginal-Cervical Factors

Vaginal fluid is acidic (pH of 4 or less), whereas cervical mucus is normally alkaline (pH of 7 or more). Ejaculation should place the sperm at or near the cervical os. The alkalinity of cervical mucus helps support sperm and permits the ascending transportation of sperm around the time of ovulation.

Endocervical mucus normally obstructs or plugs the cervix, acting as a barrier against infection, until rising estrogen levels cause the mucus to become clear, thin, and nutritionally supportive of sperm. This change occurs around the time of ovulation and lasts approximately 48 to 72 hours. The amount of cervical mucus and its characteristics are influenced by the hormone estrogen (see Teaching Guidelines, p. 184).

Vaginal-cervical infections (e.g., *Trichomoniasis vaginitis*) increase the acidity of the vaginal fluid and reduce the alkalinity of the cervical mucus. Thus vaginal infection often destroys or drastically reduces the number of viable motile sperm before they enter the cervical canal. The amount of mucus and its physical changes are influenced by the presence of blood, pathogenic bacteria, and irritants such as an intrauterine contraceptive device (IUD) or a tumor. Severe emotional stress, antibiotic therapy, and diseases such as diabetes mellitus alter the acidity of mucus.

Some infertile women have sperm antibodies. The production of antibodies by one member of a species against something that is commonly found within that species is termed **isoimmunization.** Sperm may be immobilized within the cervical mucus, or they become incapable of migration into the uterus (see postcoital test). A greater incidence of sperm agglutination occurs in women with otherwise unexplained impaired fertility. However, the true significance and reliability of tests for sperm immobilization or agglutination are uncertain.

Male Infertility

Male infertility can be caused by structural and hormonal disorders such as undescended testes, hypospadias, **varicocele** (varicose vein of the scrotum), and low testosterone levels. Mumps, especially after adolescence, can result in permanent damage to the testes. Male infertility may also be caused by factors that also affect women, such as nutrition, endocrine disorders, genetic disorders, psychologic disorders, and STIs (Bhasin et al., 1998; Hargreave & Ghosh, 1998; Liel et al., 1993). Exposure to hazards in the workplace such as radiation can also affect sperm production; exposure of the scrotum to high temperatures can both decrease and cause abnormal sperm production.

Substance abuse can be a major factor in male infertility. Alcohol consumption can cause erectile problems (impotence) (Liel et al., 1993). In addition, cigarette smoking has been associated with abnormal sperm, a decreased number of sperm, and chromosome damage. The degree of abnormality is related to the number of cigarettes smoked per day (Giwercman & Bonde, 1998). Heroin and marijuana use may depress the number and motility of sperm and increase the percentage of abnormally formed sperm. Amyl nitrate, butyl nitrate, ethyl chloride, and methaqualone (used to prolong orgasm) cause changes in spermatogenesis. Heroin, methadone, selective serotonin reuptake inhibitors (SSRIs), and barbiturates decrease libido. Monoamine oxidase (MAO), an antidepressant, adversely affects spermatogenesis. In addition, some antihypertensives may cause impotence (Liel et al., 1993).

Male fertility declines slowly after the age of 40 years. There is, however, no cessation of sperm production analogous to menopause in women.

▪ CARE MANAGEMENT

Assessment and Nursing Diagnoses

The nurse assists in the assessment by obtaining data relevant to fertility through interview and physical examination. The database needs to include information to identify whether infertility is primary or secondary. Religious, cultural, and ethnic data are noted (see Box 10-1 and the Cultural Considerations box).

▪ BOX 10-1 Religious Considerations of Infertility

Civil laws and religious proscriptions about sex must always be kept in mind by the health care provider. For example, the Orthodox Jewish husband and wife may face infertility investigation and management problems because of religious laws that govern marital relations. For example, according to Jewish law, the Orthodox couple may not engage in marital relations during menstruation and through the following 7 "preparatory days." The wife then is immersed in a ritual bath (Mikvah) before relations can resume. Fertility problems can arise when the woman has a short cycle (i.e., a cycle of 24 days or fewer; when ovulation would occur on day 10 or earlier).

The Roman Catholic Church regards the embryo as a human being from the first moment of existence and regards technical procedures such as in vitro fertilization, therapeutic donor insemination, and freezing embryos as unacceptable (Fryday, 1995). Both Orthodox Jewish and Roman Catholic women may at times question proposed diagnostic and therapeutic procedures because of religious proscriptions. These women are encouraged to consult their rabbi or priest for a ruling.

Other religious groups may also have ethical concerns about infertility tests and treatments.

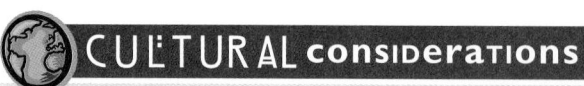

CULTURAL consiperations

Fertility/Infertility

Worldwide cultures continue to employ symbols and rites that celebrate fertility. One fertility rite that persists today is the custom of throwing rice at the bride and groom. Other fertility symbols and rites include passing out of congratulatory cigars, candy, or pencils by a new father and baby showers held in anticipation of a child's birth.

In many cultures the responsibility for infertility is usually attributed to the woman. A woman's inability to conceive may be due to her sins, to evil spirits, or to the fact that she is an inadequate person. The virility of a man in some cultures remains in question until he demonstrates his ability to reproduce by having at least one child (Geissler, 1994).

Some of the data needed to investigate impaired fertility are of a sensitive, personal nature. Obtaining these data may be viewed as an invasion of privacy. The tests and examinations are occasionally painful and intrusive and can take the romance out of lovemaking. A high level of motivation is needed to endure the investigation.

Many couples have already visited various physicians and have read extensively on the subject. Their previous experiences are recorded, and the depth and breadth of their knowledge base are explored.

Because multiple factors involving both partners are common, the investigation of impaired fertility is conducted systematically and simultaneously for both male and female partners. Both partners must be interested in the solution to the problem. The medical investigation requires time (3 to 4 months) and considerable financial expense (Box 10-2), and it causes emotional distress and strain on the couple's interpersonal relationship. Nurses can be instrumental in providing information about the latest tests and treatment.

Investigation of impaired fertility begins for the woman with a complete history and physical examination (Box 10-3). The history explores the duration of infertility and past obstetric events and contains a detailed sexual history. Medical and surgical conditions are evaluated. Exposure to reproductive hazards in the home (e.g., mutagens such as plastic-vinyl chlorides, teratogens such as alcohol, and emotional stresses) and workplace are explored.

A complete general physical examination is followed by a specific assessment of the reproductive tract. Evidence of endocrine system abnormalities is sought. Inadequate development of secondary sex characteristics (e.g., inappropriate distribution of body fat and hair) may point to problems with the hypothalamic-pituitary-ovarian axis or genetic aberrations (e.g., polycystic ovarian syndrome, Turner's syndrome).

A woman may have an abnormal uterus and tubes as a result of exposure to diethylstilbestrol (DES) in utero. Evidence of past infection of the genitourinary system is sought. Bimanual examination of internal organs may reveal lack of mobility of the uterus or abnormal contours of the uterus and adnexa. Laboratory data are assembled. Data from routine urine and blood tests are obtained along with other diagnostic tests.

Diagnostic Tests

Assessment of Female Infertility

There are several examinations and tests for impaired fertility in the woman. The basic infertility survey involves evaluation of the cervix, uterus, tubes, and peritoneum; detection of ovulation; assessment of immunologic compatibility; and evaluation of psychogenic factors (Angard, 1999; Morell, 1997). The nurse can alleviate some of the anxiety associated with diagnostic testing by explaining to clients the timing and rationale for each test (Table 10-1). Test findings that are favorable to fertility are summarized in Box 10-4.

Couples should be cautioned that everything can be normal and conception may still not occur. Unexplained infertility accounts for 10% to 15% of cases. In addition, even poor test results do not mean that pregnancy will not occur.

Detection of ovulation. All infertile women should have ovulatory function assessed, because a history of monthly menstruation is inadequate to conclude that ovulation is occurring and is optimal for conception.

Documentation of time of ovulation is important in the investigation of impaired fertility. Direct proof of ovulation is pregnancy or the retrieval of an ovum from the uterine tube. However, there are several indirect or presumptive methods for detection of ovulation. These include assessment of basal body temperature (BBT) and cervical mucus characteristics, as well as endometrial biopsy and pelvic ultrasound. A serum progesterone level may be obtained in the latter half of the menstrual cycle as part of ovulation testing. These clinical tests more or less determine whether progesterone is secreted in significant amounts to accommodate implantation and maintain pregnancy. Occurrence

BOX 10-3 **Assessment of the Woman**

HISTORY

1. Age
2. Duration of infertility: length of contraceptive and noncontraceptive exposure
3. Obstetric
   a. Number of pregnancies, miscarriages, and abortions
   b. Length of time required to initiate each pregnancy
   c. Complications of any pregnancy
   d. Duration of lactation
4. Gynecologic: detailed menstrual history, including age at onset, interruptions in regular menstruation, and any menstrual pain
5. Previous tests and therapy for infertility
6. Medical: general medical history, including chronic and hereditary disease (such as endocrine dysfunction); medications, including vitamins and over-the-counter medications; family history, especially of endocrine disorders; normal sexual development; any galactorrhea when not lactating
7. Surgical: especially abdominal or pelvic surgery
8. Sexual history: frequency of intercourse; number of lifetime sexual partners, previous history of STIs, types of sexual practices; pain or discomfort with intercourse; use of vaginal lubricants
9. Occupational and environmental exposure to chemicals or radiation; physical nature of occupation or hobbies; vacations and work habits
10. Personal: motivation for childbearing; attitude toward partner; reason for seeking advice regarding infertility at this time; support system available; amount of exercise; stress level; use of alcohol, recreational drugs, caffeine, or tobacco; weight changes

PHYSICAL EXAMINATION

1. General: complete physical examination
2. Genital tract: state of hymen (full penetration); clitoris; vaginal infection, including trichomoniasis and candidiasis; cervical tears, polyps, infection, patency of os, accessibility to insemination; uterus, including size and position, mobility; adnexae, tumors, evidence of endometriosis

LABORATORY DATA

1. *Chlamydia* test and gonorrhea culture; additional laboratory studies as indicated (e.g., urine test, complete blood cell count, serologic test for syphilis)
2. For women with irregular menstrual cycles or amenorrhea: serum prolactin level with tomographic x-rays of skull if prolactin level elevated, endometrial biopsy, FSH and LH determination. Other laboratory tests added as desired for a more complete diagnosis of endocrine problems: 17-ketosteroid assay test, 17-hydroxycorticosteroid test, glucose tolerance test
3. Rh factor and antibody titer tests—important in cases of ectopic pregnancy, abortion, and preterm birth problems
4. Sperm antibody agglutination studies: special laboratory procedure involves obtaining a fresh semen specimen from the man and a blood sample from the woman; sperm are incubated in the blood serum of the woman and checked at intervals for agglutination; the result is negative if no agglutinated sperm are found
5. Chromosome studies when indicated

TABLE 10-1 Tests for Impaired Fertility

TEST/EXAMINATION	TIMING (MENSTRUAL CYCLE DAYS)	RATIONALE
Hysterosalpingogram	7-10	Late follicular, early proliferative phase; will not disrupt a fertilized ovum; may open uterine tubes before time of ovulation
Postcoital test	1-2 days before ovulation	Ovulatory late proliferative phase; look for normal motile sperm in cervical mucus
Sperm immobilization antigen-antibody reaction	Variable, ovulation	Immunologic test to determine sperm and cervical mucus interaction
Assessment of cervical mucus	Variable, ovulation	Cervical mucus should have low viscosity, high spinnbarkeit
Ultrasound diagnosis of follicular collapse	Ovulation	Collapsed follicle is seen after ovulation
Serum assay of plasma progesterone	20-25	Midluteal midsecretory phase; check adequacy of corpus luteal production of progesterone
Basal body temperature	Chart entire cycle	Elevation occurs in response to progesterone, documents ovulation
Endometrial biopsy	21-27	Late luteal, late secretory phase; check endometrial response to progesterone and adequacy of luteal phase
Sperm penetration assay	After 2 days but no more than 1 week of abstinence	Evaluation of ability of sperm to penetrate an egg

BOX 10-4 Summary of Findings Favorable to Fertility

1. Follicular development, ovulation, and luteal development are supportive of pregnancy:
   a. BBT (presumptive evidence of ovulatory cycles) is biphasic, with temperature elevation that persists for 12 to 14 days before menstruation
   b. Cervical mucus characteristics change appropriately during phases of menstrual cycle
   c. Laparoscopic visualization of pelvic organs verifies follicular and luteal development
2. The luteal phase is supportive of pregnancy:
   a. Levels of plasma progesterone are adequate
   b. Findings from endometrial biopsy samples are consistent with day of cycle
3. Cervical factors are receptive to sperm during expected time of ovulation:
   a. Cervical os is open
   b. Cervical mucus is clear, watery, abundant, and slippery and demonstrates good spinnbarkeit and arborization (fern pattern)
   c. Cervical examination does not reveal lesions or infections
   d. Postcoital test findings are satisfactory (adequate number of live, motile, normal sperm present in cervical mucus)
   e. No immunity to sperm demonstrated

4. The uterus and uterine tubes are supportive of pregnancy:
   a. Uterine and tubal patency are documented by
      (1) Spillage of dye into peritoneal cavity
      (2) Outlines of uterine and tubal cavities of adequate size and shape, with no abnormalities
   b. Laparoscopic examination verifies normal development of internal genitals and absence of adhesions, infections, endometriosis, and other lesions
5. The male partner's reproductive structures are normal:
   a. No evidence of developmental anomalies of penis, testicular atrophy, or varicocele (varicose veins on the spermatic vein in the groin)
   b. No evidence of infection in prostate, seminal vesicles, and urethra
   c. Testes are more than 4 cm in largest diameter
6. Semen is supportive of pregnancy:
   a. Sperm (number per milliliter) are adequate in ejaculate
   b. Most sperm show normal morphology
   c. Most sperm are motile, forward moving
   d. No autoimmunity exists
   e. Seminal fluid is normal

of mittelschmerz and midcycle spotting provides unreliable presumptive evidence of ovulation.

Hormone analysis. Hormone analysis is performed to assess endocrine function of the hypothalamic-pituitary-ovarian axis when menstrual cycles are absent or irregular. Determination of blood levels of prolactin, follicle-stimulating hormone (FSH), luteinizing hormone (LH), and the thyroid hormones may be necessary to diagnose the cause of irregular or absent menstrual cycles.

Timed endometrial biopsy. Endometrial biopsy is scheduled after ovulation, during the luteal phase of the menstrual cycle. Late in the menstrual cycle, 2 to 3 days before expected menses, a small cannula is introduced into the uterus, and a small portion of the endometrium is removed for histologic evaluation. To assess the response of the endometrium to progesterone production, the tissue is dated with respect to expected normal menstrual development. Tissue that is "out of phase" with expected development signifies either abnormal function of the corpus luteum or abnormal response of the endometrium.

Findings favorable to fertility include endometrial tissue that shows no signs of tuberculosis, polyps, or inflammatory conditions and that reflects secretory changes normally seen in the presence of adequate luteal (progesterone) phase.

Hysterosalpingography. Radiographic (x-ray) film allows visualization of the uterine cavity and tubes after the instillation of radiopaque contrast material through the cervix

(Fig. 10-2). It is possible to see abnormalities of the uterus such as congenital defects or defects produced by submucous myomas and endometrial polyps. Distortions of the uterine cavity or uterine tubes can be a result of current or past pelvic inflammatory disease (PID). Scar tissue and adhesions from inflammatory processes can immobilize the uterus and tubes, kink the tubes, and surround the ovaries.

Hysterosalpingography is scheduled 2 to 5 days after menstruation to avoid flushing a potential fertilized ovum out through a uterine tube into the peritoneal cavity. Also at this time there are no open vessels, and all menstrual debris has been discharged. This decreases the risk of embolism or of forcing menstrual debris out through the tubes into the peritoneal cavity.

Referred shoulder pain may occur during this procedure. The referred pain is indicative of subphrenic irritation from the contrast media if it is spilled out of the patent uterine tubes. The discomfort can be managed with position change and mild analgesics. Pain usually subsides within 12 to 14 hours. Women with blocked tubes may have cramping up to 48 hours.

This procedure may be both therapeutic and diagnostic. The passage of contrast medium may clear tubes of mucous plugs, straighten kinked tubes, or break up adhesions within the tubes (caused by salpingitis). The procedure may stimulate cilia in the lining of the tubes to facilitate transport of the ovum. It also may aid healing as a

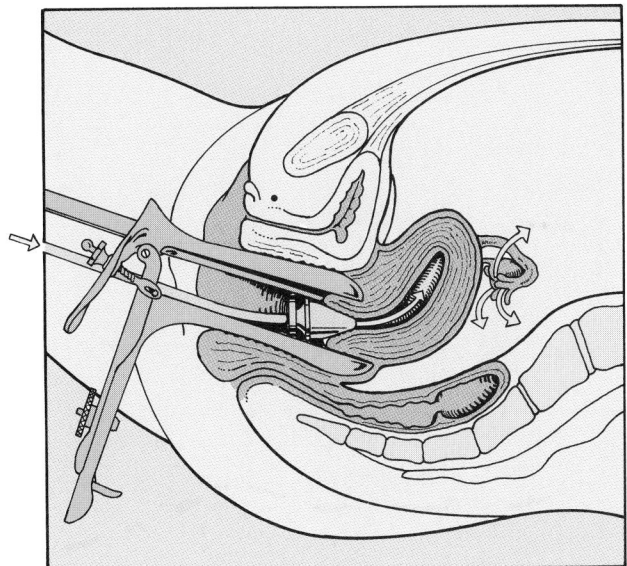

Fig. 10-2 Hysterosalpingography. Note contrast medium flows through intrauterine cannula and out through the uterine tubes.

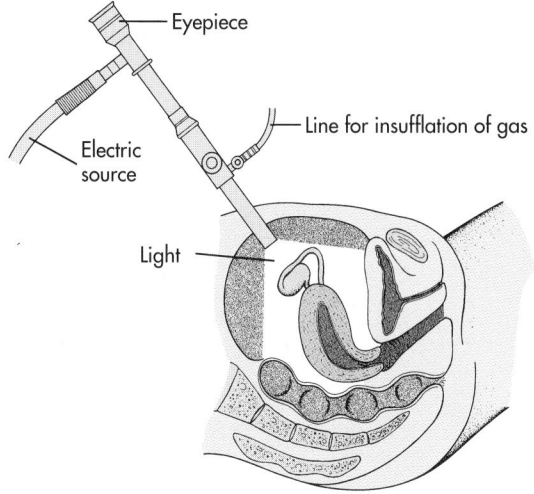

Fig. 10-3 Laparoscopy.

result of the bacteriostatic effect of the iodine within the contrast medium.

Laparoscopy. Laparoscopy is usually scheduled early in the menstrual cycle. During the procedure a small endoscope is inserted through a small incision in the anterior abdominal wall. Cold fiberoptic light sources allow for superior visualization of the internal pelvic structures (Fig. 10-3). The woman is usually admitted shortly before surgery, having taken nothing by mouth (NPO) for 8 hours. She voids before surgery. A general anesthetic is usually given, and the woman is placed in the lithotomy position. A needle is inserted, and carbon dioxide gas is pumped into the peritoneum to elevate the abdominal wall from the organs, thereby creating an empty space that permits visualization and exploration with the laparoscope. If tubal patency is being assessed, a cannula is used to instill a dye contrast medium through the cervix.

Visualization of the peritoneal cavity in infertile women may reveal endometriosis, pelvic adhesions, tubal occlusion, leiomyomas (fibroids), or polycystic ovaries. Fulguration (destruction of tissue by means of electricity) of small endometrial implants, lysis of adhesions, and taking ovarian biopsies are some of the procedures possible through the use of a laparoscope.

After surgery, deflation of most gas is done by direct expression. Trocar and needle sites are closed with a single subcuticular absorbable suture or skin clip, and an adhesive bandage is applied. Postoperative recovery requires taking vital signs, assessing level of consciousness, preventing aspiration, monitoring intravenous fluids, and reassuring the client regarding referred shoulder discomfort. Discharge from the hospital usually occurs in 4 to 6 hours.

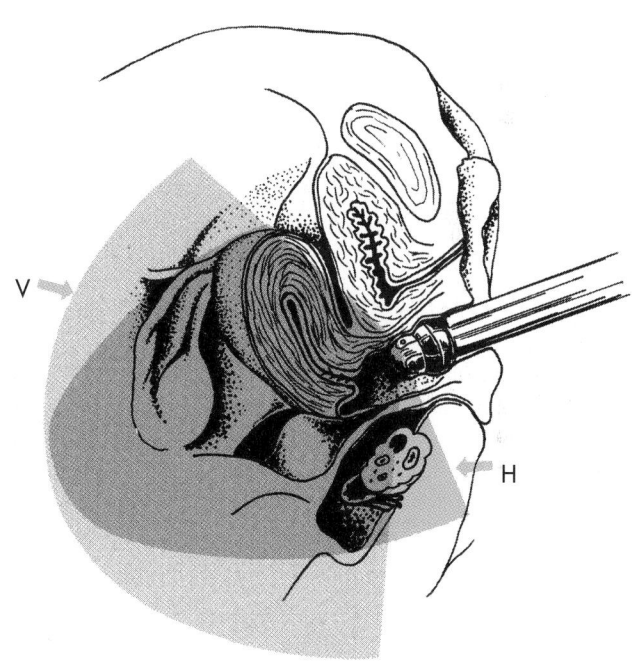

Fig. 10-4 Vaginal ultrasonography. Major scanning planes of transducer. *H,* Horizontal; *V,* vertical.

Referred shoulder pain or subcostal discomfort usually lasts only 24 hours and is relieved with a mild analgesic. Severe pain may be relieved when the woman assumes a knee-chest position. The woman must be cautioned against heavy lifting or strenuous activity for 4 to 7 days, at which time she is usually asymptomatic.

Ultrasonography. Abdominal or transvaginal ultrasound is also used to assess pelvic structures (Fig. 10-4). This procedure is used to visualize pelvic tissues for a variety of reasons (e.g., to identify abnormalities, to verify follicular development and maturity, or to confirm intrauterine versus ectopic pregnancy).

BOX 10-5 Assessment of the Man

HISTORY

1. Age
2. Fertility in this and other sexual relationships
3. Medical: general medical history, including infections (such as STIs, mononucleosis), mumps, orchitis after adolescence, chronic diseases, recent fever, medications, weight changes, undescended testes after 3 months of age, normal sexual development at puberty
4. Surgical: herniorrhaphy, injuries to genitals, or other surgery in genital area
5. Occupational and environmental exposure to chemicals or radiation, physical nature of occupation and hobbies, vacations and work habits
6. Previous tests and therapy done for study of infertility, duration of infertility in this and previous relationships
7. Sex history in detail: libido, coital history (such as frequency and ability to ejaculate), adequacy of erection, number of lifetime sex partners, attitudes toward masturbation
8. Personal: motivation for childbearing; attitude toward partner; support system available, reason for seeking advice regarding infertility at this time; amount of exercise and stress level; use of alcohol, recreational drugs, caffeine, tobacco, anabolic steroids

PHYSICAL EXAMINATION

1. General: complete physical examination, with special attention given to physical condition and fat and hair distribution

2. Genital tract: penis and urethra; scrotal size; position, size, and consistency of testes; epididymides and vasa deferentia; prostate size and consistency
3. Careful search for varicocele, with man in both supine and upright positions

LABORATORY DATA

1. Routine urine test, gonorrhea and *Chlamydia* tests; serologic test for syphilis
2. Complete semen analysis (see Box 10-6)
3. Additional laboratory studies as indicated
   a. Basic endocrine studies indicated in men with oligospermia or aspermia:
      (1) Serum FSH, LH, and testosterone levels
      (2) $T_3, T_4,$ TSH
      (3) Test for sperm antibodies, autoimmunization: autoimmune antibodies (produced by the man against his own sperm) agglutinate or immobilize sperm in fewer than 5% of men who have infertility problems
      (4) 17-hydroxycorticoids and 17-ketosteroids
      (5) Buccal smear and chromosome studies (e.g., Klinefelter's syndrome, XXY sex chromosomes)
   b. Testicular biopsy where correct interpretation is available (may give a more accurate diagnosis and prognosis in cases of azoospermia and severe oligospermia), vasography if indicated and available

Assessment of Male Infertility

The systematic investigation of infertility in the male client begins with a thorough history and physical examination (Box 10-5). Assessment of the male client proceeds in a manner similar to that of the female client, starting with noninvasive tests.

Semen analysis. The basic test for male infertility is the **semen analysis.** Examination of semen is an important part of investigation of impaired fertility, since the male is often at least partially responsible (Ross & Niederberger, 1995; Speroff, Glass, & Kase, 1994). A complete semen analysis, study of the effects of cervical mucus on sperm forward motility and survival, and evaluation of the sperm's ability to penetrate an ovum provide basic information. Sperm counts vary from day to day and are dependent on emotional and physical status and sexual activity. Therefore a single analysis may be inconclusive (Hargreave & Ghosh, 1998). Usually several specimens taken at monthly intervals are evaluated (Trantham, 1996).

Semen is collected by ejaculation into a clean container or a plastic sheath that does not contain a spermicidal agent (Speroff, Glass, & Kase, 1994). The specimen is usu-

BOX 10-6 Semen Analysis

- Liquefaction usually complete within 10 to 20 minutes
- Semen volume 2 to 5 ml (range 1 to 7 ml)
- Semen pH 7.2 to 7.8
- Sperm density 20 to 200 million cells/ml
- Normal morphology, $\geq$ 60% normal oval
- Motility (important consideration in sperm evaluation), percentage of forward-moving sperm estimated with respect to abnormally motile and nonmotile sperm $\geq$ 50%
- Ovum penetration test (may be done if further evaluation necessary)

Note: These values are not absolute, only relative to final evaluation of the couple as a single reproductive unit.

ally collected by masturbation following 2 to 5 days of abstinence from ejaculation. The semen is taken to the laboratory in a sealed container within 2 hours of ejaculation. Exposure to excessive heat or cold is avoided. Normal values for semen characteristics are given in Box 10-6.

The fertility potential of sperm is difficult to evaluate solely by semen analysis, which gives little insight into sperm survival, cervical penetration, migration to the uterine tubes, or capacity for ovum penetration and fertilization. There is insufficient knowledge regarding if or how male and female antibodies can act to inhibit fertility potential of sperm (**autoimmunization**) (Speroff, Glass, & Kase, 1994).

Seminal deficiency may be attributable to one or more of a variety of factors. The male is assessed for these factors: hypopituitarism, nutritional deficiency, debilitating or chronic disease, trauma, exposure to environmental hazards such as radiation and toxic substances, gonadotropic inadequacy, and obstructive lesions of the epididymis and vas deferens (Ross & Niederberger, 1995). Hormone analyses are done for testosterone, gonadotropin, FSH, and LH. The sperm penetration assay may be used to evaluate the ability of sperm to penetrate an egg. Because human oocytes are not readily available, hamster eggs have been used as a substitute to evaluate sperm penetration abilities (no actual fertilization occurs) (Hargreave & Ghosh, 1998). In addition, testicular biopsy may be warranted.

Assessment of the Couple

Postcoital test. The **postcoital test (PCT),** also called the Sims-Huhner test, is one method used to test for adequacy of coital technique, cervical mucus, sperm, and degree of sperm penetration through cervical mucus. The test is performed within several hours after ejaculation of semen into the vagina. A specimen of cervical mucus is obtained from the cervical os and examined under a microscope. The quality of mucus and the number of forward moving sperm are noted. A PCT with good mucus and motile sperm is associated with fertility (Hargreave & Ghosh, 1998).

Intercourse is synchronized with the expected time of ovulation (as determined from evaluation of BBT, cervical mucus changes, and usual length of menstrual cycle or use of LH detection kit to determine LH surge). It is performed only in the absence of vaginal infection. Couples may experience some difficulty abstaining from intercourse for 2 to 4 days before expected ovulation and then having intercourse with ejaculation on schedule. Sex on demand may strain the couple's interpersonal relationship. A problem may arise if the expected day of ovulation occurs when facilities or the physician is unavailable (such as over a weekend or holiday).

Nursing diagnoses are derived from the database. Examples of nursing diagnoses related to impaired fertility include the following:

▪ Nursing Diagnoses

- Anxiety related to
  - unknown outcome of diagnostic workup
- Body image or self-esteem disturbance related to
  - impaired fertility

▪ Nursing Diagnoses—cont'd

- Risk for ineffective individual/family coping related to
  - methods used in the investigation of impaired fertility
- Decisional conflict related to
  - therapies for impaired fertility
  - alternatives to therapy: childfree living or adoption
- Altered family processes related to
  - unmet expectations for pregnancy
- Anticipatory grieving related to
  - expected poor prognosis
- Pain related to
  - effects of diagnostic tests (or surgery)
- Powerlessness related to
  - lack of control over prognosis
- Altered patterns of sexuality related to
  - loss of libido secondary to medically imposed restrictions
- Risk for social isolation related to
  - impaired fertility, its investigation and management
- Knowledge deficit related to
  - preconception risk factors
  - factors surrounding ovulation
  - factors surrounding fertility
- Pain related to
  - processes of labor and birth

Expected Outcomes of Care

Planning requires sensitivity to the couple's needs. Equipped with a knowledge of impaired fertility, the nurse can help develop a plan of care for the couple with impaired fertility. The expected outcomes are phrased in client-centered terms and may include that the couple will do the following:

- Verbalize understanding of the anatomy and physiology of the reproductive system.
- Verbalize understanding of treatment for any abnormalities identified through various tests and examinations (e.g., infections, blocked uterine tubes, sperm allergy, and varicocele) and be able to make an informed decision about treatment.
- Verbalize understanding of their potential to conceive.
- Resolve guilt feelings and not need to focus blame.
- Conceive or, failing to conceive, decide on an alternative acceptable to both of them (e.g., childfree living or adoption).
- Demonstrate acceptable methods for handling pressure they may feel from peers and relatives regarding their childless state.

Plan of Care and Interventions

Psychosocial

Within the United States, feelings connected to impaired fertility are numerous and complex. The origin of some of these feelings are myths, superstitions, and misinformation

TABLE 10-2 Nursing Actions in Response to Behavior Associated with Impaired Fertility

BEHAVIORAL CHARACTERISTIC	NURSING ACTIONS
Surprise: each person assumes she or he is fertile and that pregnancy is an option	Point out resemblance to grieving process—a normal, expected reaction to loss (see Chapter 42). Refer to support group.*
	Prepare clients for length of time it may take to grieve and for types of feelings (psychologic, somatic) to expect.
	Encourage and allow time to talk of past and present feelings of sexuality, self-image, and self-esteem.
Denial: "It can't happen to me!"	Allow time for denial, because it gives the body and mind time to adjust a little at a time.
	Do not feed into the client's denial; instead say, "It must be hard to believe such a devastating report."
Anger: toward others (perhaps even at the nurse) or themselves	Explain that the reaction to loss of control and to a feeling of helplessness is often anger, which can easily be projected onto another person. Anger is a natural feeling.
	Allow time to express anger at losing their sense of control over their bodies and destinies.
	A helpful approach may be, "It's OK to be angry . . . at those who are pregnant, at people who want abortions, at self, at mate, at caregivers, and so forth."
Bargaining: "If I get pregnant, I'll dedicate the child to God."	Accept bargaining statements without comment.
Depression:	
Isolation: personal	Allow time for both woman and man to talk about how it feels whenever a sight, event, or word serves as a reminder of own state of impaired fertility.
	Develop role-playing situations to practice interactions with others under various circumstances to increase the couple's ability to cope and to solve problems (increases their self-confidence).
	The nurse may say, "You must feel so terribly alone sometimes."
Guilt or unworthiness	Allow time to identify feelings that may be related to earlier behaviors (such as abortion, premarital sex, contact with STIs).
Acceptance (resolution)	Couple or person comes to the realization that "unworthiness" and impaired fertility are unrelated.
	Clients need to know that grief feelings are never laid away forever; they may be activated by special reminders (such as anniversaries).

*RESOLVE, Inc., 1310 Broadway, Somerville, MA 02144. www.resolve.org.

about the causes of infertility. Other feelings arise from the need to undergo many tests and examinations and from being different from others.

Infertility is recognized as a major life stressor that can affect self-esteem, relations with the spouse, family and friends, and careers. Couples often need assistance in separating their concepts of success and failure related to treatment for infertility from personal success and failure. Recognizing the significance of infertility as a loss and resolving these feelings are crucial to putting infertility into perspective, even if treatment is successful (Boxer, 1996).

Nurses can help couples express and discuss their feelings as honestly as possible. Ventilation may help couples unburden themselves of negative feelings. Referral for mental health counseling may be beneficial.

The myriad of psychologic responses to a diagnosis of infertility may tax a couple's giving and receiving of physical and sexual closeness. The prescriptions and proscriptions for achieving conception may add tension to a couple's sexual functioning. Couples may report decreased desire for intercourse, orgasmic dysfunction, or midcycle erectile disorders.

To be able to deal comfortably with a couple's sexuality, nurses must be comfortable with their own sexuality so that they can better help couples understand why the private act of lovemaking needs to be shared with health care professionals. Nurses need up-to-date factual knowledge about human sexual practices and must be (1) able to accept the preferences and activities of others without being judgmental, (2) skilled in interviewing and in therapeutic use of self, sensitive to the nonverbal cues of others, and (3) knowledgeable regarding each couple's sociocultural and religious tenets (Johnson, 1996).

The woman or couple facing infertility exhibits behaviors of the grieving process that are associated with other types of loss (Table 10-2.) The loss of one's genetic continuity with the generations to come leads to a loss of self-esteem, to a sense of inadequacy as a woman or man, to a loss of control over one's destiny, and to a reduced sense of self (Schoener & Krysa, 1996). Infertile individuals have impaired self-concept and greater dissatisfaction with their marriages (Hirsch & Hirsch, 1995). The investigative process leads to a loss of spontaneity and control over the couple's marital relationship, and sometimes a loss of control over progress toward career and life goals. All people do not have all the reactions described, nor can it be predicted how long any one reaction will last for an individual.

The support systems of the couple with impaired fertility need to be explored. This exploration should include persons available to assist, their relationship to the couple, their ages, their availability, and the cultural or religious support that is available.

If the couple conceives, nurses need to be aware that the concerns and problems of the previously infertile couple may not be over. Many couples are overjoyed with the pregnancy; however, some are not. Some couples rearrange their lives, sense of self, and personal goals within their acceptance of their infertile state. The couple may feel that those who worked with them to identify and treat impaired fertility expect them to be happy with the pregnancy. The couple may be shocked to find that they themselves feel resentment because the pregnancy, once a cherished dream, now necessitates another change in goals, aspirations, and identities. The normal ambivalence toward pregnancy may be perceived as reneging on the original choice to become parents. The couple might choose to abort the pregnancy at this time. Other couples worry about miscarriage. If the couple wishes to continue with the pregnancy, they will need the care other expectant couples need. The couple may need extra preparation for the realities of pregnancy, labor, and parenthood, because they have developed fantasies about childbearing when they thought it was beyond their reach. A history of impaired fertility is considered to be a risk factor for pregnancy. If the couple does not conceive, they are assessed regarding their desire to be referred for help with adoption, therapeutic intrauterine insemination, other reproductive alternatives, or choosing a childfree state. The couple may find a list of agencies, support groups, and other resources in their community helpful (see Box 10-7 and Appendix D).

Nonmedical

Simple changes in lifestyle may be effective in the treatment of subfertile men. Only water-soluble lubricants should be used during intercourse because many commonly used lubricants contain spermicides or have spermicidal properties. High scrotal temperatures may be caused by daily hot tub bathing or saunas in which the testes are kept at temperatures too high for efficient spermatogenesis. It must be remembered that these conditions

---

BOX 10-7 Resources

1. RESOLVE, 1310 Broadway, Somerville, MA 02144. (617) 623-0744 www.resolve.org

   This national, nonprofit agency serves as a counseling, referral, and support system for infertile individuals and couples and offers education and assistance to associated professionals. RESOLVE has chapters where support groups and programs are conducted in more than 52 cities across the country.

2. American Society for Reproductive Medicine, 1209 Montgomery Hwy., Birmingham, AL 35216. (205) 978-5000 www.asrm.com

   The American Society for Reproductive Medicine is the world's largest subspecialty society devoted to infertility. Consumer literature is available.

3. International Council on Infertility Information Dissemination. (703) 379-9178 www.inciid.org

   The International Council on Infertility Information Dissemination is a clearinghouse for infertility information.

4. The American College of Obstetricians and Gynecologists (ACOG), 409 12th St., SW, Washington, DC 20024-2188. (202) 638-5577 www.acog.org

   This organization provides client information on a variety of medical conditions related to infertility, as well as obstetric and gynecologic conditions. For more information, ask for a full list of brochures and publications available for consumers.

5. www.ihr.com

   This website is an infertility organization for consumers.

---

lead only to lessened fertility and should not be employed as a means of contraception.

Treatment is available for women who have immunologic reactions to sperm. The use of condoms during genital intercourse for 6 to 12 months will reduce female antibody production in most women who have elevated antisperm antibody titers. After the serum reaction subsides, condoms are used at all times except at the expected time of ovulation. Approximately one third of couples with this problem conceive by following this course of action.

Medical

Pharmacologic therapy is often an important but expensive component of care for female infertility. Ovulatory stimulants may be warranted to induce ovulation. Clomiphene (Clomid, Serophene), an oral preparation, stimulates the ovarian follicle. It is used to treat anovulation caused by hypothalamic suppression when the hypothalamic-pituitary-ovarian axis is intact. Multifetal pregnancy rates are less than 10%, with most being twin gestations. Bromocriptine (Parlodel), a synthetic ergot alkaloid that inhibits the release of prolactin, is used to treat anovulation caused by elevated levels of prolactin. Thyroid stimulating hormone (Synthroid) is indicated if the woman has hypothyroidism.

Human menopausal gonadotropin (Pergonal) or pure FSH (Metrodin) is used when clomiphene citrate fails to induce ovulation or when pregnancy has not been achieved in 6 to 12 ovulatory cycles. These medications are extremely potent and require daily monitoring with ovarian ultrasonography and monitoring of estradiol levels to prevent hyperstimulation (Angard, 1999). The prevalence of multiple pregnancy with the use of these medications is greater than 25%. When ovulation is caused either by hypothalamic-pituitary dysfunction or failure, or failure to respond to clomiphene, gonadotropin-releasing hormone (GnRH) may be used.

Hormone replacement therapy may be indicated. The woman who has low estrogen levels is a candidate for conjugated estrogens and medroxyprogesterone. A hypoestrogenic condition may result from a high stress level or decreased percentage of body fat as a result of an eating disorder (e.g., anorexia nervosa) or excessive exercise. Hydroxyprogesterone supplementation with vaginal suppositories or intramuscular injection is used to treat luteal phase defects. The nurse may encounter other medications as well. In the presence of adrenal hyperplasia, prednisone, a glucocorticoid, is taken orally. Treatment of endometriosis may include danazol, progesterones, combined oral contraceptives, or gonadotropin-releasing hormone agonists (Session et al., 1998; Speroff, Glass, & Kase, 1994) (Table 10-3). Infections are treated with appropriate antimicrobial formulations.

Drug therapy may be indicated for male infertility. Problems with the thyroid or adrenal glands are corrected with appropriate medications. Clomiphene may be given for idiopathic subfertility, although its effectiveness in enhancing fertility rates has been poorly documented. Infections are identified and treated promptly with antimicrobials.

The primary care provider is responsible for informing clients fully about the prescribed medications. However, the nurse must be ready to answer clients' questions and to confirm their understanding of the drug, its administration, potential side effects, and expected outcomes. Because information varies with each drug, the nurse needs to consult the medication package inserts, pharmacology references, physician, and pharmacist as necessary.

Surgical

A number of surgical procedures can be used for problems causing female infertility. Ovarian tumors must be excised. Whenever possible, functional ovarian tissue is left intact. Scar tissue adhesions caused by chronic infections may cover much or all of the ovary. These adhesions usually necessitate surgery to free and expose the ovary so that ovulation can occur.

Hysterosalpingography is useful for identification of tubal obstruction and also for the release of blockage. During laparoscopy, delicate adhesions may be divided and removed and endometrial implants may be destroyed by electrocoagulation or laser. Laparotomy and even microsurgery may be required to do extensive repair of the damaged tube. Prognosis is dependent on the degree to which tubal patency and function can be restored.

A woman with a relatively small uterus may become pregnant, but the uterus may be incapable of accommodating the enlarging fetus, and a miscarriage may result. In such cases recurrent or habitual (three or more) miscarriages often occur. No medical therapy has been effective for the enlargement of an abnormally small uterus. Observation suggests that women who do become pregnant, but who miscarry, often abort at a later time with each successive pregnancy. Finally, after two or three pregnancy losses, they may give birth to a viable infant. Apparently actual growth of the uterus occurs with each pregnancy. Reconstructive surgery—for example, the unification operation for bicornuate uterus—often improves a woman's ability to conceive and carry the fetus to term.

Surgical removal of tumors or fibroids involving the endometrium or uterus often improves the woman's chance of conceiving and maintaining the pregnancy to viability. Surgical treatment of uterine tumors or maldevelopment that results in successful pregnancy usually requires birth by cesarean surgery near term gestation. The uterus may rupture as a result of weakness of the area of surgical healing.

Radial chemocautery (destruction of tissue with chemicals) or thermocautery (destruction of tissue with heat, usually electrical) of the cervix, cryosurgery (destruction of tissue by application of extreme cold, usually liquid nitrogen), or conization (excision of a cone-shaped piece of tissue from the endocervix) is effective in eliminating chronic inflammation and infection. When the cervix has been deeply cauterized or frozen or when extensive conization has been performed, extreme limitation of mucous production by the cervix may result. Therefore sperm migration may be difficult or impossible because of the absence of a mucous bridge from the vagina to the uterus. Therapeutic intrauterine insemination may be necessary to carry the sperm directly through the internal os of the cervix.

Surgical procedures may also be used for problems causing male infertility. Surgical repair of varicocele has been relatively successful in increasing sperm count but not fertility rates. A varicocele on the left side is found in a substantial number of subfertile men.

Microsurgery to reanastomose (restoration of tubal continuity) the sperm ducts can result in pregnancy rates greater than 50% (Speroff, Glass, & Kase, 1994). The rate of success decreases as the time since the procedure increases.

TABLE 10-3 Medications Used in the Treatment of Infertility

DRUG	INDICATION	MECHANISM OF ACTION	DOSE	SIDE EFFECTS
Clomiphene citrate (Clomid, Serophene)	Ovulation induction, treatment of luteal-phase inadequacy	Thought to bind to estrogen receptors in the pituitary, blocking them from detecting estrogen	Tablets, starting with 50 mg/day for 5 days, may increase to 200 mg/day	Causes hypothalamus to release more GnRH, stimulating release of FSH and LH
Human menopausal gonadotropins (Pergonal)	Ovulation induction	Pergonal, LH and FSH in 1:1 ratio, direct stimulation of ovarian follicle	Intramuscular injections, dosage regimen variable	Ovarian enlargement, ovarian hyperstimulation, local irritation at injection site, multifetal gestations
Purified FSH (Metrodin)	Treatment of polycystic ovarian disease	Direct action on ovarian follicle	Intramuscular injections, dosage regimen variable	Ovarian enlargement, ovarian hyperstimulation, local irritation at injection site, multifetal gestations
Human chorionic gonadotropin (hCG) (Profasi)	Ovulation induction	Direct action on ovarian follicle to stimulate meiosis and rupture of the follicle	2000-10,000 units intramuscularly	Local irritation at injection site
Danazol (Danocrine)	Treatment of endometriosis	Combination of estrogen and androgen suppresses ovarian activity, eliminating stimulation to endometrial glands and stroma, with resultant shrinkage and disappearance	100-800 mg/day for 6 mo	Mild hirsutism, acne, edema and weight gain, elevation of liver enzyme levels
GnRH agonists (Synarel, Lupron, Zoladex)	Treatment of endometriosis, uterine fibroids	Desensitization and downward regulation of GnRH receptors of pituitary, resulting in suppression of LH, FSH, and ovarian function	Synarel, 200 μg intranasally twice daily for 6 mo; Lupron, depot 375 mg every 28 days for 6 mo; Lupron, subcutaneously 0.1 mg daily for 6 mo	Synarel, nasal irritation, nosebleeds; Synarel and Lupron, hot flashes, vaginal dryness, myalgia and arthralgia, headaches, mild bone loss (usually reversible within 12-18 mo after treatment)
Progesterone (progesterone in oil, Progestoral)	Treatment of luteal-phase inadequacy	Direct stimulation of endometrium	Vaginal suppositories, 25-50 mg twice daily or 50 mg every night; rectal suppositories, 12.25 mg every 12 hr; progesterone capsules, 100 mg by mouth three times daily	Breast tenderness, local irritation, headaches

Adapted from Fogel, C., & Woods, N. (Eds.). (1995). *Women's health care,* Thousand Oaks, CA: Sage.

BOX 10-8 | Issues to Be Addressed by Infertile Couples Before Treatment

- Risks of multiple gestation
- Possible need for multifetal reduction
- Possible need for donor oocytes, sperm, or embryos or gestational carrier (surrogate mother)
- Freezing embryos for later use
- Possible risks of long-term effects of medications and treatment on women, children, and families

REPRODUCTIVE ALTERNATIVES

There have been remarkable developments in reproductive medicine. **Assisted reproductive therapies (ARTs)** are creating ethical and legal issues. The lack of information or misleading information about success rates and the risks and benefits of treatment alternatives prevents couples from making informed decisions. Nurses can provide information so that couples have an accurate understanding of their chances for a successful pregnancy and live birth. Nurses can also provide anticipatory guidance about the moral and ethical dilemmas regarding the use of ARTs (Box 10-8). Some of the ARTs for treatment of infertility include in vitro fertilization-embryo transfer (IVF-ET), gamete intrafallopian transfer (GIFT), zygote intrafallopian transfer (ZIFT), ovum transfer (oocyte donation), embryo adoption, embryo hosting, and surrogate parenting. Table 10-4 describes these procedures and the possible indications for the ARTs. Other options include intracytoplasmic sperm injection, assisted hatching, therapeutic donor insemination, adoption, and surrogate mothering.

LEGAL TIP Cryopreservation of Human Embryos

Couples who have excess embryos frozen for later transfer must be fully informed before consenting to the procedure, to make decisions regarding the disposal of embryos in the event of (1) death, (2) divorce, or (3) the decision that the couple no longer wants the embryos at a later time.

In Vitro Fertilization-Embryo Transfer

In vitro fertilization-embryo transfer (IVF-ET) is a common approach for women with blocked or absent uterine tubes or with unexplained infertility, and for men with very low sperm counts. As few as 560 to 1600 sperm are needed for in vitro fertilization.

Generally only three or fewer embryos are transferred, to minimize the risk of multiple pregnancy. When more than three embryos develop in the culture media, the extra embryos can be cryopreserved. If necessary, they can be thawed in a subsequent cycle for later uterine transfer.

Success rates vary widely from center to center. Each couple's physical status and age factor into their individual chances for pregnancy. Rates range from 16% frozen embryo transfer to 30% for IVF-ET per cycle and are highly individual (ASRM, 1999). Costs vary by treatment and by region of the country: IVF-ET ranges from $8,000 to $12,000 (Marrs, 1997).

Micromanipulation

Micromanipulation allows the handling of individual eggs and sperm through the use of specific instruments and controls. Techniques to improve fertilization, embryo growth, and genetic testing are improving at a rapid pace. **Intracytoplasmic sperm injection** is a technique that makes it possible to achieve fertilization or to correct abnormal fertilization by introducing sperm beneath the zona pellucida directly into the egg. Micromanipulation offers the opportunity to enhance the chances of fertilization in cases of a severe male factor (Hargreave & Ghosh, 1998).

Micromanipulation also allows removal of a single cell from a multicellular embryo for genetic study, thus advancing the possibility of genetic diagnosis at the earliest stage of development (Carcio, 1998). Blastomere analysis results in characterization of specific genes of the genome, the complete set of genes on the chromosomes of the developing embryo. These scientific advances, although exciting, open up new ethical dilemmas. For example, the gene for cystic fibrosis is known. Couples who are both carriers of this recessive gene could have blastomere analysis performed before embryo transfer. Research on the manipulation of the genetic material of embryos before their implantation is ongoing, thus potentially making it possible to "correct" a defect before embryo transfer.

Gamete intrafallopian transfer. Gamete intrafallopian tube transfer (GIFT) is similar to IVF-ET. Ovulation is induced as in IVF-ET, and the oocytes are aspirated from follicles via laparoscopy (Fig. 10-5, *A*). Semen is collected before laparoscopy, and sperm are capacitated by the same technique used for IVF-ET. The ova and sperm are then transferred to one tube (Fig. 10-5, *B*), permitting natural fertilization and cleavage, with subsequent successful pregnancies possible. About a 29% pregnancy rate per cycle has been reported for this technique (ASRM, 1999). GIFT requires women to have at least one normal uterine tube.

Zygote intrafallopian transfer. Zygote intrafallopian transfer (ZIFT) is also similar to IVF-ET. In ZIFT, after in vitro fertilization, the ova are placed in the uterine tube during the zygote stage. Success rates for ZIFT are slightly higher than for GIFT (ASRM, 1999).

Complications. Other than the established risks associated with laparoscopy and general anesthesia, few risks are associated with IVF-ET, GIFT, and ZIFT. The more common transvaginal needle aspiration requires only local or intravenous analgesia. Congenital anomalies occur no more frequently than among naturally conceived embryos. Ectopic pregnancies do occur more often, however, and these carry a significant maternal risk.

Oocyte donation. Women who have ovarian failure or oophorectomy, who have a genetic defect, or who fail

TABLE 10-4 Assisted Reproductive Therapies (ARTs)

PROCEDURE	DEFINITION	INDICATIONS
In vitro fertilization-embryo transfer (IVF-ET)	A woman's eggs are collected from her ovaries, fertilized in the laboratory with sperm, and transferred to her uterus after normal embryo development has occurred.	Tubal disease or blockage; severe male infertility; endometriosis; unexplained infertility; cervical factor; immunologic infertility
Gamete intrafallopian transfer (GIFT)	Oocytes are retrieved from the ovary, placed in a catheter with washed motile sperm, and immediately transferred into the fimbriated end of the uterine tube. Fertilization occurs in the uterine tube.	Same as for IVF-ET, *except* there must be normal tubal anatomy, patency, and absence of previous tubal disease in at least one uterine tube
IVF-ET and GIFT with donor sperm	This process is the same as described above except in cases where the husband's fertility is severely compromised and donor sperm can be used; if donor sperm are used, the wife must have indications for IVF and GIFT.	Severe male infertility; azoospermia; indications for IVF-ET or GIFT
Zygote intrafallopian transfer (ZIFT)	This process is similar to IVF-ET; after in vitro fertilization the ova are placed in one uterine tube during the zygote stage.	Same as for GIFT
Donor oocyte	Eggs are donated by an IVF procedure, and the donated eggs are inseminated. The embryos are transferred into the recipient's uterus, which is hormonally prepared with estrogen/progesterone therapy.	Early menopause; surgical removal of ovaries; congenitally absent ovaries; autosomal or sex-linked disorders; lack of fertilization in repeated IVF attempts because of subtle oocyte abnormalities or defects in oocyte/spermatozoa interaction
Donor embryo (embryo adoption)	A donated embryo is transferred to the uterus of an infertile woman at the appropriate time (normal or induced) of the menstrual cycle.	Infertility not resolved by less aggressive forms of therapy; absence of ovaries; male partner is azoospermic or is severely compromised
Gestational carrier (embryo host); surrogate mother	A couple undertakes an IVF cycle and the embryo(s) is transferred to another woman's uterus (the carrier) who has contracted with the couple to carry the baby to term. The carrier has no genetic investment in the child. Surrogate motherhood is a process by which a woman is inseminated with semen from the infertile woman's partner and then carries the baby until birth.	Congenital absence or surgical removal of uterus; a reproductively impaired uterus, myomas, uterine adhesions, or other congenital abnormalities; a medical condition that might be life-threatening during pregnancy, such as diabetes, immunologic problems, or severe heart, kidney, or liver disease
Therapeutic donor insemination (TDI)	Donor sperm are used to inseminate the female partner.	Male partner is azoospermic or has a very low sperm count; couple has a genetic defect; male partner has antisperm antibodies
Intracytoplasmic sperm injection	Selection of one sperm cell that is injected directly into the egg to achieve fertilization. Used with IVF.	Same as TDI
Assisted hatching	The zona pellucida is penetrated chemically or manually to create an opening for the dividing embryo to hatch and implant into uterine wall.	Recurrent miscarriages; to improve implantation rate in women with previously unsuccessful IVF attempts; advanced age

Data from Angard, N. (1999). Diagnosis infertility. *AWHONN Lifelines* 3(3), 22-29; Braverman, A., & English, M. (1992). Creating brave new families with advanced reproductive technologies. *NAACOG's Clin Issu Perinat Womens Health Nurs* 3(2), 353-363; Mishell, D. et al. (1997). *Comprehensive gynecology* (3rd ed.). St. Louis: Mosby; Seibel, M. (1997). *Infertility: A comprehensive text* (2nd ed.). Stamford, CT: Appleton & Lange.

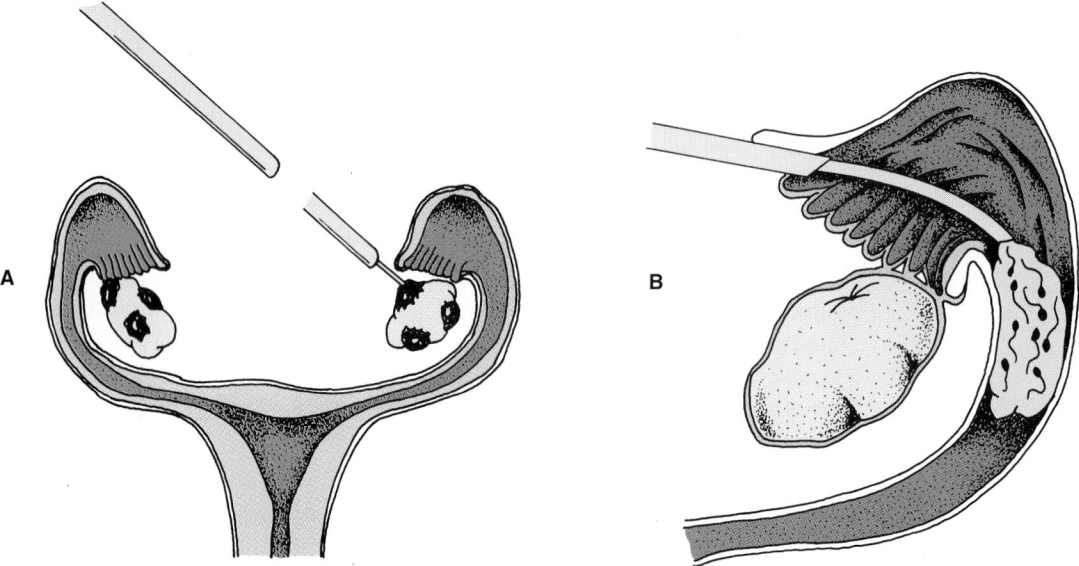

Fig. 10-5 GIFT. **A,** Through laparoscopy, a ripe follicle is located and fluid containing the egg is removed. **B,** The sperm and egg are placed separately in the uterine tube, where fertilization oc-

to achieve pregnancy with their own oocytes may be eligible for the use of donor oocytes. Donors who are younger than 35 years and healthy are recruited and paid to undergo ovarian stimulation and oocyte retrieval. The donor eggs are then fertilized in the laboratory with the male partner's sperm. The recipient woman undergoes hormonal stimulation to allow development of the uterine lining. Embryos are then transferred. Pregnancy rates vary from 5% to 20%. The psychosocial issues are similar to those in therapeutic donor insemination. Historically the courts have upheld the gestational mother as the legal mother. It is expected that the egg donor will have no rights or responsibilities in relation to the offspring.

On occasion, a couple decides that they do not want their frozen embryos, and they release these for "adoption" by other infertile couples. Infertility centers are struggling to develop guidelines and protocols to address the various legal and ethical issues associated with these procedures.

Therapeutic donor insemination. **Therapeutic donor insemination (TDI),** previously referred to as artificial insemination by donor, is used when the male partner has no sperm or a very low sperm count (less than 20 million motile sperm per milliliter), the couple has a genetic defect, or the male partner has antisperm antibodies. Couples need to be counseled extensively regarding the mutuality of their decision, their ability (particularly of the male partner) to grieve the loss of a biologic child, and long-term issues relating to parenting the child conceived through TDI (Prattke & Gass-Sternas, 1993; Van Voorhis et al., 1998). Couples also need to be aware of the legal status of TDI in their particular state.

In TDI, donor semen is subjected to laboratory testing to reduce the possibility of life-threatening illnesses for the recipient and her fetus, as well as for factors that could jeopardize the woman's future fertility or compromise the

chance of the success of the procedure. Donor semen is tested for serology, serum hepatitis B antigen, *Neisseria gonorrhoeae, Chlamydia trachomatis,* cytomegalovirus antibodies, and HIV antibodies (Speroff, Glass, & Kase, 1994; Yoshida, 1999).

The procedure is done in the physician's office or clinic, usually the day after the woman has an LH surge. The sperm are loaded into a catheter that is then inserted in the vagina, through the cervix, and placed high in the uterine cavity. The sperm are injected slowly and the catheter is removed. The woman lies flat for a few minutes and then can get up and resume her usual activities. (Seibel, 1997).

Assuming normal female fertility, intrauterine TDI at or about the time of ovulation has resulted in pregnancy in as many as 70% of cases. If pregnancy has not occurred within six cycles of well-timed insemination, further investigation of the female partner is warranted. The couple must know that there is no guarantee of pregnancy and that the miscarriage rate is approximately the same as in a control population. There is no increase in maternal or perinatal complications; the same frequencies of anomalies (about 5%) and obstetric complications (between 5% and 10%) that accompany natural insemination (through sexual intercourse) apply also to TDI.

Adoption

Couples may choose to build their family by adopting children who are not their own biologically. However, with increased availability of birth control and abortion and increasing numbers of single mothers keeping their babies, the adoption of Caucasian infants is extremely limited. Minority infants and infants with special needs, older children, and foreign adoptions are other options.

Most adults assume that they will be able to have children of their own. The discovery that they are unable to

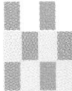

PLAN ᵒᶠ CARE   Infertility

NURSING DIAGNOSIS Knowledge deficit related to lack of understanding of the reproductive process with regard to conception as evidenced by client questions

Expected Outcome *Client and partner will verbalize understanding of the components of the reproductive process, common problems leading to infertility, usual infertility testing, and the importance of completing testing in a timely manner.*

Nursing Interventions/*Rationales*

Assess client's current level of understanding of the factors promoting conception *to identify gaps or misconceptions in knowledge base.*

Provide information in a supportive manner regarding factors promoting conception including common factors leading to infertility of either partner *to raise client's awareness and promote trust in caregiver.*

Identify and describe the basic infertility tests and the rationale for precise scheduling *to enhance completion of the diagnostic phase of the infertility workup*

NURSING DIAGNOSIS Risk for ineffective individual/family coping related to inability to conceive as evidenced by client and partner statements

Expected Outcome *Client and partner will identify situational stressors and positive coping methods to deal with testing and unknown outcomes.*

Nursing Interventions/*Rationales*

Provide opportunities through therapeutic communication to discuss feelings and concerns *to identify common feelings and perceived stressors.*

Evaluate couple's support system, including support of each other during this process *to identify any barriers to effective coping.*

Identify support groups and refer as needed *to enhance coping by sharing experiences with other couples experiencing similar problems*

do so is often accompanied by feelings of inferiority, doubts about masculinity or femininity, and feelings of guilt or blame in relation to the partner. These feelings and frustrations, combined with the anxiety of waiting for pregnancies, feelings of loss, and the endless medical procedures to investigate infertility create a unique situation for the adoptive couple who is preparing for parenthood (Hahn, 1991).

Couples who decide to adopt a child have decided that being a parent and having a child is more important than the actual process of birthing the child. The birth process is a very small aspect of having a baby and becoming a parent. So much emphasis is placed on being pregnant and having a child composed of one's own genetic makeup, that the focus of the reason to have a child becomes cloudy. The question to be answered by couples who want to adopt is, "Do you want to have a baby, or do you want to become parents?"

Hahn (1991) has proposed the following questions to aid couples in their soul searching regarding adoption as an alternative: Can you deal with having little or no information about your child's background? How will you feel if you become pregnant later? Are you willing to accept a child of school age or of different nationality or color? Can you be proud of him or her? Are you willing to tolerate differences? Is it important that your child look like you? Can

you encourage talents, skills, and preferences that are very different from your own? How do you feel about knowing the child's birth mother or father? How does your extended family feel about adopted children?

Nurses should have information on options for adoption available for couples or refer to community resources for further assistance.

Surrogate Mothers

Surrogate motherhood can be achieved by two methods. The first is to have the surrogate mother inseminated with semen from the infertile woman's partner and carry the baby until the birth. The baby is then formally adopted by the infertile couple. A less common method is to retrieve an ovum from the infertile woman, fertilize it with her partner's sperm, and place it into the uterus of a surrogate, who becomes a gestational carrier. These newer interventions raise considerable legal and ethical issues that require extensive counseling of couples and the women who choose to become pregnant.

Evaluation

Evaluation of the effectiveness of care of the couple experiencing impaired fertility is based on the previously stated outcomes (see Plan of Care).

KEY POINTS

- Infertility is the inability to conceive and carry a child to term gestation at a time the couple has chosen to do so.

- Infertility affects between 10% to 15% of otherwise healthy adults. Infertility increases in women older than 35 years.

- In the United States, about 50% of infertility is related to female causes; 35% is related to male causes; and 10% to 15% of the causes are unexplained.

- Common etiologic factors of infertility include decreased sperm production, ovulation disorders, tubal occlusion, and endometriosis.

- Reproductive alternatives for family building include IVF-ET, GIFT, ZIFT, oocyte donation, embryo donation, TDI, surrogate motherhood, and adoption.

CRITICAL THINKING EXERCISES

1 *Explore the options in your community for diagnosis, treatment alternatives, and support services for couples experiencing infertility. Discuss your findings in a clinical conference, including the ease or difficulty a couple would have in getting help with their problem.*
2 *You are assigned to the infertility clinic. A couple has arrived to begin diagnostic workup for infertility.*
  a *Interview the couple to determine how infertility has affected their lives.*
  b *Review research articles about the impact of infertility and compare findings with the couple's descriptions.*
  c *Identify ways to assist the couple in coping with the diagnostic and treatment phases of infertility.*
3 *Select one of the issues listed in Box 10-8 and examine the ethical, legal, and moral/religious implications of your selection. Discuss in a clinical conference.*

References

American Society for Reproductive Medicine. (1999). Results of joint SART/ASRM, CDC, and RESOLVE 1996 assisted reproductive technology success rate report. www.asrm.com.

Angard, N. (1999). Diagnosis infertility. *AWHONN Lifelines* 3(3), 22-29.

Bhasin, S. et al. (1998). The genetic basis of male infertility. *Endocrinol Metab Clin North Am* 27(4), 783-805.

Boxer, A. (1996). Images of infertility. *Nurse Pract Forum* 7(2), 60-63.

Braverman, A., & English, M. (1992). Creating brave new families with advanced reproductive technologies. *NAACOG's Clin Issu Perinat Womens Health Nurs* 3(2), 353-363.

Carcio, H. (1998). *Management of the infertile woman.* Philadelphia: J.B. Lippincott.

Cunningham, F. et al. (1997). *Williams obstetrics* (20th ed.). Stamford, CT: Appleton & Lange.

Fogel, C., & Woods, N. (Eds.). (1995). *Women's health care.* Thousand Oaks, CA: Sage.

Fryday, M. (1995). Treating infertility in Roman Catholics. *Nursing Standard* 10(5), 31-34.

Geissler, E. (1994). *Pocket guide to cultural assessment.* St. Louis: Mosby.

Giwercman, A., & Bonde, J. (1998). Declining male fertility and environmental factors. *Endocrinol Metab Clin North Am* 27(4), 807-830.

Hahn, S. (1991). Caring for couples considering alternatives in family building. In C. Garner (Ed.). *Principles of infertility nursing.* Boca Raton, FL: CRC Press.

Hargreave, T., & Ghosh, C. (1998). Male fertility disorders. *Endocrinol Metab Clin North Am* 27(4), 765-782.

Hatcher, R. et al. (1998). *Contraceptive technology* (17th ed.). New York: Ardent Media, Inc.

Hirsch, A., & Hirsch, S. (1995). The long-term psychosocial effects of infertility. *J Obstet Gynecol Neonatal Nurs* 24(6), 517-522.

Johnson, C. (1996). Regaining self-esteem: Strategies and interventions for the infertile woman. *J Obstet Gynecol Neonatal Nurs* 25(4), 291-295.

Liel, Y. et al. (1993). Medical conditions leading to infertility. In V. Insler, & B. Lunesfeld (Eds.). *Infertility: Male and female* (2nd ed.). Edinburgh: Churchill Livingstone.

Marrs, R. (1997). *Dr. Richard Marrs' fertility book.* New York: Delacorte Press.

Mishell, D. et al. (1997). *Comprehensive gynecology* (3rd ed.). St. Louis: Mosby.

Morell, V. (1997). Basic infertility assessment. *Prim Care* 24(1), 195-204.

Prattke, T., & Gass-Sternas, K. (1993). Appraisal, coping, and emotional health of infertile couples undergoing artificial insemination. *J Obstet Gynecol Neonatal Nurs* 22(6), 516-527.

Ross, L., & Niederberger, C. (1995). Male infertility: Diagnosis & treatment. *Compr Ther* 21(6), 276-282.

Schoener, C., & Krysa, L. (1996). The comfort and discomfort of infertility. *J Obstet Gynecol Neonatal Nurs* 25(2), 167-172.

Seibel, M. (1997). *Infertility: A comprehensive text* (2nd ed.). Stamford, CT: Appleton & Lange.

Session, D. et al. (1998). Recent advances in infertility treatment. *Minnesota Medicine* 81(10), 27-32.

Speroff, L., Glass, H., & Kase, G. (1994). *Clinical gynecologic endocrinology and infertility* (5th ed.). Baltimore: Williams & Wilkins.

Stephen, E., & Chandra, A. (1998). Updated projections of infertility in the United States, 1995-2025. *Fertil Steril* 70(1), 30-34.

Timbers, K., & Feinberg, R. (1996). Recurrent pregnancy loss: A review. *Nurse Pract Forum* 7(2), 64-75.

Trantham, P. (1996). The infertile couple. *Am Fam Physician* 54(3), 1001-1010.

Van Voorhis, B. et al. (1998). Cost-effective treatment of the infertile couple. *Fertil Steril* 70(6), 995-1005.

Yoshida, T. (1999). Infertility update: Use of assisted reproductive technology. *J Am Pharm Assoc* 39(1), 65-72.

11

Violence Against Women

Barbara C. Rynerson

LEARNING OBJECTIVES

- Define the key terms.
- Describe the historic events that have perpetuated violence against women.
- Contrast the theoretic premises underlying the victimization of women.
- Discuss the incidence of battering in pregnant women.
- Explain the cycle of violence and its use in assessment and intervention for battered women.
- Develop a plan of care for a battered woman.
- Identify behaviors associated with women who experienced sexual assault as children.

- Discuss the nursing care for a survivor of childhood sexual abuse.
- Discuss the dynamics of rape.
- Describe the rape-trauma syndrome.
- Develop a nursing plan of care for a woman in the acute phase of rape-trauma syndrome.
- Describe the resources available to women experiencing abuse.
- Identify topics of nursing research related to violence against women.

KEY TERMS

acquaintance rape	cycle of violence	rape
battered woman's syndrome	incest	rape-trauma syndrome
battering	machismo	sexual assault

he pervasiveness of violence against women is well documented. In a recent National Violence Against Women (NVAW) study sponsored by the National Institute of Justice (NIJ) and the Centers for Disease Control and Prevention (CDC), 8000 women and 8000 men were queried through a telephone survey about (1) physical assault experienced as children by adult caretakers, (2) physical assault experienced as adults by any type of perpetrator, and (3) forcible rape or stalking they experienced at any time in their life (Tjadn & Thoennes, 1998). Fifty-two percent of the women reported that they had

been physically assaulted as a child by an adult caretaker or as an adult, and almost 2% reported that they had been physically assaulted in the previous 12 months. The NVAW report estimated that 1.9 million women in the United States are assaulted annually (Tjadn & Thoennes, 1998). Thirty percent to forty percent of women who are murdered die at the hands of an intimate partner or ex-partner. Twenty-five percent to forty-five percent of women are beaten during pregnancy (Barrier, 1998).

Health care professionals should consider domestic violence a significant social problem and a major health care problem (Tjadn & Thoennes, 1998). In the United States, domestic violence is the second leading cause of injuries to women and the leading cause of injuries to women in the 15- to 44-year-old age group (Barrier, 1998). Campbell (1997) reports that $3 billion to $5 billion in direct costs and $100 billion in indirect costs are spent annually.

Women of all races and of all ethnic, educational, religious, and socioeconomic backgrounds are affected (Gelles, 1993). The NVAW survey, however, found statistically significant differences in the prevalence of women who reported rape and physical assault. Native Americans and Alaskan Natives both reported victimization by rape and physical assault, whereas Asian/Pacific Islanders were least likely to report assault victimization. Hispanic women were less inclined to report rape than non-Hispanic women (Tjadn & Thoennes, 1998). It is difficult to know the magnitude of the problem because of the variations in reporting that occur as a result of fear, lack of understanding, and the stigma surrounding violent situations.

Maternity and women's health nurses, by the very nature of their practice, are in a unique position to conduct case finding, provide sensitive care to women experiencing abusive situations, engage in prevention activities, and influence health care and public policy toward decreasing the violence. This chapter addresses battering, particularly of pregnant women; incest; sexual assault; and rape, acts usually inflicted by current or former intimate partners or people such as health care providers who are in positions that connote protection and nurturing.

HISTORICAL PERSPECTIVE

Acceptance of inhumane treatment of women is recorded throughout history. In ancient Rome, wives were chastised, divorced, or killed by husbands for adultery, public drunkenness, or attending public games (the same behaviors engaged in daily by Roman men). In the 1700s, English common law gave husbands the right to "physically chastise" an errant wife, and this legacy carried over to the United States into the nineteenth century. After 1870, wife abuse was illegal in the United States (reported in Gelles, 1995). The devaluation of women, power imbalance, viewing women as property, sex-role stereotyping, and viewing aggressive male behavior as appropriate contributed to the subordinate status of women in most of the world's societies and perpetuated dependence on the dominant male.

The power imbalance and the idea that "family matters" were private affairs kept women from publicly disclosing the numerous abuses that occurred. There was little awareness and even less response from both medical professionals and legal and justice systems to the plight of women in intimate relationships. As late as the 1960s, it was believed that violence in the family was rare and committed only by mentally ill or otherwise disturbed people. The women's movement of the 1970s first called attention to the inequality of women in all forms of interpersonal relationships; intolerance of violence then was manifested,

and public sanctions against such behavior began. Recognition of the number of both female and male injustices, including incest, rape, and elder abuse, also increased at this time.

CONCEPTUAL PERSPECTIVES ON VIOLENCE

In an attempt to conceptualize male-to-female violence, psychologic, sociologic, biologic, and feminist views are examined here. There have been many attempts in the literature to apply theoretic explanations to the causes and understanding of violence, none of which is conclusive in its evidence. Therefore, rather than the use of theory as such, this chapter focuses on a brief summary of research and theoretic premises to provide the reader sufficient data to analyze the persistent acts of violence against women that continue to prevail in society today.

Psychologic Perspective

Psychology, the study of individual behavior, places all behavior, including aggression, within the individual. Early psychoanalytic theory postulated aggression as a basic instinctual drive leading to mastery and accomplishment and, in men, as a positive force that connotes boldness, forcefulness, energy, enterprise, and so on (Hanrahan, Campbell, & Ulrich, 1993). Psychoanalytic theory promotes gender-stereotypic expectations, and thus aggression in women is viewed negatively; aggressive women are labeled as hostile and belligerent.

O'Leary (1993) posed a continuum of aggression progressing from verbal aggression (yelling, name-calling) to lesser forms of physical aggression (pushing, slapping) to true violent behavior (beating, punching) and to the extreme (murder). He contends that this model has implications for treatment as well as study, because empiric evidence indicates that the causes and the behaviors are different in each category on the continuum. Table 11-1 presents these differences.

Another psychologic stance is that abuse is committed by people who are mentally ill or deranged in some way and that the victims are innocent and defenseless (Gelles, 1993). This misconception perpetuates the notion that violence occurs among people who are not "normal." In fact, mental illness accounts for only about 10% of all violence (Gelles, 1993). Some studies suggest that borderline and antisocial personality disorders are more prevalent in men who batter (Else et al., 1993). A mental health diagnosis of alcohol abuse is frequently found in abusers but should not be misconstrued as the cause of violence.

There is no diagnostic profile of an abuser, but Box 11-1 provides some characteristics of men who batter that nurses can use to assess clients' relationships.

Women who suffer from severe and persistent mental illness may be more vulnerable to being involved in controlling and violent relationships (Fishwick, 1995). However, numerous mental health problems, such as de-

TABLE 11-1 Causes of Aggression

VERBAL AGGRESSION	PHYSICAL AGGRESSION	SEVERE PHYSICAL AGGRESSION
Need to control	Accept violence as a means of control	Personality disorder
Misuse of power	Modeling of physical aggression; abused as a child	Emotional lability
Jealousy	Alcohol abuse	Poor self-esteem
Marital discord		Aggressive personality styles

Modified from O'Leary, D. (1993). Through a psychological lens: Personality traits, personality disorders, and levels of violence. In R. Gelles & D. Loseke (Eds.). *Current controversies on family violence.* Newbury Park, CA: Sage.

pression, psychophysiologic illnesses, substance abuse, eating disorders, and anxiety reactions, experienced by women with abusive partners are more likely to be consequences of long-term abuse rather than causes (Campbell & Landenburger, 1995).

Sociologic View

The social structure and conditions in Western society provide the basis for the prevailing attitudes toward violent behavior. The United States has a long history of using violence for social control reasons, such as in wars and riots. Approval of violence in men is promoted in the double standard that women are expected to be nonviolent, whereas men are expected to be aggressive. Therefore men's violence is treated with more leniency and less stigma, particularly in the justice system. The more a culture uses physical force toward socially approved ends, the more the violence becomes generalized to other areas of social life (Hanrahan et al., 1993).

The structure of the family often sets the stage for violent behaviors: ascribed roles of family members, the ratio of time spent together, private nature of the family, intensity of emotional involvement, and stress and conflict inherent in families (Gelles, 1993). Power and violence, or even the threat of physical force, serve to maintain the patriarchal view of woman's place in the home and in the rest of society. Gender inequality, both in economic opportunities and physical strength, serves to perpetuate the power imbalance in relationships; in essence, women are dependent on men both as providers and as protectors (Hanrahan et al., 1993).

Another family issue is the intergenerational transmission of violence; both perpetuators and victims learn about violence in families of origin. Gelles (1995) cites that approximately 30% of abused children become abusers as adults, compared with 2% to 4% of nonabused children in the general population who become abusers as adults. Both lack of emotional support as children and awareness that people who love each other can be violent are prominent factors. Rynerson and Fishel (1993) found that childhood memories of more than 90% of the subjects (both men and women) in their study revealed a history of harsh physical punishment, ranging from spanking to being hit with closed fists and objects, as a means of discipline, and one third of the subjects observed violence between their parents.

BOX 11-1 Characteristics of a Potential Batterer

- Low self-esteem
- Commonly experiences problems with abandonment, loss, helplessness, dependency, insecurity, intimacy.
- Inadequate verbal skills, especially difficulty expressing feelings.
- Deficits in assertiveness.
- Frequently diagnosed as having personality disorders.
- Low frustration tolerance (loses temper easily).
- Higher incidence of growing up in an abusive or violent home.
- Denies, minimizes, blames, and lies about own actions.
- Violence is consistent with his view of himself and the world; it is an acceptable way of dealing with everyday life.
- Unable to empathize with others.
- Rigidity in male and female behaviors (sex-role stereotypes).
- Often perceives self as "special" and deserves special attention for being the provider, protector.
- Substance abuse problems are common.
- Displays an unusual amount of jealousy (e.g., expects partner to spend all of her time with him or to keep him informed of her whereabouts).

Poverty and oppression are cited as being significant factors in violent behavior (Gelles, 1993, 1995; Hanrahan et al., 1993). Low income with subsequent stress and limited resources adds to the potential for violence. Violent episodes are greater among unemployed people and those with low-prestige jobs (Gelles, 1993).

Biologic Factors

A complete biologic perspective is beyond the scope of this chapter, but evidence indicates that neurobiologic and hormonal factors influence aggression in men. Studies using imaging technology indicate that aggressive behavior is associated with the limbic structures, temporal lobes, and frontal lobes of the brain (Garza-Trevino, 1994). Changes in structural functioning of the limbic system, such as

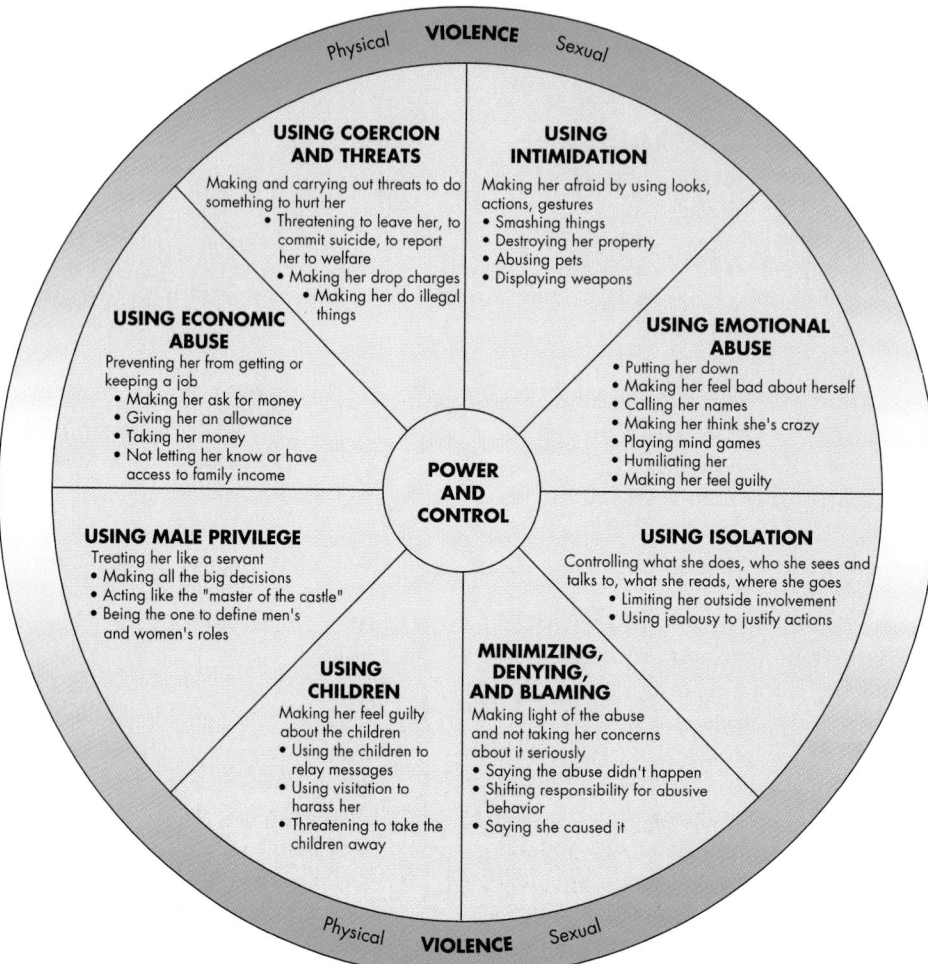

Fig. 11-1 Model of how power and control issues perpetuate battering. *(From Duluth Domestic Abuse Intervention Project. Power and control tactics of men who batter. Duluth, MN.)*

occurs with brain lesions, substance use, epilepsy, and head injuries, affect both emotional experience and behavior of the individual and thus may increase or decrease the potential for aggressive behavior (Harper-Jacques & Reimer, 1992).

Neurochemical factors also may play a role in aggressive behavior so that dysfunction or misregulation of certain neurotransmitters may result in aggression. Increased levels of both norepinephrine and L-dopa foster aggressive behavior. Lowering the levels of serotonin in animals causes aggressive behavior. The amino acid gamma-aminobutyric acid (GABA) inhibits aggressive behavior. The occurrence of violence in neurologic disorders is also reported, especially when violent reactions are out of proportion to the provoking events (Garza-Trevino, 1994).

In studies of animals, aggression is associated with abnormally high levels of testosterone. In reviewing the literature on the testosterone-aggression relationship in men, studies often report conflicting results (Garza-Trevino, 1994).

Most research indicates a combination of environmental and physical factors as resulting in violence; in essence,

aggressive behavior is an individual's response to his or her perception of the situation (Harper-Jacques & Reimer, 1992). No conclusive evidence in biologic theory, except perhaps in instances of neurologic damage, indicates that aggressive behavior cannot be controlled.

Feminist Perspective

The contemporary social view of violence is derived from feminist theory. This view, with the primary theme of male dominance and coercive control, enhances our understanding of all forms of violence against women, including wife battering, stranger and acquaintance rape, incest, and sexual harassment in the workplace. This gender and power perspective evolved from women's descriptions of their abusive experiences and from activists attempting to understand the victimization that occurred. In numerous cases, power and control tactics were central events leading to the violence (Yllo, 1993). The power and control wheel developed by the Duluth, Minnesota Domestic Abuse Intervention Project identifies the ways in which men exercise the power and control that underlie all types of intimate violence (Fig. 11-1).

Campbell and Fishwick (1993) discuss the concept of **machismo,** or compulsive masculinity, associated particularly with wife abuse. Machismo encompasses the traditional male values of "toughness" and "hardness," and thus various authors characterize male identity as a preoccupation with physical strength, athletic prowess, demonstrations of daring and valor through aggression and violence, inability to express emotions, treatment of women as commodities and conquest objects, and inability to be gentle toward and cooperate with women. This machismo framework is consistent with the feminist point of view.

Implications for Nursing

Theoretic frameworks assist the nurse to understand the dynamics and many variables in the victimization of women. This knowledge is vital in dispelling myths that prevail among professionals and their clients. The more cognizant nurses become, the more information they can share with women, who ultimately make their own decisions about the quality of their lives and relationships.

CULTURAL CONSIDERATIONS

Sociocultural characteristics of subordination of women, the objectification of women, and power inequalities in human social arrangements support the abuse of women. These are especially apparent in any social or cultural system of oppression. In assessing for abuse, nurses must note the experiences of women in the context of all the forces shaping their identities: ethnicity, race, class, language, citizenship, religion, and culture (Phillips, 1998).

The cross-cultural meaning of violence is difficult to ascertain because cultures differ in their perceptions and definitions of abuse (Hanrahan et al., 1993). Accurate data about the incidence and prevalence of violence in ethnic groups are lacking because they are infrequently represented in research studies and because violence seems to be underreported as a result of cultural norms. Some basic awareness of cultural influences on violence toward women is helpful to the nurse in being more sensitive to the needs of women whose cultural experiences differ from those of the nurse. Increasing the numbers of nurses from various ethnic groups will increase the opportunity to provide culturally appropriate care.

African-American Culture

The African-American culture supports unity among humans, nature, and the spiritual world and social connectedness and relatedness as important norms. In men, traditional sex-role socialization tends to be lower (Campbell, 1993). However, African-American men are more likely to be psychologically, socially, and economically oppressed and discriminated against, and violence may occur more frequently as a result of anger generated by environmental stresses and limited resources.

No valid evidence of greater violence seems to exist in this population, but women are more apt to report the violence. The devalued status of the female victim and racial stereotypes are barriers to African-Americans receiving help. However, their resources in extended families are greater than those for Caucasian women (Campbell, 1993).

Hispanic Culture

Hispanics in general are family oriented and have a strong family network in which unity, cooperation, respect, and loyalty are important. However, traditional families are very hierarchic, with authority given to elderly people, parents, and men. Sex roles are clearly delineated. Religion plays an important role in Hispanics' lives (Torres, 1993).

Hispanics typically seek health care from their families first, and thus women are not likely to report abuse or to seek assistance from professionals. They also are an oppressed group, and their access to health care is limited. When women do come to the nurse's attention, the nurse must be conscious of not imposing his or her own values in learning how Hispanic women handle abusive situations. Both environmental and internal factors must be addressed in their health care (Torres, 1993).

In the United States the pregnant Hispanic woman is often accompanied by her husband to the antepartum appointment if the woman does not speak English and the husband does. Unless an interpreter is available, it is difficult to interview the woman alone; in addition, asking questions about abuse through an interpreter is more difficult unless the interpreter is female and can communicate the nurse's sensitivity and concern accurately. See the Guidelines/Guías box for descriptions of abusive relationships and how a woman can recognize if she is in one.

Native American Culture

Empiric evidence about abuse in the Native American culture is lacking, but many believe that incest, sexual abuse, and domestic abuse may be the cultural norm rather than the exception. The reported prevalence rates for woman battering are 80% to 90%. It is believed that the Americanization of Native Americans has contributed to the high rate of violence. Before this oppressive process occurred, women were respected and revered, and the culture was based on communal economy and minimal class distinction. The bases of spirituality and morality were harmony with and respect for nature and all living things, sharing, cooperation, and interdependence of the sexes. Currently, lack of self-determination, disenfranchisement, poverty, isolation, racism, and high rates of substance abuse, particularly alcohol, have perpetuated violence (Bohn, 1993).

Bohn (1993) has some excellent suggestions for identifying and working with abused Native American women, including the following:

- Employ an approach that is respectful; trust takes time.
- Ask direct questions in a private setting; confidentiality is of utmost importance.
- Use open-ended questions rather than forced-choice questions to avoid further intimidation.

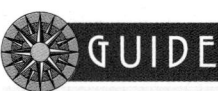 **GUIDELINES/GUÍAS**

Recognizing Violence in a Relationship

ARE YOU IN A RELATIONSHIP IN WHICH YOU ARE . . .

¿TIENES UNA RELACIÓN CON TU PAREJA EN LA QUE ESTÁS . . .

afraid of your partner's temper?
con miedo de que él pierda control?

afraid to break up because your partner has threatened to hurt someone?
con miedo de dejarlo porque él te ha amenazado con pegar o lastimar a alguien?

constantly apologizing for or defending your partner's behavior?
constantemente disculpándote por su comportameinto o defendiéndolo?

afraid to disagree with your partner?
con miedo de contradecirle?

isolated from your family or friends?
aislada de otra gente, por ejemplo, tu familia o amigas?

embarrassed in front of others because of your partner's words or actions?
avergüenzada al frente de otros por las palabras o acciones de tu pareja?

intimidated by your partner and forced into having sex?
intimidada o forzada a tener relaciones sexuales con él?

depressed and jumpy?
deprimida y/o nerviosa?

A PERSON WHO IS VIOLENT IN A RELATIONSHIP OFTEN . . .

LA PERSONA QUE TIENE UN CARÁCTER VIOLENTO A MENUDO EN SU RELACIÓN . . .

has an explosive temper.
muestra un temperamento explosivo.

is possessive or jealous of his partner's time, friends, or family.
es posesivo y tiene celos de que su pareja pase tiempo con la familia o amigos.

constantly criticizes his partner's thoughts, feelings, or appearance.
siempre critica los sentimientos, ideas, y apariencia física de su pareja.

pinches, slaps, grabs, shoves, or throws things at his partner.
pellizca, abofetea, empuja, o lanza objetos que pueden lastimar a su pareja.

forces his partner into having sex.
fuerza a su pareja ha tener relaciones sexuales.

causes his partner to be afraid.
causa que su pareja le tenga miedo.

- Speak slower and in a lower tone of voice; eye contact is very important.
- Observe posture and gestures, which may say more than words.
- Be very cognizant of the nurse's nonverbal behavior because Native American women are adept at picking up cues.

BATTERED WOMEN

Wife battering, spouse abuse, and *domestic* or *family violence* are all terms applied to a pattern of assaultive and coercive behaviors that includes physical, sexual, and psychologic attacks, as well as economic coercion inflicted by a male partner in a marriage or other heterosexual, significant, intimate relationships. The terms *domestic violence* and *spouse abuse* connote that abuse can occur by either partner against the other and do not acknowledge that women are the victims of abuse at a rate much greater than men are victimized. Campbell and Fishwick (1993) provide a much more comprehensive definition of wife (partner) **battering,** or abuse, which is "deliberate and repeated physical aggression or sexual assault inflicted on a woman by a man with whom she has had an intimate relationship" (p. 69). Relationship violence rarely consists of a single episode, but is a pattern that may start with intimidation or threats (see Fig. 11-1) and progress to more aggressive physical and sexual acts resulting in injury to the woman. Common elements of battering are economic deprivation, sexual abuse, intimidation, isolation, and stalking and terrorizing victims and their children (Yllo, 1993).

All of these elements serve to entrap a woman in a relationship in which conflicting realities exist. One reality consists of the good aspects of the partner relationship and is supported by the partner and others. The second is the reality of the abuse, which the woman may not recognize or may minimize or deny (Landenburger, 1993). Both realities may elicit the woman's hopefulness that things will change.

Characteristics of Women in Battering Relationships

Every segment of society is represented among abused women. Race, religion, social background, age, and educa-

TABLE 11-2 Comparison of Characteristics of Posttraumatic Stress Syndrome, Battered Woman's Syndrome, and Rape-Trauma Syndrome

POSTTRAUMATIC STRESS SYNDROME*	BATTERED WOMAN'S SYNDROME	RAPE-TRAUMA SYNDROME
1. The person experienced an event that involved or threatened death, a serious injury, or a threat to physical integrity of self or other.	Deliberate and repeated physical or sexual assault experienced by a woman at the hands of an intimate partner.	A violent, aggressive sexual assault on a woman without her consent from a stranger or someone she knows.
2. The person's response involved intense fear, helplessness, or horror.	The woman responds with terror, entrapment, and helplessness.	The woman responds with shock, terror, and humiliation.
3. The traumatic event is persistently reexperienced, such as through distressing recollections or dreams.	If the woman remains in the relationship, the reexperience may be real rather than recalled.	The woman relives the scene and considers what she "should have done"; she experiences a range of emotions and may feel guilty.
4. Psychologic reactivity occurs on exposure to internal or external cues symbolic of the traumatic event.	The woman feels anxious and isolated (or alone) and reacts to any expression of anger or threat by cowering or attempting to placate the abuser.	Physical symptoms such as muscle tension, hyperventilation, and flushing may occur in response to reexperiencing the rape or when approached by men, especially strangers.
5. The person persistently avoids stimuli associated with the trauma; responses are numbed.	The woman attempts to avoid arousing the anger of the abuser and tries to please him; she exerts effort to control situations to avoid abuse.	The woman avoids situations where she feels vulnerable; if in an intimate relationship, she may avoid intercourse.
6. The person has persistent symptoms of increased arousal, such as difficulty sleeping, hypervigilance, and exaggerated startle response.	The woman is alert to signs of increasing tension in the abuser during the tension-building stages; she withdraws from interaction.	The woman is afraid of being alone or in a crowd and of being attacked from behind; she takes extra precautions when going out and is suspicious.

*Modified from American Psychiatric Association. (1994). *Diagnostic and statistical manual of mental disorders* (4th ed.). Washington, DC: American Psychiatric Association.

tional level are not significant factors in differentiating women at risk. Poor and uneducated women tend to be disproportionately represented because they end up in emergency departments, they are financially more dependent, they have fewer resources and support systems, and they have fewer problem-solving skills.

Battered women may believe they are to blame for their situations because they are "not good enough wives." The woman blames herself for bringing on the violent behavior in her relationship because she believes she needs to "try harder" to please the abuser. In many cases there is a traumatic bonding with the man that hinges on loyalty, fear, terror, and learned helplessness. Many women have low self-esteem and may have histories of domestic violence in their families of origin. They fear societal rejection if they discuss their problem openly. This fear is justified in many cases because society has stereotyped these women as masochistic, which was once believed to be the case with all women in abusive relationships—they were abused because they "enjoyed" it. It is difficult for many people to comprehend why a woman would remain in a situation where she is repeatedly beaten and injured (Berlinger, 1998).

Warren and Lanning (1992) found that strong, traditional feminine characteristics of nurturing, compassion, sympathy, and yielding were more apparent in women in abusive relationships, in contrast to the traits of assertiveness, independence, and willingness to take a stand in women who were in nonviolent relationships. They also found the former group to be more willing to tolerate control from others. Social isolation seems to be another characteristic of battered women, which may result from stigma, fear, or restrictions placed on them by their partners.

Walker (1993) states that the **battered woman's syndrome** may be formally diagnosed in the fourth edition of the *Diagnostic and Statistic Manual of Mental Disorders* (DSM-IV) (American Psychiatric Association, 1994) as *posttraumatic stress disorder* (PTSD), provided that the symptoms meet the criteria. Table 11-2 compares the characteristics of PTSD with battered woman's syndrome and rape-trauma syndrome (discussed later in this chapter). Professionals making the diagnosis must guard against implying that the woman's problems are her issues alone and that she is the one who is "crazy" (Walker, 1993).

TABLE 11-3 Myths and Facts About Battering

MYTHS	FACTS
Battering occurs in a small percentage of the population.	One third to one fifth of all women experience battering by an intimate partner.
Being pregnant protects the woman from battering.	From 25% to 45% of all women who are battered are battered during pregnancy. Battering frequently begins or escalates in frequency and intensity during pregnancy. Pregnancy may be the result of forced sex or the man's control of contraception.
Battering occurs only in "problem" or lower-class families.	Domestic violence can occur in any family. Although lower-class families have a higher reported incidence of battering (Gelles, 1993), it also occurs in middle- and upper-income families. Incidence is not really known because of the tendency of middle- and upper-income families to hide their battering.
Battered women like to be beaten and deliberately provoke the attack. They are masochistic.	Women are terrified of their assailants and go to great lengths to avoid a confrontation. In some cases the woman may provoke her partner to release tension that, if left unchecked, might lead to a more severe beating and possible death.
Only men with psychologic problems abuse women.	Many batterers are successful professionals, including politicians, ministers, physicians, and lawyers. In fact, research indicates that only a small number of abusers have psychologic problems.
Only people who come from abusive families end up in abusive relationships.	Most battered women report that their partners were the first person to beat them.
Alcohol and drug abuse cause battering.	Although alcohol may be involved in abusive incidents, it is not the cause. Many batterers use alcohol as an excuse to batter and shift the blame to the alcohol.
Women would leave the relationship if the abuse were really that bad.	Those women who stay in the relationship do so out of fear and financial dependence. Shelters have long waiting lists.
Batterers and battered women cannot change.	Counseling can effectively help resocialize both batterers and battered women.

From Campbell, J. et al. (1995). The influence of abuse on pregnancy intention. *Women's Health Issues* 5(4), 214-223; Campbell, J., & Landenburger, K. (1995). Violence against women. In C. Fogel & N. Woods (Eds.). *Women's health care.* Thousand Oaks, CA: Sage; Gelles, R., & Loseke, D. (Eds.). (1993). *Current controversies on family violence.* Newbury Park, CA: Sage.

Myths About Battered Women

Many people have difficulty believing the tragedies inflicted on women and have even more trouble accepting that women stay in these harmful relationships. Health professionals often become frustrated by women they see repeatedly who have numerous signs of abuse but seem unable to liberate themselves from the battering relationships. As with other human dynamics that are not easily explained, people tend to rationalize the woman's behaviors and justify noninvolvement. A number of misconceptions have emerged to account for this perceived self-destructive behavior. If these misconceptions are believed by nurses, they result in judgments, such as blaming the victim, or in unhelpful responses to care, rather than empowering women to take control over their lives. Table 11-3 lists some myths and facts about abuse and battering.

Cycle of Violence: The Dynamics of Battering

Lenore Walker pioneered the cause of women as victims of violence in the United States when she published her research in her book *The Battered Woman* (1979). Using the

qualitative research method, she recorded results from interviews with 120 battered women. Their accounts of the progress of the abuse were remarkably similar; the resulting pattern is now recognized as the **cycle of violence.** According to this concept, battering is neither random nor constant; rather, it occurs in repeated cycles (Fig. 11-2). A three-phase cyclic pattern to the battering behavior has been described as a period of *increasing tension* leading to the *battery,* which is then followed by a period of *calm and remorse* in which the male partner displays kind, loving behavior and pleas for forgiveness. This "honeymoon" phase lasts until stress or other factors cause conflict and tension to mount again toward another episode of battering. Over time, the tension and battering phases last longer and the calm phase becomes shorter until there is no honeymoon phase (Walker, 1984).

Phase I: The Tension-Building State

Tension gradually escalates. The batterer expresses dissatisfaction and hostility without violent outbursts. He may be angered because the food is too cold, his socks can-

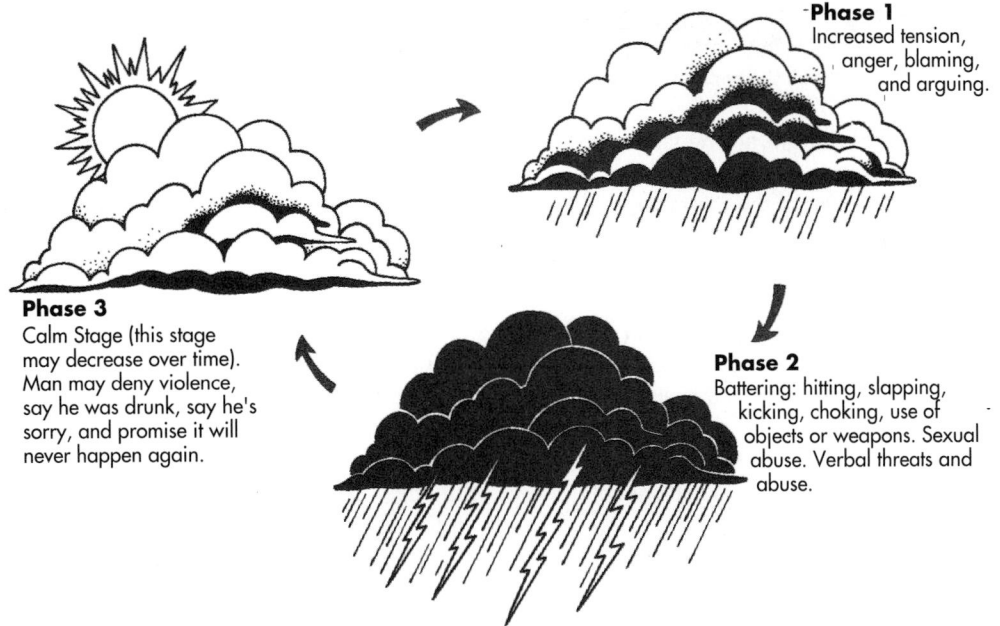

Fig. 11-2 Cycle of violence. *(From Helton, A. [1987]. A protocol of care for the battered woman. White Plains, NY: March of Dimes Birth Defects Foundation.)*

not be found, or the children are unruly. The woman senses the danger and anxiously tries to placate him. These tactics work for a time but only reinforce the woman's unrealistic belief that she can control his violent behavior. Eventually, she can no longer control his anger, and she withdraws to cope. He senses this withdrawal and becomes angrier until the violent outburst occurs. The woman suppresses the knowledge of her mate's impending abuse.

Phase II: The Acute Battering Incident

The acute battering phase is characterized by the man's uncontrollable discharge of the tension that has been building for the purpose of "teaching her a lesson." The phase can last hours to several days. The types of behaviors are slaps, punches to face and head, kicking, stomping, punching, choking, pushing, breaking of bones, burns from irons, and mutilation from knives and guns. The woman's injuries are usually to her face, buttocks, and hands and forearms as she tries to protect herself. The woman denies to herself and others the severity of the damage and may not seek medical assistance even when it is needed.

Phase III: Kindness and Contrite, Loving Behavior

This "honeymoon" phase is characterized by the batterer feeling remorseful and apologizing profusely. He may try to help her, take her to the hospital, or shower her with gifts they may not be able to afford. He promises it will never happen again, and he may believe at that time it will not. She desperately wants to believe him, and this behav-

ior restores her hope that he will change. This stage is the positive reinforcement for remaining in the relationship. The woman denies the inevitable recurrence of the abuse.

See Box 11-2 for a poem by an unknown author that graphically illustrates the cycle of violence.

Battery During Pregnancy

Studies of battered women report that 40% to 60% of pregnant women admit being battered during pregnancy (Parker & McFarlane, 1991). Pregnancy often is the beginning or escalation of violence. Furthermore, battering in teenage pregnancies ranges from 26% to 28% (Parker, McFarlane, & Soeken, 1994). McFarlane and colleagues (1999) reported on timing and severity of abuse before and during pregnancy in a group of Hispanic, African-American, and Caucasian women. They found that 51.9% of the women experienced abuse both the year before and during pregnancy. The timing and severity of the episodes were similar for the three groups.

Besides physical abuse being harmful to the mother, the risk of fetal injury is very high. Studies have demonstrated that battery during pregnancy also results in a higher rate of low-birth-weight newborns and maternal complications of low weight gain, infections, and anemia. In addition, the woman may smoke or use alcohol or other drugs as means of coping (Curry, 1998).

Pregnancy is a time of initial or increased battering episodes in violent relationships for a variety of reasons: (1) the biopsychosocial stresses of pregnancy may strain the relationship beyond the couple's ability to cope, and frustration is followed by violence; (2) the man may be

BOX 11-2 I Got Flowers Today

I got flowers today. It wasn't my birthday or any other special day.

We had our first argument last night, and he said a lot of cruel things that really hurt me.

I know he is sorry and didn't mean the things he said because he sent me flowers today.

I got flowers today. It wasn't our anniversary or any other special day.

Last night he threw me into a wall and started to choke me. It seemed like a nightmare. I couldn't believe it was real. I woke up this morning sore and bruised all over.

I know he must be sorry because he sent me flowers today and it wasn't Mother's Day or any other special day.

Last night he beat me up again. And it was much worse than all the other times. If I leave him, what will I do? How will I take care of my kids? What about money? I'm afraid of him and scared to leave.

But I know he must be sorry. Because he sent me flowers today.

I got flowers today. Today was a very special day.

It was the day of my funeral.

Last night he finally killed me. He beat me to death.

If only I had gathered enough courage and strength to leave him,

I would not have gotten flowers today.

—*Author unknown*

jealous of the fetus, resenting the intrusion into the couple's relationship and the woman's displacement of attention; (3) the man may be angry at the unborn child or the woman; and (4) the beating may be the man's conscious or subconscious attempt to end the pregnancy. After birth the mother may be so physically and emotionally drained that she may have difficulty bonding with her infant. She may be at risk of becoming an abusive mother whether or not she remains in the abusive relationship.

A recent study reports that physical and sexual abuse predicts poor health during pregnancy and the postpartum period. The authors reported an average of four medical symptoms in the abused sample, especially headaches, pain, and high levels of depression. These symptoms did not abate during the postpartum period as they did in the nonabused women (Leserman, Stewart, & Dell, 1999).

During pregnancy, the target body parts change during abusive episodes. Women report physical blows directed to the head, breasts, abdomen, and genitalia. Sexual assault is common (McFarlane, 1993). The battered pregnant woman should be treated as a high risk obstetric client because she is prone to anxiety, depression, alcohol and drug use, and inadequate and late prenatal care (Campbell et al., 1992; Curry, 1998). Physical and sexual assaults also increase the rate of miscarriages and preterm and stillborn infants.

If the pregnant woman remains with her partner, she is at additional risk for repeated physical and psychologic trauma. The potential for child abuse is great, especially if the batterer's anger is directed at the unborn child or if he is jealous of the fetus (Campbell, Oliver, & Bullock, 1993). If battering begins in pregnancy, it is likely to continue after the birth. This information is vital to share with the woman and other nurses involved in her care. Another factor in the health of both the mother and the newborn child is that the woman may expend energy on coping with the battering rather than on caring for the newborn child (Bullock, 1993).

Bullock (1993) reports that pregnant women experience the following difficulties, which may assist the nurse in identifying battering during pregnancy: consumption of an inadequate diet, lack of sleep, inadequate consumption of milk and milk products, and minimal forms of self-relaxation; in essence the battered pregnant woman may not take proper care of herself.

Battering and pregnancy in teenagers constitute a particularly difficult situation. Adolescents may be more trapped in the abusive relationship than adult women because of their inexperience. Many professionals and the adolescents themselves ignore the violence because it may not be believable, because relationships are transient, and because the jealous and controlling behavior is interpreted as love and devotion. Routine screening for abuse and sexual assault is recommended for pregnant adolescents (Parker, 1993). Because pregnancy in young adolescent girls is frequently the result of sexual abuse, the nurse should assess the desire to maintain the pregnancy.

: CARE MANAGEMENT

Care of the battered woman must begin with the nurse's self-assessment. An exploration of attitudes toward women in abusive situations, awareness of feelings that may result in judgmental communication, and knowledge about the many aspects of intimate partner violence are preparation for care. Exactly what drives a woman to seek assistance is not clear. Women who belong to any of the following three groups are more likely to seek assistance: (1) women who are beaten frequently and severely, (2) those who have not experienced or witnessed family violence in their family of origin, and (3) those who see an alternative to life in their marriages, specifically women with jobs.

Battered women are reluctant to seek help for various reasons, including the need to avoid the stigma associated with the nature of the family violence; the fear that they will not be believed; the fear of reprisal from their husbands; and in some states in which battering is a reportable crime, the desire to avoid involvement with police (see Legal Tip).

Mandatory Reporting of Domestic Violence

Forty states and the District of Columbia have laws that mandate reporting by health care providers in situations in which the woman has an injury that may be caused by a deadly weapon. Some states also require reports when there is a reason to believe the woman's injury may have resulted from an illegal act or act of violence. Only six states have mandatory reporting laws specific to domestic violence or adult abuse.

Because of the wide variation from state to state in mandatory reporting, nurses must be knowledgeable about the reporting requirements of the state in which they reside.

Assessment and Nursing Diagnoses

Clients in women's health care settings are at a high risk for abuse; therefore it is important that nurses assess all women entering the health care system for potential abuse (Campbell & Humphreys, 1993). Health care providers are often the first and only contact with someone outside the relationship that a severely isolated woman will make. Failure to identify spousal abuse and to recognize the risk of serious injury or even death further endangers the lives of women and their children.

A suspected assaulted woman should be examined and interviewed in private, and she may feel safer and more comfortable with a female health care provider. When one is taking a psychosocial history, the following information provides clues to violence or potential for violence: ways the woman and her partner resolve conflict; what happens when the woman's partner becomes angry; whether fighting occurs during disagreements; and when such fighting occurs, if it ever escalates to physical means. It may help the woman to disclose information if these events are normalized by the nurse stating, "Many people (families) have difficulty in expressing anger or expressing areas of conflict. What is that like for you and your partner?" The nurse listens for any evidence of power and control in the relationship. While inquiring about past trauma or injuries, the nurse also should ask directly if the woman has been injured by her husband or partner. At least the following two questions should be asked: (1) "Are you with a spouse or partner who physically, psychologically, or sexually hurts you?" and (2) "Are you afraid of your spouse or partner?" These questions give a woman permission to disclose sensitive information (Chez & Jones, 1995).

An assessment tool can be a part of the interview or included in a written history (see Fig. 6-10). Reports show an increase in the identification of victims of domestic violence when the nurse inquires at each visit whether a woman has been hit or threatened since her last visit (Buel & Harvard, 1995). However, if the male partner is present, the woman may not disclose experiences of abuse. Campbell and associates (1995) suggest using a question-

naire that the woman could fill out as a way for nurses to assess for abuse. Other cues to abuse are delay in seeking medical assistance (hours or days), missed appointments, vague explanation of injuries, nonspecific somatic complaints, social isolation, lack of eye contact, a husband or partner who does not want to leave the client alone with the primary health care provider, and substance abuse.

If the woman discloses information about abuse, she should be believed. One must remember that the coping mechanism most used by battered women is denial. Abused women often deny impending abuse, severity of injury, future recurrence, and death. Women may be embarrassed about their abusive relationships and believe the abuse is caused by their inadequacies. By asking a woman directly about abuse, telling her that similar injuries are common in women who have been abused, and pointing out that she is not responsible for another's violent behavior, the nurse may help her disclose the violence she is experiencing. During pregnancy, the nurse should assess for abuse at each prenatal visit and on admission to labor, although it is not appropriate to ask questions during active labor. The nurse should continue to assess for abuse after the birth (Bullock, 1993; Campbell et al., 1995).

During pregnancy particularly, the nurse should assess for injuries to the breasts, abdomen, and genitals. The woman may report a history of miscarriages, abruptio placentae, or stillbirth.

During the physical examination the nurse should observe for injuries to the face, breasts, abdomen, and buttocks. These injuries may be old or new and may range from minor bruising to serious injuries. Psychosocial assessment findings may include anxiety, insomnia, self-directed abuse, depression, and drug or alcohol abuse (Curry, 1998). Other physical signs include fractures that require significant force or that would rarely occur by accident; multiple injuries at various stages of healing; and patterns left by whatever might inflict injury, such as teeth, utensils, fists, or hot objects.

Examples of potential nursing diagnoses for battered women may include the following:

▮ Nursing Diagnoses

- Hopelessness related to
  - prolonged exposure to physical, mental, social, and sexual abuse
- Knowledge deficit related to
  - phenomenon of battering
  - cycle of violence
  - community resources
- Ineffective individual and family coping related to
  - persistence of victim-abuser relationship
- Injury related to
  - battering episode
- Situational low self-esteem related to
  - continuing victim-abuser relationship

Expected Outcomes of Care

Expected outcomes for care should be formulated in collaboration with the client. An overall outcome is to have the woman recognize the abuse she has experienced and to state all her options in making decisions about what actions to take. Specific expected outcomes are that the woman will do the following:

- Formulate a plan for safety.
- Identify her areas of strength and develop goals for herself.
- State her knowledge of alternatives, options, and choices; community resources (shelters, financial aid, child care, education, job or financial assistance); and roles of members of the health care team.
- Express a feeling of empowerment and control.
- Perceive herself as deserving of respect and not as "deserving" to be victimized.
- Express measures to protect her children or, if she is pregnant, the fetus from abuse.

Plan of Care and Interventions

Establishing a therapeutic relationship and skillful interviewing help women disclose and describe their abuse. Language is important when talking with women. For example, using the term *victim* connotes powerlessness and hopelessness (Ryan & King, 1998); a more empowering term is *survivor*. Women who have identified their abuse may appear passive, hostile, anxious, depressed, or hysterical because they may think they are at the mercy of the man's temper or they may be "out of control." In addition, they may be embarrassed, afraid, angry, sad, and shocked (Holtz & Furniss, 1993). A tool developed by Holtz and Furniss (1993) provides the following framework for sensitive nursing interventions–the *ABCDES* of caring for the abused woman:

- **A** is reassuring the woman that she is not *alone*. The isolation and denigration by the abuser keep her from knowing that others are in the same situation and that health care providers can help.
- **B** is expressing the *belief* that violence against the woman is not acceptable in any situation and that it is not her fault. This may be the first step in empowering her to think about self-protection and acceptable boundaries.
- **C** is *confidentiality*, particularly since the woman may believe that if the abuse is reported, the perpetrator will retaliate (and in reality this may happen).
- **D** is *documentation* and includes the following: (1) a clear statement by the client about the abuse that does *not* include her subjective opinion, such as "I provoked the abusive behavior"; (2) accurate descriptions of injuries and a history of the first, worst, and most recent incident of violence; and (3) with the woman's consent, evidence or photographs.
- **E** is for *education*, especially about the cycle of violence, that it is likely to recur and escalate, and about options.

- **S** is for *safety*, the most significant part of the intervention to ensure that the woman has knowledge of the resources and a plan of action should she stay with the battering partner. First, services and telephone numbers of a hotline and the battered women's shelter or other safe haven should be provided by the nurse. A safety plan includes necessities for a quick escape: a bag packed with personal items for an overnight stay (can be hidden or left with a neighbor), money or checkbook, an extra set of car keys, and any legal documents for identification. Legal options, such as those for restraining orders or arrest of the perpetrator, are also important aspects of the safety plan. If the woman chooses not to act in the throes of a violent episode, she may use the hotline or shelter for some counseling when the threat of harm is no longer present (Fishwick, 1998).

If the woman is pregnant, collaboration with maternity nurses who will be involved in her care during the pregnancy is encouraged. Each nurse can plan care that will point out the woman's strengths and raise her self-esteem. The husband or partner is welcomed to attend prenatal visits and classes and is included in other ways if the woman chooses to stay with him. Counseling services are offered to both spouses. The first days after birth are particularly crucial because the mother is physically and emotionally vulnerable and usually tired, and the baby's crying may be intolerable to both the father and the mother. The danger of abuse to mother and child is acute during this time. Facilitating the woman's establishment of a support network of maternity and pediatric staff, community health nurses, and parental crisis center personnel is important during this crucial period (see Research box). Referral to resources and provision for follow-up examination by health care providers should also be part of nursing intervention (Bullock, 1993).

Many nurses become frustrated when a battered woman returns to a previously abusive situation. It is important to remember that many victims have been abused for a long time, making it difficult for them to seek and accept help. In addition to understanding the many reasons why women stay in abusive relationships, recognizing that the most dangerous period for a battered woman is when she is in the process of leaving (Landenburger, 1998) may help nurses to be less judgmental about the woman's dilemma.

A woman indicates her readiness to leave the relationship when she indicates she is capable of planning for herself, investing in herself, recognizing that the abuse is part of a continuing pattern, and when she is able to express the desire, leaving at the moment when no abuse is occurring. She also needs some assurance that she will have economic and people resources to "make it" on her own. Although shelters provide both, shelter stays are typically limited to 30 to 90 days, and therefore a long-term plan must be in place. Women in repeated abusive situations may have lost their ability to perceive the possibility of success and be-

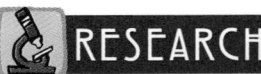

RESEARCH

Safety Behaviors of Abused Women After an Intervention During Pregnancy

Abuse during pregnancy is common and, depending on the population surveyed and instruments used, affects almost 20% of pregnant women. In addition, abuse during pregnancy is associated with significantly higher maternal rates of depression; suicide attempts; and tobacco, alcohol, and illicit drug use. Prevention of abuse to women is a national priority, and experts predict that it could be reduced by as much as 75% if identification and intervention were offered in primary care settings.

The purpose of this study was to evaluate an intervention protocol, administered during pregnancy, for increasing safety-seeking behaviors of women who are abused. A prospective, ethnically stratified cohort design was implemented. Participants included pregnant women reporting physical or sexual abuse in the year before or during the present pregnancy. One hundred thirty-two women received the intervention of three education, advocacy, and community referral sessions that included information on safety behaviors. Safety behaviors were measured before

the intervention; twice during pregnancy; and at 2, 6, and 12 months after completion of the pregnancy.

Repeated measures analysis of variance showed a significant increase in adoption of each safety behavior ($p < .0001$), with most behaviors showing a significant increase after the first intervention session. It was concluded that pregnant women who were abused and were offered an intervention protocol reported a significant increase in safety behavior adoption during and after pregnancy.

CLINICAL APPLICATION

Abuse during pregnancy is common. Nurses should implement routine screening for abuse in women. Identification of abuse victims and immediate clinical intervention that includes information about safety behaviors can result in safety behavior adoption that may prevent future abuse and increase the safety and well-being of women and infants.

Source: McFarlane, J. et al. (1998). Safety behaviors of abused women after an intervention during pregnancy. *J Obstet Gynecol Neonatal Nurs* 27(1), 64-69.

come very passive (Fishel & Rynerson, 1998). Nurses can be helpful in directing these women to sources of information, continue to be expert listeners, and offer encouragement as women struggle in their decision-making process toward freedom and control in their lives.

Prevention

Nurses can make a difference in stopping the violence and preventing further injury. Educating women that abuse is a violation of their rights and facilitating their access to protective and legal services constitute a first step. Other helpful measures for women to discourage their fall into abusive relationships are promoting assertiveness and self-defense courses; suggesting support and self-help groups that encourage positive self-regard, confidence, and empowerment; and recommending educational and skills development classes that will enhance independence or at least the ability to take care of oneself (Hadley et al., 1995).

Prevention work with children encourages and teaches them androgynous gender roles: both males and females are equal; both can be nurturing; and neither needs to dominate the other or to engage in violent behavior to have needs met. Helping children to gain problem-solving and conflict management skills may eliminate the need for violent solutions to life stresses. Encouraging schoolchildren to form and participate in Students Against Violence Everywhere (SAVE) groups, which is a nationwide pro-peace effort that promotes justice, respect, and love, gives

them an appreciation for these qualities in all facets of life. With adolescents, discussing the "macho" concept and the consequences of maintaining this image and behavior may facilitate more egalitarian relationships.

Other means of prevention are to advocate against violence in all professional arenas and to participate actively in promoting legislation and policies toward stopping violent acts.

Evaluation

Evaluation of the care of abused women must be based on expected outcomes and must be in harmony with the choices the woman has made (see Plan of Care).

SEXUAL ABUSE

It is estimated that 27% of women have experienced childhood sexual abuse (Heritage, 1998). *Childhood sexual abuse* is defined as any type of sexual exploitation that involves (1) a child younger than age 18 years at the time of the first molestation; (2) at least a 3-year age difference between the victim and perpetrator; and (3) a variety of behaviors between the victim and the perpetrator, which may include disrobing, nudity, masturbation, fondling, digital penetration, and anal, oral, or vaginal penetration (Urbanic, 1993). Childhood sexual abuse acts, according to law, are acts perpetrated by someone responsible for care of the child, such

PLAN of CARE | Battered Woman

NURSING DIAGNOSIS Risk for self-directed violence related to history of battering by partner as evidenced by physical injuries	**NURSING DIAGNOSIS** Social isolation related to stigma of battering as evidenced by behaviors of withdrawal

Expected Outcome *Client will identify factors leading to cycle of violence and develop plan for safety.*

Nursing Interventions/*Rationales*

Provide opportunity to verbalize feelings in a nonthreatening atmosphere *to give emotional support.*

Be alert for cues indicative of battering *to provide database for interventions.*

Provide information on options available to battered women (i.e., shelters, legal assistance, etc.) *to provide information in developing a future plan for safety for herself and any children.*

Refer to social services and support groups *to give further information and share experiences.*

Expected Outcome *Client will list ways to increase social contacts.*

Nursing Interventions/*Rationales*

Provide private opportunity to express feelings of aloneness *to initiate and maintain a therapeutic relationship.*

Support opportunities for social interaction *to increase feelings of self-worth and self-confidence.*

Encourage interaction with groups for socialization and support *to increase numbers of social contacts.*

---

as the parents, boyfriends, stepfathers, grandparents, day care providers, or babysitters. These childhood sexual abuse acts may include **incest,** which is any type of sexual exploitation between blood relatives or surrogate relatives before the victim reaches 18 years of age. The peak abuse ages are 7 to 12 years of age (Hunter, 1991). If a stranger commits sexual abuse, it is considered **sexual assault.**

Childhood sexual abuse continues over time and gradually escalates. The child is pressured by the adult to cooperate and maintain the relationship. The secrecy is maintained because of the child's domination by the adult, fear of punishment or of not being believed, shame, and rejection (Urbanic, 1993). This continuing victimization and accompanying feeling of helplessness, together with lack of confiding, lead to the long-term behavioral and relationship consequences seen in adult survivors of sexual assault. Common psychopathologic consequences are dissociative identity disorder, borderline personality disorder, and generalized anxiety disorder. Although clients with these diagnoses may come to the attention of maternity nurses, women who experience symptoms of PTSD, sexual dysfunctions, depression, anxiety, or substance abuse problems are more likely to be seen in obstetric and gynecologic practice. Female sexual abuse and assault victims appear to be the largest single group to experience PTSD (Silva et al., 1997).

: CARE MANAGEMENT

Clients usually do not resent or object to being asked about their sexual violence; in fact, they feel some relief because of the possibility of being relieved of the psychologic burden (Gallop et al., 1995).

The history obtained from an interview and review of medical records may reveal clues suggestive of sexual abuse. A history of dreams, flashbacks, or terror attacks may indicate PTSD (Silva et al., 1997). Hulme and Grove (1994) identify the most prominent symptoms:

- *Physical:* insomnia, sexual dysfunction, overeating, drug and alcohol abuse, severe headaches, and two or more major surgeries
- *Psychosocial:* depression, guilt, low self-esteem, inability to trust others, mood swings, suicidal thoughts, difficulty in relationships, confusion, extreme anger, and memory lapse

Clients may also exhibit feelings of self-blame, shame, body rejection, anxiety, fear, mistrust, and hatred.

Overall planning for the adult survivor of childhood sexual abuse must acknowledge that the survivor is able to recognize that the abuse occurred, to share her story, and to begin a healing process. Heritage (1998) states that disclosing must be done whenever and however the survivor chooses, that it be done with someone she trusts, and that the survivor believes she can disclose without experiencing further alienation. Either verbal or nonverbal shock and horror reactions from the nurse are particularly devastating.

Nursing Care

The survivor needs support on many different levels, and a maternity or women's health nurse may be the first person to whom she relates her story. Using therapeutic communication skills and listening are initial interventions.

Urbanic (1993) states that interventions must focus on empowering the victim in developing a sense of self-worth, mastery, competence, and control toward a resolution of the incest trauma. She also indicates that collaboration and cooperation between the nurse and the client are important in achieving goals.

Psychologic support is a necessary intervention when the survivor experiences flashbacks, learns to express feelings of anger without fear of losing control, and expresses needs without guilt. Consistently reinforcing that the adult was the responsible party is important (Urbanic, 1993).

Referral of incest survivors to appropriate support and recovery groups who assist each other in decreasing depression, anger, and guilt; reducing isolation; improving self-esteem; and developing effective coping mechanisms is an effective intervention.

RAPE

Rape is an act of violence rather than a sexual act. Rape is a legal and not a medical term and, in its strictest sense, is the penile penetration of the female sex organ or labia without her consent; it may or may not include the use of a weapon. Sexual assault, a term used interchangeably with rape, is also an act of force and has a much broader definition to include unwanted or uncomfortable touches, kisses, hugs, petting, intercourse, or other sexual acts (Orange County, N.C., Rape Crisis Center, 1995).

Hymenal penetration or ejaculation does not have to occur to qualify as rape. The key feature to establish rape is the absence of consent: threat or coercion implies the lack of consent. The victim who is mentally retarded, who is unconscious or otherwise physically unable to move, who has been drugged without her knowledge, or who is a minor (statutory rape) is not capable of giving consent. The court must prove absence of consent; thus the term *alleged rape* or *alleged sexual assault* is used in medical records.

It is vital that nurses understand the definition of rape because many people (possibly including the victim of rape) believe that the woman "invited" the rape through either seductive dress or seductive behavior (Campbell & Landenburger, 1995). The fact is that no woman deserves to be forced into any sexual behavior that she does not overtly request.

Since many reasons deter a woman from reporting the crime, accurate statistics concerning psychosocial and demographic variables relating to rape are not available. It is estimated that one in every six women will be raped during her lifetime (Petter & Whitehill, 1998). Women do not report rape because of the associated stigma; embarrassment; guilt that in some way they provoked the assault; fear of retribution from the rapist or his friends; dread of being humiliated and figuratively "raped" again by the police, the court, or the publicity; and discouragement generated by the dismally small number of convictions, among other reasons. Victims often fear the reactions of husbands, lovers, friends, family, and children and prefer to suffer alone.

The types of rape are reported as date or acquaintance rape, marital rape, gang rape, stranger rape, and psychic rape. **Acquaintance rape** involves persons who know one another, such as a classmate, neighbor, family member, or date, and is sexual assault that occurs when the trust of a relationship is violated and one person is forced by another into sexual activity (Stuart & Laraia, 1998). Victims of date and acquaintance rape are most often between 15 and 19 years of age.

Marital rape occurs partly because men may believe it is their right to engage in sex whenever they desire, regardless of the partner's desire or condition. It frequently occurs whenever there is physical abuse of the woman. Marital rape is particularly devastating to the woman because she is in a committed relationship and living with the partner (Stuart & Laraia, 1998). Most states now recognize marital rape as a legitimate, reportable crime (Humphreys & Findlater, 1993).

Gang rape occurs when one woman is raped by two or more men. *Stranger rape* is when an unknown attacker actively seeks a woman who is vulnerable. This is the type of rape most feared by women (Aguilera, 1994).

Psychic rape occurs when one's personal dignity and self-respect are assaulted (Stuart & Laraia, 1998). *Sexual harassment,* although not classified as rape, is another form of using power and control tactics to victimize women sexually, particularly in workplaces.

Dynamics of Rape

Rape is not an act of lust or an overzealous release of passion. Rape is a violent, aggressive assault on the victim's body and integrity. As one victim said, "No matter how terrible people think rape is, it's worse than they know. It's like a bomb going off at the center of your soul." Sexual assault is the use of power and control tactics and is often motivated by a desire to humiliate, defile, and dominate the victim (Stuart & Laraia, 1998).

The rapist has no regard for his victim's age, race, sexual attraction, or physical condition: 10-day-old infants as well as handicapped elderly women confined to wheelchairs have been sexually assaulted. Most rapes occur intraracially rather than interracially.

Victims of date and acquaintance rape may be less prone to recognize what is happening to them; the dynamics are different from stranger rape and may begin rather subtly. Initially, *intrusion* occurs, which may take the form of asking personal questions, invading personal space, and touching that is unwanted and uncomfortable. The woman becomes used to the perpetrator's actions, believing them to be normal and usual behavior. This is the phase of *desensitization* as one is less mindful of the uncomfortable behavior. The final stage is *isolation,* in which the victim is taken to an apartment, an isolated area in a car, or any place where the two are alone, which is where the forced act of sex frequently occurs (Orange County, N.C., Rape Crisis Center, 1995).

Rape-Trauma Syndrome

To assess and provide care to a woman who experiences rape, the nurse must first understand the **rape-trauma syndrome.** This syndrome is characterized by extreme anxiety and stress resulting in emotional and psychologic reactions and often somatic complaints in the woman. Burgess and Holmstrom (1986) have defined three phases of the syndrome.

Acute Phase: Disorganization

The assault itself marks the beginning of this phase of rape-trauma syndrome, which can last for several days or up to 3 weeks. Reactions such as shock, denial, and disbelief are similar to those described by Kübler-Ross in the process of grief and dying. In addition, the rape survivor is embarrassed, degraded, fearful, angry, and vengeful and usually blames herself. She feels unclean and wants to bathe and douche despite the fact that she may be destroying evidence. Her affect may change rapidly from crying to being calm and controlled. She relives the scene over and over in her mind and considers things she "should have done." Physiologically she may be uncomfortable, experiencing skeletal muscle pain or tension, gastrointestinal irritability, sighing respirations, hyperventilation, flushing, or a sense of feeling too hot or too cold.

Outward Adjustment Phase

During the adjustment phase the survivor may appear to have resolved her crisis. She may return to a job or to maintaining a household, or both, but she is denying and suppressing her thoughts and feelings. She needs this time to regain some control in her life. She may move, change jobs, buy a weapon to protect herself, or install an alarm system in her home. She becomes less interested in discussing the rape. She may develop specific or generalized fears that restrict her activities.

Long-Term Process: Reorganization Phase

The third phase is reorganization. Denial and suppression cannot be maintained forever. Disclosing personal thoughts and feelings has a profound effect in improving health and reducing stress. As a rape survivor's suppression of feelings and emotions starts to deteriorate, she becomes depressed and anxious. Her own healthy spirit pressures her to discuss the rape with someone. Because she is losing her control of denial, her fears start to surface; she may be afraid to be alone or in a crowd or may fear being attacked from behind. Nightmares and eating disorders are common in these last two phases.

The recovery process may take 2 years or more and can be difficult and painful (Dunn & Guilchrist, 1993). The victim has progressed through recovery when the physical distress and the constant memories of the rape have diminished. She no longer blames herself for what happened and can truly call herself a survivor.

Similar to the battered woman's syndrome, the rape-trauma syndrome may meet the criteria for PTSD and be formally diagnosed (see Table 11-2).

: CARE MANAGEMENT

Nurses in women's health care and emergency departments are most likely to see rape victims in the acute phase. However, all women who manifest any of the signs of other phases should be assessed for posttraumatic experiences.

Facilities that treat rape victims vary in protocols and resources. In its 1992 guidelines, the Joint Commission on Accreditation of Healthcare Organizations (JCAHO) requires emergency and ambulatory care departments to have protocols on physical assault, rape or sexual assault, and domestic abuse of elders, spouses, partners, and children. These protocols must address client consent, examination, and treatment guidelines and the health care facility's responsibility for collecting evidence, photographing injuries, and releasing evidence to law enforcement officials. In addition, the emergency and ambulatory care departments must provide to victims a referral list of community-based and private service agencies dealing with family violence (Limandri, 1992). The nurse interacting with the sexual assault client should be guided by the particular treatment center's protocol; Box 11-3 presents a representative protocol.

Many treatment centers have also initiated the use of the Sexual Assault Nurse Examiner (SANE). The SANE is educated in the specialty of forensic nursing and is prepared to examine clients; recognize, collect, and preserve evidence; counsel the client; link the client with vital community resources; follow up cases; and, if necessary, testify in court (Lenehan, 1991). If a SANE is not available in a particular facility, JCAHO member organizations must implement a plan for educating appropriate staff members about identifying, treating, and referring abuse victims.

Additional facility resources may include a social worker, who is usually notified the moment a rape client is admitted, or a local rape crisis center, usually staffed by specially trained volunteers on 24-hour call for just these types of emergencies. Rape counselors provide ongoing support in a variety of ways: providing emotional support; providing transportation; helping the woman interact with her family, friends, and various authorities; informing her of rape-trauma syndrome; and finding other resources for her as needed. Male volunteers may counsel male members of the victim's family and her male friends.

History

History taking is an important first step in care, and the client should be informed of all the steps involved in the rape examination and follow-up examination (Hampton, 1995). Because rape is a crime, the first nurse to see the sexually assaulted client must consider the need to preserve evidence (see Legal Tip). However, the preservation of evidence should not overshadow a survivor's rights: to be treated as a human being with respect, courtesy, and dignity.

BOX 11-3 Adult Sexual Assault Protocol: Emergency Department

PURPOSE

To outline nursing care of sexual assault (rape and/or sexual offense) clients, which includes participation in the collection of forensic evidence, and in the referral of clients for follow-up treatment.

LEVEL

Interdependent (*requires M.D. order)

SUPPORTIVE DATA

Many rape victims feel there is a stigma attached to the victim of sexual assault. As a result, only one in four cases is believed to be reported. The median age range of victims is 15 to 26 years, and the vast majority are women. Fifty to seventy-five percent of the assailants are known by their victims. The client's significant other (e.g. spouse, parent, friend), if accompanying the client, is classified as a "secondary victim."

Whenever possible, the sexual assault client will be cared for by a SANE (Sexual Assault Nurse Examiner) RN. These nurses have successfully completed a continuing education course in Forensic and Sexual Assault Evidence Collection. This course provides those nurses with the information and skills to properly care for clients following sexual assault by recognizing, collecting, and preserving evidence, interviewing the client, and linking them to vital community resources for follow-up.

RESOURCE

NORTH CAROLINA LAW: General Statutes: 14-27.2; 14-27.3; 14-27.4; 14-27.5

ASSESSMENT

1. Assess the client for any life-threatening injuries.
2. Assess the client's level of coping, coherency, and ability to control behavior.
3. Assess the client's priorities:
   - Is client seeking care for prevention of pregnancy or disease only?
   - Is client seeking forensic evidence collection?
   - Does the client want both?

     NOTE: Notify a SANE nurse to perform the examination if the client is seeking evidence collection for filing of police charges either at this time or in the future.
4. Assess the client's entire body for bruises, lacerations, and/or other skeletal/soft tissue injuries.
5. Initiate the collection of evidence using the Sexual Assault Collection Kit (SBI* Kit) if client consents:
   - *If SANE nurse is available:*
     - SANE: Complete SBI Kit.

   - SANE: Examine the vagina and rectum to include the speculum exam.

     NOTE: A toludine blue dye and culposcope may be used to collect evidence.
   - Physician performs the bimanual examination.
   - *If SANE nurse is not available:*
     - Primary nurse initiates SBI kit with the exception of vaginal, rectal, and bimanual examinations.
     - Physician performs vaginal, rectal, and bimanual examinations.
6. Ask client whether or not those who are with the client know that the client has been sexually assaulted.

   NOTE: This information cannot be given to secondary victims without the client's permission.

SAFETY

7. Notify UNC Hospitals Police when a sexual assault client presents to the ED.

   NOTE: UNC Hospitals Police will complete a risk assessment of client safety.

CARE

8. Provide care for any physical injuries. (See UNC Hospitals Trauma Protocol Manual.)
9. Provide for client privacy and nonjudgmental support.
10. Protect client confidentiality by identifying the client as "7273" rather than by name or chief complaint.
11. Assign one nurse to the client for the duration and disposition of evidence collection.
12. Telephone the Rape Crisis Center to request a rape crisis advocate.

    NOTE: The client has the right to refuse an advocate. It is the policy of the ED to allow the advocate to offer services directly to the client unless the client expressly forbids it. Notify the advocate of any secondary victims who may have accompanied the client if the secondary victim is aware that the client has been sexually assaulted.
13. Reassure the client that s/he is safe.
14. Reassure the client that the incident is not her/his fault.
15. Prepare the client for the possibility that some questions asked may be embarrassing.
16. Obtain informed consent for the physical exam, to include photographs of injuries, using UNC Hospitals' consent form for sexual assault evidence collection.

    NOTE: If the client permits the release of information to law enforcement, explain to the victim that the evidence will be turned over to the appropriate jurisdiction for processing. If the client is unwilling

Adapted with permission from University of North Carolina Hospitals, Dept. of Nursing Adult Sexual Assault Protocol, 1999 revised version.
*SBI, State Bureau of Investigation.

Continued

BOX 11-3 Adult Sexual Assault Protocol: Emergency Department—cont'd

to have law enforcement notified at this time, the client should mark "do not" on the release form so the evidence will remain in the custody of the UNC Hospitals Police. The client may later change this if the client chooses to file charges or have law enforcement involved.

17. Collect the evidence as directed in the SBI Kit and in accordance with client consent.

   NOTE: Use the UNC Hospitals forms for documentation of the evidence. Separate the forms at the completion of the exam, placing the appropriate copies in the designated areas. Each form should be addressographed with patient's identification. Any photographs taken should be labeled with the patient's information and described in the nursing notes. These photographs should then be sealed in an envelope and secured per Department of Emergency Medicine policy. The SBI Kit *must* remain in the possession of *one nurse* throughout the entire assessment procedure and treatment period, until it is released to a police agency.

18. Perform a urine pregnancy test.

19. Provide the opportunity for bathing and clean clothing following the examination.

*20. Administer medication to protect the client against pregnancy and sexually transmitted diseases.

21. Arrange for follow-up care per client preference for any medical and/or psychologic problems and/or injury.

CLIENT/SIGNIFICANT OTHER (S.O.) TEACHING

22. Explain to the client/S.O.:
   • all procedures and rationale
   • that feelings of anger, anxiety, and fear are normal
   • options for medical, legal, and emotional counseling are available to both primary and secondary victims.

NOTE: Do not assume that a friend or S.O. is aware of the assault. (See #6.)

23. Inform client/S.O. of resources available:
   • judicial system options (i.e., official police report, "blind" report)
   • financial assistance:
     — Victim's Assistance Fund if patient is UNC student *(requires a full or "blind" police report)*
     — North Carolina Victim's Compensation Fund *(requires a full police report within 72 hours and cooperation with law enforcement)*
   • other available resources:
     — Rape Crisis Center
     — Student Health Service, if victim is UNC student
     — mental health agency
     — sites and phone numbers for HIV counseling and testing
     — resource list of phone numbers (e.g., law enforcement)

DOCUMENTATION

24. Complete the UNC Hospitals forms for sexual assault evidence collection.

25. Place the original copy in the client's medical record, the appropriate copy inside the SBI Kit, and the other copy in the envelope attached to the SBI Kit (labeled for law enforcement).

26. Seal the SBI Kit as directed, and deliver it to a sworn law enforcement officer.

27. Seal all photographs in an envelope marked with patient identification, and secure per Department of Emergency Medicine policy.

28. Document care rendered, teaching done, and client response and level of understanding on ED nursing record.

LEGAL TIP Collector of Evidence

Consent forms must be signed before evidence can be collected and released to the police and before photographs can be taken. If the victim is under 16 years of age, a pediatrician is notified. A parent or guardian is required to sign the consent forms. A children's protective service may need to be called to facilitate consent.

History includes a statement of the traumatic event. Box 11-4 lists information to be collected. The woman needs privacy and assurance of confidentiality and may need a great deal of support and assistance in verbalizing the offenders' acts. For example, giving the client permission to describe the situation however she chooses and re-

stating what the client has said (without minimizing) will show empathy. It is important to tell the client that she is safe, that the incident is not her fault, and that she is not alone in what she has experienced. It is also important to obtain sexual, gynecologic, and obstetric histories (Petter & Whitehill, 1998) (see Chapter 6).

Physical Examination and Laboratory Tests

The nurse may assist with the physical examination, which is conducted after the procedure is explained to the woman. Preservation of the woman's dignity is of utmost importance during the examination. She remains clothed while her vital signs and blood pressure are determined, and her clothing is inspected for stains, tears, and foreign

- Assess the client for life-threatening injuries.
- Assess the client's level of coping, coherency, and ability to control behavior.
- Assess the client's priorities:
  Is the client seeking care for prevention of disease or pregnancy only?
  Is the client seeking forensic evidence collection?
  Does the client want both?
- Ask client to describe the event:
  Time and place of the event.
  Relationship to the assailant, if any.
  Nature of suspected physical and sexual acts.
  Time lapse between assault and current examination.
- Did the woman bathe, douche, or shower? Did she urinate or defecate?
- Ask client whether those who are with the client know that the client has been sexually assaulted.
- Ask the client if she can think of any other information that would help in her care, and inform her that it is safe and confidential to say whatever she needs to.
- Inspect the entire body for bruises, lacerations, and other injuries.
- Initiate collection of evidence using the sexual assault collection kit (or notify the Sexual Assault Nurse Examiner)

material. She is assisted to undress and is draped for the physical examination. A female attendant, rape counselor, or other person of her choice may remain with her during the examination. The physician or nurse-practitioner informs her of every step of the procedure. Her body is inspected for bruises, swelling, scratches, lacerations, stab wounds, and body lice. A head-to-toe examination is performed. Special attention is given to the area assaulted, that is, pelvic structures and genitalia. External genitals, thighs, buttocks, and lower abdomen are assessed, and if there are injuries, photographs may be taken or drawings made.

A speculum examination (without lubricant, but warm water may be used for comfort) is performed gently to detect tears or bruises and to collect appropriate specimens. The cervix may be scraped for *Neisseria gonorrhoeae*, *Chlamydia* organisms, and herpes simplex virus, and vaginal fluid is obtained for analysis. One slide is fixed and dried to be stained and examined for sperm. A swab of fluid is placed in saline solution for potential sperm serovaring (serologic variation), and a sample is assayed for acid phosphatase (an enzyme found in high concentrations in seminal fluid).

A bimanual pelvic examination is performed carefully to determine the size and position of the uterus and ad-

nexa. If a pelvic mass is palpated, it may be caused by bleeding into the broad ligament. If it is possible that the woman was pregnant when she was assaulted, a pregnancy test is done. Internal pelvic assessment ends with a rectovaginal examination.

Sexual assault kits that are intended to facilitate collection of specimens, particularly if they are to be used as evidence should the woman decide to report the rape, are available in most emergency departments. They give specific instructions on what specimens to collect from what body parts or articles of clothing and ways to preserve the evidence.

Laboratory tests obtained include a pregnancy test, as mentioned, and tests for syphilis, hepatitis B virus, and human immunodeficiency virus (Petter & Whitehill, 1998).

During the examination, the woman's emotional status is assessed and findings are recorded: what reactions she is exhibiting from the assault; her orientation to time and place; and her attention span, affect, and verbal description and feelings about the assault. The availability of family or peer support systems is assessed. She is asked about her plans to report or not report the crime to the police.

After the physical examination the woman should be allowed to shower and offered fresh clothes or a gown. She may be offered time to rest and to talk with the nurse, rape crisis counselor, family, or friends.

Nursing diagnoses for the rape victim during the immediate and later posttrauma periods include the following:

Nursing Diagnoses

Immediate posttrauma period
- Anxiety/fear related to
  - rape-trauma experience
  - interactions with police and caregivers
  - physical examination to assess injury and collect evidence
- Pain related to
  - physical injury from rape
  - examination
- Body-image disturbance related to
  - the rape
- Rape-trauma syndrome related to
  - aftermath of being sexually assaulted
  - feelings of uncleanliness and humiliation
  - silent reaction of being unable to discuss the rape
- Decisional conflict related to
  - discussing rape with family
  - possible pregnancy

Later posttrauma period
- Risk for infection with sexually transmitted diseases related to
  - sexual assault by an assailant of unknown sexual history
- Impaired social interaction related to
  - the rape

Immediate Care

Medical management includes (1) treating the physical injuries, including tetanus toxoid booster if indicated; (2) providing prophylactic antibiotic therapy for sexually transmitted infection (e.g., gonorrhea, syphilis); and (3) providing prophylaxis for pregnancy if the woman is not pregnant already. If physical trauma is life threatening, appropriate intervention takes precedence over collecting evidence.

If the victim is menarcheal, is using no contraception, and is at a time of high risk for pregnancy in her cycle, hormonal therapy may be prescribed for her. Approximately 5% of women who are raped become pregnant (Holmes et al., 1996). Emergency contraception (pregnancy prophylaxis) with combined estrogen and progestin pills must be used within 72 hours of the sexual assault (Lindberg, 1997) (see Table 9-2). The woman is told that the therapy can cause nausea and that she should expect withdrawal bleeding shortly after finishing the therapy. Antinausea therapy, such as prochlorperazine preparation (Compazine), may be prescribed to counter the side effects of high doses of estrogens. She is apprised of the availability of abortion or menstrual extraction as a backup measure. She has the option of continuing a pregnancy if pregnancy does occur but is warned, before she takes the drug, about the teratogenic effects of estrogen in these doses. If the woman is pregnant at the time of the assault, she should be observed for several hours for uterine contractility.

Discharge

The woman is discharged with medications and printed instructions about their use, printed instructions for self-care, and names and phone numbers of resource people should she require assistance. Money as needed and transportation to wherever she is staying (an alternative place may need to be found for her) add to the woman's comfort and perception of being in control. A medical follow-up examination in the gynecology or pediatric clinic is scheduled at 3 to 4 weeks for a repeat culture for gonorrhea, at 6 weeks for assessment of healing of injuries, and at 3 to 6 months for a repeat Venereal Disease Research Laboratories test and test for acquired immunodeficiency syndrome antibodies. Repeat tests are rescheduled as necessary. The woman and her counselor determine whether there is a need for an additional medical or psychologic follow-up examination between the scheduled visits. The woman has a choice of site for follow-up testing. Some women choose to continue with the health care provider who first performed the examination; others prefer their primary health care provider; and still others need referral to a clinic in the area (city, state) in which they live.

Documentation is a vital part of care. JCAHO indicates that medical records of victims of violence must include detailed documentation of the examinations, treatment, referral, and mandated reporting of known or suspected cases of abuse throughout the life cycle (Limandri, 1992).

After Discharge

Because of the phases of recovery, telephone contact by the health care provider to whom the woman is referred is continued until the woman has no further need for such help. Education in prevention strategies is often offered by community agencies or rape awareness groups. The focus of the classes is usually on increasing women's awareness of situations that put them at high risk for rape or sexual assault. Other courses may teach self-defense methods or how to change personal behaviors to reduce the risk of being victimized, such as avoiding being alone in isolated places and being alert to unusual activities or persons in one's environment. Still other courses may focus on changing societal attitudes about rape. Nurses can play a role in preventive education by offering courses or participating in courses offered by community or health care groups.

BOX 11-5 | **Resources for Violence Against Women**

Center for Women Policy Studies
2000 P St. NW, Suite 508
Washington, DC 20036
(202) 872-1770
(Publications and current federal legislation information)

National Child Abuse Hotline
(800) 422-4453

National Coalition Against Domestic Violence
(202) 544-7358
National Domestic Violence/Abuse Hotline:
 (800) 799-SAFE
(Many states have local coalitions against domestic violence.)

National Coalition Against Sexual Assault
912 North 2nd St.
Harrisburg, PA 17102
(717) 232-6771

National Organization for Women (NOW) Legal Defense and Education Fund
99 Hudson St.
New York, NY 10013-2871
(212) 925-6635

National Resource Center for Domestic Violence
(800) 537-2238

The National Center on Women and Family Law
799 Broadway, Room 402
New York, NY 10003
(212) 674-8200
(Legal information)

RESOURCES

Numerous national and local organizations provide information and assistance for women experiencing abusive situations, and both nurses and clients may find these resources helpful. All nurses who work in women's health care should become familiar with local services and legal options. See Box 11-5 for a listing of national resources and hotlines.

KEY POINTS

- Violence against women is a major social and health care problem in the United States, costing billions of dollars in direct and indirect health care costs.
- Domestic violence includes physical, sexual, emotional, psychologic, and economic abuse.
- Nurses must increase awareness of their own beliefs and values regarding victimization of women.
- Theoretic frameworks—psychologic, sociologic, biologic, and feminist perspectives—provide the foundation for understanding the complexity of victimization of women.
- Cultural influences regarding violent behaviors and relationships sensitize the nurse to the special needs of ethnic women.
- Battering affects all races; all socioeconomic, educational, and religious groups; and pregnant women.
- All states have mandatory reporting of abuse toward children and elderly people; some states have initiated mandatory reporting of wife abuse.
- *Rape* is a legal term meaning a violent, aggressive sexual assault against one's will.
- Nurses in all professional arenas must respond with sensitivity and caring toward women who experience abuse and victimization.

CRITICAL THINKING EXERCISES

1 *The adolescent daughter of a friend of the nurse asks the nurse numerous questions about how one knows if one is being abused in a dating or "steady" relationship. With some gentle probing, the nurse determines that extensive control and emotional abuse are occurring in the daughter's relationship.*
   a *What would the nurse do with this information in relation to (1) the adolescent daughter and (2) the nurse's friend, who is the daughter's mother?*

2 *Design a class or a program for adolescents on date violence and rape. What information would the nurse include? What questions would the nurse pose to engage adolescents in a discussion about their rights in dating situations? Role play how to say no in sexual encounters.*

3 *Determine dilemmas that may occur between the nurse's legal accountability and respect for the rights of a rape victim who chooses not to pursue legal action. Describe how the nurse would resolve the conflict.*

4 *Design a brochure for the Spanish-speaking population about the victimization of women to be distributed at a women's health fair in your community.*

References

Aguilera, D. (1994). *Crisis intervention: Theory and methodology* (7th ed.). St. Louis: Mosby.

American Psychiatric Association. (1994). *Diagnostic and statistical manual of mental disorders* (4th ed.). Washington, DC: American Psychiatric Association.

Barrier, P. (1998). Domestic violence. *Mayo Clin Proc* 73, 271-274.

Berlinger, J. (1998). Answers to questions about domestic violence. "Why don't you just leave him?" *Nursing 98* 28(4), 34-39.

Bohn, D. (1993). Nursing care of Native American battered women. *AWHONN Clin Issues Perinat Women's Health Nurs* 4(3), 424-436.

Buel, S., & Harvard, J. (1995). Family violence: Practical recommendations for physicians and the medical community. *Women's Health Issues* 5(4), 158-172.

Bullock, L. (1993). Nursing interventions for abused women on obstetrical units. *AWHONN Clin Issues Perinat Women's Health Nurs* 4(3), 371-377.

Burgess, A., & Holmstrom, L. (1986). *Rape, crisis, and recovery.* West Newton, MA: Awab.

Campbell, D. (1993). Nursing care of African-American battered women: Afrocentric perspectives. *AWHONN Clin Issues Perinat Women's Health Nurs* 4(3), 407-415.

Campbell, J. (1997, April). Educational seminar notes. The University of North Carolina, School of Public Health. Chapel Hill, NC.

Campbell, J., & Fishwick, N. (1993). Abuse of female partners. In J. Campbell & J. Humphreys (Eds.). *Nursing care of survivors of family violence.* St. Louis: Mosby.

Campbell, J., & Humphreys, J. (1993). *Nursing care of survivors of family violence.* St. Louis: Mosby.

Campbell, J., & Landenburger, K. (1995). Violence against women. In C. Fogel & N. Woods (Eds.). *Women's health care.* Thousand Oaks, CA: Sage.

Campbell, J., Oliver, C., & Bullock, L. (1993). Why battering during pregnancy? *AWHONN Clin Issues Perinat Women's Health Nurs* 4(3), 343-349.

Campbell, J. et al. (1992). Correlates of battering during pregnancy. *Res Nurs Health* 15, 219-226.

Campbell, J. et al. (1995). The influence of abuse on pregnancy intention. *Women's Health Issues* 5(4), 214-223.

Chez, R., & Jones, R. (1995). The battered woman. *Am J Obstet Gynecol* 173(1), 677-679.

Curry, M. (1998). The interrelationships between abuse, substance use, and psychosocial stress during pregnancy. *J Obstet Gynecol Neonatal Nurs* 27(6), 692-699.

Dunn, S., & Guilchrist, V. (1993). Sexual assault. *Prim Care* 20(2), 359-373.

Else, L. et al. (1993). Personality characteristics of men who physically abuse women. *Hosp Comm Psychiatry* 44(1), 54-58.

Fishel, A., & Rynerson, B. (1998). Domestic violence and family interdependence. *Aggression and Violent Behavior* 3(3), 295-301.

Fishwick, N. (1995). Getting to the heart of the matter: Nursing assessment and intervention with battered women in psychiatric mental health settings. *J Am Psychiatr Nurses Assoc* 1(2), 48.

Fishwick, N. (1998). Assessment of women for partner abuse. *J Obstet Gynecol Neonatal Nurs* 27(6), 661-670.

Gallop, R. et al. (1995). The impact of childhood sexual abuse on the psychological well-being and practice of nurses. *Arch Psychiatr Nurs* 9(3), 137-145.

Garza-Trevino, E. (1994). Neurobiological factors in aggressive behavior. *Hosp Comm Psychiatry* 45(7), 690-699.

Gelles, R. (1993). Through a sociological lens: Social structure and family violence. In R. Gelles & D. Loseke (Eds.). *Current controversies on family violence.* Newbury Park, CA: Sage.

Gelles, R. (1995). *Contemporary families: A sociological view.* Thousand Oaks, CA: Sage.

Gelles, R., & Loseke, D. (1993). *Current controversies on family violence.* Thousand Oaks, CA: Sage.

Hadley, S. et al. (1995). Womankind: An innovative model of health care response to domestic abuse. *Women's Health Issues* 5(4), 189-198.

Hampton, D. (1995). Care of the woman who has been raped. *N Engl J Med* 332, 234-237.

Hanrahan, P., Campbell, J., & Ulrich, Y. (1993). Theories of violence. In J. Campbell & J. Humphreys (Eds.). *Nursing care of survivors of family violence.* St. Louis: Mosby.

Harper-Jacques, S., & Reimer, M. (1992). Aggressive behavior and the brain: A different perspective for the mental health nurse. *Arch Psychiatr Nurs* 6(5), 312-320.

Helton, A. (1987). *A protocol of care for the battered woman.* White Plains, NY: March of Dimes Birth Defects Foundation.

Heritage, C. (1998). Working with childhood sexual abuse survivors during pregnancy, labor, and birth. *J Obstet Gynecol Neonatal Nurs* 27(6), 671-676.

Holmes, M., Resnick, H., Kilpatrick, D., & Best, C. (1996). Rape-related treatment: Estimates and descriptive characteristics from a national sample of women. *Am J Obstet Gynecol* 175, 320-325.

Holtz, H., & Furniss, K. (1993). The health care provider's role in domestic violence. *Trends Health Care Law Ethics* 8(2), 47-53.

Hulme, P., & Grove, S. (1994). Symptoms of female survivors of child sexual abuse. *Issues Ment Health Nurs* 15, 519-532.

Humphreys, W., & Findlater, J. (1993). The nurse and the legal system. In J. Campbell & J. Humphreys (Eds.). *Nursing care of survivors of family violence.* St. Louis: Mosby.

Hunter, J. (1991). A comparison of the psychological maladjustment of adult males and females sexually molested as children. *J Interpersonal Violence* 6(2), 205.

Landenburger, K. (1993). Exploration of women's identity: Clinical approaches with abused women. *AWHONN Clin Issues Perinat Women's Health Nurs* 4(3), 378-384.

Landenburger, K. (1998). The dynamics of leaving and recovering from an abusive relationship. *J Obstet Gynecol Neonatal Nurs* 27(6), 700-706.

Lenehan, G. (1991). Sexual assault nurse examiners: A SANE way to care for rape victims. *J Emerg Nurs* 17(1), 1-2.

Leserman, J., Stewart, J., & Dell, D. (1999). Sexual and physical abuse predicts poor health in pregnancy and postpartum. *Psychosom Med* 61, 92.

Limandri, B. (1992). Joint Commission sets abuse guidelines. *Nurs Network Violence Against Women Newslett* 3(1).

Lindberg, C. (1997). Emergency contraception: The nurse's role in providing postcoital options. *J Obstet Gynecol Neonatal Nurs* 26(2), 145-152.

McFarlane, J. (1993). Abuse during pregnancy: The horror and the hope. *AWHONN Clin Issues Perinat Women's Health Nurs* 4(3), 350-362.

McFarlane, J. et al. (1999). Severity of abuse before and during pregnancy for African-American, Hispanic, and Anglo women. *J Nurse Midwifery* 44(2), 139-144.

O'Leary, D. (1993). Through a psychological lens: Personality traits, personality disorders, and levels of violence. In R. Gelles & D. Loseke (Eds.). *Current controversies on family violence.* Newbury Park, CA: Sage.

Orange County Rape Crisis Center (1995). *Date and acquaintance rape.* Chapel Hill, NC: Author.

Parker, B. (1993). Abuse of adolescents: What can we learn from pregnant teenagers? *AWHONN Clin Issues Perinat Women's Health Nurs* 4(3), 363-370.

Parker, B., & McFarlane, J. (1991). Identifying and helping battered pregnant women. *MCN Am J Matern Child Nurs* 16, 161-164.

Parker, B., McFarlane, J., & Soeken, K. (1994). Abuse during pregnancy: Effects on maternal complications and birth weight in adult and teenage women. *Obstet Gynecol* 84(3), 323-328.

Petter, L., & Whitehill, D. (1998). Management of female sexual assault. *Am Fam Physician* 58(4), 920-926, 929-930.

Phillips, D. (1998). Culture and systems of oppression in abused women's lives. *J Obstet Gynecol Neonatal Nurs* 27(6), 678-683.

Ryan, J., & King, M. (1998). Scanning for violence. *AWHONN Lifelines* 2(3), 36-41.

Rynerson, B., & Fishel, A. (1993). Domestic violence prevention training: Participant characteristics and treatment outcomes. *J Fam Violence* 8(3), 253-266.

Silva, C. et al. (1997). Symptoms of posttraumatic stress disorder in abused women in a primary care setting. *J Womens Health* 6(5), 543-552.

Stuart G., & Laraia, M. (1998). *Stuart and Sundeen's principles and practice of psychiatric nursing* (6th ed.). St. Louis: Mosby.

Tjadn, P., & Thoennes, N. (1998). *Prevalence, incidence and consequences of violence against women: Findings from the national violence against women survey.* U.S. Department of Justice Research in Brief, November. Washington, DC: U.S. Department of Justice.

Torres, S. (1993). Nursing care of low-income battered Hispanic pregnant women. *AWHONN Clin Issues Perinat Women's Health Nurs* 4(3), 416-423.

Urbanic, J. (1993). Intrafamilial sexual abuse. In J. Campbell & J. Humphreys (Eds.). *Nursing care of survivors of family violence.* St. Louis: Mosby.

Walker, L. (1979). *The battered woman.* New York: Harper & Row.

Walker, L. (1984). *The battered woman syndrome* (Vol 6). New York: Springer.

Walker, L. (1993). The battered woman syndrome in a psychological consequence of abuse. In R. Gelles & D. Loseke (Eds.). *Current controversies on family violence.* Newbury Park, CA: Sage.

Warren, J., & Lanning, W. (1992). Sex role beliefs, control, and social isolation of battered women. *J Fam Violence* 7(1), 1.

Yllo, K. (1993). Through a feminist lens: Gender, power, and violence. In R. Gelles & D. Loseke (Eds.). *Current controversies on family violence.* Newbury Park, CA: Sage.

12

Problems of the Breast

Linda H. Snell

LEARNING OBJECTIVES

- Define the key terms.
- Discuss the pathophysiology of selected benign breast conditions and malignant neoplasms of the breast found in women.
- Discuss the emotional effect of benign and malignant neoplasms.
- Develop a nursing plan of care for the woman with a lump in her breast.

- Identify critical elements for teaching clients with selected procedures and medical-surgical management of benign or malignant neoplasms of the breast.
- Identify topics for nursing research related to breast cancer.

KEY TERMS

adjuvant chemotherapy
autologous flap reconstruction
benign tumors
cancer
fibroadenoma
fibrocystic change

galactorrhea
intraductal papilloma
lipoma
lumpectomy
malignant tumors
mammary duct ectasia

mammography
metastasis
modified radical mastectomy
neoplasm
tamoxifen

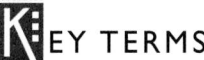

The term *neoplasia* refers to the growth of new tissue, also termed a *tumor* or **neoplasm,** that serves no physiologic function. These tumors can be either benign or malignant. **Benign tumors** usually do not endanger life, tend to grow slowly, and are not invasive. **Malignant tumors** grow rapidly in a disorganized manner and invade surrounding tissues. When this occurs, the common term used to describe this phenomenon is **cancer.**

When neoplasms occur in the female breast, there can be far-reaching effects for the woman and her family. Beyond the obvious physiologic alterations, the woman also experiences threats to her self-concept and her ability to cope. A woman's concept of herself as a sexual being can be affected by the condition and its treatments. A woman's family is also challenged in the way it responds to her diagnosis. When breast cancer occurs during or after pregnancy, it adds to the complexity of both physical and emotional responses to childbearing.

Nurses have important roles in teaching women about early detection and treatment and providing supportive care to clients and their families. This chapter presents information that will assist the nurse in providing care for women with benign breast conditions or breast cancer. Nursing care concepts related to early detection, treatment methods, and education are included. The ongoing investigations of new drug therapies to prevent breast cancer are also introduced.

BENIGN CONDITIONS OF THE BREAST

Fibrocystic Changes

Approximately 50% of women experience a breast problem at some point in their adult life. The most common benign breast problem is fibrocystic change. **Fibrocystic change** is not a disease, as previously believed, but a condition found in varying degrees in healthy women's breasts. Fibrocystic change is characterized by lumpiness, with or without tenderness, and usually occurs with changes in the menstrual cycle (Link, 1993).

Approximately 70% of fibrocystic changes are nonproliferative lesions; 26% are proliferative lesions without *atypia* (benign growing cells), and the rest are proliferative lesions with *atypical hyperplasia*. The risk of breast cancer is increased when atypical hyperplasia is present (Edge & Miller, 1994). When fibrocystic breast changes are present in a woman with a family history of breast cancer, the relative risk of breast cancer is increased (Powell & Stelling, 1994).

Etiology

No known etiologic agent is responsible for benign breast disease, although an imbalance of estrogen and progesterone may be responsible. One theory is that estrogen excess and progesterone deficiency in the luteal phase of the menstrual cycle may cause changes in breast tissue. Risk factors are associated with benign breast disease, including nulliparity, low parity, late menopause, and estrogen therapy (Powell, 1994).

Clinical Manifestations and Diagnosis

The usual clinical presentation of fibrocystic change is lumpiness in both breasts. However, single simple cysts may also occur. Symptoms usually develop about a week before menstruation begins and subside about a week after menstruation ends. When symptoms do occur, they include dull, heavy pain and a sense of fullness and tenderness that increases premenstrually (McCool, Stone-Condry, & Bradford, 1998). The woman with fibrocystic change may form cysts that manifest as painful enlarging lumps in her breasts. Cysts are common in premenopausal women who are not receiving estrogen therapy. The cysts are soft on palpation, well differentiated, and movable. Deeper cysts, especially aggregations of cysts, are indistinguishable by palpation from carcinomas, which are malignant growths that infiltrate surrounding tissue.

A first step in the workup of a breast lump is ultrasonography to determine if it is fluid filled or solid. Fluid-filled cysts are aspirated, and the woman is followed on a routine basis for development of other cysts. If the lump is solid, mammography is obtained if the woman is more

than 50 years of age. A fine-needle aspirate (FNA) is then performed, regardless of the woman's age, to determine the nature of the lump. In some cases, a core biopsy may be needed to follow FNA to harvest adequate amounts of tissue for pathologic examination (Link, 1993).

Therapeutic Management

Treatment for fibrocystic change is usually conservative and follows a two-pronged approach. Diet changes and vitamin supplements constitute the first therapy. Although still controversial, some advocate eliminating dimethylxanthines, such as caffeine and theophylline. Clients are encouraged to stop consuming coffee, cola, tea, and chocolate and discontinue certain respiratory drugs to decrease the premenstrual tenderness associated with fibrocystic changes (Love & Lindsey, 1995). Researchers have found no association among cigarette smoking, alcohol consumption, and fibrocystic changes (Powell & Stelling, 1994), although some women do report relief of symptoms by avoiding alcohol and not smoking.

Women also report decreased symptoms with such measures as taking vitamin E supplements and decreasing sodium intake or taking mild diuretics shortly before menses. Other pain relief measures include taking analgesics or nonsteroidal antiinflammatory drugs (NSAIDs) such as ibuprofen, wearing a supportive bra, and applying heat to the breasts. Some women report relief while taking oral contraceptives, but others report worsening of symptoms (Love & Lindsey, 1995).

It is important to stress that women may need to try several approaches for a number of months before improvement is noted. The recommended therapies report mostly anecdotal evidence; scientific validation of treatment strategies is lacking.

Surgical removal of nodules is attempted only in selected cases. In the presence of multiple nodules, the surgical approach involves multiple incisions and tissue manipulation and may not prevent the development of more nodules.

Fibroadenomas

The next most common benign condition of the breast that occurs is a **fibroadenoma**. Fibroadenomas occur in women from puberty through menopause. Masses are solid, encapsulated, nontender, and most often found in the upper outer quadrant of the breast.

The cause of fibroadenomas is unknown. Fibroadenomas are characterized by discrete, usually solitary lumps less than 3 cm in diameter (Link, 1993). Occasionally the woman with a fibroadenoma will experience tenderness in the tumor during the menstrual cycle (Stelling & Powell, 1994). Fibroadenomas increase in size during pregnancy and decrease in size as the woman ages. However, generally fibroadenomas do not increase in size in response to the menstrual cycle (in contrast to fibrocystic cysts). The mass tends to remain the same size or increase in size slowly over time (McCool et al., 1998).

Diagnosis is made by a review of the client history and physical examination. Mammography, ultrasonography, or magnetic resonance imaging (MRI) may be used to determine the type of lesion. FNA may be used to determine the underlying disorder. Surgical excision may be necessary if the lump is suspicious or if the symptoms are severe. Fibroadenomas do not respond to either dietary changes or hormonal therapy. Periodic observation of masses by professional physical examination or mammography may be all that is necessary for those masses not needing surgical intervention.

Lipomas

A **lipoma** is a tumor composed of fat that is soft and has discrete borders. The cause of lipoma is unknown. Lipomas are often found in women over 45 years of age. They are usually located on the chest wall and breast. They are characterized as palpable soft masses that are mobile and nontender. Mammography can be used to make a diagnosis; biopsy usually is not needed. Lipomas can be surgically excised if removal is desired (Stelling & Powell, 1994).

Nipple Discharge

Nipple discharge is a common occurrence that concerns many women. Although most nipple discharge is physiologic, each woman who has this problem must be evaluated carefully, because a small percentage will be found to have a serious endocrine disorder or malignancy. Bilateral, serous discharge expressed during nipple stimulation can be considered a normal finding. Client education and reassurance are indicated (Jardines, 1996).

Another form of breast discharge not related to malignancy is galactorrhea. **Galactorrhea** manifests as a bilaterally spontaneous, milky, sticky discharge. It is a normal finding in pregnancy. It can also occur as the result of elevated prolactin levels. Increased prolactin levels may occur as a result of a thyroid disorder, pituitary tumor, or chest wall surgery or trauma. It is essential to get a complete medication history on each client. Oral contraceptives and neuroleptic drugs are known to precipitate galactorrhea in some women. See Box 12-1 for other classes of drugs that

may be associated with galactorrhea (Hawkins, Roberto-Nichols, & Stanley-Haney, 1997; Jardines, 1996).

The optimal time to draw a prolactin level is between 8 and 10 AM. Ideally, prolactin levels should not be drawn directly after a breast examination, sexual activity, or exercise session. Other diagnostic tests that may be indicated include a microscopic analysis of the discharge from each breast, a thyroid profile, a pregnancy test, and a mammogram (Hawkins et al., 1997).

Mammary Duct Ectasia

Mammary duct ectasia is an inflammation of the ducts behind the nipple. The cause of mammary duct ectasia is unknown, although chronic inflammation and dilation of the lactiferous ducts has been suggested. It occurs most often in perimenopausal women and is characterized by a nipple discharge that is thick; sticky; and white, brown, green, or purple. Frequently the client will experience a burning pain, itching, or a palpable mass behind the nipple.

The workup includes a mammogram, aspiration of fluid, and culture of fluid. Generally, treatment is symptomatic and consists of encouraging good breast hygiene and avoidance of breast stimulation (Nettles-Carlson, 1995). Development of an infection in the inflamed area requires antibiotic therapy, and incision and drainage is necessary if an abscess develops. Treatment also may include a local excision of the affected duct or ducts if the woman has no future plans to breastfeed.

Intraductal Papilloma

Intraductal papilloma is a rare, benign condition that develops in the terminal nipple ducts. The cause is unknown. It usually occurs in women between 30 and 50 years of age. Usually too small to be palpated (less than 0.5 cm), this papilloma has the characteristic sign of nipple discharge that is serous, serosanguineous, or bloody. The discharge is unilateral and spontaneous. After the possibility of malignancy is eliminated, the affected segments of the ducts and breasts are surgically excised (McCool et al., 1998).

Table 12-1 compares common manifestations of benign breast masses.

▮ CARE MANAGEMENT

Assessment should include a careful client history and physical examination. The history should focus on risk factors for breast diseases, events related to the breast mass, and health maintenance practice. Risk factors for breast cancer are discussed later in this chapter. Information related to the breast mass should include how, when, and by whom the mass was discovered. The interval between discovery and seeking care is crucial. It is important to ask these questions because they can give clues about breast self-examination (BSE) practice and access to care. The nurse should document the following client information:

▮BOX 12-1   Drugs Associated with Galactorrhea

Estrogens, including oral contraceptives
Phenothiazines
Cimetidine
Methyldopa
Opiates
Antiemetics
Chronic use of alcohol
Marijuana

TABLE 12-1 Comparison of Common Manifestations of Benign Breast Masses

FIBROCYSTIC CHANGES	FIBROADENOMA	LIPOMA	INTRADUCTAL PAPILLOMA	MAMMARY DUCT ECTASIA
Multiple lumps	Single lump	Single lump	Single or multiple	Mass behind nipple
Nodular	Well delineated	Well delineated	Not well delineated	Not well delineated
Palpable	Palpable	Palpable	Nonpalpable	Palpable
Movable	Movable	Movable	Nonmobile	Nonmobile
Round, smooth	Round, lobular	Round, lobular	Small, ball-like	Irregular
Firm or soft	Firm	Soft	Firm or soft	Firm
Tenderness influenced by menstrual cycle	Usually asymptomatic	Nontender	Usually nontender	Painful, burning itching
Bilateral	Unilateral	Unilateral	Unilateral	Unilateral
May or may not have nipple discharge	No nipple discharge	No nipple discharge	Serous or bloody nipple discharge	Thick, sticky nipple discharge

pain, whether symptoms increase with menses, dietary habits, smoking habits, use of oral contraceptives, regular BSE, and the examination technique used. The client's emotional status, including her stress level, fears, and concerns, and her ability to cope should also be assessed.

Physical examination may include assessment of the breasts for symmetry, masses (size, number, consistency, mobility), and nipple discharge.

Nursing actions might include the following:
- Demonstrate correct BSE technique (see Chapter 6).
- Discuss the intervals for and facets of breast screening, including professional examination and mammography.
- Provide written educational materials.
- Encourage the verbalization of fears and concerns about treatment and prognosis.
- Provide specific information regarding the woman's condition and treatment, including dietary changes, drug therapy, comfort measures, stress management, and surgery.
- Describe pain-relieving strategies in detail, and collaborate with the primary health care provider to ensure effective pain control.
- Encourage discussion of feelings about body image.
- Refer to a support group or stress management resource if needed to cope with long-term consequences of benign breast conditions.

MALIGNANT CONDITIONS OF THE BREAST

The United States has one of the highest rates of breast carcinoma in the world. One in eight American women will develop breast cancer in her lifetime. Statistics released from the American Cancer Society (1999a) indicate that breast cancer incidence rose about 4% per year since 1980 and has leveled off in the 1990s to about 110 cases per 100,000 women. Rising incidence may be related to better detection of early-stage breast cancer.

The incidence of breast cancer is higher in Caucasian women than in African-American women, but the mortality rate for African-American women with breast cancer is higher. More African-American women are initially diagnosed with a later stage of breast cancer (Figs. 12-1 and 12-2) (National Cancer Institute, 1999a). African-American women have been found to practice BSE and obtain clinical breast examinations and mammograms by a professional with a frequency the same as or greater than that of Caucasian women (Douglass et al., 1995).

Etiology

Although the exact cause of breast cancer continues to elude investigators, certain factors that increase a woman's risk for developing a malignancy have been identified. These factors are listed in Box 12-2.

The most important predictor of risk for breast cancer is age. Each woman's risk of breast cancer increases as her age increases. Most of the other risk factors involve the effects of the menstrual-reproductive cycle (probably the effect of estrogen or progesterone) on the development of breast cancer. Fewer menstrual cycles and early childbearing appear to have a protective effect (McCool et al., 1998). Another important variable appears to be related to diet, weight, and exercise. Maintaining normal weight, eating a diet rich in fruits and vegetables and low in fat, and regular exercise seem to exert a protective effect against the development of breast cancer (Henderson, 1995; Nicholson, 1996; Stoll, 1996).

Although most breast cancers are not related to genetic factors, the identification of the BRCA 1 and BRCA 2 genes has demonstrated the role of heredity and genetic mutations in this disease. Only about 5% of all breast cancers are attributed to heredity, but it is believed that a higher percentage of women with breast cancer before age 40 have abnormalities in the BRCA 1 and BRCA 2 genes (Daudt, Alberg, & Helzlsouer, 1996).

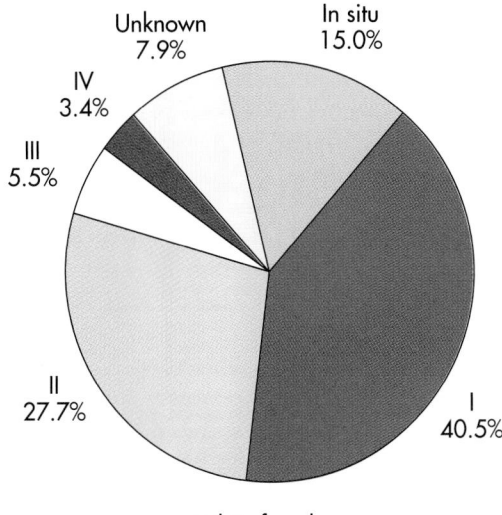

White females

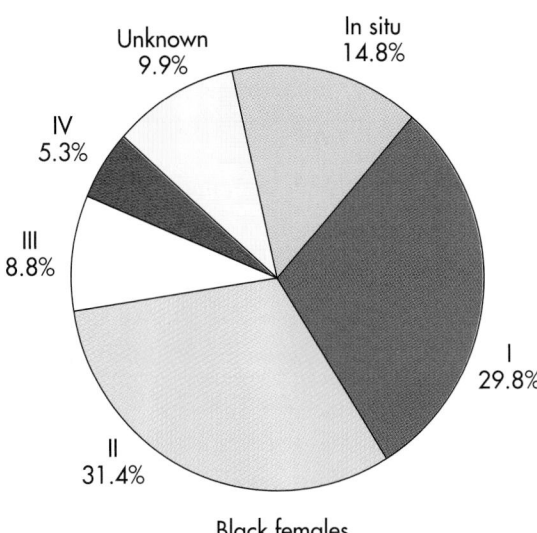

Black females

Fig. 12-1 Breast cancer stage distribution, 1995. *(Courtesy National Cancer Institute, Washington, DC.)*

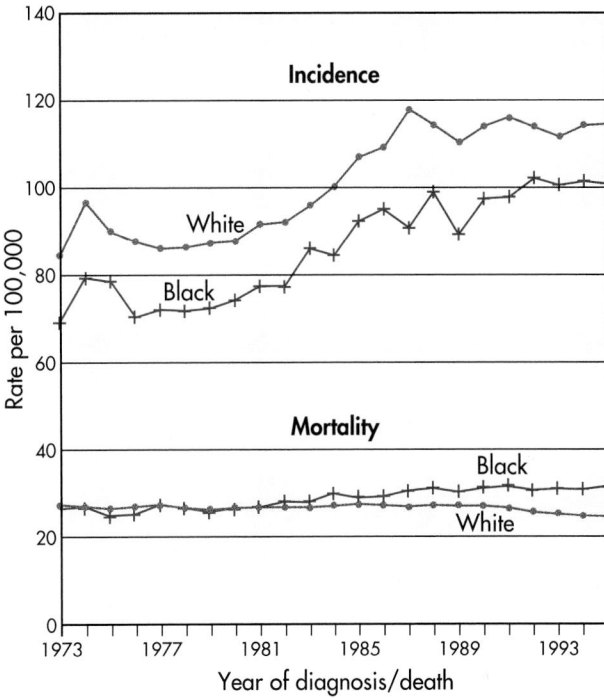

Fig. 12-2 Breast cancer incidence and mortality rates—Caucasian females vs. African-American females. *(Courtesy National Cancer Institute, Washington, DC.)*

ETHICAL CONSIDERATIONS

The ability to test for BRCA 1 and BRCA 2 has generated heated ethical debate within the health care community. Testing is expensive and often not covered by insurance. Who should be tested and who should pay for it has not been addressed adequately. What to do when a positive result is discovered is not universally agreed upon. Women and their families will most likely have increased anxiety after a positive finding. How often should screening be performed? Should prophylactic mastectomies be recommended? Will there be employment discrimination if this information is in a woman's medical record? Women requesting testing must be fully informed of the possible risks and benefits of testing before consenting to the procedure (Burke et al., 1997).

BOX 12-2 Risk Factors for Breast Cancer*

Age
Previous history of breast cancer
Family history of breast cancer, especially a mother or sister (particularly significant if premenopausally)
Previous history of ovarian, endometrial, colon, or thyroid cancer
Early menarche (before age 12)
Late menopause (after age 55)
Nulliparity or first pregnancy after age 30
Use of estrogen replacement therapy
Daily alcohol use
Obesity after menopause
Previous history of benign breast disease with epithelial hyperplasia
Race (Caucasian women have highest incidence)
High socioeconomic status
Sedentary lifestyle

*Risk factors are cumulative–the more risk factors present, the greater the likelihood of breast cancer occurring.

Research has been ongoing into the possible psychosocial risk factors for cancer. Hilakivi-Clarke and colleagues (1993) proposed that the number of stressful events a person has experienced and their significance to that person, an individual's personality characteristics, and social support all affect an ability to cope with stress. The authors suggest that stress in life, especially early in life, may influence carcinogenesis.

There has been much discussion about possible links between breast cancer and hormonal therapy. Although studies are conflicting, a number of researchers believe there may be an increased risk of breast cancer associated with the use of estrogen therapies (Helzlsouer & Couzi, 1995). Isaacs and Swain (1994) describe the reluctance to prescribe exogenous hormone therapy for healthy women as related to four factors: (1) evidence that estrogen and progesterone do help some breast tumors develop and grow, (2) the known hormonal risk factors for breast cancer, (3) the negative effect that obesity (which is common in women receiving hormone therapy) can have on breast cancer prognosis, and (4) the positive effect of ovarian ablation and tamoxifen therapy on survival of breast cancer. (*Ablation* refers to the process of stopping ovarian function through oophorectomy.) Research indicates that the safest route for women with a history of breast cancer is to avoid estrogen and progesterone replacement therapy (Isaacs & Swain, 1994).

Even with identification, risk factors help identify less than 30% of women who will eventually develop breast cancer. Two problems prevent a clear understanding of the risk factors of breast cancer. One is the long latent period, 15 to 25 years, before the development of clinically recognizable carcinoma. The other is consideration of both the duration and the intensity of factors that may induce or promote cancer. Many risk factors are additive. Although the clinical applicability of risk factors has limits, women at increased risk should be screened at more frequent intervals (McCool et al., 1998).

Pathophysiology

Breast cancer is a disease that occurs when there are genetic alterations in the deoxyribonucleic acid (DNA) of breast epithelial cells. Many types of breast cancer exist. Genetic alterations are found in the epithelial cells, compromising ductal or lobular tissue. These genetic abnormalities may have been inherited or may have developed spontaneously (Morrison, 1994). Researchers are currently investigating which oncogenes (potentially cancer-inducing genes) may cause breast cancer or change its growth pattern and how the process can be stopped.

There are ongoing studies by the National Cancer Institute of tamoxifen and raloxifene in regard to the prevention of breast cancer (National Cancer Institute, 1999b; Veronesi et al., 1998). Raloxifene prevents osteoporosis without the possible increased cancer risks of estrogen replacement. This medication may be an ideal choice for the woman at high risk for both osteoporosis and breast cancer. Tamoxifen has already been shown to reduce the recurrence of breast cancer in women with prior breast malignancies. The current prevention studies are attempting to identify which women would most benefit from preventive tamoxifen administration. Although many women may want to start tamoxifen for breast cancer prevention, the risk of occasional serious side effects demands careful consideration before prescribing tamoxifen (see later discussion).

Breast cancer begins in the epithelial cells lining the mammary ducts of the breast. The rate of breast cancer growth depends on the effect of estrogen and progesterone. These cancers can be either invasive (infiltrating) or noninvasive (in situ). Invasive or infiltrating breast cancers can grow into the wall of the mammary duct and into the surrounding tissues. By far the most frequently occurring cancer of the breast is invasive ductal carcinoma. Ductal carcinoma originates in the lactiferous ducts and forms tentacles that invade surrounding breast structures. The tumor is usually unilateral, not well delineated, solid, nonmobile, and nontender. Lobular carcinoma originates in the lobules of the breasts. It is usually bilateral and nonpalpable. Nipple carcinoma (Paget's disease) originates in the nipple. It usually occurs with invasive ductal carcinoma. Bleeding, oozing, and crusting of the nipple occur (Edge & Miller, 1994).

Breast cancer can invade surrounding tissues in such a way that the primary tumor can have tentacle-like projections. This invasive growth pattern can result in the irregular tumor border felt on palpation. As the tumor grows, fibrosis develops around it and can shorten Cooper's ligaments. When Cooper's ligaments are shortened, the result is the characteristic peau d'orange (orange skin) skin changes and edema associated with some breast cancers. If the breast cancer invades the lymphatic channels, tumors can develop in the regional lymph nodes, often occupying the axillary lymph nodes. The tumor may invade the outer layers of skin, creating ulcerations.

Metastasis results from seeding of the breast cancer cells into the blood and lymph systems, leading to tumor development in the bones, lungs, brain, and liver (Table 12-2).

Clinical Manifestations and Diagnosis

Breast cancer in its earliest form is usually detected on a mammogram before it can be felt by the woman or her health care provider. However, it is estimated that 90% of all breast lumps are detected by the client. Of this 90%, only 20% to 25% are malignant. More than half of all lumps are discovered in the upper outer quadrant of the breast (Fig. 12-3). The most common initial symptom is a lump or thickening of the breast. The lump may feel hard and fixed or soft and spongy. It may have well-defined or irregular borders. It may be fixed to the skin, thereby causing dimpling to occur. A nipple discharge that is bloody or clear also may be present.

Discharge that is unilateral and spontaneous (occurs without nipple manipulation) is associated with mastitis, intraductal papilloma, and cancer. The discharge is usually

TABLE 12-2 Stage Grouping and Stage Definitions for Breast Cancer

STAGE	PRIMARY TUMOR (T)	NODAL INVOLVEMENT (N)	DEGREE OF METASTASIS
0	T_{is}	N_0	M_0
I	T_1	N_0	M_0
IIA	T_0	N_1	M_0
	T_1	N_1	M_0
	T_2	N_0	M_0
IIB	T_2	N_1	M_0
	T_3	N_0	M_0
IIIA	T_0	N_2	M_0
	T_1	N_2	M_0
	T_2	N_2	M_0
	T_3	N_1	M_0
	T_3	N_2	M_0
IIIB	T_4	Any N	M_0
	Any T	N_3	M_0
IV	Any T	Any N	M_1

PRIMARY TUMOR (T)

T_x Primary tumor cannot be assessed

T_0 No evidence of primary tumor

T_{is} Carcinoma in situ

T_1 Tumor $\leq$ 2 cm in greatest dimension

  T_{1a} $\leq$ 0.5 cm

  T_{1b} > 0.5 cm and < 1 cm

  T_{1c} > 1 cm and < 2 cm

T_2 Tumor > 2 cm and < 5 cm

T_3 Tumor > 5 cm

T_4 Tumor of any size with direct extension to chest wall or skin

  T_{4a} Extension to chest wall

  T_{4b} Edema (including peau d'orange) or ulceration of skin or satellite skin nodules confined to same breast

  T_{4c} Both T_{4a} and T_{4b}

  T_{4d} Inflammatory carcinoma

REGIONAL LYMPH NODES (N)

N_x Regional nodes cannot be assessed

N_0 No regional node metastasis

N_1 Metastasis to movable, ipsilateral axillary lymph nodes

  N_{1a} Only micrometastasis (none larger than 0.2 cm)

  N_{1b} Metastasis to nodes larger than 0.2 cm

    N_{1bi} Metastasis in one to three nodes, > 0.2 cm and < 2 cm

    N_{1bii} Metastasis to four or more nodes, > 0.2 cm and < 2 cm

    N_{1biii} Extension of tumor beyond the capsule of a lymph node metastasis < 2 cm

    N_{1biv} Metastasis to a node $\geq$ 2 cm

N_2 Metastasis to ipsilateral axillary lymph nodes that are fixed to one another or to other structures

N_3 Metastasis to ipsilateral internal mammary lymph nodes

DISTANT METASTASIS (M)

M_x Presence of distant metastasis cannot be assessed

M_0 No distant metastasis

M_1 Distant metastasis, including metastasis to ipsilateral supraclavicular lymph nodes

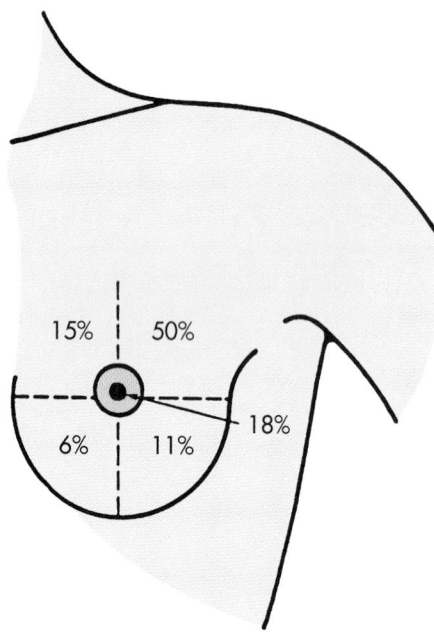

Fig. 12-3 Relative location of malignant lesions of the breast. *(Modified from DiSaia, P., & Creasman, W. [1997]. Clinical gynecologic oncology [5th ed.]. St. Louis: Mosby.)*

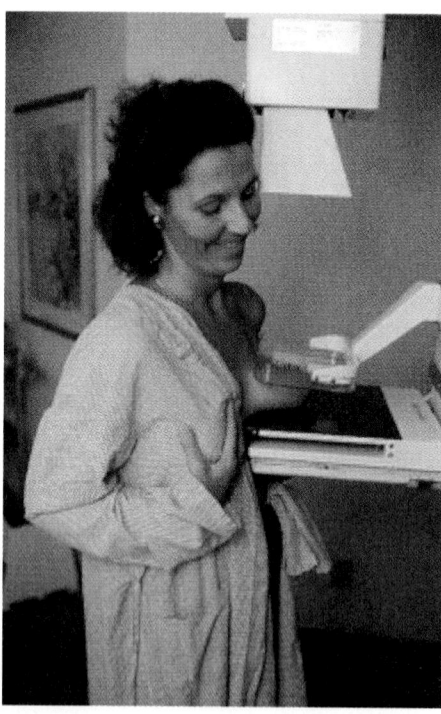

Fig. 12-4 Mammography. *(From Edge, V., & Miller, M. [1994]. Women's health care. St. Louis: Mosby.)*

intermittent and persistent. The color may be clear, serous, green-gray, purulent, serosanguineous, or sanguineous. Women with these findings need a complete diagnostic workup to determine the cause of their symptoms (Jardines, 1996; McCool et al., 1998).

TABLE 12-3	Screening Guidelines for Breast Cancer Detection in Asymptomatic Women Recommended by the American Cancer Society	
AGE	**EXAMINATION**	**FREQUENCY**
20-39	Breast self-examination (BSE)	Monthly
	Clinical breast examination	3 years
40 and older	BSE	Monthly
	Clinical breast examination	Yearly
	Mammography	Yearly

Source: American Cancer Society. (1999a). *Cancer facts and figures, 1999.* New York: American Cancer Society.

As a general principle, any breast symptom (i.e., mass, discharge, pain, or itching) that is unilateral in nature is a more ominous finding than a symptom found bilaterally. However, all findings must be carefully followed up to avoid missing a serious diagnosis such as cancer. Any delay in treatment may adversely affect the woman's subsequent prognosis and treatment options.

Early detection and diagnosis reduce the mortality rate because cancer is found when it is smaller, lesions are more localized, and there tends to be a lower percentage of positive nodes. Therefore it becomes imperative that protocols for assessment and diagnosis be established. In addition to regular BSE from midadolescence on, the use of clinical examination by a qualified health care provider and screening **mammography** (x-ray filming of the breast) (Fig. 12-4) may aid in the early detection of breast cancers. Table 12-3 lists the American Cancer Society's current recommendations for breast cancer screening.

Cultural factors may influence a woman's decision to participate in breast cancer screening. Knowledge of these factors may assist the nurse in overcoming barriers to seeking care (see Cultural Consideration box).

A number of studies have looked at factors that increase compliance with mammography guidelines. Reminder postcards, adequate insurance coverage, health care provider referral, and cancer screening interventions conducted by trained lay workers have had positive results on client breast screening activities (Sung et al., 1997; Taplin et al., 1994; Urban, Anderson, & Peacock, 1994).

In addition, it is important for a practitioner to annually assess a woman's BSE technique and frequency at the annual visit. Transillumination, thermography, and ultrasound breast imaging are being explored as methods to detect early breast carcinoma. Ultrasonography is helpful in distinguishing between solid tumors and cysts. MRI is being considered as a method of imaging to detect breast tumors in women with fibrocystic changes. It may be more effective than mammograms in detecting tumors in women with dense, fibrocystic breasts (Schneider, 1995).

Breast Screening Practices

Lower-income Hispanic women with less than a high school education were found to be more likely not to have participated in screening mammography. Reasons given by the women included fear of the test, misconceptions about cancer, embarrassment, and lack of knowledge (Fernandez, Tortolero-Luna, & Gold, 1998). Reasons African-American women report for not participating in early breast cancer screening include that breast cancer comes from "bad luck or fate," getting it is determined by a higher being, fear of gynecologic examinations, and not believing in vulnerability to cancer because no one in their family has had cancer (Lawson, 1998).

African-American women and Hispanic women were more likely to participate in clinical breast examination and mammography screening when it was offered in a mobile van in their neighborhood (Schweitzer et al., 1998). In Chinese women, a perceived lack of competence in performance of breast self-examination (BSE) may have influenced Chinese women's BSE practice (Li, 1994).

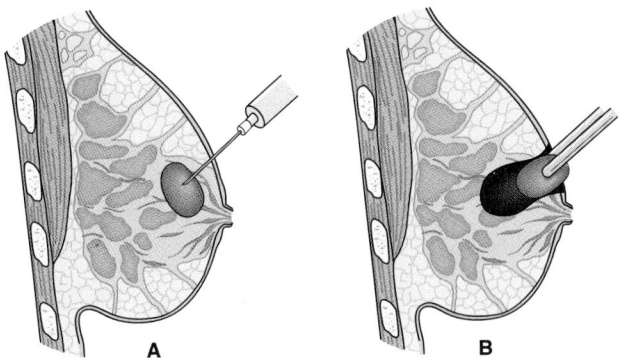

Fig. 12-5 Diagnosis. **A,** Needle aspiration. **B,** Open biopsy. *(Redrawn from National Women's Health Resource Center. [1995]. Breast health.* National Women's Health Report *13[5], 3.)*

A promising, less invasive approach to the diagnosis of breast cancer is currently being tested. On the cellular level, electrical disturbances are caused by cancer cells. Electropotential measurements of these disturbances on the skin are measured and analyzed as to whether they are consistent with those associated with cancer. After further research, it is hoped that these results will guide the health care provider in determining whether or not to proceed with a biopsy, thus saving many women from an unnecessary, painful, and upsetting procedure (Cuzick et al., 1998).

When a suspicious mammogram is noted or a lump is detected, diagnosis is confirmed by FNA or by a needle localization biopsy (Fig. 12-5). The latter procedure requires the collaborative efforts of both the radiologist and the surgeon. This often requires that the procedure take place in two different environments (radiology and surgery). Therefore clients need specific information regarding procedures, duration, and outcomes.

Analysis of cells from breast fluid offers more information to the professional. If atypical cells are present in the fluid, the lump should be removed because there is a higher chance of cancer being present (Link, 1993).

Laboratory diagnosis of breast cancer and possible cancer metastasis includes complete blood count, liver enzyme levels, serum calcium level, and alkaline phosphatase level. Elevated liver enzyme levels indicate possible liver metastasis, and increased serum calcium and alkaline phosphatase levels indicate bone metastasis.

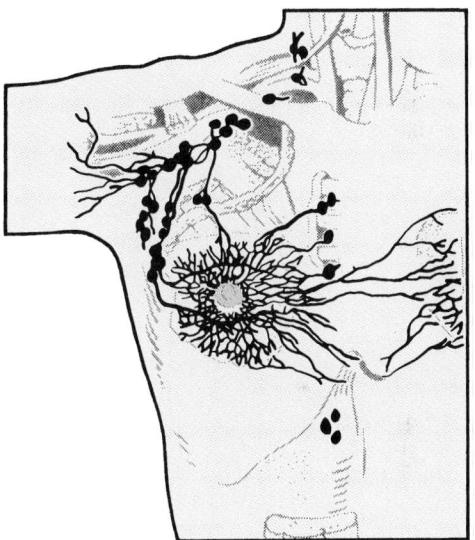

Fig. 12-6 Lymphatic spread of breast cancer.

Prognosis

Major advances in the understanding of the biology of cancer have occurred in the past 10 years. Many studies now support the theory that breast cancer is a systemic disease, which means that micrometastasis could be present at the initial presentation with or without nodal involvement (Fiorica, 1997). The area in which affected lymph nodes are located is also prognostic. The closer the lymph nodes are to the shoulder joint, the worse is the prognosis. Nodal involvement and tumor size, however, remain the most significant prognostic criteria for long-term survival (Fig. 12-6).

Other biologic factors have been shown to be helpful in predicting response to therapy or survival. These biologic factors include estrogen receptor assay, progesterone receptor assay, tumor *ploidy* (the amount of DNA in a tumor cell when compared with a normal cell), S-phase index or

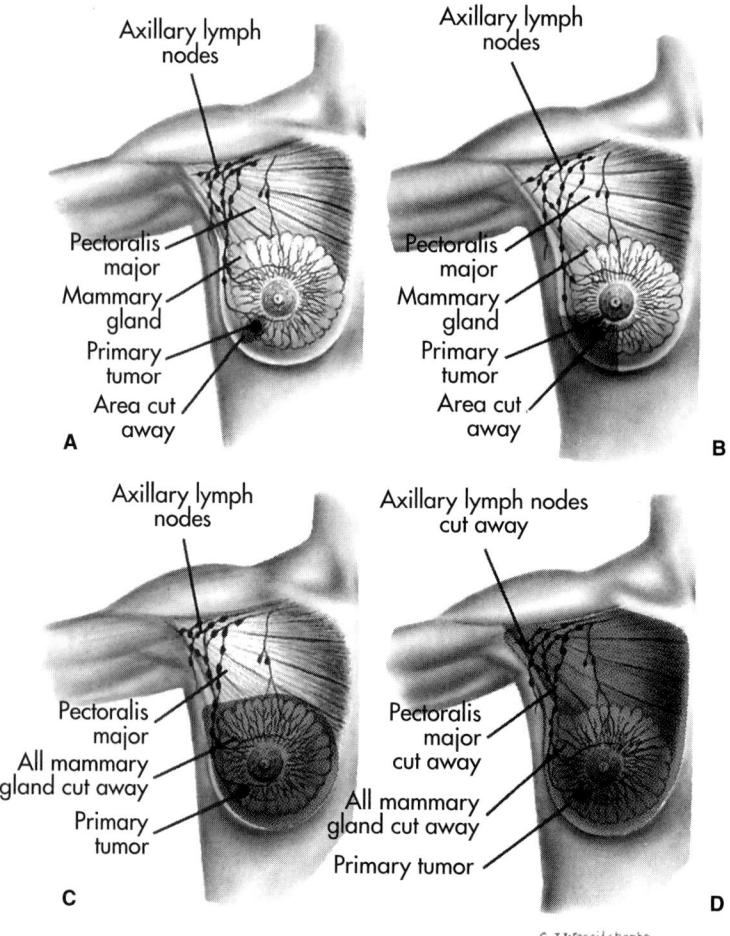

Fig. 12-7   Surgical alternatives for breast cancer. **A,** Lumpectomy (tylectomy). **B,** Quadrectomy (segmental resection). **C,** Total (simple) mastectomy. **D,** Radical mastectomy.

growth rate (done by flow cytometric determinations of the S-phase fraction), and histologic or nuclear grade (Fiorica, 1997). Estrogen and progesterone receptors are proteins in the cell cytoplasm and surface of some breast cancer cells. When these receptors are present, they bind to estrogen or progesterone, and binding promotes growth of the cancer cell. A breast cancer can have estrogen or progesterone receptors or both types. More postmenopausal women are found to be estrogen receptor (ER) positive than premenopausal women (Early Breast Cancer Trialists' Collaborative Group, 1992). Women with ER-positive tumors respond better to therapy and have higher survival rates.

Nuclear grade describes the degree of abnormalities present in the cancer cell tubules, nuclei morphology, and mitotic rates. Tumors with a high nuclear grade tend to have a large number of cells in mitosis and a high S-phase fraction. Tumors with a high S-phase fraction have a large number of cells in the synthesis phase of cell development. If a tumor has high numbers of cells in synthesis and preparing for mitosis and many cells in mitosis, it is

growing at a fast rate, is considered aggressive, and carries a poor prognosis. Cancer cells possess altered DNA content. The DNA content of breast cancer cells is analyzed to predict prognosis. Cells with a greater degree of altered DNA content are termed *aneuploid.* High nuclear grade, high S-phase fraction, and aneuploid tumor cells are all indicators of high risk for relapse (Fiorica, 1997).

Therapeutic Management

Medical management of breast cancer includes surgery, breast reconstruction, radiation therapy, and adjuvant hormone therapy and chemotherapy.

Surgery

The woman with breast cancer is usually diagnosed through the use of an FNA or incisional biopsy in an outpatient setting. After the diagnosis is made, surgical treatment options are offered to the woman. The most frequently recommended surgical approaches for the treatment of breast cancer are lumpectomy and modified radical mastectomy (Fig. 12-7). **Lumpectomy,** also termed

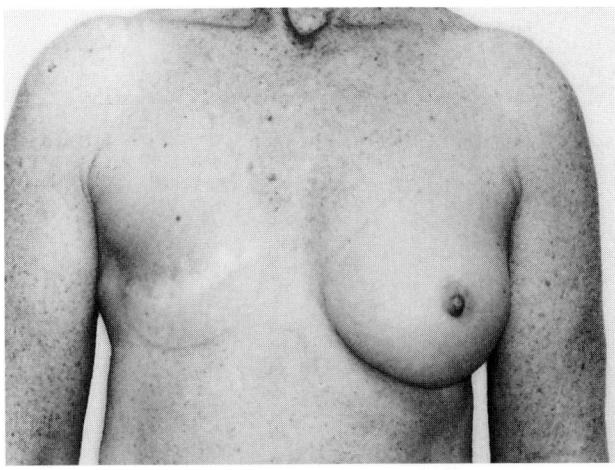

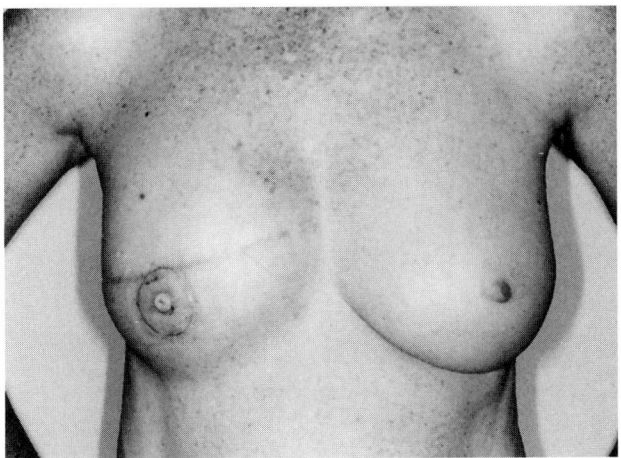

Fig. 12-8 Latissimus dorsi reconstruction after radical mastectomy.

tylectomy, partial mastectomy, or *segmental mastectomy,* involves the removal of the breast tumor, a small amount of surrounding tissue, and a sampling of axillary lymph nodes, leaving the pectoralis major muscle intact. This surgery is now used instead of the modified radical mastectomy for the primary treatment of the majority of women with early-stage (I or II) breast cancer. Lumpectomy offers survival equivalent to modified radical mastectomy and breast preservation (National Institutes of Health, 1990).

Modified radical mastectomy is the removal of the entire breast and a sample of lymph nodes, sparing the pectoral muscles. Mastectomy is used for the treatment of early-stage breast cancer when the woman fits the criteria listed in Box 12-3. Women who are found to have metastatic breast cancer at the time of diagnosis usually do not have a mastectomy because it does not offer increased chances of survival.

Women who have these surgeries experience cosmetic changes. Change in shape (because of lumpectomy) or loss of a breast results in a change in body image, which can cause significant alterations in perceptions of femininity and sexual image and interest (Fiorica, 1997).

Breast Reconstruction

The goals of surgical breast reconstruction are achievement of symmetry and preservation of body image (Fig. 12-8). Surgical reconstruction can be done immediately or at a later date. Immediate reconstruction at the time of mastectomy does not change survival rates or interfere with therapy or the treatment of recurrent disease (Hacker, 1998). It is important that women be aware of this information. Women choosing surgical reconstruction offer the following rationale for reconstructive surgery: the need to feel complete again, to avoid using an external prosthesis, to achieve symmetry, to decrease self-consciousness about appearance, and to enhance femininity (Fiorica, 1997).

Autologous flap reconstruction involves the use of the woman's own tissue to create a breast. Using the woman's own tissue results in a more natural shape. There are three types of autologous flaps: the latissimus dorsi flap, the transverse rectus abdominis myocutaneous (TRAM) flap,

and the inferior gluteus free flap. The latissimus dorsi and TRAM flaps are the most common ones used (Fig. 12-9). The latissimus flap consists of skin, fat, and muscle separated from the upper back, passed through an incision in the breast area, and attached to this area (Kroll, 1998). The TRAM flap consists of a portion of skin and fat harvested from the abdominal wall and used to reconstruct the chest area (Bostwick, 1995; Ivey & Gordon, 1994). When these flaps are used for construction, adequate blood supply to the reconstructed tissue is a major concern. For this reason, plastic surgeons are careful not to offer this option to women who may be at high risk for complications. Women at high risk for complications include those with extensive, locally invasive breast cancers, extensive chest wall disease, metastatic breast cancer, diabetes mellitus, poorly controlled pulmonary disease, or hypertension (Fiorica, 1997). Women who smoke tobacco or are obese are also at high risk for complications. After the reconstruction is done, postoperative care specific to these procedures focuses on monitoring the skin flap for signs of decreased capillary refill, hematoma, infection, and necrosis.

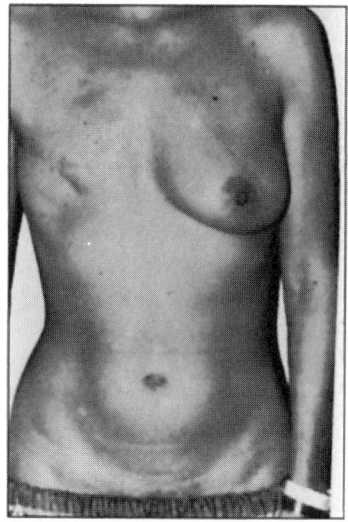 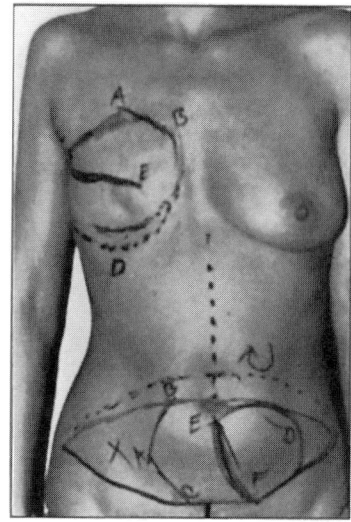 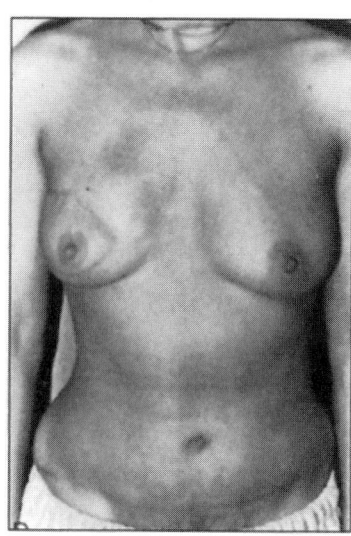

Fig. 12-9   TRAM flap reconstruction. *(From Harden, J., & Girard, N. [1994]. Breast reconstruction using an innovative flap procedure. AORN J 60[2], 184-192.)*

Standard mastectomy activity restrictions and client education points are also followed.

Another method of surgical reconstruction involves creating a breast mound with a saline-filled tissue expander implanted under the muscle or an autologous flap of the client's own tissue. Breast reconstruction using implants is not a good option for women with inadequate skin coverage, changes in muscle innervation, or a large, pendulous contralateral breast. Tissue expanders are a less often used option for breast reconstruction. The positive aspects of using tissue expanders for reconstruction include decreased time needed for insertion, ease of insertion, and no need for repeated surgeries (unless nipple reconstruction is done) (Ivey & Gordon, 1994). The tissue expander is slowly filled with saline, through an injection port, over a period of months, to stretch the skin gradually until the desired symmetry is attained (Hinojosa, 1991). Ongoing emotional support is needed for women who choose this option, because they often become impatient waiting for the implant to be totally filled or are self-conscious about the uneven appearance of their breasts. Depending on the type of implant used, the client may need to massage the implant area on a regular basis to encourage stretching of the skin and prevent firmness (Hinojosa, 1991). After each saline injection, the woman experiences mild discomfort, which is easily relieved with acetaminophen. As with all implantation procedures, risks of surgical complications such as hematoma, infection, and delayed wound healing are possible, as well as the possibility of capsular contractions from or leakage of the implant (Knopf, 1996).

The safety of silicone breast implants has been questioned. They may be used only in Food and Drug Administration protocols that are restricted mainly to reconstruction (Logothetis, 1995). Women interested in these implants should understand all the risks before making a decision (Schumann, 1994).

At the time of reconstruction or after the client has recovered from initial reconstructive surgery, she may choose to have nipple and areolar reconstruction. The three methods of nipple and areolar reconstruction are (1) removing and using the client's nipple from the affected breast, (2) using autologous tissue to construct a nipple, or (3) tattooing the client to create the appearance of a nipple (Bhatty & Berry, 1997).

Radiation

A conservative approach to treatment involves lumpectomy followed by radiation therapy. It should be noted that not all women are candidates for this approach. It is reserved for women with noninvasive or microinvasive cancer or any histologic grade, invasive ductal carcinoma, or lobular carcinoma less than 1 cm in diameter (Hortobagyi & Buzdar, 1995). For these women, the lumpectomy with radiation has demonstrated the same survival rate as other surgical techniques while preserving the breast tissue (DiSaia & Creasman, 1997).

Adjuvant Therapy

Chemotherapy administered soon after initial diagnosis and surgical removal of the tumor is referred to as **adjuvant chemotherapy.** Adjuvant chemotherapy has been found to be most useful in premenopausal women who have breast cancer with positive nodes. For these women, treatment with adjuvant chemotherapy often increases the length of time a woman with breast cancer lives and may increase the length of time she is free of disease (Early Breast Cancer Trialists' Collaborative Group, 1992; Hacker, 1998). Adjuvant chemotherapy may be given alone or with hormonal therapy.

Hormonal therapy. To determine whether a woman is a candidate for hormonal therapy, a receptor assay must be done. After the entire tumor or a portion is removed by biopsy or excision, cancer cells are examined by a pathologist for estrogen and progesterone receptors.

When a certain type of receptor is present on the cell wall, it is said that the woman is receptor positive for that type of hormone receptor. If these receptors are present, the growth of the woman's breast cancer may be influenced by estrogen, progesterone, or both. It is unknown exactly how these hormones affect breast cancer growth. Some women less than 50 years of age may undergo bilateral oophorectomy to decrease the supply of hormones available for tumor growth (Early Breast Cancer Trialists' Collaborative Group, 1992; Hacker, 1998). This is done to decrease the odds of recurrence and increase length of survival. Many physicians do not offer this procedure as a treatment option because many women's ovaries stop functioning when chemotherapy is administered. In addition to or instead of oophorectomy, medications may be given to stop tumor growth that is influenced by hormones.

Tamoxifen is an oral antiestrogen medication that mimics progesterone and estrogen. Tamoxifen attaches to the hormone receptors on cancer cells and prevents natural hormones from attaching to the receptors (McKeon, 1997). When tamoxifen fits into the receptors, the cell is unable to grow. Adjuvant hormonal therapy using tamoxifen is recommended for all women over 50 years of age. For these women, adjuvant tamoxifen therapy improves disease-free survival and in some cases length of survival. It is clear that women treated with hormonal therapy should keep receiving the therapy for at least 2 years, but it is uncertain when therapy should end (Fisher et al., 1994). Use for 5 years is current practice. Hormonal therapy for women under age 50 is still controversial. The side effects of hormonal therapy include hot flashes, nausea, vomiting, fluid retention, weight gain, and thrombocytopenia. Tamoxifen therapy also increases the risk of endometrial cancer and deep vein thrombosis (Fiorica, 1997; Pasacreta & McCorkle, 1998) (see Medication Guide).

Chemotherapy. In some cases, hormonal therapy may be combined with chemotherapy. This combination may improve or increase the disease-free survival time after therapy (Hacker, 1998). It is already known that chemotherapy drugs are most effective when used in combination. What is *not* known is the optimal type of adjuvant chemotherapy combination for low risk and high risk breast cancer. Low risk breast cancer is often defined as less than 1 cm, diploid, low S-phase fraction tumors with hormone receptors, and a low nuclear grade (Hortobagyi & Buzdar, 1995). High risk tumors are larger than 1 cm and may have the same features as low-grade tumors or have features different from low-grade tumors. Often, women at low risk for relapse of breast cancer are given a combination of Cytoxan, methotrexate, and 5-fluorouracil. Many

---

MEDICATION GUIDE

Tamoxifen (Nolvadex)

Action: Antiestrogenic effects; attaches to hormone receptors on cancer cells and prevents natural hormones from attaching to the receptors.

Indication: For treatment of metastatic breast cancer; treatment of breast cancer in postmenopausal women following breast cancer surgery and radiation therapy; to reduce the incidence of breast cancer in high risk women.

Dosage: 20 to 40 mg orally a day. Dosages over 20 mg should be given in divided doses (AM and PM).

Adverse Reactions: Common side effects include hot flashes, nausea, vomiting, vaginal bleeding or discharge, menstrual irregularities, and rash. Hair loss is an uncommon effect. Serious side effects include deep vein thrombosis, increased risk of endometrial cancer, and stroke.

Nursing Considerations: The medication may be taken on an empty stomach or with food. Missed doses should be taken as soon as possible, but taking two doses at once is not recommended. A barrier or nonhormonal form of contraception is recommended in premenopausal women because tamoxifen may be harmful to the fetus.

---

other combinations of chemotherapy agents are used for women at high risk for relapse; often cyclophosphamide, doxorubicin or epirubicin, and methotrexate are used (DiSaia & Creasman, 1997; Hortobagyi & Buzdar, 1995). New agents being tested in clinical trials of breast cancer treatment include paclitaxel (Taxol), Taxotere, vinorelbine tartrate (Navelbine), CI 941, Edatrexate, Topotecan, and Irinotecan. Some of these agents, such as paclitaxel, may sensitize breast cancer cells to radiation therapy, and thus combinations of chemotherapy and radiation therapy are being tested (Friedman, 1994). These chemotherapy drugs can cause leukopenia, neutropenia, thrombocytopenia, anemia, gastrointestinal side effects (nausea, vomiting, anorexia, mucositis), and partial or full hair loss.

Chemotherapy treatments are usually given in the ambulatory setting, once or twice per month. During the informed consent process, before the treatment is selected, the woman and her family members should be educated about the names of the medications, routes of administration, treatment schedule, timing and ordering of medications, length of time of administration, reimbursed and unreimbursed costs of therapy, potential side effects, management of side effects, possible changes in body image (e.g., full or partial hair loss), recovery time after treatment (necessitating lost work time), and need for a caregiver to transport the woman to treatment and care for her afterward. Depending on the medications used, the treatments may include intravenous, subcutaneous, and oral medications. Often a long-term central venous catheter is inserted when the women will be receiving chemotherapy for an extended period or when she will receive medications that may damage the vein. Presence of a central venous catheter, hair loss, loss of part or all of her breast, menopause, and possible infertility all have the potential to cause a change in body image for the woman with breast cancer.

Breast cancer treatment with chemotherapy, hormonal therapy, or a combination of the two often causes changes in reproductive function. The woman who has already been through menopause may have to cope with hair loss from chemotherapy and loss of part or all of her breast, both of which change her body image. The premenopausal woman may experience these changes along with symptoms of menopause and possible infertility. It is not known if hormonal therapy to ease the effects of menopause is safe for women with breast cancer; therefore it is not recommended. For this reason the nurse must use other measures to help the client cope with menopause (see Chapter 7). Often, the young woman with breast cancer is devastated by the fact that she will go through menopause and possibly be unable to have children after the diagnosis of breast cancer.

Women receiving chemotherapy and their partners must understand that chemotherapy is a *mutagen* and a *teratogen*. It is absolutely critical that any woman receiving chemotherapy who is of childbearing age, even if she is no longer menstruating, use birth control. Birth control pills are not recommended, because they contain hormones that may assist in the growth of cancer. A birth control method must be chosen with the assistance of the gynecologist and the medical oncologist, and it must be used before chemotherapy begins and continue to be used until the medical oncologist and gynecologist believe it is safe to discontinue.

With the advance in monoclonal antibody technology, it is now possible to test for residual disease with a serum tumor marker, *CA 15-3,* if it is secreted by the client's tumor. From 75% to 80% of women with breast cancer secrete this tumor marker (Stearns, Yamauchi, & Hayes, 1998). If CA 15-3 is elevated at the time of diagnosis, circulating levels of CA 15-3 can be checked periodically through the treatment course to measure response. This technology is used to determine effectiveness of therapy for cancer without the need for second-look diagnostic surgery.

⋮ CARE MANAGEMENT

Assessment and Nursing Diagnoses

The nurse takes a client history of symptoms, including timing of detection of lump, size, changes, location, nipple discharge, and breast symmetry.

In addition to taking a history and palpating the breast lump, a clinician should also compare past and present mammographic findings with physical assessment findings. The mass should be described in terms of location (using the clock-dial method), shape, size, consistency, and fixation to the surrounding tissues. Skin changes, such as dimpling, peau d'orange, increased vascularity, nipple retraction, or ulceration, may indicate advanced disease, so their presence should be recorded. Physical examination includes palpation of the infraclavicular, supraclavicular, and axillary lymph nodes. Pain and soreness in the affected breast and arm should be evaluated. Often a diagram of the breast is drawn, and findings are recorded in the client record. Psychosocial assessment should include not only the client's present emotional state, but also the reaction of her family and significant others and history of handling crises. The nurse should determine what the diagnosis of cancer means to the woman and her family.

Nursing diagnoses for women with a diagnosis of breast cancer might include the following:

⋮ Nursing Diagnoses_____

- Fear/anxiety related to
  - diagnosis of breast cancer
  - treatment choices
  - choice of reconstructive procedure
- Risk for decisional conflict related to
  - choices of and controversies about treatment options
- Risk for sexual dysfunction related to
  - altered body image
  - side effects of therapy
- Risk for ineffective family coping related to
  - diagnosis and prognosis
- Anticipatory grieving related to
  - loss of breast or diagnosis of advanced cancer
- Fatigue related to
  - cancer treatments
- Pain related to
  - incision or metastatic cancer
- Impaired skin integrity related to
  - surgery or radiation
- Body-image disturbance related to
  - loss of breast and hair loss (chemotherapy)

Expected Outcomes of Care

Planning realistic outcomes in collaboration with the woman might include that the woman will do the following:
- Experience a reasonable level of anxiety related to diagnosis that does not interfere with use of healthy coping mechanisms.
- Elicit appropriate support from significant others.
- Choose among alternative treatment options and verbalize satisfaction with the decision-making process.

- Report satisfactory sexual functioning after surgery.
- Demonstrate necessary self-care techniques correctly.
- Accept a change in body image and demonstrate a positive self-concept.
  Other expected outcomes include the following:
- The family will adapt to the diagnosis and provide appropriate support through all stages of treatment.
- The woman's skin will remain intact and will heal without complications.
- The woman will resume usual activities as tolerated during treatment.

Plan of Care and Interventions

Nursing actions that will best assist the client in achieving her expected outcomes are selected, such as the following:

- Provide time to discuss the diagnosis, answer questions, and listen to concerns.
- Encourage ventilation of feelings by client and family in a nonjudgmental atmosphere.
- Offer information about support groups or individual therapy for the client and the family members, including children.

Emotional Support After Diagnosis

When a woman is confronted with a diagnosis of cancer, she is confronted not only with the possibility of death, but also with possible major changes in appearance. The emotional reaction to the diagnosis of cancer is always intense, and the many disruptions caused by the disease challenge the woman's and family's ability to cope. Disruptions may be caused by costs of treatment, loss of role function, lack of stress-relieving activities, spouse's or child's reaction to the diagnosis, change in body image and sexual function, disability, and pain. The woman may feel despair, fear, and shame. Sexuality issues related to breast cancer include a change in body image, changes in sexual function (such as decreased vaginal lubrication caused by hormonal therapy), and relational distress. It is the nurse's responsibility to discuss the influence of breast cancer on the woman's life and to assist the woman and her family in coping effectively with these changes. Some women find that after adjusting to the diagnosis of cancer, they have a greater appreciation of the experiences of daily life. They may feel encouraged to focus on what is most important and meaningful.

It is important to realize that clients and their families often undergo a period of shock after the diagnosis of cancer. It is difficult to accept the diagnosis of cancer when the client may feel and look well. This shock period is characterized by anguish and shock followed by disbelief and denial. During this time, absorbing information and education can be difficult, and the nurse should be sensitive as to how this may affect decision-making abilities. Flexibility is the key to sensitive nursing care. As the client and family begin to come out of shock, more and more information can be shared, and care planning with full client participation can take place, including the following:

- Validate and reinforce accurate information processing by client and family.
- Suggest approaches the woman might take to deal with the sexual concerns of her significant other.
- Discuss the application of alternative therapies to alleviate stress and promote healing, such as exercise, guided imagery, meditation, and progressive muscle relaxation (Kolcaba & Fox, 1999) (see Research box).

RESEARCH

Use of Alternative Therapies Among Breast Cancer Outpatients Compared with the General Population

Cancer of the breast is the second leading cause of cancer deaths in the United States. Women are fearful of the effects of the cancer or its treatments, as well as death. Alternative therapies may be sought by breast cancer clients to augment treatments or as an alternative.

The purpose of this study was to describe the interest in and use of alternative therapies available to breast cancer clients and compare findings with a published profile of the general population. One hundred twelve women were interviewed about their interest in and use of alternative therapies and then asked to complete two questionnaires concerning their mental adjustment to and personal growth after their cancer experience.

The three most frequently used alternative therapies were prayer (76%), exercise (38%), and spiritual healing (29%). Compared with the general population, these women used 17 alternative therapies more often; use of a chiropractor was the only one used more often by the general population.

CLINICAL APPLICATION

Frequent use of religious responses to cancer have been reported by other researchers. The need for spirituality is recognized as a nursing diagnosis. Nurses working with women with breast cancer can encourage and support use of the woman's faith as a way to cope. Nurses also should recognize that alternative therapies can be used to complement conventional therapies. They must be knowledgeable about the effectiveness of different alternative therapies because client use can be influenced by the client's relationship with the health care provider.

Source: VanderCreek, L., Rogers, E., & Lester, J. (1999). Use of alternative therapies among breast cancer outpatients compared with the general population. *Alternative Therapies* 5(1), 71-76.

BOX 12-4 Decision-Making Questions to Ask

1. What kind of breast cancer is it (invasive or noninvasive)?
2. What is the stage of the cancer (i.e., how extensive is the spread)?
3. Did the cancer test positive for hormone (estrogen)? (May be slower growing.)
4. What further tests are recommended?
5. What are the treatment options? (Pros and cons of each, including side effects.)
6. If surgery is recommended, what will the scar look like?
7. If a mastectomy is done, can breast reconstruction be done (at the time of surgery or later)?
8. How long will the client be in the hospital? What kind of postoperative care will the client need?
9. How long will treatment last if radiation or chemotherapy is recommended? What effects can the client expect from these treatments?
10. What community resources are available for support?

Source: National Women's Health Resource Center. (1999). Breast health. *National Women's Health Report* 17(5), 1-11.

- Refer the client to the American Cancer Society's Reach to Recovery program.
- Refer the client to a cancer rehabilitation program, such as ENCORE, a program run by the YWCA.
- Assist in client decision making, and arrange for the client to speak with others with similar diagnoses who have chosen a variety of treatment options (Box 12-4).

The National Comprehensive Cancer Network (NCCN) and the American Cancer Society now provide specific, up-to-date recommendations on breast cancer treatments on the Internet. This is an invaluable resource for women to learn about scientifically tested treatment protocols for each stage of breast cancer (American Cancer Society, 1999b).

In addition to assisting the client with accepting the diagnosis and obtaining support, nursing care in the preoperative, postoperative, and convalescent period must be considered. The discussion that follows is pertinent to the care required by a woman who is having a modified radical mastectomy.

Preoperative Care

General preoperative teaching and care are given, including expectations regarding physical appearance, pain management, equipment to be used (e.g., intravenous therapy, drains), and emotional support. Some emotional support may be obtained by arranging for a visit from a member of an organization such as Reach for Recovery. The woman is reminded that when she awakens after surgery, her arm on the affected side will feel tight.

Immediate Postoperative Care

After recovery from anesthesia, the woman is returned to her room. Special precautions must be observed to prevent or to minimize lymphedema of the affected arm.

NURSE ALERT *When vital signs are taken, the blood pressure cuff is never applied on the affected arm.*

The affected arm is elevated with pillows above the level of her right atrium. Blood is not drawn from this arm, and parenteral fluids are not given in it. Early arm movement is encouraged. Any increase in the circumference of that arm is reported immediately.

Nursing care of the wound involves observation for signs of hemorrhage (dressing, drainage tubes, and Hemovac or Jackson-Pratt drainage reservoirs are emptied at least every 8 hours and more frequently as needed), shock, and infection. Dressings are reinforced as necessary. Because the nipple may be "stored" on another body site (abdomen) pending future reimplantation over the reconstructed breast, this site is observed for hemorrhage and infection every hour and care is given exactly as ordered.

The woman is asked to turn (alternating between unaffected side and back), cough (while the nurse or the woman applies support to the chest), and deep breathe every 2 hours. Breath sounds are auscultated every 4 hours. Active range-of-motion (ROM) exercise of legs is encouraged. Parenteral fluids are given until adequate oral intake is possible. Emotional support is continued.

Care given during the immediate postoperative period is continued as necessary. Most women who undergo lumpectomy have surgery in an ambulatory setting and return home a few hours after surgery. Women are discharged 24 to 48 hours after modified radical mastectomy. Because of the short time spent in the hospital setting, thorough teaching is important. It is best to do as much teaching as possible before surgery if the outcome is known. If this is not possible, discharge teaching should be done with the woman's caregiver present to guard against the possibility of the woman's forgetting some of the information shared because of emotional stress or recovery from anesthesia.

Women who have had breast surgery are usually seen by their surgeon within 5 days of surgery. This is important because it allows the opportunity for reinforcement of education and emotional support.

Mobility is a key subject to be addressed with women having breast surgery. Early ambulation is encouraged not only to improve circulation and ventilation and prevent loss of calcium from bone, but also for the psychologic benefits of the upright position (such as mood elevation and decreased perception of self as continuing in the sick role). Arm exercises are encouraged at least four times daily (see Client Self-Care box). Exercise is increased as tolerated and is stopped at the point of pain. Initially the woman alternately clenches and extends her fingers and then progresses to wrist and elbow exercises, gradually abducting her arm and raising it up to and over her head. She is encouraged to exercise by assisting with her care—washing her face, brushing her teeth, and eating with her hand and arm on the affected side. Physical therapy is usually prescribed. A representative of Reach to Recovery often visits, reinforces the woman's exercise efforts, assists with providing emotional support relating to her change in body image (anatomic, physiologic, sexual), and may assist with teaching wound care.

BSE of the unaffected breast, bilateral axillae, and remaining breast in women who have had a lumpectomy is another key teaching subject for the woman who has had breast surgery. Written client education materials are available from the American Cancer Society and National Cancer Institute and should be shared with the woman and her family.

It is important to discuss the appearance of the woman's breast if dressings have not been removed before discharge. Photographs can be helpful in preparing the woman and her partner, who are nervously anticipating a change in body image. In some cases the woman may not want to look at photos, but it is important to give her an opportunity.

To restore body image, some women choose an external prosthesis to replace the lost breast or portion of breast tissue. The external prosthesis is inserted into the bra. Women who choose to use a partial external prosthesis after lumpectomy or full external prosthesis after mastectomy need information about where to obtain the prosthesis and bras to place it in. Women need to be advised on how to submit the cost of the prosthesis to their insurance company. Once referred to the American Cancer Society's Reach to Recovery program, the woman with breast cancer is visited by a breast cancer survivor who has been trained in how to offer information. One of the pieces of information the Reach to Recovery volunteer offers is a list of sources for prostheses and lingerie. For some women an external prosthesis does not restore body image, but surgical reconstruction of the missing or disfigured breast may restore it (see previous discussion).

Discharge Planning and Follow-up Care

Before discharge, considerable time should be spent counseling the woman and her family about the aspects of self-care. These instructions are summarized in the Home Care box. Printed instructions should be given to the woman and her family. A referral for home nursing care

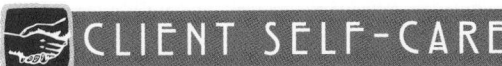

CLIENT SELF-CARE

Postmastectomy Arm Exercises

EXERCISE: CLIMBING THE WALL

1. Stand facing wall with toes close to wall.
2. Bend elbows and place palms of hands against wall at shoulder level.
3. Move both hands parallel to each other up the wall as far as possible until incisional pull or pain occurs.
4. Move both hands down to starting position.
5. Goal is complete extension with elbow straight.
6. Perform activities that use the same action: reaching top shelves, hanging out clothes, washing windows, hanging curtains, setting hair.

EXERCISE: ARM SWINGING

1. Bend forward from waist, permitting both arms to relax and hang naturally.
2. Swing arms together left to right (motion comes from shoulder).
3. Swing arms in circles parallel to floor, clockwise and counterclockwise.
4. Straighten up slowly.

EXERCISE: ROPE PULL

1. Attach a rope over a shower rod or hook.
2. Grasp each end of rope, alternately pulling on each end, raising arm on affected side to a point of incisional pull or pain.
3. Shorten rope over time until arm on affected side is raised almost directly overhead.

EXERCISE: ELBOW SPREAD

1. Clasp hands behind neck.
2. Raise elbows to chin level, holding head erect; move slowly and rest when incisional pull or pain occurs.
3. Gradually spread elbows apart; rest when pull or pain occurs.

From American Cancer Society. *Reach to recovery*. New York: The Society.

may be made if the woman needs assistance caring for her incision.

Evaluation

Evaluation is based on the client-centered expected outcomes. The nurse can be assured that care was effective to the extent that the goals for care have been achieved (see Plan of Care).

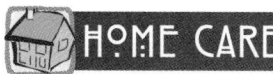

HOME CARE

After a Mastectomy

Wash hands well before and after touching incision area or drains.

Empty surgical drains twice a day and as needed, recording the date, time, drain site (if more than one drain is present), and amount of drainage in milliliters in diary you will take to each surgical checkup until your drains are removed. (Before discharge, you may receive a graduated container for emptying drains and measuring drainage.)

Avoid driving, lifting more than 10 pounds, or reaching above your head until given permission by surgeon.

Take medications for pain as soon as pain begins.

Perform arm exercises as directed.

Call physician if inflammation of incision or swelling of the incision or the arm occurs.

Avoid tight clothing, tight jewelry, and other causes of decreased circulation in the affected arm.

Until drains are removed, wear loose-fitting underwear (camisole or half-slip) and clothes, pinning surgical drains inside of clothing. (You will be taught how to do this safely.)

After drains are removed and surgical sites are healing and still tender, wear a mastectomy bra or camisole with a cotton-filled, muslin temporary prosthesis. Temporary prostheses of this type are often available from Reach to Recovery.

Avoid depilatory creams, strong deodorants, and shaving of affected chest area, axilla, and arm.

Sponge bathe until drains are removed.

Return to the surgeon's office for incision check, drain inspection, and possible drain removal as directed.

Contact Reach to Recovery for assistance obtaining external prosthesis and lingerie when dressings, drains, and staples are removed and wound is healing and nontender.

Contact insurance company for information about coverage of prosthesis and wig if needed. Obtain prescriptions for prosthesis and wig to submit with receipts of purchase for these items to the insurance company. If insurance does not pay for these items, contact hospital or agency social worker or local American Cancer Society for assistance.

Continue with monthly BSE of unaffected side and affected surgical site and axilla.

Encourage mother, sisters, and daughters (if applicable) to learn and practice monthly BSE and to have annual professional breast examinations and mammography (if appropriate).

Keep follow-up visits for professional examination, mammography, and testing to detect recurrent breast cancer.

Expect decreased sensation and tingling at incision sites and in the affected arm for weeks to months after surgery.

Resume sexual activities as desired.

PLAN °F CARE | Postmenopausal Woman with Breast Cancer

NURSING DIAGNOSIS Pain related to surgical incision and surgical drains as evidenced by client verbalizations

Expected Outcome *Client will report minimal intensity and decreased number of painful episodes.*

Nursing Interventions/*Rationales*

Utilize pain scale to assess for type and intensity of pain *to provide accurate database.*

Administer analgesics as ordered *to decrease perception of pain.*

Reposition client with affected arm elevated *to promote comfort and lymphatic channel return.*

NURSING DIAGNOSIS Risk for infection related to disruption of skin integrity and removal of lymph nodes

Expected Outcome *Client will experience no clinical manifestations of infection.*

Nursing Interventions/*Rationales*

Assess for clinical manifestations of infection at the incision and drain sites that may include redness, swelling, localized heat, fever, increasing pain, and foul-smelling drainage *to facilitate prompt treatment.*

Demonstrate the procedure for emptying and recording the amount of drainage from the Jackson-Pratt drain(s) *to provide information to the surgeon as to the appropriate removal time of drains. Drains are usually removed when 24 hours of drainage does not exceed 30 ml of fluid.*

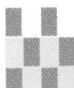

PLAN of CARE   Postmenopausal Woman with Breast Cancer—cont'd

Explain the need to avoid trauma or irritation to the affected arm *to reinforce to the client that alterations in sensation and removal of some lymph nodes may affect ability to sense irritation or prevent infection.*

Reinforce to client the need to protect arm from injury and to avoid venipunctures or blood pressures to be taken on the affected arm *to avoid trauma and infection, since decreased sensation may be present as well as decreased lymphatic return.*

Explain the importance of reporting any clinical manifestations of infection to the caregiver as soon as possible *to provide identification and treatment of problem.*

> **NURSING DIAGNOSIS** Body-image disturbance related to loss of all or part of a breast as evidenced by client statements

Expected Outcome *Client will maintain a positive body image.*

Nursing Interventions/*Rationales*

Provide opportunity through therapeutic communication to express feelings about body image changes *to clarify and validate feelings.*

Provide information about breast prostheses and other cosmetic devices *to assist in maintaining an intact body image.*

Encourage client to speak to physician about the possibility of breast reconstructive surgery *to provide additional resources for body image enhancement.*

Refer to support groups *to facilitate verbalization of feelings with women who have similar concerns.*

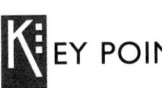

KEY POINTS

- The development of breast neoplasms, whether benign or malignant, can have a significant physical and emotional effect on the woman and her family.

- The risk of American women developing cancer of the breast is 1 in 8.

- An estimated 90% of all breast lumps are detected by the woman during breast self-examination (BSE).

- Monthly BSE, routine screening mammography, and yearly breast examinations by practitioners are recommended for early detection of breast cancer.

- The modified radical mastectomy is the most common surgical procedure for breast cancer, although lumpectomy and radiation may be an alternative for stage I and stage II disease and tumors less than or equal to 4 cm.

- Adjuvant chemotherapy is most helpful to premenopausal women with breast cancer that has spread to the lymph nodes.

- Tamoxifen, along with other promising new drug therapies currently under investigation, may provide the first real hope for the prevention of breast cancer.

CRITICAL THINKING EXERCISES

1 *Identify the similarities and differences between the BSE findings in women with fibrocystic changes and women with breast cancer. Think about how these similarities and differences might affect a woman's incentive to perform BSE. How might a woman with a history of fibrocystic changes react to finding a breast lump? Would a woman with a history of fibrocystic breast changes be more or less likely to perform BSE?*

2 *You are assigned to a woman preparing for surgery for breast cancer.*
   a. *Identify your feelings regarding breast cancer or other female reproductive malignancy. How might these feelings affect your ability to provide effective nursing care?*
   b. *What kind of support system do you believe is needed by the woman experiencing surgery for breast cancer? What might be the special needs of her family?*
   c. *Develop a plan of care for this woman and her family. Incorporate your responses to female malignancy in your plan of care.*

3 *Ask female friends or relatives age 35 or older if they have ever had a mammogram. Determine from their point of view why they did or did not take part in mammogram screening. Then use these data to brainstorm ways to encourage your female clients to follow mammography guidelines.*

References

American Cancer Society. (1999a). *Cancer facts and figures, 1999.* New York: American Cancer Society.

American Cancer Society. (1999b). Breast cancer information [Online]. Available URL: http://www.cancer.org/bottomcancinfo.html. Accessed 3/15/99.

Bhatty, M., & Berry, R. (1997). Nipple-areola reconstruction by tattooing and nipple sharing. *Br J Plastic Surg* 50(5), 331-334.

Bostwick, J. (1995). Breast reconstruction following mastectomy. *CA Cancer J Clin* 45(5), 289-304.

Burke, W. et al. (1997). Recommendations for follow-up care of individuals with an inherited predisposition to cancer: BRCA1 and BRCA2. *JAMA* 277(12), 997-1003.

Cuzick, J. et al. (1998). Electropotential measurements as a new diagnostic modality for breast cancer. *Lancet* 352, 359-363.

Daudt, A., Alberg, A., & Helzlsouer, K. (1996). Epidemiology, prevention, and early detection of breast cancer. *Curr Opin Oncol* 8, 455-461.

DiSaia, P., & Creasman, W. (1997). *Clinical gynecologic oncology* (5th ed.). St. Louis: Mosby.

Douglass, M. et al. (1995). Breast cancer early detection: Differences between African-American and white women's health beliefs and detection practices. *Oncol Nurs Forum* 22(5), 835-837.

Early Breast Cancer Trialists' Collaborative Group. (1992). Systemic treatment of early breast cancer by hormonal, cytotoxic or immune therapy: 133 randomized trials involving 31,000 recurrences and 24,000 deaths among 75,000 women. *Lancet* 339, 1-15, 71-85.

Edge, V., & Miller, M. (1994). *Women's health care.* St. Louis: Mosby.

Fernandez, M., Tortolero-Luna, G., & Gold, R. (1998). Mammography and Pap test screening among low-income foreign-born Hispanic women in USA. *Cadernos de Saude Publica* 14(suppl 3), 133-147.

Fiorica, J. (1997). Breast cancer. In P. Leppert & F. Howard (Eds.). *Primary care for women.* Philadelphia: Lippincott-Raven.

Fisher, B. et al. (1994). Endometrial cancer in tamoxifen-treated breast cancer patients: Findings from the National Surgical Adjuvant Breast and Bowel Project (NSABP) B14. *J Natl Cancer Inst* 13, 513-529.

Friedman, M. (1994). New directions for breast cancer—therapeutic research. *Hematol Oncol Clin North Am* 8(1), 113-119.

Hacker, N. (1998). Breast disease: A gynecologic perspective. In N. Hacker & J. Moore (Eds.). *Essentials of obstetrics and gynecology* (3rd ed.). Philadelphia: W.B. Saunders.

Harden, J., & Girard, N. (1994). Breast reconstruction using an innovative flap procedure. *AORN Nurs* 60(2), 184-192.

Hawkins, J., Roberto-Nichols, D., & Stanley-Haney, J. (1997). *Protocols for nurse practitioners in gynecologic settings* (6th ed.). New York: Tiresias Press.

Helzlsouer, K., & Couzi, R. (1995). Hormones and breast cancer. *Cancer Suppl* 76(10), 2059-2062.

Henderson, M. (1995). Nutritional aspects of breast cancer. *Cancer Suppl* 76(10), 2053-2062.

Hilakivi-Clarke, L. et al. (1993). Psychosocial factors in the development and progression of breast cancer. *Breast Cancer Res Treat* 29(2), 141-160.

Hinojosa, R. (1991). Breast reconstruction through tissue expansion. *Plast Surg Nurs* 11(2), 52-57.

Hortobagyi, G., & Buzdar, A. (1995). Current status of adjuvant systemic therapy for primary breast cancer: Progress and controversy. *CA Cancer J Clin* 45(4), 199-226.

Isaacs, C., & Swain, S. (1994). Hormone replacement therapy in women with a history of breast cancer. *Hematol Oncol Clin North Am* 8(1), 179-195.

Ivey, C., & Gordon, S. (1994). Breast reconstruction: New image, new hope. *RN* 57(7), 48-53.

Jardines, L. (1996). Management of nipple discharge. *American Surgeon* 62, 119-122.

Knopf, M. (1996). Breast cancers. In R. McCorkle et al. (Eds.). *Cancer nursing: A comprehensive textbook.* Philadelphia: W.B. Saunders.

Kolcaba, K., & Fox, C. (1999). The effects of guided imagery on comfort of women with early stage breast cancer undergoing radiation therapy. *Oncol Nurse Forum* 26(10), 72-76.

Kroll, S. (1998). Why autologous tissue? *Clin Plastic Surg* 25(2), 135-143.

Lawson, E. (1998). A narrative analysis: A black woman's perception of breast cancer risks and early breast cancer detection. *Cancer Nurs* 21(6), 421-429.

Li, Z. (1994). Variables associated with breast self-examination among Chinese women. *Cancer Nurs* 24(7), 96-99.

Link, J. (1993). Benign breast disease. *Nurse Pract Forum* 4(2), 96-99.

Logothetis, M. (1995). Women's reports of breast implant problems and silicone-related illness. *J Obstet Gynecol Neonatal Nurs* 24(7), 609-616.

Love, S., & Lindsey, K. (1995). *Dr. Susan Love's breast book* (2nd ed.). Indianapolis, IN: Addison-Wesley.

McCool, W., Stone-Condry, M., & Bradford, H. (1998). Breast health care: A review. *J Nurse Midwifery* 43(6), 406-430.

McKeon, V. (1997). The breast cancer prevention trial: Evaluating tamoxifen's efficacy in preventing breast cancer. *J Obstet Gynecol Neonatal Nurs* 26(1), 79-90.

Morrison, B. (1994). The genetics of breast cancer. *Hematol Oncol Clin North Am* 8(1), 15-27.

National Cancer Institute. (1999a). Breast cancer information [On-line]. Available URL: http://www.cancernet.NCI.NIH.gov. Accessed 3/15/99.

National Cancer Institute. (1999b). Cancer trials information [On-line]. Available URL: http://www.cancertrials.NCI.NIH.gov. Accessed 3/15/99.

National Institutes of Health. (1990). *Consensus development conference statement. Treatment of early-stage breast cancer.* Bethesda, MD: The Institutes.

National Women's Health Resource Center. (1999). Breast health. *National Women's Health Report* 17(5), 1-11.

National Women's Health Resource Center. (1995). Breast health. *National Women's Health Report* 13(5), 3.

Nettles-Carlson, B. (1995). Problems of the breast. In C. Fogel & N. Woods (Eds.). *Women's health care.* Thousand Oaks, CA: Sage.

Nicholson, A. (1996). Diet and the prevention and treatment of breast cancer. *Alternative Therapies* 2(6), 32-38.

Pasacreta, J., & McCorkle, R. (1998). Providing accurate information to women about tamoxifen therapy for breast cancer: Current indications, effects, and controversies. *Oncol Nurs Forum* 25, 1577-1583.

Powell, D. (1994). The normal breast: Structure, function and epidemiology. In D. Powell & C. Stelling (Eds.). *The diagnosis and detection of breast disease.* St. Louis: Mosby.

Powell, D., & Stelling, C. (1994). Fibrocystic breast changes. In D. Powell & C. Stelling (Eds.). *The diagnosis and detection of breast disease.* St. Louis: Mosby.

Schneider, D. (1995). Changing the image: Looking to MRI for diagnosing breast cancer. *Sci Am* 272(4), 42.

Schumann, D. (1994). Health risks for women with breast implants. *Nurse Pract* 19(7), 19-30.

Schweitzer, M. et al. (1998). Cost-effectiveness of detecting breast cancer in lower socioeconomic status African-American and Hispanic women through mobile mammogram services. *Medical Care Research and Review* 55(1), 99-115.

Stearns, V., Yamauchi, H., & Hayes, D. (1998). Circulating tumor markers in breast cancer: Accepted utilities and novel prospects. *Breast Cancer Res Treat* 52(13), 239-259.

Stelling, C., & Powell, D. (1994). Circumscribed breast masses. In D. Powell & C. Stelling (Eds.). *The diagnosis and detection of breast disease*. St. Louis: Mosby.

Stoll, B. (1996). Diet and exercise regimens to improve breast carcinoma prognosis. *Cancer* 78(12), 2465-2469.

Sung, J. et al. (1997). Effect of a cancer screening intervention conducted by lay health workers among inner-city women. *Am J Prev Med* 13(1), 51-57.

Taplin, S. et al. (1994). Using physician correspondence and postcard reminders to promote mammography use. *Am J Public Health* 84(4), 571-574.

Urban, N., Anderson, G., & Peacock, S. (1994). Mammography screening: How important is cost as a barrier to use? *Am J Public Health* 84(1), 50-55.

Veronesi, U. et al. (1998). Prevention of breast cancer with tamoxifen: Preliminary findings from the Italian randomised trial among hysterectomised women. *Lancet* 352, 93-97.

13

Structural Disorders and Neoplasms of the Reproductive System

Deitra Leonard Lowdermilk

LEARNING OBJECTIVES

- Define the key terms.
- Describe the various structural disorders of the uterus and vagina.
- Discuss the pathophysiology of selected benign and malignant neoplasms of the female reproductive tract.
- Identify the common medical and surgical therapies for selected conditions.
- Discuss the emotional impact of benign and malignant neoplasms.
- Develop a nursing plan of care for a woman with endometrial cancer who has had a hysterectomy.
- Explain diagnostic procedures in client-centered terms.

- Explain treatments for preinvasive and invasive conditions.
- Review health-promoting behaviors that reduce cancer risk.
- Assess the impact of benign and malignant neoplasms on pregnancy.
- Discuss the development and sequelae of gestational trophoblastic neoplasia.
- Identify critical elements for teaching clients with selected benign or malignant neoplasms.
- Identify topics for nursing research related to gynecologic neoplasia.

KEY TERMS

biopsy	gestational trophoblastic neoplasia	rectocele
cervical intraepithelial neoplasia (CIN)	hysterectomy	squamous intraepithelial lesions (SILs)
colposcopy	leiomyomas	transformation zone
conization	metastasis	urinary incontinence (UI)
cryosurgery	pelvic exenteration	uterine displacement
cystocele	pelvic relaxation	uterine prolapse
dysplasia	pessary	vulvectomy
fistula	polyps	

 omen are at risk for structural disorders and neoplastic diseases related to the reproductive system from the age of menarche through menopause and the older years. Problems that may be experienced include structural disorders of the uterus and vagina related to pelvic relax-

ation and urinary incontinence. Benign neoplasms of the reproductive organs, such as fibroids and cysts, and malignant neoplasms of the reproductive system can also occur. Benign tumors usually do not endanger life, tend to grow slowly, and are not invasive. Malignant tumors grow

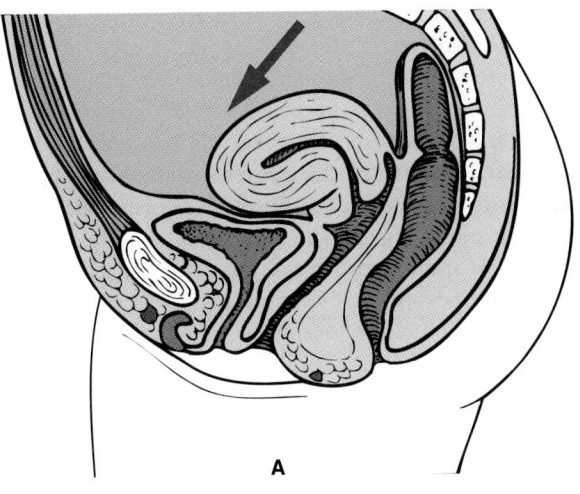

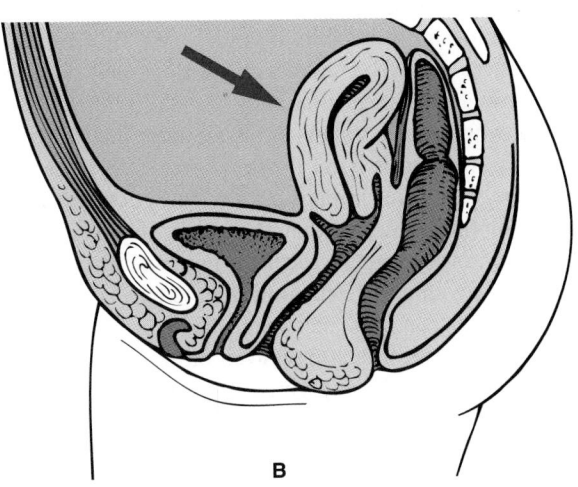

Fig. 13-1   Types of uterine displacement. **A,** Anterior displacement. **B,** Retroversion (backward displacement of uterus).

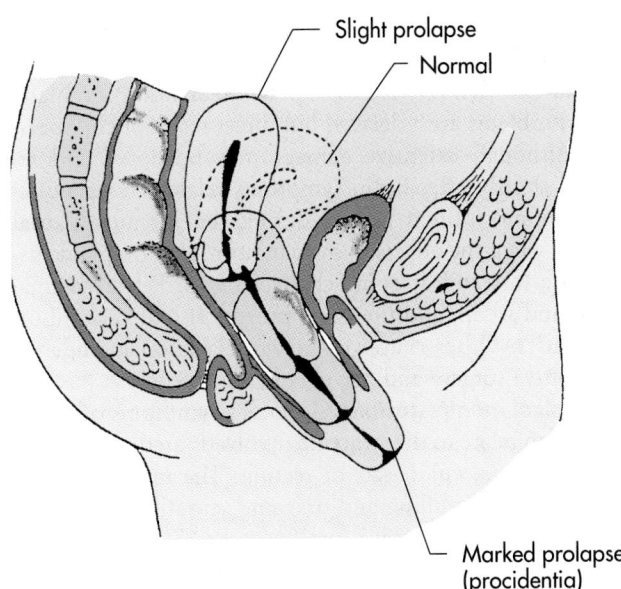

Fig. 13-2   Prolapse of uterus.

rapidly in a disorganized manner and invade surrounding tissues. When this occurs, the common term used to describe this phenomenon is *cancer.* The impact of the development of structural disorders or benign or malignant neoplasms can have far-reaching effects for the woman and her family. Beyond the obvious physiologic alterations, the woman also experiences threats to her self-concept and her ability to cope. A woman's concept of herself as a sexual being can be affected by the condition and its treatments. A woman's family is also challenged in the way it responds to her diagnosis. When neoplasia occurs with pregnancy, it adds to the complexity of both physical and emotional responses to childbearing.

Nurses have important roles in teaching women about early detection and treatment and in providing supportive care to women and their families. This chapter presents information that will assist the nurse in assessing and identi-

fying problems associated with structural problems or benign or malignant reproductive neoplasms. Nursing care concepts related to early detection, treatment methods, and education are included.

STRUCTURAL DISORDERS OF THE UTERUS AND VAGINA

Alterations in Pelvic Support

Uterine Displacement and Prolapse

Normally the round ligaments hold the uterus in anteversion, and the uterosacral ligaments pull the cervix backward and upward (see Fig. 6-2). **Uterine displacement** is a variation of this normal placement. The most common type of displacement is posterior displacement, or *retroversion,* in which the uterus is tilted posteriorly and the cervix rotates anteriorly. Other variations include retroflexion and anteflexion (Fig. 13-1).

By 2 months postpartum, the ligaments should return to normal length, but in about one third of women the uterus remains retroverted. This condition is rarely symptomatic, but conception may be difficult because the cervix points toward the anterior vaginal wall and away from the posterior fornix, where seminal fluid pools after coitus. If symptoms occur, they may include pelvic and low back pain, dyspareunia, and exaggeration of premenstrual symptoms.

Uterine prolapse is a more serious type of displacement. Degrees of prolapse can vary, from mild to complete. In complete prolapse, the cervix and body of the uterus protrude through the vagina and the vagina is inverted (Fig. 13-2).

Uterine displacement and prolapse can be caused by congenital or acquired weakness of the pelvic support structures (often referred to as **pelvic relaxation**). In many cases problems are a delayed but direct result of childbearing. Although extensive damage may be noted and repaired shortly after birth, symptoms related to pelvic relaxation most often appear during the perimenopausal period, when the effects of ovarian hormones on pelvic tissues are lost and atrophic changes begin. Pelvic trauma, stress and strain, and the aging process also are contributing causes. Other causes of pelvic relaxation include reproductive surgery and pelvic radiation.

Clinical manifestations. Generally, symptoms of pelvic relaxation relate to the structure involved: urethra, bladder, uterus, vagina, cul-de-sac, or rectum. The most common complaints are pulling and dragging sensations, pressure, protrusions, fatigue, and low backache. Symptoms may be worse after prolonged standing or deep penile penetration during intercourse. Stress urinary incontinence may be present.

Cystocele and Rectocele

Cystocele and rectocele often occur with uterine prolapse (although they can occur independently), causing the uterus to sag even further backward and downward into the vagina. **Cystocele** (Fig. 13-3) is the protrusion of the bladder downward into the vagina that develops when supporting structures in the vesicovaginal septum are injured. Anterior wall relaxation gradually develops over time, as a result of congenital defects of supports, childbearing, obesity, or advanced age. When the woman stands, the weakened anterior vaginal wall cannot support the weight of the urine in the bladder; the vesicovaginal septum is forced downward, the bladder

is stretched, and its capacity is increased. With time the cystocele enlarges until it protrudes into the vagina. Complete emptying of the bladder is difficult because the cystocele sags below the bladder neck. **Rectocele** is the herniation of the anterior rectal wall through the relaxed or ruptured vaginal fascia and rectovaginal septum; it appears as a large bulge that may be seen through the relaxed introitus (Fig. 13-4).

Clinical manifestations. Cystoceles and rectoceles often are asymptomatic. If symptoms of cystocele are present, they may include complaints of a bearing-down sensation or that "something is in my vagina." Other symptoms include urinary frequency, retention, incontinence, and possible recurrent cystitis and urinary tract infections. Pelvic examination will reveal a bulging of the anterior wall of the vagina when the woman is asked to bear down. Unless the bladder neck and urethra are damaged, urinary continence is unaffected. Women with large cystoceles complain of having to push upward on the sagging anterior vaginal wall to be able to void.

Rectoceles may be small and produce few symptoms, but some are so large that they protrude outside of the vagina when the woman stands. Symptoms are absent when the woman is lying down. A rectocele causes a disturbance in bowel function, the sensation of bearing down, or the sensation that the pelvic organs are falling out. With a very large rectocele, it may be difficult to have a bowel movement. Each time the woman strains during bowel evacuation, the feces are forced against the thinned rectovaginal wall, stretching it even more. Some women facilitate evacuation by applying digital pressure vaginally to hold up the rectal pouch.

Urinary Incontinence

About 20% of women between ages 25 and 64 years have **urinary incontinence (UI)** (uncontrollable leakage of urine). Although nulliparous women can have UI, the incidence is higher in women who have given birth and

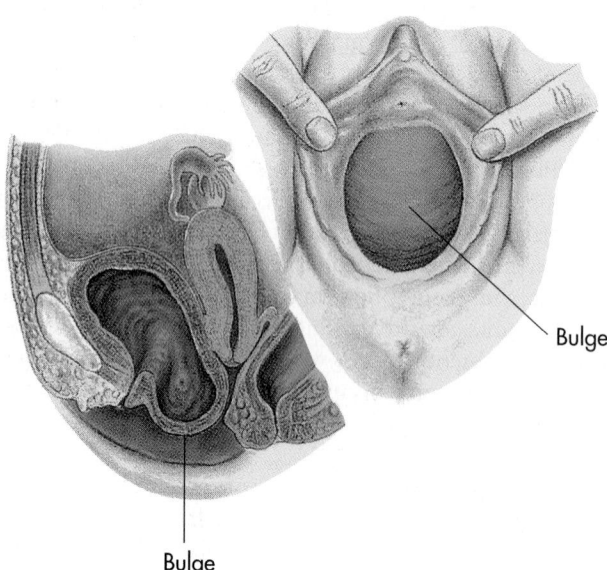

Fig. 13-3 Side and direct views of cystocele. *(From Seidel, H. et al. [1999]. Mosby's guide to physical examination [4th ed.]. St. Louis: Mosby.)*

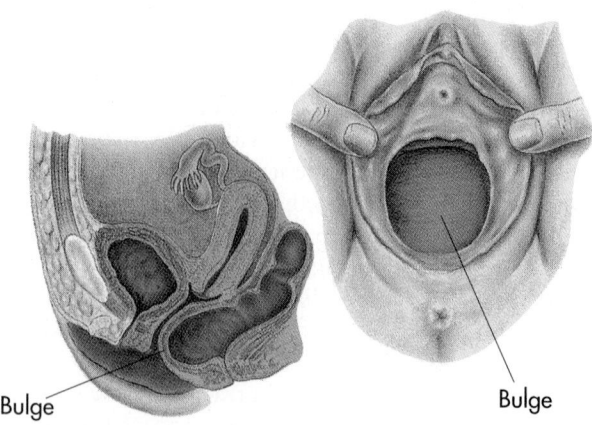

Fig. 13-4 Side and direct views of rectocele. *(From Seidel, H. et al. [1999]. Mosby's guide to physical examination [4th ed.]. St. Louis: Mosby.)*

also increases with parity (Sampselle et al., 1997). Conditions that disturb urinary control include *stress urinary incontinence,* due to sudden increases in intraabdominal pressure (such as that due to sneezing or coughing); *urge incontinence,* caused by disorders of the bladder and urethra, such as urethritis and urethral stricture, trigonitis, and cystitis; neuropathies, such as multiple sclerosis, diabetic neuritis, and pathologic conditions of the spinal cord; and congenital and acquired urinary tract abnormalities (Skoner, Thompson, & Caron, 1994).

Stress urinary incontinence may follow injury to bladder neck structures. A sphincter mechanism at the bladder neck compresses the upper urethra, pulls it upward behind the symphysis, and forms an acute angle at the junction of the posterior urethral wall and the base of the bladder (Fig. 13-5). To empty the bladder, the sphincter complex relaxes and the trigone contracts to open the internal urethral orifice and pull the contracting bladder wall upward, forcing urine out. The angle between the urethra and the base of the bladder is lost or increased if the supporting pubococcygeus muscle is injured; this change, coupled with urethrocele, causes incontinence. Urine spurts out when the woman is asked to bear down or cough while she is in the lithotomy position.

Genital Fistulas

A **fistula** is an abnormal communication between one hollow viscus and another, or from one hollow viscus to the outside. Genital fistulas may occur between the bladder and the genital tract (e.g., vesicovaginal); between the urethra and the vagina (urethrovaginal); and between the rectum or sigmoid colon and vagina (rectovaginal) (Fig. 13-6). Fistulas may be a result of a congenital anom-

aly, gynecologic surgery, obstetric trauma, cancer, radiation therapy, gynecologic trauma, or infection.

Vesicovaginal fistula, the most common urinary tract fistula, forms in the anterior vaginal wall. It is usually a result of injury near the uterovesical junction during radical hysterectomy for cancer. Urine is lost through the vagina, resulting in partial or complete incontinence.

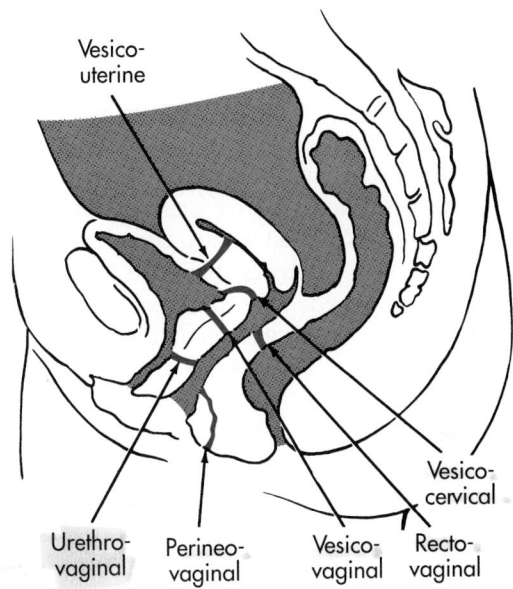

Fig. 13-6 Types of fistulas that may develop in vagina, uterus, and rectum. *(From Phipps, W., Sands, J., & Marek, J. [1999]. Medical–surgical nursing: Concepts and clinical practice [6th ed.]. St. Louis: Mosby.)*

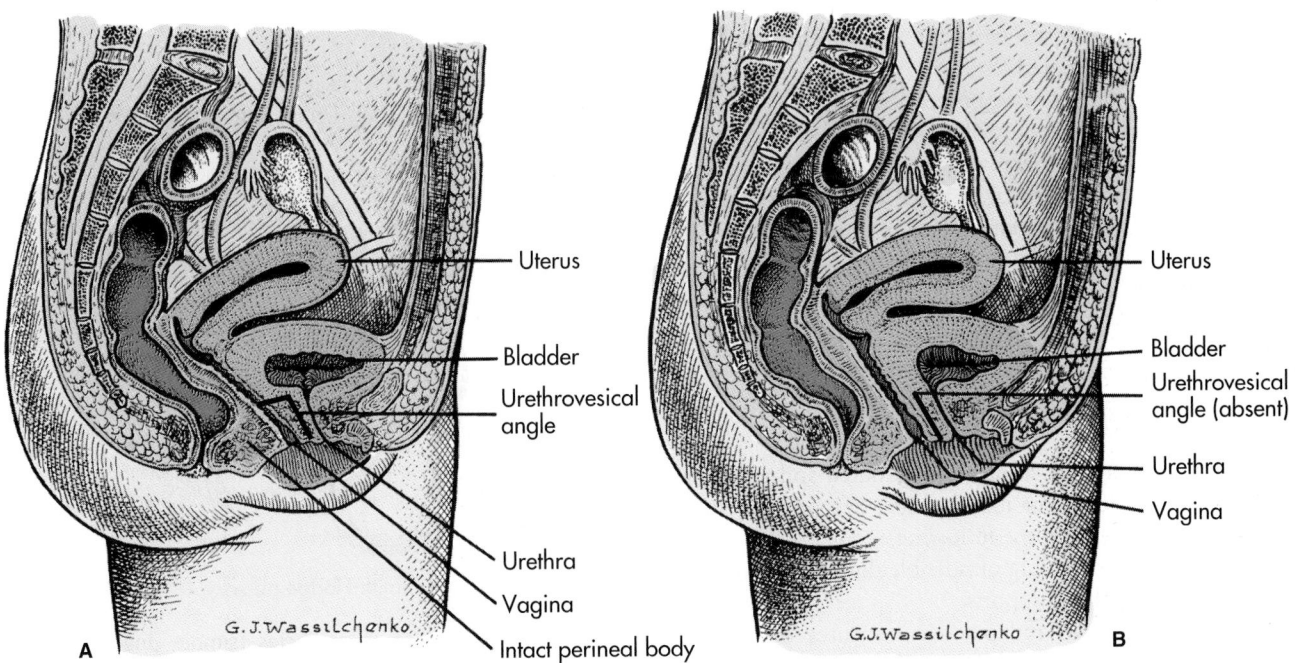

Fig. 13-5 Urethrovesical angle. **A,** Normal angle. **B,** Widening (absence) of angle.

Rectovaginal fistula is most often caused by an infection in the episiotomy, a suture placed through the rectal wall during repair, or an unrecognized rectal injury during childbirth. Rectovaginal fistulas may also be a result of extension of cervical cancer or radiation therapy.

Clinical manifestations. Signs and symptoms of vaginal fistulas depend on the site but may include presence of urine, flatus, or feces in the vagina, odors of urine or feces in the vagina, and irritation of vaginal tissues.

▐ CARE MANAGEMENT

Assessment and Nursing Diagnoses

Assessment for problems related to structural disorders of the uterus and vagina focuses primarily on the genitourinary tract, the reproductive organs, bowel elimination, and psychosocial and sexual factors. A complete health history, physical examination, and laboratory tests are done to support the appropriate medical diagnosis. The nurse should assess the woman's knowledge of the disorder, its management, and possible prognosis. Suggested nursing diagnoses for structural problems of the uterus and vagina include the following:

▐ Nursing Diagnoses _____

- Knowledge deficit related to
  - causes of structural disorders and treatment options
- Constipation or diarrhea related to
  - anatomic changes
- Pain related to
  - relaxation of pelvic support or elimination difficulties
- Ineffective coping related to
  - changes in body image
- Altered family processes or interpersonal relationships related to
  - the woman's anatomic and functional changes
- Risk for injury related to
  - lack of skill in self-care procedures
  - lack of understanding of the rationale for the need to comply with therapy
- Social isolation, spiritual distress, body-image disturbance, or low self-esteem related to
  - changes in anatomy and function
- Anxiety related to
  - surgical procedure
  - prognosis

Expected Outcomes of Care

Expected outcomes are mutually negotiated and stated in client-centered terms. Possible expected outcomes include that the woman will do the following:

- Verbalize understanding of possible disorders related to alteration in pelvic supports.
- Use good hygiene and practice measures to prevent problems related to pelvic support alterations.
- Accept change in body functions (if they occur) without loss of positive body image, self-concept, and self-esteem.
- Report less anxiety related to treatment and her prognosis.

Plan of Care and Interventions

The health care team works together to treat the disorders related to alterations in pelvic support and to assist the woman in management of her symptoms. In general, nurses working with these women can provide information and self-care education to prevent problems before they occur, to manage or reduce symptoms and to promote comfort and hygiene if symptoms are already present, and to recognize when further intervention is needed. This information can be part of all postpartum discharge teaching or can be provided at postpartum follow-up visits in clinics or in physician or midwife offices, during postpartum home visits, or during gynecologic health examinations. In addition, information on how to prevent or recognize structural problems of the uterus and vagina can be a topic for workshops for women or health fairs in community settings.

Interventions for specific problems depend on the problem and the severity of the symptoms. If discomfort related to uterine displacement is a problem, several interventions can be implemented to treat uterine displacement. Kegel exercises can be performed several times daily to increase muscle strength. A knee-chest position performed for a few minutes several times a day can correct a mildly retroverted uterus. A fitted **pessary** to support the uterus and hold it in the correct position (Fig. 13-7) may

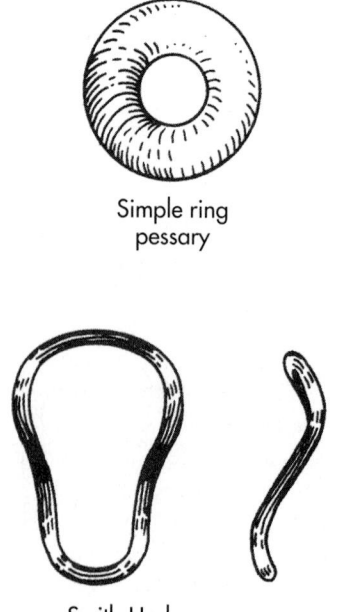

Simple ring pessary

Smith-Hodge pessary

Fig. 13-7 Examples of pessaries (simple ring and Smith-Hodge).

be inserted in the vagina. Usually a pessary is used only for a short time because it can lead to pressure necrosis and vaginitis. Good hygiene is important; some women can be taught to remove the pessary at night, cleanse it, and replace it in the morning. If the pessary is always left in place, regular douching with commercially prepared solutions or weak vinegar solutions (1 tablespoon to 1 quart of water) to remove increased secretions and to keep the vaginal pH at 4 to 4.5 is suggested. After a period of treatment, most women are free from symptoms and do not require the pessary. Surgical correction is rarely indicated.

Treatment for uterine prolapse depends on the degree of prolapse. Pessaries may be useful in mild prolapse. Estrogen therapy also may be used in the older woman to improve tone of the tissues. If these conservative treatments do not correct the problem or there is significant degree of prolapse, abdominal or vaginal hysterectomy (see p. 276) is usually recommended.

Treatment for a cystocele includes use of a vaginal pessary or surgical repair. Pessaries may not be effective. Anterior repair (colporrhaphy) is the usual surgical procedure and is usually done for large symptomatic cystoceles. This involves a surgical shortening of pelvic muscles to provide better support for the bladder. An anterior repair is often combined with a vaginal hysterectomy.

Small rectoceles may not need treatment. The woman with mild symptoms may get relief from a high-fiber diet and adequate fluid intake, stool softeners, or mild laxatives. Vaginal pessaries usually are not effective. Large rectoceles that are causing significant symptoms are usually repaired surgically. A posterior repair (colporrhaphy) is the usual procedure. This surgery is performed vaginally and involves shortening the pelvic muscles to provide better support for the rectum. Anterior and posterior repairs may be performed at the same time and with vaginal hysterectomy.

Mild to moderate urinary incontinence can be significantly decreased or relieved in many women by bladder training and pelvic muscle (Kegel) exercises (Czarapata & McKillips, 1997; Sampselle et al., 1997). Other management strategies include insertion of a bladder neck support prosthesis, estrogen therapy, and surgery (Mishell et al., 1997).

Nursing care of the woman with pelvic relaxation problems or a fistula requires great sensitivity because the woman's reactions are often intense. She may become withdrawn or, conversely, hostile because of embarrassment about odors and soiling of her clothing beyond her control. The nurse should be tactful in suggesting hygienic practices that reduce odor. Commercial deodorizing douches are available, or noncommercial solutions, such as chlorine solution (1 teaspoon of chlorine household bleach to 1 quart of water) may be used. The chlorine solution is also useful for external perineal irrigation. Sitz baths and thorough washing of the genitals with unscented, mild soap and warm water help. Sparse dusting with deodorizing powders can be useful. If a rectovaginal fistula is present, enemas given before leaving the house

may provide temporary relief from oozing of fecal material until corrective surgery is performed. Irritated skin and tissues may benefit from use of a heat lamp or application of vitamin A and D emollient ointment. Hygienic care is time consuming and may need to be repeated frequently throughout the day; protective pads or pants may need to be worn. All of these activities can be demoralizing to the woman and frustrating to her and her family.

Many of the nurse's efforts with these problems are directed toward participating in a team effort to prepare the woman for surgery. Preoperative teaching involves the primary nurse, operating room nurse, surgeon, and anesthesiologist. The nurse in the health promotion setting is usually most aware of the woman's living circumstances, physical limitations, and social problems and therefore may be best suited to coordinate continuity of care after discharge.

Evaluation

Care can be evaluated as effective if the anatomic defect is repaired and function is restored. If function cannot be fully restored through surgery, medication, or other therapy, expected outcomes are evaluated related to self-care in compliance with the medical regimen, regaining or maintaining self-esteem, and satisfactory family and interpersonal processes.

BENIGN NEOPLASMS

Benign neoplasms include a variety of nonmalignant cysts and tumors of the ovaries, uterus, vulva, and other organs of the reproductive system.

Ovarian Cysts

Functional ovarian cysts (Fig. 13-8) are cysts that are dependent on hormonal influences associated with the menstrual cycle. These cysts may be classified as follicular cysts, corpus luteum cysts, theca-lutein cysts, endometrial cysts, and polycystic ovary. Other benign ovarian neoplasms include dermoid cysts and ovarian fibromas.

Follicular Cysts

Follicular cysts develop in young women as a result of the mature graafian follicle failing to rupture or when an immature follicle does not reabsorb fluid after ovulation. A cyst is usually asymptomatic unless it ruptures, in which case it causes severe pelvic pain. If the cyst does not rupture, it usually shrinks after two or three menstrual cycles.

Corpus Luteum Cysts

Corpus luteum cysts occur after ovulation and are possibly caused by an increased secretion of progesterone that results in an increase of fluid in the corpus luteum. Clinical manifestations associated with a corpus luteum cyst include pain, tenderness over the ovary, delayed menses, and irregular or prolonged menstrual flow. A rupture can cause

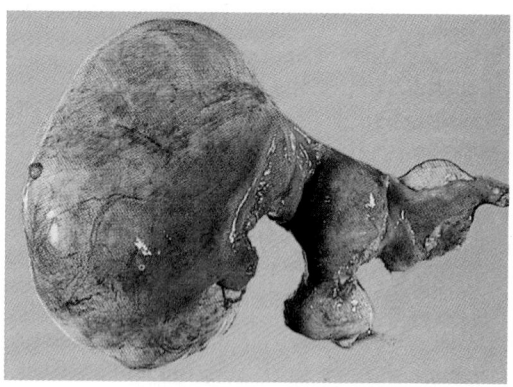
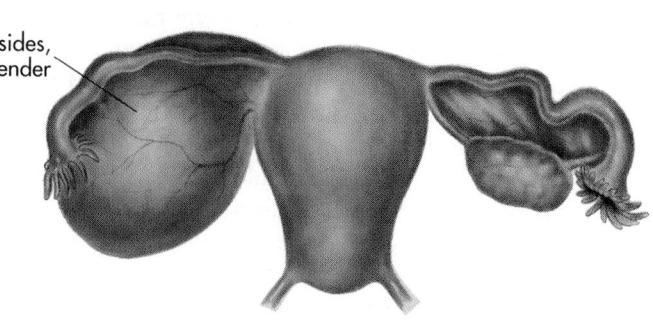

One or both sides, usually nontender

Fig. 13-8 Ovarian cyst. *(From Seidel, H. et al. [1999]. Mosby's guide to physical examination [4th ed.]. St. Louis: Mosby.)*

intraperitoneal hemorrhage. Usually corpus luteum cysts disappear without treatment within one or two menstrual cycles.

Theca-lutein Cysts

Theca-lutein cysts are uncommon and are usually associated with hydatidiform mole (see p. 300). Theca-lutein cysts develop as a result of prolonged stimulation of the ovaries by human chorionic gonadotrophin (hCG). A feeling of pelvic fullness may be noted by the woman.

Polycystic Ovary Syndrome

Polycystic ovary syndrome occurs when there is an endocrine imbalance resulting in high levels of estrogen, testosterone, and luteinizing hormone and decreased secretion of follicle-stimulating hormone. This syndrome is associated with a variety of problems in the hypothalamic-pituitary-ovarian axis and by androgen-producing tumors. The condition can be transmitted as an X-linked dominant or autosomal dominant trait (Stein-Leventhal syndrome). Multiple follicular cysts develop on one or both ovaries and produce excess estrogen. The ovaries often double in size. Clinical manifestations include obesity, hirsutism (excessive hair growth), irregular menses or amenorrhea, and infertility.

Collaborative Care

A variety of interventions may be implemented for the woman with a functional cyst. If expectant management is the treatment, the woman is advised to keep appointments for pelvic examinations to monitor the changes in size of the cyst (enlarging or shrinking). Pharmacologic interventions such as analgesics may be prescribed for pain management. Oral contraceptives may be ordered for several months for functional cysts to suppress ovulation. Large cysts (greater than 8 cm) or cysts that do not shrink may be removed surgically (cystectomy). Theca-lutein cysts are usually managed by removal of the hydatidiform mole.

Nursing care focuses on educating the woman regarding treatment options and pain management with analgesics or comfort measures such as heat to the abdomen or relaxation techniques. If surgery is performed, the nurse provides preoperative and postoperative care. Discharge

teaching includes signs of infection, postoperative incision care, and advice regarding follow-up appointments.

Other Benign Ovarian Cysts and Neoplasms

Two other ovarian neoplasms that need discussion include dermoid cysts and ovarian fibromas. *Dermoid cysts* are germ cell tumors usually occurring in childhood. These cysts contain substances such as hair, teeth, sebaceous secretions, and bones. Unless the cyst is large enough to put pressure on other organs, it is usually asymptomatic. Dermoid cysts may develop bilaterally and are often attached to the ovary. Treatment is usually surgical removal.

Ovarian fibromas are solid ovarian neoplasms developing from connective tissue and most often occurring postmenopausally. Fibromas range in size from small nodules to large masses weighing over 23 kg. Most fibromas are unilateral. They are usually asymptomatic, but if large enough they may cause ascites, feelings of pelvic pressure, or abdominal enlargement. Treatment is usually surgical removal.

Nursing care of women treated for dermoid cysts and ovarian fibromas is similar to that described for functional ovarian cysts.

Uterine Neoplasms

Polyps

Polyps may be endometrial or cervical in origin. They are tumors that are on pedicles (stalks) arising from the mucosa (Fig. 13-9). The etiology is unknown, although they may develop in response to hormonal stimulus or be due to inflammation. Polyps are the most common benign lesion of the cervix and endometrium that occur during the reproductive years. Cervical polyps are most common in multiparous women over age 40. A woman who has polyps may be asymptomatic or she may experience premenstrual or postmenstrual bleeding or postcoital bleeding.

Collaborative care. Clinical management of endometrial polyps is by surgical removal. Cervical polyps are usually removed as an office or clinic procedure without anesthesia. The polyp is grasped with a clamp and twisted or cut off. The polyp is sent for pathologic examination.

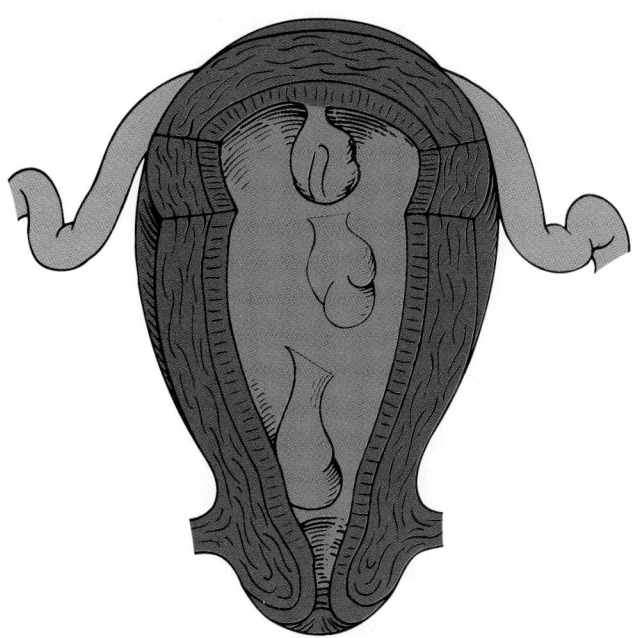

Fig. 13-9 Endometrial polyps.

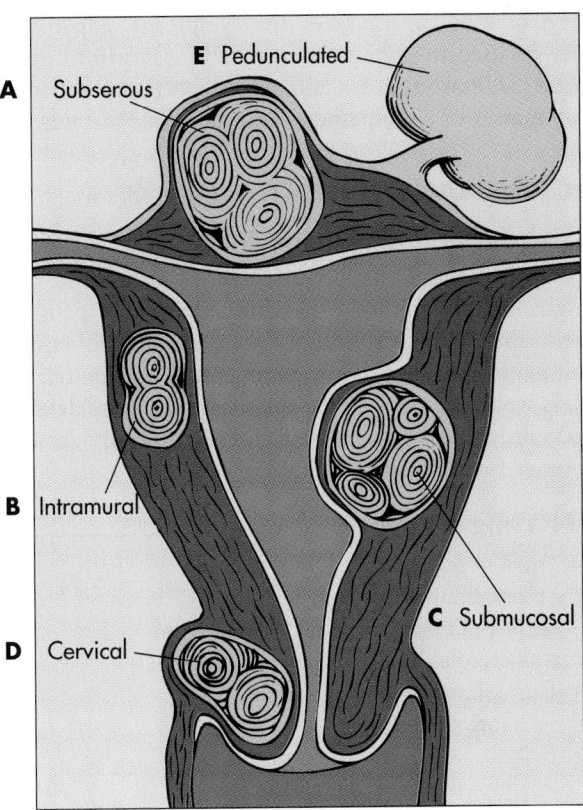

Fig. 13-10 Types of leiomyomas. **A,** Subserous. **B,** Intramural. **C,** Submucosal. **D,** Cervical. **E,** Pedunculated.

Nursing care includes preparing the woman for what to expect during the removal procedure, encouraging relaxation and breathing exercises during the procedure, and providing support during the procedure. After the procedure, the woman is advised to avoid use of tampons, sexual intercourse, and douching for up to 1 week or until the site is healed. She is taught how to identify signs of infection and to notify her health care provider if she experiences heavy bleeding (more than one pad in 1 hour).

Leiomyomas

Leiomyomas, also known as fibroid tumors, fibromas, myomas, or fibromyomas, are slow-growing benign tumors arising from the muscle tissue of the uterus (Mishell et al., 1997). They are the most common benign tumors of the reproductive system. It is estimated that 20% to 25% of women over age 30 develop uterine myomas. They tend to occur more often in African-American women, women who have never been pregnant, and women who use intrauterine devices for contraception (American College of Obstetricians and Gynecologists, 1994). They rarely become malignant. Because their growth is influenced by ovarian hormones, these benign tumors can become quite large when the woman is taking birth control pills, is pregnant, or is on hormone therapy. They spontaneously shrink after menopause when circulating ovarian hormones are diminished.

Clinical manifestations and diagnosis. The cause of leiomyomas remains unknown, although genetic factors may be involved in their development. Most of the tumors are found in the body of the uterus. Leiomyomas are classified according to the location in the uterine wall. *Subserous* leiomyomas develop beneath the peritoneal surface of the uterus and appear as small or large masses that protrude from the outer uterine surface (Fig. 13-10, *A*).

Intramural leiomyomas are tumors that develop within the wall of the uterus (Fig. 13-10, *B*). *Submucosal* leiomyomas are the least common tumors, but often they cause the most symptoms. These tumors develop in the endometrium and protrude into the uterine cavity (Fig. 13-10, *C*). Leiomyomas also can develop in the cervix and on the broad ligaments (Fig. 13-10, *D*). They also can grow on pedicles or stalks (Fig. 13-10, *E*). Occasionally these break off the pedicle and attach to other tissues (become parasitic).

Most women are asymptomatic; abnormal uterine bleeding is the most common symptom of fibroids. If the tumor is very large, pelvic circulation may be compromised, and surrounding viscera may be displaced. A woman may complain of backache, low abdominal pressure, constipation, urinary incontinence, or dysmenorrhea (painful menstruation). Nausea and vomiting may occur if the tumor is obstructing the intestines. The woman may also notice an abdominal mass if the tumor is large. Anemia may be present if the woman has excessive bleeding (Grabo et al., 1999).

The tumors appear to be influenced by the presence of estrogen; during pregnancy the tumors may produce complications such as preterm labor, miscarriage, or dystocia (difficult labor). The severity of the symptoms seems to be directly related to the size and location of the tumors.

Diagnosis is usually accomplished by a process of elimination. A pelvic examination usually identifies the presence of uterine enlargement. Pregnancy tests will rule out pregnancy as the cause of the symptoms. Laparoscopy may be used to differentiate ovarian masses from uterine masses. Ultrasound can differentiate between inflammatory masses or endometriosis and subserous fibroids.

CARE MANAGEMENT

Assessment and Nursing Diagnoses

Assessment should include a history of symptoms, which might include abnormal bleeding, abdominal pain, dysmenorrhea, pelvic fullness or heaviness, or problems with elimination, and a pelvic examination. A differential diagnosis would be made using the diagnostic tests described previously. Possible nursing diagnoses for a woman with a leiomyoma include the following:

Nursing Diagnoses

- Anxiety related to
  - uncertain diagnosis
  - fear of malignancy
  - potential surgical treatment
- Pain related to
  - leiomyomas
- Risk for sexual dysfunction related to
  - dyspareunia

Expected Outcomes of Care

Nursing diagnoses provide the direction for care. Expected outcomes are determined with the woman. Expected outcomes for the woman with a leiomyoma might include that the woman will do the following:
- Verbalize a decrease in anxiety related to the diagnosis and therapeutic regimen.
- Verbalize understanding of treatment options.
- Report no compromise in sexual functioning as a result of the therapeutic intervention.

Plan of Care and Interventions

Knowledge of the medical-surgical management of leiomyomas is essential in planning nursing care. The knowledge enables the nurse to work collaboratively with other health care providers and to meet the woman's knowledge and emotional needs. Clinical management for benign tumors of the uterus depends on the severity of the symptoms, the age of the woman, and her desire to preserve childbearing potential.

Medical Management

If symptoms are mild, regular checkups may suffice to observe for growth or changes in size. Gonadotropin-releasing hormone (GnRH) agonists such as leuprolide acetate (Lupron, Synarel) may be prescribed to reduce the size of the leiomyoma.

The woman who prefers medical treatment will need information about the different medications, their actions and side effects, and routes of administration.

NURSE ALERT *A woman who is receiving GnRH agonists to decrease the size of the fibroid needs to understand that regrowth will occur after the treatment is stopped.*

She also needs to know that a small loss in bone mass and changes in lipid levels can occur; therefore long-term use is not recommended. Amenorrhea may occur; however, women who wish to avoid pregnancy should use a nonhormonal or barrier method of contraception (Grabo et al., 1999). A discussion of administration methods for GnRH agonists, including subcutaneous and intramuscular injections, intranasal administration, and subcutaneous implantation, will assist the woman in making a decision about her preferred method of administration.

Surgical Management

If the tumor is near the outer wall of the uterus and symptoms are significant, *myomectomy* (removal of the tumor) may be performed. Myomectomy can be performed through a laparoscopic or abdominal incision approach or vaginal (hysteroscopic) approach (American College of Obstetricians and Gynecologists, 1994; Reich, 1995). Myomectomy leaves the uterine muscle walls relatively intact, thereby preserving the uterus and allowing the possibility of future pregnancies. It is usually performed in the proliferative phase of the menstrual cycle to avoid interrupting a possible pregnancy.

Laser surgery or electrocauterization can be used to destroy small fibroids through a laparoscopic (abdominal) or hysteroscopic (vaginal) approach. Myolysis is a procedure that uses laser coagulation to vaporize the fibroids and cause necrosis. Although the uterus remains in place, the vaporization process will cause scarring and adhesions in the uterine cavity and may affect future fertility. More research is needed on the safety and efficacy of this procedure (Wallach, 1997).

Hysterectomy (removal of the entire uterus) is the treatment of choice if bleeding is severe or if the fibroid is obstructing normal function of other organs. An abdominal or vaginal surgical approach depends on the size and location of the tumors. For example, abdominal hysterectomy is usually performed for leiomyomas larger than a uterus would be at 12 to 14 weeks of gestation or for multiple leiomyomas. The uterus is removed through either a vertical or transverse incision. In rare circumstances, the cervix may not be removed. Vaginal approaches can be used for smaller tumors. In both abdominal and vaginal approaches, the uterus is removed from the supporting ligaments (broad, round, and uterosacral). These ligaments are then attached to the vaginal cuff, allowing for maintenance of normal depth of the vagina (Fig. 13-11).

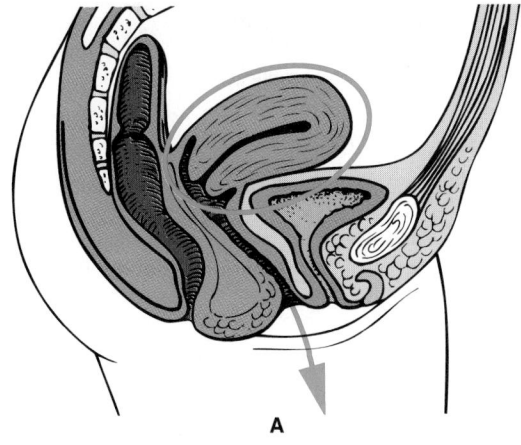

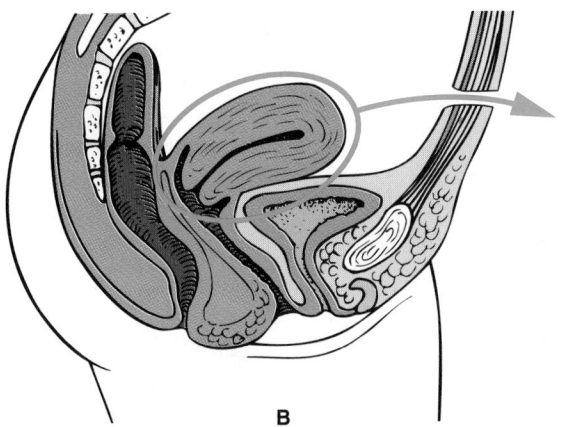

Fig. 13-11 Hysterectomy. **A,** Vaginal. **B,** Abdominal.

BOX 13-1 Preoperative Procedures for Hysterectomy

- Vaginal examination or physical examination
- Laboratory tests
  Complete blood count, type, and crossmatch
  Urinalysis
- Chest x-ray
- Electrocardiogram
- Teaching for postoperative routines
  Turning, coughing, deep breathing
  Passive and active leg exercises
  Need for early ambulation
  Pain relief options
- Nothing by mouth after midnight
- Enema if ordered
- Douche if ordered
- Abdominal—mons or perineal shave if ordered
- Removal of makeup, nail polish
- Removal of glasses, contact lenses, dentures, etc.
- Identification band in place
- Signed consent form in chart
- Have woman empty bladder immediately before surgery

Preoperative Care

Assessments needed before surgery include the woman's knowledge of treatment options, the benefits and risks of each procedure, preoperative and postoperative procedures (Box 13-1), and the recovery process. If the woman can demonstrate understanding of this information, she can make an informed decision about treatment.

Psychologic assessment is essential, particularly for a woman who is scheduled for a hysterectomy. Areas to be explored include the significance of the loss of the uterus for the woman, misconceptions about effects of surgery, and adequacy of her support system. Women who have not completed their childbearing, who believe that their self-concept is related to having a uterus (to be a complete woman), who feel that sexual functioning is related to having a uterus, or who have too little or too much anxiety about the surgery may be at risk for postoperative emotional reactions (Smith, 1997).

Postoperative Care

Postoperative assessments and care after myomectomy and abdominal hysterectomy are similar to other abdomi-

nal surgery (Box 13-2). Assessments specific to abdominal and vaginal hysterectomy include assessment for vaginal bleeding (one perineal pad saturated in less than 1 hour is excessive), urinary retention (especially after vaginal hysterectomy), perineal pain after vaginal hysterectomy, and psychologic assessments (depression is the most common emotional reaction).

Discharge Planning and Teaching

Discharge planning and teaching are similar for myomectomy and hysterectomy (see Home Care box). If a hysterectomy was performed, the woman is reminded of the physical changes that she will experience. These include cessation of menses, presence of fatigue and weakness, and possible emotional reactions such as depression (Smith, 1997). If the woman is premenopausal she will not experience menopause at this time unless her ovaries were also removed. After laser surgery the woman is instructed about the signs of infection, pain relief with analgesics or nonsteroidal antiinflammatory drugs, and resumption of normal activities within several days and informed that vaginal discharge is to be expected for 4 to 6 weeks. She should be reminded about the possible effects of ablation on her fertility, if appropriate. Vaginal intercourse may be uncomfortable at first. Use of water-soluble lubricants, relaxation exercises, and positions that control penile penetration may be beneficial (Lowdermilk, 1995b; Williamson, 1992).

BOX 13-2 Postoperative Care After Hysterectomy

- Monitor vital signs q15min until stable; then q4hr for 48 hr
- Maintain unobstructed airway
- Turn, cough, deep breathe q2hr for 24 hr
  Assist woman to splint incision with hands or pillow
- Incentive spirometry if ordered
- Leg exercises q2-4hr until ambulatory
  Assess Homan's sign
- Assess bleeding
  Abdominal—assess dressing or incision
  Vaginal—perineal pad count (one saturated pad in less than 1 hour is excessive; vaginal bleeding is usually minimal)
- Check laboratory values, especially hematocrit
- Assess lungs
- Assess bowel sounds and monitor bowel function
- Monitor intake and output
  Foley catheter may be in place for 24 hours after abdominal surgery
  After vaginal hysterectomy, urinary retention may be a problem due to manipulation of the urethra during surgery
- Assess abdominal incision or vagina for signs of infection

- Observe for signs of complications
  Abdominal hysterectomy—assess for signs of wound evisceration, pulmonary embolism, thrombophlebitis, pneumonia, bowel obstruction, bleeding (incisional or vaginal)
  Vaginal hysterectomy—assess for signs of urinary tract infection, urinary retention, wound infection, vaginal bleeding
- Pain relief
  Pharmacologic measures—Patient-controlled analgesia (PCA) or epidural narcotics may be ordered for the first 24 hours, followed by oral analgesics and nonsteroidal antiinflammatory drugs
  Nonpharmacologic measures—breathing and relaxation exercises, position changes, guided imagery, application of heat to the abdomen, and sitz baths or ice packs for the perineum; ambulation may relieve gas pains
- Psychologic assessments
  Assess for depression or other emotional reactions
  Assess support systems
  Assess sexual concerns

HOME CARE

Woman Who Has Had a Myomectomy or Hysterectomy

Eat foods high in protein, iron, and vitamin C to aid in tissue healing; include foods with high fiber content; and drink six to eight 8 oz glasses of water daily.
- Rest when tired; resume activities as comfort level permits. Avoid vigorous exercise and heavy lifting for 6 weeks. Avoid sitting for long periods. Resume driving when comfort allows or on advice from health care provider.
- Avoid tub baths, intercourse (vaginal rest), and douching until after the follow-up examination.

- When vaginal intercourse is resumed, use of water-soluble lubricants may decrease discomfort.
- Report the following symptoms to your health care provider: vaginal bleeding, gastrointestinal changes, persistent postoperative symptoms (cramping, distention, change in bowel habits), and signs of wound infection (redness, swelling, heat, or pain at incision site).
- Keep your follow-up appointment with your health care provider.

Evaluation

The nurse evaluates the care of the woman who has had treatment of uterine leiomyomas using the outcome criteria. These include that the woman states she understands her options for treatment and is satisfied with her choice, she has resumed sexual activities at her pretreatment level of satisfaction, and her anxiety about her diagnosis and treatment is minimal or relieved.

Vulvar Neoplasms

Bartholin's Cysts

Bartholin's cysts are the most common benign lesions of the vulva. The cause is obstruction of the Bartholin duct,

causing it to enlarge. Small cysts often are asymptomatic; however, large cysts or infected cysts cause symptoms such as vulvar pain, dyspareunia (painful intercourse), and a feeling of a mass in the vulvar area.

Collaborative Care

If the woman is asymptomatic, no treatment is necessary. If the cyst is symptomatic or infected, surgical incision and drainage may provide temporary relief. Cysts tend to recur; therefore a permanent opening for drainage may be recommended. This procedure is called marsupialization and is the formation of a new duct opening for drainage.

Nursing care after surgery includes teaching the woman about pain relief measures such as sitz baths, heat lamps to the perineum, and use of analgesics. The woman is taught to assess the incision site for signs of healing and infection and to take antibiotics, if prescribed, for prevention of infection.

MALIGNANT NEOPLASMS

Malignant neoplasms of the reproductive system include cancers of the endometrium, cervix, ovary, vulva, vagina, and uterine tubes.

Cancer of the Endometrium

Incidence and Etiology

Endometrial cancer is the most common malignancy of the reproductive system (American Cancer Society, 1999). It is most commonly seen in perimenopausal and postmenopausal women between 50 and 65 years of age. Certain risk factors have been associated with the development of endometrial cancer, including obesity, nulliparity, infertility, late onset of menopause, diabetes mellitus, hypertension, and family history of ovarian or breast disease. Hormone imbalance, however, seems to be the most significant risk factor. Numerous studies have correlated the use of exogenous estrogens (unopposed stimulation, i.e., absence of progesterone) in postmenopausal women with an increased incidence of uterine cancer (DiSaia & Creasman, 1997). The incidence of endometrial cancer among Caucasian women is approximately twice that among African-American women (Mishell et al., 1997).

Endometrial cancer is slow growing and for that reason has a good prognosis in 80% to 90% of cases. Most endometrial cancers are adenocarcinomas that develop from endometrial hyperplasia. The tumor usually develops in the fundus of the uterus and can spread directly to the myometrium and cervix, as well as to the reproductive organs. **Metastasis** (spread of cancer from its original site) is through the lymphatic system in the pelvis and through the blood to the liver, lungs, and brain.

⦂ CARE MANAGEMENT

Assessment and Nursing Diagnoses

Assessment includes a history of physical symptoms. The cardinal sign of endometrial cancer is abnormal uterine bleeding (e.g., postmenopausal bleeding and premenopausal recurrent metrorrhagia). Thirty percent of postmenopausal bleeding is caused by carcinoma. Late signs include a mucosanguineous vaginal discharge, low back pain, or low pelvic pain. A pelvic examination may reveal the presence of a uterine enlargement or mass.

Histologic examination is used for diagnosis. Papanicolaou smear of cellular material obtained by aspiration of the endocervix will identify only one third to one half of cases. Fractional curettage or endometrial biopsy yields the most accurate results. Fractional curettage involves scraping the endocervix and endometrium for histologic evaluation to determine the grade of neoplasm and its stage (extent). Perforation of the uterus is a possible complication of this procedure. Endometrial biopsy will identify about 90% of cases. Other diagnostic tests that may be useful include hysteroscopy (examination of the uterus through an endoscope) and vaginal ultrasonography. Other tests may be done to determine the spread of cancer. These include liver function tests, renal function tests, chest x-ray, intravenous pyelography (IVP), barium enema, computed tomography (CT), bone scans, and biopsy of suspicious tissues. The International Federation of Gynecology and Obstetrics (FIGO) classification system is used to describe the stages of endometrial carcinoma (Table 13-1). Possible nursing diagnoses that would apply to a woman with endometrial cancer include the following:

⦂ Nursing Diagnoses

- Knowledge deficit related to
  - the diagnosis, treatment, and prognosis
- Decisional conflict related to
  - treatment options
- Fear/anxiety related to
  - diagnosis of cancer, loss of uterus
- Impaired skin integrity related to
  - surgery or radiation therapy
- Pain related to
  - cancer
  - surgical procedure
- Body-image disturbance related to
  - loss of uterus
- Altered sexuality patterns related to
  - anatomic and functional changes caused by cancer or its treatment

Expected Outcomes of Care

Planning for care of the woman with endometrial cancer depends on the stage of cancer and the treatment selected. However, some outcomes can be identified for the nursing diagnoses that have been established. Examples of expected outcome criteria are that the woman will do the following:

- Demonstrate understanding of her diagnosis of endometrial cancer, the treatments available, and her prognosis.
- Make informed decisions about treatment options.
- Describe a decrease in anxiety and fear.
- Report that pain is reduced or manageable.
- Experience no skin breakdown or infection.
- State that she understands the effects of cancer and treatment on her body image and that her concerns are reduced.
- Report that she and her partner will be able to resume mutually satisfying sexual relations after treatment.

TABLE 13-1	FIGO Classification of Endometrial Carcinoma*	
Stage	IA G123	Tumor limited to endometrium
	IB G123	Invasion of less than half of the myometrium
	IC G123	Invasion of more than half of the myometrium
	IIA G123	Endocervical glandular involvement only
	IIB G123	Cervical stromal invasion
	IIIA G123	Tumor invades serosa and/or adnexae and/or positive peritoneal cytology
	IIIB G123	Vaginal metastases
	IIIC G123	Metastases to pelvic and/or paraaortic lymph nodes
	IVA G123	Tumor invasion of bladder and/or bowel mucosa
	IVB	Distant metastases, including intraabdominal and/or inguinal lymph node

Histopathology: Degree of differentiation

Cases of carcinoma of the corpus should be grouped according to the degree of differentiation of the adenocarcinoma as follows:

G1 = 5% or less of a nonsquamous or nonmorular solid growth pattern

G2 = 6% to 50% of a nonsquamous or nonmorular solid growth pattern

G3 = more than 50% of a nonsquamous or nonmorular solid growth pattern

*Approved by FIGO, October 1988, Rio de Janeiro. From DiSaia, P., & Creasman, W. (1997). *Clinical gynecologic oncology* (5th ed.). St. Louis: Mosby.

Plan of Care and Interventions

Therapeutic Management

Collaborative efforts from various health disciplines are needed to work with the woman with endometrial cancer. All must have an understanding of the treatments that may be used.

For stage I adenocarcinoma of the endometrium, total abdominal hysterectomy (TAH) and bilateral salpingo-oophorectomy (BSO) are the usual treatments of choice. A radical hysterectomy (abdominal hysterectomy plus pelvic node dissection) usually is performed for stage II endometrial cancer. Removal of the upper third of the vagina and parametrium may also be done. Surgery may be combined with radiation therapy before or after surgery. External radiation therapy to the whole pelvis (see p. 290) is usually given when there is extensive uterine disease or metastasis outside the uterus (DiSaia & Creasman, 1997). Treatment is usually 4 to 5 days a week for 6 weeks. Internal radiation

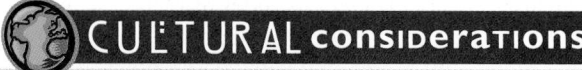

CULTURAL consideraTions

Meaning of Cancer

A woman's culture influences how she responds to the meaning of cancer. Her response must be appropriate to her cultural context for it to be acceptable to her. For example, body-image issues (e.g., loss of uterus), the meaning of death, and pain responses (e.g., stoic or expressive) are influenced by cultural beliefs and values. In making assessments about these issues the nurse takes into account the influence of culture before developing a plan of care.

therapy (placement of an applicator loaded with a radiation source into the uterine cavity) may also be used (see p. 290). Treatment is usually 1 to 3 days. Radiation therapy may cause skin ulcerations, cystitis, enteritis, and delayed complications such as genital fistulas.

Chemotherapy is used to treat advanced and recurrent disease, although no effective treatment regimen has been established (Mishell et al., 1997). Agents that have been somewhat effective include cisplatin, doxorubicin (Adriamycin), cyclophosphamide (Cytoxan), 5-fluorouracil (5-FU), and vincristine (Oncovin). Chemotherapy may cause hair loss, anemia, and bone marrow depression, as well as other side effects.

Progestational therapy—use of medroxyprogesterone (Depo-Provera) and megestrol (Megace)—may be effective for estrogen-dependent cancers. These drugs usually do not cause acute side effects. Tamoxifen (Tamofen) is an antiestrogen that is being investigated for its effectiveness against recurrent endometrial cancer. It may cause hot flashes and nausea and vomiting (DiSaia & Creasman, 1997; Mishell et al., 1997).

Nursing care. Nursing care is individualized to the woman and her specific situation and diagnosis. Interventions for the woman having surgery are directed by assessment of her perception of the anticipated surgery, her knowledge of what to expect after surgery, and any preoperative special procedures, such as cleansing enemas or douches. In today's practice of short hospital stays even for radical surgery, many of these preoperative procedures are performed at home before admission, so assessment of understanding becomes a critical nursing action (see Cultural Considerations box).

Preoperative Care

The nurse working with the woman preparing for a radical hysterectomy should explain any preoperative procedures to be done, as described on p. 277. Additional teaching is needed regarding possible postsurgical events (e.g., drainage tubes). The woman should be prepared to see a suprapubic drain that will remain in place several days to a week.

Postoperative Care

Assessment of vital signs usually follows a postanesthesia protocol, gradually decreasing in frequency to 4 times a day. IV fluids are maintained at a rate rapid enough to maintain hydration and electrolyte balance. Diet is gradually resumed as bowel sounds are heard and flatus is passed. A nasogastric tube may be in place to prevent distention. Intake and output are monitored.

The woman will need to be reminded to turn and take deep breaths, and assistance is given as needed. Breath sounds are assessed and any deviations from normal reported immediately. The most significant single cause of morbidity and prolonged hospitalization after major procedures is respiratory complications. Anesthesia and surgery alter breathing patterns and ability to cough. Atelectasis, pneumonia, and pulmonary embolus may occur.

Hemorrhage is always a possible complication after surgery. The wound drainage tube is emptied as needed or every 4 hours, and the amount and character of drainage is recorded. Drainage from any tube is assessed for bleeding. Vaginal drainage, if any, should be serosanguineous. Hematuria is noted and recorded. The primary health care provider is kept apprised of any deviations from normal expectations.

Paralytic ileus may occur after surgery in which the intestinal tract has been manipulated. A nasogastric tube, limiting oral fluids, and early ambulation all support the return of gastrointestinal function. An enema or suppository may bring relief of flatus and stimulate the return of bowel function. Oral laxatives should not be given until lower bowel function has returned.

Sitting may result in pelvic congestion, so the high Fowler's position is avoided. Pelvic congestion is discouraged by avoiding use of the knee gatch (or pillow). Nursing measures such as massages, repositioning, fresh linen, regular perineal care, and emotional support are all helpful adjuncts to pharmacologic control of discomfort.

Discharge Planning and Teaching

Because the in-hospital convalescent period is generally short, close observation by the nurse and attention to detail are critical. Nursing actions appropriate to this period include monitoring for urinary retention after the catheter is removed, monitoring the woman's appetite and diet, monitoring bowel function, and encouraging progressive ambulation and self-care.

Hormone therapy (e.g., estrogen and progesterone), if prescribed, is usually started as soon as the woman can take oral fluids. The nurse can take this opportunity to remind the woman that she will no longer have menstrual periods (if she was premenopausal) and to encourage her to verbalize questions or concerns she may have about hormonal replacement therapy.

Discharge planning and teaching is done throughout the preoperative and postoperative phases and culminates during the convalescent phase. Discharge teaching topics for the woman with a radical hysterectomy are similar to those for the woman who has had a hysterectomy for leiomyomas and can be found in the Home Care box on p. 278. (Also see Plan of Care.)

Care for the woman who has had external or internal radiation therapy is the same as described for the woman with cervical cancer (p. 291).

Nursing care for the woman undergoing chemotherapy will depend on the type of drug given. If alopecia is likely, the nurse can suggest wigs, scarves, or other kinds of head coverings. If the therapy affects the appetite or causes gastrointestinal side effects, suggestions such as those in Table 13-2 may be useful.

Psychologic care for the woman with endometrial cancer is essential. A women needs to be able to discuss her concerns about having cancer and the potential for recurrence. She may have fears of death; permanent disfigurement and change in functioning; altered feelings of self as a woman; concerns regarding her femininity, sexuality, and loss of reproductive capacity; and questions arising from things she has heard about posthysterectomy changes, radiation therapy, or chemotherapy. Significant others should be encouraged to express their questions and concerns as well. The woman may benefit from a referral to a community cancer support group.

Evaluation

The nursing care of a woman with endometrial cancer is evaluated by using the expected outcomes and measurable criteria to ascertain the degree to which the outcomes were met.

Cancer of the Ovary

Incidence and Etiology

Cancer of the ovary is the second most frequently occurring reproductive cancer and causes more deaths than any other female genital tract cancer (American Cancer Society, 1999). Because the symptoms of this type of cancer are vague and definitive screening tests do not exist, ovarian cancer is often diagnosed in an advanced stage. The 5-year survival rate for cancer diagnosed at a localized stage is about 93%; for advanced stage the rate drops to about 50% (American Cancer Society, 1999). Malignant neoplasia of the ovaries occurs at all ages, including infants and children. However, the greatest number of cases is found in women between ages 50 and 59 years.

Major histologic cell types occur in different age groups, with malignant germ cell tumors most common in women between ages 20 and 40 years and epithelial cancers occurring in the perimenopausal age groups. The spread of ovarian cancer is by direct extension to adjacent organs, but distal spread can occur through lymphatic spread to the liver and lungs.

PLAN ᴼᶠ CARE | Hysterectomy for Endometrial Cancer

NURSING DIAGNOSIS Anxiety related to lack of understanding of diagnosis, treatment, and prognosis of endometrial cancer as evidenced by client questions and concerns

Expected Outcome *Client will identify source of anxiety and verbalize understanding of diagnosis, effects of hysterectomy and prognosis.*

Nursing Interventions/*Rationales*

Assess client's level of understanding of procedure and its effects *to correct any misunderstanding, provide clarification, and identify starting point for further information.*

Provide information about cancer of the endometrium, individualizing information to client's situation *to provide clarification concerning treatment regimen.*

Provide preoperative and postoperative teaching *to give anticipatory guidance and rationales for upcoming events.*

NURSING DIAGNOSIS Fear related to diagnosis of endometrial cancer as evidenced by client questions and concerns

Expected Outcomes *Client will be able to verbalize that fears have diminished following the procedure.*

Nursing Interventions/*Rationales*

Through therapeutic communication, encourage verbalization of fears *to provide clarification and validation of feelings.*

Encourage client to identify support system *to have resources readily available as needed.*

NURSING DIAGNOSIS Pain related to surgical procedure as evidenced by client verbal and nonverbal behaviors

Expected Outcome *Client will verbalize decrease in intensity and number of painful episodes following interventions.*

Nursing Interventions/*Rationales*

Assess the location and intensity of pain using a pain scale *to utilize appropriate treatment.*

Administer prescribed analgesics *to decrease perception of pain.*

Utilize nonpharmacologic techniques such as distraction, relaxation, position changes, and heat *to decrease perception of pain.*

Evaluate effectiveness of interventions *to modify interventions if needed.*

NURSING DIAGNOSIS Risk for infection related to surgical incision and impaired skin integrity

Expected Outcome *Client will experience no infection following the procedure.*

Nursing Interventions/*Rationales*

Assess for clinical manifestations of infection—fever, drainage, redness, swelling at the incision site *to provide for prompt treatment.*

Encourage a diet high in protein, vitamin C, and calories *to promote wound healing.*

Teach client to maintain aseptic technique when performing dressing changes, such as good handwashing *to decrease chance of introducing microorganisms at the incision site.*

NURSING DIAGNOSIS Body image disturbance related to loss of uterus as evidenced by client statements of fears or concerns

Expected Outcome *Client will maintain a positive body image.*

Nursing Interventions/*Rationales*

Encourage expression of feelings through therapeutic communication *to provide clarification and validity to feelings.*

Encourage client to share feelings with significant other *to provide emotional support.*

Assist client to identify support systems *to be available in case of client need to ventilate feelings.*

NURSING DIAGNOSIS Risk for sexual dysfunction related to perceived loss of femininity

Expected Outcome *Client will maintain usual sexual relationship with partner.*

Nursing Interventions/*Rationales*

Encourage verbalization of feelings related to sexuality *to provide clarification.*

Provide opportunity for role-playing *to alleviate fears about interactions with partner.*

Refer to sexual counselor *to provide in-depth intervention as needed.*

The cause of ovarian cancer is unknown; however, a number of risk factors have been identified. These factors include nulliparity, infertility, previous breast or colon cancer, and family history of ovarian cancer. Women of North American or northern European descent have the highest incidence of ovarian cancers. Genital exposure to talc, a diet high in fat, lactose intolerance, and use of fertility drugs have been suggested as risk factors, but research findings are inconclusive (DiSaia & Creasman, 1997). Pregnancy and use of oral contraceptives seem to have some protective benefits against ovarian cancer (American Cancer Society, 1999; National Institutes of Health Consensus Conference, 1995).

Clinical Manifestations and Diagnosis

Ovarian cancer has been called a silent disease because early warning symptoms that would send a woman to her health care provider are absent (e.g., no bleeding or other discharge and no pain). Vague lower abdominal discomfort and mild digestive complaints are the early symptoms for some. An ovary enlarged 5 cm or more than normal that is found during routine examination requires careful diagnostic workup. The accompanying increase in abdominal girth (caused by ovarian enlargement or ascites) is usually attributed to an increase in weight or a shift in weight that is seen commonly in women entering their middle years. Pelvic pain, anemia, and general weakness and malnutrition are signs of late-stage disease.

Ovarian cancer is rarely diagnosed early. Seventy percent of all women have metastasis outside of the pelvis at the time of diagnosis. Attempts at early detection have not proven to be reliable so far. Taking a family history is important because it may reveal cancer of the uterus or breast. Transvaginal ultrasound, CA-125 antigen (a tumor-associated antigen) testing, and frequent pelvic examinations have all been used without a great deal of success because these tumors grow quickly and painlessly. Transvaginal ultrasound and CA-125 screening currently are not recommended for routine screening. Routine pelvic examination continues to be the only practical screening method for detecting early disease even though few cancers are detected in women without symptoms. Any ovarian enlargement should be considered highly suspicious and in need of further evaluation by laparoscopy or laparotomy. Responsibility for diagnosis rests with the pathologist. The size of the tumor is not indicative of the severity of disease. Clinical staging is done surgically and gives direction to treatment and prognosis (DiSaia & Creasman, 1997; National Institutes of Health Consensus Conference, 1995).

Collaborative Care

Treatment is dictated by the stage of the disease at the time of initial diagnosis. Surgical removal of as much of the tumor as possible is the first step in therapy. This may involve just the removal of one ovary and tube or the

TABLE 13-2 Nutritional Management for Common Problems Related to Gynecologic Cancer or Treatment

ALTERED TASTE
Mouth care after meals
Extra seasoning
Sauces and marinades for meats
Eat fish or chicken instead of red meat
Eat tart foods to stimulate taste buds

ANOREXIA
Eat with family, friends
Try new foods, recipes
Smaller servings
High calorie snacks
Protein shakes
Exercise before meals to stimulate appetite
Eat when hungry

NAUSEA AND VOMITING
Clear liquids
Avoid carbonated fluids
Avoid sweet, rich, fatty foods
Cool foods rather than hot or warm foods
Small meals
High-calorie, high-protein diet
Eat toast, bland foods
Antiemetics before meals may be needed

STOMATITIS—MILD TO MODERATE
Small meals
Eat soft, bland foods
Drink 3 L of fluids a day
Avoid citrus fruits, spicy foods
Avoid alcohol
Avoid very hot or very cold foods
Add nutritional supplements, as needed

SEVERE STOMATITIS
Eat liquid or pureed foods
Enteral or total parenteral nutrition may be needed

CONSTIPATION
Increase fiber (bran, fresh fruits and vegetables)
Increase fluid intake (3000 ml/day)
Natural laxative foods (prunes, apples)
Avoid cheese products

DIARRHEA
Avoid milk products
Avoid high fiber, spicy foods
Eat foods high in potassium
Increase fluid intake (3000 ml/day), avoid caffeine and carbonated fluids
Add nutmeg to food to decrease gastric motility
Eat a high-protein, high-carbohydrate diet

POSTOPERATIVE RECOVERY
Food high in iron
High protein foods
Foods high in vitamin C, B complex, and K
6-8 glasses of fluids a day

From Lowdermilk, D. (1995). Home care of the patient with gynecologic cancer. *J Obstet Gynecol Neonatal Nurs* 24(2), 159.

radical excision of uterus, ovaries, tubes, and omentum. Cytore-ductive surgery (the debulking of the poorly vascularized larger tumors) is also done. The smaller the volume of tumor remaining, the better the response to adjuvant therapy. Because about three fourths of women are in stage II, III, or IV disease at the time of diagnosis, surgical cure is not possible. Therefore, after tumor reduction surgery is performed, women with epithelial cell carcinoma will receive chemotherapy. Many institutions use a multiagent approach. Combinations of antineoplastic drugs such as cyclophosphamide (Cytoxan) and cisplatin or cisplatin and doxorubicin (Adriamycin) are common. Paclitaxel (Taxol) is being used in clinical trials with cisplatin and other platinum drugs in the United States. Combining immunotherapy with chemotherapy is also being investigated (DiSaia & Creasman, 1997).

Second-look surgery is a technique used to determine the response of the disease to chemotherapy and to determine whether treatment should be continued.

The efficacy of intraperitoneal installation with radioactive phosphorus (^{32}P) continues to be investigated. The role of radiation in treating advanced ovarian carcinoma is controversial. Radiation has been used as a palliative measure, and some women have had long-term survival after debulking surgery followed by radiation therapy (National Institutes of Health Consensus Conference, 1995). More research is needed regarding the role of radiation therapy in treatment of ovarian cancer.

Nursing Implications

The woman diagnosed with ovarian cancer has similar concerns as those described for the woman with endometrial and cervical cancer. Nursing interventions for the woman having surgery, chemotherapy, or external radiation therapy are described in other sections of this chapter.

Women with advanced ovarian cancer have a significant rate of recurrence. Follow-up for 5 years must be intensive. When a cure or remission cannot be achieved, palliative measures that alleviate symptoms of the progressing disease and provide comfort and maximum function are initiated. As the disease progresses, nutritional support, including enteral feedings and parenteral hyperalimentation, may be needed because of the effects of both the disease and the treatments on the gastrointestinal tract. The goal of nursing care is assisting the woman to maintain quality of life.

Because the period between a focus on cure and a focus on palliation is often prolonged, the woman with ovarian cancer is apt to experience most of the stages described by Kübler-Ross and to need support through each. After diagnosis, the woman experiences denial, then anger. As treatment begins, she may "bargain" for a cure. If treatment is successful and death is forestalled by remission or cure, the process of adjustment to terminality ceases, and the woman again focuses on life and its challenges. When treatment fails to secure a cure or remission ends, the

woman must turn again to the task of adjustment (see Legal Tip).

LEGAL TIP **Advance Directives**

Nurses who work with clients in hospitals with federal funding need to know that because of the Patient Self-Determination Act, all clients must be asked if they have knowledge of Advance Directives and be provided with the information if desired. This is important to nurses working in gynecology oncology settings, where decisions about living wills and no codes may be issues.

Family and friends also experience diverse feelings. When grieving is prolonged, as it often is when the woman has cancer, the stress can be enormous and can interfere with other interpersonal relationships. The hospital environment may further intrude on relationships, limiting privacy and access to the woman and hindering opportunities for caring gestures. Referral to a cancer support group may be useful.

Cancer of the Cervix

Incidence and Etiology

Cancer of the cervix is the third most common reproductive cancer. The accessible location of the cervix to both cell and tissue study and direct examination have led to a refinement of diagnostic techniques that have contributed to improved management of these disorders. The incidence of invasive cancer has decreased by 50% over the last 25 years, reducing mortality rates. However, the incidence of preinvasive cancer has increased, and more women in their twenties and thirties are being diagnosed with cervical neoplasia.

Cancer of the cervix begins as neoplastic changes in the cervical epithelium. Terms that have been used to describe these epithelial changes or preinvasive lesions include **dysplasia** and **cervical intraepithelial neoplasia (CIN).** Mild cervical dysplasia and CIN I refer to abnormal cellular proliferation in the lower one third of the epithelium; this dysplasia tends to be self-limiting and generally regresses to normal. Severe cervical dysplasia and CIN III involve the lower two thirds of the epithelium and often progress to carcinoma in situ. Carcinoma in situ (CIS) is diagnosed when the full thickness of epithelium shows abnormal cells (Fig. 13-12). Newer terms to describe neoplastic changes are *low grade* and *high grade* **squamous intraepithelial lesions (SILs);** however, *CIN* continues to be the most common term used in clinical practice.

Preinvasive lesions are limited to the cervix and usually originate in the squamocolumnar junction or **transformation zone** (Fig. 13-13). Intensive study of the cervix and the cellular changes that take place has shown that most cervical tumors have a gradual onset rather than an explosive one. Preinvasive conditions may exist for years before

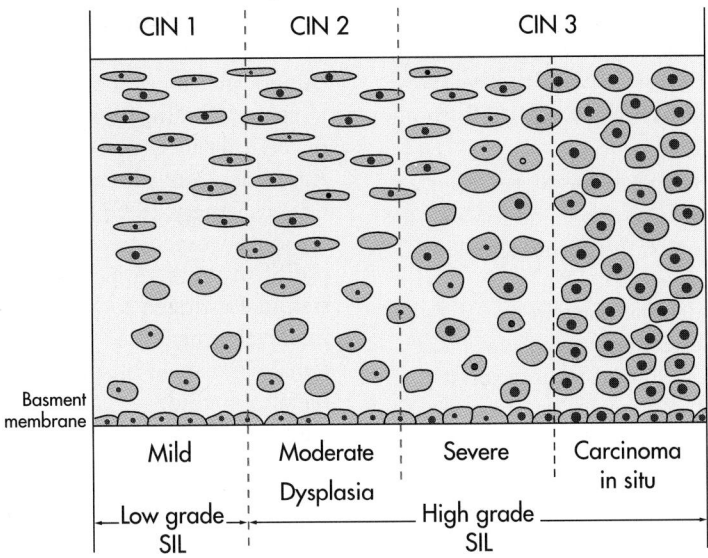

Fig. 13-12 Diagram of cervical epithelium showing progressive changes and various terminology.

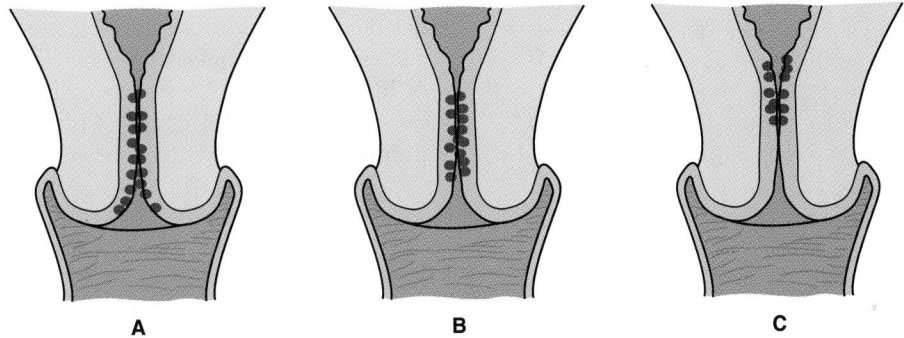

Fig. 13-13 Location of squamocolumnar junction according to age. The location where the endocervical glands meet the squamous epithelium becomes progressively higher with age. **A,** Puberty. **B,** Reproductive years. **C,** Postmenopausal. *(From Willson, J., & Carrington, E. [1991]. Obstetrics and gynecology. St. Louis: Mosby.)*

the development of invasive disease. These preinvasive conditions are highly treatable in many cases.

Invasive carcinoma is the diagnosis when abnormal cells penetrate the basement membrane and invade the stroma. Currently there are two types of invasive carcinoma of the cervix: microinvasive and invasive. *Microinvasive carcinoma* is defined as one or more lesions that penetrate no more than 3 mm into the stroma below the basement membrane with no areas of lymphatic or vascular invasion (DiSaia & Creasman, 1997). *Invasive carcinoma* is invasion that goes beyond these parameters. The staging of invasive carcinoma extends from stage 0 (carcinoma in situ) to stage IVB (distant metastasis or disease outside the true pelvis). A number of substages within each stage also exist. Clinical stages for cancer of the cervix are shown in Table 13-3.

Approximately 90% of cervical malignancies are squamous cell carcinomas; 10% are adenocarcinoma. Squamous cell carcinomas can spread by direct extension to the vaginal mucosa, pelvic wall, bowels, and bladder. Metastasis usually occurs in the pelvis, but it can spread to the lungs and brain through the lymphatic system.

The average age range for the occurrence of cervical cancer is 40 to 50 years. However, preinvasive conditions may exist for 10 to 15 years before the development of an invasive carcinoma. A strong link has been established between human papillomavirus (HPV) types 16 and 18 and cervical neoplasia. Eighteen other types have been associated with genital tract infections and may also be associated with CIN (DiSaia & Creasman, 1997; Verdon, 1997). Other sexually transmitted infections that are identified as risk factors are herpes simplex virus II and possibly cytomegalovirus. There is also a high rate of CIN in human immunodeficiency virus–positive women (DiSaia & Creasman, 1997). Other common risk factors include early age at first coitus (less than age 20); multiple sexual partners (more than two); a sexual

TABLE 13-3 FIGO Staging Classification for Cervical Carcinoma

INTERNATIONAL CLASSIFICATION OF CANCER OF THE CERVIX

Stage 0	Carcinoma in situ, intraepithelial carcinoma.
Stage I	The carcinoma is strictly confined to the cervix (extension to the corpus should be disregarded).
Stage Ia	Invasive cancer identified only microscopically; all gross lesions even with superficial invasion are stage Ib cancers. Invasion is limited to measured stromal invasion with maximum depth of 5.0 mm and no wider than 7.0 mm.
Stage Ia1	Measured invasion of stroma no greater than 3.0 mm in depth and no wider than 7.0 mm.
Stage Ia2	Measured invasion of stroma greater than 3.0 mm and no greater than 5.0 mm and no wider than 7.0 mm. The depth of invasion should not be more than 5.0 mm taken from the base of the epithelium, surface or glandular, from which it originates. Vascular space involvement, venous or lymphatic, should not alter the staging.
Stage Ib	Clinical lesions confined to the cervix or preclinical lesions greater than stage Ia.
Stage Ib1	Clinical lesions no greater than 4.0 cm in size.
Stage Ib2	Clinical lesions greater than 4.0 cm in size.
Stage II	Involvement of the vagina but not the lower third, or infiltration of the parametria but not out to the sidewall.
Stage IIa	Involvement of the vagina but no evidence of parametrial involvement.
Stage IIb	Infiltration of the parametria but not out to the sidewall.
Stage III	Involvement of the lower third of the vagina or extension to the pelvic sidewall. All cases with a hydronephrosis or nonfunctioning kidney should be included, unless they are known to be attributable to other cause.
Stage IIIa	Involvement of the lower third of the vagina but not out to the pelvic sidewall if the parametria are involved.
Stage IIIb	Extension onto the pelvic sidewall and/or hydronephrosis or nonfunctional kidney.
Stage IV	Extension outside the reproductive tract.
Stage IVa	Involvement of the mucosa of the bladder or rectum.
Stage IVb	Distant metastasis or disease outside the true pelvis.

From DiSaia, P., & Creasman, W. (1997). *Clinical gynecologic oncology* (5th ed.). St. Louis: Mosby.

partner with a history of multiple sexual partners; cigarette smoking; and belonging to a lower socioeconomic group (American Cancer Society, 1999; DiSaia & Creasman, 1997; Higgins & Smith, 1997; Mishell et al., 1997). The incidence of cervical cancer in the United States is highest in African-American and Mexican-American women (American Cancer Society, 1999; DiSaia & Creasman, 1997).

Some women have been exposed to diethylstilbestrol (DES) in utero. Administration of DES or another non-steroidal estrogen to a pregnant woman may be followed by developmental or functional genital problems in both female and male offspring. Abnormalities are rare and in females include circumferential vaginal ridges; cervical deformity, for example, "cock's comb" cervix, hooding, clefts, or pseudopolyps; hypoplastic or T-shaped uterus; constricting bands within the uterus; tubal anomalies; vaginal or cervical adenosis; dysplasia; and cervical incompetence. There appears to be an increased frequency of oligomenorrhea and a lower incidence of pregnancy in these women. Most critical is the finding that about 1 out of 1000 women exposed to DES prenatally develop vaginal or cervical clear-cell adenocarcinoma, usually during adolescence. No equivalent of female clear-cell carcinoma or increase in male genitourinary cancer has been noted; however, epididymal cysts, hydrotrophic testes, and abnormal sperm analyses have been reported.

Clinical Manifestations and Diagnosis

Preinvasive cancer of the cervix is often asymptomatic. Abnormal bleeding, especially postcoital bleeding, is the classic symptom of invasive cancer. Other late symptoms include rectal bleeding, hematuria, back pain, leg pain, and anemia. Diagnosis includes taking a history that includes menstrual and sexual activity information, particularly a history of sexually transmitted diseases and abnormal bleeding episodes. A pelvic examination usually will be normal except in late-stage cancer.

The single most reliable method to detect preinvasive cancer is the Papanicolaou (Pap) test. The Pap test will detect 90% of early cervical changes. The American College of Obstetricians and Gynecologists (ACOG) and the American Cancer Society (ACS) recommend annual Pap tests for all sexually active women and for those women who have reached 18 years of age. After three negative Pap tests, screening may be done at less frequent intervals at the discretion of the health care provider (American Cancer Society, 1999; American College of Obstetricians and Gynecologists, 1994). Women in high risk categories should have more frequent Pap tests.

Pap test results in the past have been recorded using several different classification systems. The reporting system most often used today is the Bethesda system, one that reports on gynecologic cytology as well as histology of cervical lesions (Table 13-4). Changes secondary to inflammation, treatment (e.g., radiation), and contraceptive devices can be reported, as well as changes caused by infections. Epithelial

TABLE 13-4 Comparison of Bethesda System with Other Cytology Classification Systems

DYSPLASIA/CIS	CIN	BETHESDA
Normal	Normal	Within normal limits
Benign atypia	Inflammatory atypia (organism)	Benign cellular changes Infection—specified Reactive changes Inflammation Atrophy Radiation, etc. Squamous cell abnormalities
Atypical cells	Squamous atypia	ASCUS
Mild dysplasia	CIN I	Low grade SIL { HPV, CIN I }
Moderate dysplasia	CIN II	High grade SIL { CIN II, CIN III }
Severe (marked) dysplasia } Carcinoma in situ (CIS)	CIN III	
Adenocarcinoma and CIS		Glandular cell abnormalities

From DiSaia, P., & Creasman, W. (1997). *Clinical gynecologic oncology* (5th ed.). St. Louis: Mosby.
CIN, Cervical intraepitheal neoplasia; *SIL*, squamous intraepitheleal lesion; *ASCUS*, atypical squamous cells of undetermined significance.

cell abnormalities are described in three categories–atypias, or atypical squamous cells of undetermined significance (ASCUS); low grade SILs; and high grade SILs. Low grade SILs include cellular changes associated with HPV and mild dysplasia (CIN I). A finding of ASCUS is followed with repeated Pap tests every 4 to 6 months for 2 years until there have been three negative tests; if a second ASCUS is reported within 2 years, a colposcopy may be indicated. A finding of low grade SIL is followed up with a repeated Pap test every 4 to 6 months; colposcopy and directed biopsy are indicated if repeated tests show abnormalities. High grade SILs include lesions formerly described as moderate dysplasia (CIN II), severe dysplasia (CIN III), and CIS. Follow up for a report of high grade SIL includes colposcopy and directed biopsy (Centers for Disease Control and Prevention, 1998; DiSaia & Creasman, 1997).

Colposcopy is the examination of the cervix using a stereoscopic binocular microscope that magnifies the view of the cervix. Usually a solution of 3% acetic acid is applied to the cervix for better visualization of the epithelium and to identify areas for biopsy. Colposcopy is not an invasive procedure and is well tolerated by the woman (see Research box).

Biopsy is the removal of cervical tissue for study, and several techniques can be used. An endocervical curettage is an effective diagnostic tool in about 90% of cases. It can be performed as an outpatient procedure with little or no anesthesia. It may be uncomfortable, and interventions to help the woman relax and cope with the pain may be needed.

Conization and loop electrosurgical excision procedure (LEEP) (p. 289) can be done as outpatient procedures, although neither is usually done unless the biopsy is positive or the results of the colposcopy are unsatisfactory. **Conization** involves removal of a cone of tissue from the exocervix and endocervix (Fig. 13-14). It can be done as a cold knife procedure, a laser excision, or an electrosurgical excision (see discussion on p. 289). There are two advantages to a cone biopsy. It can be used (1) to establish the diagnosis and (2) to effect a cure. If carcinoma in situ is diagnosed, and if the woman wishes to retain her childbearing capacity, conization removes the abnormal tissue; further treatment is unnecessary. The woman is monitored with Pap tests and colposcopy when indicated.

If invasive cancer is diagnosed, other diagnostic tests are done to assess the extent of spread (see previous discussion under endometrial cancer). Once the extent of the cancer is known, treatment begins.

CARE MANAGEMENT

Assessment and Nursing Diagnoses

For the woman diagnosed with invasive carcinoma of the cervix, pretherapy assessment includes physical, psychologic, and educational components, regardless of whether surgery or radiation is the method of treatment. Physical assessment includes a review of current medications, because medications for other medical problems may need to be continued. Skin is assessed to identify potential pressure points; respiratory and gastrointestinal status and state of nutrition are important factors to assess. Urinalysis and complete blood count are also commonly performed. An electrocardiogram and a chest x-ray examination may be done if use of a general anesthetic is anticipated for surgery or placement of internal applicators.

RESEARCH

Can Precolposcopy Education Increase Knowledge and Decrease Anxiety?

Standard care for women with abnormal Papanicolaou (Pap) tests is referral for colposcopy for evaluation and management. Previous research studies have indicated that women scheduled for colposcopy expressed little understanding about the reason for their referral and were not given enough information before the appointment. Because cervical cancer is more prevalent among African-Americans and Hispanics than among Caucasians, further research was indicated in this area.

The purpose of this randomized, controlled study was to investigate the impact of an educational intervention on the knowledge and anxiety levels of inner-city women scheduled for colposcopy after an abnormal Pap test. This experimental study took place in an inner-city medical school. Fifty-eight women were enrolled in the intervention group, and 55 women constituted the control group. Approximately 1 week before their appointments, the women in the intervention group received in the mail a one-page handout about colposcopy. The control group received no handout. After arriving at the clinic for their

visit, the women were asked to participate in the study and were interviewed. Knowledge of reason for visit and knowledge of colposcopy were measured by content analysis of the interview. Anxiety was measured using the Spielberger State/Trait Anxiety Inventory.

Results of this study demonstrated that 72% of the intervention group understood what a colposcopy was, compared with 42% of the control group. No significant difference in mean anxiety scores was found between the two groups. The mailing of an informational handout was shown to increase the client's knowledge about colposcopy for this population studied.

CLINICAL APPLICATION

Client education is an essential nursing function and a primary component of independent nursing practice. Although the provision of a mailed handout before a procedure, such as a colposcopy, cannot take the place of a detailed explanation by a nurse, it can provide the basis for a more educated discussion during face-to-face client education.

Source: Tomaino-Brunner, C. et al. (1998). Can precolposcopy education increase knowledge and decrease anxiety? *J Obstet Gynecol Neonatal Nurs* 27(6), 636-645.

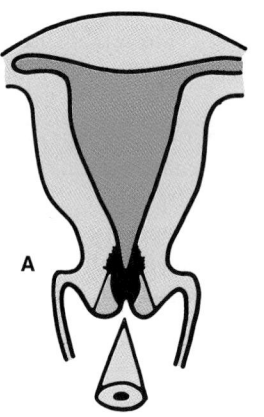 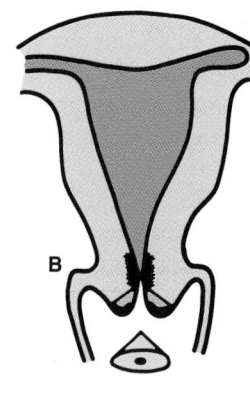

Fig. 13-14 A, Cone biopsy for endocervical disease. Limits of lesion were not seen colposcopically. **B,** Cone biopsy for CIN of the exocervix. Limits of lesion were identified colposcopically. *(From DiSaia, P., & Creasman, W. [1997]. Clinical gynecologic oncology [5th ed.]. St. Louis: Mosby.)*

Psychologic assessment is important because frequently these women are emotionally distressed about the diagnosis and anticipated treatment (i.e., fear of being radioactive and fear of pain) and fear that family or significant others will become distant.

Educational assessment involves identifying the woman's current knowledge base regarding the diagnosis and proposed therapeutic regimen. Nursing diagnoses for the

woman having surgery for cervical cancer are similar to those identified for the woman having a hysterectomy for endometrial cancer (p. 279). Nursing diagnoses that might arise from an assessment for the woman who is to have external or internal radiation therapy for treatment of cervical cancer include the following:

▪ Nursing Diagnoses

- Knowledge deficit related to
  - treatment procedures
- Fear/anxiety related to
  - diagnosis
  - anticipated pain
  - concerns about radioactivity
  - the response of the significant other or family
- Sensory deprivation related to
  - internal radiation therapy
  - restricted contact with visitors and nursing staff
- Altered skin integrity related to
  - external radiation exposure
  - immobility and bed rest (internal radiation therapy)
- Risk for injury related to
  - dislodgment of radiation source
- Risk for pain related to
  - internal applicators
- Risk for alteration of sexual function related to
  - treatment or concerns of significant other

Expected Outcomes of Care

Mutually determined outcomes for the woman undergoing radiation therapy for cervical cancer related to the identified nursing diagnoses might include that the woman will do the following:

- Verbalize an understanding of the proposed treatment and accompanying procedures.
- Verbalize her fears regarding diagnosis, treatment, and response of significant others and family.
- Maintain contact with family and friends through short visitations or by telephone if internal radiation therapy is done.
- Remain free from skin breakdown.
- Identify methods to maintain skin hygiene.
- Remain on strict bed rest on her back to prevent dislodgment of the internal applicators if internal radiation therapy is done.
- Verbalize control of pain.
- Resume a satisfactory sexual relationship with her partner.

Plan of Care and Interventions

Preinvasive Lesions

Once a diagnosis has been identified, a course of treatment is planned. For preinvasive lesions, several techniques are currently being used. As stated earlier, because many preinvasive conditions are detected in younger women who may wish to continue childbearing, treatment is geared toward eradicating abnormal cells while attempting to preserve the structure of the cervix. The techniques currently available for preinvasive lesions are cryotherapy, laser therapy, and LEEP. Treatment for invasive cancer includes surgery, radiation therapy, and chemotherapy.

Cryosurgery. Cryosurgery uses a freezing technique that freezes abnormal cells, and when sloughing occurs, regeneration of tissue is normal. Side effects occurring after treatment are usually few and not of a serious nature. A profuse watery discharge can persist for 2 to 4 weeks. Follow-up examination and a Pap test are scheduled in 4 to 6 months. Endocervical cells are thought to regenerate, leaving a normal cervical canal in most instances. Rarely, spotting or cervical stenosis are complications. Surveillance with frequent Pap tests and colposcopic examination must continue indefinitely after this type of conservative therapy. Persistent abnormal cells require reevaluation, and plans are made for repeat cryosurgery or other therapy.

Laser surgery. Laser surgery can eradicate most cases of CIN. This technique involves a laser mounted on a colposcope that allows for precise direction of a beam of light (heat) to remove diseased tissue. For treatment of the cervix (relatively insensitive tissue), the woman may need no anesthesia. Some women complain of a burning or cramping sensation that is tolerable for most women. Cervixes treated with CO_2 laser show epithelial regrowth beginning by 2 days. Cervixes are usually healed in 4 to 6 weeks. The original architecture of the cervix is preserved, and the squamocolumnar junction remains visible; how-

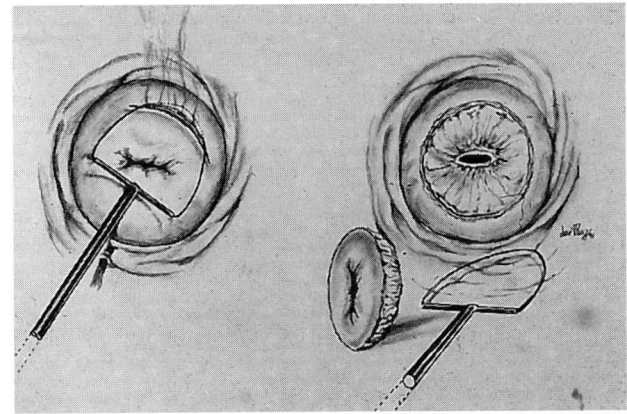

Fig. 13-15 Electrosurgical excision. The electric loop vaporizes quickly and removes cone of tissue. *(From Nichols, D. [1994]. Gynecologic and obstetric surgery. St. Louis: Mosby.)*

ever, there may be more damage to normal tissues than with other treatments. Women usually experience less vaginal discharge than with cryosurgery, but there may be more discomfort following the procedure (Mishell et al., 1997).

Electrosurgical excision. The loop electrosurgical excision procedure (LEEP) has become a standard treatment for cervical dysplasia (American College of Obstetricians and Gynecologists, 1994). This procedure uses a wire loop electrode that can excise and cauterize with minimal tissue damage (Fig. 13-15). Healing is rapid, and there is only a mild discharge afterwards. Possible complications include bleeding, cervical stenosis, infertility, and loss of cervical mucus (Mishell et al., 1997).

Invasive Cancer of the Cervix

Once the cancer is staged, treatment is begun. Microinvasive cancer is usually treated with conization, but a hysterectomy is often done if childbearing is not desired. The choice of treatment for early stage invasive cancer is by either surgery or radiation therapy because survival rates are comparable (American College of Obstetricians and Gynecologists, 1994). Locally advanced stages of cervical cancer usually are treated with radiation therapy, both external and internal. A radical hysterectomy is performed if the cancer has extended beyond the cervix but not to the pelvic wall.

Radical hysterectomy. Radical hysterectomy involves removal of the uterus, tubes, ovaries, upper third of the vagina, entire uterosacral and uterovesical ligaments, and all of the parametrium on each side, along with pelvic node dissection encompassing the four major pelvic lymph node chains: ureteral, obturator, hypogastric, and iliac. Dissection serves to preserve the bladder, rectum, and ureters while removing as much of the remaining tissue of the pelvis as is feasible. Women with positive pelvic nodes usually receive postoperative whole-pelvis irradiation, although there is little evidence that it alters the incidence of recurrence in the pelvic area (DiSaia & Creasman, 1997).

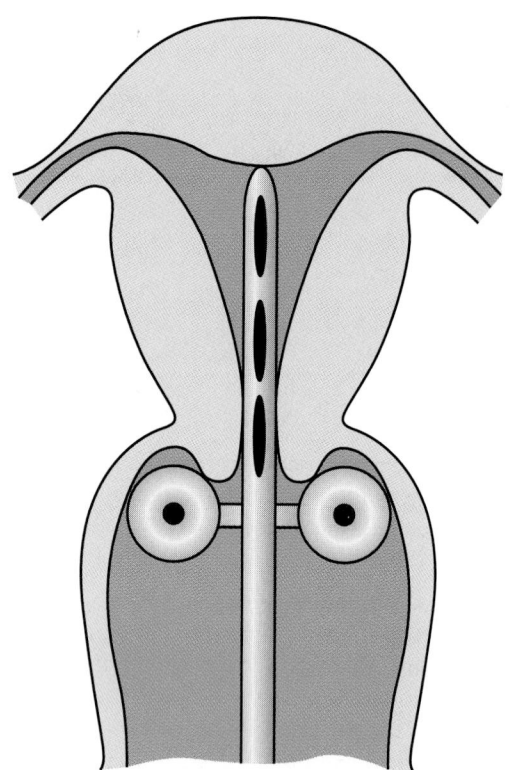

Fig. 13-16 Intracavitary implant. Applicator in place in uterus is loaded with radium source.

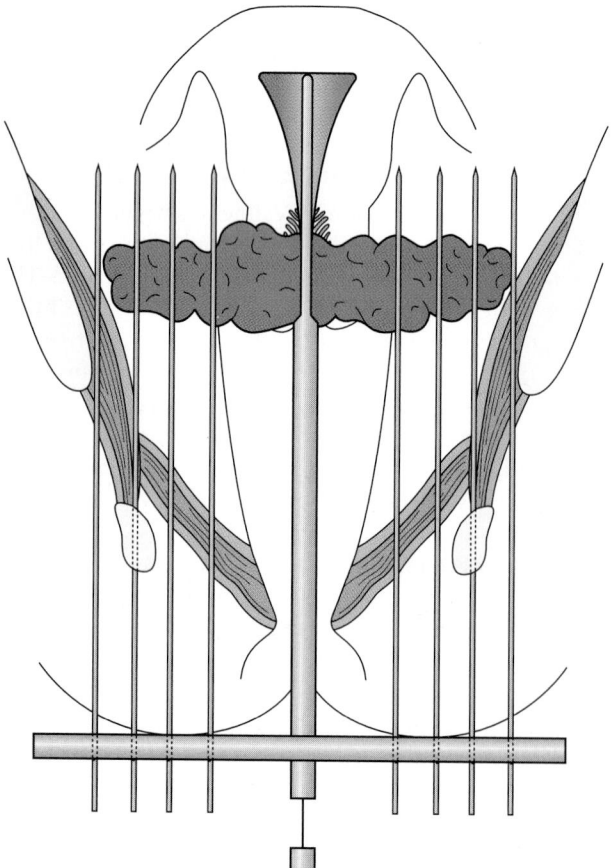

Fig. 13-17 Interstitial-intracavitary implant.

Radiation therapy. Radiation may be delivered by internal radium applications to the cervix or external radiation therapy that includes lymphatics of the pelvic side wall. In preparation for radiation therapy, the woman must maintain good nutritional status and a high-protein, high-vitamin, and high-calorie diet. Anemia, if present, should be corrected before the initiation of radiotherapy.

External irradiation and intracavitary radium therapy are used in various combinations for the best results and are tailored to each woman and her particular lesion. Megavoltage machines such as cobalt, linear accelerators, and the betatron have the distinct advantage of providing a more homogeneous dose to the pelvis. The hard, short rays of megavoltage pass through the skin without much absorption by the skin and therefore cause little dermal injury.

External radiation therapy and internal radiation therapy are given in various combinations. For example, external radiation may be given first to treat regional pelvic nodes and to shrink the tumor. External irradiation is usually an outpatient procedure given 5 days a week for 4 to 6 weeks. Internal radiation therapy consists of one or two intracavitary treatments at least 2 weeks apart (DiSaia & Creasman, 1997).

For internal radiation therapy the woman may be treated in the hospital or in a special unit in an outpatient setting. If treatment is done in the hospital, the woman is taken to the operating room, and while she is under general anesthesia, a specially designed applicator is placed into her vagina and cervix. X-rays are taken to make sure the applicator is correctly placed. The woman is returned to her room, where the radioactive source is placed into the applicator (Fig. 13-16). The source remains in place from 12 hours to 3 days. If treatment is in the outpatient setting, the applicator is inserted into the uterus in a treatment room; use of high-dose implants shortens the treatment time (Dunne-Daly, 1997).

In advanced carcinoma of the cervix, conventional intracavitary applicators are not applicable. Interstitial therapy employs a template to guide the insertion of a group of 18-gauge hollow steel needles into the lesion transperineally (Fig. 13-17). After the needles are placed, the iridium wires are inserted when the woman is returned to her room.

Complications of radiation therapy. Morbidity as a direct result from properly conducted therapy is usually minimal. Some of the morbidity seen may be caused by the uncontrolled tumor and not by the therapy. Acute treatment complications occurring during or shortly following therapy include irritation of the rectum, small bowel, and bladder; reactions in the skinfolds; and mild bone marrow suppression. Dysuria and frequency may occur. Late complications, although not common, include genital fistulas and necrosis. Symptoms of radiation proctitis may follow an asymptomatic interval of many months to years after treatment (Schlaerth, 1994).

Recurrent and Advanced Cancer of the Cervix

Approximately one third of women with invasive cervical cancer will have recurrent or persistent disease after therapy (Mishell et al., 1997). Prognosis is discouraging, with a 1-year survival rate between 10% and 15% (DiSaia & Creasman, 1997). Irradiation of metastatic areas is commonly successful in providing local control and symptomatic relief. Irradiation for recurrent disease may be considered for women who were initially treated with surgery. Further radiation may not be effective for those women who were initially treated with radiation.

Pelvic exenteration. The woman who has recurrence only within the pelvis may be considered for **pelvic exenteration** if a cure is thought to be possible. A total exenteration involves removal of the perineum, pelvic floor, levator muscles, and all reproductive organs. Additionally, pelvic lymph nodes, rectum, sigmoid colon, urinary bladder, and distal ureters are removed, and a colostomy and ileal conduit are constructed (Fig. 13-18, *A*). In very select cases, the procedure can be modified to either an anterior or a posterior exenteration. In anterior pelvic exenteration, all of the previously mentioned pelvic viscera are removed except the rectosigmoid, which is preserved. Urine is rerouted through an ileal conduit (Fig. 13-18, *B*). In the posterior pelvic exenteration procedure, all pelvic viscera with the exception of the bladder are removed. The feces is rerouted through a colostomy (Fig. 13-18, *C*). A neovagina (new vagina) may be constructed.

Women are carefully selected for this procedure; 5-year survival rates range from 20% to 62% (DiSaia & Creasman, 1997). Many of the complications that follow this surgery are those that follow any form of major surgery, for example, pulmonary embolism, pulmonary edema, myocardial infarction, and cerebrovascular accident. These complications are seen immediately after surgery. Infection originating in the pelvic cavity usually occurs later, if it occurs.

Chemotherapy. Chemotherapy may be used in advanced cancer of the cervix to reduce tumor size before surgery. In general, no long-term benefits are derived with chemotherapy, although cisplatin and 5-FU demonstrate the most effects. Chemotherapy is beneficial as a pain relief method (DiSaia & Creasman, 1997). Chemotherapy in combination with radiation treatments is being evaluated as to whether there is improvement in the results of radiation therapy (Mishell et al., 1997).

Nursing Management

Nursing care for the woman having a radical hysterectomy was discussed previously (p. 279). Nursing actions for external and internal radiation differ, so they will be discussed separately.

External radiation therapy

Pretreatment care. The woman's anxiety may be so high that information given by the radiologist may not be processed. The nurse should reinforce or fill in gaps, especially related to the following: the equipment, which is similar to that used for x-ray examination except larger; the hyperbaric oxygen chamber, which may be used to increase cellular oxygen and thus make tumor cells more radiosensitive; the radiotherapist, who will be behind a

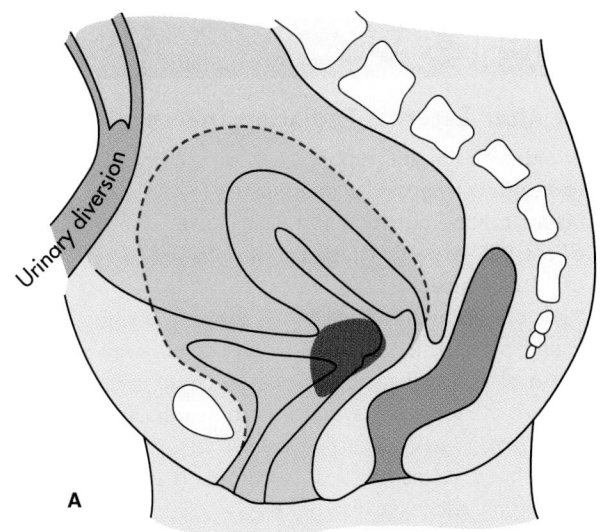

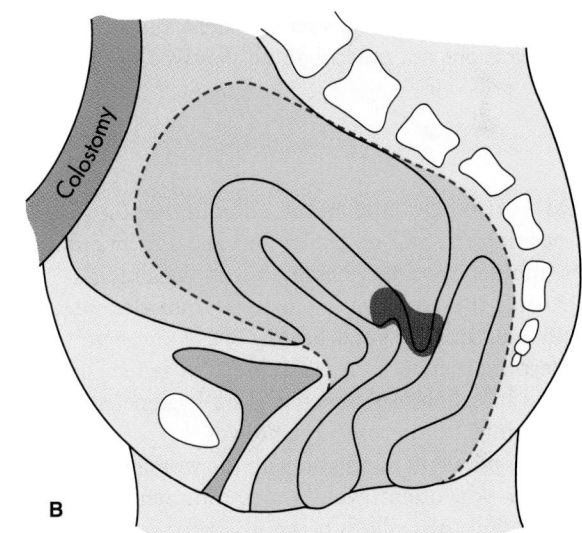

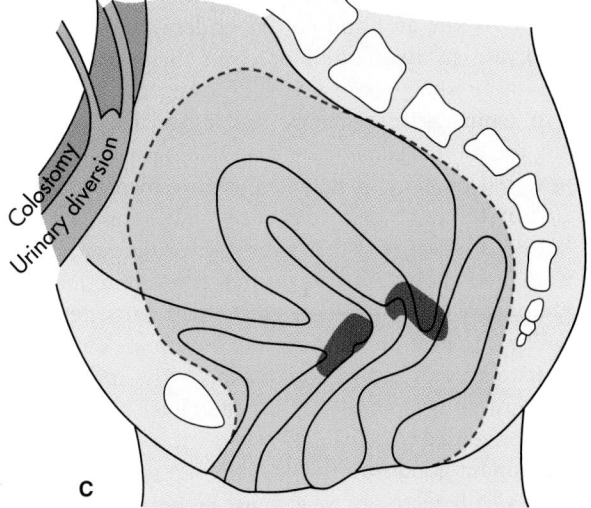

Fig. 13-18 Pelvic exenteration procedures. **A,** Anterior exenteration. **B,** Posterior exenteration. **C,** Total exenteration. *(From DiSaia, P., & Morrow, C. [1973]. Calif Med 118:13, Feb.)*

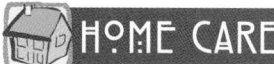

HOME CARE

Care After External Radiation Therapy

- Avoid infection and report symptoms of infection to health care provider immediately.
- Maintain good nutrition and fluid intake.
- Client may experience effects of radiation for 10 to 14 days after last treatment.
- Signs of healing should occur in about 3 weeks.
- Maintain good skin and mouth care to support a sense of well-being and prevent infection.
- Report the following symptoms to health care provider:
  - Continued gastrointestinal symptoms (nausea, vomiting, anorexia, diarrhea)
  - Increasing skin irritation at the site of therapy (redness, swelling, pain, pruritis)
- Take medications as prescribed and avoid any medications not prescribed or approved by health care provider.

shield, but still close by and in communication with her; the position she will be put in and asked to maintain for some minutes; and the therapy, which is painless.

During therapy. The woman is counseled regarding maintaining general good health. She is more vulnerable to infection; therefore she is reminded of general measures to avoid infection (e.g., practice good hygiene, avoid people with infection, avoid large crowds, keep environment clean). To maintain good skin care the woman is taught to assess her skin often; avoid soaps, ointments, cosmetics, deodorants if the axilla is being irradiated, and so on, because these may contain metals that would alter the dose she receives and could lead to skin breakdown; wear loose clothing over the area and cotton underwear (or no underwear); use an air mattress or cover the mattress with foam pads or sheep skin; avoid exposing the irradiated areas to temperature extremes; and especially avoid removing the markings made by the radiologist. If her skin becomes red or itchy, it is treated with remedies recommended by the radiologist (e.g., aloe vera lotion or warm sitz baths). To treat skin that is broken or desquamating, the woman is shown how to use remedies prescribed by the radiologist (e.g., irrigation with equal parts peroxide and saline, application of antibiotic or lanolin ointment, exposure to air, and application of a loose dressing). Use of adhesive (or any) tape directly on the target area of skin should be avoided (Mitchell, 1997).

To maintain good nutrition the woman is reminded to maintain a daily record of weight; use high-protein supplements; eat small, attractive, appetizing meals, probably bland in nature; take vitamins; and keep the environment light, airy, clean, and quiet (especially before and after

meals). If the woman is ill enough to be hospitalized, she may need total parenteral nutrition or tube feedings. Nausea interferes with adequate intake; therefore the woman may take antiemetics, as necessary. High daily fluid intake (2000 to 3000 ml) should be suggested if not contraindicated. To increase her comfort, minimize infection, and promote adequate food intake, the woman is encouraged to perform frequent oral hygiene. Table 13-2 provides other suggestions for nutritional problems associated with radiation treatment.

The nurse explains, as necessary, the need for blood studies to monitor white blood cell count (to determine degree of immunosuppression).

Posttreatment care. The woman needs information for self-care after the radiation treatment is completed. The Home Care box lists suggestions for this care.

Internal radiation therapy. Internal radiation therapy may require hospitalization or be done in a special outpatient unit. Radiation safety officers determine the precautions to be observed in each situation. This discussion focuses on treatment in the hospital setting. Printed instruction sheets are usually available stating precautions to be followed for each type of radiation substance used. A precaution sign is placed on the door of the woman's room.

> **NURSE ALERT** *Personnel who come in direct contact with anyone receiving radiation therapy should wear a film badge or other device to monitor the amount of exposure received.*

Nurses must protect themselves from overexposure to radiation. Precautions include the following behaviors (Dunne-Daly, 1997):

- Careful isolation techniques: wearing gloves while handling bodily fluids and observing good handwashing technique. These behaviors reflect knowledge that alpha and beta rays cannot pass through skin but may be in body fluids and excrement.
- Careful planning of nursing activity to limit time (to 30 minutes or less per 8 hours) spent in close proximity to the woman to avoid exposure to gamma rays, which can penetrate several inches of lead.

Exposure to radiation is controlled in three ways: distance, time, and shielding (with lead). For the woman with sealed radiotherapy, a movable lead screen is available that can be placed between the area in which the therapeutic applicator is located and the personnel. Lead aprons may also be worn while providing care at the bedside, although they are heavy. The lead screen is also used to protect visitors from radiation. Increasing the distance from the source also decreases exposure (Dunne-Daly, 1997).

Familiarity with applicators is a *must* for all nurses working with people receiving radiotherapy so that if a "strange object" is found in the linen or on the floor, it is not touched. Today most hospital protocols include having a lead container and forceps in the room for use should a radioactive implant become dislodged.

Preinsertion care. The woman is prepared for insertion with the following care, which is accompanied by an explanation for each activity. To reduce the need for an enema or attention to bowel elimination for a few days, the gastrointestinal tract is usually prepared using low-residue diet, enemas, and sometimes bowel sedation. The vaginal vault is usually prepared with an antiseptic douche such as povidone-iodine.

An indwelling urinary bladder catheter is inserted, as ordered, to prevent urinary distention that could dislodge the applicator. Nothing is taken by mouth the night before the procedure in anticipation of general anesthesia. Preoperative medications may be ordered for the morning of the procedure. Deep-breathing exercises, range-of-motion exercises, and positioning are all demonstrated before the procedure to minimize the effects of immobilization afterward. An intravenous (IV) solution will probably be started before the procedure, and IV therapy may be continued if nausea prevents good oral intake of fluids. The woman is assured that pain will be managed.

Explanations about restricted visitation of personnel and visitors are also given in the preinsertion phase. Women are often encouraged to bring reading materials or other hobbies such as crossword puzzles to the hospital to combat the boredom that isolation imposes on them (Dunne-Daly, 1997).

During therapy. The applicator is inserted in surgery with the woman under general anesthesia if necessary to facilitate vaginal examination and ease of placement. The usual postanesthesia recovery care follows, and she is returned to her room. The woman is positioned on her back. There the applicators are loaded with the radioactive substance.

A lead shield is placed next to the woman's pelvic area. Vital signs are monitored every 4 hours. Active range-of-motion and deep-breathing exercises are encouraged every 2 hours; the woman may not be permitted to turn from side to side, although logrolling may be done occasionally to relieve back pressure. The head of the bed is elevated about 15 degrees (Dunne-Daly, 1997).

The woman's diet is progressed from clear liquid to low residue, as ordered. Many women have difficulty eating while lying flat or even if the bed is elevated slightly. The nurse arranges the food so that it is easy to reach. Finger foods or liquids are generally more manageable. Parenteral or oral fluids are given up to 3000 ml daily.

The urinary catheter remains in the bladder while the implant is in place. However, no perineal or catheter care is given. Intake and output are measured. The woman is given a partial bath, washing only above her waist. Massage is restricted to her shoulders and neck. Linen is changed only as absolutely necessary. Any linen or equipment used is retained in the room until therapy is complete to prevent loss of an applicator or seed. If vaginal or

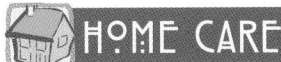

HOME CARE

Care After Internal Radiation Therapy

- Eat three balanced meals a day, and increase fluid to 3000 ml daily.
- Rest when tired, and resume normal activities as comfort permits.
- Maintain good hygiene (e.g., daily showers and daily douches until discharge stops).
- Resume sexual intercourse in 7 to 10 days or as recommended by physician. Use vaginal dilator if needed for vaginal stenosis.
- Understand that sterility and cessation of menstruation usually occur with this procedure.
- Report any of the following to your health care provider: bleeding (vaginal, rectal, or in the urine), foul-smelling vaginal discharge, fever, abdominal distention, or pain.
- Take any prescribed medications as directed.
- Do not hesitate to call health care provider or clinic if there are concerns or problems.
- Plan follow-up visits to determine emotional as well as physical recovery.

rectal bleeding or hematuria occurs, the physician is notified immediately.

Emotional support is provided by planning to be with the woman for short periods; encouraging her to verbalize concerns and needs; and encouraging family members, clergy, or others to visit for short periods daily or to communicate by phone. Pregnant women and children are not permitted to visit.

Many women undergoing internal radiation treatment are given medication to prevent complications and to promote comfort during the procedure. Such medications might include antibiotics to prevent bladder infections, heparin injections to prevent thrombophlebitis, sedatives for relaxation, antiemetics for nausea, and narcotics for pain. The woman is considered radioactive during the time the internal sources are in place (Dunne-Daly, 1997).

Posttreatment care. Posttreatment complications range from those arising from immobilization, such as thrombophlebitis, pulmonary embolism, and pneumonia, to those arising from the treatment itself, such as hemorrhage, skin reactions (rashes or inflammation), diarrhea, cramping, dysuria, and vaginal stenosis. The woman is assessed for any of these complications before discharge.

After the radium is removed, the Foley catheter is removed and the woman is assisted in getting out of bed the first time. She is usually discharged the same day. Discharge teaching can be found in the Home Care box. The woman and her family are reassured that she is not radioactive after the treatment.

The woman may experience altered patterns of sexuality related to treatment side effects. A decrease in vaginal secretions and sensation may occur, as well as vaginal stenosis. These can contribute to decreased sexual desire because pain and discomfort during intercourse can affect the desire to resume sexual activities. The nurse can initiate a discussion with the woman and her partner, offer information about the effects of radiation on the ability to have sexual intercourse, and offer suggestions for specific problems, such as using a water-based lubricant for vaginal dryness. If necessary, the couple can be referred to other resources (see Appendix D) (Mitchell, 1997).

Pelvic exenteration. Nursing care of the woman having a pelvic exenteration depends on what is removed. General preoperative considerations include assessments similar to those for a woman having a radical hysterectomy. Additionally, a thorough sexual assessment is needed because of the drastic changes that are involved. The woman needs information about the construction of a neovagina if that is an option. She will need to be assessed for stoma site selection and information about management of colostomy or ileal conduit if appropriate. Extensive preoperative bowel preparation is needed before surgery. Pain management is discussed, as is what to expect postoperatively (e.g., nasogastric tubes, arterial catheters). Significant others should be included in preoperative discussions when possible because their support is essential postoperatively.

Postoperative care usually begins in an intensive care unit until the woman's condition is stable. She is monitored for signs of complications, including shock, hemorrhage, pulmonary embolus and other pulmonary complications, fluid and electrolyte imbalance, and urinary complications (Lowdermilk, 1995b). Nursing care continues after the woman is stabilized and moved back to her room. Wound care consists of irrigation with one-half normal saline, followed by drying of the area with either a hair dryer on cool setting or a heat lamp placed at least 12 inches from the perineal area. The woman is taught how to care for her colostomy or ileal conduit when she is able to begin self-care. Assessment for psychologic reactions is important. The woman will probably experience a grief reaction over her mutilated body. She may become depressed during the long convalescence.

The woman may be discharged to a long-term care facility or to her home. She will need assistance in her physical care for at least 6 months. Teaching needed for home care includes colostomy or ureterostomy care; dietary needs for healing; perineal care, including use of perineal pads to protect clothing from discharge; range-of-motion exercises and physical activities permitted by her health care provider; and signs of complication, especially infection and bowel obstruction.

Because the woman will experience sexual disruption and the possibility of not being able to have vaginal intercourse (if the vagina is not reconstructed), counseling about sexual activity is needed. Usually even with a vaginal reconstruction, vaginal intercourse is not advised until healing has taken place, usually 12 to 18 months. Women with neovaginas may complain of decreased vaginal sensations, chronic discharge, or that the vagina is too short or too long. Women with colostomies or ureterostomies may worry about leakage or odors during sexual activities. Women may be concerned about their change in appearance. They may need counseling about alternative activities for sexual expression for themselves and their partners. The woman and her partner may need referral for further sexual counseling (Mitchell, 1997).

Evaluation

The nurse can be reasonably assured that care was effective to the extent that the expected outcomes of care for the woman who has had radiation therapy or other treatment have been achieved.

Other Pelvic Malignancies
Cancer of the Vulva

Incidence and etiology. Vulvar carcinoma accounts for about 5% of all female genital malignancies and is the fourth most commonly occurring gynecologic cancer. It appears most frequently in older women in their middle sixties to seventies. However, up to 25% of cases may be found in younger women less than 55 years of age. The disease has been linked to the presence of condylomata acuminata (genital warts) caused by HPV (types 16, 18, 31, 33, 35, 51, and possibly others).

By far the majority (90%) of vulvar carcinoma is squamous cell; other vulvar neoplasms are attributed to Paget's disease, adenocarcinoma of Bartholin's glands, fibrosarcoma and melanoma, and basal cell carcinoma. Vulvar intraepithelial neoplasia (VIN) is the first neoplastic change. VIN progresses over time to carcinoma in situ, then to invasive cancer. Metastatic spread is by direct extension and lymphatic spread.

Prognosis depends on the size of the lesion and the tumor grade at the time of diagnosis. Fifty percent of women have had symptoms for 2 to 16 months before seeking treatment. Fortunately, vulvar cancer grows slowly, extends slowly, and metastasizes fairly late. Even with a pattern of delayed diagnosis, survival rates are greater than 90% for all stages if nodes are negative. Survival rates plummet to less than 50%, however, if lymph node metastasis has occurred (DiSaia & Creasman, 1997).

Clinical manifestations and diagnosis. The most common site for vulvar lesions is on the labia majora. The vulvar lesion is usually asymptomatic until it is 1 to 2 cm in diameter. When symptomatic, women may complain of vulvar pruritis or burning or pain. Necrosis and infection of the lesion result in ulceration with bleeding or watery discharge.

Vulvar intraepithelial neoplasms are usually multifocal in young women. Unifocal lesions are associated with invasive cancer and are more common in older women. Initially, growth is superficial but later extends into the urethra, vagina, and anus. In approximately 50% of late cases, superficial inguinal and femoral lymph nodes become involved.

Simple biopsy with histologic evaluation reveals the diagnosis. The areas of pathologic involvement are identified by staining the vulva with toluidine blue (1%), allowing an absorption time of 3 to 5 minutes, and then washing with acetic acid (2% to 3%); abnormal tissue retains the dye. Biopsy is necessary to rule out such conditions as sexually transmitted diseases (e.g., chancroid, granuloma inguinale, syphilis), basal cell carcinoma, and CIS. In situ malignancies are initially small, red, white, or pigmented friable papules. In Paget's disease, the lesions are red, moist, and elevated. Melanomas appear as bluish-black, pigmented, or papillary lesions. Melanomas metastasize through the bloodstream and lymphatics.

Collaborative care

Therapeutic management. Treatment varies, depending on the extent of the disease. Laser surgery, cryosurgery, or electrosurgical excision may be used to treat VIN. A disadvantage to these treatments is that healing is slow and the treated area is painful. A local wide excision may be performed for localized lesions or a simple **vulvectomy** (removal of vulva, labia majora and minora, and possibly the clitoris). A skinning vulvectomy (Fig. 13-19, *A*) is preferred over the simple vulvectomy because it is less disfiguring. It involves removal of the superficial vulvar skin without clitoral removal, followed by split-thickness skin grafts. The fat, muscle, and glands are preserved.

For invasive disease, a radical or modified radical vulvectomy is performed. These procedures involve the removal of the entire vulva, skin, clitoris, labia, subcutaneous tissues, and the inguinal and femoral nodes (Fig. 13-19, *B*). If these nodes are positive, pelvic lymphadenectomy or pelvic lymph node irradiation is done.

External radiation therapy can be used to shrink tumors before surgery, but it is not used as the primary treatment.

Postoperative external radiation therapy may be used for women who are at risk for recurrence. Radiation treatment causes dermatitis and ulceration that are uncomfortable for the woman.

Chemotherapy has not been very effective as a treatment except for the topical application of 5-FU for CIS. This treatment is painful and not used often. Chemotherapy is being investigated in combination with radiation as an adjunct to surgery in advanced cancer of the vulva.

Nursing care. Nursing care for the woman with vulvar cancer is similar to that for the woman with other gynecologic malignancies. A history of symptoms and a physical examination should be done. An assessment of the woman's understanding of the surgical procedure and her emotional state should also be done.

Possible nursing diagnoses include the following:
- High risk for infection related to surgical incision
- Sexual dysfunction related to vulvectomy
- Body-image disturbance related to loss of sexual organ
- Altered patterns of elimination, urinary and bowel, related to surgery

Expected outcomes of care are based on the nursing diagnoses established, mutually determined, measurable, and stated in client-centered terms. A plan of care is developed based on the following outcomes:
- The woman will remain free of infection at the operative site.
- The woman will demonstrate positive adaptation to altered body image.
- The woman with a significant other will discuss altered sexuality and identify alternative means to achieve sexual satisfaction.
- The woman will maintain adequate elimination.

Interventions for the woman treated with laser therapy include applying topical steroids to the area, administering sitz baths and drying the area with a hair dryer, applying local anesthetics, or giving oral pain medication as needed.

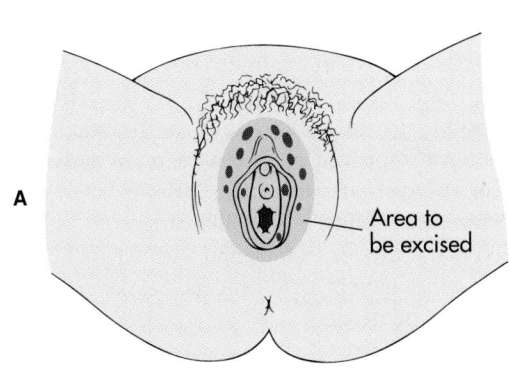
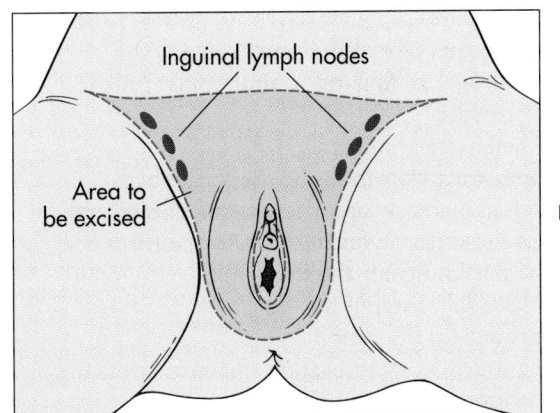

Fig. 13-19 Vulvectomy. **A,** Skinning vulvectomy. **B,** Radical vulvectomy.

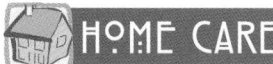

Care After Radical Vulvectomy

- Avoid sexual activity for 4 to 6 weeks or as health care provider directs.
- Rest frequently.
- Avoid crossing legs, sitting, or standing for long periods.
- Avoid tight, constricting clothing and wear cotton underwear.
- Keep perineal area clean and dry. Wash perineum with a solution of peroxide and water after each elimination, and pat dry.
- Report to your health care provider any swelling, redness, unusual tenderness, drainage, or foul odor of incision site.
- Report any temperature over 38.4° C.
- Eat a well-balanced diet to promote healing.
- Take all medications as prescribed.
- Elevate legs periodically to prevent pelvic congestion.
- Do not hesitate to call health care provider or clinic if there are concerns or problems.

Women need to be informed that pain may get worse 3 to 4 days after the treatment.

A woman undergoing radical vulvectomy requires some special nursing actions in addition to the routine postoperative care given (see Home Care box). Additional nursing actions focused on the prevention of infection would include the following:

- Irrigate the surgical site with a solution of one-half strength normal saline or other recommended solution after each elimination.
- Dry the area thoroughly, using a hair dryer on cool setting or a heat lamp.
- Give stool softeners to decrease straining and disruption of the suture line.
- Note any change in color of the surgical site.
- Note any drainage or foul odor and notify primary health care provider.
- Perform catheter care as needed.
- Provide and instruct woman in the use of sitz baths.

The woman is at high risk for sexual dysfunction related to the effects of the surgery. Nursing actions that focus on minimizing these risks include the following:

- Encouraging verbalization of feelings
- Providing privacy for discussion
- Encouraging open communication between woman and significant others
- Providing resources for counseling if necessary
- Discussing when sexual activity can be safely resumed

- Discussing alternative methods to achieve sexual satisfaction

Using the expected outcomes of care set with the woman, evaluation is based on the complete or partial achievement of those outcomes.

Cancer of the Vagina

Vaginal carcinomas account for only 1% to 2% of gynecologic malignancy, with a peak incidence between ages 50 and 70 years. About 75% to 80% are squamous cell carcinomas; nonsquamous lesions are rare. The incidence of vaginal intraepithelial neoplasia (VAIN) is increasing, probably because of earlier diagnosis resulting from better cytologic screening. Clear-cell adenocarcinoma is even rarer. It is found primarily in young women (15 to 30 years) and is related to intrauterine exposure to DES. Sarcoma botryoides (embryonal rhabdomyosarcoma) occurs in infants and children.

The etiology is unknown, but vaginal cancer may be caused by chronic vaginal irritation, vaginal trauma, and genital viruses. Vaginal lesions, usually seen in the upper one third of the vagina, often extend into the bladder and rectum in late stages. Metastasis can occur early because of the rich lymphatic drainage in the vaginal area.

Some women with vaginal cancer are asymptomatic. Diagnosis often comes after an abnormal Pap test. Symptoms that have been associated with vaginal cancer include bleeding after coitus or examination, dyspareunia, and watery discharge. Bladder involvement results in urinary frequency or urgency; rectal extension causes painful defecation. A pelvic examination may reveal a lesion.

Colposcopy examination and biopsy of Schiller-stained areas disclose the diagnosis. Therapy for vaginal cancer is directed by the extent of the lesion and the age and condition of the woman. Local excision is the preferred therapy for localized lesions. Topical application of 5-FU cream has been used with varying results. Laser surgery may be used to treat VAIN. Radical hysterectomy and removal of the upper vagina with dissection of the pelvic nodes or internal and external radiation are options for invasive cancer. Radiation therapy is the usual treatment of choice. If a vaginectomy is performed, sexual function will be lost without reconstructive surgery. Chemotherapy has not been effective in treatment of vaginal cancer, although studies are being conducted on the effectiveness of chemotherapy in combination with radiation. Survival rates have improved in recent years. In early-stage cancer 5-year survival rates approach 70% to 80%, with stage II survival rates falling in the 50% range.

Nursing care for the woman with vaginal cancer is similar to other gynecologic cancers. Sexual counseling or referral may be needed.

Cancer of the Uterine Tubes

Primary carcinoma of the uterine (fallopian) tube (usually the distal one third) is rare (less than 1%), with a peak incidence between ages 50 and 60. The cause is unknown. Most women are asymptomatic in the early stages of tubal cancer. Vaginal bleeding is the most common symptom of tubal cancer, but clear vaginal discharge and lower abdominal pain also occur frequently. An enlarging unilateral pelvic mass or ascites may occur and are often misdiagnosed as ovarian carcinoma or endometrial carcinoma. Differential diagnosis of tubal cancer is usually made postoperatively. It is currently recommended that therapy guidelines parallel those established for ovarian carcinoma. Therefore tumor-reducing surgery such as a total abdominal hysterectomy with bilateral salpingo-oophorectomy and omentectomy (removal of connective tissue covering the organs) is performed. Postoperative therapy consists of chemotherapy, using cisplatin or other platinum-based drugs, followed by second-look surgery to determine whether further treatment is needed (DiSaia & Creasman, 1997). Radiation therapy may also be used if the disease is limited to the tube, ovary, and uterus, although reports of its effectiveness vary.

Nursing care for the woman with uterine tube cancer is similar to that of the woman with ovarian cancer.

Cancer and Pregnancy

Cancer occurs with relative infrequency during the reproductive years. Approximately 1 out of every 1000 pregnant women will also have cancer (Berman, DiSaia, & Brewster, 1999). These malignancies may be responsible for up to one third of maternal deaths. Although all forms of neoplasms have been documented in conjunction with pregnancy, the most frequently occurring types are cervical cancer, breast cancer, leukemia and lymphomas, melanomas, and ovarian and tubal cancers. Bone, colorectal, vulvar, uterine, and vaginal cancers are rarely diagnosed during pregnancy. When pregnancy and cancer coincide, therapeutic issues are complex, and intense reactions occur in the woman, her family, and the health care team. Women are confronted with issues such as continuing or terminating the pregnancy. The selection and timing of therapies such as chemotherapy, radiation, and surgery are all affected by the pregnancy. Add to this the conflicting feelings the woman has (i.e., the joy of pregnancy versus the fear and anxiety associated with cancer), and the task of providing comprehensive care for the woman and her family presents a formidable challenge to the health care team. A brief discussion of the most frequent types of cancers that occur during pregnancy and the current therapies associated with them follows.

Cancer of the Cervix

The incidence of cervical cancer concurrent with pregnancy is generally reported to be around 7%, or 1 in 2000 pregnancies, making it the most common reproductive tract cancer associated with pregnancy (Berman, DiSaia, & Brewster, 1999). Birth can be accomplished by either the vaginal or cesarean route. However, there is some concern regarding vaginal birth in the presence of invasive disease because the risk of hemorrhage and metastatic seeding from local trauma may be increased (DiSaia & Creasman, 1997).

The cancer itself does not harm the pregnancy: stage for stage, the outcome for the woman with cervical cancer is roughly the same as for the nonpregnant woman (DiSaia & Creasman, 1997; Mishell et al., 1997).

Cervical abnormalities are diagnosed during pregnancy with an abnormal Pap test. If the report suggests the pregnant woman has a squamous intraepithelial lesion, a colposcopy, possibly with directed biopsy, is done. If invasive disease is not found, treatment is delayed until after the woman gives birth. Colposcopy is repeated in the third trimester and again postpartum. Cryosurgery has been performed with little effect on the pregnancy; however, conization is not advised during pregnancy unless necessary to rule out invasive cancer because it is associated with bleeding, miscarriage, and preterm birth.

The therapy of invasive carcinoma of the cervix during pregnancy is affected by many factors. The stage of the disease and the trimester in which the cancer is diagnosed are important. Equally important are the beliefs and desires of the woman and her family in terms of initiating therapy that can interrupt the pregnancy as opposed to postponing the therapy until fetal viability is achieved. If the woman chooses not to continue the pregnancy, external radiation to the pelvis is done. Miscarriage usually occurs, and then internal radiation is done. If miscarriage does not occur, a modified radical hysterectomy may be performed. If the woman desires to continue the pregnancy, treatment of early-stage invasive cervical cancer can be delayed until fetal viability is reached without harmful effects on the woman. Birth is usually by cesarean delivery followed by radiation therapy (Berman, DiSaia, & Brewster, 1999).

Cancer of the Breast

Approximately 3% to 4% of women are pregnant or lactating at the time of diagnosis of cancer of the breast (American College of Obstetricians and Gynecologists, 1994). Breast cancer complicates about 1 in 3000 pregnancies. The prognosis for women who are diagnosed with breast cancer while pregnant is some 15% to 20% below the overall survival rate because the disease is generally in the advanced stages when first diagnosed (DiSaia & Creasman, 1997). Diagnosis is often delayed because breast engorgement may obscure the mass from palpation and increased density of the tissue makes mammographic visualization more difficult. In addition, increased vascularity and lymphatic drainage in the breast of a pregnant woman may increase the speed of metastasis. Treatment is the same as for the nonpregnant woman, although surgery is usually the treatment of choice for breast cancer in pregnancy. If an invasive tumor is found, it must be determined whether the tissue is estrogen receptor (ER) positive or negative. ER-negative tumors spread more rapidly than ER-positive tumors and are more common in pregnancy.

Maternal-fetal management considers the gestational age of the fetus, extent of disease, the tumor growth potential, and the proposed treatment. Termination of the pregnancy in early stages of the disease appears to have no impact on survival. There is little evidence to suggest that pregnancy affects the malignant process. Therapeutic abortion may become an issue in the presence of advanced disease and may be deemed necessary to achieve effective palliation. For advanced disease in the second or third trimester, alkylating agents, 5-FU, and vincristine are relatively safe for the fetus (DiSaia & Creasman, 1997). Chemotherapy may significantly improve the survival of these women.

Radiation therapy is avoided if at all possible until after the birth, because even with careful shielding, the fetus may still receive sufficient radiation to produce detrimental effects.

There is no agreement about whether a postpartum woman with breast cancer should breastfeed (Berman, DiSaia, & Brewster, 1999). There are concerns that if one of the oncogens for breast cancer is a virus, as many have postulated, the remaining breast may be contaminated and the virus may be passed to the newborn, possibly acting as a latent inducer of breast carcinoma. Also lactation increases vascularity in the remaining breast, which may contain a neoplasm as well.

Pregnancy incidence after mastectomy is influenced by many factors, including prior treatment and duration of survival. About 7% of women will have one or more pregnancies within the first 5 years after mastectomy. In general, women with good prognoses (e.g., no positive nodes) are likely to be counseled to wait at least 3 years before attempting pregnancy (DiSaia & Creasman, 1997).

Hematologic Cancers

Leukemia. The average age for pregnant women with acute leukemia is 28 years; incidence during pregnancy is not specified, but the incidence in the general population in the United States is 10 in 100,000. Pregnancy seems to have no specific effect on the course of the disease except that vigorous therapy is detrimental to early gestation. Preterm labor and postpartum hemorrhage are associated with acute leukemia (DiSaia & Creasman, 1997). Acute myelocytic leukemia (90% of cases) has a more fulminant course and requires immediate therapy; in the presence of chronic myelocytic leukemia, therapy can be delayed somewhat. Some pregnant women with the chronic form of the disease who had chemotherapy and radiation therapy directed at the spleen have given birth to apparently healthy infants. The decision to terminate the pregnancy rests with the woman and her family; however, prompt, aggressive therapy is always advisable if remission is to be achieved. Decisions may be influenced by the aggressiveness of the disease.

Hodgkin's disease. Hodgkin's disease is a malignant lymphoma that affects many younger people and compli-

cates about 1 in 6000 pregnancies. Younger women (under 40 years of age) have a better prognosis.

Pregnancy appears to have no effect on the disease and vice versa, other than those effects resulting from therapy. Radiation therapy of the nodes and multiagent chemotherapy result in about a 75% cure rate. Unless gestation is well into the third trimester, delay in initiating therapy should be minimal, which brings up the dilemma of therapeutic abortion. Radiation therapy to diseased areas above the diaphragm can be initiated during the third trimester with proper shielding of the fetus. Chemotherapy is strongly contraindicated during the first trimester and is relatively contraindicated in the second and third trimesters. Termination of the pregnancy during the course of the disease is not definitely indicated (DiSaia & Creasman, 1997).

Melanoma

Malignant melanoma may be one of the rare cancers that can be affected by pregnancy. This is suggested by reports in which pregnancy has been shown to induce or exacerbate a melanoma. These suggestions are based on changes that occur naturally during pregnancy and include hyperpigmentation, an increase in melanocyte-stimulating hormone (MSH), and increased production of estrogen. Estrogen receptors have been identified in about half of all melanomas (DiSaia & Creasman, 1997).

Although pregnancy has been implicated in the more rapid metastases to regional lymph nodes, stage for stage, there does not seem to be a significant difference in the survival of pregnant and nonpregnant women. As a result, most authorities recommend that women who have histories of malignant melanoma delay pregnancy for about 3 years after surgical excision, because this is the period of highest risk for recurrence (DiSaia & Creasman, 1997).

Diagnosis is established by biopsy. Therapy consists of radical local excision. For most other malignancies, the placenta is unexplainably resistant to invasion by maternal cancer. Though melanoma accounts for few cases of malignant disease during pregnancy, almost 50% of the placental metastases and almost 90% of fetal metastases occur from maternal melanoma (DiSaia & Creasman, 1997).

Bone Tumors

Bone tumors are rare in pregnancy. Ewing's sarcoma and osteogenic sarcoma and osteocystoma are the most common primary malignant bone tumors seen in pregnancy. Usually the areas involved are the clavicle, sternum, spine, humerus, and femur. A lump or mass, local pain, and disability are characteristic manifestations.

Osteogenic sarcoma affects areas of high bone turnover (especially during growth spurts); Ewing's sarcoma is a rare condition that develops within bone marrow. Pregnancy does not affect and is not affected by the disease.

Surgical excision is usually well tolerated during pregnancy; adjuvant chemotherapy is delayed until after birth if the cancer is diagnosed near term. If the disease recurs, it usually does so within 3 years. Therefore women are counseled to defer pregnancy during this time (DiSaia & Creasman, 1997).

Other Gynecologic Cancers

Cancer of the vulva. The diagnosis of preinvasive (vulvar intraepithelial neoplasia) disease during pregnancy is uncommon. Therapy is postponed until the postpartum period.

If invasive disease (a rare occurrence) is diagnosed during the first trimester, vulvectomy with bilateral groin dissection may be done after the fourteenth week. When it is diagnosed in the third trimester, local wide excision is done, deferring definitive surgery until after birth. Pregnancy does not alter the course of the disease.

After radical vulvectomy and bilateral inguinal lymphectomy, a woman who becomes pregnant again can carry the pregnancy to term and give birth vaginally. If vaginal stenosis is present and could impede birth, cesarean birth may be more appropriate.

Cancer of the vagina. Except for clear-cell adenocarcinoma of DES-exposed women, cancer of the vagina is not common. If clear-cell adenocarcinoma of the cervix and vagina or sarcoma is found in the upper vagina, the preferred surgery is radical hysterectomy, upper vaginectomy, and bilateral pelvic lymphadenectomy, followed by chemotherapy. Radiation is usually not advocated during pregnancy. Pregnancy does not seem to affect the course of the disease or the prognosis.

Cancer of the uterus. Endometrial carcinoma during pregnancy is rare; only a few cases have been documented since 1900. Diagnosis was usually an incidental finding after therapeutic abortion or surgery, and the lesions were minimally or not invasive. Recommended therapy is total abdominal hysterectomy and bilateral salpingo-oophorectomy (TAH-BSO) and adjuvant radiotherapy (DiSaia & Creasman, 1997).

Cancer of the uterine tube. With a peak incidence between 50 and 55 years, concurrent pregnancy is only a remote possibility. Should it occur, the recommended therapy (TAH-BSO with postoperative radiotherapy or chemotherapy) is the same as for the nonpregnant woman. Removal of the uterine tube is an alternative treatment (DiSaia & Creasman, 1997).

Cancer of the ovary. Cancer of the ovary is the second most frequent reproductive cancer that occurs with pregnancy. Still, ovarian malignancy is relatively rare, being reported to occur in 1 per 20,000 to 30,000 births (Berman, DiSaia, & Brewster, 1999).

Ovarian masses occur frequently during pregnancy. Because corpus luteum cysts account for a high percentage of these masses and because 99% of these resolve by the fourteenth week, any mass less than 5 cm may simply be observed until the end of the first trimester. Any mass more than 5 cm, one that is growing, or one that does not resolve after the fourteenth week warrants further investigation. Abdominal palpation and ultrasound are the diagnostic tools of choice during pregnancy. However, in many cases laparotomy is necessary to confirm the diagnosis. Laparotomy after 16 weeks of gestation has negligible fetal wastage associated with the procedure and is therefore considered safe.

An ovarian tumor may be first diagnosed at birth or postpartum because the enlarged uterus obscured its presence. Definitive diagnosis is needed before treatment is selected. For stage I tumors treatment includes conservative surgery (unilateral oophorectomy and salpingectomy) and use of chemotherapy. If diagnosis occurs in the second or third trimester, treatment choices are difficult to make. They include interrupting the pregnancy and starting chemotherapy immediately, preserving pregnancy and starting chemotherapy with the fetus in utero (controversial), or delaying chemotherapy until the fetus is more mature and early delivery is a low risk to the fetus (DiSaia & Creasman, 1997).

Cancer Therapy and Pregnancy

Decisions about the type and timing of therapy for cancer in the pregnant woman evoke moral and philosophic dilemmas, as well as complex medical judgments and intense emotional responses. The fetus is at risk with either chemotherapy or radiation therapy. The impact of cancer therapy on the fetus can include death, miscarriage, teratogenesis, alteration in growth and development, alterations in function, and mutagenesis. The long-term effects on the fetus are unknown. However, the long-term experiences of young women exposed to DES in utero make the possibility of long-term effects associated with cancer therapy very real. These theoretic dangers must be weighed against the potential detrimental effects to the mother if treatment is withheld (see Ethical Considerations box).

ETHICAL CONSIDERATIONS

Treatment for Cancer During Pregnancy

When a pregnant woman has cancer and her survival is contingent on treatment that will harm the fetus, the health care team must work with the woman and her significant others to make decisions about how to proceed with her care. If a one-client model of ethical decision making is used, the risk-benefit analysis is applied to the maternal-fetal unit. The pregnant woman decides on what is best for her and the fetus. The woman may accept or refuse treatment. If a two-client model is used for decision making, more weight is given to fetal well-being, but the pregnant woman cannot be forced to accept harm to herself for the sake of the fetus. Thus she could elect to accept treatment.

Timing of therapy is also an important issue to discuss. Because most cancer therapy (except surgery) is geared toward having a differential and noxious effect on rapidly growing tissue, the fetus is most at risk during the first trimester, when organogenesis and rapid tissue growth occur. Surgery offers the least potential risk to the fetus. However, the risk of miscarriage and preterm labor may be increased.

Chemotherapy is avoided in the first trimester if at all possible. Although most chemotherapeutic agents have had isolated reports of fetal abnormalities associated with them, data on the agents used after the first trimester have recorded surprisingly few fetal abnormalities. The placenta may act as a barrier against the chemotherapeutic agents. Therefore, although risk still exists, the judicious use of chemotherapy after the first trimester can result in live births with few congenital abnormalities. Acute drug toxicities may occur if treatment has occurred just before birth. Breastfeeding by women who are taking cytoxic drugs is not recommended because these drugs may be excreted in breast milk.

Radiation therapy presents its own set of issues. During embryonic development, tissues are extremely radiosensitive. If cells are genetically altered or killed during this time, the child either will fail to survive or will be deformed. From a radiologic stance there are three significant periods in embryonic development:

1. Preimplantation: If irradiation does not destroy the fertilized egg, it probably does not affect it significantly.
2. Critical period of organogenesis: During this period, especially between days 18 and 38, the organism is most vulnerable; microcephaly, anencephaly, eye damage, growth restriction, spina bifida, and foot damage may occur.
3. After day 40: Large doses may still cause observable malformation and damage to the central nervous system.

Pregnancy After Cancer Treatment

If cancer therapy has not included the removal of the uterus, ovaries, or uterine (fallopian) tubes, there is a possibility that the woman may still be able to become pregnant. Although a woman's menstrual cycle may have resumed, pregnancy may be difficult to achieve. Therapy that has affected the pituitary or thyroid gland may make conception difficult. Radiation appears to have the most deleterious effects on the endocrine system. The use of chemotherapy may result in temporary or permanent sterility, depending on the drug, the dose, and the length of time since the therapy was completed. Alkylating agents are most commonly associated with infertility (Lamb, 1995).

Of growing concern is the increase in the number of childhood and adolescent cancer survivors. Long-term effects of therapy on fertility, including incidence of congenital anomalies, are not well known. The newly diagnosed client must be counseled on the potential effects of treatment on later reproductive function (Gershenson, 1997).

For recovery from the disease and treatment to be complete, a delay of at least 2 years from the end of therapy to conception is advised. An exception is the women who has had ovarian cancer, who is advised, because of a high incidence of a second primary tumor, to complete her childbearing as soon as possible (American College of Obstetricians and Gynecologists, 1994).

Before conception, women who have had cancer should have a complete physical examination to rule out complications that may place her or a fetus in jeopardy. Cardiac, pulmonary, hematologic, neurologic, renal, or gonadal function may be impaired. The woman and the potential father (if partnered) should be referred for reproductive and genetic counseling as well.

GESTATIONAL TROPHOBLASTIC DISEASE

Gestational trophoblastic disease (GTD) is a term that encompasses a spectrum of disorders arising from the placental trophoblast. It includes hydatidiform mole, invasive mole, and choriocarcinoma. **Gestational trophoblastic neoplasia** (GTN) refers to persistent trophoblastic tissue that is presumed to be malignant (DiSaia & Creasman, 1997). Table 13-5 describes the clinical classifications of GTD. Before the middle 1950s, the prognoses of these neoplasias, especially end-stage choriocarcinoma, were dismal. Today, however, GTN is recognized as the most curable gynecologic malignancy. The reason for this change in thinking is related to several factors: a sensitive marker is produced by the tumor (hCG); the tumor is extremely sensitive to various chemotherapeutic agents; high risk factors in the disease process can be identified, allowing for individualized therapy; and the aggressive use of multiple treatment methods is possible.

Malignant disease follows hydatidiform mole in about 50% of cases. Miscarriage or ectopic pregnancy precedes

TABLE 13-5 Clinical Classification of Gestational Trophoblastic Disease	
GESTATIONAL TROPHOBLASTIC DISEASE	**GESTATIONAL TROPHOBLASTIC NEOPLASIA**
Hydatidiform mole Complete (absence of fetal tissue) Incomplete (presence of fetal tissue)	Nonmetastatic (no evidence of disease outside the uterus) Metastatic (any disease outside the uterus) Low risk: good prognosis High risk: poor prognosis

about 25% of cases, and normal pregnancy precedes another 25% of cases (DiSaia & Creasman, 1997).

Continued bleeding after evacuation of a hydatidiform mole is usually the most suggestive symptom of GTN. Other clinical signs include abdominal pain and uterine and ovarian enlargement. Signs of metastasis include pulmonary symptoms (e.g., dyspnea, cough). The diagnosis is usually confirmed by rising or plateauing hCG levels following evacuation of a molar pregnancy. Once diagnosis is confirmed, other clinical studies (e.g., CT scan of lungs and brain) are done to determine the extent of the disease.

Hysterectomy with adjuvant chemotherapy is often the choice of treatment for nonmetastatic tumors in women who have completed their childbearing. For women who wish to preserve their fertility, single-agent chemotherapy is chosen. Methotrexate has been the treatment of choice for years. High-dose methotrexate followed by folinic acid "rescue" within 24 hours has also shown excellent results and causes fewer toxic effects (DiSaia & Creasman, 1997). Dactinomycin has also been used with equally good results and is used for women with liver or renal disease, both of which are contraindications for methotrexate.

Women who have metastasis are classified as having either a good or poor prognosis, depending on the absence or presence of brain or liver metastasis, unsuccessful prior chemotherapy, symptoms lasting longer than 4 months, and serum β-hCG levels greater than 40,000 mIU/ml. Treatment progresses from single-agent chemotherapy in the low risk category to multiple-agent chemotherapy and multiple methods of treatment for the high risk group. Cure rates for the low risk group are almost as good as for those with nonmetastatic disease, both approaching 100% (DiSaia & Creasman, 1997).

Therapy is continued until negative hCG levels are obtained. Follow-up after successful chemotherapy is by serum hCG levels obtained every 2 weeks for 3 months, every month for 3 months, every other month for 6 months, then every 6 months indefinitely. Physical examinations should be done yearly, and chest x-rays are done if indicated. Contraception is needed until the woman has been in remission for at least 6 months (Berman, DiSaia, & Brewster, 1999; DiSaia & Creasman, 1997). Oral contraceptives and barrier methods are acceptable methods. During a subsequent pregnancy, pelvic ultrasonography is recommended because the woman is at higher risk to develop another molar pregnancy. Serum hCG levels should be obtained 6 weeks after the birth (DiSaia & Creasman, 1997).

KEY POINTS

- Gynecologic disorders diminish the quality of life for affected women and their families.
- Pelvic relaxation and lengthening of fascial supports are most often the delayed sequelae of childbirth trauma, but they may be seen in young or childless women.
- The development of neoplasms, whether benign or malignant, can have a significant physical and emotional impact on the woman and her family.
- Abnormal uterine bleeding is the most common symptom of leiomyomas or fibroid tumors.
- Endometrial cancer is the most common reproductive system malignancy.
- Hysterectomy is the usual treatment for early-stage endometrial cancer.
- Infections such as human papillomavirus types 16 and 18 and possibly other types have been linked to subsequent cervical cancer.
- The squamocolumnar junction is an important landmark identified with neoplastic changes of the cervix.
- Preinvasive cancer of the cervix may be treated with techniques such as electrosurgical excision, cryotherapy, and laser therapy to save the structure of the cervix, particularly in women who desire to retain childbearing ability.
- External and internal radiation therapy in combination are as successful as surgery in treating early stages of cancer of the cervix.
- The Papanicolaou test will detect approximately 90% of early cervical dysplasias.
- Cancer of the ovary causes more deaths than any other female genital tract cancer.
- Nurses can control their exposure to radiation in three ways—increasing the distance from the radiation source, limiting the time of exposure, and using lead shielding.
- Cancer is relatively infrequent during pregnancy, occurring about once in every 1000 pregnancies.
- Treatment of the pregnant woman who has cancer with radiation or chemotherapy places the fetus at risk for death, miscarriage, teratogenesis, and alterations in growth and development.
- Gestational trophoblastic neoplasms are highly curable but require close monitoring of hCG levels after treatment.

CRITICAL THINKING EXERCISES

1 You are preparing a preoperative teaching class for women attending a gynecologic clinic who are to have hysterectomies.
   a. Discuss how you would differentiate information needed by women who are having a vaginal versus an abdominal procedure.
   b. How would you assess the women for possible misinformation or misconceptions about having a hysterectomy? What cultural assessments are needed?
   c. How would you include the partner in the assessment and teaching?
   d. How would you evaluate the effectiveness of your teaching?

2 You are assigned a 17-year-old adolescent who is 24 weeks pregnant. She has leukemia and is not expected to live until her fetus is full term without chemotherapy, but she does not want to take it again.
   a. Discuss how you would approach her care if you believe that she should do whatever is necessary to allow the fetus to get mature enough to be born without being too premature to survive.
   b. Discuss how you would approach her care if you support her right to not take treatment even if it means both the adolescent and her fetus will not survive.

3 Develop a poster presentation for a shopping mall or factory break room on prevention of gynecologic cancer.
   a. Discuss how you would incorporate the appropriate reading level and design strategies that will arouse the interest of women who see the poster.
   b. Identify other strategies to reduce barriers to gynecologic cancer prevention for women of different cultural backgrounds.

References

American Cancer Society. (1999). *Cancer facts and figures 1999*. New York: American Cancer Society.

American College of Obstetricians and Gynecologists. (1994). *Quality assessment and improvement in obstetrics and gynecology*. Washington, DC: ACOG.

Berman, M., DiSaia, P., & Brewster, W. (1999). Pelvic malignancies, gestational trophoblastic neoplasia, and non-pelvic malignancies. In R. Creasy & R. Resnick (Eds.). *Maternal-fetal medicine* (4th ed.). Philadelphia: W.B. Saunders.

Centers for Disease Control and Prevention. (1998). 1998 guidelines for treatment of sexually transmitted diseases. *MMWR* 47(RR-1), 96.

Czarapata, B., & McKillips, K. (1997). Silent suffering: Helping women find the path to continence. *AWHONN Lifelines* 1(2), 28-34.

DiSaia, P., &, Creasman, W. (1997). *Clinical gynecologic oncology* (5th ed.). St. Louis: Mosby.

Dunne-Daly, C. (1997). Principles of brachytherapy. In K. Dow et al. (Eds.). *Nursing care in radiation oncology* (2nd ed.). Philadelphia: W.B. Saunders.

Gershenson, D. (1997). Reproductive potential after cancer treatment. *Ob/Gyn Clinical Alert* 14(3), 22-24.

Grabo, T. et al. (1999). Uterine myomas: Treatment options. *J Obstet Gynecol Neonatal Nurs* 28(1), 23-31.

Higgins, P., & Smith, P. (1997). Assessing cervical cancer risks. *AWHONN Lifelines* 1(6), 43-47.

Lamb, M. (1995). Effects of cancer on the sexuality and fertility of women. *Semin Oncol Nurs* 11(2), 120-127.

Lowdermilk, D. (1995a). Home care of the patient with gynecologic cancer. *J Obstet Gynecol Neonatal Nurs* 24(2), 157-163.

Lowdermilk, D. (1995b). Reproductive surgery. In C. Fogel & N. Woods (Eds.). *Women's health care: A comprehensive handbook*. Thousand Oaks, CA: Sage.

Mishell, D. et al. (1997). *Comprehensive gynecology* (3rd ed.). St. Louis: Mosby.

Mitchell, S. (1997). Gynecologic cancers. In K. Dow et al. (Eds.). *Nursing care in radiation oncology* (2nd ed.). Philadelphia: W.B. Saunders.

National Institutes of Health Consensus Conference. (1995). Ovarian cancer: Screening, treatment, and follow-up. *JAMA* 273(6), 491-497.

Phipps, W., Sands, J., & Marek, J. (1999). *Medical-surgical nursing: Concepts and clinical practice* (6th ed.). St. Louis: Mosby.

Reich, H. (1995). Laparoscopic myomectomy. *Obstet Gynecol Clin North Am* 22(4), 757-780.

Sampselle, C. et al. (1997). Continence for women: Evidence-based practice. *J Obstet Gynecol Neonatal Nurs* 26(4), 375-385.

Schlaerth, J. (1994). Cancer of the cervix uteri. In D. Mishell, Jr., & P. Brenner (Eds.). *Management of common problems in obstetrics and gynecology*. Oxford: Blackwell Scientific.

Seidel, H. et al. (1999). *Mosby's guide to physical examination* (4th ed.). St. Louis: Mosby.

Skoner, M., Thompson, W., & Caron, V. (1994). Factors associated with risk of stress urinary incontinence in women. *Nurs Res* 42(5), 301-306.

Smith, K. (1997). Counseling and managing women undergoing hysterectomy/oophorectomy. In *Menopausal issues: A practical guide for nursing professionals*. Barrington, IL: The Willow Group, Inc.

Verdon, M. (1997). Issues in the management of human papillomavirus disease. *Am Fam Physician* 55(5), 1813-1819.

Wallach, E. (1997). Contemporary management of uterine leiomyomata. Paper presented at the 16th Annual Review Course in Reproductive Endocrinology, Johns Hopkins Medical Institutions, Baltimore.

Williamson, M. (1992). Sexual adjustment after hysterectomy. *J Obstet Gynecol Neonatal Nurs* 21(1), 42-47.

14

Conception, Fetal Development, and Genetics

Shannon E. Perry

LEARNING OBJECTIVES

- Define the key terms.
- Summarize the process of fertilization.
- Explain basic principles of genetics.
- Describe the development, structure, and functions of the placenta.
- Describe the composition and functions of the amniotic fluid.
- Identify three organs or tissues arising from each of the three primary germ layers.

- Summarize the significant changes in growth and development of the embryo and fetus.
- Identify the potential effects of teratogens during vulnerable periods of embryonic and fetal development.
- Describe the Human Genome Project.
- Describe the nurse's role in genetic counseling.
- Examine ethical dimensions of genetic screening.
- Identify topics for nursing research related to conception, fetal development, and genetics.

KEY TERMS

amniotic fluid	fetus	monozygotic twins
blastocyst	foramen ovale	morula
cephalocaudal development	gamete	mutation
chorionic villi	genome	placenta
chromosome	hematopoiesis	quickening
conception	human chorionic gonadotropin (hCG)	sex chromosome
decidua basalis		surfactants
dizygotic twins	implantation	teratogens
ductus arteriosus	karyotype	umbilical cord
ductus venosus	lecithin/sphingomyelin (L/S) ratio	viability
embryo	meconium	zygote
fertilization	meiosis	
fetal membranes	mitosis	

This chapter presents an overview of the process of fertilization and the development of the normal embryo and fetus. A brief discussion of genetics and genetic counseling is included.

CONCEPTION

Conception, defined as the union of a single egg and sperm, marks the beginning of a pregnancy. Conception occurs not as an isolated event, but as part of a sequential

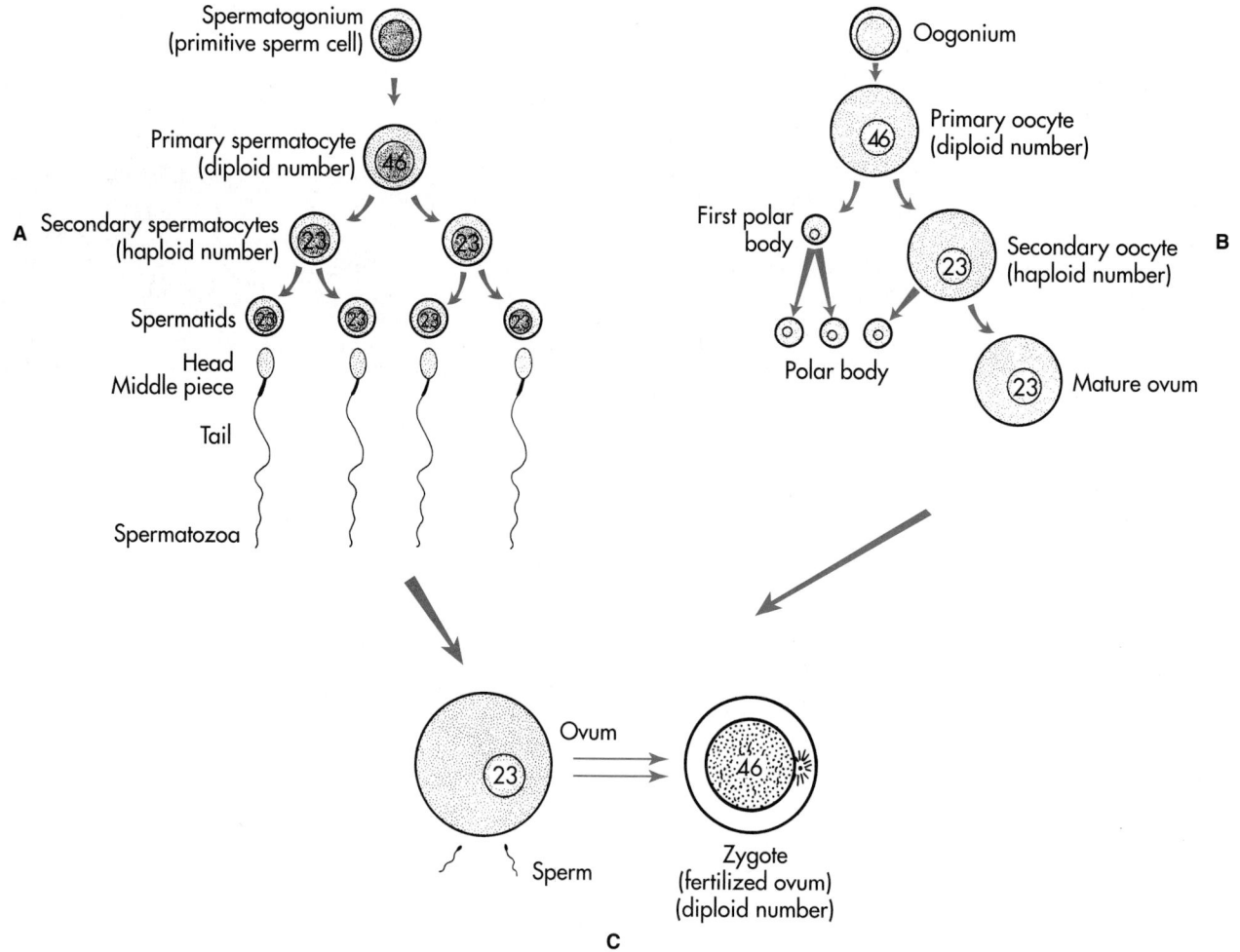

Fig. 14-1 **A,** Spermatogenesis. Gametogenesis of the male produces four mature gametes, the sperm. **B,** Oogenesis. Gametogenesis in the female produces one mature ovum and three polar bodies. Note the relative difference in overall size between the ovum and sperm. **C,** Fertilization results in the single-cell zygote and the restoration of the diploid number of chromosomes.

process. This sequential process includes **gamete** (egg and sperm) formation, ovulation (release of the egg), fertilization (union of the gametes), and implantation in the uterus.

Cell Division

Cells are reproduced by two different methods: mitosis and meiosis. In **mitosis,** body cells replicate to yield two cells with the same genetic makeup as the parent cell. First the cell makes a copy of its deoxyribonucleic acid (DNA); then it divides, and each daughter cell receives one copy of the genetic material. The purpose of mitotic division is for growth and development or cell replacement.

Meiosis produces gametes. Each homologous pair of chromosomes receives one chromosome from the mother and the other from the father; meiosis results in cells containing one of each of the 23 pairs of chromosomes. Because these germ cells contain 23 single chromosomes,

half of the genetic material of a normal somatic cell, they are called haploid. This halving of the genetic material is accomplished by replicating the DNA once and then dividing twice. In mitosis, the DNA is replicated once and followed by a single cell division. When the female gamete (egg or ovum) and the male gamete (spermatozoan) unite to form the zygote, the diploid number of human chromosomes (46 or 23 pairs) is restored.

The process of DNA replication and cell division in meiosis allows different alleles for genes to be distributed at random by each parent and then rearranged on the paired chromosomes. The chromosomes then separate and proceed to different gametes. Many combinations of genes are possible on each chromosome because parents have genotypes derived from four different grandparents. This random mixing of alleles accounts for the variation of traits seen in the offspring of the same parents (see discussion later in this chapter).

Gametogenesis

When a male reaches puberty, his testes begin the process of spermatogenesis. The cells that undergo meiosis in the male are called spermatocytes. The primary spermatocyte, which undergoes the first meiotic division, contains the diploid number of chromosomes. Remember, however, that the cell has already copied its DNA before division, so four alleles for each gene are actually present. The cell is still considered diploid because the copies are bound together—one allele plus its copy on each chromosome. During the first meiotic division, two haploid secondary spermatocytes are formed. Each secondary spermatocyte contains 22 autosomes and one sex chromosome; one contains the X chromosome (plus its copy), and the other has the Y chromosome (plus its copy). During the second meiotic division, the male produces two gametes with an X chromosome and two gametes with a Y chromosome, all of which will develop into viable sperm (Fig. 14-1, *A*).

Oogenesis, the process of egg (ovum) formation, begins in the female's fetal life. At birth, a woman's ovaries contain all of the cells that may undergo meiosis in her lifetime. The majority of the estimated 2 million primary oocytes (the cells that undergo the first meiotic division) degenerate spontaneously. Only 400 to 500 ova will mature during the approximately 35 years of a woman's reproductive life. The primary oocytes begin the first meiotic division (i.e., they replicate their DNA) during fetal life, but remain suspended at this stage until puberty (Fig. 14-1, *B*). Then usually monthly, one primary oocyte matures and completes the first meiotic division, yielding two unequal cells, the secondary oocyte and a small polar body. Both contain 22 autosomes and one X sex chromosome. At ovulation, the second meiotic division begins; however, the ovum does not complete the second meiotic division unless fertilization occurs. At fertilization, a second polar body and the zygote (the united egg and sperm) are produced (Fig. 14-1, *C*). The three polar bodies degenerate. If fertilization does not occur, the ovum also degenerates.

Ovum

Meiosis is the process by which germ cells divide and decrease their chromosomal number by half. In the female this meiotic process produces an ovum (egg) and occurs in the ovarian follicles. Each month one ovum matures with a host of surrounding supportive cells.

At ovulation the ovum is released from the ruptured ovarian follicle. High estrogen levels increase the motility of the uterine tubes so their cilia are able to capture the ovum and propel it through the tube toward the uterine cavity. An ovum cannot move by itself.

Two protective layers surround the ovum (Fig. 14-2). The inner layer is a thick, acellular layer, the zona pellucida. The outer layer, the corona radiata, is composed of elongated cells.

Ova are considered fertile for about 24 hours after ovulation. If unfertilized by a sperm, the ovum degenerates and is reabsorbed.

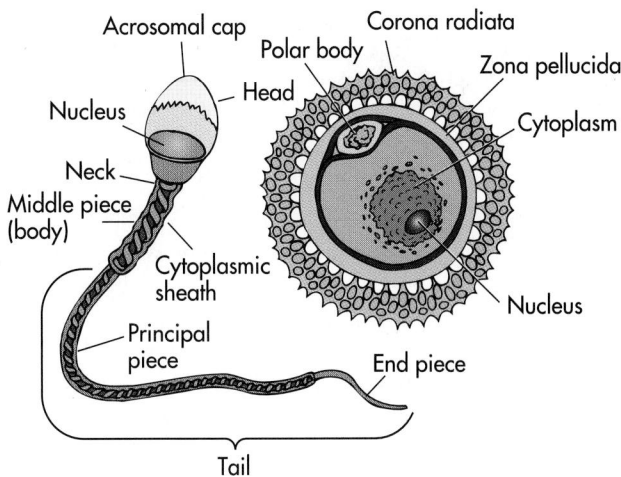

Fig. 14-2   Sperm and ovum.

Sperm

Ejaculation during sexual intercourse normally propels almost a teaspoon of semen (containing as many as 200 to 500 million sperm) into the vagina. The sperm swim with the flagellar movement of their tails. Some sperm can reach the site of fertilization within 5 minutes, but the average transit time is 4 to 6 hours. Sperm remain viable within the woman's reproductive system for an average of 2 to 3 days. Most sperm are lost in the vagina, within the cervical mucus, or in the endometrium, or they enter the uterine tube that contains no ovum.

As the sperm travel through the female reproductive tract, enzymes are produced to aid in capacitation of the sperm. Then, small perforations form in the acrosome (a cap on the sperm) and allow enzymes (e.g., hyaluronidase) to escape (see Fig. 14-2). These enzymes are necessary for the sperm to penetrate the protective layers of the ovum before fertilization.

Fertilization

Fertilization takes place in the ampulla (outer third) of the uterine (fallopian) tube. When a sperm successfully penetrates the membrane surrounding the ovum, both sperm and ovum are enclosed within the membrane, and the membrane becomes impenetrable to other sperm; this process is termed the *zona reaction.* The second meiotic division of the secondary oocyte is then completed, and the ovum nucleus becomes the female pronucleus. The head of the sperm enlarges to become the male pronucleus, and the tail degenerates. The nuclei fuse and the chromosomes combine, restoring the diploid number (46) (Fig. 14-3). Conception, the formation of the **zygote** (the first cell of the new individual), is now complete.

Mitotic cellular replication, called *cleavage,* begins as the zygote travels the length of the uterine tube into the uterus. This transit time takes 3 to 4 days. Because the

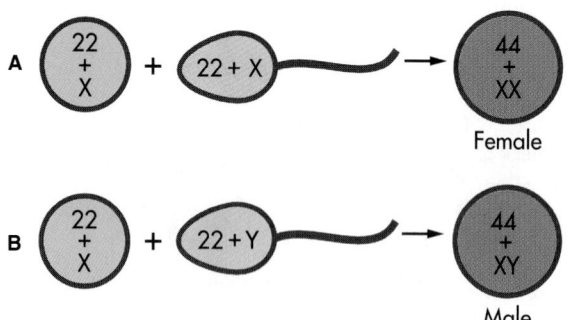

Fig. 14-3 Fertilization. **A,** Ovum fertilized by X-bearing sperm to form female zygote. **B,** Ovum fertilized by Y-bearing sperm to form male zygote.

fertilized egg divides rapidly without an increase in size, successively smaller cells, *blastomeres,* are formed with each division. A 16-cell **morula,** a solid ball of cells, is produced within 3 days still surrounded by the protective zona pellucida (Fig. 14-4, *A*). Further development occurs as the morula floats freely within the uterus. Fluid passes through the zona pellucida into the intercellular spaces between the blastomeres, separating them into two parts; the trophoblast (which gives rise to the placenta) and the embryoblast (which gives rise to the embryo). A cavity forms within the cell mass as the spaces come together, forming a structure called the *blastocyst cavity.* When the cavity becomes recognizable, the whole structure of the developing embryo is known as the **blastocyst.** The outer layer of cells surrounding the cavity is the *trophoblast* (the feeding layer).

Implantation

The zona pellucida degenerates, the trophoblast cells displace endometrial cells at the implantation site, and the blastocyst embeds in the endometrium, usually in the anterior or posterior fundal region. Between 6 and 10 days after conception, the trophoblast secretes enzymes that enable it to burrow into the endometrium until the entire blastocyst is covered. This is known as **implantation.** Endometrial blood vessels erode, and some women experience slight implantation bleeding (slight spotting or bleeding during the time of the first missed menstrual period). **Chorionic villi,** fingerlike processes or projections, develop out of the trophoblast and extend into the blood-filled spaces of the endometrium. These villi obtain oxygen and nutrients from the maternal bloodstream and dispose of carbon dioxide and waste products into the maternal blood.

After implantation, the endometrium is called the *decidua.* The portion directly under the blastocyst, where the chorionic villi tap into the maternal blood vessels, is the **decidua basalis.** The portion covering the blastocyst is the *decidua capsularis,* and the portion lining the rest of the uterus is the *decidua vera* (Fig. 14-5).

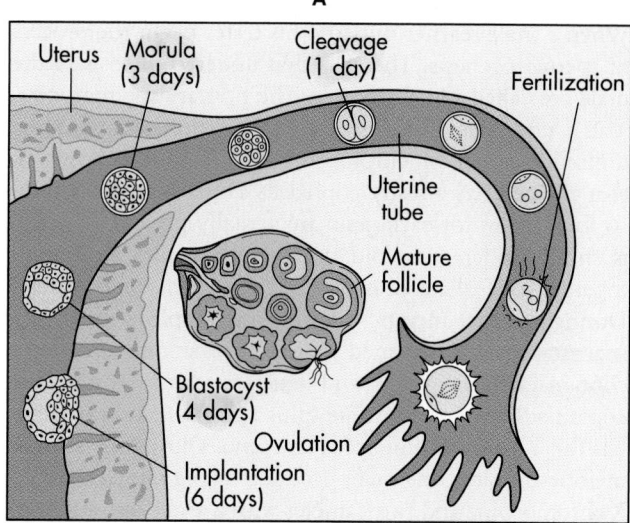

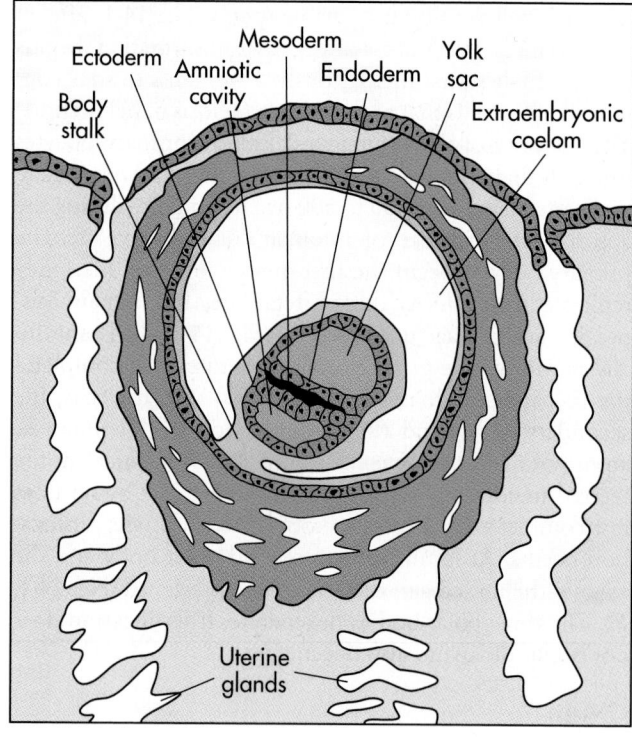

Fig. 14-4 First week of human development. **A,** Follicular development in the ovary, ovulation, fertilization, and transport of the early embryo down the uterine tube and into the uterus where implantation occurs. **B,** Blastocyst embedded in endometrium. Germ layers forming. (**A** *from Carlson, B. [1994]. Human embryology and developmental biology. St. Louis: Mosby;* **B** *adapted from Langley, L. et al. [1980]. Dynamic human anatomy and physiology [5th ed.]. New York: McGraw-Hill.)*

THE EMBRYO AND FETUS

Pregnancy lasts approximately 10 lunar months, 9 calendar months, 40 weeks, or 280 days. Length of pregnancy is computed from the first day of the last menstrual period

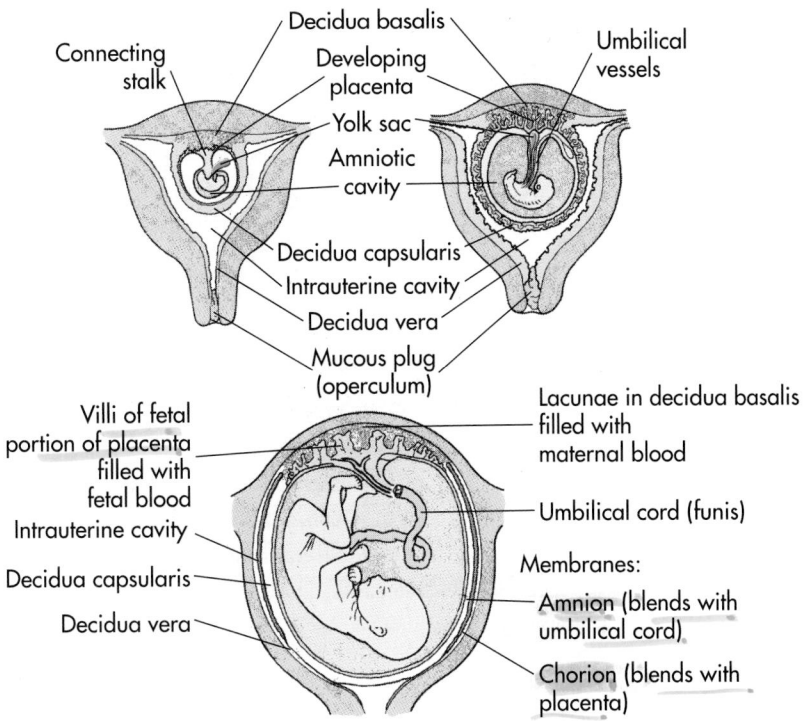

Fig. 14-5 Development of fetal membranes. Note gradual obliteration of intrauterine cavity as decidua capsularis and decidua vera meet. Also note thinning of uterine wall. Chorionic and amniotic membranes are in apposition to each other but may be peeled apart.

(LMP) until the day of birth. However, conception occurs approximately 2 weeks after the first day of the LMP. Thus the postconception age of the fetus is 2 weeks less, for a total of 266 days or 38 weeks. Postconception age is used in the discussion of fetal development.

Intrauterine development is divided into three stages: ovum or preembryonic, embryo, and fetus (Fig. 14-6). The stage of the ovum lasts from conception until day 14. This period covers cellular replication, blastocyst formation, initial development of the embryonic membranes, and establishment of the primary germ layers.

Primary Germ Layers

During the third week after conception the embryonic disk differentiates into three primary germ layers: the ectoderm, mesoderm, and endoderm (or entoderm) (Fig. 14-4, *B*). All tissues and organs of the embryo develop from these three layers.

The *ectoderm,* the upper layer of the embryonic disk, gives rise to the epidermis, glands (anterior pituitary, cutaneous, and mammary), nails and hair, the nervous system, lens of the eye, tooth enamel, and the floor of the amniotic cavity.

The middle layer, the *mesoderm,* develops into the bones and teeth, muscles (skeletal, smooth, and cardiac), dermis, and connective tissue, cardiovascular system and spleen, and urogenital system.

The lower layer, the *endoderm,* gives rise to the epithelium lining the respiratory tract, digestive tract, and glan-

dular cells of associated organs, including the oropharynx, liver and pancreas, urethra, bladder, and vagina. The endoderm forms the roof of the yolk sac.

Development of the Embryo

The embryonic stage lasts from day 15 until approximately 8 weeks after conception or until the **embryo** measures 3 cm from crown to rump. This embryonic stage is the most critical time in the development of the organ systems and the main external features. Developing areas with rapid cell division are the most vulnerable to malformation by environmental **teratogens** (a substance or exposure that causes abnormal development). At the end of the eighth week, all organ systems and external structures are present and the embryo is unmistakably human (see Fig. 14-6).

Membranes

At the time of implantation, two **fetal membranes** that will surround the developing embryo begin to form. The *chorion* develops from the trophoblast and contains the chorionic villi on its surface. The villi burrowing into the decidua basalis increase in size and complexity as the vascular processes develop into the placenta. The chorion becomes the covering of the fetal side of the placenta. It contains the major umbilical blood vessels as they branch out over the surface of the placenta. As the embryo grows, the decidua capsularis stretches. The chorionic villi on this side atrophy and degenerate, leaving a smooth chorionic membrane.

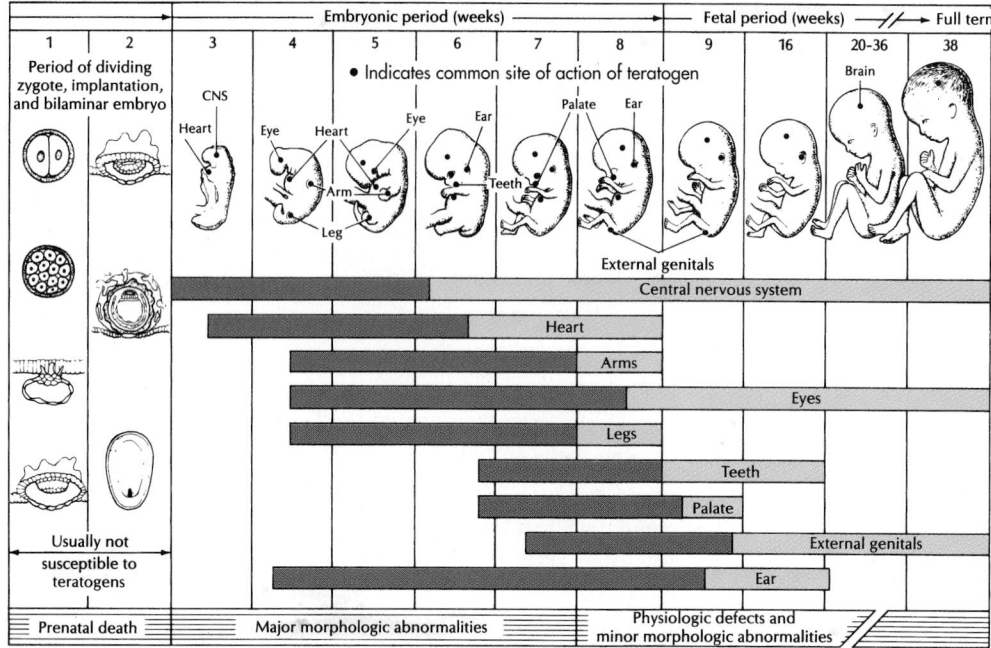

Fig. 14-6 Sensitive, or critical, periods in human development. Dark color denotes highly sensitive periods; light color indicates stages that are less sensitive to teratogens. *(From Moore, K., & Persaud, T. [1998]. Before we are born: Essentials of embryology and birth defects [5th ed.]. Philadelphia: W.B. Saunders.)*

The inner cell membrane, the *amnion*, develops from the interior cells of the blastocyst. The cavity that develops between this inner cell mass and the outer layer of cells (trophoblast) is the amniotic cavity (see Fig. 14-4, *B*). As it grows larger, the amnion forms on the side opposite the developing blastocyst (see Figs. 14-4 and 14-5). The developing embryo draws the amnion around itself, forming a fluid-filled sac. The amnion becomes the covering of the umbilical cord and covers the chorion on the fetal surface of the placenta. As the embryo grows larger, the amnion enlarges to accommodate the embryo/fetus and surrounding amniotic fluid. The amnion eventually comes in contact with the chorion surrounding the fetus.

Amniotic Fluid

Initially, the amniotic cavity derives its fluid by diffusion from the maternal blood. The amount of fluid increases weekly, so that at term, between 800 and 1200 ml of transparent liquid is normally present. The **amniotic fluid** volume changes constantly. The fetus swallows fluid, and fluid flows into and out of the fetal lungs. The fetus urinates into the fluid, greatly enhancing its volume.

Many functions are served by amniotic fluid for the embryo/fetus. Amniotic fluid helps maintain a constant body temperature. It serves as a source of oral fluid and repository for waste. It cushions the fetus from trauma by blunting and dispersing the forces. It allows freedom of movement for musculoskeletal development. The fluid keeps the embryo from tangling with the membranes, which facili-

tates symmetric growth. If the embryo does intersect with the membranes, amputations of extremities or other deformities can occur from constricting amniotic bands.

The volume of amniotic fluid is an important factor in assessing fetal well-being (Hallak et al., 1993). The presence of less than 300 ml of amniotic fluid (oligohydramnios) is associated with fetal renal abnormalities; more than 2 L (hydramnios) is associated with gastrointestinal and other malformations.

Amniotic fluid contains albumin, urea, uric acid, creatinine, lecithin, sphingomyelin, bilirubin, fructose, fat, leukocytes, proteins, epithelial cells, enzymes, and lanugo hair. Study of fetal cells in amniotic fluid through amniocentesis yields much information about the fetus. Genetic studies (karyotyping) provide knowledge about the sex and normality of chromosome number and structure. Other studies such as L/S ratio determine the health or maturity of the fetus.

Yolk Sac

At the same time the amniotic cavity and amnion are forming, another blastocyst cavity has formed on the other side of the developing embryonic disk (see Fig. 14-4, *B*). This cavity becomes surrounded by a membrane, forming the yolk sac. The yolk sac aids in transferring maternal nutrients and oxygen, which have diffused through the chorion to the embryo. Blood vessels form to aid transport. Blood cells and plasma are manufactured in the yolk sac during the second and third weeks while uteroplacental circulation is being established and forming primitive blood cells until hematopoietic activity begins. At the end of the third week, the primitive heart begins to beat and circulate the blood through the embryo, connecting stalk, chorion, and yolk sac.

The folding in of the embryo during the fourth week results in part of the yolk sac being incorporated into the embryo's body as the primitive digestive system. Primordial germ cells arise in the yolk sac and move into the embryo. The shrinking remains of the yolk sac degenerate (see Fig. 14-5). By the fifth or sixth week, the remnant has separated from the embryo.

Umbilical Cord

By day 14 after conception, the embryonic disk, amniotic sac, and yolk sac are attached to the chorionic villi by the connecting stalk. During the third week the blood vessels develop to supply the embryo with maternal nutrients and oxygen. During the fifth week, after the embryo has curved inward on itself from both ends, bringing the connecting stalk to the ventral side of the embryo, the connecting stalk becomes compressed from both sides by the amnion forming the narrower **umbilical cord** (see Fig. 14-5). Two arteries carry blood from the embryo to the chorionic villi, and one vein returns blood to the embryo. Approximately 1% of umbilical cords contain only two vessels: one artery and one vein. This occurrence is sometimes associated with congenital malformations.

The cord rapidly increases in length. At term, the cord ranges from 30 to 90 cm long (average 55 cm) and is 2 cm in diameter. It twists spirally on itself and loops around the embryo/fetus. A true knot is rare, but false knots occur as folds or kinks in the cord and may jeopardize circulation to the fetus. Connective tissue called *Wharton's jelly* prevents compression of the blood vessels to ensure continued nourishment of the embryo/fetus. Compression can occur if the cord lies between the fetal head and pelvis or is twisted around the fetal body. When the cord is wrapped around the fetal neck, it is called a nuchal cord.

As the placenta develops from the chorionic villi, the umbilical cord is usually located centrally. The blood vessels are arrayed out from the center to all parts of the placenta.

Placenta

Structure. The placenta begins to form at implantation. During the third week after conception the trophoblast cells of the chorionic villi continue to invade the decidua basalis. As the uterine capillaries are tapped, the endometrial spiral arteries fill with maternal blood. The chorionic villi grow into the spaces with two layers of cells: the outer syncytium and the inner cytotrophoblast. A third layer develops into anchoring septa, dividing the projecting decidua into separate areas called *cotyledons*. In each of the 15 to 20 cotyledons, the chorionic villi branch out and a complex system of fetal blood vessels forms. Each cotyledon is a functional unit. The whole structure is the **placenta** (Fig. 14-7).

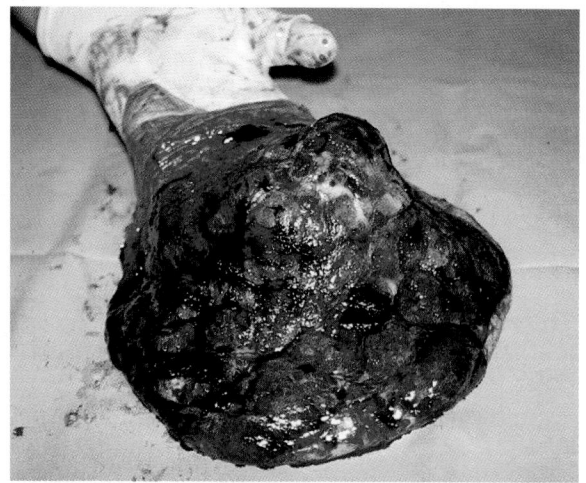

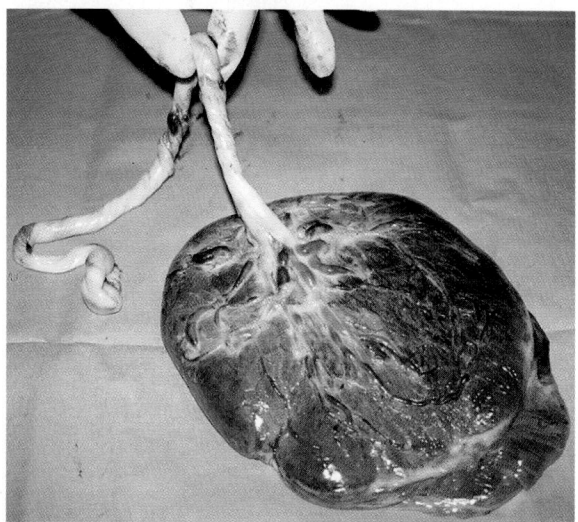

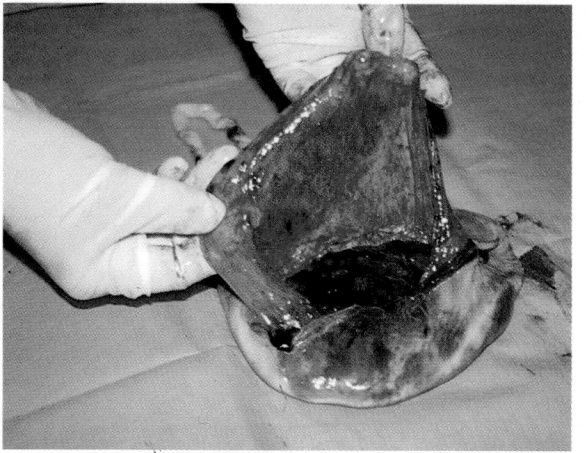

Fig. 14-7 Full-term placentas. **A,** Maternal (or uterine) surface, showing cotyledons and grooves. **B,** Fetal (or amniotic) surface, showing blood vessels running under amnion and converging to form umbilical vessels at attachment of umbilical cord. **C,** Amnion and smooth chorion are arranged to show that they are (1) fused and (2) continuous with margins of placenta. *(Courtesy Marjorie Pyle, RNC, Lifecircle, Costa Mesa, CA.)*

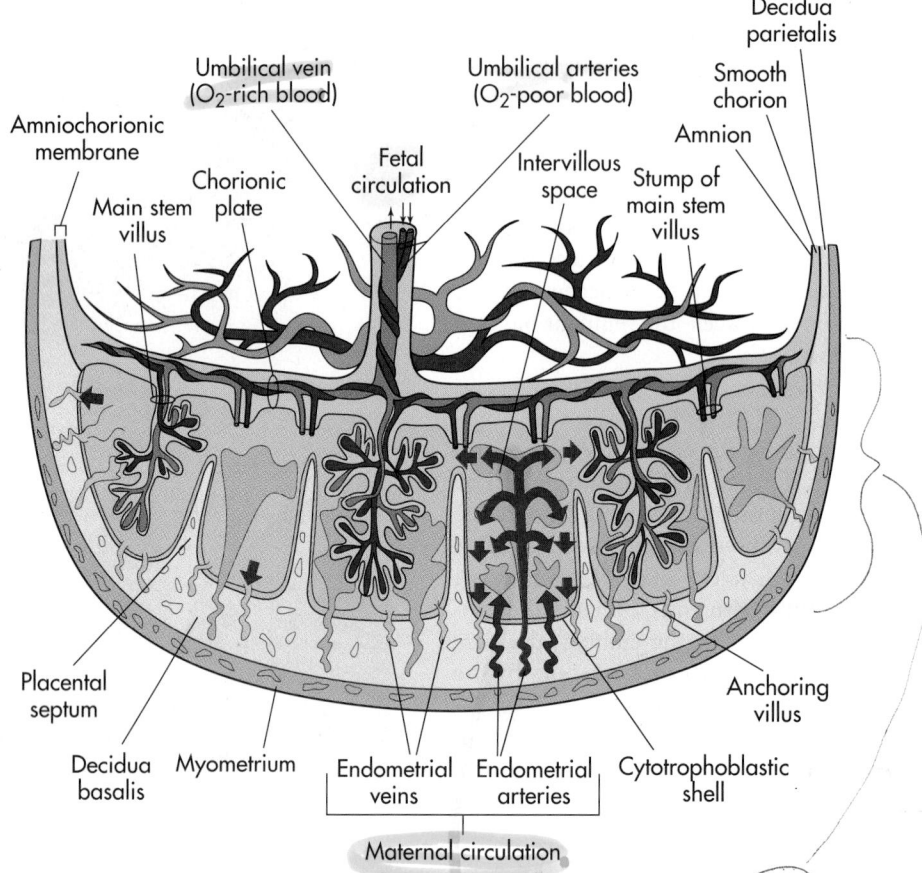

Decidua
parietalis

Umbilical vein
(O₂-rich blood)

Umbilical arteries
(O₂-poor blood)

Smooth
chorion

Amniochorionic
membrane

Chorionic
plate

Fetal
circulation

Intervillous
space

Amnion

Main stem
villus

Stump of
main stem
villus

Placental
septum

Anchoring
villus

Decidua
basalis

Myometrium

Endometrial
veins

Endometrial
arteries

Cytotrophoblastic
shell

Maternal circulation

Fig. 14-8 Schematic drawing of a transverse section through a full-term placenta, showing
(1) the relation of the villous chorion (fetal part of placenta) to the decidua basalis (maternal
part of placenta); (2) the fetal placental circulation; and (3) the maternal placental circulation.
Maternal blood flows into the intervillous spaces in funnel-shaped spurts from the spiral arteries, and exchanges occur with the fetal blood as the maternal blood flows around the branch
villi. It is through the branch villi that the main exchange of material between the mother and
embryo/fetus occurs. The inflowing arterial blood pushes venous blood out of the intervillous
space into the endometrial veins, which are scattered over the entire surface of the decidua
basalis. Note that the umbilical arteries carry poorly oxygenated fetal blood *(shown in blue)* to
the placenta and that the umbilical vein carries oxygenated blood *(shown in red)* to the fetus.
Note that the cotyledons are separated from each other by placental septa, projections of the
decidua basalis. Each cotyledon consists of two or more main stem villi and their many
branches. In this drawing, only one stem villus is shown in each cotyledon, but the stumps of
those that have been removed are indicated. *(From Moore, K., & Persaud, T. [1998].* Before we are born:
Essentials of embryology and birth defects *[5th ed.]. Philadelphia: W.B. Saunders.)*

The maternal-placental-embryonic circulation is in
place by day 17, when the embryonic heart starts beating.
By the end of the third week, embryonic blood is circulating between the embryo and chorionic villi. In the intervillous spaces, maternal blood supplies oxygen and nutrients to the embryonic capillaries in the villi (Fig. 14-8).
Waste products and carbon dioxide diffuse into the maternal blood.

The placenta functions as a means of metabolic exchange. Exchange is minimal at this time because the two

cell layers of the villous membrane are too thick. Permeability increases as the cytotrophoblast thins and disappears by the fifth month, leaving only the single layer of
syncytium between the maternal blood and fetal capillaries. The syncytium is the functional layer of the placenta.
By the eighth week, genetic testing may be done by obtaining a sample of chorionic villi by aspiration biopsy;
however, limb defects have been associated with chorionic
villus sampling done before 10 weeks (Hsieh et al., 1995).
The structure of the placenta is complete by the twelfth

Placenta Cont,

week. The placenta continues to grow wider until 20 weeks, when it covers about one half of the uterine surface. It then continues to grow thicker. The branching villi continue to develop within the body of the placenta, increasing the functional surface area.

Functions. One of the early functions of the placenta is as an endocrine gland that produces four hormones necessary to maintain the pregnancy and support the embryo/fetus. The hormones are produced in the syncytium.

The protein hormone **human chorionic gonadotropin (hCG)** can be detected in the maternal serum by 8 to 10 days after conception, shortly after implantation. This hormone is the basis for pregnancy tests. The hCG preserves the function of the ovarian corpus luteum, ensuring a continued supply of estrogen and progesterone needed to maintain the pregnancy. Miscarriage occurs if the corpus luteum stops functioning before the placenta is producing sufficient estrogen and progesterone. The amount of hCG reaches its maximum level at 50 to 70 days and then begins to decrease.

The other protein hormone produced by the placenta is human placental lactogen (hPL). This substance is similar to a growth hormone and stimulates maternal metabolism to supply needed nutrients for fetal growth. This hormone increases the resistance to insulin, facilitates glucose transport across the placental membrane, and stimulates breast development to prepare for lactation.

The placenta eventually produces more of the steroid hormone progesterone than the corpus luteum does during the first few months of pregnancy. Progesterone maintains the endometrium, decreases the contractility of the uterus, and stimulates maternal metabolism and development of breast alveoli.

By 7 weeks after fertilization, the placenta is producing most of the maternal estrogens, which are steroid hormones. The major estrogen secreted by the placenta is estriol, while the ovaries produce mostly estradiol. Measuring estriol levels is a clinical assay for placental functioning. Estrogen stimulates uterine growth and uteroplacental blood flow. It causes a proliferation of the breast glandular tissue and stimulates myometrial contractility. Placental estrogen production increases greatly toward the end of pregnancy. One theory for the cause of the onset of labor is the decrease in circulating levels of progesterone and the increased levels of estrogen.

The metabolic functions of the placenta may be summarized as respiration, nutrition, excretion, and storage. Oxygen diffuses from the maternal blood across the placental membrane into the fetal blood, and carbon dioxide diffuses in the opposite direction. In this way the placenta functions as lungs for the fetus.

Carbohydrates, proteins, calcium, and iron are stored in the placenta for ready access to meet fetal needs. Water, inorganic salts, carbohydrates, proteins, fats, and vitamins pass from the maternal blood supply across the placental membrane into the fetal blood, supplying nutrition. Water

and most electrolytes with a molecular weight less than 500 readily diffuse through the membrane. Hydrostatic and osmotic pressures aid the flow of water and some solutions. Facilitated and active transport assist in the transfer of glucose, amino acids, calcium, iron, and substances with higher molecular weight. Amino acids and calcium are transported against the concentration gradient between the maternal blood and fetal blood.

The fetal concentration of glucose is lower than the glucose level in the maternal blood because of its rapid metabolism by the fetus. This fetal requirement demands larger concentrations of glucose than simple diffusion can provide. Therefore, maternal glucose moves into the fetal circulation by active transport.

Pinocytosis is a mechanism used for transferring large molecules, such as albumin and gamma globulins, across the placental membrane. This mechanism conveys the maternal immunoglobulins that provide early passive immunity to the fetus.

Metabolic waste products of the fetus cross the placental membrane from the fetal blood into the maternal blood. The maternal kidneys then excrete them. Many viruses can cross the placental membrane and infect the fetus. Some bacteria and protozoa first infect the placenta and then infect the fetus. Drugs can also cross the placental membrane and may harm the fetus. Caffeine, alcohol, nicotine, carbon monoxide and other toxic substances in cigarette smoke, as well as prescription and recreational drugs (such as cocaine and marijuana) readily cross the placenta (Box 14-1).

Although no direct link exists between the fetal blood in the vessels of the chorionic villi and the maternal blood in the intervillous spaces, only one cell layer separates them. Breaks in the placental membrane occasionally occur. Fetal erythrocytes then leak into the maternal circulation, and the mother may develop antibodies to the fetal red blood cells. This is often the way an Rh-negative mother becomes sensitized to the erythrocytes of her Rh-positive fetus. (See discussions of isoimmunization.)

Even though the placenta and fetus are living tissue transplants, they are not destroyed by the host mother (Cunningham et al., 1997). The placental hormones suppress the immunologic response, or the tissue evokes no response (Willson & Carrington, 1991).

Placental function depends on the maternal blood pressure supplying circulation. Maternal arterial blood, under pressure in the small uterine spiral arteries, spurts into the intervillous spaces (Fig. 14-8). As long as rich arterial blood continues to be supplied, pressure is exerted on the blood already in the intervillous spaces, pushing it toward drainage by the low-pressure uterine veins. At term gestation, 10% of the maternal cardiac output goes to the uterus.

If interference with the circulation to the placenta occurs, the placenta cannot supply the embryo/fetus. Vasoconstriction, such as that caused by hypertension and

BOX 14-1 Developmentally Toxic Exposures in Humans

Aminopterin
Androgens
Angiotensin-converting enzyme inhibitors
Carbamazepine
Cigarette smoking
Cocaine
Coumarin anticoagulants
Cytomegalovirus
Diethylstilbestrol
Ethanol (>1 drink/day)
Etretinate
Hyperthermia
Iodides
Ionizing radiation (>10 rads)
Isotretinoin
Lead
Lithium
Methimazole
Methyl mercury
Parvovirus B19
Penicillamine
Phenytoin
Radioiodine
Rubella
Syphilis
Tetracycline
Thalidomide
Toxoplasmosis
Trimethadione
Valproic acid
Varicella

cocaine use, diminishes uterine blood flow. Decreased maternal blood pressure or cardiac output also diminishes uterine blood flow. When a woman lies on her back with the pressure of the uterus compressing the vena cava (vena caval syndrome), blood return to the right atrium is diminished (see discussion of supine hypotension).

Excessive maternal exercise that diverts blood to the muscles away from the uterus also compromises placental circulation. Optimal circulation is achieved when the woman is lying at rest on her side. Decreased uterine circulation may lead to intrauterine growth restriction of the fetus and infants who are small for gestational age.

Braxton Hicks contractions appear to enhance the movement of blood through the intervillous spaces, aiding placental circulation. However, prolonged contractions or too-short intervals between contractions during labor reduce blood flow to the placenta.

Fetal Maturation

The stage of the **fetus,** recognizable as a human being, lasts from 9 weeks until the pregnancy ends. Changes during the fetal period are not as dramatic, since refinement of structure and function are taking place. The fetus is less vulnerable to teratogens except for those affecting central nervous system functioning.

Viability refers to the capability of the fetus to survive outside the uterus. In the past, the earliest age at which fetal survival could be expected was 28 weeks after conception. With modern technology and advancements in maternal and neonatal care, viability is now possible at 20 weeks after conception (22 weeks since LMP, fetal weight of at least 500 g). The limitations on survival outside the uterus are based on central nervous system function and oxygenation capability of the lungs.

Fetal Circulatory System

The cardiovascular system is the first organ system to function in the developing human. Blood vessel and blood cell formation begins in the third week to supply the embryo with oxygen and nutrients from the mother. By the end of the third week the tubular heart begins to beat and the primitive cardiovascular system links the embryo, connecting stalk, chorion, and yolk sac. During the fourth and fifth weeks the heart develops into a four-chambered organ. By the end of the embryonic stage the heart is developmentally complete.

The fetal lungs do not function for respiratory gas exchange, so a special circulatory pathway, the **ductus arteriosus,** exists that bypasses the lungs. Oxygen-rich blood from the placenta flows rapidly through the umbilical vein into the fetal abdomen (Fig. 14-9). When the umbilical vein reaches the liver, it divides into two branches; one circulates some oxygenated blood through the liver. Most of the blood passes through the **ductus venosus** into the inferior vena cava. There it mixes with the deoxygenated blood from the fetal legs and abdomen on its way to the right atrium. Most of this blood passes straight through the right atrium and through the **foramen ovale,** an opening into the left atrium. There it mixes with the small amount of blood returning deoxygenated from the fetal lungs through the pulmonary veins.

The blood flows into the left ventricle and is squeezed out into the aorta, where the arteries supplying the heart, head, neck, and arms receive most of the oxygen-rich blood. This pattern of supplying the highest levels of oxygen and nutrients to the head, neck, and arms enhances the **cephalocaudal (head-to-rump) development** of the embryo/fetus.

Deoxygenated blood returning from the head and arms enters the right atrium through the superior vena cava. This blood is directed downward into the right ventricle, where it is squeezed into the pulmonary artery. A small

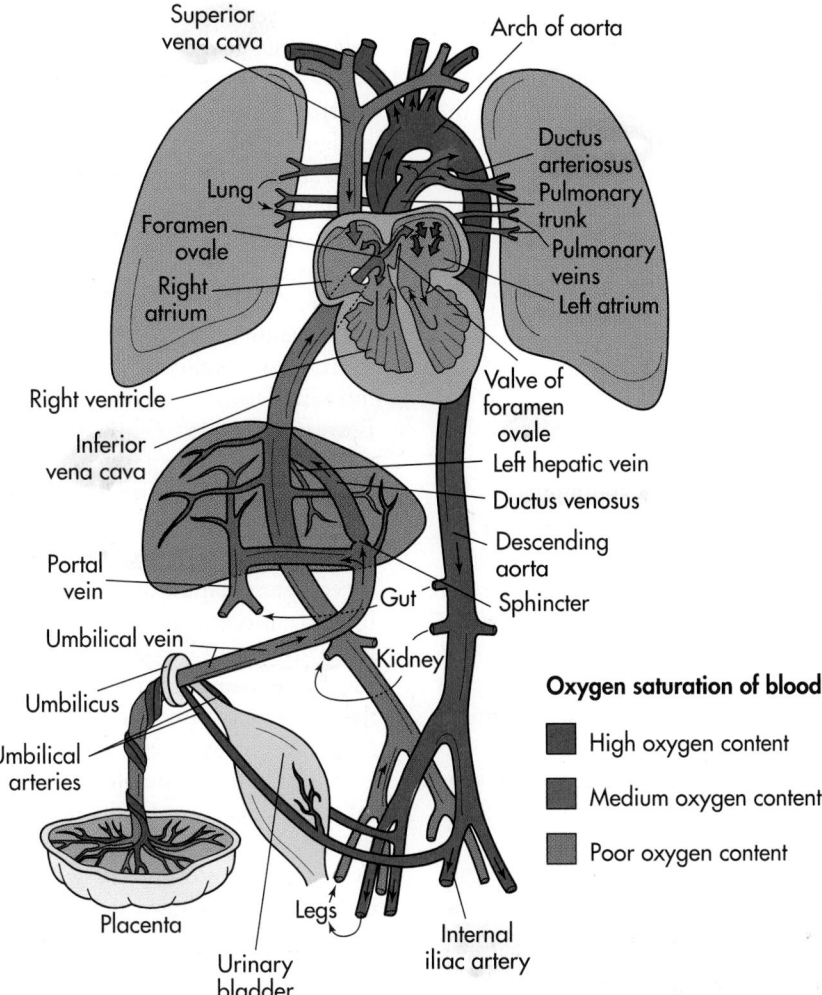

Superior
vena cava

Arch of aorta

Ductus
arteriosus
Pulmonary
trunk
Pulmonary
veins
Left atrium

Lung

Foramen
ovale
Right
atrium

Right ventricle

Valve of
foramen
ovale
Left hepatic vein
Ductus venosus
Descending
aorta
Sphincter

Inferior
vena cava

Portal
vein

Gut
Kidney

Umbilical vein

Umbilicus

Oxygen saturation of blood

Umbilical
arteries

High oxygen content

Medium oxygen content

Poor oxygen content

Placenta

Legs

Urinary
bladder

Internal
iliac artery

Fig. 14-9 Schematic illustration of the fetal circulation. The colors indicate the oxygen saturation of the blood, and the arrows show the course of the blood from the placenta to the heart.
The organs are not drawn to scale. Observe that three shunts permit most of the blood to bypass the liver and lungs: (1) ductus venosus, (2) foramen ovale, and (3) ductus arteriosus. The
poorly oxygenated blood returns to the placenta for oxygen and nutrients through the umbilical arteries. *(From Moore, K., & Persaud, T. [1998]. Before we are born: Essentials of embryology and birth
defects [5th ed.]. Philadelphia: W.B. Saunders.)*

amount of blood circulates through the resistant lung tissue, but the majority follows the path with less resistance
through the ductus arteriosus into the aorta, distal to the
point of exit of the arteries supplying the head and arms
with oxygenated blood. The oxygen-poor blood flows
through the abdominal aorta into the internal iliac arteries where the umbilical arteries direct most of it back
through the umbilical cord to the placenta. There the
blood gives up its wastes and carbon dioxide in exchange
for nutrients and oxygen. The blood remaining in the iliac arteries flows through the fetal abdomen and legs, ultimately returning through the inferior vena cava to the
heart.

The following three special characteristics enable the fetus to obtain sufficient oxygen from the maternal blood:
- Fetal hemoglobin carries 20% to 30% more oxygen
than maternal hemoglobin.
- The hemoglobin concentration of the fetus is about
50% greater than that of the mother.
- The fetal heart rate (FHR) is 120 to 160 beats/min, making the cardiac output per unit of body weight higher
than that of an adult.

Hematopoietic System

Hematopoiesis, the formation of blood, occurs in the
yolk sac (see Fig. 14-4, *B*) beginning in the third week.

Hematopoietic stem cells seed the fetal liver during the fifth week, and hematopoiesis begins there during the sixth week. This accounts for the relatively large size of the liver between the seventh and ninth weeks. Stem cells seed the fetal bone marrow, spleen and thymus, and lymph nodes between weeks 8 and 11.

The antigenic factors that determine blood type are present in the erythrocytes soon after the sixth week. For this reason, the Rh-negative woman is at risk for isoimmunization in any pregnancy that lasts longer than 6 weeks after fertilization.

Hepatic System

The liver and biliary tract develop from the foregut during the fourth week of gestation. The embryonic liver is prominent and occupies most of the abdominal cavity. Bile, a constituent of meconium, begins to form in the twelfth week.

Glycogen is stored in the fetal liver beginning at week 9 or 10. At term, glycogen stores are twice those of the adult. Glycogen is the major source of energy for the fetus and neonate who is stressed by in utero hypoxia, extrauterine loss of the maternal glucose supply, the work of breathing, or cold stress.

Iron is stored in the fetal liver. If the maternal intake is sufficient, the fetus can store enough iron to last for 5 months after birth.

During fetal life, the liver does not have to conjugate bilirubin for excretion because the unconjugated bilirubin is cleared by the placenta. Therefore the glucuronyl transferase enzyme needed for conjugation that is present in the fetal liver is less than is required after birth. This predisposes the neonate to hyperbilirubinemia.

Coagulation factors II, VII, IX, and X cannot be synthesized in the fetal liver because of the lack of vitamin K synthesis in the sterile fetal gut. This coagulation deficiency persists after birth for several days and is the rationale for the prophylactic administration of vitamin K to the newborn.

Gastrointestinal System

During the fourth week, the embryo changes from almost straight to a C shape as both ends fold in toward the ventral surface. A portion of the yolk sac is incorporated into the body from head to tail as the primitive gut (digestive system).

The foregut produces the pharynx, part of the lower respiratory tract, the esophagus, the stomach, the first half of the duodenum, the liver, the pancreas, and the gallbladder. These structures evolve over the fifth and sixth weeks. The malformations that can occur in these areas are esophageal atresia, hypertrophic pyloric stenosis, duodenal stenosis or atresia, and biliary atresia.

The midgut becomes the distal half of the duodenum, jejunum and ileum, cecum and appendix, and proximal half of the colon. The midgut loop projects into the umbilical cord between weeks 5 and 10. A malformation (omphalocele) results if the midgut fails to return to the abdominal cavity and intestines protrude from the umbilicus. Meckel's diverticulum is the most common malformation of the midgut. It occurs when a remnant of the yolk stalk that has failed to degenerate attaches to the ileum, leaving a blind sac.

The hindgut develops into the distal half of the colon, rectum and parts of the anal canal, urinary bladder, and urethra. Anorectal malformations are the most common abnormalities of the digestive system.

The fetus swallows amniotic fluid beginning in the fifth month. Gastric emptying and intestinal peristalsis occur. Fetal nutrition and elimination needs are taken care of by the placenta. As the fetus nears term, fetal waste products accumulate in the intestines as dark green to black, tarry **meconium.** Normally, this substance is passed through the rectum within 48 hours of birth. Sometimes with a breech presentation or fetal hypoxia, meconium is passed in utero into the amniotic fluid. The failure to pass meconium after birth can be indicative of atresia somewhere in the digestive tract, an imperforate anus, or a meconium ileus with a firm meconium plug blocking passage. Meconium ileus is seen in infants with cystic fibrosis.

The metabolic rate of the fetus is relatively low, but the infant has great growth and development needs. Beginning in week 9, the fetus synthesizes glycogen for storage in the liver. Between 26 and 30 weeks the fetus begins to lay down stores of brown fat in preparation for extrauterine cold stress. Thermoregulation in the neonate requires increased metabolism and adequate oxygenation.

The gastrointestinal system is mature by 36 weeks. Digestive enzymes except pancreatic amylase and lipase are present in sufficient quantity to facilitate digestion. The neonate cannot digest starches or fats efficiently. Little saliva is produced.

Respiratory System

The respiratory system begins development during embryonic life and continues through fetal life and into childhood until about 8 years of age. The development of the respiratory tract begins during week 4 and continues through week 17 with the formation of the larynx, trachea, bronchi, and lung buds. Between 16 and 24 weeks the bronchi and terminal bronchioles enlarge, and vascular structures and primitive alveoli are formed. Between 24 weeks and term birth, more alveoli form. Specialized alveolar cells, Type I and Type II cells, secrete pulmonary surfactants to line the interior of the alveoli. After 32 weeks, sufficient surfactant is present in developed alveoli to provide infants with a good chance of survival. Surfactant production peaks around 35 weeks.

Pulmonary surfactants. The detection of the presence of pulmonary **surfactants,** surface-active phospholipids, in amniotic fluid has been used to determine the degree of fetal lung maturity, or the ability of the lungs to function after birth. **Lecithin (L)** is the most critical alveolar surfactant required for postnatal lung expansion. It increases in amount after the twenty-fourth week. Another pulmonary phospholipid, **sphingomyelin (S),** remains constant in amount. Thus the measure of lecithin in relation to sphingomyelin, or the **L/S ratio,** is used to determine fetal lung maturity. When the L/S ratio reaches 2:1, the infant's lungs are considered to be mature. This occurs at approximately 35 weeks of gestation (Creasy & Resnik, 1999).

Certain maternal conditions alter the development of the fetal lungs. Those conditions that accelerate lung maturity generally cause decreased maternal placental blood flow. The resulting fetal hypoxia apparently stresses the fetus, increasing blood levels of corticosteroids that accelerate alveolar and surfactant development. Conditions such as maternal hypertension, placental dysfunction, infection, or corticosteroid use accelerate fetal lung maturity. Conditions such as gestational diabetes and chronic glomerulonephritis can retard fetal lung maturity. The use of intrabronchial synthetic surfactant in the treatment of respiratory distress syndrome in the newborn has greatly improved the chances of survival of preterm infants (see p. 1105.)

Fetal respiratory movements have been seen on ultrasound as early as the eleventh week. These fetal respiratory movements are believed to aid in development of the chest wall muscles and regulate lung fluid volume. The fetal lungs produce fluid that expands the air spaces in the lungs. The fluid drains into the amniotic fluid or is swallowed by the fetus.

Before birth, secretion of lung fluid decreases. The normal birth process squeezes out approximately one third of the fluid. Infants of cesarean births do not benefit from this squeezing process; thus they may have more respiratory difficulty at birth. The fluid remaining in the lungs at birth is usually reabsorbed into the infant's bloodstream within 2 hours of birth.

Renal System

The permanent kidneys form during the fifth week and begin to function approximately 4 weeks later. Urine formation is present during the third month. Urine is excreted into the amniotic fluid and forms a major part of the amniotic fluid volume. Oligohydramnios, an abnormally small amount of amniotic fluid, is indicative of renal dysfunction. Because the placenta acts as the organ of excretion and maintains fetal water and electrolyte balance, the fetus does not need functioning kidneys while in utero. At birth, however, the kidneys are required immediately for excretory and acid-base regulatory functions.

A fetal renal malformation can be diagnosed in utero. Corrective or palliative fetal surgery may treat the malformation successfully, or plans can be made for treatment immediately after birth (Jona, 1998).

At term, the fetus has fully developed kidneys. However, the glomerular filtration rate (GFR) is low, and the kidneys lack the ability to concentrate urine. This makes the newborn more susceptible to both overhydration and dehydration and acid-base imbalances.

Most newborns void within 24 hours of birth. With the loss of the swallowed amniotic fluid and the metabolism of nutrients provided by the placenta, voidings for the first days of life are scanty until fluid intake increases.

Neurologic System

The nervous system originates from the ectoderm (the neural plate) during the third week after fertilization. The open neural tube forms during the fourth week. It initially closes at what will be the junction of the brain and spinal cord, leaving both ends open. The embryo folds in on itself lengthwise at this time, forming a head fold in the neural tube at this junction. The cranial end of the neural tube closes, then the caudal end closes. During week 5, different growth rates cause more flexures in the neural tube, delineating three brain areas: the forebrain, midbrain, and hindbrain. Both the forebrain and hindbrain partially divide into two vesicles.

The forebrain develops into the eyes (cranial nerve II) and cerebral hemispheres. The development of all areas of the cerebral cortex continues throughout fetal life and into childhood. The olfactory system (cranial nerve I) and thalamus also develop from the forebrain. Cranial nerves III and IV (oculomotor and trochlear) form from the midbrain. The hindbrain forms the medulla, pons, cerebellum, and the remainder of the cranial nerves. Brain waves can be recorded on an electroencephalogram by week 8.

The spinal cord develops from the long end of the neural tube. Another ectodermal structure, the neural crest, develops into the peripheral nervous system. By the eighth week, nerve fibers traverse throughout the body. By week 11 or 12, the fetus makes respiratory movements, moves all extremities, and changes position in utero. The fetus can suck his or her thumb and swim in the amniotic fluid pool, turn somersaults, and sometimes tie a knot in the umbilical cord. Box 14-2 describes the major types of fetal movements. Sometime between 16 and 20 weeks, when the movements are strong enough to be perceived by the mother as "the baby moving," **quickening** has occurred. The perception of movement occurs earlier in multiparas than in primiparas. The mother also becomes aware of the sleep and wake cycles of the fetus.

Sensory awareness. Purposeful movements of the fetus have been demonstrated in response to a firm touch transmitted through the mother's abdomen. Invasive procedures to be done on a fetus require anesthesia.

Fetuses respond to sound by 24 weeks. Different types of music evoke different movements. The fetus can be soothed by the sound of the mother's voice. Acoustic stimulation can be used to evoke an FHR response (Bar-Hava & Barnhardt, 1994). The fetus becomes accustomed to noises heard repeatedly. Hearing is fully developed at birth.

BOX 14-2 Major Types of Fetal Movements

General movements. These slow gross movements involve the whole body. Their duration is from several seconds to a minute.

Startle movements. These quick (less than 1 second), generalized movements always start in the limbs and may spread to the trunk and neck.

Hiccups. These are repetitive phasic contractions of the diaphragm. A bout may last several minutes.

Fetal breathing movements. These are paradoxical movements in which the thorax moves inward and the abdomen outward with each contraction of the diaphragm.

Isolated arm or leg movements. These movements of extremities occur without movement of the trunk.

Hand-face contact. This occurs any time the moving hand makes contact with the face or mouth.

Retroflexion of the head. This is a slow to jerky backward bending of the head.

Lateral rotation of the head. This involves isolated turning of the head from side to side.

Anteflexion of the head. This is a normally slow forward bending of the head.

Opening of the mouth. This isolated movement may be accompanied by protrusion of the tongue.

Yawn. The mouth is slowly opened and rapidly closed after a few seconds.

Sucking. This burst of rhythmical jaw movements is sometimes followed by swallowing. With this movement the fetus may be drinking amniotic fluid.

Stretch. This complex movement involves overextension of the spine, retroflexion of the head, and elevation of the arms.

From Carlson, B. (1994). *Human embryology and developmental biology.* St. Louis: Mosby.

The fetus is able to distinguish taste. By the fifth month, when the fetus is swallowing amniotic fluid, a sweetener added to the fluid causes the fetus to swallow twice as fast (Poole, 1986). The fetus also reacts to temperature changes. A cold solution placed into the amniotic fluid can cause fetal hiccups.

The fetus reacts to light. Eyes have both rods and cones in the retina by the seventh month. A bright light shone on the mother's abdomen in late pregnancy causes abrupt fetal movements. During sleep time, rapid eye movements (REMs) have been observed similar to those occurring in children and adults while dreaming (Cole, 1997).

At term, the fetal brain is approximately one fourth the size of an adult brain. Neurologic development continues. Stressors on the fetus and neonate, such as chronic poor nutrition or hypoxia, drugs, environmental toxins, trauma, or disease, cause damage to the central nervous system long after the vulnerable embryonic time for malformations in other organ systems. Neurologic insult can result in cerebral palsy, neuromuscular impairment, mental retardation, and learning disabilities.

Endocrine System

The thyroid gland develops with structures in the head and neck during the third and fourth weeks. The secretion of thyroxine begins during the eighth week. Maternal thyroxine does not readily cross the placenta; therefore, the fetus who does not produce thyroid hormones will be born with congenital hypothyroidism. If untreated, hypothyroidism can result in severe mental retardation. Screening for hypothyroidism is typically included in the testing when screening for phenylketonuria (PKU) after birth.

The adrenal cortex is formed during the sixth week and produces hormones by the eighth or ninth week. As term approaches, the fetus produces more cortisol. This is believed to aid in initiation of labor by decreasing the maternal progesterone and stimulating production of prostaglandins.

The pancreas forms from the foregut during the fifth through eighth weeks. The islets of Langerhans develop during the twelfth week. Insulin is produced by the twentieth week. In infants of mothers with uncontrolled diabetes, maternal hyperglycemia produces fetal hyperglycemia, stimulating hyperinsulinemia and islet-cell hyperplasia. This results in macrosomia (large-sized fetus). The hyperinsulinemia also blocks lung maturation, placing the neonate at risk for respiratory distress and hypoglycemia when the maternal glucose source is lost at birth. Control of the maternal glucose level before and during pregnancy minimizes problems for the infant.

Reproductive System

Until the seventh week, no sex differentiation exists in the embryo. Distinguishing characteristics appear approximately the ninth week and are fully differentiated by the twelfth week. When a Y chromosome is present, testes are formed. By the end of the embryonic period, testosterone is being secreted and causes formation of the male genitalia. By week 28, the testes begin descending into the scrotum. After birth, low levels of testosterone continue to be secreted until the pubertal surge.

The female, with two X chromosomes, forms ovaries and female external genitalia. Female and male external genitalia are indistinguishable until after the ninth week. By the sixteenth week, oogenesis has been established. At birth, the ovaries contain the female's lifetime supply of ova. Most female hormone production is delayed until puberty. However, the fetal endometrium responds to maternal hormones, and withdrawal bleeding or vaginal discharge (pseudomenstruation) may occur at birth when these hormones are lost. The high level of maternal estrogen also stimulates mammary engorgement and secretion of fluid ("witch's milk") in newborn infants of both sexes.

Immunologic System

During the third trimester, albumin and globulin are present in the fetus. The only immunoglobulin that crosses the placenta is IgG, providing passive acquired immunity to specific bacterial toxins. The fetus produces IgM immunoglobulins by the end of the first trimester. These are produced in response to blood group antigens, gram-negative enteric organisms, and some viruses. IgA immunoglobulins are not produced by the fetus. However, colostrum, the precursor to breast milk, contains large amounts of IgA and can provide passive immunity to the neonate.

The normal term neonate can fight infection, but not as effectively as an older child. The preterm infant is at much greater risk for infection.

Musculoskeletal System

Bones and muscles develop from the mesoderm by the fourth week of embryonic development. At that time, the cardiac muscle is already beating. The mesoderm next to the neural tube forms the vertebral column and ribs. The parts of the vertebral column grow toward each other to enclose the developing spinal cord. Ossification, or bone formation, begins. If there is a defect in the bony fusion, various forms of spina bifida may occur. A large defect affecting several vertebrae may allow the membranes and spinal cord to pouch out from the back, producing neurologic deficits and skeletal deformity.

The flat bones of the skull develop during the embryonic period, and ossification continues throughout childhood. At birth, connective tissue sutures exist where the bones of the skull meet. The areas where more than two bones meet, called *fontanels,* are especially prominent. The sutures and fontanels allow the bones of the skull to mold, or move during birth, enabling the head to pass through the birth canal.

The bones of the shoulders, arms, hips, and legs appear in the sixth week as a continuous skeleton with no joints. Differentiation occurs, producing separate bones and joints. Ossification will continue through childhood to allow growth. Beginning during the seventh week, muscles contract spontaneously. Arm and leg movements are visible on ultrasound, although the mother does not perceive them until the sixteenth to the twentieth week.

Integumentary System

The epidermis begins as a single layer of cells derived from the ectoderm at 4 weeks. By the seventh week, there are two layers of cells. The cells of the superficial layer are sloughed and become mixed with the sebaceous gland secretions to form the white, cheesy vernix caseosa. This material protects the skin of the fetus. The vernix is thick at 24 weeks but continually decreases until term.

The basal layer of the epidermis is the germinal layer, which replaces the lost cells. Until 17 weeks the skin is very thin and wrinkled, with blood vessels visible underneath. The skin thickens, and all layers are present by term. After 32 weeks, as subcutaneous fat is deposited under the dermis, the skin becomes less wrinkled, translucent, and red in appearance.

By 16 weeks, the epidermal ridges are present on the palms of the hands, the fingers, the bottom of the feet, and the toes. This makes the hand and footprints unique to that infant.

Hairs form from hair bulbs in the epidermis, which project into the dermis. Cells in the hair bulb keratinize to form the hair shaft. As the cells at the base of the hair shaft proliferate, the hair grows to the surface of the epithelium. The very fine hairs, called *lanugo,* appear first at 12 weeks on the eyebrows and upper lip. By 20 weeks, they cover the entire body. At this time, the eyelashes, eyebrows, and scalp hair are beginning to grow. By 28 weeks, the scalp hair is longer than the lanugo, which is thinning and may disappear by term gestation.

Fingernails and toenails develop from thickened epidermis at the tips of the digits beginning during the tenth week. They grow slowly. Fingernails usually reach the fingertips by 32 weeks, and toenails reach toetips by 36 weeks. Table 14-1 summarizes embryonic and fetal development.

Multifetal Pregnancy

Twins

When two mature ova are produced in one ovarian cycle, both have the potential to be fertilized by separate sperm. This results in two zygotes or **dizygotic twins** (Fig. 14-10). There are always two amnions, two chorions, and two placentas that may be fused together. These dizygotic, or fraternal, twins may be the same sex or different sexes and are genetically no more alike than siblings born at different times. Dizygotic twinning occurs in families, more often among African-American women than among Caucasian women, and least often among Asian women. Dizygotic twinning increases in frequency with maternal age up to 35 years, with parity, and with the use of fertility drugs.

Identical twins **(monozygotic twins)** develop from one fertilized ovum, which then divides (Fig. 14-11). They are the same sex and have the same genotype. If division occurs soon after fertilization, two embryos, two amnions, two chorions, and two placentas that may be fused will develop. Most often, division occurs between 4 and 8 days after fertilization, and there are two embryos, two amnions, one chorion, and one placenta. In this case there are two embryos within a common amnion and a common chorion with one placenta. This often causes problems in circulation because the umbilical cords may tangle together, and one or both fetuses may die. If division occurs very late, cleavage may not be complete, and conjoined twins could result. Monozygotic twinning occurs in approximately 1 of 250 births (Cunningham et al., 1997).

4 WEEKS	8 WEEKS	12 WEEKS

EXTERNAL APPEARANCE

Body flexed, C-shaped; arm and leg buds present; head at right angles to body	Body fairly well formed; nose flat, eyes far apart; digits well formed; head elevating; tail almost disappeared; eyes, ears, nose, and mouth recognizable	Nails appearing, resembling a human, head erect but disproportionately large, skin pink, delicate
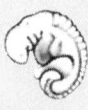	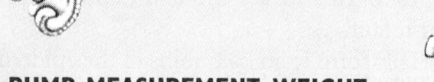	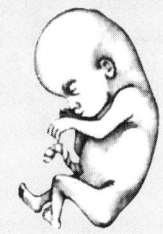

CROWN-TO-RUMP MEASUREMENT, WEIGHT

0.4-0.5 cm, 0.4 g	2.5-3 cm, 2 g	6-9 cm, 19 g

GASTROINTESTINAL SYSTEM

Stomach at midline and fusiform, conspicuous liver, esophagus short, intestine a short tube	Intestinal villi developing, small intestines coiling within umbilical cord; palatal folds present, liver very large	Bile secreted, palatal fusion complete, intestines withdrawn from cord and assume characteristic positions

MUSCULOSKELETAL SYSTEM

All somites present	First indication of ossification—occiput, mandible, and humerus; embryo capable of some movement, definitive muscles of trunk, limbs, and head well represented	Some bones well outlined, ossification spreading; upper cervical to lower sacral arches and bodies ossify; smooth muscle layers indicated in hollow viscera

CIRCULATORY SYSTEM

Heart developing; double chambers visible, beginning to beat; aortic arch and major veins completed	Main blood vessels assume final plan, enucleated red cells predominate in blood; heart beat detectable with sonography	Blood forming in marrow Heart beat audible by Doppler

RESPIRATORY SYSTEM

Primary lung buds appear	Pleural and pericardial cavities forming, branching bronchioles, nostrils closed by epithelial plugs	Lungs acquiring definite shape, vocal cords appear

RENAL SYSTEM

Rudimentary ureteral buds appear	Earliest secretory tubules differentiating, bladder-urethra separates from rectum	Kidney able to secrete urine, bladder expands as a sac

NERVOUS SYSTEM

Well-marked midbrain flexure, no hindbrain or cervical flexures, neural groove closed	Cerebral cortex begins to acquire typical cells; differentiation of cerebral cortex, meninges, ventricular foramina, cerebrospinal fluid circulation; spinal cord extends entire length of spine	Brain structural configuration roughly complete, cord showing cervical and lumbar enlargements, fourth ventricle foramina developed, sucking present

SENSORY ORGANS

Eye and ear appearing as optic vessel and otocyst	Primordial choroid plexuses develop, ventricles large relative to cortex, development progressing, eyes converging rapidly, internal ear developing	Earliest taste buds indicated, characteristic organization of eye attained

GENITAL SYSTEM

Genital ridge appearing (fifth week)	Testes and ovaries distinguishable, external genitals sexless but beginning to differentiate	Sex recognizable, internal and external sex organs specific

From Wong, D., & Perry, S. (1998). *Maternal child nursing care.* St. Louis: Mosby.

16 WEEKS	20 WEEKS	24 WEEKS

EXTERNAL APPEARANCE

Head still dominant; face looks human; eyes, ears, and nose approaching typical appearance on gross examination; arm-leg ratio proportionate; scalp hair appears	Vernix caseosa and lanugo appear, legs lengthen considerably, sebaceous glands appear	Body lean but fairly well proportioned, skin red and wrinkled, vernix caseosa present, sweat glands forming

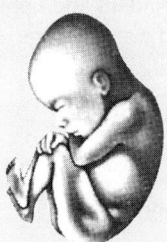 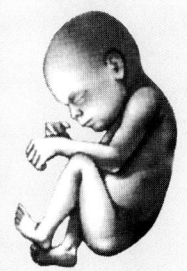 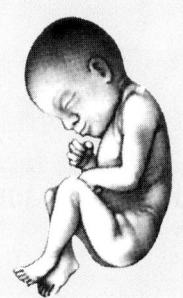

CROWN-TO-RUMP MEASUREMENT, WEIGHT

11.5-13.5 cm, 100 g	16-18.5 cm, 300 g	23 cm, 600 g

GASTROINTESTINAL SYSTEM

Meconium in bowel, some enzyme secretion, anus open	Enamel and dentine depositing, ascending colon recognizable	

MUSCULOSKELETAL SYSTEM

Most bones distinctly indicated throughout body, joint cavities appear, muscular movements detectable	Sternum ossifies, fetal movements strong enough for mother to feel	

CIRCULATORY SYSTEM

Heart muscle well-developed, blood formation active in spleen		Blood formation increases in bone marrow and decreases in liver

RESPIRATORY SYSTEM

Elastic fibers appear in lungs, terminal and respiratory bronchioles appear	Nostrils reopen, primitive respiratory-like movements begin	Alveolar ducts and sacs present, lecithin begins to appear in amniotic fluid (weeks 26-27)

RENAL SYSTEM

Kidney in position, attains typical shape and plan		

NERVOUS SYSTEM

Cerebral lobes delineated, cerebellum assumes some prominence	Brain grossly formed; cord myelination begins; spinal cord ends at level of first sacral vertebra (S1)	Cerebral cortex layered typically, neuronal proliferation in cerebral cortex ends

SENSORY ORGANS

General sense organs differentiated	Nose and ears ossifying	Ability to hear

GENITAL SYSTEM

Testes in position for descent into scrotum, vagina open		Testes at inguinal ring in descent to scrotum

Continued

28 WEEKS	30-31 WEEKS	36 AND 40 WEEKS

EXTERNAL APPEARANCE

| Lean body, less wrinkled and red; nails appear | Subcutaneous fat beginning to collect; more rounded appearance; skin pink and smooth; has assumed birth position | **36 Weeks** Skin pink, body rounded; general lanugo disappearing; body usually plump **40 Weeks** Skin smooth and pink; scant vernix caseosa; moderate to profuse hair; lanugo on shoulders and upper body only; nasal and alar cartilage apparent |

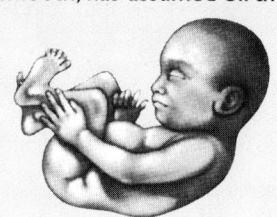

CROWN-TO-RUMP MEASUREMENT; WEIGHT

| 27 cm; 1110 g | 31 cm; 1800-2100 g | **36 Weeks** 35 cm; 2200-2900 g **40 Weeks** 40 cm; 3200+ g |

MUSCULOSKELETAL SYSTEM

| Astragalus (talus, ankle bone) ossifies; weak, fleeting movements, minimum tone | Middle fourth phalanges ossify; permanent teeth primordia seen; can turn head to side | **36 Weeks** Distal femoral ossification centers present; sustained, definite movements; fair tone; can turn and elevate head **40 Weeks** Active, sustained movement; good tone, may lift head |

RESPIRATORY SYSTEM

| Lecithin forming on alveolar surfaces | L/S ratio = 1.2:1 | **36 Weeks** L/S ratio >2:1 **40 Weeks** Pulmonary branching only two thirds complete |

RENAL SYSTEM

| | | **36 Weeks** Formation of new nephrons ceases |

NERVOUS SYSTEM

| Appearance of cerebral fissures, convolutions rapidly appearing; indefinite sleep-wake cycle; cry weak or absent; weak suck reflex | | **36 Weeks** End of spinal cord at level of third lumbar vertebra (L3); definite sleep-wake cycle **40 Weeks** Myelination of brain begins; patterned sleep-wake cycle with alert periods; cries when hungry or uncomfortable; strong suck reflex |

SENSORY ORGANS

| Eyelids reopen; retinal layers completed, light receptive; pupils capable of reacting to light | Sense of taste present; aware of sounds outside mother's body | |

GENITAL SYSTEM

| | Testes descending to scrotum | **40 Weeks** Testes in scrotum; labia majora well developed |

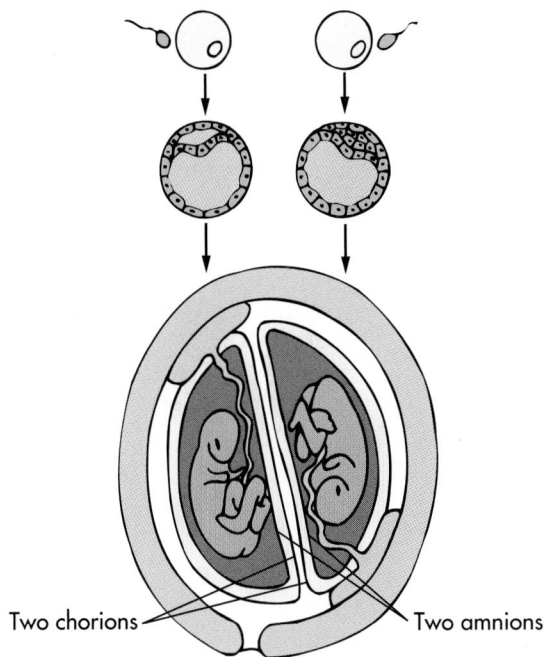

Two chorions ───── ───── Two amnions

Fig. 14-10 Formation of dizygotic twins. There is fertilization of two ova, two implantations, two placentas, two chorions, and two amnions.

There is no association with race, heredity, maternal age, or parity. Fertility drugs increase the incidence of monozygotic twinning.

Other Multifetal Pregnancies

The occurrence of multifetal pregnancies with three or more fetuses has increased with the use of fertility drugs and in vitro fertilization. Triplets occur once in about 7600 pregnancies. They can occur from the division of one zygote into two, with one of the two dividing again, producing identical triplets. Triplets can also be produced from two zygotes, one dividing into a set of identical twins and the second zygote a single fraternal sibling, or from three zygotes. Quadruplets, quintuplets, sextuplets, and so on, likewise, have similar possible derivations.

Nongenetic Factors Influencing Development

Not all congenital disorders are inherited. *Congenital* means that the condition was present at birth. Some congenital malformations may be the result of teratogens, defined as environmental substances or exposures that result in functional or structural disability. In contrast to other forms of developmental disabilities, disabilities caused by teratogens are theoretically totally preventable (Hoyme, 1990). Known human teratogens are drugs and chemicals, infections, exposure to radiation (Scialli, 1997), and certain maternal conditions such as diabetes and PKU (see Box 14-1). A teratogen has the greatest effect on the organs and

parts of an embryo during its periods of rapid growth and differentiation. This occurs during the embryonic period, specifically from days 15 to 60. During the first 2 weeks of development, teratogens either have no effect or effects so severe that they cause miscarriage. Brain growth and development continue during the fetal period, and teratogens can severely affect mental development throughout gestation (see Fig. 14-6).

Besides the genetic makeup and the influence of teratogens, the adequacy of maternal nutrition also influences development. The embryo and fetus must obtain the nutrients they need from the mother's diet; they cannot tap the maternal reserves. Malnutrition during pregnancy produces low-birth-weight (LBW) newborns who are susceptible to infection. Malnutrition also affects brain development during the latter half of gestation and may result in learning disabilities in the child.

The field of behavioral genetics is engaged in discovering links between genetics and environment in explaining normal and deviant behavior (Sherman et al., 1997). This represents a movement away from the belief that human behavior is almost completely the result of influences of the environment. For example, memory and intelligence, activity level, sociability, and shyness have some degree of genetic influence (Sherman et al., 1997).

GENETICS AND GENETIC COUNSELING

Importance of Genetics in Maternity Care

Genetic causes of disease have assumed increasing importance as the incidence of communicable diseases has decreased. Rapid expansion in the identification, understanding, and diagnosis of genetic disease has been accompanied by effective medical or surgical therapies in a small number of disorders. For most genetic conditions, therapeutic or preventive measures are nonexistent or disappointingly limited. Consequently, the most useful means of reducing the incidence of these disorders is by preventing their transmission. With the accumulation of knowledge about genetic disorders, the probability of recurrence in any given situation can be predicted with increased accuracy. At present the best means for reducing the number of children born with genetic defects is for health professionals to provide families with genetic information and services.

For all pregnancies, it is standard practice to assess for heritable disorders to identify potential problems (Creasy & Resnik, 1999). The interviewer inquires about the health status of family members, abnormal reproductive outcomes, history of maternal disorders (e.g., diabetes, PKU, cystic fibrosis), drug exposures, and illness. Advanced maternal and paternal ages are noted. Ethnic origin should be recorded, since some disorders appear more often in some groups (Creasy & Resnik, 1999). Examples include Tay-Sachs disease in Jewish individuals of Ashkenazic or Sephardic descent, β-thalassemia in Italians and Greeks, sickle cell anemia in African-Americans, α-thalassemia in

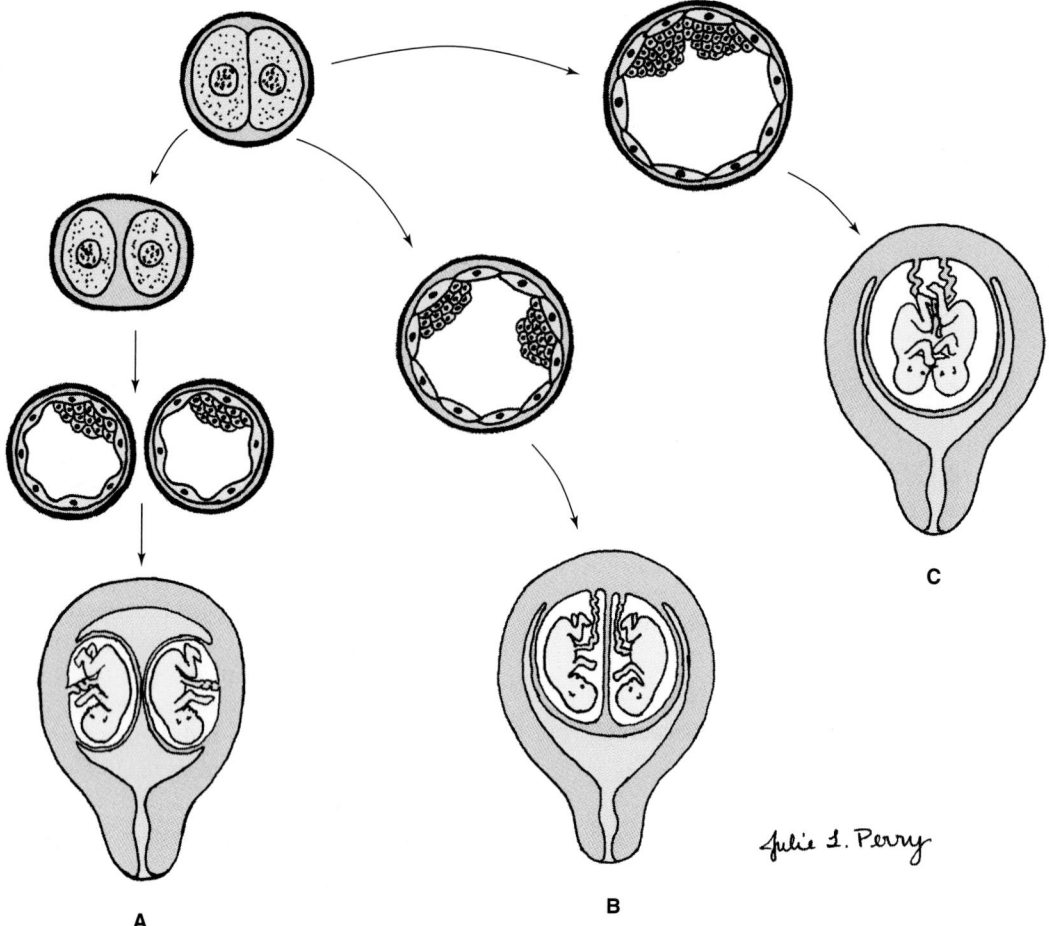

Fig. 14-11 Formation of monozygotic twins. **A,** One fertilization: blastomeres separate, result-ing in two implantations, two placentas, and two sets of membranes. **B,** One blastomere with two inner cell masses, one fused placenta, one chorion, and separate amnions. **C,** One blas-tomere with incomplete separation of cell mass resulting in conjoined twins. *(From Wong, D., & Perry, S. [1998]. Maternal child nursing care. St. Louis: Mosby.)*

Southeast Asians and Filipinos, and tyrosinemia in French Canadians from the Lac St. Jean-Chicoutimi region of Quebec.

Genetic Transmission

Human development is a complicated process that de-pends on the systematic unraveling of instructions found in the genetic material of the egg and sperm. Development from conception to birth of a normal, healthy baby occurs without incident in most cases; occasionally, however, some anomaly in the genetic code of the embryo creates a birth defect or disorder. The science of genetics seeks to ex-plain the underlying causes of congenital disorders (disor-ders present at birth) and the patterns in which inherited disorders are passed from generation to generation.

Genes and Chromosomes

The hereditary material carried in the nucleus of each of the somatic (body) cells determines an individual's physi-cal characteristics. This material, called deoxyribonucleic acid (DNA), forms threadlike strands known as **chromo-somes.** Each chromosome is composed of many smaller segments of DNA referred to as genes. Genes, or combi-nations of genes, contain coded information that deter-mines an individual's unique characteristics. The "code" is found in the specific linear order of the molecules that combine to form the strands of DNA.

All normal human somatic cells contain 46 chromo-somes arranged as 23 pairs of homologous (matched) chro-mosomes; one chromosome of each pair is inherited from each parent. There are 22 pairs of autosomes, which con-trol most traits in the body, and one pair of **sex chromo-somes,** which primarily control sex determination. The large female chromosome is called the X; the tiny male chromosome is the Y. Generally, the presence of a Y chro-mosome causes an embryo to develop as a male; in the ab-sence of a Y chromosome, the individual develops as a fe-male. Thus in a normal female the homologous pair of sex

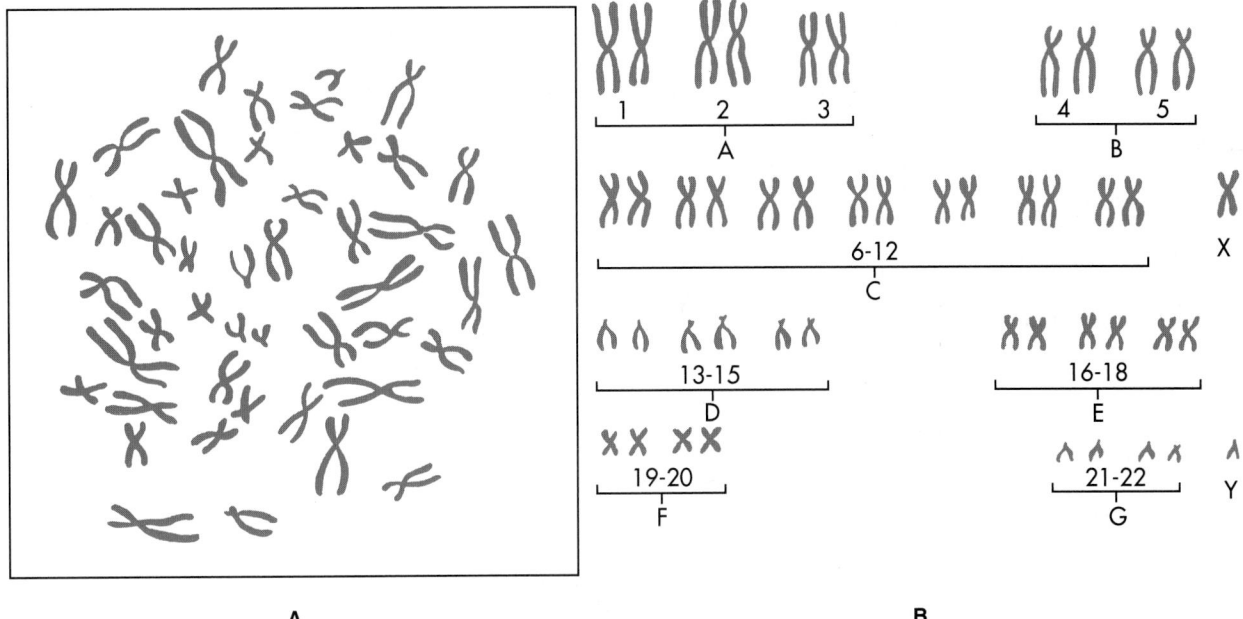

Fig. 14-12 Chromosomes during cell division. **A,** Example of photomicrograph. **B,** Chromosomes arranged in karyotype; female and male sex-determining chromosomes.

chromosomes would be XX, *female* and in a normal male the homologous pair would be XY. *Male*

Each person has two genes for every trait, because each gene occupies a specific chromosome location, and because chromosomes are inherited as homologous pairs. In other words, if an autosome has a gene for hair color, its partner will also have a gene for hair color, and they will be in the same location on the chromosome. Although both genes code for hair color, they may not code for the *same* hair color. Different genes coding for different variations of the same trait are called alleles. An individual having two copies of the same allele for a given trait is said to be homozygous for that trait; with two different alleles, the person is heterozygous for the trait.

Some genes are dominant, and their characteristics are expressed even if another allele is present on the other chromosome. Other genes are recessive, and their characteristics will be expressed only if they are carried by both homologous chromosomes. When an egg and a sperm unite, the combination of alleles becomes that individual's entire genetic makeup, or genotype, which includes all the genes that the person carries and that can be passed to offspring. The genotype determines an individual's physical appearance, or phenotype, but this determination is affected by the nature of the dominant or recessive allele.

The pictorial analysis of the number, form, and size of an individual's chromosomes is known as a **karyotype.** A karyotype can be obtained from a blood sample that has been specially treated and stained to make the replicating chromosomes visible under a microscope. The photographed chromosomes are cut out and arranged in a specific numeric order according to their length and shape.

Figure 14-12 illustrates the chromosomes in a body cell. Karyotypes can be used to determine what sex the child will be, and whether any gross chromosomal abnormalities are present.

Chromosomal Abnormalities

Errors resulting in chromosomal abnormalities can occur in mitosis or meiosis. These occur in either the autosomes or sex chromosomes. Even without the presence of obvious structural malformations, small deviations in chromosomes can cause problems in fetal development.

Autosomal Abnormalities

Autosomal abnormalities involve differences in the number or structure of chromosomes resulting from unequal distribution of the genetic material during gamete formation.

Abnormalities of chromosome number. Abnormalities of chromosome number, aneuploidy, are most often caused by nondisjunction. Nondisjunction occurs during meiosis when a pair of chromosomes fails to separate and one resulting cell contains both chromosomes and the other contains none. The product of the union of a normal gamete with a gamete containing an extra chromosome is a trisomy. The resulting individual has 47 chromosomes in each cell. The most common trisomal abnormality is Down syndrome, or trisomy 21. The affected individual has an extra chromosome 21. The clinical characteristics of Down syndrome include a broad, small skull; flat facial profile; epicanthal folds with slanted palpebral fissures in the eyes; flat, lowset ears; protruding tongue; a short neck with fat pads at the nape; short, broad

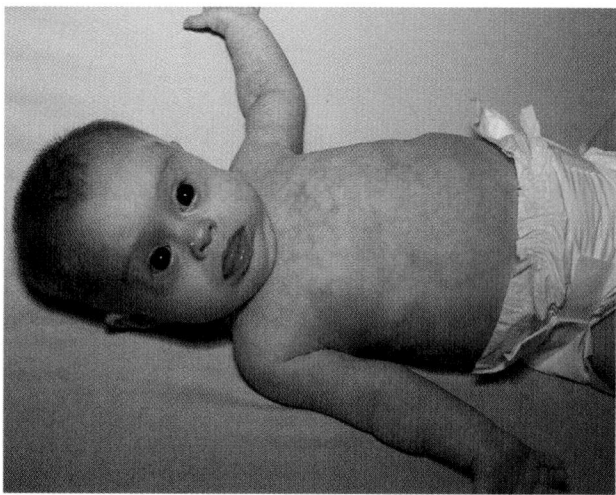

Fig. 14-13 Down syndrome in infant. Note small square head with upward slant to eyes, flat nasal bridge, protruding tongue, mottled skin, and hypotonia. *(From Wong, D. [1999]. Whaley and Wong's nursing care of infants and children [6th ed.]. St. Louis: Mosby.)*

hands with a single transverse (simian) crease, and hypotonic muscles with hypermobility of joints (Fig. 14-13).

Individuals with Down syndrome have various degrees of mental retardation. The incidence of congenital heart disease, infectious diseases, and acute childhood leukemia is increased in individuals with Down syndrome. The incidence of Down syndrome increases with maternal or paternal age. Many affected embryos miscarry spontaneously, and some affected fetuses are stillborn.

Other autosomal trisomies that have been identified are trisomy 18 and trisomy 13. Both conditions have a very poor prognosis, with most affected children dying from cardiac or respiratory complications within 6 months of birth.

The product of the union of a normal gamete (ovum or sperm) with a gamete missing a chromosome is a monosomy. This individual would have only 45 chromosomes in each cell. Missing an autosomal chromosome always results in death of the embryo.

Nondisjunction can also occur during mitosis. If this occurs early in development when cell lines are forming, the individual has a mixture of cells, some with a normal number of chromosomes and others either missing a chromosome or containing an extra chromosome. This condition is known as mosaicism.

Mosaicism in autosomes is most commonly seen as another form of Down syndrome. Depending on when the nondisjunction occurs during development, different body tissues will have different numbers of chromosomes. The clinical characteristics of Down syndrome may be present mildly or with varying degrees of severity depending on the number and location of the abnormal cells. An individual with mosaic Down syndrome may have normal intelligence.

Abnormalities of chromosome structure. Abnormalities of chromosome structure involve chromosome breakage usually resulting from one of two events: (1) translocation and (2) additions and/or deletions. Translocation occurs when genetic material is transferred from one chromosome to another different chromosome. Thus instead of two normal pairs of chromosomes, the individual has one normal chromosome of each pair and a third chromosome that is a fusion of the other two chromosomes. (As long as all genetic material is retained in the cell, the individual is unaffected but is a carrier of a balanced translocation.)

If a gamete receives the two normal chromosomes or the fused chromosome, the resulting offspring are clinically normal. If the gamete receives one of the two normal chromosomes and the fused version, the resulting offspring have an extra copy of one of the chromosomes. This condition is called an *unbalanced translocation* and often has serious clinical effects.

Whenever a portion of a chromosome is deleted from one chromosome and added to another, the gamete produced may have either extra copies of genes or too few copies. The clinical effects produced may be mild or severe depending on the amount of genetic material involved. Two of the more common conditions that have been described are the deletion of the short arm of chromosome 5 (cri du chat syndrome) and the deletion of the long arm of chromosome 18. Cri du chat syndrome, so named after the typical mewing cry of the affected infant, causes severe mental retardation with microcephaly and unusual facial appearance. Deletion of the long arm of chromosome 18 causes severe psychomotor retardation with multiple organ malformations.

Sex Chromosome Abnormalities

Several sex chromosome abnormalities have been identified that are caused by nondisjunction during gametogenesis in either parent. The most common deviation in females is Turner's syndrome, or monosomy X. The affected female is missing an X chromosome and exhibits juvenile external genitalia with undeveloped ovaries. She is usually short and has webbing of the neck. Intelligence may be impaired. Most affected embryos miscarry spontaneously.

The most common deviation in males is Klinefelter's syndrome, or trisomy XXY of the sex chromosomes. The affected male has an extra X chromosome and exhibits poorly developed secondary sexual characteristics and small testes. He is infertile, usually tall, and effeminate. Males who are mosaic for Klinefelter's syndrome may be fertile. Subnormal intelligence is usually present.

Patterns of Genetic Transmission

Heritable characteristics are those that can be passed on to offspring. The patterns by which genetic material is transmitted to the next generation are affected by the number

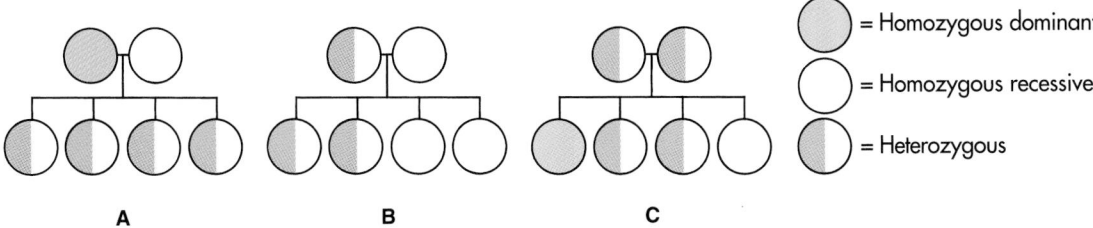

Fig. 14-14 Possible offspring in three types of matings. **A,** Homozygous-dominant parent and homozygous-recessive parent. Children all heterozygous, displaying dominant trait. **B,** Heterozygous parent and homozygous-recessive parent. Children 50% heterozygous displaying dominant trait; 50% homozygous displaying recessive trait. **C,** Both parents heterozygous. Children 25% homozygous displaying dominant trait; 25% homozygous displaying recessive trait; 50% heterozygous displaying dominant trait.

of genes involved in the expression of the trait. Many phenotypic characteristics result from two or more genes on different chromosomes acting together (referred to as *multifactorial inheritance*); others are controlled by a single gene (referred to as *unifactorial inheritance*).

Defects at the gene level cannot be determined by conventional laboratory methods such as karyotyping. Instead, genetic counselors predict the probability of the presence of an abnormal gene from the known occurrence of the trait in the individual's family and the known patterns by which the trait is inherited.

Multifactorial Inheritance

Most common congenital malformations result from multifactorial inheritance: a combination of genetic and environmental factors. Examples are cleft lip, cleft palate, congenital heart disease, neural tube defects, and pyloric stenosis. Each malformation may range from mild to severe, depending on the number of genes for the defect present or the amount of environmental influence. A neural tube defect may range from spina bifida, a bony defect in the lumbar region of the vertebrae with little or no neurologic impairment, to anencephaly, absence of brain development, which is always fatal. Some malformations occur more often in one sex. For example, pyloric stenosis and cleft lip are more common in males and cleft palate is more common in females. Multifactorial disorders also tend to occur in families.

Unifactorial Inheritance

If a single gene controls a particular trait, disorder, or defect, its pattern of inheritance is referred to as *unifactorial mendelian,* or single-gene inheritance. The number of unifactorial abnormalities far exceeds the number of chromosomal abnormalities. This is understandable considering that 50,000 to 100,000 genes in the haploid number (23) of chromosomes are passed on to an offspring from each parent.

Unifactorial or single-gene disorders follow the inheritance patterns of dominance, segregation, and independent assortment described by Mendel and include autosomal dominant, autosomal recessive, and X-linked dominant and recessive modes of inheritance.

Autosomal dominant inheritance. Autosomal dominant inheritance disorders are those in which the abnormal gene for the trait is expressed even when the other member of the pair is normal. The abnormal gene may appear as a result of a **mutation,** a spontaneous and permanent change in the normal gene structure, in which case the disorder occurs for the first time in the family. Usually, an affected individual comes from multiple generations having the disorder. An affected parent who is heterozygous for the trait has a 50% chance of passing the abnormal gene to each offspring (Fig. 14-14, *B, C*). Males and females are equally affected.

Autosomal dominant disorders are not always expressed with the same severity of symptoms. The parent may have a minor abnormality that had not been diagnosed until the birth of a more severely affected child. Predicting whether an offspring will have a minor or severe abnormality is not possible.

Examples of common autosomal dominantly inherited disorders are Marfan syndrome (a disorder of connective tissue resulting in skeletal, ocular, and cardiovascular abnormalities), achondroplasia (dwarfism), polydactyly (extra digits), Huntington's chorea, and polycystic kidney disease.

Autosomal recessive inheritance. Autosomal recessive inheritance disorders are those in which both genes of a pair must be abnormal for the disorder to be expressed. Heterozygous individuals have only one abnormal gene and are unaffected clinically because their normal gene overshadows the abnormal gene. They are known as *carriers* of the recessive trait. Because these recessive traits are inherited by generations of the same family, an increased incidence of the disorder occurs in consanguineous matings (closely related parents). For the trait to be expressed, two carriers must each contribute the abnormal gene to the offspring (see Fig. 14-14, *C*). The chance of the trait occurring in each child is 25%. A clinically normal offspring may be a carrier of the gene. Males and females are equally affected.

Most recessive disorders tend to have severe clinical manifestations, and affected offspring do not often reproduce. If they do, all their offspring will be carriers for the disorder.

Most inborn errors of metabolism, such as phenylketonuria (PKU), galactosemia, maple syrup urine disease, Tay-Sachs disease, sickle cell anemia, and cystic fibrosis, are autosomal recessive inherited disorders.

X-linked dominant inheritance. X-linked dominant inheritance disorders occur in males and heterozygous females. Because the females also have a normal gene, the effects are less severe than in affected males. Affected males transmit the abnormal gene only to their daughters on the X chromosome. Heterozygous females have a 50% chance of transmitting the abnormal gene to each offspring. An example of these extremely rare disorders is vitamin D–resistant rickets.

Fragile-X syndrome is a relatively recent diagnosis. The "fragile site" on the X chromosome was identified in a central nervous system disorder affecting males and is also seen in heterozygous carrier females. Affected individuals are mentally handicapped.

X-linked recessive inheritance. Abnormal genes for X-linked recessive inheritance disorders are carried on the X chromosome. Females may be heterozygous or homozygous for traits carried on the X chromosome because they have two X chromosomes. Males are hemizygous because they have only one X chromosome carrying genes with no alleles on the Y chromosome. Therefore X-linked recessive disorders are most commonly manifested in the male with the abnormal gene on his single X chromosome. Hemophilia, color blindness, and Duchenne muscular dystrophy are X-linked recessive disorders.

The male receives the defective gene from his carrier mother on her affected X chromosome. Female carriers (those heterozygous for the trait) have a 50% probability of transmitting the abnormal gene to each offspring. An affected male can pass the abnormal gene only to his daughters on the X chromosome but not to his sons. The daughters will be carriers of the trait if they receive a normal gene on the X chromosome from their mother. They will be affected only if they receive an abnormal gene on the X chromosome from both their mother and father.

Inborn errors of metabolism. Disorders of protein, fat, or carbohydrate metabolism reflecting absent or defective enzymes generally follow a recessive pattern of inheritance. Enzymes, the actions of which are genetically determined, are essential for all the physical and chemical processes that sustain body systems. Defective enzyme action interrupts the normal series of chemical reactions from the affected point onward. The result may be an accumulation of a damaging product such as phenylalanine or the absence of a necessary product such as thyroxin or melanin. (See Table 27-2 for screening tests for inborn errors of metabolism.)

Phenylketonuria (PKU) is an uncommon disorder caused by autosomal recessive genes. A deficiency in the liver enzyme phenylalanine hydroxylase results in failure to metabolize the amino acid phenylalanine, allowing its metabolites to accumulate in the blood. The incidence of this disorder is 1 in every 10,000 to 20,000 births. The highest incidence is found in Caucasians (from northern Europe and the United States). It is rarely seen in Jewish, African, or Japanese populations. Screening for PKU is routinely performed on all infants through a blood test.

Tay-Sachs disease, inherited as an autosomal recessive trait, results from a deficiency of hexosaminidase. It occurs primarily in Jewish families. Until 4 to 6 months of age, infants appear normal; in fact, their facial features are considered very beautiful. Then the clinical symptoms appear: apathy and regression in motor and social development and decreased vision. Death occurs between 3 and 4 years of age. No known treatment exists for Tay-Sachs disease.

Cystic fibrosis (mucoviscidosis or fibrocystic disease of the pancreas) is inherited as an autosomal recessive trait characterized by generalized involvement of exocrine glands. Clinical features are related to the altered viscosity of mucus-secreting glands throughout the body. This serious chronic disease occurs primarily in Caucasian populations but can appear in people of mixed ancestry. The overall incidence is 1 in every 2000 births. The incidence of the carrier state is estimated at 1:20 to 1:25. Advances in diagnosis and treatment have improved the prognosis, so many affected individuals now live to adulthood. Some affected women have borne children, but men are generally sterile. If the mother has cystic fibrosis and the father has no family history of the disease, the offspring have a 50% chance of inheriting the gene for cystic fibrosis.

Meconium ileus occurs in about 10% of newborns with cystic fibrosis. Although an initial stool may be passed from the rectum with none thereafter, usually no meconium is passed during the first 24 to 48 hours. The abdomen becomes increasingly distended, and eventually the newborn requires a laparotomy for diagnosis and treatment of the condition.

Human Genome Project

The Human Genome Project (Box 14-3), funded by the National Institutes of Health, is involved in mapping and sequencing the genetic makeup of humans (Kopala, 1997; Mahowald, 1997). This map will facilitate study of hereditary diseases and will provide the potential for making changes at the gene level to treat or prevent hereditary diseases (Fig. 14-15).

Genetic Counseling

It is expected that by the year 2005, the entire human **genome** (the copy of the genetic material in humans) will be mapped and that all of the 70,000 to 100,000 genes will be identified (Munro, 1999). There are more than 7000 single-gene disorders that are known (Munro, 1999). This explo-

BOX 14-3 The Human Genome Project

J JENKINS, RN, MSN, AND F COLLINS, MD, PHD

The Human Genome Project is a federally funded, co-ordinated effort to assemble data on the genetic instructions found within human DNA and within DNA of several model organisms (Collins, 1995; Guyer & Collins, 1995). The ultimate goal of the project is the complete sequencing of all 3 billion base pairs of human DNA. This includes the development of genetic and physical maps that facilitate the identification of human disease genes by positional cloning. This strategy allows the identification of human disease genes without prior information about their biologic function. The focus of genetics specialists has previously been on rare genetic disorders; however, virtually every disease (except trauma) has a genetic component. Medical genetics is now poised to uncover these genetic predispositions, opening the possibility of highly sophisticated diagnostic and therapeutic strategies.

Genes that contribute to common polygenic conditions such as diabetes, hypertension, most forms of cancer, and the major mental illnesses will be identified by this approach. These gene discoveries will lead to molecular insights that will revolutionize the treatment of disease, using gene therapy or "designer drug" strategies. For many diseases, however, health care professionals will be able to predict risks but will not be able to intervene with effective treatment for some time (Scanlon & Fibison, 1995). This creates a dilemma for all health care providers. As genetic testing becomes available for risk prediction for diseases such as cancer or Alzheimer's disease, many questions will arise. How reliable is the test? What do these results mean in terms of the actual risk of developing the disease? How useful is this information? What preventive or treatment recommendations will be available based on test results? Laboratories providing genetic testing need to be monitored for quality control of genetic test results: criteria must be established to define when a test should be done only in a research setting. DNA testing, like the administration of a drug, has potential side effects and risks that need to be studied in clinical trials and managed appropriately (Andrews et al., 1994).

Until now, most physicians and nurses have not had the opportunity to incorporate genetics into their practice. An imminent challenge is to prepare providers to be able to include components of genetic risk assessment in all health care delivery, including screening, counseling, education, surveillance, and treatment, and to use this information wisely. Because of widespread concerns about misuse of information gained through genetic testing, 5% of the Human Genome Project budget is designated for research into the Ethical, Legal, and Social Implications (ELSI) Program of the project (U.S. Department of Health and Human Services, 1995). Issues of high priority for ELSI have included genetic privacy, the safety and efficacy of genetic testing, informed consent, and the potential for genetic discrimination in health insurance and employment. A recent ruling of the Equal Employment Opportunities Commission (EEOC) renders employment discrimination on the basis of future genetic susceptibility illegal, based on the provisions of the Americans with Disabilities Act. Legislation is urgently needed to address discrimination in health insurance (Hudson et al., 1995).

All health care specialties will be required to distill this evolving body of knowledge and use the genetics information to facilitate consumer decision making. Nurses, with their long tradition of combining clinical skills and attention to the whole person, are in a critical position to lead the way.

---

sion in knowledge has implications for nurses working with mothers and infants, especially those who are involved in genetic counseling.

Purposes of Genetic Counseling

The purposes of genetic counseling are to (1) advise couples before conception of the probability of conception of an infant with a genetic disorder; (2) advise couples after conception and fetal screening of whether or not the fetus has a genetic disorder; and (3) inform the couple of the options that are available to them, including choosing not to become pregnant (Chadwick, 1993).

Genetic Counseling Services

The most efficient counseling services are associated with the larger universities and major medical centers where sup-port services are available (e.g., biochemistry and cytology laboratories) and consist of a group of specialists under the leadership of a physician trained in medical genetics. Many of these regional centers maintain satellite clinics or services in outlying areas to provide contact with both consumers and health professionals. A number of specialized groups provide clinics and services for people with a specific genetic disorder such as cystic fibrosis, muscular dystrophy, hemophilia, or diabetes. Health professionals should become familiar with people who provide genetic counseling and places in which counseling services are available to clients in their area of practice (Inati, Lazar, & Haskin-Leahy, 1994).

Ethical Considerations

Researchers have proposed using fetal neurologic, liver, and pancreatic tissues to treat adults with Parkinson's

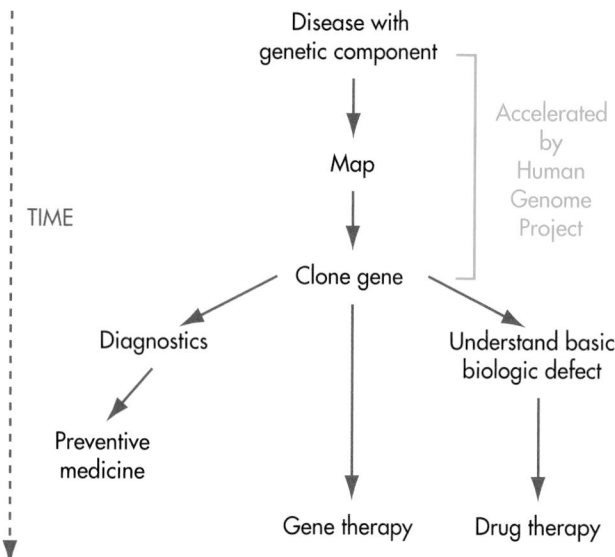

Fig. 14-15 Progress in molecular medicine. The Human Genome Project has accelerated the time required to clone a disease gene. Gene discovery often results in improved diagnostic capabilities. The timeline to develop effective drug or gene therapies is less predictable. *(From Collins, F. [1995]. Positional cloning moves from perditional to traditional. Nature Genetics 9, 347-350.)*

BOX 14-4 **Fetal Malformations Treatable by Open Fetal Surgery**

Posterior urethral valves
CCAM (congenital cystic adenomatoid malformation of the lung)
CDH (congenital diaphragmatic hernia)
Twin-twin transfusion syndrome
Sacrococcygeal teratoma
Complete heart block

From Crombleholme, T. (1994). Invasive fetal surgery: Current status and future directions. *Semin Perinatol* 18(4), 385.

---

disease, metabolic disorders, or head and spinal cord injury. The use of fetal tissue in research was banned for several years, but the ban was lifted in 1993. In part, opposition to use of fetal tissue in research was due to the belief of some that women would be encouraged or coerced to become pregnant and abort fetuses to provide material for use in this research.

Management of Genetic Disorders

At this time, there are no cures for genetic disorders, although remedies can be implemented to prevent or reduce the harmful effects of a few disorders. Structural defects can sometimes be modified to produce normal or near-normal function. Research is being conducted to devise methods to influence or change the genes directly by placing substitute DNA in the cells of those with a genetic mutation, thereby preventing or curing the disease process or relieving symptoms (Crombleholme & Bianchi, 1994). Successful treatment of adenosine deaminase deficiency and cystic fibrosis has been reported (Pickler & Munro, 1995). The major thrust in therapy is modification of the internal or external environment to minimize the effects of the disorder.

Embryonic stem cells are primitive cells that can develop into all types of body tissue, including muscles, nerves, and bones. The possibility exists that understanding these cells will lead to new medical discoveries. Thomson et al. (1998) isolated stem cells from excess embryos donated by couples undergoing *in vitro* fertilization

while Gearhart (1998) used gonads of aborted embryos. Thus, whether stem cell research falls under the ban on embryo research is being debated.

The Human Embryo Research Panel in a report to the National Institutes of Health director concluded that it is acceptable to do research on deriving embryonic stem (ES) cells provided that embryos are not expressly created for the purpose of research (Gearhart, 1998). Currently the use of federal funds for this purpose is banned. Research to date has been conducted using corporate and private funding (Gearhart, 1998).

The successful cloning of sheep, cattle, and mice; the production of rhesus monkeys through nuclear transfer of embryonic cells; and the isolation of stem cells constitute breakthroughs in technology and raise other ethical questions. The nurse involved in genetic counseling must keep abreast of such breakthroughs and be prepared to discuss ethical implications with clients and other health care providers.

Surgical therapy is employed for congenital heart defects and cosmetic defects such as cleft lip. Advances in fetal surgery are occurring (Box 14-4). Other conditions are treated with product replacement (thyroid for hereditary cretinism), diet modification (low phenylalanine diet for PKU), and corrective devices for missing limbs.

People with some disorders, such as glucose-6-phosphate dehydrogenase (G6PD) deficiency or the porphyrias, can prevent the disease simply by avoiding the specific chemical agent that precipitates the symptoms. Avoiding circumstances that reduce tissue oxygenation can reduce the sickling of red blood cells in sickle cell anemia.

Researchers continue to develop therapies for heritable diseases. Some possible methods of future management include replacement or stabilization by oral or parenteral medications or other methods, altering intracellular DNA, and other projected feats of genetic engineering. Rapid progress is evident in the field of genetic engineering (Dickler & Collier, 1994). Molecular techniques provide infinite possibilities for altering human genes through gene splicing. Thus, it will be possible to use altered genes in ova and sperm for in vitro fertilization.

Estimation of Risk

The risks of recurrence of a genetic disorder are determined by the mode of inheritance. The risk of recurrence for disorders caused by a factor that segregates during cell division (genes and chromosomes) can be estimated with a high degree of accuracy by application of the mendelian principles. In a dominant disorder the risk is 50%, or one in two, that a subsequent offspring will be affected; an autosomal-recessive disease carries a one-in-four risk of recurrence; and an X-linked disorder is related to the sex of the child. Translocation chromosomes have a high risk of recurrence.

Disorders in which a subsequent pregnancy would carry no more risk than there would be for pregnancy (estimated at 1 in 30) include those resulting from isolated incidences not likely to be present in another pregnancy. These disorders include maternal infections (e.g., rubella or toxoplasmosis), maternal ingestion of drugs, most chromosomal abnormalities, and a disorder determined to be the result of a fresh mutation.

The risk of recurrence for multifactorial conditions can be estimated empirically. An empiric risk is not based on genetic theory, but rather on experience and observation of the disorder in other families. Recurrence risks are determined by applying the frequency of a similar disorder in other families to the case under consideration.

Interpretation of Risk

Counselors explain the risk estimates to clients without making recommendations or decisions and avoid allowing their own biases to interfere. The counselor provides appropriate information about the nature of the disorder, the extent of the risks in the specific case, the probable consequences, and (if appropriate) alternative options available, but the final decision to become pregnant or to continue a pregnancy must be left to the family. An important nursing role is reinforcing the information the families are given, continuing to interpret this information on their level of understanding, and remaining nonjudgmental of the family decision.

The most important concept that must be emphasized to families is that *each pregnancy is an independent event.* For example, in monogenic disorders in which the risk factor is one in four that the child will be affected, the risk remains the same no matter how many affected children are already in the family. Families may maintain the erroneous assumption that the presence of one affected child ensures that the next three will be free of the disorder. However, "chance has no memory." The risk is one in four for each pregnancy. On the other hand, in a family with a child who has a disorder with multifactorial causes, the risk increases with each subsequent child born with the disorder.

Role of Nurse in Genetic Counseling

All nurses, especially those involved in the care of mothers and children, need to (1) have an understanding of genetic theory and the nature of more common genetic dis-

orders to recognize cues that may indicate a genetically related problem, (2) be able to help families obtain counseling services, (3) augment the counseling process (Stringer, Librizzi, & Weiner, 1991), and (4) be aware of the legal and ethical issues involved (Penticuff, 1996). Although diagnosis and treatment of genetic disorders require medical skills and, although determination of risk factors for many disorders requires the expertise of a geneticist, nurses with advanced preparation in genetics and counseling are assuming an increasingly important role in counseling people about genetically transmitted or genetically influenced conditions. Key competencies suggested for genetics nurses are that they must be able to (1) understand and communicate information on the basis of genetic disease, the patterns of inheritance, and testing options; (2) obtain an accurate family history and understand the implications of the medical history; (3) provide an environment for counseling so that clients can explore safely the condition's implications and the family's choices; and (4) be aware of their own capabilities and the need to seek guidance and refer appropriately as necessary (Skirton et al., 1997) (see Plan of Care). See Box 14-5 for information on genetic resources.

Follow-Up Care

Maintaining contact with the family after genetic counseling, testing, or therapy is one of the most important nursing responsibilities because the success of counseling is measured by the way the family uses the information presented to them. Most counseling services try to schedule at least one postdiagnostic or postcounseling visit to assess how well the family is beginning to incorporate this new information into their lives and value systems. Follow-up visits to the counseling service or visits to the home provide additional opportunities to reexplore all aspects of the situation and to answer any questions that may have occurred to the family since the previous contacts. Clarifying information is an important nursing function.

Referral to appropriate agencies is an essential part of the follow-up management. Many organizations and foundations, such as the Cystic Fibrosis Foundation and the Muscular Dystrophy Association, provide services and equipment for affected children. Early Infant Stimulation Foundation programs are available for children born with Down syndrome. There are also numerous parent groups with which the family can share experiences and derive mutual support from other families with similar problems. Nurses should become familiar with services available in their community that provide assistance and education to families with these special problems (see Appendix D).

Emotional Support

Probably the most important of all nursing functions is providing emotional support to the family during all aspects of the counseling process. Feelings that are generated under the real or imagined threat posed by a genetic

PLAN ᵒᶠ CARE | Genetic Counseling for a Woman with a Fetal Anomaly

NURSING DIAGNOSIS Decisional conflict related to whether to continue or terminate pregnancy as evidenced by client statement after confirmation of fetal anomaly diagnosis

Expected Outcome *Client will express satisfaction with decision-making process with regard to pregnancy outcome.*

Nursing Interventions/*Rationales*

Assess knowledge base of client with regard to fetal anomaly, prognosis, and possible future pregnancy outcomes *to correct any misconceptions and identify starting point for teaching.*

Provide accurate information to client in a timely fashion *to assist in decision-making efficiently in order to meet deadlines dictated by gestational age of the fetus.*

Provide emotional support through therapeutic communication *to facilitate the decision-making process in an objective manner.*

Refer client to support group focused on specific fetal anomaly if possible *to provide information and shared experiences by the group.*

NURSING DIAGNOSIS Situational low self-esteem related to diagnosis of fetal anomaly as evidenced by client statements of guilt and shame

Expected Outcome *Client will express an increased number of positive statements about herself.*

Nursing Interventions/*Rationales*

Through therapeutic communication encourage client to express feelings *to clarify and provide support.*

Assist client to identify usual effective coping mechanisms *to use during a situational crisis.*

Reinforce and clarify information regarding fetal anomaly *to provide client with objective information and increase positive feelings regarding self.*

BOX 14-5 | Resources on Genetics

THE NATIONAL SOCIETY OF GENETIC COUNSELORS
http://members.aol.com/nsgcweb/nsgchome.htm
THE INTERNATIONAL SOCIETY OF NURSES IN GENETICS (ISONG)
http://nursing.creighton.edu/ (Click on PROFESSIONAL ORGANIZATION and then ISONG.)
THE NATIONAL CENTER FOR HUMAN GENOME RESEARCH
http://www.nchgr.nih.gov

---

disorder are as varied as the people being counseled. Responses may include a variety of stress reactions, such as apathy, denial, anger, hostility, fear, embarrassment, grief, and loss of self-esteem. Guilt and self-blame are universal reactions. Many look on the disorder as a stigma, especially if the disorder is visible to others. Old wives' tales, superstitions, and long-held misconceptions are all factors that may influence a family's reaction to a genetic disorder.

The attitude of other family members and relatives can have a significant impact on some people, especially in situations where the cause can be identified (such as a dominant or an X-linked disorder). Recessive disorders are less likely to cause blaming, since both partners carry the defective gene. A genetic disorder may cause a family to alter plans for marriage or childbearing even when the probability of recurrence is no more than a random risk.

Factors such as religious beliefs, intellectual level, and prior attitudes toward the disorder affect the way in which families respond to counseling information. Sometimes counselors and other health personnel create barriers through their own attitudes toward a specific disorder. It is often difficult to be nonjudgmental and objective, and nurses may intentionally or unintentionally influence families in making decisions. Families may pressure the nurse to make decisions for them with questions such as, "What would you do if you were me?" Families and individuals need education, guidance, and support throughout the counseling process. They should be given the facts and possible consequences and all of the assistance they need in problem solving, but the final decision regarding a course of action must be their own.

Ethical Dimensions of Genetic Screening

Although genetic screening has the potential for great benefits, there is also a potential for harm. Genetic information may be used to discriminate against individuals in insurance decisions or employment. Conflicts about who will receive scarce genetic service resources may occur and some individuals may experience social stigmatization. Others may experience emotional distress when diagnosed with lethal, untreatable diseases or when the genetic information forces choices that are agonizing (Penticuff, 1996).

There is concern that prenatal screening and diagnosis will challenge our values about the kind of infants that will be born as parents with an affected fetus make the choice to continue or terminate the pregnancy (Penticuff, 1996). Some fear social pressures to make decisions contrary to personal beliefs. Newborn screening presents other dilem-

mas. The Institute of Medicine Committee on Assessing Genetic Risks "has recommended that newborn screening not be done when early detection will not alter the course of the disease, effective treatment is not available, or there is no effective treatment and testing is being done only to give information to guide their future reproductive plans" (Penticuff, 1996). Detecting carrier status can be used by parents in reproductive planning but it has the potential to result in bias or discrimination. Public demand for genetic testing is expected to increase. Principles of choice and confidentiality must be adhered to by health professionals involved (Penticuff, 1996).

KEY POINTS

- Human gestation is approximately 280 days after the last menstrual period or 266 days after conception.
- Fertilization occurs in the uterine tube within 24 hours of ovulation. The zygote undergoes mitotic divisions, creating a 16-cell morula.
- Implantation begins 6 days after fertilization.
- The organ systems and external features develop during the embryonic period, that is, the third to the eighth week after fertilization.
- Refinement of structure and function occurs during the fetal period, and the fetus becomes capable of extrauterine survival.
- There are critical periods in human development during which the embryo/fetus is vulnerable to environmental teratogens.
- Genes are the basic units of heredity responsible for all human characteristics. They comprise 23 pairs of chromosomes: 22 pairs of autosomes and 1 pair of sex chromosomes.
- Mitosis is the process by which body cells replicate for growth and development and cell replacement of the organism.
- Meiosis is the process by which gametes are formed for reproduction of the organism.
- Chromosomal abnormalities of number and structure occur in both autosomes and sex chromosomes.
- Genetic disorders follow mendelian inheritance patterns of dominance, segregation, and independent assortment of normal genetic transmission.
- Multifactorial inheritance includes genetic and environmental contributions.
- The best means for reducing the number of children born with genetic defects is to provide families with genetic information and services.
- Advances in genetics have ethical dimensions.

CRITICAL THINKING EXERCISES

1 *Sylvia Tauner confides in you that there have been several infants born into her family with serious anomalies. From previous conversations, you know that she is opposed to abortion and would never consider having one. Sylvia is currently 6 weeks pregnant, and her physician has urged her to have chorionic villus sampling (CVS). Sylvia asks you for information about CVS and the implications of a finding that her fetus has serious anomalies. Describe your response, keeping in mind genetics, the social and moral implications of genetic testing, and Sylvia's ethical and moral beliefs. What other information do you need? To whom could you refer her? What options does she have?*

2 *Select five household chemicals used in your home. Identify the purpose of the chemicals, and describe the reasons why they are hazardous to the reproductive health of women, men, and a developing embryo/fetus. List alternatives that can be substituted to accomplish the same purpose as the chemicals.*

References

Andrews, L. et al. (Eds.) (1994). *Assessing genetic risks: Implications for health and social policy.* Washington, D.C.: National Academy Press (Institute of Medicine).

Bar-Hava, I., & Barnhardt, Y. (1994). Fetal vibroacoustic stimulation. *Female Patient* 19(5), 63.

Carlson, B. (1994). *Human embryology and developmental biology.* St. Louis: Mosby.

Chadwick, R. (1993). What counts as success in genetic counseling? *J Med Ethics* 19, 43.

Cole, J. (1997). What can babies see at birth? *Mother Baby J* 2(4), 45-47.

Collins, F. (1995). Positional cloning moves from perditional to traditional. *Nature Genetics* 9, 347-350.

Creasy, R., & Resnik, J. (Eds.). (1999). *Maternal-fetal medicine* (4th ed.). Philadelphia: W.B. Saunders.

Crombleholme, T. (1994). Invasive fetal surgery: Current status and future directions. *Semin Perinatol* 18(4), 385-387.

Crombleholme, T., & Bianchi, D. (1994). In utero hematopoietic stem cell transplantation and gene therapy. *Semin Perinatol* 18(4), 376-384.

Cunningham, F. et al. (1997). *Williams obstetrics* (20th ed.). Stamford, CT: Appleton & Lange.

Dickler, H., & Collier, E. (1994). Gene therapy in the treatment of disease. *J Allergy Clin Immunol* 96, 942-951.

Gearhart, J. (1998). New potential for human embryonic stem cells. *Science* 282, 1061-1062.

Guyer, M., & Collins, F. (1995). How is the human genome project doing, and what have we learned so far? *Proc Natl Acad Sci USA* 92(24), 10841-10848.

Hallak, M. et al. (1993). Amniotic fluid index: Gestational age-specific values for normal human pregnancy. *J Reprod Med* 38, 853-856.

Hoyme, H. (1990). Teratogenically induced fetal anomalies. *Clin Perinatol* 17(3), 547-567.

Hsieh, F. et al. (1995). Limb defects after chorionic villus sampling. *Obstet Gynecol* 85(1), 84.

Hudson, K. et al. (1995). Genetic discrimination and health insurance: An urgent need for reform. *Science* 270, 391-393.

Inati, M., Lazar, E., & Haskin-Leahy, L. (1994). The role of the genetic counselor in a perinatal unit. *Semin Perinatol* 18, 133-139.

Jona, J. (1998). Advances in fetal surgery. *Pediatr Clin North Am* 45(3), 599-604.

Kopala, B. (1997). The Human Genome Project: Issues and ethics. *MCN, Am J Matern Child Nurs* 22(1), 9-15.

Langley, L. et al. (1980). *Dynamic human anatomy and physiology* (5th ed.). New York: McGraw-Hill.

Mahowald, M. (1997). An overview of the Human Genome Project and its implications for women. *Women's Health Issues* 7(4), 206-208.

Moore, K., & Persaud, T. (1998). *Before we are born: Essentials of embryology and birth defects* (5th ed.). Philadelphia: W.B. Saunders.

Munro, C. (1999). Implications for nursing of the Human Genome Project. *Neonatal Network* 18(3), 7-12.

Penticuff, J. (1996). Ethical dimensions in genetic screening: A look into the future. *J Obstet Gynecol Neonatal Nurs* 25(6), 785-789.

Pickler, R., & Munro, C. (1995). Gene therapy for inherited disorders. *J Pediatr Nurs* 10(8), 40-47.

Poole, R. (Ed.). (1986). *The incredible machine.* Washington, D.C.: National Geographic Society.

Scanlon, C., & Fibison, W. (1995). *Managing genetic information: Implications for nursing practice.* Washington, D.C.: American Nurses Association.

Scialli, A. (1997). Toxicology. *Contemp OB GYN* 42(5), 15.

Sherman, S. et al. (1997). Behavioral genetics '97: ASHG Statement. Recent developments in human behavioral genetics: Past accomplishments and future directions. *Am J Hum Genet* 60(6), 1265-1275.

Skirton, H. et al. (1997). The role and practice of the genetic nurse: Report of the AGNC working party. *J Med Genet* 34(2), 141-147.

Stringer, M., Librizzi, R., & Weiner, S. (1991). Establishing a prenatal genetic diagnosis: The nurse's role. *MCN Am J Matern Child Nurs* 16(3), 152-156.

Thomson, J. et al. (1998). Embryonic stem cell lines derived from human blastocysts. *Science* 282, 1145-1147.

U. S. Department of Health and Human Services (1995). *The Human Genome Project progress report fiscal years 1993-1994.* Washington, D.C.: National Institutes of Health.

Willson, J., & Carrington, E. (1991). *Obstetrics and gynecology* (9th ed.). St. Louis: Mosby.

Wong, D. (1999). *Whaley and Wong's nursing care of infants and children* (6th ed.). St. Louis: Mosby.

Wong, D., & Perry, S. (1998). *Maternal child nursing care.* St. Louis: Mosby.

15

Anatomy and Physiology of Pregnancy

Deitra Leonard Lowdermilk

LEARNING OBJECTIVES

- Define the key terms.
- Determine gravidity and parity using the five- and four-digit systems.
- Describe the various types of pregnancy tests.
- Explain the expected maternal anatomic and physiologic adaptations to pregnancy.
- Differentiate among presumptive, probable, and positive signs of pregnancy.

- Identify the maternal hormones produced during pregnancy, their target organs, and their major effects on pregnancy.
- Compare the characteristics of the abdomen, vulva, and cervix of the nullipara and multipara.
- Identify topics for nursing research related to the anatomy and physiology of pregnancy.

KEY TERMS

amenorrhea
ballottement
Braxton Hicks sign
carpal tunnel syndrome
Chadwick's sign
chloasma
colostrum
diastasis recti abdominis
epulis
friability
funic souffle
Goodell's sign
gravida
gravidity
Hegar's sign

human chorionic gonadotropin (hCG)
leukorrhea
lightening
linea nigra
mean arterial pressure (MAP)
Montgomery's tubercles
multigravida
multipara
nulligravida
nullipara
operculum
palmar erythema
parity
physiologic anemia

postdate or post-term
preterm
primigravida
primipara
ptyalism
pyrosis
quickening
signs and symptoms of pregnancy
  presumptive
  probable
  positive
striae gravidarum
term
uterine souffle
viability

he goal of maternity care is a healthy pregnancy with a physically safe and emotionally satisfying outcome for mother, infant, and family. Consistent health supervision and surveillance are of utmost importance in achiev-

ing this outcome. However, many maternal adaptations are unfamiliar to pregnant women and their families. Helping the pregnant woman recognize the relationship between her physical status and the plan for her care assists

TABLE 15-1 Gravidity and Parity Using Five-Digit (GTPAL) System

CONDITION	PREGNANCIES	TERM BIRTH	PRETERM BIRTH	ABORTIONS	LIVING CHILDREN
Sarah is pregnant for the first time.	1	0	0	0	0
She carries the pregnancy to term, and the infant survives.	1	1	0	0	1
She is pregnant again.	2	1	0	0	1
Her second pregnancy ends in miscarriage.	2	1	0	1	1
During her third pregnancy, she gives birth to twins at 32 weeks gestation.	3	1	1	1	3

her in making decisions and encourages her to participate in her own care.

GRAVIDITY AND PARITY

An understanding of the following terms used to describe pregnancy and the pregnant woman is essential to the study of maternity care.

- **gravida**—A woman who is pregnant
- **gravidity**—Pregnancy
- **multigravida**—A woman who has had two or more pregnancies
- **multipara**—A woman who has completed two or more pregnancies to the stage of fetal viability
- **nulligravida**—A woman who has never been pregnant
- **nullipara**—A woman who has not completed a pregnancy with a fetus or fetuses who have reached the stage of fetal viability
- **parity**—The number of pregnancies in which the fetus or fetuses have reached viability, not the number of fetuses (e.g., twins) born. Whether the fetus is born alive or is stillborn (fetus who shows no signs of life at birth) after viability is reached does not affect parity
- **postdate or post-term**—Term used to describe a pregnancy that goes beyond 42 weeks of gestation
- **preterm**—Term referring to a pregnancy that has reached 20 weeks of gestation but before completion of 37 weeks of gestation
- **primigravida**—A woman who is pregnant for the first time
- **primipara**—A woman who has completed one pregnancy with a fetus or fetuses who have reached the stage of fetal viability
- **term**—Used to describe a pregnancy from the beginning of the thirty-eighth week of gestation to the end of the forty-second week of gestation
- **viability**—Capacity to live outside the uterus; about 22 to 24 weeks since last menstrual period, or weight of fetus is greater than 500 g

Gravidity and parity information is obtained during history taking interviews and may be recorded in client records in several ways. One abbreviation commonly used in maternity centers consists of five digits separated with hy-

BOX 15-1 Using "TPAL" to Define Parity

T—term birth(s)
P—preterm birth(s)
A—abortion(s)
L—living children

phens. The first digit represents the total number of pregnancies, including the present one (gravidity); the second digit represents the total number of full-term births; the third indicates the number of preterm births; the fourth identifies the number of abortions (miscarriage or elective termination of pregnancy before viability); and the fifth is the number of children currently living. The acronym "GTPAL" may be helpful in remembering this system of notation. For example, if a woman pregnant only once with twins gives birth at the thirty-fifth week and the babies survive, the abbreviation that represents this information is "1-0-1-0-2." During her next pregnancy the abbreviation is "2-0-1-0-2." Additional examples are given in Table 15-1.

Others prefer a four-digit system. The first digit of the five-digit system, which signifies gravidity, is dropped. The acronym "TPAL" is helpful in remembering what the four digits stand for (Box 15-1).

PREGNANCY TESTS

Early detection of pregnancy allows for early initiation of care. **Human chorionic gonadotropin (hCG)** is the biologic marker on which pregnancy tests are based. Production of hCG begins as early as the day of implantation and can be detected in the blood as early as 6 days after conception, or about 20 days since the last menstrual period (LMP), and in urine about 26 days after conception (Cunningham et al., 1997). The level of hCG rises until it peaks at about 60 to 70 days of gestation and then begins to decline. The lowest level is reached between 100 to 130 days of pregnancy and remains constant until birth (Varney, 1997).

Serum and urine pregnancy tests are performed in clinics, offices, women's health centers, and laboratory settings. Both serum and urine tests provide accurate results. A 7 to 10 ml sample of venous blood is collected for serum testing. Most urine tests require a first-voided morning urine specimen because it contains levels of hCG approximately the same as those in serum. Random urine samples usually have lower levels. Urine tests are less expensive and provide more immediate results than serum tests (Hatcher et al., 1998).

Many different pregnancy tests are available, but they all depend on recognition of hCG or a beta subunit of hCG. The wide variety of tests precludes discussion of each; however, several categories of tests are described here. The nurse should read the manufacturer's directions for the test to be used.

Immunoassay or agglutination inhibition tests (AIT) depend on an antigen-antibody reaction between hCG and an antiserum. Usually the antiserum is mixed with urine and hCG-coated particles (e.g., latex or blood cells) are added. If hCG is present in the urine, agglutination does not occur because the hCG neutralizes the hCG antibody, and the test is considered positive (Cunningham et al., 1997). AIT tests are easy to do, and results are available in 2 minutes to 2 hours depending on the method used (Pagana & Pagana, 1997). Although immunologic tests are accurate from 4 to 10 days after a missed period, they are most appropriate for confirming a pregnancy at or after the sixth week of gestation (Hatcher et al., 1998).

Radioimmunoassay (RIA) pregnancy tests for the beta subunit of hCG use radioactively labeled markers and are usually performed in a laboratory. Serum or urine samples may be used. The test time ranges from 1 to 5 hours. Radioimmunoassay tests are accurate with low hCG levels and can confirm pregnancy one week after conception (Hatcher et al., 1998).

Radioreceptor assay (RRA) is a serum test that measures the ability of a blood sample to inhibit the binding of radio-labeled hCG to receptors. The test is 90% to 95% accurate from 6 to 10 days after conception. It can be completed within 1 hour (Pagana & Pagana, 1997).

Enzyme-linked immunosorbent assay (ELISA) testing is the most popular method of testing for pregnancy. It uses a specific monoclonal antibody (anti-hCG) with enzymes to bond with hCG in urine. Depending on the specific test, levels of hCG as low as 5 to 50 mIU/ml can be detected as early as 4 days after implantation (Hatcher et al., 1998). As an office or home procedure it requires minimal time and offers results in 5 minutes. A positive test is indicated by a simple color-change reaction.

ELISA technology is the basis for most over-the-counter home pregnancy tests. With these one-step tests, the woman usually applies urine to a strip and reads the results. The test kits come with directions for collection of the specimen, the testing procedure, and reading of the results. Most manufacturers of the kits provide a toll free telephone number to call if users have concerns and questions about test procedures or results (see Teaching

TEACHING guidelines

Home Pregnancy Testing

Follow the manufacturer's instructions carefully. Do not omit steps.

Review the manufacturer's list of foods, medications, and other substances that can affect the test results.

Use a first-voided morning urine specimen.

If the test done at the time of your missed period is negative, repeat the test in one week if you still have not had a period.

If you have questions about the test, contact the manufacturer.

Contact your health care provider for follow-up if the test is positive or if the test is negative and you still have not had a period.

Guidelines box). The most common error in performing home pregnancy tests is doing the test too early in pregnancy (Hatcher et al., 1998).

Interpreting the results of pregnancy tests requires some judgment. The type of pregnancy test and its degree of sensitivity (ability to detect low levels of a substance) and specificity (ability to discern the absence of a substance) have to be considered in conjunction with the woman's history. This includes the date of her last normal menstrual period (LNMP), her usual cycle length, and results of previous pregnancy tests. It is important to know if the woman is a substance abuser and what medications she is taking because drugs such as anticonvulsants and tranquilizers can cause false-positive results while diuretics and promethazine can cause false-negative results (Pagana & Pagana, 1997). Improper collection of the specimen, hormone-producing tumors, and laboratory errors also may cause false results. Whenever there is any question, further evaluation or retesting may be appropriate.

ADAPTATIONS TO PREGNANCY

Maternal physiologic adaptations are attributed to the hormones of pregnancy and to mechanical pressures arising from the enlarging uterus and other tissues. These adaptations protect the woman's normal physiologic functioning, meet the metabolic demands pregnancy imposes on her body, and provide a nurturing environment for fetal development and growth. Although pregnancy is a normal phenomenon, problems can occur. The nurse needs a foundation in normal maternal physiology to accomplish the following:

- Identify potential or actual deviation from normal adaptation to initiate care.

TABLE 15-2 Signs of Pregnancy

TIME OF OCCURRENCE (GESTATIONAL AGE)	SIGN	OTHER POSSIBLE CAUSES
PRESUMPTIVE SIGNS		
3-4 weeks	Breast changes	Premenstrual changes, oral contraceptives
4 weeks	Amenorrhea	Stress, vigorous exercise, early menopause, endocrine problems, malnutrition
4-14 weeks	Nausea, vomiting	Gastrointestinal virus, food poisoning
6-12 weeks	Urinary frequency	Infection, pelvic tumors
12 weeks	Fatigue	Stress, illness
16-20 weeks	Quickening	Gas, peristalsis
PROBABLE SIGNS		
5 weeks	Goodell's sign	Pelvic congestion
6-8 weeks	Chadwick's sign	Pelvic congestion
6-12 weeks	Hegar's sign	Pelvic congestion
4-12 weeks	Positive pregnancy test (serum)	Hydatidiform mole, choriocarcinoma
6-12 weeks	Positive pregnancy test (urine)	False-positive results may be because of pelvic infection, tumors
16 weeks	Braxton Hicks contractions	Myomas, other tumors
16-28 weeks	Ballottement	Tumors, cervical polyps
POSITIVE SIGNS		
5-6 weeks	Visualization of fetus by ultrasound examination	No other causes
16 weeks	Visualization of fetus by x-ray study	
6 weeks	Fetal heart tones detected by ultrasound examination	
8-17 weeks	Fetal heart tones detected by Doppler ultrasound, stethoscope	
17-19 weeks	Fetal heart tones detected by fetal stethoscope	
19-22 weeks	Fetal movements palpated	
Late pregnancy	Fetal movements visible	

- Help the woman understand the anatomic and physiologic changes during pregnancy.
- Allay the woman's (and family's) anxiety, possibly resulting from a lack of knowledge.
- Teach the woman (and family) signs and symptoms that should be reported to the health care provider.

Signs of Pregnancy

Some of the physiologic adaptations are recognized as signs and symptoms of pregnancy. Three commonly used categories of **signs and symptoms of pregnancy** are **presumptive**, those changes felt by the woman (e.g., amenorrhea, fatigue, nausea and vomiting, breast changes); **probable**, those changes observed by an examiner (e.g., Hegar's sign, ballottement, pregnancy tests); and **positive**, those signs that are attributed only to the presence of the fetus (e.g., hearing fetal heart tones, visualization of the fetus, and palpating fetal movements). Table 15-2 summarizes these signs of pregnancy in rela-

tion to when they might occur and other causes for their occurrence.

REPRODUCTIVE SYSTEM AND BREASTS

Uterus

Changes in Size, Shape, and Position

The phenomenal uterine growth in the first trimester is stimulated by high levels of estrogen and progesterone. Early uterine enlargement results from increased vascularity and dilation of blood vessels, hyperplasia (production of new muscle fibers and fibroelastic tissue) and hypertrophy (enlargement of preexisting muscle fibers and fibroelastic tissue), and development of the decidua. By 7 weeks gestation the uterus is the size of a large hen's egg; by 10 weeks gestation, it is the size of an orange (twice its nonpregnant size); and by 12 weeks gestation, it is the size of a grapefruit. After the third month uterine enlargement is primarily the result of mechanical pressure of the growing fetus (Varney,

TABLE 15-3	Comparison of Measurements for Nonpregnant and Pregnant Uterus at 40 Weeks*	
MEASUREMENT	NONPREGNANT	PREGNANT (40 WEEKS)
Length	6.5 cm	32 cm
Width	4 cm	24 cm
Depth	2.5 cm	22 cm
Weight	60-70 g	1100-1200 g
Volume (capacity)	≥ 10 ml	5000 ml

*Note that references vary as to the exact values, but all references agree on the magnitude of the growth of the fetus during pregnancy.

1997). Table 15-3 compares uterine measurements for the nonpregnant and pregnant uterus at 40 weeks gestation.

As the uterus enlarges, it also changes in shape and position. At conception the uterus is shaped like an upside-down pear. During the second trimester, as the muscular walls strengthen and become more elastic, the uterus becomes spherical or globular. Later, as the fetus lengthens, the uterus becomes larger and more ovoid and rises out of the pelvis into the abdominal cavity.

The pregnancy may "show" after the fourteenth week, although this depends to some degree on the woman's height and weight. Abdominal enlargement may be less apparent in the nullipara with good abdominal muscle tone (Fig. 15-1). Posture also influences the type and degree of abdominal enlargement that occurs. In normal pregnancies the uterus enlarges at a predictable rate. Uterine enlargement is determined by measuring fundal height. This measurement is commonly used to estimate the duration of pregnancy. However, variation in the position of the fundus or the fetus, variations in the amount of amniotic fluid present, the presence of more than one fetus, maternal obesity, and variation in examiner techniques can reduce the accuracy of this estimation of the duration of pregnancy.

As the uterus grows and fills the pelvic cavity, it is elevated out of the pelvic area and may be palpated above the symphysis pubis some time between the twelfth and fourteenth weeks of pregnancy (Fig. 15-2). The uterus rises gradually to the level of the umbilicus at 22 to 24 weeks gestation and nearly reaches the xiphoid process at term. Between weeks 38 and 40, fundal height drops as the fetus begins to descend and engage in the pelvis (**lightening**) (Fig. 15-2, see dashed line). Generally, lightening occurs in the nullipara about 2 weeks before the onset of labor and at the start of labor in the multipara.

Generally the uterus rotates to the right as it elevates, probably because of the presence of the rectosigmoid colon on the left side. However, the extensive hypertrophy (enlargement) of the round ligaments keeps the uterus in the midline. Eventually the growing uterus touches the anterior abdominal wall and displaces the intestines to either

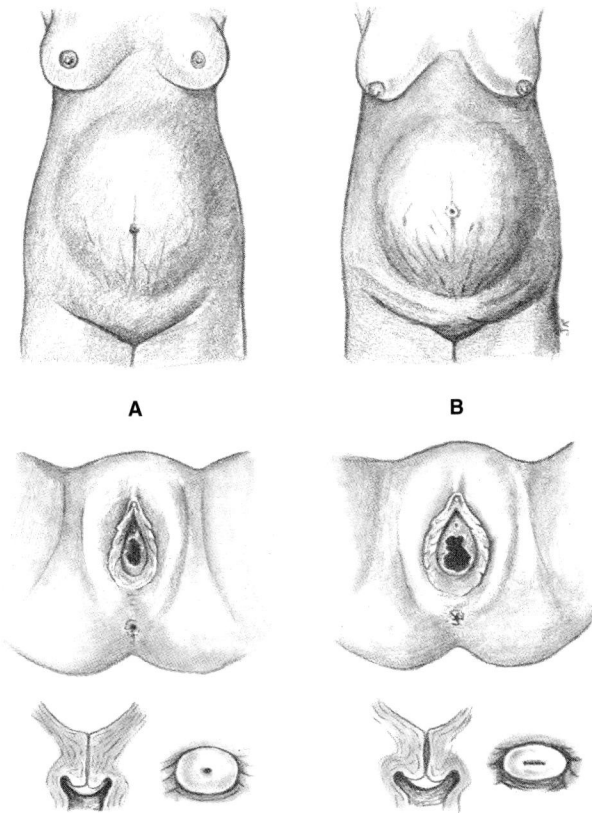

Fig. 15-1 Comparison of abdomen, vulva, and cervix in **A,** nullipara, and **B,** multipara, at the same stage of pregnancy.

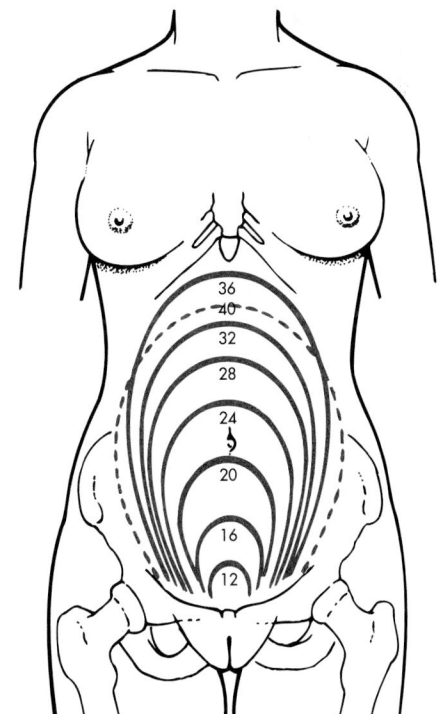

Fig. 15-2 Height of fundus by weeks of normal gestation with a single fetus. Dotted line indicates height after lightening. *(From Barkauskas, V. et al. [1994]. Health and physical assessment. St. Louis: Mosby.)*

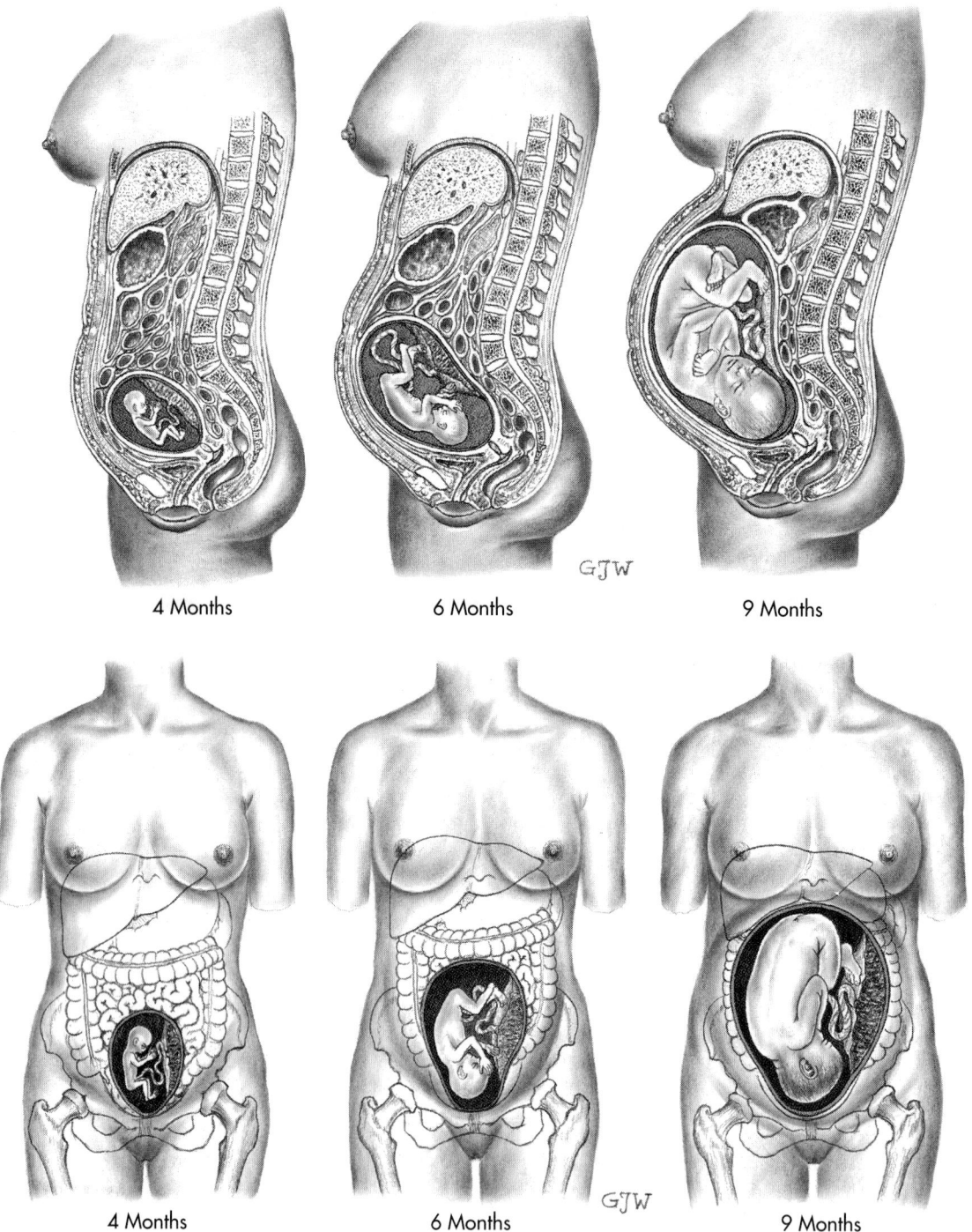

Fig. 15-3 Displacement of internal abdominal structures and diaphragm by the enlarging uterus at 4, 6, and 9 months of gestation.

4 Months   6 Months   9 Months

side of the abdomen (Fig. 15-3). Whenever a pregnant woman is standing, most of her uterus rests against the anterior abdominal wall and this contributes to altering her center of gravity.

During the early weeks of pregnancy an increase in uterine blood flow and lymph causes pelvic congestion and edema. As a result the uterus, cervix, and isthmus soften perceptibly and progressively, and the cervix takes on a bluish color (**Chadwick's sign,** a probable sign of pregnancy) (Creasy & Resnik, 1999).

At approximately 6 weeks gestation, softening and compressibility of the lower uterine segment (the uterine isthmus) occur **(Hegar's sign).** This results in exaggerated uterine anteflexion during the first 3 months of pregnancy

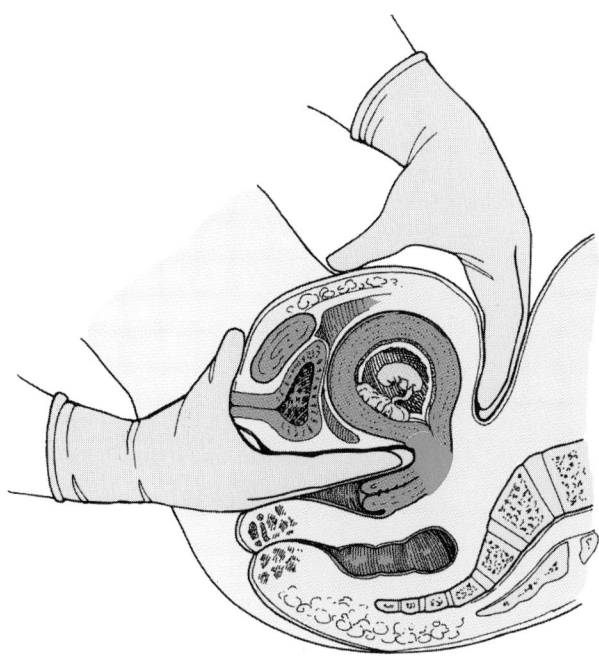

Fig. 15-4 Hegar's sign. Bimanual examination for assessing compressibility, softening of isthmus (lower uterine segment) while the cervix is still firm.

(Fig. 15-4). In this position the uterine fundus presses on the urinary bladder, causing the woman to experience urinary frequency.

Early uterine enlargement may not be symmetric, depending on the site of implantation. For example, if cornual implantation occurred, a soft, irregular bulge (Piskacek's sign) may be detected during a pelvic examination (Varney, 1997).

Changes in Contractility

Soon after the fourth month of pregnancy, uterine contractions can be felt through the abdominal wall. These contractions are referred to as the **Braxton Hicks sign,** a probable sign of pregnancy. Braxton Hicks contractions are irregular, painless contractions that occur intermittently throughout pregnancy. These contractions facilitate uterine blood flow through the intervillous spaces of the placenta and thereby promote oxygen delivery to the fetus. Although Braxton Hicks contractions are not painful, some women do complain that they are annoying. After the twenty-eighth week, these contractions become much more definite, but they usually cease with walking or exercise. Braxton Hicks contractions can be mistaken for true labor; however, they do not increase in intensity or frequency or cause cervical dilation.

Uteroplacental Blood Flow

Placental perfusion depends on the maternal blood flow to the uterus. Blood flow increases rapidly as the uterus increases in size. Although uterine blood flow increases twentyfold, the fetoplacental unit grows more rapidly. Consequently, more oxygen is extracted from the uterine blood during the latter part of pregnancy (Cunningham et al., 1997). In a normal term pregnancy, one sixth of the total maternal blood volume is within the uterine vascular system. The rate of blood flow through the uterus averages 500 ml/min, and oxygen consumption of the gravid uterus increases to meet fetal needs. A low maternal arterial pressure, contractions of the uterus, and maternal supine position are three factors known to decrease blood flow. Estrogen stimulation may increase uterine blood flow. Doppler ultrasound can be used to measure uterine blood flow velocity, especially in pregnancies at risk because of conditions associated with decreased placental perfusion such as hypertension, intrauterine growth restriction, diabetes mellitus, and multiple gestation (Creasy & Resnik, 1999).

Using an ultrasound device or a fetal stethoscope, the health care provider may hear the **uterine souffle,** or bruit, a rushing or blowing sound of maternal blood flowing through uterine arteries to the placenta that is synchronous with the maternal pulse. The **funic souffle,** which is synchronous with the fetal pulse rate and caused by fetal blood coursing through the umbilical cord, may also be heard as well as the actual fetal heart tones.

Cervical Changes

A softening of the cervical tip may be observed about the beginning of the sixth week in a normal, unscarred cervix. This probable sign of pregnancy, **Goodell's sign,** is brought about by increased vascularity, slight hypertrophy, and hyperplasia (increase in number of cells) of the muscle and its collagen-rich connective tissue, which becomes loose, edematous, highly elastic, and increased in volume. The glands near the external os proliferate beneath the stratified squamous epithelium, giving the cervix the velvety appearance characteristic of pregnancy (Fig. 15-5). **Friability** is increased; that is, the cervix bleeds easily when scraped or touched. Increased friability is the cause of the few drops of blood seen after coitus with deep penetration or after vaginal examination. These few drops are usually within normal limits. Pregnancy can also cause the squamocolumnar junction, the site for obtaining cells for cervical cancer screening to be located away from the cervix. Because of all these changes, evaluation of abnormal Papanicolaou tests during pregnancy can be complicated. However, careful assessment of all pregnant women is important because about 3% of all cervical cancers are diagnosed during pregnancy (Creasy & Resnik, 1999).

The cervix of the nullipara is rounded. Lacerations of the cervix almost always occur during the birth process. With or without lacerations, however, after childbirth the cervix becomes more oval in the horizontal plane, and the external os appears as a transverse slit (see Fig. 15-1).

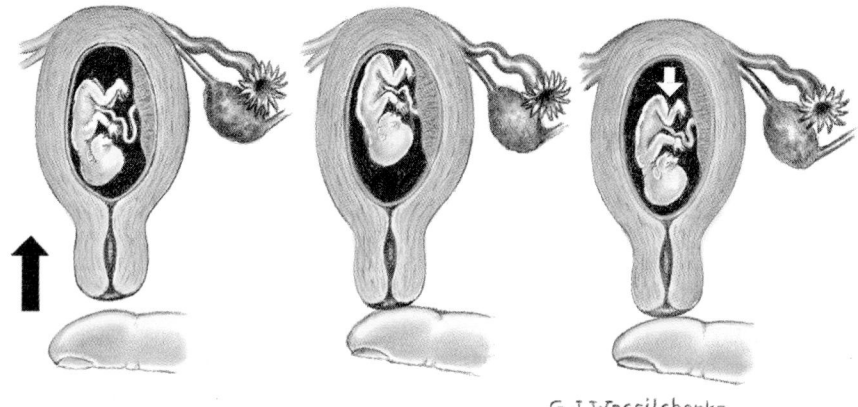

G.J. Wassilchenko

Fig. 15-5   Internal ballottement (18 weeks).

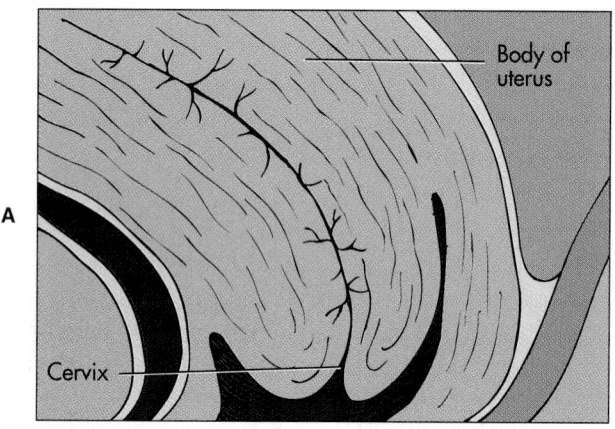

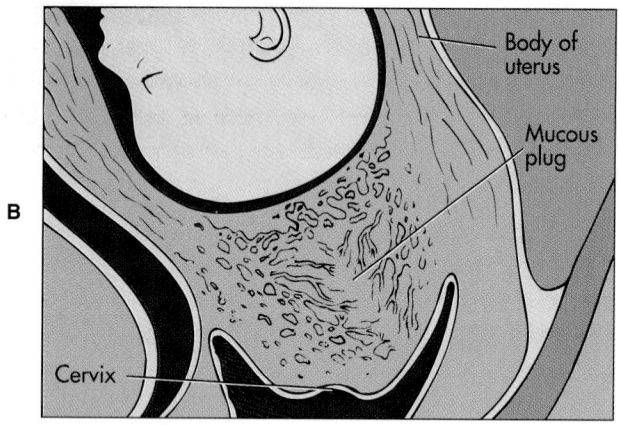

Fig. 15-6   **A,** Cervix in nonpregnant woman. **B,** Cervix during pregnancy.

Changes Related to the Presence of the Fetus

Passive movement of the unengaged fetus is called **ballottement** and can be identified generally between the sixteenth and eighteenth week. Ballottement is a technique of palpating a floating structure by bouncing it gently and feeling it rebound. In the technique used to palpate the fetus, the examiner places a finger in the vagina and taps gently upward, causing the fetus to rise. The fetus then

sinks, and a gentle tap is felt on the finger (see Fig. 15-5). Internal ballottement of a fetus within a uterus is a probable objective sign of pregnancy.

The first recognition of fetal movements, or "feeling life," by the multiparous woman may occur as early as the fourteenth to sixteenth week. The nulliparous woman may not notice these sensations until the eighteenth week or later. **Quickening,** a presumptive sign of pregnancy, is commonly described as a flutter and is difficult to distinguish from peristalsis. Gradually, fetal movements increase in intensity and frequency. The week when quickening occurs provides a tentative clue in dating the duration of gestation.

Vagina and Vulva

Pregnancy hormones prepare the vagina for stretching during labor and birth by causing the vaginal mucosa to thicken, connective tissue to loosen, smooth muscle to hypertrophy, and the vaginal vault to lengthen. Increased vascularity results in a violet-bluish color of the vaginal mucosa and cervix. The deepened color, termed Chadwick's sign, may be evident as early as the sixth week, but is easily noted at the eighth week of pregnancy.

Leukorrhea is a white or slightly gray mucoid discharge with a faint musty odor. This copious mucoid fluid occurs in response to cervical stimulation by estrogen and progesterone. The fluid is whitish because of the presence of many exfoliated vaginal epithelial cells caused by hyperplasia of normal pregnancy. This vaginal discharge is never pruritic or blood stained. Because of the progesterone effect, ferning usually does not occur in the dried cervical mucous smear, as it would in a smear of amniotic fluid. Instead, a beaded or cellular crystallizing pattern formed in the dried mucus is seen (Cunningham et al., 1997). The mucus fills the endocervical canal, resulting in the formation of the mucous plug (**operculum**) (Fig. 15-6). The operculum acts as a barrier against bacterial invasion during pregnancy.

During pregnancy, the pH of vaginal secretions ranges from about 4 to about 6.5. The acidic pH is a result of in-

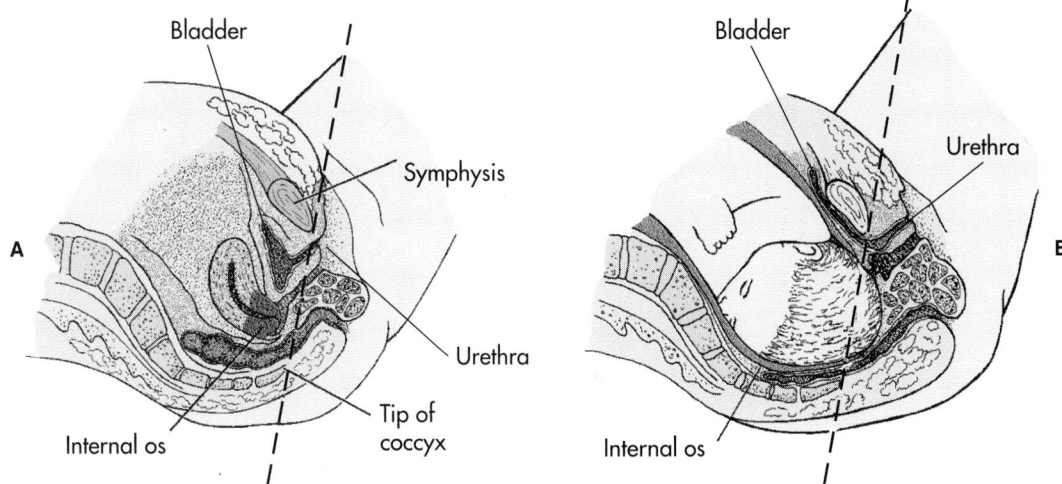

Fig. 15-7 A, Pelvic floor in nonpregnant woman. **B,** Pelvic floor at end of pregnancy. Note marked hypertrophy and hyperplasia below dotted line joining tip of coccyx and inferior margin of symphysis. Note elongation of bladder and urethra as a result of compression. Fat deposits are increased.

creased production of lactic acid in the vaginal epithelium, probably caused by increased estrogen levels. The pregnant woman is more vulnerable to vaginal infections, especially yeast infections (Mishell et al., 1997).

The increased vascularity of the vagina and other pelvic viscera results in a marked increase in sensitivity. The increased sensitivity may lead to a high degree of sexual interest and arousal, especially during the second trimester of pregnancy. The increased congestion plus the relaxed walls of the blood vessels and the heavy uterus may result in edema and varicosities of the vulva. The edema and varicosities usually resolve during the postpartum period.

External structures of the perineum are enlarged during pregnancy because of an increase in vasculature, hypertrophy of the perineal body, and deposition of fat (Fig. 15-7). The labia majora of the nullipara approximate and obscure the vaginal introitus; those of the parous woman separate and gape after childbirth and perineal or vaginal injury. Figure 15-1 compares the perineum of the nullipara and the multipara in relation to the pregnant abdomen, vulva, and cervix.

Breasts

Fullness, heightened sensitivity, tingling, and heaviness of the breasts begins in the early weeks of gestation in response to increased levels of estrogen and progesterone. These changes are considered presumptive signs of pregnancy because other factors can cause them to occur. Breast sensitivity varies from mild tingling to sharp pain. Nipples and areolae become more pigmented, secondary pinkish areolae develop, extending beyond the primary areolae, and nipples become more erectile. Hypertrophy of the sebaceous (oil) glands embedded in the primary areolae, called **Montgomery's tubercles** (see Fig. 6-6), may be

seen around the nipples. These sebaceous glands may have a protective role in that they keep the nipples lubricated for breastfeeding. Suppleness of the nipples is jeopardized if the protective oils are washed off with soap.

The richer blood supply causes the vessels beneath the skin to dilate. Once barely noticeable, the blood vessels become visible, often appearing in an intertwining blue network beneath the surface of the skin. Venous congestion in the breasts is more obvious in primigravidas. Striae gravidarum may appear at the outer aspects of the breasts.

During the second and third trimesters, growth of the mammary glands accounts for the progressive breast enlargement. The high levels of luteal and placental hormones in pregnancy promote proliferation of the lactiferous ducts and lobule-alveolar tissue, so that palpation of the breasts reveals a generalized, coarse nodularity. Glandular tissue displaces connective tissue, and as a result the tissue becomes softer and looser.

Although development of the mammary glands is functionally complete by midpregnancy, lactation is inhibited until a drop in estrogen level occurs after the birth. A thin, clear, viscous secretory material (precolostrum) can be found in the acini cells by the third month of gestation. **Colostrum,** the creamy, white-to-yellowish to orange premilk fluid, may be expressed from the nipples as early as 16 weeks of gestation (Lawrence, 1999). See Chapter 28 for discussion of lactation.

GENERAL BODY SYSTEMS

Cardiovascular System

Maternal adjustments to pregnancy involve extensive changes in the cardiovascular system, both anatomic and physiologic. Cardiovascular adaptations protect the

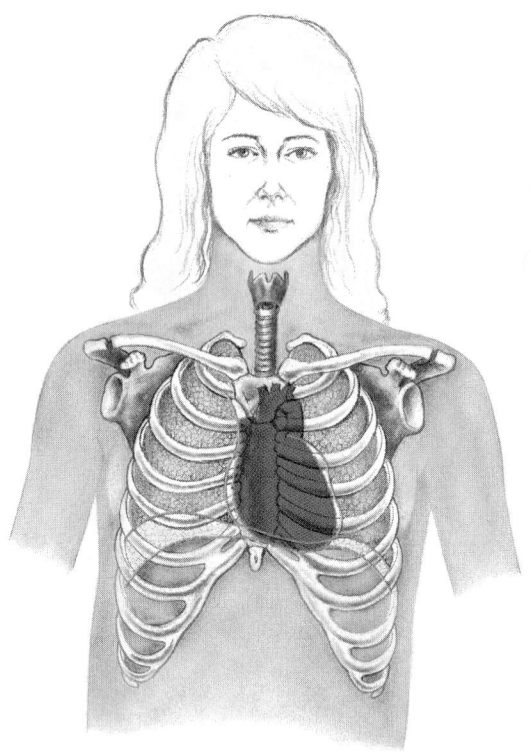

G. J. Wassilchenko

Fig. 15-8 Changes in position of heart, lungs, and thoracic cage in pregnancy. *Broken line,* nonpregnant; *solid line,* change that occurs in pregnancy.

woman's normal physiologic functioning, meet the metabolic demands pregnancy imposes on her body, and provide for fetal developmental and growth needs.

Slight cardiac hypertrophy (enlargement) is probably secondary to the increased blood volume and cardiac output that occurs. The heart returns to its normal size after childbirth. As the diaphragm is displaced upward by the enlarging uterus, the heart is elevated upward and rotated forward to the left (Fig. 15-8). The apical impulse, a point of maximum intensity (PMI), is shifted upward and laterally about 1 to 1.5 cm. The degree of shift depends on the duration of pregnancy and the size and position of the uterus.

The changes in heart size and position and increases in blood volume and cardiac output contribute to auscultatory changes common in pregnancy. There is more audible splitting of S₁ and S₂, and S₃ may be readily heard after 20 weeks of gestation. Additionally, systolic and diastolic murmurs may be heard over the pulmonic area. These are transient and disappear shortly after the woman gives birth (Cunningham et al., 1997).

Between 14 and 20 weeks gestation, the pulse increases about 10 to 15 beats/min, which then persists to term. Palpitations may occur. In twin gestations, the maternal heart rate increases significantly in the third trimester (Creasy & Resnik, 1999).

The cardiac rhythm may be disturbed. The pregnant woman may experience sinus arrhythmia, premature atrial contractions, and premature ventricular systole. In the healthy woman with no underlying heart disease, no therapy is needed; however, women with preexisting heart disease will need close medical and obstetric supervision during pregnancy (see Chapter 33).

Blood Pressure

Arterial blood pressure (brachial artery) is affected by age, activity level, and presence of health problems. Additional factors must be considered during pregnancy. These factors include maternal anxiety, maternal position, and size and type of blood pressure apparatus.

Maternal anxiety can elevate readings. If an elevated reading is found, the woman is given time to rest, and the reading is repeated.

Maternal position affects readings. Brachial blood pressure is highest when the woman is sitting, lowest when she is lying in the lateral recumbent position, and intermediate when she is supine, except for some women who experience supine hypotensive syndrome (see discussion below). Therefore at each prenatal visit the reading should be obtained in the same arm and with the woman in the same position. The position and arm used should be recorded along with the reading.

The proper size cuff is absolutely necessary for accurate readings. The cuff should be 20% wider than the diameter of the arm around which it is wrapped, or about 12 to 14 cm for average-sized individuals and 18 to 20 cm for obese persons. Too small a cuff yields a false high reading; too large a cuff yields a false low reading. Caution should also be used when comparing auscultatory and oscillatory blood pressure readings because discrepancies can occur (Green & Froman, 1996).

In the first trimester, blood pressure usually remains the same as the prepregnancy level. During the second trimester, there is a decrease in both systolic and diastolic pressure of 5 to 10 mm Hg. This decrease is probably the result of peripheral vasodilation caused by hormonal changes that occur during pregnancy. During the third trimester, maternal blood pressure should return to the first trimester levels.

Calculating the **mean arterial pressure (MAP)** (mean of the blood pressure in the arterial circulation) can increase the diagnostic value of the findings. Normal MAP readings in the nonpregnant woman are 86.4 mm Hg ±7.5 mm Hg. MAP readings for a pregnant woman are slightly higher (Creasy & Resnik, 1999). One way to calculate a MAP is illustrated in Box 15-2.

Some degree of compression of the vena cava occurs in all women who lie flat on their backs during the second half of pregnancy (see Fig. 22-4). Some women experience a fall in their systolic blood pressure of more than 30 mm Hg. After 4 to 5 minutes a reflex bradycardia is noted, cardiac output is reduced by half, and the woman feels faint.

Blood pressure: 106/70

Formula: $\dfrac{(systolic) + 2(diastolic)}{3}$

$$\dfrac{(106) + 2(70)}{3}$$

$$\dfrac{106 + 140}{3}$$

$$246/3 = 82 \text{ mm Hg}$$

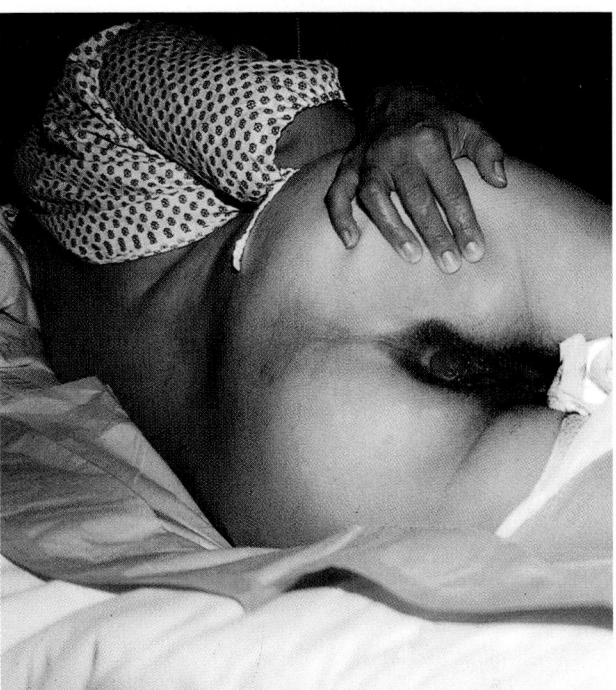

Fig. 15-9 Hemorrhoids. *(Courtesy Marjorie Pyle, RNC, Lifecircle, Costa Mesa, CA.)*

This condition is referred to as *supine hypotensive syndrome* (Cunningham et al., 1997).

Compression of the iliac veins and inferior vena cava by the uterus causes increased venous pressure and reduced blood flow in the legs (except when the woman is in the lateral position). These alterations contribute to the dependent edema, varicose veins in the legs and vulva, and hemorrhoids that develop in the latter part of term pregnancy (Fig. 15-9).

Blood Volume and Composition

The degree of blood volume expansion varies considerably. Blood volume increases by approximately 1500 ml, or 40% to 50% above nonpregnancy levels (Cunningham et al., 1997). This increase consists of 1000 ml plasma plus 450 ml red blood cells (RBCs). The blood volume starts to increase about the tenth to twelfth week, peaks about the thirty-second to thirty-fourth week, then decreases slightly at the fortieth week. The increase in volume of a multiple gestation is greater than that for a pregnancy with a single fetus (Creasy & Resnik, 1999). Increased volume is a protective mechanism. It is essential for meeting the blood needs of the hypertrophied vascular system of the enlarged uterus, adequately hydrating fetal and maternal tissues when the woman assumes an erect or supine position, and providing a fluid reserve to compensate for blood loss during birth and the puerperium. Peripheral vasodilation maintains a normal blood pressure despite the increased blood volume in pregnancy.

During pregnancy there is an accelerated production of RBCs (normal 4.2 to 5.4 million/mm³). The percentage of increase depends on the amount of iron available. The RBC mass increases by about 17% (Creasy & Resnik, 1999).

Because the plasma increase exceeds the increase in RBC production, there is a decrease in normal hemoglobin values (12 to 16 g/dl blood) and hematocrit values (37% to 47%). This state of hemodilution is referred to as **physiologic anemia**. The decrease is more noticeable during the second trimester, when rapid expansion of blood volume takes place faster than red blood cell production. If the hemoglobin value drops to 10 g/dl or less or if the hematocrit drops to 35% or less, the woman is considered anemic.

The total white cell count increases during the second trimester and peaks during the third trimester. This increase is primarily in the granulocytes; the lymphocyte count stays about the same throughout pregnancy. See Appendix A for laboratory values during pregnancy.

Cardiac Output

Cardiac output increases from 30% to 50% over the nonpregnant rate by the thirty-second week of pregnancy; it declines to about a 20% increase at 40 weeks gestation. This elevated cardiac output is largely a result of increased stroke volume and heart rate and occurs in response to increased tissue demands for oxygen (Creasy & Resnik, 1999). Cardiac output in late pregnancy is appreciably higher when the woman is in the lateral recumbent position than when she is supine. In the supine position, the large, heavy uterus often impedes venous return to the heart and affects blood pressure. Cardiac output increases with any exertion, such as labor and birth. Box 15-3 summarizes cardiovascular changes in pregnancy.

Circulation and Coagulation Times

The circulation time decreases slightly by week 32. It returns to near normal near term. There is a greater tendency for blood to coagulate (clot) during pregnancy because of increases in various clotting factors (Factors VII, VIII, IX,

BOX 15-3 Cardiovascular Changes in Pregnancy

Heart rate	Increases 10-15 beats/min
Blood pressure	Remains at prepregnancy levels in first trimester
	Slight decrease in second trimester
	Returns to prepregnancy levels in third trimester
Blood volume	Increases by 1500 ml or 40%-50% above prepregnancy level
Red blood cell mass	Increases 17%
Hemoglobin	Decreases
Hematocrit	Decreases
White blood cell count	Increases in second and third trimester
Cardiac output	Increases 30%-50%

BOX 15-4 Respiratory Changes in Pregnancy

Respiratory rate	Unchanged or slightly increased
Tidal volume	Increased 30%-40%
Vital capacity	Unchanged
Inspiratory capacity	Increased
Expiratory volume	Decreased
Total lung capacity	Unchanged to slightly decreased
Oxygen consumption	Increased 15%-20%

X, and fibrinogen). This, combined with the fact that fibrinolytic activity (the splitting up or the dissolving of a clot) is depressed during pregnancy and the postpartum period, provides a protective function to decrease the chance of bleeding but also makes the woman more vulnerable to thrombosis, especially after cesarean birth.

Respiratory System

Structural and ventilatory adaptations occur during pregnancy to provide for maternal and fetal needs. Maternal oxygen requirements increase in response to the acceleration in the metabolic rate and the need to add to the tissue mass in the uterus and breasts. In addition, the fetus requires oxygen and a way to eliminate carbon dioxide.

Elevated levels of estrogen cause the ligaments of the rib cage to relax, permitting increased chest expansion (see Fig. 15-8). The transverse diameter of the thoracic cage increases by about 2 cm, and the circumference increases by 6 cm (Cunningham et al., 1997). The costal angle increases and the lower rib cage appears to flare out. The chest may not return to its prepregnant state after birth (Seidel et al., 1999).

The diaphragm is displaced by as much as 4 cm during pregnancy. As pregnancy advances, thoracic (costal) breathing replaces abdominal breathing, and it becomes less possible for the diaphragm to descend with inspiration. Thoracic breathing is primarily accomplished by the diaphragm rather than by the costal muscles (Blackburn & Loper, 1992).

The upper respiratory tract becomes more vascular in response to elevated levels of estrogen. As the capillaries become engorged, edema and hyperemia develop within the nose, pharynx, larynx, trachea, and bronchi. This congestion within the tissues of the respiratory tract gives rise

to several conditions commonly seen during pregnancy. These conditions include nasal and sinus stuffiness, epistaxis (nosebleed), changes in the voice, and a marked inflammatory response that can develop into a mild upper respiratory infection.

Increased vascularity of the upper respiratory tract also can cause the tympanic membranes and eustachian tubes to swell, giving rise to symptoms of impaired hearing, earaches, or a sense of fullness in the ears.

Pulmonary Function

The pregnant woman breathes deeper or increases her tidal volume, which is the volume of gas moved into or out of the respiratory tract with each breath. The respiratory rate remains unchanged or is only slightly increased (about two breaths per minute). The expiratory reserve volume and residual volume decrease progressively during pregnancy. The inspiratory capacity increases slightly while the vital capacity remains unchanged. The total lung capacity decreases slightly. These changes are related to the elevation of the diaphragm and chest wall changes (Creasy & Resnik, 1999). (See Box 15-4 for respiratory changes in pregnancy.)

During pregnancy, changes in the respiratory center result in a lowered threshold for carbon dioxide. The actions of progesterone and estrogen are presumed responsible for the increased sensitivity of the respiratory center to carbon dioxide. In addition, pregnant women become more aware of the need to breathe; some may even complain of dyspnea at rest.

Although pulmonary function is not impaired by pregnancy, diseases of the respiratory tract may be more serious during this time (Cunningham et al., 1997). One important factor responsible for this may be the increased oxygen requirement.

Basal Metabolism Rate

The basal metabolism rate (BMR) varies considerably in women at the beginning and during pregnancy, although it usually increases by 15% to 20% at term (Worthington-Roberts & Williams, 1997). The BMR returns to nonpregnant levels by 5 to 6 days postpartum.

BOX 15-5 Acid-Base Values in Arterial Blood of Pregnant Women

PO$_2$	104-108 mm Hg (increased)
PCO$_2$	27-32 mm Hg (decreased)
Sodium bicarbonate (HCO$_3$)	18-31 mEq/L (decreased)
Blood pH	7.40-7.45 (slightly increased— more alkaline)

From Gabbe, S., Niebyl, J., & Simpson, J. (1996). *Obstetrics: Normal and problem pregnancies* (3rd ed.). New York: Churchill Livingstone.

The elevation in BMR during pregnancy reflects increased oxygen demands of the uterine-placental-fetal unit and greater oxygen consumption because of increased maternal cardiac work (Chamberlain & Pipkin, 1998). Peripheral vasodilation and acceleration of sweat gland activity help dissipate the excess heat resulting from the increased BMR during pregnancy. Pregnant women may experience heat intolerance, which is annoying to some women. Lassitude and fatigability after only slight exertion are experienced by many women in early pregnancy. These feelings, along with a greater need for sleep, may persist and may be caused in part by the increased metabolic activity.

Acid-Base Balance

By about the tenth week of pregnancy, there is a decrease of about 5 mm Hg in the partial pressure of carbon dioxide (PCO$_2$). Progesterone may be responsible for increasing the sensitivity of the respiratory center receptors, so that tidal volume is increased and PCO$_2$ falls, the base excess (HCO$_3$, or bicarbonate) falls, and pH increases slightly. These alterations in acid-base balance indicate that pregnancy is a state of respiratory alkalosis compensated by mild metabolic acidosis (Chamberlain & Pipkin, 1998). These changes also facilitate the transport of CO$_2$ from the fetus and O$_2$ release from the mother to the fetus. Box 15-5 lists acid-base values during pregnancy.

Renal System

The kidneys are responsible for maintaining electrolyte and acid-base balance, regulating extracellular fluid volume, excreting waste products, and conserving essential nutrients.

Anatomic Changes

Changes in renal structure during pregnancy result from hormonal activity (estrogen and progesterone), pressure from an enlarging uterus, and an increase in blood volume. As early as the tenth week of pregnancy, the renal pelvis and the ureters dilate. Dilation of the ureters is more pronounced above the pelvic brim, in part because they are compressed between the uterus and the pelvic brim. In most women the ureters below the pelvic brim are of normal size. The smooth-muscle walls of the ureters undergo hyperplasia and hypertrophy and muscle tone relaxation.

The ureters elongate, become tortuous, and form single or double curves. In the latter part of pregnancy, the renal pelvis and ureter are dilated more on the right side than on the left because the heavy uterus is displaced to the right by the sigmoid colon.

Because of these changes, a larger volume of urine is held in the pelves and ureters, and urine flow rate is slowed. The resulting urinary stasis or stagnation has the following consequences:

- There is a lag between the time urine is formed and when it reaches the bladder. Therefore clearance test results may reflect substances contained in glomerular filtrate several hours before.
- Stagnated urine is an excellent medium for the growth of microorganisms. In addition, the urine of pregnant women contains more nutrients, including glucose, thereby increasing the pH (making the urine more alkaline). This makes pregnant women more susceptible to urinary tract infection.

Bladder irritability, nocturia, and urinary frequency and urgency (without dysuria) are commonly reported in early pregnancy. Near term, bladder symptoms may return, especially after lightening occurs.

Urinary frequency results initially from increased bladder sensitivity and later from compression of the bladder (see Fig. 15-7). In the second trimester the bladder is pulled up out of the true pelvis into the abdomen. The urethra lengthens to 7.5 cm as the bladder is displaced upward. The pelvic congestion that occurs in pregnancy is reflected in hyperemia of the bladder and urethra. This increased vascularity causes the bladder mucosa to be traumatized and bleed easily. Bladder tone may decrease, which increases the bladder capacity to 1500 ml. At the same time the bladder is compressed by the enlarging uterus, resulting in the urge to void even if the bladder contains only a small amount of urine.

Functional Changes

In normal pregnancy, renal function is altered considerably. Glomerular filtration rate (GFR) and renal plasma flow (RPF) increase early in pregnancy (Cunningham et al., 1997). These changes are caused by pregnancy hormones, an increase in blood volume, the woman's posture, physical activity, and nutritional intake. The woman's kidneys must manage the increased metabolic and circulatory demands of the maternal body and also excretion of fetal waste products.

Renal function is most efficient when the woman lies in the lateral recumbent position and least efficient when the woman assumes a supine position. A side-lying position increases renal perfusion, which increases urinary output and decreases edema. When the pregnant woman is lying supine, the heavy uterus compresses the vena cava and the aorta, and cardiac output decreases. As a result, blood flow to the brain and heart is continued at the expense of other organs, including the kidneys and uterus.

Fluid and Electrolyte Balance

Selective renal tubular reabsorption maintains sodium and water balance regardless of changes in dietary intake and losses through sweat, vomitus, or diarrhea. From 500 to 900 mEq of sodium is normally retained during pregnancy to meet fetal needs. To prevent excessive sodium depletion, the maternal kidneys undergo a significant adaptation by increasing tubular reabsorption. Because of the need for increased maternal intravascular and extracellular fluid volume, additional sodium is needed to expand fluid volume and to maintain an isotonic state. As efficient as the renal system is, it can be overstressed by excessive dietary sodium intake or restriction or by use of diuretics. Severe hypovolemia and reduced placental perfusion are two consequences of using diuretics during pregnancy.

The capacity of the kidneys to excrete water during the early weeks of pregnancy is more efficient than later in pregnancy. As a result, some women feel thirsty in early pregnancy because of the greater amount of water loss. The pooling of fluid in the legs in the latter part of pregnancy decreases renal blood flow and GFR. This pooling of blood in the lower legs is sometimes referred to as *physiologic edema* or dependent edema and requires no treatment. The normal diuretic response to the water load is triggered when the woman lies down, preferably on her side, and the pooled fluid reenters general circulation.

Normally the kidney reabsorbs almost all of the glucose and other nutrients from the plasma filtrate. In pregnant women, however, tubular reabsorption of glucose is impaired so that glucosuria occurs at varying times and to varying degrees. Normal values range from 0 to 20 mg/dl, meaning that during any one day the urine is sometimes positive and sometimes negative. In nonpregnant women, blood glucose levels must be at 160 to 180 mg/dl before glucose is "spilled" into the urine (not reabsorbed). During pregnancy, glycosuria occurs when maternal glucose levels are lower than 160 mg/dl. Why glucose, as well as other nutrients such as amino acids, is wasted during pregnancy is not understood, nor has the exact mechanism been discovered. Although glycosuria may be found in normal pregnancies (1+ levels may be seen with increased anxiety states), the possibility of diabetes mellitus and gestational diabetes must be kept in mind.

Proteinuria usually does not occur in normal pregnancy except during labor or after birth (Cunningham et al., 1997). However, the increased amount of amino acids that needs to be filtered may exceed the capacity of the renal tubules to absorb it, so that small amounts of protein are then lost in the urine. Values of trace to 1+ protein (dipstick assessment) or less than 300 mg/24 hr are acceptable during pregnancy (Blackburn & Loper, 1992). The amount of protein excreted is not an indication of the severity of renal disease, nor does an increase in protein excretion in a pregnant woman with known renal disease necessarily indicate a progression in her disease. However, a pregnant woman with hypertension and proteinuria must be care-

fully evaluated because she may be at greater risk for an adverse pregnancy outcome. (See Box 15-6 for renal changes during pregnancy.)

Integumentary System

Alterations in hormonal balance and mechanical stretching are responsible for several changes in the integumentary system during pregnancy. General changes include increases in skin thickness and subdermal fat, hyperpigmentation, hair and nail growth, accelerated sweat and sebaceous gland activity, and increased circulation and vasomotor activity. Cutaneous elastic tissues are more fragile, resulting in striae gravidarum, or stretch marks. Cutaneous allergic responses are enhanced as well.

Hyperpigmentation is stimulated by the anterior pituitary hormone melanotropin, which is increased during pregnancy. Darkening of the nipples, areolae, axillae, and vulva occurs about the sixteenth week of gestation. Facial melasma, also called **chloasma** or mask of pregnancy, is a blotchy, brownish hyperpigmentation of the skin over the cheeks, nose, and forehead, especially in dark-complexioned pregnant women. Chloasma appears in 50% to 70% of pregnant women, beginning after the sixteenth week and increasing gradually until term. The sun intensifies this pigmentation in susceptible women. Chloasma caused by normal pregnancy usually fades after birth.

The **linea nigra** (Fig. 15-10) is a pigmented line extending from the symphysis pubis to the top of the fundus in the midline; this line is known as the *linea alba* before hormone-induced pigmentation. In primigravidas the exten-

---

BOX 15-6 | **Renal Changes in Pregnancy**

Bladder capacity	Increased to 1500 ml
Glomerular rate filtration (GFR)	Increased 30%-50%
Renal plasma flow (RPF)	Increased 30%

RENAL LABORATORY VALUES
Serum

Blood urea nitrogen (BUN)	Decreased (normal: 8-20 mg/dl)
Creatinine	Decreased (normal: 0.6-1.2 mg/dl)
Uric acid	Decreased first and second trimesters (normal: 4.5-5.8 mg/dl) Returns to prepregnancy levels in third trimester

Urine

Glucose	Present in urine of 20% of pregnant women (normal: 0-20 mg/dl)

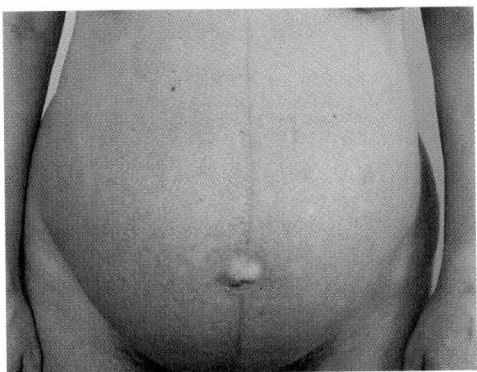

Fig. 15-10 Linea nigra. *(Seidel, H. et al. [1999]. Mosby's guide to physical examination [4th ed.]. St. Louis: Mosby.)*

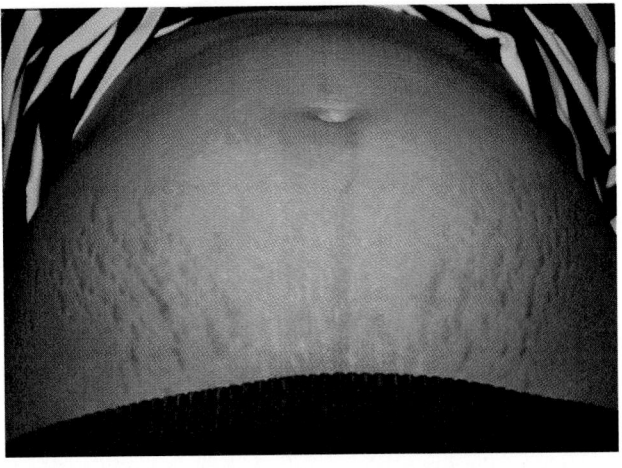

Fig. 15-11 Striae gravidarum, or "stretch marks." *(Courtesy Michael S. Clement, MD, Mesa, AZ.)*

sion of the linea nigra, beginning in the third month, keeps pace with the rising height of the fundus; in multigravidas the entire line often appears earlier than the third month. Not all pregnant women develop linea nigra.

Striae gravidarum, or stretch marks (seen over lower abdomen in Fig. 15-11), which appear in 50% to 90% of pregnant women during the second half of pregnancy, may be caused by action of adrenocorticosteroids. Striae reflect separation within the underlying connective (collagen) tissue of the skin. These slightly depressed streaks tend to occur over areas of maximum stretch (i.e., abdomen, thighs, and breasts). The stretching sometimes causes a sensation that resembles itching. The tendency to develop striae may be familial. After birth they usually fade, although they never disappear completely. Color of striae varies depending on the pregnant woman's skin color. The striae appear pinkish on a woman with light skin and are lighter than surrounding skin in dark-skinned women. In the multipara, in addition to the striae of the present pregnancy, glistening silvery lines (in light-skinned women) or purplish lines (in dark-skinned women) are commonly seen. These represent the scars of striae from previous pregnancies.

Angiomas are commonly referred to as vascular spiders. They are tiny, star-shaped or branched, slightly raised and pulsating end-arterioles usually found on the neck, thorax, face, and arms. They occur as a result of elevated levels of circulating estrogen. The spiders are bluish in color and do not blanch with pressure. Vascular spiders appear during the second to the fifth month of pregnancy in 65% of Caucasian women and 10% of African-American women. The spiders usually disappear after birth.

Pinkish-red, diffuse mottling or well-defined blotches are seen over the palmar surfaces of the hands in about 60% of Caucasian women and 35% of African-American women during pregnancy (Cunningham et al., 1997). These color changes, called **palmar erythema,** are related primarily to increased estrogen levels. (See Box 15-7 for ethnic considerations for skin assessment during pregnancy.)

BOX 15-7   Ethnic Considerations for Skin Assessment During Pregnancy

Integumentary system changes vary greatly among women of different racial backgrounds. For example, vascular spiders and palmar erythema are seen more often in Caucasian women than in African-American women. Areolar pigmentation varies by race: African-American women have the darkest areolae, Caucasian women have the lightest, and Asian women and Native American women have intermediate pigmentation. When performing physical assessments, the color of the woman's skin should be noted along with any changes that may be attributed to pregnancy.

Pruritis is a relatively common dermatologic symptom in pregnancy, with cholestasis of pregnancy being the most common cause of pruritic rash. The goal of management is to relieve the itching. Topical steroids are the usual treatment, although systemic steroids may be needed. The problem usually resolves in the postpartum period (Gordon & Landon, 1996).

Gum hypertrophy may occur. An **epulis** (gingival granuloma gravidarum) is a red, raised nodule on the gums that bleeds easily. This lesion may develop around the third month and usually continues to enlarge as pregnancy progresses. It is usually managed by avoiding trauma to the gums (e.g., using a soft toothbrush). An epulis usually regresses spontaneously after birth.

Nail growth may be accelerated. Some women may notice thinning and softening of the nails. Oily skin and acne vulgaris may occur during pregnancy. For some women the skin clears and looks radiant. Hirsutism, the excessive growth of hair or growth of hair in unusual places, is commonly reported. An increase in fine hair growth may occur but tends to disappear after pregnancy. However,

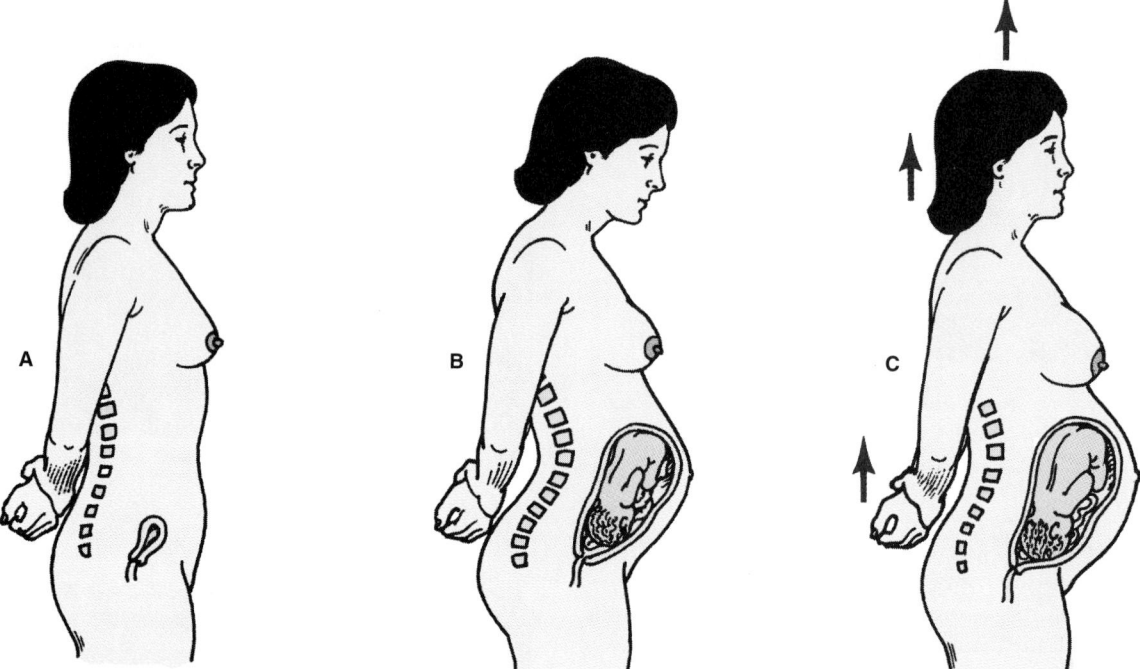

Fig. 15-12 Postural changes during pregnancy. **A,** Nonpregnant. **B,** Incorrect posture during pregnancy. **C,** Correct posture during pregnancy.

growth of coarse or bristly hair does not usually disappear after pregnancy.

Increased blood supply to the skin leads to increased perspiration. Women feel hotter during pregnancy, possibly related to a progesterone-induced increase in body temperature and the increased BMR.

Musculoskeletal System

The gradually changing body and increasing weight of the pregnant woman cause noticeable alterations in her posture (Fig. 15-12) and the way she walks. The great abdominal distention that gives the pelvis a forward tilt, decreased abdominal muscle tone, and increased weight bearing require a realignment of the spinal curvature late in pregnancy. The woman's center of gravity shifts forward. An increase in the normal lumbosacral curve (lordosis) develops, and a compensatory curvature in the cervicodorsal region (exaggerated anterior flexion of the head) develops to help her maintain her balance. Aching, numbness, and weakness of the upper extremities may result. Large breasts and a stoop-shouldered stance will further accentuate the lumbar and dorsal curves. Walking is more difficult, and the waddling gait of the pregnant woman, called "the proud walk of pregnancy" by Shakespeare, is well known. The ligamentous and muscular structures of the middle and lower spine may be severely stressed. These and related changes often cause musculoskeletal discomfort.

The young, well-muscled woman may tolerate these changes without complaint. However, older women or those with a back disorder or a faulty sense of balance may have a considerable amount of back pain during and just after pregnancy.

Slight relaxation and increased mobility of the pelvic joints are normal during pregnancy. They are secondary to the exaggerated elasticity and softening of connective and collagen tissue caused by increased circulating steroid sex hormones, especially estrogen. Relaxin, an ovarian hormone, assists in this relaxation and softening. These adaptations permit enlargement of pelvic dimensions to facilitate labor and birth. The degree of relaxation varies, but considerable separation of the symphysis pubis and the instability of the sacroiliac joints may cause pain and difficulty in walking. Obesity and multifetal pregnancy tend to increase the pelvic instability. Peripheral joint laxity also increases as pregnancy progresses, but the cause is not known (Schauberger et al., 1996).

The muscles of the abdominal wall stretch and ultimately lose some tone. During the third trimester the rectus abdominis muscles may separate (Fig. 15-13), allowing abdominal contents to protrude at the midline. The umbilicus flattens or protrudes. After birth, the muscles gradually regain tone. However, separation of the muscles (**diastasis recti abdominis**) may persist.

Neurologic System

Little is known regarding specific alterations in function of the neurologic system during pregnancy, aside from hypothalamic-pituitary neurohormonal changes. Specific phys-

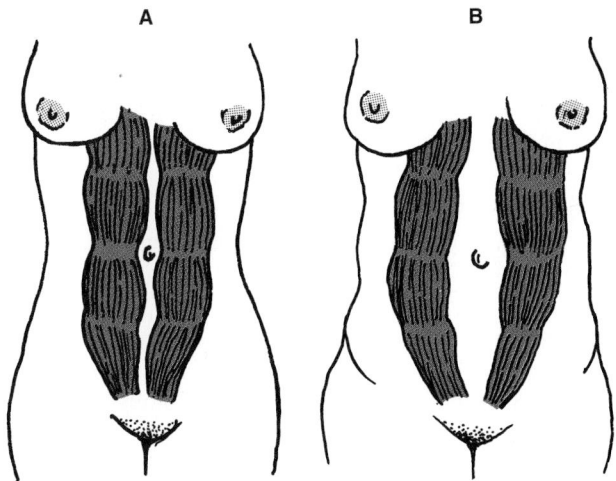

Fig. 15-13 Possible change in rectus abdominis muscles during pregnancy. **A,** Normal position in nonpregnant woman. **B,** Diastasis recti abdominis in pregnant woman.

iologic alterations resulting from pregnancy may cause the following neurologic or neuromuscular symptoms:

- Compression of pelvic nerves or vascular stasis caused by enlargement of the uterus may result in sensory changes in the legs.
- Dorsolumbar lordosis may cause pain because of traction on nerves or compression of nerve roots.
- Edema involving the peripheral nerves may result in **carpal tunnel syndrome** during the last trimester. The syndrome is characterized by paresthesia (abnormal sensation such as burning or tingling) and pain in the hand, radiating to the elbow. The sensations are caused by edema that compresses the median nerve beneath the carpal ligament of the wrist. The dominant hand is usually affected most, although as many as 80% of women experience symptoms in both hands. Symptoms usually regress after pregnancy. In some cases, surgical treatment may be necessary (Cunningham et al., 1997).
- Acroesthesia (numbness and tingling of the hands) is caused by the stoop-shouldered stance (see Fig. 15-12, *B*) assumed by some women during pregnancy. The condition is associated with traction on segments of the brachial plexus.
- Tension headache is common when anxiety or uncertainty complicates pregnancy. However, vision problems, sinusitis, or migraine may also be responsible for headaches.
- "Lightheadedness," faintness, and even syncope (fainting) are common during early pregnancy. Vasomotor instability, postural hypotension, or hypoglycemia may be responsible.
- Hypocalcemia may cause neuromuscular problems such as muscle cramps or tetany.

Gastrointestinal System

A variety of gastrointestinal system changes occur during pregnancy. The appetite fluctuates, intestinal secretion is reduced, liver function is altered, and absorption of nutrients is enhanced. The colon is displaced laterally upward and posteriorly. Peristaltic activity (motility) decreases. As a result bowel sounds are diminished, and constipation, nausea, and vomiting are common. Blood flow to the pelvis increases as does venous pressure, contributing to hemorrhoid formation in later pregnancy.

Appetite

During pregnancy, the pregnant woman's appetite and food intake fluctuate. Early in pregnancy, some women experience "morning sickness" in response to increasing levels of hCG and altered carbohydrate metabolism. *Morning sickness* refers to nausea with or without vomiting. It appears at about 4 to 6 weeks gestation and usually subsides by the end of the third month (first trimester) of pregnancy. Severity varies from mild distaste for certain foods to more severe vomiting. The condition may be triggered by the sight or odor of various foods. Fatigue may also be responsible for severe nausea, but further research is needed to determine the role of this factor (O'Brien & Zhou, 1995). By the end of the second trimester, the appetite increases in response to increasing metabolic needs. Rarely does morning sickness have harmful effects on the embryo/fetus or the woman. Whenever the vomiting is severe or persists beyond the first trimester, or when it is accompanied by fever, pain, or weight loss, further evaluation is necessary and medical intervention is likely.

Women may also experience changes in their sense of taste, leading to cravings and changes in dietary intake. Some women have non–food cravings such as ice, clay, and laundry starch. Usually these cravings, if consumed in moderation, are not harmful to the pregnancy if the woman has adequate nutrition otherwise (Cunningham et al., 1997).

Mouth

The gums become hyperemic, spongy, and swollen during pregnancy. They tend to bleed easily because the rising levels of estrogen cause selective increased vascularity and connective tissue proliferation (a nonspecific gingivitis). Epulis (discussed in the section on the integumentary system) may develop at the gumline. Some pregnant women complain of **ptyalism** (excessive salivation), which may be caused by the decrease in unconscious swallowing by the woman when nauseated or from stimulation of salivary glands by eating starch (Cunningham et al., 1997).

Esophagus, Stomach, and Intestines

Herniation of the upper portion of the stomach (hiatal hernia) occurs after the seventh or eighth month of pregnancy in about 15% to 20% of pregnant women. This condition results from upward displacement of the stomach, which causes the hiatus of the diaphragm to widen. It occurs more often in multiparas and older or obese women.

Increased estrogen production causes decreased secretion of hydrochloric acid. Therefore peptic ulcer formation or flare-up of existing peptic ulcers is uncommon during pregnancy.

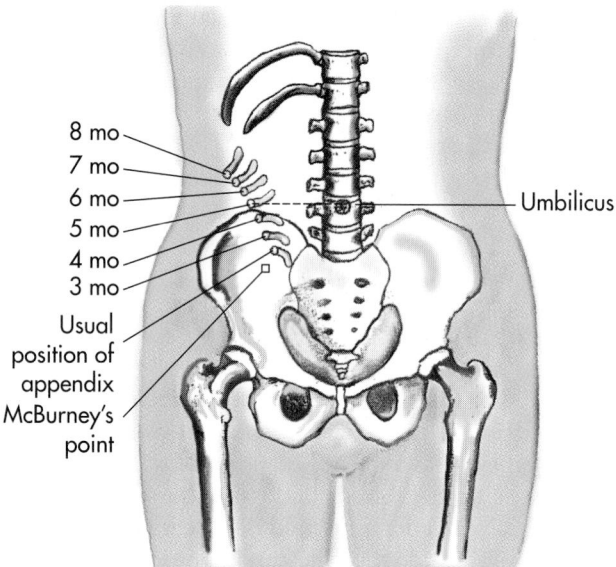

8 mo
7 mo
6 mo
5 mo
4 mo
3 mo
Usual position of appendix
McBurney's point
Umbilicus

Fig. 15-14 Change in position of appendix in pregnancy. Note McBurney's point.

Increased progesterone production causes decreased tone and motility of smooth muscles, resulting in esophageal regurgitation, slower emptying time of the stomach, and reverse peristalsis. As a result, the woman may experience "acid indigestion" or heartburn **(pyrosis).**

Iron is absorbed more readily in the small intestine in response to increased needs during pregnancy. Even when the woman is deficient in iron, it will continue to be absorbed in sufficient amounts for the fetus to have a normal hemoglobin level.

Increased progesterone (causing loss of muscle tone and decreased peristalsis) results in an increase in water absorption from the colon and may cause constipation. Constipation can also result from hypoperistalsis (sluggishness of the bowel), food choices, lack of fluids, iron supplementation, decreased activity level, abdominal distention by the pregnant uterus, and displacement and compression of the intestines. If the pregnant woman has hemorrhoids (see Fig. 15-9) and is constipated, the hemorrhoids may become everted or may bleed during straining at stool. A mild ileus (sluggishness and lack of movement resulting in obstruction) that follows birth, as well as postbirth fluid loss and perineal discomfort, contributes to continuing constipation.

Gallbladder and Liver

The gallbladder is quite often distended because of its decreased muscle tone during pregnancy. Increased emptying time and thickening of bile caused by prolonged retention are typical changes. These features, together with slight hypercholesterolemia from increased progesterone levels, may account for the development of gallstones during pregnancy.

Hepatic function is difficult to appraise during pregnancy. However, only minor changes in liver function develop. Occasionally, intrahepatic cholestasis (retention and accumulation of bile in the liver, caused by factors within the liver) occurs late in pregnancy in response to placental steroids and may result in pruritus gravidarum (severe itching) with or without jaundice. These distressing symptoms subside soon after birth.

Abdominal Discomfort

Intraabdominal alterations that can cause discomfort include pelvic heaviness or pressure, round ligament tension, flatulence, distention and bowel cramping, and uterine contractions. In addition to displacement of intestines, pressure from the expanding uterus causes an increase in venous pressure in the pelvic organs. Although most abdominal discomfort is a consequence of normal maternal alterations, the health care provider must be constantly alert to the possibility of disorders such as bowel obstruction or an inflammatory process.

Appendicitis may be difficult to diagnose in pregnancy because the appendix is displaced upward and laterally, high and to the right, away from McBurney's point (Fig. 15-14).

Endocrine System
Pituitary and Placental Hormones

During pregnancy, the elevated levels of estrogen and progesterone (produced first by the corpus luteum in the ovary until about 14 weeks gestation and then by the placenta) suppress secretion of follicle-stimulating hormone (FSH) and luteinizing hormone (LH) by the anterior pituitary. The maturation of a follicle and ovulation do not occur. Although the majority of women experience **amenorrhea** (absence of menses), at least 20% have some slight, painless spotting during early gestation. Implantation bleeding and bleeding following intercourse related to cervical friability can occur. Most of the women experiencing slight gestational bleeding continue to full term and have normal infants. However, all instances of bleeding should be reported and evaluated.

After implantation, the fertilized ovum and the chorionic villi produce human chorionic gonadotropin (hCG), which maintains the corpus luteum's production of estrogen and progesterone until the placenta takes over their production (Creasy & Resnik, 1999).

Progesterone is essential for maintaining pregnancy by relaxing smooth muscles, resulting in decreased uterine contractility and prevention of miscarriage. Progesterone and estrogen cause fat to deposit in subcutaneous tissues over the maternal abdomen, back, and upper thighs. This fat serves as an energy reserve for both pregnancy and lactation. Estrogen also promotes the enlargement of the genitals, uterus, and breasts and increases vascularity, causing vasodilation. Estrogen causes relaxation of pelvic ligaments and joints. It also alters metabolism of nutrients by interfering with folic acid metabolism, increasing the level of total body proteins, and promoting retention of sodium and water by kidney tubules. Estrogen may decrease secretion of hydrochloric acid and pepsin, which may be responsible for digestive upsets such as nausea.

Serum prolactin produced by the anterior pituitary begins to rise early in the first trimester and increases progressively to term. It is responsible for initial lactation; however, the high levels of estrogen and progesterone inhibit lactation by blocking the binding of prolactin to breast tissue until after birth (Guyton & Hall, 1997).

Oxytocin is produced by the posterior pituitary in increasing amounts as the fetus matures. This hormone can stimulate uterine contractions during pregnancy, but high levels of progesterone prevent contractions until near term. Oxytocin also stimulates the let-down or milk-ejection reflex after birth in response to the infant sucking at the mother's breast.

Human chorionic somatomammotropin (hCS), previously called human placental lactogen (hPL), produced by the placenta acts as a growth hormone and contributes to breast development. It decreases the maternal metabolism of glucose and increases the amount of fatty acids for metabolic needs (Alsat et al., 1997; Guyton & Hall, 1997).

Thyroid Gland

During pregnancy there is an increase in gland activity and hormone production. The increased activity is reflected in a moderate enlargement of the thyroid gland caused by hyperplasia of the glandular tissue and increased vascularity (Cunningham et al., 1997). Thyroxine-binding globulin (TBG) increases as a result of increased estrogen levels. This increase begins at about 20 weeks gestation. The level of total (free and bound) thyroxine (T_4) increases between 6 and 9 weeks gestation and plateaus at 18 weeks gestation. Free thyroxine (T_4) and free triiodothyronine (T_3) return to nonpregnant levels after the first trimester. Despite these changes in hormone production, the pregnant woman usually does not develop hyperthyroidism (Cunningham et al., 1997).

Parathyroid Gland

Parathyroid hormone controls calcium and magnesium metabolism. Pregnancy induces a slight hyperparathyroidism, a reflection of increased fetal requirements for calcium and vitamin D. The peak level of parathyroid hormone occurs between 15 and 35 weeks gestation when the needs for growth of the fetal skeleton are greatest. Levels return to normal after birth.

Pancreas

The fetus requires significant amounts of glucose for its growth and development. To meet its need for fuel, the fetus not only depletes the store of maternal glucose but also decreases the mother's ability to synthesize glucose by siphoning off her amino acids. Maternal blood glucose levels fall. Maternal insulin does not cross the placenta to the fetus. As a result, in early pregnancy, the pancreas decreases its production of insulin.

As pregnancy continues, the placenta grows and produces progressively larger amounts of hormones (i.e., hCS, estrogen, and progesterone). Cortisol production by the adrenals also increases. Estrogen, progesterone, hCS, and cortisol collectively decrease the mother's ability to use insulin. Cortisol stimulates increased production of insulin but also increases the mother's peripheral resistance to insulin (i.e., the tissues cannot use the insulin). Decreasing the mother's ability to use her own insulin is a protective mechanism that ensures an ample supply of glucose for the needs of the fetoplacental unit. The result is an added demand for insulin by the mother that continues to increase at a steady rate until term. The normal beta cells of the islets of Langerhans in the pancreas can meet this demand for insulin.

Adrenal Glands

The adrenal glands change little during pregnancy. Secretion of aldosterone is increased, resulting in reabsorption of excess sodium from the renal tubules. Cortisol levels are also increased (Chamberlain & Pipkin, 1998).

These profound endocrine changes are essential for pregnancy maintenance, normal fetal growth, and postpartum recovery.

KEY POINTS

- The biochemical, physiologic, and anatomic adaptations that occur during pregnancy are profound and revert back to the nonpregnant state following birth and lactation.
- Maternal adaptations are attributed to the hormones of pregnancy and to mechanical pressures exerted by the enlarging uterus and other tissues.
- The ability to recognize the beta subunit of hCG through the use of monoclonal antibody technology has revolutionized endocrine tests for pregnancy.
- Presumptive, probable, and positive signs of pregnancy aid in the diagnosis of pregnancy; only positive signs (identification of a fetal heartbeat, verification of fetal movements, and visualization of the fetus) can establish the diagnosis of pregnancy.
- Adaptations to pregnancy protect the woman's normal physiologic functioning, meet the metabolic demands pregnancy imposes, and provide for fetal development and growth needs.
- The rise in pH of the pregnant woman's vaginal secretions makes her more vulnerable to vaginal infections.
- Increased vascularity and sensitivity of the vagina and other pelvic viscera may lead to a high degree of sexual interest and arousal.
- Some adaptations to pregnancy result in discomforts such as fatigue, urinary frequency, nausea, and breast sensitivity.
- As pregnancy progresses, balance and coordination are affected by changes in the woman's joints and her center of gravity.

CRITICAL THINKING EXERCISES

1 *Interview three pregnant women (and partners, if present) at 12 weeks, 24 weeks, and 36 weeks of gestation:*
   a. *How does each pregnant woman feel about the changes in her body?*
   b. *Has her partner expressed any feelings/opinions about these changes? If so, how have these feelings/opinions affected the woman?*
   c. *Which changes do they find pleasant?*
   d. *Which changes do they find uncomfortable or troublesome?*
   e. *What is their level of understanding of these changes?*
   f. *Use your findings to develop a teaching plan for each woman's specific concerns. Provide rationales for your choices of topics to include.*

2 *Go to a local pharmacy and get information on at least three different home pregnancy test kits. (The pharmacist may be able to provide product information.) Compare the directions for use, how to interpret test results, and the costs. During a conference with others in your clinical group, discuss the pros and cons of using the different types of kits. Develop a poster presentation to guide women in decisions about use of home pregnancy tests for display in a family planning clinic.*

3 *During your experience in a prenatal clinic or physician/midwife office, survey the pregnant women that you meet about use of a home pregnancy test to confirm their pregnancies. Compare women who did home testing with those who had pregnancy tests done by their health care provider in terms of when the woman's first prenatal visit occurred. Discuss your findings with those of the other students in your clinical group. Identify researchable questions based on your discussion.*

References

Alsat, E. et al. (1997). Human placental growth hormone. *Am J Obstet Gynecol* 177(6), 526-534.

Barkauskas, V. et al. (1994). *Health and physical assessment.* St. Louis: Mosby.

Blackburn, S., & Loper, D. (1992). *Maternal, fetal, and neonatal physiology: A clinical perspective.* Philadelphia: W.B. Saunders.

Chamberlain, G., & Pipkin, F. (Eds.). (1998). *Clinical physiology in obstetrics* (3rd ed.). Oxford: Blackwell Scientific.

Creasy, R., & Resnik, R. (1999). *Maternal-fetal medicine* (4th ed.). Philadelphia: W.B. Saunders.

Cunningham, F. et al. (1997). *Williams obstetrics* (20th ed.). Stamford, CT: Appleton & Lange.

Green, L., & Froman, R. (1996). Blood pressure measurement during pregnancy: Auscultating versus oscillatory methods. *J Obstet Gynecol Neonatal Nurs* 25(2), 155-159.

Gordon, M., & Landon, M. (1996). Dermatologic disorders. In S. Gabbe, J. Niebyl, & J. Simpson. *Obstetrics: Normal and problem prgnancies (3rd ed.).* New York: Churchill Livingstone.

Guyton, A., & Hall, J. (1997). *Human physiology and mechanism of disease* (6th ed.). Philadelphia: W.B. Saunders.

Hatcher, R. et al. (1998). *Contraceptive technology* (17th ed.). New York: Ardent Media.

Lawrence, R. (1999). *Breastfeeding: A guide for the medical profession* (5th ed.). St Louis: Mosby.

Mishell, D. et al. (1997). *Comprehensive gynecology* (3rd ed.). St Louis: Mosby.

O'Brien, B., & Zhou, Q. (1995). Variables related to nausea and vomiting during pregnancy. *Birth* 22(2), 93-100.

Pagana, K., & Pagana, T. (1997). *Mosby's diagnostic and laboratory test reference* (3rd ed.). St. Louis: Mosby.

Schauberger, C. et al. (1996). Obstetrics: Peripheral joint laxity increases in pregnancy but does not correlate with serum relaxin levels. *Am J Obstet Gynecol* 174(2), 667-671.

Seidel, H. et al. (1999). *Mosby's guide to physical examination* (4th ed.). St. Louis: Mosby.

Varney, H. (1997). *Varney's midwifery* (3rd ed.). Sudbury, MA: Jones & Bartlett.

Worthington-Roberts, B., & Williams, S. (1997). *Nutrition in pregnancy and lactation* (6th ed.). Dubuque, IA: Brown & Benchmark Publishers.

Maternal and Fetal Nutrition

Mary Courtney Moore

LEARNING OBJECTIVES

- Define the key terms.
- Explain recommended maternal weight gain during pregnancy.
- State the recommended level of intake of energy sources, protein, and key vitamins and minerals during pregnancy and lactation.
- Give examples of the food sources that provide the nutrients required for optimal maternal nutrition during pregnancy and lactation.
- Examine the role of nutritional supplements during pregnancy.

- List five nutritional risk factors during pregnancy.
- Compare the dietary needs of adolescent and mature pregnant women.
- Give examples of cultural food patterns and possible dietary problems for two ethnic groups or for two alternative eating patterns.
- Assess nutritional status during pregnancy.
- Apply the nursing process to maternal and fetal nutrition.
- Identify topics for nursing research related to maternal and fetal nutrition.

KEY TERMS

Adequate Intakes (AIs)
anemia
anthropometric measurements
body mass index (BMI)
diet history
Dietary Reference Intakes (DRIs)
energy (kcal)

food cravings
intrauterine growth restriction (IUGR)
lactose intolerance
low birth weight (LBW)
neural tube defect
physiologic anemia
pica

pyrosis
Recommended Dietary Allowances (RDAs)
small for gestational age (SGA)
vegetarian diet
WIC (Women, Infants, and Children Program)

Nutrition is one of many factors that influence the outcome of pregnancy (Fig. 16-1). However, the maternal nutritional status is an especially significant factor, both because it is potentially alterable and because good nutrition before and during pregnancy is an important preventive measure for a variety of problems. These problems include birth of **low-birth-weight** (LBW; birth weight of 2500 g or less) and preterm infants. Currently at least 23 developed nations report infant mortality rates lower than those in the United States, and 64% of infant deaths in the United States occur among infants who are LBW (Guyer et al., 1998). It is essential that the importance of good nutrition be emphasized to all women of childbearing potential. Therefore the nurse must have a thorough understanding of nutrient needs before and during pregnancy, and nutrition assessment, intervention, and evaluation must be an integral part of the nursing care given to all pregnant women.

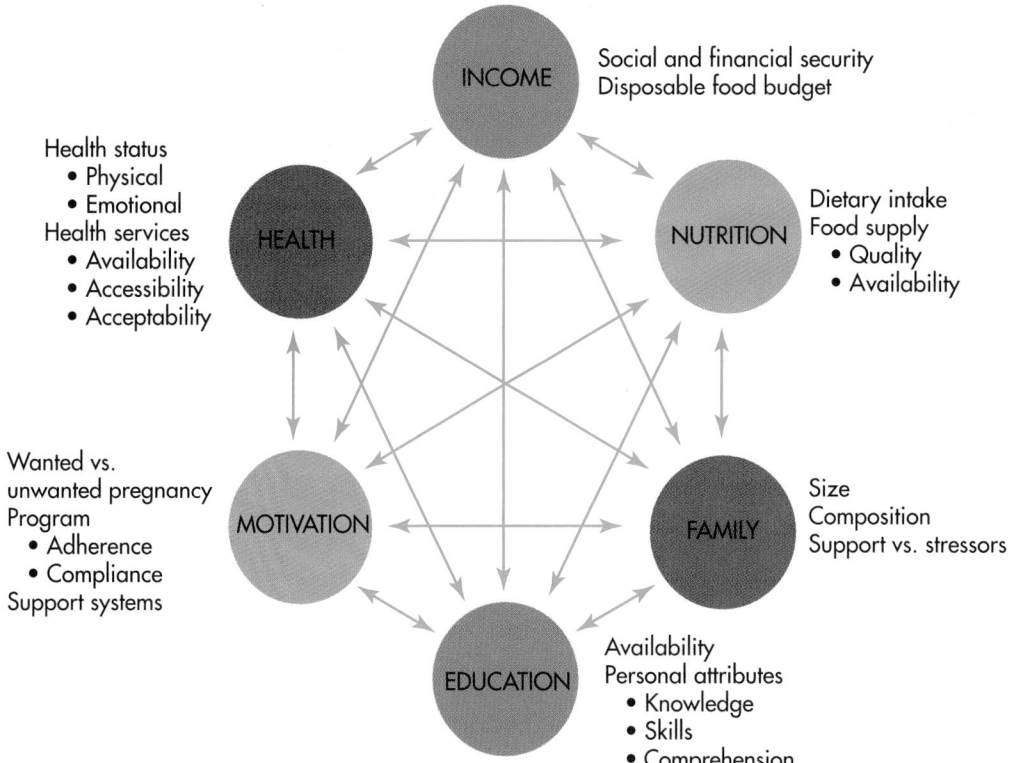

Fig. 16-1 Web of influences that can affect outcome of pregnancy. Much more than luck goes into having a healthy baby *(From Wardlaw, G., & Insel, P. [1993]. Perspectives in nutrition [2nd ed.]. St. Louis: Mosby.)*

NUTRIENT NEEDS BEFORE CONCEPTION

The first trimester of pregnancy is a crucial one in terms of embryonic/fetal organ development. A healthful diet before conception is the best way to ensure that adequate nutrients are available for the developing fetus. Folic acid (folate) intake is of particular concern in the periconceptual period, because **neural tube defects,** or failures in closure of the neural tube, are more common in infants of women with poor folic acid intake. Proper closure of the neural tube is required for normal formation of the spinal cord, and the neural tube begins to close within the first month of gestation, often before the woman realizes that she is pregnant. It is estimated that the incidence of neural tube defects could be halved if all women had an adequate folic acid intake during the periconceptual period (Butterworth & Bendich, 1996). All women capable of becoming pregnant are advised to consume 400 µg of folic acid daily in fortified foods (ready-to-eat cereals and enriched grain products) or supplements, in addition to a diet rich in folic acid–containing foods: green leafy vegetables, whole grains, and meats (Table 16-1).

Both maternal and fetal risks in pregnancy are increased when the mother is significantly underweight or overweight when pregnancy begins. Ideally all women would achieve their desirable body weights before conception.

NUTRIENT NEEDS DURING PREGNANCY

Nutrient needs are determined, at least in part, by the stage of gestation in that the amount of fetal growth varies during the different stages of pregnancy. During the first trimester the synthesis of fetal tissues places relatively few demands on maternal nutrition. Therefore during the first trimester when the embryo/fetus is very small, the needs are only slightly greater than those before pregnancy. In contrast, the last trimester is a period of noticeable fetal growth when most of the deposition of the fetal stores of energy sources and minerals occurs. Therefore as fetal growth progresses during the second and third trimesters, the pregnant woman's need for some nutrients increases greatly. Factors that contribute to the increase in nutrient needs include the following:

- The uterine-placental-fetal unit
- Maternal blood volume and constituents—During pregnancy the total blood volume increases by about 33% more than the normal volume. The plasma volume increases by 50% in women in their first pregnancies and more than this in multiparas. Although red blood cell (RBC) production is also stimulated, the expansion of RBC mass is not as great as that of plasma volume.
- Maternal mammary development
- Metabolic needs—Basal metabolic rates, when expressed as kilocalories (kcal) per minute, are approximately

TABLE 16-1 Nutritional Recommendations During Pregnancy and Lactation

NUTRIENT (UNIT)	RECOMMENDATION FOR NONPREGNANT FEMALE*	RECOMMENDATION FOR PREGNANCY*	RECOMMENDATION FOR LACTATION*	ROLE IN RELATION TO PREGNANCY AND LACTATION	FOOD SOURCES
Energy (kcal)	Variable	First trimester, same as nonpregnant; second and third trimesters, nonpregnant + 300	Nonpregnant + 500	Growth of fetal and maternal tissues; milk production	Carbohydrate, fat, and protein
Protein (g)	50	60	65	Synthesis of the products of conception; growth of maternal tissue and expansion of blood volume; secretion of milk protein during lactation	Meats, eggs, cheese, yogurt, legumes (dry beans and peas, peanuts), nuts, grains
MINERALS					
Calcium (mg)	1300/1000	1300/1000	1300/1000	Fetal and infant skeleton and tooth formation; maintenance of maternal bone and tooth mineralization	Milk, cheese, yogurt, sardines or other fish eaten with bones left in, deep green leafy vegetables except spinach or Swiss chard, tofu, baked beans
Phosphorus (mg)	1250/700	1250/700	1250/700	Fetal and infant skeleton and tooth formation	Milk, cheese, yogurt, meats, whole grains, nuts, legumes
Iron (mg)	15	30	15	Maternal hemoglobin formation, fetal liver iron storage	Liver, meats, whole or enriched breads and cereals, deep green leafy vegetables, legumes, dried fruits

Recommendations are the new Dietary Reference Intakes (RDA or AI, see text) where available (Food and Nutrition Board, National Academy of Sciences, Institute of Medicine. (1998). *Recommended levels for individual intake, B vitamins and choline.* Washington, D.C.: National Academy Press; Standing Committee on the Scientific Evaluation of Dietary Reference Intakes, Food and Nutrition Board, Institute of Medicine. (1997). *Dietary reference intakes: Calcium, phosphorus, magnesium, vitamin D, and fluoride.* Washington, D.C.: National Academy Press.) Where DRI are not yet available, the values are taken from Food and Nutrition Board (1989).
RBC, Red blood cells.
*When two values appear, separated by a diagonal slash, the first is for females <19 years and the second is for those 19 to 50 years old.

Continued

TABLE 16-1   Nutritional Recommendations During Pregnancy and Lactation—cont'd

NUTRIENT (UNIT)	RECOMMENDATION FOR NONPREGNANT FEMALE*	RECOMMENDATION FOR PREGNANCY*	RECOMMENDATION FOR LACTATION*	ROLE IN RELATION TO PREGNANCY AND LACTATION	FOOD SOURCES
Zinc (mg)	12	15	19	Component of numerous enzyme systems; possibly important in preventing congenital malformations	Liver, shellfish, meats, whole grains, milk
Iodine (µg)	150	175	200	Increased maternal metabolic rate	Iodized salt, seafood, milk and milk products, commercial yeast breads, rolls, and donuts
Magnesium (mg)	360/320	400/360	360/320	Involved in energy and protein metabolism, tissue growth, muscle action	Nuts, legumes, cocoa, meats, whole grains
FAT-SOLUBLE VITAMINS					
A (RE)	800	800	1300	Essential for cell development, tooth bud formation, bone growth	Deep green leafy vegetables, dark yellow vegetables and fruits, chili peppers, liver, fortified margarine and butter
D (µg)	5	5	5	Involved in absorption of calcium and phosphorus, improves mineralization	Fortified milk and margarine, egg yolk, butter, liver, seafood
E (mg)	8	10	12	Antioxidant (protects cell membranes from damage), especially important for preventing breakdown of RBCs	Vegetable oils, green leafy vegetables, whole grains, liver, nuts and seeds, cheese, fish

TABLE 16-1 Nutritional Recommendations During Pregnancy and Lactation—cont'd

NUTRIENT (UNIT)	RECOMMENDATION FOR NONPREGNANT FEMALE*	RECOMMENDATION FOR PREGNANCY*	RECOMMENDATION FOR LACTATION*	ROLE IN RELATION TO PREGNANCY AND LACTATION	FOOD SOURCES
WATER-SOLUBLE VITAMINS					
C (mg)	60	70	95	Tissue formation and integrity, formation of connective tissue, enhancement of iron absorption	Citrus fruits, strawberries, melons, broccoli, tomatoes, peppers, raw deep green leafy vegetables
Folic acid (µg)	400	600	500	Prevention of neural tube defects, support increased maternal RBC formation	Fortified ready-to-eat cereals and other grains, green leafy vegetables, oranges, broccoli, asparagus, artichokes, liver
Thiamin (mg)	1.0/1.1	1.4	1.5	Involved in energy metabolism	Pork, beef, liver, whole or enriched grains, legumes
Riboflavin (mg)	1.0/1.1	1.4	1.6	Involved in energy and protein metabolism	Meat, liver, deep green vegetables, whole grains
Niacin (mg)	14	18	17	Involved in energy metabolism	Meat, fish, poultry, liver, whole or enriched grains, peanuts
Pyridoxine (B_6) (mg)	1.2/1.3	1.9	2.0	Involved in protein metabolism	Meat, liver, deep green vegetables, whole grains
B_{12} (µg)	2.4	2.6	2.8	Production of nucleic acids and proteins, especially important in formation of RBC and neural functioning	Milk and milk products, egg, meat, liver, fortified soy milk

20% higher in pregnant women than in nonpregnant women. This increase includes the energy cost for tissue synthesis.

The Food and Nutrition Board of the National Academy of Sciences is preparing new nutritional recommendations for the people of the United States, the **Dietary Reference Intakes** or **DRIs** (Standing Committee, 1997). The DRIs consist of **Recommended Dietary Allowances (RDAs)** and **Adequate Intakes (AIs),** as well as guidelines for avoiding excessive nutrient intakes. "RDA" is not a

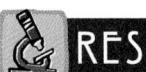

RESEARCH

Prepregnant Weight and Weight Gain During Pregnancy: Relationship to Functional Status, Symptoms, and Energy

Numerous studies have shown that both very low and excessive prepregnancy weight and weight gain during pregnancy are related to the incidence of obstetric complications during pregnancy and birth and to neonatal morbidity and mortality. Little information exists on how weight gain affects a woman's health during pregnancy as measured by her functioning, number of physical symptoms, or physical energy level. This information is essential to provide comprehensive nutritional and weight counseling during pregnancy.

The purpose of this study was to investigate the relationship of prepregnancy weight classification and weight gain during pregnancy on functional status, physical symptoms, and physical energy during each trimester, using the Roy Adaptation Model as the conceptual framework. Functional status was measured by the Inventory of Functional Status—Antepartum Period. Physical symptoms were measured by using the Symptoms Checklist. Physical energy was measured by one question. Weight and height were self-reported. Two hundred twenty-two women, whose pregnancies were low risk, comprised the study group.

The results of this study found that overweight women gained less weight on a percentage basis (M = 16.87%) than women who were of normal weight (M = 23.58%) or were underweight (M = 26.02%) ($p < .00005$). The groups did not differ in functional status, physical energy, or number or type of physical symptoms. Women who gained more than the recommended amount of weight for their prepregnant weight group had a lower level of third trimester functional status than those who did not. It was concluded that individual counseling of women regarding food intake and excessive weight gain during pregnancy needs to be reconsidered.

CLINICAL APPLICATION

Nurses need to assess functional status in women who are gaining weight above their recommended levels to determine whether performance of personal care, child care, and household activities is diminished. Nutrition and exercise counseling, an integral part of prenatal care, warrants special nursing considerations. Although dieting is not recommended during pregnancy, evaluation of the woman's nutritional intake may identify areas that require adjustment. Similarly, the nurse should evaluate the woman's level of exercise and suggest areas for improvement.

Source: Tulman, L., Morin, K., & Fawcett, J. (1998). Prepregnant weight and weight gain during pregnancy: Relationship to functional status, symptoms, and energy. *J Obstet Gynecol Neonatal Nurs* 27(6), 629-634.

new term. RDAs for some nutrients have been available for many years, and they have been revised periodically. RDAs are recommendations for daily nutritional intakes that meet the needs of almost all of the healthy members of the population. AIs, which are new, are similar to the RDAs, except that they are used when there are not enough data available to be certain that they cover the needs of the healthy population. The RDAs and AIs include a wide variety of nutrients and food components, and they are divided into age, sex, and life-stage categories (e.g., infancy, pregnancy, and lactation). They can be used as goals in planning the diets of individuals (see Table 16-1).

Energy Needs

Energy (kilocalories or kcal) needs are met by carbohydrate, fat, and protein in the diet. No specific recommendations exist for the amount of carbohydrate and fat in the diet of the pregnant woman. However, the intake of these nutrients should be adequate to support the recommended weight gain. Although protein can be used to supply energy, its primary role is to provide amino acids for the synthesis of new tissues (see discussion later in chapter). The RDA during the second and third trimesters of pregnancy is 300 kcal greater than the prepregnancy needs. Longitudinal assessment of weight gain during pregnancy is the best way to determine whether the kilocalorie intake is adequate; very underweight or active women may require more than the additional 300 kcal to sustain the desired rate of weight gain.

Weight Gain

The optimal weight gain during pregnancy is not known precisely. It is known, however, that the amount of weight gained by the mother during pregnancy has an important bearing on the course and outcome of the pregnancy. Although an adequate weight gain does not necessarily indicate that the diet is nutritionally adequate, it reduces the risk of delivering a **small-for-gestational age (SGA)** or preterm infant.

The desirable weight gain during pregnancy varies among women. The primary factor to consider in making a weight gain recommendation is the appropriateness of the prepregnancy weight for the woman's height, that is,

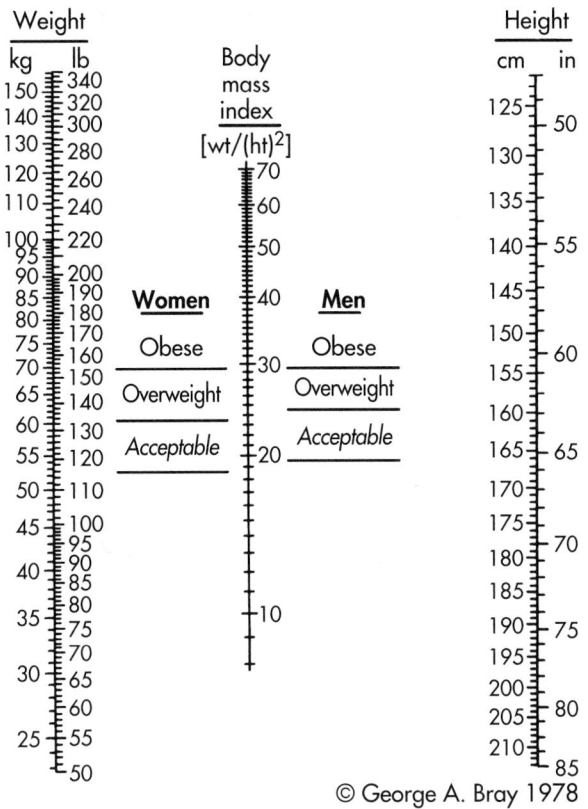

© George A. Bray 1978

Fig. 16-2 Method for determining body mass index (BMI). Use a straightedge to connect the individual's height and weight.

A commonly used method of evaluating the appropriateness of weight for height is the **body mass index (BMI),** which is calculated by the following formula:

$$BMI = Weight/height^2$$

where the weight is in kilograms and height is in meters. Thus, for a woman who weighed 51 kg before pregnancy and is 1.57 m tall:

$$BMI = 51/(1.57)^2, \text{ or } 20.7$$

The BMI can be classified into the following categories: less than 19.8, underweight or low; 19.8 to 26.0, normal; 26.0 to 29.0, overweight or high; and greater than 29.0, obese (Institute of Medicine, 1992). Figure 16-2 provides an easy way of estimating and categorizing the BMI.

For women with single fetuses, current recommendations are that women with normal BMI should gain 11.5 to 16 kg during pregnancy (Fig. 16-3), underweight women should gain 12.5 to 18 kg, overweight women should gain 7 to 11.5 kg, and obese women should gain at least 7 kg (Institute of Medicine, 1992). Adolescents are encouraged to strive for weight gains at the upper end of the recommended range for their BMI, because it appears that the fetus and the still-growing mother compete for nutrients. The risk of mechanical complications at birth is reduced if the weight gain of short adult women (<157 cm) is near the lower end of their recommended range. In twin gestations, gains of approximately 16 to 20 kg appear to be associated with the best outcomes (Ellings, Newman, & Bowers, 1998).

Pattern of Weight Gain

Weight gain should take place throughout pregnancy. The risk of delivering an SGA infant is reported to be greater when the weight gain early in pregnancy has been poor. The likelihood of preterm birth has been observed to be greater when the gains during the last half of pregnancy have been inadequate. These risks were found to exist even when the total gain for the pregnancy was in the recommended range.

The optimal rate of weight gain depends on the stage of pregnancy. During the first and second trimesters, growth takes place primarily in maternal tissues; during the third trimester, growth occurs primarily in fetal tissues. During the first trimester there is an average total weight gain of only 1 to 2.5 kg. Thereafter the recommended weight gain increases to approximately 0.4 kg per week for a woman of normal weight (see Fig. 16-3). The recommended weekly weight gain for overweight women during the second and third trimesters is 0.3 kg, and it is 0.5 kg for underweight women. The recommended caloric intake corresponds to this pattern of gain (see Table 16-1). There is no increment for the first trimester; an additional 300 kcal per day over the prepregnant intake is recommended during the second and third trimesters. The amount of food providing 300 kcal is not great. It can be provided by one additional serving from each of the following groups: milk, yogurt, or

whether the woman's weight was normal before pregnancy, or whether she was underweight or overweight (see Research box). Maternal and fetal risks in pregnancy are increased when the mother is significantly underweight or overweight before pregnancy and when weight gain during pregnancy is either too low or too high. Severely underweight women are more likely to experience preterm labor and to give birth to LBW infants. Both normal-weight and underweight women with inadequate weight gain have an increased risk of delivering an infant with **intrauterine growth restriction (IUGR).** Greater-than-expected weight gain during pregnancy may occur for many reasons, including multiple gestation, edema, pregnancy-induced hypertension (PIH), and overeating. When obesity is present (either preexisting obesity or obesity that develops during pregnancy), there is an increased likelihood of macrosomia and fetopelvic disproportion, operative birth, birth trauma, and infant mortality. Obese women are more likely than normal-weight women to have hypertension and diabetes, and their risk of giving birth to a child with a major congenital defect is double that of normal-weight women (Prentice & Goldberg, 1996). The cost of pregnancy in an obese woman has been estimated to be triple that of a normal-weight woman (Prentice & Goldberg, 1996).

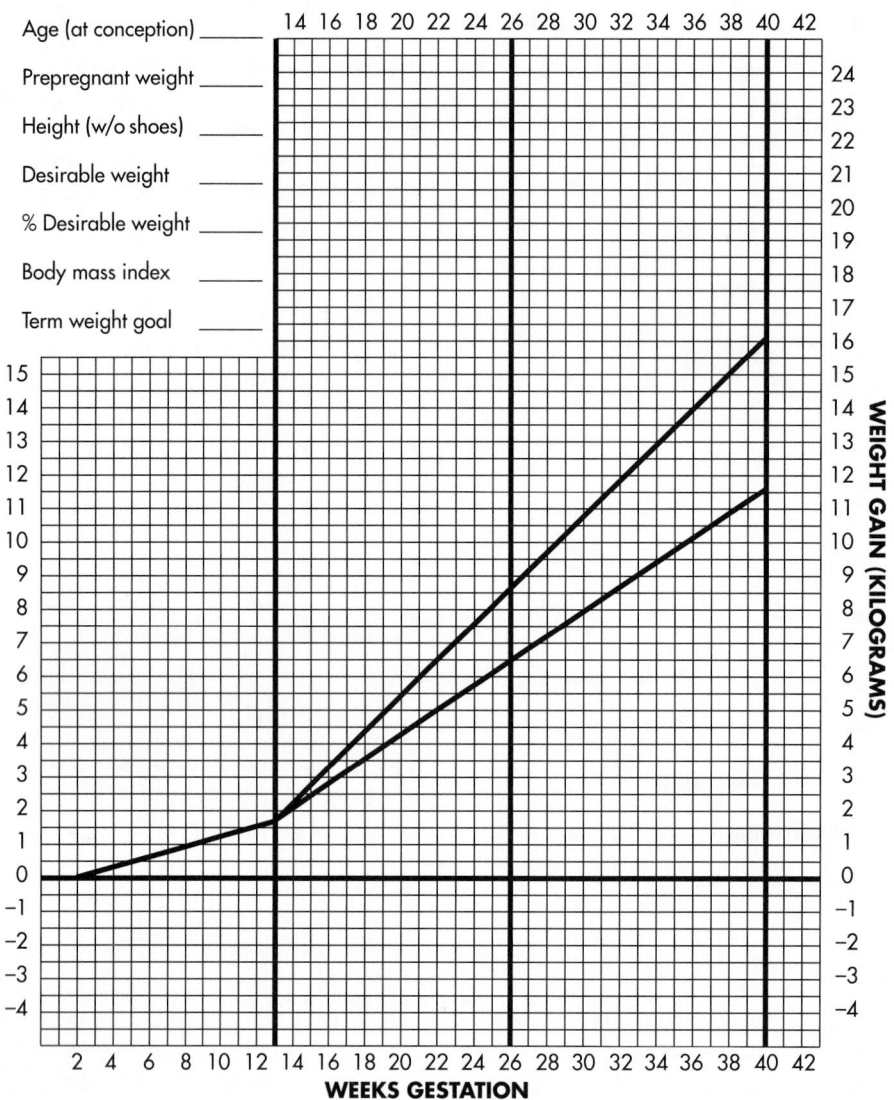

Fig. 16-3 Prenatal weight gain chart for plotting weight gain of normal weight women. *Note:* Young adolescents, African-American women, and smokers should aim for the upper end of the recommended range; short women (<157 cm) should strive for gains at the lower end of the range.

cheese (all skim milk products); fruits; vegetables; and bread, cereal, rice, or pasta.

The reasons for an inadequate weight gain (less than 1 kg per month for normal-weight women or less than 0.5 kg per month for obese women during the last two trimesters) or excessive weight gain (more than 3 kg per month) should be thoroughly evaluated. Possible reasons for deviations from the expected rate of weight gain, besides inadequate or excessive dietary intake, include measurement or recording errors, differences in the weight of clothing, the time of day, and the accumulation of fluids. An exceptionally high gain is likely to result from the accumulation of fluids, and a gain of more than 3 kg in a month, especially after the twentieth week of gestation, often heralds the development of PIH.

Hazards of Restricting Adequate Weight Gain

An obsession with thinness and dieting pervades the North American culture. Slender, figure-conscious women may find it difficult to make the transition from guarding against weight gain before pregnancy to valuing weight gain during pregnancy. In counseling these women the nurse can emphasize the positive effects of good nutrition, as well as the adverse effects of maternal malnutrition (manifested by poor weight gain) on infant growth and development. This counseling includes information on the components of weight gain during pregnancy (Fig. 16-4) and the amount of this weight that will be lost after the birth. Early in a woman's pregnancy, explaining ways to lose weight in the postpartum period helps relieve her concerns. (Because lactation can help to gradually reduce ma-

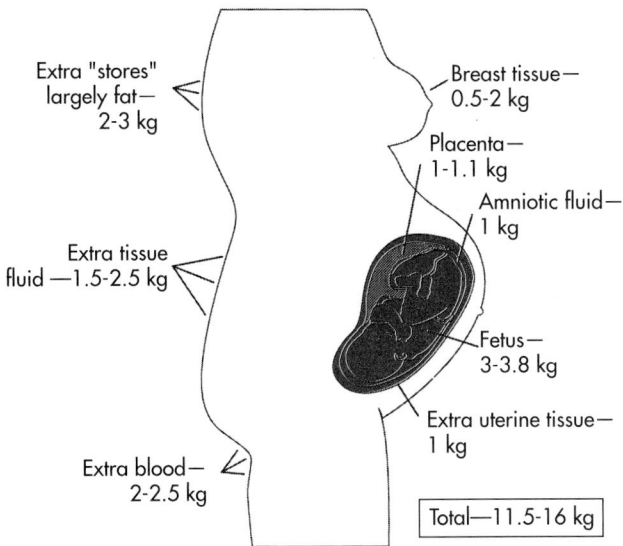

Fig. 16-4 Components of maternal weight gain at 40 weeks of gestation. *(Modified from Worthington-Roberts, B., & Williams, S. [1997]. Nutrition in pregnancy and lactation [6th ed.]. Dubuque, IA: Brown and Benchmark.)*

ternal energy stores, this also provides an opportunity to promote breastfeeding.)

Pregnancy is not a time to diet. Even overweight or obese pregnant women need to gain at least enough weight to equal the weight of the products of conception (fetus, placenta, and amniotic fluid). If they limit their caloric intake to prevent weight gain, they may also excessively limit their intake of important nutrients. Moreover, dietary restriction results in the catabolism of fat stores, which in turn augments the production of ketones. The long-term effects of mild ketonemia during pregnancy are not known, but ketonuria has been found to be correlated with the occurrence of preterm labor. It should be stressed to obese women, and all pregnant women for that matter, that the quality of the weight gain is important, with emphasis placed on the consumption of nutrient-dense foods and the avoidance of empty-calorie foods.

Weight gain is important, but pregnancy is not an excuse for uncontrolled dietary indulgence. The old saying that the pregnant woman is "eating for two" should not be interpreted to mean that the pregnant woman needs to greatly increase her food intake. Instead she should place an emphasis on the quality of her food intake as she considers her needs and those of her fetus. Excessive weight gained during pregnancy may be difficult to lose after pregnancy, thus contributing to chronic overweight or obesity, an etiologic factor in a host of chronic diseases, including hypertension, diabetes mellitus, and arteriosclerotic heart disease. The woman who gains 18 kg or more is especially at risk.

Protein

Protein, with its essential constituent nitrogen, is the nutritional element basic to growth. An adequate protein in-

take is essential to meet increasing demands in pregnancy. These demands arise from the rapid growth of the fetus; enlargement of the uterus and its supporting structures, mammary glands, and placenta; increase in the maternal circulating blood volume and the subsequent demand for increased amounts of plasma protein to maintain colloidal osmotic pressure; and formation of amniotic fluid.

Milk, meat, eggs, and cheese are complete protein foods with a high biologic value. Legumes (dried beans and peas), whole grains, and nuts are also valuable sources of protein. In addition, these protein-rich foods are a source of other nutrients such as calcium, iron, and B vitamins; plant sources of protein often provide needed dietary fiber. The recommended daily food plan (Table 16-2) is a guide to the amounts of these foods that would supply the quantities of protein needed. The recommendations provide for only a modest increase in protein intake over the prepregnant levels in adult women. Protein intake in many people in the United States is relatively high, so many women may not need to increase their protein intake at all during pregnancy. Three servings of milk, yogurt, or cheese (four for adolescents) and 5 to 6 ounces (140 to 168 g) (two servings) of meat, poultry, or fish would supply the recommended protein for the pregnant woman. Additional protein would be provided by vegetables and breads, cereals, rice, or pasta. Pregnant adolescents, women from impoverished backgrounds, and women adhering to unusual diets, such as a macrobiotic (highly restricted vegetarian) diet, are those whose protein intake is most likely to be inadequate. The use of high-protein supplements is not recommended, because they have been associated with an increased incidence of preterm births.

Fluid

Essential during the exchange of nutrients and waste products across cell membranes, water is the main substance of cells, blood, lymph, amniotic fluid, and other vital body fluids. It also aids in maintaining body temperature. A good fluid intake promotes good bowel function, which is sometimes a problem during pregnancy. The recommended daily intake is about 6 to 8 glasses (1500 to 2000 ml) of fluid. Water, milk, and fruit juices are good sources. Dehydration may increase the risk of cramping/contractions and preterm labor.

Women who consume more than 300 mg of caffeine daily (equivalent to about 500 to 750 ml of coffee) are at increased risk of miscarriage and of delivering infants with IUGR. Caffeine's ill effects have been proposed to result from vasoconstriction of the blood vessels supplying the uterus or interference with cell division in the developing fetus (Hinds et al., 1996). Consequently, caffeine-containing products, including caffeinated coffee, tea, soft drinks, and cocoa beverages, should be avoided or consumed only in limited quantities.

Aspartame (Nutrasweet, Equal) and acesulfame K (Sweet One), two artificial sweeteners commonly used in low or no-calorie beverages, have not been found to have

TABLE 16-2 Daily Food Guide for Pregnancy and Lactation

FOOD GROUP	SERVING SIZE	SUGGESTED NUMBER OF SERVINGS		
		NONPREGNANT, NONLACTATING WOMAN	PREGNANT WOMAN	LACTATING WOMAN
GRAIN PRODUCTS Include whole-grain and enriched breads, cereals, pasta, and rice.	1 slice bread; ½ bun, bagel, or English muffin; 1 oz ready-to-eat cereal; ½ c cooked grains	6-11	6-11	6-11
VEGETABLES Eat dark green leafy and deep yellow often. Eat dried beans and peas often; count ½ c cooked dried beans or peas as a serving of vegetables or 1 oz from meat group.	1 c raw leafy greens; ½ c of others	3-5	3-5	3-5
FRUITS Include citrus fruits, strawberries, or melons frequently.	1 medium apple, orange, banana, peach, etc; ½ c small or diced fruit; ¾ c juice	2-4	2-4	2-4
MILK AND MILK PRODUCTS	1 c milk or yogurt; 1½ oz cheese	2-3	3 or more	4 or more
MEAT, POULTRY, FISH, DRY BEANS, NUTS, AND EGGS Eat peanut butter or nuts rarely to avoid excessive fat intake. Limit egg intake to reduce cholesterol intake; trim fat from meat, and remove skin from poultry.	½ c cooked dried beans, 1 egg, or 1½ T peanut butter is equivalent to 1 oz of meat	Up to 6 oz total	Up to 6 oz total	Up to 6 oz total

c, Cup; *T,* tablespoon.

adverse effects on the normal mother and fetus, but aspartame use should be avoided by the mother homozygous for phenylketonuria (PKU) (Position of the ADA, 1993).

Minerals and Vitamins

In general the nutrient needs of pregnant women, with perhaps the exception of the iron needs, can be met through dietary sources. Counseling about the need for a varied diet rich in vitamins and minerals should be a part of the early prenatal care of every pregnant woman and should be reinforced throughout pregnancy. However, supplements of certain nutrients (listed in the following discussion) are recommended whenever the woman's diet is very poor or whenever significant nutritional risk factors are present. Nutritional risk factors in pregnancy are listed in Box 16-1.

Iron

Iron is needed both to allow for transfer of adequate iron to the fetus and to permit expansion of the maternal RBC mass. Beginning in the latter part of the first trimester the blood volume of the mother increases steadily, peaking at about 1500 ml more than in the nonpregnant state. In twin gestations, the increase is at least 500 ml greater than in pregnancies with single fetuses. Plasma volume increases more than RBC mass, with the difference between plasma and RBCs being greatest during the second trimester. The relative excess of plasma causes a modest decrease in the hemoglobin concentration and hematocrit, known as **physiologic anemia** of pregnancy. This is a normal adaptation during pregnancy.

However, poor iron nutriture, which can result in iron deficiency anemia, is relatively common among women in

Adolescence
Frequent pregnancies: 3 within 2 years
Poor fetal outcome in a previous pregnancy
Poverty
Poor diet habits with resistance to change
Use of tobacco, alcohol, or drugs
Weight at conception under or over normal weight
Problems with weight gain
 Any weight loss
 Weight gain of less than 1 kg/mo after the first
  trimester
 Weight gain of more than 1 kg/wk after the first
  trimester
Multifetal pregnancy
Low hemoglobin and/or hematocrit values

the childbearing years. It affects nearly one fifth of the pregnant women in industrialized countries. The maternal mortality rate is increased among anemic women, who are poorly prepared to tolerate hemorrhage at the time of birth. In addition, anemic women may have a greater likelihood of cardiac failure during labor, postpartum infections, and/or poor wound healing (Allen, 1997). The fetus is also affected by maternal anemia. The risk of preterm birth is about threefold greater in anemic women, and fetal iron stores may also be reduced by maternal anemia (Allen, 1997). Anemia is more common among adolescents and African-American women than among adult Caucasian women.

The Institute of Medicine (1992) recommends that all pregnant women receive a supplement of 30 mg of ferrous iron daily, starting by 12 weeks of gestation. (Iron supplements may be poorly tolerated during the nausea prevalent in the first trimester.) However, if iron deficiency anemia, manifested by a low hematocrit value or low serum hemoglobin and ferritin levels, is present, increased dosages (60 to 120 mg daily) are required. Certain foods taken with an iron supplement can promote or inhibit the absorption of iron from the supplement. See the Home Care box on p. 372 regarding iron supplementation. Even when a woman is taking an iron supplement, however, she should also include good food sources of iron in her daily diet (see Table 16-1).

Calcium

There is no increase in the DRI of calcium during pregnancy and lactation, in comparison to the recommendation for the nonpregnant woman (see Table 16-1). The DRI (1000 mg daily for women 19 and older and 1300 mg for those younger than 19) appears to provide sufficient calcium for fetal bone and tooth development to proceed

while maintaining maternal bone mass. Milk and yogurt are especially rich sources of calcium, providing approximately 300 mg per cup (240 ml). Nevertheless, many women do not consume these foods or do not consume adequate amounts to provide the recommended intakes of calcium. One problem that can interfere with milk consumption is **lactose intolerance,** which is the inability to digest milk sugar (lactose) because of the lack of the enzyme lactase in the small intestine. It is relatively common in adults, particularly African-Americans, Asians, Native Americans, and Eskimos. Milk consumption may cause abdominal cramping, bloating, and diarrhea in such people. Yogurt, sweet acidophilus milk, buttermilk, cheese, chocolate milk, and cocoa may be tolerated even when fresh fluid milk is not. Commercial products that contain lactase (e.g., Lactaid) are available in pharmacies and many supermarkets. The lactase in these products hydrolyzes, or digests, the lactose in the milk, making it possible for lactose-intolerant people to drink milk.

In some cultures it is uncommon for adults to drink milk. For example, Puerto Ricans and other Hispanic people may use it only as an additive in coffee. Pregnant women from these cultures may need to consume nondairy sources of calcium. Vegetarian diets may also be deficient in calcium (Box 16-2). If calcium intake appears low and the woman does not change her diet habits despite counseling, a supplement containing 600 mg of elemental calcium may be needed daily. Calcium supplements may also be recommended when a pregnant woman experiences leg cramps that are caused by an imbalance in the calcium-phosphorus ratio.

Sodium

During pregnancy the need for sodium increases slightly, primarily because the body water is expanding (e.g., the expanding blood volume). Sodium is essential for maintaining body water balance. In the past, dietary sodium was routinely restricted in an effort to control the peripheral edema that commonly occurs during pregnancy. However, it is now recognized that moderate peripheral edema is normal in pregnancy, occurring as a response to the fluid-retaining effects of elevated levels of estrogen. An excessive emphasis on sodium restriction may also make it difficult for pregnant women to achieve an adequate diet. Grain, milk, and meat products, which are good sources of the nutrients needed during pregnancy, are significant sources of sodium. In addition, sodium restriction may stress the adrenal glands and kidneys as they attempt to retain adequate sodium. In general, sodium restriction is necessary only if the woman has a medical condition such as renal or liver failure or hypertension.

Excessive intake of sodium is discouraged during pregnancy, just as it is in nonpregnant women, because it may contribute to abnormal fluid retention and edema. Table salt (sodium chloride) is the richest source of sodium. Most canned foods contain added salt, unless the label states

BOX 16-2 Calcium Sources for Women Who Do Not Drink Milk

Each of the following provides approximately the same amount of calcium as 1 cup of milk:

FISH

3 oz can of sardines
$4\frac{1}{2}$ oz can of salmon (if bones are eaten)

BEANS AND LEGUMES

3 cups of cooked dried beans
$2\frac{1}{2}$ cups of refried beans
2 cups of baked beans with molasses
1 cup of tofu (calcium added in processing)

GREENS

1 cup of collards
$1\frac{1}{2}$ cups of kale or turnip greens

BAKED PRODUCTS

3 pieces of cornbread
3 English muffins
4 slices of French toast
2 (7 inch diameter) waffles

FRUITS

11 dried figs
$1\frac{1}{8}$ cups of orange juice with calcium added

SAUCES

3 oz of pesto sauce
5 oz of cheese sauce

otherwise. Large amounts of sodium are also found in many processed foods, including meats (e.g., smoked or cured meats, cold cuts, and corned beef), baked goods, mixes for casseroles or grain products, soups, and condiments. Products low in nutritive value and excessively high in sodium include pretzels, potato and other chips, pickles, catsup, prepared mustard, steak and Worcestershire sauces, some soft drinks, and bouillon. A moderate sodium intake can usually be achieved by salting food lightly during cooking, adding no additional salt at the table, and also by avoiding low-nutrient/high-sodium foods.

Zinc

Zinc is a constituent of numerous enzymes involved in major metabolic pathways. Zinc deficiency is associated with malformations of the central nervous system in infants. When large amounts of iron and folic acid are consumed, the absorption of zinc is inhibited and the serum zinc levels are reduced as a result. Because iron and folic acid supplements are commonly prescribed during pregnancy, pregnant women should therefore be encouraged to consume good

sources of zinc daily (see Table 16-1). Women with anemia who receive high-dose iron supplements also need supplements of zinc and copper (Institute of Medicine, 1992).

Fluoride

The effect of prenatal fluoride supplementation on tooth development in the infant is not fully known. However, a prospective study of 5-year-old children whose mothers were randomized to receive prenatal fluoride supplementation or placebo suggests that prenatal fluoride supplementation has little effect on the incidence and prevalence of tooth decay (Leverett et al., 1997). No increase in fluoride intake over the nonpregnant DRI is currently recommended during pregnancy (Standing Committee, 1997).

Fat-Soluble Vitamins

Fat-soluble vitamins—A, D, E, and K—are stored in the body tissues; in the event of chronic overdoses, these vitamins can reach toxic levels. Because of the high potential for toxicity, pregnant women are therefore advised to take fat-soluble vitamin supplements only as prescribed. Vitamins A and D deserve special mention, however.

Adequate intake of vitamin A is needed so that sufficient amounts of the vitamin can be stored in the fetus. However, dietary sources can readily supply sufficient amounts. Congenital malformations have occurred in infants of mothers who took excessive amounts of vitamin A during pregnancy, and thus supplements are not recommended for pregnant women (Institute of Medicine, 1992). Vitamin A analogs (e.g., isotretinoin [Accutane]), which are prescribed for the treatment of cystic acne, are a special concern. Isotretinoin use during early pregnancy has been associated with an increased incidence of heart malformations, facial abnormalities, cleft palate, hydrocephalus, and deafness and blindness in the infant, as well as an increased risk of miscarriage. Topical agents such as tretinoin (Retin-A) do not appear to enter the circulation in any substantial amounts, but their safety in pregnancy has not been confirmed.

Vitamin D plays an important role in the absorption and metabolism of calcium. The main food sources of this vitamin are enriched or fortified foods such as milk and ready-to-eat cereals. Vitamin D is also produced in the skin by the action of ultraviolet light (in sunlight). A severe deficiency may lead to neonatal hypocalcemia and tetany, as well as to hypoplasia of the tooth enamel. Women with lactose intolerance and those who do not include milk in their diet for any reason are at risk for vitamin D deficiency. Other risk factors for deficiency are dark skin, habitual use of clothing that covers most of the skin, and living in northern latitudes where sunlight exposure is limited, especially during the winter.

Water-Soluble Vitamins

Body stores of water-soluble vitamins are much smaller than those of fat-soluble vitamins, and the water-soluble vitamins, in contrast to the fat-soluble ones, are readily excreted in the urine. Therefore good sources of these vitamins must be consumed frequently, and toxicity with overdose is less likely than it is in people taking fat-soluble vitamins.

Because of the increase in RBC production during pregnancy, as well as the nutritional requirements of the rapidly growing cells in the fetus and placenta, pregnant women should consume about 50% more folic acid than nonpregnant women, or about 600 µg daily. In the United States, all enriched grain products (which include most white breads, flour, and pasta) must contain folic acid at a level of 1.4 mg per kg flour. This level of fortification supplies approximately 0.1 mg folic acid daily in the average American diet (U.S. DHHS, FDA, 1996). All women of childbearing potential need careful counseling about including good sources of folic acid in their diet (Tinkle & Sterling, 1997).

Pyridoxine, or vitamin B$_6$, is involved in protein metabolism. Although levels of a pyridoxine-containing enzyme have been reported to be low in women with PIH, there is no evidence that supplementation prevents or eradicates the condition. No supplement is recommended routinely, but women with poor diets and those at nutritional risk (see Box 16-1) may need a supplement providing 2 mg/day (Institute of Medicine, 1992).

Vitamin C, or ascorbic acid, plays an important role in tissue formation and enhances the absorption of iron. The vitamin C needs of most women are readily met by a diet that includes at least one daily serving of citrus fruit or juice or another good source of the vitamin (see Table 16-1), but women who smoke need more. A supplement of 50 mg/day is recommended for women determined to be at nutritional risk (Institute of Medicine, 1992). However, if the mother should take excessive doses of this vitamin during pregnancy, vitamin C deficiency may develop in the infant after birth.

Nutrient Supplements

The consensus of the 1992 Institute of Medicine committee is that food can and should be the normal vehicle to meet the additional needs imposed by pregnancy, except for iron. Recall that a supplemental dose of 30 mg per day is recommended. However, some women chronically consume diets that are deficient in necessary nutrients and, for whatever reason, may be unable to change this intake. For these women a supplement should be considered. It is important that the pregnant woman understand that the use of a vitamin/mineral supplement does not lessen the need to consume a nutritious, well-balanced diet.

Other Nutritional Issues During Pregnancy

Pica and food cravings. Pica, which is the practice of consuming nonfood substances (e.g., clay, dirt, and laundry starch) or excessive amounts of foodstuffs low in nutritional value (e.g., ice or freezer frost, baking powder or soda, and cornstarch), often is influenced by the woman's cultural background. In the United States it appears to be most common among African-American women, women from rural areas, and women with a family history of pica.

The regular and heavy consumption of low-nutrient products may cause more nutritious foods to be displaced from the diet, and the items consumed may also interfere with the absorption of nutrients, especially minerals. Women with pica have been found to have lower hemoglobin levels than those without pica (Rainville, 1998). The possibility of pica must be considered when pregnant women are found to be anemic, and the nurse should provide counseling about the health risks associated with pica. The existence of pica, as well as details of the type and amounts of products ingested, is likely to be discovered only by the sensitive interviewer who has developed a relationship of trust with the woman. It has been proposed that pica and **food cravings** (i.e., the urge to have ice cream, pickles, or pizza, for example) during pregnancy are caused by an innate drive to consume nutrients missing from the diet. However, research has not supported this hypothesis.

Adolescent pregnancy. Many adolescent females have diets that fall below the recommended intakes of key nutrients, including energy, calcium, and iron. In one survey, 37% of African-American teens and 42% of Caucasian adolescents were underweight, when classified according to their BMI (Sargent et al., 1994).

Pregnant adolescents and their infants are at increased risk of complications during pregnancy and parturition. Growth of the pelvis is delayed in comparison to growth in stature, and this helps to explain why cephalopelvic disproportion and other mechanical problems associated with labor are common among young adolescents. Competition between the growing adolescent and the fetus for nutrients may also contribute to some of the poor outcomes apparent in teen pregnancies. Pregnant adolescents are encouraged to choose a weight gain goal at the upper end of the range for their BMI (Institute of Medicine, 1992). The goal is to reduce the prevalence of LBW among infants of teen mothers.

Efforts to improve the nutritional health of pregnant adolescents focus on improving the nutrition knowledge, meal planning, and food preparation/selection skills of young females; promoting access to prenatal care; developing nutrition interventions and educational programs that are effective with adolescents; and striving to understand the factors that create barriers to change in the adolescent population (Story, 1997).

Pregnancy-induced hypertension. The cause of PIH, or preeclampsia, is not known. There has been speculation that the poor intake of several nutrients, including calcium, magnesium, vitamin B$_6$, and protein, might foster its development, but there is no definite evidence that nutritional deficiencies are causes or that nutritional supplements can help prevent it. At present, a diet adequate in the recommended nutrients (see Table 16-1) appears to be the best means of reducing the risk of PIH.

Exercise during pregnancy. Moderate exercise during pregnancy yields numerous benefits, including improving muscle tone, potentially shortening the course of labor, and promoting a sense of well-being. By observing careful guidelines (ACOG, 1994), most women can safely exercise throughout pregnancy. However, two nutritional concepts are especially important for women who choose to exercise during pregnancy. First, a liberal amount of fluid should be consumed before, during, and after exercise because dehydration can trigger premature labor. Second, the calorie intake should be sufficient to meet the increased needs of pregnancy and the demands of exercise.

NUTRIENT NEEDS DURING LACTATION

Nutritional needs during lactation are similar in many ways to those during pregnancy (see Table 16-1). Needs for energy (calories), protein, calcium, iodine, zinc, the B vitamins (thiamine, riboflavin, niacin, pyridoxine, and vitamin B_{12}), and vitamin C remain elevated over nonpregnant needs. The recommendations for some of these (e.g., vitamin C, zinc, and protein) is slightly to moderately higher than during pregnancy (see Table 16-1). This allowance covers the amount of the nutrient released in the milk, as well as needs of the mother for tissue maintenance. In the case of iron and folic acid, the recommendation during lactation is lower than during pregnancy. Both of these nutrients are essential for RBC formation, and thus for maintaining the increase in the blood volume that occurs during pregnancy. With the decrease in maternal blood volume to nonpregnant levels after birth, maternal iron and folic acid needs also fall. Many lactating women experience a delay in the return of menses, and this also conserves blood cells and reduces iron and folic acid needs. It is especially important that the calcium intake be adequate; if it is not and the woman does not respond to diet counseling, a supplement of 600 mg of calcium per day may be needed.

The recommended energy intake is an increase of 500 kcal more than the woman's nonpregnant intake. The Institute of Medicine (1992) recommends that lactating women consume at least 1800 kcal per day, because it becomes difficult to obtain adequate nutrients for the maintenance of lactation at levels below that. Because of the deposition of energy stores, the woman who has gained the optimal amount of weight during pregnancy is heavier after birth than at the beginning of pregnancy. As a result of the caloric demands of lactation, however, the lactating mother usually experiences a gradual but steady weight loss. Most women rapidly lose several pounds during the first month postpartum, whether they breastfeed or not. After the first month, the average loss during lactation is 0.5 to 1.0 kg a month, and a woman who is overweight may be able to lose up to 2 kg without decreasing her milk supply (Institute of Medicine, 1992).

Fluid intake must also be adequate to maintain milk production, but the mother's level of thirst is the best guide to the right amount. There is no need to consume more fluids than that needed to satisfy thirst.

Smoking and alcohol and excessive caffeine intake should be avoided during lactation. Smoking may not only impair milk production, but also it exposes the infant to the risk of passive smoking. It is speculated that the infant's psychomotor development may be affected by maternal alcohol use, and alcoholic beverages (two drinks per day) may impair the milk ejection reflex. Coffee intake may lead to a reduced iron concentration in milk and consequently contribute to the development of anemia in the infant. The caffeine concentration in milk is only approximately 1% of the mother's plasma level, but caffeine seems to accumulate in the infant. Breastfed infants of mothers who drink large amounts of coffee or caffeine-containing soft drinks may be unusually active and wakeful.

▌ CARE MANAGEMENT

During pregnancy, nutrition plays a key role in achieving an optimal outcome for the mother and her unborn baby. The motivation to learn about nutrition is usually greater during pregnancy because parents strive to "do what's right for the baby." Optimal nutrition cannot eliminate all the problems that may arise during pregnancy, but it does establish a good foundation for supporting the needs of the mother and her unborn baby.

Assessment and Nursing Diagnoses

Assessment is based on a **diet history** (a description of the woman's usual food and beverage intake and factors affecting her nutritional status, such as medications being taken and the adequacy of income to allow her to purchase the necessary foods) obtained from an interview and review of the woman's health records, physical examination, and laboratory results. Ideally a nutritional assessment is performed before conception so that any recommended changes in diet, lifestyle, and weight can be undertaken before the woman becomes pregnant.

Diet History

Obstetric and gynecologic effects on nutrition. Nutritional reserves may be depleted in the multiparous woman or the one who has had frequent pregnancies (especially 3 pregnancies within 2 years). A history of preterm birth or birth of an LBW or SGA infant may indicate inadequate dietary intake. PIH may also be a factor in poor maternal nutrition. Birth of a large-for-gestational age (LGA) infant may indicate the existence of maternal diabetes mellitus. Previous contraceptive methods may also affect reproductive health. Increased menstrual blood loss often occurs during the first 3 to 6 months after placement of an intrauterine contraceptive device. Consequently the user may have low iron stores or even iron deficiency anemia. Oral contraceptive agents, on the other hand, are associated with decreased menstrual losses and increased iron stores; however, oral contraceptives may interfere with folic acid metabolism.

Medical history. Chronic maternal illnesses such as diabetes mellitus, renal disease, liver disease, cystic fibrosis or other malabsorptive disorders, seizure disorders and the use of anticonvulsant agents, hypertension, and PKU may affect a woman's nutritional status and dietary needs. In women with illnesses that have resulted in nutritional deficits or that require dietary treatment (e.g., diabetes mellitus or PKU), it is extremely important for nutritional care to be started and for the condition to be optimally controlled before conception. The registered dietitian can provide in-depth counseling for the woman who requires a therapeutic diet during pregnancy and lactation.

Usual maternal diet. The woman's usual food and beverage intake, the adequacy of her income and other resources to meet her nutritional needs, any dietary modifications, food allergies and intolerances, and all medications and nutrition supplements being taken, as well as pica and cultural dietary requirements, should be ascertained. In addition, the presence and severity of nutrition-related discomforts of pregnancy, such as morning sickness, constipation, and pyrosis (heartburn), should be determined. These discomforts are discussed in more detail in the section on implementation. The nurse should be alert to any evidence of eating disorders such as anorexia nervosa, bulimia, and frequent and rigorous dieting before or during pregnancy.

The impact of food allergies and intolerances on nutritional status ranges from very important to almost nil. Lactose intolerance is of special concern in pregnant and lactating women because no other food group equals milk and milk products in terms of calcium content. If a woman suffers from lactose intolerance, the interviewer should explore her intake of other calcium sources (see Box 16-2).

The assessment must include an evaluation of the woman's financial status and her knowledge of sound dietary practices. The quality of the diet increases with increasing socioeconomic status and educational level. Poor women may not have access to adequate refrigeration and cooking facilities and may find it difficult to obtain adequate nutritious food. The pregnancy rates are high among homeless women, and many such women cannot or do not take advantage of services such as food stamps.

Box 16-3 provides a simple tool for obtaining diet history information. When potential problems are identified, they should be followed up with a careful interview.

Physical Examination

Anthropometric (body) **measurements** provide short- and long-term information on a woman's nutritional status and are thus essential to the assessment. At a minimum, the woman's height and weight must be determined at the time of her first prenatal visit, and her weight should be measured at every subsequent visit (see earlier discussion of BMI).

A careful physical examination can reveal objective signs of malnutrition (Table 16-3). It is important to note, however, that some of these signs are nonspecific and the physiologic changes of pregnancy may complicate the interpretation of physical findings. For example, lower extremity edema often occurs when caloric and protein defi-

ciency are present, but it may also be a normal finding in the third trimester. The interpretation of physical findings is made easier by a thorough health history and by laboratory testing, if indicated.

Laboratory Testing

The only nutrition-related laboratory test necessary for most pregnant women is a hematocrit or hemoglobin measurement to screen for the presence of **anemia.** Because of the physiologic anemia of pregnancy, the reference values for hemoglobin and hematocrit must be adjusted during pregnancy. The lower limit of the normal range for hemoglobin during pregnancy is 11 g/dl in the first and third trimesters and 10.5 g/dl in the second trimester (compared with 12 g/dl in the nonpregnant state). The lower limit of the normal range for hematocrit is 33% during the first and third trimesters and 32% in the second trimester (compared with 36% in the nonpregnant state). Cutoff values for anemia are higher in women who smoke or live at high altitudes, because the decreased oxygen-carrying capacity of their RBCs causes them to produce more RBCs than other women (Institute of Medicine, 1992).

A woman's history or physical findings may indicate the need for additional testing, such as a complete blood cell count with a differential to identify megaloblastic or macrocytic anemia and the measurement of levels of specific vitamins or minerals believed to be lacking in the diet.

The assessment gives a basis for making appropriate nursing diagnoses.

▪ Nursing Diagnoses _____

- Nutrition, altered: less than body requirements related to
  - inadequate information about nutritional needs and weight gain during pregnancy
  - misperceptions regarding normal body changes during pregnancy and inappropriate fear of becoming fat
  - inadequate income or skills in meal planning and preparation
- Nutrition, altered: more than body requirements related to
  - excessive intake of energy (calories) or decrease in activity during pregnancy
  - use of unnecessary dietary supplements, especially supplements of fat soluble vitamins, protein (if diet is adequate in protein), and therapeutic amounts of iron (in the absence of iron deficiency anemia)
- Constipation related to
  - decrease in GI motility because of elevated progesterone levels
  - compression of intestines by enlarging uterus
  - oral iron supplementation
- Knowledge deficit related to
  - inadequate information regarding nutritional needs during pregnancy

BOX 16-3　Food Intake Questionnaire

Which of the following did you eat or drink yesterday? If the way you ate yesterday wasn't the way you usually eat, choose a recent day that was typical for you.

FOOD OR DRINK	NUMBER OF SERVINGS	FOOD OR DRINK	NUMBER OF SERVINGS
Beer, wine, other alcoholic drinks		Orange or grapefruit juice	
Tea		Fruit juice other than orange or grapefruit	
Coffee			
Fruit drink		Soft drinks	
Water		Milk	
Cheese		Cereal with milk	
Macaroni and cheese		Yogurt	
Other foods with cheese (such as lasagna, enchiladas, cheeseburgers)		Pizza	
		Melon (such as watermelon, cantaloupe, honeydew)	
Orange or grapefruit			
Bananas		Berries (kind _____)	
Peaches or apricots		Apples	
Green salad		Other fruit	
Spinach or greens		Broccoli	
Green peas		Green beans	
Sweet potatoes		Potatoes (other than fried)	
Carrots		Corn	
Meat		Other vegetables	
Fish		Chicken or turkey	
Peanut butter		Egg	
Dried beans or peas		Nuts	
Bacon or sausage		Hot dog	
Bread		Cold cuts	
Rice		Roll	
Spaghetti or other pasta		Cereal	
Tortillas		Noodles	
French fries		Chips	
Cookie		Cake	
Pie		Donut or pastry	

Are you often bothered by any of the following? (Circle all that apply.)
　Nausea　　　　　Vomiting　　　　　Heartburn　　　　　Constipation

Are you on a special diet? No____ Yes____ If yes, what kind?

Do you try to limit the amount or kind of food you eat to control your weight? No____ Yes____

Do you avoid any foods for health or religious reasons? No____ Yes____ If yes, what foods?

Do you take any prescribed drugs or medications? No____ Yes____
　If yes, what are they?

Do you take any over-the-counter medications (such as aspirin, cold medicines, Tylenol)?
No____ Yes____ If yes, what are they?

Do you ever have trouble affording the food you need? No____ Yes____

Do you have any help getting the food you need? No____ Yes____ (Circle all that apply.)
　Food stamps　　　　　WIC　　　　　School lunch or breakfast
　Food from a food pantry, soup kitchen, or food bank

Expected Outcomes of Care

An individualized nursing plan of care based on the nursing diagnoses should be developed in collaboration with the woman. For many women with uncomplicated pregnancies, the nurse can serve as the primary source of nutrition education during pregnancy. The registered dietitian, who has specialized training in diet evaluation and planning, nutritional needs during illness, and ethnic and cultural food patterns, as well as in translating nutrient needs into food patterns, frequently serves as a consultant.

TABLE 16-3 Physical Assessment of Nutritional Status

SIGNS OF GOOD NUTRITION	SIGNS OF POOR NUTRITION
GENERAL APPEARANCE	
Alert, responsive, energetic, good endurance	Listless, apathetic, cachectic, easily fatigued, looks tired
MUSCLES	
Well developed, firm, good tone, some fat under skin	Flaccid, poor tone, undeveloped, tender, "wasted" appearance
NERVOUS CONTROL	
Good attention span, not irritable or restless, normal reflexes, psychologic stability	Inattentive, irritable, confused, burning and tingling of hands and feet, loss of position and vibratory sense, weakness and tenderness of muscles, decrease or loss of ankle and knee reflexes
GASTROINTESTINAL FUNCTION	
Good appetite and digestion, normal regular elimination, no palpable organs or masses	Anorexia, indigestion, constipation or diarrhea, liver or spleen enlargement
CARDIOVASCULAR FUNCTION	
Normal heart rate and rhythm, no murmurs, normal blood pressure for age	Rapid heart rate, enlarged heart, abnormal rhythm, elevated blood pressure
HAIR	
Shiny, lustrous, firm, not easily plucked, healthy scalp	Stringy, dull, brittle, dry, thin and sparse, depigmented, can be easily plucked
SKIN (GENERAL)	
Smooth, slightly moist, good color	Rough, dry, scaly, pale, pigmented, irritated, easily bruised, petechiae
FACE AND NECK	
Skin color uniform, smooth, pink, healthy appearance; no enlargement of thyroid gland; lips not chapped or swollen	Scaly, swollen, skin dark over cheeks and under eyes, lumpiness or flakiness of skin around nose and mouth; thyroid enlarged; lips swollen, angular lesions or fissures at corners of mouth
ORAL CAVITY	
Reddish pink mucous membranes and gums; no swelling or bleeding of gums; tongue healthy pink or deep reddish in appearance, not swollen or smooth, surface papillae present; teeth bright and clean, no cavities, no pain, no discoloration	Gums spongy, bleed easily, inflamed or receding; tongue swollen, scarlet and raw, magenta color, beefy, hyperemic and hypertrophic papillae, atrophic papillae; teeth with unfilled caries, absent teeth, worn surfaces, mottled
EYES	
Bright, clear, shiny, no sores at corners of eyelids, membranes moist and healthy pink color, no prominent blood vessels or mound of tissue (Bitot's spots) on sclera, no fatigue circles beneath	Eye membranes pale, redness of membrane, dryness, signs of infection, Bitot's spots, redness and fissuring of eyelid corners, dryness of eye membrane, dull appearance of cornea, soft cornea, blue sclerae
EXTREMITIES	
No tenderness, weakness, or swelling; nails firm and pink	Edema, tender calves, tingling, weakness; nails spoon-shaped, brittle
SKELETON	
No malformations	Bowlegs, knock-knees, chest deformity at diaphragm, beaded ribs, prominent scapulas

GUIDELINES/GUÍAS

Diet and Nutrition

You need to gain weight
Usted necesita aumentar de peso.

You need to control your weight gain.
Usted necesita controlar su aumento de peso.

Eat nutritious foods.
Coma alimentos nutritivos.

Eat foods high in protein, calcium, vitamins, and iron.
Coma alimentos altos en proteínas, calcio, vitaminas, y hierro.

Eat a lot of fruits and vegetables.
Coma muchas frutas y vegetales.

Drink four glasses of milk a day.
Tome cuatro vasos de leche diariamente.

Drink low-fat instead of whole milk.
Tome la leche baja en grasa en lugar de la leche completa.

Avoid salty foods like sausage, hot dogs, and french fries.
Evite alimentos muy salados como salchichón, salchichas, y papitas fritas.

Avoid fried foods.
Evita las frituras.

Avoid caffeine.
Evita la cafeína.

There is caffeine in Coca-Cola, tea, and chocolate.
Hay cafeína en la Coca-Cola, té, y el chocolate.

Take prenatal vitamins.
Tome vitaminas prenatales.

BOX 16-4 Weight Gain During Pregnancy

- Progressive weight gain during pregnancy is essential to ensure normal fetal growth and development and the deposition of maternal stores that promote successful lactation.
- Recommended weight gain during pregnancy is determined largely by prepregnancy weight for height. Normal-weight women, 11.5-16 kg; underweight women, 12.5-18 kg; overweight women, 7-11.5 kg.
- Weight gain should be achieved through a balanced diet of regular foods chosen from all the different food groups (see Table 16-2).
- The pattern of weight gain is important: approximately 0.4 kg per week during the second and third trimesters for normal-weight women; 0.5 kg per week for underweight women; and 0.3 kg per week for overweight women

---

Pregnant women with serious nutritional problems, those with intervening illnesses such as diabetes (either preexisting or gestational), and any others requiring in-depth dietary counseling should be referred to the dietitian. The nurse, dietitian, physician, and nurse-midwife collaborate in helping the woman achieve nutrition-related expected outcomes. Some common nutrition-related outcomes require the woman to take the following actions:

- Achieve an appropriate weight gain during pregnancy—an appropriate goal for weight gain takes into account such factors as the woman's prepregnancy weight, whether she is overweight/obese or underweight, and whether the pregnancy is single or multifetal.
- Consume adequate nutrients from the diet and supplements to meet estimated needs.
- Cope successfully with the nutrition-related discomforts associated with pregnancy, such as pyrosis (heartburn), morning sickness, and constipation.
- Avoid or reduce potentially harmful practices such as smoking, alcohol consumption, and caffeine intake.
- Return to prepregnancy weight (or an appropriate weight for height) within 6 months of giving birth.

Plan of Care and Interventions

Nutritional care and teaching generally involve (1) acquainting the woman with the nutritional needs during pregnancy and the characteristics of an adequate diet, if necessary; (2) helping her to individualize her diet so that she achieves an adequate intake while conforming to her personal, cultural, financial, and health circumstances; (3) acquainting her with strategies for coping with the nutrition-related discomforts of pregnancy; (4) helping her use nutrition supplements appropriately; and (5) consulting with and making referrals to other professionals or services as indicated. Two programs that provide nutrition services are the food stamp program and the Special Supplemental Program for **Women, Infants, and Children (WIC),** which provides vouchers for selected foods to pregnant and lactating women, as well as infants and children at nutritional risk. WIC foods include eggs, cheese, milk, juice, and fortified cereals; these are chosen because they provide iron, protein, vitamin C, and other vitamins.

Adequate Dietary Intake

Diet teaching can take place in a one-on-one interview or in a group setting. In either case, teaching should emphasize the importance of choosing a varied diet composed of readily available foods (rather than specialized diet supplements). Good nutrition practices (and the avoidance of poor practices such as smoking and alcohol or drug use) are essential content for prenatal classes designed for women in early pregnancy (see Guidelines/Guías).

The food pyramid (Fig. 16-5) can be used as a guide to making daily food choices during pregnancy and lactation, just as it is during other stages of the life cycle. The pyramid places the bread, cereal, rice, and pasta group at its base.

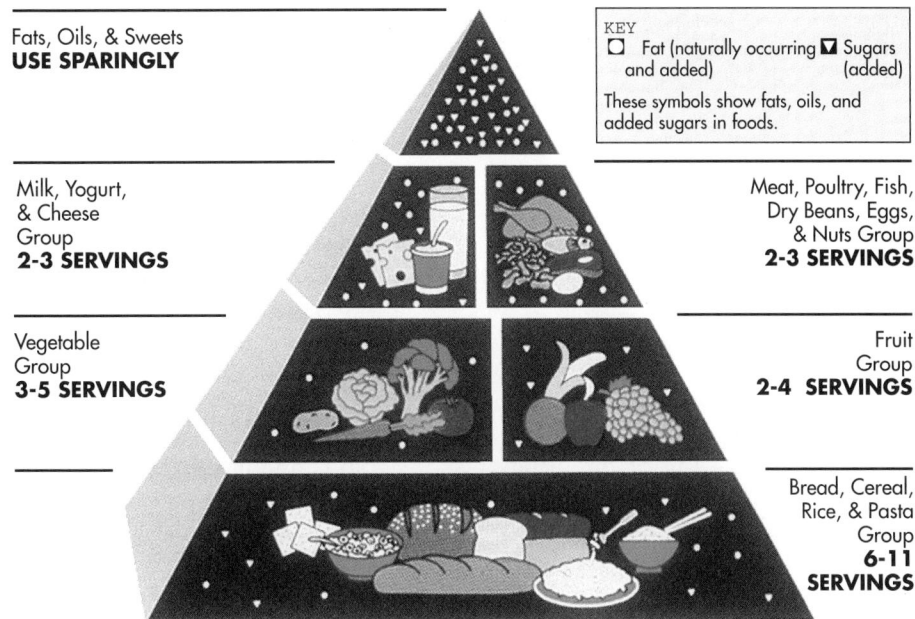

Fats, Oils, & Sweets
USE SPARINGLY

KEY
☐ Fat (naturally occurring ☑ Sugars
and added)   (added)

These symbols show fats, oils, and
added sugars in foods.

Milk, Yogurt,
& Cheese
Group
2-3 SERVINGS

Meat, Poultry, Fish,
Dry Beans, Eggs,
& Nuts Group
2-3 SERVINGS

Vegetable
Group
3-5 SERVINGS

Fruit
Group
2-4 SERVINGS

Bread, Cereal,
Rice, & Pasta
Group
**6-11
SERVINGS**

Fig. 16-5   Food guide pyramid, a guide to daily food choices. *(Courtesy U.S. Department of Agriculture, Washington, D.C.)*

This position was chosen to indicate that this group should serve as the basis for a healthy diet; six to eleven servings are recommended each day. Vegetables (three to five servings) and fruits (two to four servings) are just above the grains group. The milk, yogurt, and cheese group (two to three servings for nonpregnant adults, increasing to three to four servings for pregnant and lactating women) and the meat, poultry, fish, dried beans, eggs, and nuts group (two to three servings) form a narrow band near the top of the pyramid. At the apex are fats, oils, and sweets (not considered a food group), which are to be used sparingly. The importance of consuming adequate amounts from the milk, yogurt, and cheese group needs to be emphasized, especially for adolescents and women under 25 who are still actively adding calcium to their skeletons; adolescents need at least 1 L of milk or the equivalent daily.

Pregnancy. The pregnant woman must understand what an adequate weight gain during pregnancy means, recognize the reasons for its importance, and be able to evaluate her own gain in terms of the desirable pattern. Many women, particularly those who have worked hard to control their weight before pregnancy, may find it difficult to understand the reason the weight gain goal is so high when a newborn is so small. The nurse can explain that the maternal weight gain consists of increments in the weight of many tissues, not just the growing fetus (see Fig. 16-4).

Dietary overindulgence, on the other hand, which may result in excessive fat stores that persist after giving birth, should be discouraged. Nevertheless, it is best not to focus unduly on weight gain, which can result in feelings of stress and guilt in the woman who does not observe the preferred pattern of gain. Teaching regarding weight gain during pregnancy is summarized in Box 16-4.

Postpartum. The need for a varied diet consisting of a representation of foods from all the food groups continues throughout lactation. As mentioned previously, the lactating woman should be advised to consume at least 1800 kcal daily, and she should receive counseling if her diet appears to be inadequate in any nutrients. Special attention should be given to her zinc, vitamin B$_6$, and folic acid intake, because the recommendations for these remain higher than those for nonpregnant women (see Table 16-1). Sufficient calcium is needed to allow for both milk formation and maintenance of maternal bone mass. It may be difficult for lactating women to consume enough of these nutrients without careful diet planning.

The woman who does not breastfeed will lose weight gradually if she consumes a balanced diet that provides slightly less than her daily energy expenditure. Lactating and nonlactating women should know that fat is the most concentrated source of calories in the diet (9 kcal/g versus 4 kcal/g in carbohydrates and proteins), and fat calories are more efficiently converted into fat stores than calories from carbohydrates or proteins. Therefore the first step in weight reduction (or preventing excessive weight gain) is to evaluate the sources of fat in the diet and explore with the client ways of reducing them. Even foods such as vegetables that are originally low in fat can become high in fat when fried or sautéed, served with excessive amounts of salad dressing, consumed with high-fat dips or sauces, or seasoned with butter or bacon drippings. A reasonable weight loss goal for nonlactating women is 0.5 to 1 kg per week; a loss of 1 kg per month is recommended for most lactating women.

Daily food guide and menu planning. The daily food plan (s   16-2 and Fig. 16-5) can be used as a guide for ed   woman about nutritional needs during pregnancy and lactation. This food plan is general enough to be used by women from a wide variety of cultures, including women following a vegetarian diet. One of the more helpful teaching strategies is to help the client plan daily menus that follow the food plan and are affordable, are realistic in terms of preparation time, and are compatible with personal preferences and cultural practices. Information regarding cultural food patterns is provided later in this chapter.

Therapeutic diets. During pregnancy and lactation, the food plan for women on special therapeutic diets may have to be modified. The registered dietitian can instruct these women about their diets and assist them in meal planning. However, the nurse should understand the basic principles of the diet and be able to reinforce the diet teaching.

The nurse should be especially aware of the dietary modifications necessary for women with diabetes mellitus (gestational or preexisting) because this disease is relatively common and because fetal deformity and death occur more often in pregnancies complicated by hyperglycemia or hypoglycemia. Therefore every effort should be made to maintain blood glucose levels in the normal range throughout pregnancy. The food plan of the woman with diabetes usually includes four to six meals and snacks daily, with the daily carbohydrate intake distributed fairly evenly among the meals and snacks. The complex carbohydrates—fibers and starches—should be well represented in the diet of the diabetic woman. To maintain strict control of the blood glucose level, the pregnant diabetic woman usually must monitor her own levels daily (American Diabetes Association, 1999). Urine glucose and ketone measurements are not sensitive enough to detect hyperglycemia accurately and provide no information about hypoglycemia. The nurse must therefore teach the woman the way to monitor her own blood glucose level, unless she has already been doing this before pregnancy.

Iron Supplementation

As mentioned earlier, the nutritional supplement most commonly needed during pregnancy is iron. However, a variety of dietary factors can affect the completeness of absorption of an iron supplement. Bran, milk, egg yolks, coffee, tea, or oxalate-containing vegetables such as spinach and Swiss chard consumed at the same time as iron will inhibit iron absorption. Conversely, iron absorption is promoted by a diet rich in vitamin C (e.g., citrus fruits or melons) or "heme iron" (found in red meats, fish, and poultry). Iron supplements are best absorbed on an empty stomach; thus they can be taken between meals with beverages other than milk, tea, or coffee. Some women have gastrointestinal discomfort when they take the supplement on an empty stomach; therefore a good time for them to take the supplement is just before bedtime. Constipation is common with iron supplementation. Iron supplements should be kept away from any children in the household because their ingestion could result in acute iron poisoning and even death. The accompanying Home Care box summarizes important points regarding iron supplementation.

Coping with Nutrition-Related Discomforts of Pregnancy

The most common nutrition-related discomforts of pregnancy are nausea and vomiting or "morning sickness," constipation, and pyrosis.

Nausea and vomiting. Nausea and vomiting are most common during the first trimester. Most of the time the nausea and vomiting cause only mild to moderate problems nutritionally, although they may be a source of substantial discomfort. The pregnant woman may find the following suggestions helpful in alleviating the problems:

- Eat dry, starchy foods such as dry toast, melba toast, or crackers on awakening in the morning and at other times when nausea occurs.
- Avoid consuming excessive amounts of fluids early in the day or when nauseated (but compensate by drinking fluids at other times).
- Eat small amounts frequently (every 2 to 3 hours) and avoid large meals that distend the stomach.
- Avoid skipping meals and thus becoming extremely hungry, which may worsen nausea. Have a snack such as cereal with milk, a small sandwich, or yogurt before bedtime.
- Avoid sudden movements. Get out of bed slowly.
- Decrease intake of fried and other fatty foods. Good choices are starches such as pastas, rice, and breads and low-fat protein foods (skinless broiled or baked poultry, cooked dried beans or peas, lean meats, and broiled or canned fish).

HOME CARE

Iron Supplementation

- It is difficult to consume enough iron in the diet to meet iron needs and prevent anemia during pregnancy.
- Vitamin C (in citrus fruits, tomatoes, melons, and strawberries) and heme iron (in meats) increase the absorption of iron supplement. Therefore include these in the diet often.
- Bran, tea, coffee, milk, oxalates (in spinach and Swiss chard), and egg yolk decrease iron absorption. Avoid consuming them at the same time as the supplement.
- Iron is best absorbed if it is taken when the stomach is empty; that is, take it between meals with a beverage other than tea, coffee, or milk.
- Iron can be taken at bedtime if abdominal discomfort occurs when it is taken between meals.
- If an iron dose is missed, take it as soon as it is remembered if that is within 13 hours of the scheduled dose. Do *not* double up on the dose.
- Keep the supplement in a child-proof container and out of the reach of any children in the household.
- The iron may cause stools to be black or dark green.
- Constipation is common with iron supplementation. A diet high in fiber with adequate fluid intake is recommended.

- Fresh air may help relieve nausea. Keep the environment well ventilated (e.g., open a window), go for a walk outside, or decrease cooking odors by using an exhaust fan.
- During episodes of nausea eat foods served at cool temperatures and foods that give off little aroma.
- Avoid brushing teeth immediately after eating.
- Some women find that salty and tart foods (e.g., potato chips and lemonade) are tolerated during periods of nausea.

A sample daily food plan that follows these guidelines while providing an adequate diet for the pregnant woman is shown in Box 16-5.

Hyperemesis gravidarum, or severe and persistent vomiting causing weight loss, dehydration, and electrolyte abnormalities, occurs in up to approximately 1% of pregnant women. Intravenous fluid and electrolyte replacement is usually necessary for those women who lose 5% of their body weight. Often this is followed by improved tolerance to the oral intake of food; therapy then consists of the frequent consumption of small amounts of low-fat foods. Enteral tube feeding by means of small-bore nasogastric tubes has been successful in some women. Because the pulmonary aspiration of the feeding is a potential complica-

tion if vomiting occurs, antiemetic medications are sometimes administered in conjunction with the tube feedings. Tube feedings may be used to supplement oral intake, with the volume of the tube feeding gradually being decreased as oral intake improves. In some instances total parenteral nutrition (balanced intravenous feedings of amino acids, carbohydrates, lipids, vitamins, and minerals) has been used to nourish women with hyperemesis gravidarum when their nutritional status has been severely impaired.

Constipation. Improved bowel function generally results from increasing the intake of fiber (e.g., wheat bran and whole wheat products, popcorn, and raw or lightly steamed vegetables) in the diet, because fiber helps to retain water within the stool, creating a bulky stool that stimulates intestinal peristalsis. The recommendation for adults for fiber is 25 g to 35 g. An increase of approximately 15% would be optimal. An adequate fluid intake (at least 50 ml/kg/day) helps to hydrate the fiber and increase the bulk of the stool. Making a habit of regular exercise that uses large muscle groups (walking, swimming, cycling) also helps to stimulate bowel motility.

Pyrosis. Pyrosis, or heartburn, is usually caused by the reflux of gastric contents into the esophagus. This condition can be minimized by the consumption of small, frequent meals, rather than two or three larger meals daily. Because fluids further distend the stomach, they should not be consumed with foods. The woman needs to be sure to drink adequate amounts between meals, however. Avoiding spicy foods may help alleviate the problem. Lying down immediately after eating and wearing clothing that is tight across the abdomen can contribute to the problem of reflux.

Cultural Influences

Consideration of a woman's cultural food preferences enhances communication, providing a greater opportunity for compliance with the agreed upon pattern of intake. Women in most cultures are encouraged to eat a diet typical for them. The nurse needs to be aware of what constitutes a typical diet for each cultural or ethnic group. However, within one cultural group several variations may occur. Thus careful exploration of individual preferences is needed. Although ethnic and cultural food beliefs may seem, at first glance, to conflict with the dietary instruction provided by physicians, nurses, and dietitians, it is often possible for the empathic health care provider to identify cultural beliefs that are congruent with the modern understanding of pregnancy and fetal development. Many cultural food practices have some merit or the culture would not have survived. Food cravings during pregnancy are considered normal by many cultures, but the kinds of cravings often are culturally specific. In most cultures women crave acceptable foods, such as chicken, fish, and greens among African-Americans. Cultural influences on food intake usually lessen if the woman and her family become more integrated into the dominant culture. Nutritional beliefs and the practices of selected cultural groups are summarized in Table 16-4.

BOX 16-5 **Food Plan for Woman with Nausea and Vomiting During Early Pregnancy**

BREAKFAST
Toasted bagel, plain

MIDMORNING
Potato chips
Lemonade

LUNCH
Small turkey sub
Raw broccoli, carrots, and cherry tomatoes with ranch dip
Orange
Skim milk

AFTERNOON
Vegetable juice
Unsalted pretzels

DINNER
Bean soup
Tossed salad
Corn bread sticks
Skim milk

AFTER DINNER
Wheat bran cereal
Sliced banana
Skim milk

TABLE 16-4 **Characteristic Food Patterns of Selected Cultures**

MILK GROUP	PROTEIN GROUP	FRUITS AND VEGETABLES	BREADS AND CEREALS	POSSIBLE DIETARY PROBLEMS
NATIVE AMERICAN (MANY TRIBAL VARIATIONS; MANY "AMERICANIZED")				
Fresh milk Evaporated milk for cooking Ice cream Cream pie	Pork, beef, lamb, rabbit Fowl, fish, eggs Legumes Sunflower seeds Nuts: walnut, acorn, pine, peanut butter Game meat	Green peas, beans Beets, turnips Leafy green and other vegetables Grapes, bananas, peaches, other fresh fruits Roots	Refined bread Whole wheat Cornmeal Rice Dry cereals "Fry" bread Tortillas	Obesity, diabetes, alcoholism, nutritional deficiencies expressed in dental problems and iron deficiency anemia Inadequate amounts of all nutrients Excessive use of sugar
MIDDLE EASTERN* (ARMENIAN, GREEK, SYRIAN, TURKISH)				
Yogurt Little butter	Lamb Nuts Dried peas, beans, lentils Sesame seeds	Peppers, tomatoes, cabbage, grape leaves, cucumbers, squash Dried apricots, raisins, dates	Cracked wheat and dark bread	Fry many meats and vegetables Lack of fresh fruits Insufficient foods from milk group High consumption of sweetenings, lamb fat, and olive oil
AFRICAN-AMERICAN				
Milk† Ice cream Cheese: longhorn, American	Pork: all cuts, plus organs, chitterlings Beef, lamb Chicken, giblets Eggs Nuts Legumes Fish, game	Leafy vegetables Green and yellow vegetables Potato: white, sweet Stewed fruit Bananas and other fresh fruit	Cornmeal and hominy grits Rice Biscuits, pancakes, white breads Puddings: bread, rice	Extensive use of frying, smothering in gravy, or simmering Fats: salt pork, bacon drippings, lard, and gravies High consumption of sweets Insufficient citrus Vegetables often boiled for long periods with pork fat and much salt Limited amounts from milk group†
CHINESE (CANTONESE MOST PREVALENT)				
Milk: water buffalo	Pork sausage‡ Eggs and pigeon eggs Fish Lamb, beef, goat Fowl: chicken, duck Nuts Legumes Soybean curd (tofu)	Many vegetables Radish leaves Bean, bamboo sprouts	Rice/rice flour products Cereals, noodles Wheat, corn, millet seed	Tendency of some immigrants to use large amounts of grease in cooking Limited use of milk and milk products Often low in protein, calories, or both Soy sauce (high sodium)

MSG, Monosodium L-glutamate.
*Religious holidays may involve fasting, which is believed to increase the likelihood of preterm labor. Fasting requirement may be waived during pregnancy.
†Lactose intolerance relatively common in adults.
‡Lower in fat content than Western sausage.

MILK GROUP	PROTEIN GROUP	FRUITS AND VEGETABLES	BREADS AND CEREALS	POSSIBLE DIETARY PROBLEMS
FILIPINO (SPANISH-CHINESE INFLUENCE)				
Flavored milk Milk in coffee Cheese: gouda, cheddar	Pork, beef, goat, rabbit Chicken Fish Eggs, nuts, legumes	Many vegetables and fruits	Rice, cooked cereals Noodles: rice, wheat	Limited use of milk and milk products Tendency to prewash rice Tendency to have only small portions of protein foods
ITALIAN				
Cheese Some ice cream	Meat Eggs Dried beans	Leafy vegetables Potatoes Eggplant, tomatoes, peppers Fruits	Pasta White breads, some whole wheat Farina Cereals	Prefer expensive imported cheeses; reluctant to substitute less expensive domestic varieties Tendency to overcook vegetables Limited use of whole grains High consumption of sweets Extensive use of olive oil Insufficient servings from milk group
JAPANESE (ISEI, MORE JAPANESE INFLUENCE; NISEI, MORE WESTERNIZED)				
Increasing amounts being used by younger generations	Pork, beef, chicken Fish Eggs Legumes: soya, red, lima beans Tofu Nuts	Many vegetables and fruits Seaweed	Rice, rice cakes Wheat noodles Refined bread, noodles	Excessive sodium: pickles, salty crisp seaweed, MSG, and soy sauce Insufficient servings from milk group May use prewashed rice
HISPANIC, MEXICAN-AMERICAN				
Milk Cheese Flan, ice cream	Beef, pork, lamb, chicken, tripe, hot sausage, beef intestines Fish Eggs Nuts Dry beans: pinto, chickpeas (often eaten more than once daily)	Spinach, wild greens, tomatoes, chilies, corn, cactus leaves, cabbage, avocado, potatoes, Pumpkin, zapote, peaches, guava, papaya, citrus	Rice, cornmeal Sweet bread, pastries Tortilla: corn, flour Vermicelli (fideo)	Limited meats primarily due to cost Limited use of milk and milk products Large amounts of lard Abundant use of sugar Tendency to boil vegetables for long periods

Continued

MILK GROUP	PROTEIN GROUP	FRUITS AND VEGETABLES	BREADS AND CEREALS	POSSIBLE DIETARY PROBLEMS
POLISH				
Milk Sour cream Cheese Butter	Pork (preferred) Chicken	Vegetables—limited fresh Cabbage Roots—potatoes Fruits—limited fresh	Dark rye	Sodium in ham, sausage, pickles High consumption of sweets Tendency to over-cook vegetables Limited fruits, raw vegetables
PUERTO RICAN				
Limited use of milk products Coffee with milk (café con leche)	Pork Poultry Eggs (Fridays) Dried codfish Beans (habichuelas)	Avocado, okra Eggplant Sweet yams Starchy vegetables and fruits (viandas)	Rice Cornmeal	Small amounts of pork and poultry Extensive use of fat, lard, salt pork, and olive oil Lack of milk products
SCANDINAVIAN (DANISH, FINNISH, NORWEGIAN, SWEDISH)				
Cream Butter Cheeses	Wild game Reindeer Fish (fresh or dried) Eggs	Berries Dried fruit Vegetables: cole slaw, roots	Whole wheat, rye, barley, sweets (cookies and sweet breads)	Insufficient fresh fruits and vegetables High consumption of sweets, pickled or salted meats, and fish
SOUTHEAST ASIAN (VIETNAMESE, CAMBODIAN)				
Generally not taken Coffee with condensed cow's milk Plain yogurt Ice cream (rare) Soybean milk	Fish (daily): fresh, dried, salted Poultry/eggs: duck, chicken Pork Beef (seldom) Dry beans Tofu	Seasonal variety: fresh or preserved Green, leafy vegetables Yams Corn	Rice: grains, flour, noodles French bread "Cellophane" (bean starch) noodles	Fresh milk products generally not consumed Poultry/eggs may be limited Meat considered "unclean" is avoided Preference for a diet high in salt and pepper, as well as rice and pork High intake of MSG and soy sauce
JEWISH: ORTHODOX*				
Milk† Cheese†	Meat (bloodless; Kosher prepared): beef, lamb, goat, deer, poultry (all types), no pork Fish with fins and scales only No crustaceans	Wide variety	Wide variety	High intake of sodium in meat products

†Milk and milk products not eaten with meat, milk may be taken before the meal or 6 hours after; different sets of dishes and silverware are used to serve milk and meat products.

Vegetarian Diets

Vegetarian diets represent another cultural effect on nutritional status. Foods basic to almost all **vegetarian diets** are vegetables, fruits, legumes, nuts, seeds, and grains. However, there are many variations in vegetarian diets. Semivegetarians, who are not truly vegetarians, include fish, poultry, eggs, and dairy products in their diets but do not eat beef or pork. Such a diet can be completely adequate for pregnant women. Besides plant products, lactoovovegetarians also eat dairy products. Iron and zinc intake may not be adequate in these women, but such diets can be otherwise nutritionally sound. Strict vegetarians, or vegans, consume only plant products. Because vitamin B_{12} is found only in foods of animal origin, this diet is therefore deficient in vitamin B_{12}. As a result, strict vegetarians should take a supplement or consume vitamin B_{12} fortified foods (e.g., soy milk) regularly. Vitamin B_{12} deficiency can result in megaloblastic anemia, glossitis, and neurologic deficits in the mother. Infants born to affected mothers are likely to have megaloblastic anemia and exhibit neurodevelopmental delays. Iron, calcium, zinc, and vitamin B_6 intake may also be low in women on this diet, and some strict vegetarians have excessively low caloric intakes. The protein intake should be assessed especially carefully because plant proteins tend to be "incomplete," in that they lack one or more amino acids required for growth and the maintenance of body tissues.

However, the daily consumption of a variety of different plant proteins—grains, dried beans and peas, nuts, and seeds—helps to provide all of the essential amino acids.

Evaluation

It is essential to set concrete, measurable outcomes; evaluate the woman's progress toward these outcomes regularly; and revise the plan of care if the outcomes are not achieved. In evaluating the adequacy of nutritional intake during pregnancy, the client's weight gain can be compared with standardized grids showing recommended patterns (see Fig. 16-3). These grids are based on mean data and do not always take into account factors such as ethnic or racial variations. To evaluate the adequacy of the woman's diet, her diet can be compared with the plan in Table 16-2. Again, it is essential that individual factors affecting nutritional needs and dietary intake be considered. Physical examination and laboratory testing (see section on assessment) can be used as a means of confirming that a woman's nutritional status is adequate. If an inadequate weight gain is found or nutritional deficits appear, it is essential that the nurse reassess the woman and her understanding of her nutritional needs, reinforce teaching as needed, make referrals as indicated, and continue to reevaluate her nutritional status regularly (see Plan of Care).

PLAN OF CARE | Nutrition During Pregnancy

| **NURSING DIAGNOSIS** **Knowledge deficit related to nutritional requirements during pregnancy** |

Expected Outcomes *The client will delineate nutritional requirements and exhibit evidence of incorporating requirements into diet.*

Nursing Interventions/Rationales

Review basic nutritional requirements for a healthy diet using recommended dietary guidelines and the food guide pyramid *to provide knowledge baseline for discussion.*

Discuss increased nutrient needs (calories, protein, minerals, vitamins) that occur as a result of being pregnant *to increase knowledge needed for altered dietary requirements.*

Discuss the relationship between weight gain and fetal growth *to reinforce interdependence of fetus and mother.*

Calculate the appropriate total weight gain range during pregnancy using the woman's body mass index as a guide and discuss recommended rates of weight gain during the various trimesters of pregnancy *to provide concrete measures of dietary success.*

Review food preferences, cultural eating patterns or beliefs, and prepregnancy eating patterns *to enhance integration of new dietary needs.*

Discuss how to fit nutritional needs into usual dietary patterns and how to alter any identified nutritional deficits or excesses *to increase chances of success with dietary alterations.*

Discuss food aversions or cravings that may occur during pregnancy and strategies to deal with these if they are detrimental to fetus (e.g., pica) *to ensure well-being of fetus.*

Have woman keep a food diary delineating eating habits, dietary alterations, aversions, and cravings *to track eating habits and potential problem areas.*

| **NURSING DIAGNOSIS** **Altered nutrition: more than body requirements related to excessive intake and/or inadequate activity levels** |

Expected Outcomes *The client's weekly weight gain will be reduced to the appropriate rate using her body mass index (BMI) and recommended weight gain ranges as guidelines.*

From Wong, D., & Perry, S. (1998). *Maternal child nursing care.* St. Louis: Mosby.

Nursing Interventions/*Rationales*

Review recent diet history (including food cravings) using a food diary, 24-hour recall, or food frequency approach *to ascertain food excesses contributing to excess weight gain.*

Review normal activity and exercise routines *to determine level of energy expenditure;* discuss eating patterns and reasons that lead to increased food intake (e.g., cultural beliefs or myths, increased stress, boredom) *to identify habits that contribute to excess weight gain.*

Review optimal weight gain guidelines and their rationale *to ensure that woman is knowledgeable about healthful weight gain rates.*

Set target weight gains for the remaining weeks of the pregnancy *to establish set goals.*

Discuss with the woman what changes can be made in diet, activity, and lifestyle *to enhance chances of meeting weight gain goals and dietary needs.* (Weight reduction diets should be avoided, since they may deprive mother and fetus of needed nutrients and lead to ketonemia.)

NURSING DIAGNOSIS Altered nutrition: less than body requirements related to inadequate intake of needed nutrients

---

Expected Outcomes *The client's weekly weight gain will be increased to the appropriate rate using her BMI and recommended weight gain ranges as guidelines.*

Nursing Interventions/*Rationales*

Review recent diet history (including food aversions) using a food diary, 24-hour recall, or food frequency approach *to ascertain dietary inadequacies contributing to lack of sufficient weight gain.*

Review normal activity and exercise routines *to determine level of energy expenditure;* discuss eating patterns and reasons that lead to decreased food intake (e.g., morning sickness, pica, fear of becoming fat, stress, boredom) *to identify habits that contribute to inadequate weight gain.*

Review optimal weight gain guidelines and their rationale *to ensure that woman is knowledgeable about healthful weight gain rates.*

Set target weight gains for the remaining weeks of the pregnancy *to establish set goals.*

Review increased nutrient needs (calories, protein, minerals, vitamins) that occur as a result of being pregnant *to ensure woman is knowledgeable about altered dietary requirements.*

Review relationship between weight gain and fetal growth *to reinforce that adequate weight gain is needed to promote fetal well-being.*

Discuss with woman what changes can be made in diet, activity, and lifestyle *to enhance chances of meeting set weight gain goals and nutrient needs of mother and fetus.*

If woman has fear of being fat, if symptoms of an eating disorder are evident, or if problems in adjusting to a changing body image surface, refer woman to the appropriate mental health professional for evaluation, *since intensive treatment and follow-up may be required to ensure fetal health.*

KEY POINTS

- A woman's nutritional status before, during, and after pregnancy contributes, to a significant degree, to her well-being and that of her developing fetus.

- Many physiologic changes occurring during pregnancy influence the need for additional nutrients and the efficiency with which the body uses them.

- Both the total maternal weight gain and the pattern of weight gain are important determinants of the outcome of pregnancy.

- The appropriateness of the mother's prepregnancy weight for height (BMI) is a major determinant of her recommended weight gain during pregnancy.

- Nutritional risk factors include adolescent pregnancy; bizarre or faddish food habits; abuse of nicotine, alcohol, or drugs; a low weight for height; and frequent pregnancies.

- Iron supplementation is recommended routinely during pregnancy because it is nearly impossible to obtain adequate intakes from dietary sources alone. Other supplements may be recommended when nutritional risk factors are present.

- The nurse and client are influenced by cultural and personal values and beliefs during nutrition counseling.

- Pregnancy complications that may be nutrition related include anemia, PIH, gestational diabetes, and intrauterine growth restriction.

- Dietary adaptation can be effective interventions for some of the common discomforts of pregnancy, including nausea and vomiting, constipation, and heartburn.

CRITICAL THINKING EXERCISES

1 *Perform a nutrition assessment of a pregnant adolescent. Determine her teaching needs and outline a nutrition teaching plan for her. Include a food plan that would be appropriate for her lifestyle, yet nutritionally adequate.*

2 *Visit a prenatal clinic in the community. Interview a client from an ethnic or cultural group other than your own. Evaluate her diet, using Table 16-2. Determine the adequacy of her diet. If she uses foods or supplements unfamiliar to you, try to find information about these products from other health care workers or written sources. Identify good qualities of her diet and teaching needs that she may have.*

References

Allen, L. (1997). Pregnancy and iron deficiency: Unresolved issues. *Nutr Rev* 5(4), 91.

American College of Obstetricians and Gynecologists (ACOG). (1994). Exercise during pregnancy and the postpartum period. *Technical Bulletin #189*, Washington, D.C.: ACOG.

American Diabetes Association. (1999). Position statement: Gestational diabetes mellitus. *Diabetes Care* 22 (suppl. 1), S74-S76.

Butterworth, C., Jr., & Bendich A. (1996). Folic acid and the prevention of birth defects. *Ann Rev Nutr* 16, 73.

Ellings, J., Newman, R., & Bower, N. (1998). Prenatal care and multiple pregnancy. *J Obstet Gynecol Neonatal Nurs* 27, 457-465.

Food and Nutrition Board, National Academy of Sciences, National Research Council. (1989). *Recommended dietary allowances* (10th ed.). Washington, D.C.: National Academy Press.

Food and Nutrition Board, National Academy of Sciences, Institute of Medicine. (1998). *Recommended levels for individual intake, B vitamins and choline.* Washington, D.C.: National Academy Press.

Guyer, B. et al. (1998). Annual summary of vital statistics–1997. *Pediatrics* 102, 1333-1349.

Hinds, T. et al. (1996). The effect of caffeine on pregnancy outcome variables. *Nutr Rev* 54(7), 203.

Institute of Medicine. (1992). *Nutrition during pregnancy and lactation: An implementation guide.* Washington, D.C.: National Academy Press.

Leverett, D. et al. (1997). Randomized clinical trial of the effect of prenatal fluoride supplements in preventing dental caries. *Caries Res* 31, 174-179.

Position of the American Dietetic Association. (1993). Use of nutritive and nonnutritive sweeteners, *J Am Dietet Assoc* 93(10), 816.

Prentice, A., & Goldberg, G. (1996). Maternal obesity increases congenital malformations. *Nutr Rev* 54(5), 146.

Rainville, A. (1998). Pica practices of pregnant women are associated with lower maternal hemoglobin level at delivery. *J Am Dietet Assoc* 98, 293-296.

Sargent, R. et al. (1994). Black and white adolescent females' prepregnancy nutrition status. *Adolescence* 29, 845.

Standing Committee on the Scientific Evaluation of Dietary Reference Intakes, Food and Nutrition Board, Institute of Medicine. (1997). *Dietary Reference Intakes: Calcium, phosphorus, magnesium, vitamin D, and fluoride.* Washington, D.C.: National Academy Press.

Story, M. (1997). Promoting healthy eating and ensuring adequate weight gain in pregnant adolescents: Issues and strategies. *Ann NY Acad Sci* 817, 321.

Tinkle, M., & Sterling, B. (1997). Neural tube defects: A primary prevention role for nurses. *J Obstet Gynecol Neonatal Nurs* 26, 503-512.

U.S. Department of Agriculture. (1992). *The food guide pyramid,* Hyattsville, MD: U.S. Department of Agriculture.

U.S. Department of Health and Human Services, Food and Drug Administration. (1996). Food standards: Amendment of the standards of identity for enriched grain products to require addition of folic acid. *Federal Register* 61, 87-81.

Wardlaw, G., & Insel, P. (1993). *Perspectives in nutrition* (2nd ed.). St. Louis: Mosby.

Wong, D., & Perry, S. (1998). *Maternal child nursing care.* St. Louis: Mosby.

Worthington-Roberts, B., & Williams, S. (1997). *Nutrition in pregnancy and lactation* (6th ed.). Dubuque, IA: Brown and Benchmark.

17

Nursing Care During Pregnancy

Rebecca Burdette Saunders

LEARNING OBJECTIVES

- Define the key terms.
- Describe the process of confirming pregnancy and estimating the date of birth.
- Summarize the physical, psychosocial, and behavioral changes that usually occur as the mother and other family members adapt to pregnancy.
- Discuss the benefits of prenatal care and problems of accessibility for some women.
- Outline the patterns of health care provided to assess maternal and fetal health status at the initial and follow-up visits during pregnancy.

- Describe the nursing assessments, diagnoses, interventions, and methods of evaluation that are typical when providing care for the pregnant woman.
- Discuss education needed by pregnant women to understand physical discomforts related to pregnancy and to recognize signs and symptoms of potential complications.
- Explain the impact of culture, age, parity, and number of fetuses on the response of the family to the pregnancy and on the prenatal care provided.
- Identify topics for nursing research related to prenatal care.

KEY TERMS

ambivalence	epulis	positive indicators of pregnancy
attachment	estimated date of birth (EDB)	prenatal period
breast shells	fundal height	presumptive indicators of pregnancy
conscious relaxation	gingivitis	probable indicators of pregnancy
couvade	Kegel exercises	quickening
couvade syndrome	morning sickness	round ligament pain
cultural prescriptions	multifetal pregnancy	sonogram
cultural proscriptions	Nägele's rule	supine hypotension
effleurage	pelvic tilt (rock)	term pregnancy
emotional lability	pinch test	trimesters

he prenatal period is a time of physical and psychologic preparation for birth and parenthood. Becoming a parent is considered one of the maturational milestones of adult life, and as such it is a time of intense learning for both parents and those close to them. The prenatal period provides a unique opportunity for nurses and other members of the health care team to influence family health. During this period, essentially healthy women seek regular care and guidance. The nurse's health promotion interventions can affect the well-being of the

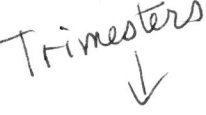

woman, her unborn child, and the rest of her family for many years.

Regular prenatal visits, ideally beginning soon after the first missed menstrual period, offer opportunities to ensure the health of the expectant mother and her infant. Prenatal health care permits diagnosis and treatment of maternal disorders that may have preexisted or may develop during the pregnancy. Care is designed to monitor the growth and development of the fetus and to identify abnormalities that may interfere with the course of normal labor. The woman and her family can seek support for stress and learn parenting skills.

Pregnancy spans 9 months, but health care providers seldom use the familiar calendar to discuss the duration of pregnancy or gestational age of the fetus. Instead, they use the concept of lunar months, which last 28 days, or 4 weeks. Normal pregnancy, then, lasts about 10 lunar months, which is the same as 40 weeks or 280 days. Health care providers also refer to early, middle, and late pregnancy as trimesters. The first trimester lasts from weeks 1 through 13; the second, from weeks 14 through 26; and the third, from weeks 27 through 40. A pregnancy is considered at term if it advances to 38 to 40 weeks. The focus of this chapter is on meeting the health needs of the expectant family over the course of pregnancy, which is known as the prenatal period.

DIAGNOSIS OF PREGNANCY

Women may suspect pregnancy when they miss a menstrual period. Many women come to the first prenatal visit after a positive home pregnancy test. However, the clinical diagnosis of pregnancy before the second missed period may be difficult in some women. Physical variations, lack of relaxation, obesity, or tumors, for example, may confound even the experienced examiner. Accuracy is important, however, because emotional, social, medical, or legal consequences of an inaccurate diagnosis, either positive or negative, can be extremely serious. A correct date for the last (normal) menstrual period (LMP), the date of intercourse, and a basal body temperature (BBT) record may be of great value in the accurate diagnosis of pregnancy (see Chapter 9).

Signs and Symptoms

Great variability is possible in the subjective and objective symptoms of pregnancy. Therefore the diagnosis of pregnancy may be uncertain for a time. Many of the indicators of pregnancy are clinically useful in the diagnosis of pregnancy, and they are classified as presumptive, probable, or positive.

Presumptive indicators of pregnancy include subjective symptoms and objective signs. Subjective symptoms are reported by the woman and may include amenorrhea, nausea and vomiting (morning sickness), breast tenderness, urinary frequency, and fatigue (Beischer, MacKay, &

Colditz, 1997). Quickening, the mother's first perception of fetal movement, may be noted between weeks 16 and 20. Objective signs that may be validated by the examiner include elevation of BBT, breast and abdominal enlargement, and changes in the uterus and vagina. Other visible changes occur in the skin, such as striae gravidarum, deeper pigmentation of the areola, chloasma (mask of pregnancy), and linea nigra (pigmented line on the abdomen) (see Chapter 15).

The presumptive indicators of pregnancy can be caused by conditions other than gestation. For example, amenorrhea may be caused by an endocrine disorder; fatigue may signify anemia or infection; a tumor may cause enlargement of the abdomen; and nausea or vomiting may be caused by a gastrointestinal upset or food allergy. Therefore these signs alone are not reliable for diagnosis.

Probable indicators of pregnancy are detected by an examiner and are mainly related to physical changes in the uterus (Hacker & Moore, 1998). Objective signs include uterine enlargement, Braxton Hicks contractions, uterine souffle, ballottement, and a positive pregnancy test. When combined with presumptive signs and symptoms, they strongly suggest pregnancy, but they are not conclusive. For example, uterine enlargement may be due to the presence of tumors; unusual bowel sounds may be misinterpreted; or positive results on a pregnancy test may be due to a malignant tumor that secretes the hormone human chorionic gonadotropin (hCG).

The positive indicators of pregnancy are directly attributed to the fetus and include the presence of a fetal heartbeat distinct from that of the mother, fetal movement felt by someone other than the mother, and visualization of the fetus with a technique such as ultrasound. The fetal heartbeat can be detected as early as 6 weeks of gestation with Doppler techniques, but ultrasound becomes 100% reliable only at 8 to 9 weeks of gestation (Beischer, MacKay, & Colditz, 1997). However, the fetal heartbeat usually cannot be detected with a stethoscope until weeks 16 to 20 (Hacker & Moore, 1998). An experienced examiner may palpate fetal movements with increasing reliability after 20 to 24 weeks.

Estimating Date of Birth

Following the diagnosis of pregnancy the woman's first question usually concerns when she will give birth. This date has traditionally been termed the estimated date of confinement (EDC). To promote a more positive perception of both pregnancy and birth, however, the term estimated date of birth (EDB) is usually used. Because the precise date of conception generally is unknown, several formulas have been suggested for calculating the EDB. None of these guides is infallible, but Nägele's rule is reasonably accurate and is the method usually used.

Nägele's rule is as follows: After determining the first day of the LMP, subtract 3 calendar months, and add 7 days and 1 year; or alternatively, add 7 days to the LMP

BOX 17-1 **Use of Nägele's Rule**

July 10, 1999, is the first day of the LMP.

	7	10	1999
	−3	+7	+1
EDB=	4	17	2000

The estimated date of birth is April 17, 2000.

and count forward 9 calendar months. Box 17-1 demonstrates use of Nägele's rule.

Nägele's rule assumes that the woman has a 28-day menstrual cycle and that pregnancy occurred on the fourteenth day. An adjustment is in order if the cycle is longer or shorter than 28 days. With the use of Nägele's rule, only about 4% to 10% of pregnant women give birth spontaneously on the EDB. Most women give birth during the period extending from 7 days before to 7 days after the EDB.

ADAPTATION TO PREGNANCY

Pregnancy affects all family members, and each family member must adapt to the pregnancy and interpret its meaning in light of his or her own needs. This process of family adaptation to pregnancy takes place within a cultural environment that is influenced by societal trends. Dramatic changes have occurred in Western society in recent years, and the nurse must be prepared to support single-parent families, reconstituted families, and dual-career families, as well as traditional families, in the childbirth experience.

Much of the investigation of family dynamics in pregnancy by scholars in the United States and Canada has been done with white, middle-class families, and findings may not apply to families who do not fit the traditional American model. Terms such as spouse, husband, and wife, for example, are used consistently in family literature but may not fit the configuration of a given family in the nurse's care. Adaptation of terms is appropriate to avoid embarrassment to the nurse and offense to the family. Additional research is needed on a variety of families to determine if research findings in traditional families are applicable to others.

Maternal Adaptation

Women of all ages use the months of pregnancy to adapt to the maternal role, a complex process of social and cognitive learning. Early in pregnancy nothing seems to be happening, and much time is spent sleeping. With the perception of fetal movement in the second trimester, the woman turns her attention inward to her pregnancy and to relationships with her mother and other women who have been or who are pregnant.

Pregnancy is a maturational milestone that can be stressful but rewarding as the woman prepares for a new level of caring and responsibility. Her self-concept changes in readiness for parenthood as she prepares for her new role. Gradually, she moves from being self-contained and independent to being committed to a lifelong concern for another human being. This growth requires mastery of certain developmental tasks: accepting the pregnancy, identifying with the role of mother, reordering the relationships between herself and her mother and between herself and her partner, establishing a relationship with the unborn child, and preparing for the birth experience (Lederman, 1996). The partner's emotional support is an important factor in the successful accomplishment of these developmental tasks. Single women with limited support may have difficulty making this adaptation.

Accepting the Pregnancy

The first step in adapting to the maternal role is accepting the idea of pregnancy and assimilating the pregnant state into the woman's way of life. Mercer (1995) described this process as cognitive restructuring and credited Reva Rubin (1984) as the nurse theorist who pioneered our understanding of maternal role attainment. The work of these scholars, Lederman (1996), and others should be studied for a deeper understanding of the complex psychosocial processes that affect behaviors of pregnant women.

The degree of acceptance is reflected in the woman's emotional responses. Many women are dismayed initially at finding themselves pregnant. However, eventual acceptance of pregnancy parallels the growing acceptance of the reality of a child. Nonacceptance of the pregnancy should not be equated with rejection of the child. A woman may dislike being pregnant but feel love for the child to be born.

Women who are happy and pleased about their pregnancy often view it as biologic fulfillment and part of their life plan. They have high self-esteem and tend to be confident about outcomes for themselves, their babies, and other family members.

Although a general state of well-being predominates, many women are surprised to experience **emotional lability**, that is, rapid and unpredictable changes in mood. These swings in emotions and increased sensitivity to others are disconcerting to the expectant mother and those around her. Increased irritability, explosions of tears and anger, and feelings of great joy and cheerfulness alternate, apparently with little or no provocation.

Profound hormonal changes that are part of the maternal response to pregnancy may be responsible for mood changes, much as they are before menstruation or during menopause. Other reasons such as concerns about finances and changed lifestyle contribute to this seemingly erratic behavior.

Pregnant women are affected emotionally by changes that occur in the physical contours and functions of their bodies. During the first trimester body shape changes little, but by the second trimester obvious bulging of the abdomen, thickening of the waist, and enlargement of the breasts proclaim the state of pregnancy. The woman develops a feeling of an overall increase in the size of her body and of occupying more space.

The woman's attitude about her body is thought to be influenced by her values and personality traits. This attitude often changes as pregnancy progresses. A positive body image usually is expressed during the first trimester. As the pregnancy advances, however, the feelings become more negative. For most women the feeling of liking or not liking their bodies in the pregnant state is temporary and does not cause permanent changes in their self-perceptions.

Most women experience ambivalent feelings during pregnancy. **Ambivalence,** having conflicting feelings simultaneously, is considered a normal response for people preparing for a new role. During pregnancy, women may, for example, feel great pleasure that they are fulfilling a lifelong dream, but they also may feel great regret that life as they now know it is ending.

Even women who are pleased to be pregnant may experience feelings of hostility toward the pregnancy or unborn child from time to time. Such things as a partner's chance remark about the attractiveness of a slim, nonpregnant woman or news of a colleague's promotion can give rise to ambivalent feelings. Body sensations, feelings of dependence, or the realization of the responsibilities of child care also can generate such feelings.

Intense feelings of ambivalence that persist through the third trimester may indicate an unresolved conflict with the motherhood role (Mercer, 1995). After the birth of a healthy child, however, memories of these ambivalent feelings usually are dismissed. If the child is born with a defect, however, a woman may look back at the times when she did not want the pregnancy and feel intensely guilty. She may believe that her ambivalence caused the birth defect. She then will need assurance that her feelings were not responsible for the problem.

Identifying with Mother Role

The process of identifying with the mother role begins early in each woman's life at the time she is being mothered as a child. Her social group's perception of what constitutes the feminine role can subsequently influence her toward choosing between motherhood or a career, being married or single, being independent rather than interdependent, or being able to manage multiple roles. Practice roles, such as playing with dolls, baby-sitting, and taking care of siblings, may increase her understanding of what being a mother entails.

Many women have always wanted a baby, liked children, and looked forward to motherhood. Their high motivation to become a parent promotes acceptance of pregnancy and eventual prenatal and parental adaptation. Other women apparently have not considered in any detail what motherhood means to them. During pregnancy conflicts such as not wanting the pregnancy and child-related or career-related decisions need to be resolved.

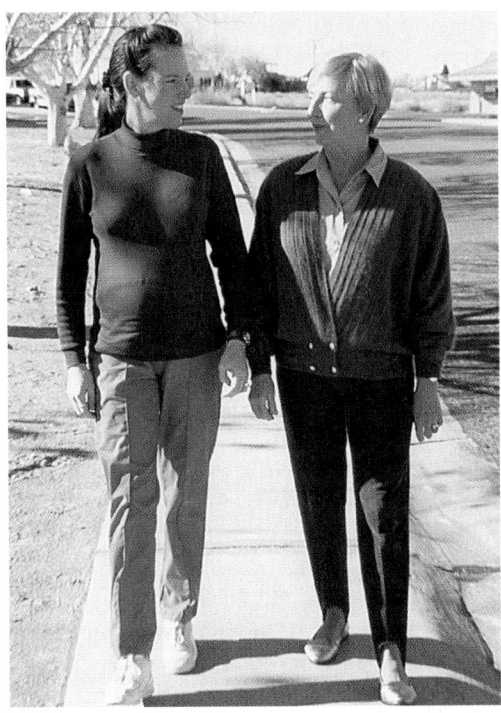

Fig. 17-1 A pregnant woman and her mother enjoying their walk together. *(Courtesy Michael S. Clement, MD, Mesa, AZ.)*

Reordering Personal Relationships

Close relationships held by the pregnant woman undergo change during pregnancy as she prepares emotionally for the new role of mother. As family members learn their new roles, periods of tension and conflict may occur. An understanding of the typical patterns of adjustment can help the nurse reassure the pregnant woman and explore issues related to social support. Promoting effective communication patterns between the expectant mother and her own mother and between the expectant mother and her partner are common nursing interventions provided during the prenatal visits.

The woman's relationship with her mother is significant in adaptation to pregnancy and motherhood. Important components in the pregnant woman's relationship with her mother are the mother's availability (past and present), her reactions to the daughter's pregnancy, respect for her daughter's autonomy, and the willingness to reminisce (Mercer, 1995).

The mother's reaction to the daughter's pregnancy signifies her acceptance of the grandchild and of her daughter. If the mother is supportive, the daughter has an opportunity to discuss pregnancy and labor and her feelings of joy or ambivalence with a knowledgeable and accepting woman (Fig. 17-1). Rubin (1975) noted that if the pregnant woman's mother is not pleased with the pregnancy, the daughter begins to have doubts about her self-worth and the eventual acceptance of her child by others.

Mothers who respect their daughters' autonomy promote feelings of self-confidence in their daughters. Parents who have helped their adult children become independent are seen as being willing to help rather than as interfering or dominating.

Reminiscing about the pregnant woman's early childhood and sharing the grandmother-to-be's account of her childbirth experience help the daughter anticipate and prepare for labor and birth. Hearing about themselves as young children makes pregnant women feel loved and wanted. They draw closer to their parents and begin to feel that, despite the errors they might make in their own mothering experiences, they will continue to be loved by their children.

Although the woman's relationship with her mother is significant in considering her adaptation in pregnancy, the most important person to the pregnant woman is usually the father of her child. A woman who is nurtured by her partner during pregnancy has fewer emotional and physical symptoms, fewer labor and childbirth complications, and an easier postpartum adjustment (Zachariah, 1994). Women express two major needs within this relationship during pregnancy: feeling loved and valued and having the child accepted by the partner.

The marital or committed relationship is not static but evolves over time. The addition of a child changes forever the nature of the bond between partners. Couples grow closer during pregnancy, and pregnancy has a maturing effect on the partners' relationship as they assume new roles and discover new aspects of one another. Partners who trust and support each other are able to share mutual-dependency needs (Mercer, 1995).

Sexual expression during pregnancy is highly individual. The sexual relationship is affected by physical, emotional, and interactional factors, including myths about sex during pregnancy, sexual dysfunction, and physical changes in the woman. Myths about body functions and fantasies about the influence of the fetus as a third party in lovemaking are commonly expressed. An individual may also inaccurately attribute anomalies, mental retardation, and other injuries to the fetus and mother to sexual relations during pregnancy. Some couples fear that the woman's genitals will be drastically changed by the birth process. Couples may not express their concerns to the health care provider because of embarrassment or because they do not want to appear foolish.

Discomfort during sexual activity may be caused by pressure on the woman's abdomen and deep penetration or thrusting. Postcoital cramping and backache may occur (see Sexual Counseling, p. 418).

As pregnancy progresses, changes in body shape, body image, and levels of discomfort influence both partners' desire for sexual expression. During the first trimester the woman's sexual desire may decrease, especially if she experiences breast tenderness, nausea, fatigue, or sleepiness. As she progresses into the second trimester, however, her sense of well-being combined with the increased pelvic congestion that occurs at this time may increase her desire for sexual release. In the third trimester, somatic complaints and physical bulkiness may increase her physical discomfort and diminish her interest in sex (Rynerson & Lowdermilk, 1993).

Partners need to feel free to discuss their sexual responses during pregnancy. Their sensitivity to each other and willingness to share concerns can strengthen their sexual relationship. Partners who do not understand the rapid physiologic and emotional changes of pregnancy can become confused by the other's behavior. By talking to each other about the changes they are experiencing, couples can define problems and then offer the needed support. Nurses can facilitate communication between partners by talking to expectant couples about possible changes in feelings and behaviors they may experience as pregnancy progresses (Rynerson & Lowdermilk, 1993).

Establishing Relationship with the Fetus

Emotional **attachment** to the child begins during the prenatal period as women use fantasizing and daydreaming to prepare themselves for motherhood (Rubin, 1975). They think of themselves as mothers and imagine maternal qualities they would like to possess. Expectant parents desire to be warm, loving, and close to their child. They try to anticipate changes that the child will bring in their lives and wonder how they will react to noise, disorder, less freedom, and caregiving activities. The mother-child relationship progresses through pregnancy as a developmental process. Three phases in the developmental pattern become apparent.

In phase 1 the woman accepts the biologic fact of pregnancy. She needs to be able to state, "I am pregnant" and incorporate the idea of a child into her body and self-image.

Early in pregnancy the mother's thoughts center around herself and the immediate reality of the pregnancy itself. The child is viewed as part of herself, and most women think of their fetus as unreal during the early period of pregnancy.

In phase 2 the woman accepts the growing fetus as distinct from herself and as a person to nurture. She can now say, "I am going to have a baby." By the fifth month, there usually is a growing awareness of the child as a separate being. This differentiation of the child from the woman's self permits the beginning of the mother-child relationship that involves not only caring but also responsibility. Attachment by a mother to her child is enhanced by experiencing a planned pregnancy, and it increases when ultrasound and quickening confirm the reality of the fetus (Smith, 1998).

With acceptance of the reality of the child (hearing the heartbeat and feeling the child move) and an overall feeling of well-being, the woman enters a quiet period and becomes more introspective. A fantasy child becomes precious to the woman. As the woman seems to withdraw and to concentrate her interest on the unborn child, her partner sometimes feels left out. If there are children in the family, they may become more demanding in their efforts to redirect the mother's attention to themselves.

During phase 3 of the attachment process, the woman prepares realistically for the birth and parenting of the child. She expresses the thought "I am going to be a mother" and defines the nature and characteristics of the child. She may, for example, speculate about the child's sex and personality traits based on patterns of fetal activity.

Although the mother alone experiences the child within, both parents and siblings believe the unborn child responds in a very individualized, personal manner. Family members may interact a great deal with the unborn child by talking to the fetus and stroking the mother's abdomen, especially when the fetus shifts position (Fig. 17-2). More research is necessary to help nurses understand the factors that promote early attachment and the benefits of those feelings (Müller, 1996).

Preparing for Childbirth

Many women actively prepare for birth. They read books, view films, attend parenting classes, and talk to other women (Lederman, 1996). They seek the best caregiver possible for advice, monitoring, and caring. The multipara has her own history of labor and birth, which influences her approach to preparation for this childbirth experience.

Anxiety can arise from concern about a safe passage for herself and her child during the birth process (Mercer, 1995; Rubin, 1975). This concern may not be expressed overtly, but cues are given as the nurse listens to plans women make for care of the new baby and other children in case "anything should happen." These feelings persist despite statistical evidence about the safe outcome of pregnancy for mothers and their infants. Many women fear the pain of childbirth or mutilation because they do not understand anatomy and the birth process. Education by the nurse can alleviate many of these fears. Women also express concern over what behaviors are appropriate during the birth process and how the persons who will be caring for them will accept them and their actions. The best preparation for labor is "a healthy sense of the realistic—an awareness of work, pain, and risk balanced by a sense of excitement and expectation of the final reward" (Lederman, 1996).

Toward the end of the third trimester breathing is difficult and fetal movements become vigorous enough to disturb the mother's sleep. Backaches, frequency and urgency of urination, constipation, and varicose veins can become troublesome. The bulkiness and awkwardness of her body interfere with the woman's ability to care for other children, perform routine work-related duties, and assume a

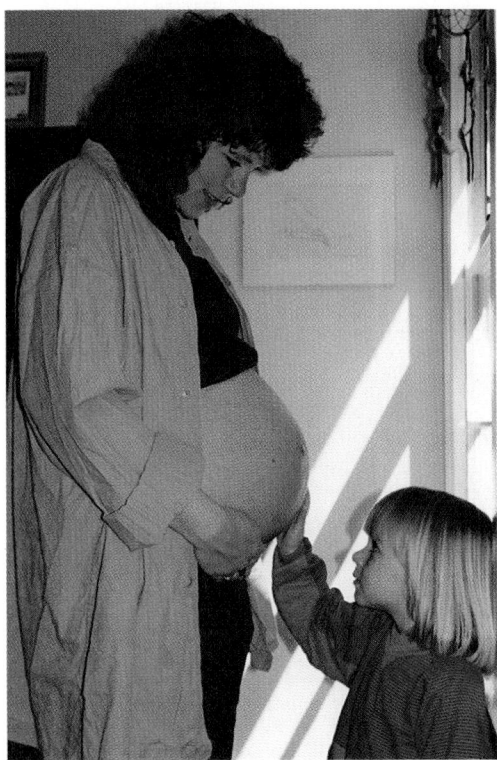

Fig. 17-2 Sibling feeling movement of fetus. *(Courtesy Kim Molloy, Knoxville, IA.)*

comfortable position for sleep and rest. By this time most women become impatient for labor to begin, whether the birth is anticipated with joy, dread, or a mixture of both. A strong desire to see the end of pregnancy, to be over and done with it, makes women at this stage ready to move on to childbirth.

Paternal Adaptation

The father's beliefs and feelings about the ideal mother and father and his cultural expectation of appropriate behavior during pregnancy affect his response to his partner's need for him. One man may engage in nurturing behavior. Another may feel lonely and alienated as the woman becomes physically and emotionally engrossed in the unborn child. He may seek comfort and understanding outside the home or become interested in a new hobby or involved with his work. Some men view pregnancy as proof of their masculinity and their dominant role. To others, pregnancy has no meaning in terms of responsibility to either mother or child. However, for most men pregnancy can be a time of preparation for the parental role with intense learning.

Accepting the Pregnancy

The ways fathers adjust to the parental role is the subject of research (Callister, 1995; Donovan, 1995; Ferketich & Mercer, 1995). In older societies the man enacted the

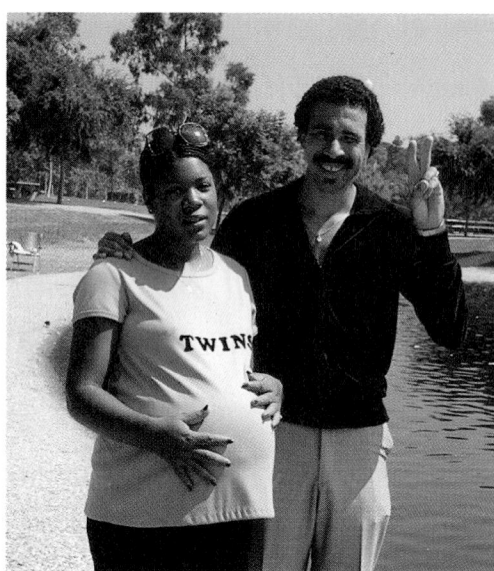

Fig. 17-3 Mother- and father-to-be walk together. Women respond positively to their partner's interest and concern. *(Courtesy Marjorie Pyle, RNC, Lifecircle, Costa Mesa, CA.)*

ritual **couvade;** that is, he behaved in specific ways and respected taboos associated with pregnancy and giving birth. In this way the man's new status was recognized and endorsed. His behavior acknowledged his psychosocial and biologic relationship to the mother and child. In Western societies the participation of fathers in childbirth has risen dramatically over the past 25 years, and the father in the role of labor coach is common.

A man's readiness for fatherhood may be reflected in the way he views the couple's relative financial security and the stability of their relationship and in the way he deals with the realization that the upcoming birth marks the end of the childless period. Many men express concern for the family's economic security. Today most young married women are employed outside the home but have a phase of unemployment for childbearing and child care. The length of unemployment is determined by the couple's economic status, the policies of the woman's employer, and the couple's value system. Some men compensate for anticipated needs by keeping their current jobs even though they had planned a change, by working overtime, or by taking on extra work. Some men acquire new or additional insurance at this time.

The man's emotional responses to becoming a father, his concerns, and informational needs change during the course of pregnancy. Phases of the developmental pattern become apparent. May (1982) described three phases characterizing the developmental tasks experienced by the expectant father: the announcement phase, the moratorium phase, and the focusing phase.

The early period, the announcement phase, may last from a few hours to a few weeks. The developmental task is to accept the biologic fact of pregnancy. Men react to the confirmation of pregnancy with joy or dismay, depending on whether the pregnancy is desired or unplanned or unwanted. Ambivalence in the early stages of pregnancy is common (Donovan, 1995).

If pregnancy is unplanned or unwanted, some men find the alterations in life plans and lifestyles difficult to accept. Some men engage in extramarital affairs for the first time during their partner's pregnancy. Others batter their partners (Gaines, 1997). Chapter 11 provides detailed information about violence against women with guidance on assessment and intervention.

The second phase, the moratorium phase, is the period when he adjusts to the reality of pregnancy. The developmental task is to accept the pregnancy. Men appear to put conscious thought of the pregnancy aside for a time. They become more introspective and engage in many discussions about their philosophy of life, religion, childbearing, and childrearing practices and their relationships with family members and friends. Depending on the man's readiness for the pregnancy, this phase may be relatively short or persist until the last trimester.

The third phase, called the focusing phase, begins in the last trimester and is characterized by the father's active involvement in both the pregnancy and his relationship with his child. The developmental task is to negotiate with his partner the role he is to play in labor and to prepare for parenthood. In this phase the man concentrates on his experience of the pregnancy and begins to think of himself as a father.

Men are involved in pregnancy in a variety of ways. May (1980, 1982) described three styles of involvement in the pregnancy exhibited by men during their wives' first pregnancy: the observer style, the expressive style, and the instrumental style.

The observer style is exhibited by those fathers who are happy about the pregnancy and supportive of their wives. However, because of cultural values or shyness, they avoid involvement in activities such as parent education classes, decisions about breastfeeding, or the choice of professional care. Other fathers who are ambivalent about pregnancy and the role of father need time to adjust to the idea of pregnancy and fatherhood. Some men cope by becoming involved in careers and resisting their wives' attempts to involve them in preparations for the coming child.

Men who show the expressive style display a strong emotional response to pregnancy and a desire to be a full partner in the project (Fig. 17-3). These men are aware of their partner's needs for support. They experience the same emotional lability and ambivalence as that experienced by pregnant women. Some expectant fathers report having nausea and other gastrointestinal complaints, fatigue, and other physical discomforts. Known as the **couvade syndrome,** the phenomenon of men's experiencing pregnancy-like symptoms has been explored by scholars in several disciplines, including nursing. Mason and Elwood

(1995) and others recommend further investigation to determine whether the basis of men's experience is physiologic or psychologic.

The instrumental style is adopted by men who see tasks they can perform in their role as manager of the pregnancy. They ask questions; are interested in the role of labor coach; and plan for photographs during pregnancy, birth, and the neonatal period. They feel responsible for the outcome of pregnancy and are protective and supportive of their wives. Changing cultural and professional attitudes have encouraged fathers' participation in the birth experience (Draper, 1997).

The three styles of involvement provide examples of the different ways men can experience pregnancy. Each man needs to feel free to define his role in pregnancy, just as the woman does. Because of cultural conditioning, personality, or a different supportive style, however, not all men are able or willing to attend childbirth classes or act as labor coaches. More research is needed to determine whether similar styles of involvement occur in the partners of multiparous women, in men from various cultural groups, and in same-sex partners, and what the effects on the relationship are when the partners' expectations do not coincide.

Identifying with Father Role

Each father brings to pregnancy attitudes that affect the way in which he adjusts to the pregnancy and parental role. His memories of the fathering he received from his own father, the experiences he has had with child care, and the perceptions of the male and father roles within his social group will guide his selection of the tasks and responsibilities he will assume. Some men are highly motivated to nurture and love a child. They may be excited and pleased about the anticipated role of father. Others may be more detached or even hostile to the idea of fatherhood.

Reordering Personal Relationships

The partner's main role in pregnancy is to nurture and respond to the pregnant woman's feelings of vulnerability. The partner must also deal with the reality of the pregnancy. The partner's support indicates involvement in the pregnancy and preparation for attachment to the child.

Some aspects of a partner's behavior indicate rivalry. Direct rivalry with the fetus may be evident, especially during sexual activity. Men may protest that fetal movements prevent sexual gratification or that they are being watched by the fetus during sexual activity.

The woman's increased introspection may cause her partner to feel uneasy as she becomes preoccupied with thoughts of the child and of her motherhood, with her growing dependence on her physician or midwife, and with her reevaluation of the couple's relationship. Couples who are told early in the pregnancy that ambivalence, anxiety, and increased tensions are common experiences for expectant couples then can devote energy towards managing the changes (Donovan, 1995).

Deciding on the infant's feeding method is of concern when the partners' preferences differ or one partner has intense opinions about a method. The recognized benefits and disadvantages of one method over another appear to be irrelevant. Some partners insist that the woman breastfeed; others are adamantly opposed to breastfeeding. If one partner refuses to voice an opinion, the other may experience uneasiness or uncertainty.

Establishing Relationship with the Fetus

The father-child attachment can be as strong as the mother-child relationship, and fathers can be as competent as mothers in nurturing their infants. The father-child attachment also begins during pregnancy. A father may rub or kiss the maternal abdomen, try to listen to the fetus, or play with the fetus as he notes fetal movement.

Men prepare for fatherhood in many of the same ways as women do for motherhood–by reading, fantasizing, and daydreaming about the baby. They may adjust work commitments or plan vacations so that they can spend time with their new family.

Daydreaming about their role as father is common in the last weeks before the birth; men rarely describe their daydreams unless they are reassured that such daydreams are normal.

Nurses can help fathers identify concerns and prepare for the reality of a baby by asking questions such as the following:
- What do you expect the baby to look and act like?
- What do you think being a father will be like?
- Have you thought about the baby's crying? Changing diapers? Burping the baby? Being awakened at night? Sharing your partner with the baby?

The father may not wish to answer such questions when he is asked but may need time to think them through or discuss them with his partner.

If an expectant father can only imagine an older child and has difficulty visualizing or talking about an infant, this situation needs to be explored. The nurse can tell the father about the unborn child's ability to respond to light, sound, and touch and encourage him to feel and talk to the fetus. Plans for seeing, holding, and examining the newborn can be made.

As the birth day approaches, fathers have more questions about fetal and newborn behaviors. Some fathers are shocked or amazed at how small the clothes and furniture for the baby are.

Some fathers become involved by picking the child's name and anticipating the child's sex, if it is not already known. Some couples select the name of the child as early as the first month of pregnancy. Family tradition, religious customs, and the continuation of the parent's name or names of relatives or friends are important in the selection process.

At the time of birth, most parents are able to accept the sex of the child, but occasionally show or voice disappointment. The parents may experience a grief reaction and sense of loss at birth as they release their fantasized image of the child and begin to accept the real child. These negative responses toward a normal, healthy baby may be difficult for nurses to understand. However, most such responses are temporary. Providing an accepting environment for parental reactions facilitates the parent's ability to move beyond disappointment to acceptance.

Preparing for Childbirth

The days and weeks immediately before the expected day of birth are characterized by anticipation and anxiety. Boredom and restlessness are common as the couple focuses on the birth process.

During the last 2 months of pregnancy, many expectant fathers experience a surge of creative energy at home and on the job. They may become dissatisfied with their present living space. If possible, they tend to act on the need to alter the environment. This activity may be overt evidence of their sharing in the childbearing experience. They are able to channel the anxiety and other feelings experienced during the final weeks before birth into productive activities. This behavior earns recognition and compliments from friends, relatives, and their partners.

The father's anxieties also may be expressed by his refusal to think about the birth, planning for other activities during his partner's labor, or sleeping and resting to the exclusion of all else. The expectant mother may become concerned about possibly being deserted physically or emotionally at a time when she is feeling most vulnerable.

The father's major concerns are getting the mother to a medical facility in time for the birth and not appearing ignorant. Many fathers want to be able to recognize labor and determine when it is appropriate to leave for the hospital or call the physician or midwife. They may fantasize different situations and plan what they will do in response to them, or they may rehearse taking various routes to the hospital, timing each route at different times of the day.

Many fathers have questions about the labor suite's furniture, nursing staff, and location, as well as the availability of the physician and anesthesiologist. Others want to know what is expected of them when their partners are in labor. The father may also have fears concerning safe passage of his partner and the mutilation or death of his partner and child. While he harbors these fears, he cannot help his mate deal with her own unspoken or overt apprehension.

With the exception of childbirth preparation classes, a father has few opportunities to learn ways to be an involved and active partner in this rite of passage into parenthood. The tensions and apprehensions of the unprepared, unsupportive father are readily transmitted to the mother and may increase her fears. His own self-doubts and fear of inadequacy may be realized if he is not supported. Self-confidence comes from achieving realistic goals and earning the approval of others.

The same fears, questions, and concerns may affect birth partners who are not the biologic fathers. Birth partners need to be kept informed, supported, and included in all activities in which the mother desires their participation.

Sibling Adaptation

Sharing the spotlight with a new brother or sister may be the first major crisis for a child. The older child often experiences a sense of loss or feels jealous at being "replaced" by the new sibling. Some of the factors that influence the child's response are age, the parents' attitudes, the role of the father, the length of separation from the mother, the hospital's visitation policy, and the way the child has been prepared for the change.

The mother with other children must devote time and effort to reorganizing her relationships with existing children. She needs to prepare siblings for the birth of the child (see Fig. 18-4 and Box 18-4) and begin the process of role transition in the family by including the children in the pregnancy and being sympathetic to older children's protests against losing their places in the family hierarchy. No child willingly gives up a familiar position.

Siblings' responses to pregnancy vary with their age and dependency needs. The 1-year-old infant seems largely unaware of the process, but the 2-year-old child notices the change in his or her mother's appearance and may comment that "Mommy's fat." The 2-year-old child's need for sameness in the environment makes the child aware of any change. Toddlers may exhibit more clinging behavior and revert to dependent behaviors in toilet training or eating.

By the third or fourth year of age children like to be told the story of their own beginning and accept its being compared to the present pregnancy. They like to listen to the fetal heartbeat and feel the baby moving in utero (see Fig. 17-2). Sometimes they worry about how the baby is being fed and what it wears.

School-age children take a more clinical interest in their mother's pregnancy. They may want to know in more detail, "How did the baby get in there?" and "How will it get out?" Children in this age group notice pregnant women in stores, churches, and schools and sometimes seem shy if they need to approach a pregnant woman directly. On the whole they look forward to the new baby, see themselves as "mothers" or "fathers," and enjoy buying baby supplies and readying a place for the baby. Because they still think in concrete terms and base judgments on the here and now, they respond positively to their mother's current good health.

Early and middle adolescents preoccupied with the establishment of their own sexual identity may have difficulty accepting the overwhelming evidence of the sexual activity of their parents. They reason that if they are too young for such activity, certainly their parents are too old. They seem to take on a critical parental role and may ask, "What will people think?" or "How can you let yourself get so fat?" Many pregnant women with teenage children will confess that the attitudes of their teenagers are the most difficult aspect in their current pregnancy.

Late adolescents do not appear to be unduly disturbed. They realize that they soon will be gone from home. Parents usually report they are comforting and act more as other adults than as children.

Grandparent Adaptation

Every pregnancy affects all family relationships. For expectant grandparents, a first pregnancy in a child is undeniable evidence that they are growing older. Many think of a grandparent as old, white-haired, and becoming feeble of mind and body; however, some people face grandparenthood while still in their 30s or 40s. A mother-to-be announcing her pregnancy to her mother may be greeted by a negative response that indicates that she is not ready to be a grandmother. Daughter and mother both may be startled and hurt by the response.

Some expectant grandparents not only are nonsupportive but also use subtle means to decrease the self-esteem of the young parents-to-be. Mothers may talk about their terrible pregnancies; fathers may discuss the endless cost of rearing children; and mothers-in-law may complain that their sons are neglecting them because their concern is now directed toward the pregnant daughters-in-law.

However, most grandparents are delighted at the prospect of a new baby in the family. It reawakens the feelings of their own youth, the excitement of giving birth, and their delight in the behavior of the parents-to-be when they were infants. They set up a memory store of the child's first smiles, first words, and first steps, which they can use later for "claiming" the newborn as a member of the family. Their and the parents' satisfaction comes with the realization that the continuity between past and present is guaranteed.

In addition, the grandparent is the historian who transmits the family history, a resource person who shares knowledge based on experience; a role model; and a support person. The grandparent's presence and support can strengthen family systems by widening the circle of support and nurturance (Fig. 17-4). Other sources of information cannot replace the unique contribution that grandparents make. The parent in turn acts as a negotiator in establishing the grandparent-grandchild relationship.

Many women report that their pregnancies bridged the final gap between them and their own mothers. The estrangement that began in adolescence disappears as the now-pregnant daughter experiences joys, concerns, and anxieties similar to those felt by her mother before her.

Expectant grandparenthood also can represent a maturational milestone for the parent of an expectant parent. To be truly family oriented, maternity care must include the grandparent in the implementation of the nursing process with childbearing families. A class for grandparents is one method of incorporating the grandparents into the

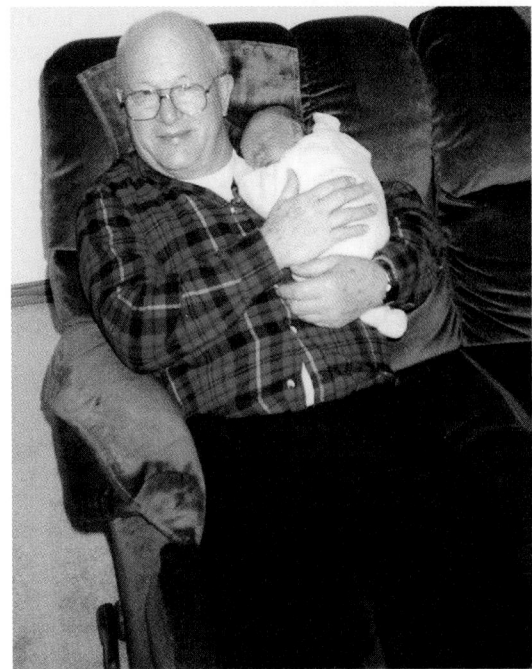

Fig. 17-4 Grandfather relaxing with grandson. *(Courtesy Kathryn Schweer, Waterloo, IA.)*

family system and encouraging communication between the generations.

Grandparents' anxieties and concerns and their relationships with expectant parents and grandchildren should be discussed during courses for expectant parents. The expectant parents may use this opportunity to begin to resolve conflicts and perceived differences with their parents, a task that can also enhance their ability to relate to their own children.

: CARE MANAGEMENT

The purpose of prenatal care is to identify existing risk factors and other deviations from normal so that pregnancy outcomes may be enhanced (Beischer, MacKay, & Colditz, 1997). Major emphasis is placed on preventive aspects of care, primarily to motivate the pregnant woman to practice optimal self-care and to report unusual changes early so that problems can be minimized or prevented. In providing holistic care, nurses also provide information and guidance about the psychosocial impact of pregnancy on the woman and members of her family. The goals of prenatal nursing care, therefore, are not only to foster a safe birth for the infant but also to promote satisfaction of the mother and family with the pregnancy and birth experience.

Prenatal care is sought routinely by women of middle or high socioeconomic status. However, women living in poverty or who lack health insurance may not be able to utilize public medical services or gain access to private care. Likewise, immigrant women who come from cultures in which prenatal care is not emphasized may not know to seek routine prenatal care. Birth outcomes in these populations are thus less positive, with higher rates of maternal and fetal or newborn complications. Problems with low birth weight (LBW) (less than 2500 g) and infant mortality have in particular been associated with lack of adequate prenatal care (Harvey, 1995). Outcomes for these women can be improved with enhanced prenatal services (Simpson, Korenbrot, & Greene, 1997).

Currently only 76% of mothers receive prenatal care (Chestnut, 1998). Barriers to obtaining health care during pregnancy include inadequate numbers of health care providers, distance from health care facilities, lack of transportation, fragmentation of services, inadequate finances, and personal attitudes. Much effort has been focused on finding ways to improve access and quality of care to ensure that all women and infants have the best opportunity for the most positive outcomes. The availability and accessibility to prenatal care may be improved by the increasing use of advanced practice nurses in collaborative practice with physicians (Mvula & Miller, 1998) or midwives (Oakley et al., 1996). The effectiveness of a regular schedule of home visiting by nurses during pregnancy also has been validated (Chestnut, 1998).

The current model for provision of prenatal care was developed more than 100 years ago (Maloni et al., 1996). The first visit usually occurs in the first trimester, with monthly visits through week 28 of pregnancy. Thereafter, visits are scheduled every 2 weeks until week 36, and then every week until birth. This model is currently being questioned, and in some practices, there is a growing tendency to have fewer visits with women who are at low risk for complications (Beischer, MacKay, & Colditz, 1997). Health care providers are challenged to create a system of prenatal care that has minimal barriers and a focus on individualized care (Maloni et al., 1996).

In recent years the concept of preconception care has become prominent (Perry, 1996). If women can be taught about the benefits of nutrition, avoidance of smoking and abuse of substances, avoidance of sexually transmitted infections (STIs) and other health hazards, a healthier pregnancy may be planned. Likewise, women who have health problems related to chronic diseases such as diabetes mellitus can be counseled regarding their special needs. This area of nursing care is not well developed, and the opportunities for health promotion services are evident.

Prenatal care is ideally a multidisciplinary activity in which nurses work with physicians or midwives, nutritionists, social workers, and others. Collaboration among these individuals is necessary to provide holistic care. The case management model, which makes use of care maps and critical pathways, is one system that promotes comprehensive care with limited overlap in services. To emphasize the nursing role, care management here is organized around the central elements of the nursing process: assessment, nursing diagnoses, expected outcomes, plan of care and interventions, and evaluation.

Assessment and Nursing Diagnoses

Once the presence of pregnancy has been confirmed and the woman's desire to continue the pregnancy has been validated, prenatal care is begun. The assessment process begins at the initial prenatal visit and is continued throughout the pregnancy. Assessment techniques include the interview, physical examination, and laboratory tests. Because the initial visit and follow-up visits are distinctly different in content and process, they are described separately below.

Initial Visit

The pregnant woman and family members who may be present should be told that the first prenatal visit is more lengthy and in-depth than future visits. The initial evaluation includes a comprehensive health history emphasizing the current pregnancy, previous pregnancies, the family, a psychosocial profile, a physical assessment, diagnostic testing, and an overall risk assessment. A prenatal history form (Fig. 17-5) is the best way to document information obtained. To be useful in communicating with other care providers, entries on the form should be made with attention to neatness and clarity.

Interview. The therapeutic relationship between the nurse and the woman is established during the initial assessment interview. It is a time for planned, purposeful communication that focuses on specific content. The data collected are of two types: the woman's subjective appraisal of her health status and the nurse's objective observations. During the interview the nurse observes the woman's affect, posture, body language, skin color, and other physical and emotional signs.

Often the pregnant woman is accompanied by one or more family members. The nurse needs to build a relationship with these people as part of the social context of the client. With her permission, those accompanying the woman can be included in the initial prenatal interview, and the observations and information about the woman's family form part of the database (Fig. 17-6). For example, if the woman is accompanied by small children, the nurse can ask about her plans for child care during the time of labor and birth. Special needs are noted at this time (e.g., wheelchair access, assistance in getting on and off the examining table, cognitive deficits).

Reason for seeking care. Although pregnant women are scheduled for "routine" prenatal visits, they often come to the health care provider seeking information or reassurance about a particular concern. When the client is asked a broad, open-ended question such as, "How have you been feeling?" she may reveal problems that could otherwise be overlooked. The woman's chief concerns should be

Patient Addressograph

Date _____

Name _____
      Last   First   Middle

ID # _____ Hospital of delivery _____

Newborn's physician _____ Referred by _____

Final EDD _____ | Primary provider group _____

Birth date Month Day Year	Age	Race	Marital status S M W D SEP	Address:		
Occupation ☐ Homemaker ☐ Outside work ☐ Student Type of work		Education (last grade completed)		Zip: Phone: (H) (O) Insurance Carrier/Medicaid #		
Husband/father of baby:			Phone:	Emergency contact: Phone:		

Total preg	Full term	Premature	AB, induced	AB, spontaneous	Ectopics	Multiple births	Living

Menstrual History

LMP	☐ Definite	☐ Approximate (month known)	Menses monthly ☐ Yes ☐ No	Frequency: Q _____ days	Menarche _____ (age onset)
	☐ Unknown	☐ Normal amount/duration	Prior menses _____ Date	On BCP at concept. ☐ Yes ☐ No	hCG + ___/___/___
	☐ Final _____				

Past Pregnancies (last six)

Date/ month/ year	GA weeks	Length of labor	Birth weight	Sex M/F	Type delivery	Anes.	Place of delivery	Preterm labor yes/no	Comments/ complications

Past Medical History

	○ Neg + Pos	Detail positive remarks Include data and treatment		○ Neg + Pos	Detail positive remarks Include data & treatment
1. Diabetes			16. D (Rh) sensitized		
2. Hypertension			17. Pulmonary (TB, asthma)		
3. Heart disease			18. Allergies (drugs)		
4. Autoimmune disorder			19. Breast		
5. Kidney disease/UTI			20. Gyn surgery		
6. Neurologic/epilepsy					
7. Psychiatric			21. Operations/hospitalizations (year and reason)		
8. Hepatitis/liver disease					
9. Varicosities/phlebitis					
10. Thyroid dysfunction			22. Anesthetic complications		
11. Trauma/domestic violence			23. History of abnormal PAP		
12. History of blood tranfus.			24. Uterine anomaly/DES		
	AMT/day Prepreg	AMT/day Preg	# Years use	25. Infertility	
13. Tobacco				26. Relevant family history	
14. Alcohol					
15. Street drugs				27. Other	

Comments: _____

ACOG ANTEPARTUM RECORD (FORM A)

The American College of Obstetricians and Gynecologists, 409 12th Street, SW, PO Box 96920, Washington, DC 20090-6920

Fig. 17-5 Prenatal history form. *(From American College of Obstetricians and Gynecologists. [1997]. Antepartum record. Washington, D.C.: ACOG. To order this publication, please call 1-800-762-2264, ext. 199.)*

Continued

recorded in her own words to alert other personnel to the priority of needs as identified by her. At the initial visit, the desire for information about what is normal in the course of pregnancy is typical (see Guideline/Guías box).

Current pregnancy. The presumptive signs of pregnancy may be of great concern to the woman. A review of symptoms she is experiencing, and how she is coping with them, helps establish a database to develop a plan of care. Some early teaching may be provided at this time.

Obstetric/gynecologic history. Data are gathered on the woman's age at menarche, menstrual history, and contraceptive history; the nature of any infertility or gynecologic conditions; her history of any STDs; her sexual history; and a detailed history of all her pregnancies,

Symptoms since LMP

Genetic Screening/Teratology Counseling
includes patient, baby's father, or anyone in either family with:

	Yes	No		Yes	No
1. Patient's age ≥35 years			12. Mental retardation/autism		
2. Thalassemia (Italian, Greek, Mediterranean, or Asian background): MCV <80			If yes, was person tested for fragile X?		
			13. Other inherited genetic or chromosomal disorder		
3. Neural tube defect (meningomyelocele, spina bifida, or anencephaly)			14. Maternal metabolic disorder (e.g., insulin-dependent diabetes, PKU)		
4. Congenital heart defect					
5. Down syndrome			15. Patient or baby's father had a child with birth defects not listed above		
6. Tay-Sachs (e.g., Jewish, Cajun, French-Canadian)			16. Recurrent pregnancy loss, or a stillbirth		
7. Sickle cell disease or trait (African)					
8. Hemophilia			17. Medications/street drugs/alcohol since last menstrual period		
9. Muscular dystrophy					
10. Cystic fibrosis			If yes, agent(s):		
11. Huntington chorea			18. Any other		

Comments/counseling: _____

Infection History	Yes	No		Yes	No
1. High risk hepatitis B/immunized?			4. Rash or viral illness since last menstrual period		
2. Live with someone with TB or exposed to TB			5. History of STD, GC, chlamydia, HPV, syphilis		
3. Patient or partner has history of genital herpes			6. Other (see comments)		

Comments: _____

Interviewer's signature: _____

Initial Physical Examination

Date ____/____/____   Prepregnancy weight _____   Height _____   BP _____

1. HEENT	☐ Normal	☐ Abnormal	12. Vulva	☐ Normal	☐ Condyloma	☐ Lesions
2. Fundi	☐ Normal	☐ Abnormal	13. Vagina	☐ Normal	☐ Inflammation	☐ Discharge
3. Teeth	☐ Normal	☐ Abnormal	14. Cervix	☐ Normal	☐ Inflammation	☐ Lesions
4. Thyroid	☐ Normal	☐ Abnormal	15. Uterus size	_____ Weeks		☐ Fibroids
5. Breasts	☐ Normal	☐ Abnormal	16. Adnexa	☐ Normal	☐ Mass	
6. Lungs	☐ Normal	☐ Abnormal	17. Rectum	☐ Normal	☐ Abnormal	
7. Heart	☐ Normal	☐ Abnormal	18. Diagonal conjugate	☐ Reached	☐ No	_____ cm
8. Abdomen	☐ Normal	☐ Abnormal	19. Spines	☐ Average	☐ Prominent	☐ Blunt
9. Extremities	☐ Normal	☐ Abnormal	20. Sacrum	☐ Concave	☐ Straight	☐ Anterior
10. Skin	☐ Normal	☐ Abnormal	21. Subpubic arch	☐ Normal	☐ Wide	☐ Narrow
11. Lymph nodes	☐ Normal	☐ Abnormal	22. Gynecoid pelvic type	☐ Yes	☐ No	

Comments (Number and explain abnormals): _____
_____ Exam by: _____

ACOG ANTEPARTUM RECORD (FORM B)

Fig. 17-5, cont'd   For legend, see p. 391.

including the present pregnancy, and their outcomes. The date of the last Papanicolaou test and the result are noted. The date of her LMP is obtained to establish the EDB. (See the Guidelines/Guías box for questions that may be used with Spanish-speaking women.)

Medical history. The medical history includes those medical or surgical conditions that may affect the pregnancy or that may be affected by the pregnancy. For example, a pregnant woman who has diabetes or epilepsy requires special care. Because most women are anxious

Patient Addressograph

Name _____
             Last   First   Middle

Drug allergy:	
Religious/cultural considerations _____	Anesthesia consult planned ☐ Yes ☐ No

Problems/plans	Medication List	Start date	Stop date
1.	1.		
2.	2.		
3.	3.		

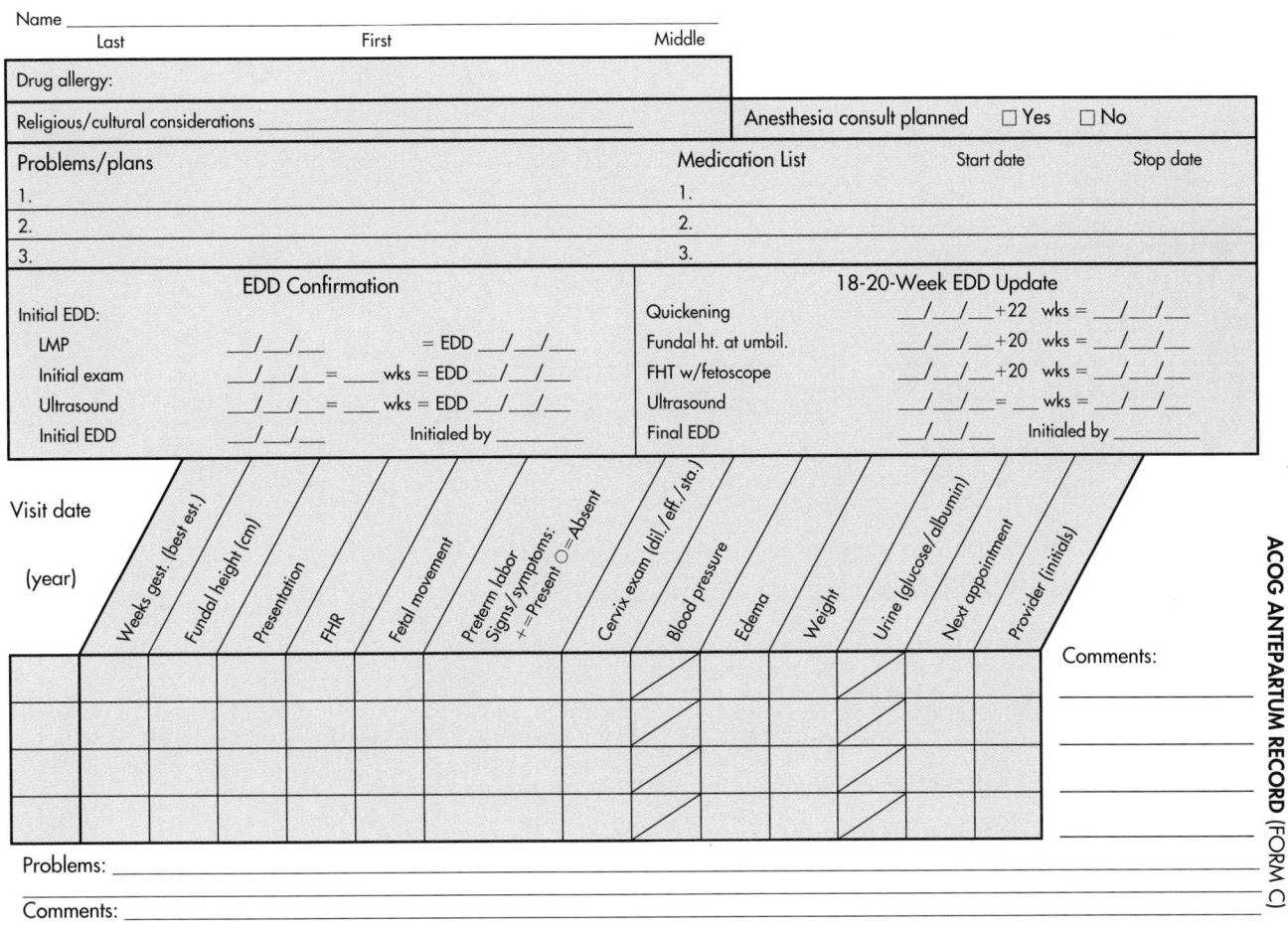

EDD Confirmation	18-20-Week EDD Update
Initial EDD:	
LMP ___/___/___ = EDD ___/___/___	Quickening ___/___/___ +22 wks = ___/___/___
Initial exam ___/___/___ = ___ wks = EDD ___/___/___	Fundal ht. at umbil. ___/___/___ +20 wks = ___/___/___
Ultrasound ___/___/___ = ___ wks = EDD ___/___/___	FHT w/fetoscope ___/___/___ +20 wks = ___/___/___
Initial EDD ___/___/___ Initialed by _____	Ultrasound ___/___/___ = ___ wks = ___/___/___
	Final EDD ___/___/___ Initialed by _____

Visit date

(year)

Weeks gest. (best est.)
Fundal height (cm)
Presentation
FHR
Fetal movement
Preterm labor Signs/symptoms: + = Present ○ = Absent
Cervix exam (dil./eff./sta.)
Blood pressure
Edema
Weight
Urine (glucose/albumin)
Next appointment
Provider (initials)

Comments:
_____
_____
_____
_____

ACOG ANTEPARTUM RECORD (FORM C)

Problems: _____

Comments: _____

Fig. 17-5, cont'd   For legend, see p. 391.

Continued

during the initial interview, the nurse's reference to cues, such as a Medic-Alert bracelet, prompts the woman to explain allergies, chronic diseases, or medications being taken (e.g., cortisone, insulin, or anticonvulsants).

The nature of previous surgical procedures should also be described. If a woman has undergone uterine surgery or extensive repair of the pelvic floor, a cesarean birth may be necessary; appendectomy rules out appendicitis as a cause of right lower quadrant pain; spinal surgery may contraindicate the use of spinal or epidural anesthesia. Any injury involving the pelvis is noted.

Often women who have chronic or handicapping conditions forget to mention them during the initial assessment because they have become so adapted to them. Special shoes or a limp may indicate the existence of a pelvic structural defect, which is an important consideration in pregnant women. The nurse who observes these special characteristics and inquires about them sensitively can obtain individualized data that will provide the basis

for a comprehensive nursing care plan. Observations are vital components of the interview process because they prompt the nurse and woman to focus on the specific needs of the woman and her family.

Nutritional history. The woman's nutritional history is an important component of the prenatal history because her nutritional status has a direct effect on the growth and development of the fetus. A dietary assessment can reveal special diet practices, food allergies, eating behaviors, and other factors related to her nutritional status. Pregnant women are usually motivated to learn about good nutrition and respond well to nutritional advice generated by this assessment.

History of drug use. A woman's past and present use of legal (over-the-counter [OTC] and prescription drugs, caffeine, alcohol, nicotine) and illegal (marijuana, cocaine, heroin) drugs needs to be assessed because many substances cross the placenta and may therefore harm the developing fetus. Periodic urine toxicology screening tests are

Patient Addressograph

Laboratory and Education

Initial Labs	Date	Result	Reviewed
Blood type	__/__/__	A B AB O	
D (Rh) type	__/__/__		
Antibody screen	__/__/__		
HCT/HGB	__/__/__	____%____ g/dl	
Pap test	__/__/__	Normal/Abnormal/___	
Rubella	__/__/__		
VDRL	__/__/__		
Urine culture/screen	__/__/__		
HBsAg	__/__/__		
HIV counseling/testing	__/__/__	☐ Pos. ☐ Neg. ☐ Declined	

Optional Labs	Date	Result	
HGB Electrophoresis	__/__/__	AA AS SS AC SC AF ↑A$_2$	
PPD	__/__/__		
Chlamydia	__/__/__		
GC	__/__/__		
Tay-Sachs	__/__/__		
Other			

8-18-Week Labs (When indicated/elected)	Date	Result	
Ultrasound	__/__/__		
MSAFP/multiple markers	__/__/__		
Amnio/CVS	__/__/__		
Karyotype	__/__/__	46, XX or 46, XY/other	
Amniotic fluid (AFP)	__/__/__	Normal ___ Abnormal ___	

24-28-Week Labs (When indicated)	Date	Result	
HCT/HGB	__/__/__	____%____ g/dl	
Diabetes screen	__/__/__	1 hour _____	
GTT (If screen abnormal)	__/__/__	____ FBS ____ 1 hour ____ 2 hour ____ 3 hour	
D (Rh) antibody screen	__/__/__		
D Immune globulin (RhIG) given (28 wks)	__/__/__	Signature _____	

32-36-Week Labs (When indicated)	Date	Result	
HCT/HGB (recommended)	__/__/__	____%____ g/dl	
Ultrasound	__/__/__		
VDRL	__/__/__		
GC	__/__/__		
Chlamydia	__/__/__		
Group B Strep (35-37 wks)	__/__/__		

Comments/Additional Labs

Plans/Education (Counseled ☐)

☐ Anesthesia plans _____
☐ Toxoplasmosis precautions (cats/raw meat) _____
☐ Childbirth classes _____
☐ Physical/sexual activity _____
☐ Labor signs _____
☐ Nutrition counseling _____
☐ Breast or bottle feeding _____
☐ Newborn car seat _____
☐ Postpartum birth control _____
☐ Environmental/work hazards _____

☐ Tubal sterilization _____
☐ VBAC counseling _____
☐ Circumcision _____
☐ Travel _____
☐ Lifestyle, tobacco, alcohol _____
Requests _____
_____

Tubal Sterilization   Date   Initials
Consent signed   __/__/__   _____

Provider signature (as required) _____

AA 128   2345/10987

ACOG ANTEPARTUM RECORD (FORM D)

Fig. 17-5, cont'd   For legend, see p. 391.

often recommended during the pregnancies of women who have a history of illegal drug use.

ETHICAL CONSIDERATIONS

Nurses may have ethical concerns if pregnant women are not informed of the possibility of random urine testing for presence of drugs. The other side of this concern is the unborn child and whether the mother has a duty not to harm him or her.

Family history. The family history provides information about the woman's immediate family, including parents, siblings, and children. These data help identify familial or genetic disorders or conditions that could affect the present health status of the woman or her fetus.

Social and experiential history. Situational factors such as the family's ethnic and cultural background and socioeconomic status are assessed while the history is obtained.

The following information may be obtained over several encounters. The woman's perception of this pregnancy is explored by asking her such questions as the following: Is this pregnancy wanted or not, planned or not? Is the woman pleased, displeased, accepting, or nonaccepting? What problems related to finances, career, or living accommodations may arise as a result of the pregnancy? The family support system is determined by asking her such questions as the following: What primary support is available to her? Are changes needed to promote adequate support? What are the existing relationships among the mother, father/partner, siblings, and in-laws? What preparations are being made for her care and that of dependent family members during labor and for the care of the infant after birth? Is financial, educational, or other support needed from the community?

What are the woman's ideas about childbearing, her expectations of the infant's behavior, and her outlook on life and the female role? Other such questions that need to be asked include: What does the woman think it will be like to have a baby in the home? How is her life going to change by having a baby? What plans does having a baby interrupt? During interviews throughout the pregnancy the nurse should remain alert to the appearance of potential parenting problems, such as depression, lack of family support, and inadequate living conditions. The nurse needs to assess the woman's attitude toward health care, particularly during childbearing, her expectations of health care providers, and her view of the relationship between herself and the nurse.

Coping mechanisms and patterns of interacting are also identified. Early in the pregnancy the nurse should determine the woman's knowledge of pregnancy; maternal changes; fetal growth; self-care; and care of the newborn, including feeding. Asking about attitudes toward unmedicated or medicated childbirth and about her knowledge of the availability of parenting skills classes is important.

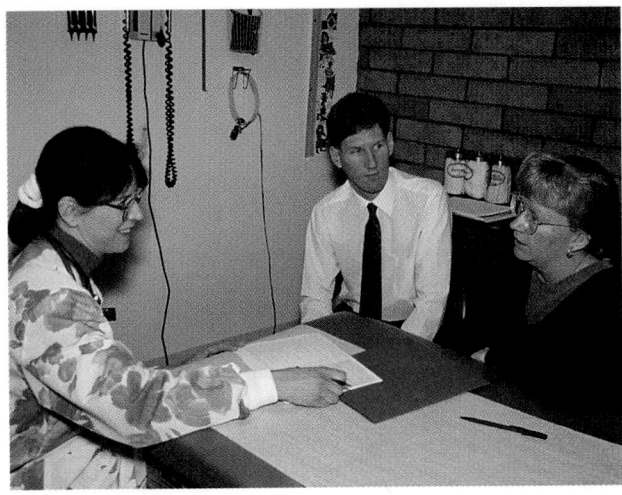

Fig. 17-6 Prenatal interview. *(Courtesy Michael S. Clement, MD, Mesa, AZ.)*

GUIDELINES/GUÍAS

Prenatal Interview

Have you had a pregnancy test?
¿Se ha hecho la prueba de embarazo?

When was your last menstrual cycle?
¿Cuándo fue su última regla?

Have you been pregnant before?
¿Estuvo embarazada antes?

How many times?
¿Cuántas veces?

How many children do you have?
¿Cuántos hijos tiene usted?

Have you ever had a miscarriage?
¿Ha tenido un aborto natural?

Have you ever had a therapeutic abortion?
¿Ha tenido un aborto provocado?

Have you ever had a stillborn?
¿Ha tenido un niño que nació muerto?

Have you ever had a cesarean?
¿Ha tenido una cesárea?

Have you had any problems with past pregnancies?
¿Ha tenido algún problema en sus embarazos previos?

Do you take drugs? Prescription medicine?
¿Usa drogas? ¿Medicina recetada?

If so, which type of medicine do you use and for what?
¿Cuál medicina usa y para qué?

Do you drink alcohol? Do you smoke?
¿Toma licor o bebidas alcohólicas? ¿Fuma?

RESEARCH

The Constipation Assessment Scale for Pregnancy

Constipation can be a problem for some women during pregnancy. In a review of the literature, no studies were found that developed or tested instruments for the assessment of the incidence or severity of constipation in pregnant women. A Constipation Assessment Scale (CAS) was developed and tested with two groups—one group of clients with cancer and a group of healthy adults—and was found to be reliable and valid. The CAS is an eight-item tool with universal characteristics of constipation and a three-point summated rating scale for constipation.

The purpose of this study was to determine the reliability and validity of the CAS during pregnancy. The assessment tool was administered first to a group of healthy women of childbearing age in a school of nursing and then to pregnant women in their physicians' offices.

An expert panel review found a calculated percentage of agreement for content validity of .75 and a Cohen's kappa of .714. Test-retest reliability based on 16 nursing students yielded high positive correlations ranging from $r = .84$ to $r = .92$. Internal consistency of the CAS for pregnancy based on the 30 surveys indicated an alpha coefficient of .82. It was concluded that the CAS for pregnancy was reliable and valid within the context of this study.

CLINICAL APPLICATION

Nurses need to include initial and ongoing assessment of bowel function during routine prenatal care or in the home setting. Assessment can include a simple inquiry about changes in bowel elimination patterns and identification of women at risk for constipation, including those with activity restrictions, with a history of problems with constipation, or who are taking constipating medications such as iron. Reliable and valid instruments such as the CAS for pregnancy can easily be included in the pregnant woman's initial visit for a baseline assessment, repeated throughout the pregnancy if she complains of symptoms of constipation, and routinely readministered during the third trimester to all pregnant women. All pregnant women stand to benefit from further research into the problem of constipation during pregnancy. Future studies designed to identify potential therapeutic interventions for constipation during pregnancy could use the CAS for pregnancy as a measurement tool.

Source: Broussard, B. (1998). The constipation assessment scale for pregnancy. *J Obstet Gynecol Neonatal Nurs* 27(3), 297-301.

Before planning for nursing care the nurse needs information about the woman's decision-making abilities and living habits (e.g., exercise, sleep, diet, diversional interests, personal hygiene, clothing). Common stressors during childbearing include the baby's welfare, labor and birth process, behaviors of the newborn, woman's relationship with the baby's father, changes in body image, and physical symptoms.

Attitudes concerning the range of acceptable sexual behavior during pregnancy should also be explored by asking questions such as the following: What has your family (partner, friends) told you about sex during pregnancy? The woman's sexual self-concept is given more emphasis by asking questions such as the following: How do you feel about the changes in your appearance? How does your partner feel about your body now? How do you feel about wearing maternity clothes?

All women should be assessed for a history or risk of physical abuse, particularly because the likelihood of abuse increases during pregnancy. Although visual cues from the woman's appearance or behavior may suggest the possibility, if questioning is limited to those women who fit the supposed profile of the battered woman, many women will be missed. Identification of abuse and immediate clinical intervention that includes information about safety can result in behaviors that may prevent future abuse and increase the safety and well-being of the woman and her infant (McFarlane et al., 1998).

Review of systems. During this portion of the interview, the woman is asked to identify and describe preexisting or concurrent problems with any of the body systems, and her mental status is assessed. The woman is questioned about physical symptoms she has experienced, such as shortness of breath or pain. Pregnancy affects and is affected by all body systems; therefore information on the present status of the body systems is important in planning care (see Research Box). For each sign or symptom described, the following additional data should be obtained: body location, quality, quantity, chronology, aggravating or alleviating factors, and associated manifestations (onset, character, course) (Seidel et al., 1999).

Physical examination. The initial physical examination provides the baseline for assessing subsequent changes. The examiner should determine the client's needs for basic information regarding reproductive anatomy and provide this information, along with a demonstration of the equipment that may be used and an explanation of the procedure itself. The interaction requires an unhurried, sensitive, and gentle approach with a matter-of-fact attitude.

The physical examination begins with assessment of vital signs including blood pressure (BP), height, and weight. The bladder should be empty before pelvic examination.

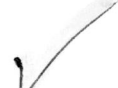

TABLE 17-1 Laboratory Tests in Prenatal Period

LABORATORY TEST	PURPOSE
Hemoglobin/hematocrit/WBC, differential	Detects anemia/detects infection
Hemoglobin electrophoresis	Identifies women with hemoglobinopathies (e.g., sickle cell anemia, thalassemia)
Blood type, Rh, and irregular antibody	Identifies those fetuses at risk for developing erythroblastosis fetalis or hyperbilirubinemia in neonatal period
Rubella titer	Determines immunity to rubella
Tuberculin skin testing; chest film after 20 weeks' gestation in women with reactive tuberculin tests	Screens for exposure to tuberculosis
Urinalysis, including microscopic examination of urinary sediment; pH, specific gravity, color, glucose, albumin, protein, RBCs, WBCs, casts, acetone; hCG	Identifies women with unsuspected diabetes mellitus, renal disease, hypertensive disease of pregnancy; infection; occult hematuria
Urine culture	Identifies women with asymptomatic bacteriuria
Renal function tests: BUN, creatinine, electrolytes, creatinine clearance, total protein excretion	Evaluates level of possible renal compromise in women with a history of diabetes, hypertension, or renal disease
Pap test	Screens for cervical intraepithelial neoplasia, herpes simplex type 2, and HPV
Vaginal or rectal smear for *Neisseria gonorrhoeae, Chlamydia,* HPV, GBS	Screens high risk population for asymptomatic infection. GBS done at 35-37 weeks
RPR/VDRL/FTA-ABS	Identifies women with untreated syphilis
HIV* antibody, hepatitis B surface antigen, toxoplasmosis	Screens for infection
1-hr glucose tolerance	Screens for gestational diabetes; done at initial visit for women with risk factors; done at 28 weeks for all pregnant women
3-hr glucose tolerance	Screens for diabetes in women with elevated glucose level after 1-hr test; must have two elevated readings for diagnosis
Cardiac evaluation: ECG, chest x-ray film, and echocardiogram	Evaluates cardiac function in women with a history of hypertension or cardiac disease

BUN, Blood urea nitrogen; *ECG,* electrocardiogram; *FTA-ABS,* fluorescent treponemal antibody absorption test; *GBS,* group B streptococcus; *hCG,* human chorionic gonadotropin; *HIV,* human immunodeficiency virus; *HPV,* human papillomavirus; *RPR,* rapid plasma reagin.
*With client permission.

This may be the opportunity to collect a specimen to test for protein, glucose, leukocytes, or other tests.

Each examiner develops a routine for proceeding with the physical examination; most choose the head-to-toe progression. Heart and breath sounds are evaluated, and extremities are examined. Distribution, amount, and quality of body hair is of particular importance because the findings reflect nutritional status, endocrine function, and attention to hygiene. The thyroid gland is assessed carefully. The height of the fundus is noted if the first examination is done after the first trimester of pregnancy. The typical basic examination is usually completed without much discomfort for the healthy woman. During the examination, the examiner needs to remain alert to the woman's cues that give direction to the remainder of the assessment and that indicate imminent untoward response such as supine hypotension. See Chapter 6 for a detailed description of the physical examination.

Whenever a pelvic examination is performed, the tone of the pelvic musculature and the need for the woman's

knowledge of Kegel exercises are assessed. Particular attention is paid to the size of the uterus because this is an indication of the timing of gestation. The nurse present during the examination can coach the woman in breathing and relaxation techniques at this time, as needed. One vaginal examination during pregnancy is recommended, but another is usually not done unless medically indicated (Bergsjo & Villar, 1997).

Laboratory tests. The laboratory data yielded by the analysis of the specimens obtained during the examination provide important information concerning the symptoms of pregnancy and the woman's health status. Such information is used for making nursing and medical diagnoses.

Specimens are collected at the initial visit so that the cause of any abnormal findings can be treated (Table 17-1). Tine or purified protein derivative (PPD) tuberculin tests are administered to assess for exposure to tuberculosis. The woman is tested for hepatitis B surface antigen (HBsAG) and hepatitis B surface antibody (HbsAB), if she has not received hepatitis B vaccine. During the pelvic examination,

BOX 17-2 HIV Screening

Pregnant women are ethically obligated to seek reasonable care during pregnancy and to avoid causing harm to the fetus. Maternity nurses should be advocates for the fetus, but not at the expense of the pregnant woman.

Mandatory HIV screening involves ethical issues related to privacy invasion, discrimination, social stigma, and reproductive risks to the pregnant woman. Incidence of perinatal transmission from an HIV-positive mother to her fetus ranges from 25% to 35%. Methods of preventing maternal-fetal transmission are not available. However, zidovudine decreases perinatal transmission with no adverse effect (Culnane et al., 1999). Until there is a change in technology that alters the diagnosis or treatment of the fetus, testing of the pregnant woman should be voluntary, although some professional groups now advocate mandatory testing. Health care providers have an obligation to make sure the pregnant woman is well informed about HIV symptoms, testing, and methods of decreasing maternal-fetal transmission.

cervical and vaginal smears are obtained for cytologic studies and for diagnosis of infection (e.g., *Chlamydia*, gonorrhea). Blood is drawn for a variety of tests: RPR/VDRL test for syphilis; complete blood cell count (CBC) with hematocrit, hemoglobin, and differential values; tests for blood type and Rh factor; antibody screen (Kell, Duffy, rubella, toxoplasmosis, and anti-Rh); test for sickle cell anemia; and measurement of the folacin level, when indicated. Urine is tested for glucose (diabetes), protein (pregnancy-induced hypertension [PIH]), and nitrites and leukocytes (urinary tract infection); culture and sensitivity tests are ordered as necessary. Testing for antibody to the human immunodeficiency virus (HIV) is strongly recommended for all pregnant women (Box 17-2).

The finding of risk factors during pregnancy may indicate the need to repeat some tests at other times. For example, exposure to tuberculosis or an STI would necessitate repeat testing. STIs are common in pregnancy and may have negative effects on mother and fetus. Careful assessment and screening is essential (Jackson & Soper, 1997).

Follow-Up Visits

Monthly visits are scheduled routinely during the first and second trimesters, although additional appointments may be made as the need arises. During the third trimester, however, the possibility for complications increases, and closer monitoring is warranted. Starting with week 28, maternity visits are scheduled every 2 weeks until week 36, and then every week until birth, unless the health care provider individualizes the schedule. Individual needs and risks of the pregnant woman may warrant visits more or

less often. The pattern of interviewing the woman first and then assessing physical changes and performing laboratory tests is maintained.

Interview

Follow-up visits are less intensive than the initial prenatal visit. At each of these follow-up visits, the woman is asked to summarize relevant events that have occurred since the previous visit. She is asked about her general emotional and physiologic well-being, complaints or problems, or questions she may have. Personal and family needs are also identified and explored.

Because the woman's emotional state affects her general well-being and that of her family, her and her family's emotional well-being is assessed at each visit. Emotional changes are common during pregnancy, and therefore it is reasonable for the nurse to ask whether the woman has experienced any mood swings; reactions to changes in her body image, bad dreams, or worries. Positive feelings (her own and those of her family) are also noted. The reactions of family members to the pregnancy and the woman's emotional changes are recorded.

How the woman is progressing through the developmental tasks of pregnancy is also assessed. By the beginning of the second trimester, most women have accepted the biologic fact of pregnancy. Usually by the fifth month, pregnant women are experiencing a growing awareness of the child as a separate being, distinct from themselves; women can say, "I am going to have a baby." With quickening, she turns her attention inward (becomes introspective) to her pregnancy and toward her relationships with others (e.g., her mother and partner).

During the third trimester, current family situations and their effect on the mother are assessed, for example, siblings' and grandparents' responses to the pregnancy and the coming child. In addition, the following questions are addressed:

- What anticipatory planning is in progress concerning new parenting responsibilities, sibling rivalry, recuperation from pregnancy and birth, and fertility management?
- What successes or frustrations with diet, rest and relaxation, sexuality, and emotional support is the mother experiencing?
- What is the mother's understanding of her family's needs in relation to the pregnancy and the unborn child?
- How well prepared are the parents for coping with an emergency? That is, does the mother know the warning signs (e.g., bleeding, abdominal pain, signs of preeclampsia), understand what they represent, and the way and to whom to report them?
- Does the mother know the signs of preterm and term labor?
- What is the mother's understanding of the labor process and expectations of herself and others during

labor? Does she know what to bring to the hospital or birthing center?

- If she is having a home birth, have all the necessary supplies been obtained?
- What plans have the mother and her family made for labor?
- What anxieties are the mother or her family experiencing regarding labor or the unborn child?
- What does the mother wish to know about the control of discomfort during labor?
- Is the mother (and her partner or support person) planning to attend any parent education classes?
- Does the mother have questions about fetal development and methods to assess fetal well-being?

A review of the woman's physical systems is appropriate at each visit, and any suspicious signs or symptoms are assessed in depth. Discomforts reflecting adaptations to pregnancy are identified. Special inquiries are made about possible infections (e.g., genitourinary tract, respiratory tract). The woman's knowledge of self-care measures is assessed, as well as the success of these and prescribed therapy.

Physical Examination

Reevaluation is a constant aspect of a pregnant woman's care (see Guidelines/Guías for phrases in Spanish for Prenatal Assessments). Each woman reacts differently to pregnancy. As a result, careful monitoring of the pregnancy and her reactions to care is vital. The database is updated at each time of contact with the pregnant woman. Physiologic changes are documented as the pregnancy progresses and reviewed for possible deviations from normal progress.

At each visit, pulse and respirations are measured. BP is taken using the same arm at every visit with the woman sitting. Her weight is determined, and the appropriateness of the weight gain is evaluated. Urine may be checked by dipstick, and the presence and degree of edema are noted. For examination of the abdomen, the woman lies comfortably on her back with her arms by her side and head supported by a pillow. The bladder should be empty. Abdominal inspection is followed by measurement of the height of the fundus. While the woman lies on her back, the nurse should be alert for the occurrence of **supine hypotension** (see Emergency box). When a woman is lying in this position, the weight of abdominal contents may compress the vena cava and aorta, causing a drop in BP and a feeling of faintness.

The findings revealed during the interview and physical examination reflect the status of maternal adaptations. When any of the findings are suspicious, an in-depth examination is performed.

Careful interpretation of BP is important in the risk factor analysis of all pregnant women. BP is evaluated on the basis of absolute values and the length of gestation and is interpreted in the light of modifying factors.

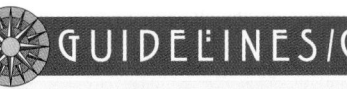

GUIDELINES/GUÍAS

Prenatal Physical Assessment

Get up on the scale, please.
Súbase a la báscula/la pesa, por favor.

I need a urine sample.
Necesito una muestra de orina.

Go to the bathroom, please.
Vaya al baño, por favor.

I need to take your blood pressure.
Necesito tomarle la presión arterial.

I am going to listen to the baby's heartbeat.
Voy a escuchar el latido del corazón del bebé.

The doctor is going to examine you.
El doctor le va hacer un examen.

Don't be afraid.
No tenga miedo.

Lie down, please.
Acuéstese, por favor.

Open your legs, please.
Separe las piernas, por favor.

Relax.
Relájese/cálmese.

Go to the laboratory for a blood test.
Vaya al laboratorio para un análisis de sangre.

Go to this office for your ultrasound.
Vaya a esta oficina para que le hagan el sonagrama.

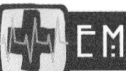

EMERGENCY

Supine Hypotension

SIGNS/SYMPTOMS
Pallor
Dizziness, faintness, breathlessness
Tachycardia
Nausea
Clammy (damp, cool) skin; sweating

INTERVENTIONS
Position woman on her side until her signs/symptoms subside and vital signs stabilize within normal limits (WNL).

SIGNS OF POTENTIAL COMPLICATIONS

First, Second, and Third Trimesters

FIRST TRIMESTER
Signs/Symptoms

Severe vomiting
Chills, fever
Burning on urination
Diarrhea
Abdominal cramping; vaginal bleeding

Possible Causes

Hyperemesis gravidarum
Infection
Infection
Infection
Miscarriage, ectopic pregnancy

SECOND AND THIRD TRIMESTERS
Signs/Symptoms

Persistent, severe vomiting

Sudden discharge of fluid from vagina before 37 weeks
Vaginal bleeding, severe abdominal pain
Chills, fever, burning on urination, diarrhea
Severe backache or flank pain
Change in fetal movements: absence of fetal movements after quickening, any unusual change in pattern or amount
Uterine contractions; pressure; cramping before 37 weeks
Visual disturbances: blurring, double vision, or spots
Swelling of face or fingers and over sacrum
Headaches: severe, frequent, or continuous
Muscular irritability or convulsions
Epigastric or abdominal pain (perceived as severe stomachache)
Glycosuria, positive glucose tolerance test reaction
Sudden weight gain 2+ kg/wk

Possible Causes

Hyperemesis gravidarum, hypertension, pregnancy-induced hypertension (PIH)
Premature rupture of membranes (PROM)
Miscarriage, placenta previa, abruptio placentae
Infection
Kidney infection or stones; preterm labor
Fetal jeopardy or intrauterine fetal death

Preterm labor
Hypertensive conditions, PIH
Hypertensive conditions, PIH
Hypertensive conditions, PIH
Hypertensive conditions, PIH
Hypertensive conditions, PIH, abruptio placentae

Gestational diabetes mellitus
PIH

An absolute systolic BP of 140 mm Hg or more and a diastolic BP of 90 mm Hg or more suggests the presence of hypertension (Helewa et al., 1997). Although the BP of 140/90 is an excellent point of reference, further investigation is needed. A rise in the systolic BP of 30 mm Hg or more than the baseline pressure or in the diastolic BP of 15 mm Hg more than the baseline pressure is also a significant finding, regardless of the absolute values. Gilbert and Harmon (1998) suggest that an increase of 20 mm Hg or more in the mean arterial pressure (MAP) also is an important indicator of hypertension (see Box 15-2).

While completing the prenatal assessments, the nurse always keeps in mind that an increase in BP could indicate the onset of PIH or preeclampsia. Investigations by Caritis et al. (1998) indicate that an absolute value MAP >80 in nulliparous women may be predictive of preeclampsia and more severe complications. See Chapter 30 for an in-depth discussion of problems associated with hypertension.

The pregnant woman is monitored continuously for a range of signs and symptoms that indicate potential complications in addition to hypertension. For example, persistent and excessive vomiting and ketonuria may indicate the

development of hyperemesis gravidarum. Uterine cramping and vaginal bleeding are signs of threatened miscarriage. Chills and fever are symptoms of infection. Discharge from the vagina may be amniotic fluid or associated with infection (see Signs of Potential Complications box.)

Fetal Assessment

Toward the end of the first trimester, before the uterus is an abdominal organ, the fetal heart tones (FHTs) can be heard with an ultrasound fetoscope or an ultrasound stethoscope. To hear the FHTs the instrument is placed in the midline, just above the symphysis pubis, and firm pressure is applied. The woman and her family should be offered the opportunity to listen to the FHTs. The health status of the fetus is assessed at each visit for the remainder of the pregnancy.

Fundal height. During the second trimester the uterus becomes an abdominal organ. The **fundal height**, measurement of the height of the uterus above the symphysis pubis, is used as one indicator of fetal growth. The measurement also provides a gross estimate of the duration of pregnancy. In addition, it may aid in the identification of high risk factors. A stable or decreased fundal height may indicate the presence of intrauterine growth restriction (IUGR); an excessive increase could indicate the presence of multifetal gestation or hydramnios.

A paper tape measure or a pelvimeter may be used to measure fundal height. To increase the reliability of the measurement, the same person could examine the pregnant woman at each of her prenatal visits, but often this is not possible because different clinicians may see the woman at prenatal visits. All clinicians who examine a particular pregnant woman should be consistent in their measurement technique. Ideally a protocol should be established for the health care setting in which the measurement technique is explicitly set forth, and the woman's position on the examining table, the measuring device, and method of measurement used are specified. Conditions under which the measurements are taken can also be described in the woman's records, including whether the bladder was empty and whether the uterus was relaxed or contracted at the time of measurement.

Various positions for measuring fundal height have been described. The woman can be supine, have her head elevated, have her knees flexed, or have both her head elevated and knees flexed. Measurements obtained with the woman in the various positions differ, making it even more important to standardize the fundal height measurement technique. The bladder must be empty before the measurement is taken. As much as 3 cm of error is possible if the bladder is full (Cunningham et al., 1997).

Placement of the tape measure can also vary. The tape can be placed in the middle of the woman's abdomen and the measurement made from the upper border of the symphysis pubis to the upper border of the fundus with the tape measure held in contact with the skin for the entire length of the uterus (Fig. 17-7, *A*). In another measurement technique, the upper curve of the fundus is not included in the measurement. Instead, one end of the tape measure is held at the upper border of the symphysis pubis with one hand and the other hand is placed at the upper border of the fundus. The tape is placed between the middle and index fingers of the other hand and the point where these fingers intercept the tape measure is taken as the measurement (Fig. 17-7, *B*).

During the second and third trimesters (weeks 18 to 30), the height of the fundus in centimeters is approximately the same as the number of weeks of gestation, if the woman's bladder is empty at the time of measurement (Cunningham et al., 1997).

Gestational age. In an uncomplicated pregnancy, fetal gestational age is estimated after the duration of pregnancy and the estimated date of birth (EDB) are determined. Fetal gestational age is determined from the menstrual history, contraceptive history, pregnancy test result, and the following findings obtained during the clinical evaluation:
- First uterine size estimate: date, size
- Fetal heart (FH) first heard: date, Doppler stethoscope, fetoscope

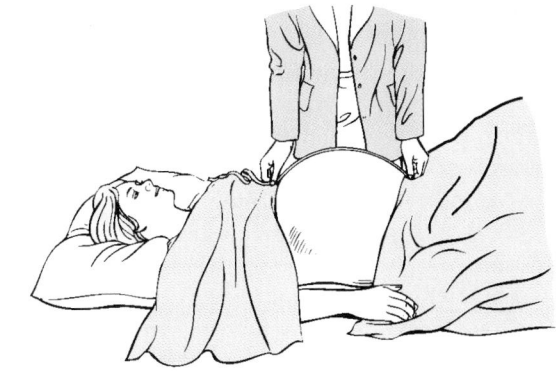

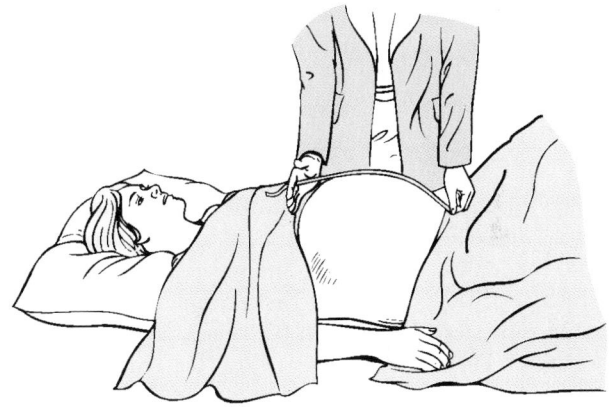

Fig. 17-7 Measurement of fundal height from symphysis that **A,** includes the upper curve of the fundus, and **B,** does not include the upper curve of the fundus. Note position of hands and measuring tape.

- Date of quickening
- Current fundal height, estimated fetal weight (EFW)
- Current week of gestation by history of LMP and/or ultrasound
- Ultrasound: date, week of gestation, biparietal diameter (BPD)
- Reliability of dates

Quickening ("feeling of life") refers to the mother's first perception of fetal movement. It usually occurs between weeks 16 through 20 of gestation and is initially experienced as a fluttering sensation.

Routine use of ultrasound examination, also called a **sonogram,** in early pregnancy has been recommended (Crowley, 1998), and many health care providers have equipment readily available in the office. This procedure may be used to establish the duration of pregnancy if the woman cannot give a precise date for her last menstrual period (LMP) or if the size of the uterus does not correspond to the EDB calculated with Nägele's rule. Ultrasound also provides information about the well-being of the fetus; however, the routine use of ultrasound has not been found to substantively improve clinical outcomes (Neilson, 1998). The debate about whether the expense justifies routine use of ultrasound examination early in pregnancy continues, but nurses who have been adequately taught to perform the ultrasound have a valuable opportunity to provide both education and support (Huffman & Sandelowski, 1997).

Health status. The assessment of fetal health status includes consideration of fetal movement, the fetal heart rate (FHR) and rhythm, and abnormal maternal or fetal symptoms.

The mother is instructed to note the extent and timing of fetal movements and to report immediately if the pattern changes or if movement ceases. Regular movement has been found to be a reliable determinant of fetal health. The FHR is checked on routine visits once it has been heard (Fig. 17-8). Early in the second trimester the heartbeat may be heard with the Doppler stethoscope (Fig. 17-8, *B*). To detect the heartbeat before the fetus can be palpated by Leopold's maneuvers (see Fig. 22-5), the scope is moved around the abdomen until the heartbeat is heard. Each nurse develops a set pattern for searching the abdomen for the heartbeat; for example, starting first in the midline about 2 to 3 cm above the symphysis, then moving to the left lower quadrant, and so on. The heartbeat is counted and the quality and rhythm noted. Later in the second trimester the FHR can be determined with the fetoscope or Pinard's stethoscope (Fig. 17-8, *A* and *C*). A normal rate and rhythm are other good indicators of fetal health. Once the heartbeat is noted, its absence is cause for immediate investigation.

Fetal health status is investigated intensively if any maternal or fetal complications arise (e.g., maternal hypertension, IUGR, premature rupture of membranes [PROM], irregular or absent FHR, or absence of fetal movements after quickening). Careful, precise, and concise recording of client responses and laboratory results contributes to the continuous supervision vital to ensuring the well-being of the mother and fetus.

Laboratory Tests

The number of routine laboratory tests done during pregnancy is limited. A clean-catch urine specimen is obtained to test for glucose, protein, and nitrites and leukocytes at each follow-up visit. Urine specimens for culture and sensitivity, as well as blood samples, are obtained only if signs and symptoms warrant. A hematocrit determination is done at each visit in some offices. A blood specimen is obtained at 16 weeks to determine the alpha-fetoprotein level.

The multiple-marker, or triple-screen, test is used to detect Down syndrome. Done between 16 and 18 weeks' gestation, it measures the maternal serum level of alpha-fetoprotein (MSAFP), hCG, and unconjugated estriol. Adjusted values are combined to yield the risk for Down syndrome. Low levels may be associated with Down syndrome and other chromosomal abnormalities (Cunningham et al., 1997).

The following blood tests are repeated as necessary: RPR/VDRL test for syphilis; complete blood cell count with hematocrit, hemoglobin, and differential values; antibody screen (Kell, Duffy, rubella, toxoplasmosis, anti-Rh, HIV; sickle cell; and level of folacin when indicated). If not done earlier in pregnancy, a glucose screen is performed in women over 25 years of age. A glucose challenge is usually done between 24 and 28 weeks' gestation. Cervical and vaginal smears are repeated as necessary to examine for *Chlamydia* organisms, gonorrhea, and herpes simplex virus Types 1 and 2. Group B streptococcus (GBS) testing is done between 35 and 37 weeks' gestation; cultures collected earlier will not accurately predict GBS status at time of birth.

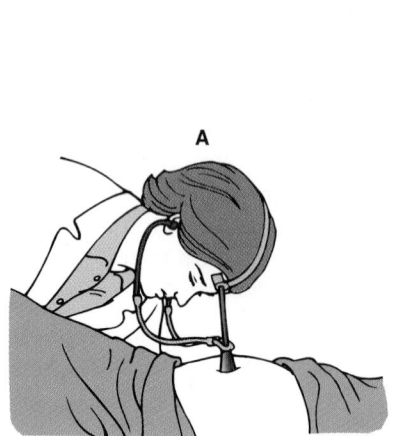
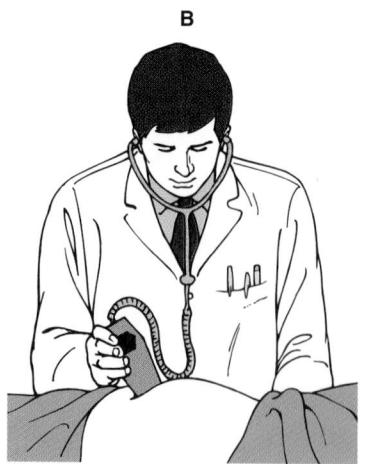
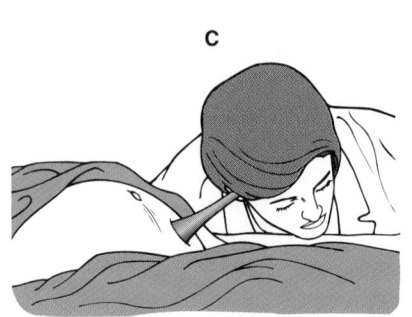

Fig. 17-8 Detecting fetal heart rate. **A,** Fetoscope (18 to 20 weeks). **B,** Doppler ultrasound stethoscope (12 weeks). **C,** Pinard's stethoscope. NOTE: Hands should not touch stethoscope while nurse is listening.

Other Tests

Other diagnostic tests are available to assess the health status of both the pregnant woman and the fetus. Ultrasonography, for example, may be performed to determine the status of the pregnancy and to confirm gestational age of the fetus. Amniocentesis, a procedure used to obtain amniotic fluid for analysis, may be needed to evaluate the fetus for genetic disorders or gestational maturity. These and other tests that are used to determine health risks for the mother and infant are described in Chapter 29.

After obtaining information through the assessment process, the data are analyzed to identify deviations from the norm and unique needs of the pregnant woman and her family. Although comprehensive health care requires collaboration among professionals from several disciplines, nurses are in an excellent position to formulate diagnoses that can be used to guide independent interventions. The diagnoses that follow are examples of the nursing diagnoses that may be appropriate in the prenatal period.

▌ Nursing Diagnoses

- Anxiety related to
  - physical discomforts of pregnancy
  - ambivalent and labile emotions
  - changes in family dynamics
  - fetal well-being
  - ability to manage anticipated labor
- Altered family processes related to
  - changing roles and responsibilities
  - inadequate understanding of physical and emotional changes in pregnancy
  - increased concern about labor
- Altered nutrition: less than body requirements related to
  - morning sickness
  - fatigue
- Body image disturbance related to
  - anatomic and physiologic changes of pregnancy
  - changes in the couple relationship
- Altered health maintenance related to knowledge deficit regarding self-care measures for
  - posture and body mechanics
  - rest and relaxation
  - personal hygiene
  - activity and exercise
  - safety
- Impaired individual coping related to knowledge deficit regarding
  - recognizing onset of complications
  - distinguishing between true and false labor
  - emergency arrangements
- Sleep pattern disturbance related to
  - discomforts of late pregnancy
  - anxiety about approaching labor

Expected Outcomes of Care

The plan of nursing care for women and their families during pregnancy is given direction by the diagnoses that have been formulated during prenatal visits. Individualized plans that are developed mutually with the pregnant woman are more likely to result in desirable outcomes than those developed by the nurse for the woman. Measured outcomes of prenatal care include not only physical outcomes but also developmental and psychosocial outcomes (Malnory, 1996).

Below are examples of outcomes that may be expected. The pregnant woman will do the following:

- Indicate decreased anxiety about the health of her fetus and herself.
- Describe improved family dynamics.
- Show appropriate weight gain patterns.
- Report increasing acceptance of changes in body image.
- Demonstrate knowledge for self-care.
- Ask for clarification of information about pregnancy and birth.
- Report signs and symptoms of complications.
- Describe appropriate measures taken to relieve physical discomforts.
- Develop a realistic birth plan.
- Indicate satisfaction with health care providers and processes.

Plan of Care and Interventions

The nurse-client relationship is critical in setting the tone for further interaction. The techniques of listening with an attentive expression, touching, and using eye contact have their place, as does recognizing the woman's feelings and her right to express these feelings. The interaction may occur in various formal or informal settings. The clinic, home visits, or telephone conversations all provide opportunities for contact and can be used effectively for this purpose. Sometimes women repeatedly seek information about a particular problem. At other times there may be another underlying problem the woman is hesitant to broach. The nurse needs to be perceptive in identifying such unvoiced needs and can help the woman by asking for a client-generated solution and a subsequent report of its effectiveness.

In supporting a client the nurse must remember that both the nurse and the woman are contributing to the relationship. The nurse has to accept the woman's responses as a factor in trying to be of help. An example of one nurse-client relationship is as follows:

> Mrs. ____ had been very forthright in saying that this pregnancy was unplanned but had countered this observation with comments such as, "All things happen for the best," and "Children bring their own love." Over time, as our relationship developed to one of mutual trust, she complained increasingly of her fear of pain, of hating to wear maternity clothes, and of having to give up helping the family. Finally I ventured to say, "Sometimes when a pregnancy is unplanned,

women resent it and are angry about it." Her relief was evident. She said, "Oh, you don't know how angry I've been." As a result, the whole tenor of support being offered changed, and the plan was adjusted to meet her real needs.

The nurse also needs to accept that the woman must be a willing partner in a purely voluntary relationship. As such, the relationship can be refused or terminated at any time by the pregnant woman or her family.

Supportive care involves developing, augmenting, or changing the mechanisms used by women and their families in coping with stress. The nurse tries to promote active participation by the people in the solution of their own problems. The nurse can help a woman gather pertinent information, explore alternative actions, decide on a course of action, and assume responsibility for the outcomes. These outcomes may include living with a problem as it is, easing the effects of a problem so that it can be accepted more readily, or eliminating the problem by effecting change.

At other times a successful outcome can be documented readily. For example, a woman who early in her pregnancy had predicted a severe depressive state in the postbirth period was elated when such a state did not materialize. She remarked to the nurse who had provided support during the pregnancy and birth, "You're the best nerve medicine I've ever had!"

Care Paths

Today there is emphasis on better coordination of prenatal care services for childbearing families. Because a large number of health care professionals are involved in care of the expectant mother, unintentional gaps or overlaps in care may occur. Care paths are used to improve the consistency of care and to reduce costs (Simon, Heaps, & Chodroff, 1997). Although the care path focuses only on prenatal education, it is one example of the type of form that might be developed to guide health care providers in carrying out the appropriate assessments and interventions in a timely way. Use of care paths may also contribute to improved satisfaction of families with the prenatal care provided, and members of the health care team may function more efficiently and effectively (see Care Path, p. 405).

Education About Maternal and Fetal Changes

Expectant parents are typically curious about the growth and development of the fetus and the consequent changes that occur in the mother's body. Mothers in particular are sometimes more tolerant of the discomforts related to the continuing pregnancy if they understand the underlying causes. Commercial literature that describes the fetal and maternal changes is often available and can be used in explaining changes as they occur. The nurse's familiarity with any reading material given to families is essential to effective client education. Table 14-1 summarizes fetal development.

Education for Self-Care

Health maintenance is an important aspect of prenatal care. Client participation in the care ensures prompt reporting of untoward responses to pregnancy. Client assumption of responsibility of health maintenance is assisted by the nurse's understanding of maternal adaptations to the growth of the unborn child and a readiness to learn. In their teacher role, nurses provide clients with the information necessary for compliance with health care guidelines.

The expectant mother needs information about many subjects. The nurse who is observant, listens, and knows typical concerns of expectant parents can anticipate questions that will be asked and prompt mothers and partners to discuss what is on their minds. Many times, printed literature can be given to supplement the individualized teaching the nurse provides, and women often avidly read books and pamphlets related to their own experience. When nurses read the literature before they distribute it, they have an opportunity to point out areas that may not correspond with local health care practices. Clients who receive conflicting advice or instruction are likely to grow increasingly frustrated with members of the health care team and the care provided. Several topics that may cause concerns in pregnant women are discussed in the following sections.

Nutrition. Proper nutrition is important in the maintenance of maternal health during pregnancy and the provision of adequate nutrients for embryonic and fetal development. The nourishment the fetus receives from its mother influences health in later life (Campbell-Brown & Hytten, 1998). Assessing a woman's nutritional status and providing information on nutrition are part of the nurse's responsibilities in providing prenatal care. In some settings, a registered dietitian conducts classes for pregnant women on the topics of nutritional status and nutrition during pregnancy or interviews them to assess their knowledge of these topics. Nurses can refer women to a registered dietitian if a need is revealed during the nursing assessment. (For detailed information concerning maternal and fetal nutritional needs and related nursing care, see Chapter 16).

Personal hygiene. During pregnancy, the sebaceous (sweat) glands are highly active because of hormonal influences, and women often perspire freely. They may be reassured that the increase is normal and that their previous patterns of perspiration will return after the postpartum period. Washing the body regularly is basic to good personal hygiene. Baths and warm showers can be therapeutic because they relax tense, tired muscles, help counter insomnia, and make the pregnant woman feel fresh. Tub bathing is permitted even in late pregnancy because little water enters the vagina unless under pressure. However, late in pregnancy, when the woman's center of gravity lowers, she is at risk for falling. Tub bathing is contraindicated after rupture of the membranes.

CARE PATH Prenatal Care Pathway

PRENATAL EDUCATION CLINICAL PATHWAY

INITIAL VISIT AND ORIENTATION: _____   SOCIAL SERVICE: _____   DIETICIAN: _____

I. EARLY PREGNANCY (WEEKS 1-20) (initial and date after education given)

Fetal growth and development   _____

Maternal changes   _____

Lifestyle: exercise/stress/nutrition   _____
  Drugs, OTC, tobacco, alcohol   _____
  STIs   _____

Psycho/social adjustments:
  FOB involved/accepts   _____
  Baby for adoption   _____

Testing: Labs _____   Ultrasound _____

Possible Complications:
  a. Threatened miscarriage   _____
  b. Diabetes   _____
  c. _____   _____

Introduction to breastfeeding   _____
Acceptance   _____
  and childbirth preparation

Dietary follow-up   _____

II. MIDPREGNANCY (WEEKS 21-27) (initial and date after education given)

Fetal growth and development   _____

Maternal changes   _____

Daily fetal movement   _____

Possible complications: _____
  a. Preterm labor prevention   _____
  b. PIH symptoms   _____
  c. _____

Breast or bottle feeding   _____

Birth plan initiated   _____

Childbirth preparation _____
_____

Dietary follow-up   _____

III. LATE PREGNANCY (WEEKS 28-40) (initial and date after education given)

Fetal growth and development   _____

Fetal evaluation: _____

Daily movement _____   NSTs _____

Kick counts _____   BPPs _____

Maternal changes   _____

Possible complications:
  a. Preterm labor prevention   _____
  b. PIH symptoms   _____
  c. _____   _____

Breastfeeding preparation:
  Nipple assessment   _____

Dietary follow-up   _____

Childbirth preparation:
  S/S of labor; labor process
  Pain management: natural childbirth,   _____
    meds, epidural
  Cesarean; VBAC   _____
  Birth plan complete   _____
  Review hospital policies   _____

Parenting preparation:
Pediatrician _____   Childcare _____
Siblings _____   Immunizations _____
Car seat/safety _____

Postpartum:
  P.P. care/check-up   _____
  Emotional changes   _____
  B.C. options   _____
  Safe sex/STDs   _____

Signature: _____   _____   _____

Prevention of urinary tract infections. Because of dramatic changes that occur in the renal system during pregnancy (see Chapter 15), urinary tract infections are common, but they may be asymptomatic. Women should be instructed to inform their health care provider if blood or pain occurs with urination. These infections pose a risk to the mother and fetus; thus, the prevention or early treatment of these infections is essential (Polivka & Nickel, 1997).

The nurse can assess the woman's understanding and use of good handwashing techniques before and after urinating and whether she knows to wipe from front to back. Soft, absorbent toilet tissue, preferably white and unscented, should be used; harsh, scented, or printed toilet paper may cause irritation. Bubble bath or other bath oils should be avoided because these may be irritating to the urethra. Women should wear underpants and panty hose with a cotton crotch and avoid wearing tight-fitting slacks or jeans for long periods; anything that allows a buildup of heat and moisture in the genital area may foster the growth of bacteria.

Some women do not consume enough fluid and food. After discovering her food preferences, the nurse should advise the woman to drink 2 to 3 L (8 to 12 glasses) of liquid a day to maintain an adequate fluid intake that ensures frequent urination. Pregnant women should not limit fluids in an effort to reduce the frequency of urination. Women need to know that if urine looks dark (concentrated), they need to increase their fluid intake. Cranberry juice may be suggested because it is more acidic than other fluids and makes the urinary tract less hospitable to bacteria by lowering the pH. The consumption of yogurt and acidophilus milk may also help prevent urinary tract and vaginal infections.

The nurse should review healthy urination practices with the woman. Women should be told not to ignore the urge to urinate because holding urine lengthens the time bacteria are in the bladder and allows them to multiply. Women should plan ahead when they are faced with situations that may normally require them to delay urination (e.g., a long car ride). They always should urinate before going to bed at night. Bacteria also can be introduced during intercourse. Therefore, women are advised to urinate before and after intercourse, then drink a large glass of water to promote additional urination.

Kegel exercises. **Kegel exercises** (exercises for the pelvic floor) strengthen the muscles around the reproductive organs and improve muscle tone. Many women are not aware of the muscles of the pelvic floor until it is pointed out that these are the muscles used during urination and sexual intercourse and therefore can be consciously controlled. Inasmuch as the muscles of the pelvic floor encircle the outlet through which the baby must pass, it is important that they be exercised, because an exercised muscle can then stretch and contract readily at the time of birth. Practice of pelvic muscle exercises during pregnancy also results in fewer complaints of urinary in-

continence in late pregnancy and postpartum (Sampselle et al., 1998).

Kegel exercises should also be done immediately after giving birth to help the pelvic floor muscles return to normal functioning. They can then strengthen these muscles and improve muscle tone. If practiced on a regular basis, the exercises can help prevent a prolapsed uterus and stress incontinence from occurring later in life.

Several ways of performing Kegel exercises have been described. The method that is suggested by nurse researchers involved in a research utilization project for continence in women is described in the Teaching Guidelines box, p. 82. The nurse can be reasonably assured that the teaching has been effective if the woman reports an increased ability to control urine flow and greater muscular control during sexual intercourse.

Preparation for breastfeeding the newborn. Pregnant women are usually eager to discuss their plans for feeding the newborn. Breast milk is the food of choice, in part because breastfeeding is associated with a decreased incidence of perinatal morbidity and mortality. The American Academy of Pediatrics recommends breastfeeding for at least a year. However, a deep-seated aversion to breastfeeding on the part of the mother or partner, the mother's need for certain medications, and certain medical complications, such as active tuberculosis, newly diagnosed breast cancer, and hepatitis C, are contraindications to breastfeeding (Lawrence, 1999). Although hepatitis B antigen has not been shown to be transmitted through breast milk, as an added precaution it is recommended that infants born to hepatitis B antigen–positive women receive the hepatitis B vaccine and hepatitis B immune globulin (HBIG) immediately after birth. Women who are HIV positive are discouraged from nursing because the risk of HIV transmission outweighs the risk of the infant dying from another cause (Lawrence, 1999).

Skinner et al. (1997) reported that a woman's decision about the method of infant feeding is made before pregnancy; thus, the education of women of childbearing age about the benefits of breastfeeding is essential. The pregnant woman and her partner are encouraged to decide which method of feeding is suitable for them; however, the benefits of breastfeeding should be emphasized. Once the couple has been given information about the advantages and disadvantages of bottle feeding and breastfeeding, they can make an informed choice. Health care providers support their decisions and provide any needed assistance.

The **pinch test** is done to determine whether the nipple is everted or inverted (Fig. 17-9). The nurse shows the woman the way to perform the pinch test. It involves having the woman place her thumb and forefinger on her areola and gently press inward. This action will cause her nipple either to stand erect or to invert. Most nipples will stand erect.

Exercises to break the adhesions that cause the nipple to invert do not work and may in fact precipitate uterine contractions (Lawrence, 1999). The use of **breast shells** by

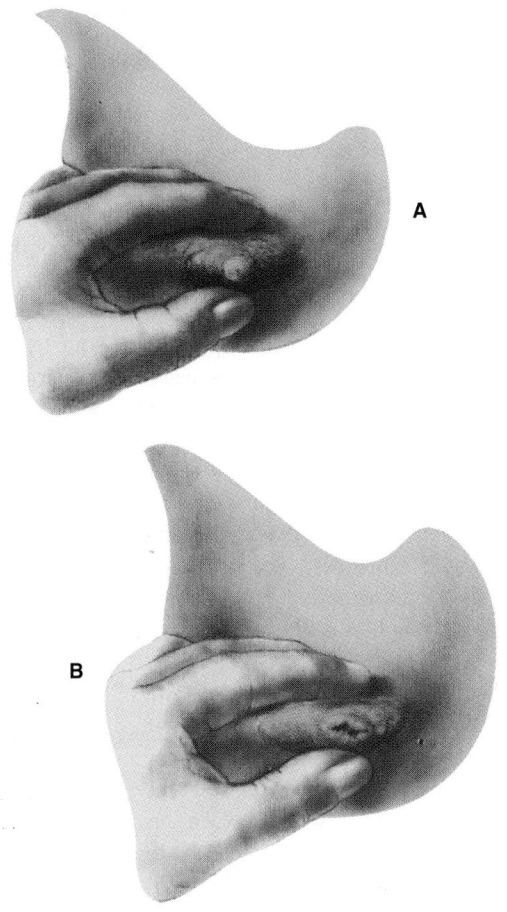

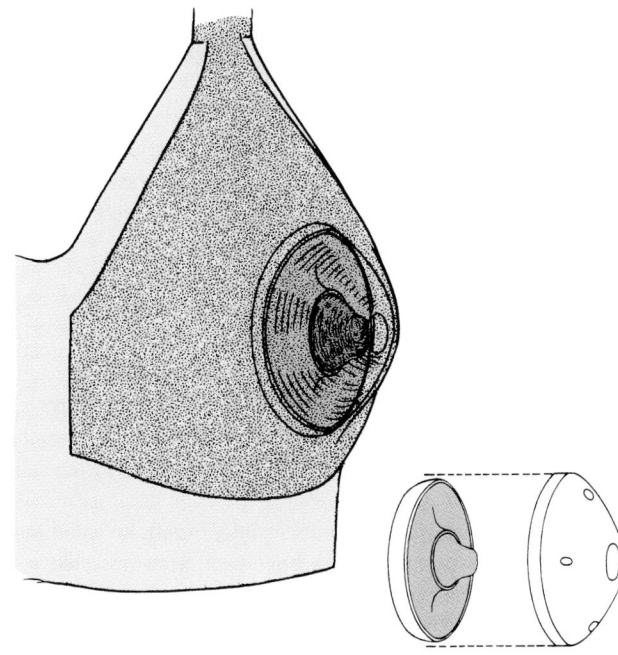

Fig. 17-10 Breast shell in place inside bra to evert nipple. *(Modified from Lawrence, R. [1999]. Breastfeeding: A guide for the medical profession. [5th ed.]. St. Louis: Mosby.)*

Fig. 17-9 **A,** Normal nipple everts with gentle pressure. **B,** Inverted nipple inverts with gentle pressure. *(Modified from Lawrence, R. [1999]. Breastfeeding: A guide for the medical profession. [5th ed.]. St. Louis: Mosby.)*

women with flat or inverted nipples is recommended (Fig. 17-10). Breast shells work by exerting a continuous, gentle pressure around the areola that pushes the nipple through a central opening in the inner shield. Breast shells should be worn for 1 to 2 hours daily during the last trimester of pregnancy. They should be worn for gradually increasing lengths of time (Lawrence, 1999). Breast stimulation is contraindicated in women at risk for preterm labor. Therefore, the decision to recommend the use of breast shells to women with flat or inverted nipples must be made judiciously. Continuous support and guidance must be given to the woman as part of the nursing care plan.

The woman is taught to cleanse the nipples with warm water to keep the ducts from being blocked with dried colostrum. Soap, ointments, alcohol, and tinctures should not be applied because they remove protective oils that keep the nipples supple. The use of these substances may cause the nipples to crack during early lactation (Lawrence, 1999).

The woman who plans to breastfeed should purchase a nursing bra that will accommodate her increased breast size during the last few months of pregnancy and during lactation. If her breasts are very heavy, or if the woman feels uncomfortable with the weight unsupported, the bra can be worn day and night.

Dental Care. Dental care during pregnancy is especially important because nausea during pregnancy may lead to poor oral hygiene, allowing dental caries to develop. No physiologic alteration during gestation can cause dental caries, however. Because calcium and phosphorus in the teeth are fixed in enamel, the old adage "for every child a tooth" is not true.

There is no scientific evidence that filling teeth or even dental extraction involving the administration of local or nitrous oxide-oxygen anesthesia precipitates miscarriage or premature labor. Antibacterial therapy should be considered for sepsis, however, especially in pregnant women who have had rheumatic heart disease or nephritis. Emergency dental surgery is not contraindicated during pregnancy. However, the risks and benefits of dental surgery need to be explained to the mother.

Physical Activity. Physical activity promotes a feeling of well-being in the pregnant woman. It improves circulation, promotes relaxation and rest, and counteracts boredom, as it does in the nonpregnant woman. Detailed exercise tips for pregnancy are presented in the Home Care box. Exercises that help relieve the low back pain that often arises during the second trimester because of the increased weight of the fetus are demonstrated in Fig. 17-11.

Posture and body mechanics. Many maternal adaptations predispose the woman to suffering backache and incurring possible injury. The pregnant woman's center of

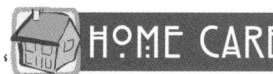

HOME CARE

Exercise Tips For Pregnant Women

Consult your health care provider when you know or suspect you are pregnant. Discuss your medical and obstetric history, your current exercise regimen, and the exercises you would like to continue throughout pregnancy.

Seek help in determining an exercise routine that is well within your limit of tolerance, especially if you have not been exercising regularly.

Consider decreasing weight-bearing exercises (jogging, running) and concentrating on non–weight-bearing activities such as swimming, cycling, or stretching. If you are a runner, starting in your seventh month, you may wish to walk instead.

Avoid risky activities such as surfing, mountain climbing, skydiving, and racquetball because such activities that require precise balance and coordination may be dangerous. Avoid activities that require holding your breath and bearing down (Valsalva's maneuver). Jerky, bouncy motions also should be avoided.

Exercise regularly at least three times a week, as long as you are healthy, to improve muscle tone and increase or maintain your stamina. If you do exercises sporadically, this may put undue strain on your muscles. Limit activity to shorter intervals. Exercise for 10 to 15 minutes, rest for 2 to 3 minutes, then exercise for another 10 to 15 minutes.

Decrease your exercise level as your pregnancy progresses. The normal alterations of advancing pregnancy, such as decreased cardiac reserve and increased respiratory effort, may produce physiologic stress if you exercise strenuously for a long time.

Take your pulse every 10 to 15 minutes while you are exercising. If it is more than 140 beats/min, slow down until it returns to a maximum of 90 beats/min. You should be able to converse easily while exercising. If you cannot, you need to slow down.

Avoid becoming overheated for extended periods of time. It is best not to exercise for more than 35 minutes, especially in hot, humid weather. As your body temperature rises, the heat is transmitted to your fetus. Prolonged or repeated elevation of fetal temperature may result in birth defects, especially during the first 3 months. Your temperature should not exceed 38° C.

Avoid the use of hot tubs and saunas.

Warm-up and stretching exercises prepare your joints for more strenuous exercise and lessen the likelihood of strain or injury to your joints. After the fourth month of gestation you should not perform exercises flat on your back.

A cool-down period of mild activity involving your legs after an exercise period will help bring your respiration, heart, and metabolic rates back to normal and prevent the pooling of blood in the exercised muscles.

Rest for 10 minutes after exercising, lying on your side. As the uterus grows, it puts pressure on a major vein in your abdomen, which carries blood to your heart. Lying on your side removes the pressure and promotes return circulation from your extremities and muscles to your heart, thereby increasing blood flow to your placenta and fetus. You should rise gradually from the floor to prevent dizziness or fainting (orthostatic hypotension).

Drink two or three 8 oz glasses of water after you exercise to replace the body fluids lost through perspiration. While exercising, drink water whenever you feel the need.

Increase your caloric intake to replace the calories burned during exercise and provide the extra energy needs of pregnancy. (Pregnancy alone requires an additional 300 kcal/day.) Choose such high-protein foods as fish, milk, cheese, eggs, or meat.

Take your time. This is not the time to be competitive or train for activities requiring speed or long endurance.

Wear a supportive bra. Your increased breast weight may cause changes in posture and put pressure on the ulnar nerve.

Wear supportive shoes. As your uterus grows, your center of gravity shifts and you compensate for this by arching your back. These natural changes may make you feel off balance and more likely to fall.

Stop exercising immediately if you experience shortness of breath, dizziness, numbness, tingling, pain of any kind, more than four uterine contractions per hour, decreased fetal activity, or vaginal bleeding, and consult your health care provider.

Modified from Artal, R, & Subak-Sharpe, G. (1992). *Pregnancy & exercise.* New York: Delacorte Press; Fishbein, E., & Phillips, M. (1990). How safe is exercise during pregnancy? *J Obstet Gynecol Neonatal Nurs* 19(1):45; ACOG.(1994). Exercise during pregnancy and the postpartum period. *Technical Bulletin* Feb, 189; Pivarnik, J. (1994). Maternal exercise in pregnancy. *Sports Med* 18:215.

gravity changes, pelvic joints soften and relax, and stress is placed on abdominal musculature as pregnancy progresses. Poor posture and body mechanics contribute to the discomfort and potential for injury. To minimize these problems, women can acquire a kinesthetic sense for good body posture (Fig. 17-12). The activities described in the

Home Care box on p. 410 can also promote greater physical comfort.

Rest and relaxation. The pregnant woman is encouraged to plan regular rest periods, particularly as pregnancy advances. The side-lying position is recommended because it promotes uterine perfusion and fetoplacental oxygena-

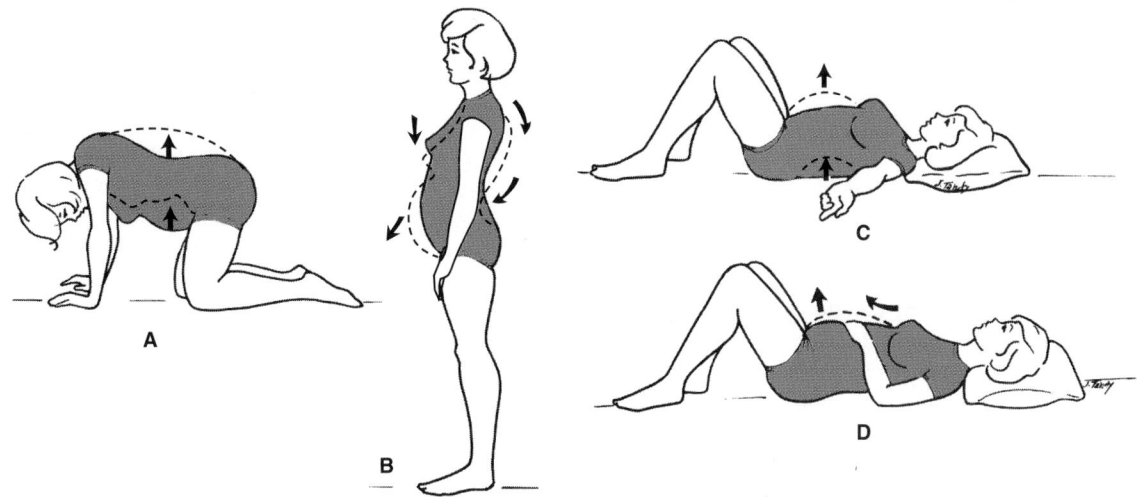

Fig. 17-11 Exercises. **A** to **C,** Pelvic rocking relieves low backache (excellent for relief of menstrual cramps as well). **D,** Abdominal breathing aids relaxation and lifts abdominal wall off uterus.

tion by eliminating pressure on the ascending vena cava and descending aorta, which can lead to supine hypotension (Fig. 17-13). The mother should also be shown the way to rise slowly from a side-lying position to prevent placing strain on the back and to minimize the orthostatic hypotension caused by changes in position common in the latter part of pregnancy. To stretch and rest back muscles at home or work, the nurse can show the woman the way to do the following exercises:

Stand behind a chair. Support and balance self using the back of the chair (Fig. 17-14). Squat for 30 seconds; stand for 15 seconds. Repeat six times, several times per day, as needed.

While sitting in a chair, lower head to knees for 30 seconds. Raise head up. Repeat six times, several times per day, as needed.

Conscious relaxation is the process of releasing tension from the mind and body through deliberate effort and practice. The ability to relax consciously and intentionally can be beneficial for the following reasons:

- It can relieve the normal discomforts related to pregnancy.
- It can reduce stress and therefore diminish pain perception during the childbearing cycle.
- It can heighten self-awareness and trust in one's own ability to control responses and functions.
- It can help the woman cope with stress in everyday life situations, whether she is pregnant or not.

The techniques for conscious relaxation are numerous and varied. The guidelines given in Box 17-3 can be used by anyone.

Employment. Employment of pregnant women usually has no adverse effects on pregnancy outcomes. Job discrimination that is based strictly on pregnancy is illegal. However, some job environments pose potential risk to the fetus (e.g., dry cleaning plants, chemistry laboratories, parking garages).

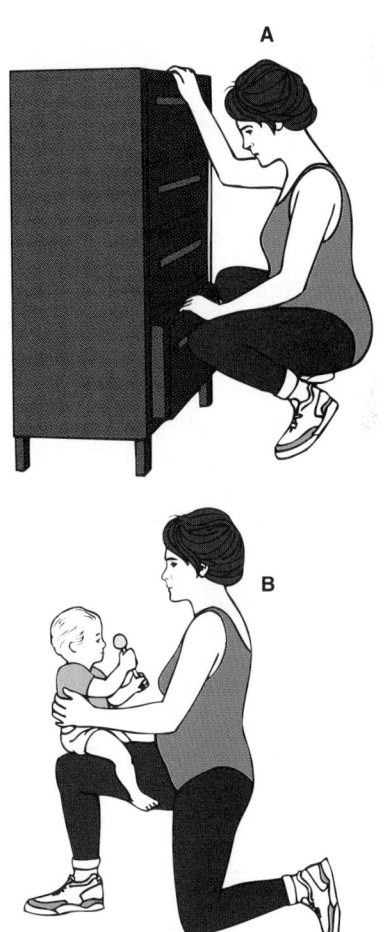

Fig. 17-12 Correct body mechanics. **A,** Squatting. **B,** Lifting.

Activities that depend on a good sense of balance should be discouraged, however, especially during the latter half of pregnancy. Commonly, excessive fatigue is the deciding factor in the termination of employment. Women in sedentary jobs need to walk around at intervals to

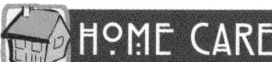

HOME CARE

Posture and Body Mechanics

To prevent or relieve backache
Do pelvic tilt:
- Pelvic tilt (rock) on hands and knees (see Fig. 17-11, A) and while sitting in straight-back chair.
- Pelvic tilt (rock) in standing position against a wall, or lying on floor (see Fig. 17-11, B and C).
- Perform abdominal muscle contractions during pelvic tilt while standing, lying, or sitting to help strengthen rectus abdominis muscle (see Fig. 17-11, D).
- Use good body mechanics.
- Use leg muscles to reach objects on or near floor. Bend at the knees, not the back. Knees are bent to lower body to squatting position. Feet are kept 12 to 18 inches apart to provide a solid base to maintain balance (see Fig. 17-12, A).
- Lift with the legs. To lift heavy object (e.g., young child), one foot is placed slightly in front of the other and kept flat as woman lowers herself onto one knee. She lifts the weight holding it close to her body and never higher than the chest. To stand up or sit down, one leg is placed slightly behind the other as she raises or lowers herself (see Fig. 17-12, B).

To restrict the lumbar curve
For prolonged standing (e.g., ironing, employment), place one foot on low footstool or box; change positions often.

Move car seat forward so that knees are bent and higher than hips. If needed, use a small pillow to support low back area.

Sit in chairs low enough to allow both feet to be placed on floor, preferably with knees higher than hips.

To prevent round ligament pain and strain on abdominal muscles
Implement suggestions given in Table 17-2.

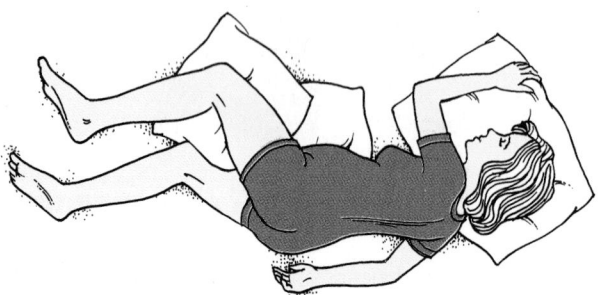

Fig. 17-13   Side-lying position for rest and relaxation. Some women prefer to support upper part of leg with pillows.

counter the usual sluggish circulation in the legs that can cause varices and thrombophlebitis to develop. They should neither sit nor stand in one position for long periods, and they should avoid crossing their legs at the knees because these activities foster such conditions. Standing for long periods of time also increases the risk of preterm labor. The pregnant woman's chair should provide adequate back support. Use of a footstool can prevent pressure on veins, relieve strain on varicosities, and minimize swelling of feet.

Clothing. Comfortable, loose clothing is best. Washable fabrics (e.g., absorbent cottons) are often preferred.

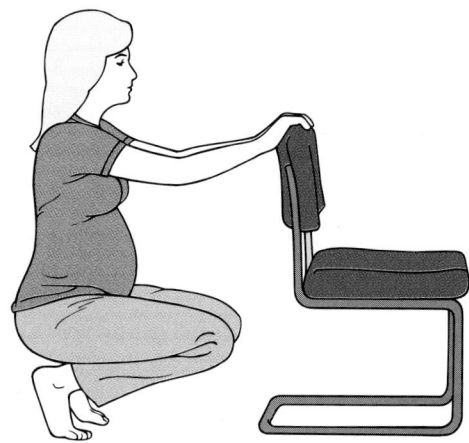

Fig. 17-14   Squatting for muscle relaxation and strengthening and keeping leg and hip joints flexible.

BOX 17-3   Conscious Relaxation Tips

Preparation: Loosen clothing, assume a comfortable sitting or side-lying position with all parts of body well supported with pillows. The use of soothing music is optional.

Beginning: Allow self to feel warm and comfortable. Inhale and exhale slowly, and imagine peaceful relaxation coming over each part of the body, starting with the neck and working down to the toes. People who learn conscious relaxation often speak of feeling relaxed even if some discomfort is present.

Maintenance: Use imagery (fantasy or daydream) to maintain the state of relaxation. Using *active imagery,* imagine yourself moving or doing some activity and experiencing its sensations. Using *passive imagery,* imagine yourself watching a scene, such as a lovely sunset.

Awakening: Return to the wakeful state gradually. Slowly begin to take in stimuli from the surrounding environment.

Further retention and development of the skill: Practice regularly for some periods each day, for example, at the same hour for 10 to 15 minutes each day, to feel refreshed, revitalized, and invigorated.

Maternity clothes may be purchased new or found at thrift shops or garage sales in good condition because they rarely wear out. Tight bras and belts, stretch pants, garters, tight-top knee socks, panty girdles, and other constrictive clothing should be avoided because tight clothing over the perineum encourages vaginitis and miliaria (heat rash), and impaired circulation in the legs can cause varicosities.

Maternity bras are constructed to accommodate the increased breast weight, chest circumference, and the size of breast tail tissue (under the arm). These bras also have drop-flaps over the nipples to facilitate breastfeeding. A good bra can help prevent neckache and backache.

Elastic hose give considerable comfort and promote greater venous emptying in women with large varicose veins. Ideally, support stockings should be put on before the woman gets out of bed in the morning. Figure 17-15 demonstrates a position for resting the legs and reducing swelling and varicosities.

Comfortable shoes that provide firm support and promote good posture and balance are also advisable. Very high heels and platform shoes are not recommended because of the woman's changed center of gravity, which can cause her to lose her balance. In addition, in the third trimester the woman's pelvis tilts forward and her lumbar curve increases. The resulting leg aches and cramps are aggravated by nonsupportive shoes.

Travel. Travel is not contraindicated in low risk pregnant women, but those with high risk pregnancies are advised to avoid long-distance travel after fetal viability has been reached so as to avert the economic and psychologic consequences of giving birth to a preterm infant far from home. Travel to areas where medical care is poor, water is untreated, or malaria is prevalent should be avoided if possible. Women who contemplate foreign travel should be aware that many health insurance carriers do not cover a birth in a foreign setting or even hospitalization for preterm labor.

Pregnant women who travel for long distances should schedule periods of activity and rest. While sitting the woman can practice deep breathing, foot circling, and alternately contracting and relaxing different muscle groups. She should avoid becoming fatigued. Although travel in itself is not a cause of adverse outcomes such as miscarriage or preterm labor, certain precautions are recommended while traveling in a car. A woman who does not wear automobile restraints risks injury to herself and her fetus. Maternal death as a result of injury is the most common cause of fetal death. The next most common cause is placental separation. This occurs because body contours change in reaction to the force of a collision. The uterus as a muscular organ can adapt its shape to that of the body, but the placenta is not resilient. At the impact of collision, placental separation can occur. A combination lap belt and shoulder harness is the most effective automobile restraint and both should be used (Fig. 17-16). The lap belt should be worn low across the pelvic bones and as snug as is comfortable. The shoulder harness should be worn above the gravid uterus and below the neck to prevent chafing. The pregnant woman should sit upright. The headrest should be used to prevent a whiplash injury.

For pregnant women traveling in high-altitude regions, lowered oxygen levels may cause fetal hypoxia, especially

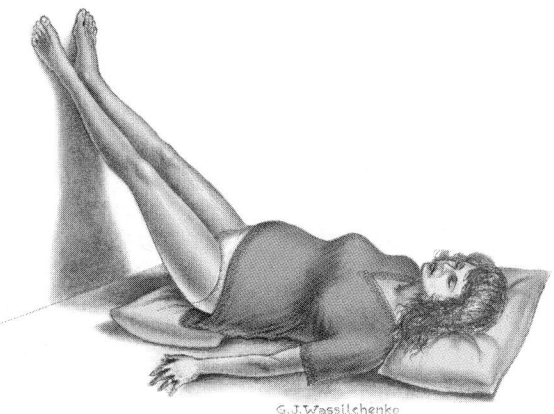

Fig. 17-15 Position for resting legs and for reducing edema and varicosities. Encourage woman with vulvar varicosities to include pillow under her hips.

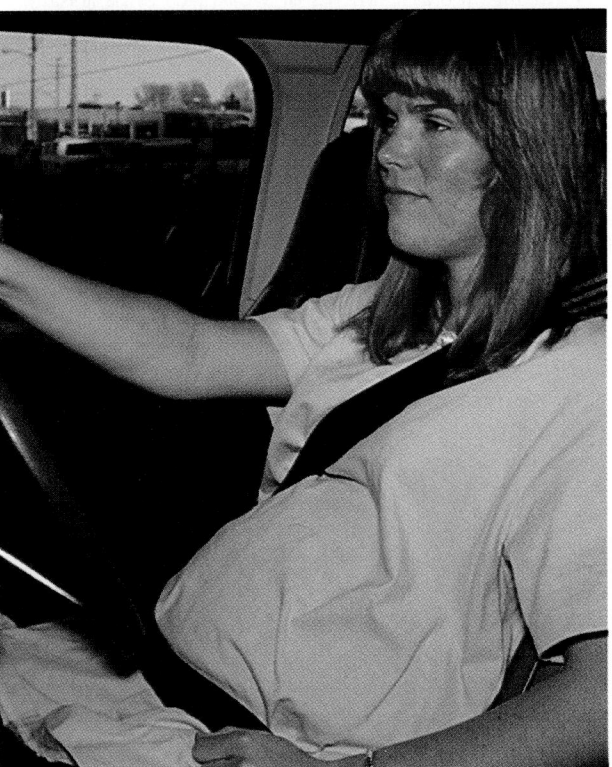

Fig. 17-16 Proper use of seat belt and head rest. *(Courtesy Michael S. Clement, MD, Mesa, AZ.)*

TEACHING guidelines

Safety During Pregnancy

Changes in the body due to pregnancy include relaxation of joints, alteration to center of gravity, faintness, and discomforts. Problems with coordination and balance are common. Therefore the woman should follow these guidelines:

- Use good body mechanics.
- Use safety features on tools/vehicles (safety seat belts, shoulder harnesses, headrests, goggles, helmets) as specified.
- Avoid activities requiring coordination, balance, and concentration.
- Take rest periods; reschedule daily activities to meet rest and relaxation needs.

Embryonic and fetal development is vulnerable to environmental teratogens. Many potentially dangerous chemicals are present in the home, yard, and workplace: cleaning agents, paints, sprays, herbicides, and pesticides. The soil and water supply may be unsafe. Therefore the woman should follow these guidelines:

- Read all labels for ingredients and proper use of product.
- Ensure adequate ventilation with clean air.
- Dispose of wastes appropriately.
- Wear gloves when handling chemicals.
- Change job assignments or workplace as necessary.
- Avoid high altitudes (not in pressurized aircraft), which could jeopardize oxygen intake.

if the pregnant woman is anemic. However, the current information on this is limited, and there are currently no set recommendations regarding the exposure of pregnant women to high altitudes.

Airline travel in large commercial jets usually poses little risk to the pregnant woman, but policies vary from airline to airline. The pregnant woman is advised to inquire about restrictions or recommendations from her carrier (Cunningham et al., 1997). Magnetometers (metal detectors) used at airport security checkpoints are not harmful to the fetus. The 8% humidity at which the cabins of commercial airlines are maintained may result in some water loss; hydration (with water) should therefore be maintained under these conditions. Sitting in the cramped seat of an airliner for prolonged periods may increase the risk of superficial and deep thrombophlebitis. A pregnant woman is encouraged to take a 15-minute walk around the aircraft during each hour of travel to minimize this risk. A seat in the nonsmoking section of flights on which smoking is permitted is advised to prevent her carboxyhemoglobin levels from becoming elevated (see the Teaching Guidelines box).

Medications. Although much has been learned in recent years about fetal drug toxicity (see Box 14-1), the possible teratogenicity of many medications, prescription and OTC, is still unknown. This is especially true for new medications and combinations of drugs. Moreover, certain subclinical errors or deficiencies in intermediate metabolism in the fetus may cause an otherwise harmless drug to be converted into a hazardous one. The greatest danger of drug-caused developmental defects in the fetus extends from the time of fertilization through the first trimester, a time when the woman may not realize she is pregnant. Self-treatment must be discouraged. The use of all drugs, including OTC medications and vitamins, should be limited and a careful record kept of all therapeutic agents used.

Immunizations. Some concern has been raised over the safety of various immunization practices during pregnancy (Cunningham et al., 1997). Immunization with live or attenuated live viruses is contraindicated during pregnancy because of its potential teratogenicity. Live-virus vaccines include those for measles (rubeola and rubella), chickenpox, and mumps, as well as the Sabin's (oral) poliomyelitis vaccine. Vaccines consisting of killed viruses may be used. Those that may be administered during pregnancy include tetanus, diphtheria, recombinant hepatitis B, and rabies vaccines.

Alcohol, cigarette smoke, and other substances. A safe level of alcohol consumption during pregnancy has not yet been established. Although the consumption of occasional alcoholic beverages may not be harmful to the mother or her developing embryo or fetus, complete abstinence is strongly advised (ACOG, 1994). Maternal alcoholism is associated with high rates of miscarriage and fetal alcohol syndrome; the risk for miscarriage in the first trimester is dose related (three or more drinks per day). Growing evidence indicates that the pattern of drinking (frequency, timing, and duration), especially in the first trimester, is more predictive of fetal damage than the amount (Abel, 1996; Wagner et al., 1998). Considerably less alcohol use is reported among pregnant women than in nonpregnant women, but a high prevalence of some alcohol use among pregnant women still exists. Such a finding underscores the need for more systematic public health efforts to educate women about the hazards of alcohol consumption in pregnancy (Ebrahim et al., 1998).

Cigarette smoking or continued exposure to a smoke-filled environment (even if the mother does not smoke) is associated with fetal growth restriction and an increase in perinatal and infant morbidity and mortality. Exposure to nicotine has been shown to have a negative effect on the growth of the fetus. Smoking is associated with an increased frequency of preterm labor, premature rupture of membranes (PROM), abruptio placentae, placenta previa, and fetal death resulting possibly from decreased placental perfusion. Laboratory studies have revealed that smoking causes fetal hypoxia.

All pregnant women who smoke should be strongly encouraged to quit or at least cut down. Pregnant women need to be told about the negative effects of even second-hand smoke on the fetus (ACOG, 1997). Nurse-managed interventions hold promise for helping pregnant smokers quit (Gebauer et al., 1998; Kilby, 1997). Better still are efforts focused on preventing girls and women from beginning to smoke (Johnson, 1998).

Most studies of human pregnancy have revealed no association between caffeine consumption and birth defects or LBW (Cunningham et al., 1997). Because other effects are unknown, however, pregnant women are advised to limit their caffeine intake.

Any drug or environmental agent that enters the pregnant woman's bloodstream has the potential to cross the placenta and harm the fetus. Marijuana, heroin, and cocaine are common examples of such substances. Although the problem of substance abuse in pregnancy is considered a major public health concern, comprehensive care of drug-addicted women improves maternal and neonatal outcomes (Jansson et al., 1996) (see Chapter 35).

Normal discomforts. Women pregnant for the first time are confronted with symptoms that would be considered abnormal in the nonpregnant state. Much of the prenatal care requested by such women is prompted by the need for explanations of the causes of the discomforts and for advice on ways to relieve the discomforts. The discomforts of the first trimester are fairly specific. Information about the physiology and prevention of and self-care for discomforts experienced during the three trimesters is given in Table 17-2. Nurses can do much to allay a first-time mother's anxiety about such symptoms by telling her about them in advance, using terminology that the woman (or couple) can understand. Women who understand the physical discomforts of pregnancy are less apt to become overly anxious about their health. In addition, understanding the rationale for treatment promotes their participation in their care. Interventions should be individualized with attention given to the woman's lifestyle and culture (Davis, 1996).

Recognizing potential complications. One of the most important responsibilities of persons involved in the care of the pregnant woman is to alert her to signs and symptoms that indicate a potential complication of pregnancy. The woman needs to know how to report such warning signs (see Potential Complications, p. 400). When one is stressed by a disturbing symptom, it is difficult to remember specifics. Therefore the pregnant woman and her family are reassured if they receive a printed form listing the signs and symptoms that warrant an investigation and the phone numbers to call in an emergency.

The nurse needs to answer questions honestly as they arise during pregnancy. Pregnant women often have difficulty deciding when to report signs and symptoms. The mother is encouraged to refer to the printed list of potential complications and to listen to her body. If she senses

Text continued on p. 418

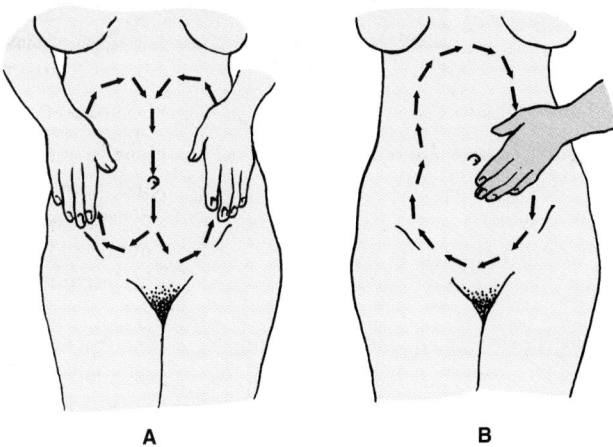

Fig. 17-17 Pattern for effleurage, a light, rhythmic stroking useful for inducing relaxation. **A,** Self-effleurage. **B,** Effleurage by another.

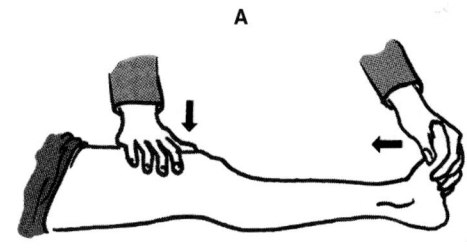

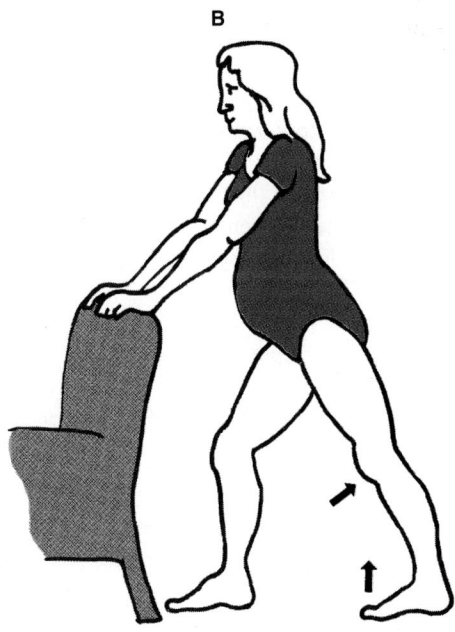

Fig. 17-18 Relief of muscle spasm (leg cramps). **A,** Another person dorsiflexes foot with knee extended. **B,** Woman stands and leans forward, thereby dorsiflexing foot of affected leg.

TABLE 17-2 Discomforts Related to Pregnancy

FIRST TRIMESTER		
DISCOMFORT	PHYSIOLOGY	EDUCATION FOR SELF-CARE
Breast changes, new sensation: pain, tingling, tenderness	Hypertrophy of mammary glandular tissue and increased vascularization, pigmentation, and size and prominence of nipples and areolae caused by hormonal stimulation	Wear supportive maternity bras with pads to absorb discharge, may be worn at night; wash with warm water and keep dry; breast tenderness may interfere with sexual expression/foreplay but is temporary
Urgency and frequency of urination	Vascular engorgement and altered bladder function caused by hormones; bladder capacity reduced by enlarging uterus and fetal presenting part	Empty bladder regularly; perform Kegel exercises; limit fluid intake before bedtime; wear perineal pad; report pain or burning sensation to primary health care provider
Languor and malaise; fatigue (early pregnancy, most commonly)	Unexplained; may be caused by increasing levels of estrogen, progesterone, and hCG or by elevated BBT; psychologic response to pregnancy and its required physical/psychologic adaptations	Rest as needed; eat well-balanced diet to prevent anemia
Nausea and vomiting, morning sickness—occurs in 50%-75% of pregnant women; starts between first and second missed periods and lasts until about fourth missed period; may occur any time during day; fathers also may have symptoms	Cause unknown; may result from hormonal changes, possibly hCG; may be partly emotional, reflecting pride in, ambivalence about, or rejection of pregnant state	Avoid empty or overloaded stomach; maintain good posture—give stomach ample room; stop smoking; eat dry carbohydrate on awakening; remain in bed until feeling subsides, or alternate dry carbohydrate 1 hour with fluids such as hot herbal decaffeinated tea, milk, or clear coffee the next hour until feeling subsides; eat five to six small meals per day; avoid fried, odorous, spicy, greasy, or gas-forming foods; consult primary health care provider if intractable vomiting occurs
Ptyalism (excessive salivation) may occur starting 2 to 3 weeks after first missed period	Possibly caused by elevated estrogen levels; may be related to reluctance to swallow because of nausea	Use astringent mouth wash, chew gum, eat hard candy as comfort measures
Gingivitis and **epulis** (hyperemia, hypertrophy, bleeding, tenderness); condition will disappear spontaneously 1 to 2 months after birth	Increased vascularity and proliferation of connective tissue from estrogen stimulation	Eat well-balanced diet with adequate protein and fresh fruits and vegetables; brush teeth gently and observe good dental hygiene; avoid infection; see dentist
Nasal stuffiness; epistaxis (nosebleed)	Hyperemia of mucous membranes related to high estrogen levels	Use humidifier; avoid trauma; normal saline nose drops or spray may be used
Leukorrhea: often noted throughout pregnancy	Hormonally stimulated cervix becomes hypertrophic and hyperactive, producing abundant amount of mucus	Not preventable; do not douche; wear perineal pads; perform hygienic practices such as wiping front to back; report to primary health care provider if accompanied by pruritus, foul odor, or change in character or color
Psychosocial dynamics, mood swings, mixed feelings	Hormonal and metabolic adaptations; feelings about female role, sexuality, timing of pregnancy, and resultant changes in life and lifestyle	Participate in pregnancy support group; communicate concerns to partner, family, and others; request referral for supportive services if needed (financial assistance)

TABLE 17-2 Discomforts Related to Pregnancy—cont'd

	SECOND TRIMESTER	
DISCOMFORT	PHYSIOLOGY	EDUCATION FOR SELF-CARE
Pigmentation deepens, acne, oily skin	Melanocyte-stimulating hormone (from anterior pituitary)	Not preventable; usually resolves during puerperium
Spider nevi (angiomas) appear over neck, thorax, face, and arms during second or third trimester	Focal networks of dilated arterioles (end-arteries) from increased concentration of estrogens	Not preventable; they fade slowly during late puerperium; rarely disappear completely
Palmar erythema occurs in 50% of pregnant women; may accompany spider nevi	Diffuse reddish mottling over palms and suffused skin over thenar eminencies and fingertips; may be caused by genetic predisposition or hyperestrogenism	Not preventable; condition will fade within 1 week after giving birth
Pruritus (noninflammatory)	Unknown cause; various types as follows: nonpapular; closely aggregated pruritic papules	Keep fingernails short and clean; contact primary health care provider for diagnosis of cause
	Increased excretory function of skin and stretching of skin possible factors	Not preventable; symptomatic; Keri baths; mild sedation
		Distraction; tepid baths with sodium bicarbonate or oatmeal added to water; lotions and oils; change of soaps or reduction in use of soap; loose clothing
Palpitations	Unknown; should not be accompanied by persistent cardiac irregularity	Not preventable; contact primary health care provider if accompanied by symptoms of cardiac decompensation
Supine hypotension (vena cava syndrome) and bradycardia	Induced by pressure of gravid uterus on ascending vena cava when woman is supine; reduces uteroplacental and renal perfusion	Side-lying position or semisitting posture, with knees slightly flexed (see supine hypotension, p. 399)
Faintness and, rarely, syncope (orthostatic hypotension) may persist throughout pregnancy	Vasomotor lability or postural hypotension from hormones; in late pregnancy may be caused by venous stasis in lower extremities	Moderate exercise, deep breathing, vigorous leg movement; avoid sudden changes in position* and warm crowded areas; move slowly and deliberately; keep environment cool; avoid hypoglycemia by eating 5 to 6 small meals per day; wear elastic hose; sit as necessary; if symptoms are serious, contact primary health care provider
Food cravings	Cause unknown; craving determined by culture or geographic area	Not preventable; satisfy craving unless it interferes with well-balanced diet; report unusual cravings to primary health care provider
Heartburn (pyrosis or acid indigestion): burning sensation, occasionally with burping and regurgitation of a little sour-tasting fluid	Progesterone slows gastrointestinal (GI) tract motility and digestion, reverses peristalsis, relaxes cardiac sphincter, and delays emptying time of stomach; stomach displaced upward and compressed by enlarging uterus	Limit or avoid gas-producing or fatty foods and large meals; maintain good posture; sip milk for temporary relief; hot herbal tea; primary health care provider may prescribe antacid between meals; contact primary health care provider for persistent symptoms

*Caution woman to rise slowly and sit on edge of bed or to assume hands-and-knee posture before rising, and to get up slowly after sitting or squatting.

Continued

TABLE 17-2 Discomforts Related to Pregnancy—cont'd

	SECOND TRIMESTER—cont'd	
DISCOMFORT	**PHYSIOLOGY**	**EDUCATION FOR SELF-CARE**
Constipation	GI tract motility slowed because of progesterone, resulting in increased resorption of water and drying of stool; intestines compressed by enlarging uterus; predisposition to constipation because of oral iron supplementation	Drink six glasses of water per day; include roughage in diet; moderate exercise; maintain regular schedule for bowel movements; use relaxation techniques and deep breathing; do not take stool softener, laxatives, mineral oil, other drugs, or enemas without first consulting primary health care provider
Flatulence with bloating and belching	Reduced GI motility because of hormones, allowing time for bacterial action that produces gas; swallowing air	Chew foods slowly and thoroughly; avoid gas-producing foods, fatty foods, large meals; exercise; maintain regular bowel habits
Varicose veins (varicosities): may be associated with aching legs and tenderness; may be present in legs and vulva; hemorrhoids are varicosities in perianal area	Hereditary predisposition; relaxation of smooth muscle walls of veins because of hormones causing tortuous dilated veins in legs and pelvic vasocongestion; condition aggravated by enlarging uterus, gravity, and bearing down for bowel movements; thrombi from leg varices rare but may be produced by hemorrhoids	Avoid obesity, lengthy standing or sitting, constrictive clothing, and constipation and bearing down with bowel movements; moderate exercises; rest with legs and hips elevated (see Fig. 17-15); wear support stocking; thrombosed hemorrhoid may be evacuated; relieve swelling and pain with warm sitz baths, local application of astringent compresses
Leukorrhea: often noted throughout pregnancy	Hormonally stimulated cervix becomes hypertrophic and hyperactive, producing abundant amount of mucus	Not preventable; do not douche; maintain good hygiene; wear perineal pads; report to primary health care provider if accompanied by pruritus, foul odor, or change in character or color
Headaches (through week 26)	Emotional tension (more common than vascular migraine headache); eye strain (refractory errors); vascular engorgement and congestion of sinuses resulting from hormone stimulation	Conscious relaxation; contact primary health care provider for constant "splitting" headache, to assess for PIH
Carpal tunnel syndrome (involves thumb, second, and third fingers, lateral side of little finger)	Compression of median nerve resulting from changes in surrounding tissues; pain, numbness, tingling, burning; loss of skilled movements (typing); dropping of objects	Not preventable; elevate affected arms; splinting of affected hand may help; regressive after pregnancy; surgery is curative
Periodic numbness, tingling of fingers (acrodysesthesia) occurs in 5% of pregnant women	Brachial plexus traction syndrome resulting from drooping of shoulders during pregnancy (occurs especially at night and early morning)	Maintain good posture; wear supportive maternity bra; condition will disappear if lifting and carrying baby does not aggravate it
Round ligament pain (tenderness)	Stretching of ligament caused by enlarging uterus	Not preventable; rest, maintain good body mechanics to avoid overstretching ligament; relieve cramping by squatting or bringing knees to chest, sometimes heat helps
Joint pain, backache, and pelvic pressure; hypermobility of joints	Relaxation of symphyseal and sacroiliac joints because of hormones, resulting in unstable pelvis; exaggerated lumbar and cervicothoracic curves caused by change in center of gravity resulting from enlarging abdomen	Maintain good posture and body mechanics; avoid fatigue; wear low-heeled shoes; abdominal supports may be useful; conscious relaxation; sleep on firm mattress; apply local heat or ice; get back rubs; do pelvic rock exercise; rest; condition will disappear 6 to 8 weeks after birth

TABLE 17-2 Discomforts Related to Pregnancy—cont'd

THIRD TRIMESTER

DISCOMFORT	PHYSIOLOGY	EDUCATION FOR SELF-CARE
Shortness of breath and dyspnea occur in 60% of pregnant women	Expansion of diaphragm limited by enlarging uterus; diaphragm is elevated about 4 cm; some relief after lightening	Good posture; sleep with extra pillows; avoid overloading stomach; stop smoking; contact health care provider if symptoms worsen to rule out anemia, emphysema, and asthma
Insomnia (later weeks of pregnancy)	Fetal movements, muscle cramping, urinary frequency, shortness of breath, or other discomforts	Reassurance; conscious relaxation; back massage or **effleurage** (Fig. 17-17); support of body parts with pillows; warm milk or warm shower before retiring
Psychosocial responses: mood swings, mixed feelings, increased anxiety	Hormonal and metabolic adaptations; feelings about impending labor, birth, and parenthood	Reassurance and support from significant other and nurse; improved communication with partner, family, and others
Gingivitis and epulis (hyperemia, hypertrophy, bleeding, tenderness): condition will disappear spontaneously 1 to 2 months after birth	Increased vascularity and proliferation of connective tissue from estrogen stimulation	Well-balanced diet with adequate protein and fresh fruits and vegetables; gentle brushing and good dental hygiene; avoid infection; see dentist for teeth cleaning
Urinary frequency and urgency return	Vascular engorgement and altered bladder function caused by hormones; bladder capacity reduced by enlarging uterus and fetal presenting part	Empty bladder regularly, Kegel exercises; limit fluid intake before bedtime; reassurance; wear perineal pad; contact health care provider for pain or burning sensation
Perineal discomfort and pressure	Pressure from enlarging uterus, especially when standing or walking; multifetal gestation	Rest, conscious relaxation, and good posture; contact health care provider for assessment and treatment if pain is present
Braxton Hicks contractions	Intensification of uterine contractions in preparation for work of labor	Reassurance; rest; change of position; practice breathing techniques when contractions are bothersome; effleurage
Leg cramps (gastrocnemius spasm), especially when reclining	Compression of nerves supplying lower extremities because of enlarging uterus; reduced level of diffusible serum calcium or elevation of serum phosphorus; aggravating factors: fatigue, poor peripheral circulation, pointing toes when stretching legs or when walking, drinking more than 1 L (1 qt) of milk per day	Check for Homans' sign; if negative, use massage and heat over affected muscle; dorsiflex foot until spasm relaxes (Fig. 17-18); stand on cold surface; oral supplementation with calcium carbonate or calcium lactate tablets; aluminum hydroxide gel, 30 ml, with each meal removes phosphorus by absorbing it
Ankle edema (nonpitting) to lower extremities	Edema aggravated by prolonged standing, sitting, poor posture, lack of exercise, constrictive clothing (e.g., garters), or by hot weather	Ample fluid intake for natural diuretic effect; put on support stockings before arising; rest periodically with legs and hips elevated (see Fig. 17-15), exercise moderately; contact health care provider if generalized edema develops; *diuretics are contraindicated*

How to Recognize Preterm Labor

Because the onset of preterm labor is subtle and often hard to recognize, it is important to know how to feel your abdomen for uterine contractions. You can feel for contractions in the following way. While lying down, place your fingertips on the top of your uterus. A contraction is the periodic tightening or hardening of your uterus. If your uterus is contracting, you will actually feel your abdomen get tight or hard and then feel it relax or soften when the contraction is over.

If you think you are having any of the other signs and symptoms of preterm labor, empty your bladder, drink three to four glasses of water for hydration, lie down tilted toward your side, and place a pillow at your back for support.

Check for contractions for 1 hour. To tell how often contractions are occurring, check the minutes that elapse from the beginning of one contraction to the beginning of the next.

It is *not normal* to have frequent uterine contractions (every 10 minutes or more often for 1 hour).

Contractions of labor are regular, frequent, and hard. They also may be felt as a tightening of the abdomen or a backache. This type of contraction causes the cervix to efface and dilate.

Call your doctor, nurse-midwife, clinic, or labor and birth unit, or go to the hospital if any of the following signs occur:

- You have uterine contractions every 10 minutes or more often for 1 hour or
- You have any of the other signs and symptoms for 1 hour or
- You have any bloody spotting or leaking of fluid from your vagina

It is often difficult to identify preterm labor. Accurate diagnosis requires assessment by the health care provider, usually in the hospital or clinic.

Post these instructions where they can be seen by everyone in the family.

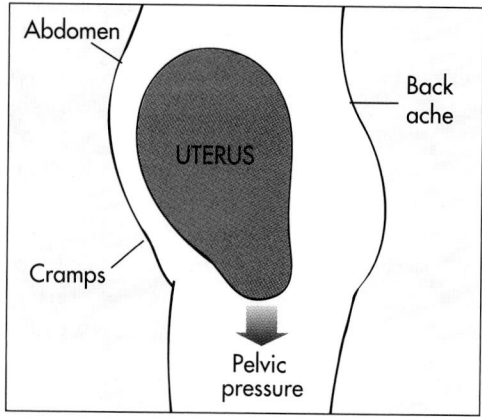

Fig. 17-19   Symptoms of preterm labor.

to come to the hospital's emergency area immediately for diagnosis and treatment if bleeding is other than one of the preceding types.

Should the pregnant woman notice cessation, noticeable diminution, or acceleration in the amount of *fetal movement,* she is to notify her health care provider.

Appearance of *edema* of the hands and around the eyes, severe *headaches, visual changes,* or feelings of *jitteriness* require immediate evaluation for PIH.

A gush or trickle of clear *watery discharge* that appears to come from the vagina may indicate rupture of membranes. The diagnosis requires a visit to the clinic or hospital for evaluation.

Recognizing preterm labor. Teaching each expectant mother to recognize preterm labor is necessary. Preterm labor is that which occurs after the twentieth week but before the thirty-seventh week of pregnancy. It is a condition in which uterine contractions cause the cervix to open earlier than normal, and it can result in preterm birth. Although certain factors, such as multifetal pregnancy, may increase a woman's chances of going into preterm labor, the specific cause (or causes) is not known. If the woman knows the warning signs and symptoms of preterm labor and seeks care early enough, should they occur, prevention of preterm birth may be possible. Warning signs and symptoms of preterm labor are given in the Home Care box. Figure 17-19 shows where in the body the symptoms of preterm labor may be located.

Sexual Counseling

The sexual counseling of expectant couples includes countering misinformation, providing reassurance of normality, and suggesting alternative behaviors. The uniqueness of each couple is considered within a biopsychosocial framework (see the Home Care box).

Counseling couples concerning sexual adjustments that must be made during pregnancy demands self-assessment

that something is wrong, she should call her care provider. Several signs and symptoms need to be discussed more extensively. These include vaginal bleeding, alteration in fetal movements, symptoms of PIH, rupture of membranes, and preterm labor.

If *vaginal bleeding* occurs in the third trimester, it is important to differentiate brownish spotting occurring during the 48 hours after vaginal examination or after intercourse from the "show" of pinkish mucus. The woman is on the part of the nurse, as well as a knowledge of the physical, social, and emotional responses to sex during pregnancy (Rynerson & Lowdermilk, 1993). Not all maternity nurses are comfortable dealing with the sexual concerns of their clients. Therefore those nurses who are aware of their personal strengths and limitations in dealing with sexual content are better prepared to make referrals if necessary.

Many women merely need permission to be sexually active during pregnancy. Many other women, however, need to be given information about the physiologic changes that occur during pregnancy and have the myths associated with sex during pregnancy dispelled. Such tasks are within the purview of the nurse and should be an integral component of the health care rendered (Alteneder & Hartzell, 1997).

Some couples need to be referred for sex therapy or family therapy. Couples with long-standing problems with sexual dysfunction that are intensified by pregnancy are candidates for sex therapy. Whenever a sexual problem is a symptom of a more serious relationship problem, the couple would benefit from family therapy.

Using the history. The couple's sexual history provides a basis for counseling, but history-taking also is an ongoing process. The couple's receptivity to changes in attitudes, body image, partner relationships, and physical status are relevant topics throughout pregnancy. Whenever changes occur, unexpected problems may arise that require intervention. The history reveals the woman's knowledge of female anatomy and physiology and her attitudes about sex during pregnancy, as well as her perceptions of the pregnancy, the health status of the couple, and the quality of their relationship. An understanding of the couple's subjective experience provides the direction and focus for sexual counseling.

Countering misinformation. Many myths and much of the misinformation related to sex and pregnancy are masked by seemingly unrelated issues. For example, a discussion about the baby's ability to hear and see in utero may be prompted by questions about the baby being an observer of lovemaking. The counselor must be extremely sensitive to the questions behind such questions when counseling in this highly charged emotional area.

Suggesting alternative behaviors. At this time research has not demonstrated conclusively that coitus and orgasm are contraindicated at any time during pregnancy for the obstetrically and medically healthy woman (Cunningham et al., 1997). However, a history of more than one miscarriage; a threatened miscarriage in the first trimester; impending miscarriage in the second trimester; and PROM, bleeding, or abdominal pain during the third trimester warrant precaution when it comes to coitus and orgasm (Rynerson & Lowdermilk, 1993).

Solitary and mutual masturbation and oral-genital intercourse may be used by couples as alternatives to penile-

HOME CARE

Sexuality in Pregnancy

- Be aware that maternal physiologic changes, such as breast enlargement, nausea, fatigue, abdominal changes, perineal enlargement, leukorrhea, pelvic vasocongestion, and orgasmic responses, may affect sexuality and sexual expression.
- Discuss responses to pregnancy with your partner.
- Keep in mind that cultural prescriptions (dos) and proscriptions (don'ts) may affect your responses.
- Although your libido may be depressed during the first trimester, it often increases during the second and third trimesters.
- Discuss and explore with your partner:
  Alternative behaviors (e.g., mutual masturbation, foot massage, cuddling)
  Alternative positions (e.g., female superior, sidelying) for sexual intercourse
- Intercourse is safe as long as it is not uncomfortable. There is no correlation between intercourse and miscarriage, but observe the following precautions:
  Abstain from intercourse if you experience uterine cramping or vaginal bleeding; report event to your caregiver as soon as possible.
  Abstain from intercourse (or any activity that results in orgasm) if you have a history of cervical incompetence, until the problem is corrected.
- Continue to use "safer sex" behaviors. Women at risk for acquiring or conveying STIs are encouraged to use condoms during sexual intercourse throughout pregnancy.

vaginal intercourse. Partners who enjoy cunnilingus (oral stimulation of the clitoris or vagina) may feel "turned off" by the normal increase in the amount and odor of vaginal discharge during pregnancy. Couples who practice cunnilingus should be cautioned against the blowing of air into the vagina, particularly during the last few weeks of pregnancy when the cervix may be slightly open. An air embolism can occur if air is forced between the uterine wall and the fetal membranes and enters the maternal vascular system through the placenta.

Showing the woman or couple pictures of possible variations of coital position often is helpful (Fig. 17-20). The female-superior, side-by-side, and rear-entry positions are possible alternative positions to the traditional male-superior position. The woman astride (superior position) allows her to control the angle and depth of penile penetration, as well as to protect her breasts and abdomen. The side-by-side

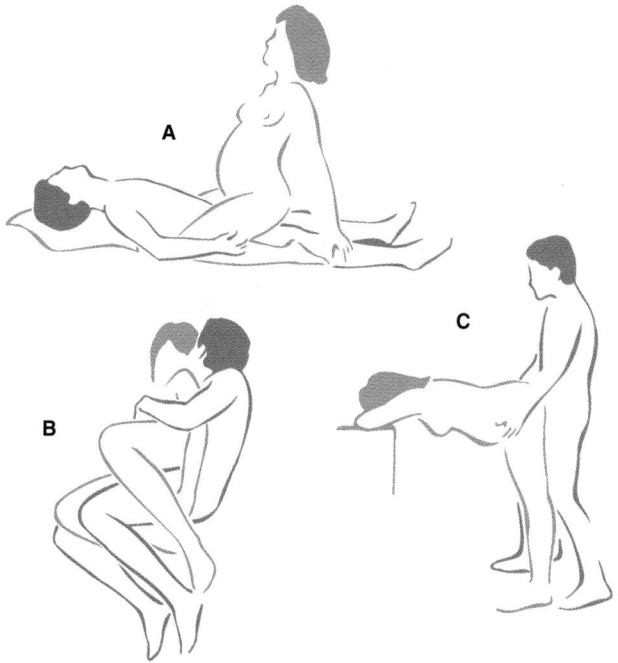

Fig. 17-20 Positions for sexual intercourse during pregnancy. **A,** Female superior. **B,** Side by side. **C,** Rear entry.

position is preferred, especially during the third trimester, because it requires less energy and places less pressure on the pregnant abdomen.

Multiparous women sometimes experience significant breast tenderness in the first trimester. A coital position that avoids direct pressure on the woman's breasts and decreased breast fondling during love play can be recommended to such couples. The woman should also be reassured that this condition is normal and temporary.

Some women complain of lower abdominal cramping and backache after orgasm during the first and third trimesters. A back rub can often relieve some of the discomfort and provide a pleasant experience. A tonic uterine contraction, often lasting up to a minute, replaces the rhythmic contractions of orgasm during the third trimester. Changes in the fetal heart rate without fetal distress have also been reported.

The objective of "safer sex" is to provide prophylaxis against the acquisition and transmission of STIs (e.g., herpes simplex virus [HSV], HIV). Because these diseases may be transmitted to the woman and her fetus, the use of condoms is recommended throughout pregnancy if the woman is at risk for acquiring an STI.

Well-informed nurses who are comfortable with their own sexuality and the sexual counseling needs of expectant couples can offer information and advice in this valuable but often neglected area. They can establish an open environment in which couples can feel free to introduce their concerns about sexual adjustment and seek support

and guidance. This intervention is as important for lesbian women and their partners as it is for women partnered by men.

Psychosocial Support

Esteem, affection, trust, concern, consideration of cultural and religious responses, and listening are all components of the emotional support given to the pregnant woman and her family. The woman's satisfaction with her relationships and support, her feeling of competence, and her sense of being in control are important issues to be addressed in the third trimester. A discussion of fetal responses to stimuli, such as sound, light, maternal posture, and tension, as well as patterns of sleeping and waking, can be helpful. Also discussed are emotional tensions that can arise in relation to the childbirth experience, such as those stemming from fear of pain, loss of control, and possible birth of the infant before reaching the hospital; anxieties about the recognized responsibilities and tasks of parenthood; parental concerns about the safety of the mother and unborn child; parental concerns about siblings and their acceptance of the new baby; parental concerns about social and economic responsibilities; and parental concerns arising from conflicts in cultural, religious, or personal value systems. Malnory (1996) has developed guidelines that identify expected behavior and appropriate nursing interventions for each stage of psychosocial development in pregnancy. Such a guide promotes thorough assessment.

The father's or partner's commitment to the pregnancy, the couple's relationship, and their concerns about sexuality and sexual expression can emerge as issues for many expectant parents. Validation, feedback, and social comparison characterize the support given.

Providing the mother- and father-to-be an opportunity to discuss their concerns, providing a listening ear, and validating the normality of their responses can meet their needs to varying degrees. Nurses must also recognize that men feel more vulnerable during their partner's pregnancy. Female partners may also have these feelings. Anticipatory guidance and health promotion strategies can help partners cope with their concerns. Nursing intervention may help them to deal with such concerns either directly through counseling or indirectly through the education of the mothers. Health care providers can stimulate and encourage open dialogue between the couple.

Evaluation

Evaluation of the effectiveness of care of the woman during pregnancy is based on the previously stated outcomes. More effort is needed in evaluating outcomes of nursing care during the prenatal period. A formal systematic follow-up on quality of care is not common but needs to be developed and incorporated in all settings (see Plan of Care).

PLAN ᴼᶠ CARE   Discomforts of Pregnancy and Warning Signs

FIRST TRIMESTER
NURSING DIAGNOSIS Knowledge deficit related to schedule of prenatal visits throughout pregnancy as evidenced by client questions and concerns

Expected Outcome:
Client will verbalize correct appointment schedule for the duration of the pregnancy.

Nursing Interventions/*Rationales*

Provide information regarding schedule of visits, tests, and other assessments and interventions that will be provided throughout the pregnancy *to empower client to function in collaboration with the caregiver.*

NURSING DIAGNOSIS Altered nutrition: less than body requirements, related to nausea and vomiting as evidenced by client report and weight loss

Expected Outcome *Client will gain 1 to 2.5 kg during the first trimester.*

Nursing Interventions/*Rationales*

Verify prepregnant weight *to plan a diet realistic according to individual client's nutritional needs.*
Obtain diet history *to identify current meal patterns and foods that may be implicated in nausea.*
Advise client to consume small frequent meals and avoid having empty stomach *to avoid further nausea episodes.*
Suggest that client eat a simple carbohydrate such as dry crackers before arising in the morning *to avoid empty stomach and decrease incidence of nausea and vomiting.*
Advise client to call health care provider if vomiting is persistent and severe *to identify possible incidence of hyperemesis gravidarum.*

NURSING DIAGNOSIS Fatigue related to hormonal changes in the first trimester as evidenced by client complaints

Expected Outcome *Client will report a decreased number of episodes of fatigue.*

Nursing Interventions/*Rationales*

Rest as needed *to avoid increasing feeling of fatigue.*
Eat a well-balanced diet *to meet increased metabolic demands and avoid anemia.*

Discuss the use of support systems to help with household responsibilities *to decrease workload at home and decrease fatigue.*

SECOND TRIMESTER
NURSING DIAGNOSIS Constipation related to progesterone influence on GI tract as evidenced by client report of altered patterns of elimination

Expected Outcome *Client will report a return to normal bowel elimination pattern following implementation of interventions.*

Nursing Interventions/*Rationales*

Provide information to client regarding pregnancy-related causes: progesterone slowing gastrointestinal motility, growing uterus compressing intestines, and influence of iron supplementation *to provide basic information for self-care during pregnancy.*
Assist client to plan a diet that will promote regular bowel movements, such as increasing amount of oral fluid intake to at least six glasses of water a day, increasing the amount of fiber in daily diet, and to maintain moderate exercise *to promote self-care.*
Reinforce for client that she should not take any laxatives, stool softeners, or enemas without first consulting the health care provider *to prevent any injuries to client or fetus.*

NURSING DIAGNOSIS Knowledge deficit related to first pregnancy as evidenced by client questions regarding possible complications of second and third trimesters

Expected Outcome *Client will correctly list signs of potential complications that can occur during the second and third trimesters.*

Nursing Interventions/*Rationales*

Provide information concerning the potential complications or warning signs that can occur during the second and third trimesters, including possible causes of signs and the importance of calling the health care provider immediately *to ensure identification and treatment of problems in a timely manner.*
Provide a written list of complications *to have a reference list for emergencies.*

Continued

PLAN ᵒᶠ CARE | Discomforts of Pregnancy and Warning Signs—cont'd

---

THIRD TRIMESTER
NURSING DIAGNOSIS Knowledge deficit regarding onset of labor and the processes of labor related to inexperience as evidenced by client questions and statement of concerns

Expected Outcome *Client will verbalize basic understanding of signs of labor onset, when to call the health care provider, and list resources for childbirth education.*

Nursing Interventions/*Rationales*

Provide information regarding signs of labor onset, when to call the health care provider, and give written information regarding local childbirth education classes *to empower and promote self-care.*

NURSING DIAGNOSIS Sleep pattern disturbance related to discomforts/insomnia of third trimester as evidenced by client report of inadequate rest

Expected Outcome *Client will report an improvement of quality and quantity of rest and sleep.*

Nursing Interventions/*Rationales*

Assess current sleep pattern and review need for increased requirement during pregnancy *to identify need for change in sleep patterns.*

Suggest change of position to side-lying with pillows between legs or to sleep in semi-Fowler's position *to increase support and decrease any problems with dyspnea or heartburn.*

Reinforce the possibility of the use of various sleep aides such as relaxation techniques, reading, and decreased activity before bedtime *to decrease the possibility of anxiety or physical discomforts before bedtime.*

VARIATIONS IN PRENATAL CARE

The course of prenatal care described thus far may seem to suggest that the experiences of childbearing women are similar and that nursing interventions are uniformly consistent across all populations. Although typical patterns of response to pregnancy are easily recognized and many aspects of prenatal care indeed are consistent, pregnant women enter the health care system with individual concerns and needs. The nurse's ability to assess unique needs and to tailor interventions to the individual are hallmarks of expertise in providing care. Variations that influence prenatal care include culture, age, and number of fetuses.

Cultural Influences

Prenatal care as we know it is a phenomenon of Western medicine. In the Western biomedical model of care, women are encouraged to seek prenatal care as early as possible in their pregnancy by visiting a physician, nurse-midwife, or office or clinic. Such visits are usually routine and, as already mentioned, follow a systematic sequence, with the initial visit followed by monthly, then semimonthly, then weekly visits. Monitoring weight and BP; testing blood and urine; teaching specific information about diet, rest, and activity; and preparing for childbirth are common components of prenatal care. This model is not only unfamiliar but seems strange to many groups. Models for providing prenatal care for women in other parts of the world, however, are being explored (Al-Qutob, Mawajdeh, & Bin-Raad, 1996).

Many cultural variations in prenatal care exist. Even if the prenatal care described is familiar to a woman, some practices may conflict with the beliefs and practices of a subculture group to which she belongs. Because of these and other factors, such as lack of money, lack of transportation, and poor communication on the part of health care providers, women from many such groups do not participate in the prenatal care system. Such behavior may be misinterpreted by nurses as uncaring, lazy, or ignorant.

A concern for modesty is also a deterrent to many women's seeking prenatal care. For some women, exposing body parts, especially to a man, is considered a major violation of their modesty. For many women, invasive procedures, such as a vaginal examination, may be so threatening that they cannot be discussed, even with their own husbands. Thus many women prefer a female to a male health care provider. Too often, health care providers assume women lose this modesty during pregnancy and labor, but actually most women value and appreciate efforts to maintain their modesty.

For numerous cultural groups a physician is deemed appropriate only in times of illness, and because pregnancy is considered a normal process and the woman is in a state of health, the services of a physician are considered inappropriate. Even if what are considered problems with pregnancy by standards of Western medicine do develop, they may not be perceived as problems by members of other cultural groups.

Although pregnancy is considered normal by many, certain practices are expected of women of all cultures to ensure a good outcome. **Cultural prescriptions** tell women what to do, and **cultural proscriptions** establish taboos. The purposes of these practices are to prevent maternal illness resulting from a pregnancy-induced imbalanced state and to protect the vulnerable fetus. Prescriptions and proscriptions regulate the woman's emotional response, clothing, activity and rest, sexual activity, and dietary practices. Exploration of the woman's beliefs, perceptions of the meaning of childbearing, and health care practices may help health care providers foster her self-actualization, promote attainment of the maternal role, and positively influence her relationship with her spouse (Callister, 1995).

To provide culturally sensitive care, the nurse must be knowledgeable about practices and customs, although it is not possible to know all there is to know about every culture and subculture, or the many lifestyles that exist. When exploring cultural beliefs and practices related to childbearing, the nurse can support and nurture those beliefs that promote physical or emotional adaptation. However, if potentially harmful beliefs or activities are identified, the nurse should carefully provide education and propose modifications.

Emotional Response

Virtually all cultures emphasize the importance of maintaining a socially harmonious and agreeable environment for a pregnant woman. An absence of stress is important in ensuring a successful outcome for the mother and baby. Harmony with other people must be fostered, and visits from extended family members may be required to demonstrate pleasant and noncontroversial relationships. If discord exists in a relationship, it is usually dealt with in culturally prescribed ways.

Besides proscriptions regarding food, other proscriptions involve imitative magic. For example, some Mexicans believe pregnant women should not witness an eclipse of the moon because it may cause a cleft palate in the infant. They also believe that exposure to an earthquake may precipitate preterm birth, miscarriage, or even a breech presentation. In some cultures a pregnant woman must not ridicule someone with an affliction for fear her child might be born with the same handicap. A mother should not hate a person lest her child resemble that person, and dental work should not be done because it may cause a baby to have a "harelip." A widely held folk belief in many cultures is that the pregnant woman should refrain from raising her arms above her head and tying knots to prevent the umbilical cord's wrapping around the baby's neck or knotting. Other cultures believe placing a knife under the bed of a laboring woman will "cut" her pain.

Clothing

Although most cultural groups do not prescribe specific clothing to be worn during pregnancy, modesty is an expectation of many. Some Mexican women of the Southwest wear a cord beneath the breast and knotted over the umbilicus. This cord, called a *muneco*, is thought to prevent morning sickness and ensure a safe birth. Amulets, medals, and beads also may be worn to ward off evil spirits (Spector, 1996).

Physical Activity and Rest

Norms that regulate the physical activity of mothers during pregnancy vary tremendously. Many groups, including Native Americans and some Asian groups, encourage women to be active, to walk, and to engage in normal although not strenuous activities to ensure that the baby is healthy and not too large. On the other hand, other groups such as Filipinos believe that any activity is dangerous, and others willingly take over the work of the pregnant woman. Some Filipinos believe that this inactivity protects the mother and child. The mother is encouraged simply to produce the succeeding generation. If health care providers do not know of this belief, they could misinterpret this behavior as laziness or noncompliance with the desired prenatal health care regimen. It is important for the nurse to find out the way each pregnant woman views activity and rest.

Sexual Activity

In most cultures, sexual activity is not prohibited until the end of pregnancy. Mexican-Americans view sexual activity as necessary to keep the birth canal lubricated. On the other hand, some Vietnamese may have definite proscriptions against sexual intercourse, requiring abstinence throughout the pregnancy because it is thought that sexual intercourse may harm the mother and fetus.

Diet

Nutritional information given by Western health care providers may also be a source of conflict for many cultural groups, but such a conflict commonly is not known by health care providers unless they understand the dietary beliefs and practices of the particular people for whom they are caring. For example, Muslims must eat meat slaughtered in accordance with Muslim law. If this is not possible, they will accept Kosher or vegetarian foods. Many cultures permit pregnant women to eat only warm foods.

Age

The age of the childbearing couple may have a significant influence on their physical and psychosocial adaptation to pregnancy. Normal developmental processes that occur in both very young and older mothers are interrupted by pregnancy and require a different type of adaptation to pregnancy than that of the woman of typical childbearing age.

Although the individuality of each pregnant woman is recognized, special needs of expectant mothers 15 years of age or younger or those 35 years or older are summarized below.

Adolescent Mothers

About one million adolescents, 4 of every 10 girls, in the United States become pregnant each year (AGI, 1998). Most of the pregnancies are unintended, and nearly 40% end in abortion. Nevertheless, adolescents are responsible for almost 500,000 births in the United States annually (Ventura et al., 1998). Hispanic adolescents currently have the highest birth rate, although the rate for African-American adolescents also is higher than that of other groups. Of girls who become pregnant, one in six will have a repeat pregnancy within 1 year (Cockey, 1997). Most of these young women are unmarried, and many are not ready for the emotional, psychological, and financial responsibilities of parenthood.

Despite these alarming statistics and the fact that the United States has the highest adolescent birth rate in the industrialized world, the birth rate for adolescents has steadily declined since 1991 (Ventura et al., 1998). Concentrated national efforts have spawned a host of adolescent pregnancy prevention programs that have had varying degrees of success. Characteristics of programs that make a difference are those that have sustained commitment to adolescents over a long period of time, involve the parents and other adults in the community, promote abstinence and personal responsibility, and assist adolescents to develop a clear strategy for reaching future goals such as a college education or a career (Cockey, 1997).

When adolescents do become pregnant and decide to give birth, they are much less likely than older women to receive adequate prenatal care, with many receiving no care at all (Ventura et al., 1998). These young women also are more likely to smoke and less likely to gain adequate weight during pregnancy. As a result of these and other factors, babies born to adolescents are at greatly increased risk of LBW, of serious and long-term disability, and of dying during the first year of life.

Delayed entry into prenatal care may be the result of late recognition of pregnancy, denial of pregnancy, or confusion about the services that are available. Such a delay in care may leave an inadequate time before birth to attend to correctable problems. The very young pregnant adolescent is at higher risk for each of the confounding variables associated with poor pregnancy outcomes (e.g., socioeconomic factors) and for those conditions associated with a first pregnancy regardless of age (e.g., PIH). However, when prenatal care is initiated early and consistently, and confounding variables are controlled, very young pregnant adolescents are at no greater risk (nor are their infants) for an adverse outcome than older pregnant women. The role of the nurse in reducing the risks and consequences of adolescent pregnancy is thus twofold: first, to encourage early and continued prenatal care and, second, to refer the adolescent, if necessary, for appropriate social support ser-

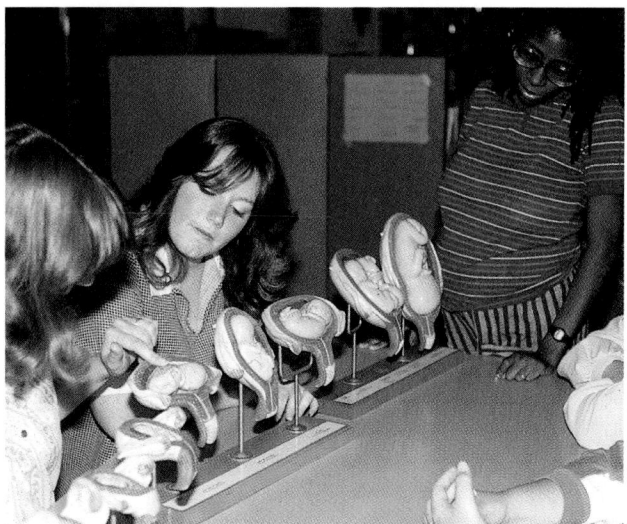

Fig. 17-21 Pregnant adolescents reviewing fetal development. *(Courtesy Marjorie Pyle, RNC, Lifecircle, Costa Mesa, CA.)*

vices, which can help reverse the effects of a negative socioeconomic environment (Fig. 17-21) (see Plan of Care).

Older Mothers

Two groups of older parents have emerged in the population of women having a child late in their childbearing years. One group consists of women who have many children or who have an additional child during the menopausal period. The other group consists of relative newcomers to maternity care. These are women who have deliberately delayed childbearing until their late 30s or early 40s.

Multiparous mothers. Multiparous women may have never used contraceptives because of personal choice or lack of knowledge concerning contraceptives. They also may be women who have used contraceptives successfully during the childbearing years but, as menopause approaches, they may cease menstruating regularly or stop using contraceptives and consequently become pregnant. The older multiparous woman may feel that pregnancy separates her from her peer group and that her age is a hindrance to close associations with young mothers. Other parents welcome the unexpected infant as evidence of continuing maternal and paternal roles.

Primiparous mothers. The number of first-time pregnancies in women between the ages of 35 and 40 years has increased significantly over the past 10 years. It is not uncommon now to see women in their late 30s or even in their early 40s pregnant for the first time. Reasons for delaying pregnancy include advanced education, career priorities, better contraceptive measures, and infertility.

These women choose parenthood as opposed to a childfree lifestyle. They often are successfully established in a career and a lifestyle with a partner that includes time for self-attention, the establishment of a home with accumulated possessions, and freedom to travel. When asked

PLAN OF CARE | Adolescent Pregnancy

NURSING DIAGNOSIS Altered nutrition: less than body requirements related to intake insufficient to meet metabolic needs of fetus and adolescent client

Expected Outcome *Client will gain weight as prescribed by age, take prenatal vitamins/iron as prescribed, and maintain normal hematocrit and hemoglobin.*

Nursing Interventions/*Rationales*

Assess current diet history/intake *to determine prescriptions for additions or changes in present dietary pattern.*

Compare prepregnancy weight with current weight *to determine if pattern is consistent with appropriate fetal growth and development.*

Provide information concerning food prescriptions for appropriate weight gain, considering preferences for "fast food" and peer influences *to correct any misconceptions and increase chances for compliance with diet.*

Include client's immediate family or support system during instruction *to ensure that person preparing family meals receives information.*

NURSING DIAGNOSIS Risk for injury, maternal or fetal, related to inadequate prenatal care and screening

Expected Outcome *Client will experience uncomplicated pregnancy and deliver a healthy fetus at term.*

Nursing Interventions/*Rationales*

Provide information, using therapeutic communication and confidentiality *to establish relationship and build trust.*

Discuss importance of ongoing prenatal and possible risks to adolescent client and fetus *to reinforce that ongoing assessment is crucial to health and well-being of client and fetus, even if client feels well. The adolescent client is more at risk for certain complications that may be avoided or managed early if prenatal visits are maintained.*

Discuss risks of alcohol, tobacco, and recreational drug use during pregnancy *to minimize risks to client and fetus, since adolescent client has a higher abuse rate than the rest of the pregnant population.*

Assess for evidence of sexually transmitted disease and provide information regarding safer sexual practice *to minimize risk to client and fetus, since adolescent is more at risk for STDs.*

Screen for PIH on an ongoing basis *to minimize risk, since adolescent population is more at risk for PIH.*

NURSING DIAGNOSIS Social isolation related to body image changes of pregnant adolescent as evidenced by client statements and concerns

Expected Outcome *Client will identify support systems and report decreased feelings of social isolation.*

Nursing Interventions/*Rationales*

Establish a therapeutic relationship *to listen objectively and establish trust.*

Discuss with client changes in relationships that have occurred as a result of the pregnancy *to determine extent of isolation from family, peers, and father of the baby.*

Provide referrals and resources appropriate for developmental stage of client *to give information for client support.*

Provide information regarding parenting classes, breastfeeding classes, and childbirth preparation classes *to give further information and group support, which lessens social isolation.*

---

the reason they choose pregnancy later in life, many reply, "because time is running out."

The dilemma of choice includes the recognition that being a parent will have positive and negative consequences. Couples need to discuss the consequences of childbearing and child rearing before committing themselves to this lifelong venture. Partners in this group seem to share the preparation for parenthood, planning for a family-centered birth, and desire to be loving and competent parents. However, the reality of child care may prove difficult for such parents.

As with mothers of all ages, the mother over 35 who is accustomed to the stimulation of the contact with other adults may find the isolation with her infant difficult to accept. Anger and resentment toward the father (or infant) can result, even with anticipatory guidance for these aspects of parenting.

First-time mothers older than 35 years select the "right time" for pregnancy; this time is influenced by their awareness of the increasing possibility of infertility or of genetic defects in the infants of older women. Such women seek information about pregnancy from books and friends. They actively try to prevent fetal disorders and are careful in searching for the best possible maternity care. They identify sources of stress in their lives. They have concerns about having enough energy and stamina to meet the demands of parenting and their new roles and relationships.

If they become pregnant after treatment for infertility, they may suddenly have negative or ambivalent feelings about the pregnancy. They may experience a multifetal pregnancy that may create emotional and physical problems. Adjusting to parenting two or more infants requires adaptability and additional resources.

During pregnancy, parents explore the possibilities and responsibilities of changing identities and new roles. They must prepare a safe and nurturing environment during pregnancy and after birth. They must integrate the child into an established family system and negotiate new roles (parent roles, sibling roles, grandparent roles) for family members.

Adverse perinatal outcomes are more common in older primiparas than in younger women even when they receive good prenatal care. Dollberg et al. (1996) reported that women 35 years of age and older are more likely than younger primiparas to have LBW infants, premature birth, IUGR, and abruptio placentae. The incidence of malpresentation also is more common in older primiparas, and they are more likely to have a cesarean birth. The occurrence of these complications is quite stressful for the new parents, and nursing interventions that provide information and psychosocial support are needed, as well as care for physical needs. In uncomplicated pregnancies, older mothers have significantly less fear of helplessness and loss of control in labor than younger women (Stark, 1997). Age and education are thought to balance the concerns of older mothers related to age.

Multifetal Pregnancy

A **multifetal pregnancy** places the mother and fetuses at risk. The maternal blood volume is increased, resulting in an increased strain on the maternal cardiovascular system. Anemia often develops because of a greater demand for iron by the fetuses. Marked uterine distention and increased pressure on the adjacent viscera and pelvic vasculature and diastasis of the two recti abdomini muscles (see Fig. 15-13) may occur. Placenta previa develops more commonly in multifetal pregnancies because of the large size or placement of the placentas (Cunningham et al., 1997). Premature separation of the placenta may occur before the second and any subsequent fetuses are born.

Twin pregnancies often end in prematurity. Spontaneous rupture of membranes before term is common. Congenital malformations are twice as common in monozygotic twins as in singletons, though there is no increase in the incidence of congenital anomalies in dizygotic twins. In addition, two-vessel cords—that is, cords with a single umbilical artery—occur more often in twins than in singletons, but this abnormality is most common in monozygotic twins. The most serious problem for the fetus is the local shunting of blood between placentas (twin-to-twin transfusion), causing the recipient twin to be larger and the donor twin to be small, pallid, dehydrated, malnourished, and hypovolemic. However, congenital heart failure may develop in the larger twin during the first 24 hours after birth.

The clinical diagnosis of multifetal pregnancy is accurate in about 90% of cases. The likelihood of a multifetal pregnancy is increased if any one or a combination of the following factors is noted during a careful assessment:

- History of dizygous twins in the female lineage
- Use of fertility drugs
- More rapid uterine growth for the number of weeks of gestation
- Hydramnios
- The palpation of a more than the expected number of small or large parts
- Asynchronous fetal heartbeats or more than one fetal electrocardiographic tracing
- Ultrasonographic evidence of more than one fetus

The diagnosis of multifetal pregnancy can come as a shock to many expectant parents, and they may need additional support and education to help them cope with the changes they face. The mother will need nutrition counseling so that she gains more weight than that needed for a singleton birth, counseling that maternal adaptations will probably be more uncomfortable, and information about the possibility of a preterm birth.

If the presence of more than three fetuses is diagnosed, the parents may receive counseling regarding selective reduction of the pregnancies to reduce the incidence of premature birth and improve the opportunities for growth to term gestation for the remaining infants (Berkowitz, 1998). This situation poses an ethical dilemma for many couples, especially those who have worked hard to overcome problems with infertility and harbor strong values regarding right to life. The nurse who is able to engage the couple in discussion to identify what resources could help the couple (e.g., a minister, priest, or mental health counselor) can make the process of making a decision somewhat less traumatic.

The prenatal care given women with multifetal pregnancies includes changes in the pattern of care and modifications in other aspects such as the amount of weight gained and the nutritional intake observed. The prenatal visits of these mothers are scheduled at least every 2 weeks in the second trimester and weekly thereafter. No specific recommendation for weight gain for women with multifetal pregnancies has been made. In twin gestations, reports of gains of 20 kg have been associated with positive outcomes. Iron and vitamin supplementation is desirable. Attempts are made to prevent preeclampsia and eclampsia, which occur more commonly during multifetal pregnancies, and vaginitis; if they cannot be prevented, they are treated.

The considerable uterine distention involved can cause the backache commonly experienced by pregnant women to be even worse. Elastic stockings or maternity tights may be worn to control leg varicosities. If there are risk factors for preterm birth (e.g., premature dilation of the cervix), abstinence from orgasm and nipple stimulation during the last trimester is recommended to help avert preterm labor. Frequent ultrasound examinations and heart rate monitoring will occur. Some practitioners recommend bed rest beginning at 20 weeks in women carrying multiple fetuses to prevent preterm labor. Other practitioners question the value of prolonged bed rest. If bed rest is recommended, the mother needs to assume a lateral position to promote increased placental perfusion. If birth is delayed until after the thirty-sixth week, the risk of morbidity and mortality decreases for the neonates.

Multiple newborns will likely place a strain on finances, space, workload, and the mother's and family's coping capability. Lifestyle changes may be necessary. Parents will need assistance in making realistic plans for the care of the babies, for example, whether to breastfeed and whether to raise them as "alike" or as separate persons. Parents should be referred to national organizations such as Parents of Twins, Mothers of Multiples, and the La Leche League for further support (see Appendix D).

KEY POINTS

- The prenatal period is a period of significant psychosocial adaptation for all members of the expectant family as they anticipate changes in roles and responsibilities.

- Prenatal care is common among women of middle and high socioeconomic status, but women living in poverty or those who lack health insurance may not be able to use public medical services or gain access to private care.

- Prenatal care is ideally a multidisciplinary activity that fosters a safe birth and promotes satisfaction of the mother and family with the pregnancy and birth experience.

- Important components of the initial prenatal visit include an in-depth interview to determine the presence of potential complications, a comprehensive physical examination, and selected laboratory tests.

- Follow-up visits are shorter than the initial visit but are important for monitoring the health of the mother and fetus and providing anticipatory guidance as needed.

- Individualized care may be implemented through the assessment process, the formulation of nursing diagnoses, and planning mutually derived outcomes with the woman and her family when appropriate; evaluation of care is an ongoing process.

- The nurse has an important role in teaching the pregnant woman and her family about the physical changes and discomforts of pregnancy and self-care measures that can be implemented.

- Each woman needs to know how to recognize and report preterm labor and other warning signs and symptoms.

- Culture, age, parity, and multiple pregnancy may have a significant impact on the course and outcome of the pregnancy.

CRITICAL THINKING EXERCISES

1 *Brenda Baer is a primigravida who comes with her husband for the first prenatal visit during her second month of pregnancy. You know that assessing family relationships is important in providing comprehensive nursing care. What observations are important? What questions might you ask? What anticipatory guidance might you provide? How would you include the partner and when would be appropriate to exclude him?*

2 *You are working in an obstetrician's office and are caring for Laurie Smith, a 26-year-old woman who is married, the mother of a 3-year-old, and working full-time as a nursing assistant. Her pregnancy is at 10 weeks, and she is complaining of unrelenting fatigue. What assessments are appropriate? What information and suggestions can you provide?*

3 *You are providing clinic care for a 15-year-old adolescent, Juanita, in her seventh month of pregnancy who has come for her first prenatal visit. Juanita is living at home with her mother and 17-year-old sister, who has a 2-year-old girl. Her mother works in the food services department of the local hospital and has told Juanita that she may live at home with her baby but that she will have to be responsible for the infant's care. Juanita describes the father of the baby as a 22-year-old who works at a fast-food restaurant, but she complains that during the past month, he has lost interest in their relationship. What are the physical risks associated with adolescent pregnancy? What are the likely psychosocial needs of Juanita? What long-term outcomes may be expected as you consider Juanita's future? How can an interdisciplinary approach to care benefit the client? What community resources should be investigated? What legal issues are involved?*

References

Abel, E. (1996). *Fetal alcohol syndrome.* Boca Raton: CRC Press.

Alan Guttmacher Institute (AGI) (1998). Teen sex and pregnancy. Retrieved 3/15/99 from www.agiusa.org/pubs/fb_teen_sex.html.

Al-Qutob, R., Mawajdeh, S., & Bin-Raad, F. (1996). The assessment of reproductive health services: A conceptual framework for prenatal care. *Health Care for Women International* 17, 423-434.

Alteneder, R., & Hartzell, D. (1997). Addressing couples' sexuality concerns during the childbearing period: Use of the PLISSIT model. *J Obstet Gynecol Neonatal Nurs* 26, 651-658.

American College of Obstetricians and Gynecologists. (1991). *Precis V: An update in obstetrics and gynecology.* Washington, DC: ACOG.

American College of Obstetricians and Gynecologists. (1994). *Precis V: An update in obstetrics and gynecology.* Washington, DC: ACOG.

American College of Obstetricians and Gynecologists. (1997). *Smoking and women's health.* Technical Bulletin 240, Washington, DC: ACOG.

Beischer, N., MacKay, E., & Colditz, P. (1997). *Obstetrics and the newborn* (3rd ed.). Philadelphia: W.B. Saunders.

Bergsjo, P., & Villar, J. (1997). Scientific basis for the content of routine antenatal care. *Acta Obstet Gynecol Scand* 76, 15-25.

Berkowitz, R. (1998). Ethical issues involving multifetal pregnancies. *Mt Sinai J Med* 65, 185-190.

Callister, L. (1995). Cultural meanings of childbirth. *J Obstet Gynecol Neonatal Nurs* 24, 327-331.

Campbell-Brown, M., & Hytten, F. (1998). Nutrition. In G. Chamberlain, & F. Broughton-Pipkin (Eds.). *Clinical physiology in obstetrics* (3rd ed.). Oxford: Blackwell Science.

Caritis, S. et al. (1998). Predictors of preeclampsia in women at high risk. *Am J Obstet Gynecol* 179, 946-951.

Chestnut, M. (1998). *High risk perinatal home care manual.* Philadelphia: Lippincott.

Cockey, C. (1997). Preventing teen pregnancy. *AWHONN Lifelines* 1(3), 32-40.

Crowley, P. (1998). Interventions to prevent, or improve outcome from, delivery at or beyond term. *Cochrane Library (Oxford)* 3, CD-ROM.

Culnane, M. et al. (1999). Lack of long-term effects of in utero exposure to zidovudine among uninfected children born to HIV-infected women. *JAMA* 281, 151-157.

Cunningham, F. et al. (1997). *Williams obstetrics* (20th ed.). Stamford, CT: Appleton & Lange.

Davis, D. (1996). The discomforts of pregnancy. *J Obstet Gynecol Neonatal Nurs* 25, 73-81.

Dollberg, S. et al. (1996). Adverse perinatal outcome in the older primipara. *J Perinatol* 16 (2 Pt l), 93-97.

Donovan, J. (1995). The process of analysis during a grounded theory study of men during their partners' pregnancies. *J Adv Nurs* 21, 708-715.

Draper, J. (1997). Whose welfare in the labour room? A discussion of the increasing trend of fathers' birth attendance. *Midwifery* 13, 132-138.

Ebrahim, S. et al. (1998). Alcohol consumption by pregnant women in the United States during 1988-1995. *Obstet Gynecol* 92, 187-192.

Ferketich, S., & Mercer, R. (1995). Paternal-infant attachment of experienced and inexperienced fathers during infancy. *Nurs Res* 44, 31-37.

Gaines, K. (1997). Part II–Abuse and pregnancy: What every childbirth educator/nurse should know. *J Perinat Educ* 6(17), 28-38.

Gebauer, C. et al. (1998). A nurse-managed smoking cessation intervention during pregnancy. *J Obstet Gynecol Neonatal Nurs* 27, 47-53.

Gilbert, E., & Harmon, J. (1998). *Manual of high risk pregnancy & delivery* (2nd ed.). St. Louis: Mosby.

Hacker, N., & Moore, J. (1998). *Essentials of obstetrics and gynecology* (3rd ed.) Philadelphia: W.B. Saunders.

Harvey, B. (1995). The economics of perinatal care in the United States. In A. Goldworth et al. (Eds.). *Ethics and perinatology.* New York: Oxford University Press.

Helewa, M. et al. (1997). Report of the Canadian Hypertension Society Consensus Conference: Definitions, evaluation and classification of hypertensive disorders in pregnancy, *Can Med Assoc J* 157, 715-725.

Huffman, C., & Sandelowski, M. (1997). The nurse-technology relationship: The case of ultrasonography. *J Obstet Gynecol Neonatal Nurse* 26, 673-682.

Jackson, S., & Soper, D. (1997). Sexually transmitted diseases in pregnancy. *Obstet Gynecol Clin North Am* 24, 631-644.

Jansson, L. et al. (1996). Pregnancy and addiction. A comprehensive care model. *J Subst Abuse Treat* 13, 321-329.

Johnson, C. (1998). Reducing smoking among women. *AWHONN Lifelines* 2(5), 16.

Kilby, J. (1997). A smoking cessation plan for pregnant women. *J Obstet Gynecol Neonatal Nurs* 26, 397-402.

Lawrence, R. (1999). *Breastfeeding: A guide for the medical profession* (5th ed.). St. Louis: Mosby.

Lederman, R. (1996). *Psychosocial adaptation in pregnancy* (2nd ed.). New York: Springer.

Maloni, J. et al. (1996). Transforming prenatal care: Reflections on the past and present with implications for the future. *J Obstet Gynecol Neonatal Nurs* 25, 17-23.

Malnory, M. (1996). Developmental care of the pregnant couple. *J Obstet Gynecol Neonatal Nurs* 25, 525-532.

Mason, C., & Elwood, R. (1995). Is there a physiological basis for the couvade and onset of paternal care? *Int J Nurs Stud* 32, 137-148.

May, K. (1980). A typology of detachment and involvement styles adopted during pregnancy by first-time expectant fathers. *West J Nurs Res* 2, 445-453.

May, K. (1982). Three phases of father involvement in pregnancy. *Nurs Res* 31, 337-342.

McFarlane, J. et al. (1998). Safety behaviors of abused women after an intervention during pregnancy. *J Obstet Gynecol Neonatal Nurs* 27, 64-69.

Mercer, R. (1995). *Becoming a mother.* New York: Springer.

Müller, M. (1996). Prenatal and postnatal attachment: A modest correlation. *J Obstet Gynecol Neonatal Nurs* 25, 161-166.

Mvula, M., & Miller, J. (1998). A comparative evaluation of collaborative prenatal care. *Obstet Gynecol* 91, 169-173.

Neilson, J. (1998). Routine ultrasound in early pregnancy. *Cochrane Library (Oxford)* 3, CD-ROM.

Oakley, D. et al. (1996). Comparison of outcomes of maternity care by obstetricians and certified nurse midwives. *Obstet Gynecol* 88, 823-829.

Perry, L. (1996). Preconception care: A health promotion opportunity. *Nurse Pract* 21(11), 24-32, 34.

Polivka, B., Nickel, J., & Wilkins, J. (1997). Urinary tract infection during pregnancy, *J Obstet Gynecol Neonatal Nurs* 26, 405-413.

Rubin, R. (1975). Maternal tasks in pregnancy. *Matern Child Nurs J* 4, 143-153.

Rubin, R. (1984). *Maternal identity and the maternal experience.* New York: Springer.

Rynerson, B., & Lowdermilk, D. (1993). Sexual intimacy in pregnancy. In R. Knuppel, & J. Drukker (Eds.). *High-risk pregnancy: A team approach* (2nd ed.). Philadelphia: W.B. Saunders.

Sampselle, C. et al. (1998). Effect of pelvic muscle exercise on transient incontinence during pregnancy and after birth. *Obstet Gynecol* 91, 406-412.

Seidel, H. et al. (1999). *Mosby's guide to physical examination* (4th ed.). St. Louis: Mosby.

Simon, N., Heaps, K., & Chodroff, C. (1997). Improving the processes of care and outcomes in obstetrics/gynecology. *Joint Commission Journal on Quality Improvement* 23, 485-497.

Simpson, L., Korenbrot, C., & Greene, J. (1997). Outcomes of enhanced prenatal services for Medicaid-eligible women in public and private settings. *Public Health Rep* 112, 122-132.

Skinner, J. et al. (1997). Transitions in infant feeding during the first year of life. *J Am Coll Nutr* 16, 209-215.

Smith, M. (1998). Professional issues: Maternal-fetal attachment. *Br J Midwifery* 6, 188-192.

Spector, R. (1996). *Cultural diversity in health and illness* (4th ed.). Stamford, CT: Appleton & Lange.

Stark, M. (1997). Psychosocial adjustment during pregnancy: The experience of mature gravidas. *J Obstet Gynecol Neonatal Nurs* 26, 206-211.

Ventura, S., Curtin, S., & Mathews, T. (1998). Teenage births in the United States: National and state trends, 1990-1996. *National Vital Statistics Reports* 47(12), 1-17.

Wagner, C. et al. (1998). The impact of prenatal drug exposure on the neonate. *Obstet Gynecol Clin North Am* 25, 169-194.

Zachariah, R. (1994). Maternal-fetal attachment: Influence of mother-daughter and husband-wife relationships. *Res Nurs Health* 17, 37-44.

18

Childbirth Education

Betty G. Harris

LEARNING OBJECTIVES

- Define the key terms.
- Explain the importance of preconception care.
- Identify the purpose of childbirth education.
- Describe the role and benefits of a doula.
- Discuss the different choices of care providers.

- Describe four birth settings.
- Compare methods of education for childbirth.
- Identify topics for nursing research in childbirth education.

KEY TERMS

birth centers
birth plan
Bradley method
doula
Grantly Dick-Read method

home birth
independent midwives
labor, delivery, recovery (LDR)
labor, delivery, recovery, postpartum (LDRP)

Lamaze method
nurse-midwives
preconception care
psychoprophylactic method (PPM)

n the broadest sense, the goal of childbirth education is to assist individuals and their family members to make informed decisions about pregnancy, birth, and parenthood. To accomplish this goal, the woman and her family need knowledge of the components of a healthy pregnancy, the process of labor and birth, and coping strategies to deal with the challenges of parenthood. Education for family members should begin before pregnancy and continue through the postpartum period.

Once a family has decided to have a baby, the next decisions involve choosing a care provider, type of care, and the place for birth; choices about infant feeding and care will follow. If a woman has had a previous cesarean birth, she may consider the possibility of a vaginal birth. This chapter discusses these considerations and the nurse's role in educating childbearing families so that family members can make informed decisions about their choices.

PRECONCEPTION CARE

Traditionally women have become pregnant without specific preconception planning with a health care provider. Today health care providers are promoting preconception care as an important component of perinatal services. **Preconception care** is designed for health maintenance. It stresses risk management and healthy behaviors that promote the health of the woman and her potential fetus. The period of greatest danger for the developing fetus is between 17 and 56 days after fertilization. By the end of the eighth week after conception and certainly by the end of the first trimester, any major structural anomalies in the fetus are already present. Because many women do not realize that they are pregnant, do not have their pregnancy confirmed, and do not seek prenatal care until well into the first trimester, the rapidly growing fetus may be exposed to many intrauterine environmental hazards during

HEALTH PROMOTION: GENERAL TEACHING

Nutrition
    Healthy diet, including folic acid
    Optimum weight
Exercise and rest
Avoidance of substance abuse (tobacco, alcohol,
    "recreational" drugs)
Use of safer sex practices
Attending to family and social needs

RISK FACTOR ASSESSMENT

Medical history
    Immune status (e.g., rubella)
    Family history (e.g., genetic disorders)
    Illnesses (e.g., infections)
    Current use of medication (prescription,
        nonprescription)
Reproductive history
    Contraceptive
    Obstetric
Psychosocial history
    Spouse/partner and family situation, including
        domestic violence
    Availability of family or other support systems
    Readiness for pregnancy (e.g., age, life goals, stress)
Financial resources
Environmental (home, workplace) conditions
    Safety hazards
    Toxic chemicals
    Radiation

INTERVENTIONS

Anticipatory guidance/teaching
Treatment of medical conditions and results
    Medications
    Cessation/reduction in substance use/abuse
    Immunizations (e.g., rubella, tuberculosis, hepatitis)
Nutrition, diet, and weight management
Exercise
Referral for genetic counseling
Referral to and use of
    Family planning services
    Family and social needs management

this vulnerable developmental phase (Cefalo & Moos, 1995).

Preconception care therefore has several purposes:
- Establish lifestyle behaviors to maintain optimal health (e.g., eating a healthy diet; getting enough rest and exercise; and cutting down or avoiding alcohol use, smoking, and drugs).

- Identify and treat risk factors before conception (e.g., medical conditions such as diabetes mellitus, substance abuse, and infections such as sexually transmitted diseases) and test for immunity from infections that could cause mental retardation or other birth defects.
- Conceive a pregnancy without unnecessary risk factors (e.g., safety of medications taken for chronic illness and health hazards in the workplace or home).
- Identify carriers of inherited diseases (e.g., Tay-Sachs disease, sickle-cell disease and thalassemia).
- Prepare psychologically for pregnancy and the responsibilities that come with parenthood.

Every woman of childbearing age should be viewed as a potential mother. Identifying and treating risk factors and providing anticipatory guidance with emphasis on a healthy lifestyle are important ways to improve the health of the next generation (Frede, 1993). The components of preconception care, such as health promotion, risk assessment, and interventions, are outlined in Box 18-1.

Preconception care is especially important for women who have had a problem with a previous pregnancy (for example, miscarriage or preterm birth). Although causes are not always identifiable, in many cases problems can be identified and treated. Preconception care is also important to minimize fetal malformations. Women with insulin-dependent diabetes mellitus who maintain excellent control of blood sugar at the time of conception could reduce the risk for congenital anomalies (malformations) in the fetus (Centers for Disease Control and Prevention, 1992). Women who have systemic lupus erythematosus are at high risk for miscarriage or preterm labor; planning a pregnancy during a remission period can increase the chances of a healthy pregnancy. An adequate maternal intake of folic acid (0.4 mg/day) before and after conception decreases the risk of having a child with a neural tube defect (Cefalo & Moos, 1995; Werler, Shipiro, & Mitchell, 1993). (A preconception assessment that identifies areas to be explored is provided in Box 18-2.)

Demographic information such as age and race are also important. Women under age 15 or over age 40 are at a higher risk during pregnancy than women ages 16 to 39. Some ethnic groups have special risks; for example, African-Americans and Southeast Asians are at risk for sickle-cell disease, and people of Jewish descent are at risk for Tay-Sachs disease (March of Dimes, 1995).

ROLE OF THE NURSE

Thoughtful assessment always provides a basis for identifying potential risks, developing outcome criteria, planning for care, and intervening. The management of preconception care is directed by findings from the interview, physical examination, and laboratory studies. If a couple is planning a pregnancy, the primary health care provider may assist them to time conception after implementing lifestyle recommendations for their health. These recommenda-

BOX 18-2 **Preconception Assessment**

INTERVIEW

Lifestyle
  Nutrition
  Exercise, rest
  Substance use: alcohol, tobacco, cocaine, other
  Occupation
  Psychosocial: stress, anxiety, depression; support from
    partner, family, friends; domestic violence
  Financial resources
Immunization status
  Rubella
  Hepatitis B
  Toxoplasmosis (not universal)
Medications
  Over-the-counter, nonprescription (e.g., aspirin)
  Herbal remedies
  Prescription
  Medical conditions: review of systems
  Hypertension, cardiovascular disease
  Seizure disorders
  Diabetes mellitus
  Renal disease
  Autoimmune disorders (e.g., lupus, rheumatoid arthritis)
  Tuberculosis, asthma, allergies
Reproductive system
  Fertility problems, endometriosis
  Contraceptive history
  Obstetric history (e.g., prior pregnancies, miscar-
    riages, child with a disorder)
  Abnormal Pap smear results
  Sexually transmitted infections (STIs)

Sexual practices
Family history, including father of baby
  Medical conditions
  Genetic conditions (e.g., sickle-cell disease, Tay-Sachs
    disease, cystic fibrosis, bleeding disorders, phenylke-
    tonuria [PKU])
  Birth defects
Treatment history
  Previous abdominal reproductive surgery
  Trauma
  Previous blood transfusion(s)
Environmental history
  Work exposures
  Home exposures

PHYSICAL EXAMINATION

General medical with emphasis on
  Thyroid gland
  Breasts
  Pelvic structures

LABORATORY STUDIES

General: CBC, urinalysis, blood type and Rh, rubella titer,
  STIs (e.g., syphilis, gonorrhea, *Chlamydia*), hepatitis B
  surface antigen, Pap smear, and cervical culture
Depending on risk:
  PPD
  HIV
  Toxicology screen
  Thalassemia

CBC, Complete blood count; *PPD,* purified protein derivative test (for tuberculosis); *HIV,* human immunodeficiency virus.

tions could include diet and weight management, physical conditioning (Ratts, 1993), immunizations, and genetic counseling. If pregnancy is not desired, the nurse can discuss the risk of unintended pregnancy, recommend the same lifestyle behaviors, and assist the couple to choose an acceptable method of contraception. Recommendations can be reinforced with videotapes or audiotapes, illustrations, and printed teaching aids (Scherger, 1993).

Prevention should be the focus of self-care in any plan of care. Preventive measures are suggested throughout the text for infection, nutrition, substance abuse, and other health-related concerns. Approximately 8% to 10% of birth defects occur as a result of environmental factors and may be amenable to nursing intervention (Pletsch, 1990). Cleanliness, ventilation, adherence to manufacturer's directions for use and disposal of materials, use of protective gear to shield against known and unknown hazards, and avoidance of exposure to radiation are examples of strategies to reduce risk. In some instances, safer materials can

be substituted for potentially hazardous ones. For example, most household cleaning needs can be met with baking soda, table salt, distilled white vinegar, lemon juice, trisodium phosphate (TSP, which does not emit fumes), a plunger, and some common sense. These substances can be used to clean drains, wash windows, degrease, prevent mold and mildew, disinfect, and scour.

Nurses must be alert to conditions in the workplace that may affect the reproductive health of workers and their partners. Stress reduction through relaxation and guided imagery and moderate exercise and rest are also useful.

As private citizens, nurses should become involved in professional and political organizations to promote and support legislation to control pollution of the environment. Nurses can teach about alternative ways to clean the home and care for yards and gardens to reduce exposure to potentially harmful substances.

Evaluation of short-term results is possible to some extent. The birth of a healthy baby with no apparent disorder or disease, the uncomplicated recovery of the new mother, continued fertility, and demonstration of a lifestyle that supports good reproductive health are some expected outcomes when preconception and pregnancy care are effective. Long-term effects may not be known for many years or generations.

CHILDBIRTH EDUCATION

Content taught in the U.S. educational system does little to prepare individuals for becoming parents. Informal preparation, especially through participation in care of younger siblings or relatives, is increasingly uncommon. As a result, many individuals facing parenthood have little information about what to expect and do not have the skills necessary to deal effectively with pregnancy and parenthood. Childbirth education classes are one way to fill this void.

Because of their knowledge, communication skills, acceptability to couples, and position in the health care system, nurses provide much of the education available for couples about reproduction, both informally and through courses focusing on aspects of the transition to parenthood. All professional nurses are prepared by their education and practice to participate in such teaching, particularly the immediate situation-based teaching needed in clinic or hospital settings. Advanced preparation for childbirth education is also available and is especially useful for the nurse teaching in group situations or in cases where a more sophisticated psychologic approach is used and involves exploration of feelings and adjustment of expectations.

History

Women have always shared information about and assisted each other in childbirth. Until the late nineteenth century, childbirth was a family and social event in which women gave birth at home, often with the help of a midwife. The Industrial Revolution, with attendant urban crowding and associated health problems, led to higher rates of maternal and infant death from puerperal fever, sepsis, and infant diarrhea (Wertz & Wertz, 1979). The associated changes of male domination of obstetrics, drugs, and medication for pain and infection control in birth, as well as the weakened family bonds consequent to industrialization, moved childbirth from being "women's work" and controlled by nature into the hospital (Lindell, 1988).

Despite these changes, women sought to have some control over the management of birth. During the late nineteenth century, women organized the National Twilight Sleep Association to promote the use of the new technique of giving morphine and scopolamine to control labor pain (Pitcock & Clark, 1992). However, by the early twentieth century most women had accepted centralized and routinized birth practices over which they had little or no control in the belief that childbirth would be safer for themselves and their babies. Not until the midtwentieth

century did women (energized by the consumer rights movement, women's movement, and increased availability of certified nurse-midwives) begin to question the rigid policies, medicalization, and routinization of birth. The parent education movement began in the 1950s and grew until prepared childbirth classes are now recommended for all families by most caregivers and by the federally appointed panel on prenatal care (Public Health Service, 1988).

Studies show that childbirth education "promotes positive attitudes towards labor and delivery and . . . fosters early maternal-infant attachment" (Lindell, 1988). A 1990 study of 800 women in England found that receipt of information and a feeling of control were important components of women's satisfaction with the birth and their subsequent emotional well-being (Hetherington, 1990). Physiologic effects of length of labor and anesthesia or analgesia on mother and infant vary; some studies found that formal preparation results in reduced use of analgesia and anesthesia (Hetherington, 1990; Lindell, 1988). However, others do not demonstrate that attendance at childbirth education classes reduces interventions during labor and birth (Lindell, 1988; Sturrock & Johnson, 1990). Slager-Earnest and colleagues (1987) demonstrated that combining a multidisciplinary team and comprehensive health services with childbirth education resulted in significantly fewer obstetric, postnatal, and neonatal complications for teenagers and their children. Thus new approaches and classes tailored to the needs of varied groups may be essential for effective outcomes.

Early Methods

An English physician, Grantly Dick-Read, published two books in which he theorized that pain in childbirth is socially conditioned and caused by a fear-tension-pain syndrome. His first book, *Natural Childbirth*, was published in 1933. Dick-Read's second book, *Childbirth Without Fear*, was published in the United States in 1944. The work of Dick-Read became the foundation for organized programs of preparation for childbirth and teacher training throughout the United States, Canada, Great Britain, and South Africa. In 1960 the nurses prepared through such programs established the International Childbirth Education Association (ICEA). The **Grantly Dick-Read method,** referred to as *childbirth without fear,* basically recommended three techniques: deep abdominal breathing during early first-stage contractions, shallow breathing for later first stage, and breath holding with pushing for the second stage of labor. As knowledge about the detrimental effects of breath holding for pushing has grown, contemporary teachers of the Dick-Read method have altered this recommendation. Relaxation is an important part of the Grantly Dick-Read method (Dick-Read, 1987). Women are taught to consciously and progressively relax different muscle groups through the entire body until a high degree of skill at relaxation is achieved. Consequently, a woman is able to relax completely between contractions and keep all muscles except the uterus relaxed during contractions.

During the 1960s the **Lamaze method,** also known as the **psychoprophylactic method (PPM),** gained popularity in the United States. PPM offered new perspectives on preparation for childbirth by emphasizing mind control. Marjorie Karmel introduced PPM to the United States in her book *Thank You, Dr. Lamaze,* which was published in the United States in 1959. PPM combines controlled muscular relaxation and breathing techniques. Active relaxation is an integral part of the Lamaze method (Lamaze, 1970). The woman is taught to contract specific muscle groups (neuromuscular control) while relaxing the remainder of her body. She thus learns to relax the uninvolved muscles in her body while her uterus contracts. Instead of tensing during uterine contractions, women respond with conditioned relaxation and breathing patterns. In 1960 the American Society for Psychoprophylaxis in Obstetrics (ASPO) was formed in New York as a national organization to promote use of the Lamaze method and prepare teachers of the method. It continues to be an active organization, known since 1998 as Lamaze International. Over 11,000 Lamaze Certified Childbirth Educators (LCCEs) have been educated and certified (Lamaze, 1999b). Their work is guided by a philosophy of birth that includes the following:

- Birth is normal, natural, and healthy.
- The experience of birth profoundly affects women and their families.
- Women's inner wisdom guides them through birth.
- Women's confidence and ability to give birth is either enhanced or diminished by the care provider and place of birth.
- Women have a right to give birth free from routine medical interventions.
- Birth can take place safely in birth centers and homes.
- Childbirth education empowers women to make informed choices in health care, to assume responsibility for their health, and to trust their inner wisdom (Lamaze, 1999a).

A Denver obstetrician, Robert Bradley, published *Husband-Coached Childbirth* in 1965. In the book he advocates what he calls true "natural" childbirth, without any form of anesthesia or analgesia and with a husband-coach and breathing techniques for labor. The American Academy of Husband-Coached Childbirth (AAHCC) was founded to make the **Bradley method** available and prepare teachers. This method of partner-coached childbirth uses breath control, abdominal breathing, and general body relaxation. Working in harmony with the body is emphasized (Bradley, 1965). Bradley's technique emphasizes environmental variables such as darkness, solitude, and quiet to make childbirth a more natural experience. Women using the Bradley method often appear to be sleeping during labor because they are in such a deep state of mental relaxation.

All three methods incorporate intellectual and physical components. In addition, all now emphasize the naturalness of childbirth, and, at least to some extent, empowering women to make choices for themselves. Each program educates women to exchange fear of the unknown for confidence and understanding. Adequate prenatal education includes information on maternal adaptation, nutrition, sexuality, basic hygiene, and labor and birth. Support for the woman in labor is provided by her husband or another support person chosen by the expectant mother.

Physiologic evidence now indicates that specific breathing techniques (such as breath holding while pushing) may be harmful to the fetus and have no advantage on progress during the second stage of labor. Appropriate changes have been incorporated into modern childbirth education classes. Other new approaches to old techniques are being proposed. These often emphasize teaching the woman to tune into and respond to her body's cues. In this holistic approach to childbirth education the emphasis is on the way the mind, body, and spirit are related and affect one another. Some specially trained professionals incorporate a variety of techniques and psychotherapeutic methods designed to promote self-awareness and identify attitudes, traumas, and anxieties that may interfere in the process of labor (Peterson, 1991; Wilberg, 1992). Dealing with these issues during pregnancy may promote more satisfying labor and assist people in becoming more effective, happier parents.

Current Practices

A variety of approaches to childbirth education have evolved as educators attempt to meet learning needs. In addition to classes designed specifically for pregnant adolescents and their partners or parents (Bachman, 1993), classes are designed for other groups with special learning needs, such as first-time mothers over age 35, single women, adoptive parents, and parents of twins. Refresher classes for parents with children review coping techniques for labor and birth and help couples prepare for sibling reactions and adjustments to a new baby. Cesarean birth classes are offered for couples who may be at risk for an operative birth. Because many women successfully give birth vaginally after a previous cesarean birth, some classes focus on vaginal birth after cesarean.

Because environmental influences and maternal behavior greatly affect newborn health, preconception and early pregnancy classes have been developed. These typically provide information about behaviors such as nutrition and exercise that promote improved pregnancy outcomes and the risks of environmental hazards, smoking, alcohol, and drugs. Women with a greater sense of self-control tend to engage in health-promoting activities during pregnancy (Lewallen, 1989; Riesch, 1988). Prenatal exercise classes taught during pregnancy should be based on American College of Obstetricians and Gynecologists exercise guidelines for pregnancy and the postpartum period (American College of Obstetricians and Gynecologists, 1994) (see box on p. 408).

Strategies

Because of the multicultural composition of the population, great diversity exists in attitudes, expectations, and behaviors judged appropriate during pregnancy and early parenthood. No one approach can meet all needs. For example, classes for new immigrants are particularly effective when taught in class members' primary language. For classes to be meaningful, childbirth educators must understand the value systems in other cultures and their influences on issues such as nutrition, early prenatal care, maternal weight gain, and infant feeding practices. Parent educators must establish rapport, be understood, and build on cultural practices, reinforcing the positive and promoting change only if a practice (for example, pica) is directly harmful (USDA and USDHHS, 1990; Waxler-Morrison, Anderson, & Richardson, 1990).

Most childbirth education classes are attended by the pregnant woman and her partner, although a friend, teenage daughter, or parent may be the selected support person. When family-centered care is practiced, other family members may be present for the birth. Classes may be offered for grandparents and siblings to prepare them for their attendance at birth or the arrival of the baby. Classes focus on preparing families intellectually, emotionally, and physically for childbirth and promoting wellness and improved lifestyle behaviors during the childbearing years.

OPTIONS FOR CARE

Birth Plan

Some expectant parents deal with decision making by developing a birth plan to help them identify options and set priorities. The **birth plan** is a natural evolution of the contemporary wellness-oriented lifestyle. It is a tool by which parents can explore their childbirth options and choose those that are most important to them. Many parents already indicate some of their preferences by the type of health care provider and birth setting (hospital, free-standing birth center, or home) they have chosen. Some pregnant women enlist the services of a health care provider only after an interview and a tour of the birth facility. Others do not give conscious thought to the conduct of their pregnancies, the labor and birth process, recovery, and early parenthood. These women may need help with decision making. After the confirmation of pregnancy, couples tend to focus on the reality of their situation and their emotional responses. However, it is acceptable for the nurse to initiate a discussion of a birth plan during the first and second prenatal visits. Some maternity clinics provide printed material describing available options and giving answers to commonly asked questions. In addition, tours of the birth setting are offered by almost all facilities that provide perinatal services.

Clients' expectations must be reasonable and in keeping with the resources available in the community. The nurse can provide couples with pertinent information so that they can make informed decisions, alerting them to various options and the advantages and consequences of each.

The nurse should assess clients' readiness to learn and avoid overloading them with information. Some health care providers provide birth plan lists. A discussion of the printed list can serve as a means of getting couples to start thinking about, discussing, and identifying what is personally important to them. However, it is important to remember that some options may be appropriate only for low risk women. The options of women with a high risk pregnancy or those in whom complications develop during labor may be severely limited.

The birth plan can serve as a means of open communication between the pregnant woman and her partner and between the couple and health care providers. An early introduction to the idea of a birth plan allows the couple time to think about events or situations that could make their childbearing experience more meaningful and those they would prefer to avoid. The nurse-client discussion of the birth plan should take place in an accepting atmosphere in which women can see themselves as unique and yet normal.

Topics for discussion and decision making may include any or all of the following:
- Partner's participation: Attend prenatal visits? Childbirth/parent education classes? Present during labor? During birth? During cesarean birth?
- Birth setting: Hospital delivery room or birthing room (if available)? A birthing center? Home?
- Labor management: Walk around during labor? Use a rocking chair? Use a shower? Use a jacuzzi, if available? Consider an electronic fetal monitor? Have music or dimmed lighting? Have older children or other people present? Is telemetry monitoring available? Consider stimulation of labor? Consider medication—what kind?
- Birth: Positions—side lying? On hands and knees, kneeling, or squatting? Use a birthing bed? Or delivery table? Will you be photographing, videotaping, or recording any of the labor or birth? Who would you like to be present—partner, older siblings, other family members, or friends? What do you know about the use of forceps? Episiotomies? Will your partner want to cut the umbilical cord?
- Immediately after birth: Do you want to hold the baby right away? Breastfeed immediately?
- Newborn care: What about circumcision for your baby (if male)? Will the baby be breastfed or bottle fed?
- Postpartum care: What kind of care do you anticipate—labor, delivery, recovery, postpartum room; mother-baby coupling; "request" coupling (newborn cared for in nursery while mother rests)? How long does your insurance company allow you to stay? Would you like to

attend self-care classes or prefer to get such information from videotapes? On which subjects?

Care Provider Options

Physicians

The nurse can provide information about the different types of health care providers and the kind of care to expect from each type. Physicians (obstetricians and family practice physicians) attend about 93% of births in the United States and Canada (National Center for Health Statistics, 1998). They see low and high risk clients. Care often includes pharmacologic and medical management of problems and the use of technologic procedures. Family practice physicians may need backup by obstetricians if a specialist is needed for a problem such as a cesarean birth. Most physicians manage births in a hospital setting.

Nurse-Midwives

Nurse-midwives are registered nurses with additional education and training in the care of obstetric clients. Throughout history, midwives have held a holistic view of childbirth (Capitulo, 1998). They provide care for about 6% of the births in the United States and Canada (National Center for Health Statistics, 1998). Certified nurse-midwives may practice with physicians or independently with an arrangement for physician backup. They usually see low risk obstetric clients. Care is often noninterventional, and the woman and family are usually encouraged to be active participants in the care. Nurse-midwives must refer clients to physicians for complications. Most births are managed in hospital settings or birth centers; a few may be managed in home settings.

Independent Midwives

Independent midwives (also called lay midwives or certified professional midwives) are nonprofessional caregivers. Their training varies greatly from formal training to self-teaching. They manage approximately 1% of births in the United States and Canada (National Center for Health Statistics, 1998). Clients who develop problems must be seen by a physician. A majority (61%) of births attended by these midwives take place in the home setting.

Doulas

Whereas the caregivers discussed previously provide medical and health supervision, manage the birth, and provide immediate and later postpartal and infant care, the doula provides a different service. A **doula** is professionally trained to provide labor support, including physical, emotional, and informational support to women and their partners during labor and birth. The doula does not get involved with clinical tasks (Doulas of North America, 1999a, 1999b, 1999c).

A doula typically meets with the mother and her husband or partner before labor. At this meeting, she ascertains the mothers' expectations and desires for the birth experience. Using this information as her guide, during labor and birth the doula focuses her efforts on assisting the woman to achieve her goals. Doulas work collaboratively with other health care providers and the husband or other supportive individuals, but their primary goal is assisting the mother. This approach has a number of positive outcomes.

Klaus and Kennell (1997) examined outcomes in eleven studies of doulas. Each study randomly assigned expectant mothers to either regular support or regular support plus a doula. Doulas provided continuous support, including praise, encouragement, reassurance, comfort measures, physical contact, and explanations regarding progress of labor. Labor outcomes for the doula-assisted group included shorter labor, less medication for pain relief, fewer operative vaginal deliveries, and in several studies a lower rate of cesarean births. Six weeks after the birth, the doula-assisted group had a higher proportion of women breast-feeding, and they had greater self-esteem and lower rates of depression, regarded their infants more positively, and were more confident of their ability to provide effective infant care. Rather than substituting for fathers, when a doula was present fathers provided more personal support to their partners. The authors concluded that although the presence of the father is important to both the father and the woman, the doula's presence is a significant factor in a positive outcome.

In a study comparing Lamaze preparation with doula instruction and support, Manning-Orenstein (1998) found that doula-supported women "were significantly less rejecting and significantly less helpless than mothers who used the Lamaze method." Four months postpartum, they had more positive moods, had higher self-esteem, and rated their infants as less fussy (see Research box).

Doulas may be found through community contacts, other health care providers, or childbirth educators. Organizations that offer information or referral services include Doulas of North America (DONA), 1100 23rd Ave. East, Seattle, WA 98112 (phone: 206-324-5440); Association of Labor Assistants and Childbirth Educators (ALACE), P.O. Box 382724, Cambridge, MA 02238 (phone: 617-441-2500); International Childbirth Education Association (ICEA), P.O. Box 20048, Minneapolis, MN 55420 (phone: 800-624-4934); and Lamaze International, 1200 19th St. NW, Suite 300, Washington, DC 20036 (phone: 202-857-1100). It is important that the expectant mother be comfortable with the doula who will be attending her. See Box 18-3 for a list of questions to ask.

Although the doula role originally developed as an assistant during labor, some women need assistance during the postpartum period. There is a small but growing number of postnatal doulas, who provide assistance to the new mother as she develops competence with infant care, feeding, and other maternal tasks.

RESEARCH

Therapeutic Effects of Doula Support on First-time Mothers' Working Models of Caregiving

Maternal competence at birth has not been promoted in Western obstetric care. Women are often dependent on technology, routines, and care providers and may view themselves as inadequate caregivers for their infants. Doulas working with women during pregnancy and labor and birth provide encouragement and support so that new mothers can be more confident in themselves and their infant caregiving skills.

This study examined whether the presence of a doula would have a beneficial effect on a first-time pregnant woman's working model of caregiving. Thirty-five first-time mothers were divided into two groups, one using a doula and the other group trained in Lamaze childbirth preparation. The women were interviewed in their third trimester and again at 4 months after giving birth. The women also completed measurement tests for mood changes and self-esteem and a postpartum self-evaluation questionnaire that assessed quality of support and evaluation of the infant's temperament. Analysis revealed that the mothers in

the doula group were significantly less rejecting and helpless in caregiving, were less emotionally stressed, had higher self-esteem, and rated their infants less fussy than women in the Lamaze group.

CLINICAL APPLICATION

Nurses in labor and birth units have always thought that they nurtured and encouraged laboring women and promoted bonding and attachment between mothers and infants. Increased use of technology in the labor and birth unit tends to take the nurse's focus away from the woman and can affect the nurse's ability to provide the level of support needed by the laboring woman. The results of this study suggest that the doula can become part of the birth team and provide a valuable function for the mother. Instead of resenting the presence of a doula, the labor and birth nurse should collaborate with her to provide the most supportive environment for birth.

Source: Manning-Orensteing, G. (1998). A birth intervention: The therapeutic effects of doula support versus Lamaze preparation on first-time mothers' working models of caregiving. *Alt Ther Health Med* 4(4), 73-81.

BOX 18-3 | Questions to Ask When Choosing a Doula

To discover the specific training, experience, and services offered by anyone who provides labor support, potential clients, nursing supervisors, physicians, midwives, and others should ask the following questions of that person:

- What training have you had?
- Tell me about your experience with birth, personally and as a doula.
- What is your philosophy about childbirth and supporting women and their partners through labor?
- May we meet to discuss our birth plans and the role you will play in supporting me through childbirth?
- May we call you with questions or concerns before and after the birth?
- When do you try to join women in labor? Do you come to our home or meet us at the hospital?
- Do you meet with us after the birth to review the labor and answer questions?
- Do you work with one or more backup doulas for times when you are not available? May we meet them?
- What is your fee?

From Simkin, P., & Way, K. (1998). *DONA position paper: The doula's contributions to modern maternity care.* Seattle, WA: Doulas of North America.

BIRTH SETTING CHOICES

With careful thought, the concept of family-centered maternity care can be implemented in any setting. The three primary options for birth settings today are the hospital, birth center, and home. Women consider several factors in choosing a setting for childbirth, including the preference of their health care provider, characteristics of the birthing unit, and preference of their third-party payer (Mackey, 1990). Approximately 99% of all births in the United States take place in a hospital setting (National Center for Health Statistics, 1998). However, the types of labor and birth services vary greatly, from the traditional labor and delivery rooms with separate postpartum and newborn units to in-hospital birthing centers where all or almost all care takes place in a single unit.

Labor, Delivery, Recovery, Postpartum (Birthing) Rooms

Labor, delivery, recovery (LDR) and **labor, delivery, recovery, postpartum (LDRP)** rooms offer families a comfortable, private space for childbirth. Women are admitted to LDR units, labor and give birth, and spend the first 1 to 2 hours there for immediate postpartum recovery and for having time with their families to bond with their newborns (Fig. 18-1, *A*). After this period of recovery, the mothers and newborns are transferred to a postpartum unit and nursery or mother-baby unit for the duration of their stay. Care is provided by different nursing staff (e.g.,

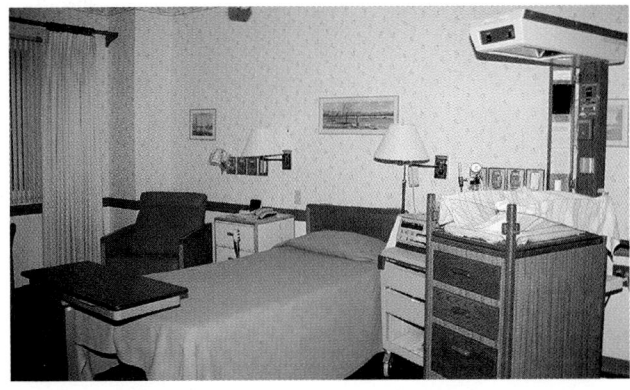

A

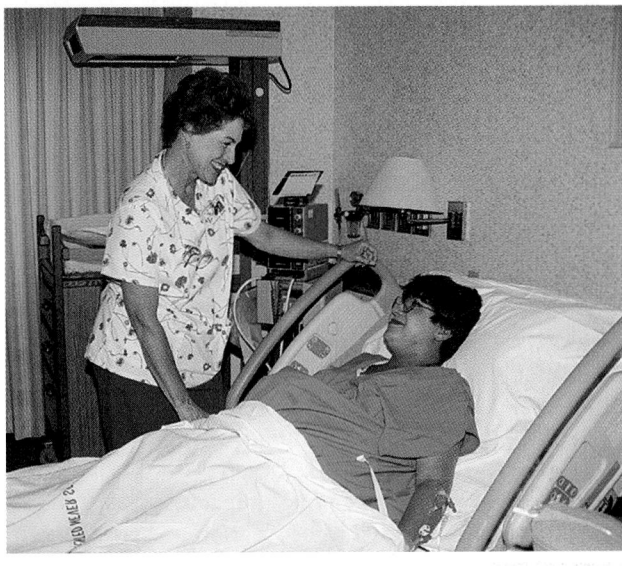

B

Fig. 18-1   **A**, LDR unit. **B**, LDRP unit. *(A, Courtesy Marjorie Pyle, RNC, Lifecircle, Costa Mesa, CA.)*

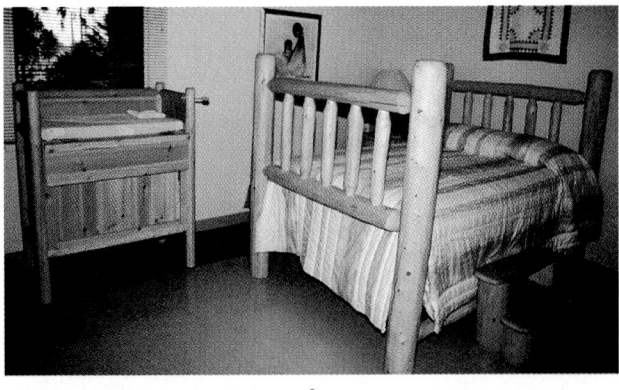

A

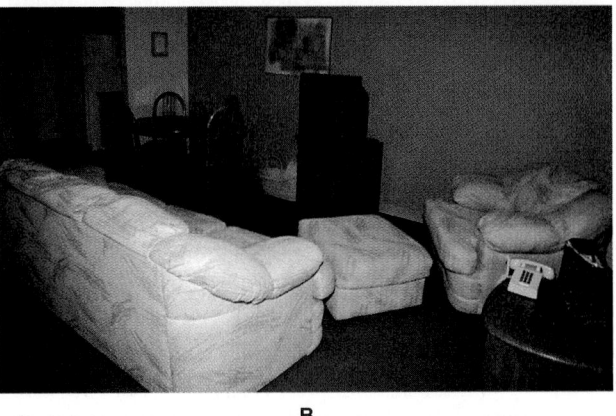

B

Fig. 18-2   Birth center. **A**, Note double bed and crib. **B**, Lounge and kitchen. *(Courtesy Michael S. Clement, MD, Mesa, AZ.)*

labor and delivery nurses, postpartum nurses, nursery nurses). In some hospitals, the same nurse provides care for both mothers and newborns.

In LDRP units, total care is provided from admission for labor through postpartum discharge in the same room, usually by the same nursing staff. The woman and her family may stay in this unit for 6 to 48 hours after giving birth. The units are furnished in a homelike atmosphere (Fig. 18-1, *B*).

Both units are equipped with fetal monitors, emergency resuscitation equipment for both mother and newborn, and heated cribs or warming units for the newborn. Often this equipment is in cabinets or closets when it is not being used.

Birth Centers

Free-standing **birth centers** are usually built in locations separate from the hospital but may be located in close proximity in case transfer of the woman or newborn is needed. These birth centers are intended to offer families an alternative to home or hospital birth, providing a third

choice that is a safe and cost-effective compromise. The centers are usually staffed by nurse-midwives or physicians who also have privileges at the local hospital. Clients are evaluated carefully as a measure to ensure that only women who are at low risk for complications are included for care (Alden & Harris, 1995).

Birth centers typically have homelike accommodations, including a double bed for the couple and a crib for the newborn (Fig. 18-2). Emergency equipment is available but often stored out of view. Many centers have an early labor lounge or a living room, and a small kitchen may be available. The family is admitted to the birth center for labor and birth and will remain there until discharge, often within 6 hours of the birth.

Other services provided by free-standing birth centers include those necessary for safe management during the childbearing cycle. In addition, attendance at childbirth and parenting classes is required of all clients. Prenatal supervision of the woman, whose nutritional and health status must be good and who must be experiencing a low-risk pregnancy, begins in the first trimester. Clients must understand when situations may require transfer to a hospital and must have agreed to abide by those guidelines. Expectant families develop birth plans, that is, the practices and procedures they would like to include in or exclude from their childbirth experience. Developing birth plans provides a means for caregivers and expectant parents to discuss options, preferences, and situations that might necessitate variation from their preferred birth method.

Birth centers may have resources such as a lending library for parents, reference files on related topics, recycled maternity clothes and baby clothes and equipment, and supplies and reference materials for childbirth educators. The centers may also have referral files for community resources that offer services related to childbirth and early parenting, including support groups (such as single parents, postbirth support group, and parents of twins), genetic counseling, women's issues, and consumer action. These centers are often close to a major hospital so that quick transfer to that institution is possible when necessary. Ambulance service and emergency procedures must be readily available. Fees vary with the services provided but typically are less than or equal to those charged by local hospitals. Some centers base fees on the ability of the family to pay (reduced-fee sliding scale). Several third-party payers, Medicaid, and TRICARE/ CHAMPUS (the armed services insurance) recognize and reimburse these centers. However, clients should check with their health care payers regarding reimbursement for prenatal care and birth in a birth center.

Home Birth

Home birth has always been popular in certain countries such as Sweden and the Netherlands. In developing countries, hospitals or adequate lying-in facilities are often unavailable to most pregnant women and home birth is a necessity. In North America, home births account for less than 1% of births (National Center for Health Statistics, 1998).

National groups supporting home birth are the Home Oriented Maternity Experience (HOME) and the National Association of Parents for Safe Alternatives in Childbirth (NAPSAC). These groups work to foster more humane childbearing practices at all levels, integrating the alternatives for childbirth to meet the needs of the total population. The literature on childbirth demonstrates that medically directed home birth services with skilled nurse-midwives and medical backup have statistically excellent outcomes (Jones, 1991).

Advantages

One advantage of home birth is that the family is in control of the experience. Another is that the birth may be more physiologically natural in familiar surroundings. The mother may be more relaxed than she would be in the hospital environment. The family can assist in and be a part of the happy event, and contact with the newborn is immediate and sustained. In addition, home birth may be less expensive than a hospital confinement. Serious infection may be less likely, assuming strict aseptic principles are followed, because people generally are relatively immune to their own home bacteria (Jones, 1991).

Disadvantages

Although some physicians, nurse-midwives, and nurses support home births that use good medical and emergency backup systems, many regard this practice as exposing the mother and fetus to unnecessary danger. Thus home births are not widely accepted by the medical community, making it difficult for a family to find a qualified health care provider to give prenatal care and attend the birth. Also, backup emergency care by a physician in a hospital may be difficult to arrange in advance. If an emergency delivery is necessary, no effective way to do this rapidly exists in the home setting.

Factors Increasing the Safety of Home Birth

Most health care providers agree that if home birth is the woman's choice, certain criteria must be met for a safe home birth experience. The woman must be comfortable with her decision to have her baby at home. She should be in good health. Home birth is not indicated for women with a high risk pregnancy, such as when the woman has diabetes, heart disease, or preeclampsia. A drive to the hospital (if needed) should take no more than 10 to 15 minutes. The woman should be attended by a well-trained physician or midwife with adequate medical supplies and resuscitation equipment, including oxygen (Jones, 1991).

Family Preparation

Facilities and supplies can approximate those available in hospitals if the family works closely with the physician, nurse, or midwife to complete preparations well in advance of the birth. Childbirth education classes should include instructions on delivery of the child without the midwife, physician, or other attendant present and should be attended by both expectant parents. Classes for siblings and grandparents are recommended if they will be present at birth. These activities add to the competence and pleasure of the parents and other family members.

Detailed descriptions for preparation are needed and may be obtained from the physician's office, the midwife, or local health agencies. Some agencies may provide some equipment and supplies. If a home birth is planned, obtaining and storing the necessary articles in advance is usually possible. In contrast, if birth in the home or elsewhere is an emergency or determined by unforeseen circumstances, considerable improvisation may be necessary.

A visit to the home by the physician or midwife who will be present during the birth is recommended well before the expected date of birth. At that time the process of birth can be discussed so that everyone is aware of the characteristics of normal labor and birth, the newborn stage, deviations from normal, and the plan of care for each stage.

Home birth is a selected alternative to hospital birth for some women and couples and a necessity for many. A physically and emotionally safe outcome can be anticipated for most women and couples and their infants, especially if they are prepared and have adequate health care support.

COMPONENTS OF CHILDBIRTH EDUCATION CLASSES

Pain Management

Fear of pain is a key issue for pregnant women and a reason many give for attending childbirth education classes. Some women do experience childbirth without pain, but most women do not. Although childbirth physicians Dick-Read and Lamaze promised "painless childbirth," numerous studies show that women who have received childbirth preparation report not less pain but less distress from and greater ability to cope with the pain than unprepared women (Nichols & Humenick, 1988). Physiologic responses to labor pain include increased respirations and sympathetic nervous system responses that lead to increased cardiac output, elevated blood pressure, and possibly respiratory alkalosis. Increased norepinephrine release blocks oxytocin, decreases contractions, and lengthens labor. Increased anxiety also correlates with increased levels of epinephrine, decreased uterine contractility, and longer labor (Simkin, 1995). These reactions may all interfere with the normal progress of labor.

Pain management strategies are an essential component of childbirth education. Some women or couples want to learn what to expect from medications (see Chapter 20). Others have a strong desire to use their own resources rather than pharmacotherapeutics to manage labor discomfort. Couples need information about the advantages and disadvantages of pain medication and other techniques for coping with labor. Although neither partner should feel guilty if pain medication is required during a particular labor experience, an emphasis on nonpharmacologic pain management strategies helps couples manage the labor and birth with dignity and increased comfort. Currently, most instructors teach a flexible approach, which helps couples learn and master many techniques that can be used during labor. Women are encouraged to incorporate their natural responses into coping with the pain of labor and birth. Couples are taught gate-control techniques such as massage, pressure on the palms or soles of the feet, hot compresses to the perineum, perineal massage, applications of heat or cold, breathing patterns, and focusing of attention on visual or other stimuli as ways to increase coping and decrease the distress from labor pain.

Other valuable tools the couple can incorporate include vocalization or "sounding" to relieve tension during pregnancy and labor, subdued lighting, warm water for showers or bathing during labor, and aromatherapy (Burns & Blamey, 1994). Some hospitals have added jacuzzi bathtubs to good effect (see Fig. 20-4). Childbearing couples are also taught to recognize labor's start and to practice coping skills such as relaxation, slow breathing, and other nonpharmacologic strategies.

Relaxation

Relaxation is a technique promoted by the three major childbirth education organizations: ICEA, Lamaze International, and AAHCC. The relaxation response counters

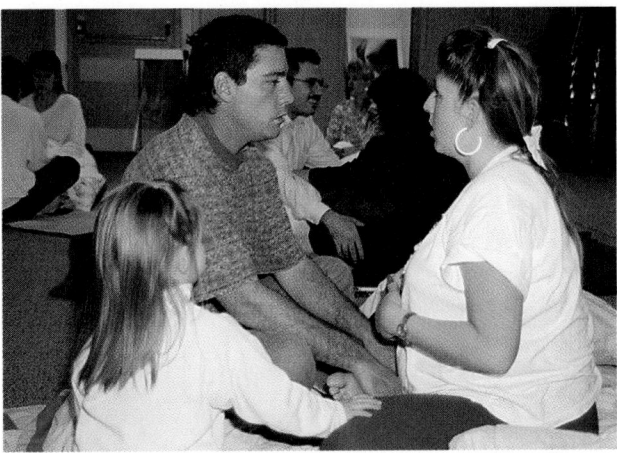

Fig. 18-3 Learning relaxation exercises with the whole family. (Courtesy Marjorie Pyle, RNC, Lifecircle, Costa Mesa, CA.)

the effects of sympathetic nervous system arousal. It also produces a balance between the sympathetic and parasympathetic systems, slows heart and breathing rates, increases uterine contractility, and produces a sense of security and tranquillity. Learning relaxation in childbirth education classes can help couples with the stresses of pregnancy, labor and birth, and adjustment to parenting and can be a form of stress management throughout life (Fig. 18-3). To be effective, varied relaxation techniques must be incorporated into every class session. When couples work together to learn relaxation, they also increase communication skills. For example, through massage with a light touch to encourage relaxation, they learn to give each other positive reinforcement and enhance their sense of being a team. The following are types of relaxation taught.

Paced Breathing

Paced breathing is the technique most associated with prepared childbirth. The Lamaze International, ICEA, and Bradley methods all encourage the couple to use breathing and relaxation patterns that work best for them. The Lamaze method involves a slow-paced, modified, and patterned breathing technique with the understanding that each labor is different and couples need to adapt breathing techniques to their individual birth experience (see Box 20-1). Nurses must be experienced in guiding couples in the application of breathing and relaxation methods during labor, adapting methods to their particular needs, and using pushing techniques for birth that avoid a Valsalva response. Such techniques often involve moaning or other noise as women push without holding their breath.

Biofeedback

Informal biofeedback helps couples develop awareness of their bodies and learn strategies to change their responses to stress. In other words, if the woman responds to pain during a contraction with tightening muscles, frowning, moaning, and breath holding, her partner uses verbal and touch feedback to help her relax (Alexander & Steeful, 1995). The electronic fetal monitor can also be a tool to help the woman know when a contraction is starting, when the peak is over, and when the contraction has eased so that she can maintain relaxation through all phases of the contraction.

Formal biofeedback, which uses machines to detect skin temperature, blood flow, or muscle tension, can also prepare women to intensify their relaxation response. With feedback from such machines, women learn to develop progressively more relaxed states and can then achieve a more relaxed state during labor.

Therapeutic Touch

Therapeutic touch is used during labor to decrease anxiety and pain and increase relaxation. Therapeutic touch requires a subjective, intuitive approach and may be taught by having the partners first experience their own energy field between their palms. They then learn the phases of centering, assessing differences of energy flow across the body, unruffling the field, and directing energy (usually over the uterus or back) to restore harmony (Mackey, 1995).

Other

Acupressure, which consists of applying pressure to various pressure points, has been correlated with relief of dizziness, headaches, back pain, leg cramps, and labor pain (Jimenez, 1992). In studies of the use of acupressure wristbands for relief of nausea in early pregnancy, researchers have reported success in treating nausea and vomiting (Belluomini et al., 1994). However, other studies report no medical benefit (O'Brien, Relyea, & Taerum, 1996).

Imagery and visualization may also be taught during preparation for birth. Although research on their use is scant, clinical reports suggest that imagery and visualization can be used to produce a sense of well-being during pregnancy, assist with cervical dilation, and decrease the experience of pain and tension during labor. Imagery involves techniques such as imagining a walk through a restful garden or breathing in light, energy, and healing color and breathing out worries and tension (Hoffart & Pross-Keene, 1998). The woman also can be taught to transform the throbbing or sensation of pain during a contraction into a pleasant, warm feeling while visualizing cervical dilation during labor (Cassidy, 1993).

Music promotes relaxation and has been known for centuries to be therapeutic. Research supports the use of music for enhancing relaxation and reducing pain responses during childbirth (Wiand, 1997). Couples who use music as a strategy often integrate it with other techniques during labor.

PROMOTING WELLNESS AND FAMILY HEALTH THROUGH EDUCATION

In addition to preparing families for childbirth, childbirth educators also promote wellness. Pregnancy is a time of growth during which most couples are open to making changes in lifestyle and habits. Information on infant care, feeding and stimulation, and couple and family adjustments are also incorporated into many prenatal classes (see Guidelines/Guías box).

Prenatal/Postnatal Nutrition and Lifestyle Management

Because most families anticipating a birth are motivated to have a healthy baby, childbirth instructors can promote good nutrition and avoidance of smoking, drinking, and taking of street drugs. Having women keep a 24-hour diet and lifestyle history and choosing foods for meals for a day from a menu and then comparing their choices with recommended foods for pregnancy are ways to stimulate healthy pregnancy choices. Pregnant women need to know expected weight gain guidelines and the way the weight gain is distributed (see Figs. 16-3 and 16-4). Expectant fathers or partners can be encouraged to help women make healthy choices for meals and snacks and can model healthy lifestyles by avoiding smoking, drugs, and alcohol during the pregnancy.

Couple Relationship and Sexuality

Pregnancy is a time when the couple relationship can be strengthened or stressed. Pregnancy, birth, and parenthood are major developmental tasks that move the couple from being a family of two to becoming a family of three. In addition to the physical changes during pregnancy, the pregnant woman and her partner face significant emotional, social, and cognitive changes. Expectant fathers or male partners often experience weight gain and nausea. They may be concerned about finances, their role as a father, sexuality, and the child's effect on the couple's relationship. Fathers or partners often worry about their role during childbirth classes and labor and birth, as well as the safety of their partner and baby during the birth. Female partners may have the same concerns, although research on lesbian partners is lacking. Both the pregnant woman and her partner need an assessment of the symptoms and changes they are experiencing and their individual coping styles. Helping couples acknowledge the many changes they are experiencing and teaching them exercises and skills to keep the lines of communication open enhance the couple's relationship.

Infant Care and Feeding

Childbearing couples who have grown up in large families or have had exposure to infants from babysitting or careers in nursing, early childhood, or medicine may be aware of the care and feeding demands of a newborn. Many couples, however, express concern about infant care and feeding techniques (Shoham-Yakubovich, Pliskin, & Carr, 1990). Although many women have already chosen a method of feeding by the third trimester, classes provide an opportunity to inform couples of the advantages and disadvantages of bottle feeding and breastfeeding, the basic techniques of each, and resources for support or information once they are home with the baby. Childbirth educators also have an opportunity to introduce issues such as the effect of disposable diapers on the environment with new families (Holaday et al., 1995). Many communities now have support or new parents' groups that are helpful to couples making the transition to parenthood. Besides the routine mother-baby classes after birth, some organizations have begun to offer father-baby classes in which new fathers spend time with their babies and a nurse educator learning about babies' unique characteristics and the basics of infant care. Fathers introduced to their newborns through the Brazelton assessment scale seem to become more aware of their infants' abilities, which sets the stage for interaction (Beal, 1989).

Infant Stimulation and Massage

Many parents still have outdated beliefs about their infants' capabilities, such as believing that babies do not see and hear until 4 to 6 weeks of age, much like newborn kittens and puppies. Because the senses are the primary source of information for babies during the first 6 months of life, childbirth educators can help parents acquire the knowledge to facilitate successful parenting (Broussard & Rich, 1990). For example, infant massage is one technique that expectant parents can learn to soothe and comfort the infant, promote relaxation and less irritability and crying, and provide a mechanism for positive interaction between parents and infants (see Chapter 25).

Family Adjustments to Parenthood

The addition of a baby brings change to all members of the family. The workload increases significantly as parents add the demands of the new infant to their other responsibilities. Childbirth educators help expectant parents anticipate these changes. One example involves working through the family workload exercise, in which parents project the way they will divide their responsibilities after birth (Starn, 1991).

Because both partners often work outside the home, a discussion about negotiating maternity and paternity leaves and plans for returning to work is important. Couples who do not have family or friends available for child care must find competent child care providers. Classes on the way to select licensed child care providers and federal and state guidelines regarding rights to maternity and paternity leaves are important sources of information. Couples also need information about the intensity and length of emotional and physiologic recovery from childbirth and the demands of adapting to parenthood. This knowledge should lead to more realistic planning for household help during the early days or weeks and more appropriate expectations of when women are typically ready to return to work.

Siblings and grandparents also experience transitions when a new baby enters the family. Parents need to know about sibling regression and ways to help older children adapt to a new brother or sister. Sibling classes that offer a tour of the birthing unit, show a birth film, and help the

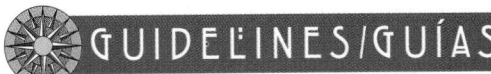

GUIDELINES/GUÍAS

Childbirth Education—General Advice

Go to childbirth education classes.
Vaya a clases prenatales.

Do preparatory exercises for labor.
Haga ejercicios preparatorios para el parto.

Avoid strenuous exercise.
Evite los ejercicios fuertes.

Sexual activity is normal during pregnancy.
La actividad sexual es normal durante el embarazo.

It is not harmful to your baby.
No hará daño a su bebé.

You may experience an increase or a decrease in your sexual interest.
Usted puede experimentar un aumento o una disminución de su interés sexual.

Rest as much as possible.
Descanse mucho.

Try to sleep 8 hours a night.
Trate de dormir ocho horas cada noche.

Don't smoke.
No fume.

Don't drink alcoholic beverages.
No tome bebidas alcohólicas.

Don't take any medications without consulting your doctor.
No tome ninguna medicina sin consultar a su doctor.

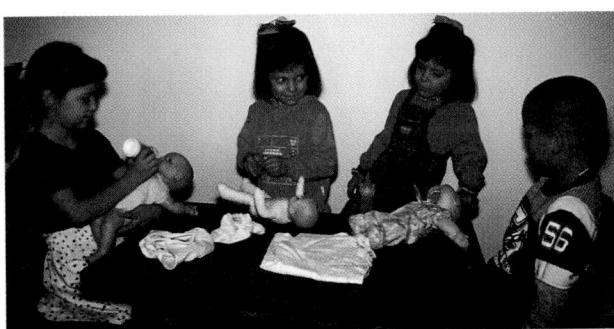

Fig. 18-4 Sibling class of preschoolers learning infant care using dolls. *(Courtesy Michael S. Clement, MD, Mesa, AZ.)*

children talk about the changes that are apt to occur, such as Mommy being busy with the baby, offer valuable interventions (Fig. 18-4). Children can also learn to cope with the adjustment to the new baby, including reduction in parental time and attention (Biasella, 1993; Spadt, Martin, & Thomas, 1990; Spero, 1993) (Box 18-4). Grandparents benefit from classes that help them learn strategies for assisting the couple's transition to parenthood. Grandparents can be a valuable asset, especially if they help with household chores and the care of older siblings and provide social support. Grandparents may be cautioned about caring for the baby instead of allowing the new parents time to develop parenting skills, criticizing the parents' caretaking, or questioning whether the baby is being adequately breastfed; these activities often undermine new parents' adjustment. Grandparents can also benefit by learning about infant stimulation and child-rearing practices that have changed since they had infants.

BOX 18-4 Tips for Sibling Preparation

PRENATAL

1. Adjust the timing and content of information about an anticipated infant to the age and understanding of the older child.
2. Take your child on a prenatal visit. Let the child listen to the fetal heartbeat and feel the baby move.
3. Involve the child in preparations for the baby, such as helping decorate the baby's room.
4. Move the child to a bed (if still sleeping in a crib) at least 2 months before the baby is due.
5. Read books, show videos, or take child to sibling preparation classes, including a hospital tour.
6. Answer your child's questions about the coming birth, what babies are like, and any other questions.
7. Take your child to the homes of friends who have babies so that the child has realistic expectations of what babies are like.

DURING THE HOSPITAL STAY

1. Have someone bring the child to the hospital to visit you and the baby (unless you plan to have the child attend the birth).
2. Don't force interactions between the child and the baby. Often the child will be more interested in seeing you and being reassured of your love.
3. Help the child explore the infant by showing how and where to touch the baby.
4. Give the child a gift (from you or from you, the father, and the baby).

GOING HOME

1. Leave the child at home with a relative or babysitter.
2. Have someone else carry the baby from the car so that you can hug the child first.

ADJUSTMENT AFTER THE BABY IS HOME

1. Arrange for a special time with the child alone with each parent.
2. Don't exclude the child during infant feeding times. The child can sit with you and the baby and feed a doll or drink juice or milk with you or sit quietly with a game.
3. Prepare small gifts for the child so that when the baby gets gifts, the sibling won't feel left out. The child can also help open the baby gifts.
4. Praise the child for acting age appropriately (so that being a baby does not seem better than being older).

KEY POINTS

- Preconception care stresses healthy behavior that promotes the health of the woman and her fetus.
- Childbirth education should be available to all pregnant women and their families in a culturally sensitive format
- Childbirth education teaches families stress and pain management strategies that enhance coping during labor and birth.
- Pain and stress management strategies are valuable family tools throughout life.
- Childbirth education strives to promote healthier pregnancies and family lifestyles.
- Childbirth education strives to support and strengthen the couple and family relationships.
- Active support during labor and birth, directed toward achieving the woman's goals, promotes personal satisfaction and adaptation to the maternal role.

CRITICAL THINKING EXERCISES

1 Role play a situation in which the nurse moderates a discussion with a woman and her husband or partner where one anticipates that an epidural will be used during labor and the other strongly advocates a "natural" birth.
2 Develop an outline for teaching a group of nonpregnant women with diabetes about preconception care.
3 Select an immigrant or other minority group and identify childbirth-related beliefs and practices that are unique. Outline ways a childbirth education program might be modified to provide essential information while incorporating cultural patterns.

References

Alden, K., & Harris, B. (1995). Choices in childbearing. In C. Fogel & N. Woods (Eds.). *Women's health care.* Thousand Oaks, CA: Sage.

Alexander, C., & Steeful, L. (1995). Biofeedback: Listen to the body. *RN* 58(8), 51-52.

American College of Obstetricians and Gynecologists. (1994). *Exercise during pregnancy and the postpartum period.* Tech Bull 189. Washington, DC: ACOG.

Bachman, J. (1993). Self-described learning needs of pregnant teen participants in an innovative university/community partnership. *Matern Child Nurs J* 21(2), 65-71.

Beal, J. (1989). The effect on father-infant interaction of demonstrating the neonatal behavioral assessment scale. *Birth* 16(1), 18-22.

Belluomini, J. et al. (1994). Acupressure for nausea and vomiting of pregnancy: A randomized, blinded study. *Obstet Gynecol* 84(2), 245-248.

Biasella, S. (1993). A comprehensive prenatal program. *AWHONNS Clin Issues Perinat Womens Health Nurs* 4(1), 5-19.

Bradley, R. (1965). *Husband-coached childbirth*. New York: HarperCollins.

Broussard, A., & Rich, S. (1990). Incorporating infant stimulation concepts into prenatal classes. *J Obstet Gynecol Neonatal Nurs* 19(5), 381-387.

Burns, E., & Blamey, C. (1994). Complementary medicine: Using aromatherapy in childbirth. *Nurs Times* 90(9), 54-60.

Capitulo, K. (1998). The rise, fall, and rise of nurse-midwifery in America. *MCN Am J Matern Child Nurs* 23(6), 314-321.

Cassidy, J. (1993). A picture perfect birth: Guided imagery interrupts the pain/anxiety cycle. *RN* 56(6), 45-46.

Cefalo, R., & Moos, M. (1995). *Preconceptional health care*. St. Louis: Mosby.

Centers for Disease Control and Prevention. (1992). Recommendation for use of folic acid to reduce numbers of spina bifida cases and other neural tube defects. *MMWR* 41(RR), 14.

Dick-Read, G. (1987). *Childbirth without fear* (5th ed.). New York: Harper & Collins.

Doulas of North America. (1999a). Do I need a doula? [On-line]. Available URL: www.dona.com.faq.html.

Doulas of North America (1999b). Doulas of North America position paper: The doula's contribution to modern maternity care [On-line]. Available URL: www.dona.com/positionpapers.html.

Doulas of North America (1999c). Mission statement [On-line]. Available URL: www.dona.com/mission.html.

Frede, D. (1993). Preconceptional education. *AWHONNS Clin Issues Perinat Womens Health Nurs* 4(1), 60-65.

Hetherington, S. (1990). A controlled study of the effect of prepared childbirth classes on obstetric outcome. *Birth* 17(2), 86-90.

Hoffart, M., & Pross-Keene, E. (1998). The benefits of visualization. *Am J Nurs* 98(12), 44-47.

Holaday, B. et al. (1995). Fecal contamination in child day care centers: Cloth vs paper diapers. *Am J Public Health* 85(1), 30-33.

Jimenez, S. (1992). Teaching acupressure for pregnancy and birth. *J Patient Education* 11(1), 58-63.

Jones, C. (1991). *Alternative birth: The complete guide*. Los Angeles: Jeremy P. Tarcher.

Klaus, M., & Kennell, J. (1997). The doula: An essential ingredient of childbirth rediscovered. *Acta Paediatr* 86, 1034-1036.

Lamaze, F. (1970). *Painless childbirth: The Lamaze method*. Chicago: Regnery Books.

Lamaze International. (1999a). About Lamaze International, Inc. [On-line]. Available URL: www.lamazechildbirth.com/fact_sheet.html.

Lamaze International. (1999b). Lamaze certified childbirth educator (LCCE) program [On-line]. Available URL: www.lamazechildbirth.com.

Lewallen, L. (1989). Health beliefs and health practices of pregnant women. *J Obstet Gynecol Neonatal Nurs* 18(3), 245-246.

Lindell, S. (1988). Education for childbirth: A time for change. *J Obstet Gynecol Neonatal Nurs* 17(2), 108-112.

Mackey, M. (1990). Women's choices of childbirth settings. *Health Care Women Int* 11(2), 175-189.

Mackey, R. (1995). Discovering the healing power of therapeutic touch. *Am J Nurs* 95(4), 26-32.

Manning-Orenstein, G. (1998). A birth intervention: The therapeutic effects of doula support versus Lamaze preparation on first-time mothers' working models of caregiving. *Alternative Therapies in Health and Medicine* 4(4), 73-81.

March of Dimes. (1995). *Prepregnancy planning, Public Health Education Information Sheet*. White Plains, NY: March of Dimes.

National Center for Health Statistics. (1998). Advance report of final natality statistics, 1996. *Monthly Vital Statistics Report* 46(11 suppl),

Nichols, F., & Humenick, A. (1988). *Childbirth education: Practice, research and theory*. Philadelphia: W.B. Saunders.

O'Brien, B., Relyea, M., & Taerum, T. (1996). Efficacy of P6 acupressure in the treatment of nausea and vomiting during pregnancy. *Am J Obstet Gynecol* 174(2), 708-715.

Peterson, G. (1991). *An easier childbirth: A mother's workbook for health and emotional well-being during pregnancy and delivery*. Los Angeles: Jeremy P. Tarcher.

Pitcock, C., & Clark, R. (1992). From Fanny to Fernand: The development of consumerism in pain control during the birth process. *Am J Obstet Gynecol* 167(3), 581-587.

Pletsch, P. (1990). Birth defect prevention: Nursing interventions. *J Obstet Gynecol Neonatal Nurs* 19(6), 482-488.

Public Health Service. (1988). *Caring for our future: The content of prenatal care*. Washington, DC: Department of Health and Human Services.

Ratts, V. (1993). Women and exercise: Effects of the reproductive system. *Female Patient* 18(7), 59.

Riesch, S. (1988). Changes in the exercise of self-care agency. *West J Nurs Res* 10(3), 257-273.

Scherger, J. (1993). Preconception care: A neglected element of prenatal services. *Female Patient* 18(7), 78.

Shoham-Yakubovich, I., Pliskin, J., & Carr, D. (1990). Infant feeding practices: An evaluation of the impact of a health education course. *Am J Public Health* 80(6), 732-734.

Simkin, P. (1995). Reducing pain and enhancing progress in labor: A guide to nonpharmacologic methods of maternity caregivers. *Birth* 22(3), 161-171.

Simkin, P., & Way, K. (1998). *DONA position paper: The doula's contributions to modern maternity care*. Seattle, WA: Doulas of North America.

Slager-Earnest, S. et al. (1987). Effects of a specialized prenatal adolescent program on maternal and infant outcomes. *J Obstet Gynecol Neonatal Nurs* 16(6), 422-429.

Spadt, S., Martin, K., & Thomas, A. (1990). Experiential classes for siblings-to-be. *MCN Am J Matern Child Nurs* 15(3), 184-186.

Spero, D. (1993). Sibling preparation classes. *AWHONNS Clin Issues Perinat Womens Health Nurs* 4(1), 122-131.

Starn, J. (1991). Childbirth classroom: Labor after birth. *Childbirth Instructor* 1, 27.

Sturrock, W., & Johnson, J. (1990). The relationship between childbirth education classes and obstetric outcome. *Birth* 17(2), 82-85.

USDA and USDHHS. (1990). *Cross-cultural counseling: A guide for nutrition and health counselors*. Washington, DC: US Government Printing Office.

Waxler-Morrison, N., Anderson, J., & Richardson, E. (Eds.). (1990). *Cross-cultural nursing*. Vancouver, Canada: University of British Columbia Press.

Werler, M., Shipiro, S., & Mitchell, A. (1993). Periconceptional folic acid exposure and risk of occurrent neural tube defects. *JAMA* 269(10), 1257-1261.

Wertz, R., & Wertz, D. (1979). *Lying in: A history of childbirth in America*. New York: Schoder.

Wiand, N. (1997). Relaxation levels achieved by Lamaze-trained pregnant women listening to music and ocean sound tapes. *J Perinatal Education* 6(4), 1-8.

Wilberg, G. (1992). *Preparing for birth and parenthood: An awareness training and teaching manual for childbirth professionals*. Boston: Butterworth-Heinemann.

19

Labor and Birth Processes

Deitra Leonard Lowdermilk

LEARNING OBJECTIVES

- Define the key terms.
- Explain the five factors that affect the labor process.
- Describe the anatomic structure of the bony pelvis.
- Recognize the normal measurements of the diameters of the pelvic inlet, cavity, and outlet.
- Review the anatomy and the normal measurements of the fetal skull.

- Explain the significance of molding of the fetal head during labor.
- Describe the cardinal movements of the mechanism of labor.
- Assess the maternal anatomic and physiologic adaptations to labor.
- Describe fetal adaptations to labor.
- Identify topics for nursing research related to factors that affect the labor process.

KEY TERMS

asynclitism
attitude
biparietal diameter
bloody show
breech presentation
cephalic presentation
dilation
effacement
engagement

Ferguson reflex
fontanels
gynecoid pelvis
labor
lie
lightening
mechanism of labor
molding
position

presentation
presenting part
shoulder presentation
station
suboccipitobregmatic diameter
Valsalva maneuver
vertex

During late pregnancy, the woman and fetus prepare for the labor process. The fetus has grown and developed in preparation for extrauterine life. The woman has undergone various physiologic adaptations during pregnancy that prepare her for birth and motherhood. Labor and birth represent the end of pregnancy, the beginning of extrauterine life for the newborn, and a change in the lives of the family.

This chapter discusses the factors affecting labor, the process involved, the normal progression of events, and the adaptations made by both the woman and fetus. This information will provide the theory base necessary for care of the laboring woman and her family.

FACTORS AFFECTING LABOR

At least five factors affect the process of labor and birth. These are easily remembered as the five *P*'s: passenger (fetus and placenta), passageway (birth canal), powers (con-

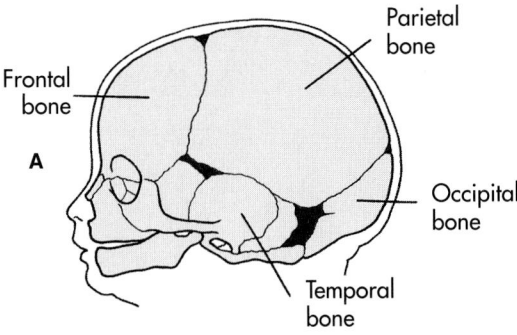

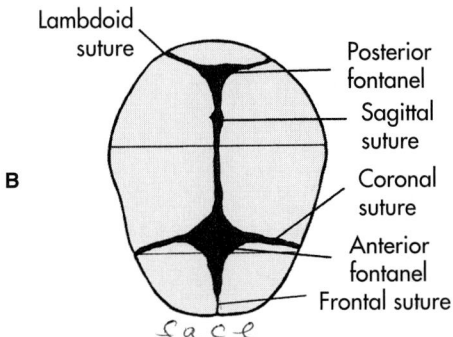

Fig. 19-1 Fetal head at term. **A,** Bones. **B,** Sutures and fontanels.

RESEARCH

The Essential Forces of Labor Revisited

Understanding the factors affecting labor progress is necessary to provide nursing care during labor. The essential forces (the 3 *P*'s) of powers (contractions), passageway (pelvis), and passenger (fetus) were first described in 1950. Later research added two more factors: position and psychologic factors. However, factors that may be part of the woman's experience and the context in which it occurred have not been identified.

The purpose of this qualitative descriptive study was to analyze birth narratives to identify factors reported by women as having exerted control during their labors. Narratives of 15 women reporting on 33 births were transcribed, and thematic and content analyses were done.

Thirteen forces (13 *P*'s) were identified, including the 5 *P*'s described in earlier research. Place of birth, preparation, professional provider, and procedures were identified as external forces. Physiology (sensations) was the only other internal force identified that was not one of the 5 *P*'s. Nurses (professional provider) were identified as having a profound impact during labor. Further research investigating essential forces of labor is recommended.

CLINICAL APPLICATION

The practice of maternity nursing can be improved by adding knowledge of the other essential forces in labor. Nurses can combine this understanding with their skills of observation, communication, and caring to provide more individualized, culturally competent care. By understanding the women's views about what impacts the labor experience, nurses can also help women and their families have a positive birth experience. ∎

Source: VandeVusse, L. (1999). The essential forces of labor revisited: 13 *P*'s reported in women's birth stories. *MCN Am J Matern Child Nurs* 24(4), 176-184.

tractions), position of the mother, and psychologic response. The first four factors are presented here as the basis of understanding the physiologic process of labor. The fifth factor is discussed in Chapter 22. Other factors may be important as well (See Research box).

Passenger

The way the passenger, or fetus, moves through the birth canal is determined by several interacting factors: the size of the fetal head, fetal presentation, fetal lie, fetal attitude, and fetal position.

Because the placenta must also pass through the birth canal, it can be considered a passenger along with the fetus. However, the placenta rarely impedes the process of labor in normal vaginal birth.

Size of the Fetal Head

Because of its size and relative rigidity, the fetal head has a major effect on the birth process. The fetal skull is composed of two parietal bones, two temporal bones, the frontal bone, and the occipital bone (Fig. 19-1, *A*). These bones are united by membranous sutures: the sagittal, lambdoidal, coronal, and frontal (Fig. 19-1, *B*). Membrane-filled spaces called **fontanels** are located where the sutures intersect. During labor, after rupture of membranes, palpation of fontanels and sutures during vaginal examination reveals fetal presentation, position, and attitude.

The two most important fontanels are the anterior and posterior ones (see Fig. 19-1, *B*). The larger of these, the anterior fontanel, is diamond shaped, about 3 cm by 2 cm in size, and lies at the junction of the sagittal, coronal, and frontal sutures. It closes by 18 months after birth. The posterior fontanel lies at the junction of the sutures of the two parietal bones and the one occipital bone, is triangular in shape, and is about 1 cm by 2 cm in size. It closes 6 to 8 weeks after birth.

Sutures and fontanels make the skull flexible to accommodate the infant brain, which continues to grow for some time after birth. Because the bones are not firmly

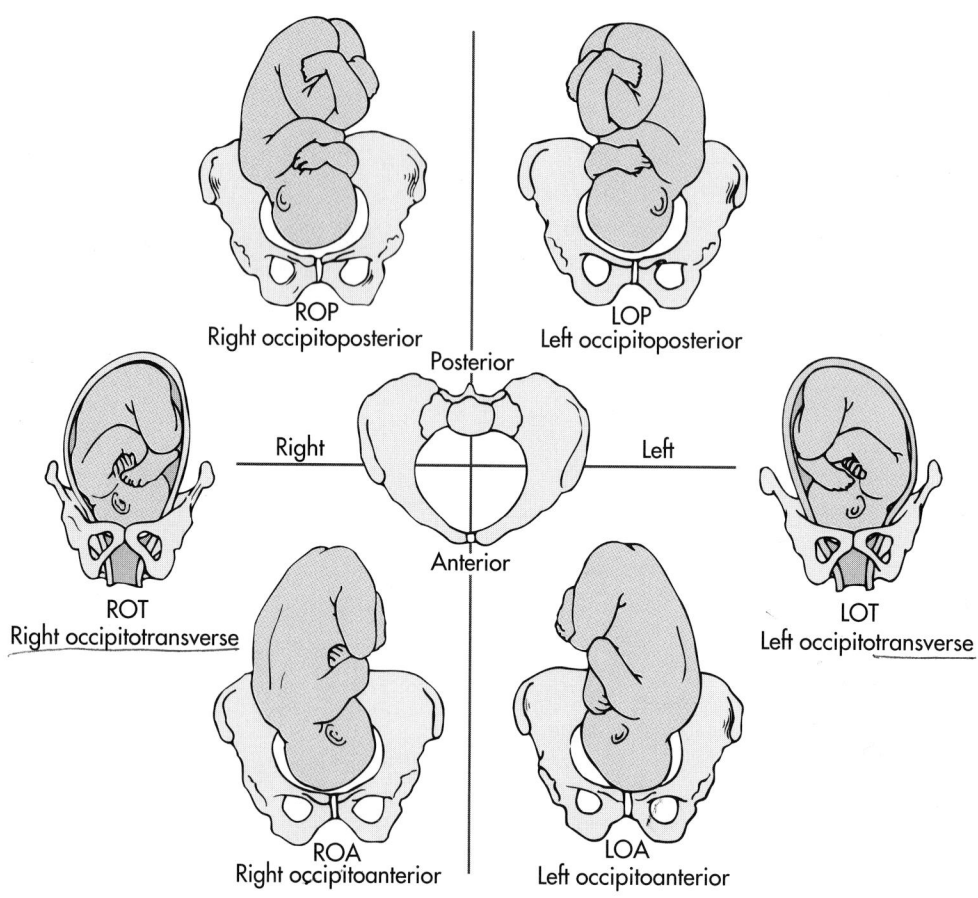

ROP
Right occipitoposterior

LOP
Left occipitoposterior

Posterior

Right

Left

Anterior

ROT
Right occipitotransverse

LOT
Left occipitotransverse

ROA
Right occipitoanterior

LOA
Left occipitoanterior

Lie: Longitudinal or vertical
Presentation: Vertex
Reference point: Occiput
Attitude: Complete flexion

Fig. 19-2 Examples of fetal vertex (occiput) presentations in relation to front, back, or side of maternal pelvis.

united, however, slight overlapping of the bones, or **molding** of the shape of the head, occurs during labor. This capacity of the bones to slide over one another also permits adaptation to the various diameters of the maternal pelvis. Molding can be extensive, but the heads of most newborns assume their normal shape within 3 days of birth.

Although the size of the fetal shoulders may affect passage, their position can be altered relatively easily during labor, so that one shoulder may occupy a lower level than the other. This creates a shoulder diameter that is smaller than the skull, facilitating passage through the birth canal. The circumference of the fetal hips is usually small enough not to create problems.

Fetal Presentation

Presentation refers to the part of the fetus that enters the pelvic inlet first and leads through the birth canal during labor at term. The three main presentations are

cephalic presentation (head first), occurring in 96% of births (Fig. 19-2); **breech presentation** (buttocks or feet first), occurring in 3% of births (Fig. 19-3, *A, B, C*); and **shoulder presentation,** seen in 1% of births (Fig. 19-3, *D*). **Presenting part** refers to that part of the fetal body first felt by the examining finger during a vaginal examination. In a cephalic presentation, the presenting part is usually the occiput; in a breech presentation, it is the sacrum; in the shoulder presentation, it is the scapula. When the presenting part is the occiput, the presentation is noted as **vertex** (see Fig. 19-2). Factors that determine the presenting part include fetal lie, fetal attitude, and extension or flexion or the fetal head.

Fetal Lie

Lie is the relationship of the long axis (spine) of the fetus to the long axis (spine) of the mother. There are two primary lies: *longitudinal,* or vertical, in which the long axis of the fetus is parallel with the long axis of the mother (see

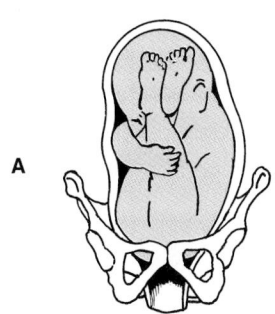

Frank breech

Lie: Longitudinal or vertical
Presentation: Breech (incomplete)
Presenting part: Sacrum
Attitude: Flexion, except for legs at knees

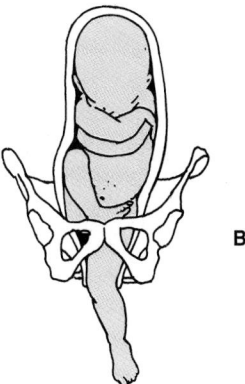

Single footling breech

Lie: Longitudinal or vertical
Presentation: Breech (incomplete)
Presenting part: Sacrum
Attitude: Flexion, except for one leg extended at hip and knee

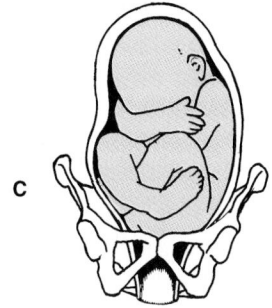

Complete breech

Lie: Longitudinal or vertical
Presentation: Breech (sacrum and feet presenting)
Presenting part: Sacrum (with feet)
Attitude: General flexion

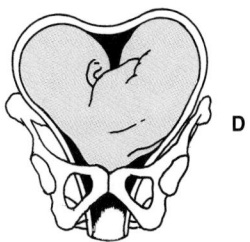

Shoulder presentation

Lie: Transverse or horizontal
Presentation: Shoulder
Presenting part: Scapula
Attitude: Flexion

Fig. 19-3 Fetal presentations. **A–C,** Breech (sacral) presentation. **D,** Shoulder presentation.

Fig. 19-2); and *transverse,* horizontal, or oblique, in which the long axis of the fetus is at a right angle diagonal to the long axis of the mother (see Fig. 19-3, *D*). Longitudinal lies are either cephalic or breech presentations, depending on the fetal structure that first enters the mother's pelvis. Vaginal birth cannot occur when the fetus stays in a transverse lie. An oblique lie is less common and usually converts to a longitudinal or transverse lie during labor (Cunningham et al., 1997).

Fetal Attitude

Attitude is the relationship of the fetal body parts to each other. The fetus assumes a characteristic posture (attitude) in utero partly because of the mode of fetal growth and partly because of the way the fetus conforms to the shape of the uterine cavity. Normally, the back of the fetus is rounded so that the chin is flexed on the chest, the thighs are flexed on the abdomen, and the legs are flexed at the knees. The arms are crossed over the thorax, and the

umbilical cord lies between the arms and the legs. This attitude is termed *general flexion* (see Fig. 19-2).

Deviations from the normal attitude may cause difficulties in childbirth. For example, in a cephalic presentation, the fetal head may be extended or flexed in a manner that presents a head diameter that exceeds the limits of the maternal pelvis, leading to prolonged labor, forceps- or vacuum-assisted birth, or cesarean birth.

Certain critical diameters of the fetal head are usually measured. The **biparietal diameter,** which is about 9.25 cm at term, is the largest transverse diameter and an important indicator of fetal head size (Fig. 19-4, *B*). In a well-flexed cephalic presentation, the biparietal diameter will be the widest part of the head entering the pelvic inlet. There are several anteroposterior diameters, but the smallest and the most critical one is the **suboccipitobregmatic diameter** (about 9.5 cm at term). When the head is in complete flexion, this diameter allows the fetal head to pass through the true pelvis easily (Fig. 19-4, *A;* Fig. 19-5, *A*). As

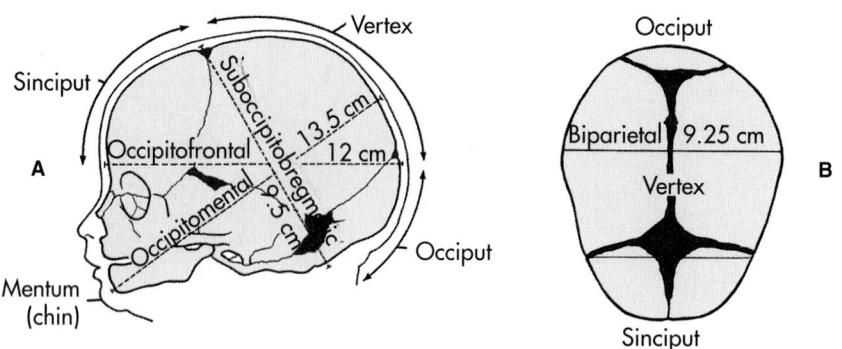

Fig. 19-4   Diameters of the fetal head at term. **A,** Cephalic presentations: occiput, vertex, and sinciput; and cephalic diameters: suboccipitobregmatic, occipitofrontal, and occipitomental. **B,** Biparietal diameter.

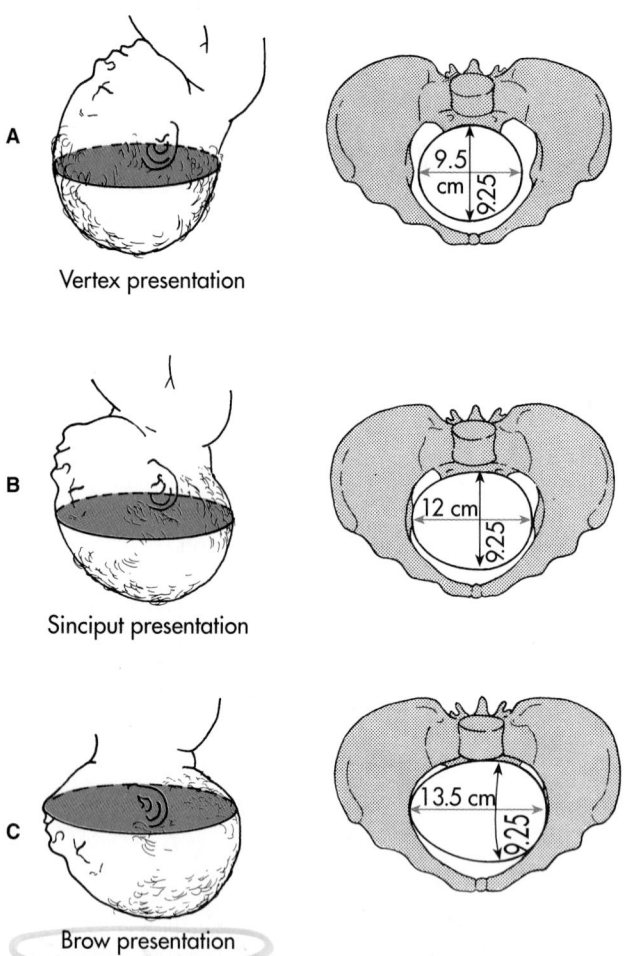

Vertex presentation

Sinciput presentation

Brow presentation

Fig. 19-5   Head entering pelvis. Biparietal diameter is indicated with shading (9.25 cm). **A,** Suboccipitobregmatic diameter: complete flexion of head on chest so that smallest diameter enters. **B,** Occipitofrontal diameter: moderate extension (military attitude) so that large diameter enters. **C,** Occipitomental diameter: marked extension (deflection) so that largest diameter, which is too large to permit head to enter pelvis, is presenting.

the head is more extended, the anteroposterior diameter widens and the head may not be able to enter the true pelvis (Fig. 19-5, *B, C*).

Fetal Position

The presentation or presenting part indicates that portion of the fetus that overlies the pelvic inlet. **Position** is the relationship of the presenting part (occiput, sacrum, mentum [chin], or sinciput [deflexed vertex]) to the four quadrants of the mother's pelvis (see Fig. 19-2). Position is denoted by a three-letter abbreviation. The first letter of the abbreviation denotes the location of the presenting part in the right (R) or left (L) side of the mother's pelvis. The middle letter stands for the specific presenting part of the fetus (O for occiput, S for sacrum, M for mentum [chin], and Sc for scapula [shoulder]). The third letter stands for the location of the presenting part in relation to the anterior (A), posterior (P), or transverse (T) portion of the maternal pelvis. For example, ROA means that the occiput is the presenting part and is located in the right anterior quadrant of the maternal pelvis (see Fig 19-2). LSP means that the sacrum is the presenting part and is located in the left posterior quadrant of the maternal pelvis (see Fig 19-3).

Station is the relationship of the presenting part of the fetus to an imaginary line drawn between the maternal ischial spines and is a measure of the degree of descent of the presenting part of the fetus through the birth canal. The placement of the presenting part is measured in centimeters above or below the ischial spines (Fig. 19-6). For example, when the lowermost portion of the presenting part is 1 cm above the spines, it is noted as being minus (−) 1. At the level of the spines, the station is referred to as 0 (zero). When the presenting part is 1 cm below the spines, the station is said to be plus (+) 1. Birth is imminent when the presenting part is at +4 to +5 cm. The station of the presenting part should be determined when labor begins so that the rate of descent of the fetus during labor can be accurately determined.

Engagement is the term used to indicate that the largest transverse diameter of the presenting part (usually the biparietal diameter) has passed through the maternal pelvic brim or inlet into the true pelvis and usually corresponds to station 0. Engagement often occurs in the weeks just be-

fore labor begins in primigravidas and may occur before labor or during labor in multigravidas. Engagement can be determined by abdominal or vaginal examination.

Passageway

The passageway, or birth canal, is composed of the mother's rigid bony pelvis and the soft tissues of the cervix, pelvic floor, vagina, and introitus (the external opening to the vagina). Although the soft tissues, particularly the muscular layers of the pelvic floor, contribute to vaginal birth of the fetus, the maternal pelvis plays a far greater role in the labor process because the fetus must successfully accommodate itself to this relatively rigid passageway. Therefore the size and shape of the pelvis must be determined before childbirth begins.

Bony Pelvis

The anatomy of the bony pelvis is described in Chapter 6. The following discussion focuses on the importance of pelvic configurations as they relate to the labor process. (It may be helpful to refer back to Fig. 6-4.)

The bony pelvis is formed by the fusion of the ilium, ischium, pubis, and sacral bones. The four pelvic joints are the symphysis pubis, the right and left sacroiliac joints, and the sacrococcygeal joint (Fig. 19-7, *A*). The bony pelvis is separated by the brim, or inlet, into two parts: the false pelvis and the true pelvis. The false pelvis is that part above the brim and plays no part in childbearing. The true pelvis, that part involved in birth, is divided into three

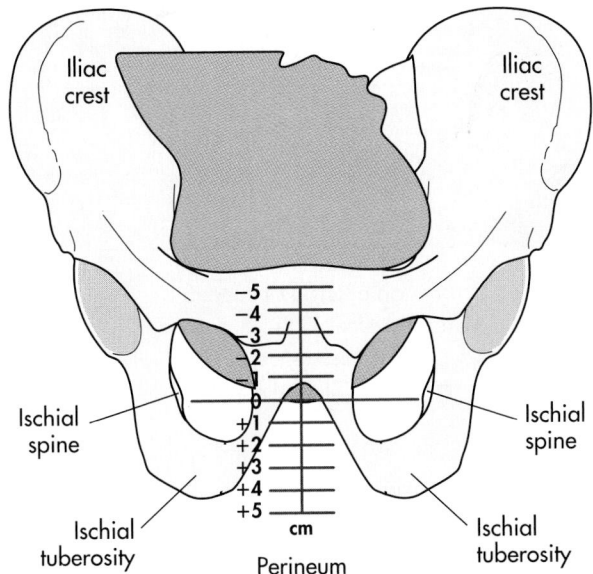

Fig. 19-6   Stations of presenting part, or degree of descent. The presenting part is just below the level of the ischial spines.

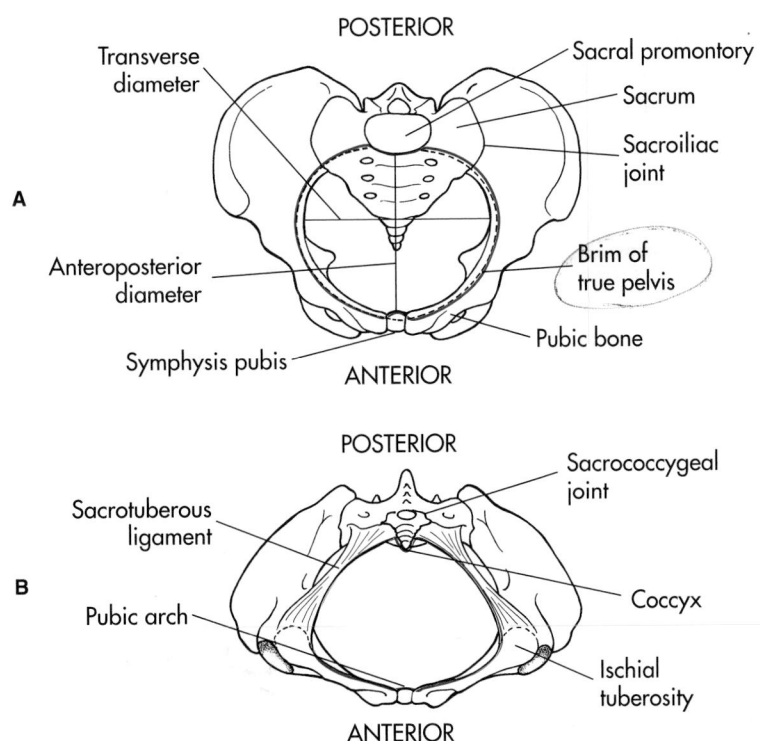

Fig. 19-7   Female pelvis. **A,** Pelvic brim above. **B,** Pelvic outlet from below.

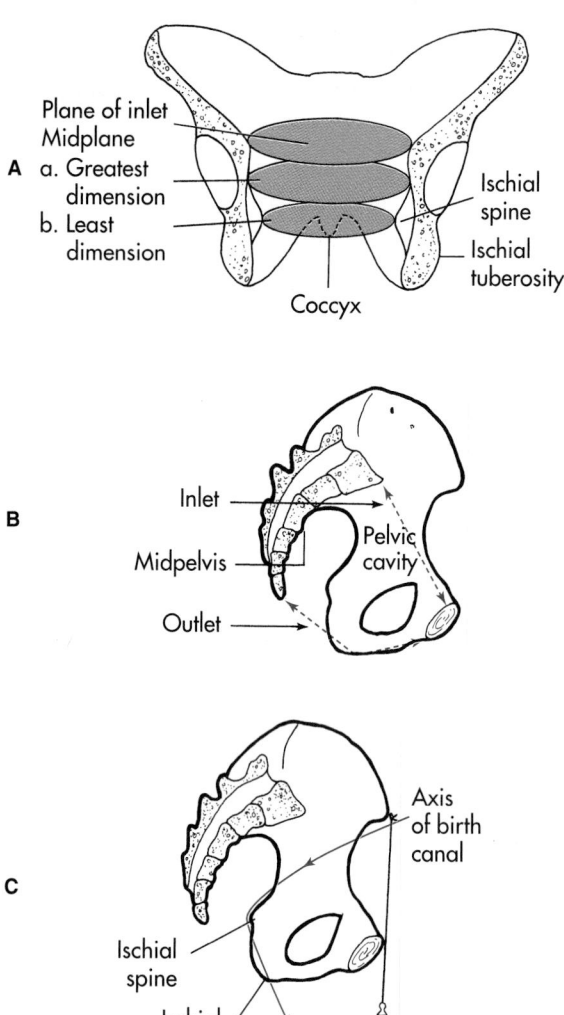

Fig. 19-8   Pelvic cavity. **A,** Inlet and midplane. Outlet now shown. **B,** Cavity of true pelvis. **C,** Note curve of sacrum and axis of birth canal.

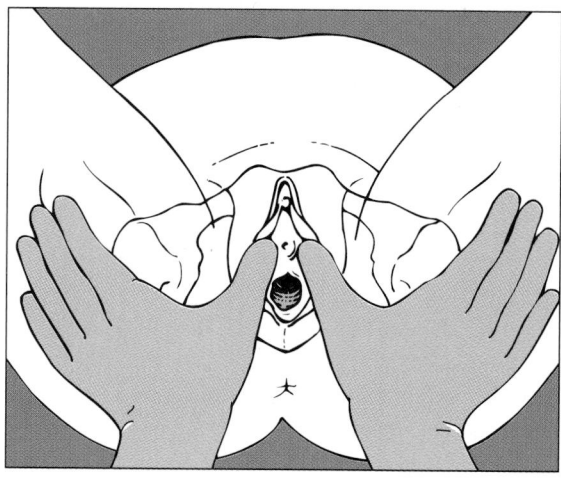

Fig. 19-9   Estimation of angle of subpubic arch. Using both thumbs, examiner externally traces descending rami down to tuberosities. *(From Barkauskas, V. et al. [1998]. Health and physical assessment [2nd ed.]. St. Louis: Mosby.)*

planes: the inlet, or brim; the midpelvis, or cavity; and the outlet.

The pelvic inlet, which is the upper border of the true pelvis, is formed anteriorly by the upper margins of the pubic bone, laterally by the iliopectineal lines along the innominate bones, and posteriorly by the anterior, upper margin of the sacrum and the sacral promontory.

The pelvic cavity, or midpelvis, is a curved passage having a short anterior wall and a much longer concave posterior wall. It is bounded by the posterior aspect of the symphysis pubis, the ischium, a portion of the ilium, the sacrum, and the coccyx.

The pelvic outlet is the lower border of the true pelvis. Viewed from below, it is ovoid, somewhat diamond shaped, bounded by the pubic arch anteriorly, the ischial tuberosities laterally, and the tip of the coccyx posteriorly (Fig. 19-7, *B*). In the latter part of pregnancy the coccyx is movable (un-

less it has been broken in a fall during skiing or skating, for example, and has fused to the sacrum during healing).

The pelvic canal varies in size and shape at various levels. The diameters at the plane of the pelvic inlet, midpelvis, and outlet, plus the axis of the birth canal (Fig. 19-8), determine whether vaginal birth is possible and the manner by which the fetus may pass down the birth canal.

The subpubic angle, which determines the type of pubic arch, together with the length of the pubic rami and the intertuberous diameter, is of great importance. Because the fetus must first pass beneath the pubic arch, a narrow subpubic angle will be less accommodating than a rounded wide arch. The method of measurement of the subpubic arch is shown in Fig. 19-9. A summary of obstetric measurements is given in Table 19-1.

The four basic types of pelvis are classified as follows:
1. Gynecoid (the classic female type)
2. Android (resembling the male pelvis)
3. Anthropoid (resembling the pelvis of anthropoid apes)
4. Platypelloid (the flat pelvis).

The **gynecoid pelvis** is the most common, with major gynecoid pelvic features present in 50% of all women. Anthropoid and android features are less common, and platypelloid pelvic features are the least common. Mixed types of pelves are more common than pure types (Cunningham et al., 1997). Examples of pelvic variations and their effects on mode of birth are given in Table 19-2.

Assessment of the bony pelvis can be performed during the first prenatal evaluation and need not be repeated if the pelvis is of adequate size and suitable shape. In the third trimester of pregnancy, the examination of the bony pelvis may be more thorough and the results more accurate because there is relaxation and increased mobility of the pelvic joints and ligaments due to hormonal influences. Widening

■ TABLE 19-1 **Obstetric Measurements**

PLANE	DIAMETER	MEASUREMENTS

Inlet (superior strait)
  Conjugates
    Diagonal
    Obstetric: measurement that
      determines whether presenting part
      can engage or enter superior strait
    True (vera) (anteroposterior)
	12.5-13 cm
	1.5-2 cm less than diagonal
	  (radiographic)
	
	≥11 cm (12.5) (radiographic)
		
		Length of diagonal conjugate (solid colored line), obstetric conjugate (broken colored line), and true conjugate (black line)*

Midplane
  Transverse diameter
    (interspinous diameter)
  The midplane of the pelvis normally
    is its largest plane and the one of
    greatest diameter.
	10.5 cm	
		Measurement of interspinous diameter*

Outlet
  Transverse diameter (intertuberous
    diameter) (biischial)
  The outlet presents the smallest
    plane of the pelvic canal.
	≥8 cm	
		Use of Thom's pelvimeter to measure intertuberous diameter*

*From Seidel, H. et al. (1999). *Mosby's guide to physical examination* (4th ed.). St. Louis: Mosby.

of the joint of the symphysis pubis and the resulting instability may cause pain in any or all of the pelvic joints.

Because the examiner does not have direct access to the bony structures and because the bones are covered with varying amounts of soft tissue, estimates of size and shape are approximate. Precise bony pelvis measurements can be determined by use of computed tomography, ultrasound, or x-ray films. However, x-ray examination is rarely done during pregnancy because the x-rays may damage the developing fetus.

TABLE 19-2 Comparison of Pelvic Types

	GYNECOID (50% OF WOMEN)	ANDROID (23% OF WOMEN)	ANTHROPOID (24% OF WOMEN)	PLATYPELLOID (3% OF WOMEN)
Brim	Slightly ovoid or transversely rounded	Heart shaped, angulated	Oval, wider anteroposteriorly	Flattened anteroposteriorly, wide transversely
	◯ Round	♡ Heart	⬭ Oval	⬭ Flat
Depth	Moderate	Deep	Deep	Shallow
Side walls	Straight	Convergent	Straight	Straight
Ischial spines	Blunt, somewhat widely separated	Prominent, narrow interspinous diameter	Prominent, often with narrow interspinous diameter	Blunted, widely separated
Sacrum	Deep, curved	Slightly curved, terminal portion often beaked	Slightly curved	Slightly curved
Subpubic arch	Wide	Narrow	Narrow	Wide
Usual mode of birth	Vaginal Spontaneous Occipitoanterior position	Cesarean Vaginal Difficult with forceps	Forceps/spontaneous occipitoposterior or occipitoanterior position	Vaginal spontaneous

Soft Tissues

The soft tissues of the passageway include the distensible lower uterine segment, cervix, pelvic floor muscles, vagina, and introitus (external opening to the vagina). Before labor begins, the uterus is composed of the uterine body (corpus) and cervix (neck). After labor has begun, uterine contractions cause the uterine body to have a thick and muscular upper segment and a thin-walled, passive, muscular lower segment. A physiologic retraction ring separates the two segments (Fig. 19-10). The lower uterine segment gradually distends to accommodate the intrauterine contents as the wall of the upper segment thickens and its accommodating capacity is reduced. The contractions of the uterine body thus exert downward pressure on the fetus, pushing it against the cervix.

The cervix effaces (thins) and dilates (opens) sufficiently to allow the first fetal portion to descend into the vagina. As the fetus descends, the cervix is actually drawn upward and over this first portion.

The pelvic floor is a muscular layer that separates the pelvic cavity above from the perineal space below. This structure helps the fetus rotate anteriorly as it passes through the birth canal. As noted earlier, the soft tissues of the vagina develop throughout pregnancy until at term the vagina can dilate to accommodate the fetus and permit passage of the fetus to the external world.

Powers

Involuntary and voluntary powers combine to expel the fetus and the placenta from the uterus. Involuntary uterine contractions, called the *primary powers*, signal the beginning of labor. Once the cervix has dilated, voluntary bearing-down efforts by the woman, called the *secondary powers*, augment the force of the involuntary contractions.

Primary Powers

The involuntary contractions originate at certain pacemaker points in the thickened muscle layers of the upper uterine segment. From the pacemaker points, contractions move downward over the uterus in waves, separated by short rest periods. Terms used to describe these involuntary contractions include *frequency* (the time from the beginning of one contraction to the beginning of the next), *duration* (length of contraction), and *intensity* (strength of contraction).

The primary powers are responsible for the effacement and dilation of the cervix and descent of the fetus. **Effacement** of the cervix means the shortening and thinning of the cervix during the first stage of labor. The cervix, normally 2 to 3 cm long and about 1 cm thick, is obliterated or "taken up" by a shortening of the uterine muscle bundles during the thinning of the lower uterine segment that occurs in advancing labor. Only a thin edge of the cervix can be palpated when effacement is complete. Effacement generally is advanced in first-time term pregnancy before more than slight dilation occurs. In subsequent pregnancies, effacement and dilation of the cervix tend to progress together. Degree of effacement is expressed in percentages from 0% to 100% (e.g., a cervix is 50% effaced) (Fig. 19-11, *A, B, C*).

Dilation of the cervix is the enlargement or widening of the cervical opening and the cervical canal that occurs once labor has begun. The diameter of the cervix increases from less than 1 cm to full dilation (approximately 10 cm)

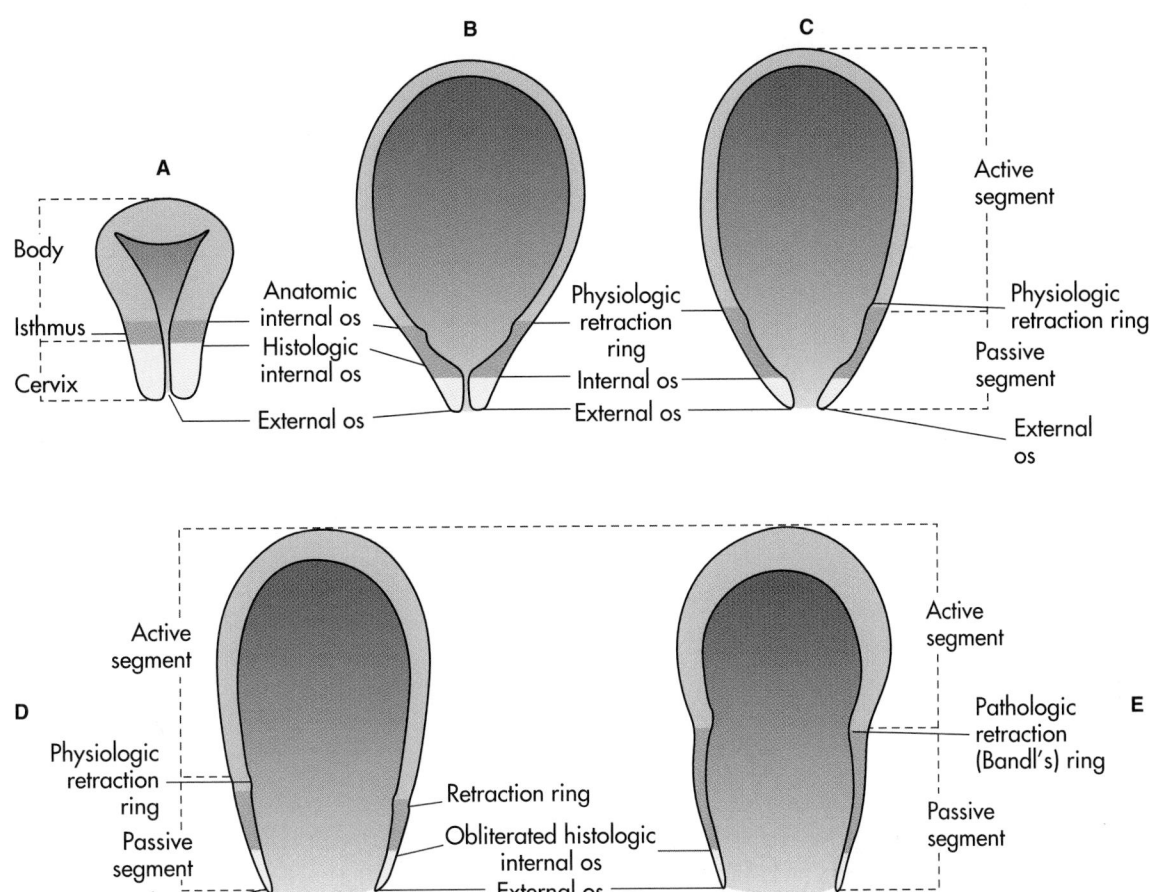

Fig. 19-10 Progressive development of segments and rings of uterus at term. Note differences in **A,** nonpregnant uterus, **B,** uterus at term, **C,** uterus in normal labor in early first stage, and **D,** in second stage. Passive segment is derived from lower uterine segment (isthmus) and cervix, and physiologic retraction ring is derived from anatomic internal os. **E,** Uterus in abnormal labor in second-stage dystocia. Pathologic retraction (Bandl's) ring that forms under abnormal conditions develops from the physiologic ring. *(Modified from Willson, J., & Carrington, E. [1991]. Obstetrics and gynecology [9th ed.]. St. Louis: Mosby.)*

to allow birth of a term fetus. When the cervix is fully dilated (and completely retracted), it can no longer be palpated (Fig. 19-11, *D*). Full cervical dilation marks the end of the first stage of labor.

Dilation of the cervix occurs by the drawing upward of the musculofibrous components of the cervix that is caused by strong uterine contractions. Pressure exerted by the amniotic fluid while the membranes are intact or by the force applied by the presenting part also can promote cervical dilation. Scarring of the cervix as a result of prior infection or surgery may slow cervical dilation.

In the first and second stages of labor, increased intrauterine pressure caused by contractions exerts pressure on the descending fetus and the cervix. When the presenting part of the fetus reaches the perineal floor, mechanical stretching of the cervix occurs. Stretch receptors in the posterior vagina cause release of endogenous oxytocin that triggers the maternal urge to bear down, or the **Ferguson reflex.**

Uterine contractions are usually independent from external forces. For example, laboring women who are paraplegic will have normal but painless uterine contractions (Cunningham et al., 1997). Uterine contractions may decrease temporarily in frequency and intensity if narcotic analgesic medication or epidural analgesia is given early in labor (Alexander et al., 1998). The exact relationship between prolonged labor and epidural analgesia continues to be investigated (Thompson et al., 1998).

Secondary Powers

As soon as the presenting part reaches the pelvic floor the contractions change in character and become expulsive. The laboring woman experiences an involuntary urge to push. She uses secondary powers (bearing-down efforts) to aid in expulsion of the fetus as she contracts her diaphragm and abdominal muscles and pushes. These bearing-down efforts result in increased intraabdominal pressure

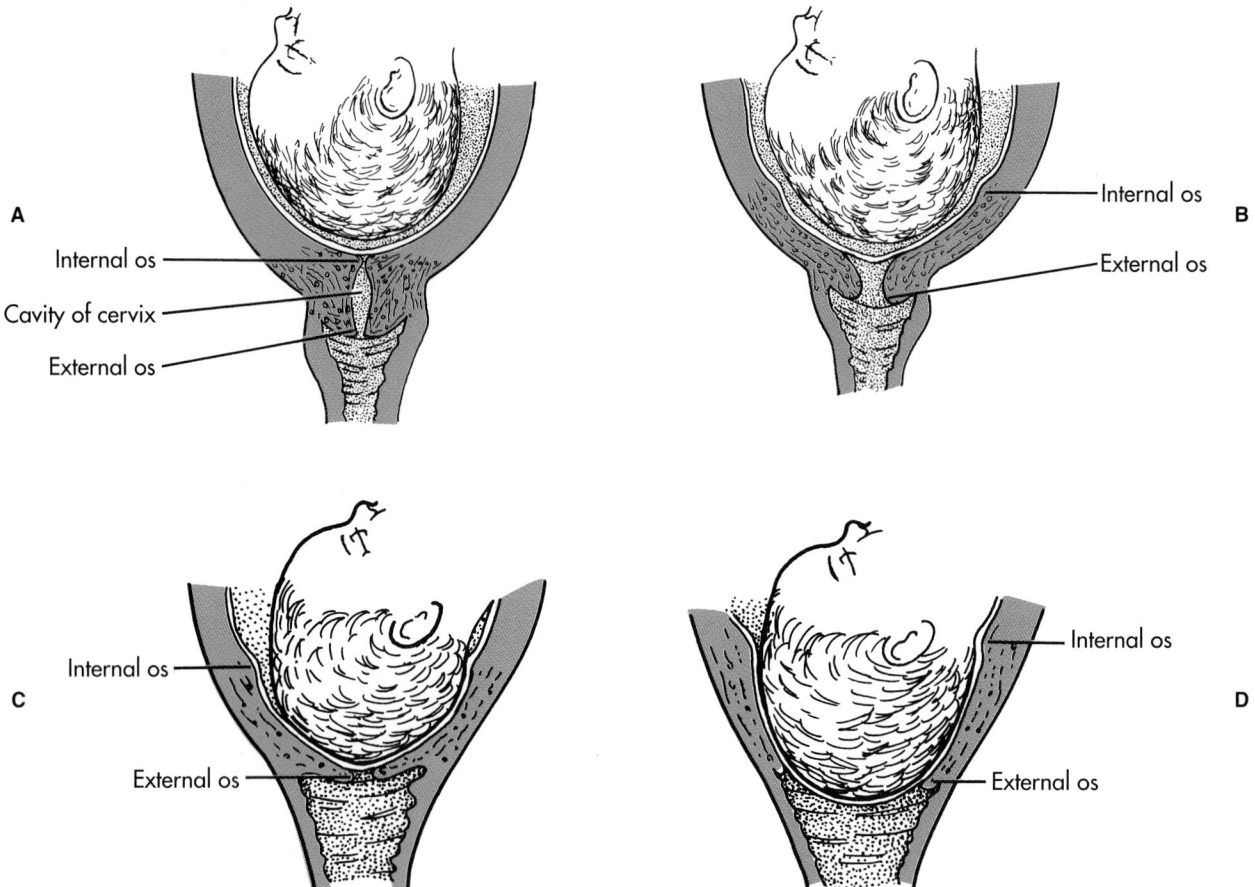

Fig. 19-11 Cervical effacement and dilation. Note how cervix is drawn up around presenting part (internal os). Membranes are intact and head is not well applied to cervix. **A,** Before labor. **B,** Early effacement. **C,** Complete effacement (100%). Head is well applied to cervix. **D,** Complete dilation (10 cm). There is some overlapping of cranial bones and membranes are still intact.

that compresses the uterus on all sides and adds to the power of the expulsive forces.

The secondary powers have no effect on cervical dilation, but they are of considerable importance in the expulsion of the infant from the uterus and vagina after the cervix is fully dilated. Studies have shown that pushing in the second stage is more effective and the woman is less fatigued when she begins to push only after she has the urge to do so rather than beginning to push without an urge to do so when she is fully dilated (Roberts & Woolley, 1996).

The way a woman pushes in second stage is a much-debated topic. Studies have investigated the effects of spontaneous bearing-down efforts, directed pushing, Valsalva (closed glottis and prolonged bearing down) pushing, open glottis pushing, "mini" pushing, and forced methods of pushing (Paine & Tinker, 1992; Thomson, 1995; Woolley & Roberts, 1995). Although no significant differences have been found in the duration of second-stage labor, adverse consequences have been reported. Fetal hypoxia and subsequent acidosis have been associated with prolonged breath holding and forceful pushing efforts. Perineal tears have been associated with directed pushing. Continued study is needed to determine the effectiveness and appro-

priateness of teaching strategies used by nurses to teach pushing techniques, the suitability and effectiveness of various pushing techniques related to nonreassuring fetal heart patterns, and the standards for length of pushing in terms of maternal and fetal outcomes (Peterson & Besuner, 1997).

Position of the Laboring Woman

Position affects the woman's anatomic and physiologic adaptations to labor. Frequent changes in position relieve fatigue, increase comfort, and improve circulation (Melzack, Belanger, & Lacroix, 1991). Therefore a laboring woman should be encouraged to find positions that are most comfortable to her (Fig. 19-12, *A*).

An upright position (walking, sitting, kneeling, or squatting) offers a number of advantages. Gravity can promote the descent of the fetus. Uterine contractions are generally stronger and more efficient in effacing and dilating the cervix, resulting in shorter labor (Golay, Vedam, & Sorger, 1993; Shermer & Raines, 1997).

An upright position is also beneficial to the mother's cardiac output, which normally increases during labor as uterine contractions return blood to the vascular bed. The increased cardiac output improves blood flow to the

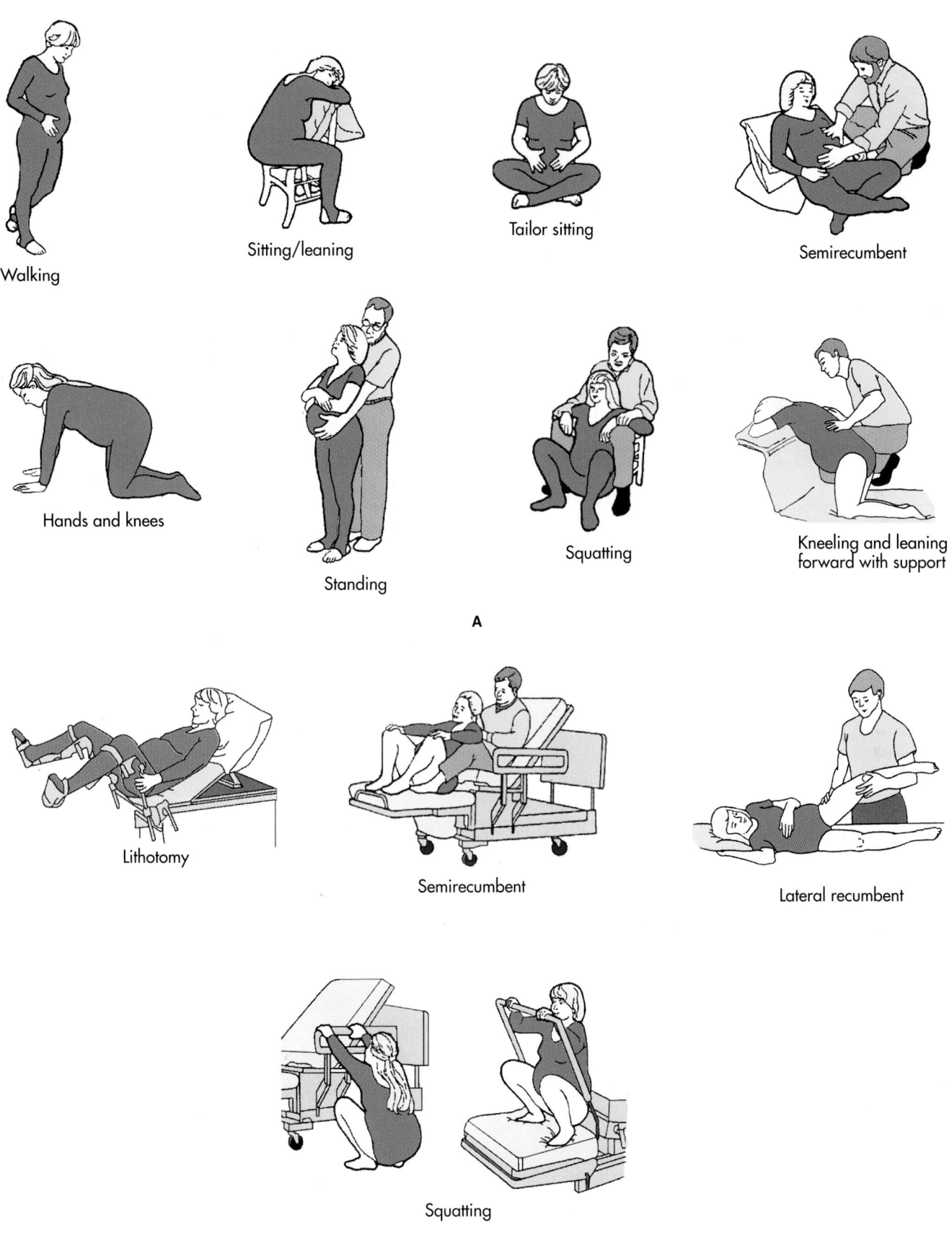

Walking

Sitting/leaning

Tailor sitting

Semirecumbent

Hands and knees

Standing

Squatting

Kneeling and leaning forward with support

A

Lithotomy

Semirecumbent

Lateral recumbent

Squatting

B

Fig. 19-12   Positions for labor and birth. **A,** Positions for labor. **B,** Positions for birth.

uteroplacental unit and the maternal kidneys. Cardiac output is compromised if the descending aorta and ascending vena cava are compressed during labor. Compression of these major vessels may result in supine hypotension that decreases placental perfusion. With the woman in an upright position pressure on the maternal vessels is reduced and compression is prevented. If the woman wishes to lie down, a lateral position is suggested (Cunningham et al., 1997).

The "all fours" position (hands and knees) may be used to relieve backache if the fetus is in an occipitoposterior position and may assist in anterior rotation of the fetus (Bennett & Brown, 1993; Simkin, 1995).

Positioning for second-stage labor (Fig. 19-12, *B*) may be determined by the woman's preference, but it is constrained by the condition of the woman or fetus, the environment, and the health care provider's confidence in assisting in a birth in a specific position (Bennett & Brown, 1993). The predominant position in the United States in physician-attended births is the lithotomy position. Alternative positions and position changes are more commonly practiced by nurse-midwives (Hanson, 1998).

A woman who pushes in a semirecumbent position needs adequate body support to push effectively because her weight will be on her sacrum, moving the coccyx forward and causing a reduction in the pelvic outlet. In a sitting or squatting position, abdominal muscles work in greater synchronicity with uterine contractions during bearing-down efforts. Kneeling or squatting moves the uterus forward and straightens the long axis of the birth canal and can facilitate the second stage of labor by increasing the pelvic outlet (Bennett & Brown, 1993).

The lateral position can be used by the woman to help rotate a fetus that is in a posterior position. It can also be used when there is a need for less force to be used during bearing down such as when there is a need to control the speed of a precipitous birth (Roberts & Woolley, 1996).

There is no evidence that any of these positions suggested for second-stage labor increase the need for use of operative techniques (e.g., forceps- or vacuum-assisted birth, cesarean birth, episiotomy) or cause perineal trauma. There is also no evidence that use of any of these positions adversely affects the newborn (Bennett & Brown, 1993; Biancuzzo, 1993; Golay, Vedam, & Sorger, 1993).

PROCESS OF LABOR

Labor is the process of moving the fetus, placenta, and membranes out of the uterus and through the birth canal. Various changes take place in the woman's reproductive system in the days and weeks before labor begins. Labor itself can be discussed in terms of the mechanisms involved in the process and the stages the woman moves through.

Signs Preceding Labor

In first-time pregnancies the uterus sinks downward and forward about 2 weeks before term, when the fetus's presenting part (usually the fetal head) descends into the true

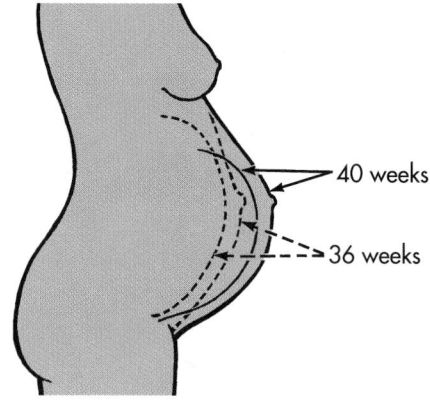

Fig. 19-13 Lightening.

pelvis. This settling is called **lightening,** or "dropping," and usually happens gradually (Fig. 19-13). After lightening, women feel less congested and breathe more easily. However, there is usually more bladder pressure as a result of this shift and consequently a return of urinary frequency. In a multiparous pregnancy, lightening may not take place until after uterine contractions are established and true labor is in progress.

The woman may complain of persistent low backache and sacroiliac distress as a result of relaxation of the pelvic joints. She may identify strong, frequent, but irregular uterine (Braxton Hicks) contractions.

The vaginal mucus becomes more profuse in response to the extreme congestion of the vaginal mucous membranes. Brownish or blood-tinged cervical mucus may be passed **(bloody show).** The cervix becomes soft (ripens) and partially effaced and may begin to dilate. The membranes may rupture spontaneously.

Other phenomena are common in the days preceding labor: (1) loss of 0.5 to 1.5 kg in weight, caused by water loss resulting from electrolyte shifts that in turn are produced by changes in estrogen and progesterone levels; and (2) a surge of energy. Women speak of having a burst of energy that they often use to clean the house and put everything in order. Less commonly, some women experience diarrhea, nausea, vomiting, and indigestion (Varney, 1997). Box 19-1 lists signs that may precede labor.

Onset of Labor

The onset of true labor cannot be ascribed to a single cause. Many factors, including changes in the maternal uterus, cervix, and pituitary gland, are involved. Hormones produced by the normal fetal hypothalamus, pituitary, and adrenal cortex probably contribute to the onset of labor. Progressive uterine distention, increasing intrauterine pressure, and aging of the placenta seem to be associated with increasing myometrial irritability. This is a result of increased concentrations of estrogen and prostaglandins, as well as decreasing progesterone levels. The mutually coordinated effects of these factors result in the occurrence of strong, regular, rhythmic uterine contractions. Normally, the outcome of these factors working together is the birth of the fetus and the expulsion of the placenta. However, it is still not completely understood how certain alterations trigger others and how proper checks and balances are maintained.

Fetal fibronectin is a protein found in plasma and cervicovaginal secretions of pregnant women before the onset of labor. Assessment for the presence of fetal fibronectin is being used to predict the likelihood of preterm labor in women who are at increased risk for this complication. The value of detection of fetal fibronectin in management of women with preterm labor has yet to be determined (Coleman et al., 1998; Lukes et al., 1997).

Stages of Labor

Labor is considered "normal" when the woman is at or near term, no complications exist, a single fetus presents by vertex, and labor is completed within 24 hours. The course of normal labor, which is remarkably constant, consists of (1) regular progression of uterine contractions, (2) effacement and progressive dilation of the cervix, and (3) progress in descent of the presenting part. Four stages of labor are recognized. These stages are discussed in greater detail, along with nursing care for the laboring woman and family, in Chapter 22.

The first stage of labor is considered to last from the onset of regular uterine contractions to full dilation of the cervix. Commonly the onset of labor is difficult to establish because the woman may be admitted to the labor unit just before birth and the beginning of labor may be only an estimate. The first stage is much longer than the second and third combined. Great variability is the rule, however, depending on the factors discussed previously in this chapter. Full dilation may occur in less than 1 hour in some multiparous pregnancies. In first-time pregnancy, complete dilation of the cervix can take up to 20 hours. There are no absolute values for the normal length of the first stage of labor (American College of Obstetricians and Gynecologists, 1995). Variations may reflect differences in the client population or in clinical practice.

The first stage of labor has been divided into three phases: a latent phase, an active phase, and a transition phase. During the latent phase there is more progress in ef-

facement of the cervix and little increase in descent. During the active phase and the transition phase there is more rapid dilation of the cervix and increased rate of descent of the presenting part.

The second stage of labor lasts from the time the cervix is fully dilated to the birth of the fetus. The second stage takes an average of 20 minutes for a multiparous woman and 50 minutes for a nulliparous woman. Labor of up to 2 hours has been considered within the normal range for the second stage, but there can be significant variations. For example, a woman who has received epidural analgesia may take up to 3 hours (Johnson & Rosenfeld, 1995). As long as there is progress and the fetal status is reassuring, the length of the second stage is usually not related to adverse perinatal outcomes (American College of Obstetricians and Gynecologists, 1995).

Three phases of the second stage have been identified and described by Simkin and associates (1991). These phases are *latent*—a period when the woman is not feeling the urge to push, is resting, or is exerting only small bearing-down efforts with contractions; *active*—a period when the woman is making strong bearing-down efforts and the fetal station is advancing; and *transition*—the time when the fetal head is crowning and the woman may be experiencing more pain and exerting either decreased or increased bearing-down efforts.

The third stage of labor lasts from the birth of the fetus until the placenta is delivered. The placenta normally separates with the third or fourth strong uterine contraction after the infant has been born. After it has separated, the placenta can be delivered with the next uterine contraction. The duration of the third stage may be as short as 3 to 5 minutes, although up to 1 hour is considered within normal limits (Bennett & Brown, 1993). The risk of hemorrhage increases as the length of the third stage increases (Cunningham et al., 1997).

The fourth stage of labor arbitrarily lasts about 2 hours after delivery of the placenta. It is the period of immediate recovery, when homeostasis is reestablished. It serves as an important period of observation for complications, such as abnormal bleeding (see Chapter 38).

Mechanism of Labor

As already discussed, the female pelvis has varied contours and diameters at different levels, and the presenting part of the passenger is large in proportion to the passage. Therefore, for vaginal birth to occur, the fetus must adapt to the birth canal during the descent. The turns and other adjustments necessary in the human birth process are termed the **mechanism of labor** (Fig. 19-14). The seven cardinal movements of the mechanism of labor that occur in a vertex presentation are engagement, descent, flexion, internal rotation, extension, external rotation (restitution), and finally birth by expulsion. Although these movements are discussed separately, in actuality a combination of movements occurs simultaneously. For example, engagement involves both descent and flexion.

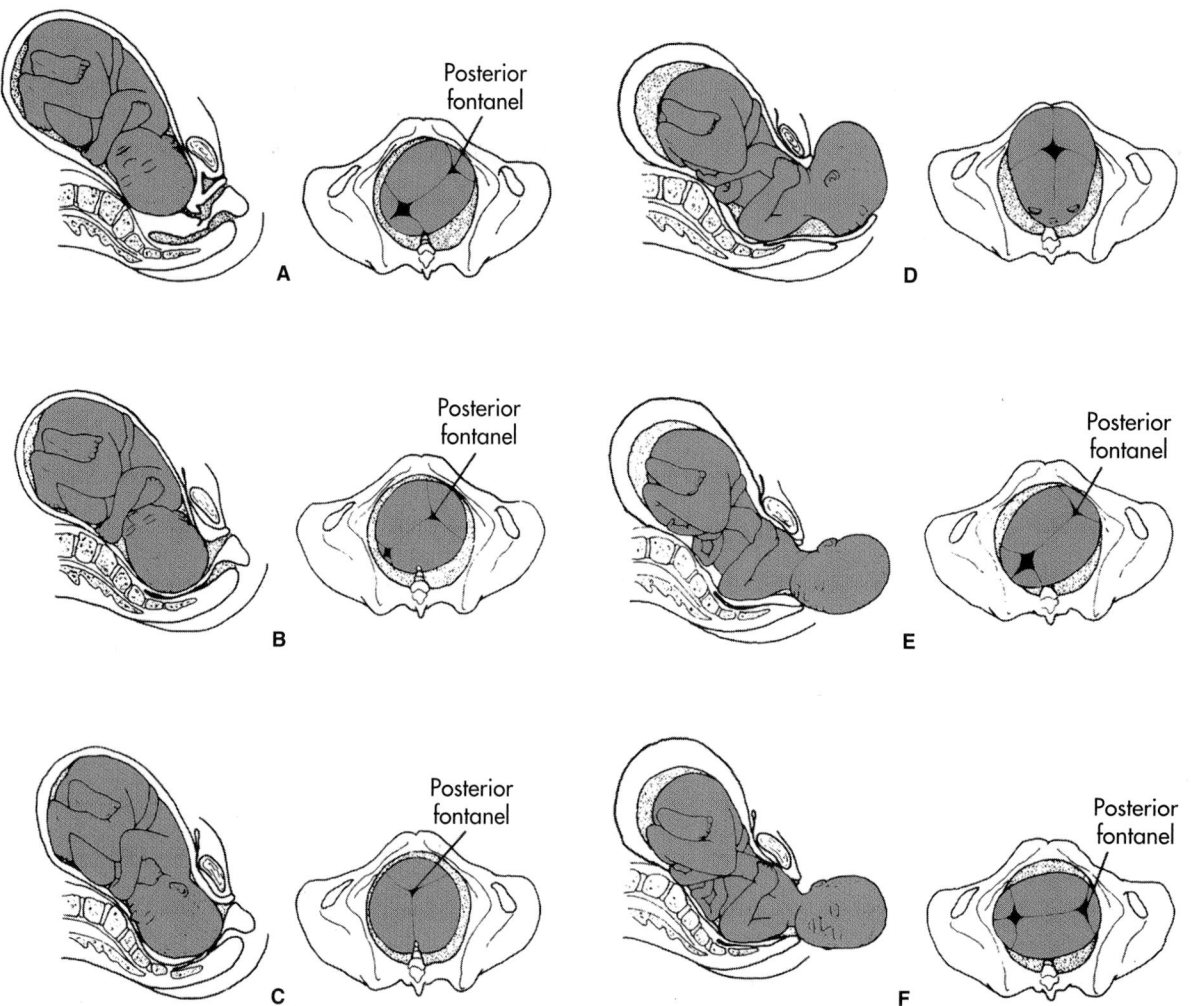

Fig. 19-14 Cardinal movements of the mechanism of labor. Left occipitoanterior (LOA) presentation. **A,** Engagement and descent. **B,** Flexion. **C,** Internal rotation to occipitoanterior position (OA). **D,** Extension. **E,** External rotation beginning (restitution). **F,** External rotation.

Engagement

When the biparietal diameter of the head passes the pelvic inlet, the head is said to be engaged in the pelvic inlet (Fig 19-14, *A*). In most nulliparous pregnancies this occurs before the onset of active labor because the firmer abdominal muscles direct the presenting part into the pelvis. However, a study by Diegmann and colleagues (1995) found almost 70% of the study participants who were nulliparas in early labor to have unengaged fetal heads. In multiparous pregnancies, in which the abdominal musculature is more relaxed, the head often remains freely movable above the pelvic brim until labor is established.

Asynclitism

The head usually engages in the pelvis in a synclitic position, one that is parallel to the anteroposterior plane of the pelvis. Frequently **asynclitism** occurs (the head is deflected anteriorly or posteriorly in the pelvis), which can facilitate descent because the head is being positioned to accommodate to the pelvic cavity (Fig. 19-15). However, extreme asynclitism can cause cephalopelvic dispropor-

tion, even in a normal-size pelvis, because the head is positioned so that it cannot descend.

Descent

Descent refers to the progress of the presenting part through the pelvis. Descent depends on at least four forces: (1) pressure exerted by the amniotic fluid, (2) direct pressure exerted by the contracting fundus on the fetus, (3) force of the contraction of the maternal diaphragm and abdominal muscles in the second stage of labor, and (4) extension and straightening of the fetal body. The effects of these forces are modified by the size and shape of the maternal pelvic planes and the size of the fetal head and its capacity to mold.

The degree of descent is measured by the station of the presenting part (see Fig. 19-9). As mentioned, little descent occurs during the latent phase of the first stage of labor. Descent accelerates in the active phase when the cervix has dilated to 5 to 7 cm. It is especially apparent when the membranes have ruptured.

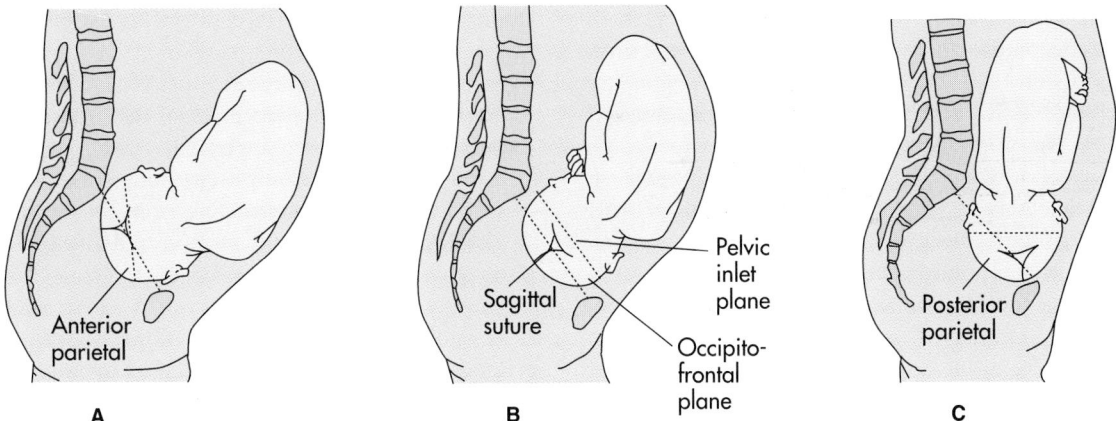

Fig. 19-15 Synclitism and asynclitism. **A,** Anterior asynclitism. **B,** Normal synclitism. **C,** Posterior asynclitism.

In a first-time pregnancy descent is usually slow but steady; in subsequent pregnancies descent may be rapid. Progress in descent of the presenting part is determined by abdominal palpation (Leopold's maneuvers) and vaginal examination until the presenting part can be seen at the introitus.

Flexion

As soon as the descending head meets resistance from the cervix, pelvic wall, or pelvic floor, it normally flexes, so that the chin is brought into closer contact with the fetal chest (see Fig. 19-14, *B*). Flexion permits the smaller suboccipitobregmatic diameter (9.5 cm) rather than the larger diameters to present to the outlet.

Internal Rotation

The maternal pelvic inlet is widest in the transverse diameter. Therefore the fetal head passes the inlet into the true pelvis in the occipitotransverse position. The outlet is widest in the anteroposterior diameter, however. Therefore, for the fetus to exit, the head must rotate. Internal rotation begins at the level of the ischial spines but is not completed until the presenting part reaches the lower pelvis. As the occiput rotates anteriorly, the face rotates posteriorly. With each contraction the fetal head is guided by the bony pelvis and the muscles of the pelvic floor. Eventually the occiput will be in the midline beneath the pubic arch. The head is almost always rotated by the time it reaches the pelvic floor (see Fig. 19-14, *C*). Both the levator ani muscles and the bony pelvis are important for achieving anterior rotation. A previous childbirth injury or regional anesthesia may compromise the function of the levator sling.

Extension

When the fetal head reaches the perineum for birth, it is deflected anteriorly by the perineum. The occiput passes under the lower border of the symphysis pubis first, then the head emerges by extension: first the occiput, then the face, and finally the chin (see Fig. 19-14, *D*).

Restitution and External Rotation

After the head is born, it rotates briefly to the position it occupied when it was engaged in the inlet. This movement is referred to as *restitution* (see Fig. 19-14, *E*). The 45-degree turn realigns the infant's head with her or his back and shoulders. The head can then be seen to rotate further. This external rotation occurs as the shoulders engage and descend in maneuvers similar to those of the head (see Fig. 19-14, *F*). As noted earlier, the anterior shoulder descends first. When it reaches the outlet, it rotates to the midline and is delivered from under the pubic arch. The posterior shoulder is guided over the perineum until it is free of the vaginal introitus.

Expulsion

After birth of the shoulders, the head and shoulders are lifted up toward the mother's pubic bone and the trunk of the baby is born by flexing it laterally in the direction of the symphysis pubis. When the baby has completely emerged, birth is complete, and the second stage of labor ends.

PHYSIOLOGIC ADAPTATION TO LABOR

In addition to the maternal and fetal anatomic adaptations that occur during birth, physiologic adaptations must also occur. Accurate assessment of the mother and fetus requires knowledge of expected adaptations.

Fetal Adaptation

Several important physiologic adaptations occur in the fetus. These changes occur in fetal heart rate, fetal circulation, respiratory movements, and other behaviors.

Fetal Heart Rate

Fetal heart rate (FHR) monitoring provides reliable and predictive information about the condition of the fetus related to oxygenation. Stresses to the uterofetoplacental unit result in characteristic FHR patterns. It is important that the nurse have a basic understanding of the factors involved in fetal oxygenation and of the fetal responses that reflect adequate fetal oxygenation. (See Chapter 21 for further discussion.)

The average FHR at term is 140 beats per minute (beats/min). The normal range is 110 to 160 beats/min. Earlier in gestation the FHR is higher, with an average of approximately 160 beats/min at 20 weeks of gestation. The rate decreases progressively as the maturing fetus reaches term. However, temporary accelerations and slight early decelerations of the FHR can be expected in response to spontaneous fetal movement, vaginal examination, fundal pressure, uterine contractions, abdominal palpation, and fetal head compression.

Fetal Circulation

Fetal circulation can be affected by many factors, including maternal position, uterine contractions, blood pressure, and umbilical cord blood flow. Uterine contractions during labor tend to decrease circulation through the spiral arterioles and subsequent perfusion through the intervillous space. Most healthy fetuses are well able to compensate for this stress and exposure to increased pressure while moving passively through the birth canal during labor. Usually umbilical cord blood flow is undisturbed by uterine contractions or fetal position (Lowe & Reiss, 1996).

Fetal Respiration

Certain changes stimulate chemoreceptors in the aorta and carotid bodies to prepare the fetus for initiating respirations immediately after birth (Lowe & Reiss, 1996). These changes include the following:

- Fetal lung fluid is cleared from the air passages during labor and birth (vaginal birth).
- Fetal oxygen pressure (PO_2) falls.
- Arterial carbon dioxide pressure (PCO_2) rises.
- Arterial pH falls.
- Bicarbonate level falls.
- Fetal respiratory movements decrease during labor.

Maternal Adaptation

Changes occur as the woman progresses through the stages of labor. Various body systems adapt to the process of labor, exhibiting both objective and subjective symptoms.

Cardiovascular Changes

The nurse can expect some changes in the woman's cardiovascular system during labor. During each contraction, 400 ml of blood is emptied from the uterus into the maternal vascular system. This increases cardiac output by about 10% to 15% in the first stage and by about 30% to 50% in the second stage. The heart rate increases slightly.

Changes in the woman's blood pressure also occur. Blood flow, which is reduced in the uterine artery by contractions, is redirected to peripheral vessels. As a result, peripheral resistance increases, and blood pressure rises (Chamberlain & Pipkin, 1998). During the first stage of labor, uterine contractions cause systolic readings to rise by

about 10 mm Hg. Therefore assessing blood pressure between contractions provides more accurate readings (Varney, 1997). During the second stage, contractions may cause systolic pressures to increase by 30 mm Hg and diastolic readings to increase by 25 mm Hg, with both systolic and diastolic pressures remaining somewhat elevated even between contractions. Therefore the woman already at risk for hypertension is at increased risk for complications such as cerebral hemorrhage.

Supine hypotension occurs when the ascending vena cava and descending aorta are compressed. The laboring woman is at greater risk for supine hypotension if the uterus is particularly large because of multifetal pregnancy, hydramnios, or obesity or if the woman is dehydrated or hypovolemic. In addition, anxiety and pain, as well as some medications, can cause hypotension.

The woman should be discouraged from using the **Valsalva maneuver** (holding one's breath and tightening abdominal muscles) for pushing during the second stage. This activity increases intrathoracic pressure, reduces venous return, and increases venous pressure. The cardiac output and blood pressure increase and the pulse slows temporarily. During the Valsalva maneuver, fetal hypoxia may occur. The process is reversed when the woman takes a breath.

The white blood cell (WBC) count can increase to 25,000/mm³, although it usually averages an increase to 14,000 to 16,000/mm³ (Cunningham et al., 1997). Although the mechanism leading to this increase in WBCs is unknown, it may be secondary to physical or emotional stress or to tissue trauma. Labor is strenuous, and physical exercise alone can increase the WBC count.

Some peripheral vascular changes occur, perhaps in response to cervical dilation or to compression of maternal vessels by the fetus passing through the birth canal. Flushed cheeks, hot or cold feet, and eversion of hemorrhoids may result (Box 19-2).

Respiratory Changes

Respiratory system adaptations also are seen. Increased physical activity with greater oxygen consumption is reflected in an increase in the respiratory rate. Hyperventilation may cause respiratory alkalosis (an increase in pH), hypoxia, and hypocapnia (decrease in carbon dioxide). In the unmedicated woman in the second stage, oxygen consumption almost doubles. Anxiety also increases oxygen consumption.

Renal Changes

Several renal system changes occur. In the second trimester, the urinary bladder becomes an abdominal organ. When filling, it is palpable above the symphysis pubis. During labor, spontaneous voiding may be difficult for various reasons: tissue edema caused by pressure from the presenting part, discomfort, analgesia, and embarrassment. Proteinuria of 1+ is a normal finding because it can occur in response to the breakdown of muscle tissue from the physical work of labor.

BOX 19-2 Maternal Physiologic Changes During Labor

Cardiac output increases 10%-15% in first stage; 30%-50% in second stage.

Heart rate increases slightly in first and second stage.

Systolic blood pressure increases during uterine contractions in first stage; systolic and diastolic pressures increase during uterine contractions in second stage.

White blood cell count increases.

Respiratory rate increases.

Temperature may be slightly elevated.

Proteinuria 1+ may occur.

Gastric motility and absorption of solid food is decreased; nausea, vomiting may occur during transition to second-stage labor.

Blood glucose level decreases.

Integumentary Changes

The integumentary system changes are evident, especially in the great distensibility (stretching) in the area of the vaginal introitus. The degree of distensibility varies with the individual. Despite this ability to stretch, even in the absence of episiotomy or lacerations, minute tears in the skin around the vaginal introitus do occur.

Musculoskeletal Changes

The musculoskeletal system is stressed during labor. Diaphoresis, fatigue, proteinuria (1+), and possibly an increased temperature accompany the marked increase in muscle activity. Backache and joint ache (unrelated to fetal position) occur as a result of increased joint laxity at term. The labor process itself and the woman's pointing her toes can cause leg cramps.

Neurologic Changes

The neurologic system reflects the stress and discomfort of labor. Sensorial changes occur as the woman moves through phases of the first stage of labor and as she moves from one stage to the next. Initially she may be euphoric. Euphoria gives way to increased seriousness, then to amnesia between contractions during the second stage, and finally to elation or fatigue after giving birth. Endogenous endorphins (a morphine-like chemical produced naturally by the body) raise the pain threshold and produce sedation. In addition, physiologic anesthesia of perineal tissues, caused by pressure of the presenting part, decreases perception of pain.

Gastrointestinal Changes

Labor affects the woman's gastrointestinal system. Dry lips and mouth may result from mouth breathing, dehydration, and emotional response to labor. During labor, gastrointestinal motility and absorption of solid foods are decreased, and stomach emptying time is slowed. Nausea and vomiting of undigested food eaten after onset of labor are common. Nausea and belching also occur as a reflex response to full cervical dilation. The woman may state that diarrhea accompanied the onset of labor, or the nurse may palpate the presence of hard or impacted stool in the rectum.

Endocrine Changes

The endocrine system is active during labor. The onset of labor may be triggered by decreasing levels of progesterone and increasing levels of estrogen, prostaglandins, and oxytocin. Metabolism increases, and blood glucose levels may decrease with the work of labor.

KEY POINTS

- Labor and birth are affected by the five *P*'s: passenger, passageway, powers, position of the woman, and psychologic responses.

- Because of its size and relative rigidity, the fetal head is a major factor in determining the course of birth.

- The diameters at the plane of the pelvic inlet, midpelvis, and outlet, plus the axis of the birth canal, determine whether vaginal birth is possible and the manner in which the fetus passes down the birth canal.

- Involuntary uterine contractions act to expel the fetus and placenta during the first stage of labor; these are augmented by voluntary bearing-down efforts during the second stage.

- The first stage of labor is from the time dilation begins to the time when the cervix is fully dilated. The second stage of labor lasts from the time of full dilation to the birth of the infant. The third stage of labor lasts from the infant's birth to the expulsion of the placenta. The fourth stage is the first 2 hours after birth.

- The cardinal movements of the mechanism of labor are engagement, descent, flexion, internal rotation, extension, restitution and external rotation, and expulsion of the infant.

- Although the events precipitating the onset of labor are unknown, many factors, including changes in the maternal uterus, cervix, and pituitary gland, are thought to be involved.

- An understanding of maternal adaptations to pregnancy is fundamental to ensuring that the pregnant woman's needs are anticipated and met.

- A healthy fetus with an adequate uterofetoplacental circulation will be able to compensate for the stress of uterine contractions.

CRITICAL THINKING EXERCISES

1 *You have been asked by the staff at the local Red Cross office to prepare a childbirth class for a group of first-time pregnant women on the process of labor.*

   a. *Identify essential content to be covered and describe how you would collect data about the group's knowledge and educational levels.*

   b. *Plan a 30-minute class, including appropriate audiovisuals. Discuss the plan with your faculty.*

   c. *Give the class and ask the group to evaluate it. Discuss this feedback with your faculty and identify modifications for future sessions.*

2 *Visit a prenatal clinic where the clients are mostly non-English speaking.*

   a. *Investigate (through an interpreter or other means) the knowledge level of women who are at least 36 weeks pregnant regarding signs of labor.*

   b. *Formulate a teaching plan that will provide the women with correct information and implement it.*

   c. *Evaluate whether your teaching was effective or ineffective.*

3 *Review nursing research on pushing in second-stage labor.*

   a. *Select a method to discuss in clinical conference.*

   b. *Try to convince the rest of the group that the method you selected is best.*

   c. *At the end of the conference develop a guide for assisting with pushing in second-stage labor based on your discussion.*

References

Alexander, J. et al. (1998). The course of labor with and without epidural analgesia. *Am J Obstet Gynecol* 178(3), 516-520.

American College of Obstetricians and Gynecologists. (1995). *Dystocia, and the augmentation of labor.* Technical Bulletin No. 218. Washington, DC: ACOG.

Barkauskas, V. et al. (1998). *Health and physical assessment* (2nd ed.). St. Louis: Mosby.

Bennet, V., & Brown, L. (1993). *Myles textbook for midwives* (12th ed.). Edinburgh: Churchill Livingstone.

Biancuzzo, M. (1993). Six myths of maternal posture during labor. *MCN Am J Matern Child Nurs* 18(5), 264-260.

Chamberlain, G., & Pipkin, F. (1998). *Clinical physiology in obstetrics* (3rd ed.). Oxford: Blackwell Scientific.

Coleman, M. et al. (1998). Fetal fibronectin detection in preterm labor: Evaluation of a prototype bedside dipstick technique and cervical assessment. *Am J Obstet Gynecol* 179(6), 1553-1558.

Cunningham, F. et al. (1997). *Williams obstetrics* (20th ed.). Stamford, CT: Appleton & Lange.

Diegmann, E., Chez, R., & Danclair, W. (1995). Stations in early labor in nulliparous women at term. *J Nurse Midwifery* 40(4), 382-385.

Golay, J., Vedam, S., & Sorger, L. (1993). The squatting position for the second stage of labor: Effects on labor and on maternal and fetal well-being. *Birth* 20(2), 73-78.

Hanson, L. (1998). Second-stage pushing in nurse-midwifery practices. Part 2. Factors affecting use. *J Nurse Midwifery* 43(5), 326-330.

Johnson, S., & Rosenfeld, J. (1995). The effect of epidural anesthesia on the length of labor. *J Fam Pract* 40(4), 244-247.

Lowe, N., & Reiss, R. (1996). Parturition and fetal adaptation. *J Obstet Gynecol Neonatal Nurs* 25(1), 339-349.

Lukes, A. et al. (1997). Predictors of positivity for fetal fibronectin in patients with symptoms of preterm labor. *Am J Obstet Gynecol* 176(3), 639-641.

Melzack, R., Belanger, E., & Lacroix, R. (1991). Labor pain: Effect of maternal position on front and back pain. *J Pain Symptom Manage* 6(8), 476-480.

Paine, L., & Tinker, D. (1992). The effect of maternal bearing-down efforts on the actual umbilical cord pH and length of second stage labor. *J Nurse Midwifery* 37(1), 61-63.

Peterson, L., & Besuner, P. (1997). Pushing techniques during labor: Issues and controversies. *J Obstet Gynecol Neonatal Nurs* 26(6), 719-726.

Roberts, J., & Woolley, D. (1996). A second look at the second stage of labor. *J Obstet Gynecol Neonatal Nurs* 25(5), 415-423.

Seidel, H. et al. (1999). *Mosby's guide to physical examination* (4th ed.). St. Louis: Mosby.

Shermer, R., & Raines, D. (1997). Positioning during the second stage of labor: Moving back to basics. *J Obstet Gynecol Neonatal Nurs* 26(6), 727-734.

Simkin, P. (1995). Reducing pain and enhancing progress in labor: A guide to nonpharmacologic methods for maternity care givers. *Birth* 22(3), 161-171.

Simkin, P., Whalley, J., & Keppler, A. (1991). *Pregnancy, childbirth and the newborn* (2nd ed.). Seattle: Childbirth Education Association of Seattle and Meadowbrook Press Inc.

Thompson, T. et al. (1998). Does epidural analgesia cause dystocia? *J Clin Anesth* 10(1), 58-65.

Thomson, A. (1995). Maternal behaviors during spontaneous and directed pushing in the second stage of labour. *J Adv Nurs* 22(6), 1027-1034.

Varney, H. (1997). *Varney's midwifery* (3rd ed.). Sudbury, MA: Jones & Bartlett.

Woolley, D., & Roberts, J. (1995). Second stage pushing: A comparison of Valsalva-style pushing with "mini" pushing. *J Perinat Educ* 4(4), 37-43.

20

Management of Discomfort

Jean A. Bachman

EARNING OBJECTIVES

- Define the key terms.
- Compare the various childbirth preparation methods.
- Describe the breathing and relaxation techniques used for each stage of labor.
- Identify nonpharmacologic strategies to enhance relaxation and decrease discomfort during labor.
- Discuss the types of analgesia and anesthesia used during labor.
- Compare the types of pharmacologic control used to relieve discomfort in the different stages of labor and for different methods of birth.
- Discuss the use of naloxone (Narcan) and naltrexone (Trexan).
- Relate each step of the nursing process to the pharmacologic management of labor discomfort.
- Describe the nursing responsibilities appropriate for a woman receiving analgesia or anesthesia during labor.
- Identify topics for nursing research related to pain management for labor and birth.

EY TERMS

agonist-antagonist compounds
analgesia
anesthesia
ataractics
Bradley method
counterpressure
Dick-Read method
effleurage
endorphins

epidural block
epidural blood patch
gate-control theory
hyperventilation
Lamaze (psychoprophylaxis) method
local infiltration anesthesia
narcotic analgesics
narcotic antagonists
neonatal narcosis

paracervical block
pudendal block
referred pain
somatic pain
spinal block
systemic analgesia
visceral pain

Pregnant women commonly worry about the pain they will experience during labor and childbirth and how they will react to and deal with that pain. A wide variety of childbirth preparation methods can provide ways to help the woman cope with the discomfort. However, the interventions selected depend on the situation and the preference of both the woman and her health care provider.

The discomforts experienced during labor are discussed in this chapter, as are the nonpharmacologic and pharmacologic interventions to relieve the discomforts that can be used during the different stages of labor. This information provides the basis for understanding the nurse's role in the management of maternal discomfort during labor.

DISCOMFORT DURING LABOR AND BIRTH

Neurologic Origins

The discomfort experienced during labor has two origins (Lowe, 1996). During the first stage of labor, uterine con-

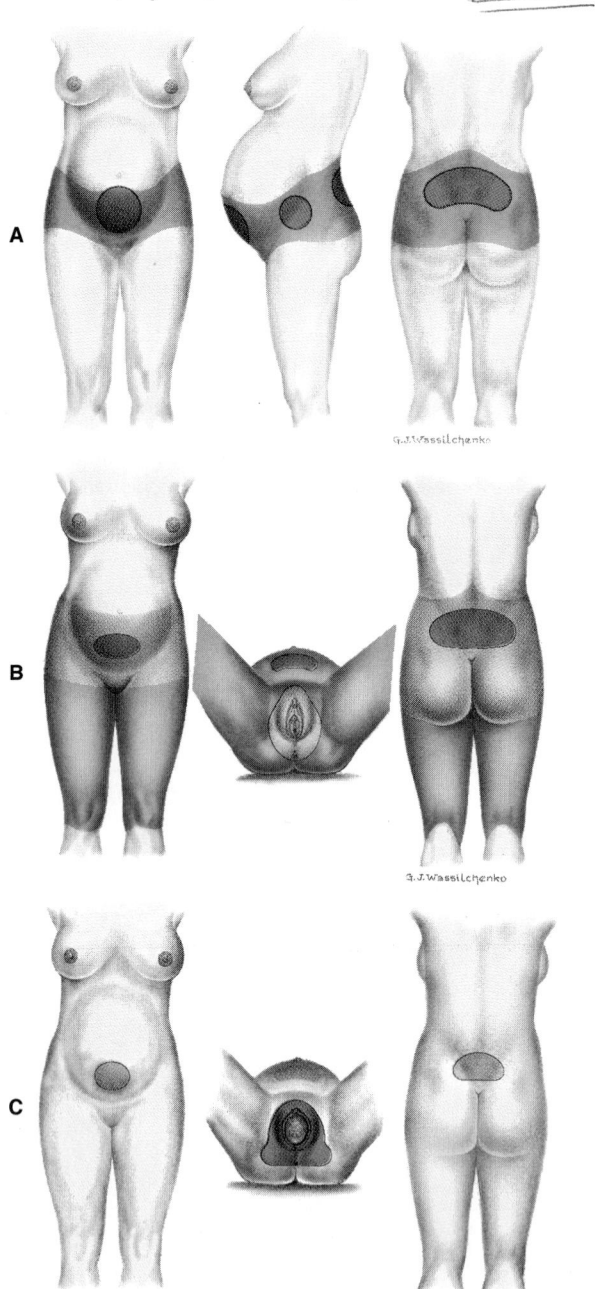

Fig. 20-1 Discomfort during labor. **A,** Distribution of labor pain during first stage. **B,** Distribution of labor pain during transition and early phase of second stage. **C,** Distribution of pain during late second stage and actual birth. *Gray areas* indicate mild discomfort; *light-colored areas* indicate moderate discomfort; *dark-colored areas* indicate intense discomfort.

tractions cause cervical dilation and effacement and uterine ischemia (decreased blood flow and therefore local oxygen deficit) resulting from contraction of the arteries supplying the myometrium. Pain impulses during the first stage of labor are transmitted via the T11–T12 spinal nerve segment and accessory lower thoracic and upper lumbar sympathetic nerves. These nerves originate in the uterine body and cervix.

The discomfort from the cervical changes and uterine ischemia is **visceral pain.** It is located over the lower portion of the abdomen and radiates to the lumbar area of the back and down the thighs. Usually the woman experiences discomfort only during contractions and is free of pain between contractions.

During the second stage of labor, the stage of expulsion of the baby, the woman experiences perineal or **somatic pain.** The perineal discomfort results from stretching of perineal tissues to allow passage of the fetus and from traction on the peritoneum and uterocervical supports during contractions. Discomfort also can be produced by expulsive forces or by pressure exerted by the presenting part on the bladder, bowel, or other sensitive pelvic structures. Pain impulses during the second stage of labor are transmitted via the S1–S4 spinal nerve segments and the parasympathetic system from perineal tissues.

Pain experienced during the third stage of labor, as well as so-called afterpains, is uterine, similar to that experienced early in the first stage of labor. Areas of discomfort during labor are shown in Fig. 20-1.

Pain may be local, with cramping and a tearing or bursting sensation resulting from distention and laceration of the cervix, vagina, or perineal tissues. This discomfort is commonly perceived as an intense burning sensation as the tissue stretches. Pain also may be referred **(referred pain),** in that the discomfort that originates in the abdominal viscera is felt in the back, flanks, or thighs.

Perception of Pain

Although the pain threshold is remarkably similar in all persons regardless of gender, social, ethnic, or cultural differences, these differences play a definite role in the individual person's perception of pain. The effects of factors such as culture, counterstimuli, and distraction in coping with pain are not fully understood. The meaning of pain and the verbal and nonverbal expressions given to pain are apparently learned from interactions within the primary social group. Cultural influences may impose unrealistic expectations. For instance, Asian women believe it shameful to scream or show pain, and they avoid verbal expression (Weber, 1996).

Expression of Pain

Pain results in psychic responses and reflex physical actions. The quality of physical pain has been described as prickling, burning, aching, throbbing, sharp, nauseating, or cramping. The pain in childbirth gives rise to symptoms that are identifiable. The activity of the sympathetic nervous system may increase in response to pain, resulting in changes in blood pressure, pulse, respiration, and skin color. Pallor and diaphoresis may be seen (Potter & Perry, 1998). Nausea and vomiting are common.

Certain affective expressions of suffering are often seen. Such changes include increasing anxiety with lessened perceptual field, writhing, crying, groaning, gesturing (hand clenching and wringing), and excessive muscular excitability throughout the body. Cultural expression of pain may vary. For example, Native American women may endure pain quietly, whereas Hispanic women may endure pain stoically, because it is expected and esteemed, but consider it acceptable to cry out (Villarruel, 1995).

FACTORS INFLUENCING PAIN RESPONSE

A woman's pain during childbirth is unique to each woman and is influenced by a variety of factors. These factors include culture, anxiety and fear, previous birth experience, childbirth preparation, and support.

Culture

The United States is increasingly becoming a multicultural society, which is reflected in the obstetric population. As nurses care for women and families from a variety of cultural backgrounds in labor and birth, they must have knowledge and understanding of how culture mediates pain (Lee & Essoka, 1998; Weber, 1996). An understanding of the beliefs, values, and practices of various cultures helps the nurse provide appropriate culturally sensitive care (see Cultural Considerations box). The nurse must take care not to have cultural blindness, an inability to see other courses of action, which may lead to cultural clashes, resulting in less than optimal care and less than satisfied women who are of a different culture than the nurse (Weber, 1996).

Anxiety and Fear

Anxiety and fear are commonly associated with increased pain during labor. Mild anxiety is considered normal for a woman during labor and birth. However, excessive anxiety and fear cause more catecholamine secretion, which increases the stimuli to the brain from the pelvis because of decreased blood flow and increased muscle tension, which in turn magnifies pain (Lowe, 1996). Thus, as fear and anxiety heighten, muscle tension increases, the effectiveness of the uterine contractions decreases, the experience of discomfort increases, and a cycle of increased fear and anxiety begins.

Previous Experience

Previous birth experiences may also influence the woman's response to pain. For women who have had a difficult and painful previous birth experience, anxiety and fear from this past experience may lead to increased pain. Conversely, a woman who has experienced a labor and birth where pain coping skills were successful may have increased anxiety because those previous coping skills no longer work because of a more difficult labor and birth.

Women with a history of substance abuse experience as much pain during labor as other women. Although it is usually unnecessary to withhold pain medications, close monitoring for complications associated with each substance is part of the nursing assessment.

Childbirth Preparation

At times, particularly intense pain stimuli can be ignored. This is possible because certain nerve cell groupings within the spinal cord, brainstem, and cerebral cortex may have the ability to modulate the pain impulse through a blocking mechanism. This **gate-control theory** helps explain the way the pain relief techniques taught in childbirth preparation classes and hypnosis work to relieve the pain of labor. According to this theory, pain sensations travel along sensory nerve pathways to the brain, but only a limited number of sensations, or messages, can travel through these nerve pathways at one time. By using distraction techniques such as massage or stroking, music, and imagery, the capacity of nerve pathways to transmit pain is reduced or

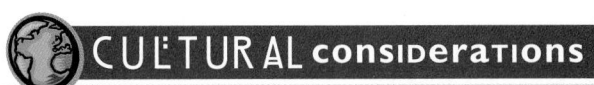

CULTURAL consideraTions

Some Cultural Beliefs About Pain

The following are only examples of how women of different cultural backgrounds may react to pain. Because they are generalizations, the nurse must assess each woman experiencing pain related to childbirth.

Chinese women may not exhibit reactions to pain, although it is acceptable to exhibit pain during childbirth. They consider it impolite to accept something when it is first offered; therefore pain interventions may need to be offered more than once. Acupuncture may be used for pain relief.

Arab or Middle Eastern women may be vocal in response to labor pain. They may prefer medication for pain relief.

Japanese women may be stoic in response to labor pain, but they may request medication when pain becomes severe.

Southeast Asian women may endure severe pain before requesting relief.

Hispanic women may be stoic until late in labor, when they may become vocal and request pain relief.

Native American women may use medications or remedies made from indigenous plants. They are often stoic in response to labor pain.

African-American women may express pain openly. Use of medication for pain relief varies.

they become completely blocked. These distractions are thought to work by closing down a hypothetic gate in the spinal cord, thus preventing pain signals from reaching the brain. The perception of pain is thereby diminished.

In addition, when the laboring woman engages in neuromuscular and motor activities, the resulting activity within the spinal cord itself further modifies the transmission of pain. Cognitive activities involving concentration on breathing and relaxation require selective and directed cortical activity that activates and closes the gating mechanism as well. This gate-control theory therefore underscores the need for a supportive birth setting that allows the laboring woman to relax and use various higher mental activities.

Support

Finally, the critical issue for the nurse is how nurse support can make a difference in the pain experience of the woman during labor and birth. The nurse must realize that the pain occurring during childbirth and the management of this pain belongs to the woman experiencing the pain, and the nurse must engage in a cooperative effort to provide whatever external tools the woman requires to manage her pain experience (Lowe, 1996). These tools include both nonpharmacologic and pharmacologic interventions.

NONPHARMACOLOGIC MANAGEMENT OF DISCOMFORT

It is important to alleviate pain, but commonly it is not the amount of pain the woman experiences but whether she meets her goals for herself in coping with the pain that influences her perception of the birth experience as "good" or "bad." The observant nurse looks for clues to the woman's desired level of control in the management of pain and its relief.

The woman who chooses to deal with childbirth pain using nonpharmacologic or a combination of nonpharmacologic and pharmacologic methods needs care and support from nurses and other care providers who are skilled in pain management. Nonpharmacologic methods for relief of discomfort are taught in many different types of prenatal preparation classes. Regardless of whether a woman or couple has attended these classes or read various books and magazines on the subject in advance, the nurse can teach the woman techniques to relieve discomfort while labor is in progress.

Childbirth Preparation Methods

Today most health care providers recommend or offer childbirth preparation classes to expectant parents. The major methods taught in the United States are the **Dick-Read method,** or natural childbirth method; the Lamaze method, or psychoprophylactic method (PPM); and the Bradley method, or husband-coached childbirth. These methods are discussed in detail in Chapter 18.

How childbirth education influences a woman's response to pain is not completely understood. Some data indicate that women who attend childbirth classes report less pain throughout labor and birth than do women who are unprepared, but other investigations have not supported this finding (Lowe, 1996). However, combined results of a number of studies suggest that not only is confidence greater after childbirth preparation but that this confidence is related to decreased pain perception and decreased analgesia during labor (Lowe, 1996).

Dick-Read Method

To replace fear of the unknown with understanding and confidence, Dick-Read's (1987) program provides information on labor and birth, as well as nutrition, hygiene, and exercise. Classes include practice in three techniques: physical exercise to prepare the body for labor, conscious relaxation, and breathing patterns.

Conscious relaxation involves progressive relaxation of muscle groups in the entire body. With practice, many women can relax on command, both during and between contractions. Some woman actually sleep between contractions.

Breathing patterns include deep abdominal respirations for most of labor, shallow breathing toward the end of the first stage, and, until recently, breath-holding for the second stage of labor.

Teachers of the Dick-Read method also contend that the weight of the abdominal musculature of the contracting uterus increases pain. The woman is taught to force her abdominal muscles to rise as the uterus rises forward during a contraction, thus lifting the abdominal muscles off the contracting uterus.

The Dick-Read method has been adapted to include labor support by the father or a support person chosen by the mother.

Lamaze Method

The **Lamaze (psychoprophylaxis) method** grew out of Pavlov's work on classical conditioning. According to Lamaze, pain is a conditioned response. Therefore women can also be conditioned not to experience pain in labor. The Lamaze method does this by conditioning women to respond to mock uterine contractions with controlled muscular relaxation and breathing patterns instead of crying out and losing control (Lamaze, 1972). Coping strategies also include concentrating on a focal point, such as a favorite picture or pattern, to keep nerve pathways occupied so they cannot respond to painful stimuli.

The woman is taught to relax uninvolved muscle groups while she contracts a specific muscle group (Fig. 20-2). She applies this during labor by relaxing uninvolved muscles while her uterus contracts. The perception of maintaining control has also been found to be closely associated with ultimate satisfaction with the birth experience.

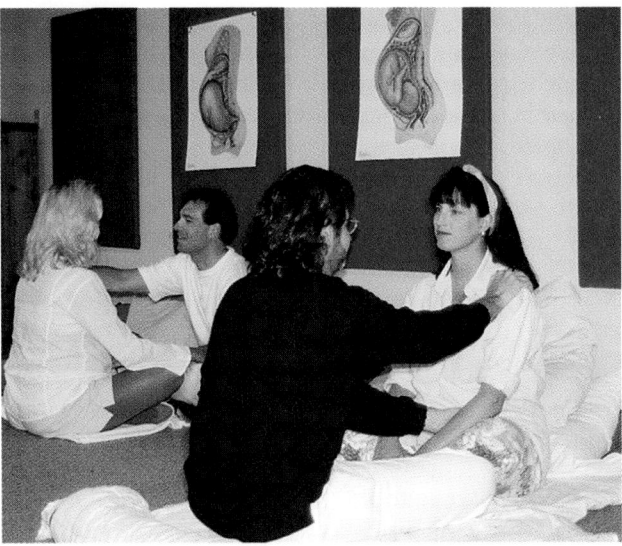

Fig. 20-2 Expectant parents learning relaxation techniques. *(Courtesy Marjorie Pyle, RNC, Lifecircle, Costa Mesa, CA.)*

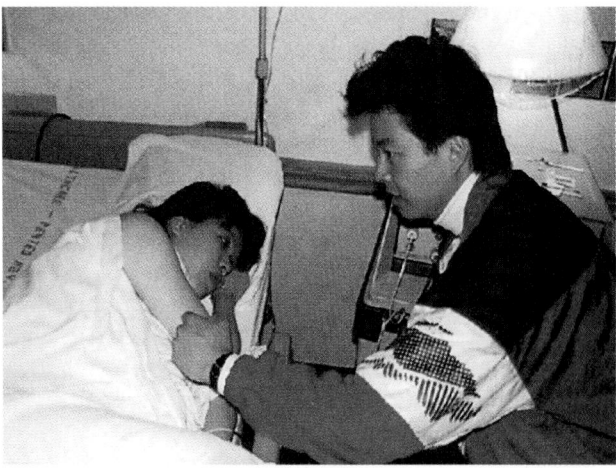

Fig. 20-3 Laboring woman using focusing and breathing techniques during contraction with coaching from her partner. *(Courtesy Marjorie Pyle, RNC, Lifecircle, Costa Mesa, CA.)*

Lamaze teachers believe that chest breathing lifts the diaphragm off the contracting uterus, thus giving it more room to expand. The chest-breathing patterns are varied according to the intensity of the contractions and the progress of labor. Teachers also seek to eliminate fear by increasing the woman's understanding of body functions and the neurophysiology of pain. Support in labor is provided by the woman's partner or other support person or by a specially trained labor attendant termed a *monitrice*.

Bradley Method

The **Bradley method,** also called husband-coached childbirth, was devised based on observations of animal behavior during birth and emphasizes working in harmony with the body, using breath control and abdominal breathing, and promoting general body relaxation (Bradley, 1981).

The husband or partner takes an active role in assisting the woman to relax and use correct breathing techniques. This method also stresses environmental factors such as darkness, solitude, and quiet to make childbirth a more natural experience.

Comparison of Childbirth Methods

Most proponents of prepared childbirth agree that the major causes of pain in labor are fear and tension. All childbirth methods attempt to reduce these two factors and eliminate pain by increasing the woman's knowledge of the labor and birth process, enhancing her self-confidence and sense of control, preparing a support person, and training the woman in physical conditioning and relaxation breathing.

There are a few fine differences in approach. For example, in the Bradley method, women are discouraged from using medication and encouraged to focus inwardly and to

take direction from their own body. In the Lamaze method, external focusing and distraction are stressed. In reality, few instructors adhere strictly to one particular method, but rather incorporate a variety of strategies aimed at increasing the woman's ability to cope with labor and minimize her need for medication.

Relaxing and Breathing Techniques

Focusing and Feedback Relaxation

Some women bring a favorite object such as a photograph to the labor room to focus their attention on during contractions. Others choose some fixed object in the labor room for this purpose. In either event, as the contraction begins, they focus on the object to reduce their perception of pain.

With imagery, the nurse encourages the woman to focus on a pleasant scene, a place where she feels relaxed, or an activity she enjoys. These techniques, coupled with feedback relaxation, help the woman work with her contractions rather than against them. The support person monitors this process, telling the woman when to begin the breathing techniques (Fig. 20-3).

In a common feedback mechanism, the woman and her coach say the word "relax" at the onset of each contraction and throughout it as needed. The nurse can assist the woman by providing a quiet environment and offering cues as needed.

Music

Music can also enhance relaxation during labor. Women should be encouraged to bring their musical preferences and tape or compact disc players to the hospital or birthing center. Use of a headset or earphones may increase the effectiveness of the music because other sounds will not be a distraction. A study of Lamaze-trained women suggested that women who listened to ocean

▪ BOX 20-1 Breathing Techniques

CLEANSING BREATH
Relaxed breath in through nose and out mouth. Used
at the beginning and end of each contraction.
SLOW-PACED BREATHING (APPROXIMATELY 6 TO
8 BREATHS PER MINUTE)
Not less than half normal breathing rate (no.
breaths/min divided by 2)
IN-2-3-4/OUT-2-3-4/IN-2-3-4/OUT-2-3-4 ...
MODIFIED-PACED BREATHING (APPROXIMATELY
32 TO 40 BREATHS PER MINUTE)
Not more than twice normal breathing rate (no.
breaths/min times 2)
IN-OUT/IN-OUT/IN-OUT/IN-OUT ...
For more flexibility and variety, the woman may com-
bine the slow and modified breathing by using the
slow breathing for beginnings and ends of contrac-
tions and modified breathing for more intense peaks.
This technique conserves energy and lessens fatigue.
PATTERNED-PACED BREATHING (SAME RATE AS
MODIFIED)
Enhances concentration
a. 3:1 Patterned breathing
IN-OUT/IN-OUT/IN-OUT/IN-BLOW
(repeat through contraction)
b. 4:1 Patterned breathing
IN-OUT/IN-OUT/IN-OUT/IN-OUT/IN-BLOW
(repeat through contraction)
You may do any pattern desired, although ratios of
5:1 or higher tend to be very tiring. Some people
like to do patterned breathing to a tune ("Yankee
Doodle," "Old McDonald"), to a repeated phrase
("I think I can, I think I can"), or in a pyramid pattern such as 1:1, 2:1, 3:1, 4:1, 5:1—5:1, 4:1, 3:1,
2:1, 1:1.
c. *Coach call:* May be used when the woman needs
more distraction and concentration (e.g., during
transition). The woman's coach signals the breathing ratio with his or her fingers or by verbal cues,
changing the ratio after each "IN-BLOW."
Example:

IN-OUT/IN-OUT/IN-BLOW

IN-OUT/IN-OUT/IN-OUT/IN-OUT/IN-BLOW

IN-OUT/IN-BLOW   ▪

From Shapiro, H. et al. (1997). *The Lamaze ready reference guide for
labor and birth* (2nd ed.). Washington, D.C.: Chapter ASPO/Lamaze.

waves and Baroque and New Age music demonstrated an
improvement in relaxation responses when compared with
women who used only progressive relaxation techniques
(Wiand, 1997).

Breathing Techniques

Different approaches to childbirth preparation stress
varying techniques for using breathing as a tool to help the
woman maintain control throughout contractions. In the
first stage of labor, such breathing techniques can promote
relaxation of the abdominal muscles and thereby enlarge
the abdominal cavity. This lessens the friction and discomfort between the uterus and abdominal wall during
contractions. Because the muscles of the genital area also
become more relaxed, they do not then interfere with descent of the fetus. In the second stage, breathing is used to
increase abdominal pressure and thereby assist in expelling
the fetus. It can also be used to relax the pudendal muscles
to prevent precipitate expulsion of the fetal head.

For those couples who have prepared for labor by practicing such relaxing and breathing techniques, occasional reminders may be all that is necessary to help them along. For
those who have had no preparation, instruction in simple
breathing and relaxation can be given early in labor and often is surprisingly successful. Motivation is high then, and
the readiness to learn is enhanced by the reality of labor.

There are various breathing techniques for controlling
pain during contractions. The nurse needs to ascertain
what, if any, techniques the laboring couple knows before
giving them instruction. Simple patterns are more easily
learned. All patterns begin with the routine cleansing
breath and end with a deep breath exhaled to "blow the
contraction away." Generally, slow abdominal breathing,
approximately half the woman's normal breathing rate, is
initiated when the woman can no longer walk or talk
through contractions (Box 20-1). As contractions increase
in frequency and intensity, the woman may need to
change to chest breathing, which is more shallow and approximately twice her normal rate of breathing.

The most difficult time to maintain control during contractions comes when the cervix dilates to 8 to 10 cm. This
period is also called the *transition period.* Even for the
woman who has prepared for labor, concentration on
breathing techniques is difficult to maintain. The type of
technique used at this stage may be the 4:1 pattern: breath,
breath, breath, breath, blow (as though blowing out a candle). This ratio may be increased to 6:1 or 8:1. However,
an undesirable side effect of this type of breathing may be
hyperventilation. The woman and her support person
must be aware of and watch for the accompanying symptoms of the resultant respiratory alkalosis: light-headedness,
dizziness, tingling of the fingers, or circumoral numbness.
Such alkalosis may be eliminated by having the woman
breathe into a paper bag held tightly around the mouth
and nose. This causes her to rebreathe carbon dioxide and
thus replace the bicarbonate ion. She can breathe into her
cupped hands if no bag is available. Maintaining the
breathing rate at no more than twice the normal rate will
lessen chances of hyperventilation. The partner can help
the mother maintain her breathing rate with visual, tactile,
or auditory means.

Effleurage and Counterpressure

Effleurage (light massage) and counterpressure are two methods that have brought relief to many women during the first stage of labor. The gate-control theory may supply the reason for the effectiveness of these measures. **Effleurage** (see Fig. 20-2), which is a light stroking of the abdomen in rhythm with breathing during contractions, is used to distract the woman from contraction pain. Often the presence of monitor belts makes it difficult to perform effleurage on the abdomen; thus a thigh or the chest may be used.

Counterpressure is steady pressure in the sacral area with the fist or heel of the hand, which may help the woman cope with the sensations of internal pressure and pain in the lower back. Although not scientifically evaluated, pressure may also be applied bilaterally to the hips or knees to reduce low back pain (Simkin, 1995).

Water Therapy

Although not universally accepted or implemented, bathing, showering, and jet hydrotherapy (whirlpool baths) using warm water are other nonpharmacologic measures that can be used to promote comfort and relaxation during labor (Fig. 20-4). Many new birthing units have baths with air jets. With or without air jets, however, the buoyancy of the warm water provides support for tense muscles.

Water therapy has several immediate benefits. The relief from discomfort and general body relaxation it produces reduce the woman's anxiety, which in turn decreases adrenaline production. This triggers an increase in the levels of oxytocin (to stimulate labor) and endorphins (to reduce pain perception). In addition, the bubbles and gentle lapping of the water stimulate the nipples, which triggers an increase in oxytocin production. This has not been observed to cause hyperstimulation. The cervix has often been observed to dilate 2 to 3 cm in 30 minutes of whirlpool therapy. In addition, it promotes diuresis and a decrease in blood pressure (Simkin, 1995). Whirlpool baths in labor have also been found to have positive effects on analgesia requirements, instrumentation rates, condition of the perineum, and personal satisfaction with labor (Rush et al., 1996).

If the woman is experiencing "back labor" secondary to an occiput posterior or transverse position, she is encouraged to assume the hands-and-knees or the side-lying position in the tub. Because this position decreases pain and increases relaxation and the production of oxytocin, the fetus can then rotate spontaneously to the occiput anterior position.

In some settings, jet hydrotherapy may need to be approved by the woman's primary health care provider. The woman's vital signs must be within normal limits, and she should be in the active phase of the first stage of labor. If she is in the latent phase, her contractions slow down. Fetal well-being must also be documented.

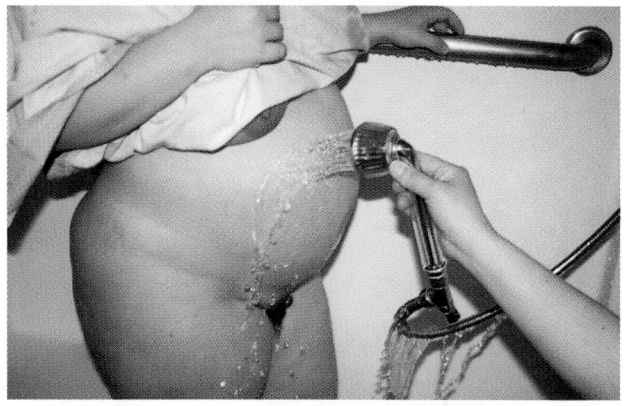

A

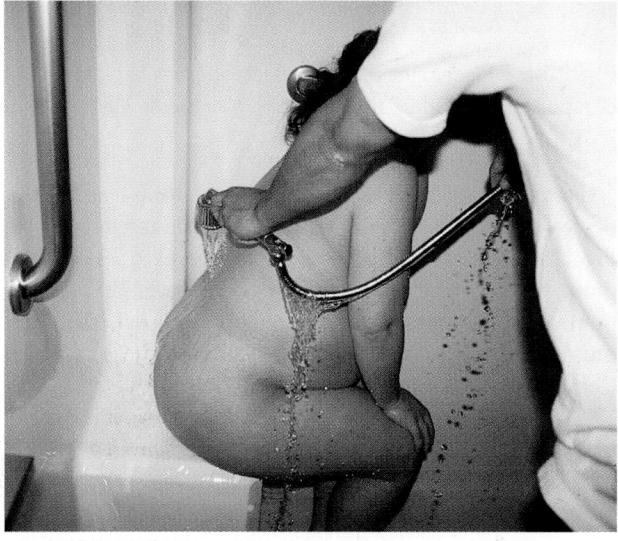

B

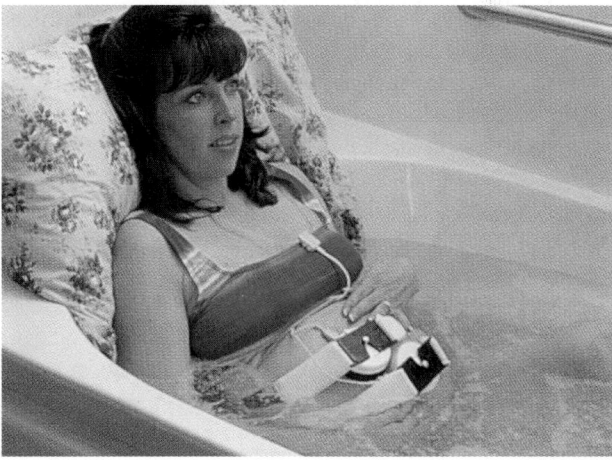

C

Fig. 20-4   Water therapy during labor. **A,** Use of shower during labor. **B,** Woman experiencing back labor relaxes as husband sprays warm water on her back. **C,** Laboring woman relaxes in jacuzzi. Note that fetal monitoring can continue during time in the jacuzzi. *(**A, B,** Courtesy Marjorie Pyle, RNC, Lifecircle, Costa Mesa, CA. **C,** Courtesy Spacelabs Medical, Redmond, WA.)*

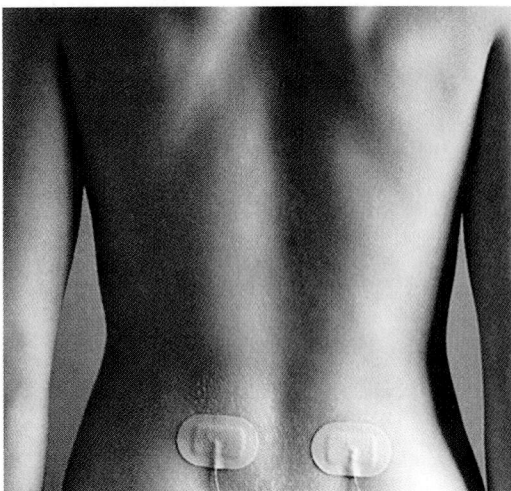

Fig. 20-5 Placement of TENS electrodes on back for relief of labor pain. *(Courtesy 3M HealthCare, Minneapolis, MN.)*

Fetal heart rate (FHR) monitoring is done by Doppler device, fetoscope, or wireless external monitor device (see Fig. 20-4, *C*). Placement of internal electrodes is contraindicated for jet hydrotherapy. The woman's membranes may be intact or ruptured. If ruptured, the fluid must be clear or only lightly stained with meconium (Simkin, 1995).

There is no limit to the time women can stay in the bath, and often women are encouraged to stay in it as long as desired. However, most women use jet hydrotherapy for 30 to 60 minutes (Schorn, McAllister, & Blanco, 1993).

During the bath, if the woman's temperature and the FHR increase, the water is cooled or she is asked to step out of the bath to cool down. The bath water is kept between 36.7° and 37.8° C (Simkin, 1995). The mother's temperature may remain slightly elevated for a short time after the bath. Fluids and ice chips and a cool face cloth are offered during the bath.

The tub must be kept meticulously clean. The cleansing solutions used vary with the institution, but household bleach (Clorox) is the one commonly used.

Transcutaneous Electrical Nerve Stimulation

Transcutaneous electrical nerve stimulation (TENS) involves the placement of two pairs of electrodes on either side of the woman's thoracic and sacral spine (Fig. 20-5) that provide continuous mild electrical currents from a battery-operated device. During a contraction the woman increases the stimulation by turning control knobs on the device. Women describe the resulting sensation as a tingling or buzzing and the pain relief as good or very good. The technique poses no risk to the mother or fetus, and it is credited with reducing or eliminating the need for analgesia and with increasing the woman's perception of control over the experience. It may be effective because of the placebo effect; that is, confidence in the effectiveness of

---

BOX 20-2 Nonpharmacologic Strategies to Encourage Relaxation and Relieve Pain

CUTANEOUS STIMULATION STRATEGIES
Counterpressure
Effleurage (light massage)
Therapeutic touch
Walking
Rocking
Changing positions
Application of heat or cold
TENS
Acupressure
Showers, baths

SENSORY STIMULATION STRATEGIES
Aromatherapy
Breathing techniques
Music
Imagery
Use of focal points

COGNITIVE STRATEGIES
Childbirth education
Hypnosis

TENS may stimulate the release of endogenous opiates (enkephalins) in the woman's body and thus alleviate the discomfort (Scott et al., 1999).

The nurse's involvement in the method consists of explaining the device and its use, carefully placing and securing the electrodes, and closely evaluating its effectiveness.

Other Nonpharmacologic Methods

There are various other nonpharmacologic methods for control of the discomfort of labor (Box 20-2). Many of these are taught in childbirth preparation classes. Most need practice for best results, although the nurse may use some of them successfully without the woman having prior knowledge.

Acupressure

Acupressure techniques can be used in pregnancy, labor, and postpartum to relieve pain and other discomforts. Pressure, heat, or cold is applied to acupuncture points called *tsubos*. These points have an increased density of neuroreceptors and increased electrical conductivity. The effectiveness of acupressure has been attributed to the gate-control theory and an increase in endorphin levels (Jimenez, 1992). Acupressure is best applied over the skin without using lubricants. Pressure is usually applied with the pads of the thumbs and fingers (Fig. 20-6). Synchronized breathing by the caregiver and the woman is

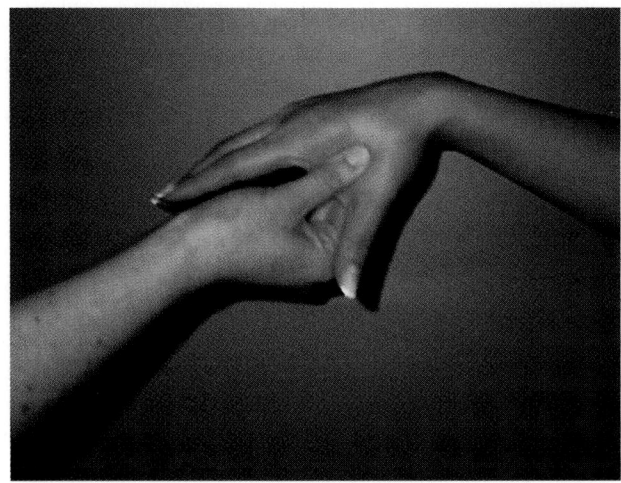

Fig. 20-6 Ho-Ku acupressure point (back of hand where thumb and index finger come together) used to enhance uterine contractions without increasing pain. *(From Dickason, E., Silverman, B., & Kaplan, J. [1998]. Maternal-infant nursing care [3rd ed.]. St. Louis: Mosby.)*

suggested for greater effectiveness. Acupressure points include shoulders, low back, hips, ankles, nails on the small toes, soles of the feet, and sacral points.

Application of Heat and Cold

Warmed blankets, warm compresses, a warm bath or shower, or use of a moist heating pad can reduce pain during labor. Heat acts to relieve muscle ischemia and increase blood flow to the area of discomfort. Heat application is effective for back pain caused by a posterior presentation or general backache from fatigue (Simkin, 1995).

Cold application such as cool cloths or ice packs may be effective to increase comfort when the woman feels warm and may be applied to areas of pain. Cooling relieves pain by lowering the muscle temperature and relieving muscle spasms (Simkin, 1995).

Heat and cold may be used alternately for a greater effect. Neither heat nor cold should be applied over ischemic or anesthetized areas because tissues can be damaged.

Therapeutic Touch

Therapeutic touch uses the concept of energy fields within the body called *prana*. Prana are thought to be deficient in people who are in pain. Therapeutic touch uses laying on of the hands of a specially trained person to redirect energy fields associated with pain (Mackey, 1995). Little is known about the use or effectiveness of therapeutic touch for relieving labor pain.

Hypnosis

Hypnosis is not commonly used for pain management in the United States, but it is associated with shorter labors and less analgesic use (Jenkins & Pritchard, 1993). Hypnosis

techniques used for labor and birth place an emphasis on relaxation. The woman may be given direct suggestions about pain relief or indirect suggestions that she is experiencing diminished sensations. The woman receives posthypnotic suggestions, such as "you will be able to push the baby out easily," to increase her confidence.

Biofeedback

Biofeedback is another relaxation technique that can be used for labor. Biofeedback is based on the theory that if a person can recognize physical signals, certain internal physiologic events can be changed (whatever signs the woman has that are associated with her pain). A woman must be educated to become aware of her body and its responses and how to relax for biofeedback to be effective (Alexander & Steeful, 1995).

Aromatherapy

Aromatherapy uses oils distilled from plants, flowers, herbs, and trees to promote health and well-being and treat illnesses. The use of herbal teas and vapors is reported to have good effects in pregnancy and labor for some women (Burns & Blamey, 1994). Lavender, clary sage, and bergamot promote relaxation and can be used by adding a few drops to a warm bath, to warm water used for soaking compresses that can be applied to the body, to an aromatherapy lamp to vaporize a room, or to oil for a back massage (Tiran, 1996).

NURSE ALERT *Caution: Never apply full-strength oils directly to the skin.*

PHARMACOLOGIC MANAGEMENT OF DISCOMFORT

Sedatives

Sedatives such as barbiturates relieve anxiety and induce sleep only in prodromal or early latent labor and in the absence of pain. If the woman is experiencing pain, sedatives given without an analgesic may only increase apprehension and cause the mother to become hyperactive and disoriented. Undesirable side effects include respiratory and vasomotor depression affecting the mother and newborn. Because of these drawbacks, barbiturates are seldom used (Scott et al., 1999).

Analgesia and Anesthesia

The use of analgesia and anesthesia was not generally accepted as part of obstetric management until Queen Victoria used chloroform during the birth of her son in 1853. Since then, much study has gone into the development of pharmacologic measures for controlling discomfort during the birth period. The goal of researchers is to develop methods that will provide adequate pain relief to women without increasing maternal or fetal risk or affecting the progress of labor.

BOX 20-3 Pharmacologic Control of Discomfort by Stage of Labor and Method of Birth

FIRST STAGE

Systemic analgesia
  Narcotic analgesic compounds
  Mixed narcotic agonist-antagonist compounds, analgesic potentiators
Nerve block analgesia/anesthesia
Lumbar epidural analgesia

SECOND STAGE

Nerve block analgesia/anesthesia
  Local infiltration anesthesia
  Pudendal block
  Subarachnoid (spinal) anesthesia
  Epidural block
  Epidural and spinal narcotics
Inhalation analgesia/anesthesia
  Nitrous oxide-oxygen
  General anesthesia

VAGINAL BIRTH

Local infiltration
Pudendal block
Lumbar epidural block
  Analgesia
  Anesthesia
Subarachnoid block
  Analgesia
  Anesthesia

CESAREAN BIRTH

Subarachnoid block
  Spinal block
  Saddle block (low spinal)
Lumbar epidural block
  Anesthesia
Inhalation
  General anesthesia

Nursing management of obstetric analgesia and anesthesia combines the nurse's expertise in maternity care with a knowledge and understanding of anatomy and physiology and of medications and their desired and undesired side effects and methods of administration.

Anesthesia encompasses analgesia, amnesia, relaxation, and reflex activity. It involves the abolition of pain perception by interrupting the nerve impulses going to the brain. The loss of sensation may be partial or complete, sometimes with the loss of consciousness.

The term **analgesia** is best reserved to describe the alleviation of the sensation of pain or the raising of the threshold for pain perception but without loss of consciousness.

The type of analgesic or anesthetic chosen is determined in part by the stage of labor the woman is in and by the method of birth planned (Box 20-3).

Systemic Analgesia

Systemic analgesia remains the major form of analgesia for relieving the pain of labor when personnel trained in administering regional analgesia are not available (Scott et al., 1999). Systemic analgesics cross the blood-brain barrier to provide central analgesic effects. However, they also cross the placental barrier. The effects on the fetus depend on the maternal dosage, the pharmacokinetics of the specific drug, and the route and timing of administration. Intravenous (IV) administration is often preferred over intramuscular (IM) administration because the onset of the drug effect is faster and more reliable. Classes of analgesic drugs used to relieve the pain of childbirth include narcotics, narcotic agonist-antagonist compounds, and tranquilizers such as analgesic-potentiating drugs (ataractics) (see Medication Guide).

Narcotic analgesic compounds. Narcotic analgesics such as meperidine (Demerol) and fentanyl (Sublimaze) are especially effective for relieving severe, persistent, or recurrent pain. They have no amnesic effect.

Meperidine is the most commonly used narcotic for women in labor (Scott et al., 1999) (see Medication Guide: Opioid Analgesics for Labor). It overcomes inhibitory factors in labor and may even relax the cervix. After IV injection, the onset of its effect is rapid (30 seconds); the maximum effect is reached in 5 to 10 minutes and lasts for about 3 hours. The peak effect after an IM injection of meperidine is reached in 40 to 50 minutes. In a randomized controlled study, women who received meperidine intravenously reported significantly lower levels of pain than those reported by women who received it intramuscularly (Isenor & Penny-MacGillivary, 1993). Ideally, birth should occur less than 1 hour or more than 4 hours after an IM injection so that neonatal central nervous system (CNS) depression resulting from meperidine is minimized. Because tachycardia is a possible side effect, meperidine is used cautiously in women with cardiac disease.

Fentanyl is a potent, short-acting narcotic analgesic (see Medication Guide). The onset of the drug effect after IV injection occurs within 2 minutes and lasts about 30 to 60 minutes. Onset of the drug effect occurs in 7 to 15 minutes after IM injection; the peak effect is reached in 20 to 30 minutes and lasts for 1 to 2 hours. Additive CNS and respiratory depression occurs if fentanyl is given with alcohol, antihistamines, antidepressants, or other sedative-hypnotics.

Mixed narcotic agonist-antagonist compounds. An *agonist* is an agent that activates something; an *antagonist* is an agent that prevents something from happening. Mixed

MEDICATION GUIDE

Opioid Analgesics for Labor

MEDICATION	Meperidine (Demerol)	Butorphanol tartrate (Stadol)	Nalbuphine (Nubain)
ACTION	Opioid agonist analgesic; decreases pain impulse transmission via opioid receptors	Mixed agonist-antagonist analgesic; mechanism of action not determined	Mixed agonist-antagonist analgesic
INDICATION	Labor pain; postoperative pain after cesarean birth	Labor pain	Labor pain; postoperative pain after cesarean birth
DOSAGE AND ROUTE	25 mg IV; 50 mg IM May repeat in 2-3 hr; use of adjunctive medications such as promethazine may potentiate the narcotic effects and decrease nausea and vomiting	1-2 mg IV/IM May repeat in 3-4 hr	10 mg IV; 10-20 mg IM q3-6 hr
ADVERSE EFFECTS	Nausea and vomiting, sedation, drowsiness, tachycardia, hypotension, dry mouth, pruritis, respiratory depression (woman and newborn), decreased FHR variability, decreased uterine activity	See meperidine; may cause transient sinusoidal-like FHR rhythm	See meperidine
NURSING CONSIDERATIONS	Assess FHR and uterine activity; observe for respiratory depression; if birth occurs within 4 hr of dose, observe newborn for respiratory depression; naloxone available as antidote; side rails up	See meperidine; may precipitate withdrawal in opiate-dependent women	See butorphanol

narcotic **agonist-antagonist compounds** such as butorphanol (Stadol) and nalbuphine (Nubain), in the doses used during labor, provide analgesia without causing respiratory depression in the mother or neonate. They are administered by either IM or IV routes. Butorphanol (1 to 3 mg IM; 0.5 to 2 mg IV) and nalbuphine (10 to 20 mg IM or IV) may be given during the first stage of labor (see Medication Guide: Opioid Analgesics for Labor).

Analgesic potentiators (ataractics). Phenothiazines, so-called tranquilizers, have the property of augmenting most of the desirable but few of the undesirable effects of analgesics or general anesthetics. These **ataractics** do not relieve pain but decrease anxiety and apprehension, as well as potentiate the narcotic effects. This potentiation effect causes the two drugs involved to work together more effectively, such that the narcotic dose can be reduced. The analgesic potentiators include promethazine (Phenergan), propiomazine (Largon), hydroxyzine (Vistaril), and promazine (Sparine).

In addition to potentiating the effects of the analgesic, the ataractic (tranquilizer) also acts as an antinauseant and antiemetic. The combination of agents can be administered

MEDICATION GUIDE

Fentanyl (Sublimaze) and Sufentanil (Sufenta)

ACTION	Opioid analgesics, rapid action with short duration (1-2 hr)
INDICATION	For epidural or intrathecal analgesia, usually in combination with a local anesthetic
DOSAGE AND ROUTE	Fentanyl—IM 50 to 100 μg; IV 25 to 50 μg Epidural—fentanyl, 1 to 2 μg with 0.125% bupivacaine at rate of 8 to 10 ml/hr; sufentanil, 1 μg with 0.125% bupivacaine at rate of 10 ml/hr
ADVERSE EFFECTS	Dizziness, drowsiness, allergic reactions, rash, respiratory depression
NURSING CONSIDERATIONS	Assess for respiratory depression; naloxone should be available as antidote

MEDICATION GUIDE

Naloxone (Narcan) and Naltrexone (Trexan)

ACTION	Opioid antagonists
INDICATION	Naloxone—reverses opioid-induced respiratory depression in woman or newborn; naltrexone—counteracts effects of epidural or intrathecal morphine; both may be used to reverse pruritis from epidural opioids
DOSAGE AND ROUTE	Naloxone—adult, 0.4 to 2 mg IV/IM/SC, repeat in 2 to 3 min up to 2 times if needed; newborn, 0.1 mg/kg IV (umbilical vein or endotracheal; repeat q2-3min up to 3 times if needed, may also be given IM or SC) Naltrexone—adult, 3 to 6 mg PO one dose
ADVERSE EFFECTS	Maternal hypotension, tachycardia, nausea and vomiting
NURSING CONSIDERATIONS	Woman should delay breast-feeding until medication is out of system; do not give if woman is using drugs of abuse—may cause abrupt withdrawal; if given to woman for reversal of respiratory depression due to opioid analgesic, pain will return

SIGNS OF POTENTIAL COMPLICATIONS

Maternal Narcotic Withdrawal

Nausea, vomiting
Headache
Irritability
Fatigue
Perspiration, chills
Tremors, weakness, restlessness
Anxiety, apprehension, jittery feeling
Convulsions (seizures)

is not completely understood. It is thought that endorphin levels increase during pregnancy and birth in humans and serve to augment the laboring woman's tolerance of acute pain.

A narcotic antagonist is especially valuable if labor is more rapid than expected and birth is anticipated when the narcotic is at its peak effect. The antagonist may be given through the woman's IV line, or it can be administered IM. Narcotic antagonists can counteract the maternal and neonatal narcotic effects. The mother must be told, however, that the pain will return with the administration of an antagonist.

NURSE ALERT *Narcotic antagonists must be administered cautiously to a substance-dependent woman because they may precipitate withdrawal symptoms (see Signs of Potential Complications).*

A narcotic antagonist can be given to the newborn to treat **neonatal narcosis,** which is a state of CNS depression in the newborn produced by a narcotic. Affected infants may exhibit respiratory depression, hypotonia, lethargy, and a delay in temperature regulation. Alterations in neurologic and behavioral responses may be evident in the newborn for 72 hours after birth. Meperidine may be present in the neonate's urine for up to 3 weeks. Some depression of attention and social responsiveness can be evident for up to 6 weeks after birth.

Nerve Block Analgesia and Anesthesia

A variety of compounds are used in obstetrics to produce regional analgesia (some pain relief and motor block) and anesthesia (pain relief and motor block). Most of these drugs are related chemically to cocaine and end with the suffix "-caine." This is a way of identifying a local anesthetic.

The principal pharmacologic effect of local anesthetics is the temporary interruption of the conduction of nerve impulses, notably pain. Examples of common agents given in 0.25% to 1% solutions are lidocaine (Xylocaine), bupivacaine (Marcaine), chloroprocaine (Nesacaine), tetracaine (Pontocaine), and mepivacaine (Carbocaine).

safely until the end of the first stage of labor. The following are the usual doses of the various agents: promethazine, 25 to 50 mg IM or 15 to 25 mg IV; promazine, 50 mg IM or 5 to 10 mg IV; and hydroxyzine, 25 to 50 mg IM. Because hydroxyzine is given only by IM injection, the onset of its effect is slower and less predictable. Fetal or neonatal problems rarely develop when the mothers are given these doses.

Narcotic antagonists. Narcotics such as meperidine and fentanyl can cause excessive CNS depression in the mother or newborn. **Narcotic antagonists** such as naloxone (Narcan) or the newer narcotic antagonist naltrexone (Trexan) can promptly reverse such narcotic effects (see Medication Guide). In addition, the antagonist also counters the effect of the stress-induced levels of endorphins. **Endorphins** are endogenous opioids secreted by the pituitary gland that act on the central and peripheral nervous systems to reduce pain. Beta-endorphin is the most potent of the endorphins. The physiologic role of endorphins

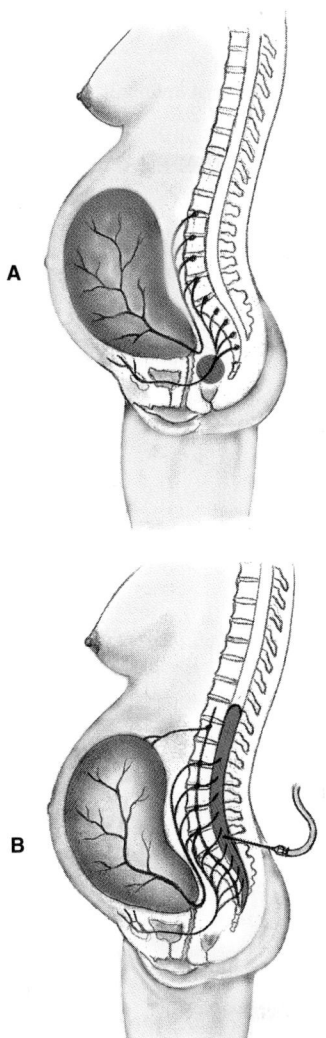

Fig. 20-7 in lower margin of left figure reads: G.J.Wassilchenko

Fig. 20-7 Pain pathways and sites of pharmacologic nerve blocks. **A,** Pudendal block; suitable during second and third stages of labor and for repair of episiotomy. **B,** Epidural block; suitable during all stages of labor and for repair of episiotomy.

Rarely, people are sensitive (allergic) to one or more local anesthetics. Such sensitivity may be identified by administering minute amounts of the drug to be used to test for an allergic reaction. Such a reaction may include respiratory depression, hypotension, and other serious adverse effects. Atropine, antihistamines, oxygen, and supportive measures should reverse these effects.

Local infiltration anesthesia. Local infiltration anesthesia of perineal tissues is commonly used when an episiotomy is to be done and when time or the fetal head position does not permit a pudendal block to be administered (Scott et al., 1999). Rapid anesthesia is produced by injecting an average of 10 to 20 ml of 1% lidocaine or 2% chloroprocaine into the skin and then subcu-

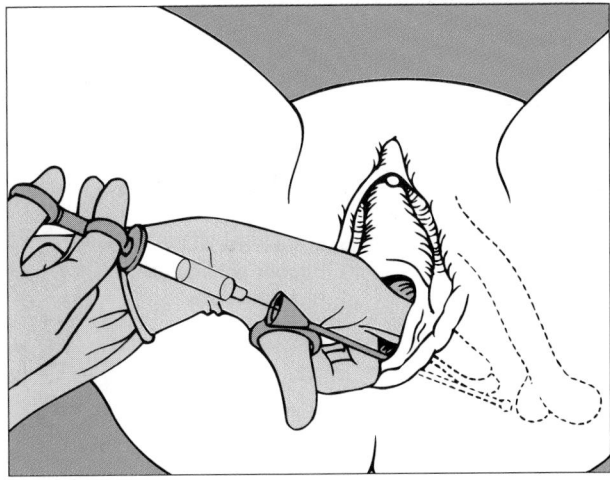

Fig. 20-8 Pudendal block. Use of needle guide (Iowa trumpet) and Luer-Lok syringe to inject medication.

taneously into the region to be anesthetized. Epinephrine often is added to the solution to intensify the anesthesia in a limited region and to prevent excessive bleeding and systemic effects by constricting local blood vessels (Clark, Queener, & Karb, 1996). Repeated injection will prolong the anesthesia as long as needed.

Pudendal block. Pudendal block is useful for the second stage of labor, episiotomy, and birth. Although it does not relieve the pain from uterine contractions, it does relieve pain in the lower vagina, vulva, and perineum (Fig. 20-7, *A*). A pudendal nerve block must be administered 10 to 20 minutes before perineal anesthesia is needed. [handwritten: only relieves Low pain no†]

The pudendal nerve traverses the sacrosciatic notch just medial to the tip of the ischial spine on each side. Injection of an anesthetic solution at or near these points anesthetizes the pudendal nerves peripherally (Fig. 20-8). The transvaginal approach is generally used because it is less painful for the woman, is more successful in blocking pain, and tends to be associated with fewer fetal complications (Chestnut, 1994). Pudendal block does not alter maternal hemodynamic or respiratory functions and vital signs or the FHR. However, it does cause the bearing-down reflex to be lessened or lost completely.

If all branches of the pudendal nerve are anesthetized, the resulting analgesia is sufficient for a spontaneous vaginal birth or an outlet (low) forceps-assisted birth. A pudendal block does not provide analgesia for uterine exploration or the manual removal of the placenta (Scott et al., 1999).

Spinal anesthesia. In a **spinal block,** local anesthetic is injected through the third, fourth, or fifth lumbar interspace into the subarachnoid space (Fig. 20-9), where the medication mixes with cerebrospinal fluid (CSF). This technique is commonly used for cesarean births. A low spinal block may be used for vaginal birth, but it is not suitable for labor. The spinal block given for cesarean birth

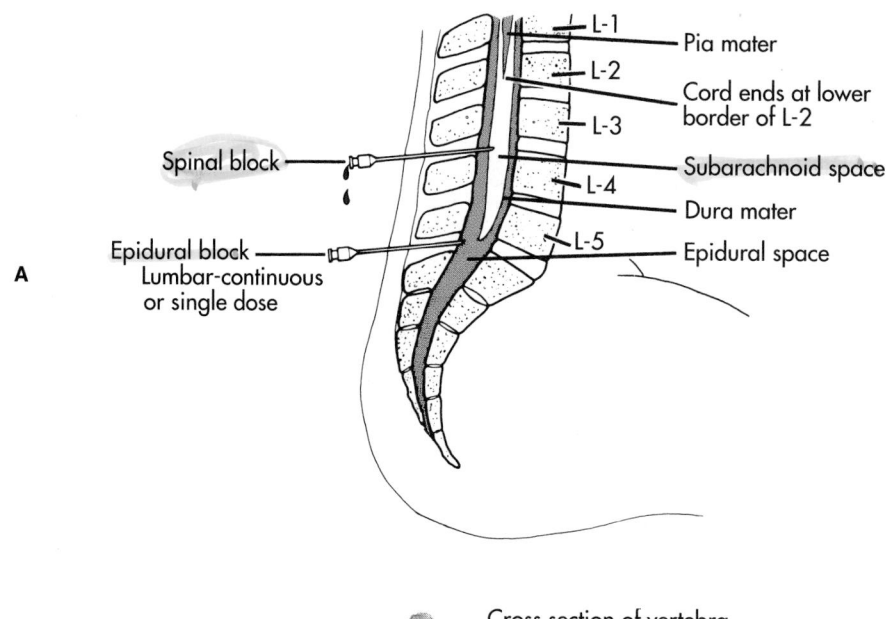

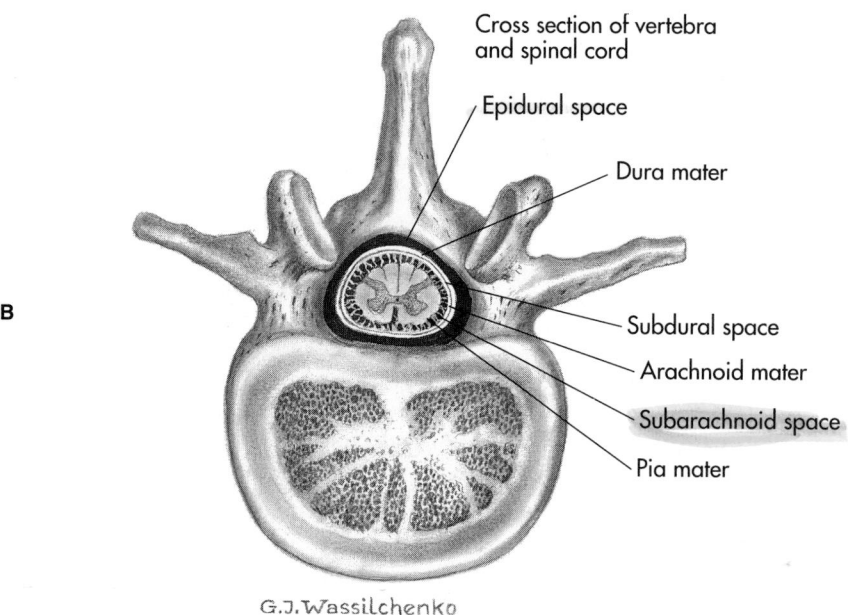

G.J. Wassilchenko

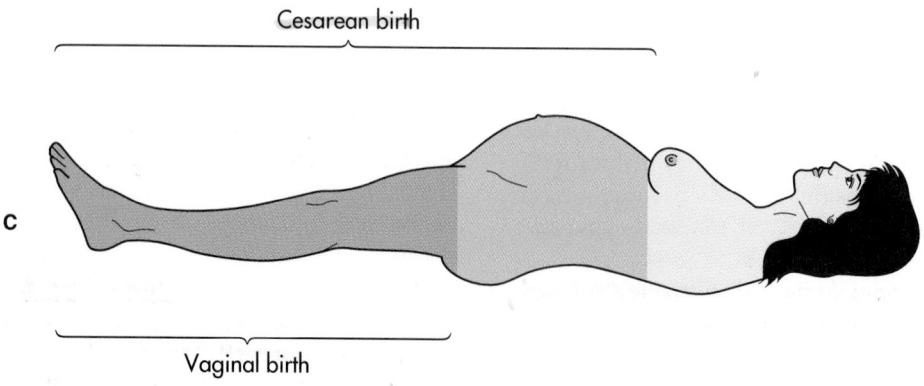

Fig. 20-9 **A,** Membranes and spaces of spinal cord and levels of sacral, lumbar, and thoracic nerves. **B,** Cross section of vertebra and spinal cord. **C,** Level of anesthesia necessary for cesarean birth and for vaginal births.

provides anesthesia from the nipple (T-6) to the feet. If used for vaginal birth the anesthesia level is from the hips (T-10) to the feet (Fig. 20-9, *C*).

For spinal block, the woman is positioned similar to that for an epidural placement so that the intervertebral space is widened. The nurse supports the woman because she must remain still during the placement of the spinal needle. The insertion is made between contractions. After the insertion, the woman may be positioned upright to get the level of anesthesia for a vaginal birth or positioned supine if the level desired is for cesarean birth. The anesthetic effect usually begins 1 to 2 minutes after the anesthetic is injected and lasts 1 to 3 hours, depending on the type of agent used (Chestnut, 1994).

Marked hypotension, decreased cardiac output and placental perfusion, and respiratory inadequacy may occur during any spinal anesthesia. If signs of serious maternal hypotension or fetal distress develop, emergency care must be instituted (see Emergency box).

Because the mother is not able to sense her contractions, she must be instructed when to bear down if having a vaginal birth. If the birth occurs in a delivery room (rather than a labor-delivery-recovery room), the mother will need assistance in being transferred to a recovery bed after delivery of the placenta.

Advantages of spinal anesthesia include ease of administration and absence of fetal hypoxia with maintenance of normotension. Maternal consciousness is maintained, excellent muscular relaxation is achieved, and blood loss is not excessive.

Disadvantages of spinal anesthesia include drug reactions (e.g., allergy), hypotension, and respiratory paralysis; cardiopulmonary resuscitation may be needed. In addition, when spinal anesthesia is given, the need for operative delivery (episiotomy, low forceps extraction) tends to be greater because the voluntary expulsive efforts are eliminated. After birth the incidence of bladder and uterine atony, as well as postspinal headache, is higher.

Leakage of cerebrospinal fluid from the site of puncture of the meninges (membranous coverings of the spinal cord) is thought to be the major causative factor in postlumbar puncture (postspinal) headache. Presumably such postural changes cause the diminished volume of CSF to exert traction on pain-sensitive CNS structures. The resulting headache, auditory, and visual problems may persist for days or weeks.

The likelihood of headache after lumbar puncture can be reduced, however, if the anesthesiologist uses a small-gauge spinal needle and avoids making multiple punctures of the meninges. Positioning the woman flat in bed (with only a small, flat pillow for her head) for at least 8 hours after spinal anesthesia has also been recommended to prevent headache, but there is no definitive evidence showing this measure is effective. Positioning the woman on her abdomen is thought to decrease the loss of CSF through the puncture site. Hydration has been claimed to be of value

 EMERGENCY

Maternal Hypotension with Decreased Placental Perfusion

SIGNS/SYMPTOMS
Maternal hypotension (20% drop from preblock level or less than 100 mm Hg systolic)
Fetal bradycardia
Decreased beat-to-beat FHR variability

INTERVENTIONS
Turn woman to left lateral position or place pillow or wedge under right hip (see Fig. 22-4) to deflect uterus.
Maintain IV infusion at rate specified, or increase prn per hospital protocol.
Administer oxygen by face mask at 10-12 L/min or per protocol.
Elevate the woman's legs.
Notify the physician/midwife/anesthesiologist/nurse anesthetist.
Administer IV vasopressor (e.g., ephedrine) per protocol.
Remain with woman; continue to monitor maternal blood pressure and FHR every 5 minutes until her condition is stable or per primary health care provider's order.

in preventing and treating headache, but there is no compelling evidence to support its use (Cunningham et al., 1997). Initial treatment for a post–lumbar puncture headache usually includes analgesics, bed rest, caffeine, and increased fluid intake (i.e., 150 ml/hr IV) (American College of Obstetricians and Gynecologists, 1996).

An autologous **epidural blood patch** (a patch repairing a tear or a hole in the dura mater around the spinal cord) is often beneficial, and such treatment may be considered if the headache does not resolve spontaneously (Scott et al., 1999). To form a patch, a few milliliters of the woman's blood without anticoagulant is injected epidurally at the site of the spinal tap (Fig. 20-10), which then forms a clot that covers the hole and prevents further fluid loss.

Epidural block. The pain of uterine contractions and birth (vaginal and abdominal) can be relieved by injecting a suitable local anesthetic into the epidural (peridural) space between the fourth and fifth lumbar vertebrae (see Figs. 20-7, *B*, and 20-9, *A*).

Complete lumbar **epidural block** for relieving the discomfort of labor and vaginal birth requires a block from T-10 to S-5. For cesarean birth, a block from at least T-8 to S-1 is essential. The diffusion of epidural anesthesia depends on the location of the catheter tip, the dose and volume of the anesthetic agent used, and the woman's position (e.g., horizontal or head-up position) (Cunningham et al., 1997).

For the induction of lumbar epidural anesthesia, the woman is positioned as for a spinal injection (i.e., sitting) or in a modified Sims position (Fig. 20-11). For this mod-

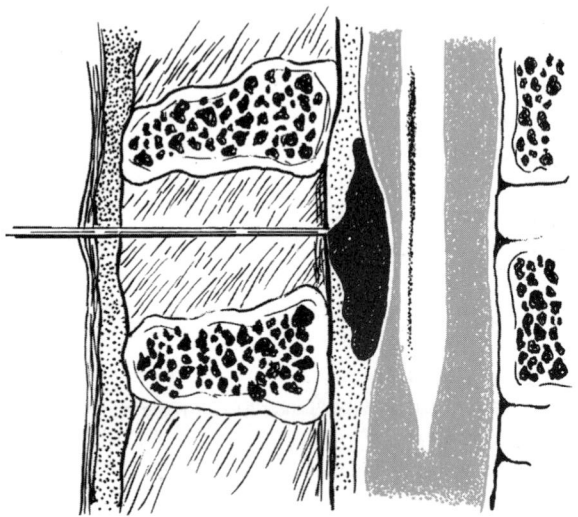

Fig. 20-10 Blood patch therapy for spinal headache.

ified lateral Sims position, the woman is placed on her side with her shoulders parallel, legs slightly flexed, and back arched.

After the epidural has been started, the woman is positioned preferably on her side so that the uterus does not compress the ascending vena cava and descending aorta, which can impair venous return and decrease placental perfusion. Oxygen should be available to treat hypotension should it occur despite maintenance of hydration with IV fluid and displacement of the uterus to the side. Ephedrine (a vasopressor used to increase maternal blood pressure) and increased IV fluid infusion may be needed (see Emergency box on p. 477). The FHR and progress in labor must be monitored carefully because the laboring woman may not be aware of changes in the strength of the uterine contractions or the descent of the presenting part.

A single injection or continuous infusion (via pump) through an indwelling plastic catheter results in excellent epidural analgesia-anesthesia. The advantages of an epidural block are numerous: the mother remains alert and cooperative, good relaxation is achieved, airway reflexes remain intact, only partial motor paralysis develops, gastric emptying is not delayed, and blood loss is not excessive. Fetal distress is rare but may occur in the event of rapid absorption or noticeable maternal hypotension. The dose, volume, and type of anesthetic can be modified to allow the mother

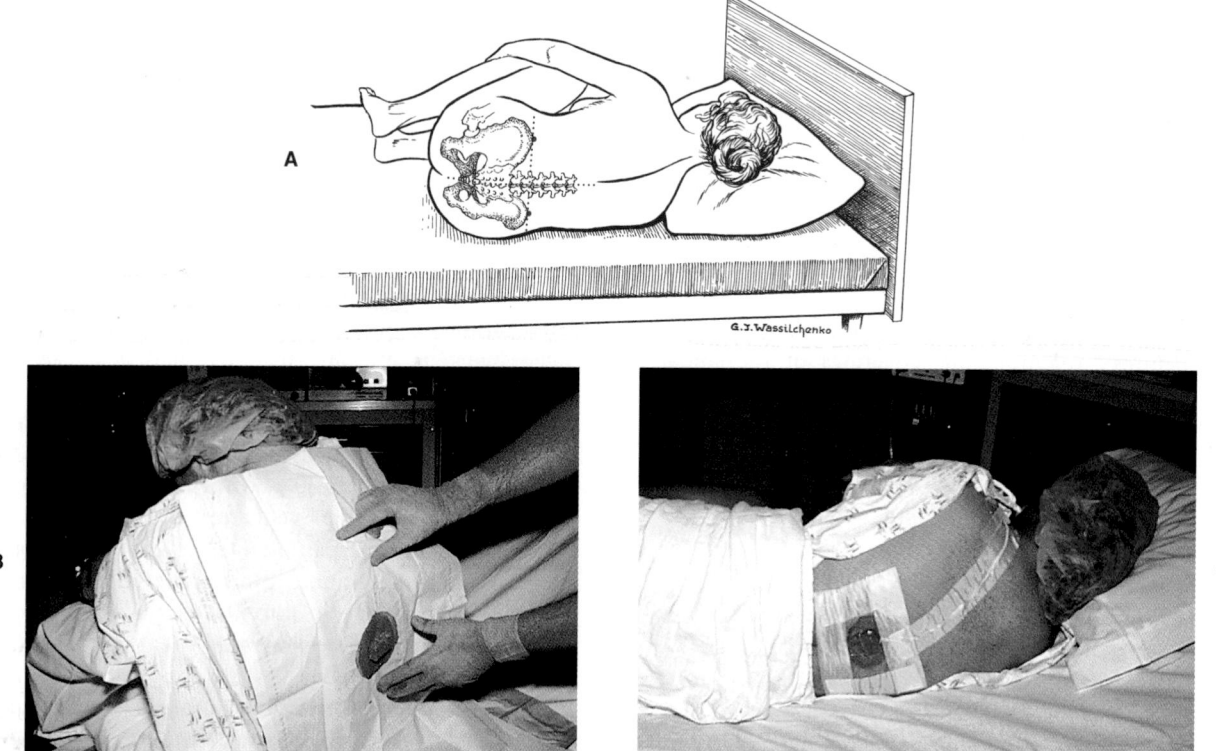

Fig. 20-11 Position for spinal and epidural blocks. **A,** Lateral position. **B,** Upright position. **C,** Catheter is taped to woman's back with port segment located near her shoulder. (**B** and **C,** *Courtesy Michael S. Clement, MD, Mesa, AZ.*)

to push, to produce perineal anesthesia, and to permit forceps or even cesarean birth if required (Cunningham et al., 1997).

The disadvantages of an epidural block for the woman include the need for an IV line, occasional dizziness, weakness of the legs, difficulty emptying the bladder, and shivering (Buggy & Bardiner, 1995; Youngstrom et al., 1996). Because a considerable amount of the drug must be used, adverse reactions or the rapid absorption of the anesthetic agent may result in maternal hypotension, convulsions, or paresthesia.

Data from retrospective studies and clinical trials suggest that there is a relationship between epidural analgesia and longer labor and increased incidence of operative birth (Howell, 1998; Thorpe & Breedlove, 1996). Occasionally, accidental high-spinal anesthesia (and later, postspinal headache) may follow inadvertent perforation of the dural membrane during the administration of lumbar epidural anesthesia.

For some women the selected anesthetic is not effective, and a second form of anesthesia is required to establish effective pain relief. For women who progress rapidly in labor, pain relief may not be obtained before birth occurs.

Epidural and intrathecal narcotics. There is a high concentration of narcotic receptors along the pain pathway in the spinal cord, in the brainstem, and in the thalamus. Because these receptors are highly sensitive to narcotics, a small quantity of narcotic produces marked analgesia lasting for several hours. The medication is injected through a catheter placed in the epidural or subarachnoid space, which communicates with these narcotic receptors, and pain transmission is blocked without compromising motor ability, thus the so-called walking epidural, which restores the woman's confidence in her ability to master labor no longer dominated by pain (Youngstrom et al., 1996) (see Research box).

The use of epidural or intrathecal narcotics during labor has several advantages. These agents do not cause maternal hypotension or affect vital signs. The woman feels contractions but not pain. Her ability to bear down during the second stage of labor is preserved because the pushing reflex is not lost and her motor power remains intact.

Fentanyl, sufentanil, or preservative-free morphine may be used. Fentanyl and sufentanil produce short-acting analgesia (1.5 to 3.5 hours), and morphine may provide pain relief for 4 to 7 hours. Morphine may be combined with fentanyl or sufentanil. The short-acting narcotics are often used with multiparous women, and the morphine may be used with nulliparous women or women with a history of long labors (Manning, 1996). For most women, intrathecal narcotics do not provide adequate analgesia for second-stage labor pain, episiotomy, or birth (Cunningham et al., 1997). Pudendal blocks or local anesthetics may be necessary.

A more common indication for the administration of epidural or intrathecal narcotics is the relief of postoperative

---

 RESEARCH

The Course of Labor With and Without Epidural Analgesia

Numerous studies suggest that epidural analgesia during labor has significant effects on the length of labor and on the method of birth. Controversy exists because study groups have not been identified and the presence of other variables such as parity, oxytocin use, and self-selection of analgesia may have affected the outcome of the studies.

This study identified inclusion criteria for subjects and conducted a randomized investigation comparing the effects of epidural analgesia on labor with effects of boluses of meperidine on a group of women with similar clinical circumstances. A total of 199 nulliparous women were included in the study. All received oxytocin before receiving the anglesic intervention and gave birth spontaneously.

The demographics of the women in the two groups, their cervical dilation at the time of admission, and their cervical dilation at the time of administration of analgesia were similar. The length of the active phase of the first stage of labor was longer in the epidural group (7.9 hr vs. 6.3 hr, $p = 0.005$); the second stage of labor was longer (60 min vs. 48 min, $p = 0.03$). The amount of oxytocin needed for each centimeter of dilation was greater in the epidural group (22 vs. 16 ml, $p = 0.009$). The researchers concluded that epidural analgesia decreased uterine performance when oxytocin was used to stimulate labor, resulting in longer labor in the first and second stages.

CLINICAL APPLICATION

Maternal movement and position changes are effective in relieving pain during labor and in augmenting slow labor. Although epidural analgesia does provide pain relief, it may also produce adverse effects. Despite these findings, if a woman chooses epidural analgesia for pain relief during labor, the nurse must be ready to make accurate assessments about labor progress and provide the needed care and support. Close observation in the active phase of the first and second stages of labor can identify slow but steady progress. Position changes should be encouraged and assistance provided as needed. Diligent care may help the woman proceed to a spontaneous vaginal birth instead of a cesarean or other operative birth.

Source: Alexander, J. et al. (1998). The course of labor with and without epidural analgesia. *Am J Obstet Gynecol* 178(3), 516-520.

pain. For example, women who give birth by cesarean receive fentanyl (Innovar) or morphine through the catheter. The catheter may then be removed, and the women are usually free of pain for 24 hours. Occasionally the catheter is left in place in case another dose is needed.

Women receiving epidurally administered morphine after the cesarean birth are up soon after surgery with surprising ease and are able to care for their babies. The early ambulation and freedom from pain afforded also facilitate bladder emptying. To those women who have had a previous cesarean birth and have experienced the usual postoperative pain, the effects of this approach seem miraculous. However, the mother may not understand why she may experience pain after the narcotic effect wears off.

Side effects of epidural and intrathecal narcotics include nausea, vomiting, pruritus (itching), urinary retention, and delayed respiratory depression. These side effects are more common when morphine is administered. Antiemetics, antipruritics, and narcotic antagonists are used to relieve these symptoms. For example, naloxone or naltrexone, nalbuphine hydrochloride (Nubain), promethazine, or metoclopramide (Reglan) may be administered. Hospital protocols should provide specific instructions for the treatment of these side effects. Use of epidural narcotics is not without risks. Respiratory depression is a serious concern; for this reason the woman's respiratory rate should be assessed and documented every hour for 24 hours, or per the timing designated by hospital protocol. Naloxone hydrochloride should be readily available for use if the respiratory rate decreases below 10 breaths per minute or if the oxygen saturation rate drops below 89%. Administration of oxygen by face mask may also be initiated, and the anesthesiologist should be notified.

Contraindications to subarachnoid and epidural blocks. Some contraindications to epidural analgesia apply equally to caudal and subarachnoid blocks (Scott et al., 1999):

- *Antepartum hemorrhage.* Acute hypovolemia leads to increased sympathetic tone to maintain the blood pressure. Any anesthetic technique that blocks the sympathetic fibers can produce significant hypotension that can endanger the mother and baby.
- *Anticoagulant therapy or bleeding disorder.* If a woman is receiving anticoagulant therapy or has a bleeding disorder, injury to a blood vessel may cause the formation of a hematoma that may compress the cauda equina or the spinal cord and lead to serious CNS sequelae.
- *Infection at the injection site.* Infection can be spread through the peridural or subarachnoid spaces if the needle traverses an infected area.
- *Allergy to the anesthetic drug.*

Drug effects on neonate. Debate persists concerning the effects of epidural anesthesia on the newborn's neurobehavioral responses. Results from studies examining associations between neurobehavioral outcome and epidural anesthesia are far from consistent. For example, studies

comparing the neonatal neurobehavioral scores for infants born to mothers who did and mothers who did not receive epidural analgesia have shown either little or no difference in the scores (Hamza, 1994; Scherer & Holzgreve, 1995) or have shown that the neonates of mothers who received epidural anesthesia did not score as well on neurobehavioral tests (Sepkoski et al., 1992).

Paracervical (uterosacral) block. Paracervical block can be used to relieve the pain from the lower uterine segment and cervix to the upper third of the vagina. It is rarely used for labor because of the potential fetal complications related to rapid absorption of the drug. Paracervical block may be used for anesthesia during abortion or other gynecologic procedures.

General Anesthesia

General anesthesia rarely is used for uncomplicated vaginal birth and is infrequently used for cesarean birth. It may be necessary if there is a contraindication to nerve block analgesia or anesthesia or if the woman is not already receiving regional analgesia when there is an emergency maternal or fetal situation.

If general anesthesia is being considered, the nurse gives the woman nothing by mouth and sees that an IV infusion is established. If time allows, the nurse premedicates the woman with a nonparticulate oral antacid such as sodium citrate (30 ml) to neutralize the acidic contents of the stomach. If there is sufficient time, some anesthesiologists and physicians also order the administration of a histamine blocker such as cimetidine to decrease the production of gastric acid and metoclopramide to increase gastric emptying (Scott et al., 1999). Before the anesthesia is given, a wedge should be placed under the woman's right hip to displace the uterus to the left. As noted, such uterine displacement prevents aortocaval compression, which interferes with placental perfusion. Sometimes the nurse is asked to assist with applying cricoid pressure (Fig. 20-12) before intubation.

Priorities for recovery room care are to maintain an open airway, maintain cardiopulmonary functions, and prevent postpartum hemorrhage. Routine postpartum care is organized around facilitating parent-child attachment as soon as possible and answering the mother's questions. Whenever appropriate, the nurse assesses the mother's readiness to see the baby, as well as her response to the anesthesia and to the event that necessitated general anesthesia (e.g., cesarean birth when vaginal birth was anticipated).

Inhalation analgesia and anesthesia. Nitrous oxide is the only inhalation agent used for obstetrics in the United States. It is rarely used for labor in the United States but may be used for this purpose in other countries.

Nitrous oxide is commonly used for cesarean births when inhalation anesthesia is needed. It is usually combined with oxygen in a 50/50 mixture. Thiopental, a short-acting barbiturate, combined with succinylcholine, a muscle relaxer, is given intravenously before tracheal intubation.

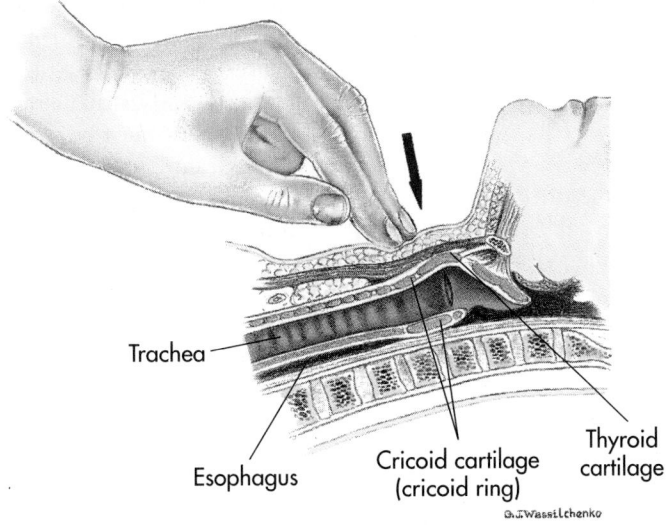

Trachea

Esophagus

Cricoid cartilage
(cricoid ring)

Thyroid
cartilage

G.J.Wassilchenko

Fig. 20-12 Technique of applying pressure on cricoid cartilage to occlude esophagus to prevent pulmonary aspiration of gastric contents during induction of general anesthesia.

Other inhalation agents include halothane, enflurane or isoflurane, and methoxyflurane. These agents relax the uterus quickly and facilitate intrauterine manipulation, version, and extraction. However, these agents cross the placenta readily and can produce narcosis in the fetus. They are rarely used today in the United States.

▍CARE MANAGEMENT

The choice of pain relief depends on a combination of factors, including the woman's special needs and wishes, the availability of the desired method, the health care provider's knowledge and expertise in nonpharmacologic and pharmacologic methods, and the phase and stage of labor. The nurse is responsible for maintaining continuous maternal and fetal assessment, establishing mutual goals with the woman (and her family), formulating nursing diagnoses, planning and implementing nursing care, and evaluating the effects of care. It is essential for the nurse to carefully document all aspects of care management.

Assessment and Nursing Diagnoses

The assessment of the woman, her fetus, and her labor is a joint effort on the part of the nurse and the primary health care providers, who consult with the woman regarding their findings and recommendations. The needs of each woman are different, and many factors must be considered whether nonpharmacologic, a combination of nonpharmacologic and pharmacologic, or pharmacologic methods of pain management are used. A self-assessment tool, such as an analog scale, allows the woman to indicate on a line how severe she perceives her pain experience to be. Self-assessment is recommended to ensure that pain management is based on the subjective nature of the woman's

GUIDELINES/GUÍAS

Pain Management

Do you want to get up and walk?
¿Desea levantarse y caminar?

Do you want pain medication?
¿Quiere medicina para el dolor?

I am going to give you the pain medicine in an injection.
Le voy a dar la medicina para el dolor en una inyección.

I am going to give you the pain medicine through an IV.
Le voy a dar la medicina para el dolor por medio del suero.

This is a pain reliever called Demerol/Stadol/Nubain.
Este es una medicina para aliviar el dolor que se llama Demerol/Stadol/Nubain.

The effects of this medicine are relatively short.
Los efectos de esta medicina son relativamente cortos.

The epidural is a stronger method of pain relief.
La anestesia espinal es un método más fuerte para aliviar el dolor.

You should not be able to feel the contraction pain.
No debe de sentir los dolores de las contracciónes.

pain rather than on just the nurse's judgment (Olden et al., 1995) (see Guidelines/Guías box).

History

The woman's prenatal record is read and relevant information identified. This includes the woman's parity, estimated date of birth, and complications and medications during pregnancy. If the woman has a history of allergies, this is noted and a warning displayed in a prominent place. A history of smoking and neurologic and spinal disorders is also noted.

Interview

Interview data consist of the time of the woman's last meal and the type of food consumed; the nature of any existing respiratory condition (cold, allergy); and unusual reactions to medications (e.g., allergy), cleansing agents, or tape. The woman is asked whether she attended childbirth preparation classes, and the extent of her preparation and her preferences for management of discomfort are noted. Her knowledge of the options for the management of discomfort is also assessed. Information on the woman's perception of discomfort and her expressed need for medication are added to the database. Relevant events that have occurred since the woman's last contact with the primary health care provider are also reviewed (e.g., infections, diarrhea, change in fetal behavior). If verbal and physical signs indicate the existence of substance abuse, the nurse should ask the woman to identify the type of drug used, the last time the drug was taken, and the method of administration.

Physical Examination

The character and status of the labor and fetal response are assessed during a physical examination. The nurse evaluates the woman's hydration status by assessing intake and output measurements, the moistness of the mucous membranes, and skin turgor. Bladder distention is noted. Any evidence of skin infection near sites of possible needle insertion is recorded and reported. Signs of apprehension such as fist clenching and restlessness are also noted.

If the woman is in labor, the status of maternal vital signs and FHR, uterine contractions, cervical effacement, and dilation; the station; and the anticipated time until birth are all considered. The length of labor and degree of fatigue are other important considerations. If pharmacologic methods are to be used, the type of analgesia or anesthesia chosen varies depending on the phase and stage of labor (see Box 20-3).

Laboratory Tests

The results of laboratory tests are reviewed to determine whether the woman is suffering from anemia (hemoglobin and hematocrit), coagulopathy or bleeding disorder (prothrombin time and platelet count), or infection (white blood cell count and differential).

Signs of Potential Problems

Any medication can cause an allergic reaction that may be minor or as severe as anaphylaxis. Severe reactions may occur suddenly and lead to shock. The most dramatic form of anaphylaxis is sudden severe bronchospasm, vasospasm, severe hypotension, and death. Signs of anaphy-

laxis are largely caused by contraction of smooth muscles, and this may be heralded by irritability, extreme weakness, nausea, and vomiting, leading to dyspnea, cyanosis, convulsions, and cardiac arrest. The acute allergic reaction—anaphylaxis—must be diagnosed and treated by the health care team immediately to prevent consequences. Treatment usually consists of 1:1000 epinephrine injected subcutaneously or intramuscularly, followed by parenteral administration of antihistamines. Supportive care is given to alleviate the symptoms, and the type of care is determined by the rapidly assessed cardiovascular and respiratory response of the woman to the primary interventions; cardiopulmonary resuscitation may be necessary. The nurse must also be alert to fetal well-being; any FHR decelerations should be noted and reported to the primary health care provider.

Minor reactions can consist of a rash, rhinitis, fever, asthma, or pruritus. Management of the less acute allergic response does not constitute an emergency. As part of the assessment for such allergic reactions, the nurse should monitor the woman's vital signs, respiratory status, cardiovascular status, platelet count, and white blood cell count. The woman is observed for side effects of drug therapy, especially drowsiness (Clark et al., 1996).

The following nursing diagnoses are relevant in the management of discomfort during labor and birth:

▪ Nursing Diagnoses _____

- Risk for altered tissue perfusion related to
  - effects of analgesia or anesthesia
  - maternal position
- Hypothermia related to
  - effects of analgesia or anesthesia
- Pain related to
  - processes of labor and birth
- Situational low self-esteem related to
  - negative perception of the woman's (or her family's) behavior
- Anxiety or fear related to knowledge deficit of
  - procedure for nerve block analgesia
  - expected sensation during nerve block analgesia
  - mother's role during nerve block analgesia
  - options for analgesia and anesthesia
- Risk for maternal injury related to
  - effects of analgesia and anesthesia on sensation and motor control
- Risk for injury to fetus related to
  - maternal hypotension
  - maternal position (aortocaval compression)

Expected Outcomes of Care

The expected outcomes of nursing care in the management of the discomfort of labor and birth include the following:

- The woman, her partner, and her family will verbalize understanding of their needs and rights with regard to the use of nonpharmacologic methods, analgesia, or anesthesia.
- The woman will experience adequate pain relief without maternal risk being increased (e.g., through the use of appropriate nonpharmacologic methods and appropriate medication, including the appropriate dose, timing, and route of administration).
- Fetal well-being will be maintained, and the newborn will adjust to extrauterine life.

Plan of Care and Interventions

A plan of care is developed for each woman and should address her particular clinical and nursing problems. The nurse collaborates with the primary health care provider and laboring woman in selecting those aspects of care relevant to the woman and her family.

Nonpharmacologic Interventions

The nurse supports and assists the woman as she uses nonpharmacologic interventions for pain relief and relaxation. During labor, the nurse should ask the woman how she feels in order to evaluate the effectiveness of the specific pain management. Appropriate interventions can then be planned or continued for effective care, such as trying other nonpharmacologic methods or combining nonpharmacologic methods with medications.

The woman's *perception* of her behavior during labor is of utmost importance. If she planned a nonmedicated birth but then needs and accepts medication, her self-esteem may falter. The nurse gives verbal and nonverbal reassurance of the acceptability of her behavior as necessary and reinforces reassurances after birth if possible. Explanations about the fetal response to maternal discomfort, the effects of maternal fatigue, and the medication itself are supportive measures. The woman may also be experiencing anxiety and stress related to the anticipated or actual pain. Stress can cause increased maternal catecholamine production. Raised levels of catecholamines have been linked to dysfunctional labor and fetal and neonatal distress and illness. Nurses must be able to implement strategies aimed at reducing this stress (Green, 1993).

Informed Consent

The primary health care provider and anesthesia care provider are responsible for informing women of the alternative methods of pharmacologic pain relief available in the hospital setting. The description of the various anesthetic techniques and what they entail is essential to the informed consent process, even if the woman has received information about analgesia and anesthesia earlier in her pregnancy. This interview should take place just before or early in labor so the woman has time to consider alternatives. Nurses play a part in the informed consent by clari-

fying and describing procedures or by acting as a client's advocate and asking the primary health care provider for further explanations. The procedure and its advantages and disadvantages must be thoroughly explained.

LEGAL TIP **Informed Consent for Anesthetic**

The Woman Receives (in an Understandable Manner):
- *Explanation of alternative methods of anesthesia and analgesia available*
- *Description of anesthetic and procedure for administration*
- *Description of the benefits, discomforts, risks, and consequences to the mother and the fetus of the anesthetic selected*
- *Explanation of how complications can be treated*
- *Information that the anesthetic is not always effective*
- *Indication that the woman may withdraw consent at any time*
- *Opportunity to answer any questions*
- *Opportunity to explain in the mother's own words components of the consent*

Consent form:
- *Written or explained in woman's primary language*
- *Woman's signature*
- *Date of consent*
- *Signature of anesthetic care provider, certifying that the woman has received and appears to understand the explanation*

Timing of Administration

It is often the nurse who notifies the primary health care provider that the woman is in need of pharmacologic measures to relieve her discomfort. Therefore the primary health care provider often writes orders for the administration of pain medication as needed based on the nurse's clinical judgment. The pharmacologic measures used to manage the discomfort of labor are summarized in Box 20-3 by stage of labor and method of birth.

Preparation for Procedures

The nurse reviews the methods of pain relief available to the woman or validates her choices and also clarifies the information for the mother as necessary. The procedure and what will be asked of her (e.g., to maintain flexed position during insertion of epidural needle) must be explained to the woman. The woman can also benefit from knowing the way that the medication is to be given, how much discomfort she is likely to experience during administration of the medication, what sensations she can expect, the way the skin is prepared, how long it will take to administer the medication, and how long it will take for the medication to take effect. The nurse also explains the reason for emptying the bladder before the analgesic or anesthetic is given and the reason for keeping the bladder empty. When an indwelling epidural catheter is to be threaded, the woman should be told that she may experience a momentary twinge down her leg, hip, or back and that this feeling is not a sign of injury. A long needle is used for pudendal blocks (see Fig. 20-8). The sight of this needle may be frightening, and the woman should be reassured that only the tip of the needle will be inserted.

Administration of Medication

Accurate monitoring of the progress of labor forms the basis for the nursing judgment of the need for pharmacologic control of discomfort. Knowledge of the medications that are used during childbirth is also essential. The most effective route of administration is selected for each woman, and then the medication is prepared and administered correctly.

Intravenous route. The preferred route of administration of medications such as meperidine or fentanyl is through IV tubing, administered into the port nearest the woman while the infusion of IV solution is stopped. The medication is given slowly in small doses at the beginning of three to five consecutive contractions. Because uterine blood vessels are constricted during contractions, the medication stays within the maternal vascular system for several seconds before the uterine blood vessels reopen. The IV infusion is then restarted slowly to prevent a bolus of medication from forming. Using this method of injection, the amount of drug crossing the placenta to the fetus is minimized. With decreased placental transfer, the mother's degree of pain relief is maximized. Use of the IV route is associated with the following advantages:

- The onset of pain relief is more predictable.
- Pain relief is obtained with small doses of the drug.
- The duration of effect is more predictable.

Intramuscular route. IM injections of analgesics, although still used, are not the preferred route for administering such agents in the laboring woman. Identified disadvantages of the IM route include the following:

- The onset of pain relief is delayed.
- Higher doses of medication are required.
- Medication is released from the muscle tissue at an unpredictable rate and is available for transfer across the placenta to the fetus.

IM injections are given in the upper portion of the arm (deltoid site) if regional anesthesia is planned later in labor. This is the preferred site because the autonomic blockade from the regional (e.g., epidural) anesthesia causes blood flow to the gluteal region to be increased and absorption of the drug to be accelerated. The maternal plasma level of the drug necessary to bring pain relief usually is reached 45 minutes after IM injection, followed by a decline in plasma levels. The maternal drug levels (after IM injections) are also unequal because of uneven distribution (maternal uptake) and metabolism. The only advantage of using the IM route is quick administration.

Nerve blocks. An IV line is established before the induction of nerve blocks such as epidural, spinal, and general anesthesia. Anesthesia protocols usually include the administration of a bolus of IV fluid before epidural and spinal anesthesia for blood volume expansion to prevent maternal hypotension.

Lactated Ringer's or Plasma-Lyte A and normal saline solutions are the preferred infusion solutions. Infusion solutions without dextrose are preferred, especially when the solution must be infused rapidly (e.g., the treatment of severe dehydration or the maintenance of blood pressure) because solutions containing dextrose raise the maternal blood glucose levels rapidly. The fetus responds to such high blood glucose levels by increasing insulin production, and this can lead to fetal or neonatal hypoglycemia. In addition, dextrose changes the osmotic pressure so that fluid is excreted from the kidneys more rapidly.

The woman needs assistance in assuming and maintaining the correct position for epidural and spinal anesthesia (see Fig 20-11).

Safety and General Care

After administration of a nerve block, the woman is protected from injury by raising the side rails and placing a call bell within easy reach when the nurse is not in attendance. Oxygen and suction should be readily available at the bedside. The nurse must make sure there is no prolonged pressure on an anesthetized part (e.g., lying on one side with weight on one leg, tight bedclothes on feet). If stirrups are to be used for birth, the nurse should place pads on them, adjust both stirrups to the same level and angle, place both of the woman's legs into them simultaneously without putting pressure on the popliteal angle, and apply restraints without restricting circulation.

The nurse monitors and records the woman's response to nonpharmacologic pain relief methods and her response to medication. This includes the level of pain relief, level of apprehension, return of sensations and perception of pain, and allergic or untoward reactions that occur (e.g., hypotension, respiratory depression, hypothermia). The nurse continues to monitor maternal vital signs, blood pressure, the strength and frequency of uterine contractions, changes in the cervix and station of the presenting part, the presence of the bearing-down reflex, bladder filling, and state of hydration. Determining the fetal response after the induction of analgesia or anesthesia is of vital importance. The woman is asked if she (or the family) has any questions. The nurse also assesses the woman's and her family's understanding of the need for ensuring her safety (e.g., keeping side rails up, calling for assistance as needed).

The time that elapses between the administration of a narcotic and the baby's birth is noted. Documentation is completed if the newborn was given any medications to reverse narcotic effects. Postpartum, the woman who has had spinal, epidural, or general anesthesia is assessed for return of sensory and motor sensations in addition to the usual postpartum assessments.

PLAN OF CARE Nonpharmacologic Management of Discomfort

NURSING DIAGNOSIS Pain related to physiologic response to labor

Expected Outcome *Woman will express decrease in intensity of discomfort and experience satisfaction with her labor and birth performance.*

Nursing Interventions/*Rationales*

Assess whether woman and significant other have attended childbirth classes, her knowledge of labor process, and her current level of anxiety *to plan supportive strategies.*

Encourage support person to remain with woman in labor *to provide support and increase probability of response to comfort measures.*

Teach or review nonpharmacologic techniques available to decrease anxiety and pain during labor (e.g., focusing and feedback, breathing techniques, effleurage, and sacral pressure) *to enhance chances of success in using techniques.*

Explore other techniques that the woman or significant other may have learned in childbirth classes (e.g., hypnosis, yoga, acupressure, biofeedback, therapeutic touch, aromatherapy, imaging, vocalizations) *to provide largest repertoire of coping strategies.*

Explore use of jet hydrotherapy if ordered by physician and if woman meets use criteria (i.e., vital signs within normal limits [WNL], cervix 4 to 5 cm dilated, active phase of first stage labor) *to aid relaxation and stimulate production of natural oxytocin.*

Explore use of transcutaneous nerve stimulation per physician order *to provide an increased perception of control over pain and an increase in release of endogenous opiates.*

Assist woman to change positions and to use pillows *to reduce stiffness, aid circulation, and promote comfort.*

Assess bladder for distention and encourage voiding often *to avoid bladder distention and subsequent discomfort.*

Encourage rest between contractions *to minimize fatigue.*

Keep woman and significant other informed about progress *to allay anxiety.*

Guide couple through the labor stages and phases, helping them use and modify comfort techniques that are appropriate to each phase *to ensure greatest effectiveness of techniques employed.*

From Wong, D., & Perry, S. (1998). *Maternal child nursing care.* St. Louis: Mosby.

Special Concerns

Two additional concerns about use of analgesia and anesthesia—the use of anesthesia in obese women and postpartum hypothermia—are discussed in the following sections.

Anesthesia in the obese woman. *Obesity* is defined as an excess of body fat causing weight to be greater than 20% over ideal weight; obesity affects 6% to 10% of pregnant women. Weight more than twice the ideal body weight is considered morbid obesity. A retrospective study of morbidly obese pregnant women covering the years 1978 to 1989 revealed that 62% underwent cesarean birth and 48% underwent emergency cesarean birth (Hood & Dewan, 1993). In a June 1, 1994, to May 31, 1995, study of 20,130 women, women who were obese before pregnancy were found to have an increased risk for cesarean delivery when compared with women who were nonobese before pregnancy (Crane et al., 1997).

As discussed in detail in Chapter 15, maternal physiologic changes are the product of hormonal influences and mechanical effects. In obese women, the weight of the fat tissue and the added metabolic demands this involves also affect maternal physiology (Endler, 1990). Both pregnancy and obesity cause blood volume and cardiac output to increase, and in the latter case, they expand in proportion to the amount of fat tissue. During labor and vaginal birth, and in the immediate postpartum period, blood values and cardiac output in obese women can reach levels 80% greater than prelabor values. The enlarged uterus and abdominal fat mass also further increase the possibility of aortocaval compression.

The respiratory system is also stressed in obese pregnant women (Endler, 1990), and the pulmonary function of an obese laboring woman is in a precarious state. Therefore the woman's oxygenation must be carefully monitored during birth and the immediate postpartum period. Monitoring by pulse oximeter has been suggested.

The gastric emptying time is delayed, tone of the cardiac sphincter decreased, and gastric contents hyperacidic in all pregnant women. However, the obese woman is also more likely to have a hiatal hernia and a marked increase in intragastric pressure and volume. Therefore these women are at great risk for regurgitation and aspiration (Endler, 1990).

Management of the obese woman during labor should focus on efforts to minimize oxygen consumption and maximize pulmonary function. Epidural analgesia administered during the first stage of labor can bring about a decreased demand on the metabolic and respiratory systems and improved oxygenation. This is because pain causes the catecholamine levels to rise, which in turn causes cardiac output to increase. Effective epidural analgesia retards this rise in catecholamine levels.

Intravenous narcotics may be used during the first stage of labor. However, the doses and the effects must be monitored carefully because obese women are extremely sensitive to the respiratory depressant effects of narcotics (Endler, 1990). An epidural block during the second stage of labor provides complete pain relief and also supports cardiovascular function.

An epidural block is preferred to general anesthesia in the obese woman who must give birth by cesarean. Problems associated with general anesthesia in obese women include potential difficulties during intubation, a hypertensive effect of laryngoscopy and intubation, and aspiration and pulmonary complications. A spinal block may be used if there is insufficient time to induce an epidural block. Uterine displacement to prevent aortocaval compression is more difficult to achieve in the obese woman in the supine position needed for cesarean birth. If the woman is extremely obese, a wedge may not be able to elevate the right hip enough to prevent compression. In this case it may be necessary to physically lift the abdominal fat pad off the abdomen until the peritoneal cavity has been entered (Endler, 1990).

Maternal hypothermia after analgesia and anesthesia. *Hypothermia* is defined as a core body temperature of less than 35° C. During labor and immediately postpartum, women are predisposed to suffering hypothermia because of the combination of the vasodilation that normally occurs during pregnancy and the effects of the analgesia and anesthesia.

Opiates/narcotics, barbiturates, tranquilizers, and antiemetics are thought to affect thermoregulation by increasing vasodilation and radiant loss; general anesthetic agents are thought to do so by depressing thermoregulation; and epidural and spinal anesthesia are thought to do so by inducing peripheral dilation (Buggy & Bardiner, 1995). During labor, during vaginal or cesarean birth, or immediately after birth women may experience shivering, hypotension, and respiratory distress. The hypothermia may result in cardiovascular, pulmonary, circulatory, hematologic, neurologic, or renal complications (Buggy & Bardiner, 1995). The nurse can minimize these complications by making sure that the birthing areas are warm, wet drapes and towels are removed, women are covered with warm blankets after birth, and hypothermia is recognized early. Explaining these effects to the woman and her support people will help allay concerns.

Evaluation

Evaluation of the effectiveness of care of the woman needing management of discomfort during labor and birth is based on the previously stated outcomes (see Plan of Care).

KEY POINTS

- The expected outcome of the preparation for childbirth and parenting is "education for choice."
- Nonpharmacologic pain and stress management strategies are valuable for managing labor discomfort alone or in combination with pharmacologic methods.
- The gate-control theory of pain and stress is the basis for many of the nonpharmacologic methods of pain relief.
- The type of analgesic or anesthetic to be used is determined in part by the stage of labor and the method of birth planned.
- Narcotic effects can be potentiated with ataractics.
- Naloxone or naltrexone are narcotic antagonists that can reverse narcotic effects, especially respiratory depression.
- Pharmacologic control of discomfort during labor requires collaboration among the health care providers and the laboring woman.
- The nurse must understand the various qualities of the medications, their expected effect, potential side effects, and methods of administration.
- An IV line and maternal hydration are essential during regional nerve blocks.
- Maternal analgesia and anesthesia potentially affect neonatal neurobehavioral response.
- The use of narcotic agonist-antagonist compounds in women with preexisting narcotic dependency may cause symptoms of narcotic withdrawal.
- General anesthesia is rarely used for vaginal birth but may be used for cesarean birth or whenever rapid anesthesia is needed in an emergency childbirth situation.

CRITICAL THINKING EXERCISES

1 *You are assigned to care for a Hispanic woman in active labor who has her fists tightly clenched and is grimacing. She does not speak English. She is not making any kind of request for anything to relieve the pain. You are convinced that discomfort should be avoided if possible.*

  a. *Examine the assumptions the nurse may have about how women of different cultures exhibit their reactions to pain.*
  b. *Examine assumptions that both the nurse and the Hispanic woman may have about pain relief.*
  c. *Analyze the arguments for and against the use of pharmacologic agents for control of discomfort.*
  d. *Propose a plan of care for pain relief in this situation, and justify your choice of interventions.*

CRITICAL THINKING EXERCISES—cont'd

2 *Talk to a woman of a different culture who has experienced childbirth. Ask her to describe her reactions to pain, how she sought relief of the pain, the atmosphere of the childbirth setting, and the attitudes of the health care providers.*

   a. Analyze the way the atmosphere of the setting and the attitudes of the health care providers might have influenced the perception of pain in such a woman from a different culture.

   b. Examine the childbirth setting where you are now assigned.

      1) What is the atmosphere of the setting, and what are the attitudes of the health care providers regarding the expression of pain by women of various cultures?

      2) Analyze the effect when the nurse's culture differs from that of the woman for whom she is caring.

References

Alexander, C., & Steeful, L. (1995). Biofeedback: Listen to the body. *RN* 58(8), 51-52.

American College of Obstetricians and Gynecologists. (1996). *Obstetric analgesia and anesthesia. Technical Bulletin No. 225.* Washington, D.C.: ACOG.

Bradley, R. (1981). *Husband-coached childbirth* (3rd ed.). New York: HarperCollins.

Buggy, D., & Bardiner, J. (1995). The space blanket and shivering during extradural anesthesia in labour. *Acta Anaesthesia Scand* 39(4), 551-553.

Burns, E., & Blamey, C. (1994). Complementary medicine: Using aromatherapy in childbirth. *Nurs Times* 90(9), 54-60.

Chestnut, D. (1994). Alternative regional anesthetic techniques: Paracervical block, lumbar sympathetic block, pudendal block and perineal infiltration. In D. Chestnut (Ed). *Obstetrics anesthesia: Principles and practice.* St. Louis: Mosby.

Clark, J., Queener, S., & Karb, V. (1996). *Pharmacological basis of nursing practice* (5th ed.). St. Louis: Mosby.

Crane, S. et al. (1997). Association between prepregnancy obesity and the risk of cesarean delivery. *Obstet Gynecol* 89(2), 213-216.

Cunningham, F. et al. (1997). *Williams obstetrics* (20th ed.). Stamford, CT: Appleton & Lange.

Dickason E., Silverman, B., & Kaplan, J. (1998). *Maternal-infant nursing care* (3rd ed.). St. Louis: Mosby.

Dick-Read, G. (1987). *Childbirth without fear* (5th ed.). New York: HarperCollins.

Endler, G. (1990). The risk of anesthesia in obese parturients. *J Perinatol* 10(2), 175-179.

Green, J. (1993). Expectations and experiences of pain in labor: Findings from a large prospective study. *Birth* 20(2), 65-72.

Hamza, J. (1994). Effect of epidural anesthesia on the fetus and the neonate. *Cahiers d Anesthesiologie* 42(2), 265-273.

Hood, D., & Dewan, D. (1993). Anesthetic and obstetric outcome in morbidly obese parturients. *Anesthesiology* 79(6), 1210-1218.

Howell, C. (1998). Epidural vs. nonepidural analgesia in labour. *The Cochrane Library* (issue 3), 110. (Oxford) CD-ROM.

Isenor, L., & Penny-MacGillivary, T. (1993). Intravenous meperidine infusion for obstetric analgesia. *J Obstet Gynecol Neonatal Nurs* 22(4), 349-356.

Jenkins, M., & Pritchard, M. (1993). Hypnosis: Practical applications and theoretical considerations. *Br J Obstet Gynecol* 100(3), 221-226.

Jimenez, S. (1992). Teaching acupressure for pregnancy and birth. *J Perinat Educ* 11(1), 58-63.

Lamaze, F. (1972). *Painless childbirth.* New York: Pocket Books.

Lee, M., & Essoka, G. (1998). Continuing education. Patient's perception of pain: Comparison between Korean-American and Euro-American obstetric patients. *Journal of Cultural Diversity* 5(1), 29-40.

Lowe, N. (1996). The pain and discomfort of labor and birth. *J Obstet Gynecol Neonatal Nurs* 25(1), 82-92.

Mackey, R. (1995). Discovering the healing power of therapeutic touch. *Am J Nurs* 95(4), 26-32.

Manning, J. (1996). Intrathecal narcotics: New approach for labor anesthesia. *J Obstet Gynecol Neonatal Nurs* 25(3), 221-224.

Olden, A. et al. (1995). Patients' versus nurses' assessments of pain and sedation after cesarean section. *J Obstet Gynecol Neonatal Nurs* 24(2), 137-141.

Potter, P., & Perry, A. (1998). *Basic nursing: A critical thinking approach* (4th ed.). St. Louis: Mosby.

Rush, J. et al. (1996). The effects of whirlpool baths in labor: A randomized, controlled trial. *Birth* 23(3), 136-143.

Scherer, R., & Holzgreve, W. (1995). Influence of epidural analgesia on fetal and neonatal well-being. *Eur J Obstet Gynecol Reprod Biol* 59(suppl), S17-S29.

Schorn, M., McAllister, J., & Blanco, J. (1993). Water immersion and the effect on labor. *J Nurse Midwifery* 38(6), 336-342.

Scott, J. et al. (Eds.). (1999). *Danforth's obstetrics and gynecology* (8th ed.). Philadelphia: Lippincott, Williams & Wilkins.

Sepkoski, C. et al. (1992). The effects of maternal epidural anesthesia on neonatal behavior during the first month. *Dev Neurol Med Child* 34(2), 1072-1080.

Shapiro, H. et al. (1997). *The Lamaze ready reference guide for labor and birth* (2nd ed.). Washington, D.C.: Chapter ASPO/Lamaze.

Simkin, P. (1995). Reducing pain and enhancing progress in labor: A guide to nonpharmacologic methods of maternity caregivers. *Birth* 22(3), 161-171.

Thorp, J., & Breedlove, G. (1996). Epidural analgesia in labor: An evaluation of risks and benefits. *Birth* 23(2), 63-83.

Tiran, D. (1996). Aromatherapy therapy in midwifery: Benefits and risks. *Complementary Therapies in Nursing and Midwifery* 2(4), 88-92.

Villarruel, A. (1995). Mexican-American cultural meanings, expressions, self-care and dependent-care actions associated with experiences of pain. *Res Nurs Health* 18, 427-436.

Weber, S. (1996). Cultural aspects of pain in childbearing women. *J Obstet Gynecol Neonatal Nurs* 25(1), 67-72.

Wiand, N. (1997). Relaxation levels achieved by Lamaze-trained pregnant women listening to music and ocean sound tapes. *J Perinat Educ* 6(4), 1-8.

Wong, D., & Perry, S. (1998). *Maternal child nursing care.* St. Louis: Mosby.

Youngstrom, P. et al. (1996). Epidurals redefined in analgesia and anesthesia: A distinction with a difference. *J Obstet Gynecol Neonatal Nurs* 25(4), 350-354.

21

Fetal Assessment

Susan M. Tucker

LEARNING OBJECTIVES

- Define the key terms.
- Identify typical signs of nonreassuring fetal heart rate (FHR) patterns.
- Compare FHR monitoring done by intermittent auscultation and external and internal electronic methods.
- Explain the baseline FHR and evaluate periodic changes.
- Describe preventive measures that can be used to maintain FHR patterns within normal limits.

- Differentiate between the nursing interventions used for managing specific FHR patterns, including tachycardia and bradycardia; increased and decreased variability; and late and variable decelerations.
- Review the application of the monitor.
- Review the documentation of the monitoring process necessary during labor.
- Identify topics for nursing research related to fetal monitoring.

KEY TERMS

acceleration
amnioinfusion
baseline fetal heart rate
bradycardia
deceleration
electronic fetal monitoring
episodic changes
head compression

hypoxemia
hypoxia
intermittent auscultation
intrauterine pressure catheter
nonreassuring FHR patterns
periodic changes
prolonged deceleration
reassuring FHR patterns

spiral electrode
tachycardia
tocolysis
tocotransducer
ultrasound transducer
uteroplacental insufficiency
Valsalva maneuver
variability

Since the 1970s, when fetal monitoring made its debut, considerable expertise has been gained in the assessment of fetal hemodynamic and oxygen status. Evaluation of the baseline fetal heart rate (FHR) remains a complex task, however, because of the number of factors that must be considered and the variations in the "normal" fetal response to labor. Ways of describing FHR patterns have been based on terminology coined by equipment manufacturers, researchers, and authors and have varied by region in the country, institution, and health care provider.

The lack of agreement on definitions and interpretations of FHR patterns has limited the study of efficacy and validity of electronic fetal monitoring (EFM). In 1995 a research-planning workshop was held to develop research guidelines for EFM interpretation. Experts in the field, including those in medicine, nursing, epidemiology, basic science, and the general public, participated. The first document to be published by the group was a proposed nomenclature system for EFM interpretation. This document presented standardized definitions for fetal heart rate monitoring (National Institute of Child Health and Human Development Research Planning Workshop, 1997). These definitions will be tested for reliability and accuracy and will be refined based on results of the tests.

Even though testing of the definitions has not yet been completed, some effect on clinical practice is likely. For that reason, this chapter includes the new definitions and discussion of the current systems of interpretation of EFM. Practitioners who continue to use the established terminology during this period of transition should continue to use guidelines developed by the Association of Women's Health, Obstetric, and Neonatal Nurses (AWHONN, 1993b) and the American College of Obstetricians and Gynecologists (1995). Practitioners who wish to use the new terminology will need to communicate with other health care providers about the use of the new terminology instead of established definitions (Harvey, 1997). They will also need to make changes in their practice as the definitions are refined through testing. All perinatal health care providers must keep abreast of the new developments in EFM technology and knowledge to ensure the best possible outcomes for mothers and newborns.

BASIS FOR MONITORING

Fetal Response

Because labor is a period of physiologic stress for the fetus, frequent monitoring of fetal health is part of the nursing care during labor. The fetal oxygen supply must be maintained during labor to prevent fetal compromise and promote newborn health after birth. The fetal oxygen supply can decrease in a number of ways:

1. Reduction of blood flow through the maternal vessels as a result of maternal hypertension (chronic hypertension or pregnancy-induced hypertension), hypotension (caused by supine maternal position, hemorrhage, or epidural analgesia or anesthesia), or hypovolemia (caused by hemorrhage)
2. Reduction of the oxygen content in the maternal blood as a result of hemorrhage or severe anemia
3. Alterations in fetal circulation, occurring with compression of the umbilical cord (transient: during uterine contractions; or prolonged: resulting from cord prolapse), placental separation or complete abruption, or head compression (head compression causes increased intracranial pressure and vagal nerve stimulation with an accompanying decrease in the FHR)

4. Reduction in blood flow to the intervillous space in the placenta secondary to uterine hypertonus (generally caused by excessive exogenous oxytocin), or secondary to deterioration of the placental vasculature associated with maternal disorders such as hypertension or diabetes mellitus

Fetal well-being during labor can be measured by the response of the FHR to uterine contractions. In general, reassuring FHR patterns are characterized by the following:

- A baseline FHR in the normal range of 110 to 160 beats per minute with no periodic changes and a moderate baseline variability
- Accelerations with fetal movement

A normal uterine activity pattern in labor is characterized by contractions occurring every 2 to 5 minutes and lasting less than 90 seconds; such contractions are moderate to strong in intensity, as evidenced by palpation, or intensity is less than 100 mm Hg, as measured by an intrauterine pressure catheter (IUPC); 30 seconds or more should elapse between the end of one contraction and the beginning of the next contraction; and between contractions uterine relaxation should be detected by palpation or by an average intrauterine pressure of 15 mm Hg or less.

Fetal Compromise

The goals of intrapartum FHR monitoring are to identify and differentiate the reassuring patterns from the nonreassuring patterns, which can be indicative of fetal compromise.

Nonreassuring FHR patterns are those associated with fetal hypoxemia, which is a deficiency of oxygen in the arterial blood. If uncorrected, hypoxemia can deteriorate to severe fetal hypoxia, which is an inadequate supply of oxygen at the cellular level. Nonreassuring FHR patterns include the following:

- Progressive increase or decrease in baseline rate
- Tachycardia of 160 beats per minute or more
- Progressive decrease in baseline variability
- Severe variable decelerations (FHR less than 60 beats per minute lasting longer than 30 to 60 seconds, with rising baseline, decreasing variability, or slow return to baseline)
- Late decelerations of any magnitude, especially those that are repetitive and uncorrectable, with decreasing variability or rising baseline FHR
- Absence of FHR variability
- Prolonged deceleration (greater than 60 to 90 seconds)
- Severe bradycardia (less than 70 beats per minute)

The nurse's role is to continually assess whether the FHR pattern is reassuring, which reflects adequate fetal oxygenation. When the pattern is nonreassuring the nurse must discriminate between those patterns that indicate mild fetal hypoxemia and other nonreassuring patterns that indicate severe fetal hypoxia. The nursing interventions to be taken when encountering nonreassuring patterns are described in detail in this chapter.

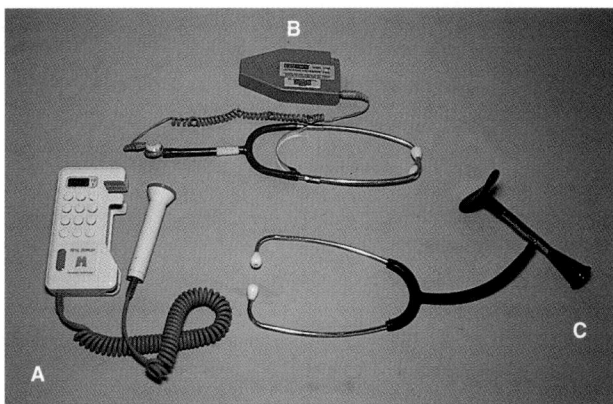

Fig. 21-1 **A,** Ultrasound fetoscope. **B,** Ultrasound stethoscope. **C,** DeLee-Hillis fetoscope. *(Courtesy Michael S. Clement, MD, Mesa, AZ.)*

MONITORING TECHNIQUES

Intermittent Auscultation

Intermittent auscultation of the fetal heart can be performed with a Leff scope, a DeLee-Hillis fetoscope, or an ultrasound device. If a Leff scope is used, the domed side should be opened to the connective tubing to the earpieces. The domed side is then applied to the maternal abdomen. The fetoscope is applied over the listener's head because bone conduction amplifies the fetal heart sounds for counting. The ultrasound device transmits ultrahigh-frequency sound waves reflecting movement of the fetal heart and converts these sounds into an electronic signal that can be counted (Fig. 21-1).

The procedure for performing auscultation is as follows:
1. Perform Leopold's maneuvers by palpating the maternal abdomen to identify fetal presentation and position.
2. Place the listening device over the area of maximum intensity and clarity of the fetal heart sounds to obtain the clearest and loudest sound, which is easiest to count.
3. Palpate the abdomen for the absence of uterine activity to be able to count the FHR between contractions.
4. Count the maternal radial pulse at the same time as listening to the FHR to differentiate it from the fetal rate.
5. Count the FHR for 30 to 60 seconds between contractions to identify the baseline rate. This rate can only be assessed during the absence of uterine activity.
6. Auscultate the FHR during a contraction and for 30 seconds after the end of the contraction to identify any increases or decreases in FHR in response to the contraction.

The method and frequency of fetal surveillance during labor will vary depending on maternal-fetal risk factors and the preference of the facility. In the absence of risk factors, the standard practice is to auscultate the FHR as follows:
- First stage
  Latent phase: every 60 minutes
  Active phase: every 30 minutes
- Second stage
  Every 15 minutes

If risk factors are present, the FHR is auscultated as follows:
- First stage
  Latent phase: every 30 minutes
  Active phase: every 15 minutes
- Second stage
  Every 5 minutes

NURSE ALERT *When the FHR is auscultated and documented, it is inappropriate to use the descriptive terms associated with electronic fetal monitoring because most of the terms are visual descriptions of the patterns produced on the monitor tracing. However, terms that are numerically defined, such as bradycardia and tachycardia, can be used.*

The ideal method of fetal assessment during labor continues to be debated. Results from multiple research studies indicate that both intermittent auscultation of the FHR at the frequencies just given and electronic FHR monitoring are associated with similar fetal outcomes (American College of Obstetricians and Gynecologists, 1995; Thacker et al., 1998). However, the advantage of intermittent auscultation is that it is a high-touch, low-technology method of assessing fetal status during labor that places less restrictions on maternal activity. Because childbirth is a natural process, most women and fetuses fare well with minimal intervention and periodic assessment.

Every effort should be made to use the method of fetal assessment the woman desires, if possible. However, auscultation of the FHR in accordance with the frequency guidelines just given may be difficult in today's busy labor and birth units. When used as the primary method of fetal assessment, auscultation requires a one-to-one nurse-to-client staffing ratio. If acuity and census change so that auscultation standards are no longer met, the nurse must inform the physician or nurse-midwife that continuous EFM will be used until staffing can be arranged to meet the standards.

The woman can become anxious if the examiner cannot readily count the fetal heartbeats. It often takes time for the inexperienced listener to locate the heartbeat and find the area of maximum intensity. To allay the mother's concerns, she can be told that the nurse is "finding the spot where the sounds are loudest." If it takes considerable time to locate the fetal heartbeats, the examiner can reassure the mother by offering her an opportunity to listen to them, too. If the examiner cannot locate the fetal heartbeat, assistance should be requested. In some cases, ultra-

TABLE 21-1   External and Internal Modes of Monitoring

EXTERNAL MODE	INTERNAL MODE
FHR	
Ultrasound transducer: High-frequency sound waves reflect mechanical action of the fetal heart. Used during the antepartum and intrapartum period. Noninvasive. Does not require rupture of membranes or cervical dilation.	*Spiral electrode:* This electrode converts the fetal ECG as obtained from the presenting part to the FHR via a cardiotachometer. This method can be used only when membranes are ruptured and the cervix is sufficiently dilated during the intrapartum period. Electrode penetrates into fetal presenting part by 1.5 mm and must be attached securely to ensure a good signal.
UTERINE ACTIVITY	
Tocotransducer: This instrument monitors frequency and duration of contractions by means of pressure-sensing device applied to the maternal abdomen. Used during both the antepartum and intrapartum periods.	*Intrauterine pressure catheter (IUPC):* This instrument monitors the frequency, duration, and intensity of contractions. There are two types of IUPCs: a fluid-filled system and a solid catheter. Both measure intrauterine pressure at the catheter tip and convert the pressure into millimeters of mercury on the uterine activity panel of the strip chart. Both can be used only when membranes are ruptured and the cervix is sufficiently dilated during the intrapartum period.

sound can be used to help locate the fetal heartbeat. Seeing the FHR on the ultrasound screen will be reassuring to the mother if there was initial difficulty in locating the best area for auscultation.

When using palpation to assess uterine activity, the examiner should keep his or her hand placed over the fundus before, during, and after contractions. The contraction intensity is usually described as mild, moderate, or strong. The contraction duration is measured in seconds, from the beginning to the end of the contraction. The frequency of contractions is measured in minutes, from the beginning of one contraction to the beginning of the next contraction. The examiner should keep his or her hand on the fundus after the contraction is over to evaluate uterine resting tone or relaxation between contractions. Resting tone between contractions is usually described as soft or relaxed.

Accurate and complete documentation of fetal status and uterine activity is especially important when intermittent auscultation and palpation are being used because there is not the paper tracing record of these assessments provided by continuous EFM. Labor flow records or computer charting systems that prompt notations of all assessments are useful for ensuring such comprehensive documentation.

Electronic Fetal Monitoring

There are two modes of **electronic fetal monitoring**. The external mode involves the use of external transducers placed on the maternal abdomen to assess FHR and uterine activity. The internal mode involves the use of a **spiral electrode** applied to the fetal presenting part to assess the fetal electrocardiogram (ECG) and an **intrauterine pressure catheter** (IUPC) to assess uterine activity and pressure. The differences between the external and internal modes of EFM are summarized in Table 21-1.

External Monitoring

Separate transducers are used to monitor the FHR and uterine contractions (Fig. 21-2). The **ultrasound transducer** works by reflecting high-frequency sound waves off a moving interface, in this case the fetal heart and valves. Therefore short-term variability and beat-to-beat changes in the FHR cannot be assessed accurately by this method. It is also difficult to reproduce a continuous and precise record of the FHR because of artifacts introduced by fetal and maternal movement. The FHR is printed on specially formatted monitor paper. The standard paper speed is 3 cm/min. Once the area of maximum intensity of the FHR has been located, conductive gel is applied to the surface of the ultrasound transducer and the transducer is then positioned over this area.

The **tocotransducer** (tocodynamometer) measures uterine activity transabdominally. The device is placed over the fundus above the umbilicus. Uterine contractions or fetal movement depress a pressure-sensitive surface on the side next to the abdomen. The tocotransducer can measure and record the frequency, regularity, and approximate duration of uterine contractions but not their intensity. This method is especially valuable for measuring uterine activity during the first stage of labor in women with intact membranes or for antepartum testing. Because the tocotransducer of most

✶ Know These

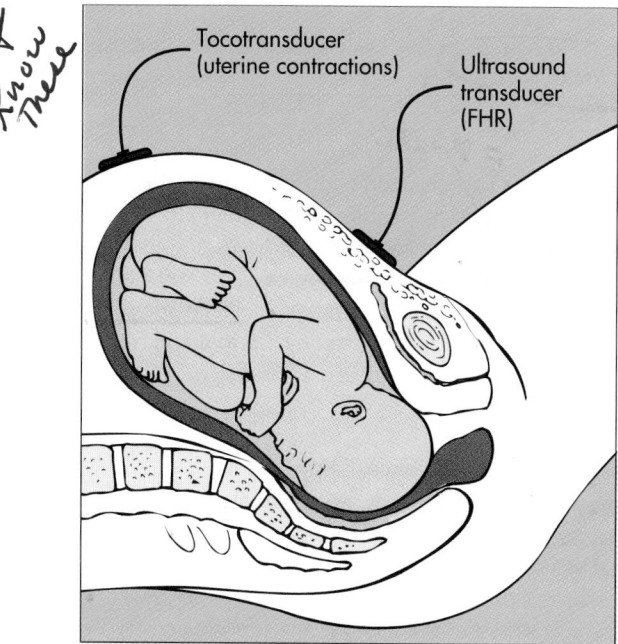

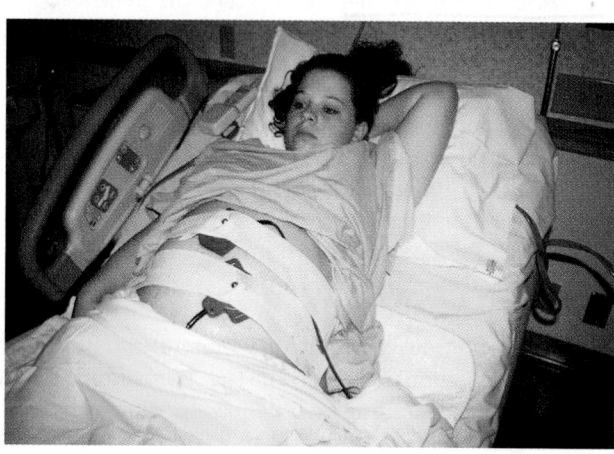

Fig. 21-2 **A,** External noninvasive fetal monitoring using tocotransducer and ultrasound transducer. **B,** Ultrasound transducer is placed below umbilicus, over the area where fetal heart rate is best heard, and tocotransducer is placed on uterine fundus. *(Courtesy Marjorie Pyle, RNC, Lifecircle, Costa Mesa, CA.)*

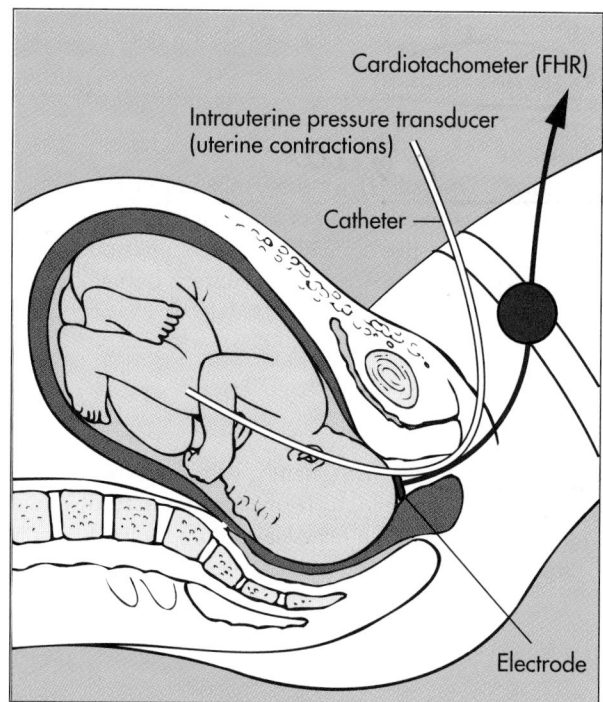

Fig. 21-3 Diagrammatic representation of internal invasive fetal monitoring with intrauterine pressure catheter and spiral electrode in place (membranes ruptured and cervix dilated).

electronic fetal monitors is designed for assessing uterine activity in the term pregnancy, it may not be sensitive enough to detect preterm uterine activity (Afriat, 1996). When monitoring the woman experiencing preterm labor, it is important to remember that the fundus may be located below the level of the umbilicus. The nurse also may need to rely on the woman to indicate when uterine activity is occurring and to use palpation as an additional way of assessing contraction frequency.

The equipment is easily applied by the nurse, but it must be repositioned as the woman or fetus changes posi-

tion (see Fig. 21-2, *B*). The woman is asked to assume a semisitting position or lateral position. The equipment is removed periodically to wash the applicator sites and to give back rubs. This type of monitoring confines the woman to bed. Portable telemetry monitors allow observation of the FHR and uterine contraction patterns by means of centrally located electronic display stations. These portable units permit the woman to walk around during electronic monitoring.

Internal Monitoring

The technique of continuous internal monitoring provides an accurate appraisal of fetal well-being during labor (Fig. 21-3). For this type of monitoring, the membranes must be ruptured, the cervix sufficiently dilated, and the presenting part low enough to allow placement of the electrode. A small spiral electrode attached to the presenting part shows a continuous FHR on the fetal monitor strip.

Internal monitoring of the FHR may be implemented without internal monitoring of uterine activity. To monitor uterine activity, a solid or fluid-filled IUPC is introduced into the uterine cavity. A solid catheter has a pressure-sensitive tip that measures changes in intrauterine pressure. A catheter filled with sterile water can also be used. As the catheter is compressed during a contraction, pressure is placed on the pressure transducer or strain gauge; this pressure is then converted into a pressure reading in millime-

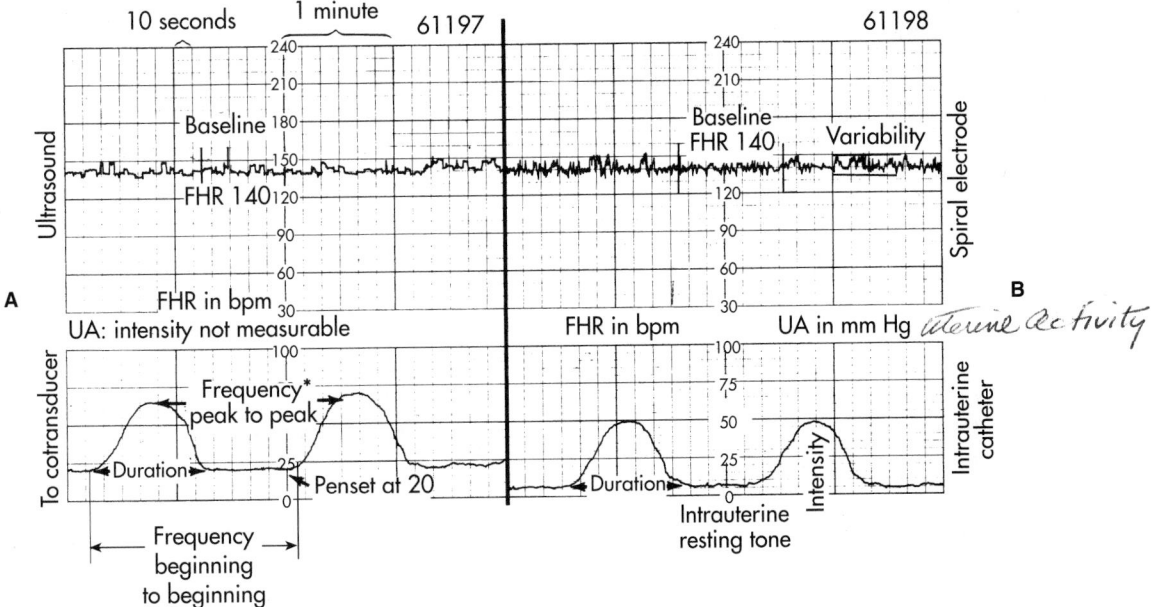

Fig. 21-4 Display of FHR and uterine activity on chart paper. **A,** External mode with ultrasound and tocotransducer as signal source. **B,** Internal mode with spiral electrode and intrauterine catheter as signal source. Frequency of contractions is measured from the beginning of one contraction to the beginning of the next. Peak-to-peak measurement is sometimes used when electronic uterine activity monitoring is done. *(From Tucker, S. [2000]. Pocket guide to fetal monitoring and assessment [4th ed.]. St. Louis: Mosby.)*

ters of mercury. The average pressure during a contraction ranges from 50 to 85 mm Hg. The IUPC can measure the frequency, duration, and intensity of uterine contractions. The way in which the FHR and uterine activity is displayed on the monitor paper differs for the two modes of electronic monitoring (Fig. 21-4). Note that each small square represents 10 seconds; each larger box of six squares equals 1 minute (when paper is moving through the monitor at 3 cm/min).

FETAL HEART RATE PATTERNS

Baseline Fetal Heart Rate

The intrinsic rhythmicity of the fetal heart and the fetal autonomic nervous system control the FHR. An increase in sympathetic response results in acceleration of the FHR. An augmentation in parasympathetic response produces a slowing of the FHR. Usually, a balanced increase of sympathetic and parasympathetic response occurs during contractions, with no observable change in the FHR.

Baseline fetal heart rate is the average rate during a 10-minute segment that excludes periodic or episodic changes, periods of marked variability, and segments of the baseline that differ by more than 25 beats per minute (National Institute, 1997). The normal range at term is 110 to 160 beats per minute.

Tachycardia is a baseline FHR above 160 beats per minute. It can be considered an early sign of fetal hypoxia

and can result from maternal or fetal infection, such as prolonged rupture of membranes with amnionitis; from maternal hyperthyroidism or fetal anemia; or in response to drugs such as atropine, hydroxyzine (Vistaril), terbutaline, or street drugs such as cocaine or methamphetamines.

Bradycardia is a baseline FHR below 110 beats per minute. (Bradycardia should be distinguished from prolonged deceleration patterns, which are periodic changes described later in this chapter.) It can be considered a later sign of fetal hypoxia and is known to occur before fetal demise. Bradycardia can result from placental transfer of drugs such as anesthetics, prolonged compression of the umbilical cord, maternal hypothermia, and maternal hypotension. Maternal supine hypotensive syndrome, caused by uterine pressure (the weight of the gravid uterus) on the vena cava, decreases the return of blood flow to the maternal heart, which then reduces maternal cardiac output and blood pressure. These responses in the mother subsequently result in a decrease in the FHR and fetal bradycardia. Table 21-2 contrasts tachycardia with bradycardia.

Variability of the FHR can be described as irregular fluctuations in the baseline FHR of 2 cycles per minute or greater (National Institute, 1997). Variability has been described as short term (beat to beat) or long term (rhythmic waves or cycles from baseline). The current definition for research does not distinguish between short-term and

TABLE 21-2 Tachycardia and Bradycardia

Normal fetal rate 120-160 (handwritten annotation)

TACHYCARDIA	BRADYCARDIA
DEFINITION	
FHR greater than 160 beats per minute lasting longer than 10 min	FHR less than 110 beats per minute lasting longer than 10 min
CAUSE	
Early fetal hypoxemia Maternal fever Parasympatholytic drugs (atropine, hydroxyzine) Beta-sympathomimetic drugs (ritodrine, isoxsuprine) Intraamniotic infection Maternal hyperthyroidism Fetal anemia Fetal heart failure Fetal cardiac dysrhythmias Street drugs (cocaine, methamphetamines)	Late fetal hypoxia/hypoxemia Beta-adrenergic blocking drugs (propranolol; anesthetics for epidural, spinal, caudal, and pudendal blocks) Maternal hypotension Prolonged umbilical cord compression Fetal congenital heart block Maternal hypothermia Prolonged maternal hypoglycemia
CLINICAL SIGNIFICANCE	
Persistent tachycardia in absence of periodic changes does not appear serious in terms of neonatal outcome (especially true if tachycardia is associated with maternal fever); tachycardia is a nonreassuring sign when associated with late decelerations, severe variable decelerations, or absence of variability.	Bradycardia with moderate variability and absence of periodic changes is not a sign of fetal compromise if FHR remains greater than 80 beats per minute; bradycardia caused by hypoxia is a nonreassuring sign when associated with loss of variability and late decelerations.
NURSING INTERVENTION	
Dependent on cause; reduce maternal fever with antipyretics as ordered and cooling measures; oxygen at 8 to 10 L/min per face mask may be of some value; carry out health care provider's orders based on alleviating cause.	Dependent on cause; intervention not warranted in fetus with heart block diagnosed by ECG; oxygen at 8 to 10 L/min per face mask may be of some value; carry out health care provider's orders based on alleviating cause. Scalp stimulation may be performed to determine whether the fetus has the ability to compensate physiologically for stress (FHR will accelerate).

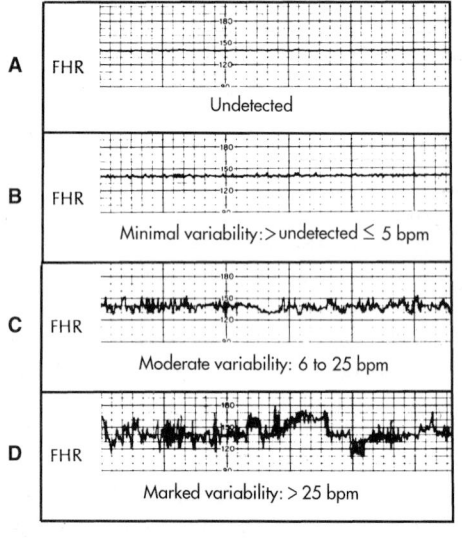

Fig. 21-5 FHR variability. **A,** Undetected. **B,** Minimal. **C,** Moderate. **D,** Marked. *(Modified from Tucker, S. [2000]. Pocket guide to fetal monitoring and assessment [4th ed.]. St. Louis: Mosby.)*

long-term variability because in actual practice, they are viewed together (National Institute, 1997). This definition does identify four ranges of variability as seen in Fig. 21-5. These are based on visualization of the amplitude in the peak-to-trough segment in beats per minute and include the following:

• Absent or undetected variability
• Minimal variability (greater than undetected but not more than 5 beats per minute)
• Moderate variability (6 to 25 beats per minute)
• Marked variability (greater than 25 beats per minute)

In clinical practice, short-term and long-term variability continue to be used to describe the FHR fluctuations.

A sinusoidal pattern, a regular smooth wavelike pattern, is not included in the current research definition of FHR variability.

Absence of or undetected variability is considered nonreassuring. Decreased variability can result from fetal hypoxemia and acidosis, as well as from certain

TABLE 21-3   Increased and Decreased Variability

INCREASED VARIABILITY	DECREASED VARIABILITY
CAUSE	
Early mild hypoxemia	Hypoxia/acidosis
Fetal stimulation by the following:	CNS depressants
Uterine palpation	Analgesics/narcotics
Uterine contractions	Meperidine (Demerol)
Fetal activity	Alphaprodine (Nisentil)
Maternal activity	Morphine
Street drugs (e.g., cocaine and methamphetamines)	Pentazocine (Talwin)
	Barbiturates
	Secobarbital (Seconal)
	Pentobarbital (Nembutal)
	Amobarbital (Amytal)
	Tranquilizers
	Diazepam (Valium)
	Ataractics
	Promethazine (Phenergan)
	Propiomazine (Largon)
	Hydroxyzine (Vistaril)
	Promazine (Sparine)
	Parasympatholytics
	Atropine
	General anesthetics
	Prematurity—less than 24 wk
	Fetal sleep cycles
	Congenital abnormalities
	Fetal cardiac dysrhythmias
CLINICAL SIGNIFICANCE	
Significance of marked variability not known; increased variability from a previous average variability is earliest FHR sign of mild hypoxemia	Benign when associated with periodic fetal sleep states, which last 20 to 30 min; if caused by drugs, variability usually increases as drugs are excreted
	Decreased variability considered nonreassuring if caused by hypoxia/asphyxia; occurring with late decelerations, decreased variability is associated with fetal acidosis and low Apgar scores
NURSING INTERVENTION	
Observe FHR tracing carefully for any nonreassuring patterns, including decreasing variability and late decelerations; if using external mode of monitoring, consider using internal mode (spiral electrode) for a more accurate tracing	Dependent on cause; intervention not warranted if associated with fetal sleep states or temporarily associated with CNS depressants; consider performing external stimulation or scalp stimulation during a vaginal examination to elicit an acceleration of FHR or return to average variability; consider application of internal mode (spiral electrode); assist health care provider with fetal blood sampling for pH if ordered; prepare for birth if so indicated by the primary health care provider

drugs that depress the central nervous system (CNS), including analgesics, narcotics (meperidine [Demerol]), barbiturates (secobarbital [Seconal] and pentobarbital [Nembutal]), tranquilizers (diazepam [Valium]), ataractics (promethazine [Phenergan]), and general anesthetics.

In addition, a temporary decrease in variability can occur when the fetus is in a sleep state. These sleep states do not usually last longer than 30 minutes. Table 21-3 contrasts key differences between increased and decreased variability.

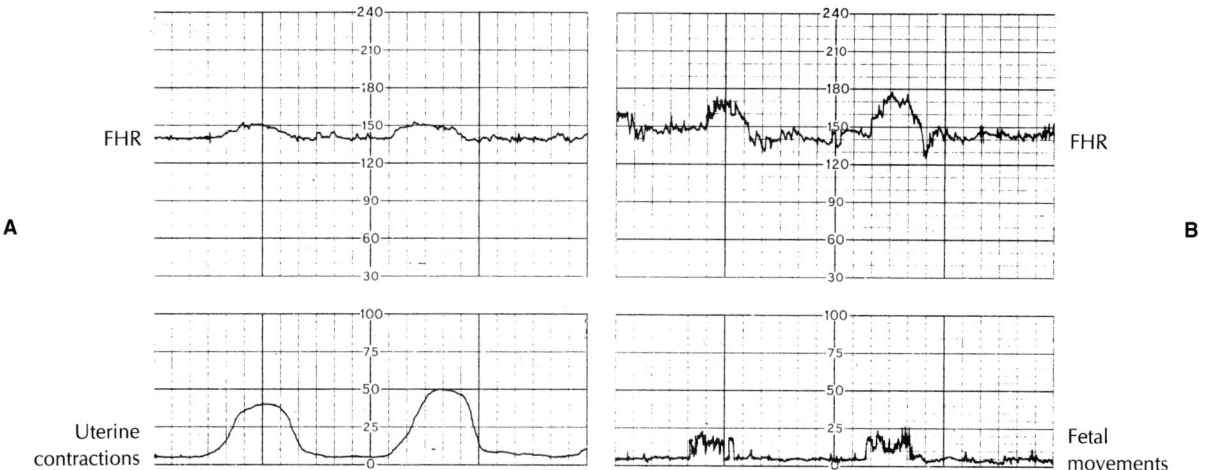

Fig. 21-6 **A,** Acceleration of FHR with uterine contractions. **B,** Acceleration of FHR with fetal movement. *(From Tucker, S. [2000]. Pocket guide to fetal monitoring and assessment [4th ed.]. St. Louis: Mosby.)*

Periodic and Episodic Changes in Fetal Heart Rate

Changes from baseline patterns in FHR are categorized as periodic or episodic. **Periodic changes** are those that occur with uterine contractions. **Episodic changes** (nonperiodic changes) are those that are not associated with uterine contractions. These patterns include accelerations and decelerations (National Institute, 1997).

Accelerations

Acceleration of the FHR is defined as a visually apparent abrupt increase in FHR above the baseline rate. The increase is 15 beats per minute or greater and lasts 15 seconds or more, with the return to baseline less than 2 minutes from the beginning of the acceleration. In preterm gestations, the definition of an acceleration is a peak of 10 beats per minute or more above baseline for at least 10 seconds. Acceleration of the FHR for more than 10 minutes is considered a baseline change.

Accelerations can be periodic or episodic. Accelerations that are periodic are caused by dominance of the sympathetic nervous response and are usually encountered with breech presentations (Fig. 21-6, *A*). Pressure of the contraction applied to the fetal buttocks results in accelerations, whereas pressure applied to the head results in decelerations. Accelerations may occur, however, during the second stage of labor in cephalic presentations. Accelerations (Fig. 21-6, *B*) of the FHR that are episodic occur during fetal movement and are indications of fetal well-being.

Decelerations

A **deceleration** (caused by dominance of parasympathetic response) may be benign or nonreassuring. The three types of decelerations that are encountered during labor are early, late, and variable. FHR decelerations are described by their relation to the onset and end of a contraction and by their shape.

Early deceleration of the FHR is a visually apparent gradual decrease in and return to baseline FHR in response to compression of the fetal head. It is a normal and usually benign finding (Fig. 21-7, *A*) (National Institute, 1997). This deceleration is characterized by a uniform shape and an early onset corresponding to the rise in intraamniotic pressure as the uterus contracts. When present, it usually occurs during the first stage of labor when the cervix is dilated 4 to 7 cm. Early decelerations sometimes are seen during the second stage when the woman is pushing. They may also occur in response to fetal **head compression** during uterine contractions, during vaginal examinations, as a result of fundal pressure, and during placement of the internal mode for fetal monitoring.

Because early decelerations are considered to be benign, interventions are not necessary. The value of identifying early decelerations is so that they can be distinguished from late or variable decelerations, which can be nonreassuring and for which interventions are appropriate. The different characteristics of accelerations of the FHR and early decelerations are contrasted in Table 21-4.

Uteroplacental insufficiency causes late decelerations. *Late deceleration* of the FHR is a visually apparent gradual decrease in and return to baseline FHR associated with uterine contractions (National Institute, 1997). The deceleration begins after the contraction has started, and the lowest point of the deceleration occurs after the peak of the contraction. Usually the deceleration does not return to baseline until after the contraction is over (Fig. 21-7, *B*).

Persistent and repetitive late decelerations usually indicate the presence of fetal hypoxemia stemming from insufficient placental perfusion. They can be associated with fetal hypoxemia progressing to hypoxia and acidemia progressing to acidosis. They should be considered an ominous sign when they are uncorrectable, especially if they are associated with decreased variability and tachycardia. Late decelerations caused by the maternal supine

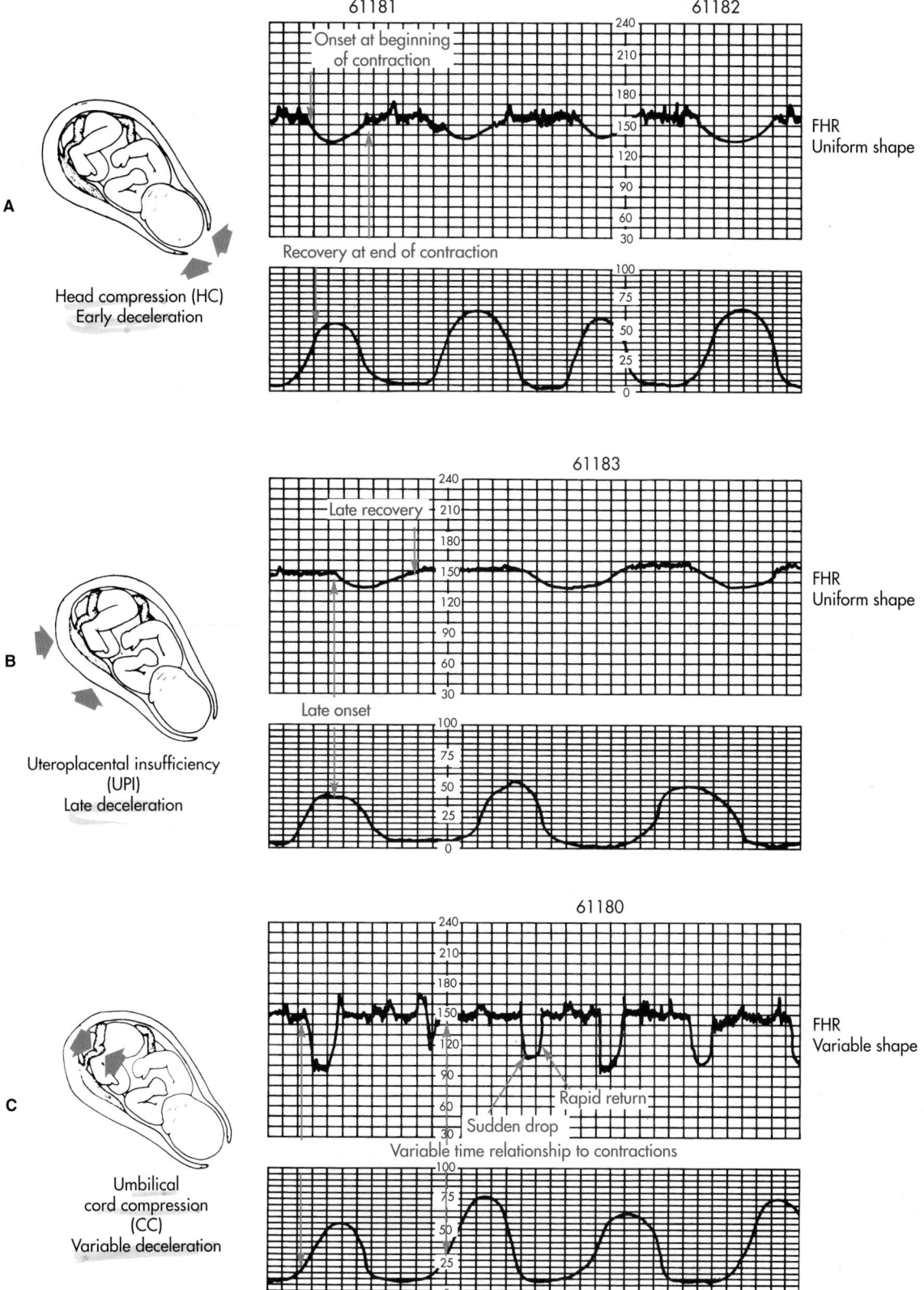

Fig. 21-7 **A,** Early decelerations caused by head compression. **B,** Late decelerations caused by uteroplacental insufficiency. **C,** Variable decelerations caused by cord compression. *(From Tucker, S. [2000]. Pocket guide to fetal monitoring and assessment [4th ed.]. St. Louis: Mosby.)*

TABLE 21-4 Acceleration and Early Deceleration

	ACCELERATION	EARLY DECELERATION
Description	Transitory increase of FHR above baseline (see Fig. 21-6)	Transitory decrease of FHR below baseline concurrent with uterine contractions (see Fig. 21-7, A)
Shape	May resemble shape of uterine contraction or be spikelike	Uniform shape; mirror image of uterine contraction
Onset	Onset to peak (30 sec; often precedes or occurs simultaneously with uterine contraction	Early in contraction phase before peak of contraction
Recovery	Less than 2 min from onset	By end of contraction as uterine pressure returns to its resting tone
Amplitude	Usually 15 beats per minute above baseline	Usually proportional to amplitude of contraction; rarely decelerates below 100 beats per minute
Baseline	Usually associated with average baseline variability	Usually associated with average baseline variability
Occurrence	Variable; may be repetitive with each contraction	Repetitious (occurs with each contraction); usually occurs between 4 and 7 cm dilation and in second stage of labor
Cause	Spontaneous fetal movement Vaginal examination Electrode application Breech presentation Occiput posterior position Uterine contractions Fundal pressure Abdominal palpation	Head compression resulting from the following: Uterine contractions Vaginal examination Fundal pressure Placement of internal mode of monitoring
Clinical significance	Acceleration with fetal movement signifies fetal well-being representing fetal alertness or arousal states	Reassuring pattern not associated with fetal hypoxemia, acidemia, or low Apgar scores
Nursing intervention	None required	None required

hypotensive syndrome are usually correctable when the woman turns on her side to displace the weight of the gravid uterus off the vena cava. Such lateral positioning allows better return of maternal blood flow to the heart, which in turn increases cardiac output and blood pressure.

Late decelerations caused by uteroplacental insufficiency can result from uterine hyperstimulation with oxytocin, pregnancy-induced hypertension, postdate or postterm pregnancy, amnionitis, small-for-gestational-age (SGA) fetus, maternal diabetes, placenta previa, abruptio placentae, conduction anesthetics (producing maternal hypotension), maternal cardiac disease, and maternal anemia.

Variable deceleration is defined as a visual abrupt decrease in FHR below baseline. The decrease is usually more than 15 beats per minute, lasts at least 15 seconds, and usually returns to baseline in less than 2 minutes from the time of onset (National Institute, 1997). Variable decelerations occur any time during the uterine contracting phase and are caused by compression of the umbilical cord. Table 21-5 contrasts late deceleration with variable deceleration.

The pattern of variable decelerations differs from that of early and late decelerations, which closely approximates the shape of the corresponding uterine contraction. Instead, variable decelerations often have a U or V shape, characterized by a rapid descent and ascent to and from the nadir (or depth) of the deceleration (Fig. 21-7, C). Some variable decelerations are preceded and followed by brief accelerations of the FHR, known as "shouldering," which is an appropriate compensatory response to compression of the umbilical cord.

Variable decelerations may be related to partial, brief compression of the cord. If encountered in the first stage of labor, they usually can be resolved by changing the mother's position, such as from one side to the other. Oxygen administration by face mask to the mother is sometimes helpful. Variable decelerations are most commonly encountered during the second stage of labor as a result of umbilical cord compression during fetal descent. If repetitive variable decelerations occur during the second stage, it is important to discourage the woman from pushing with every contraction so that the fetus has time to recover. Variable decelerations are associated with neonatal depression only when

TABLE 21-5 Late Deceleration Versus Variable Deceleration

	LATE DECELERATION	VARIABLE DECELERATION
Description	Transitory gradual decrease in FHR below baseline rate in contracting phase (see Fig. 21-7, B)	Abrupt decrease in FHR that is variable in duration, intensity, and timing related to onset of contractions (Fig. 21-7, C)
Shape	Uniform; mirror images of uterine contraction; may be deep or shallow	Variable; characterized by sudden drop in FHR in V, U, or W shape
Onset	Late in contraction phase; after peak of contraction; nadir of deceleration occurs after peak of contraction	Onset of deceleration to the beginning of nadir <30 sec; decrease in FHR baseline is ≥15 beats per minute, lasting ≥15 sec; variable times in contracting phase; often preceded by transitory acceleration
Recovery	Well after end of contraction	Return to baseline is rapid and less than 2 min from onset, sometimes with transitory acceleration or acceleration immediately preceding and following deceleration (shouldering or "overshoot"); slow return to baseline with severe variable decelerations
Deceleration	Usually proportional to amplitude of contraction; rarely decelerates below 100 beats per minute	*Mild:* decelerates to any level, less than 30 sec with abrupt return to baseline *Moderate:* decelerates no lower than 80 beats per minute, any duration with abrupt return to baseline *Severe:* decelerates below 60 beats per minute for longer than 60 sec, with slow return to baseline
Baseline	Often associated with loss of variability and increasing baseline rate	Mild variables usually associated with average baseline variability; moderate and severe variables often associated with decreasing variability and increasing baseline rate
Occurrence	Occurs with each contraction; may be observed at any time during labor	Variable; commonly observed late in labor with fetal descent and pushing
Cause	Uteroplacental insufficiency caused by the following: Uterine hyperactivity or hypertonicity Maternal supine hypotension Epidural or spinal anesthesia Placenta previa Abruptio placentae Hypertensive disorders Postmaturity Intrauterine growth restriction Diabetes mellitus Intraamniotic infection	Umbilical cord compression caused by the following: Maternal position with cord between fetus and maternal pelvis Cord around fetal neck, arm, leg, or other body part Short cord Knot in cord Prolapsed cord
Clinical significance	Nonreassuring, worrisome pattern associated with fetal hypoxemia, acidemia, and low Apgar scores; considered ominous if persistent and uncorrected, especially when associated with fetal tachycardia and loss of variability	Variable decelerations occur in about 50% of all labors and usually are transient, correctable, and not associated with low Apgar scores; mild variable decelerations are reassuring; decelerations progressing from moderate to severe are associated with fetal acidemia, hypoxemia, and low Apgar scores; severe variable decelerations with average baseline variability just before birth are usually well tolerated

Continued

TABLE 21-5   Late Deceleration Versus Variable Deceleration—cont'd

	LATE DECELERATION	VARIABLE DECELERATION
Nursing intervention	Change maternal position (lateral) Correct maternal hypotension by elevating legs Increase rate of maintenance IV; administer vasopressors Discontinue oxytocin if infusing Administer oxygen at 8 to 10 L/min with tight face mask Fetal scalp or acoustic stimulation Assist with birth (cesarean or vaginal assisted) if pattern cannot be corrected	Change maternal position (side to side); if decelerations are severe, proceed with following measures: Discontinue oxytocin if infusing Administer oxygen at 8 to 10 L/min with tight face mask Assist with vaginal or speculum examination If cord is prolapsed, examiner will elevate fetal presenting part with cord between gloved fingers until cesarean birth is accomplished Assist with amnioinfusion if ordered Assist with birth (vaginal assisted or cesarean) if pattern cannot be corrected

cord compression is severe or prolonged (i.e., tight nuchal cord, short cord, knot in cord, prolapsed cord).

Prolonged Decelerations

A **prolonged deceleration** is a visually apparent decrease in FHR below the baseline 15 beats per minute or more and lasting more than 2 minutes but less than 10 minutes. A deceleration lasting more than 10 minutes is considered a baseline change (National Institute, 1997). Generally, the benign causes are pelvic examination, application of spiral electrode, rapid fetal descent, and sustained maternal Valsalva maneuver. Other, less benign, causes are progressive severe variable decelerations, sudden umbilical cord prolapse, hypotension produced by spinal or epidural analgesia or anesthesia, paracervical anesthesia, tetanic contraction, and maternal hypoxia, which may occur during a seizure. When the deceleration lasts longer than 1 to 2 minutes, a loss of variability with rebound tachycardia usually occurs. Occasionally a period of late decelerations follows. Prolonged decelerations usually are isolated events that end spontaneously. However, when a prolonged deceleration is seen late in the course of severe variable decelerations or during a prolonged series of late decelerations, the prolonged deceleration may occur just before fetal death.

NURSE ALERT *Nurses should notify the physician or nurse-midwife immediately and initiate appropriate treatment when they see a prolonged deceleration.*

CARE MANAGEMENT

The care given to women being monitored by EFM or auscultation is the same as that given to the woman experiencing a low risk labor. Care of the woman being monitored by internal methods may vary. FHR pattern recognition and intervention may require a nurse to have additional education and clinical experience.

Assessment and Nursing Diagnoses

The assessment of the client includes the maternal temperature, pulse, respiratory rate, blood pressure, position, comfort, voiding pattern, status of membranes, uterine contraction pattern, cervical effacement and dilation, and emotional status. The fetal assessment includes the fetal presentation, fetal position, FHR, and identification of both reassuring and nonreassuring FHR patterns. A checklist may be used by the nurse to assess the FHR (Box 21-1). All of the assessment information must be documented in the client's medical record.

Evaluation of the EFM equipment must also be done to ensure that the equipment is working properly and to enable an accurate assessment of the woman and fetus. A checklist for fetal monitoring equipment can be used to evaluate the equipment functions (Box 21-2).

Nursing diagnoses for the woman who is being monitored electronically for fetal status are based on assessment findings. Possible diagnoses include the following:

Nursing Diagnoses

- Decreased maternal cardiac output related to
  - supine hypotension secondary to maternal position
- Ineffective individual coping ability related to
  - lack of knowledge concerning fetal monitoring during labor
  - restriction of mobility or movement during EFM
- Impaired fetal gas exchange related to
  - umbilical cord compression
  - placental insufficiency
- Risk for fetal injury related to
  - unrecognized hypoxemia and hypoxia or anoxia
  - infection secondary to internal monitoring or blood sampling

BOX 21-1 Fetal Heart Rate Assessment Checklist

Client's name _____

Date/time _____

1. What is the baseline fetal heart rate (FHR)?

   _____ Beats per minute

   Check one of the following as observed on the monitor strip:

   _____ Average baseline FHR (110 to 160 beats per minute)

   _____ Tachycardia (>160 beats per minute)

   _____ Bradycardia (<100 beats per minute)

2. What is the baseline variability?

   _____ Moderate variability (6 to 25 beats per minute)

   _____ Minimal variability (>5 beats per minute)

   _____ Absence of variability

   _____ Marked variability (>25 beats per minute)

3. Are there any periodic or episodic changes in FHR?

   _____ Accelerations with fetal movement

   _____ Repetitive accelerations with each contraction

   _____ Early decelerations (head compression)

   _____ Late decelerations (uteroplacental insufficiency)

   _____ Variable decelerations (cord compression)

   _____ Mild

   _____ Moderate

   _____ Severe

   _____ Prolonged deceleration

4. What does the uterine activity panel show?

   _____ Frequency (peak to peak or beginning to beginning)

   _____ Duration (beginning to end)

   _____ Intensity (in mm Hg only with intrauterine catheter)

   _____ Resting time at least 30 seconds

   _____ Resting tone (<15 mm Hg pressure)

COMMENTS: _____

_____

PANEL NUMBER _____

WHAT CAN BE OR SHOULD HAVE BEEN DONE

_____

_____

Modified from Tucker, S. (2000). *Pocket guide to fetal monitoring and assessment* (4th ed.). St. Louis: Mosby.

BOX 21-2 Checklist for Fetal Monitoring Equipment

PREPARATION OF MONITOR

1. Is the paper inserted correctly?
2. Are transducer cables plugged into the appropriate outlet of the monitor?

ULTRASOUND TRANSDUCER

1. Has ultrasound transmission gel been applied to the transducer?
2. Was the FHR tested and noted on the monitor paper?
3. Does a signal light flash or an audible beep occur with each heartbeat?
4. Is the belt secure and snug but comfortable for the laboring woman?

TOCOTRANSDUCER

1. Is the tocotransducer firmly positioned at the site of the least maternal tissue?
2. Has it been applied without gel or paste?
3. Was the pen-set knob adjusted between the 10 and 20 mm Hg marks and noted on the monitor paper?
4. Was this setting done between contractions?
5. Is the belt secure and snug but comfortable for the laboring woman?

SPIRAL ELECTRODE

1. Are the wires attached firmly to the leg plate?
2. Is the spiral electrode attached to the presenting part of the fetus?
3. Is the inner surface of the leg plate covered with electrode gel, if necessary?
4. Is the leg plate properly secured to the woman's thigh?

INTERNAL CATHETER/STRAIN GAUGE

1. Is the length line on the catheter visible at the introitus?
2. Is it noted on the monitor paper that a calibration was done?
3. Was the uterine activity tested?

Modified from Tucker, S. (2000). *Pocket guide to fetal monitoring and assessment* (4th ed.). St Louis: Mosby.

Expected Outcomes of Care

The interventions implemented are determined by the current knowledge of fetal status revealed by monitoring during labor and by standards for care. The woman's and family's concerns and questions are considered in the planning process. Expected outcomes are set for the pregnant woman and family and the fetus and include the following:

- The fetus will not suffer any hypoxemic, hypoxic, or anoxic episodes.

Nursing Diagnoses—cont'd

- Pain related to
  - use of belts to position transducers
  - maternal position
  - application of internal electrode or obtaining of blood sample

- Should fetal compromise occur, it will be identified promptly, and appropriate nursing interventions such as intrauterine resuscitation will be initiated and the physician or nurse-midwife notified.
- The pregnant woman and family will verbalize their understanding of the need for monitoring.
- The pregnant woman and the family will recognize and avoid situations that compromise maternal and fetal circulation.
- The pregnant woman and the family will achieve the type of birth experience that is both physically safe for the mother and fetus/neonate and emotionally satisfying.

Plan of Care and Interventions

It is the responsibility of the nurse providing care to women in labor to assess FHR patterns, implement independent nursing interventions, document observations and actions according to the established standard of care, and report nonreassuring patterns to the primary care provider (e.g., physician, certified nurse-midwife). (See Box 21-3 for a sample protocol for FHR monitoring.)

Summary guidelines for the care of the woman being monitored electronically for fetal status during labor are listed in Box 21-4 (see also Plan of Care).

It is important to remember that although the use of EFM can be reassuring to many parents, it can be a source of anxiety to some. Therefore the nurse must be particularly sensitive to and respond appropriately to the emotional, informational, and comfort needs of the woman in labor and those of her family (Fig. 21-8).

Electronic fetal monitoring pattern recognition

Nurses must evaluate many factors to determine whether an FHR pattern is reassuring or nonreassuring. A complete description of FHR tracings includes both qualitative and quantitative descriptions of baseline rate and variability, presence of accelerations, periodic or episodic decelerations, and changes in the FHR pattern over time (National Institute, 1997). Nurses evaluate these factors based on other obstetric complications, progress in labor, and analgesia or anesthesia. They must also consider the estimated time interval until birth. Interventions are therefore based on clinical judgment of a complex, integrated process.

LEGAL TIP Fetal Monitoring Standards

Nurses who care for women during childbirth are legally responsible for correctly interpreting FHR patterns, initiating appropriate nursing interventions based on that pattern, and documenting the outcome of those interventions. Perinatal nurses are responsible for the timely notification of the physician or nurse-midwife in the event of nonreassuring FHR patterns. Perinatal nurses are also responsible for initiating the institutional chain of command should differences in opinion arise among health care providers concerning the interpretation of the FHR pattern and the intervention required.

Nursing management of nonreassuring patterns. The term *intrauterine resuscitation* is sometimes used to refer to those interventions initiated when a nonreassuring FHR pattern is noted; they are directed primarily toward improving uterine and intervillous space blood flow and secondarily toward increasing maternal oxygenation and cardiac output (Fanaroff & Martin, 1997). The following preventive interventions are described in this chapter: avoiding the supine position and encouraging maternal position changes; encouraging spontaneous short bursts of pushing in response to involuntary bearing-down urges; and encouraging pushing with mouth open and glottis open with vocalizing. Previously it was thought that the left lateral maternal position preferentially promoted maternal cardiac output, thereby enhancing blood flow to the fetus. However, it is now known that either the right or left lateral maternal position effectively enhances uteroplacental blood flow. The key issue is to avoid positioning the laboring woman on her back to reduce the risk of supine hypotension leading to decreased placental perfusion.

Compression of the umbilical cord vessels results in variable decelerations. Amnioinfusion is an intervention that can help relieve such pressure on a nonprolapsed umbilical cord. If maternal hypotension caused by acute hemorrhage (hypovolemia) occurs, the rapid infusion of blood volume expanders may be ordered. Until the infusion is established, the nurse can elevate the woman's legs. Blood pooled in the legs, especially that occurring as the result of sympathetic blockade (e.g., epidural anesthesia), will then drain quickly into the central venous circulation, and this will augment the effective intravascular volume (Fanaroff & Martin, 1997).

Oxytocin always should be infused as a piggyback connection near the indwelling needle (AWHONN, 1993a). If FHR patterns change for any reason, oxytocin stimulation of the uterine muscle must be discontinued. This consists of turning off the IV line from the piggyback (containing oxytocin) and opening the primary infusion line.

Nurses must prioritize interventions to maximize the efficacy of the intrauterine resuscitation. The first priority is to open the maternal and fetal vascular systems; the second priority is to increase blood volume; and the third priority is to optimize oxygenation of the circulating blood volume. For example, to relieve an acute FHR deceleration, the nurse can do the following:

- Turn the woman to the side-lying position.
- Increase the maternal blood volume by increasing the rate of the primary IV infusion or by raising the woman's legs.
- Provide oxygen by face mask.

Some interventions are specific to the FHR pattern. Nursing interventions appropriate for the management of

BOX 21-3   Protocol for Fetal Heart Rate Monitoring

CLIENT/FAMILY TEACHING

Explain purpose of monitoring

Explain procedure

Provide rationale for maternal position other than supine

CARE

Assist woman to a comfortable position other than supine

Change maternal position at least every 2 hours

Change placement of external monitor belts every 2 hours when possible

Provide perineal care as needed when internal monitoring is implemented

MATERNAL/FETAL ASSESSMENTS

Obtain a 20-minute strip of EFM for all clients admitted to labor unit

Low Risk Client

Auscultate or assess tracing every 30 minutes in active phase of first stage of labor

Auscultate or assess tracing every 15 minutes in second stage

High Risk Client

Auscultate or assess tracing every 15 minutes in active phase and every 5 minutes in second stage

Auscultation—All Clients

Count baseline FHR in between contractions

Assess FHR during the contraction and for at least 30 seconds after the contraction

Note increases or decreases of FHR

Assess FHR before ambulation

Interpret FHR data, nursing interventions, and client responses

Notify primary health care provider

EFM—All Clients

Assess and interpret baseline FHR, variability of FHR (long term for external monitoring; long and short term for internal monitoring), and presence or absence of decelerations and accelerations

Assessments for All Clients

Assess uterine activity for frequency and duration, the intensity of contractions, and uterine resting tone

Assess FHR immediately after rupture of membranes, vaginal examinations, and any invasive procedure

REPORTABLE CONDITIONS

Presence of nonreassuring patterns

Worsening of any pattern

Presence of any fetal dysrhythmias

Difficulty in obtaining adequate FHR tracing or inadequate audible FHR

EMERGENCY MEASURES

Implement the following measures immediately in the event of the nonreassuring patterns:

Reposition client in lateral position to increase uteroplacental perfusion or relieve cord compression

Administer oxygen at 8 to 10 L/min or per hospital protocol via face mask

Discontinue oxytocin if infusing

Correct maternal hypovolemia by increasing IV rate per protocol or as ordered

Assess for bleeding or other cause of pattern change, such as maternal hypotension

Notify primary health care provider

Anticipate emergency preparation for surgical intervention if nonreassuring pattern continues despite interventions

DOCUMENTATION

Client Record—Auscultation

FHR baseline, rate and rhythm, increases or decreases

Client Record—EFM

Method of monitoring, change in method, and adjustments to equipment

FHR range, variability, presence of decelerations or accelerations

Uterine activity as determined by palpation or by external or internal monitoring

Interpretation of FHR data, nursing interventions, and client responses

Notification of primary health care provider

Monitor Strip

Client identification data

Assessments, procedures, and interventions (medications, etc.)

Notification of primary health care provider

Significant occurrences (sterile vaginal examination, rupture of membranes, etc.)

Adjustments of the monitor equipment

BOX 21-4 Care of Woman Using Electronic Fetal Monitoring

The following guidelines relate to client teaching and the functioning of the monitor:

Explain that fetal status can be continuously assessed by EFM, even during contractions.

Explain that the lower tracing on the monitor strip paper shows uterine activity; the upper tracing shows the FHR.

Reassure woman and partner that prepared childbirth techniques can be implemented without difficulty.

Explain that, during external monitoring, effleurage can be performed on sides of abdomen or upper portion of thighs.

Explain that breathing patterns based on the time and intensity of contractions can be enhanced by the observation of uterine activity on the monitor strip paper, which shows the onset of contractions.

Note peak of contraction; knowing that contraction will not get stronger and is half over usually is helpful.

Note diminishing intensity.

Coordinate with appropriate breathing and relaxation techniques.

Reassure woman and partner that the use of internal monitoring does not restrict movement, although she is confined to bed.*

Explain that use of external monitoring usually requires the woman's cooperation during positioning and movement.

Reassure woman and partner that use of monitoring does not imply fetal jeopardy.

Reassure her that the equipment is removed periodically to permit the applicator sites to be washed and other care to be given.

EXTERNAL MONITORING
Ultrasound Transducer
Function
Monitors FHR with high-frequency sound waves.

Nursing Care
Tap transducer before use to ensure sound transmission.

Apply ultrasound transmission gel to transducer, clean abdomen and transducer, and reapply gel q2hr and prn.

Massage reddened skin areas gently and reposition belt or adhesive device q2hr and prn.

Auscultate FHR with stethoscope or fetoscope if in doubt as to validity of tracing.

Position and reposition transducer prn to ensure receipt of clear, interpretable FHR data.

Tocotransducer
Function
Monitors uterine activity via a pressure-sensing device placed on the maternal abdomen.

Nursing Care
Position and reposition q2hr and prn on the fundus, where there is the least maternal tissue.

Keep abdominal strap snug but comfortable for the laboring woman.

Adjust pen-set between contractions to print between 10 and 20 mm Hg on the monitor strip paper.

Palpate fundus every 30 to 60 minutes to assess strength of contraction; only frequency and duration of contractions can be assessed with tocotransducer.

Do not determine woman's need for analgesia based on uterine activity displayed on monitor strip.

Gently massage reddened areas under transducer and belt qhr and prn.

INTERNAL MONITORING
Spiral Electrode
Function
Obtains fetal ECG from presenting part and converts it into FHR.

Nursing Care
Ensure that wires are appropriately attached to leg plate.

Reapply electrode paste to leg plate if needed.

Observe FHR tracing on monitor strip for variability.

Turn electrode counterclockwise to remove; never pull straight out from presenting part.

Administer perineal care after the woman voids during labor and prn.

Intrauterine Catheter
Function
Catheter (solid or fluid filled) that monitors intraamniotic pressure internally.

Nursing Care
Flush open system catheter with sterile water before insertion and prn.

Ensure that the length line on catheter is visible at introitus.

For closed system catheters, set baseline rate between uterine contractions when uterus is relaxed.

For open system catheters, turn stopcock off to woman, then with pressure valve of strain gauge released, flush strain gauge, remove syringe, and set stylus to 0 line of chart paper; test further according to manufacturer's instructions q3-4hr and prn.

Check proper functioning by tapping catheter, asking woman to cough, or applying fundal pressure; observe appropriate inflection on strip chart.

Keep catheter taped to woman's leg to prevent dislodgment.

Modified from Tucker, S. et al. (2000). *Patient care standards* (7th ed.). St. Louis: Mosby.
*Portable telemetry monitors allow the FHR and uterine contraction patterns to be observed on centrally located electronic display stations. These portable units permit ambulation during electronic monitoring.

PLAN ᵒᶠ CARE | EFM During Labor

NURSING DIAGNOSIS Maternal anxiety related to lack of knowledge about use of electronic monitor

Expected Outcomes *The client will exhibit increased understanding about fetal monitoring and signs of reduced anxiety (i.e., absence of physical indicators, absence of perceived threat, and absence of feelings of dread).*

Nursing Interventions/*Rationales*

Explain and demonstrate to woman and labor support partner how the electronic monitor (internal or external) works in assessing FHR and in detecting and assessing quality of uterine contractions *to remove fear of unknown and ensure that woman can move with the monitor.*

When making adjustment to the monitor, explain to the couple what is being done and why *because information increases understanding and allays anxiety.*

Explain that although a side-lying position or Fowler's position provides for optimum monitoring, position changes decrease discomfort; therefore encourage frequent changes in position (other than supine) and explain any monitoring adjustments that are being made as a result *to reduce discomfort and allay anxiety.*

NURSING DIAGNOSIS Risk for fetal injury related to inaccurate placement of transducers/electrodes, misinterpretation of results, or failure to use other assessment techniques to monitor fetal well-being

Expected Outcomes *Fetal well-being is adequately assessed, and any fetal compromise is identified immediately.*

Nursing Interventions/*Rationales*

Carefully follow guidelines and checklist for application and initiation of monitoring *to ensure proper placement of monitoring devices and production of accurate output from monitoring device.*

Check placement throughout monitoring process *to ensure that devices remain correctly placed.*

Regularly assess and record results of EFM (FHR and variability, decelerations, accelerations, uterine activity, contractions, uterine resting tone) *to provide consistent and timely evaluation of fetal well-being and progress of labor.*

Auscultate FHR and palpate contractions on a regular basis *to provide a cross-check on the EFM output and ensure fetal well-being.*

From Wong, D., & Perry, S. (1998). *Maternal child nursing care.* St. Louis: Mosby.

---

tachycardia and bradycardia are given in Table 21-2, and those appropriate for the management of increased or decreased variability are given in Table 21-3. No specific nursing interventions are required for the management of FHR acceleration or early deceleration (see Table 21-4). However, late and some types of variable FHR decelerations require aggressive intervention (see Table 21-5). The primary health care provider decides whether medical intervention should be instituted, what intervention is indicated, or whether immediate vaginal or cesarean birth should be performed.

Other Methods of Assessment and Intervention

Assessment techniques. Other methods of assessment are designed to be used in conjunction with EFM in an effort to identify and intervene on behalf of a fetus that is hypoxemic or acidotic. These methods include fetal blood sampling, FHR response to stimulation, and pulse oximetry monitoring of fetal oxygen saturation. Umbilical cord acid-base determination is an assessment technique that is a useful adjunct to the Apgar score in assessing the immediate condition of the newborn.

Fetal scalp blood sampling. Sampling of the fetal scalp blood was designed to assess the fetal pH, Po_2, and Pco_2. The procedure is performed by obtaining a sample of fetal

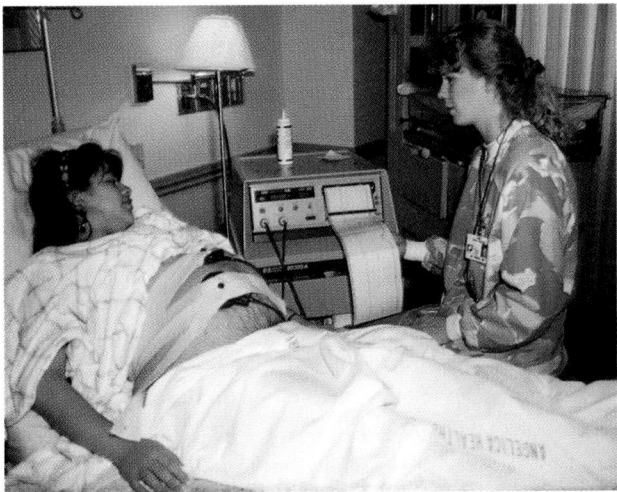

Fig. 21-8 Nurse explains EFM as ultrasound transducer monitors the FHR. *(Courtesy Marjorie Pyle, RNC, Lifecircle, Costa Mesa, CA.)*

scalp blood through the dilated cervix after the membranes have ruptured. The scalp is swabbed with a disinfecting solution before making the puncture, and the sample is then collected. However, the blood gas values vary so rapidly with transient circulatory changes that fetal blood sampling is seldom performed. When used, it is usually in tertiary centers with the capability for repetitive sampling and rapid report of results. The circulatory changes that cause the variability and thus undermine the utility of this procedure are maternal acidosis or alkalosis, caput succedaneum, the stage of labor, and the time relationship of scalp sampling to uterine contractions.

Fetal heart rate response to stimulation. Stimulation of the fetus, to elicit an acceleration of the FHR of 15 beats per minute for at least 15 seconds, is sometimes used as an alternative to fetal blood sampling (Tucker, 2000). The two methods of fetal stimulation currently in practice are scalp stimulation (using digital pressure during a vaginal examination) and vibroacoustic stimulation (using an artificial larynx or fetal acoustic stimulation device over the fetal head for 1 to 2 seconds). An FHR acceleration usually indicates fetal well-being. If the fetus does not have an acceleration, however, it does not necessarily indicate fetal compromise, but further evaluation of fetal well-being is needed.

Fetal pulse oximetry. Continuous monitoring of fetal oxygen saturation by pulse oximetry is a method of fetal assessment currently in the clinical investigation stage (Luttkus & Dudenhausen, 1998). Fetal pulse oximetry works in a similar way to the pulse oximetry used in children and adults. During a vaginal examination in a laboring woman with ruptured membranes, with the fetal head at a -2 station, a sensor is inserted next to the fetal cheek or temple area to assess oxygen saturation. The sensor is then connected to a monitor and the data are displayed on the uterine activity panel of the fetal monitor tracing. The normal range of oxygen saturation in the adult is 95% to 100%. The normal range for the healthy fetus is 30% to 70% (Lien & Garite, 1997) with the cutoff value for the critical threshold of $FSaO_2$ (fetal oxygen saturation) at 30% (Carbonne et al., 1997).

The value of fetal pulse oximetry is that in the event of nonreassuring FHR patterns, it could support the decision of whether labor should continue or whether to intervene with an expeditious assisted vaginal or cesarean delivery of the fetus. Multicenter randomized clinical trial testing is in process in the United States and Europe. The nurse's role could include the use of fetal pulse oximetry in conjunction with FHR monitoring if the device is approved for clinical use (Simpson, 1998).

Umbilical cord acid-base determination. In assessing the immediate condition of the newborn after birth, a sample of cord blood is a useful adjunct to the Apgar score. The procedure is generally done by withdrawing blood from the umbilical artery and having the blood tested for pH, Pco_2, and Po_2. Metabolic acidosis can cause a low Apgar score.

Other Interventions

In addition to the emergency measures for nonreassuring FHR patterns, amnioinfusion and tocolysis may prevent fetal compromise.

Amnioinfusion. Amnioinfusion is a procedure used during labor to either supplement inadequate amounts of amniotic fluid or dilute meconium-stained amniotic fluid with saline or lactated Ringer's solution (Schmidt, 1997). The procedure to supplement amniotic fluid is indicated for clients with oligohydramnios, secondary to uteroplacental insufficiency, premature rupture of membranes, or postmaturity, who are at risk for variable decelerations because of umbilical cord compression.

Oligohydramnios is an abnormally small amount of amniotic fluid or the absence of amniotic fluid. Without the buffer of amniotic fluid, the umbilical cord can easily become compressed during contractions or fetal movement, diminishing the flow of blood between the fetus and placenta as evidenced by variable decelerations. Amnioinfusion replaces the "cushion" for the cord and relieves both the frequency and intensity of variable decelerations.

Amnioinfusion is also indicated in the presence of moderate to thick meconium to dilute and flush out the meconium with the intent of avoiding meconium aspiration syndrome in the neonate (Strong, 1995).

Risks of amnioinfusion are overdistention of the uterine cavity and increased uterine tone. Techniques of amnioinfusion treatment vary, but usually fluid is administered through an IUPC. The woman's membranes must be ruptured for the IUPC placement. The fluid is administered by attaching plastic (intravenous) tubing to a liter of normal saline or lactated Ringer's solution through a port in the IUPC. Double-lumen IUPCs are best because the intrauterine pressure can be monitored without stopping the procedure. The fluid is usually warmed with a blood warmer before administration, especially for the preterm or small-for-gestational-age fetus (American College of Obstetricians and Gynecologists, 1995).

The flow rate can be by bolus or continuous flow or by a combination of these two methods (Wenstrom et al., 1995). The bolus method is useful for treating variable deceleration patterns. About 800 ml of fluid is infused at 10 to 15 ml per minute until the decelerations diminish. Additional boluses are given as needed. A continuous flow rate of about 3 ml per minute is useful for treating oligohydramnios (American College of Obstetricians and Gynecologists, 1995). The combination method is the most common method used. A bolus of 10 to 15 ml per minute is given for 1 hour followed by a maintenance flow rate of 3 ml per minute (Wenstrom et al., 1995). This method is useful for variable decelerations and for thick meconium-stained fluid.

Intensity and frequency of uterine contractions should be continually assessed during the procedure. The recorded uterine resting tone during amnioinfusion will appear higher than normal because of resistance to outflow and turbulence at the end of the catheter. The true resting tone can be checked by discontinuing the amnioinfusion (Afriat, 1996; Tucker, 2000).

The time needed to increase the amniotic fluid volume is about 30 minutes (Snell, 1993). Therefore the treatment for decelerations must be started before the pattern becomes ominous. If the fetal status does not improve or if it worsens, the health care team should be ready for an immediate surgical delivery.

Tocolytic therapy. Tocolysis can be achieved through the administration of drugs that inhibit uterine contractions. This therapy can be used as an adjunct to other interventions in the management of fetal compromise when the fetus is exhibiting nonreassuring patterns associated with increased uterine activity. Tocolysis improves blood flow through the placenta by inhibiting uterine contractions (Brown, 1998). Tocolysis may be considered by the primary health care provider and implemented when other interventions to reduce uterine activity, such as maternal position change and discontinuance of an oxytocin infusion, have no effect on diminishing the uterine contractions. A tocolytic drug such as magnesium sulfate or terbutaline can be administered intravenously to decrease uterine activity. If the FHR pattern improves, the woman may be allowed to continue labor; if there is no improvement, immediate surgical delivery may be needed.

Client and Family Teaching

Part of the nurse's role includes partnering with the woman to achieve a high-quality birthing experience. In addition to teaching and supporting the woman and her family with understanding of the laboring and birth process, breathing techniques, use of equipment, and pain management techniques, two factors can have an effect on fetal status: pushing and positioning. The nurse should provide information and support to the woman in regard to these two factors.

Discouraging the Valsalva maneuver. The **Valsalva maneuver** can be described as the process of making a forceful bearing down attempt while holding one's breath with a closed glottis and tightening the abdominal muscles. This process stimulates the parasympathetic division of the autonomic nervous system, producing a vagal response, and results in the decrease of the maternal heart rate and blood pressure. Prolonged pushing in this manner can decrease placental blood flow, alter maternal and fetal oxygenation, decrease the fetal pH and Po_2, increase the fetal Pco_2, and increase the likelihood of fetal hypoxemia as reflected in FHR pattern changes.

During the second stage of labor, when the woman needs to push, an alternative to breath holding with a closed glottis is to perform the open-mouth and open-glottis breathing-pushing technique. The nurse should instruct the woman to keep her mouth and glottis open and to let air escape from the lungs during the pushing process. This may result in an audible grunting sound and will serve to prevent the Valsalva maneuver.

Maternal positioning. Maternal supine hypotensive syndrome is caused by the weight and pressure of the gravid uterus on the ascending vena cava when the woman is in a supine position. This decreases venous return to the woman's heart and cardiac output and subsequently lowers her blood pressure. The low maternal blood pressure decreases intervillous space blood flow during uterine contractions and results in fetal hypoxemia. This is reflected on the fetal monitor as a nonreassuring FHR pattern, usually late decelerations. The nurse should solicit the woman's cooperation in avoiding the supine position. The woman should be encouraged to maintain a side-lying position or semi-Fowler's position with a lateral tilt to the uterus.

Documentation

Clear and complete documentation on the woman's monitor strip is started before the initiation of monitoring and consists of identifying information plus other relevant data. This documentation is continued and updated according to institutional protocol as monitoring progresses. In some institutions, observations noted and interventions implemented are recorded on the monitor strip to produce a comprehensive document that chronicles the course of labor and the care rendered. In other institutions, this documentation is confined to the labor flow record or computer chart. Advocates of documenting on both the medical record and the EFM strip cite as advantages of this approach the ease of writing directly on the strip while at the bedside and the improved accuracy in documenting critical events that occur and the interventions implemented. Others believe that charting on the EFM strip constitutes duplicate documentation of the same information noted in the medical record, and thus is unnecessary additional paperwork for the nurse.

One way of documenting that frequent maternal-fetal assessments have been done at the bedside is to either initial the EFM strip or depress the "mark" button during these assessments. Data entry devices are now available with some EFM systems; assessments are keyed in and subsequently printed on the strip. A disadvantage of documenting on both the EFM strip and the medical record is that frequently the times noted for events and interventions on the EFM strip do not correlate with what is later documented in the medical record. These inaccuracies can lead those involved in the retrospective review process carried out during litigation to infer that documentation errors have occurred. Therefore, if institutional policy mandates documentation on both the monitor strip and the medical record, it is critically important for the nurse to make sure the times and notations of events and interventions recorded in each place agree. No one method of documentation is right; rather the nurse must be aware of and follow individual institutional policies, as well as participate in formulating such policies. Many of the aspects of care and events that can be documented on the monitor strip are listed in Box 21-5.

The monitor strip, if used for documentation, is labeled with the following information: the woman's name and identification number, the date, and expected date of birth (EDB); any high risk conditions affecting the mother, such

BOX 21-5 Documentation: Monitor Strip

OBSERVATIONS

Maternal vital signs
Maternal position/repositioning
Vaginal examinations and findings
Medications (such as oxytocin); anesthesia/analgesia
Voidings; emesis
Pushing/bearing down
Fetal movement
Baseline FHR or periodic changes

ADJUSTMENTS

Relocation of transducers
Flushing or adjustment of catheter
Replacement of electrode
Replacement of catheter
Time lapsed while changing monitor strip paper
Reason for interruption/removal

INTERVENTIONS

Position change
Parenteral fluids
Discontinuance of oxytocin
Oxygen administration
Amnioinfusion
Fetal scalp stimulation
Primary health care provider notification and response

as preeclampsia and diabetes; whether membranes are intact or ruptured; the status of cervical dilation and the station of the presenting part; and the time the monitor is attached and the mode used, as well as a notation that the FHR has been reviewed and evaluated on a periodic basis.

Evaluation

Evaluation is a continuous process. The nurse can assume that care was effective when the outcomes for care have been achieved (see Plan of Care).

KEY POINTS

- Fetal well-being during labor is gauged by the response of the FHR to uterine contractions.
- FHR characteristics include the baseline FHR and periodic changes in the FHR.
- The monitoring of fetal well-being includes FHR assessment and watching for meconium-stained amniotic fluid.

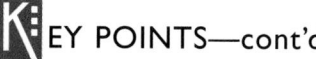

KEY POINTS—cont'd

- It is the responsibility of the nurse to assess FHR patterns, implement independent nursing interventions, and report nonreassuring patterns to the physician or nurse-midwife.
- The Association of Women's Health, Obstetric, and Neonatal Nurses and the American College of Obstetricians and Gynecologists have established and published health care provider standards and guidelines for EFM.
- The emotional, informational, and comfort needs of the woman and her family must be addressed when the mother and her fetus are being monitored.

CRITICAL THINKING EXERCISES

1 You are assigned to a woman who is in the first stage of labor. She is beginning to be uncomfortable with her contractions but notices that the tracing from the external monitor does not show them to be strong. She also wonders why the FHR is sometimes not being recorded on the monitor paper. She asks if there is "something wrong with the baby" when the FHR is not recording continuously.
   a. Based on your knowledge of how the external monitor works, how would you explain the lack of continuous tracing of the FHR and the seeming inconsistency between the mother's discomfort and the appearance of the contractions on the monitor paper?
   b. Identify nursing diagnoses based on your analysis of the situation.
   c. Develop a plan of care, including interventions, that would be reassuring and supportive, and justify your choices.
2 Review three sample or actual fetal monitor strips.
   a. For each fetal monitor strip, determine the following:
      i The baseline rate and variability of the FHR
      ii Periodic changes, if any
      iii The contraction interval, duration, and intensity, as well as the resting tone
   b. Corroborate your findings in a clinical conference.
   c. Describe appropriate nursing actions in response to each of the fetal monitor strips.
3 A woman in the first stage of labor has a birth plan that requests no electronic fetal/uterine monitoring. The labor and delivery unit's standard protocol is to monitor every woman electronically at least for baseline data. Suggest ways to provide care in this situation that considers both the woman's and care provider's viewpoints.

References

Afriat, C. (1996). Intrapartum fetal monitoring. In K. Simpson & P. Creehan (Eds.). *AWHONN perinatal nursing.* Philadelphia: Lippincott.

American College of Obstetricians and Gynecologists. (1995). *Fetal heart rate patterns: Monitoring, interpretation, and management* (ACOG Technical Bulletin No. 207). Washington, D.C.: ACOG.

Association of Women's Health, Obstetric, and Neonatal Nurses. (1993a). *Cervical ripening and induction and augmentation of labor* (Practice Resource). Washington, D.C.: AWHONN.

Association of Women's Health, Obstetric, and Neonatal Nurses. (1993b). *Didactic content and clinical skills verification for professional nurse providers of basic, high-risk, and critical-care intrapartum nursing.* Washington, D.C.: AWHONN.

Brown, C. (1998). Intrapartal tocolysis: An option for acute intrapartal fetal crisis. *J Obstet Gynecol Neonatal Nurs* 27(3), 257-261.

Carbonne, B. et al. (1997). Multicenter study on the clinical value of fetal pulse oximetry: II. Compared predictive values of pulse oximetry and fetal blood analysis. *Am J Obstet Gynecol* 177, 593-598.

Fanaroff, A., & Martin, R. (1997). *Neonatal-perinatal medicine: Diseases of the fetus and infant* (6th ed.). St. Louis: Mosby.

Harvey, C. (1997). Coming to terms: Electronic fetal monitoring update. *AWHONN Lifelines* 1(3), 49-51.

Lien, J., & Garite, T. (1997). A better way of assessing fetal oxygenation? *Contemp Ob Gyn* 4, 53-58, 62-65.

Luttkus, A., & Dudenhausen, J. (1998). Fetal pulse oximetry. *Obstet Gynecol* 10(6), 481-486.

National Institute of Child Health and Human Development Research Planning Workshop. (1997). Electronic fetal heart rate monitoring: Research guidelines for interpretation. *Am J Obstet Gynecol* 177(6), 1385-1390.

Schmidt, J. (1997). Fluid check: Making the case for intrapartum amnioinfusion. *AWHONN Lifelines* 1(5), 46-51.

Simpson, K. (1998). Intrapartum fetal oxygen saturation monitoring. *AWHONN Lifelines* 2(6), 21-24.

Snell, B. (1993). The use of amnioinfusion in nurse-midwifery procedures. *J Nurse Midwifery* 38(2), 625-715.

Strong, T. (1995). Amnioinfusion. *J Reprod Med* 49(2), 108-114.

Thacker, S., Stroup, D., & Peterson, H. (1998). Intrapartum electronic fetal monitoring data for clinical decisions. *Clinical Obstet Gynecol* 41(2), 362-368.

Tucker, S. (2000). *Pocket guide to fetal monitoring and assessment* (4th ed.). St. Louis: Mosby.

Tucker, S. et al. (2000). *Patient care standards: Collaborative practice planning guides* (7th ed.). St. Louis: Mosby.

Wenstrom, K., Andrews, W., & Maher, J. (1995). Amnioinfusion survey: Prevalence, protocols, and complications. *Obstet Gynecol* 86(4 pt 1), 572-576.

22

Nursing Care During Labor

Karen A. Piotrowski

LEARNING OBJECTIVES

- Define the key terms.
- Review the factors included in the initial assessment of the woman in labor.
- Describe the ongoing assessment of maternal progress during the first, second, and third stages of labor.
- State the physical and psychosocial findings indicative of maternal progress during labor.
- Discuss aspects of fetal assessment during labor.
- Identify signs of developing complications during the first, second, and third stages of labor.
- Develop a comprehensive plan of care relevant to each stage of labor and birth.
- Discuss the nurse's role in managing care for the woman and her significant others (support person[s], family) during each stage of labor and birth.

- Examine the influence of cultural and religious beliefs and practices on the process of labor and birth.
- Discuss the role of a woman's significant others (support person[s], family) in assisting her during labor and birth.
- Outline nursing actions in preparation for birth.
- Describe the role and responsibilities of the nurse in an emergency childbirth situation.
- Identify the impact of perineal trauma on the woman.
- Discuss the nurse's role in reducing the incidence of routine episiotomy.
- Identify topics for nursing research related to nursing care during labor.

KEY TERMS

active phase
amniotomy
artificial rupture of membranes
bloody or pink show
crowning
doula
duration of uterine contractions
episiotomy
Ferguson reflex
ferning

first stage of labor
frequency of uterine contractions
intensity of uterine contractions
latent phase
Leopold's maneuvers
lithotomy position
nitrazine test
nuchal cord
placental separation
resting tone of uterine contractions

ring of fire
Ritgen maneuver
rupture of membranes
second stage of labor
spontaneous rupture of membranes
third stage of labor
transition phase
uterine contractions
Valsalva maneuver

The labor process is an exciting and anxious time for the woman and her significant others (support persons, family). In a relatively short period of time they experience one of the most profound changes in their lives (Simkin, 1996).

To effectively and safely manage care for the laboring woman and her significant others the nurse must have comprehensive knowledge of the factors that trigger labor; the anatomic, physiologic, and emotional adaptations that occur in preparation for childbirth; the process for assessing fetal and maternal well-being in labor; the effective support measures required by the woman and her support persons and family; and the signs and symptoms of developing complications and their treatment.

For most women, labor begins with the first uterine contraction, continues with hours of hard work during cervical dilation and birth, and ends as the woman and her significant others begin the attachment process with the newborn.

FIRST STAGE OF LABOR
▪ CARE MANAGEMENT

The **first stage of labor** begins with the onset of regular uterine contractions and ends with full cervical dilation. Care begins when the woman reports one or more of the following:

- Onset of progressive, regular uterine contractions that increase in frequency, strength, and duration
- Blood-tinged vaginal discharge **(bloody or pink show)** indicating that the mucous plug has passed
- Fluid discharge from the vagina (spontaneous rupture of membranes [SROM, SRM])

The first stage of labor consists of the following three phases: the **latent phase** (up to 3 cm of dilation), the **active phase** (4 to 7 cm of dilation), and the **transition phase** (8 to 10 cm of dilation). Most nulliparous women seek admission to the hospital in the latent phase because they have not experienced labor before and are unsure of the "right" time to come in. Multiparous women usually do not come to the hospital until they are in the active phase. Even though no two labors are identical, women who have given birth before appear less anxious about the process, unless their previous experience has been negative.

The nurse uses the nursing process as a framework for managing the care of women and their significant others during all stages of labor. Nurses should involve the laboring woman as a partner in the formulation of an individualized plan of care. This helps preserve the woman's sense of control and participation in her own childbirth experience and helps enhance the woman's self-esteem and level of satisfaction (Proctor, 1998).

Fowles (1998) questioned women about the lingering impressions they had about their childbirth experience 2 months after the birth. Caregivers who were supportive, encouraging, kind, patient, professional, and comforting helped these women to remember their childbirth experience in positive terms. However, these women expressed that frustrations they felt regarding their experience stemmed from pain, lack of control, lack of knowledge, or the negative behaviors of some caregivers.

Assessment and Nursing Diagnoses

Assessment begins at the first contact with the woman, whether by telephone or in person. Many women call the hospital or birthing center first to receive validation that it is all right for them to come in for evaluation or admission. The manner in which the nurse communicates with the woman during this first contact can set the tone for a positive birth experience. A caring attitude by the nurse encourages the woman to verbalize questions and concerns. If possible, the nurse should have the woman's prenatal record in hand when speaking to her or admitting her for evaluation of labor. Copies of records are often filed on the perinatal unit at some time during the woman's third trimester.

Certain factors are assessed initially to determine whether the woman is in true or false labor and whether she should come for further assessment or admission (Varney, 1997) (see Teaching Guidelines box). When a woman calls and there is a question about whether she is in labor (or in labor advanced enough to be admitted), the nurse should suggest that she either call her primary health care provider or come to the hospital (Box 22-1).

The pregnant woman may call the primary health care provider or come to the hospital while in false labor or early in the latent phase of the first stage of labor. It can be discouraging for her and her partner to find out that the contractions that feel so strong and regular to her are not true contractions because they are not causing cervical dilation or are still not strong or frequent enough for admission.

If the woman lives near the hospital, she may be asked to stay home or return home to allow labor to progress in terms of frequency and intensity of contractions, because the ideal setting for the low risk woman at this time is the familiar environment of her home. The nurse can use the recommended approach for the telephone interview (see Box 22-1) to assess the woman's status and to give instructions regarding the optimum timing for admission and signs that require immediate notification of the primary health care provider. Measures the woman and her significant others can use to enhance the progress of labor, reduce anxiety, and maintain comfort should be described. The woman is encouraged to ambulate and asked to limit her intake of foods to either light foods and fluids or to clear liquids only, depending on the preferences of her primary health care provider.

A warm shower could be relaxing for the woman in early labor. However, warm baths should be avoided until the cervix is approximately 5 cm dilated, because water

TEACHING guidelines

How to Distinguish True Labor from False Labor

TRUE LABOR

Contractions

Occur regularly, becoming stronger, lasting longer, and occurring closer together.

Become more intense with walking.

Usually felt in lower back, radiating to lower portion of abdomen.

Continue despite use of comfort measures.

Cervix (by vaginal examination)

Shows progressive change (softening, effacement, and dilation signaled by the appearance of bloody show).

Moves to an increasingly anterior position.

Fetus

Presenting part usually becomes engaged in the pelvis. This results in increased ease of breathing; at the same time, the presenting part presses downward and compresses the bladder, resulting in urinary frequency.

FALSE LABOR

Contractions

Occur irregularly or become regular only temporarily.

Often stop with walking or position change.

Can be felt in the back or abdomen above the navel.

Often can be stopped through the use of comfort measures.

Cervix (by vaginal examination)

May be soft but there is no significant change in effacement or dilation or evidence of bloody show.

Is often in a posterior position.

Fetus

Presenting part is usually not engaged in the pelvis.

---

immersion in early labor could prolong the labor process and increase the use of oxytocin to stimulate uterine contractions and epidural analgesia for pain reduction (Eriksson, Mattsson, & Ladfors, 1997). Soothing back, foot, and hand massage or a warm drink of preferred liquids such as tea or milk can help the woman to rest and even to sleep, especially if false or early labor is occurring at night.

Diversional activities such as walking outdoors or in the house, reading, watching television, doing needlework, or talking with friends can reduce the perception of early discomfort, help the time pass, and reduce anxiety (Varney, 1997).

The woman who lives at a considerable distance from the hospital may be admitted in early labor. The same

---

BOX 22-1 Telephone Interview with Woman in Latent Phase of Labor

The perinatal nurse performs the following steps of the nursing process:

ASSESSMENT

• Gathers data regarding the woman's status, including signs and symptoms indicative of true or false labor.

• Discusses instructions given by the woman's primary health care provider regarding when to come for admission.

PLANNING AND IMPLEMENTATION

• Decides whether the woman will come for labor assessment and admission or be encouraged to stay at home until contractions increase in duration, frequency, and intensity.

• Assures the woman that she is welcome to call the perinatal unit at any time to discuss her labor status.

• Answers questions the woman and her family may have regarding labor or provides instruction as needed (e.g., which entrance of the hospital to enter).

• Suggests a variety of positions she can assume to maximally enhance uteroplacental and renal blood flow (e.g., side-lying position) and enhance the progress of labor (e.g., upright positions and ambulation).

• Suggests diversional activities, such as walking, reading, watching television, talking to friends.

• Suggests measures to maintain comfort, such as a warm shower, back or foot massage.

• Discusses the oral intake of foods and fluids appropriate for early labor (light foods or fluids or clear liquids depending on the preference of her primary health care provider).

• Instructs the woman to come in immediately if membranes rupture, bleeding occurs, or fetal movements change.

EVALUATION

• Evaluates whether instructions and information have been understood by the woman by asking her to verbalize her understanding.

---

measures used by the woman at home should be offered to the hospitalized woman in early labor.

Admission to Labor Unit

On the woman's arrival at the perinatal unit, assessment is the top priority (Fig. 22-1). The nurse first performs a screening assessment, using the techniques of interview and physical assessment, and reviews the laboratory find-

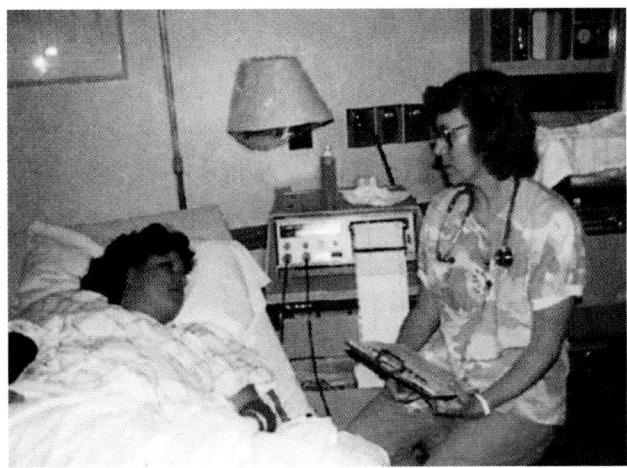

Fig. 22-1 Woman being admitted. *(Courtesy Marjorie Pyle, RNC, Lifecircle, Costa Mesa, CA.)*

ings to determine the health status of the woman and her fetus and the progress of her labor. The primary health care provider is notified, and if the woman is admitted, a detailed systems assessment is done.

When the woman is admitted, she usually is moved from an observation area to the labor room; the labor, delivery, and recovery (LDR) room; or the labor, delivery, recovery, and postpartum (LDRP) room. Because first impressions are important, the woman and her partner are welcomed by name and introduced to the staff members who will be involved in the woman's care.

If the woman wishes, her partner is included in the assessment and admission process. Significant others not participating in this process may be directed to the appropriate waiting area, if that is the policy of the unit. In many LDR and LDRP rooms, the woman may have anyone she wishes present. The woman is asked to undress and put on her own gown or a hospital gown. Her personal belongings are put away safely. If the woman prefers to wear some items of her own (e.g., socks), these are noted on her chart.

LEGAL TIP Client's Personal Items

Most hospitals have a checklist or other way of recording the woman's belongings that becomes part of her permanent record. Both the woman and the admitting nurse must sign this form. Items of value (e.g., jewelry) should be placed in the safekeeping of a family member.

The nurse orients the woman and her partner to the layout and operation of the unit and room. This includes the use of the call light and telephone system, the location of personal storage areas in the bedside and overbed tables, and how to adjust lighting in the room.

The woman is told how to notify the nurse of her wish to use the bathroom or to ambulate. An admissions bracelet is placed on the woman's wrist, as well as an al-

lergy bracelet (usually colored), when relevant. The nurse should reassure the woman that she is in competent, caring hands, that she can ask questions related to her care and status of herself and her fetus at any time during labor, and that questions will be answered.

If the woman has not already done so, she signs the necessary papers giving permission for care to be given to herself and her newborn (for example, anesthesia consent, hepatitis B vaccine consent). (Legally a permit for care must be signed before the woman can receive any medication or any procedures are instituted.)

The nurse asks whether the woman came by car and, if needed, suggests where the vehicle can be parked by the person who accompanied her to the hospital. Some women, especially those who arrive in labor unexpectedly and alone, welcome the offer of a telephone to notify their families. In some instances the nurse may have to make the calls for the woman.

The nurse can minimize the woman's anxiety by explaining terms commonly used during labor. During the review of the prenatal record, the nurse can provide short definitions of technical terms and abbreviations. The woman's interest and response guide the depth and breadth of these explanations.

Admission Data

Admission forms such as the ones in Fig. 22-2 can provide guidelines for the acquisition of important assessment information when a woman in labor is being evaluated or admitted. Additional sources of data include (1) the prenatal record, (2) the initial interview, (3) physical examination to determine baseline physiologic characteristics, (4) laboratory results, (5) expressed psychosocial and cultural factors, and (6) the clinical evaluation of labor status.

Prenatal Data

The screening nurse should review the prenatal record to identify the woman's individual needs and risks. Incomplete information regarding a woman's prenatal health status could adversely affect the quality and safety of the care provided to her during labor and after birth, to her newborn, and to her significant others. Use of standardized worksheets and flow sheets developed by health care providers and computer access to antepartal health records are strategies that can facilitate the gathering of information relevant to the safe and effective management of care during labor (Hill, Lowery, & Chez, 1998).

If the woman has not had any prenatal care, this baseline information must be obtained. If the woman is experiencing discomfort, the nurse should ask the questions between contractions when the woman can concentrate more fully on her answers.

It is important to know the woman's age so that the plan of care can be tailored to her age-group needs. For example, a 14-year-old girl and a 40-year-old woman have different but specific needs, and their ages place them at

Obstetric Admitting Record   Page 1 of 2

Basic Admission Data   Date ___ / ___ / ___ Time _____

☐ Ambulatory   ☐ Direct admit   ☐ Stretcher
☐ Wheelchair   ☐ Transfer from_____

G	T	Pt	A	L	L M P / /	E D D / /	Age
						E D By fetal D assessment / /	

Race/Ethnicity_____
Occupation_____ Education_____
Marital status S M Sep D W   Religion_____

MD/CNM Tel no	Support person/Relationship Tel no

Reasons for Admission
☐ **Onset of labor**
☐ Induction of labor
☐ Spontaneous abortion
☐ Cesarean section
    ☐ Primary ☐ Repeat
    (reason for primary_____)
☐ VBAC
☐ Tubal ligation
☐ Vaginal bleeding
☐ PROM
☐ Preterm labor
Detail reasons for admission_____
_____

Observation evaluation
☐ Fetal status
    ☐ Ultrasound
    ☐ Amniocentesis
☐ NST
☐ CST
☐ Medical complications
_____
☐ Obstetric complications
_____

Patient Triage Data

Contractions   ☐ **None**   ☐ Palpation   ☐ Tocotransducer
   Frequency_____ Duration_____ Intensity_____
   Began on___ / ___ / ___Time_____

Membranes   ☐ **Intact**   ☐ Bulging
           ☐ Ruptured (Date___ / ___ / ___ Time_____)
  Fluid   ☐ Clear   ☐ Bloody   ☐ Foul smelling
        ☐ Meconium stained   ☐ No foul odor

Vaginal bleeding ☐ **None**   ☐ Normal show
        ☐ Bleeding (describe_____)

Cervical Exam
  Station_____ Effacement_____ Dilatation_____cms
  Presentation
  ☐ Vertex   ☐ Transverse lie
  ☐ Face/Brow   ☐ Compound
  ☐ Breech (type_____) ☐ Unknown
Medication allergy/Sensitivity   ☐ **None**
  ☐ Identify_____

Other allergy/Sensitivity   = **None**
  ☐ Identify_____

Patient Care Data

Personal Effects

Item	Disposition		
	With patient	With support person	Other (describe)

Illness (≤ 14 days prior to admission) ☐ **None**
  ☐ Type/Treatment_____

Recent Exposure to Communicable Disease ☐ **None**
  ☐ Type/Date_____ ___ / ___ / ___

Last Oral Intake
  Fluids___ / ___ / ___ Time_____
  Solids___ / ___ / ___ Time_____

Medications ☐ **None**

Type/Dose	Last taken	With patient		Disposition
		No	Yes	
		☐	☐	
_____	_____			

Alcohol/Drug use   ☐ No   ☐ Yes
  Substances   Amt/Day   Last used
_____ _____ ___ / ___ / ___ Time_____
_____ _____ ___ / ___ / ___ Time_____

Plans for Birth and Hospital Stay
Support person present in L&D   ☐ No ☐ Yes_____
Other family members in L&D   ☐ No ☐ Yes_____

Anesthesia ☐ **None**
  ☐ Local   ☐ Epidural   ☐ Spinal   ☐ General

Delivery site
  ☐ DR   ☐ Birthing room   ☐ LDR   ☐ LDRP   ☐ OR
Personal requests_____

Adoption ☐ No
       ☐ Yes Contact with infant ☐ No ☐ Yes
          Adoption contact_____
Feeding preference   ☐ Breast   ☐ Bottle
Room preference   ☐ Private   ☐ Semi-Private
          ☐ Rooming-In
☐ Tubal ligation   Authorization signed   ☐ Yes   ☐ No
☐ Circumcision   Authorization signed   ☐ Yes   ☐ No

Psychosocial Data

Communication Deficit ☐ **None**
  ☐ Identify_____

Other children ☐ No ☐ Yes Age/Sex_____
_____ , _____ , _____ ,

Partner involved ☐ Yes ☐ No

Admitting signature_____ Time_____

Fig. 22-2   Obstetric admitting record. *(Permission to use and/or reproduce this copyrighted material has been granted by the owner, Hollister, Inc., Libertyville, IL.)*

Obstetric Admitting Record	Page 2 of 2	

Psychosocial Data (Cont'd.)

Basic needs met   Yes   No   If no, explain

     Housing   □   □   _____

     Clothing   □   □   _____

     Food   □   □   _____

     Transportation   □   □   _____

Free from apparent physical/emotional abuse □ Yes □ No

If no, explain_____

Life Stress   No   Yes   If no, explain

     Living   □   □   _____

     Working   □   □   _____

     Serious illness   □   □   _____

Self Care Needs   □ None   □ Needs help with_____

Emotional status   □ Happy   □ Ambivalent

                    □ Anxious   □ Depressed   □ Angry

Discharge Planning Data

Discharge planning initiated   □ Yes   □ No

Discharge needs identified_____

Social service referral □ No □ Yes ___ / ___ / ___

Planned length of stay_____ days

Significant Prenatal Data

Prenatal Records Available on Admission

□ Yes □ No

Source of prenatal data_____

First prenatal visit ___ / ___ / ___

Attended prenatal classes □ Yes □ No

Infant care provider:

Lab Findings □ None	
Blood type & Rh	_____
Rubella titer	_____
Serology	_____
HbSAg	_____

Fetal Assessment Tests   □ None

Date	Test	Result
/		
/		
/		
/		

Maternal Problems Identified   □ **None**

                               Active   Resolved

1._____ □   □

2._____ □   □

3._____ □   □

Fetal Problems Identified   □ **None**

                               Active   Resolved

1._____ □   □

2._____ □   □

3._____ □   □

Physical Assessment

Detail all abnormal findings

Height	Wt pregrav/grav

Temp	Pulse	Resp	BP

System	Normal	Abnormal
HEENT	□	□
Neurologic	□	□
Skin	□	□
Breasts	□	□
Extremities	□	□
Cardiovascular	□	□
Respiratory	□	□
Abdomen	□	□
Gastrointestinal	□	□
Urinary	□	□
Genitalia	□	□

Specimens obtained (check all that apply)

Urine test	Time	Results	Blood test	Time	Results
□ Urinalysis			□ Hgb		
□ C + S			□ Hct		
□ Glucose			□ VDRL/RPR		
□ Albumin			□ Type/Screen		
□ Ketones			□		
□ pH			□		
□ Blood			□		

Fetal Evaluation Data

Fundal height_____ cms FHR_____

Estimated

fetal weight_____

Weeks gestation (est)

By dates_____ wks

By ultrasound_____ wks

     Date ___ / ___ / ___

□ Fetoscope

□ Doppler

□ Fetal monitor

□ Other

Multiple gestation   □ **No**   □ Yes

     Infant   Presentation   Position

1. _____ _____ _____

2. _____ _____ _____

3. _____ _____ _____

Initial Problems Identified   □ **None**

1. _____

2. _____

3. _____

Physician/CNM_____

Notified by_____

           Date ___ / ___ / ___ Time_____

_____ Admitting signature

_____ Examiner signature

           Date ___ / ___ / ___ Time_____

Fig. 22-2 cont'd   For legend see p. 514.

PROCEDURE

Tests for Rupture of Membranes

NITRAZINE TEST FOR pH

Explain procedure to woman/couple.

Procedure

Wash hands.

Use **nitrazine test** paper, a dye-impregnated test paper for determining pH. (Differentiates amniotic fluid, which is slightly alkaline, from urine and purulent material [pus], which are acidic.)

Wearing a sterile glove lubricated with water, place a piece of test paper at the cervical os.

OR

Use a sterile, cotton-tipped applicator to dip deep into vagina to pick up fluid; touch applicator to test paper. (Procedure may be done during speculum examination.)

Read results:

Membranes probably intact: identifies vaginal and most body fluids that are acidic:

Yellow	pH 5.0
Olive-yellow	pH 5.5
Olive-green	pH 6.0

Membranes probably ruptured: identifies amniotic fluid that is alkaline:

Blue-green	pH 6.5
Blue-gray	pH 7.0
Deep blue	pH 7.5

Realize that false test results are possible because of presence of bloody show, insufficient amniotic fluid, or semen.

Remove gloves and wash hands.

Document Results

Positive or negative.

TEST FOR FERNING OR FERN PATTERN

Explain procedure to woman/couple.

Wash hands, apply sterile gloves, obtain specimen of fluid (usually during sterile speculum examination).

Spread a drop of fluid from vagina on a clean glass slide with a sterile, cotton-tipped applicator.

Allow fluid to dry.

Examine slide under microscope: observe for appearance of **ferning** (a frondlike crystalline pattern) (do not confuse with cervical mucus test, when high levels of estrogen are responsible for causing the ferning).

Observe for absence of ferning. (Alerts staff to possibility that amount of specimen was inadequate or that specimen was urine, vaginal discharge, or blood.)

Remove gloves and wash hands.

Document Results

Positive or negative.

---

risk for different problems. Height and weight relationships are important to determine because a weight gain greater than that recommended may place the woman at a higher risk for cephalopelvic disproportion and cesarean birth. This is especially true for women who are petite and have gained 16 kg or more. Other factors to consider are the woman's general health status, any current medical conditions or allergies she may have, her respiratory status, and previous surgical procedures she has undergone.

Her past and present obstetric and pregnancy history are carefully noted. The obstetric history includes gravidity (number of pregnancies) and parity (number of pregnancies reaching viability). Obstetric problems to consider include a history of vaginal bleeding, pregnancy-induced hypertension (PIH), anemia, gestational diabetes, infections (bacterial or sexually transmitted), and immunodeficiencies.

If this is not the woman's first labor and birth experience, it is important to note the characteristics of her previous experiences. This information includes the duration of previous labors, the type of anesthesia used, and the kind of birth (spontaneous vaginal, forceps-assisted, vacuum-assisted, or cesarean birth). The woman's perception of her previous labor and birth experiences should be explored because it may influence her attitude toward her current experience. Women can retain long-term memories of their childbirth experiences. The memory of labor and birth events can affect a woman's postpartum emotional adjustment, self-esteem, and ability to parent effectively (DiMatteo et al., 1993; Simkin, 1996).

While reviewing the data on past births, the nurse collects data related to the condition of the babies (i.e., their weight, Apgar scores, and general health at and after birth). Following is an example of such information obtained in one woman:

Mrs. Smith gained 36 pounds with her last pregnancy. Her baby was born by vacuum assistance after 3 hours of pushing, and Mrs. Smith had an extensive episiotomy. She views her experience as a difficult one, specifying that she lost control several times and her behavior was "not good." Mrs. Smith expresses fear that "the same thing will happen this time." During this pregnancy, Mrs. Smith, who is at 38 weeks of gestation, has gained 43 pounds.

Armed with such information, the nurse is then better able to anticipate the childbirth needs of this mother, her baby, and the couple. (In light of the previous birth history in this woman, it would not be surprising for her to have a long second stage or for a vacuum-assisted birth also to be needed.)

It is important to confirm that the expected date of birth (EDB) is as accurate as possible. Other data in the prenatal record include patterns of maternal weight gain, physiologic measurements such as maternal vital signs (blood pressure; temperature, pulse, respiration [TPR]); fundal height, baseline fetal heart rate (FHR), and laboratory test results. These tests include testing to determine the woman's blood type and Rh factor, a complete or partial blood cell count (hemoglobin and hematocrit), the 50 g blood glucose test, determination of the rubella titer, serologic tests (Venereal Disease Research Laboratories [VDRL] or rapid plasma reagin [RPR] test) for syphilis, surface antigen (HBsAG) for hepatitis B, culture for group B streptococci, and urinalysis. Additional tests may include a tuberculosis screen with purified protein derivative (PPD), as well as screening for the human immunodeficiency virus (HIV) or the sickle cell trait and other genetic disorders (e.g., maternal serum alpha-fetoprotein).

Interview

The woman's primary complaint or reason for coming to the hospital is determined in the interview. The primary complaint may be that her bag of waters (BOW, amniotic membranes) ruptured, with or without contractions. The woman may have come in for an obstetric check (which is a period of observation reserved for women who are unsure about the onset of their labor). If used by the hospital and approved by the woman's health insurance plan, this allows time on the unit for the diagnosis of labor without the woman's actual admission to the hospital.

Even the experienced mother may have difficulty determining the onset of labor. The woman is asked to recall the events of the previous days. She is asked to identify as best she can when regular contractions began. She is asked about the following:
- Frequency and duration of contractions
- Location and character of discomfort from contractions (e.g., back pain, suprapubic discomfort)
- Persistence of contractions despite changes in maternal position when walking or lying down
- Presence and character of vaginal discharge or show
- The status of amniotic membranes, such as whether a gush or seepage of fluid has occurred (rupture of membranes) (If there has been a discharge that may be amniotic fluid, she is asked to identify when the fluid was first noted and to describe the fluid [e.g., amount, color, unusual odor]. In many instances the findings from a sterile speculum examination and a nitrazine [pH] or fern test can confirm that the membranes are ruptured [see Procedure box]).

These descriptions of the contractions and the vaginal discharge help the nurse assess the degree of progress. Bloody or pink show is distinguished from bleeding by the fact that it is pink and feels sticky because of its mucoid nature. It is scant to begin with and increases with effacement and dilation of the cervix. A woman may report a scant brownish to bloody discharge that may be attributed to cervical trauma resulting from vaginal examination or coitus occurring within the last 48 hours.

In case general anesthesia may be required in an emergency, it is important to assess the woman's respiratory status. The nurse determines this by asking the woman if she has a "cold" or related symptoms: a "stuffy nose," sore throat, or cough. The status of allergies is rechecked, including allergies to drugs routinely used in obstetrics, such

BOX 22-2 The Birth Plan

The birth plan should include the woman's/couple's preferences related to the following:
- Presence of birth companions such as the partner, older children, parents, friends, a doula, and the role each will play
- Presence of other persons such as students, male attendants, interpreters
- Clothing to be worn
- Environmental modifications such as lighting, music, privacy, focal point, items from home such as pillows
- Labor activities such as preferred positions for labor and for birth, ambulation, birth balls, showers and whirlpool baths, oral food and fluid intake
- Repertoire of comfort and relaxation measures
- Labor and birth medical interventions such as pharmacologic pain relief measures, intravenous therapy, electronic monitoring, induction or augmentation measures, episiotomy
- Care and handling of the newborn immediately after birth such as cutting of the cord, eye care, breastfeeding
- Cultural and religious requirements related to the care of the mother, newborn, and placenta

The childbirth.org website (http://www.childbirth.org) provides couples with an interactive birth plan along with examples of birth plans.

as meperidine (Demerol) or lidocaine (Xylocaine). Some allergic responses cause swelling of the mucous membranes of the respiratory tract, which could interfere with breathing and the administration of inhalation anesthesia.

Because vomiting and subsequent aspiration into the respiratory tract can complicate an otherwise normal labor, the nurse records the time of the woman's last oral intake of food and the type of solid food and liquids consumed.

Any information not found in the prenatal record is obtained during the admission assessment. Pertinent data include the birth plan (Box 22-2), the choice of infant feeding method, the anesthesia desired (if any), and the name of the pediatrician. A client profile is obtained that identifies the woman's preparation for childbirth, the support person or family members desired during childbirth and their availability, and ethnic or cultural expectations and needs.

The woman may be scheduled for the induction of labor. This and other problems of labor, such as premature rupture of membranes, require alterations in the nursing care plan. However, even in these instances the nursing assessment process remains essentially the same.

The nurse reviews the birth plan, if available, before the woman arrives in the birthing unit. If no written plan has been prepared, the nurse helps the woman formulate a birth plan when she arrives at the hospital. The nurse describes options available and finds out the woman's wishes and preferences. The nurse also prepares the woman for the possible need to make changes in her plan as labor progresses and assures her that information will be provided as the need arises so that she can make informed decisions. The nurse uses the information in the birth plan to individualize the care given the woman during labor.

The nurse should discuss with the woman and her partner their plans for preserving childbirth memories using photography and videotaping. Health care agencies and insurance companies have begun to voice concern that this type of recording of childbirth events could be used in court should the couple sue the health care agency or health care providers. The nurse can reduce liability by assessing the couple's wishes regarding who and what will be recorded, the method that will be used, and the person who will perform this task. In addition, the client's record should reflect that the childbirth was recorded. Agency policies must be developed, including the requirement to sign a contractual agreement, use of space in the birth area, safety and infection control measures, and delineation of who and what can be recorded (Cesario, 1998).

During this initial interview, the approximate time of the onset of true labor is confirmed and information on the woman's current clinical condition is obtained.

Psychosocial Factors

The woman's general appearance and behavior (and that of her partner) provide valuable clues to the type of supportive care she will need. However, the nurse should keep in mind that general appearance and behavior may vary depending on the stage and phase of labor. Psychosocial factors to assess include the following:

Verbal interactions. Does the woman ask questions? Can she ask for what she needs? Does she talk to her support person(s)? Does she talk freely with the nurse or respond only to questions?

Body language. Is she relaxed or tense? What is her anxiety level? How does she react to being touched by the nurse or support person? Does she change positions or lie rigidly still? Does she avoid eye contact? Does she look tired? How much rest has she had during the past day?

Perceptual ability. Does she understand what the nurse says? Is there a language barrier? Are repeated explanations necessary because her anxiety level interferes with her ability to comprehend? Can she repeat what she has been told or demonstrate her understanding?

Discomfort level. To what degree does the woman describe what she is experiencing? How does she react to a contraction? Are any nonverbal pain messages seen? Does she complain to the nurse or her partner? Can she ask for comfort measures?

Women with a history of sexual abuse. Memories of sexual abuse can be triggered during labor by intrusive pro-

cedures such as vaginal examinations; loss of control; being confined to bed and "restrained" by monitors, intravenous (IV) lines, and epidurals; being watched by students; and experiencing intense sensations in the uterus and genital area, especially at the time when she must push the baby out. Women who are abuse survivors may fight the labor process by reacting in panic or anger toward care providers, may take control of every one and everything related to their childbirth, may surrender by being submissive and dependent, or may retreat by mentally dissociating themselves from the sensations of labor and birth (Rhodes & Hutchinson, 1994).

The nurse can help these women to associate the sensations they are experiencing with the process of childbirth and not their past abuse. The woman's sense of control should be maintained by explaining all procedures and why they are needed, validating her needs and paying close attention to her requests, proceeding at the woman's pace by waiting for her to give permission to touch her, accepting her often extreme reactions to labor, and protecting her privacy by limiting the amount of exposure of her body and the number of persons involved in her care. It is recommended that all laboring women be cared for in this manner, because it is not unusual for a woman to choose not to reveal a history of sexual abuse. These care measures can help a woman to perceive her childbirth experience in positive terms and to effectively parent her new baby (Heritage, 1998; Waymire, 1997).

Stress in Labor

The way in which women and their support person or family members approach labor is related to the manner in which they have been socialized to the childbearing process. Their reactions reflect their life experiences regarding childbirth—physical, social, cultural, and religious. Society communicates its expectations regarding acceptable and unacceptable maternal behaviors during labor and birth. These expectations may be used by some women as the basis for evaluating their own actions during childbirth. An idealized perception of labor and birth may be a source of guilt and a sense of failure if the woman finds the process less than joyous, especially when the pregnancy is unplanned or is the product of a shaky or terminated relationship. Often women have heard horror stories or have seen friends or relatives going through labors that appear anything but easy. Multiparous women will often base their expectations of the present labor on their previous childbirth experiences (Mackey, 1990).

High expectations for childbirth often result in greater satisfaction and a greater sense of fulfillment with the childbirth experience. On the other hand, women who have lower expectations often have less positive perceptions of their childbirth experience (Nichols, 1996).

Usually women in labor have a variety of concerns that they will voice if asked but rarely volunteer. To clear up misinformation, it is important for the nurse to ask the woman what she expects or to suggest that the woman ask her primary health care provider about an issue. The following are common concerns that women in labor have: Will my baby be all right? Will I be able to stand labor? Will my labor be long? How will I act? Will I need medication? Will it work for me? Will my partner or someone be there to support me? Do I have to have an IV?

The nurse's responsibility to the woman in labor with regard to these concerns is to answer her questions or find out the answers, to provide support for her and her support person or family, to consider the woman and her significant others as partners in the care process, and to serve as their advocate. According to McKay and Smith (1993), women equate emotional support with information giving. Nurses are perceived as supportive when they explain things in detail using positive terms and provide accurate information and specific directions. Women feel empowered when they are given information they can understand and that shows support for their efforts. This feeling of empowerment gives women the sense that they have the freedom to participate fully in their labor and birth and fosters a positive perception of the experience. In contrast, a woman's level of anxiety and fear may rise when she does not understand what is being said. The woman who is unfamiliar with expressions such as "bloody show," "the membranes ruptured," "scalp electrode," and "baby's lying on the cord" could understandably panic. Many such expressions sound violent and could conjure up thoughts of injury or pain.

The woman should understand that she is not expected to act in any particular way and that the process will yield the birth of her baby, which is the only expectation she should have. Women need to be able to behave in a manner that is natural for them and be able to "let go" (Waldenström et al., 1996). The woman's views and expectations regarding the nurse's role as caregiver should be determined. The nurse-client relationship will become increasingly important as labor progresses (Bryanton, Fraser-Davey, & Sullivan, 1994).

Women prepare themselves for labor in a variety of ways. Some go to childbirth education classes, some read books and talk to friends and relatives about childbirth, and some prepare elaborate birth plans spelling out their wishes for labor and birth. The longer the list of "wishes," however, the greater the likelihood that expectations will not be met. It is the nurse's responsibility to integrate the woman's desires into the plan of care as much as possible. The nurse can help make sure various aspects of the birth plan are observed by reviewing the plan with the physician or midwife and telling the woman to remind her primary health provider about what she wants in advance.

The father, coach, or significant other also experiences stress during labor. The nurse can assist and support these people by identifying their needs and expectations and by helping make sure they are met. The nurse can ascertain what role the support person intends to fulfill and whether he or she is prepared for that role by making observations and asking such questions as, Has the couple attended childbirth classes? What role does this person expect to play? Does he or she do all the talking? Is he or she nervous, anxious, aggressive, or hostile? Does he or she look hungry, tired, worried, or confused? Does he or she watch television, sleep, or stay out of the room instead of paying attention to the woman? Where does he or she sit? Does he or she touch the woman; what is the character of the touch? The nurse should be sensitive to the needs of support people and provide teaching and support as appropriate. Often the support this person is able to give the laboring woman is in direct proportion to the support he or she receives from the nurses and other health care providers (Nichols, 1993).

Cultural Factors

It is important to note the woman's ethnic or cultural and religious background to anticipate nursing interventions that may need to be added or eliminated from the individualized plan of care. Leininger (1991) describes two types of caregiving: generic care (caring), which involves behaviors and practices that are based on knowledge and skills transmitted through the person's culture; and professional nursing care (caring), which involves behaviors and practices that are based on knowledge and skills learned and transmitted during the education of a professional nurse. When managing the care of a laboring woman, the nurse should use an approach that blends generic and professional caregiving in order to foster the well-being of the woman and her significant others, to avert cultural conflict and stress, and to reduce anxiety and promote relaxation. Finn (1994) found that nurses do integrate generic and professional caregiving. She also identified generic and professional caring behaviors and practices that laboring women expected from their nurses. These behaviors included providing care that makes one feel protected and good (familiar, comfortable, "at home"), becoming emotionally involved and giving encouragement, being present and standing by her, using touch, involving her chosen partner (lay caregiver) in the provision of care, and explaining events and equipment. The woman should be encouraged to request specific generic caregiving behaviors and practices that are important to her. If a special request contradicts usual practices in that setting, the woman or the nurse can ask the woman's primary health care provider to write an order to accommodate the special request. For example, in many cultures having a male caregiver examine a pregnant woman is unacceptable. In some cultures it is traditional to take the placenta home; in others the woman is given only certain nourishments during labor. Some women believe that cutting her body, as with an episiotomy, allows her spirit to leave her body and that rupturing the membranes prolongs, not shortens, labor (D'Avanzo, 1992) (see Cultural Consideration box).

Cultural beliefs and values can influence a woman's reliance on her primary health care provider during labor and

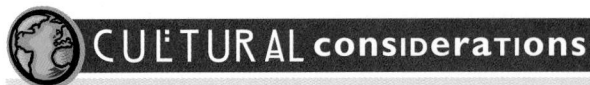

CULTURAL consiDerations

Birth Practices in Different Cultures

SOUTH KOREA
Stoic response to labor pain; fathers usually not present.

JAPAN
Natural childbirth methods practiced; may labor silently; may eat during labor; father may be present.

CHINA
Stoic response to pain; fathers usually not present; side-lying position preferred for labor and birth, because this position is thought to reduce infant trauma.

INDIA
Natural childbirth methods preferred; father is usually not present; female relatives usually present.

IRAN
Father not present; prefers female support and female caregivers.

MEXICO
May be stoic about discomfort until second stage, then may request pain relief; fathers and female relatives may be present.

LAOS
May use squatting position for birth; fathers may or may not be present; prefer female attendants.

From Geissler, E. (1994). *Pocket guide to cultural assessment.* St. Louis: Mosby.

her desire to participate in making decisions about the care she receives (Callister, Vehvilainen-Julkunen, & Lauri, 1996).

When a nurse is assessing a woman's cultural and religious preferences, Callister (1995) suggests asking questions regarding the following:
- The value and meaning placed on the childbirth experience
- The view of childbirth as a wellness or illness experience and as a private or social event
- The practices regarding diet, medications, activity, and emotional and physical support
- The appropriate maternal and paternal behaviors
- The birth companions—who they should be and what they should do
- The views regarding the newborn and the newborn's care immediately after birth

Within cultures women may have the "right" way to behave in labor instilled in them and to react to the pain experienced in that way. These behaviors can range from total silence to moaning or screaming, but they are not in and of themselves a gauge of the degree of pain. A woman who moans with contractions may not be in as much physical pain as a woman who is silent but winces during contractions (Table 22-1). Some women feel it is shameful to scream or cry out in pain if a man is present (D'Avanzo, 1992). If the woman's support person is her mother, she may perceive the need to "behave" more strongly than if her support person is the father of the baby. She will perceive herself as failing or succeeding on the basis of her ability to adhere to these "standards" of behavior. Conversely, a woman's behavior in response to pain may influence the support received from significant others. In some cultures women who lose control and cry out in pain may be scolded, whereas in other cultures support persons will become more helpful (Choudhry, 1997; Weber, 1996).

The non–English-speaking woman in labor. A woman's level of anxiety in labor rises when she does not understand what is happening to her or what is being said (McKay & Smith, 1993). Some misunderstanding may occur with English-speaking women and cause some stress, but the effect of misunderstanding on non–English-speaking women is much more dramatic because they often feel a complete loss of control over their situation if there is no health care provider present who speaks her language. They can panic and withdraw or become physically abusive when someone tries to do something they perceive might harm them or their babies. Sometimes a support person is able to serve as a translator. However, this must be done with caution because the translator may not be able to convey exactly what the nurse or others are saying or what the woman is saying and raise the woman's stress level even more.

Ideally, a bilingual nurse will care for the woman. Alternatively, an employee or volunteer translator may be contacted for assistance. If no one in the hospital is able to translate, a translation service can be called so that a translation can take place over the telephone. For some women, a female translator may be more acceptable. If no translator is available, the labor and birth unit staff can prepare a set of cards with graphic depictions that illustrate common situations that can be used to communicate with non–English-speaking women. Even when the nurse has limited ability to communicate verbally with the woman, in most instances the nurse's efforts to communicate are meaningful and appreciated by the woman (see Guidelines/Guías box).

Physical Examination
During the screening/triage process, a quick vaginal examination may be done to rule out imminent birth before proceeding with an initial examination to confirm the onset of true labor. The findings serve as a baseline for assessing the woman's progress from that point. The initial physical examination includes a general systems assessment; performance of Leopold's maneuvers to determine fetal presentation and position and the point of maximum intensity (PMI) for auscultating the FHR; assessment of

TABLE 22-1 Sociocultural Basis of Pain Experience

WOMAN IN LABOR	NURSE
PERCEPTION OF MEANING	
Origin: Cultural concept of and personal experience with pain; for example: Pain in childbirth is inevitable, something to be endured. Pain in childbirth can be avoided completely. Pain in childbirth is punishment for sin. Pain in childbirth can be controlled.	Origin: Cultural concept of and personal experience with pain; in addition, nurse becomes accustomed to working with certain "expected" pain trajectories. For example, in obstetrics, pain is expected to increase as labor progresses, be intermittent, and have an end point; relief can be derived from medications once labor is well established and fetus or newborn can cope with amount and elimination of medications; relief can also come from woman's knowledge, attitude, and support from family or friends.
COPING MECHANISMS	
Woman may exhibit the following behaviors: Be traditionally vocal or nonvocal; crying out or groaning, or both, may be part of her ritual response to pain. Use counterstimulation to minimize pain (e.g., rubbing, applying heat, or applying counterpressure). Use relaxation, distraction, or autosuggestion as pain-countering techniques. Resist any use of "needles" as modes of administering pain relief agents.	Nurse may respond by Using self effectively (e.g., using tone of voice, closeness in space, and touch as media for conveying message of interest and caring). Using avoidance, belittling, or other distracting actions as protective device for self. Using pharmacologic resources at hand judiciously. Using comfort measures. Assuming accountability for control and management of pain.
EXPECTATIONS OF OTHERS	
Nurse may be seen as someone who will accept woman's statement of pain and act as her advocate. Medical personnel may be expected to relieve woman of all pain sensations. Nurse may be expected to be interested, gentle, kind, and accepting of behavior exhibited.	Only certain verbal or nonverbal responses to pain may be accepted as appropriate responses. Couple that is prepared for childbirth may be expected to refuse medication and to wish to "do everything on their own." Woman's definition of pain may not be accepted; that is, woman may wish to experience and participate in controlling pain or may not be able to accept any pain as reasonable.

GUIDELINES/GUÍAS

Labor Assessment

What time did the contractions begin?
¿A qué hora le empezaron las contracciones?

How far apart are the contractions?
¿Con qué frecuencia tiene las contracciones?

Have the membranes ruptured? When?
¿Se le rompió la fuente? ¿Cuándo?

What color was the fluid? Red? Pink?
¿Qué color tenía el líquido? ¿Rojo? ¿Rosado?

Have you had bleeding?
¿Ha sangrado?

How much? A cupful? A tablespoonful? A teaspoonful?
¿Cuánto? ¿Una taza? ¿Una cucharada? ¿Una cucharadita?

When was the last time you ate or drank anything?
¿Cuándo fue la última vez que comió o bebió algo?

Have you had any problems with this pregnancy?
¿Ha tenido algún problema con este embarazo?

Are you taking any medications?
¿Está tomando alguna medicación?

Are you allergic to penicillin or other medicines?
¿Es alérgica a la penicilina u otras medicinas?

Please sign this consent form.
Por favor, firme esta forma de consentimiento.

▪ TABLE 22-2 Expected Maternal Progress in First Stage of Labor

PHASES MARKED BY CERVICAL DILATION*

CRITERION	0-3 CM (LATENT)	4-7 CM (ACTIVE)	8-10 CM (TRANSITION)
Duration†	About 6-8 hr	About 3-6 hr	About 20-40 min
Contractions			
Strength	Mild to moderate	Moderate to strong	Strong to very strong
Rhythm	Irregular	More regular	Regular
Frequency	5-30 min apart	3-5 min apart	2-3 min apart
Duration	30-45 sec	40-70 sec	45-90 sec
Descent			
Station of	Nulliparous: 0	Varies: +1 to +2 cm	Varies: +2 to +3 cm
presenting part	Multiparous: 0 to −2 cm	Varies: +1 to +2 cm	Varies: +2 to +3 cm
Show			
Color	Brownish discharge, mucous plug, or pale pink mucus	Pink to bloody mucus	Bloody mucus
Amount	Scant	Scant to moderate	Copious
Behavior and appearance‡	Excited; thoughts center on self, labor, and baby; may be talkative or silent, calm or tense; some apprehension; pain controlled fairly well; alert, follows directions readily; open to instructions	Becomes more serious, doubtful of control of pain, more apprehensive; desires companionship and encouragement; attention more inner directed; fatigue evidenced; malar (cheeks) flush; has some difficulty following directions	Pain described as severe; backache common; frustration, fear of loss of control, and irritability surface; vague in communications; amnesia between contractions; writhing with contractions; nausea and vomiting, especially if hyperventilating; hyperesthesia; circumoral pallor, perspiration of forehead and upper lips; shaking tremor of thighs; feeling of need to defecate, pressure on anus

*In the nullipara, effacement is often complete before dilation begins; in the multipara, it occurs simultaneously with dilation. Average total duration: nullipara–10 to 16 hr; multipara–6 to 10 hr.

†Duration of each phase is influenced by such factors as parity, maternal position, and level of activity. For example, the labor of a nullipara tends to last longer, on average, than the labor of a multipara. Women who ambulate and assume upright positions or change positions frequently during labor tend to experience a shorter first stage.

‡Women who have epidural analgesia for pain relief may not demonstrate these behaviors.

fetal status; assessment of uterine contractions; and vaginal examination to assess the status of cervical effacement and dilation, fetal descent, and amniotic membranes and fluid. The most vital aspect of the assessment is the determination of fetal status.

Women often focus on the nature of their contractions as the clearest indicator of how far advanced their labor is. However, the findings from the vaginal examination are more valid indicators of the phase of labor, especially for nulliparous women. Rupture of the membranes significantly affects the woman's plan of care because, once this occurs, the membranes can no longer protect the intrauterine cavity and fetus from infectious organisms that can travel up the birth canal. The risk of umbilical cord prolapse exists once the membranes have ruptured. Because of the bearing such information has on the care rendered, it is important to obtain as many related pieces of information as possible before planning and implementing care.

The information yielded by a complete and accurate assessment during screening serves as the basis for determin-

ing whether the woman should be admitted and what her ongoing care should be. Expected maternal progress and minimum assessment guidelines during the first stage of labor are presented in Table 22-2 and the Care Path.

The assessment procedures described in the following paragraphs can be used as a basis for teaching women and their families. The equipment needed, the nursing actions involved, and the rationale for each procedure can be shared with the woman. The nurse should thoroughly wash her hands before performing any of these procedures. Handwashing is also important after the examinations are completed. Standard Precautions should guide all assessment and care measures. The assessment findings are explained to the woman whenever possible. Throughout labor, accurate documentation is done as soon as possible after a procedure has been performed. This involves the careful noting of the findings and the time the procedure was performed on both the chart and the fetal monitoring strip, which the nurse then initials (Fig. 22-3).

Text continued on p. 528

CARE MANAGEMENT	CERVICAL DILATION		
	0-3 CM (LATENT)	**4-7 CM (ACTIVE)**	**8-10 CM (TRANSITION)**
I. ASSESSMENT MEASURES*	**Frequency**	**Frequency**	**Frequency**
• Blood pressure, pulse, respirations	Every 30-60 min	Every 30 min	Every 15-30 min
• Temperature†	Every 4 hr	Every 4 hr	Every 4 hr
• Uterine activity	Every 30-60 min	Every 15-30 min	Every 10-15 min
• Fetal heart rate (FHR)	Every 30-60 min	Every 15-30 min	Every 15-30 min
• Vaginal show	Every 30-60 min	Every 30 min	Every 15 min
• Behavior, appearance, mood, energy level of woman; condition of partner	Every 30 min	Every 15 min	Every 5 min
• Vaginal examination‡	As needed to identify progress	As needed to identify progress	As needed to identify progress
II. PHYSICAL CARE MEASURES§	Stay at home for as long as possible Relaxation measures; rest and sleep if at night Activity—ambulation; emphasize upright positions Diversional activities Nourishment—light foods and full liquids Void every 2 hr Perform basic hygiene measures	Coach breathing techniques Encourage effleurage Assist in using relaxation techniques between contractions Encourage ambulation, upright positions Assist with position changes Use comfort measures desired by woman: massage, hot/cold packs, touch, etc. Initiate hydrotherapy (shower, bath, Jacuzzi) Provide nourishment as desired Encourage voiding every 2 hr Assist with hygiene, perineal care Provide pharmacologic pain relief as indicated Provide relief for partner	Coach breathing techniques Reduce touch if increased sensitivity is noted Help to relax between contractions Assist with position changes Use comfort measures according to acceptance level Continue hydrotherapy if effective Provide clear liquids: sips, ice chips Encourage voiding every 2 hr Provide hygiene measures, emphasizing mouth and perineal care Provide pharmacologic pain relief as indicated Prepare for birth
III. EMOTIONAL SUPPORT	Review birth plan Review process of labor—what to expect, pain management techniques available Redemonstrate breathing techniques Keep informed: progress, procedures	Provide feedback about performance Reduce distractions during contractions Role model comfort measures Reassure, encourage, praise Take charge, talk through contraction until control regained Continue to keep informed	Provide continuous support Reduce distractions Role model care measures to assist partner Continue reassurance, praise, and encouragement Keep informed Take charge as needed

*Full assessment using interview, physical examination, and laboratory testing is performed on admission. Subsequently, frequency of assessment is determined by the risk status of the maternal-fetal unit. More frequent assessment is required in high risk situations. Frequency of assessment and method of documentation are also determined by agency policy, which is usually based on the recommended care standards of medical and nursing organizations.

†If membranes have ruptured, the temperature should be assessed every 1 to 2 hr; assess orally or tympanically between contractions.

‡Perform vaginal examination at admission and thereafter only when signs indicate that progress has occurred (e.g., significant increase in frequency, duration, and intensity of contractions; rupture of membranes; perineal pressure); strict aseptic technique should be used. In the presence of vaginal bleeding, the primary health care provider performs the examination under a double setup in a delivery room, or an ultrasonography is performed to determine placental location.

§Physical care measures are performed by the nurse working together with the woman's partner and significant others. The woman is capable of greater independence in the latent phase but needs more assistance during the active and transition phases.

Labor Progress Chart

Admit date __/__/__	Admit time	Blood type and Rh	Age	G	T	P	A	L	EDB __/__/__ LMP __/__/__	Membranes ☐ **Intact** ☐ Ruptured SROM AROM ☐ Bulging Date __/__/__ Time ____

Current date __/__/__	Time →																		
Vital signs	Temperature																		
Vital signs	Pulse																		
Vital signs	Respiration																		
Vital signs	Blood pressure																		
Vital signs																			
Maternal	Deep tendon reflexes (L/R)	/	/	/	/	/	/	/	/	/	/	/	/	/	/	/	/	/	/
Maternal	Urine (Protein/sugar)	/	/	/	/	/	/	/	/	/	/	/	/	/	/	/	/	/	/
Maternal	Vaginal bleeding																		
Maternal																			
Uterine activity	Monitor mode																		
Uterine activity	Frequency																		
Uterine activity	Duration																		
Uterine activity	Intensity																		
Uterine activity	Resting tone																		
Uterine activity	Peak IUP																		
Uterine activity	MVUs																		
Uterine activity																			
Fetal Assessment	Monitor mode																		
Fetal Assessment	Baseline (FHR)																		
Fetal Assessment	STV																		
Fetal Assessment	LTV																		
Fetal Assessment	Accelerations																		
Fetal Assessment	Decelerations																		
Fetal Assessment	Strip number																		
Fetal Assessment	Membranes																		
Fetal Assessment	Fluid																		
Fetal Assessment																			
Intake/Output (cc's/Hr)	IV																		
Intake/Output (cc's/Hr)	PO																		
Intake/Output (cc's/Hr)	Urine																		
Intake/Output (cc's/Hr)	Emesis																		
Cont meds	Pitocin mU/min																		
Cont meds	$MgSO_4$ gms/hr																		
Cont meds	Ritodrine mg/min																		
Cont meds	Terbutaline mg/hr																		
Cont meds																			
Intervention	Position change																		
Intervention	O_2 L/min																		
Intervention	IV bolus																		
Initials																			

Abbreviations/Key	Vaginal bleeding	Monitor mode uterine activity	MVUs montevideo units	Monitor mode fetal	STV short term variability
	NS = Normal show ABN = Frank vaginal Bleeding	P = Palpation E = External I = Internal	The sum of the peak of each uterine contraction minus resting tone, in a 10 minute period.	A = Auscultation (fetoscope) D = Doppler E = External I = Internal	STV + = Present (roughness of tracing line present) STV Ø = Absent (tracing line is smooth)

Fig. 22-3 Labor progress chart. *(Permission to use and/or reproduce this copyrighted material has been granted by the owner, Hollister, Inc., Libertyville, IL.)*

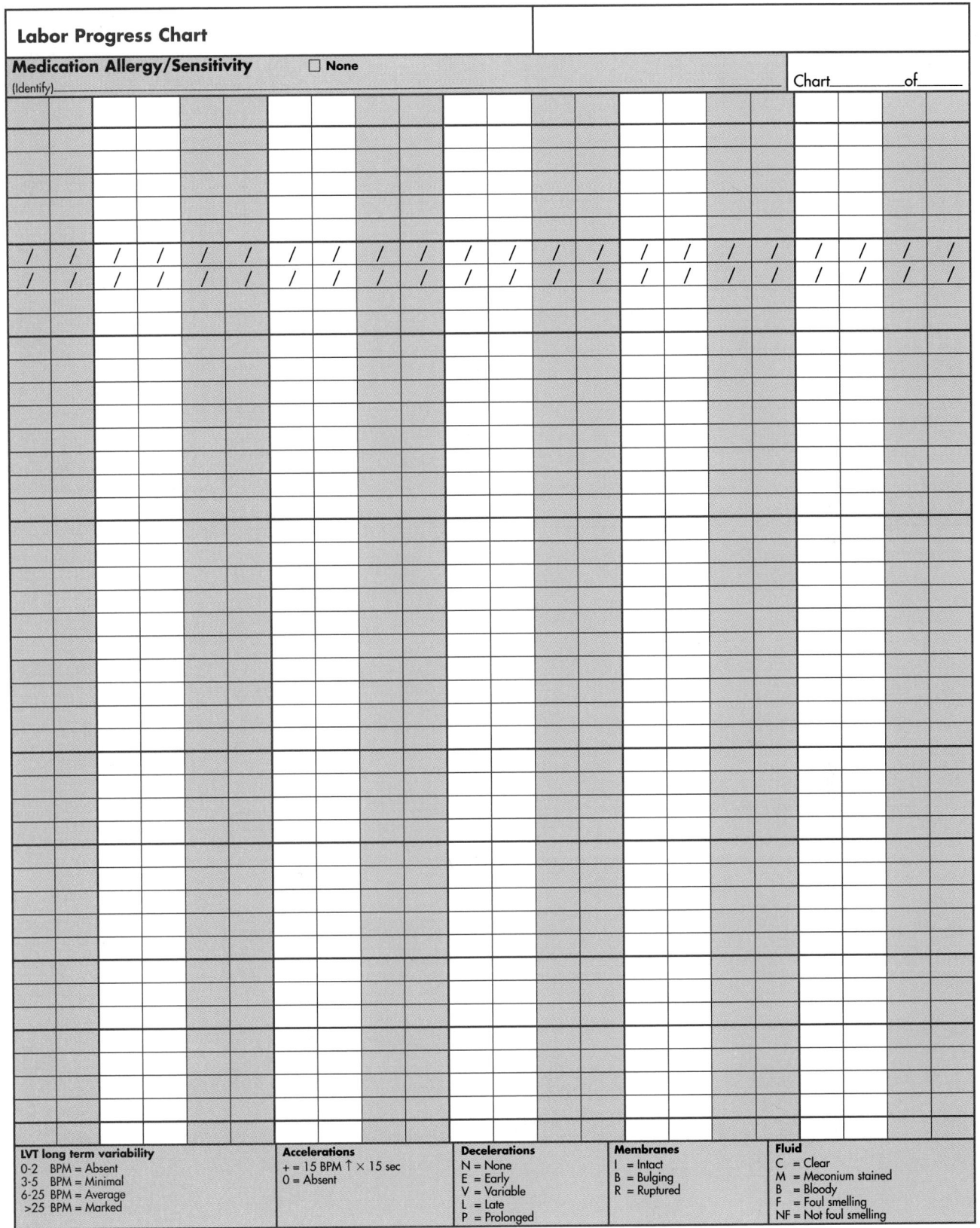

Labor Progress Chart

Medication Allergy/Sensitivity   ☐ **None**   Chart_____of_____
(Identify)

LVT long term variability
0-2   BPM = Absent
3-5   BPM = Minimal
6-25 BPM = Average
>25   BPM = Marked

Accelerations
+ = 15 BPM ↑ × 15 sec
0 = Absent

Decelerations
N = None
E = Early
V = Variable
L = Late
P = Prolonged

Membranes
I = Intact
B = Bulging
R = Ruptured

Fluid
C = Clear
M = Meconium stained
B = Bloody
F = Foul smelling
NF = Not foul smelling

Fig. 22-3, cont'd   For legend see opposite page.

Labor Progress Chart

Time →																												
Mark X • 10																												

Station: -4, -3, -2, -1, 0, +1, +2, +3
Dilatation: 10, 9, 8, 7, 6, 5, 4, 3, 2

Effacement % and/or position

Examined by:

IV Record

Start date	Time	Solution	Amount (cc's)	Medication/Dose added	Initials	Infused date	Time	Amount infused

Teaching

Topic	Date time	Comments
Oriented		
Labor review		
Support person		
Pre-Op		
Safety		

Interval Medications

Date time	Medication/Dose	Route	Site	Initials	Initials	Signature

Progress Notes

Date	Time	

Fig. 22-3, cont'd   For legend see p. 524.

Labor Progress Chart

Progress Notes (Cont'd.)

Date	Time	

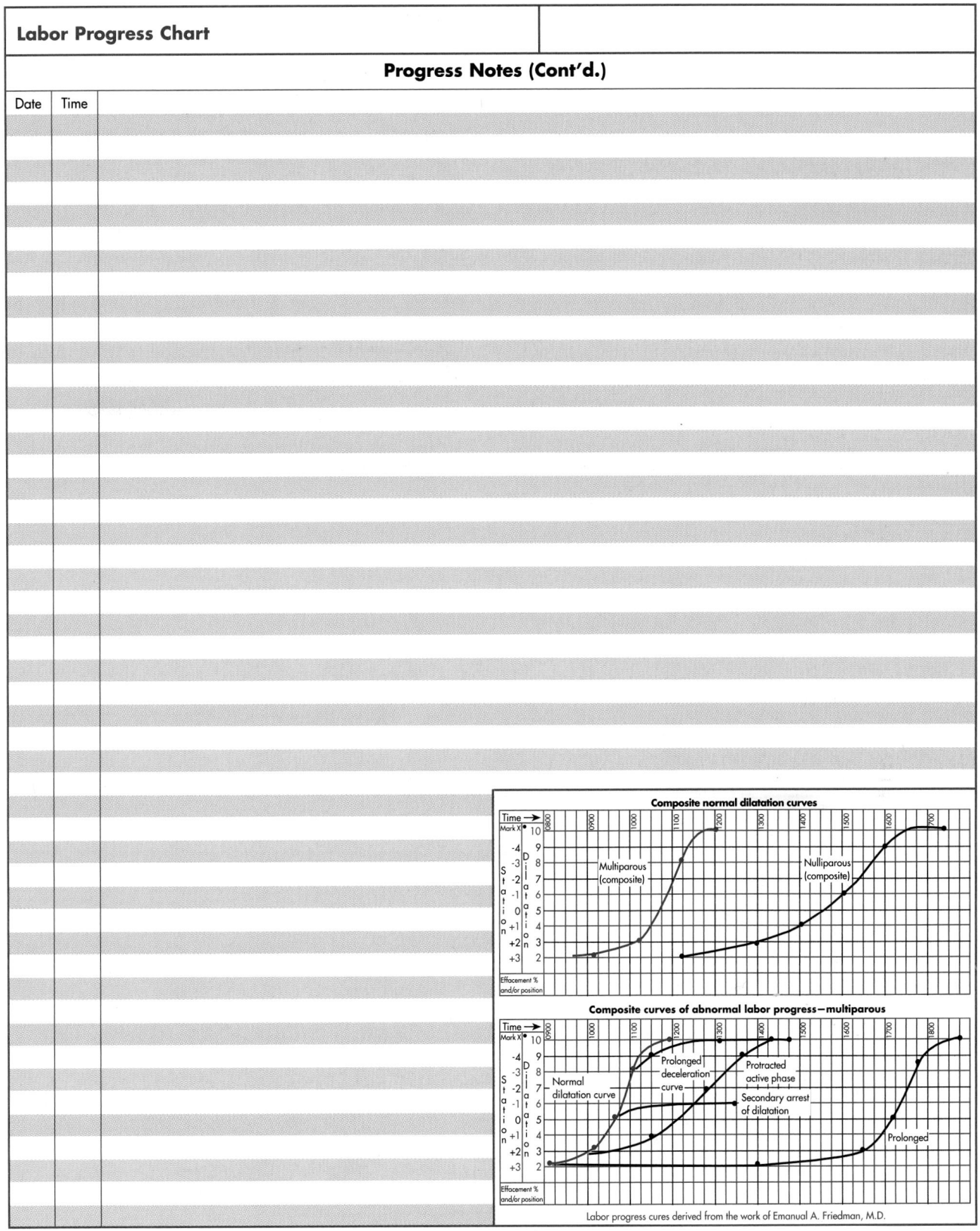

Fig. 22-3, cont'd   For legend see p. 524.

General systems assessment. A brief systems assessment is performed. This includes an assessment of the heart, lungs, and skin; an examination to determine the presence and extent of edema of the legs, face, hands, or sacrum; and testing of deep tendon reflexes and for clonus.

Vital signs (TPR and blood pressure) are assessed on admission, and the initial values are used as the baseline for comparison with subsequent values. If the blood pressure is elevated, it should be reassessed 30 minutes later, between contractions, using a correct-size blood pressure cuff to obtain a reading after the woman has relaxed. To prevent supine hypotension and fetal distress, the woman should be encouraged to lie on her side and not supine (Fig. 22-4). Her temperature is monitored so that infection or a fluid deficit (dehydration associated with inadequate intake of fluids) can be identified. The woman's intake and output should be measured at least every 8 hours. The urinary protein and the ketone levels of each voided specimen should be determined using a dipstick.

Leopold's maneuvers (abdominal palpation). **Leopold's maneuvers** are performed with the woman lying on her back for a brief period (see Procedure box and Fig. 22-5). These maneuvers help identify (1) the number of fetuses; (2) the presenting part, the fetal lie, and the fetal attitude; (3) the degree of the presenting part's descent into the pelvis; and (4) the expected location of the PMI of the FHR on the woman's abdomen.

Assessment of FHR and pattern. It is important for the nurse to understand the relationship between the location of the PMI of the FHR and fetal presentation, lie, and position. A high risk for childbirth complications may be revealed by variations in these findings. The PMI of the FHR is the location on the maternal abdomen where the FHR is heard the loudest. It is usually directly over the fetal back. The PMI is also an aid in determining the fetal presentation and position (Fig. 22-6). In a vertex presentation the FHR is heard below the mother's umbilicus in either the right or left lower quadrant of the abdomen. In a breech presentation the FHR is heard above the mother's

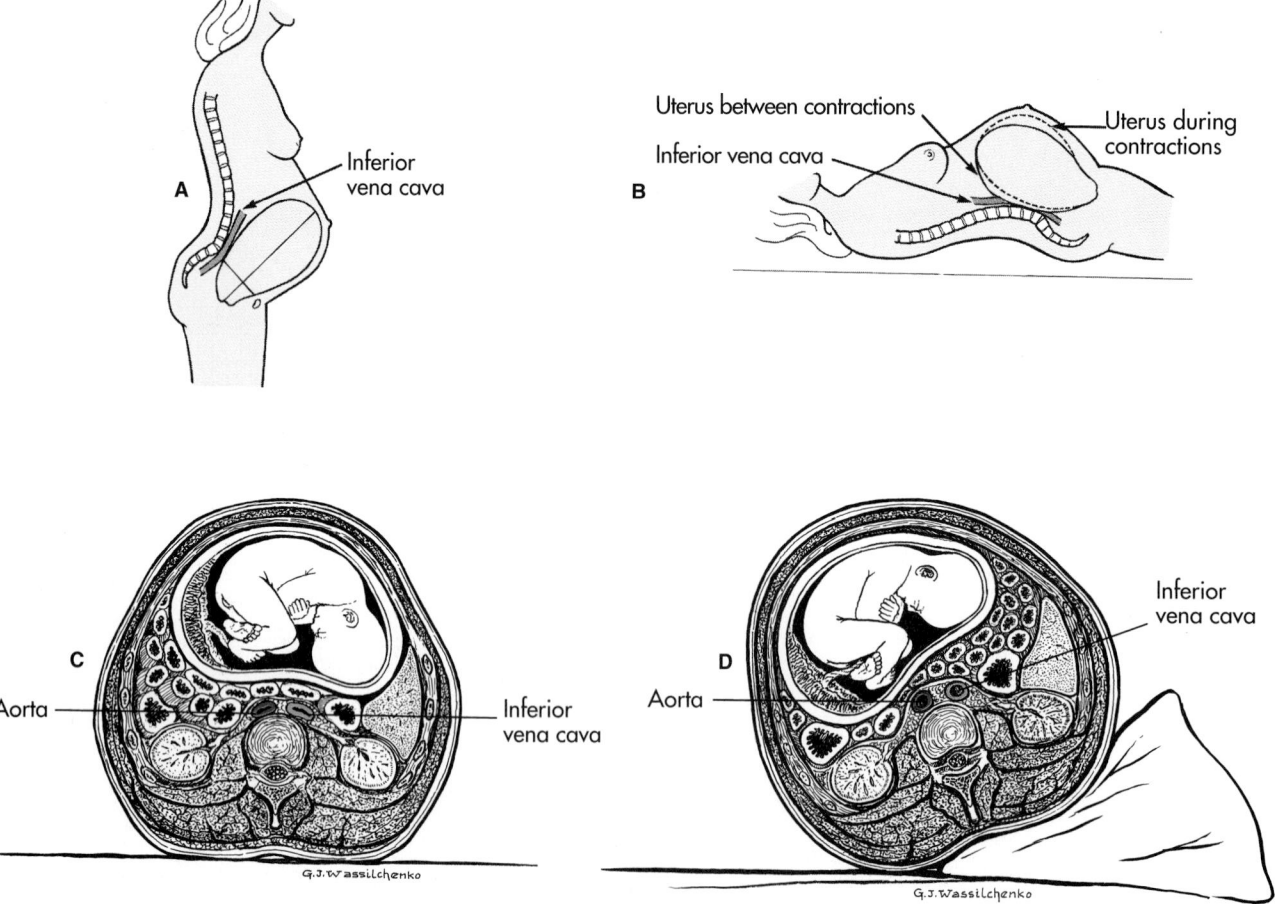

Fig. 22-4 Supine hypotension. Note relationship of pregnant uterus to ascending vena cava in **A,** standing position, and **B,** supine position. **C,** Compression of aorta and inferior vena cava with woman in supine position. **D,** Compression of these vessels is relieved by placement of a wedge pillow under the woman's right or left hip.

PROCEDURE

Leopold's Maneuvers and Determination of the Points of Maximum Intensity of the FHR

LEOPOLD'S MANEUVERS

Wash hands.

Ask woman to empty bladder.

Position woman supine with one pillow under her head and with her knees slightly flexed.

Place small rolled towel under woman's right or left hip to displace uterus off major blood vessels (prevents supine hypotensive syndrome; see Fig. 22-4).

If right-handed, stand on woman's right, facing her:

1. Identify fetal part that occupies the fundus. The head feels round, firm, freely movable, and palpable by ballottement; the breech feels less regular and softer. This maneuver identifies fetal lie (longitudinal or transverse) and presentation (cephalic or breech) (Fig. 22-5, A).

2. Using palmar surface of one hand, locate and palpate the smooth convex contour of the fetal back and the irregularities that identify the small parts (feet, hands, elbows). This maneuver helps identify fetal presentation (Fig. 22-5, B).

3. With right hand, determine which fetal part is presenting over the inlet to the true pelvis. Gently grasp the lower pole of the uterus between the thumb and fingers, pressing in slightly (Fig. 22-5, C). If the head is presenting and not engaged, determine the attitude of the head (flexed or extended).

4. Turn to face the woman's feet. Using both hands, outline the fetal head (Fig. 22-5, D) with the palmar surface of the fingertips. When the presenting part has descended deeply, only a small portion of it may be outlined. Palpation of the cephalic prominence helps identify the attitude of the head. If the cephalic prominence is found on the same side as the small parts, this means that the head must be flexed and the vertex is presenting (Fig. 22-5, D). If the cephalic prominence is on the same side as the back, this indicates that the presenting head is extended and the face is presenting (Fig. 22-5, D).

Document fetal presentation, position, and lie and whether presenting part is flexed or extended, engaged, or free floating. Use hospital's protocol for documentation (e.g., "Vtx, LOA, floating").

DETERMINATION OF PMI OF FHR *fetal ♥ Rate*

Wash hands.

Perform Leopold's maneuvers.

Auscultate FHR based on fetal presentation identified with Leopold's maneuvers. The PMI is the location where the FHR is heard the loudest, usually over the fetal back (see Figs. 22-6 and 22-7).

Chart PMI of FHR using a two-line figure to indicate the four quadrants of the maternal abdomen, as follows: right upper quadrant (RUQ), left upper quadrant (LUQ), left lower quadrant (LLQ), and right lower quadrant (RLQ):

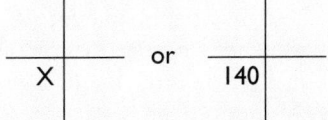

$$
\begin{array}{c|c}
\text{RUQ} & \text{LUQ} \\
\hline
\text{RLQ} & \text{LLQ}
\end{array}
$$

The umbilicus is the reference point for the quadrants (point where the lines cross). The PMI for the fetus in vertex presentation, in general flexion with the back on the mother's right side, commonly is found in the mother's right lower quadrant and is recorded with an "X" or with the FHR, as follows:

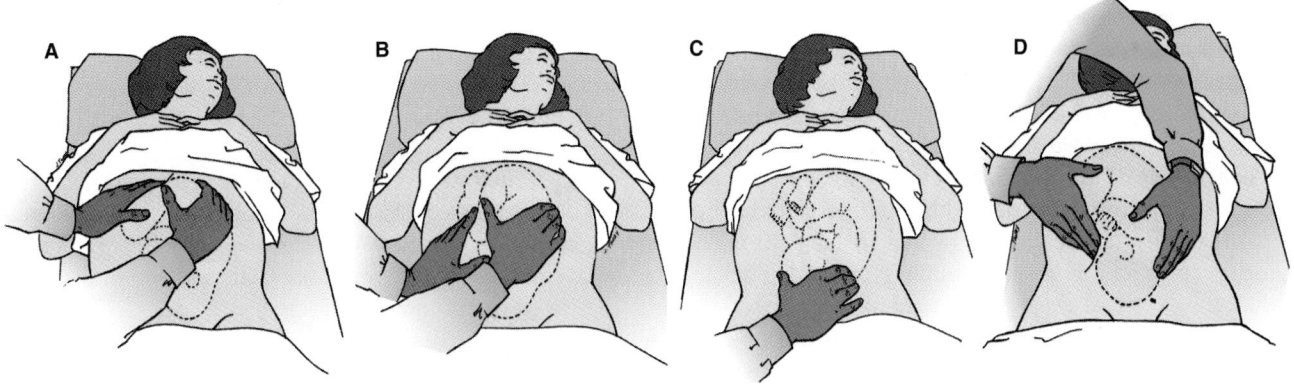

Fig. 22-5 Leopold's maneuvers.

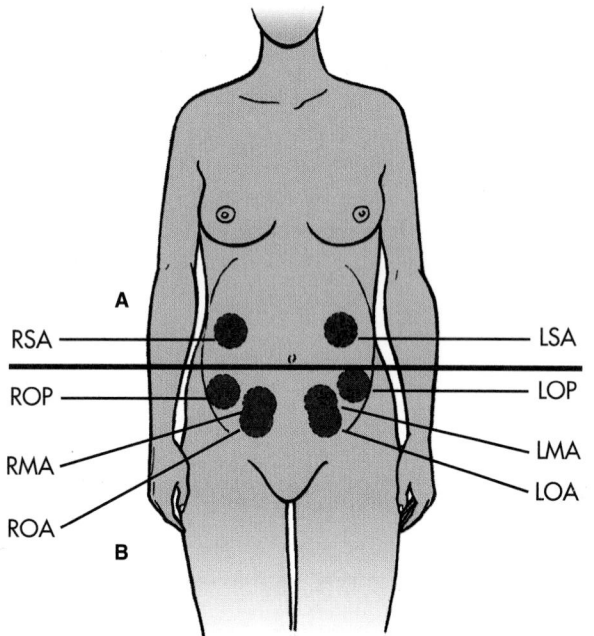

Fig. 22-6 Areas of maximum intensity of FHR for differing positions: *RSA,* right sacrum anterior; *ROP,* right occipitoposterior; *RMA,* right mentum anterior; *ROA,* right occipitoanterior; *LSA,* left sacrum anterior; *LOP,* left occipitoposterior; *LMA,* left mentum anterior; *LOA,* left occipitoanterior. **A,** Presentation is *breech* if FHR is heard *above* umbilicus. **B,** Presentation is *vertex* if FHR is heard *below* umbilicus.

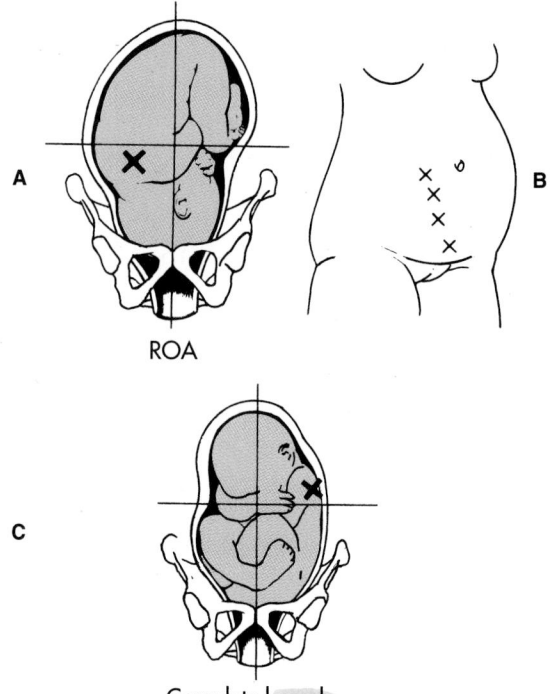

Lie: Vertical
Presentation: Breech (sacrum and feet presenting)
Reference point: Sacrum (with feet)
Attitude: General flexion

Fig. 22-7 Location of the FHR. **A,** With fetus in ROA position. **B,** Changes in location of PMI of FHR as fetus undergoes internal rotation from ROA to OA for birth. **C,** With fetus in left sacrum posterior position. *(A and C courtesy Ross Laboratories, Columbus, OH.)*

umbilicus (Fig. 22-6, *A,* and Fig. 22-7, *C*). As the fetus descends and rotates internally, the FHR is heard lower and closer to the midline of the maternal abdomen. The PMI of the fetus in the right occipitoanterior (ROA) position moves to the midline just over the symphysis pubis (Fig. 22-7, *A* and *B*). Just before birth the fetal position is occipitoanterior (OA) and the fetal back is directly above the symphysis pubis. Diagrams of the PMI for different presentations and positions are presented in Fig. 22-6. The aspects of the assessment recommended for determining fetal status in the low risk woman during each stage of labor are summarized in the Care Paths. The FHR also must be assessed (1) immediately after rupture of membranes (ROM), because this is the most common time for the umbilical cord to prolapse; (2) after any change in the contraction pattern or maternal status; and (3) before and after medicating the woman or performing a procedure.

Assessment of uterine contractions. A general characteristic of effective labor is regular uterine activity, but uterine activity is not directly related to labor progress. **Uterine contractions** are the primary powers that act involuntarily to expel the fetus and the placenta from the uterus. There are several ways of evaluating uterine contractions; these include the woman's subjective description of them, palpation and timing of the contraction by a health care provider, and electronic monitoring.

Each contraction exhibits a wavelike pattern. It begins with a slow increment (the "building up" of a contraction from its onset), gradually reaches an acme (the peak; intrauterine pressure of 50 to 75 mm Hg), and then diminishes rapidly (decrement, the "letting down" of the contraction). An interval of rest follows, during which the intrauterine pressure is 5 to 15 mm Hg; this ends when the next contraction begins. The outward appearance of the woman's abdomen during and between contractions and the pattern of a typical uterine contraction are shown in Fig. 22-8.

A uterine contraction is described in terms of the following characteristics:

- **Frequency of uterine contractions:** How often uterine contractions occur; the time that elapses from the beginning of one contraction to the beginning of the next or from the peak of one contraction to the peak of the next (if electronic monitoring)
- **Intensity of uterine contractions:** The strength of a contraction at its peak
- **Duration of uterine contractions:** The time that elapses between the onset and the end of a contraction

CARE MANAGEMENT	SECOND STAGE OF LABOR	THIRD STAGE OF LABOR
I. ASSESSMENT MEASURES*	**FREQUENCY**	**FREQUENCY**
• Blood pressure, pulse, respirations	Every 5-30 min	Every 15 min
• Uterine activity	Assess every contraction	Assess for placental separation
• Bearing-down effort	Assess each effort	
• Fetal heart rate (FHR)	Every 5-15 min	Perform Apgar at 1 and 5 min
• Vaginal show	Every 15 min	Assess bleeding until placental expulsion
• Signs of fetal descent: urge to bear down, perineal bulging, crowning	Every 10-15 min	
• Behavior, appearance, mood, energy level of woman; condition of partner	Every 10-15 min	Assess response to completion of childbirth process, reaction to newborn
II. PHYSICAL CARE MEASURES†	**Latent phase:** Assist to rest in position of comfort Encourage relaxation to conserve energy Promote urge to push; if delayed: ambulation, shower, pelvic rock, position changes **Descent phase:** Assist to bear down effectively Help to use recommended positions that facilitate descent Encourage correct breathing during bearing-down efforts Help to relax between contractions Provide comfort measures as needed Cleanse perineum immediately if fecal material is expelled **Transition phase:** Assist to pant during contraction to avoid rapid birth of head Coach to gently bear down between contractions	Assist to bear down to facilitate delivery of separated placenta Administer oxytocic as ordered Provide pain relief as needed Provide hygiene and comfort measures as needed
III. EMOTIONAL SUPPORT	Keep informed of progress of fetal descent Provide feedback for bearing-down efforts Explain purpose if medications given Role model comfort measures Provide continuous nursing presence Create a quiet, calm environment Reassure, encourage, praise Take charge as needed, until mother regains confidence in ability to birth her baby Offer mirror to watch birth	Keep informed about progress of placental separation Explain purpose if medications given Describe status of perineal tissue and inform if repair is needed Introduce parents to their baby Assess and care for newborn within view of parents; delay eye prophylaxis to facilitate eye contact Provide private time for family to bond with their new baby and help them to create memories Encourage breastfeeding if desired

*Frequency of assessment is determined by the risk status of the maternal-fetal unit. More frequent assessment is required in high risk situations. Frequency of assessment and method of documentation are also determined by agency policy, which is usually based on the recommended care standards of medical and nursing organizations.

†Physical care measures are performed by the nurse working together with the woman's partner and significant others.

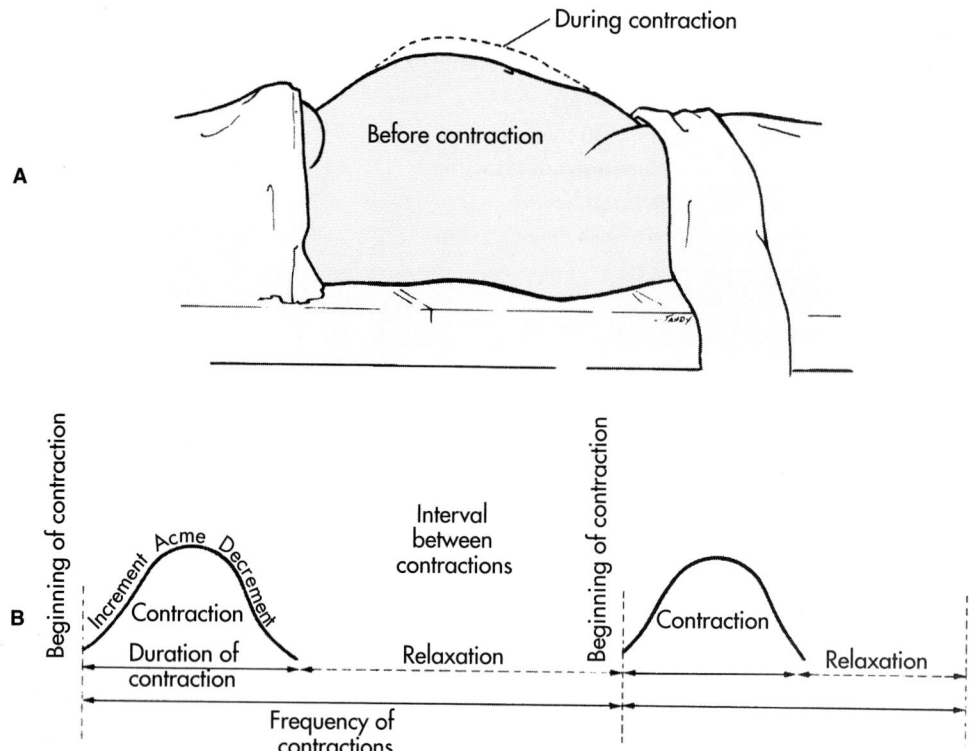

Fig. 22-8 Assessment of uterine contractions. **A,** Abdominal contour before and during uterine contraction. **B,** Wavelike pattern of contractile activity.

- **Resting tone of uterine contractions:** The tension in the uterine muscle between contractions

Uterine contractions are assessed by palpation or by an external or internal electronic monitor. Frequency and duration can be determined by all three methods of uterine activity monitoring. The accuracy of determining intensity varies by the method used. Palpation is more subjective and is a less precise way of determining the intensity of uterine contractions (Arrabal & Naegy, 1996). The following terms are used to describe what is felt on palpation:

- *Mild:* Slightly tense fundus that is easy to indent with fingertips (feels like touching finger to tip of nose)
- *Moderate:* Firm fundus that is difficult to indent with fingertips (feels like touching finger to chin)
- *Strong:* Rigid, boardlike fundus that is almost impossible to indent with fingertips (feels like touching finger to forehead)

Women in labor tend to describe the pain of contractions in terms of the sensations they are experiencing in the lower abdomen or back, which may be unrelated to the firmness of the uterine fundus. Thus their assessment of the strength of their contractions can be less valid than that of the health care provider, although the amount of discomfort reported is valid.

External electronic monitoring provides information about the relative strength of the uterine contractions. Internal electronic monitoring using an intrauterine pres-

sure catheter is the most reliable way of assessing the intensity of uterine contractions.

On the woman's admission, a 20- to 30-minute baseline monitoring of uterine contractions and the FHR usually is done (Scott et al., 1999). The minimum assessment times during the various phases of labor are given in the Care Paths, and the findings expected as labor progresses are summarized in Tables 22-2 and 22-5.

The nurse's responsibility in the monitoring of uterine contractions is to ascertain whether they are powerful and frequent enough to accomplish the work of expelling the fetus and the placenta.

NURSE ALERT *If the characteristics of contractions are found to be abnormal, either exceeding or falling below what is considered acceptable in terms of the standard characteristics, the nurse should report this to the primary health care provider.*

Cervical effacement, dilation, fetal descent. Uterine activity must be considered in the context of its effect on cervical effacement and dilation and on the degree of descent of the presenting part. The effect on the fetus also must be considered. The progress of labor can be effectively verified through the use of graphic charts (partograms) on which cervical dilation and station (descent) are plotted. This type of graphic charting helps identify early deviations from ex-

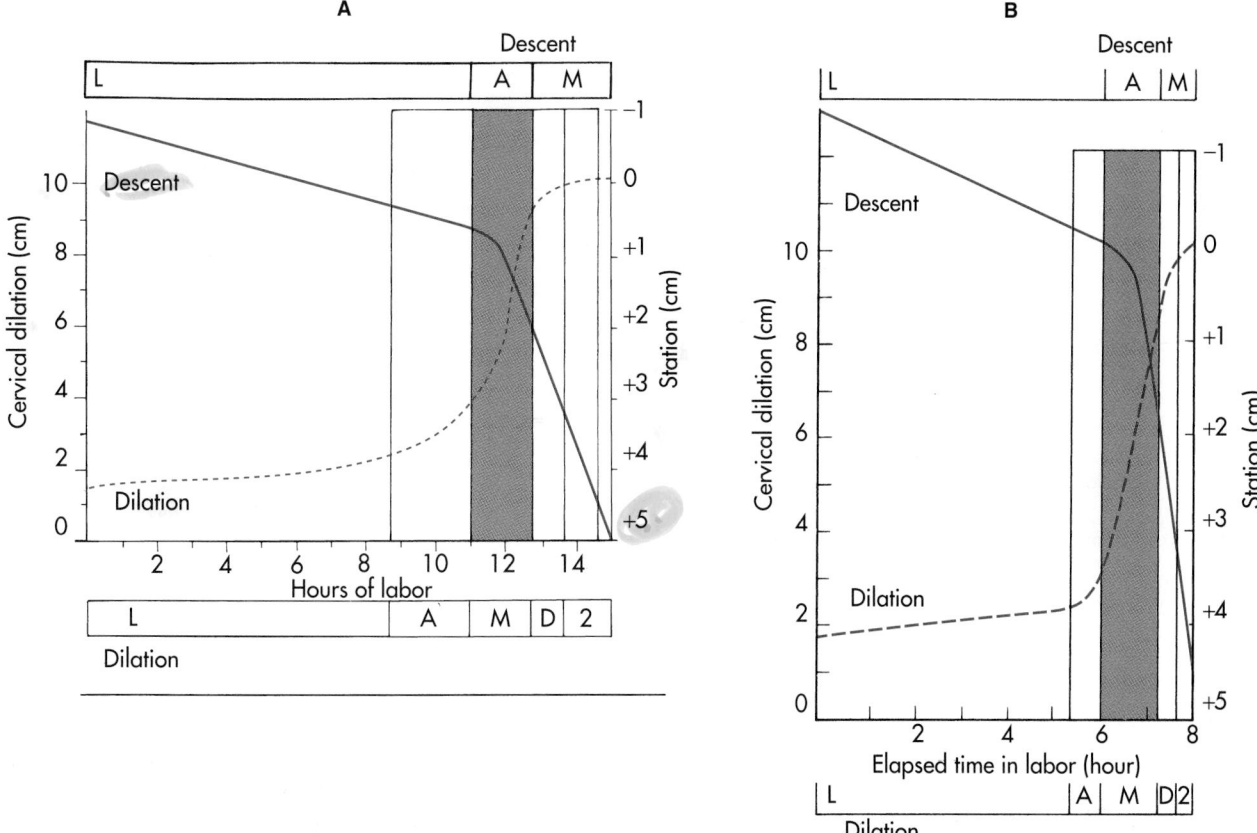

Fig. 22-9 Partograms showing relationship between cervical dilation and descent of presenting part. **A,** Labor of a nulliparous woman. **B,** Labor of a multiparous woman. The phases of cervical dilation are identified by the letters *L, A, M,* and *D.* The number *2* refers to the stage of labor. The latent phase *(L)* of the first stage of labor is the time between the onset of labor and the onset of acceleration. The active phase begins with the acceleration phase *(A)* and lasts from the onset of the upward curve of cervical dilation to the full dilation of the cervix. Freidman (1978) divides the active phase into three parts: (1) the acceleration phase *(A),* (2) the phase of maximum slope *(M),* and (3) the deceleration phase *(D).* The dotted line denotes cervical dilation. The phases of descent are identified by the letters *L, A,* and *M,* located at the top of the graph. *L* refers to the latent phase of minimum descent. Active descent *(A)* generally begins when the cervical dilation curve reaches its phase of maximum slope. The rate of descent reaches its maximum at the beginning of the deceleration phase of cervical dilation. Maximum descent *(M)* continues in a linear manner until the perineum is reached. The solid line shows the rate of descent.

pected labor patterns. Figure 22-9 shows the expected pattern of cervical dilation and descent for both nulliparous and multiparous women. Figure 22-10 provides one example of a partogram; however, hospitals and birthing centers may develop their own graphs for recording assessments. Such graphs may include not only data on dilation and descent but also on maternal vital signs, FHR, and uterine activity.

LEGAL TIP **Documentation**

Regardless of which charting format is used, complete documentation must include assessment findings, action(s) taken based on analysis of the findings, and response to the action(s) taken.

It is important for the nurse to recognize that active labor can actually last longer than the expected labor patterns. This finding should not be a cause for concern unless the maternal-fetal unit exhibits signs of distress (see Research box).

Cervical effacement. Effacement precedes significant cervical dilation in a first pregnancy and often accompanies dilation in subsequent pregnancies. The process of effacement plays a role in dilation. As the cervix is retracted upward, it becomes a part of the lower uterine segment. The "taking up" of the cervix reduces the length of the cervix from about 2 cm to a few millimeters when it is 100% effaced. This upward pull on fibers of the lower uterus and downward push on the fetus causes the presenting part to

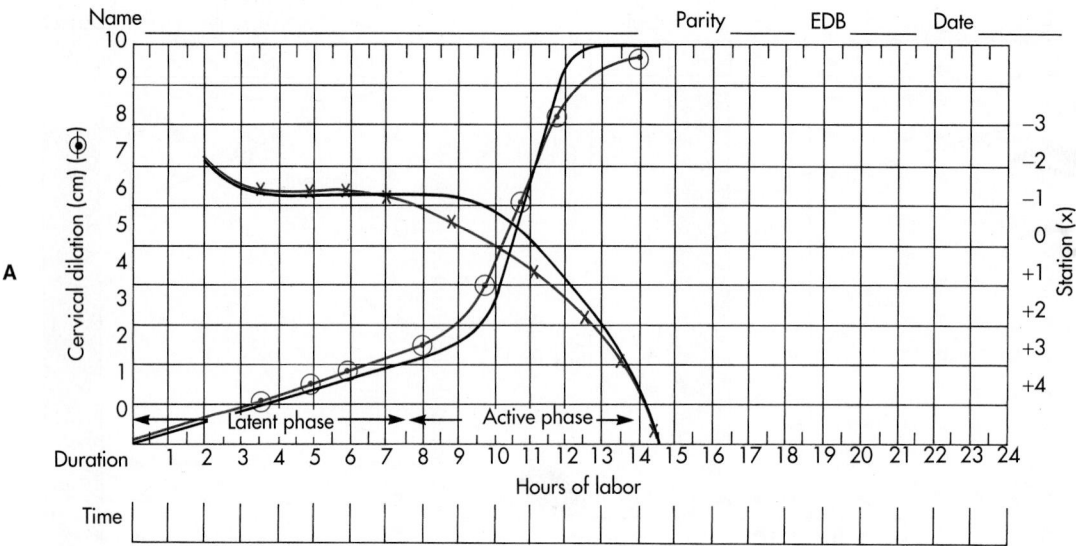

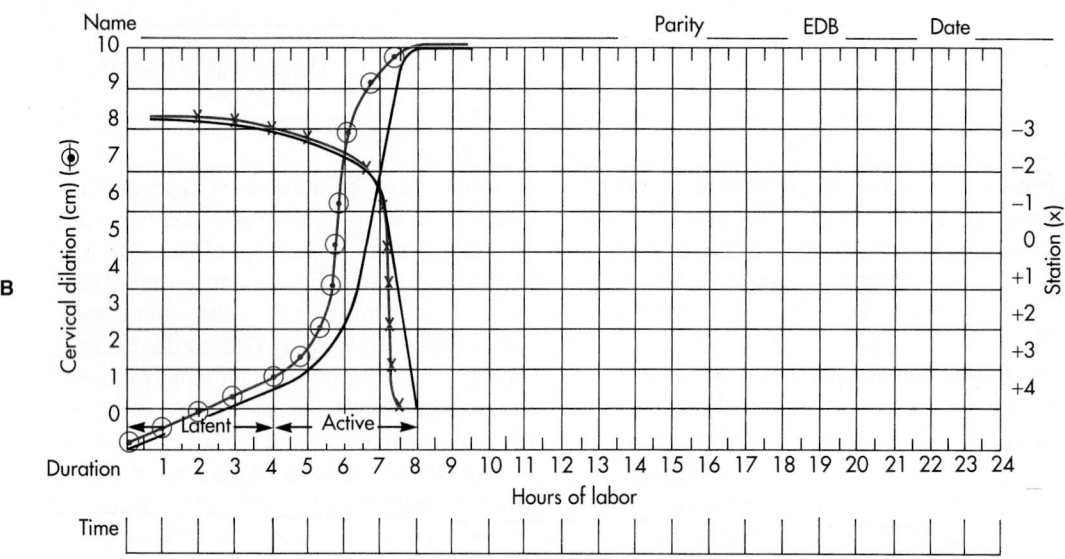

Fig. 22-10 Partogram for assessment of patterns of cervical dilation and descent. Individual woman's labor patterns *(colored)* superimposed on prepared labor graph *(black)* for comparison. **A,** Labor of a nulliparous woman. **B,** Labor of a multiparous woman. The rate of cervical dilation is plotted with the circled plot points. A line drawn through these symbols depicts the slope of the curve. Station is plotted with *X*'s. A line drawn through the *X*'s reveals the pattern of descent.

be pressed onto the cervix. As uterine contractions and retraction of the lower uterine segment continue, the cervical os dilates progressively. Effacement usually is not recorded on the partogram.

Cervical dilation. Cervical dilation is the most conclusive sign that the power of the uterine contractions is effective and labor is progressing. In a nullipara the cervix softens and thins out before it dilates. Thus, if a cervix is

long and closed, there is very little likelihood that birth will occur within a few hours. Once a cervix has completely dilated (10 cm) in a multiparous woman, it rarely will feel as closed as that of a nulliparous woman at the onset of labor. Thus it is easier to predict the duration of the latent and active phases of labor in a nulliparous woman than in one who has previously given birth. The cervix will "remember" how to dilate (tissues are more elastic), and

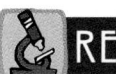

RESEARCH

The Duration of Labor in Healthy Women

Dystocia generally refers to difficult or slow labor. It is a poorly specified diagnostic category that can include prolonged labor, dysfunctional labor, and failure-to-progress labor. Inherent in these classifications is the differentiation of normal from abnormal labor based on the time spent in labor. High rates of treatment for dystocia indicate a need to reassess its definition and management.

The primary purpose of this study was to measure the length of active labor, first and second stages, in a multicultural population of low risk women who received intrapartum care in nine midwifery practices across the United States during 1996. Secondary purposes were to assess client and clinical factors associated with longer labors and identify any increased morbidity that may accompany greater time in labor.

An observational study was conducted with healthy women (N = 2511) at term who did not receive oxytocin or epidurals. Descriptive statistics were reported for the active phase, first stage (4 cm to complete cervical dilation), and second stage (complete to birth) by parity and for subgroups of women according to race/ethnicity, age, insurance, activity in labor, type of fetal monitoring, and narcotic analgesia. Logistic regression was also used to assess the contribution of each variable to longer labors with simultaneous adjustments of the other variables.

The mean length of the active phase, first stage, was 7.7 hours for nulliparas and 5.6 hours for multiparas. The mean length of second stage was 54 minutes for nulliparas and 18 minutes for multiparas. Variables associated with longer labors were electronic fetal monitoring, ambulation, maternal age over 30 years, and narcotic analgesia. Morbidity was not increased in longer labors. It was concluded that normal labor in healthy women lasted longer than many clinicians expect. The criteria for distinguishing normal labor from abnormal labor based on time must be revised.

CLINICAL APPLICATION

Dystocia is a common diagnosis in American childbearing women. The treatments are often invasive and expensive and can contribute to maternal morbidity. In view of the many changes in obstetric care and also in the childbearing population in recent decades, a fundamental reassessment of time expectations for physiologic labor would be advantageous. Nurses must increase their awareness of a wider range of "normal" for labor duration and help address the current high rates of treatment of dystocia in the United States.

Source: Albers, L. (1999). The duration of labor in healthy women. *J Perinatol* 19(2), 114-119.

this event varies with each woman and the way in which her body responds to labor. The cervix often is positioned posteriorly in early labor, particularly in nulliparous women, but moves anteriorly as labor progresses and the presenting part descends, placing pressure on the cervical rim.

Station. *Station* refers to the relationship of the lowermost portion of the presenting part to the woman's ischial spines. In early labor the presenting part often is above the level of the ischial spines, but it descends as labor progresses. If membranes are ruptured, the station is usually lower once the pelvic inlet has accommodated the presenting part. If membranes are intact, the presenting part may be floating or engaged in the inlet. If the vertex is at 0 station or below, most often engagement of the head has occurred; that is, the biparietal diameter of the head has passed through the pelvic inlet. However, if the head is unusually molded or if there is an extensive formation of a caput, or both, engagement might not have taken place even though the vertex is at 0 station or even lower (Varney, 1997).

Vaginal examination. The vaginal examination reveals whether the woman is in true labor and enables the examiner to determine whether the membranes have ruptured. Because this examination is often stressful and uncomfortable for the woman, it should be performed only when the status of the woman and her fetus indicates the need. For example, a vaginal examination should be performed on admission, when there has been significant progress in uterine activity, on maternal perception of perineal pressure or the urge to bear down, when membranes rupture, or when variable decelerations of the FHR are noted. A full explanation of the examination and support of the woman are important factors in reducing the stress and discomfort associated with the examination (Bergstrom, 1992).

Vaginal examinations should include the following steps:

1. The nurse assembles all the equipment needed, including a single sterile glove, antiseptic solution or soluble gel, and a light source. Water should be used for lubrication during the initial examination if rupture of membranes is suspected and a nitrazine test is required.
2. The nurse prepares the woman by explaining what will be done, why the examination is being performed, and how it will feel. The woman should be draped to prevent

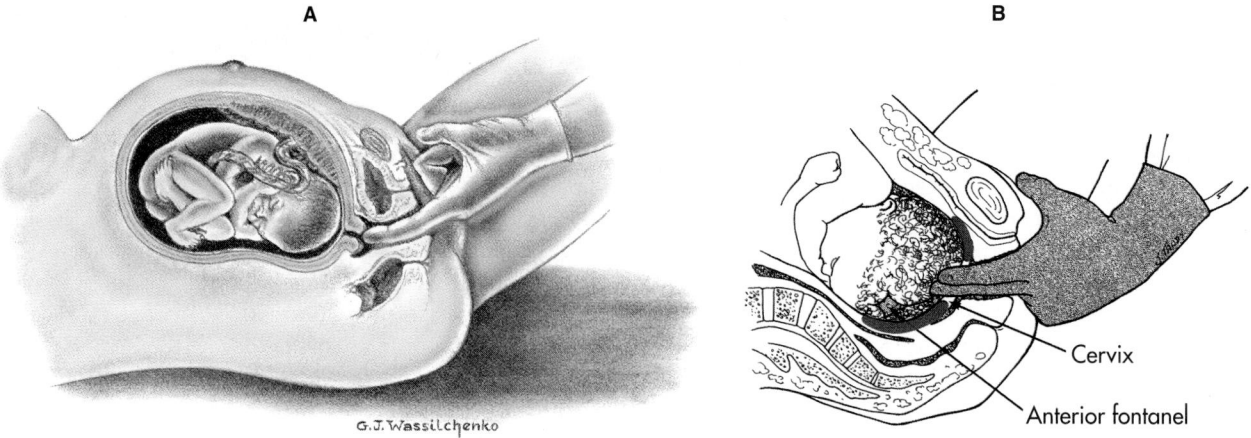

G.J. Wassilchenko

Fig. 22-11 Vaginal examination. **A,** Undilated, uneffaced cervix; membranes intact. **B,** Palpation of sagittal suture line. Cervix effaced and partially dilated.

chilling and protect her privacy and positioned to prevent supine hypotension (see Fig. 22-4). The perineum and vulva are cleansed if necessary.

3. The nurse washes her hands and puts on a sterile glove using an aseptic technique. The nurse should ask the woman for permission to touch her before proceeding (Waymire, 1997) and explains to the woman that she will feel the nurse inserting the index and middle fingers into the vagina. The examination should be performed gently, with concern for the woman's comfort. The nurse acknowledges the woman's expressions of pain or discomfort and anxiety. The woman should be encouraged to breathe slowly and relax her perineum (or gently push her perineal muscles out toward the examining finger).

4. The nurse assesses the status of the following (Fig. 22-11):
   a. Dilation and effacement of cervix
   b. Presenting part, position, station, and if vertex, any molding of the head
   c. Membranes—intact, bulging, or ruptured; amniotic fluid—color, clarity, odor, and so on
   d. Presence of stool in rectum

5. The nurse then helps the woman into a comfortable position and discusses the findings of the examination with the woman or couple.

6. The nurse documents all findings and reports them to the primary health care provider.

Laboratory and Diagnostic Tests

The nurse should anticipate the need for urinalysis, blood tests, and tests for rupture of membranes.

Analysis of urine specimen. A clean-catch urine specimen may be obtained to acquire further data about the pregnant woman's health. It is a convenient and simple procedure that can provide information about her hydration status (specific gravity, color, amount), nutritional sta-

tus (ketones), infection status (e.g., the presence of leukocytes), or the status of possible complications such as PIH (shown by finding of protein in urine). The results can be obtained quickly and help the nurse determine appropriate interventions to implement.

Blood tests. The blood tests performed vary with the hospital protocol and the woman's health status. An example of a minimum assessment is a hematocrit determination, in which the specimen is centrifuged in the perinatal unit. Blood can be obtained by a finger stick or from the hub of a catheter used to start an IV line. More comprehensive blood assessments such as white blood cell count, red blood cell count, the hemoglobin level, hematocrit, and platelet count are included in a complete blood cell count (CBC). A CBC may be ordered for women with a history of infection, anemia, PIH, and so on.

If the woman's blood type has not been verified, blood is drawn for the purpose of determining the type and Rh factor. If blood typing has already been done, the primary health care provider may choose not to repeat the test. If obvious signs of immunocompromise or substance abuse are present, other diagnostic blood tests may be ordered.

Assessment of amniotic membranes and fluid. Labor is initiated at term by **spontaneous rupture of membranes** (SROM, SRM) in approximately 25% of pregnant women. A lag period, rarely exceeding 24 hours, may precede the onset of labor. Membranes (the bag of waters) can also rupture spontaneously any time during labor.

> **NURSE ALERT** *The umbilical cord may prolapse when the membranes rupture. It is the nurse's responsibility to monitor the FHR for several minutes immediately after rupture of membranes to ascertain fetal well-being, and then to document the findings.*

Tests for assessing rupture of membranes are discussed in the Procedure box on page 516. **Artificial rupture of membranes** (AROM, ARM), or **amniotomy,** may be done to augment or induce labor or to facilitate placement of internal monitors when fetal status indicates the need for some form of direct assessment (attachment of a spiral electrode to the presenting part and insertion of an intrauterine pressure catheter). The following routine characteristics of amniotic fluid are assessed.

Color. Amniotic fluid is normally pale and straw colored and may contain white particles (flecks of vernix caseosa). If the amniotic fluid is greenish brown, the fetus has probably experienced a recent hypoxic episode, causing relaxation of the anal sphincter and the passage of meconium, the by-products of fetal ingestion, in utero. Yellow-stained amniotic fluid may indicate fetal hypoxia that occurred 36 hours or more before rupture of membranes, fetal hemolytic disease (Rh or ABO incompatibility), or intrauterine infection. Meconium-stained amniotic fluid may be a normal finding in a breech presentation and results from pressure being exerted on the fetal rectum during descent. Although meconium-stained amniotic fluid may be an ominous finding in labor, it is not always associated with fetal hypoxia and must be viewed in the context of the total clinical picture of labor. Amniotic fluid that is port wine colored may indicate the presence of bleeding associated with premature separation of the placenta (abruptio).

Viscosity and odor. Amniotic fluid normally is watery and lacks a strong odor. Infection is suspected if the fluid is thick, cloudy, or foul smelling, or a combination of these. The presence of considerable meconium can also cause amniotic fluid to have a thick consistency.

Amount. The expected amount of amniotic fluid is 500 to 1200 ml. Most of it originates from the maternal bloodstream, with fetal urine adding to it. *Hydramnios* (greater than 2000 ml of fluid) is an excessively large amount of amniotic fluid and is often associated with congenital anomalies of the fetus, in which the fetus cannot drink the fluid or in which fluid is trapped in the fetal body. *Oligohydramnios* (less than 500 ml of fluid) is an abnormally small amount of amniotic fluid and can be associated with incomplete formation or absence of the kidneys or obstruction of the urethra. If the fetus is unable to secrete and excrete urine, the volume of amniotic fluid decreases. Fetal surgical procedures can be performed to relieve some obstructive conditions.

The nurse's responsibility is to report findings promptly to the primary health care provider and to document findings in the labor record and on the monitor strip. If abnormal findings are noted, continuous electronic monitoring usually is implemented and maintained for the duration of labor. The finding of meconium-stained amniotic fluid alerts the nurse to the need to observe fetal status more closely. After birth, the newborn may also be at risk for an alteration in respiratory status if meconium is aspirated into the lungs with the first breath.

SIGNS OF POTENTIAL COMPLICATIONS

Labor

- Intrauterine pressure of more than 75 mm Hg (determined by intrauterine pressure catheter monitoring) or resting tone of more than 15 mm Hg
- Contractions consistently lasting 90 seconds or more
- Contractions consistently occurring 2 minutes or less apart
- Fetal bradycardia, tachycardia, or persistently decreased variability
- Irregular FHR; suspected fetal dysrhythmias
- Appearance of meconium-stained or bloody fluid from the vagina
- Arrest in progress of cervical dilation or effacement, descent of the fetus, or both
- Maternal temperature of 38° C or more
- Foul-smelling vaginal discharge
- Persistent bright or dark-red vaginal bleeding

Infection. When membranes rupture, microorganisms from the vagina can then ascend into the amniotic sac, causing chorioamnionitis and placentitis to develop. For this reason, maternal temperature and vaginal discharge are assessed frequently (every 1 to 2 hours) so that a developing infection after rupture of membranes can be identified early. Even when membranes are intact, however, microorganisms may ascend and cause premature rupture of membranes. There is controversy regarding whether prophylactic antibiotic therapy can protect against infection (chorioamnionitis), which involves both the maternal and fetal sides of the membrane.

Signs of Potential Problems

Assessment findings serve as a baseline for gauging the woman's subsequent progress during the first stage of labor, after she has been admitted. Although some problems of labor are anticipated, others may appear unexpectedly during the clinical course of labor. Knowledge of the physiologic and anatomic changes that occur during pregnancy, careful initial assessment, and follow-up of the woman's progress are necessary in the care of a woman experiencing normal labor and in identifying deviations from normal that could signal potential or actual problems during labor (see Signs of Potential Complications box).

Nursing diagnoses determine the types of nursing actions needed to implement a plan of care. When establishing nursing diagnoses, the nurse should analyze the significance of findings gleaned during the assessment.

▌Nursing Diagnoses _____

Initial Assessment

- Impaired verbal communication related to
  - language barrier
- Anxiety related to
  - knowledge deficit regarding physical examination procedures
  - lack of previous experience with childbirth or childbirth preparation classes
  - negative experience with previous childbirth
  - cultural differences
- Risk for injury related to
  - inadequate prenatal care
  - undiagnosed prenatal conditions
  - inadequate forces of labor

Subsequent Assessments

- Pain related to
  - intense uterine contractions
- Fluid volume deficit related to
  - decreased fluid intake
- Impaired physical mobility related to
  - advanced station of fetal presenting part
  - rupture of amniotic membranes
  - fetal monitoring
  - epidural analgesia
- Altered urinary elimination related to
  - reduced intake of oral fluids
  - bed rest
  - lack of privacy
  - diminished sensation of bladder fullness associated with epidural anesthesia or analgesia
- Risk for infection related to
  - rupture of membranes
  - placement of internal monitoring devices

Assessment of Stress During Labor

- Impaired gas exchange (fetal) related to
  - maternal position
  - maternal hyperventilation
  - maternal hypotension
  - intense, frequent uterine contractions
  - compression of umbilical cord
- Situational low self-esteem (maternal) related to
  - inability to meet self-expectations
  - loss of control during labor
- Fear related to
  - triggering of memories associated with history of sexual abuse
- Situational low self-esteem (father or partner) related to
  - unrealistic expectations regarding role as labor coach
  - perceived ineffectiveness in meeting needs of laboring woman
- Ineffective family coping, compromised, related to
  - knowledge deficit concerning comfort measures that can be used for the laboring woman

Expected Outcomes of Care

It is important for the nurse and woman to set and prioritize expected outcomes that focus on the woman, fetus, and her significant others. Appropriate nursing and client actions are then determined so that these expected outcomes can be met. This planning with the woman is essential for ensuring the implementation of expected outcomes and maintaining her sense of control over her own childbirth experience. Throughout the first stage of labor the woman will do the following:

- Demonstrate expected progression of labor.
- Express satisfaction with the assistance of her support person(s)/family and nursing staff.
- Verbalize her desires for participating in labor and participate as much as possible throughout labor.
- Continue normal progression of labor while the FHR remains within normal range and without signs of distress.
- Maintain adequate hydration status through oral or IV intake.
- Void at least every 2 hours to prevent bladder distention.
- Encourage participation of her support person(s) by verbalizing discomfort and indicating the need for measures that help reduce discomfort and promote relaxation.
- Express satisfaction with her performance during labor.

Plan of Care and Interventions

Standards of Care

Standards of care guide the nurse in preparing for and implementing procedures with the expectant mother (Box 22-3). Protocols for care based on standards include the following tasks:

- Check the primary health care provider's orders.
- Assess the primary health care provider's orders for appropriateness and correctness, for example, the analgesic to be administered to relieve discomfort.
- Check labels on IV solutions, drugs, and other materials used for nursing care.
- Check expiration date on any packs of supplies used for procedures ordered.
- Ensure that information on the woman's identification band is correct. Also check that the identification band is accurate; for example, if she has allergies, ensure that the band is the appropriate color.
- Employ an empathic approach when giving care:
  - use words the woman can understand when explaining procedures.
  - respect the woman's individual needs and behaviors.
  - establish a rapport with the woman and her significant others.
  - be kind, caring, and competent when performing necessary procedures.
  - be aware that pain and discomfort are as the woman describes them.

BOX 22-3 Client Care Plan Using Protocols and Nursing Standards

CLIENT CARE PLAN FOR LABOR

MARY JAMES
UNIT NO. 4587024

Date Initiated: _____ Time: _____ RN: _____

OUTCOME STANDARDS:

1. Client will demonstrate normal labor progress while the fetus tolerates the labor process without demonstrating nonreassuring signs. Date met: _____
2. Client will participate as desired in decisions about her care. Date met: _____
3. Client and her partner will verbalize knowledge of labor process and their expectations for the birth experience. Date met: _____

INITIATED	PROBLEM	NURSING INTERVENTIONS	DISCONTINUED
Date/RN			Date/RN
	Alteration in maternal/ fetal gas exchange	Implement fetal monitoring per protocol or orders from health care provider	
	Risk related to labor progress:	Provide nursing care per hospital procedure manual	
	• Altered pattern of urinary elimination	Implement labor care per protocol or care path	
	• Tissue trauma related to birth	Notify primary health care provider of problems (see Signs of Potential Complications box)	
		Provide care for vaginal birth per hospital procedure manual	
		Provide immediate care for newborn per hospital procedure manual	
		Implement care for fourth stage of labor per protocol or care path	
	Anxiety related to maternal/fetal status	Encourage woman and her partner to express their concerns	
		Keep couple informed of labor progress	
		Involve woman in decision making regarding her care	
	Knowledge deficit about labor/procedures	Explain procedures in terms woman can understand	
	Pain associated with labor	Promote use of relaxation techniques	
		Provide comfort measures	
		Offer pain medications as ordered	
		Evaluate response to pain relief measures	
	Other problems:		

- repeat instructions as necessary and ensure that they are understood by the woman (see Guidelines/Guías box).
- carry out appropriate comfort measures such as mouth care and back care and ensure that support person is coping.
- recognize that a woman's current childbirth experience and the actions of nurses and other health care providers can have a positive or negative effect on the woman's future childbirth experiences.
• Use Standard Precautions, including precautions appropriate to the performance of invasive procedures.

• Document care according to hospital guidelines and communicate information to the primary health care provider when indicated.

LEGAL TIP Standards of Care for Labor

1. Provide explanations of all procedures to woman and family.
2. Assess maternal and fetal status, as well as progress of labor.
   a. Continue to monitor fetal status until birth.
   b. Document all assessment findings.

GUIDELINES/GUÍAS

Care During Labor

Lie down, please.
Acuéstese, por favor.

I am going to take your vital signs.
Le voy a tomar sus signos vitales.

I'm going to listen to the baby's heartbeat.
Voy a escuchar los latidos del corazón del bebé.

This is a fetal monitor.
Este es un monitor del feto.

I need to examine you.
Necesito examinarle.

Do you need to use the bathroom?
¿Necesita usar el baño?

Would you like some pain medication?
¿Desea medicina para calmar el dolor?

Roll over on your side, please.
Póngase al lado, por favor.

Relax.
Relájese.

Breathe deeply.
Respire profundamente.

Push.
Puje.

Don't push.
No puje.

Grab your knees and push.
Agarre las rodillas y puje.

You're doing fine.
Bien. Muy bien.

Congratulations!
¡Felicidades!

You have a beautiful boy.
Usted tiene un niño precioso.

You have a beautiful girl.
Usted tiene una niña preciosa.

Physical Nursing Care During Labor

Assessment is a continuous process throughout labor. The routine for the assessment of progress and the continued well-being of the mother and fetus is usually set at a minimum level by hospital or birthing center policy (see Care Path, p. 523). Unusual findings are cause for more frequent assessments.

The signs of progress in labor are well defined (see Table 22-2). The character of uterine contractions, as well as the woman's behavior and appearance, correlate with the phase of labor. In addition, the culture the woman comes from, her level of fatigue, and other factors may affect the way in which she copes with labor.

A woman's response to labor may be reflected in her blood pressure, pulse, and respirations. Fear, anxiety, and fatigue can cause alterations from baseline findings. Continued fetal well-being is monitored through assessment of the FHR and the character of the amniotic fluid discharge.

Careful assessment provides the cues that guide the selection and implementation of nursing actions. The nurse assumes much of the responsibility for assessing the progress of labor. It is also the nurse's responsibility to keep the primary health care provider informed of the progress and of any deviations from expected findings. The prompt and accurate documentation of assessment findings is essential. A typical labor record for the ongoing documentation of assessment findings is shown in Fig. 22-3. Significant findings may also be documented on monitor strips.

The physical nursing care rendered to the woman in labor is an essential component of her care. The current emphasis on evidence-based practice has led to the following labeling of care measures used during labor and birth:

- Demonstrably beneficial (useful) or likely to be beneficial
- A trade-off between beneficial and having a potentially adverse effect or of unknown effectiveness with insufficient evidence to support use
- Unlikely to be beneficial or likely to be harmful or ineffective

Managing care using this approach will enhance the safety, effectiveness, and acceptability of the physical care measures chosen to support the woman during labor and birth (Enkin et al., 1995; Technical Working Group of the World Health Organization, 1997). The various physical needs, the requisite nursing actions, and the rationale for care are presented in Table 22-3, Plan of Care, and Care Path.

TABLE 22-3 Physical Nursing Care During Labor

NEED	NURSING ACTIONS	RATIONALE
GENERAL HYGIENE		
Showers/bed baths, Jacuzzi bath	Assess for progress in labor	Determines appropriateness of the activity
	Supervise showers closely if woman is in true labor	Prevents injury from fall; labor may be accelerated
	Suggest allowing warm water to flow over back	Aids relaxation; increases comfort
Perineum	Cleanse frequently, especially after rupture of membranes and when show increases	Enhances comfort and reduces risk of infection
Oral hygiene	Offer toothbrush or mouthwash or wash the teeth with an ice-cold, wet washcloth as needed	Refreshes mouth; improves morale; helps counteract dry, thirsty feeling
Hair	Brush, braid per woman's wishes	Improves morale; increases comfort
Handwashing	Offer washcloths before and after voiding and as needed	Maintains cleanliness; improves morale and comfort
Face	Offer cool washcloth	Improves morale; provides relief from diaphoresis
Gowns/linens	Change prn; fluff pillows	Improves morale and comfort
NUTRIENT AND FLUID INTAKE		
Oral	Offer fluids and solid foods, following orders of primary health care provider and desires of laboring woman	Provides hydration and calories; enhances positive emotional experience and maternal control
IV	Establish and maintain IV as ordered	Maintains hydration; provides venous access for medications
ELIMINATION		
Voiding	Encourage voiding at least every 2 hours	A full bladder may impede descent of presenting part; overdistention may cause bladder atony and injury, as well as postpartum voiding difficulty
Ambulatory woman	Allow ambulation to bathroom according to orders of primary health care provider, if:	
	The presenting part is engaged	Reinforces normal process of urination
	The membranes are not ruptured	Precautionary measure to protect against prolapse of umbilical cord
	The woman is not medicated	Precautionary measure to protect against injury
Woman on bed rest	Offer bedpan	Prevents complications of bladder distention and ambulation
	Allow tap water to run; pour warm water over the vulva; give positive suggestion	Encourages voiding
	Provide privacy	Shows respect for woman
	Put up side rails on bed	Prevents injury from fall
	Place call bell within reach	
	Offer washcloth for hands	Maintains cleanliness and comfort
	Wash vulvar area	Maintains standard of care
Catheterization	Catheterize according to orders of primary health care provider or hospital protocol if measures to facilitate voiding are ineffective	Prevents complications of bladder distention
	Insert catheter between contractions	Minimizes discomfort
	Avoid force if obstacle to insertion is noted	"Obstacle" may be caused by compression on urethra by presenting part
Bowel elimination—sensation of rectal pressure	Help the woman ambulate to bathroom or offer bedpan, after careful assessment	Prevents misinterpretation of rectal pressure from the presenting part as the need to defecate
	Perform vaginal examination	Determine degree of descent of presenting part
	Cleanse perineum immediately after passage of stool	Reduces risk of infection and sense of embarrassment

PLAN ᵒF CARE | First Stage of Labor

NURSING DIAGNOSIS Anxiety related to labor and the birthing process

Expected Outcome *Woman exhibits decreased signs of anxiety.*

Nursing Interventions/*Rationales*

Orient woman and significant others to labor and birth unit and explain admission protocol *to allay initial feelings of anxiety.*

Assess woman's knowledge, experience, and expectations of labor; note any signs or expressions of anxiety, nervousness, or fear *to establish a baseline for intervention.*

Discuss the expected progression of labor and describe what to expect during the process *because knowledge can allay anxiety associated with the unknown.*

Actively involve woman in care decisions during labor, interpret sights and sounds of environment (monitor sights and sounds, unit activities), and share information on progression of labor (vital signs, FHR, dilation, effacement) *to increase her sense of control and allay fears.*

Actively involve significant others in care during labor *to help woman cope with the process.*

Recognize efforts to participate in the labor process and provide positive reinforcement *to maintain her level of confidence and self-esteem.*

NURSING DIAGNOSIS Pain related to increasing frequency and intensity of contractions

Expected Outcome *Client exhibits signs of decreased discomfort.*

Nursing Interventions/*Rationales*

Assess woman's level of pain and strategies that she has used to cope with pain *to establish a baseline for intervention.*

Encourage significant other to remain as support person during labor process *to assist with support and comfort measures, because measures are often more effective when delivered by a familiar person.*

Instruct woman and support person in use of specific techniques such as conscious relaxation, focused breathing, effleurage, massage, and application of sacral pressure *to increase relaxation, decrease intensity of contractions, and promote use of controlled thought and direction of energy.*

Early in labor, use diversional activities *to provide distractions.*

Encourage regular voiding to decrease chances of distention, *which can increase discomfort during contractions and impede progress of labor.*

Provide comfort measures such as frequent mouth care to prevent dry mouth, application of damp cloth to forehead, and changing of damp gown or bed covers *to relieve discomfort associated with diaphoresis; positioning to reduce stiffness.*

Encourage conscious relaxation between contractions *to prevent fatigue, which contributes to increased pain perceptions.*

Explain what analgesics and anesthesia are available for use during labor and birth *to provide knowledge to help woman make decisions about pain control.*

NURSING DIAGNOSIS Risk for fluid volume deficit related to altered intake during labor

Expected Outcomes *Fluid balance is maintained, and there are no signs of dehydration.*

Nursing Interventions/*Rationales*

Monitor intake and output and vital signs, and inspect skin turgor and mucous membranes for dryness, *to evaluate hydration status.*

Administer oral/parenteral fluids per physician/nurse-midwife order *to maintain hydration.*

Monitor any emesis and administer antiemetic per physician/nurse-midwife order if necessary *to control emesis and prevent fluid loss.*

NURSING DIAGNOSIS Risk for infection related to rupture of membranes before or during labor

Expected Outcome *Client shows no evidence of infection.*

Nursing Interventions/*Rationales*

After rupture of membranes, assess amniotic fluid for alterations in color, odor, amount, and presence of blood and meconium, *which may be indicative of intrauterine infection.*

Monitor vital signs and FHR *to evaluate for signs of infection.*

Maintain Standard Precautions, use good handwashing technique and aseptic technique when indicated, and maintain good perineal hygiene *to prevent spread of microorganisms.*

Limit frequency of vaginal examinations *to prevent infection by reducing number of invasive procedures.*

From Wong, D., & Perry, S. (1998). *Maternal child nursing care.* St. Louis: Mosby.

NURSING DIAGNOSIS Risk for altered pattern of urinary elimination related to sensory impairment secondary to labor

Expected Outcome *Bladder does not show signs of distention.*

Nursing Interventions/Rationales

Palpate the bladder superior to the symphysis on a frequent basis *because distention may occur from increased fluid intake and inability to feel urge to void.*

Encourage frequent voiding (at least every 2 hours) and catheterize if necessary *to avoid bladder distention because it impedes progress of fetus down birth canal and may result in trauma to the bladder.*

Assist to bathroom or commode to void if appropriate and provide privacy *because an upright position (natural) and relaxation will facilitate bladder emptying.*

General hygiene. Women in labor should be offered the use of showers or Jacuzzis, if they are available, to enhance the feeling of well-being and to minimize the discomfort of contractions. Women should also be encouraged to wash their hands after voiding and to perform self-hygiene measures. Linen should be changed if it becomes wet or stained with blood, and linen savers (Chux) should be used and changed as needed.

Nutrient and fluid intake

Oral intake. Traditionally the laboring woman has been offered only clear liquids or ice chips or given nothing by mouth during the active phase of labor to minimize the risk of anesthesia complications and their sequelae should general anesthesia be required in an emergency. These sequelae include the aspiration of gastric contents and resultant compromise in oxygen perfusion, which may endanger the lives of the mother and fetus. This practice is being challenged today because regional anesthesia is used more often than general anesthesia, even for emergency cesarean births. Women are awake during regional anesthesia and are able to participate in their own care and protect their airway.

Enkin and co-workers (1995) identified the withholding of food and drink from women in labor as a form of care unlikely to be beneficial. The offering of oral fluids is demonstrably useful and should be encouraged.

Although gastric emptying is slowed as a result of labor, stress, and the use of narcotics or sedatives, fasting does not cause gastric contents to be eliminated and may even cause them to become more acidic. In addition, fasting is identified by many laboring women as a stressor with which they must cope and a source of frustration during labor related to a loss of control with regard to meeting their own nourishment needs (Fowles, 1998).

An adequate intake of fluids and calories is required to meet the energy demands and fluid losses associated with childbirth. The progress of labor slows and ketosis develops if these demands are not met and fat is metabolized. This is most likely to occur in women who begin to labor early in the morning after a night without caloric intake. When women are permitted to consume fluids and food freely, they typically regulate their own oral intake, eating light foods (e.g., eggs, yogurt, ice cream, dry toast and jelly, fruit) and drinking fluids during early labor and tapering off to the intake of clear fluids and sips of water or ice chips as labor intensifies and the second stage approaches. Common practice among health care providers, especially physicians, is to allow clear liquids (water, tea, apple juice, clear sodas, gelatin, broth) during early labor, tapering off to ice chips and sips of water as labor progresses and becomes more active. Food and fluid consumed orally during labor can meet a laboring woman's hydration and energy demands more effectively and safely than fluid administered intravenously. In addition, the woman's sense of control and level of comfort are enhanced (Ludka & Roberts, 1993; Scheepers, Essed, & Brouns, 1998; Varney, 1997). More research is needed to determine which fluids and foods should be recommended during active labor.

Nurses should follow the orders of the woman's primary health care provider when offering the woman food or fluids during labor. As advocates, however, nurses can facilitate change by informing others of the current research findings that support the safety and effectiveness of the oral intake of food and fluid during labor and by initiating such research themselves.

Intravenous intake. Fluids are administered intravenously to the laboring woman to maintain hydration, especially when a labor is long and the woman is unable to ingest a sufficient amount of fluid orally or if she is receiving epidural or intrathecal anesthesia. However, routine use of intravenous fluids during labor is a form of care that is unlikely to be beneficial and may be harmful (Enkin et al., 1995; Technical Working Group of the World Health Organization, 1997). In most cases, an electrolyte solution without glucose is adequate and does not introduce excess glucose into the bloodstream. The latter is important because an excessive maternal glucose level results in fetal hyperglycemia and fetal hyperinsulinism. After birth, the neonate's high levels of insulin will then deplete his or her glucose stores and hypoglycemia will result. Infusions containing glucose can also lower sodium levels in both the woman and the fetus, leading to transient neonatal tachypnea (Ludka & Roberts, 1993). If maternal ketosis occurs, the primary health care provider may order an IV solution containing a small amount of dextrose to provide the glucose needed to assist in fatty acid metabolism.

NURSE ALERT *Nurses should carefully monitor the intake and output of laboring women receiving IV fluids because they also face an increased danger of hypervolemia as a result of the fluid retention that occurs during pregnancy.*

Elimination
Voiding. Voiding every 2 hours should be encouraged by the nurse, especially if the bladder is distended. A distended bladder may impede descent of the presenting part, inhibit uterine contractions, and lead to decreased bladder tone or atony after birth. Women who receive epidural analgesia or anesthesia are especially at risk for the retention of urine, and the need to void should be assessed more frequently in them.

If the woman wants to walk to the bathroom, the nurse should assist her in doing so, unless the primary health care provider has ordered bed rest, the woman is receiving epidural analgesia or anesthesia, or, in the nurse's judgment, ambulation would compromise the status of the laboring woman or her fetus, or both. If external monitoring is being used and the cords will reach, monitoring can continue while the woman uses the bathroom; otherwise, the cords are unplugged from the monitor while the woman is in the bathroom and monitoring is interrupted for that time.

Catheterization. If the woman is unable to void and her bladder is obviously distended, she may need to be catheterized. Most hospitals have protocols that rely on the nurse's judgment concerning the need for catheterization. Before performing the catheterization, the nurse should clean the vulva and perineum because vaginal show and amniotic fluid may be present. If there appears to be an obstacle that prevents advancement of the catheter, this is most likely the presenting part. If the catheter cannot be advanced, the nurse should stop the procedure and notify the primary health care provider of the difficulty.

Bowel elimination. Most women do not have bowel movements during labor because of decreased intestinal motility. Stool that has formed in the large intestine often is moved downward toward the anorectal area by the pressure exerted by the fetal presenting part as it descends. This stool is often expelled during second-stage pushing and birth. However, the passage of stool with bearing-down efforts increases the risk of infection and may embarrass the woman, thereby reducing the effectiveness of these efforts. To prevent these problems, the nurse should immediately cleanse the perineal area to remove any stool, while at the same time

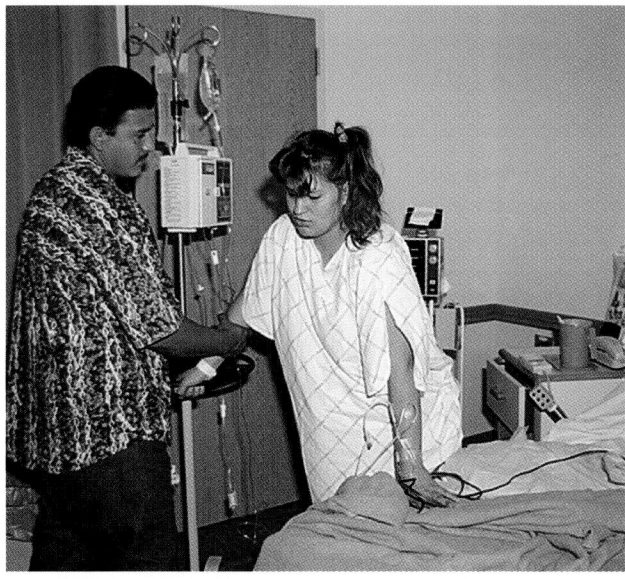

Fig. 22-12 Woman preparing to walk with partner. *(Courtesy Marjorie Pyle, RNC, Lifecircle, Costa Mesa, CA.)*

reassuring the woman that the passage of stool at this time is a normal and expected event, because the same muscles used to expel the baby also expel stool. Routine use of an enema to empty the rectum is considered to be harmful or ineffective and should be eliminated according to the Technical Working Group of the World Health Organization (1997) and Enkin and colleagues (1995).

If the presenting part is deep in the pelvis, even in the absence of stool in the anorectal area, the woman may feel rectal pressure and think she needs to defecate. The nurse should perform a vaginal examination to assess cervical dilation and station. When a multiparous woman experiences the urge to defecate, this often means birth will follow quickly.

Ambulation and positioning. Freedom of maternal movement and choice of position throughout labor are forms of care likely to be beneficial for the laboring woman and should be encouraged (Enkin et al., 1995; Technical Working Group of the World Health Organization, 1997).

The potential advantages of ambulation include enhanced uterine activity, distraction from labor's discomforts, enhanced maternal control, and an opportunity for close interaction with the woman's partner and care provider as they help her to walk. Albers and others (1997) found that ambulation is associated with a reduced rate of operative delivery (cesarean birth, use of forceps, and vacuum extraction) and less frequent use of narcotic analgesia.

Research by Bloom and colleagues (1998) found that although walking did not shorten the duration of labor, it did not impair the process or result in harm to the mother or fetus. They concluded that women should be allowed to choose to walk or not walk as they felt comfortable.

Walking, sitting, or standing during labor is more comfortable than lying down and facilitates the progress of labor (Melzack, Belanger, & Lacroix, 1991). Ambulation

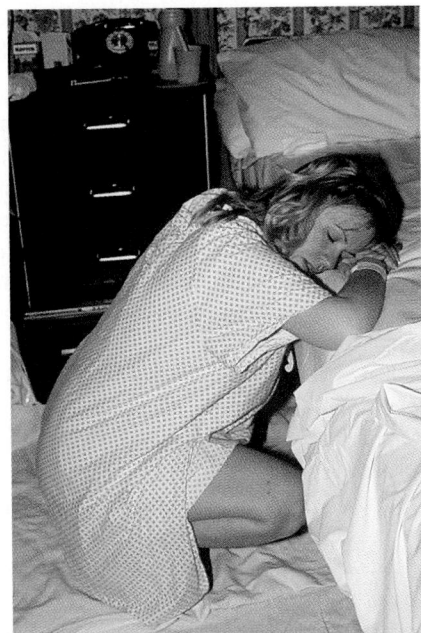

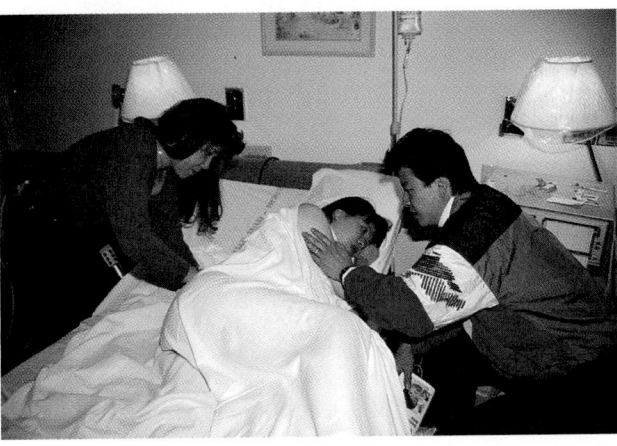

Fig. 22-13 Maternal positions for labor. **A,** Squatting. **B,** Lateral position. Support person is applying sacral pressure while partner provides encouragement. *(Courtesy Marjorie Pyle, RNC, Lifecircle, Costa Mesa, CA.)*

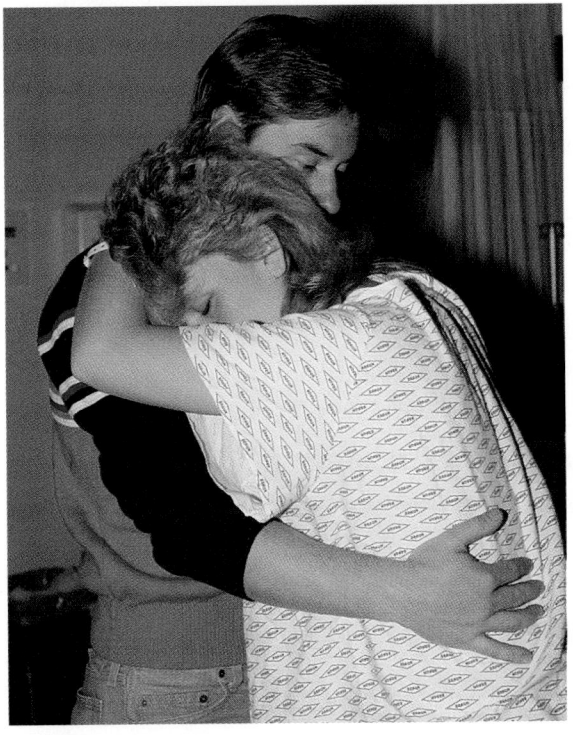

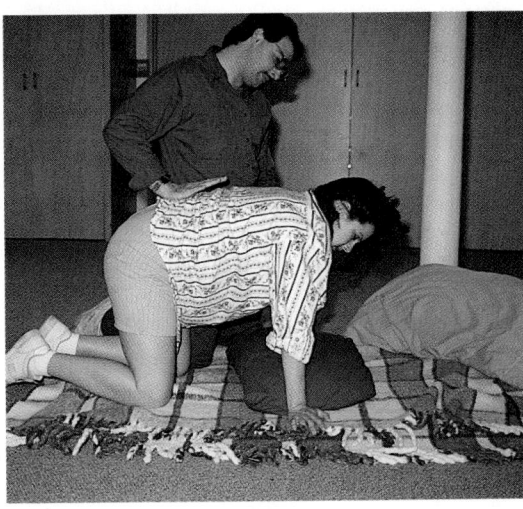

Fig. 22-14 **A,** Woman standing and leaning forward with support. **B,** Woman in hands-and-knees position. *(Courtesy Marjorie Pyle, RNC, Lifecircle, Costa Mesa, CA.)*

should be encouraged if membranes are intact, if the fetal presenting part is engaged after rupture of membranes, and if the woman has not received medication for pain (Fig. 22-12). Ambulation may be contraindicated, however, because of maternal or fetal status.

When the woman lies in bed, she will usually change her position spontaneously as labor progresses (Albers et al., 1997). If she does not change position every 30 to 60 minutes, she should be assisted to do so. The side-lying (lateral) position is preferred because it promotes optimal uteroplacental and renal blood flow and increases fetal oxygen saturation (Fig. 22-13, *B*). If the woman wants to lie supine, the nurse may place a pillow under one hip as a wedge to prevent the uterus from compressing the aorta and vena cava

(see Fig. 22-4). Sitting is not contraindicated unless it adversely affects fetal status, which can be determined by checking the FHR. If the fetus is in the occiput posterior position, it may be helpful to encourage the woman to squat during contractions, because this position increases pelvic diameter, allowing the head to rotate to a more anterior position (Fig. 22-13, *A*). A hands-and-knees position during contractions is also recommended to facilitate the rotation of the fetal occiput from a posterior to an anterior position as gravity pulls the fetal back forward (Fig. 22-14, *B*).

■BOX 22-4 Some Maternal Positions* During Labor and Birth

SEMIRECUMBENT POSITION

With woman sitting with her upper body elevated to at least a 30° angle, place wedge or small pillow under hip to prevent vena caval compression and reduce likelihood of supine hypotension (see Fig. 22-18, *B*)

- The greater the angle of elevation, the more gravity or pressure is exerted that promotes fetal descent, the progress of contractions, and the widening of pelvic dimensions.
- Convenient for rendering care measures and for external fetal monitoring.

LATERAL POSITION (SEE FIG. 22-13, *B*)

Have woman alternate between left and right side-lying position, and provide abdominal and back support as needed for comfort.

- Removes pressure from the vena cava and back; enhances uteroplacental perfusion and relieves backache.
- Makes it easier to perform back massage or counterpressure.
- Associated with less frequent, but more intense, contractions.
- Obtaining good external fetal monitor tracings may be more difficult.
- May be used as a birthing position.
- Takes pressure off perineum.

UPRIGHT POSITION

The gravity effect enhances the contraction cycle and fetal descent: the weight of the fetus places increasing pressure on the cervix; the cervix is pulled upward, facilitating effacement and dilation; impulses from the cervix to the pituitary gland increase, causing more oxytocin to be secreted; and contractions are intensified, thereby applying more forceful downward pressure on the fetus, but they are less painful.

- Fetus is aligned with pelvis, and pelvic diameters are widened slightly.
- Effective upright positions include the following:
  - Ambulation (see Fig. 22-12).
  - Standing and leaning forward with support provided by coach, end of bed, back of chair, or birth ball; relieves backache and facilitates application of counterpressure or back massage (see Fig. 22-14, A).
  - Sitting up in bed, chair, birthing chair, on toilet or bedside commode
  - Squatting (see Fig. 22-13, A).

HANDS-AND-KNEES POSITION—IDEAL POSITION FOR POSTERIOR POSITIONS OF THE PRESENTING PART (SEE FIG. 22-14, *B*)

Assume an "all fours" position in bed or on a covered floor; allows for pelvic rocking.

- Relieves backache characteristic of "back labor."
- Facilitates internal rotation of the fetus by increasing mobility of the coccyx, increasing the pelvic diameters, and using gravity to turn the fetal back and rotate the head.

*Assess the effect of each position on the laboring woman's comfort and anxiety level, progress of labor, and FHR pattern. Alternate positions every 30 to 60 minutes.

Much research is being directed toward acquiring a better understanding of the physiologic and psychologic effects of maternal position in labor. Fetal presentations and the mechanisms of labor may be helped or hindered by maternal posture (Andrews & Chrzanowski, 1990; Biancuzzo, 1993; Carbonne et al., 1996; Simkin, 1995). The variety of positions that are recommended for the laboring woman are described in Box 22-4.

A birth ball (gymnastic ball, also used in physical therapy) can be used to support a woman's body as she assumes a variety of labor and birth positions (Fig. 22-15). The woman can sit on the ball while leaning over the bed, or she can lean over the ball to support her upper body and reduce stress on her arms and hands when she assumes a hands-and-knees position. The birth ball can encourage pelvic mobility and pelvic and perineal relaxation when the woman sits on the firm yet pliable ball and rocks in rhythmic movements. Warm compresses can maximize

this relaxation effect. The birth ball should be large enough so that when the woman sits her knees are bent at a 90-degree angle and her feet are flat on the floor and approximately 2 feet apart (Perez, 1998).

Support Measures

Effective physical and emotional support provided to women during labor can result in shorter labors, reduced rates of complications and surgical or obstetric interventions (e.g., cesarean births, labor augmentations and inductions, episiotomies, forceps-assisted births), and enhanced self-esteem and satisfaction (Kennell et al., 1991; Pascoe, 1993).

The nurse can alleviate a woman's anxiety by explaining unfamiliar terms, providing information and explanations without her having to ask, and preparing her for sensations she will experience and procedures that will follow. By encouraging the woman or couple to ask questions and by providing honest, understandable answers, the nurse can play an important role in helping the woman achieve a satisfying birth experience (Proctor, 1998; Tomlinson & Bryan, 1996). The learning needs voiced by a woman in labor should be met by the nurse managing her care (Evans & Jeffery, 1995).

Supportive nursing care for a woman in labor includes (1) helping the woman maintain control and participate to the extent she wishes in the birth of her infant; (2) meeting the woman's expected outcomes for her labor; (3) acting as the woman's advocate, supporting her decisions and respecting her choices as appropriate and relating her wishes as needed to other health care providers; (4) helping the woman conserve her energy; (5) helping control the woman's discomfort; (6) acknowledging the woman's efforts, as well as those of her partner, during labor and providing positive reinforcement; and (7) protecting the woman's privacy and modesty.

The nurse serves as a coach to the woman in the absence of other support persons or as an assistant coach to the support persons present. To do this, the nurse must have a thorough knowledge of breathing and relaxation techniques.

Couples who have attended childbirth education programs that teach the psychoprophylactic approach will know something about the labor process, coaching techniques, and comfort measures. The nurse should play a supportive role and keep such a couple informed of the progress.

Couples may need a review and redemonstration of methods learned in class and practiced in the familiar environment of their home without the pain and discomfort of labor and without the anxiety of being in an unfamiliar environment. It is important that the nurse caution the woman not to begin patterned breathing techniques during the latent phase of labor because this practice has been associated with an increase in the level of fatigue the woman experiences as labor progresses (Pugh et al., 1998).

Even when expectant parents have not attended such classes, the nurse can teach them various techniques during the early phase of labor. In this case the nurse may provide more of the coaching and supportive care.

Breathing and relaxation techniques should be simple and performed with the woman until the support person feels ready to take on a more active coaching role. Comfort measures can be demonstrated by the nurse while encouraging the support person to assist and the laboring woman to express her needs and feelings.

Comfort measures vary with the situation (Fig. 22-16). The nurse can draw on the couple's repertoire of comfort measures learned during the pregnancy. Such measures include maintaining a comfortable, supportive atmosphere in the labor and birth area; using touch therapeutically (e.g., heat or cold applied to the lower back in the event of back labor, a cool cloth applied to the forehead); providing nonpharmacologic measures to relieve discomfort; administering analgesics when necessary; and most of all, just being there (Table 22-4; see also Care Paths).

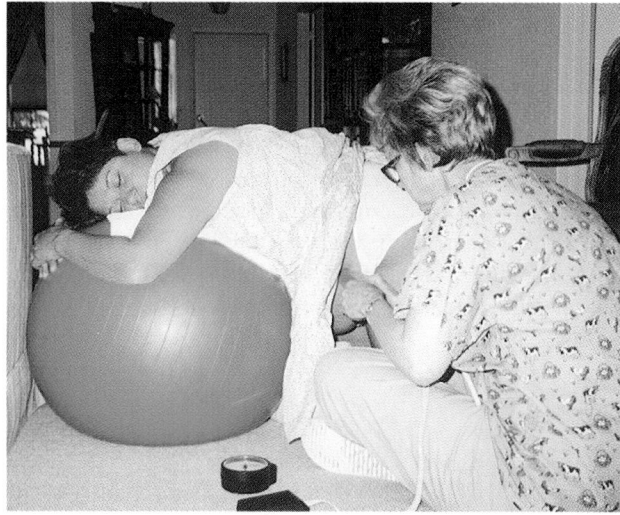

Fig. 22-15 Laboring woman using birth ball. *(Courtesy Polly Perez, Cutting Edge Press, Johnson, VT.)*

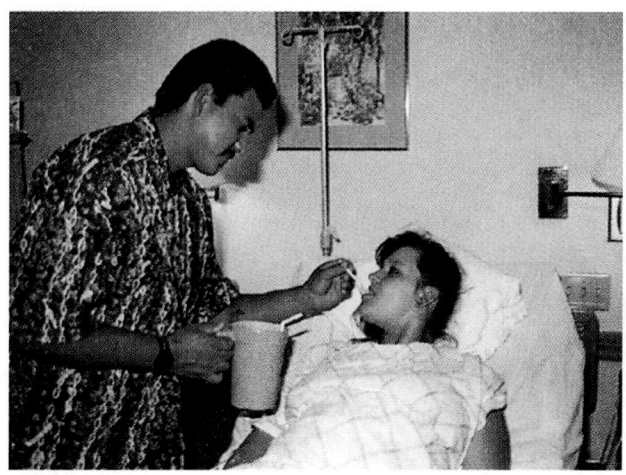

Fig. 22-16 Partner providing comfort measures. *(Courtesy Marjorie Pyle, RNC, Lifecircle, Costa Mesa, CA.)*

Labor rooms should be airy, clean, and homelike. Bright overhead lights should be turned off when not needed to enhance relaxation. The temperature is controlled to ensure the laboring woman's comfort. The room should be large enough to accommodate a comfortable chair for the woman's partner, the monitoring equipment, and hospital personnel. Couples may be encouraged to bring extra pillows to make the hospital surroundings more homelike and facilitate position changes. Women often state that this type of an environment helps them view their childbirth experience as normal and not related to illness (Proctor, 1998).

Touch. Most women in labor respond positively to touch. They appreciate gentle handling by staff members. Back rubs may be offered, especially if the woman is experiencing back labor. A support person may be taught to exert

TABLE 22-4 Woman's Responses and Support Person's Actions During First Stage of Labor

WOMAN'S RESPONSES	NURSE/SUPPORT PERSON'S ACTIONS*
DILATION OF CERVIX 0-3 CM (LATENT) (contractions 10-30 sec long, 5-30 min apart, mild to moderate)	
Mood: alert, happy, excited, mild anxiety	Provides encouragement, feedback for relaxation, companionship
Settles into labor room; selects focal point	Assists to cope with contractions
Rests or sleeps, if possible	Encourages use of focusing techniques
Uses breathing techniques	Helps to concentrate on breathing techniques
Uses effleurage, focusing, and relaxation techniques	Uses comfort measures
	Assists woman into comfortable position
	Informs woman of progress; explains procedures and routines
	Gives praise
	Offer fluids, ice chips as ordered
DILATION OF CERVIX 4-7 CM (ACTIVE) (contractions 30-45 sec long, 3-5 min apart, moderate to strong)	
Mood: seriously labor oriented, concentration and energy needed for contractions, alert, more demanding	Acts as buffer; limits assessment techniques to between contractions
	Assists with contractions
Continues relaxation, focusing techniques	Encourages woman as needed to help her maintain breathing techniques
Uses breathing techniques	Uses comfort measures
	Assists with frequent position changes, emphasizing side-lying and upright positions
	Encourages voluntary relaxation of muscles of back, buttocks, thighs, and perineum; effleurage
	Applies counterpressure to sacrococcygeal area
	Encourages and praises
	Keeps woman aware of progress
	Offers analgesics as ordered
	Checks bladder; encourages her to void
	Gives oral care; offers fluids, ice chips as ordered
DILATION OF CERVIX 8-10 CM (TRANSITION) (contractions 45-90 sec long, 2-3 min apart, strong)	
Mood: irritable, intense concentration, symptoms of transition (e.g., nausea, vomiting)	Stays with woman; provides constant support
	Assists with contractions
Continues relaxation, needs greater concentration to do this	Reminds, reassures, and encourages woman to reestablish breathing pattern and concentration as needed
Uses breathing techniques	Alerts woman to begin breathing pattern before contraction becomes too intense if she is sedated or drowsy
Uses 4:1 breathing pattern if using psychoprophylactic techniques	Prompts panting respirations if woman begins to push prematurely
Uses panting to overcome response to urge to push	Uses comfort measures
	Accepts woman's inability to comply with instructions
	Accepts irritable response to helping, such as counterpressure
	Supports woman who has nausea and vomiting; gives oral care as needed; gives reassurance regarding signs of end of first stage
	Uses relaxation techniques (effleurage and voluntary relaxation)
	Keeps woman aware of progress

*Provided by nurses and support persons in collaboration with the nurse.

counterpressure against the mother's sacrum over the occiput of the head of a fetus in a posterior position (see Fig. 22-13, *B*). The back pain is caused by the occiput pressing on spinal nerves, and counterpressure lifts the occiput off these nerves, thereby providing some relief from pain. Once counterpressure is initiated, the woman usually asks her partner to continue doing this for each following contraction. The partner will need to be relieved after a while, however, because exerting counterpressure is hard work. Hand and foot massage can be soothing and relaxing (Simkin, 1995).

The woman's perception of the soothing qualities of touch changes as labor progresses. Many women become more sensitive to touch (hyperesthesia) as labor progresses, and this is a typical finding during the transition phase (see Table 22-2). They may tell their coach to leave them alone or not to touch them. The partner who is unprepared for this normal response may feel rejected and may react by withdrawing active support. The nurse can reassure them that this response is a positive indication that the first stage is ending and the second stage is approaching. Women experiencing increased sensitivity to touch may have a positive response when touched on surfaces of the body where hair does not grow, such as the forehead, the palms of the hands, and the soles of the feet.

The woman in labor may exhibit a variety of reactions and needs support from her partner and the nurse no matter what her reactions. Critical comments directed toward the woman are unwarranted and inappropriate (see Table 22-4).

Relaxation. Relaxation measures for use during labor are often learned in childbirth classes and through life experiences. They include guided imagery, music, and soothing massage.

Music, taped or live, can cue rhythmic breathing and enhance relaxation, thereby reducing stress and anxiety and even relieving pain. Nurses can be advocates for the implementation of this complementary therapy by developing protocols for the use of music, assessing a woman's desire to use music and what type, and mobilizing the musical talents of the client, her significant others, and even health care providers (Olson, 1998).

These techniques can provide comfort, prevent fatigue, and help the woman conserve energy for the expulsive work of the second stage of labor. Today, many health care providers advocate the use of warm water (e.g., whirlpool baths or Jacuzzis, showers) for its soothing, relaxing effects and its ability to reduce discomfort and enhance the progress of labor, especially during the first 1 to 2 hours of immersion (Aderhold & Perry, 1991; Odent, 1997; Rosenthal, 1991; Simkin, 1995). Many new birthing units have baths with air jets. The buoyancy of the warm water in a bath, with or without air jets, provides support for tense muscles. The relaxing and soothing effect that the warm water has on muscles yields immediate benefits during labor and also reduces the aftereffects of tense muscles during the immediate postpartum period.

It is recommended that the use of a whirlpool bath or Jacuzzi begin when the woman is in active labor because initiation of this method in the latent phase could slow contractions or stop them temporarily (Eriksson, Mattsson, & Ladfors, 1997) (see Fig. 20-4). The temperature of the water should be maintained at 37° C or lower. Women should be encouraged to drink oral fluids while in the bath to maintain fluid balance and the beneficial effects of the hydrotherapy on the progress of the labor. After approximately 2 hours the effectiveness of hydrotherapy seems to diminish as contractions become more intense (Eriksson et al., 1997; Odent, 1997). Newborns who are born, either accidentally or intentionally, while

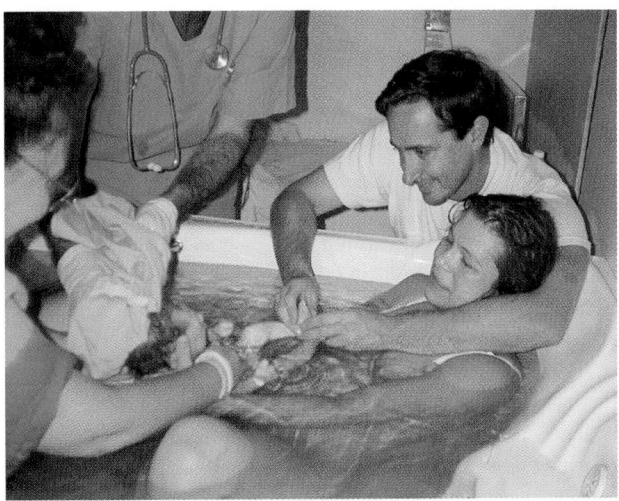

Fig. 22-17   Waterbirth. *(Courtesy Global Maternal/Child Health Association, Inc., Wilsonville, OR.)*

women are immersed in the water do not begin to breathe until removed from the water. Most authorities recommend that the birth occur out of the water; if it occurs while in the water, the newborn should be removed immediately (McCandlish & Renfrew, 1993; Odent, 1997) (Fig. 22-17). Further research is needed regarding water immersion during labor and birth to establish a protocol for its use, to validate the beneficial effects, and to determine whether detrimental effects occur and if they can be prevented. Showers can also enhance relaxation and reduce pain when warm water is directed over the laboring woman's lower back and abdomen (Simkin, 1995).

The Father or Partner During Labor

Although another woman or a man other than the father may be the woman's partner, the father of the baby is most often the support person during labor. He often is able to provide the comfort measures and touch that the laboring woman needs. When the woman becomes focused on her pain, sometimes the partner can persuade her to try nonpharmacologic variations of comfort measures. In addition, he usually is able to interpret the woman's needs and desires to staff members.

Throughout the past 20 years, childbirth preparation education has been widely available. The father's ideal role was thought to be that of labor coach, and he was expected to actively help the woman cope with labor. However, this expectation may be unrealistic, because some men have concerns about their labor-coaching abilities. Chapman (1992) reported that men assume one of at least three different roles during labor and birth—coach, teammate, or witness. As a coach, the father actively assists the woman during and after contractions. Men who are coaches express a strong need to be in control of themselves and of the labor experience. Women also express a great desire for the father to be physically involved in labor. The father who acts as the teammate assists the woman during labor and birth by responding to requests for physical or emotional support, or both. Teammates usually adopt the follower or helper role and look to the woman or nurse to tell them what to do. Women express a strong desire to have the father present and willing to help in any way. The father who acts as a witness acts as a companion, giving emotional and moral support. He watches the woman labor and give birth, but he often sleeps, watches television, or leaves the room for long periods. Witnesses believe that there is little they can do to physically help the woman and look to the nurses and health care providers to be in charge of the experience. Women do not expect more of this type of father than to just be present.

The degree of mutuality (level of interdependency and sharing) and understanding (the ability to know each other's needs) in a couple's relationship determines which role the father adopts. The coach and teammate roles are often assumed by men in couples with a high degree of mutuality. Men in couples in which mutuality is low tend to adopt the witness role. Because the father can participate in labor and birth in different ways, the nurse should encourage him to adopt the role most comfortable for him and for the woman, rather than to assume an unnatural role.

The nurse must recognize that the feelings of a first-time father change as labor progresses. Often calm at the onset of labor, feelings of fear and helplessness begin to dominate as labor becomes more active and the father realizes that labor is more work than he anticipated. The first-time father may feel excluded as birth preparations begin during the transition phase. Once the second stage begins and birth nears, the father's focus changes from the woman to the baby who is about to be born (Chandler & Field, 1997).

The father will be exposed to many sights and smells he may never before have experienced. It is therefore important to tell him what to expect and to make him comfortable about leaving the room to regain his composure should something occur that surprises him. Before he does this, provision should, of course, first be made for someone else to support the woman during his absence. Staff members should tell the father that his presence is helpful and encourage him to be involved in the care of the woman to the extent he is comfortable.

Participation in the birth is ego building. The father can be of assistance; his presence is important. The following true story illustrates this point:

> A 16-year-old single mother in labor with her first child had been thrashing about, moaning and screaming with each contraction. A nurse had remained at her bedside, coaching and comforting her, but to no avail. The adolescent father arrived and was immediately escorted into her room. Upon his appearance the young woman then continued her labor calmly and without medication through to the birth of the baby.

Supporting both the father and the woman in labor elevates the nurse's role. It is another step forward for a nurse from merely providing custodial care to enacting a therapeutic role. Support of the father reflects the nurse's orientation and commitment to each person, the family, and the community. Therapeutic nursing actions convey several important concepts to the father: first, that the father is of value as a person; second, that he can learn to be a partner in the woman's care; and third, that childbearing is a partnership.

The nurse can support the father in the following ways:

1. Regardless of the degree of involvement desired, explain the layout of the maternity unit; the location of the toilet, cafeteria, waiting room, and nursery; the visiting hours; and the names and functions of personnel present. Orient him to the woman's labor room and discuss what he can do there (e.g., sleep, use the telephone).

2. Inform him about the sights and smells he can expect to encounter. Encourage him to leave the room if he needs time to regain his composure while another person continues to coach until he returns.

3. Respect his or the couple's decisions as to his degree of involvement—whether he is to actively participate in the birthing room or just be kept informed of the progress of labor. When appropriate, provide data on which he or they can base decisions; offer them the freedom to make decisions rather than coerce them one way or another. This is their experience and their baby.

4. Tell him when his presence has been helpful and continue to reinforce this throughout labor.

5. Offer to teach him comfort measures to the extent he wants to know them. Reassure him that he is not assuming the responsibility for observation and management of his partner's labor, rather that his responsibility is to support her as the labor progresses. Suggest alternative comfort measures when the ones he is using are no longer helpful or are rejected by his partner. "Expert watching" or active role modeling can help the partner to learn effective comfort measures (Hodnett, 1996; Tomlinson & Bryan, 1996).

6. Inform him frequently of the woman's progress and her needs. Also keep him informed of procedures to be performed, what the procedures are for, and what is expected of him.

7. Prepare him for changes in the woman's behavior and physical appearance. This is especially true when the mother has just snapped at him and told him to go away. The nurse can reassure the father that this is normal behavior for a woman in transition and that, when he reenters the room after a few minutes, the woman may ask him why he was gone so long (Nichols, 1993).

8. Remind him to eat; offer him snacks and fluids if possible.

9. Relieve him of the job of support person as necessary; offer him blankets if he is to sleep in a chair by the bedside.

10. Acknowledge the stress experienced by each partner during the labor and birth and identify normal responses. The nonjudgmental attitude of staff members helps the father and mother accept their own and each other's behavior.

11. Attempt to modify or eliminate unsettling stimuli, such as extra noise and extra light.

A well-informed father can make an important contribution to the health and well-being of the mother and child, their family interrelationship, and his self-esteem.

Culture and Father Participation

A companion is an important source of support, encouragement, and comfort for women during childbirth. The nurse managing the care of pregnant women should help these women identify the person or persons they wish to be their supportive companions during childbirth. The choice of birth companion is influenced by the woman's cultural and religious background and by trends occurring within the society in which she lives. For example, in Western societies the father is being increasingly viewed as the ideal birth companion (Chalmers & Meyer, 1994). For European-American couples, attending childbirth classes together has become a traditional, expected activity–a rite of passage (Finn, 1994). Laotian (Hmong) husbands actively participate in the labor process, often by supporting their wife's position, catching the baby as it emerges, cutting the cord, and burying the placenta (D'Avanzo, 1992). A Mormon woman expects her husband to be present during her labor and to lay his hands on her head, in a blessing that imparts strength, comfort, and well-being for safe passage through childbirth (Callister, 1992, 1995). In some cultures the father may be available, but his presence in the labor room with the mother may not be considered appropriate or he may be present but resist active involvement in her care. Such behavior could be misconstrued by the nursing staff to represent a lack of concern, caring, or interest. Latina women expect their male partner to be present at their bedside during labor, to talk to them, keep them calm, and tell them everything is going to be okay and not to worry. The men are expected to show love and affection by telling the women they love them, by hugging them, and by holding their hand. However, Latino men do not become actively involved in giving their partners care during labor by performing such activities as backrubs and helping with pushing (Khazoyan & Anderson, 1994). Lantican and Corona (1992) identified the importance of the affectional bond Mexican-American and Filipina women have with their female relatives when it comes to home-related activities such as childbearing. This is also true for the women of many other cultural groups. The presence of another woman or women is highly desired at

such occasions. Women who come from some of these cultures and who give birth in the hospital like to have at least one woman present for assistance. Vietnamese, Chinese, and Indian women prefer a female companion during childbirth and are very concerned about their modesty (Choudhry, 1997; D'Avanzo, 1992). Islamic women are also very modest and would not accept the presence of a man during childbirth, not even the father (Woods, 1991). The religious beliefs of some Orthodox Jews forbid the father from touching his wife during labor or being present at the birth. Instead, while he prays, the female members of the laboring woman's family act as supportive childbirth companions (Callister, 1995; De Sevo, 1997). In India, women are attended by other women and in rural areas by a local untrained midwife or dai. Men usually are not present and in some cases may not be allowed to see the face of their child until certain prayers are said or an astrologically appropriate time is reached (Choudhry, 1997).

Support of the Grandparents

When grandparents act as labor coaches, it is especially important to support and treat them with respect. They may have a way to deal with pain relief based on their experience. They should be encouraged to help as long as their actions do not compromise the status of the mother or the fetus. Such an acceptable practice would be giving the woman herbal teas during labor. The nurse acts as a role model for clients by treating grandparents with dignity and respect, acknowledging the value of their contributions to supporting the woman, and recognizing the difficulty parents have in witnessing their child's discomfort or crisis, regardless of the child's age. If they have never witnessed a birth, the nurse may need to provide explanations of what is happening. Many of the activities used to support fathers are also appropriate for grandparents.

When possible, the nurse offers the grandparents emotional support. A nurse can show such support by offering them liquid refreshment and by initiating discussion with open-ended questions or statements, such as, "It is sometimes hard to watch a daughter in labor . . ." Nursing actions that provide support for the grandparents can have a therapeutic effect on all members of the family. In turn, a strong, supportive family unit is important for the optimal growth and development of its newest member.

Siblings During Labor

The preparation of siblings for acceptance of the new child helps promote the attachment process. Such preparation and participation during pregnancy and labor may help the older children accept this change. The older child or children who know themselves to be important to the family become active participants. Rehearsal for the event before labor is essential.

The age and developmental level of children influence their responses; therefore preparation for the children to

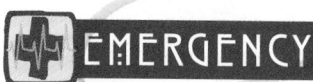

EMERGENCY

Interventions for Emergencies

SIGNS

Nonreassuring FHR Pattern

- Fetal bradycardia (FHR <110 beats/min for >10 min)†
- Fetal tachycardia (FHR >160 beats/min for >10 min in term pregnancy)§
- Irregular FHR, abnormal sinus rhythm shown by internal monitor
- Persistent decrease in baseline FHR variability without any identified cause
- Late, severe variable, and prolonged deceleration patterns
- Absence of FHR

INTERVENTIONS*

Notify primary health care provider‡
Change woman to side-lying position
Discontinue oxytocin (Pitocin) infusion, if being infused
Increase IV fluid rate, if fluid being infused per protocol order
Administer oxygen at 8 to 10 L/min by tight face mask
Check maternal temperature for elevation
Start an IV line if one is not in place
Administer amnioinfusion if ordered
Stimulate fetal scalp or use acoustic stimulation

Inadequate Uterine Relaxation

- Intrauterine pressure >75 mm Hg (shown by intrauterine pressure catheter monitoring)
- Contractions consistently lasting >90 sec
- Contraction interval <2 min

Notify primary health care provider‡
Discontinue oxytocin infusion, if being infused
Change woman to side-lying position
Increase IV fluid rate, if fluid is being infused
Administer oxygen at 8 to 10 L/min by tight face mask
Start an IV line if one is not in place
Palpate and evaluate contractions
Give tocolytics (terbutaline), as ordered

Vaginal Bleeding

- Vaginal bleeding (bright red, dark red, or in an amount in excess of that expected during normal cervical dilation)
- Continuous vaginal bleeding with FHR changes
- Pain; may or may not be present

Notify primary health care provider‡
Anticipate emergency (stat) cesarean birth
Do NOT perform a vaginal examination

*Because emergency situations are often frightening events, it is important for the nurse to explain to the woman and her support person what is happening and how it is being managed.

†Practice is to intervene within 2 to 30 min of FHR <110 beats/min.

‡In most emergency situations, nurses take immediate action, following a protocol and standards of nursing practice. Another person can notify the primary health care provider, or this can be done by the nurse as soon as possible.

§Nonreassuring sign when associated with late decelerations or absence of variability, especially of >180 beats/min.

be present during labor is adjusted to meet each child's needs. The child younger than 2 years of age shows little interest in pregnancy and labor; for the older child such preparation may reduce fears and misconceptions. Most parents have a "feel" for their children's maturational level and ability to cope. Preparation can include a description of the anticipated sights, smells, and sounds; a birth demonstration; a tour of the birthing unit; and an opportunity to be around a real newborn (Jonquil, 1993). Children must learn that their mother will be working hard during labor and birth. She will not be able to talk to them during contractions. She may groan and pant at times. They can be told that labor is uncomfortable but that their mother's body is made for the job. Storybooks about the birth process can be read to or by younger children to prepare them for the event. Films for preparing

older preschool and school-age children to participate in the birth experience are available. A specific person should be designated to watch over the children who are participating in their mother's childbirth experience, to provide them with support, explanations, diversions, and comfort as needed (Simkin, 1993).

Doulas

According to Proctor (1998), continuity of care has been cited by women as a critical component of a satisfying childbirth experience. These women expressed concern regarding a change in their caregiver when a new shift began. This need can be met by a specially trained, experienced female labor attendant called a **doula.** The doula provides a continuous, one-on-one caring presence throughout the labor and birth of the woman she is attending. The

✚ EMERGENCY—CONT'D

Interventions for Emergencies

Infection

- Foul-smelling amniotic fluid
- Maternal temperature >38° C in presence of adequate hydration (straw-colored urine)
- Fetal tachycardia >160 beats/min for >10 min

Notify primary health care provider‡
Institute cooling measures for laboring woman
Start an IV line if one is not in place
Assist with or perform collection of catheterized urine specimen and amniotic fluid sample and send to the laboratory for urinalysis and cultures

Prolapse of Cord

- Fetal bradycardia with variable deceleration during uterine contraction
- Woman reports feeling the cord after membranes rupture
- Cord lies alongside or below the presenting part of the fetus; can be seen or felt in or protruding from the vagina
- Major predisposing factors:
  - Rupture of membranes with a gush
  - Loose fit of presenting part in lower uterine segment
  - Presenting part not yet engaged

Call for assistance
Have someone notify the primary health care provider immediately
Glove the examining hand quickly and insert two fingers into the vagina to the cervix; with one finger on either side of the cord or both fingers to one side, exert upward pressure against the presenting part to relieve compression of the cord
Place a rolled towel under the woman's hip
Place woman in extreme Trendelenburg or modified Sims position or knee-chest position
Wrap the cord loosely in a sterile towel saturated with warm sterile normal saline if the cord is protruding from the vagina
Administer oxygen at 8 to 10 L/min by face mask until birth is accomplished
Start IV fluids or increase existing drip rate
Continue to monitor FHR by internal fetal scalp electrode, if possible
Do not attempt to replace cord into cervix
Prepare for immediate birth (vaginal or cesarean)

---

primary role of the doula is to focus on the laboring woman and provide physical and emotional support by using soft, reassuring words; touching, stroking, and hugging; administering comfort measures to reduce pain and enhance relaxation; and walking with the woman, helping her to change positions, and coaching her bearing-down efforts.

Another role of the doula is to support the woman's partner, who often feels unqualified to be the sole labor support. The doula can encourage and praise the partner's efforts, create a partnership as caregivers, and provide respite care. Doulas also facilitate communication between the laboring woman and her partner, as well as between the couple and the health care team (Perez & Herrick, 1998; Simkin, 1996; Simkin & Way, 1998; Zhang et al., 1996).

Based on an analysis of several research studies, Klaus and co-workers (1993) found that the continuous care provided by doulas significantly reduces the overall cesarean birth rate; duration of labor; use of oxytocin, analgesics, and forceps; and requests for epidural anesthesia. Laboring

women also reported a higher level of satisfaction with their childbirth experience and greater success with breastfeeding. More long-term benefits of doula care are reflected in more positive maternal feelings regarding their parenting ability and closer interaction with their infants up to 1 year after birth (Landry et al., 1998; Trowell, 1993).

The role of the nurse and the doula are complementary. They should work together as a team with the doula providing supportive nonmedical care measures and with the nurse focusing on monitoring the status of the maternal-fetal unit; implementing clinical care protocols, including pharmacologic interventions; and documenting assessment findings, actions, and responses.

Emergency Interventions

Emergency conditions that require immediate nursing intervention can arise with startling speed. A nonreassuring FHR, inadequate uterine relaxation, vaginal bleeding, infection, and prolapse of the cord are highlighted in the Emergency box. Interventions for immediate use are listed.

Preparation for Giving Birth

The first stage of labor ends with the complete dilation of the cervix. For many multiparous women, birth usually occurs within minutes of complete dilation, perhaps only one push later. Nulliparous women usually push for 1 to 2 hours before giving birth. If the woman has been given epidural anesthesia, pushing can last more than 2 hours. The nurse begins to prepare for birth when a multiparous woman is 6 to 8 cm dilated, because progression during the last few centimeters of dilation can occur rapidly. Factors that influence the process are fetal position and the size of the baby in relation to previous babies.

Birth Setting

Significant changes have occurred in the location where birth takes place. The most common change in birth settings is the LDRP room, where the woman stays during her entire hospitalization (see Fig. 18-1). This avoids the necessity of multiple transfers of the woman from the labor room to the delivery room to a recovery room and then to a postpartum unit. Another option is the LDR room, where the woman stays during her labor and immediate postpartum recovery period (1 to 2 hours) before her transfer to a postpartum room, where she stays for the remainder of her hospitalization. Some hospitals, however, lack birthing rooms, and transfer during the second stage is required. If birth is to occur in the delivery room, it is best to transfer the woman early enough to avoid a last-minute rush. For nulliparous women, transfer can take place when the presenting part begins to distend the perineum. For multiparous women, transfer should take place in the first stage, when the cervix is dilated 8 to 9 cm.

Birthing centers are another option. Women give birth in a homelike setting and are discharged after they and their newborn are stable (see Fig. 18-2).

The home is a safe alternative to the hospital or birth center as a site of birth for the motivated low risk woman. Prior planning is essential to ensure that the birth will be attended by an experienced home birth practitioner and that backup at a hospital is available should complications arise requiring transfer. Research indicates that women who participate in home birth use a greater variety of positions for childbirth, need fewer pharmacologic pain relief measures as a result of feeling more relaxed in their own environment, and experience less severe perineal trauma (Olsen, 1997; Wraight, 1997).

Evaluation

Evaluation of progress and outcomes is a continuous activity during the first stage of labor. The nurse must carefully evaluate each interaction with the mother-to-be and her family and critically appraise how well the formulated outcomes for care are being met.

SECOND STAGE OF LABOR

The **second stage of labor** is the stage in which the fetus is born. It begins at full cervical dilation (10 cm) and complete effacement (100%) and ends with the baby's birth. The force exerted by uterine contractions, gravity, and maternal bearing-down efforts facilitates achievement of the expected outcome of a spontaneous, uncomplicated vaginal birth.

The second stage comprises three phases: the latent, descent, and transition phases. Each phase is characterized by maternal verbal and nonverbal behaviors, uterine activity, the urge to bear down, and fetal descent. The latent phase is a period of rest and relative calm. The woman is quiet and often relaxes with her eyes closed between contractions. The urge to bear down is not well established and is experienced primarily during the acme of a contraction. The descent phase is characterized by strong urges to bear down as the **Ferguson reflex** is activated when the presenting part presses on the stretch receptors of the pelvic floor. This stimulation causes the release of oxytocin from the posterior pituitary gland, which provokes stronger expulsive uterine contractions. The woman becomes more focused on bearing-down efforts, which become rhythmic. She changes positions frequently to find a more comfortable position in which to push. The woman frequently announces the onset of contractions and becomes more vocal as she bears down. In the *transition phase*, the presenting part is on the perineum and bearing-down efforts are most effective for promoting birth. The woman may be more verbal about the pain she is experiencing; she may scream or swear and may act out of control (Aderhold & Roberts, 1991). The nurse encourages the woman to "listen" to her body as she progresses through the phases of the second stage of labor. When a woman listens to her body to tell her when to bear down, she is using an internal locus of control and often feels more satisfied with her efforts to give birth to her baby. Her sense of self-esteem and accomplishment is enhanced. The woman's trust in her own body and her ability to give birth to her baby should be fostered (Cosner & deJong, 1993; d'Entremont, 1996; Rothman, 1996).

▪ CARE MANAGEMENT

Assessment and Nursing Diagnoses

The only certain objective sign that the second stage of labor has begun is the inability to feel the cervix during vaginal examination, indicating that the cervix is fully dilated and effaced. The precise moment that this occurs is not easily determined (Bennett & Brown, 1993). Other signs that suggest the onset of the second stage include the following:

- Sudden appearance of sweat on upper lip
- An episode of vomiting
- Increased bloody show
- Shaking of extremities

- Increased restlessness; verbalization (e.g., "I can't go on")
- Involuntary bearing-down efforts

These signs commonly appear at the time the cervix reaches full dilation (Bennett & Brown, 1993; Scott et al., 1999). However, women with an epidural block may not exhibit such signs. Other indicators for each phase of the second stage are given in Table 22-5.

Women can begin to experience an irresistible urge to bear down before full dilation. For some women, this occurs as early as 5 cm dilation. An early or premature sensation of an urge to bear down is most often related to the station of the presenting part below the level of the ischial spines of the maternal pelvis. This occurrence creates a conflict between the woman, whose body is telling her to push, and her health care providers, who believe that pushing the fetal presenting part against an incompletely dilated cervix will result in cervical edema and damage, as well as a slowing down of labor progress. The premature urge to bear down must be evaluated as a phase of labor progress possibly indicating the onset of the second stage of labor. In addition, the consequences of pushing against a partially dilated cervix must be determined with research findings. When a woman pushes in relation to the degree of cervical dilation should be based on research evidence rather than tradition or routine practice (Bergstrom et al., 1997; Cosner & deJong, 1993; Varney, 1997).

TABLE 22-5 Expected Maternal Progress in Second Stage of Labor

CRITERION	LATENT PHASE (AVERAGE DURATION, 10-30 MIN)	DESCENT PHASE (AVERAGE DURATION VARIES)*	TRANSITION PHASE (AVERAGE DURATION 5-15 MIN)
Contractions Magnitude (intensity)	Period of physiologic lull for all criteria; period of peace and rest	Significant increase	Overwhelmingly strong Expulsive
Frequency		2-2.5 min	1-2 min
Duration		90 sec	90 sec
Descent, station	0 to +2	Increases and Ferguson reflex† activated, +2 to +4	Rapid, +4 to birth Fetal head visible in introitus; bloody show accompanies birth of head
Show: color and amount		Significant increase in dark red bloody show	
Spontaneous bearing-down efforts	Slight to absent, except during acme of strongest contractions	Increased urge to bear down	Greatly increased
Vocalization	Quiet; concern over progress	Grunting sounds or expiratory vocalization; announces contractions	Grunting sounds and expiratory vocalizations continue; may scream or swear
Maternal behavior	Experiences sense of relief that transition to second stage is finished Feels fatigued and sleepy Feels a sense of accomplishment and optimism, because the "worst is over" Feels in control	Senses increased urge to push Alters respiratory pattern: has short 4 to 5 sec breath holds with regular breaths in between, 5 to 7 times per contraction Makes grunting sounds or expiratory vocalizations Frequent repositioning	Describes extreme pain Expresses feelings of powerlessness Shows decreased ability to listen or concentrate on anything but giving birth Describes **ring of fire** (burning sensation of acute pain as vagina stretches and fetal head crowns) Often shows excitement immediately after birth of head

From Anderhold, K., & Roberts, J. (1991). Phases of second stage labor: four descriptive case studies. *J Nurse Midwifery* 36(5), 267-275; Mahan, C., & McKay, S. (1984). Are we overmanaging second stage labor? *Contemp OB/GYN* 24, 37-63.
*Duration of descent phase can vary depending on maternal parity, effectiveness of bearing-down effort, and presence of spinal anesthesia or epidural analgesia.
†Pressure of presenting part on stretch receptors of pelvic floor stimulates release of oxytocin from posterior pituitary, resulting in more intense uterine contractions.

Assessment is continuous during the second stage of labor. Hospital protocol determines the specific type and timing of assessments, as well as the way in which findings are documented. The Care Path for the second and third stages of labor indicates typical assessments and the recommended frequency for their performance. Signs and symptoms of impending birth (see Table 22-5) may appear unexpectedly, requiring immediate action by the nurse (Box 22-5).

Duration of Second Stage

The duration of the second stage of labor is influenced by several factors, such as the effectiveness of the primary and secondary powers of labor; the type and amount of analgesia or anesthesia used; the physical and emotional condition, position, activity level, and parity of the laboring woman; and the nature and source of support the woman receives. There is considerable controversy over the precise duration of the second stage of labor and the time limits that should be regarded as normal. Friedman's (Friedman & Sachtleben, 1965) curves for nulliparous and multiparous women are commonly used to determine the progress of the second stage. On the basis of these data the range and average duration of the second stage of labor vary with parity:

Parity	Range (min)	Average (min)
First pregnancy	25-75	57
Subsequent pregnancy	13-17	14.4

A second stage of more than 2 hours in a first pregnancy and of 1.5 hours in subsequent pregnancies may be considered prolonged in women without regional analgesia and is reported to the primary health care provider. Using assessment findings such as the FHR and pattern, the descent of the presenting part, the quality of the uterine contractions, and the status of the woman, premature intervention such as the use of episiotomies, forceps, and vacuum extraction can be avoided.

If the status of the maternal-fetal unit is reassuring and progress is continuing, interventions to end the second stage of labor are unwarranted. The duration of active pushing has been found to be more relevant to the newborn's condition at birth than the duration of the second stage of labor itself (d'Entremont, 1996; Peterson & Besuner, 1997; Roberts & Woolley, 1996).

The second stage may be prolonged in the woman who has an epidural block, which causes the urge to bear down to be lost or reduced and her ability to attain an upright position to be inhibited. By adjusting dosages to the lowest effective level, allowing the epidural to wear off, or using mixtures containing a narcotic and a local anesthetic, the woman is able to more fully perceive the urge to bear down, to move more freely, and to attain an upright position as a result of increased strength and sensation in her legs. This approach will enhance her ability to bear down effectively and achieve an uncomplicated vaginal birth (Cosner & deJong, 1993; Shermer & Raines, 1997).

Aderhold and Roberts (1991) found that encouraging the woman to assume various positions during the second stage can also help the fetus to maneuver down and out of the pelvis. The Association of Women's Health, Obstetric, and Neonatal Nurses conducted research on the way in which nurses manage second-stage labor, and findings indicate that many nurses do encourage a variety of maternal positions and spontaneous bearing-down efforts (Jordan, 1995). Nursing diagnoses that represent potential areas for concern during the second stage of labor include the following:

▌ Nursing Diagnoses _____

- Risk for injury to mother and fetus related to
  - persistent use of Valsalva maneuver during bearing-down efforts
- Situational low self-esteem related to
  - lack of knowledge regarding normal, beneficial effects of vocalization during bearing-down efforts
  - inability to carry out birth plan without medication
- Ineffective individual coping related to
  - coaching that contradicts woman's physiologic urge to push
- Pain related to
  - bearing-down efforts and distention of the perineum
- Anxiety related to
  - inability to control defecation with bearing-down efforts
  - lack of knowledge regarding and inexperience with perineal sensations associated with the urge to bear down
- Risk for maternal injury related to
  - inappropriate positioning of mother's legs in stirrups
- Risk for infection related to
  - prolonged rupture of membranes
  - perineal trauma
- Situational low self-esteem (partner or father) related to
  - inability to support mother during second stage of labor

Expected Outcomes of Care

Planning for the second and third stages of labor is done during the first stage of labor. Previously determined expected outcomes may be modified as these stages progress. Expected outcomes for the woman in the second stage of labor may include that the woman will do the following:
- Actively participate in the labor process.
- Sustain no injury during the labor process (nor will the fetus).
- Accept comfort and support measures from significant others and health care providers as needed.

1. The woman usually assumes the position most comfortable for her. A lateral position is often recommended.
2. Reassure the woman that birth is usually uncomplicated and easy in these situations. Use eye-to-eye contact and a calm, relaxed manner. If there is someone else available, such as the partner, that person could help support the woman in the position, assist with coaching, and compliment her on her efforts.
3. Wash your hands and put on gloves, if available.
4. Place under woman's buttocks whatever clean material is available.
5. Avoid touching the vaginal area to decrease the possibility of infection.
6. As the head begins to crown, you should do the following:
   a. Tear the amniotic membrane if it is still intact.
   b. Instruct the woman to pant or pant-blow, thus minimizing the urge to push.
   c. Place the flat side of your hand on the exposed fetal head and apply *gentle* pressure toward the vagina to prevent the head from "popping out." The mother may participate by placing her hand under yours on the emerging head. Note: Rapid delivery of the fetal head must be prevented because a rapid change of pressure within the molded fetal skull follows, which may result in dural or subdural tears and may cause vaginal or perineal lacerations.
7. After the birth of the head, check for the umbilical cord. If the cord is around the baby's neck, try to slip it over the baby's head or pull it *gently* to get some slack so that you can slip it over the shoulders.
8. Support the fetal head as restitution (external rotation) occurs. After restitution, with one hand on each side of the baby's head, exert *gentle* pressure downward so that the anterior shoulder emerges under the symphysis pubis and acts as a fulcrum; then, as *gentle* pressure is exerted in the opposite direction, the posterior shoulder, which has passed over the sacrum and coccyx, emerges.
9. Be alert! Hold the baby securely because the rest of the body may emerge quickly. The baby will be slippery!
10. Cradle the baby's head and back in one hand and the buttocks in the other. Keep the head down to drain away the mucus. Use a bulb syringe, if one is available, to remove mucus from the baby's mouth.
11. Dry the baby quickly to prevent rapid heat loss. Keep the baby at the same level as the mother's uterus until the end of the cord stops pulsating. Note: It is important to keep the baby at the same level as the mother's uterus to prevent the baby's blood from flowing to or from the placenta and the resultant hypovolemia or hypervolemia. Also, do not "milk" the cord.
12. Place the baby on the mother's abdomen, cover the baby (remember to keep the head warm, too) with the mother's clothing, and have her cuddle the baby. Compliment her (them) on a job well done, and on the baby, if appropriate.
13. *Wait* for the placenta to separate; *do not* tug on the cord. Note: Injudicious traction may tear the cord, separate the placenta, or invert the uterus. Signs of placental separation include a slight gush of dark blood from the introitus, lengthening of the cord, and change in the uterine contour from a discoid to globular shape.
14. Instruct the mother to push to deliver the separated placenta. Gently ease out the placental membranes using an up-and-down motion until the membranes are removed. If birth occurs outside a hospital setting, to minimize complications, do not cut the cord without proper clamps and a sterile cutting tool. Inspect the placenta for intactness. Place the baby on the placenta and wrap the two together for additional warmth.
15. Check the firmness of the uterus. Gently massage the fundus and demonstrate to the mother how she can massage her own fundus properly.
16. If supplies are available, clean the mother's perineal area and apply a peripad.
17. In addition to gentle massage of the fundus, the following measures can be taken to prevent or minimize hemorrhage:
   a. Put the baby to the mother's breast as soon as possible. Sucking or nuzzling and licking the nipple stimulates the release of oxytocin from the posterior pituitary. Note: If the baby does not or cannot nurse, manually stimulate the mother's nipples.
   b. Do not allow the mother's bladder to become distended. Assess the bladder for fullness and encourage her to void if fullness is found.
   c. Expel any clots from the mother's uterus.
18. Comfort or reassure the mother and her family or friends. Keep the mother and the baby warm. Give her fluids if available and tolerated.
19. If this is a multifetal birth, identify the infants in order of birth (using letters *A, B,* etc.).
20. Make notations regarding the following aspects of the birth:
   a. Fetal presentation and position
   b. Presence of cord around neck (nuchal cord) or other parts and number of times cord encircled part
   c. Color, character, and amount of amniotic fluid, if rupture of membranes occurs immediately before birth
   d. Time of birth
   e. Estimated time of determination of Apgar score (e.g., 1 and 5 minutes after birth), resuscitation efforts implemented, and ultimate condition of baby
   f. Sex of baby
   g. Time of placental expulsion, as well as the appearance and completeness of the placenta
   h. Maternal condition: affect, amount of bleeding, and status of uterine tonicity
   i. Any unusual occurrences during the birth (e.g., maternal or paternal response, verbalizations, or gestures in response to birth of baby)

Plan of Care and Interventions

The nurse implements plans to continuously monitor the second stage and mechanism of birth, the maternal physiologic and emotional responses to the second stage, the partner's response to the second stage, and the fetal response to the stress of the second stage.

The nurse continues to provide comfort measures for the mother, such as positioning; providing mouth care; maintaining clean, dry bedding; and keeping extraneous noise, conversation, and other distractions (e.g., laughing, talking of attending personnel in or outside the labor area) to a minimum. The woman is encouraged to indicate other support measures she would like (Table 22-6) (see also Plan of Care and Care Path, p. 531).

If the mother is to be transferred to another area for birth, the nurse accomplishes the transfer early enough to avoid rushing the woman. The birth area also is readied for the birth.

Prebirth Considerations

Maternal position. There is no single position for childbirth. Labor is a dynamic, interactive process involving the woman's uterus, pelvis, and voluntary muscles. In addition, angles between the baby and the woman's pelvis constantly change as the infant turns and flexes down the birth canal. The woman may want to assume various positions for childbirth, and she should be encouraged and assisted in attaining and maintaining her position(s) of choice. Hanson (1998a) found that sitting and side lying

TABLE 22-6	Woman's Responses and Support Person's Action During Second Stage of Labor
WOMAN'S RESPONSES	**NURSE/SUPPORT PERSON'S ACTIONS***
LATENT PHASE	
Experiences a short period of peace and rest	Encourages woman to "listen" to her body
	Continues support measures
	Suggests an upright position to encourage progression of descent if descent phase does not begin after 20 min
DESCENT PHASE	
Senses increased urgency to bear down as Ferguson reflex is activated	Encourages respiratory pattern of short breath holds
Notes increase in intensity of uterine contractions—alters respiratory pattern: short 4- to 5-sec breath holds, 5 to 7 times per contraction	Stresses normality and benefits of grunting sounds and expiratory vocalizations
Makes grunting sounds or expiratory vocalizations	Encourages bearing-down efforts with urge to push
	Encourages/suggests maternal movement and position changes (upright, if descent is not occurring)
	Encourages woman to "listen" to her body regarding movement and position change if descent is occurring
	Discourages long breath holds
	If birth is to occur in a delivery room, transfers woman to delivery room early to avoid rushing or, if permitted, offers her option of walking to delivery room
	Places woman in lateral recumbent position to slow descent if descent is too fast
TRANSITIONAL PHASE	
Behaves in manner similar to behavior during transition in first stage (8-10 cm)	Encourages slow, gentle pushing
Experiences a sense of severe pain and powerlessness	Explains that "blowing away the contraction" facilitates a slower birth of the head
Shows decreased ability to listen	Provides mirror to help woman see or touch the emerging fetal head (best to extend over two to three contractions) to help her understand the perineal sensations
Concentrates on birth of baby until head is born	
Experiences contractions as overwhelming in intensity	
Reports feeling ring of fire as head crowns	Coaches woman to relax mouth, throat, and neck to promote relaxation of pelvic floor
Maintains respiratory pattern of three to five 7-sec breath holds per contraction, followed by forced expiration	Applies warm compress to perineum to promote relaxation
Eases head out with short expirations	
Responds with excitement and relief after head is born	

*Provided by nurses and support persons in collaboration with the nurse.

are the two most common positions assumed by women for their bearing-down efforts and birth.

Birth attendants play a major role in influencing a woman's choice of positions for birth, with midwives tending to advocate the nonlithotomy positions for the second stage of labor (Hanson, 1998b). Upright positions facilitate birth in the following ways:

- Straighten the longitudinal axis of the birth canal
- Use gravity to direct the fetal head toward the pelvic inlet, thereby facilitating descent
- Enlarge pelvic dimensions and restrict the encroachment of the sacrum and coccyx into the pelvic outlet
- Increase uteroplacental circulation, resulting in more intense, efficient uterine contractions
- Enhance the woman's ability to bear down effectively, thereby minimizing maternal exhaustion (Shermer & Raines, 1997)

One upright position found to be highly effective in facilitating the descent and birth of the fetus is squatting (Andrews & Chrzanowski, 1990; Golay, Vedam, & Sorger, 1993; Roberts & Woolley, 1996). Women should assume a modified, supported squat until the fetal head is engaged, at which time a deep squat can be used. A firm surface is required for this position, and the woman will need side support. In a birthing bed a squat bar is available that she can use to help support herself.

A birth ball can help a woman maintain the squatting position. The fetus will be aligned with the birth canal, and pelvic and perineal relaxation will be facilitated as she sits on the ball or holds it in front of her for support as she squats (Perez, 1998).

When a woman uses the standing position for bearing down, her weight is borne on both femoral heads, allowing the pressure in the acetabulum to cause the transverse diameter of the pelvic outlet to increase by up to 1 cm. This can be helpful if descent of the head is delayed because the occiput has not rotated from the lateral (transverse diameter of pelvis) to the anterior position (Biancuzzo, 1993). Birthing chairs or rocking chairs may be used to provide women with a good physiologic position to enhance her bearing-down efforts during childbirth, although some women feel restricted by a chair. There is also a potential psychologic advantage to the upright position in that it allows the mother to see the birth as it occurs and also to maintain eye contact with the attendant. Most birthing chairs are designed so that if an emergency occurs, the chair can be adjusted to the horizontal or the Trendelenburg position.

PLAN OF CARE Second Stage of Labor

NURSING DIAGNOSIS Risk for ineffective individual coping related to birthing process and fatigue of labor

Expected Outcome *Woman actively participates in the birth process with no evidence of injury to her or her fetus.*

Nursing Interventions/*Rationales*

Constantly monitor events of second-stage labor and birth, including physiologic responses of woman and fetus, emotional responses of woman and partner, *to ensure maternal, partner, and fetal well-being.*

Provide ongoing feedback to woman and partner *to allay anxiety and enhance participation.*

Continue to provide comfort measures such as positioning; mouth care; clean, dry bedding; cool cloth on forehead; and minimizing distractions *to decrease discomfort and aid in focus on the birth process.*

Encourage woman to experiment with various positions *to assist downward movement of fetus.*

Ensure that woman takes deep cleansing breaths before and after each contraction *to enhance gas exchange and oxygen transport to the fetus.*

Encourage woman to push spontaneously when urge to bear down is perceived during a contraction *to aid descent and rotation of fetus.*

Teach partner about importance of spontaneous bearing down *to avoid coaching to push, which may contradict or inhibit these spontaneous urges.*

Remind woman not to hold her breath but rather exhale, taking only short breath holds while bearing down *because holding breath may trigger a Valsalva maneuver and increase intrathoracic and cardiovascular pressure and decrease perfusion of placental oxygen, placing the fetus at risk.*

Encourage woman to vocalize as she bears down *to enhance efforts.*

Have woman take deep breaths and relax between contractions *to reduce fatigue and increase effectiveness of pushing efforts.*

If woman seems reluctant to bear down, assess possible contributing factors (e.g., doubts about readiness as a mother, desire for an absent person to be present, fear of the pain of pushing, embarrassment of passing stool while pushing, fear that baby will be in danger when no longer in uterus) and address specific concern *so that woman can participate in labor process effectively.*

Have mother pant as fetal head crowns *to control birth of head.*

From Wong, D., & Perry, S. (1998). *Maternal child nursing care.* St. Louis: Mosby.

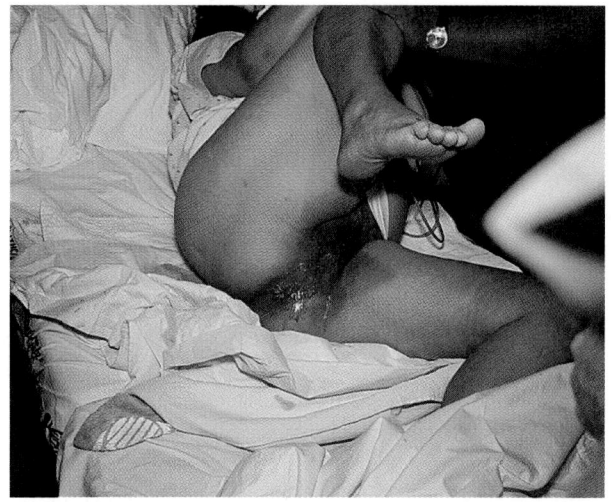

A

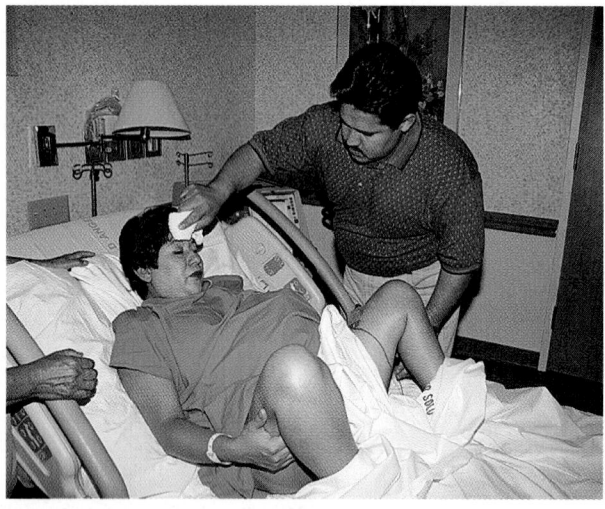

B

Fig. 22-18 **A,** Pushing, side-lying position. Perineal bulging can be seen. **B,** Pushing, semi-sitting position. Partner is wiping woman's face with cool cloth between contractions. (*A, Courtesy Michael S. Clement, MD, Mesa, AZ.* **B,** *Courtesy Marjorie Pyle, RNC, Lifecircle, Costa Mesa, CA.*)

In some hospitals, oversized beanbag chairs and large floor pillows are used for both labor and birth. They can mold around and support the mother in whatever position she selects. These chairs are of particular value for mothers who wish to be actively involved in the birth process. Birthing stools can be used to support the woman in an upright position similar to squatting (Waldenström & Gottvall, 1991).

Women may want to sit on the toilet or commode during pushing because they are concerned about stool incontinence during this stage. These women must be closely monitored, however, and removed from the toilet before birth becomes imminent.

Because sitting on chairs, stools, toilets, or commodes can increase perineal edema and blood loss, it is important

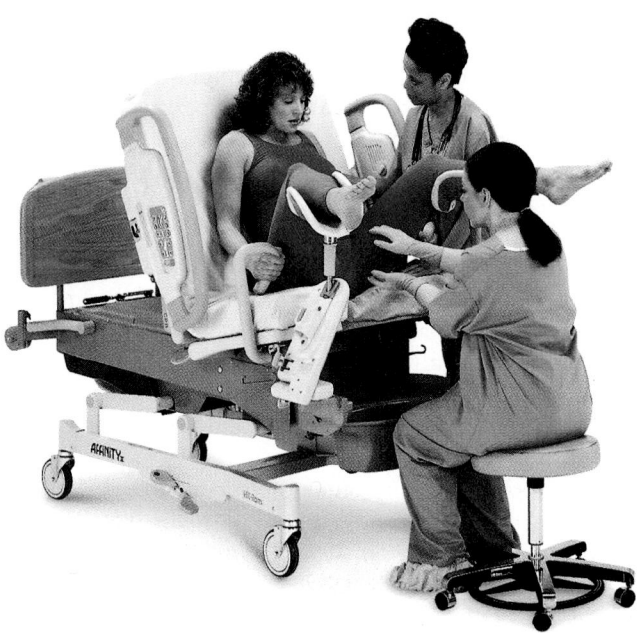

Fig. 22-19 Birth bed. (*Courtesy Hill-Rom, Batesville, IN.*)

to assist the woman to change her position every 10 to 15 minutes (Shermer & Raines, 1997; Waldenström & Gottvall, 1991).

Another second-stage position is the side-lying position, with the upper part of the woman's leg held by the nurse or coach or placed on a pillow (Fig. 22-18, *A*). Some women prefer a semi-sitting position. To maintain good uteroplacental circulation and to enhance the woman's bearing-down efforts in this position, the woman's back and shoulders should be elevated to at least a 30-degree angle and a wedge should be placed under one hip (Fig. 22-18, *B*).

The hands-and-knees position is an effective position for birth because it enhances placental perfusion, helps rotate the fetus from a posterior to an anterior position, and may facilitate the birth of the shoulders, especially if the fetus is large. Perineal trauma may also be reduced (Biancuzzo, 1991; Gannon, 1992).

The nurse should frequently assess the effect of maternal positions on fetal status. If the woman is reluctant or afraid to try different positions, the nurse should actively encourage and help the woman to do so. Information regarding the variety of effective childbirth positions should be an essential component of prepared childbirth classes.

The birthing bed is commonly used today and can be set for different positions according to the woman's needs (Figs. 22-19 and 22-20). The woman can squat, kneel, sit, recline, or lie on her side, choosing the position most comfortable for her without having to climb into bed for the birth. Squat bars, over-the-bed tables, birth balls, and pillows can be used for support. The birthing bed affords excellent exposure for the performance of examinations, the

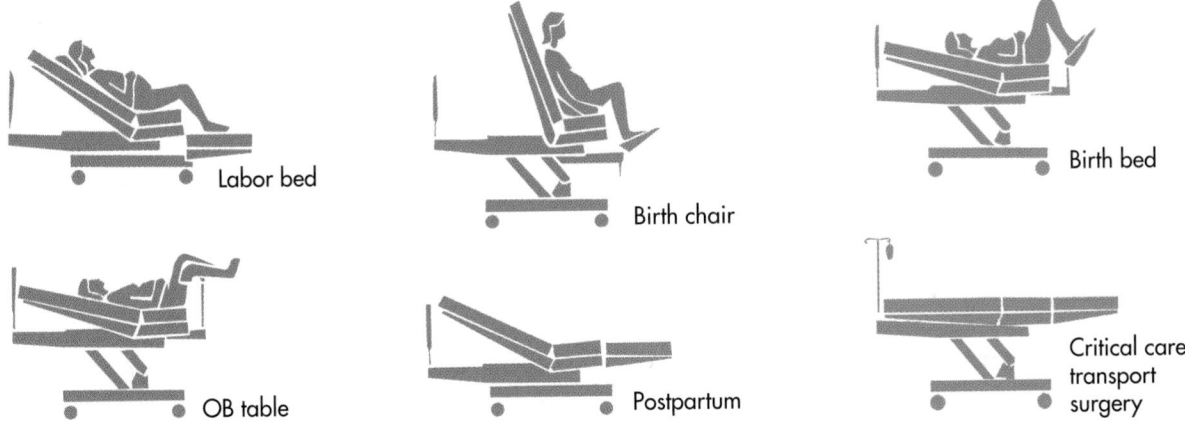

Fig. 22-20 The versatility of today's birthing bed makes it practical in a variety of settings. Note: OB table used for *lithotomy position. (Courtesy Hill-Rom, Batesville, IN.)*

placement of internal monitoring devices, and birth. By using the birthing bed, the woman has full control of both seat and back functions and can adjust her position for maximum comfort. The bed also can be positioned for the administration of anesthesia and is ideal to help women receiving an epidural to assume different positions to facilitate birth. The bed can be used to transport the woman to the operating room if a cesarean birth is necessary.

Bearing-down efforts. As the fetal head reaches the pelvic floor, most women experience the urge to bear down. Reflexively the woman will begin to exert downward pressure by contracting her abdominal muscles while relaxing her pelvic floor. This bearing down is an involuntary response to the Ferguson reflex, which is activated by the presenting part pressing on stretch receptors of the pelvic musculature.

When coaching women to push, the nurse should encourage them to push as they feel like pushing (instinctive, spontaneous pushing) rather than to give a prolonged push on command (Thomson, 1993). The nurse should watch the woman's breathing to make sure she does not hold her breath for more than 5 to 7 seconds at a time (Roberts & Woolley, 1996). Bearing down while exhaling (open-glottis pushing) and taking breaths between bearing-down efforts help maintain adequate oxygen levels for the mother and fetus and results in approximately five to six pushes during a contraction, with each push lasting about 5 seconds (d'Entremont, 1996).

A strong expiratory grunt or groan (vocalization) often accompanies pushing when the woman exhales as she pushes This natural vocalization by women during open-glottis bearing-down efforts is likely to be discouraged by nurses in part to "conserve the woman's energy" but also as a result of concern that it will seem to other nurses and clients that the woman has lost control or the nurse has lost control of her client (McKay & Roberts, 1990; Peterson & Besuner, 1997).

Prolonged breath-holding, or sustained, directed bearing down, which is still a common practice, may trigger the **Valsalva maneuver,** which occurs when the woman

closes the glottis (closed-glottis pushing), thereby increasing intrathoracic and cardiovascular pressure. This approach to bearing down is harmful or ineffective and should be discouraged (Enkin et al., 1995; Metzer & Therrien, 1990; Technical Working Group of the World Health Organization, 1997).

In addition, holding the breath for more than 5 to 7 seconds causes the perfusion of oxygen across the placenta to be diminished, resulting in fetal hypoxia. The nurse should remind the woman to take deep breaths to fully ventilate her lungs before and after each contraction (Hodnett, 1996).

A woman may reach the second stage of labor and then experience a lack of readiness to complete the process and give birth to her child. McKay and Barrows (1991) identified several factors that may cause a woman to lessen her voluntary bearing-down efforts:

- Doubts about her readiness to be a mother
- Reluctance to care for another baby
- Desire to wait for support person or primary health care provider to arrive
- Fear or anxiety regarding the unfamiliar or painful sensations of the second stage of labor and pushing
- Embarrassment regarding behaviors during pushing, including sounds made and the passage of stool
- Giving up and not wanting to proceed any further toward a vaginal birth
- Fear that the baby will be in danger once it emerges from the protective intrauterine environment

By recognizing that a woman may experience a need to hold back the birth of her baby, the nurse can then address the woman's concerns and effectively coach the woman during this stage of labor.

To ensure the slow birth of the fetal head, the nurse should encourage the woman to control the urge to bear down by coaching her to take panting breaths or to exhale slowly through pursed lips as the baby's head crowns. At this point the woman needs simple, clear directions from one person.

Amnesia between contractions often is pronounced in the second stage, and the woman may have to be roused to get her to cooperate in the bearing-down process. Parents who have attended childbirth education classes may have devised a set of verbal cues for the laboring woman to follow. It is helpful for them to have these cues printed on a card that can be attached to the head of the bed so that the nurse can better substitute as coach if the partner has to leave.

Fetal heart rate and pattern. As noted previously, the FHR must be checked. If the rate begins to slow or if there is a loss of variability, prompt treatment must be initiated. The woman can be turned on her side to reduce the pressure of the uterus against the ascending vena cava and de-

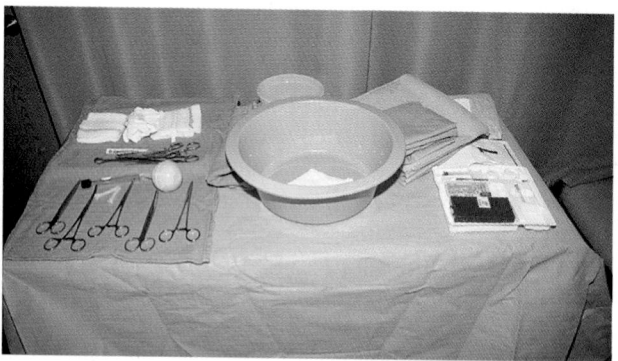

Fig. 22-21 Instrument table. *(Courtesy Marjorie Pyle, RNC, Lifecircle, Costa Mesa, CA.)*

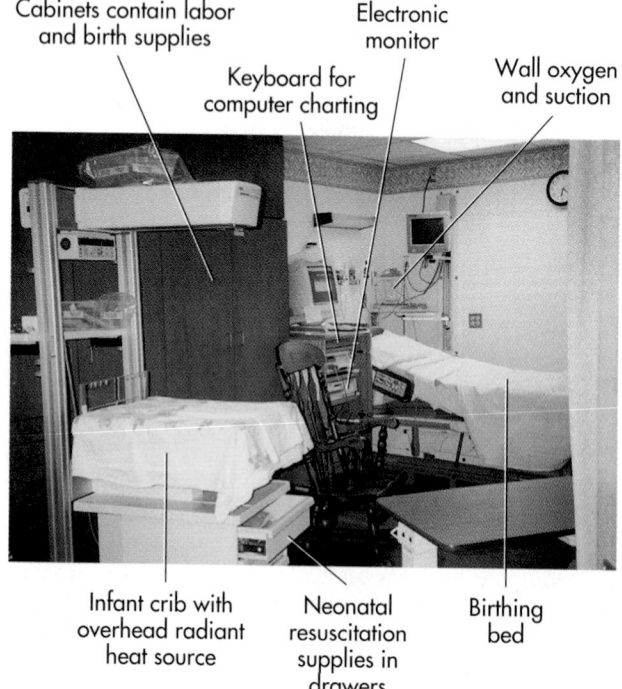

Fig. 22-22 Birthing room. *(Courtesy Dee Lowdermilk, Chapel Hill, NC.)*

scending aorta (see Fig. 22-4), and oxygen can be administered by mask at 8 to 10 L/min. This is often all that is necessary to restore the normal rate. If the FHR does not return to a normal rate immediately, the primary health care provider should be notified quickly because medical intervention may be indicated to hasten the birth.

Support of the father or coach. During the second stage the woman needs continuous support and coaching (see Table 22-6). Because the coaching process can be physically and emotionally tiring for support persons, the nurse offers them nourishment and fluids and encourages them to take short breaks. The support person who attends the birth in a delivery room is instructed to put on a cover gown or scrub clothes, mask, hat, and shoe covers, as required. The nurse also specifies support measures he or she can use for the laboring woman and points out areas of the room in which the partner can move freely. If birth occurs in an LDR or LDRP room, the partner may be allowed to wear street clothes or be required to wear a clean scrub outfit, cap, and mask (for the birth).

Partners are encouraged to be present at the birth of their infants if this is in keeping with their cultural and personal expectations and beliefs. In this way the psychologic closeness of the family unit is maintained and the partner can continue to provide the supportive care given during labor. The woman and her partner need to have an equal opportunity to initiate the attachment process with the baby.

LEGAL TIP Documentation

Documentation of all observations (e.g., maternal vital signs, FHR and pattern, progress of labor) and nursing interventions, including client response, should be done concurrently with care. The course of labor and the maternal-fetal response may change without warning. It is important that all documentation be accurate, complete, and timely. Documentation is usually done in the labor and delivery record, as well as on the monitor strip.

Supplies, instruments, and equipment. To prepare for birth in any setting, the birthing table or case cart is usually set up during the transition phase for nulliparous women and during the active phase for multiparous women.

The birthing table is prepared, and instruments are arranged on the instrument table (Fig. 22-21). Standard procedures are followed for gloving, identifying and opening sterile packages, adding sterile supplies to the instrument table, and unwrapping and handing sterile instruments to the primary health care provider. The crib and equipment are readied for the support and stabilization of the infant. A radiant warmer for the newborn is turned on when crowning begins to occur in the nulliparous woman and when the multiparous woman is 8 to 9 cm dilated (Fig. 22-22).

The items required in preparation for birth may vary among different facilities; therefore each facility's procedure manual should be consulted to determine the protocols specific to that facility. Following are suggestions for the preparation for birth:

1. The items that follow have to be collected or readied or the following tasks done.
   - Scrubbing items such as scrub brushes, cuticle sticks, and cleaning agent, as well as masks with a shield or protective glasses or goggles.
   - Sterile gowns and gloves for the primary health care provider, sterile drapes and towels for draping the woman, and sterile instruments and other supplies (e.g., bulb syringes, sutures, and anesthetic solutions). These are arranged on a sterile, draped table for convenient use.
   - A sterile basin containing water for handwashing during the birth process.
   - Supplies for cleansing the vulva (sterile basin, sterile water, and cleaning solution).
   - Birth area is warmed and free of drafts.
   - Infant identification materials.
   - Infant receiving blankets and heated crib. Also material for prophylactic care of infant's eyes and vitamin K injection.
2. The following equipment should be checked to make sure it is in working order: birthing table (bed or chair), overhead lights, and mirror.
3. Emergency equipment, anesthesia, laryngoscope, and supplies needed for the management of emergency situations such as maternal hemorrhage or fetal respiratory distress should be available and in working order.
4. Additional supplies (anesthetics, oxytocics for injection, obstetric forceps, and vacuum extractor) should be available.
5. The woman's record should be up to date and ready for use in the birth area.
6. Specific orders of the primary health care provider regarding labor and birth procedures should be ascertained.

The nurse estimates the time until the birth will occur and notifies the primary health care provider if he or she is not in the client's room. Even the most experienced nurse can miscalculate the time left before birth occurs, however. Thus every nurse who attends a woman in labor must be prepared to assist with an emergency birth if the primary health care provider is not present (see Box 22-5).

Birth in a Delivery Room or Birthing Room

The woman will need assistance if she must move from the labor bed to the delivery table (Fig. 22-23). The woman can help if this is done between contractions, but because of her awkwardness, she cannot be rushed.

The various positions assumed for birth in a delivery room are the Sims position (if this is the case, the attendant will need to support the upper part of the woman's leg), the dorsal position, and the lithotomy position.

The **lithotomy position** has been the position most commonly used for birth in Western cultures, although this practice is changing slowly. The lithotomy position is a convenient one for the primary health care provider because it enables him or her to deal with any complications that may arise (see Fig. 22-20). To place the woman in this position, her buttocks are brought to the edge of the table and her legs are placed in stirrups. Care must be taken to pad the stirrups, raise and place both legs simultaneously, and adjust the shanks of the stirrups so that the calves of the legs are supported. There should be no pressure on the popliteal space. If the stirrups are not the same height, ligaments in the woman's back can be strained as she bears down, leading to considerable discomfort in the postpartum period. The lower portion of the table may be dropped down and rolled back under the table.

It should be noted that the routine use of a supine or lithotomy position for labor and birth has been identified as a clearly harmful or ineffective practice and should be discouraged (Enkin et al., 1995; Technical Working Group of the World Health Organization, 1997)

Birth in an LDR or LDRP room. The maternal position for birth varies from a lithotomy position with the woman's legs in stirrups, to one in which her feet rest on footrests while she holds onto a squat bar, to a side-lying position with the woman's upper leg supported by the coach, nurse, or squat bar. The foot of the bed can be removed so that the primary health care provider attending the birth can gain better perineal access for performing an episiotomy, delivering a large baby, or getting access to the emerging head to facilitate suctioning. Otherwise the foot of the bed is left in place and lowered slightly to form a ledge that allows access for birth and that also serves as a place to lay the newborn.

Once the woman is positioned for birth, the vulva and perineum are cleansed. Hospital protocols and the preferences of primary health care providers for cleansing may vary and can involve washing the area thoroughly with warm, soapy water or a soapy povidone-iodine (Betadine)

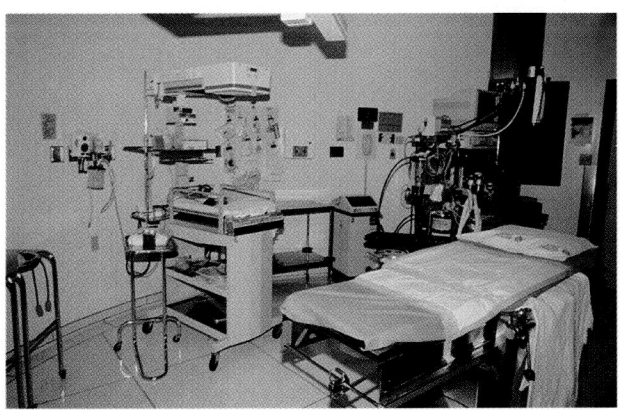

Fig. 22-23 Delivery room. *(Courtesy Michael S. Clement, MD, Mesa, AZ.)*

BOX 22-6 Standard Precautions During Childbirth

Birth is a time when nurses and other health care providers are exposed to a great deal of maternal and newborn blood and body fluids. Observation of Standard Precautions is necessary to prevent the transmission of infection. Perinatal infections most often are transmitted through contact with body fluids. The Standard Precautions applicable to childbirth include the following:

- Wash hands before and after putting on gloves and performing procedures.
- Wear gloves (clean or sterile, as appropriate) when performing procedures that require contact with the woman's genitalia and body fluids, including bloody show (e.g., during vaginal examination, amniotomy, hygienic care of the perineum, insertion of an internal scalp electrode and intrauterine pressure monitor, and catheterization).
- Wear cap, a mask that has a shield or protective eyewear, shoe covers, and cover gown during the birth. Gowns worn by the primary health care provider who is attending the birth should have a waterproof front and sleeves and should be sterile.
- Drape the woman with sterile towels and sheets as appropriate. Explain to the woman what can and cannot be touched.
- Help the woman's partner put on appropriate coverings for the birth, such as cap, mask, gown, and shoe covers. Show the partner where to stand and what can and cannot be touched.
- Wear gloves and gown when handling the newborn immediately after birth.
- Use an appropriate method to suction the newborn's airway, such as a bulb syringe, mechanical wall suction, or De Lee oral suction device that prevents the newborn's mucus from getting into the user's airway.

solution and then rinsing the area. Next the area may be sprayed with a disinfectant to prevent bacterial contamination.

The circulating nurse (usually the same nurse as the labor nurse) continues to coach and encourage the woman. She auscultates the FHR every 5 to 15 minutes, depending on whether the woman is at low or high risk for problems or per protocol of the birthing facility, or continuously monitors the FHR with electronic monitoring. She keeps the primary health care provider informed of the rate and pattern of the FHR (Tucker, 2000). The equipment for measuring blood pressure should be readied for instant use should signs of shock develop. If blood pressure readings are taken as the woman pushes, the readings will be distorted (increased) by the increase in thoracic and abdominal pressures. A reading is obtained after birth before the woman is transferred to the recovery room. An oxytocic medication such as Pitocin may be prepared so that it is ready to be administered after expulsion of the placenta. Standard Precautions should always be followed as care is administered during the process of labor and birth (Box 22-6).

The primary health care provider puts on a cap, a mask that has a shield or protective eyewear, and shoe covers. He or she must scrub his or her hands and put on a sterile gown (with waterproof front and sleeves) and gloves. Nurses attending the birth may also need to wear caps, protective eyewear, masks, gowns, and gloves. The woman may then be draped with sterile towels and sheets. The partner can help the woman remember not to touch the sterile drapes.

Nursing contact with the parents is maintained by touching, verbal comforting, explaining the reasons for care, and sharing in the parents' joy at the birth of their child.

Mechanism of Birth: Vertex Presentation

Most of the time the birth remains in the hands of the primary health care provider. At times, however, the nurse must assist the woman with giving birth. The nurse's knowledge of the birth process serves as a basis for the way

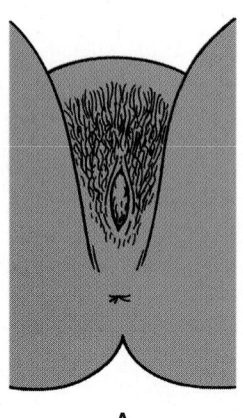 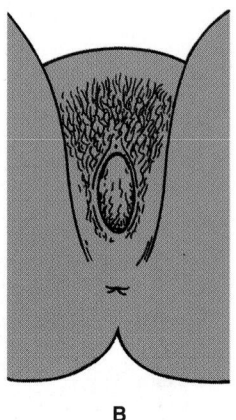 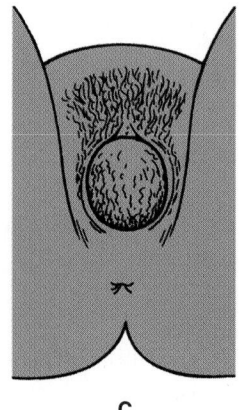 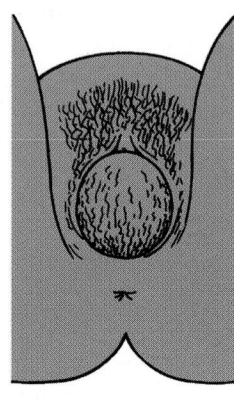

A B C D

Fig. 22-24 Beginning birth with vertex presenting. **A,** Anteroposterior slit. **B,** Oval opening. **C,** Circular shape. **D,** Crowning.

in which she prepares the woman before and during birth. This includes her reviewing with the woman or couple the cardinal movements of labor. That is, once the cervix is fully dilated, descent occurs. The presenting part (usually the vertex) advances with each contraction and recedes slightly as the contraction wanes, but descent is constant. Bulging of the perineum occurs during the descent phase, when the fetal presenting part is distending the perineum but is not yet visible at the introitus. The occiput generally rotates anteriorly, and with voluntary bearing-down efforts, the head appears at the introitus (Fig. 22-24). Although more and more head may be seen with each push, **crowning** occurs when the widest part of the head (the biparietal diameter) distends the vulva just before birth. Immediately before birth, the perineal musculature becomes greatly distended. If an **episiotomy** (incision into the perineum to enlarge vaginal outlet) is necessary, it is done at this time to minimize soft tissue damage.

The head is born by extension and after birth realigns with the shoulders (restitution). Interiorly the shoulders rotate into the anteroposterior diameter of the pelvis while the head rotates externally. The body is born by lateral flexion.

The three phases of the spontaneous birth of a fetus in a vertex presentation are (1) birth of the head, (2) birth of the shoulders, and (3) birth of the body and extremities.

Birth of head. The vertex appears first, followed by the forehead, face, chin, and neck. The speed of the birth of the head must be controlled, because sudden birth of the head may cause severe lacerations that extend through the anal sphincter or even into the woman's rectum. The primary health care provider controls the birth of the head by (1) applying pressure against the rectum, drawing it downward to aid in flexing the head as the back of the neck catches under the symphysis pubis; (2) then applying upward pressure from the coccygeal region (modified **Ritgen maneuver**) (Fig. 22-25) to extend the head during the actual birth, thereby protecting the musculature of the perineum; and (3) assisting the mother with voluntary control of the bearing-down efforts by coaching her to pant while letting uterine forces expel the fetus. Besides protecting the maternal tissues, a gradual birth may prevent fetal intracranial injury.

Occasionally the membranes may not have ruptured before birth. During the birth of the head in this situation, these membranes will look like a hood covering the head. This hood of intact amniotic membranes covering the head during birth is known as a caul.

The umbilical cord often encircles the neck **(nuchal cord)** but rarely so tightly as to cause hypoxia. After the head is born, gentle palpation is used to feel for the cord. The cord should be slipped gently over the head (Fig. 22-26). If the loop is tight or if there is a second loop, the cord is clamped twice, severed between the clamps, and unwound from around the neck before the birth is allowed to continue. Mucus, blood, or meconium in the nasal or oral passages may prevent the newborn from breathing. To eliminate this

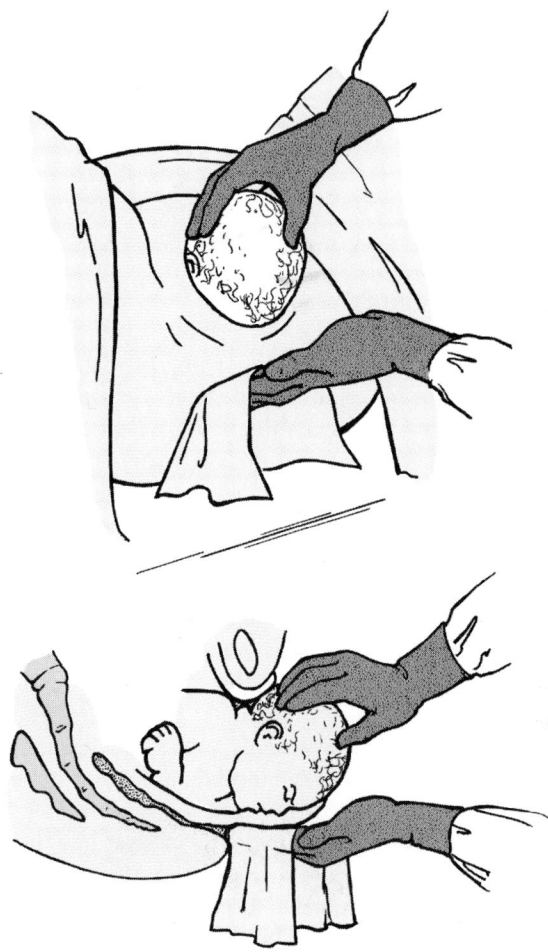

Fig. 22-25 Birth of head using modified Ritgen maneuver. Note control to prevent too rapid birth of head.

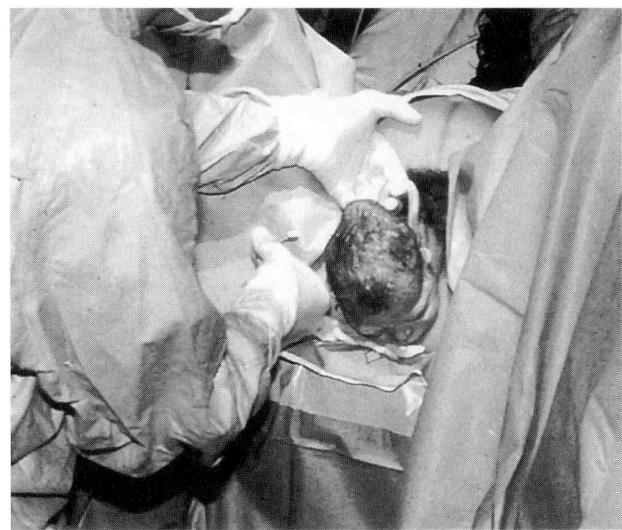

Fig. 22-26 Loosening nuchal cord (umbilical cord around neck). *(Courtesy Marjorie Pyle, RNC, Lifecircle, Costa Mesa, CA.)*

problem, moist gauze sponges are used to wipe the nose and mouth. A bulb syringe is first inserted into the mouth and oropharynx to aspirate contents and then the nares are cleared in the same fashion while the head is supported.

If meconium has been present in the amniotic fluid during labor, a De Lee suction apparatus is placed on the sterile field and preparations are made for wall suction. Thus, when the primary health care provider prepares for birth of the head, the De Lee device is connected to the suction tubing and fluids are withdrawn from the infant's mouth and nose before the first breath is taken to prevent meconium aspiration. The primary health care provider should refrain from using the De Lee device and oral suction to withdraw fluid from the infant unless the suction device is designed so that it can keep mucus from entering the user's airway.

Birth of shoulders. Before the shoulders can be born, they must engage in the pelvic inlet. For this to occur the shoulders rotate internally as the head restitutes and rotates externally, causing the shoulders to then lie in the anteroposterior diameter of the inlet. This makes it possible for the shoulders to now pass through the pelvic cavity. While awaiting rotation, the primary health care provider wipes the baby's face with sterile gauze squares and uses the bulb syringe to clear the mouth and nose of mucus in readiness for the baby's first breath.

The head is drawn downward and backward by the primary health care provider to help the anterior shoulder slide beneath the pubic arch. Normally the anterior shoulder is delivered with this slight downward traction toward the perineum. The posterior shoulder causes the perineum to distend, and to prevent perineal trauma, the head is lifted toward the symphysis pubis, resulting in the birth of the shoulder over the perineum (Bennett & Brown, 1993; Varney, 1997).

Birth of body and extremities. Expulsion of the rest of the body is controlled so that it occurs slowly. While lateral flexion is continued, the primary health care provider supports the weight of the baby to prevent perineal trauma. The body may be rotated slightly to the right or left to facilitate the birth. The time of birth is the precise time when the entire body is out of the woman. This must be recorded on the record.

If the newborn's condition is not compromised, it may be placed on the mother's abdomen immediately after birth and covered with a warm, dry blanket. The cord may be clamped at this time, and the primary health care provider may ask if the woman's partner would like to cut the cord. If so, the primary health care provider provides a sterile pair of scissors and instructs him or her to cut the cord 1 inch (2.5 cm) above the clamp.

Use of fundal pressure. Fundal pressure is the application of gentle, steady pressure against the fundus of the uterus to facilitate the vaginal birth. Historically it has been used when the administration of analgesia and anesthesia decreased the woman's ability to push during the

birth, in cases of shoulder dystocia, and when second-stage fetal bradycardia or other nonreassuring FHR pattern was present. Use of fundal pressure by nurses is not advised because there is no standard technique available for this maneuver, and no current legal, professional, or regulatory standards for its use exist. In cases of shoulder dystocia, suprapubic pressure and maternal position changes are among the recommended interventions (Cosner, 1996; Naef & Morrison, 1994; Piper & McDonald, 1994).

Immediate Assessments and Care of the Newborn

The care given immediately after the birth focuses on assessing and stabilizing the newborn. The nurse's primary responsibility at this time is the infant, because the primary health care provider is involved with the expulsion of the placenta and the care of the mother. The nurse must watch the infant for any signs of distress and initiate appropriate interventions should any appear.

A brief assessment of the newborn can be performed while the mother is holding the infant. This includes checking the infant's airway and Apgar score. Maintaining a patent airway, supporting respiratory effort, and preventing cold stress by drying the newborn and covering the newborn with a warmed blanket or placing him or her under a radiant warmer are the major priorities in terms of the newborn's immediate care. Further examination, identification procedures, and care can be postponed until later in the third stage of labor or early in the fourth stage.

Siblings During the Second Stage

Parents may wish their other children to be present during the labor and birth process. However, a young child may become frightened by the intensity of the second stage. Sights such as rupture of the membranes and sounds such as the mother's moans, screams, and grunts can be unsettling. It is not uncommon for a woman to say things during the second stage and birth that she would not say otherwise and that might scare her child, such as "I can't take any more. Take this baby out of me" or "This pain is killing me. I'm going to die." The child present during birth therefore needs someone to be close, to care just for him or her, and to give explanations in a simple and calm manner. The child may want to be held, leave the room, play, or just go to sleep.

Parents need to be prepared for birth and feel comfortable about the birth process. They know their child best and need to determine whether their child is physically and emotionally ready to observe the birth. A child who is ill or has had a recent difficult experience with health care is unlikely to be ready to view the intense event of his or her mother giving birth (Simkin, 1993).

Health care providers involved in attending women during birth must be comfortable with the presence of a child and the unpredictability of the child's questions, comments, and behaviors.

Perineal Trauma Related to Childbirth

Lacerations. Most acute injuries and lacerations of the perineum, vagina, uterus, and their support tissues occur during childbirth, and their management is an obstetric problem. Some injuries to the supporting tissues, whether they were acute or nonacute and whether they were repaired or not, may lead to gynecologic problems later in life (e.g., pelvic relaxation, uterine prolapse, cystocele, rectocele).

The soft tissues of the birth canal and adjacent structures suffer some damage during every birth. Such damage usually is more pronounced in nulliparous women because the tissues are firmer and more resistant than those in multiparous women. Besides this, the perineal skin and vaginal mucosa may appear intact, but numerous small lacerations in underlying muscle and its fascia may be obscured. Damage to pelvic supports usually is readily apparent, however, and thus is repaired after birth.

The tendency to sustain lacerations varies with each woman; that is, the soft tissue in some women may be less distensible. Heredity may be a factor in this. For example, the tissue of light-skinned women, especially those with reddish hair, is not as readily distensible as that of darker-skinned women. In addition, healing may be less efficient in these women.

Immediate repair promotes healing, limits residual damage, and decreases the possibility of infection. Immediately after birth the cervix, vagina, and perineum are inspected to look for damage. In addition, during the early postpartum period the nurse and primary health care provider continue to carefully inspect the perineum and evaluate lochia and symptoms to identify any previously missed damage.

Perineal lacerations. Perineal lacerations usually occur as the fetal head is being born. The extent of the laceration is defined in terms of its depth:

1. *First degree:* Laceration that extends through the skin and structures superficial to muscles
2. *Second degree:* Laceration that extends through muscles of the perineal body
3. *Third degree:* Laceration that continues through the anal sphincter muscle
4. *Fourth degree:* Laceration that also involves the anterior rectal wall

Perineal injury often is accompanied by small lacerations on the medial surfaces of the labia minora below the pubic rami and to the sides of the urethra and clitoris. Lacerations in this very vascular area often result in profuse bleeding. Such lacerations must be repaired with absorbable suture (Fig. 22-27).

Special attention must be paid to third- and fourth-degree lacerations so that the woman retains fecal continence. Measures are then taken to promote soft stools for a few days to increase the woman's comfort and foster healing. Antimicrobial therapy may be instituted in some cases.

When the levator ani (including the iliococcygeal and pubococcygeal muscles, which form the slinglike support of the pelvic viscera) is not involved, simple perineal injuries usually heal without permanent disability regardless of whether they were repaired. However, the vaginal introitus may gape if torn or severed (episiotomy) ends of superficial perineal muscles (e.g., the bulbocavernosus) are not well approximated during repair.

The ends of the torn or severed anal sphincter muscles must be repaired adequately to prevent fecal incontinence (Fig. 22-28). It is easier to repair a new perineal injury to prevent sequelae than it is to correct long-term damage.

Vaginal and urethral lacerations. Vaginal lacerations often occur in conjunction with perineal lacerations. Vaginal lacerations tend to extend up the lateral walls (sulci) and, if deep enough, involve the levator ani. Additional injury may occur high in the vaginal vault near the level of the ischial spines. Vaginal vault lacerations may be circular and may result from forceps rotation, especially in the presence of cephalopelvic disproportion, rapid fetal descent, or

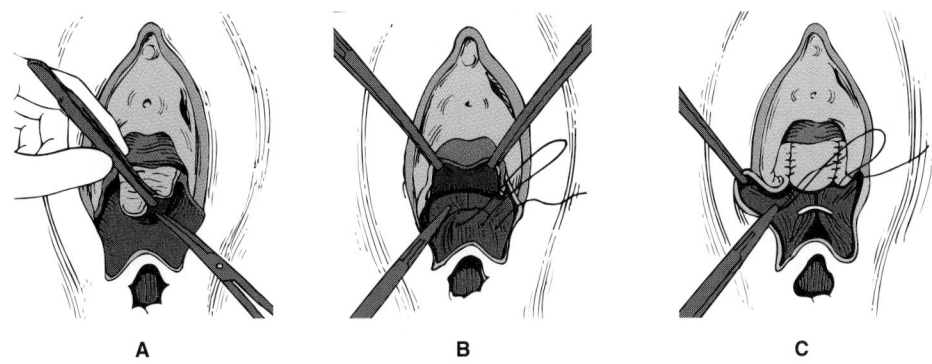

Fig. 22-27 Perineal lacerations. **A,** Bilateral sulcus tears, periurethral tear, and separation of anal sphincter. **B,** Exposure and approximation of levator ani structures. **C,** Approximation of torn bulbocavernous muscle.

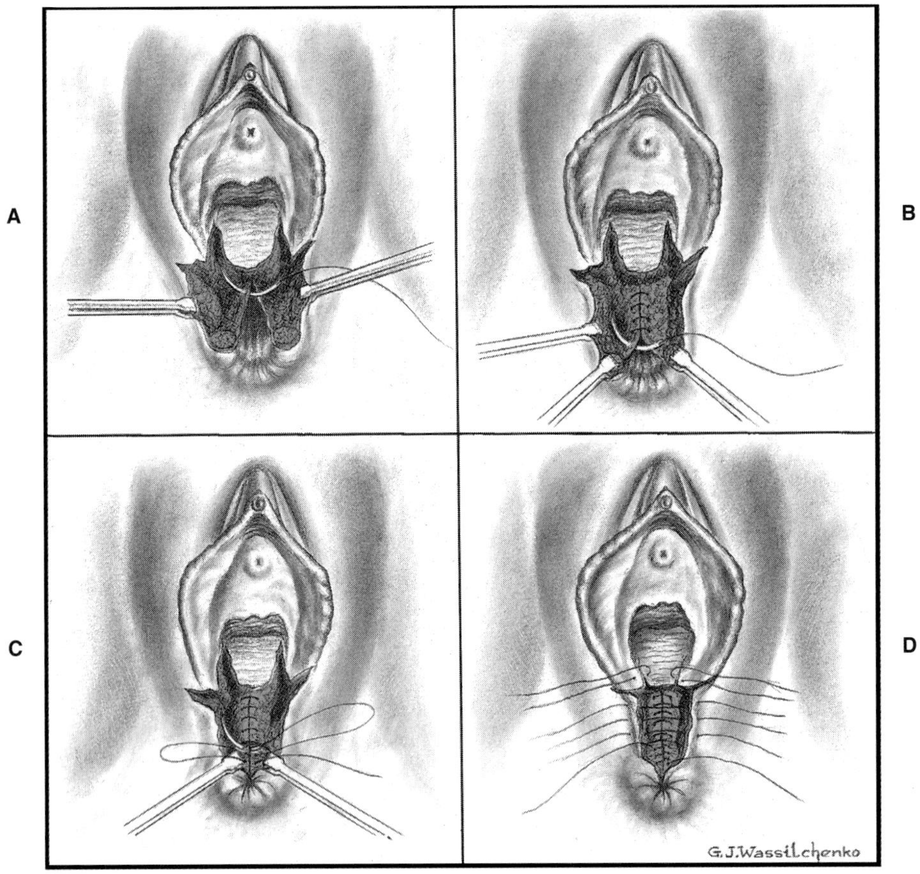

Fig. 22-28 Repair of fourth-degree laceration. **A,** Repair of rectal mucosa, with inverted sutures buried in muscles of rectal wall. **B,** Sutures of levator muscles to be buried; ends of sphincter drawn forward—first step in suturing sphincter. **C,** Second step of suturing sphincter—beginning figure-of-eight sutures. **D,** Sphincter suture completed and ready for tying. Remainder of perineal repair done in usual manner.

precipitous birth. Lacerations can also occur around the urethra (periurethral) and in the area of the clitoris.

Cervical injuries. Cervical injuries occur when the cervix retracts over the advancing fetal head. These cervical lacerations occur at the lateral angles of the external os; most are shallow, and bleeding is minimal. More extensive lacerations may extend to the vaginal vault or beyond it into the lower uterine segment and may involve serious bleeding. Extensive lacerations may be a consequence of hasty attempts to enlarge the cervical opening artificially or to deliver the fetus before the cervix is fully dilated. Injuries to the cervix can have adverse effects on future pregnancies and childbirths.

Episiotomy. An episiotomy is an incision made in the perineum to enlarge the vaginal outlet. It is performed more commonly in the United States and Canada than in Europe, probably because the side-lying position for birth is used routinely in Europe, whereas the lithotomy position is more commonly used in the United States and Canada. Because the side-lying position causes less tension on the perineum, making it possible for the perineum to

stretch gradually, with this position there are fewer indications for the use of episiotomies.

Enkin and co-workers (1995) stated that clear evidence indicates that routine or liberal performance of an episiotomy for birth is a form of care that is likely to be harmful or ineffective. In some areas of the United States, the practice of performing routine episiotomies is declining. The type of episiotomy is designated by the site and direction of the incision (Fig. 22-29).

Midline (median) episiotomy is most commonly used in the United States. It is effective, easily repaired, and generally the least painful. However, it can extend through the rectal sphincter (third-degree laceration/extension) or even into the anal canal (fourth-degree laceration/extension). Sphincter tone is usually restored following primary healing and a good repair.

Mediolateral episiotomy is used in operative births when the need for posterior extension is likely. Although a fourth-degree laceration may be prevented, a third-degree laceration may occur. Also, the blood loss is greater and the repair more difficult and painful than with mid-

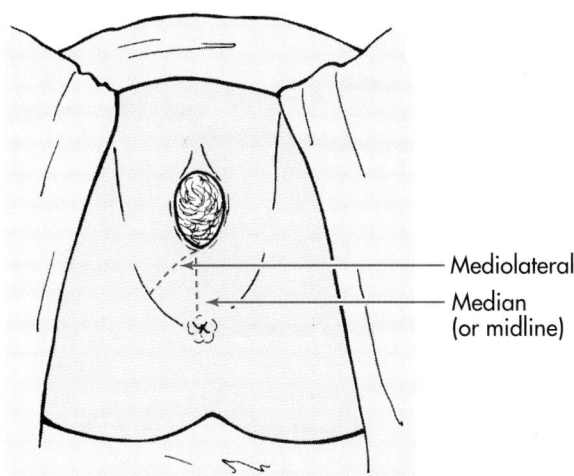

Fig. 22-29 Types of episiotomies.

Mediolateral
Median (or midline)

line episiotomies. Proponents of the use of episiotomy believe it serves the following purposes:

- Prevents tearing of the perineum. The clean and properly placed incision heals more properly than does a tear. Some conditions that predispose a woman to perineal tearing and are therefore indications for episiotomy are birth of a large infant, rapid labor in which there is insufficient time for the perineum to stretch, a narrow subpubic arch with a constricted outlet, and malpresentations of the fetus. However, McGuinness and colleagues (1991) found that women with episiotomies experienced a longer period of healing than did women without episiotomies. Midline episiotomies are also associated with a higher incidence of third- and fourth-degree lacerations (Labrecque et al., 1997; McGuinness, Norr, & Nacion, 1991; Woolley, 1995).
- Possibly minimizes prolonged and severe stretching of the muscles supporting the bladder or rectum, which may later lead to stress incontinence or to prolapse of pelvic organs (uterus, bladder, rectum). Research does not support the claim that pelvic support is protected when episiotomies are performed, however. Episiotomies and the third- and fourth-degree lacerations that can occur actually cut and extend into muscles, thereby prolonging recovery (Paciornik, 1990; Woolley, 1995).
- Reduces duration of the second stage, which may be important for maternal reasons (e.g., a hypertensive state) or fetal reasons (e.g., persistent bradycardia).
- Enlarges the vagina in case manipulation is needed to facilitate the infant's birth (e.g., in a breech presentation or for the application of forceps or a vacuum extractor).
- Shortens the second stage of labor if the well-being of the woman or fetus is in jeopardy, facilitates vacuum-assisted extraction or forceps-assisted birth, prevents cerebral hemorrhage stemming from capillary fragility during the birth of a preterm infant, facilitates the birth of a large infant (more than 4000 g), or facilitates most

forceps-assisted breech births. However, research does not support the claims that episiotomies reduce risk for fetal cerebral hemorrhage or distress or shorten the second stage of labor. Further investigation is required to determine whether episiotomies are of actual benefit in the instances cited (Woolley, 1995).

Opponents of the routine use of episiotomies believe the following:

- The perineum can be prepared for birth through the use of Kegel exercises and massage in the prenatal period. Use of Kegel exercises in the postpartum period improves and restores the tone and strength of the perineal muscles. Health practices, including good nutrition and appropriate hygienic measures, help maintain the integrity and suppleness of the perineal tissue.
- Squatting or lateral positions during childbirth, which encourage women to push as their body tells them to do so, and controlling the emergence of the fetal head while the woman pants and flexion of and counterpressure against the fetal head is accomplished increase the likelihood that the perineum will remain intact or, if lacerations occur, that they will be less severe (Albers et al., 1996; Golay, Vedam, & Sorger, 1993).
- Lacerations may occur even with an episiotomy.
- The pain and discomfort resulting from episiotomies is greater than that associated with lacerations and can interfere with mother-infant interactions and the reestablishment of parental sexual intercourse.

Risk factors associated with perineal trauma (episiotomy, lacerations) include nulliparity, occiput posterior position of the fetus, large (macrosomic) infants, use of instruments to facilitate birth, prolonged second stage of labor, and fetal distress. Research has also indicated that the rate of episiotomies is lower when nurse-midwives rather than obstetricians attend births. Socioeconomic factors associated with episiotomies include the Caucasian and Asian races and private insurance and care (Albers et al., 1996; Hueston, 1996; Lydon-Rochelle, Albers, & Teaf, 1995).

Alternative measures for perineal management, such as warm compresses, manual support, and massage, have been shown to reduce, to varying degrees, the incidence of episiotomies, but further research is recommended (Albers et al., 1996; Lydon-Rochelle, Albers, & Teaf, 1995; Renfrew et al., 1998). Nurses acting as advocates can encourage women to use alternative birthing positions that reduce pressure on the perineum and to use spontaneous bearing-down efforts. In addition, nurses can educate other health care providers about measures to preserve perineal integrity and to be more flexible in defining the maximum limit for the duration of the second stage of labor as long as the maternal-fetal unit is stable (Maier & Maloni, 1997).

Evaluation

During the second stage of labor the nurse evaluates the degree to which expected outcomes are being met, for example, the extent to which the woman has actively participated in the labor process, whether she or her fetus has sustained any injury during the labor process, the degree to which her birth plan has been fulfilled, and the extent to which she has been able to obtain comfort and support from her support person.

THIRD STAGE OF LABOR

The **third stage of labor** lasts from the time the baby is born until the placenta is delivered. The goal in the management of the third stage of labor is the prompt separation and expulsion of the placenta, achieved in the easiest, safest manner.

The placenta is attached to the decidual layer of the basal plate's thin endometrium by numerous fibrous anchor villi—much in the same way as a postage stamp is "attached" to a sheet of postage stamps. After the birth of the fetus, strong uterine contractions occur that cause the placental site to shrink markedly. This causes the anchor villi

to break and the placenta to separate from its attachments. Normally the first few strong contractions that occur 5 to 7 minutes after the baby's birth cause the placenta to be sheared away from the basal plate. A placenta cannot be detached from a flaccid (relaxed) uterus because the placental site is not then reduced in size.

¦ CARE MANAGEMENT

Assessment and Nursing Diagnoses

Placental separation is indicated by the following signs (Fig. 22-30):
- A firmly contracting fundus
- The uterus changing from a discoid to a globular ovoid shape as the placenta moves into the lower uterine segment
- A sudden gushing of dark blood from the introitus
- Apparent lengthening of the umbilical cord as the placenta gets closer to the introitus
- The finding of a vaginal fullness (the placenta) on vaginal or rectal examination or of fetal membranes at the introitus

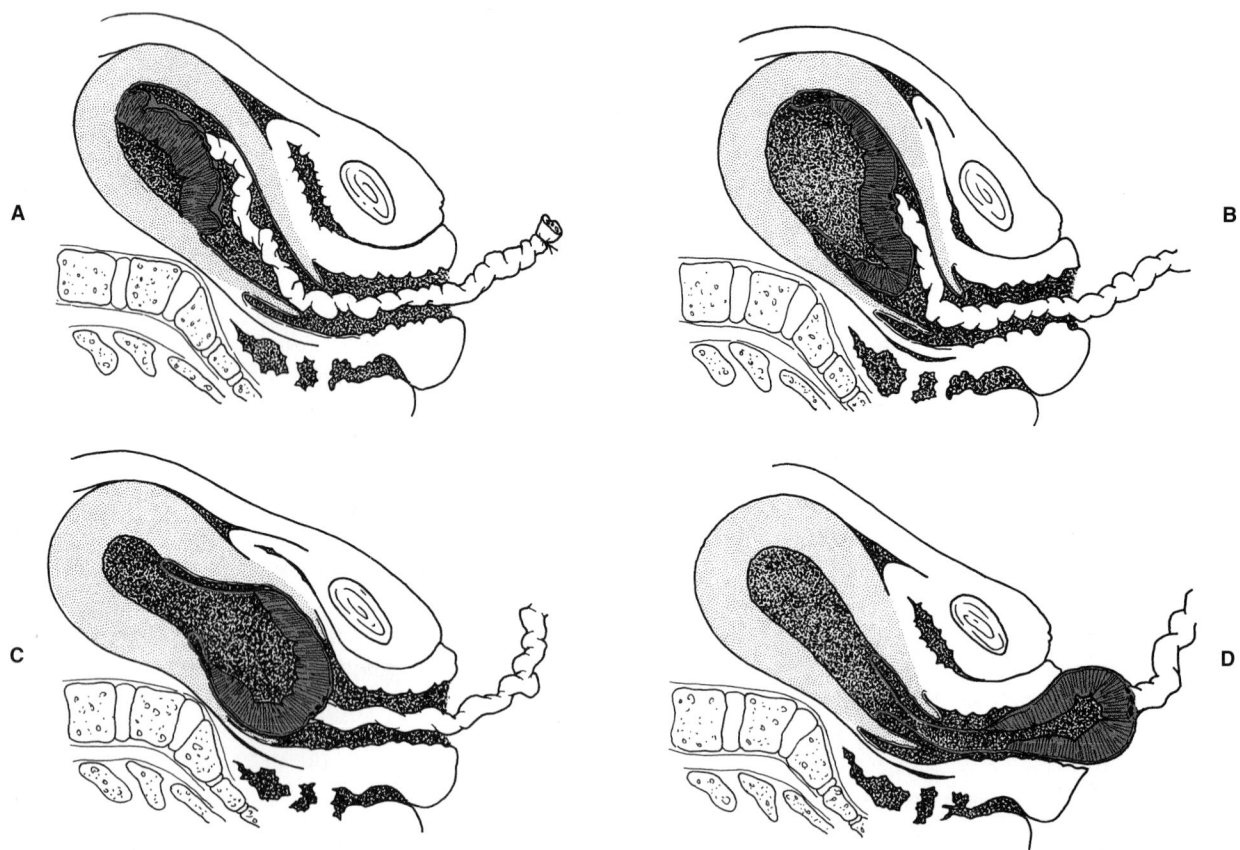

Fig. 22-30   Third stage of labor. **A,** Placenta begins to separate in central portion accompanied by retroplacental bleeding. Uterus changes from discoid to globular shape. **B,** Placenta completes separation and enters lower uterine segment. Uterus is globular in shape. **C,** Placenta enters vagina, cord is seen to lengthen, and there may be an increase in bleeding. **D,** Expulsion (delivery) of placenta and completion of third stage.

Whether the shiny fetal surface of the placenta appears first (Schultze mechanism) or the placenta turns so that its dark roughened maternal surface shows first (Duncan mechanism) is of no clinical importance. After the placenta and the amniotic membranes emerge, the primary health care provider examines it for intactness to make sure that no portion remains in the uterine cavity (i.e., no fragments of the placenta or membranes are retained) (Fig. 22-31).

LEGAL TIP Placental Examination

Examination of the placenta and its cord after birth may provide clues as to the basis for infant health problems, including mental retardation and cerebral palsy. In some instances, poor obstetric outcomes are related to preexisting problems within the placenta and cord and not to childbirth care and events. Nurses can advocate for the development of protocols regarding labor and birth events that would warrant a thorough, pathologic examination of the placenta and cord. A finding that the placenta is abnormal or diseased may play an important role in the defense of health care providers in cases of malpractice (Urbanski, 1997).

Some women and their families may have culturally based beliefs regarding the care of the placenta and the manner of its disposal after birth. Requests by the woman to take the placenta home and dispose of it according to her customs may be at odds with health care agency policies, especially those related to infection control and the disposal of biologic wastes. Many cultures follow specific rules regarding the disposal of the placenta in terms of

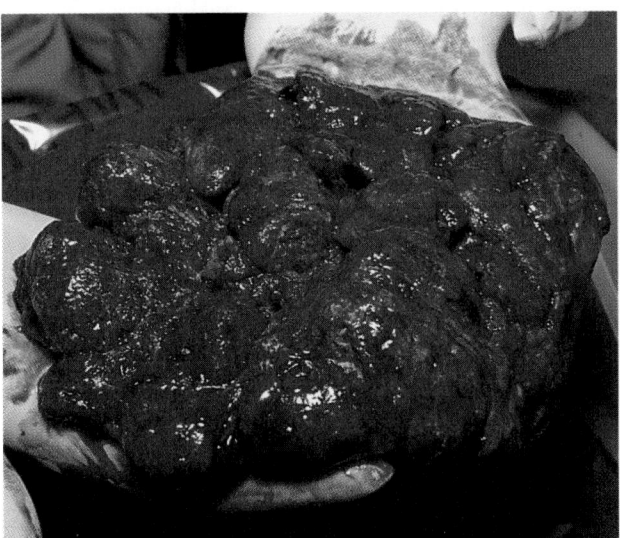

Fig. 22-31 Examination of the placenta. *(Courtesy Michael S. Clement, MD, Mesa, AZ.)*

method (burning, drying, burying, eating), site for disposal (in or near the home), and timing of disposal (immediately after birth, time of day, astrological signs). Disposal rituals may vary according to the gender of the child and the length of time before another child is desired. Many cultures view the care and disposal of the placenta as a way of protecting the newborn from bad luck and illness. If eaten, the placenta can be a means of restoring a woman's well-being after birth or ensuring quality breast milk. Health care providers can provide culturally sensitive health care by encouraging women and their families to express their wishes regarding the care and disposal of the placenta and by establishing a policy to fulfill these requests (Choudhry, 1997; Howard & Berbiglia, 1997; Schneiderman, 1998).

Maternal Physical Status

The physiologic changes in the mother after birth are profound. The cardiac output increases rapidly as maternal circulation to the placenta ceases and the pooled blood from the lower extremities is mobilized. The pulse rate slows in response to the change in cardiac output and tends to remain slightly slower than the prepregnancy rate for about 1 week.

Soon after the birth the woman's blood pressure usually returns to prepregnancy levels. Several factors contribute to an elevated blood pressure at this time: the excitement of the second stage, certain medications, and the time of day (blood pressure is highest during the late afternoon). The effects of analgesics and anesthetics that may have been administered may also cause hypotension to develop in the hour after birth.

Signs of Potential Problems

The major risk for women during the third stage of labor is postpartum hemorrhage. Even as the primary health care provider is completing the delivery of the placenta, the nurse is observing the mother for signs of excessive blood loss, including alteration in vital signs, pallor, lightheadedness, restlessness, decreased urinary output, and alteration in level of consciousness and orientation.

Because of the rapid cardiovascular changes taking place (e.g., the increased intracranial pressure during pushing and the rapid increase in cardiac output), during this period the risk of rupture of a preexisting cerebral aneurysm and the risk of formation of pulmonary emboli are greater than usual. Another dangerous, unpredictable problem that may occur is the formation of an amniotic fluid embolism (see Chapter 38).

Women with a history of cardiac disorders are at increased risk for cardiac decompensation and pulmonary edema as a result of the circulatory changes associated with the birth of the fetus and expulsion of the placenta. Nurse should carefully assess the woman's respiratory pattern and effort, especially in the early postpartum period.

Examples of nursing diagnoses relevant to the third stage of labor include the following:

Nursing Diagnoses

- Risk for fluid volume deficit related to
  - blood loss occurring following placental separation and expulsion
  - inadequate contraction of the uterus
- Ineffective individual coping (mother) related to
  - lack of preparation for sensations that occur during third stage of labor
- Anxiety related to
  - lack of knowledge regarding birth of the placenta
  - occurrence of perineal trauma and the need for repair
- Fatigue related to
  - energy expenditure associated with childbirth and the bearing-down efforts of the second stage
- Ineffective family coping related to
  - unexpected birth of an infant with serious congenital anomalies
  - birth of an infant whose sex was not preferred by the parents
  - situational low self-esteem related to perceived inability to meet personal expectations regarding performance during childbirth.

Expected Outcomes of Care

Planning for this stage of labor focuses on the rapid physiologic changes taking place in the woman and the timely delivery of an intact placenta. At the same time, the emotional environment of the family is also maintained. Expected outcomes for the third stage of labor may include the following:

- The placenta is expelled, and maternal blood loss is less than 500 ml or less than 1% of body weight.
- The mother is prepared for the sensations she will experience.
- The mother, father or partner, and family initiate the processes of bonding and attachment with the newborn.

Plan of Care and Interventions

To assist the woman in the delivery of the placenta, the nurse or primary health care provider has the woman push when signs of separation have occurred. If possible, the placenta should be expelled by maternal effort during a uterine contraction, but alternate compression and elevation of the fundus, plus minimum, controlled traction on the umbilical cord, may be used to facilitate delivery of the placenta and amniotic membranes. Oxytocics may be administered because they stimulate the uterus to contract, thereby helping to prevent hemorrhage after the placenta is removed.

NURSE ALERT *If an oxytocic medication is ordered (e.g., 10 to 20 units of Pitocin diluted in an IV solution, 10 units of Pitocin given as an intramuscular injection, or 0.2 mg of methylergonovine maleate [Methergine] injected intramuscularly), the nurse administers the medication in the dose and by the route indicated by the primary health care provider only after the placenta has been expelled.*

Rogers and associates (1998) compared the effectiveness of active versus expectant management of the third stage of labor in reducing the incidence of postpartum hemorrhage. Active management involved the administration of one or more oxytocic (uterotonic) medications after emergence of the anterior shoulder of the fetus, clamping and cutting of the cord immediately, before the cessation of pulsation, and delivery of the placenta by controlled cord traction when signs of placental separation were noted. Conversely, expectant management involved the natural expulsion of the placenta by efforts of the mother, with clamping and cutting of the cord after pulsation ceased. No oxytocic (uterotonic) medications were given. Findings indicated a significantly lower incidence of postpartum hemorrhage when active management was the approach followed during the third stage of labor. Further research was recommended.

When the third stage is complete and any lacerations are repaired or an episiotomy is sutured, the vulvar area is gently cleansed with warm sterile water or normal saline. The nurse or primary health care provider does the following:

- Applies a sterile perineal pad or ice pack.
- Removes any drapes or places dry linen under the woman's buttocks.
- Repositions the birthing table or bed.
- Lowers the mother's legs simultaneously from the stirrups if she is in a lithotomy position.
- Assists the woman onto her bed if she is to be transferred from the birthing area to the recovery area; assistance is also necessary to move the woman from the birthing table onto a bed if the woman has had anesthesia and does not have full use of her lower extremities.
- Provides the woman with a clean gown and covers her with a warmed blanket.
- Raises the side rails of the bed during the transfer. In some hospitals, the mother is given the baby to hold during the transfer; in other hospitals, the father or partner carries the baby or the nurse or partner transports the baby in a crib, either to the nursery or to the recovery area for the duration of the mother's recovery period.

If the woman labors, gives birth, and recovers in the same bed and room, she is refreshed following the protocol already described (see Plan of Care: Third Stage of Labor). Maternal and neonatal assessments for the fourth stage of labor are instituted. Box 22-7 summarizes normal vaginal childbirth.

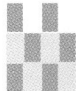

PLAN °ᶠ CARE | Third Stage of Labor

NURSING DIAGNOSIS Ineffective individual coping related to sense that labor process is over with emergence of neonate and lack of experience with sensations of third stage of labor

Expected Outcome *Client will actively participate in expulsion of the placenta.*

Nursing Interventions/Rationales

Explain to woman and labor partner what is expected in the third stage of labor *to enlist cooperation.*

Have woman maintain her position *to facilitate delivery of the placenta.*

Ask mother if she wishes to dispose of the placenta in any specific manner *to comply with certain cultural customs.*

NURSING DIAGNOSIS Fatigue related to energy expenditure required during labor and birth

Expected Outcome *Mother's energy levels are restored.*

Nursing Interventions/Rationales

Educate mother and partner about need for rest and help them plan strategies (e.g., restricting visitors, increasing role of support systems performing functions associated with daily routines) that allow specific times for rest and sleep *to ensure that woman can restore depleted energy levels in preparation for caring for a new infant.*

Monitor woman's fatigue level and the amount of rest received *to ensure restoration of energy.*

NURSING DIAGNOSIS Risk for fluid volume deficit related to decreased fluid intake and blood loss during the birth

Expected Outcomes *Fluid balance is maintained, and there are no signs of dehydration.*

Nursing Interventions/Rationales

Monitor fluid loss (i.e., blood, urine, perspiration) and vital signs; inspect skin turgor and mucous membranes for dryness *to evaluate hydration status.*

Administer oral/parenteral fluids per physician/nurse-midwife orders *to maintain hydration.*

Monitor the fundus for firmness after placental separation *to ensure adequate contraction and prevent further blood loss.*

Administer medications per physician/nurse-midwife orders *to aid contraction of the uterus.*

From Wong, D., & Perry, S. (1998). *Maternal child nursing care.* St. Louis: Mosby.

The Family During the Third Stage

Most parents enjoy being able to handle, hold, explore, and examine the baby immediately after birth. Both parents can assist with the thorough drying of the infant. The infant may be wrapped in a receiving blanket and placed on the woman's abdomen. If skin-to-skin contact is desired, the unwrapped infant may be placed on the woman's abdomen and then covered with a warm blanket.

Holding the newborn next to her skin helps the mother maintain the baby's body heat and provides skin-to-skin contact; care must be taken to keep the head warm. Stockinette caps are sometimes used to cover the newborn's head. It is the nurse's responsibility to make sure the infant stays warm and is in no danger of slipping from the parent's grasp.

Many women wish to begin breastfeeding their newborns at this time to take advantage of the infant's alert state (first period of reactivity) and to stimulate the production of oxytocin that promotes contraction of the uterus. Others prefer to wait until the newborn, parents, and older siblings are together in the recovery area. In some cultures, breastfeeding is not considered acceptable until the milk comes in.

The woman usually feels some discomfort while the primary health care provider carries out the postbirth vaginal examination. The nurse can assist the woman to use relaxation techniques. Because the woman may be focusing on herself, the nurse can use this time to assess the newborn's physical condition; the infant can be weighed and measured, given eye prophylaxis and a vitamin K injection, given an identification bracelet, wrapped in warm blankets, and then given to the partner or back to the mother to hold when she is ready.

Parent-Newborn Relationships

The woman's reaction to the sight of her newborn may range from excited outbursts of laughing, talking, and even crying to apparent apathy. A polite smile and nod may be her only acknowledgment of the comments of nurses and the primary health care provider. Occasionally the reaction

BOX 22-7 | Normal Vaginal Childbirth

FIRST STAGE

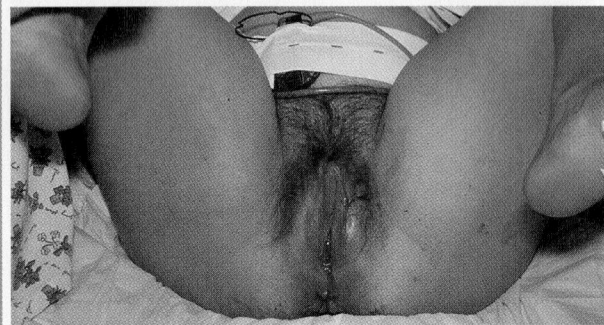

Anteroposterior slit. Vertex visible during contraction.

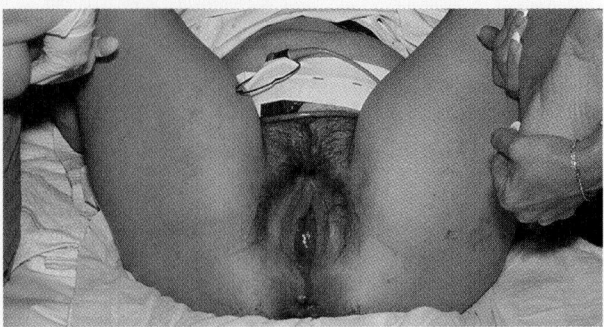

Oval opening. Vertex presenting. Note: nurse (on left) is wearing gloves but support person (on right) is not.

SECOND STAGE

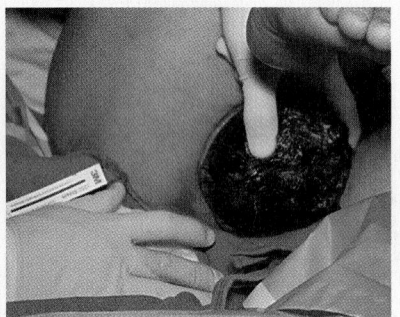

Crowning.

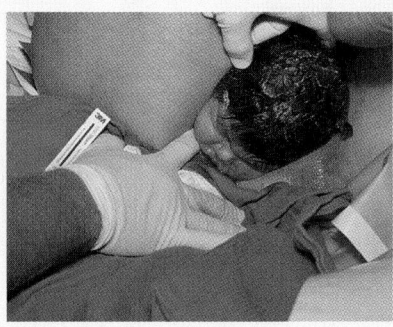

Nurse-midwife using Ritgen maneuver as head is born by extension.

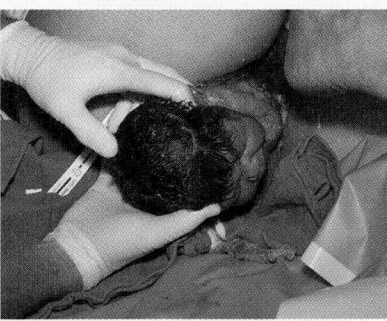

After nurse-midwife checks for nuchal cord, she supports head during external rotation and restitution.

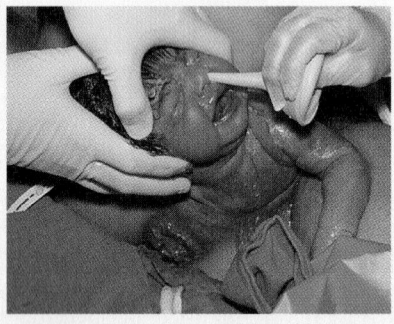

Use of bulb syringe to suction mucus.

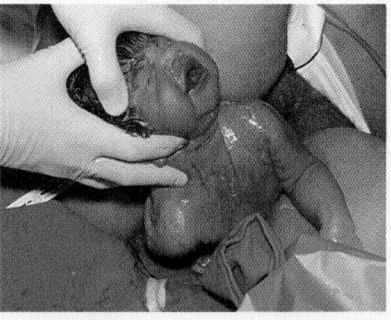

Birth of posterior shoulder.

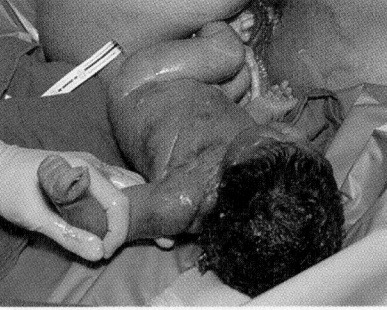

Birth of newborn by slow expulsion.

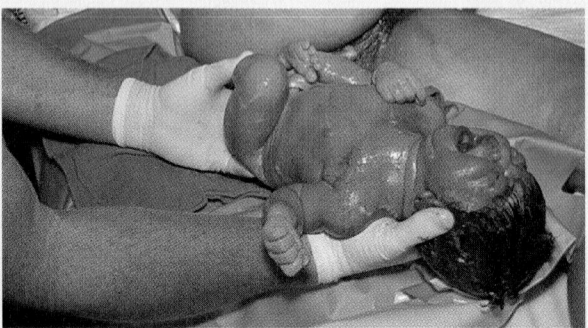

Second stage complete. Note that newborn is not completely pink yet.

Courtesy Michael S. Clement, MD, Mesa, AZ.

BOX 22-7 Normal Vaginal Childbirth—cont'd

THIRD STAGE

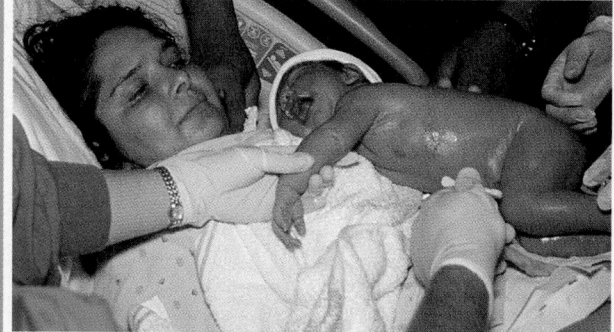

Newborn placed on mother's abdomen while cord is clamped and cut.

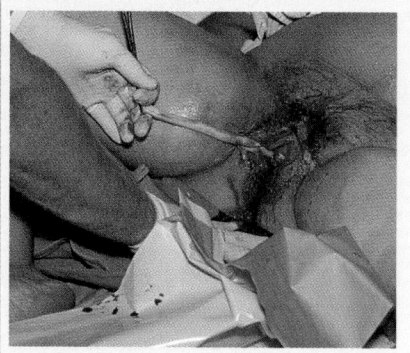

Note increased bleeding as placenta separates.

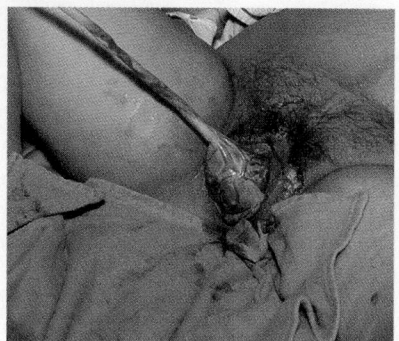

Expulsion of placenta.

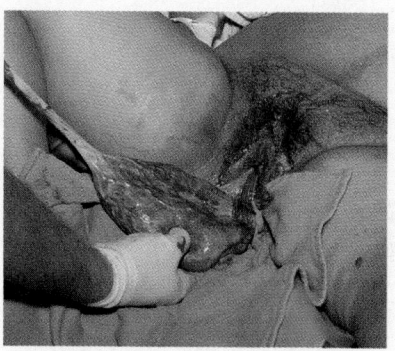

Expulsion is complete, marking the end of the third stage.

THE NEWBORN

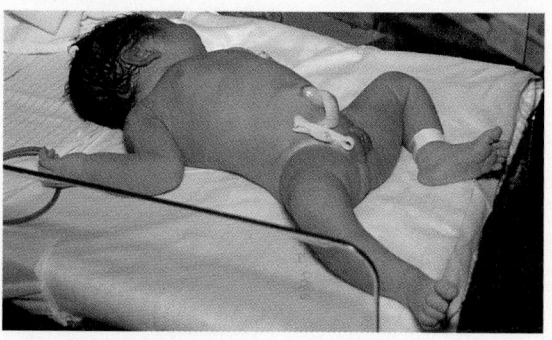

Newborn awaiting assessment. Note that color is almost completely pink.

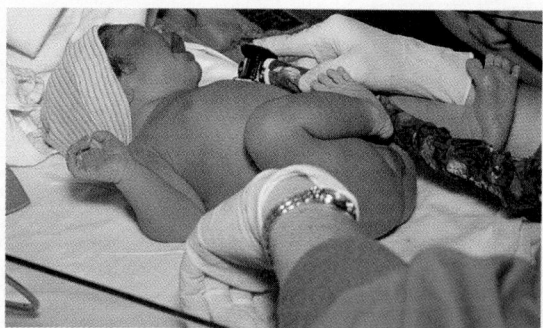

Newborn assessment under radiant warmer.

Parents admiring their newborn.

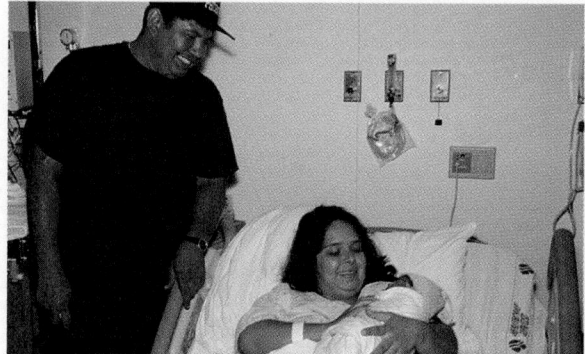

is one of anger or indifference; the woman turns away from the baby, concentrates on her own pain, and sometimes makes hostile comments. These varied reactions can arise from pleasure, exhaustion, or deep disappointment. When evaluating parent-newborn interactions after birth, the nurse should also consider the cultural characteristics of the woman and her family and the expected behaviors of that culture. In some cultures, the birth of a male child is preferred and women may grieve when a female child is born (Choudhry, 1997).

Whatever the reaction and its cause may be, the woman needs continuing acceptance and support from all staff. Notation regarding the parents' reaction to the newborn can be made in the recovery record. Nurses can assess this reaction by asking themselves such questions as, How do the parents look? What do they say? What do they do? The parent-newborn relationship can be further assessed as care is given during the period of recovery. This is especially important if warning signs (e.g., passive or hostile reactions to the newborn, disappointment with sex or appearance of the newborn, absence of eye contact, limited interaction of parents with each other) were noted immediately after birth. The nurse may find it helpful to discuss any warning signs that may have been noted with the woman's primary health care provider.

Siblings, who may have appeared only remotely interested in the final phases of the second stage, tend to experience renewed interest and excitement and can be encouraged to hold the new baby (Fig. 22-32).

Parents usually respond to praise of their newborn. Many need to be reassured that the dusky appearance of their baby's extremities immediately after birth is normal until circulation is well established. If appropriate, the nurse should explain the reason for the molding of the newborn's head. Information about hospital routine can be communicated. It is important, however, for nurses to recognize that the cultural background of the parents may influence their expectations regarding the care and handling of their newborn immediately after birth. For example, some traditional Southeast Asians believe that the head should not be touched because it is the most sacred part of a person's body. They also believe that praise of the baby is dangerous because jealous spirits may then cause the baby harm or take it away (D'Avanzo, 1992). Hospital staff members, by their interest and concern, can provide the environment for making this a satisfying experience for parents, family, and significant others.

Evaluation

Evaluation is ongoing. During each encounter with the new mother during the third stage of labor, the nurse evaluates the degree to which expected outcomes are being met.

The evaluation process should also include a review, with the woman and her significant others present at the birth, of the entire childbirth experience. A health care provider such as the midwife or a nurse who supported the woman and her family during the childbirth process should conduct the review. In addition, the woman can describe the quality of her care by completing a discharge questionnaire or interview before or just after discharge. Determining a woman's satisfaction with and impressions of her childbirth experience is a critical component in the provision of high-quality maternal-newborn health care that meets the individual needs of women and families using these services (Fowles, 1998; Young, 1998). In addition, reviewing the childbirth experience with someone who will listen, support, and explain has been found to reduce the degree of postpartum depression experienced by many women during the first week or so following birth (Wessely, 1998).

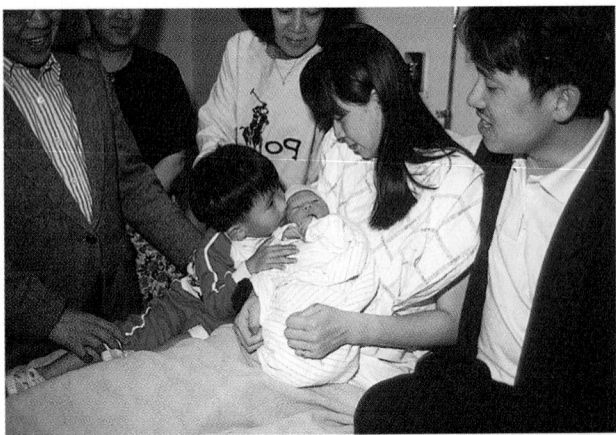

Fig. 22-32 Big brother becomes acquainted with new baby sister. *(Courtesy Marjorie Pyle, RNC, Lifecircle, Costa Mesa, CA.)*

K EY POINTS

- The onset of labor may be difficult to determine for both the nulliparous and multiparous woman.

- The familiar environment of her home is most often the ideal place for a woman during the latent phase of the first stage of labor.

- The nurse assumes much of the responsibility for assessing the progress of labor and for keeping the primary health care provider informed about progress in labor and deviations from expected findings.

- The fetal heart rate and pattern reveal how the fetus is responding to the stress of the labor process.

- Although meconium-stained amniotic fluid may be associated with fetal asphyxia, it is not always an indication of nonreassuring fetal status.

KEY POINTS—cont'd

- Assessment of the laboring woman's urinary output and bladder is critical to ensure her progress and to prevent injury to the bladder.

- Regardless of the actual labor and birth experience, the woman's or couple's perception of the birth experience is most likely to be positive when events and performances are consistent with expectations, especially in terms of maintaining control and adequacy of pain relief.

- The woman's level of anxiety may rise when she does not understand what is being said to her about her labor because of the medical terminology used or because of a language barrier.

- Coaching, emotional support, and comfort measures help the woman to use her energy constructively in relaxing and working with the contractions.

- The progress of labor is enhanced when a woman changes her position frequently during the first stage of labor.

- Doulas provide a continuous supportive presence during labor that can have a positive effect on the process of childbirth and its outcome.

- The cultural beliefs and practices of a woman and her significant others, including her partner, can have a profound influence on their approach to labor and birth.

- The nurse who is aware of particular sociocultural aspects of helping and coping that pertain to a woman or couple acts as an advocate or protective agent for her or them during labor.

- The quality of the nurse-client relationship is a factor in the woman's ability to cope with the stressors of the labor process.

- Women with a history of sexual abuse often experience profound stress and anxiety during childbirth.

- Inability to palpate the cervix during vaginal examination indicates that complete effacement and full dilation have occurred and is the only certain, objective sign that the second stage has begun.

- Women may experience an urge to bear down at various times during labor; for some it may be experienced before the cervix is fully dilated and for others it may not be experienced until the active phase of the second stage of labor.

- When allowed to respond to the rhythmic nature of the second stage of labor, the woman normally changes body positions, bears down spontaneously, and vocalizes (open-glottis pushing) when she perceives the urge to push (Ferguson reflex).

KEY POINTS—cont'd

- Women should bear down several times during a contraction using the open-glottis pushing method; sustained closed-glottis pushing should be avoided because oxygen transport to the fetus will be inhibited.

- Episiotomies may be performed and lacerations may occur even during "normal" childbirth, and their appropriate and prompt repair is essential.

- Nurses can use the role of advocate to prevent routine use of episiotomy and to reduce the incidence of lacerations by empowering women to take an active role in their birth and educating health care providers about approaches to managing childbirth that reduce the incidence of perineal trauma.

- Objective signs indicate that the placenta has separated and is ready to be expelled; excessive traction (pulling) on the umbilical cord, before the placenta has separated, can result in maternal injury.

- Most parents and families enjoy being able to handle, hold, explore, and examine the baby immediately after the birth.

- Siblings present for labor and birth need preparation and support for the event.

- After an emergency childbirth, postpartum hemorrhage can be prevented by stimulating the mother's nipple manually or by the infant's suckling. This can stimulate the release of natural oxytocin from the maternal posterior pituitary gland, which, by stimulating the uterus to contract, prevents such hemorrhage.

- A woman benefits from reviewing her childbirth experience with the nurse who managed her care during the process of labor and birth.

CRITICAL THINKING EXERCISES

1 *An 18-year-old nulliparous woman at 39 weeks of gestation is in the latent phase of the first stage of labor. She and her 19-year-old boyfriend, who is the father of the baby, arrive for admission to the labor and birth unit after her membranes ruptured during a routine prenatal visit. During the admission interview, the couple report that they were too shy to go to childbirth classes because they were not married but they want to work together to have their baby. Outline the approach the nurse should use to support this couple during the labor and birth process.*

Continued

CRITICAL THINKING EXERCISES cont'd

2 A nulliparous woman calls the birthing center and anxiously tells the nurse, "I am in labor. My husband is going to bring me in right now for admission." Role play the approach the nurse should take in responding to this woman's report.

3 A couple pregnant with their third baby tell the nurse during an expectant childbirth class that they would like their 8-year-old daughter and 5-year-old son to participate in the labor of their mother and birth of their sibling. How can the nurse assist this couple to fulfill their goal?

4 A nurse is conducting a special childbirth class to address the concerns of expectant fathers who plan to coach their partners during labor and birth. One of the fathers tells the nurse that his partner wants to have a doula present during childbirth along with him. "I want to help her but what am I going to do if she has a doula there to give her support? Maybe I should just stay home or in the waiting room until it's time for the baby to be born." How should the nurse respond to this father's concern?

5 You are the nurse manager of a labor and birth unit of a hospital. After attending a national nursing educational meeting regarding evidence-based approaches to enhance the progress of childbirth, you determine that these measures should be implemented on your unit. Acting as an advocate for your clients and a catalyst for change on your unit, outline the approach you would use to convince the nursing and medical staff to include these approaches when managing the care of laboring women.

References

Aderhold, K., & Perry, L. (1991). Jet hydrotherapy for labor and postpartum pain relief. *MCN Am J Matern Child Nurs* 16(2), 97-99.

Aderhold, K., & Roberts, J. (1991). Phases of second stage labor: Four descriptive care studies. *J Nurse Midwifery* 36(5), 267-275.

Albers, L. et al. (1996). Factors related to perineal trauma in childbirth. *J Nurse Midwifery* 41(4), 269-276.

Albers, L. et al. (1997). The relationship of ambulation in labor to operative delivery. *J Nurse Midwifery* 42(1), 4-8.

Andrews, C., & Chrzanowski, M. (1990). Maternal position, labor, and comfort. *Appl Nurs Res* 3(1), 7-13.

Arrabal, P., & Naegy, D. (1996). Is manual palpation of uterine contractions accurate? *Am J Obstet Gynecol* 114(1 pt 1), 217-219.

Bennett, B. & Brown, L. (1993). *Myles textbook for midwives* (12th ed.). Edinburgh: Churchill Livingstone.

Bergstrom, L. et al. (1992). "You'll feel me touching you, sweetie": Vaginal examination during the second stage of labor. *Birth* 19(1), 10-20.

Bergstrom, L. et al. (1997). "I gotta push. Please let me push." Social interactions during the change from first to second stage of labor. *Birth* 24(3), 173-180.

Biancuzzo, M. (1991). The patient observer: Does the hand-and-knees posture during labor help to rotate the occiput posterior fetus? *Birth* 18(1), 40-47.

Biancuzzo, M. (1993). Six myths of maternal posture during labor. *MCN Am J Matern Child Nurs* 18(5), 264-269.

Bloom, S. et al. (1998). Lack of effect of walking on labor and delivery. *N Engl J Med* 339(2), 76-79.

Bryanton, J., Fraser-Davey, H., & Sullivan, P. (1994). Women's perception of nursing support during labor. *J Obstet Gynecol Neonatal Nurs* 23(8), 638-644.

Callister, L. (1992). The meaning of the childbirth experience to the Mormon woman. *J Perinat Educ* 1(1), 50-57.

Callister, L. (1995). Cultural meanings of childbirth. *J Obstet Gynecol Neonatal Nurs* 24(4), 327-331.

Callister, L., Vehvilainen-Julkunen, K., & Lauri, S. (1996). Cultural perceptions of childbirth. *J Holistic Nurs* 14(1), 66-78.

Carbonne, B. et al. (1996). Maternal position during labor: Effects on fetal oxygen saturation measured by pulse oximetry. *Obstet Gynecol* 88(5), 797-800.

Cesario, S. (1998). Should cameras be allowed in the delivery room? *MCN Am J Matern Child Nurs* 23(2), 87-91.

Chalmers, B., & Meyer, D. (1994). Companionship in the perinatal period: A cross-cultural survey of women's experiences. *J Nurse Midwifery* 39(4), 265-272.

Chandler, S., & Field, P. (1997). Becoming a father—First-time fathers' experience of labor and delivery. *J Nurse Midwifery* 42(1), 17-24.

Chapman, L. (1992). Expectant father's roles during labor and birth. *J Obstet Gynecol Neonatal Nurs* 21(2), 114-120.

Choudhry, U. (1997). Traditional practices of women from India: Pregnancy, childbirth, and newborn care. *J Obstet Gynecol Neonatal Nurs* 26(5), 533-539.

Cosner, K. (1996). Use of fundal pressure during second-stage labor: A pilot study. *J Nurse Midwifery* 41(4), 334-337.

Cosner, K., & deJong, E. (1993). Physiologic second-stage labor. *MCN Am J Matern Child Nurs* 18(1), 38-43.

D'Avanzo, C. (1992). Bridging the cultural gap with Southeast Asians. *MCN Am J Matern Child Nurs* 17(4), 204-208.

d'Entremont, M. (1996). Directed pushing in the second stage of labour. *Modern Midwife* 6(6), 12-16.

De Sevo, M. (1997). Keeping the faith: Jewish traditions in pregnancy and childbirth. *AWHONN Lifelines* 1(4), 46-49.

DiMatteo, M. et al. (1993). Narratives of birth and the postpartum: Analysis of the focus group responses of new mothers. *Birth* 20(4), 204-211.

Enkin, M. et al. (1995). Effective care in pregnancy and childbirth: A synopsis. *Birth*, 22(2), 101-110.

Eriksson, M., Mattsson, L., & Ladfors, L. (1997). Early or late bath during the first stage of labour: A randomized study of 200 women. *Midwifery* 13(3), 146-148.

Evans, S., & Jeffery, J. (1995). Maternal learning needs during labor and delivery. *J Obstet Gynecol Neonatal Nurs* 24(3), 235-240.

Finn, J. (1994). Culture care of Euro-American women during childbirth: Using Leininger's theory. *Transcultural Nursing*, 5(2), 25-37.

Fowles, E. (1998). Labor concerns of women 2 months after delivery. *Birth* 25(4), 235-240.

Friedman, E. (1978). *Labor: Evaluation and management* (2nd ed.). New York: Appleton-Century-Crofts.

Friedman, E., & Sachtleben, M. (1965). Station of the presenting part. *Am J Obstet Gynecol* 93(4), 522-529.

Gannon, J. (1992). Delivery on the hands and knees: A case study approach. *J Nurse Midwifery* 37(1), 48-52.

Geissler, E. (1994). *Pocket guide to cultural assessment.* St. Louis: Mosby.

Golay, J., Vedam, S., & Sorger, L. (1993). The squatting position for the second stage of labor: Effects on labor and on maternal and fetal well-being. *Birth* 20(2), 73-78.

Hanson, L. (1998a). Second stage positioning in nurse midwifery practices. Part 1: Position use and preferences. *J Nurse Midwifery* 43(5), 320-324.

Hanson, L. (1998b). Second stage positioning in nurse midwifery practices. Part 2: Factors affecting use. *J Nurse Midwifery* 43(5), 326-330.

Heritage, C. (1998). Working with childhood sexual abuse survivors during pregnancy, labor, and birth. *J Obstet Gynecol Neonatal Nurs* 27(6), 671-677.

Hill, V., Lowery, L., & Chez, R. (1998). Charting progress: Taking steps toward better documentation in the L&D. *AWHONN Lifelines* 2(1), 43-46.

Hodnett, E. (1996). Nursing support of the laboring woman. *J Obstet Gynecol Neonatal Nurs* 25(3), 257-264.

Howard, J., & Berbiglia, V. (1997). Caring for childbearing Korean women. *J Obstet Gynecol Neonatal Nurs* 26(6), 665-671.

Hueston, W. (1996). Factors associated with the use of episiotomy during vaginal delivery. *Obstet Gynecol* 87(6), 1001-1005.

Jonquil, S. (1993). Preparing siblings. *Midwifery Today Childbirth Education* 28(Winter), 34-35.

Jordan, E. (1995). Second stage labor nursing management. Presented at District IV AWHONN Conference, Washington, DC, October 8, 1995.

Kennell, J. et al. (1991). Continuous emotional support during labor in a US hospital. A randomized controlled trial. *JAMA* 265(17), 2197-2201.

Khazoyan, C., & Anderson, N. (1994). Latina's expectations for their partners during childbirth. *MCN Am J Matern Child Nurs* 19(4), 226-229.

Klaus, M., Kennell, J., & Klaus, P. (1993). *Mothering the mother.* Redwood City, CA: Addison-Wesley.

Labrecque, M. et al. (1997). Association between median episiotomy and severe perineal lacerations in primiparous women. *CMAJ* 156(6), 797-802.

Landry, S. et al. (1998). The effects of doula support during labor on mother-infant interaction at 2 months. *Pediatric Res* 43, 13A.

Lantican, L., & Corona, D. (1992). Comparison of the social support networks of Filipinos and Mexican American primigravidas. *Health Care Women Int* 13(4), 329-338.

Leininger, M. (1991). *Cultural care diversity and universality: A theory of nursing.* New York: National League of Nursing.

Ludka, L., & Roberts, C. (1993). Eating and drinking in labor, a literature review. *J Nurse Midwifery* 38(4), 199-207.

Lydon-Rochelle, M., Albers, L., & Teaf, D. (1995). Perineal outcomes and nurse-midwifery management. *J Nurse Midwifery* 40(1), 13-18.

Mackey, M. (1990). Women's preparation for the childbirth experience. *Matern Child Nurs J* 19(2), 143-173.

Maier, J., & Maloni, J. (1997). Nurse advocacy for selective versus routine episiotomy. *J Obstet Gynecol Neonatal Nurs* 26(2), 155-161.

McCandlish, R., & Renfrew, M. (1993). Immersion in water during labor and birth: The need for evaluation. *Birth* 20(2), 79-85.

McGuinnes, M., Norr, K., & Nacion, K. (1991). Comparison between different perineal outcomes on tissue healing. *J Nurse Midwifery* 36(3), 192-198.

McKay, S., & Barrows, T. (1991). Holding back: Maternal readiness to give birth. *MCN Am J Matern Child Nurs* 16(5), 250-254.

McKay, S., & Roberts, J. (1990). Obstetrics by ear. Maternal and caregiver perceptions of the meaning of maternal sounds during second stage labor. *J Nurse Midwifery* 35(5), 266-273.

McKay, S., & Smith, S. (1993). "What are they talking about? Is something wrong?" Information sharing during the second stage of labor. *Birth* 20(3), 142-147.

Melzack, R., Belanger, E., & Lacroix, R. (1991). Labor pain: Effects of maternal position on front and back pain. *J Pain Symptom Manage* 6(8), 476-480.

Metzger, B., & Therrien, B. (1990). Effect of position on cardiovascular response during the Valsalva maneuver. *Nurs Res* 39(4), 198-202.

Naef, R., & Morrison, J. (1994). Guidelines for the management of shoulder dystocia. *J Perinatol* 14(6), 435-441.

Nichols, F. (1996). The meaning of the childbirth experience: A review of the literature. *J Perinat Educ* 5(4), 71-77.

Nichols, M. (1993). Paternal perspectives of the childbirth experience. *Matern Child Nurs J* 21(3), 99-108.

Odent, M. (1997). Can water immersion stop labor? *J Nurse Midwifery* 42(5), 414-416.

Olsen, O. (1997). Meta-analysis of the safety of home birth. *Birth* 24(1), 4-16.

Olsen, S. (1998). Bedside musical care: Applications in pregnancy, childbirth, and neonatal care. *J Obstet Gynecol Neonatal Nurs* 27(5), 569-575.

Paciornik, M. (1990). Commentary: Arguments against episiotomy and in favor of squatting for birth. *Birth* 17(2), 104-105.

Pascoe, J. (1993). Social support during labor and duration of labor: A community-based study. *Public Health Nurs* 10(2), 97-99.

Perez, P. (1998). *Using the Gymnastik Ball in pregnancy, labor, birth, and postpartum.* Katy, TX: Cutting Edge Press.

Perez, P., & Herrick, L. (1998). Doulas: Exploring their roles with parents, hospitals, and nurses. *AWHONN Lifelines* 2(2), 54-55.

Peterson, L., & Besuner, P. (1997). Pushing techniques during labor: Issues and controversies. *J Obstet Gynecol Neonatal Nurs* 26(6), 719-726.

Piper, D., & McDonald, P. (1994). Management of anticipated and actual shoulder dystocia. *J Nurse Midwifery* 39(2 suppl), 91S-105S.

Proctor, S. (1998). What determines quality in maternity care? Comparing the perceptions of childbearing women and midwives. *Birth* 25(2), 85-93.

Pugh, L. et al. (1998). First stage of labor management: An examination of patterned breathing and fatigue. *Birth* 25(4), 241-245.

Renfrew, M. et al. (1998). Practices that minimize trauma to the genital tract in childbirth: A systematic review of the literature. *Birth* 25(3), 143-160.

Rhodes, N., & Hutchinson, S. (1994). Labor experiences of childhood sexual abuse survivors. *Birth* 21(4), 213-220.

Roberts, J., & Woolley, D. (1996). A second look at the second stage of labor. *J Obstet Gynecol Neonatal Nurs* 25(5), 415-423.

Rogers, J. et al. (1998). Active versus expectant management of third stage labour: The Hinchingbrooke randomized controlled trial. *Lancet* 351(9104), 693-699.

Rosenthal, M. (1991). Warm-water immersion in labor and birth. *Female Patient* 16(8), 35-47.

Rothman, B. (1996). Women, providers, and control. *J Obstet Gynecol Neonatal Nurs* 25(3), 253-256.

Scheepers, H., Essed, G., & Brouns, F. (1998). Aspects of food and fluid intake during labour: Policies of midwives and obstetricians in the Netherlands. *Eur J Obstet Gynecol Reprod Biol* 78(1), 37-40.

Schneiderman, J. (1998). Rituals of placenta disposal. *MCN Am J Matern Child Nurs* 23(3), 142-143.

Scott, J. et al. (1999). *Danforth's obstetrics and gynecology* (8th ed.). Philadelphia: Lippincott/Williams & Wilkins.

Shermer, R., & Raines, D. (1997). Positioning during the second stage of labor: Moving back to basics. *J Obstet Gynecol Neonatal Nurs* 26(6), 727-734.

Simkin, P. (1993). When should a child attend a sibling's birth? *Midwifery Today Childbirth Education* 28(Winter), 37.

Simkin, P. (1995). Reducing pain and enhancing progress in labor: A guide to nonpharmacologic methods for maternity caregivers. *Birth* 22(3), 161-171.

Simkin, P. (1996). The experience of maternity in a woman's life. *J Obstet Gynecol Neonatal Nurs* 25(3), 247-252.

Simkin, P., & Way, K. (1998). *Doulas of North America Position Paper: The doula's contribution to modern maternity care.* Seattle: DONA.

Technical Working Group, World Health Organization. (1997). Care in normal birth: A practical guide. *Birth* 24(2), 121-123.

Thomson, A. (1993). Pushing techniques in the second stage of labour. *J Adv Nurs* 18(2), 171-177.

Tomlinson, P., & Bryan, A. (1996). Family centered intrapartum care: Revisiting an old concept. *J Obstet Gynecol Neonatal Nurs* 25(4), 331-337.

Trowell, J. (1993). Emergency cesarean section: A research study of the mother/child relationship of a group of women admitted expecting a normal vaginal delivery. *Child Abuse and Neglect* 7, 387-394.

Tucker, S. (2000). *Pocket guide to fetal monitoring* (4th ed.). St. Louis: Mosby.

Urbanski, P. (1997). Placental evaluation: Pregnancy's black box? *AWHONN Lifelines* 1(2), 54-55.

Varney, H. (1997). *Varney's midwifery* (3rd ed.). Sudberry, MA: Jones & Bartlett.

Waldenström, U., & Gottvall, K. (1991). A randomized trial of birthing stool or conventional semirecumbent position for second stage labor. *Birth* 18(1), 5-10.

Waldenström, U. et al. (1996). The childbirth experience: A study of 295 new mothers. *Birth* 23(3), 144-153.

Waymire, V. (1997). A triggering time: Childbirth may recall sexual abuse memories. *AWHONN Lifelines* 1(2), 47-50.

Weber, S. (1996). Cultural aspects of pain in childbearing women. *J Obstet Gynecol Neonatal Nurs* 25(1), 67-72.

Wessely, S. (1998). Commentary: Reducing distress after normal childbirth. *Birth* 25(4), 220-221.

Willson, J., & Carrington, E. (1991). *Obstetrics and gynecology* (9th ed.). St. Louis: Mosby.

Wong, D., & Perry, S. (1998). *Maternal child nursing care.* St. Louis: Mosby.

Woods, A. (1991). Nurse midwifery in rural Pakistan. *J Nurse Midwifery* 36(4), 249-252.

Woolley, R. (1995). Benefits and risks of episiotomy: A review of the English-language literature since 1980. Part I and part II. *Obstet Gynecol Surv* 50(11), 806-835.

Wraight, A. (1997). Home births. *Midwives* 110(1312), 104-106.

Young, D. (1998). First class delivery: The importance of asking women what they think about their maternity care. *Birth* 25(2), 71-72.

Zhang, J. et al. (1996). Continuous labor support from labor attendant for primiparous women: A meta-analysis. *Obstet Gynecol* 88(4), 739-744.

23

Postpartum Physiology

Kitty Cashion

LEARNING OBJECTIVES

- Define the key terms.
- Describe the anatomic and physiologic changes that occur during the postpartum period.
- Identify characteristics of uterine involution and lochial flow and describe ways to measure them.

- List expected values for vital signs and blood pressure, deviations from normal findings, and probable causes of the deviations.
- Identify research topics on postpartum physiology.

KEY TERMS

colostrum	fourth trimester of pregnancy	lochia serosa
diaphoresis	hemorrhoids	pelvic relaxation
diastasis recti abdominis	involution	puerperium
diuresis	lochia alba	subinvolution
engorgement	lochia rubra	thromboembolism

The postpartum period is the 6-week interval between the birth of the newborn and the return of the reproductive organs to their normal nonpregnant state. This period is sometimes referred to as the **puerperium,** or **fourth trimester of pregnancy.** The physiologic changes that occur as the processes of pregnancy are reversed, though distinctive, are considered normal. Many factors, including the mother's energy level and degree of comfort, the health of the newborn, and the care and encouragement given by health professionals, contribute to the mother's response to her infant during this time. To provide care during the recovery period that is beneficial to the mother, her infant, and her family, the nurse must synthesize knowledge of maternal anatomy and physiology, the newborn's physical and behavioral characteristics, infant care activities, and the family response to the birth of the child. This chapter focuses on anatomic and physio-

logic changes that occur in the woman during the postpartum period.

REPRODUCTIVE SYSTEM AND ASSOCIATED STRUCTURES

Uterus

Involution Process

The return of the uterus to a nonpregnant state after birth is known as **involution.** This process begins immediately after expulsion of the placenta with contraction of the uterine smooth muscle.

At the end of the third stage of labor, the uterus is in the midline, about 2 cm below the level of the umbilicus, with the fundus resting on the sacral promontory. At this time, the uterus is approximately the size it was at 16 weeks of gestation (about the size of a grapefruit) and it weighs about 1000 g.

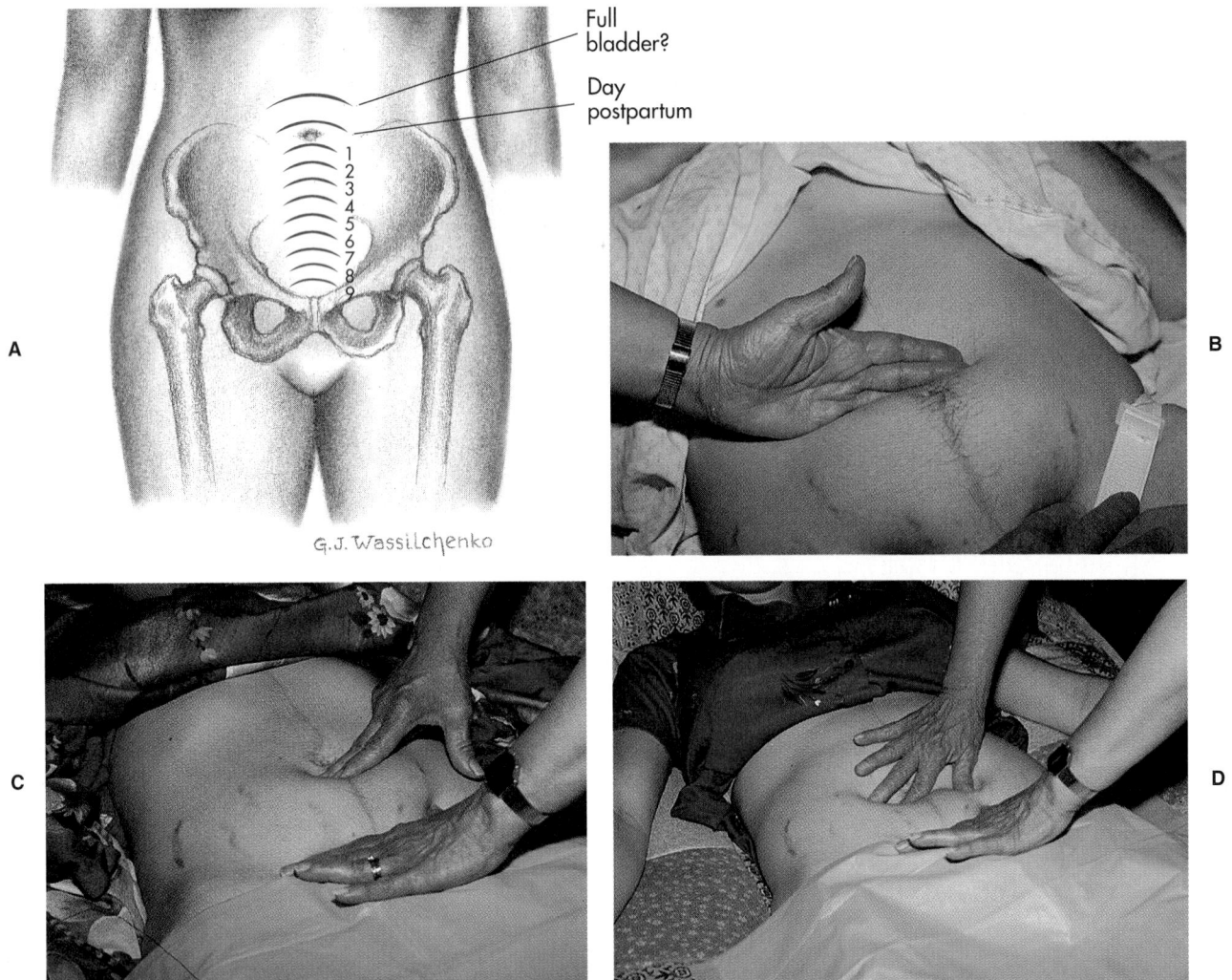

G.J. Wassilchenko

Fig. 23-1. Assessment of involution of uterus after childbirth. **A,** Normal progress, days 1 through 9. **B,** Size and position of uterus 2 hours after childbirth. **C,** Two days after childbirth. **D,** Four days after childbirth. *(B, C, and D courtesy Marjorie Pyle, RNC, Lifecircle, Costa Mesa, CA.)*

Within 12 hours the fundus may be approximately 1 cm above the umbilicus (Fig. 23-1). Involution progresses rapidly during the next few days. The fundus descends about 1 to 2 cm every 24 hours. By the sixth postpartum day the fundus is normally located halfway between the symphysis pubis and the umbilicus. A week after childbirth the uterus once again lies in the true pelvis. The uterus should not be palpable abdominally after the ninth postpartum day.

The uterus, which at full term weighs approximately 11 times its prepregnancy weight, involutes to about 500 g by 1 week after birth and 350 g by 2 weeks after birth. At 6 weeks it weighs 50 to 60 g (see Fig. 23-1).

Increased estrogen and progesterone levels are responsible for stimulating the massive growth of the uterus during pregnancy. Prenatal uterine growth is the result of both *hyperplasia,* an increase in the number of muscle cells, and *hypertrophy,* enlargement of the existing cells. Postpartally the decrease in the secretion of these hormones causes *autolysis,* which is the self-destruction of excess hypertrophied tissue. The additional cells laid down during pregnancy remain, however, and account for the fact that uterine size increases slightly after each pregnancy.

Subinvolution is the failure of the uterus to return to a nonpregnant state. The most common causes of subinvolution are retained placental fragments and infection.

Contractions

Postpartum hemostasis is achieved primarily by compression of intramyometrial blood vessels as the uterine muscle contracts, rather than by platelet aggregation and clot formation. The hormone oxytocin, which is released from the pituitary gland, strengthens and coordinates these uterine contractions, which compress blood vessels and thereby promote hemostasis. During the first 1 to 2 postpartum hours, uterine contractions may decrease in intensity and become uncoordinated. Because it is vital that the uterus remain firm and well contracted, exogenous oxytocin (Pitocin) is usually administered intravenously or intramuscularly immediately after expulsion of the placenta. Mothers who plan to breastfeed may be encouraged to put the baby to breast immediately after birth as well, because suckling stimulates the release of oxytocin.

Afterpains

In first-time mothers, uterine tone is increased, so the fundus generally remains firm. Periodic relaxation and vigorous contraction are more common in subsequent pregnancies and may cause uncomfortable cramping called *afterpains* that persist throughout the early puerperium. Afterpains are more noticeable after births in which the uterus was overdistended (for example, a large baby, multifetal gestation). Breastfeeding and exogenous oxytocin medication usually cause these afterpains to intensify, because both stimulate uterine contractions.

Placental Site

Immediately after the placenta and membranes are expelled, vascular constriction and thrombosis cause the placental site to be reduced to an irregular nodular and elevated area. Upward growth of the endometrium causes the sloughing of necrotic tissue and prevents the scar formation that is characteristic of normal wound healing. This unique healing process enables the endometrium to resume its usual cycle of changes and to permit implantation and placentation in future pregnancies. Endometrial regeneration is completed by the end of the third postpartum week, except at the placental site. Regeneration at the placental site usually is not complete until 6 weeks after birth.

Lochia

Postchildbirth uterine discharge, commonly called lochia, is initially bright red, changing later to a pinkish red or reddish brown. It may contain small clots of blood.

For the first 2 hours after birth the amount of uterine discharge should be about that of a heavy menstrual period. After that time, the lochial flow should steadily decrease.

Lochia rubra consists mainly of blood and decidual and trophoblastic debris. The flow pales, becoming pink or brown after 3 to 4 days (lochia serosa). **Lochia serosa** consists of old blood, serum, leukocytes, and tissue debris. About 10 days after childbirth the drainage becomes yellow to white (lochia alba). **Lochia alba** consists of leukocytes, decidua, epithelial cells, mucus, serum, and bacteria. Lochia alba may continue to drain from the vaginal opening for up to and beyond 6 weeks after childbirth (Visness, Kennedy, & Ramos, 1997).

It is difficult to judge the amount of lochial flow based only on observation of perineal pads. Luegenbiehl and

colleagues (1990) suggested one method for subjectively estimating postpartal blood loss, which entails gauging the extent of staining on a perineal pad (see Fig. 24-7). Weighing perineal pads before and after use provides a more objective measurement of lochial flow but is not common in practice. Each 1 g increase in weight is roughly equivalent to 1 ml of blood loss. Any estimation of lochial flow is inaccurate and incomplete, however, without considering the time factor. For example, the woman who saturates a peripad in 1 hour or less is bleeding much more than the woman who saturates a peripad in 8 hours.

If the woman receives an oxytocic medication, regardless of the route of administration, the flow of lochia is usually scant until the effects of the medication wear off. Also, the amount of lochia is usually less after cesarean births. The flow of lochia usually increases with ambulation and breastfeeding. Lochia tends to pool in the vagina when the woman is lying in bed; the woman may then experience a gush of blood when she stands. This gush should not be confused with hemorrhage.

Persistence of lochia rubra early in the postpartum period suggests continued bleeding as a result of retained fragments of the placenta or membranes. Recurrence of bleeding about 10 days after birth is from the healing placental site. However, any bleeding occurring 3 to 4 weeks after birth may be caused by infection or subinvolution. The continued flow of lochia serosa or lochia alba may indicate endometritis, particularly if this is accompanied by fever, pain, or abdominal tenderness. Lochia should smell like normal menstrual flow; an offensive odor usually indicates infection.

It is important to remember that not all postpartal vaginal bleeding is necessarily lochia. Another common source of vaginal bleeding after birth is unrepaired vaginal or cervical lacerations. Table 23-1 distinguishes between lochial and nonlochial bleeding.

TABLE 23-1 Lochial and Nonlochial Bleeding

LOCHIA	NONLOCHIAL BLEEDING
Lochia usually trickles from the vaginal opening. The steady flow is greater as the uterus contracts.	If the bloody discharge spurts from the vagina, there may be cervical or vaginal tears in addition to the normal lochia.
A gush of lochia may result as the uterus is massaged. If it is dark, it has been pooled in the relaxed vagina; the amount soon lessens to a trickle of bright red lochia (in the early puerperium).	If the amount of bleeding continues to be excessive and bright red, a cervical or vaginal tear may be the source.

Cervix

The cervix is soft immediately after birth. By 18 hours postpartum, however, it has shortened, become firm, and regained its form. The cervix up to the lower uterine segment remains edematous, thin, and fragile for several days after birth. The ectocervix (that portion of the cervix that protrudes into the vagina) appears bruised and has some small lacerations, constituting an optimal condition for the development of infection. The cervical os, which is dilated to 10 cm during labor, closes gradually. It may still be possible to introduce two fingers into the cervical os for the first 4 to 6 days postpartum; however, only the smallest curette may be introduced by the end of 2 weeks. The external cervical os never regains its prepregnancy appearance; it is no longer shaped like a circle but appears as a jagged slit often described as a "fish mouth." Lactation delays the production of cervical and other estrogen-influenced mucus and mucosal characteristics.

Vagina and Perineum

The estrogen deprivation that occurs postpartum is responsible for causing the thinness of the vaginal mucosa and the absence of rugae. The greatly distended, smooth-walled vagina gradually returns to its prepregnancy size by 6 to 8 weeks after childbirth. Rugae reappear by about the fourth week, although they are never as prominent as they are in the nulliparous woman. Most rugae may be permanently flattened. The mucosa remains atrophic in the lactating woman, at least until menstruation begins again. Thickening of the vaginal mucosa occurs with the return of ovarian function. The reduced estrogen levels are also responsible for causing a decreased amount of vaginal lubrication. Localized dryness and coital discomfort (dyspareunia) may persist until ovarian function returns and menstruation resumes. Use of a water-soluble lubricant that can help reduce discomfort during intercourse is usually recommended.

Initially the *introitus* is erythematous and edematous, especially in the area of the episiotomy or laceration repair. However, it is usually barely distinguishable from that of a nulliparous woman if lacerations and an episiotomy have been carefully repaired, hematomas are prevented or treated early, and the woman observes good hygiene during the first 2 weeks after birth.

Most *episiotomies* are visible only if the woman is lying on her side with her buttock raised or if she is placed in the lithotomy position. A good light source is essential for visualization of some episiotomies. An episiotomy heals the same way as any surgical incision. Signs of infection (pain, redness, warmth, swelling, or discharge) or the loss of approximation (separation of the incision edges) may occur. Healing should occur within 2 to 3 weeks.

Hemorrhoids (anal varicosities) are commonly seen. Women often experience associated symptoms such as itching, discomfort, and bright red bleeding with defecation. Hemorrhoids usually decrease in size within 6 weeks of childbirth.

Pelvic Muscular Support

The supporting structure of the uterus and vagina may be injured during childbirth and may contribute to gynecologic problems later. The supportive tissues of the pelvic floor that are torn or stretched during childbirth may require up to 6 months to regain tone. Women are often encouraged to do Kegel exercises after birth to help strengthen perineal muscles and promote healing. The term **pelvic relaxation** refers to the lengthening and weakening of the fascial supports of pelvic structures. These structures include the uterus, upper posterior vaginal wall, urethra, bladder, and rectum. Although pelvic relaxation can occur in any woman, it is usually a direct but delayed complication of childbirth.

ENDOCRINE SYSTEM

Placental Hormones

Significant hormonal changes occur during the postpartal period. Expulsion of the placenta results in dramatic decreases of the hormones produced by that organ. Decreases in human placental lactogen (hPL), estrogens, cortisol, and the placental enzyme insulinase cause the diabetogenic effects of pregnancy to be reversed, resulting in significantly lower blood sugar levels in the immediate puerperium. Mothers with type 1 diabetes will thus be likely to require much less insulin for several days after birth. Because these normal hormonal changes make the puerperium a transitional period for carbohydrate metabolism, it is more difficult to interpret the results of glucose tolerance tests at this time.

Estrogen and progesterone levels drop markedly following expulsion of the placenta, reaching their lowest levels 1 week into the postpartum period. Decreased estrogen levels are associated with breast engorgement and with the diuresis of excess extracellular fluid that has accumulated during pregnancy. The estrogen levels in nonlactating women begin to rise by 2 weeks after birth and are higher by postpartum day 17 than in women who breastfeed (Bowes, 1996).

Pituitary Hormones and Ovarian Function

Lactating and nonlactating women differ considerably in the time when the first ovulation occurs and when menstruation is reestablished. The persistence of elevated serum prolactin levels in breastfeeding women appears to be responsible for suppressing ovulation. Because levels of follicle-stimulating hormone (FSH) have been shown to be identical in lactating and nonlactating women, it is thought that ovulation is suppressed in lactating women because the ovary does not respond to FSH stimulation when increased prolactin levels are present (Bowes, 1996).

Prolactin levels in blood rise progressively throughout pregnancy. In women who breastfeed, however, prolactin levels remain elevated into the sixth week after birth (Bowes, 1996). Serum prolactin levels are influenced by the frequency of breastfeeding, the duration of each feeding, and the degree to which supplementary feedings are used. The individual differences in the strength of the infant's sucking stimulus probably also affect prolactin levels. This emphasizes the fact that breastfeeding is not a reliable form of birth control. After birth, prolactin levels decline in nonlactating women, reaching the prepregnant range in 4 to 6 weeks (Rebar, 1999).

Ovulation occurs as early as 27 days after birth in nonlactating women, with a mean time of about 70 to 75 days. Ovulation resumes by 2 months postpartum in most nonbreastfeeding women (Bowes, 1996). About 70% of nonbreastfeeding women resume menstruating by 3 months after birth (Resnik, 1999). The mean time to ovulation in women who breastfeed is about 190 days (Bowes, 1996). In lactating women, both the resumption of ovulation and the return of menses are determined in large part by breastfeeding patterns (Resnik, 1999). The fact that many women ovulate before their first postpartum menstrual period occurs reemphasizes the need for discussion of contraceptive options early in the puerperium (Rebar, 1999).

The first menstrual flow after childbirth is usually heavier than normal. Within three to four cycles the amount of menstrual flow has returned to the woman's prepregnant volume.

ABDOMEN

When the woman stands up during the first days after birth, her abdominal muscles protrude and give her a still-pregnant appearance. During the first 2 weeks after birth the abdominal wall is relaxed. It takes approximately 6 weeks for the abdominal wall to return almost to its prepregnancy state. The skin regains most of its previous elasticity, but some striae may persist. The return of muscle tone depends on previous tone, proper exercise, and the amount of adipose tissue. Occasionally, with or without overdistention because of a large fetus or multiple fetuses, the abdominal wall muscles separate, a condition termed **diastasis recti abdominis** (see Fig. 15-3). Persistence of this defect may be disturbing to the woman, but surgical correction is rarely necessary. With time, the defect becomes less apparent.

URINARY SYSTEM

The hormonal changes of pregnancy (high steroid levels) may be partly responsible for causing an increase in renal function, whereas the diminishing steroid levels after birth may partly explain the reduced renal function that occurs during the puerperium. Kidney function returns to normal within a month after birth. About 2 to 8 weeks are required for the pregnancy-induced hypotonia and dilation of the ureters and renal pelves to return to the prepregnant state (Cunningham et al., 1997). In a small percentage of women, dilation of the urinary tract may persist for 3 months, which increases the chance for the development of a urinary tract infection.

Urine Components

The renal glycosuria induced by pregnancy disappears, but lactosuria may occur in lactating women. The blood urea nitrogen (BUN) level increases during the puerperium as autolysis of the involuting uterus occurs. This breakdown of excess protein in the uterine muscle cells also results in a mild (+1) proteinuria for 1 to 2 days after childbirth in about 50% of women (Simpson & Creehan, 1996). Ketonuria may occur in women with an uncomplicated birth or after a prolonged labor with dehydration.

Postpartal Diuresis

Within 12 hours of birth, women begin to lose the excess tissue fluid that has accumulated during pregnancy. One mechanism responsible for reducing these retained fluids of pregnancy is the profuse **diaphoresis** that often occurs, especially at night, for the first 2 or 3 days after childbirth. Postpartal **diuresis,** caused by decreased estrogen levels, removal of increased venous pressure in the lower extremities, and loss of the remaining pregnancy-induced increase in blood volume, is another mechanism by which the body rids itself of excess fluid. The fluid loss through perspiration and the increased urinary output accounts for a weight loss of approximately 2.25 kg during the puerperium. This elimination of excess fluid accumulated during pregnancy is sometimes referred to as *reversal of the water metabolism of pregnancy.*

Urethra and Bladder

Trauma to the urethra and bladder may occur during the birth process as the infant passes through the pelvis. As a result the bladder wall may be hyperemic and edematous, often with small areas of hemorrhage. Clean-catch or catheterized urine specimens after birth often reveal hematuria from bladder trauma. The urethra and urinary meatus may also be edematous.

Birth-induced trauma, increased bladder capacity following childbirth, and the effects of conduction anesthesia combine to cause a decrease in the urge to void. In addition, pelvic soreness from the forces of labor, vaginal lacerations, or the episiotomy reduces or alters the voiding reflex. Decreased voiding, along with postpartal diuresis, may result in bladder distention. Immediately after birth, excessive bleeding can occur if the bladder becomes distended because this pushes the uterus up and to the side and prevents the uterus from firmly contracting. Later in the puerperium overdistention can make the bladder more susceptible to infection and impede the resumption of normal voiding (Cunningham et al., 1997). With adequate emptying of the bladder, bladder tone is usually restored 5 to 7 days after childbirth.

GASTROINTESTINAL SYSTEM

Appetite

The mother is usually hungry shortly after giving birth and can tolerate a light diet. Most new mothers are ravenously hungry after full recovery from analgesia, anesthesia, and fatigue. Requests for extra portions of food and frequent snacks are not uncommon.

Bowel Evacuation

A spontaneous bowel evacuation may be delayed until 2 to 3 days after childbirth. This can be explained by decreased muscle tone in the intestines during labor and the immediate puerperium, prelabor diarrhea, lack of food, or dehydration. The mother often anticipates discomfort during the bowel movement because of perineal tenderness as a result of episiotomy, lacerations, or hemorrhoids and therefore resists the urge to defecate. Regular bowel habits should be reestablished when bowel tone returns.

Obstetric trauma (e.g., direct injury to the sphincter muscle, damage to the innervation of the pelvic floor) is perhaps the leading cause of anal incontinence in otherwise healthy women (Toglia, 1996). Women should be taught during pregnancy about episiotomy and its possible sequelae. Pelvic floor (Kegel) exercises should be encouraged.

BREASTS

Promptly after childbirth there is a reduction in the concentrations of hormones that stimulated breast development during pregnancy (estrogen, progesterone, human chorionic gonadotropin, prolactin, cortisol, and insulin). The time it takes for these hormones to return to prepregnancy levels is determined in part by whether the mother breastfeeds her infant.

Breastfeeding Mothers

As lactation is established, a mass (lump) may be felt in the breast. Unlike the lumps associated with fibrocystic breast changes or cancer, which may be consistently palpated in the same location, a filled milk sac will shift position from day to day. Before lactation begins, the breasts feel soft and a yellowish fluid, **colostrum,** can be expressed from the nipples. After lactation begins, the breasts feel warm and firm. Tenderness may persist for about 48 hours after the start of lactation. Bluish-white milk with a skim milk appearance (true milk) can be expressed from the nipples. The nipples are examined for erectility and signs of irritation, such as cracks, blisters, or reddening.

Nonbreastfeeding Mothers

Generally the breasts feel nodular (in nonpregnant women they feel granular). The nodularity is bilateral and diffuse.

Prolactin levels drop rapidly. Colostrum is excreted for the first few days after childbirth. Palpation of the breast on the second or third day, as milk production begins, may reveal tissue tenderness in some women. On the third or fourth postpartum day, **engorgement** may occur. The breasts become distended (swollen), firm, tender, and warm to the touch (caused by vasocongestion). Breast distention is primarily caused by the temporary congestion of veins and lymphatics rather than from an accumulation of milk. Milk is present but should not be expressed. Axillary breast tissue (the tail of Spence) and any accessory breast or nipple tissue along the milk line may also be involved. Engorgement resolves spontaneously, and discomfort usually decreases within 24 to 36 hours. A breast binder or tight bra, ice packs, or mild analgesics may be used to relieve discomfort. Nipple stimulation is avoided. If suckling is never begun (or is discontinued), lactation ceases within a few days to a week.

CARDIOVASCULAR SYSTEM

Blood Volume

The changes in blood volume after birth depend on several factors, such as blood loss during childbirth and the amount of extravascular water (physiologic edema) mobilized and subsequently excreted. Blood loss results in an immediate but limited decrease in total blood volume. Thereafter most of the blood volume increase during pregnancy (1000 to 1500 ml) is eliminated within the first 2 weeks after birth, with return to nonpregnant values by 6 months postpartum (Simpson & Creehan, 1996).

Pregnancy-induced hypervolemia (an increase in blood volume of at least 40% more than prepregnancy values near term) allows most women to tolerate a considerable blood loss during childbirth. Many women lose approximately 300 to 400 ml of blood during vaginal birth of a single fetus and about twice this amount during cesarean birth.

The readjustments in the maternal vasculature after childbirth are dramatic and rapid. The woman's response to blood loss during the early puerperium differs from that in a nonpregnant woman. Three postpartum physiologic changes help protect the woman from excessive blood loss: (1) elimination of uteroplacental circulation reduces the size of the maternal vascular bed by 10% to 15%, (2) loss of placental endocrine function removes the stimulus for vasodilation, and (3) mobilization of extravascular water stored during pregnancy increases blood volume. Thus hypovolemic shock usually does not occur in women who experience a normal blood loss during the early puerperium.

Cardiac Output

The pulse rate, stroke volume, and cardiac output increase throughout pregnancy. Immediately after the birth, they remain elevated or rise even higher for 30 to 60 minutes as the blood that was shunted through the uteroplacental circuit suddenly returns to the maternal systemic venous circulation. These values increase regardless of the type of birth or use of conduction anesthesia (Bowes, 1996). Data regarding the exact return of cardiac hemodynamic levels to normal are not available, but cardiac output values remain elevated for at least 48 hours after birth, decrease rapidly in the first 2 weeks postpartum, and return to prepregnancy level by 24 weeks postpartum (Simpson & Creehan, 1996). Recently, stroke volume, cardiac output, end-diastolic volume, and systemic vascular resistance values have been shown to remain greatly elevated for as long as 12 weeks postpartum (Resnik, 1999).

Vital Signs

Few alterations in vital signs are seen under normal circumstances. There may be a small, transient rise in both systolic and diastolic blood pressure lasting about 4 days after the birth (Bowes, 1996) (Table 23-2). Respiratory function returns to the nonpregnant state by 6 to 8 weeks after birth. After the uterus is emptied, the diaphragm descends, the normal cardiac axis is restored, and the point of maximum impulse (PMI) and the electrocardiogram (ECG) are normalized.

Blood Components

Hematocrit and Hemoglobin

During the first 72 hours after childbirth there is a greater loss in plasma volume than in the number of blood cells. This results in a rise in the hematocrit and hemoglobin levels by the seventh day after birth. There is no accelerated red blood cell (RBC) destruction during the puerperium, but any excess will disappear gradually in accordance with the life span of the RBC. The exact time when the RBC volume returns to nonpregnant values is not known, but it is within normal limits when measured 8 weeks after childbirth (Bowes, 1996).

White Blood Cell Count

Normal leukocytosis of pregnancy averages about $12,000/mm^3$. During the first 10 to 12 days after childbirth,

TABLE 23-2   Vital Signs After Childbirth

NORMAL FINDINGS	DEVIATIONS FROM NORMAL FINDINGS AND PROBABLE CAUSES
TEMPERATURE During first 24 hours may rise to 38° C as a result of dehydrating effects of labor. After 24 hours the woman should be afebrile.	A diagnosis of puerperal sepsis is suggested if a rise in maternal temperature to 38° C is noted after the first 24 hours after childbirth and recurs or persists for 2 days. Other possibilities are mastitis, endometritis, urinary tract infections, and other systemic infections.
PULSE Pulse, along with stroke volume and cardiac output, remains elevated for the first hour or so after childbirth. It then begins to decrease at an unknown rate. By 8 to 10 weeks after childbirth the pulse has returned to a nonpregnant rate.	A rapid pulse rate or one that is increasing may indicate hypovolemia as a result of hemorrhage.
RESPIRATIONS The respiratory rate should decrease to within the woman's normal prebirth range by 6 to 8 weeks after childbirth.	Hypoventilation may occur after an unusually high subarachnoid (spinal) block or epidural narcotic after a cesarean birth.
BLOOD PRESSURE Blood pressure is altered *slightly* if at all. Orthostatic hypotension, as indicated by feelings of faintness or dizziness immediately after standing up, can develop in the first 48 hours as a result of the splanchnic engorgement that may occur after birth.	A low or decreasing blood pressure may indicate the existence of hypovolemia secondary to hemorrhage. However, it is a late sign, and other symptoms of hemorrhage usually alert the staff. An increased reading may result from excessive use of vasopressor or oxytocic medications. Because pregnancy-induced hypertension can persist into or occur first in the postpartum period, routine evaluation of blood pressure is needed. If a woman complains of headache, hypertension must be ruled out as a cause before analgesics are administered.

however, values of between 20,000 to 25,000/mm^3 are common. Neutrophils are the most numerous white blood cells (WBCs). This leukocytosis coupled with the normal increase in erythrocyte sedimentation rate that occurs may obscure the diagnosis of acute infections at this time.

Coagulation Factors

Clotting factors and fibrinogen levels are normally increased during pregnancy and remain elevated in the immediate puerperium. This hypercoagulable state, when combined with the vessel damage that occurs during childbirth and the immobility of the woman during recovery, increases the risk of **thromboembolism** (blood clots), especially after cesarean birth. Fibrinolytic activity also increases during the first few days after childbirth (Bowes, 1996). Levels of factors I, II, VIII, IX, and X decrease to nonpregnant levels within a few days. Fibrin split products, probably released from the placental site, can also be found in maternal blood.

Varicosities

Varicosities (varices) of the legs and around the anus (hemorrhoids) are common during pregnancy. Varices, even the less common vulvar varices, regress (empty) rapidly immediately after childbirth. Surgical repair of varicosities is not considered during pregnancy. Total or near-total regression of the varices is expected after childbirth.

NEUROLOGIC SYSTEM

Neurologic changes during the puerperium are those resulting from a reversal of maternal adaptations to pregnancy and those resulting from trauma during labor and childbirth.

Pregnancy-induced neurologic discomforts abate after birth. The elimination of physiologic edema through the diuresis that occurs after childbirth relieves carpal tunnel syndrome by easing the compression of the median nerve. The periodic numbness and tingling of fingers that afflict 5% of pregnant women usually disappear after childbirth unless lifting and carrying the baby aggravates the condition. Headache requires careful assessment. Postpartum headaches may be caused by various conditions, including pregnancy-induced hypertension (PIH), stress, and the leakage of cerebrospinal fluid into the extradural space during placement of the needle for administration of epidural or spinal anesthesia. Headaches last from 1 to 3 days to several weeks, depending on the cause and effectiveness of the treatment.

MUSCULOSKELETAL SYSTEM

Adaptations of the mother's musculoskeletal system that occur during pregnancy are reversed in the puerperium. These adaptations include the relaxation and subsequent hypermobility of the joints and the change in the mother's center of gravity in response to the enlarging uterus. The joints are completely stabilized by 6 to 8 weeks after birth. However, although all other joints return to their normal prepregnancy state, those in the parous woman's feet do not. The new mother may notice a permanent increase in her shoe size.

INTEGUMENTARY SYSTEM

Chloasma of pregnancy usually disappears at the end of pregnancy. Hyperpigmentation of the areolae and linea nigra may not regress completely after childbirth. These changes in pigmentation may be permanent in some women. Stretch marks on breasts, abdomen, hips, and thighs may fade but usually do not disappear.

Vascular abnormalities such as spider angiomas (nevi), palmar erythema, and epulis generally regress in response to the rapid decline in estrogens after the end of pregnancy. For some women, spider nevi persist indefinitely.

The abundance of fine hair seen during pregnancy usually disappears after birth; however, any coarse or bristly hair that appears during pregnancy usually remains. Fingernails return to their nonpregnant consistency and strength.

The profuse diaphoresis that occurs in the immediate postpartum period is the most noticeable change in the integumentary system.

IMMUNE SYSTEM

No significant changes in the maternal immune system occur during the postpartum period. The mother's need for rubella vaccination or for prevention of Rh isoimmunization is determined.

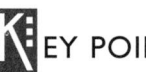 EY POINTS

- The uterus involutes rapidly after birth, returning to the true pelvis within 1 week.
- The rapid drop in estrogen and progesterone after expulsion of the placenta is responsible for triggering many of the anatomic and physiologic changes in the puerperium.
- Assessment of lochia and fundal height is essential to monitor the progress of normal involution and to identify potential problems.
- Breastfeeding is *not* a reliable form of birth control.
- Under normal circumstances, few alterations in vital signs are seen after childbirth.
- Activation of blood-clotting factors, immobility, and sepsis predispose the woman to thromboembolism.
- Marked diuresis, decreased bladder sensitivity, and overdistention of the bladder can lead to problems with urinary elimination.
- Postpartum physiologic changes allow the woman to tolerate considerable blood loss at birth.

CRITICAL THINKING EXERCISES

1 *What aspects of the normal postpartum physiologic changes would you explain to a new mother who is going home in 24 hours after birth?*

   a. *How would your explanation be different if the woman had given birth to other children?*

   b. *How would you explain these changes to a woman who does not speak English?*

2 *Assess the accuracy of subjective estimates of blood loss.*

   a. *Pour measured amounts of a red fluid (or expired blood from the blood bank, if available) on perineal pads or on plastic-backed underpads.*

   b. *Ask nursing students, maternity nurses, medical students, obstetricians, nurse-midwives, and anesthesiologists to make independent assessments of the volume.*

   c. *Calculate the percentage of correct responses among the total group and within each category of observer.*

   d. *Compare the results. Do profession, area of specialization, or years of experience correlate with more reliable estimates? Were people more likely to overestimate or underestimate the amount? Were the estimates for perineal pads or for underpads different? Were the errors in judgment large enough to raise concern about the accuracy of estimates of blood loss?*

References

Bowes, W. (1996). Postpartum care. In S. Gabbe, J. Niebyl, & J. Simpson (Eds.). *Obstetrics: Normal and problem pregnancies* (3rd ed.). New York: Churchill Livingstone.

Cunningham, F. et al. (1997). *Williams obstetrics* (20th ed.). Stamford, CT: Appleton & Lange.

Luegenbiehl, D. et al. (1990). Standardized assessment of blood loss. *MCN Am J Matern Child Nurs* 15(4), 241-244.

Rebar, R. (1999). The breast and the physiology of lactation. In R. Creasy & R. Resnik (Eds.). *Maternal-fetal medicine* (4th ed.). Philadelphia: WB Saunders.

Resnik, R. (1999). The puerperium. In R. Creasy & R. Resnik (Eds.). *Maternal-fetal medicine* (4th ed.). Philadelphia: W.B. Saunders.

Simpson, K., & Creehan, P. (1996). *AWHONN's perinatal nursing.* Philadelphia: J.B. Lippincott.

Toglia, M. (1996). Anal incontinence: An underrecognized, undertreated problem. *The Female Patient* 21(1), 17-30.

Visness, C., Kennedy, K., & Ramos, R. (1997). The duration and character of postpartum bleeding among breast-feeding women. *Obstet Gynecol* 89(2), 159-163.

24

Assessment and Care During the Postpartum Period

Kitty Cashion

LEARNING OBJECTIVES

- Define the key terms.
- Identify the priorities of maternal care given during the fourth stage of labor.
- Identify common selection criteria for safe early postpartum discharge.
- List the pros and cons of early postpartum discharge.
- Give examples of physical and psychosocial nursing diagnoses pertaining to women in the postpartum period.
- Identify expected outcomes for postpartum physical and psychosocial care.
- Summarize nursing interventions to prevent infection and excessive bleeding.

- Summarize nursing interventions to promote normal bladder and bowel patterns and care for the breasts of women who are breastfeeding or bottle-feeding.
- Explain the influence of cultural expectations on postpartum adjustment.
- Discuss the nurse's responsibilities related to discharge teaching and preparation for home care.
- Describe the nurse's role in these postpartum follow-up strategies: home visits, telephone follow-up, warm lines and help lines, support groups, and referrals to community resources.
- Identify topics for nursing research related to postpartum care.

KEY TERMS

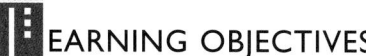

afterbirth pains	Homans' sign	rubella vaccine
couplet care	Kegel exercises	thrombus
early postpartum discharge	Kleihauer-Betke test	uterine atony
engorgement	oxytocic medications	warm line
fourth stage of labor	Rh immune globulin	

The goal of nursing care in the immediate postpartum period is to assist women and their partners during their initial transition to parenting. The approach to the care of women after birth has changed from one modeled on sick care to one that is wellness oriented. Consequently, in the United States most women remain hospitalized as few as 1 or 2 days after giving birth and some for as few as

6 hours. Because there is so much important information to be shared with these women in a very short time, it is vital that their care be thoughtfully planned and provided. The nurse provides care that focuses on the woman's physiologic recovery, her psychologic well-being, and her ability to care for herself and her new baby. In addition, the nurse considers the needs of other family members and includes

strategies in the plan of care to assist the family in adjusting to the new baby.

To provide quality care, the nurse must be knowledgeable about physical changes in the mother and psychosocial and emotional changes in the entire family. This chapter focuses on using the nursing process to meet both the mother's and the family's needs during this crucial time.

THE FOURTH STAGE OF LABOR

The first 1 to 2 hours after birth, sometimes referred to as the **fourth stage of labor,** is a crucial time for the mother and newborn. Both are not only recovering from the physical process of birth but also are becoming acquainted with each other and with additional family members. During this time, maternal organs start to undergo readjustment to the nonpregnant state, and the functions of body systems begin to stabilize. Meanwhile, the newborn continues to make the transition from an intrauterine to extrauterine existence.

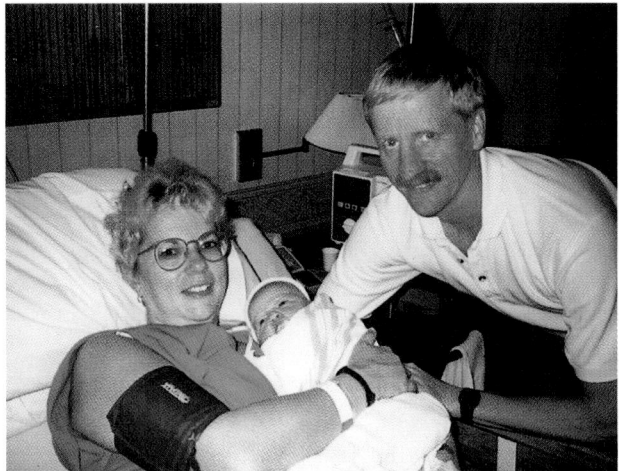

Fig. 24-1 Parents becoming acquainted with daughter. *(Courtesy Jan Harmon, St. Louis.)*

NURSE ALERT

The nurse's role during the fourth stage of labor is to monitor the recovery of the new mother and infant and to promptly identify and manage any deviations from the normal processes that may occur.

The fourth stage of labor is an excellent time to begin breastfeeding because the infant is in an alert state and ready to nurse. Breastfeeding at this time also promotes the contraction of the uterus and the prevention of maternal hemorrhage. Getting breastfeeding off to a good start is not just encouraging for the mother; it is also physiologically vital for the infant. Colostrum loosens mucus and acts as a laxative, thus promoting the rapid elimination of meconium. It also decreases the likelihood of hypoglycemia, reduces the severity of physiologic hyperbilirubinemia, and provides important immunologic benefits.

In most centers, the mother remains in the labor and birth area during this recovery time. In an institution where labor, delivery, and recovery (LDR) rooms are used, the woman stays in the same room where she gave birth. In traditional settings, women are taken from the delivery room to a separate recovery area for observation. Arrangements for the care of the newborn vary during the fourth stage of labor. In many settings, the baby remains at the mother's bedside and the labor or birth nurse cares for both of them. In other institutions, the baby is taken to the nursery for several hours of observation after an initial bonding period with the parents (Fig. 24-1).

Assessment

If the recovery nurse has not previously cared for the new mother, her assessment begins with an oral report from the nurse who attended the woman during labor and birth and

a review of the prenatal, labor, and birth records. Of primary importance are conditions that could predispose the mother to hemorrhage, such as precipitous labor, a large baby, grand multiparity, or induced labor. For healthy women, hemorrhage is probably the most dangerous potential complication that can occur.

To help the nurse provide comprehensive care, use of a worksheet or recovery record is suggested. Figure 24-2 illustrates an easy-to-use flow sheet that has the essential immediate postpartum and anesthesia recovery assessments. During the first hour in the recovery room, physical assessments of the mother are frequent. All factors except temperature are assessed every 15 minutes for 1 hour. Temperature is assessed at the beginning and end of the recovery period. After the fourth 15-minute assessment, if all parameters have stabilized within the normal range, the process is usually repeated every 30 minutes during the second hour. Box 24-1 and Fig. 24-3 describe the physical assessment of the mother during the fourth stage.

During the fourth stage of labor, many postpartum women experience intense tremors that resemble shivering from a chill. They are commonly seen after birth and are not related to infection. Several theories have been offered to explain these tremors or shivering, such as their being the result of a sudden release of pressure on pelvic nerves after birth, a response from a fetus-to-mother transfusion that occurred during placental separation, a reaction to maternal adrenaline production during labor and birth, or a reaction to epidural anesthesia. The nurse can help women who experience these chills by providing warm blankets and reassurance that the chills or tremors are common, self-limiting, and last only a short while.

The nutritional status of the woman is assessed. Restriction of food and fluid intake and the loss of fluids (blood, perspiration, or emesis) during labor cause many women to express a strong desire to eat or drink soon after birth.

Procedure: _____
Diagnosis: _____
Physician: _____
Anesthesia: _____
Anesthetist: _____
Armbands: _____ mother _____ infant
Clothing: _____ c̄ family _____ c̄ patient

Maternity Recovery Room Record

Admission note:

Activity	
Able to move 4 extremities voluntarily or on command	2
Able to move 2 extremities voluntarily or on command	1
Able to move 0 extremities voluntarily or on command	0
Respiration	
Able to deep breathe and cough freely	2
Dyspnea or limited breathing	1
Apneic	0
Blood pressure	
BP ± mm Hg of preanesthetic level	2
BP ± 25-50 mm Hg of preanesthetic level	1
BP ± Greater than 50 mm Hg of preanesthetic level	0
Conscious level	
Fully aware	2
Arousable on calling	1
Not responding	0
Color	
Pink	2
Pale, dusky, blotchy, jaundiced, other	1
Cyanotic	0

Par score: ADM: _____ DC: _____   Homan's Sign   Pos☐ Neg☐

	Bonding	Teaching
Activity	☐Appropriate	☐Fundal massage
Respiration	☐Inappropriate	☐TC & DB
Blood pressure	☐NA (explain)	☐Breastfeeding
Conscious level		☐Assistance on
Color		1st ambulation
Total		☐_____

Vital signs: Initial hour: q 15 min then Routine: q 4 other per protocol Tox: *q 1	Time											Meds / IV / Rate	Time / Initial
	BP												
	Pulse												
	Resp / O₂Sat												
Fundus FB-Fingerbreath B-Boggy FM-Firm MD-Midline	Fundus												
Lochia CL-Clots MOD-Moderate SM-Small LG-Large	Lochia												
Bladder D-Distended F-Foley ND-Nondistended	Bladder												
Episiotomy/Incision NL-Normal D-Dry ABNL-Abnormal I-Intact	Epis / Inc												
q 4°	Temp												
Clear CL Wheezing W Diminished	Breath sounds												
q 1° / q 4°	DTR / Protein												
Admission intake Total													
Admission output Total											Intake total Shift 7A 3P 11P	Signature
Initials													
Discharge note											Output total Shift 7A 3P 11P	
Report called to:												
Anesthesia D/C: Epidural catheter: In Out NA											IV ____cc LTC @ D/C	

*Toxemia (preeclampsia) LTC, left to count.

Fig. 24-2 An example of a maternity recovery room record. *(Courtesy The Regional Medical Center at Memphis [The Med], Memphis, TN.)*

BOX 24-1 Assessment During Fourth Stage of Labor

Before beginning the assessment, wash hands thoroughly, assemble necessary equipment, and explain the procedure to the woman.

BLOOD PRESSURE

Measure blood pressure per assessment schedule.

PULSE

Assess rate and regularity.

TEMPERATURE

Determine temperature.

FUNDUS

Put on clean examination gloves.
Position woman with knees flexed and head flat.
Just below the umbilicus, cup hand and press firmly into abdomen. At the same time, stabilize the uterus at the symphysis with the opposite hand.
If fundus is firm (and bladder is empty), with uterus in midline, measure its position relative to woman's umbilicus. Lay fingers flat on abdomen under umbilicus; measure how many fingerbreadths (fb) or centimeters (cm) fit between the umbilicus and top of fundus. If the fundus is above the umbilicus, this is recorded as plus fb or cm; if below, as minus fb or cm.
If the fundus is *not* firm, massage it gently to help it contract and expel any clots before measuring the distance from the umbilicus.
Place hands appropriately; massage gently *only until firm.*
Expel clots while keeping hands placed as shown in Fig. 24-3. With upper hand, apply firm pressure downward toward vagina; observe perineum for amount and size of expelled clots.

BLADDER

Assess distention by noting location and firmness of uterine fundus and by observing and palpating bladder. A distended bladder is seen as a rounded suprapubic bulge that is dull to percussion and fluctuates like a water-filled balloon. When the bladder is distended, the uterus is usually boggy in consistency, well above the umbilicus, and to the woman's right side.
Assist woman to void spontaneously. *Measure amount of urine voided.*
Catheterize as necessary.
Reassess after voiding or catheterization to make sure the bladder is not palpable and the fundus is firm and in the midline.

LOCHIA

Observe lochia on perineal pads and on linen under the woman's buttocks. Determine amount and color; note size and number of clots and odor.
Observe perineum for source of bleeding (e.g., episiotomy, lacerations).

PERINEUM

Ask or assist woman to turn on her side and flex upper leg on hip.
Lift upper buttock.
Observe perineum in good lighting.
Assess episiotomy site or laceration repair for intactness, hematoma, edema, bruising, redness, and drainage.
Assess for presence of hemorrhoids.

In the absence of complications, a woman who has given birth vaginally, has recovered from the effects of the anesthetic, and has stable vital signs, a firm uterus, and small to moderate lochial flow may have fluids and a regular diet as desired (American Academy of Pediatrics & American College of Obstetricians and Gynecologists, 1997).

Postanesthesia Recovery

The woman who has given birth by cesarean or has received regional anesthesia for a vaginal birth requires special attention during the recovery period. In fact, obstetric recovery areas are held to the same standard of care that would be expected of any other postanesthesia recovery room. A recovery from anesthesia requires the nurse to have available cardiopulmonary support and emergency supplies (e.g., resuscitation bag, face mask) (Johnson & Johnson, 1996). A postanesthesia recovery (PAR) score is

determined for each client upon her arrival and is updated as part of every 15 minute assessment. Components of the PAR score include activity, respirations, blood pressure, level of consciousness, and color.

NURSE ALERT

Regardless of her obstetric status, no woman should be discharged from the recovery area until she has completely recovered from the effects of anesthesia.

If the woman received general anesthesia, she should be awake and alert, oriented to time, place, and person. Her respiratory rate should be within normal limits, and her oxygen saturation levels at least 95%, as measured by a pulse oximeter. If the woman received epidural or spinal anesthesia, she should be able to raise her legs, extended at

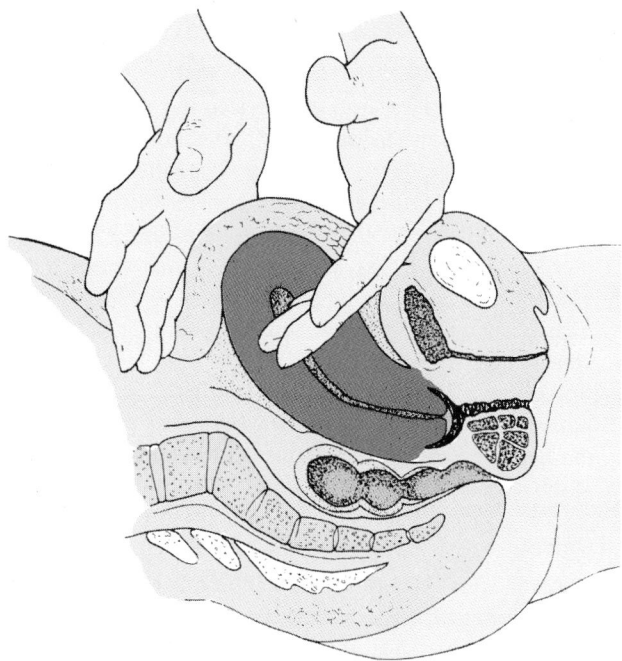

Fig. 24-3 Palpating fundus of uterus during the fourth stage of labor. Note that upper hand is cupped over fundus; lower hand dips in above symphysis pubis and supports uterus while it is massaged gently.

the knees, off the bed, or to flex her knees, place her feet flat on the bed, and raise her buttocks well off the bed. The numb or tingling, prickly sensation should be entirely gone from her legs. Often it takes 1½ to 2 hours for these anesthetic effects to disappear.

Transfer from the Recovery Area

After the initial recovery period of 1 to 2 hours has been completed, the woman may be transferred to a postpartum room in the same or another nursing unit. In facilities with labor, delivery, recovery, postpartum (LDRP) rooms, the nurse who provides care during the recovery period usually continues the care for the woman. Women who have received general or regional anesthesia must be cleared for transfer from the recovery area by a member of the anesthesia care team.

In preparing the transfer report, the recovery nurse uses information from the records of admission, birth record, and recovery. Information that must be communicated to the postpartum nurse includes identity of the primary health care provider; gravidity and parity; age; anesthetic used; any medications given; duration of labor and time of rupture of membranes; oxytocin induction or augmentation; type of birth and repair; blood type and Rh status; GBS status; status of rubella immunity; syphilis and hepatitis serology test results; intravenous infusion of any fluids; physiologic status since birth; description of the fundus, lochia, bladder, and perineum; sex and weight of the infant; time of birth; pediatrician; chosen method of feeding; any abnormalities noted; and assessment of initial parent-infant interaction.

Most of this information is also documented for the nursing staff in the newborn nursery. In addition, specific information should be provided regarding the infant's Apgar scores, weight, voiding, and whether fed since birth. Nursing interventions that have been completed (e.g., eye prophylaxis, vitamin K injection) must also be recorded.

Table 24-1 gives examples for documenting this information before the transfer of the woman from the recovery area.

Women who give birth in birthing centers may go home within a few hours after the woman's and infant's conditions are stable.

DISCHARGE—BEFORE 24 HOURS AND AFTER 48 HOURS

Postpartum home care has been an area of significant growth and interest because of the shortening hospital stay and the need of women, newborns, and family for ongoing care in the home. **Early postpartum discharge,** *shortened hospital stay,* and *1-day maternity stays* are all terms for the decreasing length of hospital stays of mothers and their babies after a low risk birth.

In years past it was common for maternity stays to be set at a predetermined duration (usually counted in days) after birth. For example, the usual length of stay was 3 days after a vaginal birth and 5 days after a cesarean birth. Knowing the number of days enabled the health care team and family to plan care accordingly. Then for several years, it was common for the length of stay to be 24 hours or less for women who experienced a normal vaginal birth and approximately 72 hours for women who experienced a cesarean birth.

This trend of shortened hospital stay was based largely on efforts to reduce health care costs (economic factors) coupled with consumer demands to have less medical intervention and more family-centered experiences (Ferguson & Engelhard, 1997; Wilkerson, 1996), all of which has increasingly affected numbers of maternity clients and the nurses who provide their care.

Laws Relating to Discharge

Health care providers expressed concern that some medical problems do not show up in the first 24 hours after birth and that new mothers have not sufficiently learned how to care for their newborns and identify newborn health problems such as jaundice and dehydration related to breastfeeding difficulties (Havens & Hannan, 1996). The first day after birth is not a time conducive to learning for many women (Barnes, 1996; Brown & Johnson, 1998). There has also been concern that shortened hospital stays will increase maternal hospital readmission for infection, hypertension, and hemorrhage of women who delivered vaginally.

TABLE 24-1 Recovery Nurse's Report

ITEM	EXAMPLE OF DOCUMENTATION OF MOTHER	EXAMPLE OF DOCUMENTATION OF NEWBORN
Type of labor and birth: unusual observations, if any, of the placenta	Spontaneous or assisted (forceps) vaginal birth; vertex presentation	Spontaneous or assisted (forceps, vacuum extractor) vaginal birth in vertex presentation; time of ROM
Gravidity and parity, age	G1, P1, 22 years old; 39 weeks of gestation	G1, P1, 22 years old; 39 weeks of gestation
Anesthesia and analgesia used	None; epidural, low spinal, local	None; epidural, low spinal, or local
Condition of perineum	Episiotomy; repair of lacerations; intact	
Events since birth	Vital signs, BP, fundus, lochia, intake and output, medications (dosage, time of administration, and results), response to newborn, observation of family interactions, including siblings, if present	Nursed at breast Voided × 1; meconium stool × 1 Eye prophylaxis given Vitamin K injection given Held by siblings who are happy (or have other response to newborn)
Condition and sex of newborn; other information	Time of birth; Apgar at 1 and 5 min; weight; whether breastfeeding or bottle feeding; sex of the baby	Time of birth; Apgar scores at 1 and 5 min Sex; weight; name of pediatrician; breastfeeding or bottle feeding; mother's hepatitis B status and GBS status; whether mother received MgSO₄; time of last systemic analgesia
Relevant information from prenatal record	Need for rubella vaccination; presence of infections; hepatitis B status; HIV status; blood type; Rh status; GBS status and treatment if positive	Unremarkable pregnancy
Miscellaneous information IV drip	If IV drip is infusing, rate of infusion, medications added (e.g., Pitocin), whether to keep open or discontinue after completion of bag that is hung	
Social factors	If woman is releasing baby for adoption, whether she wants to see baby, breastfeed, allow visitors, or other preferences she may have	Baby up for adoption; to stay in NBN until discharge

BP, Blood pressure; *GBS*, group B streptococcus; *NBN*, newborn nursery; *ROM*, rupture of membranes.

Parents are experiencing a major life transition during the immediate days and weeks of the fourth trimester. They are recovering from the events surrounding birth, adjusting to the demands of a newborn, parenting, applying their postdischarge instructions, shifting priorities, and realigning some roles while assuming new ones. An additional challenge occurs when there are other children at home who must be helped to adjust in sharing their home and parents with the newborn. The stress inherent in such profound transitions is the source of a tremendous potential for crisis and growth during the early postpartum period.

The widespread concern for the potential increase in adverse maternal-child outcomes from hospital early discharge practices led the American College of Obstetricians and Gynecologists (ACOG), the American Academy of Pediatrics (AAP), and other professional health care organizations to promote the enactment of federal and various state maternity length-of-stay bills to ensure adequate care for both the mother and the newborn. The passage of the landmark Newborns' and Mothers' Health Protection Act of 1996 provides minimum federal standards for health plan coverage for mothers and their newborns (Ferguson & Engelhard, 1997). Under the Act, all health plans are required to allow the new mother and newborn to remain in the hospital for a minimum of 48 hours after a normal vaginal birth and for 96 hours after a cesarean birth unless the attending provider, in consultation with the mother, decides upon early discharge.

Research studies to determine the appropriate length of hospital stay for newborns seem to support this legislation. One large study (Liu et al., 1997) found that newborns discharged early (less than 30 hours after birth) were more likely to be rehospitalized for jaundice, dehydration, and infection within 1 month of life than newborns discharged later (30 to 72 hours after birth). Edmonson, Stoddard, and Owens (1997) were unable to find any significant reason for newborn readmission; however, they concluded that readmission was more likely among babies who were firstborn, breastfed, or born to unmarried and poorly educated women.

Several early postpartum hospital discharge programs that provided extensive prenatal preparation and postpartum follow-up found it generally safe for mothers who gave birth vaginally and their newborns to be discharged less than 48 hours after birth (Fishbein & Burggraf, 1998; Williams & Cooper, 1996).

Proponents of early postpartum discharge cite the following advantages of the practice:
- Reinforces the concept of childbirth as a normal physiologic event.
- Allows shorter separations between mothers and other children.
- Extends a couple's sense of control and participation beyond the birth itself.
- Capitalizes on the security of the home environment during the stressors of early parenting.
- Decreases unnecessary exposure to the pathogens in the hospital environment.
- Allows beds on the maternity service to be used more effectively (that is, quick turnover in clients or greater availability for clients with a complication).
- Allows more time for mother/father/partner/infant and other family members to bond (Fig. 24-4).
- Creates less disruption in the daily life of the family.
- Promotes active involvement of family and support persons in assisting the mother and newborn.

Opponents of early postpartum discharge cite the following disadvantages of the practice:
- Complications (maternal or newborn) may go unrecognized.
- Families may be or feel unprepared for the reality they face once the baby is at home.
- The mother is fatigued from the labor and childbirth process.
- The mother is experiencing postpartum pain or discomfort.
- The length of time for learning after the birth in the hospital setting is decreased.
- A vulnerability and crisis potential exists for both women and families.

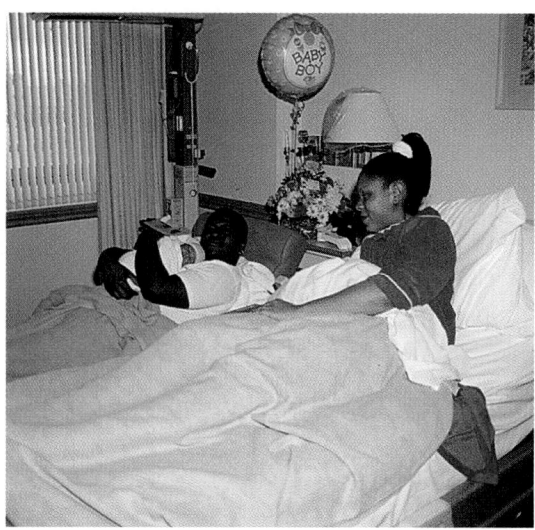

Fig. 24-4 Bonding and attachment begun early after birth are fostered in the postpartum period. *(Courtesy Marjorie Pyle, RNC, Lifecircle, Costa Mesa, CA.)*

The protest against early discharge becomes more powerful in the conventional health care arena in which care does not include a home care visit and there is a long interval between discharge and the first follow-up examination.

The Future of Early Postpartum Discharge

There has been much debate about the best practice for women, newborns, and their families in terms of the length of hospitalization. All components of health care systems (that is, hospitals, physicians, nurses, nurse-midwives, home health care, managed care, and health maintenance organizations [HMOs]) are exploring models that ensure the delivery of safe, effective care.

The specialty of postpartum home care has emerged as increased numbers of clients are being referred for home follow-up after a short maternity stay or for follow-up after a cesarean birth. With this trend, new and existing home care programs are likely to extend their services and service area to a greater number of clients. In addition, common problems such as maternal infection and infant hyperbilirubinemia, identified after discharge, can be treated in the home (Brown & Johnson, 1998).

Criteria for Discharge

Early discharge and postpartum home care can be a safe and satisfying option for women and their families when it is comprehensive and based on individual needs (Wilkerson, 1996). However, early discharge is not appropriate for every mother and newborn (AAP & ACOG, 1997). Hospital stays need to be long enough to identify problems and to ensure that the woman is sufficiently recovered and prepared to care for herself and the baby at home.

It is essential that nurses consider the medical needs of the woman and her baby and provide care that is coordi-

▪ BOX 24-2 Criteria for Early Discharge

MOTHER

Uncomplicated pregnancy, labor, vaginal birth, and post-partum course

No evidence of premature rupture of membranes

Blood pressure, temperature stable and within normal limits

Ambulating unassisted

Voiding adequate amounts without difficulty

Hemoglobin >10 g

No significant vaginal bleeding; perineum intact or no more than second-degree episiotomy or laceration repair; uterus is firm

Received instructions on postpartum self-care

INFANT

Term infant (38 to 42 weeks) with weight appropriate for gestational age

Normal findings on physical assessment

Temperature, respirations, and heart rate within normal limits and stable for the 12 hours preceding discharge

At least two successful feedings completed (normal sucking and swallowing)

Urination and stooling have occurred at least once

No evidence of significant jaundice in the first 24 hours after the birth

No excessive bleeding at the circumcision site for at least 2 hours

Screening tests performed according to state regulations; tests to be repeated at follow-up visit if done before the infant is 24 hours old

Initial hepatitis B vaccine given or scheduled for first follow-up visit

Laboratory data reviewed: maternal syphilis and hepatitis B status; infant or cord blood type and Coombs' test results if indicated

GENERAL

No social, family, or environmental risk factors identified

Family or support person available to assist mother and infant at home

Follow-up scheduled within 1 week if discharged before 48 hours after the birth

Documentation of skill of mother in feeding (breast or bottle), cord care, skin care, perineal care, infant safety (use of car seat, sleeping positions), and recognizing signs of illness and common infant problems

Source: American Academy of Pediatrics. (1995). Hospital stay for healthy term infants. *Pediatrics* 96(4), 788-790; Weekly, S., & Neumann, M. (1997). Speaking up for baby: The case for individualized neonatal discharge plans. *AWHONN Lifelines* 1(1), 24-29.

nated to meet those needs in order to provide timely physiologic interventions and treatment to prevent morbidity and hospital readmission. With predetermined criteria for identifying low risk in the mothers and newborns (Box 24-2), the length of hospitalization can be based on the medical need for care in an acute care setting or in consideration of the ongoing care needed in the home environment (AAP & ACOG, 1997; Weekly & Neumann, 1997).

In conjunction with the attending physician or nurse-midwife and family, the hospital-based maternity nurse is instrumental in determining the readiness of a woman for home care and in preparing the woman and the family for the home care plan of treatment. An example of a care path for the progression of postpartum physical, psychosocial, and self-care changes and for the teaching needs of women after uncomplicated, vaginal birth within a 24-hour time frame is found on p. 598. A similar format can be used for a cesarean birth care path with time frame adjustments accounting for a longer hospital stay (e.g., 3 to 4 days) (Simpson & Creehan, 1996).

Care paths provide the nurse with an organized approach toward meeting essential maternal-newborn care and teaching goals within a limited time frame. Other methods such as postpartum order sets and maternal-

newborn teaching checklists (Fig. 24-5) can also be used to accomplish designated client care and educational outcomes. By determining what is most appropriate for the individual woman and newborn, the length of stay and care coordinated by the health care team can be adjusted to ensure the delivery of safe and effective care.

Hospital-based maternity nurses continue to play invaluable roles as caregivers, teachers, and client and family advocates in developing and implementing effective home care strategies. It is imperative that nurses adapt their care to meet the needs of their clients and families in the acute care setting (Brown & Johnson, 1998). In collaboration with other health care providers, the nurse is instrumental in determining whether the mother and newborn meet the criteria for early discharge. With coordination, clinical care and education can be planned and provided throughout pregnancy, during the hospital stay, and in the home after discharge to ensure the family's continued well-being.

▪ CARE MANAGEMENT: PHYSICAL NEEDS
Assessment and Nursing Diagnoses

A complete physical assessment, including measurement of vital signs, is performed upon admission to the postpartum

Date of Birth: _____
Hour of Birth: _____

The uncomplicated vaginal birth client's admission/discharge is based on a 24-hour length of stay postbirth based on individual needs.

*IHSP denotes a test done to determine whether follow-up is needed in the Infant Hearing Screening Program (IHSP).

Time: _____

		RECOVERY	ADM. TO PP UNIT—8 HOUR	9-16 HOURS	17-24 HOURS/DISCHARGE
PRIMARY PHYSIOLOGIC FOCUS		Woman will have normal vital signs as documented on flowsheet.	Woman will have normal VS and moderate lochia rubra.	Woman will have normal VS and minimal lochia rubra.	Woman will have normal VS and minimal lochia rubra.
		NA MET VARIANCE	**NA MET VARIANCE**	**NA MET VARIANCE**	**NA MET VARIANCE**
		Vital signs every 15 min × 1 hour, then every 4 hours. Assess perineum/ episiotomy. Ice pack prn. Assess lochia.	Vital signs every 4 hours. Assess perineum/ episiotomy. Ice pack prn. Assess lochia.	Vital signs every shift. Assess perineum/ episiotomy. Ice pack prn. Assess lochia.	Vital signs every shift. Assess perineum/ episiotomy. Ice pack prn. Assess lochia.
IVs/LABWORK/ MEDICATIONS		**RECOVERY**	**ADM. TO PP UNIT—8 HOURS**	**9-16 HOURS**	**17-24 HOURS/DISCHARGE**
		Woman will have appropriate lab work done and medication given by time of transfer to Mother/ Baby Unit.	Woman will begin to verbalize understanding of hepatitis status and medication requirements.	Woman will have appropriate lab work done by 16 hours PP.	Woman will have appropriate lab work done and appropriate meds initiated.
		NA MET VARIANCE	**NA MET VARIANCE**	**NA MET VARIANCE**	**NA MET VARIANCE**
		CBC, if not done before birth. Urine drug screen if ordered. U/A—dipstick. (Send to lab, if abnormal.)	Review hepatitis B status. Medication regimen initiated	CBC. Review Rubella status. Review Hgb and Hct.	Fe Tab. Prenatal Vitamin. Rubella vaccine, if appropriate. RhoGAM, if indicated. Laxative.
NUTRITION/ ELIMINATION		**RECOVERY**	**ADM. TO PP UNIT—8 HOURS**	**9-16 HOURS**	**17-24 HOURS/DISCHARGE**
		Patient will be up to bathroom before transfer.	Woman will resume normal nutritional status and bladder function.	Woman will resume normal nutritional status and bladder function.	Woman will have normal bowel and bladder function.
		NA MET VARIANCE	**NA MET VARIANCE**	**NA MET VARIANCE**	**NA MET VARIANCE**
		Assess bladder fullness. Assist to bathroom. Assess for tolerance of PO intake.	Encourage ambulation. Encourage PO fluids. Assist to bathroom as needed. Assess bladder function. Encourage PO intake.	Encourage ambulation. Encourage PO fluids. Assist to bathroom as needed. Assess bladder function. Encourage PO intake.	Encourage ambulation. Encourage PO fluids. Assist to bathroom as needed. Laxative prn.
PSYCHOSOCIAL		**RECOVERY**	**ADM. TO PP UNIT—8 HOURS**	**9-16 HOURS**	**17-24 HOURS/DISCHARGE**
		Woman/family will begin attachment behaviors with newborn.	Woman/family will demonstrate appropriate attachment behaviors.	Family will verbalize comfort with new infant.	Family will verbalize comfort with new infant.
		NA MET VARIANCE	**NA MET VARIANCE**	**NA MET VARIANCE**	**NA MET VARIANCE**
		Encourage mother/family members to hold and touch infant. Provide skin-to-skin contact of mother/infant. Provide mother the opportunity to breastfeed, if applicable.	Offer flexible rooming-in with infant. Allow for verbalization of woman's feelings. Assess discharge needs and need for Social Service consult.	Reinforce interventions.	Reinforce interventions. Completion of birth certificate. Arrange for home visit.

	RECOVERY	ADM. TO PP UNIT—8 HOURS	9-16 HOURS	17-24 HOUR/DISCHARGE
SELF-CARE ACTIVITY	Woman will begin self-care activities as tolerated.	Woman will be up to bathroom/shower with assistance.	Woman will be up to bathroom/shower independently.	Woman will be up to bathroom/shower independently.
	NA MET VARIANCE	NA MET VARIANCE	NA MET VARIANCE	NA MET VARIANCE
	Instruct woman in pericare and pad changes.	Reinforce proper pericare. Instruct on use of Sitz bath. Encourage woman to shower.	Reinforce proper pericare. Reinforce use of Sitz bath.	Reinforce proper pericare. Reinforce use of Sitz bath.

	RECOVERY	ADM. TO PP UNIT—8 HOURS	9-16 HOURS	17-24 HOURS/DISCHARGE
TEACHING/ DISCHARGE PLANNING	Woman will begin to verbalize and/or demonstrate self-care and infant care activities.	Woman will begin to verbalize and/or demonstrate infant and self-care activities.	Woman/family will demonstrate appropriate infant care activities.	Woman/family will demonstrate appropriate infant care activities.
	NA MET VARIANCE	NA MET VARIANCE	NA MET VARIANCE	NA MET VARIANCE
	Date:			
	Initials:			
	Teaching to include: Breastfeeding latch-on and positioning, if applicable. Appropriate handwashing techniques. Cough and deep breathing exercises. Instruct in pain relief techniques/medication.	Teaching to include: Breastfeeding/formula initial feeding information. Breast care. Perineal care. Proper nutrition. Safety issues reviewed.	Teaching to include: Attendance at mother/baby care class. Breast care or formula information. Newborn channel. Lactation consult prn. Appropriate handwashing techniques.	Teaching to include: Reinforcement of teaching from mother/baby class. Plans for self/infant follow-up. Review IHSP.* Review Baby Net program. Telephone number for follow-up questions. Home-going meds and purposes.
	1.	1.	1.	1.
	2.	2.	2.	2.
	3.	3.	3.	3.
	4.	4.	4.	4.

Variance Documentation: _____

_____

_____

_____

_____

_____

unit. If the woman's vital signs are within normal limits, they will likely be assessed every 4 to 8 hours for the remainder of her hospitalization. Other components of the initial assessment include the mother's emotional status, energy level, degree of physical discomfort, hunger, and thirst. Intake and output assessments should always be done if an intravenous infusion or a urinary catheter is in place. If the woman gave birth by cesarean, the incisional dressing should be assessed as well. To some degree, her knowledge level concerning self-care and infant care can also be determined at this time.

Ongoing Physical Assessment

The postpartum woman should be evaluated thoroughly during each nursing shift throughout hospitalization (see Guidelines/Guías box). Physical assessments include evaluation of the breasts, uterine fundus, lochia, perineum, bladder and bowel function, vital signs, and legs. If a woman has an intravenous (IV) line in place, her fluid and hematologic status should be evaluated before it is removed. Signs of potential problems that may be identified during the assessment process are listed in the Signs of Potential Complications box.

Routine Laboratory Tests

Several laboratory tests may be performed in the immediate postpartum period. Hemoglobin and hematocrit values are often requested on the first postpartum day to assess effects of blood loss during childbirth, especially after cesarean birth. In some hospitals a clean-catch or catheterized urine specimen may be obtained and sent for routine urinalysis or culture and sensitivity, especially if an indwelling urinary catheter was inserted during the intrapartum period. In addition, if the woman's rubella and Rh status are unknown, tests to determine her status and need for possible treatment should be performed at this time.

Although all women experience similar physiologic changes during the postpartum period, certain factors act to make each woman's experience unique. From a physiologic standpoint, the length and difficulty of the labor, type of birth (vaginal or cesarean), presence of episiotomy or lacerations, and whether the mother plans to breastfeed or bottle feed are important factors to be investigated with each woman. After analyzing the data obtained during the assessment process, the nurse establishes nursing diagnoses that will guide the plan of care. Examples of nursing diagnoses commonly established for the postpartum client include the following:

▋ Nursing Diagnoses _____

- Risk for infection related to
  - childbirth trauma to tissues
- Constipation or urinary retention related to
  - postchildbirth discomfort
  - childbirth trauma to tissues

▋ Nursing Diagnoses—cont'd _____

- Sleep pattern disturbance related to
  - discomforts of postpartum period
  - long labor process
  - infant care and hospital routine
- Pain related to
  - involution of uterus
  - trauma to perineum
  - episiotomy
  - hemorrhoids
  - engorged breasts
- Risk for injury related to
  - postpartum hemorrhage
  - effects of anesthesia
- Ineffective breastfeeding related to
  - maternal discomfort
  - infant positioning

Expected Outcomes of Care

The nursing plan of care includes both the postpartum woman and her infant, even if the nursery nurse retains primary responsibility for the infant. In many hospitals, **couplet care** (also called mother and baby care or single room maternity care) is practiced. Nurses in these settings have been educated in both mother and infant care and function as the primary nurse for both mother and infant, even if the infant is kept in the nursery. This approach is a variation of rooming-in, in which the mother and child room together and mother and nurse share the care of the infant. The organization of the mother's care must take the newborn into consideration. The day actually revolves around the baby's feeding and care times.

Once the nursing diagnoses are formulated, the nurse plans with the woman what nursing measures will be appropriate and which are to be given priority. During her hospital stay the mother is encouraged to assume increasing responsibility for her self-care and her infant's care. As the woman and her partner provide more care for herself and the baby, the nurse's role changes from one of providing direct care to one of teaching, encouragement, and support.

The nursing plan of care will include periodic assessments to detect deviations from normal physical changes, measures to relieve discomfort or pain, safety measures to prevent injury or infection, and teaching and counseling measures designed to promote the woman's feelings of competence in self-care and baby care. Family members are included in the teaching. The nurse evaluates continuously and is ready to change the plan if indicated. Almost all hospitals use standardized care plans as a base. The nurse's ability to adapt the standardized plan to specific medical and nursing diagnoses results in individualized

Abbott Northwestern Hospital
A HealthSpan™ Organization

SELF/FAMILY LEARNING CHECKLIST

Patient Name, Social Security #, Date of Birth

I learn best by: ☐ *Group classes* ☐ *Individual instruction* ☐ *Video instruction* ☐ *Reading it myself*

Please indicate your desired learning needs by placing a check in one of the columns next to each topic.

KEY	1 = Most important to learn before I go home 2 = I already know

(Please DATE when learning need is met.)

CARING FOR YOURSELF	1	2	DATE	CARING FOR BABY	1	2	DATE
Episiotomy and perineal care				Diapering			
Vaginal discharge				Baby bath, skin and cord care			
Hemorrhoids/Constipation				Circumcised/uncircumcised care			
Breast care				Burping			
Nutrition				Bowel movements/wet diapers			
Activity				Sleeping habits			
Post partal exercises				Newborn behavior			
Return of menstruation				Jaundice			
Family planning				Signs of illness			
Blood clots				Car seat safety			
Post partum emotions				General infant safety/poison control			
Post partum warning signs				Signs/symptoms of dehydration			
				Bulb syringe			
Cesarean Birth							
Incisional care				**BREAST FEEDING**			
				Sore nipples			
				Positioning			
				Frequency of feedings			
AFTER DISCHARGE				Expressing/storing milk			
When to call health care provider				Engorgement			
				Feeding water			
				Nursing while working			
OTHER				Weaning			
Working mothers							
Day care				**BOTTLE FEEDING**			
Sibling adjustment				Types of formula			
Single parent support				Preparing formula			
Time out for parents				Frequency of feedings			
Infant safety and security							
Infant As A Person Class							
New Parent Connection							

MEDICATIONS AT HOME

MEDICATIONS	STRENGTH	DOSAGE	FREQUENCY	PURPOSE/SPECIAL INSTRUCTIONS
			times per day	
			times per day	
			times per day	

RESOURCES REFERRALS
☐ Physician Discharge Instructions _____
☐ Home Care Agency _____
☐ Other Referrals _____

VALUABLES: ☐ Returned ☐ None   **MEDICATIONS:** ☐ Returned ☐ None   ☐ Room checked for belongings

Patient verbalized understanding of discharge information received.

PATIENT OR
SUPPORT PERSON _____   NURSE'S
SIGNATURE _____   DATE _____

SELF/FAMILY LEARNING CHECKLIST

SELF/FAMILY LEARNING CHECKLIST

Fig. 24-5 Self/family learning checklist. *(Copyright Abbott Northwestern Hospital of Allina Health System, Minneapolis and St. Paul, MN.)*

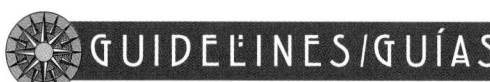

GUIDELINES/GUÍAS

Postpartum Physical Assessment

Are you planning to breastfeed or bottle feed?
¿Piensa darle pecho o biberón al bebé?

Lie down.
Acuéstese.

I am going to take your vital signs.
Le voy a tomar sus signos vitales.

I need to take your blood pressure.
Necesito tomarle la presión de sangre.

Do you need to use the bathroom?
¿Necesita usar el baño?

I need to examine you.
Necesito examinarle.

Spread your knees and legs apart.
Abra las rodillas y las piernas.

Roll over on your side.
Póngase al lado.

Would you like some pain medication?
¿Desea medicina para calmar el dolor?

Would you like to take a sitz bath?
¿Desea tomar un baño de asiento?

SIGNS OF POTENTIAL COMPLICATIONS

Physiologic Problems

TEMPERATURE
More than 38° C after the first 24 hr

PULSE
Tachycardia or marked bradycardia

BLOOD PRESSURE
Hypotension or hypertension

ENERGY LEVEL
Lethargy, extreme fatigue

UTERUS
Deviated from the midline, boggy consistency, remains above the umbilicus after 24 hr

LOCHIA
Heavy, foul odor, bright red bleeding that is not lochia

PERINEUM
Pronounced edema, not intact, signs of infection, marked discomfort

LEGS
Homans' sign positive; painful, reddened area; warmth on posterior aspect of calf

BREASTS
Redness, heat, pain, cracked and fissured nipples, inverted nipples, palpable mass

APPETITE
Lack of appetite

ELIMINATION
Urine: inability to void, urgency, frequency, dysuria; bowel: constipation, diarrhea

REST
Inability to rest or sleep

---

client care. Caution is advised against total reliance on a standardized plan; by doing so the uniqueness of the individual may be overlooked.

Expected outcomes for the postpartum period are based on the nursing diagnoses identified for the individual woman. Examples of common expected outcomes for physiologic needs are that the woman will do the following:
- Remain free from infection.
- Demonstrate normal involution and lochial characteristics.
- Remain comfortable and injury free.
- Demonstrate normal bladder and bowel patterns.
- Demonstrate knowledge of breast care for breastfeeding and bottle feeding, as appropriate.
- Protect the health of future pregnancies and children.
- Integrate the newborn into the family.

Plan of Care and Interventions

Nurses assume many roles while implementing the nursing plan of care. They provide direct physical care, teach mother and baby care, and provide anticipatory guidance and counseling. Perhaps most important of all they nurture the client by providing encouragement and support as the woman begins to assume the many tasks of motherhood. Nurses who take the time to "mother the mother" do much to increase feelings of self-confidence in new mothers.

The first step in providing individualized care is to confirm the woman's identity by checking her wristband. At the same time, the infant's identification number is matched with the corresponding band on the mother's and, in some instances, the father's wrist. The nurse demonstrates caring and respect by determining how the mother wishes to be addressed and then notes her preference in her record and in her nursing plan of care.

The woman and her family are oriented to their surroundings. Familiarity with the unit, routines, resources, and personnel reduces one potential source of anxiety–the unknown. The mother is reassured by knowing whom and how she can call for assistance and what she can expect in the way of supplies and services. If the woman's usual daily routine before admission differs from the facility's routine, the nurse works with the woman to develop a mutually acceptable routine.

Infant abduction from hospitals in the United States has increased in the past few years. The mother should be taught to check the identity of any person who comes to remove the baby from her room. Hospital personnel usually wear picture identification badges. On some units, all staff members wear matching scrubs or special badges. Other units use closed circuit television, computer monitoring systems or fingerprint identification pads. As a rule, the baby is never carried in a staff member's arms between the mother's room and the nursery but is always wheeled in a bassinet, which also contains baby care supplies. Clients and nurses must work together to ensure the safety of newborns in the hospital environment.

PLAN ᴼᶠ CARE   A Woman Who Has Had a Spontaneous Vaginal Birth

> **NURSING DIAGNOSIS** Risk for fluid volume deficit related to uterine atony

Expected Outcomes *Woman's fundus will remain firm and lochia rubra moderate.*

Nursing Interventions/Rationales

Review woman's history for risk factors, such as uterine overdistention, *to identify and assess women who may be more at risk for postpartum hemorrhage.*

Assess fundal character and location frequently as well as response to gentle massage *to promote contraction of the uterus.*

Express clots. Demonstrate to woman how to assess and massage her own fundus *to promote self-care.*

Evaluate bladder character and promote voiding if full *to avoid uterine relaxation and displacement of uterine fundus.*

Assess amount and color of lochia *to indicate amount of blood loss.*

Monitor vital signs *to determine extent of fluid loss.*

Administer medications to enhance uterine contractility as prescribed, such as Pitocin and Methergine, *to prevent hemorrhage.*

Initiate or increase IV therapy *to replace fluid loss.*

> **NURSING DIAGNOSIS** Pain related to perineal trauma and hormonal influences as evidenced by client report

Expected Outcomes *Woman will report lessening of discomfort and identify methods effective in decreasing discomfort.*

Nursing Interventions/Rationales

Assess character, location, and pain scale as reported by woman *to identify appropriate interventions.*

Inspect perineum for redness, edema, ecchymoses, discharge, and approximation (REEDA scale) *to identify any complications.*

Apply ice pack to perineum during the first 12 to 24 hours postbirth *to decrease edema and promote comfort by local anesthesia.*

Administer analgesics as prescribed *to decrease perception of painful impulses.*

Teach woman to contract gluteal muscles when sitting *to avoid direct pressure on perineum.*

> **NURSING DIAGNOSIS** Risk for altered urinary elimination related to perineal trauma and effects of anesthesia

Expected Outcomes *Woman will void within 6 to 8 hours postbirth and empty bladder completely.*

Nursing Interventions/Rationales

Assess position and character of uterine fundus and bladder *to ascertain if any further interventions are indicated because of displacement of the fundus or distension of the bladder.*

Measure intake and output *to assess any evidence of dehydration and subsequent decreased anticipated urine output.*

Encourage voiding by walking woman to bathroom, running water over perineum, running water in sink, providing privacy *to use a variety of interventions to encourage voiding.*

Encourage oral intake *to replace any fluids lost at delivery and prevent dehydration.*

Catheterize as necessary with indwelling or straight method *to ensure bladder emptying and allow for uterine involution.*

Implementation of the nursing plan of care involves putting into practice specific activities that should result in achieving the expected outcomes planned for each individual woman (see Plan of Care).

Prevention of Infection

One important means of preventing infection is maintenance of a clean environment. Bed linens should be changed as needed. Disposable pads and draw sheets may need to be changed frequently. Women should avoid walking about barefoot to avoid contaminating bed linens when they return to bed. Supervision of use of equipment to prevent cross-contamination is also necessary. For example, a common sitz bath or heat lamp must be scrubbed after each woman's use. Staff members are another important part of the hospital environment. Personnel must be conscientious about their handwashing techniques to prevent cross-infection. Standard Precautions must be practiced. Staff members with colds, coughs, or skin infections (e.g., a cold sore on the lip [herpes simplex virus, type 1]) must follow hospital protocol when in contact with postpartum women. In many hospitals, staff with open herpetic lesions, strep throat, conjunctivitis, upper respiratory infections, or diarrhea are encouraged to avoid contact with mothers and infants by staying home until the condition is no longer contagious.

Proper care of the episiotomy site and any perineal lacerations prevents infection in the genitourinary area and aids the healing process. Educating the woman to wipe from front to back (urethra to anus) after voiding or defecating is a simple first step. In many hospitals a squeeze bottle filled with warm water or other antiseptic solutions is used after each voiding to cleanse the perineal area (Box 24-3). The woman should also be taught to change her perineal pad from front to back each time she voids or defecates and to wash her hands thoroughly before and after doing so.

Prevention of Excessive Bleeding

The most frequent cause of excessive bleeding following childbirth is **uterine atony,** failure of the uterine muscle to contract firmly. The two most important interventions for preventing excessive bleeding, therefore, are maintaining good uterine tone and preventing bladder distention.

NURSE ALERT

If uterine atony occurs, the relaxed uterus distends with blood and clots, and blood vessels in the placental site are not clamped off, thus excessive bleeding results.

Excessive blood loss following childbirth may also be caused by vaginal or vulvar hematomas, unrepaired lacerations of the vagina or cervix, and retained placental fragments.

NURSE ALERT

A perineal pad saturated in 15 minutes or less or pooling of blood under the buttocks are indications of excessive blood loss, requiring immediate notification of the primary health care provider.

Accurate visual estimation of blood loss is an important nursing responsibility. Blood loss is usually described subjectively as scant, light, moderate, or heavy (profuse). Figure 24-7 shows examples of perineal pad saturation corresponding to each of these descriptions.

Luegenbiehl (1997) studied the ability of nurses to accurately assess blood loss visually. She found that nurses in general are inaccurate and tend to overestimate, rather than underestimate, blood loss. Luegenbiehl also found that different brands of peripads vary in their saturation volume and soaking appearance. For example, blood placed on some brands tends to soak down into the pad, whereas blood tends to spread outward on other brands. She strongly recommends that nurses determine saturation volume and soaking appearance for the peripad brands used at their institution in order to improve accuracy of blood loss estimation.

More objective estimates of blood loss include weighing blood clots and items saturated with blood (1 ml blood equals 1 g), using devices that catch and measure blood flowing from the vagina, and establishing the milliliters of blood it takes to saturate perineal pads being used (Johnson & Johnson, 1996; Luegenbiehl, 1997).

NURSE ALERT

The nurse always checks under the mother's buttocks as well as on the perineal pad. Blood may flow between the buttocks onto the linens under the mother while the amount on the perineal pad is slight, and thus excessive bleeding goes undetected.

Blood pressure is not a reliable indicator of impending shock from early hemorrhage. More sensitive means of identifying shock are provided by respirations, pulse, skin condition, urinary output, and level of consciousness (Johnson & Johnson, 1996). The frequent physical assessments performed during the fourth stage of labor are designed to provide prompt identification of excessive bleeding (see Emergency box.)

Maintenance of uterine tone. A major intervention to restore good tone is stimulation by gently massaging the uterine fundus until firm (see Fig. 24-3). Fundal massage may cause a temporary increase in the amount of vaginal bleeding seen as pooled blood leaves the uterus.

BOX 24-3 Interventions for Episiotomy, Lacerations, and Hemorrhoids

Explain both procedure and rationale before implementation.

CLEANSING

Wash hands before and after cleansing perineum and changing pads.
Wash perineum with mild soap and warm water at least once daily.
Cleanse from symphysis pubis to anal area.
Apply peripad from front to back, protecting inner surface of pad from contamination.
Wrap soiled pad and place in covered waste container.
Change pad with each void or defecation or at least 4 times per day.
Assess amount and character of lochia with each pad change.

ICE PACK

Apply a covered ice pack to perineum from front to back.
1. During first 2 hours to decrease edema formation and increase comfort
2. After the first 2 hours following the birth to provide anesthetic effect

SQUEEZE BOTTLE

Demonstrate for and assist woman; explain rationale.
Fill bottle with tap water warmed to approximately 38° C (comfortably warm on the wrist).
Instruct woman to position nozzle between her legs so that squirts of water reach perineum as she sits on toilet seat. Explain that it will take whole bottle of water to cleanse perineum.
Remind her to blot dry with toilet paper or clean wipes.
Remind her to avoid contamination from anal area.
Apply clean pad.

SITZ BATH
Built-in Type

Prepare bath by thoroughly scrubbing with cleaning agent and rinsing.
Pad with towel before filling.
Fill one-half to one-third full with water of correct temperature: 38° to 40.6° C. Some women prefer cool sitz baths. Ice is added to water to lower the temperature to the level comfortable for the woman.

Encourage woman to use at least twice a day for 20 minutes.
Place call bell within easy reach.
Teach woman to enter bath by tightening gluteal muscles and keeping them tightened and then relaxing them after she is in the bath.
Place dry towels within reach.
Ensure privacy.
Check woman in 15 minutes; assess pulse as needed.

Disposable Type

Clamp tubing and fill bag with warm water.
Raise toilet seat, place bath in bowl with overflow opening directed toward back of toilet.
Place container above toilet bowl.
Attach tube into groove at front of bath.
Loosen tube clamp to regulate rate of flow: fill bath to about one-half full; continue as above for built-in sitz bath.

SURGI-GATOR

Assemble Surgi-Gator (Fig. 24-6).
Instruct woman regarding use and rationale.
Follow package directions.
Instruct woman to sit on toilet with legs apart and to put nozzle so tip is just past the perineum, adjusting placement as needed.
Remind her to return her applicator to her bedside stand.

DRY HEAT

Inspect lamp for defects.
Cover lamp with towels.
Position lamp 50 cm from perineum; use 3 times a day for 20-minute periods.
Teach regarding use of 40-W bulb at home.
Provide draping over woman.
If same lamp is being used by several women, clean it carefully between uses.

TOPICAL APPLICATIONS

Apply anesthetic cream or spray: use sparingly 3 to 4 times per day.
Offer witch hazel pads (Tucks) after voiding or defecating; woman pats perineum dry from front to back, then applies witch hazel pads.

Clots may also be expelled. Client education is extremely important in maintaining uterine tone. Fundal massage can be a very uncomfortable procedure. Understanding the causes and dangers of uterine atony and the purpose of fundal massage can help the woman to be more cooperative. Teaching the woman to do self-fundal massage enables her to maintain some control and decreases her anxiety. The uterus may remain boggy even after massage and

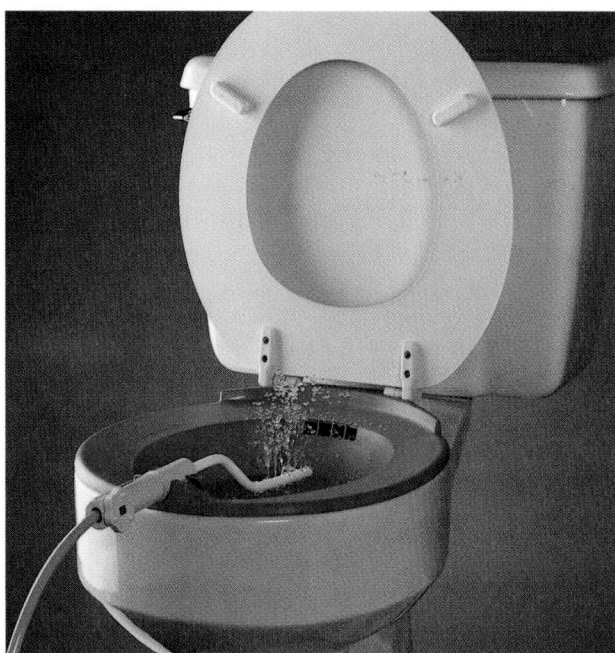

Fig. 24-6 Hygienic sitz bath (Surgi-Gator) for perineal care. *(Courtesy Andermac, Inc., Yuba City, CA.)*

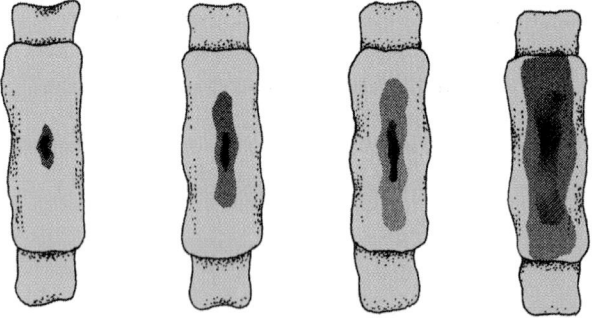

Fig. 24-7 Blood loss after birth is assessed by the extent of perineal pad saturation as (from left to right) scant (<2.5 cm); light (<10 cm); or heavy (one pad saturated within 2 hours).

expulsion of clots. If this occurs, it is a major warning sign of uterine atony. The nurse must remain with the client and summon help, including notifying the primary health care provider immediately. Additional interventions likely to be employed are administration of intravenous fluids and **oxytocic medications** (drugs that stimulate contraction of the uterine smooth muscle). Table 38-1 contains information about common oxytocic medications.

LEGAL TIP Client Abandonment

In an emergency situation the nurse must remain with the client and call for help. Leaving the client can lead to a charge of client abandonment.

Prevention of bladder distention. A full bladder causes the uterus to be displaced above the umbilicus and well to one side of midline in the abdomen. It also prevents the uterus from contracting normally. Nursing interventions focus on helping the woman spontaneously empty her bladder as soon as possible. The first priority is to assist the woman to the bathroom or onto a bedpan if she is unable to ambulate. Having the woman listen to running water, placing her hands in warm water, or pouring water from a squeeze bottle over her perineum may stimulate voiding. Other techniques include assisting the woman into the shower or sitz bath and encouraging her to void or placing spirits of peppermint in a bedpan under the woman. The vapors may relax the urinary meatus and trigger spontaneous voiding. Administering analgesics, if ordered, may be indicated because some women may fear voiding because of the anticipated pain. If these measures are unsuccessful, a sterile catheter may be inserted to drain the urine.

Evaluation of the woman's responses to intervention is an ongoing part of the nursing process. All responses to interventions should be carefully recorded. If the expected outcomes are not met or new needs emerge, the plan of care is modified accordingly. For example, if the uterus is firm and the bladder empty, something other than uterine atony is causing the excessive bleeding. Further assessment is necessary to determine the cause and correct the problem. See Chapter 38 for further discussion of postpartum hemorrhage.

Promotion of Comfort, Rest, Ambulation, and Exercise

Comfort. Most women experience some degree of discomfort during the immediate postpartum period. Common causes of discomfort include afterbirth pains, episiotomy or perineal lacerations, hemorrhoids, and breast engorgement. The woman's description of the type and severity of her pain is the nurse's best guide in choosing an appropriate intervention. To confirm the location and extent of discomfort, the nurse inspects and palpates areas of pain as appropriate for redness, swelling, discharge, and heat and observes for body tension, guarded movements, and facial tension. Blood pressure, pulse, and respirations may be elevated in response to acute pain. Diaphoresis may accompany severe pain. A lack of objective symptoms does not necessarily mean there is no pain because there may also be a cultural component to the expression of pain. Nursing interventions are intended to eliminate the pain sensation entirely or reduce it to a tolerable level that allows the woman to care for herself and her baby. Nurses may employ both nonpharmacologic and pharmacologic interventions to promote comfort. Depending on reported severity, nonpharmacologic measures should be employed either alone or in combination with pharmacologic interventions. Pain relief is enhanced by using more than one method or route.

Nonpharmacologic interventions. Afterbirth pains are the menstrual-like cramps experienced by many women as the uterus contracts following childbirth. Warmth, distraction, deep breathing, imagery, therapeutic touch, relaxation, and interaction with the infant may decrease the discomfort associated with these uterine contractions.

Simple interventions that can decrease the discomfort associated with an episiotomy or perineal lacerations include encouraging the woman to lie on her side whenever possible and to use a pillow when sitting. Other interventions include application of an ice pack; topical applications (if ordered); dry heat; cleansing with a squeeze bottle; and a cleansing shower, tub bath, or sitz bath. Many of these interventions are also effective for hemorrhoids, especially ice packs, sitz baths, and topical applications (such as witch hazel pads). Box 24-3 gives more specific information about these interventions.

The discomfort associated with engorged breasts may be lessened by the application of either ice or heat to the breasts and the wearing of a well-fitted support bra. Decisions about specific interventions for relieving engorgement are based on whether the woman chooses to breastfeed or bottle feed (see Chapter 28).

Pharmacologic interventions. Most primary health care providers routinely order a variety of analgesics to be administered as needed, including both narcotic and nonnarcotic (nonsteroidal antiinflammatory medications) choices, with their dosage and time frequency ranges. Topical application of antiseptic or anesthetic ointment or sprays is a common pharmacologic intervention. Patient-controlled analgesia (PCA) pumps and continuous epidural analgesia infusions are technologies frequently used to provide postpartum pain relief after cesarean birth. The nurse should carefully monitor all women receiving opioids because respiratory depression and decreased intestinal motility are side effects. Many women want to participate in decisions about analgesia. Severe pain, however, may interfere with active participation in choosing pain relief measures. If an analgesic is to be given, the nurse must make a clinical judgment of the type, dosage, and frequency from the medications ordered. The woman is informed of the prescribed analgesic and its common side effects; this teaching is documented.

Breastfeeding mothers often have concerns about the effects on the infant of taking an analgesic. Although nearly all medications present in maternal circulation are also found in breast milk, many analgesics commonly used during the postpartum period are considered relatively safe for breastfeeding mothers (see Appendix C). Often the timing of medications can be adjusted to minimize infant exposure. A mother may be given pain medication immediately after breastfeeding, for example, so that the interval between medication administration and the next nursing period is as long as possible. The decision to administer medications of any kind to a breastfeeding mother must

always be made by carefully weighing the woman's need for the medication against actual or potential risks to the infant.

If acceptable pain relief has not been obtained in 1 hour and there has been no change in the initial assessment, the nurse may need to contact the primary care provider for additional pain relief orders or further directions. Unrelieved pain results in fatigue, anxiety, and a worsening perception of the pain. It might also indicate the presence of a previously unknown or untreated problem. Further assessment

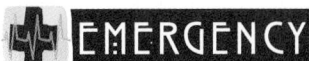

EMERGENCY

Hypovolemic Shock

SIGNS AND SYMPTOMS

Persistent significant bleeding—perineal pad soaked within 15 minutes; *may not be accompanied by a change in vital signs or maternal color or behavior.*

Woman states she feels weak, light-headed, "funny," "sick to my stomach," or "sees stars."

Woman begins to act anxious or exhibits air hunger.

Woman's skin turns ashen or grayish.

Skin feels cool and clammy.

Pulse rate increases.

Blood pressure declines.

INTERVENTIONS

Notify primary health care provider.

If uterus is atonic, massage gently and expel clots to cause uterus to contract; compress uterus manually, as needed, using two hands. Add oxytocic agent to IV drip, as ordered.

Give oxygen by face mask or nasal prongs at 8 to 10 L/min.

Tilt the woman to her side or elevate the right hip; elevate her legs to at least a 30-degree angle.

Provide additional or maintain existing IV infusion of lactated Ringer's solution or normal saline solution to restore circulatory volume.

Administer blood or blood products, as ordered.

Monitor vital signs.

Insert an indwelling urinary catheter to monitor perfusion of kidneys.

Administer emergency drugs, as ordered.

Prepare for possible surgery or other emergency treatments or procedures.

Chart incident, medical and nursing interventions instituted, and results of treatments.

and treatment will likely be necessary to determine the cause of the pain and correct it.

Rest. The excitement and exhilaration experienced after the birth of the infant may make rest difficult. The new mother, who is often anxious about her ability to care for her infant or is uncomfortable, may also have difficulty sleeping. In the days that follow, the demands of the infant, along with the influence of the hospital environment and routines, contribute to alterations in her sleep pattern.

Fatigue. Fatigue is common in the postpartum period (Pugh et al., 1999) and involves both physiologic components associated with long labors, cesarean birth, anemia, and breastfeeding and psychologic components related to depression and anxiety. Infant behavior can also be related to fatigue, particularly with mothers of more difficult infants.

Interventions must be planned to meet the woman's individual needs for sleep and rest. Backrubs, other comfort measures, and medication for sleep for the first few nights may be necessary. Support and encouragement in mothering behaviors help reduce anxiety. Hospital and nursing routines may also be adjusted to meet individual needs. In addition, the nurse can help the family limit visitors and provide a comfortable chair or bed for the partner.

Ambulation. Early ambulation is successful in reducing the incidence of thromboembolism and in promoting the woman's more rapid recovery of strength. Confinement to bed is not required for the woman who had general anesthesia, epidural or spinal anesthesia, or local anesthesia such as a pudendal block. Free movement is permitted once the anesthetic wears off unless an analgesic has been administered. After the initial recovery period is over, the mother is encouraged to ambulate frequently.

NURSE ALERT

Having a hospital staff or family member present the first time the woman gets out of bed after childbirth is wise because she may feel weak, dizzy, faint, or light-headed.

The rapid decrease in intraabdominal pressure after birth results in a dilation of blood vessels supplying the intestines, which is known as splanchnic engorgement, and causes blood to pool in the viscera. This condition contributes to the development of orthostatic hypotension and may occur when the woman who has recently given birth sits or stands up, first ambulates, or takes a warm shower or sitz bath (Johnson & Johnson, 1996). The nurse needs to also consider several factors, such as the baseline blood pressure; amount of blood loss; and type, amount, and timing of analgesic or anesthetic medications administered when assisting a woman to ambulate.

Prevention of **thrombus** (clot formation) is part of the nursing plan of care. Women who must remain in bed after giving birth are at an increased risk for the develop-

ment of thrombus. If a woman remains in bed longer than 8 hours (e.g., postpartum $MgSO_4$ therapy for preeclampsia), exercise to promote circulation in the legs is indicated using the following routine:

1. Alternate flexion and extension of feet.
2. Rotate ankle in circular motion.
3. Alternate flexion and extension of legs.
4. Press back of knee to bed surface; relax.

If the woman is susceptible to thromboembolism, she is encouraged to walk about actively and discouraged from sitting immobile in a chair. Women with varicosities are encouraged to wear support hose. If a thrombus is suspected—as evidenced by a positive **Homans' sign** (complaint of pain in calf muscles when the foot is dorsiflexed) or warmth, redness, or tenderness in the suspected leg—the primary health care provider should be notified immediately; meanwhile the woman should be confined to bed, with the affected limb elevated on pillows.

Exercise. Most women who have just given birth are extremely interested in regaining their nonpregnant figure. Postpartum exercise can begin soon after birth, although the woman should be encouraged to start with simple exercises and gradually progress to more strenuous ones (see Research box). Figure 24-8 illustrates a number of exercises appropriate for the new mother. Abdominal exercises are postponed until about 4 weeks after cesarean birth.

Kegel pelvic exercises to strengthen muscle tone are extremely important, particularly after vaginal birth. To perform them, the woman consciously contracts and relaxes the muscles around the vagina. **Kegel exercises** help women to regain the muscle tone that is often lost as pelvic tissues are stretched and torn during pregnancy and birth. Women who maintain muscle strength may benefit years later by maintaining urinary continence.

However, it is essential that women learn to perform the Kegel exercises correctly (see Teaching Guidelines box in Chapter 5). Studies have shown that approximately one fourth of all women who learn Kegel exercises are doing them incorrectly and may increase their risk of incontinence (Sampselle & Miller, 1996). This may occur when women inadvertently bear down on the pelvic floor muscles (Valsalva effort), thrusting the perineum outward. The health care provider can teach and assess the woman's technique during the pelvic examination at the 6-week check-up, inserting two fingers intravaginally and checking whether the pelvic floor muscles correctly contract and relax.

Promotion of Nutrition

During the hospital stay, most women display a good appetite and eat well; nutritious snacks are usually welcomed. Women may request that family members bring to the hospital favorite or culturally appropriate foods. Cultural dietary preferences must be respected. This interest in food presents an ideal opportunity for nutritional counseling on dietary needs after pregnancy, such as for breastfeeding, preventing constipation and anemia, weight loss, and promoting healing and well-being (see Chapter 16). Prenatal vitamins and iron supplements are often continued until 6 weeks postpartum or the ordered supply has been used.

Promotion of Normal Bladder and Bowel Patterns

Bladder. After giving birth the mother should void spontaneously within 6 to 8 hours. The first several voidings should be measured to document adequate emptying of the bladder. A volume of at least 150 ml is expected for each voiding. Some women experience difficulty in emptying the bladder, possibly as a result of diminished bladder tone, edema from trauma, or fear of discomfort. Nursing interventions for inability to void and bladder distention are discussed on p. 606.

Bowel. Nursing interventions to promote normal bowel elimination include educating the woman about measures to avoid constipation. These interventions include ensuring adequate roughage and fluid intake and promoting exercise. Alerting the woman to side effects of medications such as narcotic analgesics (i.e., decreased gastrointestinal tract motility) may encourage her to implement measures to reduce the risk of constipation. Stool softeners or laxatives are often routinely ordered and may be necessary during the early postpartum period. With early discharge, a new mother is often home before having a bowel movement.

Breastfeeding Promotion and Lactation Suppression

Breastfeeding promotion. The first 2 hours after birth are an excellent time to encourage the mother to breastfeed. The infant is in an alert state and ready to breastfeed. Breastfeeding aids in the contraction of the uterus and prevention of maternal hemorrhage. This is a wonderful opportunity for the nurse to instruct the mother in breastfeeding and to assess the physical appearance of the breasts. (See Chapter 28 for further information on assisting the breastfeeding woman.)

Lactation suppression. Suppression of lactation is necessary when the woman has decided not to breastfeed or in the event of neonatal death. One very important nonpharmacologic intervention is wearing a well-fitted support bra or breast binder continuously for at least the first 72 hours after giving birth. Women should also avoid any breast stimulation, including running warm water over the breasts, newborn suckling, or pumping of the breasts. A few nonbreastfeeding mothers experience severe breast **engorgement** (swelling of breast tissue caused by increased blood and lymph supply to the breasts preceding lactation). If breast engorgement occurs, it can usually be managed satisfactorily with nonpharmacologic interventions.

RESEARCH

Physical Activity and Postpartum Well-Being

Regular physical activity is a recognized factor in the promotion of lifelong health. Health care providers rarely incorporate women's exercise goals into the postpartum care plan, and little information is available to guide postpartum fitness activities. Knowledge about the effect of childbearing on levels of physical activity and about potential physical and psychosocial benefits of exercise to postpartum women is also sparse.

The purposes of this exploratory investigation were to describe reported patterns of postpartum physical activity and to identify associated benefits or risks. Secondary analyses of longitudinal data on 1200 women were collected prenatally and postpartum in a study of obstetric outcomes at a Midwestern tertiary-care center and its ambulatory satellite and hospital clinics. Nearly 35% of the sample reported doing vigorous exercise with a modal frequency of three times per week. More active women had retained significantly less weight (3.9 kg) than their less active counterparts (5.1 kg).

Vigorous exercisers demonstrated a consistent pattern of better scores on measures of postpartum adaptation and were more likely than nonexercisers to participate in fun activities, such as socializing, hobbies, and entertainment. Breastfeeding was not adversely affected by vigorous exercise. These exploratory results indicate that physical and psychological benefits may accrue to postpartum women who are able to exercise vigorously and avoid decreasing their usual level of activity.

CLINICAL APPLICATION

Exercise has rarely been an element in postpartum care plans. Nurses who care for women after childbirth should assess women's exercise goals, incorporate these goals into the plan of care, and support the women in their desired activities. All postpartum women should be informed of the benefits of exercise and encouraged to resume or extend their current level of physical activity. ∎

Source: Sampselle, C. et al. (1999). Physical activity and postpartum well-being. *J Obstet Gynecol Neonatal Nurs* 28(1), 41-49.

Ice packs to the breasts are helpful in decreasing the discomfort associated with engorgement. The woman should use a 15 minutes on, 45 minutes off schedule to prevent the rebound swelling that can occur if ice is used continuously, or she can place fresh cabbage leaves inside

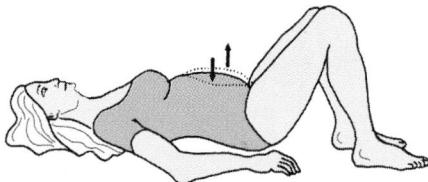

Abdominal Breathing. Lie on back with knees bent. Inhale deeply through nose. Keep ribs stationary and allow abdomen to expand upward. Exhale slowly but forcefully while contracting the abdominal muscles; hold for 3 to 5 seconds while exhaling. Relax.

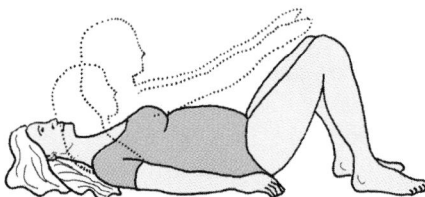

Reach for the Knees. Lie on back with knees bent. While inhaling, deeply lower chin onto chest. While exhaling, raise head and shoulders slowly and smoothly and reach for knees with arms outstretched. The body should only rise as far as the back will naturally bend while waist remains on floor or bed (about 6 to 8 inches). Slowly and smoothly lower head and shoulders back to starting position. Relax.

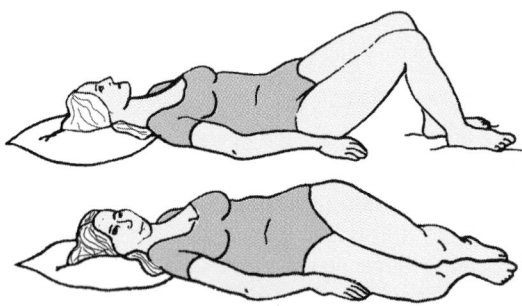

Double Knee Roll. Lie on back with knees bent. Keeping shoulders flat and feet stationary, slowly and smoothly roll knees over to the left to touch floor or bed. Maintaining a smooth motion, roll knees back over to the right until they touch floor or bed. Return to starting position and relax.

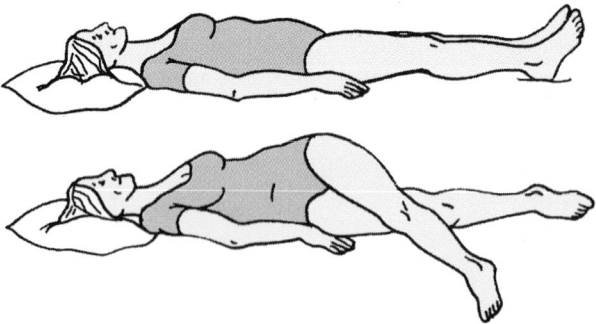

Leg Roll. Lie on back with legs straight. Keeping shoulders flat and legs straight, slowly and smoothly lift left leg and roll it over to touch the right side of floor or bed and return to starting position. Repeat, rolling right leg over to touch left side of floor or bed. Relax.

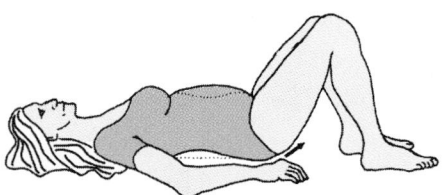

Combined Abdominal Breathing and Supine Pelvic Tilt (Pelvic Rock). Lie on back with knees bent. While inhaling deeply, roll pelvis back by flattening lower back on floor or bed. Exhale slowly but forcefully while contracting abdominal muscles and tightening buttocks. Hold for 3 to 5 seconds while exhaling. Relax.

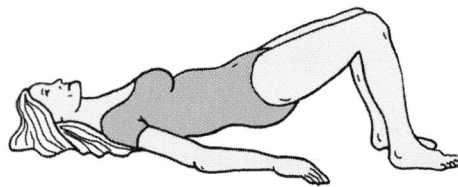

Buttocks Lift. Lie on back with arms at sides, knees bent, and feet flat. Slowly raise buttocks and arch back. Return slowly to starting position.

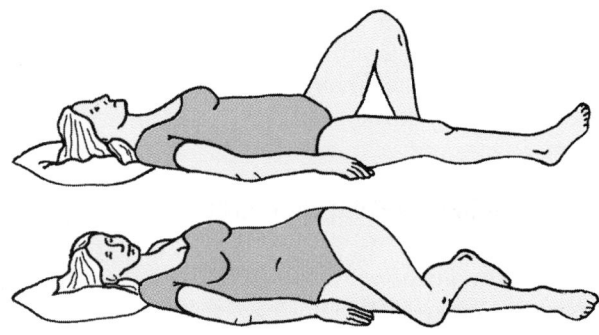

Single Knee Roll. Lie on back with right leg straight and left leg bent at the knee. Keeping shoulders flat, slowly and smoothly roll left knee over to the right to touch floor or bed and then back to starting position. Reverse position of legs. Roll right knee over to the left to touch floor or bed and return to starting position. Relax.

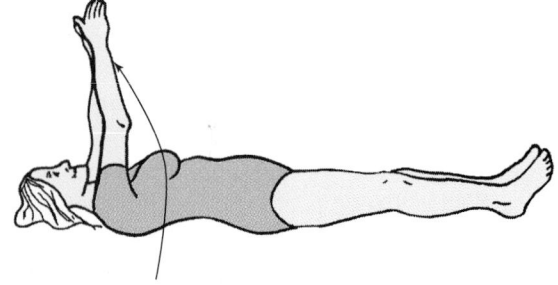

Arm Raises. Lie on back with arms extended at 90 degree-angle from body. Raise arms so they are perpendicular and hands touch. Lower slowly.

Fig. 24-8 Postpartum exercise should begin as soon as possible. The woman should start with simple exercises and gradually progress to more strenuous ones.

her bra. Cabbage leaves have been used to treat swelling in other cultures for years (Roberts, 1995). The exact mechanism of action is not known, but it is thought that naturally occurring plant estrogens or salicylates may be responsible for the effects. The leaves are replaced each time they wilt. A mild analgesic may also be necessary to help the mother through this uncomfortable time. Medications that were once prescribed for lactation suppression (estrogen, estrogen and testosterone, and bromocriptine) are no longer used.

Health Promotion of Future Pregnancies and Children

If the assessment data indicate the need, rubella vaccination and Rh immune globulin (RhoGAM) are administered during the puerperium. Failure to administer these products to women at risk of contracting rubella or developing Rh isoimmunization can seriously jeopardize the health of any future pregnancies and children.

Rubella vaccination. For women who have not had rubella (10% to 20% of all women) or women who are serologically not immune (titer of 1:8 or enzyme immunoassay [EIA] level <0.8) a subcutaneous injection of **rubella vaccine** is recommended in the immediate postbirth period to prevent fetal anomalies in future pregnancies. Seroconversion occurs in approximately 90% of women vaccinated after birth. The live attenuated rubella virus is not communicable; therefore breastfeeding mothers can be vaccinated. However, because the virus is shed in urine and other body fluids, the vaccine should not be given if the mother or other household members are immunocompromised. Rubella vaccine is made from duck eggs, so women who have allergies to these eggs may develop a hypersensitivity reaction to the vaccine for which they will need adrenaline. A transient arthralgia or rash is common in vaccinated women but is benign. Because the vaccine may be teratogenic, the client must be informed about the vaccine (see Legal Tip).

LEGAL TIP Rubella Vaccination

Informed consent for rubella vaccination in the postpartum period includes information about the possible side effects and the risk of teratogenic effects. Women must understand that they must practice contraception to avoid pregnancy for 2 to 3 months after being vaccinated.

Prevention of Rh isoimmunization. Injection of **Rh immune globulin** (a solution of gamma globulin that contains Rh antibodies) within 72 hours after birth prevents sensitization in the Rh-negative woman who has had a fetomaternal transfusion of Rh-positive red blood cells (RBCs) (see Medication Guide). The Rh immune globulin promotes lysis of the fetal Rh-positive blood cells before the mother forms her own antibodies against them.

NURSE ALERT

Postpartally, Rh immune globulin is administered to all Rh-negative, antibody (Coombs') negative women who give birth to Rh-positive infants.

The administration of 300 μg (1 vial) of Rh immune globulin is usually sufficient to prevent maternal sensitization. If a large fetomaternal transfusion is suspected, however, the dosage needed should be determined by performing a **Kleihauer-Betke test,** which detects the amount of fetal blood in the maternal circulation. If more than 15 ml of fetal blood is present in maternal circulation, the dosage of Rh immune globulin must be increased.

A 1:1000 dilution of Rh immune globulin is crossmatched to the mother's RBCs to ensure compatibility. Because Rh immune globulin is usually considered to be a blood product, precautions similar to those used for transfusing blood are necessary when it is given. The identification number on the client's hospital wristband should correspond to the identification number found on the laboratory slip. The nurse must also check to see that the lot number on the laboratory slip corresponds to the lot number on the vial. Finally, the expiration date on the vial should be checked to ensure a usable product.

NURSE ALERT *Rh immune globulin is administered to the mother intramuscularly. It should never be given to an infant.*

Rh immune globulin suppresses the immune response. Therefore the woman who receives both Rh immune globulin and rubella vaccine must be tested at 3 months to see if she has developed rubella immunity. If not, the woman will need another dose of rubella vaccine.

There is some disagreement about whether Rh immune globulin should be considered a blood product. Health care providers need to discuss the most current information about this issue with women whose religious beliefs conflict with having blood products administered to them.

Evaluation

The nurse can be reasonably assured that care was effective when the expected outcomes of care for physical needs have been achieved.

▌CARE MANAGEMENT: PSYCHOSOCIAL NEEDS

Meeting the psychosocial needs of new mothers involves planning care that considers the composition and functioning of the entire family. Nurses assess the parents' reactions to the birth experience, feelings about themselves, and interactions with the new baby and other family members. Specific interventions are then planned

MEDICATION GUIDE

Rh Immune Globulin, RhoGAM, Gamulin Rh, HypRho-D

ACTION

Suppression of immune response in nonsensitized women with Rh-negative blood who receive Rh-positive blood cells because of fetomaternal hemorrhage, transfusion, or accident

INDICATIONS

Suppress antibody formation in women with Rh-negative blood after birth, miscarriage/pregnancy termination, abdominal trauma, ectopic pregnancy, amniocentesis, version, or chorionic villi sampling

DOSAGE/ROUTE

Standard dose 1 vial (300 μg) IM in deltoid or gluteal muscle; microdose 1 vial (50 μg) IM in deltoid muscle

ADVERSE EFFECTS

Myalgia, lethargy, localized tenderness and stiffness at injection site, possible allergic response

NURSING CONSIDERATIONS

- Give standard dose to mother within 72 hours after birth if baby is Rh positive, at 28 weeks of gestation as prophylaxis, or after an incident or exposure risk that occurs after 28 weeks of gestation (e.g., amniocentesis, second trimester miscarriage or abortion, after version).
- Give microdose for first trimester miscarriage or abortion, ectopic pregnancy, chorionic villi sampling.
- Verify that the woman is Rh negative and has not been sensitized, that Coombs test is negative, and that baby is Rh positive. Provide explanation to the woman about procedure, including the purpose, possible side effects, and effect on future pregnancies. Have the woman sign a consent form if required by agency. Verify correct dosage and confirm lot number and woman's identity before giving injection (verify with another RN or other procedure per agency policy); document administration per agency policy.

to increase the parents' knowledge and self-confidence as they assume the care and responsibility of the new baby and integrate a new member into their existing family structure in a way that meets their cultural expectations.

Assessment and Nursing Diagnoses

Impact of the Birth Experience

Many women indicate a need to examine the birth process itself and look at their own intrapartal behavior in retrospect. Their partners may express similar desires. During pregnancy the woman and her partner may have developed a specific birth plan that included a vaginal birth and very little medical intervention. If their birth experience was quite different (e.g., labor induction, epidural anesthesia, cesarean birth), both partners may need to mourn the loss of their expectations before they can adjust to the reality of their birth experience. Inviting them to review the events and describe how they feel helps the nurse assess how well they understand what happened and how well they have been able to put their childbirth experience into perspective.

Maternal Self-Image

An important assessment concerns the woman's self-concept, body image, and sexuality. How this new mother feels about herself and her body during the puerperium may affect her behavior and adaptation to parenting. The woman's self-concept and body image may also affect her sexuality.

Feelings related to sexual adjustment after childbirth are often a cause of concern for new parents. Women who have recently given birth may be reluctant to resume sexual intercourse for fear of pain or may worry that coitus could damage healing perineal tissue. Because many new parents are anxious for information but reluctant to bring up the subject, postpartum nurses should matter-of-factly include the topic of postpartum sexuality during their routine physical assessment. While examining the episiotomy site, for example, the nurse can say, "I know you're sore right now, but it probably won't be long until you (or you and your partner) are ready to make love again. Have you thought about what that might be like? Would you like to ask me questions?" This approach assures the woman and her partner that resuming sexual activity is a legitimate concern for new parents and indicates the nurse's willingness to answer questions and share information.

Adaptation to Parenthood/Parent-Infant Interactions

The psychosocial assessment also includes evaluating adaptation to parenthood, as evidenced by the mother's and father's reactions to and interactions with the new baby. Clues indicating successful adaptation begin to appear early in the postbirth period as parents react positively to the newborn infant and continue the process of establishing a relationship with him or her.

Parents are adapting well to their new role when they exhibit a realistic perception and acceptance of their newborn's needs and his or her limited abilities, immature social responses, and helplessness. Examples of positive parent-infant interactions include taking pleasure in their infant and in the tasks done for and with him or her, understanding their infant's emotional states and providing comfort, and reading their infant's cues for new experiences and sensing his/her fatigue level. See Chapter 25 for a more in-depth discussion of parenting.

Family Structure and Functioning

Another important component of the psychosocial assessment is examining the family composition and functioning. A woman's adjustment to her role as mother is affected greatly by her relationships with her partner, her mother and other relatives, and any other children. Nurses can help to ease the new mother's return home by identifying possible conflicts among family members and helping the woman plan strategies for dealing with these problems before discharge. Such a conflict could arise when couples have very different ideas about parenting. Dealing with the stresses of sibling rivalry and unsolicited grandparent advice can also affect the woman's transition to motherhood. Only by asking about the woman's relationship with other nuclear and extended family members can the nurse discover potential problems in such relationships and help to plan workable solutions for them.

Impact of Cultural Diversity

The final component of a complete psychosocial assessment is the client's cultural beliefs and values. Much of a woman's behavior during the postpartum period is strongly influenced by her cultural background. In today's world, where travel is commonplace, nurses are likely to come in contact with women from many different countries and cultures. The nurse must remember that all cultures have developed safe and satisfying methods of caring for new mothers and babies. Only by understanding and respecting the values and beliefs of each woman can the nurse design a plan of care to meet their individual needs.

Following is an example of one "clash of cultures." The nurse in this case was able to take this information and modify her plan of care to make it culturally relevant, and therefore more satisfying, for the woman.

> A Vietnamese woman who had been in the United States for 4 years requested rooming-in facilities following childbirth. Instead of participating in the care of her infant, she refused to do so, remained in bed, wore a woolen cap, and appeared distressed and angry. The staff were puzzled and upset by her behavior. One nurse decided to put newly learned concepts concerning cross-cultural nursing into effect. She began by praising the woman's ability to speak English and, after eliciting a smile, remarked, "Every country has developed good ways to look after mothers and babies. Would you tell me about the care in Vietnam?" There was an immediate response. The woman explained that in her country women remained in bed for 10 days after birth, and the biggest danger to their health was getting a cold. The baby was kept in the room with his mother, but either a grandmother or nurse took complete charge of the care.

Sometimes the psychosocial assessment indicates serious actual or potential problems that must be addressed. The Signs of Potential Complications box lists several psychosocial needs that, at a minimum, warrant ongoing evaluation following hospital discharge. Clients exhibiting these needs should be referred to appropriate community resources for assessment and management.

After analyzing the data obtained during the assessment process, the nurse establishes nursing diagnoses to provide a guide for planning care. Nursing diagnoses related to psychosocial issues that are frequently established for the postpartum woman include the following:

SIGNS OF POTENTIAL COMPLICATIONS

Psychosocial Needs

Unable or unwilling to discuss labor and birth experience.
Refers to self as ugly and useless.
Excessively preoccupied with self (body image).
Markedly depressed.
Lacks a support system.
Partner and/or other family members react negatively to the baby.
Refuses to interact with or care for baby. For example, does not name baby, does not want to hold or feed baby, is upset by vomiting and wet or dirty diapers. (Cultural appropriateness of actions needs to be considered.)
Expresses disappointment over baby's sex.
Sees baby as messy or unattractive.
Baby reminds mother of family member or friend she doesn't like.

▮ Nursing Diagnoses _____

* Altered family processes related to
  – unexpected birth of twins
* Impaired verbal communication related to
  – woman's hearing impairment
  – woman's language not the same as nurse's
* Altered parenting related to
  – long, difficult labor
  – unmet expectations of labor and the birth
* Anxiety related to
  – newness of parenting role
* Risk for situational low self-esteem related to
  – body image changes

Expected Outcomes of Care

The psychosocial plan of care for the postpartum woman includes all family members. The postnatal period is a crucial one for the family because it contains the potential for crisis in family adjustment. Developing a plan of care that recognizes family strengths and provides support for family weaknesses does much to help family members take on new tasks and responsibilities.

Expected psychosocial outcomes during the postpartum period are based on the nursing diagnoses identified for the individual woman and her family. Examples of common expected outcomes include that the woman (family) will do the following:

- Identify measures that promote a healthy personal adjustment in the postpartum period.
- Maintain healthy family functioning based on cultural norms and personal expectations.

Plan of Care and Interventions

The nurse functions in the roles of teacher, encourager, and supporter rather than doer while implementing the psychosocial plan of care for a postpartum woman. Implementation of the psychosocial care plan involves carrying out specific activities to achieve the expected outcomes of care planned for each individual woman. Several topics that should be included in the psychosocial plan of care include promotion of parenting skills and family member adjustment to the newest member. Chapter 25 discusses these topics.

Cultural issues must also be considered when planning care. In contrast with Allopathic medicine, there are many traditional health beliefs and practices among the different cultures within the American population. Traditional health practices that are used to maintain health or to avoid illnesses deal with the whole person (body, mind, and spirit) and tend to be culturally based. There is increasing scientific information about the effect of these traditional health practices on maintaining a person's health (Spector, 1995).

Women from various cultures may view health as a balance between opposing forces (e.g., yin versus yang), being in harmony with nature, or just "feeling good." Traditional practices may include the observance of certain dietary restrictions, clothing, or taboos for balancing the body; participation in certain activities such as sports and art for maintaining mental health; and use of silence, prayer, or meditation for developing spiritually. Practices (e.g., using religious objects, eating garlic) are used to protect oneself from illness and may involve avoiding people who are believed to create hexes, spells, or who have an evil eye. Restoration of health may involve a person taking folk medicines (e.g., herbs, animal substances) or using a traditional healer.

Childbirth occurs within this sociocultural context. Rest, seclusion, dietary restraints, and ceremonies honoring the mother are all common traditional practices that are followed for the promotion of the health and well-being of the mother and baby (D'Avanzo, 1992; Horn, 1990; Jambunathan, 1995; Jiménez, 1995; Lipson et al., 1996; Schneiderman, 1996; Spector, 1995).

There are several common traditional health practices used and beliefs held by women and their families during the postpartum period. In Asia, for example, pregnancy is considered to be a hot (yang) condition, then childbirth results in a sudden loss of yang forces (Mattson, 1995). Therefore balance needs to be restored by increasing the return of yang forces present physically or symbolically in hot food, hot water, and warm air (Jambunathan, 1995; Schneiderman, 1996). Hmong women reported that if they did not follow the traditional diet after childbirth, they would not be able to bear another child and would have "sagging and shaking legs" in old age (Jambunathan, 1995; Schneiderman, 1996).

Another common belief is that the mother and baby remain in a weak and vulnerable state for a period of several weeks following birth (Jambunathan, 1995; Jiménez, 1995; Schneiderman, 1996). During this time the mother may remain in a passive role, not take baths or showers, and stay in bed to prevent cold air from entering her body.

Women who have immigrated to the United States or other Western nations without their extended family may not have much help at home, thus making it extremely difficult for them to observe these activity restrictions (Park & Peterson, 1991). Box 24-4 lists some common cultural beliefs about the postpartum period.

It is important that nurses consider all cultural aspects when planning care and not use their own cultural beliefs as the framework for that care. A nursing diagnosis of noncompliance is not appropriate for a client who has a language barrier or behaves culturally different than what is generally expected by nurses during postpartum care. Although the beliefs and behaviors of other cultures may seem different or strange, they should be encouraged as long as the mother wants to conform to them and she and the baby suffer no ill effects. The nurse needs to determine whether a woman is using any folk medicine during the postpartum period because active ingredients in folk medicine may have adverse physiologic effects on the woman when ingested with prescribed medicines (Lea, 1994). Also, the nurse should not assume that a mother desires to use traditional health practices that represent a particular cultural group merely because she is a member of that culture. Many young women who are first-generation or second-generation Americans follow their cultural traditions only when older family members are present or not at all.

BOX 24-4 Some Cultural Beliefs About the Postpartum Period and Contraception

POSTPARTUM CARE

Chinese, Mexican, Korean, and Southeast Asian women may wish to eat only warm foods and drink hot drinks to replace blood loss and to restore the balance of hot and cold in their bodies. These women may also wish to stay warm and avoid bathing, exercises, and hair washing for 7 to 30 days after childbirth. Self-care may not be a priority; care by family members is preferred. The woman has respect for elders and authority. These women may wear abdominal binders. They may prefer not to give their babies colostrum.

Haitian women may request to take the placenta home to bury or burn.

Muslim women follow strict religious laws on modesty and diet. A Muslim woman must keep her hair, body, arms to the wrist, and legs to the ankles covered at all times. She cannot be alone in the presence of a man other than her husband or a male relative. Observant Muslims will not eat pork or pork products and are obligated to eat meat slaughtered according to Islamic laws (halal meat). If halal meat is not available, kosher meat, seafood, or a vegetarian diet is usually accepted.

CONTRACEPTION

Birth control is government mandated in mainland *China*. Most *Chinese women* will have an IUD inserted after the birth of their first child. Women do not want hormonal methods of contraception because they fear putting these medications in their bodies.

Saudi Arabian and Hispanic women will likely choose the rhythm method because most are Catholic.

(East) Indian men are encouraged to have voluntary sterilization by vasectomy.

Muslim couples may practice contraception by mutual consent as long as its use is not harmful to the woman. Acceptable contraceptive methods include foam and condoms, the diaphragm, and natural family planning.

Hmong women highly value and desire large families, which limits birth control practices.

Nursing needs to be culturally relevant. As in planning care to meet physiologic needs, standardized care plans must be adapted to meet the specific needs of the individual families. The nurse needs to be open and to continue to learn about how best to meet the health needs of childbearing women with diverse cultural backgrounds.

Evaluation

The nurse can be reasonably assured that care was effective if expected outcomes for care for psychosocial needs have been met.

DISCHARGE TEACHING

Self-Care, Signs of Complications

Bridging the gap between hospital and home care requires sensitive and knowledgeable nursing care. Discharge planning begins at the time of admission to the unit and should be reflected in the plan of care developed for each individual woman. For example, a great deal of time during the hospital stay is usually spent in teaching about maternal and newborn care because all women must be capable of providing basic care for themselves and their infants at the time of discharge (see Research Box). It is also crucial that every woman be taught to recognize physical signs and symptoms that might indicate problems and how to obtain advice and assistance quickly if these signs appear. The Signs of Potential Complications boxes on pp. 602 and 613 list several common indications of maternal physical and psychosocial problems in the postpartum period. Before discharge, women also need basic instruction regarding the resumption of intercourse, prescribed medications, routine mother-baby checkups, and contraception (see Guidelines/Guías box).

Just before the time of discharge, the nurse reviews the woman's chart (audits the chart) to see that laboratory reports, medications, signatures, and so on are in order. Some hospitals have a checklist to follow before the woman's discharge. The nurse verifies that medications, if ordered, have arrived on the unit, that any valuables kept secured during the woman's stay have been returned to her and that she has signed a receipt for them, and that the infant is ready to be discharged.

The nurse is careful not to administer any medication that would make the mother sleepy if she is the one who will be holding the baby on the way out of the hospital. In most instances the woman is seated in a wheelchair and is usually given the baby to hold. Some families leave unescorted and ambulatory, depending on hospital protocol. The woman's possessions are gathered and taken out with her and her family. *The woman's and the baby's identification bands are carefully checked.* As the woman and the baby are assisted into the car, the nurse should make sure that there is a car seat in which to secure the baby.

LEGAL TIP Early Discharge

Whether or not the woman and her family have chosen early discharge, the nurse and the primary care provider are held responsible if the woman is discharged before her condition has stabilized within normal limits. If complications occur, the medical and nursing staff could be sued for abandonment.

RESEARCH

Postpartum Teaching Priorities: The Viewpoint of Nurses and Mothers

Health education is an important part of maternal-child nursing care. During the postpartum period, nurses educate mothers about health behaviors that enhance positive maternal-infant outcomes, especially those related to infant and self-care. Nurses and clients set goals together and plan the process of implementation to maximize goal achievement and mutual satisfaction. Mothers tend to be eager learners who can identify their own learning needs. This often results in misalignment of teaching priorities. Literature suggests that perceptions of maternal learning needs differ between mothers and nurses. In this study, mothers' and nurses' perceptions of postpartum learning needs and effective teaching modalities were compared. A convenience sample of 236 mothers and 82 nurses were asked to complete a 44-item questionnaire to assess perceived learning needs of mother and infant care topics. Mothers were given a questionnaire during their postpartum stay before discharge and nurses rated similar items on the basis of their perception of what is most important

for mothers to learn during their postpartum stay. Mothers and nurses agreed that topics related to immediate physical health needs were most important. Unmarried mothers considered topics related to personal care and mobility as most important. First-time mothers rated more topics as important than did experienced mothers. Individual teaching was rated most effective by both groups. The study supports postpartum education that focuses on the physical needs of mothers and infants, as well as individual teaching models.

PRIORITIES

Nurses cannot teach mothers about every topic of interest during the postpartum hospital stay. The immediate physical health needs of mothers and infants, as well as signs of illness, need to be addressed first. Nurses should assess individual learning needs of different groups of mothers and accommodate these needs whenever possible.

Source: Berger, D., & Loveland Cook, C. (1998). Postpartum teaching priorities: The viewpoints of nurses and mothers. *J Obstet Gynecol Neonatal Nurs* 27(2), 161.

Sexual Activity/Contraception

Many couples resume sexual activity before the traditional postpartum checkup 6 weeks after childbirth. Risk of hemorrhage and infection are minimal approximately 2 weeks postpartum. Couples may be anxious about the topic but feel uncomfortable and unwilling to bring it up. It is important that the nurse discuss the physical and psychologic effects that giving birth can have on lovemaking. The Home Care box contains helpful information about the resumption of sexual intercourse. Contraceptive options should also be discussed with women (and their partners if present) before discharge so that they can make informed decisions about fertility management before resuming sexual activity. Waiting to discuss contraception at the 6-week checkup may be too late. It is possible, particularly in women who bottle feed, for ovulation to occur as soon as 1 month after birth. A woman who engages in unprotected sex risks becoming pregnant much sooner than she planned. Current contraceptive options are discussed in detail in Chapter 9. Women who are undecided about contraception at the time of discharge need information about using condoms with foam or creams until the 6-week checkup.

Prescribed Medications

Most women have at least one medication prescribed for their use after discharge. Many health care providers routinely have women continue to take their prenatal vitamins and iron during the 6-week postpartum period. It is especially important that women who are breastfeeding or who are discharged with a lower than normal hematocrit level take these medications as ordered. Women with extensive episiotomies (third or fourth degree) or vaginal lacerations are usually given stool softeners to take at home. Pain relief medications (analgesics or nonsteroidal antiinflammatory medications) may be prescribed, especially for women who had cesarean birth. The nurse should make certain that the woman knows the route, dosage, and frequency of all ordered medications and the common side effects.

Routine Mother and Baby Checkups

Women who have experienced uncomplicated vaginal births are still commonly scheduled for the traditional 6-week postpartum examination. Women who have had a cesarean birth are often seen in the health care provider's office or clinic 2 weeks after hospital discharge. The date and time for the follow-up appointment should be included in the discharge orders. If an appointment has not been made before the woman leaves the hospital, she should be encouraged to call the health care provider's office or clinic immediately and schedule an appointment herself.

Parents who have not already done so need to make plans for newborn follow-up at the time of discharge. Most offices and clinics like to see newborns for an initial

GUIDELINES/GUÍAS

Discharge Teaching

When you go to the bathroom, always wipe from front to back.
Cuando vaya al baño, séquese siempre de adelante hacia atrás.

Sit in a warm tub to relieve discomfort.
Siéntese en una bañera con agua tibia para aliviarse.

You will have moderate amounts of vaginal discharge.
Usted tendrá cantidades moderadas de sangrado vaginal.

It may last from 4 to 6 weeks.
Puede durar desde 4 a 6 semanas.

The color may vary from dark brown to red to pink.
El color puede variar entre café oscuro a rojo a rosado.

It may contain blood clots.
Es probable que contenga coágulos.

Use a sanitary pad instead of a tampon.
Use una toalla sanitaria en vez de un tampón.

Your menstrual period will not resume for 4 to 10 weeks.
Su periodo menstrual no regresará hasta 4 a 10 semanas más tarde.

If you are breastfeeding, it may take a little longer.
Si está amamantando, puede demorar un poco más.

It is possible to become pregnant while you are breast-feeding.
Es posible quedar embarazada mientras amamanta.

Avoid having sexual relations for 2 to 4 weeks after birth.
Evite las relaciones sexuales por 2 a 4 semanas después del parto.

Gradually increase activity to incorporate everyday routines.
Aumente las actividades gradualmente hasta llegar a su rutina normal.

Do your Kegel exercises.
Haga sus ejercicios Kegel.

Do not lift heavy objects (over 10 pounds).
No levante objetos pesados (de más de diez libras).

Rest as often as possible.
Descanse mucho.

Rest when your baby sleeps.
Descanse cuando duerma su bebé.

Eat daily:
Diariamente comase:

4 servings of bread/cereals, fruits/vegetables (green), milk or foods made from milk, and 2 servings of meat. You need to drink 8 glasses of fluids a day to support breastfeeding.
4 porciones de pan/cereal, frutas/vegetales (verduras), leche o comidas del grupo de leche, y 2 porciones de carne. Tiene que beber 8 vasos de líquidos diariamente para soportar el dar de pecho.

Call your doctor (obstetrician) if you have:
Llame al médico de obstetricas si tenga cualquier de lo siguiente:

* Fever >38° C
  Fiebre de 38° o más

* Increased vaginal bleeding (more than a regular period)
  Aumento de desangre vaginal (más que una regla normal)

* Chills
  Escalofrío

* Painful, burning urination
  Orin que le duele o le quema

* Foul-smelling vaginal discharge
  Desangre vaginal de muy mal olor

* Increased pain or swelling
  Aumento de dolor o hinchazón

* Drainage or separation of incision (cesarean)
  Desangre o deshecho de la herida

examination within the first week or by 2 weeks of age. Again, if an appointment for a specific date and time was not made for the infant before leaving the hospital, the parents should be encouraged to call the office or clinic right away.

Follow-Up After Discharge
Home Visits

The Association of Women's Health, Obstetric, and Neonatal Nurses (AWHONN) (1994) has published guidelines for postpartum home care that describe comprehensive perinatal home care follow-up services. Although these services may be offered by hospitals, maternity centers, home care agencies, public health agencies, private physicians, or entrepreneurs, it is the nursing profession that is a constant presence in this care. The common goal of these services is to ensure that the mother, newborn, and family have an optimal opportunity to prepare for and enjoy safe, comprehensive, and quality perinatal care.

HOME CARE

RESUMPTION OF SEXUAL INTERCOURSE

You can safely resume sexual intercourse by the second to fourth week after birth when bleeding has stopped and the episiotomy has healed. For the first 6 weeks to 6 months, the vagina does not lubricate well.

Your physiologic reactions to sexual stimulation for the first 3 months after birth will be slower and less intense. The strength of the orgasm is reduced.

A water-soluble gel, cocoa butter, or a contraceptive cream or jelly might be recommended for lubrication. If some vaginal tenderness is present, your partner can be instructed to insert one or more clean, lubricated fingers into the vagina and rotate them within the vagina to help relax it and to identify possible areas of discomfort. A position in which you have control of the depth of the insertion of the penis also is useful. The side-by-side or female-on-top position may be more comfortable.

The presence of the baby influences postbirth lovemaking. Parents hear every sound made by the baby; conversely you may be concerned that the baby hears every sound you make. In either case, any phase of the sexual response cycle may be interrupted by hearing the baby cry or move, leaving both of you frustrated and unsatisfied. In addition, the amount of psychologic energy expended by you in child care activities may lead to fatigue. Newborns require a great deal of attention and time.

Some women have reported feeling sexual stimulation and orgasms when nursing their babies. Nursing mothers often are interested in returning to sexual activity before nonnursing mothers.

You should be instructed to correctly perform the Kegel exercises to strengthen your pubococcygeal muscle. This muscle is associated with bowel and bladder function and with vaginal feeling during intercourse.

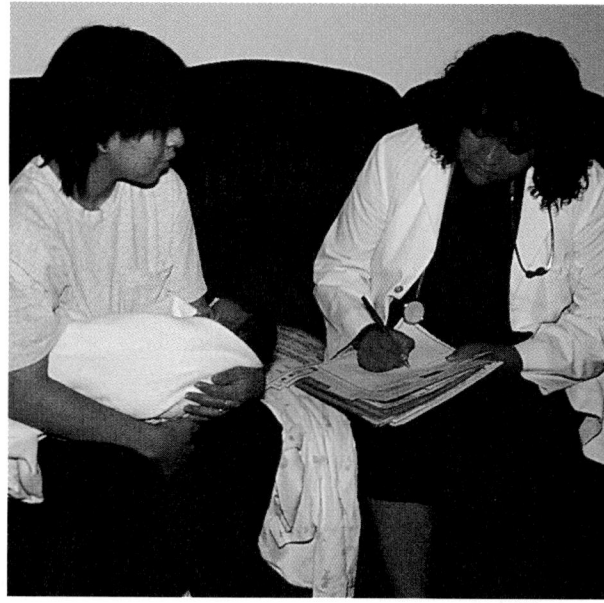

Fig. 24-9 Home care nurse visiting with woman and her infant. *(Courtesy Michael S. Clement, MD, Mesa, AZ.)*

Home visits to new mothers and babies within a few days of discharge can help bridge the gap between hospital care and routine visits to health care providers. Nurses are able to assess the mother, infant, and home environment; answer questions and provide education; and make referrals to community resources if necessary (Fig. 24-9). Home visits may also help reduce the need for more expensive health care, such as nonroutine health care visits and rehospitalization, and decrease stress in new families (Brown & Johnson, 1998).

A referral form containing information about both mother and baby should be completed at hospital discharge and sent immediately to the home care agency. Figure 24-10 is an example of such a referral form.

The home visit is most commonly scheduled on the woman's second day home from the hospital, but it may be scheduled on the first, third, or fourth day home, depending on the individual family's situation and needs. Additional visits are planned throughout the first week, as needed. The home visits may be extended beyond that time if the family's needs warrant it and if a home visit is the most appropriate option for carrying out the follow-up care required to meet the specific needs identified.

A home visit progresses more effectively if it is preplanned and well organized. In advance, the nurse reviews the hospital's discharge summary, teaching plan, and any other records, including the physician's orders; this serves to structure the interview and physical assessment and hence provide continuity of care. Before the visit, the nurse also obtains directions to the family's home and gets a map, if necessary.

Telephone Follow-Up

As part of the routine follow-up of a woman and her infant after discharge from the hospital, many providers are implementing one or more postpartum telephone follow-up calls to their clients for assessment, health teaching, identification of complications to effect timely intervention, and referrals. Telephone follow-up may be part of the services offered by the hospital, private physician or clinic, or a private agency and may be either a separate service or combined with other strategies for extending postpartum care. If no home care follow-up is provided, then telephone follow-up may take its place. If the family has a home care visit, this follow-up is incorporated into that care. Telephonic nursing assessments are frequently used

OB Homecare

Phone: 612-863-4478

Fax: 612-863-4568

POSTPARTUM HOME CARE REFERRAL

☐PHN Referral Made to _____ County _____

Mother's Name:_____

Address/Phone where mother will be staying:

Address: _____

City: _____

Phone #:(_____)_____

☐ **Address & Phone Verified**

Language Spoken: ☐ English   ☐ Other:_____

Understands English: ☐ Well   ☐ Poor

☐ Mother Needs Interpreter   ☐ Hearing Impaired

Who interpreted in hospital: _____

Phone: (_____)_____

Mom's MD/Midwife: (Full Name)_____

Phone #: (_____)_____

Next Appt: _____

MOTHER:

Gravida _____ T____ P____ A____ L____

Marital Status: S   M   W   D   Sep

Normal Maternal Exam: ☐Yes ☐No (explain below)

☐ Vaginal Birth   ☐ C/Birth

Epis/Incision:_____

Meds: _____

Allergies: _____

☐ Needs Large BP Cuff

OTHER ISSUES:

Diabetic: _____

Hgb pp, if abnormal: _____

Psycho/Social Issues:

☐ Parent/Child Interaction   ☐ Limited Support System

☐ Mental Health Status   ☐ Drug Use/Dependency

☐ Previous Losses   ☐ Hx of Domestic Violence

☐ Other: _____

Husband/Significant Other: _____

Baby's Name: _____   ☐ M   ☐ F

Delivery Date/Time:_____@_____

Mother's Discharge Date/Time: _____@_____

Baby's MD (Full Name):_____

Phone #: (_____)_____

Next Appt: _____

BABY: _____

Gestation: _____weeks   ☐ Fetal Loss

Birth Weight:_____   Discharge wt: _____

Apgars: 1"_____   5"_____

Feedings: ☐ Breast   ☐ Bottle   ☐ Both

Feeding Issues:_____

_____

Normal Infant Exam: ☐ Yes   ☐ No (explain below)

Circumcised: ☐ Yes   ☐ No

Additional Order:

☐ Home care to draw newborn screen

**Must send lab-slip home with family.

**ADDITIONAL COMMENTS or
ABNORMAL FINDINGS FOR MOTHER OR BABY:**

_____

_____

_____

_____

_____

_____

_____

_____

_____

Mom aware of referral: ☐Yes ☐No   **REFERRAL COMPLETED BY:** _____

☐ *Faxed to OB Homecare @-612-863-4568:* ☐ *Facesheet*   ☐ *Referral*

☐ *Faxed to PHN* _____ *County:* ☐ *Facesheet*   ☐ *Referral*

Currently being seen by PHN: ☐ Yes ☐ No

Fig. 24-10 Referral form. *(Courtesy OB Homecare of Allina Hospitals and Clinics, Minneapolis, MN.)*

after a postpartum home care visit to reassess a woman's knowledge about the signs and symptoms of adequate hydration in breastfeeding or, after initiating home phototherapy, to assess the caregiver's knowledge regarding equipment complications.

Warm Lines

The warm line represents another type of telephone link between the new family and concerned caregivers or experienced parent volunteers. Warm line services sometimes are best understood in contrast to hot lines, which may be more familiar to new parents. For example, they might have seen advertisements of hot lines in their area that provide emergency help to prevent suicide or child abuse.

In contrast, a **warm line** is a helpline or consultation service, not a crisis intervention line. The warm line is appropriately used for dealing with less extreme concerns that may seem urgent at the time the call is placed but are not actual emergencies. Calls to warm lines commonly relate to infant feeding, prolonged crying, or sibling rivalry. Warm line services may extend beyond the fourth trimester. Families need to call when concerns arise and be given phone numbers for easy access for answers to their questions.

Support Groups

Humans are inherently social beings, involved on a daily basis in some kind of group—groups of family members, classmates, co-workers, and friends. Education, work, worship, and leisure time often take place in groups. Thus, at times of difficult transitions, it seems reasonable for people to turn to groups for support.

A special group experience is sometimes sought by the woman adjusting to motherhood. On occasion, postpartum women who have met earlier in prenatal clinics or on the hospital unit may begin to associate for mutual support. Members of Lamaze classes who attend a postpartum reunion may decide to extend their relationship during the fourth trimester. Realizing the value of group support, nurses may wish to make postpartum support groups available as a strategy for bridging the hospital and home experience.

A postpartum support group enables mothers and fathers to share with and support each other as they adjust to parenting. Many new parents find it reassuring to discover that they are not alone in their feelings of confusion and uncertainty. Often in a postpartum support group an experienced parent can impart concrete information that can be valuable to other group members. Inexperienced parents may find themselves imitating the behavior of others in the group whom they perceive as particularly capable.

Referral to Community Resources

To develop an effective referral system, it is important that the nurse have an understanding of the needs of the woman and family and of the organization and community resources that are available for meeting those needs. Locating and compiling information about available community services contributes to the development of a referral system. It is important for the nurse to develop his or her own resource file of services that are frequently used by health care providers.

The nurse can begin by gathering existing information from community resources such as the local health department, library, or church; local resource agencies such as Planned Parenthood, HAND, or La Leche League; and major service organizations such as March of Dimes, American Red Cross, and WIC Supplemental Nutrition Program. Also, national perinatal organizations such as Nursing Mothers Counsel, Depression After Delivery–National, Postpartum Support, International, Positive Pregnancy and Parenting Fitness, National Perinatal Association, and Child Welfare League of America can be helpful. These services can provide published resource guides and lists of community service agencies specific to the group or condition that they represent (Clemen-Stone, McGuire, & Eigsti, 1998; Perinatal resources, 1997).

KEY POINTS

- Postpartum care is modeled on the concept of health.
- Cultural beliefs and practices affect the client's response to the puerperium.
- The nursing plan of care includes assessments to detect deviations from normal, comfort measures to relieve discomfort or pain, and safety measures to prevent injury or infection.
- The nurse provides teaching and counseling measures designed to promote the woman's feelings of competence in self-care and baby care.
- The nurse must exhibit both clinical and decision-making skills to provide safe and effective physical care. Common nursing interventions include evaluating and treating the boggy uterus and the full urinary bladder, providing for pharmacologic and nonpharmacologic relief of pain and discomfort associated with the episiotomy or lacerations, and instituting measures to promote or suppress lactation.
- Nurses can help promote the health of the woman's future pregnancies and children by administering rubella vaccine and Rh immune globulin if indicated.
- Meeting the psychosocial needs of new mothers involves planning care that takes into consideration the composition and functioning of the entire family.
- Early postpartum discharge will continue to be the trend as a result of consumer demand, medical necessity, discharge criteria for low risk childbirth, and cost-containment measures.

KEY POINTS—cont'd

▪ The short-stay option in perinatal care is safer when selection criteria are used to determine a woman's eligibility for early discharge and when home care follow-up is available.

▪ Home visits, telephone follow-up, warm lines, support groups, and referral to community resources—used either individually or in combination—are effective means of preventing crisis and facilitating physiologic and psychologic adjustments in the postpartum period.

CRITICAL THINKING EXERCISES

1 Tina is a primigravida, 15 years old, and she gave birth to an 8 pound girl 24 hours ago. Physically, she is meeting all expected outcomes. However, Tina is having difficulty breastfeeding and is uncertain about how to bathe and care for the baby. She seems to have difficulty recognizing the baby's cues. Tina is also in need of baby clothes and equipment (e.g., car seat). Tina plans to stay with her parents while she continues her high school education and is eager to go home as soon as possible to see her friends.

   a. Determine whether Tina would be eligible for early home discharge and explain why.

   b. Develop a home care discharge plan for Tina.

   c. Discuss the type of follow-up postpartum home care services needed to ensure a continuum of comprehensive postpartum care for Tina.

   d. Identify existing community resources that you would suggest to Tina and explain your rationale.

   e. What does the nurse need to consider in order to make the referral with Tina more successful?

2 Mrs. Chow is a Chinese primipara who has a temperature of 37.8° C 12 hours after birth. The nurse noticed that Mrs. Chow has not gotten up, is covered with several blankets and a robe, and has not taken any liquids or eaten much food on her food tray. The nursing staff members tell you to make her follow the physician's order for activity, that is, to get out of bed as needed and to perform self-care activities.

   a. Identify five cultural issues that are in conflict in this situation.

   b. List several culturally sensitive nursing diagnoses.

   c. Discuss how the nurse could approach and communicate with Mrs. Chow to facilitate understanding and modification of care.

   d. List several nursing interventions that incorporate Mrs. Chow's cultural practices and promote safe, postpartum recovery.

References

American Academy of Pediatrics. (1995). Hospital stay for healthy term infants. *Pediatrics* 96(4), 788-790.

American Academy of Pediatrics & American College of Obstetricians and Gynecologists. (1997). *Guidelines for perinatal care* (3rd ed.). Elk Grove Village, IL: American Academy of Pediatrics.

Association of Women's Health, Obstetric, and Neonatal Nurses (AWHONN). (1994). *Didactic content and clinical skills verification for professional nurse providers of perinatal home care.* Washington, DC: AWHONN.

Barnes, L. (1996). Meeting the challenge of early postpartum discharge. *MCN: Am J Matern Child Nurs* 21(3), 129.

Beger, D., & Loveland Cook, C. (1998). Postpartum teaching priorities: The viewpoints of nurses and mothers. *J Obstet Gynecol Neonatal Nurs* 27(2), 161-168.

Brown, S., & Johnson, B. (1998). Enhancing early discharge with home follow-up: A pilot project. *J Obstet Gynecol Neonatal Nurs* 27(1), 33-38.

Clemen-Stone, S., McGuire, S., & Eigsti, D. (1998). *Comprehensive community health nursing* (5th ed.). St. Louis: Mosby.

D'Avanzo, C. (1992). Bridging the cultural gap with Southeast Asians. *MCN Am J Matern Child Nurs* (17(4), 204-208.

Edmonson, M., Stoddard, J., & Owens, L. (1997). Hospital readmission with feeding-related problems after early postpartum discharge of normal newborns. *JAMA* 278(4), 299-303.

Ferguson, S., & Engelhard, C. (1997). Short stay: The art of legislating quality and economy. *AWHONN Lifelines* 1(1), 17-23.

Fishbein, E., & Burggraf E. (1998). Early postpartum discharge: How are mothers managing? *J Obstet Gynecol Neonatal Nurs* 27(2), 142-148.

Havens, D., & Hannan, C. (1996). Legislation to mandate maternal and newborn length of stay. *J Pediatr Health Care* 10(3), 141-144.

Horn, B. (1990). Cultural concepts and postpartal care. *J Transcult Nurs* 2(1), 48-51.

Hutchinson, M., & Baqi-Aziz, M. (1994). Nursing care of the childbearing Muslim family. *J Obstet Gynecol Neonatal Nurs* 23(9), 767-777.

Jambunathan, J. (1995). Hmong cultural practices and beliefs: The postpartum period. *Clin Nurs Res* 4(3), 335-345.

Jiménez, S. (1995). The Hispanic culture, folklore, and perinatal health. *J Perinatal Educ* 4(1), 9.

Johnson & Johnson. (1996). *Compendium of postpartum care.* Skillman, NJ: Johnson & Johnson Consumer Products, Inc.

Lea, A. (1994). Nursing in today's multicultural society: A transcultural perspective. *J Adv Nurs* 20(2), 307-313.

Lipson, J., Dibble, S., & Minarik, P. (1996). *Culture & nursing care: A pocket guide.* San Francisco: UCSF Nursing Press.

Liu, L. et al. (1997). The safety of newborn early discharge. The Washington State Experience. *JAMA* 278(4), 293-298.

Luegenbiehl, D. (1997). Improving visual estimation of blood volume on peripads. *MCN Am J Matern Child Nurs* 22(6), 294-298.

Mattson, S. (1995). Culturally sensitive perinatal care for Southeast Asians. *J Obstet Gynecol Neonatal Nurs* 24(4), 335-341.

Park, K., & Peterson, L. (1991). Beliefs, practices, and experiences of Korean women in relation to childbirth. *Health Care Women Int* 12, 261-269.

Perinatal resources: Publications and organizations. (1997). *J Perinatal Educ* 6(2), 61-68.

Pugh, L. et al. (1999). Clinical approaches in the assessment of childbearing fatigue. *J Obstet Gynecol Neonatal Nurs* 28(1), 74-80.

Roberts, K. (1995). A comparison of chilled cabbage leaves and chilled gel-paks in reducing breast engorgement. *J Hum Lact* 11(1), 17-20.

Sampselle, C., & Miller, J. (1996). Pelvic muscle exercise: Effective patient teaching. *The Female Patient* 21(5), 29-36.

Schneiderman, J. (1996). Postpartum nursing for Korean mothers. *MCN Am J Matern Child Nurs* 21(3), 155-158.

Simpson, K., & Creehan, P. (1996). *AWHONN's perinatal nursing.* Philadelphia: J.B. Lippincott.

Spector, R. (1995). Cultural concepts of women's health and health-promoting behaviors. *J Obstet Gynecol Neonatal Nurs* 24(3), 241-245.

Weekly, S., & Neumann, M. (1997). Speaking up for baby: The case for individualized neonatal discharge plans. *AWHONN Lifelines* 1(1), 24-29.

Wilkerson, N. (1996). Appraisal of early discharge programs. *J Perinatal Educ* 5(2), 1.

Williams, L., & Cooper, M. (1996). A new paradigm for postpartum care. *J Obstet Gynecol Neonatal Nurs* 25(9), 745-749.

25

Transition to Parenthood

Lienne D. Edwards

EARNING OBJECTIVES

- Define the key terms.
- Discuss transition as a concept central to the discipline of nursing.
- Describe the two components of the parenting process.
- Discuss five preconditions that influence attachment.
- Describe sensual responses that strengthen attachment.
- Differentiate the three periods in parental role change after childbirth.
- Discuss the six parental tasks and responsibilities.
- Identify infant behaviors that facilitate and inhibit parental attachment.
- Identify behaviors of the three phases of maternal adjustment.

- Discuss paternal adjustment.
- Discuss ways to facilitate parent-infant adjustment.
- Discuss the effects of the following on parental response: parental age (adolescence and over 35 years), social support, culture, socioeconomic conditions, personal aspirations, and sensory impairment.
- Describe sibling adjustment.
- Describe grandparent adaptation.
- Discuss nursing care management for assisting transition to parenthood.
- Identify topics for nursing research related to family dynamics during the transition to parenthood.

EY TERMS

acquaintance	fourth trimester	postpartum blues
attachment	infant-parent interaction	reciprocity
biorhythmicity	rhythm	sibling rivalry
bonding	repertoire of behaviors	synchrony
claiming process	responsivity	taking-hold phase
en face	letting-go phase	taking-in phase
engrossment	maternal adjustment	transition
entrainment	paternal adjustment	transition to parenthood

ecoming a parent creates a period of change and instability for all men and women who decide to have children. This holds true whether parenthood is biologic or adoptive and whether the parents are married husband-wife couples, cohabiting couples, single mothers, single fathers, lesbian couples with one woman as biologic mother, or gay

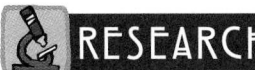

RESEARCH

Labor Concerns of Women Two Months After Birth

The transition from being a childless woman to becoming a mother requires complex cognitive, affective, and behavioral changes. Women strive to incorporate their labor and birth experiences into their self-image. It is important to understand a woman's expectations and satisfaction with the birthing experience, since her perceptions of the birth contribute to her self-image as a mother. Examining a woman's satisfaction with the birth experience is also an important step in providing quality nursing care and maternity service.

The purpose of this research study was to explore the discrepancies that women may have felt between their expectations of labor and birth and their realities. A descriptive, qualitative design was applied to examine responses to an open-ended question from a convenience sample of 77 women who were nine weeks postpartum. The women were from three geographically diverse Midwestern hospitals. Responses were subjected to content analysis to identify major categories of concern related to labor and birth.

The women expressed positive responses relating to who helped them in labor and to the context of the experience, frustrations relating to pain, negative reactions to health caregivers, lack of control, and lack of knowledge. It was concluded that these findings offer direction to health care professionals for making labor and childbirth a positive experience, thus easing the transition to motherhood.

CLINICAL APPLICATION

Assessing childbirth outcomes, such as satisfaction with the birth experience, is necessary to ensure that a family-centered approach to maternity care is being followed. Evaluation of these outcomes helps identify topics for staff education programs, such as proper use of labor coping techniques, that would enhance the maternity caregiver's ability to meet the expectations of the woman in labor.

A woman's feelings of frustration with the experience of birth are clearly remembered long after giving birth and often result from her feeling a lack of control and having unmet expectations during the birth process. Health care professionals and hospital administrators caring for the childbearing family must strive to meet the expectations and return control of labor to the woman and her partner as much as possible. Adhering to the principles of family-centered care enhances satisfaction with the birth experience and promotes a successful transition to motherhood.

Source: Fowles, E. (1998). Labor concerns of women two months after delivery. *Birth* 25(4), 235-240.

male couples who adopt a child. This period of developmental change is referred to as the **transition to parenthood.**

Transition is a concept central to the discipline of nursing. **Transition** is defined as a passage or process occurring over time involving development; flow; or movement from one state, condition, or place to another (Meleis, 1991; Schumacher & Meleis, 1994). Nurses often encounter clients during times of transition that occur because of developmental, situational, or health-illness events. The transition to parenthood is one such time.

Transition often entails profound change, such as changes in identities, roles, relationships, abilities, and patterns of behavior, and may have dramatic effects on the lives of the individuals and significant others involved (Schumacher & Meleis, 1994; Vehvilainen-Julkunen, 1995). Wide variation occurs in how individuals and families experience transition. Schumacher and Meleis (1994), in an extensive review of nursing literature on transition, identified six conditions that influence the transition experience:

1. Meanings: Understanding the meaning of a transition from the perspective of those experiencing it is essential.
2. Expectations: People may or may not know what to expect of a transition, just as their expectations may or may not be realistic. Knowing what to expect realistically may help alleviate some of the stress associated with transitions (see Research box).
3. Level of knowledge: Transitions often require new knowledge or skills. Individuals involved experience degrees of uncertainty as they progress to increased levels of knowledge.
4. Environment: Facilitative resources external to the person are important for successful transition. Such resources include social support from spouse, partner, family, friends, and colleagues; effective communication; institutional support; and flexibility. Understanding the sociocultural context is important.
5. Level of planning: Success of a transition depends in part on the level of planning that occurs before and during the transition. Effective planning involves identification of needs, problems, and issues that may arise during the transition.
6. Emotional and physical well-being: A wide range of emotions accompanies transition, the more distressful ones attesting to the difficulties encountered during transition. As individuals and families work through the transition, they report feeling overwhelmed, anxious, insecure, frustrated, depressed, ambivalent, isolated, and lonely. Role conflict and low self-esteem may also be experienced. Physical discomfort and bodily unpredictability can interfere with the assimilation of new information.

Indicators of healthy transition outcomes include:
1. Subjective well-being: As successful transition occurs, emotional distress gives way to a sense of well-being. Individuals experience effective coping, managing one's emotions, personal integrity, increased self-esteem, growth, and role satisfaction.

2. Role mastery: People achieve skilled role performance, empowerment, and comfort with the behaviors required in the new situation. When role mastery is reached, they feel competent and self-confident.

3. Well-being of interpersonal relationships: Transitions involving one or more family members must be evaluated in terms of the whole family. Disagreements or family disruption may occur. As members move toward successful conclusion to the transition, family relationship well-being is restored or promoted. Outcomes include family adaptation, enhanced appreciation and closeness, meaningful interaction, and integration with the broader social networks and community.

A thorough understanding of the process parents go through during their transition to parenthood guides the nurse in helping family members adapt. This chapter reviews the transition to parenthood, including the parenting process and the adjustment of parents, siblings, and grandparents.

PARENTING PROCESS

Biologic parenthood begins with the union of ovum and sperm. During the prenatal period the mother provides an environment in which the unborn child develops and grows. This close symbiotic union ends with birth. At this point, other people assume partial or complete involvement in the infant's care. The biologic or substitute woman or man parent then enters into a crucial relationship with the child that persists throughout the life of each. Men and women, of course, may live without a child; thus parenthood is optional. Parenthood can serve as a maturation factor for women and men regardless of whether it is biologically based. For children, parenthood is all important; their continued existence depends on the quality of care they receive.

Sank (1991) described parenting as a process of role attainment and role transition that begins during pregnancy. The transition ends when the parent develops a sense of comfort and confidence in performing the parental role. The parenting process has two components. The first, skill and knowledge, is more practical and mechanical and involves cognitive and motor skills. The second component, valuing and comfort, is emotional and involves cognitive and affective skills. The infant's well-being and development depend on both components.

Skill and Knowledge Component

The first component in the process of parenting includes knowledge of and skill in child care activities such as feeding, holding, clothing, and bathing the infant and protecting the baby from harm. The ability to competently and confidently perform these task-oriented activities does not appear automatically with the birth of a child. Many parents must learn to do these tasks, and this learning process can be difficult. However, almost all parents become adept in caregiving activities when they have the desire to learn and the support of others.

Valuing and Comfort Component

The psychologic component in the parenting process probably stems from the parents' earliest experiences with a loving, accepting parent or parental figure, during which a sense of trust in and concern for others developed. In essence, parents "inherit" the ability to show concern and tenderness and then pass this ability to the next generation by providing for their children the kind of parent-child relationship they experienced. The valuing and comfort component of the parenting process includes an attitude of tenderness, awareness, and concern for the infant's needs and desires. This component of parenting profoundly affects the manner in which the practical aspects of child care are performed and the emotional response of the child to the care. A positive parent-child relationship is mutually rewarding. This relationship helps a person develop confidence in the expectations that others will be willing to help and that the person is worth helping.

Nurses can help inexperienced parents feel confident and competent in their new roles. They can provide opportunities for parents to practice child care tasks in the hospital, birth setting, or in the home, where assistance and feedback are available. Nursing approaches and strategies can enhance parents' self-concept by helping them feel more comfortable and confident in their parenting skills.

PARENTAL ATTACHMENT, BONDING, AND ACQUAINTANCE

Although much research has been directed toward unraveling the process by which a parent comes to love and accept a child and a child comes to love and accept a parent, researchers still do not know what motivates and commits parents and children to decades of supportive and nurturing care of each other. This process is referred to as **attachment**. The research and writings of Klaus and Kennell have exerted great influence on nursing practice, writings, and research about parental attachment.

Using the terms *attachment* and *bonding*, Klaus and Kennell proposed that "There is a period shortly after birth that is uniquely important to mother-to-infant attachment in the human being" (Klaus et al., 1972). They defined the phenomenon of **bonding** as a sensitive period in the first minutes and hours after birth when mothers and fathers must have close contact with their infants for "later development to be optimal" (Klaus & Kennell, 1976). Subsequently, Klaus and Kennell (1982) revised their theory of parent-infant bonding, modifying their claim of the critical nature of immediate contact with the infant after birth. They acknowledged the adaptability of human parents, stating it took longer than minutes or hours for parents to form an emotional relationship with their infants. Nurse researchers of that time integrated both concepts of attachment and acquaintance into a conceptual framework of the bonding process.

The terms *attachment* and *bonding* continue to be used interchangeably. In an extensive review and critique of nursing research on attachment, Walker (1992) identified two key components of definitions of attachment: (1) an affective tie to another and (2) a specificity and an enduring nature of the tie. Walker also found little agreement about the way to conduct or measure the concepts of attachment and bonding.

The process of attachment has been described as linear–beginning during pregnancy, intensifying during the early postpartum period, having developmental periods of progress and regression, and being constant and consistent once established. Components of the attachment process frequently observed in parents include favorable preconditions and identification and claiming of the infant by the parent (Mercer, 1983).

Favorable preconditions for attachment to begin and progress without unusual difficulty include the following:

- A parent's emotional health (including the ability to trust another person)
- A social support system encompassing mate, friends, and family
- A competent level of communication and caregiving skills
- Parental proximity to the infant
- Parent-infant fit (including infant state, temperament, and sex)

If any of these preconditions are not present or are distorted, nurses must intervene to facilitate the attachment process.

Attachment is developed and maintained by proximity and interaction with the infant, through which the parent becomes acquainted with the infant, identifies the infant as an individual, and claims the infant as a member of the family. Attachment is facilitated by positive feedback (i.e.,

social, verbal, and nonverbal responses, whether real or perceived, that indicate acceptance of one partner by the other). Attachment occurs through a mutually satisfying experience. A mother commented on her son's grasp reflex, "I put my finger in his hand, and he grabbed right on. It is just a reflex, I know, but it felt good anyway" (Fig. 25-1).

The concept of attachment has been extended to include mutuality; that is, the infant's behaviors and characteristics call forth a corresponding set of maternal behaviors and characteristics. The infant displays signaling behaviors such as crying, smiling, and cooing that initiate the contact and bring the caregiver to the child. These behaviors are followed by executive behaviors such as rooting, grasping,

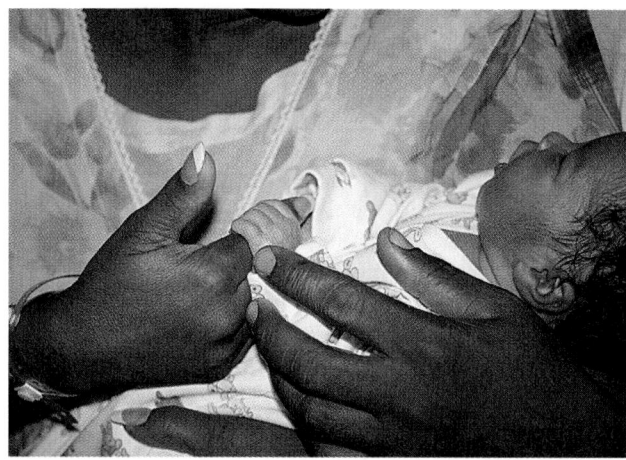

Fig. 25-1 Hands. *(Courtesy Marjorie Pyle, RNC, Lifecircle, Costa Mesa, CA.)*

▪ TABLE 25-1 Infant Behaviors Affecting Parental Attachment

FACILITATING BEHAVIORS	INHIBITING BEHAVIORS
Visually alert; eye-to-eye contact; tracking or following of parent's face	Sleepy; eyes closed most of the time; gaze aversion
Appealing facial appearance; randomness of body movements reflecting helplessness	Resemblance to person parent dislikes; hyperirritability or jerky body movements when touched
Smiles	Bland facial expression; infrequent smiles
Vocalization; crying only when hungry or wet	Crying for hours on end; colicky
Grasp reflex	Exaggerated motor reflex
Anticipatory approach behaviors for feedings; sucks well; feeds easily	Feeds poorly; regurgitates; vomits often
Enjoys being cuddled, held	Resists holding and cuddling by crying, stiffening body
Easily consolable	Inconsolable; unresponsive to parenting, caretaking tasks
Activity and regularity somewhat predictable	Unpredictable feeding and sleeping schedule
Attention span sufficient to focus on parents	Inability to attend to parent's face or offered stimulation
Differential crying, smiling, and vocalizing; recognizes and prefers parents	Shows no preference for parents over others
Approaches through locomotion	Unresponsive to parent's approaches
Clings to parent; puts arms around parent's neck	Seeks attention from any adult in room
Lifts arms to parents in greeting	Ignores parents

From Gerson, E. (1973). *Infant behavior in the first year of life.* New York: Raven Press.

and postural adjustments that maintain the contact. The caregiver is attracted to an alert, responsive, cuddly infant and repelled by an irritable, apparently disinterested infant. Attachment occurs more readily with the infant whose temperament, social capabilities, appearance, and sex fit the parent's expectations. If the child does not meet these expectations, resolution of the parent's disappointment can delay the attachment process. A list of infant behaviors affecting parental attachment that continues to be a classic comprehensive reference is presented in Table 25-1. A corresponding list of parental behaviors that affect infant attachment is presented in Table 25-2.

An important part of attachment is **acquaintance** (Klaus & Kennell, 1983). Parents use eye contact (Fig. 25-2), touching, talking, and exploring to become acquainted with their infant during the immediate postpartum period. Adoptive parents undergo the same process when they first meet their new child. During this period families engage in the **claiming process,** which is the identification of the new baby (Fig. 25-3). The child is first identified in terms of "likeness" to other family members, then in terms of "differences," and finally in terms of "uniqueness." The unique newcomer is thus incorporated into the family. Mothers and fathers scrutinize their infant carefully and point out characteristics that the child shares with other family members and that are indicative of a relationship between them. The claiming process is revealed by maternal comments such as the following: "Russ held him close and said, 'He's the image of his father,' but I found one part like me—his toes are shaped like mine."

On the other hand, some mothers react negatively. They "claim" the infant in terms of the discomfort or pain the baby causes. The mother interprets the infant's normal responses as being negative toward her and reacts to her child with dislike or indifference. She does not hold

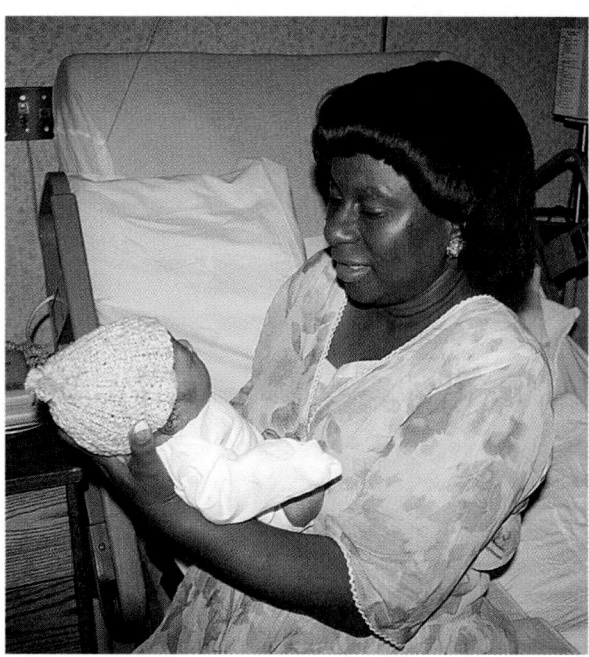

Fig. 25-2 Mother and baby make eye contact in *en face* position. *(Courtesy Marjorie Pyle, RNC, Lifecircle, Costa Mesa, CA.)*

TABLE 25-2 Parental Behaviors Affecting Infant Attachment

FACILITATING BEHAVIORS	INHIBITING BEHAVIORS
Looks; gazes; takes in physical characteristics of infant; assumes en face position; eye contact	Turns away from infant; ignores infant's presence
Hovers; maintains proximity; directs attention to, points to infant	Avoids infant; does not seek proximity; refuses to hold infant when given opportunity
Identifies infant as unique individual	Identifies infant with someone parent dislikes; fails to discern any of infant's unique features
Claims infant as family member; names infant	Fails to place infant in family context or identify infant with family member; has difficulty naming
Touches; progresses from fingertip to fingers to palms to encompassing contact	Fails to move from fingertip touch to palmar contact and holding
Smiles at infant	Maintains bland countenance or frowns at infant
Talks to, coos, or sings to infant	Wakes infant when infant is sleeping; handles roughly; hurries feeding by moving nipple continuously
Expresses pride in infant	Expresses disappointment, displeasure in infant
Relates infant's behavior to familiar events	Does not incorporate infant into life
Assigns meaning to infant's actions and sensitively interprets infant's needs	Makes no effort to interpret infant's actions or needs
Views infant's behaviors and appearance in positive light	Views infant's behavior as exploiting, deliberately uncooperative; views appearance as distasteful, ugly

From Mercer, R. (1983). Parent-infant attachment. In L. Sonstegard, K. Kowalski, & B. Jennings (Eds.). *Women's health,* vol. 2, *Childbearing.* New York: Grune & Stratton.

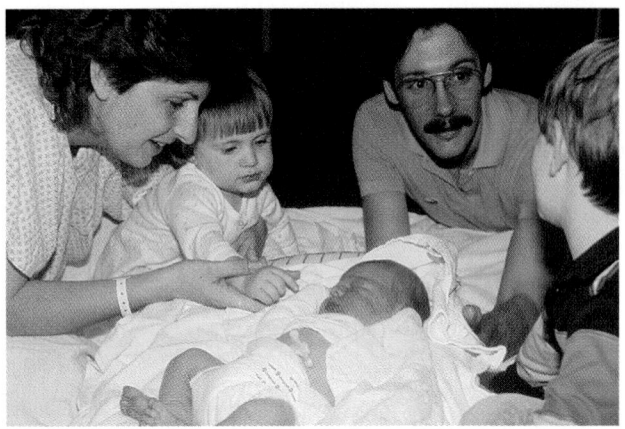

Fig. 25-3 Family members examine the new baby. They discuss how she resembles them and other family members. *(Courtesy Marjorie Pyle, RNC, Lifecircle, Costa Mesa, CA.)*

the child close or touch the child to be comforting; for example, "The nurse put the baby into Marie's arms. She promptly laid him across her knees and glanced up at the television. 'Stay still until I finish watching—you've been enough trouble already.'"

Bonding research in years past demonstrated that neither the type of birth (vaginal, planned cesarean, unplanned cesarean) nor type of infant feeding were related to parental attachment. Parents' perception of their own competence was found to be an important predictor of parental attachment for mothers and fathers in low risk and high risk pregnancies and births (Mercer & Ferketich, 1990). Müller (1996) demonstrated a positive correlation between prenatal and postnatal attachment for mothers; however, because the correlation was modest, Müller advises caution in promoting increased prenatal attachment in hopes of improving postnatal attachment. Nurses can

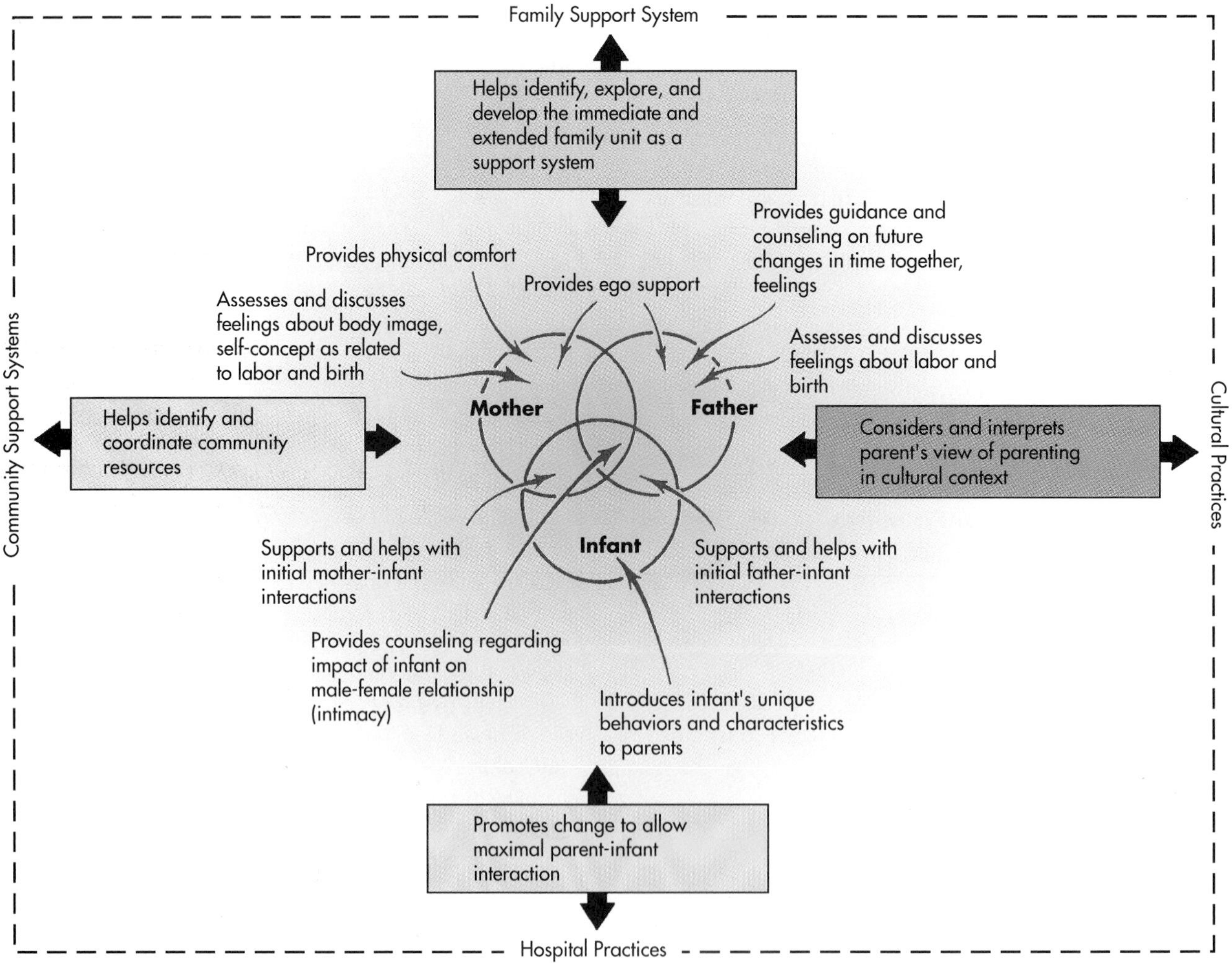

Family Support System

Helps identify, explore, and develop the immediate and extended family unit as a support system

Provides physical comfort

Provides ego support

Provides guidance and counseling on future changes in time together, feelings

Assesses and discusses feelings about body image, self-concept as related to labor and birth

Assesses and discusses feelings about labor and birth

Mother

Father

Community Support Systems

Helps identify and coordinate community resources

Cultural Practices

Considers and interprets parent's view of parenting in cultural context

Supports and helps with initial mother-infant interactions

Infant

Supports and helps with initial father-infant interactions

Provides counseling regarding impact of infant on male-female relationship (intimacy)

Introduces infant's unique behaviors and characteristics to parents

Promotes change to allow maximal parent-infant interaction

Hospital Practices

Fig. 25-4 The role of the nurse in facilitating parental attachment to the infant. *(Modified from Mercer, R. [1983]. Parent-infant attachment. In L. Sonstegard, K. Kowalski, & B. Jennings [Eds.]. Women's health, vol. 2, Childbearing. New York: Grune & Stratton.)*

use these findings to reassure mothers who have had unplanned cesarean births that they can bond as successfully with their infants as if they had had vaginal births. Through teaching and positive reinforcement, nurses can strengthen parents' sense of competence.

Nurses play an important role in facilitating parental attachment (Fig. 25-4). They can enhance positive parent-infant contacts by heightening parental awareness of an infant's responses and ability to communicate. As parents attempt to become competent and loving in their role, nurses can bolster the parents' self-confidence and egos. Nurses are in prime positions to identify actual and potential problems and collaborate with other health care professionals who will provide care for the parents after discharge. Nursing considerations for fostering maternal-infant bonding among special populations may vary (see Cultural Considerations box).

Nursing interventions related to the promotion of parent-infant attachment are numerous and varied. In an attempt to better define such nursing interventions, Denehy (1992) surveyed neonatal nurse-practitioners who were practicing in a variety of inpatient, outpatient, and educational settings. Six attachment-promotion intervention labels with critical and supporting activities were identified. Table 25-3 lists current activities for these interventions.

 CULTURAL considerations

Nursing Considerations to Foster Bonding Among Specific Populations

WOMEN IN ECONOMICALLY DISADVANTAGED SITUATIONS

Low-income mothers may have to contend with stressors that distract them from developing a relationship with their babies. Inability to pay for infant supplies or child care, chaotic home situations, and worry over eligibility for social and health care services deplete these women's psychologic energy.

Nurses need to conduct nonjudgmental, individual assessments of resources and social networks to avoid inaccurate and stereotypical assumptions. Nurses can help economically disadvantaged mothers access social services, such as the Women, Infants, and Children (WIC) program and Medicaid. For mothers whose home environments provide little or no support and multiple stressors, early discharge may not be optimal. Nurses can advocate for longer hospital stays for these mothers when the hospital environment is more conducive to bonding.

Economically disadvantaged mothers, especially adolescents, are not as likely to be aware of the benefits of bonding or to be knowledgeable of normal infant behaviors. These women may not be aware of maternity care options, such as rooming-in, or may be less assertive in asking for such options. The nurse needs to be a client educator and advocate, explaining the choices and the potential benefits. The nurse should ensure a supportive, encouraging environment that will help mothers engage in positive interactions with their infants. By use of the Brazelton Neonatal Behavioral Assessment Scale, the nurse can capture the mother's attention with a mother-infant interactional experience and, at the same time, increase the mother's knowledge of infant behavior. Written material can be provided after the assessment to reinforce the behavioral concepts.

Examples, from sections of an individualized handout written as if from the baby, include "My strengths: great motor maturity—I stretch my arms way up over my head" and "How you can help: swaddle my arms so I can suck on my hands" (Tedder, 1991).

WOMEN OF VARYING ETHNIC AND CULTURAL GROUPS

Childbearing practices and rituals of other cultures may not be congruent with standard practices associated with bonding in the Anglo-American culture. For example, Chinese families traditionally use extended family members to care for the newborn so that the mother can rest and recover, especially after a cesarean birth. Some Native American, Asian, and Hispanic women do not initiate breastfeeding until their breast milk comes in. Haitian families do not name their babies until after the confinement month. Amount of eye contact varies among cultures, too. Yup'ik Eskimo mothers almost always position their babies so that eye contact can be made.

Nurses should become knowledgeable of the childbearing beliefs and practices of diverse cultural and ethnic groups. Because individual cultural variations exist within groups, nurses need to clarify with the client and family members or friends what cultural norms the client follows. Incorrect judgments may be made about mother-infant bonding if nurses do not practice culturally sensitive care. ▪

Modified from Geissler, E. (1994). *Pocket guide to cultural assessment.* St. Louis: Mosby; Symanski, M. (1992). Maternal-infant bonding. Practice issues for the 1990s. *J Nurse Midwifery* 37(2 Suppl),67S-73S; Tedder, J. (1991). Using the Brazelton Neonatal Assessment Scale to facilitate the parent-infant relationship in a primary care setting. *Nurse Pract* 16(3), 26-30, 35-36.

TABLE 25-3 Examples of Parent-Infant Attachment Interventions

INTERVENTION LABEL/DEFINITION	CRITICAL ACTIVITIES	SUPPORTING ACTIVITIES
ATTACHMENT PROMOTION		
Facilitation of development of parent-infant relationship	Give parents opportunity to hold infant soon after birth Keep infant with parents after birth when possible	Provide rooming-in in hospital Provide pain relief for mother Provide opportunity for parents to see, hold, and examine newborn immediately after birth
ENVIRONMENTAL MANAGEMENT: ATTACHMENT PROCESS		
Manipulation of environment that facilitates development of parent-infant relationship	Allow for family visitation as desired Create environment that fosters privacy	Permit father/significant other to sleep in room with mother Provide rocking chair
FAMILY INTEGRITY PROMOTION: CHILDBEARING FAMILY		
Facilitation of growth of individuals or families who are adding infant to family	Convey accepting attitude (for non-threatening environment for family to express feelings) Reinforce parenting behaviors	Offer to be listener for significant other Discuss sibling's reaction to newborn, as appropriate
LACTATION COUNSELING		
Use of interactive helping process to assist in maintenance of successful breastfeeding	Educate parents about infant feeding for informed decision making Give parents recommended education material, as needed	Provide information about advantages and disadvantages of breastfeeding Inform parents about appropriate classes or groups for breastfeeding
PARENT EDUCATION: CHILDBEARING FAMILY		
Preparation of individuals to perform their role as parents	Reinforce skills parent does well in caring for infant to promote confidence Assist parents in interpreting infant cues	Monitor learning needs of family Appraise parents' learning styles (how they learn best)
RISK IDENTIFICATION: CHILDBEARING FAMILY		
Identification of individuals or families who are likely to have difficulties in parenting and prioritization of strategies to prevent parenting problems	Review maternal history of chemical dependency, noting duration, type of drug(s), and time and strength of last dose before birth Monitor behaviors indicative of problem with attachment	Determine parents' feelings about unplanned pregnancy Determine economic, marital, and educational status of parents

Modified from McCloskey, J., & Bulechek, G. (1996). *Nursing interventions classification* (2nd ed.). St. Louis: Mosby.

Assessment of Attachment Behaviors

One of the most important areas of assessment is careful observation of those behaviors thought to indicate the formation of emotional bonds between the newborn and family, especially the mother. Although the words "bonding" and "attachment" are sometimes referred to as separate phenomena, with bonding representing the development of emotional ties from parent to infant and attachment representing the emotional ties from infant to parent, in this discussion the words are used interchangeably to denote both processes.

Unlike physical assessment of the neonate, which has concrete guidelines to follow, assessment of parent-infant attachment requires much more skill in terms of observation and interviewing. Rooming-in of mother and infant and liberal visiting privileges for father, siblings, and grandparents facilitate recognition of behaviors that demonstrate positive or negative attachment. Guidelines for assessment of bonding behaviors are presented in the accompanying Teaching Guidelines box.

Talking to the parents uncovers many variables that can affect the development of attachment and parenting. What expectations do they have for this child? In other words, how similar are their predictions of the fantasy child and their realizations about the real child? Encourage them to talk about their relationship with their own parents, since the type of parenting that parents received as a child influences their child-rearing practices. Was this a planned pregnancy? How do they see the addition of a dependent family member affecting their lifestyle? What arrangements have they made in terms of such changes in lifestyle? What support system or significant others are available for assistance? What are their views regarding child rearing?

The labor process also significantly affects the immediate attachment of mothers to their newborn children. Factors such as a long labor, feeling tired or "drugged" after birth, and problems with breastfeeding can delay the development of initial positive feelings toward the newborn.

During pregnancy, and often even before conception occurs, parents develop an image of the "ideal" or "fantasy" infant. At birth the fantasy infant becomes the real infant. How closely the dream child resembles the real child influences the bonding process. Assessing such expectations during pregnancy and at the time of the infant's birth allows identification of discrepancies in the parents' view of the fantasy child versus the real child.

Because attachment involves a mutually reciprocal interchange, observing the interaction between parent and infant is very important. An excellent opportunity exists during feeding. A useful instrument for systematically describing the parent's and infant's behaviors is the Nursing Child Assessment Feeding Scale (NCAFS) (Barnard, 1994). It consists of 76 behavioral items; 50 items describe the parent's behavior regarding sensitivity to cues, response to child's distress, social-emotional growth fosterings, and cognitive growth fostering. Twenty-six items focus on the child's behavior in terms of clarity of cues and responsiveness to parent. The results can also be shared with the parent to encourage discussion of feelings about the infant and to highlight behaviors of the dyad that foster successful interaction. The NCAFS is appropriate for use with infants during the first year.

PARENT-INFANT CONTACT

Since the early 1970s consumers have strived for childbirth practices that promote the family as the focus of care. The alternatives of home birth, birthing centers, and family-centered maternity care units reflect parents' desires to share in the birth process and have more contact with their infants.

Early Contact

Research with mammals other than humans indicates that early contact between the mother and her offspring is important in developing future relationships. The first hours or days after birth may be a sensitive time for parent-infant interaction. Early close contact may facilitate the attachment process between parent and child. This does not

TEACHING guiDeLines

Assessing Attachment Behavior

When the infant is brought to the parents, do they reach out for the infant and call the infant by name? (Recognize that in some cultures, parents may not name the infant in the early newborn period.)

Do the parents speak about the infant in terms of identification—whom the infant looks like; what appears special about their infant over other infants?

When parents are holding the infant, what kind of body contact is there—do parents feel at ease in changing the infant's position; are fingertips or whole hands used; are there parts of the body they avoid touching or parts of the body they investigate and scrutinize?

When the infant is awake, what kinds of stimulation do the parents provide—do they talk to the infant, to each other, or to no one; how do they look at the infant—direct visual contact, avoidance of eye contact, or looking at other people or objects?

How comfortable do the parents appear in terms of caring for the infant? Do they express any concern regarding their ability or disgust for certain activities, such as changing diapers?

What type of affection do they demonstrate to the newborn, such as smiling, stroking, kissing, or rocking?

If the infant is fussy, what kinds of comforting techniques do the parents use, such as rocking, swaddling, talking, or stroking?

mean that a delay will inhibit this process (humans are too resilient for that), but additional psychologic energy may be needed to achieve the same effect. To date, no scientific evidence has demonstrated that immediate contact after birth is essential for the human parent-child relationship. In fact, research evidence is conflicting.

In the 1980s Siegel (1982) documented the positive effect of early contact on early maternal affectional behavior. In the 1990s Mercer and Ferketich (1990) found that, for low risk, as well as high risk, mothers and fathers, early contact was not predictive of parent-infant attachment during the first postpartum day. More recently Prodromidis and colleagues (1995) studied early and extended contact for young, unmarried, predominantly African-American, low socioeconomic mothers. They found that mothers who had early and extended contact (rooming-in) with their infants during the first 18 hours after birth looked at, talked to, and touched their newborns more than did mothers who had minimal contact (infant feedings only).

Two studies by Troy (1993, 1995) produced conflicting results regarding time of first holding of the infant and the development of maternal attachment feelings. In one study, Troy (1993) demonstrated that feelings of attachment began when the infant was first held regardless of how long after birth the holding occurred. In the second study, Troy (1995) found that the earlier after birth that the mother holds her infant, the sooner she develops feelings of maternal attachment.

In a study of the timing of parents' first holding (also being skin-to-skin) of small preterm infants, Gloppestad (1996) found that fathers held their infants later than did the mothers even though fathers saw their infants before the mothers did. Both mothers and fathers rated their experience of love significantly higher when holding their preterm infants skin-to-skin than when holding them wrapped in blankets (Gloppestad, 1998).

Women who have had a long, difficult labor are often too exhausted to respond other than in a superficial way to the newborn. They may welcome the attention of others and be grateful that the infant is healthy, but their primary need centers on recovery from the physical and emotional aspects of pregnancy and childbirth. Infants born at risk as a result of either fetal or maternal disabilities are usually transferred to the intensive care nursery as quickly as possible. Concerns for their need for intensive medical and nursing interventions take priority over the need for close contact with the parents. Opportunities for parents to be with the infant in the intensive care nursery, to touch or hold the baby if at all possible, and to receive reports of the infant's progress must be part of the nursing plan of care.

Parents who desire but are unable to have early contact with their newborn can be reassured that such contact is not essential for optimal parent-infant interactions. Otherwise, adopted infants would not form the usual affectional ties with their parents. Nor does the mode of infant-mother contact after birth (skin-to-skin versus wrapped) appear to have any important effect. Nurses need to counsel parents to assure them that the emotional bond to the infant is not necessarily weaker because they missed early contact or the contact was not skin-to-skin. Nurses need to stress that the parent-infant relationship is a process that occurs over time.

Extended Contact

The provision of rooming-in facilities for the mother and her baby is a prevalent aspect of family-centered care. The infant is transferred to the area from the transitional nursery (if the facility uses one) after showing satisfactory extrauterine adjustment. The father is encouraged to participate in the care of the infant, and siblings and grandparents are also encouraged to visit and become acquainted with the infant. Many hospitals have established family birth units such as labor-delivery-recovery (LDR) rooms; labor-delivery-recovery-postpartum (LDRP) rooms; and single room maternity care (SRMC). The mother is accompanied by her partner during the birth of the infant, and all three may remain together until discharged around 48 hours after birth. Whether rooming-in or a family birth unit is the method of family-centered care, mothers and their partners are considered equal and integral parts of the developing family. Partners are encouraged to take as active a role as they wish. Some hospitals arrange for the discharge of the mother and infant any time from 2 to 24 hours after the birth if the condition of the mother and that of the child warrant it. Follow-up care with nursing personnel from a home health care agency is usually part of this plan.

Mother-baby care, also called couplet care, is another form of family-centered care. Care and teaching for the mother and baby are provided by a primary nurse, fostering family unity. Parents involved in this approach are likely to be more self-confident in care, and maternal attachment and role attainment are promoted.

Extended contact with the infant should be available for all parents but especially for those at risk for parenting inadequacies, such as adolescents and low-income women. Any activity that optimizes family-centered care is worthy of serious consideration by postpartum nurses.

COMMUNICATION BETWEEN PARENT AND INFANT

The parent-infant relationship is strengthened through the use of sensual responses and abilities by both partners in the interaction. The nurse should keep in mind that there may be cultural variations in these interactive behaviors used in communications between parent and infant that are described below.

Touch

Touch, or the tactile sense, is used extensively by parents and other caregivers as a means of becoming acquainted with the newborn. Many mothers reach out for their infants as soon as they are born and the cord is cut. They lift them to their breasts, enfold them in their arms, and cradle them. Once the infant is close to them, they begin the exploration process with their fingertips, one of the most touch-sensitive areas of the body. For some mothers and other caregivers (fathers, nursing and medical students) studies have depicted a predictable pattern of touch behavior (Klaus & Kennell, 1982; Rubin, 1963; Tulman, 1985). The caregiver begins with a fingertip exploration of the infant's head and extremities. Within a short time the caregiver uses the palm to caress the baby's trunk and eventually enfolds the infant. Gentle stroking motions are used to soothe and quiet the infant; patting or gently rubbing the infant's back is a comfort after feedings. Infants also pat the mother's breast as they nurse. Both seem to enjoy sharing each other's body warmth. There is a desire in parents to touch, pick up, and hold the infant (Fig. 25-5). They comment on the softness of the baby's skin and are aware of milia and rashes. As parents become increasingly sensitive to the infant's like or dislike of different types of touch, they draw closer to their baby.

Variations in touching behaviors have been noted in mothers from different cultural groups (Galanti, 1991;

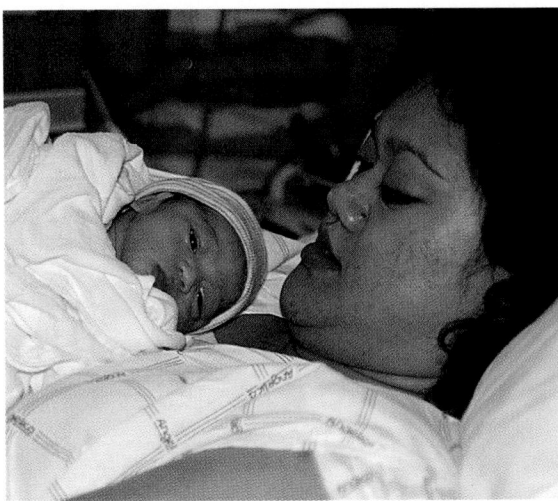

Fig. 25-5 Mother interacts with newborn. *(Courtesy Judy Bamber, San Jose, CA.)*

Inman, 1996; Jambunathan & Stewart, 1995; Jiménez, 1995). For example, minimal touching and cuddling is a traditional Southeast Asian practice thought to protect the infant from evil spirits. Because of tradition and spiritual beliefs, women in India and Bali have practiced infant massage since ancient times.

Eye-to-Eye Contact

Interest in having eye contact with the baby has been demonstrated repeatedly by parents. Some mothers remark that once their babies have looked at them, they feel much closer to them. Parents spend much time getting their babies to open their eyes and look at them. In American culture, eye contact appears to have a cementing effect on the development of a trusting relationship and is an important factor in human relationships at all ages. In other cultures, eye-to-eye contact may be perceived differently. For example, in Mexican culture, sustained direct eye contact is considered to be rude, immodest, and dangerous for some. This danger may arise from the *mal ojo* (evil eye), resulting from excessive admiration. Women and children are thought to be more susceptible to the *mal ojo* (Geissler, 1994).

As newborns become functionally able to sustain eye contact with their parents, time is spent in mutual gazing, often in the *en face* position (Fig. 25-6). **En face,** "face-to-face," is a position in which the parent's face and the infant's face are approximately 8 inches apart and on the same plane. Nursing and medical practices need to be implemented that encourage this interaction. Immediately after birth, for example, the infant can be positioned on the mother's abdomen or breasts with the mother's and the infant's faces on the same plane so that they can easily make eye contact. This would not be accomplished well with the infant lying in the mother's arms at her side. Lights can be dimmed so that the infant's eyes will open. Instillation of

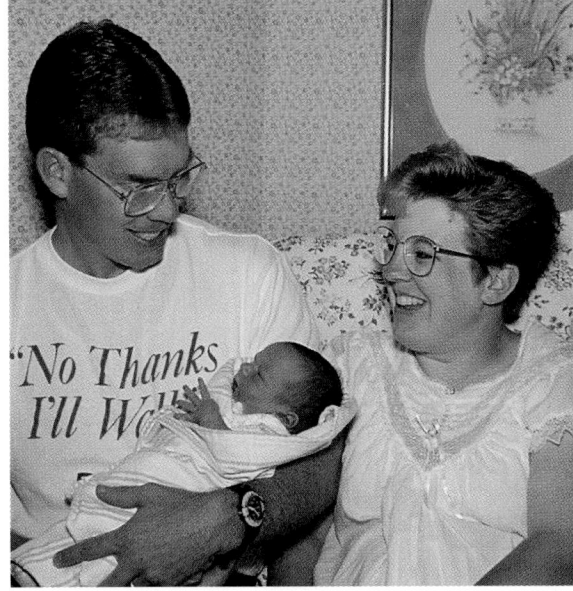

Fig. 25-6 Father, mother, and newborn getting to know each other. *(Courtesy Michael S. Clement, MD, Mesa, AZ.)*

prophylactic antibiotic ointment in the infant's eyes can be delayed until the infant and parents have had some time together in the first hour after birth.

Voice

The shared response of parents and infants to each other's voices is also remarkable. Parents wait tensely for the first cry. Once that cry has reassured them of the baby's health, they begin comforting behaviors. As the parents talk in high-pitched voices, the infant is alerted and turns toward them.

Infants respond to higher-pitched voices and can distinguish their mother's voice from others soon after birth. Infants use their cries to signal hunger, pain, boredom, and tiredness. With experience, parents learn to distinguish such cries.

Odor

Another behavior shared by parents and infants is a response to each other's odor. Mothers comment on the smell of their babies when first born and have noted that each infant has a unique odor. Infants learn rapidly to distinguish the odor of their mother's breast milk.

Entrainment

Newborns move in time with the structure of adult speech. They wave their arms, lift their heads, and kick their legs, seemingly "dancing in tune" to a parent's voice. This means that culturally determined rhythms of speech have been ingrained in the infant long before spoken language is used to communicate. Carryover, or **entrainment,** occurs once the child begins to talk. This shared rhythm also gives the parent positive feedback and establishes a positive setting for effective communication.

Biorhythmicity

The fetus is in tune with the mother's natural rhythms, such as heartbeats. After birth a crying infant may be soothed by being held in a position where the mother's heartbeat can be heard or by hearing a recording of a heartbeat. One of the newborn's tasks is to establish a personal rhythm, or **biorhythmicity.** Parents can help in this process by giving consistent loving care and using their infant's alert state to develop responsive behavior and thereby increase social interactions and opportunities for learning. The more quickly parents become competent in child care activities, the more quickly their psychologic energy can be directed toward observing the communication cues the infant gives them.

Reciprocity and Synchrony

Reciprocity is a type of body movement or behavior that provides the observer with cues. The observer or receiver interprets those cues and responds to them. Reciprocity often takes several weeks to develop with a new baby. For example, when the newborn fusses and cries, the mother responds by picking up and cradling the infant; the baby becomes quiet and alert and establishes eye contact; the mother verbalizes, sings, and coos while the baby maintains eye contact. The baby then averts the eyes and yawns; the mother decreases her active response. If the parent continues to stimulate the infant, the baby may become fussy.

Synchrony refers to the "fit" between the infant's cues and the parent's response. When parent and infant experience a synchronous interaction, it is mutually rewarding (Fig. 25-7). Parents need time to interpret the infant's cues correctly. For example, after a certain time the infant develops a specific cry in response to different situations such as boredom, loneliness, hunger, and discomfort. The

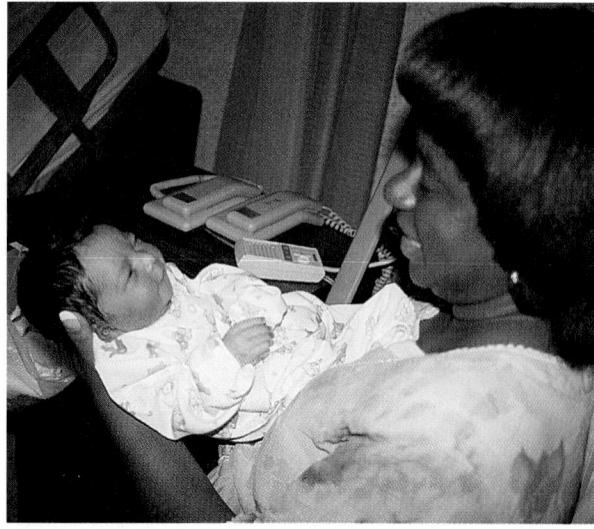

Fig. 25-7 Sharing a smile: example of synchrony. *(Courtesy Marjorie Pyle, RNC, Lifecircle, Costa Mesa, CA.)*

parent may need assistance in deciphering these cries, along with trial and error interventions, before synchrony develops.

PARENTAL ROLE AFTER CHILDBIRTH

For the biologic parent the parental role is enlarged and intensified at birth. The care and nurturing of the child were initiated well before birth. The mother who carried out the dictates of health (e.g., diet, rest, and exercise) for the "good of her baby," the partner who supported and sheltered her, and the parents who became aware of and attached to their unborn child were already functioning in the parental role before the birth. Even preconception decisions about whether and when to have a child influence mothers' and fathers' adjustment to the parental role.

The 6 weeks after birth form what is called the **fourth trimester.** During the postpartum period, new tasks and responsibilities arise and old behaviors need to be modified or new ones added. The responses of mothers and their partners to the parental role change over time and tend to follow a predictable course. During the first 3 to 4 weeks of the fourth trimester, parents have to reorganize their relationship with the newborn. What was accomplished through the biologic process of pregnancy now requires an array of caregiving activities. The infant's needs for shelter, nourishment, protection, and socializing must be met. These early weeks are characterized by intense learning and need for nurturing.

The next few weeks represent a time of drawing together and uniting the family unit. This period of consolidation involves negotiations as to roles (wife-husband, mother-father, mother-partner, parent-child, sibling-sibling). Family integrity and adaptation occur when transactions between spouses regarding roles and role relationships are successful (Tomlinson & Irwin, 1993).

Adaptation involves a stabilizing of tasks, a coming to terms with commitments. Parents demonstrate growing competence in child care activities and are more attuned to their infant's behavior. Typically, the period from the decision to conceive through the first months of having a child is termed the transition to parenthood.

Transition to Parenthood

The transition to parenthood is frequently described as a time of disorder and disequilibrium, as well as satisfaction, for mothers and their partners (Rogan et al., 1997; Sethi, 1995; Tomlinson, 1996). Usual methods of coping often seem ineffective. For example, some parents can be so distressed that they are unable to be supportive of each other. Men typically identify their spouses as their primary or only source of support. The transition can be harder for the fathers, who feel deprived because the mothers, who are also experiencing stress, cannot provide the usual level of support. Strong emotions such as helplessness, inadequacy, and anger that arise when dealing with a crying infant catch many parents unprepared. On the other hand, parenthood allows adults to develop and display a selfless, warm, and caring side of themselves, which may not be expressed in other adult roles. To view the world through the eyes of a child and to be childlike (not childish) are two rich rewards of parenthood.

Historically, the transition to parenthood was viewed as a crisis. The current perspective is that parenthood is a developmental transition (Tomlinson, 1996) rather than a major life crisis for the majority of families. A concept that is derived from the developmental crisis perspective but that has relevance for the developmental transition theory is that at the point of crisis a moment occurs when a person is mentally and physically prepared for, the culture is pushing for, and the person is reaching out to achieve some developmental change. Because of this, the person is motivated for change. For the majority of mothers and their partners, the transition to parenthood represents such a period and is viewed as an opportunity rather than a time of danger. Parents are stimulated to try new coping strategies as they work to master their new roles and reach new developmental levels. As they work through the transition, personal strength and resourcefulness are revealed (Rogan et al., 1997).

Parental Tasks and Responsibilities

Parents need to reconcile the actual child with the fantasy and dream child. This means coming to terms with the infant's physical appearance, sex, innate temperament, and physical status. If the real child differs greatly from the fantasy child, parents may delay acceptance of the child. In some instances, they may never accept the child.

Some parents are startled by the normal appearance of the neonate—size, color, molding of the head, or bowed appearance of the legs. Many fathers have commented that they thought the odd shape of the infant's head (molding) meant the infant would be mentally retarded.

Although many parents know the sex of the infant before birth because of the use of ultrasound assessments, for those who do not have this information, disappointment over the sex of the infant can take time to resolve. The parents may provide adequate physical care but find it difficult to be sincerely involved with the infant until this internal conflict has been resolved. As one mother remarked, "I really wanted a boy. I know it is silly and irrational, but when they said, 'She's a lovely little girl,' I was so disappointed and angry—yes, angry—I could hardly look at her. Oh, I looked after her okay, her feedings and baths and things, but I couldn't feel excited. To tell the truth, I felt like a monster not liking my child. Then one day she was lying there and she turned her head and looked right at me. I felt a flooding of love for her come over me, and we looked at each other a long time. It's okay now. I wouldn't change her for all the boys in the world."

Nursing care plans need to include discussion about reconciliation of the real versus the fantasy child. Nurses need to provide opportunities for parents to discuss their lack of parental feelings without fear of censure or ridicule. Often the expression of doubts and concerns provides relief and makes it easier for parents to deal with and resolve such feelings.

Parents need to establish the newborn as a person separate from themselves, that is, as someone having many dependency needs and requiring much nurturing. Nurses can discuss with parents that this acceptance of the infant as a separate being with many needs evolves over time. Parents who see the baby by ultrasound assessments during pregnancy may begin to appreciate earlier that the baby is a real—and separate—human being.

Parents need to become adept in the care of the infant, including caregiving activities, noting the communication cues given by the infant to indicate needs, and responding appropriately to the infant's needs.

Parents need to establish reasonable evaluative criteria for assessing the success or failure of the care given the infant. Parents are surprisingly sensitive to infant responses. One father spoke about his first attempt to give his infant a kiss. At that moment the infant turned her head. The father felt hurt, although he understood that the baby was totally unaware of her own movements. The infant's response to the parental care and attention may be interpreted by the parent as a comment on the quality of that care. Examples of infant behaviors that are interpreted by parents as positive responses to their care include being consoled easily, enjoying being cuddled, and making eye contact. Spitting frequently after feedings, crying, and being unpredictable may be perceived as negative responses to parental care. Continuation of these infant responses that are viewed as negative by the parent can result in alienation of parent and infant to the detriment of the infant.

Self-esteem grows with competence. Mothers of preterm infants have noted that their own efforts appear inadequate after the skillful handling of their infants by nurses. Breastfeeding makes mothers feel they are contributing in a unique way to the welfare of the infant.

Assistance, including advice by husbands, partners, wives, mothers, mothers-in-law, and professional workers, can either be seen as supportive or an indication of how inept these people have judged the new parents to be. Criticism, real or imagined, of the new parents' ability to provide adequate physical care, nutrition, or social stimulation for the infant can prove devastating. By providing encouragement and praise for parenting efforts, nurses can bolster the new parents' confidence. Parents should feel safe discussing concerns about other peoples' criticisms with the nurses who can help them practice assertiveness techniques to use with unwanted "critics." The nurses, as client advocates, can also use positive, nonjudgmental approaches to help critics direct their advice constructively.

Parents must establish a place for the newborn within the family group. Whether the infant is the firstborn or the last born, all family members must adjust their roles to accommodate the newcomer. The firstborn child needs support to accept a rival for parental affections. An older child needs help dealing with losing a favored position in the family hierarchy. The parents are expected to negotiate these changes.

Parents need to establish the primacy of their adult relationships to maintain the family as a group. Because this includes reorganizing many roles—for example, sexual, child care, career, and community roles—time and energy must be provided for this vital task.

Maternal Adjustment

Three phases are evident as the mother adjusts to her parental role. These phases of **maternal adjustment** are characterized by dependent behavior, dependent-independent behavior, and interdependent behavior (Table 25-4).

TABLE 25-4 Phases of Maternal Postpartum Adjustment

PHASE	CHARACTERISTICS
Dependent: taking-in*	• First 24 hours (range of 1 to 2 days) • Focus: self and meeting of basic needs • Reliance on others to meet needs for comfort, rest, closeness, and nourishment • Excited and talkative • Desire to review birth experience
Dependent-independent: taking-hold*	• Starts second or third day; lasts 10 days to several weeks • Focus: care of baby and competent mothering • Desire to take charge • Still need for nurturing and acceptance by others • Eagerness to learn and practice—optimal period for teaching by nurses • Handling of physical discomforts and emotional changes • Possible experience with "blues"
Interdependent: letting go*	• Focus: forward movement of family as unit with interacting members • Reassertion of relationship with partner • Resumption of sexual intimacy • Resolution of individual roles

*From Rubin, R. (1961). Basic maternal behavior. *Nurs Outlook 9*, 683-686.

Dependent Phase

During the first 24 to 48 hours after childbirth the mother's dependency needs predominate. To the extent that these needs are met by others, the mother is able to divert her psychologic energy to her infant rather than to focus them on herself. She needs "mothering" herself to "mother." Rubin (1961) aptly described these few days as the **taking-in phase:** a time when nurturing and protective care are required by the new mother. In Rubin's classic description the taking-in phase lasted 2 to 3 days. Later studies by Ament (1990) and Wrasper (1996) supported Rubin's work, except that women were now found to move more rapidly through the taking-in phase. A strong taking-in phase was noted only in the first 24 hours after birth. Evans and colleagues (1998), in a study of women giving birth vaginally, found that both taking-in and taking-hold were present on the evening of birth. There were small decreases in taking-in and small increases in taking-hold between the evening of birth and the first morning.

For 24 hours after the birth, mature and apparently healthy women appear to suspend their involvement in everyday responsibilities. They rely on others to satisfy their needs for comfort, rest, nourishment, and closeness to their families and newborn.

This dependent phase is a time of great excitement during which parents need to verbalize their experience of pregnancy and birth. Focusing on, analyzing, and accepting these experiences help the parents move on to the next phase. Some parents use staff members or other mothers as an "audience," whereas others are more comfortable talking with family and friends about the pregnancy and birth experience.

Because anxiety and preoccupation with her new role often narrow a mother's perceptions, information may have to be repeated. The new mother may require reminders to rest or, conversely, to ambulate enough to promote recovery. Hospital or birth center routines may not necessarily be an important priority to the new mother; she may take showers when examinations are scheduled and be involved in a telephone conversation rather than "being ready" for the baby. Regulations seem cumbersome, and sometimes mothers and their families have difficulty accepting rules that interfere with their need to share reactions about their infant.

Physical discomfort from an episiotomy, sore nipples, hemorrhoids, afterpains, and occasionally a sprained coccygeal joint can interfere with the mother's need for rest and relaxation. The selective use of comfort measures and medication depends on the nurse. Many women hesitate to ask for medication, believing that any pain they experience is normal and to be expected; breastfeeding mothers may fear the effects of medication on the infant. Few have a knowledge of the use of heat or cold to relieve local pain.

Dependent-Independent Phase

If the mother has received adequate nurturing in the first few hours or days, by the second or third day, her desire for independent action reasserts itself. In the dependent-independent phase, the mother alternates between a need for extensive nurturing and acceptance by others and the desire to "take charge" once again. She responds enthusiastically to opportunities to learn and practice baby care or, if she is an accomplished mother, to carry out or direct this care (Mercer & Ferketich, 1995). Rubin (1961) described this phase as the **taking-hold phase,** noting that it lasts approximately 10 days. Several studies (Evans et al., 1998; Martell, 1996; Wrasper, 1996) have found that contemporary women exhibit taking-hold behaviors sooner than did the women in Rubin's study; however, the peak and duration of the taking-hold phase were not determined. In a study by Martell (1996) women exhibited some taking-in and taking-hold behaviors but not in the sequence of postpartum phases described originally by Rubin. Evans and associates (1998) found that taking-hold behaviors began increasing between the evening of birth and the first morning despite high levels of sleep disturbance.

Childbirth preparation classes, early contact with the newborn, rooming-in, and early discharge are some of the current obstetric practices that seem to enhance taking-hold behaviors (Martell, 1996; Wrasper, 1996). Given these changes in health care and in women's lives, more research is needed to evaluate the effect of such changes on patterns of women's behaviors during the postpartum period.

Most mothers are discharged home during this dependent-independent phase. Contemporary mothers have short hospital stays, ranging from 6 to 48 hours for low risk, uncomplicated births and from 48 to 96 hours for a cesarean birth. Once home, mothers must continue to cope with physical adaptations and psychologic adjustments.

In a study of the experience of low risk mothers (25 multiparas and 25 primiparas) during the first 2 weeks postpartum, the majority of mothers identified fatigue as their major physical concern (Ruchala & Halstead, 1994; Smith-Hanrahan & Deblois, 1995). This fatigue affected various aspects of their lives, such as their relationships with their husbands and other family members and household responsibilities.

Some studies indicate that primiparas experience more sleep disturbance and fatigue than do multiparas (Waters & Lee, 1996) and that this higher level of fatigue, especially in the morning, continues for several weeks (Troy & Dalgas-Pelish, 1997).

Because fatigue continues to be a major concern of women during the early weeks of parenthood, nurses need to provide anticipatory guidance regarding sleep disturbance and fatigue, as well as suggestions for dealing with the fatigue. Another strategy for helping new mothers cope with fatigue is a self-care guide for postpartum fatigue such as the "Tiredness Management Guide" developed by Troy and Dalgas-Pelish (1995). This guide provides a list of eight sources of postpartum fatigue: infection; no chance to rest; inability to get everything done; interrupted sleep; feeling stressed, anxious, or other psychological changes from demands placed on the mother; low hemoglobin; and social activities. For each source of fatigue, there is a list of techniques for the mother to use. Two of the techniques, suggested for no chance to rest are (1) sit or lie in a comfortable position when you feed your baby and (2) organize your day for rest between tiring activities. The self-care guide is grounded on the principle that adult learners are self-directed, oriented to tasks specific to their social roles, and motivated to learn when immediate application is needed, all of which fits the postpartum woman.

Other physical concerns were loss of weight or figure, pain from the episiotomy or cesarean incision, sexual relations, and hemorrhoids. Most women described the early postpartum period as hectic and a time of adjustment. Several also said it was an enjoyable time. Primiparas reported feeling uncertain, trapped, and overwhelmed by fatigue and lack of experience in infant care. Many of the multiparas described their experience as being better than with previous births, primarily because of their comfort with caring for an infant.

Emotional concerns were a recurring theme, with mothers reporting feeling "down," being tense and irritable, and being depressed. All who reported feeling depressed said that it was transient, lasting less than a week. Crying was the most frequently reported emotional symptom. A primipara said, "It bothers me being so easily depressed . . . when I cry so easily. . . . It goes with the territory, though, I guess. It won't last forever" (Ruchala & Halstead, 1994). All mothers said that they realized the emotional changes were normal and ascribed them to fatigue, physical discomfort, the condition of their bodies, the infants' temperaments, and the impact of the infant on their freedom. Those mothers who reported feeling confident in caring for their infants identified someone, usually their own mothers, who had influenced them or been a role model for infant care.

These findings have implications for nursing care. Prenatally and postnatally, nurses can discuss the usual postpartal concerns that mothers experience and provide anticipatory guidance on coping strategies, such as resting when the infant sleeps and planning with an extended family member or friend to do the housework for the first week or two after the baby is born. Once a mother is home, periodic phone calls from a nurse who cared for her in the birth setting can provide the mother with an opportunity to vent her concerns and get support and advice from "her nurse." Nurses should plan additional supportive counseling for first-time mothers inexperienced in child care, women whose careers had provided outside stimulation, women who lack friends or family members with whom to share delights and concerns, and adoles-

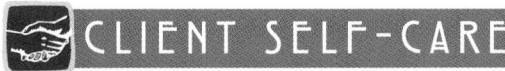

CLIENT SELF-CARE

Coping with Postpartum Blues

- Remember that the "blues" are normal.
- Get plenty of rest; nap when the baby does if possible. Go to bed early, and let friends know when to visit.
- Use relaxation techniques learned in childbirth classes (or ask the nurse to teach you and your partner some techniques).
- Do something for yourself. Take advantage of the time your partner or family members care for the baby—soak in the tub or go for a walk.
- Plan a day out of the house—go to the mall with the baby, being sure to take a stroller or carriage, or go out to eat with friends without the baby. Many communities have churches or other agencies that provide child care programs such as Mothers' Morning Out.
- Talk to your partner about the way you feel—for example, about feeling tied down, how the birth met your expectations, and things that will help you.
- If you are breastfeeding, give yourself and your baby time to learn.
- Seek out and use community resources such as La Leche League or community mental health centers. Some nationally recognized resources are as follows:
  Postpartum Support International
  927 North Kellogg Avenue
  Santa Barbara, CA 93111
  (805) 967-7636

cent mothers. When possible, postpartum home visits are included in the plan of care.

Postpartum "Blues"

The "pink" period surrounding the first day or two after birth, characterized by heightened joy and feelings of well-being, is often followed by a "blue" period. Approximately 75% to 80% of women experience the **postpartum blues** or "baby blues" (Albright, 1993; Wood et al., 1997) that occur in women of all ethnic and racial groups (Campbell, 1992). During the blues, women are emotionally labile, often crying easily and for no apparent reason. This lability seems to peak around the fifth day, subsiding by the tenth day. Other symptoms of postpartum blues include depression, a let-down feeling, restlessness, fatigue, insomnia, headache, anxiety, sadness, and anger. Biochemical, psychologic, social, and cultural factors have been explored as possible causes of the postpartum depressive state; however, the etiology remains unknown. Whatever the cause, the early postpartum period appears to be one

of emotional and physical vulnerability for new mothers, who may be psychologically overwhelmed by the reality of parental responsibilities. The mother may feel deprived of the supportive care she received from family members and friends during pregnancy. Some mothers regret the loss of the mother-unborn child relationship and mourn its passing. Still others experience a let-down feeling when labor and birth are complete. Fatigue after childbirth is compounded by the around-the-clock demands of the new baby and can accentuate the feelings of depression. A lowered level of circulating glucocorticoids or a subclinical hypothyroidism may exist during the puerperium. Postpartum depressive symptoms can have a negative effect on maternal role attainment (Fowles, 1998). To help mothers cope with postpartum blues, nurses can suggest various strategies (see Client Self-Care box).

"Am I Blue?" (Johnson & Johnson, 1996), a self-administered questionnaire, can help mothers to assess their level of "blues" and to decide when to seek advice from their nurse, nurse-midwife, or physician (Fig. 25-8). Nurse home visits and telephone follow-up calls to assess the mother's pattern of "blue" feelings and behavior over time are important.

Although the postpartum blues are usually mild and short lived, approximately 10% to 15% of women experience a more severe syndrome called postpartum depression (PPD) (Wood et al., 1997) (see Chapter 35). The symptoms can range from mild to severe, with women having "good days" and "bad days." All symptoms can be equally distressing and make the woman feel as if she is "going mad." PPD leaves the woman with feelings of failure, overwhelming guilt, loneliness, and low self-esteem.

Nurses need to teach women how to differentiate symptoms of the "blues" and PPD and to urge women to report depressive symptoms promptly if they occur. Indicators that distinguish PPD from postpartum blues include the following (Herz, 1992; Wood et al., 1997):

- Worsening of sleep disturbances and an inability to go back to sleep after infant feedings, despite extreme fatigue
- Appetite change; eating problems
- Increased intensity and duration of depressed feelings, irritability, especially if unrelated to events; preoccupation with self-deprecatory thoughts (e.g., about her conduct during childbirth and competence as a mother), increasing discomfort with the maternal role, fears for the child, and even suicidal thoughts
- Lack of compensatory measures to deal with fatigue and exhaustion to the point that energy loss interferes with functioning
- Withdrawal and social isolation while complaining about lack of emotional support, especially from her partner
- Faulty interaction with the baby, including perception of the infant as demanding and burdensome

Am I Blue?

Many new mothers feel anxious, sad, or angry about the changes in their lives after the birth of their new baby. It is perfectly normal to feel this way, but sometimes the feelings grow so strong that they make life difficult. This quiz lists many feelings and experiences of "blue" or depressed mothers. Mark how strong each of these feelings or experiences is for you, compared with what is normal for you. For example: Do you feel no anger [0]; mild (very little) anger [1]; moderate (some) anger [2]; or severe (very strong) anger [3] compared with the way you usually feel? Add up your total score when you are finished, and discuss the results with your health care provider.

0 = Not there at all 1 = Mild 2 = Moderate 3 = Severe	0	1	2	3
Anger				
Anxiety attacks: periods of very strong fear, shortness of breath, rapid heartbeat				
Increased or decreased appetite and/or weight gain or loss that doesn't seem normal				
Strong feeling that you need to get away, need more time for your own interests				
Problems in a relationship with a family member, lover, close friend, etc.				
Crying spells				
Less interest in your personal appearance				
Less motivation—less energy or interest in accomplishing goals				
Depression				
Fatigue—feeling tired or exhausted				
Fear of harming yourself or your baby				
Loss of your sense of humor				
Nervousness, feeling tense or edgy				
Feelings of guilt				
Feelings of panic				
Feeling alone or lonely; without the support of others				
Feeling no love, or not enough love, for your baby				
Feeling forgetful, distracted, absent-minded—having trouble concentrating				
Frustration				
Hopelessness				
Insomnia				
Feeling irritable, bad-tempered				
Loss of sexual desire and/or pleasure in sex				
Loss of self-respect or confidence—feeling like you don't count or can't do anything right				
Feeling confused, uncertain				
Mood swings—your moods and emotions change all the time				
Obsessive thoughts—ideas or feelings you can't stop from repeating in your mind				
Odd or frightening thoughts—thoughts or images that scare you or that you can't control				
Thoughts of suicide, feeling like you want to die				
Feeling sad, unhappy				
	TOTAL			

SCORE:

0 – 31 = MILD BLUES

This will probably pass, but pay attention to your feelings and needs.

32 – 64 = MODERATE BLUES

You may want to ask for help from a close friend or family member, or ask the advice of your health care provider.

65 – 98 = SEVERE BLUES

You could be depressed; see your health care provider for a check-up and advice as soon as possible.

If you are afraid you might harm yourself or your baby—ask a health care provider you trust for help— you don't have to be alone!

Fig. 25-8 Am I Blue? *(Courtesy Johnson & Johnson Consumer Products, Skillman, NJ.)*

BOX 25-1 Risk Factors for Postpartum Depression (PPD)

- High anxiety throughout pregnancy
- Ambivalence about maintaining the pregnancy
- Presence of marital discord
- Absence of confidant or extended family members
- Previously diagnosed PPD after 8 weeks postpartum
- History of severe premenstrual syndrome
- History of thyroid problems
- Family history of physical or sexual abuse, alcoholism, and/or neglect
- Recent stressful life events, especially death of her mother
- Mismatch between mother's and infant's temperaments
- Low income level
- Frequent use of avoidance coping.
- Combination of maternal concerns with short maternity leave.

From Hamilton, J., & Harberger, P. (1992). *Postpartum psychiatric illness: A picture puzzle*. Philadelphia: University of Pennsylvania Press; Herz, E. (1992). Prediction, recognition, and prevention. In J. Hamilton, & P. Harberger (Eds.). *Postpartum psychiatric illness: A picture puzzle*. Philadelphia: University of Pennsylvania Press; Hunt, D. (1995). A beautiful baby: Why am I so sad? Paper presented at the 25th Annual Conference of North Carolina AWHONN. April 1, 1995. Winston-Salem, NC; Wood, A. et al. (1997). The downward spiral of postpartum depression. *MCN Am J Matern Child Nurs 22*, 308-316.

PPD can go undetected because new mothers generally do not voluntarily admit to this kind of emotional distress out of embarrassment, guilt, or fear. The focus of the postpartum check-up is usually on the woman's reproductive system, with little or no time spent assessing her psychologic state and needs. A woman voicing concern for such symptoms often has them brushed aside as normal and temporary. No further assessment is done because many of the symptoms, such as mood fluctuations and sleep disturbances, are common during the postpartum period. Such false reassurance from health care professionals not only belittles a woman's concerns, increases her self-doubt, and deprives her of a safe opportunity to discuss her feelings but also reinforces the woman's silence, perpetuates her isolation, and stimulates deterioration of her condition. Nurses need to be active listeners and compassionate intermediaries in interactions with new mothers so that symptoms of PPD can be recognized early, assessed, and treated. Through careful attention to holistic health histories, nurses can identify women who are at high risk for PPD (Box 25-1). Nurses can use screening tools in assessing whether the depressive symptoms have progressed from postpartum blues to PPD (see Chapter 35). Examples are the Postpartum Depression Checklist developed by Beck (1995) and the Edinburgh Postnatal Depression Scale

developed by Cox, Holden, and Sagovshy (1989). Nurses can also educate women about normal newborn/infant growth and development and help the women develop realistic expectations about infant behavioral cues (Wood et al., 1997).

Interdependent Phase

In this phase, interdependent behavior reasserts itself, and the mother and her family move forward as a unit with interacting members. The relationship of the partners, although altered by the introduction of a baby, resumes many of its former characteristics. A primary need is to establish a lifestyle that includes but in some respects also excludes the baby. The couple must share interests and activities that are adult in scope.

The couple may begin to engage in sexual intercourse by the third or fourth week after the baby is born. Some couples begin earlier, as soon as it can be accomplished without discomfort, depending on factors such as timing, amount of vaginal dryness, and breastfeeding status. Sexual intimacy enhances the adult aspect of the family, and the adult pair shares a closeness denied to other family members. Many new fathers speak of the alienation experienced when they observe the intimate mother-infant relationship, and some are frank in expressing feelings of jealousy toward the infant. The resumption of sexual intimacy seems to bring the parents' relationship back into focus.

The interdependent phase, termed the **letting-go phase,** is often stressful for the parental pair. Interests and needs often diverge during this time. Women and their partners must resolve the effects on their relationship of their individual roles related to child rearing, homemaking, and careers. Mothers (and partners) may take a more traditional role in an effort to adapt to parenthood; however, traditional women have reported more family disorganization months into parenthood (Tomlinson & Irwin, 1993). A special continuing effort has to be undertaken to strengthen the adult-adult relationship as a basis for the family unit.

Little is known about postpartum maternal adjustment in the lesbian couple. Relationship satisfaction in first-time lesbian parent couples appears related to egalitarianism, commitment, sexual compatibility, and communication skills, as well as the birth mother's decision for insemination by an anonymous sperm donor (Osterwell, 1991). Similar to heterosexual parent couples, most lesbian parent couples voice concern about less time and energy for their relationship after the arrival of the baby (Gartrell et al., 1996). Both partners consider themselves to be equal parents of the baby who share actively in child rearing (Brewaeys et al., 1995).

Lesbian couples face strong social sanctions regarding pregnancy and parenting. Their families may not have resolved the initial dismay and guilt over learning of their daughters' homosexuality or they may disagree with the lesbian couple's decision to parent. In situations where family

TABLE 25-5	Transition to Fatherhood: A Three-Stage Process
STAGES	**CHARACTERISTICS**
Stage 1: expectations	Father has preconceptions about what life will be like after baby comes home
Stage 2: reality	Father realizes that expectations are not always based on fact
	Common feelings experienced are as follows:
	Sadness
	Ambivalence
	Jealousy
	Frustration
	Overwhelming desire to be more involved
	Some fathers are pleasantly surprised at ease and fun of parenting
Stage 3: transition to mastery	Father makes conscious decision to take control and become more actively involved with infant

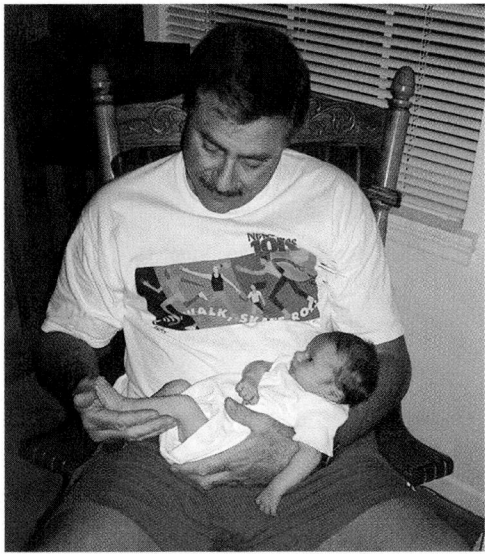

Fig. 25-9 Engrossment. Father absorbed in looking at his newborn. *(Courtesy Leslie Canerday, Phoenix, AZ.)*

support is limited or absent, the nurse can help the couple locate more supportive social groups, lesbian or heterosexual.

Paternal Adjustment

Research on **paternal adjustment** to parenthood indicates that fathers go through a predictable three-stage process during the first 3 weeks of their transition to parenthood (Henderson & Brouse, 1991) (Table 25-5). During this period, fathers experience intense emotions. Stage 1 (expectations) involves approaching the experience with preconceptions about what it will be like when the baby is home. In stage 2 (reality) some fathers realize that their expectations are not based on fact. Many fathers acknowledge that their expectations were of limited value once they were immersed in the reality of parenthood. Feelings that often accompany this reality are sadness, ambivalence, jealousy, frustration at not being able to participate in breastfeeding, and an overwhelming desire to be more involved, most of which are different from the feelings mothers report. On the other hand, some fathers are pleasantly surprised at the ease and fun of parenting. Stage 3 (transition to mastery) involves a conscious decision to take control and become more actively involved in the infant's life.

First-time fathers perceive the first 4 to 10 weeks of parenthood in much the same way that mothers do, that is, as a period characterized by uncertainty, increased responsibility, disruption of sleep, and inability to control time needed to care for the infant and reestablish the marital dyad. Fathers express concern about (1) decreased attention from their partners relative to their personal relationship, (2) the mother's lack of recognition of the father's desire to participate in decision making for the infant, and (3) limited time available to establish a relationship with their infants. These concerns can precipitate feelings of jealousy of the infant. Discussing their needs with the partner and becoming more involved with their infants and partner can help alleviate such feelings of jealousy. A consistent finding in the literature is that fathers who feel affection and support in the relationships with their partners or mates are more involved with infant care and their involvement is more responsive, affectionate, and developmentally stimulating (Anderson, 1996a, 1996b; Broom, 1994; Ferketich & Mercer, 1995).

Father-Infant Relationship

In American culture, neonates have a powerful impact on their fathers, who become intensely involved with their babies (Fig. 25-9). The term used for the father's absorption, preoccupation, and interest in the infant is **engrossment.** Characteristics of engrossment include some of the sensual responses relating to touch and eye-to-eye contact that have been discussed earlier and also the father's keen awareness of features both unique and similar to himself that validate his claim to the infant. An outstanding response is one of strong attraction to the newborn. Fathers spend considerable time "communicating" with the infant and taking delight in the infant's response to them. A sense of increased self-esteem and a sense of being proud, bigger, more mature, and older are all experienced by fathers after seeing their baby for the first time.

Anderson (1996a, 1996b) analyzed first-time Caucasian fathers' experiences in developing a relationship with their infants. Three major categories were identified as operative in the development process: making a commitment, becoming connected, and making room for baby. "Commitment" is the father's willingness to invest in and take responsibility for nurturing the relationship with his infant despite difficulties in parenting and other life demands. Fathers felt the reality of commitment when the pregnancy was confirmed, during the pregnancy or birth, when they assumed responsibility for infant care, and when the infant responded to them. Because of the helpless nature of the infant, fathers felt a duty to nurture and protect their infants. Fathers also wanted to get to know and be psychologically involved with their infants. Rewards of the father-infant relationship identified by the fathers included the infant's smile, increased self-esteem, gaining a new dimension in life, and finding the child within themselves.

"Becoming connected" appears to be the basic psychological process in the development of the father-infant relationship (Anderson, 1996a). When meeting their infant for the first time, fathers experienced feelings of joy, elation, awe, and wonderment. Some fathers felt an immediate bond, while others felt it once they touched and held their infants. For others, the feelings of love and engrossment did not occur quickly, but gradually increased during the first 2 months of the infant's life. A turning point in the relationship development was when fathers perceived their infants as more responsive, predictable, and familiar.

In "making room for baby," fathers made changes in their work and social/personal time, in relationships with their wives, and within themselves so that they might be physically and emotionally available to their infants (Anderson, 1996a). In describing the qualities that fathers should have, fathers identified the following: to love, protect, and be emotionally present for the infant; to be supportive of their partners in the mothering role; and to use good communication skills. These fathers did not focus on the more traditional roles of provider and disciplinarian.

Many studies on fathers of infants have focused on the amount of time fathers spend with their infants and what they do when they are with their infants. Two consistent findings are that (1) fathers spend less time than mothers with infants and (2) fathers' interactions with infants tend to be characterized by stimulating social play rather than caretaking. In the United States, fathers tend to take the lead in initiating play and to play in a rougher manner, whereas mothers tend to take the lead in caregiving activities. In India, fathers are not characterized as vigorous, playful partners. They appear to use more affectional display than very rough play with infants. The subtle and more open differences in stimulation from two sources,

mother and father, provide a wider social experience for the infant.

Research has demonstrated that fathers can be sensitive and competent in caring for infants (Anderson, 1996a; Broom 1994), yet few studies have tried to identify factors that influence fathers' parental competence with infants. Some identified factors associated with fathers' parental competence are family functioning, partner relationships, and a sense of mastery (Ferketich & Mercer, 1995); relationship with own father and emotional and informational support from wives (Anderson, 1996b); and knowledge of infant development and an infant with an "easier" temperament (Edwards, 1990).

One way nurses can help fathers feel more competent in the parental role is to teach and provide information. Men entering parenthood with knowledge and realistic expectations may cope more successfully with the demands of a young infant and develop nurturing relationships with their infants. For nurses, dissemination of information can be a cost-effective intervention. Use of videos on infant cognitive and social capabilities and on early infant care and stimulation, as well as direct parent teaching methods such as exposure to newborn assessments and classes on parenting skills and infant behavioral cues, has been successful (Lawhon, 1994; Vehvilainen-Julkunen, 1995).

Impact of Fatherhood

The impact of first-time fatherhood on men has been investigated (Anderson, 1996a, 1996b). For Caucasian, middle-class American husbands, first-time fatherhood is seen as a maturing event during which increased responsibility is assumed. Fathers report taking their work more seriously while at the same time trying to balance work and family demands. These men experience an identity change, developing an image of themselves as a father. Over time, they develop strong bonds with their infants and feel a sense of fulfillment and purpose in life.

Studies investigating the impact of fatherhood on African-American men are sparse. One study on parental role attainment by African-American parents (Sank, 1991) provides nurses with some understanding of the father's experience. Self-concept was found to be the best predictor of these fathers' parental role attainment during the postpartum period. Fathers felt less competent with the skill and knowledge component of parenting than did the mothers but were at ease with the valuing and comfort component. Although these fathers did not see themselves as skillful as their partners in caring for infants, they valued parenthood and felt comfortable in the father role.

Despite their active involvement in the perinatal period, fathers tend to gravitate toward a more traditional division of family responsibilities. One reason for this return to more traditional roles may be the new father's concerns about his ability to support his new family financially. As a first-time father explained: "[Child care] costs much more than I expected. The cost was amazing. I would have never guessed how much of a drain child care could put on our income" (Leventhal-Belfer, Cowan, & Cowan, 1992).

Fathers can benefit from nursing interventions during the postpartum period just as mothers can. Nurses can arrange to teach infant care when the father is present and provide anticipatory guidance for fathers about the transition to parenthood. Separate prenatal and parenting classes and parenting support groups for fathers can provide them with an opportunity to discuss their concerns and have some of their needs met. Postpartum phone calls and home visits by the nurse need to include time for assessment of the father's adjustment and needs.

Infant-Parent Adjustment

It has long been recognized that newborns participate actively in shaping their parents' reaction to them. Research has demonstrated that the behavioral characteristics of the infant influence parenting behaviors (Anderson, 1996a; Vehvilainen-Julkunen, 1995). The infant and the parent each have unique rhythms, behaviors, and response styles that are brought to every interaction. **Infant-parent interactions** can be facilitated in any of three ways: (1) modulation of rhythm, (2) modification of behavioral repertoires, and (3) mutual responsivity. Nurses can teach parents about these three aspects of infant-parent interaction through

discussions, written materials, and videotapes on infant capabilities (e.g., *The Amazing Newborn*). A creative approach is to videotape the parent-infant pair during an interaction and then use the individualized tape to discuss the pair's rhythm, behavioral repertoire, and responsivity.

Rhythm

To modulate **rhythm,** both parent and infant must be able to interact. Therefore the infant must be in the alert state, one of the most difficult of the sleep-wake states to maintain. The alert state occurs most often during a feeding or in face-to-face play (Fig. 25-10, *A*). The parent must work hard to help the infant maintain the alert state long enough and often enough for interactions to take place. The en face position (the parent's face is positioned in the same plane as that of the newborn) is usually assumed (Fig. 25-10, *D*). Multiparous mothers in particular are very sensitive and responsive to the infant's feeding rhythms. Mothers learn to reserve stimulation for pauses in sucking activity and not to talk or smile excessively while the infant is sucking because the infant will stop feeding to interact with her. With maturity the infant can sustain longer interactions by modulating activity rhythms, that is, limb movement, sucking, gaze alternation, and habituation (Fig. 25-11). Meanwhile, the parent becomes more attuned to the infant's rhythms and learns to

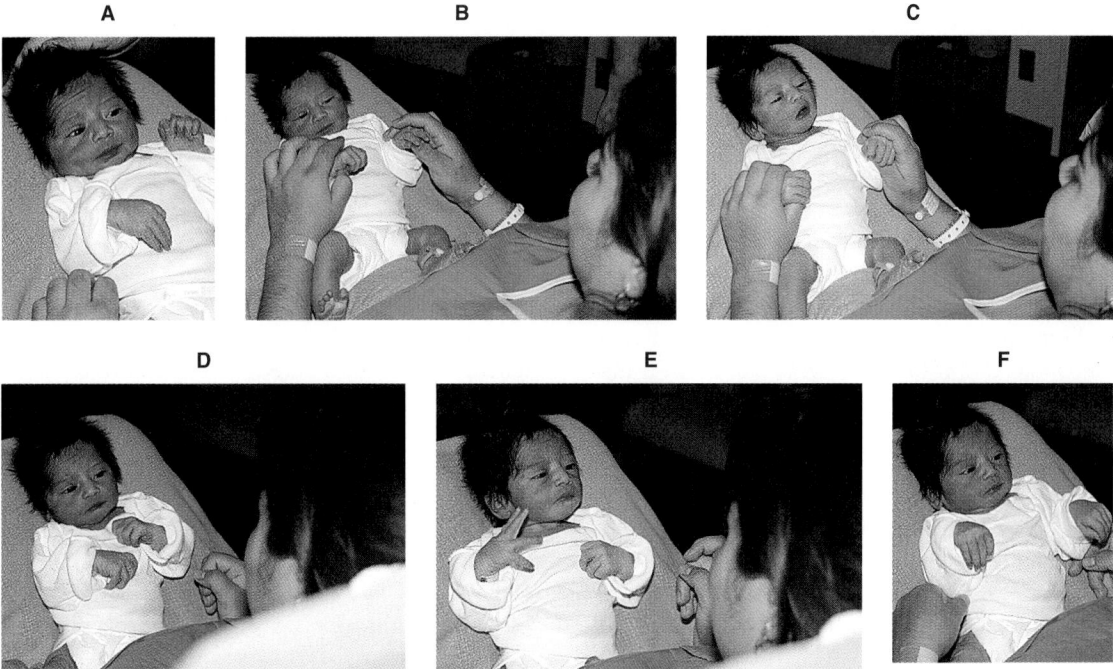

Fig. 25-10   Holding newborn in *en face* position, mother works to alert her daughter, 6 hours old. **A,** Infant is quiet and alert. **B,** Mother begins talking to daughter. **C,** Infant responds, opens mouth like her mother. **D,** Infant gazes at her mother. **E,** Infant waves hand. **F,** Infant glances away, resting. Hand relaxes. *(Courtesy Marjorie Pyle, RNC, Lifecircle, Costa Mesa, CA.)*

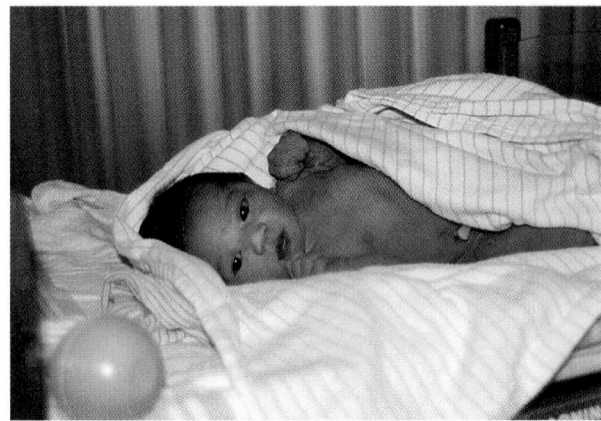

Fig. 25-11 Infant in alert state. *(Courtesy Marjorie Pyle, RNC, Lifecircle, Costa Mesa, CA.)*

modulate the rhythms, facilitating a rhythmic turn-taking interaction.

Behavioral Repertoires

Both the infant and the parent have a **repertoire of behaviors** they can use to facilitate interactions. Fathers and mothers engage in these behaviors depending on the extent of contact and caregiving of the infant.

The infant's behavioral repertoire includes gazing, vocalizing, and facial expressions. The infant is able to focus and follow the human face from birth and is also able to alternate the gaze voluntarily, looking away from the parent's face when understimulated or overstimulated (Fig. 25-10, F). Brazelton and associates (1974) suggest that one of the key responses for the parents to learn is to be sensitive to the infant's capacity for attention and inattention. Developing this sensitivity is especially important when interacting with preterm infants.

Body gestures form a part of the infant's "early language." Babies greet parents with waving hands (Fig. 25-10, E) or a reaching out of hands. They can raise an eyebrow or soften their expression to elicit loving attention. Game playing can stimulate them to smile or laugh. Pouting or crying, arching of the back, and general squirming usually signal the end of an interaction.

The parents' repertoire includes various types of interactive behaviors such as constantly looking at the infant and noting the infant's response. New parents often remark that they are exhausted from looking at the baby and smiling. Adults also "infantilize" their speech to help the infant "listen." They do this by slowing the tempo, speaking loudly and rhythmically, and emphasizing key words. Phrases are repeated frequently. Infantilizing does not mean using "baby talk," which involves distortion of sounds.

Facial expressions such as slow and exaggerated looks of surprise, happiness, and confusion are often used by par-

ents to communicate these emotions to the infant. Games such as "peek-a-boo" and imitation of the infant's behaviors are other means of interaction. For example, if the baby smiles, so does the parent; if the baby frowns, the parent responds in kind.

Responsivity

Contingent responses **(responsivity)** are those that occur within a specific time and are similar in form to a stimulus behavior. The adult has the feeling of having an influence on the interaction. Infant behaviors such as smiling, cooing, and sustained eye contact, usually in en face position, are viewed as contingent responses. The infant's responses act as rewards to the initiator and encourage the adult to continue with the game when the infant responds positively. When the adult imitates the infant, the infant appears to enjoy it. There is a progression in the types of behaviors that parents present for the baby to imitate; for example, in early interactions the parent will grimace rather than laugh, which is in keeping with the infant's developmental level. Such "turnabout" behaviors sustain interactions and promote harmony in the relationship.

FACTORS INFLUENCING PARENTAL RESPONSES

How parents respond to the birth of their child is influenced by various factors, including age, social networks, socioeconomic conditions, and personal aspirations of the future.

Age

Maternal age has a definite effect on the outcome of pregnancy. The mother and fetus are both at highest risk when the mother is an adolescent or is more than 35 years old.

The Adolescent Mother

Although it is biologically possible for the adolescent female to become a parent, her egocentricity and concrete thinking interfere with her ability to parent effectively. The very young adolescent mother is inexperienced and unprepared to recognize the early signs of illness, potential danger, or household hazards. She may inadvertently neglect her child. The higher mortality rates among the infants of adolescent mothers are attributed to the inexperience, lack of knowledge, and immaturity of the mothers, causing them to be unable to recognize a problem and obtain the necessary resources to rectify the situation. Nevertheless, in most instances, with adequate support and developmentally appropriate teaching, adolescents can learn effective parenting skills.

The developmental tasks of parenthood include (1) reconciling the imagined infant with the actual infant, (2) becoming adept at caregiving activities, (3) being aware of the infant's needs, and (4) establishing oneself and one's infant as a family.

The transition to parenthood may be difficult for adolescent parents. Coping with the developmental tasks of parenthood is often complicated by the unmet developmental needs and tasks of adolescence. Some young parents may experience difficulty accepting a changing self-image and adjusting to new roles related to the responsibilities of infant care. Other adolescent parents, however, may have higher self-concepts than their nonparenting peers (Alpers, 1998). Self-concept of pregnant and parenting teens appears to vary in relation to age, years of schooling, types of schools attended, income sources, and receipt of public assistance (Alpers, 1998). Nurses developing or implementing teen parenting programs need to have occasional checkpoints in place throughout their programs to reassess the self-concept of adolescent parents and the types of socioeconomic supports these teens use.

As adolescent parents move through the transition to parenthood, they may feel "different" from their peers, excluded from "fun" activities, and prematurely forced to enter an adult social role. The conflict between their own desires and the infant's demands, in addition to the low tolerance for frustration that is typical of adolescence, further contribute to the normal psychosocial stress of childbirth. Lower maternal education is associated with less favorable maternal responses to distress and infant behavior (Diehl, 1997).

Maintaining a relationship with the baby's father is beneficial for the teen mother and her infant. A close and satisfying relationship is positively correlated with maternal-fetal and maternal-infant attachment (Bloom, 1998). The involvement of the baby's father is related to appropriate maternal behaviors and positive mother-infant relationship (Diehl, 1997).

Some differences between adolescent and adult mothers have been observed. For example, adolescent mothers provide warm and attentive physical care; however, they use less verbal interaction than do older parents, and adolescents tend to be less responsive and to interact less positively with their infants than older mothers (Barratt & Roach, 1995). Thompson and others (1995) found that adolescent mothers were at risk for nonnurturing behaviors with their infant. Interventions emphasizing verbal and nonverbal communication skills between mother and infant are important. Such intervention strategies must be concrete and specific because of the cognitive level of adolescents. Although some observers suggest that some adolescents may use more aggressive behaviors, a higher incidence of child abuse has not been documented. In comparison with adult mothers, teenage mothers have a limited knowledge of child development. They tend to expect too much of their children too soon and often characterize their infants as being fussy. This limited

knowledge may cause teenagers to respond to their infants inappropriately.

Many young mothers pattern their maternal role on what they themselves experienced. Therefore nurses need to determine the kind of support that people close to the young mother are able and prepared to give, as well as the kinds of community aid available to supplement this support. The majority of adolescent mothers can identify at least one source of social support, with their own mother being their predominant source of support (Thompson et al., 1995). Rural adolescent mothers who reported firm encouragement and resources to pursue their life aspirations had more resilient adjustments to parenthood than adolescent mothers who did not have this type of support (Camarena et al., 1998).

The need for continued assessment of the new mother's parenting abilities during this postbirth period is essential. In addition, continued support should also be provided by involving the grandparents and other family members, as well as through home visits and group sessions for discussion of infant care and parenting problems. Outreach programs concerned with self-care, parent-child interactions, child injuries, and failure to thrive, in addition to programs that provide prompt and effective community intervention, prevent more serious problems from occurring. As the adolescent performs her mothering role within the framework of her family, she may need to address dependency versus independency issues. The adolescent's family members may also need help adapting to their new roles.

The Adolescent Father

As with the adolescent mother, the nurse must be aware of the male adolescent's cognitive-developmental levels, values, and culture. The more successful outreach programs also address cultural diversity in teenage fathers.

The adolescent father and mother face immediate developmental crises, which include completing the developmental tasks of adolescence, making a transition to parenthood, and sometimes adapting to marriage. These transitions can be stressful. The nurse may initiate interaction with the adolescent father by asking him to be present when postpartum home visits are made and to accompany the mother and the baby to well-baby checks at the clinic or pediatrician's office. With the adolescent mother's agreement, the nurse may contact the father directly. The decision to include the young father in all aspects of the care is based on assessment in the following four areas: (1) the couple's relationship; (2) levels of stress, concern, and coping; (3) educational and vocational goals; and (4) the level of health education knowledge. Adolescent fathers need support to discuss their emotional responses to the pregnancy. The nurse's nonjudgmental attitude is essential for open communication. The father's feelings of guilt, powerlessness, or bravado should be recognized because of their negative consequences for both the parents and the child. Counseling of adolescent fathers needs to be reality oriented. Topics such as finances, child care, parenting skills, and the father's role in the birth experience need to be discussed. Teenage fathers also need to know about reproductive physiology and birth control options.

The adolescent father may continue to be involved in an ongoing relationship with the young mother and his baby. In many instances he also plays an important role in the decisions about child care and raising the child. The nurse supports the young father by helping him develop realistic perceptions of his role as "father to a child." The nurse encourages him to use coping mechanisms that are not detrimental to his own, his partner's, or his child's well-being. The nurse enlists support systems, parents, and professional agencies on his behalf. The father is encouraged to be involved in decisions regarding future contraception and safer sex practices.

Maternal Age Greater Than 35 Years

Issues and concerns related to women with a maternal age over 35 years have become increasingly more prominent in the last decade. There have always been women older than 35 years who have continued their childbearing either by choice or because of a lack or failure of contraception during the perimenopausal years. Added to this group are women who have postponed pregnancy because of careers or other reasons and women with infertility problems who have become pregnant because of technologic advances that have increased the alternatives for couples desiring children.

Older mothers have unique needs related to increased biologic risk. Higher rates of gestational diabetes, pregnancy-induced hypertension, gestational bleeding, abruptio placentae, and intrapartal fetal distress have been reported (Berkowitz et al., 1990; Fretts et al., 1995; Gilbert, Nesbitt, & Danielson, 1999). Many of these mothers, because they are less physically resilient than younger women, may need to stay in the hospital longer.

Researchers have examined the adjustment of midlife mothers to parenthood. Many older mothers reported having a hard time coping, especially with irregular sleep patterns and the fussy periods babies have in the late afternoon and early evening. Mothers admitted to unrealistic preconceptions about parenting. As one mother said, "I was surviving, not living, for the first 3 months. I couldn't get over how dramatically my life changed. I had thought the baby would adjust to our lifestyle. I didn't understand that everyone had to adapt" (Cain, 1994).

Adjusting to the enormity of the change was a pervading theme in these studies. A factor that helped these older mothers adjust and see themselves as competent parents was support from their partners. Support from other family members and friends was also important for positive

self-evaluation of parenting, a sense of well-being and satisfaction, and help in dealing with stress. Positive self-evaluation of parenting early in the transition to parenthood was associated with greater confidence and support in mothering at 1 year (Reece, 1993; Reese, 1995; Reese & Harkless, 1996).

Older mothers reported having to adjust to changes in the relationships with their partners. Some women regarded the changes as negative (e.g., having less time together), whereas others saw the changes as positive (e.g., feeling closer to their partners). Because many of these couples had been together for many years before the baby was born, the loss of the "just-the-two-of-us" aspect of the relationship was stressful (Cain, 1994). One mother stated, "We were by ourselves for so long, it was a hard adjustment—very, very difficult."

Changes in the sexual aspect of a relationship can be a stressor for new midlife parents. Mothers reported that finding time and energy for a romantic rendezvous was more difficult. They attributed much of this to the reality of caring for an infant but also mentioned the decreasing libido that normally accompanies getting older. Many of today's midlife mothers spent their late adolescence and early adulthood in the late 1960s and early 1970s, when youth spoke openly about sex and participated actively in the sexual revolution (Cain, 1994). As one woman so aptly expressed it, having no sex life along with a decreased libido was "more than an adjustment. It's practically an identity crisis. Now that our mid-life conservatism has taken over, there seems to be no one with whom to discuss our fears and changes. We're all seemingly back in the closet."

Work/career issues are sources of conflict for older mothers (Reese & Harkless, 1996). Conflicts emerge over being disinterested, worrying about giving enough attention to work with the distractions of a new baby, and anticipating what it will be like to return to work. A major factor causing stress about work is child care.

Another major issue for older mothers with careers is the perception of loss of control (Reese & Harkless, 1996). Mothers older than 35, compared with younger mothers, are at a different stage in their careers, having attained high levels of education, career, and income. The loss of control experienced when going from the consistency of a work role to the inconsistency of the parent role, comes as a surprise to many. Perhaps this is because of the women's previous achievements and high expectations of themselves (Reese & Harkless, 1996). Nurses should be aware of the older mother's sense of loss of control and of the pre-occupation with juggling career and family. Nurses can provide anticipatory guidance during pregnancy and early parenthood, with special attention to the issues of career women. Helping the older mother have realistic expectations of herself and of parenthood is essential.

BOX 25-2 Resources for Older Parents

FEMALE (Formerly Employed Mother at the Leading Edge)
P.O. Box 31
Elmhurst, IL 60126
(630) 941-3553

Mothers at Home
8310A Old Courthouse Road
Vienna, VA 22182
(703) 827-5903

National Council for Adoption
(202) 328-8072

New mothers who are also perimenopausal may find it hard to distinguish fatigue, loss of sleep, decreased libido, or other physiologic symptoms as the cause of the changes in their sex lives. Although many women view menopause as a natural stage of life, for midlife mothers this cessation of menstruation coincides with the state of parenthood. The changes of midlife and menopause can add more emotional and physical stress to older mothers' lives because of the time- and energy-consuming aspects of raising a young child (Cain, 1994). Resources that older parents may find helpful are listed in Box 25-2.

Paternal Age Greater Than 35 Years

Literature on the experiences of first-time fathers with a paternal age over 35 years is sparse. However, in the available literature, older fathers described their experience of midlife parenting as wonderful but not without drawbacks. What they saw as positive aspects of parenthood in older years included increased love and commitment between the spouses, a reinforcement of why one married in the first place, a feeling of being complete, experiencing of "the child" again in oneself, more financial stability than in younger years, and more freedom to focus on parenting rather than on career. A common theme expressed was sharing: sharing joy, sharing in raising the child, sharing as a family. The main drawback of midlife parenting that these men reported was the change that it made in the relationships with their partners. They missed the deeper and more selfish couple relationship and looked forward to the time when they could have that again (Cain, 1994). Some fathers mentioned age as a disadvantage: "Some-times I think I'm the oldest father in [the group]. I can't do quite as many physical things as I used to when I was younger." All fathers seemed to qualify statements about the less desirable side of parenting with positive statements such as ". . . but, I would not change it for the world!" or "I can't imagine life not being a parent now."

Social Support

Social support is strongly related to positive adaptation by new parents during the transition to parenthood (Reece, 1993; Susman, 1996). Social support is multidimensional and includes the number of members in a person's social network, types of support, perceived general support, actual support received, and satisfaction with support available and received. The type and satisfaction of support seem to be more important than the total number of support network members.

A type of social support that has become popular in the United States within the last couple of years is the doula. A doula is a person other than the father of the baby who is trained to provide emotional and physical support to the mother during labor. Postpartum women who have received social support from a doula, compared to women who did not have a doula, demonstrate a stronger self-esteem, less depression, more positive feelings for their infant, and increased ability to care for their infant during the transition to parenthood (Klaus & Kennell, 1997).

Across cultural groups, families and friends of new parents form an important dimension of the parent's social network. For example, the extended family unit is the single strongest unit in the lives of most Asians. Extended family are also relied on heavily after childbirth by Jordanians (Geissler, 1994). Through helpseeking within the social network, new mothers learn practices that are culturally valued and develop role competency (Pridham, 1997).

Social networks provide a support system on which parents can rely for assistance (Reece, 1993), but they can also be a source of conflict. Sometimes a large network can cause problems because it results in conflicting advice from numerous people. Grandparents or in-laws are most appreciated when they assist with household responsibilities and do not intrude into the parents' privacy or judge them critically (Hansen & Jacob, 1992).

Women who have given birth before may have different support needs than first-time mothers. First-time mothers may need more follow-up for parenting skills, including referral to community resources. Women with other children may be more realistic in anticipating physical limitations and the changes in roles and relationships. However, these experienced mothers express concerns over separation from their firstborn, loss of the exclusive relationship with the older child or children, and the challenge of caring for two or more children.

Because of the extent of restructuring and reorganization that occurs in a family with the birth of another child, the mothers' moods and fatigue in the postpartum period can be helped more by situation-specific support from family and friends than from general support (Gottlieb & Mendelson, 1995). General support addresses feeling loved, respected, and valued. Situation-specific support relates to practical concerns such as physical needs and child care. For example, the practical support of a grandparent bathing the infant can help lessen a second-time mother's feelings of loss by providing her time to be with her firstborn child. Second-time mothers report that practical support is the most useful and desirable type of support during the postpartum period.

Nurses need to be aware that not all types of support are equally beneficial to mothers postpartum, and therefore, need to assess the presence and types of practical help available to new mothers. The assumption that second-time (experienced) mothers are "old pros" and therefore do not need help should be avoided. Because second-time mothers may expect this of themselves, nurses can help these mothers explore the differences associated with adding another child to the family and identify the types of support that they need the most. As Gottlieb and Mendelson (1995) suggest, there must be a "fit" between the availability of support and a parent's needs for the support to be effective, and support may change with changing situations.

Culture

Cultural beliefs and practices are important determinants of parenting behaviors. Culture defines what is socially acceptable in terms of eye contact, touch, and space (Lipson, Dibble, & Minarik, 1996). Culture influences the interactions with the baby as well as the parent's or family's caregiving style. For example, the provision for a period of rest and recuperation for the mother after birth is prominent in several cultures. Asian mothers must remain at home with the baby at least 30 days after birth and are not supposed to engage in household chores, including care of the baby. Many times the grandmother takes over the baby's care immediately, even before discharge from the hospital (Geissler, 1994). Likewise, Jordanian mothers have a 40-day lying-in after birth during which their mothers or sisters care for the baby (Geissler, 1994). Hispanics practice an intergenerational family ritual, la cuarentena. For 40 days after birth, the mother is expected to recuperate and get acquainted with her infant. Traditionally this involves many restrictions concerning food (spicy or cold foods, fish, pork, and citrus are avoided; tortillas and chicken soup are encouraged), exercise, and activities, including sexual intercourse. Abdominal binding is a traditional practice, and many women avoid tub bathing and washing their hair. Traditional Hispanic husbands do not expect to see their wives or infants until both have been cleaned and dressed after birth. La cuarentena incorporates individuals into the family, instills parental responsibility, and integrates the family during a critical life event (Geissler, 1994; Niska, Snyder, & Lia-Hoagberg, 1998).

Desire for and valuing of children is salient in all cultures. In Asian families, children are valued as a source of family strength and stability, are perceived as wealth, and are objects of parental love and affection. Infants almost always are given an affectionate "cradle" name that is used during the first years of life; for example, a Filipino girl might be called "Ling-Ling" and a boy "Bong-Bong." In the Yup'ik culture of the Alaskan Eskimos, where sharing has been necessary for survival throughout their history, children are looked on as security. There is no concept of illegitimacy; whether parents are married does not matter. Every child is welcomed and loved. Adoption is common and is usually within the extended family, for example, by grandparents (MacDonald-Clark & Boffman, 1995).

Differing cultural values can influence parents' interactions with health care professionals. For example, Asians are taught to be humble and obedient; to be outspoken is frowned on. They are brought up not to question authority figures (such as a nurse), to avoid confrontation, and to respect the yin/yang balance in nature. Because of these learned values, an Asian mother might not confront the nurse about the length of time it has taken to receive the medication requested for her episiotomy pain. A mother may nod and say "Yes" in response to the nurse's directions for using an iced sitz bath but then will not use the sitz bath. The "yes," in this case, is a gesture of courtesy, meaning "I'm listening"; it is not an indication of agreement to comply. The mother does not use the iced sitz bath because of her traditional avoidance of bathing and cold in the puerperium. Because all members of a cultural group do not necessarily adhere to traditional practices, validating which cultural practices are important to individual parents is important. Also refer to Table 2-2 for examples of some traditional cultural beliefs that may be important to parents from African-American, Asian, and Hispanic cultures.

Knowledge of cultural beliefs can help the nurse make more accurate assessments and diagnoses of observed parenting behaviors (see Cultural Considerations box). For example, nurses may become concerned when they observe cultural practices that appear to reflect poor maternal-infant bonding. Algerian mothers may not unwrap and explore their infants as part of the acquaintance process because in Algeria, babies are wrapped tightly in swaddling clothes to protect them physically and psychologically (Geissler, 1994). The nurse may observe a Vietnamese woman who gives minimal care to her infant but refuses to cuddle or further interact with her baby. This apparent lack of interest in the newborn is this cultural group's attempt to ward off "evil spirits" and actually reflects an intense love and concern for the infant (Galanti, 1991). An Asian mother might be criticized for almost immediately relinquishing the care of the infant to the grandmother and not even attempting to hold her baby when it is brought to her room. However, in Asian extended families, members show their support for a new mother's rest and recuperation by assisting with the care of the baby. Contrary to the guidance given to mothers in the United States about "nipple confusion," a mix of breastfeeding and bottle feeding is standard practice for Japanese mothers. This is out of concern for the mother's rest during the first 2 to 3 months and does not lead to any problems with lactation; breastfeeding is widespread and successful among Japanese women (Sharts-Hopko, 1995).

Cultural beliefs and values give perspective to the meaning of childbirth for a new mother. Nurses can provide an opportunity for a new mother to talk about her perception of the meaning of childbearing. This may foster self-actualization, promote maternal role attainment, improve her relationship with her partner, and enrich the family perspective (Callister, 1995).

An example of a culture in which the norm of maternal behaviors with infants parallels what is expected in the United States is the Yup'ik culture of the Alaskan Eskimos. New Yup'ik mothers typically are observed to be quiet, loving, and gentle with their newborns, almost always holding their infants in a position where eye contact can be made. They are keenly aware of and responsive to their infants' cues. In one study, Yup'ik mothers scored higher on measures of responsiveness to infant cues, especially distress cues, than did the normative group (Caucasian, African-American, and Hispanic mothers) (MacDonald-Clark & Boffman, 1995).

Discontinuities of culture and related traditions may be problematic for some families during the transition to parenthood. Hansen and Jacob (1992) found that when the couples' backgrounds diverged ethnically, religiously, or socioeconomically, the differences had a major impact on intergenerational relationships. Some couples were unable to integrate the differences and chose either the maternal or paternal family for support, thus magnifying the conflict between generations. Some couples broke completely with both families.

In helping new families adjust to parenthood, nurses must provide culturally sensitive care by following principles that facilitate nursing practice within transcultural situations (see Cultural Considerations box).

Socioeconomic Conditions

Socioeconomic conditions often determine access to available resources. Parents whose economic condition is made worse with the birth of each child and who are unable to use an effective method of fertility management may find childbirth complicated by concern for their own health and a sense of helplessness. Mothers who are single, separated, or divorced from their husbands or without a partner, family, and friends for whatever reason may view the birth of a child with dread. Serious financial problems may override any desire for mothering the infant. Nurses need to be sensitive to the stressors that economically disadvantaged mothers have to contend with and consider these in efforts to foster mother-infant bonding (Sharts-Hopko, 1995) (see Cultural Considerations). Nursing measures designed to help mothers in trying socioeconomic circumstances involve referral to social and economic community service agencies, as well as health care agencies. A

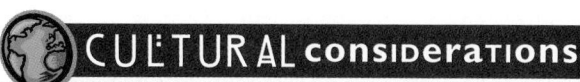

CULTURAL consiperations

Principles for Facilitating Nursing Practice Within Transcultural Situations

1. *The stress of new parenthood overlies the stressors of transcultural migration.* It is exacerbated to the extent that clients do not speak the dominant language. Because of emigration, the client may also be experiencing altered socioeconomic status and isolation from loved ones, and it may have resulted from war, famine, or other great suffering.

2. *Nurses may be able to foster connections with networks of specific cultural groups,* although with the awareness that intracultural differences, like religion, can create important barriers. Bilingual volunteers can be a great help in easing hospital stays for non–English-speaking clients and their families.

3. *Nurses can enhance their ability to care for large immigrant populations by learning about those cultures* through reading, talking with representatives of the groups, attending educational programs, or viewing films.

4. *Nurses will serve as more effective interpreters of the childbearing experience to transcultural clients if they operate on the assumptions that clients (1) do not know what will be done to them, (2) may not convey their needs or may express them differently, and (3) may not know how they are expected to respond in the situation.* Caring behaviors are culture specific. For example, informed consent is an American issue that has no meaning in some other cultures. Withholding food from a Japanese woman in labor, to her, undermines her energy for effective pushing. Expecting new mothers to assume child care within a day after birth can seem callous to people in cultures who place a high value on recuperation. Devaluing traditional practices of the mother's cultural group devalues her as a person.

5. *Differing practices must be evaluated from the standpoint of safety as understood by health care professionals in the United States,* but a healthy measure of humility is warranted.

satisfactory outcome for such problems often requires long-term commitments from both the woman or couple and the community. Adequate situational supports need to be instituted in the prenatal period.

Personal Aspirations

For some women, parenthood interferes with or blocks their plans for personal freedom or advancement in their career. Resentment concerning this loss may not have been resolved during the prenatal period, and if it remains unresolved, it will spill over into caregiving activities. This may result in indifference and neglect of the infant, or in excessive concern and the setting of impossibly high standards by the mother for her own behavior or the child's performance.

In a study of first-time mothers with career commitments, Leonard (1993) found that the meaning and content of work and of motherhood, and the timing of return to work had a powerful influence in shaping the career woman's experience with the transition to parenthood. Women expected that having a baby would add a role to their repertoire of roles; however, the women experienced motherhood as "world-transforming," not simply additive. Returning to work was especially stressful to these career women, particularly if the work setting did not recognize the needs and responsibilities the women now had as mothers. If the women viewed their work as meaningful and if their income was economically important for their family, the stress they experienced was mitigated.

Role models that assist women in integrating work role and motherhood role may be helpful for new mothers; however, these role models are lacking (Hartrick, 1997; Miller, 1996). Mothers returning to work who do not identify with such role models appear to improvise and negotiate relationships in order to manage their careers and the care of their infants (Miller, 1996). Over time, new mothers progress to where they can nurture themselves and make new connections, to a time of reclaiming and discovery (Hartrick, 1997). Not all new mothers experience role conflict. Some have less role conflict because their careers provide a sense of self-fulfillment and self-worth, especially when they feel supported by their family and confident in child care arrangements.

Nursing intervention includes providing opportunities for mothers to express their feelings freely to an objective listener; to discuss measures to permit personal growth and to learn about the care of their infant.

Nurses can also be proactive in influencing changes in work policies related to maternity and paternity leaves, varying models of work sharing, and "family friendly" work environments. Some corporations already structure their work sites to support new mothers, for example by providing on-site day care facilities and breastfeeding rooms.

PARENTAL SENSORY IMPAIRMENT

In the early dialogue between the parent and child, all senses—sight, hearing, touch, taste, and smell—are used by each to initiate and sustain the attachment process. A parent who has an impairment of one of the senses needs to maximize use of the remaining senses.

Visually Impaired Parent

Although parents who are visually impaired need the presence and the support of another responsible person, they can become adept in many child care activities, as the following report indicates:

> We had always planned to have a child. My family and Dick's both wanted us to have the happiness of children and were willing to help us with the baby care. First I bathed and changed a doll; then I practiced caring for my sister's baby. I would feel in all the creases with my finger to see if they were clean and dry. We used disposable diapers that do not need pins. My mother made baby clothes with fastenings of press cloth (Velcro) so I would not have to fiddle with buttons. I feel really confident now. I know I can't do everything for her, but I can do enough to feel like a mother, and I know she will have all the love she needs.

A strength that visually impaired people have is a heightened sensitivity to other sensory outputs. A blind mother can tell when her infant is facing her because she can feel the baby's breath on her face.

One of the major difficulties that visually impaired parents experience is the skepticism, open or hidden, of health care professionals. Blind people sense a reluctance on the part of others to acknowledge that they have a right to be parents. All too often, nurses and doctors lack the experience to deal with the childbearing and child-rearing needs of visually impaired mothers, as well as mothers with other disabilities (such as hearing impaired, physically impaired, and mentally challenged). Shyness, fear, or reluctance on the part of nurses can result in visually impaired parents being left alone or being involved in awkward conversations. The best approach by the nurse is to assess the mother's capabilities. From that basis, the nurse can make plans to assist the woman, often in much the same way as for a mother with sight. Visually impaired mothers have made suggestions for providing care for women such as themselves during childbearing (Box 25-3). Such approaches by the nurse can help avoid a sense of increased vulnerability on the mother's part.

Eye-to-eye contact is considered important in American culture. With a parent who is visually impaired, this critical factor in the parent-child attachment process is obviously missing. However, the blind parent, who may never have experienced this method of strengthening relationships, does not miss it. The infant will need other sensory input from that parent. An infant looking into the eyes of a mother who is blind may not be aware that the eyes are unseeing. Other people in the newborn's environment can also participate in active eye-to-eye contact to supply this need. A problem may arise, however, if the visually impaired parent has an impassive facial expression. Her infant, making repeated unsuccessful attempts to engage in face play with the mother, will abandon the behavior with her and intensify it with the father or other people in the household. Nurses can provide anticipatory guidance regarding this situation and help the mother learn to nod and smile while talking and cooing to the infant.

BOX 25-3 Nursing Approaches for Working with Visually Impaired Parents

1. Parents who are blind need verbal teaching by health care providers because maternity information is not accessible to blind people.
2. A visually impaired parent needs an orientation to the hospital room that allows the parent to move about the room independently. For example, "Go to the left of the bed and trail the wall until you feel the first door. That is the bathroom."
3. Parents who are blind need explanations of routines.
4. Parents who are blind need to feel devices (e.g., monitors, pelvic models) and to hear descriptions of the devices.
5. Visually impaired parents need "a chance to ask questions."
6. Visually impaired parents need the opportunity to hold and touch the baby after birth.
7. Nurses need to demonstrate baby care by touch and to follow with, "Now let me see you do it."
8. Nurses need to give instructions such as, "I'm going to give you the baby. The head is to your left side."

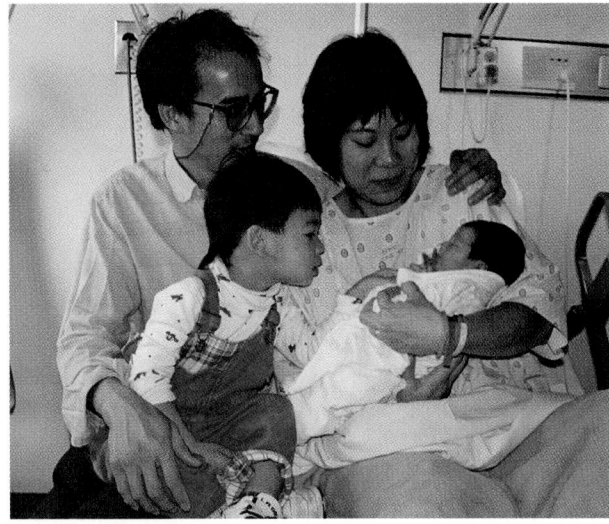

Fig. 25-12 Parents introducing "big" brother to infant daughter. *(Courtesy Kim Molloy, Knoxville, IA.)*

Hearing-Impaired Parent

The parent who has a hearing impairment faces another set of problems, particularly if the deafness dates from birth or early childhood. The mother and her partner are likely to have established an independent household. A number of devices that transform sound into light flashes are now marketed and can be fitted into the infant's room to permit immediate detection of crying. Even if the parent is not speech trained, vocalizing can serve as both a stimulus and a response to the infant's early vocalizing. Deaf parents can provide additional vocal training by use of recordings and television so that from birth the child is aware of the full range of the human voice. Sign language is acquired readily by young children, and the first sign used is as varied as the first word.

Section 504 of the Rehabilitation Act of 1973 requires that hospitals and other institutions receiving funds from the U.S. Department of Health and Human Services use various communication techniques and resources with the deaf, including having staff members or certified interpreters who are proficient in sign language. For example, provision of written materials with demonstrations and having nurses stand where the parent can read their lips (if the parent practices lip reading) are two techniques that can be used. A creative approach is for the nursing unit to develop videotapes in which information on postpartum care, infant care, and parenting issues is signed by an interpreter and spoken by a nurse. A videotape in which a nurse signs while speaking would be ideal.

SIBLING ADAPTATION

Because the family is an interactive, open unit, the addition of a new family member affects everyone in the family. Siblings are no exception. Older children have to assume new positions within the family hierarchy. The older child's goal is to maintain the lead position. Parents are faced with the task of caring for a new child while not neglecting the others. Parents need to distribute their attention in an equitable manner.

Reactions of siblings may result from temporary separation from the mother, changes in the mother's or father's behavior, or the siblings' response to the infant's coming home. Sibling reactions are manifested in behavioral changes. Positive behavioral changes include interest in and concern for the baby and increased independence. Regression in toileting and sleep habits, aggression toward the baby, and increased seeking of attention and whining are examples of negative behaviors.

The introduction of a baby into a family with one or more children challenges parents to promote acceptance of the baby by siblings (Fig. 25-12). The parents' attitudes toward the arrival of the baby can set the stage for the other children's reactions. In some families, parental support promoted sibling adjustment; in others the needs of the sibling shaped the parental support.

Because the baby absorbs the time and attention of the important people in the other children's lives, jealousy is to be expected once the initial excitement of having a new baby in the home is over. However, more recent research suggests that the expectation of **sibling rivalry,** or negative behaviors in siblings, may have been overemphasized. Gullicks and Crase (1993) studied the difference between parental expectations for sibling behavior and actual sibling

BOX 25-4 **Strategies for Facilitating Sibling Acceptance of a New Baby**

1. Take your firstborn child on a tour of your hospital room and point out similarities to his or her birth. This is like the room I was in with you, and the baby is in the same kind of bassinet that you were in.
2. Have a small gift from the baby to give to your older child each day.
3. Give the older child a T-shirt that says "I'm a big brother" (or "sister").
4. Arrange for your children to be in the first group (grandparents, sister) to see the newborn. Let them hold the baby in the hospital. One mother and father arranged for their firstborn son to be present at the births of his three brothers and to be the first one to hold them.
5. Plan time for both children. "When I get home, I'll arrange my day so that I can have the baby's care done in the morning while Sam (first child) is at school. Maybe the baby will sleep part of the afternoon and I can spend some time with Sam."
6. Fathers can spend time with the older sibling while mothers are taking care of the baby and vice versa. Siblings like to have time and attention from both parents.
7. Give preschool and early school-age siblings a newborn doll as "their baby" to care for. Give sibling a photograph of the new baby to take to school to show off "his" or "her" baby. Older siblings may enjoy the responsibility of helping care for the newborn, such as learning how to give the baby a bottle or change a diaper. One mother let her preschooler help burp the new baby by patting on the baby's back. She figured her son could pat the baby fairly firmly without harming him and at the same time get out some pent-up aggressive feelings.

behavior 4 weeks after the birth of a second child. They found that parents expected more negative behaviors toward the infant than they observed. The firstborn children continued their usual routines, were more pleased with the newborns, and were more understanding of the infants' need for care than the parents predicted. Parents also reported that the levels of developmentally appropriate behaviors in siblings were similar prenatally and postnatally.

Parents, especially mothers, spend much time and energy promoting sibling acceptance of a new baby. Participating in sibling preparation classes makes a difference in the ability of mothers to cope with sibling behavior. Older children are actively involved in preparing for the infant, and this involvement intensifies after the birth of the child. Parents face a number of tasks related to sibling rivalry and adjustment. For example, parents have to man-

age the feeling of guilt that the older children are being deprived of parental time and attention. They also have to monitor the behavior of older children toward the more vulnerable infant and divert aggressive behavior. Strategies that parents have used to facilitate acceptance of a new baby by siblings are presented in Box 25-4.

Siblings demonstrate acquaintance behaviors with the newborn. The acquaintance process depends on the information given to the child before the baby is born and on the child's cognitive development level. The initial behaviors of siblings with the newborn include looking at the infant and touching the head (Fig. 25-13). The initial adjustment of older children to a newborn takes time, and children should be allowed to interact at their own pace rather than being forced to do so. To expect a young child to accept and love a rival for the parents' affection assumes an unrealistic level of maturity. Sibling love grows as does other love, that is, by being with another person and sharing experiences (Fig. 25-14). The relationship that develops between siblings has been conceptualized as sibling attachment. This bond between siblings involves a secure base in which one child provides support for the other, is missed when absent, and is looked to for comfort and security.

Direct sibling contact does not place healthy newborns at risk for exposure to pathogenic organisms. Therefore separation of newborns and older siblings does not appear to be justified.

GRANDPARENT ADAPTATION

Grandparents are unique. They contribute to a sense of family continuity and provide maintenance of cultural traditions. They can educate their grandchildren about their roots and relate anecdotes about their parents. In turn, the presence of grandchildren often helps relieve the grandparents' loneliness and boredom. Grandparents who are free to love the grandchild can have a significant positive influence on the child's life (Fig. 25-15).

Just as the new parents go through a transition to parenthood, so do grandparents experience a transition to grandparenthood. Intergenerational relationships shift and grandparents must deal with changes in practices and attitudes toward childbirth, child rearing, and men's and women's roles at home and in the workplace. The degree to which grandparents understand and accept current practices can influence how supportive they are perceived to be by their adult children (Hansen & Jacob, 1992).

At the same time that they are adjusting to grandparenthood, the majority of grandparents are experiencing normative middle- and old-age life transition issues, such as retirement and a move to smaller housing, and need support from their adult children. Some may feel regret about their limited involvement because of poor health or geographic distance. Maternal grandmothers, more so than the other three grandparents, may have high expecta-

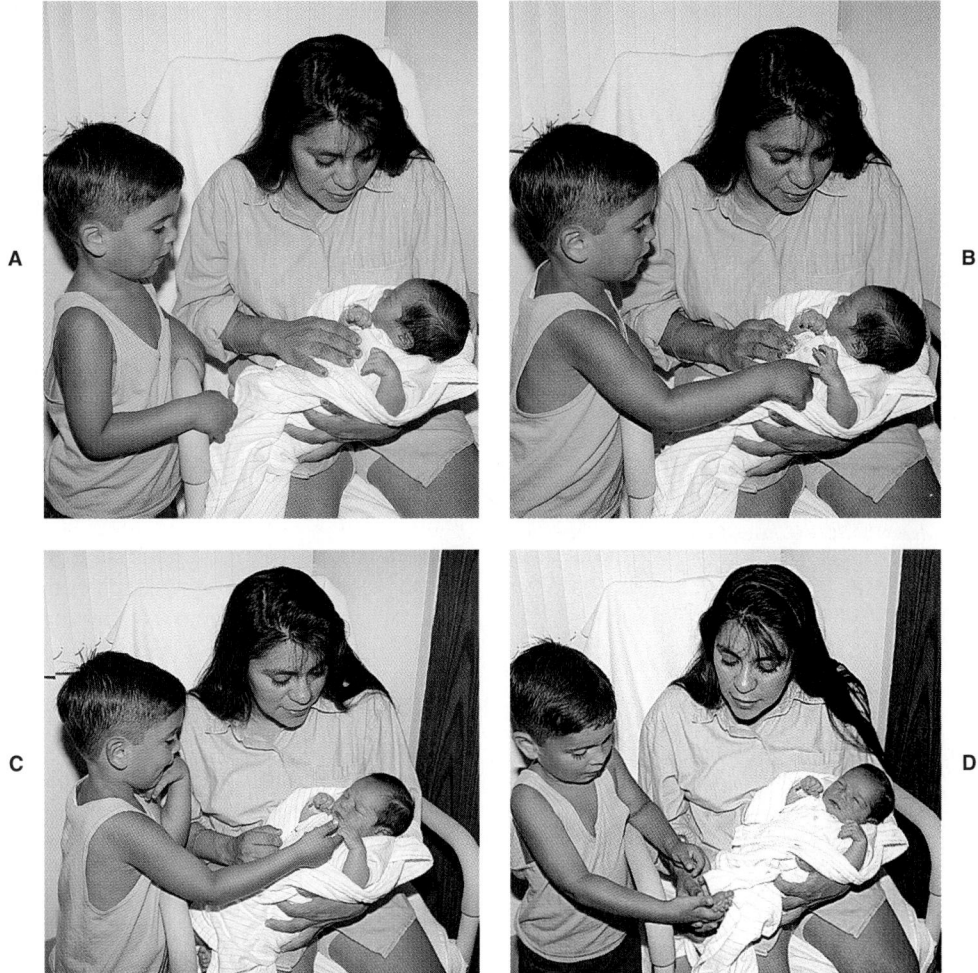

Fig. 25-13 First meeting. **A,** Boy with mother during first meeting with new sibling. **B,** First tentative touch. **C,** Testing with fingertip. **D,** Relationship more secure: it is now okay to hold with whole hand. *(Courtesy Marjorie Pyle, RNC, Lifecircle, Costa Mesa, CA.)*

tions of themselves that cause them to be very self-critical (Hansen & Jacob, 1992).

The extent of involvement of grandparents in the care of the newborn depends on many factors, for example, the willingness of the grandparents to become involved, the proximity of the grandparents, and ethnic and cultural expectations of the grandparents' role. If the new parents live in the United States, Asian grandparents, for example, typically are asked to come to the United States to care for the baby and the mother after birth and to care for the children once the parents return to work. In the United States, paternal grandparents, in contrast to those in other cultures, frequently consider themselves secondary to the maternal grandparents. Less seems expected of them and they are initially less involved. Nevertheless, these grandparents are eager to help and express great pleasure in their son's

fatherhood and his involvement with the baby. Support that they provide for their son has been shown to be positively related to his support of the new mother and to a smoother parental adjustment for the new parents (Hansen & Jacob, 1992).

For first-time parents, pregnancy and parenthood can reawaken old issues related to dependence versus independence. From interviews with expectant parents, Hansen and Jacob (1992) found that the couples did not plan on their parents' help immediately after the baby arrived. They wanted time "to be a family," inferring a couple-baby unit, not the intergenerational family network. Intergenerational help was perceived to be interference. Contrary to their expectations, however, these new parents did call on their parents for help. The majority of maternal grandmothers were present soon after the birth, being called in on short notice by the parents af-

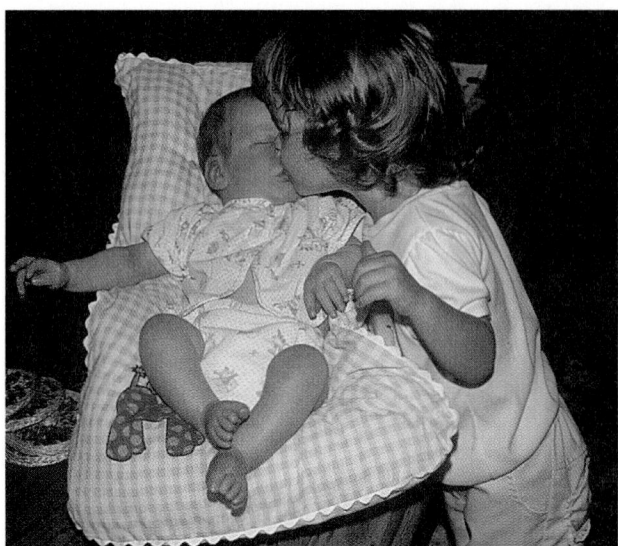

Fig. 25-14 Sister kisses her new brother. Family contacts are important for newborn and siblings. *(Courtesy Marjorie Pyle, RNC, Lifecircle, Costa Mesa, CA.)*

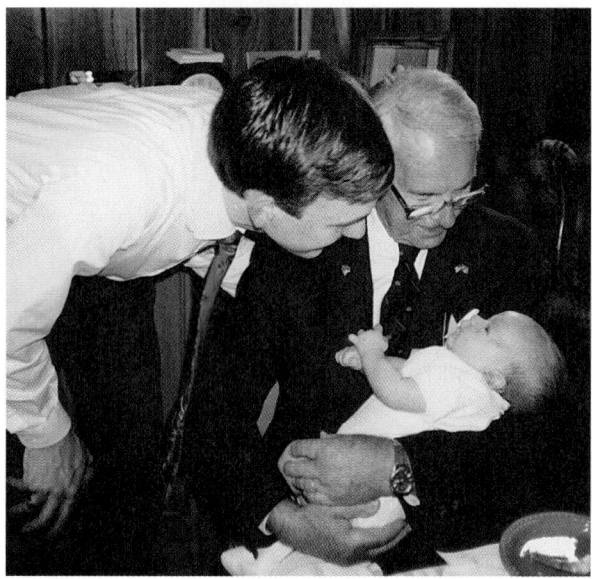

Fig. 25-15 Father, grandfather, and new grandson get acquainted. *(Courtesy Eric Schult.)*

ter several nights with a crying baby. Grandparents, respecting their children's wishes for autonomy while remaining available, provided most of the support.

As parents are assisted in working through differing opinions and unresolved conflicts (e.g., feelings of dependency and control) between themselves and their parents, they can move toward mastery of the developmental tasks of adulthood. The support of grandparents can be a stabilizing influence for families undergoing developmental transitions such as childbearing and new

parenthood (Hansen & Jacob, 1992; Strom et al., 1992-1993). Grandparents can foster the learning of parental skills and preserve tradition. The maternal grandmother is an important model for child-rearing practices, a source of knowledge, and a support person. In the case of teenage mothers, the regular assistance of grandparents with child care has allowed these young mothers to continue their educations (Unger & Cooley, 1992).

Nurses should be aware that the transition to parenthood and grandparenthood offers and demands new intergenerational adaptations. Rather than taking for granted intergenerational support between adult children and their parents, nurses must acknowledge the wide range of dynamic issues that enhance or mitigate experiences of intergenerational support. Early in pregnancy, a family assessment that includes an intergenerational perspective can identify whether grandparents are included in the couple's social support network and whether their support is wanted and helpful.

One simple technique to help people span the generation gap is through a printed "letter to new parents" (written from the grandparents' perspective), which can be included in prenatal kits distributed in childbirth preparation classes and made available to all family members on the postpartum unit. Another way to help grandparents bridge the generation gap and understand their adult children's parenting concepts is to offer classes. Included in these classes would be information about up-to-date childbearing practices (especially family-centered care); infant care, feeding, and safety (car seats); and exploration of roles that grandparents play in the family unit. Both techniques can foster open discussion between the generations about the feelings and needs of parents and grandparents.

CARE MANAGEMENT: PRACTICAL SUGGESTIONS FOR THE FIRST WEEKS AT HOME

Numerous changes occur during the first weeks of parenthood. Care management should be directed toward helping parents cope with infant care, role changes, altered lifestyle, and change in family structure resulting from the addition of a new baby. Parents may have inadequate or incorrect understanding of what to expect in the early postpartum weeks. Developing skill and confidence in caring for an infant can be especially anxiety provoking.

Nurses, especially those making postpartum visits to parents' homes, are in a prime position to help new families. The nurse's role becomes primarily one of teacher-supporter, focusing on enabling new parents to become capable of self-care and infant care and of meeting the needs of the family unit.

Assessment and Nursing Diagnoses

Assessment should include a psychosocial assessment focusing on parent-infant attachment, adjustment to the parental role, sibling adjustment, social support, and education needs, as well as mother's and baby's physical adaptation. Early home visits are an excellent opportunity for the nurse to assess beginnings of successful or harmful parenting behaviors. Parents demonstrating loving and nurturing behaviors with their infant need to be given positive reinforcement. Parents who interact in inappropriate or abusive ways with their infant should be followed more closely, and an appropriate mental health practitioner or professional social worker should be notified (Johnson & Johnson, 1996).

Home visits often offer an opportunity to involve all family members. The mother, father, siblings, and even grandparents may ask questions and express concerns. The nurse can share her assessments and observations and develop a plan of care collaboratively with the family. Nursing diagnoses pertinent to the period of transition to parenthood include the following:

▮ Nursing Diagnoses

- Family coping: potential for growth related to
  - positive attitude and realistic expectations for newborn and adapting to parenthood
  - nurturing behaviors with newborn
  - verbalizing positive, joyous factors in lifestyle change; perceived strong and satisfying social support system
- Ineffective family coping; ineffective individual coping related to
  - disorganization and role change during assumption of parent role and adaptation to parenthood
  - unrealistic expectations of newborn/infant and family life changes
  - lack of social support system or perceived dissatisfaction with social support system
  - fatigue and interrupted sleep
- Risk for altered parenting related to
  - lack of knowledge of infant care
  - feelings of incompetence and/or lack of confidence
  - unrealistic expectations of newborn/infant
  - lack of satisfying social support systems
  - fatigue from interrupted sleep
- Parental role conflict related to
  - role transition and role attainment
  - unwanted pregnancy
  - lack of resources to support parenting (e.g., hourly wage earner without paid leave)
  - unplanned pregnancy interfering with professional career
- Risk for altered parent-infant attachment related to
  - difficult labor and birth
  - postpartum complications
  - neonatal complications/anomalies
  - unrealistic expectations of newborn
  - lack of knowledge
  - lack of satisfying social support system

Expected Outcomes of Care

A plan of care is formulated in collaboration with the family, incorporating their priorities and preferences, to meet their specific needs. Goals are set and prioritized. Expected outcomes for effective transition to parenthood include that the parents will do the following:

- Interact with the newborn in a loving and nurturing way.
- Demonstrate behaviors that reflect appreciation of sensory and behavioral capacities of the infant.
- Respond appropriately to infant cues.
- Verbalize increasing confidence and competence in feeding, diapering, dressing, and sensory stimulation of the infant.
- Identify deviations from normal in the infant that should be brought to the immediate attention of the primary health care provider.
- Relate not only stressful or challenging factors in lifestyle change, but also positive and joyous ones.
- Describe or demonstrate emergency procedures and verbalize ways of getting emergency help.
- Interact in a supportive manner.
- Collaborate effectively with each other in caring for the newborn and other children.
- Relate effectively to the newborn's grandparents and siblings.

Plan of Care and Interventions

Instructions for the First Days at Home

Parents, especially first-time parents, must be helped to anticipate what the transition from hospital to home will be like. Anticipatory guidance can help prevent a shock of reality that might negate the parents' joy or cause them undue stress. Even the simplest strategies can provide enormous support. Written information reinforcing education topics is helpful to provide to parents, as is a list of available community resources, both local and national (Box 25-5). An excellent resource for the nurse is the *Compendium of Postpartum Care*, developed by Johnson and Johnson Products, Inc., in association with the Association of Women's Health, Obstetric, and Neonatal Nurses (1996). Postpartum nurses will find the "Patient Handouts" section especially useful. It includes handouts on topics such as rest and exercise, emotional well-being during adaptation to parenthood, understanding the blues, and what to expect and do regarding the infant's health. Classes in the prenatal period or during the postpartum stay are helpful. Instructions for the first days at home should minimally include activities of daily living, dealing with visitors, and activity and rest.

Activities of daily living. Given the demands of a newborn, the mother's discomfort or fatigue associated with giving birth, and a busy homecoming day, even small details of daily life can become stressful. Such things as using disposable diapers, preparing frozen and/or microwave dinners, or getting takeout meals, can decrease stress by

The Fatherhood Project at the Families and Work Institute
330 Seventh Avenue
New York, NY 10001
(212) 465-2044

The Institute for Responsible Fatherhood and Family Revitalization
1146 19th Street NW
Suite 800
Washington, DC 20036
(800) 7-FATHER or (800) 732-8437

At-Home Dad (newsletter for fathers who stay at home)
61 Brightwood Avenue
North Andover, MA 01845-1702
E-mail: athomedad@aol.com

Postpartum Support International
927 North Kellogg Avenue
Santa Barbara, CA 93111
(805) 967-7636

La Leche League International
1400 North Meacham Road
Schaumburg, IL 60173
(847) 519-7730
(Local La Leche League groups are usually listed in city and town phone books)

Motherhood Maternity Health and Fitness Program
SBI Corporation
1106 Stratford Drive
Carlisle, PA 17013
(717) 258-4641

Single Parent Resource Center
141 West 28th Street
Suite 302
New York, NY 10001
(212) 947-0221

Pink Inc.! Publishing
P.O. Box 866
Atlantic Beach, FL 32233-0866
(904) 731-7120

eliminating at least one or two parental responsibilities during the first few days at home.

Visitors. New parents are often inadequately prepared for the reality of bringing a new infant home because they romanticize the homecoming. One mother stated, "By the time we drove an hour through traffic, my stitches were hurting and all I wanted was a warm sitz bath and some private time with Bill and the baby, in that order. Instead, a carload of visitors pulled into the driveway as we were unbuckling the baby from his car seat. I thought I would surely cry."

The nurse can help parents explore ways, in advance, to assert their need to limit visitors. When family and friends ask what they can do to help, new parents can suggest they prepare and bring them a meal or pick up items at the store. Parents can work out a signal for alerting the partner that the mother is getting tired or uncomfortable and needs the partner to invite the visitors to another room or to leave. Some mothers find that wearing a robe and not appearing ready for company leads visitors to stay a shorter time. A sign on the front door saying, "Mother and baby resting. . . . Please do not disturb" may be useful.

Activity and rest. Because mothers have reported fatigue as a major problem during the first few weeks after giving birth, mothers need to be encouraged to limit their activities and be realistic about their level of fatigue. Activities should not be sustained for long periods of time. Family, friends, and neighbors can be solicited for support and help with meals, housecleaning, picking up other children, etc. Rest periods throughout the day are important. Mothers can nap when the baby sleeps. Adequate nutrition is also important for postpartum recovery and in dealing with fatigue.

On postpartum days 1 through 3, mothers can begin a regimen of light exercise, especially Kegel and isometric abdominal muscle-toning exercises. Many new mothers have concerns about body image. The nurse can help new mothers develop realistic expectations of how quickly and to what extent their bodies will return to the nonpregnant state.

New parents also need to develop realistic expectations about resumption of their sexual life. Nurses need to let couples know that it is normal to feel that their sex life is somewhat limited by fatigue, the baby's needs, and the woman's physical recovery and emotional changes. It is helpful for the nurse to bring up the subject, since many couples are reluctant to do so.

Infant Care

Providing practical suggestions for infant care can help parents adjust to parenthood. Mothers and fathers want to feel capable and confident in the physical care of their infant. The nurse should assess each parent's need for instruction on care such as bathing, clothing, and safety (see Guidelines/Guías box).

Infant bathing. The infant bath time provides a wonderful opportunity for parent-infant social interaction. Some fathers consider this their own special time with their babies. While bathing their baby, parents can talk to the infant, caress and cuddle the infant, and engage in arousal and imitation of facial expressions and smiling (Fig. 25-16).

GUIDELINES/GUÍAS

Daily Care

BATHING

Bathing two or three times a week is enough, using a mild soap like Johnson's, Dove, Tone, or Purpose. Sponge bathe the baby until the umbilical cord falls off and the belly button looks healed. Never leave the baby alone in the tub or sink!

Necesita bañar a su bebé dos o tres veces a la semana. Use un jabón suave como Johnson's, Dove, Tone, o Purpose. Lávelo con un paño o con una esponja de cuerpo suave hasta que se caiga el cordón umbilical y parece ser curado y seco el ombligo. ¡Nunca deje al bebé solo el la bañera o en el lavabo!

CLOTHING

The best clothing is soft and made of cotton. Dress your baby lightly when indoors and on hot days. Too many layers of clothing or blankets can make the baby too hot. On cold days, cover the baby's head when you go outdoors.

La mejor ropa para su bebé debe ser suave y hecha de algodón. No le ponga mucha ropa al bebé cuando esté dentro de la casa o en los días calientes. Demasiada ropa o mantas puede darle calor al bebé. En los días de frio, póngale una capa en la cabeza.

CAR SEATS

Use a real car seat (not a baby carrier for the house). It should face the rear of the car until the baby is 1 year old. Always place the car seat in the back seat of the car. Make sure the shoulder straps are snug enough that they don't fall off the baby's shoulders. Car seats are required until age 4.

Use un asiento de coche que está hecho para un coche. El asiento debe mirar hacia la parte atrás del coche hasta que el bebé tenga un año. Siempre ponga el bebé en el asiento atrás del coche. Los cinturones deben estar apretados pero no deben limitar los movimientos del bebé. Se requiere por ley usar los asientos de coche hasta que el bebé tenga cuatro años.

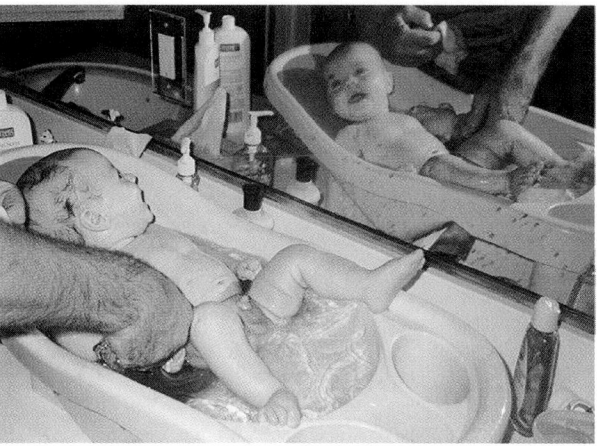

A

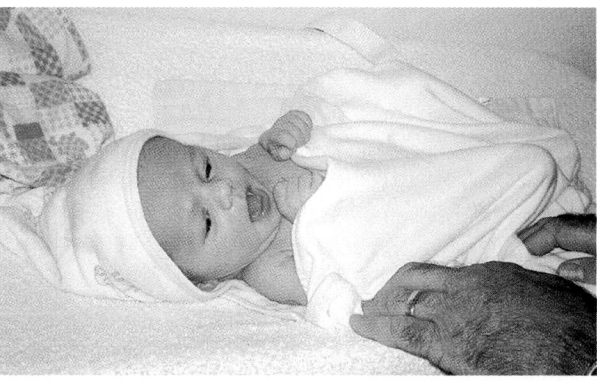

B

Fig. 25-16 A, Baths can be special times for babies and parents. **B,** After the bath, the baby is gently dried to minimize heat loss. *(Courtesy Leslie Canerday, Phoenix, AZ.)*

BOX 25-6 Tub Bathing

See guidelines for sponge bathing (see Chapter 27).

Place liner on bottom of tub to prevent infant from slipping.

Add 3 inches of comfortably warm water (36.6° to 37.2° C—pleasantly warm to your inner wrist).

Wash face and shampoo hair as for sponge bath. Undress baby. Lower infant slowly into water.

Hold baby safely with fingers under the baby's armpit, with your thumb around the shoulder. The other hand supports the baby's bottom and legs.

Wash the front of the baby.

Go from front to back between the legs. Rinse with a wet washcloth.

Wash the baby's back with your free hand lathered with soap.

Rinse well with the wet washcloth.

Remove infant from the water and gently pat dry.

Sponge baths are used until the infant's umbilical cord falls off and the umbilicus is healed (see Chapter 27 for the Home Care box on sponge baths). At about 10 to 14 days, tub baths can be started (Box 25-6). Newborns do not need a bath every day. The diaper area and creases under the arms and neck need more attention. Parents can pick a time that is easy for them and when the baby is awake, usually before a feeding.

Questions have arisen about some routine practices: use of soap, lotion, oil, and powder. An important consideration in skin cleansing is preservation of the skin's acid mantle. The acid mantle is formed from the uppermost horny layer of the epidermis, sweat, superficial fat, metabolic products, and external substances such as amniotic fluid, microorganisms, and cosmetics. By 4 days of age, the newborn skin surface becomes more acidic, falling to within the bacteriostatic range (pH 5). Thus only plain, warm water should be used. Alkaline soaps (such as Ivory), oils, powders, and many lotions alter the acid mantle and provide a medium for bacterial growth. Powders are not recommended, because the infant can inhale powder.

Infant clothing. Parents commonly ask how warmly they should dress their infant. A simple rule of thumb is to dress the child as the parents would dress themselves, adding or subtracting clothes and wraps for the infant as necessary. A shirt and diaper may be sufficient clothing for the young infant. A bonnet is needed to protect the scalp and to minimize heat loss if it is cool or to protect against sunburn and to shade the infant's eyes if it is sunny and hot. Sunglasses for infants are available. Wrapping the infant snugly in a blanket maintains body temperature and promotes a feeling of security. Overdressing in warm temperatures can cause discomfort and prickly heat rash. Underdressing in cold weather also can cause discomfort; cheeks, fingers, and toes can easily become frostbitten.

Infants have sensitive skin; therefore new clothes should be washed before putting them on the infant. Baby clothes should be washed with a mild detergent and hot water. A double rinse usually removes traces of the potentially irritating cleansing agent or acid residue from urine or stool. If possible, the clothing and bed linens are dried in the sun to neutralize residue. Parents who have to use coin-operated machines in laundromats to wash and dry clothes may find it expensive or impossible to wash and rinse the baby's clothes well.

Bedding requires frequent changing. The top of a plastic-coated mattress should be washed frequently, and the crib or bassinet should be dusted with a damp cloth. The infant's toilet articles may be kept convenient for use in a box, basket, or plastic carrier.

Infant safety. Providing for the safety of an infant is not a matter of common sense. There are many things new parents may not be aware of that are potential dangers to their infant (e.g., window blind cords near the crib or a parent throwing an infant in the air during play). Nurses should provide parents with concrete instructions on infant safety (Box 25-7). An excellent resource for the nurse is *Protecting Your Newborn, Video and Instructor's Guide,* produced in 1997 by the Ford Motor Company and the U.S.

Department of Transportation National Highway Traffic Safety Administration (NHTSA). This guide includes a pamphlet with color pictures demonstrating the correct use of infant and child car seats and a set of handouts on child passenger safety tips (see Fig. 27-26 and 27-27). The NHTSA also has a toll-free Auto Safety Hotline (800-424-9393) and a Web page (www.nhtsa.dot.gov) for parents to use.

Anticipatory Guidance Regarding the Newborn

Anticipatory guidance helps prepare new parents for what to expect as their newborn grows and develops. Parents with realistic expectations of infant needs and behavior are prepared better to adjust to the demands of a new baby and to parenthood itself.

In giving anticipatory guidance, the nurse should not try to cover all content at one time. New parents can be overwhelmed by a large volume of information and become anxious. Printed materials and audiotapes and/or videotapes for parents to take home are helpful as well. These resources (1) reinforce content discussed in the hospital, (2) allow parents another chance to review the material in private and at their own pace, and (3) provide new information not covered in the hospital. Anticipatory guidance needs to include the following: newborn sleep-wake cycles, interpretation of crying and quieting techniques, infant developmental milestones, sensory enrichment/infant stimulation, recognizing signs of illness, and well-baby follow-up and immunizations.

Development of day-night routines. Nurses can help prepare new parents for the fact that most newborns cannot tell the difference between night and day and must learn the rhythm of day-night routines. Nurses should provide basic suggestions for settling a newborn and for helping him or her develop a predictable routine. Examples of such suggestions include:

- In the late afternoon, bring the baby out to the center of family activity. Keep the baby there for the rest of the evening. If the baby falls asleep, let the baby do so in the infant seat or in someone's arms. Save the crib or bassinet for nighttime sleep.
- Give the baby a bath right before bedtime. This soothes the baby and helps him or her expend energy.
- Feed the baby for the last evening time around 11 PM and put him or her to bed in the crib or bassinet.
- For nighttime feedings and diaper changes, keep a small night-light on to avoid turning on bright lights. Talk in soft whispers (if at all) and handle the baby gently and only as absolutely necessary to feed and diaper. Night-time feedings should be all business and no play! Babies usually go back to sleep if the room is quiet and dark.

A predictable, stable routine gradually develops for most babies; however, there will be some babies who never develop one. New parents will find it easier if they are will-

BOX 25-7 Tips for Keeping Your Baby Safe

- Never leave your baby alone on a bed, couch, or table. Even newborns can move enough to eventually reach the edge and fall off.
- Never put your baby on a cushion, pillow, beanbag, or waterbed to sleep. Your baby may suffocate. Also, do not keep pillows, large floppy toys, or loose plastic sheeting in the crib.
- Do not place your infant on his or her stomach to sleep during the first few months of life. The American Academy of Pediatrics advises against this prone position because it has been associated with an increased incidence of sudden infant death syndrome (SIDS). The side-lying or back-lying position is preferable.
- When using an infant carrier, stay within arm's reach when the carrier is on a high place, such as a table, sofa, or store counter. If at all possible, place the carrier on the floor near you.
- Infant carriers do not keep your baby safe in a car. Always place your baby in an approved car safety seat when traveling in a motor vehicle (car, truck, bus, or van). Car safety seats are recommended for travel on trains and airplanes as well. Use the car seat for *every* ride. Your baby should be in a rear-facing infant car seat from birth to 20 pounds, and the car seat should be in the back seat of the car (see Fig. 27-26). This is especially important in vehicles with front passenger air bags, because when air bags inflate they can be fatal for infants and toddlers (see Fig. 27-27).

- When bathing your baby, never leave him or her alone. Newborns and infants can drown in 1 to 2 inches of water.
- Be sure that your hot water heater is set at 49° C or less. Always check bathwater temperature with your elbow before putting your baby in the bath.
- Do not tie anything around your baby's neck. Pacifiers, for example, tied around the neck with a ribbon or string may strangle your baby.
- Check your baby's crib for safety. Slats should be no more than $2\frac{1}{2}$ inches apart. The space between the mattress and sides should be less than 2 finger widths. There should be no decorative knobs on the bedposts.
- Keep crib or playpen away from window blind and drapery cords; your baby could strangle on them.
- Keep crib and playpen well away from radiators, heat vents, and portable heaters. Linens in crib or playpen could catch fire if in contact with these heat sources.
- Install smoke detectors on every floor of your home. Check them once a month to be sure they work. Change batteries once a year.
- Avoid exposing your baby to cigarette or cigar smoke in your home or other places. Passive exposure to tobacco smoke greatly increases the likelihood that your infant will have respiratory symptoms and illnesses.
- Be gentle with your baby. Do not pick your baby up or swing your baby by the arms or throw him or her up in the air.

---

ing to be flexible and to give up some control during those early weeks.

Interpretation of crying and quieting techniques. Crying is an infant's first social communication. Some babies cry more than others, but all babies cry. They cry to communicate that they are hungry, uncomfortable, wet, ill, or bored, and sometimes for no apparent reason at all. The longer parents are around their infants, the easier it becomes to interpret what a cry means. Many infants have a fussy period during the day, often in the late afternoon or early evening when everyone is naturally tired. Environmental tension adds to the length and intensity of crying spells. Babies also have periods of vigorous crying where no comforting can help. These periods of crying may last for long stretches until the infants seem to cry themselves to sleep. Possibly the infants are trying to discharge enough energy so that they can settle themselves down. The nurse needs to reinforce for new parents that time and infant maturation will take care of these types of cries.

Crying because of colic is a common concern of new parents. Babies with colic cry inconsolably for several

hours, pull their legs up to their stomach, and pass large amounts of gas. No one really knows what colic is or why babies get it. Parents can be encouraged to contact their nurse-practitioner or pediatrician if they are concerned that their baby has colic.

Developmentalists studying the roots of human behavior have long recognized that certain types of sensory stimulation can calm and quiet infants and help them get to sleep. Important characteristics of this sensory stimulation—whether tactile, vestibular, auditory, or visual—appear to be that the stimulation is mild, slow, and rhythmic, and consistently and regularly presented. Tactile stimulation can include warmth, patting, back rubbing, and covering the skin with textured cloth. Swaddling to keep arms and legs close to the body (as in utero) provides widespread and constant tactile stimulation and a sense of security. Vestibular stimulation is especially effective and can be accomplished by mild rhythmic movement such as rocking or by holding the infant upright, as on the parent's shoulder.

The nurse can teach parents a number of strategies that help quiet a fussy baby, prevent crying, and induce quiet attention or sleep (Boxes 25-8 and 25-9).

BOX 25-8 | How to Swaddle an Infant

1. Fold down the top corner of the blanket. Position the infant on the blanket with the infant's neck near the fold.
2. Bring the blanket around the infant's right side and across the infant, tucking the corner under the left side.
3. Bring the bottom of the blanket up to the infant's chest.
4. Bring the remaining corner of the blanket across the infant, tucking the corner under the infant's right side. The infant should be wrapped securely but not tightly; some room should be left for the infant to move.

Developmental milestones. Knowledge of infant growth and development helps parents have realistic expectations of what an infant can do. When parents understand and appreciate the limitations and developing abilities of their infant, adjustment to parenthood can go more smoothly. Emphasizing the individuality of the infant enhances the capacity of the family to offer their infant an optimally nurturing environment (Brazelton, 1995).

Nurses can play a crucial role in the success of a family system through efforts to enable new parents to understand and enhance their baby's development. For this role, Brazelton (1995) suggests the concept of "touch-points" for intervention, that is, points at which a change in the system (baby, parent, and family) is brought about by the baby's spurts in development (cognitive, motor, or emotional).

Immediately before each spurt in development, there is a predictable short period of disorganization in the baby. Parents are likely to feel disorganized and stressed as well. Because these periods of disorganization are predictable, nurses can offer parents anticipatory guidance to help them understand what happens with infant development and to prepare them for the subsequent spurts in development (see Guidelines/Guías box).

Two touchpoints occur during the early postpartum-newborn period: one soon after birth and another at 2 to 3 weeks (Brazelton, 1995). In the hospital or at a home visit during the first week, the nurse can use Brazelton's Neonatal Behavioral Assessment Scale (Brazelton & Nugent, 1996) to demonstrate to parents their baby's amazing repertoire of abilities. In this way, parents begin to appreciate their baby's individuality and become more sensitive to their baby's behavioral cues. At 2 to 3 weeks, the home care nurse or pediatric office nurse should assess for the regular end-of-the-day fussy period that most infants have between 3 and 12 weeks of age. Helpful topics to include in the anticipatory guidance are (1) the normalcy and positive value of the fussy period, (2) how to settle a fussy baby, and (3) ways to help a baby develop a predictable schedule.

BOX 25-9 | Infant Quieting Techniques

- Many newborns feel insecure in the center of a large crib. They prefer a small, warm, soft space that reminds them of intrauterine life. Try a smaller bed, such as a bassinet, portable crib, buggy, or cradle, or use a rolled-up blanket to turn a corner of the big crib into a smaller place.
- Carry your baby in a frontpack or backpack.
- Swaddle your newborn snugly in a receiving blanket. Swaddling keeps your newborn's arms and legs close to his or her body, similar to the intrauterine position. It makes the newborn feel more secure.
- Prewarm the crib sheets with a hot water bottle or heating pad that you remove before putting your baby to bed. Some babies startle when placed on a cold sheet.
- Some newborns need extra sucking to soothe themselves to sleep. Breastfeeding mothers may prefer to let their infant suckle at the breast as a soothing technique. Other mothers choose to use a pacifier. Stroke the pacifier against the roof of the baby's mouth to encourage him or her to suck it during the first 2 weeks. Around 3 months of age, infants become able to consistently find and suck their thumbs as a way of self-consoling.
- A rhythmic, monotonous noise simulating the intrauterine sounds of your heartbeat and blood flow may help your infant settle down. Some parents have found that putting the baby in a portable crib beside the dishwasher or washing machine helps settle a fussy baby.
- Movement often helps quiet a baby. Take your baby for a ride in the car, or take your baby for an outing in a stroller or carriage. Rock your baby in a rocking chair or cradle.
- Place your baby on his or her stomach across your lap; pat and rub his or her back while gently bouncing your legs or swaying them from left to right.
- Babies enjoy close skin-to-skin contact. A combination of this and warm water often helps soothe a fussy baby. Fill your tub with warm water. Get in and let the baby lie on your chest so that the baby is immersed in the water up to his or her neck. Cuddle the baby close.
- Let your baby see your face. Talk to your baby in a soothing voice.
- Your baby may simply be bored. Bring him or her into the room where you and the rest of the family are. Change your baby's position; many babies like to be upright, such as being held up on your shoulder.

It is also helpful for nurses to provide parents with information on month-by-month infant growth and development. Written information that parents can refer to later is especially helpful. See Table 25-6 for a summary of

✳ GUIDELINES/GUÍAS

General Advice

CRYING

Babies cry when they are hungry; need to burp; have a wet diaper; feel cold, hot, tired, bored, or overstimulated; and (rarely) when they are sick or in pain. After a while you will learn the meaning of your baby's different cries. Be careful not to feed him every time he cries, since overfeeding causes tummy aches. Check to see if he needs burping or a new diaper. It is not harmful to let a baby cry for short periods (5 to 10 minutes). This may be what he needs to fall asleep.

Todos los bebés lloran cuando tienen hambre; cuando necesitan eructar; cuando necesitan que le cambia el pañal; cuando tienen calor o frío; cuando están cansados, aburridos, o sobreestimulados; y cuando están enfermos o tienen un dolor. Después de un tiempo, usted aprenderá los modos varios que tiene su bebé de llorar y podrá distinguir entre cada uno de ellos para saber lo que necesita. No le dé de comer cada vez que llore porque si come demasiado le puede dar dolor de estómago. Mire a ver si está mojado el pañal o si necesita eructar. No le hará ningún daño al bebé si llora por cinco o diez minutos. Puede ser que esto sea justo lo que necesita para quedarse dormido.

SLEEPING

Most babies can sleep through most of the night without a feeding by 4 to 5 months of age. You can help your baby sleep by keeping things quiet and dark at night. Both you and he will usually sleep better and wake up less often if he is sleeping in a separate bed. If your baby stirs at night but doesn't fully wake up, give him a chance to fall back asleep by himself. Only get him up if he stays wide awake and seems hungry. The baby should sleep on his side or back for safety. Babies sleeping on their tummies seem to be more prone to crib death.

La mayoría de los bebés pueden dormir la noche entera sin comer cuando tienen algunos meses de edad. Un domicilio quieto y calmo ayuda a su bebé dormir tranquilo. Se duermen mejor (y se despiertan menos) si usted y el bebé están en camas separadas. Si se despierta el bebé durante la noche, dele la oportunidad de dormirse de nuevo. Pero si se queda despierto y tiene hambre, atiéndalo. La posición de dormir más segura para los infantes es en la espalda con la boca para arriba. Los bebés que duermen en los estómagos con la boca para abajo tienen un riesgo más grande de morir en la camita de niño.

SPITTING UP

Most babies spit up a little after feedings. If your baby is gaining weight, this is normal. It helps to keep your baby upright and quiet for a few minutes after feedings. If your baby seems to be spitting up a lot, bring him to your doctor for a weight check.

La mayoría de los bebés echan a fuera un poco de la leche después de comer o cuando eructan. Esto es normal si su bebé está aumentando de peso. Es bueno mantenerlo recto y quieto por unos minutos después de darle de comer. Si parece que está echando mucha leche o si lo hace con mucha frecuencia, llévelo al doctor para que lo pese.

---

infant growth and development during the first 2 to 3 months.

Infant stimulation. Interacting with their parents is an important way in which infants learn about themselves and their environment. Nurses can teach parents a variety of ways to stimulate their infant's development and to enrich the infant's learning environment. Home health nurses are in a prime position to evaluate the home environment and to make suggestions to parents for promotion of their baby's physical, cognitive, and emotional development. Suggestions for teaching infants during the first few months are presented in Boxes 25-10 and 25-11. Table 25-7 presents suggestions for visual, auditory, tactile, and kinetic stimulation.

Another method of sensory enrichment that parents can learn to use is infant massage. This type of nurturing touch can help create a loving bond between the infant and parent and has been shown to contribute to the physical and emotional well-being of the massage giver and receiver (Schneider, 1996, 1997). Infant massage is not manipulative, but a gentle, warm communication. It is done with the infant, not to the infant, the focus being on reciprocal interaction between infant and parent. The parent talks to the infant, asks permission to start the massage, questions the infant, and facilitates dialogue.

Schneider (1997) outlines the many benefits of infant massage (Box 25-12); one of the most important for the parents is the improved ability to read their infant's cues. Positive cues include eye contact, smiling, looking at the parent's face, babbling or cooing, and smooth movements of arms and legs. Negative cues from the infant include pulling away, frowning,

Text continued on p. 664

TABLE 25-6 Growth and Development During Infancy

1 MONTH	2 MONTHS	3 MONTHS
PHYSICAL		
Weight gain of 150 to 210 g weekly for first 6 mo	Posterior fontanel closed	Primitive reflexes fading
Height gain of 2.5 cm monthly for first 6 mo	Crawling reflex disappears	
Head circumference increases by 1.5 cm monthly for first 6 mo		
Primitive reflexes present and strong		
Doll's eye reflex and dance reflex fading		
Preferential nose breathing (most infants)		
GROSS MOTOR		
• Assumes flexed position with pelvis high but knees not under abdomen when prone (at birth, knees flexed under abdomen)	• Assumes less flexed position when prone—hips flat, legs extended, arms flexed, head to side	Able to hold head more erect when sitting, but still bobs forward
• Can turn head from side to side when prone, lifts head momentarily from bed	Less head lag when pulled to sitting position	Has only slight head lag when pulled to sitting position
Has marked head lag, especially when pulled from lying to sitting position	Can maintain head in same plane as rest of body when held in ventral suspension	Assumes symmetric body positioning
Holds head momentarily parallel and in midline when suspended in prone position	When prone, can lift head almost 45 degrees off table	Able to raise head and shoulders from prone position to a 45- to 90-degree angle from table; bears weight on forearms
Assumes asymmetric tonic neck reflex position when supine	When held in sitting position, head is held up but bobs forward	When held in standing position, able to bear slight fraction of weight on legs
When held in standing position, body limp at knees and hips	Assumes asymmetric tonic neck reflex position intermittently	Regards own hand
In sitting position back is uniformly rounded, absence of head control		
FINE MOTOR		
Hands predominantly closed	Hands often open	• Actively holds rattle but will not reach for it
Grasp reflex strong	Grasp reflex fading	Grasp reflex absent
Hand clenches on contact with rattle		Hands kept loosely open
		Clutches own hand; pulls at blanket and clothes
SENSORY		
• Able to fixate on moving object in range of 45 degrees when held at a distance of 20-25 cm	Binocular fixation and convergence to near objects beginning	• Follows object to periphery (180 degrees)
Visual acuity approaches 20/100*	When supine, follows dangling toy from side to point beyond midline	• Locates sound by turning head to side and looking in same direction
Follows light to midline	Visually searches to locate sounds	Begins to have ability to coordinate stimuli from various sense organs
Quiets when hears a voice	Turns head to side when sound is made at level of ear	

From Wong, D. (1999). *Whaley & Wong's nursing care of infants and children* (6th ed.). St. Louis: Mosby.
•Milestones that represent essential integrative aspects of development that lay the foundation for the achievement of more advanced skills.
*Degree of visual acuity varies according to vision measurement procedure used.

TABLE 25-6 Growth and Development During Infancy—cont'd

I MONTH	2 MONTHS	3 MONTHS
VOCALIZATION		
Cries to express displeasure	• Vocalizes, distinct from crying	• Squeals aloud to show pleasure
Makes small throaty sounds	Crying becomes differentiated	Coos, babbles, chuckles
	Coos	Vocalizes when smiling
		"Talks" a great deal when spoken to
Makes comfort sounds during feeding	Vocalizes to familiar voice	Less crying during periods of wakefulness
SOCIALIZATION/COGNITION		
Is in sensorimotor phase—stage I, use of reflexes (birth-1 mo), and stage II, primary circular reactions (1-4 mo)	• Demonstrates social smile in response to various stimuli	Displays considerable interest in surroundings
Watches parent's face intently as she or he talks to infant		Ceases crying when parent enters room
		Can recognize familiar faces and objects, such as feeding bottle
		Shows awareness of strange situations

BOX 25-10 Teaching Your Newborn

- Newborns learn things every day. You can teach your newborn by playing with him or her and giving your newborn toys that help him or her to learn.
- Talk to your baby a lot. Tell your baby what is going on in the room ("Listen to the dog barking."). Label objects that you see or use ("Here's the washcloth.") and describe things you are doing ("Let's put the shirt over Kerry's head!").
- Look at your baby's face and make eye contact. Play face-making games: smile, stick out your tongue, open your eyes wide. As your baby gets older, he or she will try to imitate these facial expressions.
- Babies like music and rhythmic movement. Rock or swing your baby as you sing to him or her in a gentle voice.

- Acknowledge your baby's attempts to "answer" your talking and singing. He or she will respond to you by looking in your direction, making eye contact, moving his or her arms and legs, and/or making sounds.
- Babies like bright colors and vivid contrasts. Show your baby pictures and objects that are black and white, bright primary colors (red, blue, yellow, green), and/or large patterns. Keep colorful mobiles and toys where your baby can see them.
- Babies like to be held upright. Holding your newborn on your shoulder lets your baby look around his or her world and provides vestibular stimulation. Let your baby lift his or her head for a few seconds. Keep your hand ready to support your baby's head.

BOX 25-11 Teaching Your 1- to 2-Month-Old Infant

At 1 to 2 months of age, your infant is gaining more control of his or her movements: more head control, even holding an object briefly in his or her hand. Your baby also is becoming more social. He or she demonstrates behaviors to engage you in interaction: smiling, cooing, making longer eye contact, and following you with his or her eyes.

During these months you can help your baby learn if you:

- Put your baby on his or her stomach on a blanket on the floor. Lie on your stomach facing your baby. Talk to your baby to get him or her to raise his or her head to see you.
- Roll your baby onto his or her back and play with your baby's legs. Move the legs in a bicycle-riding motion. Try to get your baby to kick his or her legs.
- Play hand games, such as pat-a-cake, with your baby; kiss your baby's fingers; place your baby's hands on

your face. Bring your baby's hands in front of his or her eyes as you play; get your baby to look at his or her hands.
- Encourage your baby to watch and follow things with his or her eyes. Use a noise-making toy, such as a rattle or a chime, or a brightly colored object about 12 inches from his or her eyes; move it slowly to one side and then the other. Objects hanging from a play frame are good for your baby to watch while he or she is on his or her back or sitting in an infant seat.
- Continue to talk and sing a lot to your baby. Continue to tell your baby what you are doing with him or her and what is going on in the immediate environment.
- Keep your baby near you during times when the family usually is together, such as at mealtimes. Infant seats, especially ones that bounce or rock, and infant swings are good to use at these times.

grimacing, turning the head away, arching the back, crying, squirming, and flailing the arms and legs. Increased ability to read their infant's cues can increase parental confidence and self-esteem, thereby assisting adaptation to parenthood.

Optimally, parents can learn infant massage from a certified infant massage instructor (CIMI). Nurses can provide parents with names, addresses, and phone numbers of CIMIs in their community, as well as contact information for the International Association of Infant Massage (IAIM;

TABLE 25-7 **Play During Infancy: From Birth Through 3 Months**

AGE (MONTHS)	VISUAL STIMULATION	AUDITORY STIMULATION	TACTILE STIMULATION	KINETIC STIMULATION
SUGGESTED ACTIVITIES				
Birth-1	Look at infant at close range Hang bright, shiny object within 20-25 cm of infant's face and in midline Hang mobiles with black-and-white contrast designs	Talk to infant, sing in soft voice Play music box, radio, television Have ticking clock or metronome nearby	Hold, caress, cuddle Keep infant warm May like to be swaddled	Rock infant, place in cradle Use carriage for walks
2-3	Provide bright objects Make room bright with pictures or mirrors on walls Take infant to various rooms while doing chores Place infant in infant seat for vertical view of environment	Talk to infant Include in family gatherings Expose to various environmental noises other than those of home Use rattles, wind chimes	Caress infant while bathing, at diaper change Comb hair with a soft brush	Use infant swing Take in car for rides Exercise body by moving extremities in swimming motion Use cradle gym

From Wong, D. (1999). *Whaley & Wong's nursing care of infants and children* (6th ed.). St. Louis: Mosby.

BOX 25-12 **Benefits of Infant Massage**

IN THE PSYCHOSOCIAL DOMAIN

Benefits to the Infant of Receiving Massage
• Promotes bonding and attachment
• Promotes body/mind/spirit connection
• Increases self-esteem
• Increases sense of love, acceptance, respect, and trust
• Enhances communication

Benefits to the Parent of Giving Massage
• Improves ability to read infant cues
• Improves synchrony between caregiver and infant
• Promotes bonding
• Increases confidence in parenting
• Increases communication—verbal and nonverbal
• Improves relaxation
• Provides time to share and quality time
• Promotes parenting skills

IN THE PHYSIOLOGIC/PHYSICAL GROWTH DOMAIN

Benefits to the Infant of Receiving Massage
• Improves relaxation and release of accumulated stress
• Stimulates circulation
• Strengthens digestive, circulatory, and gastrointestinal systems, which can lead to weight gain
• Reduces discomfort from teething, congestion, gas, colic, and emotional stress
• Improves muscle tone/coordination
• Increases elimination, circulation, and respiration
• Improves sleep patterns
• Increases hormonal function

Benefits to the Parent of Giving Massage
• Improves sense of well-being
• Reduces blood pressure
• Reduces stress
• Improves overall health

From Schneider, E. (1997). Touch communication: The power of infant massage, *Massage Magazine* 68, 40.

800-248-5432). Parents may find helpful the book *Infant Massage: A Handbook for Loving Parents* by Vimala McClure. Also, nurses can consider becoming CIMIs through the certification program offered by IAIM and thus provide this service to their community.

Well-baby follow-up and immunizations. Parents should be advised to plan for their infant's health follow-up care at the following ages: 2 to 4 weeks of age, then every 2 months until 6 to 7 months, then every 3 months until 18 months, at 2 years, at 3 years, at preschool, and every 2 years thereafter. These well-baby follow-up visits with a nurse-practitioner or pediatrician are important for the parents, as well as the infant. They provide a time for parents to have questions answered, to get reassurance about their adaptation to parenthood, and to receive anticipatory guidance for the ensuing weeks before the next well-baby visit.

The schedule for immunizations should be reviewed with parents (Table 25-8). An infant's ability to protect himself or herself against antigens by the formation of antibodies develops sequentially; therefore the infant must be developmentally capable of responding to these antibodies. This is the reason for planning sequential immunizations for infants.

A form of passive immunity is already present in colostrum and breast milk. However, these antibodies are specific for microbes present in the mother's gastrointestinal tract and protect against overgrowth as fresh colonization occurs in the newborn.

The active ingredients in immunizations for diphtheria-pertussis-tetanus (DPT), hepatitis B, rubella, measles, and mumps, as well as the oral poliovirus vaccine (OPV), do not appear to be altered by breast milk and should be given according to the regular recommended schedule (Lawrence, 1999).

Recognizing signs of illness. As well as explaining the need for well-baby follow-up visits, the nurse should discuss with parents the signs of illness in newborns (Box 25-13).

Parents should be advised to call their nurse-practitioner or pediatrician immediately if they notice such signs and to ask about over-the-counter medications, such as Tylenol for infants, to keep at home. (See Plan of Care.)

Evaluation

Evaluation is based on the expected outcomes of care. The plan is revised as needed based on the evaluation findings.

TABLE 25-8 Immunizations

IMMUNIZATION	AGE OF ORIGINAL IMMUNIZATION
DTP (diphtheria, tetanus, pertussis)	2, 4, 6 mo
HIB (*Haemophilus influenzae* b conjugate vaccine)	2, 4, 6 mo (HIBTITER vaccine); 2, 4 mo (PedvaxHIB vaccine)
TOPV (trivalent oral poliovirus vaccine)	2, 4 mo
MMR (measles, mumps, rubella)	15 mo (12 mo if community outbreak)
HBIG (if mother is HBsAg positive)	Within 12 hr of birth
HBV (hepatitis B)*	Before hospital discharge, 1-2 mo, 6-18 mo, or 1-2 mo, 4 mo, 6-18 mo
Tuberculin skin test (not an immunization)	12-15 mo
Varicella	12-18 mo

*First dose within 12 hr of birth if mother is HBsAg positive.

BOX 25-13 Signs of Illness to Report Immediately

- Fever: temperature above 38° C axillary (under arm for 3 to 4 minutes); also, a continual rise in temperature
- Hypothermia: temperature below 36.6° C axillary
- Poor feeding or little interest in food: refusal to eat for two feedings in a row
- Vomiting: more than one episode of forceful vomiting or frequent vomiting (over a 6-hour period)
- Diarrhea: two consecutive green, watery stools (Note: Stools of breastfed infants are normally looser than stools of formula-fed infants. Diarrhea will leave a water ring around the stool, whereas breastfed stools will not.)
- Decreased bowel movement: less than two soiled diapers per day after 48 hours or less than three soiled diapers per day by the fifth day of life
- Decreased urination: no wet diapers for 18 to 24 hours or less than six to eight wet diapers per day
- Breathing difficulties: labored breathing with flared nostrils or absence of breathing for more than 15 seconds (Note: A newborn's breathing is normally irregular and between 30 to 40 breaths per minute. Count the breaths for a full minute.)
- Cyanosis whether accompanying a feeding or not
- Lethargy: sleepiness, difficulty waking, or periods of sleep longer than 6 hours (Most newborns sleep for short periods, usually from 1 to 4 hours, and wake to be fed.)
- Inconsolable crying (attempts to quiet not effective) or continuous high-pitched cry
- Bleeding or purulent drainage from umbilical cord or circumcision
- Drainage developing in the eyes

PLAN ᵒᶠ CARE | Home Care Follow-Up: Transition to Parenthood

> **NURSING DIAGNOSIS** Risk for ineffective breast-feeding related to frustration with the process

Expected Outcomes *Woman expresses physical and psychologic comfort with the feeding process, and infant feeds successfully and appears satisfied for at least 1 hour after feeding.*

Nursing Interventions/Rationales

Explore woman's knowledge of breastfeeding, assess for presence of flat or inverted nipples, determine level of ambivalence and anxiety tied to breastfeeding, and observe the technique being used *to evaluate the process and direct nursing interventions.*

If a problem area is identified, refer to the nursing care plan in Chapter 28 on breastfeeding.

> **NURSING DIAGNOSIS** Risk for infant care deficit related to lack of experience/lack of support

Expected Outcomes *Infant care routines are adequate, and infant appears healthy.*

Nursing Interventions/Rationales

Observe infant care routines (bathing, diapering, feeding, play) *to evaluate parental ease with care and adequacy of techniques.*

Discuss parental concerns about care issues and infant response *to assess for possible problem areas.*

Observe infant appearance (height-weight ratio, head circumference, fontanels, skin tone and turgor); assess infant's vital signs, overall tone, reflexes, and age-appropriate developmental skills *to evaluate for signs indicative of inadequate care.*

Explore available support systems for infant care *to determine adequacy of existing system.*

Help parents identify and address areas of care that need improvement *to ensure infant safety and health.*

Demonstrate troublesome care routines and have involved family members return demonstration *to facilitate improvements in care.*

Provide ongoing follow-up as needed *to ensure amelioration of identified potential and actual care deficits.*

> **NURSING DIAGNOSIS** Sleep pattern disturbance related to infant demands and environmental interruptions

Expected Outcomes *Woman sleeps for uninterrupted periods and feels rested on waking.*

Nursing Interventions/Rationales

Discuss woman's routine and specify things that interfere with sleep *to determine scope of problem and direct interventions.*

Explore ways woman and significant others can make environment more conducive to sleep (i.e., privacy, darkness, quiet, back rubs, soothing music, warm milk); teach use of guided imagery and relaxation techniques *to promote optimal conditions for sleep.*

Avoid things or routines (i.e., caffeine, foods that induce heartburn, strenuous mental/physical activity) *that may interfere with sleep.*

Advise family to limit visitors and activities *to avoid further taxation and fatigue.*

Have family plan specific times to care for the newborn to allow mother time to sleep; have mother learn to use infant nap time as a time for her to nap as well *to replenish energy and decrease fatigue.*

> **NURSING DIAGNOSIS** Risk for impaired home maintenance management related to addition of new family member/inadequate resources/inadequate support systems

Expected Outcome *Home exhibits signs of safe and functional environment.*

Nursing Interventions/Rationales

Observe the home environment (i.e., available living space and sleeping arrangements; adequacy of facilities for food preparation and storage, hygiene and toileting; overall state of repair; cleanliness; presence of safety hazards) *to determine adequacy and effective use of resources.*

Observe arrangements for the newborn, such as sleeping space, care equipment and supplies (bathing, changing, feeding, transportation) *to determine adequacy of resources.*

From Wong, D., & Perry, S. (1998). *Maternal child nursing care.* St. Louis: Mosby.

PLAN ᴼᶠ CARE | Home Care Follow-up: Transition to Parenthood—cont'd

Explore who is responsible for cooking, cleaning, child care, and newborn care and determine whether the mother seems adequately rested *to determine adequacy of support systems.*

Collaborate with family to remedy identified safety issues immediately *to prevent physical injury.*

Identify and arrange referrals to needed social agencies (i.e., Aid to Families with Dependent Children [AFDC], Women, Infants, and Children [WIC] program, food pantries) *to ameliorate resource deficits (finances, supplies, equipment).*

Identify and arrange referrals if needed for additional support (i.e., housekeeper, child care, postpartum support groups, "warm lines") *to supplement existing support systems.*

Continue home visitation as needed and provide coordination with referral services *to facilitate successful adaptation of environment.*

NURSING DIAGNOSIS Risk for altered family processes related to inclusion of new family member

---

Expected Outcome *Infant is successfully assimilated into family structure.*

Nursing Interventions/Rationales

Explore with family the ways that the birth and neonate have changed family structure and function *to evaluate functional and role adjustment.*

Observe family interaction with the newborn and note degree of bonding, evidence of sibling rivalry, and involvement in newborn care *to evaluate acceptance of newest family member.*

Assist family in reframing any perceived negative outcomes in a more positive light *to promote constructive interaction.*

Clarify identified misinformation and misperceptions *to promote clear communication.*

Assist family to explore options for solutions to identified problems *to promote effective problem resolution.*

Support family efforts as they move toward adjusting and incorporating the new member *to reinforce new functions and roles.*

If needed, make referrals to appropriate social services or community agencies *to ensure ongoing support and care.*

KEY POINTS

- The birth of a child necessitates changes in the existing interactional structure of a family.
- Either parent may exhibit "motherliness."
- Attachment is the process by which the parent and infant come to love and accept each other.
- Attachment is strengthened through the use of sensual responses or interactions by both partners in the parent-infant interaction.
- Early contact with the newborn is not essential for attachment to occur.
- For the biologic parent, the parental role does not begin at birth but rather enlarges and intensifies from the preconception decision to have a child.
- The father is considered an equal and integral part of the developing family.
- In adjusting to the parental role, the mother moves from a dependent state (taking in) to an interdependent state (letting go).
- Mothers may exhibit signs of postpartum blues (baby blues).

KEY POINTS—cont'd

- Fathers experience emotions and adjustments during the transition to parenthood that are similar to, and also distinctly different from, those of mothers.
- Modulation of rhythm, modification of behavioral repertoires, and mutual responsivity facilitate infant-parent adjustment.
- A primary need of parents is to establish a lifestyle that includes, but in some respects excludes, the baby.
- Many factors influence adaptation to parenthood (e.g., age, culture, socioeconomic level, and expectations of what the child will be like).
- Parents face a number of tasks related to sibling adjustment that require creative parental interventions.
- Grandparents can be a source of knowledge and support and can have a positive influence on the postpartum family.
- Anticipatory guidance helps prepare new parents for what to expect.

CRITICAL THINKING EXERCISES

1 You are assigned to care for Melissa (38 years old) and Doug (40 years old), who are first-time parents. They postponed parenthood because of Melissa's career. They plan to go home from the birth center tomorrow. While you are talking with them about their birth experience, Doug comments, "Yeah, I was glad I was there. The birth was easier than we thought it might be. But . . . I guess tomorrow we'll find out what it's really going to be like. I mean . . . with a new baby and having Melissa home all the time now."

a. How would you respond to Doug's comment? Justify your answer.

b. What does the literature tell us about new parents' adjustment during the transition to parenthood?

c. How are mothers' and fathers' adjustments to the parental role similar? Different?

d. Identify factors that help parents have a smoother transition to parenthood.

e. Given that Melissa has a career, how might her transition to parenthood be different from a non-career woman's?

f. Develop a teaching plan to use in discussing the transition to parenthood with mothers who are career women.

2 You are the nurse in a neighborhood health clinic that has a partnership with three communities: two whose residents are blue collar and one whose residents are of a low socioeconomic level, living in subsidized housing. At a regular meeting with the neighborhood advisory group, a priority identified is the need for a support group and parenting classes for the adolescent mothers and fathers. These adolescent parents have children between the ages of 2 weeks and 14 months.

a. What are the common concerns/needs of these parents of newborns and infants?

b. How will you determine what content to include in the classes? Outline the content for the parenting classes: state a rationale to justify each area of content. How will you design the support group? What should be the goal/purpose of the support group?

c. Identify community resources you will use for the support group and the parenting classes.

d. How will the demographic characteristics of the residents of these communities influence the design and content of the support group and parenting classes?

References

Albright, A. (1993). Postpartum depression: An overview. *Journal of Counseling Development* 71, 316.

Alpers, R. (1998). The changing self-concept of pregnant and parenting teens. *J Prof Nurs* 14(2), 111-118.

Ament, L. (1990). Maternal tasks of the puerperium re-identified. *J Obstet Gynecol Neonatal Nurs* 19(4), 330-335.

Anderson, A. (1996a). The father-infant relationship: Becoming connected. *J Soc Pediatr Nurs* 1(2), 83-92.

Anderson, A. (1996b). Factors influencing the father-infant relationship. *J Fam Nurs* 2(3), 306-324.

Barnard, K. (1994). *NCAST feeding manual.* Seattle: University of Washington.

Barratt, M., & Roach, M. (1995). Early interactive processes: Parenting by adolescent and adult single mothers. *Infant Behavior and Development* 18, 97-109.

Beck, C. (1995). Screening methods for postpartum depression. *J Obstet Gynecol Neonatal Nurs* 24(4), 308-312.

Berkowitz, G. et al. (1990). Delayed childbearing and the outcome of pregnancy. *N Engl J Med* 322, 659-664.

Bloom, K. (1998). Perceived relationship with the father of the baby and maternal attachment in adolescents. *J Obstet Gynecol Neonatal Nurs* 27(4), 420-430.

Brazelton, T. (1995). Working with families: Opportunities for early intervention. *Pediatr Clin North Am* 42(1), 1.

Brazelton, T., & Nugent, J. (1996). *Neonatal behavioural assessment scale* (3rd ed.). London: MacKeith.

Brazelton, T. et al. (1974). The origins of reciprocity: The early mother-infant interaction. In M. Lewis, & L. Rosenblum (Eds.). *The effect of the infant on its caregiver.* New York: John Wiley & Sons.

Brewaeys, A. et al. (1995). Lesbian mothers who conceived after donor insemination: A follow-up study. *Hum Reprod* 10(10), 2731-2735.

Broom, B. (1994). Impact of marital quality and psychological well-being on parental sensitivity. *Nurs Res* 43(3), 138-143.

Cain, M. (1994). *First time mothers, last chance babies: Parenting at 35+.* Far Hills, NJ: New Horizon Press.

Camarena, P. et al. (1998). The nature and support of adolescent mothers' life aspirations. *Family Relations* 47(2), 129-137.

Callister, L. (1995). Cultural meanings of childbirth. *J Obstet Gynecol Neonatal Nurs* 24(4), 327-331.

Campbell, J. (1992). Maternity blues: A model for biological research. In J. Hamilton, & P. Harberger (Eds.). *Postpartum psychiatric illness: A picture puzzle.* Philadelphia: University of Pennsylvania Press.

Cox, J., Holden, J., & Sagovshy, R. (1989). Edinburgh Postnatal Depression Scale. *Br J Psychol* 150, 782-786.

Diehl, K. (1997). Adolescent mothers: What produces positive mother-infant interaction? *MCN Am J Matern Child Nurs* 22, 89-95.

Denehy, J. (1992). Interventions related to parent-infant attachment. *Nurs Clin North Am* 27(2), 425-433.

Edwards, L. (1990). *Paternal, infant, and social contextual characteristics as determinants of competent parental functioning by fathers with young infants.* Doctoral dissertation, The University of North Carolina at Greensboro.

Evans, M. et al. (1998). Postpartum sleep in the hospital: Relationship to taking-in and taking-hold. *Clin Nurs Res* 7(4), 379-389.

Ferketich, S., & Mercer, R. (1995). Predictors of role competence for experienced and inexperienced fathers. *Nurs Res* 44(2), 89-95.

Fowles, E. (1998). The relationship between maternal role attainment and postpartum depression. *Health Care for Women International* 19(1), 83-94.

Fretts, R. et al. (1995). Increased maternal age and the risk of fetal death. *N Engl J Med* 333, 953-957.

Galanti, G. (1991). *Caring for patients from different cultures.* Philadelphia: University of Pennsylvania Press.

Gartrell, N. et al. (1996). The National Lesbian Family Study: Interview with prospective mothers. *Am J Orthopsychiatry* 66(2), 272-281.

Geissler, E. (1994). *Pocket guide to cultural assessment.* St. Louis: Mosby.

Gerson, E. (1973). *Infant behavior in the first year of life.* New York: Raven Press.

Gilbert, W., Nesbitt, T., & Danielsen, B. (1999). Childbearing beyond age 40: Pregnancy outcome in 24,032 cases. *Obstet Gynecol* 93, 9-14.

Gloppestad, K. (1996). Parents' skin to skin holding of small premature infants: Differences between fathers and mothers. *Nursing Science and Research in the Nordic Countries* 16(1), 22-27.

Gloppestad, K. (1998). Experiences of maternal love and paternal love when preterm infants were held skin to skin and wrapped in blankets. *Nursing Science and Research in the Nordic Countries* 18(1), 23-30.

Gottlieb, L., & Mendelson, M. (1995). Mothers' moods and social support when a second child is born. *Matern Child Nurs J* 23, 3.

Gullicks, J., & Crase, S. (1993). Sibling behavior with a newborn: Parents' expectations and observations. *J Obstet Gynecol Neonatal Nurs* 22(5), 438-444.

Hamilton, J., & Harberger, P. (1992). *Postpartum psychiatric illness: A picture puzzle.* Philadelphia: University of Pennsylvania Press.

Hansen, L., & Jacob, E. (1992). Intergenerational support during the transition to parenthood: Issues for new parents and grandparents. *Families in Society: The Journal of Contemporary Human Services* 73(8), 471-479.

Hartrick, G. (1997). Women who are mothers: The experience of defining self. *Health Care for Women International* 18, 263-277.

Henderson, A., & Brouse, A. (1991). The experiences of new fathers during the first three weeks of life. *J Adv Nurs* 16(3), 293-298.

Herz, E. (1992). Prediction, recognition, and prevention. In J. Hamilton, & P. Harberger (Eds.). *Postpartum psychiatric illness: A picture puzzle.* Philadelphia: University of Pennsylvania Press.

Hunt, D. (1995). A beautiful baby: Why am I so sad? Paper presented at the 25th Annual Conference of North Carolina AWHONN, Winston-Salem, NC, April 1, 1995.

Inman, M. (1996). The power of touch: Infant massage therapy. *Childbirth Instructor Magazine* 4th quarter.

Jambunathan, J., & Stewart, S. (1995). Hmong women in Wisconsin: What are their concerns in pregnancy and childbirth? *Birth* 22(4), 204-210.

Jiménez, S. (1995). The Hispanic culture, folklore, and perinatal health. *J Perinatal Educ* 4(1), 9.

Johnson and Johnson. (1996). *Compendium of postpartum care.* Skillman, NJ: Johnson and Johnson Consumer Products.

Klaus, M. et al. (1972). Maternal attachment: Importance of first post-partum days. *N Engl J Med* 286, 460-463.

Klaus, M., & Kennell, J. (1983). *Bonding: The beginnings of parent-infant attachment.* St. Louis: Mosby.

Klaus, M., & Kennell, J. (1997). The doula: An essential ingredient of childbirth rediscovered. *Acta Pediatrica* 86, 1034-1036.

Klaus, M., & Kennell, J. (1976). *Maternal-infant bonding.* St. Louis: Mosby.

Klaus, M., & Kennell, J. (1982). *Parent-infant bonding* (2nd ed.). St. Louis: Mosby.

Lawhon, G. (1994). *Facilitation of parenting within the newborn intensive care unit.* Doctoral dissertation, University of Washington.

Lawrence, R. (1999). *Breastfeeding: A guide for the medical profession* (5th ed.). St. Louis: Mosby.

Leventhal-Belfer, L., Cowan, P., & Cowan, C. (1992). Satisfaction with child care arrangements: Effects on adaptation to parenthood. *J Orthopsychiatry* 62(2), 165-177.

Leonard, V. (1993). *Stress and coping in the transition to parenthood of first-time mothers with career commitments: An interpretive study.* Doctoral dissertation. University of California, San Francisco.

Lipson, J., Dibble, S., & Minarik, P. (1996). *Culture and nursing care: A pocket guide.* San Francisco: UCSF Nursing Press.

MacDonald-Clark, N., & Boffman, J. (1995). Mother-child interaction among the Alaskan Eskimos. *J Obstet Gynecol Neonatal Nurs* 24(5), 450-457.

Martell, L. (1996). Is Rubin's "taking-in" and "taking-hold" a useful paradigm? *Health Care of Women International* 17(1), 1-13.

McCloskey, J., & Bulechek, G. (1996). *Nursing interventions classification* (2nd ed.). St. Louis: Mosby.

Meleis, A. (1991). *Theoretical nursing: Development and progress* (2nd ed.). Philadelphia: J.B. Lippincott.

Mercer, R. (1983). Parent-infant attachment. In L. Sonstegard, K. Kowalski, & B. Jennings (Eds.). *Women's health,* vol 2, *Childbearing.* New York: Grune & Stratton.

Mercer, R., & Ferketich, S. (1995). Experienced and inexperienced mothers maternal competence during infancy. *Res Nurs Health* 18, 333-343.

Mercer, R., & Ferketich, S. (1990). Predictors of parental attachment during early parenthood. *J Adv Nurs* 15, 268-280.

Miller, S. (1996). Questioning, resisting, acquiescing, balancing: New mothers' career reentry strategies. *Health Care for Women International* 17, 109-131.

Müller, M. (1996). Prenatal and postnatal attachment: A modest correlation. *J Obstet Gynecol Neonatal Nurs* 25(2), 161-166.

Niska, K., Snyder, M., & Lia-Hoagberg, B. (1998). Family ritual facilitates adaptation to parenthood. *Public Health Nurs* 15(5), 329-337.

Osterwell, D. (1991). *Correlates of relationship satisfaction in lesbian couples who are parenting their first child together.* Doctoral dissertation, Berkeley, California School of Professional Psychology.

Pridham, K. (1997). Mothers' help seeking as care initiated in a social context. *Image J Nurs Sch* 29(1), 65-70.

Prodromidis, M. et al. (1995). Mothers touching newborns: A comparison of rooming-in versus minimal contact. *Birth* 22(4), 196.

Reece, J. (1993). Social support and the early maternal experience of primiparas over 35. *Matern Child Nurs J* 21(3), 91-98.

Reese, S. (1995). Stress and maternal adaptation in first-time mothers more than 35 years old. *Appl Nurs Res* 8(2), 61-66.

Reese, S., & Harkless, G. (1996). Divergent themes in maternal experience in women older than 35 years of age. *Appl Nurs Res* 9(3), 148-153.

Rogan, F. et al. (1997). 'Becoming a mother'–Developing a new theory of early motherhood. *J Adv Nurs* 25, 877-885.

Rubin, R. (1961). Basic maternal behavior. *Nurs Outlook* 9, 683-686.

Rubin, R. (1963). Maternal touch at first contact with the newborn infant. *Nurs Outlook* 11, 828.

Ruchala, P., & Halstead, L. (1994). The postpartum experience of low-risk women: A time of adjustment and change. *Matern Child Nurs J* 22(3), 83-89.

Sank, J. (1991). *Factors in the prenatal period that affect parental role attainment during the postpartum period in Black American mothers and fathers.* Doctoral dissertation, University of Texas at Austin.

Schneider, E. (1997). Touch communication: The power of infant massage. *Massage Magazine* 68, 40.

Schneider, E. (1996). The power of touch: Massage for infants. *Infants and Young Children* 8(3), 40-55.

Schumacher, K., & Meleis, A. (1994). Transitions: A central concept in nursing. *Image J Nurs Sch* 26(2), 119-127.

Sethi, S. (1995). The dialectic in becoming a mother: Experiencing a postpartum phenomenon. *Scandinavian Journal of Caring Sciences* 9(4), 235-244.

Sharts-Hopko, N. (1995). Birth in the Japanese context. *J Obstet Gynecol Neonatal Nurs* 24(14), 343-351.

Siegel, E. (1982). A critical examination of studies of parent-infant bonding. In M. Klaus, & M. Robertson (Eds.). *Birth interaction and attachment.* Evansville, IL: Johnson & Johnson Baby Products.

Smith-Hanrahan, C., & Deblois, D. (1995). Postpartum early discharge. *Clin Nurs Res* 4(1), 50-66.

Strom, R. et al. (1992-1993). Strengths and needs of Black grandparents. *Int J Aging Hum Dev* 36(4), 255-268.

Susman, J. (1996). Postpartum depressive disorders. *J Fam Pract* 43, S17-S24.

Symanski, M. (1992). Maternal-infant bonding. Practice issues for the 1990s. *J Nurse Midwifery* 37(2 Suppl), 67S-73S.

Tedder, J. (1991). Using the Brazelton neonatal assessment scale to facilitate the parent-infant relationship in a primary care setting. *Nurse Pract* 16(3), 26-30, 35-36.

Thompson, P. et al. (1995). Adolescent parenting: Outcomes and maternal perceptions. *J Obstet Gynecol Neonatal Nurs* 24, 713-718.

Tomlinson, P. (1996). Marital relationship change in the transition to parenthood: A reexamination as interpreted through transition theory. *J Fam Nurs* 2(3), 286-305.

Tomlinson, P., & Irwin, B. (1993). Qualitative study of women's reports of family adaptation pattern four years following transition to parenthood. *Issues in Men Health Nursing* 14, 119-139.

Troy, N. (1995). The time of first holding of the infant and maternal self-esteem related to feelings of maternal attachment. *Women Health* 22(3), 59-72.

Troy, N. (1993). Early contact and maternal attachment among women using public health care facilities. *Appl Nurs Res* 6(4), 161-166.

Troy, N., & Dalgas-Pelish, P. (1995). Development of a self-care guide for postpartum fatigue. *Appl Nurs Res* 8(2), 92-101.

Troy, N., & Dalgas-Pelish, P. (1997). The natural evolution of postpartum fatigue among a group of primiparous women. *Clin Nurs Res* 6(2), 126-141.

Tulman, L. (1985). Mothers and unrelated persons' initial handling of newborn infants. *Nurs Res* 34(4), 205-210.

Unger, D., & Cooley, M. (1992). Partner and grandmother contact in Black and White teen parent families. *J Adolesc Health* 13, 546-552.

Vehvilainen-Julkunen, K. (1995). Family training: Supporting mothers and fathers in the transition to parenthood. *J Adv Nurs* 22, 731-737.

Walker, L. (1992). *Parent-infant nursing science: Paradigms, phenomena, methods.* Philadelphia: F.A. Davis.

Waters, M., & Lee, K. (1996). Differences between primigravidae and multigravidae mothers in sleep disturbances, fatigue, and functional status. *J Nurse Midwifery* 41(5), 364-367.

Wood, A. et al. (1997). The downward spiral of postpartum depression. *MCN Am J Matern Child Nurs* 22, 308-316.

Wong, D. (1999). *Whaley and Wong's nursing care of infants and children* (6th ed.). St. Louis: Mosby.

Wong, D., & Perry, S. (1998). *Maternal child nursing care.* St. Louis: Mosby.

Wrasper, C. (1996). Discharge timing and Rubin's concept of puerperal change. *J Perinatal Educ* 5(2), 13-23.

26

Physiology and Physical Adaptations of the Newborn

Bette B. Hammond

EARNING OBJECTIVES

- Define the key terms.
- Describe the changes in the biologic system of the neonate during the transition to extrauterine life.
- Identify the sequence to follow in assessment of the newborn.
- Gather appropriate neonatal health history information from the prenatal and intrapartal periods.
- Recognize deviations from normal physiologic findings during examination of the newborn.

- Compare and contrast the four types of heat loss in a neonate and describe how to prevent heat loss.
- Describe the behavioral adaptations of the newborn, including sleep-wake states and periods of reactivity.
- Identify the sensory/perceptual functioning of the neonate.

KEY TERMS

acrocyanosis	cold stress	sleep-wake states
Brazelton Neonatal Behavioral Assessment Scale (BNBAS)	habituation	state-related behavior
	hyperbilirubinemia	surfactant
brown fat	mongolian spot	thermoregulation
caput succedaneum	physiologic jaundice	transition period
cephalhematoma	sensory capability	

The neonatal period includes the time from birth through the twenty-eighth day of life. During this time the neonate must make many adjustments to extrauterine life. Many of these developmental tasks occur shortly after birth. Biologic tasks are those that involve (1) establishing and maintaining respirations; (2) adjusting to circulatory changes; (3) regulating temperature; (4) ingesting, retaining, and digesting nutrients; (5) eliminating waste; and (6) regulating weight. Behavioral tasks include (1) establishing a regulated behavioral tempo independent of the mother, which involves self-regulation of arousal, self-monitoring of changes in state, and patterning of sleep; (2) processing,

storing, and organizing multiple stimuli; and (3) establishing a relationship with caregivers and the environment. The infant at term (an infant between 38 and 42 weeks of gestation) normally makes these adjustments with little or no difficulty.

Infants undergo phases of instability during the first 6 to 8 hours after birth. These phases collectively are termed the **transition period** between intrauterine and extrauterine existence (Fig. 26-1). To detect disorders in adaptation soon after birth, nurses must be aware of normal features of the transition period. Labor and immediate neonatal events stimulate a sympathetic response reflected by changes in heart rate, color,

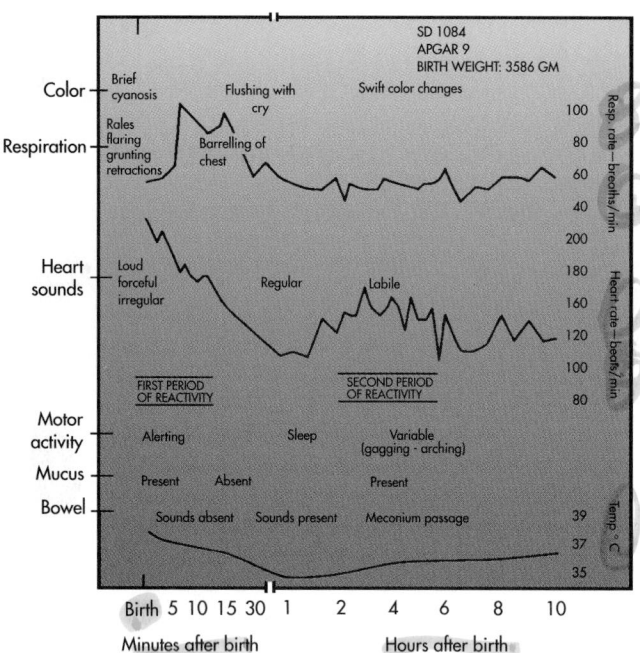

Fig. 26-1 Normal transition period.

respiration, motor activity, gastrointestinal function, and temperature of the infant (Fanaroff & Martin, 1997). Behavioral characteristics also change during this transitional period.

The first phase of the transition period lasts up to 30 minutes after birth and is called the *first period of reactivity*. The newborn's heart rate increases rapidly to 160 to 180 beats/min but gradually falls by 30 minutes to a baseline rate of between 100 and 120 beats/min. Respirations are irregular, with a rate between 60 and 80 breaths/min. Crackles may be present on auscultation; audible grunting, nasal flaring, and retractions of the chest may also be noted. In addition, brief periods of apnea (periodic breathing) may occur. Coincident with these changes in heart rate and respiratory rate, the infant is alert. The infant's behavior is marked by spontaneous startle reactions, tremors, crying, and movement of the head from side to side. This characteristic exploratory behavior is accompanied by a decrease in body temperature and generalized increase in motor activity, with an increase in muscle tone (Fanaroff & Martin, 1997). Gastrointestinal manifestations of this first period of reactivity include the onset of bowel sounds, passage of meconium, and production of saliva.

After the first period of reactivity, the newborn either sleeps or has a marked decrease in motor activity. This period of unresponsiveness, frequently accompanied by sleep, lasts for 60 to 100 minutes and is followed by a second period of reactivity.

The second period of reactivity occurs roughly between the fourth and eighth hours after birth. This period of reactivity lasts from 10 minutes to several hours. Periods of tachycardia and tachypnea occur, associated with increased muscle tone, skin color, and mucus production. Meconium is frequently passed at this time.

This sequence occurs in all newborns, regardless of gestational age or type of birth. The length of time the periods last will vary depending on the amount and kind of stress experienced by the fetus.

BIOLOGIC CHARACTERISTICS

With the cutting of the umbilical cord, the infant must undergo rapid and complex changes. Many biologic adaptations occur that make it possible for the infant to adapt to extrauterine life. All the systems of the infant change their functions or become established during the neonatal period (Lowe & Reiss, 1996). Because an understanding of these changes in the various systems is essential for analyzing physical and behavioral assessment data, this chapter discusses these changes first and then proceeds to describe the physical assessment and behavioral characteristics of the newborn.

Respiratory System

The most critical adjustment a newborn must make at birth is the establishment of respirations. At term the lungs hold approximately 20 ml fluid/kg (Blackburn & Loper, 1992). Air must be substituted for the fluid that filled the respiratory tract. During normal vaginal birth some lung fluid is squeezed or drained from the newborn's trachea and lungs. With the first breath of air, the newborn begins a sequence of cardiopulmonary changes.

Initiation of Breathing

Initial breathing is probably the result of a reflex triggered by pressure changes, chilling, noise, light, and other sensations related to the birth process. In addition, the chemoreceptors in the aorta and carotid bodies initiate neurologic reflexes when arterial oxygen pressure (Po_2) falls from 80 to 15 mm Hg, arterial carbon dioxide pressure (Pco_2) rises from 40 to 70 mm Hg, and arterial pH falls below 7.35. When these changes are extreme, respiratory depression can occur. In most cases an exaggerated respiratory reaction follows within 1 minute of birth, and the infant takes a first gasping breath and cries.

Certain respiratory patterns are characteristic of the normal term newborn. After respirations are established, breaths are shallow and irregular, ranging from 30 to 60 breaths/min, with short periods of apnea (less than 15 seconds). These short periods of apnea occur most often during the active (rapid eye movement [REM]) sleep cycle and decrease in frequency and duration with age. Apneic periods over 15 seconds in duration should be evaluated.

NURSE ALERT

Newborn infants are preferential nose breathers. The reflex response to nasal obstruction is to open the mouth to maintain an airway. This response is not present in most infants until 3 weeks after birth. Therefore cyanosis or asphyxia may occur with nasal blockage.

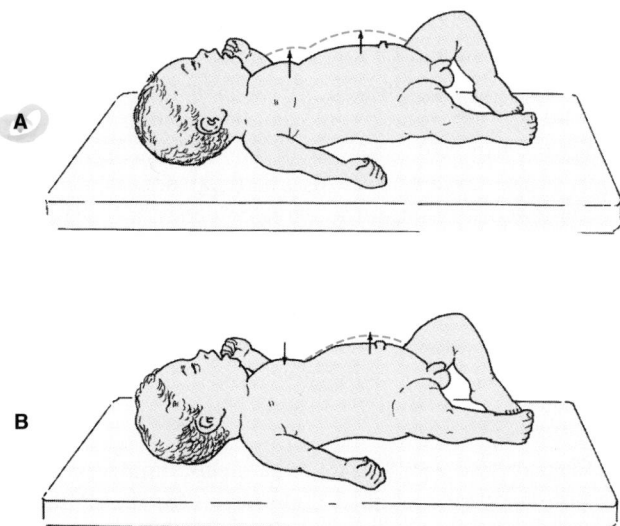

Fig. 26-2 Comparison of normal and seesaw respirations. **A,** Normal respiration. Chest and abdomen rise with inspiration. **B,** Seesaw respiration. Chest wall retracts and abdomen rises with inspiration. *(Courtesy Mead Johnson & Co., Evansville, IN.)*

Signs of Respiratory Distress

Most term infants breathe spontaneously and continue to have normal respirations. However, infants can manifest other problems through respiratory distress. Signs of respiratory distress may include nasal flaring, retractions (indrawing of tissue between the ribs, below the rib cage, or above the sternum and clavicles), or grunting with expirations. Any increased use of the intercostal muscles may be a sign of distress. Seesaw respirations instead of normal abdominal respirations are not normal and should be reported (Fig. 26-2, *B*). A respiratory rate that is less than 30 or greater than 60 breaths/min with the infant at rest needs to be reported to the pediatrician. The respiratory rate of the infant is negatively influenced (slowed or depressed) by the analgesics or anesthetics administered to the mother during labor and birth. Apneic episodes also can be related to rapid warming or cooling of the infant, whereas tachypnea may result from aspiration or a diaphragmatic hernia. Apneic periods longer than 15 seconds must be reported to the pediatrician for evaluation. Even a normal-appearing infant requires close observation because changes in the respiratory system can occur very rapidly.

Maintaining Adequate Oxygen Supply

During the first hour of life the pulmonary lymphatics continue to remove large amounts of fluid. Removal of fluid is also a result of the pressure gradient from alveoli to interstitial tissue to blood capillary. Reduced vascular resistance accommodates this flow of lung fluid.

Abnormal respiration and failure to completely expand the lungs retard the movement of fetal lung fluid from alveoli and interstices into the pulmonary circulation.

Retention of fluid interferes with the infant's ability to maintain adequate oxygenation.

The chest circumference is approximately 30 to 33 cm at birth. Auscultation of the chest of a newborn infant reveals loud, clear breath sounds that seem very near, because little chest tissue intervenes. The ribs of the infant articulate with the spine at a horizontal rather than a downward slope; consequently, the rib cage cannot expand with inspiration as readily as an adult's. Neonatal respiratory function is largely a matter of diaphragmatic contraction. The negative intrathoracic pressure is created by the descent of the diaphragm, much like negative pressure is created in the barrel of a syringe when medication is drawn up by retracting the plunger. The newborn infant's chest and abdomen rise simultaneously with inspiration. (Fig. 26-2, *A*).

The alveoli of the infant's lungs are lined with **surfactant.** Lung expansion augments surfactant secretion. Surfactant functions (1) to lower surface tension, therefore requiring less pressure to keep the alveolus open, and (2) to maintain alveolar stability by changing surface tension as the size of the alveolus changes. The surfactant system develops as the infant develops in utero. Fetal pulmonary maturity can be determined by examining amniotic fluid for lecithin/sphingomyelin ratio (L/S) and other phospholipid levels. Phosphatidylglycerol appears at 35 to 36 weeks; its presence is a more predictable indicator of lung maturity.

The ratio of lecithin to sphingomyelin increases with gestational age. Mature fetal lungs have an L/S ratio greater than 2:1. Infants born before the L/S ratio is 2:1 will have varying degrees of respiratory distress. Characteristics of the respiratory system of the neonate and the effects of these characteristics on respiratory function are listed in Table 26-1.

Circulatory System

The circulatory system changes markedly after birth. The foramen ovale, ductus arteriosus, and ductus venosus close. The umbilical arteries, umbilical vein, and hepatic arteries become ligaments (see Fig. 14-9).

The infant's first breath inflates the lungs and reduces pulmonary vascular resistance to the pulmonary blood flow. The pulmonary artery pressure drops. This sequence is the major mechanism by which pressure in the *right atrium declines.* The increased pulmonary blood flow returned to the left side of the heart *increases* the pressure in the *left atrium.* This change in pressures causes a functional closure of the foramen ovale. During the first few days of life, crying may reverse the flow through the foramen ovale temporarily and lead to mild cyanosis.

When the P_{O_2} level in the arterial blood approximates 50 mm Hg, the ductus arteriosus constricts (fetal $P_{O_2} \sim$ 27 mm Hg). Later, the ductus arteriosus occludes and becomes a ligament. With the clamping and severing of the cord, the umbilical arteries, umbilical vein, and ductus venosus close immediately and are converted into ligaments. The hypogastric arteries also occlude and become

TABLE 26-1	Characteristics of the Respiratory System of the Neonate	
CHARACTERISTIC	**EFFECT ON FUNCTION**
Lung elastic tissue and recoil is decreased	Lung compliance is decreased; more work and higher pressure are required to expand; risk of atelectasis
Limited movement of diaphragm	Respiratory movement less effective; risk of atelectasis
Preferential nose breather; larynx and epiglottis high	Can breathe and swallow at the same time; risk of airway obstruction; difficulty intubating
Airway passages small and compliant; high airway resistance; weak cough reflex	Risk of obstruction of airway and apnea
Surfactant system altered in immature infants	Atelectatic areas; work of breathing increased; risk of respiratory distress syndrome (RDS)
Respiratory control immature	Respirations irregular; unable to increase rate and depth of respirations rapidly

From Blackburn, S. (1992). Alterations of the respiratory system in the neonate: Implications for clinical practice. *J Perinat Neonatal Nurs* 6(2), 46-58.

ligaments. Table 26-2 summarizes the cardiovascular changes at birth.

Heart Rate and Sounds

The heart rate averages 140 beats/min at birth, with variations noted during sleeping and waking states. Shortly after the first cry the infant's heart rate may accelerate to 175 to 180 beats/min. The range of the heart rate in the full-term infant is about 100 beats/min during deep sleep and 120 to 160 beats/min while awake. A heart rate of 180 beats/min is not unusual when the infant cries. A heart rate that is either high (>160 beats/min) or low (<120 beats/min) should be reevaluated within an hour or when the activity of the infant changes. Immediately after birth the heart rate can be palpated by grasping the base of the umbilical cord.

By term the infant's heart lies midway between the crown of the head and the buttocks, and the axis is more transverse than in an adult (Fig. 26-3). The apical impulse (point of maximal impulse [PMI]) in the newborn is at the fourth intercostal space and to the left of the midclavicular line. The PMI is often visible.

Apical pulse rates should be obtained on all infants. Auscultation should be for a full minute, preferably when the infant is asleep. Sinus dysrhythmia (irregular heart rate) may be considered a physiologic phenomenon in infancy and an indication of good heart function. Detecting irregular heart rates in normal newborns is therefore not uncommon.

Heart sounds during the neonatal period are of higher pitch, shorter duration, and greater intensity than during adult life. The first sound is typically louder and duller than the second sound, which is sharp. Most heart murmurs heard during the neonatal period have no pathologic significance, and more than half of the murmurs disappear by 6 months.

Blood Pressure

Blood pressure (BP) tends to be highest immediately after birth and lowest about 3 hours later. Overall, BP during the neonatal period is the lowest BP over an individual's life span because the left ventricle is underdeveloped and the heart muscle is immature, as are all other muscles. This underdevelopment of the left ventricle leads to low output, and therefore the BP is low. BP in infants varies daily. A drop in systolic BP (about 15 mm Hg) within the first hour after birth is common. Average values for BP measured several hours after birth through the neonatal period are 60 to 80 mm Hg systolic pressure and 40 to 50 mm Hg diastolic pressure. Crying and movement result in changes in BP, especially in the systolic pressure. BP is also sensitive to the changes in blood volume that occur with the adaptations in circulation. The measurement of BP is best accomplished with a Doppler device and while the infant is at rest. The correct size BP cuff must be used for accurate measurement of an infant's BP. When arm BP measurement is followed by leg BP measurement, different-sized cuffs may be needed because arms and legs are rarely the same size.

Blood Volume

The blood volume of the newborn depends on the amount of blood transferred placentally. The blood volume of the full-term infant is about 80 to 85 ml per kilogram of body weight. Immediately after birth the total blood volume averages 300 ml, but this volume can increase by as much as 100 ml, depending on the length of time the infant is attached to the placenta (Wong, 1999). The preterm infant has a proportionally greater blood volume than the infant born at term. This occurs because the preterm infant has a greater plasma volume, not a greater red blood cell (RBC) mass.

A number of differences in the circulatory dynamics of the newborn result from early or delayed clamping of the cord. Holding the newborn below the level of the placenta and delaying clamping for several minutes after birth result in an expansion of blood volume from 40% to 60%, the so-called placental transfusion. This in turn causes an increase in heart size, higher systolic BP, and an increased respiratory rate. Pulmonary crackles and transient cyanosis are also encountered after delayed clamping. To date, the

▪ TABLE 26-2 Cardiovascular Changes at Birth

PRENATAL STATUS	POSTBIRTH STATUS	ASSOCIATED FACTORS
PRIMARY CHANGES		
Pulmonary circulation: high pulmonary vascular resistance, increased pressure in right ventricle and pulmonary arteries	Low pulmonary vascular resistance; decreased pressure in right atrium, ventricle, and pulmonary arteries	Expansion of collapsed fetal lung with air
Systemic circulation: low pressures in left atrium, ventricle, and aorta	High systemic vascular resistance; increased pressure in left atrium, ventricle, and aorta	Loss of placental blood flow
SECONDARY CHANGES		
Umbilical arteries: patent, carrying of blood from hypogastric arteries to placenta	Functionally closed at birth, obliteration by fibrous proliferation possibly taking 2-3 months, distal portions becoming lateral vesico-umbilical ligaments, proximal portions remaining open as superior vesicle arteries	Closure preceding that of umbilical vein, probably accomplished by smooth muscle contraction in response to thermal and mechanical stimuli and alteration in oxygen tension, mechanically severed with cord at birth
Umbilical vein: patent, carrying of blood from placenta to ductus venosus and liver	Closed, becoming ligamentum teres hepatis after obliteration	Closure shortly after umbilical arteries, hence blood from placenta possibly entering neonate for short period after birth, mechanically severed with cord at birth
Ductus venosus: patent, connection of umbilical vein to inferior vena cava	Closed, becoming ligamentum venosum after obliteration	Loss of blood flow from umbilical vein
Ductus arteriosus: patent, shunting of blood from pulmonary artery to descending aorta	Functionally closed almost immediately after birth, anatomic obliteration of lumen by fibrous proliferation requiring 1-3 months, becoming ligamentum arteriosum	High systemic resistance increasing aortic pressure, low pulmonary resistance reducing pulmonary arterial pressure Increased oxygen content of blood in ductus arteriosus creating vasospasm of its muscular wall
Foramen ovale: formation of a valve opening that allows blood to flow directly to left atrium (shunting of blood from right to left atrium)	Functionally closed at birth, constant apposition gradually leading to fusion and permanent closure within a few months or years in majority of persons	Increased pressure in left atrium and decreased pressure in right atrium causing closure of valve over foramen

Modified from Wong D. (1995). *Whaley and Wong's nursing care of infants and children* (5th ed.). St. Louis: Mosby.

value of early or delayed clamping of the cord has not been determined. Although the increased blood volume may stress the heart and pulmonary vasculature, a decrease in the incidence of neonatal respiratory distress has been reported in infants in whom cord clamping was delayed. Furthermore, breakdown of the additional RBCs increases the storage supply of iron; 80 ml of placental blood yields 50 mg of iron (Seidel, Rosenstein, & Pathak, 1993). On the other hand, breakdown of excess RBCs may contribute to hyperbilirubinemia (Fanaroff & Martin, 1997).

Hematopoietic System

The hematopoietic system of the newborn exhibits certain variations from that of the adult. Levels of RBCs and leukocytes differ, but platelet levels are relatively the same.

Red Blood Cells and Hemoglobin

Because fetal circulation is less efficient at oxygen exchange than the lungs, the fetus needs additional RBCs for transport of oxygen in utero. Therefore at birth the average levels of RBCs and hemoglobin are higher than at the adult stage. Cord blood of the term newborn may have a hemoglobin concentration of 14 to 24 g/dl, with a mean of 17 g/dl. The hematocrit ranges from 44% to 64% (mean, 55%). The RBC count is correspondingly elevated, ranging from 4.8 to 7.1/mm³. By the end of the first month these values decrease to average levels of 11 to 17 g/dl and 4.2 to 5.2/mm³, respectively. The blood values may be affected by delayed clamping of the cord, which results in a rise in hemoglobin level, RBC count, and hematocrit value. The source of the sample is another important factor because

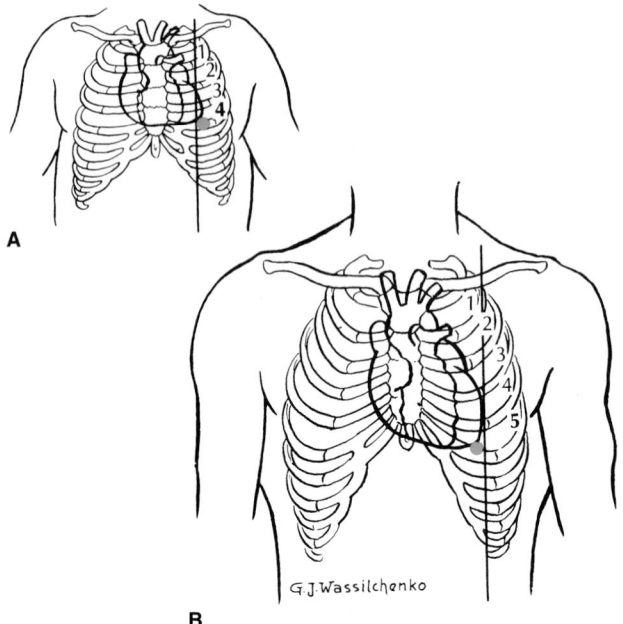

G.J.Wassilchenko

Fig. 26-3   Differences in locations of apical pulse in newborn from that of adult. **A**, Neonate. **B**, Adult.

capillary blood yields higher values than venous blood. The time after birth when the blood sample was obtained is also significant; the slight rise in RBC numbers after birth is followed by a substantial drop. At birth, 80% of the infant's blood contains fetal hemoglobin, but because of the shorter life span of the cells containing fetal hemoglobin, the percentage falls to 55% by 5 weeks and to 5% by 20 weeks. Iron stores are generally sufficient to sustain normal RBC production for 5 months, and thus mild, brief anemia is not serious.

Leukocytes

Leukocytosis, with a white blood cell (WBC) count of approximately 18,000/mm^3 (range, 9000 to 30,000/mm^3), is normal at birth. The number of WBCs, predominantly polymorphonuclear leukocytes, increases to 23,000 to 24,000/mm^3 during the first day after birth. This early high WBC count of the newborn decreases rapidly, and a resting level of 11,500/mm^3 is normally maintained during the neonatal period. Serious infection is not well tolerated by the newborn, and a marked increase in the WBC count is unlikely, even in critical sepsis (infection). In most instances, sepsis is accompanied by a decline in WBCs, particularly in neutrophils. The activity of the bone marrow is accurately reflected by the number of circulating cells—both erythrocytes and leukocytes. Leukopenia found in African-American children and adults is apparent by 1 year of age and is caused primarily by a decrease in the number of neutrophils. By 6 years of age, in all children, the peripheral blood makeup is approximately the same as that of an adult.

Platelets

The platelet count ranges between 150,000 and 350,000/mm^3 and is essentially the same in newborns as in adults. The level of factors II, VII, IX, and X, found in the liver, is decreased during the first few days of life because the newborn cannot synthesize vitamin K. However, bleeding tendencies in the newborn are rare, and unless the vitamin K deficiency is great, clotting is sufficient to prevent hemorrhage.

Blood Groups

The infant's blood group is genetically determined and established early in fetal life. However, during the neonatal period the strength of the agglutinogens present in the membrane of the RBCs gradually increases. Samples of cord blood may be drawn after birth, especially if the mother's blood is type O or Rh factor negative. Cord blood samples are usually sent to the laboratory for identification of the infant's blood type and determination of the Rh factor.

Signs of Risk for Cardiovascular Problems

Close monitoring of the infant's vital signs is important for early detection of impending problems. Persistent tachycardia (≥170 beats/min) may indicate respiratory distress syndrome (RDS), whereas persistent bradycardia (≤120 beats/min) may be a sign of a congenital heart block. Any prolonged cyanosis other than in the hands or feet may indicate respiratory and/or cardiac problems. A difference between upper and lower extremity BP may be an early sign of coarctation of the aorta. The presence of jaundice may indicate ABO or Rh factor problems.

Thermogenic System

Heat regulation is second to the establishment of respirations and circulation as a factor critical to an infant's survival. **Thermoregulation** is the maintenance of balance between heat loss and heat production (Sheeran, 1996). Newborns are homeothermic; that is, they attempt to stabilize their internal body temperatures within a narrow range. Hypothermia from excessive heat loss is a common and dangerous problem in neonates. The infant's ability to produce heat often approaches the capacity of the adult. However, the tendency toward rapid heat loss in a cold environment is increased in the newborn and poses a hazard.

Thermogenesis

Heat production is often referred to as *thermogenesis* (*thermo,* "heat"; *genesis,* "origin"). The shivering mechanism of heat production is rarely operable in the newborn. Nonshivering thermogenesis is accomplished primarily by **brown fat,** which is unique to the newborn (Fanaroff & Martin, 1997), and secondarily by increased metabolic activity in the brain, heart, and liver. Brown fat is located in superficial deposits in the interscapular region and axillae, as well as in deep deposits at the thoracic inlet, along the vertebral column, and around the kidneys. Brown fat has a richer vascular and nerve supply than ordinary fat. Heat produced by intense lipid metabolic activity in brown fat can warm the newborn by increasing heat production as much as 100%. Reserves of brown fat, usually present for several weeks after birth, are rapidly depleted with cold stress. The less mature the infant, the less reserve of this essential fat is available at birth.

Heat Loss

Heat loss in the newborn occurs by four modes:

1. *Convection* is the flow of heat from the body surface to cooler ambient air. Because of heat loss by convection, the ambient temperatures in the nursery are kept at 24° C, and newborns are wrapped to protect them from the cold.
2. *Radiation* is the loss of heat from the body surface to a cooler solid surface not in direct contact but in relative proximity. Nursery cribs and examining tables are placed away from outside windows to prevent this type of heat loss.
3. *Evaporation* is the loss of heat that occurs when a liquid is converted to a vapor. In the newborn, heat loss by evaporation occurs as a result of vaporization of moisture from the skin. The process is invisible and is known as *insensible water loss (IWL)*. This heat loss can be intensified by failure to dry the newborn directly after birth or by too-slow drying of the infant after a bath.
4. *Conduction* is the loss of heat from the body surface to cooler surfaces in direct contact. When admitted to the nursery, the newborn is placed in a warmed crib to minimize heat loss. Loss of heat must be controlled to protect the infant.

As already noted, control of such modes of heat loss is the basis of caregiving policies and techniques.

Temperature Regulation

Anatomic and physiologic differences among the newborn, child, and adult are notable. The newborn's thermal insulation is less than that of an adult. The blood vessels are closer to the surface of the skin. Changes in environmental temperature alter the temperature of the blood, thereby influencing temperature-regulation centers in the hypothalamus. Newborns have larger body surface to body weight (mass) ratios than children and adults. The flexed position of the newborn helps guard against heat loss because it diminishes the amount of body surface exposed to the environment. Infants can also reduce the loss of internal heat via the body surface by constricting peripheral blood vessels.

Signs of Risk for Thermogenic Problems

Changes in environmental temperature can disturb body temperature. This may lead to serious consequences in the newborn. Brown fat metabolism is activated in response to changes in environmental temperature that are perceived by the thermal sensors in the newborn's skin, even when the temperature of the newborn is unchanged. Unlike adults, newborns cannot change body posture to decrease the amount of skin surface exposed (e.g., by flexion of the extremities) in response to cold. When exposed to cold, the newborn may cry, become restless, and increase muscular activity to generate heat. However, crying increases workload and energy is expended. Newborns may also increase their respiratory rates to attempt stimulation of muscular activity.

Cold stress imposes metabolic and physiologic demands in all infants, regardless of gestational age and condition. The respiratory rate increases in response to the increased need for oxygen. In the cold-stressed infant, oxygen consumption and energy are diverted from maintaining normal brain and cardiac function and growth to thermogenesis for survival. If the infant cannot maintain an adequate oxygen tension, vasoconstriction occurs and jeopardizes pulmonary perfusion. As a consequence, the partial pressure of arterial oxygen (Pao_2) is decreased, and the blood pH drops. These changes aggravate existing respiratory distress syndrome (RDS). Moreover, decreased pulmonary perfusion and oxygen tension may maintain or reopen the right-to-left shunt across the patent ductus arteriosus.

The basal metabolic rate increases with cold stress. If cold stress is protracted, anaerobic glycolysis occurs, resulting in increased production of acids. Metabolic acidosis develops (Fig. 26-4), and if a defect in respiratory function is present, respiratory acidosis also develops. Excessive fatty acids displace the bilirubin from the albumin-binding sites. The resulting increased level of circulating unbound bilirubin heightens the risk of kernicterus even at serum bilirubin levels of 10 mg/dl or less.

Hyperthermia develops more rapidly in the newborn than in the adult because of the larger surface area of an infant. Although newborns have 6 times as many sweat glands per unit area as adults, these glands do not function. Serious overheating of the newborn can cause cerebral damage from dehydration or heat stroke and death.

Renal System

The kidneys are formed by the fourth month of fetal life. In utero, urine is produced in the kidneys and excreted into the amniotic fluid. A small quantity (approximately 40 ml) of urine is usually present at birth in the bladder of a full-term infant.

At term the kidneys occupy a large portion of the posterior abdominal wall. The bladder lies close to the anterior abdominal wall and is an abdominal as well as a pelvic organ. In the newborn almost all palpable masses in the abdomen are renal in origin.

Kidney function comparable to that of the adult is not approached until the second year of life. The newborn has a minimal range of chemical balance and safety. Diarrhea, infection, and improper feeding can lead rapidly to acidosis

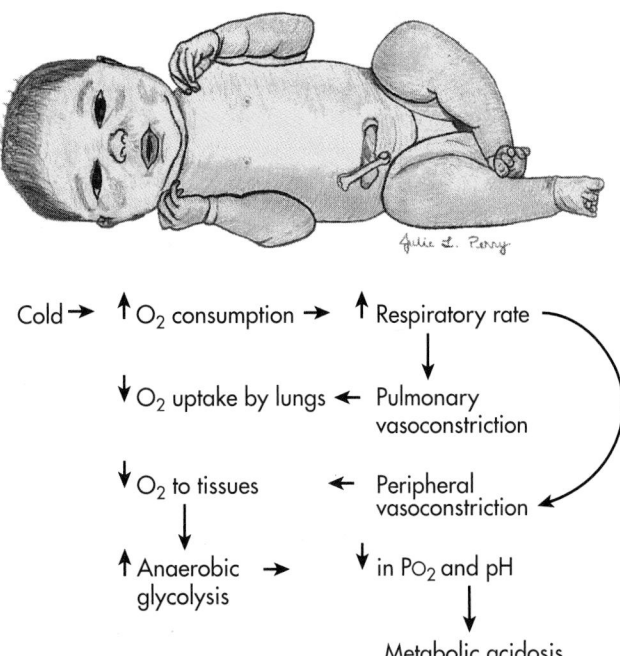

Cold → ↑O₂ consumption → ↑Respiratory rate

↓O₂ uptake by lungs ← Pulmonary vasoconstriction

↓O₂ to tissues ← Peripheral vasoconstriction

↑Anaerobic glycolysis → ↓in PO₂ and pH

Metabolic acidosis

Fig. 26-4 Effects of cold stress. When an infant is stressed by cold, oxygen consumption increases and pulmonary and peripheral vasoconstriction occur, thereby decreasing oxygen uptake by the lungs and oxygen to the tissues; anaerobic glycolysis increases; and there is a decrease in PO₂ and pH, leading to metabolic acidosis.

and fluid imbalances (dehydration or edema). Renal immaturity also limits the newborn's ability to excrete drugs.

About 17% of newborns void at the time of birth, 92% by 24 hours, and 99% within 48 hours (Fanaroff & Martin, 1997).

NURSE ALERT

Noting and recording first voidings is important. An infant who has not voided after 24 hours should be assessed for adequacy of fluid intake, bladder distention, restlessness, and symptoms of pain. If the infant has not voided within 24 hours, the pediatrician must be notified.

The frequency of voiding ranges from 2 to 6 times during the first and second days of life and from 5 to 25 times during the subsequent 24 hours. About 6 to 10 voidings per day of pale straw-colored urine are indicative of adequate fluid intake. Generally, term infants void 15 to 60 ml/kg/day (Blackburn & Loper, 1992; Fanaroff & Martin, 1997). In addition to excretion of urine, infants lose additional water through insensible fluid loss (70% of the water evaporates from the skin and 35% from the respiratory tract). Stool water loss is estimated at 5 to 10 ml/kg/day.

Full-term infants are unable to concentrate urine; therefore, the specific gravity of the urine may range from 1.001 to 1.020 (Pagana & Pagana, 1998). The ability to concentrate

urine fully is attained by about 3 months of age. After the first voiding the infant's urine may appear cloudy (because of mucous content) and have a much higher specific gravity. This decreases as fluid intake increases. Normal urine during early infancy is usually straw colored and almost odorless. Sometimes pink-tinged stains (brick dust) appear on the diaper. These stains are caused by uric acid crystals and are normal. Blood may be found on a diaper of a female infant. This pseudomenstruation is caused by the withdrawal of maternal hormones. Males may have some bloody spotting from a circumcision. If there is no apparent cause of bleeding, the physician should be notified.

Loss of fluid through urine, feces, lungs, increased metabolic rate, and limited fluid intake results in a 5% to 10% loss of the birth weight. This usually occurs during the first 3 to 5 days of life. If the mother is breastfeeding and her milk supply has not come in yet (which happens on the third or fourth day after birth) the neonate is protected from dehydration by its increased extracellular fluid volume. The neonate should regain the birth weight within 10 days.

Because renal thresholds are low in the infant, bicarbonate concentration and buffering capacity are decreased. This may lead to acidosis and electrolyte imbalance.

Fluid and Electrolyte Balance

Differences in the newborn's fluid and electrolyte balance from adult physiologic response include the following:
- Distribution of extracellular and intracellular fluid. About 40% of the body weight of the newborn is extracellular fluid, whereas in the adult it is 20%.
- Rate of exchange of extracellular fluid. Each day the newborn takes in and excretes 600 to 700 ml of water, which is 20% of the total body fluid, or 50% of the extracellular fluid. In comparison, the adult exchanges 2000 ml of water, which is 5% of the total body fluid and 14% of the extracellular fluid.
- Composition of body fluids. There is a higher concentration of sodium, phosphates, chloride, and organic acids and a lower concentration of bicarbonate ions in the newborn. These findings mean that the newborn is in a compensated acidotic state.
- The glomerular filtration rate is about 30% in the newborn, compared with 50% in the adult. This results in a decreased ability to remove nitrogenous and other waste products from the blood. However, the newborn's ingested protein is almost totally metabolized for growth.
- The decreased ability to excrete excessive sodium results in hypotonic urine, compared with plasma.
- The sodium reabsorption decreases as a result of lowered sodium-potassium–activated adenosine-triphosphatase (ATPase) activity.
- The newborn can dilute urine down to 50 milliosmols (mOsm). The capacity to dilute urine exceeds the capacity to concentrate it. There is some limitation in the ability to increase urinary volume.

- The newborn can concentrate urine from 600 to 700 mOsm, compared with the adult's capacity of 1400 mOsm. The inability to concentrate urine is not absolute, but in terms of adult function, it is somewhat limited. See Appendix B for newborn laboratory values.
- The newborn has a higher renal threshold for glucose.

Signs of Risk for Renal System Problems

The renal system has a wide range of functions, and dysfunction can result from physiologic abnormalities ranging from the lack of a steady stream of urine to gross anomalies. Gross anomalies such as hypospadias and exstrophy of the bladder can be identified easily at birth. Enlarged or cystic kidneys may be identified as masses during abdominal palpation. Some kidney anomalies can also be detected by ultrasound during pregnancy.

Gastrointestinal System

The infant's gastrointestinal system is not mature at birth, but reaches adult maturity levels in 2 to 3 years. The full-term newborn is capable of swallowing, digesting, metabolizing, absorbing proteins and simple carbohydrates, and emulsifying fats. With the exception of pancreatic amylase, the characteristic enzymes and digestive juices are present even in low-birth-weight neonates.

In the adequately hydrated infant, the mucous membrane of the mouth is moist and pink. The hard and soft palates are intact. Drooling of mucus is common in the first few hours after birth. Retention cysts, small whitish areas (Epstein's pearls), may be found on the gum margins and at the juncture of the hard and soft palate. The cheeks are full because of well-developed sucking pads. These, like the labial tubercles (sucking calluses) on the upper lip, disappear when the sucking period is over, around the age of 12 months.

Even though sucking motions in utero have been recorded by ultrasound, these motions are not coordinated in any infant who is less than 1500 grams at birth or born before 32 weeks of gestation. Sucking behavior is influenced by neuromuscular maturity, maternal medications received during labor and birth, and the type of initial feeding.

A special mechanism present in normal newborns coordinates the breathing, sucking, and swallowing reflexes necessary for oral feeding. Sucking in the newborn takes place in small bursts of three or four sucks at a time. In the term newborn, longer and more efficient sucking attempts occur a few hours after birth. The infant is unable to move food from the lips to the pharynx; therefore placing the nipple (breast or bottle) well inside the baby's mouth is necessary. Peristaltic activity in the esophagus is uncoordinated in the first few days of life. It quickly becomes a coordinated pattern in normal infants, and they swallow easily.

Teeth begin developing in utero, with enamel formation continuing until about 10 years of age. Tooth development is influenced by neonatal or infant illnesses, medications, and illnesses of or medications taken by the mother during pregnancy. The fluoride level in the water supply also influences tooth development. Occasionally an infant may be born with one or more teeth. Native American infants are commonly born with teeth.

Bacteria are not present in the infant's gastrointestinal tract at birth. Soon after birth, oral and anal orifices permit entry of bacteria and air. Generally the highest bacterial concentration is found in the lower portion of the intestine, particularly in the large intestine. Normal colonic bacteria are established within the first week after birth, and normal intestinal flora help synthesize vitamin K, folate, and biotin. Bowel sounds can usually be heard 1 hour after birth.

The capacity of the stomach varies from 30 to 90 ml depending on the size of the infant. The emptying time for the stomach is highly variable. Several factors, such as time and volume of feedings, type and temperature of food, and psychologic stress, may affect emptying time. The cardiac sphincter is immature, and nervous control of the stomach is not well established, so some regurgitation may occur. Regurgitation during the first day or two of life can be decreased by avoiding overfeeding, burping the infant, and positioning the infant with the head slightly elevated.

Digestion

The infant's gastric acidity at birth normally equals the adult level but is reduced within a week and may remain reduced for 2 to 3 months. The reduction in gastric acidity may lead to "colic." Infants with colic usually remain awake, crying in apparent distress between feedings, often between the same two feedings every day. Nothing seems to appease them. They appear to "grow out" of this behavior by 3 months of age.

Further digestion and absorption of nutrients occur in the small intestine. This complex process is made possible by secretions from the pancreas, liver (through the common bile duct), and duodenal portion of the small intestine.

The infant's ability to digest carbohydrates, fats, and proteins is regulated by the presence of certain enzymes. Most of these enzymes are functional at birth. One exception is amylase, produced by the salivary glands after about 3 months and by the pancreas at about 6 months of age. This enzyme is necessary to convert starch into maltose. The other exception is lipase, also secreted by the pancreas; it is necessary for the digestion of fat. Thus the normal newborn is capable of digesting simple carbohydrates and proteins but has a limited ability to digest fats.

Stools

Newborn stools consist of meconium and are replaced by transitional stools. At birth the lower intestine is filled with meconium. Meconium is formed during fetal life from the amniotic fluid and its constituents, intestinal secretions (including bilirubin), and cells (shed from the mucosa). Meconium is greenish black and viscous and contains occult blood. The first meconium passed is sterile, but within hours, all meconium passed contains bacteria. About 69% of normal-term infants pass meconium within 12 hours of life, 94% by 24 hours, and 99.8% in 48 hours (Blackburn & Loper, 1992).

The number of stools passed varies during the first week, being most numerous between the third and sixth days. Newborns fed early pass stools sooner. Transitional stools (thin, slimy, and brown to green because of the continued presence of meconium) are passed from the third to sixth day. The stools of the breastfed infant are loose and golden yellow and are nonirritating to the infant's skin. The breastfed baby should have at least two bowel movements every 24 hours during the first several weeks. Fewer stools are an indication of insufficient intake. The stools of the formula-fed baby are formed but soft and pale yellow and have a typical stool odor. They tend to be irritating to the infant's skin. The number of stools decreases in the first 2 weeks from five or six each day (after every feeding) to one or two per day.

The infant develops an elimination pattern by the second week of life. With the addition of solid food (around 6 months of age), the baby's stool gradually assumes the characteristics of an adult's stool.

Feeding Behaviors

Variations occur among infants regarding interest in food, symptoms of hunger, and amount ingested at one time. The amount of food that the infant takes in at any feeding depends on the size, hunger level, and alertness of the infant. When an infant is put to breast, some feed immediately, whereas others require a learning period of up to 48 hours before breastfeeding is completely effective. Random hand-to-mouth movement and sucking of fingers are actions that are well developed at birth and intensified when the infant is hungry. Caregivers should be alert to these hunger cues.

Signs of Risk for Gastrointestinal Problems

The time, color, and character of the infant's first stool should be noted. A lack of passage of stool could indicate an inborn error of metabolism (e.g., cystic fibrosis) or a congenital disorder (e.g., Hirschsprung's disease or an imperforate anus). An active rectal "wink" reflex (contraction of the anal sphincter muscle in response to touch) usually is a good sign of sphincter tone.

Some infants do not digest specific formulas well. If an infant is allergic to or unable to digest a formula, the stools may become very soft with a high water content that is seen as a distinct water ring around the stool on the diaper. Forceful ejection of stool and a water ring around the stool are signs of diarrhea. Care must be taken to avoid misinterpreting transitional stools for diarrhea. The loss of fluid in diarrhea can rapidly lead to fluid and electrolyte imbalance. Passage of meconium from the vagina or urinary meatus is a sign of a possible fistulous tract from the rectum.

Abdominal distention at birth usually indicates a serious disorder such as a ruptured viscus (from abdominal wall defects) or tumors. Distention that occurs later may be the result of overfeeding or may signal gastrointestinal disorders. A scaphoid (sunken) abdomen with bowel sounds heard in the chest and signs of respiratory distress indicate a diaphragmatic hernia.

The amount and frequency of regurgitation ("spitting up") after feedings need to be recorded. Color change, gagging, and projectile (very forceful) vomiting occur in association with esophageal and tracheoesophageal anomalies.

Hepatic System

The liver and gallbladder are formed by the fourth week of gestation. In the newborn the liver can be palpated about 1 cm below the right costal margin because it is enlarged and occupies about 40% of the abdominal cavity. The infant's liver plays an important role in iron storage, carbohydrate metabolism, conjugation of bilirubin, and coagulation.

Iron Storage

The fetal liver (which serves as the site for production of hemoglobin after birth) begins storing iron in utero. The infant's iron store is proportional to the total body hemoglobin content and length of gestation. At birth the term neonate has approximately 270 mg of iron (depending on gestational age and birth weight), of which approximately 140 to 170 mg is in hemoglobin (Blackburn & Loper, 1992). If the mother had an adequate iron intake during pregnancy, the infant will have an iron store that will last until the fifth month of life.

Carbohydrate Metabolism

The infant's carbohydrate reserves are low, with one third of this reserve in the form of liver glycogen. The infant's liver may not be mature enough to form glucose from protein; therefore newborns are susceptible to hypoglycemia. Glucose is the main source of energy during the first 4 to 6 hours of life. Blood glucose levels fall rapidly and then stabilize at about 50 to 60 mg/dl. By the time the infant is 3 days old, blood glucose levels should be approximately 60 to 70 mg/dl. If the infant appears to be jittery or has tremors, the blood glucose level should be determined to rule out hypoglycemia.

Conjugation of Bilirubin

The fetal liver begins to metabolize bilirubin at a gestational age of 12 weeks but loses this ability by 36 weeks. The fetus does not conjugate bilirubin, thereby allowing it to cross the placenta and be excreted by the mother.

Bilirubin is a yellow pigment derived from the hemoglobin released with the breakdown of RBCs and the myoglobin in muscle cells. The hemoglobin is phagocytized by the reticuloendothelial cells, converted to bilirubin, and released in an unconjugated form. Unconjugated bilirubin,

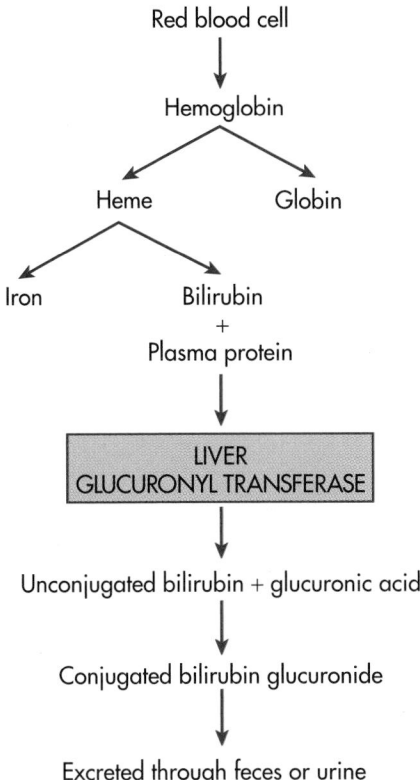

Fig. 26-5 Formation and excretion of bilirubin. *(From Wong, D. [1999]. Whaley and Wong's nursing care of infants and children [6th ed.]. St. Louis: Mosby.)*

termed *indirect bilirubin,* is relatively insoluble and almost entirely bound to circulating albumin, a plasma protein. The unbound bilirubin can leave the vascular system and permeate other extravascular tissues (e.g., the skin, sclera, and oral mucous membranes). The resultant yellow coloring is termed *jaundice.*

The liver controls the amount of circulating unbound bilirubin. In the liver the unbound bilirubin is conjugated with glucuronide in the presence of the enzyme glucuronyl transferase. The conjugated form of bilirubin is excreted from liver cells as a constituent of bile. This form is termed *direct bilirubin* and is soluble. Along with other components of bile, direct bilirubin is excreted into the biliary tract system that carries the bile into the duodenum. Bilirubin is converted to urobilinogen and stercobilin within the duodenum by the action of the bacterial flora. Urobilinogen is excreted in urine and feces; stercobilin is excreted in the feces (Fig. 26-5). The total serum bilirubin level is the sum of the levels of both conjugated (direct) and unconjugated (indirect) bilirubin.

Adequate serum albumin–binding sites are available unless the infant experiences asphyxia neonatorum (respiratory failure in the newborn), cold stress, or hypoglycemia. A mother's prebirth ingestion of medications such as sulfa drugs and aspirin can reduce the amount of serum albumin–binding sites in the newborn. Although the neonate

has the functional capacity to convert bilirubin, physiologic hyperbilirubinemia commonly occurs in infants.

Physiologic Hyperbilirubinemia

Physiologic jaundice or neonatal **hyperbilirubinemia** normally occurs in 50% of full-term and 80% of preterm newborns. The incidence and severity of physiologic jaundice is increased in Asian, Native American, and Eskimo infants (Merenstein & Gardner, 1998). Although neonatal jaundice is considered benign, bilirubin may accumulate to hazardous levels and lead to a pathologic condition. Guyton and Hall (1995) noted that neonatal jaundice occurs for the following reasons:

- The newborn has a higher rate of bilirubin production. In the newborn the number of fetal RBCs per kilogram of weight is greater than in an adult. Fetal RBCs have a shorter survival time—40 to 90 days—compared with 120 days for adult RBCs.
- The reabsorption of bilirubin from the neonatal small intestine is considerable.

Physiologic jaundice fulfills the following specific criteria (Korones, 1995):

- The infant is otherwise well.
- In term infants, jaundice first appears after 24 hours and disappears by the end of the seventh day.
- In premature infants, jaundice is first evident after 48 hours and disappears by the ninth or tenth day.
- The serum concentration of unconjugated bilirubin usually does not exceed 12 mg/100 dl in term and 15 mg/100 dl in preterm infants.
- Hyperbilirubinemia is almost exclusively of the unconjugated variety, and conjugated (direct) bilirubin does not exceed 1 to 1.5 mg/100 dl.
- Daily increments of bilirubin concentration should not surpass 5 mg/100 dl. Bilirubin levels in excess of 12 mg/100 dl may indicate an exaggeration of the physiologic handicap or the presence of disease.

> **NURSE ALERT**
>
> *At any serum bilirubin level the appearance of jaundice during the first day of life or persistence beyond the ages previously delineated usually indicates a pathologic process.*

Jaundice is generally first noticed in the head, especially the sclera and mucous membranes, and then progresses gradually to the thorax, abdomen, and extremities.

Feeding practices may influence the appearance and degree of physiologic hyperbilirubinemia. Early feeding (within the first hour) tends to keep the serum bilirubin level low by stimulating intestinal activity (the gastrocolic reflex) and passage of meconium.

Cold stress of the newborn may result in acidosis and raise the level of free fatty acids. In the presence of acidosis, albumin binding of bilirubin is weakened and bilirubin is freed.

Kernicterus, the most serious complication of neonatal hyperbilirubinemia, is caused by the precipitation of bilirubin in neuronal cells, resulting in their destruction. Cerebral palsy, epilepsy, and mental retardation may occur if the infant survives kernicterus.

In cases where the infant is discharged from the hospital before 48 hours after birth or the infant is born at home, a professional attendant may not be available to assess pathologic rises in circulating unbound bilirubin. Therefore all parents need instruction in how to assess jaundice and to whom to report the findings.

Breast Milk Jaundice

Breast milk jaundice has been defined as a progressive indirect hyperbilirubinemia beyond the first week of life. (See Chapter 28 for a discussion of this topic.)

Breastfeeding Jaundice

Breastfeeding jaundice is associated with the breastfeeding pattern and occurs earlier than breast milk jaundice. (See Chapter 28 for a discussion of this topic.)

Coagulation

The liver plays an important role in blood coagulation. Coagulation factors, which are synthesized in the liver, are activated by vitamin K. The lack of intestinal bacteria needed to synthesize vitamin K results in a transient blood coagulation deficiency between the second and fifth days of life. The levels of coagulation factors slowly rise to reach adult levels by 9 months of age. An injection of vitamin K on the day of birth helps prevent clotting problems. Any bleeding problems noted in an infant should be reported immediately and tests for clotting ordered.

Signs of Risk for Hepatic System Problems

Some problems such as kernicterus and hypoglycemia have already been discussed. The infant's hemoglobin levels must be assessed for anemia. Because infants may develop a coagulation deficiency, a male child who has been circumcised needs to be observed closely for signs of hemorrhage. Hemorrhage also could be caused by a clotting defect, indicating a serious problem such as hemophilia.

Immune System

The cells that provide the infant with immunity are developed early in fetal life; however, they are not activated for several months. For the first 3 months of life, the infant is protected by passive immunity received from the mother. Natural barriers such as the acidity of the stomach and the production of pepsin and trypsin, which maintain sterility of the small intestine, are not fully developed until 3 to 4 weeks of age (Guyton & Hall, 1995). The membrane-protective IgA is missing from the respiratory and urinary tracts, and unless the newborn is breastfed, it is also absent from the gastrointestinal tract. The infant begins to synthesize IgG, and about 40% of adult levels are reached by 1 year of age (Guyton & Hall, 1995). Significant concentrations of IgM are produced at birth, and adult levels are reached by 9 months of age. The production of IgA, IgD, and IgE is much more gradual, and maximum levels are not attained until early childhood. The infant who is breastfed receives passive immunity through the colostrum and breast milk. The protection provided varies with the age and maturity of the infant and the mother's level of immunity (Lawrence, 1999).

Signs of Risk for Immune System Problems

All newborns and preterm newborns especially are at high risk for infection during the first several months of life. During this period, infection represents one of the leading causes of morbidity and mortality. The newborn cannot limit the invading pathogen to the portal of entry because of the generalized hypofunctioning of the inflammatory and immune mechanisms. Any unusual discharges from the infant's eyes, nose, mouth, or other orifice must be investigated. If a rash appears, it must be evaluated closely; many normal rashes in the newborn are not associated with any infection. When an infant is septic, the usual response is respiratory distress. Infants need to be protected from infections by the use of good handwashing techniques.

Integumentary System

All skin structures are present at birth. The epidermis and dermis are loosely bound and extremely thin. Vernix caseosa (a cheeselike, whitish substance) is also fused with the epidermis and serves as a protective covering. The infant's skin is very sensitive and can be easily damaged. The term infant has an erythematous (red) skin for a few hours after birth, after which it fades to its normal color. The skin often appears blotchy or mottled, especially over the extremities. The hands and feet appear slightly cyanotic. This bluish discoloration, **acrocyanosis,** is caused by vasomotor instability, capillary stasis, and a high hemoglobin level. This is normal and appears intermittently over the first 7 to 10 days, especially with exposure to cold.

The healthy term newborn is plump. Subcutaneous fat accumulated during the last trimester acts as insulation. The newborn's skin may be slightly tight, suggesting fluid retention. Fine lanugo hair may be noted over the face, shoulders, and back. Actual edema of the face and ecchymosis (bruising) may be noted as a result of face presentation or forceps-assisted birth.

Creases can be found on the palms of the hands. The simian line, a single palmar crease, is often found in Asian infants or Down syndrome. The soles of the feet should be inspected for the number of creases. Premature newborns have few if any creases. Increasing numbers of creases correlate with a greater maturity rating.

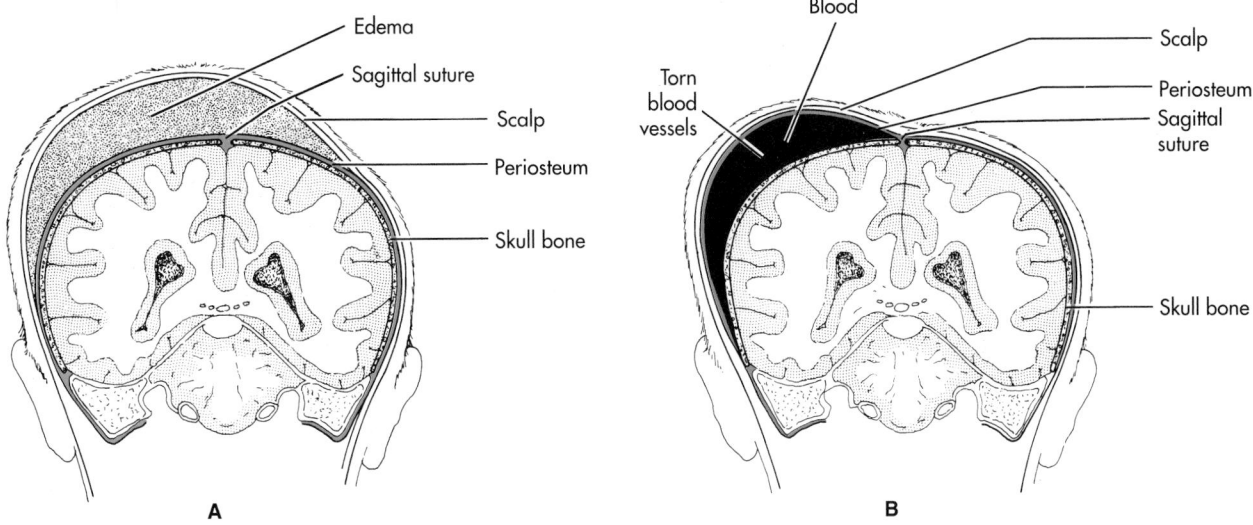

Fig. 26-6 Differences between caput succedaneum and cephalhematoma. **A,** Caput succedaneum: edema of scalp noted at birth; crosses suture lines. **B,** Cephalhematoma: bleeding between periosteum and skull bone appearing within first 2 days; does not cross suture lines.

Caput Succedaneum

Caput succedaneum is a generalized, easily identifiable edematous area of the scalp, most commonly found on the occiput area (Fig. 26-6, *A*). The sustained pressure of the presenting vertex against the cervix results in compression of local vessels, thereby slowing venous return. The slower venous return causes an increase in tissue fluids within the skin of the scalp, and an edematous swelling develops. This boggy edematous swelling, present at birth, extends across suture lines of the fetal skull and disappears spontaneously within 3 to 4 days. Infants who are delivered with the assistance of vacuum extraction usually have a caput in the area of application of the cup.

Cephalhematoma

Cephalhematoma is a collection of blood between a skull bone and its periosteum. Therefore a cephalhematoma does not cross a cranial suture line (Fig. 26-6, *B*). Often, caput succedaneum and cephalhematoma occur simultaneously.

Bleeding may occur with spontaneous birth from pressure against the maternal bony pelvis. Low forceps birth and difficult forceps rotation and extraction may also cause bleeding. This soft, fluctuating, irreducible fullness does not pulsate or bulge when the infant cries. It appears several hours or the day after birth and may not become apparent until a caput succedaneum is absorbed. A cephalhematoma is usually largest on the second or third day, by which time the bleeding stops. The fullness of a cephalhematoma spontaneously resolves in 3 to 6 weeks. It is not aspirated because infection may develop if the skin is punctured.

As the hematoma resolves, hemolysis of RBCs occurs. Hyperbilirubinemia (jaundice) may result after the newborn is home. Therefore the parents are instructed to observe the newborn for jaundice and may be asked to bring the infant in to be rechecked before the usual 2- to 4-week visit.

Desquamation

Desquamation (peeling) of the skin of the term infant does not occur until a few days after birth. Its presence at birth is an indication of postmaturity.

Sweat and Oil Glands

Sweat glands are present at birth but do not respond to increases in ambient or body temperature. Some fetal sebaceous (oil) gland hyperplasia and secretion of sebum result from the hormonal influences of pregnancy. Vernix caseosa is a product of the sebaceous glands. Removal of the vernix is followed by desquamation of the epidermis in most infants (Fanaroff & Martin, 1997). Distended, small, white sebaceous glands, noticeable on the newborn face, are known as *milia*. Although sebaceous glands are well developed at birth, they are only minimally active during childhood. They become more active as androgen production increases before puberty.

Mongolian Spots

Mongolian spots, bluish-black areas of pigmentation, may appear over any part of the exterior surface of the body, including the extremities. They are more commonly noted on the back and buttocks (Fig. 26-7). These pigmented areas are most frequently noted in babies

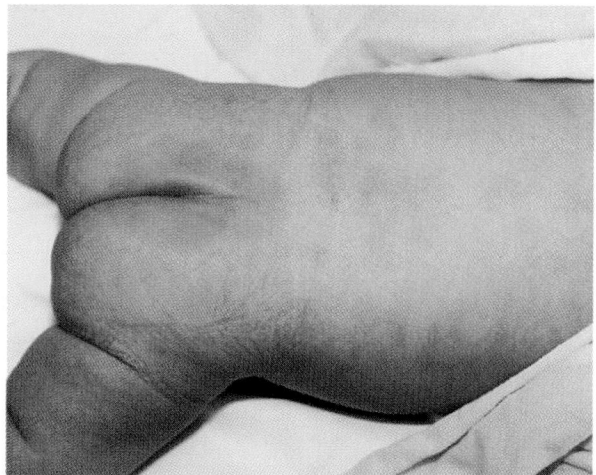

Fig. 26-7 Mongolian spot. *(From Wong, D. [1999]. Whaley and Wong's nursing care of infants and children [6th ed.]. St. Louis: Mosby.)*

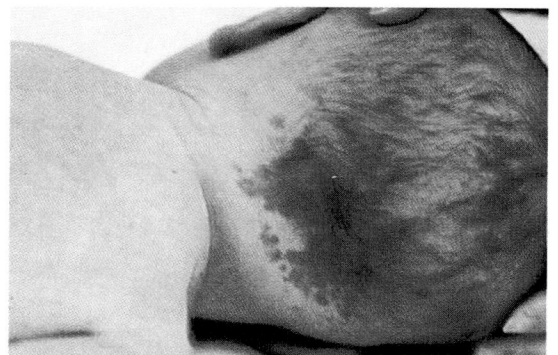

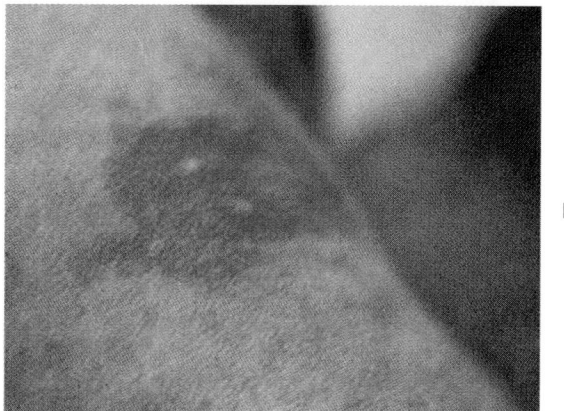

Fig. 26-8 **A,** Telangiectatic nevi (stork bite). **B,** Erythema toxicum (flea bite). *(Courtesy Mead Johnson & Co., Evansville, IN.)*

whose ethnic origins are in the Mediterranean area, Latin America, Asia, or Africa. They are more common in dark-skinned individuals, regardless of race. They fade gradually over months or years.

Nevi

Known as "stork bites," telangiectatic nevi are pink and easily blanched (Fig. 26-8, *A*). They appear on the upper eyelids, nose, upper lip, lower occiput bone, and nape of the neck. They have no clinical significance and fade between the first and second year of life.

The strawberry mark, or nevus vasculosus, is a common type of capillary hemangioma. It consists of dilated, newly formed capillaries occupying the entire dermal and subdermal layers with associated connective tissue hypertrophy. The typical lesion is a raised, sharply demarcated, bright or dark red, rough-surfaced swelling that resembles a strawberry. Lesions usually are single but may be multiple, with 75% occurring on the head. These lesions can remain until the child is of school age or sometimes even longer.

A port-wine stain, or nevus flammeus, is usually observed at birth and is composed of a plexus of newly formed capillaries in the papillary layer of the corium. It is red to purple; varies in size, shape, and location; and is not elevated. True port-wine stains do not blanch on pressure or disappear. They are most frequently found on the face.

Erythema Toxicum

A transient rash, erythema toxicum, is also called erythema neonatorum, "newborn rash" or "flea bite" dermatitis. It has lesions in different stages: erythematous maculas, papules, and small vesicles (Fig. 26-8, *B*). The lesions may appear suddenly anywhere on the body. The

rash is thought to be an inflammatory response. Eosinophils, which help decrease inflammation, are found in the vesicles. The rash is found in term neonates (gestational age of 36 weeks or more) during the first 3 weeks of age (Seidel, Rosenstein, & Pathak, 1993). Although the appearance is alarming, the rash has no clinical significance and requires no treatment.

Signs of Risk for Integumentary Problems

Close observation of the newborn's skin color can lead to early detection of potential problems. Any pallor, plethora (deep purplish color from increased circulating RBCs), petechiae, cyanosis, or jaundice should be noted and described. The skin should be examined for signs of birth injuries, such as forceps marks and lesions related to fetal monitoring. Ecchymosis may be present on the head, neck, and face of an infant born with a nuchal cord (cord around the neck). When bruises are present, the infant's bilirubin levels may be elevated. Petechiae may be present if increased pressure was applied to an area. Petechiae scattered over the infant's body should be reported to the pediatrician because their presence may indicate underlying problems such as low platelet count or infection. Unilateral or bilateral periauricular papillomas (skin tags) occur fairly frequently. Their occurrence is usually a family trait and of no consequence.

Reproductive System

Female

At birth the ovaries contain thousands of primitive germ cells. These represent the full complement of potential ova; no oogonia form after birth in term infants. The ovarian cortex, which is made up primarily of primordial follicles, occupies a larger portion of the ovary in the female newborn than in the female adult. From birth to sexual maturity, the number of ova decreases by approximately 90%.

An increase of estrogen during pregnancy followed by a drop after birth results in a mucoid vaginal discharge and even some slight bloody spotting (pseudomenstruation). External genitals are usually edematous with increased pigmentation. In term newborn infants the labia majora and minora cover the vestibule (Fig. 26-9, *A*). In preterm infants the clitoris is prominent and the labia majora are small and widely separated. Vaginal or hymenal tags are common findings and have no clinical significance. Vernix caseosa may be present between the labia.

If the female was born in the breech position, the labia may be very edematous. Bruising commonly appears because of the trauma of the breech birth. These two problems usually correct themselves within a few days, and no further treatment is needed.

Male

The testes descend into the scrotum by birth in 90% of newborn boys. Although this percentage drops with premature birth, by 1 year of age the incidence of undescended testes in all males is less than 1%. Spermatogenesis does not occur until puberty.

A tight prepuce (foreskin) is common in newborns. The urethral opening may be completely covered by the prepuce, which may not be retractable for 3 to 4 years. Smegma, a white, cheesy substance, is commonly found under the foreskin. Small, white, firm lesions called *epithelial pearls* may be seen at the tip of the prepuce. At 36 to 40 weeks of gestation, the testes are palpable in the upper scrotum and rugae appear on the anterior portion. After 40 weeks the testes can be palpated in the scrotum, and rugae cover the scrotal sac. The postterm neonate has deep rugae and a pendulous scrotum. The scrotum is usually more deeply pigmented than the rest of the skin (Fig. 26-9, *B*) and is especially apparent in darker-skinned infants. This pigmentation is a response to maternal estrogen. Hydroceles, caused by an accumulation of fluid around the testes, may be found. They can be easily transilluminated with a light and usually decrease in size without treatment.

If the male infant was born in a breech presentation, the scrotum will appear very edematous. Often the scrotum is also bruised from the trauma of the breech birth. The swelling and discoloration subside within a few days.

Swelling of Breast Tissue

Swelling of the breast tissue in infants of both sexes is caused by the hyperestrogenism of pregnancy. In a few in-

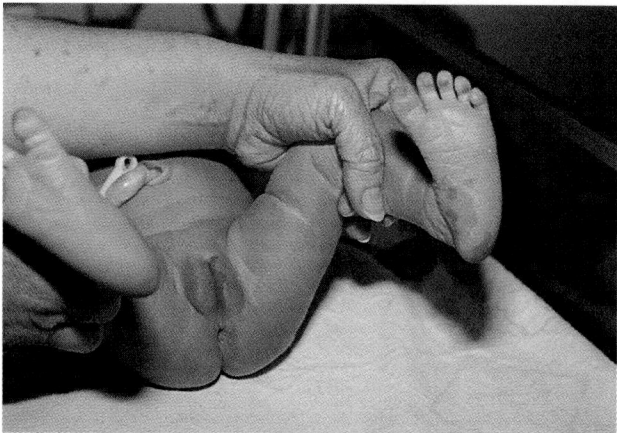

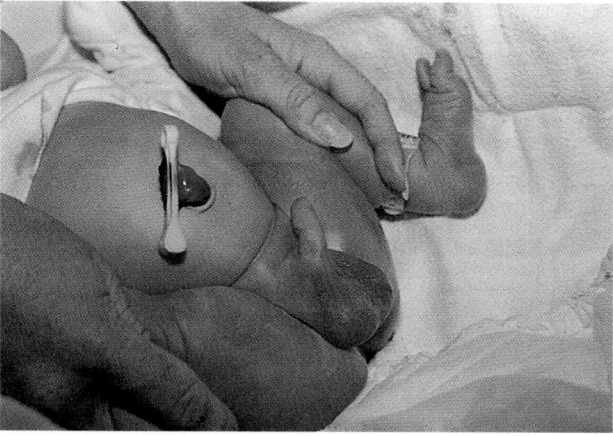

Fig. 26-9 External genitalia. **A,** Genitals in female term infant. Note mucoid vaginal discharge. **B,** Genitals in male infant. Uncircumcised penis. Rugae cover scrotum, indicating term gestation. Cord has been swabbed with ethylene blue to prevent infection. *(Courtesy Marjorie Pyle, RNC, Lifecircle, Costa Mesa, CA.)*

fants a thin discharge (witch's milk) can be seen. This condition has no clinical significance, requires no treatment, and subsides as the maternal hormones are eliminated from the infant's body within a few days. The nipples should be symmetric on the chest.

Breast tissue and areola size increase with gestation. The areola appears slightly elevated at 34 weeks of gestation. By 36 weeks a breast bud of 1 to 2 mm is palpable and increases to 12 mm by 42 weeks. Increased breast tissue may indicate subcutaneous fat in larger babies. However, a greater quantity of breast tissue generally indicates a higher maturity rating (Seidel, Rosenstein, & Pathak, 1993).

Signs of Risk for Reproductive Problems

The infant must be closely inspected for ambiguous genitalia and other abnormalities. Normally in a female the urethral opening is located behind the clitoris. Any deviation from this may mistakenly suggest that the clitoris

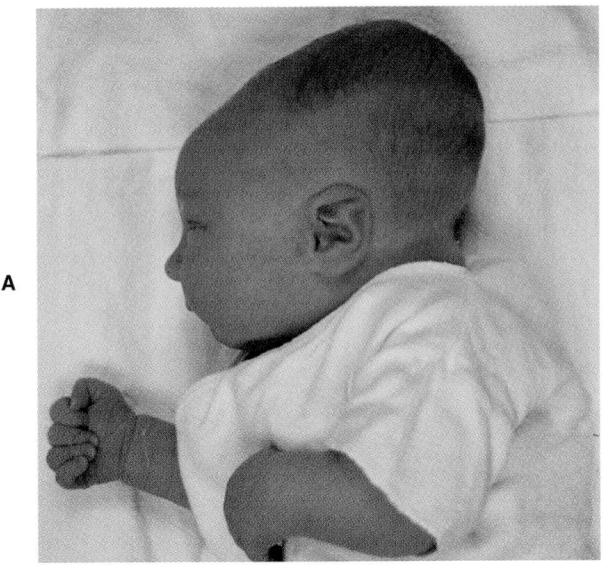

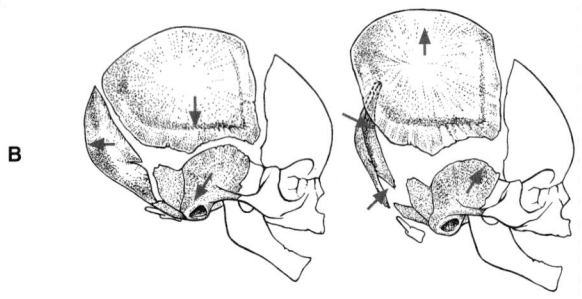

Fig. 26-10 Molding. **A,** Significant molding, soon after birth. **B,** Schematic of bones of skull when molding is present. (**A,** *Courtesy Kim Molloy, Knoxville, IA.*)

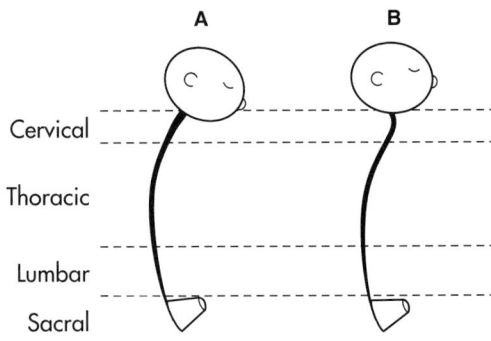

Fig. 26-11 Development of spinal curvatures. **A,** Newborn. **B,** Cervical secondary curvature. *(From Wong, D. [1999]. Whaley and Wong's nursing care of infants and children [6th ed.]. St. Louis: Mosby.)*

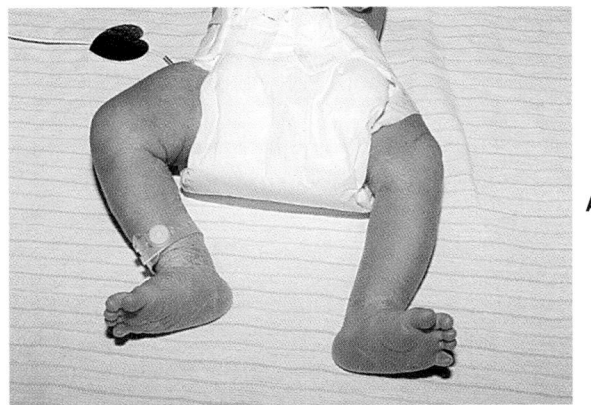

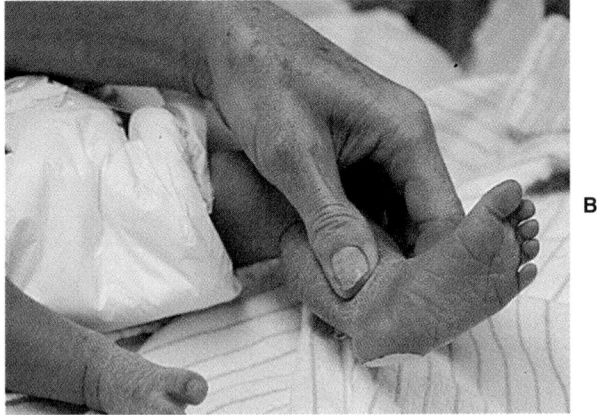

Fig. 26-12 Extremities. **A,** Bowed appearance of legs. **B,** Normal absence of arch in newborn's foot. *(Courtesy Marjorie Pyle, RNC, Lifecircle, Costa Mesa, CA.)*

is a small penis, which can occur in conditions such as adrenal hyperplasia. Nearly all females are born with hymenal tags. Absence of such could indicate vaginal agenesis. Fecal discharge from the vagina indicates a rectovaginal fistula. Any of these findings needs to be reported to the physician for further evaluation.

The male infant's scrotum should always be palpated for the presence of testes. Inguinal hernias may be present and become more obvious when the infant cries. If the urinary meatus is not at the tip of the glans penis, hypospadias (urethral meatus opening on the underside of the penis) or epispadias (urethral meatus opening on the top of the penis) may be present. These problems are usually associated with other anomalies.

Skeletal System

The infant's skeletal system undergoes rapid development during the first year of life. At birth, more cartilage is present than ossified bone. Because of cephalocaudal (head-to-tail) development, the newborn looks somewhat out of proportion.

At term the head is one-fourth the total body length. The arms are slightly longer than the legs. In the newborn the legs are one-third the total body length but only 15% of the total body weight. In the adult the legs make up half the total body height and 30% of the total body weight. As

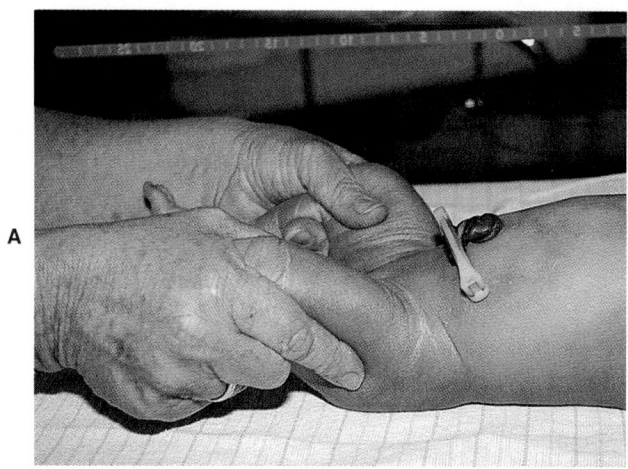 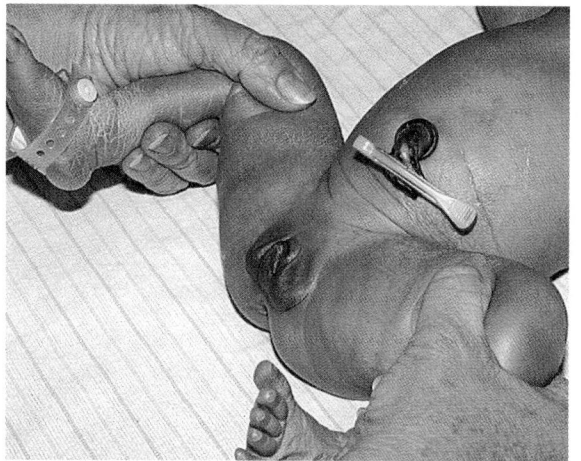

Fig. 26-13 Method of assessing for hip dysplasia or dislocation using Ortolani's maneuver. **A,** Examiner's middle fingers are placed over greater trochanter, and thumbs are placed over inner thigh opposite lesser trochanter. **B,** Gentle pressure is exerted to further flex thigh on hip, and thighs are rotated outward. If hip dysplasia is present, head of femur can be felt to slip forward in acetabulum and flip back when pressure is released and legs are returned to their original position. A click is sometimes heard *(Ortolani's sign)*. *(Courtesy Marjorie Pyle, RNC, Lifecircle, Costa Mesa, CA.)*

growth proceeds, the midpoint in head-to-toe measurements gradually descends from the level of the umbilicus at birth to the level of the symphysis pubis at maturity.

The face appears small in relation to the skull. The skull appears large and heavy. Cranial size and shape can be distorted by molding. Molding is the shaping of the fetal head by the overlapping of cranial bones to facilitate movement through the birth canal during labor (Fig. 26-10). Shaping makes the head appear conelike (see Fig. 26-10, *A*).

The bones in the vertebral column of the newborn form two primary curvatures, one in the thoracic region and one in the sacral region (Fig. 26-11, *A*). Both are forward, concave curvatures. As the infant gains head control at approximately 3 months of age, a secondary curvature appears in the cervical region (Fig. 26-11, *B*).

In some newborns a significant separation of the knees occurs when the ankles are held together, resulting in an appearance of bowlegs (Fig. 26-12, *A*). If the infant's presentation was breech, the knees may remain extended, and the infant will maintain the in utero position for several weeks. What sometimes appears as a gross anomaly may simply be a result of in utero positioning. These conditions are self-limiting. The newborn is also very flat footed because no clearly apparent arch to the foot is present (Fig. 26-12, *B*).

The infant's extremities should be symmetric and of equal length. Fingers and toes should be equal in count and should have nails present. Extra digits (polydactyly) are sometimes found on hands or feet. Fingers or toes may be fused (syndactyly).

The infant's hips should be inspected for symmetry. Skin folds should be equal and symmetric. Hip integrity is assessed by using Ortolani's maneuver (Fig. 26-13). The ex-

aminer places the index and middle fingers of each hand over the greater trochanters of the hips at the same time. Downward pressure is exerted on the hips while the neonate's knees are flexed. The hips are flexed at least 70 degrees and then abducted. The motion should be smooth without any unusual clicks. The presence of a click, an unequal movement, or extra skin folds is considered a positive response, indicating that the hip is dislocated, and the physician should be notified.

The newborn's spine appears straight and can be easily flexed. The newborn can lift the head and turn it from side to side when prone. The vertebrae should appear straight and flat. The base of the spine should not have a dimple. If a dimple is noted, further inspection is required to determine whether a sinus is present. A pilonidal dimple, especially with a sinus and nevus pilosis (hairy nevus), is significant because it can be associated with spina bifida.

Signs of Risk for Skeletal Problems

Skeletal deformities may be congenital or drug induced. Clubfoot (talipes equinovarus), a deformity in which the foot turns inward and is fixed in a plantar flexion position, and any absence of a limb or digit should be recorded and reported. Additional digits or webbing of digits must also be recorded and reported.

Neuromuscular System

Unlike the skeletal system, the neuromuscular system is almost completely developed at birth. The term newborn is recognized to be a vital, responsive, and reactive being. The newborn shows remarkable sensory development and an amazing ability for self-organization and social interaction (Fanaroff & Martin, 1997).

Postbirth growth of the brain follows a predictable pattern: rapid during infancy and early childhood, more gradual during the remainder of the first decade, and minimal during adolescence. The cerebellum ends its growth spurt, which began at about 30 gestational weeks, by the end of the first year. This may be the reason the brain is vulnerable to nutritional deficiencies and trauma in early infancy.

The brain requires glucose as a source of energy and a relatively large supply of oxygen for adequate metabolism. Such requirements signal a need for careful assessment of the infant's respiratory status. The necessity for glucose requires attentiveness to those neonates who may have hypoglycemic episodes.

Spontaneous motor activity may be seen as transient tremors of the mouth and chin, especially during crying episodes, and of the extremities, notably the arms and hands. The transient tremors are normal and can be observed in nearly every newborn. These tremors should not be present when the infant is quiet and should not persist beyond 1 month of age. Persistent tremors or tremors involving the total body may indicate pathologic conditions. Marked tonicity, clonicity, and twitching of facial muscles are signs of convulsions. The physician needs to differentiate among normal tremors, tremors of hypoglycemia, and central nervous system (CNS) disorders so that diagnostic workups and corrective care can be instituted as necessary (Carey, 1996).

Neuromuscular control in the newborn, although still very limited, can be noted. If newborns are placed face down on a firm surface, they will turn their heads to the side to maintain an airway. They attempt to hold their heads in line with their bodies if they are raised by their arms. Various reflexes serve to promote safety and adequate food intake.

Newborn Reflexes

The newborn has many primitive reflexes. The times at which these reflexes appear and disappear reflect the maturity and intactness of the developing nervous system. The most common reflexes found in the normal newborn are described in Table 26-3.

Signs of Risk for Neuromuscular Problems

Any absence of a newborn reflex could indicate major neurologic problems. Birth trauma may cause nerve damage that results in facial asymmetry and paralysis. CNS depression, because of maternal medications received during labor and birth, will also influence neuromuscular functioning. Observation of the neonate for any abnormalities must be made and documented. A thorough physical examination of the newborn assists in detecting any potential complications.

PHYSICAL ASSESSMENT

The assessment of the newborn should progress systematically from head to toe, with evaluation and assessment of each system, that is, cardiovascular, respiratory, and so on. The findings provide a database for implementing the nursing process with newborns and providing anticipatory guidance for the parents. An immediate assessment of the newborn is carried out in the room where the birth occurred. The Apgar score (see Chapter 27), determined at 1 and 5 minutes, provides information that must be considered in the context of data from the total assessment.

A complete physical examination should be done within 24 hours after birth, after the newborn's temperature stabilizes or under a radiant warmer. The area used for the examination should be well-lighted, warm, and free from drafts. The infant is undressed as needed and placed on a firm, warmed flat surface or under a radiant warmer. The physical assessment should begin with a review of the maternal history and prenatal and intrapartal records. This provides a background for the recognition of any potential problems.

This assessment includes appearance, behavior, cardiorespiratory function, skin, vital signs, and maternal-infant interactions. Descriptions of any variations from normal and all abnormal findings are included. (Table 26-4 summarizes the newborn assessment.) After the birth, ongoing assessments of the newborn are made and an evaluation is performed before discharge. After initial stabilization is effected, the steps that follow are included in a newborn assessment.

General Appearance

The neonate's maturity level can be gauged by assessment of general appearance. Features to assess in the general survey include posture, head size, lanugo, vernix caseosa, breast tissue, sole creases, cry, and state of alertness. The normal resting position of the neonate is one of general flexion. The umbilicus is the center of the newborn's body. The neck is short and the abdomen is prominent.

Vital Signs

The temperature, heart rate, and respiratory rate are always obtained. BP may not be routinely assessed unless cardiac problems are possible. An irregular, very slow, or very fast heart rate may indicate a need for BP measurements.

The axillary temperature is a safe, accurate substitute for the rectal temperature. Temperature should therefore be measured by the axillary route. Electronic thermometers have expedited this task and provide a reading within 1 minute. If standard mercury thermometers are used, they should be held in place for at least 3 minutes. Taking an infant's temperature may cause the infant to cry and struggle against the placement of the thermometer in the axilla. Tympanic thermometers may be used after the newborn's ear canals are free of vernix. Before taking the temperature, the examiner may want to determine the heart and respiratory rates while the infant is quiet and at rest.

The normal axillary temperature averages 37° C with a range from 36.5° to 37.2° C.

Text continued on p. 705

TABLE 26-3 · Assessment of Newborn's Reflexes

REFLEX	ELICITING THE REFLEX	CHARACTERISTIC RESPONSE	COMMENTS
Sucking and rooting	Touch infant's lip, cheek, or corner of mouth with nipple	Infant turns head toward stimulus, opens mouth, takes hold, and sucks	Response is difficult if not impossible to elicit after infant has been fed; if response weak or absent, consider prematurity or neurologic defect Parental guidance: Avoid trying to turn head toward breast or nipple, allow infant to root; response disappears after 3 to 4* mo but may persist up to 1 yr
Swallowing	Feed infant; swallowing usually follows sucking and obtaining fluids	Swallowing is usually coordinated with sucking and usually occurs without gagging, coughing, or vomiting	If response is weak or absent, this may indicate prematurity or neurologic defect Sucking and swallowing are often uncoordinated in preterm infant
Grasp 　Palmar 　Plantar	Place finger in palm of hand Place finger at base of toes	Infant's fingers curl around examiner's fingers, toes curl downward	Palmar response lessens by 3 to 4 mo, parents enjoy this contact with infant, plantar response lessens by 8 mo
Extrusion	Touch or depress tip of tongue	Newborn forces tongue outward	Response disappears about fourth month of life
Glabellar (Myerson's)	Tap over forehead, bridge of nose, or maxilla of newborn whose eyes are open	Newborn blinks for first four or five taps	Continued blinking with repeated taps is consistent with extrapyramidal disorder
Tonic neck or "fencing"	With infant falling asleep or sleeping, turn head quickly to one side	With infant facing left side, arm and leg on that side extend; opposite arm and leg flex (turn head to right, and extremities assume opposite postures)	Responses in leg are more consistent Complete response disappears by 3 to 4 mo, incomplete response may be seen until third or fourth year After 6 wk, persistent response is sign of possible cerebral palsy

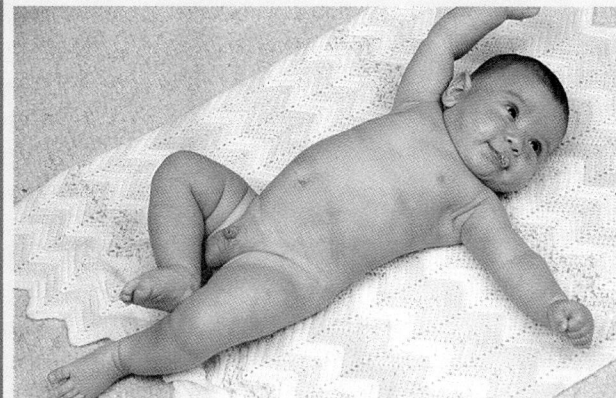

Classic pose in spontaneous tonic neck reflex. *(Courtesy Marjorie Pyle, RNC, Lifecircle, Costa Mesa, CA.)*

*All durations for persistence of reflexes are based on time elapsed after 40 weeks of gestation, that is, if this newborn was born at 36 weeks of gestation, add 1 month to all time limits given.

Continued

■ TABLE 26-3 Assessment of Newborn's Reflexes—cont'd

REFLEX	ELICITING THE REFLEX	CHARACTERISTIC RESPONSE	COMMENTS
Moro's	Hold infant in semisitting position, allow head and trunk to fall backward to an angle of at least 30 degrees Place infant on flat surface, strike surface to startle infant	Symmetric abduction and extension of arms are seen; fingers fan out and form a C with thumb and forefinger; slight tremor may be noted; arms are adducted in embracing motion and return to relaxed flexion and movement Legs may follow similar pattern of response Preterm infant does not complete "embrace"; instead, arms fall backward because of weakness	Response is present at birth; complete response may be seen until 8 wk; body jerk only is seen between 8 and 18 wk; response is absent by 6 mo if neurologic maturation is not delayed; response may be incomplete if infant is deeply asleep; give parental guidance about normal response Asymmetric response may connote injury to brachial plexus, clavicle, or humerus Persistent response after 6 mo indicates possible brain damage

A, Moro's reflex.

Stepping or "walking"	Hold infant vertically, allowing one foot to touch table surface	Infant will simulate walking, alternating flexion and extension of feet; term infants walk on soles of their feet, and preterm infants walk on their toes	Response is normally present for 3 to 4 wk

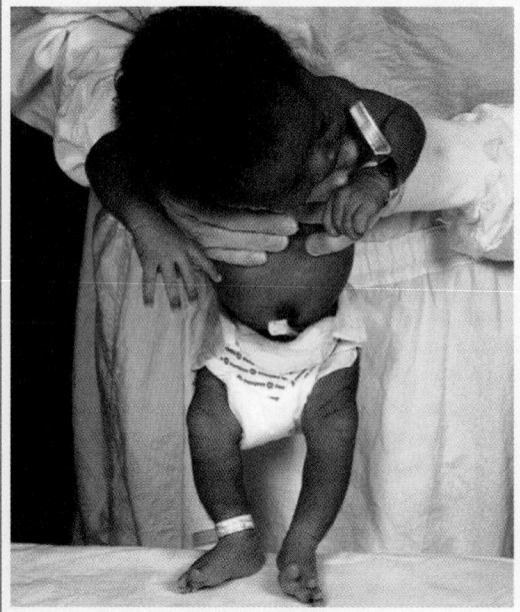

B, Stepping reflex. *(From Dickason, E., Silverman, B., & Kaplan, J. [1998]. Maternal-infant nursing care [3rd ed.]. St. Louis: Mosby.)*

■ **TABLE 26-3** **Assessment of Newborn's Reflexes—cont'd**

REFLEX	ELICITING THE REFLEX	CHARACTERISTIC RESPONSE	COMMENTS
Crawling	Place newborn on abdomen	Newborn makes crawling movements with arms and legs	Response should disappear about 6 wk of age
Deep tendon	Use finger instead of percussion hammer to elicit patellar, or knee jerk, reflex; newborn must be relaxed	Reflex jerk is present; even with newborn relaxed, nonselective overall reaction may occur	
Crossed extension	Infant should be supine; extend one leg, press knee downward, stimulate bottom of foot; observe opposite leg	Opposite leg flexes, adducts, and then extends	

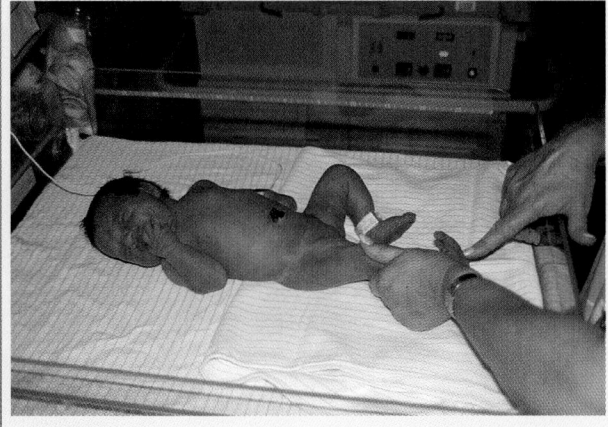

Crossed extension reflex. With the infant in supine position, examiner extends one leg of the infant and presses the knee down. Stimulation of sole of foot of fixated limb should cause free leg to flex, adduct, and extend as if attempting to push away stimulating agent. This reflex should be present during newborn period. *(Courtesy Marjorie Pyle, RNC, Lifecircle, Costa Mesa, CA.)*

REFLEX	ELICITING THE REFLEX	CHARACTERISTIC RESPONSE	COMMENTS
Startle	Perform sharp hand clap; best elicited if newborn is 24 to 36 hr old or older	Arms abduct with flexion of elbows, hands stay clenched	Response should disappear by 4 mo of age Response is elicited more readily in preterm newborn (inform parents of this characteristic)
Babinski's sign (plantar)	On sole of foot, beginning at heel, stroke upward along lateral aspect of sole, then move finger across ball of foot	All toes hyperextend, with dorsiflexion of big toe—recorded as a positive sign	Absence requires neurologic evaluation, should disappear after 1 yr of age

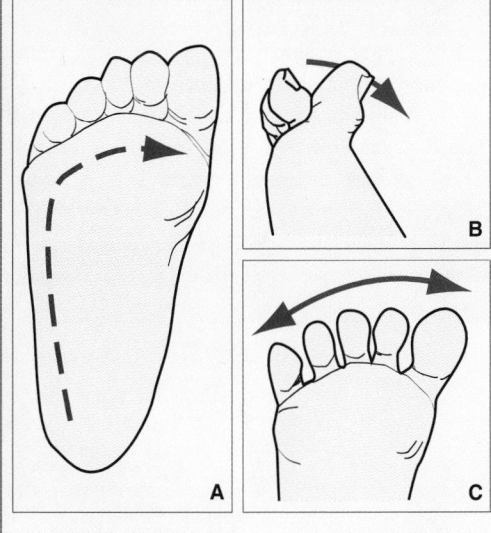

Babinski's reflex. **A,** Direction of stroke. **B,** Dorsiflexion of big toe. **C,** Fanning of toes. *(From Wong, D. [1999]. Whaley and Wong's nursing care of infants and children [6th ed.]. St. Louis: Mosby.)*

Continued

■ **TABLE 26-3** **Assessment of Newborn's Reflexes—cont'd**

REFLEX	ELICITING THE REFLEX	CHARACTERISTIC RESPONSE	COMMENTS
Pull-to-sit (traction)	Pull infant up by wrists from supine position with head in midline	Head will lag until infant is in upright position, then head will be held in same plane with chest and shoulder momentarily before falling forward; infant will attempt to right head	Response depends on general muscle tone and maturity and condition of infant
Trunk incurvation (Galant)	Place infant prone on flat surface, run finger down back about 4 to 5 cm lateral to spine, first on one side and then down other	Trunk is flexed and pelvis is swung toward stimulated side	Response disappears by fourth week Absence suggests general depression of nervous system

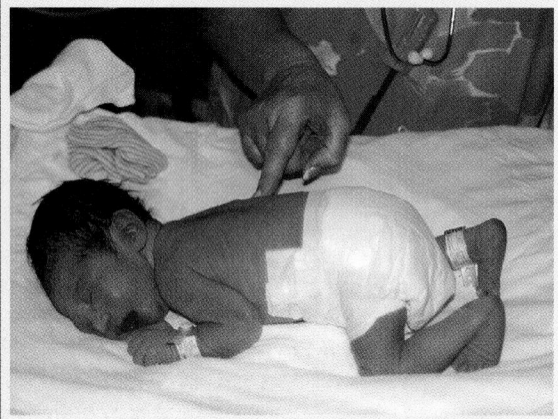

Trunk incurvation reflex. In prone position, infant responds to linear skin stimulus (blunt end of pin or finger) along paravertebral area by flexing the trunk and swinging the pelvis toward stimulus. With transverse lesions of cord, no response below the level of the lesion is present. Response may vary but should be obtainable in all infants, including preterm ones. If not seen in the first few days, it is usually apparent by 5 to 6 days. *(Courtesy Marjorie Pyle, RNC, Lifecircle, Costa Mesa, CA.)*

REFLEX	ELICITING THE REFLEX	CHARACTERISTIC RESPONSE	COMMENTS
Magnet	Place infant in supine position, partially flex both lower extremities and apply pressure to soles of feet	Both lower limbs should extend against examiner's pressure	Absence suggests damage to spinal cord or malformation Reflex may be weak or exaggerated after breech birth.

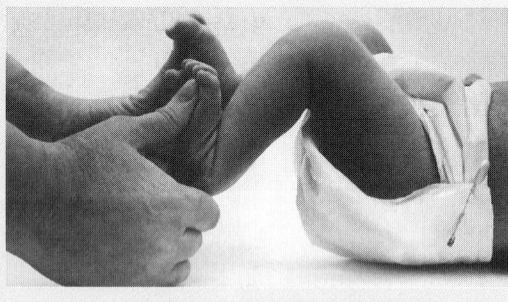

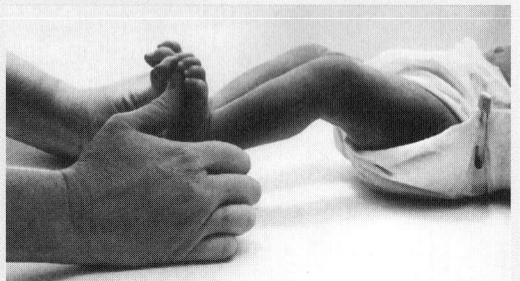

Magnet reflex. With child in supine position and lower limbs semi-flexed, light pressure is applied with fingers to both feet. Normally, while the examiner's fingers maintain contact with the soles of the feet, the lower limbs extend. Weak reflex may be seen after breech presentation *without* extended legs or may indicate sciatic nerve stretch syndrome. Breech presentation *with* extended legs may evoke exaggerated response. *(Courtesy Mead Johnson & Co., Evansville, IN.)*

TABLE 26-3 Assessment of Newborn's Reflexes—cont'd

REFLEX	ELICITING THE REFLEX	CHARACTERISTIC RESPONSE	COMMENTS
Additional newborn responses Yawn, stretch, burp, hiccup, sneeze	These are spontaneous behaviors	May be slightly depressed temporarily because of maternal analgesia or anesthesia, fetal hypoxia, or infection	Parental guidance: Most of these behaviors are pleasurable to parents Parents need to be assured that behaviors are normal Sneeze is usually response to lint, etc., in nose and not an indicator of a cold No treatment is needed for hiccups, sucking may help

TABLE 26-4 Physical Assessment of Newborn

AREA ASSESSED AND APPRAISAL PROCEDURE	NORMAL FINDINGS		DEVIATIONS FROM NORMAL RANGE: POSSIBLE PROBLEMS (ETIOLOGY)
	AVERAGE FINDINGS	NORMAL VARIATONS	
POSTURE			
Inspect newborn before disturbing for assessment Refer to maternal chart for fetal presentation, position, and type of birth (vaginal, surgical), since newborn readily assumes prenatal position	Vertex: arms, legs in moderate flexion; fists clenched Resistance to having extremities extended for examination or measurement, crying possible when attempted Cessation of crying when allowed to reassume curled-up fetal position Normal spontaneous movement bilaterally asynchronous (legs moving in bicycle fashion) but equal extension in all extremities	Frank breech: legs straighter and stiff, newborn assuming intrauterine position in repose for a few days Prenatal pressure on limb or shoulder possibly causing temporary facial asymmetry or resistance to extension of extremities	Hypotonia, relaxed posture while awake (prematurity or hypoxia in utero, maternal medications) Hypertonia (drug dependence, central nervous system [CNS] disorder) Opisthotonos (CNS disturbance) Limitation of motion in any of extremities (see Skeletal System, p. 686)
VITAL SIGNS			
Check heart rate and pulses: Thorax (chest) Inspection Palpation Auscultation Apex: mitral valve Second interspace, left of sternum: pulmonic valve Second interspace, right of sternum: aortic valve Junction of xiphoid process and sternum: tricuspid valve	Visible pulsations in left mid-clavicular line, fifth intercostal space Apical pulse, fourth intercostal space 120-160 beats/min Quality: *first sound* (closure of mitral and tricuspid valves) and *second sound* (closure of aortic and pulmonic valves) sharp and clear	100 beats/min (sleeping) to 160 beats/min (crying); possibly irregular for brief periods, especially after crying Murmurs, especially over base or at left sternal border in interspace 3 or 4 (foramen ovale anatomically closing at about 1 yr)	Tachycardia: persistent, ≥160 beats/min (respiratory distress syndrome [RDS]) Bradycardia: persistent, ≤120 beats/min (congenital heart block) Murmurs (possibly functional) Arrhythmias: irregular rate Sounds Distant (pneumomediastinum) Poor quality Extra Heart on right side of chest: Dextrocardia, often accompanied by reversal of intestines

Continued

■ **TABLE 26-4** Physical Assessment of Newborn—cont'd

AREA ASSESSED AND APPRAISAL PROCEDURE	NORMAL FINDINGS		DEVIATIONS FROM NORMAL RANGE: POSSIBLE PROBLEMS (ETIOLOGY)
	AVERAGE FINDINGS	NORMAL VARIATONS	
VITAL SIGNS—cont'd			
For femoral pulse palpation, place fingers along inguinal ligament about midway between symphysis pubis and iliac crest; feel bilaterally simultaneously	Femoral pulses equal and strong		Weak or absent femoral pulses (hip dysplasia, coarctation of aorta, thrombophlebitis)
Attain temperature: Axillary: method of choice until 6 yr of age Electronic: thermistor probe (avoid taping over bony area)	Axillary: 37° C Temperature stabilized by 8-10 hr of age Undeveloped shivering mechanism	36.5°-37.2° C Heat loss: 200 kcal/kg/min from evaporation, conduction, convection, radiation	Subnormal (prematurity, infection, low environmental temperature, inadequate clothing, dehydration) Increased (infection, high environmental temperature, excessive clothing, proximity to heating unit or in direct sunshine, drug addiction, diarrhea and dehydration) Temperature not stabilized by 10 hr after birth (if mother received magnesium sulfate, newborn less able to conserve heat by vasoconstriction; maternal analgesics possibly reducing thermal stability in newborn)
Check respiratory rate and effort: Observe respirations when infant is at rest Count respirations for full minute Check apnea monitor Listen for sounds audible without stethoscope Observe respiratory effort	40/min Tendency to be shallow and irregular in rate, rhythm, and depth when infant is awake No sounds audible on inspiration or expiration Breath sounds: bronchial; loud, clear, near	30-60/min Possibly appearing to be Cheyne-Stokes with short periods of apnea and no evidence of respiratory distress First period (reactivity): 50-60/min Second period: 50-70/min Stabilization (1-2 days): 30-40/min	Apneic episodes: >15 sec (preterm infant: "periodic breathing," rapid warming or cooling of infant) Bradypnea: <25/min (maternal narcosis from analgesics or anesthetics, birth trauma) Tachypnea: >60/min (RDS, aspiration syndrome, diaphragmatic hernia) Sounds Crackles, rhonchi, wheezes (fluid in lungs) Expiratory grunt (narrowing of bronchi) Distress evidenced by nasal flaring, retractions, chin tug, labored breathing (RDS, fluid in lungs)

▌TABLE 26-4 **Physical Assessment of Newborn—cont'd**

AREA ASSESSED AND APPRAISAL PROCEDURE	NORMAL FINDINGS		DEVIATIONS FROM NORMAL RANGE: POSSIBLE PROBLEMS (ETIOLOGY)
	AVERAGE FINDINGS	NORMAL VARIATONS	
VITAL SIGNS—cont'd			
Attain blood pressure (BP) (usually assessed only if a problem is suspected) Check electronic monitor BP cuff: BP cuff width affects readings, use cuff 2.5 cm wide and palpate radial pulse	78/42 (approximately) At birth Systolic: 60-80 mm Hg Diastolic: 40-50 mm Hg At 10 days Systolic: 95-100 mm Hg Diastolic: slight increase	Variation with change in activity level: awake, crying, sleeping	Difference between upper and lower extremity pressures (coarctation of aorta) Hypotension (sepsis, hypovolemia) Hypertension (coarctation of aorta)
WEIGHT*			
Put protective liner cloth or paper in place and adjust scale to 0 (see Fig. 26-14) Weigh at same time each day Protect newborn from heat loss	Female 3400 g Male 3500 g Regaining of birth weight within first 2 weeks	2500-4000 g Acceptable weight loss: 10% or less Second baby weighing more than first	Weight ≤2500 g (prematurity, small for gestational age, rubella syndrome) Weight ≥4000 g (large for gestational age, maternal diabetes, heredity—normal for these parents) Weight loss over 10% (dehydration)
LENGTH			
Measure length from top of head to heel, measuring is difficult in term infant because of presence of molding, incomplete extension of knees (see Fig. 26-15, D)	50 cm	45-55 cm	<45cm or >55 cm (chromosomal aberration, heredity—normal for these parents)
HEAD CIRCUMFERENCE			
Measure head at greatest diameter: occipitofrontal circumference (see Fig. 26-15, A) May need to remeasure on second or third day after resolution of molding and caput succedaneum	33-35 cm Circumference of head and chest approximately the same for first 1 or 2 days after birth	32-36.8 cm	Small head ≤32 cm: microcephaly (rubella, toxoplasmosis, cytomegalic inclusion disease) Hydrocephaly: sutures widely separated, circumference ≥4 cm more than chest circumference Increased intracranial pressure (hemorrhage, space-occupying lesion)
CHEST CIRCUMFERENCE			
Measure at nipple line (see Fig. 26-15, B)	2-3 cm less than head circumference, averages between 30 and 33 cm		≤30 cm (prematurity)

*Note: Weight, length, and head circumference should all be close to same percentile for any child.

Continued

TABLE 26-4   Physical Assessment of Newborn—cont'd

AREA ASSESSED AND APPRAISAL PROCEDURE	NORMAL FINDINGS		DEVIATIONS FROM NORMAL RANGE: POSSIBLE PROBLEMS (ETIOLOGY)
	AVERAGE FINDINGS	NORMAL VARIATONS	
ABDOMINAL CIRCUMFERENCE			
Measure below umbilicus (see Fig. 26-15, C) (not usually measured unless specific indication)	Abdomen enlargement after feeding because of lax abdominal muscles Same size as chest		Enlarging abdomen between feedings (abdominal mass or blockage in intestinal tract)
SKIN			

Check color:
Inspect and palpate
  Inspect naked newborn in well-lit, warm area without drafts; natural daylight provides best lighting
  Inspect newborn when quiet and when active
	Generally pink
	Varying with ethnic origin, skin pigmentation beginning to deepen right after birth in basal layer of epidermis
	Acrocyanosis, especially if chilled
		Mottling
		Harlequin sign
		Plethora
		Telangiectases ("stork bites" or capillary hemangiomas)
		Erythema toxicum/neonatorum ("newborn rash")
		Milia
		
		Petechiae over presenting part
		
		Ecchymoses from forceps in vertex births or over buttocks, genitalia, and legs in breech births
			Dark red (prematurity, polycythemia)
			Pallor (cardiovascular problem, CNS damage, blood dyscrasia, blood loss, twin-to-twin transfusion, nosocomial infection)
			Cyanosis (hypothermia, infection, hypoglycemia, cardiopulmonary diseases, cardiac, neurologic, or respiratory malformations)
			Petechiae over any other area (clotting factor deficiency, infection)
			Ecchymoses in any other area (hemorrhagic disease, traumatic birth)

Check for jaundice	None at birth	Physiologic jaundice in 50% of term infants after first 24 hr	Gray (hypotension, poor perfusion) Jaundice within first 24 hr (Rh isoimmunization)
Check birthmarks: Inspect and palpate for location, size, distribution, characteristics, color	Transient hyperpigmentation Areolae Genitals Linea nigra	Mongolian spotting Infants of African-American, Asian, and Native American origin: 70% Infants of Caucasian origin: 9%	Hemangiomas Nevus flammeus: port-wine stain Nevus vasculosus: strawberry mark Cavernous hemangiomas
Check condition: Inspect and palpate for intactness, smoothness, texture, edema	No skin edema Opacity: few large blood vessels visible indistinctly over abdomen	Slightly thick; superficial cracking, peeling, especially of hands, feet No visible blood vessels, a few large vessels clearly visible over abdomen Some fingernail scratches	Edema on hands, feet; pitting over tibia Texture thin, smooth, or of medium thickness; rash or superficial peeling visible Numerous vessels very visible over abdomen (prematurity) Texture thick, parchmentlike; cracking, peeling (postmaturity)

■ TABLE 26-4 **Physical Assessment of Newborn—cont'd**

AREA ASSESSED AND APPRAISAL PROCEDURE	NORMAL FINDINGS		DEVIATIONS FROM NORMAL RANGE: POSSIBLE PROBLEMS (ETIOLOGY)
	AVERAGE FINDINGS	NORMAL VARIATONS	
SKIN—cont'd			
Check condition:—cont'd			Skin tags, webbing Papules, pustules, vesicles, ulcers, maceration (impetigo, candidiasis, herpes, diaper rash)
Assess hydration and consistency Weigh infant routinely Inspect and palpate Gently pinch skin between thumb and forefinger over abdomen and inner thigh to check for turgor Check subcutaneous fat deposits (adipose pads) over cheeks, buttocks	Dehydration: loss of weight best indicator After pinch released, skin returning to original state immediately	Normal weight loss after birth: up to 10% of birth weight Possibly puffy Variation in amount of subcutaneous fat	Loose, wrinkled skin (prematurity, postmaturity, dehydration: fold of skin persisting after release of pinch) Tense, tight, shiny skin (edema, extreme cold, shock, infection) Lack of subcutaneous fat, prominence of clavicle or ribs (prematurity, malnutrition)
Check voiding	Voiding within 24 hours of birth Voiding 6 to 10 times per day		
Check vernix caseosa: Observe amount		Variation in amount; usually more found in creases, folds	Absent or minimal (postmaturity) Excessive (prematurity)
Observe its color and odor before bath or wiping	Whitish, cheesy, odorless		Yellow color (possible fetal anoxia more than 36 hr before birth, Rh or ABO incompatibility) Green color (possible in utero release of meconium or presence of bilirubin) Odor (possible intrauterine infection)
Assess lanugo: Inspect for this fine, downy hair, including its amount, distribution	Over shoulders, pinnas of ears, forehead	Variation in amount	Absent (postmaturity) Excessive (prematurity, especially if lanugo abundant and long and thick over back)
HEAD			
Palpate skin	See Skin	Caput succedaneum, possibly showing some ecchymosis	Cephalhematoma

Continued

TABLE 26-4 Physical Assessment of Newborn—cont'd

AREA ASSESSED AND APPRAISAL PROCEDURE	NORMAL FINDINGS		DEVIATIONS FROM NORMAL RANGE: POSSIBLE PROBLEMS (ETIOLOGY)
	AVERAGE FINDINGS	NORMAL VARIATONS	
HEAD—cont'd			
Inspect shape, size	Making up one fourth of body length Molding (see Fig. 26-10)	Slight asymmetry from intrauterine position Lack of molding (prematurity, breech presentation, cesarean birth)	Molding Severe molding (birth trauma) Indentation (fracture from trauma)
Palpate, inspect, measure fontanels	Anterior fontanel 5-cm diamond, increasing as molding resolves Posterior fontanel triangle, smaller than anterior	Variation in fontanel size with degree of molding Difficulty in feeling fontanels possible because of molding	Fontanels Full, bulging (tumor, hemorrhage, infection) Large, flat, soft (malnutrition, hydrocephaly, retarded bone age, hypothyroidism) Depressed (dehydration)
Palpate sutures	Palpable and unjoined sutures	Possible overlap of sutures with molding	Sutures Widely spaced (hydrocephaly) Premature closure
Inspect pattern, distribution, amount of hair; feel texture	Silky, single strands lying flat; growth pattern toward face and neck	Variation in amount	Fine, woolly (prematurity) Unusual swirls, patterns, hairline or coarse, brittle (endocrine or genetic disorders)
EYES			
Check placement on face	Eyes and space between eyes each one third the distance from outer-to-outer canthus	Epicanthal folds: normal racial characteristic	Epicanthal folds when present with other signs (chromosomal disorders such as Down, cri-du-chat syndromes)
Check for symmetry in size, shape	Symmetric in size, shape		
Check eyelids for size, movements, blink	Blink reflex	Edema if silver nitrate instilled; also may occur with instillation of erythromycin and tetracycline	
Assess for discharge	None	Some discharge if silver nitrate used	Discharge: purulent (infection)
Evaluate eyeballs for presence, size, shape	No tears Both present and of equal size, both round, firm	Occasional presence of some tears Subconjunctival hemorrhage	Agenesis or absence of one or both eyeballs Small eyeball size (rubella syndrome) Lens opacity or absence of red reflex (congenital cataracts, possibly from rubella) Lesions: coloboma, absence of part of iris (congenital) Pink color of iris (albinism) Jaundiced sclera (hyperbilirubinemia)

■ TABLE 26-4 **Physical Assessment of Newborn—cont'd**

AREA ASSESSED AND APPRAISAL PROCEDURE	NORMAL FINDINGS		DEVIATIONS FROM NORMAL RANGE: POSSIBLE PROBLEMS (ETIOLOGY)
	AVERAGE FINDINGS	NORMAL VARIATONS	
EYES—cont'd			
Check pupils	Present, equal in size, reactive to light		Pupils: unequal, constricted, dilated, fixed (intracranial pressure, medications, tumors)
Evaluate eyeball movement	Random, jerky, uneven, focus possible briefly, following to midline	Transient strabismus or nystagmus until third or fourth month	Persistent strabismus Doll's eyes (increased intracranial pressure) Sunset (increased intracranial pressure)
Assess eyebrows: amount of hair, pattern	Distinct (not connected in midline)		Connection in midline (Cornelia de Lange's syndrome)
NOSE			
Observe shape, placement, patency, configuration of bridge of nose	Midline Apparent lack of bridge, flat, broad Some mucus but no drainage Preferential nose breather Sneezing to clear nose	Slight deformity from passage through birth canal	Copious drainage, with or without regular periods of cyanosis at rest and return of pink color with crying (choanal atresia, congenital syphilis) Malformed (congenital syphilis, chromosomal disorder) Flaring of nares (respiratory distress)
EARS			
Observe size, placement on head, amount of cartilage, open auditory canal	Correct placement: line drawn through inner and outer canthi of eyes reaching to top notch of ears (at junction with scalp) Well-formed, firm cartilage	Size: small, large, floppy Darwin's tubercle (nodule on posterior helix)	Agenesis Lack of cartilage (prematurity) Low placement (chromosomal disorder, mental retardation, kidney disorder) Preauricular tags Size: possibly overly prominent or protruding ears
Assess hearing	Responses to voice and other sounds	State (e.g., alert, asleep) influencing response	Deaf: no response to sound
FACIES			
Observe overall appearance of face	"Normal" appearance, well-placed, proportionate, symmetric features	Positional deformities	Infant appearance "odd" or "funny" Usually accompanied by other features such as low-set cars, other structural disorders (hereditary, chromosomal aberration)

Continued

TABLE 26-4 **Physical Assessment of Newborn—cont'd**

AREA ASSESSED AND APPRAISAL PROCEDURE	NORMAL FINDINGS		DEVIATIONS FROM NORMAL RANGE: POSSIBLE PROBLEMS (ETIOLOGY)
	AVERAGE FINDINGS	NORMAL VARIATONS	
MOUTH			
Inspect and palpate Check placement on face Assess lips for color, configuration, movement	Symmetry of lip movement	Transient circumoral cyanosis	Gross anomalies in placement, size, shape (cleft lip and/or palate, gums) Cyanosis, circumoral pallor (respiratory distress, hypothermia) Asymmetry in movement of lips (seventh cranial nerve paralysis)
Check gums	Pink gums	Inclusion cysts (Epstein's pearls—Bohn's nodules, whitish, hard nodules on gums or roof of mouth)	Teeth: predeciduous or deciduous (hereditary)
Assess tongue for attachment, mobility, movement, size	Tongue not protruding, freely movable, symmetric in shape, movement	Short frenulum	Macroglossia (prematurity, chromosomal disorder)
Evaluate cheeks	Sucking pads inside cheeks		Thrush: white plaques on cheeks or tongue that bleed if touched (Candida albicans)
Assess palate (soft, hard): Arch Uvula	Soft and hard palates intact Uvula in midline	Anatomic groove in palate to accommodate nipple, disappearance by 3 to 4 yr of age Epstein's pearls	Cleft hard or soft palate
Assess chin	Distinct chin		Micrognathia (Pierre Robin or other syndrome)
Evaluate saliva for amount, character	Mouth moist		Excessive saliva (esophageal atresia, tracheoesophageal fistula)
Check reflexes: Rooting Sucking Extrusion	Reflexes present	Reflex response dependent on state of wakefulness and hunger	Absent (prematurity)
NECK			
Inspect and palpate length Check sternocleidomastoid muscles, movement and position of head	Short, thick, surrounded by skin folds; no webbing Head held in midline (sternocleidomastoid muscles equal), no masses Freedom of movement from side to side and flexion and extension, no movement of chin past shoulder	Transient positional deformity apparent when newborn is at rest: passive movement of head possible	Webbing (Turner's syndrome) Restricted movement, holding of head at angle (torticollis [wryneck], opisthotonos) Absence of head control (prematurity, Down syndrome)
Assess trachea for position and thyroid gland	Thyroid not palpable		Masses (enlarged thyroid) Distended veins (cardiopulmonary disorder) Skin tags

■ **TABLE 26-4**   **Physical Assessment of Newborn—cont'd**

AREA ASSESSED AND APPRAISAL PROCEDURE	NORMAL FINDINGS		DEVIATIONS FROM NORMAL RANGE: POSSIBLE PROBLEMS (ETIOLOGY)
	AVERAGE FINDINGS	NORMAL VARIATONS	
CHEST			
Inspect and palpate Shape	Almost circular, barrel shaped	Tip of sternum possibly prominent	Bulging of chest, unequal movement (pneumothorax, pneumomediastinum) Malformation (funnel chest—pectus excavatum)
Check respiratory movements	Symmetric chest movements, chest and abdominal movements synchronized during respirations	Occasional retractions, especially when crying	Retractions with or without respiratory distress (prematurity, RDS)
Evaluate clavicles	Clavicles intact		Fracture of clavicle (trauma); crepitus
Assess ribs	Rib cage symmetrical, intact; moves with respirations		Poor development of rib cage and musculature (prematurity)
Assess nipples for size, placement, number	Nipples prominent, well formed; symmetrically placed		Nipples Supernumerary, along nipple line Malpositioned or widely spaced
Check breast tissue	Breast nodule: approximately 6 mm in term infant	Breast nodule: 3-10 mm Secretion of witch's milk	Lack of breast tissue (prematurity)
Auscultate: Heart sounds and rate and breath sounds (see Vital signs).			Sounds: bowel sounds (see Abdomen, below)
ABDOMEN			
Inspect, palpate, and smell umbilical cord	Two arteries, one vein Whitish gray Definite demarcation between cord and skin, no intestinal structures within cord Dry around base, drying Odorless Cord clamp in place for 24 hr	Reducible umbilical herniation	One artery (renal anomalies) Meconium stained (intrauterine distress) Bleeding or oozing around cord (hemorrhagic disease) Redness or drainage around cord (infection, possible persistence of urachus) Hernia: herniation of abdominal contents into area of cord (e.g., omphalocele); defect covered with thin, friable membrane, possibly extensive
Inspect size of abdomen and palpate contour (see Fig. 26-15, C).	Rounded, prominent, dome shaped because abdominal musculature not fully developed Liver possibly palpable 1-2 cm below right costal margin	Some diastasis of abdominal musculature	Gastroschisis: fissure of abdominal cavity Distention at birth (ruptured viscus, genitourinary masses or malformations: hydronephrosis, teratomas, abdominal tumors)

Continued

▪ TABLE 26-4   Physical Assessment of Newborn—cont'd

AREA ASSESSED AND APPRAISAL PROCEDURE	NORMAL FINDINGS		DEVIATIONS FROM NORMAL RANGE: POSSIBLE PROBLEMS (ETIOLOGY)
	AVERAGE FINDINGS	NORMAL VARIATONS	
ABDOMEN—cont'd			
	No other masses palpable		Mild (overfeeding, high gastrointestinal tract obstruction)
	No distention		Marked (lower gastrointestinal tract obstruction, imperforate anus)
			Intermittent or transient (overfeeding)
			Partial intestinal obstruction (stenosis of bowel)
			Visible peristalsis (obstruction)
			Malrotation of bowel or adhesions
			Sepsis (infection)
Auscultate bowel sounds and note number, amount, and character of stools; note behavior—crying, fussiness—before or during elimination	Sounds present within 1-2 hr after birth		Scaphoid, with bowel sounds in chest and respiratory distress (diaphragmatic hernia)
	Meconium stool passing within 24-48 hr after birth		
Assess color		Linea nigra possibly apparent and caused by hormone influence during pregnancy	
Check movement with respiration	Respirations primarily diaphragmatic, abdominal and chest movement synchronous		Decreased abdominal breathing (intrathoracic disease, diaphragmatic hernia)
			"Seesaw" (respiratory distress)
GENITALIA			
Female (see Fig. 26-9, A)			
Inspect and palpate			
General appearance	Female genitals	Increased pigmentation caused by pregnancy hormones	Ambiguous genitals—enlarged clitoris with urinary meatus on tip, fused labia (chromosomal disorder, maternal drug ingestion)
Clitoris	Usually edematous		
Labia majora	Usually edematous, covering labia minora in term newborns	Edema and ecchymosis after breech birth	Stenosed meatus
Labia minora	Possible protrusion over labia majora	Blood-tinged discharge from pseudomenstruation caused by pregnancy hormones	
Discharge	Smegma		
Vagina	Open orifice	Some vernix caseosa between labia possible	Labia majora widely separated and labia minora prominent (prematurity)
	Mucoid discharge		Absence of vaginal orifice or imperforate hymen
	Hymenal/vaginal tag		Fecal discharge (fistula)
Urinary meatus	Beneath clitoris, difficult to see—to watch for voiding	Rust-stained urine (uric acid crystals)*	

*To determine whether rust color is caused by uric acid or blood, wash urine under running warm tap water; uric acid washes out, blood does not.

TABLE 26-4 Physical Assessment of Newborn—cont'd

AREA ASSESSED AND APPRAISAL PROCEDURE	NORMAL FINDINGS		DEVIATIONS FROM NORMAL RANGE: POSSIBLE PROBLEMS (ETIOLOGY)
	AVERAGE FINDINGS	NORMAL VARIATONS	
GENITALIA—cont'd			
Male (see Fig. 26-9 B)			
Inspect and palpate			
General appearance	Male genitals	Increased size and pigmentation caused by pregnancy hormones	Ambiguous genitals
Penis	Meatus at tip of penis		Urinary meatus not on tip of glans penis (hypospadias, epispadias)
Urinary meatus as slit			Round meatal opening
Prepuce	Prepuce (foreskin) covering glans penis and not retractable	Prepuce removed if circumcised	
		Wide variation in size of genitals	
Scrotum	Large, edematous, pendulous in term infant; covered with rugae	Scrotal edema and ecchymosis if breech birth	Scrotum smooth and testes undescended (prematurity, cryptorchidism)
Rugae (wrinkles)		Hydrocele, small, noncommunicating	Hydrocele
			Inguinal hernia
Testes	Palpable on each side	Bulge palpable in inguinal canal	Undescended (prematurity)
Check urination	Voiding within 24 hr, stream adequate, amount adequate	Rust-stained urine (uric acid crystals)	
Check reflexes:			
Erection	Erection possibly occurring spontaneously and when genitals touched		
Cremasteric	Testes retracted, especially when newborn is chilled		
EXTREMITIES			
Make a general check:			
Inspect and palpate	Assuming of position maintained in utero	Transient (positional) deformities	Limited motion (malformations)
Degree of flexion	Attitude of general flexion		Poor muscle tone (prematurity, maternal medications, CNS anomalies)
Range of motion	Full range of motion, spontaneous movements		Positive scarf sign
Symmetry of motion			
Muscle tone			
Check arms and hands:			
Inspect and palpate	Longer than legs in newborn period	Slight tremors sometimes apparent	Asymmetry of movement (fracture/crepitus, brachial nerve trauma, malformations)
Color	Contours and movement symmetric	Some acrocyanosis, especially when chilled	Asymmetry of contour (malformations, fracture)
Intactness			Amelia or phocomelia (teratogens)
Appropriate placement			Palmar creases
			Simian line with short, incurved little fingers (Down syndrome)

Continued

TABLE 26-4 Physical Assessment of Newborn—cont'd

AREA ASSESSED AND APPRAISAL PROCEDURE	NORMAL FINDINGS		DEVIATIONS FROM NORMAL RANGE: POSSIBLE PROBLEMS (ETIOLOGY)
	AVERAGE FINDINGS	NORMAL VARIATONS	
EXTREMITIES—cont'd			
Check number of fingers	Five on each hand		Webbing of fingers: syndactyly
	Fist often clenched with thumb under fingers		Absence or excess of fingers
			Strong, rigid flexion; persistent fists; positioning of fists in front of mouth constantly (CNS disorder)
Palpate humerus	Intact		Fractured humerus
Evaluate joints	Full range of motion, symmetric contour		Increased tonicity, clonicity, prolonged tremors (CNS disorder)
Shoulder			
Elbow			
Wrist			
Fingers			
Check reflex: grasp			
Check legs and feet:			
Inspect and palpate	Appearance of bowing because lateral muscles more developed than medial muscles	Feet appearing to turn in but can be easily rotated externally, positional defects tending to correct while infant is crying	Amelia, phocomelia (chromosomal defect, teratogenic effect)
Color			
Intactness			
Length in relation to arms and body and to each other		Acrocyanosis	
Number of toes	Five on each foot		Webbing, syndactyly (chromosomal defect)
			Absence or excess of digits (chromosomal defect, familial trait)
Femur	Intact femur		Femoral fracture (difficult breech birth)
Head of femur as legs are flexed and abducted, placement in acetabulum (see Fig. 26-13)	No click heard, femoral head not overriding acetabulum		Congenital hip dysplasia/dislocation
Major gluteal folds	Major gluteal folds even		
Soles of feet	Soles well lined (or wrinkled) over two thirds of foot in term infants		Soles of feet
			Few lines (prematurity)
			Covered with lines (postmaturity)
	Planter fat pad giving flat-footed effect		Congenital clubfoot
			Hypermobility of joints (Down syndrome)
Evaluate joints	Full range of motion, symmetric contour		Yellowed nail beds (meconium staining)
Hip			
Knee			Temperature of one leg differing from that of the other (circulatory deficiency, CNS disorder)
Ankle			
Toes			
Check reflexes			Asymmetric movement (trauma, CNS disorder)

TABLE 26-4 Physical Assessment of Newborn—cont'd

AREA ASSESSED AND APPRAISAL PROCEDURE	NORMAL FINDINGS		DEVIATIONS FROM NORMAL RANGE: POSSIBLE PROBLEMS (ETIOLOGY)
	AVERAGE FINDINGS	NORMAL VARIATONS	
BACK			
Assess anatomy:			
Inspect and palpate Spine Shoulders Scapulae Iliac crests Base of spine—pilonidal area	Spine straight and easily flexed Infant able to raise and support head momentarily when prone Shoulders, scapulae, and iliac crests lining up in same plane	Temporary minor positional deformities, correction with passive manipulation	Limitation of movement (fusion or deformity of vertebra) Pigmented nevus with tuft of hair, location anywhere along the spine, often associated with spina bifida occulta Spina bifida cystica (meningocele, myelomeningocele)
Check reflexes (spinal related) Test trunk incurvation reflex	Trunk flexed and pelvis swings to stimulated side	May not be apparent in first few days but is usually present in 5-6 days	If transverse lesion is present, no response below lesion; absence of response: nervous system abnormality or general depression
Test magnet reflex	Lower limbs extend as pressure applied to feet with legs in semiflexed position	Weak or exaggerated response with breech presentation	Absence: suggestive of spinal cord damage or malformation
ANUS			
Inspect and palpate Placement Number Patency Test for sphincter response (active "wink" reflex) Observe for following: Abdominal distention Passage of meconium Passage of fecal drainage from surrounding orifices	One anus with good sphincter tone Passage of meconium within 24 hr after birth Good "wink" reflex of anal sphincter	Passage of meconium within 48 hr of birth	Low obstruction: anal membrane High obstruction: anal or rectal atresia Drainage of fecal material from vagina in female or urinary meatus in male (rectal fistula)
STOOLS			
Observe frequency, color, consistency	Meconium followed by transitional and soft yellow stools		No stool (obstruction) Frequent watery stools (infection, phototherapy)

The respiratory rate varies with the state of alertness after birth. Respirations are abdominal and can easily be counted by observing or lightly feeling the rise and fall of the abdomen.

Neonatal respirations are shallow and irregular. It is important to count the respirations for a full minute to obtain an accurate count because of normal short periods of apnea. The examiner should also observe for symmetry of chest movements. See Table 26-4 for normal respiratory rates.

Because of variations, counting the heart rate for a full minute is important. Apical pulse rates are always taken to rule out dysrhythmias and murmurs. Heart and respiratory

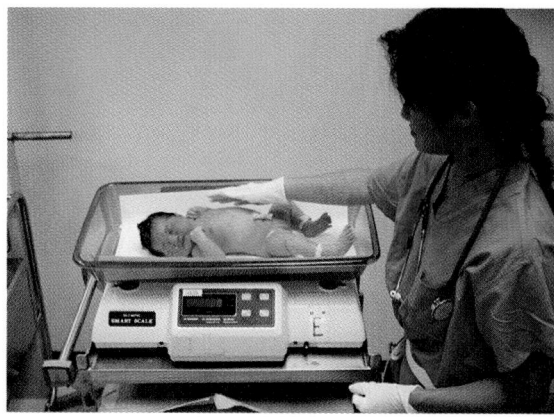

Fig. 26-14 Weighing the infant. Note that a hand is held over infant as a safety measure. The scale is covered to protect against cross infection. *(Courtesy Kim Molloy, Knoxville, IA.)*

rates are taken when the infant is not crying. The infant may need to be held and comforted during assessment. See Table 26-4 for normal heart rates.

If BP is measured, a Doppler (electronic) monitor facilitates this procedure. Neonatal BP usually is highest immediately after birth and falls to a minimum by 3 hours after birth. It then begins to rise steadily and reaches a plateau between 4 and 6 days after birth. This measurement is usually equal to that of the immediate postbirth BP. The BP reading varies with the neonate's activity.

BP may be measured in both arms and legs to detect any discrepancy between the two sides or between the upper and lower body. A discrepancy of 10 mm Hg or more between the arms and legs may signal a cardiac defect such as coarctation of the aorta.

Baseline Measurements of Physical Growth

The examiner takes and records baseline measurements to help assess the progress of the neonate. Measurements are used to determine the neonate's growth patterns. These may be recorded on growth charts. The following measurements are made when the neonate is assessed.

Weight

The newborn is usually weighed shortly after birth. The totally unclothed neonate is placed in the center of the scale, which is usually covered with a disposable pad or diaper to prevent heat loss from conduction. The nurse should place one hand over (but not touching) the neonate to prevent the infant from falling off the scales (Fig. 26-14). The infant is commonly weighed at the same time every day during the hospital stay.

The birth weight of a term infant ranges from 2500 to 4000 g. Neonates lose about 10% or less of their birth weight after birth. This is caused by the excretion of fluids through the lungs, urinary bladder, and bowels, and the low level of intake during the first few days of life. They usually regain their birth weight by 10 to 14 days of age.

Circumferences and Length

The head is measured at the widest part, which is the occipitofrontal diameter (Fig. 26-15, *A*). The tape measure is placed around the head at the infant's eyebrows.

The chest circumference usually measures about 2 cm less than the head circumference. Frequently the chest is the same size as the head but should not exceed it. The tape is placed around the infant's chest at the nipple line (Fig. 26-15, *B*).

Abdominal circumference is measured by placing the tape around the abdomen just below the umbilicus (Fig. 26-15, *C*). Measurements vary with the size of the infant. The abdomen should be cylindrical and protrude slightly. Abdominal measurements are not always taken but should be made when abdominal distention is suspected.

The length may be difficult to measure because of the flexed posture of the newborn (Fig. 26-15, *D*). The examiner places the newborn on a flat surface and extends the leg until the knee is flat against the surface. Placing the head against a perpendicular surface and extending the leg may assist with this measurement (see Research box).

Skin Texture, Color, Opacity

Observations should include color and color changes during activity, familial and racial features, rashes, milia, anomalies or deformities, birthmarks, jaundice, petechiae, forceps marks, tone, and hydration status. Any of these characteristics should be noted and recorded.

Color varies with racial background, pigmentation, and physiologic changes. Acrocyanosis is characterized by bluish discoloration of the hands and feet. This normal condition is caused by vasomotor instability and poor peripheral circulation. To distinguish between true cyanosis and acrocyanosis, the examiner vigorously rubs the sole of the infant's foot. If the sole turns pink, the discoloration is caused by acrocyanosis. It will not turn pink with true cyanosis. In addition, acrocyanosis should disappear when the infant cries.

The newborn's skin often appears mottled, which is a response to temperature changes. Harlequin color changes may be seen. This occurs when one side of the body develops a deep red color. Harlequin color is a response to a normal vasomotor disturbance causing the blood vessels on one side of the body to constrict while those on the other side dilate. Although a common occurrence, it should be recorded and reported.

The skin should be inspected for any signs of lesions or birthmarks. Location, size, color, characteristics, and distribution should be noted and recorded. The examiner should inspect the scalp for any sign of a lesion from an internal scalp electrode. Forceps or vacuum cup marks should also be recorded.

Head and Neck

Molding may give the neonate's head an asymmetric appearance (see Fig. 26-10). Parents should be reassured that this will go away and that nothing need be done to the head.

RESEARCH

Reliability of Length Measurements in Full-Term Neonates

Length measurements are a routine part of the physical assessment performed on newborns at birth and throughout infancy. At birth, length measurements are used to assess fetal growth and to establish a baseline to assess future growth. Accurate length measurements are essential for safe clinical practice because inaccurate measurements may cause clinicians to perform unnecessary testing on healthy infants or overlook potentially serious health problems. Despite the importance, infant length measurement has not been studied adequately.

The purpose of this study was to describe and compare the intra- and interexaminer reliability of length measurements in full-term newborns obtained using four measurement techniques: crown-heel, supine, paper barrier, and Neo-infantometer. An additional purpose of this study was to determine whether the measurements obtained by the four techniques differed significantly. Two experienced nurses measured thirty-two healthy full-term newborns twice using the four different length techniques.

Results found that intra- and interexaminer differences were significantly larger when examiners used the crown-heel measurement technique. Although the intra- and interexaminer reliability of length measurements obtained with the supine, paper barrier, and Neo-infantometer techniques did not differ significantly, the amount of error in these measurements was large. It was concluded that crown-heel measurements were significantly less reliable than the other techniques tested.

CLINICAL APPLICATION

Until further research studies document the reliability of crown-heel measurements, nurses should interpret any results obtained with this technique with caution and use another measurement technique in their practice. Nurses should use one measurement technique consistently in their practice, and all nurses in the same setting should use the same technique.

Source: Johnson, T. et al. (1998). Reliability of length measurements in full-term neonates. *J Obstet Gynecol Neonatal Nurs* 27(3), 270-276.

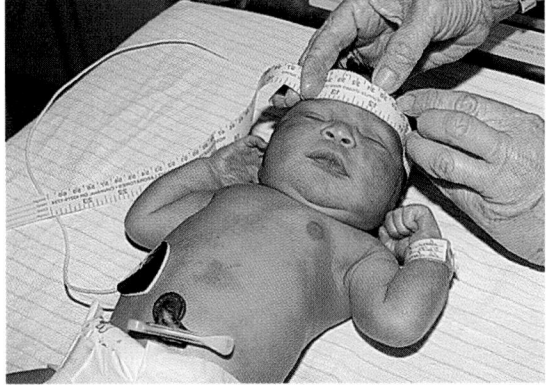
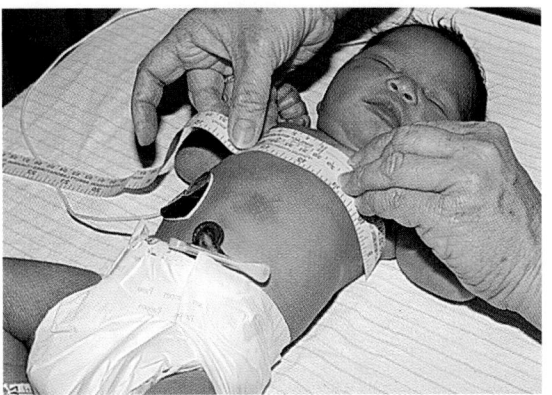
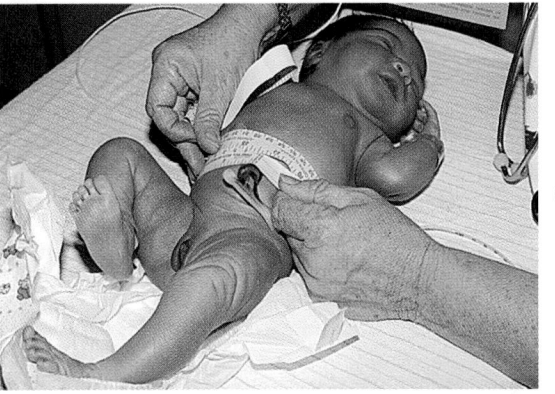
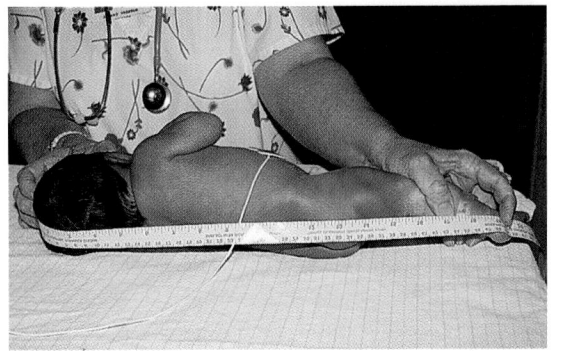

Fig. 26-15 Measurements. **A,** Circumference of head. **B,** Circumference of chest. **C,** Abdominal circumference. **D,** Length, crown to rump. To determine total length, include length of legs. If measurements are taken before infant's initial bath, the nurse must wear gloves. *(Courtesy Marjorie Pyle, RNC, Lifecircle, Costa Mesa, CA.)*

The fontanels are palpated and measured. The anterior fontanel is located at the junction of the sagittal and coronal sutures and is diamond shaped. The fontanel usually feels soft and may pulsate. The posterior fontanel is a triangular depression located at the junction of the lambdoidal and sagittal sutures. The posterior fontanel is often not palpable.

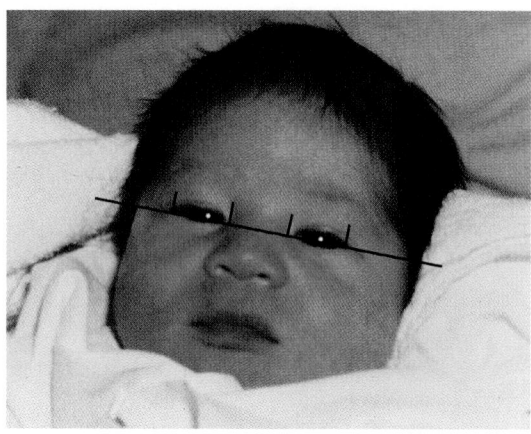

Fig. 26-16 Eyes. Pseudostrabismus: inner epicanthal folds cause the eyes to appear misaligned; however, corneal light reflexes are perfectly symmetric. Eyes are symmetric in size and shape and are well placed.

The examiner inspects the neonate's face for symmetry of features. Facial asymmetry may occur from in utero pressure, and the lopsided appearance disappears spontaneously in time. The mouth should appear at the midline, and its size should be appropriate for the face. Movement of the mouth should be symmetric. The chin normally is slightly receding. The examiner touches the tongue lightly to check for the normal reaction–a forward tongue thrust. The oral cavity should never be inspected just after a feeding because the gag reflex could be stimulated, causing vomiting and subsequent aspiration. The examiner inserts the little finger into the infant's mouth, allowing assessment of the hard and soft palates. This also stimulates the suck reflex, and the intensity of the reflex can be evaluated (Tappero & Honeyfield, 1996).

The sclerae should be clear and white. They may appear slightly yellow in dark-skinned infants. The conjunctivae should be clear and may be somewhat bluish. The iris color should be distributed evenly (Tappero & Honeyfield, 1996). Occasionally, subconjunctival hemorrhage, a result of the pressure the infant experiences while traversing the birth canal during labor and birth, may be seen. Tears are not usually produced until 2 months of age.

The pupils are examined with a penlight or flashlight and with room lights dim. The retina should be transparent and intact and the pupils round and centered in the iris. When exposed to light in a darkened room, the pupils should constrict equally bilaterally. A newborn's eyes do not accommodate. To assess for the red reflex, the examiner places the penlight or ophthalmoscope directly in front of the pupil and turns on the light. The pupils should appear red bilaterally (Tappero & Honeyfield, 1996).

Occasionally the eyes may appear crossed, a condition known as *strabismus.* In the neonate, however, transient strabismus (pseudostrabismus) and nystagmus (constant, involuntary cyclic movement of the eyeball) may be seen

until the third or fourth month; it persists until the eye muscles develop sufficiently to act in coordination (Fig. 26-16). When the neonate's head is rotated from side to side, the eyes do not follow in response to head movements. This doll's-eye phenomenon persists for about 10 days.

The ears are inspected for symmetric shape and size. The top of the ear should align with the inner and outer canthi of the eyes (Fig. 26-17). Skin tags, pinpoint holes, and sinus tracts along the helix or preauricular surface may represent minor abnormalities. The neonate's hearing should be checked. A loud noise should elicit the startle reflex or crying. At 36 weeks of gestation the upper two thirds of the pinna are incurved and the pinna recoils instantly. In the term neonate the pinna has well-defined incurving (Tappero & Honeyfield, 1996). Old blood and vernix may be in the ear canal for several days, and therefore the tympanic membrane may not be visible.

Because the neonate cannot coordinate tongue movements well, the tongue often falls backward, occluding the oral airway. Consequently, the neonate is a preferential nose breather who depends on patent nares (nostrils). To assess the nares for patency, the examiner occludes them one at a time and holds the mouth closed. The neonate should be able to breathe through the open naris. To check for the sneeze reflex, the examiner occludes both nares for 1 to 2 seconds, which should trigger sneezing (Tappero & Honeyfield, 1996). The neonate's nose is also examined for size, shape, mucous membrane integrity, and discharge. The nose should be midline on the face. The mucous membranes will appear pink and moist with no copious drainage.

The mouth should be inspected and palpated with gloved fingers. The examiner strokes the corner of the neonate's mouth to check the rooting reflex.

The tongue should be freely movable and symmetric in shape and movement. Occasionally a neonate may have a shortened frenulum ("tongue tie"). The neonate has moist oral mucous membranes but does not drool constantly.

The posterior pharynx is easiest to see when the neonate is crying. Saliva is usually scant because the salivary glands are immature. The presence of excessive saliva in a neonate should alert the nurse to the possibility of tracheoesophageal fistula or esophageal atresia.

The neck should appear symmetric and without webbing; it should also be flexible enough to allow the head to move freely and equally to each side.

Chest

The thoracic cavity should be cylindric and symmetric. Normally, chest wall excursion is equal bilaterally.

The ribs should be flexible and symmetric, with no palpable masses. The xiphoid process may be palpable at the bottom of the sternum and may be visible in a thin neonate.

When palpating the clavicles, the examiner moves the fingers slowly over the anterior clavicular surface. If a mass

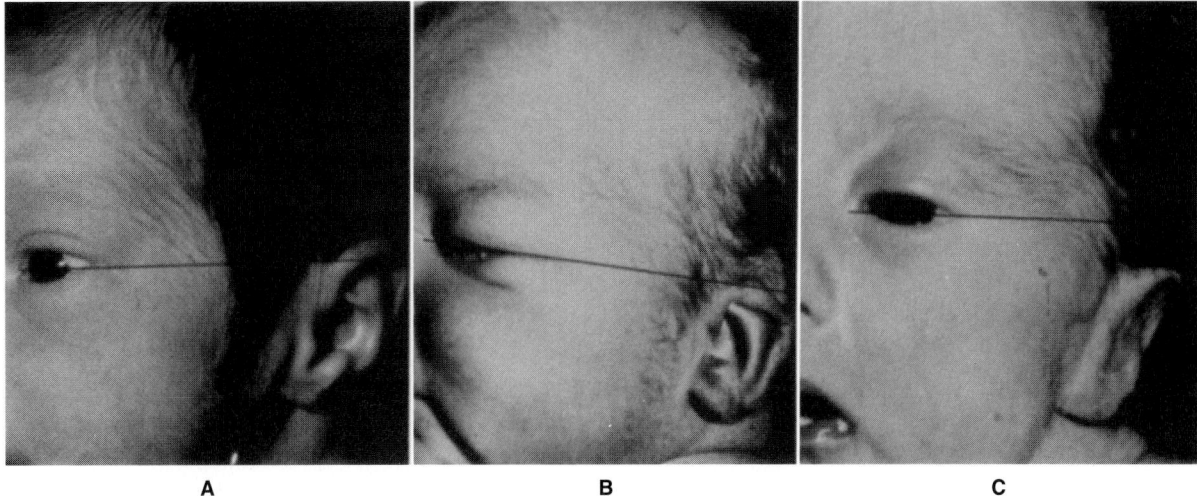

Fig. 26-17 Placement of ear on head in relation to line drawn from inner to outer canthus of eye. **A,** Normal position. **B,** Abnormally angled ear. **C,** True low-set ear. *(Courtesy Mead Johnson & Co., Evansville, IN.)*

or lump is detected, the examiner tries to move the neonate's arm gently while palpating with the other hand. A grating sensation and uneven movement of two juxtaposed bone fragments indicate a fracture (Tappero & Honeyfield, 1996).

Breast Size

The examiner assesses breast tissue through observation and palpation. To measure breast tissue, the examiner palpates the nipple gently with one finger or places the second and third fingers on either side of the nipple. The amount of breast tissue is measured between the two fingers.

Breast tissue and areola size increase with gestational age. The nipples are inspected for spacing and number. Supernumerary nipples may appear as darkened spots just below or beside natural nipples (Tappero & Honeyfield, 1996). Any discharge must be noted and documented.

Abdomen

The abdomen should have a symmetric, slightly rounded contour. Peristaltic waves normally are not visible; however, the abdomen should move visibly during breathing. The umbilical cord remnant should appear bluish-white, and contain two arteries and one vein.

The umbilical cord is clamped or tied at birth and the clamp or tie is usually removed when the cord is dry in approximately 24 hours. The umbilical cord begins to dry, shrivels, and blackens by the second or third day of life. The umbilicus should be inspected frequently for signs of infection (foul odor, redness, and purulent drainage), granuloma (small, red, raw-appearing polyp where the umbilical cord separates), bleeding, and discharge. The cord normally falls off by 2 weeks after birth. By the time the neonate is 1 month old, the umbilicus should be healed.

Auscultation of the abdomen is performed before palpation and percussion. To promote relaxation and comfort during palpation, the examiner flexes the neonate's legs in the fetal position. If the neonate has an asymmetric abdomen, which suggests an internal mass, great caution must be used during the assessment.

The posterior position of the kidneys makes them less accessible to palpation. If they cannot be palpated with one hand, bimanual palpation is used. In this technique, the examiner places one hand behind the neonate's back while palpating the abdomen with the fingertips of the other hand. The kidney should be felt between the hands (Tappero & Honeyfield, 1996).

Unless the bladder is distended, it should not be visible (Tappero & Honeyfield, 1996). The bladder may be percussed just above the symphysis pubis. The presence of urine will produce a tympanic sound. Pressing on the bladder may induce voiding or expression of urine. The time of the first voiding should be noted.

The abdomen should be percussed just after the neonate voids to prevent misleading findings. Percussion should reveal tympany (a clear, hollow note like that of a drum) below the left costal margin, reflecting a gastric bubble. Most other abdominal areas should also be tympanic. However, dullness should be percussed over the liver, spleen, and bladder. Percussion delineates the borders of these organs to detect enlargement, indicated by increased areas of dullness. Decreased areas of dullness suggest fluid or air where solid tissue is expected.

Back and Anus

To assess the back the examiner positions the neonate prone and inspects for spinal alignment, enlargement, and masses. The back should be straight. The sacrum is examined for dimpling, a tuft of hair, or bulges. The vertebral column is palpated for enlargement and signs of pain (Kenner, Lott, & Flendermeyer, 1997).

The perineum should be smooth and without dimpling or extra orifices. The anus should be midline and patent. The anal sphincter is assessed by lightly stroking the anus with a cotton-tipped applicator and observing anal constriction—a reaction called the anal wink. Passage of meconium indicates patency of the rectum, which should be noted.

Genitalia

In the male neonate the genitalia should be assessed for testicular descent, scrotal size, and number of rugae (skin folds). Hydroceles are a common finding and usually decrease without intervention.

If the male neonate is circumcised, he must be observed for signs of bleeding and ability to void.

The female genitalia should be assessed for signs of gestational maturity. The degree to which the labia majora and minora have come together and reduced the visual prominence of the labia minora and clitoris reflects the stage of the infant's maturity (Tappero & Honeyfield, 1996). Any discharge or abnormalities should be recorded and reported.

Extremities

The extremities are inspected for length, symmetry relative to each other and to the body as a whole, equality, muscle tone, and range of motion. Normally, the term neonate has a full range of motion, which can be tested either actively or passively. The examiner inspects the hands and feet for the number of digits, palmar and plantar creases, and abnormalities such as webbing (Tappero & Honeyfield, 1996).

Movement of the arms should be assessed. Trauma to the brachial plexus during a difficult birth may result in brachial palsy. The most common type, Duchenne-Erb paralysis, involves the fifth and sixth cervical nerve roots. The affected arm is held in a position of tight adduction and internal rotation at the shoulder. The grasp reflex on the affected side may be intact; however, Moro's reflex is absent on that side. With treatment most neonates have complete recovery.

To assess leg length, the examiner extends the legs simultaneously. The legs should be equal length, with symmetric skin folds. The examiner inspects the legs in both the prone and supine positions.

Plantar (sole) creases should be assessed immediately after birth because the drying effect of environmental exposure causes additional creases to form.

Neurologic Assessment

The physical assessment includes a neurologic assessment of the newborn's reflexes (see Table 26-3). This provides useful information about the infant's nervous system and state of neurologic maturation. Many reflex behaviors are

---

▪ BOX 26-1 Clusters of Neonatal Behaviors in BNBAS

Habituation—ability to respond to and then inhibit responding to discrete stimulus (light, rattle, bell, pinprick) while asleep.

Orientation—quality of alert states and ability to attend to visual and auditory stimuli while alert

Motor performance—quality of movement and tone

Range of state—measure of general arousal level or arousability of infant

Regulation of state—how infant responds when aroused

Autonomic stability—signs of stress (tremors, startles, skin color) related to homeostatic (self-regulator) adjustment of the nervous system

Reflexes—assessment of several neonatal reflexes

---

important for survival, for example, sucking and rooting. Other reflexes act as safety mechanisms, for instance, gagging, coughing, and sneezing. The assessment needs to be carried out as early as possible because abnormal signs present in the early neonatal period may disappear. They may reappear months or years later as abnormal functions.

BEHAVIORAL CHARACTERISTICS

The healthy infant must achieve behavioral and biologic tasks to develop normally. Behavioral characteristics form the basis of the social capabilities of the infant. The behavioral characteristics of the newborn represent a second phase in human development. The first phase, the fetal phase, indicates that the individual personalities and behavioral characteristics of infants play a major role in the ultimate relationship between infants and their parents.

Normal newborns differ in their activity levels, feeding patterns, sleeping patterns, and responsiveness. Parents' reactions to their newborns are often determined by these differences. Showing parents the unique characteristics of their infant assists parents to develop a more positive perception of the infant with increased interaction between infant and parent.

Behavioral characteristics, as well as physical characteristics, change during the period of transition. **The Brazelton Neonatal Behavioral Assessment Scale (BNBAS)** can be used to systematically assess the infant's behavior (Brazelton & Nugent, 1996). The BNBAS is an interactive examination that assesses the infant's response to 28 areas organized according to the clusters in Box 26-1. It is generally used as a research or diagnostic tool and requires special training.

In addition to use as initial and ongoing tools to assess neurologic and behavioral responses, the scales can be used to assess initial parent-infant relationships and as a guide

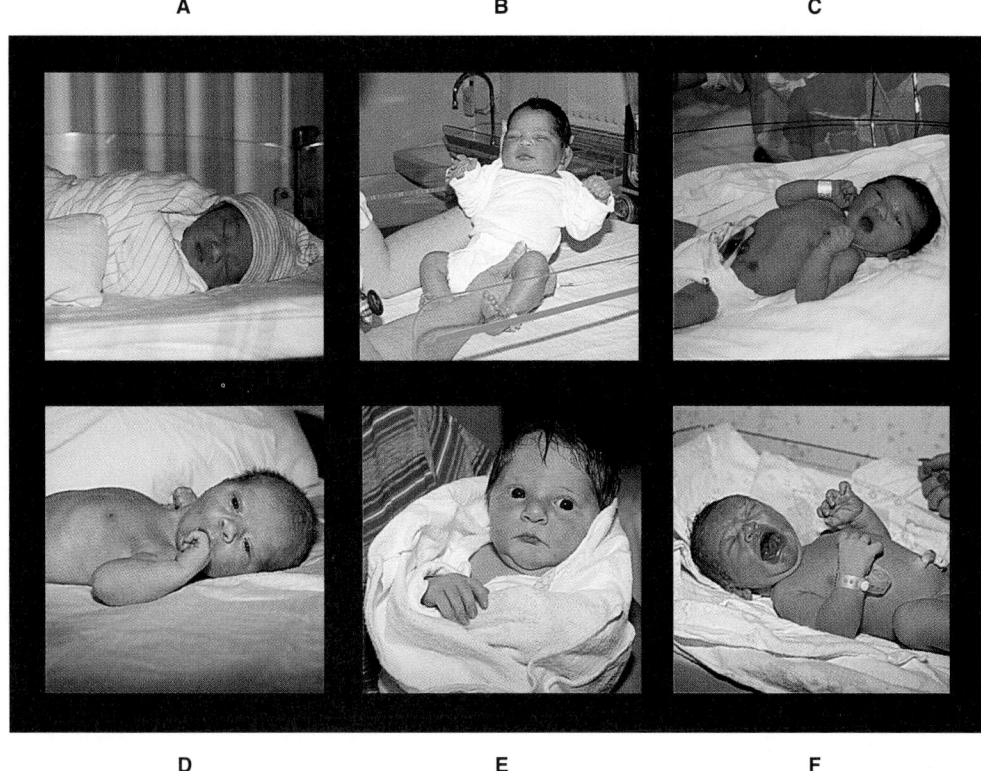

Fig. 26-18 Summary of newborn sleep-wake states. States of consciousness: **A,** Deep sleep, **B,** Light sleep. **C,** Drowsy. **D,** Quiet alert. **E,** Active alert. **F,** Crying. *(Courtesy Marjorie Pyle, RNC, Lifecircle, Costa Mesa, CA.)*

for parents to help them focus on their infant's individuality and to develop a deeper attachment to their child. See Chapter 25 for further discussion of attachment.

Sleep-Wake States

Variations in the state of consciousness of infants are called **sleep-wake states** (Brazelton & Nugent, 1996). The six states form a continuum from deep sleep to extreme irritability (Fig. 26-18). There are two sleep states—deep sleep and light sleep—and four wake states—drowsy, quiet alert, active alert, and crying. Each state has specific characteristics and **state-related behaviors.** The optimum state of arousal is the quiet alert state. During this state infants may be seen as smiling, vocalizing, moving in synchrony with speech, watching their parents' faces, and responding to people speaking to them. The infants' reaction to internal and external stimuli and ability to control their responses while in these sleep-wake states reflect their ability to organize behavior.

Infants use purposeful behavior to maintain the optimal arousal state: (1) actively withdrawing by increasing physical distance, (2) rejecting by pushing away with hands and feet, (3) decreasing sensitivity by falling asleep or breaking eye contact by turning head, or (4) using signaling behaviors, such as fussing and crying (Brazelton, 1984).

These behaviors permit infants to quiet themselves and reinstate readiness to interact.

The first 6 weeks of life involve a steady decrease in the proportion of active REM sleep to total sleep. A steady increase in the proportion of quiet sleep to total sleep also occurs. Periods of wakefulness increase 25% over the first 3 or 4 weeks of life. For the first few weeks the wakeful periods seem dictated by hunger, but soon thereafter a need for socializing appears as well. The newborn sleeps approximately 17 hours a day, with periods of wakefulness gradually increasing. By the fourth week of life, some infants stay awake from one feeding to the next. Children do not achieve the adult sleeping pattern until 4 to 5 years of age.

Other Factors Influencing Behavior of Newborns

Other variables in addition to the sleep-wake state affect the newborn's responses. Several factors are discussed below.

Gestational Age

The gestational age of the infant and level of CNS maturity affect the observed behavior. In an infant with an immature CNS the entire body responds to a pinprick of the foot. The mature infant withdraws only the foot. CNS immaturity is reflected in reflex development and sleep-wake cycles. Preterm infants have brief periods of alertness but have difficulty maintaining this state. Premature or sick infants show fatigue or stress sooner than full-term healthy infants (Tappero & Honeyfield, 1996).

Time

The time it takes for infants to recuperate from labor and birth affects the behavior of infants as they attempt to become organized initially. Time elapsed since the previous feeding and time of day may also influence infants' responses.

Stimuli

Environmental events and stimuli affect the behavioral responses of infants. Nurses in intensive care nurseries observe that infants respond to loud noises, bright lights, monitor alarms, and tension in the unit. If a mother is tense and has a fast heart beat while feeding an infant, the infant will have an increase in heart rate that is similar to the mother's. In addition, the newborn responds differently to animate and inanimate stimulation.

Medication

Controversy surrounds the effects of maternal medication (analgesia, anesthesia) during labor on infant behavior. Some researchers note that infants of mothers given medications may continue to demonstrate poor state organization after the fifth day. Others maintain that the effect can be beneficial or nonexistent (Dixon & Stein, 1992).

Ethnicity

Some of the most interesting research findings have been regarding the ethnic differences in infant behavior (Chitty & Winter, 1989; Freedman, 1979). Freedman (1979) found that Chinese-American infants had more self-quieting activities, fewer state changes, and more rapid responses to consoling activities than Caucasian American infants. The results from a study of Navajo newborns reinforced the stereotype of the stoic, impassive Native American (Freedman, 1979). Among Navajo babies, crying was rare and limb movements reduced, and calming was almost immediate after tests for Moro's reflex. In Freedman's study (1979), Japanese newborns were more sensitive and irritable than either Chinese or Navajo newborns. Mexican mothers use tactile stimulation more often than vocalizations to quiet their newborns (Garcia-Coll, 1990). These studies suggest that neonatal behavior represents a behavioral phenotype, which expresses a complex relationship among genetic endowment, intrauterine environment, and maternal obstetric history (Garcia-Coll, 1990). Because these studies occurred 10 to 20 years ago, they need to be replicated.

Sensory Behaviors

From birth, infants possess **sensory capabilities** that indicate a state of readiness for social interaction. Infants effectively use behavioral responses in establishing their first di-

alogues. These responses, coupled with the newborns' "baby appearance" (with the face being proportioned such that the forehead and eyes are larger than the lower portion of the face) and their smallness and helplessness, rouse feelings of wanting to hold, protect, and interact with them.

Vision

At birth the eye is structurally incomplete and the muscles are immature. The pupils react to light, the blink reflex is easily stimulated, and the corneal reflex is activated by light touch. The clearest visual distance is 17 to 20 cm, which is about the distance the infant's face is from the mother's face as she breastfeeds or cuddles. Infants are sensitive to light. They will frown if a bright light is flashed in their eyes and will turn toward a soft, red light. If the room is darkened, they will open their eyes wide and look about. This is noticeable when the birthing area is darkened after birth. By 2 months of age, they can detect color but seem more attracted by black-and-white patterns at 5 days of age and younger (Kenner, Lott, & Flandermeyer, 1997).

Response to movement is noticeable. If a bright object is shown to newborns (even at 15 minutes of age), they will follow it visually and some will even turn their heads to do so. Because human eyes are bright, shiny objects, newborns will track their parents' eyes. Parents often comment on how exciting this behavior is.

Visual acuity is surprising; even at 2 weeks of age, infants can distinguish patterns with stripes 3 mm apart. By 6 months their vision is as acute as that of an adult. They prefer to look at patterns rather than plain surfaces, even if the latter are brightly colored. They prefer more complex patterns to simple ones. They prefer novelty (changes in pattern) by 2 months of age. The infant of a few weeks of age is therefore capable of responding actively to an enriched environment.

Hearing

As soon as the amniotic fluid drains from the ear, the infant's hearing is similar to an adult's. This may occur as early as 1 minute of age. Loud sounds of about 90 decibels cause the infant to respond with a startle reflex. The newborn responds to low-frequency sounds such as a heartbeat or lullaby by decreasing motor activity or stopping crying. The response to a high-frequency sound elicits an alerting reaction.

Studies indicate that the infant responds readily to the mother's voice (Brazelton & Nugent, 1996). This may be a response to having heard or felt sound waves from the mother's voice while in utero.

These studies indicate a selective listening to maternal voice sounds and rhythms during intrauterine life that prepares newborns for recognition and interaction with their primary caregivers—their mothers. Newborns are accustomed in the uterus to hearing the regular rhythm of the mother's heartbeat. As a result, they respond by relaxing and ceasing to fuss and cry if a regular heartbeat simulator is placed in their cribs.

The internal and middle portions of the ear are larger at birth, but the external canal is small. The mastoid process and bony parts of the external canal have not developed. Therefore the tympanic membrane and facial nerve are very close to the surface and can be easily damaged.

Touch

The infant is responsive to touch on all parts of the body. The face (especially the mouth), the hands, and the soles of the feet appear to be the most sensitive. Reflexes can be elicited by stroking the infant. The newborn's responses to touch suggest this sensory system is well prepared to receive and process tactile messages. Touch and motion are essential to normal growth and development. However, each infant is unique, and variations can be seen in newborns' responses to touch. Birth trauma or stress and depressant drugs taken by the mother decrease the infant's sensitivity to touch or painful stimuli.

Taste

The newborn has a well-developed taste system, and different solutions elicit different facial expressions. A tasteless solution produces no response, whereas a sweet solution causes eager sucking. A sour solution results in puckering of the lips, and a bitter solution causes a grimace. Newborns prefer glucose water over plain water (Lawrence, 1999). These studies demonstrate not only the newborn's response to various tastes but also the strength of the taste response and its independence from cortical levels of the nervous system.

Young infants are particularly oriented toward the use of their mouths, both for meeting their nutritional needs for rapid growth and for releasing tension through sucking. The early development of circumoral sensation, muscle activity, and taste would seem to be preparation for survival in the extrauterine environment.

Smell

The newborn's sense of smell has been reported to be well developed at birth. Newborns appear to react similarly to adults when exposed to strong or pleasant odors. Breastfed infants are able to smell breast milk and can differentiate their mother from other lactating women (Lawrence, 1999).

Response to Environmental Stimuli

Infants respond to the environment in a number of ways. Classic studies have identified individual variations in the primary reaction pattern of newborns and described them as temperament (Dixon & Stein, 1992; Thomas et al., 1961, 1970). Their style of behavioral response to stimuli is guided by the temperament affecting the newborn's sensory threshold, ability to habituate, and response to maternal behaviors.

The human newborn possesses sensory receptors capable of responding selectively to various stimuli present in the internal and external environment. The infant also possesses individual characteristics that affect the response.

Temperament

The behavioral styles of infants and children "show distinct individuality in temperament in the first weeks of life, independently of their parents' handling or personality style." In addition, "the original characteristics of temperament tend to persist in most children over the years" (Chess, 1969; Chess & Thomas, 1977).

Chess' classical work (1969) led to the development of nine categories of primary reactivity to evaluate behavioral style:
1. Activity level—the diurnal proportion of active to inactive periods
2. Rhythmicity—the regularity and predictability of bodily function and sleep-wake cycle
3. Approach or withdrawal—the response to a new stimulus
4. Adaptability—the speed and ease with which current behavior is modified in response to environmental changes
5. Intensity of reaction—the energy in a response regardless of its quality or direction
6. Threshold of responsiveness—the intensity of stimuli required to evoke a response
7. Quality of mood—the proportion of happy to unhappy behavior
8. Distractibility—the efficacy of external stimuli in changing the direction of ongoing behavior
9. Attention span and persistence—the duration one activity is pursued and effect of distraction

These nine categories were then grouped into three major patterns of behavioral style or temperament:
1. The easy child who demonstrates regularity in bodily functions, readily adapts to change, has a predominantly positive mood and moderate sensory threshold, and approaches new situations or objects with a moderate response
2. The slow-to-warm-up child who has a low activity level, withdraws on first exposure to new stimuli, is slow to adapt and low in intensity of response, and is somewhat negative in mood
3. The difficult child who is irregular in bodily functions, intense in reactions, generally negative in mood, and resistant to change or new stimuli and often cries loudly for long periods

The human newborn possesses sensory receptors capable of responding selectively to various stimuli present in the internal and external environment. The infant also possesses individual characteristics that affect the response. The range of responses may impress the parent with the newborn's formidable neurologic capacity.

Habituation

Habituation is a protective mechanism that allows the infant to become accustomed to environmental stimuli. Habituation is a psychologic and physiologic phenomenon whereby the response to a constant or repetitive stimulus is decreased. In the term newborn this can be demonstrated in several ways. Shining a bright light into a newborn's eyes will cause a startle or squinting the first 2 to 3 times. The third or fourth flash will elicit a diminished response, and by the fifth or sixth flash, the infant ceases to respond (Brazelton & Nugent, 1996). The same response pattern holds true for the sounds of a rattle or a pinprick to the heel. A newborn presented with new stimuli becomes wide eyed and alters its gaze for a time but will eventually show a diminished interest.

The ability to habituate also allows the newborn to select stimuli that promote continued learning about the social world, thus avoiding overload. The intrauterine experience seems to have programmed the newborn to be especially responsive to human voices, soft lights, soft sounds, and sweet tastes.

The newborn quickly learns the sounds in a newborn nursery and the home and is able to sleep in their midst. The selective responses of the newborn indicate cerebral organization capable of remembering and making choices. The ability to habituate depends on state of consciousness, hunger, fatigue, and temperament. These factors also affect consolability, cuddliness, irritability, and crying.

Consolability

Barr (1990) described variations in the ability of newborns to console themselves or to be consoled. In the crying state, most newborns initiate one of several ways to reduce their distress. Hand-to-mouth movements are common, with or without sucking, as well as alerting to voices, noises, or visual stimuli.

Cuddliness

Cuddliness is especially important to parents because they often gauge their ability to care for the child by the child's responses to their actions. The degree to which newborns will mold into the contours of the persons holding them varies. Barr (1990) tested the effect of body contact and vestibular stimulation in both soothing babies and creating alertness. The vestibular stimulation of being picked up and moved had the greater effect.

Irritability

Some newborns cry longer and harder than others. For some the sensory threshold seems low. They are readily upset by unusual noises, hunger, wetness, or new experiences, and thus respond intensely. Others with a high sensory threshold require a great deal more stimulation and variation to reach the active, alert state (Barr, 1990).

Crying

Crying in an infant may signal hunger, pain, desire for attention, or fussiness. Some mothers state that they are eventually able to distinguish the reasons for crying. This is a means of communication.

Barr (1990) reported five characteristics of crying. (1) Crying progressively increases to a peak in the second month and then gradually decreases. (2) A diurnal rhythm is present, with more crying occurring in the evening hours. (3) Babies vary considerably in the amount and timing of crying. (4) Individual day-to-day variations seem to occur. (5) The crying does not seem to differ with different caretakers.

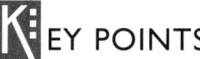

KEY POINTS

- By term the infant's various anatomic and physiologic systems have reached a level of development and functioning that permits a physical existence apart from the mother. The infant has sensory capabilities that indicate a state of readiness for social interaction.

- There are several significant differences between the respiratory, renal, and thermogenic systems in the newborn and those of an adult.

- At any serum bilirubin level the appearance of jaundice during the first day of life or persistence of jaundice for more than 7 days usually indicates a pathologic process in term infants.

- Loss of heat in a newborn, even a healthy newborn, may result in acidosis and raise the level of free fatty acids, leading to cold stress.

- Assessment of the newborn requires data from the prenatal, intrapartal, and postpartal periods.

- The newborn assessment should proceed systematically so that each system is thoroughly evaluated.

- Many reflex behaviors are important for the newborn's survival.

- Individual personalities and behavioral characteristics of infants play a major role in their ultimate relationships with their parents.

- Sleep-wake states and other factors influence the newborn's behavior.

- Each newborn has a predisposed capacity to handle the multitude of stimuli in the external world.

CRITICAL THINKING EXERCISES

1 *Observe and record findings of normal term infants of at least two ethnic groups immediately after birth and in a follow-up period. Include both physiologic and behavioral data and compare findings. Explain the way this information can be used in planning care.*

2 *Use the newborn's sensory abilities and social responses to design a nursery for the new baby (in the home). Incorporate these abilities into a list of suggestions for appropriate parent-child interactions.*

3 *Prepare a discharge teaching guide for parents on normal physical findings of a newborn and how to recognize deviations from normal that need intervention. Include information on the interventions that parents can implement. Identify deviations that parents should report to their pediatric care provider.*

References

Barr, R. (1990). The normal crying curve: What do we really know? *Dev Med Child Neurol* 32, 356-362.

Blackburn, S. (1992). Alterations of the respiratory system in the neonate: Implications for clinical practice. *J Perinat Neonatal Nurs* 6(2), 46-58.

Blackburn, S., & Loper, D. (1992). *Maternal, fetal and neonatal physiology: A clinical perspective.* Philadelphia: W.B. Saunders.

Brazelton, T. (1984). *Neonatal behavioral assessment scale* (2nd ed.). Philadelphia: J.B. Lippincott.

Brazelton, T., & Nugent, K. (1996). *Neonatal behavioral assessment scale* (3rd ed.). London: MacKeith.

Carey, B. (1996). Physical assessment of the newborn: A comprehensive approach to the art of assessment-neurologic assessment. *Mother Baby J* 1(3), 33-38.

Chess, S. (1969). Individuality and baby care. *Dev Med Neurol* 11, 749-754.

Chess, S., & Thomas, A. (1977). Temperament and the parent-child interaction. *Pediatr Ann* 6(9), 574-582.

Chitty, L., & Winter, R. (1989). Perinatal morbidity in different ethnic groups. *Arch Dis Child* 64, 1036-1041.

Dickason, E., Silverman, B., & Kaplan, J. (1998). *Maternal-infant nursing care* (3rd ed.). St. Louis: Mosby.

Dixon, S., & Stein, M. (1992). *Encounters with children: Pediatric behavior and development* (2nd ed.). St. Louis: Mosby.

Fanaroff, A., & Martin, R. (1997). *Neonatal-perinatal medicine: Diseases of the fetus and infant* (6th ed.). St. Louis: Mosby.

Freedman, D. (1979, Jan). Ethnic differences in babies. *Hum Nature*, 36.

Garcia-Coll, C. (1990). Developmental outcome of minority infants: A process-oriented look into our beginnings. *Child Dev* 61, 270-289.

Guyton, A., & Hall, J. (1995). *Textbook of medical physiology* (9th ed.). Philadelphia: W.B. Saunders.

Johnson, T. et al. (1998). Reliability of length measurements in full-term neonates. *J Obstet Gynecol Neonatal Nurs* 27(3), 270-276.

Kenner, C., Lott, J., & Flandermeyer, A. (1997). *Comprehensive neonatal nursing* (2nd ed.). Philadelphia: W.B. Saunders.

Korones, S. (1995). *High-risk newborn infants: The basis for intensive care* (5th ed.). St. Louis: Mosby.

Lawrence, R. (1999). *Breastfeeding: A guide for the medical profession* (5th ed.). St. Louis: Mosby.

Lowe, N., & Reiss, R. (1996). Parturition and fetal adaptation. *J Obstet Gynecol Neonatal Nurs* 25(4), 339-349.

Merenstein, G., & Gardner, S. (1998). *Handbook of neonatal intensive care* (4th ed.). St. Louis: Mosby.

Pagana, K., & Pagana, T. (1998). *Mosby's manual of diagnostic and laboratory tests.* St. Louis: Mosby.

Seidel, H., Rosenstein, G., & Pathak, A. (1993). *Care of the full-term newborn.* St. Louis: Mosby.

Sheeran, M. (1996). Thermoregulation in neonates: Obtaining an accurate axillary temperature measurement. *J Neonatal Nurs* 2(4), 6-9.

Tappero, E., & Honeyfield, M. (1996). Physical assessment of the newborn: A comprehensive approach to the art of physical examination. *Mother Baby J* 1(1), 39-45.

Thomas, A. et al. (1961). Individuality in responses of children to similar environmental situations. *Am J Psychiatry* 117, 798.

Thomas, A. et al. (1970). The origin of personality. *Sci Am* 223, 102-109.

Wong, D. (1999). *Whaley and Wong's nursing care of infants and children* (6th ed.). St. Louis: Mosby.

Assessment and Care of the Newborn

Bette B. Hammond
Shannon E. Perry

LEARNING OBJECTIVES

- Define the key terms.
- Identify purpose and components of the Apgar score.
- Compare and contrast the characteristics of preterm, term, postterm, and postmature neonates.
- Assess the gestational age and birth weight of newborns.
- Rate infants using the physical maturity scale and neuromuscular maturity scale.
- Explain what is meant by a safe environment.
- Discuss phototherapy and the guidelines for teaching parents about this treatment.

- Explain purposes for and methods of circumcision, the postoperative care of the circumcised infant, and parent teaching information regarding circumcision.
- Review procedures for doing a heel stick, collecting urine specimens, assisting with venipuncture, and restraining the newborn.
- Review the anticipatory guidance nurses provide the parents before discharge.
- Identify topics for nursing research related to assessment and care of the newborn.

KEY TERMS

acid mantle	large for gestational age (LGA)	premature
Apgar score	low birth weight (LBW)	preterm
appropriate for gestational age (AGA)	ophthalmia neonatorum	protective environment
circumcision	phimosis	small for gestational age (SGA)
hypothermia	phototherapy	term
intrauterine growth restriction (IUGR)	postmature	very low birth weight (VLBW)
	postterm (postdate)	

Although most infants make the necessary biopsychosocial adjustment to extrauterine existence without undue difficulty, their well-being depends on the care they receive from others. This chapter describes assessment and care of the infant immediately after birth until discharge. Assessment of gestational age and birth weight are emphasized because of the bearing these factors have on perinatal morbidity and mortality and infants' long-term developmental outcomes.

CARE MANAGEMENT: FROM BIRTH THROUGH THE FIRST 2 HOURS

Care begins immediately after the birth and focuses on assessing and stabilizing the newborn's condition. The nurse has primary responsibility for the infant during this period, because the physician or midwife is involved with delivery of the placenta and caring for the mother. The nurse must be alert for any signs of distress and initiate appropriate interventions.

TABLE 27-1 Apgar Score

SIGN	SCORE		
	0	1	2
Heart rate	Absent	Slow (<100)	Over 100
Respiratory rate	Absent	Slow, weak cry	Good cry
Muscle tone	Flaccid	Some flexion of extremities	Well flexed
Reflex irritability	No response	Grimace	Cry
Color	Blue, pale	Body pink, extremities blue	Completely pink

Initial Assessment and Nursing Diagnoses

The initial assessment of the neonate is done at birth and uses the Apgar score (Letko, 1996) (Table 27-1) and a brief physical examination (Box 27-1). A gestational age assessment is done within 2 hours of birth (Fig. 27-1), and a more comprehensive physical assessment may be completed within 24 hours of birth (Tappero & Honeyfield, 1996) (see Table 26-4).

Apgar Score

The **Apgar score** permits a rapid assessment of the need for resuscitation based on five signs that indicate the physiologic state of the neonate (see Table 27-1): *heart rate*, based on auscultation with a stethoscope; *respiration*, based on observed movement of the chest wall; *muscle tone*, based on degree of flexion and movement of the extremities; *reflex irritability*, based on response to gentle slaps on the soles of the feet; and *color*, described as pallid, cyanotic, or pink. Each item is scored as a 0, 1, or 2. Evaluations are made 1 and 5 minutes after birth. Scores of 0 to 3 indicate severe distress, scores of 4 to 6 indicate moderate difficulty, and scores of 7 to 10 indicate that the infant should have no difficulty adjusting to extrauterine life (Letko, 1996). Apgar scores do not predict future neurologic outcome but the 5-minute score does correlate with the degree of risk for neonatal morbidity and mortality.

Initial Physical Assessment

The *initial physical assessment* includes a brief review of systems (see Box 27-1). For this initial brief examination, the nurse assesses the following:

1. *External:* Notes skin color, staining, peeling, or wasting (dysmaturity); notes length of nails and creases on soles of feet; checks for presence of breast tissue; assesses nasal patency by covering one nostril at a time while observing respirations and color; notes meconium staining of cord, skin, fingernails, or amniotic fluid (staining may indicate fetal hypoxia; offensive odor may indicate intrauterine infection)

2. *Chest:* Palpates for site of PMI and auscultates for rate and quality of heart tones and murmurs; notes character of respirations and presence of crackles or rhonchi; notes equality of breath sounds on each side of chest by holding stethoscope in each axilla

BOX 27-1 Initial Physical Assessment by Body System

CNS [ ] moves extremities, muscle tone good
[ ] symmetric features, movement
[ ] suck, rooting, Moro response, grasp reflexes good
[ ] anterior fontanel soft and flat
CV [ ] heart auscultation, strong and regular
[ ] no murmurs heard
[ ] pulses strong/equal bilaterally
RESP [ ] lungs auscultated, clear bilaterally
[ ] respiratory rate <60 breaths/min
[ ] chest expansion symmetric
[ ] no upper airway congestion
GU [ ] male: urethral opening at tip of penis; testes descended bilaterally
female: vaginal opening apparent
GI [ ] abdomen soft, no distention
[ ] cord attached and clamped
[ ] anus appears patent
ENT [ ] eyes clear
[ ] palates intact
[ ] nares patent
SKIN Color [ ] pink [ ] acrocyanotic
[ ] no lesions or abrasions
[ ] no peeling
[ ] birthmarks _____
[ ] caput/molding
[ ] vacuum "cap"
[ ] forceps marks
[ ] other
Comments: _____
_____
_____
_____

3. *Abdomen:* Verifies presence of a domed abdomen and absence of anomalies; notes number of vessels in cord

4. *Neurologic:* Checks muscle tone and reflex reaction; assesses Moro reflex; palpates anterior fontanel for

NEUROMUSCULAR MATURITY

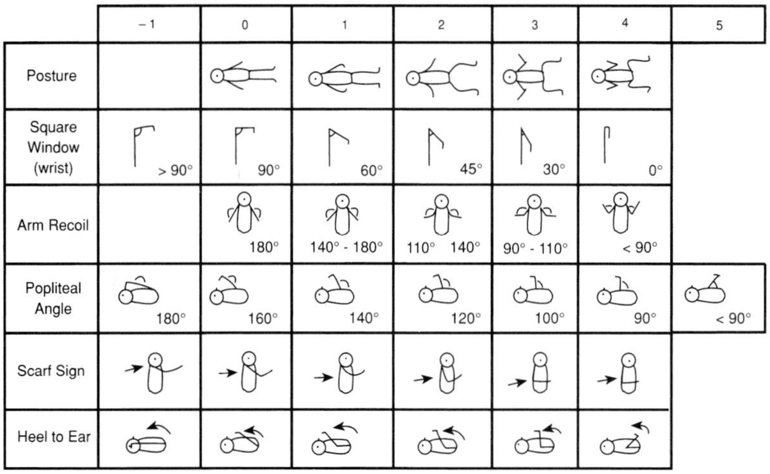

	-1	0	1	2	3	4	5
Posture							
Square Window (wrist)	> 90°	90°	60°	45°	30°	0°	
Arm Recoil		180°	140° - 180°	110° 140°	90° - 110°	< 90°	
Popliteal Angle	180°	160°	140°	120°	100°	90°	< 90°
Scarf Sign							
Heel to Ear							

PHYSICAL MATURITY

Skin	sticky friable transparent	gelatinous red, translucent	smooth pink, visible veins	superficial peeling or rash, few veins	cracking pale areas rare veins	parchment deep cracking no vessels	leathery cracked wrinkled
Lanugo	none	sparse	abundant	thinning	bald areas	mostly bald	
Plantar Surface	heel-toe 40-50 mm: -1 <40 mm: -2	>50 mm no crease	faint red marks	anterior transverse crease only	creases ant. 2/3	creases over entire sole	
Breast	imperceptible	barely perceptible	flat areola no bud	stippled areola 1-2 mm bud	raised areola 3-4 mm bud	full areola 5-10 mm bud	
Eye/Ear	lids fused loosely: -1 tightly: -2	lids open pinna flat stays folded	sl. curved pinna; soft; slow recoil	well-curved pinna; soft but ready recoil	formed & firm instant recoil	thick cartilage ear stiff	
Genitals (male)	scrotum flat, smooth	scrotum empty faint rugae	testes in upper canal rare rugae	testes descending few rugae	testes down good rugae	testes pendulous deep rugae	
Genitals (female)	clitoris prominent labia flat	prominent clitoris small labia minora	prominent clitoris enlarging minora	majora & minora equally prominent	majora large minora small	majora cover clitoris & minora	

MATURITY RATING

score	weeks
-10	20
-5	22
0	24
5	26
10	28
15	30
20	32
25	34
30	36
35	38
40	40
45	42
50	44

Fig. 27-1 Estimation of gestational age. **A,** New Ballard Scale for newborn maturity rating. Expanded scale includes extremely premature infants and has been refined to improve accuracy in more mature infants. (**A** from Ballard, J. et al. [1991]. *New Ballard Score, expanded to include extremely premature infants.* J Pediatr 119[3], 417.)

fullness or bulge; notes by palpation the presence and size of the fontanels and sutures

5. *Other observations:* Notes gross structural malformations obvious at birth

The nurse responsible for the care of the newborn immediately after birth verifies that respirations have been established, dries the infant, assesses temperature, and places identical identification bracelets on the infant and the mother. In some settings, the father also wears an identification bracelet. The infant may be wrapped in a warm blanket and placed in the arms of the mother, given to the father to hold, or kept undressed under a radiant warmer. In some settings, immediately after birth the infant is placed on the mother's abdomen to allow skin-to-skin contact, which contributes to maintenance of the infant's optimum temperature and parental bonding. The infant may be admitted to a nursery or remain with the parents throughout the hospital stay.

The initial examination of the newborn can occur while the nurse is drying and wrapping the infant, or observa-

CLASSIFICATION OF NEWBORNS—
BASED ON MATURITY AND INTRAUTERINE GROWTH
Symbols: X - 1st Examination O - 2nd Examination

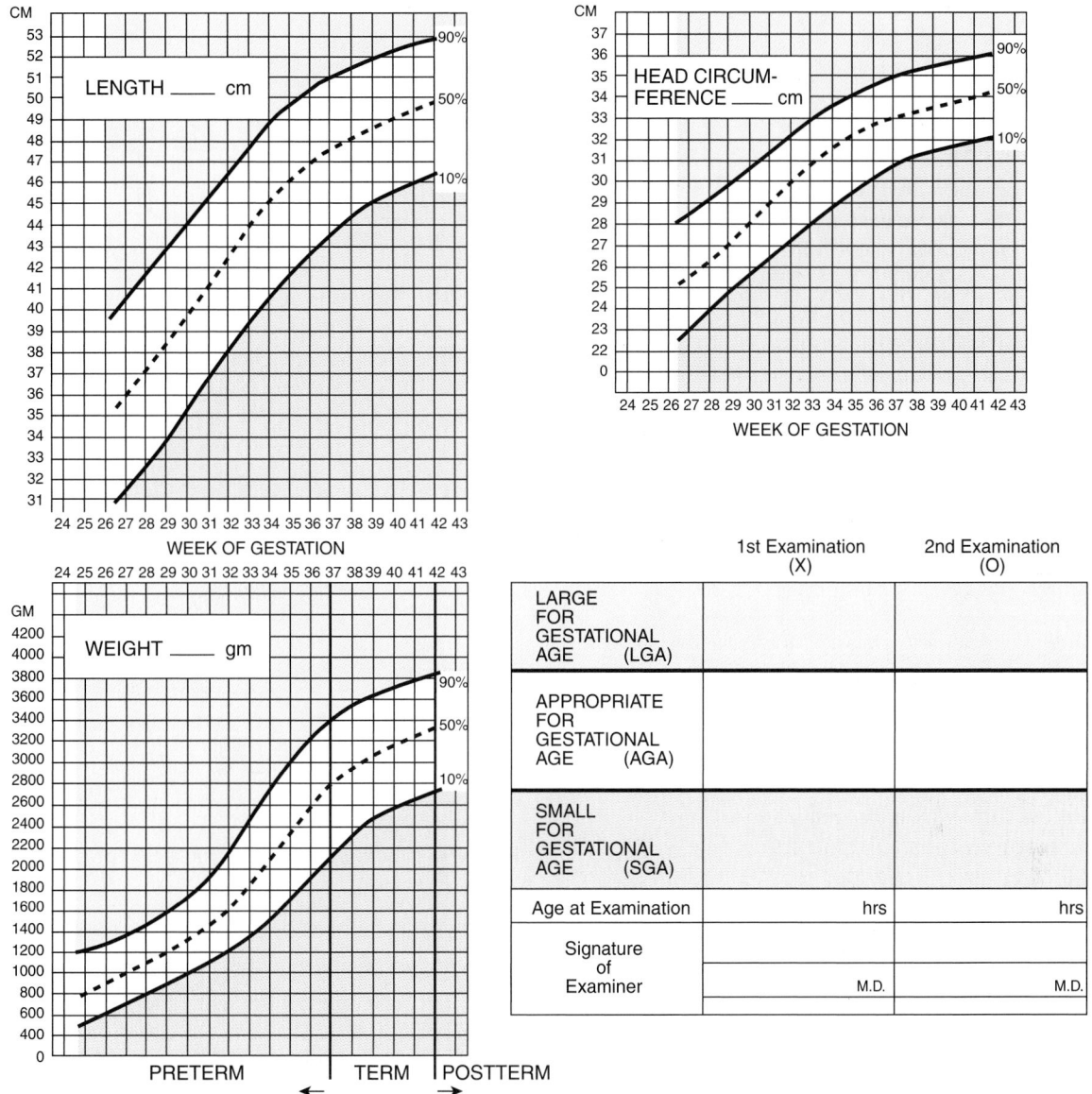

Fig. 27-1, cont'd   Estimation of gestational age. **B,** Newborn classification based on maturity and intrauterine growth. (*B modified from Lubchenco, L., Hansman, C., & Boyd, E. [1966]. Intrauterine growth in length and head circumference as estimated from live births at gestational ages from 26 to 42 weeks. J Pediatr 37[3], 403; and Battaglia, F., & Lubchenco, L. [1967]. A practical classification of newborn infants by weight and gestational age. J Pediatr 71[2], 159.*)

tions can be made while the infant is lying on the mother's abdomen or in her arms immediately after birth. Efforts should be directed to minimizing interference in the initial parent-infant acquaintance process. If the infant is breathing easily, has good color, and is normal in appearance, then further examination can be delayed until after the parents have had an opportunity to interact with the infant.

Routine procedures and the admission process can be carried out in the mother's room or in a separate nursery. Box 27-2 shows an example of newborn routine orders.

BOX 27-2 Routine Admission Orders

Vital signs: on admission and q30min × 2, q1hr × 2, then q8hr

Weight, length, and head and chest circumference on admission; then weigh daily

Tetracycline or erythromycin ophthalmic ointment 5 mg/g 1½- to 2-cm line in lower conjunctiva of each eye (ou)

Vitamin K 1 mg IM

Hematocrit by warm heel stick within 3 to 8 hours of age; call health care provider if <44 or >72

Dextrostix prn; notify health care provider if <40 mg/dl; offer early D_5W PO

Feedings: sterile water × 1 by nurse within first 4 hr of life; if tolerated, begin formula q3-4hr on demand (Breastfeeding on demand may be initiated immediately after birth without initial sterile water feeding.)

Rooming-in as desired and infant's condition permits

Newborn screen for phenylketonuria (PKU), thyroxine (T_4), and galactosemia or other screening tests as ordered at least 24 hr after first feeding

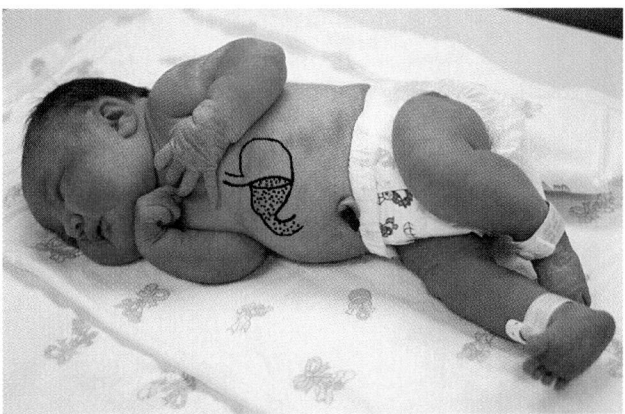

Fig. 27-2 Side-lying position. Infant is turned to right side and supported in this position to facilitate drainage from mouth and promote emptying of stomach contents into the small intestine. *(From Wong, D. [1999]. Whaley & Wong's nursing care of infants and children. [6th ed.]. St. Louis: Mosby.)*

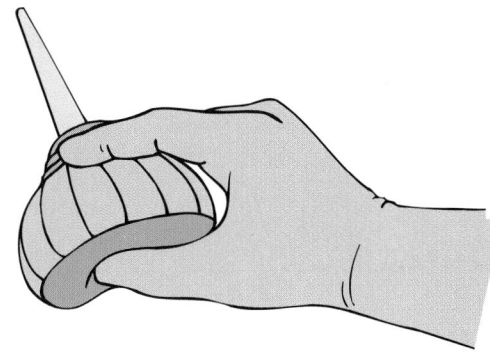

Fig. 27-3 Bulb syringe. Bulb must be compressed before insertion.

Nursing diagnoses are established after analysis of the findings of the physical assessment. Nursing diagnoses for the newborn include the following:

Nursing Diagnoses

- Ineffective airway clearance related to
  - airway obstruction with mucus
- Impaired gas exchange related to
  - hypothermia
- Ineffective thermoregulation related to
  - heat loss to the environment
- Risk for infection related to
  - umbilical cord stump
  - circumcision
  - fetal scalp electrode sites
- Risk for injury related to
  - helplessness
- Pain related to
  - procedures such as heel sticks and circumcision

Expected Outcomes of Care

The expected outcomes for newborn care apply both to the infant and to the caregiver. The expected outcomes for the infant include that the infant will achieve the following:

- Maintain effective breathing patterns.
- Maintain effective thermoregulation.
- Remain free from infection.
- Receive the necessary nutrition for growth.

- Establish adequate elimination patterns.
- Experience minimal pain related to circumcision (if performed).

Expected outcomes for the parents include that they will do the following:

- Attain knowledge, skill, and confidence relevant to infant care activities.
- State understanding of biologic and behavioral characteristics of the newborn.
- Have opportunities to intensify relationships with their newborn.
- Begin to integrate the infant into the family.
- Demonstrate behavior and lifestyle changes that reduce the potential for problems to develop.

Plan of Care and Interventions

Events can occur rapidly in newborns immediately after birth. Assessment must therefore be followed quickly by the implementation of appropriate care.

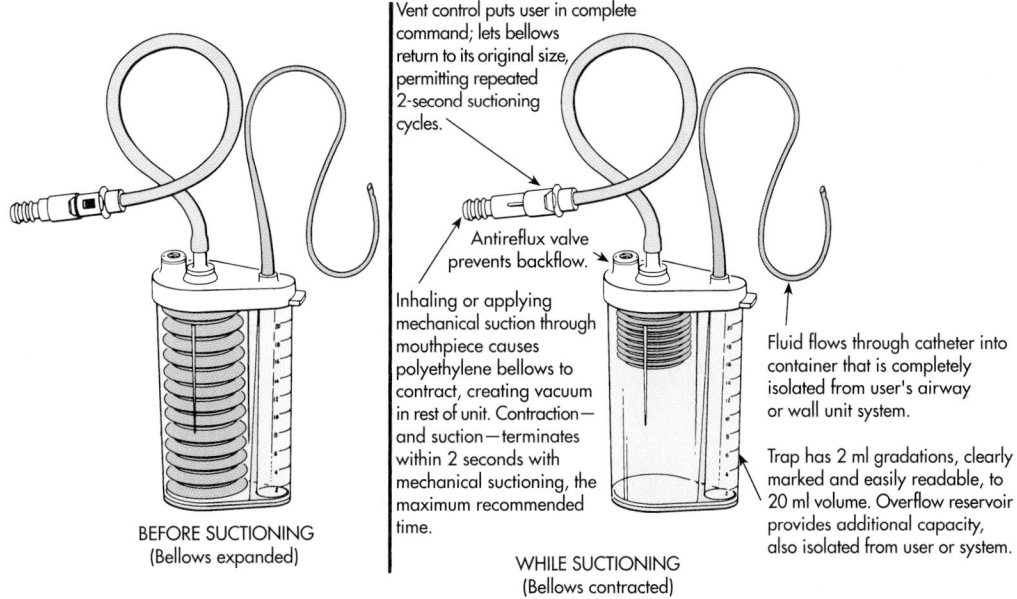

Vent control puts user in complete command; lets bellows return to its original size, permitting repeated 2-second suctioning cycles.

Antireflux valve prevents backflow.

Inhaling or applying mechanical suction through mouthpiece causes polyethylene bellows to contract, creating vacuum in rest of unit. Contraction— and suction—terminates within 2 seconds with mechanical suctioning, the maximum recommended time.

Fluid flows through catheter into container that is completely isolated from user's airway or wall unit system.

Trap has 2 ml gradations, clearly marked and easily readable, to 20 ml volume. Overflow reservoir provides additional capacity, also isolated from user or system.

BEFORE SUCTIONING
(Bellows expanded)

WHILE SUCTIONING
(Bellows contracted)

Fig. 27-4 Isolated DeLee suction method with catheter and mucous trap. *(Courtesy Busse Hospital Disposables, Hauppauge, NY.)*

Stabilization and Resuscitation

Generally, the normal term infant born vaginally has little difficulty clearing the air passages. Most secretions are moved by gravity and brought to the oropharynx by the cough reflex to be drained or swallowed. The infant is maintained in a side-lying position with a rolled blanket at the back to facilitate drainage (Fig. 27-2).

If the infant has excess mucus in the respiratory tract, the mouth and nasal passages may be suctioned with a bulb syringe (Fig. 27-3) or a DeLee mucous trap suction catheter (Fig. 27-4). The nurse may perform gentle percussion over the chest wall using a soft circular mask or a percussion cup to aid in loosening secretions before suctioning (Fig. 27-5). "Milking" the trachea is ineffective, may injure cartilage, and often delays effective suctioning. The infant who is coughing and choking on the secretions should be supported with the head downward. The infant should never be suspended by the ankles. First, the mouth is suctioned. This prevents the infant from inhaling pharyngeal secretions by gasping as the nares are touched. The bulb is compressed and inserted into one side of the mouth. The center of the infant's mouth is avoided because this could stimulate the gag reflex. The nasal passages are suctioned one nostril at a time. When the infant's cry does not sound as though it is through mucus or a bubble, suctioning can be stopped. The bulb syringe should always be kept in the infant's crib. The parents should be given demonstrations on how to use the bulb syringe and asked to perform a return demonstration.

The DeLee mucous trap suction apparatus is used most commonly during the birth process. The isolated DeLee suction method (Busse bac/shield) provides safe oral or

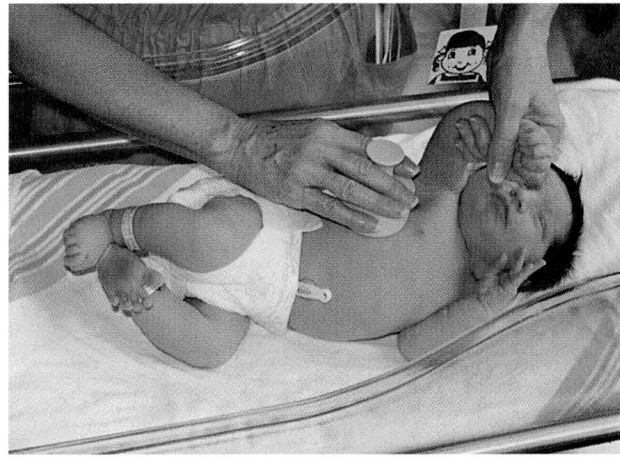

Fig. 27-5 Chest percussion. Nurse performs gentle percussion over the chest wall using a percussion cup to aid in loosening secretions before suctioning.

mechanical suctioning of newborns while preventing the transmission of bacteria, viruses, and other infectious material from the newborn to the user.

Use of a nasopharyngeal catheter with mechanical suction apparatus. Deeper suctioning may be necessary to remove excessive or tenacious mucus from the infant's nasopharynx. Proper tube insertion and suctioning for 10 seconds or less per tube insertion helps prevent laryngospasms and oxygen depletion. If wall suction is used, the pressure should be adjusted to less than 80 mm Hg. The catheter is lubricated in sterile water. The catheter is inserted either orally along the base of the tongue or up and

EMERGENCY

Relieving Airway Obstruction

Back blow and chest thrusts are used to clear an airway obstructed by a foreign body.

BACK BLOWS (FIG. 27-6, A)

Position the infant prone over forearm with the head down and the infant's jaw firmly supported.

Rest the supporting arm on the thigh.

Deliver four back blows forcefully between the infant's shoulder blades with the heel of the free hand.

TURN INFANT

Place the free hand on the infant's back to sandwich the baby between both hands; one hand supports the neck, jaw, and chest while the other supports the back.

Turn the infant over and place the head lower than the chest, supporting the head and neck.

Alternative position: Place the infant face down on your lap with the head lower than the trunk; firmly support the head. Apply back blows and then turn the infant as a unit.

CHEST THRUSTS (FIG. 27-6, B)

Provide four downward chest thrusts on the lower third of the sternum.

Remove foreign body, if it is visible.

OPEN AIRWAY

Open airway with the head tilt–chin lift maneuver and attempt to ventilate.

Repeat the sequence of back blows, turning, and chest thrusts.

Continue these emergency procedures until signs of recovery occur:

Palpable peripheral pulses return.

The pupils become normal in size and are responsive to light.

Mottling and cyanosis disappear.

Record the time and duration of the procedure and the effects of this intervention.

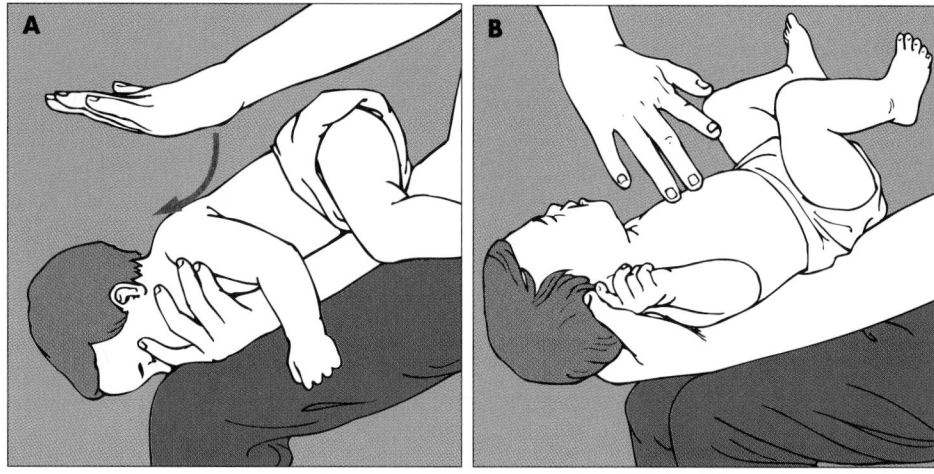

Fig. 27-6 Back blows and chest thrust in infant to clear airway obstruction. **A,** Back blow. **B,** Chest thrust.

back into the nares. After the catheter is properly placed, suction is created by placing a thumb over the control as the catheter is carefully rotated and gently withdrawn. This procedure may need to be repeated until the infant's cry sounds clear and air entry into the lungs is heard by stethoscope.

Relieving airway obstruction. A choking infant needs immediate attention. Often, simply repositioning the infant and suctioning the mouth and nose with the bulb syringe eliminates the problem. The infant should be posi-

tioned with the head slightly lower than the body to facilitate gravity drainage. The nurse should also listen to the infant's respiration and lung sounds with a stethoscope to determine whether there are crackles and wheezes. If the lungs are clear, the bulb syringe is used to clear the mouth and nose. If the bulb syringe does not provide relief, mechanical suction can be used.

If these measures do not relieve the obstruction, the nurse gives the infant back blows and chest thrusts (see Emergency box). To do this, the nurse places the infant face down over the arm with the head lower than the trunk and supported. The nurse can additionally support the infant by supporting his or her own arm firmly against his or her own thigh. The nurse then delivers four quick, sharp back blows between the infant's shoulder blades with the heel of the hand (Fig 27-6, *A*). After this, the nurse places his or her free hand on the infant's back so that the infant is "sandwiched" between the nurse's two hands, making certain that the neck and chin are well supported. While the nurse maintains support with the infant's head lower than the trunk, the nurse turns the infant and places the infant supine on his or her thigh, and then applies four chest thrusts in rapid succession in the same way as the external chest compressions are performed for cardiopulmonary resuscitation (see Emergency box and Figs. 27-6, *B*, and 27-9).

All personnel working with infants must have current infant CPR certification. Many institutions offer infant CPR courses to new parents (Donaher-Wagner & Braun, 1992). Because cardiac and respiratory arrest can occur in infants, careful monitoring is necessary so that rapid treatment can be instituted.

Maintaining an adequate oxygen supply. Four conditions are essential for maintaining an adequate oxygen supply:
- A clear airway
- Respiratory efforts
- A functioning cardiopulmonary system
- Heat support (exposure to cold stress increases oxygen needs)

Signs of potential complications related to abnormal breathing are shown in the Signs of Potential Complications box.

Maintenance of Body Temperature

Effective neonatal care is based on the maintenance of an optimal thermal environment. Cold stress is detrimental to the newborn. It increases the need for oxygen and can upset the acid-base balance. The infant may react by increasing his or her respiratory rate and may become cyanotic. Several ways to stabilize the newborn's body temperature are by placing the infant directly on the mother's abdomen and covering the infant with a warm blanket; drying and wrapping the newborn in warmed blankets immediately after birth, taking care to keep the head well covered while the parent is holding the newborn; and keeping the ambient temperature of the nursery at 24° C.

If the infant does not remain with the parents during the first 1 to 2 hours after birth, the thoroughly dried, unclothed infant can be placed under a radiant heat panel or warmer until the body temperature stabilizes. The infant's skin temperature is used as the point of control when using a warmer with a servocontrolled mechanism. The control panel usually is maintained between 36° and 37° C. This setting should maintain the infant's skin temperature around 36.5° C. A thermistor probe (automatic sensor) is

---

SIGNS OF POTENTIAL COMPLICATIONS

Abnormal Newborn Breathing
- Bradypnea: respirations (≤25/min)
- Tachypnea: respirations (≥60/min)
- Abnormal breath sounds: crackles, rhonchi, wheezes, expiratory grunt
- Respiratory distress: nasal flaring, retractions, chin tug, labored breathing

---

taped to the right upper quadrant of the abdomen immediately below the right intercostal margin, never over a bone. This will ensure detection of minor changes resulting from peripheral vasoconstriction, vasodilation, or increased metabolism long before a change in deep (core) body temperature develops. The other end of the probe cord is attached to the control panel. The sensor needs to be checked periodically to make sure it is securely attached to the infant's skin. An axillary temperature should be taken every hour until the newborn's temperature stabilizes. Initial temperatures as low as 36° C are not uncommon. By the twelfth hour, the newborn's temperature should stabilize within the normal range.

During all procedures, heat loss must be avoided or minimized for the newborn; therefore examinations and activities are performed with the newborn under a heat panel. The initial bath is postponed until the newborn's skin temperature reaches 36.5° C (Penny-MacGillavary, 1996).

Even a normal term infant in good health can become hypothermic. Birth in a car on the way to the hospital, a cold birthing room, or inadequate drying and wrapping immediately after birth may cause the infant's temperature to fall below the normal range **(hypothermia).** Warming the hypothermic infant is accomplished with care. Rapid warming or cooling may cause apneic spells and acidosis in an infant. Therefore the warming process is monitored to progress slowly over a period of 2 to 4 hours.

Immediate Interventions

It is the nurse's responsibility to perform certain interventions immediately after birth to provide for the safety of the newborn.

Identification. The nurse applies matching identification bracelets to the newborn and mother immediately after birth. Information on the bracelets should include name, sex, date and time of birth, and identification number, according to hospital protocol. In some institutions the father or significant other also wears a matching identification bracelet. Infants are also foot printed using a form that includes the mother's fingerprints, name, and date and time of birth. These identification procedures must be performed before the mother and infant are separated.

Cardiopulmonary Resuscitation

Wash hands before and after touching infant and equipment. Wear gloves, if possible.

ASSESS RESPONSIVENESS

Observe color; tap or gently shake shoulders.
Yell for help; if alone, perform CPR for 1 min before calling for help again.

POSITION INFANT

Turn the infant onto back, supporting the head and neck.
Place the infant on firm, flat surface.

AIRWAY

Open the airway with the head tilt–chin lift method (Fig. 27-7).
Place one hand on the infant's forehead and tilt the head back.
Place the fingers of other hand under the bone of the lower jaw at the chin.

BREATHING

Assess for evidence of breathing:
  Observe for chest movement.
  Listen for exhaled air.
  Feel for exhaled air flow.
To breathe for infant:
  Take a breath.
  Place mouth over the infant's nose and mouth to create a seal.
NOTE: When available, a mask with a one-way valve should be used.
Give two slow breaths (1 to 1.5 sec/breath), pausing to inhale between breaths.
NOTE: Gently puff the volume of air in your cheeks into infant. Do not force air.
The infant's chest should rise slightly with each puff; keep fingers on the chest wall to sense air entry.

CIRCULATION

Assess circulation:
Check pulse of the brachial artery (Fig. 27-8) while maintaining the head tilt.
If the pulse is present, initiate rescue breathing. Continue doing once every 3 sec or 20 times/min until spontaneous breathing resumes.
If the pulse is absent, initiate chest compressions and coordinate them with breathing.
Chest compression. There are two systems of chest compression. Nurses should know both methods.
Maintain the head tilt and:
  1. Place thumbs side-by-side in the middle third of the sternum with fingers around the chest and supporting the back (Fig. 27-9).
     – Compress the sternum 1.25 to 2 cm.
  2. Place index finger of hand just under an imaginary line drawn between the nipples. Place the middle and ring fingers on the sternum adjacent to the index finger.
     – Using the middle and ring fingers, compress the sternum approximately 1.25 to 2.5 cm.
Avoid compressing the xiphoid process.
Release the pressure without moving the thumbs/fingers from the chest.
Repeat at least 100 times/min, doing five compressions in 3 sec or less.
Perform 10 cycles of five compressions and one ventilation.
After the cycles, check the brachial artery to determine whether there is a pulse.
Discontinue compressions when the infant's spontaneous heart rate reaches or exceeds 80 beats/min.
Record the time and duration of the procedure and the effects of intervention.

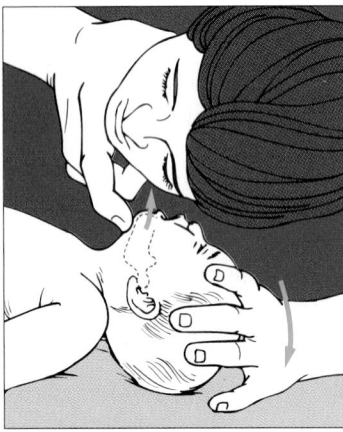

Fig. 27-7 Opening airway with head tilt-chin lift method.

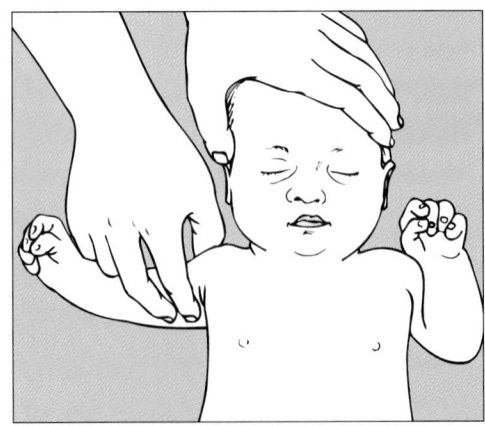

Fig. 27-8 Checking pulse of brachial artery.

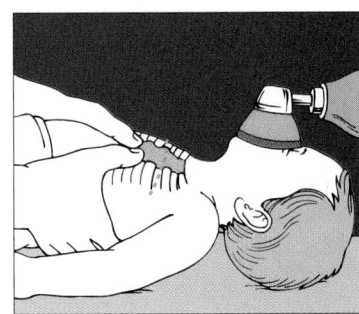

Fig. 27-9 Side-by-side thumb placement for chest compressions in newborn.

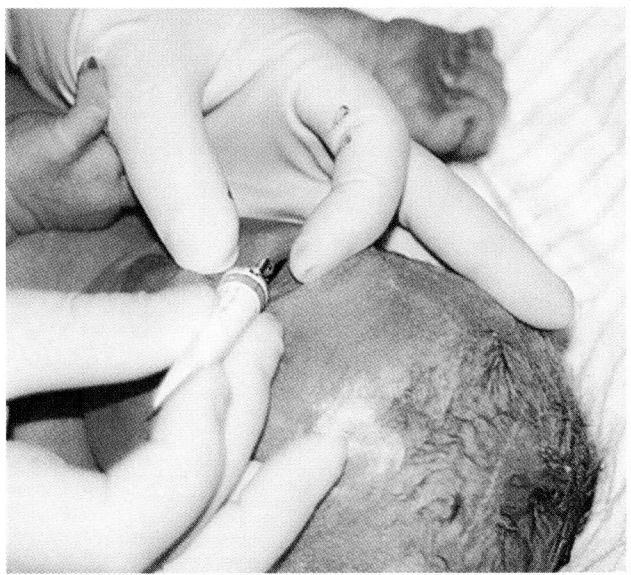

Fig. 27-10 Instillation of medication into eye of newborn. Thumb and forefinger are used to open the eye; medication is placed in the lower conjunctiva from the inner to the outer canthus. *(Courtesy Marjorie Pyle, RNC, Lifecircle, Costa Mesa, CA.)*

Therapeutic Interventions

Eye prophylaxis. The instillation of a prophylactic agent in the eyes of all neonates is mandatory in the United States as a precaution against **ophthalmia neonatorum** (Fig. 27-10). This is an inflammation of the eyes resulting from gonorrheal or chlamydial infection contracted as the newborn passes through the mother's infected birth canal. In some Canadian institutions the parents may sign a form refusing such eye prophylaxis. In the United States, if the family objects to this treatment, the primary care provider asks the parents to sign an informed consent form, and their refusal is noted in the neonate's record. The agent used for prophylaxis varies according to hospital protocols, but the usual agents are forms of erythromycin and tetracycline. Canadian hospitals have not recommended the use of silver nitrate since 1986. Its use in the United States is minimal because silver nitrate does not protect against chlamydial infection and can cause chemical conjunctivitis. In some institutions, eye prophylaxis is delayed until an hour or so after birth so that eye contact and parent-infant attachment and bonding are facilitated. The Centers for Disease Control and Prevention specify that a delay of up to 2 hours is safe (see Medication Guide box).

Vitamin K administration. Administering vitamin K intramuscularly is routine in the newborn period. A single parenteral dose of 0.5 to 1 mg of vitamin K is given soon after birth to prevent hemorrhagic disorders (Snapp, 1996). Vitamin K is produced in the gastrointestinal (GI) tract starting soon after microorganisms are introduced. By day 8, normal newborns are able to produce their own vitamin K (see Medication Guide box).

MEDICATION GUIDE

Eye Prophylaxis: Erythromycin Ophthalmic Ointment 0.5% and Tetracycline Ophthalmic Ointment 1%

ACTION
These antibiotic ointments are both bacteriostatic and bactericidal. They provide prophylaxis against *Neisseria gonorrhoeae* and *Chlamydia trachomatis*.

INDICATION
These medications are for the prevention of ophthalmia neonatorum in newborns of mothers who are infected with gonorrhea and conjunctivitis in newborns of mothers infected with chlamydia.

NEONATAL DOSAGE
Apply a 1- to 2-cm ribbon of ointment to the lower conjunctival sac of each eye; may also be used in drop form.

ADVERSE REACTIONS
May cause chemical conjunctivitis that lasts 24 to 48 hours; vision may be blurred temporarily.

NURSING CONSIDERATIONS
Administer within 1 to 2 hours of birth. Wear gloves. Cleanse eyes if necessary before administration. Open eyes by putting a thumb and finger at the corner of each lid and gently pressing on the periorbital ridges. Squeeze the tube and spread the ointment from the inner canthus of the eye to the outer canthus. Do not touch the tube to the eye. After 1 minute, excess ointment may be wiped off. Observe eyes for irritation. Explain treatment to parents.

Eye prophylaxis for ophthalmia neonatorum is required by law in all states of the United States.

Umbilical cord care. The care of the umbilical cord is the same as that for any surgical wound (Krebs, 1998). The goal of care is prevention and early identification of hemorrhage or infection. The umbilical cord stump is an excellent medium for bacterial growth and can easily become infected.

NURSE ALERT *If bleeding from the blood vessels of the cord is noted, the nurse checks the clamp (or tie) and applies a second clamp next to the first one. If bleeding is not stopped immediately, the nurse calls for assistance.*

Hospital protocol directs the time and technique for routine cord care. The stump and base of the cord should be assessed for edema, redness, and purulent drainage with each diaper change. The nurse cleanses the cord and skin

MEDICATION GUIDE

Vitamin K: Phytonadione (AquaMEPHYTON, Konakion)

ACTION

This intervention provides vitamin K because the newborn does not have the intestinal flora to produce this vitamin in the first week after birth. It also promotes formation of clotting factors (II, VII, IX, X) in the liver.

INDICATION

Vitamin K is used for prevention and treatment of hemorrhagic disease in the newborn.

NEONATAL DOSAGE

Administer a 0.5- to 1-mg (0.25- to 0.5-ml) dose intramuscularly within 2 hours of birth; may be repeated if newborn shows bleeding tendencies.

ADVERSE REACTIONS

Edema, erythema, and pain at injection site may occur rarely; hemolysis, jaundice, and hyperbilirubinemia have been reported, particularly in preterm infants.

NURSING CONSIDERATIONS

Wear gloves. Administer in the middle third of the vastus lateralis muscle using a 25-gauge, ⅝-inch needle. Inject into skin that has been cleaned, or allow alcohol to dry on puncture site for 1 minute to remove organisms and prevent infection. Stabilize leg firmly and grasp muscle between the thumb and fingers. Insert the needle at a 90-degree angle; aspirate and inject medication slowly if there is no blood return. Massage the site with a dry gauze square after removing needle to increase absorption. Observe for signs of bleeding from the site.

area around the cord with the prescribed preparation (e.g., erythromycin solution, triple blue dye, or alcohol). Dore and co-workers (1998) found that the cord separated earlier with natural drying when compared to cleansing with 70% isopropyl alcohol and that no infants in either group developed cord infections. The cord clamp is removed after 24 hours when the cord is dry.

Promote Parent-Infant Bonding

Today's childbirth practices strive to promote the family as the focus of care. Parents generally desire to share in the birth process and have early contact with their infants. Early contact between mother and newborn can be important in developing future relationships. It also has a positive effect on the duration of breastfeeding. There are physiologic benefits of early mother-infant contact. Oxy-

tocin and prolactin levels rise in the mother while sucking reflexes are activated early in the infant. The process of developing active immunity begins as the infant ingests flora from the mother's skin. The nurse should encourage early contact between the newborn and the parents if the condition of both mother and infant allow it. The infant is often placed on the mother's abdomen or at breast. During the first 30 to 60 minutes after birth, when the newborn is in the first period of reactivity, the family unit should be provided privacy to allow for development of the parent-infant relationship.

Evaluation

Evaluation of the effectiveness of care of the newborn is based on the previously stated outcomes.

CARE MANAGEMENT: FROM 2 HOURS AFTER BIRTH UNTIL DISCHARGE

The infant's admission to the nursery may be delayed, or it may never actually occur. Depending on the routine of the hospital, the infant frequently remains in the labor area and is then transferred to either the nursery or the postpartum unit with the mother. Many hospitals have adopted variations of single-room maternity care (SRMC) in which one nurse provides care for the mother and newborn. SRMC allows the infant to remain with the parents after the birth. Many of the procedures, such as weighing and measuring the infant, instilling eye medications, administering the intramuscular (IM) injection of vitamin K, and physically assessing the infant, may be carried out in the labor and birth unit. Nurses who work in an SRMC unit; labor, delivery, and recovery (LDR) room; or labor, delivery, recovery, and postpartum (LDRP) room need to be educated in obstetric, neonatal, and postpartum nursing care and competent in providing it. If an infant is transferred to the nursery, the infant's identification is verified by the nurse receiving the infant, who places the baby in a warm environment and begins the admission process.

Regardless of the way in which care is physically organized, many hospitals have a small holding nursery, which is available for the performance of procedures or on the request of the mother who wishes her infant to be placed there. This setup promotes parent-infant bonding while still allowing the new parents some time to be alone.

Assessment and Nursing Diagnoses
Assessment of Gestational Age

The assessment of physical and neurologic findings to determine gestational age is based on the method devised by Dubowitz, Dubowitz and Goldberg (1970). Ideally the tests are performed when the infant is between 2 and 8 hours of age. If the tests are done earlier while the infant is recovering from the stress of birth, muscle movements may reflect fatigue; for example, the arm recoil is slower. After 48 hours, there are some significant changes. For instance, the plantar creases on the soles of the feet appear to become more numerous and visible as the skin loses fluid and dries.

Assessment of gestational age is important because perinatal morbidity and mortality are related to gestational age and birth weight. A commonly used method of determining gestational age is the simplified *Assessment of Gestational Age* by Ballard, Novak, and Driver (1979). The Ballard scale can be used to measure gestational ages of infants between 35 and 42 weeks. It assesses six external physical and six neuromuscular signs. Each sign has a number score, and the cumulative score correlates with a maturity rating of 26 to 44 weeks of gestation. The score is accurate to plus or minus 2 weeks and is accurate for infants of all races (Stevens-Simon et al., 1989).

The *New Ballard Scale,* a revision of the original scale, can be used with newborns as young as 20 weeks of gestation. The tool has the same physical and neuromuscular sections but includes −1 to −2 scores that reflect signs of extremely premature infants, such as fused eyelids; imperceptible breast tissue; sticky, friable, transparent skin; no lanugo; and square-window (flexion of wrist) angle greater than 90 degrees (see Fig. 27-1, *A*). The examination of infants with a gestational age of 20 weeks or less should be performed at a postnatal age of less than 12 hours. For infants with a gestational age of at least 26 weeks, the examination can be performed up to 96 hours after birth. The scale overestimates gestational age by 2 to 4 days in infants younger than 37 weeks of gestation, especially at gestational ages of 32 to 37 weeks (Ballard et al., 1991).

Classification of Newborns by Gestational Age and Birth Weight

There is a normal range of birth weights for each gestational week (see Fig. 27-1, *B*), but the birth weights of preterm, term, postdate, or postmature newborns may also be outside these normal ranges. Birth weights are classified in the following ways:

- **Large for gestational age (LGA).** Weight is above the 90th percentile (or two or more standard deviations above the norm) at any week.
- **Appropriate for gestational age (AGA).** Weight falls between the 10th and 90th percentile for infant's age.
- **Small for gestational age (SGA).** Weight is below the 10th percentile (or two or more standard deviations below the norm).
- **Low birth weight (LBW).** Weight of 2500 g or less at birth. These newborns have had either less than the expected rate of intrauterine growth or a shortened gestation period. Preterm birth and LBW commonly occur together (e.g., less than 32 weeks of gestation and birth weight less than 1200 g).
- **Very low birth weight (VLBW).** Weight of 1500 g or less at birth.

- **Intrauterine growth restriction (IUGR)** is the term applied to the fetus whose rate of growth does not meet expected norms.

Newborns are classified according to their gestational age in the following ways:
- **Preterm or premature.** Born before completion of 37 weeks of gestation, regardless of birth weight.
- **Term.** Born between the beginning of week 38 and the end of week 42 of gestation.
- **Postterm (postdate).** Born after completion of week 42 of gestation.
- **Postmature.** Born after completion of week 42 of gestation and showing the effects of progressive placental insufficiency.

Maternal Effects on Gestational Age Assessment and Birth Weight

Some maternal conditions can affect the results of the gestational assessment. For instance, any infant who has experienced oxygen deprivation during labor will show poor muscle tone. Infants in respiratory distress tend to be flaccid and assume a "frog-leg" posture. Even though an infant may look large, such as the infant of a diabetic mother, it may respond more like a premature infant. The infant of a mother who has been on magnesium sulfate will tend to be somewhat lethargic.

The causes of preterm and postdate birth are largely unknown. It is known, however, that the incidence of preterm birth is highest among women from low socioeconomic groups. The lack of comprehensive prenatal health care in such women is a likely contributing factor. Other social factors associated with preterm birth include African-American race, single marriage status, low maternal age, low prepregnancy weight, stress, standing for long periods, short stature, and less than 12 years of education. Obstetric events associated with preterm birth include previous fetal or neonatal death, previous preterm birth or miscarriage, incompetent cervix, maternal genital abnormality, maternal in utero exposure to diethylstilbestrol, short interpregnancy interval, premature rupture of membranes, late or no prenatal care, preeclampsia or eclampsia, hyperemesis, placental accidents, multifetal pregnancy, and fetal congenital anomalies (Cloherty & Stark, 1997; Witter & Keith, 1993).

Common causes of LGA newborns include glucose intolerance of pregnancy, true maternal diabetes mellitus, maternal overnutrition, parity, heredity, and certain congenital anomalies. Causes of SGA newborns may be maternal smoking, hypertensive states, undernutrition, anemia, or nephritis. In addition, the birth of an SGA newborn may be associated with multifetal gestation, a discordant twin pregnancy, or congenital anomalies. Living at a high altitude, infection with the rubella virus, or intrauterine infection may also predispose a woman to giving birth to an SGA newborn. Fetal malnutrition, IUGR, and chronic fetal stress are other conditions associated with the birth of SGA infants.

INFANT MORTALITY AND MORBIDITY

Preterm birth is responsible for causing almost two thirds of infant deaths. The reason for infants born before term being at greater risk for dying is that they have not grown and developed enough to be able to make an uncomplicated adjustment to extrauterine life. As a result, the prospects for survival or good health in these infants may be severely diminished. Infants weighing more than 2500 g and born after 37 weeks of gestation have the best prospects of survival. There is a dramatic reduction in the mortality rate of infants, regardless of weight, born after week 36 of gestation. The mortality rate is less than 5% if the pregnancy has progressed to 35 weeks and the fetus weighs more than 2000 g.

Children and adults who were LBW infants are also more likely to have major problems such as cerebral palsy, mental retardation, and sensory and cognitive disabilities and are also more likely to have difficulty successfully adapting socially, psychologically, and physically to an increasingly complex environment (Fanaroff & Martin, 1997). In addition to the potential alterations in the lifestyles of such people and their families, the cost of the care required by LBW infants is estimated to be in the billions of dollars each year.

High Risk Infants Based on Gestational Age and Birth Weight

Preterm Infants

Preterm infants are at a distinct disadvantage when trying to make the transition from intrauterine to extrauterine life. They are at risk because their organ systems are immature and they lack adequate reserves of body nutrients. The degree of this disadvantage depends primarily on their level of maturity. If these infants have physiologic disorders and anomalies as well, these also affect the infant's response to treatment. In general, the closer infants are to term from the standpoint of both gestational age and birth weight, the easier their adjustment to the external environment.

Postmature or Postterm Infants

A pregnancy that is prolonged beyond 42 weeks is a postterm pregnancy, and the infant who is born is called postmature. Postmaturity can be associated with placental insufficiency, resulting in a fetus who has a wasted appearance (dysmaturity) at birth due to loss of subcutaneous fat and muscle mass. However, not all postmature infants show signs of dysmaturity; some continue to grow in utero and are large at birth.

The perinatal mortality rate is significantly higher in the postmature fetus and neonate. One reason for this is that during labor and birth the increased oxygen demands of the postmature fetus may not be met. Insufficient gas exchange in the postmature placenta also increases the likelihood of intrauterine hypoxia, which may result in the passage of meconium in utero, thereby increasing the risk for meconium aspiration syndrome. Of all the deaths that occur in postmature newborns, one half occur during labor and birth, about one third occur before the onset of labor, and one sixth occur during the postpartum period.

Large-for-Gestational-Age Infants

The LGA, or oversized, infant traditionally has been regarded as one weighing 4000 g or more at birth. An infant is considered LGA despite gestation when the weight falls above the 90th percentile on growth charts or two standard deviations above the mean weight for gestational age. About 10% of newborns weigh this much and about 0.4% to 0.9% weigh 4500 g or more (Korones, 1995). Most of these newborns also have other proportionately larger measurements. Many are born well after the estimated date of birth.

Maternal pelvic diameters have not kept pace with better maternal health and nutrition resulting in larger babies. As a result, fetopelvic disproportion often occurs with LGA babies, particularly in obese women, women who gain 16 kg or more during gestation, and women with undiagnosed or uncontrolled diabetes, who are prone to having large babies. Birth trauma, especially in infants presenting in a breech or shoulder presentation, is a serious hazard for the oversized neonate. Asphyxia or central nervous system (CNS) injury, or both, may occur.

Small for Gestational Age and Intrauterine Growth Restriction

Infants whose birth weight falls below the 10th percentile expected at term or who fall two standard deviations below the mean for gestational age, for reasons other than heredity, are considered at high risk, with the perinatal mortality rate four to eight times greater than that for the normal term infant.

Various conditions can affect and impede growth in the developing fetus. The cause, severity, and gestational age at which the insult occurs determine the way in which fetal growth is affected and what problems affect the newborn. Conditions occurring in the first trimester that affect all aspects of fetal growth (infections, teratogens, and chromosomal abnormalities) or extrinsic conditions occurring early in pregnancy result in a symmetric IUGR (head circumference, length, and weight all fall below the 10th percentile). Conditions causing symmetric IUGR result in a short SGA infant, usually with a smaller head circumference and reduced brain capacity.

There is an array of maternal, fetal, and placental prenatal factors associated with IUGR. The maternal factors include socioeconomic factors, preeclampsia, advanced diabetes, malnutrition, cigarette smoking, alcohol consumption, narcotic addiction, and living at a high altitude. Fetal factors include multifetal pregnancy, chromosomal and nonchromosomal congenital anomalies, and chronic infection (rubella and cytomegalovirus). Placental factors consist of placental insufficiency and arteriovenous anastomosis (Korones, 1995).

Growth restriction in the later stages of pregnancy results in asymmetric IUGR (with respect to gestational age, weight falls below the 10th percentile, whereas length and head circumference fall above the 10th percentile). Asymmetric IUGR occurs as a result of maternal, fetal, and placental conditions (Korones, 1995). Such infants can grow and develop normally. Abnormal fetal size may also indicate an adaptive response with diminished fetal weight–sparing brain growth (Fanaroff & Martin, 1997).

Common problems that affect SGA, IUGR, and dysmature infants are perinatal asphyxia, meconium aspiration, hypoglycemia, and heat loss. Care of infants with specific problems related to gestational age and birth weight are discussed in Chapter 41.

ASSESSMENT OF COMMON PROBLEMS IN THE NEWBORN

Physical Examination

A complete physical examination is done within 24 hours, after the infant's temperature has stabilized. See Chapter 26 for a detailed description of this examination.

Physical Injuries

Birth trauma constitutes any physical injury sustained by a newborn during labor and birth. Many injuries are minor and readily resolve in the neonatal period without treatment. Other types of trauma require some form of intervention. A few are serious enough to be fatal. Several factors predispose an infant to birth trauma (Fanaroff & Martin, 1997). *Maternal factors* include uterine dysfunction that leads to prolonged or precipitous labor, preterm or postterm labor, and cephalopelvic disproportion. Injury may result from dystocia caused by fetal macrosomia, multifetal gestation, abnormal or difficult presentation, and congenital anomalies. *Intrapartum events* that can result in scalp injury include the use of intrapartum monitoring of the fetal heart rate (FHR) and fetal scalp sampling. *Obstetric birth techniques* can also cause injury. These include forceps-assisted birth, vacuum extraction, version and extraction, and cesarean birth.

Soft-Tissue Injuries

Caput succedaneum and *cephalhematoma* are described in Chapter 26 (see Fig. 26-6).

Subconjunctival and *retinal hemorrhages* occur when capillaries rupture because of the increased intracranial pressure during birth. These hemorrhages clear within 5 days after birth and usually present no further problems. However, parents need to have these injuries explained and be reassured that they are harmless.

There may be *erythema, ecchymoses, petechiae, abrasions, lacerations,* or *edema* involving the buttocks and extremities. A localized discoloration may appear over presenting or dependent parts; it is caused by the application of forceps or the vacuum extractor. Ecchymoses and edema may appear anywhere on the body. Petechiae, or pinpoint hemorrhagic areas, acquired during birth may extend over the upper trunk and face. These lesions are benign if they disappear within 2 days of birth and no new lesions appear. Ecchymoses and petechiae may be signs of a more serious disorder, such as *thrombocytopenic purpura*. To differentiate hemorrhagic areas from skin rashes and discolorations, try to blanch the skin with two fingers. Petechiae and ecchymoses do not blanch because extravasated blood remains within the tissues, whereas skin rashes and discolorations do.

Trauma secondary to dystocia occurs to the presenting part. Forceps injury and bruising from the vacuum cup occur at the site where the instruments were applied. In a forceps injury there is commonly a linear mark across both sides of the face that is in the shape of the forceps blades. The affected areas are kept clean to minimize the risk of infection. With the increased use of the vacuum extractor and the use of padded forceps blades, the incidence of these lesions may be significantly reduced (Fanaroff & Martin, 1997).

Accidental lacerations may be inflicted with a scalpel during a cesarean birth. These cuts may occur on any part of the body but are most often found on the scalp, buttocks, and thighs. Usually they are superficial and only need to be kept clean. Butterfly adhesive strips can hold together the edges of more serious lacerations. Rarely are sutures needed.

Skeletal Injuries

The clavicle is the bone most often fractured during birth, and usually the break occurs in the middle third of the bone (Fig. 27-11). Dystocia, particularly shoulder dystocia, may be the predisposing problem. Limitation of

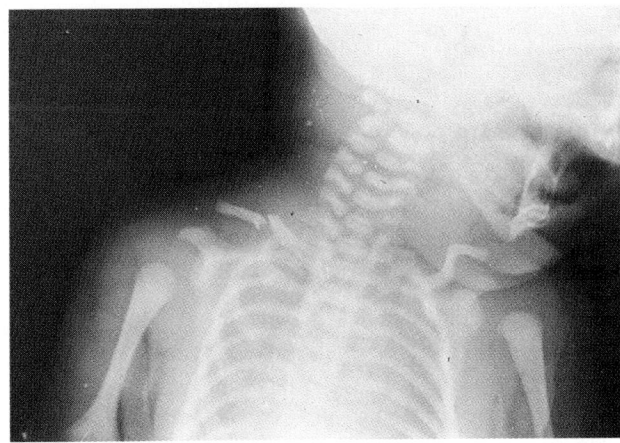

Fig. 27-11 Fractured clavicle after shoulder dystocia. *(From O'Doherty, N. [1986]. Neonatology: Micro atlas of the newborn. Nutley, NJ: Hoffmann-La Roche.)*

motion of the arm, crepitus of the bone, and an absent Moro's reflex on the affected side are diagnostic findings. Except for the use of gentle rather than rigorous handling of the infant, there is no accepted treatment for a fractured clavicle. The infant may be positioned in bed with the fractured side up. The figure-of-eight bandage, which is appropriate for the older child with a fractured clavicle, should not be used for the newborn. The prognosis is good.

The *humerus* and *femur* are other bones that may be fractured during a difficult birth, but such fractures in newborns generally heal rapidly. Immobilization is accomplished with slings, splints, swaddling, and other devices.

The infant's immature, flexible skull can withstand a great deal of molding before fracture results. The location of a skull fracture determines whether it is insignificant or fatal. Unless a blood vessel is involved, linear fractures heal without special treatment. These fractures account for 70% of all fractures in this age group. Depressed skull fractures may occur without laceration of either the skin or the dural membrane (Fig. 27-12). These fractures may occur during difficult births and result from the head pressing on the bony pelvis or from the injudicious application of forceps. Spontaneous or nonsurgical elevation of the indentation using a hand breast pump or vacuum extractor has been reported (Fanaroff & Martin, 1997).

Congenital dislocation of the hip, or *congenital hip dysplasia*, is often a hereditary disorder and occurs more commonly in girls because of the structure of the female pelvis. In this condition, the acetabulum is abnormally shallow and this allows the head of the femur to become dislocated upward and backward so that it lies on the dorsal aspect of the ilium. The pressure of the displaced femoral head may then form a false acetabulum on the ilium. A stretched joint capsule results, and ossification of the femoral head is delayed.

Reduced movement, splinting of the affected hip, limited abduction, and asymmetry of the hip may be noted before dislocation occurs. After dislocation, all of these signs are present, together with external rotation and shortening of the leg. A clicking sound may be heard on gentle forced abduction of the leg (Ortolani's sign; see Fig. 26-13 on p. 687), and a bulge of the femoral head is felt or seen. Congenital dysplasia of the hip can be seen on x-ray examination.

Treatment involves pressing the femoral head into the acetabulum to form an adequate socket before ossification is complete. Thick diapers may be applied to abduct and externally rotate the leg and flex the hip; the anterior flaps of the diapers are pinned under the posterior flaps. Alternatively, a Frejka pillow may be applied over a diaper and plastic pants. A Pavlik harness is also used frequently in the treatment of congenital hip dislocation (see Fig. 40-12). Later a spica cast may be applied to maintain abduction, plus extension and internal rotation, usually with the infant in a "frog-leg" position.

Parents need emotional support when it comes to handling a newborn with skeletal injuries because they are often fearful of hurting it. Parents are encouraged to practice handling, changing, and feeding the injured newborn under the guidance of the nursing staff. This increases the parents' knowledge and confidence, in addition to facilitating attachment. A plan for follow-up therapy is developed with the parents so that the times and arrangements for therapy are convenient for them.

Physiologic Problems

Physiologic Jaundice

Approximately 50% of all full-term newborns are visibly jaundiced (yellowish) during the first 3 days of life. Visible skin jaundice does not usually occur if serum bilirubin levels are less than 5 mg/dl. Physiologic jaundice is characterized by a progressive increase in the serum levels of unconjugated bilirubin from 2 mg/dl in cord blood to a mean peak of 6 mg/dl by 72 hours of age, followed by a decline to 5 mg/dl by day 5, and not exceeding 12 mg/dl. These serum values are considered to represent the normal physiologic limits for the healthy term newborn who has not been exposed to perinatal complications such as hypoxia. No bilirubin toxicity develops under these conditions. For the normal full-term newborn, a serum bilirubin level of 12 to 15 mg/dl is usually the cut-off point for the use of phototherapy and 20 mg/dl is the cut-off point for exchange transfusion.

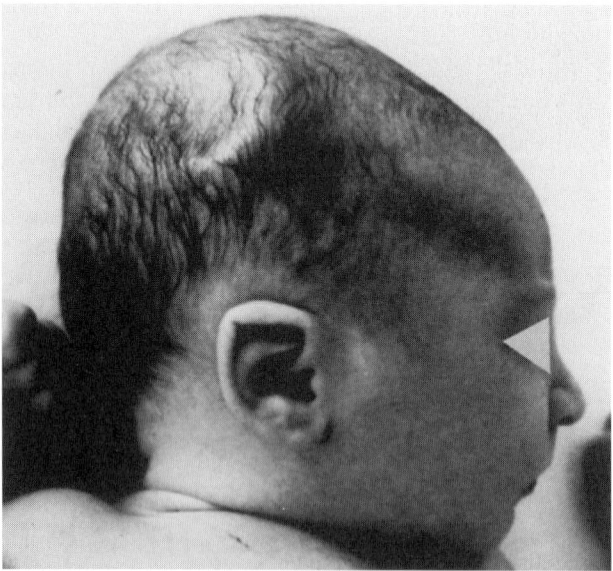

Fig. 27-12 Depressed skull fracture in a full-term male after rapid (1-hour) labor. The infant was delivered by occiput-anterior presentation after rotation from occiput-posterior position. *(From Fanaroff, A., & Martin, R. [1997]. Neonatal-perinatal medicine: Diseases of the fetus and infant. [6th ed.]. St. Louis: Mosby.)*

Every newborn is assessed for jaundice. The blanch test helps differentiate cutaneous jaundice from skin color. To do the test, apply pressure with a finger over a bony area (e.g., the nose, forehead, sternum) for several seconds to empty all the capillaries in that spot. If jaundice is present, the blanched area will look yellow before the capillaries refill. The conjunctival sacs and buccal mucosa are also assessed, especially in darker-skinned infants. It is better to assess for jaundice in daylight, because artificial lighting and reflection from nursery walls can distort the actual skin color.

Jaundice is noticeable first in the head and then progresses gradually toward the abdomen and extremities because of the newborn infant's circulatory pattern (cephalocaudal developmental progression).

Hypoglycemia

Hypoglycemia during the early newborn period of a term infant is defined as a blood glucose concentration of less than 35 mg/dl or as a plasma concentration of less than 40 mg/dl. It occurs because at birth when the cord is cut the newborn abruptly loses its glucose supply. The glucose level normally declines during the first hours after birth. Because hypoglycemia may be asymptomatic, a blood glucose test is often done soon after birth and repeated at 4 hours of age. More frequent testing is required if the newborn is in an at-risk group (i.e., LGA, SGA, or LBW) or has been exposed to stressors such as cold, perinatal asphyxia, or tocolysis to inhibit preterm labor.

Signs of hypoglycemia include jitteriness; an irregular respiratory effort; cyanosis; apnea; a weak, high-pitched cry; feeding difficulty; hunger; lethargy; twitching; eye-rolling; and seizures. The signs may be transient and recurrent.

Hypoglycemia in the low risk term infant is usually eliminated by feeding the infant. Occasionally the intravenous administration of glucose is required.

Hypocalcemia

Hypocalcemia (less than 7 mg/dl) may occur in newborns of diabetic mothers or in those who suffered perinatal asphyxia or trauma, and in LBW and preterm infants. Early-onset hypocalcemia occurs within the first 72 hours after birth. Signs of hypocalcemia include jitteriness, edema, apnea, intermittent cyanosis, and abdominal distention.

In most instances, early-onset hypocalcemia is self-limiting and resolves within 1 to 3 days. Treatment includes early feeding and, occasionally, the administration of calcium supplements.

Jitteriness is a symptom of both hypoglycemia and hypocalcemia. Therefore hypocalcemia must be considered if the therapy for hypoglycemia proves ineffective. In many newborns, jitteriness remains despite therapy and cannot be explained by hypoglycemia or hypocalcemia (Fanaroff & Martin, 1997).

BOX 27-3	Standard Laboratory Values in a Term Newborn
Hemoglobin	14-24 g/dl
Hematocrit	44%-64%
Glucose	40-60 mg/dl
Bilirubin, direct	0-1 mg/dl
Blood gases	
Arterial	pH 7.32-7.49
	PCO_2 26-41 mm Hg
	PO_2 60-70 mm Hg
Venous	pH 7.31-7.41
	PCO_2 40-50 mm Hg
	PO_2 40-50 mm Hg

LABORATORY AND DIAGNOSTIC TESTS

The measurement of blood glucose levels and urinalysis are commonly performed in newborns. Other tests may be performed as needed, including the measurement of bilirubin levels, newborn screening tests (e.g., phenylketonuria [PKU]), hematocrits, and drug tests. Standard laboratory values for a term newborn are given in Box 27-3.

Some states require that newborns be tested for up to nine disorders. Information about the tests required in a particular state can be obtained from state health departments. About 30 states require testing for sickle cell anemia, and some locations now require testing for cystic fibrosis (March of Dimes, 1994) and HIV (Frank, Esch, & Margeson, 1998). Some of the major disorders for which infants are screened are described in Table 27-2.

Collection of Specimens

The ongoing evaluation of a newborn often requires the acquisition of blood by the heel stick or venipuncture method or the collection of a urine specimen.

Heel Stick

Most blood specimens are drawn by laboratory technicians. Nurses, however, may be required to perform heel sticks to obtain blood for glucose monitoring and to measure hematocrit levels. The same technique is needed to complete the PKU form or to test for galactosemia and hypothyroidism or other inborn errors of metabolism (see Table 27-2).

It may be helpful to warm the heel before the sample is taken, because the application of heat for 5 to 10 minutes helps dilate the vessels in the area.

A cloth soaked with warm water and wrapped loosely around the foot can effectively warm the foot (Fig. 27-13, A). Disposable heel warmers are also available from a variety of companies but should be used with care to prevent burns. Nurses should wear gloves when collecting any

TABLE 27-2 Newborn Screening Summary

DISORDER/EVIDENCE	SYMPTOMS	SCREENING INCIDENCE	TREATMENT
PKU (classic) Elevated phenylalanine	Severe mental retardation, eczema, seizures, behavior disorders, decreased pigmentation, distinctive "mousey" odor	1:10,000 to 1:15,000 More common in Caucasians	Lifelong dietary management with low-phenylalanine diet; possible tyrosine supplementation
Congenital hypothyroidism (primary) Low T_4, elevated TSH	Mental and motor retardation, short stature, coarse, dry skin and hair, hoarse cry, constipation	Overall 1:4,000 with ethnic variation 1:12,000 African-American 1:1,000 Native American	Maintain l-thyroxine levels in upper half of normal range; periodic bone age to monitor growth
Galactosemia (transferase deficiency) Elevated galactose; low or absent fluorescence	Neonatal death from severe dehydration, sepsis, or liver pathology; mental retardation, jaundice, blindness, cataracts	1:10,000 to 1:90,000	Eliminate galactose and lactose from the diet; soy formulas in infancy; lactose-free solid foods
Maple syrup urine disease (MSUD) Elevated leucine	Acidosis; hypertonicity and seizures, vomiting, drowsiness, apnea, coma; infant death or severe mental retardation and neurologic impairment; behavioral disorders	1:90,000 to 1:200,000	Diet low in leucine, isoleucine, and valine; thiamine supplement if responsive
Homocystinuria Elevated methionine	Mental retardation, seizures, behavioral disorders, early-onset thromboses, dislocated lenses, tall lanky body habitus	1:200,000	Methionine-restricted diet; cystine supplement; vitamin B_6 supplement if responsive
Congenital adrenal hyperplasia (CAH) Elevated 17-hydroxyprogesterone; abnormal electrolytes	Hyponatremia, hypokalemia, hypoglycemia, dehydration, and early death; ambiguous genitalia in females; progressive virilization in both sexes	1:15,000 to 1:3,000 native Eskimos	Replace corticosteroids; plastic surgery to correct ambiguous genitalia
Biotinidase deficiency Deficient or absent activity of biotinidase on colorimetric assay	Mental retardation, seizures, ataxia, skin rash, hearing loss, alopecia, optic nerve atrophy, coma, and death	1:60,000 to 1:100,000	10 mg biotin daily

Data from Wright, L., Brown, A., & Davidson-Mundt, A. (1992). Newborn screening: The miracle and the challenge. *J Pediatr Nurs* 7(1), 26-42.

specimen. The nurse first cleanses the area with alcohol, restrains the infant's foot with her free hand, and then punctures the site. A spring-loaded automatic puncture device causes less pain and requires fewer punctures than a manual lance blade (Paes et al., 1993).

The most serious complication of an infant heel stick is necrotizing osteochondritis resulting from lancet penetration of the bone (Meehan, 1998). To prevent this, the stick should be made at the outer aspect of the heel and should penetrate no deeper than 2.4 mm (Wong, 1999). To identify the appro-priate puncture site, the nurse should draw an imaginary line from between the fourth and fifth toes that runs parallel to the lateral aspect of the heel, where the stick should be made; a line can also be drawn running from the great toe that runs parallel to the medial aspect of the heel, another site for a stick (Fig. 27-13, *B*). Repeated trauma to the walking surface of the heel can cause fibrosis and scarring that may lead to problems with walking later in life.

After the specimen has been collected, pressure should be applied with a dry gauze square, but no further alcohol

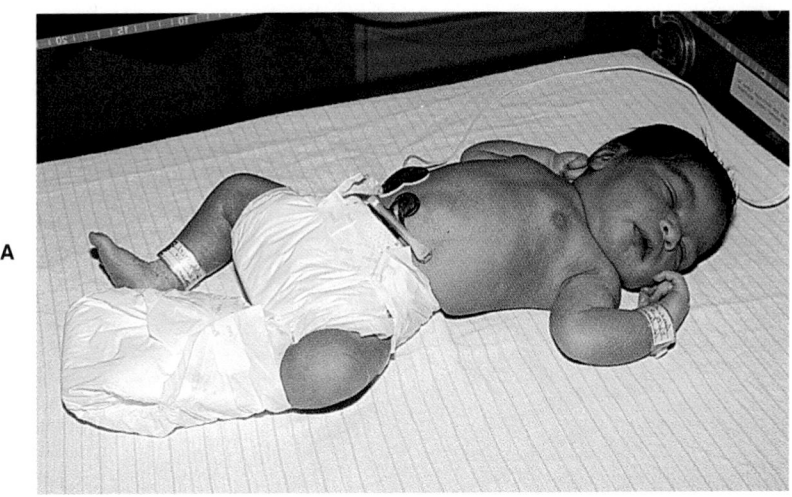

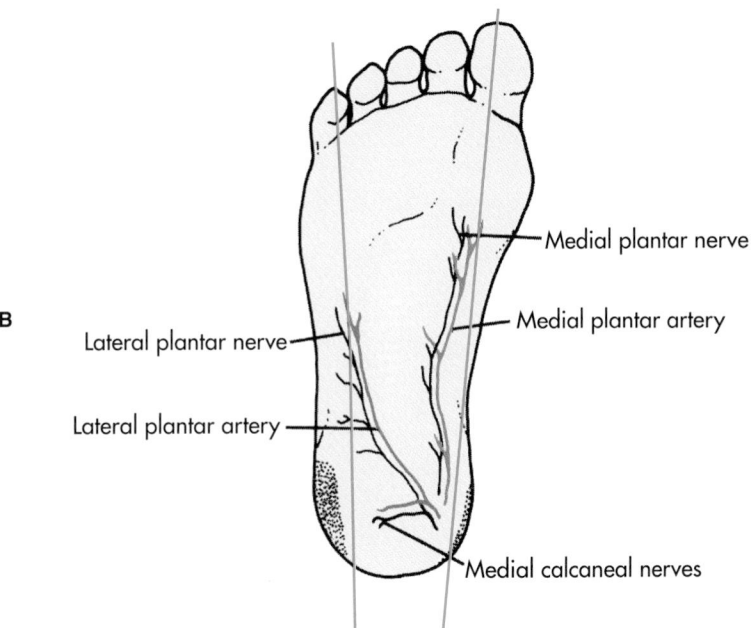

Medial plantar nerve

Medial plantar artery

Lateral plantar nerve

Lateral plantar artery

Medial calcaneal nerves

Fig. 27-13 Heel stick. **A,** Newborn with foot wrapped for warmth to increase blood flow to extremity before heel stick. **B,** Heel stick sites (shaded areas) on infant's foot for obtaining samples of capillary blood. (**A** *courtesy Marjorie Pyle, RNC, Lifecircle, Costa Mesa, CA.*)

should be applied because this will cause the site to continue to bleed. The site is then covered with an adhesive bandage. The nurse makes sure the equipment used is properly disposed of, reviews the laboratory slip for correct identification, and checks the specimen to make sure the labeling and routing information is adequate.

A heel stick can be traumatic for the infant and, because pain pathways are present and functional in the infant, can cause pain. After several heel sticks, infants have been observed to withdraw their feet when they are touched. Therefore, to reassure the infant and promote feelings of safety, the neonate should be cuddled and comforted when the procedure is complete.

Obtaining Urine Specimen

Examination of urine is a valuable laboratory tool for infant assessment, but the way in which the urine specimen is collected may influence the results. In addition, the urine sample should be fresh and examined within 1 hour of collection.

A variety of urine collection bags are available, including the Hollister U-Bag (Fig. 27-14). These are clear plastic, single-use bags with an adhesive material around the opening at the point of attachment.

To prepare the infant, the nurse removes the diaper and places the infant supine. The genitalia, perineum, and surrounding skin are washed and thoroughly dried because

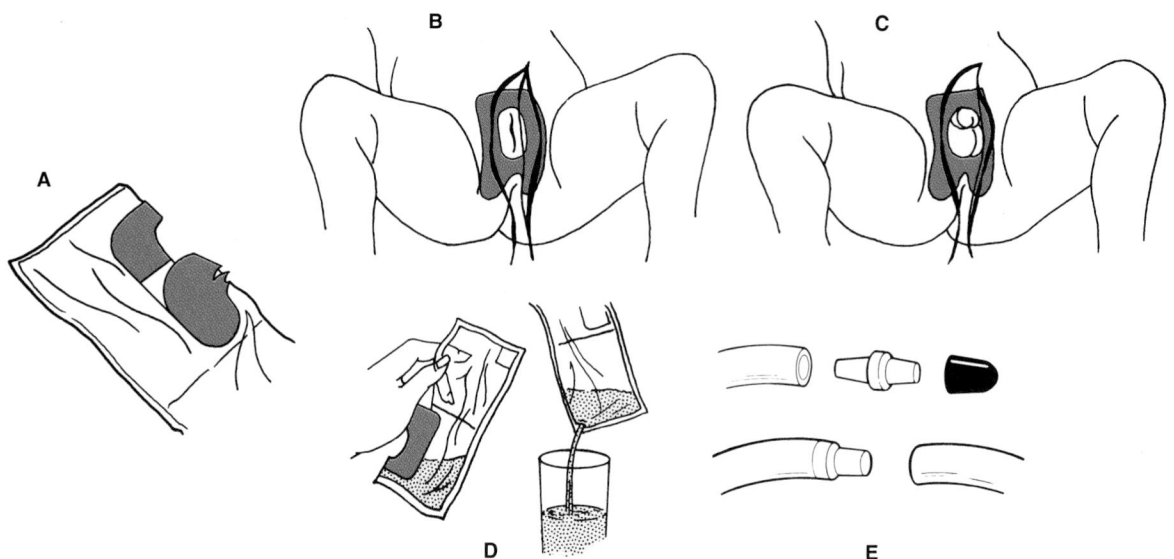

Fig. 27-14 Collection of urine specimen. **A,** Protective paper is removed from the adhesive surface. **B,** Applied to females. **C,** Applied to males. **D,** Cut to drain urine. **E,** Collection tube. *(Permission to use and/or reproduce this copyrighted material has been granted by the owner, Hollister, Inc., Libertyville, IL.)*

the adhesive on the bag will not stick to moist, powdered, or oily skin surfaces. The protective paper is removed to expose the adhesive (Fig. 27-14, *A*). In female infants the perineum is first stretched to flatten skin folds, and then the adhesive area on the bag is pressed firmly onto the skin all around the urinary meatus and vagina. (NOTE: Start with the narrow portion of the butterfly-shaped adhesive patch.) The nurse must be sure to start at the bridge of skin separating the rectum from the vagina and work upward (Fig. 27-14, *B*). In male infants the penis and scrotum are tucked through the opening into the collection bag before the nurse removes the protective paper from the adhesive and presses it firmly onto the perineum, making sure the entire adhesive is firmly attached to skin and the edges of the opening do not pucker (Fig. 27-14, *C*). This helps ensure a leak-proof seal and decreases the chance of contamination from stool. Cutting a slit in the diaper and pulling the bag through the slit may also help prevent leaking.

The diaper is carefully replaced, and the bag is checked frequently. The bag is removed when 1 to 2 ml of urine have been obtained. The infant's skin is observed for signs of irritation while the bag is in place. The specimen can be aspirated with a syringe or drained directly from the bag. To drain the bag, the bag is held in the one hand and tilted to keep urine away from the tab. The tab is then removed and the urine drained into a clean receptacle (Fig. 27-14, *D*).

Collection of a 24-hour specimen can be a challenge. To do this the infant may need to be restrained. The 24-hour U-Bag is applied in the same manner as that just described, and the urine collected is drained into a receptacle. The collection tube can be shortened or capped (Fig.

27-14, *E*). During the collection the infant's skin is watched closely for signs of irritation and lack of a proper seal.

For some types of urine tests, urine can be aspirated directly from the diaper by means of a syringe without a needle. If the diaper has absorbent gelling material that traps urine, a small gauze dressing or some cotton balls can be placed inside the diaper and the urine aspirated from them (Wong, 1999).

Venipuncture

Venous blood samples can be drawn from radial veins, jugular veins, or femoral veins, or they can be drawn through heparin lock devices. However, use of a heparin lock device is not very successful and may only shorten the use of the device as an IV site (Wong, 1999). If an IV site is used to obtain a blood specimen, it is important to consider the type of fluid being infused, because contamination of the blood with the fluid can alter the results.

When venipuncture is required, positioning of the needle is extremely important. Although regular venipuncture needles may be used for this purpose, some personnel prefer to use scalp vein needles. It is necessary to be very patient during the procedure, because the blood return in small veins is slow, meaning also that the small needle must remain in place longer.

The mummy restraint frequently is used to help secure the infant during venipuncture of the head and neck (Fig. 27-15).

For *external jugular venipuncture,* "mummy" the infant as necessary, then lower the infant's head over a rolled towel, the edge of a table, or your knee, and stabilize. For *femoral venipuncture,* place your hands over the infant's knees, but avoid pressing your fingers over the inner aspect of the

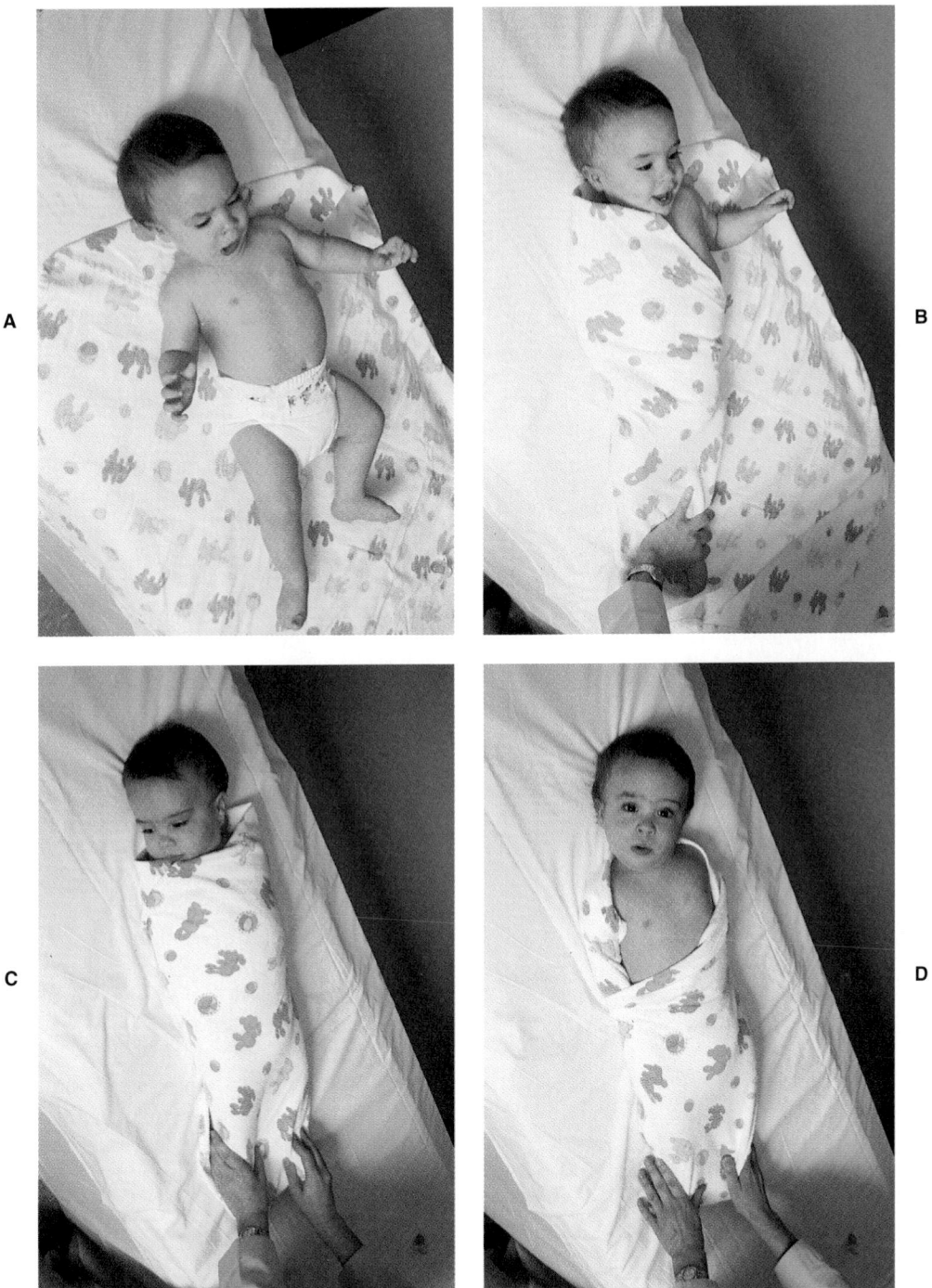

Fig. 27-15 Application of mummy restraint. **A,** Infant is placed on folded corner of blanket. **B,** One corner of blanket is brought across body and secured beneath the body. **C,** Second corner is brought across body and secured, and lower corner is folded and tucked or pinned in place. **D,** Modified mummy restraint with chest uncovered. *(From Wong, D. [1999].* Whaley & Wong's nursing care of infants and children *[6th ed.]. St. Louis: Mosby.)*

thigh. Both of these positions ensure the safety of the infant and exposure of the puncture sites (Fig. 27-16). If the radial vein is used, the infant's arm is exposed and held securely in place. The nurse may also restrain the infant (see Restraining the Infant in the following text).

If venipuncture or arterial puncture is being performed for blood gas studies, crying, fear, and agitation will affect the values. Therefore every effort must be made to keep the infant quiet during the procedure. For blood gas studies the blood sample tubes are packed in ice to reduce

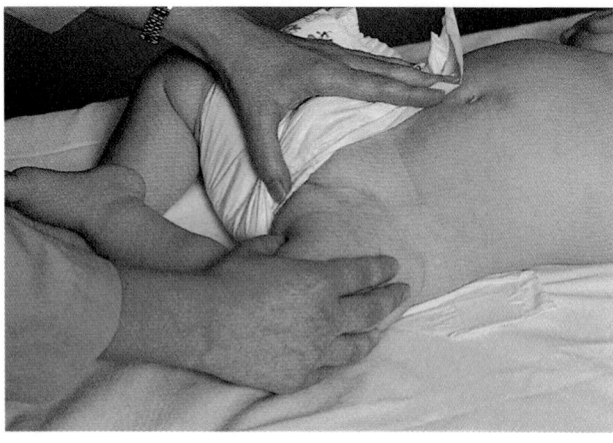

A

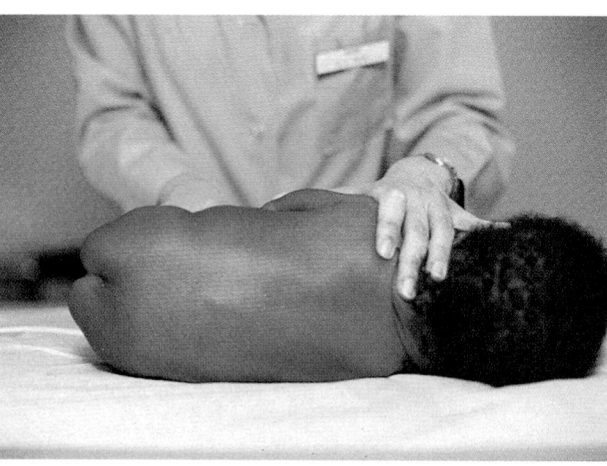

B

Fig. 27-16 **A,** Restraining infant for femoral vein puncture. **B,** Modified side-lying position for lumbar puncture. *(From Wong, D. [1999]. Whaley & Wong's nursing care of infants and children [6th ed.]. St. Louis: Mosby.)*

blood cell metabolism and are taken immediately to the laboratory for analysis.

Pressure must be maintained over an arterial or femoral vein puncture with a dry gauze square for at least 3 to 5 minutes to prevent bleeding from the site. The nurse should then observe the infant frequently for evidence of bleeding or hematoma formation at the puncture site for an hour after any venipuncture. The infant's tolerance of the procedure should also be noted and recorded. The infant should be cuddled and comforted (e.g., rocked, given a pacifier) when the procedure is completed.

Restraining the Infant

Infants may be restrained to (1) protect the infant from injury, (2) facilitate examinations, and (3) limit discomfort during tests, procedures, and specimen collections. Following are special considerations that must be kept in mind when restraining an infant:

• Check the infant hourly, or more frequently if indicated.

• Apply restraints and check them to make sure they are not irritating the skin or impairing circulation.
• Maintain proper body alignment.
• Apply restraints without using knots or pins, if possible. If knots are necessary, make the kind that can be released quickly. Use pins with care so that there is no danger of their puncturing or pressing against the infant's skin—and also no danger of the infant's swallowing one of them.
• If the infant is in an isolette, secure the infant to the mattress to protect its extremities, especially whenever the lid is raised or the mattress moved.

Restraint Without Appliance

The nurse may restrain the infant by using her hands and body. Figure 27-16, *B*, illustrates the way in which to restrain an infant for lumbar puncture.

PAIN PHYSIOLOGY

Pain has been defined physiologically and psychologically. The psychologic component of pain and the diffuse total body response to pain exhibited by the neonate led many health care providers to believe that infants, especially premature infants, do not experience pain (Franck & Gregory, 1993; McLaughlin et al., 1993). It is now known, however, that the CNS of fetuses is well developed as early as 24 weeks. The peripheral and spinal structure that transmits pain information is present and functional between the first and second trimester. Synaptic development begins in the cortex and achieves functional maturity by 20 to 24 weeks of gestation. The pituitary-adrenal axis is also well developed at this time, and a fight-or-flight reaction is observed in response to the catecholamines released in response to stress (Franck, 1998; Lawrence et al., 1993).

The physiologic response to pain in neonates can be life threatening because it can involve a decrease in the tidal volume, an increase in the demands on the cardiovascular system, an increase in metabolism, and neuroendocrine imbalance. The hormonal-metabolic response to pain in a term infant is also of a greater magnitude and shorter duration than that of adults. In addition, the newborn's sympathetic response to pain is less mature and thus less predictable than an adult's (Franck & Gregory, 1993).

Assessment

Three components to the response to pain must be considered in the pain assessment of newborns: behavioral, physiologic and autonomic, and metabolic (Franck & Gregory, 1993). Each component is reviewed separately.

Behavioral Responses

The most common behavioral sign of pain is a vocalization or cry. Through acoustical analysis the pain cry has been found to be distinctive (Craig & Grunau, 1993). It has been described as being high pitched and shrill (Lynam, 1995). A cry face is also characteristic of an infant experiencing pain. Such infants also flex and adduct their upper body and lower limbs in an attempt to withdraw from the painful stimulus. Other facial features exhibited during pain include eye squeeze, brow contraction, deepened nasolabial furrows, a taut and quivering tongue, and open mouth (Fig. 27-17). The extremities and body exhibit withdrawal, thrashing, jerking, and rigid posture (Anand, Grunau, & Oberlander, 1997; Craig & Grunau, 1993; Hadjistavropoulos et al., 1997).

Physiologic and Autonomic Responses

Significant changes in heart rate, blood pressure (increased or decreased), intracranial pressure, vagal tone, respiratory rate, and oxygen saturation occur during noxious stimuli (Franck & Gregory, 1993; Lynam, 1995).

Metabolic Responses

Epinephrine, norepinephrine, glucagon, corticosterone, cortisol, 11-deoxycorticosterone, lactate, pyruvate, and glucose are released in infants in response to pain (Franck & Gregory, 1993; Lynam, 1995). Box 27-4 lists the infant's physiologic and behavioral responses to pain.

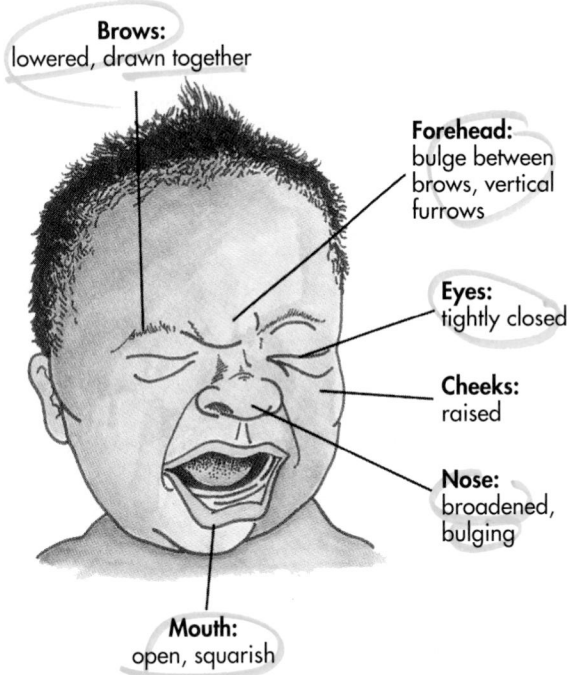

Brows: lowered, drawn together

Forehead: bulge between brows, vertical furrows

Eyes: tightly closed

Cheeks: raised

Nose: broadened, bulging

Mouth: open, squarish

Fig. 27-17 Facial expression of physical distress is the most salient behavioral indicator of pain in infants. *(From Wong, D. [1999]. Whaley & Wong's nursing care of infants and children [6th ed.]. St. Louis: Mosby.)*

BOX 27-4 Manifestations of Acute Pain in the Neonate

PHYSIOLOGIC RESPONSES

Vital signs: observe for variations
  Increased heart rate
  Increased blood pressure
  Rapid, shallow respirations
Oxygenation
  Decreased transcutaneous O_2 saturation (tcPO$_2$)
  Decreased arterial O_2 saturation (SaO$_2$)
Skin: Observe color and character
  Pallor or flushing
  Diaphoresis
  Palmar sweating
Other observations
  Increased muscle tone
  Dilated pupils
  Decreased vagal tone
  Increased intracranial pressure
Laboratory evidence of metabolic or endocrine changes
  Hyperglycemia
  Lowered pH
  Elevated corticosteroids

BEHAVIORAL RESPONSES

Vocalizations: observe quality, timing, and duration
  Crying
  Whimpering
  Groaning
Facial expressions: observe characteristics, timing, orientation of eyes and mouth (see Fig. 27-17)
  Grimaces
  Brow furrowed
  Chin quivering
  Eyes tightly closed
  Mouth open and squarish
Body movements and posture: observe type, quality, and amount of movement or lack of movement; relationship to other factors
  Limb withdrawal
  Thrashing
  Rigidity
  Flaccidity
  Fist clenching
Changes in state: observe sleep, appetite, activity level
  Changes in sleep/wake cycles
  Changes in feeding behavior
  Changes in activity level
  Fussiness, irritability
  Listlessness

Pain Management

The goals of the management of neonatal pain are (1) to minimize the intensity, duration, and physiologic cost of the pain and (2) to maximize the neonate's ability to cope and recover from the pain (Franck & Gregory, 1993). Nonpharmacologic and pharmacologic strategies are used.

Nonpharmacologic Management

Containment, also known as swaddling, is effective in reducing excessive immature motor responses. This may also provide comfort through other senses, such as the thermal, tactile, and proprioceptive senses (Franck & Gregory, 1993; Lynam, 1995). Nonnutritive sucking is the most common comfort measure used. However, the effectiveness of nonnutritive sucking in reducing the pain response has been found to be limited and confined to the pain caused by certain procedures (Lynam, 1995; Mohan et al., 1998). Distraction with visual, oral, auditory, or tactile stimulation may be helpful in term or older infants (Franck & Gregory, 1993).

Pharmacologic Management

Pharmacologic agents are routinely used for adults during painful procedures. These same agents are also now becoming routinely used in neonates to alleviate such pain. Local anesthesia may be used for circumcision and has also become a routine measure during certain invasive procedures such as chest tube insertion. Topical anesthesia has been used for circumcision, lumbar puncture, venipuncture, and heel sticks (Franck, 1998; Mohan et al., 1998; Taddio et al. 1998). Opioids have been used as preprocedural analgesia. However, if the infant is not ventilated, the use of opioids is of concern because of the potential for these agents to cause respiratory depression (Franck, 1998; Franck & Gregory, 1993). For further discussion of pain management, see Chapter 41.

Nursing diagnoses are established once the significance of assessment findings is analyzed. Possible nursing diagnoses for the newborn include the following:

▪ Nursing Diagnoses _____

- Ineffective breathing pattern related to
  - obstructed airway
- Impaired gas exchange related to
  - hypothermia (cold stress)
- Risk for ineffective thermoregulation related to
  - heat loss to environment
- Risk for infection related to
  - environmental factors
- Pain related to
  - circumcision
  - heel sticks, venipuncture

Possible nursing diagnoses for the parent or parents of a newborn include the following:

▪ Nursing Diagnoses _____

- Family coping, potential for growth related to
  - knowledge of newborn's social capabilities
  - knowledge of newborn's dependency needs
  - knowledge of biologic characteristics of newborn
- Situational low self-esteem related to
  - misinterpretation of newborn's responses

The Plan of Care on p. 739 provides examples of ways of formulating nursing diagnoses on the basis of specific assessment findings.

Expected Outcomes

The expected outcomes for newborn care relate to the infant and parents. The expected outcomes for the infant include that the infant will do the following:

- Make the transition from intrauterine to extrauterine life.
- Maintain effective breathing patterns.
- Maintain effective thermoregulation.
- Remain free from infection.
- Receive measures to relieve pain.

For the parents, expected outcomes will include the following:

- Attain knowledge, skill, and confidence relevant to infant-care activities.
- State understanding of biologic and behavioral characteristics of their newborn.
- Demonstrate interactional/lifestyle behaviors that promote healthy family functioning.
- Have opportunities to intensify their relationship with the infant.
- Begin to integrate the infant into the family.

Plan of Care and Interventions

In the inpatient setting, priorities of care must be established and a systematic teaching plan for infant care devised. One way to accomplish this is to use critical path case management. A care path may also be developed that covers the changes expected in the infant during the first several days. Such a care path is shown on p. 741. When variations from the care path occur, further assessment and intervention may be necessary.

Protective Environment

The provision of a **protective environment** is basic to the care of the newborn. The construction, maintenance, and operation of nurseries in accredited hospitals are monitored by national professional organizations such as the American Academy of Pediatrics and local or state governing bodies. In addition, hospital personnel develop their own policies and procedures for protecting the newborns

NURSING DIAGNOSIS Risk for ineffective airway clearance related to excess mucus production/improper positioning

Expected Outcomes *Neonate's airway remains patent; breath sounds are clear and no respiratory distress is evident.*

Nursing Interventions/*Rationales*

Suction mouth and nasopharynx with bulb syringe as needed; clean nares of crusted secretions *to clear airway and prevent aspiration and airway obstruction.*

Position neonate on right side after feeding *to prevent aspiration* and on back or side when sleeping *to prevent suffocation.*

Keep diapers, clothing, and covers loose enough *to allow for maximum lung expansion.*

Teach parents that gagging, coughing, and sneezing are normal neonatal responses *that assist the neonate in clearing airways.*

Teach parents how to hold, suction, and position the neonate with return demonstration *to ensure parental skill at airway clearance and maintenance.*

Teach parents feeding techniques that prevent overfeeding and distention of the abdomen and to burp neonate frequently *to prevent regurgitation and aspiration.*

NURSING DIAGNOSIS Risk for altered body temperature related to larger body surface in relationship to mass

Expected Outcome *Neonate temperature remains in range of 36.5° to 37.2° C.*

Nursing Interventions/*Rationales*

Maintain neutral thermal environment *to identify any changes in neonate's temperature that may be related to other causes.*

Monitor neonate's temperature frequently *to identify any changes promptly and ensure early interventions.*

Bathe neonate efficiently when temperature is stable, using warm water, drying carefully, and avoiding exposing neonate to drafts *to avoid heat losses from evaporation and convection.*

Report any alterations in temperature findings promptly *to assess and treat for possible infection.*

NURSING DIAGNOSIS Risk for infection related to immature immunologic defenses/environmental exposure

Expected Outcome *The neonate will be free from signs of infection.*

Nursing Interventions/*Rationales*

Review maternal record for evidence of any risk factors *to ascertain whether the neonate may be predisposed to infection.*

Monitor vital signs *to identify early possible evidence of infection, especially temperature instability.*

Have all care providers, including parents, practice good handwashing techniques before handling newborn *to prevent spread of infection.*

Monitor and instruct parents to also monitor visitors and personnel for evidence of infection and limit contact as needed *to prevent spread of infection.*

Keep eyes and eyelashes clean and free of mucus; provide prescribed eye prophylaxis *to prevent infection.*

Keep genital area clean and dry using proper cleansing techniques *to prevent skin irritation, cross-contamination, and infection.*

Teach parents to bathe neonate using mild soap and patting dry and to inspect skin for rashes *to avoid disturbing protective acid mantle of skin and treat any infections promptly.*

Keep umbilical stump clean and dry and keep exposed to air *to allow to dry and minimize chance of infection.*

If circumcised, keep site clean and dressed with prescribed ointment and diaper applied loosely *to prevent trauma and infection and to promote healing.*

Administer topical, oral, and parenteral antibiotics as prescribed *to eradicate pathogens.*

Teach parents to keep neonate away from crowds and environmental irritants *to reduce potential sources of infection.*

NURSING DIAGNOSIS Risk for injury related to sole dependence on caregiver

Expected Outcome *Neonate remains free of injury.*

Nursing Interventions/*Rationales*

Monitor environment for hazards such as sharp objects, long fingernails of caretaker and neonate, and jewelry of caretaker that may be sharp *to prevent injury*

Handle neonate gently and support head, transport only in crib, ensure use of car seat by parents, teach parents never to place neonate on high surface unsupervised, and to supervise pet and sibling interactions *to prevent injury.*

Assess neonate thoroughly for possible evidence of injury or congenital anomalies *to detect injury or defects promptly and promote early treatment.*

Assess neonate frequently for any evidence of jaundice *to identify rising bilirubin levels, treat promptly, and prevent kernicterus.*

Continued

PLAN ᵒᶠ CARE | Normal Newborn—cont'd

> **NURSING DIAGNOSIS** Coping, family; potential for growth related to anticipatory guidance regarding responses to neonate's crying

Expected Outcome *Parents will verbalize understanding of methods of coping with neonate's crying and describe increased success in interpreting neonate's cries.*

Nursing Interventions/*Rationales*

Alert parents to crying as neonate's form of communication and that cries can be differentiated to indicate hunger, wetness, pain, and loneliness *to provide reassurance that crying is not indicative of neonate's rejection of parents and that parents will soon be able to interpret the different cries of their child.*

Differentiate self-consoling behaviors from fussing/crying *to give parents concrete examples of interventions.*

Discuss methods of consoling a neonate who has been crying, such as checking and changing diapers; showing parent's face to neonate; talking softly to neonate; holding neonate's arms close to body; swaddling; picking neonate up; rocking; using a pacifier, feeding, or burping; using mechanical swing; or going for a car ride *to provide anticipatory guidance.*

---

under their care. Prescribed standards cover areas such as the following:

- Environmental factors include adequate lighting, elimination of potential fire hazards, safety of electrical appliances, adequate ventilation, and controlled temperature (warm and free of drafts) and humidity (lower than 50%).
- Measures to control infection include adequate floor space to permit the positioning of bassinets at least 60 cm apart, handwashing facilities, and areas for the cleaning and storage of equipment and supplies.

Only those personnel directly involved in the care of mothers and infants are allowed in this area, thereby reducing the opportunities for the transmission of pathogenic organisms.

> **NURSE ALERT** *Personnel are instructed to use good handwashing techniques, with handwashing between each infant handling being the single most important measure in the prevention of neonatal infection.*

Health care personnel must wear gloves when handling the infant until blood and amniotic fluid have been removed from its skin, when drawing blood (e.g., heel stick), when caring for a fresh wound (e.g., circumcision), and when changing diapers.

Visitors and health care providers such as nurses, physicians, parents, brothers and sisters, department supervisors, electricians, and housekeepers are expected to wash their hands before coming in contact with infants or equipment. Cover gowns are not necessary.

Persons with infectious conditions are excluded from contact with newborns, or the infected persons must take special precautions when working with the infants. This includes persons with upper respiratory tract infections, GI tract infections, and infectious skin conditions. Most agencies have now coupled this day-to-day self-screening of personnel with yearly health examinations.

- *Safety factors.* Security measures have been implemented in many agencies in response to the infant abductions from nurseries that have been occurring with greater frequency. Some examples of the measures that have been instituted are placing identical identification bracelets on infants and their parents, and footprinting or taking identification pictures after birth before the infant leaves the mother's side.

Personnel wear picture identification badges or other badges that identify them as newborn personnel. There may be infant tracking systems in mother-baby units that set off an alarm if a baby is left alone or is with unauthorized personnel. Mothers are also instructed to be certain they know the identity of anyone who cares for the infant and never to release the infant to anyone who is not wearing the appropriate identification.

SUPPORTING PARENTS IN THE CARE OF THEIR INFANT

The sensitivity of the caregiver to the social responses of the infant is basic to the development of a mutually satisfying parent-child relationship. Such sensitivity increases over time as parents become more aware of their infant's social capabilities (see Cultural Considerations box).

Social Interactions

The activities of daily care during the neonatal period present the best times for infant and family interactions. While caring for their baby, the mother and father can talk to the infant, play baby games, and caress and cuddle the child. In Fig. 27-18, a mother, father, and infant are shown engaging in arousal, imitation of facial expression, and

CARE PATH — Neonatal Adaptation to Extrauterine Life

	DAY 1	DAY 2	DAY 3	DAY 4	DAY 7	DAY 14
WEIGHT		Loss of 5%-10% of birth weight	Gain of 150-300 g per day			Birth weight regained
TEMPERATURE	Stabilized at 37° C					
FEEDINGS						
VOLUME						
Formula	15-60 ml	60-90 ml	60-90 ml	60-90 ml	60-90 ml	60-90 ml
Breast		Softening of at least one breast at each feeding				
FREQUENCY						
Formula	6-10 times/ 24 hr		6-10 times/ 24 hr		6-10 times/ 24 hr	
Breast	8-12 times/ 24 hr		8-12 times/ 24 hr		8-12 times/ 24 hr	
VOIDING	At least 1 time in first 24 hr	2-6 times/ 24 hr	6-10 times/ 24 hr			6-10 times/ 24 hr
STOOLS		Meconium; at least 1 time in first 48 hr	Transitional stool: 1-5/day	Yellow stool: 1-5/day		Yellow stool: 1-2/day
SLEEP	16-20 hr/24 hr					16-20 hr/24 hr
UMBILICAL CORD	Moist; clamped	Dry; clamp removed				Cord off
CIRCUMCISION	Red; sore	Yellow exudate covers glans	Healing	Healing		Healed
COLOR	Pink; acrocyanotic	Pink; slight jaundice	Peak of jaundice		Pink	
BILIRUBIN LEVEL	0-6 mg/dl	≤ 8 mg/dl	≤12 mg/dl		≤2 mg/dl	
LABORATORY TESTS	Glucose when required; HCT	PKU, T$_4$, galactose				Repeat PKU, if needed
MEDICATIONS	Eye prophylaxis and vitamin K within 2 hr of birth; HBV within 12 hr of birth					

HBV, Hepatitis B vaccine; *HCT*, hematocrit, *PKU*, phenylketonuria.

smiling. However, too much stimulation should be avoided after feeding and before a sleep period. Older children's contact with a newborn needs to be supervised in terms of the strength of hugs, the exploring of eyes and nose, and attempts to feed the baby. Parents often keep baby books that record their infant's progress.

Infant Feeding

The infant may be put to breast shortly after birth or at least within 4 hours of birth. If the infant is to be bottle fed, a nurse may first offer it a few sips of sterile water to make certain its sucking and swallowing reflexes are intact and that there are no anomalies such as a tracheo-esophageal fistula. Most infants are on *demand-feeding schedules* and are allowed to feed when they awaken. Ordinarily, mothers are encouraged to feed their infants every 3 to 4 hours during the day and only when the infant awakens during the night in the first few days after birth. Breastfed babies nurse more often than bottle-fed babies because breast milk is digested faster than formulas made from cow's milk and the stomach empties sooner as a result. Water supplements are usually not recommended. For a thorough discussion of infant feeding, see Chapter 28.

THERAPEUTIC AND SURGICAL PROCEDURES

Intramuscular Injection

As previously mentioned, it is routine to administer a single parenteral dose of 0.5 to 1 mg of vitamin K intramuscularly to an infant soon after birth to prevent hemorrhagic disorders because normal newborns are not able to produce their own vitamin K until about 8 days after birth (see Medication Guide box on p. 726). Vitamin K is produced in the gastrointestinal tract starting soon after microorganisms are introduced.

Hepatitis B vaccination (Hep B) is recommended for all infants. Infants at highest risk of contracting hepatitis B are those born to women who come from Asia, Africa, South America, the South Pacific, or southern or eastern Europe (Medication Guide box). If the infant is born to an infected mother or to a mother who is a chronic carrier, hepatitis vaccine and hepatitis B immune globulin (HBIG) should be administered within 12 hours of birth (see Medication Guide box). The hepatitis vaccine is given in one site and the HBIG in another. The first dose of the vaccine for infants born to healthy women may be given at birth or at 1 or 2 months of age. Parental consent should be obtained before administering these medications.

In most cases a 25-gauge, $^5/_8$-inch needle should be used for the vitamin K and hepatitis vaccine injections. A 22-gauge needle may be necessary if thicker medications such as some penicillins are to be given.

Selection of the injection site is important. Injections must be given in muscles large enough to accommodate the medication, but major nerves and blood vessels avoided. The muscles of newborns may not tolerate more than a 0.5 ml IM injection. The injection site for newborns is the vastus lateralis (Fig. 27-19). Except for the femoral artery on the medial aspect of the thigh, this muscle is free of important nerves and blood vessels. The vastus lateralis muscle is well developed in the newborn. The posterior gluteal muscle is very small and poorly developed in infants; it is also dangerously close to the sciatic nerve, which occupies a larger space in infants than in older children. Therefore it is not recommended that it be used as an injection site until the child has been walking for at least 1 year.

CULTURAL consiperations

Cultural Beliefs and Practices

Nurses working with childbearing families from other cultures and ethnic groups must be aware of cultural beliefs and practices that are important to individual families. People with a strong sense of heritage may hold on to traditional health beliefs long after adopting other American lifestyle practices. These health beliefs may involve practices regarding the newborn. For example, some Asians, Hispanics, eastern Europeans, and Native Americans delay breastfeeding because they believe that colostrum is "bad." Some Hispanics and African-Americans place a belly band over the infant's navel. The birth of a male child is generally preferred by Asians and Indians, and some Asians and Haitians delay naming their infant (Geissler, 1994).

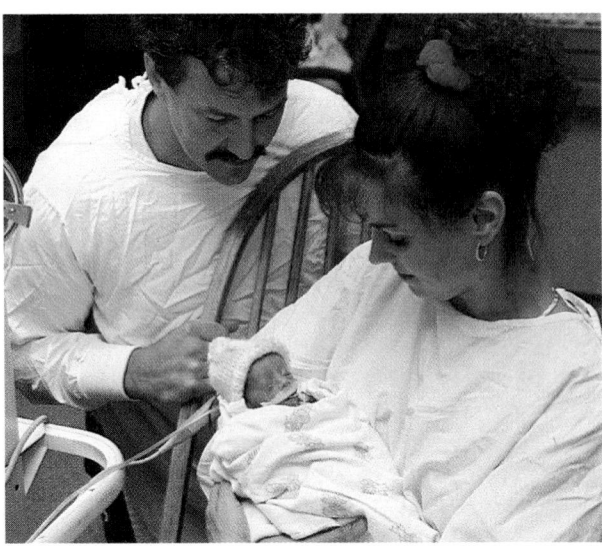

Fig. 27-18   Mother-father-baby interaction. *(From Wong, D. [1999]. Whaley & Wong's nursing care of infants and children [6th ed.]. St. Louis: Mosby.)*

Newborn infants offer little, if any, resistance to injections. Although they squirm and may be difficult to hold in position if they are awake, they can usually be restrained without the need for assistance from a second person if the nurse is experienced.

The neonate's leg should be stabilized, and gloves should be worn by the person giving the injection. The nurse cleanses the injection site with alcohol and then pinches up the infant's muscle between her thumb and first finger. The needle is inserted into the vastus lateralis at a 90-degree angle. The muscle is then released and the plunger of the syringe gently withdrawn. If no blood is aspirated, the medication is injected. If blood is aspirated, the needle is withdrawn and the injection is given in another site. After the injection has been given, the needle is withdrawn quickly and the site massaged with a gauze square to hasten absorption unless contraindicated. It is not uncommon for blood to ooze from the injection site, but it is not necessary to cover the site with an adhesive bandage. Pressure should be applied until oozing stops.

The nurse should always remember to comfort the infant after an injection and to properly discard equipment. It is important to record the name of the medication, the date and time of administration, the amount, the route, the site of injection, and the infant's tolerance of injection.

Therapy for Hyperbilirubinemia

The best therapy for hyperbilirubinemia is prevention. This is done by feeding the newborn soon after birth because this stimulates the gastrocolic reflex and the passage of meconium in which bilirubin is excreted. However, even despite this, the term infant may have trouble conjugating the increased amount of bilirubin derived from disintegrating fetal red blood cells. As a result, the serum

---

MEDICATION GUIDE

Hepatitis B Vaccine (Recombivax HB, Engerix-B)

ACTION

Hepatitis B vaccine induces protective anti–hepatitis B antibodies in 95% to 99% of healthy infants who receive the recommended three doses. The duration of protection of the vaccine is unknown.

INDICATION

HBV is for immunization against infection caused by all known subtypes of hepatitis B virus.

NEONATAL DOSAGE

The usual dosage is Recombivax HB 5 μg/0.5 ml or Engerix-B 10 μg/0.5 ml at 0, 1, and 6 months. An alternate dosing schedule is 0, 1, 2, and 12 months and is usually for newborns whose mothers were HBsAg positive.

ADVERSE REACTIONS

Common adverse reactions are rash, fever, erythema, swelling, and pain at injection site.

NURSING CONSIDERATIONS

Parental consent must be obtained before administration. Wear gloves. Administer in the middle third of the vastus lateralis muscle using a 25-gauge, ⅝-inch needle. Inject into skin that has been cleaned, or allow alcohol to dry on puncture site for 1 minute to remove organisms and prevent infection. Stabilize leg firmly and grasp muscle between the thumb and fingers. Insert the needle at a 90-degree angle; aspirate and inject medication slowly if there is no blood return. Massage the site with a dry gauze square after removing needle to increase absorption. If the infant was born to HBsAg-positive mother, hepatitis B immune globulin (HBIG) should be given within 12 hours of birth in addition to the HB vaccine. Separate sites must be used.

MEDICATION GUIDE

Hepatitis B Immune Globulin (HBIG)

ACTION

HBIG provides a high titer of antibody to hepatitis B surface antigen (HBsAg).

INDICATION

The HBIG vaccine provides prophylaxis against infection in infants born of HBsAg-positive mothers.

NEONATAL DOSAGE

Administer one 0.5 ml dose intramuscularly within 12 hours of birth.

ADVERSE REACTIONS

Hypersensitivity may occur.

NURSING CONSIDERATIONS

Must be given within 12 hours of birth. Wear gloves. Administer in the middle third of the vastus lateralis muscle using a 25-gauge, ⅝-inch needle. Inject into skin that has been cleaned, or allow alcohol to dry on puncture site for 1 minute to remove organisms and prevent infection. Stabilize leg firmly and grasp muscle between the thumb and fingers. Insert the needle at a 90-degree angle; aspirate and inject medication slowly if there is no blood return. Massage the site with a dry gauze square after removing needle to increase absorption. May be given at same time as hepatitis B vaccine, but at a different site.

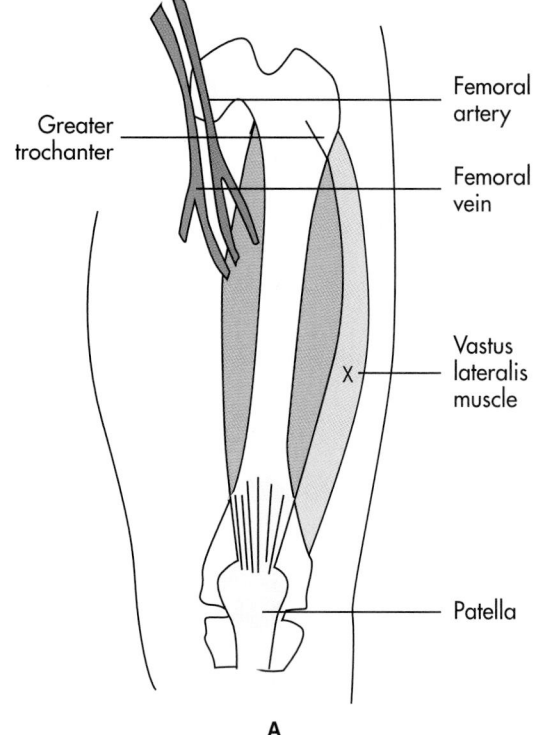

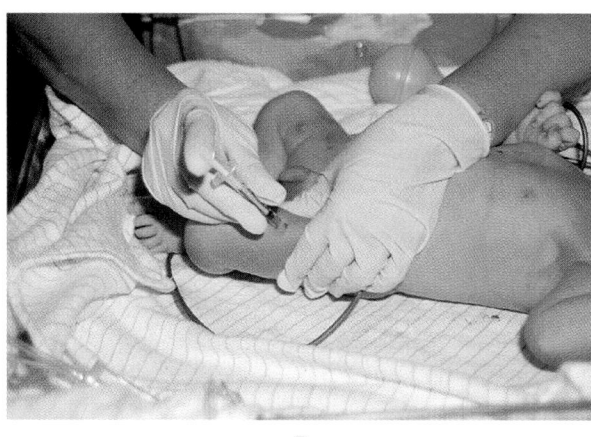

Fig. 27-19 Intramuscular injection. **A,** Acceptable intramuscular injection site for newborn infant. X, Injection site. **B,** Infant's leg stabilized for intramuscular injection. Nurse is wearing gloves to give injection. (**B** *courtesy Marjorie Pyle, RNC, Lifecircle, Costa Mesa, CA.*)

levels of unconjugated bilirubin may rise beyond normal limits, causing hyperbilirubinemia (see Chapter 26). If this goes untreated, the levels can continue to rise, and with this the risk of kernicterus. The goal of hyperbilirubinemia treatment therefore is to help reduce the newborn's serum levels of unconjugated bilirubin. There are two principal ways of doing this: phototherapy and exchange blood transfusion. Exchange transfusion is used to treat those infants whose raised bilirubin levels cannot be controlled by phototherapy.

Phototherapy

During **phototherapy** the unclothed infant is placed approximately 45 to 50 cm away from a bank of lights. The distance may vary based on unit protocol and type of light used. The infant is turned every 2 hours to expose all body surfaces to the light. This is done for several hours or days until the infant's serum bilirubin level decreases to within an acceptable range. The decision to discontinue therapy is based on the observation of a definite downward trend in the bilirubin values. After therapy has been terminated, the infant may have a rebound in bilirubin levels, which is usually harmless.

Several precautions must be taken while the infant is undergoing phototherapy. The lamp energy output should be monitored routinely during treatment with a photometer (Fanaroff & Martin, 1997). The infant's eyes must be protected by an opaque mask to prevent overexposure to the light, and the eye shield should completely cover the eyes but not occlude the nares. In addition, before the mask is applied, the infant's eyes should be closed gently to prevent excoriation of the corneas. The mask should be removed during infant feedings so that the eyes can be checked and the parents can have visual contact with the infant (Fig. 27-20, *A* and *B*).

To promote optimal skin exposure, yet sufficient protection of the genitals and bedding, often a "string bikini" made from a disposable face mask is used instead of a diaper. Before its application, the metal strip must be removed from the mask so that the infant is not burned. Lotions and ointments should not be applied to the infant because they absorb heat and this can cause burns.

Phototherapy may cause the infant to sleep for longer than the usual 4-hour periods, but the infant needs to be kept on a regular feeding schedule. The number and consistency of stools are monitored. Because bilirubin breakdown increases gastric motility, which results in the formation of loose stools that can cause skin excoriation and breakdown, the infant's buttocks are cleaned after each stool to help maintain skin integrity.

Because the infant is unclothed and the lights produce heat, the infant's temperature may become elevated, and for this reason needs to be monitored at least every 4 hours. The lights also accelerate the rate of insensible water loss, making it possible for fluid loss and dehydration to occur. Therefore it is important that the infant be adequately hydrated. All aspects of the phototherapy rendered should be accurately recorded in the infant's chart.

An alternative device for phototherapy that is as safe and effective as traditional phototherapy is a fiberoptic panel attached to an illuminator. This fiberoptic blanket, which essentially wraps light around the newborn's torso, delivers continuous phototherapy. While wearing it the newborn can remain in the mother's room in an open crib or in her arms; follow unit protocol for the use of eye patches (Fig. 27-20, *C*). The blanket may also be used for home phototherapy.

Parent Education

Serum levels of bilirubin in the newborn continue to rise until the fifth day of life. However, because most parents leave the hospital within 48 hours and some as early as 6 hours after birth, parents must be able to assess the newborn's degree of jaundice. They should therefore have written instructions for assessing the infant's condition that include the name of the person they should contact to report their findings. Some hospitals have a nurse make a home visit to evaluate the infant's condition. If it proves necessary to measure the infant's bilirubin levels after discharge from the hospital, either the home care nurse may draw the blood specimen or the parents may take the baby to a laboratory for the determination (see Teaching Guidelines box).

Circumcision

Circumcision is commonly performed in the United States. Although there is controversy over its value the American Academy of Pediatrics (AAP) Task Force on Circumcision (1989) stated that a properly performed newborn circumcision prevents **phimosis** (a constriction of the prepuce that prevents retraction of the foreskin, may impede urine flow, and predisposes males to penile infection) and may reduce the risk of urinary tract infections. In addition, the incidence of penile cancer has been found to be lower in American men who are circumcised. However, there is still conflicting evidence regarding the association between circumcision and sexually transmitted infections. Because newborn circumcision has potential medical benefits and advantages, as well as disadvantages and risks, and because of the continuing controversy about these advantages and disadvantages, the decision to perform this elective surgical procedure is left to the parents.

Circumcision is a matter of personal parental choice. Parents usually decide to have their newborn circumcised for one or more of the following reasons: hygiene, religious conviction, tradition, culture, or social norms. Regardless of the reason for the decision, it should be made only after parents have been given the available facts and have sufficient time to review their options.

Expectant parents need to begin learning about circumcision during the prenatal period, but circumcision often is not discussed with the parents before labor. In many instances, it is only when the mother is being admitted to the hospital or birth unit that she is first confronted with the decision regarding circumcision. Because the stress of the intrapartal period makes this a difficult time for parental decision making, this is not an ideal time to broach the topic of circumcision and expect a well-thought-out decision. The mother may be asked to sign a circumcision permit form during the admission process, but usually this request is made after the birth. Some hospitals require parents to sign a different form stating they do not wish their male infant to be circumcised, if that is their desire.

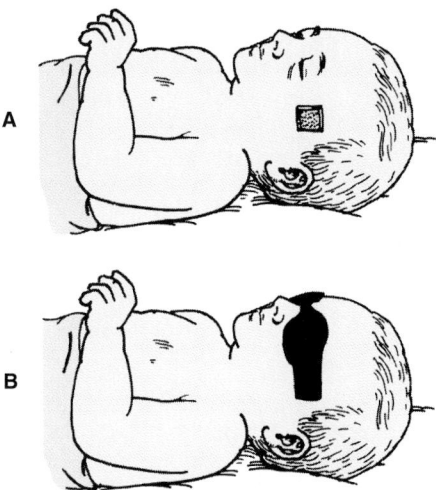

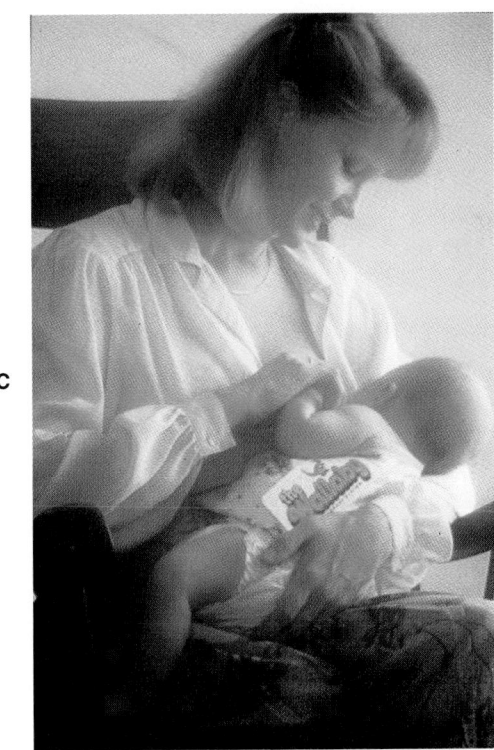

Fig. 27-20 Eye patches for newborns receiving phototherapy. **A,** Small Velcro patch stuck to both sides of head. **B,** Eye cover sticks to Velcro patch, which reduces movement of eye cover and facilitates removal for feedings. **C,** A mother can breastfeed her baby without interrupting phototherapy. *(Courtesy Respironics, Inc., Pittsburgh, PA.)*

Procedure

Circumcision involves removing the prepuce (foreskin) of the glans. The procedure is usually not done immediately after birth because of the danger of cold stress but is performed in the hospital before the infant's discharge. The circumcision of a Jewish male is performed on the eighth day after birth and is done at home, in a ceremony

TEACHING guidelines

Hyperbilirubinemia

DEFINITIONS

Hyperbilirubinemia: higher levels of bilirubin than normal

Bilirubin: end product of RBCs when they mature and break down

RBCs: red blood cells

Jaundice: yellow skin, sclerae, and mucous membranes caused by circulating bilirubin

Phototherapy: the use of fluorescent light to break down the bilirubin in the skin into substances that can be excreted in the feces (stool) and urine

Bililites: fluorescent lights used for phototherapy

HOW JAUNDICE HAPPENS

When RBCs break down, they release bilirubin, which then circulates in the blood. The bilirubin combines with another substance in the liver. This combined substance moves through the blood to the kidneys and the intestines, where it is eliminated in the urine and the stool. The bilirubin gives the yellow color to urine and the brown color to the stool.

Before birth, babies have more RBCs in each ounce of blood than adults have. The RBCs of the unborn infant also have a shorter life span (70 to 90 days) than RBCs formed after birth (120 days). When the RBCs of a fetus break down, the bilirubin produced by this is carried by the fetus's blood, through the placenta, and to the mother's liver to be excreted.

After birth, the infant's liver must get rid of the bilirubin. Even though a baby's liver functions well, it may not be able to get rid of all the bilirubin produced by breakdown of RBCs. Bilirubin then seeps out of the blood and into the tissues, coloring them yellow (jaundice). The blood level of bilirubin rises quickly up to the fifth day and then it declines; the jaundice usually clears up by the end of the week.

THE DANGER OF EXCESS BILIRUBIN

Some newborns seem to have extra bilirubin to excrete. High levels of bilirubin may cause damage to the brain.

According to the American Academy of Pediatrics guidelines (1994), phototherapy is considered in a healthy term infant who is 1 to 2 days old if the total bilirubin level is 12 mg/dl or more, or it is instituted if the bilirubin level is 15 mg/dl or more. The infant is placed under phototherapy lights or on a bili blanket. This helps the infant eliminate the extra bilirubin and prevents damage to the brain.

CARING FOR THE INFANT

The newborn is placed in an incubator under phototherapy lights so that it can be kept warm and the nurse can observe it.

The infant wears an eye mask to keep the light out of the eyes.

The infant is undressed so that as much light as possible can reach the skin. The newborn may wear a "string bikini" as a small diaper, which is made out of a paper diaper or a face mask.

The infant's temperature is taken often so that any changes in temperature can be noted and the infant is not allowed to become too hot or too cold.

The infant may be given extra water to drink or extra breastfeedings because infants have watery, green stools resulting from excretion of the extra bilirubin, and this can lead to dehydration.

The newborn is taken out from under the lights for feedings and cuddling unless a bili blanket is being used. There is no need to remove the bili blanket for feeding.

Blood is taken from the heel to check the amount of bilirubin still in the newborn's blood, and the nurse updates the parents about the results.

AFTER THE NEWBORN GOES HOME

The parents should be encouraged to ask any questions that they might have. The nurse gives them a telephone number to call at any hour with their questions. If therapy is continued at home, referral is made to home care.

---

called a bris, unless the infant is unwell. This is logical from a physiologic standpoint because clotting factors drop somewhat immediately after birth and do not return to prebirth levels until the end of the first week.

Feedings are usually withheld up to 4 hours before the circumcision to prevent vomiting and aspiration. To prepare the infant for the circumcision, he is positioned on a plastic restraint form (Fig. 27-21) and his penis is cleansed with soap and water or a preparatory solution such as povidone-

iodine. The infant is draped to provide warmth and a sterile field, and the sterile equipment is readied for use.

Although some circumcision procedures require no special equipment or appliances (Fig. 27-22), numerous instruments have been designed for this purpose. Use of the Yellen or Mogen clamp (Fig. 27-23) may make this an almost bloodless operation. The procedure itself takes only a few minutes to perform. After it is completed, a small petrolatum gauze dressing or a generous amount of

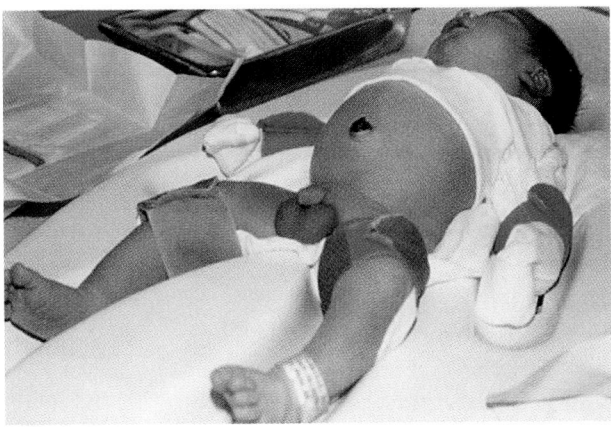

Fig. 27-21 "Circ board" restrains infant during circumcision. (*Courtesy Marjorie Pyle, RNC, Lifecircle, Costa Mesa, CA.*)

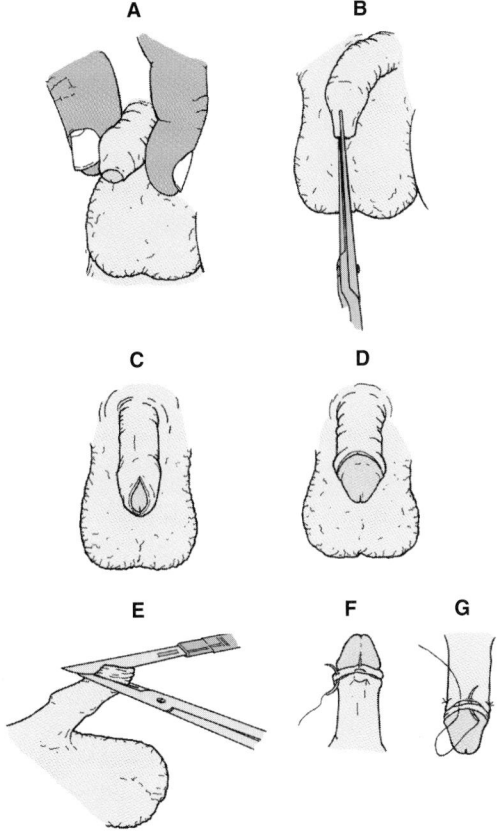

Fig. 27-22 Technique of circumcision. **A** to **D,** Prepuce is stripped and slit to facilitate its retraction behind glans penis. **E,** Prepuce is now clamped and excessive prepuce cut off. **F** and **G,** A very small needle and plain 2-0 or 3-0 catgut are used for suture material; some physicians prefer silk.

petrolatum or A & D ointment may be applied for the first day to keep a diaper from adhering to the site. A Plastibell may also be used for the circumcision. The advantages to its use are that it applies constant direct pressure to prevent hemorrhage during the procedure and afterwards protects

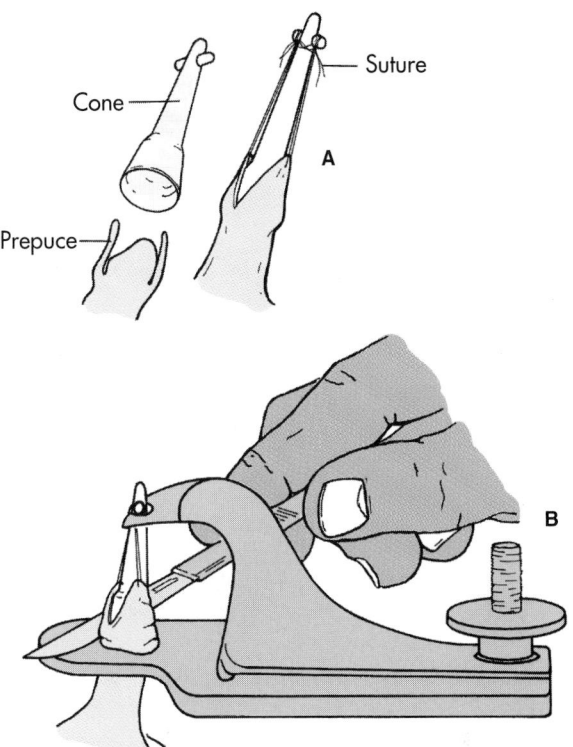

Fig. 27-23 Circumcision with Yellen clamp. **A,** Prepuce drawn over cone. **B,** Yellen clamp is applied, hemostasis occurs, then prepuce (over cone) is cut away.

against infection, keeps the site from sticking to the diaper, and prevents pain with urination. When using the bell for circumcision, it is first fitted over the glans, the suture is tied around the rim of the bell, and excess prepuce is then cut away. The plastic rim remains in place for about a week until it falls off, after healing has taken place (Fig. 27-24). Petrolatum does not need to be applied when the bell is used.

Discomfort

Circumcision is painful and the pain is manifested by both physiologic and behavioral changes in the infant. Three types of anesthesia/analgesia are used in newborns who undergo circumcisions. These include (from most effective to less effective) ring block, dorsal penile nerve block (DPNB), and topical anesthetic (Williamson, 1997).

A ring block is the injection of buffered lidocaine administered subcutaneously on each side of the penile shaft. A DPNB includes subcutaneous injections of buffered lidocaine at the 2 o'clock and 10 o'clock positions at the base of the penis. The circumcision should not be done for at least 5 minutes after these injections.

A topical cream containing prilocaine-lidocaine such as EMLA can be applied to the base of the penis at least 1 hour before the circumcision. The area where the prepuce attaches to the glans is well coated with the cream and then covered with a transparent occlusive dressing or

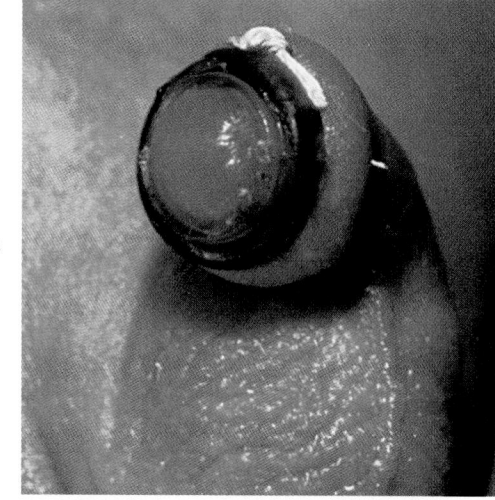

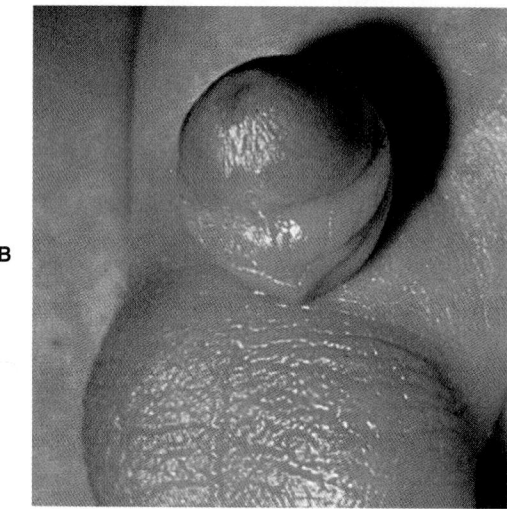

Fig. 27-24 Circumcision using Hollister Plastibell. **A,** Suture around rim of Plastibell controls bleeding. **B,** Plastic rim and suture drop off in 7 to 10 days. *(Permission to use and/or reproduce this copyrighted material has been granted by the owner, Hollister, Incorporated, Libertyville, IL.)*

finger cot. After the procedure, the cream is removed. Blanching or redness of the skin may occur.

Oral acetaminophen and comfort measures such as the infant sucking on a pacifier and talking to the infant in a soothing voice have not proven to be effective in pain reduction (Williamson, 1997). However pacifiers dipped in a concentrated glucose solution have been used during procedures with varied levels of effectiveness. More research is needed to determine what interventions are effective for pain reduction.

In the Jewish ritual the newborn is given a few drops of wine to relax him in preparation for the procedure.

After the circumcision, the infant is comforted until he is quieted. If the parents were not present during the procedure, the infant is returned to them. The infant may be fussy for several hours or may refuse a feeding.

Care of the Newly Circumcised Penis

The nurse checks the penis hourly for the next 12 hours to make sure no bleeding is occurring and voiding is normal. If bleeding is noted from the circumcision, the nurse applies gentle pressure to the site of bleeding with a folded sterile gauze square or sprinkles powdered gel foam on it. If bleeding is not easily controlled, a blood vessel may need to be ligated. In this event, one nurse notifies the physician and prepares the necessary equipment (circumcision tray and suture material), while another nurse maintains intermittent pressure until the physician arrives. If the parents take the baby home before the end of the 12-hour observation period, they have to be taught the proper home care (Home Care box). Before the infant is discharged, the nurse checks to see that the parents have the physician's telephone number.

Nursing actions are planned and implemented to prevent infection. Prepackaged wipes for cleaning the diaper area should not be used because they contain alcohol, which delays healing and causes discomfort. Instead the nurse washes the penis gently with water to remove urine and feces and, if necessary, reapplies fresh petrolatum around the glans after each diaper change. The glans penis, which is normally dark red during healing, becomes covered with a yellow exudate in 24 hours. This is part of normal healing, not an infective process. No attempt is made to remove the exudate, which persists for 2 to 3 days. Parents should be taught to fanfold the diaper so that it does not press on the circumcised area. They should also be encouraged to change the diaper at least every 4 hours to prevent it from sticking to the penis.

DISCHARGE PLANNING AND TEACHING

Infant care activities can cause much anxiety for the new parent (see Plan of Care). The kind of support given by the nursing staff members can be an important factor in determining whether new mothers seek and accept help in the future. Whether this is the woman's or parents' first baby, or an adolescent whose mother will be the primary caregiver, or whether they attended parenthood preparation classes, parents appreciate anticipatory guidance in the care of their infant. The nurse should not try to cover all the content at one time because the parents can be overwhelmed by too much information and become anxious. However, because of the early discharge of new mothers that is currently common practice, it may be a problem for the nurse to impart all of the information necessary. As a result, many institutions have developed home visitation programs that take the necessary teaching to the new parents (see Chapter 25), although the hospital nurse still provides most of the essential information for newborn care.

The care of the newborn is shared by the nurse and the parents, with the nurse acting as teacher and support person. As soon as the mother feels physically able, she is encouraged to participate in her infant's care. The care given the infant is supervised, and the parents are encouraged to ask questions. The mother's need for knowledge and the factors that may hinder her learning are determined through questioning and observation. The content taught and teaching aids used should be in keeping with the mother's level of understanding. Films and tapes can be valuable time-savers as teaching tools. Most hospitals also provide parents with written instructions for infant care.

To set priorities for teaching, the nurse follows parental cues. Knowledge deficits should be identified before teaching begins. Normal growth and development and the changing needs of the infant (e.g., for stimulation, exercise, and social contacts), as well as the following topics should be included during the discharge planning session with parents.

Temperature

The following topics should be reviewed:

- The causes of an elevated body temperature (e.g., exercise, cold stress with resultant vasoconstriction, minimum response to infection) and the body's response to extremes in environmental temperature
- Signs to be reported, such as high or low temperatures with accompanying fussiness, stuffy nose, lethargy, irritability, poor feeding, and crying
- Ways to promote normal body temperature, such as giving a warm tub bath, dressing the infant appropriately for the air temperature, and protecting the infant from long exposure to sunlight
- The use of warm wraps or extra blankets in cold weather
- The method for taking the baby's axillary temperature

Feeding Schedules

Feeding practices and schedules for newborns are discussed in Chapter 28.

Elimination

A review includes the following reminders:

- Changes to be expected in the color of the stool (meconium to transitional to soft yellow/golden yellow) and the number of bowel evacuations, plus the odor of stools for breastfed and bottle-fed infants (see Chapter 28).
- The color of normal urine and the number of voidings (6 to 10) to expect each day.

Positioning and Holding

Positioning the infant on the right side after feeding promotes gastric emptying into the small intestine (see Fig. 27-2). Placing the infant in the crib in a side-lying position also promotes the drainage of mucus from the mouth and applies no pressure to the cord or the sensitive circumcised penis. The American Academy of Pediatrics

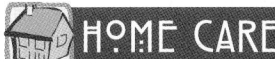
HOME CARE

Circumcision

- Wash hands before touching the newly circumcised penis.

CHECK FOR BLEEDING

- Check circumcision for bleeding every hour for the first 12 hours after the procedure.
- If bleeding occurs, apply gentle pressure with a folded sterile gauze square. If bleeding does not stop with pressure, notify primary health care provider.

OBSERVE FOR URINATION

- Check to see that the infant urinates after being circumcised.
- Infant should have a wet diaper 6 to 10 times per 24 hours.

KEEP AREA CLEAN

- Change diaper and inspect circumcision at least every 4 hours.
- Wash penis gently with warm water to remove urine and feces. Apply petrolatum to the glans with each diaper change (omit petrolatum if Plastibell was used).
- Use soap only after circumcision is healed.
- Fanfold diaper to prevent pressure on the circumcised area.

CHECK FOR INFECTION

- Glans penis is dark red after circumcision, then becomes covered with yellow exudate in 24 hours. This is normal and will persist for 2 to 3 days. Do not attempt to remove it.
- Redness, swelling, or discharge indicate infection. Notify primary health care provider if you think the circumcision area is infected.

PROVIDE COMFORT

- Circumcision is painful. Handle the area gently.
- Provide extra holding, feeding, and opportunities for nonnutritive sucking for a day or two.

advises against placing an infant in the prone position during the first few months of life; the supine position is recommended (AAP, 1996). The placement of infants in prone positions has been associated with an increased incidence of sudden infant death syndrome (SIDS).

Anatomically the infant's shape—barrel chest and flat, curveless spine—makes it easy for the child to roll when startled. The placement of a folded or rolled blanket against the infant's spine will keep it from rolling to the supine position and promote a feeling of security. Care must be taken to prevent the infant from rolling off of flat, unguarded surfaces. When an infant is on such a surface, the parent or nurse who must turn away from the infant even for a moment should always keep one hand placed securely on the infant.

The infant is always held securely with its head supported because newborns are unable to maintain an erect head posture for more than a few moments. Fig. 27-25 illustrates various positions for holding an infant with adequate support.

Using the Bulb Syringe

The parents should be shown the way to use the bulb syringe and asked to demonstrate the technique back to the nurse. If the infant has excess mucus in the respiratory tract, the nurse or parent may need to aspirate the mouth and nasal passages with a bulb syringe. The infant who is coughing and choking on the secretions should be supported with its head downward. The mouth is suctioned first because, if the nasal passages are suctioned first, the infant may inhale the pharyngeal secretions by gasping when the nares are touched. The bulb is compressed and inserted into one side of the mouth (see Fig. 27-3). The center of the

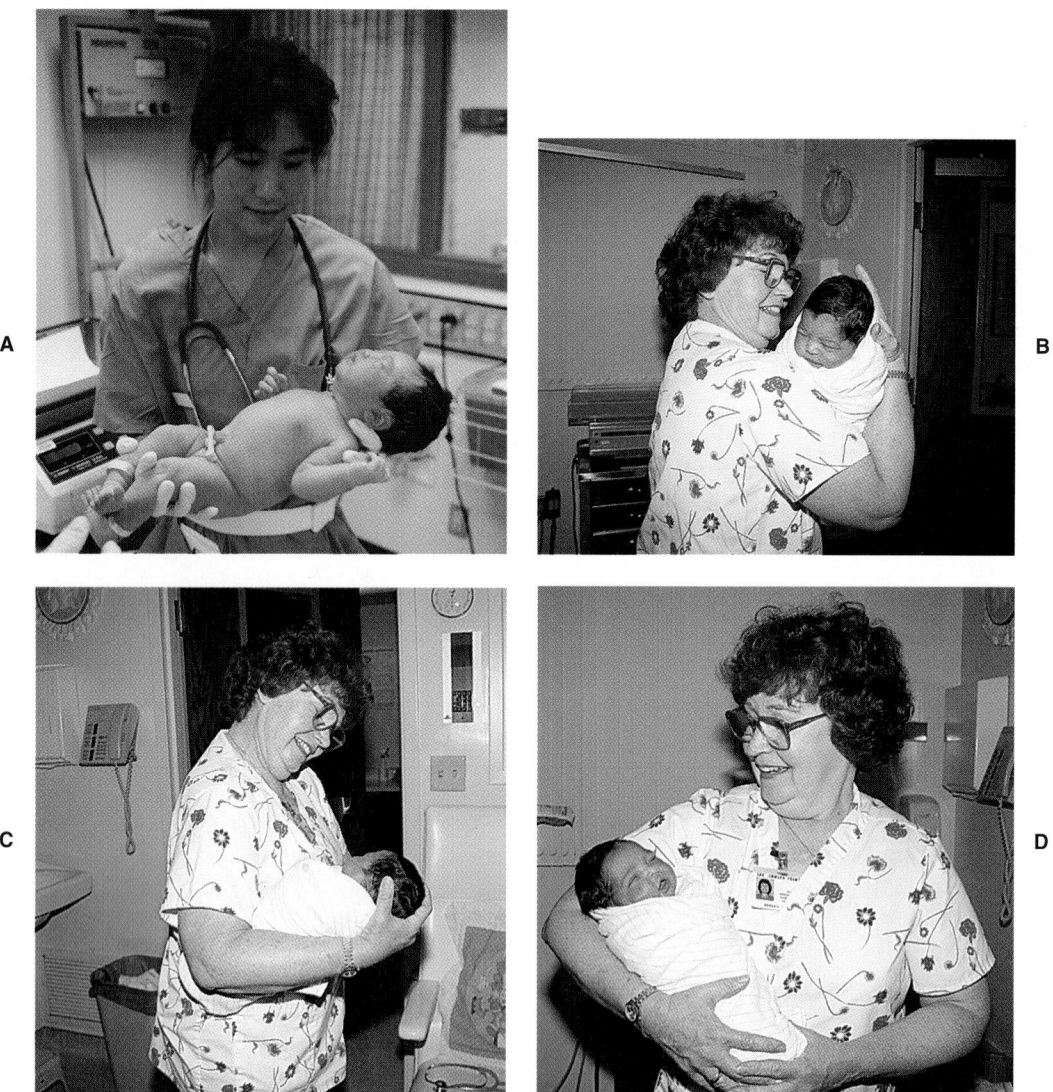

Fig. 27-25 Holding baby securely with support for head. **A,** Holding infant while moving infant from one place to another. Baby is undressed to show posture. **B,** Holding baby upright in "burping" position. **C,** "Football" hold. **D,** Cradling hold. (*A courtesy Kim Molloy, Knoxville, IA; **B, C,** and **D** courtesy Marjorie Pyle, RNC, Lifecircle, Costa Mesa, CA.*)

infant's mouth should be avoided, however, because this could stimulate the gag reflex. The nasal passages are then suctioned one nostril at a time. When the infant's cry does not sound as though it were coming through mucus or a bubble, suctioning can be stopped. It is current practice to keep the bulb syringe in the infant's crib.

Safety: Use of Car Seat

Infants should travel only in federally approved rear-facing safety seats secured in the rear seat (Fig. 27-26). The safest area of the car is in the back seat. A car seat that faces the rear gives the best protection for the disproportionately weak neck and heavy head of an infant. In this position, the force of a frontal crash is spread over the head, neck, and back; the back of the car seat supports the spine.

NURSE ALERT *Infants should use a rear-facing car seat from birth to 20 pounds and to 1 year of age.*

The car seat is secured using the vehicle seat belt; the infant is secured using the harness system in the car seat. If the infant must ride in the front seat, the air bag must be turned off to prevent injury from the air bag.

NURSE ALERT *In cars equipped with air bags, rear-facing infant seats must not be placed in the front seat. Serious injury can occur if the air bag inflates because these types of infant seats fit closer to the dashboard (Fig. 27-27).**

Infants less than 37 weeks of gestation should be observed in a car seat for a period of time before discharge. The infant is monitored for apnea, bradycardia and a decrease in SaO₂. It may be necessary to place blanket rolls on either side of the infant for support of the head and trunk. To prevent slumping, the back-to-crotch strap distance should be 14 cm. In addition, a rolled blanket can be placed between the infant and the crotch strap.

Nonnutritive Sucking

Sucking is the infant's chief pleasure. However, sucking may not be satisfied by breastfeeding or formula-feeding alone (Wong, 1999). In fact, it is such a strong need that infants who are deprived of sucking, such as those with a cleft lip, will suck on their tongue. Some newborns are born with sucking pads on their fingers that developed during in utero sucking. Several benefits of nonnutritive sucking have been documented, such as an increased weight gain in premature infants and decreased crying (Treloar, 1994).

*Air bag safety sheets are available from the American Academy of Pediatrics, 141 Northwest Point Blvd., Elk Grove Village, IL 60007; 800-433-9016; fax (847) 228-1281; www.aap.org.

Problems arise when parents are concerned about the sucking of fingers, thumb, or pacifier and try to restrain this natural tendency. Before giving advice, nurses should investigate the parents' feelings and base the guidance they give on the information elicited. For example, some parents may see no problem with the use of a finger but may find the use of a pacifier objectionable. In general, there is no need to restrain either practice, unless thumb sucking persists past 4 years of age or past the time when the permanent

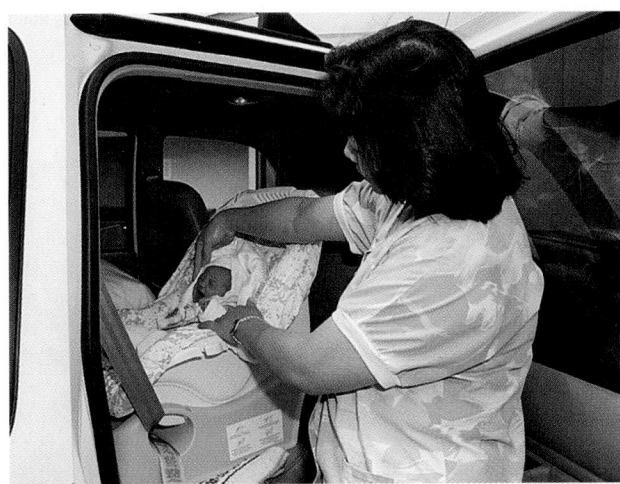

Fig. 27-26 Rear-facing infant seat in rear seat of car. Infant is placed in seat when going home from hospital. *(Courtesy Marjorie Pyle, RNC, Lifecircle, Costa Mesa, CA.)*

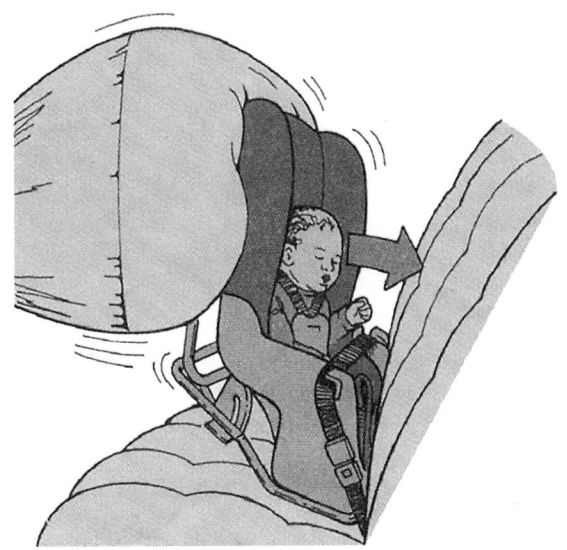

Fig. 27-27 An airbag could strike a child safety seat causing serious injury to the child. *(Redrawn from Health Alert. [1994]. AAP News 10[4], 22. In Wong, D. [1999]. Whaley & Wong's nursing care of infants and children [6th ed.]. St. Louis: Mosby.)*

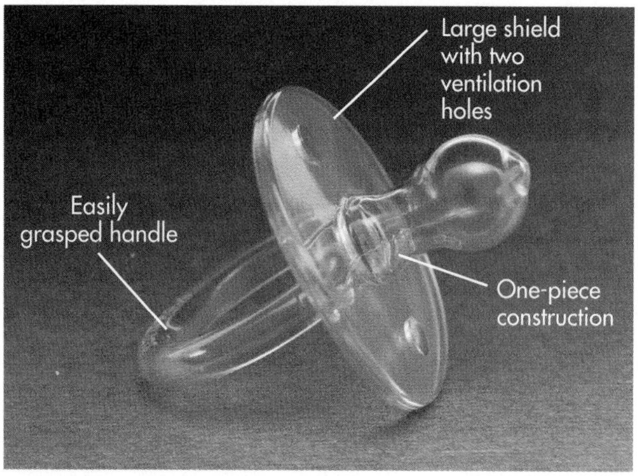

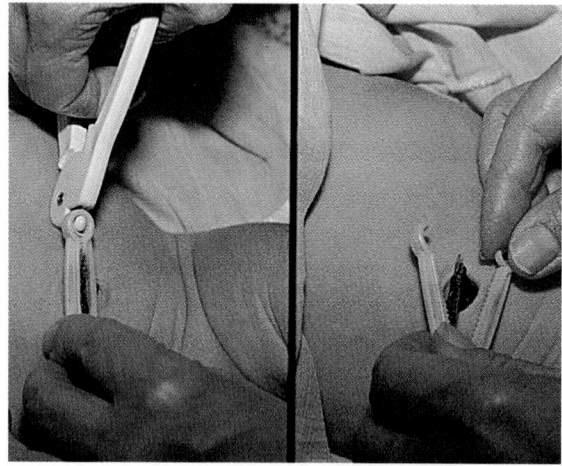

Fig. 27-28 Design of safe pacifier. *(From Wong, D. [1999]. Whaley & Wong's nursing care of infants and children [6th ed.]. St. Louis: Mosby.)*

Fig. 27-29 Using special scissors, remove clamp after cord dries (about 24 hours). *(Courtesy Marjorie Pyle, RNC, Lifecircle, Costa Mesa, CA.)*

teeth erupt. Parents are advised to consult with their pediatrician and pediatric nurse-practitioner about this topic.

To decrease an infant's dependence on nonnutritive sucking, the feeding time can be prolonged. One way of doing this in bottle-fed infants is to use a small-holed, firm nipple because this necessitates stronger sucking and slows the feeding. A parent's excessive use of the pacifier to calm the child should also be explored, however. It is not unusual for parents to place a pacifier in their infant's mouth as soon as it begins to cry, thus only reinforcing a pattern of distress-relief.

If parents choose to let their child use a pacifier, they need to be made aware of certain safety considerations before purchasing one. A homemade or poorly designed pacifier can be dangerous because the entire object may be aspirated if it is small or a portion may become lodged in the pharynx. Improvised pacifiers, such as those commonly made in hospitals from a padded nipple, also pose dangers because the nipple may separate from the plastic collar and be aspirated. In addition, parents may continue to offer this pacifier to the infant at home rather than obtaining a more appropriate one. Safe pacifiers should be made of one piece that includes a shield or flange that is large enough to prevent entry into the mouth and a handle that can be grasped (Fig. 27-28).

Sponge Bathing, Cord Care, and Skin Care
Bathing

Bathing serves a number of purposes. It provides opportunities for (1) completely cleansing the infant, (2) observing the infant's condition, (3) promoting comfort, and (4) parent-child-family socializing.

An important consideration in skin cleansing is the preservation of the skin's **acid mantle,** which is formed from the uppermost horny layer of the epidermis, sweat, superficial fat, metabolic products, and external substances such as amniotic fluid, and microorganisms. At birth the skin has a pH of 6.34. Within 4 days, however, the pH of the newborn's skin surface falls to within the bacteriostatic range (pH <5) (Krebs, 1998). Consequently, only plain warm water should be used for the bath during that 4-day period. Alkaline soaps such as Ivory, oils, powder, and lotions should not be used during this time because they alter the acid mantle, thus creating a medium for bacterial growth. Although the sponging technique is generally used, bathing the newborn by immersion has been found to allow less heat loss and provoke less crying but is not advised until the umbilical cord falls off.

Until the initial bath is completed, personnel must wear gloves whenever they handle the newborn.

The umbilical cord begins to dry, shrivel, and blacken by the second or third day of life. The umbilicus should be inspected frequently for signs of infection (foul odor, redness, and purulent drainage), granuloma (small, red, raw-appearing polyp where the umbilical cord separates), bleeding, and discharge. The cord clamp is removed when the cord is dry, in about 24 hours (Fig. 27-29). The cord normally falls off in 10 to 14 days after birth.

In the hospital the umbilical cord is usually cleaned with alcohol or other designated solution with each assessment and with diaper changes if the cord is moist (see Research box).

See the accompanying Home Care box for information regarding sponge bathing, skin care, cord care, cutting nails, and dressing the infant.

Infant Follow-up Care

With shorter hospital stays, the focus and site of infant care is changing. Home care may either be provided by a nurse as part of the follow-up of clients or be rendered through a visiting nurse or community health nurse referral service. For infants discharged early, newborn home care is essential (see Home Care box) (see also Chapter 25).

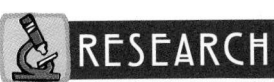

RESEARCH

Alcohol Versus Natural Drying for Newborn Cord Care

Historically, the practice of cleaning the newborn cord with alcohol has been observed throughout North America and stemmed from the belief that alcohol protected the cord from infection and helped it fall off faster. No evidence supported this belief. While moving forward to a more natural, family-centered approach, health care providers have continued some historical practices without scientific justification. The current research study compared infection rates, cord separation time, maternal comfort, and cost of alcohol cleaning with those of the nonintervention of natural drying.

One thousand eight hundred eleven newborns, from birth until separation of the cord, were randomized to either (1) umbilical cleansing with 70% isopropyl alcohol at each diaper change or (2) natural drying of the umbilical site without special treatment.

No newborn in either group developed a cord infection. Primary care providers obtained cultures for cord concerns in 32 newborns (1.8%), with colonization for normal flora, *Staphylococcus aureus,* and group B *Streptococcus* proportionately equal in alcohol and air dry groups. Cord separation time was statistically significant (alcohol group, 9.8 days; natural drying group, 8.16 days; t = 8.9; p = <.001).

Mothers described comfort with cord care and relief with cord separation. Costs of alcohol drying while in the hospital were greater than that of natural drying.

In conclusion, evidence from this research study does not support continued use of alcohol for newborn cord care. Health care providers need to explain the normal process of cord separation, including appearance and possible odor, to all parents. Nurses should also continue to develop evidence to support or eliminate unproven historical practices.

CLINICAL APPLICATION

The results of this study support discontinuing the use of alcohol for newborn cord care. The evaluation and possible elimination of such historically accepted practices must continue to be the focus of nursing research. Moving from intervention to nonintervention, particularly in a healthy population, speaks to the healthy, naturalistic approach to care supported by nurses. Only through continued efforts to examine our assumptions about historic health care routines will we be able to demonstrate evidence-based practice and to advance nursing care.

Source: Dore, S. et al. (1998). Alcohol versus natural drying for newborn cord care. *J Obstet Gynecol Neonatal Nurs* 27(6), 621-627.

HOME CARE

Sponge Bathing

FITTING BATHS INTO FAMILY'S SCHEDULE

Give a bath at any time convenient to you but not immediately after a feeding period because the increased handling may cause regurgitation.

PREVENTING HEAT LOSS

The temperature of the room should be 24° C (75° F), and the bathing area should be free of drafts.

Control heat loss during the bath to conserve the infant's energy. Bathing the infant quickly, exposing only a portion of the body at a time, and thorough drying are all parts of the bathing technique.

GATHERING SUPPLIES AND CLOTHING BEFORE STARTING

Clothing suitable for wearing indoors: diaper, shirt; stretch suit or nightgown optional
Unscented, mild soap
Pins, if needed for diaper, closed and placed well out of baby's reach
Cotton balls
Towels for drying infant and a clean washcloth
Receiving blanket
Tub for water or use a sink

BATHING THE BABY

Bring infant to bathing area when all supplies are ready. *Never leave the infant alone on bath table or in bath water, not even for a second!* If you have to leave, take the infant with you or put back into crib.

Test temperature of the water. It should feel pleasantly warm to the inner wrist 36.6° to 37.2° C (98° to 99° F).

Do not hold infant under running water—water temperature may change, and infant may be scalded or chilled rapidly.

Wash infant's head before unwrapping and undressing to prevent heat loss.

Cleanse the eyes from the inner canthus outward, using separate parts of a clean washcloth for each eye. For the first 2 to 3 days there may be a discharge resulting from the reaction of the conjunctiva to the substance (erythromycin) used as a prophylactic measure against infection. Any discharge should be considered abnormal and reported to the health care provider.

Wash the scalp with water and mild soap; rinse well and dry thoroughly (Fig. 27-30). Scalp desquamation, called *cradle cap,* often can be prevented by removing any scales with a fine-toothed comb or brush after washing. If condition persists, the health care provider may prescribe an ointment to massage into the scalp.

Continued

HOME CARE—CONT'D

Sponge Bathing—cont'd

Creases under the chin and arms and in the groin may need daily cleansing. The crease under the chin may be exposed by elevating the infant's shoulders 5 cm and letting the head drop back.

Cleanse ears and nose with twists of moistened cotton or a corner of the washcloth. Do not use cotton-tipped swabs because they may cause injury.

Undress baby and wash body and arms and legs. Pat dry gently. Baby may be tub bathed after the cord drops off and umbilicus and circumcised penis are completely healed.

PREVENTING SKIN TRAUMA

The fragile skin can be injured by too vigorous cleansing.

If stool or other debris has dried and caked on the skin, soak the area to remove it. Do not attempt to rub it off, because abrasion may result. Gentleness, patting dry rather than rubbing, and use of a mild soap without perfumes or coloring are recommended. Chemicals in the coloring and perfume can cause rashes on sensitive skin.

CARE OF THE CORD

Use a cotton swab. Dip swab in solution the health care provider has ordered and cleanse around base of the cord where it joins the skin. Notify the health care provider of any odor, discharge, or skin inflammation around the cord. The clamp is removed when the cord is dry (approximately 24 hours). The diaper should not cover the cord because a wet or soiled diaper will slow or prevent drying of the cord and foster infection. When the cord drops off after a week to 10 days, small drops of blood may be seen when the baby cries. This will heal by itself. It is not dangerous.

CARE OF HANDS AND FEET

Wash and dry between the fingers and toes.

Do not cut fingernails and toenails immediately after birth. The nails have to grow out far enough from the skin so that the skin is not cut by mistake. If the baby scratches himself or herself, apply loosely fitted mitts over each of the baby's hands. Do so as a last resort, however, because it interferes with the baby's ability for self-consolation sucking on thumb or finger. When the nails have grown, the fingernails and toenails can be cut more easily with manicure scissors (preferably scissors with rounded tips) when the infant is asleep. Nails should be kept short.

CLEANSING GENITALS

Cleanse the genitals of infants daily and after voiding or defecating. For girls, the genitals may be cleansed by separating the labia and gently washing from the pubic area to the anus. For uncircumcised boys, gently pull back (retract) the foreskin. Stop when resistance is felt. Wash and rinse the tip (glans) with soap and warm water and replace the foreskin. The foreskin must be returned to its original position to prevent constriction and swelling. In most newborns the inner layer of the foreskin adheres to the glans and the foreskin cannot be retracted. By the age of 3 years in 90% of boys, the foreskin can be retracted easily without causing pain or trauma. For others, the foreskin is not retractable until adolescence. As soon as the foreskin is partly retractable and the child is old enough, he can be taught self-care. Once healed, the circumcised penis does not require any special care other than cleansing with diaper changes.

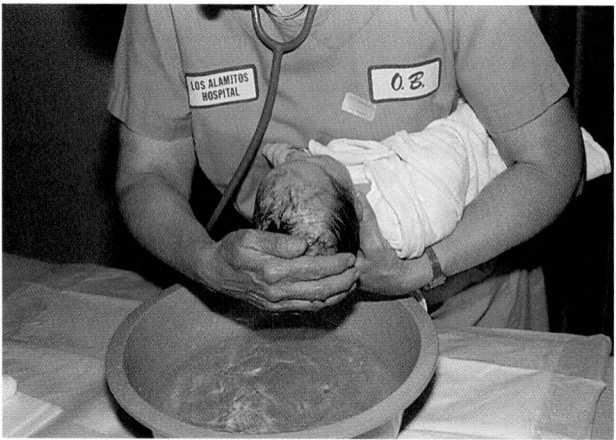

Fig. 27-30 Wash hair with baby wrapped to prevent heat loss from wet scalp. *(Courtesy Marjorie Pyle, RNC, Lifecircle, Costa Mesa, CA.)*

Parents should plan for their infant's health follow-up care at the following ages: 2 to 4 weeks of age, then every 2 months until 6 to 7 months of age, then every 3 months until 18 months, at 2 years, at 3 years, at preschool, and every 2 years thereafter.

Immunizations

The schedule for immunizations should be reviewed with the parents. HBV (hepatitis B) vaccine is currently administered to newborns before hospital discharge with parental permission. Please refer to Chapter 25 for a complete discussion of infant immunizations.

Evaluation

The nurse can be reasonably assured that care was effective to the extent that the expected outcomes for care have been achieved.

HOME CARE

Newborn Home Care Following Early Discharge

Wet diapers: 6 to 10 per day

Breastfeeding: Successful latch-on and feeding every 1½ to 3 hr daily

Formula feeding: Successfully, voiding as noted above, taking 3 to 4 oz every 3 to 4 hr daily

Circumcision: Wash with warm water only; yellow exudate forming, nonbleeding, Plastibell intact 48 hr

Stools: At least one every 48 hr (bottle-feeding) or two to three per day (breastfeeding)

Color: Pink to ruddy when crying; pink centrally when at rest or asleep

Activity: Has four to five wakeful periods per day and alerts to environmental sounds and voices.

Jaundice: Physiologic jaundice (not appearing in first 24 hr), feeding, voiding, and stooling as noted above or practitioner notification for suspicion of pathologic jaundice (appears within 24 hr of birth, ABO/Rh problem suspected); decreased activity; poor feeding; dark orange skin color persisting beyond fifth day in light-skinned newborn

Cord: Kept above diaper line; nonodorous; drying

Vital signs: Heart rate 120 to 140 beats/min at rest; respiratory rate 30 to 55 at rest without evidence of sternal retractions, grunting, or nasal flaring; temperature 36.5° to 37.2° C (97.3° to 98.6° F) axillary

Position of sleep: Back

From Wong, D. (1999). *Whaley & Wong's nursing care of infants and children* (6th ed.). St. Louis: Mosby.
*Any deviation from the above and/or suspicion of poor newborn adaptation should be reported to the practitioner at once.

KEY POINTS

- SGA infants are considered at risk because of fetal growth restriction.

- The high incidence of nonreassuring fetal status among postmature infants is related to the progressive placental insufficiency that occurs in a postdate pregnancy.

- Providing a protective environment is a key responsibility of the nurse and includes such measures as careful identification procedures, restraining techniques, ways to prevent infection, and support of physiologic functions.

- Maintenance of adequate ventilation includes ensuring an adequate airway and body temperature within the normal range.

- Parent education is a major responsibility of the nurse and includes the involvement of parents in all phases of the nursing process.

- Circumcision is an elective surgical procedure.

- The newborn has social, as well as physical, needs.

- Parent education is a major responsibility of the nurse and includes involvement of parents in all phases of the nursing process.

- Parents appreciate being given anticipatory guidance in the care of their newborn, whether or not it is their first child.

CRITICAL THINKING EXERCISES

1 *Prepare and conduct one 20-minute class in infant care for parents. Before the class, prepare a written teaching plan that includes an assessment of clients' learning needs, a teaching-learning diagnosis, a plan with prioritized client-centered goals, content and teaching methods with rationale, and evaluative criteria.*

2 *Prepare a display on SIDS and infant sleep position for a local pediatric or well-baby clinic. Decide how you will incorporate information, keeping in mind the level of education and ethnicity of parents who use the clinic.*

References

American Academy of Pediatrics (AAP). (1989). Report of the task force on circumcision. *Pediatrics 84*(4), 388-391.

American Academy of Pediatrics (AAP). (1996). Task force on infant positioning: Positioning and sudden infant death syndrome (SIDS) update. *Pediatrics 98*(6), 1216-1218.

American Academy of Pediatrics Provisional Committee for Quality Improvement and Subcommittee on Hyperbilirubinemia. (1994). Practice parameter: Management of hyperbilirubinemia in the healthy term newborn. *Pediatrics 94*(4 Pt. 1), 558.

Anand, K., Grunau, R., & Oberlander, T. (1997). Developmental character and long-term consequences of pain in infants and children. *Child and Adolescent Psychiatric Clinics of North America 6*(4), 703-724.

Ballard, J., Novak, K., & Driver, M. (1979). A simplified score for assessment of fetal maturity of newly born infants. *J Pediatr 95*(5 Pt. 1), 769-774.

Ballard, J. et al. (1991). New Ballard score, expanded to include extremely premature infants. *J Pediatr* 119(3), 417-423.

Battaglia, F., & Lubchenco, L. (1967). A practical classification of newborn infants by weight and gestational age. *J Pediatr* 71(2), 159-163.

Cloherty, J., & Stark, A. (1997). *Manual of neonatal care* (4th ed.). Boston: Little, Brown.

Craig, K., & Grunau, R. (1993). Neonatal pain perception and behavioral measurement. In K. Anand & P. McGrath (Eds). *Pain in neonates*. Amsterdam: Elsevier.

Donaher-Wagner, B., & Braun, D. (1992). Infant cardiopulmonary resuscitation for expectant and new parents, *MCN Am J Matern Child Nurs* 17(1), 27-28.

Dore, A. et al. (1998). Alcohol versus natural drying for newborn cord care. *J Obstet Gynecol Neonatal Nurs* 27(6), 621-627.

Dubowitz, L., Dubowitz, V., & Goldberg, C. (1970). Gestational age of the newborn. *J Pedatr* 77(1), 1-10.

Fanaroff, A., & Martin, R. (1997). *Neonatal-perinatal medicine: Diseases of the fetus and infant* (6th ed.). St. Louis: Mosby.

Franck, L. (1998). Identification, management, and prevention of pain in the neonate. In C. Kenner, J.W. Lott, & A.A. Flandermeyer (Eds.). *Comprehensive neonatal nursing: A physiologic perspective (2nd ed.)*. Philadelphia: W.B. Saunders.

Franck, L., & Gregory, G. (1993). Clinical evaluation and treatment of infant pain in the neonatal intensive care unit. In M. Schechter, C. Berde, & M. Yaster (Eds.). *Pain in infants, children and adolescents*. Baltimore: Williams & Wilkins.

Frank, S., Esch, J., & Margeson, N. (1998). Mandatory HIV testing of newborns: The impact on women. *Am J Nurs* 98(10), 49-51.

Geissler, E. (1994). *Pocket guide to cultural assessment*. St. Louis: Mosby.

Hadjistavropoulos, H. et al. (1997). Judging pain in infants: Behavioural, contextual, and developmental determinants. *Pain* 73(3), 319-324.

Korones, S. (1995). *High-risk newborn infants: The basis for intensive care* (5th ed.). St. Louis: Mosby.

Krebs, T. (1998). Cord care: Is it necessary? *Mother Baby J* 3(2), 5-12, 18-20.

Lawrence, J. et al. (1993). The development of a tool to assess neonatal pain. *Neonatal Netw* 12(6), 59.

Letko, M. (1996). Understanding the Apgar score. *J Obstet Gynecol Neonatal Nurs* 25(4), 299-303.

Lubchenco, L., Hansman, C., & Boyd, E. (1966). Intrauterine growth in length and head circumference as estimated from live births at gestational ages from 26-42 weeks. *J Pediatr* 37(3), 403-408.

Lynam, L. (1995). Research utilization: Nonpharmacological management of pain in neonates. *Neonatal Netw* 14(5), 59-62.

March of Dimes (1994). *Public health information sheet: Newborn screening tests*. White Plains, NY: March of Dimes.

McLaughlin, C. et al. (1993). Neonatal pain: A comprehensive survey of attitudes and practices. *Journal of Pain and Symptom Management* 8(1), 7-16.

Meehan, R. (1998). Heelsticks in neonates for capillary blood sampling. *Neonatal Netw* 17(1), 17-24.

Mohan, C. et al. (1998). Comparison of analgesics in ameliorating the pain of circumcision. *J Perinat* 18(1), 13-14.

O'Doherty, N. (1986). *Neonatology: Micro atlas of the newborn*. Nutley, NJ: Hoffman-La Roche.

Paes, B. et al. (1993). A comparative study of heelstick devices for infant blood collection. *Am J Dis Child* 147, 346-348.

Penny-MacGillivary, T. (1996). A newborn's first bath: When? *J Obstet Gynecol Neonatal Nurs* 25(6), 481-487.

Snapp, B. (1996). Hemorrhagic disease of the newborn and vitamin K. *Mother Baby J* 1(4), 17-23.

Stevens-Simon, C. et al. (1989). Effects of race on validity of clinical estimates of gestational age. *J Pediatr* 115(6), 1000-1002.

Taddio, A. et al. (1998). A systematic review of lidocaine-prilocaine cream (EMLA) in the treatment of acute pain in neonates. *Pediatrics* 101(2), E1.

Tappero, E., & Honeyfield, M. (1996). Physical assessment of the newborn: A comprehensive approach to the art of physical examination. *Mother Baby J* 1(1), 39-45.

Treloar, D. (1994). The effect of nonnutritive sucking on oxygenation in healthy, crying full-term infants. *Appl Nurs Res* 7, 52-58.

Williamson, M. (1997). Circumcision anesthesia: A study of nursing implications for dorsal penile nerve block. *Pediatr Nurs* 23, 59-63.

Witter, F., & Keith, L. (1993). *Textbook of prematurity: Antecedents, treatment and outcome*. Boston: Little, Brown.

Wong, D. (1999). *Whaley and Wong's nursing care of infants and children* (6th ed.). St. Louis: Mosby.

Wright, I., Brown, A., & Davidson-Mundt, A. (1992). Newborn screening: The miracle and the challenge. *J Pediatr Nurs* 7(1), 26-42.

28

www.mosby.com/Merlin/Lowdermilk/MatWmnHlth

Newborn Nutrition and Feeding

Kathryn Rhodes Alden

LEARNING OBJECTIVES

- Define the key terms.
- List newborn feeding-readiness cues.
- Describe current recommendations for feeding infants.
- Discuss benefits of breastfeeding for infants, mothers, families, and society.
- Explain the nurse's role in helping families to choose an infant feeding method.
- Describe nutritional needs of infants.
- Describe the anatomy and physiology of breastfeeding.
- Explain the species specificity of human breast milk and its uniqueness for the infant.

- Identify nursing interventions to facilitate and promote successful breastfeeding.
- List signs of adequate intake in the breastfed infant.
- Develop a nursing plan of care for the breastfeeding mother and infant.
- Identify common problems associated with breastfeeding and nursing interventions to help resolve them.
- List the types of commercial infant formula, advantages of each, and appropriate methods of preparation.
- Discuss client teaching for the formula-feeding family.
- Identify topics for nursing research related to newborn nutrition and feeding.

KEY TERMS

colostrum
demand feeding
engorgement
feeding-readiness cues
growth spurts
inverted nipples
lactation consultant
lactiferous ducts

lactiferous sinuses
lactogenesis
latch-on
let-down reflex
mastitis
milk ejection reflex (MER)
monilial infection
nipple confusion

nipple erection reflex
oxytocin
physiologic jaundice
plugged milk duct
prolactin
rooting
supply-meets-demand system

 In the minds of many, nutrition and nurturing are synonymous. One's effectiveness as a parent is often judged on the growth and development of the infant, which is largely dependent on proper nutrition. Infant feeding is more than the provision of nutrition; it represents opportunity for social, psychologic, and even educational interaction between parent and infant. Thus the selection of an infant feeding method is an emotion-laden decision for most prospective parents who are seeking optimal health and well-being for their offspring.

Through preconception and prenatal education and counseling, nurses play an instrumental role in assisting parents with the selection of an infant feeding method. They should be aware that this decision is influenced by a variety of physical, psychologic, social, cultural, and economic factors. In addition, nurses must be knowledgeable about the advantages and disadvantages of breastfeeding and formula feeding as they provide information to expectant parents. Whether the parents choose to breastfeed or formula feed, nurses provide support and ongoing education. Education of parents is necessarily based on current research findings and standards of practice.

Skillful health supervision of infants requires that the nurse be knowledgeable about nutritional needs and expectations for normal growth and development. This chapter focuses on infant nutrition during the first 6 months of life with emphasis on the neonatal period, when feeding practices and patterns are being established.

RECOMMENDED INFANT NUTRITION

In 1997 the American Academy of Pediatrics (AAP) Work Group on Breastfeeding published the following recommendations for infant nutrition:

"Exclusive breastfeeding is ideal nutrition and sufficient to support optimal growth and development for approximately the first 6 months after birth. Infants weaned before 12 months of age should not receive cow's milk feedings but should receive iron-fortified infant formulas. Gradual introduction of iron-enriched solid foods in the second half of the first year should complement the breast milk diet. It is recommended that breastfeeding continue for at least 12 months, and thereafter for as long as mutually desired."

BREASTFEEDING RATES

Based on the AAP's recommendation, it is surprising that just over half of the babies born in the United States are breastfed. We are currently experiencing a resurgence in breastfeeding initiation rates, as well as in continuance of breastfeeding through the first 6 months. This increase has been gradual, but certain. After a low of 26.5% in 1970, breastfeeding initiation rates climbed to 58% in 1985, only to gradually decline to 51.5% in 1990. Since that time, breastfeeding rates have steadily risen to 59.4% in 1995. Likewise, the number of infants still breastfeeding at 6 months has increased from 14.1% in 1970 to 20.8% in 1995 (Ryan, 1997).

Breastfeeding rates have increased across all demographic groups, although the most significant increases are seen among women who have historically been less likely to breastfeed. These individuals are typically young (younger than 25 years of age), lower-income, African-American primiparas with grade school education or less, employed full time outside the home, residing in the South Atlantic region of the United States, mothers of low-birth-weight infants, and enrolled in the Women, Infants, and Children (WIC) program (Ryan, 1997).

The characteristics of women most likely to breastfeed have remained consistent over the years. These women are multiparas, college educated, with higher incomes, not employed outside the home, residents of western states, not participating in the WIC program, and mothers of newborns with normal birth weights (Ryan, 1997).

BENEFITS OF BREASTFEEDING

Human milk is designed specifically for human infants and is nutritionally superior to any alternative. Breast milk is considered a living tissue because it contains almost as many live cells as blood. It is bacteriologically safe and always fresh. The nutrients in breast milk are more easily absorbed than those in formula.

Numerous research studies have identified the beneficial effects of human milk for infants during the first year of life. Long-term epidemiologic studies have shown that these benefits do not cease when the infant is weaned, but instead extend into childhood and beyond. Breastfeeding has many advantages for mothers, for families, and for society in general. In discussing the benefits of breastfeeding with parents, it is critical that nurses and other health care professionals have a thorough understanding of these benefits from both a physiologic and a psychosocial perspective. Benefits for the infant include the following:

- Breast milk enhances maturation of the gastrointestinal (GI) tract and contains immune factors that contribute to a lower incidence of diarrheal illness, necrotizing enterocolitis, Crohn's disease, and celiac disease (Barnard, 1997; Dewey, Heinig, & Nommsen-Rivers, 1995; Fuchs, Victoria, & Martines, 1996; Lopez-Alarcon, Villalpando, & Fajardo, 1997; Scariati, Grummer-Strawn, & Fein, 1997).
- Breastfed infants receive specific antibodies and cell-mediated immunologic factors that help protect against otitis media, respiratory illnesses such as respiratory syncytial virus (RSV) and pneumonia, urinary tract infections, bacteremia, and bacterial meningitis (Cushing et al., 1998; Dewey et al., 1995; Lopez-Alarcon et al., 1997; Sassen, Brand, & Grote, 1994).
- There is a lower incidence of allergies among infants from families at high risk. Allergic manifestations occur at a greater rate and are more severe in formula-fed infants (Halken & Host, 1996; Saarinen & Kajosaari, 1995).
- Breastfed infants are less likely to die from sudden infant death syndrome (SIDS) (Ford et al., 1993).
- Breast milk may have a protective effect against childhood lymphoma and insulin-dependent diabetes (Davis, 1998; Gerstein, 1994; Shu et al., 1995).
- Breast milk may enhance cognitive development

(Lucas et al., 1992; Lucas et al., 1994; Wang & Wu, 1996).

Maternal benefits include the following:

- Women who have breastfed have a decreased risk of ovarian, uterine, and breast cancer (Enger et al., 1998; Hirose et al., 1995; Rosenblatt & Thomas, 1995).
- Breastfeeding promotes uterine involution and is associated with a decreased risk of postpartum hemorrhage (Chua et al., 1994; Lawrence, 1999).
- Mothers who are breastfeeding tend to return to their prepregnancy weight more quickly (Dewey, Heinig, & Nommsen, 1993).
- Breastfeeding may provide some protection against the development of osteoporosis (Eisman, 1998; Melton et al., 1993).
- Breastfeeding provides a unique bonding experience and increases maternal role attainment (Lawrence, 1999).

Benefits to families and society include the following:

- Breastfeeding represents lower costs to families. The cost of formula far exceeds the cost of extra food for the lactating mother.
- Breastfeeding is convenient; there are no bottles or other necessary equipment to purchase or clean. Breastfed babies are portable; when traveling, there are fewer supplies to take along.
- Because breastfed infants have a lower incidence of illness and infection, health care costs are lower for families and federal, state, and local governments. Billions of dollars could be saved each year if more infants were breastfed. Less time is lost from work by parents who must stay home with sick infants, which is a benefit to employers (Riordan, 1997).
- Breastfeeding families who are eligible for WIC represent a cost savings to the government. It has been estimated that if 75% of infants within the United States WIC program were breastfed for 3 months, $4 million would be saved (Montgomery & Splett, 1997).
- Intangible benefits for families and society include increased quality of life through psychologic benefits for mothers and infants, increased mothering behaviors, and more free time for interaction with family and friends.

CHOOSING AN INFANT FEEDING METHOD

Women who elect to breastfeed their infants most often do so because they are aware of the benefits to the infant. Many are seeking the unique bonding experience between mother and infant that is characteristic of breastfeeding. The support of the partner and family is a major factor in the mother's decision to breastfeed and in her ability to do so successfully. Prenatal preparation ideally includes the

father of the baby, with information about benefits of breastfeeding and how he can participate in infant care and nurturing (Bar-Yam & Darby, 1997).

Parents who elect to formula feed often make this decision without complete information and understanding of the benefits of breastfeeding and the potential hazards of formula feeding. Numerous myths and misconceptions about breastfeeding influence women's decision making. Many women see bottle feeding as more convenient or less embarrassing than breastfeeding. Some lack confidence in their ability to produce an adequate quantity or quality of breast milk. Breastfeeding is seen by some women as incompatible with an active social life, or they think that it will prevent them from going back to work. There are significant societal barriers against breastfeeding in public. A major barrier for many women is the influence of family and friends; this is especially true for lower-income mothers, where bottle feeding is the norm.

To make an informed decision about an infant feeding method, parents must be presented with factual information about the nutritional and immunologic needs of the infant that *are* met by human milk, the potential benefits to the infant and the mother, and the inherent risks associated with infant formulas. The nurse must provide this information to parents in a nonjudgmental manner and respect their decision. Some health care professionals may attempt to avoid this responsibility with the rationalization that they do not want parents to feel guilty if they choose not to breastfeed. However, the nurse is required to give complete information about infant feeding to parents and to document having done so (see Research box).

The key to encouraging mothers to breastfeed is education, beginning as early as possible during pregnancy and even before pregnancy. Prenatal breastfeeding classes are an excellent vehicle to relay important information to expectant parents. Each encounter with an expectant mother is an opportunity to dispel myths, clarify misinformation, and address personal concerns. Connecting expectant mothers with women who are breastfeeding or have successfully breastfed and are from similar backgrounds may be helpful. Peer counseling programs, such as those instituted by WIC programs, are beneficial, particularly in lower socioeconomic groups, where bottle feeding is common (Arlotti et al., 1998).

The postnatal period is not too late to educate parents about the benefits of breastfeeding. For those women with limited access to health care, the postpartum period may provide the first opportunity for education about breastfeeding. Even women who have indicated the desire to bottle feed may benefit from information about the differences in formula and breast milk for their infants. Offering these women the chance to try breastfeeding with the assistance of a nurse may influence a change in infant feeding practices.

RESEARCH

Lactation Duration: Influences of Human Milk Replacements and Formula Samples on Women Planning Postpartum Employment

Although breastfeeding is recognized as the best method of infant feeding and offers multiple benefits to mother and child, only 54% of American women start breastfeeding and only 21% continue to breastfeed 5 to 6 months postpartum. Numerous research studies have shown that the use of pacifiers, feeding fluids other than breast milk, and receipt of formula samples are associated with shortened breastfeeding duration. Although distribution of formula samples and early oral supplemental feeding of the infant may shorten the length of lactation, there has been little research on the effects of these practices in working women, a group particularly vulnerable to premature cessation of lactation.

The purpose of this research was to examine the influences of human milk replacement and formula samples on duration of lactation in women planning employment during the first postpartum year. Fifty-three participants completed telephone interviews prenatally, at 6 weeks, 3 months, and 6 months postpartum.

During hospitalization, 19% of infants received formula; the incidence of breastfeeding at 6 weeks and duration of breastfeeding were significantly shorter in these infants compared with infants who were not fed formula. Fifty-nine percent of participants received formula samples from the hospital, 30% received samples from a physician's office, and 51% received samples by mail. Receipt of formula samples by mail was associated with reduced incidence of breastfeeding at 6 weeks and shortened duration of lactation. It was concluded that both early formula feeding and receipt of formula samples by mail are barriers to lactation in women employed outside the home.

CLINICAL APPLICATION

Some mothers perceived that formula offered to their newborns indicated that medical professionals prefer formula feeding over breastfeeding. Also, commercial hospital packs given to new mothers may negatively influence breastfeeding outcomes. Ethical concerns about administering oral fluids other than breast milk when no medical indication exists must also be explored by nurses. Providing similar lactation education programs for all health care professionals caring for expectant and breastfeeding mothers, both within and outside the hospital setting, may be useful in the protection, support, and promotion of breastfeeding.

Source: Chezem, J. et al. (1998). Lactation duration: Influences of human milk replacements and formula samples on women planning postpartum employment. *J Obstet Gynecol Neonatal Nurs* 27(6), 646-651.

It is the responsibility of the nurse and other health care professionals to promote feelings of competence and confidence in the breastfeeding mother and to reinforce the unequaled contribution she is making toward the health and well-being of her infant. To provide effective support for the mother, health care professionals must necessarily be knowledgeable about benefits of breastfeeding, the basic process of breastfeeding, breastfeeding management, and interventions for common problems (Box 28-1).

Cultural Influences on Infant Feeding

Cultural beliefs and practices are significant influences on infant feeding methods. While there are recognized cultural norms, one cannot assume that generalized observations about any cultural group hold true for all members of that group. Within the United States there are many regional and ethnic cultures. Dealing effectively with these groups requires that the nurse be knowledgeable about and sensitive to the cultural factors influencing infant feeding practices.

Persons who have immigrated to the United States from poorer countries often choose to formula feed their infants because they believe it is a better, more "modern" method.

Others adopt formula feeding because they want to adapt to American culture and perceive that it is the custom to bottle feed (Rassin et al., 1994).

As many as 50 of 120 cultures studied by Morse, Jehle, and Gamble (1990) typically do not give colostrum to newborns and begin breastfeeding after the milk has "come in." This is true for some Filipinos, Mexican-Americans, Vietnamese, Hmong, Koreans, and Nigerians. When breastfeeding is delayed until the milk is in, babies are given prelacteal food. In India, infants may be fed such liquids as honey, tea, water, or sugar water before the initiation of breastfeeding (Choudhry, 1997). Other cultures begin breastfeeding immediately and offer the breast each time the infant cries. Cultural attitudes regarding modesty and breastfeeding are important considerations.

Some cultures have specific beliefs and practices related to the mother's intake of foods that foster milk production. Korean mothers often eat seaweed soup and rice to enhance milk production. Hmong women believe that boiled chicken, rice, and hot water is the only appropriate nourishment during the first postpartum month. The balance between energy forces, hot and cold, or yin and yang is integral to the diet of the lactating mother. Hispanics,

BOX 28-1 **AWHONN's Guidelines for Breastfeeding Support**

- During pregnancy a breast assessment is performed that includes a breastfeeding history, a breast examination, and a medication use history.
- A prenatal plan of care is developed to prepare the woman for lactation.
- Immediately after birth, the newborn is kept with the mother when possible so that breastfeeding can be initiated when the newborn is most receptive.
- After birth:
  - Assistance with latch-on and positioning are given as needed.
  - Encouragement of frequent feedings is reinforced.
  - Discharge instructions for knowing criteria for successful breastfeeding are given.
  - Information about community resources for breastfeeding is given.
- Especially for premature and low-birth-weight infants, breastfeeding is encouraged.

From AWHONN. (1998). *Standards and guidelines for professional nursing practice in the care of women and newborns* (5th ed.). Washington, D.C.: The Association.

Vietnamese, Chinese, East Indians, and Arabs often use this belief in choosing foods. "Hot" foods are considered best for new mothers; this does not necessarily relate to the temperature or spiciness of foods. For example, chicken and broccoli are considered "hot," whereas many fresh fruits and vegetables are considered "cold." Families often bring desired foods into the health care setting.

In Kenya, mothers feed preterm infants only by breast and often begin feeding earlier than the practice in other countries. Kenyans never use gavage tubes. Preterm babies are cup fed until they are able to suck.

FEEDING READINESS

Term neonates are born with reflexes that facilitate feeding: **rooting**, sucking, and swallowing. Healthy newborns have experience with sucking on fingers and swallowing amniotic fluid for several weeks in utero but have made no connection between sucking and satiation. Neither have they needed to suck, swallow, and breathe before they emerged from the uterus. While the majority of newborns do not experience hunger or thirst in the first hours after birth, they will suckle when given the opportunity. Newborns of mothers who experienced an unmedicated labor have been noted to crawl to the breast when laid on the mother's abdomen, seek out the nipple, and begin to suckle (Widstrom, Ransjo-Arvidsson, & Christensson, 1993).

Physical assessment of the newborn reveals signs that the baby is physiologically ready to begin feeding:
- Vital signs (temperature, respirations, heart rate) within normal limits
- Unlabored respirations; nares patent; no cyanosis
- Active bowel sounds
- No abdominal distention

When newborns experience hunger, they usually cry vigorously until their needs are met. Some infants, however, will withdraw into sleep because of discomfort associated with hunger. Babies exhibit **feeding-readiness cues** that can be recognized by a knowledgeable caregiver. Instead of waiting to feed until the infant is crying distraughtly or withdraws into sleep, it is better to begin a feeding when the baby exhibits some of these cues (even during light sleep):
- Hand-to-mouth or hand-to-hand movements
- Sucking motions
- Rooting
- Mouthing

Babies normally consume small amounts of milk during the first 3 days of life. The breastfed infant receives colostrum, which is very concentrated and high in protein. Similarly, bottle-fed infants initially require small feedings. However, as the baby adjusts to extrauterine life and the digestive tract is cleared of meconium, milk intake increases from 15 to 30 ml per feeding in the first 24 hours to 60 to 90 ml or more per feeding thereafter.

At birth and for several months thereafter, all of the secretions of the infant's digestive tract contain enzymes especially suited to the digestion of human milk. The ability to digest foods other than milk depends on the physiologic development of the infant. The capacities for salivary, gastric, pancreatic, and intestinal digestion increase with age, indicating that the natural time for introduction of solid foods may be around 6 months of age.

Babies are born with a tongue extrusion reflex that causes them to push out of the mouth anything placed on the tongue. This reflex disappears by 6 months—another indication of physiologic readiness for solids.

Early introduction of solids may make the infant more prone to food allergies. Regular feeding of solids can lead to decreased intake of breast milk or formula and may be associated with early cessation of breastfeeding.

NUTRIENT NEEDS

Fluids

The fluid requirement for normal infants is 80 to 100 ml of water per kilogram of body weight per 24 hours (Behrman, Kliegman, & Arvin, 1996). In general, neither breastfed nor formula-fed infants need to be fed water, not even those living in very hot climates. Breast milk contains 87% water, which easily meets fluid requirements. Feeding water to infants may only decrease caloric consumption at a time when infants are growing rapidly.

Infants have room for little fluctuation in fluid balance and should be monitored closely for fluid intake and water loss. Infants lose water through excretion of urine and through insensible losses such as respiration. Under normal circumstances, infants are born with some fluid reserve and some of the weight loss during the first few days is related to fluid loss. In some cases, however, infants do not have this fluid reserve, possibly because of inadequate maternal hydration during labor or birth.

Energy

Infants require adequate caloric intake to provide energy for growth, digestion, physical activity, and maintenance of organ metabolic function. For the first 3 months, the infant needs 110 kcal/kg/day. From 3 months to 6 months, the requirement is 100 kcal/kg/day. This decreases slightly to 95 kcal/kg/day from 6 to 9 months and increases to 100 kcal/kg/day from 9 months to 1 year (AAP, 1998).

Human milk provides 67 kcal/100 ml or 20 kcal/oz; the greatest amount of energy is provided by the fat content of breast milk. Infant formulas are made to simulate the caloric content of human milk; standard formulas contain 20 kcal/oz.

Carbohydrate

Because newborns have only small hepatic glycogen stores, carbohydrates should provide at least 40% to 45% of the total calories in the diet. Moreover, newborns may have a limited ability to carry out gluconeogenesis (the formation of glucose from amino acids and other substrates) and ketogenesis (the formation of ketone bodies from fat), which are mechanisms that provide alternative sources of energy.

As the primary carbohydrate in human milk, lactose is the most abundant carbohydrate in the diet of infants up to 6 months of age. It provides calories in an easily available form. Its slow breakdown and absorption probably also increase calcium absorption. Corn syrup solids or glucose polymers have been added to infant formulas to supplement the lactose in the cow's milk and thereby provide sufficient carbohydrates.

Fat

For infants to acquire adequate calories from the limited amount of human milk or formula they are able to consume, at least 15% of the calories provided must come from fat (triglycerides). This fat must therefore be easily digestible. The fat in human milk is easier to digest and absorb than that in cow's milk because of the arrangement of the fatty acids on the glycerol molecule. Fat absorption is also related to the natural lipase activity present in human milk.

Cow's milk is used in most infant formulas, but the milk fat is removed, and another fat source such as corn oil, which can be digested and absorbed by the infant, is added in its place. If whole milk or evaporated milk without added carbohydrate is fed to infants, the resulting fecal loss of fat and therefore loss of energy may be excessive because the milk moves through the infant's intestines too quickly for adequate absorption to take place. This can lead to poor weight gain.

In addition to its energy contributions, fat also furnishes essential fatty acids (EFAs), which are required for growth and tissue maintenance. EFAs are components of cell membranes and precursors of some hormones. An inadequate intake of EFAs results in eczema and growth failure. The lack of EFAs in skim and low-fat milk is another reason for not feeding these products to infants.

Protein

The protein requirement per unit of body weight is greater in the newborn than at any other time of life. The recommended daily allowance (RDA) for protein during the first 6 months is 2.2 g/kg.

The protein content of human milk, which is lower than that of unmodified cow's milk, is ideal for the newborn. Human milk contains far more lactalbumin in relation to casein than does cow's milk, and lactalbumin is more easily digested than casein. In addition, the amino acid composition of human milk is suited to the newborn's metabolic capabilities. For example, the phenylalanine and methionine levels are low, and cystine and taurine levels are high. The protein in some commercial formulas is modified so that the amount of lactalbumin, or whey, protein is increased and the relative proportion of casein is decreased to more closely approximate the protein composition of human milk.

Vitamins

Human milk contains all of the vitamins required for infant nutrition, with individual variations based on maternal diet and genetic differences. Vitamins are added to cow's milk formulas to resemble levels found in breast milk. While cow's milk contains adequate amounts of vitamin A and vitamin B complex, vitamin C (ascorbic acid) and vitamin E must be added.

Vitamin D is also added to commercial infant formulas. While human milk may be somewhat deficient in vitamin D, supplementation may not be necessary provided that the infant is exposed to sunlight for 30 minutes per week wearing only a diaper, or for 2 hours per week fully clothed but without a hat. To prevent rickets, supplementation may be recommended for preterm or dark-skinned infants with limited exposure to the sun, as well as infants whose mothers eat vegetarian diets that exclude meat, fish, and dairy products.

Vitamin K, required for blood coagulation, is produced by intestinal bacteria. However, the gut is sterile at birth, and a few days are needed for intestinal flora to become established and produce vitamin K. To prevent hemorrhagic problems in the newborn, an injection of vitamin K is given at birth.

Minerals

The mineral content of commercial infant formula is designed to reflect that of breast milk. Unmodified cow's milk is much higher in mineral content than human milk, providing evidence of its unsuitability for infants during the first year of life. Minerals are typically highest in human milk during the first few days after birth and decrease slightly throughout lactation.

The ratio of calcium to phosphorus in human milk is 2:1, a proportion optimal for bone mineralization. Although cow's milk is high in calcium, the calcium-to-phosphorus ratio is low, resulting in decreased calcium absorption. Consequently, young infants fed unmodified cow's milk are at risk for hypocalcemia, seizures, and tetany. The calcium-to-phosphorus ratio in commercial infant formula is between that of human milk and cow's milk.

Iron levels are low in all types of milk; however, iron from human milk is better absorbed (50%) than from cow's milk, iron-fortified formula, or infant cereals. Breastfed infants draw on iron reserves deposited in utero and benefit from the high lactose and vitamin C levels in human milk that facilitate iron absorption. The infant who is entirely breastfed normally maintains adequate hemoglobin levels for the first 6 months. After that time, iron-fortified cereals and other iron-rich foods are added to the diet. Infants who are weaned from the breast before 6 months of age and all formula-fed infants should receive an iron-fortified commercial infant formula until 12 months of age.

Fluoride levels in human milk and commercial formulas are low. This mineral, which is important in the prevention of dental caries, may cause spotting of the permanent teeth (fluorosis) in excess amounts. It is recommended that a fluoride supplement be given only to those infants not receiving fluoridated water after the age of 6 months (AAP, 1997).

OVERVIEW OF LACTATION

Milk Production

Each female breast is composed of approximately 15 to 20 segments (lobes) embedded in fat and connective tissues and lavishly supplied with blood vessels, lymphatic vessels, and nerves (Fig. 28-1). Within each lobe are alveoli, the milk-producing cells, surrounded by myoepithelial cells, which contract to send the milk forward into the ductules. Each ductule enlarges into **lactiferous ducts** and **sinuses** where milk collects just behind the nipple. Each nipple has 15 to 20 pores through which milk is transferred to the suckling infant. The size of the breast is not an accurate indicator of its ability to produce milk. Because of the effects of estrogen and progesterone during pregnancy, the lobular components of the breast enlarge while the ductal system proliferates and differentiates. The nipples become more erect, and pigmentation of the areola in-

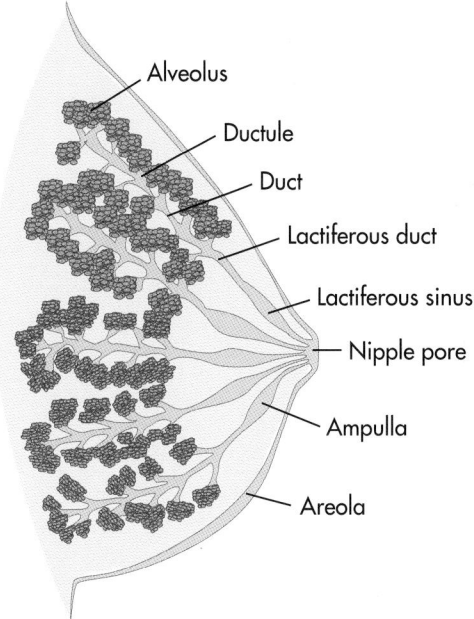

Fig. 28-1 Detailed structural features of human mammary gland.

creases. Nipples and areola may enlarge. The breasts increase in size and sensitivity and exhibit more prominent veins. Around the sixteenth week of gestation the alveoli begin producing colostrum (early milk) in response to human placental lactogen.

After birth of the neonate, there is a precipitous drop in the mother's estrogen and progesterone levels, which triggers the release of prolactin from the anterior pituitary. During pregnancy, prolactin prepares the breasts to secrete milk and, during lactation, to synthesize and secrete milk. **Prolactin**, one of the two hormones necessary for milk production, is subsequently produced in response to infant suckling and emptying of the breasts (note that lactating breasts are never completely empty; milk is constantly being produced by the alveoli as the infant feeds) (Fig. 28-2, *A*). Milk production is a **supply-meets-demand system;** that is, as milk is removed from the breast, more is produced. Incomplete emptying of the breasts with feedings can lead to a decreased milk supply. Prolactin levels are highest during the first 10 days after birth, gradually declining over time, but remaining above baseline levels for the duration of lactation.

Oxytocin is the other hormone essential to lactation. As the nipple is stimulated by the suckling infant, the posterior pituitary is prompted by the hypothalamus to produce oxytocin. This hormone is responsible for the **milk ejection reflex (MER)**, or **let-down reflex** (Fig. 28-2, *B*). The myoepithelial cells surrounding the alveoli respond to oxytocin by contracting and sending the milk forward through the ducts to the nipple. Many "let-downs" can occur with each feeding session. The milk ejection reflex can

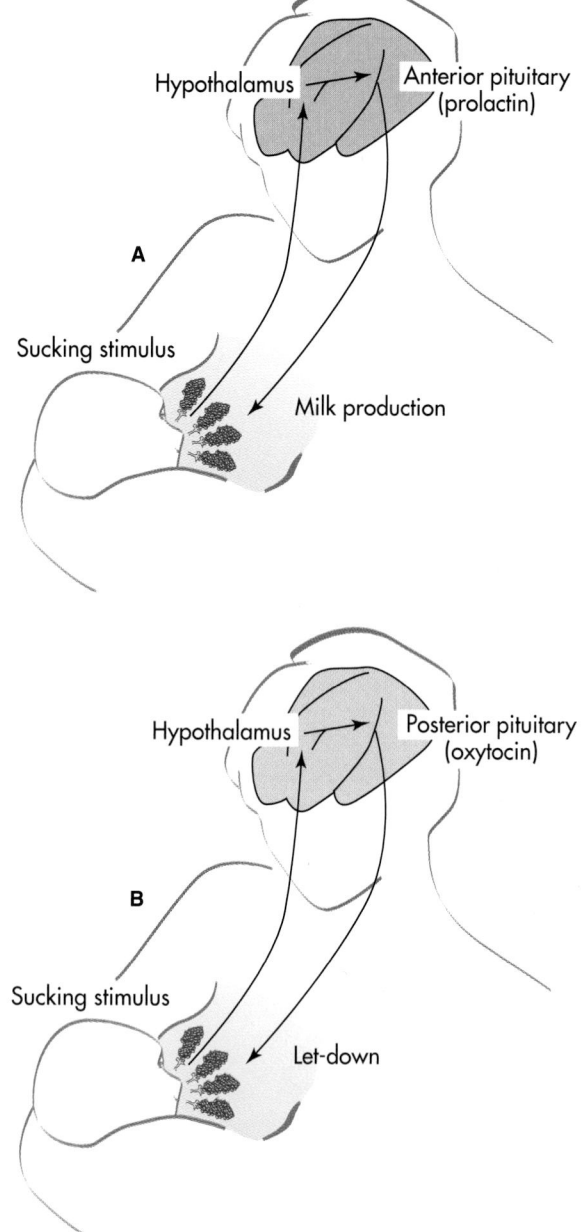

Fig. 28-2 Maternal breastfeeding reflexes. **A,** Milk production. **B,** Let-down.

be triggered by thoughts, sights, sounds, or odors that the mother associates with her baby (or other babies), such as hearing the baby cry. Many women report a tingling "pins and needles" sensation in the breasts as let-down occurs, although some mothers can detect milk ejection only by observing the sucking and swallowing of the infant. Let-down may also occur during sexual activity, since oxytocin is released during orgasm.

Oxytocin is the same hormone that stimulates uterine contractions during labor. Consequently, the laboring woman can experience let-downs that may be evidenced

by leakage of colostrum. This readies the breast for immediate feeding by the infant after birth. Oxytocin has the important function of contracting the mother's uterus after birth to control postpartum bleeding and promote uterine involution. Thus mothers who breastfeed are at decreased risk for postpartum hemorrhage. These uterine contractions that occur with breastfeeding can be painful during and after the feeding, particularly in multiparas. The "afterpains" usually subside within 3 to 5 days after giving birth.

Prolactin and oxytocin have been referred to as the "mothering hormones," since they are known to affect the postpartum woman's physical state, as well as her emotions. Many women report feeling thirsty or very relaxed during breastfeeding, probably as a result of these hormones.

The **nipple erection reflex** is an integral part of lactation. When the infant cries, suckles, or rubs against the breast, the nipple becomes erect. This assists in the propulsion of milk through the lactiferous sinuses to the nipple pores. Nipple sizes, shapes, and ability to become erect vary with individuals. Some women have flat or **inverted nipples** that do not become erect with stimulation. Babies are usually able to learn to successfully breastfeed with any nipple. It is important that these infants are not offered bottles or pacifiers until breastfeeding is well established.

Uniqueness of Human Milk

Human milk is a highly complex species-specific fluid uniquely designed to meet the needs of the human infant. It is a dynamic substance whose composition changes to meet the changing nutritional and immunologic needs of the infant. It is specific to the needs of each newborn; for example, the milk of preterm mothers differs in composition from that of mothers who give birth at term.

The components of human milk are continually being investigated. Human milk contains antimicrobial factors (antibodies) that provide some protection against a broad spectrum of bacterial, viral, and protozoan infections. Secretory IgA is the major antibody in human milk. Other factors in human milk that help protect against infection include lactoferrin, the bifidus factor, oligosaccharides, milk lipids, and milk leukocytes. There are antiinflammatory agents, growth factors, hormones, and enzymes in human milk, many of which contribute to the maturation of the infant's intestine. Immunomodulating agents found in human milk are instrumental in preventing disease after infancy (Goldman, 1993) (Table 28-1).

Human milk composition and volumes vary according to the stage of lactation. In **lactogenesis** stage I, beginning in pregnancy, the breasts are preparing for milk production. Colostrum is present in the breasts at this time. **Colostrum,** a clear yellowish fluid, is more concentrated than mature milk and is extremely rich in immunoglobulins. It has higher concentrations of protein and minerals, but less fat than mature milk. The high protein level of

TABLE 28-1 Summary of Immune Properties of Breast Milk

COMPONENT	ACTION
WHITE BLOOD CELLS	
B lymphocytes	Give rise to antibodies targeted against specific microbes.
Macrophages	Kill microbes outright in baby's gut, produce lysozyme, and activate other components of the immune system.
Neutrophils	May act as phagocytes, ingesting bacteria in baby's digestive system.
T lymphocytes	Kill infected cells directly or send out chemical messages to mobilize other defenses. They proliferate in the presence of organisms that cause serious illness in infants. They also manufacture compounds that can strengthen an infant's own immune response.
MOLECULES	
Antibodies of secretory IgA class	Bind to microbes in infant's digestive tract and thereby prevent them from passing through walls of the gut into body's tissues.
B_{12}-binding protein	Reduces amount of vitamin B_{12}, which bacteria need to grow.
Bifidus factor	Promotes growth of *Lactobacillus bifidus,* a harmless bacterium, in infant's gut. Growth of such nonpathogenic bacteria helps crowd out dangerous varieties.
Fatty acids	Disrupt membranes surrounding certain viruses and destroy them.
Fibronectin	Increases antimicrobial activity of macrophages; helps repair tissues that have been damaged by immune reactions in infant's gut.
Gamma-interferon	Enhances antimicrobial activity of immune cells.
Hormones and growth factors	Stimulate infant's digestive tract to mature more quickly. Once the initially "leaky" membranes lining the gut mature, infants become less vulnerable to microorganisms.
Lactoferrin	Binds to iron, a mineral many bacteria need to survive. By reducing the available amount of iron, lactoferrin thwarts growth of pathogenic bacteria.
Lysozyme	Kills bacteria by disrupting their cell walls.
Mucins	Adhere to bacteria and viruses, thus keeping such microorganisms from attaching to mucosal surfaces.
Oligosaccharides	Bind to microorganisms and bar them from attaching to mucosal surfaces.

From Newman, J. (1995). How breast milk protects newborns. *Sci Am* 273(6):76-79.

colostrum facilitates binding of bilirubin, and the laxative action of colostrum promotes early passage of meconium. Colostrum gradually changes to mature milk; this is referred to as "the milk coming in" or as lactogenesis stage II. By the third to fifth day after birth, most women have experienced this onset of copious milk secretion. Breast milk continues to change in composition for approximately 10 days, when the mature milk is established. This is considered stage III of lactogenesis (Lawrence, 1999).

The composition of mature milk changes during each feeding. As the infant nurses, the fat content of breast milk increases. Initially, a bluish-white foremilk is released that is part skim milk (about 60% of the volume) and part whole milk (about 35% of the volume). It provides primarily lactose, protein, and water-soluble vitamins. The hindmilk, or cream (about 5%), is usually let down 10 to 20 minutes into the feeding, although it may occur sooner. It contains the denser calories from fat necessary for ensuring optimal growth and contentment between feedings. Because of this changing composition of human milk during each feeding, it is important to breastfeed the infant long enough to supply a balanced feeding.

Milk production gradually increases, so that by the time her infant is 2 weeks old, the mother produces 720 to 900 ml of milk every 24 hours. Babies experience fairly predictable **growth spurts** (at about 10 days, 3 weeks, 6 weeks, 3 months, and 4 to 6 months), when more frequent feedings stimulate increased milk production. These growth spurts usually last 24 to 48 hours, and then the infants resume their usual feeding pattern.

Although nearly every woman can lactate, there are some mothers who have insufficient glandular development to exclusively breastfeed their infants. Breasts may appear immature or tubular, with or without asymmetry. Women with insufficient glandular tissue experience little or no change in breast size during pregnancy. In some cases, women may still be able to breastfeed and offer supplemental nutrition to support optimal infant growth. There are devices available to allow mothers to offer supplements while the baby is at the breast (Fig. 28-3).

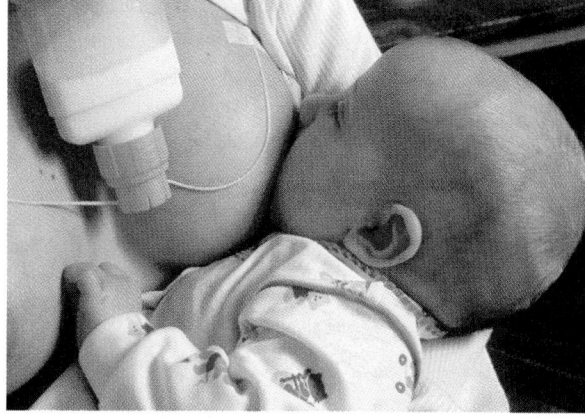

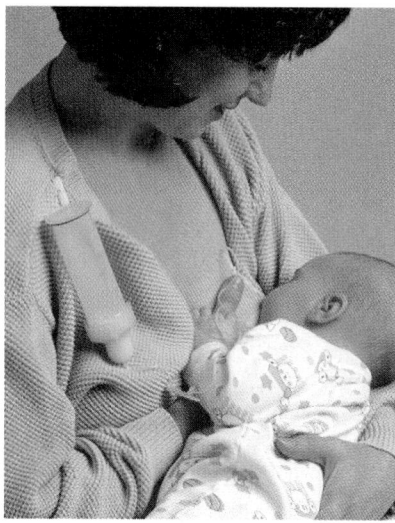

Fig. 28-3 Supplemental nursing system. *(Courtesy Medela, Inc., McHenry, IL.)*

▪ CARE MANAGEMENT: THE BREASTFEEDING MOTHER AND INFANT

Effective management of the breastfeeding mother and infant requires that the caregivers be knowledgeable about the benefits of breastfeeding, as well as about basic anatomy and the physiology of breastfeeding, how to assist the mother with feeding, and interventions for common problems. Ongoing support of the mother enhances her self-confidence and promotes a satisfying and successful breastfeeding experience. Planning care for the breastfeeding couple is based on thorough assessment of both the mother and infant.

Assessment and Nursing Diagnoses

Infant

Before the initiation of breastfeeding, the nurse needs to consider the following in preparing to effectively assist the breastfeeding infant:

- Maturity level: gestational age, term or preterm, birth weight (small for gestational age [SGA], large for gestational age [LGA])
- Labor and birth: length of labor, maternal medications (narcotics, magnesium sulfate [MgSO₄]); type of birth: vaginal with or without use of vacuum extraction or forceps; cesarean; type of anesthesia
- Birth trauma: fractured clavicle, bruising of face or head
- Maternal risk factors: diabetes, preeclampsia, infection, human immunodeficiency virus (HIV), herpes
- Congenital defects: cleft lip or palate, cardiac anomalies, Down syndrome or other genetic anomalies
- Physical stability: vital signs within normal limits, unlabored respirations, bowel sounds present
- State of alertness: awake, sleepy, crying

Assessment during feeding: the infant is assessed for the following by direct observation while breastfeeding:

- **Latch-on** (attachment of the infant to the breast for feeding)
- Position, alignment
- Sucking/swallowing

Assessment of the infant:

- Behavior after/between feedings: contented, sleepy
- Elimination patterns: within 24 hours after birth, at least 1 wet diaper and 1 stool; by day 3, 3 to 4 wet diapers and 1 or 2 stools that are beginning to change from meconium to yellowish; after day 4 (and mother's milk has "come in"), 6 to 8 wet diapers and at least 3 stools per 24 hours (AAP, 1998).
- General assessment: presence of jaundice; weight loss <10%; regain birth weight by 10 to 14 days of age.

Mother

Before breastfeeding is begun, it is important that the nurse carefully assess the mother's knowledge of breastfeeding, as well as her physical and psychologic readiness to breastfeed. This assessment can be accomplished through interviews, discussion, and direct observation. Factors to consider include:

- Previous experience with breastfeeding: first baby; unsuccessful breastfeeding with previous infants
- Knowledge about breastfeeding: prenatal classes, support groups, books/pamphlets, videos, friends/relatives who breastfed; knowledge about positioning, latch-on, frequency/duration of feedings, etc.
- Cultural factors: belief that colostrum is bad, modesty issues, language barrier
- Feelings about breastfeeding: anxious, fear of failure; confident–expects to succeed
- Physical features: development of breast tissue, protractility of nipples (flat or inverted), previous breast surgery, chronic illness, carpal tunnel syndrome, visual or hearing impairment, physical limitations
- Physical/psychologic readiness: risk factors, time since giving birth, type of birth, complications, perineal discomfort, level of pain, medications, mood (eager, cheerful), energy level (tired, exhausted)

- Support: father of baby or family members/friends present and their level of knowledge about breastfeeding

As breastfeeding is becoming established, the nurse performs ongoing assessment of the mother and infant to determine appropriate interventions. During the time in the hospital, the nurse can help the mother to view each breastfeeding session as a "feeding lesson" or "practice session" that will foster maternal confidence and a satisfying breastfeeding experience for mother and baby. Items that need to be assessed are:

- Condition of nipples: during feeding, mother feels a "tugging" sensation, but no pain after the initial latch-on; presence of soreness, redness, cracking, bleeding
- Transition to mature milk: milk is "in" by day 4 or 5
- Breasts feel softer or lighter after feedings
- Mother states she feels relaxed or sleepy during feedings
- Mother reports uterine cramping and/or increased lochia flow during/after feeding
- Mother appears comfortable with breastfeeding techniques, including positioning and latch-on

Nursing diagnoses for the breastfeeding woman include the following:

▌ Nursing Diagnoses

- Effective breastfeeding related to
  - mother's knowledge of breastfeeding techniques
  - mother's appropriate response to infant's feeding-readiness cues
  - mother's ability to facilitate efficient breastfeeding
- Risk for ineffective breastfeeding related to
  - insufficient knowledge regarding newborn's reflexes and breastfeeding techniques
  - lack of support by father of baby, family, friends
  - lack of maternal self-confidence; anxiety, fear of failure
  - poor infant sucking reflex
  - difficulty waking sleepy baby
- Risk for altered nutrition: less than body requirements related to
  - increased caloric and nutrient needs for breastfeeding (mother)
  - incorrect latch-on and inability to transfer milk (infant)
- Risk for fluid volume deficit related to
  - ineffective sucking (infant)

Expected Outcomes of Care

In planning care, the nurse discusses the desired outcomes with the parents. The expected outcomes include that the infant will do the following:

- Latch on and feed effectively at least eight times per day.
- Gain weight appropriately.
- Remain well hydrated (have 6 to 8 wet diapers and at least 3 bowel movements every 24 hours after day 4).

- Sleep or seem contented between feedings.

Examples of expected outcomes for the mother include that she will do the following:

- Verbalize/demonstrate understanding of breastfeeding techniques, including positioning and latch-on, signs of adequate feeding, self-care.
- Report no nipple discomfort with breastfeeding.
- Express satisfaction with the breastfeeding experience.
- Consume a nutritionally balanced diet with appropriate caloric and fluid intake to support breastfeeding.

Plan of Care and Interventions

Interventions are based on the expected outcomes and are influenced by the resources and time available to achieve the desired goals. In the early days after birth, interventions focus on helping the mother and the newborn initiate breastfeeding and achieve some degree of success/satisfaction before discharge from the hospital. Interventions to promote breastfeeding progress from basics such as latch-on and positioning to signs of adequate feeding and self-care measures such as prevention of engorgement. An important intervention is to provide the parents with a list of resources that they may contact after discharge from the hospital. Guidelines for Spanish-speaking clients are in the accompanying Guidelines/Guías box.

The ideal time to begin breastfeeding is within 1 hour after birth (AAP, 1997) when the infant is in the quiet, alert state. If this is not possible because of the effects of labor medications or anesthesia, it is advantageous to place the infant in skin-to-skin contact on the mother's chest for the first hour after birth. Each mother should receive instruction, assistance, and support in positioning and latching on until she is able to do so independently.

Positioning

There are four basic positions for breastfeeding: football hold, cradle, modified cradle or across-the-lap, and side-lying position (Fig. 28-4). Initially, it is advantageous to use the position that most easily facilitates latch-on while allowing maximum comfort for the mother. The football hold is often recommended for early feedings because the mother can easily visualize the baby's mouth as she guides the infant on to the nipple. The football hold is usually preferred by mothers who gave birth by cesarean. The modified cradle or across-the-lap hold also works well for early feedings. The side-lying position allows the mother to rest while breastfeeding and is often preferred by women experiencing perineal pain and swelling. Cradling is the most common breastfeeding position for infants who have learned to latch on easily and feed effectively. Before discharge from the hospital, the mother should be assisted in trying all of the positions so that she will feel confident in her ability to vary positions at home.

✸ GUIDELINES/GUÍAS

Breastfeeding: Latching On

Do you want to breastfeed your baby?
¿Desea amamantar a su bebé?

I will help you.
Yo le ayudo.

Hold your baby's head close to your breast.
Sostenga la cabeza del bebé cerca del pecho.

Lightly touch your nipple to the baby's lower lip until he opens his mouth.
Con el pezón, toque ligeramente el labio inferior del bebé hasta que abra la boca.

Lift your breast to the baby's mouth.
Levante el seno hasta la boca del bebé.

Center your nipple and areola as far in the baby's mouth as possible.
Centre el pezón y la areola lo más que se pueda dentro de la boca del bebé.

Make sure the baby's tongue is under the nipple and the gums close around the areola.
Asegurese que la lengua del bebé está debajo del pezón y sus encías se cierren sobre la areola.

To change breasts, push one of your fingers into the corner of the baby's mouth.
Para cambiar al otro seno, introduzca un dedo en el ángulo de la boca del bebé.

This will break the suction and prevent the baby from biting the nipple.
Esto rompe la succión y impide que el bebé muerda el pezón.

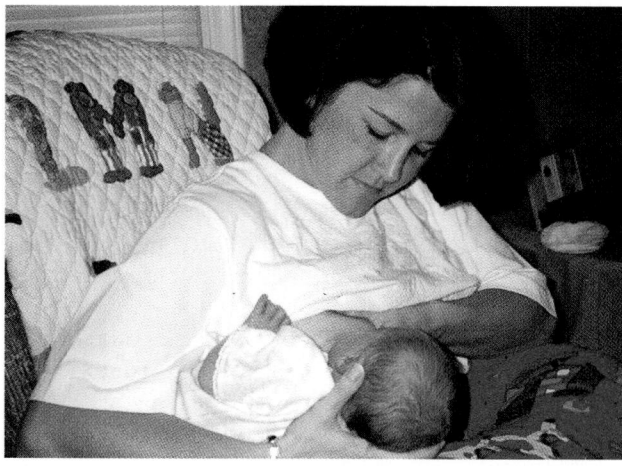

A

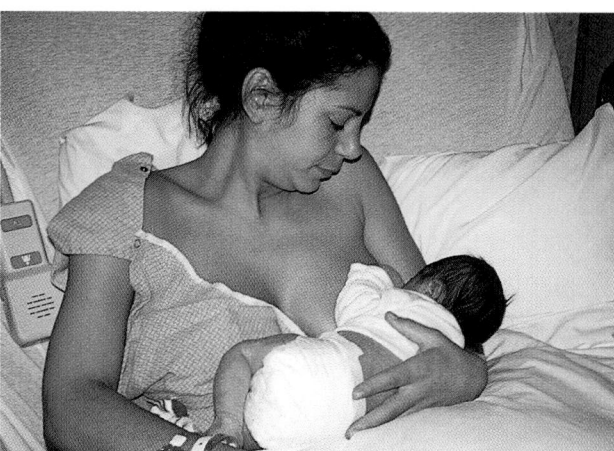

B

Whichever position is used, the mother should be comfortable, with pillows used as needed to provide support for her back and arms. The infant is placed at the level of the breast, supported by pillows or folded blankets, turned completely on his or her side, and facing the mother so that the infant is "belly to belly," with the arms "hugging" the breast. The baby's mouth is directly in front of the nipple. It is important that the mother support the baby's neck and shoulders with her hand and not push on the occiput. Pushing on the back of the head may result in biting, extension of the neck, or an aversion to being brought near the breast. The baby's body is held in correct alignment (ears, shoulders, and hips are in a straight line) during latch-on and feeding (Fig. 28-5).

Latch-On

In preparation for latch-on, it may be helpful for the mother to manually express a few drops of colostrum or

C

Fig. 28-4 Breastfeeding positions. **A,** Football hold. **B,** Cradling. **C,** Lying down. (*B* and *C* *courtesy Marjorie Pyle, RNC, Lifecircle, Costa Mesa, CA.*)

milk and spread it over the nipple. This lubricates the nipple and may entice the baby to open the mouth as the milk is tasted.

To facilitate latch-on, the mother supports her breast in one hand with the thumb on top and four fingers underneath at the back edge of the areola. The breast is compressed slightly, as one might compress a large sandwich in preparing to take a bite, so that an adequate amount of breast tissue is taken into the mouth with latch-on (Weissinger, 1998). Most mothers need to support the breast during feeding for at least the first few weeks until the infant is adept at feeding.

With the baby held close to the breast with the mouth directly in front of the nipple, the mother tickles the baby's lower lip with the tip of her nipple, stimulating the mouth to open. When the mouth is open wide and the tongue is down, the mother quickly pulls the baby onto the nipple. She brings the baby to the breast, not the breast to the baby. If the breast is pushed into the baby's mouth, the typical response is for the baby to close the mouth too soon, which precludes correct latch-on (see Fig. 28-5).

The amount of areola in the baby's mouth with correct latch-on depends on the size of the baby's mouth and the size of the areola and the nipple. In general, the baby's mouth should cover the nipple and an areolar radius of approximately 2 to 3 cm all around the nipple.

When the baby is latched on correctly, the nose, cheeks, and chin should all be touching the breast (Fig. 28-6). It is important for the mother not to pull the nipple out of the mouth when trying to create a breathing space for the baby's nose. Depressing the breast tissue around the baby's nose is not necessary. If she is worried about the baby's breathing, the mother can raise the baby's hips slightly to change the angle of the baby's head at the breast. The nurse should reassure the mother that if the baby cannot breathe, innate reflexes will prompt the baby to move the head and pull back to breathe.

Sucking creates a vacuum in the intraoral cavity as the breast is compressed between the tongue and the palate. If the mother experiences pinching or pain after the initial sucks or does not feel a strong tugging sensation on the nipple, the latch-on and positioning should be evaluated. The baby's body should be in straight alignment (ears, shoulders, and hips in a straight line), the back and hips well supported, and no pressure on the back of the head.

If each suck is painful, the baby may be having difficulty keeping the tongue out over the lower gum ridge. Clicking or smacking may be audible when this occurs. The nurse can place a finger on the side of the baby's lower jaw, pulling down gently but firmly as the baby sucks, to help stabilize the jaw so that the tongue stays in place.

When the baby is latched on correctly and sucking appropriately, (1) the mother reports a firm tugging sensation on her nipples, but no pinching or pain; (2) the baby sucks with cheeks rounded, not dimpled; (3) the baby's jaw glides smoothly with sucking; and (4) swallowing is audible.

Any time the signs of adequate latch-on and sucking are not present, the baby should be taken off the breast and latch-on attempted again. To prevent nipple trauma as the baby is taken off the breast, the mother is instructed to break

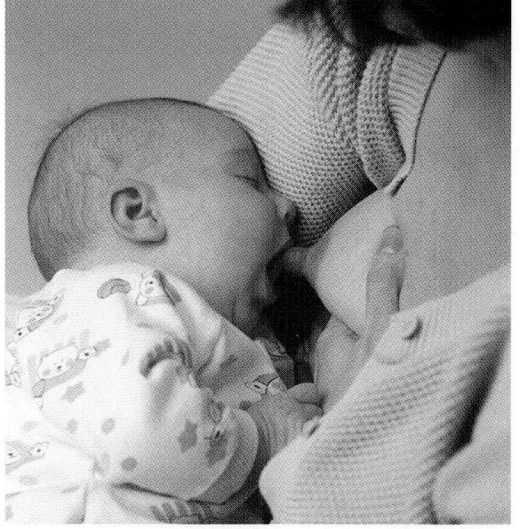

A

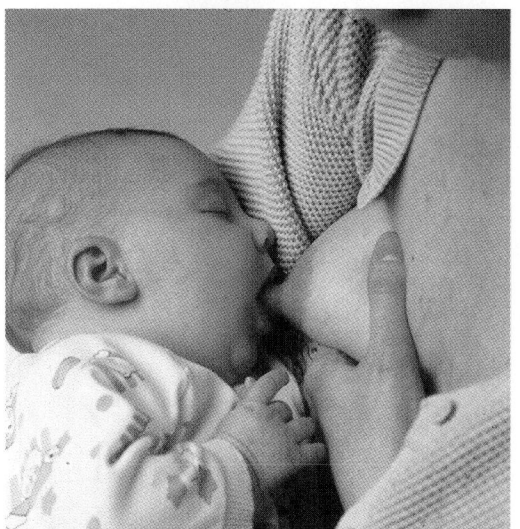

B

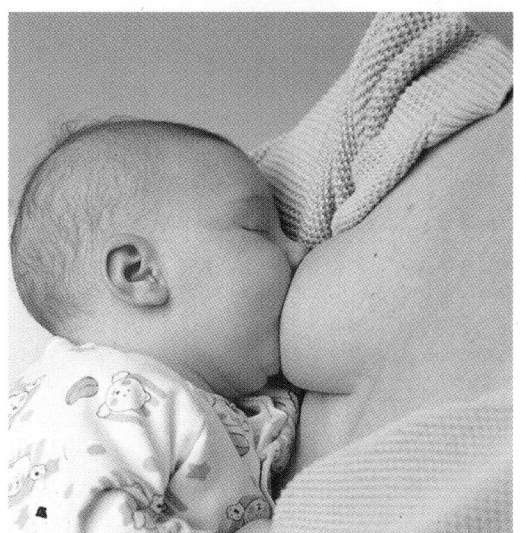

C

Fig. 28-5 Latching on. **A,** Tickle baby's lower lip with your nipple until he or she opens wide. **B,** Once baby's mouth is opened wide, quickly pull baby onto breast. **C,** Baby should have as much areola (dark area around nipple) in his or her mouth as possible, not just the nipple. *(Courtesy Medela, Inc., McHenry, IL.)*

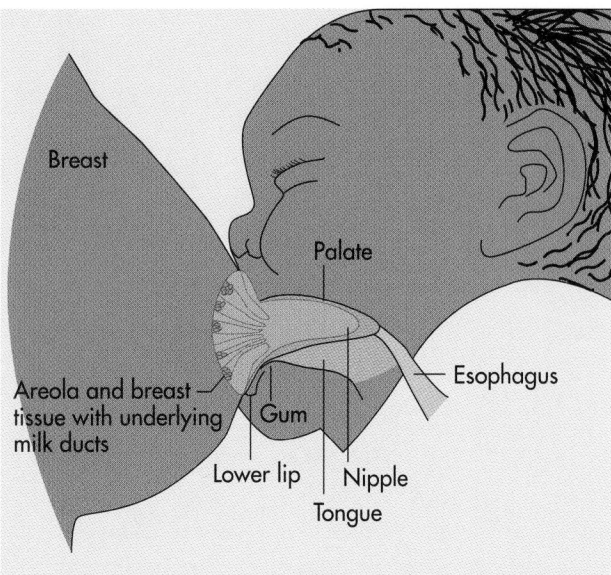

Fig. 28-6 Correct attachment (latch-on) of infant at breast.

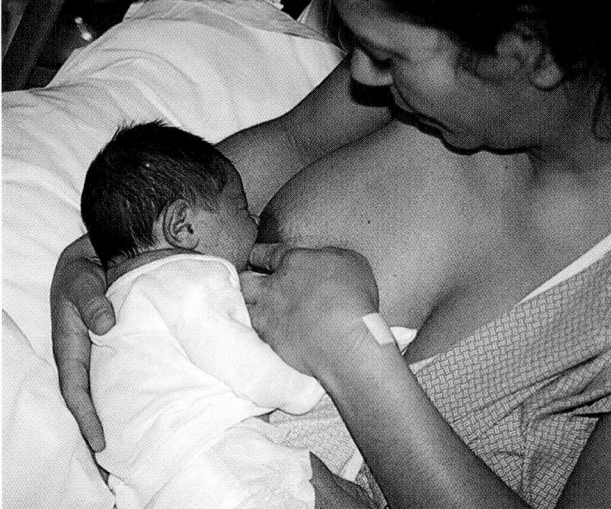

Fig. 28-7 Removing infant from the breast. *(Courtesy Marjorie Pyle, RNC, Lifecircle, Costa Mesa, CA.)*

the suction by inserting a finger in the side of the baby's mouth between the gums and leaving it there until the nipple is completely out of the baby's mouth (Fig. 28-7).

Milk Ejection or Let-Down

As the baby begins sucking on the nipple, the let-down, or milk ejection, reflex is stimulated. The hormone oxytocin causes milk to be sent forward from the milk ducts to the nipple. The following signs indicate that let-down has occurred:

- The mother may feel a tingling sensation in the nipples, although many women never feel their milk let down.

- The baby's suck changes from quick, shallow sucks to a slower, more drawing, sucking pattern.
- Swallowing is heard as the baby sucks.
- The mother experiences uterine cramping and may have increased lochia during and after feedings.
- The mother feels relaxed, even sleepy, during feedings.
- The opposite breast may leak.

Frequency of Feedings

Newborns need to breastfeed 8 to 12 times in a 24-hour period (AAP, 1997). During the first 24 to 48 hours after birth, most babies do not awaken this often to feed. It is important that parents understand that they should awaken the baby to feed at least every 3 hours during the day and at least every 4 hours at night. (Feeding frequency is determined by counting from the beginning of one feeding to the beginning of the next.) Once the infant is feeding well and gaining weight adequately, it is more appropriate to go to **demand feeding** when the infant determines the frequency of feedings.

Parents should be cautioned about attempting to place newborn infants on strict feeding schedules that are recommended by some contemporary child-rearing experts. There have been incidences of dehydration, poor weight gain, and failure to thrive in infants whose parents adhered to a strict feeding schedule.

NURSE ALERT *Newborns have no concept of time and respond to the messages and cues they receive from their bodies about hunger and thirst. They should be fed whenever they exhibit feeding cues such as hand-to-mouth movements and mouth and tongue movements. Crying is a late sign of hunger and babies may become frantic when they have to wait too long to feed. Some infants will shut down or go into a deep sleep when their needs are not met.*

Keeping the baby close is the best way to observe and respond to infant feeding cues. Newborns should remain with mothers during the recovery period after birth and room in during the hospital stay. At home, babies should be kept nearby so that parents can observe signs that the baby is ready to feed.

Duration of Feedings

The duration of breastfeeding sessions is highly variable, since the timing of milk transfer differs for each mother-baby pair. While some infants may complete a feeding in 5 to 10 minutes, others may require 45 minutes or longer. The average time for feeding is 30 minutes, or approximately 15 minutes per breast; this is a common recommendation. In reality, instructing mothers to feed for a set number of minutes is inappropriate. It is better to teach mothers how to determine when a baby has finished a feeding: the baby's suck/swallow pattern has slowed, the breast is softened, and the baby appears content and may fall asleep or release the nipple.

If a baby seems to be feeding effectively and the urine output is adequate but the weight gain is not, this may be due to the mother's switching to the second breast too soon. She may have been told to feed the baby for 10 minutes on each breast. Consequently, the baby is drinking only the foremilk (skim milk) and never reaches the rich, calorie-dense hindmilk. The foremilk is high in lactose and may cause the baby to have explosive stools, gas pains, and inconsolable crying. Feeding on the first breast until it softens ensures that the baby will receive the hindmilk and gain weight properly.

Indicators of Effective Breastfeeding

In the newborn period when breastfeeding is becoming established, it is important to teach parents the signs that breastfeeding is going well (Box 28-2). When they understand these signs, they will be more likely to recognize when problems arise and know when to seek assistance.

Supplements, Bottles, and Pacifiers

"No supplements (water, glucose water, formula, and so forth) should be given to breastfeeding newborns unless a medical indication exists. With sound breastfeeding knowledge and practice, supplements rarely are needed. Supplements and pacifiers should be avoided whenever possible, and if used at all, only after breastfeeding is well established" (AAP, 1997, p. 1036) (see Research Box on p. 760).

There are few reasons for offering supplemental feedings to breastfeeding newborns. Situations that may necessitate feeding include such things as low birth weight, hypoglycemia, dehydration, or inborn errors of metabolism. Mothers may be unable to breastfeed because of severe illness such as eclampsia or shock, or they may be on medications incompatible with breastfeeding.

The practice of offering formula to a baby after breastfeeding just to "make sure the baby is getting enough" is neither necessary nor advisable. This can foster **nipple confusion** (difficulty knowing how to latch on to the breast) and can lead to a decreased milk supply because the baby becomes overfull and does not breastfeed enough. Supplementation interferes with the supply-meets-demand system of milk production. The parents may interpret the baby's willingness to take a bottle to mean that the mother's milk supply is inadequate. They need to know that a baby will automatically suck from a bottle as the nipple triggers the suck/swallow reflex.

Babies can become confused going from breast to bottle or bottle to breast. Breastfeeding and bottle feeding require different skills. The way babies use their tongues, cheeks, and lips, as well as the sucking and swallowing patterns, are very different. While some babies can transition easily between breast and bottle, some experience considerable

BOX 28-2 Indicators of Effective Breastfeeding During the First Week

INFANT
Physical Assessment

The baby is alert when awake and appears well hydrated, with normal skin turgor and moist mucous membranes. The fontanels are soft and flat, and the baby demonstrates a strong and coordinated suck. Periods of wakefulness and hunger alternate with periods of contentment/sleeping. Weight loss is less than 8% before discharge, and the infant gains 15 to 30 g/day after milk is "in." Birth weight should be regained by 10 to 14 days.

Feeding Frequency

The infant should eat 8 to 12 times per 24 hours.

Feeding Behavior

Baby latches on easily and sucks with gliding jaw movements in bursts of 10 to 12 sucks/swallows at beginning of feeding, slowing to bursts of 2 to 3 sucks/swallows at end of feeding. Swallowing is audible. Baby appears relaxed during feeding and contented when finished.

Output

After milk is in, the baby should have 6 to 8 wet diapers per 24 hours. The baby may stool with every feeding, but should minimally have 3 bowel movements per 24 hours. Stools transition from meconium to milk stools by 3 to 5 days of age.

MOTHER
Physical Assessment

Nipples are intact (no redness, cracking, scabs, or bleeding), and nipple tenderness is minimal. Breasts are full, soft, and without engorgement, with no redness and minimal tenderness to palpation. The mother should have no fever.

Nursing Behavior

Milk is "in" by the third or fourth day. Breasts are full at beginning of feeding and soften as baby breastfeeds. Baby softens at least one breast per feeding. There should be no pinching or nipple pain with sucking, and the mother should feel a strong tugging sensation as the baby sucks.

Mother easily positions and latches baby on and experiences let-down with feeding. She may have a tingling sensation in the breast as the milk lets down. During the first 4 or 5 days after birth, she may feel uterine cramping and have increased lochia. As she breastfeeds, the mother may be thirsty and experience leaking from the opposite breast. She should feel relaxed during feeding.

▪ **BOX 28-3** Waking the Sleepy Newborn

- Lay the baby down and unwrap.
- Remove clothing except for diaper.
- Change the diaper.
- Hold the baby upright, turn from side to side.
- Talk to the baby.
- Gently, but firmly massage the chest and back.
- Carefully elicit "doll's eye" reflex.
- Apply cool cloth to face.

▪ **BOX 28-4** Calming the Fussy Baby

- Swaddle the baby.
- Hold closely.
- Gently move or rock.
- Talk soothingly.
- Reduce environmental stimuli.
- Allow baby to suck on adult finger.
- Place baby skin-to-skin with mother.

difficulty. It is impossible to predict which babies will adapt well and which ones will not. Therefore, it is best to avoid bottles until breastfeeding is well established, usually after 3 to 4 weeks. If supplementation is needed, there are mechanisms such as supplemental nursing systems, where the baby can be supplemented while breastfeeding (see Fig. 28-3). Although some parents combine breastfeeding and bottle feeding, many babies never take a bottle and go directly from the breast to a cup as they grow.

Pacifiers are not recommended until breastfeeding is well established. Their use has been associated with early termination of breastfeeding (Righard & Alade, 1997; Victora et al., 1997). Newborns need to learn the association between sucking and satiation. Although some infants have nonnutritive sucking needs between feedings, it is best to wait to introduce a pacifier until the infant is proficient at breastfeeding.

Special Considerations

Sleepy baby. During the first few days of life, some babies need to be awakened for feedings. Parents are instructed to be alert for behavioral signs or feeding cues such as rapid eye movements under the eyelids, sucking movements, or hand-to-mouth motions. When these signs are present, it is a good time to attempt breastfeeding. If the infant is awakened from a sound sleep, attempts at feeding are more likely to be unsuccessful. Helpful hints for parents as they try to bring the baby to an alert state for feeding are unwrapping the baby, changing the diaper, sitting the baby upright, talking to the baby with variable pitch, gently massaging the baby's chest or back, and stroking the palms or soles (Box 28-3).

Fussy baby. Babies sometimes awaken from sleep crying frantically. Although they may be hungry, they cannot focus on feeding until they are calmed. The nurse can encourage parents to swaddle the baby, hold the baby close, talk soothingly, and allow the baby to suck on a clean finger until calm enough to latch on to the breast (Box 28-4).

Babies sometimes cry as soon as they are positioned for feeding. This may be due to a bruised head or previously undetected fractured clavicle. Changing the feeding position may solve such a problem.

If an infant required extensive suctioning at birth, there may be an aversion to oral stimulation and the baby may scream and stiffen if anything approaches the mouth. Parents may need to spend time holding and cuddling the baby before attempting to breastfeed.

An infant may become fussy and appear discontent when sucking if the nipple does not extend far enough into the mouth. The feeding may begin with well-organized sucks and swallows, but the infant soon begins to pull off the breast and cry. It may be helpful for the mother to support her breast throughout the feeding so that the nipple stays in the same position as the feeding proceeds and the breast softens.

Fussiness may be related to gastrointestinal distress—cramping and gas pains. This may occur in response to an occasional feeding of infant formula or it may be related to something the mother has ingested. Although most mothers can consume their normal diet without affecting the baby, some foods may aggravate some babies. It may be cabbage and broccoli for one mother or onions for another. There are no standard foods that all mothers should avoid when breastfeeding; each mother/baby couple responds individually. The baby may have simply inherited food intolerances from the parents. Usually only one or two foods bother a baby. It may be helpful to give the baby liquid simethicone drops before feeding if gas is a problem.

Occasionally, infants develop gastrointestinal distress if mothers ingest dairy products. The baby is reacting to the cow's milk protein. In this case, the mother should eliminate all dairy products from her diet until the baby is older, making certain she receives adequate calcium from other sources. These infants should not receive any cow's milk–based formulas.

Parents should be taught that persistent crying or refusing to breastfeed can indicate illness, and the health care provider should be notified. Ear infections, sore throat, or oral thrush may cause the infant to be fussy and not breastfeed well.

Slow weight gain. It is not unusual for newborns to lose 8% to 10% of their birth weight during the first 3 to 5 days after birth because they are eliminating amniotic fluid and meconium. Thereafter, they should begin to show a weight gain of 110 to 200 g per week or 20 to 28 g per day. If an infant continues to lose weight after 5 days or does not regain birth weight by 14 days, or his weight is below the 10th percentile by 1 month, he should be evaluated and closely monitored by a health care provider.

Most often, slow weight gain is related to inadequate breastfeeding. Feedings may be short or infrequent, or the infant may be latching on incorrectly or sucking ineffectively or inefficiently. Other possibilities are illness/infection, malabsorption, or circumstances that increase the baby's energy needs such as congenital heart disease, cystic fibrosis, or simply being small for gestational age (SGA).

Maternal factors may be the cause of slow weight gain. There may be a problem with inadequate emptying of the breasts, pain with feeding, or inappropriate timing of feedings. Inadequate glandular breast tissue or previous breast surgery may affect milk supply. Severe intrapartum or postpartum hemorrhage (Sheehan's syndrome), illness, or medications may decrease milk supply. Stress and fatigue may also negatively affect milk production.

Usually, the solution to slow weight gain is to improve the feeding technique. Positioning and latch-on are evaluated and adjustments made. It may help to squeeze in another feeding or two in 24 hours. If the problem is a sleepy baby, parents are taught waking techniques.

Alternate breast massage, used during feedings, may help increase the amount of milk going to the infant. With this technique, the mother massages her breast from the chest wall to the nipple whenever the baby has sucking pauses. Some think this technique may also increase the fat content of the milk, which aids in weight gain.

When babies are calorie-deprived and need supplementation, it can be given with a spoon or cup, a nursing supplementer, or a bottle. If there are latch-on problems, it is best to avoid bottles. In most cases, supplementation is needed only for a short time until the baby gains weight and is feeding adequately.

If the problem is related to the mother's milk supply, it must be determined if this is an actual or perceived problem and whether it is related to milk production or milk transfer to the infant. Maternal health habits should be assessed because such things as smoking, stress, fatigue, or infection can decrease milk supply.

Jaundice. Jaundice (hyperbilirubinemia) in the newborn is discussed in detail in Chapter 26. **Physiologic jaundice** usually occurs after 24 hours of age and peaks by the third day. This has been referred to as early-onset jaundice, which in the breastfed infant may be associated with insufficient feeding and infrequent stooling. Colostrum has a natural laxative effect and promotes early passage of meconium. Bilirubin is excreted from the body primarily (98%) through the intestines. Infrequent stooling allows bilirubin in the stool to be reabsorbed into the infant's system, thus promoting hyperbilirubinemia. Infants who receive water or glucose water supplements are more likely to have hyperbilirubinemia, since only 2% of bilirubin is excreted through the kidneys. Decreased caloric intake (less milk) is associated with decreased stooling and increased jaundice.

To prevent early-onset breastfeeding jaundice from occurring, babies should be breastfed early and frequently during the first several days of life. More frequent feedings are associated with lower bilirubin levels.

To treat early-onset jaundice, breastfeeding is evaluated in terms of frequency and length of feedings, positioning and latch-on, and the infant's ability to empty the breast. Factors such as a sleepy or lethargic baby or breast engorgement may interfere with effective breastfeeding and should be corrected. If the infant's intake of milk needs to be increased, a supplemental feeding device may be used to deliver additional breast milk or formula while the infant is nursing. Hyperbilirubinemia may reach levels that require treatment with phototherapy administered with light or a blanket (see Chapter 27).

Late-onset jaundice affects few breastfed infants and develops in the second week of life, peaking at about 10 days of age. These infants are typically thriving, gaining weight, and stooling normally, and all pathologic causes of jaundice have been ruled out. It was once postulated that an enzyme in the milk of some mothers caused the bilirubin level to increase. It now appears that a factor in human milk increases the intestinal absorption of bilirubin. In most cases no intervention is necessary, although some experts recommend temporary interruption of breastfeeding for 12 to 24 hours to allow bilirubin levels to decrease. During this time, the mother pumps her breasts and the baby is offered alternative nutrition, usually formula (Lawrence, 1999).

Preterm infants. Human milk is the ideal food for preterm infants, with benefits that are unique and in addition to those received by term, healthy infants. Benefits include protection against infection, necrotizing enterocolitis, and atopic disease. Breast milk enhances retinal maturation in the preterm infant and improves neurocognitive outcome. There is also greater physiologic stability with breastfeeding as compared with bottle feeding (Brown et al., 1996; Meier & Brown, 1996).

In addition, the mothers of preterm infants receive specific emotional benefits in breastfeeding or providing breast milk for their babies. They report rewards in knowing they can provide the healthiest nutrition for the infant and believe that breastfeeding enhances feelings of closeness to the infant (Kavanaugh et al., 1997).

Mothers of preterm infants should begin pumping their breasts as soon as possible after birth with a hospital-grade electric pump. To establish an optimal milk supply, the mother should use a dual collection kit and pump 8 to 10 times daily for 10 to 15 minutes and/or until the milk flow has ceased for a few minutes (Meier, 1997). These women are taught proper handling and storage of breast milk to minimize bacterial contamination and growth.

Nurses in neonatal intensive care units provide essential support to mothers of preterm infants as the babies progress from being held in skin-to-skin contact by their mothers to learning how to latch on and suck effectively. Clinical specialists and lactation consultants assigned to

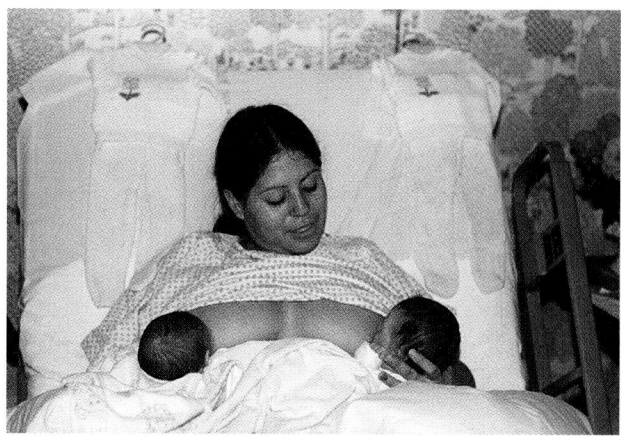

Fig. 28-8 Breastfeeding twins. *(Courtesy Marjorie Pyle, RNC, Lifecircle, Costa Mesa, CA.)*

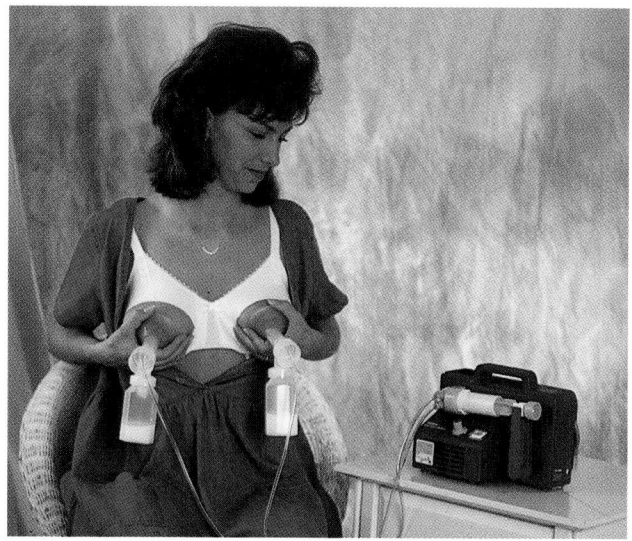

Fig. 28-9 Bilateral breast pumping. *(Courtesy Medela, Inc., McHenry, IL.)*

these units often prove invaluable in promoting effective breastfeeding by preterm infants.

Breastfeeding twins. Caring for twins takes some planning, but breastfeeding twins means that feedings are always ready instantly and no one has to wash bottles and fix formula. Some mothers are able to feed both babies at once. However, the mother of twins may need extra nourishment (200 to 500 kcal per day for each baby).

Each baby feeds from one breast per feeding, usually for about 20 to 30 minutes. Some mothers assign each baby a breast; others switch babies from one breast to the other, either on a schedule or randomly. The mother may find it easiest to use a modified demand feeding schedule. This involves feeding the first baby who wakes up and then waking the second baby for feeding.

During the early weeks, parents may find it helpful to keep a record of feeding times and which breast was used first by which baby. If one twin nurses more vigorously than the other, that twin should be alternated between breasts in order to equalize breast stimulation.

If the mother wants to feed the babies simultaneously, she may wish to experiment with positions. For example, one baby could be held in the football hold and the other in the cradle hold, or the babies could each be held in a cradling position. In another approach, each baby could be supported on firm pillows while in the football hold (Fig. 28-8), although, at first, some mothers who use this position may require help getting the babies off the breasts.

Expressing and Storing Breast Milk

There are situations when expression of breast milk is necessary or desirable, such as when:
- Engorgement occurs.
- The mother and baby are separated (e.g., preterm or sick infant is in neonatal intensive care).
- The mother is employed outside the home and needs to maintain her milk supply.
- The nipples are severely sore or cracked.

- The mother is leaving the infant in the care of the father or other caregiver and will not be available to breastfeed.

Because pumping and hand expression are rarely as efficient as a baby in removing milk from the breast, the milk supply should never be judged based on the volume expressed.

Hand expression. After her hands are thoroughly washed, the mother places one hand on her breast at the edge of the areola. With her thumb above and fingers below, she presses in toward her chest wall and gently compresses the breast while rolling her thumb and fingers forward. These motions are repeated rhythmically until the milk begins to flow. The mother simply maintains steady, light pressure while the milk is flowing easily. The thumb and fingers should not pinch the breast or slip down to the nipple, and the mother should rotate her hand to reach all sections of the breast. After expressing milk from the second breast, she should return and express milk from the first breast, then repeat the second breast until all readily available milk is expressed.

Pumping. For most women, it is advisable to initiate pumping only after the milk supply is well established and the infant is latching on and breastfeeding well. When breastfeeding is delayed after birth, pumping is started as soon as possible and continued regularly until the infant is able to breastfeed effectively.

There are numerous ways to approach pumping. Some women pump on awakening in the morning, or when the baby has fed but did not completely empty the breast. Others choose to pump after feedings or may pump one breast while the baby is feeding from the other. Double pumping (pumping both breasts at the same time) saves time and may stimulate the milk supply more effectively than single pumping (Fig. 28-9).

The amount of milk obtained when pumping depends on the type of pump being used, the time of day, how long it has been since the baby breastfed, the mother's milk supply, how practiced she is at pumping, and her comfort level (pumping is uncomfortable for some women). Breast milk may vary in color and consistency, depending on the time of day, the age of the baby, and foods the mother has eaten (e.g., the milk may appear green after the mother eats a spinach salad).

Types of pumps. Numerous breast pumps are available, with wide variation in cost, effectiveness, and ease of operation. Before purchasing or renting a breast pump, the mother would benefit from counseling by a nurse or lactation consultant to determine which pump best suits her needs.

Full-service electric pumps, or hospital-grade pumps, are most similar to the sucking action and pressure of the breastfeeding infant. These are expensive and therefore are usually rented. When breastfeeding is delayed after birth (e.g., the newborn is preterm or ill), or when mother and baby are separated for lengthy periods, these pumps are most appropriate (Fig. 28-10, *A*). Electric, self-cycling double pumps are efficient and easy to use. These pumps were designed for working mothers. Some of these pumps come with carry bags containing coolers to store pumped milk (see Fig. 28-9).

Smaller electric or battery-operated pumps are also available. Some have automatic suck/release cycling and others require use of a finger to regulate strength and speed of suction. These are typically used when pumping is done occasionally, but some models are satisfactory for working mothers or others who pump on a regular basis.

Manual or hand pumps are least expensive and most portable. These are most often used by mothers who are pumping for an occasional bottle (Fig. 28-10, *B*).

Storage of breast milk. Breast milk can be safely stored in any clean glass or plastic container. Disposable bottle liners are easy and inexpensive to use when storing milk. When using bottle liners, double bagging is recommended to protect the milk most effectively.

Breast milk can be refrigerated safely for 48 hours after it is expressed. If it is not used within that time, it can be frozen (0° C) for up to 6 months; it should be kept in the middle or toward the back of the freezer to avoid variations in temperature. Milk can be stored for 1 year in a −20° C freezer. When storing breast milk, the container should be dated, and the oldest milk should be used first.

Frozen milk is thawed by placing the container in warm water or in the refrigerator. It cannot be refrozen, and it should be used within 24 hours. After thawing, the container should be shaken to mix the layers that have separated.

NURSE ALERT *Frozen milk is never thawed or heated in a microwave oven. Microwaving does not heat evenly and can cause encapsulated boiling bubbles to form in the center of the liquid. This may not be detected when*

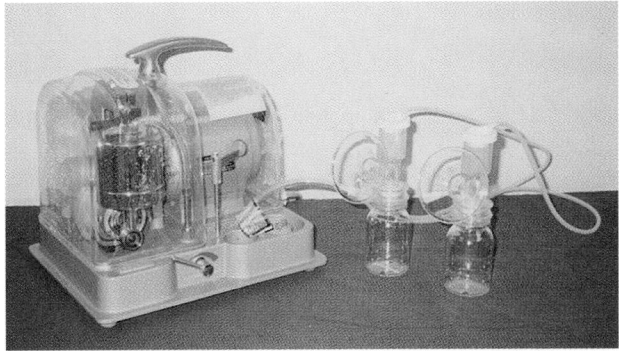

A

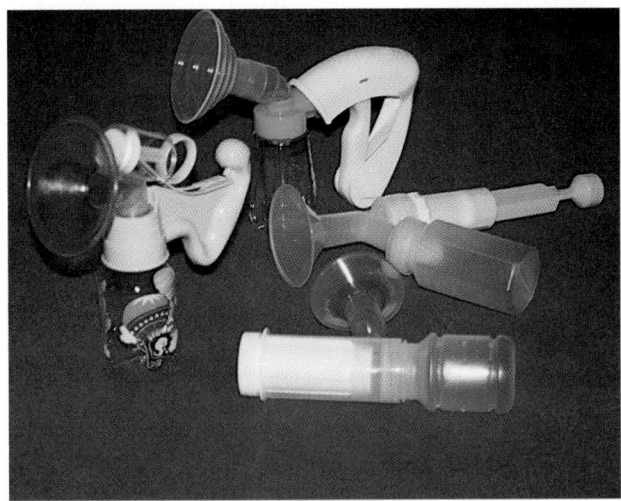

B

Fig. 28-10 A, Hospital-grade electric breast pump. **B,** Manual breast pumps. (**B** *courtesy Marjorie Pyle, RNC, Lifecircle, Costa Mesa, CA.*)

drops of milk are checked for temperature. Babies have sustained severe burns to the mouth, throat, and upper GI tract as a result of microwaved milk (Lawrence, 1999).

Being Away From the Baby

Many women are able to successfully combine breastfeeding with employment, attending school, or other commitments. If feedings are missed, the milk supply may be affected. Some women's bodies adjust the milk supply to the times she is with the baby for feedings, whereas others find they must pump or the supply diminishes quickly. Businesses are increasingly making available rooms where mothers can nurse their infants or use breast pumps (Fig. 28-11).

Breastfeeding mothers who work outside the home often feel a special connection to their babies even when they are separated. It is easy to continue breastfeeding while working. Planning ahead makes the transition back to work after birth much smoother and easier for both mother and baby. Breastfed babies are healthier, and mothers are less likely to miss work; this is an added benefit for the family and the employer.

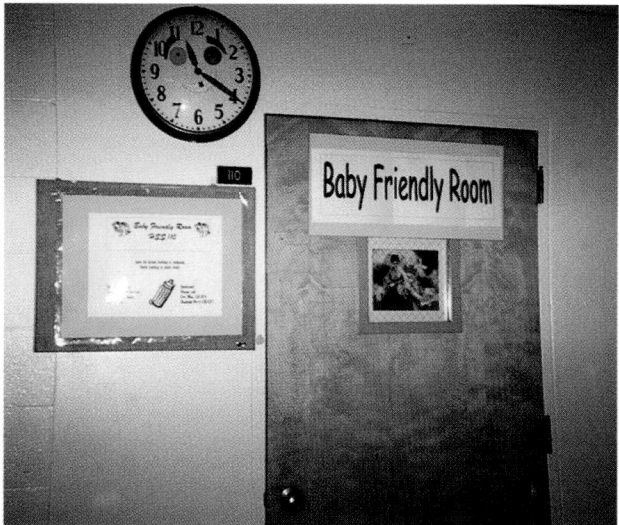

Fig. 28-11 Room on a university campus dedicated to parents and infants. The room contains comfortable furniture, a breast pump, a refrigerator, a baby changing table, and a television and VCR for instructional purposes. The room is available to students, faculty, and staff. (*Courtesy Shannon Perry, San Jose, CA.*)

Weaning

Typically, weaning is initiated at a time chosen by the mother or the infant. Weaning can be accomplished with little effort and no discomfort when it is done gradually. Abrupt weaning is likely to be distressing for both mother and baby, as well as physically uncomfortable for the mother.

Infant-led weaning means that the infant moves at his or her own pace in omitting feedings. Drinking from a cup and increasing the amount of solid foods substitute for breastfeeding.

Mother-led weaning means that the mother decides which feedings to drop. This is most easily done by omitting the feeding of least interest to the baby or the one the infant is most likely to sleep through. It can also be the feeding most convenient for the mother to omit. After a week or more, another feeding is dropped, and so on, until the infant is weaned from the breast. Allowing time for the milk supply to adjust before omitting another feeding prevents discomfort for the mother as her supply gradually decreases.

Infants can be weaned directly from the breast to a cup. Bottles are usually offered to infants less than 6 months of age. If the infant is weaned before 1 year of age, formula should be offered instead of cow's milk.

If abrupt weaning is necessary, breast engorgement often occurs. The mother is instructed to take mild analgesics, wear a supportive bra, apply ice packs or cabbage leaves to the breasts, and pump if needed to increase comfort. The pump should not be used to empty the breasts,

since they should remain full enough to promote a decrease in the milk supply.

Many women feel that weaning is the end to a special, satisfying relationship with the infant and benefit from time to adapt to the changes. Sudden weaning may evoke feelings of guilt and disappointment; some women go through a grieving period after weaning. The nurse can assist the mother by discussing other ways to continue this nurturing relationship with the infant, such as skin-to-skin contact while bottle feeding, or holding and cuddling the baby. Support from the father of the baby and other family members is essential at this time.

Milk Banking

For those infants who cannot be breastfed but who also cannot survive except on human milk, banked donor milk is critically important. Because of the antiinfective and growth-promoting properties of human milk, as well as its superior nutrition, donor milk is used in many neonatal intensive care units for preterm or sick infants when the mother's own milk is not available. Donor milk is also being used therapeutically for some medical purposes, such as in transplant recipients who are immunocompromised.

The Human Milk Banking Association of North America (HMBANA) has established annually reviewed guidelines for the operation of donor human milk banks (Arnold & Tully, 1996). Donor milk banks collect, screen, process, and distribute the milk donated by breastfeeding mothers who are feeding their own infants and pumping a few ounces extra each day for the milk bank. All donors are screened both by interview and serologically for communicable diseases. Donor milk is stored frozen until it is heat processed to kill potential pathogens; then it is refrozen for storage until it is dispensed for use. The heat processing adds a level of protection for the recipient that is not possible with any other donor tissue or organ. Banked milk is dispensed only by prescription. There is a per-ounce fee charged by the bank to pay for the processing costs, but the HMBANA guidelines prohibit payment to donors (see Appendix D).

Care of the Mother

Diet. The composition of human milk varies slightly among women, regardless of their diets. The mother's milk automatically contains everything the baby needs, except in rare cases of maternal nutrient deficiencies. For most women, only 200 to 500 extra calories per day need to be added to the diet to provide adequate nutrients for the infant while also protecting the mother's body stores.

There are no specific foods or drinks that all breastfeeding mothers must either consume or avoid. Lactating mothers should ideally consume a balanced diet of nutrient-dense foods. Adequate amounts of calcium, minerals, and fat-soluble vitamins are important.

If the breastfeeding mother is drinking enough fluids to quench her thirst, she is likely drinking enough to support lactation. Typically, women find that they are drinking as much as 2 to 3 quarts of fluid each day, with the choice of fluid depending on the mother's preference. Because of her increased need for fluids, the breastfeeding mother may wish to keep a drink within reach during feedings. An indicator of adequate fluid intake is the color of the mother's urine. If she is drinking enough fluids, her urine should be clear to light yellow throughout the day.

Weight loss. Because it takes energy to produce milk, many mothers experience a gradual weight loss while breastfeeding as fat stores deposited during pregnancy are used. This fact can be an added incentive for breastfeeding in the mother who is overweight. However, the mother who wants to diet while lactating should avoid losing large amounts of weight quickly because fat-soluble environmental contaminants to which she has been exposed are stored in her body's fat reserves and these may be released into her milk. In addition, some mothers find that their milk supply decreases when their caloric intake is severely restricted. Most mothers find that they can lose about 1 kg per week without affecting their milk supply.

Exercise. There is no reason for a breastfeeding woman to restrict her physical activity. Women can continue to engage in activities such as hiking, jogging, swimming, and aerobics with no detrimental effect on the milk supply or composition (Dewey et al., 1994). For comfort, mothers may find it beneficial to engage in exercise soon after breastfeeding, when their breasts are as empty as possible. Wearing a well-designed, supportive bra may also be helpful.

Rest. It is important for the breastfeeding mother to rest as much as possible, especially in the first 1 or 2 weeks after birth. Fatigue, stress, and worry can negatively affect milk production and let-down. The nurse can encourage the mother to sleep when the baby sleeps. Breastfeeding in a side-lying position promotes rest for the mother. Assistance with household chores and caring for other children can be done by the father, grandparents or other relatives, and friends.

Breast care. The breastfeeding mother's normal routine bathing is all that is necessary to keep her breasts clean. Soap can have a drying effect on nipples, so she should be instructed to avoid washing the nipples with soap. The small amount of soap that runs down her breasts while washing her face and neck or shampooing her hair is of no concern.

Breast creams should not be used routinely because they may block the natural oil secreted by the Montgomery glands on the areola. Some breast creams contain alcohol, which may dry the nipples. Vitamin E oil or cream is not recommended for use on nipples because it is a fat-soluble vitamin and a breastfeeding infant might consume enough vitamin E from the nipple to reach toxic levels. In addition, some people are allergic to vitamin E oil.

Modified lanolin with reduced allergens can be used safely on dry or sore nipples. Research has shown that

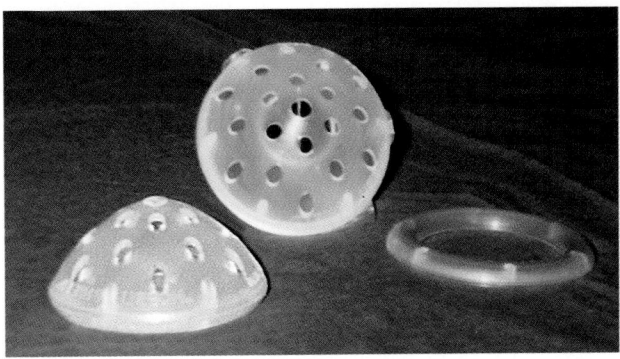

Fig. 28-12   Breast shells.

lanolin is beneficial in moist wound healing of sore nipples (Brent et al., 1998; Huml, 1995). Because lanolin is made from sheep's wool, the nurse should ask the mother if she is allergic to wool before applying the lanolin. Lanolin is not recommended if it is suspected that nipple soreness may be due to a monilial infection. Antifungal creams are used to treat yeast infections on nipples.

The mother with flat or inverted nipples will likely benefit from wearing breast shells in her bra. These hard plastic devices exert mild pressure around the base of the nipple to encourage nipple eversion. They are also useful for sore nipples to keep the mother's bra or clothing from touching the nipples (Fig. 28-12).

If a mother needs breast support, she will be uncomfortable unless she wears a bra, because the ligament that supports the breast (Cooper's ligament) will otherwise stretch and be painful. If she is comfortable without a bra, there is no reason for her to wear one. If a women prefers to wear a bra, it should fit well, offer nonbinding support, and feel comfortable. Underwire bras or improperly fitting bras may contribute to clogged milk ducts. Mothers should be encouraged to breastfeed at least once daily without a bra on so that all milk ducts can empty well.

Leakage of milk between feedings is a problem for some women. Using breast pads (disposable or washable) inside a bra and wearing layered or printed tops can help camouflage the leakage. Plastic-lined breast pads are not recommended because they trap moisture and may contribute to sore nipples. To stop leakage, the mother can be alert to any sensation, such as tingling, that her milk is letting down. If this happens, she can usually stop the letdown by pressing straight back on her nipples. In public, she can fold her arms across her chest to apply pressure unobtrusively.

Although only 1% to 2% of cases of breast cancer are diagnosed during pregnancy or lactation, the breastfeeding woman should perform monthly breast self-examination (BSE) (see Chapter 6). Before the resumption of menstrual periods, the woman needs to choose a convenient date on which to do her BSE each month. She needs to become familiar with the normal nodularity of her lactating breasts so that she can detect anything unusual on examination. Nodules that match in location in both breasts are likely breast tissue. Nodules that increase and decrease in size are probably milk glands or ducts. Because lactating breasts are very dense, mammography is of limited diagnostic value. Should a suspicious nodule be discovered, a biopsy can usually be done without interrupting breastfeeding.

Effect of menstruation. The return of menstrual periods varies among lactating women. The majority will resume menstruation by 6 months postpartum. Menstruation has no effect on breastfeeding. There are no hormonal effects on the infant, although some babies may seem fussy for the first day. The quality of the milk is not affected (Lawrence, 1999).

Sexual sensations. Some women experience rhythmic uterine contractions during breastfeeding. Such sensations are not unusual because uterine contractions and milk ejection are both triggered by oxytocin, but they may be disturbing to some mothers who perceive them to be similar to orgasm.

Breastfeeding and contraception. Although breastfeeding confers a period of infertility, it is not considered an effective method of contraception. Breastfeeding delays the return of ovulation and menstruation; however, ovulation may occur even before the first menstrual period after childbirth. Thus the breastfeeding woman who is relying on the lactational amenorrhea (LAM) method of birth control needs to be knowledgeable about ways to determine when ovulation occurs (basal body temperature, cervical mucus, cervical position). Hormonal contraceptives, including pills, injectables, and implants, may cause a decrease in the milk supply and are best avoided during the first 6 weeks after birth. Oral contraceptives containing estrogen are not recommended for breastfeeding mothers. Progestin-only birth control pills are less likely to interfere with the milk supply. Some women find that the progestin-only injection (Depo-Provera) or the implantable Norplant interferes with milk production, although others notice no alteration in the milk supply. Nonhormonal contraceptive methods (foam, condoms, nonhormonal intrauterine device [IUD], natural family planning, sterilization) are least likely to have a detrimental effect on breastfeeding (Kelsey, 1996).

Breastfeeding during pregnancy. It is possible for a breastfeeding woman to conceive and continue breastfeeding throughout the pregnancy if there are no medical contraindications (e.g., risk of preterm labor). Interestingly, when the baby is born, colostrum is produced. The practice of breastfeeding a newborn and an older child is called *tandem nursing.* The nurse should remind the mother to always feed the infant first to ensure that the newborn is receiving adequate nutrition. The supply-meets-demand principle works in this situation just as in the feeding of twins or triplets.

Diabetic mother. The diabetic mother is encouraged to breastfeed. In addition to benefits for the infant, and maternal satisfaction, breastfeeding has an antidiabetogenic effect. Blood glucose levels and insulin requirements are lower because of the carbohydrate used in milk production. During lactation, the diabetic woman may be able to eat more food and still take less insulin. However, insulin dosage must be adjusted as the baby is weaned. Some diabetic women are at increased risk for sore nipples caused by monilial infections and may have an increased risk for mastitis (Lawrence, 1999).

Drugs and breastfeeding. Although there is much concern about the compatibility of drugs and breastfeeding, there are in fact few drugs that are contraindicated during lactation. In evaluating the safety of a specific medication during breastfeeding, the health care provider considers the pharmacokinetics of the drug in the maternal system, as well as the absorption, metabolism, distribution, storage, and excretion in the infant. The gestational and chronologic age of the infant, body weight, and breastfeeding pattern are also considered (Lawrence, 1997).

The AAP (1994) has categorized commonly used medications according to their safety during breastfeeding (see Appendix C).

Drugs of abuse are contraindicated during lactation. These include amphetamine, cocaine, heroin, marijuana, nicotine, and phencyclidine hydrochloride ("angel dust," PCP) (AAP, 1994).

Nicotine can cause a decrease in the milk supply over time because of its effect on the milk ejection reflex. Mothers who continue to smoke tobacco when lactating should be advised not to smoke within 2 hours before breastfeeding and to never smoke in the same room with the infant (Lawrence, 1997).

Consumption of alcohol during lactation is approached with caution. Excessive amounts can have serious effects on the infant and can adversely affect the mother's milk ejection reflex. The level of alcohol in breast milk decreases over time, unlike the levels of many drugs that remain in milk until it is removed from the breasts. If a mother chooses to consume alcohol, she should be advised to minimize its effects by having only one drink, and to consume the drink immediately after breastfeeding. The mother who is pumping for a sick or preterm infant should avoid alcohol until her infant is healthy.

Although only 1% of the caffeine ingested by the mother is passed into her breast milk, the infant's immature system limits the ability to excrete the caffeine. Caffeine accumulates in the infant's system and can cause irritability and poor sleeping patterns. Some infants are sensitive to even small amounts of caffeine. Mothers of such infants should limit caffeine intake. Caffeine is found in coffee, tea, chocolate, and many soft drinks (Lawrence, 1999).

Herbs and herbal teas are becoming more widely used during lactation. Although some are considered safe, others contain pharmacologically active compounds that may have detrimental effects. A thorough history should include the consumption of any herbal remedies. Each remedy should then be evaluated for its compatibility with breastfeeding. The regional poison control center may provide information on the active properties of herbs (Lawrence, 1997).

Environmental contaminants. Chemicals that are lipophilic (dissolve in fat) are found in the lipid components of human milk. The amount depends on the mother's exposure to chemicals. Except under unusual circumstances, breastfeeding is not contraindicated because of exposure to environmental contaminants such as DDT (an insecticide) and tetrachloroethylene (used in dry cleaning plants) (Lawrence, 1997).

Special Considerations

The breastfeeding mother may experience some common problems. In the majority of cases, these complications are preventable if the mother receives appropriate education about breastfeeding. Early recognition and resolution of these problems is important to prevent interruption of breastfeeding and to promote the mother's comfort and sense of well-being. The nurse or lactation consultant is likely to be the first contact the mother makes when these problems arise. Using astute interview and assessment skills, the nurse can gather essential data related to these problems, make necessary referrals to the physician or nurse practitioner, and assist the mother in initiating the appropriate treatment plan. Emotional support provided by the nurse or lactation consultant is essential to help allay the mother's frustration and anxiety and to prevent early cessation of breastfeeding.

Engorgement. **Engorgement** usually occurs 3 to 5 days after birth when the milk "comes in" and lasts about 24 hours. It is a common response of the breasts to the sudden change in hormones and the presence of an increased volume of milk. Blood supply to the breasts increases and causes swelling of tissues surrounding the milk ducts. The ducts may be pinched shut, so that the milk does not flow. The breasts are firm, tender, hot, and may appear shiny and taut. The tenderness and swelling extends into the axilla. The areola are firm and the nipples may flatten. The unyielding areola make it difficult for the infant to latch on. Because back pressure on full milk glands inhibits milk production, if milk is not removed from the breasts, the milk supply may suffer.

Preparing the mother for what to expect when the milk comes in may help prevent engorgement or minimize its severity. Breastfeeding the baby frequently, at least every 2 to 3 hours, as the milk is coming in may help prevent engorgement. The baby should be encouraged to feed at least 15 to 20 minutes on each breast or until one breast softens per feeding.

When engorgement occurs, the nurse should reassure the mother that this a temporary condition usually resolved within 24 hours. The mother is instructed to feed every 2 hours, softening at least one breast, and pumping

the other breast to soften. Pumping during engorgement will not cause a problematic increase in milk supply.

Because of the swelling of breast tissue surrounding the milk glands' ducts, ice packs are recommended in a 15 to 20 minutes on, 45 minutes off rotation, in between feedings. The ice packs should cover both breasts. Large bags of frozen peas or corn make easy packs and can be refrozen between uses.

Raw cabbage leaves placed over the breasts in between feedings may help reduce the swelling (Roberts, 1995). The mother washes the cabbage leaves and places them in her freezer until they are cold, then places them over her breasts. The leaves are replaced when they begin to wilt. Although the exact mechanism of action of cabbage leaves in treatment of engorgement is not understood, it is thought that continuous application might decrease milk supply. (They are often very effective for formula-feeding mothers who want their milk to "dry up.")

Anti-inflammatory medications, such as ibuprofen, may help reduce the pain and swelling associated with engorgement. Mothers often run a low grade fever with engorgement and experience achiness in their breasts, which ibuprofen can help remedy.

Because heat increases blood flow, the application of heat to an already congested breast is usually counterproductive. Occasionally, however, standing in a warm shower will start the milk leaking, or the mother may be able to manually express enough milk to soften the areola so that the baby is able to latch on and feed.

Sore nipples. Mild nipple discomfort at the beginning of feedings or mild nipple tenderness during the first few days of breastfeeding is not abnormal. Severe soreness and abraded, cracked, or bleeding nipples are not normal and most often result from poor positioning, incorrect latch-on, improper suck, or a monilial infection. Many women expect breastfeeding to be painful based on stories they have heard from family and friends. The nurse or lactation consultant needs to emphasize that breastfeeding is not supposed to be a painful experience and that limiting the time at the breast will not prevent sore nipples. The key to preventing sore nipples is correct breastfeeding technique.

For the first few days after birth, the mother may experience some tenderness with the infant's initial sucks. This should quickly dissipate as the milk begins to flow and acts as a lubricant. To make the initial sucks less painful, the mother can express a few drops of milk to moisten the nipple and areola before latch-on.

If the mother continues to experience nipple pain or discomfort after the first few sucks, it is necessary to help the mother evaluate the baby's position at the breast to determine if the baby is well-supported, is in straight body-alignment, and has no pressure on the back of his or her head. The baby's nose, cheeks, and chin should be touching the breast, and the mother should be supporting the breast with her hand during the early feedings. The nurse helps the mother to reposition as necessary to try to resolve the nipple discomfort.

If the mother reports a pinching sensation on the nipple as the baby sucks, it may be helpful to gently pull down on the side of the baby's jaw while sucking to increase the amount of breast tissue in the baby's mouth. If the nipple pain continues, the mother needs to remove the baby from the breast, breaking suction with her finger in the baby's mouth. She then proceeds to attempt latch-on again, making sure the baby's mouth is open wide before the baby is pulled quickly to the breast (see Fig. 28-5). Often, sore nipples are the result of the mother latching the baby onto the breast before the mouth is open wide.

The infant's suck can be assessed by the nurse or lactation consultant simply by inserting a clean gloved finger in the baby's mouth and stimulating the baby to suck. If the baby is not extruding his tongue over the lower gum, and the mother reports pain or pinching with sucking, the baby may have a short frenulum (commonly referred to as being "tongue-tied"). Sometimes this is corrected surgically to free the tongue for less painful, more effective breastfeeding.

The treatment for sore nipples is first to correct the cause. Once the problem is identified and corrected, sore nipples should heal within a few days, even though the baby continues to breastfeed regularly.

When sore nipples occur, it is more comfortable to start the feeding on the least sore nipple. Applying ice to the nipple for 2 to 3 minutes provides a numbing effect that increases comfort with latch-on. After feeding, the nipples are wiped with water to remove the baby's saliva. A few drops of milk can be expressed, rubbed into the nipple, and allowed to air dry. It is usually soothing to apply a cooled, steeped caffeinated tea bag to sore nipples (tannic acid may help promote healing). The tea bag is "dabbed" on the nipples, and should not be left in place for longer than 1 to 2 minutes. Warm water compresses may also be comforting (Lavergne, 1997).

If nipples are extremely sore or damaged and the mother cannot tolerate breastfeeding, she may be advised to use an electric breast pump for 24 to 48 hours to allow the nipples to begin healing before resuming breastfeeding. It is important that the mother use a pump that will effectively empty the breasts; a rental pump is likely the best choice (see Fig. 28-10, *A*).

Sore nipples should be open to air as much as possible. Breast shells worn inside the bra allow for air to circulate, while keeping clothing off sore nipples (see Fig. 28-12).

Flexible nipple shields have been marketed as a treatment for sore nipples; however, it does not protect the nipple and can actually chafe the nipple as the baby sucks. There is also the danger of the baby not receiving adequate milk flow through the shield because it is difficult for most infants to get far enough back on the breast to adequately compress the lactiferous sinuses and get the milk to flow. There are special situations in which nipple shields are use-

ful; however, they should be used only by trained lactation consultants who closely monitor the infant's intake of milk and growth.

Monilial infections. Nipple soreness that is not resolved by the previously mentioned methods may be due to a **monilial** (yeast) **infection.** Sore nipples that occur after the newborn period are often due to a yeast infection. The mother usually reports severe nipple pain and tenderness, burning or stinging, and may have sharp, shooting, burning pains into the breasts during and after feedings. The nipples appear somewhat pink and shiny or may be scaly or flaky; there may be a visible rash, small blisters, or thrush. Most often, the pain is out of proportion to the appearance of the nipple. Yeast infections of the nipples and breast can be excruciatingly painful and can lead to early cessation of breastfeeding if not recognized and treated promptly.

Babies may or may not exhibit symptoms of monilial infection. Oral thrush and a red, raised diaper rash are common indications of a yeast infection. An affected infant is often very fussy and gassy. When feeding, the baby is likely to pull off the breast soon after starting to feed, crying with apparent pain. The infant may be biting or gumming at the breast.

The most common predisposing factors for yeast infection of the breast include previous antibiotic use, vaginal yeast infections, and nipple damage.

Mothers and babies must be treated simultaneously, even if the infant has no visible signs of infection. Treatment for mother is typically an antifungal cream applied to the nipples after feedings. Most pediatricians prescribe an oral antifungal medication, such as Nystatin, for infants. Treatment of mother and baby should continue for at least 7 days after symptoms begin to improve. Careful handwashing is essential to prevent the spread of yeast.

Family members may have symptoms of yeast infections and should receive appropriate treatment. Jock itch and finger or toenail fungus are types of yeast infections. Other children in the family may have diaper rash due to yeast (Amir, Hoover, & Mulford, 1995).

Plugged milk ducts. A milk duct may become plugged or clogged, causing an area of the breast to become swollen and tender. This area typically does not empty or soften with feeding or pumping. There may also be a small white pearl on the tip of the nipple; this is the curd of milk blocking the flow. The mother is afebrile and has no generalized symptoms.

Plugged ducts are most often the result of inadequate emptying of the breast. This may be due to clothing that is too tight, a poorly fitting or underwire bra, or always using the same position for feeding.

Application of warm compresses to the affected area and to the nipple before feeding helps promote emptying of the breast and release of the plug. (A disposable diaper filled with warm water makes an easy compress.) Soaking in a warm bath before feeding may be helpful.

Frequent feeding is recommended, with the baby beginning the feeding on the affected side to foster more complete emptying. The mother is advised to massage the affected area while the baby nurses or while she is pumping. Varying feeding positions and feeding without wearing a bra may be useful in resolving a plugged duct.

If the mother develops fever or flulike symptoms, she may have developed mastitis and should notify her health care provider. Plugged milk ducts do not necessarily cause mastitis, but milk stasis may increase the susceptibility to a breast infection.

Mastitis. A breast infection, or **mastitis,** is characterized by the sudden onset of flulike symptoms such as fever, chills, body aches, and headache. (Flulike symptoms in a breastfeeding mother should be considered indicative of mastitis, until proven otherwise.) There is localized breast pain and tenderness and a hot, reddened area on the breast, often resembling the shape of a pie wedge. Mastitis most commonly occurs in the upper outer quadrant of the breast; it may affect one or both breasts.

There are certain factors that may predispose a woman to mastitis. Inadequate emptying of the breasts is common, related to engorgement, plugged ducts, a sudden decrease in the number of feedings, abrupt weaning, or wearing underwire bras. Sore, cracked nipples may lead to mastitis by providing a portal of entry for causative organisms (*Staphylococcus, Streptococcus,* and *E. coli* are most common). Sore nipples often preclude complete emptying of the breast during feeding because of maternal discomfort. Stress and fatigue, ill family members, breast trauma, and poor maternal nutrition are also predisposing factors for mastitis (Fetherston, 1998).

Breastfeeding mothers should be taught the signs of mastitis before they are discharged from the hospital after birth and they need to know to call the health care provider promptly if the symptoms occur. Treatment includes antibiotics such as cephalexin or dicloxacillin, and analgesics/antipyretic medications such as ibuprofen. Rest is extremely important; the mother is advised to sleep whenever the baby sleeps. The mother should feed the baby or pump frequently, striving to adequately empty the affected side. Warm compresses to the breast before feeding or pumping may be useful. Adequate fluid intake and a balanced diet are important for the mother with mastitis.

Complications of mastitis include breast abscess, chronic mastitis, or fungal infections of the breast. Most complications can be prevented by early recognition and treatment.

ROLE OF THE NURSE IN PROMOTING SUCCESSFUL LACTATION

Nurses play a major role in breastfeeding education and support for new parents. Nurses often work in collaboration with lactation consultants in hospitals, physician offices, or community settings. Although the vast majority

are registered nurses, lactation consultants come from a variety of backgrounds such as nutrition, physical or occupational therapy, home economics, psychology, social work, education, or the basic sciences. **Lactation consultants** have had specialized postbaccalaureate education, training, and clinical experience related to breastfeeding. Most lactation consultants are certified by the International Board of Lactation Consultant Examiners, having met specific criteria for academic and clinical experience and having passed the certifying examination. The professional organization for lactation consultants is the International Lactation Consultant Association (ILCA) and is open to anyone interested in breastfeeding. The organization publishes the *Journal of Human Lactation,* which includes research and clinical articles related to breastfeeding.

Nurses who deal with women in prenatal settings are often the first to inquire about the mother's plans regarding infant feeding. It is the role of the nurse to educate the mother and her partner about the advantages of breastfeeding and to explore reasons why they may prefer formula feeding. Current reading materials and information about prenatal classes are made available to expectant parents. At each encounter the nurse offers to answer questions and provide additional information as needed.

Assessment of the mother's breasts and nipples during pregnancy are important. The nurse should inquire about breast changes during pregnancy, such as enlargement of the breasts. Flat or inverted nipples are identified, and the mother is offered breast shells (see Fig. 28-12) to wear during the last trimester of pregnancy to encourage eversion of the nipples, although antepartal use may be ineffective. These breast shells can also be worn postpartum between feedings.

Prenatal education of the mother who plans to breastfeed includes information about nipple preparation. There is no special nipple preparation necessary. The mother is advised to avoid using soap directly on her nipples. In previous years, women were told to pull on nipples and to rub them with a towel to "toughen" nipples for breastfeeding; women should be cautioned against these practices. The stimulation associated with pulling on nipples can prompt the release of oxytocin and result in preterm labor. Rubbing nipples with a towel can damage the outer layer of protective skin cells, which may increase the risk of sore nipples.

Through interviewing the pregnant woman and assessing the breasts, the nurse should determine if there have been any previous breast surgeries. Breast reduction or augmentation may interfere with the ability to produce milk and transfer it successfully to the baby. Interruption of milk ducts, and the blood and nerve supply associated with various surgical techniques can impact the woman's ability to breastfeed. It is important to discuss concerns about previous breast surgery with the woman and to stress the need to monitor the breastfeeding baby carefully for signs of adequate intake.

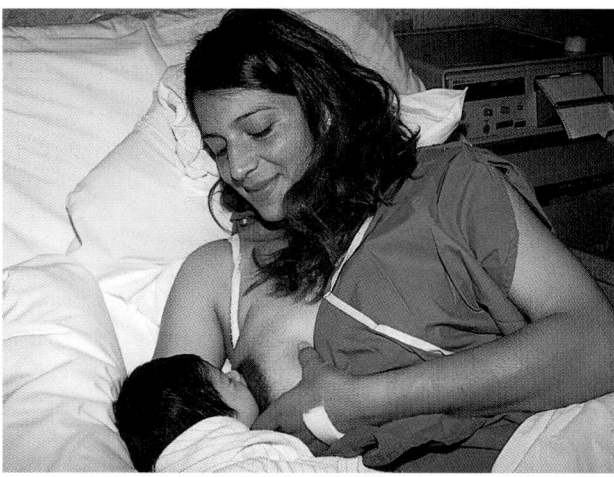

Fig. 28-13 Mother and infant enjoying breastfeeding. *(Courtesy Marjorie Pyle, RNC, Lifecircle, Costa Mesa, CA.)*

In the immediate postpartum period, the nurse is instrumental in helping the mother initiate breastfeeding as soon as possible after birth. Encouraging parents to keep the baby in the mother's room (rooming in) allows the opportunity for the mother to learn to recognize feeding cues and to feed the baby when these cues are present. The nurse provides help with positioning and latch-on until the mother can do so independently. Explanations are given early on regarding frequency and duration of feedings, how to wake a sleepy baby, and how to determine if the baby is getting enough milk. Before discharge, the nurse verifies that the parents are knowledgeable about breastfeeding and are prepared for what to expect in the days ahead. For example, information about the transition to mature milk (milk coming in) and how to prevent engorgement is needed. The mother is also informed about prevention and treatment of sore nipples and about signs of mastitis (including the importance of contacting the health care provider if these occur).

Parents often expect that because breastfeeding is "natural," it comes naturally for both mother and baby. This misconception needs to be clarified early on so that parents may view breastfeeding as a learning process. Then they are able to give themselves and their baby permission to learn, without unrealistic expectations. Nurses, physicians, and other health care providers who are knowledgeable about breastfeeding can offer needed support and encouragement to parents, helping to instill a sense of confidence (Fig. 28-13).

Follow-Up After Hospital Discharge

The hospital nurse is instrumental in assisting mothers with positioning, latch-on, waking a sleepy baby, and establishing a feeding routine. Problems with sore nipples, engorgement, and jaundice are likely to occur after discharge. Thus it is the role of the hospital nurse to educate

and prepare the mother for problems she may encounter once she is home. It is critical that the mother be given a list of resources for help with breastfeeding concerns and that she realizes when to call for assistance. Community resources for breastfeeding mothers include lactation consultants in hospitals, physicians' offices, or in private practice; nurses in pediatric or obstetric offices; support groups such as La Leche League; and peer counseling programs (e.g., those offered through WIC).

Telephone follow-up by hospital or office nurses within the first day or two after discharge can provide a means to identify any problems and offer needed advice and support. The AAP recommends that infants discharged before 48 hours of age be seen by a health care provider within 48 hours and have an office visit within 7 days after discharge. In some settings and circumstances, home care follow-up is available for mothers after hospital discharge.

Evaluation

Evaluation is based on the expected outcomes, and the plan of care is revised as needed based on the evaluation (see Plan of Care).

FORMULA FEEDING

Reasons for Formula Feeding

The decision to feed a baby infant formula may be the result of the mother's or partner's personal preference, the influence of other significant family members, or simply a lack of familiarity with breastfeeding. Occasionally there is no other option: the mother may have extensive breast scarring or may have had a bilateral mastectomy; the mother may be on medications that preclude breastfeeding; or the baby may be adopted. Some mothers are able to induce lactation for an adopted baby. Rarely, an infant may have galactosemia and must be fed a lactose-free formula.

Infant formula may be used to supplement breastfeeding if the mother's milk supply is inadequate. It may also be fed to the baby if the mother will be away and wishes to leave a bottle of formula instead of expressed breast milk.

Formula feeding is also recommended for mothers who are infected with the human immunodeficiency virus (HIV).

Parent Education

Inexperienced mothers and fathers who are formula feeding their infants usually need teaching, counseling, and support. They may need assistance with the feeding process and with any problems they may experience. Some parents who are formula feeding express concern that the baby will suffer as a result of their decision. Emphasis on the beneficial use of feeding times for close contact and socializing with the infant can help relieve some of this concern.

PLAN ᵒᶠ CARE | Newborn—Insufficient Intake of Nutrients

NURSING DIAGNOSIS Ineffective breastfeeding related to knowledge deficit of mother as evidenced by ongoing incorrect latch-on technique

---

Expected Outcome *Client will express increased satisfaction with breastfeeding, and neonate will exhibit satisfaction of hunger and sucking needs.*

Nursing Interventions/*Rationales*

Assess client's knowledge and motivation for breastfeeding *to acknowledge client's desire for effective outcome and provide starting point for teaching.*

Observe a breastfeeding session *to provide database for positive reinforcement and problem identification.*

Describe and demonstrate ways to stimulate the sucking reflex, various positions for breastfeeding, and the use of pillows during a session *to promote client and neonatal comfort and effective latch-on.*

Monitor neonatal position of mouth on areola and position of head and body *to give positive reinforcement for correct latch-on position or to correct poor latch-on position.*

Teach client ways to stimulate neonate to maintain an awake state by diapering, unwrapping, massaging, or burping *to complete a breastfeeding thoroughly and satisfactorily.*

Give client information regarding lactation diet, expression of milk by hand or pump, and storage of expressed breast milk *to provide basic information.*

Make sure client has written information on all aspects of breastfeeding *to reinforce verbal instructions and demonstrations.*

Refer to support groups and lactation consultant if needed *to provide further information and group support.*

Readiness for Feeding

The first feeding of formula is ideally given after the initial transition to extrauterine life is made. Feeding readiness cues include such things as stability of vital signs, presence of bowel sounds, and an active sucking reflex.

Before the first formula feeding, some institutions have the policy of offering sips of water to the newborn to assess patency of the GI tract and absence of tracheoesophageal fistula. If the infant sucks and swallows the water without difficulty, formula is then offered.

Feeding Patterns

Typically, a newborn will drink 7.5 to 15 ml of formula at a feeding at first, with the intake gradually increasing during the first week of life. Most babies are drinking 90 to 150 ml at a feeding by the end of the second week, or sooner. Generally, a baby who weighs less than 4.5 kg takes in about 840 ml of formula every 24 hours after the newborn period. A baby who weighs more than 4.5 kg ingests about 960 ml in 24 hours.

The newborn infant should be fed at least every 3 to 4 hours, even if that requires waking the baby for the feedings. The infant showing an adequate weight gain can be allowed to sleep at night and fed only on awakening. Most newborns need 6 to 8 feedings in 24 hours, and the number of feedings decreases as the infant matures. Usually by 3 to 4 weeks after birth, a fairly predictable feeding pattern has developed. Scheduling feedings arbitrarily at predetermined intervals may not meet a baby's needs, but initiating feedings at convenient times often moves the baby's feedings to times that work for the family.

Mothers will usually notice increases in the infant's appetite at 7 to 10 days, 3 weeks, 6 weeks, 3 months, and 6 months. These appetite spurts correspond to growth spurts. The amount of formula per feeding should be increased by about 30 ml to meet the baby's needs at these times.

Feeding Technique

Parents who choose formula feeding often need education regarding feeding techniques. During feedings they should be encouraged to sit comfortably, holding the infant closely in a semiupright position. Feedings provide opportunities to bond with the baby through touching, talking, singing, or reading to the infant. Parents should consider feedings as a time of peaceful relaxation with the baby (Fig. 28-14).

A bottle should never be propped with a pillow or other inanimate object and left with the infant. This practice may result in choking, and it deprives the infant of important interaction during feeding. Moreover, propping the bottle has been implicated in causing nursing bottle caries, or decay of the first teeth resulting from continuous bathing of the teeth with carbohydrate-containing fluid as the infant sporadically sucks the nipple.

The bottle should be held so that fluid fills the nipple and none of the air in the bottle is allowed to enter the nipple (Fig. 28-15). After the newborn period the infant who falls asleep, turns aside the head, or ceases to suck usually is signaling that enough formula has been taken. Parents should be taught to look for these cues and avoid overfeeding, which could contribute to obesity.

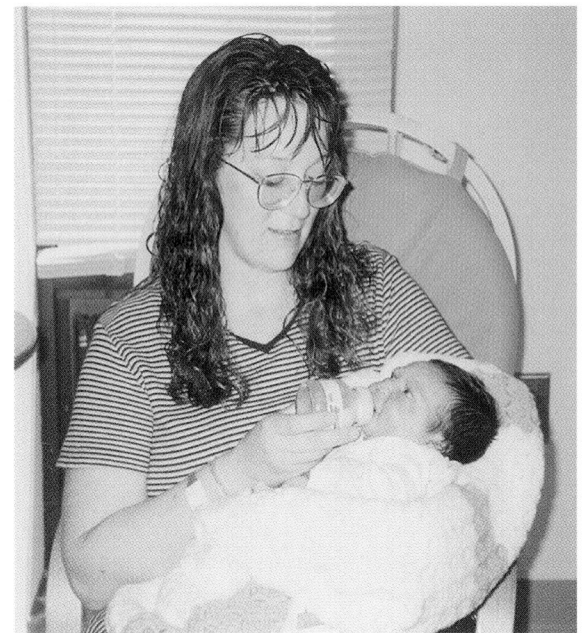

Fig. 28-14 Mother bottle feeding her 1-day-old infant.

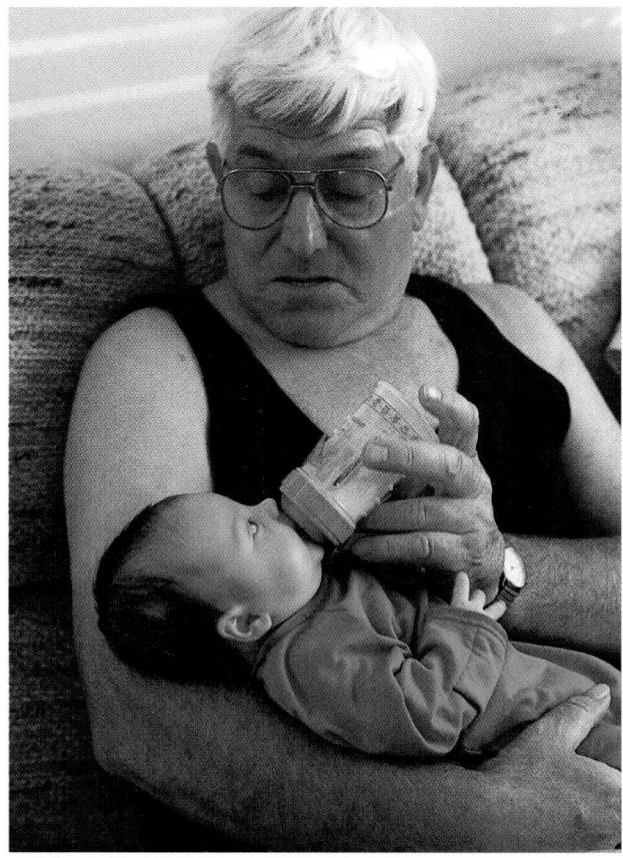

Fig. 28-15 Grandfather feeding infant granddaughter. Note angle of bottle that ensures milk covers nipple area. *(Courtesy Kim Molloy, Knoxville, IA.)*

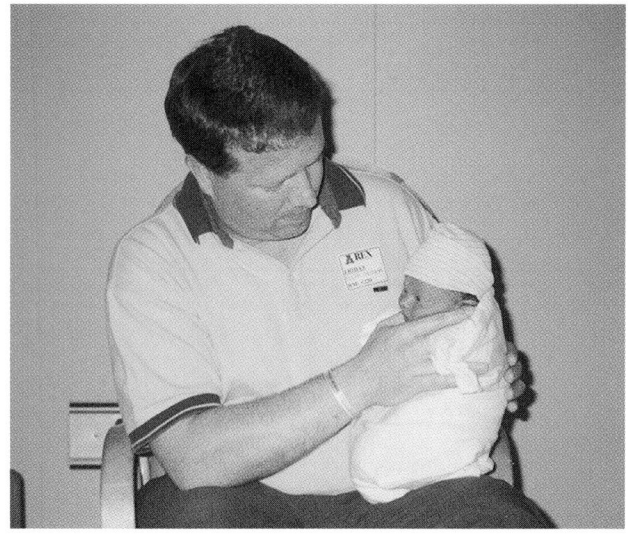

A

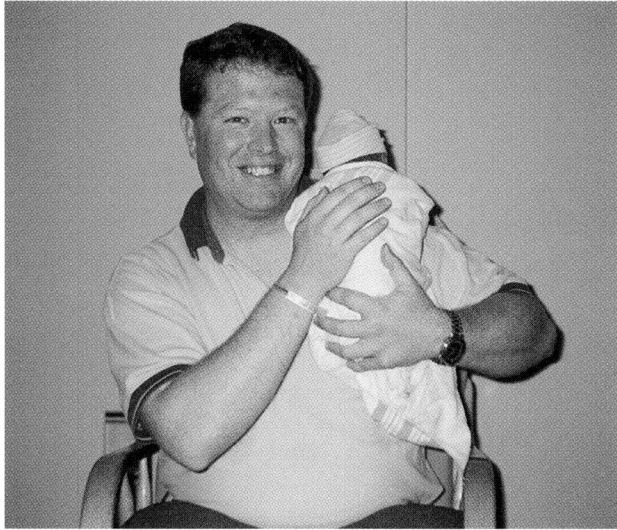

B

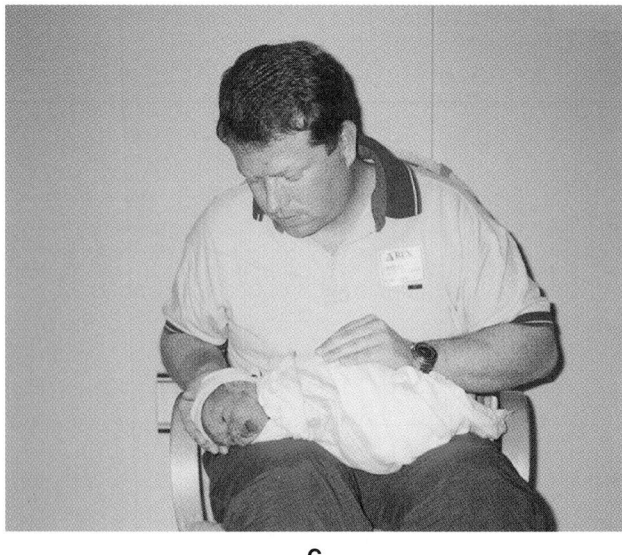

C

Fig. 28-16 Positions for burping an infant. **A,** Sitting. **B,** On the shoulder. **C,** Across the lap.

Most infants swallow air when fed from a bottle and should be given a chance to burp several times during a feeding (Fig. 28-16) (see Guidelines/Guías box).

Bottles and Nipples

There are various brands and styles of bottles and nipples available to parents. Most babies will feed well with any bottle and nipple. It is important that the bottles and nipples be washed in warm soapy water, using a bottle and nipple brush to facilitate thorough cleansing. Careful rinsing is necessary. Boiling of bottles and nipples is not needed unless there is some question about the safety of the water supply.

Infant Formulas

Commercial formulas. Because human milk is species specific to meet the needs of the human infant, it is used as the standard for all infant formulas. Commercial infant formulas are designed to resemble human milk as closely as possible, although none has ever duplicated it.

Infants who are not breastfed should be given commercial formulas. If this is too expensive, the family would likely be eligible for services through the WIC program, which provides iron-fortified infant formula. Cow's milk is the basis for most infant formulas, although soy-based and other specialized formulas are available for the infant who cannot tolerate cow's milk.

Commercial formulas are available in three forms: powder, concentrate, and ready-to-feed. All are equivalent in terms of nutritional content, but they vary considerably in cost:

- Powdered formula is the least expensive type. It is easily mixed by using one scoop for every 60 ml of water.
- Concentrated formula is more expensive than powder. It is diluted with equal parts of water and can be stored in the refrigerator for 24 hours after opening.
- Ready-to-feed formula is the most expensive but easiest to use. The desired amount is poured into the bottle. The opened can is safely refrigerated for 24 hours. This type of formula can be purchased in individual disposable bottles for the most convenient feeding.

Special formulas. Some infants have an allergic reaction to cow's milk formula. They may experience diarrhea, rash, colic, or vomiting, and, in extreme cases, fail to thrive. Some of these infants may better tolerate a soy milk formula; however, some then prove to be allergic to soy protein. If hypersensitivity to cow's milk protein is suspected, a hydrolyzed casein formula may be effective. Special formulas are very expensive. Some women may be able to begin breastfeeding or, in life-threatening cases, obtain human milk through a milk bank, at least temporarily.

Evaporated milk. Although evaporated milk is concentrated and less expensive than commercial formula, the mixing of evaporated milk and water to feed a baby is no longer recommended because evaporated milk does not provide adequate nutrition for an infant.

Unmodified cow's milk. Unmodified cow's milk is not suited to the nutritional needs of the human infant in the first year of life. Specific concerns include the excessive

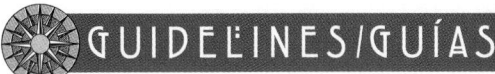

GUIDELINES/GUÍAS

Burping

Position #1 (Fig. 28-16, B)
Posición #1

Hold your baby up, head on your shoulder.
Ponga su bebé con la cabeza muy alta sobre su hombro.

Put one arm under the baby's bottom.
Ponga un brazo debajo de las nalgas del bebé.

With the other hand, pat or rub the baby's back.
Con la otra mano, dé leves palmaditas o sobe la espalda del bebé.

Position #2 (Fig. 28-16, A)
Posición #2

Sit your baby up in your lap.
Siente al bebé sobre su regazo.

Hold the head and back with one hand.
Con una mano, sostenga la cabeza y la espalda del bebé.

Hold the chin and front with the other.
Con la otra mano, sostenga la barbilla y la parte delantera del bebé.

Rock the baby's upper body back and forth.
Mueva la parte superior del bebé hacia adelante y hacia atrás.

Or pat the baby's back.
O dé suaves palmaditas a la espalda del bebé.

Position #3 (Fig. 28-16, C)
Posición #3

Lay your baby face down on your lap.
Coloque al bebé boca abajo sobre su regazo.

Hold the baby's head with one hand.
Con una mano, sostenga la cabeza del bebé.

Rub or pat the baby's back.
Sobe o dé suaves palmaditas a la espalda del bebé.

amounts of calcium, phosphorus, and other minerals it contains; an imbalance of calcium and phosphorus; its excessive protein content; the poor absorption of the fat it contains; and its low iron concentration. In addition, its use in infants is apt to cause microscopic hemorrhages that lead to GI blood loss. This blood loss, as well as the low levels of iron in the milk, increases the likelihood of iron deficiency anemia.

Formula Preparation

Recent recommendations for the labeling of commercial infant formulas require that the directions for the preparation and use of the formula be communicated with pictures and symbols for the benefit of nonliterate people. In addition, manufacturers are translating the directions into

HOME CARE

Formula Preparation and Feeding

Your newborn baby will be hungry about every $2\frac{1}{2}$ to 3 hours but sometimes may go 3 to 4 hours between feedings. The newborn should not go longer than 4 hours between feedings until a weight gain pattern is established—usually in about 2 weeks. Your baby needs to be awake before being fed. If your baby is sleepy, massage the baby's back and chest and talk to him or her.

Your baby's feedings will change a lot in the first week after birth. The first day, most babies only drink 7.5 to 15 ml of formula at a feeding. By the time they are a week old, most babies drink 30 to 60 ml at a feeding and then gradually increase their intake as they grow. If you do not use all of the formula at a feeding, throw away what is left, because it spoils once it has mixed with the baby's saliva.

You may want to write down how many milliliters your baby drinks each day. When you take the baby in for a checkup, the physician or nurse will ask you about how much formula the baby drinks. By 1 week of age, most babies who weigh 3 to 4.5 kg are drinking about 840 ml in 24 hours. Smaller babies drink a little less. Babies weighing more than 4.5 kg drink about 960 ml each day.

To feed your baby, place the nipple in the baby's mouth on the tongue. It should touch the roof of the mouth to stimulate the baby's sucking reflex. Hold the bottle like a pencil. Keep the bottle tipped so that the nipple stays filled with milk and the baby does not suck in air.

Hold your baby close for feedings. This should be a pleasant time for social interaction and cuddling. Some newborns take longer to feed than others. Be patient. It may be necessary to keep the baby awake and encourage continued sucking. Moving the nipple gently in the baby's mouth may stimulate more sucking.

Some newborns swallow air when sucking. Give your baby a chance to burp several times during early feedings. As your baby gets older and you get more experienced, you will know when to stop for burping.

If your baby fusses or cries in between feedings, check the diaper to see if he or she needs to be changed and see if the baby needs to be picked up and cuddled. If the baby continues to cry and acts hungry, then he or she needs to be fed. Babies do not get hungry on a schedule.

Place your baby on the right side after feedings so that air bubbles can come up easily. A rolled-up receiving blanket or small towel against the baby's back will keep him or her in the side-lying position. Some babies sleep better on their backs. To decrease the risk of SIDS, however, it is important not to put your baby to sleep stomach down.

The stools (bowel movements) of a formula-fed newborn are yellow and soft but formed. The baby will probably have a stool during or after each feeding in the first 2 weeks, but this will then gradually decrease to one to two stools each day.

SAFETY TIPS

- Babies should be held and never left alone while feeding. Do not prop the bottle. The baby could inhale formula or choke on any that was spit up.
- Know how to use the bulb syringe in case your baby should choke.
- Drinking bottles of formula or juice while falling asleep can cause tooth decay in young children (nursing bottle caries).

FORMULA PREPARATION

- Wash your hands and clean the bottle, nipple, and can opener carefully before preparing formula.
- If new nipples seem too hard, they can be softened by boiling them in water for 5 minutes before use.
- Read the label on the container of formula and mix it exactly according to the directions.
- Use tap water to mix concentrated or powdered formula unless directed otherwise by your baby's physician or nurse.
- Test the size of the nipple hole by holding a prepared bottle upside down. The formula should drip from the nipple. If it runs in a stream, the hole is too big and should not be used. If it has to be shaken for the formula to come out, the hole is too small. You can either buy a new nipple or enlarge the hole by boiling the nipple for 5 minutes with a sewing needle inserted in the hole.
- If a nipple collapses when your baby sucks, loosen the nipple ring a little to let in air.
- Opened cans of ready-to-feed or concentrated formula should be covered and refrigerated. Any unused portions must be discarded after 48 hours.
- Bottles or cans of unopened formula can be stored at room temperature.
- If the formula is refrigerated, warm it by placing the bottle in a pan of hot water. Never use a microwave to warm any food to be given to a baby. Test the temperature of the formula by letting a few drops fall on the inside of your wrist. If the formula feels comfortably warm to you, it is the correct temperature.

various languages, such as Spanish, French, Vietnamese, Chinese, and Arabic, to prevent misunderstanding and errors in formula preparation. It is important to impress on families that the proportions must not be altered—neither diluted to expand the amount of formula nor concentrated to provide more calories.

Although manufacturers of commercial formula include directions for preparing their products, the nurse should review formula preparation with the mother. It is especially important that formula be mixed properly. The newborn's kidneys are immature, and giving the infant overly concentrated formula may provide protein and minerals in amounts that exceed the kidney's excretory ability. In contrast, if the formula is diluted too much (sometimes done in an effort to save money), the infant does not consume enough calories and does not grow well.

Sterilization of formula rarely is recommended for those families with access to a safe public water supply. Instead, the formula is prepared with attention to cleanliness. When water from a private well is used, parents should be advised to contact the health department to have a chemical and bacteriologic analysis of the water done before using the water in formula preparation. The presence of nitrates, excess fluoride, or bacteria may be harmful to the infant.

In addition, if the sanitary conditions in the home appear unsafe, it would be better to recommend the use of ready-to-feed formula or to teach the mother to sterilize the formula. The two traditional methods for sterilization are terminal heating and the aseptic method. In the terminal heating method, the prepared formula is placed in the bottles, which are topped with the nipples placed upside down and covered with the caps, and then sealed loosely with the rings. The bottles are then boiled together in a water bath for 25 minutes. In the aseptic method, the bottles, rings, caps, nipples, and any other necessary equipment, such as a funnel, are boiled separately, after which the formula is poured into the bottles. Any formula left in the bottle after the feeding should be discarded because the baby's saliva has mixed with it. (Instructions for formula preparation and feeding are provided in the Home Care box.)

Vitamin and Mineral Supplementation

Commercial iron-fortified formula has all of the nutrients the infant needs for the first 6 months of life. After 6 months, the only mineral supplementation required is 0.25 mg of fluoride daily if the local water supply is not fluoridated (AAP, 1997).

Weaning

The bottle-fed infant will gradually learn to use a cup, and the parents will find that they are preparing fewer bottles. Often the bottle feeding before bedtime is the last one to remain. Babies have a strong need to suck, and the baby who has the bottle taken away too early or abruptly will compensate with nonnutritive sucking on his or her fingers, thumb, a pacifier, or even his or her own tongue. Weaning

from a bottle should therefore be done gradually because the baby has learned to rely on the comfort that sucking provides. This comfort helps a baby to cope with other events, such as toilet training or the birth of a sibling.

Introducing Solid Foods

The infant receives the right balance of nutrients from breast milk or formula during the first 4 to 6 months. It is not true that the feeding of solids will help the infant sleep through the night. Introduction of solid foods before the infant is 4 to 6 months of age may result in overfeeding and decreased intake of breast milk or formula. The infant cannot communicate feeling full as can an older child, who is able to turn the head away. The proper balance of carbohydrate, protein, and fat for an infant to grow properly is in the breast milk or formula.

The infant's individual growth pattern should help determine the right time to start solids. The primary health care provider will advise when to introduce solid foods. The schedule for introducing solid foods and the type of foods to serve will be discussed during well-baby supervision visits with the pediatrician or pediatric nurse-practitioner.

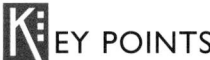

KEY POINTS

- Human breast milk is species specific and is the recommended form of nutrition for infants, providing immunologic protection against many infections and diseases.
- Breast milk changes in composition with each stage of lactation, during each feeding, and as the infant grows.
- During the prenatal period, parents should be informed of the benefits of breastfeeding for infants, mothers, families, and society.
- Infants should be breastfed as soon as possible after birth and at least 8 to 12 times per day thereafter.
- There are specific, measurable indications that the infant is breastfeeding effectively.
- Breast milk production is based on a supply-meets-demand principle: the more the infant nurses, the greater the milk supply.
- Commercial infant formulas provide satisfactory nutrition for most infants.
- All infants should be held for feedings.
- Parents should be instructed about the types of commercial infant formulas, proper preparation for feeding, and correct feeding technique.
- Unmodified cow's milk is inappropriate for infants during the first year of life.
- Solid foods should be started after 6 months of age.
- Nurses must be knowledgeable about feeding methods and provide education and support for families.

CRITICAL THINKING EXERCISES

I As the postpartum home care nurse, you arrive at the residence of Jane and Jim Taylor, first-time parents of 3-day-old Michael. Jane and Michael were discharged from the hospital at 36 hours after an uncomplicated vaginal birth. Jim greets you at the door, "I am so glad to see you. The baby is screaming; Jane is in tears. She's so full that he can't latch on." You find Jane looking very tired and frustrated; baby Michael appears frantic. Jane says, "I feel like a failure. Breastfeeding looked so easy in the videos." Describe how you would approach this situation, including client education and follow-up.

2 Nakesha is a 19-year-old single African-American who has come to the prenatal clinic for her 36-week visit. You inquire about how she plans to feed her infant, because she has not yet decided, according to the prenatal record. She says she would like to breastfeed, but thinks it will be too embarrassing. Devise a teaching plan to help Nakesha make her decision about whether to breastfeed or formula feed. What community resources might be useful to her if she chooses to breastfeed?

3 You are assisting Pamela in positioning her 1-day-old daughter at the breast. The baby has been very sleepy and difficult to arouse for feedings, but is now awake and alert. The baby latches on, but Pamela reports that it feels like she is pinching the nipple and it is very painful. What assessments should you make? What interventions are appropriate?

References

American Academy of Pediatrics (AAP). (1994). The transfer of drugs and other chemicals into human breast milk. *Pediatrics* 93(1), 137-150.

American Academy of Pediatrics (AAP). (1998). *Pediatric nutrition handbook* (4th ed.). Elk Grove Village, IL: American Academy of Pediatrics.

American Academy of Pediatrics Work Group on Breastfeeding. (1997). Breastfeeding and the use of human milk. *Pediatrics* 100(6), 1035-1039.

Amir, L., Hoover, K., & Mulford, C. (1995). *Candidiasis and breastfeeding (Unit 18). Lactation consultant series.* New York: Avery Publishing.

Arlotti, J. et al. (1998). Breastfeeding among low-income women with and without peer support. *J Community Health Nurs* 15(3), 163-178.

Arnold, L., & Tully, M. (1996). *Guidelines for the establishment and operation of a donor human milk bank* (6th ed.). West Hartford, CT: Human Milk Banking Association of North America.

Association of Women's Health, Obstetric, and Neonatal Nurses (AWHONN). (1998). *Standards and guidelines for professional nursing practice in the care of women and newborns* (5th ed.). Washington, D.C.: The Association.

Barnard, J. (1997). Gastrointestinal disorders due to cow's milk consumption. *Pediatr Ann* 26(4), 244-250.

Bar-Yam, N., & Darby, L. (1997). Fathers and breastfeeding: A review of the literature. *J Hum Lact* 13(1), 45-50.

Behrman, R., Kliegman, R., & Arvin, A. (Eds.). (1996). *Nelson's textbook of pediatrics* (15th ed.). Philadelphia: W.B. Saunders.

Brent, N. et al. (1998). Sore nipples in breastfeeding women: A clinical trial of wound dressings vs. conventional care. *Arch Pediatr Adolesc Med* 152(11), 1077-1082.

Brown, L. et al. (1996). Use of human milk for low-birth-weight infants. *Online J Know Synth Nurs* 3(27), 1-9.

Choudhry, U. (1997). Traditional practices of women from India: Pregnancy, childbirth, and newborn care. *J Obstet Gynecol Neonatal Nurs* 26(5), 533-539.

Chua, S. et al. (1994). Influences of breastfeeding and nipple stimulation on postpartum uterine activity. *Br J Obstet Gynaecol* 101, 804-805.

Cushing, A. et al. (1998). Breastfeeding reduces risk of respiratory illness in infants. *Am J Epidemiol* 147(9), 863-870.

Davis, M. (1998). Review of the evidence for an association between infant feeding and childhood cancer. *Int J Cancer* (Suppl)11, 29-33.

Dewey, K. et al. (1994). A randomized study of the effects of aerobic exercise by lactating women on breast-milk volume and composition. *N Engl J Med* 330(7), 449-453.

Dewey, K., Heinig, M., & Nommsen, L. (1993). Maternal weight-loss patterns during prolonged lactation. *Am J Clin Nutr* 58, 162-166.

Dewey, K., Heinig, M., & Nommsen-Rivers, L. (1995). Differences in morbidity between breastfed and formula-fed infants. *J Pediatr* 126(5 pt 1), 696-702.

Eisman, J. (1998). Relevance of pregnancy and lactation to osteoporosis. *Clin Perinatol* 25(2), 303-326.

Enger, S. et al. (1998). Breastfeeding experience and breast cancer risk among postmenopausal women. *Cancer Epidemiol Biomarkers Prev* 7(5), 365-369.

Fetherston, C. (1998). Risk factors for lactational mastitis. *J Hum Lact* 14(2), 101-109.

Ford, R. et al. (1993). Breastfeeding and the risk of sudden infant death syndrome. *Int J Epidemiol* 22(5), 885-890.

Fuchs, S., Victoria, C., & Martines, J. (1996). Case-control study of risk of dehydrating diarrhea in infant in the vulnerable period after full weaning. *Br Med J* 313(7054), 391-394.

Gerstein, H. (1994). Cow's milk exposure and type I diabetes mellitus. *Diabetes Care* 17, 13-19.

Goldman, A. (1993). The immune system of human milk: Antimicrobial, antiinflammatory and immunomodulating properties. *Pediatr Infect Dis J* 12(8), 664-671.

Halken, S., & Host, A. (1996). Prevention of allergic disease: Exposure to food allergens and dietetic intervention. *Pediatr Allergy Immunol* 7(9 suppl), 102-107.

Hirose, K. et al. (1995). A large-scale, hospital-based case-control study of risk factors of breast cancer according to menopausal status. *Jpn J Cancer Res* 86(2), 146-154.

Huml, S. (April 1995). Cracked nipples in the breastfeeding mother. *Adv Nurs Pract*, 1.

Kavanaugh, K. et al. (1997). The rewards outweigh the efforts: Breastfeeding outcomes for mothers of preterm infants. *J Hum Lact* 13(1), 15-21.

Kelsey, J. (1996). Hormonal contraception and lactation. *J Hum Lact* 12(4), 315-318.

Lavergne, N. (1997). Does application of tea bags to sore nipples while breastfeeding provide effective relief? *J Obstet Gynecol Neonatal Nurs* 26(1), 53-58.

Lawrence, R. (1997). A review of the medical benefits and contraindications to breastfeeding in the United States. *Maternal and child health technical information bulletin.* Arlington, VA: National Center for Education in Maternal and Child Health.

Lawrence, R. (1999). *Breastfeeding: A guide for the medical profession* (5th ed.). St. Louis: Mosby.

Lopez-Alarcon, M., Villalpando, S., & Fajardo, A. (1997). Breastfeeding lowers the frequency and duration of acute respiratory infections and diarrhea in infants under six months of age. *J Nutr* 127(3), 436-443.

Lucas, A. et al. (1992). Breast milk and subsequent intelligence quotient in children born preterm. *Lancet* 339(8788), 261-264.

Lucas, A. et al. (1994). A randomised multicentre study of human milk versus formula and later development in preterm infants. *Arch Dis Child Fetal Neonatal Ed.* 70(2), F141-F146.

Meier, P. (1997). *Professional guide to breastfeeding premature infants.* Columbus, OH: Ross Products Division, Abbott Laboratories.

Meier, P. & Brown, L. (1996). State of the science: Breastfeeding for mothers and low-birth-weight infants. *Nurs Clin North Am* 31(2), 351-365.

Melton, L. et al. (1993). Influence of breastfeeding and other reproductive factors on bone mass later in life. *Osteoporosis Int* 3(2), 76-83.

Mohrbacher, N., & Stock, J. (1997). *The breastfeeding answer book* (2nd ed.). Schaumburg, IL: La Leche League International.

Montgomery, D., & Splett, P. (1997). Economic benefit of breastfeeding infants enrolled in WIC. *J Am Diet Assoc* 97(4), 379-385.

Morse, J., Jehle, C., & Gamble, D. (1990). Initiating breastfeeding: A world survey of the timing of postpartum breastfeeding. *Int J Nurs Stud* 27(3), 303-313.

Newman, J. (1995). How breast milk protects newborns. *Sci Am* 273(6), 76-79.

Rassin, D. et al. (1994). Acculturation and the initiation of breastfeeding. *Clin Epidemiol* 47(7), 739-746.

Righard, L., & Alade, M. (1997). Breastfeeding and the use of pacifiers. *Birth* 24, 116-120.

Riordan, J. (1997). The cost of not breastfeeding: A commentary. *J Hum Lact* 13(2), 93-97.

Roberts, K. (1995). A comparison of chilled cabbage leaves and chilled gel-paks in reducing breast engorgement. *J Hum Lact* 11(1), 17-20.

Rosenblatt, K., & Thomas, D. (1995). Prolonged lactation and endometrial cancer. WHO collaborative study of neoplasia and steroid contraceptives. *Int J Epidemiol* 24, 499-503.

Ryan, A. (1997). The resurgence of breastfeeding in the United States. *Pediatrics* 99(4), E12.

Saarinen, U., & Kajosaari, M. (1995). Breastfeeding as prophylaxis against atopic disease: Prospective follow-up study until 17 years old. *Lancet* 346(8982), 1065-1069.

Sassen, M., Brand, R., & Grote, J. (1994). Breastfeeding and acute otitis media. *Am J Otolaryngol* 15(5), 351-357.

Scariati, P., Grummer-Strawn, L., & Fein, S. (1997). A longitudinal analysis of infant morbidity and the extent of breastfeeding in the United States. *Pediatrics* 99(6), E5.

Shu, X. et al. (1995). Infant breastfeeding and the risk of childhood lymphoma and leukemia. *Int J Epidemiol* 24(1), 27-32.

Victora, C. et al. (1997). Pacifier use and short breastfeeding duration: Cause, consequence, or coincidence? *Pediatrics* 99, 445-453.

Wang, Y., & Wu, S. (1996). The effect of exclusive breastfeeding on development and incidence of infection in infants. *J Hum Lact* 12, 27-30.

Weissinger, D. (1998). A breastfeeding teaching tool using a sandwich analogy for latch-on. *J Hum Lact* 14(1), 51-56.

Widstrom, A., Ransjo-Arvidsson, A., & Christensson, K. (1993). *Breastfeeding is the baby's choice.* Richmond, VA: BGK Enterprises Production.

29

Assessment for Risk Factors

Cynthia Garrett

LEARNING OBJECTIVES

- Define the key terms.
- Explore the scope of high risk pregnancy.
- Discuss regionalization of health care services.
- Examine risk factors identified through history, physical examination, and diagnostic techniques.
- Describe diagnostic techniques and the implications of findings.

- Explain diagnostic techniques to clients and their families.
- Identify topics for nursing research related to assessment of high risk pregnancy.

KEY TERMS

acoustic stimulation test
alpha-fetoprotein (AFP)
amniocentesis
amniotic fluid index (AFI)
amniotic fluid volume (AFV)
biophysical profile (BPP)
biparietal diameter (BPD)

chorionic villus sampling (CVS)
contraction stress test (CST)
daily fetal movement count (DFMC)
Doppler ultrasound
fetal activity determination (FAD)
magnetic resonance imaging (MRI)
nonstress test (NST)

percutaneous umbilical blood
  sampling (PUBS)
triple marker test
ultrasound
uteroplacental insufficiency (UPI)

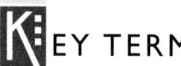

pproximately 500,000 of the 4 million births that occur in the United States each year will be categorized as high risk because of maternal or fetal complications. Identification of the risks, together with appropriate and timely intervention during the perinatal period, can prevent morbidity and mortality among mothers and infants.

With the changing demographics in the United States, more women and families can be identified as at risk because of factors other than biophysical criteria. The increasing numbers of homeless, single, or uninsured pregnant women who have no access to prenatal care during any stage of pregnancy and the behaviors and lifestyles

that pose a risk to the health of the mother and fetus contribute to the problem (Fogel & Lewallen, 1995).

Care of these high risk clients requires the unified efforts of medical and nursing personnel. The high risk client and the factors associated with a diagnosis of high risk are identified in this chapter; diagnostic techniques used to monitor the maternal-fetal unit are emphasized.

DEFINITION AND SCOPE OF THE PROBLEM

A high risk pregnancy is one in which the life or health of the mother or fetus is jeopardized by a disorder coincidental with or unique to pregnancy. For the mother the high risk status arbitrarily extends through the puerperium (30 days after childbirth). Postbirth maternal complications are usually resolved within 1 month of birth, but perinatal morbidity may continue for months or years.

Advances in the management of disorders that affect pregnant women have resulted in a significant decrease in maternal mortality and morbidity rates. In the United States, maternal mortality rates have remained the same between 1982 and 1996 at approximately 7.5 per 100,000 (National Center for Health Statistics, 1998a).

However, the decline in perinatal mortality and morbidity is not as significant and needs to be examined when the scope of high risk pregnancy is being considered. Infant mortality rates have shown improvement, dropping from 10 per 1000 live births in 1970 to 7.1 per 1000 live births in 1997, the lowest ever recorded in the United States. Yet, compared with other developed countries the United States ranks twenty-third in infant mortality (Guyer et al., 1998).

High risk pregnancy represents a critical problem of modern medical and nursing care. The new social emphasis on the quality of life and the wanted child has resulted in a reduction of family size and the number of unwanted pregnancies. At the same time, technologic advances have enabled pregnancies in previously infertile couples. As a consequence, emphasis is on the safe birth of normal infants who can develop to their potential. Scientific and technologic advances have allowed perinatal health care to reach a level far beyond that previously available.

Although pregnancy is often referred to as a maturational crisis, the diagnosis of high risk imposes another crisis, a situational one (e.g., loss of pregnancy before the anticipated date, development of gestational diabetes mellitus with its potential complications, or birth of a neonate who does not meet cultural, societal, or familial norms and expectations).

Maternal Health Problems

The leading causes of maternal death attributable to pregnancy differ over the world. In general, three major causes have persisted for the last 40 years: hypertensive disorders, infection, and hemorrhage. The three leading causes of maternal mortality today are pregnancy-induced hypertension, pulmonary embolism, and hemorrhage (National Center for Health Statistics, 1997).

Even though the maternal death rate has remained at about 7.5 per 100,000 live births (National Center for Health Statistics, 1998a), the goal set by Healthy People 2000: National Health Promotion and Disease Prevention Objectives was no more than 3.3 maternal deaths per 100,000 live births (Koonin et al., 1997). This goal will not be attained by the year 2000. Factors that are strongly related to maternal death include age (less than 20 years and 35 years or greater), lack of prenatal care, low educational attainment, unmarried status, and nonwhite race. African-American maternal mortality rates are three to four times higher than those for Caucasian women (Koonin et al., 1997).

Although the overall number of maternal deaths is small, maternal mortality remains a significant problem because a high proportion of deaths are preventable, primarily through improving the access to and use of prenatal care services. Educating the public about the importance of obtaining early and regular care during pregnancy is a function that nurses are well positioned to perform.

Fetal and Neonatal Health Problems

Fetal and neonatal health problems are described under certain categories: fetal death (demise), neonatal death, perinatal death, perinatal death rate, and infant mortality. (Definitions for these terms are found in Chapter 1.) The incidence of each disorder that results in infant mortality is expressed as the number of deaths per 1000 live births. The infant mortality rate includes neonatal deaths.

The leading cause of death in the neonatal period is congenital anomalies (National Center for Health Statistics, 1998b). Other causes of neonatal death include disorders related to short gestation and low birth weight, sudden infant death, respiratory distress syndrome, and the effects of maternal complications. Increased rates of survival during the neonatal period have resulted largely from high quality prenatal care and the improvement in perinatal services, including technologic advances in neonatal intensive care and obstetrics. These factors may account for at least a 50% reduction in mortality in neonates weighing less than 1500 g (Richardson et al., 1998).

Commitment at national, state, and local levels is required to reduce the infant mortality rate. More research is needed to identify the extent to which financial, educational, sociocultural, and behavioral factors impact perinatal morbidity and mortality. Barriers to care must be removed and perinatal services modified to meet contemporary health care needs (Dooley, Freels, & Turnock, 1997).

Regionalization of Health Care Services

Early and ongoing risk assessment is a crucial component of perinatal care. Conditions associated with perinatal morbidity and mortality can be prevented, treated, or referred to more skilled health care providers. Factors to consider when determining a client's risk status include resources available locally to treat the condition, availability of appropriate facilities for transport if needed, and determination of the best match for the client's needs.

Not all facilities develop and maintain the full spectrum of services required for high risk perinatal clients. As a consequence, the concept of regionalization of health care services—facilities within a geographic region organized to provide different levels of care—emerged.

However, regionalization alone has not consistently improved perinatal outcomes (Dooley, Freels, & Turnock, 1997). Furthermore, managed care markets and other financial pressures have forced some providers to be more competitive. In order to meet this challenge, facilities began to extend the kind of perinatal services offered. Perinatal

GUIDELINES/GUÍAS

HIGH RISK ASSESSMENT	POTENTIAL PROBLEM
Have you had blurred vision? *¿Ha tenido la vista borrosa?*	PIH
Have you had severe headaches? *¿Ha tenido dolores fuertes de cabeza?*	PIH
Have you had difficulty breathing? *¿Ha tenido dificultad para respirar?*	Cardiac disease
Have you had heart palpitations? *¿Ha tenido palpitaciones del corazón?*	Cardiac disease
Have you been vomiting? *¿Ha estado vomitando?*	Hyperemesis gravidarum
Have you had any problems with this pregnancy? *¿Ha tenido algún problema con este embarazo?*	
Have you had any infections? *¿Ha tenido alguna infección?*	STIs/vaginal infections
Have you had swelling? *¿Ha tenido hinchazón?*	PIH
Were all your pregnancies term? *¿Llegaron a las cuarenta semanas todos sus embarazos?*	Preterm labor
Have you ever had diabetes? *¿Ha tenido diabetes?*	Diabetes
Have you ever had high blood pressure? *¿Ha tenido presión alta?*	PIH
Have you ever had anemia? *¿Ha tenido anemia?*	Anemia
Do you take drugs? Prescription medicine? *¿Toma drogas? ¿Medicina recetada?*	Substance abuse
Do you drink alcohol? Smoke? *¿Toma alcohol? ¿Fuma?*	Substance abuse

services in some areas were duplicated, creating an imbalance in the provision of services within a geographic area.

Clearer guidelines were established regarding the level of care that could be expected at any given facility. In ambulatory settings, providers must distinguish themselves by the level of care they provide. *Basic care* is provided by obstetricians, family physicians, certified nurse midwives, and other advanced practice clinicians approved by local governance. Routine risk-oriented prenatal care, education, and support is provided. Providers offering *specialty care* are obstetricians who must provide fetal diagnostic testing and management of obstetric and medical complications in addition to basic care. *Subspecialty care* is provided by maternal-fetal medicine specialists and includes the aforementioned in addition to genetic testing, advanced fetal therapies, and management of severe maternal and fetal complications (American Academy of Pediatrics/American College of Obstetricians and Gynecologists [AAP/ACOG], 1997).

In hospital settings, perinatal services are also designated as basic, specialty, or subspecialty. Criteria for basic perinatal services include care of all clients admitted to the service, with an established triage system for high risk clients who should be transferred to a higher level of care; ability to perform a cesarean birth within 30 minutes of a decision to do so; availability of blood and blood products; availability of radiology, anesthesia, and laboratory services on a 24-hour basis; presence of nursery and postpartum care; resuscitation and stabilization of all neonates born in hospital; availability of transport for all sick neonates; family visitation; and data collection and retrieval (AAP/ACOG, 1997).

Specialty hospital care includes the above requirements in addition to care of high-risk mothers and fetuses, stabilization of ill neonates before transfer, and care of preterm infants with a birth weight of 1500 g or more. Preterm labor or impending births of 32 weeks of gestation or less should be transferred for subspecialty care. Other criteria for subspecialty care include comprehensive prenatal services, research and educational support, and utilization of high-risk technologies. Collaboration among providers to meet the client's needs is key in reducing perinatal morbidity and mortality (AAP/ACOG, 1997).

Assessment of Risk Factors

Pregnancies can be designated as high risk for any of several undesirable outcomes. Those considered to be at risk for uteroplacental insufficiency carry a serious threat for fetal growth restriction, intrauterine fetal death, intrapartum death, intrapartum fetal distress, and various types of neonatal morbidity.

In the past, risk factors were evaluated only from a medical viewpoint; thus only adverse medical, obstetric, or physiologic conditions were considered to place the client at risk. Today, a more comprehensive approach to high risk pregnancy is used, and the factors associated with high risk childbearing are grouped into broad categories based on threats to health and pregnancy outcome (see Guidelines/Guías box).

BOX 29-1 Categories of High Risk Factors

BIOPHYSICAL FACTORS

1. *Genetic considerations.* Genetic factors may interfere with normal fetal or neonatal development, result in congenital anomalies, or create difficulties for the mother. These factors include defective genes, transmissible inherited disorders and chromosome anomalies, multiple pregnancy, large fetal size, and ABO incompatibility.
2. *Nutritional status.* Adequate nutrition, without which fetal growth and development cannot proceed normally, is one of the most important determinants of pregnancy outcome. Conditions that influence nutritional status include the following: young age; three pregnancies in the previous 2 years; tobacco, alcohol, or drug use; inadequate dietary intake because of chronic illness or food fads; inadequate or excessive weight gain; and hematocrit value less than 33%.
3. *Medical and obstetric disorders.* Complications of current and past pregnancies, obstetric-related illnesses, and pregnancy losses put the client at risk (see Box 29-3).

PSYCHOSOCIAL FACTORS

1. *Smoking.* A strong, consistent, causal relationship has been established between maternal smoking and reduced birth weight. Risks include low birth weight infants, higher neonatal mortality rates, increased miscarriages, and increased incidence of premature rupture of membranes. These risks are aggravated by low socioeconomic status, poor nutritional status, and concurrent use of alcohol.
2. *Caffeine.* Birth defects in humans have not been related to caffeine consumption. High intake (three or more cups of coffee per day) has been related to a slight decrease in birth weight.
3. *Alcohol.* Although its exact effects in pregnancy have not been quantified and its mode of action is largely unexplained, alcohol exerts adverse effects on the fetus, resulting in fetal alcohol syndrome, fetal alcohol effects, learning disabilities, and hyperactivity.
4. *Drugs.* The developing fetus may be adversely affected by drugs through several mechanisms. They can be teratogenic, cause metabolic disturbances, produce chemical effects, or cause depression or alteration of CNS function. This category includes medications prescribed by a health care provider or bought over the counter, as well as commonly abused drugs such as heroin, cocaine, and marijuana. (See Chapter 35 for more information about drug and alcohol abuse.)
5. *Psychologic status.* Childbearing triggers profound and complex physiologic, psychologic, and social changes, with evidence to suggest a relationship between emotional distress and birth complications. This risk factor includes conditions such as specific intrapsychic disturbances and addictive lifestyles; a history of child or spouse abuse; inadequate support systems; family disruption or dissolution; maternal role changes or conflicts; noncompliance with cultural norms; unsafe cultural, ethnic, or religious practices; and situational crises.

SOCIODEMOGRAPHIC FACTORS

1. *Low income.* Poverty underlies many other risk factors and leads to inadequate financial resources for food and prenatal care, poor general health, increased risk of medical complications of pregnancy, and greater prevalence of adverse environmental influences.
2. *Lack of prenatal care.* Failure to diagnose and treat complications early is a major risk factor arising from financial barriers or lack of access to care; depersonalization of the system resulting in long waits, routine visits, variability in health care personnel, and unpleasant physical surroundings; lack of understanding of the need for early and continued care or cultural beliefs that do not support the need; and fear of the health care system and its providers.
3. *Age.* Women at both ends of the childbearing age spectrum have a higher incidence of poor outcomes; however, age may not be a risk factor in all cases. Both physiologic and psychologic risks should be evaluated.
   Adolescents—More complications are seen in young mothers (less than 15 years old), who have a 60% higher mortality rate than those over age 20, and in pregnancies occurring less than 6 years after menarche. Complications include anemia, pregnancy-induced hypertension (PIH), prolonged labor, and contracted pelvis and cephalopelvic disproportion. Long-term social implications of early motherhood are lower educational status, lower income, increased dependence on government support programs, higher divorce rates, and higher parity.
   Mature mothers—The risks to older mothers are not from age alone but from other considerations such as number and spacing of previous pregnancies; genetic disposition of the parents; and medical history, lifestyle, nutrition, and prenatal care. The increased likelihood of chronic diseases and complications that arises from more invasive medical management of a pregnancy and labor combined with demographic characteristics put an older woman at risk. Medical conditions more likely to be experienced by mature women include hypertension and PIH, diabetes, extended labor, cesarean birth, placenta previa, abruptio placentae, and mortality. Her fetus is at greater risk for low birth weight and macrosomia, chromosomal abnormalities, congenital malformations, and neonatal mortality.

Continued

BOX 29-1   **Categories of High Risk Factors—cont'd**

4. *Parity.* The number of previous pregnancies is a risk factor that is associated with age and includes all first pregnancies, especially a first pregnancy at either end of the childbearing age continuum. The incidence of PIH and dystocia is higher with a first birth.

5. *Marital status.* The increased mortality and morbidity rates for nonmarried women, including a greater risk for PIH, are often related to inadequate prenatal care and a younger childbearing age.

6. *Residence.* The availability and quality of prenatal care varies widely with geographic residence. Women in metropolitan areas have more prenatal visits than those in rural areas, who have fewer opportunities for specialized care and consequently a higher incidence of maternal mortality. Health care in the inner city, where residents are usually poorer and begin childbearing earlier and continue for longer, may be of lower quality than in a more affluent neighborhood.

7. *Ethnicity.* Although ethnicity by itself is not a major risk, race is an indicator of other sociodemographic risk factors. Nonwhite women are more than 3 times as likely as Caucasian women to die of pregnancy-related causes. African-American babies have the highest rates of prematurity and low birth weight, with the infant mortality rate among African-Americans being more than double that for Caucasians.

ENVIRONMENTAL FACTORS

Various environmental substances can affect fertility and fetal development, the chance of a live birth, and the child's subsequent mental and physical development. Environmental influences include infections, radiation, chemicals such as pesticides, therapeutic drugs, illicit drugs, industrial pollutants, cigarette smoke, stress, and diet. Paternal exposure to mutagenic agents in the workplace has been associated with an increased risk of miscarriage.

Categories of risk are biophysical, psychosocial, sociodemographic, and environmental (Fogel & Lewallen, 1995) (Box 29-1).

Biophysical risks include factors that originate within the mother or fetus and affect the development or functioning of either one or both.

Psychosocial risks are comprised of maternal behaviors and adverse lifestyles that have a negative effect on the health of the mother or fetus. These risks may include emotional distress and disturbed interpersonal relationships, as well as inadequate social support and unsafe cultural practices (Box 29-2).

Sociodemographic risks arise from the mother and her family. These risks may place the mother and fetus at risk (Box 29-3).

Environmental factors include hazards in the workplace and the woman's general environment (see Research box).

Risk factors are interrelated and cumulative in their effects and are shown in Fig. 29-1. Risk factors of the postpartum woman and newborn are shown in Box 29-4. The development of a comprehensive database for pregnancy risk assessment will help generate appropriate nursing diagnoses. For example, use of functional health patterns can be the basis for an assessment tool (Box 29-5).

ANTEPARTUM TESTING/BIOPHYSICAL ASSESSMENT

The major expected outcome of antepartum testing is the detection of potential fetal compromise. Ideally, the technique used identifies fetal compromise before intrauterine

BOX 29-2   **Antepartum Cultural Assessment**

All cultures recognize pregnancy as a special transitional period and have particular customs and beliefs that dictate behavior during this time. In the antepartum period the nurse should assess the following:

• Beliefs of whether pregnancy is a state of illness or health
• Behavioral expectations of the mother and of the health care provider
• Dietary prescriptions or restrictions (e.g., hot/cold balance theory, pica)
• Activity restrictions or prescriptions (e.g., use of massage)
• Availability of advice (e.g., from whom and at what time advice will be sought and when prenatal care will begin [if at all])
• Considerations of modesty

---

asphyxia of the fetus so that the health care provider can take measures to prevent or minimize adverse perinatal outcomes. No single test can provide this information. Assessment tests should be selected based on their effectiveness, and the results must be interpreted in light of the complete clinical picture. The most reliable evidence for effectiveness is provided by randomized controlled trials. Nurses can be informed about the most recent research on fetal assessment by using an up-to-date systematic review such as the Cochrane Database of Systematic Reviews (Enkin et al., 1995). Table 29-1 (p. 798) lists the evidence

BOX 29-3 Specific Pregnancy Problems and Related Risk Factors

PRETERM LABOR

Age less than 16 or more than 35 years
Low socioeconomic status
Maternal weight below 50 kg
Poor nutrition
Previous preterm birth
Incompetent cervix
Uterine anomalies
Smoking
Drug addiction and alcohol abuse
Pyelonephritis, pneumonia
Multiple gestation
Anemia
Abnormal fetal presentation
Preterm rupture of membranes
Placental abnormalities
Infection
Abdominal surgery in current pregnancy
History of cervical surgery

POLYHYDRAMNIOS

Diabetes mellitus
Multiple gestation
Fetal congenital anomalies
Isoimmunization (Rh or ABO)
Nonimmune hydrops
Abnormal fetal presentation

INTRAUTERINE GROWTH RESTRICTION (IUGR)

Multiple gestation
Poor nutrition

Maternal cyanotic heart disease
Prior pregnancy with IUGR
Maternal collagen diseases
Chronic hypertension
Pregnancy-induced hypertension
Recurrent antepartum hemorrhage
Smoking
Maternal diabetes with vascular problems
Fetal infections
Fetal cardiovascular anomalies
Drug addiction and alcohol abuse
Fetal congenital anomalies
Hemoglobinopathies

OLIGOHYDRAMNIOS

Renal agenesis (Potter's syndrome)
Prolonged rupture of membranes
IUGR
Intrauterine fetal death

POSTTERM PREGNANCY

Anencephaly
Placental sulfatase deficiency
Perinatal hypoxia, acidosis
Placental insufficiency

CHROMOSOMAL ABNORMALITIES

Maternal age 35 years or more
Balanced translocation (maternal and paternal)

From DeCherney, A., & Pernoll, M. (Eds.). (1994). *Current obstetric and gynecologic diagnosis and treatment* (8th ed.). Norwalk, CT: Appleton & Lange.

RESEARCH

Risk of Adverse Outcomes in Pregnant Women Exposed to Solvents

Although large numbers of women and men of reproductive age are employed, benefits and risks associated with employment and exposure to reproductive hazards in the workplace are not well-defined. The purpose of the study was to compare maternal and live birth outcomes of women who received consultation services between 1990 and 1993 from the Wisconsin occupational reproductive health nurse consultant, 76% of whom were exposed to solvent, and a sample of women and their offspring selected randomly from birth certificate records from the same years.

Confounded data by race, prenatal care, and gestational diabetes were controlled by stratification. Logistic regression was used to control for age differences. Clients had elevated relative risk (RR) estimates for pregnancy-induced hypertension (RR = 2.4) and hydramnios (RR = 5.2), and their offspring were more likely to have 5-minute Apgar scores less than 8 (RR = 3.6). All other outcomes that were examined, including prematurity, low birth weight, and birth defects, were similar between groups.

Most maternal and live birth outcomes were similar between the clients who sought consultation and the

Source: Hewitt, J., & Tellier, L. (1998). Risk of adverse outcomes in pregnant women exposed to solvents. *J Obstet Gynecol Neonatal Nurs* 27(5), 521-531.

Continued

RESEARCH

Risk of Adverse Outcomes in Pregnant Women Exposed to Solvents—cont'd

random sample of women. This research study supported previous research, which showed an elevated risk of pregnancy-induced hypertension associated with solvent exposure in women. The increased risk of hydramnios found in this largely solvent-exposed cohort was not previously found in the literature.

CLINICAL APPLICATION

It is imperative that clinicians take thorough health histories, including information on workplace exposures to hazardous chemicals such as solvents, before conception and during pregnancy. Perinatal nurses and others increasingly are being exhorted to incorporate occupational and environmental health into their practices. Assessment and

documentation of occupational health in medical records and on birth records are crucial for communicating assessment and intervention data.

A related implication for perinatal nursing practice of this study's findings is the need to standardize the procedures to achieve greater validity in recording birth certificate data. Uniform criteria and procedures are needed to document maternal and birth outcomes and to elicit and record information about occupation and place of employment on the birth certificate. Perinatal nurses have a significant role in determining the quality of birth certificate data used for formal studies and health surveillance activities and are urged to take an active part in improving these vital statistics.

---

for recommending care for fetal assessment screening based on this database.

Daily Fetal Movement Count

Assessment of fetal activity by the mother is a simple yet valuable method for monitoring the condition of the fetus. The **daily fetal movement count (DFMC)** can be done at home, is noninvasive, is simple to understand, and usually does not interfere with a daily routine. The presence of movements is generally a reassuring sign of fetal health.

Several protocols are used for counting. Except for establishing a very low number of daily fetal movements or a trend toward decreased motion, the clinical value of the absolute number of fetal movements has not been established, except in the situation in which fetal movements cease entirely for 12 hours (the fetal alarm signal). Generally, a count of less than three fetal movements within 1 hour warrants further evaluation by nonstress or contraction stress testing, biophysical profile, or a combination of these. Clients should be taught the significance of fetal movements, the procedure for counting that is to be used, and how to record findings on a daily fetal movement record.

> **NURSE ALERT** *In assessing fetal movements it is important to remember that they are usually not present during the fetal sleep cycle; they may be temporarily reduced if the woman is taking depressant medications, drinking alcohol, or smoking a cigarette; and they do not decrease as the woman nears term.*

Ultrasonography

Sound is a form of wave energy that causes small particles in a medium to oscillate. The frequency of sound, which refers to the number of peaks or waves that traverse a given point per unit of time, is expressed in hertz (Hz). Sound with a frequency of one cycle, or one peak per second, has

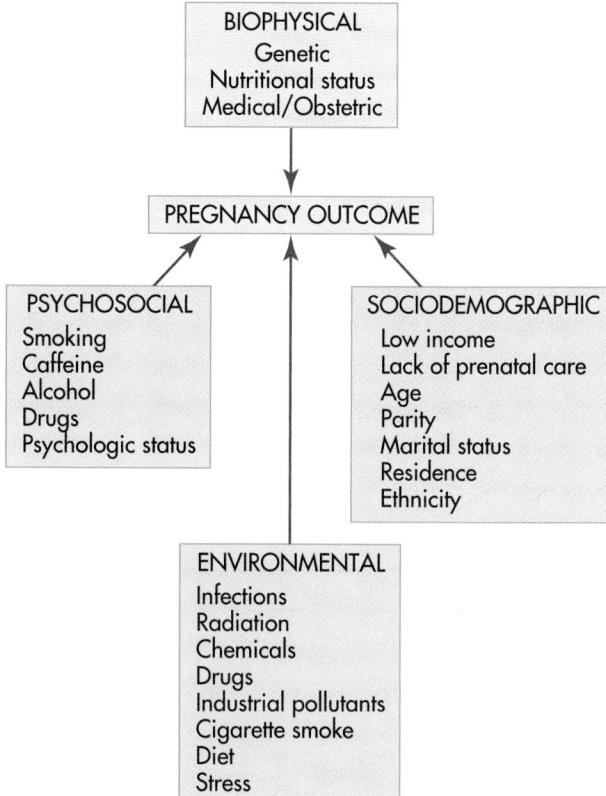

Fig. 29-1 Interrelationship of risk factors that may affect pregnancy outcome. *(Modified from Fogel, C., & Woods, N. [1995]. Health care of women. Thousand Oaks, CA: Sage.)*

a frequency of 1 Hz. When directional beams of sound strike an object, an echo is returned. The time delay between the emission of the sound and the return of the echo and the direction of the echo are noted. From these data the distance and location of an object can be calculated.

BOX 29-4   Factors That Place the Postpartum Woman and Neonate at High Risk

THE MOTHER
Hemorrhage
Infection
Abnormal vital signs
Traumatic labor or birth
Psychosocial factors

THE INFANT (FOR ADMISSION TO NICU)
High Risk Category
Infants who continue with or develop signs of RDS or other respiratory distress
Asphyxiated infants (Apgar score <6 at 5 min), resuscitation required at birth
Preterm infants, dysmature infants
Infants with cyanosis or suspected cardiovascular disease, persistent cyanosis
Infants with major congenital malformations requiring surgery, chromosomal anomalies
Infants with convulsions, sepsis, hemorrhagic diathesis, or shock
Meconium aspiration syndrome

CNS depression for >24 hr
Hypoglycemia
Hypocalcemia
Hyperbilirubinemia

Moderate Risk
Dysmaturity
Prematurity (weight between 2000 and 2500 g)
Apgar score <5 at 1 min
Feeding problems
Multifetal birth
Transient tachypnea
Hypomagnesemia or hypermagnesemia
Hypoparathyroidism
Failure to gain weight
Jitteriness or hyperactivity
Cardiac anomalies not requiring immediate catheterization
Heart murmur
Anemia
CNS depression for <24 hr

CNS, Central nervous system; *NICU,* neonatal intensive care unit; *RDS,* respiratory distress syndrome.

BOX 29-5   Assessment for High Risk Pregnancy Using Functional Health Patterns

For each of the following functional health patterns the nurse includes questions that will provide data about the individual woman, her family, her community, and her cultural practices and beliefs:
• Health-perception/health management pattern
  Current health, past medical history, family medical history, environmental/chemical exposure, family decision making about health, community resources, beliefs about health care during pregnancy
• Nutritional-metabolic pattern
  Nutritional status, knowledge of pregnancy needs, pregnancy discomforts, community resources (WIC), cultural eating practices
• Elimination pattern
  Urinary and bowel patterns, family or cultural practices (laxatives), community waste/sanitation services
• Activity-exercise pattern
  Usual exercise, recreation, community resources, cultural practices or taboos for activities during pregnancy
• Sleep-rest pattern
  Usual sleep patterns, use of remedies, family sleep arrangements, cultural beliefs about sleep and rest in pregnancy

• Cognitive-perceptual pattern
  Communication problems, knowledge deficits about pregnancy and birth (individual and family), community resources for support for high risk pregnant clients, cultural beliefs about pain and its management
• Self-perception/self-concept pattern
  Body image, responses of family to high risk pregnancy, housing conditions, cultural practices about parenting
• Role-relationship pattern
  Feelings of security, occupation, hobbies, family living arrangements, community resources
• Sexuality-reproductive pattern
  Sexual activities, problems, restrictions, previous obstetric history, current obstetric status, cultural beliefs about sexual practices during pregnancy
• Coping-stress pattern
  Life stressors, losses experienced, coping mechanisms, support systems, community resources, spiritual or religious practices or beliefs that are important

Data from Gilbert, E., & Harmon, J. (1998). *Manual of high risk pregnancy and delivery* (2nd ed.). St Louis: Mosby; Gordon, M. (1994). *Nursing diagnosis: Process and application* (3rd ed.). St. Louis: Mosby.

TABLE 29-1 Fetal Assessment Screening: Recommendations for Care

FETAL ASSESSMENT TEST	RECOMMENDATION/CONCLUSION
• Doppler ultrasound use in pregnancy at high risk for fetal compromise	Beneficial effects Effects likely to be beneficial
• Ultrasound use to estimate gestational age in first and early second trimesters • Ultrasound use to confirm multiple pregnancy • Ultrasound use for placental location in placenta previa • Early second trimester amniocentesis for identification of chromosomal abnormalities • Transabdominal instead of transvaginal chorionic villus sampling (CVS)	
• Formal systems of risk scoring • Routine use of early ultrasound • CVS versus amniocentesis for diagnosing chromosomal abnormalities • Serum alpha feto-protein screening for neural tube defects • Routine fetal movement counts to improve perinatal outcome	There is a trade-off between beneficial and adverse effects
• Placental grading by ultrasound to improve perinatal outcome • Biophysical profile for fetal surveillance	Unknown effectiveness
• Routine use of ultrasound for fetal anthropometry (body measurements) in late pregnancy • Use of Doppler ultrasound in all pregnancies • Measurement of placental hormones (estriol)	Unlikely to be beneficial
• Nipple stimulation test to improve perinatal outcome • Nonstress test to improve perinatal outcome • Contraction stress test to improve perinatal outcome	Likely to be ineffective or harmful

Source: Enkin, M. et al. (1995). Effective care in pregnancy and childbirth. *Birth* 22(2):101-110.

Diagnostic ultrasonography is an important technique in antepartum fetal surveillance. **Ultrasound** is sound having a frequency higher than that detectable by humans, namely greater than 20,000 Hz. Diagnostic ultrasound instruments operate within a frequency range of 2 to 10 million Hz (or 2 to 10 MHz), which is below the range used by sonar and radar equipment.

Ultrasound can be done abdominally or transvaginally during pregnancy. Both produce a three-dimensional view from which a pictorial image is obtained. Abdominal ultrasonography is more useful after the first trimester when the pregnant uterus becomes an abdominal organ. For the procedure the woman usually needs to have a full bladder to get a better image of the fetus. Transmission gel or paste is applied to the abdomen before a transducer is moved over the skin to enhance transmission and reception of the sound waves.

Transvaginal ultrasonography, in which the probe is inserted into the vagina, allows pelvic anatomy to be evaluated in greater detail and intrauterine pregnancy to be diagnosed earlier (Cunningham et al., 1997). A transvaginal ultrasound examination is well tolerated by most clients because it alleviates the need for a full bladder. It is especially useful in obese clients whose thick abdominal layers cannot be penetrated adequately by an abdominal approach. Transvaginal ultrasonography is optimally used in the first trimester to detect ectopic pregnancies, monitor the developing embryo, help identify abnormalities, and help establish gestational age. In some instances, it may be used as an adjunct to abdominal scanning to evaluate preterm labor in second- and third-trimester pregnancies (Guzman et al., 1998).

Levels of Ultrasonography

Perinatal care providers and ultrasonographers have come to a tentative agreement on terminology describing two different levels of ultrasonography. The basic screening or limited examination is used most frequently and can be performed by ultrasonographers or other health care professionals, including nurses, who have had special training. Indications for limited ultrasonography are described in detail in the next section; its primary use is to detect fetal viability, determine the presentation of the fetus, assess gestational age, locate the placenta, and determine amniotic fluid volume. Targeted or comprehensive examinations are performed if a client is suspected of carrying an anatomically or a physiologically abnormal fetus. Indications for a comprehensive examination include abnormal findings on clinical examination, especially with polyhydramnios or oligohydramnios, elevated alpha-fetoprotein (AFP) levels, and a history of offspring with anomalies that can be de-

TABLE 29-2 Major Uses of Ultrasonography During Pregnancy

FIRST TRIMESTER	SECOND TRIMESTER	THIRD TRIMESTER
Confirm pregnancy	Establish or confirm dates	Confirm gestational age
Confirm viability	Confirm viability	Confirm viability
Determine gestational age	Detect polyhydramnios, oligohydramnios	Detect macrosomia
Rule out ectopic pregnancy		Detect congenital anomalies
Detect multiple gestation	Detect congenital anomalies	Detect IUGR
Visualization during chorionic villus sampling	Detect intrauterine growth restriction (IUGR)	Determine fetal position
Detect maternal abnormalities such as bicornuate uterus, ovarian cysts, fibroids	Confirm placenta placement	Detect placenta previa or abruptio placentae
	Visualization during amniocentesis	Visualization during amniocentesis, external version
		Biophysical profile
		Amniotic fluid volume assessment
		Doppler flow studies
		Detect placental maturity

tected by ultrasound. Comprehensive ultrasonography is performed by highly trained and experienced personnel.

Indications for Use

Major indications for obstetric sonography appear by trimester in Table 29-2. During the first trimester, ultrasound examination is performed to obtain information on (1) number, size, and location of gestational sacs; (2) presence or absence of fetal cardiac and body movements; (3) presence or absence of uterine abnormalities (e.g., bicornuate uterus or fibroids) or adnexal masses (e.g., ovarian cysts or an ectopic pregnancy); (4) date of pregnancy (by measuring the crown-rump length); and (5) presence and location of an intrauterine contraceptive device.

During the second and third trimesters, information on the following conditions is sought: (1) fetal viability, number, position, gestational age, growth pattern, and anomalies; (2) amniotic fluid volume; (3) placental location and maturity; (4) uterine fibroids and anomalies; (5) adnexal masses; and (6) cervical length (Fig. 29-2, *A*).

Findings

Ultrasonography has led to earlier diagnoses, allowing therapy to be instituted early in the pregnancy and thereby decreasing the severity and duration of morbidity, both physical and emotional, for the family. For instance, early diagnosis of a fetal anomaly gives the family choices such as (1) intrauterine surgery or other therapy for the fetus, (2) termination of the pregnancy, or (3) preparation for the care of an infant with a disorder.

Fetal heart activity. Fetal heart activity can be demonstrated as early as 6 to 7 weeks by real-time echo scanners and at 10 to 12 weeks by Doppler mode. By 9 to 10 weeks, gestational trophoblastic disease can be diagnosed. Fetal death can be confirmed by lack of heart motion, the presence of fetal scalp edema, and maceration and overlap of the cranial bones.

Gestational age. Gestational dating by ultrasonography is indicated for conditions such as (1) uncertain dates

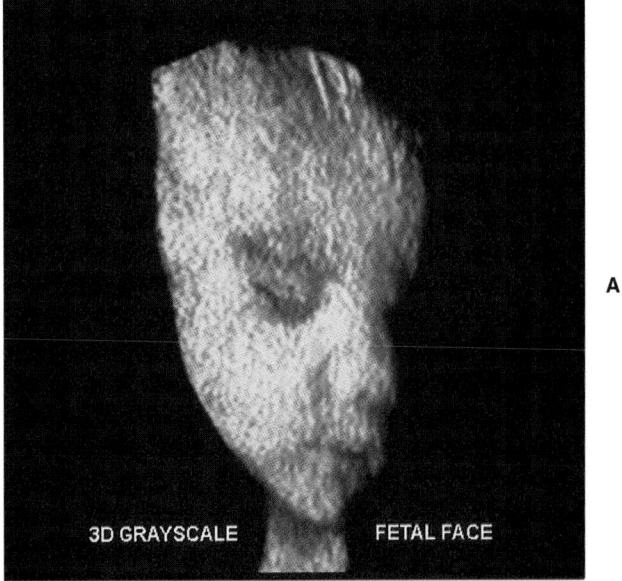

A

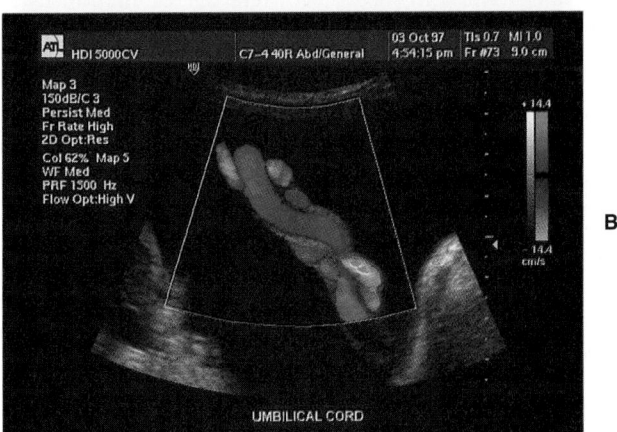

B

Fig. 29-2 Two views of the fetus during ultrasonography. **A,** Fetal face (20 weeks). **B,** Umbilical cord (26 weeks). *(Courtesy Advanced Technology Laboratories, Bothell, WA.)*

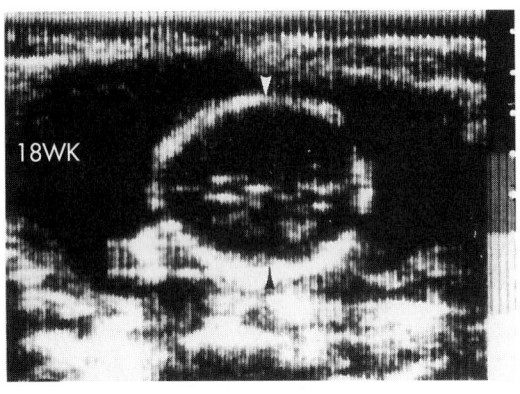

Fig. 29-3 Real-time image of fetal biparietal diameters at 18 weeks. *(From Athay, P., & Haddock, F. [1985]. Ultrasound in obstetrics and gynecology [2nd ed.]. St. Louis: Mosby.)*

TABLE 29-3	Correlation of Fetal Weight and BPD	
BPD (CM)	**ESTIMATED FETAL WEIGHT**	
8.2	2290 g	
8.5	2500 g	
8.8	2730 g	
9.4	3180 g	
10.0	3630 g	
10.6	4070 g	

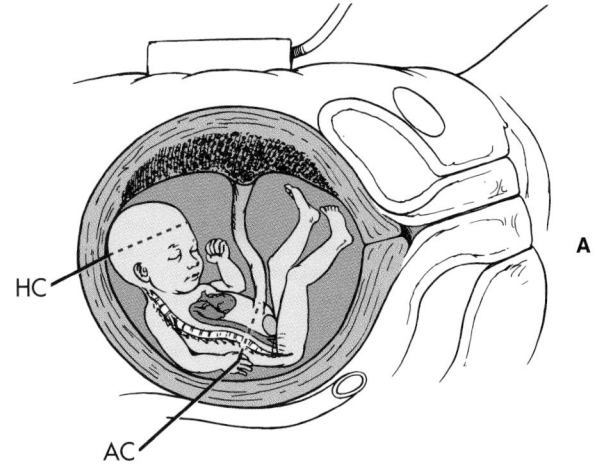

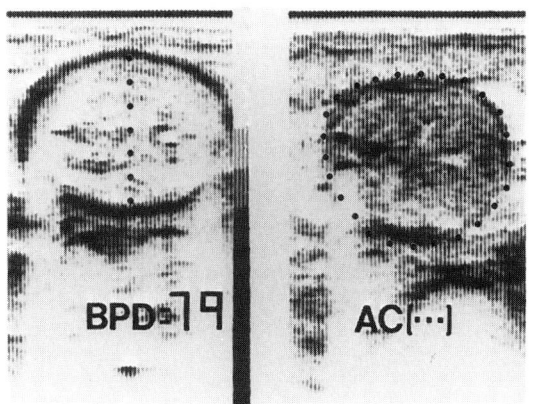

Fig. 29-4 A, Appropriate planes of sections *(dotted lines)* for BPD, head circumference *(HC)*, and abdominal circumference *(AC)*. **B,** Real-time ultrasound image demonstrates typical head and body images that correspond to planes in **A.** By use of these two images, BPD (7.9 cm), head circumference (30 cm), abdominal circumference (28 cm), and estimated fetal weight (1840 g) in this normal 32-week fetus can be determined. *(From Athay, P., & Haddock, F. [1985]. Ultrasound in obstetrics and gynecology [2nd ed.]. St. Louis: Mosby.)*

for the last normal menstrual period, (2) recent discontinuation of oral contraceptives, (3) bleeding episode during the first trimester, (4) uterine size that does not agree with dates, and (5) other high risk conditions.

During the first 20 weeks of gestation, ultrasonography provides an accurate assessment of gestational age because most normal fetuses grow at the same rate. Accuracy is increased as the fetus ages because more than one variable is measured. The four methods of fetal age estimation used include: (1) determination of gestational sac dimensions (at about 8 weeks), (2) measurement of crown-rump length (between 7 and 14 weeks), (3) measurement of the **biparietal diameter (BPD)** (after 12 weeks), and (4) measurement of femur length (after 12 weeks). Fetal BPD at 36 weeks should be approximately 8.7 cm. Term pregnancy and fetal maturity can be diagnosed with some confidence if the biparietal measurement by ultrasound examination is greater than 9.8 cm (Fig. 29-3 and Table 29-3), especially when this is combined with appropriate femur length measurement.

In later gestational periods, serial measurements can provide a more accurate determination of fetal age. Two and preferably three composite measurements are recommended, at least 2 weeks apart, and these are plotted against standard fetal growth curves. This method, when applied between 24 and 32 weeks of gestation, yields an estimation error of 10 days more or less than the actual age (Manning, 1999).

Fetal growth. Fetal growth is determined by both intrinsic growth potential and environmental factors. Conditions that require ultrasound assessment of fetal growth include (1) poor maternal weight gain or pattern of weight gain, (2) previous intrauterine growth restriction (IUGR), (3) chronic infections, (4) ingestion of drugs (tobacco, alcohol, over-the-counter, and street drugs), (5) maternal diabetes mellitus, (6) hypertension, (7) multifetal pregnancy, and (8) other medical or surgical complications.

Serial evaluations of BPD and limb length can differentiate between size discrepancy resulting from inaccurate dates and true IUGR. IUGR may be symmetric (the fetus being small in all parameters) or asymmetric (head and body growth varying). Symmetric IUGR reflects a chronic or long-standing insult and may be caused by low genetic growth potential, intrauterine infection, undernutrition, heavy smoking, or chromosomal aberration. Asymmetric growth suggests an acute or late-occurring deprivation, such as placental insufficiency resulting from hypertension, renal disease, or cardiovascular disease. Reduced fetal growth is still one of the most frequent conditions associated with stillbirth (Fig. 29-4). Macrosomic infants (those weighing >4000 g) are at increased risk for trauma during birth. In addition, fetal macrosomia associated with maternal glucose intolerance carries an increased risk of intrauterine fetal death.

Adjunct to amniocentesis, percutaneous umbilical blood sampling, and chorionic villus sampling. The safety of amniocentesis is increased when the positions of the fetus, placenta, and pockets of amniotic fluid can be identified accurately. Ultrasound scanning has reduced risks previously associated with amniocentesis, such as fetomaternal hemorrhage from a pierced placenta. Percutaneous umbilical blood sampling and chorionic villus sampling are also guided by ultrasonography to identify the cord and chorion frondosum accurately (see Fig. 29-2, *B*).

Fetal anatomy. Anatomic structures that may be identified by ultrasonography (depending on the gestational age) include the following: head (including ventricles and blood vessels), neck, spine, heart, stomach, small bowel, liver, kidneys, bladder, and limbs. Ultrasonography permits the confirmation of normal anatomy, as well as the detection of major fetal malformations. The presence of an anomaly may influence the location of birth (e.g., a delivery room versus a labor-delivery-recovery room or a subspecialty center versus a basic care center) and the method of birth to optimize neonatal outcomes.

The number of fetuses and their presentations may also be assessed by ultrasonography, allowing plans for therapy and mode of birth to be made in advance.

Placental position and function. The pattern of uterine and placental growth and the fullness of the maternal bladder influence the apparent location of the placenta by ultrasonography. During the first trimester, differentiation between the endometrium and small placenta is difficult. By 14 to 16 weeks the placenta is clearly defined, but if it is seen to be low lying, its relationship to the internal cervical os can sometimes be dramatically altered by varying the fullness of the maternal bladder. In approximately 15% to 20% of all pregnancies in which ultrasound scanning is performed during the second trimester, the placenta seems to be overlying the os, but the incidence of placenta previa at term is only 0.5%. Thus the diagnosis of placenta previa can seldom be confirmed before 27 weeks, primarily because of the elongation of the lower uterine segment as pregnancy advances.

Another use for ultrasonography is grading of placental maturation (Box 29-6). Calcium deposits are of signifi-

BOX 29-6 Placental Grading

Third-trimester grading of placental maturation can be accomplished by ultrasound scanning. The placenta undergoes detectable maturational changes throughout gestation; a relationship has been noted between advancing placental grade and fetal pulmonary maturity. Placentas are graded as 0, I, II, and III (with grade III placentas being the most mature) on the basis of the identification and distribution of calcium deposits within the fetal portion (Manning, 1999). Ultrasound examination can identify changes in the chorionic plate, placental substance, and basal layer of the placenta that correspond to the various grades: (1) grade 0 placentas are seen in the first and second trimesters, (2) grade I placentas appear between 30 and 32 weeks and may even persist until term, (3) grade II placentas are observed at around 36 weeks and persist until term in 45% of pregnancies, and (4) grade III placentas are seen at 38 weeks and reflect the greatest maturation. However, only a small number of placentas are grade III.

cance in postterm pregnancies because as they increase, the available surface area that can be adequately bathed by maternal blood decreases. The point at which this results in fetal wastage and hypoxia cannot be determined precisely; however, the effects are usually observable by 42 weeks and are progressive (Gilbert & Harmon, 1998).

Fetal well-being. Physiologic parameters of the fetus that can be assessed with ultrasound scanning include amniotic fluid volume, vascular waveforms from the fetal circulation, heart motion, fetal breathing movements, fetal urine production, and fetal limb and head movements. Assessment of these parameters, singly or in combination, yields a fairly reliable picture of fetal well-being. The significance of these findings is discussed in the following sections.

Amniotic fluid volume. Abnormalities of **amniotic fluid volume (AFV)** are frequently associated with fetal disorders. Subjective determinants of oligohydramnios (decreased fluid) include the absence of fluid pockets in the uterine cavity and the impression of crowding of small fetal parts. An objective criterion of decreased AFV is met if the largest pocket of fluid measured in two perpendicular planes is less than 1 cm. In the case of polyhydramnios (increased fluid), subjective criteria include multiple large pockets of fluid, the impression of a floating fetus, and free movement of fetal limbs. The diagnosis may be made when the largest pocket of fluid exceeds 8 cm in two perpendicular planes (Fischer & Depp, 1995). The total AFV can be evaluated by a method developed in which the depths (in centimeters) of the amniotic fluid in all four quadrants surrounding the maternal umbilicus are totaled, providing an **amniotic fluid index (AFI)**. An AFI less than

5 cm indicates oligohydramnios, 5 to 19 cm is considered a normal measurement, and a measurement greater than 20 cm reflects polyhydramnios (Chervenak & Gabbe, 1996).

Oligohydramnios is associated with congenital anomalies (such as renal agenesis), growth restriction, and fetal distress during labor. Polyhydramnios is associated with neural tube defects, obstruction of the fetal gastrointestinal tract, multiple fetuses, and fetal hydrops.

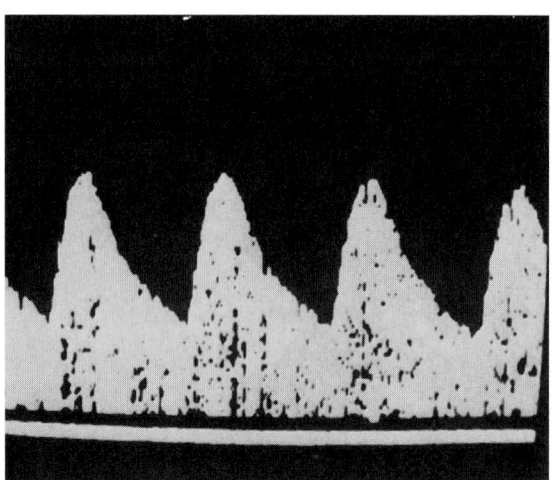

Fig. 29-5 Normal umbilical artery velocity waveforms and measurements from systole and end-diastole. *(From Schulman, H. [1990]. Doppler ultrasound. In R. Eden, & F. Boehm [Eds.]. Assessment and care of the fetus: Physiological, clinical and medicolegal principles. Norwalk, CT: Appleton & Lange.)*

Doppler blood flow analysis. One of the major advances in perinatal medicine is the ability to study blood flow noninvasively in the fetus and placenta. **Doppler ultrasound** is a helpful adjunct in the management of pregnancies at risk because of hypertension, IUGR, diabetes mellitus, multiple fetuses, or preterm labor (Miller, 1998).

When a sound wave is reflected from a moving target, there is a change in frequency of the reflected wave relative to the transmitted wave. This is called the *Doppler effect*. An ultrasound beam scattered by a group of red blood cells (RBCs) is an example of this effect. The velocity of the RBCs can be determined by measuring the change in the frequency of the sound wave reflected off the cells.

The shifted frequencies can be displayed as a plot of velocity versus time, and the shape of these waveforms can be analyzed to give information about blood flow and resistance in a given circulation. Velocity waveforms from umbilical and uterine arteries, reported as systolic/diastolic (S/D) ratios, can be first detected at 15 weeks of pregnancy. Because of the progressive decline in resistance in both the umbilical and uterine arteries, this ratio decreases as pregnancy advances. Most fetuses will achieve an S/D ratio of 3 or less by 30 weeks (Fig. 29-5). Persistent elevation of S/D ratios after 30 weeks is associated with IUGR, usually resulting from uteroplacental insufficiency (UPI). In postterm pregnancies evaluated by Doppler umbilical flow studies, an elevated S/D ratio indicates a poorly perfused placenta. Abnormal results are also seen with certain chromosome abnormalities (trisomy 13 and 18) in the fetus and with lupus erythematosus in the mother (Farmakides et al., 1994). Exposure to nicotine from maternal smoking has also been reported to increase the S/D ratio (Fig. 29-6).

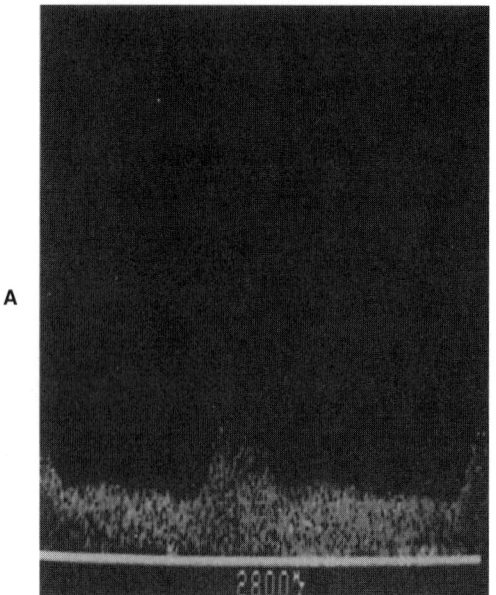
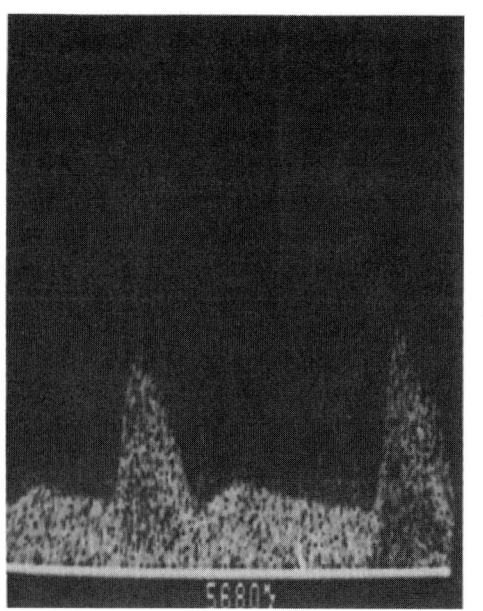

Fig. 29-6 Normal and abnormal uteroplacental vessels at 34 weeks. **A,** Normal S/D ratio of 2.1. **B,** S/D ratio of 3.4. *(From Schulman, H. [1990]. Doppler ultrasound. In R. Eden, & F. Boehm [Eds.]. Assessment and care of the fetus: Physiological, clinical, and medicolegal principles. Norwalk, CT: Appleton & Lange.)*

Biophysical profile. Real-time ultrasound permits detailed assessment of the physical and physiologic characteristics of the developing fetus and cataloging of normal and abnormal biophysical responses to stimuli. The **biophysical profile (BPP)** is a noninvasive dynamic assessment of a fetus and its environment by ultrasonography and external fetal monitoring.

BPP scoring is a method of fetal risk surveillance based on the assessment of both acute and chronic markers of fetal disease. The BPP includes fetal breathing movements, fetal movements, fetal tone, fetal heart rate patterns by means of a nonstress test, and AFV, and the procedure may therefore be considered a physical examination of the fetus, including determination of vital signs. The fetal response to central hypoxia is alteration in movement, muscle tone, breathing, and heart rate patterns. The presence of normal fetal biophysical activities indicates that the central nervous system (CNS) is functional and the fetus therefore is not hypoxemic (Manning, 1995). BPP variables and scoring are detailed in Table 29-4.

The BPP is an accurate indicator of impending fetal death. Fetal acidosis can be diagnosed early with a nonreactive nonstress test and absent fetal breathing movements (FBM). An abnormal BPP score and oligohydramnios are indications that labor should be induced (Manning, 1995). Fetal infection in women whose membranes rupture prematurely (at less than 37 weeks of gestation) can be diagnosed early by changes in biophysical activity that precede the clinical signs of infection and indicate the necessity for immediate birth. When the BPP score is normal and the risk of fetal death low, intervention is indicated only for obstetric or maternal factors.

Nursing Role

Although a growing number of nurses perform ultrasound scans and BPPs in certain centers, the main role of nurses is in counseling and educating women about the procedure.

LEGAL TIP **Performance of Limited Ultrasound Examinations**

Nurses who have the training and competence may perform limited ultrasound examinations if it is within the scope of practice in their state or area and consistent with regulations of the agencies in which they practice (Treanor, 1998). Limited ultrasound examinations include identification of fetal number, fetal presentation, fetal cardiac activity, location of the placenta, and BPP, including amniotic fluid volume assessment. Clients should be informed about the limited information provided by these examinations. They are not meant to evaluate or identify fetal anomalies, assess fetal age, or estimate fetal weight. The obstetric health care provider is responsible for

TABLE 29-4 **Biophysical Profile**

VARIABLES	NORMAL (SCORE = 2)	ABNORMAL (SCORE = 0)
Fetal breathing movements	One or more episodes in 30 min, each lasting ≥30 sec	Episodes absent or no episode ≥30 sec in 30 min
Gross body movements	Three or more discrete body or limb movements in 30 min (episodes of active continuous movement being considered as a single movement)	Less than three episodes of body or limb movements in 30 min
Fetal tone	One or more episodes of active extension with return to flexion of fetal limb(s) or trunk, opening and closing of hand being considered normal tone	Slow extension with return to flexion, movement of limb in full extension, or fetal movement absent
Reactive fetal heart rate	Two or more episodes of acceleration (≥15 beats/min) in 20 min, each lasting ≥15 sec and associated with fetal movement	Less than two episodes of acceleration or acceleration of <15 beats/min in 20 min
Qualitative amniotic fluid volume	One or more pockets of fluid measuring ≥1 cm in two perpendicular planes	Pockets absent or pocket <1cm in two perpendicular planes

SCORE

Normal	8-10 (if Amniotic Fluid Index is adequate)
Equivocal	6
Abnormal	<4

Data from Manning, F. (1995). Dynamic ultrasound-based fetal assessment: The fetal biophysical profile score. *Clin Obstet Gynecol* 38(1), 26-44.

obtaining a more comprehensive ultrasound examination when complete client assessment is necessary (AWHONN, 1998).

Providing accurate information regarding the procedure is imperative to allay the mother's anxiety. Although ultrasound scanning has become a widely used diagnostic tool, recommendations for the procedure are based on expectations of a fetal problem and therefore may cause concern. Clients should be provided ample opportunity to ask questions and be reassured that the procedure is safe.

For an abdominal ultrasound the woman is usually directed to come for the examination with a full bladder because it supports the uterus in position for the imaging. She is then positioned comfortably with small pillows under her head and knees. The display panel is positioned so that the woman and/or her partner can observe the images on the screen if they desire.

A transvaginal ultrasound may be performed with the woman in a lithotomy position or with her pelvis elevated by towels, cushions, or a folded pillow. This pelvis tilt is optimal to image the pelvic structures. A protective cover such as a condom, the finger of a clean rubber surgical glove, or a special probe cover provided by the manufacturer is used to cover the transducer probe. The probe is lubricated with a water-soluble gel and placed in the vagina either by the examiner or by the woman herself. During the examination the position of the probe or the tilt of the examining table may be changed so that the complete pelvis is in view. The procedure is not physically painful, although the woman will feel pressure as the probe is moved.

Safety of Diagnostic Ultrasonography

In the 30 years that diagnostic ultrasonography has been used, no conclusive evidence of any harmful effects on humans has emerged. Although the possibility of unidentified biologic effects exists, the benefits to the client of prudent use of diagnostic ultrasonography appear to outweigh any possible risk (Anthony, 1996).

Magnetic Resonance Imaging

Magnetic resonance imaging (MRI) is a noninvasive radiologic technique used for obstetric and gynecologic diagnosis. Like computerized tomography (CT), MRI provides excellent pictures of soft tissue. Unlike CT, ionizing radiation is not used; thus vascular structures within the body can be visualized and evaluated without injection of an iodinated contrast medium, thus eliminating any known biologic risk. Like sonography, MRI is noninvasive and can provide images in multiple planes, but there is no interference from skeletal, fatty, or gas-filled structures and imaging of deep pelvic structures does not require a full bladder.

MRI can evaluate (1) fetal structure (CNS, thorax, abdomen, genitourinary tract, musculoskeletal system) and overall growth, (2) placenta (position, density, and presence of gestational trophoblastic disease), (3) quantity of amniotic fluid, (4) maternal structures (uterus, cervix, adnexa, and pelvis), (5) biochemical status (pH, adenosine triphosphate content) of tissues and organs, and (6) soft tissue, metabolic, or functional anomalies.

The woman is placed on a table in the supine position and slid into the bore of the main magnet, which is similar in appearance to a CT scanner. Depending on the reason for the study, the procedure may take from 20 to 60 minutes during which time the woman must be perfectly still except for short respites. Because of the long time needed to produce magnetic resonance images, the fetus will probably move, which will obscure anatomic details. The only way to ensure that this does not occur is to administer a sedative to the mother, but this approach should be reserved for selected cases in which visualization of fetal detail is critical.

MRI has little effect on the fetus; concerns that the fetal heart rate or fetal movement would decrease have not been supported (Poutamo et al., 1998).

BIOCHEMICAL ASSESSMENT

Biochemical assessment involves biologic examination (e.g., as chromosomes in exfoliated cells) and chemical determinations (e.g., L/S ratio and bilirubin level). Procedures used to obtain the needed specimens include amniocentesis, percutaneous umbilical blood sampling, chorionic villus sampling, and maternal sampling (Table 29-5).

Amniocentesis

Amniocentesis is performed to obtain amniotic fluid, which contains fetal cells. Under direct ultrasonographic visualization, a needle is inserted transabdominally into the uterus, amniotic fluid is withdrawn into a syringe, and the various assessments are performed. Amniocentesis is possible after week 14 of pregnancy, when the uterus becomes an abdominal organ and sufficient amniotic fluid is available for testing (Fig. 29-7). Indications for the procedure include prenatal diagnosis of genetic disorders or congenital anomalies (neural tube defects in particular), assessment of pulmonary maturity, and diagnosis of fetal hemolytic disease.

Complications in the mother and fetus occur in fewer than 1% of the cases and include the following:

Maternal—Hemorrhage, fetomaternal hemorrhage with possible maternal Rh isoimmunization, infection, labor, abruptio placentae, inadvertent damage to the intestines or bladder, and amniotic fluid embolism. Because of the possibility of fetomaternal hemorrhage, it is standard practice after an amniocentesis to administer Rh$_0$ D immune globulin (RhoGAM) to the woman who is Rh negative.

Fetal—Death, hemorrhage, infection (amnionitis), direct injury from the needle, miscarriage or preterm labor, and leakage of amniotic fluid.

Many of the complications have been minimized or eliminated by using ultrasonography to direct the procedure.

TABLE 29-5   Summary of Biochemical Monitoring Techniques

TEST	POSSIBLE FINDINGS	CLINICAL SIGNIFICANCE
MATERNAL BLOOD		
Coombs' test	Titer of 1:8 and rising	Significant Rh incompatibility
AFP	See below	See below
AMNIOTIC FLUID ANALYSIS		
Color	Meconium	Possible hypoxia or asphyxia
Lung profile		Fetal lung maturity
L/S ratio	>2	
Phosphatidylglycerol	Present	
Creatinine	>2 mg/dl	Gestational age >36 weeks
Bilirubin (ΔOD 450/nm)	<0.015	Gestational age >36 weeks, normal pregnancy
	High levels	Fetal hemolytic disease in Rh isoimmunized pregnancies
Lipid cells	>10%	Gestational age >35 weeks
AFP	High levels after 15-week gestation	Open neural tube or other defect
Osmolality	Decline after 20-week gestation	Advancing nonspecific gestational age
Genetic disorders	Dependent on cultured cells for karyotype and enzymatic activity	Counseling possibly required
Sex-linked		
Chromosomal		
Metabolic		

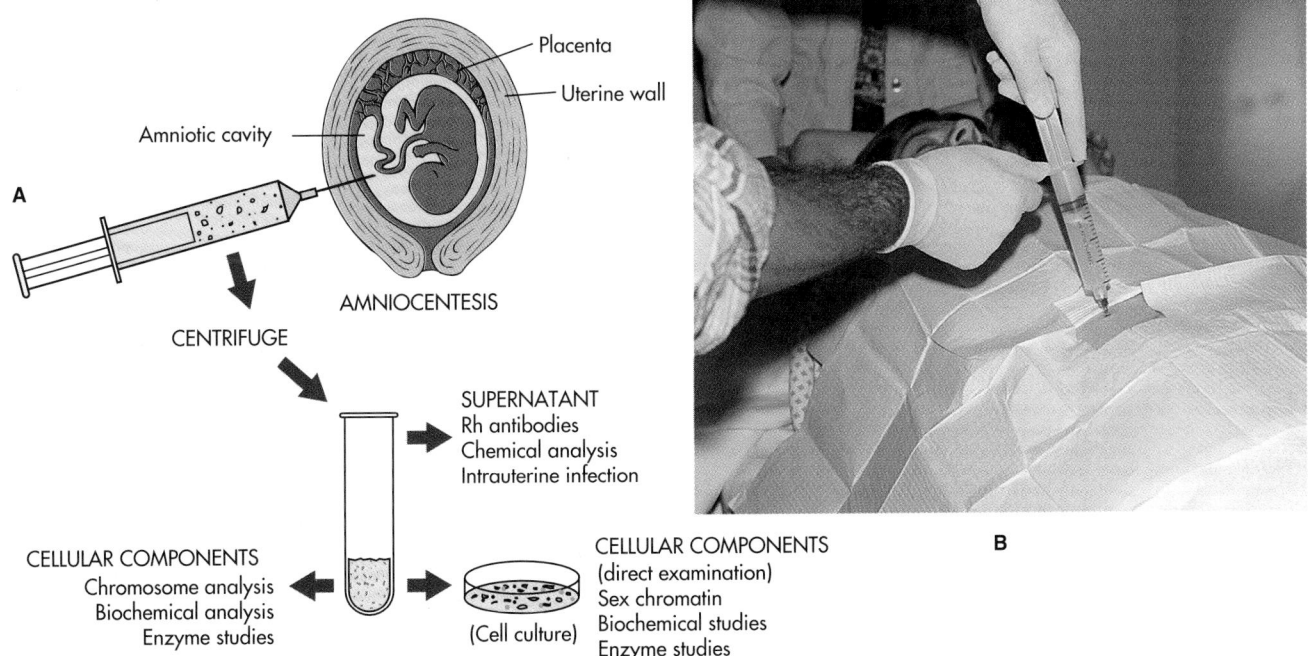

Fig. 29-7   A, Amniocentesis and laboratory use of amniotic fluid aspirant. **B,** Transabdominal amniocentesis. *(Courtesy Marjorie Pyle, RNC, Lifecircle, Costa Mesa, CA.)*

Genetic Problems

Prenatal assessment of genetic disorders is indicated in women more than 35 years old, with a previous child with a chromosomal abnormality, or with a family history of chromosomal anomalies. Inherited errors of metabolism (such as Tay-Sachs disease, hemophilia, and thalassemia) and other disorders for which marker genes are known may also be detected.

Karyotyping of cultured fetal cells (see Chapter 14) reveals fetal chromosomal aberrations in 1% to 2% of women between 35 and 38 years old, 2% of women between 39 and 44 years old, and 10% of women more than 45 years old. Karyotyping also permits determination of fetal sex, which is important if an X-linked disorder (occurring almost always in a male fetus) is suspected.

Biochemical analysis of enzymes in amniotic fluid can detect inborn errors of metabolism. For example, **alpha-fetoprotein (AFP)** levels in amniotic fluid are assessed as a follow-up for elevated levels in maternal serum. High AFP levels in amniotic fluid help confirm the diagnosis of a neural tube defect such as spina bifida or anencephaly or an abdominal wall defect such as omphalocele. The elevation results from the increased leakage of cerebrospinal fluid into the amniotic fluid through the closure defect. In normal fetuses, circulatory levels of AFP are high but amniotic fluid levels decrease to 18.5 g/ml at 15 weeks and 0.26 g/ml at term. AFP levels may also be elevated in a normal multifetal pregnancy and with intestinal atresia, presumably caused by lack of fetal swallowing.

A concurrent test for the presence of acetylcholinesterase almost always indicates a fetal defect (Scioscia, 1999). In such instances, concurrent ultrasound examination is recommended.

Fetal Maturity

Accurate assessment of fetal maturity is possible through examination of amniotic fluid or its exfoliated cellular contents. The laboratory tests described are determinants of term pregnancy and fetal maturity (see Table 29-4).

Fetal Hemolytic Disease

Another indication for amniocentesis is the identification and follow-up of fetal hemolytic disease in cases of isoimmunization. The procedure is usually not done until the mother's antibody titer reaches 1:8 and is rising. However, percutaneous umbilical blood sampling is now the procedure of choice to evaluate and treat fetal hemolytic disease.

Meconium

The presence of meconium in the amniotic fluid is usually determined by visual inspection of the sample.

Antepartal period. Meconium in the amniotic fluid before the beginning of labor is not usually associated with an adverse fetal outcome. The finding may be the result of acute and subsequently corrected fetal stress, chronic con-tinuing stress, or simply the physiologic passage of meconium. Because there has been some association between meconium in amniotic fluid in the third trimester and hypertensive disorders and postmaturity, the fetus should undergo further antepartum evaluation if the birth is not imminent (Glantz & Woods, 1999).

Intrapartal period. Intrapartal meconium-stained amniotic fluid is an indication for more careful evaluation by electronic fetal monitoring (EFM) and perhaps fetal scalp blood sampling. The presence of meconium, however, should not be the sole indicator for intervention.

Three possible reasons for the passage of meconium during the intrapartal period are as follows: (1) it is a normal physiologic function that occurs with maturity (meconium passage being infrequent before weeks 23 or 24, with an increased incidence after 38 weeks), (2) it is the result of hypoxia-induced peristalsis and sphincter relaxation, and (3) it may be a sequela to umbilical cord compression-induced vagal stimulation in mature fetuses.

The following criteria have been proposed for evaluating meconium-stained amniotic fluid during the intrapartal period (Scott et al., 1999):

1. *Consistency.* A thick, fresh consistency is more likely to be the result of fetal stress.
2. *Timing.* Thick, fresh meconium passed for the first time in late labor and in association with nonremediable severe variable or late fetal heart rate (FHR) decelerations is an ominous sign. The presence of meconium alone, however, is not necessarily a sign of fetal distress.
3. *Presence of other indicators.* Meconium passage and nonremediable severe variable or late FHR decelerations (especially with poor baseline variability), with or without acidosis confirmed by scalp-blood sampling, are ominous signs of fetal distress.

The birth team should be ready to suction the nasopharynx of the neonate carefully at the time of birth, ideally before the first breath is taken. Suctioning at this time effectively reduces the incidence and severity of meconium aspiration in the neonate.

Percutaneous Umbilical Blood Sampling

Direct access to the fetal circulation during the second and third trimesters is possible through **percutaneous umbilical blood sampling (PUBS)**, or cordocentesis, which is the most widely used method for fetal blood sampling and transfusion (Baumann & McFarland, 1994). PUBS involves the insertion of a needle directly into a fetal umbilical vessel under ultrasound guidance. Ideally, the umbilical cord is punctured 1 to 2 cm from its insertion into the placenta (Fig. 29-8). At this point the cord is well anchored and will not move, and the risk of maternal blood contamination (from the placenta) is slight. Generally, 1 to 4 ml of blood is removed and tested immediately by the Kleihauer-Betke procedure to ensure that it is fetal in origin. Indications for use of PUBS include prenatal diagnosis of inherited blood disorders, karyotyping of malformed fetuses, detection of fetal infection, determination of the acid-base status of fetuses with IUGR, and assessment and treatment of isoimmunization and thrombocytopenia in the fetus (Harmon, 1999). Complications that can occur include leaking of blood from the puncture site, cord laceration, thromboembolism, preterm labor, premature rupture of membranes, and infection.

In fetuses at risk for isoimmune hemolytic anemia, PUBS permits precise identification of fetal blood type and RBC count and may prevent further intervention. If the fetus is positive for the presence of maternal antibodies, a direct blood test can confirm the degree of anemia resulting from hemolysis. Intrauterine transfusion of severely anemic fetuses can be done 4 to 5 weeks earlier than through the intraperitoneal route.

Follow-up includes continuous FHR monitoring for several minutes to 1 hour and a repeat ultrasound examination 1 hour later to ensure that no further bleeding or hematoma formation has occurred.

Chorionic Villus Sampling

The combined advantages of earlier diagnosis and rapid results have made **chorionic villus sampling (CVS)** a popular technique for genetic studies, although some risks to the fetus exist.

The procedure is performed between 10 and 12 weeks of gestation and involves the removal of a small tissue specimen from the fetal portion of the placenta (Fig. 29-9). Because chorionic villi originate in the zygote, this tissue reflects the genetic makeup of the fetus (ACOG, 1995).

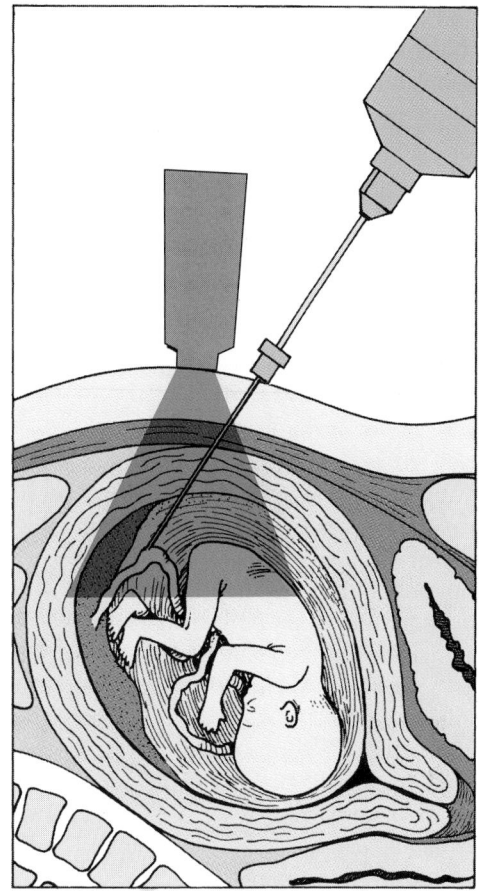

Fig. 29-8   Technique for PUBS guided by ultrasound.

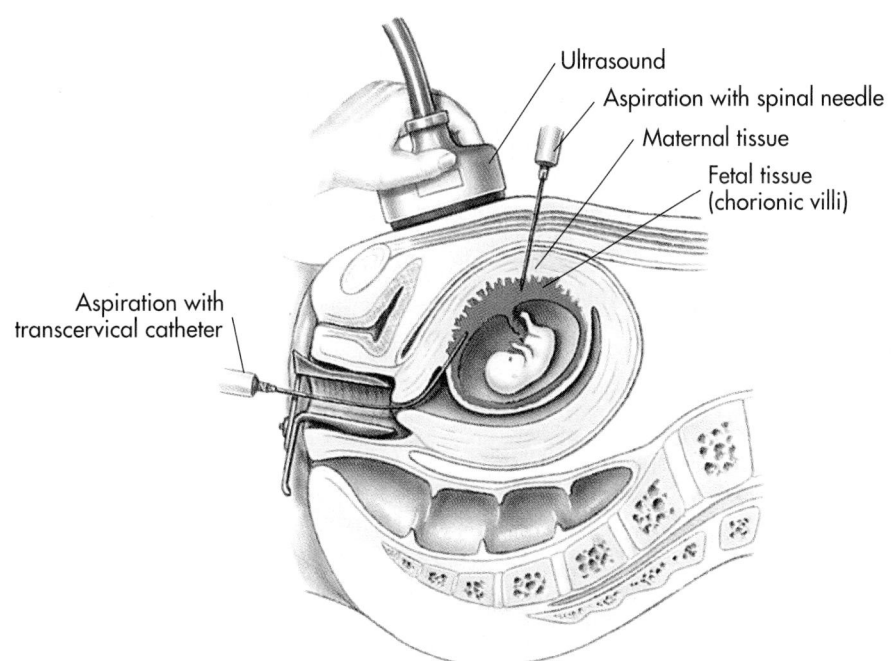

Fig. 29-9   Chorionic villus sampling. (Courtesy Medical and Scientific Illustration, Crozet, VA.)

CVS procedures can be accomplished either transcervically or transabdominally. In transcervical sampling, a sterile catheter is introduced into the cervix under continuous ultrasonographic guidance and a small portion of the chorionic villi is aspirated with a syringe. The aspiration cannula and obturator must be placed at a suitable site, and rupture of the amniotic sac must be avoided.

If the abdominal approach is used, an 18-gauge spinal needle with stylet is inserted under sterile conditions through the abdominal wall into the chorion frondosum under ultrasound guidance. The stylet is then withdrawn and the chorionic tissue is aspirated into a syringe (see Fig. 29-9).

Complications of the procedure include vaginal spotting or bleeding immediately afterward, miscarriage (in 0.3% of cases), rupture of membranes (in 0.1% of cases), and chorioamnionitis (in 0.5% of cases). Because of the possibility of fetomaternal hemorrhage, women who are Rh negative should receive immune globulin (RhoGAM) to avoid isoimmunization (Gilbert & Harmon, 1998). An increased risk of limb anomalies (transverse digital anomalies) has been noted when CVS is done before 10 weeks of gestation (ACOG, 1995).

Indications for CVS are similar to those for amniocentesis. About 90% of the procedures are performed because of advanced maternal age (over age 35 years) (Scioscia, 1999). Other indications include biochemical and molecular assays for infections or metabolic disorders (Box 29-7).

Maternal Assays

AFP

Maternal serum AFP (MSAFP) levels have been used as a screening tool for neural tube defects (NTDs) in pregnancy. Through this technique, approximately 80% to 85% of all open NTDs and open abdominal wall defects can be detected early in pregnancy. Screening is recommended for all pregnant women (ACOG, 1996).

The cause of NTDs is not well understood, but 95% of all affected infants are born to women with no previous family history of similar anomalies. The defect occurs in 1 to 2 per 1000 births in most parts of the United States. The birth of one affected child increases the risk of NTD recurrence in future pregnancies to 1% to 5% (Cunningham et al., 1997; Scioscia, 1999).

BOX 29-7 Fetal Rights

Amniocentesis, PUBS, and CVS are prenatal tests used for diagnosing fetal defects in pregnancy. They are invasive and carry risks to the mother and fetus. A consideration of abortion is linked to the performance of these tests because there is no treatment for genetically affected fetuses. Thus the issue of fetal rights is a key ethical concern in prenatal testing for fetal defects.

AFP is produced by the fetal liver and increasing levels are detectable in the serum of pregnant women from 14 to 34 weeks. Although amniotic fluid AFP is diagnostic for NTD, MSAFP is a screening tool only and identifies candidates for the more definitive procedures of amniocentesis and ultrasound examination. MSAFP screening can be done with reasonable reliability any time between 15 and 22 weeks of gestation (16 to 18 weeks being ideal) (ACOG, 1996).

Once the maternal level of AFP is determined, it is compared with normal values for each week of gestation. Values should also be correlated with maternal age, weight, race, and whether the woman is an insulin-dependent diabetic (Covington et al., 1996). If findings are abnormal, follow-up procedures include genetic counseling for families with a history of NTD, repeat AFP, ultrasound examination, and possibly, amniocentesis.

Down syndrome and probably other autosomal trisomies are associated with lower-than-normal levels of MSAFP and amniotic fluid AFP. The **triple-marker test,** is also performed at 16 to 18 weeks of gestation and uses the levels of three markers, MSAFP, unconjugated estriol, and human chorionic gonadotropin (hCG), in combination with maternal age to calculate a new risk. In the presence of a fetus with Down syndrome, the MSAFP and unconjugated estriol levels are low, whereas the hCG level is elevated. With the two additional screening tests, approximately 60% of cases of Down syndrome can be identified (Ross & Elias, 1997).

As with MSAFP, these tests are screening procedures only and are not diagnostic. A definitive examination of amniotic fluid for AFP and chromosomal analysis combined with ultrasound visualization of the fetus is necessary for diagnosis.

Estriols

The steroid precursor produced by the fetal adrenal glands is synthesized into estriols in the placenta and is excreted by the mother's healthy kidneys. Estriol levels may also be assayed in maternal serum, which is the preferred method. At this time, unconjugated estriol levels are determined only as part of the triple-marker test described earlier.

Coombs' Test

Coombs' test for Rh incompatibility is discussed in Chapter 40. If the maternal titer for Rh antibodies is greater than 1:8, amniocentesis for determination of bilirubin in amniotic fluid is indicated to establish the severity of fetal hemolytic anemia. Coombs' test can also detect other antibodies that may place the fetus at risk for incompatibility with maternal antigens.

ELECTRONIC FETAL MONITORING

Indications

First- and second-trimester antepartal assessment is directed primarily at the diagnosis of fetal anomalies. The goal of third-trimester testing is to determine whether the intrauterine environment continues to be supportive to the fetus. The testing is often used to determine the timing of childbirth for clients at risk for **uteroplacental insufficiency (UPI)** (the gradual decline in delivery of needed substances by the placenta to the fetus). Gradual loss of placental function results first in inadequate nutrient delivery to the fetus, leading to IUGR. Subsequently, respiratory function is also compromised, resulting in fetal hypoxia. Indications for both the **nonstress test (NST)** (or **fetal activity determination [FAD]**) and the **contraction stress test (CST)** include but are not limited to the following:

Maternal diabetes mellitus
Chronic hypertension
Pregnancy-induced hypertension (PIH)
IUGR
Maternal asthma
Sickle cell disease
Maternal cyanotic heart disease
Postmaturity
History of previous stillbirth
Maternal trauma
Decreased fetal movement
Isoimmunization
Meconium-stained amniotic fluid at third-trimester amniocentesis
Hyperthyroidism
Collagen disease
Older pregnant woman
Chronic renal disease

No clinical contraindications exist for the NST, but results may not be conclusive if gestation is 26 weeks or less. Absolute contraindications for the CST are the following: rupture of membranes, previous classic incision for cesarean birth, preterm labor, placenta previa, and abruptio placentae. Other conditions in which CST may be contraindicated are multifetal pregnancy, previous preterm labor, hydramnios, more than 36 weeks of gestation, and incompetent cervix. As a rule, reactive patterns with the NST or negative results with the CST are associated with favorable outcomes.

Fetal Responses to Hypoxia or Asphyxia

Hypoxia or asphyxia elicits a number of responses in the fetus. There is a redistribution of blood flow to certain vital organs. This series of responses (redistribution of blood flow favoring vital organs, decrease in total oxygen consumption, and switch to anaerobic glycolysis) is a temporary mechanism that enables the fetus to survive up to 30 minutes of limited oxygen supply without decompensation of vital organs. However, during more severe asphyxia or sustained hypoxemia, these compensatory responses are no longer maintained, and a decrease in the cardiac output, arterial blood pressure, and blood flow to the brain and heart occurs (Parer, 1999), with characteristic FHR patterns reflecting these changes.

Variability

Considerable evidence supports the clinical belief that FHR variability indicates an intact nervous pathway through the cerebral cortex, midbrain, vagus nerve, and cardiac conduction system. With a 98% accuracy in predicting fetal well-being, the presence of normal FHR variability is a reassuring indicator. Inputs from various areas of the brain decrease after cerebral asphyxia, leading to a decrease in variability after failure of the fetal hemodynamic compensatory mechanisms to maintain cerebral oxygenation (Parer, 1999).

NONSTRESS TEST (FETAL ACTIVITY DETERMINATION)

The NST is the most widely applied technique for antepartum evaluation of the fetus. The basis for the NST, or FAD, is that the normal fetus will produce characteristic heart rate patterns in response to fetal movement. In the healthy fetus with an intact CNS, 90% of gross fetal body movements are associated with accelerations of the FHR. This response can be blunted by hypoxia, acidosis, drugs (analgesics, barbiturates, and β-blockers), fetal sleep, and some congenital anomalies (Tucker, 2000).

Advantages

NST can be performed easily in an outpatient setting because it is noninvasive. It is also relatively inexpensive and has no known contraindications.

Disadvantages

Disadvantages center around the high rate of false-positive results for nonreactivity as a result of fetal sleep cycles, medications, and fetal immaturity. The test is also slightly less sensitive in detecting fetal compromise than are the CST or BPP.

Procedure

The woman is seated in a reclining chair (or in semi-Fowler's position) to avoid supine hypotension. The FHR is recorded by a Doppler transducer, and a tocotransducer is applied to detect uterine contractions or fetal movements. The strip chart is observed for signs of fetal activity and a concurrent acceleration of FHR. If evidence of fetal movement is not apparent on the strip, the woman may be asked to depress a button on a hand-held event marker connected to the monitor when she feels fetal movement. The movement is then noted on the strip. Because almost all accelerations are accompanied by fetal movement, the movements need not be recorded for the test to be considered reactive. The test is usually completed within 20 to 30 minutes, but it may take longer if the fetus needs to be awakened from a sleep state.

It has been suggested that the woman drink orange juice or be given glucose to raise her blood sugar and thereby stimulate fetal movements. In fact this practice is common; however, research has not proven this practice to be effective (McCarthy & Narrigan, 1995). Other methods that have been used to stimulate fetal activity, such as manipulating the woman's abdomen or using a transvaginal light, have not been very effective either. Only acoustic stimulation has had some impact (Marden et al., 1997).

Interpretation

Generally accepted criteria for a reactive tracing are as follows:
- Two or more accelerations of 15 beats/min lasting for 15 seconds over a 20-minute period
- Normal baseline rate
- Long-term variability amplitude of 10 or more beats per minute

If the test does not meet the criteria after 40 minutes, it is considered nonreactive (Fig. 29-10 and Table 29-6), in which case further assessments are needed with a CST or BPP. The current recommendation is that the NST be performed twice weekly (after 28 weeks of gestation) with clients who are diabetic or at risk for fetal death.

Fetal Acoustic Stimulation

The **acoustic stimulation test** is another method of testing antepartum FHR response. The test takes approximately 15 minutes to complete, with the fetus monitored for 5 to 10 minutes before stimulation to obtain a baseline FHR. The sound source (usually a laryngeal stimulator) is then activated for 3 seconds on the maternal abdomen over the fetal head. Monitoring continues for another 5 minutes, after which the monitor tracing is assessed. A test is considered reactive if there is an immediate and sustained increase in long-term variability and heart rate accelerations. The accelerations produced may have a significant increase in duration. The test may be repeated at 1-minute intervals up to three times when there is no response. Further evaluation is needed with BPP or CST if the pattern is still nonreactive.

Marden and associates (1997) found that fetuses who were exposed to vibroacoustic stimulation exhibited significantly more movement than controls and therefore were more likely to have reactive NSTs.

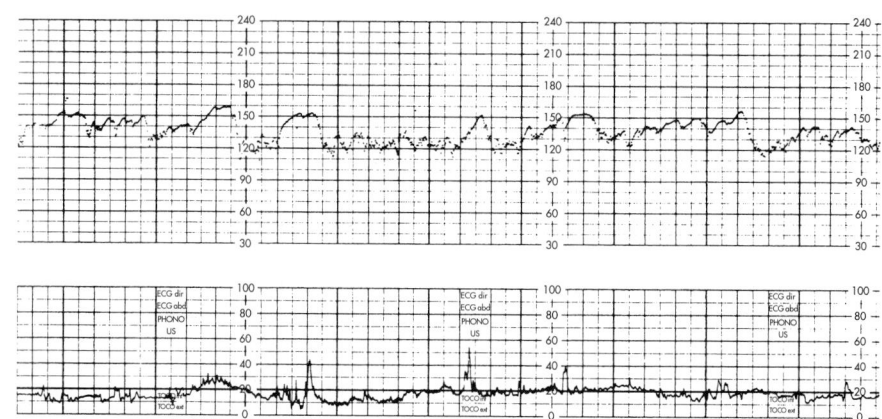

Fig. 29-10 Reactive NST (fetal heart rate acceleration with movement). *(From Tucker, S. [2000]. Pocket guide to fetal monitoring and assessment [4th ed.]. St. Louis: Mosby.)*

TABLE 29-6	**Interpretation of the Nonstress Test**	
RESULT	**INTERPRETATION**	**CLINICAL SIGNIFICANCE**
Reactive	Two or more accelerations of FHR of 15 beats/min lasting 15 sec or more, associated with each fetal movement in 20 min period	As long as twice-weekly NSTs remain reactive, most high risk pregnancies are allowed to continue
Nonreactive	Any tracing with either no FHR accelerations or accelerations <15 beats/min or lasting less than 15 sec throughout any fetal movement during testing period	Further indirect monitoring may be attempted with abdominal fetal electrocardiography in effort to clarify FHR pattern and quantitate variability; external monitoring should continue, and CST or BPP should be done
Unsatisfactory	Quality of FHR recording not adequate for interpretation	Test is repeated in 24 hr or CST is done depending on clinical situation

BPP, Biophysical profile; *CST,* contraction stress test; *FHR,* fetal heart rate; *NST,* nonstress test.

Contraction Stress Test

The CST is one of the first electronic methods to be developed for assessment of fetal health. It was devised as a graded stress test of the fetus, and its purpose was to identify the jeopardized fetus that was stable at rest but showed evidence of compromise after stress. Uterine contractions decrease uterine blood flow and placental perfusion. If this decrease is sufficient to produce hypoxia in the fetus, a deceleration in FHR will result, beginning at the peak of the contraction and persisting after its conclusion (late deceleration).

NURSE ALERT *In a healthy fetoplacental unit, uterine contractions usually do not produce late decelerations, whereas if there is underlying uteroplacental insufficiency, contractions will produce late decelerations.*

Advantages

The CST provides an earlier warning of fetal compromise than the NST and with fewer false-positive results.

Disadvantages

In addition to the contraindications described earlier, the CST is more time consuming and expensive than the NST. It is also an invasive procedure if oxytocin stimulation is required.

Procedure

The woman is placed in semi-Fowler's position or sits in a reclining chair. She is monitored indirectly, and the strip is observed for 10 minutes for baseline rate, long-term variability, and the possible occurrence of spontaneous contractions. The two methods of CST are the nipple-stimulated contraction test and the oxytocin-stimulated contraction test.

Nipple-stimulated contraction test. After the procedure is explained to the woman, warm, moist washcloths are applied to both breasts for several minutes. The woman is then asked to massage one nipple for 10 minutes. Massaging the nipples causes a release of oxytocin from the posterior pituitary. An alternative approach is for her to massage the nipple for 2 minutes, rest for 2 minutes, and continue for four cycles of massage and rest. If unilateral stimulation does not achieve adequate contractions (three occurring within a 10-minute window), unilateral continuous stimulation should be tried (if the intermittent approach was used), followed by bilateral stimulation for 10 minutes. When adequate contractions or hyperstimulation occurs, stimulation should be stopped. If the stimulation and rest cycle method is used, it can be performed indefinitely until considered unsuccessful (Devoe, 1995).

Oxytocin-stimulated contraction test. If nipple stimulation is not successful, an exogenous oxytocin-stimulated CST should be performed. An intravenous (IV) infusion is begun with a scalp needle. The oxytocin is diluted in an IV solution (usually 10 U to 1000 ml fluid), infused into the tubing of the main IV device via a piggy-back port, and delivered by an infusion pump to ensure accurate dosage. The oxytocin infusion is usually begun at 0.5 mU/min and increased by 0.5 mU/min at 15- to 30-minute intervals until three uterine contractions of good quality are observed within a 10-minute period. The typical rate of oxytocin infusion used to elicit uterine contractions is 4 to 5 mU/min and rarely is more than 8 mU/min required. The infusion rate should probably not be increased to more than 20 mU/min; however, each case should be assessed individually (Devoe, 1995).

Interpretation

If no late decelerations are observed with the contractions, the findings are considered negative (Fig. 29-11, *A*). Repetitive late decelerations, render the test results positive (Fig. 29-11, *B* and Table 29-7).

After interpretation of the FHR pattern, the oxytocin infusion is halted and the maintenance IV solution infused until uterine activity has returned to the prestimulation level. If the CST is negative, the IV device is removed and the fetal monitor disconnected. If the CST is positive, continued monitoring and further evaluation of fetal well-being are indicated.

NURSING ROLE IN ANTEPARTAL ASSESSMENT FOR RISK

The nurse's role is that of educator and support person when the woman is undergoing such examinations as ultrasonography, MRI, CVS, PUBS, and amniocentesis. In some instances the nurse may assist the physician with the procedure. In many antepartal settings, nurses perform NSTs, CSTs, and BPPs; conduct an initial assessment; and begin necessary interventions for nonreassuring patterns. These nursing procedures are accomplished after additional education and training, under guidance of established protocols, and in collaboration with physicians (Treanor, 1998). Client teaching, which is an integral component of this role, involves preparing the client for the procedure, interpreting the findings, and providing psychosocial support when needed.

All women who undergo antepartal assessments are at risk for real and potential problems and may be in an anxious frame of mind. In most instances the tests are ordered because of suspected fetal compromise, deterioration of a maternal condition, or both. In the third trimester, pregnant women are most concerned about protecting themselves and their fetuses and consider themselves most vulnerable to outside influences. The label of high risk will increase this sense of vulnerability (Wright, 1994).

Most clients have incomplete knowledge of the assessment, whether it is regarding the procedure itself, the implications of findings, or the need for further evaluation or counseling. Perinatal nurses can provide the required education and, by keeping the clients well informed, can also promote a positive parental self-image in these high risk individuals.

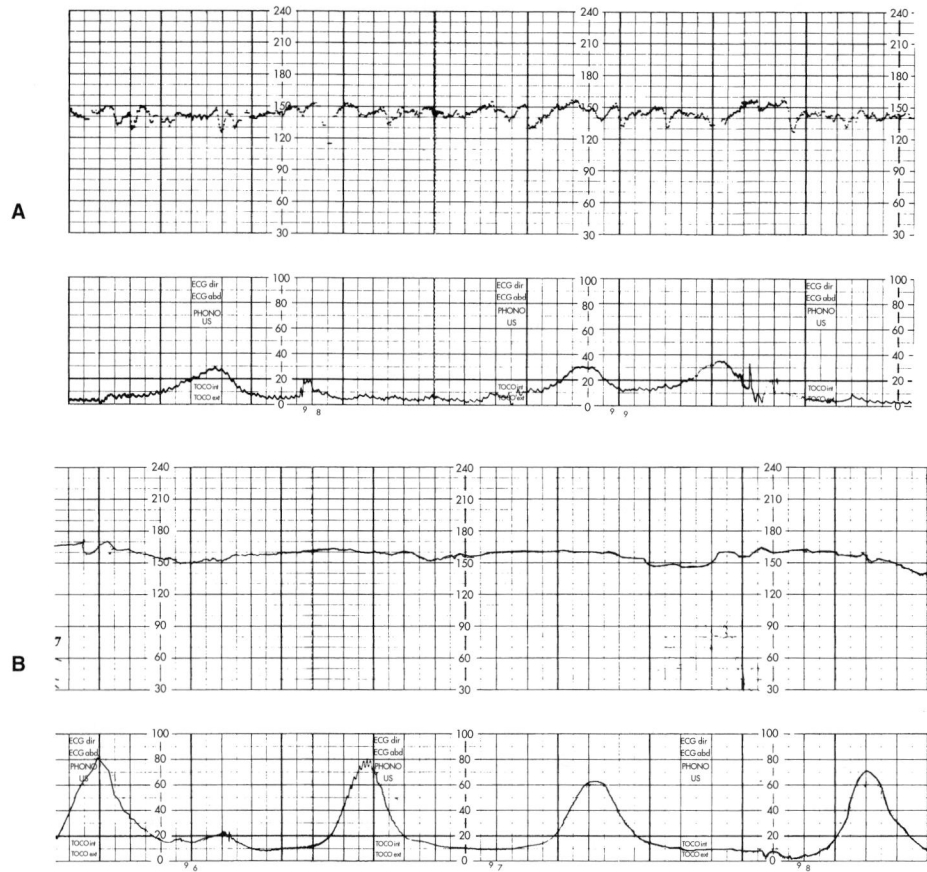

Fig. 29-11   CST. **A,** Negative CST. **B,** Positive CST. *(From Tucker, S. [2000]. Pocket guide to fetal monitoring and assessment [4th ed.]. St. Louis: Mosby.)*

TABLE 29-7	Guide for Interpretation of the CST
INTERPRETATION	**CLINICAL SIGNIFICANCE**
Negative No late decelerations, with minimum of three uterine contractions lasting 40 to 60 sec within 10 min period (see Fig. 29-11, A)	Reassurance that the fetus is likely to survive labor should it occur within 1 wk; more frequent testing may be indicated by clinical situation
Positive Persistent and consistent late decelerations occurring with more than half of contractions (Fig. 29-11, B)	Management lies between use of other tools of fetal assessment such as BPP and termination of pregnancy; a positive test result indicates that fetus is at increased risk for perinatal morbidity and mortality; physician may perform expeditious vaginal birth after successful induction or may proceed directly to cesarean birth; decision to intervene is determined by fetal monitoring and presence of FHR reactivity

TABLE 29-7   Guide for Interpretation of the CST—cont'd

INTERPRETATION	CLINICAL SIGNIFICANCE
Suspicious Late decelerations occurring in less than half of uterine contractions once adequate contraction pattern established	NST and CST should be repeated within 24 hr; if interpretable data cannot be achieved, other methods of fetal assessment must be used*
Hyperstimulation Late decelerations occurring with excessive uterine activity (contractions more often than every 2 min or lasting longer than 90 sec) or persistent increase in uterine tone	
Unsatisfactory Inadequate uterine contraction pattern or tracing too poor to interpret	

*Applies to results noted as suspicious, hyperstimulation, or unsatisfactory.

KEY POINTS

- A high risk pregnancy is one in which the life or well-being of the mother or infant is jeopardized by a biophysical or psychosocial disorder coincidental with or unique to pregnancy.

- Factors that place the pregnancy and fetus or neonate at risk include biophysical, sociodemographic, psychosocial, and environmental ones.

- Psychosocial perinatal warning indicators include characteristics of the parents, the child, their support systems, and family circumstances.

- Maternal and perinatal mortality rates for Caucasians are considerably lower than for other ethnic groups in the United States.

- Mortality rate decreases when risk is identified early and intensive care is applied.

- Biophysical assessment techniques include fetal movement counts, ultrasonography, and MRI.

- Biochemical monitoring techniques include amniocentesis, PUBS, CVS, and MSAFP.

- Reactive NSTs and negative CSTs suggest fetal well-being.

- Most assessment tests have some degree of risk for the mother and fetus, and usually cause some anxiety for the woman and her family.

CRITICAL THINKING EXERCISES

1 *Ms. Brown has been sent from the antepartum testing center to the labor and birth unit for a CST to be performed after a nonreactive NST. She is frightened of this test and its implications for the rest of her pregnancy and the health of her fetus. Explain the procedure and the rationale for doing the CST.*

2 *Formulate a teaching plan for a woman who has been advised to monitor fetal activity at home. Include the times monitoring is to take place and instruct her on the way to count movements and when to notify her health care provider.*

3 *Review several pregnant clients' charts. Identify risk factors (biophysical, psychosocial, sociodemographic, and environmental) and give your rationale for each choice.*

4 *Identify resources in your community for families who are experiencing a high risk pregnancy, including support groups, home care agencies, and counseling facilities. Make a list for the antepartal clinic, including accessibility by public transportation and costs.*

References

American Academy of Pediatrics/American College of Obstetricians and Gynecologists (AAP/ACOG). (1997). *Guidelines for perinatal care* (4th ed.). Elk Grove Village, IL: AAP/ACOG.

American College of Obstetricians and Gynecologists (ACOG) Committee on Genetics. (1995). Chorionic villi sampling. *Committee Opinion* 160. Washington, D.C.: ACOG.

American College of Obstetricians and Gynecologists (ACOG) Committee Opinion. (1996). Chorionic villi sampling. *Int J Gynaecol Obstet* 52(2), 206-208.

American College of Obstetricians and Gynecologists (ACOG). (1996). Management of isoimmunization in pregnancy. *Educ Bull* 227. Washington, D.C.: ACOG.

Anthony, A. (1996). Biologic effects and safety. In T. Dubose (Ed.). *Fetal sonography.* Philadelphia: W.B. Saunders.

Association of Women's Health, Obstetric and Neonatal Nurses (AWHONN). (1998). *Nursing practice competencies and educational guidelines for limited ultrasound examination in obstetric and gynecology/infertility settings* (2nd ed.). Washington, D.C.: AWHONN.

Athay, P., & Haddock, F. (1985). *Ultrasound in obstetrics and gynecology* (2nd ed.). St. Louis: Mosby.

Baumann, P., & McFarland, B. (1994). Prenatal diagnosis. *J Nurse Midwifery* 39(2 Suppl), 35S-51S.

Chervenak, F., & Gabbe, S. (1996). Obstetric ultrasound: Assessment of fetal growth and anatomy. In S. Gabbe, J. Niebyl, & J. Simpson (Eds.). *Obstetrics: Normal and problem pregnancies* (3rd ed.). New York: Churchill Livingstone.

Covington, C. et al. (1996). Family care related to alpha-fetoprotein screening. *J Obstet Gynecol Neonatal Nurs* 25(2), 125-130.

Cunningham, F. et al. (1997). *Williams obstetrics* (20th ed.). Stamford, CT: Appleton & Lange.

DeCherney, A., & Pernoll, M. (Eds.). (1994). *Current obstetric and gynecologic diagnosis and treatment* (8th ed.). Norwalk, CT: Appleton & Lange.

Devoe, L. (1995). Nonstress and contraction stress testing. In J. Sciarra (Ed.). *Gynecology and obstetrics,* vol 3. *Maternal and fetal medicine.* Philadelphia: J.B. Lippincott.

Dooley, S., Freels, S., & Turnock, B. (1997). Quality assessment of perinatal regionalization by multivariate analysis: Illinois, 1991-1993. *Obstet Gynecol* 89, 193-198.

Enkin, M. et al. (1995). Effective care in pregnancy and childbirth. *Birth* 22(2):101-110.

Farmakides, G. et al. (1994). Doppler velocity. Where does it belong in evaluation of fetal status? *Clin Perinat* 21(4), 848-861.

Fischer, R., & Depp, R. (1995). Amniotic fluid: Physiology and assessment. In J. Sciarra (Ed.). *Gynecology and obstetrics,* vol 3. *Maternal and fetal medicine.* Philadelphia: J.B. Lippincott.

Fogel, C., & Lewallen, L. (1995). High risk childbearing. In C. Fogel, & N. Woods (Eds.). *Women's health care: A comprehensive handbook.* Thousand Oaks, CA: Sage.

Gilbert, E., & Harmon, J. (1998). *Manual of high risk pregnancy and delivery* (2nd ed.). St. Louis: Mosby.

Glantz, J., & Woods, J. (1999). Significance of amniotic fluid meconium. In R. Creasy, & R. Resnik (Eds.). *Maternal-fetal medicine* (4th ed.). Philadelphia: W.B. Saunders.

Gordon, M. (1994). *Nursing diagnosis: Process and application* (3rd ed.). St. Louis: Mosby.

Guyer, B. et al. (1998). Annual summary of vital statistics, 1997. *Pediatrics* 102(6), 1333-1347.

Guzman, E. et al. (1998). Longitudinal assessment of endocervical canal length between 15 and 24 weeks' gestation in women at risk for pregnancy loss or preterm birth. *Obstet Gynecol* 92, 31-37.

Harmon, C. (1999). Percutaneous fetal blood sampling. In R. Creasy, & R. Resnik (Eds.). *Maternal-fetal medicine* (4th ed.). Philadelphia: W.B. Saunders.

Koonin, L. et al. (1997). Pregnancy-related mortality surveillance–United States, 1987-1990. *MMWR* 46, 17-36.

Manning, F. (1995). Dynamic ultrasound-based fetal assessment: The fetal biophysical profile score. *Clin Obstet Gynecol* 38(1), 26-44.

Manning, F. (1999). General principles and applications of ultrasound. In R. Creasy, & R. Resnik (Eds.). *Maternal-fetal medicine* (4th ed.). Philadelphia: W.B. Saunders.

Marden, D. et al. (1997). A randomized controlled trial of a new fetal acoustic stimulation test for fetal well-being. *Am J Obstet Gynecol* 176(6), 1386-1388.

McCarthy, K., & Narrigan, D. (1995). Is there scientific support for the use of juice to facilitate the nonstress test? *J Obstet Gynecol Neonatal Nurs* 24(4), 303-306.

Miller, D. (1998). Antepartum testing. *Clin Obstet Gynecol* 41(3), 647-653.

National Center for Health Statistics. (1997). Pregnancy-related mortality surveillance–United States, 1987-1990. *MMWR: CDC Surveillance Summaries* 46, 17-36.

National Center for Health Statistics. (1998a). Maternal mortality–United States, 1982-1996. *MMWR* 47, 705-707.

National Center for Health Statistics. (1988b). Trends in infant mortality attributable to birth defects–United States, 1980-1995. *MMWR* 47, 773-778.

Parer, J. (1999). Fetal heart rate. In R. Creasy, & R. Resnik (Eds.). *Maternal-fetal medicine* (4th ed.). Philadelphia: W.B. Saunders.

Poutamo, J. et al. (1998). MRI does not change fetal cardiotocographic parameters. *Prenat Diagn* 18, 1149-1154.

Richardson, D. et al. (1998). Declining severity adjusted mortality: Evidence of improving neonatal intensive care. *Pediatrics* 102, 893-899.

Ross, H., & Elias, S. (1997). Maternal serum screening for fetal genetic disorders. *Obstet Gynecol Clin North Am* 24(1), 33-47.

Schulman, H. (1990). Doppler ultrasound. In R. Eden, & F. Boehm (Eds.). *Assessment and care of the fetus: Physiological, clinical, and medicolegal principles.* Norwalk, CT: Appleton & Lange.

Scioscia, A. (1999). Prenatal genetic diagnosis. In R. Creasy, & R. Resnik (Eds.). *Maternal-fetal medicine* (4th ed.). Philadelphia: W.B. Saunders.

Scott, J. et al. (Eds.). (1999). *Danforth's obstetrics and gynecology* (8th ed.). Philadelphia: Lippincott Williams & Wilkins.

Treanor, C. (1998). Exploring nurses' roles in limited ultrasound. *AWHONN Lifelines* 2, 13-14.

Tucker, S. (2000). *Pocket guide to fetal monitoring and assessment* (4th ed.). St. Louis: Mosby.

Wright, L. (1994). Prenatal diagnosis in the 1990s. *J Obstet Gynecol Neonatal Nurs* 23(6), 506-515.

30

Hypertensive Disorders in Pregnancy

Judith H. Poole

EARNING OBJECTIVES

- Define the key terms.
- Differentiate between pregnancy-induced hypertension (PIH) and chronic hypertension.
- Review etiologic theories of PIH.
- Describe the pathophysiology of PIH.
- Evaluate maternal, fetal, and newborn morbidity and mortality attributable to PIH.
- Identify assessment techniques for PIH.
- Differentiate between the management of the woman with mild preeclampsia and the woman with severe preeclampsia.

- Describe HELLP syndrome, including appropriate nursing actions.
- Identify the priorities for management of eclamptic seizures.
- Evaluate the use of anticonvulsant and antihypertensive therapies.
- Identify topics for nursing research related to hypertensive disorders in pregnancy.

EY TERMS

arteriolar vasospasm	dependent edema	pitting edema
chronic hypertension	eclampsia	preeclampsia
clonus	edema	pregnancy-induced hypertension
deep tendon reflexes	HELLP syndrome	proteinuria

roviding safe and effective care for the high risk client requires a joint effort from all members of the health care team, with each member contributing unique skills and talents to provide optimal outcomes for mother and infant. This chapter focuses on the classification and theories of hypertensive disorders of pregnancy and their associated sequelae. Gestational hypertensive disorders are also referred to as **pregnancy-induced hypertension** (PIH). **Preeclampsia** and **eclampsia** are the primary focus of the chapter. Pathophysiology is discussed as it affects maternal organ systems and the pregnancy. This background pro-

vides a working basis for early identification of the onset or worsening of the hypertensive condition and helps guide nurses in selecting timely and appropriate nursing interventions for preventing injury to the woman and fetus.

SIGNIFICANCE AND INCIDENCE

Hypertension is the most common medical complication of pregnancy, with the incidence ranging from 1% to 5% (Ventura et al., 1999). A significant contributor to maternal and perinatal morbidity and mortality, preeclampsia complicates approximately 5% to 8% of all pregnancies not terminating in first-trimester abortions (American College of Obstetricians and Gynecologists, 1996; Sibai et al., 1997). In women with a history of chronic hypertension or renal disease predating pregnancy, the occurrence of preeclampsia is 25% (Jones & Hayslett, 1996). The prevalence rate for pregnancy-associated hypertension has risen in recent years. The rate has risen among all age, racial, and ethnic groups since the early 1990s (Ventura et al., 1999). Based on 1997 birth certificate data, the rate of pregnancy-associated hypertension was 36.8 per 1000 births. The rates for chronic hypertension and eclampsia have remained essentially unchanged during the 1990s—6.9 and 3.3 per 1000 births, respectively (Ventura et al., 1999).

MORBIDITY AND MORTALITY

In the United States, when maternal deaths related to ruptured ectopic pregnancy are excluded, preeclampsia ranks second only to embolic events as a cause of maternal mortality. Preeclampsia predisposes the woman to potentially lethal complications, including eclampsia, abruptio placentae, disseminated intravascular coagulation (DIC), acute renal failure, hepatic failure, adult respiratory distress syndrome (ARDS), and cerebral hemorrhage (American College of Obstetricians and Gynecologists, 1996; Cunningham et al., 1997; Roberts, 1999; Working Group on High Blood Pressure in Pregnancy, 1990). Hypertension (chronic and pregnancy induced) complicating pregnancy increases the woman's risk for a cesarean birth, which further increases the risk of morbidity and mortality.

Preeclampsia occurs primarily after the second trimester of pregnancy, representing a great danger to the fetus and neonate. Preeclampsia contributes significantly to intrauterine fetal death (IUFD) and perinatal mortality (Sibai, 1996a, 1996b). Causes of perinatal death related to preeclampsia are uteroplacental insufficiency (UPI) and abruptio placentae, which lead to intrauterine death, preterm birth, and low birth weight (Roberts, 1999).

Eclampsia (characterized by seizures) from profound cerebral effects of preeclampsia is the major maternal hazard. As a rule, maternal and perinatal morbidity and mortality are highest among cases in which eclampsia is seen early in gestation (before 28 weeks), maternal age is greater than 25 years, the woman is a multigravida, and chronic hypertension or renal disease is present. The fetus of the eclamptic woman is at increased risk from abruptio placentae, preterm birth, intrauterine growth restriction (IUGR), and acute hypoxia (Gilbert & Harmon, 1998).

CLASSIFICATION

Current terminology used to describe the hypertensive disorders of pregnancy is associated with imprecise usage, causing confusion for health care providers caring for women with hypertensive complications during pregnancy

TABLE 30-1	Classification of Hypertensive States of Pregnancy
TYPE	**DESCRIPTION**
GESTATIONAL HYPERTENSIVE DISORDERS: PREGNANCY-INDUCED HYPERTENSION (PIH)	
Transient hypertension	Development of mild hypertension during pregnancy in previously normotensive client without proteinuria or pathologic edema
Gestational proteinuria	Development of proteinuria after 20 weeks of gestation in previously nonproteinuric client without hypertension
Preeclampsia	Development of hypertension and proteinuria in previously normotensive client after 20 weeks of gestation or in early postpartum period; in presence of trophoblastic disease it can develop before 20 weeks of gestation
Eclampsia	Development of convulsions or coma in preeclamptic client
CHRONIC HYPERTENSIVE DISORDERS	
Chronic hypertension	Hypertension or proteinuria in pregnant client with chronic hypertension
Superimposed preeclampsia/eclampsia	Development of preeclampsia or eclampsia in client with chronic hypertension

From Gilbert, E., & Harmon, J. (1998). *Manual of high risk pregnancy and delivery* (2nd ed.). St. Louis: Mosby.

and childbirth. The two classification systems most commonly used in the United States today are based on reports from the American College of Obstetricians and Gynecologists (1996) and the Working Group on High Blood Pressure in Pregnancy (1990). These classification systems are summarized in Table 30-1.

Clinically, there are two basic types of hypertension during pregnancy—chronic hypertension and PIH—with the distinction based on the onset of hypertension in relation to pregnancy. Chronic hypertension is hypertension that predates the pregnancy or hypertension continuing beyond

█ TABLE 30-2 Differentiation Between Mild and Severe Preeclampsia

	MILD PREECLAMPSIA	SEVERE PREECLAMPSIA
MATERNAL EFFECTS		
Blood pressure	BP reading of 140/90 mm Hg ×2, 4-6 hr apart	Rise to ≥160/110 mm Hg on two separate occasions 4-6 hr apart with pregnant woman on bed rest
Mean arterial pressure (MAP)	>105 mm Hg	>105 mm/Hg
Weight gain	Weight gain of more than 0.5 kg/wk during the second and third trimesters or sudden weight gain of 2 kg/wk at any time	Same as mild preeclampsia
Proteinuria – Qualitative dipstick – Quantitative 24 hr analysis	Proteinuria of 0.3 g/L in a 24 hr specimen or >0.1 g/L in a random daytime specimen on two or more occasions 6 hr apart (because protein loss is variable); with dipstick, values varying from 2+ to 3+	Proteinuria of >5 g/L in 24 hr or >4+ protein on dipstick
Edema	Dependent edema, some puffiness of eyes, face, fingers; pulmonary edema absent	Generalized edema, noticeable puffiness; eyes, face, fingers; pulmonary edema possibly present
Reflexes	May be normal	Hyperreflexia ≥3+, possible ankle clonus
Urine output	Output matching intake, ≥30 ml/hr or <650 ml/24 hr	<20 ml/hr or <400 ml to 500 ml/24 hr
Headache	Absent/transient	Severe
Visual problems	Absent	Blurred, photophobia, blind spots on funduscopy
Irritability/changes in affect	Transient	Severe
Epigastric pain	Absent	Present
Serum creatinine	Normal	Elevated
Thrombocytopenia	Absent	Present
AST elevation	Normal or minimal	Marked
FETAL EFFECTS		
Placental perfusion	Reduced	Decreased perfusion expressing as IUGR in fetus; FHR: late decelerations
Premature placental aging	Not apparent	At birth placenta appearing smaller than normal for duration of pregnancy, premature aging apparent with numerous areas of broken syncytia, ischemic necroses (white infarcts) numerous, intervillous fibrin deposition (red infarcts)

AST, Aspartate aminotransferase; *FHR,* fetal heart rate.

42 days postpartum (American College of Obstetricians and Gynecologists, 1996). Pregnancy-induced hypertension is the onset of hypertension, generally after the twentieth week of pregnancy, appearing as a marker of a pregnancy-specific vasospastic condition (American College of Obstetricians and Gynecologists, 1996; Roberts, 1999). Chronic hypertension and PIH may occur independently or simultaneously. PIH is further classified according to the maternal organ systems affected.

Preeclampsia

Preeclampsia, a pregnancy-specific condition in which hypertension develops after 20 weeks of gestation in a previously normotensive woman, is a multisystem, vasospastic disease process characterized by the presence of hypertension and proteinuria (American College of Obstetricians and Gynecologists, 1996). Preeclampsia is usually categorized as mild or severe in terms of management (Table 30-2).

BOX 30-1 | **Protocol for Blood Pressure Measurement**

1. Measure blood pressure with the woman seated (ambulatory) or in a 30-degree tilt on her left side.
2. After positioning, allow the woman at least 5 minutes of quiet rest before blood pressure measurement, to encourage relaxation.
3. Use the right arm for blood pressure measurement.
4. Hold the arm in a roughly horizontal position at heart level.
5. Use the proper-sized cuff (cuff should cover approximately 80% of the upper arm).
6. Maintain a slow, steady deflation rate.
7. Take the average of two readings at least 6 hours apart to minimize recorded blood pressure variations across time.
8. Use Korotkoff phase V (disappearance of sound) for recording the diastolic value (some sources recommend recording both phase IV [the muffled sound] and phase V).
9. Use accurate equipment.
10. If interchanging manual and electronic devices, use caution in interpreting different blood pressure values.

An elevated blood pressure is often the first sign of preeclampsia to develop. Hypertension is defined as a blood pressure greater than or equal to 140/90 mm Hg. The Committee on Terminology of the American College of Obstetricians and Gynecologists has also defined hypertension as a mean arterial pressure (MAP) of 105 mm Hg or more.

Elevations over prepregnancy values are no longer considered diagnostic for hypertension. The blood pressure elevation must be present on two occasions at least 4 to 6 hours apart (Fairlie & Sibai, 1999). One of the difficulties in diagnosing hypertension has been a lack of standardization in blood pressure measurement. Box 30-1 presents recommendations for standardizing this procedure.

Proteinuria is defined as a concentration of 0.1 g/L (1+ to 2+ on dipstick measurement) or more in at least two random urine specimens collected at least 6 hours apart. In a 24-hour specimen, *proteinuria* is defined as a concentration of 0.3 g/L per 24 hours.

Pathologic **edema** is clinically evident, generalized accumulation of fluid of the face, hands, or abdomen that is not responsive to 12 hours of bed rest. It may also be manifested as a rapid weight gain of more than 2 kg in 1 week. Presence of edema is no longer considered necessary for the diagnosis of preeclampsia (Sibai & Rodriguez, 1999).

Severe Preeclampsia

Severe preeclampsia is the presence of any one of the following in the woman diagnosed with preeclampsia: (1) systolic blood pressure of at least 160 mm Hg or a diastolic blood pressure of at least 110 mm Hg; (2) proteinuria of greater than 5 g protein excreted in a 24-hour specimen, or greater than 3+ to 4+ on dipstick measurement; (3) oliguria, less than 400 to 500 ml of urine output over 24 hours; (4) cerebral or visual disturbances, such as altered level of consciousness, headache, scotomata, or blurred vision; (5) hepatic involvement; (6) thrombocytopenia with a platelet count less than $150,000/mm^3$; (7) pulmonary or cardiac involvement; (8) development of eclampsia; (9) development of the HELLP syndrome; or (10) certain cases of severe fetal growth restriction (American College of Obstetricians and Gynecologists, 1996; Roberts, 1999; Sibai, 1996b; Working Group on High Blood Pressure in Pregnancy, 1990).

Eclampsia

Eclampsia is the onset of seizure activity or coma in the woman diagnosed with PIH, with no history of preexisting neurologic pathology (American College of Obstetricians and Gynecologists, 1996). A seizure can be the initial sign for a pregnancy complicated by PIH.

HELLP Syndrome

HELLP syndrome is a laboratory diagnosis for a variant of severe preeclampsia characterized by hemolysis (H), elevated liver enzymes (EL), and low platelets (LP) (Stone, 1998).

Chronic Hypertension

Chronic hypertension is defined as hypertension present before the pregnancy or diagnosed before the twentieth week of gestation. Hypertension that persists longer than 6 weeks postpartum is also classified as chronic hypertension. There is no widely accepted definition of mild hypertension. Severe hypertension is usually defined as a diastolic blood pressure of <110 mm Hg or higher (Sibai, 1996a). Preconception counseling is recommended for women with respect to the increased risk of superimposed preeclampsia and lifestyle adjustments that may be necessary.

Chronic Hypertension with Superimposed Preeclampsia

Women with chronic hypertension may acquire preeclampsia or eclampsia. *Superimposed preeclampsia* is defined as an increase in blood pressure (30 mm Hg systolic or 15 mm Hg diastolic or <105 mm Hg MAP) along with proteinuria or generalized edema in women with chronic hypertension (Sibai, 1996b).

Transient Hypertension

Transient hypertension is the development of hypertension during pregnancy or the first 24 hours postpartum

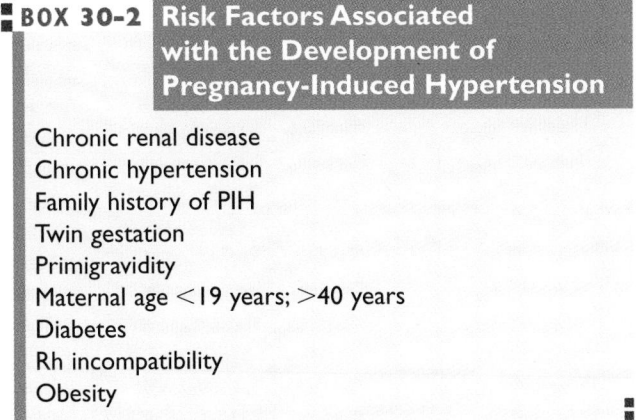

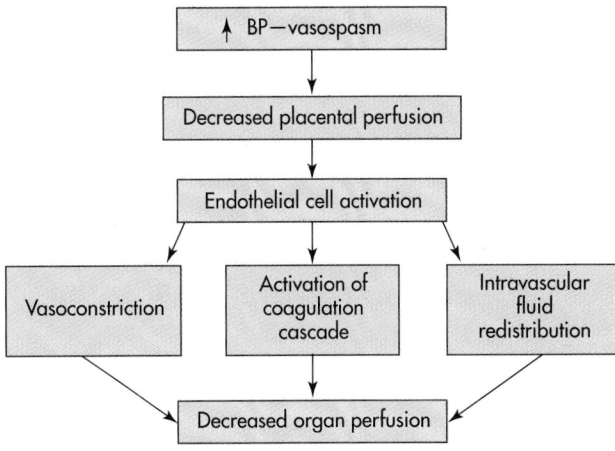

Fig. 30-1 Etiology of PIH. Endothelial cell dysfunction and preeclampsia.

without other signs of preeclampsia or preexisting hypertension. Blood pressure must return to normal levels by the tenth postpartum day (Sibai, 1996b). The presence of transient hypertension may be predictive of the eventual development of essential hypertension.

ETIOLOGY

Proposed causes of hypertension in pregnancy are multiple and have been the subject of extensive research and much speculation. The ultimate cause remains unknown.

Preeclampsia is a condition unique to human pregnancy; signs and symptoms develop only during pregnancy and disappear quickly after birth of the fetus and placenta. No single client profile identifies the woman who will have preeclampsia. However, certain high risk factors are associated with development of the disease: primigravidity, multifetal pregnancy, and morbid obesity (Box 30-2).

Several major concepts that contribute to current theories regarding the etiology of PIH are increased vasoconstrictor tone (Gilstrap & Gant, 1990), abnormal prostaglandin action (Friedman, 1988), and endothelial cell activation (Dekker & Sibai, 1998; Friedman, 1995). Immunologic factors may play an important role (Dekker & Sibai, 1999).

In part, vasospasms are the underlying mechanism for the signs and symptoms of preeclampsia. Vasospasms result from an increased sensitivity to circulating pressors, such as angiotensin II, and possibly an imbalance between the prostaglandins prostacyclin and thromboxane A_2 (Cunningham & Lindheimer, 1992; Magness & Gant, 1994; Working Group on High Blood Pressure in Pregnancy, 1990).

Endothelial cell dysfunction, believed to result from decreased placental perfusion, may account for many preeclampsia changes, as depicted in Fig. 30-1. In addition to endothelial damage, arteriolar vasospasm may contribute to an increased capillary permeability. This increases edema and further decreases intravascular volume, predisposing the woman with preeclampsia to pulmonary edema (Roberts, Taylor, & Goldfien, 1991).

The relationship of the immune system to preeclampsia suggests that immunologic factors play an important role in the development of preeclampsia (Sibai, 1991). The presence of foreign protein, the placenta, or the fetus may trigger an adverse immunologic response. This theory is supported by the increased incidence of preeclampsia or eclampsia in first-time mothers (first exposure to fetal tissue) and multiparous women pregnant by a new partner (different genetic material) (Trupin, Simon, & Eskanazi, 1996) (Fig. 30-2). The protective role of the immunologic response is poorly understood. Preeclampsia may be an immune complex disease in which the maternal antibody system is overwhelmed from excessive fetal antigens in the maternal circulation. This theory seems compatible with the high incidence of preeclampsia among women exposed to a large mass of trophoblastic tissue as seen in twins and hydatidiform moles.

Genetic predisposition may be another immunologic factor. Cooper, Brennecke, and Wilton (1993) found a greater frequency of preeclampsia and eclampsia among daughters and granddaughters of women with a history of eclampsia, which suggests an autosomal recessive gene controlling the maternal immune response. Paternal factors are also being examined (Robillard et al., 1993).

Diets inadequate in nutrients, especially protein, calcium, sodium, magnesium, and vitamins E and A, may be an etiologic factor in PIH. Proponents of this theory prescribe high-protein diets without caloric or sodium restriction in prevention and treatment of this disorder (Stone,

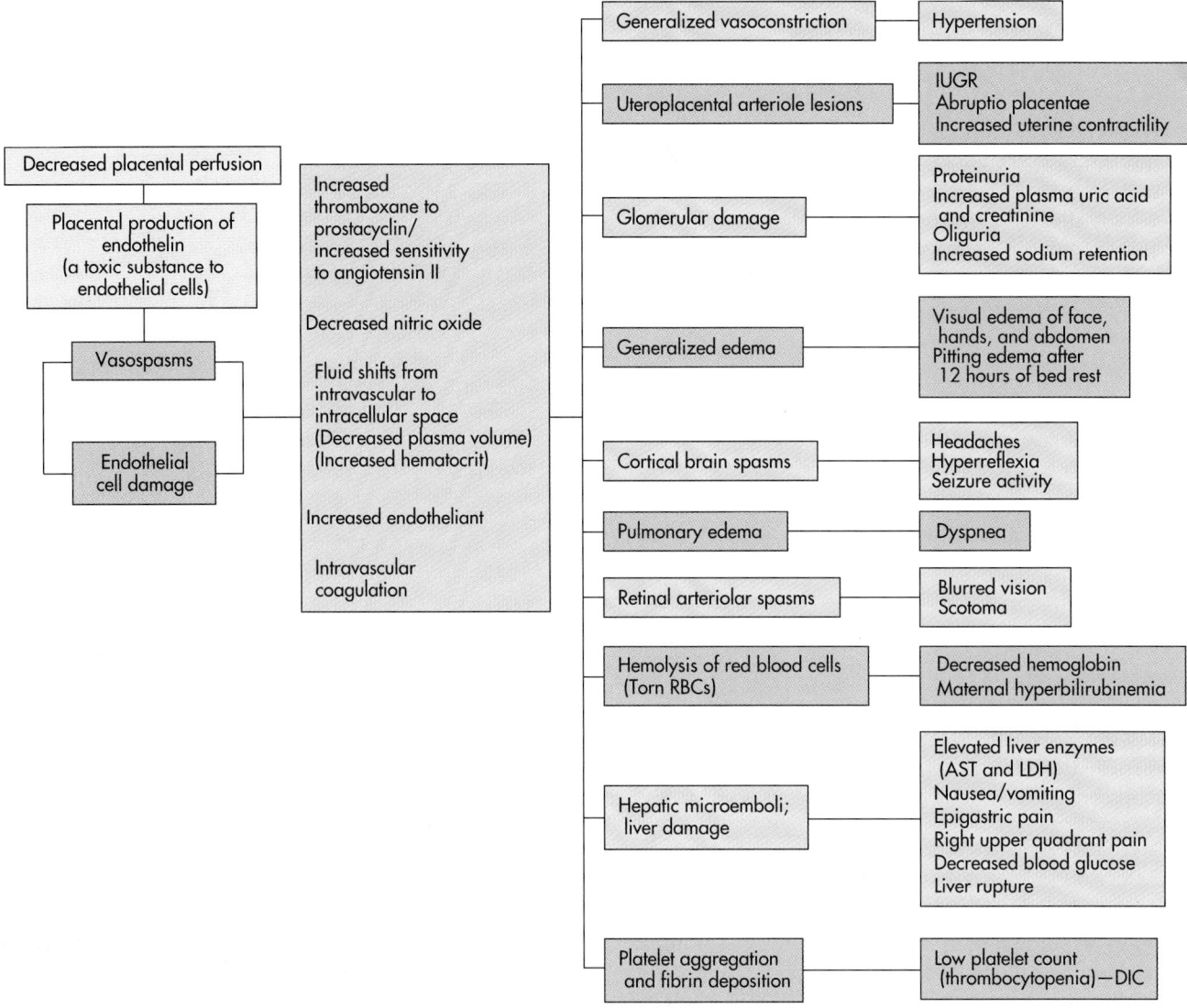

Fig. 30-2 Pathophysiology of PIH. *(Modified from Gilbert, E., & Harmon, J. [1998]. Manual of high risk pregnancy and delivery [2nd ed.]. St. Louis: Mosby.)*

1998). However, data are inconclusive for an association between diet and the development of preeclampsia.

PATHOPHYSIOLOGY

Preeclampsia progresses along a continuum from mild disease to severe preeclampsia, HELLP syndrome, or eclampsia. The pathophysiology of preeclampsia reflects alterations in the normal adaptations of pregnancy. Normal physiologic adaptations to pregnancy include increased blood plasma volume, vasodilation, decreased systemic vascular resistance, elevated cardiac output, and decreased colloid osmotic pressure (Box 30-3).

Preeclampsia is quite different from chronic hypertension. Pathologic changes in the endothelial cells of the glomeruli (glomeruloendotheliosis) are uniquely characteristic of preeclampsia, particularly in nulliparous women

(85%). The main pathogenic factor is not an increase in blood pressure but poor perfusion as a result of vasospasm. **Arteriolar vasospasm** diminishes the diameter of blood vessels, which impedes blood flow to all organs and raises blood pressure (Working Group on High Blood Pressure in Pregnancy, 1990). Function in organs such as the placenta, kidneys, liver, and brain is depressed by as much as 40% to 60%. The pathophysiologic sequelae are shown in Fig. 30-2.

Impaired placental perfusion leads to early degenerative aging of the placenta and possible IUGR of the fetus. Reduced kidney perfusion decreases the glomerular filtration rate and leads to degenerative glomerular changes and oliguria. Protein, primarily albumin, is lost in the urine. Uric acid clearance is decreased; however, blood urea nitrogen (BUN), serum creatinine, and serum uric acid levels increase (Dildy et al., 1991). Sodium and water are re-

BOX 30-3 Normal Physiologic Adaptations to Pregnancy

CARDIOVASCULAR

↑ Blood volume; plasma volume expansion greater than red cell mass expansion, leading to physiologic anemia of pregnancy

↓ Total peripheral resistance, decreases in blood pressure readings and MAP

↑ Cardiac output resulting from increased blood volume, slight increase in heart rate to compensate for peripheral relaxation

↑ Oxygen consumption

Physiologic edema related to ↓ plasma colloid osmotic pressure and ↑ venous capillary hydrostatic pressure

HEMATOLOGIC

↑ Clotting factors, predisposing to DIC and clotting

↓ Serum albumin resulting in decreases in colloid osmotic pressure, predisposing toward pulmonary edema

RENAL

↑ Renal plasma flow and glomerular filtration rate

ENDOCRINE

↑ Estrogen production resulting in ↑ renin–angiotensin II–aldosterone secretion

↑ Progesterone production blocking aldosterone effect (slight ↓ Na)

↑ Vasodilator prostaglandins resulting in resistance to angiotensin II (slight ↓ blood pressure)

tained. Plasma colloid osmotic pressure decreases as serum albumin levels decrease. Intravascular volume is reduced as fluid moves out of the intravascular compartment, resulting in hemoconcentration, increased blood viscosity, and tissue edema. The hematocrit value increases as fluid leaves the intravascular space (Cunningham et al., 1997). In severe preeclampsia, blood volume may fall to or below nonpregnancy levels; severe edema develops and rapid weight gain is seen.

Decreased liver perfusion causes impaired function. Hepatic edema and subcapsular hemorrhage, felt by the pregnant woman as epigastric or right upper quadrant pain, is one sign of impending eclampsia (convulsion). Liver enzyme levels (e.g., aspartate aminotransferase [AST]) rise in the wake of liver damage.

Arteriolar vasospasms and decreased blood flow to the retina lead to visual symptoms such as scotomata (blind spots) and blurring. The same pathologic condition leads to cerebral edema and hemorrhages, as well as to increased central nervous system (CNS) irritability (Dildy et al., 1991). CNS irritability manifests as headache, hyper-

reflexia, positive ankle clonus, and occasionally the development of eclampsia. Changes in affect (changes in emotion, mood, and consciousness) are typical symptoms of cerebral edema and increasing intercranial pressure (Scott et al., 1999).

If the hypertension is difficult to bring under control, cardiac and pulmonary complications can occur. Heart failure, a common cause of maternal death attributed to preeclampsia, is rare among young, otherwise healthy women (Scott et al., 1999). Sudden circulatory collapse and shock may occur in women with a history of repeated hypertensive pregnancies.

Typically, pulmonary edema caused by preeclampsia is associated with severe generalizable edema. Intravenous (IV) fluid infusion is an iatrogenic cause of fluid overload. A weak, rapid pulse; increased respiratory rate; lowered blood pressure; and pulmonary crackles suggest circulatory failure. Pulmonary edema and congestive heart failure are the only accepted indications for diuretic therapy during pregnancy (Scott et al., 1999). Diuretic therapy further reduces intervillous blood flow (placental perfusion), which may lead to serious fetal jeopardy. Impaired intervillous perfusion is the main cause of perinatal morbidity and mortality associated with hypertension (Scott et al., 1999).

HELLP SYNDROME

HELLP syndrome appears in only 2% to 12% of severely preeclamptic women, or about 1 in 1000 pregnancies (Stone, 1998). Although the exact mechanism is unknown, HELLP syndrome is thought to arise as a result of changes occurring with preeclampsia (see Fig. 30-2). Arteriolar vasospasm, endothelial damage, and platelet aggregation with resultant tissue hypoxia are the underlying mechanisms for the pathophysiology of HELLP syndrome (Poole, 1993, 1997). A circulating immunologic component may be the underlying cause. Maternal mortality rates have been reported as high as 24%. Perinatal mortality rates range from 79 to 367 per 1000 live births (Portis et al., 1997).

Most commonly, HELLP syndrome is seen in older, Caucasian, multiparous women. About 90% of women report a history of malaise for several days. Many women (65%) experience epigastric or right upper quadrant abdominal pain (possibly related to hepatic ischemia), and approximately half develop nausea and vomiting. It is extremely important to understand that many women with HELLP syndrome may not have signs or symptoms of severe preeclampsia. For example, many of these women are normotensive or have only slight elevations in blood pressure. Proteinuria also may be absent. As a result, women with HELLP syndrome are often misdiagnosed with a variety of other medical or surgical disorders (Sibai, 1996b).

HELLP syndrome is a laboratory, not a clinical, diagnosis. To make a diagnosis of HELLP syndrome, a woman's platelet count must be less than 100,000/mm³,

TABLE 30-3 Common Laboratory Changes in Preeclampsia

	NORMAL	PIH	HELLP
Hemoglobin/hematocrit	12-16 g/dl 37% to 47%	May increase	Decreased
Platelets	150,000-400,000/mm³	Unchanged	<100,000/mm³
PT/PTT	12-14 sec/60-70 sec	Unchanged	Unchanged
Fibrinogen	150-400 mg/dl	300-600 mg/dl	Decreased
Fibrin split products (FSP)	Absent	Absent	Present
Blood urea nitrogen	10-20 mg/dl	<10 mg/dl	Increased
Creatinine	0.5-1.1 mg/dl	<1 mg/dl	Increased
Lactate dehydrogenase (LDH)	45-90 U/L	Unchanged	Increased
Aspartate aminotransferase (AST)	4-20 U/L	Unchanged	Increased
Alanine aminotransferase (ALT)	3-21 U/L	Unchanged	Increased
Creatinine clearance	80-125 ml/min	130-180 ml/min	Decreased
Burr cells/schistocytes	Absent	Absent	Present
Uric acid	2-6.6 mg/dl	4.5-6 mg/dl	>10 mg/dl
Bilirubin (total)	0.1-1 mg/dl	Unchanged or increased	Increased

her liver enzyme levels (AST and alanine aminotransferase [ALT]) must be elevated, and there must be some evidence of intravascular hemolysis (burr cells on peripheral smear or elevated bilirubin level) (Stone, 1998). A unique form of coagulopathy (not DIC) occurs with HELLP syndrome. The platelet count is low, but coagulation factor assays, prothrombin time (PT), partial thromboplastin time (PTT), and bleeding time remain normal (Stone, 1998).

Recognition of the clinical and laboratory findings associated with HELLP syndrome is important if early, aggressive therapy is to be initiated to prevent maternal and neonatal mortality. Complications reported with HELLP syndrome include renal failure, pulmonary edema, ruptured liver hematoma, DIC, and placental abruption (Sibai, 1996b). Common laboratory findings in preeclampsia are listed in Table 30-3.

CARE MANAGEMENT

Assessment and Nursing Diagnoses

Hypertensive disorders of pregnancy can occur without warning or with the gradual development of symptoms. Because the cause is unknown and proven methods to prevent the illness are nonexistent, a key goal is early detection of the disease to prevent the catastrophic maternal and fetal sequelae that can occur. One strategy to meet this goal is the identification of high risk individuals at the initial prenatal visit (see Box 30-1). During each subsequent visit the woman is assessed for signs or symptoms that suggest the onset or presence of preeclampsia.

Obstetric conditions associated with increased placental mass, such as multifetal gestation and hydatidiform moles, and chronic medical disorders, such as hypertension, collagen vascular disease, and diabetes mellitus, lead to a greater risk of preeclampsia (Roberts et al., 1999).

Interview

The nurse reviews the woman's admission form and prenatal record. When the nurse and client are comfortable, the nurse begins with the interview to clarify, expand, or complete the form. Medical history is reviewed, especially the presence of diabetes mellitus, renal disease, and hypertension. Family history is explored for occurrence of preeclamptic or hypertensive conditions, diabetes mellitus, and other chronic conditions. The social and experiential history provides information about the woman's marital status, nutritional status, cultural beliefs, activity level, and health habits such as smoking and alcohol consumption.

A review of systems adds to the database for detecting blood pressure changes from baseline, abnormal weight gain and pattern of weight gain, increased signs of edema, and presence of proteinuria. Noting whether the woman is having unusual, frequent, or severe headaches; visual disturbances; or epigastric pain is also important.

Physical Examination

Accurate and consistent blood pressure assessment is important for establishing a baseline and monitoring subtle changes throughout pregnancy. Many variables can influence blood pressure measurements, such as position, cuff size, arm used, and emotional state of the client. Personnel caring for pregnant women must be consistent in taking and recording blood pressure measurements in the standardized manner (see p. 818). If electronic blood pressure devices are used, a manual reading should be taken to validate the electronic device reading. Electronic blood pressure devices show a widening of the pulse pressure as compared to manual readings; the MAP, however, remains unchanged (Marx et al., 1993). Also, it must be kept in mind that electronic blood pressure devices are less accurate in high-flow states such as pregnancy.

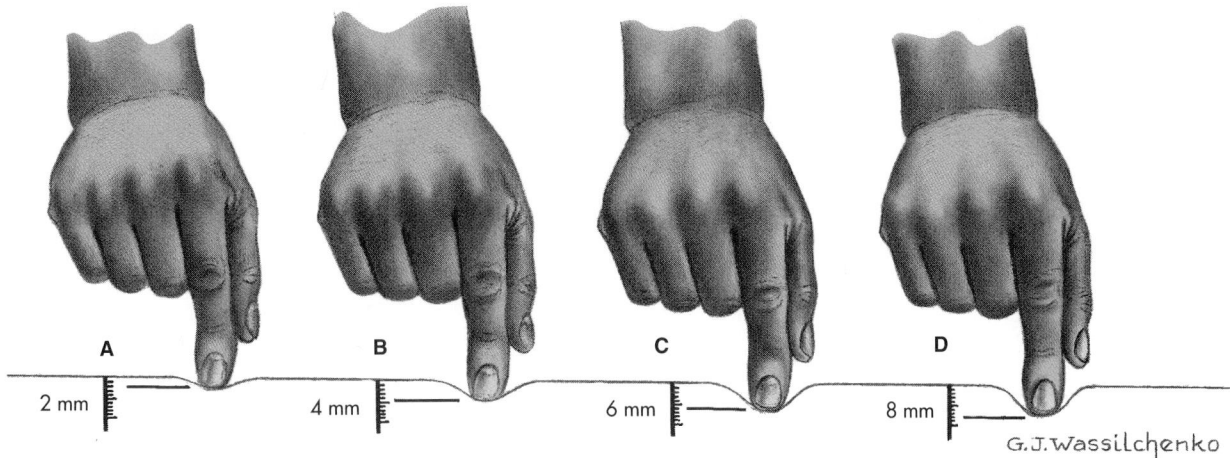

Fig. 30-3 Assessment of pitting edema of lower extremities. **A,** +1; **B,** +2; **C,** +3; **D,** +4.

Observation of edema in addition to hypertension warrants additional investigation. Edema is assessed for distribution, degree, and pitting. If periorbital or facial edema is not obvious, the pregnant woman is asked whether it was present when she awoke. Edema may be described as dependent or pitting.

Dependent edema is edema of the lowest or most dependent parts of the body, where hydrostatic pressure is greatest. If a pregnant woman is ambulatory, this edema may first be evident in the feet and ankles. If the pregnant woman is confined to bed, the edema is more likely to occur in the sacral region.

Pitting edema is edema that leaves a small depression or pit after finger pressure is applied to the swollen area. The pit, which is caused by movement of fluid to adjacent tissue away from the point of pressure, normally disappears within 10 to 30 seconds. Although the amount of edema is difficult to quantitate, the method described in Fig. 30-3 may be used to record relative degrees of edema formation.

Symptoms reflecting CNS and visual system involvement usually accompany facial edema. Although it is not a routine assessment during the prenatal period, evaluation of the fundus of the eye yields valuable data. An initial baseline finding of normal eye grounds assists in differentiating preexisting disease from a new disease process (Fig. 30-4). The woman may be unable to relate other symptoms such as epigastric pain or oliguria. Respirations are assessed for crackles, which may indicate pulmonary edema.

Deep tendon reflexes (DTRs) are evaluated if preeclampsia is suspected. The biceps and patellar reflexes and ankle clonus are assessed, and the findings recorded (Fig. 30-5, Table 30-4). The evaluation of DTRs is especially important if the woman is being treated with magnesium sulfate; absence of DTRs is an early indication of impending magnesium toxicity. To elicit the biceps reflex,

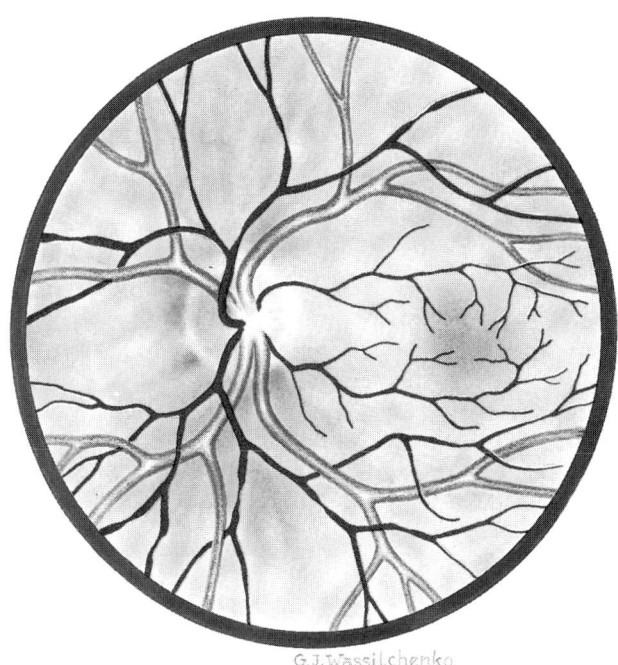

Fig. 30-4 Funduscopic evidence of severe pregnancy-induced hypertension: arteriospasm, edema, hemorrhages, arteriovenous nicking, and exudates.

the examiner strikes a downward blow over the thumb, which is situated over the biceps tendon. Normal response is flexion of the arm at the elbow, described as a 2+ response (see Table 30-4). The patellar reflex is elicited with the woman's legs hanging freely over the end of the examining table or with the woman lying on her left side with the knee slightly flexed. A blow with a percussion hammer is dealt directly to the patellar tendon, inferior to the patella. Normal response is the extension or kicking out of the leg. To assess for hyperactive reflexes (**clonus**) at

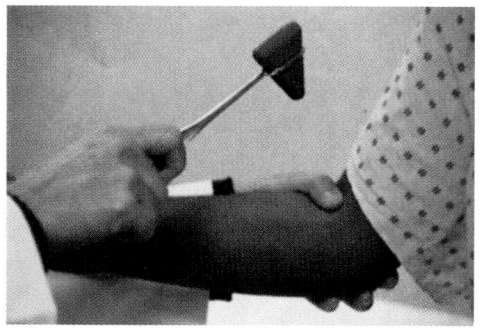 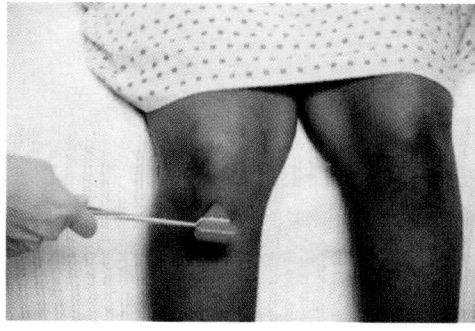 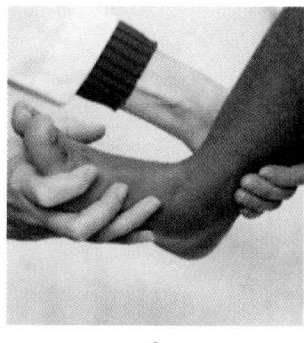

A   B   C

Fig. 30-5 **A,** Biceps reflex. **B,** Patellar reflex with client's legs hanging freely over end of examining table. **C,** Test for ankle clonus. *(From Seidel, H. et al. [1999]. Mosby's guide to physical examination [4th ed.]. St. Louis: Mosby.)*

█ TABLE 30-4 Assessing Deep Tendon Reflexes

GRADE	DEEP TENDON REFLEX RESPONSE
0	No response
1+	Sluggish or diminished
2+	Active or expected response
3+	More brisk than expected, slightly hyperactive
4+	Brisk, hyperactive, with intermittent or transient clonus

From Seidel, H. et al. (1999). *Mosby's guide to physical examination* (4th ed.). St. Louis: Mosby.

the ankle joint, the examiner supports the leg with the knee flexed. With one hand, the examiner sharply dorsiflexes the foot, maintains the position for a moment, and then releases the foot. Normal *(negative clonus)* response is elicited when no rhythmic oscillations (jerks) are felt while the foot is held in dorsiflexion. When the foot is released, no oscillations are seen as the foot drops to the plantarflexed position. Abnormal *(positive clonus)* response is recognized by rhythmic oscillations of one or more "beats" felt when the foot is in dorsiflexion and seen as the foot drops to the plantar-flexed position.

An important assessment is determination of fetal status. Uteroplacental perfusion is decreased in women with preeclampsia, placing the fetus in jeopardy. The fetal heart rate (FHR) is assessed for baseline rate and variability and accelerations, which indicate an intact, oxygenated fetal CNS. Abnormal baseline rate, decreased or absent variability, and late or variable decelerations are indications of fetal intolerance to the intrauterine environment. Biophysical or biochemical monitoring, such as nonstress testing, contraction stress testing, biophysical profile, and serial ultrasonography, is used to assess fetal status.

Doppler flow velocimetry studies are now being used to evaluate maternal and fetal well-being (see Chapter 29). Uteroplacental perfusion is assessed by measuring the ve-

locity of blood flow through the uterine artery, umbilical artery, or both. A systolic/diastolic ratio greater than 3 after 26 weeks of gestation is considered abnormal, and ratios of 3.8 have been associated with preeclampsia and IUGR (Farmakides et al., 1994).

Uterine tonicity is evaluated for signs of labor and abruptio placentae. If labor is suspected, a vaginal examination for cervical changes is indicated. Women with hypertension are at increased risk for an abruption.

NURSE ALERT *Uterine tenderness in the presence of increasing tone may be the earliest finding of an abruption. Idiopathic preterm contractions may also be an early sign.*

During the physical examination, the pregnant woman is examined for signs of progression of mild preeclampsia to severe preeclampsia or eclampsia. Signs of worsening liver involvement, renal failure, worsening hypertension, cerebral involvement, and developing coagulopathies must be assessed and documented. Respirations are assessed for crackles or diminished breath sounds, which may indicate pulmonary edema. Warning signs of preeclampsia and the differentiation of mild from severe preeclampsia are summarized in Table 30-2. Noninvasive assessment parameters include level of consciousness, blood pressure, hemoglobin oxygen saturation (pulse oximetry), electrocardiographic findings, and urine output. Invasive hemodynamic monitoring may be indicated in selected clients (American College of Obstetricians and Gynecologists, 1992). Eclampsia is usually preceded by various premonitory symptoms and signs, including headache, severe epigastric pain, hyperreflexia, and hemoconcentration. However, convulsions can appear suddenly and without warning in a woman in seemingly stable condition who has only minimum blood pressure elevation (Sibai, 1996b).

The convulsions that occur in eclampsia are frightening to observe. Increased hypertension and tonic contraction

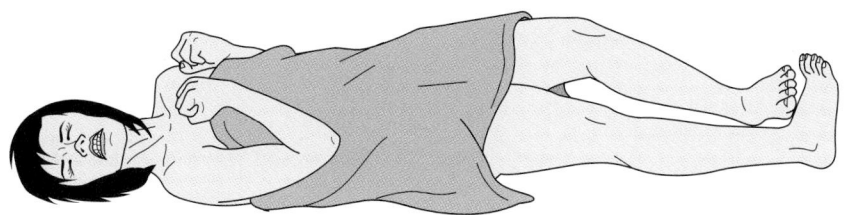

Fig. 30-6 Eclampsia (convulsions or seizures).

of all body muscles (seen as arms flexed, hands clenched, legs inverted) precede the tonic-clonic convulsions (Fig. 30-6). During this stage, muscles alternately relax and contract. Respirations are halted and then begin again with long, deep, stertorous inhalation. Hypotension follows, and coma ensues. Nystagmus and muscular twitching persist for a time. Disorientation and amnesia cloud the immediate recovery. Oliguria and anuria are notable. Seizures may recur within minutes of the first convulsion, or the woman may never have another. During the convulsion the mother and fetus are not receiving oxygen, so eclamptic seizures produce a marked metabolic insult to both mother and fetus.

Laboratory Tests

The nurse assists in obtaining a number of blood and urine specimens to aid in the diagnosis and treatment of preeclampsia, HELLP syndrome, and chronic hypertension. Baseline laboratory test information is useful in cases of early diagnosis of preeclampsia because it can be compared with later results to evaluate progression and severity of disease (see Table 30-3). An initial blood specimen is obtained for the following tests to assess the disease process and its effect on renal and hepatic functioning:

- Complete blood cell count (including a platelet count)
- Clotting studies (including bleeding time, prothrombin time, partial prothrombin time, and fibrinogen)
- Liver enzymes (lactate dehydrogenase [LDH], AST, ALT)
- Chemistry panel (BUN, creatinine, glucose, uric acid)
- Type and screen, possible crossmatch

The hematocrit, hemoglobin, and platelet levels are monitored closely for changes indicating a worsening of client status. Because hepatic involvement is a possible complication, serum glucose levels are monitored if liver function tests indicate elevated liver enzymes. Once the platelet count drops below 100,000/mm³, coagulation profiles are needed to identify developing DIC (Leduc et al., 1992).

Proteinuria is determined from dipstick testing of a clean-catch or catheterized urine specimen. A reading of 2+ on two or more occasions at least 6 hours apart should be followed by a 24-hour urine collection (Gilbert & Harmon, 1998). A 24-hour collection for protein and creatinine clearance is more reflective of true renal status.

Proteinuria is usually a late sign in the course of preeclampsia (Working Group on High Blood Pressure in Pregnancy, 1990). Protein readings are designated as follows:

0	Negative
Trace	Trace
+1	30 mg/dl (equivalent to 300 mg/L)
+2	100 mg/dl
+3	300 mg/dl
+4	>1000 mg (1 g)/dl

Urine output is assessed for volume of at least 30 ml/hr or 120 ml/4 hr.

Renal laboratory assessments include monitoring trends in serum creatine and BUN levels. As renal function becomes compromised, renal excretion of creatinine and other waste products, including magnesium sulfate, decreases. As renal excretion decreases, serum levels for creatinine, BUN, uric acid, and magnesium rise.

Nursing diagnoses for the woman with hypertensive disorders in pregnancy may include the following:

▪ Nursing Diagnoses

- Anxiety related to
  - preeclampsia and its effect on woman and infant
- Knowledge deficit related to
  - management (diet, medications, activity restrictions)
- Ineffective individual/family coping related to
  - woman's restricted activity and concern over a complicated pregnancy
  - woman's inability to work outside the home
  - transfer of the woman to a tertiary center for more intensive management
- Powerlessness related to
  - inability to prevent or control condition and outcomes
- Altered tissue perfusion related to
  - hypertension
  - cyclic vasospasms
  - cerebral edema
  - hemorrhage
- Risk for impaired gas exchange related to
  - magnesium sulfate therapy
  - pulmonary edema

Continued

▌ Nursing Diagnoses—cont'd _____

- Risk for alteration in cardiac output, decreased, related to
  - excessive hypertensive therapy
  - cardiac involvement of the disease process
- Risk for injury to fetus related to
  - uteroplacental insufficiency
  - preterm birth
  - abruptio placentae
- Risk for injury to mother related to
  - CNS irritability secondary to cerebral edema, vasospasm, decreased renal perfusion
  - magnesium sulfate and antihypertensive therapies
  - abruptio placentae

Expected Outcomes of Care

Planning of care follows medical diagnosis, choice of home or hospital management, and the woman's and family's resources. A plan is developed mutually with the woman if possible and should be individually tailored and related specifically to the needs of the client and her family. Expected outcomes for care of clients with hypertensive disorders of pregnancy include that the woman will do the following:

- Recognize and immediately report signs and symptoms indicative of worsening condition.
- Adhere to the medical regimen to minimize risk to herself and her fetus.
- Identify and use available support systems.
- Verbalize her fears and concerns to cope with the condition and situation.
- Develop no signs of eclampsia and its complications.
- Give birth to healthy infant.
- Develop no sequelae to her condition or its management.

Plan of Care and Interventions
Preeclampsia

Nursing actions are derived from medical management, health care provider directives, and nursing diagnoses. The most effective therapy is prevention. Early prenatal care, identification of pregnant women at risk for preeclampsia, and recognition and reporting of physical warning signs are essential components in the optimization of maternal and perinatal outcomes. The role of the nurse's skills in assessing the client for factors and symptoms of preeclampsia cannot be overestimated.

Nurses can do much in the advocacy role. Measurements should be taken to improve public education and access to antepartal care. Counseling, referral to community resources, mobilization of support systems, nutrition counseling, and information about normal adaptation to pregnancy are essential preventive components of care. The nurse's role as educator is important in informing the woman about her condition and responsibilities in preeclampsia management, whether in the home or hospital.

The goals of therapy are (1) to ensure maternal safety and (2) to deliver a healthy newborn, as close to term as possible, who will not require prolonged intensive care (Sibai, 1996b). At or near term, the plan of care for a woman with preeclampsia is most likely to be induction of labor, preceded, if necessary, by cervical ripening.

When preeclampsia is diagnosed in a woman who is at less than 37 weeks of gestation, however, immediate delivery may not be in the best interest of the fetus. In this situation, the initial intervention is usually a thorough evaluation of both the maternal and fetal condition. Women may be hospitalized during this initial evaluation, or the evaluation may be done in a high risk clinic or the physician's office. A multidisciplinary plan of care is then developed, based on the assessment findings. Whenever possible, the plan should take into account the wishes of the woman and her family.

Emotional and psychologic support are essential in assisting the woman and her family to cope. Their perception of the disease process, the reasons for it, and the care received will affect their compliance with and participation in therapy. The family will need to use coping mechanisms and support systems to help them through this crisis. A plan of care specifically designed for the woman with preeclampsia is superimposed on the nursing care all women need during labor and the birth process.

Mild preeclampsia and home care. If the woman has mild preeclampsia (blood pressure is stable, urine protein is less than 500 mg in a 24-hour collection, and no subjective complaints), she may be managed expectantly, usually at home. The maternal-fetal condition should be assessed two to three times per week. Many agencies are available to provide this assessment in the home. Arrangements for this service may be made, depending on the woman's insurance coverage. If home nursing care is not possible, the woman may be asked to perform self-assessment daily, including weight, urine dipstick protein determinations, blood pressure measurement, and fetal movement counting (Lowdermilk & Grohar, 1999). In addition, she will be asked to immediately report the development of any subjective symptoms (see Home Care box). In this case, she will probably return to the physician's office or high risk clinic at least twice each week for continued fetal assessment.

The fetal condition is also closely monitored because the only reason for expectant management of preeclampsia is to allow additional time for fetal growth and maturation. An ultrasound for evaluation of fetal growth should be obtained every 3 weeks. Fetal movement is counted daily. Other fetal assessment tests include a nonstress test once or twice a week and a biophysical profile as needed. Fetal jeopardy as evidenced by inappropriate growth or abnormal testing necessitates immediate delivery (Sibai, 1996b).

Activity restriction. Bed rest in the lateral recumbent position is a traditional therapy for preeclampsia that may improve uteroplacental blood flow during pregnancy. However, bed rest recommendations for all high risk pregnant women are becoming more controversial. Maloni

HOME CARE

Assessing and Reporting Clinical Signs of Preeclampsia

Report immediately any increase in your blood pressure, protein in urine, weight gain greater than I lb/wk, or edema.

Take your blood pressure on the same arm in a sitting position each time for consistent and accurate readings. Support arm on a table in a horizontal position at heart level.

Use the same scale, wearing the same clothes, at the same time each day, after voiding, before breakfast, for reliable daily weights.

Dipstick test your clean-catch urine sample to assess proteinuria; report frequency or burning on urination.

Report to your health care provider if proteinuria is +2 or more or if you have a decrease in urine output.

Assess your baby's activity daily. Decreased activity (three or fewer movements per hour) may indicate fetal compromise.

It is important to keep your scheduled prenatal appointments so that any changes in your or your baby's condition can be detected immediately.

Keep a daily log or diary of your assessments for your home health care nurse, or bring it with you to your next prenatal visit.

 HOME CARE

Coping with Bed Rest

In bed, lie on your side. This allows more blood to get to your uterus (womb) and baby. The bed or sofa should be near a window and a bathroom.

Increase your fluid intake to 8 glasses/day and add roughage (bran, fruits, leafy vegetables) to your diet to decrease constipation. Keep a bowl of fruit and a large container full of water close by.

Include diversionary activities, such as puzzles, reading, and crafts, to reduce boredom. Place a box or table within reach to store magazines, books, telephone, etc.

Do gentle exercises, such as circling your hands and feet or gently tensing and relaxing arm and leg muscles. This improves muscle tone, circulation, and sense of well-being.

Encourage family participation in your care.

Have significant others assist you with care of the house, children, etc.

Use relaxation to help cope with stress. Relax your body one muscle at a time, or imagine some pleasant scene, word, or image. Soothing music can also help you relax.

HOME CARE

Nutrition

Eat a nutritious, balanced diet (60 to 70 g protein; 1200 mg calcium; and adequate zinc, magnesium, and vitamins). Consult with registered dietitian on the diet best suited for you as an individual.

There is no sodium restriction; however, consider limiting excessively salty foods (luncheon meats, pretzels, potato chips, pickles, sauerkraut).

Eat foods with roughage (whole grains, raw fruits, and vegetables).

Drink six to eight 8-oz glasses of water per day.

Avoid alcohol and limit caffeine intake.

(1994) documented adverse physiologic outcomes related to complete bed rest, including cardiovascular deconditioning; diuresis with accompanying fluid, electrolyte, and weight loss; muscle atrophy; and psychologic stress. These changes begin on the first day of bed rest and continue for the duration of therapy. Sibai (1996b) recommends rest at home, rather than strict bed rest, and allows women hospitalized with mild preeclampsia to be out of bed.

Bed rest has been shown to be beneficial in decreasing blood pressure and promoting diuresis. Women with mild preeclampsia feel reasonably well; boredom from the restriction is therefore common. Diversionary activities, visits from friends, telephone conversations, and creation of a comfortable and convenient environment are just a few ways of coping with this boredom (see Home Care box). Gentle exercise (e.g., range of motion, stretching, Kegel, pelvic tilts) is important in maintaining muscle tone, blood flow, regularity of bowel function, and a sense of well-being (Grohar, 1994; Maloni, 1998).

Relaxation techniques can help reduce the stress associated with the high risk condition and prepare the woman for labor and birth.

Diet. Diet and fluid recommendations are much the same as for healthy pregnant women. The efficacy of a high-protein diet, avoidance of foods high in sodium, and forgoing additional salt at the table have not been proven.

Sibai (1996a) recommends a regular diet with no salt restriction. Because pregnant women with hypertension have a lower plasma volume than do normotensive women, sodium restriction is not necessary. Women need salt for maintenance of blood volume and placental perfusion. The exception may be the woman with chronic hypertension that was successfully controlled with a low-salt diet before the pregnancy. Adequate fluid intake helps maintain optimum fluid volume and aids in renal perfusion and filtration. The nurse uses assessment data regarding the woman's diet to counsel her as needed in areas of deficiency (see Home Care box).

Successful home care requires the woman to be well educated about preeclampsia and motivated to follow the plan of care. She must also be reliable about keeping appointments. For home care to be effective, the home environment must be assessed and the woman's ability to assume responsibility determined. In addition, the effects of illness, language, age, culture, beliefs, and support systems must be considered. The woman's support systems must be mobilized and involved in planning and implementing her care. During the period of instruction for the woman and her family, time must be allowed for assimilation of information, questions, and concerns. A client's understanding is usually directly associated with compliance with the prescribed treatment program. Methods for enhancing learning include visual aids, videotapes, handouts, and demonstrations with return demonstrations (see Plan of Care).

PLAN OF CARE | Mild Preeclampsia: Home Care

NURSING DIAGNOSIS Risk for injury related to signs of preeclampsia

Expected Outcomes *Client will demonstrate ability to assess self and fetus for signs of worsening preeclampsia; no adverse sequelae will occur as result of preeclamptic condition.*

Nursing Interventions/Rationales

Review warning signs/symptoms of preeclampsia *to ensure adequate knowledge base exists for decision making.*

Assess home environment, including woman's ability to assume self-care responsibilities, support systems, language, age, culture, beliefs, and effects of illness, *to determine if home care is viable option.*

Teach woman how to do a self-assessment for clinical signs of preeclampsia (take and record blood pressure, measure urine protein, maintain daily weight log, assess edema formation, assess fetal activity) *to provide immediate evidence of a worsening condition.*

Teach woman to report any increases in blood pressure, +2 proteinuria, weight gain greater than 1 lb per week, presence of edema, and decreased fetal activity to her health care provider immediately *to prevent worsening of preeclamptic condition.*

Teach woman about use of rest and relaxation as palliative treatment options *to decrease blood pressure and promote diuresis.*

NURSING DIAGNOSIS Fear/anxiety related to preeclampsia and its effect on the fetus

Expected Outcomes *Client's feelings and symptoms of fear/anxiety will decrease/ease.*

Nursing Interventions/Rationales

Provide a calm, soothing atmosphere and teach family to provide emotional support *to facilitate coping.*

Encourage verbalization of fears *to decrease intensity of emotional response.*

Involve woman and family in the management of her preeclamptic condition *to promote a greater sense of control.*

Help woman identify and use appropriate coping strategies and support systems *to reduce fear/anxiety.*

Explore use of desensitization strategies such as progressive muscle relaxation, visual imagery, or thought stopping *to reduce fear-related emotions and related physical symptoms.*

NURSING DIAGNOSIS Diversional activity deficit related to imposed bed rest

Expected Outcomes *Client will verbalize diminished feelings of boredom.*

Nursing Interventions/Rationales

Assist woman to creatively explore personally meaningful activities that can be pursued from the bed *to ensure activities that have meaning, purpose, and value to the individual.*

Maintain emphasis on personal choices of woman *to promote control and minimize imposition of routines by others.*

Evaluate what support and system resources are available in the environment *to assist in providing diversional activities.*

Explore ways for woman to remain an active participant in home management and decision making *to promote control.*

Engage support of family and friends in carrying out chosen activities and making necessary environmental alterations *to ensure success.*

Teach woman about stress management and relaxation techniques *to help manage tension of confinement.*

From Wong, D., & Perry, S. (1998). *Maternal child nursing care.* St. Louis: Mosby.

Severe Preeclampsia and HELLP Syndrome

If the woman's condition worsens or she already has severe preeclampsia or HELLP syndrome and is critically ill, she should receive appropriate management (usually in a tertiary care center), ranging from immediate birth to conservative management of the pregnancy (Leicht & Harvey, 1999; Sibai, 1991). Recognition of the clinical and laboratory findings of severe preeclampsia or HELLP syndrome is important if early, aggressive therapy is to be initiated to prevent maternal and perinatal mortality. An unfavorable (uneffaced and undilated) cervix, resulting from the gestational age and the aggressive nature of this disorder, support cesarean birth. Prolonged induction of labor could increase maternal morbidity.

Important components of management include the administration of magnesium sulfate as prophylaxis against seizures and an antihypertensive agent if diastolic blood pressure is higher than 100 to 110 mm Hg.

Hospital care. The woman with severe preeclampsia or HELLP syndrome has multiple problems and provides a complex challenge for the health care team. Nursing care must focus on both mother and fetus.

Antepartum care focuses on stabilization and preparation for birth. The woman may be admitted to an antepartum or a labor and birth unit, depending on the hospital. If the woman's condition is severe, she may be placed in an intensive care unit for any necessary hemodynamic monitoring. Maternal and fetal surveillance, client education regarding the disease process, and supportive measures directed toward the woman and her family are initiated. Assessments include review of the cardiovascular system, pulmonary system, renal system, hematologic system, and CNS. Fetal assessments for well-being (e.g., nonstress test, biophysical profile, Doppler velocimetry) are important because of the potential for hypoxia related to uteroplacental insufficiency. Baseline laboratory assessments include metabolic studies for liver enzyme (AST, ALT, LDH) determination, complete blood count with platelets, coagulation profile to assess for DIC, and electrolyte studies to establish renal functioning.

Weight is measured on admission and every day thereafter. An indwelling urinary catheter facilitates monitoring of renal function and effectiveness of therapy. If appropriate, vaginal examination may be done to check for cervical changes. Abdominal palpation establishes uterine tonicity and fetal size, activity, and position. Electronic monitoring to determine fetal status is initiated at least once a day. The nurse's skill in implementing the techniques described here can be reassuring to the woman and her family. The woman's room must be close to staff and emergency drugs, supplies, and equipment. Noise and external stimuli must be minimized. Seizure precautions are taken (Box 30-4).

Bed rest is commonly ordered. The nurse's ingenuity may be called on to help the woman cope physically and psychologically with the side effects of immobility and an environment limited in stimuli and support. Thrombo-

embolic events, a risk factor during normal pregnancy, pose an even greater risk with preeclampsia (see Plan of Care, p. 830).

Intrapartum nursing care of the woman with severe preeclampsia or HELLP syndrome involves continuous monitoring of maternal and fetal status as labor progresses. The assessment and prevention of tissue hypoxemia and hemorrhage, both of which can lead to permanent compromise of vital organs, continue throughout the intrapartum and postpartum periods (Leicht & Harvey, 1999).

Magnesium sulfate. One of the important goals of care for the woman with severe preeclampsia is prevention or control of convulsions. Magnesium sulfate (MgSO$_4$) is the drug of choice in the prevention and treatment of convulsions caused by preeclampsia or eclampsia (American College of Obstetricians and Gynecologists, 1996). Benefits of magnesium sulfate therapy include an increase in uterine blood flow to protect the fetus and an increase in prostacyclins to prevent uterine vasoconstriction (Gilbert & Harmon, 1998).

Magnesium sulfate is administered as a secondary infusion to the main IV line by volumetric infusion pump. An initial loading dose of 4 to 6 g magnesium sulfate per protocol or physician's order is infused over 15 to 30 minutes. This dose is followed by a maintenance dose of magnesium sulfate that is diluted in an IV solution per physician's order (e.g., 40 g magnesium sulfate in 1000 ml lactated Ringer's solution) and administered by infusion pump at 1 to 3 g/hr (Gilbert & Harmon, 1998; Mandeville & Troiano, 1999). This dose should maintain a therapeutic serum magnesium level of 4 to 8 mg/dl. Serum magnesium levels are obtained after the client has received magnesium sulfate for 4 to 6 hours. The infusion rate is adjusted to maintain the therapeutic level (Sisson & Sauer, 1996) (Box 30-5).

After the loading dose, there may be a transient lowering of the arterial blood pressure as a result of relaxation of smooth muscle.

■ BOX 30-4 Hospital Precautionary Measures

Environment
- Quiet
- Nonstimulating
- Lighting subdued

Seizure precautions
- Suction equipment tested and ready to use
- Oxygen administration equipment tested and ready to use

Call button within easy reach

Emergency medication tray immediately accessible
- Hydralazine or other antihypertensive medication and magnesium sulfate in or adjacent to woman's room
- Calcium gluconate immediately available

Emergency birth pack accessible

PLAN ᵒᶠ CARE   Severe Preeclampsia: Hospital Care

NURSING DIAGNOSIS Risk for injury to mother and fetus related to **CNS irritability**

Expected Outcomes *Client will show diminished signs of CNS irritability (e.g., DTRs 2+, absence of clonus) and have no convulsions.*

Nursing Interventions/*Rationales*

Establish baseline data (e.g., DTRs, clonus) *to use as basis for evaluating effectiveness of treatment.*

Administer IV MgSO₄ per physician's orders *to decrease hyperreflexia and minimize risk of convulsions.*

Monitor maternal vital signs, FHR, urine output, DTRs, IV flow rate, and serum levels of MgSO₄ *to assess for and prevent MgSO₄ toxicity (e.g., depressed respirations, oliguria, sudden drop in blood pressure, hyporeflexia, fetal distress).*

Have calcium gluconate at bedside if needed *as antidote for MgSO₄ toxicity.*

Maintain a quiet, darkened environment *to avoid stimuli that may precipitate seizure activity.*

NURSING DIAGNOSIS Altered tissue perfusion related to preeclampsia secondary to arteriolar vasospasm

Expected Outcomes *Client will exhibit signs of increased vasodilation (diuresis, decreased edema, weight loss).*

Nursing Interventions/*Rationales*

Establish baseline data (weight, degree of edema) *to use as basis for evaluating effectiveness of treatment.*

Administer intravenous magnesium sulfate per physician order, *which serves to relax vasospasms and increase renal perfusion.*

Place woman on bed rest in a side-lying position *to maximize uteroplacental blood flow, reduce blood pressure, and promote diuresis.*

Monitor intake and output, edema, and weight *to assess for evidence of vasodilation and increased tissue perfusion.*

NURSING DIAGNOSIS Risk for
- **Fluid volume excess related to increased sodium retention secondary to administration of MgSO₄**
- **Impaired gas exchange related to pulmonary edema secondary to increased vascular resistance**
- **Decreased cardiac output related to use of anti-hypertensive drugs**
- **Injury to fetus related to uteroplacental insufficiency secondary to use of antihypertensive medications**

Expected Outcomes *Client will exhibit signs of normal fluid volume (balanced intake and output, normal serum creatinine levels, normal breath sounds); adequate oxygenation (normal respirations; fully oriented to person, time, and place); normal range of cardiac output (normal pulse rate and rhythm); and fetal well-being (adequate fetal movement, normal FHR).*

Nursing Interventions/*Rationales*

Monitor woman for signs of fluid volume excess (increased edema, decreased urine output, elevated serum creatinine level, weight gain, dyspnea, crackles) *to prevent complications.*

Monitor woman for signs of impaired gas exchange (increased respirations, dyspnea, altered blood gases, hypoxemia) *to prevent complications.*

Monitor woman for signs of decreased cardiac output (altered pulse rate and rhythm) *to prevent complications.*

Monitor fetus for signs of difficulty (decreased fetal activity, decreased FHR) *to prevent complications.*

Record findings and report signs of increasing problems to physician *to enable timely interventions.*

From Wong, D., & Perry, S. (1998). *Maternal child nursing care.* St. Louis: Mosby.

NURSE ALERT *The woman's blood pressure, pulse, and respiratory status should be monitored closely while the loading dose is being administered IV and every 15 to 30 minutes at other times, depending on the stability of the woman's condition. Administration of magnesium sulfate is continued for at least the first 12 to 24 hours postpartum to prevent the occurrence of seizures.*

Intramuscular (IM) magnesium sulfate is rarely used because the absorption rate cannot be controlled, injections are painful, and tissue necrosis may occur. The IM route may be used with some women who are being transported to a tertiary care center. The IM dose is 4 to 5 g given in each buttock, a total of 10 g (with 1% procaine possibly being added to the solution to reduce injection pain), and

BOX 30-5 Protocol for Care of Client with Preeclampsia Receiving Magnesium Sulfate

MAGNESIUM SULFATE ADMINISTRATION
Client and Family Teaching
Explain technique, rationale, and reactions to expect
- Route and rate
- Purpose of "piggyback"

Reasons for use
- Tailor information to client's readiness to learn
- Explain that it is to prevent disease progression
- Explain that it is to prevent seizures

Reactions to expect from medication
- Initially client will feel flushed, hot, sedated, especially during the bolus
- Sedation will continue

Monitoring to anticipate
- Maternal: blood pressure, pulse, DTRs, level of consciousness, urine output (indwelling catheter likely), presence of headache, visual disturbances, epigastric pain
- Fetal: FHR and activity

Administration
- Verify physician order
- Position woman in side-lying position
- Prepare solution and administer with an infusion control device (pump)
- Piggyback a solution of 40 g magnesium sulfate in 1000 ml of lactated Ringer's solution with an infusion control device at the ordered rates: loading dose—initial bolus of 4-6 g over 15 to 30 min; maintenance dose—1-3 g/hr

Maternal and Fetal Assessments
- Monitor blood pressure, pulse, respiratory rate, FHR, and contractions every 15-30 min, depending on client condition

- Monitor intake and output, proteinuria, DTRs, presence of headache, visual disturbances, and epigastric pain at least hourly
- Restrict hourly fluid intake to a total of 100 to 125 ml/hr; urinary output should be at least 30 ml/hr

Reportable Conditions
- Blood pressure: systolic 160 mm Hg, diastolic 110 mm Hg, or both
- Respiratory rate: 12 breaths/min
- Urinary output <30 ml/hr
- Presence of headache, visual disturbances, or epigastric pain
- Increasing severity or loss of DTRs, increasing edema, proteinuria
- Any abnormal laboratory values (magnesium levels, platelet count, creatinine clearance, levels of uric acid, AST, ALT, prothrombin time, partial thromboplastin time, fibrinogen, fibrin split products)
- Any other significant change in maternal or fetal status

Emergency Measures
- Keep emergency drug tray at bedside with calcium gluconate and intubation equipment
- Keep side rails up
- Keep lights dimmed and maintain a quiet environment

Documentation
- All of the above

---

can be repeated at 4-hour intervals. Z-track technique should be used for the deep IM injection, followed by gentle massage at the site.

Magnesium sulfate interferes with the release of acetylcholine at the synapses, decreasing neuromuscular irritability, depressing cardiac conduction, and decreasing CNS irritability (Dildy et al., 1991). Because magnesium circulates free and unbound to protein and is excreted in the urine, accurate recordings of maternal urine output must be obtained.

Diuresis within 24 to 48 hours is an excellent prognostic sign. It is considered evidence that perfusion of the kidney has improved as a result of relaxation of arteriolar spasm. With improved perfusion, fluid moves from interstitial spaces to the intravascular bed and edema is re-

duced. Diuresis results in weight loss. Although diuresis generally indicates improvement, diuresis in the presence of worsening clinical status may indicate impending renal failure. As renal function declines and serum creatinine levels rise, renal filtration is compromised. The woman can excrete large volumes of urine (>200 ml/hr) but will not excrete magnesium sulfate.

Because magnesium sulfate is a CNS depressant, the nurse assesses for signs and symptoms of magnesium toxicity (see Box 30-5). Serum magnesium levels are obtained on the basis of the woman's response and if any signs of toxicity are present. Early symptoms of toxicity include nausea, a feeling of warmth, flushing, muscle weakness, decreased reflexes, and slurred speech.

NURSE ALERT *Loss of patellar reflexes, respiratory depression, oliguria, and decreased level of consciousness are signs of magnesium toxicity. Actions are needed to prevent respiratory or cardiac arrest. If magnesium toxicity is suspected, the infusion should be discontinued immediately. Calcium gluconate, the antidote for magnesium sulfate, may also be ordered (10 ml of a 10% solution, or 1 g) and given by slow IV push (usually by the physician) over at least 3 minutes (Sibai, 1996b) to avoid undesirable reactions such as dysrhythmias, bradycardia, and ventricular fibrillation.*

Because magnesium sulfate is also a tocolytic agent, its use may increase the duration of labor.

NURSE ALERT *A preeclamptic woman receiving magnesium sulfate may need augmentation with oxytocin during labor. The amount of oxytocin needed to stimulate labor may be more than that needed for a woman who is not on magnesium sulfate.*

Magnesium sulfate is not thought to affect FHR variability in a healthy term fetus and is rarely toxic in the healthy term neonate whose weight is within normal range for gestational age. Toxic levels in the fetus can, however, cause marked slowing of respirations and hyporeflexia after birth (Sibai, 1988). Neonatal hypermagnesemia can be treated with calcium and exchange transfusion with citrated blood, or the neonate may require assisted mechanical ventilation until serum levels have normalized.

If eclampsia develops after the initiation of magnesium sulfate therapy, the treatment of choice is to administer an additional 2 g of magnesium sulfate IV push over 3 to 5 minutes (Leicht & Harvey, 1999) (see Emergency box). Occasionally, it is necessary to repeat the dose because the woman will experience additional seizures. Rarely, the woman will continue to experience seizures despite adequate blood magnesium levels. In that case, 250 mg of sodium amobarbital may be administered by slow IV push over 3 to 5 minutes (Sibai, 1996b). Diazepam is sometimes used to treat eclamptic seizures. However, this drug can cause phlebitis and venous thrombosis. If administered too rapidly, it can also lead to apnea or cardiac arrest (Sibai, 1996b).

Both sodium amobarbital and diazepam have fetal and neonatal effects as well. FHR demonstrates a loss of variability, a reflection of fetal oxygenation. High levels of these drugs in the neonate depress sucking ability, cause hypotonia, and may result in temperature instability. The neonate's respiratory rate may be decreased. Careful surveillance of both maternal and fetal or neonatal status is warranted.

Control of blood pressure. For the severely hypertensive preeclamptic woman, antihypertensive medications are usually ordered to lower the blood pressure (systolic BP 160 to 180 mm Hg; diastolic BP 100 to 110 mm Hg). Initiation of antihypertensive therapy reduces maternal morbidity and mortality associated with left ventricular

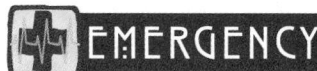

EMERGENCY

Eclampsia

TONIC-CLONIC CONVULSION SIGNS

Stage of invasion: 2-3 sec, eyes are fixed, twitching of facial muscles occurs

Stage of contraction: 15-20 sec, eyes protrude and are bloodshot, all body muscles are in tonic contraction

Stage of convulsion: muscles relax and contract alternately (clonic), respirations are halted and then begin again with long, deep, stertorous inhalation, coma ensues

INTERVENTION

Keep airway patent: turn head to one side, place pillow under one shoulder or back if possible

Call for assistance

Protect with side rails up

Observe and record convulsion activity

AFTER CONVULSION OR SEIZURE

Do not leave unattended until fully alert

Observe for postconvulsion coma, incontinence

Use suction as needed

Administer oxygen via face mask at 10 L/min

Start IV fluids and monitor for potential fluid overload

Give magnesium sulfate or anticonvulsant drug as ordered

Insert indwelling urinary catheter

Monitor blood pressure

Monitor fetal and uterine status

Expedite laboratory work as ordered to monitor kidney function, liver function, coagulation system, and drug levels

Provide hygiene and a quiet environment

Support and keep woman and family informed

Be prepared for delivery when woman is in stable condition

failure and cerebral hemorrhage. Because a degree of maternal hypertension is necessary to maintain uteroplacental perfusion, antihypertensive therapy must not decrease the arterial pressure too much or too rapidly. The target range for the diastolic pressure is therefore 90 to 100 mm Hg (Leicht & Harvey, 1999).

Intravenous hydralazine remains the antihypertensive agent of choice for the treatment of hypertension in severe preeclampsia. Intravenous labetalol hydrochloride and oral methyldopa and nifedipine are also used (Cunningham et al., 1997; Sibai, 1996b; Sisson & Sauer, 1996). The choice of agent used depends on client response and physician preference. Table 30-5 compares antihypertensive agents used to treat hypertension in pregnancy.

TABLE 30-5 Pharmacologic Control of Hypertension in Pregnancy

ACTION	TARGET TISSUE	EFFECTS		NURSING ACTIONS
		MATERNAL	FETAL	
HYDRALAZINE (APRESOLINE, NEOPRESOL)				
Arteriolar vasodilator	Peripheral arterioles: to decrease muscle tone, decrease peripheral resistance; hypothalamus and medullary vasomotor center for minor decrease in sympathetic tone	Headache, flushing, palpitation, tachycardia, some decrease in uteroplacental blood flow, increase in heart rate and cardiac output, increase in oxygen consumption, nausea and vomiting	Tachycardia; late decelerations and bradycardia if maternal diastolic pressure <90 mm Hg	Assess for effects of medications, alert mother (family) to expected effects of medications, assess blood pressure frequently because precipitous drop can lead to shock and perhaps abruptio placentae; assess urinary output; maintain bed rest in a lateral position with side rails up; use with caution in presence of maternal tachycardia
LABETALOL HYDROCHLORIDE (NORMODYNE)				
β-blocking agent causing vasodilation without significant change in cardiac output	Peripheral arterioles (see hydralazine)	Minimal: flushing, tremulousness; minimal change in pulse rate	Minimal, if any	See hydralazine; less likely to cause excessive hypotension and tachycardia; less rebound hypertension than hydralazine
METHYLDOPA (ALDOMET)				
Maintenance therapy if needed: 250-500 mg orally every 8 hr (α_2-receptor agonist)	Postganglionic nerve endings: interferes with chemical neurotransmission to reduce peripheral vascular resistance, causes CNS sedation	Sleepiness, postural hypotension, constipation; rare: drug-induced fever in 1% of women and positive Coombs' test result in 20%	After 4 mo maternal therapy, positive Coombs' test result in infant	See hydralazine
NIFEDIPINE (PROCARDIA)				
Calcium-channel blocker	Arterioles: to reduce systemic vascular resistance by relaxation of arterial smooth muscle	Headache, flushing; possible potentiation of effects on CNS if administered concurrently with magnesium sulfate, may interfere with labor	Minimal	See hydralazine; use caution if client also getting magnesium sulfate

NURSE ALERT *When administering antihypertensive therapy, the nurse must remember that the drug effects are dependent on intravascular volume. Because preeclampsia is associated with contracted intravascular volume, initial doses should be given with caution and maternal response monitored closely.*

Eclampsia

Immediate care. The immediate care during a convulsion is to ensure a patent airway (see Emergency box). When convulsions occur, the woman is turned onto her side to prevent aspiration of vomitus and supine hypotension syndrome. After the convulsion ceases, food and fluid are suctioned from the glottis or trachea, and oxygen is administered by face mask. Magnesium sulfate or other anticonvulsant is given as ordered (Sibai, 1996b). If an IV infusion is not in place, one is begun with a large-bore needle. Time, duration, and description of convulsions are recorded, and any urinary or fecal incontinence is noted. The fetus is monitored for adverse effects. Transient fetal bradycardia and decreased FHR variability are common.

Aspiration is a leading cause of maternal morbidity and mortality after eclamptic seizure. After initial stabilization and airway management, the nurse should anticipate orders for a chest radiograph and possibly arterial blood gases to rule out the possibility of aspiration.

A rapid assessment of uterine activity, cervical status, and fetal status is performed after a convulsion. During the convulsion, membranes may have ruptured; the cervix may have dilated, because the uterus becomes hypercontractile and hypertonic; and birth may be imminent. If not, once a woman's seizure activity and blood pressure are controlled, a decision should be made regarding whether birth should take place. The more serious the condition of the woman, the greater the need to proceed to birth. The route of birth—that is, induction of labor versus cesarean birth—depends on maternal and fetal condition. If fetal lungs are not mature and the birth can be delayed for 48 hours, steroids such as betamethasone may be given.

The woman may have been incontinent of urine and stool during the convulsion; she will need assistance with hygiene and a change of gown. Oral care with a soft toothbrush may be of comfort.

Immediately following a seizure, the woman may be very confused and can be combative, necessitating the temporary use of restraints. It may take several hours for the woman to regain her usual level of mental functioning. The health care provider explains procedures briefly and quietly. The woman is never left alone. The family is also kept informed of management, rationale for treatment, and the woman's progress.

Determination of central venous pressure or pulmonary arterial wedge pressure (Swan-Ganz catheter) may occasionally be required for accurate fluid monitoring in the presence of pulmonary edema or acute renal failure

(American College of Obstetricians and Gynecologists, 1996) (see Chapter 34). No oral intake is permitted if the woman is convulsing or has symptoms of severe preeclampsia. An indwelling catheter is required for accurate measurement of urinary output. For correction of hypovolemia, crystalloids (0.9% saline solution or lactated Ringer's solution) are infused IV at a rate that maintains a urine output of at least 30 ml/hr, and the maternal response is recorded.

Medications (e.g., magnesium sulfate) are given as directed. The woman's response is monitored and recorded, and all drugs, dosages, and times are noted. Laboratory tests are ordered to assess for HELLP syndrome and to have blood typed and crossmatched for administration of packed red blood cells as needed. Blood is kept available for emergency transfusion; abruptio placentae, with accompanying hemorrhage and shock, often occurs in women with eclampsia. Other tests include determination of electrolyte levels, liver function battery, and complete hemogram and clotting profile, including platelet count and fibrin split product levels (to assess for DIC).

Postpartum nursing care. After birth the symptoms of preeclampsia or eclampsia resolve quickly, usually within 48 hours; however, symptoms have been reported up to several weeks postpartum (see Research box). The hematopoietic and hepatic complications of HELLP syndrome may persist longer. These clients often show an abrupt decrease in platelet count, with a concomitant increase in LDH and AST levels, after a trend toward normalization of values has begun. Generally the laboratory abnormalities seen with HELLP syndrome resolve in 72 to 96 hours.

The nursing care of the woman with hypertensive disease differs from that required in the usual postpartum period in a number of respects. The following variations in the nursing process are described.

Careful assessment of the woman with a hypertensive disorder continues throughout the postpartum period. Blood pressure is measured at least every 4 hours for 48 hours or more frequently as the woman's condition warrants. Even if no convulsions occurred before the birth, they may occur within this period. Magnesium sulfate infusion is usually continued 12 to 24 hours after the birth. The same assessments continue until the medication is discontinued.

NURSE ALERT *The woman is at risk for a boggy uterus and a large lochia flow as a result of the magnesium sulfate therapy. Assessments of uterine tone and lochia flow must be monitored closely.*

The preeclamptic woman is hemoconcentrated and unable to tolerate excessive postpartum blood loss. Oxytocin or prostaglandin products are used to control bleeding. Ergot products (e.g., Ergotrate and Methergine) are contraindicated because they can increase blood pressure. The

in the care of the neonate are encouraged to the extent that the woman and her family desire. In addition, the woman and her family need opportunities to discuss their emotional response to complications. The nurse provides information concerning the prognosis. Preeclampsia and eclampsia do not necessarily recur in subsequent pregnancies (recurrence rate is approximately 30%), but careful prenatal care is essential.

Prevention. There have been numerous clinical trials describing various methods to prevent preeclampsia. The etiology continues to be unknown. Some of the strategies to prevent preeclampsia that have been or are being studied are described in the following paragraph. However, until a cause is discovered, prevention remains elusive.

Efforts to prevent or reduce the incidence of preeclampsia have used dietary supplementation and pharmacologic interventions. Large randomized clinical trials have not proven the use of low-dose aspirin to be a beneficial form of care (Caritis et al., 1998a). Mattar and Sibai (1999) reviewed more than 70 studies of interventions for the prevention of preeclampsia. These studies included the use of calcium, magnesium, zinc, and fish oil dietary supplementation. None of these interventions demonstrated a benefit in reducing the incidence or severity of preeclampsia in healthy pregnant women. Antihypertensive agents, diuretics, and low-salt diets have also been studied in numerous clinical trials with no beneficial results related to prevention reported (Sibai, 1998). Continued research in prevention is needed because no strategies have been proven to have beneficial effects. Most are of unknown effectiveness or are not likely to be beneficial. Nurses should be aware of what strategies are being studied and use the most reliable evidence about the results so that they can counsel pregnant women about interventions that are likely to be beneficial. One resource is the Cochrane Pregnancy and Childbirth Database (Enkin et al., 1995).

Evaluation

Evaluation of the effectiveness of care of the woman with preeclampsia is based on the expected outcomes.

woman is asked to report symptoms such as headaches and blurred vision. The nurse assesses affect, level of consciousness, blood pressure, pulse, and respiratory status before an analgesic is given for headache. Magnesium sulfate potentiates the action of narcotics, CNS depressants, and calcium-channel blockers; these drugs must be administered with caution. The woman may need to continue an antihypertensive medication regimen if her diastolic blood pressure exceeds 100 mm Hg at discharge.

The woman's and family's responses to labor, birth, and the neonate are monitored. Interactions and involvement

KEY POINTS

- Hypertensive disorders during pregnancy are a leading cause of infant and maternal morbidity and mortality worldwide.
- The cause of PIH is unknown, and there are no known reliable tests for predicting which women are at risk for preeclampsia.
- Preeclampsia is a multisystem disease rather than only an increase in blood pressure.

Continued

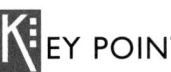

KEY POINTS—cont'd

- Failure of trophoblastic invasion of spiral arterioles is proposed as the triggering mechanism that eventually leads to vasospasm and organ ischemia; the cure is delivery of the fetus and placenta.

- The pathologic changes of preeclampsia, involving every organ system in the body, are present long before clinical manifestations are evident.

- Historical risk factors (e.g., first pregnancy or pregnancy of new genetic makeup, history of vascular disease, and multiple gestation) are associated with a higher incidence of preeclampsia.

- Progression of hypertensive disorders during pregnancy is unpredictable; mild hypertension must therefore be taken seriously and managed for preeclampsia.

- Once preeclampsia becomes clinically evident, therapeutic intervention is palliative (bed rest, diet); this may slow the progression of the disease and allow the pregnancy to continue.

- Home care management is an option only for women whose condition is stable and who are able to comply with the medical regimen, reliably perform self-monitoring, and immediately recognize and report abnormal signs and symptoms.

- HELLP syndrome can occur in women with severe preeclampsia and is considered life threatening.

- Magnesium sulfate, the anticonvulsive agent of choice for preventing eclampsia, requires careful monitoring of reflexes, respirations, and urinary output; its antidote, calcium gluconate, should be available at the bedside.

- The intent of emergency interventions for eclampsia is to prevent self-injury, ensure adequate oxygenation, reduce aspiration risk, establish seizure control with magnesium sulfate, and correct maternal acidemia.

CRITICAL THINKING EXERCISES

1 Angie T., a 16-year-old G2 P0 A1, comes into clinic for a routine prenatal visit at 32 weeks of gestation. You find that her blood pressure is 150/96, she has 1+ proteinuria on a urine dipstick, and she has gained 6 pounds since her last clinic visit 10 days ago.
   a. During your initial assessment, what other signs and symptoms of preeclampsia might you find?
   b. Develop a plan for Angie's care at home.
   c. What would you teach her about diet, rest, self-assessment, and fetal assessment?
   d. What danger signs should Angie be told to report immediately?

2 Angie talks daily on the phone with the clinic nurse and is seen twice-weekly at the clinic for evaluation. At her visit 2 weeks later, she reports a "blinding headache," "terrible heartburn," and blurred vision. Her blood pressure is 190/115. She is immediately admitted to the labor and delivery unit.
   a. What other assessment tests will most likely be performed on Angie and her fetus on admission to the hospital?
   b. Discuss MgSO₄ administration: dosage, route, aim of therapy, side effects, indications for discontinuing.
   c. What other medications might this client receive?

3 Marie has a diagnosis of severe preeclampsia. She is in labor in her labor-delivery-recovery-postpartum (LDRP) room with four family members present. The family members are conversing loudly while watching a ball game on television and taking bets. The woman states that she wishes that these people would leave and let her rest, but she is unwilling to confront them. Role play a nurse attempting to provide teaching to family members who resist changes in the labor plan. Ask the group to suggest different strategies.

4 Evaluate the interventions described in this chapter in terms of benefit to the client according to evidence documented in the Cochrane Pregnancy and Childbirth Database. Discuss in a clinical conference how nursing practice could be changed to be more effective.

References

American College of Obstetricians and Gynecologists. (1992). Invasive hemodynamic monitoring in obstetrics and gynecology. *ACOG Tech Bull* 175. Washington, DC: ACOG.

American College of Obstetricians and Gynecologists. (1996). Hypertension in pregnancy. *ACOG Tech Bull* 219. Washington, DC: ACOG.

Caritis, S. et al. (1998a). Low-dose aspirin to prevent preeclampsia in women at high risk. *N Engl J Med* 338(11), 7011-7015.

Caritis, S. et al. (1998b). Predictors of preeclampsia in women at high risk. *Am J Obstet Gynecol* 179(4), 946-951.

Cooper, D., Brennecke, S., & Wilton, A. (1993). Genetics of preeclampsia. *Hypertens Pregn* 12, 1-23.

Cunningham, F., & Lindheimer, M. (1992). Hypertension in pregnancy. *N Engl J Med* 326(14), 927-932.

Cunningham, F. et al. (1997). *Williams obstetrics* (20th ed.). Stamford, CT: Appleton & Lange.

Dekker, G., & Sibai, B. (1998). Etiology and pathogenesis of preeclampsia: Current concepts. *Am J Obstet Gynecol* 179(5), 1359-1375.

Dekker, G., & Sibai, B. (1999). The immunology of preeclampsia. *Semin Perinat* 23(1), 24-33.

Dildy, N. et al. (1991). Complications in pregnancy-induced hypertension. In S. Clark et al. (Eds.). *Critical care obstetrics* (2nd ed.). Boston: Blackwell Scientific.

Enkin, M. et al. (1995). Effective care in pregnancy and childbirth: A synopsis. *Birth* 22(2), 101-110.

Fairlie, F., & Sibai, B. (1999). Hypertensive diseases in pregnancy. In E. Reece et al. (Eds.). *Medicine of the fetus and mother* (2nd ed.). Philadelphia: J.B. Lippincott.

Farmakides, G. et al. (1994). Doppler velocimetry. Where does it belong in evaluation of fetal status? *Clin Perinatol* 21(4), 849-861.

Friedman, S. (1988). Preeclampsia: A review of the role of prostaglandins. *Obstet Gynecol* 71(1), 122-137.

Friedman, S. et al. (1995). Biochemical corroboration of endothelial involvement in severe preeclampsia. *Am J Obstet Gynecol* 172, 202-203.

Gilbert, E., & Harmon, J. (1998). *Manual of high risk pregnancy and delivery* (2nd ed.). St. Louis: Mosby.

Gilstrap, L., & Gant, N. (1990). Pathophysiology of preeclampsia. *Semin Perinatol* 14(2), 147-151.

Grohar, J. (1994). Nursing protocols for antepartum home care. *J Obstet Gynecol Neonatal Nurs* 23(8), 687-694.

Jones, D., & Hayslett, J. (1996). Outcome of pregnancy in women with moderate or severe renal insufficiency. *N Engl J Med* 335, 226-232.

Leduc, L. et al. (1992). Coagulation profile in severe preeclampsia. *Obstet Gynecol* 79(1), 14-18.

Leicht, T., & Harvey, C. (1999). Hypertensive disorders in pregnancy. In L. Mandeville & C. Harvey (Eds.). *AWHONN's high risk and critical care intrapartum nursing* (2nd ed.). Philadelphia: J.B. Lippincott.

Lowdermilk, D., & Grohar, J. (1999). *High risk antepartal home care.* White Plains, NY: March of Dimes.

Magness, R., & Gant, N. (1994). Control of vascular reactivity in pregnancy: The basis for therapeutic approaches to prevent pregnancy-induced hypertension. *Semin Perinatol* 18(2), 45-69.

Maloni, J. (1994). Home care of the high risk pregnant woman requiring bed rest. *J Obstet Gynecol Neonatal Nurs* 23(8), 696-706.

Maloni, J. (1998). *Antepartum bed rest: Case studies, research and nursing care.* Washington, DC: AWHONN.

Mandeville, L., & Troiano, N. (1999). *AWHONN's high risk and critical care intrapartum nursing* (2nd ed.). Philadelphia: J.B. Lippincott.

Marx, G. et al. (1993). Automated blood pressure measurements in laboring women: Are they reliable? *Am J Obstet Gynecol* 168, 796-798.

Mattar, F., & Sibai, B. (1999). Prevention of preeclampsia. *Semin Perinatol* 23(1), 58-64.

Poole, J. (1993). HELLP syndrome and coagulopathies of pregnancy. *Crit Care Nurs Clin North Am* 5(3), 457-487.

Poole, J. (1997). Aggressive management of HELLP syndrome and preeclampsia. *AACN Clin Issues* 8(4), 646-648.

Portis, R. et al. (1997). HELLP syndrome (hemolysis, elevated liver enzymes, and low platelets) pathophysiology and anesthetic considerations. *AANA J* 65(1), 37-47.

Roberts, J. (1999). Pregnancy-related hypertension. In R. Creasy & R. Resnik (Eds.). *Maternal-fetal medicine* (4th ed.). Philadelphia: W.B. Saunders.

Roberts, J., Taylor, R., & Goldfien, A. (1991). Endothelial cell activation as a pathogenic factor in preeclampsia. *Semin Perinatol* 15, 86-93.

Robillard, P. et al. (1993). Paternity patterns and risk of preeclampsia in the last pregnancy in multiparae. *J Reprod Immunol* 24, 1-12.

Scott, J. et al. (1999). *Danforth's obstetrics and gynecology* (8th ed.). Philadelphia: J.B. Lippincott.

Seidel, H. et al. (1999). *Mosby's guide to physical examination* (4th ed.). St. Louis: Mosby.

Sibai, B. (1988). Pitfalls in diagnosis and management of preeclampsia. *Am J Obstet Gynecol* 159(1), 1-5.

Sibai, B. (1991). Management of preeclampsia. *Clin Perinatol* 18(4), 793-808.

Sibai, B. (1996a). Drug therapy: Treatment of hypertension in pregnant women. *N Engl J Med* 335(4), 257-265.

Sibai, B. (1996b). Hypertension in pregnancy. In S. Gabbe, J. Niebyl, & J. Simpson (Eds.). *Obstetrics: Normal and problem pregnancies* (3rd ed.) New York: Churchill Livingstone.

Sibai, B. (1998). Prevention of preeclampsia: A big disappointment. *Am J Obstet Gynecol* 179(5), 1275-1278.

Sibai, B. et al. (1997). Risk factors associated with preeclampsia in healthy nulliparous women. *Am J Obstet Gynecol* 177(5), 1003-1010.

Sibai, B., & Rodrigues, J. (1999). Preeclampsia: Diagnosis and management. In E. Reece et al. (Eds.). *Medicine of the fetus and mother.* Philadelphia: J.B. Lippincott.

Sisson, M., & Sauer, P. (1996). Pharmacologic therapy for pregnancy-induced hypertension. *J Perinat Neonatal Nurs* 9(4), 1-12.

Stone, J. (1998). HELLP syndrome: Hemolysis, elevated liver enzymes, and low platelets. *JAMA* 280(6), 559-562.

Trupin, L., Simon, L., & Eskenazi, B. (1996). Change in paternity: A risk factor for preeclampsia in multiparas. *Epidemiology* 7, 240-244.

Ventura, S. et al. (1999). *Births: Final data for 1997. National Vital Statistics Reports,* vol 47, no 18. Hyattsville, MD: National Center for Health Statistics.

Wong, D., & Perry, S. (1998). *Maternal child nursing care.* St. Louis: Mosby.

Working Group on High Blood Pressure in Pregnancy. Consensus Report (1990). National high blood pressure education program working group report on high blood pressure in pregnancy. *Am J Obstet Gynecol* 163(5 pt 1), 1689-1712.

31

Antepartal Hemorrhagic Disorders

S. Kim Genovese

LEARNING OBJECTIVES

- Define the key terms.
- Compare and differentiate abruptio placentae and placenta previa.
- Discuss clotting disorders in pregnancy, with emphasis on disseminated intravascular coagulation.
- Discuss differences in plans of care for the woman with an unruptured ectopic pregnancy versus a ruptured ectopic pregnancy.
- Review the physiology of a hydatidiform mole and the risk factors for the woman's immediate health future.
- Summarize the role of the nurse in the health care team approach to the treatment of bleeding disorders.
- Identify topics for nursing research related to antepartal maternal hemorrhagic disorders.

KEY TERMS

abruptio placentae
cerclage
cervical funneling
Couvelaire uterus
Cullen sign
disseminated intravascular coagulation

ectopic pregnancy
hydatidiform mole (molar pregnancy)
incompetent cervix (premature dilation of the cervix)
miscarriage
placenta previa

spontaneous abortion
succenturiate placenta
velamentous insertion of the cord

aternal adaptations in the hematologic and cardiovascular systems during pregnancy result in a hypervolemic state, with concomitant decreases in systemic and pulmonary vascular resistance. Increases in plasma volume and red blood cell mass occur as early as 4 to 8 weeks of gestation and serve (1) to meet the metabolic demands of the mother and fetus, (2) to protect against the potentially deleterious impairment in venous return caused by the pressure of an enlarging uterus, and (3) to safeguard the mother against the effects of blood loss at birth (Knuppel & Hatangadi, 1995). Any bleeding in pregnancy may therefore jeopardize both maternal and fetal well-being.

Maternal blood loss decreases oxygen-carrying capacity, which predisposes the woman to increased risk for hypovolemia, anemia, infection, preterm labor, and preterm birth and adversely affects oxygen delivery to the fetus. Fetal risks from maternal hemorrhage include blood loss or anemia, hypoxemia, hypoxia, anoxia, and preterm birth. If the bleeding involves fetal blood loss, the effects are exponential because of the smaller fetal blood volume.

Hemorrhagic disorders in pregnancy are medical emergencies. It is estimated that one in every five pregnancies is complicated by bleeding; the incidence and type of bleeding vary by trimester (Thorp, 1993). In the first trimester most bleeding is a result of miscarriage and ectopic pregnancy. Approximately 50% of bleeding in the third trimester is caused by placenta previa and abruptio placentae (Cunningham et al., 1997). Antepartal hemorrhage is a leading cause of maternal death, with ectopic pregnancy rupture and abruptio placentae being responsible for most maternal deaths (Koonin et al., 1997). Prompt assessment and intervention by the health care team is essential to save the life of the mother and fetus.

EARLY PREGNANCY BLEEDING

Bleeding during early pregnancy is alarming to the woman and of concern to health care providers. The common bleeding disorders of early pregnancy include spontaneous abortion/miscarriage, incompetent cervix, ectopic pregnancy, and hydatidiform mole (molar pregnancy).

Spontaneous Abortion (Miscarriage)

A pregnancy that ends before 20 weeks of gestation is defined as an abortion. This 20-week marker is considered to be the

point of viability, when a fetus may survive in an extrauterine environment. A fetal weight less than 500 g may also be used to define an abortion (Cunningham et al., 1997).

A **spontaneous abortion**, commonly called a miscarriage, results from natural causes. **Miscarriage** is suggested as a more appropriate term to use with clients because abortion may be an insensitive term to use with families who are grieving a pregnancy loss (Freda, 1999). The term *miscarriage* is used throughout this discussion. The term *abortion* is used when discussing therapeutic or elective induced abortion (see Chapter 9).

Incidence and Etiology

Approximately 10% to 15% of all clinically recognized pregnancies end in miscarriage (Simpson, 1996). An early miscarriage is one that occurs before 12 weeks of gestation.

At least 50% of all clinically recognized pregnancy losses result from chromosomal abnormalities (Simpson, 1996). The majority (more than 90%) of miscarriages occur early, before 8 weeks of gestation (Simpson, 1996). Possible causes include endocrine imbalance (as in women who

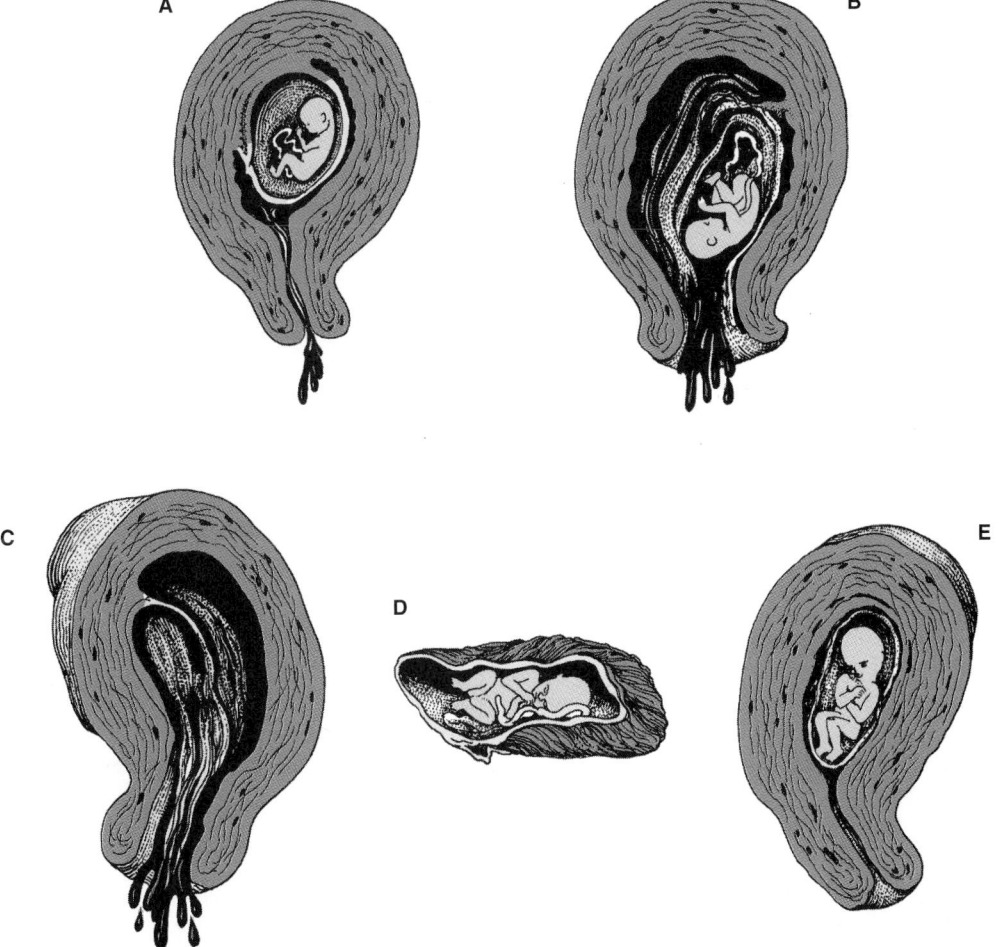

Fig. 31-1 Miscarriage. **A,** Threatened. **B,** Inevitable. **C,** Incomplete. **D,** Complete. **E,** Missed.

TABLE 31-1 Assessing Miscarriage and the Usual Management

TYPE OF MISCARRIAGE	AMOUNT OF BLEEDING	UTERINE CRAMPING	PASSAGE OF TISSUE	CERVICAL DILATION	MANAGEMENT
Threatened	Slight, spotting	Mild	No	No	Bed rest, sedation, and avoidance of stress and orgasm usually recommended. Further treatment depends on woman's response to treatment.
Inevitable	Moderate	Mild to severe	No	Yes	Prompt termination of pregnancy is accomplished, usually by dilation and curettage.
Incomplete	Heavy, profuse	Severe	Yes	Yes, with tissue in cervix	
Complete	Slight	Mild	Yes	No	No further intervention may be needed if uterine contractions are adequate to prevent hemorrhage and there is no infection.
Missed	None, spotting	None	No	No	If spontaneous evacuation of the uterus does not occur within 1 month, pregnancy is terminated by method appropriate to duration of pregnancy. Blood clotting factors are monitored until uterus is empty. DIC and incoagulability of blood with uncontrolled hemorrhage may develop in cases of fetal death after the twelfth week, if products of conception are retained for longer than 5 weeks.
Septic	Varies, usually malodorous	Varies	Varies	Yes, usually	Immediate termination of pregnancy by method appropriate to duration of pregnancy. Cervical culture and sensitivity studies are done, and broad-spectrum antibiotic therapy (e.g., ampicillin) is started. Treatment for septic shock is initiated if necessary.
Recurrent	Varies	Varies	Yes	Yes, usually	Varies depends on type. Prophylactic cerclage may be done if premature cervical dilation is the cause.

From Gilbert, E., & Harmon, J. (1998). *Manual of high risk pregnancy and delivery* (2nd ed.). St. Louis: Mosby.

have luteal phase defects or insulin-dependent diabetes mellitus with high blood glucose levels in the first trimester), immunologic factors (e.g., antiphospholipid antibodies), infections (e.g., bacteriuria and *Chlamydia trachomatis*), systemic disorders (e.g., lupus erythematosus), and genetic factors (American College of Obstetricians and Gynecologists [ACOG], 1995; Gilbert & Harmon, 1998).

A late miscarriage is one that occurs between 12 and 20 weeks of gestation. It usually results from maternal causes, such as advancing maternal age and parity, chronic infections, premature dilation of the cervix and other anomalies of the reproductive tract, chronic debilitating

diseases, inadequate nutrition, and recreational drug use (Cunningham et al., 1997). Little can be done to avoid genetically caused pregnancy loss, but correction of maternal disorders, immunization against infectious diseases, adequate early prenatal care, and treatment of pregnancy complications can do much to prevent miscarriage.

Types

The types of miscarriage include threatened, inevitable, incomplete, complete, and missed. Miscarriage (both early and late) can recur; all but the threatened miscarriage can lead to infection (Fig. 31-1).

Clinical Manifestations

Signs and symptoms of miscarriage depend on the duration of pregnancy. The presence of uterine bleeding, uterine contractions, or uterine pain is an ominous sign during early pregnancy that must be considered a threatened miscarriage until proven otherwise.

If miscarriage occurs before the sixth week of pregnancy, the woman may report a heavy menstrual flow. Miscarriage that occurs between the sixth and twelfth weeks of pregnancy causes moderate discomfort and blood loss. After the twelfth week, miscarriage is typified by more severe pain, similar to that of labor, because the fetus must be expelled. Diagnosis of the type of miscarriage is based on the signs and symptoms present (Table 31-1 and Fig. 31-1).

Symptoms of a threatened miscarriage (see Fig. 31-1, *A*) include spotting of blood but with the cervical os closed. Mild uterine cramping may be present.

Inevitable (see Fig. 31-1, *B*) and incomplete (see Fig. 31-1, *C*) miscarriages involve a moderate to heavy amount of bleeding with an open cervical os. Tissue may be present with the bleeding. Mild to severe uterine cramping may be present. An inevitable miscarriage is often accompanied by rupture of membranes (ROM) and cervical dilation; passage of the products of conception will occur. An incomplete miscarriage involves the expulsion of the fetus with retention of the placenta (Cunningham et al., 1997).

In a complete miscarriage (see Fig. 32-1, *D*), all fetal tissue is passed, the cervix is closed, and there may be slight bleeding. Mild uterine cramping may be present.

The term *missed abortion* (see Fig. 32-1, *E*) refers to a pregnancy in which the fetus has died but miscarriage does not occur. It may be diagnosed by ultrasonic examination after the uterus stops increasing in size or even decreases in size. There may be no bleeding or cramping, and the cervical os remains closed. If the products of conception are retained after a missed abortion, they may calcify, forming a uterine lithopedion, or "womb stone" (see Fig. 32-1, *E*).

Recurrent early (habitual) miscarriage is the loss of three or more previable pregnancies.

Miscarriage can become septic, although this is not a common occurrence. Symptoms include fever and abdominal tenderness. Vaginal bleeding, which may be slight to heavy, is usually malodorous.

CARE MANAGEMENT

Assessment and Nursing Diagnoses

A thorough assessment should be performed on the prenatal client with vaginal bleeding in early pregnancy (Box 31-1). The data to be collected include pain, bleeding, and last menstrual period (LMP) to determine the approximate length of gestation. The initial database includes vital signs (a temperature higher than 38° C may indicate infection), previous pregnancies, previous pregnancy losses, type and location of pain, quantity and nature of bleeding, allergies, and emotional status (see Box 31-1). It is not uncommon

---

BOX 31-1 Assessment of Bleeding in Pregnancy

INITIAL DATABASE

Chief complaint
Vital signs
Gravidity, parity
Last menstrual period/estimated date of birth
Pregnancy history (previous and current)
Allergies
Nausea and vomiting
Pain (onset, quality, precipitating event, location)
Bleeding or coagulation problems
Level of consciousness
Emotional status

EARLY PREGNANCY

Confirmation of pregnancy
Bleeding (bright or dark, intermittent or continuous)
Pain (type, intensity, persistence)
Vaginal discharge

LATE PREGNANCY

Estimated date of birth
Bleeding (quantity, associated pain)
Vaginal discharge
Amniotic membrane status
Uterine activity
Abdominal pain
Fetal status/viability

---

for the client to be anxious and fearful regarding what may happen to her and to her pregnancy.

Various laboratory findings are characteristic of miscarriage. Evaluation of human chorionic gonadotropin (hCG), a placental hormone, is used in the diagnosis of pregnancy and pregnancy loss. Human chorionic gonadotropin is produced by the syncytiotrophoblast, and the β-subunit of hCG (β-hCG) can be detected in maternal plasma and urine 8 to 9 days after ovulation if the woman is pregnant. In early pregnancy, the concentration of β-hCG should double every 1.4 to 2.0 days until about 60 or 70 days of gestation (Cunningham et al., 1997). Before 8 weeks of gestation, if miscarriage is suspected, two serum quantitative β-hCG levels are drawn 48 hours apart. If a normal pregnancy is present, the β-hCG level doubles in this time frame. Ultrasonography can then be used to determine the presence of a viable gestational sac. With considerable or persistent blood loss, anemia is likely (hemoglobin level less than 10.5 g/dl). If infection is present, the white blood cell count (WBC) is greater than 12,000/mm³. Sedimentation rate is not helpful for differential diagnostic purposes because an increased sedimentation rate occurs with pregnancy, anemia, or infection.

The following nursing diagnoses are appropriate for the woman experiencing a miscarriage:

▪ Nursing Diagnoses

- Anxiety/fear related to
  - unknown outcome and unfamiliarity with medical procedures
- Fluid volume deficit related to
  - excessive bleeding secondary to miscarriage
- Acute pain related to
  - uterine contractions
- Anticipatory grieving related to
  - unexpected pregnancy outcome
- Situational low self-esteem related to
  - inability to successfully carry a pregnancy to term gestation
- Risk for altered health maintenance related to
  - lack of knowledge of risk factors and preventive measures for early miscarriage and incompetent cervix
- Risk for infection related to
  - surgical treatment
  - dilated cervix

Expected Outcomes of Care

Expected outcomes of care for the woman experiencing miscarriage may include that the woman will do the following:
- Discuss the impact of the loss on her and her family.
- Identify and use available support systems.
- Display no signs or symptoms of complications (e.g., hemorrhage or infection).
- Identify health promotion measures that decrease her risk of miscarriage and state understanding of reasons for diagnostic and genetic follow-up if needed.
- Report relief from pain.

Plan of Care and Interventions

Immediate nursing care focuses on physiologic stabilization. Typical orders to be followed would be initiation of an intravenous line, request for blood testing of hemoglobin and hematocrit, blood type and Rh, and indirect Coombs screen. An ultrasound is performed for diagnostic confirmation.

Medical Management

Medical management (see Table 31-1) depends on the classification and on signs and symptoms. Traditionally, threatened miscarriages have been managed with bed rest and supportive care. Follow-up treatment depends on whether the threatened miscarriage progresses to actual miscarriage or symptoms subside and the pregnancy remains intact. Dilation and curettage (D&C) is a surgical procedure in which the cervix is dilated and a curette is in-

serted to scrape the uterine walls and remove uterine contents. A D&C is commonly performed to treat inevitable and incomplete miscarriage. The nurse reinforces explanations, answers any questions or concerns, and prepares the woman for surgery.

Dilation and evacuation, performed after 16 weeks of gestation, consists of wide cervical dilation followed by instrumental removal of the uterine contents.

Before either surgical procedure is performed, a full history should be obtained and general and pelvic examinations should be performed. General preoperative and postoperative care are appropriate for the woman requiring surgical intervention. Analgesics and anesthesia appropriate to the procedure are used.

For late incomplete or inevitable miscarriages (16 to 20 weeks) and missed abortions, prostaglandins may be administered into the amniotic sac or by vaginal suppository to induce or augment labor and cause the products of conception to be expelled. Intravenous oxytocin may also be used.

Nursing care is similar to care for any woman whose labor is being induced (see Chapter 37). Special care may be needed for management of side effects of prostaglandin such as nausea and vomiting and diarrhea. If the products of conception are not passed in entirety, the woman may be prepared for manual or surgical evacuation of the uterus.

After evacuation of the uterus, 10 to 20 U of oxytocin in 1000 ml of fluids may be given to prevent hemorrhage. For excessive bleeding, ergot products such as ergonovine or a prostaglandin derivative such as carboprost tromethamine may be given to contract the uterus. Three or four doses of ergonovine, 0.2 mg orally or intramuscularly every 4 hours, may be given if the woman is normotensive. A 25 mg dose of carboprost may be given intramuscularly every 15 to 90 minutes for as many as eight doses (Cunningham et al., 1997). Antibiotics are given as necessary. Analgesics, such as antiprostaglandin agents, may decrease discomfort from cramping. Transfusion therapy may be required for shock or anemia. The woman who is Rh negative and does not have isoimmunization is given an intramuscular injection of $Rh_0(D)$ immune globulin ▪▪ within 72 hours of the miscarriage.

Psychosocial aspects of care focus on what the pregnancy loss means to the woman and her family. After miscarriage, Hutti (1992) found that responses of women ranged from no grief to intense long-lasting grief. Prediction of who will have which reaction would assist nurses in providing individualized care (see Research box). Explanations are provided regarding the nature of the miscarriage, expected procedures, and possible future implications for childbearing.

As with the other fetal or neonatal losses, the woman should be offered the option of seeing the products of conception. She may also want to know what the hospital does with the products of conception or whether she needs to make a decision about final disposition.

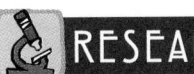

RESEARCH

A Study of Miscarriage: Development and Validation of the Perinatal Grief Intensity Scale

Perinatal grief has been studied since the 1960s, and differences in how people react to pregnancy loss have been reported. How to predict who will have intense grief and need intervention has yet to be identified. The purpose of this study was to develop and test the Perinatal Grief Intensity Scale (PGIS), a test based on a theoretic model designed to predict the intensity of grief responses to early pregnancy loss. A convenience sample of 186 women who had experienced miscarriage before 16 weeks of gestation in the preceding 12 to 16 months completed the 36-item PGIS by mail. Factor analysis was used to evaluate the responses. Fourteen of the 36 items were retained after the analysis. The 14 items loaded on a three-factor solution and accounted for 65% of the variance. The three factors that were found to influence the intensity of grieving were Reality of the Pregnancy and the Baby Within, the Ability to Confront Others, and Congruence Between the Actual Experience and the Standard of the Desirable. All three subscales were found to be significantly correlated to self-report of grief intensity and length of grieving. Moderate to intense grief responses were reported by almost 75% of the sample, but only 39% reported grieving over 6 months.

CLINICAL APPLICATION

Although the researchers suggest further testing of the PGIS, nursing interventions can be planned using the theoretic framework of the PGIS. How real the pregnancy and the baby within are to the woman is thought to determine the intensity of grief responses. Factors such as infertility, previous pregnancy loss, previous pregnancy success, and maternal age may influence grieving by altering the parents' perception of the miscarriage. Because grief responses after a miscarriage can vary on a continuum from no response to an intense, long-lasting grief response, nurses should assess the significance of the loss before intervening. This assessment would lead to a more individualized plan of care for the woman and her family.

Source: Hutti, M., dePacheco, M., & Smith, M. (1998). A study of miscarriage: Development and validation of the Perinatal Grief Intensity Scale. *J Obstet Gynecol Neonatal Nurs* 27(5), 547-555.

Home Care

The woman will be discharged to home postoperatively after a D&C when vital signs are stable, vaginal bleeding remains minimal, and she is alert after anesthesia. Discharge teaching emphasizes the need for rest. If significant blood loss has occurred, iron supplementation may be ordered. Teaching includes information about normal physical findings, such as cramping, type and amount of bleeding, resumption of sexual activity, and family planning. Follow-up care should assess the woman's physical and emotional recovery. Referrals to local support groups should be provided as needed (see the Teaching Guidelines box).

Follow-up phone calls after a loss are important. The woman may appreciate a phone call on what would have been her due date. These calls provide opportunities for the woman to ask questions, seek advice, and receive information to help process her grief.

Evaluation

Evaluation is based on the predetermined client-centered outcomes.

Incompetent Cervix (Premature Dilation of the Cervix)

Another cause of late miscarriage is **incompetent cervix (premature dilation of the cervix),** which has traditionally been defined as passive and painless dilation of the cervix during the second trimester. This definition assumes

TEACHING guidelines

Discharge Teaching for the Woman After Early Miscarriage

- Advise the woman to report any heavy, profuse, or bright red bleeding to health care provider.
- Reassure the woman that a scant, dark discharge may persist for 1 to 2 weeks.
- To reduce the risk of infection, remind the woman not to put anything into the vagina until bleeding has stopped (e.g., no tampons, no vaginal intercourse). She should take antibiotics as prescribed.
- Acknowledge that the woman has experienced a loss and that time is required for recovery. She may have mood swings and depression.
- Refer the woman to support groups, clergy, or professional counseling as needed.
- Advise the woman that attempts at pregnancy should be postponed for at least 2 months to allow her body to recover.

From Gilbert, E., & Harmon, J. (1998). *Manual of high risk pregnancy and delivery* (2nd ed.). St. Louis: Mosby.

an "all or nothing" role for the cervix; it is either "competent" or "incompetent." Current research contends that cervical competence is variable and exists as a continuum that is determined in part by cervical length. Other related factors include composition of the cervical tissue and the individual circumstances associated with the pregnancy in terms of maternal stress and lifestyle. Iams (1996) refers to this condition as abnormal or reduced cervical competence. Freda (1995) suggests the term *premature dilation of the cervix.*

Etiology

Etiologic factors include a history of previous cervical lacerations during childbirth, excessive cervical dilation for curettage or biopsy, or the woman's mother's ingestion of diethylstilbestrol during pregnancy with the woman. Other instances may result from a congenitally short cervix or cervical or uterine anomalies. Reduced cervical competence is a clinical diagnosis, based on history. Short labors and recurring loss of the pregnancy at progressively earlier gestational ages are characteristics of reduced cervical competence. Ultrasound is used to diagnose this condition. A short cervix (less than 20 mm in length) is indicative of reduced cervical competence. Often, but not always, the short cervix is accompanied by **cervical funneling,** or effacement of the internal cervical os (Iams, 1996).

Collaborative Care

The nurse assesses the woman's feelings about her pregnancy and her understanding of reduced cervical competence. It is also important to evaluate the woman's support systems. Because the diagnosis of reduced cervical competence is usually not made until the woman has lost one or two pregnancies, she may feel guilty or to blame for this impending loss. It is therefore important to assess for previous reactions to stresses and appropriateness of coping responses. The woman needs the support of her health care providers, as well as that of her family.

Medical management. Conservative management consists of bed rest, hydration, and tocolysis (inhibition of uterine contractions). A cervical **cerclage** may be performed. During gestation, a McDonald cerclage, band of homologous fascia, or nonabsorbable ribbon (Mersilene) may be placed around the cervix beneath the mucosa to constrict the internal os of the cervix (Fig. 31-2).

Prophylactic cerclage is placed at 10 to 14 weeks of gestation, after which the woman is told to refrain from intercourse, prolonged (more than 90 minutes) standing, and heavy lifting. She is followed during the course of her pregnancy with ultrasound scans to assess for cervical shortening and funneling. The cerclage is electively removed (usually an office or a clinic procedure) when the woman reaches 37 weeks of gestation, or it may be left in place and a cesarean birth performed. Approximately 80% to 90% of pregnancies treated with cerclage result in live, viable births (Iams, 1996). If removed, cerclage placement must be repeated with each successive pregnancy.

A woman whose reduced cervical competence is diagnosed during the current pregnancy may undergo emer-

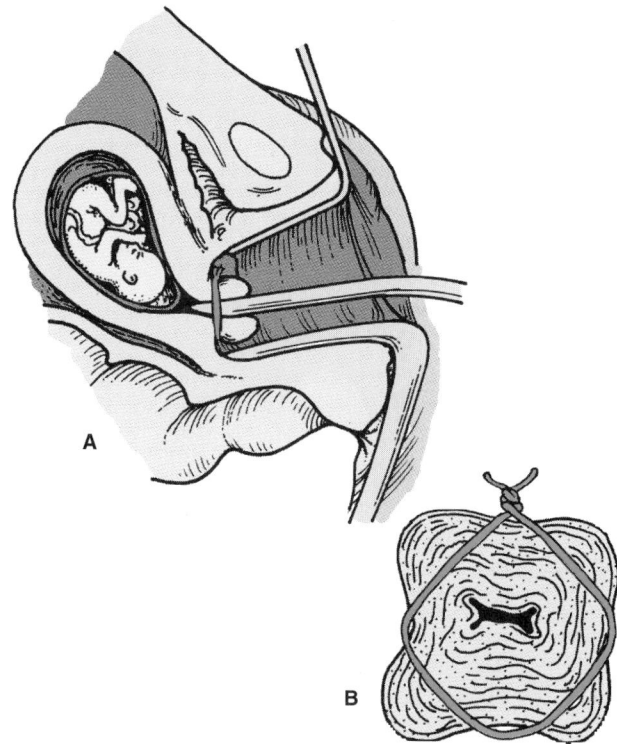

Fig. 31-2 **A,** Cerclage correction of premature dilation of the cervical os. **B,** Cross-sectional view of closed internal os.

gency cerclage placement. Risks of the procedure include premature rupture of membranes, preterm labor, and chorioamnionitis. Because of these risks, and because bed rest and tocolytic therapy can be used to prolong the pregnancy, cerclage is rarely performed after 26 weeks of gestation (Iams, 1996).

Nursing management. If a cervical cerclage is performed, the nurse monitors the woman postoperatively for contractions, ROM, and signs of infection. Discharge teaching focuses on continued monitoring of these aspects at home. Home uterine monitoring may be indicated with follow-up from a home health agency.

Antepartal home care. The woman must understand the importance of activity restriction at home and the need for close observation and supervision. Instruction includes the rationale for bed rest or activity restriction and warning signs of preterm labor, ROM, and infection to report (Lowdermilk & Grohar, 1999). The woman must be instructed on the importance of taking oral tocolytic medication if prescribed, the expected response, and possible side effects. Tocolytics may be given prophylactically to prevent uterine contractions and further dilation of the cervix. If home uterine monitoring is implemented, the woman is taught how to apply a uterine contraction monitor and transmit the monitor tracing by telephone to the monitoring center. Nurses at the monitoring center assess the tracing for contractions, answer questions, provide emotional support and education, and report information to the

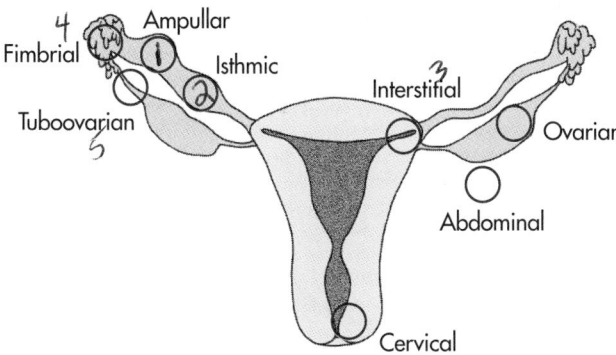

Fig. 31-3 Sites of implantation of ectopic pregnancies. Order of frequency of occurrence is ampulla, isthmus, interstitium, fimbria, tuboovarian ligament, ovary, abdominal cavity, and cervix (external os).

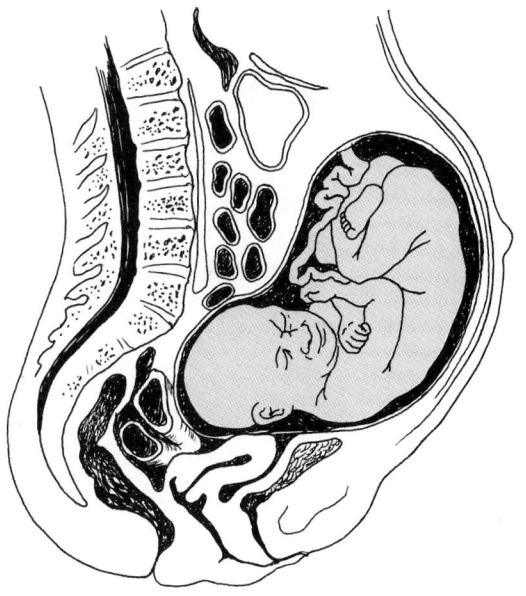

Fig. 31-4 Ectopic pregnancy, abdominal.

woman's physician or nurse-midwife. The woman should know the signs that would warrant immediate transfer to the hospital, including strong contractions less than 5 minutes apart, rupture of membranes, severe perineal pressure, and an urge to push (Health Care Resources, 1997). If management is unsuccessful and the fetus is born before viability, appropriate grief support should be provided. If the fetus is born prematurely, appropriate anticipatory guidance and support will be necessary.

Ectopic Pregnancy
Incidence and Etiology

Ectopic pregnancy is one in which the fertilized ovum is implanted outside the uterine cavity (Fig. 31-3). It accounts for 2% of all pregnancies in the United States (Flystra, 1998).

Approximately 95% of ectopic pregnancies occur in the uterine (fallopian) tube, with most located on the ampullar or largest portion of the tube. Other sites include the abdominal cavity (3% to 4%), ovary (1%), and cervix (1%).

Ectopic pregnancy is responsible for 10% of all maternal mortality, and it is the leading pregnancy-related cause of first trimester maternal mortality (Powell & Spellman, 1996; Simpson, 1996). Moreover, ectopic pregnancy is a leading cause of infertility. Only about 60% of women who have been treated for ectopic pregnancy are able to conceive afterward, and approximately 40% of those pregnancies are ectopic (Powell & Spellman, 1996).

The incidence of ectopic pregnancy is increasing. In part, this increase is due to improved diagnostic techniques, such as more sensitive β-hCG assays and the availability of transvaginal ultrasound. Other reasons include an increased incidence of sexually transmitted infections, better treatment of pelvic inflammatory disease (which formerly would have caused sterility), increased numbers of tubal sterilizations, and surgical reversal of tubal sterilizations (Simpson, 1996).

Ectopic pregnancy is classified according to site of implantation (e.g., tubal or ovarian). The uterus is the only organ capable of containing and sustaining a term pregnancy. However, abdominal pregnancy with birth by laparotomy may result in a living infant in 5% to 25% of such pregnancies (Fig. 31-4); the risk of deformity is as high as 40% (Gilbert & Harmon, 1998).

Clinical Manifestations

A missed period, adnexal fullness, and tenderness may suggest an unruptured tubal pregnancy. The tenderness can progress from a dull pain to a colicky pain when the tube stretches. Pain may be unilateral, bilateral, or diffuse over the abdomen. Abnormal vaginal bleeding occurs in 50% to 80% of women. If the ectopic pregnancy ruptures, pain increases. This pain may be generalized, unilateral, or acute deep lower quadrant pain caused by blood irritating the peritoneum. Referred shoulder pain can occur as a result of diaphragmatic irritation caused by blood in the peritoneal cavity. The woman may exhibit signs of shock related to the amount of bleeding in the abdominal cavity and not necessarily related to obvious vaginal bleeding. An ecchymotic blueness around the umbilicus **(Cullen sign),** indicating hematoperitoneum, may develop in an undiagnosed ruptured intraabdominal ectopic pregnancy.

Diagnosis

The differential diagnosis of ectopic pregnancy involves consideration of numerous disorders that share many signs and symptoms. The physician, nurse-midwife, or nurse-practitioner must consider miscarriage, ruptured corpus luteum cyst, appendicitis, salpingitis, ovarian cysts, torsion of the ovary, and urinary tract infection (Table 31-2).

TABLE 31-2   Differential Diagnosis of Ectopic Pregnancy

	ECTOPIC PREGNANCY	APPENDICITIS	SALPINGITIS	RUPTURED OVARIAN CYST	MISCARRIAGE
Pain	Unilateral cramps and tenderness before rupture May be colicky after rupture Sudden sharp abdominal pelvic pain Abdominal tenderness	Epigastric, periumbilical, then right lower quadrant pain, tenderness localizing at McBurney's point, rebound tenderness	Usually in both lower quadrants with or without rebound Mild to severe pelvic pressure	Unilateral, becoming general with progressive bleeding, dull cramping	Mild uterine cramps to severe uterine pain
Nausea and vomiting	Occasionally before, frequently after rupture	Usual, precedes shift of pain to right lower quadrant	Infrequent	Rare	Almost never
Menstruation	Some aberration, missed period, spotting	Unrelated to menses	Hypermenorrhea, metrorrhagia, or both	Period delayed, then bleeding, often with pain	Amenorrhea, then spotting, then brisk bleeding
Temperature, pulse, and blood pressure	37.2°-37.8° C, pulse variable, normal before and rapid after rupture, ↓BP after rupture	37.2°-37.8° C, pulse rapid	37.2°-40° C: pulse elevated in proportion to fever	Not over 37.2° C, pulse normal unless blood loss marked, then rapid	To 37.2° C Signs of shock related to obvious bleeding
Pelvic examination	Unilateral tenderness, especially on movement of cervix, crepitant mass on one side or in cul-de-sac; dark red or brown vaginal discharge	No masses, rectal tenderness high on right side No vaginal discharge	Bilateral tenderness on movement of cervix Purulent discharge	Tenderness over affected ovary, no masses	Cervix open or closed, uterus slightly enlarged, irregularly softened, tender with infection, vaginal bleeding
Laboratory findings	White blood cell count (WBC) to 15,000/mm³ Pregnancy test positive Ultrasound to rule out pregnancy after 6 weeks	WBC 10,000-18,000/mm³ (rarely normal) Pregnancy test negative	WBC 15,000-30,000/mm³ Pregnancy test negative	WBC normal to 10,000/mm³ Pregnancy test negative unless also pregnant Ultrasound will show ovarian cyst	WBC normal Pregnancy test positive

Modified from Gilbert, E., & Harmon, J. (1998). *Manual of high risk pregnancy and delivery* (2nd ed.). St. Louis: Mosby.

Diagnostic evaluation for an ectopic pregnancy includes laboratory testing and vaginal sonography.

Most ectopic pregnancies occur in the uterine tube. In the past, these tubal pregnancies were usually diagnosed at the time of rupture, when the major management problem was hemorrhage. Often, laparotomy, followed by removal of the entire uterine tube, was the treatment necessary to control bleeding and save the woman's life.

Removal of the ectopic pregnancy by salpingostomy is possible before rupture. Residual tissue is dissolved with a dose of methotrexate postoperatively. Methotrexate is a folic acid analogue that destroys the rapidly dividing cells (DeLoia, Stewart-Akers, & Cremin, 1998). It may also be used in a single-dose intramuscular injection to treat unruptured pregnancies (Lipscomb et al., 1998). It has been shown to produce results similar to those of surgical therapy, in terms of high success rate, low complication rate, and good reproductive potential (Simpson, 1996).

Advanced ectopic abdominal pregnancy requires laparotomy as soon as the woman has been stabilized for operation. If the placenta of a second- or third-trimester abdominal pregnancy is attached to a vital organ, such as the liver, separation is usually not attempted because of the risk of hemorrhage. The cord is cut flush with the placenta and the abdomen is closed, with the placenta left in place. Degeneration and absorption of the placenta usually occur without complication, although infection and intestinal obstruction may occur. Methotrexate may be given to dissolve the residual tissue (Cunningham et al., 1997).

Collaborative Care

The key to early detection of ectopic pregnancy is having a high index of suspicion for this condition. Any woman with complaints of abdominal pain, vaginal spotting or bleeding, and a positive pregnancy test should undergo screening for ectopic pregnancy. Laboratory screening includes determination of serum progesterone and β-hCG levels. If either of these values is lower than would be expected for a normal pregnancy, the woman is asked to return within 48 hours for serial measurements. At this time, the woman will also undergo transvaginal ultrasound to confirm intrauterine or tubal pregnancy (Powell & Spellman, 1996).

The woman should also be assessed for the presence of active bleeding, which is associated with tubal rupture. If internal bleeding is present, assessment may reveal vertigo, shoulder pain, hypotension, and tachycardia. A vaginal examination should be performed only once, and then with great caution. Approximately half of clients with a tubal pregnancy have a palpable mass on examination. It is possible to rupture the mass during a bimanual examination, so gentleness is critical (Simpson, 1996).

Hospital care. Once an ectopic pregnancy is suspected, the physician is notified of assessment findings. Vital signs (pulse, respirations, and blood pressure) are assessed every 15 minutes or as needed, according to severity of the bleeding and the woman's condition. Laboratory tests include determination of blood type and Rh factor, complete blood cell count, and serum quantitative β-hCG assay. Ultrasonography is used to confirm an extrauterine pregnancy. General preoperative and postoperative care is appropriate for the woman requiring surgical intervention for an ectopic pregnancy. Blood replacement may be necessary. The nurse verifies the woman's Rh and antibody status and administers $Rh_0(D)$ immune globulin if appropriate. The woman should be encouraged to verbalize her

feelings related to the loss. Referral to community resources may be appropriate.

Home care. Hemodynamically stable women with ectopic pregnancies are eligible for methotrexate therapy if the mass is unruptured and measures less than 4 cm in diameter by ultrasound (Simpson, 1996). Methotrexate therapy avoids surgery and is a safe, effective, and cost-conscious way of managing many cases of tubal pregnancy. Management is almost always accomplished on an outpatient basis.

The woman is informed how the medication works, what adverse effects are possible, who to call if she has concerns or problems develop, and the importance of follow-up care. After receiving the single methotrexate injection, the woman must return at least weekly for follow-up laboratory studies for an average of 2 to 8 weeks. A repeat dose may be necessary if hCG titers do not drop to 15% by day 7 (Maiolatesi & Petticord, 1996). Multiple-dose regimens may also be given (Minnick-Smith & Cook, 1997). During that time, she is instructed to put nothing in the vagina (no tampons, douches, or intercourse) and to avoid sun exposure because the drug will make her more photosensitive (Powell & Spellman, 1996).

NURSE ALERT *The woman on methotrexate therapy who drinks alcohol and takes vitamins containing folic acid (e.g., prenatal vitamins) increases her risk of experiencing side effects of the drug or exacerbating the ectopic rupture.*

The issue of future fertility should be discussed. Any woman who has been diagnosed with an ectopic pregnancy should be told to contact her health care provider as soon as she suspects that she might be pregnant, because of the increased risk for recurrent ectopic pregnancy. These women may need referral to grief or infertility support groups. In addition to the loss of the current pregnancy, they are faced with the possibility of future pregnancy losses and infertility.

Hydatidiform Mole (Molar Pregnancy)

Hydatidiform mole (molar pregnancy) is a gestational trophoblastic disease. There are two distinct types of hydatidiform moles: complete (or classic) mole and partial mole.

Incidence and Etiology

Hydatidiform mole occurs in 1 in 1200 pregnancies in the United States, but a higher incidence has been reported in Asian countries (Berman, DiSaia, & Brewster, 1999). The etiology is unknown, although there may be an ovular defect or nutritional deficiency. Women at higher risk for hydatidiform mole formation are those who have undergone ovulation stimulation with clomiphene (Clomid) and those who are in their early teens or older than 40 years of age. The risk of a second mole is 1% to 2%.

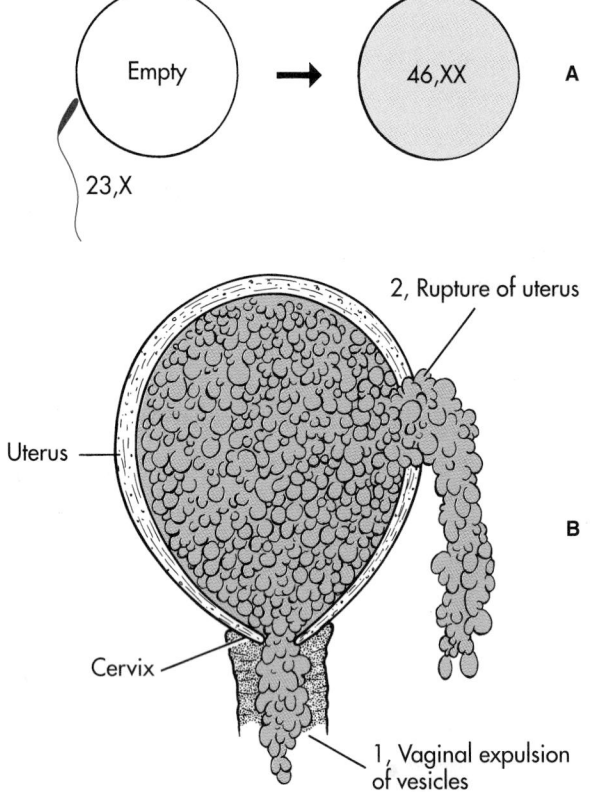

Fig. 31-5 **A,** Chromosomal origin of complete mole. Single sperm (color) fertilizes an "empty" ovum. Reduplication of sperm's 23,X set gives completely homozygous diploid 46,XX. Similar process follows fertilization of empty ovum by two sperm with two independently drawn sets of 23,X or 23,Y; both karyotypes of 46,XX and 46,XY can therefore result. **B,** Uterine rupture with hydatidiform mole. *1,* Evacuation of mole through cervix. *2,* Rupture of uterus and spillage of mole into peritoneal cavity (rare).

Types

The complete mole results from fertilization of an egg whose nucleus has been lost or inactivated (Fig. 31-5, *A*). The nucleus of a sperm (23,X) duplicates itself (resulting in the diploid number, 46,XX) because the ovum has no genetic material or the material is inactive. The mole resembles a bunch of white grapes (Fig. 31-5, *B*). The hydropic (fluid-filled) vesicles grow rapidly, causing the uterus to be larger than expected for the duration of the pregnancy. Usually the complete mole contains no fetus, placenta, amniotic membranes, or fluid. Maternal blood has no placenta to receive it; hemorrhage into the uterine cavity and vaginal bleeding therefore occur. In about 20% of cases of complete mole, progression toward choriocarcinoma occurs.

For a partial mole, chromosomal studies often show a karyotype of 69,XXY; 69,XXX; or 69,XYY. This occurs as a result of two sperm fertilizing an apparently normal ovum (Fig. 31-6). Partial moles often have embryonic or fetal parts and an amniotic sac present. Congenital anomalies are usually present. The potential for malignant transformation is about 2% to 6% (Copeland & Landon, 1996).

Clinical Manifestations

The clinical manifestations of a complete hydatidiform mole in the early stages cannot be distinguished from those of normal pregnancy. Later, vaginal bleeding occurs in almost 95% of cases. The vaginal discharge may be dark brown (resembling prune juice) or bright red, either scant or profuse. It may continue for only a few days or intermittently for weeks. Early in pregnancy the uterus in about half of affected women is significantly larger than expected from menstrual dates. The percentage of women with an excessively enlarged uterus increases as length of time since LMP increases. Approximately 25% of affected women have a uterus smaller than would be expected from menstrual dates.

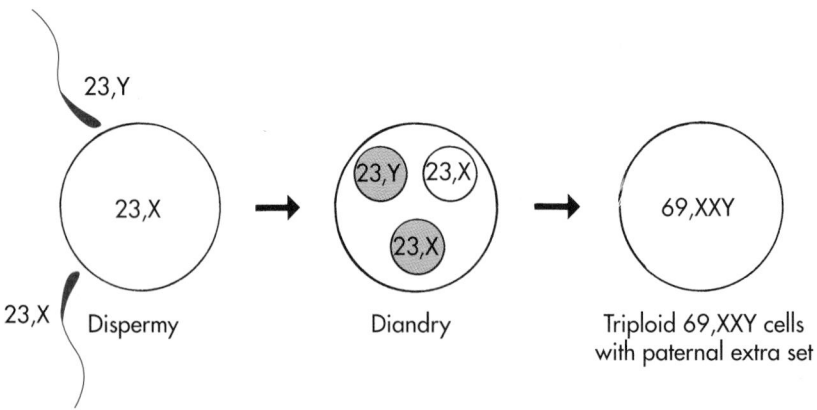

Fig. 31-6 Chromosomal origin of triploid, partial mole. Normal ovum with 23,X haploid set is fertilized by two sperms to give total of 69 chromosomes. Sex configuration of XXY, XXX, or XYY is possible.

Anemia from blood loss, excessive nausea and vomiting (hyperemesis gravidarum), and abdominal cramps caused by uterine distention are relatively common findings. Preeclampsia occurs in about 15% of cases, usually between 9 and 12 weeks of gestation, but any symptoms of pregnancy-induced hypertension before 24 weeks of gestation may suggest hydatidiform mole. Hyperthyroidism and pulmonary embolization of trophoblastic elements occur less commonly but are serious complications of hydatidiform mole. Partial moles cause few of these symptoms and may be mistaken for an incomplete or missed abortion.

Passage of vesicles may occur around 16 weeks of gestation. There is no fetal movement, fetal heart rate, or palpable fetal parts. Some women have signs and symptoms of hyperthyroidism. A trophoblastic pulmonary embolus may develop in about 20% of women with hydatidiform mole (Berkowitz, Goldstein, & Bernstein, 1996).

Collaborative Care

Nursing assessments during prenatal visits should include observation for signs of molar pregnancy during the first 24 weeks. If hydatidiform mole is suspected, ultrasonography and serial β-hCG immunoassays will be used to confirm the diagnosis. The sonographic pattern of a molar pregnancy is characterized by a diffuse "snowstorm" pattern. A β-hCG titer will remain high or rise above normal peak after the time at which it normally drops (70 to 100 days) (Cunningham et al., 1997).

Medical-surgical management. Although most moles pass spontaneously, suction curettage offers a safe, rapid, and effective method of evacuation of hydatidiform mole if necessary (Gilbert & Harmon, 1998). Induction of labor with oxytocic agents or prostaglandins is not recommended because of the increased risk of embolization of trophoblastic tissue (Copeland & Landon, 1996). Administration of $Rh_0(D)$ immune globulin to women who are Rh negative is necessary to prevent isoimmunization.

Nursing care. The nurse provides the woman and her family with information about the disease process, the necessity for a long course of follow-up, and the possible consequences of the disease. The nurse helps the woman understand and cope with pregnancy loss and recognize that the pregnancy was abnormal. The woman and her family are encouraged to express their feelings, and information is provided about support groups or counseling resources if needed. Explanations about the importance of the need to postpone a subsequent pregnancy and contraceptive counseling are provided to emphasize the importance of consistent and reliable use of the method chosen.

NURSE ALERT *To avoid confusion with signs of pregnancy, pregnancy should be avoided for 1 year. Any contraceptive method except an intrauterine device is acceptable. Oral contraceptives are highly effective.*

Home care. Follow-up management includes frequent physical and pelvic examinations along with biweekly measurements of β-hCG level until the level drops to normal and remains normal for 3 weeks. Monthly measurements are taken for 6 months, then every 2 months for a total of 1 year. A rising titer and an enlarging uterus may indicate choriocarcinoma (see Chapter 13). Referral to community support resources may be needed.

LATE PREGNANCY BLEEDING

Late pregnancy bleeding disorders include placenta previa, premature separation of placenta (abruptio placentae), and variations in the cord insertion and the placenta. Expedient assessment for and diagnosis of the cause of bleeding are essential to reduce maternal and perinatal morbidity and mortality (Fig. 31-7).

Placenta Previa

In **placenta previa,** the placenta is implanted in the lower uterine segment near or over the internal cervical os. The degree to which the internal cervical os is covered by the placenta has traditionally been used to classify three types of placenta previa (Fig. 31-8). Placenta previa often is described as total if the internal os is entirely covered by the placenta when the cervix is fully dilated. Partial placenta previa implies incomplete coverage of the internal os. Marginal placenta previa indicates that only an edge of the placenta extends to the internal os but may extend onto the os during dilation of the cervix during labor. The term *low-lying placenta* is used when the placenta is implanted in the lower uterine segment but does not reach the os.

Vasa previa is the result of a velamentous insertion (see Cord Insertion and Placental Variations, later in this chapter) of the umbilical cord. With vasa previa, the umbilical vein and arteries are not surrounded by Wharton's jelly and have no supportive tissue. The umbilical blood vessels are thus at risk for laceration at any time, but laceration occurs most frequently during ROM (Clark, 1999). The sudden appearance of bright red blood at the time of ROM (spontaneous or artificial) and a sudden change in the fetal heart rate without other known risk factors should immediately alert the nurse to the possibility of vasa previa.

Although it occurs rarely (fewer than 1 in 3000 pregnancies), vasa previa is associated with high incidence of fetal morbidity and mortality because of the potential for fetal exsanguination (Thorp, 1993). Diagnosis before birth is unusual, although there are reports of examiners palpating a pulsing vessel. Vasa previa may also be noted on ultrasonographic examination or by direct visualization (Cunningham et al., 1997).

Incidence and Etiology

The incidence of placenta previa is approximately 0.5% of births (Clark, 1999). The most important risk factors are

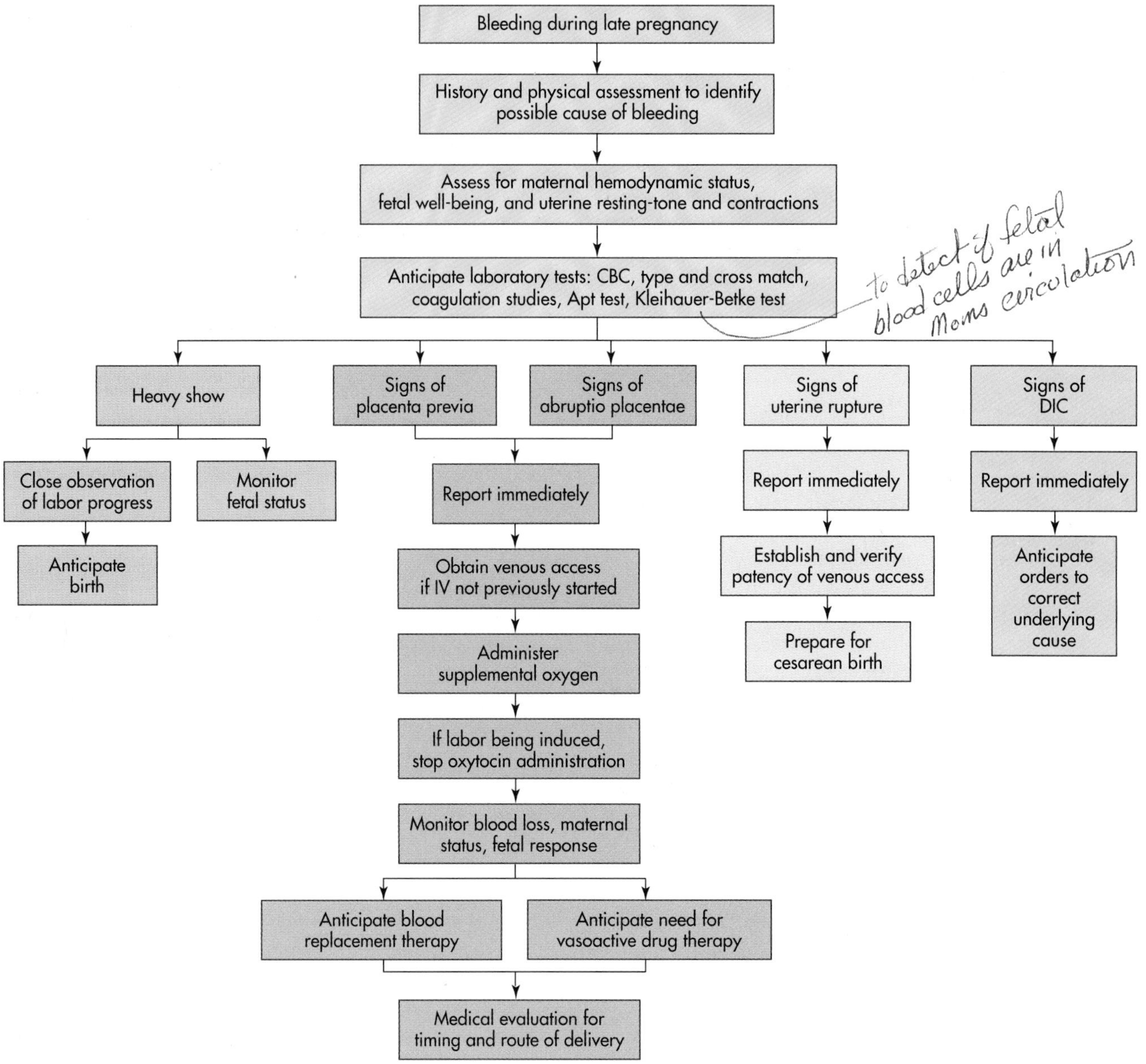

Bleeding during late pregnancy

↓

History and physical assessment to identify possible cause of bleeding

↓

Assess for maternal hemodynamic status, fetal well-being, and uterine resting-tone and contractions

↓

Anticipate laboratory tests: CBC, type and cross match, coagulation studies, Apt test, Kleihauer-Betke test

to detect if fetal blood cells are in Moms circulation

Heavy show
- Close observation of labor progress → Anticipate birth
- Monitor fetal status

Signs of placenta previa / **Signs of abruptio placentae**
- Report immediately
- Obtain venous access if IV not previously started
- Administer supplemental oxygen
- If labor being induced, stop oxytocin administration
- Monitor blood loss, maternal status, fetal response
  - Anticipate blood replacement therapy
  - Anticipate need for vasoactive drug therapy
- Medical evaluation for timing and route of delivery

Signs of uterine rupture
- Report immediately
- Establish and verify patency of venous access
- Prepare for cesarean birth

Signs of DIC
- Report immediately
- Anticipate orders to correct underlying cause

Fig. 31-7 Bleeding during late pregnancy. *CBC,* Complete blood count; *IV,* intravenous.

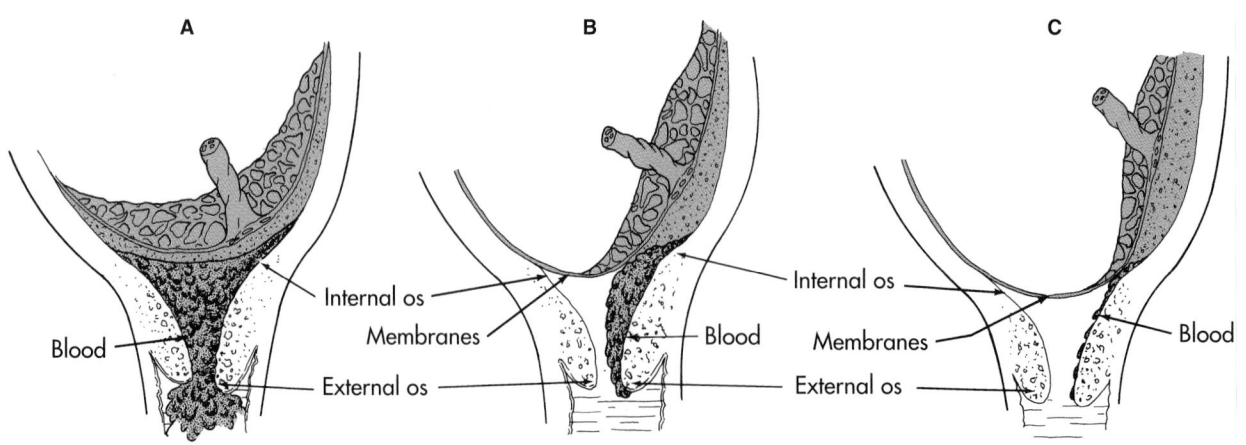

Fig. 31-8 Types of placenta previa after onset of labor. **A,** Complete, or total. **B,** Incomplete, or partial. **C,** Marginal, or low lying.

previous placenta previa, previous cesarean birth, and induced abortion, possibly related to endometrial scarring (Ananth et al., 1997). The risk also increases with multiple gestation (because of the larger placental area), closely spaced pregnancies, advanced maternal age (older than 35 years), African or Asian ethnicity, smoking, and cocaine use (Clark, 1999).

Clinical Manifestations

About 70% of women with placenta previa have painless vaginal bleeding; 20% have vaginal bleeding associated with uterine activity. Previa should be suspected whenever vaginal bleeding occurs after 24 weeks of gestation. This bleeding is associated with the stretching and thinning of the lower uterine segment that occurs during the third trimester. Placental attachment is gradually disrupted and bleeding occurs when the uterus is not able to adequately contract and stop blood flow from open vessels (Benedetti, 1996). The initial bleeding is usually a small amount and stops as clots form; however, it can recur at any time (Table 31-3). It is bright red in color.

Vital signs may be normal, even with heavy blood loss, because a pregnant woman can lose up to 40% of blood volume without showing signs of shock. Clinical presentation and decreasing urinary output may be better indicators of acute blood loss than vital signs alone. The fetal heart rate will be reassuring unless there is a major detachment of the placenta (Gilbert & Harmon, 1998).

Abdominal examination usually reveals a soft, relaxed, nontender uterus with normal tone. If the fetus is lying

TABLE 31-3 Summary of Findings: Abruptio Placentae and Placenta Previa

	ABRUPTIO PLACENTAE			
	GRADE 1 MILD SEPARATION (10% TO 20%)	GRADE 2 MODERATE SEPARATION (20% TO 50%)	GRADE 3 SEVERE SEPARATION (>50%)	PLACENTA PREVIA
Bleeding, external, vaginal	Minimal	Absent or moderate	Absent to moderate	Minimal to severe and life-threatening
Total amount of blood loss	<500 ml	1000-1500 ml	>1500 ml	Varies
Color of blood	Dark red	Dark red	Dark red	Bright red
Shock	Rare; none	Mild shock	Common, often sudden, profound	Uncommon
Coagulopathy	Rare, none	Occasional DIC	Frequent DIC	None
Uterine tonicity	Normal	Increased, may be localized to one region or diffuse over uterus, uterus fails to relax between contractions	Tetanic, persistent uterine contraction, boardlike uterus	Normal
Tenderness (pain)	Usually absent	Present	Agonizing, unremitting uterine pain	Absent
Ultrasonographic findings				
Location of placenta	Normal, upper uterine segment	Normal, upper uterine segment	Normal, upper uterine segment	Abnormal, lower uterine segment
Station of presenting part	Variable to engaged	Variable to engaged	Variable to engaged	High, not engaged
Fetal position	Usual distribution*	Usual distribution*	Usual distribution*	Commonly transverse, breech, or oblique
Pregnancy-induced or chronic hypertension	Usual distribution*	Commonly present	Commonly present	Usual distribution*
Fetal effects	Normal fetal heart rate pattern	Nonreassuring fetal heart rate pattern	Nonreassuring fetal heart rate pattern, death can occur	Normal fetal heart rate pattern

Usual distribution refers to the usual variations of incidence seen when there is no concurrent problem.

longitudinally, the fundal height is usually greater than expected for gestational age because the low placenta hinders descent of the presenting fetal part. Leopold's maneuvers may reveal a fetus in an oblique or breech position or lying transverse because of the abnormal site of placental implantation.

Diagnosis and Medical Management

The standard for the diagnosis of placenta previa is a transabdominal ultrasonographic examination. This study is accurate 93% to 97% of the time, with false-negative and false-positive results occurring as a result of factors such as an engaged cephalic presentation, a posteriorly implanted placenta, maternal obesity, and compression of the lower uterine segment by an overdistended bladder. Transvaginal ultrasound is also used for placental location, particularly when the exact relationship of the lower placental margin to the internal os is not clearly seen with transabdominal examination (Clark, 1999). If ultrasonographic scanning reveals a normally implanted placenta, a speculum examination is performed to rule out local causes of bleeding (e.g., cervicitis, polyps, or carcinoma of the cervix), and a coagulation profile is obtained to rule out other causes of bleeding. If expectant management is to be implemented, a vaginal speculum examination by the health care provider is postponed until fetal viability has been reached (preferably after 34 weeks of gestation). If a pelvic examination is needed before that time, anticipate the possibility that an immediate cesarean birth may be required. The woman is taken to a delivery or operating room set up for cesarean birth because profound hemorrhage can occur during the examination. This type of vaginal examination, known as the double-setup procedure, is not done often.

Management of placenta previa includes expectant management and cesarean birth depending on the gestational age of the fetus and the amount of bleeding present. Expectant management (observation and bed rest) is usually implemented when the fetus is not mature. Women may be placed in the hospital for complete bed rest, or this care may be managed at home. If a woman is bleeding, she is usually placed in the labor and birth unit where she and the fetus can be closely monitored.

If the woman's condition stabilizes and the fetus is less than 36 weeks of gestation, the woman may remain in the hospital for bed rest with bathroom privileges and perhaps limited activity (e.g., rides in a wheelchair). Ultrasonographic examinations are done every 2 to 3 weeks. Fetal surveillance may include nonstress testing (NST) or a biophysical profile once or twice a week. Outpatient management (home care) is a possibility if the woman lives close to the hospital, has transportation available, and understands the risks and the need to follow medical advice with respect to activities (Lowdermilk & Grohar, 1999).

If the fetus is 36 weeks of gestation or more, if the bleeding continues, or if labor begins, a cesarean birth is usually performed. Ideally the cesarean is performed after fetal maturity is determined (as with lecithin-sphingomyelin ratio of 2:1 or positive phosphatidylglycerol result on amniocentesis), but an emergency cesarean birth may be necessary at any time.

Vaginal birth is usually not performed unless the placenta previa is minor. If vaginal birth is attempted, the nurse caring for the woman should be aware of the possibility of acute hemorrhage, necessitating an emergency cesarean procedure.

Blood loss may not cease with the birth of the infant. The large vascular channels in the lower uterine segment may continue to bleed because of that segment's diminished muscle content. The natural mechanism to control bleeding so characteristic of the upper part of the uterus—the interlacing muscle bundles, the "living ligature" contracting around open vessels—is absent in the lower part of the uterus. Postpartum hemorrhage may therefore occur even if the fundus is contracted firmly. If uterine bleeding cannot be controlled with oxytocic drugs, ligation of the hypogastric (internal iliac) arteries or even hysterectomy may be necessary.

Hypovolemia must be treated without overtransfusion or overinfusion. Precise control of blood and fluid replacement may necessitate continuous hemodynamic monitoring (see Chapter 34).

Maternal and Fetal Outcome

Maternal morbidity is about 5% and mortality is less than 1% with placenta previa (Clark, 1999). Complications associated with placenta previa include preterm ROM, preterm birth, surgery-related trauma to structures adjacent to the uterus, anesthesia complications, blood transfusion reactions, overinfusion of fluids, other placental problems, postpartum hemorrhage, anemia, and infection.

The greatest risk of fetal mortality is caused by preterm birth. Other fetal risks include malpresentation and congenital anomalies (Gilbert & Harmon, 1998). Infants who are small for gestational age or have intrauterine growth restriction also have been associated with placenta previa; this association may be related to poor placental exchange or hypovolemia resulting from maternal blood loss and maternal anemia (Clark, 1999).

▪ CARE MANAGEMENT
Assessment and Nursing Diagnoses

A woman with third-trimester vaginal bleeding requires immediate evaluation. Necessary history data include gravidity, parity, estimated date of birth, general status, bleeding (quantity, precipitating event, associated pain), vital signs, and fetal status. Abdominal assessment reveals a soft, relaxed, nontender uterus with normal tone. Laboratory studies include a complete blood cell count, determination of blood type and Rh factor, coagulation profile, and possible type and crossmatch.

Potential nursing diagnoses for the woman with a placenta previa are listed below:

▪ Nursing Diagnoses

- Decreased cardiac output related to
  - excessive blood loss secondary to placenta previa
- Fluid volume deficit related to
  - excessive blood loss secondary to placenta previa
- Risk for fluid volume excess related to
  - fluid resuscitation
- Altered peripheral tissue perfusion related to
  - hypovolemia and shunting of blood to central circulation
- Risk for injury (fetal) related to
  - decreased placental perfusion secondary to placenta previa
- Anxiety/fear related to
  - maternal condition and pregnancy outcome
- Knowledge deficit related to
  - hospitalization and treatment regimens
- Altered family processes related to
  - mother's condition and hospitalization
- Anticipatory grieving related to
  - actual/perceived threat to self, pregnancy, or infant
- Risk for infection related to
  - anemia, hemorrhage, placenta previa, and transfusions
- Risk for injury (mother) related to
  - invasive monitoring procedures and treatment

Expected Outcomes of Care

Expected outcomes for the woman experiencing placenta previa may include the following. The woman will:
- Verbalize understanding of her condition and its management.
- Identify and use available support systems.
- Demonstrate compliance with prescribed activity limitations.
- Develop no complications related to bleeding.
- Carry the pregnancy to term or near term.
- Give birth to a healthy infant.

Plan of Care and Interventions

Hospital Care

Active management. Once placenta previa has been diagnosed, a management plan is developed based on gestational age, amount of bleeding, and fetal condition. If the woman is at term (greater than or equal to 37 weeks of gestation) and in labor or bleeding persistently, immediate delivery by cesarean is almost always indicated. In women with partial or marginal previas who have minimal bleeding, vaginal birth may be attempted. Vaginal birth may

also be indicated for previable gestations or births involving intrauterine fetal demise (Benedetti, 1996).

If cesarean birth is undertaken, the nurse continuously assesses maternal and fetal status while preparing the woman for surgery. Maternal vital signs are assessed frequently for decreasing blood pressure, rising pulse rate, changes in level of consciousness (LOC), and oliguria. Fetal assessment is maintained by continuous electronic fetal monitoring to assess for signs of hypoxia.

Emotional support for the woman and her family is extremely important. The actively bleeding woman is concerned not only for her own well-being but for the well-being of her fetus. All procedures should be explained, and a support person should be present. The woman should be encouraged to express her concerns and feelings. If the woman and her support person or family desire pastoral support, the nurse can notify the hospital chaplain service or provide information about other supportive resources.

Expectant management. If the woman is less than 36 weeks of gestation, not in labor, and the bleeding is mild or has stopped, expectant management is generally the treatment of choice to give the fetus time to mature in utero.

Expectant management consists of rest and close observation. The woman is usually placed on bed rest, although she may be allowed bathroom privileges and limited activity (up in a wheelchair for an hour or so daily). Bleeding is assessed by checking the amount of bleeding on perineal pads, bed pads, and linens. Weighing pads, although not often used, is one way to more accurately assess blood loss: 1 g represents 1 ml blood.

Ultrasonographic examinations may be done every 2 to 3 weeks. Fetal surveillance may include nonstress testing or biophysical profiles once or twice weekly. Serial laboratory values are evaluated for falling hemoglobin and hematocrit levels and changes in coagulation values. Venous access with an IV infusion or heparin lock may be placed in case blood or blood component therapy is needed. Antepartum steroids (betamethasone) may be ordered to promote fetal lung maturity if the woman is less than 34 weeks of gestation.

No vaginal or rectal examinations are performed, and the woman is placed on pelvic rest (nothing in the vagina). Once she reaches 37 weeks of gestation and fetal lung maturity is documented, cesarean birth can be scheduled. During her hospitalization, the woman with placenta previa should always be considered a potential emergency because massive blood loss with resulting hypovolemic shock can occur quickly if bleeding resumes. The possibility that she may require an emergency cesarean for birth always exists. Placenta previa in a preterm gestation may be an indication for transfer to a tertiary perinatal center because many community hospitals are not equipped to perform emergency cesarean births 24 hours per day, 7 days per week.

Home Care

Criteria for home care management vary among primary perinatal providers and home care agencies and are usually determined on a case-by-case basis. To be considered for home care referral, the woman must be in stable condition with no evidence of active bleeding and must have resources to be able to return to the hospital immediately if active bleeding resumes (Lowdermilk & Grohar, 1999).

She must have close supervision by family or friends in the home. The woman should be taught how to assess fetal and uterine activity and bleeding and told to avoid intercourse, douching, and enemas. She should limit her activities according to the advice of her physician and be advised to keep all appointments for fetal testing, laboratory assessments, and prenatal care. Visits by a perinatal home care nurse may be arranged (Lowdermilk & Grohar, 1999).

If hospitalization or home care with activity restriction is prolonged, the woman may have concerns about her work- or family-related responsibilities or may become bored with inactivity. She should be encouraged to participate in her own care and decisions about care as much as possible. Provision of diversionary activities or encourage-

---

PLAN OF CARE | Placenta Previa

NURSING DIAGNOSIS Decreased cardiac output related to bleeding secondary to placenta previa

Expected Outcome *Client will exhibit signs of increased blood volume and restoration of cardiac output (i.e., normal pulse and blood pressure; normal heart and breath sounds; normal skin color, tone, and turgor; normal capillary refill).*

Nursing Interventions/*Rationales*

Palpate uterus for tenderness and tone; assess bleeding rate, amount, color, degree of bleeding, CBC values, and coagulation profile *to determine severity of situation.* Do not perform vaginal examination *because it may stimulate further bleeding.*

Establish baseline data for cardiac output (vital signs; heart and breath sounds; skin color, tone, turgor; capillary refill; level of consciousness; urinary output; pulse oximetry) *to use as basis for evaluating effectiveness of treatment.*

Initiate intravenous therapy or blood transfusions and medications per physician order *to restore blood volume and prevent organ compromise to mother and fetus.*

Place woman on bed rest *to decrease oxygen demands.*

Monitor vital signs, intake and output, hemodynamic status, and laboratory values *to evaluate treatment response.*

Provide emotional support to woman and her family (e.g., explain procedures and their rationale; explain what is happening and what to expect; keep support person present) *to allay fears and provide the family with some sense of control.*

After stabilization, teach woman home management, including bed rest, watching for spotting/bleeding, close follow-up with her health care provider, and preparation for immediate return to hospital if needed *to prevent or stem further complications.*

NURSING DIAGNOSIS Risk for injury to the fetus related to decreased uterine/placental perfusion secondary to bleeding

Expected Outcome *Client will exhibit ongoing signs of fetal well-being (i.e., adequate fetal movement, normal fetal heart rate, reactive NST, normal biophysical profile [BPP]).*

Nursing Interventions/*Rationales*

Monitor fetus daily for signs of tachycardia, decreased movement, loss of reactivity on NST *to identify and treat changes in fetal status early.*

Obtain BPP per physician order to assess for signs of chronic asphyxia.

Maintain maternal side-lying position *to prevent compression of aorta and vena cava.*

NURSING DIAGNOSIS Risk for infection related to anemia and bleeding secondary to placenta previa

Expected Outcome *Client will show no signs of intrauterine infection.*

Nursing Interventions/*Rationales*

Monitor vital signs for elevated temperature, pulse, and blood pressure; monitor laboratory results for elevated white blood cell count, differential shift; check for uterine tenderness and malodorous vaginal discharge *to detect early signs of infection resulting from exposure of placental tissue.*

Provide/teach perineal hygiene *to decrease the risk of ascending infection.*

From Wong, D., & Perry, S. (1998). *Maternal child nursing care.* St. Louis: Mosby.

ment to participate in activities she enjoys and can do during bed rest is needed (see suggestions for activities in the box on p. 970).

Evaluation

The expected outcomes of care are used to evaluate the care for the woman with placenta previa (see Plan of Care).

Premature Separation of Placenta

Premature separation of the placenta, also termed **abruptio placentae,** is the detachment of part or all of the placenta from its implantation site (Fig. 31-9). Separation occurs in the area of the decidua basalis after 20 weeks of pregnancy and before the birth of the baby.

Incidence and Etiology

Premature separation of the placenta is a serious event that accounts for significant maternal and fetal morbidity and mortality. Current literature reports that 1% of all pregnancies are complicated by abruption. Approximately 10% of cases of abruption are severe enough to threaten fetal viability (Hunter & Weiner, 1996), and premature separation of the placenta accounts for about 15% of all perinatal deaths. Approximately one third of infants born to women with premature separation of the placenta die. More than 50% of these deaths are the result of preterm birth; many others are the result of intrauterine hypoxia.

Maternal hypertension is probably the most consistently identified risk factor for abruption (Benedetti, 1996). Cocaine is also a risk factor, which is likely in part because cocaine use is associated with the development of hypertension (Abu-Heija, al-Chalabi, & el-Iloubani, 1998). Blunt external abdominal trauma, most often the result of motor vehicle accidents or maternal battering, is an increasingly significant cause of placental abruption (Benedetti, 1996). Maternal smoking and poor nutrition

may be associated with an increased risk (Kramer et al., 1997). In the past, advanced maternal age and parity, short umbilical cord, and folic acid deficiency were all thought to cause increased risk; however, more recent research has failed to confirm this (Benedetti, 1996). There is a significant (5% to 17%) recurrence risk for placental abruption. A woman who has had two previous premature separations has a recurrence risk of 25% in the next pregnancy (Benedetti, 1996).

Classification Systems

The most common classification of placental abruption is according to type and severity. This classification system grades an abruption as follows (Clark, 1999; Hunter & Weiner, 1996).

Grade I. The woman has vaginal bleeding perhaps with uterine tenderness and mild tetany, but neither mother nor baby is in distress. Approximately 10% to 20% of the total placental surface area is detached.

Grade 2. The woman has uterine tenderness and tetany, with or without external evidence of bleeding. The mother is not in shock, but there is fetal distress. Approximately 20% to 50% of the total surface area is detached.

Grade 3. Uterine tetany is severe, the woman is in shock (although the bleeding may not be obvious), and the fetus is dead. Often the woman has coagulopathy. Greater than 50% of the placental surface area detaches (Gilbert & Harmon, 1998).

These grades are often classified as mild (grade 1), moderate (grade 2), and severe (grade 3) (Hunter & Weiner, 1996).

Clinical Manifestations

The separation may be partial or complete, or only the margin of the placenta may be involved. Bleeding from the placental site may dissect (separate) the membranes

Abruptio placentae (premature separation)

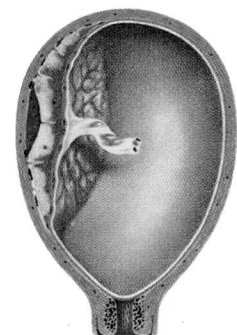
Partial separation
(concealed hemorrhage)

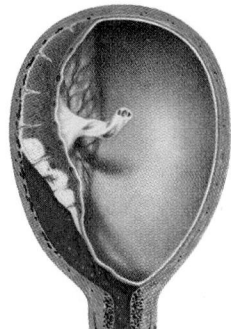
Partial separation
(apparent hemorrhage)

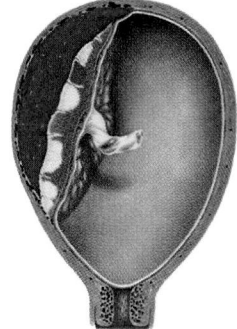
Complete separation
(concealed hemorrhage)

Fig. 31-9 Abruptio placentae. Premature separation of normally implanted placenta.

from the decidua basalis and flow out through the vagina, it may remain concealed (retroplacental hemorrhage), or it may do both (see Fig. 31-9). Clinical symptoms vary with degree of separation (see Table 31-3).

Classically, abruptio placentae is seen with vaginal bleeding, abdominal pain, and uterine tenderness and contractions. Vaginal bleeding is present in as many as 70% to 80% of women with abruption (Clark, 1999). It should be remembered that although abdominal pain and uterine tenderness are characteristic for this complication, either finding may be absent in the presence of a silent abruption (Konje & Walley, 1995). Bleeding may result in maternal hypovolemia (shock, oliguria, anuria) and coagulopathy. Mild to severe uterine hypertonicity is present. Pain is mild to severe and localized over one region of the uterus or diffuse over the uterus with a boardlike abdomen.

Extensive myometrial bleeding damages the uterine muscle. If blood accumulates between the separated placenta and the uterine wall, it may produce a **Couvelaire uterus.** The uterus appears purplish and copper colored, it is ecchymotic, and contractility is lost. Shock may occur and is out of proportion to blood loss. Laboratory findings include a positive Apt test result (blood in amniotic fluid); a drop in hemoglobin and hematocrit levels (which may appear later); and a drop in coagulation factor levels. Clotting defects (e.g., disseminated intravascular coagulation [DIC]) develop in 10% to 30% of clients (most within 8 hours of hospital admission), as does increased clot retraction. A Kleihauer-Betke stain may be ordered to determine the presence of fetal-to-maternal bleeding (transplacental hemorrhage).

Maternal, fetal, and neonatal outcomes. The maternal mortality rate approaches 1% for abruptio placentae; this condition remains a leading cause of maternal death. The mother's prognosis depends on the extent of placental detachment, overall blood loss, degree of DIC, and time between placental detachment and birth.

Maternal complications are associated with the abruption or its treatment. Hemorrhage, hypovolemic shock, hypofibrinogenemia, and thrombocytopenia are associated with severe abruption. Couvelaire uterus, DIC, and infection may occur. Renal failure and pituitary necrosis (Sheehan syndrome) may result from ischemia. In rare cases, women who are Rh negative can become sensitized if fetal-to-maternal hemorrhage occurs and the fetal blood type is Rh positive.

Perinatal mortality rates range from 15% to 30%, and mortality occurs as a result of fetal hypoxia, preterm birth, and status as small for gestational age. Risks of neurologic defects are increased (Cunningham et al., 1997).

Collaborative Care

Abruptio placentae should be strongly suspected in the woman who has a sudden onset of intense, usually localized, uterine pain, with or without vaginal bleeding. Initial assessment is much the same as for placenta previa. Physical examination usually reveals abdominal pain, uterine tenderness, and contractions. The fundal height may be measured over time, because increasing fundal height indicates concealed bleeding. Vaginal bleeding is present in about 80% of cases (Benedetti, 1996). Approximately 60% of live fetuses exhibit nonreassuring signs on the electronic fetal heart monitor, such as loss of variability and late decelerations; uterine hyperstimulation and increased resting tone may also be noted on the monitor tracing (Benedetti, 1996). Many women demonstrate coagulopathy, as evidenced by abnormal clotting studies (fibrinogen, platelet count, prothrombin time [PT], partial thromboplastin time [PTT], fibrin split products). Sonographic examination is used to rule out placenta previa; however, it is not always diagnostic for abruption. A retroplacental mass may be detected by ultrasonographic examination, but negative findings do not rule out a life-threatening abruption (Clark, 1999; Cunningham et al., 1997). Better imaging technology has made it possible to demonstrate ultrasonographic evidence of hemorrhage in more than 50% of cases of confirmed placental abruption (Benedetti, 1996).

Nursing diagnoses and expected outcomes of care are similar to those described for placenta previa.

Hospital care. Once abruption has been diagnosed, a management plan is developed. Treatment depends on the severity of blood loss and fetal maturity and status. If the abruption is mild and the fetus is less than 36 weeks of gestation and not in distress, expectant management may be implemented. The woman is hospitalized and observed closely for signs of bleeding and labor. The fetal status is also monitored with intermittent fetal heart rate monitoring and NST or biophysical profiles until fetal maturity is determined or until the woman's condition deteriorates and immediate birth is indicated. Use of corticosteroids to accelerate fetal lung maturity is appropriately included in the plan of care for expectant management (ACOG, 1994; Hunter & Weiner, 1996). Women who are Rh negative may be given Rh$_0$(D) immune globulin if fetal-to-maternal hemorrhage occurs and the fetal blood is Rh positive.

Delivery is the treatment of choice if the fetus is at term gestation or if the bleeding is moderate to severe and mother or fetus is in jeopardy. At least one large-bore (16-gauge) intravenous line should be started. Maternal vital signs are monitored frequently to observe for signs of declining hemodynamic status, such as increasing pulse rate and decreasing blood pressure. Serial laboratory studies include hematocrit or hemoglobin determinations and clotting studies. Continuous electronic fetal monitoring is mandatory. An indwelling Foley catheter is inserted for continuous assessment of urine output, an excellent indirect measure of maternal organ perfusion (Benedetti, 1996).

Blood and fluid volume replacement will most likely be ordered, with a goal of maintaining the urine output at greater than or equal to 30 ml/hr and the hematocrit at greater than or equal to 30%. If this goal is not reached despite vigorous attempts at replacement, hemodynamic monitoring may be necessary (Benedetti, 1996). Fresh frozen plasma or cryoprecipitate may be given to maintain the fibrinogen level at a minimum of 100 to 150 mg/dl.

Vaginal birth is usually feasible and is especially desirable in cases of fetal demise. Cesarean birth should be reserved for cases of fetal distress or other obstetric indications. Cesarean birth should not be attempted when the woman has severe and uncorrected coagulopathy because it may result in surgically uncontrollable bleeding (Benedetti, 1996).

Nursing care of clients experiencing moderate-to-severe abruption is demanding because it requires meticulous assessment of maternal and fetal condition, as described previously. Information about abruptio placentae, including cause, treatment, and expected outcome, is given to the woman and her family. Emotional support is also extremely important because the woman and her family may be experiencing fetal loss in addition to the mother's critical illness.

Home care. Women with abruptio placentae are usually not managed out of the hospital because the placenta can separate further at any time and immediate intervention or delivery may be necessary.

Cord Insertion and Placental Variations

Velamentous insertion of the cord is a rare placental anomaly associated with placenta previa and multiple gestation. The cord vessels begin to branch at the membranes and then course onto the placenta (Fig. 31-10, *A*). ROM or traction on the cord may tear one or more of the fetal vessels. As a result the fetus may rapidly bleed to death. Battledore (marginal) (Fig. 31-10, *B*) insertion of the cord increases the risk of fetal hemorrhage, especially after marginal separation of the placenta.

Rarely, the placenta may be divided into two or more separate lobes, resulting in **succenturiate placenta** (Fig. 31-10, *C*). Each lobe has a distinct circulation; the vessels collect at the periphery, and the main trunks eventually unite to form the vessels of the cord. Blood vessels joining the lobes may be supported only by the fetal membranes and are therefore in danger of tearing during labor, birth, or expulsion of the placenta. During recovery of the placenta, one or more of the separate lobes may remain attached to the decidua basalis, preventing uterine contraction and increasing the risk of postpartum hemorrhage.

Clotting Disorders in Pregnancy

Normal Clotting

Normally, there is a delicate balance (homeostasis) between the opposing hemostatic and fibrinolytic systems. The hemostatic system is involved in the lifesaving

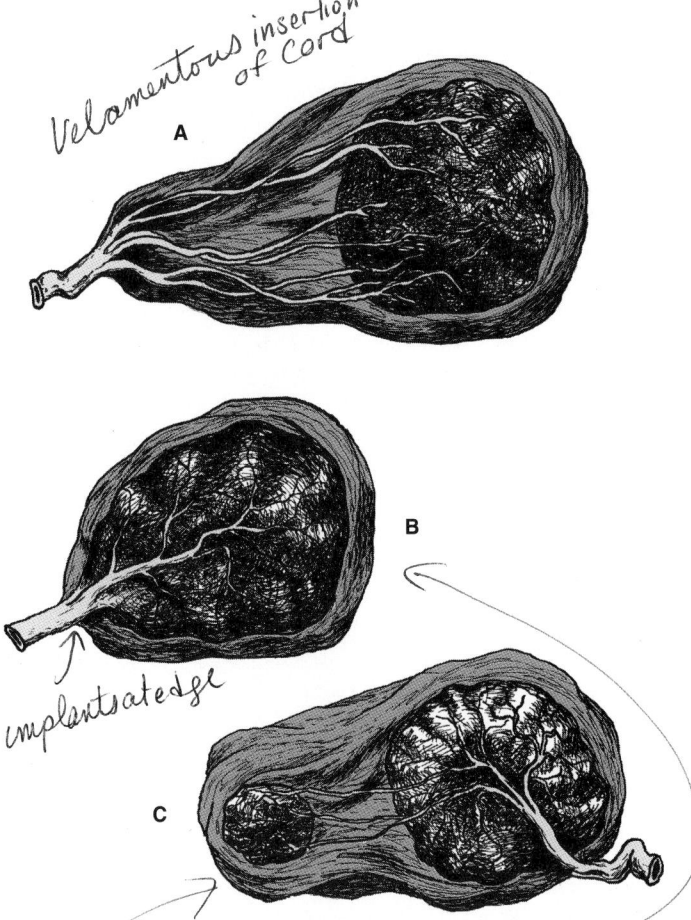

Fig. 31-10 Cord insertion and placental variations. **A,** Velamentous insertion of cord. **B,** Battledore placenta. **C,** Placenta succenturiate.

process. This system stops the flow of blood from injured vessels, in part through the formation of insoluble fibrin, which acts as a hemostatic platelet plug. The phases of the coagulation process involve an interaction of the coagulation factors in which each factor sequentially activates the factor next in line, the "cascade effect" sequence. The fibrinolytic system is the process through which the fibrin is split into fibrinolytic degradation products and circulation is restored.

Clotting Problems

A history of abnormal bleeding, inheritance of unusual bleeding tendencies, and a report of significant aberrations of laboratory findings indicate a bleeding or clotting problem. For the pregnant woman, bleeding disorders are suspected if the woman has pregnancy-induced hypertension, HELLP syndrome, retained dead fetus syndrome, amniotic fluid embolism, sepsis, or hemorrhage. Determination of hemostasis is made by testing the usual mechanisms for the control of bleeding, the function of platelets, and the necessary clotting factors.

Disseminated intravascular coagulation. **Disseminated intravascular coagulation** is a pathologic form of clotting that is diffuse and consumes large amounts of clotting factors, causing widespread external bleeding, internal bleeding, or both. DIC is an overactivation of the clotting cascade and the fibrinolytic system that results in depletion of platelets and clotting factors. This results in the formation of multiple fibrin clots throughout the body's vasculature, even in the microcirculation. Blood cells are destroyed as they pass through these fibrin-choked vessels. Thus DIC results in a clinical picture of hemorrhage, anemia, and ischemia.

It is important to understand that DIC is always a secondary diagnosis. In the obstetric population, DIC is most often triggered by the release of large amounts of tissue thromboplastin, which occurs, for example, in abruptio placentae, retained dead fetus, and amniotic fluid embolus. Severe preeclampsia, HELLP syndrome, and gram-negative sepsis are examples of conditions that can also trigger DIC because of widespread damage to vascular integrity.

Medical management. The diagnosis of DIC is made according to clinical findings and laboratory markers. Physical examination reveals unusual bleeding; spontaneous bleeding from the woman's gums or nose may be noted. Petechiae may appear around a blood pressure cuff placed on the woman's arm. Excessive bleeding may occur from the site of a slight trauma (e.g., venipuncture sites, intramuscular or subcutaneous injection sites, and injury from insertion of urinary catheter). Maternal symptoms may include tachycardia and diaphoresis.

Laboratory assessment includes a battery of tests often termed *clotting studies.* These tests evaluate both the clotting and lysing systems and include PT, PTT, platelet count, fibrinogen level, and presence of fibrin split (or degradation) products. The clot retraction test, which is often performed when blood is drawn for clotting studies, provides a quick assessment of the body's ability to clot. Blood placed in a plain (red top) Vacutainer tube should form a solid clot within 10 minutes. A positive clot retraction test indicates a fibrinogen level of at least 100 mg/dl. The clot retraction test can assist in clinical decision making while awaiting the results of laboratory tests.

In DIC, usually all of the clotting studies are abnormal. Both the PT and PTT are prolonged. The platelet count and the fibrinogen level are decreased. Fibrin split products are present.

Primary management in all cases of DIC involves correction of the underlying cause, which may be removal of the dead fetus, treatment of existing infection or of preeclampsia or eclampsia, or removal of a placental abruption. Other treatment is aimed at supporting physiologic functioning and replacing essential factors faster than the body can consume them. Intravenous fluids are given to replace volume lost through severe bleeding. Packed red blood cells are administered to maintain enough circulating red blood cells to ensure tissue oxygenation. Fresh frozen plasma or cryoprecipitate is given to replace fibrinogen and coagulation factors. Platelets may also be administered.

Clotting studies are repeated every couple of hours to determine the effects of therapy on the coagulation process. The aim of replacement therapy is to maintain a urine output of greater than or equal to 30 ml/hr, a hematocrit of greater than or equal to 30%, a fibrinogen level of greater than or equal to 150 mg/dl, and a platelet count of greater than or equal to 100,000 cells/mm³ (Benedetti, 1996).

Nursing care. The nurse caring for the pregnant woman at risk for DIC must be aware of risk factors. Careful and thorough assessment is required, with particular attention to signs of bleeding (petechiae, oozing from injection sites, and hematuria). Because renal failure is one consequence of DIC, urinary output is carefully monitored, using an indwelling Foley catheter. Vital signs are assessed frequently.

The pregnant woman should be maintained in a side-lying tilt to maximize blood flow to the uterus. Oxygen may be administered through a tight-fitting rebreathing mask at 8 to 10 L/min, or per hospital protocol or physician order. Blood and blood products must be administered safely. Fetal assessments are done to identify fetal well-being.

The educational and emotional needs of the woman and her family must be recognized and supported. They need information about her condition and explanations of unfamiliar equipment and procedures and will most likely be very anxious about the health of mother and baby.

von Willebrand disease. von Willebrand disease, a type of hemophilia, is probably the most common of all hereditary bleeding disorders (Cunningham et al., 1997). It results from a factor VIII deficiency and platelet dysfunction that is transmitted as an incomplete autosomal dominant trait to both sexes. Although von Willebrand disease is rare, it is among the most common congenital clotting defects in American women of childbearing age. Symptoms include a familial bleeding tendency, previous bleeding episodes, prolonged bleeding time (the most important test), factor VIII deficiency (mild to moderate), and bleeding from mucous membranes. Factor VIII increases during pregnancy, and this increase may be sufficient to offset danger from hemorrhage during childbirth. von Willebrand disease is variable in its clinical course, severity, and laboratory values, so it is possible for this condition to go undetected throughout pregnancy until bleeding problems develop following birth. If the woman is known to have von Willebrand disease before labor, factor VIII levels should be monitored and cryoprecipitate given as needed to maintain activity at 40% of normal near term gestation (Benedetti, 1996) (see also Chapter 38).

KEY POINTS

- Blood loss during pregnancy should always be regarded as a warning sign until the cause is determined.

- Some miscarriages occur for unknown reasons, but fetal or placental maldevelopment and maternal factors account for many others.

- The type of spontaneous abortion or miscarriage directs care management.

- Ectopic pregnancy is a significant cause of maternal morbidity and mortality, even in developed countries.

- There are two distinctive types of hydatidiform mole, complete and partial.

- Premature separation of the placenta and placenta previa are differentiated by type of bleeding, uterine tonicity, and presence or absence of pain.

- Clotting disorders are associated with many obstetric complications.

CRITICAL THINKING EXERCISES

1 A 21-year-old woman is seen in the emergency department complaining of abdominal pain and nausea. Discuss immediate assessment, lab work, and differential diagnosis for this client. After diagnosis, 50 mg of methotrexate is ordered to be given to the woman intramuscularly. List discharge instructions for the woman receiving this medication.

2 You are assigned to a woman who has come into the labor unit with vaginal bleeding at 35 weeks of gestation. Abruptio placentae is suspected. You note on her admission history that the woman is a Jehovah's Witness and is against having any blood transfusions. Discuss different management strategies that the health care providers could implement that would consider the woman's beliefs.

3 Develop a teaching plan for a woman at 32 weeks of gestation who has a diagnosis of placenta previa and who is going to be managed at home. Include strategies and activities she can engage in to deal with her restricted activities, specifically pelvic rest.

References

Abu-Heija, A., al-Chalabi, H., & el-Iloubani, N. (1998). Abruptio placentae: Risk factors and perinatal outcome. *J Obstet Gynaecol Res* 24(2), 141-144.

American College of Obstetricians and Gynecologists. (1994). Antenatal cortecosteroid therapy for fetal maturation. *ACOG Tech Bull* No. 147. Washington, D.C.: ACOG.

American College of Obstetricians and Gynecologists. (1995). Early pregnancy loss. *ACOG Tech Bull* No. 212. Washington, D.C.: ACOG.

Ananth, C., Smulian, J., & Vintzileos, A. (1997). The association of placenta previa with history of cesarean delivery and abortion: A meta-analysis. *Obstet Gynecol* 177(5), 1071-1078.

Benedetti, T. (1996). Obstetric hemorrhage. In S. Gabbe, J. Niebyl, & J. Simpson (Eds.). *Obstetrics: Normal and problem pregnancies* (3rd ed.). New York: Churchill Livingstone.

Berkowitz, R. Goldstein, D., & Bernstein, M. (1996). Update on gestational trophoblastic disease. *Contemp Ob/Gyn* 40(4), 21-29.

Berman, M., DiSaia, P., & Brewster, W. (1999). Pelvic malignancy, gestational trophoblastic neoplasm, and nonpelvic malignancies. In R. Creasy & R. Resnik (Eds.). *Maternal-fetal medicine* (4th ed.). Philadelphia: W.B. Saunders.

Clark, S. (1999). Placenta previa and abruptio placenta. In R. Creasy & R. Resnik (Eds.). *Maternal-fetal medicine* (4th ed.). Philadelphia: W.B. Saunders.

Copeland, L., & Landon, M. (1996). Malignant diseases and pregnancy. In S. Gabbe, J. Niebyl, & J. Simpson (Eds.). *Obstetrics: Normal and problem pregnancies* (3rd ed.). New York: Churchill Livingstone.

Cunningham, F. et al. (1997). *Williams obstetrics* (20th ed.). Stamford, CT: Appleton & Lange.

DeLoia, J., Stewart-Akers, A., & Creinin, M. (1998). Effects of methotrexate on trophoblast proliferation and local immune responses. *Hum Reprod* 13(4), 1063-1069.

Flystra, D. (1998). Tubal pregnancy: A review of current diagnosis and treatment. *Obstet Gynecol Surv* 53(5), 320-328.

Freda, M. (1995). Arrest, trial, and failure. *J Obstet Gynecol Neonatal Nurs* 24(5), 393-394.

Freda, M. (1999). The power of words. *MCN Am J Matern Child Nurs* 24(2), 63.

Gilbert, E., & Harmon, J. (1998). *Manual of high risk pregnancy and delivery* (2nd ed.). St. Louis: Mosby.

Health Care Resources. (1997). *Handbook of high risk prenatal home care.* St. Louis: Mosby.

Hunter, S., & Weiner, C. (1996). Obstetric hemorrhage. In J. Repke (Ed.). *Intrapartum obstetrics.* New York: Churchill Livingstone.

Hutti, M. (1992). Parent's perceptions of the miscarriage experience. *Death Studies* 16(5), 401-415.

Iams, J. (1996). Preterm birth. In S. Gabbe, J. Niebyl, & J. Simpson (Eds.). *Obstetrics: Normal and problem pregnancies* (3rd ed.). New York: Churchill Livingstone.

Knuppel, R., & Hatangadi, S. (1995). Acute hypotension related to hemorrhage in the obstetric patient. *Obstet Gynecol Clin North Am* 22(1), 111-129.

Konje, J., & Walley, R. (1995). Bleeding in late pregnancy. In D. James et al. (Eds.). *High risk pregnancy: Management options.* Philadelphia: W.B. Saunders.

Koonin, L. et al. (1997). Pregnancy-related mortality surveillance—United States 1987-1990. *MMWR* 46(4), 17-36.

Kramer, M. et al. (1997). Etiologic determinants of abruptio placentae. *Obstet Gynecol* 89(2), 221-226.

Lipscomb, G. et al. (1998). Analysis of three hundred fifteen ectopic pregnancies treated with single-dose methotrexate. *Am J Obstet Gynecol* 178(6), 1354-1358.

Lowdermilk, D., & Grohar, J. (1999). *High risk antepartal home care.* White Plains, NY: March of Dimes.

Maiolatesi, C., & Petticord, K. (1996). Methotrexate for nonsurgical treatment of ectopic pregnancy: Nursing implications. *J Obstet Gynecol Neonatal Nurs* 25(2), 205-208.

Minnick-Smith, K., & Cook, F. (1997). Current treatment options for ectopic pregnancy. *MCN Am J Matern Child Nurs* 22(10), 21-25.

Powell, W., & Spellman, J. (1996). Medical management of the patient with an ectopic pregnancy. *J Perinat Neonatal Nurs* 9(4), 31-43.

Simpson, J. (1996). Fetal wastage. In S. Gabbe, J. Niebyl, & J. Simpson (Eds.). *Obstetrics: Normal and problem pregnancies* (3rd ed.). New York: Churchill Livingstone.

Thorp, J. (1993). Third-trimester bleeding. In T. Moore et al. (Eds.). *Gynecology and obstetrics: A longitudinal approach.* New York: Churchill Livingstone.

Wong, D., & Perry, S. (1998). *Maternal child nursing care.* St. Louis: Mosby.

Endocrine and Metabolic Disorders

Kitty Cashion

LEARNING OBJECTIVES

- Define the key terms.
- Differentiate the types of diabetes mellitus and their respective risk factors in pregnancy.
- Summarize the effects of pregnancy on insulin requirements.
- Discuss maternal and fetal risks or complications associated with diabetes in pregnancy.
- Discuss care management for the pregnant woman with pregestational or gestational diabetes.
- Discuss care management for the woman with hyperemesis gravidarum.
- Discuss care management for the woman with thyroid dysfunction.
- Describe the effects of maternal phenylketonuria on pregnancy outcome.
- Identify topics for nursing research related to diabetes in pregnancy and other endocrine disorders.

KEY TERMS

diabetes mellitus
euglycemia
gestational diabetes mellitus
glycosylated hemoglobin A1$_c$
hyperemesis gravidarum

hyperglycemia
hyperthyroidism
hypoglycemia
hypothyroidism
ketoacidosis

macrosomia
oral glucose tolerance test
phenylketonuria
pregestational diabetes mellitus

Endocrine and metabolic disorders, which often complicate pregnancy, require careful management to promote maternal and fetal well-being and a positive pregnancy outcome. Diabetes mellitus is the most common endocrine disorder associated with pregnancy. Hyperemesis gravidarum and disorders of the thyroid, although encountered less often, also require careful planning for care. Phenylketonuria, an inborn error of metabolism, is a relatively new disorder of women of reproductive age, and it has significant implications for pregnancy outcome.

Providing sound, effective nursing care that meets the unique maternal and fetal needs prompted by these endocrine and metabolic conditions can be challenging. The primary objective of nursing care must be to guide and support the woman and her family in achieving the optimal outcome for both the pregnant woman and the fetus. The nurse serves as teacher, counselor, and support person to assist the woman and her family in achieving the best possible outcome and to deal with the problems and disappointments that may arise.

DIABETES MELLITUS

Before the discovery of insulin in 1922, it was uncommon for a woman with diabetes to give birth to a healthy baby. Many women of childbearing age were infertile or sterile, and the majority of those who became pregnant were unable to carry a fetus to term. The perinatal mortality rate was approximately 65%, with stillbirth being the largest cause of fetal death (Landon, 1996).

Advances in medicine have greatly improved perinatal outcome. Today, the perinatal mortality rate for well-managed diabetic pregnancies, excluding major congenital malformations, is about the same as for any other pregnancy (Landon, 1996). The incidence of major congenital malformations in infants born to women with diabetes has not changed significantly over time. Experts have concluded that the key to an optimal pregnancy outcome is strict maternal glucose control before conception, as well as throughout the gestational period. Consequently, much emphasis is placed on preconceptional counseling for women with diabetes.

Despite the advances in care, pregnancy complicated by diabetes is still considered high risk. It is most successfully managed by a multidisciplinary approach involving the obstetrician, internist or diabetologist, neonatologist, nurse, nutritionist, and social worker. A favorable outcome of diabetic pregnancy requires commitment and active participation by the woman and her family. The woman must comply with a schedule of frequent prenatal visits, strict adherence to the dietary regimen, regular self-monitoring of her blood glucose level, frequent laboratory evaluation, intensive fetal surveillance, and possible hospitalization.

Care of the pregnant woman with diabetes requires that the nurse fully understand the normal physiologic responses to pregnancy and the altered metabolism of diabetes. Furthermore, the nurse must understand the relationship between pregnancy and diabetes, including psychosocial implications, to assess the woman accurately, plan for her care, and intervene appropriately.

Pathogenesis

Diabetes mellitus is a group of metabolic diseases characterized by hyperglycemia resulting from defects in insulin secretion, insulin action, or both (Expert Committee on the Diagnosis and Classification of Diabetes Mellitus, 1997). Insulin, produced by the beta cells in the islets of Langerhans in the pancreas, regulates blood glucose levels by enabling glucose to enter adipose and muscle cells, where it is used for energy. Insulin also stimulates protein synthesis and storage of free fatty acids. When insulin is insufficient or ineffective in promoting glucose uptake by the muscle and adipose cells, glucose accumulates in the bloodstream, and hyperglycemia results. Hyperglycemia causes hyperosmolarity of the blood, which attracts intracellular fluid into the vascular system, resulting in cellular dehydration and expanded blood volume. Consequently, the kidneys function to excrete large volumes of urine (polyuria) in an attempt to regulate excess vascular volume and to excrete the unusable glucose (glycosuria). Polyuria, along with cellular dehydration, causes excessive thirst (polydipsia).

The body compensates for its inability to convert carbohydrate (glucose) into energy by burning proteins (muscle) and fats. However, the end products of this metabolism are ketones and fatty acids, which, in excess quantities, produce ketoacidosis and acetonuria. Weight loss occurs as a result of the breakdown of fat and muscle tissue. This tissue breakdown causes a state of starvation that compels the individual to eat excessive amounts of food (polyphagia).

Over time, diabetes causes significant changes in both the microvascular and macrovascular circulations. These structural changes affect a variety of organ systems, particularly the heart, eyes, kidneys, and nerves. Complications resulting from diabetes include premature atherosclerosis, retinopathy, nephropathy, and neuropathy.

Diabetes may be caused by either impaired insulin secretion, when the beta cells of the pancreas are destroyed by an autoimmune process, or by inadequate insulin action in target tissues at one or more points along the metabolic pathway. Both of these conditions are frequently present in the same person, and it is unclear which, if either, abnormality is the primary cause of the disease (Expert Committee on the Diagnosis and Classification of Diabetes Mellitus, 1997).

Classification

The classification and diagnosis of diabetes have been revised by an international Expert Committee working under the sponsorship of the American Diabetes Association (ADA). The Expert Committee report, published in July 1997, recommended that the old classification system developed by the National Diabetes Data Group in 1979 be revised to reflect current knowledge of the disease. The revised classification system includes four groups: type 1 diabetes, type 2 diabetes, other specific types (e.g., diabetes caused by infection or drug-induced diabetes), and gestational diabetes mellitus. A major change proposed by the Expert Committee is a move away from a system that classifies the disease by its pharmacologic management to one based on disease etiology. Therefore the terms insulin-dependent diabetes mellitus and non–insulin-dependent diabetes mellitus have been eliminated (Expert Committee on the Diagnosis and Classification of Diabetes Mellitus, 1997).

Type 1 diabetes includes those cases that are primarily due to pancreatic islet beta cell destruction and that are prone to ketoacidosis. People with type 1 diabetes usually have an absolute insulin deficiency. Type 1 diabetes includes cases currently thought to be caused by an autoimmune process, as well as those for which the cause is unknown (Expert Committee on the Diagnosis and Classification of Diabetes Mellitus, 1997).

Type 2 diabetes is the most prevalent form of the disease and includes individuals who have insulin resistance and usually relative (rather than absolute) insulin deficiency. Specific etiologies for type 2 diabetes are unknown at this time. Type 2 diabetes often goes undiagnosed for years because hyperglycemia develops gradually and often is not severe enough for the person to recognize the classic signs of polyuria, polydipsia, and polyphagia. Many people who develop type 2 diabetes are obese or have an increased amount of body fat distributed primarily in the abdominal area. Other risk factors for the development of type 2 diabetes include aging, a sedentary lifestyle, hypertension, and prior gestational diabetes. Type 2 diabetes often has a strong genetic predisposition (Expert Committee on the Diagnosis and Classification of Diabetes Mellitus, 1997).

Pregestational diabetes mellitus is the label sometimes given to type 1 or type 2 diabetes that existed before pregnancy.

Gestational diabetes mellitus (GDM) is any degree of glucose intolerance with the onset or first recognition occurring during pregnancy. This definition is appropriate whether or not insulin is used for treatment or the diabetes persists after pregnancy. It does not exclude the possibility that the glucose intolerance preceded the pregnancy. Women experiencing gestational diabetes should be reclassified 6 weeks or more after the pregnancy ends (Expert Committee on the Diagnosis and Classification of Diabetes Mellitus, 1997).

Metabolic Changes Associated with Pregnancy

Normal pregnancy is characterized by complex alterations in maternal glucose metabolism, insulin production, and metabolic homeostasis. During normal pregnancy, adjustments in maternal metabolism allow for adequate nutrition for both the mother and the developing fetus. Glucose, the primary fuel used by the fetus, is transported across the placenta through the process of carrier-mediated facilitated diffusion. This means that the glucose levels in the fetus are directly proportional to maternal levels. Although glucose crosses the placenta, insulin does not. By the tenth week of gestation the embryo or fetus secretes its own insulin at levels adequate to use the glucose obtained from the mother. Thus as maternal glucose levels rise, fetal glucose levels are increased, resulting in increased fetal insulin secretion.

During the first trimester of pregnancy the pregnant woman's metabolic status is significantly influenced by the rising levels of estrogen and progesterone. These hormones stimulate the beta cells in the pancreas to increase insulin production, which promotes increased peripheral use of glucose and decreased blood glucose, with fasting levels being reduced by approximately 10% (Fig. 32-1, *A*). There is a concomitant increase in tissue glycogen stores and a decrease in hepatic glucose production, which further encourage lower fasting glucose levels. As a result of these normal metabolic changes of pregnancy, women who are diabetic and are insulin dependent are prone to hypoglycemia during the first trimester.

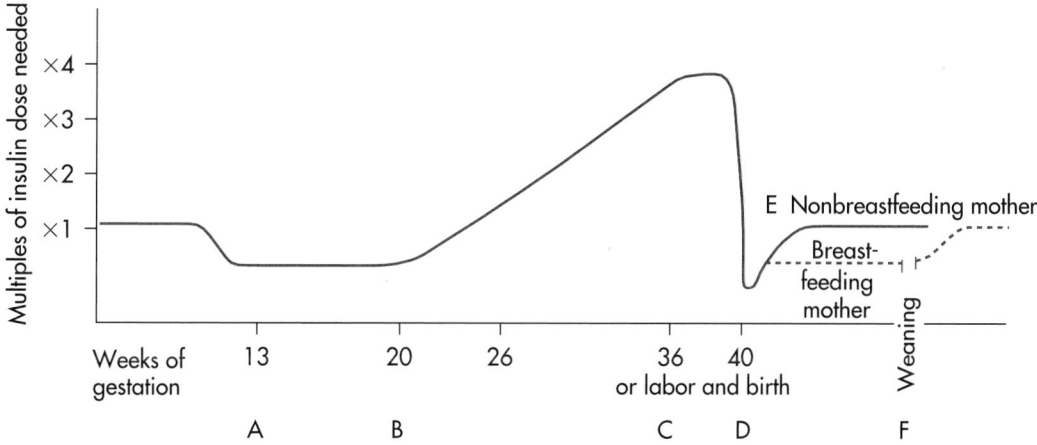

Fig. 32-1 Changing insulin needs during pregnancy. **A,** First trimester: insulin need is reduced because of increased insulin production by pancreas and increased peripheral sensitivity to insulin; nausea, vomiting, and decreased food intake by mother and glucose transfer to embryo or fetus contribute to hypoglycemia. **B,** Second trimester: insulin needs begin to increase as placental hormones, cortisol, and insulinase act as insulin antagonists, decreasing insulin's effectiveness. **C,** Third trimester: insulin needs may double or even quadruple but usually level off after 36 weeks of gestation. **D,** Day of birth: maternal insulin requirements drop drastically to approach prepregnancy levels. **E,** Breastfeeding mother maintains lower insulin requirements, as much as 25% less than prepregnancy; insulin needs of nonbreastfeeding mother return to prepregnancy levels in 7 to 10 days. **F,** Weaning of breastfeeding infant causes mother's insulin needs to return to prepregnancy levels.

During the second and third trimesters, pregnancy exerts a "diabetogenic" effect on the maternal metabolic status. Because of the major hormonal changes, there is a decreased tolerance to glucose, an increased insulin resistance, decreased hepatic glycogen stores, and an increased hepatic production of glucose. Rising levels of human placental lactogen, estrogen, progesterone, prolactin, cortisol, and insulinase increase insulin resistance through their actions as insulin antagonists. Insulin resistance is a glucose-sparing mechanism that ensures an abundant supply of glucose for the fetus. Maternal insulin requirements may double or quadruple by the end of the pregnancy, usually leveling off or declining slightly after 36 weeks (Fig. 32-1, *B* and *C*).

At birth, expulsion of the placenta prompts an abrupt drop in levels of circulating placental hormones, cortisol, and insulinase (Fig. 32-1, *D*). Maternal tissues quickly regain their prepregnancy sensitivity to insulin. For the nonbreast-feeding mother the prepregnancy insulin-carbohydrate balance usually returns in about 7 to 10 days (Fig. 32-1, *E*). Lactation uses maternal glucose; thus the breastfeeding mother's insulin requirements will remain low for up to 6 to 9 months. On completion of weaning, the prepregnancy insulin requirement is reestablished (Fig. 32-1, *F*).

Pregestational Diabetes Mellitus

Women who have pregestational diabetes may have either type 1 or type 2 diabetes, which may or may not be complicated by vascular disease, retinopathy, nephropathy, or other diabetic sequelae. Almost all women with pregestational diabetes are insulin dependent during pregnancy.

The diabetogenic state of pregnancy imposed on the compromised metabolic system of the woman with pregestational diabetes has significant implications. The normal hormonal adaptations of pregnancy affect glycemic control, and pregnancy may accelerate the progress of vascular complications.

During the first trimester, when maternal blood glucose levels are normally reduced and the insulin response to glucose is enhanced, glycemic control is improved. The insulin dosage for the woman with well-controlled diabetes may need to be reduced to avoid **hypoglycemia** (low blood glucose levels). There is an increased incidence of hypoglycemic episodes in those with type 1 diabetes during early pregnancy. Nausea, vomiting, and cravings typical of early pregnancy result in dietary fluctuations, which influence maternal glucose levels and necessitate a reduction in insulin dosage.

Because insulin requirements steadily increase after the first trimester, insulin dosage must be adjusted accordingly to prevent **hyperglycemia** (high blood glucose levels). Insulin resistance begins as early as 14 to 16 weeks and continues to rise until it stabilizes during the last few weeks of pregnancy.

In the past it was believed that pregnancy worsened microvascular complications. In fact, women who had diabetes and had vascular disease such as retinopathy or nephropathy were often encouraged to avoid or terminate pregnancy. With current management practices, however, women with vasculopathy other than coronary artery disease can achieve good pregnancy outcomes (Moore, 1999; Reece & Homko, 1994).

Diabetic nephropathy has more impact on perinatal outcome than any other vascular complication. Increased risks of preeclampsia, preterm labor, intrauterine growth restriction (IUGR), fetal distress, stillbirth, and neonatal death are associated with this condition (Moore, 1999).

Although neuropathic complications are common in type 1 and type 2 diabetes, little information exists about the effect of pregnancy on diabetic neuropathy. An autonomic neuropathy such as gastroparesis (e.g., anorexia, vomiting of undigested food, belching, early satiety, and weight loss) may affect diabetic control because of its effects on intake and absorption of adequate nutrition (Reece & Homko, 1993).

Preconceptional Counseling

Preconceptional counseling, which is recommended for all women of reproductive age with diabetes, is associated with an improved pregnancy outcome (Landon, 1996; Moore, 1999). Under ideal circumstances the pregestational diabetic woman is counseled before the time of conception to plan the optimal time for pregnancy, establish glycemic control before conception, and diagnose any vascular complications of diabetes. Unfortunately, it has been estimated that fewer than 20% of women with diabetes in the United States participate in preconceptional counseling (Landon, 1996).

The woman's partner should be included in the counseling to assess the couple's level of understanding related to the effects of pregnancy on the diabetic condition and of the potential complications of pregnancy as a result of diabetes. The couple should also be informed of the anticipated alterations in management of diabetes during pregnancy and the need for a multidisciplinary team approach to health care. Financial implications of diabetic pregnancy and other demands related to frequent maternal and fetal surveillance should be discussed. Contraception is another important aspect of preconceptional counseling to assist the couple in planning effectively for pregnancy.

Preconceptional counseling is particularly important because strict metabolic control before conception and in the early weeks of gestation is instrumental in decreasing the risk of congenital anomalies (Moore, 1999).

Some types of oral hypoglycemic agents (sulfonylureas such as tolbutamide) may have teratogenic effects on the fetus; they should be discontinued in the preconceptional period in women with type 2 diabetes (Hagay & Reece, 1999). These women are started on insulin before pregnancy when the pregnancy is planned, or as soon as the pregnancy is diagnosed when it is unplanned.

Maternal Risks and Complications

Although maternal morbidity and mortality rates have improved significantly, the pregnant woman with diabetes remains at risk for the development of complications during pregnancy. Research has repeatedly demonstrated that the best predictor of pregnancy outcome for the woman and her neonate is the degree of maternal glycemic control during pregnancy.

Poor glycemic control around the time of conception and in the early weeks of pregnancy is associated with an increased incidence of miscarriage in women with diabetes. Those women with good glycemic control before conception and in the first trimester are no more likely than women who do not have diabetes to have a miscarriage (Moore, 1999).

Poor glycemic control later in pregnancy, particularly in women without vascular disease, increases the rate of fetal macrosomia. Macrosomia occurs in 20% to 25% of diabetic pregnancies. These large infants tend to have a disproportionate increase in shoulder and trunk size. Because of this, the risk of shoulder dystocia is greater in these babies than in other macrosomic infants. Thus women with diabetes face an increased likelihood of cesarean birth because of failure to progress or descend, or operative vaginal birth (delivery using episiotomy, forceps, or vacuum extractor) (Landon, 1996; Moore, 1999).

Pregnancy-induced hypertension (PIH), or preeclampsia, occurs more frequently during diabetic pregnancy. The highest incidence occurs in women with preexisting vascular changes related to diabetes (Cunningham et al., 1997).

Hydramnios (polyhydramnios) occurs about 10 times more often in diabetic than in nondiabetic pregnancies. Hydramnios—amniotic fluid more than 2000 ml—increases the possibility of compression of maternal abdominal blood vessels (vena cava and aorta), causing supine hypotension. Maternal dyspnea may result from upward pressure on the diaphragm by the distended uterus. Premature rupture of membranes (PROM) and the onset of preterm labor are associated with hydramnios. Overdistention of the uterus caused by hydramnios may increase the incidence of postpartum hemorrhage.

Infections are more common and more serious in pregnant women with diabetes. Disorders of carbohydrate metabolism alter the body's normal resistance to infection. The inflammatory response, leukocyte function, and vaginal pH are all affected. Vaginal infections, particularly monilial vaginitis, are more common. Urinary tract infections (UTIs) are also more prevalent. Infection is serious because it causes increased insulin resistance and may result in ketoacidosis. Postpartum infection is more common among women who are insulin dependent.

Ketoacidosis occurs most often during the second and third trimesters, when the diabetogenic effect of pregnancy is the greatest. When the maternal metabolism is stressed by illness or infection, the woman is at increased

risk for diabetic ketoacidosis (DKA). The use of beta-sympathomimetic drugs (e.g., terbutaline [Brethine]) may also contribute to the risk for hyperglycemia and subsequent DKA (Hagay & Reece, 1999). DKA may also occur because of the woman's failure to take insulin appropriately. The onset of previously undiagnosed diabetes during pregnancy is another cause of DKA. DKA may occur with blood glucose levels barely exceeding 200 mg/dl, compared with 300 to 350 mg/dl in the nonpregnant state. In response to stress factors such as infection or illness, hyperglycemia occurs as a result of increased hepatic glucose production and decreased peripheral glucose use. Stress hormones, which act to impair insulin action and further contribute to insulin deficiency, are released. Fatty acids are mobilized from fat stores to enter into the circulation, and as they are oxidized, ketone bodies are released into the peripheral circulation. The woman's buffering system is unable to compensate, and metabolic acidosis develops. The excessive blood glucose and ketone bodies result in osmotic diuresis with subsequent loss of fluid and electrolytes, volume depletion, and cellular dehydration. Prompt treatment of DKA is necessary to prevent maternal coma and death. Ketoacidosis occurring at any time during pregnancy can lead to intrauterine fetal death and is also a cause of preterm labor. The perinatal mortality rate is about 20% with maternal ketoacidosis (Cunningham et al., 1997) (Table 32-1).

The risk of hypoglycemia is also increased. Early in pregnancy, when hepatic production of glucose is diminished and peripheral use of glucose is enhanced, hypoglycemia occurs frequently, often during sleep. Later in pregnancy, as insulin doses are adjusted to maintain normoglycemia, hypoglycemia may also result. Women with a prepregnancy history of severe hypoglycemia are at increased risk for severe hypoglycemia during gestation. Mild to moderate hypoglycemic episodes do not appear to have significant deleterious effects on fetal well-being. The long-term fetal effects of severe maternal hypoglycemia are as yet uncertain (Hagay & Reece, 1999) (see Table 32-1).

Fetal and Neonatal Risks and Complications

From the moment of conception, the infant of a woman with diabetes faces an increased risk of complications that may occur during the antepartum, intrapartum, and neonatal periods. These complications may be mild and transient but are often life-threatening and may result in the infant's death. Infant morbidity and mortality rates associated with diabetic pregnancy are significantly reduced with strict control of maternal glucose levels before and during pregnancy.

Despite the improvements in care of diabetic pregnancy, sudden and unexplained stillbirth is still a major concern. Typically, this is observed in pregnancies after 36 weeks in women with vascular disease or poor glycemic control. It may also be associated with DKA, preeclampsia, hydramnios, or macrosomia. Although the exact cause

TABLE 32-1 Differentiation of Hypoglycemia (Insulin Shock) and Hyperglycemia (Diabetic Ketoacidosis)

CAUSES	ONSET	SYMPTOMS	INTERVENTIONS
HYPOGLYCEMIA (INSULIN SHOCK)			
Excess insulin	Rapid (regular insulin)	Irritability	Check blood glucose level when
Insufficient food (delayed or missed meals)	Gradual (modified insulin or oral hypoglycemic agents)	Hunger	symptoms first appear
		Sweating	Eat or drink 10-15 g simple
		Nervousness	carbohydrate immediately
Excessive exercise or work		Personality change	Recheck blood glucose level in 15 min
		Weakness	and eat or drink another 10-15 g
Indigestion, diarrhea, vomiting		Fatigue	simple carbohydrate if glucose
		Blurred or double vision	remains low
		Dizziness	Recheck blood glucose level in 15 min
		Headache	Notify primary health care provider if
		Pallor; clammy skin	no change in glucose level
		Shallow respirations	If woman is unconscious, administer
		Rapid pulse	50% dextrose IV push, 5%-10%
		Laboratory values	dextrose in water IV drip, or
		Urine: negative for sugar and acetone	glucagon
		Blood glucose: ≤60 mg/dl	Obtain blood and urine specimens for laboratory testing
HYPERGLYCEMIA (DKA)			
Insufficient insulin	Slow (hours to days)	Thirst	Notify primary health care provider
Excess or wrong kind of food		Nausea or vomiting	Administer insulin in accordance with
		Abdominal pain	blood glucose levels
Infection, injuries, illness		Constipation	Give IV fluids such as normal saline
		Drowsiness	solution or one-half normal saline
Emotional stress		Dim vision	solution; potassium when urinary
Insufficient exercise		Increased urination	output is adequate; bicarbonate for
		Headache	pH <7
		Flushed, dry skin	Monitor lab testing of blood and urine
		Rapid breathing	
		Weak, rapid pulse	
		Acetone (fruity) breath odor	
		Laboratory values	
		Urine: positive for sugar and acetone	
		Blood glucose: ≥200 mg/dl	

of stillbirth is unknown, it may be related to chronic intrauterine hypoxia.

The most important cause of perinatal deaths in diabetic pregnancy is congenital anomalies. The incidence of congenital anomalies in infants born to diabetic women is 6% to 10%, a twofold to fivefold increase over that of the general population. Up to 40% of all perinatal deaths among infants of women with diabetes are caused by congenital malformations (Hagay & Reece, 1999). The incidence of congenital malformations is related to the severity and duration of the diabetes. In addition to hyperglycemia, hyperketonemia and hypoglycemia may also

play a role in the development of congenital anomalies (Landon, 1996). Cardiac defects are the most common anomalies seen, followed by central nervous system and skeletal defects (Hagay & Reece, 1999).

Macrosomia, excessive growth, is often defined as a weight of 4000 to 4500 g or greater. Macrosomia may also be defined as large for gestational age (LGA), wherein the fetus or newborn is bigger than 90% of similar babies the same age (Landon, 1996). The fetal pancreas begins to secrete insulin at 10 to 14 weeks of gestation. The fetus responds to maternal hyperglycemia by secreting large amounts of insulin (hyperinsulinism). Insulin acts as a growth hormone, causing the fetus to produce excess stores of glycogen, protein, and adipose tissue, leading to increased fetal size. During birth, the macrosomic infant is at risk for a fractured clavicle, liver or spleen laceration, brachial plexus injury, facial palsy, phrenic nerve injury, or subdural hemorrhage (Hagay & Reece, 1999; Moore, 1999) (see Chapter 39).

Intrauterine growth restriction is often seen in infants of women with diabetes with vascular disease. It is related to compromised uteroplacental circulation and may be worsened in the presence of ketoacidosis and preeclampsia. The amount of oxygen available to the fetus is decreased as a result of maternal vascular changes (Bernstein & Gabbe, 1996).

Infants are at increased risk for respiratory distress syndrome (RDS). Hyperglycemia and hyperinsulinemia may be instrumental in delaying pulmonary maturation in the fetus (Hagay & Reece, 1999).

For infants of a diabetic pregnancy the transition to extrauterine life is often beset with metabolic abnormalities. Within the first 30 to 60 minutes after birth, neonatal hypoglycemia often occurs. This is caused by the effects of fetal hyperinsulinism and the rapid use of glucose after birth. The incidence of neonatal hypoglycemia is related to the mother's glycemic control during pregnancy and to her glucose levels during labor and birth. Hypocalcemia, hypomagnesemia, hyperbilirubinemia, and polycythemia occur more frequently in infants of women with diabetes, which places these neonates at increased risk (Landon, 1996).

▪ CARE MANAGEMENT
Assessment and Nursing Diagnoses
Interview

When a pregnant woman with diabetes initiates prenatal care, a thorough evaluation of her health status is completed. In addition to the routine prenatal assessment, a detailed history regarding the onset and course of the diabetes and its management and the degree of glycemic control before pregnancy is obtained. Effective management of the diabetic pregnancy depends on the woman's adherence to a plan of care. For the woman to care for her diabetes on a daily basis, she must have an adequate understanding of her disease and the prescribed regimen. Thus with the initial prenatal visit the woman's knowledge regarding diabetes and pregnancy, potential maternal and fetal complications, and the plan of care are thoroughly assessed. With subsequent visits follow-up assessments are completed. Data from these assessments are used to identify the woman's specific learning needs. The support person's knowledge of diabetes is also assessed, and teaching needs are identified.

The woman's emotional status is assessed to determine how she is coping with pregnancy superimposed on preexisting diabetes. Although normal pregnancy typically evokes some degree of stress and anxiety, pregnancy designated as "high risk" serves to compound anxiety and stress levels. Fear of maternal and fetal complications is a major concern. Strict adherence to the plan of care necessitates alterations in patterns of daily living and may be an additional source of stress.

The woman's support system is assessed to identify those people significant to the pregnant woman and their role in her life. It is important to assess reactions of the family members and significant other to the pregnancy and to the strict management plan and their involvement in the treatment regimen. Socioeconomic factors are also reviewed. Any area of emotional stress is identified because such stress can precipitate complications.

Physical Examination

At the initial visit a thorough physical examination is performed to assess the woman's current health status. In addition to the routine prenatal examination, specific efforts are made to assess the effects of the diabetes. A baseline electrocardiogram (ECG) may be done to assess cardiovascular status. Evaluation for retinopathy is done, with follow-up by an ophthalmologist each trimester and more frequently if retinopathy is diagnosed. Blood pressure is monitored carefully throughout pregnancy because of the increased risk for preeclampsia. The woman's weight gain is also monitored at each visit. Fundal height is measured, noting any abnormal increase in size for dates, which may indicate hydramnios or fetal macrosomia. Leopold's maneuvers may be performed to check for fetal size and possible hydramnios.

Laboratory Tests

Routine prenatal laboratory examinations are performed. In addition, baseline renal function may be assessed with a 24-hour urine collection for total protein excretion and creatinine clearance. Urinalysis and culture are performed on the initial prenatal visit and throughout the pregnancy to assess for the presence of UTI, which is common in diabetic pregnancy. At each visit urine is also tested for the presence of glucose and ketones. Because of the risk of coexisting thyroid disease, thyroid function tests may also be performed (see later discussion of thyroid disorders).

For the woman with pregestational type 1 or type 2 diabetes, laboratory tests may be done to assess past glycemic control. At the initial prenatal visit, **glycosylated hemoglobin A1$_C$** level may be measured. With prolonged hyperglycemia some of the hemoglobin remains saturated with glucose for the life of the red blood cell (RBC). Therefore a test for glycosylated hemoglobin provides a measurement of glycemic control over time, specifically over the previous 4 to 6 weeks. Regular measurements of glycosylated hemoglobin provide data for altering the treatment plan and lead to improvement of glycemic control. Values for the measurement of hemoglobin A1$_C$, the

most commonly used index of glycosylated hemoglobin, are as follows (Pagana & Pagana, 1997):
Adult/elderly: 4% to 8%
Good diabetic control: 7%
Fair diabetic control: 10%
Poor diabetic control: 13% to 20%

Fasting blood glucose and/or random (1 to 2 hours after eating) glucose levels may be assessed during antepartum visits (Fig. 32-2). Blood glucose self-monitoring records may also be reviewed. Nursing diagnoses for the woman with pregestational diabetes include the following:

Nursing Diagnoses

- Knowledge deficit related to
  - diabetic pregnancy, management, and potential effects on pregnant woman and fetus
  - insulin administration and its effects
  - hypoglycemia and hyperglycemia
  - diabetic diet
- Risk for ineffective individual coping related to
  - woman's responsibility in managing her diabetes during her pregnancy
- Anxiety, fear, dysfunctional grieving, powerlessness, body image disturbance, situational low self-esteem, spiritual distress, altered role performance, altered family processes related to
  - stigma of being labeled "diabetic"
  - effects of diabetes and its potential sequelae on the pregnant woman and the fetus
- Risk for noncompliance related to
  - lack of understanding of diabetes and pregnancy and requirements of treatment plan
  - lack of financial resources to purchase blood glucose monitoring supplies or insulin and necessary supplies
  - insufficient funds or lack of transportation to grocery store to follow dietary regimen
- Risk for injury to fetus related to
  - uteroplacental insufficiency
  - birth trauma
- Risk for injury to mother related to
  - improper insulin administration
  - hypoglycemia and hyperglycemia
  - cesarean or operative vaginal birth
  - postpartum infection
- Altered nutrition: less or more than body requirements related to
  - noncompliance with dietary regimen
  - knowledge deficit regarding increased nutritional needs during pregnancy

Expected Outcomes of Care

Expected outcomes of care for the pregnant woman with pregestational diabetes include that she will do the following:

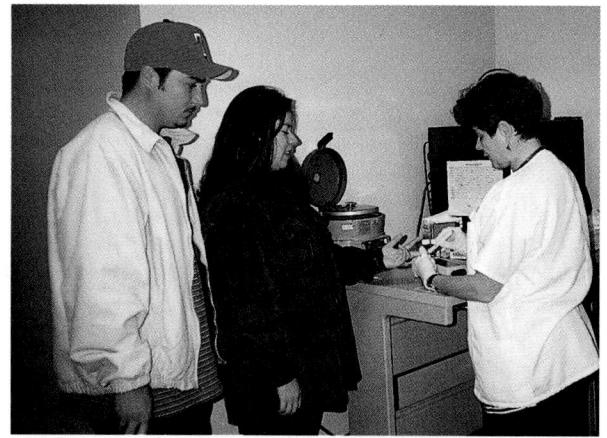

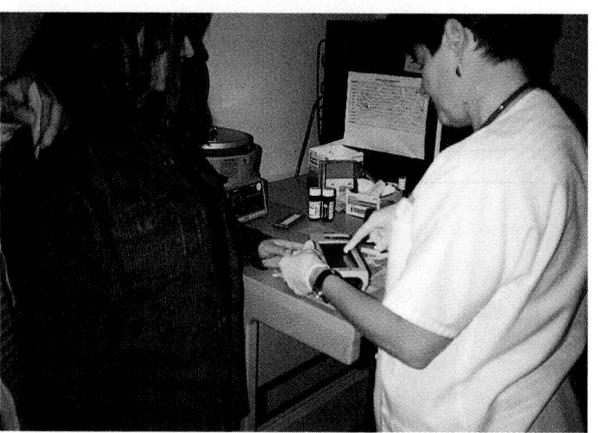

Fig. 32-2 **A,** Clinic nurse collects blood to determine glucose level. **B,** Nurse interprets glucose value displayed by monitor. *(Courtesy Dee Lowdermilk, UNC Ambulatory Care Clinics, Chapel Hill, NC.)*

- Demonstrate/verbalize understanding of diabetic pregnancy, the plan of care, and the importance of glycemic control.
- Follow the plan of care.
- Achieve and maintain glycemic control.
- Demonstrate effective coping.
- Experience no complications (maternal morbidity or mortality).
- Give birth to a healthy infant at term.

Plan of Care and Interventions

Antepartum

Because of her high risk status, the woman with diabetes is monitored much more frequently and thoroughly than other pregnant women. During the first and second trimesters of pregnancy her routine prenatal care visits will be scheduled every 1 to 2 weeks. Throughout the last trimester she will probably be seen one to two times each week. In the past, routine hospitalization for management of the diabetes, such as insulin dose changes, was common

RESEARCH

Frequency, Timing, and Diagnoses of Antenatal Hospitalizations in Women with High Risk Pregnancies

National strategies to control health care costs have resulted in reduced hospitalizations and increased use of home services for many high risk, high-cost client groups. Preventing or minimizing hospitalizations for high risk pregnant women can significantly decrease consumption of health care resources.

The purpose of this study was to examine the frequency, time of gestation, and reasons for antenatal hospitalizations in women with medically high risk pregnancies. Subjects (N=150) included women with pregestational and gestational diabetes, women with chronic hypertension, and women diagnosed or at high risk for preterm labor.

The study found that 83% (n=125) of the women had one or more antenatal hospitalizations with a mean length of stay of 123 hours. All women with diabetes were hospitalized at least once. Women with pregestational diabetes had the greatest number of hospitalizations, whereas those with gestational diabetes had the least. Major reasons for hospitalizations were preterm labor, glucose control, premature cervical dilation, and preeclampsia.

CLINICAL APPLICATION

The study findings have important implications for defining resource requirements to prevent or minimize hospitalizations in women with high risk pregnancies. Hospitalization for glucose control can potentially be avoided through client education that emphasizes the importance of adhering to diet, problem solving, and making lifestyle changes where needed. Education of monitoring of blood pressure, signs and symptoms of impending preeclampsia, and dietary restrictions could also reduce hospitalizations for those women prone to hypertensive events.

Nurses may be able to reduce the frequency of hospitalizations for some women through expanded client education, improved screening, and more targeted provider and client monitoring for early signs and symptoms of impending complications in the groups most frequently hospitalized.

Source: Brooten, D. et al. (1998). Frequency, timing, and diagnoses of antenatal hospitalizations in women with high risk pregnancies. *J Perinatol* 18(5), 372-376.

(see Research box). With the availability of better home glucose monitoring and the growing reluctance of third-party payers to reimburse for hospitalization, pregnant women with diabetes are now generally managed as outpatients. Some client and family education and maternal and fetal assessment may be done in the home, depending on the woman's insurance coverage and care provider preference.

Achieving and maintaining constant **euglycemia,** with blood glucose levels in the range of 65 to 130 mg/dl (Table 32-2), is the primary goal of medical therapy for the pregnant woman with diabetes. Euglycemia is achieved through a combination of diet, insulin, exercise, and blood glucose determinations. Providing the woman with the knowledge, skill, and motivation she needs to achieve and maintain excellent blood glucose control is the primary nursing goal.

Achieving euglycemia requires commitment on the part of the woman and her family to make the necessary lifestyle changes, which can sometimes seem overwhelming. Maintaining tight blood glucose control necessitates that the woman follow a consistent daily schedule. She must get up and go to bed, eat, exercise, and take insulin at the same time each day. Blood glucose measurements are done frequently to determine how well the major com-

TABLE 32-2 Target Blood Glucose Levels During Pregnancy

TIME OF DAY	TARGET GLUCOSE LEVEL (MG/DL)
Premeal	>65 but <95
Postmeal (1 hour)	<130
Postmeal (2 hours)	<120
During hours of sleep	No less than 70

Source: Moore, T. (1999). Diabetes in pregnancy. In R. Creasy & R. Resnik (Eds.). *Maternal-fetal medicine* (4th ed.). Philadelphia: W.B. Saunders.

ponents of therapy—diet, insulin, and exercise—are working together to control blood glucose levels.

In addition to the routine prenatal care provided to all pregnant women, the woman with diabetes will receive additional counseling. She should wear an identification bracelet at all times and should carry insulin, syringes, and "glucose boosters" with her whenever she is away from home. She should also be given written instructions for reporting the development of problems such as nausea, vomiting, and infections, including directions for reaching her health care provider by phone at night and on weekends and holidays. (See Home Care box below.)

Because the diabetic woman is at risk for infections, eye problems, and neurologic changes, foot care and general skin care are important. A daily bath that includes good perineal care and foot care is important. For dry skin, lotions, creams, or oils can be applied. Tight clothing should be avoided. Shoes or slippers should be worn at all times, should fit properly, and are best worn with socks or stockings. Feet should be inspected regularly; toenails should be cut straight across, and professional help should be sought for any foot problems. Extremes of temperature should be avoided.

Diet. The woman with pregestational diabetes has probably been previously exposed to nutritional counseling regarding management of the diabetes. Because pregnancy precipitates special nutritional concerns and needs, the woman must be educated to incorporate these changes into dietary planning. Nutritional counseling is usually provided by a registered dietitian.

Dietary management during diabetic pregnancy must be based on blood (not urine) glucose levels. The diet is individualized to allow for increased fetal and metabolic requirements, with consideration of such factors as prepreg-

nancy weight and dietary habits, overall health, ethnic background, lifestyle, stage of pregnancy, knowledge of nutrition, and insulin therapy. The dietary goal is to provide weight gain consistent with a normal pregnancy, to prevent ketoacidosis, and to minimize widely fluctuating blood glucose levels.

Energy needs are usually calculated on the basis of 30 to 35 calories per kilogram of ideal body weight, with the average diet including 2200 (first trimester) to 2500 calories (second and third trimesters). Total calories may be distributed among three meals and one evening snack, or more commonly, three meals and at least two snacks. Meals should be eaten on time and never skipped. Snacks must be carefully planned in accordance with insulin therapy to avoid fluctuations in blood glucose levels. A large bedtime snack of at least 25 g of carbohydrate with some protein is recommended to help prevent hypoglycemia and starvation ketosis during the night.

The ratio of carbohydrate, protein, and fat is important to meet the metabolic needs of the woman and the fetus. Approximately 50% to 60% of the total calories should be carbohydrate, with a minimum of 250 g per day. Simple carbohydrates are limited; complex carbohydrates that are high in fiber content are recommended because the starch and protein in such foods help regulate the blood glucose level as a result of more sustained glucose release. Protein intake should constitute 12% to 20% of the total kilocalories, and 20% to 30% of the daily caloric intake should come from fat, with no more than 10% saturated fats (see Home Care box below). Weight gain for most women should be about 12 kg during the pregnancy (Gilbert & Harmon, 1998).

🏠 HOME CARE

Treatment for Hypoglycemia

- Be familiar with signs and symptoms of hypoglycemia (nervousness, headache, shaking, irritability, personality change, hunger, blurred vision, sweaty skin, tingling of mouth or extremities).
- Check blood glucose level immediately when hypoglycemic symptoms occur.
- If blood glucose is <60 mg/dl, immediately eat or drink something that contains 10 to 15 g of simple carbohydrate. Examples:
    ½ cup (4 ounces) unsweetened fruit juice
    ½ cup (4 ounces) regular (not diet) soda
    5 to 6 Life Savers candies
    1 tablespoon honey or corn (Karo) syrup
    1 cup (8 ounces) milk
    2 to 3 glucose tablets
- Rest for 15 minutes, then recheck blood glucose.
- If glucose level is still <60 mg/dl, eat or drink another serving of one of the "glucose boosters" listed above.
- Wait 15 minutes, then recheck blood glucose. If it is still <60 mg/dl, notify health care provider immediately.

Source: American Diabetes Association. (1995). *Medical management of pregnancy complicated by diabetes* (2nd ed.). Alexandria, VA: The Association; Becton Dickinson & Co. (1997). *Controlling low blood sugar reactions.* Franklin Lakes, NJ: Becton Dickinson.

🏠 HOME CARE

Dietary Management of Diabetic Pregnancy

- Follow the prescribed diet plan.
- Eat a well-balanced diet, including daily food requirements for a normal pregnancy.
- Divide daily food intake between three meals and two to four snacks, depending on individual needs.
- Eat a substantial bedtime snack to prevent a severe drop in blood glucose level during the night.
- Limit the intake of fats if weight gain occurs too rapidly.
- Take daily vitamins and iron as prescribed by the health care provider.
- Avoid foods high in refined sugar.
- Eat consistently each day; never skip meals or snacks.
- Reduce the intake of saturated fat and cholesterol.
- Eat foods high in dietary fiber.
- Avoid alcohol and caffeine.

Exercise. Although it has been shown that exercise enhances the use of glucose and decreases insulin need in nonpregnant women with diabetes, there are limited data regarding exercise in pregnancy. Any prescription of exercise during diabetic pregnancy should be done by the primary health care provider and should be closely monitored to prevent complications. For those women with vasculopathy, only mild exercise is recommended because exercise causes a redistribution of blood flow, which increases the potential for ischemic injury to the placenta and already compromised organs. Also, women with vasculopathy typically depend completely on exogenous insulin and are at greater risk for wide fluctuations in blood glucose levels and ketoacidosis, which can be worsened by exercise.

When exercise is prescribed by the health care provider as part of the treatment plan, careful instructions are given to the woman. She should be told that exercise need not be vigorous to be beneficial: 15 to 30 minutes of walking four to six times a week is satisfactory for most pregnant women. Other exercises that may be recommended are non–weight-bearing activities such as arm ergometry or use of a recumbent bicycle. The best time for exercise is after meals, when the blood glucose level is rising. If the woman exercises at a time when the insulin is peaking or engages in prolonged exercise without carbohydrate intake, hypoglycemia may result. Hyperglycemia may occur when exercise is done at a time when insulin action is waning. To monitor the effect of insulin on blood glucose levels, the woman can measure blood glucose before, during, and after exercise.

NURSE ALERT *The woman should be aware of the possibility of uterine contractions occurring during exercise and stop immediately if they are detected.*

Insulin therapy. Adequate insulinization of the pregnant woman is the primary factor in the maintenance of normoglycemia during pregnancy, thus ensuring proper glucose metabolism of the mother and fetus. Insulin requirements during pregnancy change dramatically as the pregnancy progresses, necessitating frequent adjustments in insulin dosage. In the first trimester there is little or no change in prepregnancy insulin requirements; however, insulin dosage may need to be decreased because of hypoglycemia. During the second and third trimester, because of insulin resistance, dosage must be increased to maintain target glucose levels.

For the woman with type 1 pregestational diabetes who has typically been accustomed to one injection per day of intermediate-acting insulin, multiple daily injections of mixed insulin are a new experience. The woman with type 2 diabetes previously treated with oral hypoglycemics is faced with the task of learning to self-administer injections of insulin. The nurse is instrumental in education and support with regard to insulin administration and adjustment

of insulin dosage to maintain normoglycemia (see Client Self-Care box).

More types of insulin are available today than ever before. Beef and pork insulin have largely been replaced by biosynthetic human insulin preparations (Humulin or Novolin), which are less likely to cause antibody formation. Clients with new onset of diabetes are almost always started on this type of insulin. Lispro (Humalog), a new rapid-acting insulin, is now available. It has a faster onset and shorter duration of action than regular insulin.

CLIENT SELF-CARE

Administration of Insulin

PROCEDURE FOR MIXING NPH (INTERMEDIATE-ACTING) AND REGULAR (SHORT-ACTING) INSULIN

- Wash hands thoroughly and gather supplies. Be sure the insulin syringe corresponds to the concentration of insulin you are using.
- Check insulin bottle to be certain it is the appropriate type and check the expiration date.
- Gently rotate (do not shake) the insulin vial to mix the insulin.
- Wipe off rubber stopper of each vial with alcohol.
- Draw into syringe the amount of air equal to total dose.
- Inject air equal to NPH (intermediate-acting) dose into NPH vial. Remove syringe from vial.
- Inject air equal to regular insulin dose into regular insulin vial.
- Invert regular insulin bottle and withdraw regular insulin dose.
- Without adding more air to NPH vial, carefully withdraw NPH dose.

PROCEDURE FOR SELF-INJECTION OF INSULIN

- Select proper injection site (remember to rotate sites).
- Injection site should be clean. Use of alcohol is not necessary. If alcohol is used, let it dry before injecting.
- Pinch the skin up to form a subcutaneous pocket and, holding the syringe like a pencil, puncture the skin at a 45- to 90-degree angle. If there is a great deal of fatty tissue at the site, spread the skin taut and inject the syringe at a 90-degree angle.
- Slowly inject the insulin.
- As you withdraw the needle, cover the injection site with sterile gauze and apply gentle pressure to prevent bleeding.
- Record insulin dosage and time of injection.

TABLE 32-3	**Insulin Administration During Pregnancy: Expected Time of Action**		
TYPE OF INSULIN	**ONSET**	**PEAK**	**DURATION**
Lispro (rapid acting)	Within 15 min	30-90 min	3 hr
Regular (rapid acting)	30 min-1 hr	2-4 hr	5-8 hr
Intermediate acting	2-4 hr	5-10 hr	12-24 hr
Long acting	3-4 hr	14-24 hr	24-36 hr

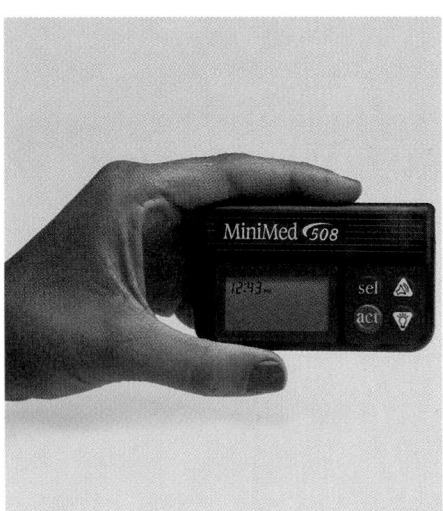

Fig. 32-3 Insulin pump shows basal rate for pregnant women with diabetes. *(Courtesy MiniMed, Inc., Sylmar, CA.)*

Advantages of lispro include convenience, because it is injected immediately before mealtime; less hyperglycemia following meals; and fewer hypoglycemic episodes in some clients. Because its effects last 5 hours, most clients require a longer-acting insulin along with lispro to maintain optimal blood glucose levels (Eli Lilly & Co., 1996; Hoffmeister & Haines, 1996; Moore, 1999) (Table 32-3). Lispro can be used safely in pregnancy, but unlike other insulins, it is available only with a prescription.

Most women with insulin-dependent diabetes are managed with two to three injections per day. Usually, two thirds of the daily insulin dose, with longer-acting (NPH) and short-acting (regular or lispro) insulin combined in a 2:1 ratio, is given before breakfast. Sometimes the remaining one third, again a combination of longer- and short-acting insulin, is administered in the evening before dinner. To reduce the risk of hypoglycemia during the night, often separate injections are administered, with short-acting insulin given before dinner, followed by longer-acting insulin at bedtime. Another alternative insulin regimen that works well for some women is to administer short-acting insulin before each meal and longer-acting insulin at bedtime (Hagay & Reece, 1999).

Although subcutaneous insulin injections are most commonly used, continuous insulin infusion systems may be used during pregnancy. The insulin "pump" is designed to mimic more closely the function of the pancreas in secreting insulin (Fig. 32-3). This portable, battery-powered device infuses regular insulin at a set basal rate and has the capacity to deliver up to four different basal rates in 24 hours. The pump also delivers bolus doses of insulin before meals to control postmeal blood glucose levels. The infusion tubing from the insulin pump can be left in place for several weeks without local complications. Although the insulin pump is convenient and generally provides good glycemic control, complications such as DKA, infection, or hypoglycemic coma can still develop. Use of the insulin pump requires a knowledgeable, motivated client, skilled health care providers, and 24-hour availability of emergency assistance (Hagay & Reece, 1999; Moore, 1999).

Monitoring blood glucose levels. Blood glucose testing at home is the commonly accepted method for monitoring blood glucose levels and the most important tool available to the woman to assess her degree of glycemic control. In addition, this monitoring provides motivation to continue the prescribed treatment plan, and the data obtained facilitate interaction with the health care team in maintaining glycemic control and minimizing fetal risk.

Women with pregestational diabetes are often familiar with self-monitoring of blood glucose levels because it is typically included in the management plan for type 1 and some cases of type 2 diabetes. However, a thorough assessment of the woman's knowledge and skill related to blood glucose testing is essential to ensure accurate monitoring of glucose levels during pregnancy. The nurse observes the woman performing blood glucose monitoring to determine her accuracy and comfort with the system. The family is also included in the assessment and in subsequent instruction.

Pregnancy demands more frequent and judicious monitoring than many women have practiced previously. Willingness to comply with the monitoring schedule is essential to the management plan. Home glucose monitoring should be done using a glucose reflectance meter, which is battery powered and determines the blood glucose level by the amount of light reflected from a reacted test strip. Most insurance companies will cover the cost of a meter and necessary supplies. To perform blood glucose monitoring, a drop of blood is obtained by a finger stick and placed on a test strip. After a specified amount of time, the glucose level can be read by the meter (see Client Self-Care box).

CLIENT SELF-CARE

Testing Blood Glucose Level

- Gather supplies, check expiration date, and read instructions on testing materials. Prepare glucose reflectance meter for use according to manufacturer's directions.
- Wash hands in warm water (warmth increases circulation).
- Select site on side of any finger (all fingers should be used in rotation).
- Pierce site with lancet (may use automatic, spring-loaded, puncturing device). Cleaning the site with alcohol is not necessary.
- Drop hand down to side; with other hand gently squeeze finger from hand to fingertip.
- Allow blood to drop onto testing strip. Be sure to cover entire reagent area.
- Determine blood glucose value using the glucose reflectance meter, following manufacturer's instructions.
- Record results.
- Repeat daily as instructed by health care provider and as needed for signs of hypoglycemia or hyperglycemia.

Source: American Diabetes Association. (1995). *Medical management of pregnancy complicated by diabetes* (2nd ed.). Alexandria, VA: The Association.

Meters that incorporate memory to store a large number of readings are available; however, the woman is still encouraged to keep written records of glucose levels. She should bring her written records, her meter containing stored test results, or both with her to each appointment. It is important that the monitoring equipment be checked for accuracy at intervals by comparing the woman's results on her machine with the results of a laboratory test done at the same time on a capillary whole blood sample.

Blood glucose levels are routinely measured at various times throughout the day, such as before breakfast, lunch, and dinner; 2 hours after each meal; at bedtime; and in the middle of the night. Because hyperglycemia is to be avoided, postprandial measurements are often performed. Hyperglycemia will most likely be identified in 2-hour postprandial values, because blood glucose levels peak about 2 hours after a meal. The health care provider will determine for each individual woman the number and timing of routine blood glucose determinations.

Special circumstances may necessitate more frequent testing. Women are instructed to check glucose levels at any sign of hypoglycemia or hyperglycemia. When there is any readjustment in insulin dosage or diet, more frequent measurement of blood glucose is warranted. If nausea,

vomiting, or diarrhea occur, or if any infection is present, the woman will probably be asked to monitor her blood glucose levels more closely.

Target levels of blood glucose during pregnancy are lower than nonpregnant values. Acceptable fasting levels are generally between 65 and 95 mg/dl, and 2-hour postprandial levels should be less than 120 mg/dl (see Table 32-2) (Moore, 1999). The woman should be told to immediately report episodes of hypoglycemia (less than 60 mg/dl) and hyperglycemia (greater than 200 mg/dl) to her health care provider so that adjustments in diet or insulin therapy can be made (ADA, 1994).

Pregnant women with diabetes are much more likely to develop hypoglycemia than hyperglycemia, because the goal of therapy is to maintain the blood glucose in a narrow, low-normal range of 65 to 130 mg/dl. Although a blood glucose level greater than 130 mg/dl is considered too high for a pregnant woman, it will not produce the classic signs and symptoms of hyperglycemia. On the other hand, many women will experience signs and symptoms of hypoglycemia with blood glucose levels below 65 mg/dl (see Table 32-1).

Most episodes of mild or moderate hypoglycemia can be treated with oral intake of 10 to 15 g of simple carbohydrate (see Home Care box, on p. 870). If severe hypoglycemia occurs, in which the woman experiences a decrease or loss of consciousness or an inability to swallow, she will require a parenteral injection of glucagon or intravenous (IV) glucose (ADA, 1994; Becton Dickinson & Co., 1997). Because hypoglycemia can develop rapidly and because impaired judgment can be associated with even moderate episodes, it is vital that family members, friends, and work colleagues be able to quickly recognize signs and symptoms and initiate proper treatment if necessary (Becton Dickinson & Co., 1997).

Although hyperglycemia is less likely to occur in compliant clients, it is still a dangerous complication. Hyperglycemia can rapidly progress to diabetic ketoacidosis. Women and family members should be particularly alert for signs and symptoms of hyperglycemia, especially when infections or other illnesses occur (see Table 32-1 and Home Care box, p. 874).

Urine testing. Urine testing for ketones continues to have a place in diabetic management, because it may provide vital information for the pregnant woman, such as the onset of DKA. Women may be taught to perform urine testing daily with the first morning urine. Testing may also be done if a meal is missed or delayed, when illness occurs, or when the blood glucose level is greater than 200 mg/dl.

Spilling a trace or a small amount of ketones requires no treatment. However, if ketones appear repeatedly at the same time each day, some adjustment in diet may be needed. If testing shows a large amount of ketones, the health care provider should be contacted immediately (ADA, 1995).

Fetal surveillance. Diagnostic techniques for fetal surveillance are often performed to assess fetal growth and

HOME CARE

What to Do When Illness Occurs

- Be sure to take insulin even though appetite and food intake may be less than normal. (Insulin needs are increased with illness or infection.)
- Call the health care provider and relay the following information:
  - Symptoms of illness (e.g., nausea, vomiting, diarrhea)
  - Fever
  - Most recent blood glucose level
  - Urine ketones
  - Time and amount of last insulin dose
- Increase oral intake of fluids to prevent dehydration.
- Rest as much as possible.
- If unable to reach health care provider and blood glucose exceeds 200 mg/dl with urine ketones present, seek emergency treatment at the nearest health care facility. Do not attempt to self-treat for this.

well-being. The goals of fetal surveillance are to detect fetal compromise as early as possible and to prevent intrauterine fetal death or unnecessary preterm birth. The majority of fetal surveillance measures are concentrated in the third trimester, when the risk of fetal compromise is greatest.

Early in pregnancy, efforts are made to determine the estimated date of birth. A baseline sonogram is done during the first trimester to assess gestational age. Follow-up ultrasound examinations are usually performed during the pregnancy, as often as every 4 to 6 weeks, to monitor fetal growth; estimate fetal weight; and detect hydramnios, macrosomia, and congenital anomalies.

Because diabetic pregnancies are at greater risk for neural tube defects (e.g., spina bifida, anencephaly, microcephaly), measurement of maternal serum alpha-fetoprotein is performed between 16 and 18 weeks of gestation. This is often done in conjunction with a detailed ultrasound study to examine the fetus for neural tube defects.

Fetal echocardiography may be performed between 18 and 22 weeks of gestation to detect cardiac anomalies. Some practitioners repeat this fetal surveillance test at 34 weeks. Doppler studies of the umbilical artery may be performed in women with vascular disease to detect placental compromise.

Maternal evaluation of fetal movements (kick counts) is used primarily as a screening technique in fetal surveillance. Few research studies have investigated the use of this method in diabetic pregnancies.

A commonly used measure of fetal well-being is the nonstress test, typically beginning around 28 to 32 weeks

of gestation (see Chapter 29). After 32 weeks, testing may be done twice weekly. For the woman with vascular disease, testing may begin earlier and continue more frequently. In the presence of a nonreactive nonstress test, a contraction stress test or fetal biophysical profile may be used to evaluate fetal well-being (Hagay & Reece, 1999; Landon, 1996; Moore, 1999).

Complications requiring hospitalization. Occasionally it becomes necessary to hospitalize a woman with diabetes during pregnancy. A few days in the hospital early in pregnancy may be required to complete baseline cardiovascular, renal, and ophthalmologic evaluations and balance diet and insulin to achieve satisfactory glucose control. Infection, which can lead to hyperglycemia and diabetic ketoacidosis, is an indication for hospitalization, regardless of gestational age. At any time during the pregnancy, women who fail to maintain acceptable blood glucose levels may be hospitalized. A few days in a controlled environment often greatly increases compliance with diet and insulin therapy, resulting in marked improvement in blood glucose levels. Hospitalization during the third trimester for closer maternal and fetal observation may be indicated for women with vasculopathy because of the increased risk for renal impairment, hypertensive disorders, and fetal compromise (ADA, 1994).

Determination of birth date and mode of birth. Today the majority of diabetic pregnancies are allowed to progress to term (38 to 40 weeks of gestation), as long as good metabolic control is maintained and all parameters of antepartum fetal surveillance remain within normal limits. Reasons to proceed with delivery before term include poor metabolic control, worsening hypertensive disorders, fetal macrosomia, or fetal growth restriction (Hagay & Reece, 1999; Moore, 1999).

Many practitioners plan for elective labor induction between 38 and 40 weeks provided that maternal glucose levels are well controlled. To confirm fetal lung maturity before birth, an amniocentesis may be performed in pregnancies earlier than 39 weeks. For the pregnancy complicated by diabetes, fetal lung maturation is better predicted by the amniotic fluid phosphatidylglycerol than by the lecithin/sphingomyelin ratio. If the fetal lungs are still immature, birth should be postponed as long as the results of fetal assessment remain reassuring. Amniocentesis may be repeated to monitor lung maturity. Delivery despite poor fetal lung maturity may be essential when testing suggests fetal compromise or if preeclampsia (PIH), rapidly worsening retinopathy, or renal failure develops (Landon, 1996).

The mode of birth for women with pregestational diabetes is a subject of controversy among practitioners. The cesarean rate for these women is exceedingly high, around 45%. Cesarean birth is often performed when antepartum testing suggests fetal distress or the estimated fetal weight is 4000 to 4500 g. Also, when induction of labor is desired and the cervix fails to respond, cesarean birth is often necessary (Hagay & Reece, 1999; Landon, 1996; Moore, 1999).

Intrapartum

During the intrapartum period the woman with pregestational diabetes must be monitored closely to prevent complications related to dehydration, hypoglycemia, and hyperglycemia. Most women use large amounts of energy (calories) to accomplish the work and manage the stress of labor and birth; however, this calorie expenditure varies with the individual. Blood glucose levels and hydration must be carefully controlled during labor. An IV line is inserted for infusion of a maintenance fluid, such as lactated Ringer's or 5% dextrose in lactated Ringer's solution. Insulin may be administered by continuous infusion or intermittent subcutaneous injection. Determinations of blood glucose levels are made every hour, and fluids and insulin are adjusted to maintain blood glucose levels at 70 to 90 mg/dl. It is essential that these target glucose levels be maintained because hyperglycemia during labor can precipitate metabolic problems, particularly hypoglycemia, in the neonate (Hagay & Reece, 1999).

During labor, continuous fetal heart monitoring is necessary to observe for uteroplacental insufficiency. The mother should assume a side-lying position during bed rest in labor to prevent supine hypotension because of a large fetus or polyhydramnios. Labor is allowed to progress provided normal rates of cervical dilation, fetal descent, and fetal well-being are maintained. Failure to progress may indicate a macrosomic infant.

NURSE ALERT *The nurse should be alert for shoulder dystocia if vaginal birth of a macrosomic infant is attempted.*

Cephalopelvic disproportion necessitates cesarean birth. The woman is observed and treated during labor for diabetic complications such as hyperglycemia, ketosis, ketoacidosis, and glycosuria. A neonatologist, pediatrician, or neonatal nurse-practitioner may be present at the birth to initiate assessment and neonatal care.

If a cesarean birth is planned, it should be scheduled in the early morning to facilitate glycemic control. The morning dose of insulin should be withheld and the woman given nothing by mouth. Epidural anesthesia is recommended because hypoglycemia can be detected earlier if the woman is awake (Hagay & Reece, 1999).

Postpartum

In the immediate postpartum period, insulin requirements decrease substantially because the major source of insulin resistance, the placenta, has been removed. Women with type 1 diabetes may require only one half the prenatal insulin dose on the first postpartum day, provided that they are eating a full diet. It takes several days after birth to reestablish carbohydrate homeostasis (see Fig. 32-1, *D, E*). Blood glucose levels are monitored in the postpartum period, and insulin dosage is adjusted accordingly. Blood glucose levels do not need to be as tightly controlled after birth. Usually insulin is not given until the blood glucose level is greater than 200 mg/dl (Hagay & Reece, 1999). The woman who is insulin dependent must realize the importance of eating on time even if the baby needs feeding or other pressing demands exist. Women with type 2 diabetes often require no insulin in the postpartum period and are able to maintain normoglycemia through diet alone or with oral hypoglycemics.

Possible postpartum complications include preeclampsia-eclampsia, hemorrhage, and infection. Hemorrhage is a possibility if the mother's uterus was overdistended (hydramnios, macrosomic fetus) or overstimulated (oxytocin induction). Postpartum infections such as endometritis are more likely to occur in a woman with diabetes.

Postpartum thyroid dysfunction is more common among women with diabetes (see later discussion of thyroid disorders). Routine thyroid screening may be performed during postpartum visits (Alvarez-Marfany et al., 1994; Gerstein, 1993).

Mothers are encouraged to breastfeed. In addition to the advantages of maternal satisfaction and pleasure, breastfeeding has an antidiabetogenic effect. Many mothers with diabetes find that their glucose levels are easier to control. Insulin requirements may be half the prepregnancy levels because of the carbohydrate used in human milk production. Because glucose levels are lower, breastfeeding women are at increased risk for hypoglycemia, especially in the early postpartum period and after breastfeeding sessions (Hagay & Reece, 1999; Moore, 1999). It is important to remind the mother that continued dietary modification is needed to ensure adequate nutrition during lactation. Breastfeeding mothers with diabetes may be at increased risk for mastitis and yeast infections of the breast, particularly if glucose levels are not well controlled. Insulin dosage, which is decreased during lactation, must be recalculated at weaning (Landon, 1996) (see Fig. 23-1, *F*).

The mother may have early breastfeeding difficulties. Poor metabolic control may delay lactogenesis and contribute to decreased milk production (Moore, 1999). Because many women give birth by cesarean, the effects of anesthesia and postoperative discomfort may delay maternal attachment and make breastfeeding more difficult. In addition, initial contact and opportunity to breastfeed the infant are often delayed because many institutions place infants of mothers with diabetes in neonatal intensive care units or special care nurseries for observation during the first few hours after birth. Support and assistance from nursing staff and lactation specialists can facilitate the mother's early experience with breastfeeding and encourage her to continue.

Recent evidence suggests that infants who are exclusively breastfed are less likely to develop diabetes and that exposure to cow's milk products before 8 days of age is an important risk factor for the disease. Because children born to diabetic women are at increased risk to develop diabetes, this information further supports the importance of encouraging all women with diabetes to breastfeed (Moore, 1999).

The new mother needs information about family planning and contraception. Although family planning is important for all women, it is essential for the woman with diabetes to safeguard her own health and to promote optimal outcomes in future pregnancies. The woman and her partner should be informed that the risks associated with pregnancy increase with the duration and severity of the diabetic condition and that pregnancy may contribute to vascular changes associated with diabetes.

The risks and benefits of contraceptive methods should be discussed with the mother and her partner before discharge from the hospital. The barrier method is the preferred method of contraception for the woman who is insulin dependent. Barrier methods such as the diaphragm or condom and spermicide pose the least risk. The problem with these methods, however, is the inconsistency of use, which often leads to unplanned pregnancy (Landon, 1996).

Use of oral contraceptives is controversial because of the risk of thromboembolic and vascular complications and the effect on carbohydrate metabolism. In women without vascular disease or other risk factors, low-dose oral contraceptives may be prescribed. Close monitoring of blood pressure and glucose levels is necessary to detect complications (Kjos, 1996; Landon & Gabbe, 1995).

Intrauterine contraceptive devices increase the risk of infection, especially during the first 4 months after insertion. However, they may be used for women who are older or who have hypertension or other vascular disease. Such an individual should be parous, in a monogamous relationship, and at low risk for sexually transmitted infections (STIs), with no history of pelvic infection. These women must be able to recognize the signs of pelvic infection and STIs and notify their health care providers promptly if these signs occur (Kjos, 1996).

There is no contraindication to use of the Norplant system in women with diabetes who have no cardiovascular complications (Jovanovic-Peterson, 1993).

Sterilization should be discussed with the woman who has completed her family or who has significant vasculopathy (ADA, 1994).

Evaluation

Evaluation of the care of the pregnant woman with pregestational diabetes is based on the previously stated expected outcomes of care, which are closely associated with the degree of maternal metabolic control during pregnancy (see Plan of Care).

Gestational Diabetes Mellitus

Gestational diabetes mellitus (GDM) complicates approximately 4% of all pregnancies in the United States and accounts for 90% of all cases of diabetic pregnancy. Prevalence varies by racial and ethnic groups. GDM is more likely to occur among Hispanic, Native American, Asian, and African-American populations than in Caucasians (Expert Committee on the Diagnosis and Classification of Diabetes Mellitus, 1997). Persons with GDM are at significant risk of developing glucose intolerance later in life; about 50% will be diagnosed as diabetic within 22 to 28 years. This is especially true of women whose GDM is diagnosed early in pregnancy or who manifest fasting hyperglycemia (Landon, 1996). Classic risk factors for GDM include maternal age greater than 30 years; obesity; family history of type 2 diabetes; and an obstetric history of an infant weighing more than 9 pounds, hydramnios, unexplained stillbirth, miscarriage, or an infant with congenital anomalies. Women at high risk for GDM are often screened at their initial prenatal visit and then rescreened later in pregnancy if the initial screen is negative.

The diagnosis of gestational diabetes is usually made during the second half of pregnancy. Because fetal nutrient demands rise during the late second and the third trimester, maternal nutrient ingestion induces greater and more sustained levels of blood glucose. At the same time, maternal insulin resistance is also increasing because of the insulin antagonistic effects of the placental hormones, cortisol, and insulinase. Consequently, maternal insulin demands rise as much as threefold. The majority of pregnant women are capable of increasing insulin production to compensate for insulin resistance and to maintain normoglycemia. When the pancreas is unable to produce sufficient insulin or the insulin is not used effectively, gestational diabetes can result.

Maternal-Fetal Risks

Women with GDM have twice the risk of developing hypertensive disorders compared with normal pregnant women (Metzger & Coustan, 1998). They also have increased risk for fetal macrosomia, which can lead to increased rates of perineal lacerations, episiotomy, and cesarean delivery (Jones & Stone, 1998). Infants born to women with GDM are at risk for macrosomia with associated shoulder dystocia and birth trauma. GDM also places the neonate at increased risk for hypoglycemia, hypocalcemia, hyperbilirubinemia, thrombocytopenia, polycythemia, and respiratory distress syndrome (Jones & Stone, 1998; Metzger & Coustan, 1998).

The overall incidence of congenital anomalies among infants of women with gestational diabetes approaches that of the general population because gestational diabetes usually develops after the twentieth week of pregnancy—after the critical period of organogenesis (first trimester) has passed.

PLAN of CARE · Pregnancy Complicated by Insulin-Dependent Diabetes

NURSING DIAGNOSIS Knowledge deficit related to lack of recall of information as evidenced by client questions and concerns

Expected Outcomes *Client will be able to verbalize important information regarding diabetes, its management, and potential effects on the pregnant woman and fetus.*

Nursing Interventions/*Rationales*

Assess client's current knowledge base regarding disease process, management, effects on pregnancy and fetus, and potential complications *to provide database for further teaching.*

Review the pathophysiology of diabetes, effects on pregnancy and fetus, and potential complications *to promote client recall of information and compliance with treatment plan.*

Review procedure for insulin administration, demonstrate procedure for blood glucose monitoring and insulin measurement and administration, and obtain return demonstration *to establish client comfort and competence with procedures.*

Discuss diet and exercise as prescribed by diabetologist *to promote self-care.*

Review signs and symptoms of complications of hypoglycemia and hyperglycemia and appropriate interventions *to promote prompt recognition of complications and self-care.*

Provide contact numbers for health care team for prompt interventions and answers to questions on an ongoing basis *to promote client comfort.*

NURSING DIAGNOSIS Risk for fetal injury related to elevated maternal glucose levels

Expected Outcome *Fetus will remain free of injury and be delivered at term in a healthy state.*

Nursing Interventions/*Rationales*

Assess client's current diabetic control *to identify risk for fetal mortality and congenital anomalies.*

Monitor fundal height during each prenatal visit *to identify appropriate fetal growth.*

Monitor for signs and symptoms of pregnancy-induced hypertension *to identify early manifestations because diabetic pregnant women are more at risk.*

Assess fetal movement and heart rate during each prenatal visit and perform weekly nonstress tests during the last 4 weeks of pregnancy *to assess for fetal well-being.*

Review procedure for blood glucose testing and insulin administration *to promote self-care.*

NURSING DIAGNOSIS Anxiety related to threat to maternal and fetal well-being as evidenced by client verbal expressions of concern

Expected Outcomes *Client will identify sources of anxiety and report feeling less anxious.*

Nursing Interventions/*Rationales*

Through therapeutic communication, promote an open relationship with client *to promote client trust.*

Listen to client's feelings and concerns *to assess for any misconception or misinformation that may be contributing to anxiety.*

Review potential dangers by providing factual information *to correct any misconceptions or misinformation.*

Encourage client to share concerns with her health care team *to promote client and team collaboration in her care.*

CARE MANAGEMENT

Nurses involved in prenatal care delivery can be instrumental in the identification of women with GDM. Although protocols regarding which women will undergo screening and exactly how the screening will be done vary among care providers, nurses are often responsible for ensuring that the screen is performed on the identified group of women at the proper gestational age. Careful adherence

to screening protocols is crucial in order to correctly identify women with GDM.

Assessment

Screening for Gestational Diabetes Mellitus

Earlier recommendations from the ADA were that all pregnant women should be screened for the development of GDM. However, the Expert Committee on the Diagnosis and Classification of Diabetes Mellitus stated in its 1997 report that it is neither cost-effective nor necessary to screen certain women who are at low risk for GDM. This low risk group includes normal-weight women younger than 25 years of age who have no family history of diabetes and are not members of an ethnic or a racial group known to have a high prevalence of the disease. The American College of Obstetricians and Gynecologists (ACOG) (1994) has stated that selective screening may be appropriate in some low risk settings (e.g., teen clinics), but that universal screening might be more appropriate for high risk populations. ACOG also states that screening is unnecessary in certain populations with a high prevalence of GDM. Women in these groups may be considered to have an abnormal screen and proceed directly to diagnostic testing.

The screening test (Glucola screening) most often used in North America consists of a 50 g oral glucose load, followed by a plasma glucose determination 1 hour later. Screening should be performed at 24 to 28 weeks of gestation. It is not necessary that the woman be fasting. A glucose value of 140 mg/dl is considered a positive screen.

A positive Glucola screen requires follow-up with a 3-hour **oral glucose tolerance test** (OGTT). The 3-hour OGTT is administered after an overnight fast and at least 3 days of unrestricted diet (at least 150 g of carbohydrate) and physical activity. The woman is instructed to avoid caffeine because it tends to increase glucose levels and to abstain from smoking for 12 hours before and during the test. A fasting blood glucose level is drawn before giving a 100 g glucose load. Blood glucose levels are then drawn 1, 2, and 3 hours later. The woman is diagnosed with gestational diabetes if two or more values are met or exceeded (Fig. 32-4).

Controversy exists over the management of women with only one abnormal OGTT value. Many experts believe that these women are at increased risk for fetal macrosomia. Some experts immediately diagnose and treat these women as if they had gestational diabetes. Other authorities prefer to retest them with another 3-hour OGTT 1 month later (Landon, 1996). Often women with one abnormal OGTT value will be placed on a modified diabetic diet that contains no concentrated sweets (candy, cookies, cake, pie, sugar-sweetened drinks) for the remainder of the pregnancy.

Nursing diagnoses are similar to those identified for women with pregestational diabetes (see p. 868).

Expected outcomes of care for the woman with GDM are basically the same as for women with pregestational diabetes except that the time frame for planning may be shortened with GDM because the diagnosis is usually made later in pregnancy.

Interventions

Antepartum

When the diagnosis of gestational diabetes is made, treatment begins immediately, allowing little or no time for the woman and her family to adjust to the diagnosis before they are expected to participate in the treatment plan. This is in contrast to the woman with pregestational diabetes, who may have had years to learn about the disease and to adapt to dietary modifications, self-monitoring of glucose, and insulin administration. With each step of the treatment plan, the nurse and other health care providers should educate the woman and her family, providing detailed and comprehensive explanations to ensure understanding, participation, and adherence to the necessary interventions. Potential complications should be dis-

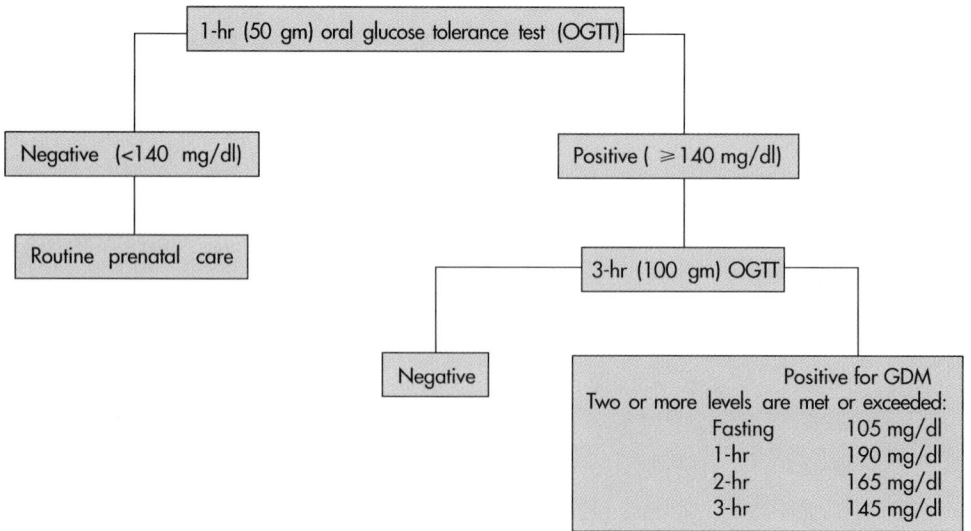

Fig. 32-4 Screening and diagnosis for gestational diabetes. *(From American Diabetes Association. [1997]. Position statement: Gestational diabetes mellitus. Diabetes Care 20[suppl 1], S44.)*

cussed, and the need for maintenance of normoglycemia throughout the remainder of the pregnancy is reinforced. It may be reassuring for the woman and her family to know that gestational diabetes typically disappears when the pregnancy is over.

As with pregestational diabetes, the aim of therapy in women with GDM is meticulous blood glucose control. Fasting blood glucose levels should be less than 105 mg/dl, and 2-hour postprandial blood levels should be less than 120 mg/dl (Hagay & Reece, 1999; Landon, 1996).

Diet. Dietary modification is the mainstay of treatment for GDM. The woman with GDM is placed on a standard diabetic diet immediately on diagnosis. The usual prescription is for 30 to 35 kcal/kg of present pregnancy weight, which translates into 2000 to 2500 calories per day for most women. Some authorities recommend fewer calories for overweight or morbidly obese women, believing that such a diet will cause less hyperglycemia and reduce the need for insulin (Landon, 1996; Metzger & Coustan, 1998). Dietary counseling by a nutritionist is recommended. Most women with GDM do not require hospitalization for dietary instruction and management.

Exercise. Exercise in women with GDM appears to be safe. It helps lower blood glucose levels and may be instrumental in eliminating the need for insulin. Women with GDM who already have an active lifestyle should be encouraged to continue an exercise program. Brisk walking, use of a recumbent bicycle, and swimming are often recommended; exercises that use the upper body are ideal for most women because they are not associated with increased uterine contractions. Sedentary women may also be encouraged to increase their physical activity. They may be advised to begin by exercising three or four times a week for 15 to 30 minutes, gradually increasing intensity and duration (Jones & Stone, 1998). Of course, any exercise program should always be initiated or continued with the knowledge and consent of the primary health care provider.

Monitoring blood glucose levels. Continuous blood glucose monitoring is necessary to determine if euglycemia can be maintained by diet and exercise. Fasting and postprandial glucose levels should be monitored at least weekly (ACOG, 1994). Some women with GDM are provided with reflectance meters and encouraged to perform frequent self-monitoring at home, or monitoring may be done only at the clinic or office visit.

Insulin therapy. It is important to understand that many women with GDM will require insulin during the pregnancy to maintain adequate blood glucose levels, despite compliance with the prescribed diet. This is true because as pregnancy progresses, placental hormones increase blood glucose levels and cause insulin to work less effectively. Depending on the diet prescribed and the blood glucose thresholds used by the practitioner, as many as half of all women with GDM may require insulin at some point during pregnancy (Landon, 1996). Therefore

the nurse should never assume that increased blood glucose levels in the woman with GDM have been caused by dietary indiscretion alone without first taking a thorough history.

ACOG (1994) recommends that women who repetitively exceed the glucose thresholds of 105 mg/dl fasting and 120 mg/dl 2 hours postprandial be started on insulin therapy. In practice, however, many health care providers use either lower or higher thresholds for initiating insulin (Landon, 1996). The woman and her family should be taught the necessary skills to manage insulin administration (see previous discussion). Sometimes hospitalization may be required to regulate blood glucose levels and to educate the woman about glycemic control through insulin therapy in conjunction with dietary modification.

Fetal surveillance. There is no standard recommendation for fetal surveillance in pregnancies complicated by GDM. Women whose blood glucose levels are well controlled by diet are at low risk for fetal death. Many practitioners do not routinely perform antepartum fetal testing on them so long as their fasting and 2-hour postprandial blood glucose levels remain within normal limits and they have no other risk factors. More research must be done to determine if routine antepartum monitoring in this group of low risk clients would be of benefit. Usually these women are allowed to progress to term and spontaneous labor without intervention. Once the woman reaches 40 weeks of gestation, fetal surveillance once or twice weekly is usually instituted (ACOG, 1994; Landon, 1996; Metzger & Coustan, 1998).

Women with GDM whose blood glucose levels are not well controlled or who require insulin therapy, have hypertension, or have a history of previous stillbirth generally receive more intensive fetal biophysical monitoring. There is no standard recommendation regarding initiation of testing. Nonstress tests and biophysical profiles are often performed weekly, beginning anywhere from 32 to 36 weeks of gestation (ACOG, 1994; Landon, 1996; Metzger & Coustan, 1998).

Intrapartum

During the labor and birth process, blood glucose levels are monitored at least every 2 hours to maintain levels at 100 mg/dl or less. Glucose levels within this range will decrease the severity of neonatal hypoglycemia. IV fluids containing glucose are not given as a bolus to the woman who has gestational diabetes, although they may be necessary as maintenance fluids. Routine uterine activity and fetal heart rate assessments are done. Although gestational diabetes is not an indication for cesarean birth, it may be necessary in the presence of problems, such as preeclampsia or macrosomia.

Postpartum

Most women with GDM will return to normal glucose levels after childbirth (Metzger & Coustan, 1998). However,

GDM is likely to recur in future pregnancies. Of women with previous GDM, 50% to 60% will develop overt diabetes later in life, many within 10 years of the pregnancy complicated by GDM (Jones & Stone, 1998). Assessment for carbohydrate intolerance can be initiated 6 to 12 weeks postpartum or after breastfeeding has stopped and should be repeated at regular intervals throughout the woman's life (Metzger & Coustan, 1998). Obesity is a major risk factor for the later development of diabetes. Thus women with a history of GDM, particularly those who are overweight, should be encouraged to make lifestyle changes that include weight loss and exercise to reduce this risk (Hagay & Reece, 1999; Metzger & Coustan, 1998). Because offspring of women with GDM are at risk to develop obesity and diabetes in childhood or adolescence (Metzger & Coustan, 1998), regular health care for these children is essential.

Evaluation

Care of the woman with GDM is evaluated using the expected outcomes previously described for the woman with pregestational diabetes.

HYPEREMESIS GRAVIDARUM

Nausea and vomiting complicate approximately 70% of all pregnancies and are usually confined to the first trimester (Cruikshank et al., 1996). Although these manifestations are distressing, they are typically benign, with no significant metabolic alterations or risks to the mother or fetus.

When vomiting during pregnancy becomes excessive enough to cause weight loss of at least 5% of prepregnancy weight and is accompanied by dehydration, electrolyte imbalance, ketosis, and acetonuria, the disorder is termed **hyperemesis gravidarum.** The estimated incidence varies from 0.5 to 10 per 1000 births (Snell et al., 1998). Hyperemesis gravidarum usually begins during the first 10 weeks of pregnancy. Women with hyperemesis tend to be younger than 20 years of age, obese, and nonsmokers. They are also more likely to have multifetal or molar pregnancies (Riely, 1999).

Several researchers have found that vomiting during pregnancy has been shown to be associated with a decreased risk of miscarriage, but they could find no consistent association with perinatal mortality. Other studies have reported an association between multiple hospital admissions for severe nausea and vomiting and decreased maternal weight gain and neonatal birth weight (Hill & Fleming, 1999; Snell et al., 1998).

Etiology

The etiology of hyperemesis gravidarum remains obscure. Several theories have been proposed as to the cause, although none of them adequately explains the disorder. Hyperemesis gravidarum may be related to high levels of estrogen or human chorionic gonadotropin (hCG) and may be associated with transient hyperthyroidism during pregnancy. It may be accompanied by liver disfunction manifested by elevated transaminase and abnormal bilirubin level and prothrombin time. Other possible causes include vitamin B deficiencies and increased sensitivity to circulating sex steroid hormones (Hill & Fleming, 1999; Riely, 1999; Snell et al., 1998).

Psychologic factors may also play a part in the development of hyperemesis gravidarum, at least in some women. Ambivalence toward the pregnancy and difficult relationships with mothers or partners have been identified as causative factors. High stress levels are probably also associated with this condition (Hill & Fleming, 1999; Snell et al., 1998). Conflicting feelings regarding prospective motherhood, body changes, and lifestyle alterations may contribute to episodes of vomiting, particularly if these feelings are excessive or unresolved.

Clinical Manifestations

The woman with hyperemesis usually has significant weight loss and dehydration. She may have a decreased blood pressure, increased pulse rate, and poor skin turgor (Snell et al., 1998). She is almost always unable to keep down even clear liquids taken by mouth. Laboratory tests may reveal electrolyte imbalances.

Collaborative Care

Whenever a pregnant woman has a complaint of nausea and vomiting, the first priority is a thorough assessment to determine the severity of the problem. In most cases, the woman should be told to come immediately to the health care provider's office or to the emergency department, because the severity of the illness is often difficult to determine by phone conversation.

The history includes information about the frequency, severity, and duration of episodes of nausea and vomiting. Other symptoms such as diarrhea, indigestion, and abdominal pain or distention are also identified. The woman is asked to report any precipitating factors relating to the onset of her symptoms. Any pharmacologic or nonpharmacologic treatment measures should be recorded. Prepregnancy weight and documented weight gain or loss during pregnancy are important to note.

The woman's weight and vital signs are measured, and a complete physical examination is performed, with attention to signs of fluid and electrolyte imbalance and nutritional status. The most important initial laboratory test to be obtained is a dipstick determination of ketonuria. Other laboratory tests that may be ordered are a urinalysis, a complete blood cell count, electrolytes, liver enzymes, and bilirubin levels. These tests help rule out the presence of underlying diseases such as pyelonephritis, pancreatitis, cholecystitis, and hepatitis (Cruikshank et al., 1996). Because of the recognized association between hyperemesis gravidarum and hyperthyroidism, thyroid function may also be assessed.

Psychosocial assessment includes asking the woman about anxiety, fears, and concerns related to her own health and the effects on pregnancy outcome. Family members should be assessed both for anxiety and in regard to their role in providing support for the woman.

Initial Care

Initially the woman who is unable to keep down clear liquids by mouth will require IV therapy for correction of fluid and electrolyte imbalances. She should be kept on nothing-by-mouth (NPO) status until dehydration has been resolved and for at least 48 hours after vomiting has stopped to prevent rapid recurrence of the problem (Cruikshank et al., 1996). In the past, women requiring IV therapy were admitted to the hospital. Today, however, they may be, and often are, successfully managed at home. Antiemetic medications may be used if nausea and vomiting are uncontrolled; commonly used drugs include pyridoxine, droperidol, diphenhydramine, and metoclopramide. Corticosteroids have also been used successfully to treat refractory hyperemesis gravidarum. In addition to medical management, some women can also benefit from psychotherapy or stress reduction techniques (Hill & Fleming, 1999; Snell et al., 1998). Once the vomiting has stopped, feedings are started in small amounts at frequent intervals, and the diet is slowly advanced as tolerated.

In severe cases of hyperemesis gravidarum, enteral nutrition via a feeding tube or parenteral nutrition may be necessary to correct maternal nutritional deprivation. Total parenteral nutrition has also been used successfully (Hill & Fleming, 1999; Snell et al., 1998).

Initial care of the hyperemetic woman involves implementing the medical plan of care, whether in the hospital or home setting. Interventions may include initiating and monitoring IV therapy, administering drugs and nutritional supplements, and monitoring the woman's response to interventions. The nurse observes the woman for any signs of complications such as metabolic acidosis, jaundice, or hemorrhage and alerts the physician should these occur.

Accurate measurement of intake and output, including the amount of emesis, is an important aspect of care. Oral hygiene while the woman is receiving nothing by mouth, and after episodes of vomiting, helps allay associated discomforts. Assistance with positioning and providing a quiet, restful environment that is free from odors may increase the woman's comfort. When the woman begins responding to therapy, limited amounts of oral fluids and bland foods such as crackers or toast are begun. The diet is progressed slowly as tolerated by the woman until she is able to consume a nutritionally sound diet. Because sleep disturbances may accompany hyperemesis gravidarum, promoting adequate rest is important. The nurse can assist in coordinating treatment measures and periods of visitation to provide opportunity for rest periods (see Plan of Care).

Home Care

After several days of treatment, whether in the hospital or at home, most women are able to take nourishment by mouth. Education at this time is important to prevent rapid recurrence of nausea and vomiting. Women should be encouraged to eat small, frequent meals and low-fat protein foods, to avoid greasy and highly seasoned foods, and to increase their dietary intake of potassium and magnesium. Herbal teas such as chamomile or raspberry leaf may decrease nausea. Taking fluids between meals rather than with them sometimes helps decrease nausea. Many pregnant women find exposure to cooking odors nauseating. If other family members can take over cooking chores, even temporarily, the woman's nausea and vomiting may decrease. Finally, the woman should be told to contact her health care provider immediately if the nausea and vomiting recurs, especially if accompanied by abdominal pain, dehydration, or significant weight loss (e.g., greater than 11 kg in 1 week) (Lowdermilk & Grohar, 1999).

A few women will continue to experience intractable nausea and vomiting throughout pregnancy. Rarely, it may be necessary to maintain a woman on enteral, parenteral, or total parenteral nutrition in order to provide adequate nutrition for the mother and fetus. Many home health agencies are able to provide these services, and arrangements for service may be made depending on the woman's insurance coverage.

Regardless of the site of care, the nurse must remain calm, compassionate, and sympathetic, recognizing that the manifestations of hyperemesis can be physically and emotionally debilitating. Irritability, tearfulness, and mood changes are often consistent with this disorder. Fetal well-being is a primary concern of the woman. The nurse can provide an environment conducive to discussion of those concerns and assist the woman in identifying and mobilizing sources of support. The family members should be included in the plan of care whenever possible. Encouraging their participation may help alleviate some of the emotional stress associated with this disorder. Psychologic counseling may be needed, as well as referral to a social worker. Education of the woman and her family about hyperemesis, its causes, potential complications, and a management plan is necessary at the onset because understanding enhances adherence to the treatment plan and influences maternal and fetal outcomes.

THYROID DISORDERS

Hyperthyroidism

Hyperthyroidism occurs in approximately 2 of every 1000 pregnancies (Landon, 1996; Seely & Burrow, 1999). In 90% to 95% of pregnant women, it is caused by Graves' disease. Other rare but possible causes are toxic nodular goiter and thyroiditis (Inzucchi & Burrow, 1999; Seely & Burrow, 1999). Clinical manifestations of hyperthyroidism are associated with an increased basal metabolism rate and

PLAN ᵒᶠ CARE | Hyperemesis Gravidarum

NURSING DIAGNOSIS Altered nutrition: less than body requirements, related to nausea and persistent vomiting as evidenced by weight decrease as compared with prepregnant weight

---

Expected Outcomes *Client will exhibit no further weight losses and weight will stabilize. Client will tolerate regular diet with adequate nutrients for pregnancy with no further nausea and vomiting.*

Nursing Interventions/*Rationales*

Ascertain client's prepregnant weight and monitor client's current weight and intake and output *to provide a database for care planning.*

Resume oral diet as tolerated and prescribed by caregiver *to provide oral nutrition at optimum time.*

Provide small, frequent bland meals as client tolerates *to assess client's response to limited oral intake.*

Administer antiemetic medications as prescribed *to decrease or eliminate episodes of vomiting.*

Provide a quiet, restful environment *to decrease associated discomforts.*

Teach client the importance of a low-fat, high-protein diet with fluids between meals *to provide optimum nutrition for fetal growth and keep nausea to a minimum.*

Refer to dietitian to develop optimum diet plan that is individualized to client's current preferences, culture, and lifestyle *to encourage ongoing compliance.*

Discuss with client the importance of contacting health care provider if intractable nausea and vomiting recur *to provide prompt treatment and avoid complications.*

NURSING DIAGNOSIS Fluid volume deficit related to excessive vomiting as evidenced by fluid and electrolyte imbalance

---

Expected Outcome *Client's fluid and electrolyte balance will be restored.*

Nursing Interventions/*Rationales*

Assess and document skin turgor, condition of mucous membranes, vital signs, and urine specific gravity *to provide database for planning care.*

Obtain daily weight *to provide ongoing evaluation of care.*

Monitor laboratory values and report deviations from normal *to prevent complications.*

Maintain accurate intake and output record *to assess for evidence of fluid deficit.*

Initiate and maintain IV therapy carefully *to maintain fluid balance.*

Administer antiemetics as prescribed *to inhibit nausea and vomiting.*

Begin oral fluids slowly and carefully *to slowly increase tolerance and restore fluid balance.*

NURSING DIAGNOSIS Anxiety related to effects of hyperemesis on fetal well-being as evidenced by client statements of concern

---

Expected Outcome *Client will exhibit decreased incidence of anxiety.*

Nursing Interventions/*Rationales*

Use therapeutic communication to listen to client concerns *to maintain a relationship and feeling of trust.*

Provide information regarding any potential risks to the fetus *to alleviate anxiety.*

Assist client to identify personal strengths and previous coping mechanisms *to reinforce to client those strengths and coping mechanisms that may be of assistance during this illness.*

Help client identify sources of support and mobilize support person or group of her choice *to provide support as needed.*

Refer to social services as needed *for ongoing evaluation and assistance.*

---

increased sympathetic nervous system activity. Typical symptoms include fatigue, heat intolerance, warm skin, diaphoresis, emotional lability, tremulousness, and a wide pulse pressure. Many of these symptoms also occur with pregnancy, so the disorder can be difficult to diagnose. Signs that may help differentiate hyperthyroidism from normal pregnancy include unplanned weight loss, onycholysis (loose nails), and a pulse rate greater than 100 beats per minute that does not decrease with the Valsalva ma-

neuver (Diehl, 1998; Seely & Burrow, 1999). Laboratory findings include an elevated free thyroxine (T_4) level and a suppressed serum thyroid-stimulating hormone (TSH) level (Diehl, 1998; Seely & Burrow, 1999). Mild hyperthyroidism is not thought to impair fertility, although it is rare to find severe disease in early pregnancy. Hyperthyroidism should be treated during pregnancy; untreated or inadequately treated women give birth to infants with low birth weight and more minor fetal anomalies. Women with hyperthyroidism are also at increased risk to develop severe preeclampsia (Diehl, 1998; Seely & Burrow, 1999). Hyperemesis gravidarum is often associated with elevated thyroid hormone levels (Landon, 1996; Seely & Burrow, 1999).

The primary treatment of hyperthyroidism during pregnancy is drug therapy; the medication of choice is propylthiouracil (PTU). The usual starting dose is 100 to 150 mg every 8 hours. Clients generally show clinical improvement within 2 weeks of beginning therapy, but the medication requires 6 to 8 weeks to reach full effectiveness. During therapy the woman's free T_4 levels are measured monthly and the results used to taper the drug to the smallest effective dosage to prevent unnecessary fetal hypothyroidism (Diehl, 1998; Seely & Burrow, 1999). PTU is well tolerated by most clients. Rare side effects include pruritus, skin rash, fever, a metallic taste, nausea, bronchospasm, oral ulcerations, hepatitis, and a lupus-like syndrome (Seely & Burrow, 1999). The most severe side effect is agranulocytosis, which is more common in women over 40 years of age and in those taking high doses of PTU (Seely & Burrow, 1999). Symptoms of agranulocytosis are fever and sore throat; these symptoms should be reported immediately to the health care provider, and the woman should stop taking the PTU. Transient, benign leukopenia may occur as a result of PTU therapy. PTU readily crosses the placenta and may induce fetal hypothyroidism and goiter, although these complications rarely occur (Landon, 1996; Seely & Burrow, 1999).

Beta-adrenergic blockers such as propranolol may be used in severe hyperthyroidism. Long-term use is not recommended because of the potential for IUGR and altered response to anoxic stress, postnatal bradycardia, and hypoglycemia (Seely & Burrow, 1999).

Radioactive iodine must not be used in diagnosis or treatment of hyperthyroidism in pregnancy because it may compromise the fetal thyroid. If a mother taking hyperthyroid medication chooses to breastfeed, she should be aware that physiologically significant doses of the drug are passed to the infant through the breast milk. The infant's thyroid status should be monitored periodically so that hypothyroidism can be prevented (Cunningham et al., 1997; Seely & Burrow, 1999).

In severe cases surgical treatment of hyperthyroidism, subtotal thyroidectomy, may be performed during the second or third trimester. Because of the increased risk of miscarriage and preterm labor associated with major surgery, this treatment is usually reserved for women with severe disease, those for whom drug therapy proves toxic, and those who are unable to adhere to the prescribed medical regimen. Postoperative hypothyroidism is common, occurring in at least 20% of women who were previously hyperthyroid.

A serious but uncommon complication of undiagnosed or partially treated hyperthyroidism is thyroid storm, which may occur in response to stress such as infection, birth, or surgery. A woman with this emergency disorder may have fever, restlessness, tachycardia, vomiting, hypotension, or stupor. Prompt treatment is essential; IV fluids and oxygen are administered along with high doses of PTU. Potassium iodide, antipyretics, dexamethasone, and beta-adrenergic blockers may also be given; sedation may be necessary for extreme restlessness (Inzucchi & Burrow, 1999; Landon, 1996).

Hypothyroidism

Hypothyroidism during pregnancy is a rare phenomenon because women with this disorder are often infertile. Hypothyroidism is usually caused by Hashimoto's disease, thyroid gland ablation by radiation, previous surgery, or antithyroid medications. Reduced thyroid function resulting from hypothalamic or pituitary failure is rare, with only a few reported cases. Iodine deficiency in the United States is also rare (Diehl, 1998; Landon, 1996).

Characteristic symptoms of hypothyroidism include weight gain; fatigue; cold intolerance; constipation; cool, dry skin; coarsened hair; and muscle weakness. Laboratory values in pregnancy include low or low-normal T_3 and T_4 levels and elevated levels of TSH (Diehl, 1998; Inzucchi & Burrow, 1999).

Pregnant women with untreated hypothyroidism are at risk for preeclampsia, placental abruption, and stillbirth. Infants born to mothers with hypothyroidism may be of low birth weight, but for the most part are healthy and without evidence of thyroid dysfunction (Diehl, 1998; Inzucchi & Burrow, 1999).

Thyroid hormone supplements are used to treat hypothyroidism. Levothyroxine (e.g., L-thyroxine [Synthroid]) is most often prescribed during pregnancy. The usual beginning dosage is 0.10 mg to 0.15 mg per day, in a single daily dose.

NURSE ALERT *Pregnant women should be told to take L-thyroxine 2 hours before or after iron tablets, because ferrous sulfate lowers the effectiveness of the medication (Diehl, 1998).*

As pregnancy progresses, the woman usually requires increased amounts of L-thyroxine. The aim of drug therapy is to maintain the woman's TSH level within the normal range for pregnant women. Dosage adjustments are made as necessary by measuring her TSH levels periodically throughout pregnancy. Each dosage change should be followed by determining the TSH level 4 to 6 weeks later. Any known hypothyroid woman with hypothyroidism who becomes pregnant should have her thyroid status checked immediately. If her TSH level is normal, no dosage adjustment is necessary, although periodic determinations throughout pregnancy are recommended (Diehl, 1998; Inzucchi & Burrow, 1999).

The fetus depends on maternal thyroid hormones until 12 weeks of gestation, when fetal production begins. Thus maternal hypothyroidism does not cause fetal hypothyroidism. However, maternal treatment of hypothyroidism may result in increased fetal levels of thyroid hormones. Careful monitoring of the neonate's thyroid status is important to detect any abnormalities.

Collaborative Care

The pregnant woman with thyroid dysfunction often needs assistance from the nurse in coping with the discomforts and frustrations associated with symptoms of the disorder. For example, the woman with hyperthyroidism who has nervousness and hyperactivity concomitantly with weakness and fatigue may benefit from suggestions to channel excess energies into quiet diversional activities such as reading or crafts. Discomfort associated with hypersensitivity to heat (hyperthyroidism) or cold intolerance (hypothyroidism) can be minimized by appropriate clothing and regulation of environmental temperatures, when possible, and by avoidance of temperature extremes.

Nutritional counseling with a registered dietitian may provide guidance in selecting a well-balanced diet. The woman with hyperthyroidism who has increased appetite and poor weight gain and the hypothyroid woman with hypothyroidism who has anorexia and lethargy need counseling to ensure adequate intake of nutritionally sound foods to meet both maternal and fetal needs.

Education of these women is essential to promote compliance with the plan of treatment. The woman is instructed regarding the disorder and its potential impact on herself and her fetus, the medication regimen and possible side effects, the need for continuing medical supervision, and the importance of compliance.

Psychologic and emotional implications of pregnancy complicated by thyroid dysfunction are similar to those of any high risk pregnancy. The woman is encouraged to verbalize feelings, concerns, and frustrations and is assisted in identifying support systems. The family is incorporated into the plan of care to foster mutuality and support among the members.

MATERNAL PHENYLKETONURIA

Phenylketonuria (PKU), a recognized cause of mental retardation, is an inborn error of metabolism caused by an autosomal recessive trait that creates a deficiency in the enzyme phenylalanine hydrolase. Absence of this enzyme impairs the body's ability to metabolize the amino acid phenylalanine, found in all protein foods. Consequently, there is toxic accumulation of phenylalanine in the blood, which interferes with brain development and function. PKU affects 1 in every 10,000 live births in the United States.

PKU was the first inborn error of metabolism to be universally screened for in the United States. Beginning in 1961, all newborns were tested soon after birth for this disorder. Prompt diagnosis and therapy with a phenylalanine-restricted diet significantly decreased the incidence of mental retardation. Children with PKU were treated with the special diet up to age 6; after that time further treatment was thought to be unnecessary (Luke, 1999). However, subtle but detrimental effects of elevated levels of phenylalanine on neurologic, behavioral, and intellectual function have been found in women who discontinued treatment in childhood. Dietary therapy for PKU has been recommended for continuation throughout adulthood (Acosta, 1995).

Now many of these women with PKU have reached their childbearing years and are starting families. To have the best possible pregnancy outcomes, they must resume special dietary therapy before conception, although even then a normal child cannot be guaranteed (Aminoff, 1999). Women with untreated PKU have an increased risk of miscarriage, and their children are more likely to be born with mental retardation, microcephaly, congenital heart disease, and low birth weight. These problems result from high maternal PKU levels, which cross the placenta and are teratogenic to the developing fetus (Aminoff, 1999; Luke, 1999).

The key to prevention of fetal anomalies caused by PKU is the identification of women in their reproductive years who have the disorder. Screening programs in the premarital period and even earlier, such as during school physical examinations, may help identify those individuals with PKU so that dietary therapy can be instituted before conception occurs. Before conception these women and their families should be educated about the potential risks to the fetus if phenylalanine levels are not controlled.

Screening for undiagnosed maternal PKU at the first prenatal visit may be warranted, especially in individuals with a family history of the disorder, with low intelligence of uncertain etiology, or who have given birth to microcephalic infants. Ultrasound scans may be used to monitor fetal growth and identify anomalies. Although it may be too late to improve the current pregnancy outcome through diet therapy, the woman and her family will be aware of the problem and the necessary treatment should future pregnancies occur (Aminoff, 1999).

Infants born to women with PKU will either be homozygous or heterozygous for the trait. Homozygous infants definitely need phenylalanine-restricted diet therapy. Proper nutritional management of heterozygous infants is less clear. Women with PKU have been discouraged from breastfeeding because their milk contains a high concentration of phenylalanine (Aminoff, 1999). However, breastfeeding can be done safely if the amount of breast milk ingested is monitored so that phenylalanine levels do not get too high. Mothers who choose to breastfeed must still supplement the infant's diet with a special milk preparation that contains little or no phenylalanine. Monitoring amounts of phenylalanine can be tedious and frustrating. Health care providers can help parents in their decision making about how to feed their infant (Kirby, 1999).

KEY POINTS

- Lack of maternal glycemic control before conception and in the first trimester of pregnancy may be responsible for fetal congenital malformations.

- Maternal insulin requirements increase as the pregnancy progresses and may quadruple by term as a result of insulin resistance created by placental hormones, insulinase, and cortisol.

- Poor glycemic control before and during pregnancy can lead to maternal complications such as miscarriage, infection, and dystocia (difficult labor) caused by fetal macrosomia.

- Careful glucose monitoring, insulin administration when necessary, and dietary counseling are used to create a normal intrauterine environment for fetal growth and development in the pregnancy complicated by diabetes mellitus.

- Because gestational diabetes mellitus is asymptomatic in most cases, many women undergo routine screening during pregnancy.

- Hyperemesis gravidarum is frequently managed at home. The woman should receive intravenous fluids and electrolytes and remain on NPO status until nausea and vomiting have stopped. She can then slowly advance her diet as tolerated.

- Thyroid dysfunction during pregnancy requires close monitoring of thyroid hormone levels to regulate therapy and prevent fetal insult.

- High levels of PKU in the maternal bloodstream cross the placenta and are teratogenic to the developing fetus. Damage can be prevented or minimized by dietary restriction of phenylalanine before and during pregnancy.

CRITICAL THINKING EXERCISES

1 Carmelita Hershey is admitted to the antepartum unit. She is a type 1 diabetic who is 30 weeks pregnant. She receives insulin twice a day. Her blood glucose level on admission is 220 mg/dl. This admission is to control her blood glucose and assess both her status and that of her fetus.
   a. What assessment would you need to do in order to determine why Carmelita's blood glucose levels are out of control?
   b. How would Carmelita's fetus respond to increased maternal glucose levels? What complications might this cause in the fetus?
   c. Carmelita is from Mexico, and she likes to eat tortillas and beans and spicy foods. Prepare a diet exchange list for a 2200-calorie ADA diet that would incorporate foods that she prefers.

2 Attend a high risk prenatal clinic on a day when women with diabetes are scheduled. Interview several women with gestational diabetes and talk with their significant others. Ask them the following questions, and then analyze your interview data and present a clinical conference on the impact of gestational diabetes.
   a. How did you feel when you were first told that you had gestational diabetes?
   b. What changes in your lifestyle have you made as a result of being a gestational diabetic? Which change has been the hardest to make?
   c. What was the best thing that your health care provider did to help you adjust to being a gestational diabetic?
   d. What could your health care providers have done differently that might have helped you adjust more quickly or easily to having gestational diabetes?

3 Tammy H., a 19-year-old G1 P0, is at the clinic today for her initial prenatal visit at approximately 8 weeks of gestation. As you take her history, Tammy tells you that she followed a special diet when she was a small child "for high PKU." However, she has been eating "anything I want" for many years now.
   a. Plan a phenylalanine-restricted diet for Tammy to follow during pregnancy. What types of foods does she need to avoid? How would you motivate Tammy to follow her diet carefully?
   b. Because Tammy is still early in her pregnancy, should she be concerned about the health of her fetus?
   c. What advice would you give Tammy in regard to future pregnancies?

References

Acosta, P. (1995). Nutrition support of maternal phenylketonuria. *Semin Perinat* 19(3), 182-190.

Alvarez-Marfany, M. et al. (1994). Long-term prospective study of postpartum thyroid dysfunction in women with insulin dependent diabetes mellitus. *J Clin Endocrinol Metab* 79(1), 10-16.

American College of Obstetricians and Gynecologists. (1994). Diabetes and pregnancy. *ACOG Tech Bull* 200. Washington, D.C.: ACOG.

American Diabetes Association. (1994). *Medical management of insulin-dependent (type 1) diabetes* (2nd ed.). Alexandria, VA: The Association.

American Diabetes Association. (1995). *Medical management of pregnancy complicated by diabetes* (2nd ed.). Alexandria, VA: The Association.

American Diabetes Association. (1997). Position statement: Gestational diabetes mellitus. *Diabetes Care* 20(suppl 1), S44.

Aminoff, M. (1999). Neurologic disorders. In R. Creasy & R. Resnik (Eds.). *Maternal-fetal medicine* (4th ed.). Philadelphia: W.B. Saunders.

Becton Dickinson & Co. (1997). *Controlling low blood sugar reactions.* Franklin Lakes, NJ: Becton Dickinson & Co.

Bernstein, I., & Gabbe, S. (1996). Intrauterine growth restriction. In S. Gabbe, J. Niebyl, & J. Simpson (Eds.). *Obstetrics: Normal and problem pregnancies* (3rd ed.). New York: Churchill Livingstone.

Cruikshank, D. et al. (1996). Maternal physiology in pregnancy. In S. Gabbe, J. Niebyl, & J. Simpson (Eds.). *Obstetrics: Normal and problem pregnancies* (3rd ed.). New York: Churchill Livingstone.

Cunningham, F. et al. (1997). *Williams obstetrics* (20th ed.). Stamford, CT: Appleton & Lange.

Diehl, K. (1998). Thyroid dysfunction in pregnancy. *J Perinat Neonatal Nurs* 11(4), 1-12.

Eli Lilly & Co. (1996). *Humalog.* Indianapolis: Eli Lilly & Co.

Expert Committee on the Diagnosis and Classification of Diabetes Mellitus. (1997). Report of the Expert Committee on the Diagnosis and Classification of Diabetes Mellitus. *Diabetes Care* 20(7), 1183-1187.

Gerstein, H. (1993). Incidence of postpartum thyroid dysfunction in patients with type 1 diabetes mellitus. *Ann Intern Med* 118(6), 419-423.

Gilbert, E., & Harmon, J. (1998). *Manual of high risk pregnancy and delivery* (2nd ed.). St. Louis: Mosby.

Hagay, A., & Reece, E. (1999). Diabetes mellitus in pregnancy. In E. Reece & J. Hobbins (Eds.). *Medicine of the fetus and mother* (2nd ed.). Philadelphia: Lippincott-Raven.

Hill, W., & Fleming, A. (1999). Gastrointestinal diseases complicating pregnancy. In E. Reece & J. Hobbins (Eds.). *Medicine of the fetus and mother* (2nd ed.). Philadelphia: Lippincott-Raven.

Hoffmeister, A., & Haines, S. (1996). The newest insulin: Lispro. *Diabetes Wellness Lett* 2(12), 1.

Inzucchi, S., & Burrow, G. (1999). Endocrine disorders in pregnancy. In E. Reece & J. Hobbins (Eds.). *Medicine of the fetus and mother* (2nd ed.). Philadelphia: Lippincott-Raven.

Jones, M., & Stone, L. (1998). Management of the woman with gestational diabetes mellitus. *J Perinat Neonatal Nurs* 11(4), 13-24.

Jovanovic-Peterson, L. (Ed.). (1993). *Medical management of pregnancy complicated by diabetes.* Alexandria, VA: American Diabetes Association.

Kirby, R. (1999). Maternal phenylketonuria: A new cause for concern. *J Obstet Gynecol Neonatal Nurs* 28(3), 227-234.

Kjos, S. (1996). Contraception in the diabetic woman. *Obstet Gynecol Clin North Am* 23(1), 243-258.

Landon, M. (1996). Diabetes mellitus and other endocrine disorders. In S. Gabbe, J. Niebyl, & J. Simpson (Eds.). *Obstetrics: Normal and problem pregnancies* (3rd ed.). New York: Churchill Livingstone.

Landon, M., & Gabbe, S. (1995). Diabetes mellitus. In W. Barron & M. Lindheimer (Eds.). *Medical disorders during pregnancy* (2nd ed.). St. Louis: Mosby.

Lowdermilk, D., & Grohar, J. (1999). *High risk antepartal home care.* White Plains, NY: March of Dimes.

Luke, B. (1999). Maternal nutrition. In E. Reece & J. Hobbins (Eds.). *Medicine of the fetus and mother* (2nd ed.). Philadelphia: Lippincott-Raven.

Metzger, B., & Coustan, D. (1998). Summary and recommendations of the fourth international workshop-conference on gestational diabetes mellitus. *Diabetes Care* 21(suppl 2), B161-B167.

Moore, T. (1999). Diabetes in pregnancy. In R. Creasy & R. Resnik (Eds.). *Maternal-fetal medicine* (4th ed.). Philadelphia: WB Saunders.

Pagana, K., & Pagana, T. (1997). *Mosby's diagnostic and laboratory test reference* (3rd ed.). St. Louis: Mosby.

Reece, E., & Homko, C. (1993). Diabetes-related complications of pregnancy. *J Natl Med Assoc* 85(7), 537-545.

Reece, E., & Homko, C. (1994). Assessment and management of pregnancies complicated by pregestational and gestational diabetes mellitus. *J Assoc Acad Minority Phys* 5(3), 87-97.

Riely, C. (1999). Liver diseases in pregnancy. In E. Reece & J. Hobbins (Eds.). *Medicine of the fetus and mother* (2nd ed.). Philadelphia: Lippincott-Raven.

Seely, L., & Burrow, G. (1999). Thyroid disease and pregnancy. In R. Creasy & R. Resnik (Eds.). *Maternal-fetal medicine* (4th ed.). Philadelphia: WB Saunders.

Snell, L. et al. (1998). Metabolic crisis: Hyperemesis gravidarum. *J Perinat Neonatal Nurs* 12(2), 26-37.

33

Medical-Surgical Problems in Pregnancy

Shannon E. Perry

 EARNING OBJECTIVES

- Define the key terms.
- Describe the management of cardiovascular disorders in pregnant women.
- Identify nursing interventions for the pregnant woman with a cardiovascular disorder.
- Discuss anemia during pregnancy.
- Explain the care of pregnant women with pulmonary disorders.
- Review the effect of gastrointestinal disorders on gastrointestinal function during pregnancy.

- Review the effects of neurologic disorders on pregnancy.
- Describe the care of women whose pregnancies are complicated by autoimmune disorders.
- Explain the basic principles of care for a pregnant woman having abdominal surgery.
- Identify topics for nursing research on medical-surgical problems in pregnancy.

 EY TERMS

adult respiratory distress syndrome (ARDS)
autoimmune disorders
cardiac decompensation
cholecystitis
cholelithiasis

Eisenmenger's syndrome
infective endocarditis
Marfan's syndrome
mitral valve prolapse (MVP)
mitral valve stenosis
peripartum cardiomyopathy

reflex bradycardia
rheumatic heart disease (RHD)
sickle cell hemoglobinopathy
systemic lupus erythematosus

The effects of selected preexisting medical disorders on pregnancy and the nursing care that can lead to their effective management are presented in this chapter. These disorders, including cardiovascular, respiratory, gastrointestinal (GI), integumentary, and central nervous system (CNS) disorders, are sometimes first diagnosed during pregnancy. Abdominal surgery and the related nursing roles are discussed.

CARDIOVASCULAR DISORDERS

During a normal pregnancy the maternal cardiovascular system undergoes many changes that put a physiologic strain on the heart. The major cardiovascular changes that occur during a normal pregnancy and that affect the client with cardiac disease are increased intravascular volume, decreased systemic vascular resistance, cardiac output changes occurring during labor and birth, and the intravascular volume changes that occur just after childbirth. The strain is present during pregnancy and continues for a few weeks after birth. The normal heart can compensate for the increased workload so that pregnancy, labor, and birth are generally well tolerated, but the diseased heart is hemodynamically challenged.

If the cardiovascular changes are not well tolerated, cardiac failure can develop during pregnancy, labor, or the postpartum period. In addition, if myocardial disease develops, valvular disease exists, or a congenital heart defect is present, **cardiac decompensation** (inability of the heart to maintain a sufficient cardiac output) is anticipated.

About 1% of pregnancies are complicated by heart disease (Cunningham et al., 1997), the leading cause of nonobstetric maternal mortality. It ranks fourth overall as a cause of maternal death. A perinatal mortality of up to 50% is anticipated with persistent cardiac decompensation. See Box 33-1 for maternal cardiac disease risk groups.

The degree of disability experienced by the woman with cardiac disease is often more important in the treatment and prognosis of cardiac disease complicating pregnancy than is the diagnosis of cardiovascular disease. The New York Heart Association's (NYHA) (1964) functional classi-

fication of organic heart disease, a widely accepted standard, is as follows:

Class I: Asymptomatic at normal levels of activity
Class II: Symptomatic with increased activity
Class III: Symptomatic with ordinary activity
Class IV: Symptomatic at rest

No classification of heart disease can be considered rigid or absolute, but the NYHA classification offers a basic practical guide for treatment, assuming that frequent prenatal visits, good client cooperation, and appropriate obstetric care occur. Medical therapy is conducted by a team approach, including the cardiologist, obstetrician, and nurses. The functional classification may change for the pregnant woman because of the hemodynamic changes that occur in the cardiovascular system. There is a 30% to 50% increase in cardiac output compared with nonpregnancy resting values, with most of the increase in the first trimester and the peak at 20 to 24 weeks of gestation (Cunningham et al., 1997). The functional classification of the disease is determined at 3 months and again at 7 or 8 months of gestation.

There are contraindications to pregnancy in women with heart disease (Box 33-2). The incidence of miscarriage is increased, and preterm labor and birth are more prevalent in the pregnant woman with cardiac problems. In addition, intrauterine growth restriction (IUGR) (impeded or delayed development of the fetus) is common, probably because of low oxygen pressure (PO_2) in the mother.

The incidence (4% to 16%) of congenital heart lesions is increased in children of mothers with congenital heart disease; thus preconception counseling is important (Mendelson, 1997).

A diagnosis of cardiac disease depends on the history, physical examination, x-ray findings, and, if indicated, ultrasonogram results. The differential diagnosis of heart disease also involves ruling out respiratory problems and other potential causes of chest pain.

Maternal mortality of more than 50% during pregnancy has been associated with pulmonary hypertension; it is vital that the woman with cardiac disease be assessed and the diagnosis established as soon as possible (Mendelson, 1997).

BOX 33-1 Maternal Cardiac Disease Risk Groups

GROUP I (MORTALITY 1%)

Corrected tetralogy of Fallot
Pulmonic/tricuspid disease
Mitral stenosis (classes I, II)
Patent ductus
Ventricular septal defect
Atrial septal defect
Porcine valve

GROUP II (MORTALITY 5%-15%)

Mitral stenosis with atrial fibrillation
Artificial heart valves
Mitral stenosis (classes III, IV)
Uncorrected tetralogy
Aortic coarctation (uncomplicated)
Aortic stenosis

GROUP III (MORTALITY 25%-50%)

Aortic coarctation (complicated)
Myocardial infarction
Marfan's syndrome
True cardiomyopathy
Pulmonary hypertension

From Gilbert, E., & Harmon, J. (1998). *Manual of high risk pregnancy and delivery* (2nd ed.). St. Louis: Mosby.

BOX 33-2 Contraindications to Pregnancy in a Woman with Heart Disease

Pulmonary hypertension
Shunt lesions associated with Eisenmenger's syndrome
Complex cyanotic congenital heart disease
Aortic coarctation complicated by aortic dissection
Poor ventricular function
Marfan's syndrome with marked aortic dilation

Adapted from Mendelson, M. (1997). Congenital cardiac disease and pregnancy. *Clin Perinatol* 24(2), 467-482.

▪ CARE MANAGEMENT: ANTEPARTUM

The presence of cardiac disease makes the decision to become pregnant more difficult (see Box 33-2). Planned pregnancy requires that the woman understand the peripartum risks. If the pregnancy is unplanned, the nurse needs to explore the woman's desire to continue the pregnancy after examining the risks in relation to the status of her cardiac condition. The nurse should review with the woman options for pregnancy termination if her cardiac status is tenuous and abortion is an acceptable alternative. The woman's significant other and family should be included in the discussion. Teaching sessions for the woman and her support people should be offered as indicated by their learning needs.

Care of these high risk women requires a multidisciplinary approach. The multidisciplinary team includes a cardiologist who is familiar with expected cardiovascular changes in pregnancy; a perinatologist; an anesthesiologist (Mendelson, 1997); and nurses expert in labor, fetal, and hemodynamic monitoring.

Assessment and Nursing Diagnosis

The pregnant woman with cardiac disease requires detailed assessment throughout the peripartum period to determine the potential for optimal maternal health and a viable fetus. If she chooses to continue the pregnancy, the high risk pregnant woman's condition may be assessed as often as weekly.

Interview

The nurse solicits information from the woman regarding her personal medical history and that of her family. Special notation is made of diseases of cardiovascular significance, including congenital heart disease, streptococcal infections, rheumatic fever, valvular disease, endocarditis, congestive heart failure, angina, or myocardial infarction.

The nurse assesses for factors that would increase stress on the heart, such as anemia (see p. 901), infection, and edema. In reviewing for symptoms, the nurse should assess how the woman is adapting to the physiologic changes of pregnancy.

In assessing the pregnant woman with a cardiovascular disorder, special attention is given to the review of the cardiovascular and pulmonary systems. The nurse should determine whether the client has experienced chest pain at rest or on exertion; edema of the face, hands, or feet; hypertension; heart murmurs; palpitations; paroxysmal nocturnal dyspnea; diaphoresis; pallor; or syncope. Pulmonary symptoms such as cough, hemoptysis, shortness of breath, and orthopnea also can be signs of cardiac disease. See Table 33-1 for normal and abnormal cardiovascular signs and symptoms during pregnancy.

The nurse documents all medication taken by the client—including over-the-counter (OTC) medications such as supplemental iron—and is alert to their potential side effects and interactions. The woman is also assessed

for undue emotional stress that might further compromise cardiac status. Examples of emotional stress are depression, anxiety or fear of morbidity or mortality for herself and the fetus, financial concerns related to extended hospitalization, anger because of impaired social interaction, and feelings of inadequacy regarding her inability to meet family and household demands.

The woman's cultural background may affect the amount of support that she is able to receive from significant others. Family size (number of children and extended family members in the home) and role expectations within the family may be dictated by cultural norms. For the woman with cardiac impairment, family expectations may be a cause of major stress if she is unable to bear the expected number of children or if it is unacceptable to receive help with domestic chores. The nurse should be aware of the cultural customs of the pregnant woman and her family.

Physical Examination

Routine assessments continue during the prenatal period, including monitoring the amount and pattern of edema, vital signs, discomforts of pregnancy, and amount and pattern of weight gain.

▪ **TABLE 33-1** **Cardiovascular Signs and Symptoms During Pregnancy**

NORMAL	ABNORMAL
SIGNS	
Neck vein pulsation	Neck vein distention
Diffuse/displaced apical pulse	Cardiomegaly; heave
Split S_1, accentuated S_2	Loud P_2; wide split of S_2
Third heart sound	Summation gallop
Systolic murmur (1-2/6)	Loud systolic murmur (4-6/6)
Venous hum	Diastolic murmur
Sinus dysrhythmia	Sustained dysrhythmia
Peripheral edema	Clubbing/cyanosis
SYMPTOMS	
Fatigue	Symptoms at rest
Chest pain	Exertional chest pain
Dyspnea	Exertional, severe dyspnea
Orthopnea	Orthopnea (progressive)
Hyperpnea	Paroxysmal nocturnal dyspnea
Palpitations	Tachycardia (>120 beats/min); dysrhythmia
Syncope (vasovagal)	Exertional syncope

Adapted from Mendelson, M. (1997). Congenital cardiac disease and pregnancy. *Clin Perinatol* 24(2), 467-482.

SIGNS of POTENTIAL COMPLICATIONS

Cardiac Decompensation

PREGNANT WOMAN: SUBJECTIVE SYMPTOMS
- Increasing fatigue or difficulty breathing, or both, with usual activities
- Feeling of smothering
- Frequent cough
- Palpitations; feeling that her heart is racing
- Swelling of face, feet, legs, fingers (e.g., rings do not fit anymore)

NURSE: OBJECTIVE SIGNS
- Irregular weak, rapid pulse ($\geq$100 beats/min)
- Progressive, generalized edema
- Crackles at base of lungs after two inspirations and exhalations
- Orthopnea; increasing dyspnea
- Rapid respirations ($\geq$25 breaths/min)
- Moist, frequent cough
- Increasing fatigue
- Cyanosis of lips and nail beds

The woman is observed for signs of cardiac decompensation, that is, progressive generalized edema, crackles at the base of the lungs, or pulse irregularity (Signs of Potential Complications box). Symptoms of cardiac decompensation may appear abruptly or gradually. Medical intervention must be instituted immediately to maintain optimal cardiac status. Dyspnea, palpitations, syncope, and edema occur commonly in pregnant women and can mask the symptoms of a developing or worsening cardiovascular disorder. A woman's sudden inability to perform activities that she previously was comfortable doing may indicate cardiovascular decompensation.

Laboratory and Diagnostic Tests

Routine urinalysis and blood work (complete blood cell count and blood chemistry) are done during the initial visit. The woman with cardiac impairment requires a baseline electrocardiogram (ECG) at the beginning of her pregnancy, if not before pregnancy, which permits vital diagnostic comparisons of subsequent ECGs. Echocardiograms and pulse oximetry studies may be performed as indicated. Chest films may be necessary during late pregnancy, provided the abdomen is carefully shielded. In addition, fetal ultrasound, fetal movement studies, or fetal nonstress tests may be used to determine fetal well-being.

The following lists nursing diagnoses that may be formulated. As always, individualization of diagnoses is vital.

▮ Nursing Diagnoses

- Fear related to
  - increased peripartum risk
- Risk for ineffective individual/family coping related to
  - woman's cardiac condition
  - changes in relationships
- Risk for altered tissue perfusion related to
  - hypotensive syndrome
- Activity intolerance related to
  - cardiac condition
- Knowledge deficit related to
  - cardiac condition
  - pregnancy and how it affects cardiac condition
  - requirements to alter self-care activities
- Risk for self-care deficit (bathing, grooming, dressing) related to
  - fatigue or activity intolerance
  - need for bedrest
- Impaired home maintenance management related to
  - mother's confinement to bed and/or limited activity level

Expected Outcomes of Care

The mother with cardiovascular problems faces curtailment of her activities. These restrictions can have physical and emotional implications. The community health nurse, social worker, and physical or occupational therapist are some of the resource people whose services may need to be incorporated into the plan of care. Expected outcomes such as the following might be appropriate.

The pregnant woman (and family, if appropriate) will do the following:
- Verbalize understanding of the disorder, management, and probable outcome.
- Describe her role in management, including when and how to take medication, adjust diet, and prepare for and participate in treatment.
- Cope with emotional reactions to pregnancy and infant at risk.
- Adapt to the physiologic stressors of pregnancy and labor and birth.
- Carry her fetus to viability or to term.
- Identify and use support systems.
- Develop no complications in the postpartum period.

Plan of Care and Interventions

The nursing diagnoses derived from analyses of clinical findings act as guides to the development of a plan of care individualized for each client. Therapy for the pregnant woman with heart disease is focused on minimizing stress on the heart, which is greatest between 28 and 32 weeks as the he-

TEACHING guidelines

The Pregnant Woman at Risk for Cardiac Decompensation

- Assess lifestyle patterns, emotional status, and environment of woman.
- Arrange for consultations as needed (i.e., dietitian, home care, child care, social work).
- Determine woman's and her family's understanding of her heart disease and how the disease affects her pregnancy.
- Determine stressors in the woman's life. Assist woman in identifying effective coping strategies.
- Instruct woman to report signs of cardiac decompensation or congestive heart failure: generalized edema, distention of neck veins, dyspnea, pulmonary crackles, cough, palpitations, weight gain of 4.4 kg in 1 day.
- Instruct woman to be watchful for signs of thromboembolism, such as redness, tenderness, pain or swelling of the legs. Instruct woman to seek medical help immediately if such symptoms occur.
- Instruct woman to avoid constipation and thus straining with bowel movements (Valsalva maneuver) by taking in adequate fluids and fiber. A stool softener may be ordered.
- Explore with woman ways to obtain the needed rest throughout the day. Depending on the level of her cardiac disease, she may need to sleep 10 hours per night and rest 30 minutes after meals (class I or II) or rest for most of the day (class III or IV).
- Help woman make use of community resources, including support groups, as indicated.
- Emphasize the importance of keeping her prenatal visits.

From Gilbert, E., & Harmon, J. (1998). *Manual of high risk pregnancy and delivery* (2nd ed.). St. Louis: Mosby; Grohar, J. (1994). Nursing protocols for antepartum home care. *J Obstet Gynecol Neonatal Nurs* 23(8), 687-694; Health Care Resources. (1997). *Handbook of high risk perinatal home care.* St. Louis: Mosby.

modynamic changes reach their maximum. Factors that increase the risk of cardiac decompensation are avoided. The workload of the cardiovascular system is reduced by appropriate treatment of any coexisting emotional stress, hypertension, anemia, hyperthyroidism, or obesity.

Signs and symptoms of cardiac decompensation are reviewed during the prenatal period. The woman with class I or II heart disease requires 8 to 10 hours of sleep every day and should take 30-minute naps after eating. Her activities are restricted, with housework, shopping, and exer-

BOX 33-3 Prophylaxis for Bacterial Endocarditis

DURING PREGNANCY FOR MINOR PROCEDURES

Low Risk Clients

Amoxicillin 3 g PO 1 hr before procedure; 1.5 g PO 6 hr after procedure

High Risk Clients

Vancomycin 1 g IV (over 1 hr) plus gentamicin 1.5 mg/kg (up to 80 mg) IM or IV 1 hr before procedure; repeat dose 8 hr after procedure

DURING LABOR AND BIRTH

Ampicillin 2 g IM or IV plus gentamicin 1.5 mg/kg (up to 80 mg) IM or IV during active labor and repeated 8 hr later and postpartum

Penicillin-Allergic Clients

Vancomycin 1 g IV may be substituted for the ampicillin

From Jackson, G., & Clark, S. (1993). Cardiac and pulmonary disorders and pregnancy. In T. Moore et al. (Eds.). *Gynecology and obstetrics: A longitudinal approach.* New York: Churchill Livingstone; Landon, M. (1996). Cardiac and pulmonary disease. In S. Gabbe, J. Niebyl, & J. Simpson (Eds.). *Obstetrics: Normal and problem pregnancies* (3rd ed.). New York: Churchill Livingstone.

cise limited to the amount allowed for the functional classification of her heart disease.

The pregnant woman with class II cardiac disease should avoid heavy exertion and should stop any activity that causes even minor signs and symptoms of cardiac decompensation. She should also be admitted to the hospital near term (earlier if signs of cardiac overload or dysrhythmia develop) for evaluation and treatment.

Bed rest for much of each day is necessary for pregnant women with class III cardiac disease. About 30% of these women experience cardiac decompensation during pregnancy. With this possibility the woman may require hospitalization for the remainder of the pregnancy.

Because decompensation occurs even at rest in persons with class IV cardiac disease, a major initial effort must be made to improve the cardiac status of the pregnant woman in this category who chooses to continue her pregnancy (see Teaching Guidelines box).

Infections are treated promptly because respiratory, urinary, or GI tract infections can complicate the condition by accelerating the heart rate and by direct spread of organisms (e.g., streptococci) to the heart structure. The woman should notify her physician at the first sign of infection or exposure to an infection. Hospitalization may be required until the infection is cured. Women who have valvular disorders should receive prophylactic antibiotics against bacterial endocarditis during gestation (Box 33-3).

TABLE 33-2   Selected Drugs Used in Treatment of Cardiac Disorders in the Pregnant Woman

CROSSES PLACENTA	CONSIDERATIONS	REFERENCES
DIGITALIS		
Yes	Fetal concentration of the drug is determined to avoid fetal toxicity (fetal toxicity existing with maternal overdose)	Briggs & Garite, 1991
	Possible need to increase maternal dose because of increased blood volume while keeping in therapeutic range	Gilbert & Harmon, 1998
	Uterine contractility possibly affected, leading to preterm labor	Jackson & Clark, 1993
	Used successfully to treat fetal cardiac dysrhythmias	James et al., 1994
PROCAINAMIDE		
Yes	No known teratogenic effects	Briggs & Garite, 1991
	Slow elimination from fetus, possible accumulation of drug	Jackson & Clark, 1993
	Caution needed with use	James et al., 1994
		Kulb, 1990
		Mendelson & Lang, 1995
VERAPAMIL		
Yes	Considered safe for use in pregnancy but can produce maternal hypotension with decreased uterine blood flow	Jackson & Clark, 1993
	Effects on infant unclear, caution needed with use	
PROPRANOLOL		
Yes	Considered safe for use in pregnancy	Jackson & Clark, 1993
	No known teratogenic effects	James et al., 1994
	Associated with fetal bradycardia, diminished uterine blood flow, IUGR, increased uterine irritability, and premature labor	
	Necessary to monitor newborn for 24-48 hr for bradycardia and hypoglycemia if woman receiving propranolol at time of birth	
HEPARIN		
No	If anticoagulant therapy needed, heparin used	Hurst & Alpert, 1994
	Risk of maternal hemorrhage, preterm birth, stillbirth	James et al., 1994
	Prolonged IV use possibly inducing osteopenia in woman	
WARFARIN		
Yes	Fetal anomalies and hemorrhage, mental retardation, blindness, deafness	Kulb, 1990

Nutrition counseling is necessary, optimally with the woman's family present. The pregnant woman needs a well-balanced diet high in iron and protein and adequate in calories to gain weight. Iron supplements tend to cause constipation. The pregnant woman should increase her intake of fluids and fiber. A stool softener may be prescribed. It is important that the woman with a cardiac disorder avoid straining during defecation, thus causing Valsalva maneuver (forced expiration against a closed airway, which when released causes blood to rush to the heart and overload the cardiac system). Sodium intake may be restricted; careful monitoring for hyponatremia is necessary. The sodium ion, with its ability to attract and hold fluid, affects the quality and the amount of the circulating blood volume. The woman's intake of potassium is monitored to prevent hypokalemia, which is associated with heart and other muscular weakness and dysfunction.

Cardiac medications are prescribed as needed for the pregnant woman, with attention to fetal well-being. The hemodynamic changes that occur during pregnancy, such as increased plasma volume and increased renal clearance of drugs, can alter the amount of medication

TABLE 33-2 Selected Drugs Used in Treatment of Cardiac Disorders in the Pregnant Woman—cont'd

CROSSES PLACENTA	CONSIDERATIONS	REFERENCES
FUROSEMIDE		
Yes	Fetal levels estimated to be equal to maternal levels	Briggs & Garite, 1991
	Newborns have increased diuresis, thus sodium and potassium excretion	
	No known teratogenic effects	
	Uncommon to be used in first trimester	
	Necessary to monitor for decreased plasma volume, which could lead to decreased placental perfusion	
THIAZIDES		
Yes	Neonatal jaundice, thrombocytopenia, fluid and electrolyte depletion	Kulb, 1990
LIDOCAINE		
Yes	Safe as long as toxic levels avoided	James et al., 1994
	Toxic dose—fetal CNS and cardiac toxicity	
QUINIDINE		
Yes	No known teratogenic effects	Jackson & Clark, 1993
		James et al., 1994
		Mendelson & Lang, 1995
NIFEDIPINE		
Yes	No adverse effects on fetus as long as the woman's blood pressure not too low	Briggs & Garite, 1991
	Used with caution until potential fetal toxicity evaluated further	Fenakel et al., 1991
	Adverse interaction with magnesium	
DIAZOXIDE		
Yes	Fetal and maternal hyperglycemia possible	Barron, 1995
	Reserved for severe hypertension unresponsive to other medications	Wasserstrum, 1991
	Potent relaxant of uterine smooth muscle	
SODIUM NITROPRUSSIDE		
Yes	Use only in critical care unit for brief time with lowest possible therapeutic dose	Barron, 1995
	Low dose does not appear to cause toxic cyanide levels (fetal cyanide toxicity possibly occurring with higher doses)	Briggs & Garite, 1991
	No congenital defects found	Wasserstrum, 1991

needed to establish and maintain a therapeutic drug level (Jackson & Clark, 1993). The woman's size and ethnic background must also be taken into consideration. For example, women of short stature or of Asian descent require less medication for the desired physiologic response. Therefore the nurse must monitor the pregnant woman for adverse side effects and the blood level of the medication.

Research on the effects of cardiovascular drugs on the fetus and pregnant woman has been limited. The nurse should review current pharmacologic literature, especially when administering any medication to a woman and her unborn child (Table 33-2).

If anticoagulant therapy is required during pregnancy, heparin should be used because this large-molecule drug does not cross the placenta (James et al., 1994). The nurse should closely monitor the woman's blood tests, including clotting factors. The woman may need to learn to self-administer heparin. She also requires specific nutritional teaching to avoid foods high in vitamin K, such as raw, dark green, and leafy vegetables, which counteract the effects of the heparin. In addition,

EMERGENCY

CPR for the Pregnant Woman

AIRWAY

Determine unresponsiveness.
Activate emergency medical system.
Position woman on flat, firm surface with uterus displaced laterally with a wedge (e.g., a rolled towel placed under her hip) or manually.
Open airway with head tilt–chin lift maneuver.

BREATHING

Determine breathlessness (look, listen, feel).
If the woman is not breathing, give two slow breaths.

CIRCULATION

Determine pulselessness by feeling carotid pulse.
If there is no pulse, begin chest compressions at rate of 80 to 100/min.
After 4 cycles of 15 compressions and 2 breaths, check her pulse. If pulse is not present, continue CPR.

Source: American Heart Association (AHA). (1997). *Basic life support, heart saver guide*. Dallas: AHA.

she will require a substitute source for folic acid in her diet.

Tests for fetal maturity and well-being and placental sufficiency may be necessary. Other therapy is directly related to the functional classification of heart disease. The nurse may need to reinforce the need for close medical supervision. Information about management of labor and birth and the postpartum period allows the woman time to plan for necessary extra care (Legal Tip).

LEGAL TIP Cardiac and Metabolic Emergencies

The management of emergencies such as maternal cardiopulmonary distress or arrest or maternal metabolic crisis should be documented in policies, procedures, and protocols. Any independent nursing actions appropriate to the emergency should be clearly identified.

Cardiopulmonary Resuscitation of the Pregnant Woman

Trauma, pulmonary embolism, anesthesia complications, drug overdose, hypovolemia, or septic shock may result in cardiopulmonary arrest. Preexisting disorders such as heart or pulmonary disease, hypertension, or autoimmune collagen vascular disease increase this risk (Luppi, 1999). Some modifications of the procedure for cardiopulmonary resuscitation (CPR) (see Emergency box) are needed during pregnancy (Fig. 33-1).

Various protocols exist for CPR during pregnancy. The most widely used guide is the American Heart Association (AHA) ACLS Protocol (AHA, 1992). This protocol recommends 5 to 10 minutes of standard CPR with the uterus displaced laterally, fluid volume restoration, and defibrillation if indicated. If these measures are not successful within 15 minutes of the arrest, open chest heart massage is recommended if the fetus is viable. If there is still no change in maternal status after 15 minutes of open chest cardiac massage or there is fetal distress, immediate cesarean birth is recommended. Other protocols recommend cesarean birth within 5 minutes while still others recommend cesarean birth based on the gestational age of the fetus (Luppi, 1999). No matter what protocol is used, nurses and other health care providers must be prepared if CPR is to be successful.

NURSE ALERT *In the event of cardiac arrest, standard resuscitative efforts with a few modifications are implemented. To prevent supine hypotension, the woman is placed on a firm surface with the uterus displaced to the left laterally either manually or with a wedge or rolled blanket or towel under the right hip (Association of Women's Health, Obstetric, and Neonatal Nurses [AWHONN], 1998; Bajo, 1997). If defibrillation is needed, the paddles need to be placed one rib interspace higher than usual because the heart is displaced slightly by the enlarged uterus. If possible, the fetus should be monitored during the cardiac arrest (Bajo, 1997).*

Complications may be associated with CPR of a pregnant woman. These complications may include laceration of the liver, rupture of the uterus, hemothorax, or hemoperitoneum. Fetal complications also may occur. These include cardiac dysrhythmia or asystole related to maternal defibrillation and medications, CNS depression related to antidysrhythmic drugs and inadequate uteroplacental perfusion, and onset of preterm labor.

If there is successful resuscitation, the woman and her fetus must receive careful monitoring. The woman remains at increased risk for recurrent pulmonary arrest and dysrhythmias (ventricular tachycardia, supraventricular tachycardia, bradycardia). Therefore her cardiovascular, pulmonary, and neurologic status should be assessed continuously. Uterine activity and resting tone must be monitored. Fetal status and gestational age should be determined and used in decision making regarding the continuation of the pregnancy or the timing and route of birth. All assessment data influence both the medical and nursing plans of care.

Heart Surgery During Pregnancy

If possible, operations for the correction of congenital or acquired heart disease should be performed before pregnancy, especially in women with cyanotic heart disease. Pregnancy after open heart surgery is often possible if the congenital cardiac disorder was improved significantly. Cardiac disease may have different signs and symptoms in pregnancy than in the nonpregnant state. When medical therapy for a pregnant woman fails, cardiac surgery should be performed (Mendelson & Lang, 1995). The early second trimester is the best time for surgery. The client, fetus, and uterus must be monitored carefully during surgery. Closed cardiac surgery, such as release of a stenotic mitral orifice, can be accomplished with little risk to mother or fetus. Open heart surgery requires extracorporeal circulation, and under these circumstances hypoxia, fetal bradycardia, and increased uterine contractions may develop (Strickland et al., 1991). As a result, the risk of fetal damage or loss rises to 10% to 20% and is thought to result from the nonpulsatile circulation created by the extracorporeal pump (Kulb, 1990).

Some women who are free of symptoms after earlier cardiac surgery have significant deterioration during pregnancy. The normal hemodynamic demands of pregnancy compromise their cardiac status. For these clients, therapeutic abortion, if acceptable to the client and her family, is advised before the hemodynamic demands are fully manifested. An increased incidence of miscarriage, stillbirth, low-birth-weight infants, and malformed fetuses occurs in women with valvular heart disease.

Evaluation

The nurse knows that care was effective if expected outcomes of care have been met. See the Plan of Care for the Pregnant Woman with Cardiac Disease.

Intrapartum

For all pregnant women the intrapartum period is the one that evokes the most apprehension in clients and caregivers. The woman with impaired cardiac function has additional reasons to be anxious because labor and giving birth place an additional burden on her already compromised cardiovascular system.

Cesarean birth is not routinely recommended for women who have cardiovascular disease; there is risk of dramatic fluid shifts, hemodynamic changes that are sustained, and increased blood loss. There is increased mortality in women with Eisenmenger's syndrome who have cesarean birth (Mendelson, 1997). In Class IV disease, maternal mortality approaches 50%; perinatal mortality is even higher. One of the roles of the nurse is to decrease the anxiety of the client and her family. Anxiety is minimized by maintaining a calm atmosphere in the labor and birth rooms. The nurse provides anticipatory guidance by keeping the woman and her family informed of labor progress and events that will likely occur and by answering any questions they have. The woman's childbirth preparation method should be supported to the degree it is feasible for her cardiac condition. Nursing techniques that promote comfort, such as back massage, are used.

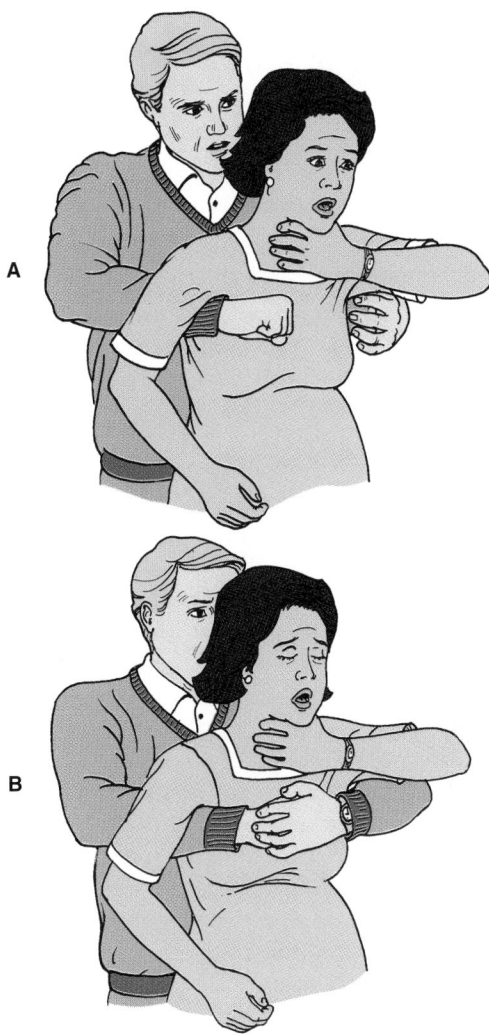

Fig. 33-1 Heimlich maneuver. Clearing airway obstruction in woman in late stages of pregnancy (can also be used in markedly obese victim). **A,** Standing behind victim, place your arms under woman's armpits and across chest. Place thumb side of your clenched fist against middle of sternum, and place other hand over fist. **B,** Perform backward chest thrusts until foreign body is expelled or woman becomes unconscious. If pregnant woman becomes unconscious because of foreign-body airway obstruction, place her on her back and kneel close to victim's side. (Be sure uterus is displaced laterally by using, for example, a rolled blanket under her hip.) Open mouth with tongue-jaw lift, perform finger sweep, and attempt rescue breathing. If unable to ventilate, position hands as for chest compression. Deliver five chest thrusts firmly to remove obstruction. Repeat above sequence of Heimlich maneuver, finger sweep, and attempt to ventilate. Continue above sequence until pregnant woman's airway is clear of obstruction or help has arrived to relieve you (Chandra & Hazinski, 1994). If woman is unconscious, give chest compressions as for woman without pulse.

PLAN ᵒᶠ CARE | The Pregnant Woman with Cardiac Disease

> **NURSING DIAGNOSIS** Activity intolerance related to effects of pregnant state on underlying cardiac condition

Expected Outcome *Client will show no evidence of cardiac decompensation (i.e., no fatigue, shortness of breath, palpitations, edema, rapid irregular pulse, crackles, rapid respirations, cyanosis of nail beds and lips).*

Nursing Interventions/*Rationales*

Assist woman in identifying factors that decrease activity tolerance and explore extent of limitations *to establish a baseline for evaluation.*

Help woman to develop an individualized program of activity and rest *that maintains sufficient cardiac output.*

Teach woman to monitor physiologic response to activity (i.e., pulse rate, respiratory rate) and reduce activity that provokes fatigue and/or pain *to maintain sufficient cardiac output and prevent harm to fetus.*

Enlist significant others to assist woman in pacing activities and to provide support in performing role functions and self-care activities that are too strenuous *to increase chances of compliance with activity restrictions.*

Have woman maintain an activity log that records activities, time, duration, intensity, and physiologic response *to evaluate effectiveness of and adherence to activity program.*

> **NURSING DIAGNOSIS** Risk for altered tissue perfusion related to cardiac condition secondary to increased circulatory needs during pregnancy

Expected Outcomes *The mother will exhibit signs of hemodynamic stability (i.e., blood pressure, pulse, ABGs, and WBC counts are within normal limits). The fetus will exhibit signs of well-being (i.e., fetal activity and fetal heart rate [FHR] are within normal limits).*

Nursing Interventions/*Rationales*

Monitor heart rate and rhythm, blood pressure, skin color and temperature, WBCs, hemoglobin and hematocrit, and ABGs *to detect early signs of cardiac failure/hypoxia.*

Monitor fetal activity and FHR, and perform nonstress testing as indicated *to assess fetal status and detect uteroplacental insufficiency.*

Teach woman how to detect and report early signs of cardiac decompensation *to prevent maternal/fetal complications.*

> **NURSING DIAGNOSIS** Decreased cardiac output related to increased circulatory volume secondary to pregnancy and cardiac condition

Expected Outcome *The client will exhibit signs of adequate cardiac output (i.e., normal pulse and blood pressure; normal heart and breath sounds; normal skin color, tone, and turgor; normal capillary refill; normal urine output; no evidence of edema).*

Nursing Interventions/*Rationales*

Reinforce importance of use of activity/rest cycles *to prevent cardiac complications.*

Teach woman to lie in lateral position *to increase uterine blood flow* and to elevate legs while sitting *to promote venous return.*

Monitor intake and output and check for edema *to assess for renal complications or venous return problems.*

Monitor fetal activity and FHR, and perform nonstress testing as indicated *to assess fetal status and detect uteroplacental insufficiency.*

From Wong, D., & Perry, S. (1998). *Maternal child nursing care.* St. Louis: Mosby.

Physical Examination

The woman with Class III or Class IV disease will likely be hospitalized before the onset of labor.

During the intrapartum period routine assessments for all laboring women and assessments for cardiac decompensation should be made because labor and birth place an additional burden on an already compromised cardiovascular system. The latter include taking vital signs at least every 10 to 30 minutes or according to institutional protocol or physi-

cian's orders. The color and temperature of the skin are noted. The woman is carefully watched for signs of emotional stress.

NURSE ALERT *The physician is alerted if the pulse rate is 100 beats per minute or greater or if respirations are 25 breaths per minute or greater. Respiratory status is checked frequently for developing dyspnea, coughing, or crackles at the base of the lungs. Pale, cool, clammy skin may indicate cardiac shock.*

To decrease the hemodynamic burden on the heart, pain and anxiety need to be minimized and the second stage of labor should be shortened (e.g., forceps- or vacuum-assisted birth). The client is placed on a heart monitor to identify the presence of disturbances in rhythm.

Cardiac function is supported by keeping the woman's head and shoulders elevated and her body parts resting on pillows. The side-lying position usually facilitates hemodynamics during labor.

Arterial blood gases (ABGs) may be needed to assess for adequate oxygenation. A Swan-Ganz catheter may be inserted to accurately monitor hemodynamic status during labor and birth (see Chapter 34). ECG monitoring and continuous monitoring of blood pressure should be instituted. Continuous fetal monitoring during labor is also implemented in high risk cases.

Discomfort is relieved with medication and supportive care. For birth the nurse will assist in the administration of drugs to relieve discomfort. Epidural regional analgesia provides better pain relief than do narcotics and it causes fewer alterations in hemodynamics (Cunningham et al., 1997). Hypotension must be avoided. Epidural analgesia is controversial in Eisenmenger's syndrome and pulmonary hypertension because it causes a decrease in cardiac output. Epidural analgesia is avoided in idiopathic hypertrophic subaortic stenosis (IHSS) because it causes severe bradycardia (Thornhill & Camann, 1994). Epidural analgesia can be administered slowly for clients with ischemic heart disease and valvular disease.

The woman may require other types of medication (e.g., anticoagulants, prophylactic antibiotics). If evidence of cardiac decompensation appears, the physician may order deslanoside (Cedilanid-D) for rapid digitalization, furosemide (Lasix) for rapid diuresis, and oxygen by intermittent positive pressure to decrease the development of pulmonary edema.

β-Adrenergic agents (i.e., ritodrine and terbutaline) should not be used for tocolysis. These medications are associated with myocardial ischemia. A synthetic oxytocin (Syntocinon) can be used for induction of labor. This drug does not appear to cause significant coronary artery constriction in doses prescribed for labor induction or control of postpartum uterine atony. Cervical ripening agents containing prostaglandin are not contraindicated, but reports of use in pregnant women with cardiac disease are not available.

Vaginal birth is recommended and may be accomplished with the woman in the side-lying position to facilitate uterine perfusion. If the supine position is used, a pad is positioned under the hip to laterally displace the uterus and minimize the danger of supine hypotension. The knees are flexed, and the feet are flat on the bed. To prevent compression of popliteal veins and an increase in blood volume in the chest and trunk as a result of the effects of gravity, stirrups are not used. Open-glottis pushing is recommended and the Valsalva maneuver must be avoided during pushing in the second stage of labor because it reduces diastolic ventricular filling and obstructs

left ventricular outflow. Mask oxygen is important. Episiotomy and outlet forceps may be used because these procedures decrease the work of the heart.

Penicillin prophylaxis may be ordered for nonallergic pregnant women with class II or higher cardiac disease to protect against bacterial endocarditis in labor and during the early puerperium (see Box 33-3). Dilute IV oxytocin immediately after birth may be employed to prevent postbirth hemorrhage. Ergot products should not be used because they can cause transient hypertension. If tubal sterilization is desired, surgery is delayed at least several days to ensure homeostasis.

Postpartum

Monitoring for cardiac decompensation in the postpartum period is essential. The first 24 to 48 hours postpartum are the most hemodynamically difficult for the woman. Monitoring for cardiac decompensation continues through the first week after birth because of hormonal shifts that affect hemodynamics. These shifts have been known to occur as late as the seventh postpartum day.

Routine postpartum assessments are included in the review of systems. Assessments for postpartum women with cardiac disease include vital signs, amount and character of bleeding, uterine contractility, urinary output, pain, the activity-rest pattern, diet, and daily weights.

NURSE ALERT *The immediate postbirth period is hazardous for a woman whose heart function is compromised. Cardiac output increases rapidly as extravascular fluid is remobilized into the vascular compartment. At the moment of birth intraabdominal pressure is reduced drastically; pressure on veins is removed, the splanchnic vessels engorge, and blood flow to the heart is increased. When blood flow increases to the heart, a **reflex bradycardia** (slowing of the heart in response to the increased blood flow) may result.*

Special attention is given to the woman who is at risk for cardiac decompensation. The increased intravascular fluid can cause fluid volume excess in these women. Hemorrhage or infection, or both, may worsen the cardiac condition. The woman with a cardiac disorder may continue to require a Swan-Ganz catheter and arterial blood gas monitoring.

Nursing diagnoses appropriate for the postpartum period include the following:

⦂ Nursing Diagnoses _____

- Anxiety related to
  - fear for infant's safety
- Fear of dying related to
  - perceived physiologic inability to cope with stress of labor
- Risk for impaired gas exchange related to
  - cardiac condition

Continued

▪ Nursing Diagnoses—cont'd _____

- Risk for fluid volume excess related to
  - extravascular fluid shifts
- Situational low self-esteem related to
  - restriction placed on involvement in care of infant
  - ineffective (compromised) family coping
- Ineffective breastfeeding (class I or II cardiac disease) related to
  - fatigue from cardiac condition
- Risk for altered mother/infant attachment related to
  - separation due to prematurity
  - fatigue from cardiac condition

Care in the postpartum period is tailored to the woman's functional capacity. Postpartum positioning of the woman with cardiac disease is the same as that for labor; that is, the head of the bed is elevated and the woman is encouraged to lie on her side. Bed rest may be ordered, with or without bathroom privileges. The nurse assesses the woman's affect; pulse rate; breath sounds; coughing; edema; and skin color, temperature, and dryness (e.g., pink, warm, and dry; or pale, cool, and clammy) before and after walking. The nurse may need to help the woman meet her grooming and hygiene needs and even help her with turning in bed, eating, and other activities. Respiratory and cardiovascular sequelae to immobility, as well as boredom, must be addressed. Progressive ambulation may be permitted as tolerated. Bowel movements without stress or strain are promoted with stool softeners, diet, and fluids, plus mild analgesia and local anesthetic spray.

Overdistention of the bladder should be prevented; a distended bladder can result in an atonic uterus and hemorrhage.

Anemia from hemorrhage may result and add additional stress to cardiac function. The woman must be protected from infection. A private room is one method to restrict traffic into her room.

The woman may direct a designated family member in the care of the infant. Breastfeeding is not contraindicated, but not all women with heart disease (particularly those with life-threatening disease) will be able to do it (Lawrence, 1999). The woman who chooses to breastfeed will need the support of her family and the nursing staff to be successful. For example, the woman may need assistance in positioning herself and/or the infant for feeding. To further conserve the woman's energy, the infant may need to be brought to the mother and taken from her after the feeding.

NURSE ALERT *Women who breastfeed may need less medication for their cardiac condition, especially diuretics. Because diuretics can cause neonatal diuresis that can lead to dehydration, lactating women need to be monitored closely to determine if medications' doses can be reduced and still be effective.*

If the woman is unable to breastfeed and her energies do not allow her to bottle feed the infant, the fed baby can be brought regularly to the mother. The infant should be held at the mother's eye level and near her lips and brought to her fingers so she can establish an emotional bond with her baby with a low expenditure of energy. At the same time, involving the mother passively in her infant's care helps the mother feel vitally important—as she is—to the infant's well-being (e.g., "You can offer something no one else can: provide your baby with your sounds, touch, and rhythms that are so comforting"). Perhaps the woman can be encouraged to make a tape recording of her talking, singing, or whispering, which can be played for the baby in the nursery to help the infant feel her presence and be in contact with her voice. This also enhances maternal-infant bonding.

Preparation for discharge is carefully planned with the woman and family. Provision of help for the woman in the home by relatives, friends, and others must be addressed. If necessary, the nurse refers the family to community resources (e.g., for homemaking services). Rest and sleep periods, activity, and diet must be planned. The couple may need information about reestablishing sexual relations and contraception or sterilization (especially if the woman's condition is classified as class II, III, or IV).

ASSOCIATED CARDIOVASCULAR DISORDERS

Nursing care of the woman with a cardiovascular disorder combines routine peripartum care with care specific for the cardiac diagnosis. Cardiac diseases vary in their impact on pregnancy because of acuteness or chronicity. The following discussion focuses on peripartum cardiomyopathy, rheumatic heart disease, infective endocarditis, Eisenmenger's syndrome, mitral valve prolapse, Marfan's syndrome, and cerebrovascular accidents.

Peripartum Cardiomyopathy

The classical definition of **peripartum cardiomyopathy** is "congestive heart failure with cardiomyopathy found in the last month of pregnancy or in the first five months postpartum" (Landon, 1996). The etiology of the disease is unknown; theories suggest genetic predisposition, autoimmunity, and viral infections.

Peripartum cardiomyopathy is more likely to occur in African-Americans, in a woman who is 30 years old or more with a twin pregnancy, and in the presence of preeclampsia (Mendelson & Lang, 1995). Maternal mortality has been estimated in the range of 25% to 50%, whereas infant mortality is approximately 10% (Jackson & Clark, 1993). Clinical findings are those of congestive heart failure (left ventricular failure). Signs include breathlessness, tachydysrhythmias, and edema with radiologic findings of cardiomegaly (Fig. 33-2). The prognosis is good if cardiomegaly does not persist for 6 months postpartum. Women whose hearts remain enlarged 6 months postpar-

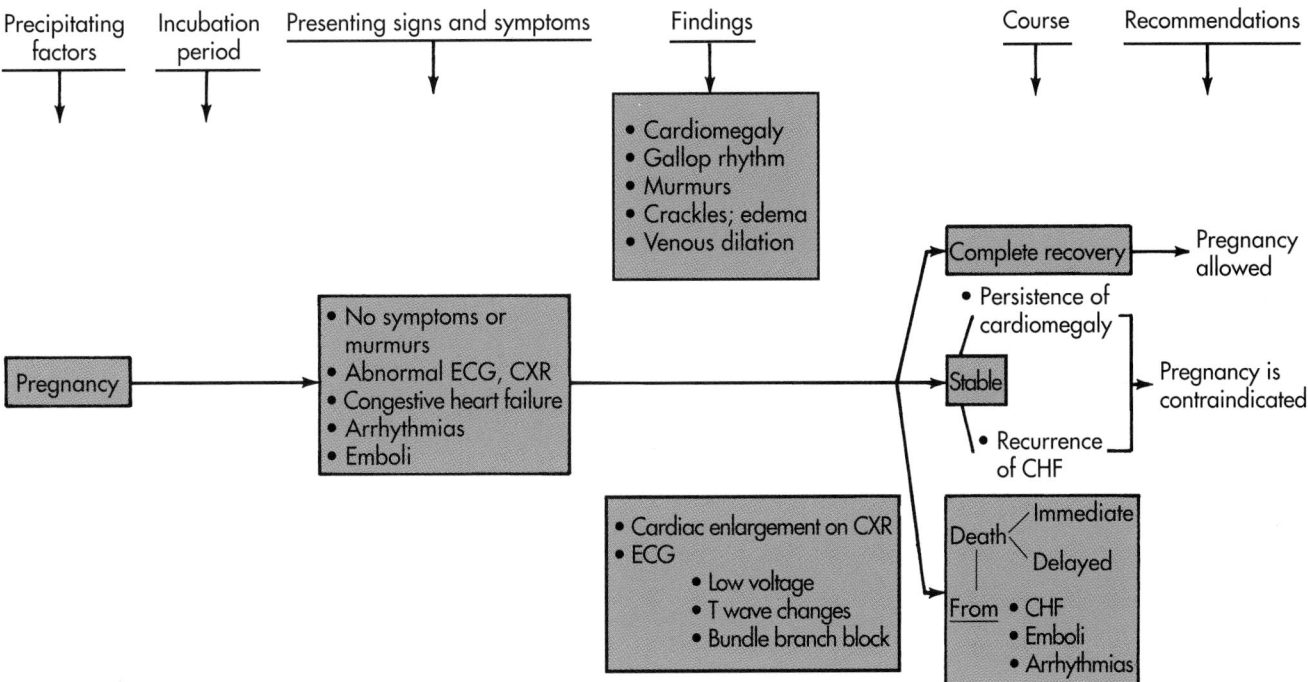

Fig. 33-2 Summary of course of peripartum cardiomyopathy.

tum will have peripartum cardiomyopathy in future pregnancies (Jackson & Clark, 1993). Sterilization should be considered because the mortality rate approaches 100%. Oral contraceptives are contraindicated because of the risk of thromboembolism.

Medical management of cardiomyopathy during pregnancy includes diuretics, potassium, anticoagulants, and digitalis. Bed rest is generally recommended, but its benefit is unclear (Jackson & Clark, 1993; Landon, 1996).

The nursing care of clients with peripartum cardiomyopathy is essentially the same as for those with other types of cardiac problems. Trendelenburg's position has been demonstrated to relieve syncope. The necessity for prolonged bed rest can pose social and economic hardships for the family; therefore referral to community resources for assistance may be necessary. Because sudden death is a feature of this condition, the family needs to be trained in CPR. Clients need to have ready access to emergency care.

Rheumatic Heart Disease

Rheumatic fever usually develops suddenly several symptom-free weeks after an inadequately treated group A β-hemolytic streptococcal infection of the throat. Episodes of rheumatic fever create an autoimmune reaction in the heart tissue, leading to permanent damage of heart valves (usually the mitral valve) and the chorda tendineae cordis. This damage is referred to as **rheumatic heart disease (RHD).** RHD may be evident during acute rheumatic fever or discovered years later. Recurrences of rheumatic fever are common, each with the potential to increase the severity of heart damage. If a woman has had rheumatic fever in the past, a recurrence can occur during pregnancy,

most likely early in the pregnancy. The American Heart Association recommends lifelong prophylaxis with benzathine penicillin, even during pregnancy. For those with penicillin allergies, erythromycin is an acceptable alternative during pregnancy. Heart murmurs resulting from stenosis, valvular insufficiency, or thickening of the walls of the heart characterize RHD. Abnormal pulse rate and rhythm and congestive heart failure are common.

Mitral Valve Stenosis

Mitral valve stenosis (narrowing of the opening of the mitral valve caused by stiffening of valve leaflets, which obstructs blood flow from the atrium to the ventricles) accounts for 90% of RHD seen in pregnancy (McAnulty, Metcalfe, & Ueland, 1995). Even though a history of rheumatic fever may be absent, it remains the most likely cause of mitral stenosis. As the mitral valve narrows, dyspnea worsens, occurring first on exertion and eventually at rest. A tight stenosis plus the increase in blood volume and thus cardiac output of normal pregnancy may cause ventricular failure and pulmonary edema; hemoptysis may occur.

Atrial fibrillation can precipitate a drop in the cardiac output. IV verapamil, cardioversion, and digitalis therapy may be used to treat atrial fibrillation (McAnulty, Metcalfe, & Ueland, 1995). Cardiac failure occurs for the first time during pregnancy in 25% of women with mitral valve stenosis. The care of the woman with mitral stenosis typically is managed by reducing her activity, restricting dietary sodium, and increasing bed rest. The pregnant woman with mitral stenosis should be followed clinically for symptoms and by echocardiograms to monitor the atrial and ventricular size, as well as heart valve function. Prophylaxis for intrapartum endocarditis and pulmonary infections is provided (see Box 33-3).

β-Blockers may be used to blunt heart rate response to exercise and anxiety. Adverse fetal and neonatal effects include IUGR, delayed neonatal breathing, and bradycardia. Epidural analgesia for labor and avoidance of IV fluid overload are appropriate (Cunningham et al., 1997). Even with close monitoring, the woman with moderate to severe mitral stenosis will commonly have pulmonary edema for the first 1 to 2 days after giving birth because of volume shifts after birth (Mendelson & Lang, 1995).

For clients with NYHA class III or IV cardiac disease, closed valvotomy can be considered. Closed mitral valvotomy has been successful with low maternal mortality (2%) and fetal mortality (10%) in one study and zero in another (Mendelson & Lang, 1995). Mitral valvotomy during pregnancy often brings dramatic relief of congestive heart failure that has been unresponsive to medical treatment. An alternative and safer therapeutic procedure is percutaneous, transseptal, mitral balloon valvotomy with transesophageal echocardiography.

Infective Endocarditis

Infective endocarditis (inflammation of the innermost lining–endocardium–of the heart caused by invasion of microorganism) is an uncommon disorder during pregnancy (Mendelson & Lang, 1995). It may be seen in women taking street drugs intravenously. Bacterial endocarditis, leading to incompetence of heart valves and thus congestive heart failure and cerebral emboli, can result in death. Treatment is the same as for the nonpregnant woman, that is, antibiotics.

Eisenmenger's Syndrome

Eisenmenger's syndrome is a "right-to-left or bidirectional shunting at either the atrial or ventricular level, combined with elevated pulmonary vascular resistance" (Landon, 1996). The syndrome is associated with high mortality: 12% to 70% in mothers and 50% in fetuses; thus, pregnancy is contraindicated. Contraception is essential and tubal ligation should be considered; oral contraceptives and intrauterine devices carry considerable risk (Mendelson & Lang, 1995). If pregnancy occurs, termination may be recommended if the woman has significant pulmonary hypertension (Landon, 1996).

The amount of right-to-left shunting depends on the degree of pulmonary hypertension present. Pulmonary and systemic vascular resistance also affect the amount of shunting. Right ventricular failure limits pulmonary blood flow and can increase shunting. The physical signs of the syndrome include cyanosis and clubbing of the fingers. Symptoms associated with a poor prognosis include chest pain, hemoptysis, and syncope (Landon, 1996).

During pregnancy, physical activity should be limited and the supine position avoided; prophylactic anticoagu-

lation is considered (Mendelson & Lang, 1995). During labor and birth, Swan-Ganz monitoring is essential. Central hypovolemia should be avoided. If epidural analgesia is used, serial determinations of arterial oxygen concentrations should be done.

Mitral Valve Prolapse

Mitral valve prolapse (MVP) is a common, usually benign, condition occurring in nearly 10% of women of reproductive age (Cunningham et al., 1997). The mitral valve leaflets prolapse into the left atrium during ventricular systole, allowing some backflow of blood. Midsystolic click and late systolic murmur are hallmarks of this syndrome. Most cases are asymptomatic. A few women have atypical chest pain (sharp and located in the left side of the chest) that occurs at rest, unrelated to exercise, and does not respond to nitrates. They may also have anxiety, palpitations, dyspnea on exertion, and syncope. Clients usually are treated with β-blockers such as propranolol (Inderal). Pregnancy and its associated hemodynamic changes may change or alleviate the murmur and click of MVP, as well as the symptoms. Pregnancy usually is well tolerated unless bacterial endocarditis occurs. As with RHD, antibiotic prophylaxis is given before invasive procedures for at-risk clients and for complicated vaginal births in clients with MVP.

Marfan's Syndrome

Marfan's syndrome is an autosomal-dominant disorder characterized by generalized weakness of the connective tissue, resulting in joint deformities, ocular lens dislocation, and weakness of the aortic wall and root (McAnulty, Metcalfe, & Ueland, 1995). About 90% of individuals with this syndrome have MVP, and 25% have aortic insufficiency. There is an increased risk of aortic dissection and rupture during pregnancy (McAnulty, Metcalfe, & Ueland, 1995). Excruciating chest pain is the most common symptom of aortic dissection. Preconceptional genetic counseling is recommended to make clients aware of the risks of pregnancy with this condition. The woman should have baseline data gathered about the aortic root before pregnancy or at the first prenatal visit by noninvasive imaging with transesophageal echocardiography, computed tomography, or magnetic resonance imaging (MRI). Management during pregnancy includes restricted activity and β-blockers; surgery may be indicated in some women. Antibiotic prophylaxis is suggested for labor; regional anesthesia is well tolerated. Mortality rates may be as high as 50% in women who have significant cardiac disease.

Cerebrovascular Accidents

Ischemia of the brain tissues, or a *cerebrovascular accident (CVA)* or *stroke*, occurs from occlusion of blood vessels that normally perfuse the area. A stroke may result from a cerebral hemorrhage or an embolus. Though uncommon during pregnancy, stroke is still a significant cause of maternal deaths in the United States (Cunningham et al., 1997).

Cerebral hemorrhages are associated with hypertension, preeclampsia-eclampsia, aneurysm, and thrombosis (Cunningham et al., 1997). The incidence of CVAs varies according to population studies ranging from 1:7000 to 1:11,000 (Cunningham et al., 1997). The extent of damage depends on the location and extent of ischemia. Symptomatic treatment may include corticosteroids for cerebral edema or anticoagulants for emboli. Rehabilitation should be started as soon after the event as possible.

ANEMIA

Anemia is the most common medical disorder of pregnancy affecting at least 20% of pregnant women. Women with anemia have a higher incidence of puerperal complications such as infection than do pregnant women with normal hematologic values.

Anemia results in reduction of the oxygen-carrying capacity of the blood, and the heart tries to compensate by increasing the cardiac output. This effort increases the workload of the heart and stresses ventricular function. Therefore anemia that occurs with any other complication (e.g., preeclampsia) may result in congestive heart failure.

An indirect index of the oxygen-carrying capacity is the packed red blood cell (RBC) volume, or hematocrit level. The normal hematocrit range in nonpregnant women is 38% to 45%. However, normal values for pregnant women with adequate iron stores may be as low as 34%. This has been explained by hydremia (dilution of blood), or the physiologic anemia of pregnancy.

At or near sea level, the pregnant woman is anemic when her hemoglobin level is less than 10 g/dl or the hematocrit is less than 33%. At high altitudes much higher values indicate anemia; for example, at 1500 m (5000 ft) above sea level a hemoglobin level less than 14 g/dl indicates anemia (Pagana & Pagana, 1997).

When a woman has anemia during pregnancy, the loss of blood at birth, even if minimal, is not well tolerated. She is at an increased risk for requiring blood transfusions. About 90% of cases of anemia in pregnancy are of the iron deficiency type. The remaining 10% embrace a considerable variety of acquired and hereditary anemias, including folic acid deficiency, sickle cell anemia, and thalassemia.

Nursing care of the anemic pregnant woman requires that the nurse be able to distinguish between the normal physiologic anemia of pregnancy and the disease states. During prenatal visits the nurse should take a diet history and provide dietary teaching as appropriate. Pregnancy may cause increased fatigue, stress, and financial difficulties for a woman with anemia as she copes with her activities of daily living. The nurse should assess the woman's needs and provide her with appropriate resources or referral.

Iron Deficiency Anemia

Pathologic anemia of pregnancy is primarily caused by iron deficiency (James et al., 1994). Without iron therapy

even pregnant women who have excellent nutrition will end pregnancy with an iron deficit. Iron for the fetus comes from the maternal serum (Duffy, 1995). Diet alone cannot replace gestational iron losses. Inadequate nutrition without therapy will certainly mean iron deficiency anemia during late pregnancy and the puerperium.

Successful iron therapy during pregnancy can be carried out in most cases with oral iron supplements (e.g., ferrous sulfate, 30 to 60 mg per day). It is important to teach the woman the significance of the iron therapy (see Home Care box on p. 372). In addition, the woman should be instructed in dietary ways to decrease the GI side effects of iron therapy. Some pregnant women cannot tolerate the prescribed oral iron because of nausea and vomiting. In such cases the woman should receive parenteral iron such as an iron-dextran complex (Imferon) (Duffy, 1995).

Folic Acid Deficiency Anemia

Folic acid deficiency during conception and early pregnancy increases the incidence of neural tube defects, cleft lip, and cleft palate (Letsky, 1995). It is common in multiple gestations. During pregnancy the recommended daily intake is 400 μg per day of folic acid, although women who have a deficiency may need 1 mg or more per day.

Poor diet, cooking with large volumes of water, or home canning of food (especially vegetables) may lead to folate deficiency. Malabsorption may also play a part in the development of anemia caused by a lack of folic acid.

Since 1998, the U.S. Food and Drug Administration has required the addition of folic acid to cereals, pasta, breads, and other foods that are labeled "enriched." However, the amount added is small and most pregnant women will need a supplement.

Sickle Cell Hemoglobinopathy

Sickle cell hemoglobinopathy is a disease caused by the presence of abnormal hemoglobin in the blood. Sickle cell trait (SA hemoglobin pattern), sickling of the RBCs but with a normal RBC life span, usually causes only mild clinical symptoms. Sickle cell anemia (sickle cell disease) is a recessive, hereditary, familial hemolytic anemia that affects those of African-American or Mediterranean ancestry. These individuals usually have abnormal hemoglobin types (SS or SC). People with sickle cell anemia have recurrent attacks (crises) of fever and pain in the abdomen or extremities. These attacks are attributed to vascular occlusion (from abnormal cells), tissue hypoxia, edema, and RBC destruction. Crises are associated with normochromic anemia, jaundice, reticulocytosis, a positive sickle cell test, and the demonstration of abnormal hemoglobin (usually SS or SC).

Almost 10% of African-Americans in North America have the sickle cell trait, but fewer than 1% have sickle cell anemia. The anemia is often complicated by iron and folic acid deficiency.

Nurses working in women's health clinics should encourage clients with sickle cell trait to undergo genetic counseling before pregnancy is undertaken because pregnancy usually results in a worsening of most aspects of the disease (Scott et al., 1999). The anemia that occurs in normal pregnancies may aggravate sickle cell anemia and bring on more crises. Fetal loss is high because of impaired oxygen supply, sickling, and infarcts in the placental circulation (James et al., 1994). Pregnant women with sickle cell anemia are prone to pyelonephritis, leg ulcers, bone abnormalities, strokes, cardiopathy, congestive heart failure, and preeclampsia. Urinary tract infections (UTI) and hematuria are common. An aplastic crisis may follow serious infection. Medical therapy may include prophylactic transfusions to the mother to decrease sickle cells and increase hemoglobin (Duffy, 1995). Cesarean birth is warranted only for obstetric indications. Oral contraceptives are contraindicated.

Table 33-3 identifies some potential problems faced by the woman with sickle cell disease and some preventive and maintenance interventions.

■ TABLE 33-3 Sickle Cell Anemia: Potential Problems, Prevention, and Maintenance

POTENTIAL PROBLEM	PREVENTION AND MAINTENANCE
1. Inadequate oxygen to meet needs of labor and prevent sickling	1. a. Monitor Hb level and HCT to maintain Hb at ≥8 g and HCT at ≥20% b. Have typed and crossmatched blood available c. Assist with transfusions d. Administer oxygen continuously during labor e. Coach for relaxation and to lessen anxiety
2. Infection: UTI, pyelonephritis, pneumonia	2. a. Continue actions as under No. 1 b. Maintain adequate hydration c. Administer antibiotics as ordered d. Maintain strict asepsis e. Encourage frequent voiding to keep bladder empty
3. Sequestration crisis caused by need for and destruction of RBCs	3. Administer folic acid supplement (1 mg/day) to decrease erythropoietic demands and reduce probability of capillary stasis
4. Crisis caused by hypoxia, hypotension, acidosis, dehydration, exertion, sudden cooling, low-grade fever	4. a. Continue actions as under No. 1 b. Avoid supine hypotension c. Maintain adequate hydration d. Maintain comfortable room temperature: use warm blankets or cool cloths as needed e. Assist with analgesia and anesthesia
5. Pseudotoxemia (hypertension, proteinuria, no large weight gain); often accompanying bone pain crisis	5. a. If true PIH occurs, care is the same as for PIH b. Monitor blood pressure and urine
6. Thromboembolism (from increased blood viscosity)	6. a. Monitor for positive Homans' sign b. Initiate bed rest if Homans' sign is positive or if reddened, warm areas, or lump appears in the calf c. Maintain adequate hydration d. Administer heparin as ordered e. Apply warm compresses f. Apply antiembolism stockings
7. Congestive heart failure	7. a. Assess pulse, respiratory rate b. Place in semirecumbent position; lateral position for labor c. Auscultate for crackles in the lungs frequently d. Administer oxygen and medications (e.g., digitalis, antibiotics, diuretics, analgesics) e. Regional analgesia for pain relief in labor
8. Pulmonary infarction (hemoptysis, cough, temperature to 38.9° C, friction rub)	8. Assess for this possible complication to facilitate early diagnosis
9. Postpartum hemorrhage (resulting from heparin therapy)	9. Administer ordered oxytocic medication

Hb, Hemoglobin; *HCT,* hematocrit; *PIH,* pregnancy-induced hypertension; *RBCs,* red blood cells; *UTI,* urinary tract infection.

Thalassemia

Thalassemia (Mediterranean or Cooley's anemia) is a relatively common anemia in which an insufficient amount of hemoglobin is produced to fill the RBCs. The condition eventually manifests itself in severe bone deformities caused by massive marrow tissue expansion. For the infant born with severe thalassemia, death from cardiac failure is common (Letsky, 1995). Thalassemia is a hereditary disorder that involves the abnormal synthesis of the alpha or beta chains of hemoglobin. β-Thalassemia is the more common variety in the United States and often is diagnosed in persons of Italian, Greek, southern Chinese, Mediterranean, North African, African-American, Middle Eastern, southern Asian, or Indo-Pakistani descent. The unbalanced synthesis of hemoglobin leads to premature RBC death, resulting in severe anemia. Thalassemia major is the homozygous form of this disorder; thalassemia minor is the heterozygous form. Couples with the thalassemia trait should seek genetic counseling.

Thalassemia major complicates pregnancy. Preeclampsia is more common in women with thalassemia major. It may be associated with low-birth-weight infants and increased fetal death. Placental weight often is increased, perhaps secondary to maternal anemia. The frequency of fetal distress from hypoxia is greater than in women without thalassemia major.

Pregnant clients are managed similarly to those who have sickle cell disease. Folic acid should be given to avoid folate deficiency. The anemia will not respond to iron therapy. Prolonged parenteral iron can lead to harmful, excessive iron storage. Regular transfusion may be necessary.

Splenectomy may be necessary if enlargement and pain occur. Women with thalassemia major may die of chronic infection or progressive hepatic or cardiac failure—the result of excessive iron deposition—because much of the hemoglobin that is present is precipitated in the form of hard crystals. Iron in any form is contraindicated.

People with *thalassemia minor* have a mild, persistent anemia, but the RBC level may be normal or even elevated. However, no systemic problems are caused by the anemia. Thalassemia minor must be distinguished from iron deficiency anemia.

Pregnancy will neither worsen thalassemia minor nor be compromised by the disease. The anemia will not respond to iron therapy, and prolonged parenteral iron therapy can lead to harmful, excessive iron storage. People with thalassemia minor should have a normal life span despite a moderately reduced hemoglobin level.

PULMONARY DISORDERS

As pregnancy advances and the uterus impinges on the thoracic cavity, any pregnant woman may have increased respiratory difficulty. This difficulty will be compounded by pulmonary disease.

A pulmonary disorder in pregnancy requires assessment, planning, and interventions specific to the disease process, in addition to routine peripartum care. The nurse also must be alert to pulmonary complications precipitated by pregnancy.

Asthma

Bronchial asthma is an acute respiratory illness caused by allergens, marked change in ambient temperature, or emotional tension. In many cases the actual cause may be unknown. A family history of allergy is common in people with asthma. In response to stimuli, there is widespread but reversible narrowing of the hyperreactive airways, making it difficult to breathe. The clinical manifestations are expiratory wheezing, productive cough, thick sputum, and/or dyspnea.

From 1% to 4% of pregnant women have asthma (Mabie, 1996). The effect of pregnancy on asthma is unpredictable. About one half will improve, one third will stay the same, and one third will worsen (Jackson & Clark, 1993). Physiologic alterations induced by pregnancy do not make the pregnant women more prone to asthmatic attacks. However, some adverse events are associated with asthma.

Mabie (1996) reviewed studies of asthma in pregnancy and reported that the incidence of low birth weight, preterm labor, perinatal mortality, preeclampsia, chronic hypertension, hyperemesis gravidarum, and complicated labor was higher in pregnancy complicated by asthma. Adverse outcomes among studies were variable; however, differences in study population characteristics likely account for the differences that were observed (Mabie, 1996). With good care, the morbidity and mortality rate of the woman with asthma is equivalent to that of the general population of pregnant women (ACOG, 1996; Niswander & Evans, 1995).

Therapy for asthma has three objectives: (1) relief of the acute attack, (2) prevention or limitation of later attacks, and (3) adequate maternal and fetal oxygenation. In all persons with asthma, known allergens should be eliminated and a comfortable home temperature maintained.

Respiratory infections should be treated and mist or steam inhalation used to aid expectoration of mucus. Bronchial asthma therapy is initiated. Acute episodes may require albuterol, steroids, aminophylline, oxygen, β-adrenergic agents, and correction of fluid-electrolyte imbalance.

Asthma attacks can occur in labor; thus medications for asthma are continued in labor and postpartum. Some medications are to be avoided in pregnancy because they may precipitate or exacerbate an asthma attack. See Table 33-4 for medications that are preferred or are to be avoided in pregnancy.

Adult Respiratory Distress Syndrome

Adult respiratory distress syndrome (ARDS), or shock lung, occurs when the lungs are unable to maintain levels of oxygen and carbon dioxide within normal limits.

There is an increase in pulmonary capillary permeability, decrease of lung volume, and shunting, which results in arterial hypoxemia.

TABLE 33-4 Medications Used In Pregnancy in Clients with Asthma

STAGE/CONDITION OF PREGNANCY	PREFERRED MEDICATION	MEDICATION(S) TO AVOID (RATIONALE)
Labor	Continue asthma medications	
Induction	Oxytocin	Prostaglandins (may cause bronchoconstriction or bronchospasm)
Pain relief	Fentanyl Epidural anesthesia	Morphine and Demerol (release histamine)
Preterm labor	Magnesium sulfate, nifedipine, β-agonist	β-Agonist if client is already taking one for her asthma (may cause respiratory distress) NSAIDs (may exacerbate asthma)
Postpartum hemorrhage	Oxytocin	Methylergonovine and 15-methyl prostaglandin $F_{2\alpha}$ (may worsen asthma)

NSAIDs, Nonsteroidal antiinflammatory drugs.
Data from Mabie, W. (1996). Asthma in pregnancy. *Clin Obstet Gynecol* 39(1), 56-69.

Marked tachycardia, dyspnea, and cyanosis that do not respond to nasal oxygen or intermittent positive pressure breathing are the most noted signs. ARDS is not specific to pregnancy; it also can result from chest trauma, drug ingestion, or pneumonia. When ARDS is associated with pregnancy, pulmonary embolism, disseminated intravascular coagulation (DIC), and aspiration pneumonia are the precipitators.

To provide the best fetal environment, early intubation and mechanical ventilation is recommended (Cunningham et al., 1997). With severe lung injury, positive end-expiratory pressure (PEEP) may be necessary.

Artificial surfactant has been used to try to improve outcomes in ARDS; however, no significant improvement was noted (Anzeuto et al., 1996).

The postpartum incidence of ARDS is not affected by the method of birth but by the amount of trauma occurring during pregnancy and birth. It may also occur after miscarriage or medically induced abortion.

Laboratory reports are important in identifying the origin of acute pulmonary problems. The important observations for the nurse to note are vital signs, signs of thrombophlebitis, and hemorrhage. During the postpartum period apprehension, distended neck veins, cyanosis, diaphoresis, or pallor provide clues. Mental confusion or disorientation may also be noted.

The pulse rate increases to compensate for respiratory insufficiency of any origin. The severity of the pulmonary problem increases as the pulse rate rises. An initial rise in blood pressure occurs as cardiac output increases in an attempt to supply the tissue with oxygen. When lung damage is severe, blood pressure drops.

Respiratory changes are the most important indicators of ARDS. The rate, depth, respiratory pattern, symmetry of chest movement, and use of accessory muscles should be noted; therefore observation of respiratory characteristics after activity is important.

NURSE ALERT *If there is any indication of abnormality, respirations are counted for a full minute; an error in rate of plus or minus four respirations per minute may be highly significant.*

On auscultation, crackles, rhonchi, wheezes, or a pleural friction rub should be reported, especially when they have occurred following an earlier assessment with normal findings. The pregnant woman should be positioned for breathing comfort. Oxygen and emergency equipment should be available. The woman should be reassured and coached in relaxation techniques to lessen her anxiety.

Attention to fluid balance is critical; fluid overload further compromises pulmonary status. A client who is mechanically ventilated retains an added liter of fluid each day (Cunningham et al., 1997). In addition, in ARDS, fluid leads into the interstitium of the lungs at normal pressures because of a pulmonary permeability defect. The lowest pulmonary capillary wedge pressures possible that do not decrease cardiac output should be maintained (Cunningham et al., 1997).

This syndrome has a high mortality rate. The prognosis is good if the woman is otherwise healthy and if ventilatory support can be maintained until the underlying disease can be treated (Cunningham et al., 1997).

Cystic Fibrosis

Cystic fibrosis is a common autosomal-recessive genetic disorder in which the exocrine glands produce excessive viscous secretions, which causes problems with both respiratory and digestive functions.

There is an increase in pulmonary capillary permeability, decrease of lung volume, and shunting, which results in arterial hypoxemia. Respiratory failure and early death (early 20s) may occur.

Since the gene for cystic fibrosis was identified in 1989, better understanding of the disorder has occurred (Hilman,

Aitken, & Constantinescu, 1996). Improvements in diagnosis and treatment have allowed an increasing number of women with cystic fibrosis to survive to adulthood. Preconception counseling is essential for women with cystic fibrosis.

In women with good nutrition, mild obstructive lung disease, and good chest x-rays, pregnancy is tolerated well (Hilman, Aitken, & Constantinescu, 1996). In those with severe disease, the pregnancy is often complicated by chronic hypoxia and frequent pulmonary infections. Women with cystic fibrosis show a decrease in their residual volume during pregnancy, as do normal pregnant women, and are unable to maintain vital capacity. Presumably the pulmonary vasculature cannot accommodate the increased cardiac output of pregnancy. The results are decreased oxygen to the myocardium, decreased cardiac output, and increased hypoxemia. A pregnant woman with less than 50% of expected vital capacity usually has a difficult pregnancy.

Indications for termination of pregnancy should be addressed with women for whom this option is acceptable (Hilman, Aitken, & Constantinescu, 1996).

Weight and symptoms of malabsorption should be monitored at each prenatal visit and pancreatic enzymes adjusted as necessary. Oral supplements, including nasogastric feedings, may be necessary to maintain nutritional status (Hilman, Aitken, & Constantinescu, 1996).

Increased maternal and perinatal mortality is related to severe pulmonary infection.

During labor monitoring for fluid and electrolyte balance is required. The amount of sodium lost through sweat can be significant, and hypovolemia can occur. Conversely, if any degree of cor pulmonale is present, fluid overload is a concern. Oxygen is freely given during labor and monitoring by pulse oximetry is recommended (Hilman, Aitken, & Constantinescu, 1996). Epidural or local analgesia is the preferred analgesic for birth.

Preterm birth is a significant risk factor; approximately 35% of infants are born before term. Neonates with cystic fibrosis may be born with meconium ileus. The neonate may also "taste salty" when kissed and have a positive sweat test result.

Breastfeeding appears to be safe as long as the sodium content of the milk is not abnormal (Lawrence, 1999). Pumping and discarding the milk is done until the sodium content has been determined.

INTEGUMENTARY DISORDERS

The skin surface may exhibit many physiologic and pathologic conditions during pregnancy. Dermatologic disorders induced by pregnancy include melasma (chloasma), herpes gestationis, noninflammatory pruritus of pregnancy, vascular "spiders," palmar erythema, and pregnancy granuloma (including epulides). Skin problems generally aggravated by pregnancy are acne vulgaris (acne) (in the first trimester),

erythema multiforme, herpetiform dermatitis (fever blisters and genital herpes), granuloma inguinale (Donovan bodies), condylomata acuminata (genital warts), neurofibromatosis (von Recklinghausen's disease), and pemphigus. Dermatologic disorders usually improved by pregnancy include acne vulgaris (in the third trimester), seborrheic dermatitis (dandruff), and psoriasis. An unpredictable course during pregnancy may be expected in atopic dermatitis, lupus erythematosus, and herpes simplex.

NURSE ALERT *Isotretinoin (Accutane), commonly prescribed for cystic acne, is highly teratogenic. There is a risk for craniofacial, cardiac, and CNS malformations in exposed fetuses. This drug should not be taken during pregnancy.*

Explanation, reassurance, and commonsense measures should suffice for normal skin changes. Disease processes during and soon after pregnancy may be extremely difficult to diagnose and treat.

NEUROLOGIC DISORDERS

The pregnant woman with a neurologic disorder needs to deal with potential teratogenic effects of prescribed medications, changes of mobility during pregnancy, and ability to care for the baby. The nurse should be aware of all drugs the client is taking and the associated potential for producing congenital anomalies. As the pregnancy progresses, the woman's center of gravity shifts and causes balance and gait changes. The nurse needs to advise the woman of these expected changes and to suggest safety measures as appropriate. Familial and community resources should be assessed to provide child care for the neurologically impaired woman.

Epilepsy

Epilepsy is a disorder of the brain causing recurrent seizures and is the most common neurologic disorder accompanying pregnancy (Cartlidge, 1995). Epilepsy may result from developmental abnormalities or injury, as well as having no known cause. Convulsive seizures may be more frequent or severe during complications of pregnancy, such as edema, alkalosis, fluid-electrolyte imbalance, cerebral hypoxia, hypoglycemia, and hypocalcemia.

The effect of epilepsy on pregnancy is unpredictable. Up to 80% of women have no change in seizure activity during pregnancy, while 20% have an increase and up to 25% have a decrease in seizures (Gilmore, Pennell, & Stern, 1998).

The differential diagnosis between epilepsy and eclampsia may pose a problem. Epilepsy and eclampsia can coexist. However, a history of seizures and a normal plasma uric acid level, as well as the absence of hypertension, generalized edema, or proteinuria, point to epilepsy. Electroencephalography rarely is diagnostic.

During pregnancy, the risk of vaginal bleeding is doubled, and there is a threefold risk of abruptio placentae. Abnormal presentations are more common in labor and birth, and the possibility that the fetus will experience seizures in utero is increased (Mishell & Brenner, 1994).

Metabolic changes in pregnancy usually alter pharmacokinetics. In addition, nausea and vomiting may interfere with ingestion and absorption of medication.

Failure to take medications is a common factor leading to worsening of seizure activity during pregnancy. This is largely due to the message that drugs are harmful to the fetus (Gilmore, Pennell, & Stern, 1998). Teratogenicity of antiepileptic drugs (AED) has been described thoroughly but the risks to the fetus have been exaggerated. Congenital anomalies associated with AED include cleft lip or palate, congenital heart disease, urogenital defects and neural tube defects (Gilmore, Pennell, & Stern, 1998).

Antiepileptic drugs should be monotherapeutic and should be used in the smallest therapeutic dose with the least side effects. Daily folic acid supplementation is important because of the depletion that occurs when taking anticonvulsants (Cartlidge, 1995).

During the neonatal period, infants can experience a hemorrhagic disorder associated with AED-induced vitamin K deficiency. Prophylaxis consists of administering vitamin K 20 mg orally daily during the last month of pregnancy and administering 1 mg IM to the newborn at birth (Gilmore, Pennell, & Stern, 1998).

Multiple Sclerosis

Multiple sclerosis (MS), a patchy demyelinization of the spinal cord and CNS, may be a viral disorder. MS has a greater prevalence in females and is more common during the childbearing years, between the ages of 20 and 40 years (Cartlidge, 1995). Infertility, miscarriage, stillbirth, and fetal anomalies do not appear to be increased in women with MS; however, most women with MS choose not to become pregnant (James et al., 1994).

MS may occasionally complicate pregnancy, but exacerbations and remissions are unrelated to the pregnant state. Steroids are commonly used to treat acute exacerbations. Nursing care of the pregnant woman with MS is similar to the care of the normal pregnant woman. Women with MS occasionally may have an almost painless labor. The character of uterine contractions is unaffected by the disease, however.

Bell's Palsy

An association between Bell's palsy (idiopathic facial paralysis) and pregnancy was first cited by Bell in 1830. The incidence of Bell's palsy in pregnancy is about 57 per 100,000 per year. The incidence usually peaks during the third trimester and the puerperium (Cartlidge, 1995). Blinking is impaired; eye pain is often the presenting symptom (Gleicher, 1992). A causative relationship does not seem to exist between the appearance of Bell's palsy and any complications of pregnancy.

No effects of maternal Bell's palsy have been observed in infants. Maternal outcome is generally good unless there is a complete block in nerve conduction. Steroids sometimes are prescribed for the condition, but they do not hasten recovery. In most affected women, 90% or more of facial function can be expected to return (Cunningham et al., 1997). Supportive care includes prevention of injury to the exposed cornea, facial muscle massage, careful chewing and manual removal of food from inside the affected cheek, and reassurance that return of total neurologic function is likely.

AUTOIMMUNE DISORDERS

Autoimmune disorders make up a large group of diseases that disrupt the function of the immune system of the body. In these types of disorders the body develops antibodies that attack its normally present antigens, causing tissue damage. Autoimmune disorders have a predilection for women in their reproductive years; therefore associations with pregnancy are not uncommon. Pregnancy may affect the disease process. Some disorders adversely affect the course of pregnancy or are detrimental to the fetus. Autoimmune disorders include rheumatoid arthritis, systemic lupus erythematosus, hyperthyroidism, myasthenia gravis, and immunologic thrombocytopenic purpura.

Rheumatoid Arthritis

Rheumatoid arthritis is a chronic polyarthritis with symptoms of synovitis, anorexia, weakness, fatigue, and vague musculoskeletal symptoms (Cunningham et al., 1997). The wrists, hands, knees, and feet are often involved. There is significant pain upon movement, which is associated with swelling.

The peak age of onset of rheumatoid arthritis (RA) is between 35 and 40 years. RA affects women more often than men (Gilbert & Harmon, 1998). During pregnancy, women with RA experience an increase in α_2-glycoprotein. In addition, total plasma and free cortisol (especially estrogens and progesterone) show an increase. Two thirds of women with RA find that the severity of symptoms decreases during pregnancy, but in many women exacerbation often follows childbirth (Lockshin & Druzin, 1995).

Management of RA during pregnancy includes an appropriate balance of rest and exercise, heat and physical therapy, salicylates, and low-dose steroids (Scott et al., 1999). Low-dose aspirin probably remains the safest and most useful antiinflammatory drug for these women.

Systemic Lupus Erythematosus

One of the most common serious disorders of childbearing age, **systemic lupus erythematosus (SLE)** is a chronic, multisystem inflammatory disease characterized by autoimmune antibody production that affects the skin, joints, kidneys, lungs, CNS, liver, and other body organs

(James et al., 1994). More than 250,000 persons are known to have SLE, with an estimated 50,000 new cases per year. The exact cause is unknown, but viral infection and hormonal and genetic factors may be related.

Early symptoms, such as fatigue, weight loss, skin rashes, and arthralgias may be overlooked. Pericarditis is often the presenting symptom. Eventually all organs become involved. The condition is characterized by a series of exacerbations and remissions.

If the diagnosis has been established and the woman desires a child, she is advised to wait until she has been in remission for at least 6 months before attempting to get pregnant (Gilbert & Harmon, 1998). An exacerbation of SLE during pregnancy or postpartum occurs in 15% to 60% of women (James et al., 1994).

SLE during pregnancy is associated with increased rates of preterm deliveries, IUGR, stillbirth, and perinatal mortality (Cunningham et al., 1997). Complications such as preeclampsia and HELLP syndrome are common.

Medical therapy is kept to a minimum in women who are in remission or who have a mild form of SLE. Antiinflammatory drugs such as prednisone and aspirin may be used. Immunosuppressive drugs are not recommended during pregnancy but may be used in some situations. Nursing care focuses on early recognition of signs of SLE exacerbation and pregnancy complications, education and support of the woman and her family, and assessment of fetal well-being.

Women with SLE should limit their number of pregnancies because of increased adverse perinatal outcomes as well as the guarded maternal prognosis (Cunningham et al., 1997). Family planning is important; oral contraceptives are used with caution because vascular disease commonly accompanies SLE; tubal ligation may be the optimum means of managing fertility. Progestin implants have no known effects on flare-ups of lupus; intrauterine devices are prescribed cautiously (Cunningham et al., 1997).

Myasthenia Gravis

Myasthenia gravis (MG), an autoimmune motor (muscle) end-plate disorder that involves acetylcholine use, affects the motor function at the myoneural junction. Muscle weakness, particularly of the eyes, face, tongue, neck, limbs, and respiratory muscles, results. Myasthenia gravis occurs at the rate of 1 in 10,000 and in women twice as often as in men (Cunningham et al., 1997).

The response of women with MG to pregnancy is unpredictable; remission, exacerbation, or remaining stable during pregnancy may occur. Some maternal deaths due to complications of MG have been reported (Plauché, 1991).

The nurse and physician should be alert to symptoms, which include easy fatigue, intermittent double vision, upper eyelid drooping, and facial muscle weakness. Clients may have easy fatigability; diplopia; and difficulty speaking, swallowing, and clearing secretions (James et al., 1994).

In more serious cases upper arm weakness and breathing difficulty occur. Infections may precipitate onset or relapse and must be treated aggressively during pregnancy.

Women with MG usually tolerate labor well because they already have some degree of muscle relaxation. Meperidine is the obstetric analgesic of choice. Local anesthesia is preferred. Oxytocin may be given, but scopolamine and muscle relaxants (e.g., magnesium sulfate) are contraindicated because they worsen the neuromuscular blockade. Some women are unable to push effectively in second stage labor and may need a forceps-assisted birth. After birth, women must be carefully supervised because relapses often occur during the puerperium.

Approximately 15% of infants develop symptoms: feeble cry, respiratory distress, and weak suck. These symptoms are treated with parenteral neostigmine. With proper management complete recovery of the infant is usual.

GASTROINTESTINAL DISORDERS

Compromise of GI function during pregnancy is a concern. Obvious physiologic alterations, such as the greatly enlarged uterus, and less apparent changes, such as hormonal differences and hypochlorhydria (deficiency of hydrochloric acid in the stomach's gastric juice), require understanding for proper diagnosis and treatment. Gallbladder disease and inflammatory bowel disease are two GI disorders that may occur during pregnancy.

Cholelithiasis and Cholecystitis

Women are twice as likely to have **cholelithiasis** (presence of gallstones in the gallbladder) as men (Baker, 1995), and pregnancy seems to make the woman more vulnerable to gallstone formation (Home Care box). Decreased muscle tone allows gallbladder distention, thickening of the bile, and prolonged emptying time. Increased progesterone levels result in a slight hypercholesterolemia.

Cholecystitis (inflammation of the gallbladder) is also more common in pregnancy, probably because pressure of

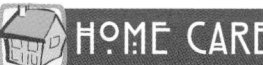
HOME CARE

Nutritional Counseling for the Pregnant Woman with Cholecystitis or Cholelithiasis

- Assess your diet for foods that cause discomfort and flatulence and omit foods that trigger episodes.
- Reduce dietary fat intake to 40 to 50 g per day.
- Limit protein to 10% to 12% of total calories.
- Choose foods so that most of the calories come from carbohydrates.
- Prepare food without adding fats or oils as much as possible.
- Avoid fried foods.

the enlarged uterus interferes with the normal circulation and drainage of the gallbladder. Acute cholecystitis occurs in about 1 in 4000 pregnancies, most often in older women who have been pregnant several times and who have a history of previous attacks (Depp, 1996).

Women with acute cholecystitis usually present with colicky abdominal pain, nausea, and vomiting. Fever and an increased leukocyte count may also be present. Ultrasound is often used to detect the presence of stones or dilation of the common bile duct (Depp, 1996).

Generally, gallbladder surgery should be postponed until the puerperium. Usually the woman can be treated with medical therapy, consisting of antibiotics, antispasmodics, intravenous fluids, bowel rest, and nasogastric suctioning (Depp, 1996; Gleicher, 1992). Morphine should not be used as an analgesic because it may cause ductal spasm (Gleicher, 1992). The woman's condition should improve significantly within 48 hours of beginning treatment. Impaction of a stone in the cystic or common bile duct or development of pancreatitis may necessitate immediate cholecystectomy or cholecystotomy. If surgery is necessary, there is significant risk of subsequent preterm labor (Depp, 1996).

Inflammatory Bowel Disease

Inflammatory bowel disease can be acute or chronic. Infection or antibiotic therapy can induce acute inflammation of the bowel. Chronic inflammatory bowel disease can be classified as regional enteritis (Crohn's disease) or ulcerative colitis.

Chronic inflammatory bowel diseases are prone to periods of exacerbation and remission. The cause is unknown. The clinical manifestations for this chronic disorder are liquid diarrhea, urgency of defecation, and crampy lower abdominal pain. Blood, mucus, and/or pus may be seen in the stool.

Treatment and therapy are the same for the pregnant woman as for the nonpregnant woman. Medications include sulfasalazine and prednisone. Folic acid and vitamin supplementation is especially important because of the problems with malabsorption and malnutrition associated with chronic inflammatory bowel disease.

The effect of inflammatory bowel disease on pregnancy is minimal unless there is marked debilitation, whereupon miscarriage, fetal death, or preterm birth may occur. In general, when pregnancy coincides with active ulcerative colitis, most women will experience a severe exacerbation of the disease. When pregnancy occurs during a period of inactivity of the disorder, a flare-up is unlikely.

Appendicitis

Appendicitis is the most common acute surgical condition seen in pregnancy, occurring approximately once in 2000 pregnancies. This condition occurs in approximately the same frequency during each trimester of pregnancy and the postpartum period (Depp, 1996). The diagnosis of appendicitis is often delayed because the usual signs and symptoms mimic some normal changes of pregnancy such as nausea and vomiting and increased WBC count. As pregnancy progresses, the appendix is pushed upward and to the right from its usual anatomic location (see Fig. 15-14). Because of these changes, appendiceal rupture and peritonitis occur two to three times more often in pregnant women than in nonpregnant women.

The woman with appendicitis most commonly presents with abdominal pain, nausea and vomiting, and loss of appetite. Approximately half of these affected women have muscle guarding. Moving the uterus tends to increase the pain. Temperature may be normal or mildly increased (to 38.3° C). Because of the physiologic increase in WBCs that occurs in pregnancy, significant increases associated with appendicitis must be documented either by rising levels on serial samples or by an increasing left shift.

The diagnosis of appendicitis requires a high level of suspicion because the typical signs and symptoms are similar to those found in many other conditions, including pyelonephritis, round ligament pain, placental abruption, torsion of an ovarian cyst, cholecystitis, and preterm labor (Depp, 1996).

The likelihood of miscarriage or preterm labor increases in the presence of appendicitis (Cunningham et al., 1997). Diagnostic errors may lead to removal of a normal appendix. However, it is better to operate unnecessarily than to wait until generalized peritonitis develops (Cunningham et al., 1997).

Appendectomy before rupture usually does not require either antibiotic or tocolytic therapy. If surgery is delayed until after rupture, multiple antibiotics are ordered. Rupture is likely to result in preterm labor, perhaps necessitating the use of tocolytic agents. However, the value of prophylactic tocolytic therapy in cases of rupture has not been proven (Depp, 1996).

Intestinal Obstruction

The second most common nonobstetric abdominal emergency in pregnancy is intestinal obstruction (Gleicher, 1992). Any woman with a laparotomy scar is more likely to have an intestinal obstruction (adynamic ileus) during pregnancy. Adhesions as a result of previous surgery or pelvic inflammatory disease, an enlarging uterus, and displacement of the intestines are etiologic factors.

Constipation, persistent cramplike abdominal pain, vomiting, auscultatory rushes within the abdomen, and "laddering" of the intestinal shadows on x-ray films aid in the diagnosis of intestinal obstruction. Immediate surgical intervention is required for release of the obstruction. Pregnancy is rarely affected by the surgery, assuming the absence of complications such as peritonitis. Intestinal obstruction is not an indication for cesarean birth.

Abdominal Hernias

The incidence of abdominal hernias and related incarceration of the bowel is reduced during pregnancy despite permanent enlargement of umbilical or incisional hernial rings. Displacement of a nonadherent bowel by the enlarging uterus and its shielding of so-called weak areas of the abdominal wall are responsible. In fact, temporary spontaneous reduction of some abdominal wall hernias occurs during gestation. In contrast, however, the uncommon irreducible or adherent hernias may become incarcerated as pregnancy progresses.

Straining or bearing down during the second stage of labor may be contraindicated for women with hernias. Therefore low forceps-assisted birth may be planned. Abdominal hernia is not an indication for cesarean birth; herniorrhaphy should be performed between pregnancies.

SURGERY DURING PREGNANCY

The incidence of surgery requiring anesthesia during pregnancy ranges from 0.2% to 2.2%, affecting an estimated 50,000 pregnant women each year. It is difficult to determine the true incidence because many surgeries may occur very early in gestation, before women recognize the pregnancy (Kendrick, 1994). The need for abdominal surgery occurs as frequently among pregnant women as among nonpregnant women of comparable age. However, pregnancy may make diagnosis more difficult. An enlarged uterus and displaced internal organs may make abdominal palpation more difficult, alter the position of an affected organ, and/or change the usual signs and symptoms associated with a particular disorder.

▋ CARE MANAGEMENT

Initial assessment of the pregnant woman requiring surgery focuses on her presenting signs and symptoms. A thorough history and physical examination are performed. Laboratory testing includes, at a minimum, a complete blood count with differential and a urinalysis. Additional laboratory and other diagnostic tests may well be necessary to reach a diagnosis. In addition, fetal heart rate and activity, along with uterine activity, should be monitored and constant vigilance for symptoms of impending obstetric complications maintained. The extent of presurgery assessment is determined by the immediacy of surgical intervention and the specific disorder that requires surgery.

Hospital Care

When surgery becomes necessary during pregnancy, the woman and her family are concerned about the effects of the procedure and medication on fetal well-being and the course of pregnancy. Kendrick (1994) reported that every participant in her study of women undergoing surgery during pregnancy described her greatest fear related to surgery as the fear of losing her baby. An important part of preoperative nursing care is encouraging the woman to express her fears, concerns, and questions.

Preoperative care for a pregnant woman differs from that for a nonpregnant woman in one significant aspect: the presence of at least one other person, the fetus. Continuous FHR and uterine contraction monitoring should be performed if the fetus is considered viable. Procedures such as preparation of the operative site and time of insertion of IV lines and urinary retention catheters vary with the physician and the facility. However, in every instance there is a total restriction of solid foods and liquids or a clear specification of the type, amount, and time at which clear liquids may be taken before surgery. Food by mouth is restricted for several hours before a scheduled procedure. Even if she has had nothing by mouth—but more important, if surgery is unexpected—the woman is in danger of vomiting and aspirating, and special precautions are taken before anesthetic is administered (e.g., administering an antacid).

Intraoperatively, perinatal nurses may collaborate with the surgical staff to increase their knowledge about the special needs of pregnant women undergoing surgery. One intervention to improve fetal oxygenation is positioning the woman on the operating table with a lateral tilt to avoid maternal compression of the vena cava (Kendrick, 1994). Perinatal nurses may also recommend continuous fetal and uterine monitoring during the procedure because the risk of preterm labor, especially following abdominal surgery, is great. Monitoring may be accomplished using sterile aquasonic gel and a sterile sleeve for the transducer. During abdominal surgery, uterine contractions may be manually palpated (Kendrick, 1994).

In the immediate recovery period, general observations and care pertinent to postoperative recovery are initiated. Frequent assessments are carried out for several hours following surgery. Whether the woman is cared for in the surgical postanesthesia recovery area or in labor and delivery, continuous fetal and uterine monitoring will likely be initiated or resumed because of the increased risk of preterm labor. Tocolysis may be necessary if preterm labor occurs (see Chapter 36).

Home Care

Plans for the woman's return home and for convalescent care should be completed as early as possible before discharge. Depending on her insurance coverage, nursing care may be provided through a home health agency. If not, the woman and other support persons need to be taught necessary skills and procedures, such as care of the incision and/or dressing changes. Ideally, the woman and other caregivers should have opportunities for supervised practice before discharge so that they can feel comfortable with their knowledge and ability before being totally responsible for providing care. Box 33-4 lists information that should be included in discharge teaching for the postoperative client. The woman may also need referrals to various community agencies for evaluation of the home situation, child care, home health care, and financial or other assistance.

BOX 33-4 | **Discharge Teaching for Home Care**

- Care of incision site
- Diet and elimination related to GI function
- Signs and symptoms of developing complications; wound infection, thrombophlebitis, pneumonia
- Equipment needed and technique for assessing temperature
- Recommended schedule for resumption of activities of daily living
- Treatments and medications ordered
- List of resource persons and their telephone numbers
- Schedule of follow-up visits

If birth has not occurred:
  - Assessment of fetal activity (kick counts)
  - Signs of preterm labor

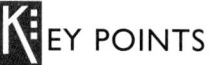

KEY POINTS

- The stress of the normal maternal adaptations to pregnancy on a heart whose function is already taxed may cause cardiac decompensation.

- In the case of a cardiac arrest in a pregnant woman, the standard advanced cardiac life support guidelines should be implemented without modification.

- Maternal morbidity and mortality is a significant risk in a pregnancy complicated by mitral stenosis.

- The chance of ARDS developing increases with the amount of trauma occurring during pregnancy or birth.

- The normal hemodynamic values are significantly altered as a result of pregnancy.

- Anemia, the most common medical disorder of pregnancy, affects at least 20% of pregnant women.

- Autoimmune disorders (e.g., systemic lupus erythematosus, myasthenia gravis) show a predilection for women in their reproductive years; therefore associations with pregnancy are not uncommon.

- In the pregnant woman an enlarged uterus, displaced internal organs, and altered laboratory values may confound differential diagnosis when the need for immediate abdominal surgery occurs.

- Preoperative care for a pregnant woman differs from that for a nonpregnant woman in one significant aspect: the presence of at least one other person, the fetus.

CRITICAL THINKING EXERCISES

1 *You are assigned to admit a woman with abdominal pain. She is in the third trimester of pregnancy. She is complaining of fatigue, right-sided pain, and nausea.*
   a. *What questions will you ask her?*
   b. *List three medical diagnoses that might be relevant. What questions can you ask to help make the differential diagnosis? What laboratory tests will likely be ordered?*
   c. *Given a medical diagnosis of cholecystitis, what are your nursing diagnoses? Formulate your plan of care. Begin discharge planning.*

2 *A 32-year-old woman, pregnant with her second child, is admitted with respiratory distress. She has a history of rheumatic disease as an adolescent.*
   a. *What is the likely origin of her respiratory distress? What are nursing diagnoses that are relevant?*
   b. *Antibiotics are ordered for her. What is the usual antibiotic regimen for someone with her history?*
   c. *Clients in respiratory distress are often anxious. Give examples of interventions to reduce her anxiety. How can you involve her family in her care?*

3 *Your neighbor has been diagnosed as having anemia due to folic acid deficiency. She has asked you to help her understand what caused her problem and to assist her in planning menus that would correct the deficiency. She asked you if her 5-year-old daughter should be checked for this deficiency.*
   a. *What are signs and symptoms of this type of anemia? Who is most at risk for the deficiency? What foods contain folic acid? What are sequelae of folic acid deficiency?*
   b. *Plan a 7-day menu of foods high in folic acid. Can a folic acid deficiency be corrected with diet alone?*
   c. *What are the ethical considerations of providing such information to a neighbor?*

References

American College of Obstetricians and Gynecologists (ACOG). (1996). Pulmonary disease in pregnancy. *ACOG Tech Bull* 224. Washington, D.C.: ACOG.

American Heart Association (AHA). (1992). Subcommittee on Emergency Cardiac Care. Standards and guidelines for cardiopulmonary resuscitation and emergency cardiac care. *JAMA* 268, 2172, 2249.

American Heart Association (AHA). (1997). *Basic life support, heart saver guide.* Dallas: The Association.

Anzueto, A. et al. (1996). Aerosolized surfactant in adults with sepsis-induced acute respiratory distress syndrome. *N Engl J Med* 334, 1417-1421.

Association of Women's Health, Obstetric, and Neonatal Nurses (1998). *Standards and guidelines for professional nursing practice in the care of women and newborns* (5th ed.). Washington, D.C.: The Association.

Bajo, T. (1997). Cardiopulmonary resuscitation of the pregnant patient. In M. Foley, & T. Strong (Eds.). *Obstetric intensive care.* Philadelphia: W.B. Saunders.

Baker, A. (1995). Liver and biliary tract disease. In W. Barron, & M. Lindheimer (Eds.) *Medical disorders during pregnancy* (2nd ed.). St. Louis: Mosby.

Barron, W. (1995). Hypertension. In W. Barron, & M. Lindheimer (Eds). *Medical disorders during pregnancy.* St. Louis: Mosby.

Briggs, G. & Garite, T. (1991). Effects on the fetus of drugs used in critical care. In S. Clark et al. (Eds). *Critical care obstetrics* (2nd ed.). Boston: Blackwell Scientific.

Cartlidge, N. (1995). Neurologic disorders. In W. Barron, & M. Lindheimer (Eds). *Medical disorders during pregnancy.* St. Louis: Mosby.

Chandra, N., & Hazinski, M. (Eds.). (1994). *American Heart Association textbook of basic life support for healthcare providers.* Dallas: AHA.

Cunningham, F. et al. (1997). *Williams' obstetrics* (20th ed.). Stamford, CT: Appleton & Lange.

Depp, R. (1996). Cesarean delivery. In S. Gabbe, J. Niebyl, & J. Simpson (Eds). *Obstetrics: Normal and problem pregnancies* (3rd ed.). New York: Churchill Livingstone.

Duffy, T. (1995). Hematologic aspects of pregnancy. In G. Burrow, & T. Ferris (Eds). *Medical complications during pregnancy.* Philadelphia: W.B. Saunders.

Fenakel, K. et al. (1991). Nifedipine in the treatment of severe preeclampsia. *Obstet Gynecol 77,* 331-337.

Gilbert, E., & Harmon, J. (1998). *Manual of high risk pregnancy and delivery* (2nd ed.). St. Louis: Mosby.

Gilmore, J., Pennell, P., & Stern, B. (1998). Medication use during pregnancy for neurologic conditions. *Neurol Clin North Am 16,* 189-206.

Gleicher, N. (Eds.). (1992). *Principles and practice of medical therapy in pregnancy* (2nd ed.). Norwalk, CT: Appleton & Lange.

Grohar, J. (1994). Nursing protocols for antepartum home care. *J Obstet Gynecol Neonatal Nurs 23(8),* 687-694.

Health Care Resources (1997). *Handbook of high risk perinatal home care.* St. Louis: Mosby.

Hilman, B., Aitken, M., & Constantinescu, M. (1996). Pregnancy in patients with cystic fibrosis. *Clin Obstet Gynecol 39,* 70-86.

Hurst, J., & Alpert, J. (1994). *Diagnostic atlas of the heart.* New York: Raven Press.

Jackson, G., & Clark, S. (1993). Cardiac and pulmonary disorders and pregnancy. In T. Moore et al. (Eds.). *Gynecology and obstetrics: A longitudinal approach.* New York: Churchill Livingstone.

James, D. et al. (Eds.). (1994). *High risk pregnancy: Management options.* Philadelphia: W.B. Saunders.

Kendrick, J. (1994). Fetal and uterine response during maternal surgery. *MCN Am J Matern Child Nurs 19(3),* 165-170.

Kulb, N. (1990). Cardiac disorders. In K. Buckley, & N. Kulb (Eds.). *High risk maternity nursing manual.* Baltimore: Williams & Wilkins.

Landon, M. (1996). Cardiac and pulmonary disease. In S. Gabbe, J. Niebyl, & J. Simpson (Eds.). *Obstetrics: Normal and problem pregnancies* (3rd ed.). New York: Churchill Livingstone.

Lawrence, R. (1999). *Breastfeeding: A guide for the medical profession* (5th ed.). St. Louis: Mosby.

Letsky, E. (1995). Hematologic disorders. In W. Barron, & M. Lindheimer (Eds.). *Medical disorders during pregnancy* (2nd ed.). St. Louis: Mosby.

Lockshin, M., & Druzin, M. (1995). Rheumatic disease. In W. Barron, & M. Lindheimer (Eds.). *Medical disorders during pregnancy* (2nd ed.). St. Louis: Mosby.

Luppi, C. (1999). Cardiopulmonary resuscitation in pregnancy. *AWHONN's Lifelines 3(3),* 41-45.

Mabie, W. (1996). Asthma in pregnancy. *Clin Obstet Gynecol 39(1),* 56-69.

McAnulty, J. Metcalfe, J., & Ueland, K. (1995). Cardiovascular disease. In G. Burrow, & T. Ferris (Eds.). *Medical complications during pregnancy.* Philadelphia: W.B. Saunders.

Mendelson, M. (1997). Congenital cardiac disease and pregnancy. *Clin Perinatol 24(2),* 467-482.

Mendelson, M., & Lang, R. (1995). Pregnancy and heart disease. In W. Barron, & M. Lindheimer (Eds.). *Medical disorders during pregnancy* (2nd ed.). St. Louis: Mosby.

Mishell, D., & Brenner, P. (Eds.). (1994). *Management of common problems in obstetrics and gynecology* (3rd ed.). Boston: Blackwell Scientific.

Muller, J., & Goldman, M. (1991). Cardiovascular disease in pregnancy. In S. Cherry, & I. Merkatz (Eds.). *Complications of pregnancy: Medical, surgical, gynecologic, psychosocial, and perinatal* (4th ed.). Baltimore: Williams & Wilkins.

New York Heart Association (NYHA). (1964). *Diseases of the heart and blood vessels—Nomenclature and criteria for diagnosis* (6th ed.). Boston: Little, Brown.

Niswander, K., & Evans, S. (1995). *Manual of obstetrics.* Boston: Little, Brown.

Pagana, K., & Pagana, T. (1997). *Mosby's diagnostic and laboratory test reference* (3rd ed.). St. Louis: Mosby.

Plauché, W. (1991). Myasthenia gravis in mothers and their newborns. *Clin Obstet Gynecol 34,* 82.

Scott, J. et al. (Eds.). (1999). *Danforth's obstetrics and gynecology* (8th ed.). Philadelphia: J.B. Lippincott, Williams & Wilkins.

Strickland, R. et al. (1991). Anesthesia, cardiopulmonary bypass and the pregnant client. *Mayo Clin Proc 66,* 411-429.

Thornhill, M., & Camann, W. (1994). Cardiovascular disease. In D. Chestnut (Ed.). *Obstetric anesthesia: Principles and practice.* St. Louis: Mosby.

Wasserstrum, N. (1991). Nitroprusside in preeclampsia: Circulatory distress and paradoxical bradycardia. *Hypertension 18,* 79.

Wong, D., & Perry, S. (1998). *Maternal child nursing care.* St. Louis: Mosby.

34

Obstetric Critical Care

Mildred G. Harvey

EARNING OBJECTIVES

- Define the key terms.
- Discuss factors that have contributed to the development of the specialty of critical care obstetrics.
- Describe conditions that may place a pregnant woman in a critically ill state.
- Discuss factors that affect the provision of obstetric critical care when a pregnant woman becomes critically ill.
- Describe significant cardiovascular, pulmonary, and hematologic alterations during pregnancy that affect critical care for the pregnant woman.
- Review cardiac anatomy and physiologic features, including location of chambers, valves, major vessels, and path of circulation.
- List the four determinants of cardiac output and relate the clinical significance of each.
- Describe the parameters measured and normal values for pulmonary artery monitoring.

- Describe the parameters measured and normal values for arterial pressure monitoring.
- Discuss treatment strategies based on interpretation of hemodynamic profiles.
- Discuss implications of trauma on mother and fetus during pregnancy.
- Identify physiologic alterations of pregnancy that affect stabilization and treatment of the pregnant woman who has undergone trauma.
- Describe immediate assessment and stabilization measures for the pregnant victim of trauma.
- Describe components of the primary and secondary surveys for the pregnant woman who has undergone trauma.
- Discuss inclusion of the components of family-centered maternity care for the critically ill pregnant woman.
- Identify topics for nursing research about critical care obstetrics.

EY TERMS

afterload	perimortem cesarean delivery	pulmonary vascular resistance
arterial pressure catheter	preload	secondary survey
capillary hydrostatic pressure	primary survey	stroke volume
cardiac output	pulmonary artery catheter	SvO_2 monitoring
colloid osmotic pressure	pulmonary artery pressure	systemic vascular resistance
contractility	pulmonary capillary wedge pressure	

bstetric and critical care units are equally challenged whenever presented with the multiple, complex needs of a critically ill pregnant woman and her fetus. Optimal outcome for mother and fetus depends on (1) swift recognition of severe complications and (2) delivery of critical care therapies adjusted for the physiologic alterations of pregnancy. Fetal effects of therapies must also be considered. Management of the critically ill pregnant woman includes measures to continually assess both maternal and fetal status, selection of therapeutic interventions appropriate for both mother and fetus, and careful management for the timing of birth.

The provision of critical care and hemodynamic monitoring for the seriously ill pregnant woman has developed slowly in many institutions. This seems to have been the result of two factors: (1) obstetric nurses and physicians, expert in the care of pregnant women, feel threatened by pressure transducers, alarms, hemodynamic monitoring, and ventilators; and (2) critical care nurses and physicians, expert in hemodynamic monitoring and mechanical ventilation, feel threatened by the pregnant uterus, labor, birth, the fetus, and fetal monitoring. The result is that few institutions have been able to provide optimum care whenever a sudden, acute, life-threatening complication has occurred in a pregnant woman.

A critical care unit, or intensive care unit, provides the setting where advanced care necessary to support life is immediately available. An expert medical, nursing, and technical staff uses sophisticated, state-of-the-art techniques and equipment for invasive hemodynamic monitoring and immediate lifesaving interventions. The development of specialized critical care units has evolved in parallel with advances in invasive surgical and medical procedures and techniques.

Critical care obstetrics evolved as a subspecialty of perinatal medicine in response to the need for optimum care for the critically ill pregnant woman and her fetus. This subspecialty prepares the obstetric team, which has in-depth knowledge of pregnancy, to use critical care techniques in the management of the critically ill pregnant woman and her fetus. Obstetric intensive care units (OBICUs) have been developed so that expensive, specific equipment and individuals with special training and expertise in obstetric care and critical care are available to provide this care.

OBSTETRIC INTENSIVE CARE UNIT

Complications may develop during pregnancy that are so severe and life threatening that optimum maternal and fetal outcome, and many times survival, depends on the woman receiving critical care that meets her specific needs. Maternal adaptations that are normal for the pregnancy state alter physiologic status and make the pregnant woman hemodynamically different from the nonpregnant woman. Before the development of OBICUs, care for the

critically ill pregnant woman was usually provided in an intensive care unit for adults, where management modalities were based on hemodynamic values that are normal for the nonpregnant individual. Less than desirable outcomes in many cases led to studies that resulted in the development and establishment of OBICUs, which are set up to meet the specific needs of the critically ill pregnant woman.

Research in some of the first OBICUs reported on physical and hemodynamic differences during the pregnant state. Normal hemodynamic values for pregnancy were identified. Maternal and fetal outcomes improved when management of care was based on the enhanced hemodynamic state that accompanies normal pregnancy and care was provided in the specialized units (Mabie & Sibai, 1990).

PROVISION OF OBSTETRIC CRITICAL CARE

Anyone providing care for pregnant women may encounter the pregnant woman with a life-threatening complication and be challenged to recognize the need for immediate, critical care and to provide such care. This care may be delivered in a variety of ways.

Development of a viable plan to provide care for the critically ill pregnant woman; adequate education of nursing, medical, and ancillary staff; provision of necessary equipment at the bedside; and liberal consultation between the obstetric and critical care units can decrease problems and provide solutions to provide optimum care for critically ill pregnant women.

The most practical, efficient, economic way to provide care for the critically ill obstetric client who requires invasive hemodynamic monitoring, mechanical ventilation, or both depends primarily on the numbers of pregnant women cared for annually and the referral patterns in a specific facility (Hankins & Harvey, 1993). The ideal method to provide care for the pregnancy would be a specially trained team of obstetricians and obstetric nurses in an OBICU, augmented by anesthesiologists, pulmonologists, cardiologists, and intensivists as needed. The larger tertiary center is more likely to have this type of unit because the census of pregnant clients cared for annually in the referral center would support development of the service.

Other institutions may have an obstetric service established to provide care during the low risk pregnancy or have such a small census of pregnant clients per year that the numbers do not financially support development of such an OBICU in the obstetric suite. The plan for the smaller unit or the low risk unit may be for the nursing and medical team to immediately recognize the critical illness, stabilize the woman, and initiate measures for transport to the tertiary center and OBICU. The level II, or intermediate, institution caring for a moderate number of pregnant women annually may have a plan for the obstetric team that includes immediate recognition of the critical illness, stabilization of the pregnant woman, preparation for transport to the adult or trauma intensive care unit, and assisting the intensive care unit or trauma staff after transport by providing continuous fetal monitoring and obstetric consultation. In some intermediate settings the intensive care team may bring their skills and techniques to the labor and birth unit. The institution must develop policies and procedures so that care is provided where it is most advantageous to the pregnant woman.

Standards and Guidelines for Professional Nursing Practice in the Care of Women and Newborns (Association of Women's Health, Obstetric, and Neonatal Nurses [AWHONN], 1998) includes guidelines on the care of the pregnant woman requiring critical care.

LEGAL TIP **Nursing Assignments**

Continuous assignment of an obstetric and an intensive care nurse, or one nurse experienced in both specialities, is required in the care of the critically ill woman with a viable pregnancy.

LEGAL TIP **Client Care Standards**

Client care standards established for both obstetric care and intensive care must be met within the plan developed by an institution to provide complex, critical care for the critically ill pregnant woman. Standards of care from both specialties must be followed.

Obstetric clients requiring critical care are at increased risk for undesirable outcomes of the pregnancy because of the severity of complications, including decreased oxygen transport and multiple system organ failure and the possibility of long-term residual physical effects of the illness (Hankins & Harvey, 1993). It is important that the medical and nursing care administered to this woman and her fetus or neonate meet the standards for care established for obstetrics and critical care.

LEGAL TIP **Legal Review**

Because an optimal outcome is uncertain when the pregnant woman is critically ill, the medical records, with documentation of the medical and nursing care that mother, fetus, and neonate received, are more likely to be subjected to legal review than are medical records of other clients.

EQUIPMENT AND EXPERTISE

Appropriate care of the critically ill pregnant woman and her fetus depends on the availability of adequate, appropriate equipment and the presence of individuals educated in their use. The usual equipment for a labor, delivery, and recovery suite is mandatory for an intensive care unit or surgical suite where this client may be placed for care. Staff and equipment for neonatal resuscitation must also be available. Likewise, the usual equipment for intensive care, including hemodynamic monitoring and mechanical ventilation, is equally necessary whenever the critically ill client is in the labor and birth unit.

Obstetric critical care may be delivered according to individual plans developed by individual institutions on the basis of a needs assessment. However, it is imperative that all institutions providing care for pregnant women have a plan and staff educated to care for the occasional woman who has a life-threatening complication during pregnancy. Pregnant women with a critical complication must receive the care needed; critical care must not be denied to pregnant women. Pregnancy is not a contraindication for invasive hemodynamic monitoring.

INDICATIONS FOR OBSTETRIC CRITICAL CARE

A severe complication of pregnancy may prompt the need for obstetric critical care with hemodynamic monitoring or mechanical ventilation. See Box 34-1 for a list of complications that indicate a need for critical care.

The number of pregnant women who need obstetric critical care has increased in recent years. This apparently is the result of women surviving childhood illnesses because of advances in pediatric care. These include the development of pediatric intensive care units; improved surgical procedures for infants with congenital defects, such

---

█ BOX 34-1 **Complications of Pregnancy That Indicate the Need for Critical Care**

1. Severe preeclampsia-eclampsia with complications
   a. Refractory pulmonary edema
   b. Refractory oliguria
   c. Hypertensive crisis
   d. Severe hemorrhage or disseminated intravascular coagulation (DIC)
   e. Renal failure
2. Hemorrhage or DIC that requires multiple transfusions
3. Cardiac problems
4. Chronic health problems
   a. Systemic lupus erythematosus
   b. Diabetic ketoacidosis
   c. Sickle cell disease
   d. Diabetes complicated by vascular changes
   e. Others
5. Trauma victim
   a. Motor vehicle crash
   b. Violence, battering

as cardiac lesions; and advanced knowledge in pediatric care for children with chronic health problems, including diabetes, cystic fibrosis, and pulmonary disorders. The wish to become a parent is not eliminated by a chronic health problem, and many women each year risk their lives to have a baby (Harvey, 1994). Women have had successful pregnancies after kidney transplants (Maurer & Abriola, 1994), after heart transplants (Jordan & Pugh, 1996), and after liver transplants (Laifer et al., 1990). More pregnant women with chronic health problems are predicted as graduates of neonatal intensive care units reach adulthood.

Other pregnant women need critical care because of trauma resulting from automobile crashes or violence and battering. These causes account for most of the traumatic injuries during pregnancy.

The most common diagnosis for admission to an OBICU is severe pregnancy-induced hypertension (PIH) with complications, including refractory pulmonary edema, refractory oliguria, hypertensive crisis, severe hemorrhage or disseminated intravascular coagulation (DIC), and renal failure. Massive hemorrhage or DIC is reported as the second most common reason for admission (Austin et al., 1994). OBICUs are often small and may consist of one bed. Admissions may be limited only to the very sickest women and may not include all women eligible for a bed in the OBICU.

Conditions that classify the parturient as critically ill and indicate the need for a pulmonary artery catheter include the following (American College of Obstetricians and Gynecologists [ACOG], 1992):

- Sepsis with refractory hypotension or oliguria
- Unexplained or refractory pulmonary edema, congestive heart failure, or oliguria
- Severe PIH with pulmonary edema or refractory oliguria
- Intraoperative or intrapartum cardiovascular decompensation
- Massive blood loss or volume replacement needs
- Adult respiratory distress syndrome
- Shock of undefined source
- Chronic disease, particularly when associated with labor or major surgery

The identification of women needing OBICU services merits careful consideration. It is important not to visualize just the "sickest client scenario"—that dramatic case, never to be forgotten. Instead, the typical picture of a critically ill pregnant woman is one with severe preeclampsia, whose condition has worsened and today has headache, high blood pressure, oliguria, and low platelets. Or the woman may be sent in for referral from the level I center with a preexisting cardiac lesion exacerbated by pregnancy and that has gradually deteriorated from class I to class III cardiac disease. Her presenting complaint may be "feeling extremely tired."

Approximately 0.9% to 1% of pregnant women giving birth in an institution require care in an OBICU. The percentage and numbers of pregnant women needing care in an OBICU are higher in an institution that receives referrals from a large area. As the number of high risk pregnant women served in an institution increases, the number of women likely to become critically ill also increases. It is also interesting to note that more seriously ill pregnant women receive immediate critical care when an institution has an OBICU than when the pregnant woman must be transported to a medical-surgical intensive care unit to receive care (Kilpatrick & Matthay, 1992; Mabie & Sibai, 1990).

CARDIORESPIRATORY CHANGES OF PREGNANCY

The normal physiologic adaptations that accompany pregnancy and produce profound hemodynamic changes are the primary factors that make the pregnant woman a different type of critical care client and merit a separate critical care facility. Knowledge of the effects of the physiologic alterations during pregnancy is essential for optimum critical care management. Normal maternal alterations during pregnancy affect the major systems: the cardiovascular, pulmonary, renal, and hematologic systems (Harvey, 1999; Harvey & Moretti, 1993).

Cardiovascular Changes

The cardiovascular system changes dramatically during pregnancy. Pregnancy is a state of high flow, low resistance so that pregnancy is hemodynamically similar to early sepsis. Hypervolemia is the result of the influence of estrogen and progesterone on aldosterone, which produces an increase in circulating blood volume. The increase in maternal blood volume begins with a 22% increase by 8 weeks of gestation. Total expansion increases progressively to a maximum of 45% by 32 to 34 weeks of gestation. This represents an increase of approximately 1570 ml for the singleton gestation. This includes a 40% to 50% increase in plasma volume and a 20% to 30% increase in red blood cell mass, a disproportional increase that results in a state of hemodilution. An increase in total body water of 6 to 8 L in the extravascular compartment, accompanied by an accumulation of 500 to 900 mEq of sodium, also occurs during pregnancy. Heart rate increases 20% (10 to 15 beats/min) with the major increase in the third trimester, and stroke volume increases to accommodate the increased circulating volume. See Table 34-1 for a summary of cardiovascular adaptations.

Colloid Osmotic Pressure

Colloid osmotic pressure (COP) is the gradient controlling whether fluid remains inside the capillary or moves into the interstitial space. The force to keep the fluid inside the vessel is the pulling pressure of the colloids, or proteins, present in the plasma. The most important plasma proteins are albumin, globulin, and fibrinogen. Pregnancy

TABLE 34-1 Cardiovascular Changes During Pregnancy

PARAMETER	CHANGE
Blood volume	40%-50% increase
Plasma volume	45%-50% increase (1200-1300 ml)
Red blood cell mass	20%-30% increase (250-450 ml)
Heart	Displaced to left and upward
PMI	Fourth intercostal space and lateral
Rate	20% increase (10-15 beats/min)
Sounds	Exaggerated splitting first sound
	Systolic murmur usually present
	Third sound present
Stroke volume	32% increase by 20-24 weeks
Cardiac output	Increases 30%-50%
	22% increase by 28 weeks
	43% increase by term
	Increases during labor
	≤3 cm, 17% increase
	4-7 cm, 23% increase
	≥8 cm, 34% increase

Source: Harvey, M. (1999). Physiologic changes during pregnancy. In L. Mandeville & N. Troiano (Eds.). *AWHONN's high risk and critical care intrapartum nursing* (2nd ed.). Philadelphia: J.B. Lippincott.

TABLE 34-2 Colloid Osmotic (Oncotic) Pressure Values

Nonpregnant	25.4 ± 2.3 mm Hg
Pregnant, antepartum	22.4 ± 0.54 mm Hg
Pregnant, postpartum	15.4 ± 2.1 mm Hg
PIH, antepartum	17.9 ± 0.68 mm Hg
PIH, postpartum	13.7 ± 0.46 mm Hg

TABLE 34-3 Arterial Blood Gas (ABG) Values

ABGS	NONPREGNANT	PREGNANT
pH	7.35-7.45	7.40-7.45
PO_2 (mm Hg)	80-100	104-108
PCO_2 (mm Hg)	35-42	27-32
Bicarbonate (HCO_3) (mEq/L)	26	18-31

produces a decrease in COP values resulting from the hemodilution state that reduces the concentration of plasma proteins. Severe preeclampsia-eclampsia (PIH) usually produces renal damage, with a subsequent loss of proteins in the urine, further reducing the COP. The force exerted to push fluids through the membrane is the **capillary hydrostatic pressure** and is measured as the **pulmonary capillary wedge pressure** (PCWP). COP is measured with an oncometer. Colloid osmotic (oncotic) values in pregnancy are shown in Table 34-2.

The lower the COP and the higher the PCWP, the more likely pulmonary edema is to develop, as reflected by a lower COP-PCWP gradient. COP-PCWP gradient values are as follows:

Nonpregnant: 14.5 ± 2.5

Pregnancy: 10.5 ± 2.7

Pulmonary edema is more likely to develop in pregnancy. For example, the normal PCWP is 6 to 10 mm Hg during pregnancy and 4 to 9 mm Hg in the nonpregnant state (Clark et al., 1989). With a PCWP of 8, calculations of the COP-PCWP gradient show

Nonpregnant: COP of 25 − PCWP of 8 = 17 mm Hg

Pregnant woman with severe preeclampsia:

COP of 13 − PCWP of 8 = 5 mm Hg

Lower COP-PCWP gradients during pregnancy are usually caused by lower COP values occurring during pregnancy.

Respiratory Changes

Anatomic and physiologic alterations during pregnancy are necessary to supply adequate oxygenation to mother and fetus. A relative hyperventilation of pregnancy begins in the first trimester and increases 42% by term. Respiratory rate increases only slightly. Tidal volume and minute ventilations increase about 50% by term to meet increased oxygen consumption needs. The enlarging uterus pushes the diaphragm upward approximately 4 to 7 cm, reducing lung volume. Compensation is necessary to meet increased ventilatory demands, and the transverse diameter of the thorax increases 2 to 4 cm as the rib cage flares out. The functional residual capacity decreases 25% as more of the inhaled air is used. The hyperventilation of pregnancy is associated with a resting arterial carbon dioxide tension below 30 mm Hg. Maternal alkalosis is prevented by the compensatory decrease in serum bicarbonate of about 4 mEq/L, from 26 to 22 mEq. During gestation respiratory acidosis and metabolic acidosis develop more rapidly than in the nonpregnant state.

Normal arterial blood gas values for pregnancy reflect a chronic state of compensated respiratory alkalosis, represented by a right shift in the oxyhemoglobin dissociation curve caused by the increased levels of 2,3-diphosphoglycerate from the high progesterone and estrogen levels present. Normal pregnancy values in comparison with the nonpregnant state are listed in Table 34-3.

Hematologic Changes

Pregnancy is a hypercoagulable state, as preparation is made for blood loss that accompanies childbirth. Table 34-4 gives a summary of alterations that enhance coagulation.

Bleeding and clotting times remain unchanged even when hypervolemia and hemodilution are present. The critically ill pregnant woman is at increased risk for throm-

TABLE 34-4	**Gestational Changes That Enhance Coagulation**
Fibrinogen	Increased 30%-50% (from 300 to 480 mg/dl)
Coagulation factors VII-X	Increased
Fibrinolysis	Depressed

bus formation whenever hemoconcentration develops, as occurs with preeclampsia-eclampsia or dehydration.

Systemic Vascular Resistance

Systemic vascular resistance (SVR) is a measure of the tension required for the ejection of blood into the circulation (afterload). To describe the physiologic relationships between pressure and flow, measurements are made by the following formula as a ratio of pressure to flow:

$$SVR = [(MAP - CVP)/CO] \times 80$$

where MAP is mean arterial pressure (in millimeters of mercury), CVP is central venous pressure (in millimeters of mercury), and CO is cardiac output (in liters per minute).

Vasodilation of arterial vessels, a result of hormonal influences, and development of the uteroplacental circulation result in a decrease in SVR of 20% to 25% and a decrease in pulmonary vascular resistance of 40% during pregnancy. Systolic and diastolic blood pressures decrease during pregnancy, reaching the nadir at midtrimester, with a gradual return to prepregnancy values by term.

HEMODYNAMIC MONITORING

Anatomic and Physiologic Characteristics of Circulation

An in-depth knowledge of normal functioning and hemodynamics of the cardiovascular system is the basis for understanding hemodynamic monitoring; therefore a review of these functions is included. The purpose of the cardiopulmonary system is to deliver oxygenated blood to the tissues throughout the body and to remove waste products through the dynamics of normal circulation as follows (Fig. 34-1).

Deoxygenated blood flows from the capillaries into the veins and the right side of the heart through the superior vena cava, draining the upper part of the body, and from the inferior vena cava, draining the lower part of the body. Venous blood flows into the right atrium, a holding chamber for the right side of the heart. When the atrium is filled, the tricuspid valve opens and blood flows through this valve into the right ventricle.

When the right ventricle is filled, its muscles (myocardium) contract, and blood is ejected through the pulmonic valve into the pulmonary artery. Blood is pushed through the pulmonary artery through its branches to the capillary beds (pulmonary beds) in both lungs. Gas ex-

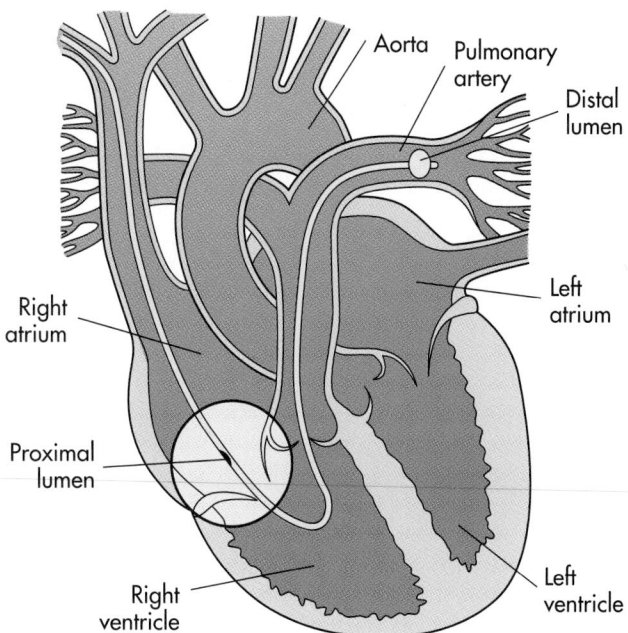

Fig. 34-1   Diagram of heart with position of pulmonary artery catheter.

change occurs in the capillary beds as carbon dioxide is released and oxygen enters the circulation across the alveolar membrane.

Oxygenated blood drains from the pulmonary beds into the pulmonary veins, two from each lung, into the left atrium, the holding chamber for the left side of the heart. When the left atrium is filled, the mitral valve opens and blood flows through this valve into the left ventricle. After the left ventricle is filled, the muscles of the left ventricle contract and the oxygenated blood is ejected through the aortic valve into the aorta and then pumped throughout the systemic arterial system so that oxygen is supplied to the organs and tissues of the body.

Synchronization by the electrical conduction system of the myocardium causes the right and left atrial and ventricular contractions to occur simultaneously. The period of the cardiac cycle when both ventricles are relaxed and filling is termed *diastole*, and the period of the cardiac cycle when both ventricles contract is termed *systole*.

Left ventricle contractions must generate enough force to pump blood throughout the systemic circulation. Force required for right ventricular work is less because the right ventricle has to exert only enough force for blood to flow through the pulmonary circulation. Therefore the left ventricle is referred to as the *hemodynamic ventricle* and the left side of the heart is referred to as the *hemodynamic heart*. Hemodynamic monitoring with a PAC provides left heart values, and during a critical illness values of left heart function are more significant than values of right heart function.

Cardiac Output

Cardiac output (CO) is the volume of blood ejected from the left ventricle in 1 minute; it is measured in liters per

TABLE 34-5	Effect of Maternal Position on Cardiac Output
Knee chest	6.9 (±2.1)
Right lateral	6.8 (±1.3)
Left lateral	6.6 (±1.4)
Sitting	6.2 (±2.0)
Supine	6.0 (±1.4)
Standing	5.4 (±2.0)

minute. CO is the product of **stroke volume** (SV), the volume of blood ejected from the left ventricle during one cardiac cycle, and heart rate (HR) (CO = HR × SV). Because HR and SV increase during pregnancy, CO increases. The normal prepregnancy range of CO is 3 to 5 L per minute. CO increases 40% to 50% during pregnancy, to produce a normal CO in the last trimester of 6 to 7 L per minute at rest. Labor produces an additional 40% increase in CO because of catecholamine release in response to pain perception and the shunting of blood from the placental-fetal unit with uterine contractions, for a CO range during labor of 8 to 10 L per minute. CO increases further after birth because of significant hemodynamic fluctuations that reflect the net effect of blood loss at birth and the autotransfusion with approximately 1000 ml of blood that occurs after the uterus is emptied. Soon after birth the accumulated 6 to 8 L of extravascular fluid is mobilized into the intravascular compartment. The large increase in CO remains for 7 to 10 days after birth in the healthy woman but will continue longer if usual diuresis fails to occur because of a complication.

Positional Changes

Maternal CO in the last trimester is position dependent. Clark and co-workers (1991b) showed the effect of maternal position on CO output (Table 34-5).

The right lateral recumbent or the left lateral recumbent position provides optimum CO for the critically ill pregnant woman. Any time maternal CO is decreased, compensatory mechanisms are initiated. The first compensatory response is to shunt blood away from the peripheral circulation to the central circulation, to save the heart and brain. Peripheral circulation includes circulation to the skin, renal system, gastrointestinal system, lung beds, and reproductive system. Enhancing maternal CO enhances fetal perfusion.

NURSE ALERT *During the last trimester CO drops so significantly when the woman is supine that a hip wedge under one hip or manual displacement of the uterus to one side is necessary to prevent a sudden decrease in CO and a subsequent decrease in fetal perfusion.*

Cardiac Output Determinants

The four determinants of cardiac output are reflected in the calculation for cardiac output (CO = HR × SV) because SV is the result of preload, afterload, and contractility.

Preload is defined as the volume of blood in the ventricles at the end of diastole; preload is determined by intraventricular pressure and volume. Right preload is assessed by right atrial or central venous pressure, and left preload is assessed by pulmonary capillary wedge pressure. The volume of blood in the ventricles stretches the myocardial muscle fibers and produces the intraventricular pressure. Measurements are made at end-diastole, the time immediately preceding systole when the ventricles reach maximum stretch because of the extra amount of blood delivered into the ventricles when the tricuspid and mitral valves snap closed.

Right preload reflects the blood circulating through the right side of the heart, and left preload reflects the amount of blood circulating in the left side of the heart. The two sides of the heart are not equal when cardiac or pulmonary complications are present; therefore they are measured separately.

Preload must be adequate to maintain CO, and plotting of CO against preload gives a cardiac function curve (Fig. 34-2). As preload increases, CO increases up to the point of failure. The cardiac function curve shows that a heart in failure will require a higher preload than the healthy heart to produce the same CO. Bedside manipulations of preload are possible with continuous hemodynamic monitoring to determine effects on CO. A low preload can be increased by the administration of fluids, including crystalloid, colloid, or blood, and by positioning with legs elevated. A high preload can be decreased by the administration of a vasodilator or diuretic or by phlebotomy and positioning in an upright position.

Afterload is defined as the ventricular wall tension during systole, or the resistance the blood meets as blood is ejected from the ventricles. Afterload is dependent on the end-diastolic radius of the ventricle, the aortic pressure, and the thickness of the ventricle wall. As afterload increases, CO decreases, and bedside manipulation of afterload is possible to achieve optimum cardiac output (Fig. 34-3). Right afterload is assessed by the **pulmonary vascular resistance** (PVR), and left afterload is assessed by the SVR. Arterial blood pressure measurement does not give as accurate an indication of left ventricular work as the SVR but is used clinically as reflecting left afterload. The formula to calculate blood pressure (BP) is BP = CO × SVR. Therefore control of the client's blood pressure is used to control left afterload.

Afterload must be adequate for circulation and CO; extremes of afterload may decrease CO. Increased left afterload occurs with hypertensive disease caused by the systemic arterial vasoconstriction. Increased right afterload occurs with pulmonary hypertension resulting from vasoconstriction in the pulmonary circulation.

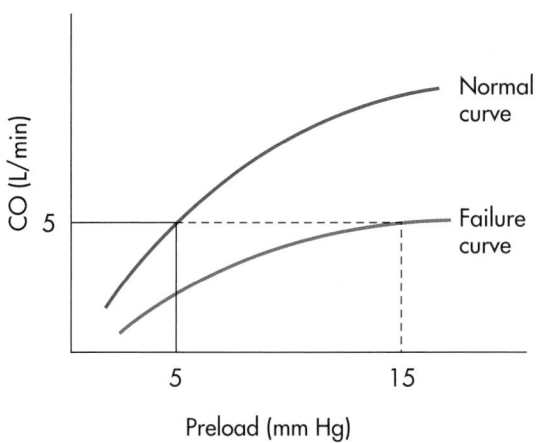

Fig. 34-2 Relation of preload to CO. Ventricular function (Starling) curve for heart showing both normal function and during failure.

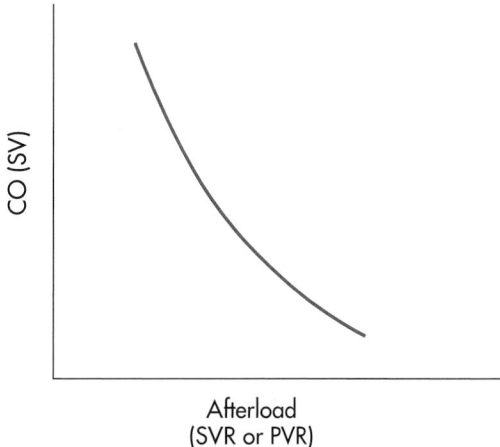

Fig. 34-3 Relation of afterload to CO when preload is maintained constant. As afterload increases, cardiac output decreases.

Increased afterload can be corrected by the administration of vasodilator drugs. Hydralazine is an arterial vasodilator that is used most commonly in intermittent intravenous doses for obstetric clients. The administration of hydralazine has proved safe for mother and fetus (Hankins & Harvey, 1993) and is the first-line drug of choice for hypertensive crisis during pregnancy. Sodium nitroprusside has the potential to produce such immediate changes in SVR that continuous intraarterial blood pressure monitoring is required. Sodium nitroprusside produces cyanide as a metabolite; fetal cyanide toxicity must be a concern if this drug is administered during pregnancy.

NURSE ALERT *The continuous intravenous infusion of sodium nitroprusside is the vasodilator drug used most commonly in the adult intensive care setting, but it is saved for emergency use for pregnant women.*

Severe vasodilation and loss of arterial resistance with a decreased afterload impedes venous return of blood to the right side of the heart and decreases CO. This situation is seen with septic shock. Decreased afterload can be corrected by fluid administration to fill the vascular space or by the administration of alpha-adrenergic drugs such as phenylephrine (Mandeville & Troiano, 1999).

Contractility (inotropic state of the heart) is defined as the force and velocity of ventricular contractions when preload and afterload are held constant. Contractility is governed by the Frank-Starling law, which states that the greater the length of the muscle fibers before contraction, the greater will be the contraction of the fibers, up to the point of failure. Fiber length is related to the maximum stretch of preload, because as more blood volume enters the ventricles the more the fibers in the myocardium stretch to accommodate the increased volume.

Decreased contractility results in decreased CO. The first response to correct this problem is bedside manipulation to optimize both preload and afterload. If this fails to increase CO to the desired level, medications to increase myocardial contractility are indicated. Inotropic drugs such as dopamine hydrochloride or dobutamine are administered. Digitalis therapy may also be necessary.

Heart rate is the fourth determinant of cardiac output. The rate at which the ventricles fill and contract affects CO. Extremes of heart rate may decrease CO.

Sustained tachycardia can decrease CO as a result of myocardial ischemia or the decreased time for adequate filling of the ventricles during diastole and shortened systolic ejection times. The cause, such as fever, hypoxia, pain, hypovolemia, or hyperthyroidism, should be determined and treated. Drugs to correct tachycardia are seldom necessary for obstetric clients. However, propranolol, digoxin, or calcium-channel blockers such as verapamil are effective agents to decrease heart rate if needed.

Bradycardia can compromise CO when there is an inadequate number of ventricular contractions per minute to deliver the circulating volume needed to perfuse and oxygenate the body. If treatment is necessary for this problem, atropine or cardiac pacing is used.

Invasive Hemodynamic Monitoring

Invasive hemodynamic monitoring provides continuous measurements of preload, afterload, myocardial contractility, and heart rate in the critically ill pregnant woman so that therapeutic manipulations may be made quickly at the bedside in response to changes in client status. Monitoring may be done by use of a **pulmonary artery catheter** (PAC) (a balloon-tipped, multilumen catheter) or by central venous pressure (CVP).

Although there is a lack of adequate clinical studies at this time to demonstrate the benefit of pulmonary artery catheterization for the critically ill client, most critical care bedside clinicians use the PAC to direct their therapy modalities and believe that use of the PAC does improve outcomes in selected critically ill clients (Troiano, 1999). Conners and associates (1996) reported no benefit to right heart catheterization in the initial care of critically ill clients, and they even questioned whether the Food and Drug Administration should stop its use. The Society of Critical Care Medicine quickly held a consensus development conference and issued a consensus statement regarding the use of the PAC in critical care environments (Society of Critical Care Medicine, 1997). The consensus statement then issued reiterated that, as with all other technology, the clinical usefulness of the PAC is dependent on correct interpretation of the data by clinicians. With respect to pregnancy, the ACOG guidelines (1992) for invasive hemodynamic monitoring were referenced. The statement also included a recommendation for additional research.

Use of a PAC allows the management of care to be based on immediate recognition of changes in hemodynamic values from the left ventricle. Immediate information is obtained, calculations are made, and management is adjusted quickly as needed. Results of therapeutic strategies can be calculated and evaluated (ACOG, 1992). The continuous hemodynamic measurements obtained will reinforce therapies in use or show that therapy should be changed. Use of a PAC or Swan-Ganz catheter in combination with an arterial pressure catheter and a pulse oximeter provides adequate data to continuously assess cardiac, fluid, and pulmonary status of the client. Indications for the use of invasive hemodynamic monitoring are the same in obstetrics as in any other area of medicine.

It is essential to evaluate risks and benefits of any procedure before use, especially because there are associated risks with invasive techniques. The information obtained from hemodynamic monitoring is essential for management of critical, complex cases and is unavailable by other means; thus the benefits outweigh the risks in most cases.

The overall complication rate in the obstetric population is low, approximately 1%. This low rate of complications is related to three factors: (1) the pregnant woman usually needs the device because of an acute event, (2) the duration of use is usually short, and (3) the majority of pregnant women requiring its use were young and healthy before the acute event.

It is essential that meticulous attention be paid to each step and detail of all procedures to decrease problems with the technique itself. Thorough, detailed care by the knowledgeable and skilled physician and nurse can decrease the risks associated with invasive hemodynamic monitoring and make the procedures much safer for the pregnant woman (Baumgartner, 1991).

Pulmonary Artery Catheter

A pulmonary artery catheter, commonly called the Swan-Ganz catheter, provides continuous measurements of **pulmonary artery pressure** (PAP) and right atrial pressure (RAP) or CVP. Intermittent measurements of PCWP and CO are also possible. The standard flow-directed thermodilution PAC has three lumina and a thermistor connector (Fig. 34-4). The distal lumen or port is located in the pulmonary artery after insertion. It is connected to a transducer with a heparinized pressure line to measure a continuous PAP when the balloon is deflated and intermittent PCWP when the balloon is inflated. A continuous flush of 3 ml per hour of heparinized solution maintains patency of the lumen.

The proximal lumen or port exits approximately 30 cm from the tip of the catheter and is located in the right atrium after insertion. This port is also connected to a transducer with a heparinized line and it can be used to measure continuous RAP, which is comparable to the CVP, or to administer fluid or drugs. Both the proximal and distal lumina of the catheter can be used to withdraw blood samples for laboratory studies.

The balloon lumen ends in a small latex balloon, located 0.5 inch from the tip of the PAC. Inflation of the balloon is used to assist in the insertion of the catheter and to obtain PCWP readings.

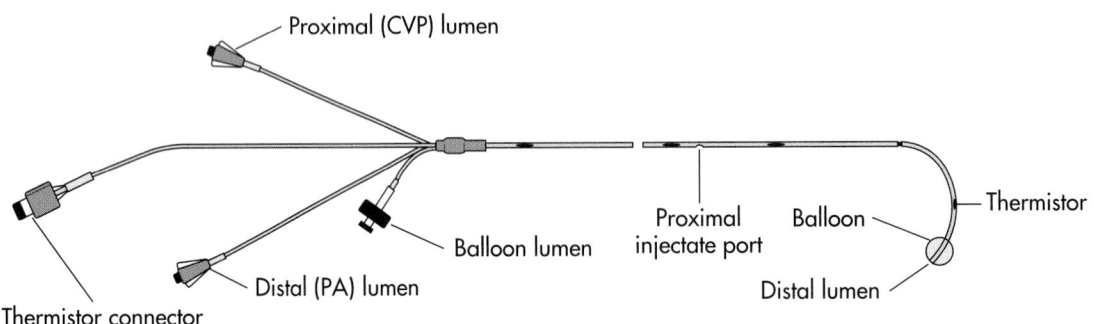

Fig. 34-4 Standard triple-lumen flow-directed pulmonary artery catheter.

The thermodilution port is connected to a thermistor, a temperature sensor, located 5 cm proximal to the tip of the PAC. The thermistor continuously measures the temperature of the blood in the pulmonary artery.

Other types of PACs are available in addition to the standard PAC. Some have an extra right atrial port for intracardiac infusions. The small size of the ports make them more effective for the administration of vasopressors or drugs such as antibiotics, rather than for the use of rapid administration of large volumes of blood or fluids. A fiberoptic PAC includes a sensor to measure the hemoglobin saturation of mixed venous blood, the SvO_2, in the pulmonary artery continuously and is useful in cases of decreased oxygen transport, such as with preeclampsia-eclampsia (Hankins & Harvey, 1993). Another type for selected cases is modified PAC with a heated filament to provide continuous CO values (Boldt et al., 1994).

Venous Access

The internal or external jugular vein or the subclavian vein is most commonly used for venous access for invasive hemodynamic monitoring during pregnancy. Access with femoral or antecubital veins is not used as frequently for pregnant women because of the greater difficulty in positioning the catheter when this route is accessed. Furthermore, with use of a vein in the inguinal area, birth of the infant at a critical time can limit access to and manipulation of the catheter. However, with certain disorders, such as a coagulopathy, antecubital access may be preferred to decrease the possibility of intrathoracic bleeding (Hankins & Harvey, 1993).

The flow-directed PAC is usually inserted at the bedside after preparations are complete. Meticulous attention to detail is critical when the equipment is prepared. Flushing the pressure tubing to eliminate any air, establishing a zero reference point, and both zeroing and calibrating the pressure transducer are done carefully before insertion. The Procedure box explains how to set up a pressure line and how to zero-reference and calibrate a pressure transducer. Box 34-2 describes nursing care during insertion and continuing care for a PAC.

Hemodynamic monitoring systems have three major components: (1) a pressure transducer that converts physiologic pressures into electrical energy, (2) an amplifier to magnify the volume of the signal being measured, and (3) a monitor screen to display in digital and graphic form the converted physiologic signal (Fig. 34-5).

Waveforms and Pressure Readings

The basis of interpretation of assessments obtained by hemodynamic monitoring is to understand the relationship of the waveforms observed on the monitor screen and the pressure readings obtained to cardiovascular status.

Specific chambers in the heart have different pressures that are reflected by changing waveform patterns, and

---

PROCEDURE

How to Set Up, Calibrate, and Zero-Reference Pressure Lines

1. Connect pressure tubing to sterile disposable pressure transducer.
2. Check all connections for a tight fit to prevent leakage.
3. Heparinize flush solution of normal saline solution. Heparin is necessary for the pregnant client to prevent thrombus formation.
4. Connect the pressure tubing to the intravenous bag of heparinized solution.
5. Gently flush both pressure tubing and transducer to remove all air. Cap stopcocks with nonvented covers.
6. Connect transducer to hemodynamic monitor.
7. Place a pressure bag on the heparinized solution. Inflate to 300 mm Hg of pressure. (This allows a continuous rate of 3 ml/hr of heparinized solution to flow as a flush solution.) The heparinized solution and continuous flow of fluid prevent clot formation on the tip of the catheter.
8. Calibrate the pressure transducer by zeroing the line.
9. Zero-reference the transducer by positioning the woman supine with a hip wedge under the right hip, locating the phlebostatic axis at the fourth intercostal space at the midaxillary line, and marking on the chest wall.
10. Open stopcock to air. Push zero button on the monitor to identify zero. The transducer negates atmospheric pressure and establishes a baseline for subsequent readings. Close the stopcock to air.

NOTE: The phlebostatic axis is the physiologic reference point used when measuring pulmonary and arterial line pressures (see Fig. 34-7 for an illustration of this procedure).

---

placement of the PAC is evaluated through the pressure and waveform changes that appear on the monitor screen to reflect the position of the catheter. Figure 34-6 displays pressure waveforms in different chambers of the heart.

Because the right atrium is a holding chamber with relatively small muscle mass, the waveform pattern for this chamber has a low amplitude. Right atrium pressures reflect intravascular volume and compliance of the right ventricle. Mean right atrium pressures in pregnancy are relatively low, 0 to 7 mm Hg.

When the catheter flows into the right ventricle, pressures change and a distinct spiking waveform appears. The low-amplitude waveform of the right atrium converts to a high-amplitude waveform with distinct systolic and diastolic components in the right ventricle with a baseline

BOX 34-2 Pulmonary Artery Catheter Protocol

SETUP

- Prepare two pressure lines for the distal and proximal ports as described in the Procedure box on how to set up, calibrate, and zero-reference pressure lines.
- Connect an intravenous line of normal saline solution, per infusion pump, to the introducer.
- Check PAC balloon for symmetric inflation, absence of air leak, and ease of spontaneous deflation.

CLIENT PREPARATION FOR INSERTION

- Assess client's knowledge level and explain procedure to ensure her understanding, cooperation, and acceptance of the procedure.
- Confirm that informed consent form is signed and attached to chart.
- Provide support and encouragement throughout the procedure.
- Initiate electrocardiographic (ECG) monitoring. Obtain baseline ECG pattern.

NURSING MANAGEMENT DURING INSERTION

- Monitor ECG continuously as catheter passes through right ventricle to recognize any ventricular ectopy present.
- Use a slight Trendelenburg position with a hip wedge. This position engorges the neck veins and facilitates placement of the catheter. When the internal jugular approach is used, tilt head to the side away from the site of cannulation.
- Be available to provide assistance to the operator throughout the procedure.
- Adjust intravenous line connected to the introducer to maintain patency.
- Observe waveform patterns on the monitor screen and record pressures as the catheter advances through the chambers in the heart.
- Have lidocaine hydrochloride available for arrhythmias.
- Ensure balloon is deflated. Deflate balloon passively.
- Anticipate orders for chest x-ray film to verify catheter placement.
- Apply dressing after physician secures introducer.
- Observe monitor screen for continuous tracing of pulmonary artery pressures.

NURSING ASSESSMENTS

- Verify that alarms are set at all times.
- Observe monitor screen closely for pressures and waveforms that denote placement of catheter. Be prepared to intervene when necessary (see Box 34-3).

- Record hemodynamic parameters according to client status and unit care protocols. Follow the procedure for obtaining a pulmonary capillary wedge pressure reading (see Procedure box).
- Inspect all connection sites every 2 hours and entire monitor system for presence of air or blood clots.
- Examine insertion site frequently for bleeding or signs of infection. Perform site care every shift or daily, as indicated by unit infection control policy.
- Change pressure and intravenous lines every 24 to 48 hours, as indicated by unit infection control policy.
- Monitor heparinized pressure flush for continuous correct pressure (300 mm Hg).
- Rezero and calibrate transducer every shift and as necessary.

NURSING MANAGEMENT FOR CATHETER REMOVAL

- Document vital signs and ECG pattern.
- Monitor for ECG arrhythmias during removal.
- After catheter removal, pressure to site must be applied for 5 minutes or more. Anticipate that physician may request application of pressure. Ensure that bleeding has stopped completely before pressure is removed.
- Apply pressure dressing to site, per unit protocol. Keep pressure dressing in place for 8 hours.

DOCUMENTATION

- Presence of signed informed consent form on chart.
- Date, time, site of insertion, type of introducer, and name of operator who performed procedure.
- Type of pulmonary catheter, number of attempts, confirmation of placement by x-ray studies, and any ventricular ectopy.
- Client's tolerance of procedure.
- Zeroing and calibration of transducers and verification of alarm settings.
- Hemodynamic parameters obtained according to client status.
- Pertinent nursing assessments and medical and nursing care.
- Site assessments and care.
- Changes of pressure and intravenous lines.
- Date and time of removal of intact catheter, date and removal of introducer.
- Nursing care and assessments after catheter removal.

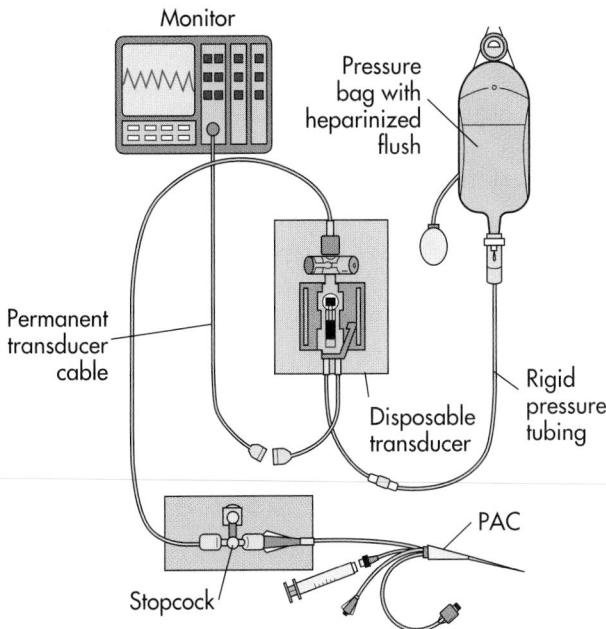

Fig. 34-5 Components of hemodynamic monitoring system: pressurized tubing, pressure transducer, and hemodynamic monitor.

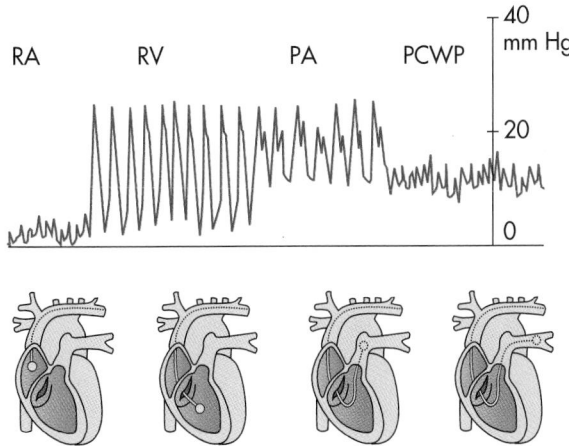

Fig. 34-6 Pressure waveforms in relation to catheter position from right atrium *(RA)*, to right ventricle *(RV)*, to pulmonary artery *(PA)*, to pulmonary capillary wedge pressure *(PCWP)*.

pressure of 0 mm Hg. Right ventricular pressures are measured as systolic and diastolic. Normal right ventricle systolic pressure is 18 to 30 mm Hg and the normal diastolic pressure is 0 to 7 mm Hg.

The catheter is then advanced into the pulmonary artery. This is reflected by a different spiking waveform with baseline pressures above 0 mm Hg. Pulmonary artery systolic pressures are equal to the systolic pressures in the

right ventricle, but pulmonary artery diastolic pressures abruptly increase to the range of 6 to 10 mm Hg.

The catheter advances through the pulmonary artery as far as possible and becomes "wedged" in the vessel. This wedging is reflected by a distinct waveform of a dampened tracing with respiratory variation. This relatively low amplitude reflects the low pressures in the capillary beds of the lungs.

The PCWP is obtained when the balloon is inflated, with all pressures from the right side of the heart obstructed, so that the distal port now reads pressures from the left side of the heart across the lungs, because there are no valves in the pulmonary circulation. The PCWP measures left atrial filling pressures or left-sided preload. During right ventricular diastole, the pulmonic valve is closed, with the mitral valve open; the diastolic PAP is measured. In the absence of a problem, such as mitral valve disease or pulmonary edema, PAP diastolic readings reflect PCWP or left ventricular preload. The diastolic PAP is therefore used clinically to reflect left preload (Lipp-Ziff & Kawanishi, 1991). See the Procedure box for obtaining a PCWP reading.

The normal PCWP during pregnancy is 6 to 10 mm Hg. Pressures higher than 20 mm Hg are usually caused by abnormal left ventricular performance, such as left ventricular failure, mitral valve stenosis, or fluid volume overload. Lower-than-normal readings are seen usually with hypovolemia (Fig. 34-7).

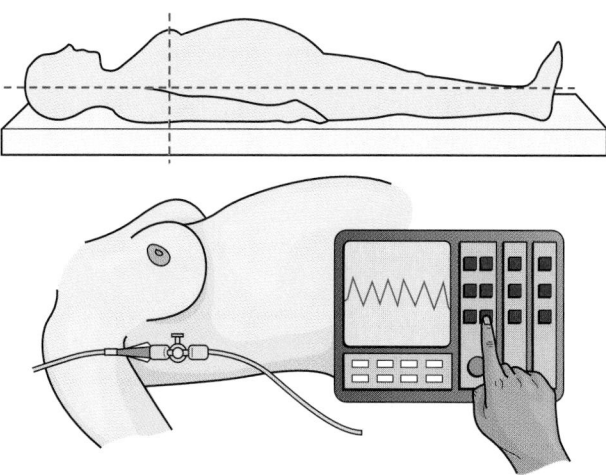

Fig. 34-7 Location of phlebostatic axis and zeroing.

Box 34-3 describes nursing measures for managing selected problems that may arise with a pulmonary artery catheter.

Arterial Pressure Catheter

Percutaneous arterial catheterization, in which a Teflon intravenous catheter, usually 20 gauge, is placed in an artery and connected to a hemodynamic monitor by a pressure line, provides continuous measurements of the systolic, diastolic, and mean arterial blood pressures. The **arterial pressure catheter** produces a waveform and also provides access for arterial blood gas sampling and analysis.

Indications for use of this type of hemodynamic monitoring include situations where frequent and accurate blood pressure measurements are needed, such as the administration of potent drugs (e.g., dopamine to treat septic shock or nitroprusside to treat severe hypertensive disease) or when frequent arterial blood gas determinations are needed. Characteristics of desirable arteries for an arterial line are (1) a vessel that has a diameter large enough for accurate measurement of pressure without occlusion of the artery by the catheter, (2) adequate collateral circulation, (3) ease of access to the site for care, and (4) a site not prone to infection. The most common vessels used in the pregnant woman are the radial, axillary, and pedal arteries, in that order.

In preparation for insertion of the arterial line into the radial artery, the procedure should be explained to the woman in simple terms, informed consent obtained, and Allen's test performed to validate collateral circulation into the hand by demonstrating a patent ulnar artery. Box 34-4 describes the steps to perform Allen's test.

The most common risk associated with an intraarterial line is infection. More serious, but less common, risks include hemorrhage, thrombus formation, and embolization. The heparinized continuous flush solution of the pressure line helps prevent thrombus formation. Once the

---

BOX 34-3   Nursing Interventions Protocol: Trouble-Shooting Pulmonary Artery Catheter Problems

SPONTANEOUS WEDGING: PCWP WAVEFORM APPEARS ON MONITOR SCREEN

- Assess syringe. Determine if balloon is inflated or deflated.
- Have woman turn her head, cough deeply 2 to 3 times, and then take a few deep breaths while observing monitor screen for return of pulmonary artery waveform.
- If wedgeform continues, call physician immediately to the bedside to reposition catheter. (Catheter will need to be pulled back into larger-diameter vessel.)
- Monitor screen for return of pulmonary artery waveform.

MIGRATION OF CATHETER BACKWARD: RIGHT VENTRICULAR WAVEFORM ON SCREEN

- Call physician immediately to bedside to reposition catheter. (Balloon will need to be reinflated for catheter to flow back into the pulmonary artery.)
- Monitor ECG pattern for ventricle ectopy, especially premature ventricle contractions if catheter tip irritates wall of right ventricle.
- Have lidocaine hydrochloride available.

SUSPECTED BALLOON RUPTURE: ABSENCE OF RESISTANCE FELT WHEN INFLATING BALLOON OR INABILITY TO OBTAIN PCWP READING

- Confirm tight attachment of syringe. Do NOT inject air. Slowly withdraw plunger.
- If able to aspirate blood or fluid, balloon rupture is confirmed. Do NOT inject any air. Tape closed and label balloon inflation port, "balloon rupture."
- Rupture may be assumed if unable to aspirate blood or fluid because of absence of resistance in syringe. Do NOT inject any air. Tape closed and label balloon inflation port, "balloon rupture."
- Notify physician.
- Usually does not necessitate change of catheter, especially if diastolic PAP and PCWP readings have been similar. Diastolic PAP will be monitored to reflect left preload values.

---

line is in place, a transparent occlusive dressing is applied. The transducer is then rezeroed. An arm board is used to prevent movement of the wrist (Harvey, 1994).

The hemodynamic monitor displays an arterial waveform and the systolic, diastolic, and mean arterial pressures for the health care team to interpret. Normal versus abnormal waveforms must be recognized at the bedside, and

1. Determine handedness of woman. Use opposite extremity.
2. Elevate woman's hand and occlude both radial and ulnar arteries.
3. Have woman clench and unclench fist to facilitate venous drainage.
4. Observe that palm is blanched.
5. Release pressure on the ulnar artery only. Radial artery remains occluded.
6. Observe and time the palm for capillary refill (normal time is 5 seconds or less).
7. If it takes more than 5 seconds, collateral circulation may be impaired.

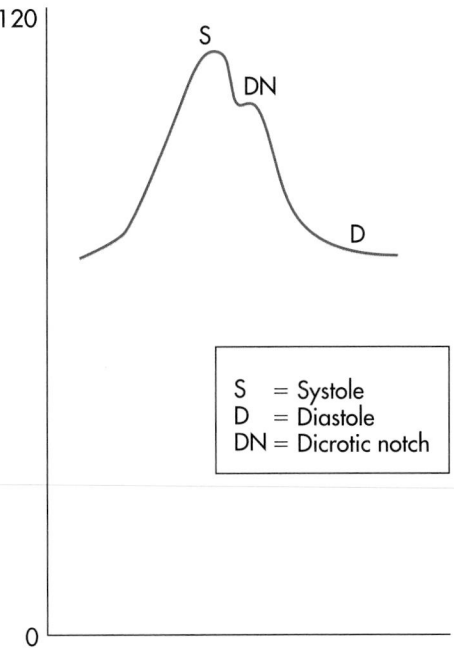

S = Systole
D = Diastole
DN = Dicrotic notch

Fig. 34-8   Arterial waveform.

immediate intervention must be available as needed. The normal waveform should include the following (Fig. 34-8):
- Rapid upstroke to systole
- Clear dicrotic notch, which denotes closure of the aortic valve
- Definite end-diastolic wave

A blood pressure taken with a sphygmomanometer should be ascertained periodically to verify accuracy of the hemodynamic monitor.

Continuing assessments and documentation should include the following:
- Systolic and diastolic arterial pressures
- Cuff pressure readings
- Intraarterial strip recording
- Site care
- Dressing and line changes
- Transducer zeroing and calibration
- Description of the circulation in the extremity

Pressure Lines

All pressure lines use a specialized high-pressure tubing to transmit the physiologic signal to the transducer and monitor. The pressure tubing is rigid to prevent the dampening or absorption of pressure itself, so that the physiologic pressures are transmitted directly from the catheter tip to the transducer through the fluid that fills the length of the tubing. The line includes a continuous flushing mechanism to ensure patency (see Fig. 34-5).

Data Collection

Continuous measurements of the central venous and pulmonary artery pressures and intermittent PCWPs are obtained from the PAC. CO is also calculated intermittently by the use of a PAC with the thermodilution technique. ECG monitoring permits continuous evaluation of heart rate and rhythm. Newer ECG monitors with sensitive leads connected to the chest wall also monitor respiratory rate. Systemic arterial blood pressure can be evaluated by a manual or an automatic sphygmomanometer or by an arterial pressure line. Placement of an arterial pressure line also permits ready access for frequent arterial blood sampling and analysis, especially for arterial blood gases.

Mean pressure values are used to evaluate client status. They can be determined for the pulmonary arterial and systemic circulations by electronic dampening of the respective tracing or by use of the following calculation formula (Hankins & Harvey, 1993):

$$\text{Mean arterial pressure} = \frac{\text{Systolic pressure} + 2\,(\text{Diastolic pressure})}{3}$$

The PCWP, a dampened pressure tracing, is reported as a mean value, determined by the average of its maximum and minimum deflections on the monitor screen or oscilloscope. Reading values from the oscilloscope is usually adequate for clinical management at the bedside; however, for complex cases strip chart recordings are recommended. See the Procedure box for making and recording hemodynamic assessments.

When the thermodilution procedure to calculate cardiac output in a pregnant woman is performed, the injectate should be chilled to obtain an accurate reading because of the high cardiac outputs normal for pregnancy (Wallace & Winslow, 1993). The thermistor at the tip of the PAC measures the speed with which the blood temperature cools and returns to normal after the chilled fluid is injected. The time required for the temperature changes is computed and a CO readout is given. The Procedure box describes the thermodilution procedure for measuring CO.

PROCEDURE

Making and Recording Hemodynamic Assessments

1. Position woman in supine position with a hip wedge.
2. Rezero all pressure transducers.
3. Print a strip recording of the PAC and arterial line blood pressures. Observe oscilloscope for mean values.
4. Record findings of the PAP, central venous pressure, and arterial blood pressure.
5. Calibrate PCWP according to the Procedure box for obtaining a PCWP reading. Record the mean determination.
6. Calibrate cardiac output according to the Procedure box outlining the thermodilution procedure for measuring CO.
7. Document all findings and client's tolerance of procedures.

PROCEDURE

Thermodilution Procedure for Measuring Cardiac Output

1. Enter the CO coefficient into the computer.
2. Chill injectate per ice bath.
3. Use insulated syringe.
4. Flush coiled tubing with injectate solution to remove all air.
5. Connect syringe to three-way stopcock at the proximal port.
6. Draw injectate (5 or 10 ml per unit protocol) into insulated syringe.
7. Depress the CO control on the computer.
8. Inject the injectate as rapidly as possible with both hands. Observe oscilloscope for a smooth curve.
9. Repeat the procedure twice. Calculate results. If readings are within 15% of each other, average the three to determine CO. If not, omit the highest and lowest.

Oxygenation

Oxygen delivery to and use by the peripheral tissues must be adequate. Determination of oxygen transport is essential in the care of the critically ill pregnant woman. Oxygen delivery is directly proportional to cardiac output; if CO decreases 50%, oxygen delivery decreases 50%. Conversely, increasing CO 50% doubles oxygen delivery. Oxygen delivery can also be improved by improving the hemoglobin value, which can be accomplished by the administration of red blood cells.

SaO_2 Monitoring

Oxygen is transported to the tissues in two ways: dissolved in plasma and bound to hemoglobin. The oxygen dissolved in plasma (PaO_2) makes up only 1% to 2% of the total oxygen content, whereas the oxygen bound to hemoglobin (SaO_2) makes up 98% to 99% of the total oxygen content. Results of arterial blood gas determination reflect the dissolved oxygen according to the PaO_2 value. The PaO_2 reflects the partial pressure that oxygen exerts when it is dissolved in blood; it is measured in millimeters of mercury. The normal PaO_2 for the pregnant state is 100 to 106 mm Hg, and it must be at least 60 mm Hg for fetal survival (Clark et al., 1991). The partial pressure of the oxygen tension is important because circulation transports the higher PaO_2 blood to organs with a lower PaO_2, and gas exchange occurs as gases move from the higher concentration to the lower concentration. The higher tension (PaO_2) pushes the oxygen molecule off the hemoglobin molecule through the cell membrane so that tissues receive a supply of oxygen.

The oxygen that cells are able to use are the oxygen molecules bound to hemoglobin (SaO_2). Each molecule of hemoglobin has four binding sites for oxygen; when all four sites are bound, an oxyhemoglobin molecule results. The saturation of hemoglobin with oxygen (SaO_2) is evaluated with the pulse oximeter. The normal range for SaO_2 is 95% to 100%, and normal SaO_2 values for pregnancy are 97% to 100%. Critically ill pregnant women benefit from continuous SaO_2 monitoring.

SvO_2 Monitoring

The percentage of saturation of hemoglobin with oxygen in mixed venous and arterial blood is reflected as an SvO_2 value. **SvO_2 monitoring** involves insertion of a fiberoptic PAC that is connected to a bedside microprocessor to give a continuous SvO_2 value. Mixed venous blood saturation reflects the balance between oxygen delivery and oxygen use. It reflects tissue perfusion, the variation in oxygen requirements for different organs, and the affinity of hemoglobin to accept and then release oxygen (Hankins & Harvey, 1993). Average SvO_2 is 73%. SvO_2 levels below 60% are interpreted as abnormally low.

Fiberoptic pulmonary artery catheters and bedside microprocessors provide the technology to continuously plot the mixed venous blood oxygen saturation. Plotting of mixed venous oxygen content is used as an early warning system because values may fall before any other evidence of hemodynamic instability is seen (Hankins & Harvey, 1993).

Use of pulse oximetry permits evaluation of the SaO_2, arterial blood saturation. Arterial blood usually has a saturation of 90% or greater. Because of the shape of the oxyhemoglobin dissociation curve, fluctuations at the high levels of oxygen tension, 90% and higher, are reflected by a small change in arterial oxygen saturation (SaO_2). However, the lower levels of oxygen tension in mixed venous blood (40% or less) produce a linear relationship between saturation and tension, resulting in the SvO₂ becoming a sensitive alarm to detect physiologic instability.

Arterial blood analysis evaluates pulmonary oxygen exchange and ventilation but does not evaluate overall adequacy of oxygen delivery to the peripheral tissues. However, mixed venous blood analysis (SvO₂) reflects the end product of supply and demand and is used to evaluate overall adequacy of oxygen delivery to the peripheral tissues. This technique provides additional data and can be especially useful to support or change management strategies when used in conjunction with thermodilution CO calculations.

NURSE ALERT *Stable CO measurements in conjunction with an improvement in SvO₂ readings are associated with clinical improvement and is a good prognostic sign. The same improved SvO₂ readings in conjunction with a 100% increase in CO is a common first sign of the development of sepsis.*

Continuous monitoring of SvO₂ is recommended for titration of vasoactive or inotropic drugs; during adjustments of positive end-expiratory pressure, evaluation of fluid administration, and routine care of critically ill pregnant women; and as an early warning system for changes in cardiopulmonary status (Hankins & Harvey, 1993).

Central Venous Pressure Lines

Before the development of the flow-directed PAC in the early 1970s, CVP lines were used for the critically ill. Two primary problems with the use of CVP lines became apparent. First, CVP monitoring provides right-sided heart information only, the right preload. When a cardiac or pulmonary complication is present, right- and left-sided values are not equal. CVP monitoring gives no information about left ventricular function. Second, changes in CVP values occur much later with left ventricular dysfunction. This type of monitoring does not permit rapid calculation of effects of treatment modalities. Critically ill clients need a PAC monitoring that provides a continuous PAP, intermittent PCWP and CO calculations; therefore CVP monitoring is seldom used (Clark et al., 1994).

Interpretation of Hemodynamic Data

Data obtained with hemodynamic monitoring techniques include values that reflect blood volume in the pulmonary and systemic circulations, which profoundly affect cardiac performance, in the following ways:
- Right atrial pressure or CVP indicates right end-diastolic pressure and reflects right preload.
- PAP. PVR is the calculation for right afterload. Clinically, PAP reflects right afterload.
  - Systolic PAP.
  - Diastolic PAP approximates PCWP and reflects left preload.
- PCWP indicates left end-diastolic pressure and reflects left preload.

TABLE 34-6	Normal Hemodynamic Values in Pregnancy
Right atrial pressure or CVP	0-7 mm Hg
PAP	18-30 mm Hg (systolic)
	6-10 mm Hg (diastolic)
PCWP	6-10 mm Hg
CO	6-7 L/min
SVR	1210 ± 266
PVR	78 ± 22

TABLE 34-7	Central Hemodynamic Normal Values	
PARAMETER	NONPREGNANT	PREGNANT
CO (L/min)	4.3 ± 0.9	6.2 ± 1.0
Heart rate (beats/min)	71 ± 10.0	83 ± 10.0
SVR (dyne/cm/sec⁻⁵)	1530 ± 520	1210 ± 266
PVR (dyne/cm/sec⁻⁵)	119 ± 47.0	78 ± 22
PCWP (mm Hg)	6.3 ± 2.1	7.5 ± 1.8
CVP (mm Hg)	3.7 ± 2.6	3.6 ± 2.5
Left ventricular work index	41 ± 8	48 ± 6

- CO refers to the volume of blood ejected from the left ventricle in liters per minute.
- SVR is the calculation for left afterload; arterial blood pressure reflects left afterload.

Hemodynamic profiles provide valuable data for evaluating status of the client and changing treatment strategies as needed. Normal hemodynamic values for calculation in the cases below are shown in Table 34-6. Table 34-7 compares normal nonpregnant hemodynamic values with normal values during pregnancy.

Oliguria is diagnosed if urine output falls below 25 to 30 ml for 2 consecutive hours. It may indicate severe renal dysfunction (Dildy, Phelan, & Cotton, 1991). If oliguria is not corrected with fluid challenge, the woman is diagnosed as having oliguria refractory to conservative therapy.

Refractory oliguria caused by preeclampsia may be associated with three different hemodynamic subsets: hypovolemia, hypervolemia, and renal artery spasm. Treatment strategies for correction of oliguria are different for each hemodynamic subset. Noninvasive assessments are not able to differentiate the type of treatment that would be appropriate for the pregnant woman. Recognition of which hemodynamic subset has produced the refractory oliguria is obtained only by the use of a PAC. Failure to use pulmonary artery catheterization when refractory oliguria is present can result in inappropriate treatment.

Examples of three different pregnant women with preeclampsia complicated by refractory oliguria are included in Box 34-5 to demonstrate how useful hemodynamic monitoring is to identify the appropriate care for the individual woman with this complication. These three women, all with severe preeclampsia-eclampsia with similar noninvasive assessment findings, illustrate the need for use of a PAC when the pregnant woman with hypertensive disease and oliguria fails a fluid challenge test. Noninvasive parameters do not reflect volume status. Completely different treatment modalities to correct oliguria are indicated for each of these three women.

Pulmonary Edema

One of the most common uses of pulmonary artery catheterization during pregnancy is the differentiation of cardiogenic (heart failure or hydrostatic) pulmonary edema from noncardiogenic (permeability or lung failure) pulmonary edema (Hankins & Harvey, 1993). Optimum therapy for the two types of pulmonary edema are dramatically different; however, the correct diagnosis can be determined only by evaluation of the hemodynamic profile.

Cardiogenic or heart failure pulmonary edema develops as a result of left ventricular failure or acute fluid overload. The PCWP will be elevated because of the volume of fluid in the pulmonary circulation. Therapy is focused on improvement of myocardial contractility with an inotropic drug, decreasing left afterload, if elevated, with an arterial vasodilator and reducing preload with a diuretic drug to a normal range. This type of pulmonary edema usually responds to therapy within a few hours, and a normal PCWP is restored.

Pulmonary edema may also result from damage to the pulmonary alveolar capillary membrane by numerous factors, the most common being sepsis. Disturbance of membrane permeability results in the leakage of both protein and fluid into the pulmonary interstitium and alveoli, in the presence of normal cardiac function and ventricular filling pressures (Hankins & Harvey, 1993). The PCWP is normal. Alveolar membranes require days to heal, and adult respiratory distress disease may develop if the source of injury is not found and eradicated. The focus of therapy is to maintain the PCWP in the low-normal range to minimize transudation of protein and fluid into the lung and to eliminate the source of injury.

When radiography reveals pulmonary edema, evaluation of the hemodynamic profile is the only way to correctly diagnose the type of pulmonary edema present, as illustrated in the following two hemodynamic profiles:

Case I

CVP	4 mm Hg
PAP	44/21 mm Hg
PCWP	20 mm Hg
CO	6.1 L/min

The high wedge pressure reflects a high left preload and correlates with cardiogenic pulmonary edema. Treatment would include an inotropic drug such as dobutamine, a vasodilator such as hydralazine if hypertension is present,

and a diuretic such as furosemide (Lasix) because cardiac output is adequate.

Case II

CVP	2 mm Hg
PAP	23/8 mm Hg
PCWP	7 mm Hg
CO	7.1 L/min

All readings are in the normal range, although pulmonary edema is present. This correlates with noncardiogenic pulmonary edema. A diuretic should not be administered. Preload is in the low-normal range. Lowering the preload with a diuretic drug could decrease CO and jeopardize the client's status. Instead, sepsis should be suspected and treatment should focus on antibiotic therapy and elimination of foci of infection, continuing assessments, and support of vital systems while lung membranes heal.

TRAUMA DURING PREGNANCY

Trauma continues to be a common complication during pregnancy because of the continuation of usual activities by the majority of pregnant women in the United States.

Significance

Approximately 8% of pregnancies have been reported to be complicated by physical trauma (Lavery & Staten-McCormick, 1995). As pregnancy progresses, the risk of trauma seems to increase because more cases of trauma are reported in the third trimester than earlier in gestation. Approximately 8% of injuries are reported in the first trimester, 40% during the second, and 52% during the third (Clark et al., 1994).

Most maternal injuries are a result of motor vehicle accidents. Falls, burns, gunshot wounds, and assault are other major sources (Daddario, 1998).

Acts of violence are a significant health problem in the United States. The risk of trauma caused by battering and abuse is increased during pregnancy, and rates of recurrence are high. The incidence of physical abuse during pregnancy ranges from 25% to 40% (Barrier, 1998).

Reports show that up to 45% of women subject to domestic violence before pregnancy continue to be abused during the pregnancy. Abuse may also have its onset with the pregnant state (Biester et al., 1997).

Trauma is the leading nonobstetric cause of maternal mortality and accounts for 20% of maternal deaths each year (Clark et al., 1994). More than 70% of these fatal injuries result from motor vehicle accidents. Maternal death caused by trauma is usually the result of head injury or hemorrhagic shock (Harvey & Troiano, 1992). Fetal death usually occurs as a sequela to maternal death or as a result of placental abruption (see Research box).

Fortunately, the majority of trauma injuries during pregnancy are minor and have no impact on pregnancy

▪ BOX 34-5   Case Studies

CASE 1

J.W.G. is a 24-year-old woman, gravida 4, para 2, at 35 weeks of gestation, diagnosed with severe preeclampsia-eclampsia. She is scheduled for labor induction today because of the increasing severity of the disease.

Everything went well for the first 5 hours after admission. However, this hour urine output is only 22 ml. The physician orders a fluid challenge of 1000 ml of lactated Ringer's solution (LR); 1 hour after this fluid infusion is completed, urine output is 24 ml.

This is a failed fluid challenge. A Swan-Ganz catheter (PAC) is inserted to determine volume status and to help determine why the kidneys are not excreting urine. The woman's hemodynamic profile was determined to be the following:

CVP	2 mm Hg
PAP	15/5 mm Hg
PCWP	4 mm Hg
CO	6.1 L/min

Evaluation

Evaluation of this profile shows a low PCWP of 4 mm Hg, which denotes decreased left preload and reflects hypovolemia. The low PAP reflects the decreased pulmonary circulating volume. CO is low for a laboring woman, probably as a result of the decreased preload. Her CO at 6.1 L/min is probably being maintained by her elevated heart rate; however, she is not in danger of dying with a CO of 6 L/min or greater. This hemodynamic profile correlates with hypovolemia as the reason for oliguria. Urine is not being produced because the renal system is not adequately perfused. Additional fluids are needed rapidly. The oliguria is due to compensatory mechanisms that shunt the blood from the peripheral circulation to the central circulation in response to the extremely low preload. The 1000 ml of fluid given in the fluid challenge was not adequate to correct the hypovolemia. Additional fluid should be administered until left preload is adequate.

CASE 2

S.L.C. is an 18-year-old primigravid woman at 34 weeks of gestation with a diagnosis of severe preeclampsia-eclampsia. She is scheduled for induction of labor today because of increasing severity of disease.

Everything went well for the first 5 hours after admission. However, this hour urine output is only 23 ml. The physician orders a fluid challenge of 1000 ml of LR. One hour after this fluid is infused, urine output is 24 ml.

This is a failed fluid challenge. A Swan-Ganz catheter is inserted to determine volume status and to help determine the cause of the oliguria. Hemodynamic profile is determined to be the following:

CVP	2 mm Hg
PAP	22/9 mm Hg
PCWP	8 mm Hg
CO	7.8 L/min

Evaluation

Evaluation of this profile shows a normal PCWP of 8 mm Hg, a normal PAP, and a CO of 7.8 L/min. A normal hemodynamic profile in conjunction with refractory oliguria is associated with renal artery spasm that decreases perfusion and oxygenation to the kidneys and results in decreased urine output. Renal dose (low-dose) dopamine is used as the first-line management strategy to correct this type of oliguria. An arterial pressure line will be used during administration of the drug to monitor blood pressure closely. Relaxation of the renal artery will improve renal system perfusion and correct the oliguria.

CASE 3

B.J.S. is a 32-year-old woman, gravida 5, para 4, at 36 weeks of gestation with a diagnosis of severe preeclampsia-eclampsia. She is scheduled for labor induction today because of increasing severity of disease.

Everything went well for the first 5 hours after admission. However, this hour urine output is only 20 ml. The physician orders a fluid challenge of 1000 ml of LR. One hour after this fluid is completed, urine output is 22 ml.

This is a failed fluid challenge. A Swan-Ganz catheter is inserted to determine volume status and to help determine the cause of the oliguria. Hemodynamic profile is determined to be the following:

CVP	2 mm Hg
PAP	44/20 mm Hg
PCWP	18 mm Hg
CO	6.6 L/min

Evaluation

Evaluation of this profile shows a high PCWP of 18 mm Hg, which denotes an increased left preload. CO is adequate. This profile correlates with oliguria in the hypervolemic pregnant woman. Lack of urine excretion is probably due to renal damage from the ischemia accompanying the severe hypertensive disease. Intravenous fluids should be restricted to 50 ml per hour. The high wedge pressure correlates with pulmonary edema during pregnancy. With such severe preeclampsia, pulmonary edema is usually a combined cardiogenic and noncardiogenic type. Cardiogenic pulmonary edema is a result of the increased SVR, which increased the resistance that the left ventricle must overcome to eject blood. This can lead to congestive heart failure. The noncardiogenic pulmonary edema is a result of an extremely low COP, a result of renal disease and protein excretion. Reduction of left afterload with hydralazine is the initial management strategy to correct the pulmonary edema. CO is adequate, probably because of the increased HR and circulating volume. The high PAP reflects the increased pressures in the pulmonary circulation because of the excessive fluid that is present, produced by the increased left afterload. Immediate delivery will permit further renal studies to evaluate renal function. Dialysis may be indicated.

RESEARCH

Trauma in Pregnancy: Maternal and Fetal Outcomes

Trauma occurs in approximately 6% to 7% of all pregnancies and necessitates hospital admission in 0.3% to 0.4% of all pregnancies. The more active lifestyles led by pregnant women in today's society may put them at increased risk of injury, although the exact nature of these risks and the population at risk must be better defined.

Fetal loss after trauma is often difficult to predict. This has led to the common practice of prolonged observation and monitoring of pregnant women even after apparently trivial trauma. The purpose of this study was to determine (1) the demographic, physiologic, and injury characteristics of injured pregnant women; (2) whether pregnancy increased morbidity and mortality rates after trauma; and (3) the risk factors associated with fetal loss.

A retrospective, case-control analysis of all injured pregnant women admitted to the Trauma Service at the University of California San Diego Medical Center from 1985 to 1995 was performed. One hundred fourteen pregnant clients were identified. Motor vehicle crashes accounted for 70% of injuries, and of these, 46% of clients were not using seat belts or helmets. Violence accounted for 12% of injuries. Injured pregnant women with Injury Severity Scores greater than 8 demonstrated similar mortality, morbidity, and length of stay to matched nonpregnant control clients. Pregnant women were more likely to sustain serious abdominal injury and were less likely to

sustain severe head injury. Identified risk factors for fetal loss included maternal death, overall maternal injury severity, the presence of severe abdominal injury, and the presence of hemorrhagic shock.

It was concluded that there appears to be a group of pregnant women in San Diego at high risk for traumatic injury who should be targeted for preventive strategies, including improved seat belt use. Pregnancy does not increase morbidity or mortality rates after trauma but does influence the pattern of injury. Maternal death, high Injury Severity Score, serious abdominal injury, and hemorrhagic shock are risk factors for fetal loss.

CLINICAL APPLICATION

Preventive strategies for prenatal clients should be developed and implemented, including improved seat belt use and better identification of victims of physical abuse. Nurses working in emergency facilities and trauma units must be aware that pregnancy imposes significant physiologic demands that may confuse and complicate the evaluation, resuscitation, and definitive management of pregnant women who sustain trauma. The usefulness of prolonged tocodynamic and tocographic monitoring of the otherwise stable client is unclear from this study and requires further investigation.

Source: Shah, K. et al. (1998). Trauma in pregnancy: Maternal and fetal outcomes. *J Trauma* 45(1), 83-86.

---

outcome. However, each case of trauma during pregnancy must be evaluated carefully because pregnancy can mask signs of severe injury. Research has not yet revealed an accurate "trauma score" to predict risk of adverse pregnancy outcome from the initial physical assessment (Biester et al., 1997). Therefore prolonged assessments are usually completed before discharge from the unit in seemingly "mild" cases of trauma (Anquist et al., 1994).

Multisystem trauma during pregnancy is usually the result of a serious motor vehicle crash, especially if the woman is not wearing a seat belt with a shoulder harness and is ejected from the vehicle. Failure to wear restraining devices during pregnancy increases maternal and fetal risks. ACOG (1991b) recommends that pregnant women wear properly positioned restraints at all times when in a motor vehicle.

Trauma increases the incidence of miscarriage, preterm labor, abruptio placentae, and stillbirth (Pearlman & Tintinalli, 1991). The effect of trauma on pregnancy is influenced by the length of gestation, type and severity of the trauma, and degree of disruption of uterine and fetal physiologic features. Fetal death as a result of trauma is more common than the occurrence of both maternal and

fetal death (Pearlman & Tintinalli, 1991). Less serious trauma is associated with numerous complications for pregnancy, including fetomaternal hemorrhage, abruptio placentae, intrauterine fetal death, and preterm labor and birth (Pearlman & Tintinalli, 1991). Careful evaluation of mother and fetus after all types of trauma is imperative (AAP & ACOG, 1997).

Special considerations for mother and fetus are necessary when trauma occurs during pregnancy because of the physiologic alterations that accompany pregnancy and because of the presence of the fetus. Fetal survival depends on maternal survival. Therefore the pregnant woman must receive immediate stabilization and appropriate care for optimum fetal outcome.

Maternal Physiologic Characteristics

Optimum care for the pregnant woman after trauma is dependent on understanding the physiologic state of pregnancy and its effects on trauma. The pregnant woman's body will exhibit responses different from those of a nonpregnant person to the same traumatic insults. Because of the different responses to injury during pregnancy, man-

TABLE 34-8 Maternal Adaptations During Pregnancy and Relationship to Trauma

SYSTEM	ALTERATION	CLINICAL RESPONSES
Respiratory	↑Oxygen consumption	↑ Risk of acidosis
	↑ Tidal volume	
	↓ Functional residual capacity	
	Chronic compensated alkalosis	↑ Risk of respiratory mismanagement
	↓ $PaCO_2$	↓ Blood buffering capacity
	↓ Serum bicarbonate	
Cardiovascular	↑ Circulating volume 1600 ml	Can lose 1000 ml blood
	↑ CO	No signs of shock until blood loss >30% total
	↑ Heart rate	blood volume
	↓ SVR	↓ Placental perfusion in supine position
	↓ Arterial blood pressure	Point of maximal impulse, fourth intercostal
	Heart displaced upward to left	space
Renal	↑ Renal plasma flow	
	Dilation of ureters and urethra	↑ Risk of stasis, infection
	Bladder displaced forward	↑ Risk of bladder trauma
Gastrointestinal	↓ Gastric motility	↑ Risk of aspiration
	↑ Hydrochloric acid production	
	↓ Competency of gastroesophageal sphincter	Passive regurgitation of stomach acids if head
		lower than stomach
Reproductive	↑ Blood flow to organs	Source of ↑ blood loss
	Uterine enlargement	Vena caval compression in supine position
Musculoskeletal	Displacement of abdominal viscera	↑ Risk of injury, altered rebound response
	Pelvic venous congestion	Altered pain referral
	Cartilage softened	↑ Risk for pelvic fracture
		Center of gravity changed
	Fetal head in pelvis	↑ Risk of fetal injury
Hematologic	↑ Clotting factors	↑ Risk of thrombus formation
	↓ Fibrinolytic activity	

agement strategies must be adapted for appropriate resuscitation, fluid therapy, positioning, assessments, and most other interventions. Significant maternal adaptations and the relationship to trauma are summarized in Table 34-8.

The uterus and bladder are confined to the bony pelvis during the first trimester of pregnancy and are at reduced risk for injury in cases of abdominal trauma. After pregnancy progresses beyond the fourteenth week, the uterus becomes an abdominal organ and the risk for injury increases in cases of abdominal trauma. During the second and third trimesters the distended bladder becomes an abdominal organ and is at increased risk for injury and rupture. Bowel injuries occur less often during pregnancy because of the protection provided by the enlarged uterus.

The elevated levels of progesterone that accompany pregnancy relax smooth muscle and profoundly affect the gastrointestinal tract. Gastrointestinal motility decreases, with a resultant increased time required for gastric emptying, whereas the production of hydrochloric acid increases in the last trimester, and the gastroesophageal sphincter relaxes (Harvey & Moretti, 1993). Airway management of the unconscious pregnant woman is of critical importance.

NURSE ALERT *The unconscious pregnant woman is at increased risk for regurgitation of gastric contents and aspiration whenever her head is positioned lower than her stomach or if abdominal pressure is applied.*

A pregnant woman has decreased tolerance for hypoxia and apnea because of her decreased functional residual capacity and increased renal loss of bicarbonate. Acidosis develops more quickly in the pregnant than in the nonpregnant state.

CO increases 44% to 50% over prepregnancy values and is positionally dependent in the third trimester. Because of compression of the inferior vena cava and descending aorta by the pregnant uterus, CO will drop dramatically if the woman is placed in the supine position. The supine position must be avoided, even in women with cervical spine injuries. It is a primary priority that lateral uterine displacement be accomplished without any head movement. As soon as the neck is immobilized, the stretcher should be tilted laterally.

Circulating blood volume increases 50% during gestation, and pregnant women can tolerate a 1000 ml blood loss readily without demonstrating clinical signs. Hemodynamic instability that indicates the need for transfusion may not be apparent until blood loss nears 1500 to 2000 ml (Clark et al., 1994). Clinical signs of hemorrhage do not appear until after a 30% loss of circulating volume occurs. Although heart rate increases with pregnancy, a maternal heart rate greater than 100 beats per minute should be considered abnormal.

Fetal Physiologic Characteristics

Perfusion of the uterine arteries, which provide the primary blood supply to the uteroplacental unit, depends on adequate maternal arterial pressure because these vessels lack autoregulation. Therefore maternal hypotension decreases uterine and fetal perfusion (Pearlman & Tintinalli, 1991). Maternal shock results in splanchnic and uterine artery vasoconstriction (Rice, 1991), which decreases blood flow and oxygen transport to the fetus. Electronic fetal monitoring (EFM) tracings can assist in the evaluation of maternal status after trauma. EFM tracings reflect fetal cardiac responses to hypoxia and hypoperfusion, including tachycardia or bradycardia, decreased or absent baseline variability, and late decelerations.

Careful monitoring of fetal status assists greatly in maternal assessment, because the fetal monitor tracing works as an "oximeter" of internal maternal well-being. Hypoperfusion may be present in the pregnant woman before the onset of clinical signs of shock. The EFM tracings show the first signs of maternal compromise, such as when maternal HR, BP, and color appear normal, yet the EFM printout shows signs of fetal hypoxia (Pearlman & Tintinalli, 1991).

Mechanisms of Trauma

Blunt Abdominal Trauma

Blunt abdominal trauma is most commonly the result of motor vehicle crashes but may also be the result of battering or falls. Maternal and fetal mortality and morbidity rates are directly correlated with whether the mother remains inside the vehicle or is ejected. Death is usually the result of a head injury or exsanguination from a major vessel rupture. The most common fetal injury in severe trauma is skull fracture with subsequent intracranial hemorrhage (Pearlman & Tintinalli, 1991). Serious retroperitoneal hemorrhage after lower abdominal and pelvic trauma is reported more frequently during pregnancy. Serious maternal abdominal injuries are usually the result of splenic rupture or liver or renal injury.

When maternal survival of trauma occurs, fetal death is usually the result of abruptio placentae occurring within 48 hours of the accident (Pearlman & Tintinalli, 1991). Placental separation is thought to be a result of deformation of the elastic myometrium around the relatively inelastic placenta. Shearing of the placental edge from the underlying decidua basalis results and is worsened by the increased intrauterine pressure resulting from the impact.

It is critical that all pregnant victims be carefully evaluated for signs and symptoms of abruptio placentae after even minor blunt abdominal trauma.

NURSE ALERT *Signs and symptoms of abruptio placentae include uterine tenderness or pain, uterine irritability, uterine contractions, vaginal bleeding, leaking of amniotic fluid, or a change in fetal heart rate characteristics.*

Pelvic fracture may result from severe injury and may produce bladder trauma or retroperitoneal bleeding with the two-point displacement of pelvic bones that usually occurs. One point of displacement is commonly at the symphysis pubis and the second point is posterior, because of the structure of the pelvis. Careful evaluation for clinical signs of internal hemorrhage is indicated.

Direct fetal injury as a complication of trauma during pregnancy most often involves the fetal skull and brain. Most commonly this injury accompanies maternal pelvic fracture in late gestation, after the fetal head becomes engaged. When the force of the impact is great enough to fracture the maternal pelvis, the fetus will often sustain a skull fracture. Evaluation for fetal skull fracture or intracranial hemorrhage is indicated.

Uterine rupture as a result of trauma is rare, occurring in only 0.6% of all reported cases of trauma during pregnancy. Uterine rupture depends on numerous factors, including gestational age and the intensity of the impact and the presence of a predisposing factor such as a distended uterus caused by polyhydramnios or multiple gestation or the presence of a uterine scar resulting from previous uterine surgery (Pearlman, Tintinalli, & Lorenz, 1990a). When uterine rupture occurs, the force responsible is usually a direct, high-energy blow. Fetal death is common with traumatic uterine rupture. However, maternal death occurs less than 10% of the time, and when it occurs it is usually the result of massive injuries sustained from an impact severe enough to rupture the uterus.

Penetrating Abdominal Trauma

Bullet wounds are the most frequent cause of penetrating abdominal injury, followed by stab wounds. Penetrating abdominal wounds have disparate prognoses for mother and fetus in almost 66% of cases. The enlarged uterus may protect other maternal organs, but the fetus is more vulnerable (Hinkle & Belts, 1995).

Numerous factors determine the extent and severity of maternal and fetal injury from a bullet wound, including size and velocity of the bullet, anatomic region penetrated, angle of entry, path of the bullet, organs damaged, gestational age, and exit wound. Once the bullet enters the body, it may ricochet several times as it encounters organs or bone, or it may sever a large blood vessel. During the second half of pregnancy the fetus usually sustains a direct injury from the bullet. Gunshot wounds require surgical exploration to determine the extent of injury and repair damage as needed (ACOG, 1991a).

Stab wounds are limited by the length and width of the penetrating object and are usually confined to the pathway of the weapon. Maternal and fetal injury are less if the stab wound is located in the upper abdomen and from movement of the penetrating object from above the head downward toward the abdomen than from movement of the penetrating object from the ground upward toward the lower abdomen. Stab wounds usually require surgical exploration to clean out debris, determine extent of injury, and repair damage.

Thoracic Trauma

Thoracic trauma is reported to produce 25% of all trauma deaths. Pulmonary contusion results from nearly 75% of blunt thoracic trauma and is a potentially life-threatening condition (Ruth-Sahd, 1991). Pulmonary contusion can be difficult to recognize, especially if flail chest is also present or if there is no evidence of thoracic injury. Pulmonary contusion should be suspected in cases of thoracic injury, especially after blunt acceleration or deceleration trauma, such as that occurring when a rapidly moving vehicle crashes into an immovable object.

Penetrating wounds into the chest can result in pneumothorax or hemothorax. This type of injury is usually caused by a vehicular crash that results in impalement by the steering column or a loose article in the vehicle that became projectile with the force of impact. Stab wounds into the chest may also occur as a result of violence.

Immediate Stabilization

Immediate priorities for stabilization of the pregnant woman after trauma should be identical to those of the nonpregnant trauma client. Pregnancy should not result in any restriction of the usual diagnostic, pharmacologic, or resuscitative procedures or maneuvers (ACOG, 1991a). The initial response of many trauma team members when caring for the pregnant woman is to assess fetal status first because of the concern for a healthy neonate. The trauma team should follow a methodical evaluation of maternal status to ensure complete assessment and stabilization of the mother. Fetal survival depends on maternal survival, and stabilization of the mother improves fetal chance of survival.

NURSE ALERT *Priorities of care for the pregnant woman after trauma must be to resuscitate the woman and stabilize her condition first and then consider fetal needs.*

Primary Survey

The systematic evaluation begins with a **primary survey** and the initial *ABCs* of resuscitation: establishment of and maintaining an *airway,* ensuring adequate *breathing,* and maintenance of an adequate *circulatory volume.*

Increased oxygen needs during gestation necessitate a rapid response, using jaw thrust rather than neck hyperextension to establish an airway. The presence of a cervical spine injury is always assumed. Once an airway is established, assessment should focus on adequacy of oxygenation. The chest wall is observed for movement. If breathing is absent, ventilations and endotracheal intubation are initiated. Supplemental oxygen should be administered with a tight-fitting, nonrebreathing face mask at 10 to 12 L per minute to maintain a maternal arterial oxygen tension (PaO_2) greater than 60 mm Hg and a hemoglobin saturation greater than 90% to maintain fetal status (Troiano, 1991). The chest wall is assessed for penetrating chest wound or flail chest. Breathing with a flail chest will be rapid and labored; chest wall movements will be uncoordinated and asymmetric; crepitus from bony fragments may be palpated.

NURSE ALERT *Hyperextension of the neck is avoided; instead jaw thrust is used to establish an airway for the trauma victim.*

Rapid placement of two large-bore (14- to 16-gauge) intravenous lines is necessary in most seriously injured clients. It is important to place the lines while veins are still distended. Cardiac arrest during the immediate stabilization period is usually the result of profound hypovolemia; massive fluid resuscitation is necessary when arrest is caused by hypovolemia. Infusion of crystalloids such as Ringer's solution or normal saline solution should be given as a 3:1 ratio; that is, 3 ml of crystalloid replacement to 1 ml of the estimated blood loss is given over the first 30 to 60 minutes of acute resuscitation (ACOG, 1991a). Because of the 50% increase in blood volume during pregnancy, published formulas for nonpregnant adults used for estimating crystalloid and blood replacement to counter blood loss must be adjusted upward for pregnancy.

Replacement of red blood cells and other blood components is anticipated, and blood is drawn for type, cross-match, complete blood cell count, and platelet count (Harvey & Troiano, 1992). Infusion of type-specific whole blood or packed red blood cells is usually necessary to improve fetal oxygenation status and to replace blood loss. During an extreme emergency, type O Rh-negative blood may be administered without matching (Troiano, 1991).

Vasopressor drugs to restore maternal arterial blood pressure should be avoided, if possible, until volume replacement is administered. Although vasopressor agents result in decreased perfusion to the uterus, they should be given, and not withheld, if needed for successful resuscitation of the mother (ACOG, 1991a).

After 20 weeks of gestation, venous return to the heart is best accomplished by positioning the uterus to one side to eliminate the weight of the uterus compressing the inferior vena cava or the descending aorta. This facilitates efforts to establish the forward flow of blood through resuscitation and stabilization. If a lateral position is not possible because of resuscitative efforts or cervical spine immobilization, the uterus can be manually deflected to the left or a wedge should be inserted underneath the right side of the backboard or stretcher.

Signs of bleeding may be more difficult to recognize in the pregnant woman because a 30% to 35% loss of maternal blood volume may produce only a minimal change in maternal mean arterial pressure. Hypovolemia can be detrimental for the fetus because the vascular bed of the uterus is a low-resistance system that depends on adequate maternal arterial pressure to maintain uterine and fetal perfusion. Maternal hypovolemia can be fatal for the fetus.

Establishing a baseline neurologic status (level of consciousness, pupil size and reactivity) is essential. The Glasgow Coma Scale is commonly used at the scene of the accident to help determine the extent of the head injury. The scale is simple and easy to use (Box 34-6).

Secondary Survey

After immediate resuscitation and successful stabilization measures, a more detailed **secondary survey** of the mother and fetus should be accomplished. A complete physical assessment including all body systems is performed.

The maternal abdomen should be evaluated carefully, because a large percentage of serious injuries involves the uterus, intraperitoneal structures, and retroperitoneum. The pregnant client's stomach is assumed to be full. A nasogastric tube can be used to empty the stomach to help prevent acid aspiration syndrome. An empty stomach facilitates respiratory efforts. The uterus should be evaluated for evidence of gross deformity, tenderness, irritability, or contractions (ACOG, 1991a).

The greatest clinical concern after vehicular crashes is abruptio placentae. Assessments should focus on recogni-tion of this complication, with careful evaluation of fetal monitor tracings, uterine tenderness, labor, or vaginal bleeding. Ultrasound may be performed to determine gestational age, viability of fetus, and placental location. However, ultrasound studies cannot exclude abruptio placentae (Smith & Phelan, 1991).

Peritoneal lavage for the pregnant woman after blunt abdominal trauma has proved to be a safe procedure and can be helpful in the early diagnosis of intraperitoneal injury or hemorrhage. An open technique rather than blind paracentesis is recommended. Under direct visualization the peritoneum is incised, and a peritoneal dialysis catheter is positioned. If aspiration yields free-flowing blood, the test is considered positive and a laparotomy should be performed. If no blood is aspirated, a liter of warmed Ringer's solution is infused through the catheter and allowed to drain. The returning fluid is then analyzed for cell count and amylase (Smith & Phelan, 1991). This procedure is not necessary before laparotomy if intraperitoneal bleeding is clinically apparent. Indications for peritoneal lavage include abdominal symptoms or signs suggestive of intraperitoneal bleeding, alteration in mental status, unexplained shock, and severe multiple injury.

If trauma is the result of a penetrating wound, the woman should be completely undressed and carefully examined for all entrance and exit wounds. A bullet may be located on x-ray films. Exploratory laparotomy is necessary after a gunshot wound to explore the abdominal cavity for organ damage and to repair any damage present, with careful examination of all organs, the entire bowel, and posterior vessels. If uterine injury is determined, a careful evaluation of the risks and benefits of cesarean birth is quickly accomplished. A cesarean birth is desirable if the fetus is alive and near term and may be necessary for the preterm fetus because of the high incidence of fetal in-

BOX 34-6	**Glasgow Coma Scale**			
Eyes	Open	Spontaneously	4
		To verbal command	3
		To pain	2
		No response	1
Best motor response	To verbal command	Obeys	6
	To painful stimulus	Localizes pain	5
		Flexion-withdrawal	4
		Flexion-abnormal (decorticate rigidity)	3
		Extension (decerebrate rigidity)	2
		No response	1
Best verbal response		Oriented and converses	5
		Disoriented and converses	4
		Inappropriate words	3
		Incomprehensible sounds	2
		No response	1
TOTAL			3-15

jury in these cases. Tetanus prophylaxis guidelines are not changed by pregnancy. The fetus usually tolerates surgery and anesthesia if adequate uterine perfusion and oxygenation are maintained.

Electronic Fetal Monitoring

Use of EFM may be predictive of abruptio placentae in pregnant trauma victims beyond the twentieth week of gestation (ACOG, 1991a). Continuous EFM may show early signs of abruptio placentae, including a change in baseline rate, loss of accelerations, or the presence of late decelerations. Reports show that abnormal fetal heart rate tracings, including tachycardia and late decelerations, were seen frequently in cases of abruptio placentae, and no cases were seen in women without uterine contractions (Pearlman, Tintinalli, & Lorenz, 1990b).

Fetal monitoring should be initiated soon after the woman is stable because abruptio placentae usually becomes apparent shortly after the injury. Fetal monitoring should be continued and further evaluation initiated if any of the aforementioned signs occur. The external device to monitor uterine activity, the tocodynamometer, is unable to measure pressures, and the pattern made with this device shows the frequency and duration of contractions only. Palpation is required to evaluate the intensity of contractions and the uterine resting tone. It is important to palpate between contractions to verify that the uterus is well relaxed. If the uterus does not relax between contractions, abruptio placentae could be present.

Abruptio placentae occurring after trauma may be delayed up to 48 hours after the incident (Smith & Phelan, 1991). Reports show that EFM periods of 2 to 6 hours after minor trauma are adequate if there are no uterine contractions, uterine tenderness, or bleeding (ACOG, 1991a; Goodwin & Breen, 1990). However, fetal reassurance must be established after minor trauma before fetal monitoring is discontinued and the woman is discharged.

LEGAL TIP Care of Pregnant Woman Involved in Minor Trauma Situation

After minor trauma the pregnant woman may be discharged after an adequate period of EFM that demonstrates fetal reassurance and absence of uterine contractions. However, clear instructions must be given for immediate return if vaginal bleeding, leaking of amniotic fluid, decreased fetal movement, or abdominal pain occurs (ACOG, 1991a).

Fetal-Maternal Hemorrhage

The potential for fetal-maternal hemorrhage exists after trauma; hemorrhage can lead to fetal anemia, distress, or even death. If the pregnant trauma victim is Rh negative, fetal-maternal hemorrhage can result in sensitization and hemolytic disease of the neonate. The routine use of the Kleihauer-Betke assay in clients with blunt abdominal trauma or multiple trauma helps identify cases with a hemorrhage of more than 30 ml (ACOG, 1991a). Because most cases have less than 30 ml of hemorrhage, the routine administration of 300 g (one ampule) of $Rh_0(D)$ immunoglobulin is appropriate because this practice would protect almost all pregnant trauma clients negative for $Rh_0(D)$ from isoimmunization (ACOG, 1991a).

Ultrasound

Ultrasonography after trauma is not as sensitive as EFM for diagnosing abruptio placentae. Ultrasound may be useful to help establish gestational age, locate the placenta, evaluate cardiac activity (to determine whether the fetus is alive), and determine amniotic fluid volume (ACOG, 1991a). Ultrasound may also be used to evaluate the presence of intraabdominal fluid that would suggest the presence of intraabdominal hemorrhage.

Radiation Exposure

If the pregnant woman has sustained serious injuries, any necessary radiographic examination should be performed, regardless of fetal exposure. If radiographic examination would be performed for the nonpregnant trauma victim, it should also be performed for the pregnant woman. Special efforts can minimize the dose to the lower abdomen. Shielding the uterus during irradiation procedures and eliminating duplicate films usually exposes the fetus to a radiation dose of less than 1 rad (ACOG, 1991a).

In some victims with blunt abdominal trauma, abdominal-pelvic computed tomography is preferred to visualize extraperitoneal and retroperitoneal structures and the genitourinary tract. This procedure, in general, exposes the fetus to 5 to 10 rad and should not be withheld for the pregnant woman.

Blunt head trauma and loss of consciousness necessitate skull films and computed tomographic assessment with neurosurgical consultation (Smith & Phelan, 1991). Magnetic resonance imaging may also be used to assess injuries (ACOG, 1991a).

Perimortem Cesarean Delivery

In the presence of multisystem trauma, **perimortem cesarean delivery** may be indicated. Removal of the stressor of pregnancy early in the process of resuscitation may increase the chance for maternal survival. Fetal survival is unlikely if cesarean delivery is accomplished more than 20 minutes after maternal death. Therefore, to facilitate resuscitative efforts, consideration may be given to cesarean delivery for maternal benefit after 5 minutes of resuscitative efforts that produce no response in the mother (Clark et al., 1994; Luppi, 1999).

Physical Assessment

Trauma may affect numerous systems in the maternal body and may affect more than the pregnancy. External signs of maternal trauma should suggest the possibility of internal trauma. Back and neck pain suggest spine injury, abrasions on the chest suggest chest injury, and limb pain and malposition suggest limb fractures. If head injury results in nonresponsiveness, suspect spinal, thoracic, and abdominal injuries. Hypovolemic shock can occur with internal hemorrhage, fracture of long bones, ruptured liver or spleen, hemothorax, or arterial dissection. Military antishock trousers (MAST), a pneumatic antishock garment, may be used for severe hypotension if the abdominal compartment is not inflated and the stretcher is tilted to the side to prevent vena cava syndrome.

Once immediate stabilization is achieved, obstetric clients with severe trauma and massive blood loss that merits vigorous fluid resuscitation will usually benefit from the use of hemodynamic monitoring with a fiberoptic pulmonary catheter to determine cardiac and pulmonary function more precisely and to calculate volume and oxygen needs. The hemodynamic profile will permit precise fluid resuscitation volumes. Oxygenation status calculations, including oxygen content, delivery, and consumption, will demonstrate which fluids are needed to enhance oxygen transport. Precise determinations can help prevent the potential sequelae of too little or too much fluid administration. With massive trauma this care may be best provided in a regional trauma center with the obstetric team, working closely with the trauma team, providing the obstetric care, while the trauma team provides the trauma care.

All female trauma victims of childbearing age should be considered pregnant until proved otherwise. Determination of the health history and a history of the events preceding the trauma are important components of care. If the pregnant woman was involved in a vehicular crash, it should be determined whether she was the driver or a passenger and if she was ejected from the vehicle or used a restraining device and remained within the vehicle.

The physical examination should be performed in a systematic manner (Box 34-7).

BOX 34-7 Physical Examination of the Pregnant Trauma Victim

HEAD

Check scalp for signs of cuts, bruises, or edema. Examine skull for deformities, depressions, or lumps. Examine eyes and eyelids. Evaluate pupils for size, equality, and reaction to light. If contact lenses are present, remove them. Examine nose and ears and observe for serous or bloody fluid. Open the mouth and look for blood, vomitus, loose teeth, and dentures.

Neurologic function should be evaluated frequently because the most frequent cause of death in women not using seat belts is head trauma (Smith & Phelan, 1991). If neurologic checks show a possible head trauma, a complete neurologic consultation and examination should be obtained quickly, including skull films and computed tomographic examination.

NECK

Palpate for tenderness over the cervical spine area. Immobilize with a cervical collar and backboard if complaints of tenderness are present or any injury is suspected. Tilt backboard to side as soon as the pregnant woman is placed on backboard.

CHEST

Observe for lacerations, contusions, wounds, or impaled objects. Observe chest wall movement for symmetry and equal expansion. Assess breath sounds and quality and rate of respirations. Observe for deviated trachea, sounds of sucking wounds, and flail chest. Palpate ribs, sternum, and clavicle.

ABDOMEN

Observe for lacerations, contusions, wounds, or impaled objects. Perform light and then deep palpation. Apply external EFM devices, both the ultrasound Doppler device and tocodynamometer. Palpate for intensity of uterine contractions and determine uterine resting tone. Observe fetal heart rate tracing for signs of fetal reassurance or compromise.

LOWER BACK

Palpate for tenderness. Observe for contusions, deformities, or other signs of injury.

EXTREMITIES

Examine for deformities, edema, dislocation, bleeding, contusions, and fractures. Palpate for tenderness. Assess radial and pedal pulses. Request pregnant woman to move extremities; observe response.

VAGINA

Use digital examination for term gestation without vaginal bleeding; use sterile speculum examination for preterm gestation or if vaginal bleeding is present. Assess for signs of labor, injuries to tissues, or evidence of ruptured membranes.

URINARY TRACT

Observe for the presence of blood in the urine. Trauma to the lower urinary tract is usually accompanied by a fractured pelvis, requiring use of a Foley catheter. Rupture of the bladder may occur in late pregnancy without a pelvic fracture because the full bladder becomes an abdominal organ. Maintain accurate intake and output and observe color of urine.

FAMILY-CENTERED OBSTETRIC CRITICAL CARE

Obstetric critical care should include the components of family-centered maternity care because this critically ill woman is also experiencing pregnancy and birth.

Components of family-centered critical care include the following elements:

1. Open visitation so that spouse, significant other, or family members are present and provide support during labor, birth, and postpartum period.
2. Facilitation of parent-infant contact and attachment. The neonate should be brought to the bedside frequently if the condition permits. When the infant's condition does not permit leaving the neonatal intensive care unit, pictures of the infant should be placed within focus of the mother's eyes. Staff and family can talk about the infant and keep her updated on the infant's condition.
3. Sibling visitation, reassuring the mother that the older child is included in the experience.
4. Family visitation as the mother desires. This can be arranged around necessary care procedures. The critically ill mother needs this care, perhaps even more than the healthy mother does.

Obstetric nurses have become accustomed to family-centered maternity care. When the critically ill mother receives care in an OBICU, there seem to be fewer problems for inclusion of the components of family-centered care than when the mother has to be transported to the adult intensive care unit, probably because the obstetric staff is accustomed to this care and the nursery is more readily available to the labor suite than to the intensive care unit. However, obstetric and critical care nurses can work together to include the components of family-centered care. Critical care nurses are supportive of these components.

Never assume that the mother is too ill to see and hold her infant. Encourage this and observe her body language to determine how much contact with the infant she desires. If perinatal loss occurs as a result of severe illness, provide grief support. Initiate all the components of grief support as usual for the institution. Burial plans can be delayed until the mother's condition improves so that her concerns are addressed.

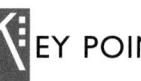

KEY POINTS

- The numbers of critically ill pregnant women are increasing, paralleling improvements in pediatric and neonatal care. Any nurse providing care for pregnant women may encounter the critically ill pregnant woman and must be able to initiate appropriate care.
- Nurses must recognize early signs of severe complications and expedite the institution's plan for the critically ill pregnant woman to receive necessary complex care.

KEY POINTS—cont'd

- The institutional plan may consist of actual implementation of critical care procedures in a labor and birth unit, stabilization, and preparation for transport to a tertiary center or adult intensive care unit, with obstetric consultation after transport.
- Normal physiologic alterations during pregnancy produce profound hemodynamic changes. The critical care team should base care on knowledge of normal hemodynamic values for the pregnant state.
- Pregnancy is not a contraindication for hemodynamic monitoring.
- Invasive hemodynamic monitoring is associated with potential complications. However, the benefits usually outweigh the risks when the woman is critically ill.
- Pulmonary artery catheterization provides continuous information about left ventricle function; this information is not available from any other method.
- Use of a pulmonary artery catheter in combination with an arterial pressure catheter and pulse oximeter provides adequate data to continuously assess both cardiac and pulmonary status.
- The fiberoptic pulmonary artery catheter provides a continuous SvO_2, which is a sensitive marker of physiologic instability because it reflects overall adequacy of oxygen delivery to the tissues.
- The active roles assumed by most pregnant women today place them at risk for vehicular crashes, falls, violence, and other injuries.
- Domestic violence and battering increase during pregnancy.
- Pregnancy does not limit or restrict resuscitative, diagnostic, or pharmacologic treatment after trauma.
- Fetal survival depends on maternal survival. After trauma the first priority is resuscitation and stabilization of the mother before consideration of fetal concerns.
- Optimum care for the pregnant victim of trauma depends on knowledge of the physiologic state of pregnancy.
- Minor trauma is associated with major complications for the pregnancy, including abruptio placentae, fetomaternal hemorrhage, preterm labor and birth, and fetal death.
- Trauma from accidents is the most common cause of death in women of childbearing age.
- Care of the critically ill pregnant woman should include the components of family-centered childbirth.

CRITICAL THINKING EXERCISES

1 Evaluate the plan in your institution for providing appropriate care for the critically ill pregnant woman. Compare your policies and procedures for hemodynamic monitoring with those outlined in this chapter.

   a. Will critically ill women receive care in your institution, or will they need to be transported to a tertiary care center?

   b. Are guidelines clear for immediate stabilization procedures?

   c. If care is to be provided in your institution, is the location an OBICU or an adult intensive care unit? If transport to the intensive care unit is necessary, are clear guidelines written for the obstetric nurse and fetal monitor to accompany the pregnant woman?

   d. Is the procedure for performing Allen's test before insertion of an arterial pressure line in the radial artery included in your policy and procedure manual?

   e. Are hemodynamic values for pregnancy readily available for all team members?

2 D.L., a 26-year-old primigravida at 36 weeks of gestation, is brought to the labor and delivery suite by ambulance stretcher after a motor vehicle crash. Her blood pressure is 90/50 mm Hg, heart rate 156 beats per minute, and respirations 30 per minute. Mucous membranes are pale, and skin is clammy. A hard, boardlike uterus is palpated. Intravenous access is obtained with two large-bore catheters, and fluid resuscitation with 3 L of lactated Ringer's solution and 6 U of type O, Rh-negative packed red blood cells is rapidly administered. No fetal heart tones are present. Bright red vaginal bleeding is present. The diagnosis is abruptio placentae. A PAC is inserted and the woman's hemodynamic profile reveals the following information:

CVP	2 mm Hg
PAP	13/4 mm Hg
PCWP	3 mm Hg
CO	4.8 L/min

   a. Is the CO adequate? Is the client in danger of dying?

   b. Was the volume of fluid resuscitation adequate? Would it be safe to rapidly administer more volume?

   c. Is pulmonary edema developing from the massive fluid load?

   d. Should a β-blocker be given to slow the heart rate?

3 N.A.J., a woman with class II cardiac disease with mitral valve stenosis, is 28 years old, gravida 2, para 0 at 35 weeks of gestation. She has tolerated pregnancy fairly well to this point with reduction in physical activity. Fetal lung maturity is present, and she is admitted for induction of labor. Assessments reveal normal findings on admission, and breath sounds are clear. Medical orders are to start a primary intravenous infusion of lactated Ringer's solution, limit intake to 50 ml per hour, and start low-dose

CRITICAL THINKING EXERCISES—cont'd

oxytocin induction. Five hours into induction the woman requires the head of the bed elevated "to breathe." Her blood pressure is 122/74 mm Hg, heart rate 146 beats per minute, and respirations 33 per minute. Breath sounds include crackles bilaterally. Chest x-ray films show pulmonary edema. A PAC is inserted. The client's hemodynamic profile reveals the following data:

CVP	5 mm Hg
PAP	38/21 mm Hg
PCWP	20 mm Hg
CO	6.4 L/min

   a. Is the CO adequate? Is the woman in danger of dying?

   b. Does this profile correlate with pulmonary edema? If yes, which type? With the fluid restriction of only 50 ml per hour, did noncardiogenic pulmonary edema develop? Why?

   c. According to a positive chest x-ray report of pulmonary edema, if furosemide (Lasix) had been given without benefit of a hemodynamic profile, what would be the potential effects?

References

American College of Obstetricians and Gynecologists. (1991a). Trauma during pregnancy. *ACOG Tech Bull* No. 161. Washington, D.C.: ACOG.

American College of Obstetricians and Gynecologists. (1991b). Automobile passenger restraints for children and pregnant women. *ACOG Tech Bull* No. 151. Washington, D.C.: ACOG.

American College of Obstetricians and Gynecologists. (1992). Invasive hemodynamic monitoring in obstetrics and gynecology. *ACOG Tech Bull* No. 175. Washington, D.C.: ACOG.

American Academy of Pediatrics & American College of Obstetricians and Gynecologists. (1997). *Guidelines for perinatal care* (4th ed.). Elk Grove Village, IL: AAP/ACOG.

Anquist, K. et al. (1994). An unexpected fetal outcome following a severe maternal motor vehicle accident. *Obstet Gynecol* 84(4, pt 2), 656-659.

Association of Women's Health, Obstetric, and Neonatal Nurses. (1998). *Standards and guidelines for professional nursing practice in the care of women and newborns* (5th ed.). Washington, D.C.: AWHONN.

Austin, D. et al. (1994). Critical care obstetrics expert's round table discussion. *J Perinat Neonatal Nurs* 8(2), 1-14.

Barrier, P. (1998). Domestic violence. *Mayo Clin Proc* 73, 271-274.

Baumgartner, R. (1991). Invasive hemodynamic monitoring in the critically ill or high risk obstetric patient. In C. Harvey (Ed.). *Critical care obstetrical nursing*. Gaithersburg, MD: Aspen.

Biester, E. et al. (1997). Trauma in pregnancy: Normal revised trauma score in relation to other markers of maternofetal status—a preliminary study. *Am J Obstet Gynecol* 176, 1206-1212.

Boldt, J. et al. (1994). Is continuous cardiac output measurement using thermodilution reliable in the critically ill patient? *Crit Care Med* 22(12), 1913-1918.

Clark, S. et al. (1989). Central hemodynamic assessment of normal term pregnancy. *Am J Obstet Gynecol* 161(6), 1439-1442.

Clark, S. et al. (1991). Position change and central hemodynamic profile during normal third-trimester pregnancy and postpartum. *Am J Obstet Gynecol* 164(3), 883-887.

Clark, S. et al. (Eds.). (1994). *Handbook of critical care obstetrics.* Boston: Blackwell Scientific.

Conners, A. et al. (1996). The effectiveness of right heart catheterization in the initial care of critically ill patients. *JAMA* 18, 889-897.

Daddario, J. (1999). Trauma in pregnancy. In L. Mandeville & N. Troiano (Eds.). *AWHONN's high risk and critical care intrapartum nursing* (2nd ed.). Philadelphia: J.B. Lippincott.

Dildy, G., Phelan, J., & Cotton, D. (1991). Complications of pregnancy induced hypertension. In S. Clark et al. (Eds.). *Critical care obstetrics* (2nd ed.). Boston: Blackwell Scientific.

Goodwin, T., & Breen, M. (1990). Pregnancy outcome and fetomaternal hemorrhage after noncatastrophic trauma. *Am J Obstet Gynecol* 162, 665-671.

Hankins, G., & Harvey, C. (1993). Critical care of the pregnant patient. In R. Knuppel & J. Drukker (Eds.). *High-risk pregnancy: A team approach* (2nd ed.). Philadelphia: WB Saunders.

Harvey, M. (1994). *Hemodynamic monitoring of the critically ill obstetric patient.* White Plains, NY: March of Dimes Birth Defects Foundation.

Harvey, M. (1999). Physiologic changes during pregnancy. In L. Mandeville & N. Troiano (Eds.). *AWHONN's high risk and critical care intrapartum nursing* (2nd ed.). Philadelphia: J.B. Lippincott.

Harvey, M., & Moretti, M. (1993). Maternal adaptations to pregnancy. In R. Knuppel & J. Drukker (Eds.). *High-risk pregnancy: A team approach* (2nd ed.). Philadelphia: W.B. Saunders.

Harvey, M., & Troiano, N. (1992). Trauma during pregnancy. *NAACOG's Clin Issues Perinat Women's Health Nurs* 3(3), 521-529.

Hinkle, J., & Betz, S. (1995). Gunshot injuries. *AACN Clin Issues* 6(2), 175-186.

Jordan, E., & Pugh, L. (1996). Pregnancy after cardiac transplantation: Principles of nursing care. *J Obstet Gynecol Neonatal Nurs* 25(2), 131-135.

Kilpatrick, S., & Matthay, M. (1992). Obstetric patients requiring critical care: A five-year review. *Chest* 101, 1407-1412.

Laifer, S. et al. (1990). Pregnancy and liver transplantation. *Obstet Gynecol* 76, 1083-1088.

Lavery, J., & Staten-McCormick, M. (1995). Management of moderate to severe trauma in pregnancy. *Obstet Gynecol Clin North Am* 22(1), 69-90.

Lipp-Ziff, E., & Kawanishi, D. (1991). A technique for improving accuracy of the pulmonary artery diastolic pressure as an estimate of left ventricular end-diastolic pressure. *Heart Lung* 20(2), 107-115.

Luppi, C. (1999). Cardiopulmonary resuscitation in pregnancy. In L. Mandeville & N. Troiano (Eds.). *AWHONN's high risk and critical care intrapartum nursing* (2nd ed.). Philadelphia: J.B. Lippincott.

Mabie, W., & Sibai, B. (1990). Treatment in an obstetric intensive care unit. *Am J Obstet Gynecol* 162(1), 1-4.

Mandeville, L., & Troiano, N. (Eds.). (1999). *AWHONN's high risk and critical care intrapartum nursing* (2nd ed.). Philadelphia: J.B. Lippincott.

Mauer, G., & Abriola, D. (1994). Pregnancy following renal transplant. *J Perinat Neonatal Nurs* 8(1), 28-36.

Pearlman, M., & Tintinalli, J. (1991). Evaluation and treatment of the gravida and fetus following trauma during pregnancy. *Obstet Gynecol Clin North Am* 18, 371-381.

Pearlman, M., Tintinalli, J., & Lorenz, R. (1990a). Blunt trauma during pregnancy. *N Engl J Med* 323, 1609-1613.

Pearlman, M., Tintinalli, J., & Lorenz, R. (1990b). A prospective controlled study of outcome after trauma during pregnancy. *Am J Obstet Gynecol* 162, 1505-1510.

Rice, V. (1991). Shock, a clinical syndrome: An update. Part 4. Nursing care of the shock patient. *Crit Care Nurse* 11, 28-32, 35-40.

Ruth-Sahd, L. (1991). Pulmonary contusion: The hidden danger in blunt chest trauma. *Crit Care Nurs* 11, 46-57.

Smith, C., & Phelan, J. (1991). Trauma in pregnancy. In S. Clark et al. (Eds.). *Critical care obstetrics* (2nd ed.). Boston: Blackwell Scientific.

Society of Critical Care Medicine Consensus Development Conference. (1997). Pulmonary artery catheter consensus conference: Consensus statement. *New Horizons* 5(3), 175-193.

Troiano, N. (1991). Trauma during pregnancy. In C. Harvey (Ed.). *Critical care obstetrical nursing.* Gaithersburg, MD: Aspen.

Troiano, N. (1999). Invasive hemodynamic monitoring in obstetrics. In L. Mandeville & N. Troiano (Eds.). *AWHONN's high risk and critical care intrapartum nursing* (2nd ed.). Philadelphia: J.B. Lippincott.

Wallace, D., & Winslow, E. (1993). Effects of iced and room temperature injectate on cardiac output measurements in critically ill patients with low and high cardiac outputs. *Heart Lung* 32(1), 2-12.

35

Mental Health Disorders and Substance Abuse

Anne Hopkins Fishel

EARNING OBJECTIVES

- Define the key terms.
- Discuss emotional complications during pregnancy, including management of anxiety disorders and mood disorders.
- Discuss substance abuse during pregnancy, including dual diagnosis, prevalence, risk factors, legal considerations, treatment programs, barriers to treatment, and care management.

- Differentiate among postpartum emotional complications, including incidence, risk factors, signs and symptoms, and management.
- Summarize the role of the nurse in assessing and managing care of women with emotional complications during pregnancy and postpartum.
- Identify topics for nursing research on mental health disorders and substance abuse in pregnancy.

EY TERMS

anxiety disorder
bipolar disorder
dual diagnosis
mood disorders

obsessive-compulsive disorder
panic disorder
phobias
postpartum depression

postpartum psychosis
posttraumatic stress disorder
substance abuse

anagement of mental health disorders takes place primarily in community settings. Women who have serious mental disorders have an opportunity for engaging in sexual activities that can result in pregnancy. Mental health disorders have implications for the pregnant woman, the fetus, the newborn, and the entire family. Between 10% and 15% of women suffer from these disorders. The symptoms and treatment can complicate pregnancy, childbirth, and the postpartum period (Wintz, 1999).

MENTAL HEALTH DISORDERS DURING PREGNANCY

The pregnant woman may have a history of anxiety disorder, mood disorder, substance use disorder, schizophrenia,

personality disorder, or developmental disorder. If she is currently not in treatment, assessment throughout pregnancy and postpartum is critical to the mother's and the baby's health. With a previous history of mental illness, referral to a mental health specialist for evaluation is recommended.

Anxiety Disorders

Anxiety disorder symptoms often subside completely during pregnancy and reappear in the postpartum period (National Women's Health Resource Center, 1998). Anxiety disorders are the most common mental disorder. They include **phobias** (irrational fears that lead a person to avoid common objects, events, or situations), **panic disorder** (repeated, unprovoked episodes of intense fear, which develop without warning and are not related to any specific event), generalized anxiety disorder (constant worry unrelated to any event), obsessive-compulsive disorder, and posttraumatic stress disorder (American Psychiatric Association [APA], 1994).

Obsessive-compulsive disorder (OCD) is more likely to begin when a woman is pregnant, even if she has never experienced OCD symptoms. Symptoms of OCD include recurrent, persistent, and intrusive thoughts that cause anxiety that a person tries to control by performing repetitive behaviors or "compulsions" (APA, 1994). The pregnant woman may experience persistent thoughts that something is wrong with the baby, or she may become very preoccupied with checking and rechecking to make sure the baby is all right. Although she recognizes that these rituals are excessive, she will still perform them because of the fear that harm will come to her or the baby if she does not. Treatment usually includes antidepressant medication such as fluvoxamine (Luvox), cognitive-behavioral therapy, and education about the illness and how to manage the symptoms (Fishel, 1998).

Posttraumatic stress disorder (PTSD) can occur as a result of rape (see Chapter 11). Symptoms include re-experiencing the traumatic event, persistent avoidance of stimuli, and numbing, as well as difficulty sleeping, irritability or angry outbursts, difficulty concentrating, hypervigilance, and exaggerated startle response (APA, 1994). Nurses can support the healing process of persons with PTSD by being alert to what the woman is experiencing during pregnancy and labor (Clark, 1997).

If the current pregnancy is a result of rape, the woman may be extremely ambivalent about the baby. If the rape occurred some time ago, the whole experience of pregnancy with prenatal examinations can trigger memories of the original trauma. She may avoid prenatal examinations because of the anxiety triggered by bodily touch and vaginal examinations. Some pregnant women with PTSD may feel more comfortable with a female nurse-midwife or female physician. Giving birth can trigger memories of being out of control, and she may lose contact with reality. The nurse can verbalize understanding of the anxiety and orient to current reality by saying, "You're having an examination to make sure the baby is okay" or "You're in labor preparing to give birth to your baby. I am your nurse. You're in the hospital. I will stay with you. You are safe here." Treatment usually includes psychotherapy and referral to support groups.

Collaborative Care

Although antidepressant medications may be used to help control the symptoms of anxiety and panic, some women would prefer to avoid medications during their pregnancy. Other women who have been using benzodiazepines for "anxiety," nervousness," or insomnia may not realize that these medications are teratogenic and that their use during pregnancy is not advised (Kaplan &

BOX 35-1	Commonly Used Benzodiazepines

Alprazolam (Xanax)
Chlordiazepoxide (Librium)
Clonazepam (Lonopin)
Clorazepate (Tranxene)
Diazepam (Valium)
Flurazepam (Dalmane)
Lorazepam (Ativan)
Midazolam (Versed)
Temazepam (Restoril)
Triazolam (Halcion)

Sadack, 1998). The use of benzodiazepines in the third trimester can precipitate a withdrawal syndrome in newborns. Nurses should educate women about the dangers of benzodiazepines during pregnancy, assess for use during pregnancy, and help pregnant women find other ways to handle their anxiety, or refer them to a psychiatrist who specializes in psychiatric disorders in pregnancy. Nursing strategies to reduce anxiety include empowerment through education; sensory interventions such as music therapy and aromatherapy; behavioral interventions such as breathing exercises, progressive muscle relaxation, guided imagery, and medication; and cognitive strategies such as encouraging positive self-talk and questioning negative thinking (Fishel, 1998) (Box 35-1).

Mood Disorders

Women who are being treated for depression may get pregnant, either intentionally or accidentally. **Mood disorders** are defined as disorders that have as their dominant feature a disturbance in the prevailing emotional state. To be diagnosed with major depression, at least five of the following must be present nearly every day: depressed mood, often with spontaneous crying; markedly diminished interest in all activities; insomnia or hypersomnia; weight changes (increases and decreases); psychomotor retardation or agitation; fatigue or loss of energy; feelings of worthlessness or inappropriate guilt; diminished ability to concentrate; and suicidal ideation with or without a suicidal plan (Fishel, 1995).

Approximately 6% of women develop depression for the first time during their pregnancy. Depressive symptoms may be evident during the first trimester of pregnancy, as early as 10 to 14 weeks, in women who have no history of depression (Pederson, 1998). This finding dispels the myth that early pregnancy is a pleasant and happy event for all women.

NURSE ALERT *Diagnostic assessment for depression in pregnant women is difficult because many of the symptoms of pregnancy mimic depression. Critical cues are the presence of psychologic symptoms, a suicide plan,* *and major disruptions in sleep pattern. Risk factors for developing depression in pregnancy include a prior history in self or family, a lack of social support, stressful life events, partner discord, and history of PMS.*

Collaborative Care

Medical management of depression is usually a combination of antidepressants, cognitive-behavioral or interpersonal psychotherapy, and self-help strategies such as exercise, respite from caregiving, self-help groups, and making time for self (Fishel, 1999). Nursing strategies include educating the woman about depression as an illness, about treatment success, and about antidepressant medications. For the woman who refuses medications during pregnancy, the nurse should discuss alternative treatments and respect her choice. The nurse also can be effective by maintaining a caring relationship, which includes being hopeful. The nurse can ask about a time when the woman was coping well and how she was able to combat the depression then.

If a woman becomes psychotic during pregnancy, usually because she has quit taking mood stabilizers or antipsychotics, or because she has a history of schizophrenia, this is a medical emergency. To treat a psychotic state, antipsychotic medication or electroconvulsive therapy is preferable to lithium or anticonvulsant medications (Kaplan & Sadock, 1998).

Antidepressant medications. There is no consensus about safety in the use of antidepressant medications with pregnant women. If possible, the medications should be stopped preconception through the first trimester (Schatzberg & Nemeroff, 1998). For women with severe depression who would be at risk of suicide without medication, clinical judgment usually dictates continued use of antidepressants. The commonly used antidepressant drugs are often divided into four groups: selective serotonin reuptake inhibitors (SSRIs), heterocyclics (including tricyclic antidepressants [TCAs]), monoamine oxidase inhibitors (MAOIs), and other antidepressant agents not in the above classifications (Keltner & Folks, 1997) (Box 35-2). None of these medications is rated for use in pregnancy as a Food and Drug Administration (FDA) Category A drug (controlled studies show no risk to the fetus). The only ones classified as Category B (no evidence of risk in humans) are maprotiline (Ludiomil), bupropion (Wellbutrin), fluoxetine (Prozac), fluvoxamine (Luvox), paroxetine (Paxil), and sertraline (Zoloft). The remaining antidepressant medications are rated as Category C (risk cannot be ruled out, but potential benefits may justify potential risk) or D (positive evidence of risk to the fetus but potential benefits may outweigh risk). Many scientists are reluctant to do research on the effects of psychotropic medications on fetuses. Minimal research appears in the literature; however, two recent studies reported no harm to the fetus who was exposed to antidepressants. Nulman and others (1997) found no effect from TCAs and fluoxetine on global IQ, language development, or behavioral develop-

---

BOX 35-2 Antidepressant Medications

SELECTIVE SEROTONIN REUPTAKE INHIBITORS
Fluoxetine (Prozac)
Fluvoxamine (Luvox)
Paroxetine (Paxil)
Sertraline (Zoloft)

HETEROCYCLICS/TRICYCLICS
Amitriptyline (Elavil)
Amoxapine (Asendin)
Clomipramine (Anafranil)
Desipramine (Norpramin)
Doxepin (Sinequan)
Imipramine (Tofranil)
Nortriptyline (Pamelor)
Maprotiline (Ludiomil)
Protriptyline (Vivactil)

MONOAMINE OXIDASE INHIBITORS
Phenelzine (Nardil)
Tranylcypromine (Parnate)

OTHER AGENTS
Bupropion (Wellbutrin)
Mirtazepine (Remeron)
Nefazodone (Serzone)
Trazodone (Desyrel)
Venlafaxine (Effexor)

---

ment. Kulin and others (1998) reported that fluvoxamine, paroxetine, and sertraline do not appear to increase the teratogenic risk when used in correct doses.

The SSRIs are prescribed more frequently today than other groups of antidepressant medications. They are relatively safe and carry fewer side effects than the TCAs. However, if an SSRI is taken with dextromethorphan, an agent found in cough syrup, the combination could trigger the serotonin syndrome (mental status changes, agitation, hyperreflexia, shivering, diarrhea, etc.) (Keltner & Folks, 1997). The most frequent side effects with the SSRIs are gastrointestinal (GI) disturbances (nausea, diarrhea), headache, and insomnia. In about one third of patients, the SSRIs reduce libido, arousal, or orgasmic function. SSRIs can also inhibit specific P-450 isoenzymes, resulting in marked elevations in drug concentrations and reduction in drug clearance.

The TCAs cause many central nervous system (CNS) and peripheral nervous system (PNS) side effects. Although some are simply annoying, others are significant or even dangerous (Keltner & Folks, 1997). In overdose, these medications can cause death. A common CNS effect is sedation, and this could easily interfere with mothers caring for their babies. A mother could doze off while holding the baby and drop him or her, or she could have trouble getting fully awake during the night to care for the baby. Other side effects include weight gain, tremors, grand mal seizures, nightmares, agitation or mania, and extrapyramidal side effects. Anticholinergic side effects include dry mouth, blurred vision (usually temporary), difficulty voiding, constipation, sweating, and orgasm difficulty (Keltner & Folks, 1997).

Medications to avoid during pregnancy. If the pregnant woman is receiving pharmacologic treatment, the nurse must make sure that the woman is being followed by a psychiatrist or an advanced practice psychiatric nurse. The basic rule is to avoid administering any medication to a woman who is pregnant, particularly during the first trimester (Kaplan & Sadock, 1998). Medications that must be avoided are mood stabilizers such as lithium carbonate; anticonvulsants such as carbamazepine (Tegretol) and divalproex sodium (Depakote); and the benzodiazepines (Kaplan & Sadock, 1998; Schatzberg & Nemeroff, 1998). Mood stabilizers (including the anticonvulsants) are often taken over the lifetime by women with bipolar disorder. Lithium administration during pregnancy is associated with a high incidence of birth abnormalities, including Ebstein's anomaly, a serious abnormality in cardiac development (Kaplan & Sadock, 1998). Anticonvulsants used during pregnancy are associated with fetal craniofacial and neural tube abnormalities in less than 10% of infants. The administration of psychotherapeutic medications at or near birth may cause a baby to be overly sedated at birth and need a respirator, or to be physically dependent on the drug and to require detoxification and treatment of a withdrawal syndrome.

SUBSTANCE ABUSE DURING PREGNANCY

The damaging effects of alcohol and illicit drugs on pregnant women and their unborn babies are well documented (National Women's Health Resource Center, 1998). Alcohol and other drugs easily pass from a mother to her baby through the placenta. Smoking during pregnancy has serious health risks, including bleeding complications, miscarriage, stillbirth, prematurity, low birth weight, and sudden infant death syndrome (National Women's Health Resource Center, 1998). Congenital abnormalities have occurred in infants of mothers who have taken drugs (Stuart & Laraia, 1998). The safest pregnancy is one in which the mother is totally drug and alcohol free, with one exception: for pregnant women addicted to heroin, methadone maintenance is safer for the fetus than acute opiate detoxification (Stuart & Laraia, 1998).

Substance abuse refers to the continued use of substances despite related problems in physical, social, or interpersonal areas (APA, 1994). Recurrent abuse results in failure to fulfill major role obligations, and there may be substance-related legal problems. Any use of alcohol or illicit drugs during pregnancy is considered abuse (APA, 1994).

Dual diagnosis is the coexistence of substance abuse and psychiatric disorders within the same person. Approximately 4.7% of the population has dual diagnosis (Naegle, 1997). Major depression and anxiety disorders are the psychiatric disorders that commonly occur with substance abuse.

Prevalence

Because many pregnant women are reluctant to reveal their use of substances or to reveal the extent of their use, data on prevalence are highly variable. One study of North Carolina prenatal clients reported that before pregnancy, 62% of the women had used one or more substances (cigarettes, alcohol, or illegal drugs); and during pregnancy, 31% had used one or more substances. This study is significant in that half of the women stopped using during their pregnancy (Finkelstein, 1999). Out of 4 million pregnant women in the United States, 820,000 used tobacco, 757,000 used alcohol, and 50,000 women used illicit drugs (Finkelstein, 1999). Although tobacco and alcohol were most often reported, public opinion seems to view illicit drugs as the bigger problem.

Risk Factors

Women have a clearer pattern of self-medication and are more likely than men to use a combination of alcohol and prescription drugs. Women begin to use following depression, to relax on dates, to feel more adequate, to lose weight, to decrease stress, or to help them sleep at night (National Women's Health Resource Center, 1998). Poor self-esteem is a major issue for most women who develop problems with drugs and alcohol. A history of psychiatric illness or a history of physical or sexual abuse greatly increases a woman's risk for developing substance abuse problems (National Women's Health Resource Center, 1998).

Research on 80 mothers of children with fetal alcohol syndrome (FAS) revealed that as a group, the mothers were found to be extremely fragile. Eighty percent had a major mental illness; 100% had been seriously sexually, physically, or emotionally abused; 80% lived with men who did not want them to stop drinking; and 60% had phobias that caused them to be reluctant to leave home and seek help (Clarren, 1999). In a study of 2000 prenatal clients in North Carolina, 26% had been victims of violence during their lives (Martin et al., 1996). Both before and during pregnancy, victims of violence were significantly more likely to use multiple substances than were nonvictims. Continuation of substance use during pregnancy was significantly more likely among victims of violence than among nonvictims.

Barriers to Treatment

Pregnant women who abuse substances commonly have little understanding of the ways in which these substances affect them, their pregnancies, or their babies. Pregnant

RESEARCH

Knowledge and Attitudes of Registered Nurses Toward Perinatal Substance Abuse

The problem of perinatal substance abuse is a continuing one in today's society. There continues to be significant morbidity and mortality among women, their infants, and their children who are exposed to these substances prenatally. However, nurses and other health care professionals receive little content on substance abuse in their education.

The purposes of this descriptive study were to explore the knowledge and attitudes of registered nurses toward perinatal substance abuse and determine the relationships between registered nurses' knowledge of and attitudes toward perinatal substance abuse. Three hundred ninety-two registered nurses employed at Florida perinatal units completed the 34-item adapted Attitudes About Drug Abuse in Pregnancy (AADAP) questionnaire. Knowledge scores for this sample ranged from 6 to 18 (mean: 12.144) out of a possible score of 20. Attitude scores ranged from 16 to 56 (mean: 35.81) out of a possible range of 14 to 70. Scores at the lower end of the scale indicate punitive, negative attitudes.

It was concluded that registered nurses demonstrated limited knowledge about substance exposure, addiction, and its effects. Nurses were also found to hold attitudes that were more punitive and negative than positive or supportive toward women who abused substances during the perinatal period. Nurses in this study demonstrated increased knowledge and more positive attitudes if substance abuse information was included in their nursing curricula.

CLINICAL APPLICATION

Pregnancy presents an opportunity to motivate women to stop their abuse of substances. To do so, nurses must be armed with knowledge and information necessary to screen and identify women who abuse substances while pregnant. They must also maintain a nonjudgmental, nonpunitive attitude. It is with this knowledge and understanding that nurses are most likely to exhibit positive behaviors and attitudes while they provide support for women needing substance abuse treatment. A two-pronged approach is needed to provide the substance abuse education necessary for the nursing profession: expansion of content in nursing curricula and education of practicing nurses.

Source: Selleck, C., & Redding, B. (1998). Knowledge and attitudes of registered nurses toward perinatal substance abuse. *J Obstet Gynecol Neonatal Nurs* 27(1), 70-77.

women who are substance abusers often do not seek prenatal care until labor begins. Often, pregnant mothers who use psychoactive substances receive negative feedback from society, as well as from health care providers, who may not only condemn them for endangering the life of their fetus, but may even withhold support as a result (see Research box). Substance-abusing women are often viewed as sexually promiscuous, weak willed, negligent of their children, and irresponsible in their decisions to bear more children (Finkelstein, 1994). Stigma, shame, and guilt lead to high denial of drinking or drug problems both by the woman herself and by family members and friends, who conceal the abuse from outsiders to protect the abuser (Finkelstein, 1994). In addition, numerous studies have reported that lack of services for mothers and children together and lack of child care and children's treatment are major barriers to treatment for substance-abusing mothers (Finkelstein, 1994).

Legal Considerations

Because of the risks to the unborn children, pregnant women who abuse substances may now face criminal charges under expanded interpretations of child abuse and drug-trafficking statutes. Some states are prosecuting pregnant women on charges of child abuse because they be-

came pregnant while addicted to drugs. Some policymakers have proposed that pregnant women who abuse substances should be jailed, placed under house arrest, or committed to psychiatric hospitals for the remainder of their pregnancies (Stuart & Laraia, 1998). Nurses can play a positive role by advocating primary prevention programs and counseling and treatment programs for those already addicted.

LEGAL TIP Drug Testing During Pregnancy

There is no state requirement for a health care provider to test either the mother or the newborn for the presence of drugs. However, nurses need to know the practices of the states in which they are working. In some states a woman whose urine drug screen test is positive at the time of labor and birth must be referred to child protective services. If the mother is not in a drug treatment program or is judged unable to provide care, the infant may be placed in foster care.

Cigarette Smoking and Caffeine Consumption

Cigarette smoking and caffeine consumption are two examples of legal substances that can be addicting or harm-

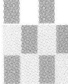

PLAN of CARE | Substance Abuse During Pregnancy

NURSING DIAGNOSIS Altered nutrition: less than body requirements related to insufficient intake for prenatal metabolic needs as evidenced by insufficient weight gain for gestational age of fetus

Expected Outcome *Client will maintain steady weight gain appropriate for trimester of pregnancy.*

Nursing Interventions/*Rationales*

Compare current client weight to prepregnant weight *to assess if weight is appropriate for trimester of pregnancy.*

Assess client's current diet plan and caloric intake *to identify where modifications are necessary.*

Provide client with information regarding nutritional requirements during pregnancy *to assist client to provide modifications to diet and promote self-care.*

Weigh client frequently *to establish client compliance and effectiveness of plan.*

NURSING DIAGNOSIS Ineffective individual coping related to lack of support system as evidenced by client verbalization of concerns

Expected Outcome *Client will express satisfaction with identified effective coping methods.*

Nursing Interventions/*Rationales*

Remain nonjudgmental while listening to client express feelings and concerns *to promote trust.*

Assist client to identify positive coping methods and strengths *to promote involvement in self-care.*

Encourage client to take responsibility for activities leading to recovery *to promote self-care, self-esteem, and responsibility for self and fetus's well-being.*

Refer to appropriate health professionals and support groups *to promote involvement and responsibility in health and well-being of self and fetus.*

---

ful to the pregnant woman and her fetus and the newborn. Effects of nicotine and caffeine on the woman are discussed in Chapter 5. Effects on the fetus and newborn are discussed in Chapter 39.

Alcohol

Prenatal alcohol exposure is the single greatest preventable cause of mental retardation (National Women's Health Resource Center, 1998). One of the greatest risks of alcohol use during pregnancy is FAS, as well as fetal alcohol effects (FAE). Low birth weight, mental retardation, behavioral problems, and learning and physical problems are some of the symptoms of FAS babies (Clarren, 1999) (see Chapter 39). Severe facial deformities of FAS occur at day 20 of conception (Clarren, 1999)—a time when women may not even suspect they are pregnant. Alcohol use during pregnancy can cause high blood pressure, miscarriage, premature birth, stillbirth, and anemia (National Women's Health Resource Center, 1998). In addition, women may experience nutritional deficiencies, pancreatitis, alcoholic hepatitis, deficient milk ejection, and cirrhosis (Center for Substance Abuse Treatment, 1993).

Approximately 1% to 5% of pregnant women meet the diagnostic criteria for alcoholism (Thorpe, 1995). Accurate data are difficult to obtain because alcohol is rapidly absorbed in the small intestine and metabolized in the liver, so it is difficult to test for its presence in blood. The underdiagnosing and underreporting of alcohol use in pregnancy is a major concern of health care providers.

Symptoms occurring during alcohol withdrawal can be managed with short-acting barbiturates or benzodiazepines; however, they are potentially teratogenic. Some clinicians recommend avoiding their use if at all possible. Disulfiram (Antabuse), a medication that acts as a deterrent to alcohol ingestion because it produces a dramatic, unpleasant reaction when small amounts of alcohol are consumed, is contraindicated during pregnancy. Its use has been associated with clubfoot and other problems (Center for Substance Abuse Treatment, 1993). Two medications that have been proven efficacious for decreasing alcohol intake, Naltrexone and Acamprosate (http://www.ahcpr.gov/clinic/alcosumm.htm), have not been tested in pregnant women and therefore should be avoided (see Plan of Care).

Marijuana

Marijuana is a substance derived from the cannabis plant. It is usually rolled into a cigarette and smoked, but it may also be mixed into food and eaten. Marijuana produces an altered state of awareness, relaxation, mild euphoria, and reduced inhibition (Stuart & Laraia, 1998). Prolonged use may lead to apathy, lack of energy, loss of desire to work or be productive, diminished concentration, poor personal hygiene, and preoccupation with marijuana—the amotivational syndrome (Stuart & Laraia, 1998). Marijuana readily crosses the placenta and causes increased carbon monoxide levels in the mother's blood, which reduces the oxygen supply to the fetus. Research findings regarding the effects of marijuana on pregnancy are inconsistent; however, it may cause fetal abnormalities (Stuart & Laraia, 1998).

Cocaine

Cocaine is a powerful CNS stimulant that blocks the reuptake of norepinephrine and dopamine at the nerve endings. Because more neurotransmitter is present at the synapse, the receptors are continuously activated. It is believed that this causes the euphoria. At the same time, presynaptic supplies of dopamine and norepinephrine are depleted. This causes the "crash" that happens when the effect of the drug wears off (Stuart & Laraia, 1998). The euphoria caused by cocaine is short acting, starting with a 10- to 20-second rush and followed by 15 to 20 minutes of less intense euphoria (Stuart & Laraia, 1998). A person who is high on cocaine feels euphoric, energetic, self-confident, and sociable. The relapse rate for clients who try to discontinue cocaine use is very high (Stuart & Laraia, 1998).

The smokable form of cocaine is produced by a process called freebasing. Crack is cocaine mixed with baking soda and heated until it reaches its purest form. It is sold in the form of "rocks," which are smoked in pipes. Crack is used by people from all cultures, and the low cost and availability make it the drug of choice among the economically disadvantaged. Because crack is highly addictive, it poses new problems for health care providers who care for pregnant addicts. In the United States, approximately 10% to 15% of all pregnant women use cocaine (Glantz & Woods, 1993).

Predisposing factors and problems associated with cocaine use in pregnancy are polydrug use, poor nutrition, poverty, sexually transmitted infections, hepatitis B infection, dysfunctional family systems, employment difficulties, stress, anger, poor self-esteem, and previous or present physical, emotional, and sexual abuse (Fox, 1994). The clinical manifestations of cocaine use include tachycardia, pupillary dilation, and hypertension.

Medical complications of cocaine use in pregnancy range from mild to severe. Some of the less serious medical problems are lack of energy, insomnia, sinusitis, nose bleeds, sore throat, and decreased libido. More serious problems develop as the person's general health deteriorates. These include perforation of the nasal septum, increased cardiovascular stress, tachycardia, systemic hypertension, ventricular dysrhythmias, sudden coronary artery spasm, and myocardial infarction. Cocaine-associated complications also include liver damage, intestinal ischemia, pulmonary disease with acute pulmonary edema, seizures, hemorrhagic bronchitis, headache, and death. Needle-borne diseases such as hepatitis B and acquired immunodeficiency syndrome (AIDS) are common among cocaine users. Needle tracks, septic phlebitis, cellulitis, and superficial abscesses are seen in intravenous drug users. The tachycardia and subsequent rise in blood pressure is caused by the increasing levels of catecholamines produced by the cocaine. During pregnancy, uterine blood vessels are normally maximally dilated, but they vasoconstrict in the presence of catecholamines. The separation of the placenta (abruption) or the acute onset of preterm labor with long, hard contractions and precipitous birth seen in pregnant women after the intravenous administration of cocaine probably is secondary to acute spasm of uterine blood vessels (Chisum, 1990). Maternal cocaine use also has been identified as a risk factor for abdominal pregnancy (Audain et al., 1999).

With consequences such as these, one wonders why pregnant women use cocaine. To begin to answer this question, a nurse researcher interviewed 60 women who reported using crack cocaine at least once a week during pregnancy (Kearney, 1997). A basic social psychologic process, "salvaging self," was identified. Threats that the pregnancy created led the women to delay acknowledging their pregnancies. As pregnancy progressed, women felt guilt, fear, and the need to take action. They used "facing the situation" and "evading harm" to salvage themselves and "maximize well-being" within their social worlds. They tried to reduce harm and manage stigma to decrease damage to the fetus and to their identities.

One of the newer and promising treatments for cocaine abuse in pregnancy is acupuncture. A component of traditional Chinese medicine, acupuncture is used to redirect energy flow (chi) within the body, reduce cravings, and enhance well-being. The pace and location of the flow of chi can be influenced by the insertion of needles at certain points along the meridians to facilitate harmony (Bennett, 1995). Studies of acupuncture alone or in combination with other therapies have had mixed results. In two studies, acupuncture reduced drug use more rapidly than did standard therapy and improved treatment retention during the initial stages of treatment (Konefal, Duncan, & Clemence, 1994; Richard et al., 1995). In a comparison case study of two pregnant women, one treated with acupuncture and the other treated with traditional therapies, the results were clearly better for the acupuncture-treated client (Bennett, 1995). She had only one relapse and delivered a full-term, healthy baby. The pregnant woman treated with traditional Western methods continued to use substances and delivered a premature baby (1474 kg) following abruptio placentae. Treatment costs were estimated at $133,800 for the traditionally treated woman and $4050 for the woman receiving acupuncture (Bennett, 1995).

Opiates

The opiates include opium, heroin, meperidine, morphine, codeine, and methadone. Methadone is used to treat addiction to other opiates. It can be used either to aid withdrawal or to provide maintenance at a stable dose. Clients taking methadone may work and live normally, although still addicted to narcotics. Heroin is one of the most commonly abused drugs of this class. It is usually taken by intravenous injection but can be smoked or "snorted." The signs and symptoms of heroin use are euphoria, relaxation, relief from pain, "nodding out" (apathy, detachment from reality, impaired judgment, and drowsiness), constricted pupils, nausea, constipation, slurred speech, and respiratory depression (APA, 1994).

The incidence of heroin use among pregnant women is unknown; however, those women with a dependency on heroin may use multiple drugs. Possible effects on pregnancy include preeclampsia, intrauterine growth restriction, miscarriage, premature rupture of membranes, infections, breech presentation, and preterm labor (Center for Substance Abuse Treatment, 1993). Possible effects on the mother include poor nourishment with vitamin, iron, and folic acid deficiencies; medical complications from frequent use of dirty needles; sexually transmitted infections; and hypertension (Center for Substance Abuse Treatment, 1993).

The recommended treatment is methadone maintenance combined with psychotherapy. This is a well-documented approach to improve outcomes for both the woman and her fetus (Center for Substance Abuse Treatment, 1993). The other approach is slow medical withdrawal with methadone, but the safety of this second approach is questionable. In pregnancy, methadone is metabolized more rapidly, leading to withdrawal symptoms in less than 24 hours in many women. Withdrawal symptoms can include fetal hyperactivity and if severe, preterm labor or fetal death. Women may resort to heroin to alleviate these uncomfortable symptoms. Doses of methadone that increase during the course of pregnancy and are delivered in split doses (morning and evening) are most effective in preventing withdrawal and subsequent heroin use (Kearney, 1997).

Methamphetamine

The active metabolite of methamphetamine is amphetamine, a CNS stimulant known as "speed" and "meth." Agents used as appetite suppressants or diet pills are closely related substances. The crystalline form of methamphetamine is known as "ice." When smoked, it produces a long, steady high and is more addictive than heroin. Ice enables a person to go without rest or food for 24 hours, only to "crash" for the next 24 hours.

Approximately 2% of the adult population has used methamphetamine at some time during their lives (APA, 1994). It is used by people from all levels of society, but its use is most common in the 18- to 30-year-old age group.

Clinical manifestations of methamphetamine use are euphoria, abrupt awakening, increased energy, talkativeness, agitation, tachycardia, tachypnea, hyperactivity, irritability, grandiosity, diaphoresis, weight loss, insomnia, hypertension, increased temperature, ectopic heartbeat, urinary retention, constipation, dry mouth, paranoid delusions, and violent behavior. Seizures, cardiac shock, and death may occur as a result of overdose (Stuart & Laraia, 1998). Most of the effects of amphetamines are similar to those of cocaine.

Although fewer maternal and neonatal complications have been attributed to this class of substances than to cocaine (APA, 1994), the rates of preterm births and of intrauterine growth restriction with smaller head circumference are higher in methamphetamine-exposed pregnant women than in pregnant women who abuse other substances.

Phencyclidine

Phencyclidine (PCP) is a synthetic drug known by various names (peace pill, elephant, angel dust, hog). Its use is more prevalent among ethnic minorities and in people between the ages of 18 and 40. Its effects are unpredictable and include hostility, aggressiveness, and other bizarre behavior (Cook, Peterson, & Moore, 1994). Signs and symptoms of PCP use include confusion, disorientation, euphoria, hallucinations, paranoia, grandiosity, agitation, a tendency toward violence, and antisocial behavior, but the severity of these symptoms depends on the dose. Clinical manifestations include red, dry skin; dilated pupils; nystagmus; ataxia; hypertension; rigidity; and seizures (Stuart & Laraia, 1998). Because some effects mimic the signs and symptoms of schizophrenia, a user may be admitted to a psychiatric unit.

After use, PCP persists in the brain and body fat for an extended period. In pregnant women it crosses the placenta, and its concentration in fetal tissue tends to be higher than that in maternal tissue. In fact, fetal levels may be as much as 10 times higher than maternal levels (Glantz & Woods, 1993). However, an appreciation of the specific effects of PCP on pregnancy, the fetus, and the neonate has been limited by the fact that it tends to be used in various combinations with alcohol, cocaine, and marijuana (Cook et al., 1994). The major concerns regarding PCP use in pregnant women are its association with polydrug abuse and the neurobehavioral effects on the neonate (Glantz & Woods, 1993). See Table 35-1 for psychologic and physiologic effects of selected illicit drugs.

▋ CARE MANAGEMENT

Assessment and Nursing Diagnoses

The care of the substance-dependent pregnant woman is based on historical data, symptoms, physical findings, and laboratory results. The nurse should include screening questions for alcohol and drug abuse in the overall assessment of the first prenatal visit of all women. Any judgmental attitude on the part of the nurse will be evident to the client and will interfere with the development of trust and with an accurate report of consumption (Cefalo & Moos, 1995). Information about drug use should be obtained by first asking about the woman's intake of over-the-counter and prescribed medications. Next, her usage of legal drugs, such as caffeine, nicotine, and alcohol, should be ascertained. Finally, the woman should be questioned about her use of illicit drugs, such as cocaine,

TABLE 35-1 Psychoactive Substance Effects

DRUG	PSYCHOLOGIC SIGNS	PHYSIOLOGIC SIGNS
ALCOHOL		
Intoxication	Labile mood	Slurred speech
	Impaired attention	Flushed face
	Irritability	Unsteady gait
	Talkativeness	Nystagmus
Withdrawal	Anxiety	Nausea and vomiting
	Depressed mood	Malaise or weakness
	Maladaptive behavior	Hyperactivity
		Coarse tremor of hands, tongue, eyelids
		Orthostatic hypertension
COCAINE		
Intoxication	Psychomotor agitation	Tachycardia
	Elation	Pupillary dilation
	Grandiosity	Hypertension
	Hypervigilance	Perspiration, chills
	Maladaptive behaviors	Nausea; vomiting
Withdrawal	Depressed mood	Fatigue
	Disturbed sleep	Headache
	Increased dreaming	Convulsions
HEROIN		
Intoxication	Euphoria	Pupillary constriction
	Psychomotor retardation	Drowsiness
	Apathy	Slurred speech
	Maladaptive behavior	
	Impaired attention	
Withdrawal	Insomnia	Lacrimation
		Rhinorrhea
		Pupillary dilation
		Sweating
		Diarrhea
		Yawning
		Mild hypertension
		Tachycardia
		Fever
METHAMPHETAMINE		
Intoxication	Hyperactivity	Tachycardia, palpitations
	Insomnia	Tachypnea
	Restlessness	Nausea, vomiting
	Irritability	Constipation
	Aggressiveness	Impotence
Withdrawal	Depression	Headache
	Increased sleeping	Nausea, vomiting
	Lethargy	Muscle pain
		Weakness
PHENCYCLIDINE (PCP)	Euphoria	Vertical or horizontal nystagmus
	Psychomotor agitation	Hypertension
	Increased anxiety	Increased heart rate
	Emotional lability	Numbness
	Grandiosity	Decreased response to pain
	Sensation of slowed time	Ataxia, dysarthria
	Synesthesias	
	Maladaptive behaviors	

heroin, and marijuana. The approximate frequency and amount should be documented for each drug used (Redding & Selleck, 1993).

The CAGE Questionnaire (Ewing, 1984) (Box 35-3) and the Brief Michigan Alcoholism Screening Test (MAST) (Pokorny, Miller, & Kaplan, 1972) are two well-known screens for alcohol use that are often administered by the nurse or included in the written previsit questionnaire. On the CAGE, if the woman answers yes to even one question, that is considered positive for substance abuse. One of the problems with these questionnaires is that they have not been tested for reliability with pregnant women. Two screening tests, the T-ACE (Hankin & Sokol, 1995) (Box 35-4) and the TWEAK (Russell, 1994), have been developed to screen specifically for alcohol abuse during pregnancy. Urine screening is unreliable because alcohol is undetectable within a few hours following ingestion (Redding & Selleck, 1993). Abnormal liver function studies can provide diagnostic data about physical effects of alcohol abuse.

Urine toxicology testing is often performed to screen for illicit drug use. Drugs may be found in urine days to weeks after ingestion, depending on how quickly they are metabolized and excreted from the body (Gilbert & Harmon, 1998).

In addition to screening for alcohol and drug abuse, the nurse should also screen for physical and sexual abuse and history of psychiatric illness, because these are risk factors in women who abuse substances. Substance-abusing women feel much stigma, shame, and guilt, which leads to denial of the abuse. If the nurse can help reduce those feelings, the woman will be more apt to confide in the nurse, and that is the first step in receiving help. Also, asking about how their spouses or partners feel about using substances can reveal whether there are family supports or barriers.

Initial and serial ultrasound studies may be performed to determine the gestational age, because amenorrhea, which is common among drug users, precludes dating on the basis of the history of the last menstrual period. Because of concerns about stillbirth and increased frequency of the birth of small-for-gestational-age infants, and the potential for hypoxia, nonstress testing may be performed, at least in the third trimester, in those pregnant women who are known substance abusers (Glantz & Woods, 1993).

All states mandate that nurses report suspected child abuse or neglect, and these reports must be made in a timely manner and for each separate incident. Nurses who have filed a report with Children's Protective Services because of a mother's perinatal substance abuse have shared feelings of being torn between the mandated reporting law and trying to maintain some connectedness with the mother (Kovalesky & Flagler, 1997). Child custody loss can elicit feelings of grief, anger, or hopelessness in women and can promote or inhibit recovery from their addiction. Recurrent pregnancies in women who have lost custody of one or more children and who are not in recovery also are

BOX 35-3 CAGE Questionnaire

C	Have you ever felt you ought to CUT DOWN on your drinking?
A	Have people ANNOYED you by criticizing your drinking?
G	Have you ever felt bad or GUILTY about your drinking?
E	Have you ever had a drink first thing in the morning to steady your nerves or get rid of a hangover? EYE-OPENER

BOX 35-4 T-ACE Test

- How many drinks can you hold before getting sleepy or passing out? (TOLERANCE)
- Have people ANNOYED you by criticizing your drinking?
- Have you ever felt you ought to CUT DOWN on your drinking?
- Have you ever had a drink first thing in the morning to steady your nerves or get rid of a hangover? (EYE-OPENER)

Scoring: Two points are given for the TOLERANCE question for the ability to hold at least a six pack of beer or a bottle of wine. A "yes" answer to any of the other questions receives one point. An overall score of ≥ 2 indicates a high probability that the woman is a risk drinker.

Source: Hankin, J., & Sokol, R. (1995). Identification and care of problems associated with alcohol ingestion in pregnancy. *Semin Perinatol* 19(4), 286.

common. Information about the women's experiences and the various types of out-of-home placements for children can assist nurses in planning interventions that help mothers process their feelings about custody loss (Kovalesky & Flagler, 1997). Nursing diagnoses for the woman who is a substance abuser may include the following:

Nursing Diagnoses

- Risk for fluid volume deficit related to
  - effects of excessive use of psychoactive drugs
- Risk for altered nutrition: less than body requirements related to
  - effects of excessive use of psychoactive drugs
- Risk for injury to self, fetus, or newborn related to
  - sensory effects of drug
- Risk of infection related to
  - lifestyle
  - dehydration and malnutrition
  - method of administration of drug

Continued

⁞ Nursing Diagnoses—cont'd_____

- Self-care deficit, bathing or hygiene, related to
  - effects of substance used
- Denial related to
  - stigma
  - shame
  - guilt
- Ineffective individual coping related to
  - lack of support system
  - low self-esteem
  - lack of anger management techniques
- Risk for violence related to
  - maintenance of drug habit
  - effects of substance used
  - lifestyle
- Hopelessness related to
  - inability to stop using substances
- Powerlessness related to
  - lack of resources
  - relationship with abusive partners
- Risk for suicide related to
  - depression
  - impulsivity while on substances

Expected Outcomes of Care

Planning the care for a pregnant woman who is a substance abuser must take into consideration the woman's lifestyle and habits. The ideal long-term outcome would be total abstinence, but the woman may be unable to face that level of commitment at that time. The thought of giving up the substance forever only provokes anxiety. A realistic goal may be to cut down on the use of substances. Short-term outcomes are necessary, and the woman must participate in the formulation of these expected outcomes. The outcomes must be stated in clear behavioral expectations. The expected outcomes may be written as a contract that is then signed by the woman and the nurse, and a copy is given to the woman. Short-term outcomes for the woman and her family may include the following:

- The woman will keep appointments for prenatal and postpartum care for herself and the well baby care for the infant.
- Fetal effects will be minimized; baby will be safe.
- The woman's physiologic symptoms will stabilize and she will be able to care for herself and her infant.
- The woman will become involved in a substance abuse treatment program.

Plan of Care and Interventions

An interdisciplinary model is essential when planning the care for women who abuse substances. Major issues that must be addressed in treatment for women that generally are not part of treatment for men are low self-esteem, stigmatization, high probability of sexual abuse and physi-

cal abuse, lack of social support, need for social services and child care, need for women's health services, and need for support and education in the mothering role (Kearney, 1997). Drug-free public housing or residential communities may offer an ideal route to stabilization in a safe environment. Treatment must demonstrate cultural sensitivity and responsiveness to recognize ethnicity and culture as an important part of her identity. Other needs of many women include relationship counseling, coping skills training, and vocational and legal assistance (Kearney, 1997).

Women for Sobriety may be a more helpful organization for women than Alcoholics Anonymous or Narcotics Anonymous, which are based on the 12-step program. The emphasis on powerlessness over addiction and avoidance of codependency found in 12-step programs may disempower and isolate women, particularly women of color (Saulnier, 1996). The confrontational techniques of the 12-step program, developed to break down denial in men, may be especially threatening to women who often feel unworthy and full of shame and guilt.

Pregnancy presents a window of opportunity for motivating women to stop their abuse of substances (Selleck & Redding, 1997). But what specifically can the nurse do?

First, nurses must be knowledgeable about how to screen and identify women who abuse substances while pregnant. They also must maintain a nonjudgmental, nonpunitive attitude. Nurses can advocate for access to woman-centered drug treatment and harm reduction measures to minimize the damage caused by alcohol and drugs (Kearney, 1997). Collaboration with advanced practice psychiatric nurses will enable nurses to deal with their feelings and provide better care for this challenging group of women. Until the nurse can approach the patient with caring and concern, the therapeutic alliance, which is so important for any change to take place, will not occur. The nurse's role is aimed not only at promoting abstinence, but also at providing a caring, nurturing, and empowering environment in which women can rediscover their values and become authentic, independent decision makers (Kearney, 1997).

Second, the nurse should determine the individual's readiness for change. One model for doing this was developed by Prochaska and DiClemente (1992). The five stages illustrate the readiness of women to change. *Precontemplation* is the earliest stage, in which individuals are unaware, unwilling, or discouraged about changing substance use behavior. They will be least responsive to interventions focused on change activities. First they need to take ownership of the problem. *Contemplation* involves an active consideration of the prospects of change. They engage in information seeking and begin to reevaluate themselves in light of their substance abuse behavior. *Preparation* indicates a readiness to change. They intend to change in the near future and have learned valuable lessons from past change attempts and failures. *Action* involves the overt modification of the problem behavior, and individuals must have the skills to carry out the changes. *Maintenance* is the final stage, and environmental supports are particularly important here, as well as supportive relationships with health care providers (Prochaska & DiClemente, 1992).

When working with pregnant adolescents with addictions, the nurse must also consider their developmental stage. A part of normal adolescence often includes experimenting with drugs or alcohol, so how does the nurse know when alcohol or drug use is a problem? Certain patterns, such as drinking to escape reality or drinking to "get wasted," are more dangerous than others (Bragg, 1997). Drinking alone and being secretive about drugs and alcohol also are unhealthy patterns.

Third, the nurse uses supportive nursing interventions such as mutuality and avoidance of confrontation. In mutuality, the nurse conveys to women drug users that their perspective on their life situation is as valid as that of the nurse. Women should be encouraged to describe their views on the role of drug use in their lives, the degree of impairment they are experiencing, and the feasibility of change at this point in time (Kearney, 1997). Avoidance of confrontation is important because it can be damaging to the nurse-client relationship. The likely consequences of continued drug use can be presented in a warmly concerned, factual manner rather than as threats.

Fourth, the nurse uses principles of motivational interviewing (Miller & Rollnick, 1991) to effect change. These principles include the following:
- Displaying empathy
- Developing discrepancy between individuals' perceptions of where they are and where they want to be
- Avoiding argumentation
- Rolling with resistance
- Supporting the client's sense of self-efficacy

When problematic drug use is suspected, the nurse might ask in a noncritical way, "Are drugs or alcohol any part of this situation you have been describing?" By asking about the role of drugs in self-medication of stressors, the nurse can help the woman reflect on the degree of the problem and avenues for change. The woman can be helped to express the positive aspects of drug use that lead her to continue using and the harmful consequences that she has observed. She can be asked about times she tried to reduce or quit using her drug of choice. What interfered with her success? What times was she successful? What enabled her to succeed at those times? Praise can be given for being able to be successful at some time and optimism expressed that she can be successful again.

Treatment Programs for Alcohol- and Drug-Dependent Women

National concern regarding the problem of alcohol and drug use during pregnancy has brought to the forefront the lack of treatment programs specifically targeted to pregnant women. Traditional frameworks for substance abuse treatment include the psychodynamic model, cognitive-behavioral model, relapse prevention model, 12-step self-help model, and medical model with medication treatment (Kearney, 1997). However, newer programs that provide comprehensive, coordinated, and "holistic" treatment are better able to draw pregnant women into care, as well as provide more effective treatment (Finkelstein, 1993). Any discussion of treatment programs must start with the understanding that substance abuse in women is a complex problem surrounded by multiple individual, familial, and social issues that require many levels of intervention and treatment (Finkelstein, 1994). The powerlessness of the alcoholic condition and the powerlessness of the female condition act on each other, reinforcing the impotence and hopelessness of both, leaving the woman with few resources to regain a grip on her life.

Whereas the treatment approach of male substance abusers tends to be oriented toward the individual, substance-abusing women should be viewed within the context of their relationships to others. Women tend to find satisfaction, pleasure, and a sense of worth if they experience their life activities as arising from and leading back to a sense of connection with others (Finkelstein, 1994). Alcohol- and drug-abusing women experience multiple social and personal disconnections in their lives, and they may turn to alcohol or other drugs to relieve the pain and anxiety caused by these disconnections. Many alcoholic and drug-abusing women are involved in intimate relationships with other substance abusers. In fact, their use is frequently dependent on the initiation, assistance, and encouragement of other people (Finkelstein, 1994). Women who use illicit drugs are likely to be introduced to and supplied with these drugs by men as part of an intimate or sexual relationship.

Finkelstein (1993) identified a number of principles for providing care for substance-abusing pregnant women:
- Services should be family focused.
- Services should promote competency building and empowerment.
- Services should be community based (i.e., in the local community).
- Services should be multidisciplinary, comprehensive, and coordinated.
- A program should offer services that address the multiplicity of needs such as child care, physical health problems, homelessness, unemployment, mental illness, and dual diagnosis.
- Service interventions should be individually tailored and long term.
- A continuum of care from outpatient to day treatment to inpatient and long-term residential care should be provided.

Evaluation

Evaluation is difficult in pregnant women with substance-abuse problems because the long-range effects cannot be projected. If the goals are realistic and short term, evaluation is easier. Short-term positive achievements are indicators of some success. Complete abstinence from drugs and assumption of mature adult behaviors within a short time are unrealistic. Long-term care is usually necessary.

POSTPARTUM PSYCHOLOGIC COMPLICATIONS

Mental health disorders in the postpartum period have implications for the mother, the newborn, and the entire family. Such conditions can interfere with attachment to the newborn and family integration, and some may threaten the safety and well-being of the mother, newborn, and other children. Because birth is usually thought to be a happy event, a new mother's emotional distress may puzzle and immobilize family and friends. At a time when she most needs the caring attention of loved ones, they may either criticize or withdraw because of their own anxiety.

Mood Disorders

Mood disorders are the predominant mental health disorder in the postpartum period, typically occurring within 4 weeks of childbirth (APA, 1994). The majority of women experience a mild depression or "baby blues" following the birth of a child. Others can have more serious depressions that can eventually incapacitate them to the point of being unable to care for themselves or their babies. Postpartum depression exerts a moderate to large effect on the interaction of mothers and infants (Beck, 1995a), and disturbances in early mother-infant interactions are found to be predictive of poorer infant cognitive outcome (Murray, Fiori-Crowley, & Hooper, 1996). Male babies seem to be especially vulnerable. In one study, 3-year-old boys with depressed mothers scored approximately 1 standard deviation lower on standardized tests of intellectual attainment than boys whose mothers were well (Sharp et al., 1995). In the rarest of cases, a disturbed mother may kill her infant, other family members, or herself. Nurses are strategically positioned to offer anticipatory guidance, to assess the mental health of new mothers, to offer therapeutic interventions, and to refer when necessary. Failure to do so may result in tragic consequences.

Clinical Manifestations

The Diagnostic and Statistical Manual of Mental Disorders contains the official guidelines for the assessment and diagnosis of psychiatric illness (APA, 1994). From less severe to most severe, the disorders are categorized as postpartum blues (discussed in Chapter 25), postpartum depression without psychotic features, and postpartum depression with psychotic features (postpartum psychosis).

Postpartum Depression Without Psychotic Features

Postpartum depression (PPD) is an intense and pervasive sadness with severe and labile mood swings and is more serious and persistent than postpartum blues. Intense fears, anger, anxiety, and despondency that persist past the baby's first few weeks are not a normal part of postpartum blues (Shrock, 1994). Occurring in approximately 10% to 15% of new mothers, these symptoms rarely disappear without outside help. Wickberg and

Hwang (1997) reported a prevalence of depression of 12.5% at 8 weeks and 8.3% at 12 weeks postpartum in a Swedish population.

The symptoms of postpartum major depression do not differ from the symptoms of nonpostpartum mood disorders except that the mother's ruminations of guilt and inadequacy feed her worries about being an incompetent and inadequate parent (Kumar, 1990). In PPD, there may be odd food cravings (often sweet desserts) and binges with abnormal appetite and weight gain (Shrock, 1994). New mothers report an increased yearning for sleep, sleeping heavily, but awakening instantly with any infant noise, and an inability to go back to sleep after infant feedings (Herz, 1992).

A distinguishing feature of PPD is irritability (Shrock, 1994). These episodes of irritability may flare up with little provocation, and they may sometimes escalate to violent outbursts or dissolve into uncontrollable sobbing (Shrock, 1994). Many of these outbursts are directed against significant others ("He never helps me") or the baby ("She cries all the time and I feel like hitting her"). Women with postpartum major depressive episodes often have severe anxiety, panic attacks, and spontaneous crying long after the usual duration of baby blues.

Many women feel especially guilty about having depressive feelings at a time when they believe they should be happy (APA, 1994). They may be reluctant to discuss their symptoms or their negative feelings toward the child. A prominent feature of PPD is rejection of the infant, often caused by abnormal jealousy. The mother may be obsessed by the notion that the offspring may take her place in her partner's affections. Attitudes toward the infant may include disinterest, annoyance with care demands, and blaming because of her lack of maternal feeling. When observed, she may appear awkward in her responses to the baby. Obsessive thoughts about harming the child are very frightening to her. Often she does not share these thoughts because of embarrassment, but when she does, other family members become very frightened.

Medical management. The natural course is one of gradual improvement over the 6 months after birth. Support treatment alone is not efficacious for major postpartum depression. Pharmacologic intervention is needed in most instances. Treatment options include antidepressants, anxiolytic agents, and electroconvulsive therapy. Psychotherapy focuses on her fears and concerns regarding her new responsibilities and roles, as well as monitoring for suicidal or homicidal thoughts. For some women, hospitalization is necessary.

Postpartum Depression with Psychotic Features

Postpartum psychosis is a syndrome most often characterized by depression (as described previously), delusions, and thoughts by the mother of harming either the infant or herself (Kaplan & Sadock, 1998).

A postpartum mood disorder with psychotic features occurs in 1 to 2 per 1000 births (Kaplan & Sadock, 1998). Once a woman has had one postpartum episode with psychotic features, there is a 35% to 60% likelihood of recurrence with each subsequent birth (APA, 1994). Research, however, reported that women with histories of postpartum depression (both with and without psychotic features) who were treated with high-dose oral estrogen immediately following birth had a low relapse rate—9% (Sichel et al., 1995). The authors hypothesized that the low rate of relapse suggests that oral estrogen may stem the rapid rate of change in estrogen following birth, thereby preventing the potential impact on dopaminergic and serotonergic neuroreceptors, which trigger depression.

Symptoms often begin within days after the birth, although the mean time to onset is 2 to 3 weeks and almost always within 8 weeks of birth (Kaplan & Sadock, 1998). Characteristically, the woman begins to complain of fatigue, insomnia, and restlessness and may have episodes of tearfulness and emotional lability. Complaints regarding the inability to move, stand, or work are also common. Later, suspiciousness, confusion, incoherence, irrational statements, and obsessive concerns about the baby's health and welfare may be present (Kaplan & Sadock, 1998). Delusions may be present in 50% of all women and hallucinations in about 25%. Auditory hallucinations that command the mother to kill the infant can also occur in severe cases. When delusions are present, they are often related to the infant. The mother may think the infant is possessed by the devil, has special powers, or is destined for a terrible fate (APA, 1994). Grossly disorganized behavior may be manifested as a disinterest in the infant or an inability to provide care. Some will insist that something is wrong with the baby or accuse nurses or family of hurting or poisoning their child (Shrock, 1994). Nurses are advised to be alert for mothers who are agitated, overactive, confused, complaining, or suspicious.

A specific illness included in depression with psychotic features is **bipolar disorder** (formerly called manic depressive illness). This mood disorder is preceded or accompanied by manic episodes, characterized by elevated, expansive, or irritable moods. Bipolar disorders occur in approximately 0.6% to 0.88% of the population (APA, 1994). Clinical manifestations of a manic episode include at least three of the following symptoms that have been significantly present for at least 1 week: grandiosity, decreased need for sleep, pressured speech, flight of ideas, distractibility, psychomotor agitation, and excessive involvement in pleasurable activities without regard for negative consequences (APA, 1994). Because clients are hyperactive, they may not take the time to eat or sleep, which leads to inadequate nutrition, dehydration, and sleep deprivation. While in a manic state, mothers will need constant supervision when caring for their infant. Mostly they will be too preoccupied to provide child care.

Medical management. A favorable outcome is associated with a good premorbid adjustment (before the onset of the disorder) and a supportive family network (Kaplan & Sadock, 1998). The course of the syndrome is similar to that seen in clients with mood disorders. Because mood disorders are usually episodic, women may experience another episode of symptoms within a year or two of the birth. Postpartum psychosis is a psychiatric emergency. In one study 5% of the patients committed suicide, and 4% committed infanticide (Kaplan & Sadock, 1998). Antidepressants and lithium are the treatments of choice. If the mother is breastfeeding, some sources say no pharmacologic agents should be prescribed (Kaplan & Sadock, 1998), but other sources advise caution while prescribing some agents (Schatzberg & Nemeroff, 1998) (see later discussion). The mother will probably need psychiatric hospitalization. It is usually advantageous for the mother to have contact with her baby if she so desires, but visits must be closely supervised. Psychotherapy is indicated after the period of acute psychosis is past.

Etiology

A multidisciplinary approach is needed to understand the causes of PPD, including biologic (hormonal, neurotransmitter, and genetic theories), psychologic (personality and attributional theories), and sociocultural (social support, life stress, culture, preparation for childbearing) (Boyer, 1990). Each of these theories will be explained by at least one research study illustrating the significance of that particular approach.

Biologic Theories

Some factors unique to the reproductive process play a major role. Alterations in hypothalamic-pituitary-adrenal (HPA) axis function attributable to childbearing show remarkable similarity to those observed in depressed women (Wisner & Stowe, 1997). Postpartum women are also at increased risk for hypothalamic-pituitary-thyroidal (HPT) axis dysfunction that may increase affective-disorder vulnerability. Women with a history of major depression who relapsed during postpartum were found to have a significantly greater growth hormone response to apomorphine than those who remained well. The development of increased sensitivity of hypothalamic dopamine D_2 receptors in the postpartum period appears to predict the onset of depression (McIvor et al., 1996).

Psychologic Theories

Theories that predict risk factors for PPD include poor marital relationship (Shrock, 1994), family stress (Gotlib, 1991), fewer support systems, more stressful life events, and fewer personal resources (Logsdon, McBride, & Birkimer, 1994). One study of Portuguese women reported that aside from a history of depression, the only other powerful predictor of PPD was the negative impact score of life events (Areias et al., 1996). Women who feel close to their husbands report fewer depressive symptoms; women with psychiatric histories who did not relapse in the postpartum period had partners who were more positive about them than partners of high risk women who relapsed (Marks et al., 1996). Postnatal depression in fathers was associated with PPD in their wives (Areias et al., 1996). Low self-esteem was found to be a reliable contributing factor to PPD in several studies (Chen, 1996; Fontaine & Jones, 1997). Mothers with low self-esteem were 39 times more likely to have high depressive symptoms than those with high self-esteem (Hall et al., 1996).

Sociocultural Theories

Theories about contributing causes of PPD are also reported from sociology. Stress (Chen, 1996), labeling, and feminist models have been hypothesized to contribute to PPD (Thurtle, 1995). Leathers, Kelley, and Richman (1997) reported that low levels of self-reported social gratification, support, and control at work and in the parenting role were related to postpartum depression.

CARE MANAGEMENT

Even though the prevalence of PPD is fairly well established, only 2 to 3 out of 100 are referred to a mental health care provider; of the remainder, only about half are identified by family doctors, nurse-practitioners, or other persons (Kumar, 1990). Those identified are often treated inappropriately with benzodiazepines or subtherapeutic doses of antidepressants.

Assessment and Nursing Diagnoses

In order to recognize symptoms of PPD as early as possible, the nurse should be an active listener and demonstrate a caring attitude. In one research study (Whitton, Warner, & Appleby, 1996), British women suffering from postpartum depression were interviewed about their symptoms, help-seeking behavior, and treatment. Over 90% recognized that there was something wrong, but only one third believed they were suffering from postpartum depression. Over 80% had not reported their symptoms to any health professional. Nurses cannot depend on women volunteering unsolicited information about their depression or asking for help. The nurse should observe for signs of depression and ask appropriate questions to determine moods, appetite, sleep, energy and fatigue levels, and ability to concentrate. Examples of ways to initiate conversation include the following: "How is your life going now that you have a baby (or another child)? . . . Have you changed much since having the baby?" (Shrock, 1994) and "How much time do you spend crying?" If the nurse assesses that the new mother is depressed, she or he must ask if the mother has thought about hurting herself or the baby. The woman may be more willing to answer honestly if the nurse says, "Lots of women feel depressed after having a baby, and some feel so badly that they think about hurting themselves or the baby. Have you had these thoughts?"

NURSE ALERT *Recalling risk factors for postpartum depression can alert the nurse to identify those postpartum women at greatest risk. Risk factors include prenatal depression, a history of previous depression, child care stress, meager or absent social support, stressful life events, prenatal anxiety, maternity blues, and poor marital relationship (Beck, 1998a).*

Nurses can use screening tools in assessing whether the depressive symptoms have progressed from postpartum blues to PPD. Examples are the Postpartum Depression Checklist developed by Beck (1995a) (Box 35-5) and the Edinburgh Postnatal Depression Scale (EPDS) (Cox, Holden, & Savogsky, 1989) (Box 35-6). The EPDS, with a cutoff point of 11.5, was found to identify all but two women with major depression, giving it a sensitivity of 96% (Wickberg & Hwang, 1996b). Particularly if the initial interaction reveals some question that the patient might be depressed, a formal screening is helpful in determining the urgency of the referral and the type of provider. Also important is the need to assess the woman's family because they may be able to offer valuable information, as well as have a need to express how they have been affected by the woman's emotional disorder.

Planning is based on the following nursing diagnoses and is focused on meeting the individualized needs of the family to ensure safety, especially for the mother and infant and any other children, and to facilitate functional family coping.

Nursing Diagnoses

- Risk for injury to newborn related to
  - mother's depression (inattention to infant's needs for hygiene, nutrition, safety) and psychotropic medications via breast milk
- Ineffective family coping related to
  - increased care needs of mother and infant
- Risk for altered parenting related to
  - inability of depressed mother to attach to infant
- Risk for altered growth and development of infant related to
  - lack of stimulation and inadequate loving care
- Anxiety in the mother related to
  - postpartum hormonal fluctuation
- Self-esteem disturbance in the mother related to
  - stresses associated with role changes
- Risk for violence toward self (mother) or children related to
  - postpartum depression

Expected Outcomes of Care

Specific measurable criteria can be developed based on the following general outcomes:
- The mother will no longer be depressed.
- The mother's and infant's physical well-being will be maintained.
- The family will cope effectively.

BOX 35-5 Suggested Questions to Elicit Responses from the Postpartum Depression Checklist

LACK OF CONCENTRATION

Are you experiencing difficulty concentrating?
Does your mind seem to be filled with cobwebs?
Does it seem at times like fogginess sets in?

LOSS OF INTERESTS

Do you feel your life is empty of your previous interests and goals?
Have you lost interest in your hobbies that used to bring you pleasure and enjoyment?

LONELINESS

Are you experiencing feelings of loneliness?
Do you feel as though no one really understands what you are experiencing?
Do you feel uncomfortable around other people?
Have you been isolating yourself from other people?

INSECURITY

Have you been feeling insecure, fragile, or vulnerable?
Does the responsibility of motherhood seem overwhelming?

OBSESSIVE THINKING

Is your mind constantly filled with obsessive thinking, such as "What's wrong with me?" "Am I going crazy?" "Why can't I enjoy being with my baby?"
When trying to fall asleep at night, is your mind still racing with repetitive thoughts?

LACK OF POSITIVE EMOTIONS

Are you experiencing feelings of emptiness?
Do you feel like a robot just going through the motions?
When caring for your infant/child, do you feel any joy or love?

LOSS OF SELF

Do you feel as though you are not the same person you used to be?
Are you afraid that your life will never be normal again?

ANXIETY ATTACKS

Are you experiencing uncontrollable anxiety attacks?
Are you experiencing periods of palpitations, chest pains, sweating, or tingling hands?
When going through an anxiety attack, do you feel as though you're losing your mind?

LOSS OF CONTROL

Do you feel you are in control of your emotions and thoughts?
Are you experiencing loss of control in any aspects of your life?

GUILT

Are you feeling guilty because you are not giving your infant/child the love and attention he or she needs?
Are you experiencing guilt over thoughts of harming your infant/child?
Do you feel you are a good mother?

CONTEMPLATING DEATH

Have you ever experienced thoughts of harming yourself?
Have you been feeling so low that the thought of leaving this world is appealing to you?

Source: Beck, C. (1995). Screening methods for postpartum depression. *J Obstet Gynecol Neonatal Nurs* 24(4), 308-312.

- Family members will demonstrate continued healthy growth and development.
- The infant will be fully integrated into the family.

Plan of Care and Interventions

On the Postpartum Unit

The astute postpartum nurse must observe the new mother carefully for any signs of teariness, and conduct further assessments as necessary. Information about PPD must be discussed by nurses to prepare new parents for potential problems in the postpartum period. The family must be able to recognize the symptoms and know where to go for help. In addition, a teaching brochure that explains what the woman can do to prevent depression could be used as part of discharge planning (Boyer, 1990). This brochure might include an elaboration of the ideas listed in the Home Care box.

In these days of early discharge, postpartum moms usually leave the hospital before the blues or depression hits (Shrock, 1994). If the postpartum nurse is concerned about the mother, a mental health consult should be requested before the mother leaves the hospital. All clients should be urged to maintain contact with the postpartum staff for urgent referrals or resources. Routine instructions regarding PPD should be given to whomever comes to take the patient home; for example, "If you notice that your wife (or daughter) is upset or crying a lot, please call the postpartum care provider immediately–don't wait for the routine postpartum appointment."

BOX 35-6 Edinburgh Postnatal Depression Scale (EPDS)

Name:

Address:

Baby's age:

As you have recently had a baby, we would like to know how you are feeling. Please UNDERLINE the answer which comes closest to how you have felt IN THE PAST 7 DAYS, not just how you feel today.

Here is an example, already completed.

I have felt happy

    Yes, all the time

    <u>Yes, most of the time</u>

    No, not very often

    No, not at all

This would mean: "I have felt happy most of the time" during the past week. Please complete the other questions in the same way.

IN THE PAST 7 DAYS:

1. I have been able to laugh and see the funny side of things

    As much as I always could

    Not quite as much now

    Definitely not so much now

    Not at all

2. I have looked forward with enjoyment to things

    As much as I ever did

    Rather less than I used to

    Definitely less than I used to

    Hardly at all

*3. I have blamed myself unnecessarily when things went wrong

    Yes, most of the time

    Yes, some of the time

    Not very often

    No, never

4. I have been anxious or worried for no good reason

    No, not at all

    Hardly ever

    Yes, sometimes

    Yes, very often

*5. I have felt scared or panicky for no very good reason

    Yes, quite a lot

    Yes, sometimes

    No, not much

    No, not at all

*6. Things have been getting on top of me

    Yes, most of the time I haven't been able to cope at all

    Yes, sometimes I haven't been coping as well as usual

    No, most of the time I have coped quite well

    No, I have been coping as well as ever

*7. I have been so unhappy that I have had difficulty sleeping

    Yes, most of the time

    Yes, sometimes

    Not very often

    No, not at all

*8. I have felt sad or miserable

    Yes, most of the time

    Yes, quite often

    Not very often

    No, not at all

*9. I have been so unhappy that I have been crying

    Yes, most of the time

    Yes, quite often

    Only occasionally

    No, never

*10. The thought of harming myself has occurred to me

    Yes, quite often

    Sometimes

    Hardly ever

    Never

Scoring: Response categories are scored 0, 1, 2, and 3 according to increased severity of the symptom.

Items marked with an asterisk are reverse scored (i.e., 3, 2, 1, and 0). The total score is calculated by adding together the scores for each of the 10 items.

Source: Cox, J., Holden, J., & Sagovsky, M. (1989). Edinburgh Postnatal Depression Scale. *Br J Psychiatry* 150, 782-786.

 HOME CARE

Activities to Prevent Postpartum Depression

- Share knowledge about postpartum emotional problems with close family and friends.
- Take care of yourself—eat a balanced diet, exercise on a regular basis, and get enough sleep. Ask someone to take care of the baby so that you can get a full night's sleep.
- Share your feelings with someone close to you; don't isolate yourself at home with the TV.

- Don't overcommit yourself or feel like you need to be a superwoman.
- Don't place unrealistic expectations on yourself.
- Don't be ashamed of having emotional problems after your baby is born—it happens to approximately 15% of women.

In the Home and Community

Postpartum home visits can reduce the incidence of or complications from depression. A brief home visit or phone call at least once a week until the new mother returns for her postpartum visit may save the life of a mother and her infant. In a Swedish research project, 41 postpartum depressed women were randomly allocated to a study and a control group (Wickberg & Hwang, 1996a). The women in the study group received six weekly counseling visits by the Child Health Clinic nurse and the control group received routine primary care. Twelve (80%) postpartum women with major depression in the study group were fully recovered after the intervention compared with four (25%) in the control group. More research about the effectiveness of home visits as an intervention for PPD is needed.

Supervision of the mother with emotional complications may become a prime concern. Because depression can greatly interfere with her mothering functions, family and friends may need to participate in the infant's care. This supervision can be planned by the collaborative efforts of the nurse and family members. This is a time for the extended family and friends to determine what they can do to help, and the nurse can work with them to ensure adequate supervision and their understanding of the woman's mental illness.

Caring is one of the nurse's most powerful tools. Using a phenomenologic research methodology, interviews with 10 mothers who had experienced postpartum depression were analyzed. Seven themes emerged that illustrated nurses' caring for mothers experiencing PPD: having sufficient knowledge about PPD; using astute observation and intuition to make quick, correct diagnoses; providing hope that the mothers' living nightmares will come to an end; readily sharing their time; making appropriate referrals for the right path to recovery; providing continuity of care; and understanding what the mothers were experiencing (Beck, 1995b).

Facilitating relationship with partner. The woman with PPD may not be able to attend to her partner's needs. The nurse can guide the woman and her partner in working together to cope with this stressful time. Depression can make a woman overly observant of a loved one's unhelpful behavior while failing to recognize loving, helpful gestures. The health care provider must not agree that the partner is nonsupportive, even when the postpartum woman is being critical. The nurse can say, "It seems right now that you feel he is not being supportive of you," or "You feel like your needs are not being met even though he may be doing the best he knows how." The nurse can also encourage the postpartum woman to identify several specific requests for her partner, such as asking for a hug or asking him to watch the baby so that she can take a walk outside.

When the woman has PPD, a partner often reacts with confusion, shock, denial, and anger and feels neglected and blamed. The nurse can talk with the woman about how her condition is hard for him too, and that he is probably very worried about her. Men oftentimes withdraw or criticize when they are deeply worried about their significant others. The nurse can provide nonjudgmental opportunities for the partner to verbalize feelings and concerns, help the partner identify positive coping strategies, and be a source of encouragement for the partner to continue supporting the woman. Both the woman and her partner need an opportunity to express their needs, fears, thoughts, and feelings in a nonjudgmental environment (Shrock, 1994).

Suggesting changes and resources. Even if the mother is severely depressed, if adequate resources can be mobilized to ensure safety for both mother and infant, hospitalization can be avoided. Whether the mother has private insurance or is referred to state-supported agencies, the nurse in home health will need to make frequent phone calls or home visits to do assessment and counseling. Some parents may need to reassess their daily routines, their expectations of parenthood, and the concept of "good mothering." Postpartum women may need rest, household help, or a prescription for medication (Shrock, 1994). Other community resources that may be helpful are temporary child care or foster care, homemaker service, meals on wheels, parenting guidance centers, mother's-day-out programs, and telephone support groups. Mild cases of postpartum depression can be referred to support groups (Berchtold & Burrough, 1990) such as Postpartum Support International Hotline (425-881-6580) or Depression After Delivery (DAD) (P.O. Box 1282, Morrisville, PA 19067; 908-575-9121).

Providing safety. When depression is suspected, the nurse asks, "Have you thought about hurting yourself?" If delusional thinking about the baby is suspected, the nurse asks, "Have you thought about hurting your baby?" There are four criteria to measure in assessing the seriousness of a suicidal plan: method, availability, specificity, and lethality. Has the woman specified a method? Is the method of choice available? How specific is the plan? If the method is concrete and detailed, with access to it right at hand, the suicide risk increases. How lethal is the method? The most lethal method is shooting, with hanging a close second. The least lethal is slashing one's wrists.

> **NURSE ALERT** *Suicidal thoughts or attempts are one of the most serious symptoms of PPD and require immediate assessment and intervention (Fishel, 1995).*

Referral. Women with moderate to severe cases of PPD should be referred to a mental health therapist, such as an advanced practice psychiatric nurse, for evaluation and therapy so as to avoid the effects that postpartum depression can have on the woman and on her relationships with her partner, baby, and other children (Shrock, 1994). Inpatient psychiatric hospitalization may be necessary. This decision is made when the safety needs of the mother or children are threatened.

Psychiatric Hospitalization

Women with postpartum psychosis are a psychiatric emergency and must be referred immediately to a psychiatrist, who can prescribe medication and other forms of therapy and assess the need for hospitalization.

LEGAL TIP *If a woman with PPD is experiencing active suicidal ideation or harmful delusions about the baby and is unwilling to seek treatment, legal intervention may be necessary to commit the woman to an inpatient setting for treatment.*

To review the question of whether an infant should be admitted to psychiatric services when a severe psychiatric disorder necessitates admission of the mother, Barnett and Morgan (1996) reviewed all available literature on mother-infant admission. Early reports favored joint admission; however, this has changed, possibly for economic reasons. Recent research data indicate longer-term adverse effects of postnatal depression on the children and the finding of psychologic and psychiatric morbidity in many of the fathers. Joint admission to designated special units can be valuable, but such facilities are cost-efficient and effective only if established as part of an appropriate, broader plan for managing postpartum psychiatric disorder.

Within the hospital setting, the reintroduction of the baby to the mother can occur at the mother's own pace. A schedule is set for increasing the hours of the mother's caring for the baby over several days, culminating in the infant staying overnight in the mother's room. This allows the mother to experience meeting the infant's needs and giving up sleep for the baby, a situation difficult for new mothers even under ideal conditions. The mother's readiness for discharge and caring for the baby is assessed. Her interactions with her baby are also carefully supervised and guided.

Nurses should also observe the mother for signs of bonding with the baby. Attachment behaviors are defined as eye-to-eye contact; physical contact that involves holding, touching, cuddling, and talking to the baby and calling the baby by name; and the initiation of appropriate care. A staff member is assigned to keep the baby in sight at all times. Indirect teaching, praise, and encouragement are designed to bolster the mother's self-esteem and self-confidence. The Bethlem Mother-Infant Interaction Scale can be used by inpatient nurses to aid clinical decisions about the safety of parenting by individual mothers with severe mental illness in the postpartum period (Hipwell & Kumar, 1996).

Psychotropic Medications

PPD is usually treated with antidepressant medications. If the woman with PPD is not breastfeeding, antidepressants can be prescribed without special precautions. In addition to the SSRIs and TCAs discussed previously, MAOIs, mood stabilizers, and antipsychotic medications may be prescribed for nonbreastfeeding women with postpartum depression.

Hypertensive crisis is the main reason that MAOIs are not prescribed more frequently, even though they are effective. The woman should be taught to watch for signs of hypertensive crisis–throbbing, occipital headache, stiff neck, chills, nausea, flushing, retroorbital pain, apprehension, pallor, sweating, chest pain, and palpitations (Keltner & Folks, 1997). This crisis is brought on by the client taking any of a large variety of over-the-counter medications or eating foods that contain tyramine, a sympathomimetic pressor amine, which normally is broken down by the enzyme monoamine oxidase. The nurse must do extensive teaching about foods and medications to avoid that contain tyramine.

The woman taking mood stabilizers (Box 35-7) must be taught about the many side effects, and especially, for those on lithium, the need to have serum lithium levels drawn every 6 months. Women with severe psychiatric syndromes such as schizophrenia, bipolar disorder, or psychotic depression will probably require antipsychotic medications (Box 35-8).

Client education is especially important when caring for people who are taking antipsychotic medications. The nurse should use discretion in selecting the content to be shared because clients may become anxious about the potential side effects. The nurse may choose to do more extensive education with a close family member. Most of these medications can cause sedation and orthostatic hypotension–both

---

BOX 35-7 Mood Stabilizers

Carbamazepine (Tegretol)
Clonazepam (Klonopin)
Divalproex (Depakote)
Lithium carbonate (Eskalith)

BOX 35-8 Commonly Used Antipsychotic Medications

PHENOTHIAZINES

Chlorpromazine (Thorazine)
Fluphenazine (Prolixin)
Perphenazine (Trilafon)
Thioridazine (Mellaril)
Trifluoperazine (Stelazine)

OTHER

Clozapine (Clozaril)
Haloperidol (Haldol)
Loxapine (Loxitane)
Olanzapine (Zyprexa)
Pimozide (Orap)
Quetiapine (Seroquel)
Risperidone (Risperdal)
Thiothixene (Navane)

of which could interfere with the mother being able to safely care for her baby. They can also cause PNS effects such as constipation, dry mouth, blurred vision, tachycardia, urinary retention, weight gain, and agranulocytosis. CNS effects may include akathisia, dystonias, parkinsonism-like symptoms, tardive dyskinesia (irreversible), and neuroleptic malignant syndrome (potentially fatal).

Psychotropic Medications and Lactation

About one half of all new mothers breastfeed. A major clinical dilemma is the antidepressant treatment of women suffering from PPD who want to breastfeed their infants. In the past, women were told to discontinue lactation. To date, the FDA has not approved any psychotropic medication for use during lactation. However, the American Academy of Pediatrics (AAP) (1994) published a report on excretion of medications into human breast milk. Their classification includes medications that are contraindicated during breastfeeding, medications whose effects on nursing infants are unknown but may be of concern because they could alter CNS development, and medications usually compatible with breastfeeding. Because all psychotropic medications pass through breast milk to the infant, the risks associated with the use of such medication must be weighed against the risks associated with maternal agitation and potentially self-destructive behavior.

In PPD with psychotic features, the mother may need to discontinue breastfeeding in order to take antipsychotic and antimanic medications without fearing harm to the baby. This loss, however, can intensify the mother's depression. It has been recommended that nonpharmacologic interventions be used before medications; however, in today's managed care climate, interventions such as frequent psychotherapy sessions, constant supervision by home health nurses and family, and inpatient hospitalizations for mother and infant may not be readily available (Schatzberg & Nemeroff, 1998).

To date, breast milk excretion studies have demonstrated that antidepressants are present in breast milk, with a milk-to-serum ratio that is typically greater than 1:1 (Schatzberg & Nemeroff, 1998). For amitriptyline and desipramine, there is a peak increase in breast milk concentrations 4 to 6 hours after an oral dose. Adjusting both the schedule of dosing of the antidepressant and the infant's feeding schedule may considerably reduce the concentration of the drug to which the infant is exposed. The majority of investigators recommend using the secondary amine TCAs (nortriptyline and desipramine) (Schatzberg & Nemeroff, 1998). Typically MAOIs are avoided; minimal data are available concerning the SSRIs. No human data have been published on the newer antidepressants. Most of the drugs listed in Boxes 35-2, 35-7, and 35-8 are classified as drugs whose effects on infants are unknown but may be of concern (see Appendix C).

Wisner, Perel, and Findling (1996) reviewed 15 studies that systematically investigated the antidepressant effects during the postpartum period. The results revealed that sertraline and several tricyclics, including amitriptyline, nortriptyline, desipramine, and clomipramine, fail to exert significant adverse effects and do not increase infant antidepressant levels. In contrast, colic and increased blood levels have been reported in breastfed infants whose mothers took fluoxetine, and respiratory depression occurred in those treated with doxepin. The data to date suggest that no documented developmental delays are evident in 9- to 36-month-old infants of antidepressant-treated mothers (Wisner, Perel, & Findling, 1996).

Antipsychotic medications are excreted into breast milk. With the exception of clozapine (Clozaril), which is Category B, all of the other antipsychotic medications are Category C. The most widely studied is chlorpromazine; seven infants did not demonstrate any developmental deficits at 16-month and 5-year follow-ups. The breast milk concentrations of several other antipsychotics have been measured; the milk-to-serum ratio is less than or equal to 1.0 (Schatzberg & Nemeroff, 1998). The older antipsychotic medications have been widely used for three decades, and risks are minimal for nursing infants; even so, their use should be avoided during the first trimester of pregnancy (Schatzberg & Nemeroff, 1998). None of these medications has been proven safe during lactation; the AAP does not rate any of the antipsychotic medications as compatible with breastfeeding.

Mood-stabilizing and antimanic medications are present in breast milk. Carbamazepine and clonazepam are Category C, and lithium and divalproex are Category D. Nursing infants can achieve serum lithium concentrations that are 40% to 50% of maternal levels (Schatzberg & Nemeroff, 1998); lithium is contraindicated in breastfeeding. In contrast, both carbamazepine and divalproex appear in low concentrations in human milk, and both are considered compatible with breastfeeding levels; however, the benefits of breastfeeding and the potential risks must be carefully considered (AAP, 1994).

Nursing Implications

When breastfeeding women have emotional complications and need psychotropic medications, referral to a psychiatrist who specializes in postpartum disorders is preferred. Depressed women who are not breastfeeding will need the nurse to reinforce the need to take antidepressants as ordered. Because they do not exert any effect before about 2 weeks and usually do not reach full effect before 4 to 6 weeks, many women discontinue taking the medication on their own. Women taking any of the antidepressants should be cautioned about combining them with alcohol or over-the-counter medications. (For additional information, see Fishel, 1995) (see Plan of Care).

Postpartum Onset of Panic Disorder

Approximately 3% to 5% of women develop panic disorder or obsessive-compulsive disorder in the postpartum period.

PLAN OF CARE | Postpartum Depression

NURSING DIAGNOSIS Risk for injury to the newborn and client related to client's emotional state as evidenced by maternal behaviors and increased score on a postpartum depression scale

Expected Outcome *The client and newborn will remain free of injury.*

Nursing Interventions/*Rationales*

Assess the postpartum client for risk factors for depression; use assessment scale to determine which clients may be most at risk *to identify clients needing prompt interventions.*

Maintain frequent contact with client by telephone calls and home visits *to determine if further interventions are necessary because most clients are discharged early from the inpatient setting.*

Advise client and family to telephone health care provider if behaviors indicating depression, such as crying, increase *to provide prompt care and referral if necessary and avoid injury to newborn and client.*

Provide opportunities for client and family to verbalize feelings and concerns in a nonjudgmental setting *to promote a trusting relationship.*

Assess client for any suicidal thoughts or plans *to provide for safety of client and neonate.*

Refer mild cases of depression to support groups *to provide group interaction with women having similar problems.*

Refer moderate to severe cases of depression to mental health therapist *to provide for individualized psychiatric care.*

Refer breastfeeding mother to lactation consultant *for information regarding effects of antidepressant and antipsychotic medications.*

NURSING DIAGNOSIS Ineffective family coping, disabling, related to postpartum maternal depression as evidenced by family members' denial of client's illness

Expected Outcomes *Family will identify positive coping mechanisms and initiate a plan to cope with the client's depression.*

Nursing Interventions/*Rationales*

Provide opportunity for family and significant others to verbalize feelings and concerns *to establish a trusting relationship.*

Give information to the family regarding postpartum depression *to clarify any misconceptions or misinformation.*

Assist family to identify positive coping mechanisms that have been effective during past crises *to promote active participation in care.*

Assist family to identify community sources of support *to provide additional resources as needed.*

Refer family to mental health counselor as needed *to provide further expertise from a mental health professional.*

Panic attacks are discrete periods in which there is the sudden onset of intense apprehension, fearfulness, or terror (APA, 1994). During these attacks, symptoms such as shortness of breath, palpitations, chest pain, choking, smothering sensations, and fear of losing control are present. They have intrusive thoughts about terrible injury done to the infant, such as stabbing or burns, sometimes by themselves (Pederson, 1998). Rarely do they harm the baby.

Clinical Characteristics

From an analysis of interviews of mothers' experiences of panic during the postpartum period, the following themes were identified that described the essence of the experiences (Beck, 1998b):

- The terrifying physical and emotional components of panic paralyzed women, leaving them feeling totally out of control.
- During panic attacks women's cognitive functioning abruptly diminished, and between these attacks women experienced a more insidious decrease in their cognitive functioning.
- During the panic attacks, women feverishly struggled to maintain their composure, leading to exhaustion.
- Because of the terrifying nature of panic, preventing further panic attacks was paramount in the lives of the women. They sought to discover specific panic triggers particular to their own lives. At times, being away from their babies triggered a panic attack.

- As a result of recurring panic attacks, negative changes in women's lifestyles ensued—lowering of their self-esteem and leaving them to bear the burden of disappointing not only themselves but also their families.
- Mothers were haunted by the prospect that their panic could have residual effects on themselves and their babies. Some others wondered if they had been so preoccupied with the panic that they missed their children's cues for help.

Nurses need only to listen to hear symptoms of panic disorder. Usually these women are so distraught that they will share with whomever will listen. Oftentimes the family has tried to tell them that what they are experiencing is normal, but they know differently. The major nursing diagnoses are as follows:

⫶ Nursing Diagnoses

- Anxiety related to
  - postpartum adaptations and expectations
- Fear of harming others related to
  - obsessions
- Powerlessness related to
  - feelings of losing control
- Knowledge deficit related to
  - postpartum mental health problems

⫶ CARE MANAGEMENT

Treatment is usually a combination of medications, education, psychotherapy, and cognitive behavioral interventions. Antidepressants such as SSRIs may be prescribed, and sertraline (Zoloft) is currently the drug of choice with panic disorder; fluvoxamine (Luvox) may be especially helpful with obsessions. In addition, the following nursing interventions are suggested.

- Education is a crucial nursing intervention. New mothers should be provided with anticipatory guidance concerning the possibility of panic attacks during the postpartum period. Preparing for the attacks may help decrease their unexpected, terrifying nature (Beck, 1998b).
- Empowerment conveys to the woman that she can sort through her fears and expectations and take charge of her life. Women can be reassured that it is common to feel a sense of impending doom and fear of insanity during panic attacks. These fears are temporary and disappear once the panic attack is over (Beck, 1998b). Nurses can help women identify panic triggers that are particular to their own lives. Keeping a diary can help identify the triggers (Beck, 1998b).
- Family and social supports are helpful. The new mother is encouraged to put usual chores on hold and to ask for and accept help.
- Support groups allow these mothers to experience comfort in seeing others like themselves.

- Sensory interventions such as music therapy and aromatherapy are nonintrusive and inexpensive.
- Behavioral interventions such as breathing exercises and progressive muscle relaxation can be helpful (Fishel, 1998).
- Cognitive interventions such as positive self-talk training, reframing and redefining, and reassurance can alter the negative thinking (Fishel, 1998).

Evaluation

The nurse can be assured that care has been effective if the physical well-being of the mother and infant is maintained, the mother and family are able to cope effectively, and each family member continues to show a healthy adaptation to the presence of the new member of the family.

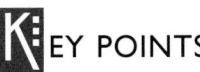

KEY POINTS

- ⫶ Because pregnant women may have a history of mental disorder or substance abuse, careful assessment is extremely important at the first and each subsequent prenatal and postnatal visit.
- ⫶ Values clarification for health care workers may be necessary to assist them in providing nonjudgmental care for substance abusers.
- ⫶ Alcohol abuse during pregnancy is the leading cause of mental retardation in the United States, and it is entirely preventable.
- ⫶ Treatment programs must start with an understanding that substance abuse in women is a complex problem surrounded by multiple individual, familial, and social issues that require many levels of intervention and treatment.
- ⫶ Mood disorders account for most mental health disorders in the postpartum period.
- ⫶ Identification of women at greatest risk for substance abuse during pregnancy and depression in the postpartum period can be facilitated by use of various screening tools.
- ⫶ Suicidal thoughts or attempts are one of the most serious symptoms of postpartum depression.
- ⫶ Antidepressant medications are the usual treatment for postpartum depression; however, specific precautions are needed for breastfeeding women.
- ⫶ Treatment of postpartum onset of panic disorder requires a combination of medication, education, supportive measures, and psychotherapy.

CRITICAL THINKING EXERCISES

1 *Identify resources in your community for women with substance abuse, postpartum depression, and postpartum panic disorder. Develop criteria to evaluate these resources and compare these resources according to the criteria.*

2 *Develop an information packet that could be distributed to postpartum clients during discharge teaching on how to find a resource for postpartum depression and include the strengths and weaknesses (or pros and cons) of each.*

3 *You are assigned to a clinic to take maternal histories at the first prenatal visit. A 16-year-old gives the following history. She was date-raped at a party 8 weeks ago. She has missed one menstrual period and her pregnancy test was positive. She smokes a half pack of cigarettes a day and drinks beer every weekend. She has experimented with marijuana occasionally and tried cocaine twice in the past month. Her parents are divorced, and she currently lives with her mother, who is unaware of the pregnancy. She states that she plans to keep the baby and raise it by herself. She does not have a boyfriend at this time.*

   a. Formulate nursing diagnoses.

   b. Prioritize the nursing diagnoses.

   c. Plan goals and expected outcomes of care.

   d. Plan interventions and give the rationale for each. Include referrals and community resources.

References

American Academy of Pediatrics Committee on Drugs. (1994). The transfer of drugs and other chemicals into human milk. *Pediatrics* 93(1), 137-150.

American Psychiatric Association. (1994). *Diagnostic and statistical manual of mental disorders* (4th ed.). Washington, D.C.: American Psychiatric Association Press.

Areias, M. et al. (1996). Correlates of postnatal depression in mothers and fathers. *Br J Psychiatry* 169(1), 36-41.

Audain, L. et al. (1999). Cocaine and pregnancy: A deadly mix. *Epikrisis* 10(1), 1-2.

Barnett B., & Morgan M. (1996). Postpartum psychiatric disorder: Who should be admitted and to which hospital? *Aust N Z J Psychiatry* 30(6), 709-714.

Beck, C. (1998a). A checklist to identify women at risk for developing postpartum depression. *J Obstet Gynecol Neonatal Nurs* 27, 39-46.

Beck, C. (1998b). Postpartum onset of panic disorder. *Image J Nurs Sch* 30(2), 131-135.

Beck, C. (1995a). Screening methods for postpartum depression. *J Obstet Gynecol Neonatal Nurs* 24(4), 308-312.

Beck, C. (1995b). Perceptions of nurses' caring by mothers experiencing postpartum depression. *J Obstet Gynecol Neonatal Nurs* 24(9), 819-825.

Bennett, C. (1995). The tao, acupuncture, and crack cocaine. *Capsules and Comments in Psychiatric Nursing* 1(4), 2-8.

Berchtold, N., & Burrough, M. (1990). Reaching out: Depression after delivery support group network. *NAACOG's Clin Issues Perinat Women Health Nurs* 1(3), 385-394.

Boyer, D. (1990). Prediction of postpartum depression. *NAACOG's Clin Issues Perin Women Health Nurs* 1(3), 359-368.

Bragg, E. (1997). Pregnant adolescents with addictions. *J Obstet Gynecol Neonatal Nurs* 26, 577-584.

Cefalo, R., & Moos, M. (1995). *Preconceptional health care, a practical guide* (2nd ed.). St. Louis: Mosby.

Center for Substance Abuse Treatment. (1993). *Pregnant substance-using women*. Rockville, MD: U.S. Department of Health and Human Services.

Chen, C. (1996). Postpartum depression among adolescent mothers and adult mothers. *Kaohsiung J Med Sci* 12(2), 104-113.

Chisum, T. (1990). Nursing interventions with the antepartum substance abuser. *J Perinat Neonatal Nurs* 3(4), 26-33.

Clark, C. (1997). PTSD: How to support healing. *Am J Nurs* 97(8), 27-32.

Clarren, S. (1999). FAS: A diagnosis for two. Presentation at the 8th Annual Statewide Conference of the NC Governor's Institute on Alcohol and Substance Abuse, Greensboro, NC.

Cook, P., Peterson, R., & Moore, D. (1994). *Alcohol, tobacco, and other drugs may harm the unborn*. Rockville, MD: U.S. Department of Health and Human Services.

Cox, J., Holden, J., & Sagovsky, R. (1989). Edinburgh Postnatal Depression Scale. *Br J Psychiatry* 150, 782-786.

Ewing, J. (1984). Detecting alcoholism: The CAGE questionnaire. *J Am Med Assoc* 22(14), 1905-1907.

Finkelstein, N. (1993). Treatment programming for alcohol- and drug-dependent pregnant women. *Int J Addict* 28(13), 1275-1309.

Finkelstein, N. (1994). Treatment issues for alcohol- and drug-dependent pregnant and parenting women. *Health Soc Work* 19(1), 7-15.

Finkelstein, N. (1999). Substance abuse and women. Keynote address for the 8th Annual Statewide Conference of the NC Governor's Institute on Alcohol an Substance Abuse, Greensboro, NC.

Fishel, A. (1995). Mental health. In C. Fogel & N. Woods (Eds). *Women's health care*. Thousand Oaks, CA: Sage.

Fishel, A. (1998). Nursing management of anxiety and panic. *Nurs Clin North Am* 33(1), 135-151.

Fishel, A. (1999). Evidenced-based psychosocial therapies. In C. Shea (Ed.). *Advanced practice nursing in psychiatric and mental health care*. St. Louis: Mosby.

Fontaine, K., & Jones, L. (1997). Self-esteem, optimism, and postpartum depression. *J Clin Psych* 53(1), 9-63.

Fox, C. (1994). Cocaine use in pregnancy. *J Am Board Fam Pract* 7, 225-228.

Gilbert, E., & Harmon, J. (1998). *Manual of high risk pregnancy & delivery* (2nd ed.). St. Louis: Mosby.

Glantz, J., & Woods, J. (1993). Cocaine, heroin and phencyclidine: Obstetric perspectives. *Clin Obstet Gynecol* 36(2), 279-301.

Gotlib, I. (1991). Prospective investigation of postpartum depression: Factors involved in onset and recovery. *J Abnorm Psychol* 100(2), 122-132.

Hall, L. et al. (1996). Self-esteem as a mediator of the effects of stressors and resources on depressive symptoms in postpartum mothers. *Nurs Res* 45(4), 231-238.

Hankin, J., & Sokol, R. (1995). Identification and care of problems associated with alcohol ingestion in pregnancy. *Semin Perinatol* 19(4), 286-292.

Herz, E. (1992). Prediction, recognition, and prevention. In F. Hamilton & P. Harberger (Eds.). *Postpartum psychiatric illness: A picture puzzle*. Philadelphia: University of Pennsylvania Press.

Hipwell, A., & Kumar, R. (1996). Maternal psychopathology and prediction of outcome based on mother-infant interaction ratings. *Br J Psychiatry* 169(5), 655-661.

Kaplan, H., & Sadock, B. (1998). *Synopsis of psychiatry* (8th ed.). Baltimore: Williams & Wilkins.

Kearney, M. (1997). Drug treatment for women: Traditional modes and new directions. *J Obstet Gynecol Neonatal Nurs* 26(4), 459-468.

Keltner, N., & Folks, D. (1997). *Psychotropic drugs*. St. Louis: Mosby.

Konefal, J., Duncan, R., & Clemence, C. (1994). The impact of an acupuncture treatment program to an existing Metro-Dade County outpatient substance abuse treatment facility. *J Addict Dis* 13(3), 71-99.

Kovalesky, A., & Flagler, S. (1997). Child placement issues of women with addictions. *J Obstet Gynecol Neonatal Nurs* 26, 585-592.

Kulin, N. et al. (1998). Pregnancy outcome following maternal use of the new selective serotonin reuptake inhibitors: A prospective controlled multicenter study. *JAMA* 279(8), 609-610.

Kumar, R. (1990). An overview of postpartum psychiatric disorders. *NAACOG's Clin Issue Perinat Women Health Nurs* 1(3), 351-358.

Leathers, S., Kelley, M. & Richman, J. (1997). Postpartum depressive symptomatology in new mothers and fathers: Parenting, work, and support. *J Nerv Ment Dis* 185(3), 129-139.

Logsdon, M., McBride, A., & Birkimer, J. (1994). Social support and postpartum depression. *Res Nurs Health* 17(6), 449-457.

Marks, M. et al. (1996). How does marriage protect women with histories of affective disorder from postpartum relapse? *Br J Med Psychol* 69(pt 4): 329-342.

Martin, S. et al. (1996). Violence and substance use among North Carolina pregnant women. *Am J Public Health* 86(7), 991-998.

McIvor, R. et al. (1996). The growth hormone response to aporphine at 4 days postpartum in women with a history of major depression, *J Affect Disord* 40(3), 131-136.

Miller, W., & Rollnick, S. (1991). *Motivational interviewing: Preparing people to change addictive behaviour*. New York: Guilford Press.

Murray, L., Fiori-Crowley, A., & Hooper, R. (1996). The impact of postnatal depression and associated adversity on early mother-infant interactions and later infant outcome. *Child Dev* 67(5), 2512-2526.

Naegle, M. (1997). Understanding women with dual diagnoses. *J Obstet Gynecol Neonatal Nurs* 26, 567-575.

National Women's Health Resource Center. (1998). Anxiety disorders and women' health. *Natl Womens Health Rep* 20(5), 1-6.

Nulman, I. et al. (1997). Neurodevelopment of children exposed in utero to antidepressant drugs. *N Engl J Med* 336(4), 258-262.

Pederson, C. (1998). *Medical management of postpartum psychiatric disorders*. Psychiatric Nursing Institute Presentation. Chapel Hill, NC.

Pokorny, A., Miller, B., & Kaplan, H. (1972). The Brief MAST: A shortened version of the Michigan Alcoholism Screening Test. *Am J Psychiatry* 129(3), 342-345.

Prochaska, J., & DiClemente, C. (1992). Stages of change in the modification of problem behaviors. In M. Hersen, R. Eisler, & P. Miller (Eds.). *Progress in behavior modification*. Sycamore, IL: Sycamore.

Redding, B., & Selleck, C. (1993). Perinatal substance abuse: Assessment and management of the pregnant woman and her children. *Nurs Pract Forum* 4(4), 216-223.

Richard, A. et al. (1995). Effectiveness of adjunct therapies in crack cocaine treatment. *J Subst Abuse Treat* 12, 401-413.

Russell, M. (1994). New assessment tools for risk drinking during pregnancy: T-ACE, TWEAK, and others. *Alcohol Health Res World* 18(1), 55.

Saulnier, C. (1996). Images of the twelve-step model and sex and love addiction in an alcohol intervention group for black women. *J Drug Issues* 26, 95-123.

Schatzberg, A., & Nemeroff, C. (1998). *The American psychiatric press textbook of psychopharmacology* (2nd ed). Washington, D.C.: American Psychiatric Press.

Selleck, C., & Redding, B. (1998). Knowledge and attitudes of registered nurses toward perinatal substance abuse. *J Obstet Gynecol Neonatal Nurs* 27(1), 70-77.

Sharp, D. et al. (1995). The impact of postnatal depression on boys' intellectual development. *J Child Psychol Psychiatry* 36(8), 1315-1336.

Shrock, P. (1994). More than baby blues. *Adv Nurse Pract* 2(6), 24-26.

Sichel, D. et al. (1995). Prophylactic estrogen in recurrent postpartum affective disorder. *Biol Psychiatry* 38(1), 814-818.

Stuart, G., & Laraia, M. (1998). *Stuart and Sundeen's principles and practice of psychiatric nursing* (6th ed.). St. Louis: Mosby.

Thorpe, J. (1995). Management of drug dependency, overdose and withdrawal in the obstetric patient. *Obstet Gynecol Clin North Am* 22(1), 131-142.

Thurtle, V. (1995). Post-natal depression: The relevance of sociological approaches. *J Adv Nurs* 22(3), 416-424.

Whitton, A., Warner, R., & Appleby, L. (1996). The pathway to care in post-natal depression: Women's attitudes to post-natal depression and its treatment. *Br J Gen Pract* 46(408), 427-428.

Wickberg, B., & Hwang, C. (1996a). Counselling of postnatal depression: A controlled study on a population based Swedish sample. *J Affect Disord* 39(3), 209-216.

Wickberg, B., & Hwang, C. (1996b). The Edinburgh Postnatal Depression Scale: Validation on a Swedish community sample. *Acta Psychiatr Scand* 94(3), 181-184.

Wickberg, B., & Hwang, C. (1997). Screening for postnatal depression in a population-based Swedish sample. *Acta Psychiatr Scand* 95(1), 62-66.

Wintz, C. (1999). Difficult decisions: Women of childbearing age, mental illness, and psychopharmacologic therapy. *J Am Psychiatr Nurses Assoc* 5(1), 5-14.

Wisner, K., Perel, J., & Findling, R. (1996). Antidepressant treatment during breastfeeding. *Am J Psychiatry* 153, 1132-1137.

Wisner, K., & Stowe, Z. (1997). Psychobiology of postpartum mood disorders. *Semin Reprod Endocrinol* 15(1), 77-89.

36

Preterm Labor and Birth

Margaret Comerford Freda

LEARNING OBJECTIVES

- Define the key terms.
- Understand the difference between preterm birth and low birth weight.
- Identify the risk factors for preterm birth.
- Understand current interventions to prevent preterm birth.
- Describe the appropriate client education for pregnant women regarding preterm birth.
- Discuss the use of tocolytics and antenatal glucocorticoids in preterm prevention.

- Discuss the nursing care of women confined to home for prevention of preterm birth.
- Describe the deleterious effects of bed rest on pregnant women.
- Define preterm premature rupture of membranes.
- Identify the nursing care strategies for women with preterm premature rupture of membranes.
- Identify topics for nursing research related to preterm labor and birth.

KEY TERMS

antenatal glucocorticoids
chorioamnionitis
intrauterine growth restriction (IUGR)

low birth weight
premature rupture of membranes (PROM)
preterm birth

preterm labor
preterm premature rupture of membranes (PPROM)
tocolytic therapy

PRETERM LABOR AND BIRTH

Preterm birth is any birth that occurs before the completion of 37 weeks of pregnancy. **Preterm labor** is defined as cervical change and uterine contractions occurring between 20 weeks and 37 weeks of pregnancy (ACOG/AAP, 1997). Preterm labor and birth are the most serious complications of pregnancy because they lead to about 75% of the perinatal mortality today (March of Dimes, 1997). Preterm labor and birth also affect infant mortality rates and are second only to congenital anomalies as leading causes of infant mortality in the United States (March of Dimes, 1997). Despite the fact that infant mortality rates in the United States have dropped precipitously since 1950

(29.2% in 1950 versus 7.1% in 1997), preterm birth rates have continued to rise. In 1996, the preterm birth rate in the United States was 11%, having steadily risen over a 15-year period from 7.5% in 1982 (March of Dimes, 1997).

Preterm Birth Versus Low Birth Weight

Although they have distinctly different meanings, the terms "preterm birth" and "low birth weight" are frequently used interchangeably. Preterm birth, however, describes length of gestation (<37 weeks of gestation), whereas **low birth weight** describes only weight at the time of birth (≤2500 g at birth). Low birth weight is far easier to measure than preterm birth, and thus in many settings and publications, low birth weight has been used as a substitute term for preterm birth. Preterm birth, however, is a more dangerous health condition for an infant because length of time in the uterus correlates with immaturity of body systems. Low-birth-weight babies can be preterm, but are not necessarily preterm; low birth weight can be caused by conditions other than preterm labor, such as **intrauterine growth restriction (IUGR),** a condition of fetal growth not necessarily correlated with initiation of labor. Pregnant women who suffer from various complications of pregnancy, such as pregnancy-induced hypertension (PIH), may give birth to a baby at term who is low birth weight because of IUGR. Preterm birth, conversely, simply means birth before 37 completed weeks of pregnancy, no matter the birth weight of the infant.

Incidence and Etiology

The incidence of preterm birth in the United States varies considerably according to race. The rate for African-Americans is almost double the rate for Caucasians (Box 36-1).

Although research has not led us to a real understanding of why there are race-based differences in preterm birth, anecdotal evidence suggests that sociodemographics may play a part (Institute of Medicine, 1985). Preterm birth rates are higher among socially disadvantaged populations, including minorities, women with low levels of education, and women who receive late or no prenatal care.

Predicting Preterm Labor and Birth

Since the early 1970s, researchers have attempted to determine who might be at highest risk for preterm birth in order to target those women for specialized interventions. The known risk factors for preterm birth were compiled by the Institute of Medicine in 1985 and are shown in Box 36-2.

Using the risk factors contained in Box 36-2, much research has taken place over the past 20 years to determine which women might go into labor prematurely. Risk assessment schema were developed, risk scoring systems were used, and specialized interventions were developed for women considered at highest risk (Collaborative Group on Preterm Birth Prevention, 1993; Freda et al., 1990a; Herron, Katz, & Creasy, 1982; Papiernik, 1989). None of these risk scoring systems, however, have resulted in lowering the preterm birth rate in the United States (Main et al., 1989).

Decades of research have demonstrated that risk scoring systems do not predict who will go into labor prematurely because at least 50% of all women who ultimately give birth prematurely have no identifiable risk factors (U.S. Public Health Service, 1989). This fact is one that nurses need to keep in mind when caring for pregnant women. If programs are developed with the aim of decreasing rates of preterm birth, program components must be implemented for both the women labeled as "high risk for preterm birth" and those not so labeled in order to ultimately

---

BOX 36-1 Preterm Birth by Race in the United States, 1996

Total	11%
African-American	18.1%
Caucasian	9.6%

Source: March of Dimes. (1997). *Stat book.* White Plains, NY: March of Dimes Birth Defects Foundation.

BOX 36-2 Risk Factors for Preterm Labor and Birth

DEMOGRAPHIC RISKS
African-American race (doubles the risk)
Below 17 or above 34 years
Low socioeconomic status
Unmarried
Low level of education

MEDICAL RISKS PREDATING THIS PREGNANCY
History of previous preterm birth (triples the risk)
Multiple abortions (miscarriage or elective)
Uterine anomalies
Low prepregnancy weight for height
Parity (0 or >4)
Diabetes
Hypertension

MEDICAL RISKS IN CURRENT PREGNANCY
Multiple gestation
Infection (e.g., bacterial vaginosis)
Incompetent cervix
Short interpregnancy interval
Urinary tract infection
Bleeding in first trimester
Placenta previa or abruptio placentae
Anemia
Fetal anomalies
Premature rupture of membranes (PROM)

BEHAVIORAL AND ENVIRONMENTAL RISKS
Diethylstilbestrol (DES) exposure
Smoking
Poor nutrition
Alcohol or other substance use, especially cocaine
Late or no prenatal care

OTHER RISKS
Stress
Uterine irritability
Long working hours
Inability to rest

Data from Institute of Medicine. (1985). *Preventing low birthweight.* Washington, D.C.: National Academy Press.

BOX 36-3 Multifactorial Etiology of Preterm Labor and Birth

MATERNAL BEHAVIORS

Smoking
Substance use (alcohol or illegal drugs)
Poor nutrition
Work/fatigue
Short interpregnancy interval
Sexual activity

MATERNAL CHARACTERISTICS

Young or old age
Previous preterm birth
Short stature
Short cervix
Uterine anomalies
DES exposure
Incompetent cervix
Low prepregnancy weight
African-American race
Unmarried
Low socioeconomic status
Victim of domestic violence

OTHER FACTORS

Inadequate support systems
Stress
Uterine irritability
Multiple gestation
Late or no prenatal care
Preterm premature rupture of membranes (PPROM)
Anemia
Infection
Catecholamine release
Decreased progesterone production
Decidual cell disruption
Prostaglandin synthesis
Cytokine release

BOX 36-4 Infections and Risk of Preterm Labor

Bacterial vaginosis	40% increased risk
Syphilis and gonorrhea	50% increased risk
Asymptomatic bacteriuria	50% increased risk

Source: Fiscella, K. (1996). Racial disparity in preterm births: The role of urogenital infections. *Public Health Rep* 111, 104-113; Hillier S. et al. (1995). Association between bacterial vaginosis and preterm delivery of a low birthweight infant. *N Engl J Med* 333, 1732-1742.

---

include the 50% of women without known risk factors who deliver preterm. Unless all women are included in prevention efforts, the widespread reduction of preterm birth rates cannot be expected (U.S. Public Health Service, 1989).

Biochemical markers. Biochemical markers have been used in the recent past in an effort to predict who might experience preterm labor. The two most commonly used markers are fetal fibronectin and salivary estriol.

Fetal fibronectins are glycoproteins found in plasma and produced during fetal life. They appear in the cervical canal early in pregnancy, and then again in late pregnancy. Lockwood and associates (1991) found that their appearance between 24 and 34 weeks of gestation could predict preterm labor. As Moore (1999) has documented, the negative predictive value of fetal fibronectins is high (up to 95%). The positive predictive value of the fetal fibronectin test is lower (25% to 40%). This means that it may be possible to predict who will *not* go into preterm labor, but not who will. The test is done during a vaginal examination. The cost of the test ($180 to $215) limits the usefulness of this marker for the general public.

Salivary estriol, the other biochemical marker, is a form of estrogen produced by the fetus that is present in plasma at 9 weeks of gestation. Levels of salivary estriol have been shown to increase before preterm birth. Specimens of salivary estriol are collected by the woman in the home, at a cost of about $90/test, with the testing done every 2 weeks for about 10 weeks for a total of about $450 per woman. This marker also has a high negative predictive value (98%) and a lower positive predictive value (7% to 25%) (Moore, 1999). More research is needed before it will be known if these biochemical markers offer valuable assistance in the risk assessment for preterm labor.

Endocervical length. Another possible predictor of imminent preterm labor is endocervical length as measured by transvaginal ultrasound. Some studies have suggested that a shortened cervix precedes preterm labor and can be determined by ultrasound measurement (Crane et al., 1997). Although the association has not been shown for multiple gestations, it seems that shortened cervical length (<30 mm) in singleton pregnancies, when measured by transvaginal ultrasound, can predict some instances of preterm labor.

Causes of Preterm Labor and Birth

The cause of preterm labor is unknown and is assumed to be multifactorial (Goldenberg & Rouse, 1998) (Box 36-3). The list of possible causes of preterm labor and birth, however, is exhaustive (Goldenberg & Rouse, 1998; Hauth et al., 1995; Hillier et al., 1995). Infection is thought to be a major culprit in the etiology of some preterm labor, but trials of antibiotic therapy for all women at risk have not resulted in statistically significant reductions in preterm births (Fiscella, 1995; Gibbs et al., 1992; Goldenberg & Williams, 1996; Mercer & Lewis, 1997). We know that when cervical, bacterial, or urinary tract infections are present, however, risk of preterm birth is increased (Box 36-4). Thus, early, continuous, and comprehensive prenatal care during which infection can be detected and treated is essential in dealing with this aspect of preterm birth prevention.

Not all preterm births can or even should be prevented. About 25% of all preterm births are iatrogenic, that is, babies are intentionally delivered prematurely because of pregnancy complications that put the fetus' or the mother's life or health in danger and not because of preterm labor. Another 25% of all preterm births are preceded by spontaneous rupture of the membranes followed by labor. These preterm births are not known to be preventable. About 50% of preterm births, therefore, are possibly amenable to prevention efforts, and are considered idiopathic preterm births (Goldenberg & Rouse, 1998).

Sociodemographic factors such as poverty, low educational level, lack of social support, smoking, little or no prenatal care, domestic violence, and stress are thought to contribute to the 50% of possibly preventable preterm births (Bullock & McFarlane, 1989; Copper et al., 1996; Curry, Perrin, & Wall, 1998; McFarlane & Gondolf, 1998; Moore et al., 1995; Moore & Freda, 1998; Parker, McFarlane, & Soeken, 1994; Paarlburg et al., 1996; Vitoratos et al., 1997). Some of these factors, such as domestic violence, have received little attention in the preterm birth prevention literature and are not represented on the usual risk assessment forms used when assessing for high risk for preterm birth.

Physiology of Preterm Labor

Despite 100 years of active biomedical research programs in the United States, the cause of spontaneous labor has not been discovered. Hypotheses including prostaglandin release and uterine stretching, among many others, have not been proven. Science has yet to discover why term labor begins, and therefore why preterm labor begins.

It is known from animal models that many substances contribute to the initiation of preterm labor. Some hypotheses include increased sensitivity of the myometrium to oxytocin (Lopez-Bernal et al., 1993); estrogen and progesterone action on smooth muscle (Valenzuela, Germain, & Foster, 1993); cytokine release and prostaglandin effects on myometrial contractility (Lockwood, 1994; Lopez-Bernal et al., 1993); and corticotropin-releasing hormone activation due to fetal or maternal stress (Lockwood, 1994; Wadhwa et al., 1998). Research continues in this important arena.

▌ CARE MANAGEMENT
Assessment and Nursing Diagnoses

Because it is clear that all pregnant women must be considered at risk for preterm labor (as they are for any other pregnancy complication), nursing assessment begins at the time of entry to prenatal care. In addition, because the onset of preterm labor is often insidious and can be easily

---

▌ BOX 36-5   Symptoms of Preterm Labor (Occurring Between 20 and 37 Weeks of Pregnancy)

Pelvic pressure (feels like the baby is pushing down)
Low, dull backache
Menstrual-like cramps
Change or increase in vaginal discharge
Uterine contractions (hardness) occurring every 10 minutes or more often, with or without pain
Intestinal cramping, with or without diarrhea

---

mistaken for normal discomforts of pregnancy, it is essential that nurses teach pregnant women how to detect the early symptoms of preterm labor (Box 36-5) (Freda, Damus, & Merkatz, 1991; Freston et al., 1997).

The nurse caring for women in the antenatal setting should use known successful modalities for teaching the pregnant woman about early recognition of preterm symptoms, and then reassess the woman at each prenatal visit for the symptoms of early preterm labor. Pregnant women also need to be taught what to do if the symptoms of preterm labor occur (Guidelines/Guías box). Research has shown that some women wait hours or days before contacting a provider after preterm labor symptoms have begun (Freston et al., 1997; Iams et al., 1990). Waiting too long to see a health care provider could result in inevitable preterm birth without the added benefit of the administration of **antenatal glucocorticoids** (medication given to accelerate fetal lung maturity) and ultimately result in a neonate being born at higher risk for respiratory distress syndrome and intraventricular hemorrhage.

One important nursing intervention that could be helpful in helping women learn about preterm labor is the elimination of the term "Braxton-Hicks contractions" in teaching about pregnancy expectations. Nursing research has shown that women are often confused by early symptoms of preterm labor and suffer from "diagnostic confusion" in attempting to decide whether to notify their health care provider (Patterson et al., 1992).

The use of the term "Braxton-Hicks contractions" contributes to this confusion, for it tells women that there are "normal contractions" (Braxton-Hicks) that should cause them no worry. Since no one can discriminate between Braxton-Hicks contractions and the contractions of early preterm labor, nurses who use this terminology unduly contribute to this diagnostic confusion (Hill & Lambertz, 1990). Client education regarding any symptoms of contractions or cramping between 20 and 36 weeks of gestation should be directed toward telling the woman that these symptoms are not normal discomforts in pregnancy, and contractions or cramping that do not go away should prompt the woman to contact her primary health care provider (Freda & Patterson, 1995).

GUIDELINES/GUÍAS

What to Do if Symptoms of Preterm Labor Occur

Lie down on your left side for 1 hour.
Acuéstese de lado izquierdo por una hora.

Drink 2 to 3 glasses of water or juice.
Bebase de 2 o 3 vasos de agua o jugo.

Palpate for contractions like this.
Palpe por contracciones así.

If symptoms continue, call your health care provider or go to the hospital.
Si le continuen los síntomas, llame a su proveedor de salud o vaya al hospital.

If symptoms abate, resume light activity, but not what you were doing when the symptoms began.
Si se alivien los síntomas, resuma actividades leves, pero no lo que hacía cuando le empezaron los síntomas.

If symptoms come back, call your health care provider or go to the hospital.
Si le regresen los síntomas, llame a su proveedor de salud o vaya al hospital.

If any of the following symptoms occur, call your health care provider immediately:
Si le continue cualquier de los síntomas siguientes, llame a su proveedor de salud inmediatamente:

Uterine contractions every 5 minutes or less
Contracciones uterinas cada 5 minutos o menos

Vaginal bleeding
Sangrimiento vaginal

Odorous vaginal discharge
Desangre vaginal de muy mal olor

Fluid leaking from the vagina
Flujo que le gotea vaginal

Since the use of videotapes for teaching women about preterm symptoms has been shown by nursing research to be effective in teaching women this information (Freda et al., 1990a), nurses can feel confident in using client education materials that have been scientifically evaluated, such as the March of Dimes videotape "Helpful Hints: Some Ideas to Help Prevent Preterm Labor" and its accompanying client education booklet (Freda et al., 1990b). No matter which method of client education is used, it is imperative that nurses in prenatal settings make concerted efforts to teach all pregnant women about how to recognize early preterm labor.

Pregnant women who have risk factors for preterm birth, however, are often offered special care with more frequent visits. Although we have no evidence in the literature that this enhanced care results in better outcomes, clinically it makes sense to evaluate at-risk women on a more frequent basis. The U.S. Public Health Service's Expert Panel on the Content of Prenatal Care has endorsed this clinical intervention (U.S. Public Health Service, 1989). Moore and coworkers (1998) have demonstrated through nursing research and a randomized controlled trial that a program that offers nursing telephone support to at-risk women can result in a 26% decrease in low-birth-weight births and a 27% decrease in preterm births in African-American women. This study demonstrates the power of nursing care, nursing support, and client education in the care of women at highest risk for preterm birth. Nursing diagnoses relevant for women at risk for preterm birth include the following:

Nursing Diagnoses

- Knowledge deficit related to
  - recognition of preterm symptoms
- Risk for maternal or fetal injury related to
  - preterm labor and birth
- Anxiety related to
  - preterm birth and family consequences
- Impaired mobility related to
  - prescribed bed rest
- Anticipatory grieving related to
  - preterm labor and birth

Expected Outcomes of Care

The nurse develops a plan of care based on each individual woman's needs. Assessment of each pregnant woman's knowledge of the dangers of preterm birth, symptoms of preterm labor, and what to do if symptoms should occur is the first step in working toward a positive outcome of pregnancy.

Expected outcomes include that the woman will do the following:
- Learn the symptoms of preterm labor and be able to assess herself and her need for intervention.
- Comply with teaching suggestions and call her provider if symptoms occur.
- Not experience preterm symptoms, or if she does, she will take appropriate action.
- Maintain her pregnancy for at least 37 completed weeks.
- Give birth to a healthy, full-term infant.

Plan of Care and Interventions

Prevention

It is not known whether preterm labor and birth can truly be prevented, but nursing efforts toward this goal continue. The most important nursing intervention aimed at preventing preterm birth is the education of pregnant women about the early symptoms of preterm labor, so that

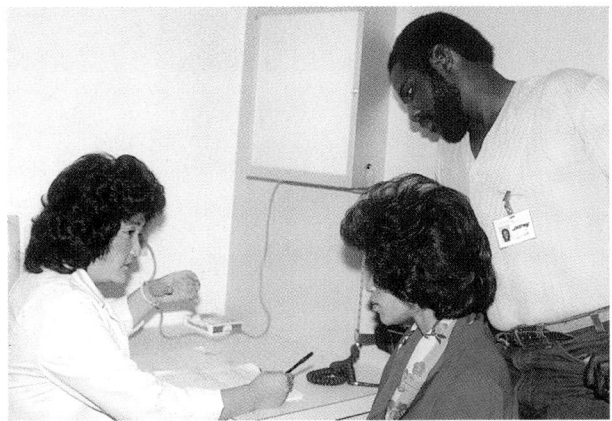

Fig. 36-1   Nurse teaching woman signs and symptoms of preterm labor. *(Courtesy Marjorie Pyle, RNC, Lifecircle, Costa Mesa, CA.)*

---

if the symptoms occur the women can be referred promptly to their provider of care for more intensive care. Box 36-5 and the Guidelines/Guías box describe the symptoms of preterm labor and what the woman should do if the symptoms appear. All pregnant women should be taught this information and told to act on it if they are between 20 weeks and 37 weeks of pregnancy (Fig. 36-1).

Lifestyle Modifications

Some research has shown that pregnant women who exhibit symptoms of preterm labor can decrease those symptoms by modifying some factors in their lifestyle (Freda et al., 1990b; Herron et al., 1982; Katz, Goodyear, & Creasy, 1990; Lynam & Miller, 1992; Papiernik, 1989). Nurses caring for women who exhibit symptoms of preterm labor should question the women about whether they have symptoms when they are engaged in any of the following activities:

- Sexual activity
- Riding long distances in automobiles, trains, buses
- Carrying heavy loads such as laundry, groceries, or a small child
- Standing more than 50% of the time
- Heavy housework
- Climbing stairs
- Hard physical work
- Being unable to stop and rest when tired

If symptoms occur when the woman is engaged in any of these activities, the woman should consider what she was doing when the symptoms began, and then consider stopping those activities until 37 weeks of pregnancy when preterm birth is no longer a risk. Counseling about lifestyle modification should be individualized for each pregnant woman. Because pregnancy is not an illness, but rather a normal function, it is important for nurses to remember that only women who have symptoms of preterm labor when they are engaged in certain activities need to alter their lifestyle. There are no specific rules about which

---

BOX 36-6   Adverse Effects of Bed Rest

MATERNAL EFFECTS (PHYSICAL)

- Weight loss
- Muscle wasting, weakness
- Bone demineralization and calcium loss
- Decreased plasma volume and cardiac output
- Increased clotting tendency; risk for thrombophlebitis
- Alteration in bowel function
- Sleep disturbance, fatigue
- Prolonged postpartum recovery

MATERNAL EFFECTS (PSYCHOSOCIAL)

- Loss of control associated with role reversals
- Dysphoria—anxiety, depression, hostility, and anger
- Guilt associated with difficulty complying with activity restriction and inability to meet role responsibilities
- Boredom, loneliness
- Emotional lability (mood swings)

EFFECTS ON SUPPORT SYSTEM

- Stress associated with role reversals, increased responsibilities, and disruption of family routines
- Financial strain associated with loss of maternal income and cost of treatment
- Fear and anxiety regarding the well-being of the mother and fetus

---

activities are safe for pregnant women and which are not. Each pregnant woman must understand which lifestyle factors might be contributing to her symptoms and be taught to modify only those factors. Sexual activity, for instance, is not prohibited during pregnancy. If, however, symptoms of preterm labor occur after sexual activity, then that activity may need to be curtailed until 37 weeks of gestation.

Bed rest.   Bed rest is a frequently used intervention for the prevention of preterm birth. There is no evidence in the literature to support the efficacy of this intervention, however. Maloni and others (1993) have shown that there are deleterious effects of bed rest on women: after 3 days there is decreased muscle tone, weight loss, calcium loss, and glucose intolerance. Weeks of bed rest lead to bone demineralization, constipation, fatigue, isolation, anxiety, and depression (Maloni et al., 1993) (see Research box). May (1994) has also documented the father's sense of constant worry when bed rest is prescribed for their wives. Bed rest has also been examined for its costs to society; the economic costs were estimated to be $1,417 for each woman, based on lost wages, household and child care help expenses, and hospital costs (Goldenberg et al., 1994). Bed rest, therefore, although frequently prescribed, is not a benign intervention and has furthermore never been shown to decrease preterm birth rates (Maloni, 1998) (Box 36-6).

RESEARCH

Strategies Women Engage in When Managing Preterm Labor at Home

Despite widespread efforts to prevent preterm birth in the United States, greater than 10% of the more than 4 million births that occur each year are preterm. Up to 75% of morbidity and mortality in infants is linked to preterm labor and birth. Bed rest, which may have adverse physical and psychologic effects, is commonly prescribed to manage preterm labor. This study describes the experiences of women in programs of home management for preterm labor. Interview data from 25 women treated at home for preterm labor was analyzed using the grounded theory method.

Findings from this study indicate that the process of home management of preterm labor involves managing activity restriction. Women employed certain strategies when demands from relationships, households, and careers competed with the prescription of bed rest. These strategies included cheating, piggybacking, and testing the limits of their activity restriction. It was concluded that realistic expectations from the health care provider may assist these women in staying within the overall guidelines of their medical prescription and avoiding feelings of cheating and its associated guilt.

Clinical Application

Awareness of the strategies women use to manage preterm labor at home can assist health care providers to counsel women on managing bed rest and to direct care to the client's specific concerns. Exploring with clients the realities of their daily lives may help nurses work with their clients to set realistic guidelines they can follow to limit their activity. Nurses also need to improve communication with women to address the context of their lives and enhance perinatal outcomes. ∎

Source: Durham, R. (1998). Strategies women engage in when managing preterm labor at home. *J Perinat* 18(1), 61-64.

Women who are asked to maintain bed rest at home require expert nursing care and may benefit from the suggested activities described in the Home Care box (Fig. 36-2). Family needs must also be considered; suggested activities for children of women on bed rest are listed in the Home Care box.

Early Recognition and Diagnosis

If interventions such as tocolytic therapy and administration of antenatal glucocorticoids (discussed later in this chapter) are to be implemented successfully, then early recognition of preterm labor is essential. Nursing actions to promote early recognition include educating the pregnant women about symptoms (see Box 36-5 and the Guidelines/Guías box).

 HOME CARE

Suggested Activities for Women on Bed Rest

- Set a routine for daily activities (e.g., getting dressed, moving from the bedroom to a "day bed rest place," [see Fig. 36-2] having social time, eating meals, self-monitoring fetal and uterine activity).
- Do passive exercises as allowed.
- Review childbirth education information or have a childbirth class at home, if this can be arranged.
- Plan menus and make up grocery shopping lists.
- Shop by phone.
- Read books about high risk pregnancy or other topics.
- Keep a journal of the pregnancy.
- Keep a calendar of your progress.
- Reorganize files, recipes, household budget.
- Update address book.
- Do mending, sewing.
- Listen to audiotapes, watch videos or TV.
- Do crossword puzzles, jigsaw puzzles, etc.
- Do craft projects; make something for the baby.
- Put pictures in photo albums.
- Call a friend, family member, or support person each day or use e-mail.
- Treat yourself to a facial, manicure, neck massage, or other special treat when you need a lift. ∎

From Gilbert, E., & Harmon, J. (1998). *Manual of high risk pregnancy and delivery* (2nd ed.). St. Louis: Mosby; Isennock, P. (1992). *Bed rest before baby: What's a mother to do?* Perry Hall, MD: Mustard Seed Publications; and Maloni, J. (1998). *Antepartum bedrest. Case studies, research, & nursing care.* Washington, D.C.: AWHONN

HOME CARE

Activities for Children of Women on Bed Rest

- Schedule brief play periods throughout the day.
- Keep a few favorite toys in a box or basket close to the bed or couch.
- Read to the child(ren).
- Put puzzles together.
- Watch videos, play video games (remote control for TV is ideal).
- Play cards or board games.
- Color in coloring books.
- Cut out pictures from magazines and paste on cardboard.
- Play bed basketball with a soft (sponge) ball or rolled up sock and a trash can or empty laundry basket. ∎

Adapted from Isennock, P. (1992). *Bed rest before baby: What's a mother to do?* Perry Hall, MD: Mustard Seed Publications; Bolane, J., & Furlong, J. (1994). *Coping with bedrest in pregnancy,* Waco, TX: Childbirth Graphics.

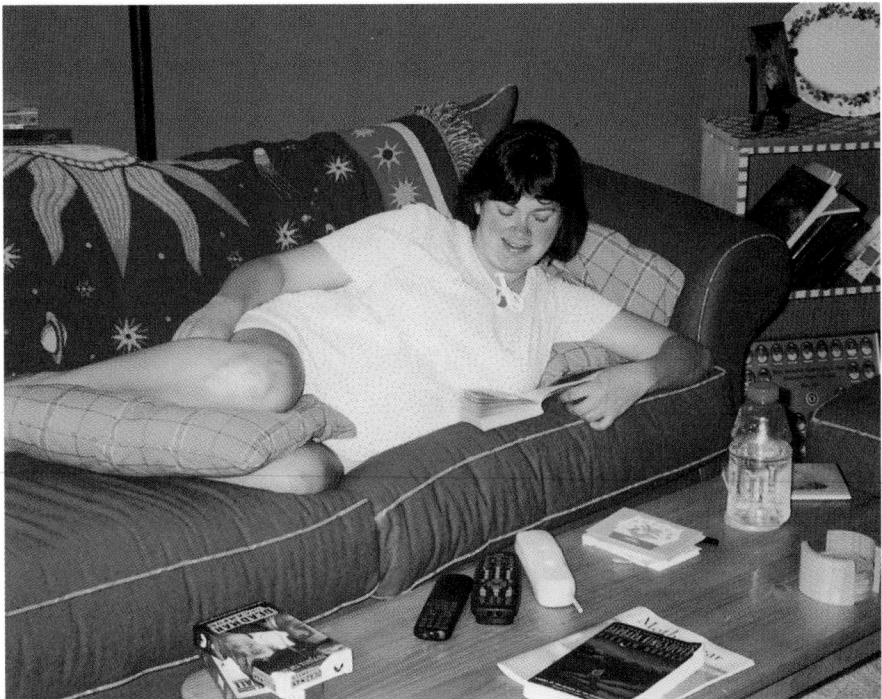

Fig. 36-2 Woman at home on restricted activity for preterm labor prevention. Note how she has arranged her daytime resting area so that needed items are close at hand. *(Courtesy Amy Turner, Cary, NC.)*

The diagnosis of preterm labor is sometimes difficult to make. According to the ACOG/AAP Guidelines for Perinatal Care (1997), the diagnostic criteria for preterm labor are
- 20 to 36 weeks of gestation; and
- documented uterine contractions; and either
- documented cervical change, cervical effacement of 80%, or cervical dilation of greater than 1 cm

Therefore, the pregnant woman at 30 weeks with an irritable uterus but no documented cervical change or effacement is not in preterm labor.

Nurses caring for women who have been diagnosed with preterm labor should be aware of the official diagnostic criteria in order to assist the others on the health care team with in-service education concerning appropriate diagnosis. Misdiagnosis of preterm labor can lead to inappropriate use of pharmacologic agents that can be dangerous to the woman's and fetus' health.

Home uterine activity monitoring. Research in the 1980s suggested that monitoring of uterine activity at home combined with telephone counseling from a nurse could prevent preterm birth by assisting women to access care early in preterm labor (Katz, Gill, & Newman, 1986; Morrison et al., 1987). Although the early research studies showed promising results, the body of research done in the past 15 years has concluded that home uterine activity monitoring does not prevent preterm birth, and its prohibitive cost makes it an unacceptably expensive intervention in the larger scheme of prenatal care (Dyson et al., 1998). This topic remains controversial however (Roberts & Morrison, 1998).

Many companies provide home uterine monitoring services for women diagnosed with preterm labor (Fig. 36-3), and nurses are usually an integral part of the system developed by the companies to educate the clients they serve. While the technology involved in monitoring may not be preventing preterm birth, some research suggests that it is the nursing care offered by the home care nurses that helps the women the most (Iams, Johnson, & O'Shaughnessy, 1988; Moore et al., 1998).

Suppression of Uterine Activity

Tocolytics. Should preterm labor occur, women are usually admitted to the hospital for assessment, fetal monitoring, cervical/vaginal cultures, assessment of cervical status, assessment of amniotic fluid leakage, and assessment of maternal temperature (an early symptom of chorioamnionitis). It is at this time that initiation of tocolytic therapy might be considered. **Tocolytic therapy,** the administration of pharmaceutical agents that suppress uterine activity, has been the subject of research since the late 1970s (Viamantes, 1996). Although before the 1990s it was thought that use of tocolytic therapy could prolong a threatened pregnancy indefinitely, research has since demonstrated that a gain of 24 hours to several days is the best outcome that can be expected (Goldenberg & Rouse, 1998). It is now thought that the best reason to use tocolytics is that it affords the opportunity to begin administering antenatal glucocorticoids, a strategy that can accelerate fetal lung maturity and reduce the severity of sequelae in infants born preterm (Goldenberg & Rouse, 1998).

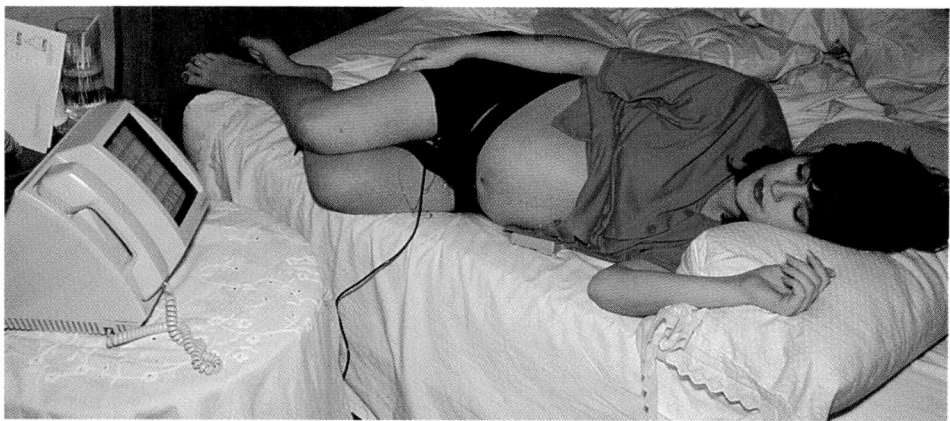

Fig. 36-3 Home uterine activity monitoring. Recording unit and transmitter are on bedside table. *(Courtesy Michael S. Clement, MD, Mesa, AZ.)*

BOX 36-7 Contraindications to Tocolysis

MATERNAL

Severe PIH or eclampsia
Active vaginal bleeding
Intrauterine infection
Cardiac disease
Medical or obstetric condition that contraindicates
 continuation of pregnancy

FETAL

Estimated gestational age over 37 weeks
Dilation over 4 cm
Estimated birth weight greater than 2500 g
Fetal demise
Lethal fetal anomaly
Chorioamnionitis
Acute fetal distress
Chronic IUGR

BOX 36-8 Nursing Care for Women Receiving Tocolytic Therapy

Position woman on side for better placental perfusion.
Explain the purpose, side effects, and contraindications
 of the drug.
Assess blood pressure, pulse, and respirations regu-
 larly, according to institution's policies (in many insti-
 tutions q15 min).
Notify provider if maternal pulse exceeds 120.
Assess for signs of pulmonary edema (chest pain,
 shortness of breath, crackles, rhonchi).
Assess urinary output q1 hr; monitor for ketonuria.
Limit fluid intake to 2500 to 3000 ml/day.
Provide psychosocial support and opportunities for
 woman to express anxiety.
Monitor electrolytes, blood glucose levels.

The drugs most commonly used for this purpose are ritodrine, terbutaline, magnesium sulfate, indomethacin, and nifedipine. There are important contraindications to the use of all tocolytics (Box 36-7).

Ritodrine and terbutaline, the most commonly used betamimetic drugs for tocolysis, work by relaxing smooth muscle (King et al., 1988). Ritodrine is the only drug approved by the Food and Drug Administration (FDA) specifically for the purpose of cessation of uterine contractions. However, other drugs are used for this purpose on an "unlabeled" basis (i.e., drugs known to be effective for a specific purpose though not specifically developed and tested for this purpose). Betamimetics have many maternal and fetal side effects and must always be used with extreme caution and careful, conscientious nursing care. Major maternal side effects of betamimetics are pulmonary edema, myocardial ischemia, cardiac dysrhythmias, hypotension, hyperglycemia, hypokalemia, jitteriness, apprehension, and headache. Fetal side effects can include tachycardia, myocardial ischemia, hyperglycemia, hyperinsulinemia, and heart failure. Medication administration and nursing care when the pregnant woman is receiving betamimetic medication in the hospital setting is aimed at maintaining a therapeutic level of medication and avoiding the most serious side effects while maintaining optimal health of the fetus (Box 36-8 and the Medication Guide). Terbutaline is also given in the home setting using pump therapy, although whether this therapy is effective in prolonging gestation is controversial (Guinn et al., 1998).

NURSE ALERT *Caution must be used when administering intravenous fluids to women in preterm labor because this practice can increase the risk for tocolytic-induced pulmonary edema. It is recommended that the total oral and intravenous fluid intake in 24 hours should be restricted to 2400 to 3000 ml. Strict intake and output measurement, daily weight determination, and assessment of pulmonary function should be instituted (ACOG, 1995; Freda & DeVore; 1996; Hill, 1995).*

TOCOLYTIC THERAPY FOR PRETERM LABOR

MEDICATION	ACTION	INDICATION	DOSAGE AND ROUTE	ADVERSE REACTIONS	NURSING CONSIDERATIONS
Ritodrine (Yutopar)	β-Adrenergic receptor stimulant; relaxes smooth muscles, inhibiting uterine activity and causing bronchodilation	Stop preterm labor	0.1 mg/min (IV); increase by 0.05 mg q10 min until contractions stop; maximum dose: 0.35 mg/min; PO dose: 5-10 mg q4 hr	Tachycardia, dysrhythmias, tremors, headache, nausea and vomiting, hyperglycemia, hypokalemia, fetal tachycardia, hypoxia	Close supervision necessary See Box 37-9. Women should be screened with ECG before therapy begins. Start PO dose 30 min before IV dose is discontinued
Terbutaline (Brethine)	See ritodrine	Stop preterm labor May also be used to reduce hypertonic contractions	0.25 mg SC q30 min for 2 hr; maximum dose: 0.5 mg q4-6 hr; PO dose: 2.5-5 mg q4-6 hr	Tachycardia, flushing, palpitations, tremors, headache, nausea and vomiting, hypokalemia, ketonuria, altered glucose metabolism, fetal tachycardia	Close supervision necessary See Box 37-9. Caution: not FDA approved for use in preterm labor (unlabeled use) Subcutaneous pump may be used for continuous SC therapy
Magnesium sulfate	CNS depressant, relaxes smooth muscles; competes with calcium entry into muscles and decreases intensity	Stop preterm labor	Initially 4-6 g IV over 20 min; then 1-3 g/hr until contractions stop	Hot flushes, sweating, nausea and vomiting, drowsiness, ↓ respirations, ↓ DTRs, ↓ urine output, ↓ BP	Assess for side effects; monitor magnesium levels; assess BP, respirations, urine output, DTRs; monitor FHR and uterine activity; antidote is calcium gluconate
Nifedipine (Procardia, Adalat)	Calcium channel blocker, relaxes smooth muscles	Stop preterm labor	Initially 10 mg (sublingual), then 10-20 mg q6 hr PO	Dizziness, headache, nervousness, nausea, palpitations, peripheral edema, hypotension	Do not use with magnesium sulfate; assess BP, pulse before giving; assess for signs of PTL Caution: not FDA approved for PTL (unlabeled use)
Indomethacin	Prostaglandin inhibition, relaxes smooth muscles	Stop preterm labor	100 mg (rectally), then 25-50 mg q4-6 hr (PO) up to 48 hr	Nausea and vomiting; dyspepsia, dizziness; fetal: premature closure of ductus arteriosus, oligohydramnios	Uncommon use Do not use for woman with any bleeding potential; fetal assessment includes serial ultrasound to determine amniotic fluid levels and any change in ductus arteriosus; may cause hyperbilirubinemia in neonate Caution: not FDA approved for PTL (unlabeled use)

BP, Blood pressure; *DTRs*, deep tendon reflexes; *ECG*, electrocardiogram; *FHR*, fetal heart rate; *PTL*, preterm labor.

Magnesium sulfate is a commonly used tocolytic agent, although its exact mechanism of action on uterine muscle is unclear. It has been used for decades for seizure control in women with preeclampsia, and began to be used for tocolysis in the 1970s (Iams, 1996). Maternal side effects include flushing, nausea and vomiting, headache, muscle weakness and diplopia, shortness of breath, chest pain, and pulmonary edema. Administration and nursing care for the woman receiving magnesium sulfate is in Box 36-8 and the Medication Guide.

Indomethacin, a nonsteroidal antiinflammatory (NSAID) medication, has been shown in some trials to cause a cessation of uterine contractions (Besinger et al., 1991). Maternal side effects of indomethacin include nausea and vomiting, GI bleeding, thrombocytopenia, and acute hypertensive episodes in women with hypertension, and alterations in coagulation. Maternal contraindications to the use of indomethacin include renal disease, peptic ulcer, hypertension, asthma and coagulation disorders. Fetal contraindications to the use of indomethacin include IUGR, renal anomalies, chorioamnionitis, cardiac disease, and twin-to-twin transfusion syndrome. The fetal side effects of indomethacin can be serious. The most common are constriction of the fetal ductus arteriosus, oligohydramnios, and neonatal pulmonary hypertension. The severity of these fetal side effects has made the use of indomethacin for tocolysis less common than other classes of tocolytic drugs. Macones and Robinson (1998) studied the risk of using indomethacin versus the benefit of delayed birth in 1000 women, however, and found that it was more beneficial to the fetus to have received indomethacin and gained gestational age than was preterm birth at 32 weeks.

Nifedipine, a calcium channel blocker, is another tocolytic agent that can suppress contractions (Read & Wellby, 1986). It works by inhibiting calcium from entering smooth muscle cells, thus reducing uterine contractions. Maternal side effects include mild hypotension, increased pulse, headache, occasional flushing, dizziness, nausea, and vomiting. Despite the mild maternal side effects, this medication might be used less than other tocolytic agents because of the common fetal side effects of decreased uteroplacental blood flow, fetal bradycardia, and fetal hypoxia. Garcia-Velasco and Gonzalez-Gonzalez (1998) compared the tocolytic effects and maternal tolerance of nifedipine and ritodrine, and found no significant differences in length of delay of birth, but significantly fewer maternal side effects with nifedipine (see the Medication Guide)

Promotion of Fetal Lung Maturity

Antenatal glucocorticoids. Since the 1970s, the use of antenatal glucocorticoids given as intramuscular injections to the mother has been known to accelerate fetal lung maturity. Widespread use of these drugs did not begin, however, until recently when the National Institutes

of Health convened a Consensus Panel on the topic (National Institutes of Health, 1995). In addition to affecting fetal lung maturity, this class of drugs also seems to decrease rates of intraventricular hemorrhage in preterm infants (Goldenberg & Rouse, 1998). The Consensus Conference's recommendations were that all women between 24 and 34 weeks of gestation be given antenatal glucocorticoids by injection when preterm birth is threatened, unless there is a medical indication for immediate delivery such as cord prolapse, chorioamnionitis, or abruptio placentae (National Institutes of Health, 1995). They also supported and encouraged use of antenatal glucocorticoids even in women with preterm premature rupture of membranes, provided that chorioamnionitis is not present. In an effort to increase the use of antenatal glucocorticoids, the Agency for Health Care Policy and Research recently conducted a multicenter randomized study to learn how best to encourage providers to use this class of drugs, resulting in a 108% increase in usage among providers in the experimental group (Leviton et al., 1999).

NURSE ALERT *Nurses need to know that when any woman is admitted to the hospital and is 24 to 34 weeks pregnant, she should receive antenatal glucocorticoids unless she has chorioamnionitis. These drugs require a 24-hour period to become effective, so timely administration is essential.*

The regimen for administration of antenatal glucocorticoids is given in the Medication Guide.

Home Care

Despite the fact that bed rest has not been shown in randomized controlled trials to reduce preterm birth, it is still commonly prescribed, and women who are at high risk for preterm birth still find themselves told it would be best if they were at home on bed rest for weeks or months. The home care of the woman at risk for preterm birth is a challenge for the nurse, who needs to assist the woman and her family in dealing with the many difficulties faced by families in which one member must be incapacitated. Nurses might be working for a perinatal home care company that provides nursing care in the home, or a public health department that provides visiting nurse service for women and families in need. The scope of care given to women in their homes could range from occasional visits to monitor the maternal and fetal condition, to daily telephone consultation and reading of uterine monitoring strips.

Regardless of the frequency of visits, nursing care for the woman and family in the home demands organization and a sense of just how this family's life has been disrupted by the loss of activity of this essential family member. Families might need help from the nurse in learning how to organize time and space or restructuring family routines so that the pregnant woman can be a part of the family

MEDICATION GUIDE

ANTENATAL GLUCOCORTICOID THERAPY: BETAMETHASONE, DEXAMETHASONE

ACTION

Stimulates fetal lung maturation by promoting release of enzymes that induce production and/or release of lung surfactant. Note: The FDA has not approved these medications for this use (i.e., this is an unlabeled use for obstetrics).

INDICATION

To prevent or reduce the severity of respiratory distress syndrome in preterm infants between 24 and 34 weeks of gestation

DOSAGE AND ROUTE

Betamethasone: 12 mg IM × 2 doses 12 hr apart
Dexamethasone: 6 mg IM × 2 doses 12 hr apart
May be repeated in 7 days if birth has not occurred.

ADVERSE REACTIONS

Possible maternal infection, pulmonary edema (if given with β-adrenergic medications), may worsen maternal condition (diabetes, hypertension)

NURSING CONSIDERATIONS

Give deep IM in gluteal muscle. Teach signs of pulmonary edema. Assess blood glucose levels and lung sounds. Do not give if woman has infection. Use in women with PPROM not universally recommended.

---

activity while still maintaining bed rest. It is also important for the nurse to work toward assisting all the family members to explore their feelings regarding the anxieties of preterm labor and help them to share their feelings with each other.

Management of Inevitable Preterm Birth

Labor that has progressed to a cervical dilation of 4 cm is likely to lead to inevitable preterm birth. It has been demonstrated that preterm birth that occurs in a tertiary care center leads to better neonatal and maternal outcomes (Lubchenco et al., 1989). Women considered at risk for inevitable preterm birth, therefore, should be transferred quickly to such a facility to ensure the best possible outcome. The first dose of antenatal glucocorticoids should be given before the transfer because these drugs require 24 hours to take effect.

Maternal transport, while helping to ensure a better health outcome for the mother and baby, is not without its complications. Sometimes women are transported to ter-

tiary centers far from home, making visiting by the family difficult, and increasing the anxiety levels of the woman and her family members. Attention to the needs of the woman and her family before, during, and after the transport is essential to comprehensive nursing care for these families.

Evaluation

Evaluation of the nursing care provided for a woman at risk for preterm birth includes consideration of whether nursing goals have been met. Evaluation might include:

- The woman has learned the signs of preterm labor.
- The woman with symptoms of preterm labor knows which lifestyle factors might be contributing to those symptoms.
- The woman understands when to contact her provider if symptoms occur.
- The woman being cared for at home understands how to alter her activities so she can be a part of the family while maintaining altered ambulation.
- The family members of the woman being cared for at home verbalize their feelings and anxieties.
- The woman admitted to the hospital for preterm labor receives the appropriate treatment and suffers no complications from tocolysis.
- Antenatal glucocorticoids are administered in a timely manner to the woman with threatened preterm labor.
- The woman with threatened preterm labor is transferred to a tertiary center (see Plan of Care).

PRETERM PREMATURE RUPTURE OF MEMBRANES

Incidence and Etiology

Premature rupture of membranes (PROM) is the rupture of the amniotic sac and leakage of amniotic fluid beginning at least 1 hour before the onset of labor at any gestational age. **Preterm premature rupture of the membranes (PPROM)** (membranes rupture before 37 weeks of gestation) occurs in up to 25% of all cases of preterm labor. Infection often precedes PPROM, but the etiology of PPROM remains unknown. PPROM is diagnosed after the woman complains of either a sudden gush of fluid from the vagina, or a slow leak of fluid from the vagina.

Infection is the serious side effect of PPROM that makes it a major complication of pregnancy. **Chorioamnionitis** is an intraamniotic infection of the chorion and amnion that is potentially life-threatening for the fetus and the woman. It is ultimately diagnosed in 10% of women with PPROM (range 3% to 30%), but 25% to 30% of women with PPROM eventually have a positive amniotic fluid culture (Iams, 1996). Moretti and Sibai (1988) report that most cases of intrauterine infection respond well to antibiotics, yet sepsis can occur and can lead to maternal death. Fetal complications from chorioamnionitis include congenital pneumonia, sepsis, and meningitis (Mercer et al., 1997).

NURSING DIAGNOSIS Knowledge deficit related to recognition of preterm labor

Expected Outcome *Woman and significant other delineate the signs and symptoms of preterm labor.*

Nursing Interventions/*Rationales*

Assess what the partners know about abnormal signs and symptoms during pregnancy *to identify areas of deficit.*

Discuss signs and symptoms that serve as warning signs of preterm labor *so that the woman or her partner has adequate information to identify problems early.*

Provide written supplemental materials that include a list of warning signs and instructions regarding what to do if any of the listed signs occur *so that the couple can reinforce and review learning and act swiftly and appropriately should a sign occur.*

Discuss and demonstrate how to assess and time the contractions *to provide needed skills to assess the signs of labor.*

NURSING DIAGNOSIS Risk for maternal/fetal injury related to recurrence of preterm labor

Expected outcomes *Woman demonstrates ability to assess self and fetus for signs of recurring labor; maternal-fetal well-being is maintained.*

Nursing Interventions/*Rationales*

Teach woman/partner how to monitor fetal and uterine contraction activity daily *to provide immediate evidence of a worsening condition.*

Have woman/partner report rupture of membranes, vaginal bleeding, cramping, pelvic pressure, or low backache to appropriate health care resource immediately *because such symptoms are signs of labor.*

If home uterine activity monitoring is to be used, teach woman/partner how to use the monitoring device and how to transmit the data to the health care provider via telephone *to enhance correct use of monitoring device and increase the accuracy of detection of early labor.*

Have woman monitor her weight, diet, fluid intake, and vital signs on a daily basis *to evaluate for potential problems.*

Limit activities to bed rest with bathroom privileges *to decrease the likelihood of onset of labor.*

Use a side-lying position *to enhance placental perfusion.*

Abstain from sexual intercourse and nipple stimulation *because such activities may stimulate uterine contractions.*

Practice relaxation techniques *to decrease uterine tone and decrease anxiety and stress.*

Take tocolytic or other medications per physician's orders *to inhibit uterine contractions.*

Teach woman/partner about and have them report any medication side effects immediately *to prevent medication-induced complications.*

Have family arrange for alternative strategies in carrying out the woman's usual roles and functions *to decrease stress and limit temptations to increase activity.*

If small children are part of the household, encourage family to make alternative arrangements for child care *to enhance woman's adherence to bed rest protocol.*

NURSING DIAGNOSIS Fear/anxiety related to preterm labor and potentially premature neonate

Expected outcome *Feelings and symptoms of fear/anxiety abate.*

Nursing Interventions/*Rationales*

Provide a calm, soothing atmosphere and teach family to provide emotional support *to facilitate coping.*

Encourage verbalization of fears *to decrease intensity of emotional response.*

Involve woman and family in the home management of her condition *to promote a greater sense of control.*

Help the woman identify and use appropriate coping strategies and support systems *to reduce fear/anxiety.*

Explore the use of desensitization strategies such as progressive muscle relaxation, visual imagery, or thought stopping *to reduce fear-related emotions and related physical symptoms.*

NURSING DIAGNOSIS Diversional activity deficit related to imposed bed rest

Expected outcome *Verbalization of diminished feelings of boredom.*

Nursing Interventions/*Rationales*

Assist woman to creatively explore personally meaningful activities that can be pursued from the bed *to ensure activities that have meaning, purpose, and value to the individual.*

Maintain emphasis on personal choices of the woman *because doing so promotes control and minimizes imposition of routines by others.*

Evaluate what support and system resources are available in the environment *to assist in providing diversional activities.*

Explore ways for the woman to remain an active participant in home management and decision making *to promote control.*

Engage support of family and friends in carrying out chosen activities and making necessary environmental alterations *to ensure success.*

Teach woman about stress management and relaxation techniques *to help manage tension of confinement.*

From Wong, D., & Perry, S. (1998). *Maternal child nursing care.* St. Louis: Mosby.

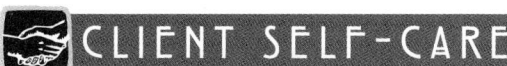

BOX 36-9   Criteria for Home Care of the Woman with PPROM

Documented PPROM >72 hr
Cervical dilation ≤3 cm
No signs or symptoms of chorioamnionitis/pyelonephritis
No signs or symptoms of preterm labor
Client willingness to comply with strict pelvic rest
No breech or transverse presentation (chance of prolapsed cord)

From Lowdermilk, D., & Grohar, J. (1999). *High risk antepartal home care.* White Plains, NY: March of Dimes.

CLIENT SELF-CARE

The Woman with PPROM

Take your temp q4hr when awake
Report temp of more than 38°C
Remain on modified bed rest
Insert nothing in the vagina
No sexual activity
Assess for uterine contractions
Do fetal movement counts daily
No tub baths
Watch for foul-smelling vaginal discharge
Wipe front to back after urinating or having a bowel movement
Take antibiotics if prescribed
See primary health care provider as scheduled

Pregnancy threats due to PPROM are not just infectious in nature. Even in the absence of infection, PPROM can precipitate cord prolapse, a potentially life-threatening complication for the fetus.

CARE MANAGEMENT: HOME VERSUS HOSPITAL

Whenever PPROM is suspected, strict sterile technique should be used in any vaginal examination to avoid introduction of infection. In an era of managed care, long-term hospitalization due to PPROM is unlikely. Women with this diagnosis are often cared for at home, with more frequent visits to the provider (Box 36-9).

Vigilance for signs of infection is a major part of the nursing care and client education for women with PPROM (Client Self-Care Box). Women need to be taught that nothing should be introduced into the vagina and that any signs of foul-smelling vaginal discharge or elevation of temperature should be reported to the provider of care immediately.

HOME CARE

Instructions for Self-Care Counting Fetal Movements (Kick Counts)

Choose a time of day when you can sit or lie quietly
Choices for counting strategies:
- Starting at 9 AM, count the baby's movements until you have counted 10. If you have not counted 10 movements in 12 hours, notify your primary health care provider immediately.
- Count 4 movements, three times a day after meals. Most people count 4 movements in 1 hour. If you don't, then count for 1 more hour. If at the end of 2 hours you still haven't felt 4 movements, call your primary health care provider immediately.

Women with PPROM should also be taught how to count fetal movements daily because a slowing of fetal movement has been shown to be a precursor to severe fetal compromise. If a woman feels less than 10 fetal movements in a 12-hour period, she needs to be evaluated immediately for fetal status (Freda et al., 1993). Fetal movement counting has also been demonstrated to improve maternal-fetal attachment (Mihkail et al., 1991). Several methods are commonly used to count fetal movements, but no one method has been shown to be more effective than another or more acceptable to pregnant women (Freda et al., 1993). One method for fetal movement counting is in the Home Care Box.

Expectant management of the woman continues as long as there are no signs of infection or fetal distress. This care includes all the assessments previously described, as well as other tests of fetal well-being, such as biophysical profile, especially measurement of amniotic fluid index.

KEY POINTS

- Preterm birth is any birth that occurs before the completion of 37 weeks of pregnancy.
- Preterm labor is cervical change and uterine contractions occurring between 20 weeks and 37 weeks of pregnancy.
- The incidence of preterm birth in the United States varies considerably according to race.
- It is not possible to predict which women will go into preterm labor.
- The cause of preterm labor is unknown, and is assumed to be multifactorial.
- Because the onset of preterm labor is often insidious and can be easily mistaken for normal

Continued

KEY POINTS—cont'd

discomforts of pregnancy, it is essential that nurses teach all pregnant women how to detect the early symptoms of preterm labor and to call their primary health care provider when symptoms occur.

- Bed rest, although a frequently prescribed intervention for women experiencing preterm labor symptoms, is not benign, has many deleterious side effects, and has never been shown to decrease preterm birth rates.

- Should preterm labor occur, women are usually admitted to the hospital for assessment, fetal monitoring, cervical/vaginal cultures, assessment of cervical status, assessment of amniotic fluid leakage, and assessment of maternal temperature (an early symptom of chorioamnionitis), and possible initiation of tocolytic therapy.

- Although in previous decades it was thought that use of tocolytic therapy could prolong a threatened pregnancy indefinitely, research has since demonstrated that a gain of 24 hours to several days is the best outcome that can be expected. It is now thought that the best reason to use tocolytic therapy is that it affords the opportunity to begin administration of antenatal glucocorticoids, a strategy that can accelerate fetal lung maturity and reduce the severity of sequelae in infants born preterm.

- Betamimetics are a class of drugs that have many maternal and fetal side effects and must always be used with extreme caution and conscientious, careful nursing care.

- All women between 24 and 34 weeks of gestation should be given antenatal glucocorticoids by injection when preterm birth is threatened unless there is a medical indication for immediate delivery such as chorioamnionitis or bleeding.

- The home care of the woman at risk for preterm birth is a challenge for the nurse, who needs to assist the woman and her family to deal with the many difficulties faced by families in which one member must be incapacitated.

- It has been demonstrated that preterm birth that occurs in a tertiary care center leads to better neonatal and maternal outcomes. Women considered at risk for inevitable preterm birth, therefore, should be transferred to such a facility quickly to ensure the best outcome possible.

- Whenever PPROM is suspected, any vaginal examinations done should use strict sterile technique in order to avoid introduction of infection.

- Vigilance for signs of infection is a major part of the nursing care and client education for women with PPROM.

CRITICAL THINKING EXERCISES

1 You are working for a public health nursing agency, and are assigned to visit a woman who is 28 weeks pregnant and has threatened preterm labor. Her physician has ordered bed rest at home. She has 2 other children, ages 3 and 7.
 a. What are the strategies you might use for assisting this family to cope with this situation?
 b. Discuss the scientific basis for the bed rest order.
 c. What is the nursing care plan for this woman at home?

2 A woman is admitted to a community hospital to the labor floor with contractions every 10 minutes. She is 30 weeks pregnant. You are the labor nurse. The physician has written orders for magnesium sulfate, but no other medications. The woman is to be transported to a tertiary care hospital.
 a. What are the issues concerning transport that you must be aware of in planning your nursing care for this woman?
 b. Discuss the various medications that might be ordered for this woman, their side effects, the nursing care involved, and the precautions that must be taken.
 c. What important medication has not yet been ordered for this woman who is at risk of delivering preterm? Using your knowledge of the literature, what will you ask the physician about this oversight?

3 Mrs. Jones, your next door neighbor, is 27 weeks pregnant and calls you to tell you that she thinks she has been leaking some fluid from her vagina, but she isn't sure what to do.
 a. What is your first and best advice to her?
 b. Discuss the client education necessary when caring for a woman with PPROM.

References

American College of Obstetricians and Gynecologists & American Academy of Pediatrics (ACOG/AAP). (1997). *Guidelines for perinatal care* (4th ed.). Washington, D.C.: ACOG.

American College of Obstetricians and Gynecologists. (1995). Preterm labor. *Technical Bulletin* 206, Washington, D.C.: ACOG.

Besinger, R. et al. (1991). A randomized comparative trial of indomethacin and ritodrine for the long term treatment of preterm labor. *Am J Obstet Gynecol* 164, 981-986.

Bolane, J., & Furlong, J. (1994). *Coping with bedrest in pregnancy.* Waco, TX: Childbirth Graphics.

Bullock, L., & McFarlane, J. (1989). The birth weight/battering connection. *Am J Nurs* 89, 1153-1155.

Collaborative Group on Preterm Birth Prevention (1993). Multicenter randomized controlled trial of a preterm birth prevention program. *Am J Obstet Gynecol* 169, 352-366.

Copper, R. et al. & the National Institute of Child Health and Human Development Maternal Fetal Medicine Units Network. (1996). The preterm prediction study: Maternal stress is associated with spontaneous preterm birth at less than thirty-five weeks' gestation. *Am J Obstet Gynecol* 175, 1286-1292.

Crane, J. et al. (1997). Transvaginal ultrasound in the prediction of preterm delivery: Singleton and twin gestations. *Obstet Gynecol* 90(3), 357-363

Curry, M., Perrin, N., & Wall, E. (1998). Effects of abuse on maternal complications and birthweight in adult and adolescent women. *Obstet Gynecol* 92, 530-534.

Dyson, D. et al. (1998). Monitoring women at risk for preterm labor. *N Engl J Med* 338, 15-19.

Fiscella, K. (1996). Racial disparity in preterm births: The role of urogenital infections. *Public Health Rep* 111, 104-113.

Fiscella, K. (1995). Does prenatal care improve birth outcomes? A critical review. *Obstet Gynecol* 85, 468-479.

Freda, M., Damus, K., & Merkatz, I. (1991). What do pregnant women know about the prevention of preterm birth? *J Obstet Gynecol Neonatal Nurs* 20(2), 140-145.

Freda, M., & DeVore, N. (1996). Should intravenous hydration be the first line of defense with threatened preterm labor? A critical review of the literature. *J Perinatol* 16(5), 385-389.

Freda, M., & Patterson, E. (1995). *Preterm birth: Prevention and nursing management. Nursing module.* New York: March of Dimes.

Freda, M. et al. (1990a). A "PROPP" for the Bronx: Preterm birth prevention education in the inner city. *Obstet Gynecol* 76, 93-96.

Freda, M. et al. (1990b). Lifestyle modification as an intervention in the prevention of preterm birth. *J Adv Nurs* 15, 364-372.

Freda, M. et al. (1993). Fetal movement counting: Which method? *MCN Am J Matern Child Nurs* 18, 314-321.

Freston, M. et al. (1997). Responses of pregnant women to potential preterm labor symptoms. *J Obstet Gynecol Neonatal Nurs* 26, 35-41.

Garcia-Velasco, J., & Gonzalez-Gonzalez, A. (1998). A prospective, randomized trial of nifedipine vs. ritodrine in threatened preterm labor. *Int J Gynecol Obstet* 61, 239-244.

Gibbs, R. et al. (1992). A review of premature birth and subclinical infection. *Am J Obstet Gynecol* 166, 1515-1528.

Gilbert, E., & Harmon, J.(1998). *Manual of high risk pregnancy and delivery* (2nd ed.). St. Louis: Mosby.

Goldenberg, R., & Rouse, D. (1998). Prevention of premature birth. *N Engl J Med* 339, 313-320.

Goldenberg, R., & Williams, W. (1996). Intrauterine infection and why preterm prevention programs have failed. Editorial. *Am J Public Health* 86, 781-782.

Goldenberg, R. et al. (1994). Bed rest in pregnancy. *Obstet Gynecol* 84, 131-136.

Guinn, D. et al. (1998). Terbutaline pump maintenance therapy for prevention of preterm delivery: A double-blind trial. *Am J Obstet Gynecol* 179, 874-878.

Hauth, J. et al. (1995). Reduced incidence of preterm delivery with metronidazole and erythromycin in women with bacterial vaginosis. *N Engl J Med* 333, 1732-1736.

Herron, M., Katz, M., & Creasy, R. (1982). Evaluation of a preterm birth prevention program: A preliminary report. *Obstet Gynecol* 59, 442-445.

Hill, W. (1995). Risks and complications of tocolysis. *Clin Obstet Gynecol* 38(4), 725-745.

Hill, W., & Lambertz, E. (1990). Let's get rid of the term "Braxton-Hicks contractions." *Obstet Gynecol* 75, 709-710.

Hillier, S. et al. (1995). Association between bacterial vaginosis and preterm delivery of a low birth-weight infant. *N Engl J Med* 333, 1737-1742.

Iams, J. (1996). Preterm birth. In S. Gabbe, J. Niebyl, & J. Simpson (Eds.). *Obstetrics: Normal and problem pregnancies* (3rd ed.). New York: Churchill Livingstone.

Iams, J., Johnson, F., & O'Shaughnessy, R. (1988). A prospective randomized trial of home uterine monitoring in pregnancies at increased risk of preterm labor. *Am J Obstet Gynecol* 159, 595-603.

Iams, J. et al. (1990). Symptoms that precede preterm labor and preterm premature rupture of membranes. *Am J Obstet Gynecol* 162, 486-490.

Institute of Medicine (1985). *Preventing low birthweight.* Washington, D.C.: National Academy Press.

Isennock, P. (1992). *Bed rest before baby: What's a mother to do?* Perry Hall, MD: Mustard Seed Publications.

Katz, M., Gill, P., & Newman, R. (1986). Detection of preterm labor by ambulatory monitoring of uterine activity: A preliminary report. *Obstet Gynecol* 65, 773-778.

Katz, M., Goodyear, K., & Creasy, R. (1990). Early signs and symptoms of preterm labor. *Am J Obstet Gynecol* 162, 1150-1153.

King, J. et al. (1988). Betamimetics in preterm labor: An overview of randomized controlled trials. *Br J Obstet Gynaecol* 95, 211-222.

Leviton, L. (1999). A randomized controlled trial of methods to encourage the use of antenatal corticosteroid therapy for fetal maturation. *JAMA* 281(1), 46-52.

Lockwood, C. (1994). Recent advances in elucidating the pathogenesis of preterm delivery: The detection of patients at risk, and preventive therapies. *Curr Opin Obstet Gynecol* 6, 7-18.

Lockwood, C. et al. (1991). Fetal fibronectin in cervical and vaginal secretions as a predictor of preterm delivery. *N Engl J Med* 325, 669-674.

Lopez-Bernal, A. et al. (1993). Biochemistry and physiology of preterm labor and delivery. *Balliere's Clin Obstet Gynecol* 7, 523-552.

Lowdermilk, D., & Grohar, J. (1999). *High risk antepartal home care.* White Plains, NY: March of Dimes.

Lubchenco, L. et al. (1989). Outcome of very low birth weight infants: Does antepartum versus neonatal referral have a better impact on mortality, morbidity, or long term outcome? *Am J Obstet Gynecol* 160, 539-545.

Lynam, L. & Miller, M. (1992). Mothers' and nurses' perceptions of the needs of women experiencing preterm labor. *J Obstet Gynecol Neonatal Nurs* 21, 126-136.

Macones, G., & Robinson, C. (1998). Is there justification for using indomethacin in preterm labor? An analysis of neonatal risks and benefits. *Am J Obstet Gynecol* 178, 873-874.

Main, D. et al. (1989). Risk scoring for preterm labor: Where do we go from here? *Am J Obstet Gynecol* 157, 789-793.

Maloni, J. (1998). *Antepartum bedrest: Case studies, research, & nursing care.* Washington, D.C.: AWHONN.

Maloni, J. et al. (1993). Physical and psychosocial side effects of antepartum bed rest. *Nurs Res* 42(4), 197-203.

March of Dimes (1997). *Stat Book.* White Plains, NY: March of Dimes Birth Defects Foundation.

May, K. (1994). Impact of maternal activity restriction for preterm labor on the expectant father. *J Obstet Gynecol Neonatal Nurs* 23, 246-251.

McFarlane, J. & Gondolf, E. Preventing abuse during pregnancy: A clinical protocol. (1998). *MCN Am J Matern Child Nurs* 23, 22-26.

Mercer, B., & Lewis, R. (1997). Preterm labor and preterm premature rupture of the membranes: Diagnosis and management. *Infect Dis Clin North Am* 11, 177-201.

Mercer, B. et al. (1997). Antibiotic therapy for reduction of infant morbidity after preterm premature rupture of the membranes. *JAMA* 278(12), 989-995.

Mikhail, M. et al. (1991). The effect of fetal movement counting on maternal attachment to the fetus. *Am J Obstet Gynecol* 165, 988-991.

Moore, M. (1999). Biochemical markers for preterm birth. *MCN Am J Matern Child Nurs* 24, 66-74.

Moore, M., & Freda, M. (1998). Reducing preterm and low birth-weight births: Still a nursing challenge. *MCN Am J Matern Child Nurs* 23, 200-208.

Moore, M. et al. (1995). Reduction and cessation of smoking in pregnant women: The effect of a telephone intervention. *J Perinat Educ* 4(1), 35-39.

Moore, M. et al. (1998). A randomized trial of nurse intervention to reduce preterm and low birthweight births. *Obstet Gynecol* 91, 656-661.

Morretti, M., & Sibai, B. (1988). Maternal and perinatal outcome of expectant management of premature rupture of membranes in the midtrimester. *Am J Obstet Gynecol* 159, 390-396.

Morrison, J. et al. (1987). Prevention of preterm birth by ambulatory assessment of uterine activity: A randomized study. *Am J Obstet Gynecol* 156, 536-543.

National Institutes of Health Consensus Development Conference Group. (1995). Effect of corticosteroids for fetal maturation on perinatal outcomes. *Am J Obstet Gynecol* 173, 246-252.

Paarlburg, K. et al. (1996). Psychosocial factors as predictors of low birth weight and preterm delivery. *Am J Obstet Gynecol* 174, 381.

Papiernik, E. (1989). *Effective prevention of preterm birth: The French experience at Hagenau.* New York: March of Dimes.

Parker, B., McFarlane, J., & Soeken, K. (1994). Abuse during pregnancy: Effects on maternal complications and birthweight in adult and teenage women. *Obstet Gynecol* 84, 323-328.

Patterson, E. et al. (1992). Symptoms of preterm labor and self-diagnostic confusion. *Nurs Res* 41, 367-372.

Read, M., & Wellby, D. (1986). The use of a calcium antagonist (nifedipine) to suppress preterm labor. *Br J Obstet Gynaecol* 93, 933-937.

Roberts, W., & Morrison, J. (1998). Has the use of home monitors, fetal fibronectin, and measurement of cervical length helped predict labor and/or prevent preterm delivery in twins? *Clin Obstet Gynecol* 41, 94-102.

U.S. Public Health Service. (1989). *Caring for our future: The content of prenatal care.* Washington, D.C.

Valenzuela, G., Germain, A., & Foster, T. (1993). Physiology of uterine activity in pregnancy. *Curr Opin Obstet Gynecol* 5, 640-646.

Viamantes, C. (1996). Pharmacologic intervention in the management of preterm labor: An update. *J Perinat Neonatal Nurs* 9(4), 13-30.

Vitoratos, N. et al. (1997). Smoking and preterm labor. *Clin Exp Obstet Gynecol* 24, 220-222.

Wadhwa, P. et al. (1998). Maternal corticotropin-releasing hormone levels in the early third trimester predict length of gestation in human pregnancy. *Am J Obstet Gynecol* 179, 1079-1085.

Wong, D. & Perry, S. (1998). *Maternal child nursing care.* St. Louis: Mosby.

37

www.mosby.com/Merlin/Lowdermilk/MatWmnHlth

Labor and Birth Complications

Karen A. Piotrowski

LEARNING OBJECTIVES

- Define the key terms.
- Identify the assessments for women experiencing different types of abnormal labor.
- Formulate nursing diagnoses based on the assessment of abnormal labor.
- Describe the nursing management of a trial of labor, the induction and augmentation of labor, forceps-assisted birth, vacuum-assisted birth, cesarean birth, and vaginal birth after a cesarean birth.

- Discuss the criteria for evaluating the nursing care of women experiencing labor and birth complications.
- Describe the care management of women experiencing a postterm pregnancy.
- Discuss obstetric emergencies and their appropriate management.
- Identify topics for nursing research related to labor and birth complications.

KEY TERMS

amniotic fluid embolism (AFE)
amniotomy
artificial rupture of membranes (AROM)
augmentation of labor
Bishop score
cephalopelvic disproportion (CPD)
cesarean birth
dysfunctional labor
dystocia

external cephalic version (ECV)
forceps-assisted birth
hypertonic uterine dysfunction
hypotonic uterine dysfunction
induction of labor
multifetal pregnancy
oxytocin
postterm pregnancy
precipitous labor
prolapse of the umbilical cord

prolonged labor
prostaglandins
rupture of the uterus
shoulder dystocia
therapeutic rest
trial of labor (TOL)
vacuum-assisted birth
vaginal birth after cesarean (VBAC)

The development of complications during labor and birth is associated with an increase in perinatal morbidity and mortality. Some complications are anticipated, especially if the mother is identified as being at risk for a particular complication during the antepartum period; others are unexpected or unforeseen. The woman, her family, and the health care team can feel devastated when things go wrong. Nurses must recognize these feelings if they are to provide effective support. It is crucial for nurses to understand the normal birth process in order to be able to prevent and detect deviations from normal labor and birth and to implement appropriate nursing measures if complications arise. Optimal care of the laboring woman experiencing complications, as well as of her fetus and family, is possible only when the nurse and other members of the obstetric team use their knowledge and skills in a concerted effort to provide competent and compassionate care.

DYSTOCIA

Dystocia is defined as long, difficult, or abnormal labor and is caused by various conditions associated with the five factors affecting labor. It is estimated that dystocia occurs in approximately 8% to 11% of women during the first stage of labor when the fetus is in a vertex presentation. Second-stage dystocia is equally as common (Wiznitzer, 1995). Dystocia can be caused by any of the following:

1. *Dysfunctional labor,* resulting in ineffective uterine contractions or maternal bearing-down efforts (the powers). It is the most common cause of dystocia (Cunningham et al., 1997).
2. *Alterations in the pelvic structure* (the passage).
3. *Fetal causes,* including abnormal presentation or position, anomalies, excessive size, and number of fetuses (the passenger).
4. *Maternal position* during labor and birth.
5. *Psychologic responses* of the mother to labor related to past experiences, preparation, culture and heritage, and support system.

These five factors are interdependent. In assessing the woman for an abnormal labor pattern, the nurse must consider the way in which these factors interact and influence labor progress. Dystocia is suspected when there is an alteration in the characteristics of uterine contractions, a lack of progress in the rate of cervical dilation, or a lack of progress in fetal descent and expulsion.

Dysfunctional Labor

Dysfunctional labor is described as abnormal uterine contractions that prevent the normal progress of cervical dilation, effacement (primary powers), or descent (secondary powers), or a combination of these. Dysfunction of uterine contractions can be further described as being hypertonic or hypotonic.

In 1996, dysfunctional labor occurred in more than 27 of 1000 live births, with the highest rate occurring in women between 40 and 49 years of age (Ventura et al., 1998). Gilbert and Harmon (1998) cite several factors that seem to increase a woman's risk for uterine dystocia. These factors include:

- Body build: 30 pounds or more overweight, short stature
- Uterine abnormalities: congenital malformations, overdistension as with multiple gestation or hydramnios
- Malpresentations and positions of the fetus
- Cephalopelvic disproportion (CPD)
- Overstimulation with oxytocin
- Maternal fatigue, dehydration and electrolyte imbalance, fear
- Inappropriate timing of analgesic or anesthetic administration

A recent study found a familial occurrence of dystocia. Laboring women whose mothers or sisters experienced dystocia during their labors had an increased risk for experiencing dystocia themselves, possibly related to a genetic factor affecting uterine activity (Berg-Lekas, Hogberg, & Winkvist, 1998).

Hypertonic Uterine Dysfunction

The woman who is experiencing **hypertonic uterine dysfunction,** or primary dysfunctional labor, often is an anxious first-time mother who is having painful and frequent contractions that are ineffective in causing cervical dilation or effacement to progress. These contractions usually occur in the latent stage (cervical dilation of < 4 cm) and are uncoordinated (Fig. 37-1). The force of the contractions may be in the midsection of the uterus rather than in the fundus, and the uterus is therefore unable to apply downward pressure to push the presenting part against the cervix. The uterus may not relax completely between contractions (Gilbert & Harmon, 1998; Varney, 1997).

Women experiencing hypertonic uterine dysfunction may be exhausted and express concern about loss of control because of the intense pain they are experiencing and the lack of progress. **Therapeutic rest,** which is achieved with a warm bath or shower and the administration of analgesics such as morphine, meperidine, or nubain to inhibit uterine contractions, reduce pain, and encourage sleep, is usually prescribed for the management of hypertonic uterine dysfunction. After a 4- to 6-hour rest period these women are likely to awaken in active labor with a normal uterine contraction pattern (Gilbert & Harmon, 1998).

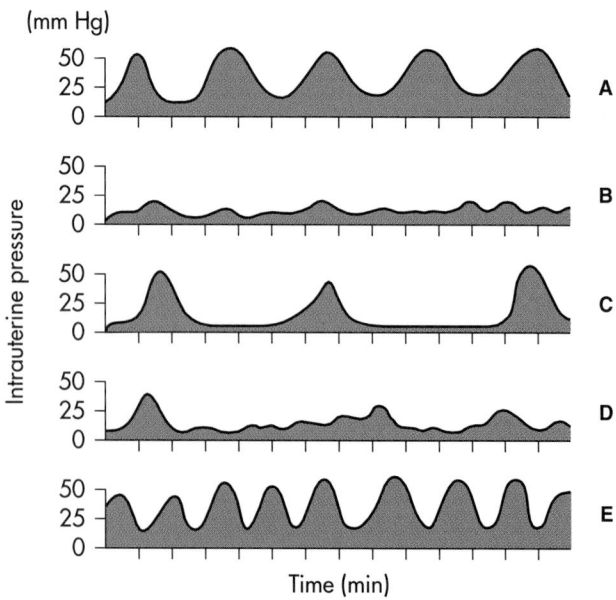

Fig. 37-1 Uterine contractility patterns in labor. **A,** Typical normal labor. **B,** Subnormal intensity, with frequency greater than needed for optimum performance. **C,** Normal contractions but too infrequent for efficient labor. **D,** Incoordinate activity. **E,** Hypercontractility.

Hypotonic Uterine Dysfunction

The second and more common type of uterine dysfunction is **hypotonic uterine dysfunction,** or secondary uterine inertia. In this form of uterine dysfunction, the woman initially makes normal progress into the active stage of labor, then the contractions become weak and inefficient or stop altogether (see Fig. 37-1). The uterus is easily indented, even at the peak of contractions. Intrauterine pressure (IUP) during the contraction (<25 mm Hg) is insufficient for progress of cervical effacement and dilation (Gilbert & Harmon, 1998). Cephalopelvic disproportion and malpositions are common causes of this type of uterine dysfunction.

A woman experiencing hypotonic uterine dysfunction may be in either her first or subsequent pregnancy. She may become exhausted and is at increased risk for infection. Management usually consists of performing an ultrasound or x-ray examination to rule out cephalopelvic disproportion and assessing the fetal heart rate (FHR) pattern, characteristics of amniotic fluid if membranes are ruptured, and maternal well-being. If findings are normal, then measures can be used to augment the progress of labor, including ambulation, hydrotherapy, enema, stripping or rupture of membranes, nipple stimulation, and oxytocin infusion (Varney, 1997).

Secondary Powers

Secondary powers, or bearing-down efforts, are compromised when large amounts of analgesic are given. Anesthesia may also block the bearing-down reflex and, as a result, alter the effectiveness of voluntary efforts (see Research box). Exhaustion resulting from lack of sleep or long labor and fatigue resulting from inadequate hydration and food intake also affect the woman's voluntary efforts. In addition, maternal position can work against the forces of gravity, as well as decrease the strength and efficacy of contractions. The characteristics of dysfunctional labor are summarized in Table 37-1.

Alterations in Pelvic Structure

Pelvic Dystocia

Pelvic dystocia can occur whenever there are contractures of the pelvic diameters that reduce the capacity of the bony pelvis, including the inlet, midpelvis, outlet, or any combination of these planes.

Disproportion of the pelvis is the least common cause of dystocia (Cunningham et al., 1997). Pelvic contractures may be caused by congenital abnormalities, maternal malnutrition, neoplasms, or lower spinal disorders. An immature pelvic size predisposes some adolescent mothers to pelvic dystocia. Pelvic deformities may also be the result of automobile or other accidents.

An inlet contracture occurs in 1% to 2% of term births and is diagnosed whenever the diagonal conjugate is less than 11.5 cm. The incidence of face and shoulder presentation is increased. Because these presentations prevent engagement and fetal descent, the risk of prolapse of the umbilical cord is increased during such births. Inlet contracture is associated with maternal rickets and a flat pelvis. Weak uterine contractions may be noted during the first stage of labor in affected women.

Midplane contracture, the most common cause of pelvic dystocia, is diagnosed whenever the sum of the interischial spinous and posterior sagittal diameters of the midpelvis is 13.5 cm or less. Fetal descent is arrested (transverse arrest of the fetal head) in such births because the head cannot rotate internally. These infants are usually born by cesarean, but vacuum-assisted birth has been used safely when the cervix is fully dilated. Midforceps-assisted birth usually is not done because of the increased perinatal morbidity associated with this intervention.

Outlet contracture occurs when the interischial diameter is 8 cm or less. It rarely occurs in the absence of midplane contracture. Women with outlet contracture have a long, narrow pubic arch and an android pelvis, and this causes fetal descent to be arrested. Maternal complications include extensive perineal lacerations during vaginal birth because the fetal head is pushed posteriorly.

Soft-Tissue Dystocia

Soft-tissue dystocia results from obstruction of the birth passage by an anatomic abnormality other than that involving the bony pelvis. The obstruction may result from placenta previa (low-lying placenta) that partially or completely obstructs the internal os of the cervix. Other causes, such as leiomyomas (uterine fibroids) in the lower uterine segment, ovarian tumors, and a full bladder or rectum, may prevent the fetus from entering the pelvis. Occasionally, cervical edema occurs during labor when the cervix is caught between the presenting part and the symphysis pubis or when the woman begins bearing-down efforts prematurely, thereby inhibiting complete dilation.

Bandl's ring, a pathologic retraction ring, is associated with prolonged rupture of membranes and protracted labor (Cunningham et al., 1997).

Fetal Causes

Dystocia of fetal origin may be caused by anomalies, excessive fetal size and malpresentation, malposition, or multifetal pregnancy. Complications associated with dystocia of fetal origin include neonatal asphyxia, fetal injuries or fractures, and maternal vaginal lacerations. Although spontaneous vaginal birth is possible in these instances, a low-forceps or vacuum-assisted birth or cesarean birth often is necessary.

Anomalies

Gross ascites, abnormal tumors, open neural tube defects such as myelomeningocele, and hydrocephalus are fetal anomalies that can also cause dystocia. The anomalies affect the relationship of the fetal anatomy to the maternal pelvic capacity, with the result that the fetus is unable to descend through the birth canal.

Cephalopelvic Disproportion

Cephalopelvic disproportion (CPD), also called *fetopelvic disproportion (FPD),* is related to excessive fetal size

TABLE 37-1 Dysfunctional Labor: Primary and Secondary Powers

HYPERTONIC UTERINE DYSFUNCTION	HYPOTONIC UTERINE DYSFUNCTION	INADEQUATE VOLUNTARY EXPULSIVE FORCES
DESCRIPTION		
Usually occurs before 4 cm dilation; cause unknown, may be related to fear and tension (primary powers)	Cause may be contracture and fetal malposition, overdistention of uterus (e.g., twins), or unknown (primary powers)	Involves abdominal and levator ani muscles Occurs in second stage of labor; cause may be related to conduction anesthetic, heavy analgesic, exhaustion
CHANGE IN PATTERN OF PROGRESS		
Pain out of proportion to intensity of contraction Pain out of proportion to effectiveness of contraction in effacing and dilating the cervix Contractions increase in frequency Contractions uncoordinated Uterus is contracted between contractions, cannot be indented	Contractions decrease in frequency and intensity Uterus easily indentable even at peak of contraction Uterus relaxed between contractions (normal)	No voluntary urge to push or bear down or inadequate/ineffective pushing
POTENTIAL MATERNAL EFFECTS		
Loss of control related to intensity of pain and lack of progress Exhaustion	Infection Exhaustion Psychologic trauma	Spontaneous vaginal birth prevented
POTENTIAL FETAL EFFECTS		
Fetal asphyxia with meconium aspiration	Fetal infection Fetal and neonatal death	Fetal asphyxia
CARE MANAGEMENT		
Initiate therapeutic rest measures • Administer analgesic (e.g., morphine, nubain, meperidine) if membranes not ruptured or cephalopelvic disproportion not present • Relieve pain to permit mother to rest • Assist with measures to enhance rest and relaxation (e.g., hydrotherapy)	Rule out cephalopelvic disproportion Stimulate labor with oxytocin (augmentation) Perform amniotomy Assist with measures to enhance the progress of labor (e.g., position changes, ambulation, hydrotherapy)	Coach mother in bearing down with contractions; assist with relaxation between contractions Position mother in favorable position for pushing Reduce epidural infusion rate Apply low forceps or vacuum if assistance is needed Schedule cesarean birth only if nonreassuring fetal status occurs

(4000 g or more) and occurred at a rate of 23 per 1000 live births in 1996 (Ventura et al., 1998).

When CPD is present, the fetus cannot fit through the maternal pelvis to be born vaginally. Excessive fetal size, or macrosomia, is associated with maternal diabetes mellitus, obesity, multiparity, or the large size of one or both parents. If the maternal pelvis is too small, abnormally shaped, or deformed, CPD may be of maternal origin. In this case the fetus may be of average size or even smaller.

Malposition

The most common fetal malposition is the persistent occipitoposterior position (right occipitoposterior [ROP] or left occipitoposterior [LOP]; see Fig. 19-2), occurring in

RESEARCH

Use of Delayed Pushing with Epidural Anesthesia: Findings from a Randomized, Controlled Trial

Women receiving epidural anesthesia are thought to experience prolonged labor. Conventional care management for anesthetized women typically includes promotion of strong, sustained, and directed Valsalva or closed-glottis pushing efforts. Recently, it has been recommended that pushing be delayed and rest be promoted. In terms of minimizing adverse maternal and neonatal outcomes, the benefits of a delayed pushing approach provided the support for further investigation of second stage labor management for women receiving epidural anesthesia.

The purpose of this study was to compare outcomes between women receiving epidural anesthesia assigned to a group either following a 1-hour delayed pushing protocol or directed to initiate pushing at full cervical dilation. A sample of 153 subjects from 4 Level III labor and birth units comprised the study group.

A 13.68-minute difference occurred in second stage labor length ($p = 0.225$). No differences were found in Apgar scores ($p > 0.09$). An estimated odds ratio, that progress in terms of one fetal station unit would occur for control group subjects as compared with subjects with similar progress in the experimental group, was 1.51 (95% confidence interval: 1.16, 1.95). It was concluded that second stage labor was not significantly lengthened, and a similar rate of fetal descent occurred in the absence of directed pushing. Findings support further research on the potential advantages of minimizing the duration of pushing in labor.

CLINICAL APPLICATION

Although women who delayed pushing for 1 hour after complete cervical dilation experienced approximately a 14-minute longer second stage, the clinical significance of this outcome should be questioned. Continued nursing research designed to evaluate improvements in labor management guidelines may be warranted based on the potential for contributing data relevant to the long-term health of women.

Source: Mayberry, L. et al. (1999). Use of delayed pushing with epidural anesthesia: Findings from a randomized, controlled trial. *J Perinatol* 19(1), 26-30.

BOX 37-1   Back Labor—Occiput Posterior Position

MEASURES TO RELIEVE BACK PAIN AND FACILITATE ROTATION OF FETAL HEAD

Measures to Reduce Back Pain During a Contraction

- *Counterpressure:* apply fist or heel of hand to sacral area
- *Heat or cold applications:* apply to sacral area
- *Double hip squeeze:*
  Woman assumes a position with hip joints flexed such as knee-chest
  Partner, nurse, or doula places hands over gluteal muscles and presses with palms of hands up and inward toward the center of the pelvis
- *Knee press:*
  Woman assumes a sitting position with knees a few inches apart and feet flat on the floor or on a stool
  Partner, nurse, or doula cups a knee in each hand with heels of hands on top of tibia then presses the knees straight back toward the woman's hips while leaning forward toward the woman

Measures to Facilitate the Rotation of the Fetal Head (May Also Relieve Back Pain)

- *Lateral abdominal stroking:* stoke the abdomen in direction that the fetal head should rotate
- *Hands-and-knees position* (all-fours); can also be accomplished by kneeling while leaning forward over a birth ball, padded chair seat, bed, or over-the-bed table
- *Squatting*
- *Pelvic rocking*
- *Stair climbing*
- *Lateral position:* lie on side toward which the fetus should turn
- *Lunges:* widens pelvis on side toward which woman lunges
  Woman stands, facing forward, next to/alongside a chair so that she can lunge toward the side the fetal back is on or in the direction of the fetal occiput
  Places foot on seat of chair with toes pointed toward the back of the chair then lunges
  Alternative position for lunge: kneeling

---

about 25% of all labors. Labor in these women, especially the second stage, is prolonged.

This type of labor is often referred to as back labor because the woman typically complains of severe back pain resulting from the fetal head (occiput) pressing against her sacrum. Box 37-1 describes suggested measures to relieve back pain and facilitate rotation of the fetal occiput to an anterior position, which will facilitate birth (Gilbert & Harmon, 1998; Simkin, 1995).

Malpresentation

Breech presentation is the most common form of malpresentation, occurring in 3% to 4% of all births and in up to 25% of preterm births.

In 1996, it was the third most commonly reported complication of labor and birth. There are four main types of breech presentation: frank breech (thighs flexed, knees extended), complete breech (thighs and knees flexed), and two types of incomplete breech, one in which the knee extends below the buttocks and the other in which the foot extends below the buttocks (Fig. 37-2). Breech presentations are associated with multifetal gestation, preterm birth, fetal and maternal anomalies, hydramnios, and oligohydramnios. Diagnosis is made on the basis of the findings yielded by abdominal palpation and vaginal examination and usually is confirmed by ultrasound scan (Laros, Flanagan, & Kilpatrick, 1995; Lydon-Rochelle et al., 1993; Ventura et al., 1998).

During labor, the descent of the fetus in a breech presentation may be slow because the breech is not as good a dilating wedge as the fetal head, but the labor itself usually is not prolonged. There is risk of the cord prolapsing if the membranes rupture in early labor. The presence of meconium in amniotic fluid is not necessarily a sign of fetal distress, however, because it results from the pressure being exerted on the fetal abdominal wall as it traverses the birth canal. Assessment of FHR and pattern should be used to determine if the passage of meconium is an expected finding associated with breech presentation or is a nonreassuring sign associated with fetal hypoxia.

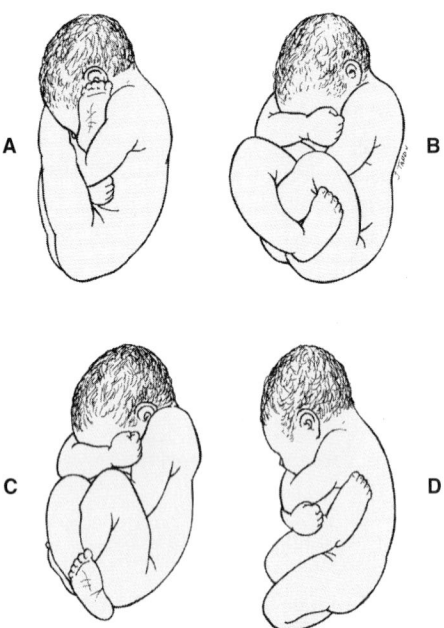

Fig. 37-2 Types of breech presentation. **A,** Frank breech: thighs are flexed on hips; knees are extended. **B,** Complete breech: thighs and knees are flexed. **C,** Incomplete breech: foot extends below buttocks. **D,** Incomplete breech: knee extends below buttocks.

The fetal heart tones of infants in a breech position are best heard at or above the umbilicus. Vaginal birth is accomplished by mechanisms of labor that manipulate the buttocks and lower extremities as they emerge from the birth canal (Varney, 1997) (Fig. 37-3). Piper forceps sometimes are used to deliver the head (see Fig. 37-9).

Besides the vaginal birth of the fetus in breech presentation, external cephalic version (ECV) may be tried to turn the fetus to a vertex presentation. Cesarean birth may also prove necessary (Laros et al., 1995).

Although opinions vary regarding the conditions calling for cesarean birth, it is commonly performed for nulliparas, women with fetuses estimated to be larger than 3800 g or smaller than 1500 g if labor is ineffective or complications occur (Scott, 1999). Although cesarean birth reduces the risks to the fetus, the maternal risks are increased. ECV also poses risks and is not always successful. Women whose breech presentation occurs late in pregnancy need to be informed of the options for birth, as well as the risks associated with each.

Face and brow presentations (Fig. 37-4) are uncommon and are associated with fetal anomalies, pelvic contractures, and CPD. Vaginal birth is possible if the fetus flexes to a vertex presentation, although forceps often are used. Cesarean birth is indicated if the presentation persists, there is fetal distress, or labor stops progressing.

Cesarean birth is usually necessary for a fetus in a shoulder presentation (the fetus is in a transverse lie), although ECV may be attempted after 38 weeks of gestation (Cunningham et al., 1997; Varney, 1997).

Multifetal Pregnancy

Multifetal pregnancy is the gestation of twins, triplets, quadruplets, or more infants.

The multiple birth rate, which primarily measures the birth of twins, was 27.4 in 1996 representing an increase of 5% from the rate in 1995. Since 1980, the twin birth rate has increased by 37% and the higher order multiple rate has quadrupled (Ventura et al., 1998). It is speculated that this trend is related to use of fertility-enhancing drugs and procedures. Their births are associated with more complications, including dysfunctional labor, than are single births. This high incidence of complications and risk of perinatal mortality primarily stems from the birth of low-birth-weight infants resulting from preterm birth or intrauterine growth restriction (IUGR) in part related to placental dysfunction and twin-to-twin transfusion. Fetuses may experience distress and asphyxia during the birth process as a result of cord prolapse and the onset of placental separation with the birth of the first fetus.

In addition, fetal complications such as congenital anomalies and abnormal presentations can result in dystocia and cause the incidence of cesarean birth to be increased. For example, in only half of all twin pregnancies do both fetuses present in the vertex position, the most favorable for vaginal birth; in one third of the pregnancies, one twin may present in the vertex position and one in the breech (Cunningham et al., 1997; Ellings, Newman, & Bowers, 1998; Varney, 1997).

The health status of the mother may be compromised by an increased risk for hypertension, anemia, and hemorrhage associated with uterine atony, abruptio placentae, and multiple or adherent placentas. Duration of the phases and stages of labor may vary from the duration experienced with singleton births. The latent phase of the first stage of labor is usually shorter as a result of early cervical changes while the active phase and the second stage are often longer.

Teamwork and planning are essential components of the management of childbirth in multiple pregnancies, especially those of the higher order multiples. The nurse plays a key role in coordinating the activities of many highly skilled health care professionals. Early detection and care of the maternal/fetal/newborn complications associated with multiple births are essential to achieve a positive outcome for mother and babies. Maternal positioning and active support are used to enhance labor progress and placental perfusion. Stimulation of labor with oxytocin, epidural anesthesia, forceps and vacuum assistance, and internal or external cephalic version may be used to accomplish the vaginal birth of twins. Cesarean birth is most likely with higher order multiple births. Emotional support that includes expres-sion of feelings and full explanations of events as they occur and of the status of the mother and the fetuses/newborns is important to reduce the anxiety and stress the mother and her family experience (Ellings et al., 1998).

Position of the Mother

The functional relationships between the uterine contractions, the fetus, and the mother's pelvis are altered by the maternal position. In addition, the position can have either a mechanically advantageous or disadvantageous effect on

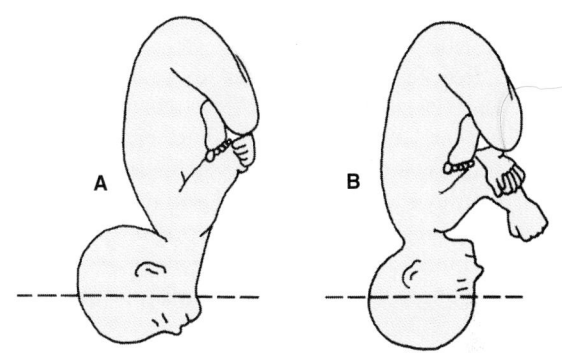

Fig. 37-4 Extension of normally flexed head. Face (**A**) and brow (**B**) presentations.

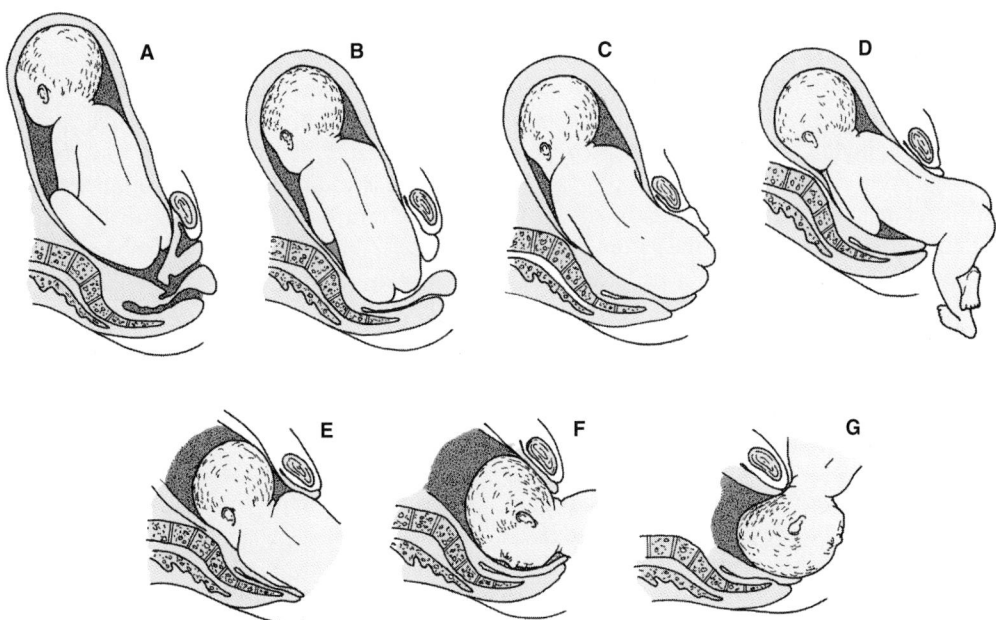

Fig. 37-3 Mechanism of labor in breech presentation. **A,** Breech before onset of labor. **B,** Engagement and internal rotation. **C,** Lateral flexion. **D,** External rotation or restitution. **E,** Internal rotation of shoulders and head. **F,** Face rotates to sacrum when occiput is anterior. **G,** Head is born by gradual flexion during elevation of fetal body.

the mechanisms of labor by altering the effects of gravity and the relationships among body parts that are important to the progress of labor. For example, the hands-and-knees position more effectively facilitates rotation of the fetus from a posterior occiput position than does the lateral position. Sitting and squatting facilitate fetal descent during pushing and shorten the second stage of labor (Biancuzzo, 1993). In addition, discouraging maternal movement or restricting the woman's position during labor to the recumbent or lithotomy position may compromise labor. The incidence of dystocia is also increased in women confined to these positions, resulting in an increased need for augmentation of labor, the use of forceps or vacuum-assisted or cesarean birth (Andrews & Chrzanowski, 1990).

Psychologic Responses

Hormones released in response to stress can also bring about dystocia. Sources of stress vary for each woman, but pain and the absence of a support person are two accepted factors. Confinement to bed and the restriction of maternal movement can also be a source of psychologic stress that compounds the physiologic stress caused by immobility in the unmedicated laboring woman. If the woman's anxiety is excessive, it can cause normal cervical dilation to be inhibited, resulting in **prolonged labor** and increased pain perception. Anxiety also causes an increase in the levels of stress-related hormones (β-endorphin, adrenocorticotropic hormone, cortisol, and epinephrine). These hormones act on the smooth muscles of the uterus; increased levels can lead to dystocia by reducing uterine contractility (Biancuzzo, 1993).

Abnormal Labor Patterns

In 1996, prolonged labor patterns occurred at a rate of 8.9 per 1000 live births. The incidence of prolonged labor patterns was slightly higher among women who were 40 to 49 years of age (Ventura et al., 1998).

Six abnormal labor patterns have been identified and classified by Friedman (1989) according to the nature of the cervical dilation and fetal descent. The labor patterns seen in normal and abnormal labor are described in Table 37-2.

These patterns may result from a variety of causes, including ineffective uterine contractions, pelvic contractures, CPD, abnormal fetal presentations or position, early use of analgesics, conduction anesthesia, and anxiety and stress. In these women, progress in either the first or second stage of labor can be either protracted (prolonged) or arrested (stopped). Abnormal progress can be identified by plotting cervical dilation on a labor graph at various intervals after the onset of labor and comparing the resulting curve with a normal labor curve. Figure 37-5, *A*, is a labor graph showing a normal labor progress in a first-time mother. Figure 37-5, *B*, shows major types of deviation from the normal progress of labor. If a woman exhibits an abnormal labor pattern, as depicted by the broken lines, the primary health care provider is notified.

TABLE 37-2 Labor Patterns in Normal and Abnormal Labor

NORMAL LABOR

1. Dilation: continues
   a. Latent phase: <4 cm and low slope
   b. Active phase: >5 cm or high slope
   c. Deceleration phase: ≥9 cm
2. Descent: active at ≥9 cm dilation

ABNORMAL LABOR

PATTERN	NULLIPARAS	MULTIPARAS
Prolonged latent phase	>20 hr	>14 hr
Protracted active phase dilation	<1.2 cm/hr	<1.5 cm/hr
Secondary arrest: no change	≥2 hr	≥2 hr
Protracted descent	<1 cm/hr	<2 cm/hr
Arrest of descent	≥1 hr	≥½ hr
Failure of descent	No change during deceleration phase and second stage	
Precipitous labor	>5 cm/hr	10 cm/hr

Health care providers must be careful when diagnosing a labor pattern as prolonged and when intervening based on this diagnosis. Criteria defining the differences between false, latent, and active labor should be established. Using admission areas to evaluate a woman's labor status has been found to be helpful in preventing the premature implementation of labor interventions such as induction of epidural anesthesia, administration of analgesics, stimulation of labor, and use of operative interventions such as forceps- and vacuum-assisted and cesarean birth. If a woman is found to be in false or latent (early) labor she can be sent home or remain in the admissions area until labor becomes active. However, women in active labor are admitted to the labor and birth unit (McNiven et al., 1998).

The risk of fetal death increases sharply whenever the active first stage of labor lasts for more than 15 hours. Maternal morbidity and death may occur as a result of uterine rupture, infection, serious dehydration, and postpartum hemorrhage. A long and difficult labor also can have an adverse psychologic effect on the mother, father, and family.

Precipitous Labor

Precipitous labor is defined as labor that lasts less than 3 hours from the onset of contractions to the time of birth. This abnormal labor pattern occurred at a rate of 20.2 per 1000 live births in 1996. As with prolonged labor patterns, precipitous labor occurred at a slightly higher rate among women aged 40 to 49 (Ventura et. al., 1998).

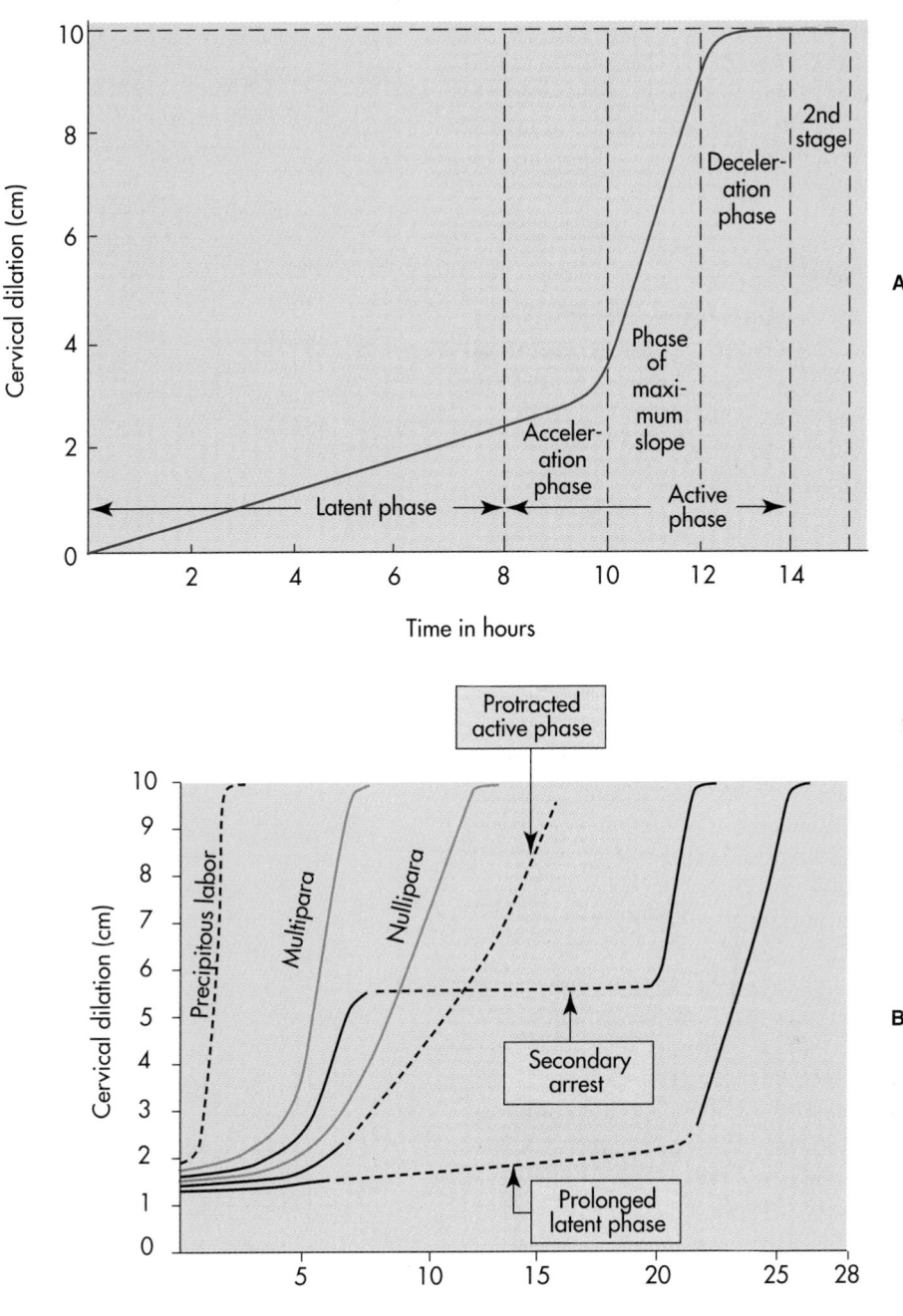

Fig. 37-5 **A,** Depiction of a normal labor for a primigravida. **B,** Major types of deviation from normal progress of labor may be detected by noting dilation of cervix at various intervals after labor begins. If a woman exhibits an abnormal labor pattern, as depicted by broken lines, primary health care provider should be notified.

Precipitous labor may result from hypertonic uterine contractions that are tetanic-like in intensity. Maternal and fetal complications can occur as a result. Maternal complications include uterine rupture, lacerations of the birth canal, amniotic fluid embolism, and postpartum hemorrhage. Fetal complications include hypoxia resulting from decreased periods of uterine relaxation between contrac-

tions and intracranial hemorrhage related to rapid birth (Cunningham et al., 1997).

Women who have experienced precipitous labor often describe feelings of disbelief that their labor began so quickly, alarm that their labor progressed so rapidly, panic about the possibility they would not make it to the hospital on time to give birth, and finally, relief when they arrived at the hospital. In addition, women have expressed frustration when nurses would not believe them when they reported their readiness to push. Some women have difficulty remembering the details of their labor and birth and require others, including caregivers, to help them to fill in the gaps in their memory (Rippin-Sisler, 1996).

▪ CARE MANAGEMENT

The care management of the woman at risk for problems related to abnormal labor or birth, or both, involves all members of the health care team. Nursing care is facilitated through the use of the nursing process.

Assessment and Nursing Diagnoses

Risk assessment is a continuous process in the laboring woman. Review of the findings obtained during the initial interview conducted at the woman's admission to the labor unit and ongoing observations of her psychologic response to labor may reveal factors that can be a source of dysfunctional labor, for example, anxiety or fear, a complication of pregnancy, or previous labor complications. The initial physical assessment and ongoing assessments provide information about maternal well-being; status of labor in terms of the characteristics of uterine contractions and progress of cervical effacement and dilation; fetal well-being in terms of FHR and pattern, presentation, station, and position; and status of the amniotic membranes.

Laboratory data such as the scalp pH can be used to identify fetal distress and ultrasound scanning can identify potential dysfunctional labor problems related to the fetus or maternal pelvis. All these assessments help in the accurate identification of potential and actual nursing diagnoses related to dystocia and maternal-fetal compromise and should serve as the rationale for labor interventions.

Nursing diagnoses vary with the type of dystocia, as well as with the individual needs of the woman and her family. Potential or actual nursing diagnoses that might be identified in women experiencing dystocia include the following:

▪ Nursing Diagnoses _____

- Anxiety related to
  - slowed labor progress
  - perceived threat to well-being of self or fetus
- Pain related to
  - dystocia
  - obstetric procedures
- Risk for fetal injury related to
  - obstetric procedures
- Risk for maternal injury related to
  - interventions implemented for dystocia
- Risk for infection related to
  - rupture of membranes
  - invasive procedures

▪ Nursing Diagnoses—cont'd _____

- Fatigue related to
  - prolonged labor
- Risk for altered parent-infant attachment related to
  - unplanned cesarean birth
- Ineffective individual coping related to
  - lack of knowledge regarding measures to enhance labor and facilitate birth
  - pain
  - fatigue
  - inadequate support system
- Situational low self-esteem related to
  - inability to labor and give birth as expected

Expected Outcomes of Care

Expected outcomes for the woman who is experiencing dystocia include that she will do the following:
- Verbalize understanding of the causes and treatment of dysfunctional labor.
- Use measures recommended by the health care team to enhance the progress of labor and birth.
- Use positive patterns of coping to maintain a positive self-concept.
- Demonstrate diminished or minimal anxiety.
- Verbalize relief of pain.
- Experience labor and birth with minimal or no complications, such as infection, injury, or hemorrhage.
- Give birth to a healthy infant who has not experienced fetal distress or birth injury.

Plan of Care and Interventions

Nurses assume many caregiving roles when labor is complicated. They also collaborate and work with other health care providers such as nurse-midwives, anesthesiologists, obstetricians, and other physicians in providing care. Interventions that the nurse may implement or assist with implementing include external cephalic version, trial of labor, induction or augmentation with oxytocin, amniotomy, and operative procedures. The nursing role is identified with each of the procedures described.

LEGAL TIP **Standard of Care—Labor and Birth Complications**

- *Document all assessment findings, interventions, and client responses on client record, and monitor strips according to unit protocols, procedures, and/or policies and professional standards.*
- *Assess whether the woman, and her family as appropriate, is fully informed about procedures to which she is consenting.*
- *Maintain safety in administering medications and treatments correctly.*

*   *Have verbal orders signed as soon as possible.*
*   *Provide care at the acceptable standard (e.g., according to hospital protocols, professional standards).*
*   *If short staffing occurs in the unit and the nurse is assigned additional clients, the nurse should document that rejecting these assignments would have placed the woman in danger as a result of abandonment.*
*   *Maternal and fetal monitoring continues until birth according to the policies, procedures, and/or protocols of the birthing facility, even when a decision to carry out cesarean birth is made.*

Version

Version is the turning of the fetus artificially from one presentation to another and may be done either externally or internally.

External cephalic version. **External cephalic version (ECV)** is used to attempt to turn the fetus from a breech or shoulder presentation to a vertex presentation for birth. It may be attempted in a labor and birth setting after 37 weeks of gestation. Before it is attempted, however, ultrasound scanning is done to determine the fetal position, to locate the umbilical cord, to rule out placenta previa, and to assess the amount of amniotic fluid, the fetal age, and the presence of any anomalies. A nonstress test is also performed to confirm fetal well-being or the FHR pattern is monitored for a period of time, usually 10 to 20 minutes. Informed consent must be obtained for the maneuver to be done. Contraindications to its use include uterine anomalies, previous cesarean birth, CPD, placenta previa, multifetal gestation, and oligohydramnios (Cunningham et al., 1997; Laros et al., 1995).

ECV is accomplished by the exertion of gentle, constant pressure on the abdomen (Fig. 37-6). A tocolytic agent, such as magnesium sulfate or terbutaline often is given to relax the uterus and facilitate the maneuver. Ultrasound scanning is done to identify potential problems, such as cord entanglement and placental separation (Cunningham et al., 1997; Laros et al., 1995).

During an attempted ECV, the nurse continuously monitors the FHR, especially for bradycardia; frequently checks the maternal vital signs; and assesses the woman's level of comfort because the procedure may cause discomfort. After the procedure is completed, the nurse continues to monitor maternal vital signs, uterine activity, and FHR and watches for vaginal bleeding until the woman's condition is stable. Women who are Rh negative should receive Rh immune globulin because the manipulation can cause fetomaternal bleeding (Cunningham et al., 1997; Laros et al., 1995).

Internal version. With internal version, the fetus is turned by the physician who inserts a hand into the uterus and changes the presentation to a cephalic (head) or podalic (foot) one. Internal version may be used in multifetal pregnancies to deliver the second fetus. The safety of this procedure has not been documented; maternal and fetal injury are possible. Cesarean birth is the usual method

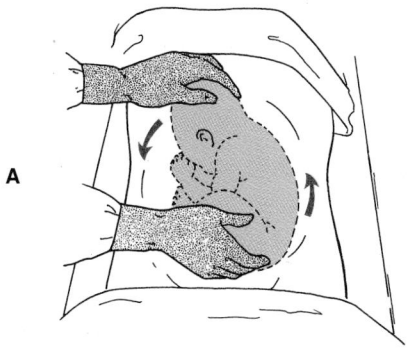

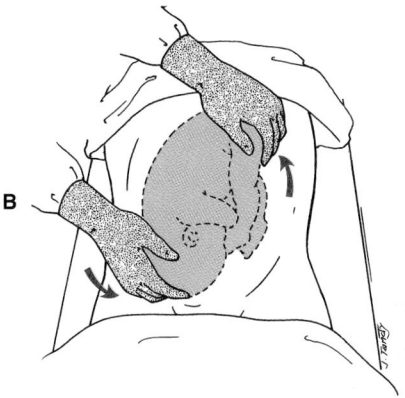

Fig. 37-6 External version of fetus from breech to vertex presentation. This must be achieved without force. **A,** Breech is pushed up out of pelvic inlet while head is pulled toward inlet. **B,** Head is pushed toward inlet while breech is pulled upward.

for managing malpresentation in multifetal pregnancies. The nurse's role is to monitor the status of the fetus and to provide support to the woman.

Trial of Labor

A **trial of labor (TOL)** is the allowance of a reasonable period (4 to 6 hours) of spontaneous active labor so that the safety of a vaginal birth for the mother and infant can be assessed. TOL may be initiated if the mother's pelvis is of questionable size or shape, if she wishes to give birth vaginally after a previous cesarean birth, or if the fetus is in an abnormal presentation. Fetal sonography or maternal pelvimetry, or both, may be done before a TOL to rule out CPD. The cervix must be soft and dilatable. During TOL, the woman is evaluated for the occurrence of active labor, including adequate contractions, engagement and descent of the presenting part, and effacement and dilation of the cervix.

During a TOL the nurse assesses uterine activity, cervical changes, maternal vital signs, and fetal status. If maternal or fetal complications are identified, the nurse is responsible for initiating appropriate actions, including notifying the primary health care provider, and for evaluating and documenting the maternal or fetal response to the interventions. Nurses must recognize that the woman and her partner are often anxious about her health and well-being and that of their baby. Supporting and encouraging the woman and her partner and providing information regarding progress can reduce stress and enhance the labor process and facilitate a successful outcome.

Induction of Labor

Induction of labor is the chemical or mechanical initiation of uterine contractions before their spontaneous onset for the purpose of bringing about the birth (see Guidelines/Guías box). In 1996, the rate of labor induction was estimated to be 169 per 1000 live births, representing an increase of approximately 6% from 1995. The rates of both induction and stimulation of labor have been increasing every year since 1989 (Ventura et al., 1998). Labor induction should be used in circumstances in which the risk of labor stimulation and birth to the mother and fetus is less than the risk of continuing the pregnancy (Mathews, 1998).

Labor can be induced by both chemical and mechanical methods. Intravenous oxytocin and amniotomy are the most common methods used in the United States. Less commonly used methods include nipple stimulation (manual or with a breastpump), the ingestion of castor oil or herbal preparations, a soap-suds enema, stripping of the membranes, and acupuncture (Summers, 1997). Prosta-

glandins are also used for inducing labor, but their use for this purpose continues to be investigated (Day & Snell, 1993; Mastrogiannis & Knuppel, 1995; Summers, 1997).

The success of the induction of labor is greater if the condition of the cervix is favorable, or inducible. A rating system such as the **Bishop score** (Table 37-3) can be used to evaluate inducibility. For example, a score of 9 or more on this 13-point scale indicates that the cervix is soft, anterior, 50% or more effaced, and dilated 2 cm or more, and that the presenting part is engaged. Induction of labor is likely to be more successful if the score for nulliparas is 9 or more and the score for multiparas is 5 or more (Gilbert & Harmon, 1998).

Cervical Ripening Methods

Chemical agents. Various **prostaglandins** (hormones) have been applied to the cervix before induction to "ripen" (soften and thin) the cervix. This treatment usually results in a higher success rate for the induction of labor, the need for lower dosages of oxytocin during the induction, and shorter induction times. In some cases, women will go into labor after the application of prostaglandin, thereby eliminating the need to administer oxytocin to induce labor. Since 1993, a prostaglandin gel has been approved by the FDA for use as a cervical ripening agent (ACOG, 1995a) The gel is available in a 2.5-ml syringe that contains 0.5 mg of dinoprostone (Prepidil), which is a form of prostaglandin E_2. After being brought to room temperature, the gel is inserted into the cervical canal just below the internal os using a soft, plastic catheter. A warm water bath or microwave oven should not be used to speed up the warming process because inactivation of prostaglandin can occur.

The woman is instructed to remain in the supine position with a hip tilt or in a lateral position for 30 to 60 minutes after administration to minimize leakage. The dose may be repeated in 6 hours if there is no cervical response. A maximum of 1.5 mg of dinoprostone can be given in a 24-hour period. Induction of labor using an intravenous infusion of oxytocin can begin in 6 to 12 hours after the instillation if cervical ripening has occurred (ACOG, 1995a; Simpson & Poole, 1998; Summers, 1997).

GUIDELINES/GUÍAS

Labor and Birth Complications

INDUCTION OF LABOR

Your labor is not progressing.
Su trabajo de parto no está progresando.

We need to stimulate the contractions.
Necesitamos provocar las contracciones.

I'm going to give you some medication to make your contractions stronger.
Le voy a dar una medicina para hacerle mas fuertes las contracciones.

I'm going to give you pitocin through your IV.
Le voy a dar pitufina por medio del suero.

CESAREAN BIRTH

You need a cesarean.
Necesita una operación cesárea.

Do you understand why you need a cesarean?
¿Entiende usted por qué necesita una operación cesárea?

Please sign this consent form.
Por favor, firme esta forma de consentimiento.

TABLE 37-3 Bishop Score

	SCORE			
	0	1	2	3
Dilation (cm)	0	1-2	3-4	5-6
Effacement (%)	0-30	40-50	60-70	80
Station (cm)	−3	−2	−1	−1
Cervical consistency	Firm	Medium	Soft	
Cervix position	Posterior	Midline	Anterior	

Prostaglandin E$_2$ may also be administered in the form of a vaginal insert (Cervidil), which contains 10 mg of dinoprostone. The insert is placed in the posterior fornix of the vagina where it absorbs moisture, swells, and slowly releases the dinoprostone.

Cervidil does not need warming, is simple to insert, and it can be easily removed by pulling its string after 12 hours, when active labor begins, or if hyperstimulation of the uterus occurs. The manufacturer recommends that the woman remain in a supine position for 2 hours after insertion. Labor induction can begin 30 minutes after the insert is removed.

Systemic maternal side effects related to prostaglandin use, which include vomiting, fever, and diarrhea, are usually mild. Hyperstimulation of the uterus with or without fetal distress can occur, usually within 1 hour of administration. Terbutaline 0.25 mg can be given subcutaneously or intravenously to reduce uterine activity if hyperstimulation occurs. Prostaglandin E$_2$ should be used with caution in women who have a history of asthma, reactive airway disease, glaucoma, renal disease, hepatic disease, and cardiovascular disease. Contraindications include active pelvic infection, vaginal bleeding, and hypersensitivity (ACOG, 1995a, Gilbert & Harmon, 1998). Before application of prostaglandin gel or insert, the woman needs to be given a full explanation of the procedure. It is upon this explanation that her informed consent is based. Baseline data regarding the health and well-being of the maternal-fetal unit should be obtained. Condition of the cervix (Bishop score) and uterine activity need to be assessed and documented. It should be determined that vaginal bleeding, fever, regular uterine contractions, and fetal distress are absent.

After the gel or insert has been administered, the nurse monitors uterine activity and the FHR pattern continuously for 30 minutes to 2 hours and periodically thereafter. Maternal vital signs are taken every hour for 2 hours or for 4 hours if uterine contractions occur and continue. The woman should remain in the supine position with her hips elevated for the recommended length of time. Then the woman may be ambulatory and allowed to go home if no signs of labor or fetal distress are exhibited. She is instructed to return the next day for oxytocin induction of her labor. If contractions are still occurring, the oxytocin infusion should be postponed or used with great caution in a very low dose (ACOG, 1995a; Gilbert & Harmon, 1998; Simpson & Poole, 1998) (Medication Guide). Measures to treat uterine hyperstimulation may need to be implemented (Emergency box).

Misoprostol (Cytotec) is a synthetic prostaglandin analog that can be administered orally or intravaginally at a relatively low cost when compared with dinoprostone. The vaginal route is preferred because it seems to reduce the incidence of gastrointestinal side effects. Cytotec is not approved by the FDA for cervical ripening (unlabeled use) but it is effective, especially when membranes are ruptured, and it compares favorably with dinoprostone prepa-

rations. Dosages range from 25 mg to 100 mg (Mundle & Young, 1996; Simpson & Poole, 1998) (Medication Guide).

Mechanical methods. Hydroscopic dilators (substances that absorb fluid from surrounding tissues and then enlarge) also can be used for cervical ripening, especially if contraindications to prostaglandins exist. These consist of laminaria tents (natural cervical dilators made from seaweed) and synthetic dilators containing magnesium sulfate (Lamicel), which are inserted into the endocervix without rupturing the membranes. As they absorb fluid, they expand and cause the cervix to dilate. These dilators are left in place for 6 to 12 hours before being removed to assess cervical dilation. Fresh dilators are inserted if further cervical dilation is necessary. Synthetic dilators swell faster than natural dilators and become larger with less discomfort (ACOG, 1995a; Simpson & Poole, 1998; Summers, 1997).

Hydroscopic dilators compare favorably with prostaglandins in terms of their effectiveness in ripening the cervix but are associated with a higher incidence of postpartum maternal and newborn infections, especially with the use of natural dilators. Cervical lubrication with a bacteriostatic cream or jelly and saturation of the sponges (used to hold the dilators in place) with povidone-iodine or a bacteriostatic cream or jelly can help to decrease the risk for infection.

Nursing responsibilities for women who have dilators inserted include documenting the number of dilators and sponges inserted during the procedure, as well as the number removed, and assessment for urinary retention, rupture of membranes, uterine tenderness/pain, contractions, vaginal bleeding, and fetal distress (Gilbert & Harmon, 1998; Simpson & Poole, 1998).

Other methods that can be used to ripen the cervix include stripping of the amniotic membranes and insertion of a balloon catheter (e.g., a Foley catheter) into the cervical os.

Amniotomy (artificial rupture of membranes [AROM]) can be used to induce labor when the condition of the cervix is favorable (ripe) or to augment labor if progress begins to slow. Labor usually begins within 12 hours of the rupture; however, if amniotomy does not stimulate labor, the resulting prolonged rupture may lead to infection. Once an amniotomy is performed, the woman is committed to giving birth. For this reason, amniotomy often is used in combination with oxytocin induction. Before the procedure, the woman should be told what to expect; she should also be assured that the actual rupture of the membranes is painless for her and the fetus though she may experience some discomfort when the Amnihook or other sharp instrument is inserted through the vagina and cervix (Procedure box).

The presenting part of the fetus should be engaged and well applied to the cervix to reduce the risk of cord prolapse (ACOG, 1995a; Summers, 1997). The membranes are ruptured with an Amnihook or other sharp instrument, and the amniotic fluid allowed to drain slowly. The color, odor, and consistency of the fluid is assessed (i.e., for the

MEDICATION GUIDE

Cervical Ripening Using Prostaglandin E$_2$ (PGE$_2$): Dinoprostone (Cervidil Insert; Prepidil Gel)

ACTION
PGE$_2$ ripens the cervix, making it softer and causing it to begin to dilate and efface; stimulates uterine contractions.

INDICATIONS
PGE$_2$ is used for preinduction cervical ripening (ripen cervix before oxytocin induction of labor when the Bishop score is 4 or less), and to induce labor or abortion (abortifacient agent)

DOSAGE
Place Cervidil insert (10 mg dinoprostone gradually released over 12 hours) intravaginally into the posterior fornix. Insert Prepidil gel (2.5-ml syringe containing 0.5 mg of dinoprostone) into cervical canal just below internal cervical os. Repeat gel insertion in 6 hours as needed to a maximum of 1.5 mg in a 24-hour period. Continue treatment until maximum dosage is administered or until an effective contraction pattern is established (3 or more uterine contractions in 10 minutes), cervix ripens (Bishop score of 8 or greater), or significant adverse reactions occur.

ADVERSE REACTIONS
Potential adverse reactions include headache, nausea and vomiting, diarrhea, fever, hypotension, tachysystole (12 or more uterine contractions in 20 minutes without alteration of FHR pattern), hyperstimulation of the uterus (tachysystole with nonreassuring FHR patterns), or fetal passage of meconium.

NURSING CONSIDERATIONS
- Explain procedure to woman and her family. Ensure that an informed consent has been obtained as per agency policy.
- Assess maternal-fetal unit, before each insertion and during treatment following agency protocol for frequency. Assess maternal vital signs and health status, FHR pattern, and status of pregnancy, including indications for cervical ripening or induction of labor, signs of labor or impending labor, and the Bishop score. Recognize that a nonreassuring FHR pattern; maternal fever, infection, vaginal bleeding, or hypersensitivity; and regular, progressive uterine contractions contraindicate the use of dinoprostone.
- Use caution if the woman has a history of asthma; glaucoma; or renal, hepatic, or cardiovascular disorders.
- Bring gel to room temperature before administration. Do not force warming process by using a warm water bath or other source of external heat (e.g., microwave).
- Assist woman to maintain a supine position with lateral tilt or a side-lying position for 30 to 60 minutes after insertion of gel or for 2 hours after placement of insert.
- Prepare to swab vagina to remove remaining gel using a saline-soaked gauze wrapped around fingers or pull string to remove insert and to administer terbutaline 0.25 mg subcutaneously or intravenously if significant adverse reactions occur.
- Initiate oxytocin for induction of labor within 6 to 12 hours after last instillation of gel or within 30 minutes after removal of the insert.
- Follow agency protocol for induction if ripening has occurred and labor has not begun.
- Document all assessment findings and administration procedures.

Dinoprostone is the only FDA-approved medication for cervical ripening or labor induction.

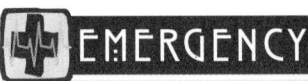 EMERGENCY

Uterine Hyperstimulation with Oxytocin

SIGNS
Uterine contractions lasting more than 90 seconds and occurring more frequently than every 2 minutes
Uterine resting tone greater than 20 mm Hg
Nonreassuring FHR:
 Abnormal baseline (<110 or >160 beats/min)
 Absent variability
 Repeated late decelerations or prolonged decelerations

INTERVENTIONS
Maintain woman in side-lying position
Turn off oxytocin infusion; keep maintenance IV line open; increase rate
Start administering oxygen by face mask, per protocol or physician's order
Notify primary health care provider
Prepare to administer terbutaline (Brethine) 0.25 mg subcutaneously if ordered to decrease uterine activity
Continue monitoring FHR and uterine activity
Document responses to actions

MEDICATION GUIDE

Cervical Ripening Using Prostaglandin E₁ (PGE₁): Misoprostol (Cytotec)

ACTION

PGE₁ ripens the cervix, making it softer and causing it to begin to dilate and efface; stimulates uterine contractions.

INDICATIONS

PGE₁ is used for preinduction cervical ripening (ripen cervix before oxytocin induction of labor when the Bishop score is 4 or less) and to induce labor or abortion (abortifacient agent).

DOSAGE

Insert 25 to 50 μg ($\frac{1}{4}$ to $\frac{1}{2}$ of a 100-μg tablet) intravaginally into the posterior fornix using the tips of index and middle fingers without the use of a lubricant. Repeat every 3 to 6 hours as needed to a maximum of 300 to 400 μg in a 24-hour period or until an effective contraction pattern is established (3 or more uterine contractions in 10 minutes), cervix ripens (Bishop score of 8 or greater), or significant adverse reactions occur.

ADVERSE REACTIONS

Higher dosages are more likely to result in adverse reactions such as nausea and vomiting, diarrhea, fever, tachysystole (12 or more uterine contractions in 20 minutes without alteration of FHR pattern), hyperstimulation of the uterus (tachysystole with nonreassuring FHR patterns), or fetal passage of meconium.

NURSING CONSIDERATIONS

- Explain procedure to woman and her family. Ensure that an informed consent has been obtained as per agency policy.
- Assess maternal-fetal unit, before each insertion and during treatment following agency protocol for frequency. Assess maternal vital signs and health status, FHR pattern, and status of pregnancy, including indications for cervical ripening or induction of labor, signs of labor or impending labor, and the Bishop score. Recognize that a nonreassuring FHR pattern; maternal fever, infection, vaginal bleeding, or hypersensitivity; and regular, progressive uterine contractions contraindicate the use of misoprostol.
- Use caution if the woman has a history of asthma, glaucoma, or renal, hepatic, or cardiovascular disorders.
- Assist woman to maintain a supine position with lateral tilt or a side-lying position for 30 to 40 minutes after insertion.
- Prepare to swab vagina to remove unabsorbed medication using a saline soaked gauze wrapped around fingers and to administer terbutaline 0.25 mg subcutaneously or intravenously if significant adverse reactions occur.
- Initiate oxytocin for induction of labor no sooner than 4 hours after last dose of misoprostol was administered, following agency protocol, if ripening has occurred and labor has not begun.
- Document all assessment findings and administration procedures.

Misoprostol (Cytotec) has not yet been approved by the FDA for cervical ripening or labor induction.

PROCEDURE

Assisting with Amniotomy

PROCEDURE

Explain to the woman what will be done.

Assess FHR before procedure begins to obtain a baseline reading.

Place several underpads under the woman's buttocks to absorb the fluid.

Position the woman on a padded bed pan, fracture pan, or rolled up towel to elevate her hips.

Assist the health care provider who is performing the procedure by providing sterile gloves and lubricant for the vaginal examination.

Unwrap sterile package containing Amnihook or Allis clamp and pass instrument to the primary health care provider, who inserts it alongside the fingers and then hooks and tears the membranes.

Reassess the FHR.

Assess the color, consistency, and odor of the fluid.

Assess the woman's temperature every 2 hours or per protocol.

Evaluate the woman for signs and symptoms of infection.

DOCUMENTATION

Record the following:

Time of rupture

Color, odor, and consistency of the fluid

FHR before and after the procedure

Maternal status (how well procedure was tolerated)

BOX 37-2 Protocol: Induction of Labor with Oxytocin

CLIENT/FAMILY TEACHING

Explain technique, rationale, and reactions to expect:
- Route and rate for administration of medication
- What "piggyback" is for
- Reasons for use:
  Induce labor, improve labor
- Reactions to expect concerning the nature of contractions: the intensity of contraction increases more rapidly, holds the peak longer, and ends more quickly; contractions will come regularly and more often
- Monitoring to anticipate:
  Maternal: blood pressure, pulse, uterine contractions, uterine tone
  Fetal: heart rate, activity
- Success to expect: a favorable outcome will depend on inducibility of the cervix (Bishop score of 9 for nulliparas and 5 for multiparas)
- Keep woman and support person informed of progress

ADMINISTRATION

Position woman in side-lying or upright position
Assess status of maternal fetal unit
Prepare solutions and administer with pump delivery system according to prescribed orders:
- Infusion pump and solution are set up (e.g., 10 U/1000 ml isotonic electrolyte solution)
- Piggyback solution is connected to IV line at proximal port (port nearest point of venous insertion)
- Solution with oxytocin is flagged with a medication label
- Begin induction at 0.5 to 2 mU/min
- Increase dose 1 to 2 mU/min at intervals of 15 to 60 minutes until either a dose of up to 20-40 mU/min or 300 Montevideo units (MVUs) is reached (see Box 37-3)

MAINTAIN DOSE IF

- Intensity of contractions results in intrauterine pressures of 40 to 90 mm Hg (shown by internal monitor)
- Duration of contractions is 40 to 90 seconds
- Frequency of contractions is 2- to 3-minute intervals
- Cervical dilation of 1 cm/hr in the active phase

MATERNAL/FETAL ASSESSMENTS

- Monitor blood pressure, pulse, and respirations every 30 to 60 minutes and with every increment in dose
- Monitor contraction pattern and uterine resting tone every 15 minutes and with every increment in dose
- Assess intake and output; limit IV intake to 1000 ml/8 hr; output should be 120 ml or more every 4 hours
- Perform vaginal examination as indicated
- Monitor for nausea, vomiting, headache, hypotension
- Assess fetal status using electronic fetal monitoring; evaluate tracing every 15 minutes and with every increment in dose
- Observe emotional responses of woman and her partner

REPORTABLE CONDITIONS

- Uterine hyperstimulation
- Nonreassuring FHR pattern
- Suspected uterine rupture
- Inadequate uterine response at 20 mU/min

EMERGENCY MEASURES

Discontinue use of oxytocin per hospital protocol:
- Turn woman on her side
- Increase primary IV rate up to 200 ml/hr, unless client has water intoxication, in which case, the rate is decreased to one that keeps the vein open
- Give woman oxygen by face mask at 8 to 10 L/min or per protocol or physician's order

DOCUMENTATION

- Medication: kind, amount, time of beginning, increasing dose, maintaining dose, and discontinuing medication in client record and on monitor strip
- Reactions of mother and fetus
  Pattern of labor
  Progress of labor
  FHR
  Maternal vital signs
  Nursing interventions and woman's response
- Notification of primary health care provider

From American College of Obstetricians and Gynecologists (ACOG). (1995a). Induction of labor. *Technical Bulletin* 217, Washington, D.C.: ACOG; Pozaic, S. (1999). Induction and augmentation of labor. In L. Mandeville, & N. Troiano (Eds.). *High-risk and critical care intrapartum nursing* (2nd ed.). Philadelphia: Lippincott; Simpson, K., & Poole, J. (1998). *Cervical ripening and induction and augmentation of labor.* Washington, D.C.: AWHONN; Summers, L. (1997). Methods of cervical ripening and labor induction. *J Nurse Midwifery* 42(2), 71-85.

presence or absence of meconium or blood). The time of rupture is recorded.

NURSE ALERT *The FHR is assessed before and immediately after the procedure to detect any changes (e.g., decelerations) that may indicate cord compression or prolapse.*

The woman's temperature should be checked at least every 2 hours to rule out possible infection. The primary health care provider is notified if her temperature is found to be 38° C or higher. The nurse also assesses for other signs and symptoms of infection, such as maternal chills, fetal tachycardia, uterine tenderness on palpation, and foul-smelling vaginal drainage (Simpson & Poole, 1998). Comfort measures, such as frequently changing the woman's underpads, and perineal cleansing are implemented.

Oxytocin

Oxytocin is a hormone normally produced by the posterior pituitary gland that stimulates uterine contractions. It may be used either to induce the labor process or to augment a labor that is progressing slowly because of inadequate uterine contractions.

The indications for oxytocin induction or augmentation of labor may include, but are not limited to, the following:
- Suspected fetal jeopardy (e.g., intrauterine growth restriction)
- Inadequate uterine contractions; dystocia
- Premature rupture of membranes
- Postterm pregnancy
- Chorioamnionitis
- Maternal medical problems (e.g., woman with severe Rh isoimmunization, diabetes, renal disease, or chronic pulmonary disease)
- Pregnancy-induced hypertension
- Fetal demise (death)
- Multiparous women with a history of precipitous labor or who live far from the hospital

The management of stimulation of labor is the same regardless of the indication. Because of the potential dangers associated with the injection of oxytocin in the prenatal and intrapartal periods, however, the FDA has issued certain restrictions to its use.

Contraindications to oxytocin stimulation of labor include, but are not limited to, the following:
- CPD, prolapsed cord, transverse lie
- Nonreassuring FHR
- Placenta previa or vasa previa
- Prior classic uterine incision or uterine surgery
- Active genital herpes infection
- Invasive cancer of the cervix

Certain maternal and fetal conditions, although not contraindications to the use of oxytocin to stimulate labor, do require special caution during its administration. These conditions include the following:
- Multifetal presentation
- Breech presentation
- Presenting part above the pelvic inlet
- Abnormal FHR pattern not requiring emergency birth
- Polyhydramnios
- Grand multiparity
- Maternal cardiac disease; hypertension

Oxytocin use can pose hazards to the mother and fetus. These hazards are primarily dose related, with high doses given rapidly creating the most problems. Maternal hazards include water intoxication and tumultuous labor with tetanic contractions, which may cause premature separation of the placenta, rupture of the uterus, lacerations of the cervix, or postbirth hemorrhage. These complications can lead to infection, disseminated intravascular coagula-

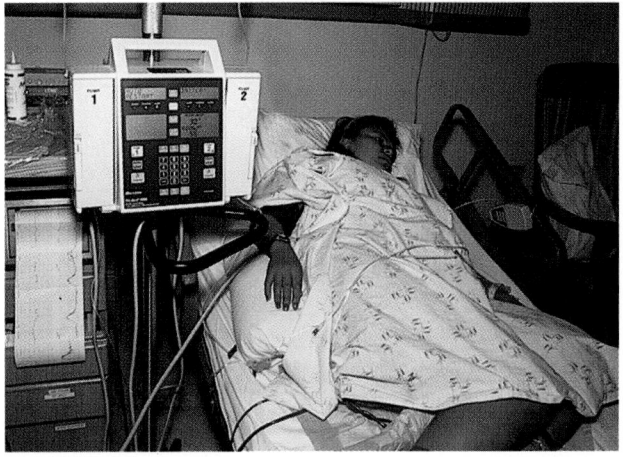

Fig. 37-7 Woman in side-lying position receiving oxytocin. (*Courtesy Michael S. Clement, MD, Mesa, AZ.*)

tion, or amniotic fluid embolism. Women also may become anxious or fearful if the induction is not successful because of concerns they may then have about the method of birth.

Uterine hyperstimulation reduces the blood flow through the placenta and results in FHR decelerations (bradycardia, diminished variability, late decelerations), fetal asphyxia, and neonatal hypoxia. If the estimated date of birth is inaccurate, physical injury, neonatal hyperbilirubinemia, and prematurity are other hazards.

It is the primary health care provider who is responsible for ordering the induction or augmentation of labor with oxytocin and the nurse who initiates the IV infusion through a secondary line and implements appropriate assessment and care measures following agency protocol and professional standards (Fig. 37-7; Box 37-2).

In the past the aim of induction has been to achieve a contraction pattern that simulates the active phase of labor as quickly as possible. However, research on uterine tolerance to oxytocin has now shown that lower doses given over a longer time are as effective as previous protocols and are less likely to cause uterine hyperstimulation and dysfunctional labor (ACOG, 1995a; Simpson & Poole, 1998; Summers, 1997)

Nursing considerations. A written protocol for the preparation and administration of oxytocin should be established by the obstetric department (physicians, nurses) at each institution. Procedures that are recommended for a woman who is eligible for induction of labor are discussed in Boxes 37-2 and 37-3. Policies, protocols, and procedures of individual institutions will also dictate set-up and administration, the frequency of administration, and documentation.

NURSE ALERT *Oxytocin is discontinued immediately and the primary health care provider notified if uterine hyperstimulation or a nonreassuring FHR occurs.*

Other nursing interventions, such as administering oxygen by face mask, positioning the woman on her side, and infusing more intravenous fluids are implemented immediately (see Emergency box on p. 994). Based on the status of the maternal-fetal unit, the primary health care provider may restart the infusion once the FHR and uterine activity return to acceptable levels (ACOG, 1995a).

Augmentation of labor is the stimulation of uterine contractions after labor has started spontaneously but progress is unsatisfactory. Common augmentation methods include oxytocin infusion, amniotomy, and nipple stimulation. Augmentation is usually implemented for the management of hypotonic uterine dysfunction resulting in a slowing of the labor process (protracted active phase). Noninvasive methods such as emptying of the bladder, ambulation and position changes, relaxation measures, nourishment and hydration, and hydrotherapy should be attempted before invasive interventions are initiated. Augmentation of labor using oxytocin is similar to induction of labor; however, protocols for dosage and increments may vary somewhat (Gilbert & Harmon, 1998; Pozaic, 1999; Simpson & Poole, 1998) (see Plan of Care).

Some physicians advocate the active management of labor, that is, the augmentation of labor to establish efficient labor so that the woman gives birth within 12 hours of admission (ACOG, 1995b). Advocates of active management believe that intervening early (as soon as a nulliparous labor is not progressing at least 1 cm/hr) with the aggressive use of oxytocin (e.g., a starting dose of 6 mU/min with increases of 6 mU/min every 15 minutes to a maximum dose of 40 mU/min) shortens labor and is associated with a lower incidence of cesarean birth (ACOG, 1995b).

Additional components of the active management of labor include strict criteria to diagnose that the woman is in active labor with 100% effacement, amniotomy within 1 hour of admission of a woman in labor if spontaneous rupture of the membranes has not occurred, and the con-

tinuous presence of a personal nurse who provides one-on-one care for the woman while she is in labor. Active management of labor continues to be under study in the United States to determine effectiveness and impact on perinatal morbidity and mortality. To date results have been disappointing, especially in terms of a lack of reduction in the rate of cesarean births. The disappointing results have been attributed, in part, to a greater than one-to-one nurse client ratio and the high rate of epidural anesthesia (Gilbert & Harmon, 1998; Simpson & Poole, 1998) (see Research Box on p. 985).

Forceps-Assisted Birth

A **forceps-assisted birth** is one in which an instrument with two curved blades is used to assist in the birth of the fetal head. The cephalic-like curve of the forceps commonly used is similar to the shape of the fetal head, with a pelvic curve to the blades conforming to the curve of the pelvic axis. The blades are joined by a pin, screw, or groove arrangement. These locks prevent the forceps from compressing the fetal skull. Maternal indications for forceps-assisted birth include the need to shorten the second stage of labor in the event of dystocia (difficult labor) or to compensate for the woman's deficient expulsive efforts (e.g., if she is tired or has been given spinal or epidural anesthesia), as well as to reverse a dangerous condition (e.g., cardiac decompensation).

The use of forceps during childbirth has been decreasing. In 1996, forceps were used to assist 3.2% of births compared with 5.5% in 1989. This represents a decline of 42% (Ventura et al., 1998).

Fetal indications include birth of a fetus in distress, in certain abnormal presentations, or in arrest of rotation, as well as to deliver an aftercoming head in a breech presentation.

Certain conditions are required for a forceps-assisted birth to be successful. The woman's cervix must be fully dilated to avert lacerations and hemorrhage. The bladder should be empty. The presenting part must be engaged, and a vertex presentation is desired. Membranes must be ruptured so that the position of the fetal head can be determined and the forceps can firmly grasp the head during birth. In addition, CPD should not be present.

There are different definitions of forceps applications. According to ACOG (1994a), it is appropriate to use *outlet* forceps if the fetal scalp is visible on the perineum without manually separating the labia (Fig. 37-8). Outlet forceps are used to shorten the second stage of labor. *Low forceps* refers to the application of forceps to the fetal head that is at least at the +2 cm station. *Midforceps* refers to the application of forceps to the fetal head that is engaged (no higher than station 0) but above the +2 cm station. There are no instances in which forceps should be applied to an unengaged presenting part.

Nursing considerations. When a forceps-assisted birth is deemed necessary, the nurse obtains the type of forceps requested by the physician (Fig. 37-9). The FHR is

PLAN ᵒꜰ CARE   Dysfunctional Labor: Secondary Inertia

> **NURSING DIAGNOSIS** Risk for injury to mother and/or fetus related to oxytocin stimulation secondary to dysfunctional labor

Expected Outcomes *Maternal-fetal well-being is maintained; labor progresses and birth occurs.*

Nursing Interventions/*Rationales*

Explain oxytocin protocol to woman and her labor partner *to allay apprehension and enhance participation.*

Encourage woman to void before beginning protocol *to prevent discomfort and remove a barrier to labor progress.*

Apply the electronic fetal monitor per hospital protocol and obtain a 15- to 20-minute baseline strip *to ensure adequate assessment of FHR and contractions.*

Position woman in a side-lying position and administer the oxytocin per physician order using an IV infusion pump *to stimulate uterine activity and provide adequate control of the flow rate.*

Regulate the oxytocin per protocol and advancing the dose in increments of 1 to 2 mU/min every 15 to 60 minutes *to allow adequate evaluation of the woman's response to stimulation and to prevent hyperstimulation and fetal hypoxia.*

Maintain oxytocin dose and rate when contractions occur every 2 to 3 minutes with a duration of 40 to 90 seconds and intrauterine pressures of 40 to 90 mm Hg *to produce effective uterine stimulation without risk of hyperstimulation.*

If infusion rate is advanced to 20 mU/min without achieving the desired contractility pattern, notify physician *because woman is at risk for hyperstimulation and water intoxication.*

Monitor maternal vital signs every 30 to 60 minutes *to assess for oxytocin-induced hypertension.*

Monitor contractility pattern and FHR pattern every 15 minutes *to assess uterine activity for possible hypertonicity or ineffective uterine response to oxytocin and to detect evidence of fetal distress.*

Monitor intake, output, and specific gravity (limit intake to 1000 ml/8 hr; output should be at least 120 ml/4 hr) *to assess for urinary retention and prevent water intoxication.*

Monitor cervical dilation, effacement, and station *to assess progress of labor.*

If hypertonicity or signs of fetal distress are detected, discontinue oxytocin immediately *to arrest the progress of hypertonicity;* turn woman on her side *to increase placental blood flow;* increase primary IV rate to 200 ml/hr (unless signs of water toxicity are present); administer oxygen per face mask *to enhance placental perfusion;* notify physician; and continuously monitor maternal vital signs and FHR *to provide ongoing assessment of maternal/fetal status.*

> **NURSING DIAGNOSIS** Pain related to increasing frequency, regularity, intensity, and prolonged peak of contractions

Expected Outcome *The woman exhibits signs of decreased discomfort.*

Nursing Interventions/*Rationales*

Prepare woman and labor partner for the change in the nature of the contractions once the oxytocin drip is initiated *to prepare them and allow for more effective coping.*

Remind woman and labor partner that analgesics are available for use during labor *to provide knowledge to help them make decisions about pain control.*

Review the use of specific techniques such as conscious relaxation, focused breathing, effleurage, massage, and application of sacral pressure *to increase relaxation, decrease intensity of pain of contractions, and promote use of controlled thought and direction of energy.*

Provide comfort measures such as frequent mouth care *to prevent dry mouth,* application of damp cloth to forehead and changing of damp gown or bed covers *to relieve discomfort of diaphoresis,* and positioning *to reduce stiffness.*

Encourage conscious relaxation between contractions *to prevent fatigue, which contributes to increased pain perceptions.*

> **NURSING DIAGNOSIS** Anxiety/ineffective coping related to prolonged labor, increased pain, and fatigue

Expected Outcomes *Woman's anxiety is reduced; woman actively participates in the labor process.*

Nursing Interventions/*Rationales*

Provide ongoing feedback to woman and partner *to allay anxiety and enhance participation.*

Present care options when possible *to increase feelings of control.*

Continue to provide comfort measures *to maintain a posture of support and caring and to aid woman in focusing on the labor process.*

Encourage woman and partner to continue to use those mechanisms that promote effective labor (e.g., breathing, positioning) *to keep woman and partner actively involved in process.*

From Wong, D., & Perry, S. (1998). *Maternal child nursing care.* St. Louis: Mosby.

Continued

PLAN ᵒᶠ CARE · Dysfunctional Labor: Secondary Inertia—cont'd

NURSING DIAGNOSIS Risk for maternal/fetal infection related to prolonged rupture of membranes or possible invasive procedures (e.g., use of fetal scalp electrodes, use of forceps, episiotomy, cesarean birth)

Expected Outcome *There is no evidence of infection.*

Nursing Interventions/*Rationales*

Monitor temperature *because elevation is early indicator of infection.*

Monitor FHR/variability *because rates greater than 160 beats/min and minimal variability may be indicative of maternal fever and infection.*

Monitor intake and output for dehydration *because signs of infection closely resemble those of dehydration, and differentiation is needed.*

Maintain Standard Precautions and use scrupulous handwashing techniques when providing care *to prevent spread of infection.*

Use strict aseptic technique when performing invasive procedures such as urinary catheterization, insertion of intravenous lines, or application of scalp electrodes *to reduce risk of nosocomial infection.*

Monitor IV sites, electrode sites, and incision sites for signs such as pain, redness, edema, heat, and drainage, *which are indicative of infection.*

Monitor urine for color, concentration, odor, clouding, casts, and sediment, *which may indicate a urinary tract infection.*

When membranes rupture, assess fluid for color, amount, and odor, and for the presence of meconium stain *because alterations may be indicative of intrauterine infection.*

After membrane rupture, keep vaginal examinations to a minimum and use sterile gloves *to decrease risk of uterine infection.*

Assist woman to maintain good personal hygiene habits (e.g., wiping perineal region from front to back, keeping area dry *to reduce introduction of bacteria.*

Monitor laboratory values (e.g., white blood cell count, culture) *for indicators of infection.*

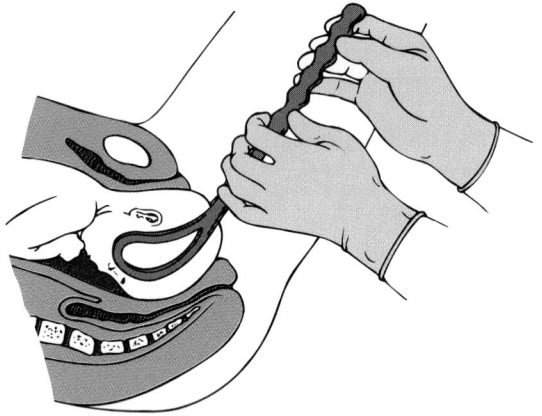

Fig. 37-8 Outlet forceps-assisted extraction of the head.

checked, reported, and recorded *before* the forceps are applied. The nurse may explain to the mother that the forceps blades fit like two tablespoons around an egg, with the blades coming over the baby's ears.

NURSE ALERT *Because compression of the cord between the fetal head and the forceps would cause a drop in FHR, the FHR is rechecked, reported, and recorded* before *and after* application of the forceps.

If a drop in FHR occurs, the physician would then remove and reapply the forceps. Ordinarily traction is applied during contractions.

After birth, the mother is assessed for vaginal and cervical lacerations (bleeding that occurs even with a contracted uterus) and urine retention, which may result from bladder injuries. The infant should be assessed for bruising or abrasions at the site of the blade applications, facial palsy resulting from pressure of the blades on the facial nerve (cranial nerve VII), and subdural hematoma. Newborn and postpartum caregivers should be told that forceps-assisted birth has been performed.

Vacuum-Assisted Birth

Vacuum-assisted birth, or vacuum extraction, is a birth method involving the attachment of a vacuum cup to the fetal head, using negative pressure. Indications for its use are similar to those for the use of outlet forceps. Prerequisites for use include a vertex presentation, ruptured membranes, and absence of CPD (Cunningham et al., 1997).

While the use of forceps to assist birth has been declining, the use of the vacuum extractor has been increasing. In 1996, 6.2% of births were vacuum-assisted compared with 3.5% in 1989 (Ventura et al., 1998).

When vacuum extraction is to be done, the woman is prepared for a vaginal birth in the lithotomy position to allow for sufficient traction. The cup is applied to the fetal head, and a caput develops inside the cup as the pressure is initiated (Fig. 37-10). Traction is then applied to facilitate descent of the fetal head, and the woman is encouraged to push as suction is applied. As the head crowns, an episiotomy is performed if necessary. The vacuum cup is released and removed after birth of the head. If vacuum extraction is not successful, a forceps-assisted or cesarean birth is then performed.

Risks to the newborn include cephalhematoma, scalp lacerations, and subdural hematoma. Fetal complications can be reduced by strict adherence to the manufacturer's recommendations for method of application, degree of suction, and duration of application. Maternal complications are uncommon but can include perineal, vaginal, or cervical lacerations.

Nursing considerations. The nurse's role in the care of the woman who has given birth with the assistance of vacuum extraction is one of support person and educator. The nurse can prepare the woman for birth and encourage her to remain active in the birth process by pushing during contractions. In addition, the nurse assesses the FHR frequently during the procedure. After birth, the newborn should be observed for signs of trauma at the application site and for cerebral irritation (e.g., poor sucking, listlessness). The newborn may be at risk for cephalhematoma and neonatal jaundice as bruising resolves, as well as infection at the application site. The parents may need to be reassured that the caput succedaneum will begin to disappear in a few hours. Neonatal caregivers should be alerted that the birth was assisted by vacuum extraction.

Cesarean Birth

Cesarean birth is the birth of a fetus through a transabdominal incision of the uterus. Although the myth persists that Julius Caesar was born in this manner, the name is more likely derived from the Latin word *caedo*, meaning "to cut." Whether cesarean birth is planned (scheduled) or unplanned (emergency), the loss of the experience of giving birth to a child in the traditional manner may have a negative effect on a woman's self-concept. An effort is therefore made to maintain the focus on the birth of a child rather than on the operative procedure.

The basic aim of cesarean birth is to preserve the life or health of the mother and her fetus and may be the best choice for birth when there is evidence of maternal or fetal complications. Since the advent of modern surgical methods and care, there has been a decrease in the maternal and fetal morbidity and mortality associated with cesarean birth. In addition, today incisions are made into the lower uterine segment rather than into the muscular body of the uterus to promote more effective healing. However, despite these advances, cesarean birth still poses threats to the health of the mother and infant.

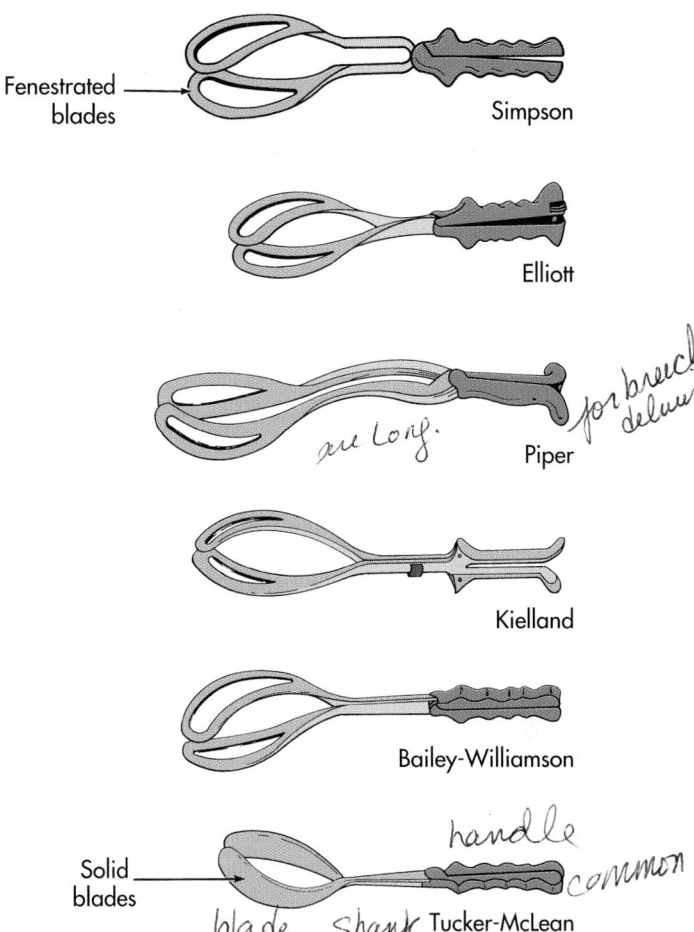

Fig. 37-9 Types of forceps. Piper forceps are used to assist delivery of the head in a breech birth.

ETHICAL CONSIDERATIONS

Forced Cesarean Birth

A woman's refusal to undergo cesarean birth for fetal reasons is often described as a maternal-fetal conflict. Health care providers are ethically obliged to protect the well-being of both the mother and the fetus; a decision for one affects the other. If a woman refuses a cesarean birth that is recommended because of fetal jeopardy, health care providers need to make every effort to find out why she is refusing and provide information that may persuade her to change her mind. If the woman continues to refuse surgery, then health care providers must decide if it is ethical to get a court order for the surgery. Every effort should be made to avoid this legal step, however.

The incidence of cesarean births has increased from less than 5% in 1965 to more than 20% in 1997 (Guyer et al., 1998). Factors cited as sources of this increase include use of electronic fetal monitoring and epidural anesthesia; an increase in the number of first-time pregnancies, as well as

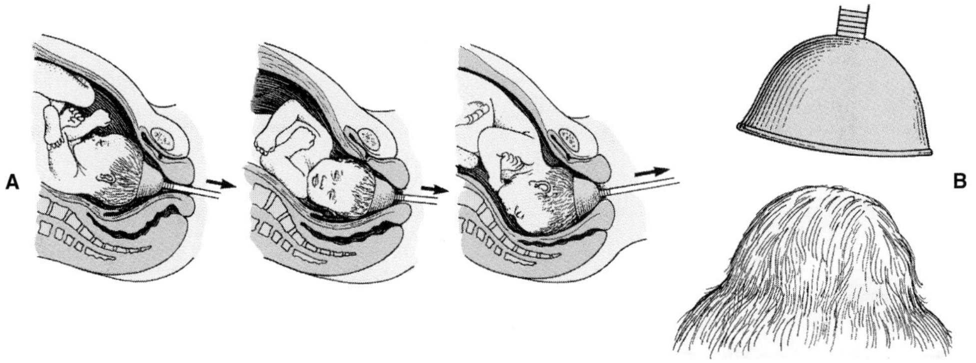

Fig. 37-10 Use of vacuum extraction to rotate fetal head and assist with descent. **A,** Arrow indicates direction of traction on the vacuum cup. **B,** Caput succedaneum formed by the vacuum cup.

BOX 37-4 **Selected Measures to Reduce Cesarean Birth Rate and Increase Rate of VBACs**

Educate women regarding
- Advantages and safety of the home environment for early or latent labor
- Indicators for hospital admission
- Management techniques to use during labor to enhance progress
- Nonpharmacologic measures to reduce pain and discomfort and enhance relaxation
- Safety and effectiveness of TOLs and VBACs

Establish admission criteria for women in labor
- Distinguish clinical manifestations for false labor, latent/early labor, and active labor
- Conduct admission assessments in a separate admissions area
- Send women in false or early/latent labor home or keep them in the admissions area
- Admit women in active labor to the labor and birth unit

Use appropriate assessment techniques to
- Determine status of the maternal-fetal unit
- Establish an individualized rationale for initiating labor interventions such as epidural anesthesia, induction/augmentation, amniotomy, cesarean birth

Initiate a doula program that provides one-to-one support for women in labor

Develop a philosophy of labor management that
- Schedules admission during active labor
- Avoids automatic interventions such as routine induction for spontaneous rupture of membranes at term or postterm pregnancy and cesarean birth for breech presentation, twin gestation, genital herpes, or failure to progress
- Relies on assessment findings reflective of the status of the maternal-fetal unit rather than strict adherence to set ranges for the duration of the stages and phases of labor
- Employs intermittent rather than continuous electronic fetal monitoring of low risk pregnant women
- Focuses on measures that are known to enhance the progress of labor such as upright positions, frequent position changes, ambulation, oral nutrition and hydration, relaxation techniques, hydrotherapy
- Emphasizes nonpharmacologic measures to relieve pain
- Uses pharmacologic measures in a manner that reduces their labor-inhibiting effects
- Establishes criteria for elective cesarean birth and TOL
- Encourages women who have had a previous cesarean birth to participate in a trial of labor to attempt a vaginal birth.

---

pregnancy at an older age; and the high incidence of repeat cesarean births.

Women 35 years of age and older have a total cesarean birth rate that, at 30%, is almost twice the rate for teenage women (15.7%) (Curtin & Kozak, 1998).

Women who have private insurance, are of a higher socioeconomic status, or deliver in a private hospital are more likely to experience cesarean birth than are women who are poor, have no insurance, are receiving public assistance

(e.g., Medicaid), or deliver in public hospitals (DiMatteo et al., 1996; Porreco & Thorp, 1996; Scott, 1999).

While the rate of cesarean birth has declined slightly since 1990, it is still the most common major surgery performed in the United States. The decline in rate may be attributed, in part, to more attempts at vaginal births in mothers who have previously given birth by cesarean. From 1989 to 1996, the rate of vaginal births after cesarean increased 50% (Ventura et al., 1998).

Several approaches for the management of labor and birth have been recommended for reducing the rate of cesarean births, while increasing the rate of vaginal births after cesarean (VBAC) (Box 37-4). These management approaches involve the combined efforts of health care professionals and pregnant women and their families (Flamm, Berwick, & Kabcenell, 1998; McNiven et al., 1998).

The type of nursing care given may also influence the rate of cesarean births. Radin, Harmon, and Hanson (1993) found that cesarean rates were lower for women whose nurses provided supportive care during labor. A labor management approach that uses one-to-one support and emphasizes ambulation, maternal position changes, relaxation measures, oral fluids and nutrition, hydrotherapy, and nonpharmacologic pain relief facilitates the progress of labor and reduces the incidence of dystocia, a major cause for cesarean birth, especially in first-time labors (Albers, Lydon-Rochelle, & Krulewitch, 1995; Porreco & Thorp, 1996). The labor management approach that most consistently reduced cesarean birth rates was one-to-one support of the laboring woman by another female such as a nurse, nurse-midwife, or doula (Cefalo & Bowes, 1998; Gabay & Wolfe, 1997).

Indications. There are few absolute indications for cesarean birth. Today most are performed primarily for the benefit of the fetus. The most common indications for cesarean birth are related to labor and birth complications. The complications most closely associated with cesarean birth include fetal distress, CPD, malpresentations such as breech and shoulder, placental abnormalities (previa, abruptio), umbilical cord prolapse, dysfunctional labor pattern, and multiple gestation. Maternal health problems that complicate pregnancy may also be indications for cesarean birth. Medical risk factors most closely associated with cesarean birth include hypertensive disorders, active genital herpes, and diabetes (Porreco & Thorpe, 1996; Ventura et al., 1998).

Surgical techniques. There are two main types of cesarean operation: classic and lower-segment cesarean births. Classic cesarean birth is rarely performed today, although it may be used when rapid birth is necessary and in some cases of shoulder presentation and placenta previa. The incision is made vertically into the upper body of the uterus (Fig. 37-11, *A*). Because the procedure is associated with a higher incidence of blood loss, infection, and uterine rupture in subsequent pregnancies than is lower-segment cesarean birth, vaginal birth after a classic cesarean birth is contraindicated.

Lower-segment cesarean birth can be achieved through a vertical or transverse incision into the uterus (Fig. 37-11, *B* and *C*). The transverse incision is more popular, however, because it is easier to perform, is associated with less blood loss and fewer postoperative infections, and is less likely to rupture in subsequent pregnancies (Cunningham et al., 1997; Scott, 1999).

Complications and risks. Cesarean births are not without complications, either for the mother or the fetus.

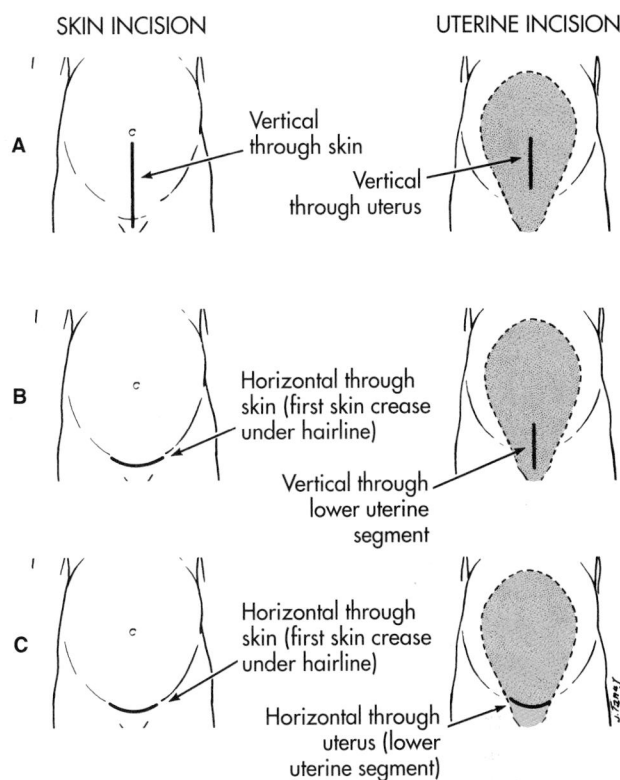

Fig. 37-11 Cesarean birth: skin and uterine incisions. **A,** Classic: vertical incisions of skin and uterus. **B,** Low cervical: horizontal incision of skin; vertical incision of uterus. **C,** Low cervical: horizontal incisions of skin and uterus.

Maternal complications occur in 25% to 50% of births and include aspiration, pulmonary embolism, wound infection, wound dehiscence, thrombophlebitis, hemorrhage, urinary tract infection, injuries to the bladder or bowel, and complications related to anesthesia. There also is a risk that the fetus will be born prematurely if the gestational age has not been accurately determined; in addition, fetal injuries can occur during the surgery (Scott, 1999). Besides these risks, the woman is at economic risk because the cost of cesarean birth is higher than that of vaginal birth and a longer recovery period may necessitate additional expenditures.

Many women who experience a cesarean birth speak of having feelings that interfere with their maintaining an adequate self-concept. These feelings include fear, disappointment, frustration at losing control, anger (the "why me" syndrome), and loss of self-esteem related to a change in body image and perceived inability to give birth as they had expected and hoped. Often the ability to interact with their newborns after birth is delayed. Women who experience cesarean birth are less likely to breastfeed and may even have some difficulty expressing positive feeling about their newborns for some time after birth. They are often less satisfied with their childbirth experience and report more fatigue and poor physical functioning during the first few weeks after discharge. These reactions are more pronounced among women who had unplanned or emergency cesarean birth (DiMatteo et al., 1996). Success at mothering and in the recovery process can do much to restore the self-esteem of these women. Some women see the scar as mutilating, and worries concerning sexual attractiveness may surface. Some men are fearful of resuming intercourse because of the fear of hurting their partners. Parents may wonder if a cesarean birth was absolutely necessary, and such feelings may surface even years later. They should therefore be given opportunities to discuss the experience to try to understand and resolve concerns after the birth.

Anesthesia. Spinal, epidural, and general anesthetics are used for cesarean births. Epidural blocks are popular because women want to be awake for and aware of the birth experience. However, the choice of anesthetic depends on several factors. The mother's medical history or present condition, such as a spinal injury or hemorrhage, may rule out the use of regional anesthesia. Time is another factor, especially if there is an emergency and the life of the mother or infant is at stake. In this event, general anesthesia will most likely be used, unless the woman already has an epidural block in effect. The woman herself is a factor. Either she may not know all the options or she may have fears about having "a needle in her back" or about being awake and feeling pain. The woman needs to be fully informed about the risks and benefits of the different types of anesthesia so that she can participate in the decision whenever there is a choice.

Scheduled cesarean birth. Cesarean birth is scheduled or planned if labor is contraindicated (e.g., complete placenta previa), if birth is necessary but labor is not inducible (e.g., hypertensive states, which cause a poor intrauterine environment that threatens the fetus), or if this has been decided upon by the primary health care provider and the woman (e.g., a repeat cesarean birth).

Women who are scheduled to have a cesarean birth have time to prepare for it psychologically. However, the psychologic responses of these women may differ. Those having a repeat cesarean birth may have disturbing memories of the conditions preceding the initial surgical birth and of their experiences in the postoperative recovery period. They may be very concerned about the added burdens of caring for an infant and perhaps other children while recovering from a surgical operation. Others may feel glad that they have been relieved of the uncertainty about the date and time of the birth and of the pain of labor.

Unplanned cesarean birth. The psychosocial outcomes of unplanned or emergency cesarean birth are usually more pronounced and negative in nature when compared with the outcomes associated with a scheduled or planned cesarean birth (DiMatteo et al., 1996). Women and their families experience abrupt changes in their expectations for birth, postbirth care, and the care of the new baby at home. This may be an extremely traumatic experience for all.

The woman usually approaches the procedure tired and discouraged after an ineffective and difficult labor. Fear predominates as the woman worries about her own safety and well-being and that of her fetus. The woman may be dehydrated, with low glycogen reserves. Because preoperative procedures must be done quickly and competently, the time for an explanation of the procedures and the operation is often short. Because maternal and family anxiety levels are high at this time, much of what is said may be forgotten or perhaps misunderstood. The woman may experience feelings of anger or guilt in the postpartum period. Fatigue is often noticeable in these women, and they need much supportive care.

After surgery, therefore, time must be spent reviewing the events preceding the operation and the operation itself to ensure that the woman understands what has happened and that gaps in her recollections are filled. This approach will help create more realistic memories of the childbirth experience, thereby having a more positive influence on future pregnancies and labors (Ryding, Wijma, & Wijma, 1998).

Prenatal preparation. Concerned professional and lay groups in the community have established councils for cesarean birth to meet the needs of these women and their families. Such groups advocate that a discussion of cesarean birth be included in all parenthood preparation classes. No woman can be guaranteed a vaginal birth, even if she is in good health and there is no indication of danger to the fetus before the onset of labor. For this reason, every woman needs to be aware of and prepared for this eventuality.

Childbirth educators stress the importance of emphasizing the similarities as well as the differences between cesarean and vaginal birth. In support of the philosophy of family-centered birth, many hospitals have instituted policies that permit fathers and other partners and family members to share in these births as they do in vaginal ones. Women who have undergone cesarean birth agree that the continued presence and support of their partners helped them respond positively to the entire experience. In addition to preparing women for the possibility of cesarean birth, childbirth educators should empower women to believe in their ability to give birth vaginally and to seek care measures during labor that will enhance the progress of their labors and reduce their risk for cesarean birth.

Preoperative care. Family-centered care is the goal for the woman who is to undergo cesarean birth and for her family. The preparation of the woman for cesarean birth is the same as that done for other elective or emergency surgery. The primary health care provider discusses the need for the cesarean birth and the prognosis for the mother and infant with the woman and her family. The anesthesiologist assesses the woman's cardiopulmonary system and describes the options for anesthesia. Informed consent is obtained for the procedure.

Maternal vital signs and blood pressure and FHR continue to be assessed per the hospital routine until the operation begins. Physical preoperative preparation usually includes the insertion of a retention catheter to keep the bladder empty and the administration of prescribed preoperative medications. Additionally, the abdominal-mons area may be shaved or pubic hair clipped. An antacid is administered orally as a precautionary measure if general anesthesia is anticipated to neutralize gastric secretions in case of aspiration. Intravenous fluids are started to maintain hydration and to provide an open line for the administration of blood or medications as necessary. Blood and urine samples are collected and sent to the laboratory for analysis. Laboratory tests, which are usually ordered to establish baseline data, include a complete blood cell count and chemistry, blood typing and cross-matching, and urinalysis.

Removal of dentures, nail polish, and jewelry may be optional, depending on hospital policies. If the woman wears glasses and is going to be awake, the nurse should make sure her glasses accompany her to the operating room so she can see her infant. If the woman wears contact lenses, the nurse can find out whether they can be worn for the birth.

During the preoperative preparation the support person is encouraged to remain with the woman as much as possible to provide continuing emotional support if this action is culturally acceptable to the woman and support person.

The nurse also provides essential information about the preoperative procedures during this time. Although the nursing actions may be carried out quickly if a cesarean birth is unplanned, verbal communication, particularly explanations, is important. Silence can be frightening to the woman and her support person. The nurse's use of touch can communicate feelings of care and concern for the woman.

The nurse can assess the woman's and her partner's perceptions about cesarean birth. For example, the woman may feel that she is a failure because she did not have a vaginal birth. As the woman expresses her feelings, the nurse may identify a potential for a disturbance in self-concept during the postpartum period that may need to be addressed.

If there is time before the birth, the nurse can teach the woman about postoperative expectations, as well as pain relief, turning, coughing, and deep breathing measures.

Intraoperative care. Cesarean births occur in operating rooms in the surgical unit or in the labor and birth unit. Once the woman has been taken to the operating room, her care becomes the responsibility of the obstetric team, surgeon, anesthesiologist, pediatrician, and surgical nursing staff (Fig. 37-12). If possible, the partner, who is gowned appropriately, accompanies the mother to the surgical unit and remains close to her so that he or she can provide continued support and comfort.

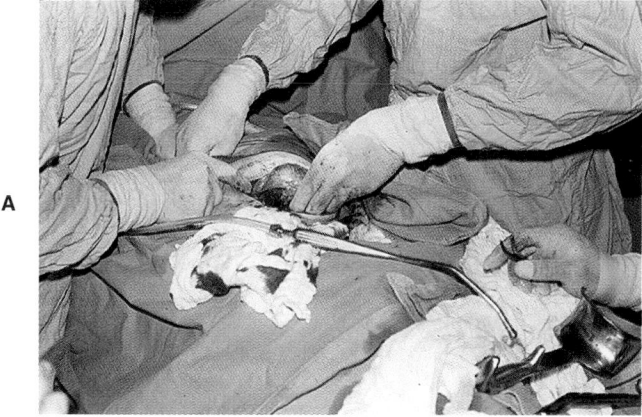

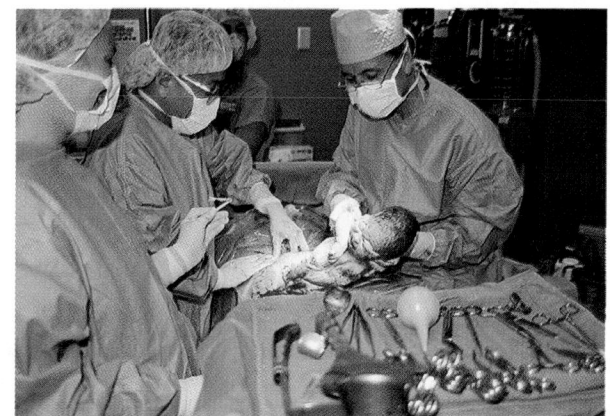

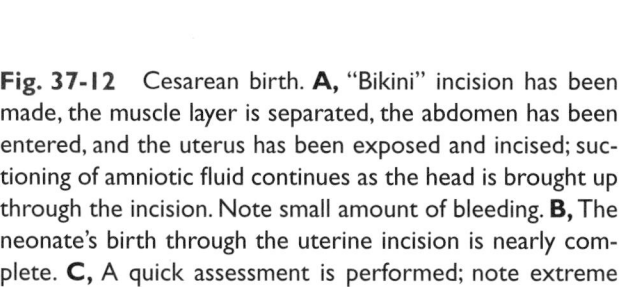

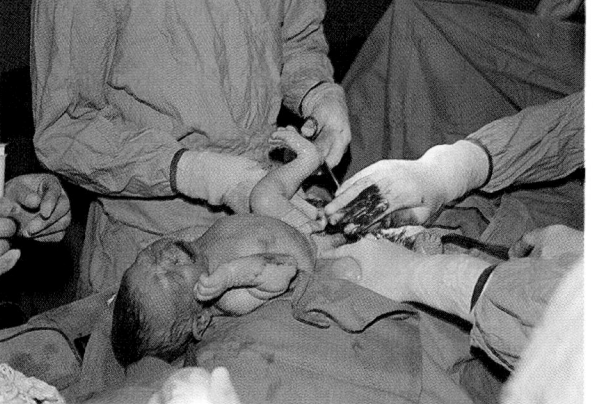

Fig. 37-12 Cesarean birth. **A,** "Bikini" incision has been made, the muscle layer is separated, the abdomen has been entered, and the uterus has been exposed and incised; suctioning of amniotic fluid continues as the head is brought up through the incision. Note small amount of bleeding. **B,** The neonate's birth through the uterine incision is nearly complete. **C,** A quick assessment is performed; note extreme molding of head resulting from cephalopelvic disproportion. *(Courtesy Marjorie Pyle, RNC, Lifecircle, Costa Mesa, CA.)*

The nurse who is circulating may assist with positioning the woman on the birth (surgical) table. It is important to position her so that the uterus is displaced laterally to prevent compression of the inferior vena cava, which causes placental perfusion to decrease. This is usually accomplished by placing a wedge under the hip. A Foley catheter is inserted into the bladder at this time if one is not already in place.

If the partner is not allowed or chooses not to be present, the nurse can stay in communication with him or her and give progress reports whenever possible. If the mother is awake during the birth, the nurse and/or anesthesiologist can tell her what is happening and provide support. The mother may be anxious about the sensations she is experiencing, such as the coldness of solutions used to prepare the abdomen and pressure or pulling during the actual birth of the infant. She also may be apprehensive because of the bright lights and the presence of unfamiliar equipment and masked and gowned personnel in the room. Anticipatory guidance by the nurse can help decrease the woman's anxiety.

Care of the infant usually is delegated to a pediatrician or a nurse team skilled at neonatal resuscitation, because these infants are considered to be at risk until there is evidence of physiologic stability after the birth.

A crib with resuscitation equipment is readied before the birth. Those responsible for care are expert not only in resuscitative techniques but also in their ability to detect normal and abnormal infant responses. After birth, if the infant's condition permits, the baby can be given to the woman's partner to hold. If the mother is awake, she can see and touch the baby (Fig. 37-13). The infant whose condition is compromised is transported after initial stabilization to the nursery for observation and the implementation of appropriate interventions. In some institutions the partner may accompany the infant; if not, personnel keep

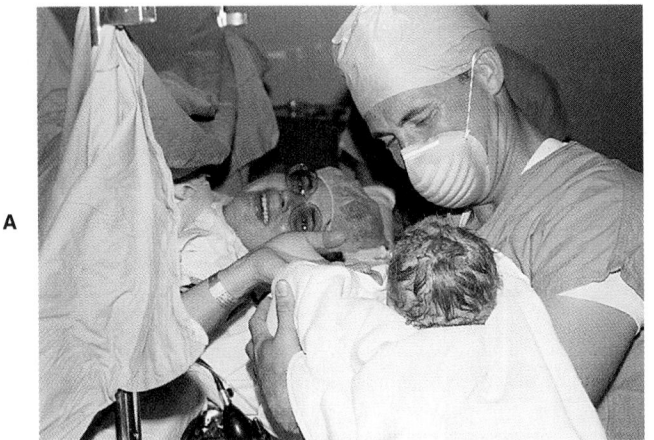

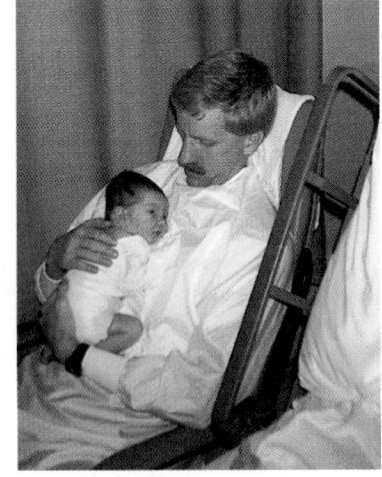

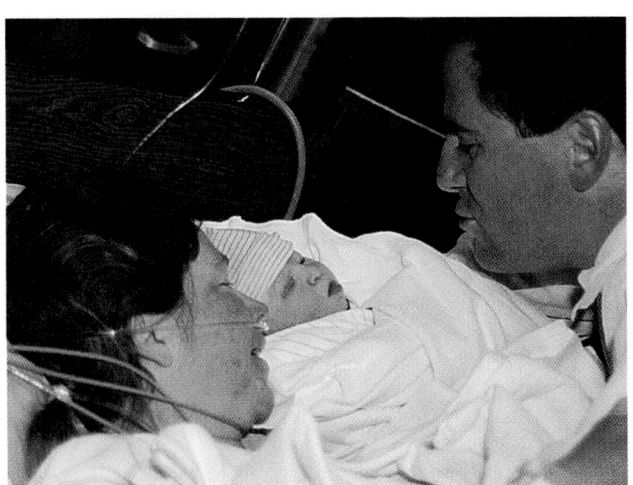

Fig. 37-13 **A,** Parents and their newborn. The physician manually removes the placenta, suctions the remaining amniotic fluid and blood from the uterine cavity, and closes the uterine incision, peritoneum, muscle layer, fatty tissue, and finally the skin, while the new family shares some private time. **B,** Father holding newborn son. **C,** Parents become better acquainted with their newborn while mother rests after surgery. (**A** and **C** courtesy Marjorie Pyle, RNC, Lifecircle, Costa Mesa, CA; **B** courtesy Jan Harmon, St. Louis.)

the family informed of the infant's progress and parent-infant contacts are initiated as soon as possible.

If the family cannot accompany the woman during surgery, the family is directed to the surgical or obstetric waiting room. The physician then reports on the condition of the mother and child to the family members after the birth is completed. Family members may accompany the infant as she or he is transferred to the nursery, giving the family an opportunity to see and admire the new baby.

Immediate postoperative care. Once surgery is completed, the mother is transferred to a recovery room or back to her labor room. Women who have experienced a cesarean birth have both postoperative and postpartum needs that must be addressed. They are surgical clients as well as new mothers (Eakes & Brown, 1998). Nursing assessments in this immediate postbirth period include the degree of recovery from the effects of anesthesia, the postoperative and postbirth status, and the degree of pain. A patent airway is maintained, and the woman is positioned to prevent possible aspiration. Vital signs are taken every 15 minutes for 1 to 2 hours, or until stable. The condition of the incisional dressing, the fundus, and the amount of lochia are assessed, as well as the intravenous intake and the urine output through the Foley catheter. The woman is helped to turn and do coughing, deep-breathing, and leg exercises. Medications to relieve pain may be administered.

If the baby is present, the mother and her partner are given some time alone with him or her to facilitate bonding and attachment. Breastfeeding can be initiated if the mother feels like trying. The woman usually is transferred to the postpartum unit after 1 to 2 hours, or once her condition is stable and the effects of anesthesia have worn off (i.e., alert, oriented, able to feel and move extremities) (see Care Path).

Postpartum care. The attitude of the nurse and other health team members can influence the perception the woman has of herself after a cesarean birth. The caregivers should stress that the woman is a new mother as well as a surgical client. This will help the woman perceive herself as having the same problems and needs as other new mothers while at the same time requiring supportive postoperative care.

The women's physiologic concerns for the first few days may be dominated by pain at the incision site and pain resulting from intestinal gas, and hence the need for pain relief. If epidural anesthesia was used for the surgery, epidural narcotics can be given in the recovery period to provide pain relief for approximately 24 hours. Otherwise, pain medications usually are given every 3 to 4 hours, or patient-controlled analgesia may be ordered instead. Other comfort measures such as position changes, splinting of the incision with pillows, and relaxation techniques may be implemented. Women are often the best judges of what their bodies need and can tolerate, including the ingestion of foods and fluids postoperatively. If desired by the woman, the early introduction of solid food is safe.

Women who eat early have been found to require less analgesia. Gastrointestinal problems do not occur (Burrows et al., 1995). Ambulation and rocking in a rocking chair may relieve gas pains, and avoiding the consumption of gas-forming foods and carbonated beverages may help minimize them (Thomas et al., 1990) (see Client Self-Care Box).

Other physiologic concerns of women after cesarean birth may include fatigue, activity intolerance, and incisional problems (Miovech et al., 1994). Nurses need to be alert to a woman's physiologic needs, managing care to ensure adequate rest and pain relief. Mother-baby care (couplet care) for a cesarean birth mother needs to be modified according to her physiologic limitations as a surgical client (Eakes & Brown, 1998).

Daily care includes perineal care, breast care, and routine hygienic care, including showering after the dressing has been removed (if showering is acceptable according to the women's cultural prescriptions). The nurse assesses the woman's vital signs, incision, fundus, and lochia in accordance with hospital policies, procedures, or protocols. Breath sounds, bowel sounds, circulatory status of lower extremities, and urinary and bowel elimination also are assessed.

During the postpartum period the nurse can also provide care that meets the psychologic and teaching needs of mothers who have had cesarean births. For instance, the nurse can explain postpartum procedures to the woman to help elicit her cooperation in her recovery from surgery. The nurse can help the woman plan care and visits from family and friends that will allow for adequate rest periods. In addition, the nurse can give her information on infant care and assist her with infant care to facilitate her adjustment to the mothering role. The woman should be encouraged to breastfeed her baby by receiving one-to-one assistance to comfortably hold and position the baby at her breast. The partner can be included in infant care teaching sessions, as well as explanations about the woman's recovery. The couple should also be encouraged to express their feelings about the birth experience. Some parents are angry, frustrated, or disappointed that a vaginal birth was not possible. Some women express feelings of low self-esteem or a negative self-image. Others express relief and gratitude that the baby is healthy and was born safely. It may be helpful for them to have the nurse who was present during the birth visit and help fill in "gaps" about the experience. Other psychologic and lifestyle concerns that have been reported include depression, feeling limited in activities, and changes in family interactions (Miovech et al., 1994; Ryding et al., 1998).

Discharge after cesarean birth is usually by the third postoperative day compared to the second postpartum day for vaginal births (Curtin & Kozak, 1998). The time is often determined by criteria established by the woman's insurance carrier or the federal government (e.g., diagnosis-related groups).

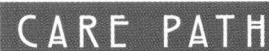

	IMMEDIATE POST-OP CESAREAN	BY 4TH HOUR AFTER ADMISSION TO PP UNIT	5 TO 24 HOURS	25 TO 48 HOURS	BY DISCHARGE
ASSESSMENTS	Recovery room/PACU admission assessment completed	PP admission assessment and care plan completed			
Vital Signs	q15min × 1 hr; q30min × 4 hr, WNL	q1hr × 3, WNL	q4-8hr, WNL	q8hr, WNL	q8hr, WNL
Postpartum Assessment	q15min × 1 hr, WNL	q1hr × 3, WNL	q8hr, WNL	q8-12hr, WNL	q8-12hr, WNL
Abdominal Incision	Dressing dry and intact	Dressing dry and intact	Dressing dry and intact	Dressing off or changed, incision intact	Incision intact; staples may be removed and steri-strips in place, incision WNL
Genitourinary	Retention catheter output >30 ml/hr	Retention catheter output >30 ml/hr	Retention catheter output >30 ml/hr	Catheter discontinued, output >100 ml/void or 240 ml/8 hr	Urine output >240 ml/8 hr
Gastrointestinal		Absent or hypoactive BS	Hypoactive to active BS	Active BS + flatus	Active BS + flatus; may or may not have BM
Musculoskeletal	Alert or easily aroused, can move legs	Alert and oriented, moving all extremities	Ambulating with help	Ambulating unassisted	Ambulating ad lib
Bonding	Evidence of parent-infant bonding; first breastfeeding if desired		Parent-infant bonding continues	Parent-infant bonding progressing	
Laboratory Tests			Intrapartal CBC results on chart/computer; determine Rh status and need for anti-Rh globulin; check for rubella immunity	PP HCT WNL, all lab results on chart, give anti-Rh globulin if indicated	Give rubella vaccine if indicated
INTERVENTIONS					
IV	IV continues	IV continues	IV continues	IV may be discontinued	
Diet	NPO	Ice chips, sips of clear liquids	Clear liquids	Regular diet or as tolerated	Regular diet
Perineal Care		Peri-care by nurse	Peri-care with help	Self-pericare	
Activity	Bed rest	Bed rest	OOB × 3 with help, ADLs assisted, assisted to comfortable position to hold and feed baby	Holds baby comfortably, ambulates without assistance, ADLs unassisted	Activity ad lib

ADLs, Activities of daily living; *BM,* bowel movement: *BS,* bowel sounds; *CBC,* complete blood count; *HCT,* hematocrit; *IV,* intravenous; *NPO,* nothing by mouth; *NSAIDs,* nonsteroidal antiinflammatory agents; *OOB,* out of bed; *PCA,* patient-controlled analgesia; *PNV,* prenatal vitamins; *PP,* postpartum: *TCDB,* turn, cough, deep breathe; *WNL,* within normal limits.

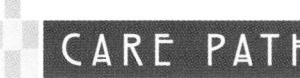

	IMMEDIATE POST-OP CESAREAN	BY 4TH HOUR AFTER ADMISSION TO PP UNIT	5 TO 24 HOURS	25 TO 48 HOURS	BY DISCHARGE
INTERVENTIONS—cont'd					
Pulmonary Care	Patent airway; O₂ discontinued	TCDB q2hr with splinting, incentive spirometry q1hr if ordered, lungs clear	TCDB q2hr while awake; lungs clear	TCDB as needed; lungs clear	
Medications	Oxytocin added to IV Pain control: analgesics, IV, or epidural narcotic	Oxytocin continued Pain control: analgesics—PCA, IM, PO, or epidural narcotic	Oxytocin may be discontinued Pain control: IM, PO, PCA narcotics or analgesics	Oxytocin discontinued Pain control: PO analgesics, NSAIDs; PCA discontinued; stool softener, PNV	Rx filled or given to take home
Teaching, Discharge Plan	Breastfeeding, positioning, leg exercises	Verbalize understanding/unit routines, how to achieve rest, TCDB, involution, pain control	*Self:* comfort measures and care; reinforce TCDB and positioning; introduce teaching videos, lactation promotion or suppression *Infant:* Handwashing, infant safety, positioning for feeding and burping; if breastfeeding, then positioning baby, latching on, timing, removing from breast	*Self:* diet; activity/rest; bowel/bladder function *Infant:* bonding; parent concerns; feeding; infant bath, cord care; need for car seat; newborn characteristics; circumcision, if requested; answer questions	*Self:* home care, signs of complications (infections, bleeding), normal psychologic adjustments, normal ADLs; resumption of sexual activities; contraception; identification of support system at home; self-concept issues related to cesarean birth. Inform whom to call if problems; review need to keep follow-up appointment; provide information about community resources; provide copy of home care *Infant:* parents to demonstrate infant care; reinforce use of booklets for infant care, whom to call if problems; discuss immunization needs; review need to keep follow-up appointments

O₂ discontinued

CLIENT SELF-CARE

Postpartum Pain Relief After Cesarean Birth

INCISIONAL

Splint incision with a pillow when moving or coughing.
Use relaxation techniques such as music, breathing, and dim lights.
Apply a heating pad to the abdomen.

GAS

Walk as often as you can.
Do not eat or drink gas-forming foods, carbonated beverages, or whole milk.
Do not use straws for drinking fluids.
Take antiflatulence medication if prescribed.
Lie on your left side to expel gas.
Rock in a rocking chair.

HOME CARE

Signs of Postoperative Complications After Discharge

Report the following signs to your health care provider:
Temperature exceeding 38° C
Painful urination
Lochia heavier than a normal period
Wound separation
Redness or oozing at the incision site
Severe abdominal pain

The Newborn's and Mother's Health Protection Act of 1996 provides for a length of stay of up to 96 hours for cesarean births. Some states have added home-care provisions for mothers who meet appropriate criteria for discharge and choose to leave sooner than the allowed length of stay. This policy recognizes that home care is less costly than hospital care and in most cases is more beneficial for recovery (Carpenter, 1998). These criteria may not coincide with the woman's physical or psychosocial readiness for discharge.

Eakes and Brown (1998) studied the expressed postdischarge needs of women who experienced planned and unplanned cesarean births. Findings revealed that the three predominant needs expressed by both groups of women were for rest and sleep; relief of pain and discomfort; and assistance with household chores, infant care and feeding, and self-care. Women who experienced planned cesarean births also expressed a need for help with depression, socialization, and family closeness, especially with regard to the limited amount of time they had to spend with their other children.

The nurse must provide discharge teaching to prepare women for self-care and newborn care in a limited time, while trying to ensure that the woman is comfortable and able to rest. The nurse needs to assess the woman's information needs and coordinate the health care team's efforts to meet them.

Discharge teaching and planning should include information about nutrition, measures to relieve pain and discomfort, exercise and specific activity restrictions, time management that includes periods of uninterrupted rest and sleep, hygiene, breast and incisional care measures, timing for resumption of sexual activity and contraception, signs of complications, and infant care. See the Client Self-Care box for postpartum pain relief and the Home Care box for signs of postpartum complications after discharge. The nurse also assesses the woman's need for continued support or counseling to facilitate her physical, psychosocial, and emotional recovery from the birth.

The woman's family and friends should be educated regarding her needs during the recovery process and their assistance should be coordinated before discharge. Referral to support groups or to community agencies may be indicated to further promote the recovery process. A postdischarge program of telephone follow-up and home visits can facilitate the woman's full recovery following cesarean birth.

Vaginal Birth After Cesarean

Indications for primary cesarean birth, such as dystocia, breech presentation, or fetal distress, often are nonrecurring. Therefore a woman who has had a cesarean birth may not have any contraindications to labor and vaginal birth at a subsequent pregnancy.

Most obstetricians no longer adhere to the belief that "once a cesarean, always a cesarean." ACOG (1994b) recommends that a TOL and **vaginal birth after cesarean (VBAC)** be routinely attempted in women who have had one previous cesarean birth by low transverse incision. As proof of the merits of this approach, vaginal births after previous cesarean birth increased 46% from 1989 to 1995. In 1996, the rate of vaginal births after previous cesarean birth (VBAC) was 28.3 per 1000 live births. In contrast, the rate was 18.9 in 1983.

Studies have shown that such a vaginal birth is relatively safe, with only a 0.5% risk of uterine rupture through a lower uterine segment scar (Knuppel & Drukker, 1993). Labor and vaginal birth are not recommended if there are contraindications, such as a previous fundal classic cesarean scar or evidence of CPD.

According to Scott (1999), 60% to 88% of women can give birth vaginally after a TOL. Women are most often the primary decision makers with regard to choice of birth method. During the antepartal period, the women should be given information about VBAC and encouraged to choose it as an alternative to repeat cesarean birth, as long as no contraindications occur. VBAC support groups and prenatal classes can help prepare the woman psychologically for labor and vaginal birth.

Women need to believe not only that their efforts during a TOL will be successful but also that they are fully capable of doing what is necessary to give birth vaginally (self-efficacy). They need to be given the opportunity to discuss their previous labor experience, including feelings of failure and loss of control and to express any uncertainty and concern they may have about how they will manage during their upcoming labor and birth (Dilks & Beal, 1997).

This labor should occur in a hospital facility that has the equipment and personnel available to begin the surgery within 30 minutes from the time a decision is made to perform cesarean birth. Ideally the woman is admitted to the labor and birth unit at the onset of spontaneous labor. In the latent phase of labor, the nurse encourages her to engage in normal activities such as ambulation. In the active phase of labor, FHR and uterine activity usually are monitored electronically and intravenous access such as a heparin lock may be established. Collaboration among the woman in labor, the nurse, and other health care providers often results in a successful VBAC.

There is no evidence that administering oxytocin to induce or augment labor or the use of epidural anesthesia is contraindicated, although some physicians may elect not to use these measures (Cunningham et al., 1997).

Attention should be paid to the woman's psychologic, as well as physical, needs during the TOL. Anxiety can inhibit the release of oxytocin, thus delaying the progress of labor and possibly leading to a repeat cesarean birth. To alleviate such anxiety, the nurse can encourage the woman to use breathing and relaxation techniques and to change positions to promote labor progress. The woman's partner can be encouraged to provide comfort measures and emotional support (Fawcett, Tulman, & Spedden, 1994). If a TOL does not proceed to vaginal birth, the woman will need support and encouragement to express her feelings about having another cesarean birth.

Evaluation

To evaluate the effectiveness of nursing care for a woman experiencing dystocia, the nurse reviews the expected outcomes that were met and assesses the woman's and the family's level of satisfaction with the care received.

POSTTERM PREGNANCY, LABOR, AND BIRTH

A **postterm** or postdate **pregnancy** is one that extends beyond the end of week 42 of gestation, or 294 days from the first day of the last menstrual period. The incidence of postterm pregnancy is estimated to be between 4% and 14% with an average of 10% (Cunningham et al., 1997).

Many pregnancies are misdiagnosed as prolonged. This can occur because (1) the pregnancy is inaccurately dated because the woman has an irregular menstrual cycle pattern, (2) an accurate date of the last menstrual period is unknown, or (3) entry into prenatal care was delayed or did not occur. When dating histories and assessment techniques are used to pinpoint gestational age more accurately, the true incidence of postterm pregnancy appears to be approximately 1% to 2% (Wood, 1994). A woman who experiences one postterm pregnancy is 30% to 40% more likely to experience it again in subsequent pregnancies (Arulkumarian, 1997).

Although the exact cause of postterm pregnancy is still unknown, a possible cause may be a deficiency of placental estrogen and continued secretion of progesterone. Low levels of estrogen may result in a decrease in prostaglandin precursors and reduced formation of oxytocin receptors in the myometrium (Gilbert & Harmon, 1998).

Clinical manifestations of a postterm pregnancy after 42 weeks include maternal weight loss (>1.4 kg/wk), decreased uterine size, meconium in the amniotic fluid, and advanced bone maturation of the fetal skeleton with an exceptionally hard fetal skull (Gilbert & Harmon, 1998).

Maternal and Fetal Risks

Maternal risks are often related to the birth of an excessively large infant. The woman is at increased risk for dysfunctional labor; birth canal trauma, including lacerations and extension of episiotomy related to vaginal birth; postpartum hemorrhage; and infection. Interventions such as induction of labor with oxytocin, forceps- or vacuum-assisted birth, and cesarean birth are more likely to be necessary. The woman also may experience fatigue and psychological reactions such as depression, frustration, and feelings of inadequacy as she passes her estimated date of birth (Arulkumarian, 1997; Freeman & Lagrew, 1996; Gilbert & Harmon, 1998).

Fetal risks appear to be twofold. The first is the possibility of prolonged labor, shoulder dystocia, birth trauma, and asphyxia from macrosomia. Macrosomia occurs when the placenta continues to provide adequate nutrients to support fetal growth after 40 weeks of gestation. It is estimated to occur in approximately 25% of prolonged pregnancies (Freeman & Lagrew, 1996). The second risk is the compromising effects an "aging" placenta is believed to have on the fetus. Spellacy (1999) notes that placental function gradually decreases after 37 weeks of gestation. Amniotic fluid volume (AFV) declines to approximately 800 ml by 40 weeks of gestation and to about 400 ml by 42 weeks of gestation. The resulting oligohydramnios can lead to fetal hypoxia related to cord compression. If placental insufficiency is present, there is a high likelihood of fetal distress occurring during labor. Neonatal problems related to placental insufficiency include asphyxia, meconium aspiration syndrome, dysmaturity syndrome, hypoglycemia, polycythemia, and respiratory distress (Gilbert & Harmon, 1998). Whether an infant born after a postterm pregnancy has neurologic, behavioral, or intellectual development problems needs to be further investigated.

CARE MANAGEMENT

The management of postterm pregnancy is still controversial. The induction of labor at 41 to 42 weeks is suggested by some authorities as a means of reducing the rate of cesarean birth and stillbirth or neonatal death (Hannah et al., 1996). Others follow a more individualized approach, allowing the pregnancy to proceed to 43 weeks of gestation as long as assessment of fetal well-being using a combination of tests is performed and the results of the tests are normal. Tests are usually performed on a weekly or twice-weekly basis.

LEGAL TIP **Informed Consent Regarding Care During Postterm Pregnancy**

The woman with a postterm pregnancy should be informed of the risks and benefits of both treatment and nontreatment. The standard of practice for postterm pregnancy is to begin antepartal surveillance (maternal assessments and tests of fetal well-being) by 14 days after the EDB, no matter how the date was derived. A plan of care should be mutually agreed upon by the woman and her primary health care provider (Wood, 1994).

Antepartum assessments for postterm pregnancy may include daily fetal movement counts, nonstress tests, amniotic fluid volume assessments, contraction stress tests, biophysical profiles, and Doppler flow measurements.

The amniotic fluid volume (AFV) should be greater than 8 with at least one pocket of amniotic fluid greater than 2 cm and amniotic fluid should be present throughout the uterine cavity (Gilbert & Harmon, 1998, Schmidt, 1999). The biophysical profile may be the best way of gauging fetal well-being because it combines nonstress testing with real-time ultrasound scanning to assess fetal movements, fetal breathing movements, and the AFV. Determining the AFV is critical in women with postterm pregnancies because a decreased AFV has been associated with fetal stress.

Cervical checks usually are performed weekly after 40 weeks of gestation to determine whether the condition of the cervix is favorable for induction (>5 on the Bishop score for multiparas and 9 for nulliparas) (see Table 37-3). Vaginal secretions may be assessed for the amount of fetal fibronectin (FFN) because a low concentration may predict increased risk for prolonged pregnancy (Gilbert & Harmon, 1998). Amniocentesis or amnioscopy may be performed to detect meconium in the amniotic fluid (Spellacy, 1999).

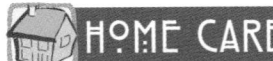 **HOME CARE**

Postterm Pregnancy

Perform daily fetal movement counts.
Assess for signs of labor.
Call your primary health care provider if your membranes rupture, or if you perceive a decrease in or no fetal movement.
Keep appointments for fetal assessment tests or cervical checks.
Come to the hospital soon after labor begins.

During the postterm period the woman is encouraged to assess fetal activity daily, assess for signs of labor, and keep appointments with her primary health care provider (Home Care box).

Providing the woman and her family with information about the tests that are required and why they are performed as well as progress reports about the health status of the maternal-fetal unit is important to reduce the stress and anxiety often experienced when the expected date of birth passes and pregnancy is prolonged. The woman and her family should be encouraged to express their feelings of frustration, impatience, anger, and fear and should be helped to recognize that these feelings are normal. The emotional and physical strain of a postterm pregnancy may seem insurmountable. Referral to a support group or another supportive resource may be needed (Schmidt, 1999).

If the woman's cervix is ripe, labor is usually induced with oxytocin. If her cervix is not ripe, continued fetal surveillance or a cervical ripening agent such as a prostaglandin insert or gel may be administered followed by oxytocin induction (Gilbert & Harmon, 1998; Hannah et al., 1996; Schmidt, 1999).

During the labor of a woman with a postterm pregnancy, the fetus should be monitored electronically for a more accurate assessment of the FHR pattern. Fetal scalp pH sampling may be done to determine whether there is acidosis. If oligohydramnios is present, amnioinfusion may be implemented to restore amniotic fluid volume in order to maintain a cushioning of the cord. Inadequate fluid leads to compression of the cord, which results in fetal hypoxia that is reflected in variable or prolonged FHR deceleration patterns and passage of meconium. Amnioinfusion may also be used to prevent or minimize meconium aspiration syndrome (MAS) by diluting amniotic fluid thickened with meconium passed by a hypoxic fetus. Maternal-fetal risks related to amnioinfusion, although rare, can result from infection and overdistention of the uterine cavity with infused fluid (Folsom, 1997; Gilbert & Harmon, 1998; Schmidt, 1997). Accurate assessment of the woman's labor pattern also is important because dysfunctional labor is common (Spellacy, 1999).

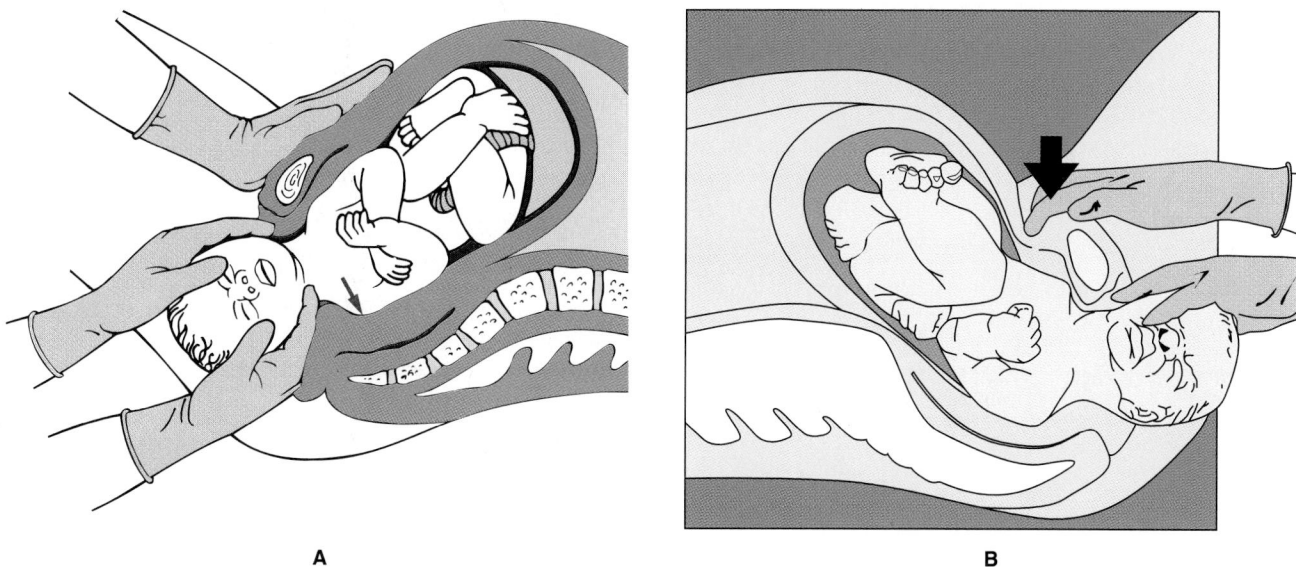

Fig. 37-14 Application of suprapubic pressure. **A,** Mazzanti technique. Pressure is applied directly posteriorly and laterally above the symphysis pubis. **B,** Rubin technique. Pressure is applied obliquely posteriorly against the anterior shoulder.

Emotional support is essential for the woman with a postterm pregnancy and her family. Although a vaginal birth is anticipated, the couple should be prepared for the possibility of an induction of labor, a forceps- or vacuum-assisted birth, or a cesarean birth if complications arise.

Expected outcomes include that the woman and her family use appropriate coping mechanisms to deal with the emotional aspects of her postterm pregnancy and that the woman and her newborn experience no injury during the birth.

OBSTETRIC EMERGENCIES

Shoulder Dystocia

Etiologic Factors and Clinical Manifestations

Shoulder dystocia is a rare emergency that increases the risk for fetal/neonatal and maternal morbidity and mortality during the attempt to deliver the fetus vaginally. The fetus/newborn is more likely to experience birth injuries related to asphyxia, brachial plexus damage, and fracture, especially of the humerus or clavicle. The mother's primary risk stems from excessive blood loss as a result of uterine atony or rupture, lacerations, extension of the episiotomy, or endometritis. It is estimated that 0.23% to 2.09% of all vaginal births are complicated by shoulder dystocia (Bruner et al., 1998; Naef & Martin, 1995).

In this condition, the head is born, but the anterior shoulder cannot pass under the pubic arch. Fetopelvic disproportion related to excessive fetal size (macrosomia) or maternal pelvic abnormalities may be a cause (Hall, 1997; Wiznitzer, 1995), although shoulder dystocia can occur in the absence of any known risk factors. The nurse should be

observant for signs that could indicate the presence of shoulder dystocia, including slowing of the progress of labor and formation of a caput succedaneum that increases in size. When the head emerges, it retracts against the perineum (turtle sign) and external rotation does not occur (Hall, 1997; Wiznitzer, 1995).

CARE MANAGEMENT

Many maneuvers such as suprapubic pressure and maternal position changes have been suggested and tried to free the anterior shoulder, although no one maneuver has been found to be most effective (Naef & Morrison, 1994). Suprapubic pressure can be applied to the anterior shoulder using the Mazzanti or Ruben technique (Fig. 37-14) in an attempt to push the shoulder under the symphysis pubis (Naef & Morrison, 1994). Having the woman move to a hands-and-knees position, a squatting position, or lateral recumbent position has also resolved shoulder dystocia (Hall, 1997; Piper & McDonald, 1994).

In the McRoberts maneuver (Fig. 37-15), the woman's legs are flexed apart, with her knees on her abdomen (Piper & McDonald, 1994). This causes the sacrum to straighten and the symphysis pubis to rotate toward the mother's head; the angle of pelvic inclination is thereby decreased, freeing the shoulder. Suprapubic pressure can be applied at this time. The McRoberts maneuver is the preferred method when a woman is receiving epidural anesthesia. The Gaskin maneuver requires that the woman assume an all-fours position on her hands and knees (Bruner et al., 1998). Although the exact reason this maneuver works is unknown, it is proposed that the effect of a change in position along with the force of gravity and slight increase in pelvic diameters may play a role. Fundal pressure is usually not advised as a method of relieving shoulder dystocia (Naef & Morrison, 1994; Piper & McDonald, 1994).

The nurse helps the woman to assume the position(s) that may facilitate birth of the shoulders and provides encouragement and support to reduce anxiety and fear. In addition the nurse assists the primary health care provider with these maneuvers and techniques during birth and documents the maneuvers and techniques used and the results.

Newborn assessment should include examination for fracture of the clavicle or humerus as well as brachial plexus injuries, and asphyxia (Hall, 1997). Maternal assessment should focus on early detection of hemorrhage.

Prolapsed Umbilical Cord

Etiologic Factors and Clinical Manifestations

Prolapse of the **umbilical cord** occurs when the cord lies below the presenting part of the fetus. Umbilical cord prolapse may be occult (hidden, not visible) at any time during labor whether or not the membranes are ruptured (Fig. 37-16, *A* and *B*). It is most common to see frank (visible) prolapse directly after rupture of membranes, when gravity washes the cord in front of the presenting part (Fig. 37-16, *C* and *D*). This occurs in 1 of 400 births. Contributing factors are a long cord (>100 cm), malpresentation (breech), transverse lie, or unengaged presenting part.

When the presenting part does not fit snugly into the lower uterine segment, as can occur in hydramnios or rupture of membranes, a sudden gush of amniotic fluid may cause the cord to be displaced downward. Similarly the cord may prolapse during amniotomy if the presenting part is high. A small fetus may not fit snugly into the lower uterine segment; as a result, cord prolapse is more likely to occur. Other factors predisposing to cord prolapse that are associated with a high presenting part are multiparity, CPD, and placenta previa.

CARE MANAGEMENT

Prompt recognition of a prolapsed umbilical cord is important because fetal hypoxia resulting from prolonged

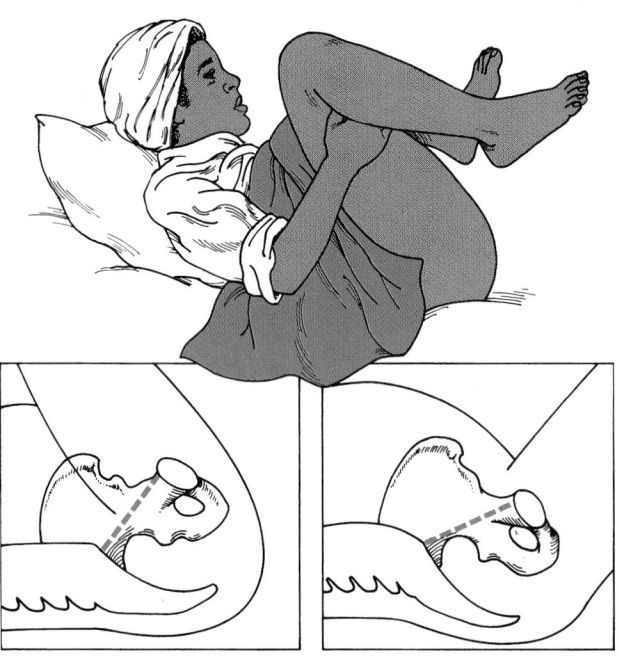

Fig. 37-15 McRoberts maneuver. *(Modified from Gabbe, S., Niebyl, J., & Simpson, J. [1996]. Obstetrics: Normal and problem pregnancies [3rd ed.]. New York: Churchill Livingstone.)*

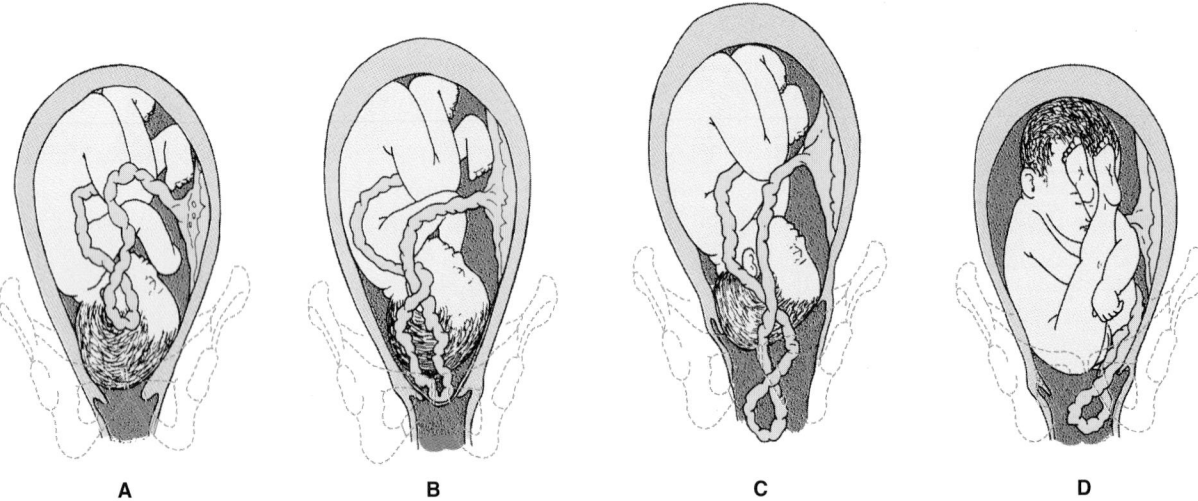

A	**B**	**C**	**D**

Fig. 37-16 Prolapse of umbilical cord. Note pressure of presenting part on umbilical cord, which endangers fetal circulation. **A,** Occult (hidden) prolapse of cord. **B,** Complete prolapse of cord. Note membranes are intact. **C,** Cord presenting in front of fetal head may be seen in vagina. **D,** Frank breech presentation with prolapsed cord.

cord compression (occlusion of blood flow to and from the fetus for more than 5 minutes) usually results in central nervous system damage or death of the fetus. Pressure on the cord may be relieved by the examiner putting a sterile gloved hand into the vagina and holding the presenting part off of the umbilical cord (Fig. 37-17, *A* and *B*). The woman is assisted into a position such as a modified Sims' (Fig. 37-17, *C*), Trendelenburg, or knee-chest (Fig. 37-17, *D*) position, in which gravity keeps the pressure of the presenting part off of the cord. If the cervix is fully dilated, forceps- or vacuum-assisted birth can be performed for the fetus in a cephalic presentation; otherwise a cesarean birth is likely to be performed. Nonreassuring fetal status, inadequate uterine relaxation, and bleeding can also occur as a result of a prolapsed umbilical cord. Indications for immediate interventions are presented in the Emergency box.

Rupture of the Uterus

Etiologic Factors and Clinical Manifestations

Rupture of the uterus is a rare but very serious obstetric injury that occurs in 1 to 1500 to 2000 births. The most frequent causes of uterine rupture during pregnancy are separation of the scar of a previous classic cesarean birth, uterine trauma (e.g., accidents, surgery), and a congenital uterine anomaly. During labor and birth, uterine rupture may be caused by intense spontaneous uterine contractions, labor stimulation (e.g., oxytocin), an overdistended uterus (e.g., multifetal gestation), malpresentation, external or internal version, or a difficult forceps-assisted birth. It occurs more frequently in multigravidas than in primigravidas (Varney, 1997).

A uterine rupture is classified as either complete or incomplete. A complete rupture extends through the entire uterine wall into the peritoneal cavity or broad ligament. An incomplete rupture extends into the peritoneum but not into the peritoneal cavity or broad ligament. Bleeding is usually internal. An incomplete rupture may also be a partial separation at an old cesarean scar and may go unnoticed unless the woman undergoes a subsequent cesarean birth or other uterine surgery.

Signs and symptoms vary with the extent of the rupture and may therefore be silent or dramatic. In an incomplete rupture, pain may not be present. The fetus may or may not show late decelerations, decreased variability, an increased or decreased heart rate, or other nonreassuring signs. The woman may experience vomiting, faintness, increased abdominal tenderness, hypotonic uterine contractions, and lack of progress. Eventually, bleeding and the effects of blood loss will be noted. Fetal heart tones may be lost. In a complete rupture the woman may complain of sudden, sharp shooting pain in her lower abdomen and may state that "something tore" or "gave way." If she is in labor, her contractions will cease and pain is relieved. She may exhibit signs of hypovolemic shock caused by hemorrhage (hypotension, tachypnea, pallor, cool, clammy skin). If the placenta separates, the FHR will be absent.

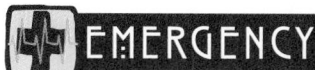

EMERGENCY

Prolapsed Cord

SIGNS

Fetal bradycardia with variable deceleration during uterine contraction.

Woman reports feeling the cord after membranes rupture.

Cord is seen or felt in or protruding from the vagina.

INTERVENTIONS

Call for assistance.

Notify primary health care provider immediately.

Glove the examining hand quickly and insert two fingers into the vagina to the cervix. With one finger on either side of the cord or both fingers to one side, exert upward pressure against the presenting part to relieve compression of the cord (Fig. 37-17, *A* and *B*). Place a rolled towel under the woman's right or left hip.

Place woman into the extreme Trendelenburg or a modified Sims' position (Fig. 37-17, *C*), or a knee-chest position (Fig. 37-17, *D*).

If cord is protruding from vagina, wrap loosely in a sterile towel saturated with warm sterile normal saline solution.

Administer oxygen to the woman by mask at 8 to 10 L/min until birth is accomplished.

Start IV fluids or increase existing drip rate.

Continue to monitor FHR by internal fetal scalp electrode, if possible.

Explain to woman and support person what is happening and the way it is being managed.

Prepare for immediate vaginal delivery if cervix is fully dilated or cesarean birth if it is not.

Fetal parts may be palpable through the abdomen. The nurse should suspect pulmonary embolism if the woman complains of chest pain (Varney, 1997).

:CARE MANAGEMENT

Prevention is the best treatment. Women who have undergone a classic cesarean birth are advised not to attempt vaginal birth in subsequent pregnancies. Women at risk for uterine rupture are assessed closely during labor. In addition, women whose labor is induced with oxytocin are monitored for signs of uterine hyperstimulation, because this also can precipitate uterine rupture. If hyperstimulation occurs, the oxytocin infusion is discontinued or decreased and a tocolytic drug may be given to decrease the intensity of the uterine contractions. After giving birth,

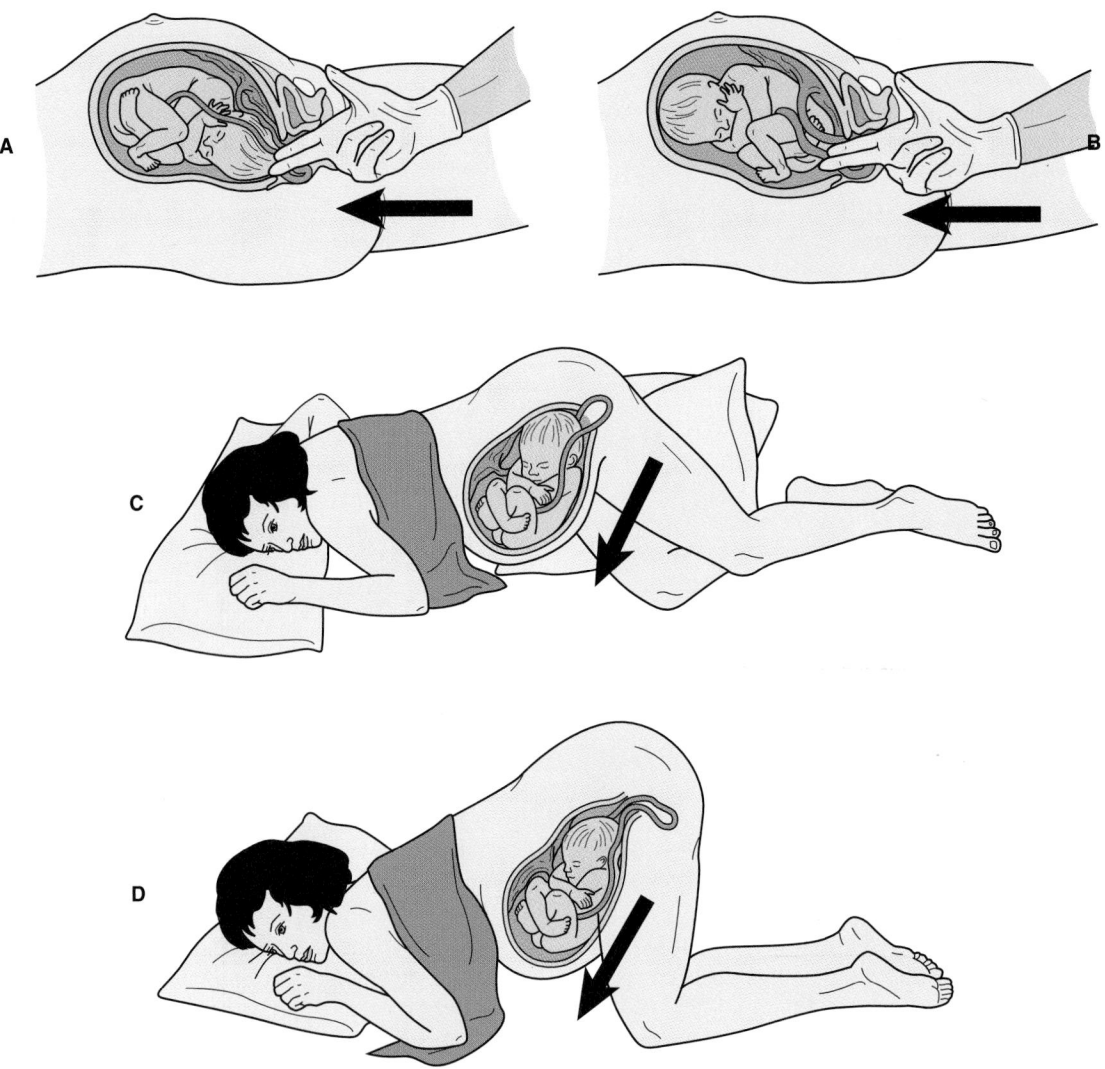

Fig. 37-17 Arrows indicate direction of pressure against presenting part to relieve compression of prolapsed umbilical cord. Pressure exerted by examiner's fingers in **A,** vertex presentation, and **B,** breech presentation. **C,** Gravity relieves pressure when woman is in modified Sims' position with hips elevated as high as possible with pillows. **D,** Knee-chest position.

women are assessed for excessive bleeding, especially if the fundus is firm and there are signs of hemorrhagic shock.

If rupture occurs, the type of medical management implemented depends on the severity. A small rupture may be managed with a laparotomy and birth of the infant, repair of the laceration, and blood transfusions, if needed. In the event of complete rupture, hysterectomy and blood replacement is the usual treatment.

The nurse's role may include starting intravenous fluids, transfusing blood products, administering oxygen and assisting with the preparation for immediate surgery. Supporting the woman's family and giving them information about the treatment are also important during this emergency (Varney, 1997). The associated fetal mortality rate is high (>80%), and the maternal mortality rate may be as high as 50% to 75% (Cunningham et al., 1997). Providing information about spiritual support services or suggesting that the family contact their own support system may therefore be warranted.

Amniotic Fluid Embolism

Etiologic Factors and Clinical Manifestations

An **amniotic fluid embolism (AFE)** occurs when amniotic fluid containing particles of debris (e.g., vernix, hair, skin cells, meconium) enters the maternal circulation and obstructs pulmonary vessels, causing respiratory distress and circulatory collapse. This can happen because fluid can enter the maternal circulation any time there is an opening in the amniotic sac or an opening in the maternal uterine veins, accompanied by enough intrauterine pres-

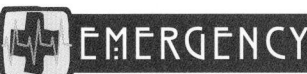

EMERGENCY

Amniotic Fluid Embolism

SIGNS
Respiratory Distress
- Restlessness
- Dyspnea
- Cyanosis
- Pulmonary edema
- Respiratory arrest

Circulatory Collapse
- Hypotension
- Tachycardia
- Shock
- Cardiac arrest

Hemorrhage
- Coagulation failure: bleeding from incisions, venipuncture sites, trauma (lacerations); petechiae, ecchymoses, purpura
- Uterine atony

INTERVENTIONS
Oxygenate
- Administer oxygen by face mask (8 to 10 L/min) or resuscitation bag delivering 100% oxygen
- Prepare for intubation and mechanical ventilation
- Initiate or assist with cardiopulmonary resuscitation. Tilt pregnant woman 30 degrees to side to displace uterus

Maintain Cardiac Output and Replace Fluid Losses
- Position woman on her side
- Administer IV fluids
- Administer blood: packed cells, fresh frozen plasma
- Insert indwelling catheter, and measure hourly urine output

Correct Coagulation Failure
Monitor Fetal and Maternal Status
Prepare for Emergency Birth once Woman's Condition Is Stabilized
Provide Emotional Support to Woman, Her Partner, and Family

sure to force the amniotic fluid into the veins (e.g., if the placenta separates or if there are rapid or strong contractions that cause the uterus to rupture or lacerate). This complication is estimated to be associated with a maternal mortality rate as high as 86% and a fetal mortality rate of 50% (Martin, 1996).

Amniotic fluid is more damaging if it contains meconium and other particulate matter such as mucus, fat globules, lanugo, bacterial products, or debris from a dead fetus because emboli can then form more readily. Maternal death occurs most often, however, if thick meconium is present in the amniotic fluid because it clogs the pulmonary veins more completely than other debris. Even if death does not occur immediately, serious coagulation problems such as disseminated intravascular coagulopathy usually occur. The substances in the amniotic fluid can also adversely affect pulmonary blood vessels, by causing venospasm or pulmonary hypertension, and cardiac function, by causing left ventricular failure. Hemorrhage is an additional problem that often accompanies AFE.

Maternal factors, including multiparity, tumultuous labor, abruptio placentae, and oxytocin induction of labor, and fetal problems, including macrosomia, death, and meconium passage, have been associated with an increased risk for the development of AFE (Clark, 1995; Cunningham et al., 1997; Martin, 1996).

▪ CARE MANAGEMENT

The immediate interventions for AFE are summarized in the Emergency box. Such medical management must be instituted immediately. Cardiopulmonary resuscitation is often necessary. The woman is usually placed on mechanical ventilation, and blood replacement is initiated and coagulation defects treated. Although the incidence of possible complications is small, their immediate recognition and the prompt initiation of treatment is important.

The nurse's immediate responsibility is to assist with the resuscitation efforts. If the woman survives, she is usually moved to a critical care unit, where hemodynamic monitoring and blood replacement and coagulopathy treatment are implemented.

Support of the woman's partner and family is needed because they will be anxious and distressed. Brief explanations of what is happening are important during the emergency, with reexplanation and further explanation given after the immediate crisis. If the woman dies, emotional support and involvement of the perinatal loss support team or other resource is needed (see Chapter 42).

KEY POINTS

- ▪ Dystocia occurs if there are differences in the normal relationships among any of the five factors affecting labor.
- ▪ Dystocia and normal labor are characterized by differences in the pattern of progress in labor.
- ▪ Dysfunctional labor occurs as a result of hypertonic uterine dysfunction, hypotonic uterine dysfunction, or inadequate voluntary expulsive forces.

Continued

KEY POINTS—cont'd

- The functional relationships among the uterine contractions, the fetus, and the mother's pelvis are altered by maternal positioning.
- Uterine contractility is stimulated by the effects of oxytocin and prostaglandin.
- Cervical ripening using chemical or mechanical measures can increase the success of labor induction.
- Expectant parents benefit from learning about operative obstetrics (e.g., forceps-assisted and cesarean birth) during the prenatal period.
- The basic purpose of cesarean birth is to preserve the life or health of the mother and her fetus.
- Unless contraindicated, vaginal birth is possible after a cesarean birth. Women must be empowered to recognize their ability to give birth vaginally and to choose a trial of labor (TOL) when appropriate.
- Labor management that emphasizes one-to-one support of the laboring woman by another female (doula, nurse, nurse-midwife) can reduce the rate of cesarean birth and increase the rate of VBACs.
- A postterm pregnancy poses a risk to both the mother and the fetus.
- Obstetric emergencies (e.g., shoulder dystocia, prolapsed cord, rupture of the uterus, and amniotic fluid embolism) occur rarely but require immediate intervention to preserve the health or life of the mother and newborn.

CRITICAL THINKING EXERCISES

1 You have been invited to present a class to a group of pregnant women and their partners who are beginning their second trimester. The topic of the class is *Reducing the Rate of Labor Interventions and Cesarean Birth: Measures You Can Use to Enhance the Progress of Your Labor.*
   a. What factors that can increase the rate of labor interventions, including stimulation of uterine contractions, use of forceps- and vacuum-assists, and cesarean birth would you emphasize in your class?
   b. Describe three measures you would recommend to the couples to enhance the progress of labor and reduce the possibility of unwanted interventions, including cesarean birth.
   c. Discuss the role of the partner in terms of assisting the laboring woman to use appropriate measures to enhance the progress of labor.

CRITICAL THINKING EXERCISES—cont'd

2 You are preparing a woman and her partner for an unplanned cesarean birth necessitated by nonreassuring fetal status.
   a. Describe the possible reaction of the woman and her partner to this situation and how these reactions should influence the nursing care provided.
   b. Describe the feelings you might have regarding this situation and how these feelings could influence the care you administer.
   c. How would your preparation of this couple differ from the way in which you would prepare a couple for a planned cesarean birth?
   d. Discuss how this woman's postpartum care would differ from a woman who experienced a vaginal birth.
   e. How would you involve the woman's partner and other members of her support group in assisting with her care after discharge, especially if she chooses an early discharge?

3 A woman (2-0-0-1-0) is determined to be at 43 weeks of gestation and has been admitted for induction of her labor. You are the nurse assigned to manage her care.
   a. What assessment measures are critical before the initiation of the induction protocol?
   b. Dinoprostone insert (Cervidil) has been ordered if needed. Why is this medication used and what protocol would you follow in implementing the order?
   c. What guidelines should be followed in preparing the oxytocin infusion?
   d. The woman becomes very anxious as she begins to feel pain from her contractions. She tells you that she is sure her labor will be awful because induced labors are very hard. "Why can't my doctor just do a cesarean?" How would you respond to this woman's concern and support her during labor?
   e. Outline the assessment protocol you would follow to determine the response of the maternal-fetal unit to the oxytocin infusion.

4 You are assigned to care for a woman whose fetus is in a left occiput posterior position (LOP). Outline the care management approach you would use to help relieve this woman's pain and facilitate the progress of her labor.

References

Albers, L., Lydon-Rochelle, M., & Krulewitch, C. (1995). Maternal age and labor complications in healthy primigravidas at term. *J Nurse Midwifery* 40(1), 4-11.

American College of Obstetricians and Gynecologists (ACOG). (1994a). Operative vaginal delivery. *Technical Bulletin* 196, Washington, D.C.: ACOG.

American College of Obstetricians and Gynecologists (ACOG). (1994b). Committee Opinion: Vaginal delivery after a previous cesarean birth. *Committee on Obstetrics Practice* 143, Washington, D.C.: ACOG.

American College of Obstetricians and Gynecologists (ACOG). (1995a). Induction of labor. *Technical Bulletin* 217, Washington, D.C.: ACOG.

American College of Obstetricians and Gynecologists (ACOG). (1995b). Dystocia and the augmentation of labor. *Technical Bulletin* 218, Washington, D.C.: ACOG.

Andrews, C., & Chrzanowski, M. (1990). Maternal position, labor, and comfort. *Appl Nurs Res* 3(1), 7-13.

Arulkumarian, S. (1997). Prolonged pregnancy. In D. James et al. (Eds.). *High risk pregnancy management options.* London: W.B. Saunders.

Berg-Lekas, M., Hogberg, U., & Winkvist, A. (1998). Familial occurrence of dystocia. *Am J Obstet Gynecol* 179(1), 117-121.

Biancuzzo, M. (1993). Six myths of maternal position during labor. *MCN Am J Matern Child Nurs* 18(5), 264-269.

Bruner, J. et al. (1998). All-fours maneuver for reducing shoulder dystocia during labor. *J Reprod Med* 43(5), 439-443.

Burrows, W. et al. (1995). Safety and efficacy of early postoperative solid food consumption after cesarean section. *J Reprod Med* 40(6), 463-467.

Carpenter, J. (1998). Shortening the short stay. *AWHONN Lifelines* 2(1), 28-34.

Cefalo, R., & Bowes, W. (1998). Managing labor—Never walk alone. *N Engl J Med* 339, 117-119.

Clark, S. (1995). Amniotic fluid embolism: Analysis of the national registry. *Am J Obstet Gynecol* 172(4 pt 1), 1158-1167.

Cunningham, F. et al. (1997). *William's obstetrics* (20th ed.). Stamford, CT: Appleton & Lange.

Curtin, S., & Kozak, L. (1998). Decline in U.S. cesarean delivery rate appears to stall. *Birth* 25(4), 259-262.

Day, M., & Snell, B. (1993). Use of prostaglandin for induction of labor. *J Nurse Midwifery.* 38(2) (suppl), 42S-48S.

Dilks, F., & Beal, J. (1997). Role of self-efficacy in birth choice. *J Perinat Neonatal Nurs* 11(1), 1-9.

DiMatteo, M. et al. (1996). Cesarean childbirth and psychosocial outcomes: A meta-analysis. *Health Psychol* 15(4), 303-314.

Eakes, M., & Brown, H. (1998). Home alone—Meeting the needs of mothers after cesarean birth. *AWHONN Lifelines* 2(1), 36-40.

Ellings, J., Newman, R., & Bowers, N. (1998). Intrapartum care for women with multiple pregnancy. *J Obstet Gynecol Neonatal Nurs* 27(4), 466-472.

Fawcett, J., Tulman, L., & Spedden, J. (1994). Responses to vaginal birth after cesarean section. *J Obstet Gynecol Neonatal Nurs* 23(3), 253-259.

Flamm, B., Berwick, D., & Kabcenell, A. (1998). Reducing cesarean section rates safely: Lessons from a "Breakthrough Series" Collaborative. *Birth* 25(2), 117-124.

Folsom, M. (1997). Amnioinfusion for meconium staining: Does it help? *MCN Am J Matern Child Nurs* 22(2), 74-79.

Freeman, R., & Lagrew, D. (1996), Post date pregnancy. In S. Gabbe, J. Niebyl, & J. Simpson (Eds.). *Obstetrics: Normal and problem pregnancies* (3rd ed.). New York: Churchill Livingstone.

Friedman, E. (1989). Normal and dysfunctional labor. In W. Cohen et. al. (Eds.). *Management of labor* (2nd ed.). Rockville, MD: Aspen.

Gabay, M., & Wolfe, S. (1997). The beneficial alternative. *Public Health Rep* 112, 386-394.

Gabbe, S., Niebyl, J., & Simpson, G. (1996). *Obstetrics: Normal and problem pregnancies* (3rd ed.). New York: Churchill Livingstone.

Gilbert, E., & Harmon, J. (1998). *Manual of high risk pregnancy and delivery* (2nd ed.). St. Louis: Mosby.

Guyer, B. et al. (1998). Annual summary of vital statistics, 1997. *Pediatrics* 102(6), 333-349.

Hall, S. (1997). The nurse's role in the identification of risks and treatment of shoulder dystocia. *J Obstet Gynecol Neonatal Nurs* 26(1), 25-32.

Hannah, M. et al. (1996). Postterm pregnancy: Putting the merits of a policy of induction of labor into perspective. *Birth* 23(1), 13-19.

Knuppel, R., & Drukker, J. (1993). *High-risk pregnancy: A team approach* (2nd ed.). Philadelphia: W.B. Saunders.

Laros, R., Flanagan, T., & Kilpatrick, J. (1995). Management of term breech presentation: A protocol of external cephalic version and selective trial of labor. *Am J Obstet Gynecol* 172(6), 1916-1923.

Lydon-Rochelle, M. et. al. (1993). Accuracy of Leopold maneuvers in screening for malpresentation: A prospective study. *Birth* 20(3), 132-135.

Martin, R. (1996). Amniotic fluid embolism. *Clin Obstet Gynecol* 39(1), 101-106.

Mastrogiannis, D., & Knuppel, R. (1995). Labor induced using methods that do not involve oxytocin. *Clin Obstet Gynecol* 38(2), 259-266.

Mathews, T. (1998). Trends in stimulation and induction of labor, 1989-1995. *Stat Bull* 78(4), 20-26.

Mayberry, L. et al. (1999). Use of delayed pushing with epidural anesthesia: Findings from a randomized, controlled trial. *J Perinatol* 19(1), 26-30.

McNiven, P. et al. (1998). An early labor assessment program: A randomized, controlled trial. *Birth* 25(1), 5-10.

Miovech, S. et al. (1994). Major concerns of women after cesarean delivery. *J Obstet Gynecol Neonatal Nurs* 23(1), 53-59.

Mundle, W., & Young, D. (1996). Vaginal misoprostol for induction of labor: A randomized, controlled trial. *Obstet Gynecol* 88(4 pt 1), 521-525.

Naef, R., & Martin, J. (1995). Emergent management of shoulder dystocia. *Obstet Gynecol Clin North Am* 22(2), 247-259.

Naef, R., & Morrison, J. (1994). Guidelines for the management of shoulder dystocia. *J Perinatol* 14(6), 435-41.

Piper, D., & McDonald, P. (1994). Management of anticipated and actual shoulder dystocia: Interpreting the literature. *J Nurse Midwifery* 39(suppl 2), 91S-105S.

Porreco, R., & Thorp, J. (1996). The cesarean birth epidemic: Trends, causes, and solutions. *Am J Obstet Gynecol* 175(2), 369-374.

Pozaic, S. (1999). Induction and augmentation of labor. In L. Mandeville, & N. Troiano (Eds.). *High-risk and critical care intrapartum nursing* (2nd ed.). Philadelphia: Lippincott.

Radin, T., Harmon, J., & Hanson, D. (1993). Nurses' care during labor: Its effects on the cesarean birth rate of healthy nulliparous women. *Birth* 20(1), 14-21.

Rippin-Sisler, C. (1996). The experience of precipitate labor. *Birth* 23(4), 224-228.

Ryding, E., Wijma, K., & Wijma, B. (1998). Experiences of emergency cesarean section: A phenomenological study of 53 women. *Birth* 25(4), 246-251.

Schmidt, J. (1997). Fluid check—Making the case for intrapartum amnioinfusion. *AWHONN Lifelines* 1(5), 46-51.

Schmidt, J. (1999). Prolonged pregnancy. In L. Mandeville, & N. Troiano (Eds.). *High-risk and critical care intrapartum nursing* (2nd ed.). Philadelphia: Lippincott.

Scott, J. (1999). Cesarean delivery. In Scott, J. et al. (Eds.). *Danforth's obstetrics and gynecology* (8th ed.). Philadelphia: Lippincott, Williams & Wilkins.

Simkin, P. (1995). Reducing pain and enhancing the progress of labor: A guide to nonpharmacologic methods for maternity caregivers. *Birth* 22(3), 161-171.

Simpson, K., & Poole, J. (1998). *Cervical ripening and induction and augmentation of labor.* Washington, D.C.: AWHONN.

Spellacy, W. (1999). Postdate pregnancy. In J. Scott et. al. (Eds.). *Danforth's obstetrics and gynecology* (8th ed.). Philadelphia: Lippincott, Williams & Wilkins.

Summers, L. (1997). Methods of cervical ripening and labor induction. *J Nurse Midwifery* 42(2), 71-85.

Thomas, L. et al. (1990). The effects of rocking, diet modifications, and antiflatulent medication on postcesarean section gas pain. *J Perinat Neonatal Nurs* 4(3), 12-24.

Varney, H. (1997). *Varney's textbook for midwives* (3rd ed.). Sudberry, MA: Jones & Bartlett.

Ventura, J. et al. (1998). Report of Final Natality Statistics, 1996. *Monthly Vital Statistics Report* 46(11 suppl), 1-100.

Wiznitzer, A. (1995). Obstructed labor and shoulder dystocia. *Curr Opin Obstet Gynecol* 7(6), 486-491.

Wood, C. (1994). Postdate pregnancy update. *J Nurse Midwifery* 39(suppl 2), 110S-122S.

38

Postpartum Complications

Deitra Leonard Lowdermilk

LEARNING OBJECTIVES

- Define the key terms.
- Identify postpartum hemorrhage causes, signs and symptoms, possible complications, and medical and nursing management.
- Describe hemorrhagic shock, including management and hazards of therapy.
- Differentiate the causes of postpartum infection
- Apply the nursing process to care of women with postpartum infection.

- Describe thromboembolic disorders including incidence, etiology, signs and symptoms, and management.
- Summarize the role of the nurse in the home setting in assessing potential problems and managing care of women with postpartum complications.
- Identify topics for nursing research related to postpartum complications.

KEY TERMS

disseminated intravascular coagulation (DIC)
endometritis
hematoma

hemorrhagic (hypovolemic) shock
inversion of the uterus
mastitis
postpartum hemorrhage (PPH)

puerperal infection
subinvolution
thrombophlebitis
uterine atony

ollaborative efforts of the health care team are needed to provide safe and effective care to the woman and family experiencing postpartum complications. This chapter focuses on hemorrhage and infection. Psychologic complications are discussed in Chapter 35.

POSTPARTUM HEMORRHAGE

Definition and Incidence

Postpartum hemorrhage (PPH) continues to be a leading cause of maternal morbidity and mortality in the United States today (Anderson, Kochanek, & Murphy, 1997). It is

a life-threatening event that can occur with little warning and is often unrecognized until the mother has profound symptoms (Grimes, 1994; Norris, 1997). PPH has been traditionally defined as the loss of greater than 500 ml of blood after vaginal birth and 1000 ml after cesarean birth. A 10% change in hematocrit between admission for labor and postpartum or the need for erythrocyte transfusion also has been used to define PPH (ACOG, 1998). However, defining PPH is not a clear-cut issue. The American College of Obstetricians and Gynecologists (ACOG) states that hemorrhage is difficult to define clinically (ACOG, 1998). Diagnosis is often based on subjective observations

BOX 38-1 Risk Factors and Causes of Postpartum Hemorrhage

Uterine atony
- Overdistended uterus
  Large fetus
  Multiple fetuses
  Hydramnios
  Distention with clots
- Anesthesia and analgesia
  Conduction anesthesia
- Previous history of uterine atony
- High parity
- Prolonged labor, oxytocin-induced labor
- Trauma during labor and birth
  Forceps-assisted birth
  Vacuum-assisted birth
  Cesarean birth
Lacerations of the birth canal
Retained placental fragments
Ruptured uterus
Inversion of the uterus
Placenta accreta
Coagulation disorders
Placental abruption
Placenta previa
Manual removal of a retained placenta
Magnesium sulfate administration during labor or postpartum
Endometritis
Uterine subinvolution

with blood loss often being underestimated by as much as 50%.

Traditionally, PPH has been classified as early or late with respect to the birth. Early, acute, or primary PPH occurs within 24 hours of the birth. Late or secondary PPH occurs more than 24 hours but less than 6 weeks postpartum (ACOG, 1998). Today's health care environment encourages shortened stays after birth, thereby increasing the potential for acute episodes of PPH to occur outside the traditional hospital or birth center setting.

Etiology and Risk Factors

The most common cause of PPH is uterine atony, which complicates approximately 1 in 20 births (Gonik, 1999). Less common causes include retained placenta, placenta accreta, cervical or vaginal lacerations, uterine rupture or inversion, lower genital tract lacerations and hematomas, infection, and coagulopathies (ACOG, 1998; Varner, 1998).

Several factors predispose the woman to PPH, although many instances of PPH occur with no predisposing factor (Akins, 1994). Research studies have identified antepartal factors including an association with nulliparity, previous

history of PPH, and Asian or Hispanic ethnicity (Combs, Murphy, & Laros, 1991). Intrapartal risk factors include prolonged labor, cesarean birth, oxytocin induction of labor, uterine infection, and overdistention of the uterus (ACOG, 1998; Benedetti, 1996). Box 38-1 lists these and other predisposing factors for PPH that have been identified in research studies.

It is helpful to consider the problem of excessive bleeding with reference to the stages of labor. From birth of the infant until separation of the placenta, the character and quantity of blood passed may suggest excessive bleeding. For example, dark blood is probably of venous origin, perhaps from varices or superficial lacerations of the birth canal. Bright blood is arterial and may indicate deep lacerations of the cervix. Spurts of blood with clots may indicate partial placental separation. Failure of blood to clot or remain clotted indicates a pathologic condition or coagulopathy such as disseminated intravascular coagulation.

Excessive bleeding may occur during the period from the separation of the placenta to its expulsion or removal. Commonly, such excessive bleeding is the result of incomplete placental separation, undue manipulation of the fundus, or excessive traction on the cord. After the placenta has been expelled or removed, persistent or excessive blood loss usually is the result of atony of the uterus (failure to contract well or maintain contraction) or prolapse of the uterus into the vagina. Late PPH may be the result of subinvolution of the uterus, endometritis, or retained placental fragments (ACOG, 1998).

Uterine Atony

Uterine atony is marked hypotonia of the uterus. Normally, placental separation and expulsion are facilitated by contraction of the uterus, which also prevents hemorrhage from the placental site. The corpus is in essence a basket weave of strong, interdigitating smooth muscle bundles through which many large maternal blood vessels pass. If the uterus is flaccid after detachment of all or part of the placenta, brisk venous bleeding occurs and normal coagulation of the open vasculature is impaired and continues until the uterine muscle is contracted.

Uterine atony is the leading cause of PPH, accounting for greater than 90% of all cases of PPH (Norris, 1997). It is associated with high parity, hydramnios, a macrosomic fetus, and multifetal gestation. In such conditions the uterus is "overstretched" and contracts poorly after the birth. Other causes of atony include traumatic birth, use of halogenated anesthesia (e.g., halothane) or magnesium sulfate, rapid or prolonged labor, chorioamnionitis, and use of oxytocin for labor induction or augmentation (ACOG, 1998; Varner, 1998).

Lacerations of the Genital Tract

Lacerations of the cervix, vagina, and perineum are also causes of PPH. Hemorrhage related to lacerations should be suspected if bleeding continues despite a firm, contracted uterine fundus. This bleeding can be a slow trickle, an oozing, or frank hemorrhage.

Factors that influence the causes and incidence of obstetric lacerations of the lower genital tract include operative birth, precipitous birth, congenital abnormalities of the maternal soft parts, and contracted pelvis. Size, abnormal presentation, and position of the fetus; relative size of the presenting part and the birth canal; previous scarring from infection, injury or operation; and vulvar, perineal, and vaginal varicosities can also cause lacerations.

Extreme vascularity in the labial and periclitoral areas often results in profuse bleeding if laceration occurs. Hematomas may also be present.

Lacerations of the perineum are the most common of all injuries in the lower portion of the genital tract. These are classified as first, second, third, and fourth degree (see Chapter 22). An episiotomy may extend to become either third- or fourth-degree laceration.

Prolonged pressure of the fetal head on the vaginal mucosa ultimately interferes with the circulation and may produce ischemic or pressure necrosis. The state of the tissues in combination with the type of birth may result in deep vaginal lacerations, with consequent predisposition toward vaginal hematomas.

Pelvic **hematomas** (a collection of blood in the connective tissue) may be vulvar, vaginal, or retroperitoneal in origin. Vulvar hematomas are the most common. Pain is the most common symptom and most vulvar hematomas will be visible. Vaginal hematomas occur more commonly in association with a forceps-assisted birth, an episiotomy, or primigravidity (Ridgeway, 1995). Retroperitoneal hematomas are the least common but are life threatening. They are caused by laceration of one of the vessels attached to the hypogastric artery, usually associated with rupture of a cesarean scar during labor (Benedetti, 1996). During the postpartum period, if the woman reports a persistent perineal or rectal pain or a feeling of pressure in the vagina, a careful examination is made. However, a subperitoneal hematoma may cause minimal pain, and the initial symptoms may be signs of shock (Ridgeway, 1995).

Cervical lacerations usually occur at the lateral angles of the external os. Most are shallow, and bleeding is minimal. More extensive lacerations may extend into the vaginal vault or into the lower uterine segment.

Retained Placenta

Nonadherent Retained Placenta

The normally implanted placenta separates with the first or second strong uterine contraction after birth of the infant. Placental separation occurs within 15 minutes in about 90% of women; within 30 minutes after birth, about 95% of women will have a separated placenta. About 98% achieve placental separation 45 minutes after birth. However, if the placenta has not been recovered within 30 minutes of birth, most health care providers will attempt to remove it manually.

Retained placenta may result from partial separation of a normal placenta, entrapment of the partially or completely separated placenta by an hourglass constriction ring of the uterus, mismanagement of the third stage of labor, or abnormal adherence of the entire placenta or a portion of the placenta to the uterine wall. Placental retention because of poor separation is common in very preterm births (20 to 24 weeks of gestation).

Management of nonadherent retained placenta is by manual separation and removal by the primary health care provider. Supplementary anesthesia is not usually needed for women who have had regional anesthesia for birth. For other women, administration of light nitrous oxide and oxygen inhalation anesthesia or intravenous thiopental facilitates uterine exploration and placental removal. After this removal, the woman is at continued risk for PPH or for infection.

Adherent Retained Placenta

Abnormal adherence of the placenta occurs for reasons unknown, but it is thought to result from zygotic implantation in an area of defective endometrium so that there is no zone of separation between the placenta and the decidua. Attempts to remove the placenta in the usual manner are unsuccessful, and laceration or perforation of the uterine wall may result, putting the woman at great risk for severe PPH and infection (Cunningham et al., 1997).

Predisposing factors for abnormal placental attachment include scarring of the uterus resulting from high parity, cesarean birth, myomectomy, or vigorous curettage; abnormal site of implantation, such as the cervix or lower uterine segment where the muscle configuration is not as effective for keeping the uterus contracted to prevent bleeding; and malformation of the placenta (ACOG, 1998).

Unusual placental adherence may be partial or complete. The following degrees of attachment are recognized:
- *Placenta accreta,* slight penetration of myometrium by placental trophoblast
- *Placenta increta,* deep penetration of myometrium by placenta
- *Placenta percreta,* perforation of uterus by placenta

Bleeding with complete or total placenta accreta may not occur unless separation of the placenta is attempted. With more extensive involvement, bleeding will become profuse when delivery of the placenta is attempted. Treatment includes blood component replacement therapy and hysterectomy may be indicated (Cunningham et al., 1997).

Inversion of the Uterus

Inversion of the uterus (turning inside out) after birth is a potentially life-threatening complication. The incidence of uterine inversion is approximately 1 in 2000 to 2500 births (ACOG, 1998), and may recur with a subsequent birth.

Uterine inversion may be partial or complete. Complete inversion of the uterus is obvious; a large, red, rounded mass (perhaps with the placenta attached) protrudes 20 to

30 cm outside the introitus. Incomplete inversion cannot be seen but must be felt; a smooth mass will be palpated through the dilated cervix.

Contributing factors to uterine inversion include fundal implantation of the placenta, vigorous fundal pressure, excessive traction applied to the cord, uterine atony, leiomyomas, and abnormally adherent placental tissue (Bowes,

1999; Cunningham et al., 1997). Uterine inversion occurs most often in multiparous women and with placenta accreta or increta. Although proper management of the third stage of labor prevents most cases of uterine inversion, some are unavoidable.

The primary presenting signs of uterine inversion are hemorrhage, shock, and pain. Hemorrhage is the primary

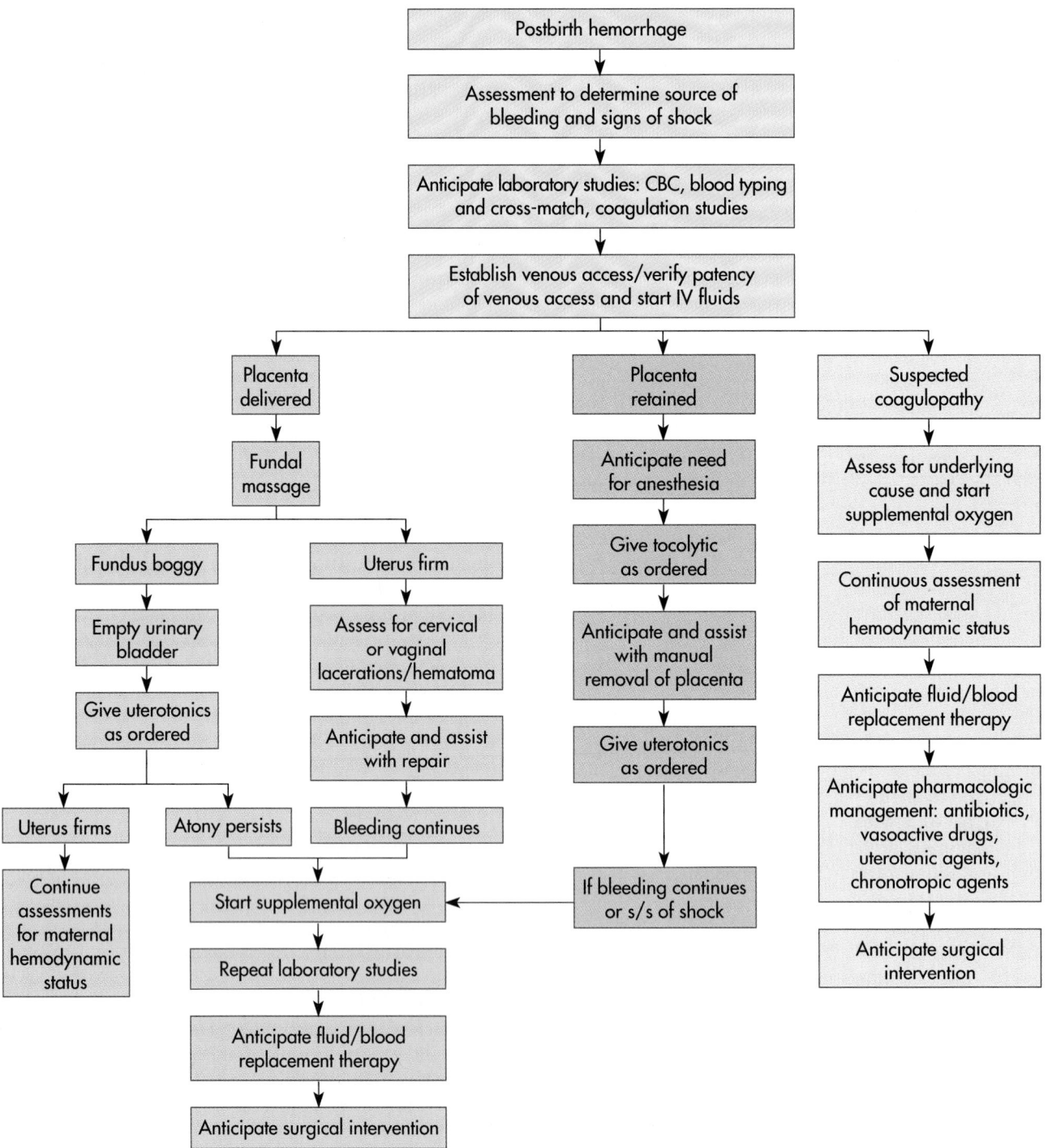

Fig. 38-1 Nursing assessments for postpartum bleeding. *CBC,* Complete blood count; *IV,* intravenous; *s/s,* signs and symptoms; *uterotonics,* medications to contract the uterus.

presenting sign in as many as 94% of women with uterine inversion, with blood loss estimated to range from 800 to 1800 ml. As many as 40% of these women may also have shock (Wendel & Cox, 1995).

Prevention—always the easiest, cheapest, and most effective therapy—is especially appropriate for uterine inversion. *The umbilical cord should not be pulled on strongly unless the placenta has definitely separated.*

Subinvolution of the Uterus

Late postpartum bleeding may occur as a result of subinvolution of the uterus. **Subinvolution** is defined as the delayed return of the enlarged uterus to normal size and function. Recognized causes of subinvolution include retained placental fragments and pelvic infection.

Signs and symptoms include prolonged lochial discharge, irregular or excessive bleeding, and sometimes hemorrhage. A pelvic examination usually reveals a uterus that is larger than normal and one that may be boggy.

▋ CARE MANAGEMENT
Assessment and Nursing Diagnoses

PPH may be sudden and even exsanguinating. With blood flow of approximately 650 ml/min to the uterine vasculature and placenta, disruption of vascular integrity has the potential for maternal exsanguination within a matter of minutes (Knuppel & Hatangadi, 1995). The nurse must therefore be alert to the symptoms of hemorrhage and hypovolemic shock and be prepared to act quickly to minimize blood loss (Fig. 38-1 and Box 38-2).

The woman's history should be reviewed for factors that cause predisposition to PPH (see Box 38-1). The fundus is assessed to determine whether it is firmly contracted at or near the level of the umbilicus. Bleeding should be

---

BOX 38-2 Noninvasive Assessments of Cardiac Output in Postpartum Clients Who Are Bleeding

Palpation of pulses (rate, quality, equality)
• Arterial
• Blood pressure
Auscultation
• Heart sounds/murmurs
• Breath sounds
Inspection
• Skin color, temperature, turgor
• Level of consciousness
• Capillary refill
• Urinary output
• Neck veins
• Pulse oximetry
• Mucous membranes
Presence or absence of anxiety, apprehension, restlessness, disorientation

---

assessed for color and amount. The perineum is inspected for signs of lacerations or hematomas to determine the possible source of bleeding.

Vital signs may not be reliable indicators of shock immediately postpartum because of the physiologic adaptations of this period. However, frequent vital sign measurements during the first 2 hours after birth may identify trends related to blood loss (e.g., tachycardia, tachypnea, falling blood pressure).

Assessment for bladder distention is important because a distended bladder can displace the uterus and prevent contraction. The skin is assessed for warmth and dryness; nail beds are checked for color and promptness of capillary refill. Laboratory studies include evaluation of hemoglobin and hematocrit levels.

Late PPH may develop within 24 hours of birth or later in the postpartum period. The woman may be at home when the symptoms occur. Discharge teaching should emphasize the signs of normal involution, as well as potential complications. Nursing diagnoses for women experiencing PPH include the following:

▋ Nursing Diagnoses
• Fluid volume deficit (immediate) related to
  – excessive blood loss secondary to uterine atony, lacerations, or uterine inversion
• Risk for fluid volume excess related to
  – blood and fluid volume replacement therapy
• Risk for infection related to
  – excessive blood loss or exposed placental attachment site
• Risk for injury (maternal) related to
  – attempted manual removal of retained placenta
  – administration of blood products
  – operative procedures
• Fear/anxiety related to
  – threat to self
  – knowledge deficit regarding procedures and operative management
• Risk for altered parenting related to
  – separation from infant secondary to treatment regimen
• Altered peripheral tissue perfusion related to
  – excessive blood loss and shunting of blood to central circulation

Expected Outcomes of Care

Expected outcomes of care for the woman experiencing postpartum hemorrhage may include that the woman will do the following:
• Identify and use available support systems.
• Maintain normal vital signs and laboratory values.
• Develop no complications related to excessive bleeding.
• Express understanding of her condition, its management, and discharge instructions.

Plan of Care and Interventions

Medical Management

Early recognition and acknowledgment of the diagnosis of PPH are critical to care management. The first step is to evaluate the contractility of the uterus. If the uterus is hypotonic, management is directed toward increasing contractility and minimizing blood loss.

Hypotonic uterus. If hemorrhage occurs, oxygen can be given to enhance oxygen delivery to the cells. A urinary catheter is usually inserted to monitor urine output as a measure of intravascular volume. Laboratory studies usually include a complete blood count with platelet count, fibrinogen, fibrin split products, prothrombin time and partial thromboplastin time. Blood type and antibody screen are done if not previously performed (ACOG, 1998).

The initial management of excessive postpartum bleeding is firm massage of the uterine fundus, expression of any clots in the uterus, eliminating any bladder distention, and continuous intravenous infusion of 10 to 40 units of oxytocin in 1000 ml lactated Ringer's or normal saline solution. If the uterus fails to respond to oxytocin, a 0.2 mg dose of ergonovine (Ergotrate) or methylergonovine (Methergine) may be given intramuscularly to produce sustained uterine contractions. If these first-line drugs are not effective, a derivative of prostaglandin $F_{2\alpha}$ (carboprost tromethamine) 0.25 mg is given intramuscularly. It can also be given intramyometrially at cesarean birth or intraabdominally after vaginal birth. Most hemorrhage can be controlled after one or two injections of 0.25 mg intramuscularly (ACOG, 1998). See Table 38-1 for a comparison of drugs used to manage PPH. In addition to the medications used to contract the uterus, rapid administration of crystalloid solutions and or blood will be needed to restore the woman's intravascular volume.

> **NURSE ALERT** *Use of ergonovine or methylergonovine is contraindicated in the presence of hypertension or cardiovascular disease. Prostaglandin $F_{2\alpha}$ should be used cautiously in women with cardiovascular disease or asthma (Bowes, 1999).*

If bleeding persists, bimanual compression may be considered by the obstetrician or nurse midwife. This procedure involves inserting a fist into the vagina and pressing the knuckles against the anterior side of the uterus, then placing the other hand on the abdomen and massaging the posterior uterus with it. If the uterus still does not become firm, manual exploration of the uterine cavity for retained placental fragments is implemented. If the preceding procedures are ineffective, surgical management may be the only alternative. Surgical management options include vessel ligation (uteroovarian, uterine, hypogastric), angiographic embolization, and hysterectomy (ACOG, 1998; Roberts, 1995).

Bleeding with a contracted uterus. If the uterus is firmly contracted and bleeding continues, the source of bleeding still needs to be identified and treated. Assessment may include visual or manual inspection of the perineum, vagina, uterus, cervix, or rectum and laboratory studies (e.g., hemoglobin, hematocrit, coagulation studies, platelet count) (ACOG, 1998). Treatment depends on the source of the bleeding. Lacerations are usually sutured.

TABLE 38-1 Drugs Used to Manage Postpartum Hemorrhage

	OXYTOCIN (PITOCIN)	METHYLERGONOVINE (METHERGINE)	PROSTAGLANDIN $F_{2\alpha}$ (PROSTIN/15M; HEMABATE)
ACTION	Contraction of uterus; decreases bleeding	Contraction of uterus	Contraction of uterus
SIDE EFFECT	Infrequent; water intoxication; nausea and vomiting	Hypertension, nausea, vomiting, headache	Headache, nausea, vomiting, fever
CONTRAINDICATIONS	None for PPH	Hypertension, cardiac disease	Asthma, hypersensitivity
DOSAGE; ROUTE	10-40 U/L diluted in lactated Ringer's solution or normal saline at 125-200 mU/min IV or 10-20 U IM	0.2 mg IM q2-4 hr up to 5 doses; 0.2 mg IV only for emergency	0.25 mg IM or intramyometrially q15-90 min up to 8 doses
NURSING CONSIDERATIONS	Continue to monitor vaginal bleeding and uterine tone	Check blood pressure before giving and do not give if >140/90; continue monitoring vaginal bleeding and uterine tone	Continue to monitor vaginal bleeding and uterine tone

Hematomas may be managed with observation, application of cold therapy, or ligation of the bleeding vessel. Fluids and or blood replacement may be needed (Akins, 1994; Druelinger, 1994; Roberts, 1995).

Uterine inversion. Uterine inversion is an emergency situation requiring immediate recognition, replacement of the uterus within the pelvic cavity, and correction of associated clinical conditions. Medical management of this condition involves all of the following interventions (Benedetti, 1996; Bowes, 1999; Wendel & Cox, 1995):
- Shock is treated. Usually lactated Ringer's solution is infused intravenously; blood component products may also be transfused.
- The fundus of the uterus is repositioned. This is often accomplished manually after the placenta has already separated. However, tocolytic agents such as terbutaline or magnesium sulfate or general anesthesia may be needed to relax the uterus for repositioning. As soon as the uterus is repositioned, these relaxing agents are discontinued.
- Oxytocic agents are given only after the uterus is repositioned. These may include oxytocin, prostaglandin $F_{2\alpha}$ or Prostin/15M (0.25 mg intramuscularly or intramyometrially). Bimanual compression may be effective in controlling bleeding until these oxytocic drugs take effect.
- Vaginal manual replacement is usually successful in about 75% of women who experience uterine inversion. If it is not successful, abdominal or vaginal surgery may be necessary to reposition or even remove the uterus.
- Broad-spectrum antibiotic therapy may be initiated to prevent infection and a nasogastric tube may be inserted to minimize the risk of paralytic ileus.

Subinvolution. Treatment of subinvolution depends on the cause. Ergonovine 0.2 mg every 4 hours for 2 or 3 days and antibiotic therapy are the most common medications used (Cunningham et al., 1997). Dilation and curettage (D&C) may be needed to remove retained placental fragments or to debride the placental site.

Herbal Remedies

Herbal remedies have been used with some success to control PPH in some settings. Some herbs have homeostatic actions, while others work as oxytocic agents to contract the uterus (Akins, 1994; Weed, 1986). Box 38-3 lists herbs that have been used and their actions. However, published evidence of the safety and efficacy of herbal therapy is lacking. Evidence from well-controlled studies is needed before recommendation for practice should be made (Enkin et al., 1995).

Nursing Interventions

Immediate nursing care of the woman with PPH includes assessment of vital signs and uterine consistency and ad-

ministration of oxytocin or other drugs to stimulate uterine contraction. The primary health care provider is notified if not present. Labor and birth units have standing orders or protocols for the nurse to implement interventions, such as starting intravenous infusions and administering medications and oxygen. If bleeding is not controlled, the nurse may be responsible for preparing the woman for operative intervention.

The woman and her family will be anxious about her condition. The nurse can intervene by calmly providing explanations about interventions being performed and the need to act quickly.

After the bleeding has been controlled, the care of the woman with lacerations of the perineum is similar to that for women with episiotomies (analgesia as needed for pain and hot or cold applications as necessary). The need for increased roughage in the diet and increased intake of fluids is emphasized. Stool softeners may be used to assist the woman in reestablishing bowel habits without straining and putting stress on the suture lines.

> **NURSE ALERT** *To avoid injury to the suture line, a woman with third- or fourth-degree lacerations is not given rectal suppositories or enemas.*

The care of the woman who has experienced an inversion of the uterus focuses on immediate stabilization of hemodynamic status. This requires close observation of her response to treatment to prevent shock or fluid overload. If the uterus has been repositioned manually, care must be taken after the birth to avoid aggressive fundal massage.

BOX 38-3 Herbal Remedies for Postpartum Hemorrhage

HERBS	ACTION
Witch hazel	Homeostatic
Lady's mantle	Homeostatic
Blue cohosh	Oxytocic
Cotton root bark	Oxytocic
Motherwort	Promotes uterine contraction; vasoconstrictive
Shepherd's purse	Promotes uterine contraction
Alfalfa leaf	Increases availability of vitamin K; increases hemoglobin
Nettle	Increases availability of vitamin K; increases hemoglobin
Red raspberry leaves	Homeostatic, promotes uterine contraction

Source: Schirmer, G. (1998). *Herbal medicine.* Bedford TX: MED2000; Weed, S. (1986). *Wise woman herbal for the childbearing year,* Woodstock, NY: Ash Tree Publishing Co.

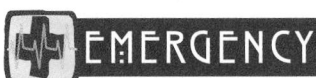

EMERGENCY

Hemorrhagic Shock

ASSESSMENTS	CHARACTERISTICS
Respirations	Rapid and shallow
Pulse	Rapid, weak, irregular
Blood pressure	Decreasing (late sign)
Skin	Cool, pale, clammy
Urinary output	Decreasing
Level of consciousness	Lethargy → coma
Mental status	Anxiety → coma
Central venous pressure	Decreased

INTERVENTION

Summon assistance and equipment.
Start IV infusion per standing orders.
Ensure patent airway; administer oxygen.
Continue to monitor status.

From Wong, D. & Perry, S. (1998). *Maternal child nursing care.* St. Louis: Mosby.

Discharge instructions for the woman who has had PPH are similar to those for any postpartum woman. In addition, she should be told that she will probably feel fatigue, even exhaustion, and will need to limit her physical activities to conserve her strength. She may need instructions in increasing her dietary iron and protein intake and iron supplementation to rebuild lost red cell volume. She may need assistance with infant care and household activities until she has regained strength. Some women have problems with delayed or insufficient lactation and postpartum depression (Akins, 1994). Referrals for home care follow-up or to community resources may be needed.

Evaluation

The nurse can be reasonably assured that care was effective to the extent that the expected outcomes were achieved.

HEMORRHAGIC (HYPOVOLEMIC) SHOCK

Hemorrhage may result in **hemorrhagic (hypovolemic) shock.** Shock is an emergency situation in which the perfusion of body organs may become severely compromised and death may occur. Physiologic compensatory mechanisms are activated in response to hemorrhage. The adrenal glands release catecholamines, causing arterioles and venules in the skin, lungs, gastrointestinal tract, liver, and kidneys to constrict. The available blood flow is diverted to the brain and heart and away from other organs, including the uterus. If shock is prolonged, the continued reduction in cellular oxygenation results in an accumulation of lactic acid and acidosis (from anaerobic glucose metabolism). Acidosis (lowered serum pH) causes arteriolar vasodilation; venule vasoconstriction persists. A circular pattern is established; that is, decreased perfusion, increased tissue anoxia and acidosis, edema formation, and pooling of blood further decrease the perfusion. Cellular death occurs. See the Emergency Box for assessments and interventions for hemorrhagic shock.

Medical Management

Vigorous treatment is necessary to prevent adverse sequelae. Medical management of hypovolemic shock involves restoring circulating blood volume and treating the cause of the hemorrhage (e.g., lacerations, uterine atony, or inversion). To restore circulating blood volume, a rapid intravenous infusion of crystalloid solution is given at a rate of 3 ml infused for every 1 ml of estimated blood loss (e.g., 3000 ml infused for 1000 ml of blood loss). Packed RBCs are usually infused if the woman is still actively bleeding and no improvement in her condition is noted after the initial crystalloid infusion (Roberts, 1995). Infusion of fresh-frozen plasma may be needed if clotting factors and platelet counts are below normal values (Cunningham et al., 1997).

Nursing Interventions

Hemorrhagic shock can occur rapidly, but the classic signs of shock may not appear until the postpartum woman has lost 30% to 40% of blood volume. The nurse needs to continue to reassess the woman's condition, as evidenced by the degree of measurable and anticipated blood loss, and mobilize appropriate resources.

Most interventions are instituted to improve or monitor tissue perfusion. The nurse continues to monitor the woman's pulse and blood pressure. If invasive hemodynamic monitoring is ordered, the nurse may assist with the placement of the central venous pressure (CVP) or pulmonary artery (Swan-Ganz) catheter and monitor CVP, pulmonary artery pressure, or pulmonary artery wedge pressure as ordered (Clark et al., 1994; White & Poole, 1996).

Additional assessments to be made include evaluation of skin temperature, color, and turgor, as well as assessment of the woman's mucous membranes. Breath sounds should be auscultated before fluid volume replacement, if possible, to provide a baseline for future assessment. Inspection for oozing at the sites of incisions or injections and assessment of the presence of petechiae or ecchymosis in areas not associated with surgery or trauma are critical in the evaluation for disseminated intravascular coagulopathy.

Oxygen is administered, preferably by nonrebreathing face mask, at 10 to 12 L/min to maintain oxygen saturation. Oxygen saturation should be monitored with a pulse oximeter, although measurements may not always be accurate in a client with hypovolemia or decreased perfusion. Level of consciousness is assessed frequently and provides additional indications of blood volume and oxygen saturation. In early stages of decreased blood flow, the woman may report "seeing stars" or feeling dizzy or nauseated. She may become restless and orthopneic. As cerebral hypoxia increases, she may become confused and react slowly or not at all to stimuli. Some women complain of headaches. An improved sensorium is an indicator of improved perfusion.

Continuous electrocardiographic monitoring may be indicated for the woman who is hypotensive or tachycardic, continues to bleed profusely, or is in shock. A Foley catheter with a urometer is inserted to allow hourly assessment of urinary output. The most objective and least invasive assessment of adequate organ perfusion and oxygenation is urinary output of at least 30 ml/hr (White & Poole, 1996). Blood may need to be drawn and sent to the laboratory for studies that include hemoglobin and hematocrit levels, platelet count, and coagulation profile.

Fluid or Blood Replacement Therapy

Critical to successful management of the woman with a hemorrhagic complication is establishment of venous access, preferably with a large-bore IV catheter. The establishment of two IV lines facilitates fluid resuscitation. Vigorous fluid resuscitation includes the administration of crystalloids (lactated Ringer's, normal saline solutions), colloids (albumin), blood, and blood components. Fluid resuscitation must be carefully monitored because fluid overload may occur. Intravascular fluid overload occurs more frequently with colloid therapy.

Transfusion therapy is used to restore oxygen-carrying capacity and intravascular volume. Packed red blood cells (250 to 300 ml/unit) may be administered to increase vascular volume and improve oxygen-carrying capacity. Each unit of packed red blood cells increases the hematocrit by 3%. Fresh-frozen plasma contains clotting factors and fibrinogen and is the only source of factors V, XI, and XII. Each unit (250 ml/unit) of fresh-frozen plasma increases intravascular volume and fibrinogen (10 mg/dl per unit). Platelets increase platelet count by 5000 to 10,000 cells/unit and provide limited volume expansion. Cryoprecipitate is used to correct specific clotting disorders; it contains factor VIII, von Willebrand's factor, and fibrinogen. Administration of cryoprecipitate increases fibrinogen 10 mg/dl per unit (Gonik, 1999).

Administration of blood and blood components is not without risk. Banked blood is cold (4° C) and has an acid pH (6.6 to 6.8), which can result in hypothermia, dysrhythmias, and acidosis. In addition, banked blood can result in electrolyte imbalances because of the electrolyte composition of the blood (sodium 150 to 160 mEq/L, potassium 10 to 15 mEq/L, no ionized calcium, and low levels of 2,3-diphosphoglyceric acid). Coagulopathies may result from massive transfusion therapies because banked blood is deficient in platelets and clotting factors.

Transfusion reactions may follow administration of blood or blood components, including cryoprecipitates. Even in an emergency, each unit should be checked per hospital protocol (Legal Tip). Complications include hemolytic reactions, febrile reactions, allergic reactions, circulatory overloading, and air embolism.

LEGAL TIP Standard of Care for Bleeding Emergencies

The standard of care for obstetric emergency situations such as postpartum hemorrhage or hypovolemic shock is that provision should be made for the nurse to implement actions independently. Policies, procedures, standing orders or protocols, and clinical guides should be established by each health care facility in which births occur and should be agreed upon by health care providers involved in the care of obstetric clients.

COAGULOPATHIES

When bleeding is continuous and there is no identifiable source, a coagulopathy may be the cause. The woman's coagulation status needs to be assessed quickly and continuously. The nurse may draw and send blood to the laboratory for studies. Abnormal results depend on the cause and may include increased prothrombin time, increased partial prothrombin time, decreased platelets, decreased fibrinogen level, increased fibrin degradation products, and prolonged bleeding time (Druelinger, 1994). Causes of coagulopathies may be pregnancy complications such as idiopathic thrombocytopenic purpura or von Willebrand's disease.

Idiopathic Thrombocytopenic Purpura

Idiopathic or *immune thrombocytopenic purpura (ITP)* is an autoimmune disorder in which antiplatelet antibodies decrease the life span of the platelets. Thrombocytopenia, capillary fragility, and increased bleeding time are diagnostic findings. ITP may cause severe hemorrhage after cesarean birth or from cervical or vaginal lacerations. Incidences of postpartum uterine bleeding and vaginal hematomas are also increased.

Medical management focuses on control of platelet stability. If ITP was diagnosed during pregnancy, the woman likely was treated with corticosteroids or intravenous immunoglobulin. Platelet transfusions are usually given when there is significant bleeding. A splenectomy may be needed if the ITP does not respond to medical management. Neonatal thrombocytopenia, a result of the maternal disease process, occurs in about 50% of cases and is associated with high mortality (Kilpatrick & Laros, 1999).

von Willebrand's Disease

von Willebrand's disease, a type of hemophilia, is probably the most common of all hereditary bleeding disorders (Kleinert et al., 1997). It results from a factor VIII deficiency and platelet dysfunction that is transmitted as an incomplete autosomal dominant trait to both sexes. Although von Willebrand's disease is rare, it is among the most common congenital clotting defects in American women of childbearing age. Symptoms include a familial bleeding tendency, previous bleeding episodes, prolonged bleeding time (the most important test), factor VIII deficiency (mild to moderate), and bleeding from mucous membranes. Factor VIII increases during pregnancy, and this increase may be sufficient to offset danger from hemorrhage during childbirth. However, the woman's condition should be observed for at least 1 week after childbirth. Treatment of von Willebrand's disease may include replacement of factor VIII if it is at less than 30% of normal levels and administration of cryoprecipitate or fresh frozen plasma.

Disseminated Intravascular Coagulation

Disseminated intravascular coagulation (DIC) is a pathologic form of clotting that is diffuse and consumes large amounts of clotting factors, including platelets, fibrinogen, prothrombin, and factors V and VII. Widespread external bleeding, internal bleeding, or both can result. DIC also causes vascular occlusion of small vessels resulting from small clots forming in the microcirculation. In the obstetric population, DIC may occur as a result of abruptio placentae, amniotic fluid embolism, dead fetus syndrome (fetus has died but is retained in utero for at least 6 weeks), severe preeclampsia, septicemia, cardiopulmonary arrest, and hemorrhage.

The diagnosis of DIC is made according to clinical findings and laboratory markers. Physical examination reveals unusual bleeding; spontaneous bleeding from the woman's gums or nose may be noted. Petechiae may appear around a blood pressure cuff placed on the woman's arm. Excessive bleeding may occur from the site of a slight trauma (e.g., venipuncture sites, intramuscular or subcutaneous injection sites, nicks from shaving of perineum or abdomen, and injury from insertion of a urinary catheter). Symptoms may also include tachycardia and diaphoresis.

Laboratory tests reveal decreased levels of platelets, fibrinogen, proaccelerin, antihemophilic factor, and prothrombin (the factors consumed during coagulation). Levels of other factors should be normal. Fibrinolysis is increased at first but is later severely depressed. Degradation of fibrin leads to the accumulation of fibrin-split products in the blood. Fibrin-split products have anticoagulant properties and prolong the prothrombin time. Bleeding time is normal, coagulation time shows no clot, clot retraction time shows no clot, and partial thromboplastin time is increased. DIC must be distinguished from other clotting disorders before therapy is initiated.

Primary medical management in all cases of DIC involves correction of the underlying cause (e.g., removal of the dead fetus, treatment of existing infection or of preeclampsia or eclampsia, or removal of a placental abruption). Volume replacement, blood component therapy, optimization of oxygenation and perfusion status and continued reassessment of laboratory parameters are the usual forms of treatment (Clark et al., 1994; Richey, Gilstrap, & Ramin, 1995). Plasma levels usually return to normal within 24 hours after birth. Platelet counts usually return to normal within 7 days (Kilpatrick & Laros, 1999).

Nursing interventions include assessment for signs of bleeding and signs of complications from the administration of blood and blood products. Because renal failure is one consequence of DIC, urinary output is monitored, usually by insertion of an indwelling urinary catheter. Urinary output must be maintained at more than 30 ml/hr.

The woman and her family will be anxious or concerned about her condition and prognosis. The nurse offers explanations about care and provides emotional support to the woman and her family through this critical time.

THROMBOEMBOLIC DISEASE

A thrombosis is the formation of a blood clot or clots inside a blood vessel and is caused by inflammation (**thrombophlebitis**) or partial obstruction of the vessel. Three thromboembolic conditions are of concern in the postpartum period:

- *Superficial venous thrombosis:* Involvement of the superficial saphenous venous system
- *Deep venous thrombosis*: Involvement varies but can extend from the foot to the iliofemoral region
- *Pulmonary embolism*: Complication of deep venous thrombosis occurring when part of a blood clot dislodges and is carried to the pulmonary artery where it occludes the vessel and obstructs blood flow to the lungs

Incidence and Etiology

The incidence of thromboembolic disease in the postpartum period varies from about 1 in 1000 to 1 in 2000 women (Cunningham et al., 1997). The incidence has declined in the last 20 years because early ambulation after childbirth has become the standard practice. The major causes of thromboembolic disease are venous stasis and hypercoagulation, both of which are present in pregnancy and continue into the postpartum period. Other risk factors include cesarean birth, history of venous thrombosis or varicosities, obesity, maternal age over 35, multiparity, and smoking (Falter, 1997).

Clinical Manifestations

Superficial venous thrombosis is the most frequent form of postpartum thrombophlebitis. It is characterized by pain and tenderness in the lower extremity. Physical examination may reveal warmth, redness, and an enlarged, hardened vein over the site of the thrombosis. Deep vein thrombosis is more common in pregnancy and is characterized by unilateral leg pain, calf tenderness, and swelling (Fig. 38-2). Physical examination may reveal redness and warmth, but women may also have a large amount of clot and have few symptoms (Mishell et al., 1997). A positive Homans' sign may be present, but further evaluation is needed because the calf pain may be attributed to other causes such as a strained muscle resulting from the birthing position. Pulmonary embolism is characterized by dyspnea and tachypnea. Other signs and symptoms frequently seen include apprehension, cough, tachycardia, hemoptysis, elevated temperature, and pleuritic chest pain (Laros, 1999).

Physical examination is not a sensitive diagnostic indicator for thrombosis. Venography is the most accurate method for diagnosing deep venous thrombosis, but it is associated with serious complications. It is an invasive procedure that exposes the woman and fetus to ionizing radiation. Noninvasive diagnostic methods are more commonly used; these include real time and color Doppler ultrasound (Cunningham et al., 1997). Cardiac auscultation may reveal murmurs with pulmonary embolism. Electrocardiograms are usually normal. Arterial P_{O_2} may be lower than normal. A ventilation/perfusion scan, Doppler ultrasound, and pulmonary arteriogram may be used for diagnosis (Laros, 1999).

Medical Management

Superficial venous thrombosis is treated with analgesia (nonsteroidal antiinflammatory agents), rest with elevation of the affected leg, and elastic stockings (Falter, 1997). Local application of heat may also be used. Deep venous thrombosis is initially treated with anticoagulant (usually continuous intravenous heparin) therapy, bed rest with the affected leg elevated, and analgesia. After the symptoms have decreased, the woman may be fitted with elastic stockings to use when she is allowed to ambulate. Intravenous heparin therapy continues for 5 to 7 days. Oral anticoagulant therapy (warfarin) is started during this time and will be continued for about 3 months. Continuous intravenous heparin therapy is used for pulmonary embolism until symptoms have resolved. Intermittent subcutaneous heparin or oral anticoagulant therapy is usually continued for 6 months.

Nursing Interventions

In the hospital setting nursing care of the woman with a thrombosis consists of continued assessments: inspection and palpation of the affected area; palpation of peripheral pulses; checking Homans' sign; measurement and comparison of leg circumferences; inspection for signs of bleeding; monitoring for signs of pulmonary embolism including chest pain, coughing, dyspnea, and tachypnea; and respiratory status for presence of crackles. Laboratory reports are monitored for prothrombin or partial pro-

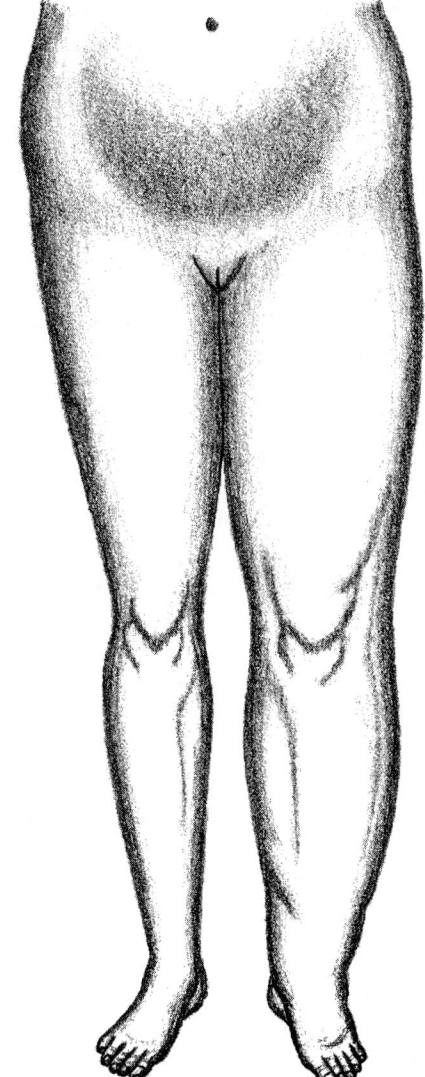

Fig. 38-2   Deep vein thrombophlebitis. *(Courtesy Julie L. Perry.)*

thrombin times. The woman and her family are assessed for their level of understanding about the diagnosis and their ability to cope during the unexpected extended period of recovery.

Interventions include explanations and education about the diagnosis and the treatment. The woman will need assistance with personal care as long as she is on bed rest; the family should be encouraged to participate in the care if that is what they wish. While the woman is on bed rest, she should be encouraged to change positions frequently, but not to place the knees in a sharply flexed position that could cause pooling of blood in the lower extremities. She should also be cautioned not to rub the affected area as this action could cause the clot to dislodge. Once the woman is allowed to ambulate, she is taught how to prevent venous congestion by putting on the elastic stockings before getting out of bed.

The nurse administers heparin and warfarin as ordered and notifies the physician if clotting times are outside the therapeutic level. If the woman is breastfeeding, she is assured that neither heparin nor warfarin is excreted in significant quantities in breastmilk. (If the infant has been discharged, the family is encouraged to bring the infant for feedings as permitted by hospital policy; the mother can also express milk to be sent home.)

Pain can be managed with a variety of measures. Position changes, elevating the leg, and application of moist warm heat may decrease discomfort. Administration of analgesics and antiinflammatory medications may be needed.

NURSE ALERT *Drugs containing aspirin are not given to women on anticoagulant therapy because aspirin inhibits synthesis of clotting factors and can lead to prolonged clotting time and increased risk of bleeding.*

The woman is usually discharged home on oral anticoagulants and will need explanations about the treatment schedule and possible side effects. If subcutaneous injections are to be given, the woman and family are taught how to administer the medication and about site rotation. The woman and her family should also be given information about safe care practices to prevent bleeding and injury while she is on anticoagulant therapy, such as using a soft toothbrush and using an electric razor. She will also need information about the need for follow-up with her health care provider to monitor clotting times and to make sure the correct dose of anticoagulant therapy is maintained. The woman should also use a reliable method of contraception if taking warfarin because this medication is considered teratogenic (Toglia & Nolan, 1997).

POSTPARTUM INFECTIONS

Postpartum or **puerperal infection** (puerperal sepsis or childbed fever) is any clinical infection of the genital canal that occurs within 28 days after miscarriage, induced abortion, or childbirth. The first symptom of postpartum infection is usually a fever of 38° C or more on 2 successive days of the first 10 postpartum days (not counting the first 24 hours after birth) (Hamedel, Dedmon, & Mozeley, 1995). Puerperal infection is probably the major cause of maternal morbidity and mortality throughout the world; however, it occurs after only 6% of births in the United States (3% after vaginal births; 5 to 10 times higher after cesarean births) (Gibbs & Sweet, 1999). Common postpartum infections include endometritis, wound infections, mastitis, urinary tract infections, and respiratory tract infections.

The most common infecting organisms are the numerous streptococcal and anaerobic organisms. *Staphylococcus aureus,* gonococci, coliform bacteria, and clostridia are less common but serious pathogenic organisms that also cause

> **BOX 38-4 Predisposing Factors for Postpartum Infection**
>
> **PRECONCEPTION OR ANTEPARTAL FACTORS**
> History of previous venous thrombosis, urinary tract infection, mastitis, pneumonia
> Diabetes mellitus
> Alcoholism
> Drug abuse
> Immunosuppression
> Anemia
> Malnutrition
>
> **INTRAPARTAL FACTORS**
> Cesarean birth
> Prolonged rupture of membranes
> Chorioamnionitis
> Prolonged labor
> Bladder catheterization
> Internal fetal/uterine pressure monitoring
> Multiple vaginal examinations after rupture of membranes
> Epidural anesthesia
> Retained placental fragments
> Postpartum hemorrhage
> Episiotomy or lacerations
> Hematomas

puerperal infection (Clark, 1995). Postpartum infections are more common in women who have concurrent medical or immunosuppressive conditions or who had a cesarean or other operative delivery. Intrapartal factors such as prolonged rupture of membranes, prolonged labor, and internal maternal or fetal monitoring also increase the risk of infection (Varner, 1998). Factors that predispose the woman to postpartum infection are listed in Box 38-4.

Endometritis

Endometritis (uterine infection) is the most common cause of postpartum infection. It usually begins as a localized infection at the placental site (Fig. 38-3), but can spread to involve the entire endometrium. Incidence is higher after cesarean birth. Assessment for signs of endometritis may reveal a fever (usually greater than 38° C); increased pulse; chills; anorexia; nausea; fatigue and lethargy; pelvic pain; uterine tenderness; or foul-smelling, profuse lochia (Calhoun & Brost, 1995). Leukocytosis and a markedly increased red blood cell (RBC) sedimentation rate are typical laboratory findings of postpartum infections. Anemia may also be present. Blood cultures or intracervical or intrauterine bacterial cultures (aerobic and anaerobic) should reveal the offending pathogens within 36 to 48 hours.

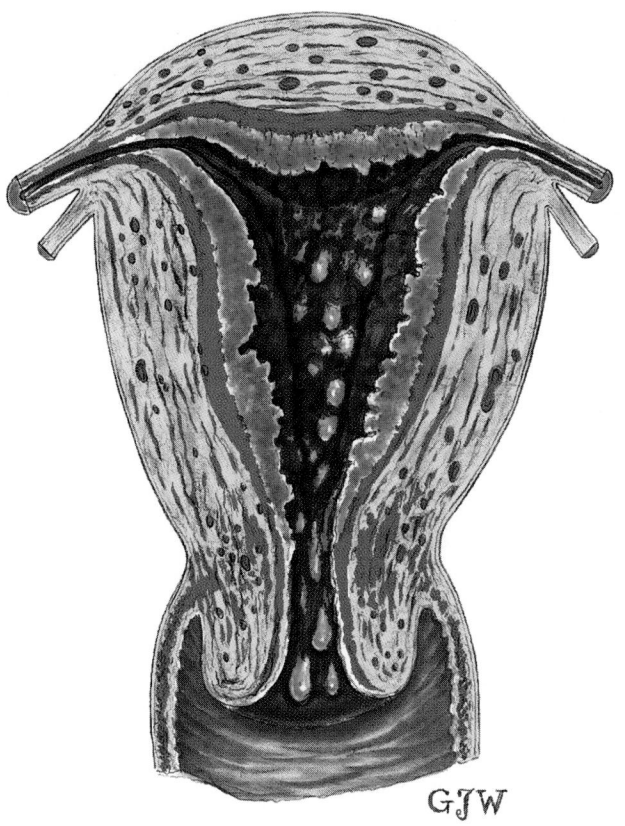

Fig. 38-3 Postpartum infection—endometritis.

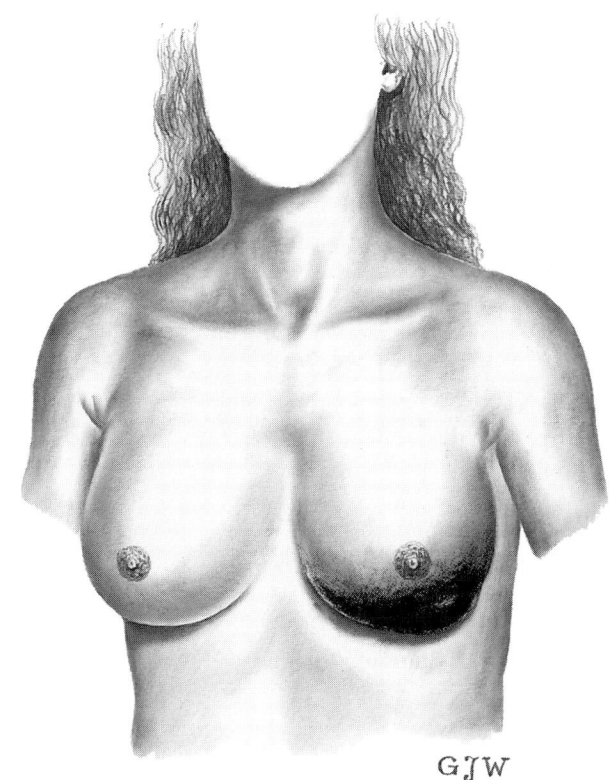

Fig. 38-4 Mastitis.

Wound Infections

Wound infections are also common postpartum infections but often develop after the woman is at home. Sites of infection include the cesarean incision and the episiotomy or repaired laceration site. Predisposing factors are similar to those for endometritis (see Box 38-4). Signs of wound infection include erythema, edema, warmth, tenderness, seropurulent drainage, and wound separation. Fever and pain may also be present.

Urinary Tract Infections

Urinary tract infections (UTIs) occur in 2% to 4% of postpartum women. Risk factors include urinary catheterization, frequent pelvic examinations, epidural anesthesia, genital tract injury, history of UTI, and cesarean birth (Clark, 1995). Signs and symptoms include dysuria, frequency and urgency, low grade fever, urinary retention, hematuria, and pyuria. Costovertebral angle (CVA) tenderness or flank pain may indicate upper UTI. Urinalysis results may reveal *Escherichia coli,* although other gram-negative aerobic bacilli may also cause UTIs.

Mastitis

Mastitis, or breast infection, affects about 1% of women soon after childbirth, most of whom are first-time mothers who are breastfeeding. Mastitis almost always is unilateral and develops well after the flow of milk has been established (Fig. 38-4). The infecting organism generally is the hemolytic *S. aureus.* An infected nipple fissure usually is the initial lesion, but the ductal system is involved next. Inflammatory edema and engorgement of the breast soon obstruct the flow of milk in a lobe; regional, then generalized, mastitis follows. If treatment is not prompt, mastitis may progress to a breast abscess.

Symptoms rarely appear before the end of the first postpartum week and are more common in the second to fourth weeks. Chills, fever, malaise, and local breast tenderness are noted first. Localized breast tenderness, pain, swelling, redness, and axillary adenopathy may also occur. Antibiotics are prescribed. Lactation is maintained (if desired) by emptying the breasts every 2 to 4 hours by breastfeeding, manual expression, or breast pump.

▪ CARE MANAGEMENT

Assessment and Nursing Diagnoses

Prenatal and intrapartal factors that can predispose a woman to postpartum infection were listed in Box 38-4. Signs and symptoms associated with postpartum infection have been discussed with each infection. Laboratory tests usually performed include a complete blood count, venous blood cultures, and uterine tissue cultures. Nursing diagnoses for women experiencing postpartum infection include the following:

▌ Nursing Diagnoses

- Knowledge deficit related to
  - etiology, management, course of infection
  - transmission and prevention of infection
- Impaired tissue integrity related to
  - effects of infection process
- Pain related to
  - mastitis
  - puerperal infection
  - urinary tract infection
- Altered family processes related to
  - unexpected complication to expected postpartum recovery
  - possible separation from newborn
  - interruption in process of realigning relationships after the addition of the new family member
- Risk of altered parenting related to
  - fear of spread of infection to newborn.

Expected Outcomes of Care

A plan of care is formulated that relates specifically to the needs of the woman and her family. Expected outcomes are determined in collaboration with the woman and her family and include that the woman will do the following:

- State the etiology, management, and sequelae of infection; she will identify measures to prevent reinfection.
- Describe a reduction or elimination of pain.
- With her family, verbalize acceptance of the unexpected events; they will verbalize positive coping measures (e.g., arrangement for home health care).

Plan of Care and Interventions

The most effective and cheapest treatment of postpartum infection is prevention. Preventive measures include good prenatal nutrition to control anemia and intrapartal hemorrhage. Good maternal perineal hygiene is emphasized. Strict adherence by all health care personnel to aseptic techniques during childbirth and the postpartum period is very important.

Management of endometritis consists of intravenous broad-spectrum antibiotic therapy (cephalosporins, penicillins, or clindamycin and gentamicin) and supportive care, including hydration, rest, and pain relief (Duff, 1996). Antibiotic therapy is usually discontinued 24 hours after the woman is asymptomatic (Gibbs & Sweet, 1999). Assessments of lochia, vital signs, and changes in the woman's condition continue during treatment. Comfort

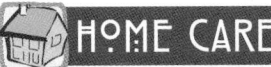

HOME CARE

Prevention of Genital Tract Infections

- Practice genital hygiene.
- Choose underwear or hosiery with a cotton crotch.
- Avoid tight-fitting clothing (especially tight jeans).
- Select cloth car seat covers instead of vinyl.
- Limit time spent in damp exercise clothes (especially swimsuits and leotards or tights).
- Limit exposure to bath salts or bubble bath.
- Avoid colored or scented toilet tissue.
- If sensitive, discontinue use of feminine hygiene deodorant sprays.
- Use condoms.
- Void before and after intercourse.
- Decrease dietary sugar.
- Drink yeast-active milk and eat yogurt (with lactobacilli).
- Avoid douching.

measures depend on the symptoms and may include cool compresses, warm blankets, perineal care, and sitz baths. Teaching should include side effects of therapy, prevention of spread of infection (see Home Care Box), signs and symptoms of worsening condition, and adherence to the treatment plan and the need for follow-up care. Women may need to be encouraged or assisted to maintain mother-infant interactions and breastfeeding (if allowed during treatment).

Postpartum women are usually discharged to home by 48 hours after birth. This is often before signs of infection are evident. Nurses in birth centers and hospital settings need to be able to identify women at risk for postpartum infection and to provide anticipatory teaching and counseling before discharge. After discharge, telephone follow-up, hot lines, support groups, lactation counselors, home visits by nurses, and teaching materials (videos, written materials) are all interventions that can be implemented to decrease the risk of postpartum infections. Home care nurses need to be able to recognize signs and symptoms of postpartum infection so that the woman can contact her primary health care provider. These nurses must also be able to provide the appropriate nursing care for women who need follow-up home care. See Plan of Care for a woman with a postpartum infection.

Treatment of wound infections may combine antibiotic therapy with wound debridement. Wounds may be opened and drained. Nursing care includes frequent wound and vital sign assessments and wound care. Comfort measures include sitz baths, warm compresses, and perineal care. Teaching includes good hygiene techniques (i.e., changing perineal pads front to back, handwashing after perineal care), self-care measures, and signs of worsening conditions

PLAN ᵒᶠ CARE | Postpartum Infection

> **NURSING DIAGNOSIS** Infection of genital canal related to retained placental fragments

Expected Outcome *Infection is resolved with no adverse effects.*

Nursing Interventions/*Rationales*

Administer and monitor broad-spectrum antibiotics per physician order *to stem invading pathogens and prevent systemic infection until specific pathogen can be identified.*

Assist with collection of intrauterine cultures for laboratory analysis *to identify specific causative organism.*

Maintain Standard Precautions and use good handwashing technique when providing care *to prevent spread of infection.*

Monitor vital signs *to assess client's response to treatment and status of infection.*

Monitor level of fatigue and lethargy, evidence of chills, loss of appetite, nausea and vomiting, and abdominal pain, *which are indicative of extent of infection and serve as indicators of status of infection.*

Monitor lochia for foul smell and profusion *as indicators of infection state.*

Monitor laboratory values (i.e., WBC count, cultures) *for indicators of type and status of infection.*

Help client maintain good handwashing technique (particularly before handling her newborn) and to maintain scrupulous perineal care with frequent change and careful disposal of perineal pads *to avoid spread of infection.* Avoid use of communal sitz baths.

Ensure adequate fluid and nutritional intake *to fight infection;* administer antiemetics as needed per physician order.

Monitor intake and output and electrolyte laboratory values *to evaluate fluid and electrolyte balance.*

From Wong, D. & Perry, S. (1998). *Maternal child nursing care.* St. Louis: Mosby.

---

to report to the health care provider. The woman is usually discharged to home for self-care or home nursing care after treatment is initiated in the inpatient setting.

Medical management for UTIs consists of antibiotic therapy, analgesia, and hydration. Postpartum women are usually treated on an outpatient basis; therefore teaching should include instructions on how to monitor temperature, bladder function, and appearance of urine. The woman should also be taught about signs of potential complications and the importance of taking all antibiotics as prescribed. Other suggestions for prevention of UTIs include proper perineal care, wiping from front to back after urinating or having a bowel movement, and increasing fluid intake (Clark, 1995).

Because mastitis rarely occurs before the postpartum woman is discharged, teaching should include warning signs of mastitis and counseling about prevention of cracked nipples. Management includes intensive antibiotic therapy (e.g., cephalosporins and vancomycin, which are particularly useful in staphylococcal infections), support of breasts, local heat (or cold), adequate hydration, and analgesics.

Almost all instances of acute mastitis can be avoided by proper breastfeeding technique to prevent cracked nipples. Missed feedings, waiting too long between feedings, and abrupt weaning may lead to clogged nipples and mastitis. Cleanliness practiced by all who have contact with the newborn and new mother also reduces the incidence of mastitis. See Chapter 28 for further information.

KEY POINTS

- Postpartum hemorrhage (PPH) is the most common and most serious type of excessive obstetric blood loss.
- Uterine atony is the leading cause of PPH.
- Inversion of the uterus is a rare but life-threatening complication that is usually preventable.
- Hemorrhagic (hypovolemic) shock is an emergency situation in which the perfusion of body organs may become severely compromised, leading to significant morbidity or mortality for the mother.
- The potential hazards of the therapeutic interventions may further compromise the woman with a hemorrhagic disorder.
- Clotting disorders are associated with many obstetric complications.
- Postpartum infection is usually diagnosed by the presence of a temperature greater than 38° C on 2 consecutive days in the first 10 postpartum days.
- Prevention is the most effective and inexpensive treatment of postpartum infection.

CRITICAL THINKING EXERCISES

1 *Two objectives of the Healthy People 2000: National Health Promotion and Disease Prevention Objectives are to reduce the maternal mortality rate to no more than 3.3 per 100,000 live births and to reduce severe complications of pregnancy to no more than 15 per 100 births. What is the maternal mortality rate in the state in which you live? Discuss the potential impact of current health care reform initiatives in achieving these goals in your state.*

2 *As part of a clinical group discussion, identify needs of families who have experienced a maternal death. Investigate community resources and support groups to determine if there is assistance available for families who have experienced a maternal death. Develop one resource to be used by nursing students who have been in a clinical situation in which there was a maternal death.*

3 *Review protocols in your labor and birth units for care of obstetric clients during emergency situations such as PPH or pulmonary embolism. Interview labor and delivery nurses about their roles during these emergencies. Evaluate whether the protocols allow the nurses to function as needed in the emergency. Suggest changes in the protocols based on your interviews.*

4 *Develop a protocol for nursing management of postpartum infection using Fig. 38-1 as a guide.*

References

Akins, S. (1994). Postpartum hemorrhage: A 90s approach to an age-old problem. *J Nurse Midwifery* 39(2 suppl), 123S-134S.

American College of Obstetricians and Gynecologists (ACOG). (1998). *Postpartum hemorrhage, AGOG Educational Bulletin* 243. Washington, D.C.: ACOG.

Anderson, R., Kochanek, K., & Murphy, S. (1997). Report of final mortality statistics, 1995. *Monthly Vital Statistics Report* 45(11). Hyattsville, MD: National Center for Health Statistics.

Benedetti, T. (1996). Obstetric hemorrhage. In S. Gabbe, J. Niebyl, & J. Simpson (Eds.). *Obstetrics: Normal and problem pregnancies* (3rd ed.). New York: Churchill Livingstone.

Bowes, W. (1999). Clinical aspects of normal and abnormal labor. In R. Creasy, & R. Resnick (Eds.). *Maternal-fetal medicine* (4th ed.). Philadelphia: W.B. Saunders.

Calhoun, B., & Brost, B. (1995). Emergency management of sudden puerperal fever. *Obstet Gynecol Clin North Am* 22(2), 357-367.

Clark, R. (1995). Infection during the postpartum period. *J Obstet Gynecol Neonatal Nurs* 24(6), 542-548.

Clark, S. et al. (Eds.). (1994). *Handbook of critical care obstetrics.* Boston: Blackwell Scientific.

Combs, A., Murphy, E., & Laros, R. (1991). Factors associated with postpartum hemorrhage with vaginal birth. *Obstet Gynecol* 77(1), 69-76.

Cunningham, F. et al. (1997). *Williams obstetrics* (20th ed.). Stamford, CT: Appleton & Lange.

Druelinger, L. (1994). Postpartum emergencies. *Emerg Med Clin North Am* 12(1), 219-237.

Duff, P. (1996). Maternal and perinatal infections. In S. Gabbe, J. Niebyl, & J. Simpson (Eds.). *Obstetrics: Normal and problem pregnancies* (3rd ed.). New York: Churchill Livingstone.

Enkin, M. et al. (1995). Effective care in pregnancy and childbirth. *Birth* 22(2), 101-110.

Falter, H. (1997). Deep vein thrombosis in pregnancy and the puerperium: A comprehensive review. *J Vasc Nurs* 15(2), 58-62.

Gibbs, R. & Sweet, R. (1999). Maternal and fetal infectious disorders. In R. Creasy, & R. Resnick (Eds.). *Maternal-fetal medicine* (4th ed.). Philadelphia: W.B. Saunders.

Gonik, B. (1999). Intensive care monitoring of the critically ill pregnant patient. In R. Creasy, & R. Resnick (Eds.). *Maternal-fetal medicine* (4th ed.). Philadelphia: W.B. Saunders.

Grimes, D. (1994). The morbidity and mortality of pregnancy: Still risky business. *Am J Obstet Gynecol,* 170(5 pt 2), 1489-1494.

Hamedel, G., Dedmon, C., & Mozeley, P. (1995). Postpartum fever. *Am Fam Physician* 52(2), 531-538.

Kilpatrick, S., & Laros, R. (1999). Maternal hematologic disorders. In R. Creasy, & R. Resnick (Eds.). *Maternal-fetal medicine* (4th ed.). Philadelphia: W.B. Saunders.

Kleinert, D. et al. (1997). von Willebrand disease: A nursing perspective. *J Obstet Gynecol Neonatal Nurs* 26(3), 271-276.

Knuppel, R., & Hatangadi, S. (1995). Acute hypotension related to hemorrhage in the obstetric patient. *Obstet Gynecol Clin North Am* 22(1), 111-129.

Laros, R. (1999). Thromboembolitic disease. In R. Creasy, & R. Resnick (Eds.). *Maternal-fetal medicine* (4th ed.). Philadelphia: W.B. Saunders.

Mishell, D. et al. (1997). *Comprehensive gynecology.* (3rd ed.). St. Louis: Mosby.

Norris, T. (1997). Management of postpartum hemorrhage. *Am Fam Physician* 55(2), 635-640.

Richey, M., Gilstrap, L., & Ramin, S. (1995). Management of disseminated intravascular coagulopathy. *Clin Obstet Gynecol* 38(3), 514-520.

Ridgeway, L. (1995). Puerperal emergency: Vaginal and vulvar hematomas. *Obstet Gynecol Clin North Am* 22(2), 275-282.

Roberts, W. (1995). Emergent obstetric management of postpartum hemorrhage. *Obstet Gynecol Clin North Am* 22(2), 283-302.

Schirmer, G. (1998). *Herbal medicine.* Bedford, TX: MED2000 Inc.

Toglia, M., & Nolan, T. (1997). Venous thromboembolism during pregnancy: A review of diagnosis and management. *Obstet Gynecol Survey* 52(1), 60-72.

Varner, M. (1998). Medical conditions of the puerperium. *Clin Perinatol* 25(2), 403-416.

Weed, S. (1986). *Wise woman herbal for the childbearing year.* Woodstock, NY: Ash Tree Publishing Co.

Wendel, P., & Cox, S. (1995). Emergent obstetric management of uterine inversion. *Obstet Gynecol Clin North Am* 22(2), 261-274.

White, D., & Poole, J. (Eds.). (1996). *Obstetrical emergencies for the perinatal nurse.* White Plains, NY: Education & Health Promotion Dept., March of Dimes Birth Defects Foundation.

Wong, D., & Perry, S. (1998). *Maternal child nursing care.* St. Louis: Mosby.

39

Acquired Problems of the Newborn

Debbie Fraser Askin

LEARNING OBJECTIVES

- Define the key terms.
- Describe assessment of infants for birth trauma and for sequelae of a diabetic pregnancy.
- Develop nursing care plans for complications typically seen in infants of diabetic mothers.
- Summarize the care of the newborn with soft tissue, skeletal, and nervous system injuries.
- Describe in detail the assessment of a newborn for infection.
- Formulate nursing diagnoses for the infant and family for common bacterial and viral infections.

- Review implementation and evaluation of care of infants with infections, including their families.
- Assess the effects of maternal use of alcohol, heroin, methadone, marijuana, cocaine, and smoking on the fetus and newborn.
- Describe the assessment of a newborn experiencing drug withdrawal.
- Develop a care plan for the newborn experiencing drug withdrawal, including the infant's family.
- Identify topics for nursing research related to acquired problems of the newborn.

KEY TERMS

birth trauma (injury)
brachial paralysis
caput succedaneum
cardiomyopathy
cephalhematoma
congenital rubella infection
facial paralysis (palsy)
fetal alcohol effects
fetal alcohol syndrome

hyperinsulinemia
infants of diabetic mothers
infants of gestational diabetic
   mothers
intracranial hemorrhage
macrosomia
meningitis
neonatal abstinence syndrome
opportunistic infections

phosphatidylglycerol
phrenic nerve injury
sepsis
septic shock
septicemia
subconjunctival (scleral) and retinal
   hemorrhages
thrush
TORCH

This chapter deals with acquired problems of the newborn. *Acquired problems* refer to those conditions resulting from environmental factors rather than genetic circumstances. The focus is on birth trauma, the infant of a diabetic mother, neonatal infections, and effects of maternal substance abuse.

BIRTH TRAUMA

Birth trauma (injury) is physical injury sustained by a neonate during labor and birth. The significance of birth injuries is assessed most accurately by review of recent mortality data. These data show a decline in fatal birth injuries. In 1981 birth injuries ranked sixth among major causes of infant mortality in the United States, resulting in 23.8 deaths per 100,000 live births. In 1997 birth injuries ranked eighth and caused 19.3 deaths per 100,000 live births (Guyer et al., 1998). This improvement is attributed to refinements in obstetric techniques, increased use of cesarean birth for births that would be difficult vaginally, and decreased use of vacuum extraction and version and extraction. Despite this decrease, birth injuries still are an important source of neonatal morbidity. Therefore the clinician should consider the broad range of birth injuries in the differential diagnosis of neonatal clinical disorders (Fanaroff & Martin, 1997).

In theory, most birth injuries may be avoidable, especially if careful assessment of risk factors and appropriate planning of birth occur. The use of ultrasonography allows antepartum diagnosis of macrosomia, hydrocephalus, and unusual presentations. Elective cesarean birth can be chosen for some pregnancies to prevent significant birth injury (Merenstein & Gardner, 1998). A small percentage of significant birth injuries are unavoidable despite skilled and competent obstetric care, as in especially difficult or prolonged labor or when the infant is in an abnormal presentation (Fanaroff & Martin, 1997). Some injuries cannot be anticipated until the specific circumstances are encountered during childbirth. Emergency cesarean birth may provide a last-minute salvage, but in these circumstances the injury may be truly unavoidable. The same injury might be caused in several ways. For example, a cephalhematoma could result from an obstetric technique such as forceps birth or vacuum extraction or from pressure of the fetal skull against the maternal pelvis.

Many injuries are minor and resolve readily in the neonatal period without treatment. Other traumas require some degree of intervention. A few are serious enough to be fatal. The nurse's contributions to the welfare of the newborn begin with early observation and accurate recording. The prompt reporting of signs that indicate deviations from normal permits early initiation of appropriate therapy. Table 39-1 provides an overview of neurologic birth injuries and the sites in which they occur.

CARE MANAGEMENT

Assessment and Nursing Diagnoses

Several factors predispose an infant to birth injuries (Fanaroff & Martin, 1997; Merenstein & Gardner, 1998). Maternal factors include uterine dysfunction that leads to prolonged or precipitous labor, preterm or postterm labor, and cephalopelvic disproportion. Injury may result from dystocia caused by fetal macrosomia, multifetal gestation, abnormal or difficult presentation (not caused by maternal uterine or pelvic conditions), and congenital anomalies. Intrapartum events that can result in scalp injury include the use of intrapartum monitoring of fetal heart rate (FHR) and collection of fetal scalp blood for acid-base assessment. Obstetric birth techniques can cause injury. Forceps birth,

TABLE 39-1 Types of Birth Injuries

SITE OF INJURY	TYPE OF INJURY
Scalp	Caput succedaneum
	Subgaleal hemorrhage
	Cephalhematoma
Skull	Linear fracture
	Depressed fracture
	Occipital osteodiastasis
Intracranial	Epidural hematoma
	Subdural hematoma (laceration of falx, tentorium, or superficial veins)
	Subarachnoid hemorrhage
	Cerebral contusion
	Cerebellar contusion
	Intracerebellar hematoma
Spinal cord (cervical)	Vertebral artery injury
	Intraspinal hemorrhage
	Spinal cord transection or injury
Plexus	Erb's palsy
	Klumpke's paralysis
	Total (mixed) brachial plexus injury
	Horner syndrome
	Diaphragmatic paralysis
	Lumbosacral plexus injury
Cranial and peripheral nerve	Radial nerve palsy
	Medial nerve palsy
	Sciatic nerve palsy
	Laryngeal nerve palsy
	Diaphragmatic paralysis
	Facial nerve palsy

Source: Moe, P., & Paige, L. (1998). Neurologic disorders. In G. Merenstein & S. Gardner (Eds.). *Handbook of neonatal intensive care* (4th ed.). St. Louis: Mosby.

vacuum extraction, version and extraction, and cesarean birth are potential contributory factors. Often more than one factor is present, and multiple predisposing factors may be related to a single maternal disease.

The Apgar score may alert the caregiver to birth injuries and help in identifying infants in need of immediate resuscitation. Flaccid muscle tone, regardless of cause, increases the risk of joint dislocations and separation during the birth process. Flaccid tone in extremities may be traced to nerve plexus injuries or long-bone fractures. A weak or hoarse cry is characteristic of laryngeal nerve palsy as a result of excessive traction on the neck during birth. Pronounced bruising of the skin may preclude accurate assessment for color.

A complete physical assessment of the newborn is performed soon after birth. Because evidence of birth injury may not be apparent at the initial examination, assessment continues during each contact with the neonate. The nursing diagnoses depend on the particular injury incurred. Thus the following list represents examples only.

▪ Nursing Diagnoses

Infant

- Impaired physical mobility related to
  - brachial plexus injury
- Impaired gas exchange related to
  - diaphragmatic paralysis (partial or complete)
- Pain related to
  - injury
- Injury related to
  - bruising, cephalhematoma, hyperbilirubinemia

Parents and Family

- Anxiety related to knowledge deficit regarding
  - injury and its cause
  - management and therapy
  - prognosis
- Anticipatory grieving related to
  - possible sequelae of the birth injury

Expected Outcomes of Care

Meeting the unique needs of the birth-injured newborn requires constant vigilance. Expected outcomes are established and prioritized. Nursing actions are selected in terms of the particular disorder and individual needs of the infant and family. The overall outcomes for care of infants with birth trauma include the following:

- The newborn will suffer minimal or no sequelae of trauma.
- The infant will receive prompt and appropriate treatment.
- The parents will initiate and maintain a positive parent-child relationship.
- The parents' and family's educational needs regarding the injury and its management will be met.

Plan of Care and Interventions

Soft Tissue Injuries

Caput succedaneum is a localized edematous swelling of the scalp that is not confined within the suture lines of the skull. The swelling persists for a few days after birth and then disappears without treatment. It is most often seen after vertex vaginal births and has no pathologic significance (see Fig. 26-6, *A*).

Cephalhematoma is a collection of blood from ruptured blood vessels between the periosteum and the surface of the skull. Because blood collects beneath the periosteum, it does not cross the cranial suture lines (see Fig. 26-6, *B*). The swelling may appear unilaterally or bilaterally, usually is minimal or absent at birth, increases over the first 3 days of life, and disappears gradually in 2 to 3 weeks. Occasionally, hyperbilirubinemia may result from breakdown of the accumulated blood.

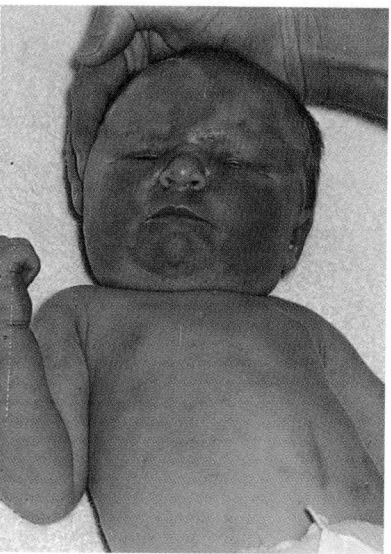

Fig. 39-1   Marked bruising on the entire face of an infant born vaginally after face presentation. Less severe ecchymoses were present on the extremities. Phototherapy was required for treatment of jaundice resulting from the breakdown of accumulated blood. *(From O'Doherty, N. [1986]. Neonatology: Micro atlas of the newborn. Nutley, NJ: Hoffmann-La Roche.)*

Subconjunctival (scleral) and retinal hemorrhages result from rupture of capillaries caused by increased intracranial pressure (ICP) during birth. They clear within 5 days after birth and usually present no problems. However, parents need reassurance about their presence.

Erythema, ecchymoses, petechiae, abrasions, lacerations, and edema of buttocks and extremities may be present. Localized discoloration may appear over presenting or dependent parts. Ecchymoses and edema may appear anywhere on the body and on the presenting body part from the application of forceps. They also may result from manipulation of the infant's body during birth.

Bruises over the face may be the result of face presentation (Fig. 39-1). In a breech presentation, bruising and swelling may be seen over the buttocks or genitalia (Fig. 39-2). The skin over the entire head may be ecchymotic and covered with petechiae caused by a tight nuchal cord. Petechiae, or pinpoint hemorrhagic areas, acquired during birth may extend over the upper portion of the trunk and face. These lesions are benign if they disappear within 2 days of birth and no new lesions appear. Ecchymoses and petechiae may be signs of a more serious disorder, such as thrombocytopenic purpura. If the hemorrhagic areas do not disappear spontaneously in 2 days, the physician is notified. To differentiate hemorrhagic areas from skin rashes and discolorations such as mongolian spots, the nurse blanches the skin with two fingers. Because extravasated blood remains within the tissues, petechiae and ecchymoses do not blanch.

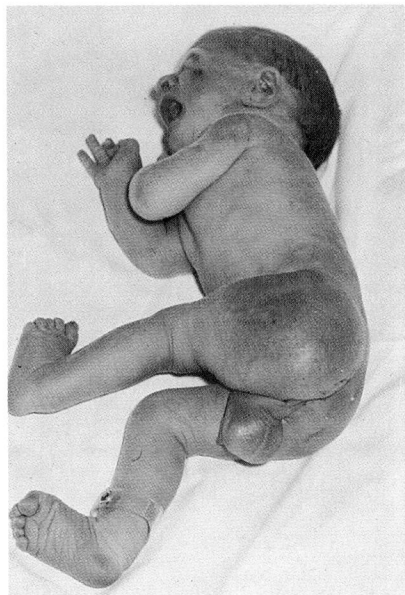

Fig. 39-2 Swelling of the genitals and bruising of the buttocks after a breech delivery. *(From O'Doherty, N. [1986]. Neonatology: Micro atlas of the newborn. Nutley, NJ: Hoffmann-La Roche.)*

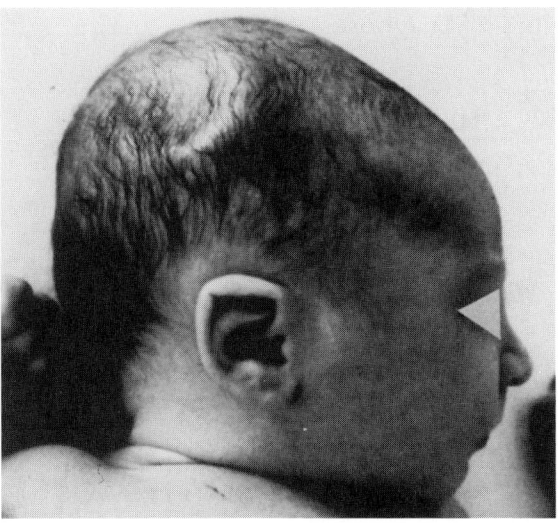

Fig. 39-3 Depressed skull fracture in a full-term male born after rapid (1-hour) labor. The infant was delivered by occiput-anterior presentation after rotation from occiput-posterior position. *(From Fanaroff, A., & Martin, R. [1997]. Neonatal-perinatal medicine: Diseases of the fetus and infant [6th ed.]. St. Louis: Mosby.)*

Forceps injury occurs at the site of application of the instrument. Forceps injury typically has a linear configuration across both sides of the face, outlining the placement of the forceps. The affected areas are kept clean to minimize the risk of secondary infection. These injuries usually resolve spontaneously within several days with no specific therapy. The increased use of padded forceps blades and vacuum-assisted birth may reduce the incidence of these lesions (Fanaroff & Martin, 1997).

Accidental lacerations may be inflicted with a scalpel during cesarean birth or with scissors during an episiotomy. These cuts may occur on any part of the body but most often are found on the scalp, buttocks, and thighs. Usually they are superficial, needing only to be kept clean. Butterfly adhesive strips will hold the edges of more serious lacerations together. Rarely, sutures are needed.

Skeletal Injuries

The newborn's immature, flexible skull can withstand a great degree of deformation (molding) before fracture results. Considerable force is required to fracture the newborn's skull. Two types of skull fractures typically are identified in the newborn: linear fractures and depressed fractures. The location of the fracture and involvement of underlying structures determine its significance.

If an artery lying in a groove on the undersurface of the skull is torn as a result of the fracture, increased ICP will ensue. Unless a blood vessel is involved, linear fractures (which account for 70% of all fractures for this age group)

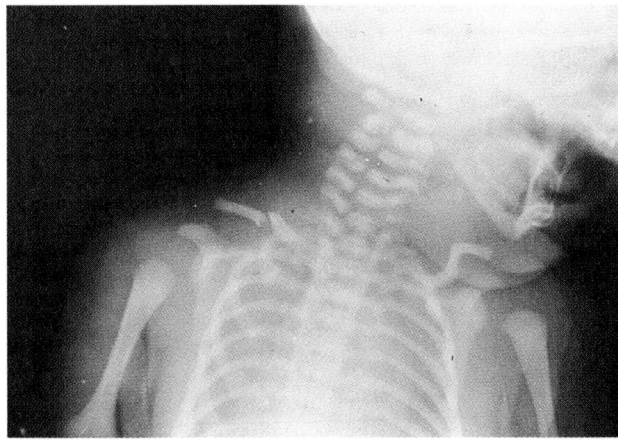

Fig. 39-4 Fractured clavicle after shoulder dystocia. *(From O'Doherty, N. [1986]. Neonatology: Micro atlas of the newborn. Nutley, NJ: Hoffmann-La Roche.)*

heal without special treatment. The soft skull may become indented without laceration of either the skin or the dural membrane. These depressed fractures, or "ping-pong ball" indentations, may occur during difficult births from pressure of the head on the bony pelvis (Fig. 39-3). They also can occur as a result of injudicious application of forceps.

The clavicle is the bone most often fractured during birth. Generally the break is in the middle third of the bone (Fig. 39-4). Dystocia, particularly shoulder impaction, may be the predisposing problem. Limitation of motion of the arm, crepitus over the bone, and the absence of Moro's reflex on the affected side are diagnostic. Except for use of gentle rather than vigorous handling, no accepted treatment for fractured clavicle exists, and the prognosis is good. The figure-of-eight bandage appropriate for the older child should not be used for the newborn.

The humerus and femur are other bones that may be fractured during a difficult birth. Fractures in newborns generally heal rapidly. Immobilization is accomplished with slings, splints, swaddling, and other devices.

The parents need support in handling these infants because they often are fearful of hurting them. Parents are encouraged to practice handling, changing, and feeding the affected neonate under the guidance of nursery personnel. This increases their confidence and knowledge and facilitates attachment. A plan for follow-up therapy is developed with the parents so that the times and arrangements for therapy are acceptable to them.

Peripheral Nervous System Injuries

Erb-Duchenne paralysis (**brachial paralysis** of the upper portion of the arm) is the most common type of paralysis associated with a difficult birth, occurring at rates of 0.5 to 1.9 per 1000 live births (Moe & Paige, 1998) (Fig. 39-5). Injury to the upper plexus results from stretching or pulling the head away from the shoulder during the difficult birth. Typical symptoms are a flaccid arm with the elbow extended and the hand rotated inward, absence of Moro's reflex on the affected side, sensory loss over the lateral aspect of the arm, and an intact grasp reflex.

Treatment is by intermittent immobilization, proper positioning, and range-of-motion (ROM) exercises. Gentle manipulation and ROM exercises are delayed until about the tenth day to prevent additional injury to the brachial plexus.

Immobilization may be accomplished with a brace or splint or by pinning the infant's sleeve to the mattress. The infant should be positioned for 2 or 3 hours at a time as follows:
- Abduct the arm 90 degrees.
- Externally rotate the shoulder.
- Flex the elbow 90 degrees.
- Supinate the wrist with the palm directed slightly toward the face (Fig. 39-6).

Damage to the lower plexus, *Klumpke's palsy*, is less common. With lower arm paralysis, the wrist and hand are flaccid, the grasp reflex is absent, deep tendon reflexes are present, and dependent edema and cyanosis may be apparent (in the affected hand). Treatment consists of placing the hand in a neutral position, padding the fist, and gently exercising the wrist and fingers.

Parents are taught to position and immobilize the arm or wrist or both. They can gently massage and manipulate the muscles to prevent contractures while the arm is healing. If edema or hemorrhage is responsible for the paralysis, the prognosis is good and recovery may be expected in a few weeks. If laceration of the nerves has occurred and

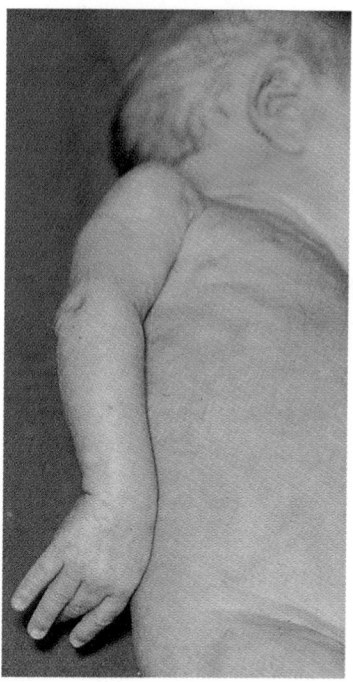

Fig. 39-5 Erb-Duchenne paralysis in newborn infant. Moro's reflex was absent in right upper extremity. Recovery was complete. *(From O'Doherty, N. [1986]. Neonatology: Micro atlas of the newborn. Nutley, NJ: Hoffmann-La Roche.)*

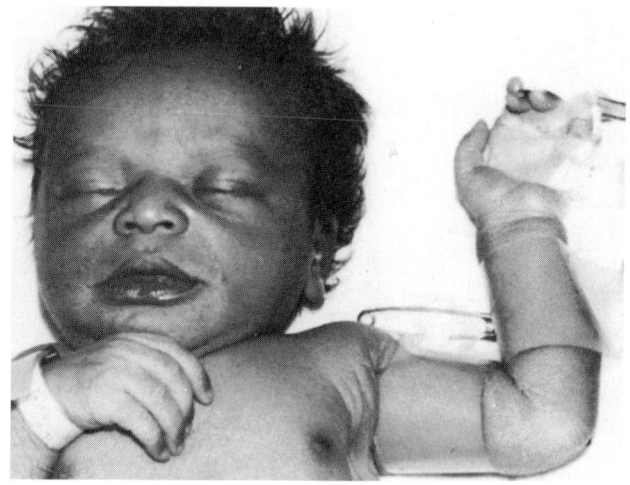

Fig. 39-6 Recommended corrective positioning for treatment of Erb-Duchenne paralysis. Notice abduction and external rotation at shoulder, flexion at elbow, supination of forearm, and slight dorsiflexion at wrist. *(From Behrmann, R. [1973]. Neonatology: Diseases of the fetus and infant. St. Louis: Mosby.)*

healing does not result in return of function within a few months (3 to 6 months or 2 years at the most), surgery may be indicated; however, little or no function will develop. Full recovery is expected in 88% to 92% of infants (Moe & Paige, 1998).

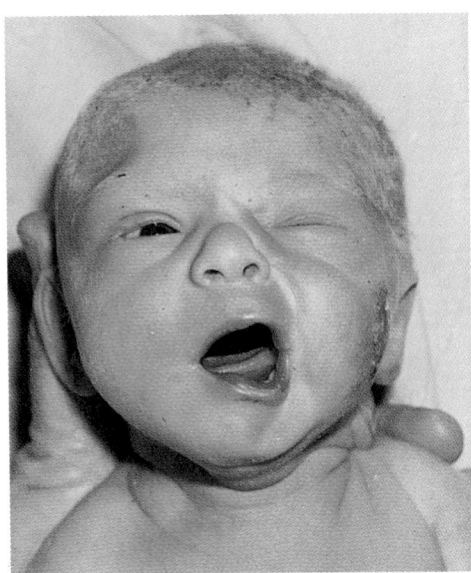

Fig. 39-7 Facial paralysis 15 minutes after forceps birth. Absence of movement on affected side is especially noticeable when infant cries. *(From O'Doherty, N. [1986]. Neonatology: Micro atlas of the newborn. Nutley, NJ: Hoffmann-La Roche.)*

Facial paralysis (palsy) (Fig. 39-7) generally is caused by pressure on the facial nerve during birth. The face on the affected side is flattened and unresponsive to the grimace that accompanies crying or stimulation, and the eye will remain open. Moreover, the forehead will not wrinkle. Often the condition is transitory, resolving within hours or days of birth. Permanent paralysis is rare.

Treatment involves assistance with feeding, prevention of damage to the cornea of the open eye, and supportive care of the parents. Usually the infant's face appears distorted, especially when crying. Feeding may be prolonged, with the milk flowing out the newborn's mouth around the nipple on the affected side. The mother will need understanding and sympathetic encouragement while learning how to feed and care for the infant, as well as how to hold and cuddle the baby.

Phrenic nerve injury almost always occurs as a component of brachial plexus injury rather than as an isolated problem. Injury to the phrenic nerve results in diaphragmatic paralysis. Cyanosis and irregular thoracic respirations, with no abdominal movement on inspiration, are characteristic of paralysis of the diaphragm. Babies with diaphragmatic paralysis usually require mechanical ventilatory support, at least for the first few days after birth. Other treatments include diaphragmatic pacing or surgical correction.

Central Nervous System Injuries

All types of **intracranial hemorrhage** (ICH) occur in newborns. ICH as a result of birth trauma is more likely to occur in the full-term, large infant. The frequency and degree of severity of ICH are different in the newborn than in older children or adults. In the newborn more than one type of hemorrhage can and frequently does occur (Fanaroff & Martin, 1997; Wong, 1999).

Subdural hemorrhages (hematomas), life-threatening collections of blood in the subdural space, most often are produced by the stretching and tearing of the large veins in the tentorium of the cerebellum, the dural membrane that separates the cerebrum from the cerebellum. When this type of bleeding occurs, the typical history includes a nulliparous mother, with the total labor and birth occurring in less than 2 or 3 hours, a difficult birth involving high forceps or midforceps application, or a large-for-gestational-age (LGA) infant. Subdural hematoma occurs infrequently today because of improvements in obstetric care. However, it is especially serious because of its inaccessibility to aspiration by subdural tap (Fanaroff & Martin, 1997; Wong, 1999).

Subarachnoid hemorrhage, the most common type of ICH, occurs in term infants as a result of trauma and in preterm infants as a result of hypoxia. Small hemorrhages are the most common. Bleeding is of venous origin, and underlying contusion also may occur (Wong, 1999).

The clinical presentation of hemorrhage in the full-term infant can vary considerably. In many infants, signs are absent, and hemorrhaging is diagnosed only because of abnormal findings on lumbar puncture, for example, red blood cells in the cerebrospinal fluid (CSF). The initial clinical manifestations of neonatal subarachnoid hemorrhage may be the early onset of alternating depression and irritability, with refractory seizures (Fanaroff & Martin, 1997). Occasionally the infant appears normal initially and then has seizures on the second or third day of life, followed by no apparent sequelae.

Intracerebellar hemorrhage, although infrequent, may occur in low-birth-weight (LBW) infants in association with perinatal trauma and asphyxia. At present the exact causes are not fully understood. The clinical picture is characterized by severe progressive apnea, a falling hematocrit level, and death (Fanaroff & Martin, 1997).

In general, nursing care of an infant with ICH is supportive and includes monitoring of ventilatory and intravenous therapy, observation and management of seizures, and prevention of increased ICP. Minimal handling to promote rest and reduce stress should guide nursing care (Wong, 1999).

Spinal cord injuries almost always result from breech births, especially difficult ones in which version and extraction are used. Brow and face presentations, dystocia, preterm birth, maternal nulliparity, and precipitous birth have also been identified as predisposing factors in these types of injuries. Stretching of the spinal cord, usually by forceful longitudinal traction on the trunk while the head is still firmly engaged in the pelvis, is the most common mechanism of injury. This injury is rarely seen today because cesarean birth is often used for breech presentation (Fanaroff & Martin, 1997).

Clinical manifestations depend on the severity and location of the injury. High cervical cord injuries are more likely to cause stillbirths or rapid death of the neonate. Lower lesions cause an acute spinal cord syndrome. Common signs of spinal shock include flaccid extremities, diaphragmatic breathing, paralyzed abdominal movements, atonic anal sphincter, and distended bladder. Therapy is supportive and usually unsatisfactory. Infants who survive present a therapeutic challenge that requires combined treatment from many health care providers, including the pediatrician, neurologist, neurosurgeon, urologist, orthopedist, nurse, physical therapist, and occupational therapist. Parents need to understand fully the implications of severe injury to the spinal cord and the overwhelming implications it presents for the family (Fanaroff & Martin, 1997; Merenstein & Gardner, 1998).

Evaluation

The nurse can be assured that care has been effective if the outcomes for care have been achieved. That is, the injury receives prompt and appropriate therapy, the newborn suffers no or minimal sequelae of trauma, and the parents understand how to care for the infant.

INFANTS OF DIABETIC MOTHERS

No single physiologic or biochemical event can explain the diverse clinical manifestations seen in the **infants of diabetic mothers** (IDMs) or **infants of gestational diabetic mothers** (IGDMs). A better understanding of maternal and fetal metabolism, resulting in stricter control of maternal diabetes and improved obstetric and neonatal intensive care, has led to a decrease in the perinatal mortality rate in diabetic pregnancy from more than 10% to less than 4% in the last 25 years (Fanaroff & Martin, 1997). However, maternal diabetes continues to play a significant role in neonatal morbidity and mortality. IDMs make up 5% of all admissions to neonatal intensive care units (Tyrala, 1996).

All infants born to mothers with diabetes are at some risk for complications. The degree of risk is affected by the severity and duration of maternal disease. Problems seen in IDMs include congenital anomalies, macrosomia, birth trauma and perinatal asphyxia, respiratory distress syndrome (RDS), hypoglycemia, hypocalcemia and hypomagnesemia, cardiomyopathy, and hyperbilirubinemia and polycythemia.

Pathophysiology

The mechanisms responsible for the problems seen in IDMs are not fully understood. In early pregnancy, fluctuations in blood glucose levels and episodes of ketoacidosis are believed to cause congenital anomalies. Later in pregnancy, when the mother's pancreas cannot release sufficient insulin to meet increased demands, maternal hyperglycemia results. The high levels of glucose cross the placenta and stimulate the fetal pancreas to release insulin. The combination of the increased supply of maternal glucose and other nutrients and increased fetal insulin results in excessive fetal growth called macrosomia (see later discussion).

Hyperinsulinemia accounts for many of the problems the fetus or infant develops. In addition to fluctuating glucose levels, maternal vascular involvement or superimposed maternal infection adversely affects the fetus. Normally, maternal blood has a more alkaline pH than carbon dioxide–rich fetal blood does. This phenomenon encourages the exchange of oxygen and carbon dioxide across the placental membrane. When the maternal blood is more acidotic than the fetal blood, such as during ketoacidosis, little carbon dioxide or oxygen exchange occurs at the level of the placenta. The mortality rate for unborn babies resulting from an episode of maternal ketoacidosis may be as high as 50% or more (Fanaroff & Martin, 1997).

There are indications that some neonatal conditions—macrosomia, hypoglycemia, polyhydramnios, preterm birth, and perhaps fetal lung immaturity—may be eliminated or the incidence decreased by maintaining control over maternal glucose levels within narrow limits (Reece et al., 1998). *Good control* is defined as the maintenance of maternal blood glucose between 100 and 120 mg/dl.

Congenital Anomalies

Congenital anomalies occur in about 7% to 10% of IDMs. Their incidence is two to three times that for infants born to mothers without diabetes (Tyrala, 1996). The incidence is greatest among small-for-gestational-age (SGA) newborns. Intrauterine growth restriction (IUGR) leading to SGA infants is seen in IDMs with severe vascular disease. The most frequently occurring anomalies involve the cardiac, musculoskeletal, and central nervous systems. In most defects associated with diabetic pregnancies, the structural abnormality occurs before the eighth week after conception. This reinforces the importance of control of blood glucose both before conception and in the early stages of pregnancy.

The incidence of congenital heart lesions in these infants is five times higher than that in the general population. Coarctation of the aorta, transposition of the great vessels, and atrial or ventricular septal defects are the most common lesions encountered in the IDM. Maternal diabetic control is correlated with the incidence of lesions; that is, the better the control, the fewer the lesions.

Central nervous system anomalies include anencephaly, encephalocele, meningomyelocele, and hydrocephalus. The musculoskeletal system may be affected by *caudal regression syndrome* (*sacral agenesis*, with weakness or deformities of the lower extremities, malformation and fixation of the hip joints, and shortening or deformity of the femurs). Hypertrichosis on the pinnae (excessive hair growth on the external ear) has been added to the list of

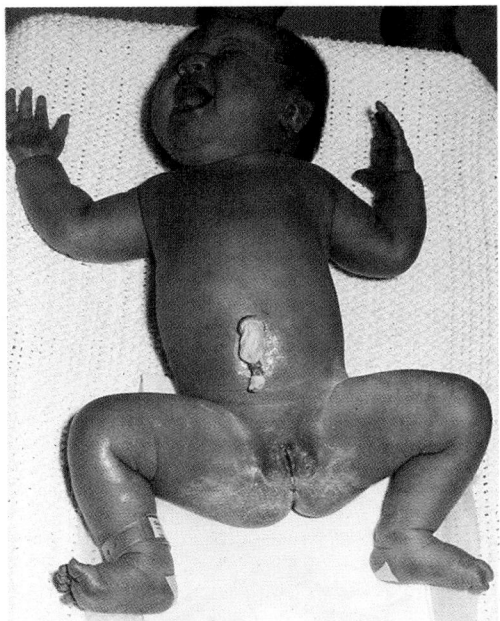

Fig. 39-8 Macrosomia. *(From O'Doherty, N. [1986]. Neonatology: Micro atlas of the newborn. Nutley, NJ: Hoffmann-La Roche.)*

characteristic clinical features (Fanaroff & Martin, 1997). Other defects noted in this population include gastrointestinal atresia and urinary tract malformations.

Neonatal small left colon syndrome, also called lazy colon syndrome, occurs in some IDMs and IGDMs. This syndrome is suspected when failure to pass meconium, abdominal distention, and bile-stained vomitus are noted. Contrast enemas show a greatly diminished caliber of the left colon from the splenic flexure. The syndrome is transient, with normal bowel function developing early in infancy (Fanaroff & Martin, 1997).

Macrosomia

Despite improvements in the control of maternal blood sugar levels, the incidence of **macrosomia** in the insulin-dependent diabetic is 20% to 30% (Ogata, 1994). At birth the typical LGA infant has a round, cherubic ("tomato" or cushingoid) face, a chubby body, and a plethoric or flushed complexion (Fig. 39-8). These are the characteristics of macrosomia. The infant has enlarged internal organs (hepatosplenomegaly, splanchnomegaly, cardiomegaly) and increased body fat, especially around the shoulders. The placenta and umbilical cord are larger than average. The brain is the only organ that is not enlarged. IDMs may be LGA but physiologically immature.

Insulin has been implicated as the primary growth hormone for intrauterine development. Maternal diabetes results in elevated maternal levels of amino acids and free fatty acids along with hyperglycemia. As the nutrients cross the placenta, the fetal pancreas responds by producing in-

sulin to match the fuel supply. The resulting accelerated protein synthesis, together with a deposition of excessive glycogen and fat stores, is responsible for the typical macrosomic infant. This is the infant most at risk for the neonatal complications of hypoglycemia, hypocalcemia, hyperviscosity, and hyperbilirubinemia. The excessive amounts of metabolic fuels presented to the fetus from the mother and the consequent fetal hyperinsulinism are now understood to represent the basic pathologic mechanism in the diabetic pregnancy (Fanaroff & Martin, 1997).

The excessive shoulder size in these infants often leads to dystocia, particularly because the head may be smaller in proportion to the shoulders than in a nonmacrosomic infant. Macrosomic infants, born vaginally or by cesarean birth after a trial of labor, may incur birth trauma.

Birth Trauma and Perinatal Hypoxia

Birth injury (resulting from macrosomia or method of birth) and perinatal hypoxia occur in 20% of IGDMs and 35% of IDMs. Examples of birth trauma include cephalhematoma; paralysis of the facial nerve (seventh cranial nerve) (see Fig. 39-7); fracture of the clavicle or humerus; brachial plexus paralysis, usually Erb-Duchenne (right upper arm) palsy (see Fig. 39-5); and phrenic nerve paralysis, invariably associated with diaphragmatic paralysis.

Respiratory Distress Syndrome

IDMs and IGDMs are four to six times more likely than normal infants to develop RDS. With improved maternal glucose control, this risk has been substantially reduced.

In the fetus exposed to high levels of maternal glucose, synthesis of surfactant may be delayed because of the high fetal serum level of insulin (Tyrala, 1996). Fetal lung maturity, as evidenced by a lecithin/sphingomyelin (L/S) ratio of 2:1, is not reassuring if the mother has diabetes mellitus or gestation-induced diabetes mellitus. For the infants of such mothers, an L/S ratio of 3:1 or more or the presence of **phosphatidylglycerol** in the amniotic fluid is more indicative of adequate lung maturity.

Hypoglycemia

Hypoglycemia (blood glucose levels less than 40 mg/dl in term infants) affects many IDMs, with a reported incidence of 25% to 40%. LGA and preterm infants have the highest risk (Tyrala, 1996). After constant exposure to high circulating levels of glucose, hyperplasia of the fetal pancreas occurs, resulting in hyperinsulinemia. Disruption of the fetal glucose supply occurs with the clamping of the umbilical cord, and the neonate's blood glucose level falls rapidly in the presence of fetal hyperinsulinism. Hypoglycemia is most common in the macrosomic infant, but blood glucose levels should be monitored in all infants of known or suspected diabetic mothers.

Asymptomatic or symptomatic hypoglycemia most frequently manifests within the first 1 to 3 hours after birth.

Signs of hypoglycemia include jitteriness, apnea, tachypnea, and cyanosis. Significant hypoglycemia may result in seizures. Hypoglycemia is worsened by the presence of hypothermia or respiratory distress.

Hypocalcemia and Hypomagnesemia

Hypocalcemia has been reported to occur in as many as 50% of IDMs. A number of these cases are related to hypoxia or prematurity; however, the overall incidence of hypocalcemia is higher than in nondiabetic pregnancies (Tyrala, 1996). Hypomagnesemia is believed to develop because of maternal renal losses that occur in diabetes. Hypocalcemia is associated with preterm birth, birth trauma, and perinatal asphyxia. Signs of hypocalcemia, a prevalent finding in IDMs and IGDMs, are similar to those of hypoglycemia, but they occur between 24 and 36 hours of age. However, hypocalcemia must be considered if therapy for hypoglycemia is ineffective.

Cardiomyopathy

All IDMs need careful observation for **cardiomyopathy** because an increased heart size is often found in this client population. Two types of cardiomyopathy can occur. Clinicians must be alert to correctly identify the type of lesion so that appropriate therapy is instituted. Both types of lesions are associated with respiratory symptoms and congestive heart failure.

Hypertrophic cardiomyopathy (HCM) is characterized by a hypercontractile and thickened myocardium. The ventricular walls are thickened, as is the septum, which in severe cases results in outflow tract obstructions. The mitral valve is poorly functioning. In nonhypertrophic cardiomyopathy (non-HCM) the myocardium is poorly contractile and overstretched. The ventricles are increased in size, and there is no outflow obstruction. Most infants are asymptomatic, but severe outflow obstruction may cause left ventricular heart failure. HCM may be treated with a beta-adrenergic blocker (such as propranolol to decrease contractility and heart rate). A cardiotonic agent is used to treat non-HCM (such as digoxin to increase contractility and decrease heart rate). The abnormality usually resolves in 3 to 12 months (Fanaroff & Martin, 1997).

Hyperbilirubinemia and Polycythemia

IDMs are at increased risk of developing hyperbilirubinemia. Many IDMs are also polycythemic. Polycythemia increases blood viscosity, thereby impairing circulation. In addition, this increased number of red blood cells to be hemolyzed increases the potential bilirubin load that the neonate must clear. The excessive red blood cells are produced in extramedullary foci (liver and spleen) in addition to the usual sites in bone marrow. Therefore both liver function and bilirubin clearance may be adversely affected. Bruising associated with birth of a macrosomic infant will contribute further to high bilirubin levels.

Nursing Care

Nursing care depends on the neonate's particular problems. General care of the compromised infant is addressed in Chapter 41. If the maternal blood glucose level was well controlled throughout the pregnancy, the infant may require only monitoring. Because euglycemia (normal blood glucose levels) is not always possible, the nurse must promptly recognize and treat any consequences of maternal diabetes that arise. The most common problems IDMs experience that require intervention include birth trauma and perinatal asphyxia; RDS; difficult metabolic transition, including hypoglycemia and hypocalcemia; and congenital anomalies (see previous sections and Plan of Care).

NEONATAL INFECTIONS

Sepsis

Sepsis (presence of microorganisms or their toxins in blood or other tissues) continues to be one of the most significant causes of neonatal morbidity and mortality. The newborn infant is susceptible to infection. Maternal immunoglobulin (IgM) does not cross the placenta. IgA and IgM require time to reach optimum levels after birth. Phagocytosis is less efficient. Serum complement levels are inadequate; serum complement (C1 through C6) is involved in immunologic reactions, some of which kill or lyse bacteria and enhance phagocytosis. Dysmaturity seen with IUGR and preterm and postdate birth further compromises the neonate's immune system.

Table 39-2 outlines risk factors for neonatal sepsis. Special precautions for preventing infection, as well as prompt recognition when it occurs, are necessary for optimum newborn care. Neonatal infections may be acquired in utero, during birth, during resuscitation, and nosocomially (Fanaroff & Martin, 1997).

Prenatal acquisition of infection occurs by organisms placentally transferred directly into the fetal circulatory system and from infected amniotic fluid, such as with herpes simplex virus (HSV), cytomegalovirus (CMV), and rubella. Microorganisms ascend from the vagina and pass through the cervix. The membranes become infected and may rupture. Infection of the fetal skin and respiratory or gastrointestinal tract may result.

During birth, contact with an infected birth canal can result in generalized or local infection. The upper airway and gastrointestinal tract are again the principal pathways for generalized infections. The conjunctiva and oral cavity are the usual sites of local infection.

Postnatal infection may be acquired during resuscitation or through the introduction of foreign objects such as indwelling catheters or endotracheal tubes. Nursery-acquired infections may be transferred to the infant by the hands of the parents or health care personnel or spread from contaminated equipment. The umbilicus is a

PLAN °ᶠ CARE | Infant of Mother with Gestational Diabetes

NURSING DIAGNOSIS Risk for injury related to hypoglycemia, hypocalcemia, polycythemia, or hyperbilirubinemia secondary to maternal gestational diabetes

Expected Outcome *Infant will exhibit blood glucose, serum calcium, hematocrit, and serum bilirubin levels that are within normal limits.*

Nursing Interventions/*Rationales*

Monitor blood glucose levels (less than 40 mg/dl indicative of hypoglycemia); and serum calcium levels (less than 7 mg/dl indicative of hypocalcemia); and serum bilirubin levels (over 15 mg/dl indicative of hyperbilirubinemia) *to assess and detect early onset to prevent complications.*

Observe for signs of hypoglycemia (jitteriness, twitching, lethargy, apathy, convulsions, cyanosis, sweating, eye rolling, refusal to eat); hypocalcemia (jitters, apnea, high-pitched cry, abdominal distention); polycythemia (plethora); and hyperbilirubinemia (jaundice) *to assess and detect signs of onset to prevent complications.*

Early feeding of infant, glucose supplements as prescribed *to prevent or treat early hypoglycemia;* increased milk feedings/calcium supplements per physician order *to prevent or treat early hypocalcemia;* early and frequent feedings *to reduce hematocrit and enhance excretion of bilirubin in stool;* phototherapy *for bilirubin over 12 to 15 mg/dl.*

Reduce adverse environmental factors (e.g., stimuli such as jarring or shaking, cold stress, and respiratory distress), *which can predispose infant to hypoglycemia or precipitate a seizure.*

NURSING DIAGNOSIS Risk for impaired gas exchange related to lung immaturity or cardiomyopathy secondary to maternal gestational diabetes

Expected Outcome *Infant will exhibit signs of adequate oxygen supply (respiratory rate, rhythm, and amplitude and blood gas levels within normal limits).*

Nursing Interventions/*Rationales*

Monitor infant vital signs, blood gas levels per order, patency of airway *to evaluate pulmonary and circulatory status.*

Avoid activities that may lower body temperature and lead to cold stress, *which can induce respiratory distress.*

Suction as needed *to keep airway patent and prevent aspiration.*

Position infant on side *to facilitate mucus drainage.*

Have resuscitation equipment and oxygen available *for quick treatment of respiratory distress.*

NURSING DIAGNOSIS Risk for ineffective thermoregulation related to physiologic immaturity; potential for infection related to immature immunologic defenses/environmental exposure

See the Nursing Plan of Care for the normal newborn in Chapter 27.

NURSING DIAGNOSIS Anxiety (risk for powerlessness, situational low self-esteem, ineffective coping) related to neonate's condition, management, and prognosis

Expected Outcome *Parents demonstrate understanding of prognosis and therapy for infant.*

Nursing Interventions/*Rationales*

Explain potential effects of maternal diabetic condition on newborn *to relieve fear of unknown and support ability to cope.*

Encourage open communication (e.g., inform parents of ongoing condition, procedures, and treatment; answer questions; correct misperceptions; actively listen to parental concerns) *to provide support and help provide sense of control.*

Encourage parents to interact with infant and to become involved in care routines *to foster emotional connection.*

From Wong, D., & Perry, S. (1998). *Maternal child nursing care.* St. Louis: Mosby.

receptive site for cutaneous infection leading to sepsis (Fanaroff & Martin, 1997).

Neonatal bacterial infection is classified into two patterns according to the time of presentation. Early-onset or congenital sepsis usually manifests within 24 hours of birth, progresses more rapidly than later-onset infection, and carries a mortality rate of 10% to 25% (Klein & Marcy, 1995). Early-onset infection is usually caused by microorganisms from the normal flora of the maternal vaginal tract, including group B streptococci, *Haemophilus influen-*

zae, Listeria monocytogenes, Escherichia coli, and *Streptococcus pneumoniae* (Merenstein, Adams, & Weisman, 1998). It is associated with a history of obstetric complications, such as preterm labor, premature rupture of membranes, maternal fever during labor, and chorioamnionitis (Klein & Marcy, 1995).

Acquired infection is most frequently seen after 2 weeks of age and is slower in progression. Bacteria responsible for late-onset sepsis are varied, may be acquired from the birth canal or from the external environment, and include *Staphylococcus aureus, Staphylococcus epidermidis, Pseudomonas* organisms, and group B streptococci.

Viral infections may cause miscarriage, stillbirth, intrauterine infection, congenital malformations, and acute disease. These pathogens also may cause chronic infection, with subtle manifestations that may be recognized only after a prolonged period. It is important to recognize the manifestations of infections in the neonatal period to treat the acute infection and to prevent nosocomial infections in other infants, and to anticipate effects on the infant's subsequent growth and development.

Fungal infections are of greatest concern in the immunocompromised or premature infant. Occasionally, fungal infections such as thrush are found in otherwise healthy term infants.

Septicemia refers to a generalized infection in the bloodstream. Pneumonia, the most common form of neonatal infection, is one of the leading causes of perinatal death (Fanaroff & Martin, 1997). Bacterial **meningitis** affects 1 in 2500 live-born infants. Gastroenteritis is sporadic, depending on epidemic outbreaks. Local infections such as conjunctivitis and omphalitis occur frequently, but incidence rates are unavailable. Infection continues to be a significant factor in fetal and neonatal morbidity and mortality.

CARE MANAGEMENT

Assessment and Nursing Diagnoses

The prenatal record is reviewed for risk factors associated with infection and signs and symptoms suggestive of it. Maternal vaginal or perineal infection may be transmitted directly to the infant during passage through the birth canal. Psychosocial history and history of sexually transmitted infections (STIs) may indicate possible human immunodeficiency virus (HIV), hepatitis B virus (HBV), or CMV infection.

The perinatal events also are reviewed. Premature rupture of membranes (PROM) may be caused by maternal or intrauterine infection. Ascending infection may occur after prolonged PROM, prolonged labor, or intrauterine fetal monitoring. A maternal history of fever during labor or the presence of foul-smelling amniotic fluid may also indicate the presence of infection. Antibiotic therapy initiated during labor should be noted. Resuscitation that re-

TABLE 39-2	Risk Factors for Neonatal Sepsis
SOURCE	**RISK FACTORS**
Maternal	Low socioeconomic status
	Poor prenatal care
	Poor nutrition
	Substance abuse
Intrapartum	Premature rupture of fetal membranes
	Maternal fever
	Chorioamnionitis
	Prolonged labor
	Premature labor
	Maternal urinary tract infection
Neonatal	Twin gestation
	Male
	Birth asphyxia
	Meconium aspiration
	Congenital anomalies of skin or mucous membranes
	Galactosemia
	Absence of spleen
	Low birth weight or prematurity
	Malnourishment
	Prolonged hospitalization

From Askin, D. (1995). Bacterial and fungal sepsis in the neonate. *J Obstet Gynecol Neonatal Nurs* 24(7), 635-643.

quires intubation and deep suctioning may result in infection. The neonate's gestational age, maturity, birth weight, and sex all affect the incidence of infection. Sepsis occurs about twice as often and results in a higher mortality rate in male than in female infants. The neonate is assessed for respiratory distress, skin abscesses, rashes, and other indications of infection.

During the postnatal period the time of onset of suspicious signs is noted. Onset within the first 48 hours of life is more often associated with prenatal or perinatal predisposing factors. Onset after 2 or 3 days more frequently reflects disease acquired at or subsequent to birth (Fanaroff & Martin, 1997).

The earliest clinical signs of neonatal sepsis are characterized by a lack of specificity. The nonspecific signs include lethargy, poor feeding, poor weight gain, and irritability. The nurse or parent may simply note that the infant is just not doing as well as before. Differential diagnosis may be difficult because signs of sepsis are similar to signs of noninfectious neonatal problems such as anemia or hypoglycemia. Additional clinical and laboratory information and appropriate cultures supplement the findings described. Table 39-3 outlines signs of sepsis.

TABLE 39-3 Signs of Sepsis*

SYSTEM	SIGNS
Respiratory	Apnea, bradycardia
	Tachypnea
	Grunting, nasal flaring
	Retractions
	Decreased oxygen saturation
	Acidosis
Cardiovascular	Decreased cardiac output
	Tachycardia
	Hypotension
	Decreased perfusion
Central nervous	Temperature instability
	Lethargy
	Hypotonia
	Irritability, seizures
Gastrointestinal	Feeding intolerance
	Abdominal distention
	Vomiting, diarrhea
Integumentary	Jaundice
	Pallor
	Petechiae

From Askin, D. (1995). Bacterial and fungal sepsis in the neonate. *J Obstet Gynecol Neonatal Nurs* 24(7), 635-643.
*Laboratory findings include neutropenia, increased bands, hypoglycemia or hyperglycemia, metabolic acidosis, and thrombocytopenia.

Laboratory studies are performed. Specimens for cultures include blood, nasopharyngeal or oropharyngeal, CSF, stool, and urine. Increased direct (conjugated) bilirubin levels may be found, especially if the infecting microorganism is gram negative. Complete blood cell count with differential is performed to determine the presence of anemia, increased white blood cell count, or decreased white blood cell count (an ominous sign). C-reactive protein may or may not be elevated.

Vigilant assessment continues during and after treatment. The newborn continues to be assessed for sequelae to septicemia. Before the advent of antibiotics, 90% of newborns with sepsis died. Antibiotic therapy decreased mortality rates to between 13% and 45% depending on the causative organism.

Sequelae to septicemia include meningitis, disseminated intravascular coagulation (DIC), and septic shock.

Septic shock results from the toxins released into the bloodstream. The most common sign is a drop in blood pressure, a vital sign often overlooked in the care of the neonate. Other signs are rapid, irregular respirations and pulse (similar to septicemia in general).

Any number of nursing diagnoses are possible, depending on the infant's gestational age and birth weight, the organ systems involved, and the nature of the infection. Examples of nursing diagnoses related to neonatal infections include the following:

Nursing Diagnoses

Newborn
- Infection related to
  - maternal vaginal (or other) infection
  - need for resuscitation or ventilation therapy
  - need for indwelling umbilical catheters, total parenteral nutrition (TPN), parenteral fluids
  - intrauterine electronic fetal monitoring
  - male sex
  - dysmaturity, IUGR, gestational age
- Ineffective thermoregulation related to
  - infection
- Impaired tissue integrity related to
  - need for multiple supportive measures (e.g., biometric monitoring, TPN, inhalation therapy)
- Pain related to
  - need for multiple supportive measures

Parents and family
- Anxiety, fear, or anticipatory grieving related to
  - uncertainty about infant's prognosis
  - poor prognosis
- Risk for altered parent-infant attachment related to
  - separation of parent and newborn
  - feelings of inadequacy in caring for infant
- Powerlessness or spiritual distress related to
  - perinatal events or newborn's condition
- Anxiety related to knowledge deficit regarding
  - newborn's condition, its course, and its management

Expected Outcomes of Care

Planning begins with the development of standards for preventive measures in nurseries and protocols for diagnosis and treatment of infections. Individual assessment findings are used to plan care for each infant. Parents and family are encouraged to participate in planning. Expected outcomes include the following:
- The newborn will remain free of sepsis.
- The newborn's early signs of sepsis will be recognized, and appropriate therapy will be instituted.
- If therapy is necessary, the newborn will suffer no harmful sequelae.
- Parents will begin bonding and attachment to newborn.
- Parents will maintain self-esteem.
- Staff members will establish caring relationship with parents to foster their trust and to encourage continuing, active, positive interactions of family with members of health care system.

Plan of Care and Interventions

Preventive Measures

Virtually all controlled clinical trials have demonstrated that effective handwashing is responsible for the prevention of nosocomial infection in nursery units (Fanaroff & Martin, 1997). Nursing is directly or indirectly responsible for minimizing or eliminating environmental sources of infectious agents in the nursery. Measures to be taken include standard precautions, careful and thorough cleaning, frequent replacement of used equipment (e.g., changing intravenous tubing per hospital protocol, cleaning resuscitation and ventilation equipment), and disposal of excrement and linens in an appropriate manner. Overcrowding must be avoided in nurseries.

Instillation of antibiotic in newborns' eyes 1 to 2 hours after birth is done to prevent infection, such as gonorrhea and chlamydiosis. The skin, its secretions, and its normal flora are natural defenses that protect against invading pathogens. Warm water may be used to remove blood and meconium from the neonate's face, head, and body. A mild nonmedicated soap (in single-use container or in a small bar reserved for a single newborn) can be used with careful water rinsing. The vernix caseosa is left in place. No single method of cord care has been shown to prevent colonization and subsequent disease. Alcohol, triple dye, or an antimicrobial agent is typically used. Recent research has demonstrated that cords cleaned with sterile water or those left to dry naturally separate more quickly than those cleaned with alcohol. No cord care or cord care with sterile water did not result in increased numbers of infections (Dores et al., 1998; Medves & O'Brien, 1997). Nurses must follow agency protocols for cord care.

Curative Measures

Breastfeeding or feeding the newborn breast milk from the mother is encouraged. Protective mechanisms exist in breast milk. Colostrum contains immunoglobulin A (IgA), which offers protection against infection in the gastrointestinal tract. Human milk contains iron-binding protein that exerts a bacteriostatic effect on *E. coli*. Human milk also contains macrophages and lymphocytes. The vulnerability of infants to common mucosal pathogens such as respiratory syncytial virus (RSV) may be reduced by passive transfer of maternal immunity in the colostrum and breast milk.

Administering medications, taking precautions when performing treatments, and following isolation procedures are also interventions to be considered when a newborn has an infection.

Monitoring the intravenous infusion rate and administering antibiotics are the nurse's responsibility. It is important to administer the prescribed dose of antibiotic within 1 hour after it is prepared to avoid loss of drug stability. If the intravenous fluid the infant is receiving contains electrolytes, vitamins, or other medications, the nurse should check with the hospital pharmacy before adding antibiotics. The antibiotic (or other medication) may be deactivated or may form a precipitate when combined with other substances. In that case a piggyback solution of the prescribed fluid is attached with a three-way stopcock at the infusion site.

Care must be taken in suctioning secretions from any newborn's oropharynx or trachea. These secretions may be infected.

Isolation procedures are implemented according to hospital policy as indicated. Isolation protocols are changing rapidly, and the nurse is urged to participate in continuing education and in-service programs to remain up to date.

Rehabilitative Measures

Rehabilitative measures vary with the individual needs of the neonate. Some neonates will need to be weaned from ventilatory support systems. Those who suffer sequelae such as mental retardation and epilepsy will require a knowledgeable family and supportive community resources. Some children will require corrective care for problems with dentition, vision, and hearing.

Evaluation

The nurse can be reasonably assured that care was effective if the outcomes for care are achieved: the newborn remains free of sepsis or the newborn's early signs of sepsis are recognized and appropriately treated (see Care Path).

TORCH Infections

The occurrence of certain maternal infections during early pregnancy is known to be associated with various congenital malformations and disorders. The most common and best understood infections are represented by the acronym **TORCH,** for *t*oxoplasmosis, *o*ther (gonorrhea, syphilis, varicella, HBV, and HIV), *r*ubella, *c*ytomegalovirus, and *h*erpes simplex virus (Box 39-1). HSV may result in a severe, often fatal systemic illness in neonates. Survivors of herpetic infection may have residual neurologic defects and chorioretinitis. The other congenital infections also may result in encephalopathy with various anomalies, including microcephaly, chorioretinitis, intracranial calcifications, microphthalmos, and cataracts. To a certain extent the varied clinical manifestations of these infections overlap, but a specific diagnosis can be made by the clustering of clinical findings, as well as specific antibody studies (Fanaroff & Martin, 1997).

Toxoplasmosis

Toxoplasmosis is a multisystem disease caused by the protozoan *Toxoplasma gondii*. About 30% of women who contract toxoplasmosis during gestation transmit the disease to their offspring (Lynfield & Guerina, 1997). Fetal infection occurs in 0.07% to 0.11% of all pregnancies

CARE PATH | Suspected Neonatal Sepsis

Assessments	1. Potential maternal risk factors and unstable vital signs, especially temperature instability. 2. Sepsis screen in first hour (CBC with differential, platelets, and CRP level) if there are significant maternal risk factors (prolonged rupture of membranes, maternal temperature) or if infant demonstrates physiologic signs of sepsis.
Treatment	1. Start IV administration of antibiotics by peripheral IV. 2. Provide other treatments as needed for additional physiologic problems (ventilator for respiratory distress, incubator for temperature instability).
Possible Consultations	1. Neonatologists and advanced practice nurses for care of unstable infants. 2. Medical specialists for care of infants with additional problems (congenital deformities). 3. Lactation consultant, interpreter, social worker, and chaplain as needed or requested.
Additional Assessments	1. Weight and measurements. 2. Blood culture, chest x-ray study, urinalysis, and lumbar puncture, if infant is symptomatic or CRP level is positive. 3. Repeat determination of CRP level in the morning for 2 days. If negative and infant not symptomatic, stop antibiotic treatment. 4. Continuous cardiac and saturation monitor assessment if infant's condition is unstable.
Direct Infant Care	1. Vital signs every 1 to 2 hours for the first 4 hours, then every 4 hours. 2. Advance oral feedings as tolerated (infant NPO only if condition is physiologically unstable). 3. Bath and cord care done per unit protocols.
Teaching and Discharge Planning	1. Initiate on admission. Provide parents with written and oral information on suspected sepsis. 2. Reinforce information and determine parents' understanding of information before discharge. Include information on well-baby care and community follow-up with the family's primary health care provider.

Courtesy Lucile Salter Packard Children's Hospital at Stanford, California.

BOX 39-1 | TORCH Infections Affecting Newborns

T Toxoplasmosis
O Other: gonorrhea, syphilis, varicella, hepatitis B virus (HBV), human immunodeficiency virus (HIV)
R Rubella
C Cytomegalovirus (CMV) infections or cytomegalic inclusion disease (CMID)
H Herpes simplex virus (HSV) infection

(Beazley & Egerman, 1998; Boyer, 1996). The diagnosis of toxoplasmosis in the neonate is supported by elevated levels of cord blood serum IgM.

More than 70% of affected infants are free of symptoms. The clinical features of toxoplasmosis resemble cytomegalic inclusion disease (CMID) in the infant. Both diseases are responsible for serious perinatal mortality and morbidity: 10% to 15% die, 85% have severe psychomotor problems or mental retardation by 2 to 4 years, and 50% have visual problems by 1 year. Transmission of toxoplasmosis from an infected mother to her fetus can be significantly reduced by maternal treatment with spiramycin (Lynfield & Guerina, 1997).

Severe toxoplasmosis is associated with preterm birth, growth restriction, microcephaly or hydrocephaly, microphthalmos, chorioretinitis, central nervous system (CNS) calcification, thrombocytopenia, jaundice, and fever. Petechiae or a maculopapular rash may also be evident. Some clinical manifestations do not develop until later in life. The affected infant may be treated with pyrimethamine, as well as oral sulfadiazine, but folic acid supplement will be required to prevent anemia.

Gonorrhea

The incidence of gonococcal infection in pregnant women has ranged from 2.5% to 7.3% (Fanaroff & Martin,

1997). With this high incidence, it is not surprising that neonatal infection with *Neisseria gonorrhoeae* occurs frequently. After rupture of membranes, ascending infection can result in orogastric contamination of the fetus. The organism also may invade mucosal surfaces such as the conjunctiva (ophthalmia neonatorum), rectal mucosa, and pharynx. Contamination may occur as the infant passes through the birth canal, or it may occur postnatally from an infected adult. Neonatal gonococcal arthritis, septicemia, meningitis, vaginitis, and scalp abscesses also can develop.

Eye prophylaxis (e.g., with 0.5% erythromycin ointment) is administered at or shortly after birth to prevent ophthalmia neonatorum. The infant with a mild infection often recovers completely with appropriate treatment, such as neonatal ceftriaxone. Occasionally, infants die of overwhelming infection in the early neonatal period.

Syphilis

Congenital and neonatal syphilis have reemerged in recent years as significant health problems. It is estimated that for every 100 women diagnosed with primary or secondary disease, 2 to 5 infants will contract congenital syphilis. If syphilis during pregnancy is untreated, 40% to 50% of neonates born to these women will have symptomatic congenital syphilis. Treatment failure can occur, particularly when treatment is given in the third trimester; therefore infants born to women treated within 4 weeks of delivery should be investigated for congenital syphilis. The following factors have been identified as placing the neonate at high risk for exposure to syphilis: inadequate prenatal care, single or teenage mother, substance abuse in mother or partner, multiple sexual partners or partner with known STI, past history of STI, poverty, homelessness, and HIV infection (Cloherty, 1998).

Fetal infestation with the spirochete *Treponema pallidum* is blocked by Langhans' layer in the chorion until this layer begins to atrophy between 16 and 18 weeks of gestation. If spirochetemia is untreated, it will result in fetal death by midtrimester miscarriage or stillbirth in one in four cases. All neonates in whom the infection occurs before 7 months of gestation are affected. Only 60% are affected if the infection occurs late in pregnancy. If maternal infection is treated adequately before the eighteenth week, neonates seldom demonstrate signs of the disease. Although treatment after the eighteenth week may cure fetal spirochetemia, pathologic changes may not be prevented completely.

Because the fetus becomes infected after the period of organogenesis (first trimester), maldevelopment of organs does not result. Congenital syphilis may stimulate preterm labor, but no evidence indicates that it causes IUGR. Stigmas of congenital syphilis may include inflammatory and destructive changes in the placenta; in organs such as the liver, spleen, kidneys, and adrenal glands; and in bone covering and marrow. Disorders of the CNS, teeth, and cornea may not become evident until several months after birth.

Clinical manifestations. The most severely affected infants may be hydropic (edematous) and anemic, with enlarged liver and spleen. Hepatosplenomegaly probably is the result of extramedullary hematopoietic activity stimulated by the severe anemia.

In some infants, signs of congenital syphilis do not appear until late in the neonatal period. In these newborns, early signs, such as poor feeding, slight hyperthermia, and snuffles, may be nonspecific. *Snuffles* refers to the copious, clear, serosanguineous mucous discharge from the obstructed nose. A mucopurulent discharge indicates secondary infection, usually by streptococci or staphylococci.

By the end of the first week of life, a copper-colored maculopapular dermal rash appears in untreated newborn cases. The rash is characteristically first noticeable on the palms of the hands, soles of the feet, the diaper area, and around the mouth and anus. The maculopapular lesions may become vesicular and confluent and extend over the trunk and extremities. *Condylomata* (elevated wartlike lesions) may be seen around the anus. Rough, cracked, mucocutaneous lesions of the lips heal to form circumoral radiating scars known as *rhagades*.

Other involvement results in exfoliation (separation, flaking) of nails and loss of hair. Iritis and choroiditis are characteristic of infection of the eyes. Nephrotic syndrome secondary to renal infection; hepatitis with jaundice, lymphadenopathy, and inflammation of the pancreas, testes, and colon; and a pseudoparalysis of the extremities may be noted. Laboratory tests may show a pleocytosis (usually lymphocytosis) and elevated CSF protein levels.

By 3 months of age, in 90% of infants (treated or untreated), periostitis and metaphyseal osteochondritis may be demonstrated by roentgenographic studies. These bone lesions generally disappear by 10 months of age whether or not the infant receives antibiotic treatment.

Medical management. If the mother was adequately treated before giving birth and serologic testing of the infant does not show syphilis, generally the infant is not treated with antibiotics. The infant is checked for antibody titer (received from the mother through the placenta) every 2 weeks for 3 months, at which time the test result should be negative. Some physicians recommend antibiotic therapy for asymptomatic or inconclusive cases.

Treatment should be carried out in the following situations: when the diagnosis of congenital syphilis is confirmed or suspected, when maternal treatment status is unknown, when the mother is treated within 4 weeks of giving birth or does not respond to treatment, when medications other than penicillin are used to treat the mother, and when inadequate neonatal follow-up is anticipated (Hollier & Cox, 1998).

For antibiotic treatment to be effective, an "adequate" blood level must be maintained for an "adequate" period. The suggested medication protocol in the presence of symptomatic systemic disease differs from author to author and from physician to physician. Penicillin is the usual treatment (Hollier & Cox 1998). After 12 hours of antibiotic therapy, the child's condition is not considered contagious. It generally is accepted that erythromycin is the substitute antibiotic of choice for infants sensitive to penicillin.

Prognosis. In general, treatment of syphilis is more effective if it is begun early rather than late in the course of the disease. However, a recurrence rate of 5% can be expected. Even adequate treatment of congenital syphilis after birth does not always prevent late (5 to 15 years after initial infection) complications. Potential complications include neurosyphilis, deafness, Hutchinson's teeth (notched incisors), saber shins, joint involvement, saddle nose (depressed bridge), gummas (soft, gummy tumors) over the skin and other organs, and interstitial keratitis (inflammation of the cornea).

Varicella-Zoster

The varicella-zoster virus responsible for chickenpox and shingles is a member of the herpes family. Approximately 90% of women in the childbearing years are immune; therefore the risk of infection in pregnancy is low, 0.7 to 3 per 1000 deliveries (Birthistle & Carrington, 1998; Chapman, 1998).

Varicella transmission to the fetus may occur across the placenta when the disease is contracted in the first half of pregnancy, but this is relatively infrequent. When transmission to the fetus does occur in the early part of pregnancy, the effects on the fetus include limb atrophy, neurologic abnormalities, eye abnormalities, and IUGR.

When maternal infection occurs in the last 3 weeks of pregnancy, 25% of infants born to these mothers will develop clinical varicella (Nathwani et al., 1998). The severity of the infant's illness will increase greatly if maternal infection occurred within 5 days before or 2 days after birth. The mortality rate in severe illness is 30% (Chapman, 1998).

Seroimmune pregnant women exposed to active chickenpox can be given varicella-zoster immune globulin (VZIG), which does not reduce the incidence of infection but should decrease the effects of the virus on the fetus. The immunoglobulin must be given within 72 hours of exposure to be effective.

Infants born to mothers who develop chickenpox between 5 days before birth and 48 hours after should be given VZIG at birth because of the risk of severe disease. Acyclovir can be used to treat infants with generalized involvement and pneumonia (Chapman, 1998; Nathwani et al., 1998).

Term infants exposed to chickenpox after birth will have a mild or no infection if they are born to immune mothers. Those born to nonimmune mothers may develop chickenpox, but the course is not usually severe. Experts are divided as to whether this group of infants should receive VZIG. Infants less than 28 weeks are at risk regardless of their mother's status and probably benefit from VZIG if exposed to chickenpox.

Hepatitis B Virus

Hepatitis B virus (HBV) infection during pregnancy is not associated with an increase in malformations, stillbirths, or IUGR; however, approximately a 32% increase in risk exists for preterm birth (Fanaroff & Martin, 1997). The transmission rate of HBV to the newborn is as high as 90% when the mother is seropositive for both hepatitis B surface antigen (HBsAg) and hepatitis B e antigen (HBeAg) (Duff, 1998). Transmission occurs transplacentally, serum to serum, and by contact with contaminated urine, feces, saliva, semen, or vaginal secretions during birth. Infants are most frequently infected during birth or in the first few days of life. The rate of transmission is highest when the mother contracts the virus immediately before birth. These mothers will be positive for HBsAg. Transmission may possibly occur through breast milk, but antigens also develop in formula-fed infants at the same or higher rate. Diagnosis is made by viral culture of amniotic fluid, as well as the presence of HBsAg and IgM in the cord or baby's serum.

Neonatal and fetal effects are serious. Preterm birth exposes the neonate to the problems of prematurity. Infants may be symptom free at birth or show evidence of acute hepatitis with changes in liver function. The mortality rate for full-blown hepatitis is 75%. Infants who become carriers are at high risk for chronic hepatitis, cirrhosis of the liver, or liver cancer even years later (Fanaroff & Martin, 1997).

Infants whose mothers have antibodies for HBsAg or who have developed hepatitis during pregnancy or the postpartum period should be treated with hepatitis B immunoglobulin (HBIG), 0.5 ml intramuscularly, as soon as possible after birth—within the first 12 hours of life. Concurrently, but at a different site, the vaccine also should be given (Fanaroff & Martin, 1997). The second dose of vaccine is given at 1 month and the third dose at 6 months. The vaccine should protect the child for up to 9 years. After the infant has been cleansed thoroughly and has received the vaccine, breastfeeding may be initiated. Vaccination for infants not exposed to HBV is recommended before discharge; breastfeeding for these infants may begin before the vaccine is given (Corrarino, 1998).

Human Immunodeficiency Virus and Acquired Immunodeficiency Syndrome

Maternal infection with the retrovirus HIV is discussed in Chapter 8. The focus of this discussion is the neonate at risk for infection with HIV. It is estimated that globally, more than 1 million children born to HIV-infected women will acquire the virus (Mofenson, 1997). The majority of cases of pediatric AIDS result from maternal-to-fetal transmission. Since 1994, when research demonstrated that prenatal treatment of HIV-positive women reduced the vertical transmission of the HIV virus to the fetus, there has been an almost 70% drop in the risk of transmission, from 25% to 8% (Minkoff, 1998). Universal counseling and screening of pregnant women is recommended in the United States and Canada (American College of Obstetricians and Gynecologists, 1997; Centers for Disease Control and Prevention, 1998).

Transmission of HIV from the mother to the infant may occur transplacentally at various gestational ages. Transmission early in gestation is assumed when the virus is detected by polymerase chain reaction (PCR) within 48 hours after birth (Scarlatti, 1996). Transmission close to or at the time of birth is thought to account for 50% to 80% of cases (Franck & Johnson, 1998; Mofenson, 1997; Scarlatti, 1996). Postnatal transmission through breastfeeding may also occur with an additional risk of 14% attributed to breast milk contact (Scarlatti, 1996).

Prevention. A number of factors have been identified that increase the risk of HIV transmission from mother to fetus. A high viral load correlates strongly with increased transmission, as does a low maternal CD4 T-lymphocyte count indicative of severe disease. Asymptomatic women can transmit infection but are less likely than symptomatic women to do so. Chorioamnionitis, rupture of membranes more than 4 hours before birth, and preterm birth have also been shown to increase the risk of HIV transmission to the fetus (Franck & Johnson, 1998; Minkoff, 1998; Mofenson, 1997).

Strategies to prevent HIV acquisition in the fetus and newborn should address these risk factors. Antenatal and postnatal treatment with antiretroviral agents such as zidovudine has been shown to reduce the infant's risk of acquiring HIV. More recently, it has been shown that combination therapy with several anti-HIV medications is of additional benefit in lowering transmission rates and preventing the development of drug resistance (Newshan & Hoyt, 1998). Vaginal birth within 4 hours of rupture of membranes and cesarean birth have been shown to reduce contact with maternal virus; however, the elective use of cesarean birth remains controversial (Tuomala, 1997). HIV-positive women should be counseled to avoid breastfeeding.

Diagnosis. Diagnosis of HIV infection in the neonate is complicated by the presence of maternal IgG antibodies, which cross the placenta after 32 weeks of gestation. Three methods to detect HIV virus or its components are available for use in neonates. Viral cultures detect the presence of HIV in the neonate's blood. This is a sensitive but expensive test that requires 4 to 6 weeks for a result. Detection of core protein antigen p24 is less expensive but also less sensitive in neonates. PCR detects HIV DNA or RNA in peripheral blood. This test is highly sensitive and results are available in 24 to 48 hours.

The accuracy of all HIV tests varies according to the infant's age and is dependent on the viral load in the blood.

The Centers for Disease Control and Prevention (CDC) recommends that at least two PCR assays or viral cultures be done before a definitive diagnosis is made (Franck & Johnson, 1998). Testing should be done in the first 48 hours of life, at age 1 to 2 months, and at age 3 to 6 months (CDC, 1998).

Typically the HIV-infected neonate is asymptomatic at birth. These infants tend to be of lower birth weight than those born to noninfected mothers. Some will have physical stigma from concurrent exposure to injectable drugs or other STIs. Early-onset HIV disease (virus detected within 48 hours of birth) is attributed to prenatal infection and occurs in 10% to 15% of infected infants (Franck & Johnson, 1998). These babies develop **opportunistic infections** (caused by an organism that usually does not cause illness) and rapid progression of immunodeficiency, which progresses to death in the first 1 to 2 years of life (Franck & Johnson, 1998).

The remainder of infants develop AIDS more slowly. Eighty to ninety percent of perinatally infected infants show signs by 1 year of life. Some children infected at birth are still showing no signs of disease 8 to 10 years later (Scarlatti, 1996). The age of onset of symptoms predicts the length of survival. Children with late-onset infection receiving treatment may live into adolescence.

The presenting signs and symptoms of HIV infection vary from severe immunodeficiency to nonspecific findings such as failure to thrive, parotitis, and recurrent or persistent upper respiratory infections. In the first year of life, lymphadenopathy and hepatosplenomegaly are observed in more than 50% of infants with HIV infection (Scarlatti, 1996). The infant may have fever, chronic diarrhea, chronic dermatitis, persistent thrush, interstitial pneumonitis, and AIDS-defining secondary infections. Common secondary infections include *Pneumocystis carinii* pneumonia, candidiasis, CMV infection, cryptosporidiosis, herpes simplex or herpes zoster, and disseminated varicella.

Care management. Although it is rare for an infant to be born with symptoms of HIV infection, all infants born to seropositive mothers should be presumed to be HIV positive. Management begins by implementing Standard Precautions. Measures should be undertaken to protect the infant from further exposure to maternal blood and body fluids. The infant's skin should be cleansed with soap and water and alcohol before invasive procedures such as vitamin K administration or heel punctures. Umbilical cord stumps are cleaned meticulously every day until healing is complete. Isolation is not required, and the infant can usually be cared for in the normal nursery. The use of gloves is not required for routine care activities such as dressing or feeding the infant.

Regimens for the prevention of HIV transmission include treatment of the neonate for 6 weeks following delivery with zidovudine until the infant's HIV status is determined (CDC, 1998; Tuomala, 1997). If a diagnosis of

HIV infection in the infant is made, the family should be counseled about conventional and investigational treatment options. The Pediatric AIDS Clinical Trials group sponsors research studies that allow infants to receive the latest investigational treatments and follow-up care (Franck & Johnson, 1998). The efficacy of treating asymptomatic infants with antiretroviral drugs has not yet been demonstrated in clinical trials; however, early initiation of treatment is thought to be advantageous (CDC, 1998). Aggressive therapy using a combination of antiretroviral drugs is currently being investigated. Monotherapy is no longer recommended for the treatment of known HIV infection regardless of the age of the client.

Counseling regarding the care of the mothers themselves, the family's care of the infant, and future pregnancies challenges the caregiver. Some parents opt to place the infected infants in foster homes despite the low risk for transmission among members of the same household. Social services are required in these cases. If the parent chooses to keep the infant, home health care may be arranged. For more information and updated information, parents are offered the following resource: the National AIDS hotline, 1-800-342-AIDS.

The family must be counseled about vaccinations. Children with symptomatic or asymptomatic HIV infection should receive all routine vaccines except oral poliovirus and varicella vaccines. The family should be advised that household contacts should not receive oral polio vaccine because the virus can be transmitted to the immunocompromised child. Inactivated poliomyelitis vaccine can be given (Franck & Johnson, 1998; Wong, 1999).

Rubella Infection

Since the rubella vaccination program was begun in 1969, cases of **congenital rubella infection** have been reduced dramatically; however, it is still seen occasionally in the newborn. Vaccination failures, lack of compliance, and the migration of nonimmunized persons result in periodic outbreaks of rubella, also known as German measles.

The risk of a congenitally infected infant varies with the gestational age of the fetus when maternal infection occurs. Abnormalities are most severe if the mother contracts the virus during the first trimester.

More than two thirds of infected infants show no apparent symptoms at birth, but sequelae may develop years later. Hearing loss, the most common result, appears to be progressive after birth. Congenital rubella syndrome comprises cataracts or glaucoma, hearing loss, and cardiac defects (pulmonary artery stenosis, patent ductus arteriosus, or coarctation of the aorta) (Rosa, 1998). Multiple other abnormalities are also present, including IUGR, microphthalmia, hypotonia, hepatosplenomegaly, thrombocytopenic purpura (Fig. 39-9), dermatoglyphic abnormalities, bony radiolucencies, and brain wave abnormalities (Burchett, 1998). Severe infection may result in fetal death.

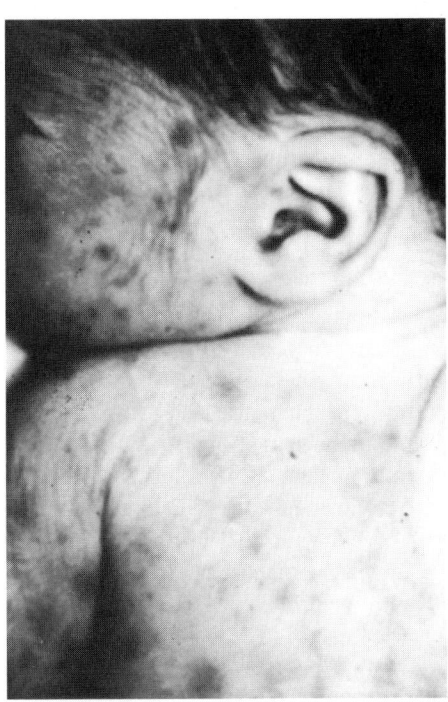

Fig. 39-9 Newborn with congenital rubella syndrome, showing multiple purpuric lesions over face and trunk. *(Courtesy Donald C. Anderson, Baylor College of Medicine, Houston, TX.)*

Delayed effects of infection manifest as thyroid dysfunction, diabetes mellitus, growth hormone deficiency, myocarditis, glaucoma, microcephaly, and polycystic kidney disease (Fanaroff & Martin, 1997).

The rubella virus has been cultured in infants for up to 18 months after their birth. These infants are a serious source of infection to susceptible individuals, particularly women in the childbearing years. Extended pediatric isolation is mandatory until the noncontagious stage of rubella has been reached. (The infant should be isolated until pharyngeal mucus and urine are free of virus.)

Cytomegalovirus Infection

CMV infection during pregnancy may result in miscarriage, stillbirth, or congenital or neonatal cytomegalic inclusion disease (CMID). It is the most common cause of congenital viral infections in humans, occurring in 1% of all newborns (Fanaroff & Martin, 1997). Most (90% to 95%) of the affected infants are asymptomatic at birth; however, hearing loss and learning disabilities have been reported in previously asymptomatic infants (Brown & Abernathy, 1998).

The neonate with classic, full-blown CMID displays IUGR and has microcephaly. The neonate also has a rash, jaundice, and hepatosplenomegaly (Fig. 39-10). Anemia, thrombocytopenia, and hyperbilirubinemia are to be expected. Intracranial, periventricular calcification often is noted on x-ray films. Inclusion bodies ("owl's eye" figures)

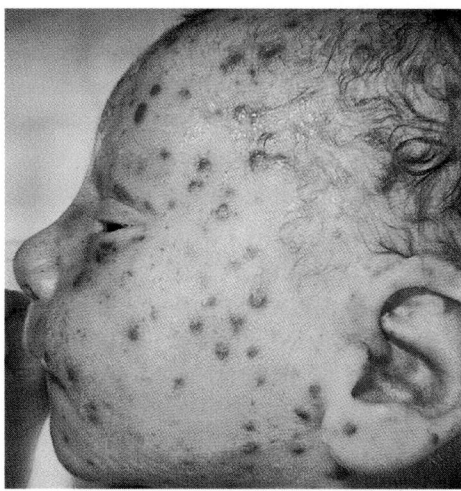

Fig. 39-10 Neonatal cytomegalovirus (CMV) infection. Typical rash seen in a severely affected infant. *(Courtesy David A. Clarke, Philadelphia, PA.)*

in cells sedimented from freshly voided urine or in liver biopsy specimens are typical.

Elevated levels of cord blood IgM are suggestive of disease. The virus may be isolated from urine or saliva of the newborn. Differential diagnosis includes other causes of jaundice, syphilis (positive Venereal Disease Research Laboratories [VDRL] findings), toxoplasmosis (positive Sabin-Feldman dye test result), hemolytic disease of the newborn (positive Coombs' test reaction), or coxsackievirus infection (positive culture).

Despite the extensive, endemic nature of the disease in women and men and its potential for havoc in perinatal life, critically affected newborns are born only occasionally. Milder forms of the disease often may result when the fetus is affected late in pregnancy. CMV can be transmitted through breast milk while the mother is experiencing acute CMV syndrome. CMV infections acquired after birth are often asymptomatic and have no sequelae. Exceptions to this occur in preterm infants in whom postnatal acquisition of CMV can result in pneumonia, hepatitis, thrombocytopenia, and long-term neurologic sequelae.

Antenatally infected infants who are asymptomatic at birth are at risk for late sequelae. Hearing loss may not be apparent until after the first year of life. Chorioretinitis, microcephaly, mental retardation, and neuromuscular deficits may occur by 2 years of age. Some children are at risk for a defect in tooth enamel, resulting in severe caries.

Herpes Simplex Virus

HSV infections among newborns are being diagnosed more frequently. HSV infection is estimated to occur in as many as 1 in 2000 to 1 in 5000 births (Fanaroff & Martin, 1997).

The neonate may acquire the virus by any of four modes of transmission:

- Transplacental infection (5%)
- Ascending infection by way of the birth canal
- Direct contamination during passage through an infected birth canal
- Direct transmission from infected personnel or family (5%) (Riley, 1998)

Transplacental transmission of HSV infection to the neonate may occur during maternal viremia. However, an ascending transcervical infection first involves the intact fetal membranes, causing chorioamnionitis. This infection then is likely to be the cause of rupture of membranes rather than the sequela to their rupture. Ascending transcervical infection of intact membranes may account for an increased rate of miscarriages in the first 20 weeks of gestation with genital HSV infections, the development of neonatal infections despite cesarean births with intact membranes, and the high rate of preterm births (Brown et al., 1997). Transcervical infection can be accelerated by fetal monitoring scalp electrodes. The electrodes break the fetal skin barrier and increase the risk of infection; however, most infants show no evidence of infection in utero.

Congenital infection is rare and characterized by in utero destruction of normally formed organs. Affected infants are growth restricted. They have severe psychomotor restriction, with intracranial calcifications, microcephaly, hypertonicity, and seizures. They suffer eye involvement, including microphthalmos, cataracts, chorioretinitis, blindness, and retinal dysplasia. Some infants have patent ductus arteriosus, limb anomalies, and recurrent skin vesicles, with a short life expectancy.

Most infants are infected directly during passage through the birth canal. The risk of infection during vaginal birth in the presence of genital herpes has not been clearly delineated. It may be as high as 40% to 60%, with active primary infection at term. Primary maternal infections after 32 weeks of gestation carry a higher risk for the fetus and newborn than do recurrent infections (Fanaroff & Martin, 1997). The transmission rate of chronic vaginal herpes from the pregnant woman to her newborn is low, 8% or less (Toltzis, 1991). Passive intrauterine immunity to herpes may be responsible.

Postnatal acquisition of the virus and spread within a nursery have been documented by DNA analysis. Both mother and father, as well as maternal breast lesions, have been implicated in neonatal infections. There also is concern regarding symptomatic and asymptomatic shedding among hospital personnel. Nursery personnel with cold sores should practice strict handwashing and wear a mask, but no evidence indicates that they should be removed from the nursery unless they have a herpetic whitlow (primary HSV infection of the terminal segment of a finger) (Fanaroff & Martin, 1997).

Clinically, neonatal HSV infections are classified as disseminated infection; encephalitis; or localized infection of the skin, eye, or mouth. Disseminated infections may involve virtually every organ system, but the liver, adrenal glands, and lungs are primarily involved. Affected infants exhibit initial symptoms usually in the first week of life but sometimes in the second week, with signs of bacterial sepsis or shock. Clinical manifestations include skin vesicles in about 50% of infants (Fig. 39-11). Death results from progression of CNS involvement, respiratory distress and pneumonitis, shock, DIC, and bleeding. Overall, the mortality rate without antiviral therapy is 57% (Riley, 1998).

Encephalitis may occur as a component of disseminated disease. Blood-borne seeding of the brain results in multiple lesions of cortical hemorrhagic necrosis. It also can occur alone or in association with oral, eye, or skin lesions. In the second to fourth week of life, brain involvement usually manifests. Only 60% of the infants have skin lesions, and the CSF of fewer than 50% will reveal the virus. Lethargy, poor feeding, irritability, and local or generalized seizures may be the presenting manifestations. Almost half of the infants die of neurologic deterioration as late as 6 months after onset, and virtually all survivors have severe sequelae, including microcephaly and blindness (Fanaroff & Martin, 1997).

Localized HSV infections most often occur with skin findings or rarely with isolated oral cavity lesions (Fig. 39-12). CNS or disseminated disease develops in 70% of the infants with skin vesicles. Ocular involvement, which can occur alone, may be secondary to either HSV-1 or HSV-2. Ocular disease may not be discovered for months. Microphthalmos, cataracts, optic atrophy, and corneal scarring may result from chorioretinitis, keratitis, and retinal hemorrhage (Fanaroff & Martin, 1997).

Care management. Gloves should be worn when caregivers are in contact with these infants. The neonate's eyes, oral cavity, and skin are inspected carefully for the presence of any lesions. Cultures are obtained from the mouth, the eyes, and any possible lesions. Circumcision, if performed, is delayed until the infant is ready to be discharged. The infant may be discharged with the mother if the infant's cultures are negative for the virus. As long as no suspicious lesions are on the mother's breasts, breastfeeding is allowed. For the infant at risk, prophylactic topical eye ointment (vidarabine) is administered for 5 days for prevention of keratoconjunctivitis. No current recommendations exist for prophylactic systemic therapy; each case should be considered individually. Blood, urine, and CSF specimens should be cultured when indicated clinically. If herpetic lesions first occur after 6 weeks of life, the risk of dissemination and severe illness is very low (Fanaroff & Martin, 1997).

Therapy includes general supportive measures, as well as treatment with vidarabine or acyclovir. Acyclovir is the most frequently used drug. It is considered safe because only viral replication is inhibited, although long-term sequelae are not yet known. Acyclovir is easier to administer; however, a randomized controlled trial has shown no difference between vidarabine and acyclovir for treatment of HSV (Jacobs, 1998). The current recommended dose of acyclovir is 10 mg/kg/day intravenously every 8 hours for at least 14 days. Continuing therapy may be required in case of recurrence. Ophthalmic ointment should be administered simultaneously (Fanaroff & Martin, 1997).

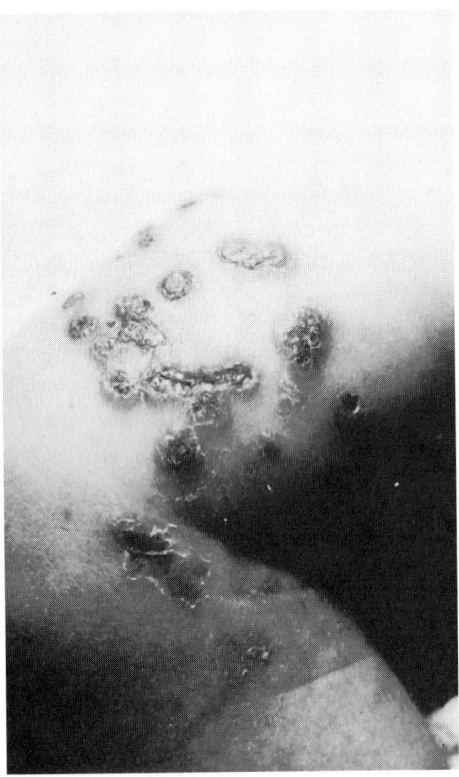

Fig. 39-11 Neonatal herpes simplex virus (HSV) skin infection. *(From Fanaroff, A., & Martin, R. [1995]. Neonatal-perinatal medicine: Diseases of the fetus and infant [5th ed.]. St. Louis: Mosby.)*

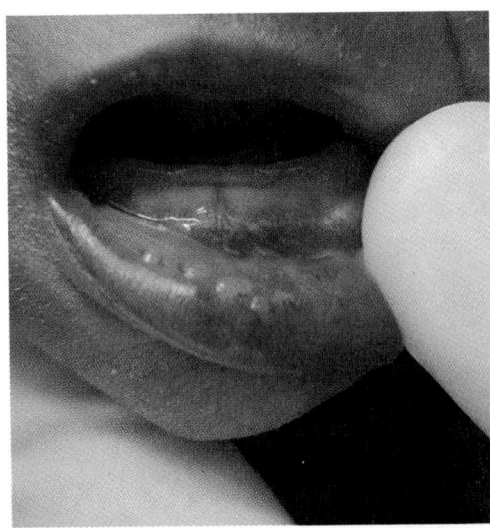

Fig. 39-12 Neonatal HSV oral lesions. *(Courtesy David A. Clarke, Philadelphia, PA.)*

Bacterial Infections

Group B Streptococcus

The most common cause of neonatal sepsis and meningitis in the United States is group B streptococcus (GBS) (Lieu et al., 1998; Philipson & Herson, 1996). Between 15% and 20% of pregnant women are colonized with GBS (Guerina, 1998). The incidence of early-onset GBS infection is 0.7 to 4 per 1000 live births (Adriaanse et al., 1996; Guerina, 1998). Early-onset GBS infection in the neonate occurs in the first 7 days of life but most commonly manifests in the first 24 hours following birth. Risk factors for the development of early-onset GBS include low birth weight, preterm birth, rupture of membranes of more than 18 hours, maternal fever, previous GBS infant, maternal GBS bacteriuria, and multiple gestation (Adriaanse et al., 1996; Guerina, 1998). Usually resulting from vertical transmission from the birth canal, early-onset disease results in a respiratory illness that mimics the symptoms of severe respiratory distress. The infant may rapidly develop septic shock, which carries a significant mortality rate. In recent years, prophylactic antibiotics given to mothers with risk factors during labor significantly reduced the incidence and severity of early-onset GBS infection in the newborn (CDC, 1996; Lieu et al., 1998).

Late-onset GBS infections occur between 1 week and 3 months of age with an average age of onset of 24 days. Eighty-five percent of infants with late-onset GBS have meningitis and have a mortality rate of 0% to 23%. Fifty percent of the survivors develop neurologic damage (Adriaanse et al., 1996).

Escherichia Coli

E. coli is the second most common cause of neonatal sepsis and meningitis in the United States (Guerina, 1998). *E. coli* is found in the gastrointestinal tract soon after birth and makes up the bulk of human fecal flora. In addition to meningitis, *E. coli* can also cause infections in other body systems, including the urinary tract. There is concern that increasing use of ampicillin in labor as prophylaxis against GBS disease will result in more virulent *E. coli* disease resulting from ampicillin-resistant organisms (Joseph, Pyati, & Jacobs, 1998).

Tuberculosis

The incidence of tuberculosis (TB), caused by *Mycobacterium tuberculosis*, is once again increasing in Canada and the United States. Congenitally acquired TB, although rare, can cause otitis media, pneumonia, hepatosplenomegaly, enlarged lymph glands, or disseminated disease. After birth, exposed infants contract TB through droplets expelled by infected individuals, which results in pneumonia and necrosis of lung tissue. Untreated neonatal tuberculosis is almost always fatal. When maternal treatment is initiated early in pregnancy, however, neonatal morbidity and mortality rates are similar to those in pregnancies unaffected by TB (Figueroa-Damian & Arredondo-Garcia, 1998).

Listeriosis

Listeria monocytogenes is a bacterium capable of producing significant intrapartum illness. Prenatal infection causes chorioamnionitis or endometritis and should be suspected in cases of meconium-stained amniotic fluid in infants less than 37 weeks of gestation. It has also been implicated as a cause of miscarriage and stillbirth (Guerina, 1998; Nolla-Salas et al., 1998). With disseminated fetal infection, microabscesses have been reported in the liver, lungs, and adrenal glands of stillborn infants. Live-born infants demonstrate granulomas on the skin and posterior pharyngeal wall. Listeriosis can also manifest as meningitis in a late-onset infection (Bortolussi & Schlech, 1995).

Chlamydia Infection

Chlamydia trachomatis is an intracellular bacterium that causes neonatal conjunctivitis and pneumonia. The conjunctivitis (congestion and edema), with minimal discharge, develops 5 days to 2 weeks after birth. Inclusion conjunctivitis is usually self-limiting, but if untreated, chronic follicular conjunctivitis, with conjunctival scarring and corneal microgranulations (Schachter & Grossman, 1995), has been reported.

The neonate also is treated with oral erythromycin for 2 to 3 weeks. Silver nitrate is not effective against *C. trachomatis*, but erythromycin or tetracycline ointment may prevent ophthalmic infection (Fanaroff & Martin, 1997). Eye prophylaxis is not sufficient to prevent the development of chlamydial pneumonia; therefore infants at risk should also be treated with systemic antibiotics such as oral erythromycin syrup.

Fungal Infections

Candidiasis

Candida infections, formerly known as moniliasis, may occur in the newborn. *Candida albicans*, the organism usually responsible, may cause disease in any organ system. It is a yeastlike fungus (producing yeast cells and spores) that can be acquired from a maternal vaginal infection during birth, by person-to-person transmission, or from contaminated hands, bottles, nipples, or other articles. It usually is a benign disorder in the neonate, often confined to the oral and diaper regions (Wong, 1999).

Candidal diaper dermatitis appears on the perianal area, inguinal folds, and lower portion of the abdomen. The affected area is intensely erythematous, with a sharply demarcated, scalloped edge, frequently with numerous satellite lesions that extend beyond the larger lesion. The source of the infection is through the gastrointestinal tract. Treatment is with applications of an anticandidal ointment, such as nystatin (Mycostatin) or miconazole 2% (Monistat), with each diaper change. The infant also may be given an oral antifungal preparation to eliminate any gastrointestinal source of infection (Wong, 1999).

Oral candidiasis (**thrush,** or mycotic stomatitis) is characterized by the appearance of white plaques on the oral

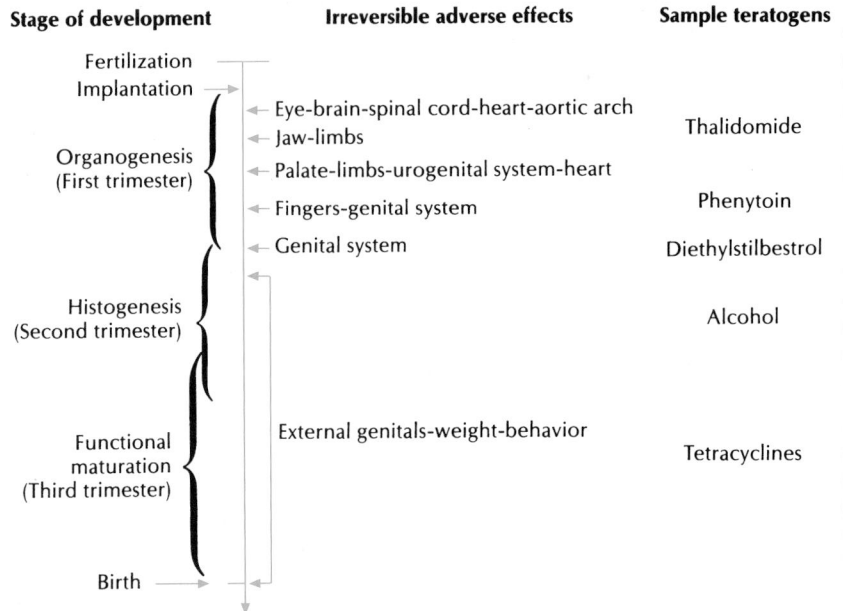

Fig. 39-13 Critical periods in human embryogenesis. *(From Fanaroff, A., & Martin, R. [1995]. Neonatal-perinatal medicine: Diseases of the fetus and infant [5th ed.]. St. Louis: Mosby.)*

mucosa, gums, and tongue. The white patches are easily differentiated from milk curds; the patches cannot be removed and tend to bleed when touched. In most cases the infant does not seem to be in discomfort from the infection. A few infants seem to have some difficulty swallowing.

Infants who are sick, debilitated, or receiving antibiotic therapy are more susceptible to thrush. Those with conditions such as cleft lip or palate, neoplasms, and hyperparathyroidism seem to be more vulnerable to mycotic infection.

The objectives of management are to eradicate the causative organism, to control exposure to *C. albicans,* and to improve the infant's resistance. Interventions include maintenance of scrupulous cleanliness to prevent reinfection (nursing personnel, parents, others). Good handwashing technique is always essential. Clean surfaces should be provided for neonates. Proper cleanliness of the equipment and environment is ensured. If the infant is breastfeeding, the mother also is treated with topical nystatin.

Medications are administered as ordered. Nystatin is instilled into the newborn's mouth with a medicine dropper after the infant is given sterile water to wash out any residual milk. Nystatin also may be swabbed over mucosa, gums, or tongue. Less frequently, an aqueous solution of gentian violet (1% to 2%) is applied with a swab to oral mucosa, gums, and tongue. The nurse should guard against staining the skin, clothes, and equipment and should warn parents about the purple staining of the baby's mouth.

SUBSTANCE ABUSE

Certain maternal behaviors result in perinatal risk. Maternal habits hazardous to the fetus and neonate include drug addiction, smoking, and alcohol abuse. Occasional withdrawal reactions have been reported in neonates of mothers who use to excess such drugs as barbiturates, alcohol, or amphetamines. Serious reactions are seen in neonates whose mothers abuse psychoactive drugs or are treated with methadone. Almost 50% of pregnancies of women addicted to opioids result in low-birth-weight (LBW) infants who are not necessarily preterm. Alcohol is a teratogen. Maternal ethanol abuse during gestation can lead to a readily identifiable fetal alcohol syndrome. Maternal substance abuse is discussed in Chapter 35.

The adverse effects of exposure of the fetus to drugs are varied. They include transient behavioral changes such as fetal breathing movements or irreversible effects such as fetal death, IUGR, structural malformations, or mental retardation. Critical determinants of the effect of the drug on the fetus include the specific drug, the dosage, the route of administration, the genotype of the mother or fetus, and the timing of the drug exposure. Fig. 39-13 shows critical periods in human embryogenesis and the teratogenic effects of drugs. Table 39-4 summarizes the effects of commonly abused substances on the fetus and neonate.

Alcohol

Documentation of the **fetal alcohol syndrome** (FAS) can be found in the literature since the early part of the eigh-

TABLE 39-4	Summary of Neonatal Effects of Commonly Abused Substances
SUBSTANCE	**NEONATAL EFFECTS**
Alcohol	*Fetal alcohol syndrome* (FAS): craniofacial anomalies, including short eyelid opening, flat midface, flat upper lip groove, thin upper lip; microcephaly; hyperactivity; developmental delays; attention deficits *Fetal alcohol effects:* milder forms of FAS, cardiac anomalies, failure to thrive
Cocaine	Prematurity, small for gestational age, microcephaly, poor feeding, irregular sleep pattern, diarrhea, visual attention problems, hyperactivity, difficult to console, hypersensitivity to noise and external stimuli, irritability, developmental delays, congenital anomalies such as prune belly syndrome (distended, flabby, wrinkled abdomen caused by lack of abdominal muscles)
Heroin	Low birth weight, small for gestational age, neonatal abstinence syndrome (see Table 39-6)
Amphetamines	Small for gestational age, prematurity, poor weight gain, lethargy
Tobacco	Prematurity, low birth weight, increased risk for sudden infant death syndrome, increased risk for bronchitis, pneumonia, developmental delays
Marijuana	Possible neonatal tremors, possible low birth weight

teenth century. The incidence of FAS in the United States is about 2 per 1000 population (Church & Abel, 1998).

According to Abel (1997), FAS is based on minimum criteria of signs in each of three categories: prenatal and postnatal growth restriction; CNS malfunctions, including mental retardation; and craniofacial features such as microcephaly, small eyes or short palpebral fissures, thin upper lip, flat midface, and an indistinct philtrum. Neurologic problems in FAS children include some degree of IQ deficit, attention deficit disorder, diminished fine motor skills, and poor speech. These children have been shown to lack inhibition, have no stranger anxiety, and lack appropriate judgment skills (D'Apolito, 1998). Infants exposed prenatally to alcohol who are affected but do not meet the criteria for FAS may be said to have **fetal alcohol effects** (FAEs) (D'Apolito, 1998). These effects run the gamut from learning disabilities and behavioral problems to speech or language problems and hyperactivity. Often these problems are not detected until the child goes to school and learning problems become evident. FAEs can be seen with other disorders, such as fetal hydantoin syndrome; therefore a careful history is needed.

Predictable abnormal patterns of fetal and neonatal morphogenesis are attributed to severe, chronic alcoholism in women who continue to drink heavily during pregnancy. The pattern of growth deficiency begun in prenatal life persists after birth, especially in the linear growth rate, rate of weight gain, and growth of head circumferences.

Ocular structural anomalies are common findings (Fig. 39-14). Limb anomalies and a variety of cardiocirculatory anomalies, especially ventricular septal defects, pose problems for the child. Table 39-5 outlines physical findings in FAS. Mental retardation (IQ of 79 or below at 7 years of age), hyperactivity, and fine motor dysfunction (poor hand-to-mouth coordination, weak grasp) add to the handicapping problems that maternal alcoholism can impose. Genital abnormalities are seen in daughters of alcohol-ad-

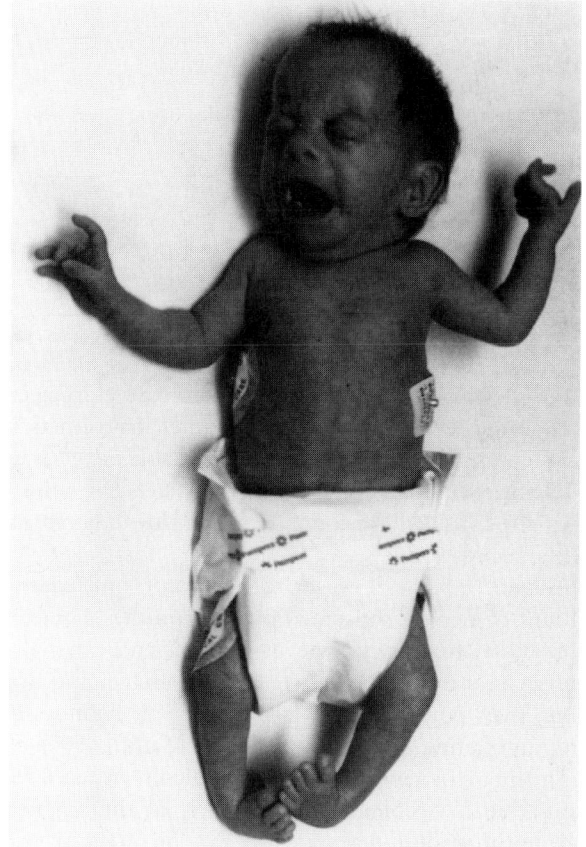

Fig. 39-14 Infant with fetal alcohol syndrome. *(From Wong, D. [1999]. Whaley and Wong's nursing care of infants and children [6th ed.]. St. Louis: Mosby.)*

dicted mothers. Two thirds of newborns with FAS are girls; the cause of this altered fetal sex ratio is unknown. Severe and chronic alcoholism (ethanol toxicity), not maternal malnutrition, is responsible for the severity and consistency of postnatal performance problems (Fanaroff & Martin,

TABLE 39-5 **Features of Fetal Alcohol Syndrome**

AFFECTED PART	CHARACTERISTICS
Eyes	Epicanthal folds, strabismus, ptosis, hypoplastic retinal vessels
Mouth	Poor suck, cleft lip, cleft palate, small teeth
Ears	Deafness
Skeleton	Radioulnar synostosis, fusion of cervical vertebrae, restricted bone growth
Heart	Atrial and ventricular septal defects, tetralogy of Fallot, patent ductus arteriosus
Kidney	Renal hypoplasia, hydronephrosis, urogenital sinus
Liver	Extrahepatic biliary atresia, hepatic fibrosis
Immune system	Increased infections: otitis media, upper respiratory infections, immune deficiencies
Tumors	Nonspecific neoplasms
Skin	Abnormal palmar creases, irregular hair, whorls

From Weiner, L., & Morse, B. (1991). FAS: Clinical perspectives and prevention. In I. Chasnoff (Ed.). *Drugs, alcohol, pregnancy and parenting.* Boston: Kluwer.

1997). High alcohol levels are lethal to the developing embryo. Lower levels cause brain and other malformations. Long-term prognosis (no studies are available as yet) is discouraging even in an optimum psychosocial environment, when one considers the combination of growth failure and mental retardation.

Alcohol effects, however, depend not only on the amount of alcohol consumed but also on the interaction of quantity, frequency, type of alcohol, and other drug abuse. Other drugs, such as cigarettes, caffeine, and marijuana, may potentiate the fetal effects of alcohol consumption during gestation (Fanaroff & Martin, 1997).

The infant of a mother who abuses alcohol is faced with many clinical problems. Identification of the problems leads to the medical diagnosis of FAS. The infant may suffer respiratory distress related to preterm birth, neurologic damage, and a "floppy" epiglottis and small trachea. Tracheoepiglottal anomalies may cause cardiopulmonary arrest. Other disorders include recurrent otitis media and hearing loss. Craniofacial features may be important in diagnosing craniofacial and oral anomalies, dental development abnormalities, and long-term body growth patterns. Feeding difficulties are related to preterm birth, poor sucking ability, and possible cleft palate. The infant may exhibit brain dysfunction, microcephaly, and grand mal seizures.

Long-term effects into childhood may include impaired visuomotor perception and performance, lowered IQ scores, and delayed receptive and expressive language, as well as reduced capacity to process and store factual data (Church & Abel, 1998). It is now recognized as one of the leading causes of mental retardation in the United States. Although the distinctive facial features of the infant tend to become less evident, the mental capacities never become normal.

Nursing care involves many of the same strategies used for the care of preterm infants (see Chapter 41). Special efforts are made to involve the parents in their child's care and to encourage opportunities for parent-child attachment.

Placing infants in a warm, caring environment with understanding caregivers who can deal with the infant's hyperirritability can lead to improved emotional development and social functioning (D'Apolito, 1998; Wagner et al., 1998). These caregivers provide extensive cuddling and human contact and can deal with the eating problems that typically lead to a diagnosis of failure to thrive. However, these infants may not go home to such an environment. Often the family is dysfunctional.

Heroin

Heroin crosses the placenta and frequently results in IUGR. Heroin may have a direct growth-inhibiting effect on the fetus, but the exact mechanisms of growth inhibition are not clear. There is an increased rate of stillbirths but not of congenital anomalies.

Many of the medical complications attributed to heroin result from prematurity. Other risks include physical dependence in the fetus and the risk of exposure to infections, including hepatitis B and C virus and HIV. Drug withdrawal in the mother is accompanied by fetal withdrawal, which can lead to fetal death (Kaltenbach, Berghella, & Finnegan, 1998; Wagner et al., 1998).

Maternal detoxification in the first trimester carries an increased risk of miscarriage. Detoxification is not recommended after the thirty-second week because of possible withdrawal-induced fetal distress (Kaltenbach et al., 1998).

Heroin withdrawal occurs in 50% to 80% of infants born to addicted mothers, usually within the first 48 to 72 hours of life (Wagner et al., 1998). The signs depend on the length of maternal addiction, the amount of drug taken, and the time of injection before birth. The infant whose mother is taking methadone may not demonstrate signs of withdrawal until a week or so after birth. The symptoms of infants whose mothers used heroin or methadone are similar in nature. Initially the infant may be depressed. The withdrawal syndrome may manifest as a combination of any of the following signs. The infant may be jittery and hyperactive. Usually the infant's cry is shrill and persistent. The infant may yawn or sneeze frequently. The tendon reflexes are increased, but Moro's reflex is decreased. The neonate may exhibit poor feeding and sucking, tachypnea, vomiting, diarrhea, hypothermia or hyperthermia, and sweating. In addition, an abnormal sleep cycle, with absence of quiet sleep and disturbance of active sleep, has been described in these infants (Fanaroff & Martin, 1997).

If withdrawal is not treated, vomiting, diarrhea, dehydration, apnea, and convulsions may develop. Death may follow. Therapy is individualized. Dehydration and electrolyte imbalance are prevented or treated. Usually one of the following drugs is ordered: phenobarbital, paregoric (compound tincture of opium), or diazepam, singly or in combination.

> **NURSE ALERT** *The use of naloxone (Narcan) is contraindicated in infants born to narcotic addicts because it may cause severe signs and symptoms of narcotic abstinence syndrome and seizures.*

The long-term effect on these infants is now being studied. The risk of sudden infant death syndrome (SIDS) is 5 to 10 times higher for infants with significant withdrawal problems than for infants in the general population.

Methadone

Methadone, a synthetic opiate, has been the therapy of choice for heroin addiction since 1965. Methadone crosses the placenta. An increasing number of infants have been born to methadone-maintained mothers, who seem to have better prenatal care and a somewhat better lifestyle than those taking heroin (Fanaroff & Martin, 1997).

Some question exists concerning the benefits of methadone therapy during pregnancy because of its effect on the fetus. In one study (Levine & Rebarber, 1995), nonstress tests performed on women receiving methadone were found to be significantly less reactive than nonstress tests reported in the general population of pregnant women. These findings question the benefits of methadone treatment for pregnant heroin abusers and the related ethical issues. Methadone withdrawal occurs in about 80% to 95% of infants born to these women.

Methadone withdrawal resembles heroin withdrawal but tends to be more severe and prolonged. In addition, the incidence of seizures is higher. Seizures usually occur between days 7 and 10. The infants exhibit a disturbed sleep pattern similar to that seen in heroin withdrawal. The infants have a higher birth weight than that in heroin withdrawal, usually appropriate for gestational age. No increased incidence of congenital anomalies is seen.

Late-onset withdrawal occurs at 2 to 4 weeks and may continue for weeks or months. A higher incidence of SIDS also has been reported in these infants (Wagner et al., 1998). This factor is important for perinatal nurses who coordinate follow-up care for the infant and education for the mother or other caregiver. Community health nurses must know about the potential for withdrawal symptoms to occur.

Therapy for methadone withdrawal is similar to that for heroin withdrawal. The few available follow-up studies of these infants reveal a high incidence of hyperactivity, learning and behavior disorders, and poor social adjustment (Fanaroff & Martin, 1997).

Marijuana

Marijuana crosses the placenta. Its use during pregnancy may result in a shortened gestation and a higher incidence of IUGR (Wagner et al., 1998). Some investigators have found a higher incidence of meconium staining (Fanaroff & Martin, 1997). Some association has been reported between the use of marijuana and a decrease in infant birth weight and length and the occurrence of congenital anomalies; however, the findings have been inconsistent (Lee, 1998). A longitudinal study by Fried (1993) followed infants of marijuana users for 2 years and found no association between marijuana use and cognitive abilities at 12, 24, or 36 months but at 48 months found memory and verbal measures of cognitive ability affected in the infants of heavy marijuana users. Compounding the issue of the effects of marijuana is multidrug use, especially among adolescents, thus combining the harmful effects of marijuana, tobacco, alcohol, and cocaine. Long-term follow-up studies on exposed infants are needed.

Cocaine

Cocaine crosses the placenta and is found in breast milk. Approximately 20% to 30% of cocaine-exposed infants have resulting physical abnormalities (Chasnoff, 1992).

Antenatal effects of maternal cocaine ingestion include infarctions to developing organs, resulting in defects such as hydronephrosis, hypospadias, prune belly syndrome (distended flabby abdomen and renal anomalies), congenital heart disease, skull defects, ileal atresia, and limb reduction. Infants born to cocaine-abusing mothers show a high rate of perinatal morbidity, IUGR, preterm birth, and placental or cerebral infarction (Plessinger & Woods, 1998).

Cocaine-dependent neonates do not experience a process of withdrawal seen in narcotic-exposed infants but rather suffer from neurotoxic effects of the drug. Signs of exposure have some of the same characteristics as heroin withdrawal but can be highly varied. There may be an increased risk for SIDS (Plessinger & Woods, 1998). The effects of prenatal exposure to cocaine on neonatal behavior have been studied extensively. Findings indicate that cocaine-exposed infants have limited ability to habituate to stimuli. As these children enter school they demonstrate a reduced capacity for verbal reasoning and difficulties maintaining attention (Plessinger & Woods, 1998). Box 39-2 summarizes neonatal effects of maternal cocaine use.

Phencyclidine ("Angel Dust")

Phencyclidine (PCP) increases the risk of injury to the pregnant woman and therefore also to her passively dependent fetus. The user may be unaware that she is ingesting PCP because it frequently is misrepresented as another drug of abuse or mixed with other drugs (Carroll, 1990).

PCP crosses the placenta and is found in breast milk. Literature about the effects on infants is limited. The infants exposed to PCP may exhibit abnormal motor behavior such as irritability, jitteriness, and hypertonicity (D'Apolito, 1998).

Miscellaneous Substances

The fetal and neonatal effects of maternal use of methamphetamines in pregnancy are not well known. The effects appear to be dose related. LBW, preterm birth, and perinatal mortality may be consequences of higher doses used throughout pregnancy. A higher incidence of cleft lip and palate and cardiac defects has been reported in infants exposed to amphetamines in utero (Plessinger, 1998). Following birth infants may experience bradycardia or tachycardia that resolves as the drug is cleared from the infant's system. Lethargy may continue for several months, along with frequent infections and poor weight gain. Emotional disturbances and delays in gross and fine motor coordination may be seen during early childhood.

Phenobarbital crosses the placenta readily and is subsequently found in high levels in the fetal liver and brain. Because of its slow metabolic rate, when withdrawal does occur, onset is generally at 2 to 14 days after birth and duration is about 2 to 4 months. Irritability, crying, hiccoughs, and sleepiness mark the initial response. During the second stage the infant is extremely hungry, regurgitates and gags frequently, and demonstrates episodic irritability, sweating, and a disturbed sleep pattern.

Treatment consists of swaddling, frequent feedings, and protection from noxious external stimuli. If no improvement occurs, the neonate should be given phenobarbital and then slowly withdrawn from this drug after control of symptoms (Fanaroff & Martin, 1995).

Caffeine has not been implicated as a teratogen in humans. Fernandes and colleagues (1998) reported that caffeine consumption of greater than 150 mg per day was associated with IUGR and LBW. Santos and co-workers (1998) reported no adverse effects in the fetus with consumption of less than 300 mg of caffeine per day.

Tobacco

Cigarette smoking in pregnancy has been found to be associated with birth-weight deficits of up to 250 g for a full-term neonate (Fanaroff & Martin, 1997). Maternal cigarette smoking is implicated in 21% to 39% of LBW infants. Passive exposure to secondhand smoke by a pregnant woman may also result in the birth of an LBW infant. Also, if pregnant smokers drink five or more cups of coffee and one or more drinks of alcohol per day, the risk of IUGR is increased considerably (Fried, 1993).

The rate of miscarriage and preterm birth is increased in the smoking population. When other variables have been controlled for, no clear association has been found between maternal smoking and congenital anomalies (Lee, 1998). Nicotine and cotinine, the two pharmacologically active substances in tobacco, are found in higher concentrations in infants whose mothers smoke. These substances can be secreted in breast milk for up to 2 hours after the mother has smoked. Cigarette smoke contains more than 2000 compounds, including carbon monoxide, dioxin, cyanide, and cadmium. Long-term studies show residual effects beyond the neonatal period (Floyd et al., 1993). Deficits in growth, in intellectual and emotional development, and in behavior have been documented. These include poor auditory responsiveness, increased fine motor tremors, hypertonicity, and decreased verbal comprehension.

Pregnant women need to be aware of the harmful effects of smoking on their unborn baby's health. These include IUGR, miscarriage, PROM, placenta previa, and SIDS (Lee, 1998). Increasing concern surrounds secondhand smoke and its potential effects on infants and siblings. Mothers and all others should refrain from smoking near the infant. Several studies have reported a positive as-

---

BOX 39-2 | **Neonatal Effects of Maternal Cocaine Use**

PHYSICAL

Preterm birth
Decreased length
Decreased head circumference
Intrauterine growth restriction
Ileal atresia
Prune belly syndrome
Cryptorchidism
Hypospadias
Hydronephrosis
Seizures
Fever
Congenital heart disease
Skull defects
Hypertension
Cerebral infarction
Vomiting
Diarrhea
SIDS
Tachypnea

BEHAVIORAL

Irritability
Tremors
Poor feeding
Abnormal sleep patterns
Increased startles
Disorganized behavior
Lability
Poor visual processing
Difficult to console

sociation between maternal smoking and SIDS (Floyd et al., 1993; Lee, 1998; Milerad et al., 1998). It is not clear whether this association reflects in utero exposure or passive exposure postnatally, or both.

CARE MANAGEMENT

Assessment of the newborn requires a review of the mother's prenatal record. A medical and social history of drug abuse and detoxification is noted. The infant may have IUGR or be preterm with LBW.

The woman who is addicted to narcotics may have infections that compound the risk to the infant, including hepatitis, septicemia, and STIs, including AIDS (Wagner et al., 1998).

The nurse often is the first to observe the signs of drug dependence in the infant. The nurse's observations help the physician differentiate between drug dependence and other conditions, such as tracheoesophageal fistula, CNS disorder, sepsis, hypoglycemia, and electrolyte imbalance.

The infant is assessed by means of the guidelines discussed in Chapter 26. The infant's gestational age and maturity are noted. In utero exposure to some drugs results in observable malformations or dysmorphism (abnormality of shape). Neonatal behavior may arouse suspicion. **Neonatal abstinence syndrome** is the term given to the group of signs and symptoms associated with drug withdrawal in the neonate (Table 39-6). Figure 39-15 provides an example of a scoring system for assessing withdrawal symptoms. Because many women are multidrug users, the newborn initially may exhibit a confusing complex of signs.

Urine or meconium screening may be used to identify substances abused by the mother. Initially costly and of limited availability, tests of meconium collected on day 1 or 2 of life have been shown to be both sensitive and reliable in detecting the metabolites of several street drugs, including cocaine (Buchi, 1998; Kwong & Shearer, 1998).

Neonatal Drug Screening

Testing of neonatal urine or meconium for the presence of drug metabolites is a sensitive and reliable means of identifying neonates at risk for withdrawal symptoms. Controversy arises over whether universal drug screening should be instituted and whether informed consent is needed for screening neonates. Ethical issues include the cost versus benefit of universal testing and the rights of parents versus the medical need to diagnose withdrawal.

Nursing diagnoses, which depend on the assessment findings, are tailored to the individual needs of the neonate and the family.

Nursing Diagnoses

Neonate

- Risk for infection related to
  - maternal risk behaviors
  - PROM
- Altered growth and development related to
  - effects of maternal substance abuse
- Sleep pattern disturbance related to
  - drug withdrawal
- Disorganized infant behavior related to
  - effects of maternal substance abuse

Parents

- Altered parenting related to
  - continuation of substance abuse or detoxification program
  - guilt about infant's condition
  - inability to cope with care needs of a special infant
- Anxiety related to knowledge deficit regarding
  - care needs of an affected infant
- Violence: self-directed or directed toward infant related to
  - drug-dependent lifestyle

TABLE 39-6 Signs of Neonatal Abstinence Syndrome

SYSTEM	SIGNS
Gastrointestinal	Poor feeding, vomiting, regurgitation, diarrhea, excessive sucking
Central nervous	Irritability, tremors, shrill cry, incessant crying, hyperactivity, little sleep, excoriations on knees and face, convulsions
Metabolic, vasomotor, respiratory	Nasal congestion, tachypnea, sweating, frequent yawning, increased respiratory rate >60/min, fever >37.2° C

Nursing Care

Planning for care of the infant born to a substance-abusing mother presents a challenge to the health care team. Parents are included in the planning for the newborn's care and also are encouraged to plan for their own care. A multidisciplinary approach is needed that includes home health or community resource personnel (e.g., regulatory agencies such as child protective services).

Education and social support to prevent the abuse of drugs provide the ideal approach. However, given the scope of the drug abuse problem, total prevention is unrealistic.

Nursing care of the drug-dependent neonate involves supportive therapy for fluid and electrolyte balance, nutrition, infection control, and respiratory care. Swaddling, holding, reducing stimuli, and feeding as necessary may be helpful in easing withdrawal (see Plan of Care). Specific

NEONATAL ABSTINENCE SCORING SYSTEM

SYSTEM	SIGNS AND SYMPTOMS	SCORE	AM						PM					COMMENTS
CENTRAL NERVOUS SYSTEM DISTURBANCES	Excessive High Pitched (Or other) Cry	2												Daily Weight:
	Continuous High Pitched (Or other) Cry	3												
	Sleeps <1 Hour After Feeding	3												
	Sleeps <2 Hours After Feeding	2												
	Sleeps <3 Hours After Feeding	1												
	Hyperactive Moro Reflex	2												
	Markedly Hyperactive Moro Reflex	3												
	Mild Tremors Disturbed	1												
	Moderate-Severe Tremors Disturbed	2												
	Mild Tremors Undisturbed	3												
	Moderate-Severe Tremors Undisturbed	4												
	Increased Muscle Tone	2												
	Excoriation (Specific Area)	1												
	Myoclonic Jerks	3												
	Generalized Convulsions	5												
METABOLIC/VASOMOTOR/RESPIRATORY DISTURBANCES	Sweating	1												
	Fever <101 (99-100.8 F./37.2-38.2C.)	1												
	Fever >101 (38.4C. and Higher)	2												
	Frequent Yawning (>3-4 Times/Interval)	1												
	Mottling	1												
	Nasal Stuffiness	1												
	Sneezing (>3-4 Times/Interval)	1												
	Nasal Flaring	2												
	Respiratory Rate >60/min	1												
	Respiratory Rate >60/min with Retractions	2												
GASTROINTESTINAL DISTURBANCES	Excessive Sucking	1												
	Poor Feeding	2												
	Regurgitation	2												
	Projectile Vomiting	3												
	Loose Stools	2												
	Watery Stools	3												
	TOTAL SCORE													
	INITIALS OF SCORER													

Fig. 39-15 Neonatal Abstinence Scoring (NAS) system, developed by L. Finnegan. *(From Nelson, N. [1990]. Current therapy in neonatal-perinatal medicine [2nd ed.]. St. Louis: Mosby.)*

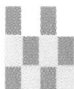

PLAN ᵒᶠ CARE | Infant Undergoing Drug Withdrawal

NURSING DIAGNOSIS Risk for injury related to hyperactivity, seizures secondary to passive narcotic addiction resulting from maternal substance abuse during pregnancy

Expected Outcome *Infant exhibits no signs of seizure activity.*

Nursing Interventions/*Rationales*

Administer phenobarbital, diazepam per physician order *to decrease CNS irritability and control seizure activity.*

Decrease environmental stimuli *that may trigger irritability and hyperactive behaviors.*

Plan care activities carefully *to allow for minimum stimulation.*

Wrap infant snugly and hold infant tightly *to reduce self-stimulation behaviors and protect skin from abrasions.*

If infant is cocaine addicted, position to avoid eye contact, swaddle infant, use vertical rocking techniques, and use a pacifier *to counter poor organizational response to stimuli and depressed interactive behaviors.*

Monitor activity level, note the relationship between activity level and external stimulation, and stop external stimulation *if it causes activity increase.*

NURSING DIAGNOSIS Altered nutrition, less than body requirements related to CNS irritability, poor suck reflex, vomiting, and diarrhea

Expected Outcome *Infant exhibits ingestion and retention of adequate nutrients and appropriate weight gain.*

Nursing Interventions/*Rationales*

Feed in frequent small amounts, elevate head during and after feeding, and burp well *to diminish vomiting and aspiration.*

Experiment with various nipples *to find one most effective in compensating for poor suck reflex.*

Monitor weight daily and maintain strict intake and output *to evaluate success of feeding.*

If intake is insufficient, feed by oral gavage per physician order *to ensure ingestion of needed nutrients.*

Have suction available as required *to reduce chances of aspiration.*

NURSING DIAGNOSIS Risk for fluid volume deficit related to diarrhea and vomiting

Expected Outcome *Infant exhibits evidence of fluid homeostasis.*

Nursing Interventions/*Rationales*

Administer oral and parenteral fluids per physician order and regulate *to maintain fluid balance.*

Monitor hydration status (skin turgor, weight, mucous membranes, fontanels, urine specific gravity, electrolytes) and intake and output *to evaluate for evidence of dehydration.*

NURSING DIAGNOSIS Ineffective maternal coping, anxiety, powerlessness related to drug use, infant distress during withdrawal, and single-parent status

Expected Outcomes *Woman will accept newborn's condition and participate in care activities, showing evidence of maternal-infant bonding process.*

Nursing Interventions/*Rationales*

Explain effects of maternal drug use on newborn and the withdrawal process *to provide understanding and reality concerning effects of drug use.*

Encourage open communication (e.g., inform mother of ongoing condition, procedures, and treatment; answer questions; correct misperceptions; actively listen to her concerns) *to provide a sense of respect, provide support, and encourage a sense of control.*

Encourage mother to interact with infant and to become involved in care routines *to foster emotional connection.*

Explain how to do care procedures, how to avoid excess stimulation, and how to hold and rock infant *to enhance mother's care abilities and her sense of confidence and control.*

If the mother is addicted to cocaine, explain infant's inability to interact, gaze aversion, arching back, and lack of response to cuddling *to enhance understanding of infant behaviors.*

Make appropriate referrals to social agencies for treatment of maternal drug addiction, infant development programs, and other needed support services *to ensure adequate resources for care of self and infant.*

From Wong, D., & Perry, S. (1998). *Maternal child nursing care.* St. Louis: Mosby.

TEACHING guidelines

Care of Infant Experiencing Withdrawal

- Place the infant in a side-lying position with the spine and legs flexed.
- Position the infant's hands in midline with the arms at the side.
- Carry the infant in a flexed position.
- When interacting with the infant, introduce one stimulus at a time when the infant is in a quiet, alert state.

Watch for time-out or distress signals (gaze aversion, yawning, sneezing, hiccoughs, arching, mottled color).
- When the infant is distressed, swaddle in a flexed position and rock in a slow, rhythmic fashion.
- Put the infant in a sitting position with chin tucked down for feeding.

RESEARCH

Improving Interactions Between Substance-Abusing Mothers and Their Substance-Exposed Newborns

Between 500,000 and 700,000 infants annually are exposed in utero to illicit drugs. When mother, infant, or both are exposed to stressors (e.g., substance abuse and its concomitant medical problems), the quality and quantity of mother-infant interactions are at risk. If nurses can ascertain which couplets are in need of additional assistance, they can work to provide that aid. The purpose of this study was to determine whether teaching comforting and interacting techniques within 24 hours of birth to substance-abusing mothers would improve mother-newborn interactions 48 to 72 hours after hospital discharge, as measured by the Nursing Child Assessment Feeding Scale (NCAFS).

Sixty mother-newborn couplets completed the study. Two observers, blind to the mother's drug history, completed the NCAFS of all participants within 24 hours of birth. Mothers in the experimental group were given the intervention (teaching comforting and interacting techniques). The observers completed the NCAFS in the mothers' homes 48 to 72 hours after discharge.

At the home visit, couplets in the treatment group showed significant improvement in their total NCAFS score ($F = 5.18$; $p = .008$). When analyzed separately, only maternal scores showed a significant difference between the treatment and control groups at the home visit ($F = 6.48$; $p = .0029$). It was concluded that by demonstrating caregiving behavior, nurses can help mothers recognize and respond to newborns' behavior cues, thus enhancing mother-newborn interactions.

CLINICAL APPLICATION

Results of this study indicate that the nurse's teaching of comforting and interacting techniques was an important factor in improving mother-newborn interactions. Having programs available concerning the effects of substance use on pregnancy, the developing fetus, and couplet interaction may help the mother develop a beginning attachment to her fetus. Following up on missed appointments may bring the mother back into the health care system, thereby improving mother and infant outcomes and promoting a positive, interactive environment after birth.

Source: French, E. et al. (1998). Improving interactions between substance-abusing mothers and their substance-exposed newborns. *J Obstet Gynecol Neonatal Nurs* 27(3), 262-269.

suggestions for providing care to infants experiencing withdrawal are listed in the Teaching Guidelines box.

Pharmacologic treatment is usually based on the severity of withdrawal symptoms, as determined by an assessment tool (see Fig. 39-15). When indicated, medications are given as ordered. Neonatal morphine solution (0.4 mg/ml) is given at a dose of 0.05 ml/kg every 4 hours with the dose increased by 0.05 mg at the end of each 4-hour period un-

til withdrawal symptoms are controlled. Dosing may also be determined according to the abstinence score (Schechner, 1998). The dosage of phenobarbital is as follows: 20 mg/kg IM or IV loading dose followed by 10 mg/kg IM or IV every 12 hours until symptoms are under control; and then 2.5 mg/kg every 12 hours orally for 3 or 4 days. The dose is reduced by one third every 2 days for about 2 weeks, at which time treatment is discontinued.

TABLE 39-7	Drugs of Abuse Contraindicated During Breastfeeding*	
DRUG	**REPORTED EFFECT OR REASONS FOR CONCERN**	
Amphetamine†	Irritability, poor sleeping pattern	
Cocaine	Cocaine intoxication	
Heroin	Tremors, restlessness, vomiting, poor feeding	
Marijuana	Only one report in literature; no effect mentioned; at risk for inhaling smoke	
Nicotine (smoking)	Shock, vomiting, diarrhea, rapid heart rate, restlessness; decreased milk production	
Phencyclidine	Potent hallucinogen	

Modified from American Academy of Pediatrics. (1994). The transfer of drugs and other chemicals into human milk. *Pediatrics* 93(1), 137-150; also in Lawrence, R. (1999). *Breastfeeding: A guide for the medical profession* (5th ed.). St. Louis: Mosby.

*AAP Committee on Drugs strongly believes that breastfeeding mothers should not ingest any substances listed here. Not only are they hazardous to the nursing infant, but they are also detrimental to the physical and emotional health of the mother. This list is obviously not complete; no drug of abuse should be ingested by breastfeeding mothers even though adverse reports are not in the literature.
†Drug is concentrated in human milk.

Although less common, paregoric may be ordered: 0.8 ml/kg/day in 6 divided doses initially with increments of 0.4 ml/kg/day until symptom control is achieved. The dose is then decreased by 10% per day.

Drug dependence in the neonate is physiologic, not psychologic. Thus a predisposition to dependence later in life is not believed to be a factor. However, the psychosocial environment in which the infant may be raised may create a tendency to addiction.

The mother requires considerable support. Her need for and her abuse of drugs result in a decreased capacity to cope. The infant's withdrawal signs and decreased consolability stress her coping abilities even further. Home health care, treatment for addiction, and education are important considerations. Sensitive exploration of the woman's options for the care of her infant and herself and for future fertility management may help her see that she has choices. This approach helps communicate respect for the new mother as a person who can make responsible decisions (see Research box).

The issue of breastfeeding in this population is a difficult one. Although breast milk remains the optimum source of nutrition for these infants, care must be taken to avoid exposing the infant to additional drugs through the breast milk. The American Academy of Pediatrics has compiled a list of drugs contraindicated in breastfeeding (Table 39-7).

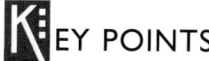

KEY POINTS

- A small percentage of significant birth injuries may occur despite skilled and competent obstetric care.
- The same birth injury may be caused in several ways.
- The nurse's primary contribution to the welfare of the neonate begins with early observation, accurate recording, and prompt reporting of abnormal signs.
- Metabolic abnormalities of diabetes mellitus in pregnancy adversely affect embryonic and fetal development.
- Prepregnancy planning and good diabetic control, coupled with strict diabetic control during pregnancy, may prevent the embryonic, fetal, and neonatal conditions associated with pregnancies complicated by diabetes mellitus.
- Regardless of the infant's disorder or condition, the care provider must remember that the infant belongs to a family that also has many needs.
- Infection in the neonate may be acquired in utero, during birth, during resuscitation, and from within the nursery.
- The most common maternal infections during early pregnancy that are associated with various congenital malformations are represented by the acronym TORCH.
- HIV transmission from mother to infant occurs transplacentally at various gestational ages, perinatally by maternal blood and secretions, and by breast milk.
- The nurse often first observes signs of newborn drug withdrawal and acquires information from the maternal history.
- Providing high-quality perinatal care to a varied population with multiple conditions is complicated by the special needs of high risk drug-dependent clients.
- Signs and symptoms of infant withdrawal vary in time of onset depending on the drug involved.
- Rehabilitative measures must be included in the plan for care for the infant and parents to offer the infant an opportunity for optimum development after discharge.

CRITICAL THINKING EXERCISES

1 Identify the resources available in your community for the drug-exposed infant. Discuss costs and ease of use (location, hours of service).

2 Develop a follow-up plan of care for an infant with HIV being discharged home.

3 Observe care of infants of substance-abusing mothers. Describe nursing care given to calm the infant experiencing withdrawal. Are these interventions evidence based? Suggest research-based interventions that could be implemented.

References

Abel, E. (1997). *Fetal alcohol abuse syndrome revisited.* New York: Plenum Press.

Adriaanse, A. et al. (1996). Neonatal early onset group B streptococcal infection. A nine-year retrospective study in a tertiary care hospital. *J Perinat Med* 24(5), 531-538.

American Academy of Pediatrics Committee on Drugs. (1994). The transfer of drugs and other chemicals into human milk. *Pediatrics* 93(1), 137-150.

American College of Obstetricians and Gynecologists. (1997). Human immunodeficiency virus infection in pregnancy. *Int J Gynecol Obstet* 57, 73-80.

Askin, D. (1995). Bacterial and fungal sepsis in the neonate. *J Obstet Gynecol Neonatal Nurs* 24(7), 635-643.

Beazley, D., & Egerman, R. (1998). Toxoplasmosis. *Semin Perinatol* 22(4), 332-338.

Behrmann, R. (1973). *Neonatology: Diseases of the fetus and infant.* St. Louis: Mosby.

Birthhistle, K., & Carrington, D. (1998). Fetal varicella syndrome—A reappraisal of the literature. *J Infect* 36(S1), 25-29.

Bortolussi, R., & Schlech, W. (1995). Listeriosis. In S. Remington & J. Klein (Eds.). *Infectious diseases of the fetus and newborn infant.* Philadelphia: W.B. Saunders.

Boyer, K. (1996). Diagnosis and treatment of congenital toxoplasmosis. *Adv Pediatr Infect Dis* 11, 449-457.

Brown, H., & Abernathy, M. (1998). Cytomegalovirus infection. *Semin Perinatol* 22(4), 260-266.

Brown, Z. et al. (1997). The acquisition of herpes simplex virus during pregnancy. *N Engl J Med* 337(8), 509-515.

Buchi, K. (1998). The drug exposed infant in the well baby nursery. *Clin Perinatol* 25(2), 335-348.

Burchett, S. (1998). Viral infections. In J. Cloherty & A. Stark (Eds.). *Manual of neonatal care* (4th ed.). Boston: Little, Brown.

Carroll, M. (1990). PCP and hallucinogens. *Adv Alcohol Substance Abuse* 9(1-2), 167-190.

Centers for Disease Control and Prevention. (1996). Prevention of perinatal group B streptococcal disease: A public health perspective. *MMWR* 45(RR-7), 1-24.

Centers for Disease Control and Prevention. (1998). CDC working group on antiretroviral therapy and medical management of HIV-infected children: Guidelines for the use of antiretroviral agents in pediatric HIV infection [On-line]. Available URL: www.cdc.gov/epo/mmwr/preview.

Chapman, S. (1998). Varicella in pregnancy. *Semin Perinatol* 22(4), 339-346.

Chasnoff, I. (1992). Cocaine, pregnancy and the growing child. *Curr Probl Pediatr* 22(7), 302-321.

Church, M., & Abel, E. (1998). Fetal alcohol syndrome: Hearing, speech and vestibular disorders. *Obstet Gynecol Clin North Am* 25(1), 85-97.

Cloherty, J. (1998). Syphilis. In J. Cloherty & A. Stark (Eds.). *Manual of neonatal care* (4th ed.). Boston: Little, Brown.

Corrarino, J. (1998). Perinatal hepatitis B: Update and recommendations. *MCN Am J Matern Child Nurs* 23(5), 246-252.

D'Apolito, K. (1998). Substance abuse: Infant and childhood outcomes. *J Pediatr Nurs* 13(5), 307-316.

Dores, S. et al. (1998). Alcohol versus natural drying for newborn cord care. *J Obstet Gynecol Neonatal Nurs* 27(6), 621-627.

Duff, P. (1998). Hepatitis in pregnancy. *Semin Perinatol* 22(4), 277-283.

Fanaroff, A. & Martin, R. (1995). *Neonatal-perinatal medicine: Diseases of the fetus and infant* (5th ed.). St. Louis: Mosby.

Fanaroff, A., & Martin, R. (1997). *Neonatal-perinatal medicine: Diseases of the fetus and infant* (6th ed.). St. Louis: Mosby.

Fernandes, O. et al. (1998). Moderate to heavy caffeine consumption during pregnancy and relationship to spontaneous abortion and abnormal fetal growth: A meta-analysis. *Reprod Toxicol* 12(4), 435-444.

Figueroa-Damian, R., & Arredondo-Garcia, J. (1998). Pregnancy and tuberculosis: Influence of treatment on perinatal outcome. *Am J Perinatol* 15(5):303-306.

Finnegan, L. (1991). Drug addiction and pregnancy: The newborn. In I. Chasnoff (Ed.). *Drugs, alcohol, pregnancy and parenting.* Boston: Kluwer.

Floyd, R. et al. (1993). A review of smoking in pregnancy: Effect on pregnancy outcome and cessation efforts. *Ann Rev Public Health* 14, 379-411.

Franck, L., & Johnson, L. (1998). Recognition and management of neonates at risk for perinatally acquired infection with human immunodeficiency virus. *Crit Care Nurse* 18(4), 74-85.

Fried, P. (1993). Prenatal exposure to tobacco and marijuana: Effects during pregnancy, infancy and early childhood. *Clin Obstet Gynecol* 36(2), 319-337.

Guerina, N. (1998). Bacterial and fungal infections. In J. Cloherty & A. Stark (Eds.). *Manual of neonatal care* (4th ed.). Boston: Little, Brown.

Guyer, B. et al. (1998). Annual summary of vital statistics—1997. *Pediatrics* 102(6), 1333-1349.

Hollier, L., & Cox, S. (1998). Syphilis. *Semin Perinatol* 22(4), 323-331.

Jacobs, R. (1998). Neonatal herpes simplex virus infections. *Semin Perinatol* 22(1), 64-71.

Joseph, T., Pyati, S., & Jacobs, N. (1998). Neonatal early-onset *Escherichia coli* disease. *Arch Pediatr Adolesc Med* 152(1), 35-40.

Kaltenbach, K., Berghella, V., & Finnegan, L. (1998). Opioid dependence during pregnancy. Effects and management. *Obstet Gynecol Clin North Am* 25(1), 139-151.

Klein, J., & Marcy, S. (1995). Bacterial sepsis and meningitis. In S. Remington & J. Klein (Eds.). *Infectious diseases of the fetus and newborn infant.* Philadelphia: W.B. Saunders.

Kwong, T., & Shearer, D. (1998). Detection of drug use during pregnancy. *Obstet Gynecol Clin North Am* 25(1), 43-64.

Lawrence, R. (1999). *Breastfeeding: A guide for the medical profession* (5th ed.). St. Louis: Mosby.

Lee, M. (1998). Marihuana and tobacco use in pregnancy. *Obstet Gynecol Clin North Am* 25(1), 65-83.

Levine, A., & Rebarber, A. (1995). Methadone maintenance, treatment and the nonstress test. *J Perinatol* 15(3), 229-231.

Lieu, T. et al. (1998). Neonatal group B streptococcal infection in a managed care population. *Obstet Gynecol* 92(1), 21-27.

Lynfield, R., & Guerina, N. (1997). Toxoplasmosis. *Pediatr Rev* 18(3), 75-83.

Medves, J., & O'Brien, B. (1997). Cleaning solutions and bacterial colonization in promoting healing and early separation of the umbilical cord in healthy newborns. *Can J Public Health* 88(6), 380-382.

Merenstein, G., Adams, K., & Weisman, L. (1998). Infection in the neonate. In G. Merenstein & S. Gardner (Eds.). *Handbook of neonatal intensive care* (4th ed.). St. Louis: Mosby.

Merenstein, G., & Gardner, S. (Eds.). (1998). *Handbook of neonatal intensive care* (4th ed.). St. Louis: Mosby.

Milerad, J. et al. (1998). Objective measurements of nicotine exposure in victims of sudden infant death syndrome and in other unexpected child deaths. *J Pediatr* 133(2), 232-236.

Minkoff, H. (1998). Human immunodeficiency virus infection in pregnancy. *Semin Perinatol* 22(4), 293-308.

Moe, P., & Paige, L. (1998). Neurologic disorders. In G. Merenstein & S. Gardner (Eds.). *Handbook of neonatal intensive care* (4th ed.). St. Louis: Mosby.

Mofenson, L. (1997). Mother-child HIV-1 transmission: Timing and determinants. *Obstet Gynecol Clin North Am* 24(4), 759-784.

Nathwani, D., McLean, A., Conway, S., & Carrington, D. (1998). Varicella infections in pregnancy and the newborn. *J Infect* 36(S1), 59-71.

Nelson, N. (1990). *Current therapy in neonatal-perinatal medicine* (2nd ed.). St. Louis: Mosby.

Newshan, G., & Hoyt, J. (1998). Use of combination antiretroviral therapy in pregnant women with HIV disease. *MCN Am J Matern Child Nurs* 23(6), 307-312.

Nolla-Salas, J. et al. (1998). Perinatal listeriosis: A population based multicenter study in Barcelona, Spain. *Am J Perinatol* 15(8), 461-467.

O'Doherty, N. (1986). *Neonatology: Micro atlas of the newborn.* Nutley, NJ: Hoffmann-La Roche.

Ogata, E. (1994). Carbohydrate homeostasis. In G. Avery, M. Fletcher, & M. MacDonald (Eds.). *Pathophysiology and management of the newborn.* Philadelphia: J.B. Lippincott.

Philipson, E., & Herson, V. (1996). Intrapartum chemoprophylaxis for group B streptococcus infection to prevent neonatal disease: Who should be treated? *Am J Perinatol* 13(8), 487-490.

Plessinger, M. (1998). Prenatal exposure to amphetamines. *Obstet Gynecol Clin North Am* 25(1), 119-138.

Plessinger, M., & Woods, J. (1998). Cocaine in pregnancy. *Obstet Gynecol Clin North Am* 25(1), 99-118.

Reece, E. et al. (1998). Pregnancy outcomes among women with and without diabetic microvascular disease (White's classes B to FR) versus nondiabetic controls. *Am J Perinatol* 15(9), 549-555.

Riley, L. (1998). Herpes simplex virus. *Semin Perinatol* 22(4), 284-292.

Rosa, C. (1998). Rubella and rubeola. *Semin Perinatol* 22(4), 318-322.

Santos, I. et al. (1998). Caffeine intake and low birth weight: A population-based case-control study. *Am J Epidemiol* 147(7), 620-627.

Scarlatti, G. (1996). Pediatric HIV infection. *Lancet* 348(9031), 863-867.

Schachter, J., & Grossman, M. (1995). Chlamydia. In J. Remington & J. Klein (Eds.). *Infectious diseases of the fetus and newborn.* Philadelphia: W.B. Saunders.

Schechner, S. (1998). Drug abuse and withdrawal. In J. Cloherty & A. Stark (Eds.). *Manual of neonatal care* (4th ed.). Boston: Little, Brown.

Toltzis, P. (1991). Current issues in neonatal herpes simplex virus infection. *Clin Perinatol* 18(2), 193-208.

Tuomala, R. (1997). Prevention of transmission. *Obstet Gynecol Clin North Am* 24(4), 785-795.

Tyrala, E. (1996). The infant of the diabetic mother. *Obstet Gynecol Clin North Am* 23(1), 221-240.

Wagner, C. et al. (1998). The impact of prenatal drug exposure on the neonate. *Obstet Gynecol Clin North Am* 25(1), 169-194.

Weiner, L., & Morse, B. (1991). FAS: Clinical perspectives and prevention. In I. Chasnoff (Ed.). *Drugs, alcohol, pregnancy and parenting.* Boston: Kluwer.

Wong, D. (1999). *Whaley and Wong's nursing care of infants and children* (6th ed.). St. Louis: Mosby.

Wong, D. & Perry, S. (1998). *Maternal child nursing care.* St. Louis: Mosby.

40

Hemolytic Disorders and Congenital Anomalies

Gayle Tart Davis

LEARNING OBJECTIVES

- Define the key terms.
- Discuss assessment of the newborn for hyperbilirubinemia.
- Develop a nursing plan of care for the prevention, identification, and management of hyperbilirubinemia in a newborn.
- Compare Rh and ABO incompatibility.
- Explain nursing management to prevent the pathologic consequences of hyperbilirubinemia.
- Review prenatal diagnosis of neonatal disorders.
- Present assessment strategies during the postnatal period to aid in diagnosis of congenital disorders.

- Describe preoperative and postoperative nursing care of the newborn.
- Develop a nursing plan of care for parents of a newborn with a defect or disorder.
- Describe each congenital disorder presented in this chapter and identify the priority of nursing care for each.
- Identify topics for nursing research related to developmental problems.

KEY TERMS

ABO incompatibility	erythroblastosis fetalis	intrauterine transfusion
anencephaly	esophageal atresia	isoimmunization
choanal atresia	exchange transfusions	jaundice
choreoathetoid cerebral palsy	gastroschisis	kernicterus
cleft lip or palate	hydramnios	microcephaly
clubfoot	hydrocephalus	myelomeningocele
congenital	hydrops fetalis	neural tube defects
Coombs' test	hyperbilirubinemia	omphalocele
developmental dysplasia of the hip	hypospadias	$Rh_0(D)$ immune globulin
diaphragmatic hernia	imperforate anus	teratoma
epispadias	inborn errors of metabolism	

The physiologic alterations that occur in infants during the newborn period can differ and have varying effects. The nurse must be alert to the presence of any deviations from normal, ranging from an obvious congenital anomaly, such as myelomeningocele, to a less obvious deviation such as an increase in the bilirubin level or a congenital heart defect, neither of which may be immediately symptomatic. The nurse must therefore possess the assessment skills necessary to detect any deviation from normal, as well as the knowledge base necessary to participate in the skilled care called for in such affected infants. The nurse must also be cognizant of the special needs of the family with a child who is born with or acquires an abnormal condition.

The complications that affect newborns can stem from three basic problems: problems relating to gestational age or intrauterine growth that does not follow normal patterns, such as a preterm birth; acquired problems resulting from maternal or newborn physiologic factors, such as ABO incompatibility or respiratory distress syndrome; and physical problems, such as congenital anomalies or birth defects.

HYPERBILIRUBINEMIA

Hyperbilirubinemia is the name for the condition in which the bilirubin level in the blood is increased. It is characterized by a yellow discoloration of the skin, mucous membranes, sclera, and various organs. This yellow discoloration is referred to as **jaundice,** or *icterus.* Jaundice is caused primarily by the accumulation in the skin of unconjugated bilirubin, a breakdown product of hemoglobin forming after its release from hemolyzed red blood cells. Physiologic jaundice, discussed in Chapters 26 and 27, is the most common abnormal finding in newborns and is usually benign. The challenge in the care of neonates with hyperbilirubinemia is to distinguish physiologic jaundice from a serious clinical pathologic condition.

Physiologic Jaundice

Physiologic jaundice occurs in about half of all healthy full-term newborns and typically arises more than 24 hours after birth. In both Caucasian and African-American infants it is manifested by a progressive increase in the unconjugated bilirubin level in cord blood of from 2 mg/dl to a mean peak of 5 to 6 mg/dl between 60 and 72 hours of age. In Asian and Native American infants the level may increase to 10 to 14 mg/dl between 72 and 120 hours of age. Resolution in Caucasian and African-American newborns is evidenced by a rapid decline in the unconjugated bilirubin level to 2 mg/dl by 5 days after birth; in Asian and Native American infants this takes 7 to 10 days.

Physiologic jaundice is more common and typically more severe in preterm infants, in whom the serum bilirubin level typically reaches a mean peak of 10 to 12 mg/dl by the fifth day of life. The primary reason why it takes longer for the maximum concentration to be reached in preterm than in full-term infants is that the livers of preterm infants are immature, and hence liver function is not fully developed.

Pathologic Jaundice

Pathologic jaundice, or hyperbilirubinemia, is not defined solely in terms of the serum concentrations of unconju-

gated bilirubin. It also refers to that level of serum bilirubin which, if left untreated, can result in kernicterus, or the deposition of bilirubin in the brain and in other body cells. Following are the findings that support a diagnosis of pathologic jaundice and that, if encountered in an infant, warrant further investigation (Fanaroff & Martin, 1997):

- Serum bilirubin concentrations of greater than 4 mg/dl in cord blood
- Clinical jaundice evident within 24 hours of birth
- Total serum bilirubin levels increasing by more than 5 mg/dl in 24 hours or increasing at a rate of 0.5 mg/dl or greater over a 4- to 8-hour period
- A serum bilirubin level in a full-term newborn that exceeds 15 mg/dl at any time or clinical jaundice lasting more than 10 days
- A serum bilirubin level in a preterm newborn that exceeds 10 mg/dl at any time
- Any case of visible jaundice that persists for more than 10 days of life in a full-term infant or 21 days in a preterm infant, unless the infant is receiving breast milk

There are many potential causes of pathologic hyperbilirubinemia in neonates. The most common is incompatibility between the maternal and fetal blood, specifically Rh and ABO incompatibility, and these are discussed later in this chapter. Other, less common, conditions that may be associated with pathologic jaundice in the neonate are bacterial or nonbacterial maternal infections and maternal medical conditions such as diabetes. In addition, oxytocin administration and the maternal ingestion of sulfonamides, diazepam, or salicylates near the time of birth can affect the neonate's ability to excrete bilirubin.

There are also neonatal conditions that can predispose to the development of pathologic hyperbilirubinemia. One of these is the decreased ability of preterm or low-birth-weight neonates to conjugate bilirubin because of an ineffective glucuronyl transferase enzyme system. Hepatic cell damage caused by infection or drugs also interferes with the functioning of this enzyme system. Other conditions that can result in pathologic jaundice include neonatal hypothyroidism or other metabolic abnormalities; polycythemia resulting from twin-to-twin transfusion or the transfusion of a large volume of blood by means of the placenta; and an intestinal obstruction such as meconium ileus (the most common manifestation of cystic fibrosis in the neonate) or pyloric stenosis or that resulting from such disorders as Hirschsprung disease. Biliary atresia may also cause jaundice, but such jaundice usually occurs after the neonatal period.

Sequestered blood can also be responsible for causing pathologic jaundice. Such an increase in the serum bilirubin level occurs when the blood in cephalhematomas, ecchymosis, or hemangiomas or the blood that becomes trapped during bleeding into internal organs is hemolyzed. Maternal blood swallowed by the neonate during birth may also be responsible for causing the bilirubin levels to increase as the blood is absorbed and broken down in the neonate's intestinal mucosa.

Kernicterus

The goal of the care given the infant with hyperbilirubinemia is the prevention of kernicterus. **Kernicterus,** or bilirubin encephalopathy, is caused by the deposition of bilirubin in the brain, especially within the basal ganglia, cerebellum, and hippocampus. This deposition can occur because unconjugated bilirubin is highly lipid soluble, making it capable of crossing the blood-brain barrier if it is not bound to protein. It results in the yellowish staining of the brain tissue and the necrosis of neurons and occurs if the concentration of unconjugated bilirubin reaches toxic levels. Kernicterus, which can develop in newborns who show no apparent signs of clinical jaundice, is generally considered to be directly related to the total serum bilirubin level, although these levels alone do not predict the risk of brain injury. In a full-term infant, a serum bilirubin level of 25 mg/dl is considered the upper limit beyond which the risk for kernicterus increases, although the condition may occur at much lower levels in premature infants or infants with other complications. In some high risk, low-birthweight infants, a mean peak level of unconjugated bilirubin of even 10 to 12 mg/dl may be associated with the development of kernicterus (Fanaroff & Martin, 1997). Some of the perinatal events that increase the likelihood of kernicterus developing, even at these lower bilirubin levels, include hypoxia, asphyxia, acidosis, hypothermia, hypoglycemia, sepsis, treatment with certain medications, and hypoalbuminemia. These conditions cause kernicterus by interfering with the conjugation of bilirubin or by competing for albumin-binding sites. The resulting unconjugated bilirubin can then pass through the blood-brain barrier and enter the brain, resulting in kernicterus.

Kernicterus has been associated with acute and long-term symptoms of neurologic damage; it is never present at birth. The clinical manifestations typically appear between 2 and 6 days after birth and go through several phases as the disease progresses, generally beginning after the bilirubin level has peaked. During the first phase, the newborn is hypotonic and lethargic and shows a poor suck and depressed or absent Moro reflex. These more subtle signs are followed by the appearance of a high-pitched cry, opisthotonos (severe muscle spasm that causes the back to arch acutely), spasticity, hyperreflexia, and often by fever and seizures. All of this occurs over a period of about 24 hours. About half of the affected infants survive, although they often suffer permanent neurologic sequelae, such as choreoathetoid cerebral palsy or ataxia, sensorineural hearing loss, perceptual problems, mental retardation, or an attention deficit disorder.

Choreoathetoid cerebral palsy is a chronic condition characterized by both choreiform (jerky, ticlike twitching) and athetoid (slow, writhing) movements. Fortunately, because it is now possible to identify the problem early and institute timely treatment with phototherapy and exchange transfusions, the classic bilirubin encephalopathy just described is not as prevalent as it once was.

NURSE ALERT *There have been reports of several cases of kernicterus in infants of mothers who were discharged early after birth. The discharge teaching for and follow-up of infants who are discharged early is therefore imperative.*

Hemolytic Disease of the Newborn

The most common causes of pathologic hyperbilirubinemia are hemolytic diseases of the newborn. These occur most often if the blood groups of the mother and baby are different, and the most frequent of these are ABO and Rh factor incompatibilities.

The four major blood groups in the ABO system are A, B, AB, and O. People with type A blood have A antigen, those with type B have B antigen, those with type AB have both A and B antigens, and those with type O have no antigen. In turn, people with type A blood have plasma antibodies to type B blood, those with type B blood have antibodies to type A blood, those with type AB blood have no antibodies, and those with type O blood have antibodies to type A and B blood. If a person is administered or exposed to an incompatible blood type, he or she will form antibodies against the antigen in that blood, with an agglutination, or clumping, occurring as the antibodies in the plasma mix with the antigens of the different blood group.

The Rh factor, which is a genetically determined factor present on red blood cells, can be a major source of incompatibility. There are several forms of the Rh antigen, with the D antigen the most significant one because it causes the most antibody production in a person who is Rh negative. Rh positivity is a dominant trait, so one must inherit the recessive gene from both parents to be Rh negative. A person who has the Rh factor is considered Rh positive; a person without it is considered Rh negative. As an illustration of the foregoing discussion, a mother who has A-negative blood has the A antigen, plasma antibodies to the B antigen, and no Rh factor on her red blood cells.

Hemolytic disorders occur because maternal antibodies are present naturally or form in response to an antigen from the fetal blood crossing the placenta and entering the maternal circulation. The maternal antibodies of the IgG class in turn cross the placenta, causing hemolysis of the fetal red blood cells, resulting in hyperbilirubinemia and jaundice.

ABO incompatibility. **ABO incompatibility** is more common than Rh incompatibility but causes less severe problems in the affected infant. It occurs if the fetal blood type is A, B, or AB and the maternal type is O. It occurs rarely in infants with type B blood born to mothers with type A blood. The incompatibility arises because naturally occurring anti-A and anti-B antibodies are transferred across the placenta to the fetus. Unlike the situation that pertains to Rh incompatibility (discussed in the next section), firstborn infants may be affected, because mothers with type O blood already have anti-A and anti-B antibodies in their blood. Such a newborn may show a weakly positive result to a direct Coombs' test. The cord bilirubin level usually is less than 4 mg/dl, and any resulting hyperbilirubinemia usually can be treated with phototherapy. Exchange transfusions are required only occasionally. Although jaundice is frequently observed during the first 24 hours of the neonate's life and ABO incompatibility is a frequent cause of hyperbilirubinemia, it rarely precipitates significant anemia resulting from the hemolysis of red blood cells.

Rh incompatibility. Rh incompatibility, or **isoimmunization,** occurs when an Rh-negative mother has an Rh-positive fetus who inherits the dominant Rh-positive gene from the father. If the mother is Rh negative and the father is Rh positive and homozygous for the Rh factor, all the offspring will be Rh positive. If the father is heterozygous for the factor, there is a 50% chance that each infant born of the union will be Rh positive and a 50% chance that each will be born Rh negative (see Fig. 14-14). An Rh-negative fetus is in no danger because it has the same Rh factor as the mother. An Rh-negative fetus with an Rh-positive mother is also in no danger. It is only the Rh-positive offspring of an Rh-negative mother who is at risk. From 10% to 15% of all Caucasian couples and about 5% of African-American couples have Rh incompatibility. It is rare in Asian couples. The incidence of Rh sensitization and resulting hemolytic disease of the newborn has decreased dramatically since the development of $Rh_0(D)$ immune globulin in 1968.

New treatment modalities, including early detection and fetal blood transfusions, have improved the outcome of affected fetuses. However, hemolytic disease of the fetus or newborn resulting from isoimmunization continues to be a significant problem in the United States.

The pathogenesis of Rh incompatibility is as follows. Hematopoiesis in the fetus, or the formation of blood cells, begins as early as the eighth week of gestation and, in up to 40% of pregnancies, these cells pass through the placenta into the maternal circulation. Whenever the fetus is Rh positive and the mother Rh negative, the mother forms antibodies against the fetal blood cells—first IgM antibodies that are too large to pass through the placenta, and then later, IgG antibodies that can cross the placenta. The process of antibody formation is called *maternal sensitization.* Sensitization may occur during pregnancy, birth, abortion, or amniocentesis. Usually women become sensitized in their first pregnancy with an Rh-positive fetus but do not produce enough antibodies to cause lysis of fetal blood cells. During subsequent pregnancies, antibodies form in response to repeated contact with the antigen from the fetal blood, resulting in lysis or destruction of fetal red blood cells.

Severe Rh incompatibility results in marked fetal hemolytic anemia, because the fetal erythrocytes are destroyed by maternal Rh-positive antibodies. Although the placenta usually clears the bilirubin generated by the red blood cell breakdown, in extreme cases fetal bilirubin levels increase. This results in fetal jaundice, also known as *icterus gravis.*

The fetus compensates for the anemia by producing large numbers of immature erythrocytes to replace those hemolyzed, thus the name for this condition—**erythroblastosis fetalis.** In the most severe form of this disease, **hydrops fetalis,** the fetus has marked anemia, together with cardiac decompensation, cardiomegaly, and hepatosplenomegaly. Hypoxia results from the severe anemia. In addition, because of the decreased intravascular oncotic pressure involved, fluid leaks out of the intravascular space, resulting in generalized edema, as well as effusions into the peritoneal (ascites), pericardial, and pleural (hydrothorax) spaces. The placenta is often edematous, which, along with the edematous fetus, can cause the uterus to rupture.

Intrauterine or early neonatal death may occur as a result of hydrops fetalis, although intrauterine exchange transfusions and early birth of the fetus may avert this. **Intrauterine transfusion** involves the infusion of Rh-negative, type O blood into the umbilical vein. Such transfusions are administered as needed until birth.

▪ CARE MANAGEMENT

Assessment and Nursing Diagnoses

It is important to determine the blood type and Rh factor of the pregnant woman prenatally. A thorough history must then be obtained in the Rh-negative pregnant woman to assess for the existence of events that could have caused her to develop antibodies to the Rh factor. Such events include previous pregnancy with an Rh-positive fetus; transfusion with Rh-positive blood, which causes immediate sensitization; miscarriage or induced abortion after 8 or more gestational weeks; amniocentesis performed for any reason; premature separation of the placenta; and trauma.

Because hematopoiesis begins in the fetus during the eighth gestational week, a woman who has experienced a miscarriage or induced abortion after this time or has previously given birth to a child may have been inoculated with fetal blood at the time of placental separation. During amniocentesis, the needle may cause localized damage to the single layer of cells that separates the maternal and fetal circulation in the placenta, thereby allowing fetal red blood cells to enter the maternal circulation.

If any of these events have occurred, the woman's record is checked to determine whether she has received $Rh_0(D)$ **immune globulin,** such as Rhogam, which is a commercial preparation of passive antibodies against the Rh factor. This injection of anti-Rh antibodies destroys any fetal red blood cells that are in the maternal circulation by causing the cells to be phagocytosed before the woman's immune system is activated to produce antibodies.

An indirect **Coombs' test** should be done at the first prenatal visit of an Rh-negative woman with a fetus who may be Rh-positive to determine whether she has antibodies to the Rh antigen. In this test the maternal blood serum is mixed with Rh-positive red blood cells. If the Rh-positive red blood cells agglutinate or clump, this indicates that maternal antibodies are present. The dilution of the specimen of blood at which clumping occurs determines the titer, or level, of maternal antibodies. This titer indicates the degree of maternal sensitization. A level of 1:8 rarely results in fetal jeopardy. If the titer reaches 1:16, amniocentesis is performed to determine optical density (delta OD) of amniotic fluid to estimate the fetal hemolytic process (see Chapter 29). Bilirubin discolors the amniotic fluid. Rising bilirubin levels may indicate the need for an intrauterine transfusion.

The indirect Coombs' test is repeated at 28 weeks and, if the result remains negative, indicating that sensitization has not occurred, the woman is given an intramuscular injection of $Rh_0(D)$ immune globulin. If the test result is positive, showing that sensitization has occurred, it is then repeated every 4 to 6 weeks to monitor the maternal antibody titer, as just described. Examples of nursing diagnoses pertinent to newborns at risk because of hyperbilirubinemia include the following:

Nursing Diagnoses

* Risk for injury to neurons and cells in the kidney, pancreas, and intestine related to
  - hyperbilirubinemia
* Impaired gas exchange related to
  - hemolytic anemia
* Risk for fluid volume deficit related to
  - phototherapy
* Risk for parental anxiety related to
  - hyperbilirubinemia, its management, and potential sequelae
* Risk for impaired skin integrity related to
  - increased stooling while undergoing phototherapy
* Risk for ineffective thermoregulation (increased or decreased) related to
  - phototherapy

Expected Outcomes of Care

Hospital protocols for the care of infants with hyperbilirubinemia are developed as a collaborative effort of the health care team. These protocols are then used in individualizing care for the infant and parents. Expected outcomes for care are stated in client-centered terms, as in the following:

* The infant's prenatal and perinatal risk factors will be identified, and intervention will be implemented when appropriate.

* The infant will not develop hyperbilirubinemia or its sequela, kernicterus.
* The infant will have minimal or no sequelae from hyperbilirubinemia and its treatment.
* The infant will tolerate the treatment for hyperbilirubinemia without complications.
* The infant's serum bilirubin levels will return to normal.
* The infant's parents will demonstrate an understanding of the infant's condition, the therapies, and the possible sequelae of the condition.

Plan of Care and Interventions

Prenatally the prevention of hyperbilirubinemia is the primary focus of care. The implementation of interventions focused on the care of the woman whose fetus is considered at risk for hyperbilirubinemia is essential to prevent problems in the newborn. Prenatal control of diabetes mellitus, prevention of maternal infection, avoidance of drugs such as diazepam and salicylates near the time of birth, and prevention of preterm birth reduce the risk.

There must be early identification of the Rh-negative woman, and care must be taken to prevent sensitization. The Rh-negative woman should be asked about any blood transfusion or any of the other factors already cited that would predispose her to sensitization. $Rh_0(D)$ immune globulin is administered in the following amounts to Rh-negative women whose Coombs' tests are negative (Fanaroff & Martin, 1997; Wandstrat, 1997):

* 50 μg
  After chorionic villus sampling, ectopic pregnancy, or abortion before 13 weeks of gestation
* 300 μg
  After miscarriage or elective abortion after 13 weeks of gestation
  After percutaneous umbilical sampling
  After amniocentesis
  After abruptio placentae or placenta previa
  After trauma
  At 28 weeks of gestation
  Within 72 hours of the preterm or term birth of an Rh-positive infant
* More than 300 μg
  After large transplacental hemorrhage
  After mismatched blood transfusion

The fetus and maternal antibody titers are monitored prenatally. If amniocentesis reveals that the delta OD is high and the fetus is in jeopardy, intrauterine transfusion may be done every 1 to 2 weeks between 26 and 32 weeks. If the endangered fetus is at more than 32 weeks of gestation, a preterm birth may be indicated, usually by cesarean.

Postpartum interventions focus on preventing sensitization in the mother, if it has not occurred already, and treating any complications in the neonate resulting from the hemolysis of red blood cells (see Plan of Care). The un-

PLAN of CARE | Infant with Hyperbilirubinemia

NURSING DIAGNOSIS Risk for injury related to hemolytic disease and treatment effects

Expected Outcomes *Bilirubin levels decrease with treatment, there is no evidence of harmful effects from phototherapy (i.e., no eye irritation, dehydration, temperature instability, or skin breakdown), and there are no complications from exchange transfusions.*

Nursing Interventions/*Rationales*

Initiate early feedings *to enhance excretion of bilirubin in stools.*

Observe skin and mucous membranes for signs of jaundice, *indicative of rising bilirubin levels;* monitor serum bilirubin levels *to determine rate of rise and treatment response.*

Note time of jaundice onset *to help distinguish physiologic from other causes of jaundice.*

Observe for signs of hypoxia, hypothermia, hypoglycemia, and metabolic acidosis, *which occur as a result of hyperbilirubinemia and increase the risk of brain damage.*

Initiate phototherapy per physician order *to decrease bilirubin levels.*

During phototherapy, shield infant's eyes *to prevent damage to corneas and retinas;* keep infant nude and change positions frequently *for maximum body surface exposure;* cleanse skin frequently *to prevent irritation;* maintain adequate fluid intake *to prevent dehydration;* monitor body temperature *to prevent hyperthermia.*

Before exchange transfusion, keep infant on nothing-by-mouth (NPO) status (2 to 4 hours) *to prevent aspiration;* check donor blood for compatibility *to prevent transfusion reaction;* have resuscitation equipment (oxygen, Ambu bag, endotracheal tubes, laryngoscope) at bedside *in preparation for emergency action.*

Assist physician with exchange transfusion procedure; track amounts of blood withdrawn and transfused *to*

maintain balanced blood volume; maintain body temperature *to avoid hypothermia and cold stress;* monitor vital signs and observe for rash *for indicators of transfusion reaction.*

After transfusion, continue to monitor vital signs *for transfusion reaction or other complications;* check umbilical cord *for bleeding or signs of infection.*

NURSING DIAGNOSIS Risk for knowledge deficit related to administration of home phototherapy

Expected Outcome *Family demonstrates ability to provide home therapy.*

Nursing Interventions/*Rationales*

Explore family's willingness to try home phototherapy *to evaluate feasibility of home therapy option.*

Explore family's understanding of jaundice and proposed therapy *to establish baseline for teaching.*

Teach family with demonstration–return demonstration, allowing for several practice sessions, and supplement with written materials with pictorial representations *to ensure safe and optimum results.*

Include the following in your instructions: placement of lamp or fiberoptic unit; proper eye care and patching; proper skin care; proper positioning under lamp; provision of increased fluid intake; monitoring of time under lamp; monitoring of vital signs, skin, eyes, feeding patterns, stooling and voiding patterns; observation for complications.

Stress importance of obtaining the prescribed bilirubin tests on schedule *as a way of tracking success of therapy.*

Give parents a contact if they have any questions while carrying out therapy *to offer ongoing support and increase parent comfort.*

From Wong, D., & Perry, S. (1998). *Maternal child nursing care.* St. Louis: Mosby.

---

sensitized Rh-negative mother whose baby is Rh positive should receive 300 g of $Rh_0(D)$ immune globulin within 72 hours of birth. This should prevent her from producing antibodies to the fetal blood cells that entered her bloodstream during the birth.

The neonate's cord blood is sent to the laboratory to determine the infant's blood type and Rh status. A direct Coombs' test is performed on this cord blood to determine whether there are maternal antibodies in the fetal blood. If antibodies are found to be present, the titer, in-

dicating the degree of maternal sensitization, is measured. If the titer is 1:64, an exchange transfusion is indicated. In addition, the prevention of or prompt therapy for perinatal asphyxia, acidosis, cold stress, sepsis, and hypoglycemia will decrease the newborn's risk for severe hemolytic disease and his or her susceptibility to kernicterus. Early feeding is also initiated to stimulate the gastrocolic reflex and thus facilitate the removal of bilirubin through stooling.

If pathologic jaundice is present, the cause is determined and therapeutic management begun. This includes monitoring and reducing the raised bilirubin level. The bilirubin level can also be measured noninvasively using transcutaneous bilirubinometry. This is a screening test for neonatal jaundice that uses as its basis the relationship between the yellow color of the skin and the total serum bilirubin level.

Phototherapy is used to reduce the serum bilirubin levels, particularly if the jaundice is physiologic rather than pathologic, the jaundice occurs past the 24-hour period after birth, and the bilirubin levels are generally less than 15 mg/dl. Phototherapy using bili-lights or a phototherapy blanket is carried out in the normal newborn nursery (see Chapter 27 and Fig. 27-16).

Exchange transfusions are needed less frequently today because of the decrease in the incidence of hemolytic disease in newborns resulting from isoimmunization. However, it is still the treatment of choice for some infants, with recommendations for treatment based on the total serum bilirubin and the age of the infant. For example, it is recommended that a healthy term newborn between 25 and 48 hours old receive an exchange transfusion after intensive phototherapy has failed to produce a decrease in total serum bilirubin of 1 to 2 mg/dl within 4 to 6 hours, with the total serum bilirubin continuing to fall and remaining below 20 mg/dl (Frank, Cooper, & Merenstein, 1998). Other indications for transfusion include a positive direct Coombs' test performed on cord blood; a hemoglobin concentration of less than 12 g/dl, indicating hemolytic disease in the newborn; hydrops fetalis; or signs of cardiac failure. In addition, because premature infants are thought to be more susceptible to bilirubin toxicity than term infants, treatment strategies have been aimed at keeping serum bilirubin levels lower in these infants (Bratlid, 1996). Other factors must always be considered as well, particularly the clinical condition of the infant, because it is a procedure with many potential complications and a mortality risk of about 0.5% (Frank et al., 1998).

An exchange transfusion reduces the serum bilirubin level in infants who have severe hyperbilirubinemia resulting from any cause. In infants with Rh incompatibility, it removes the red blood cells that would otherwise be hemolyzed by circulating maternal antibodies, removes the antibodies responsible for hemolysis, and corrects the anemia caused by hemolysis of the infant's sensitized red blood cells. It also reduces the serum bilirubin level in infants who have severe hyperbilirubinemia resulting from any cause.

Exchange transfusion is accomplished by alternately removing a small amount of the infant's blood and replacing it with an equal amount of donor blood. If the infant has Rh incompatibility, type O Rh-negative blood is used for transfusion, so the maternal antibodies still present in the infant do not hemolyze the transfused blood. Depending on the infant's size, maturity, and condition, amounts of from 5 to 20 ml of the infant's blood are removed at one time and replaced with donor blood. The total amount of blood exchanged approximates 170 ml/kg of body weight, or 75% to 85% of the infant's total blood volume. The amount exchanged is limited to no more than 500 ml. During the procedure the health care team members observe the infection control precautions for invasive procedures. The infant is monitored closely during and after the procedure, including the heart rate and rhythm, respirations, blood pressure, temperature, pedal pulses, and the presence of edema. Hypervolemia or hypovolemia, as well as air emboli, may be a complication of the procedure. Symptoms of hypocalcemia, such as jitteriness, irritability, convulsions, tachycardia, and electrocardiogram changes, may be triggered by preservatives in the donor blood that lower the infant's serum calcium level. This may necessitate an infusion of calcium gluconate to correct the deficit. The nurse also monitors the infusion site for hemorrhage and is constantly alert for any other complications that may occur, such as embolization or thrombosis, volume overload and cardiac arrest, other electrolyte abnormalities, and overheparinization and bleeding (Frank et al., 1998).

Ongoing clinical trials are studying the treatment of hyperbilirubinemia by a modality that involves using a drug to decrease bilirubin production. Heme oxygenase (HO) is the first enzyme in the heme catabolic sequence that results in bilirubin. Inhibition of HO activity therefore prevents the production of bilirubin. A metalloporphyrin, such as tin mesoporphyrin (SnMP), is a compound that is an HO inhibitor. When bilirubin production is suppressed by the administration of SnMP, heme is excreted directly into bile. Infants receiving a single dose of SnMP have lower peak bilirubin levels and a decreased need for phototherapy. Clinical studies have shown that side effects have been minimal and that dosages used in the studies appear to be safe for administration to newborns for the management of hyperbilirubinemia. Metalloporphyrins are not approved by the Food and Drug Administration for use in humans, and much work remains to be done with regard to safety, efficacy, and clinical dosing (Dixit & Gartner, 1999). Additional studies are ongoing (Dennery & Rodgers, 1996; Drummond, Valaes, & Kappas, 1996; Frank et al., 1998).

Phenobarbital is effective in reducing serum bilirubin levels in newborns. It is not commonly used, however, primarily because it requires up to 6 days of treatment for maximum effect (Dixit & Gartner, 1999).

A device that measures carbon monoxide production, which is an index of bilirubin production, is being evaluated. This noninvasive device measures carbon monoxide by sampling expired air with a small nasal catheter. Hemolysis can be identified before anemia and hyperbilirubinemia develop (Augustine, 1999).

Planning for rehabilitative measures is necessary if kernicterus occurs. The family will need the services of many community resources to care for the affected child. An interdisciplinary approach that includes social services must be taken (see Home Care box).

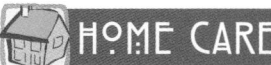

HOME CARE

Monitoring for Jaundice After Early Discharge

If the infant is discharged from the hospital before 48 hours of age, the parents should receive teaching regarding adequate hydration and assessment of the infant for the appearance of jaundice. Appropriate testing and follow-up of the infant should be available. A program of home phototherapy, where available, allows infants to receive treatment of uncomplicated hyperbilirubinemia following discharge from the hospital. For these infants, nurses provide monitoring of treatment and of serum bilirubin levels as outlined by hospital or agency policy.

Evaluation

On a short-term basis, the nurse can consider nursing care to be effective to the degree that the following outcomes for care are achieved.

CONGENITAL ANOMALIES

The desired and expected outcome of every wanted pregnancy is a normal, functioning infant with a good intellectual potential. Fulfillment of this hope depends on numerous hereditary and environmental factors. Probably all human characteristics have a genetic component, including those that produce symptoms or physical abnormalities that impair the fitness of the person. Some disorders or diseases occur through the influence of a single gene or the combined action of many genes inherited from the parents; others result from the action of the intrauterine environment. Many defects appear to occur as the result of multifactorial inheritance, which is the interaction of multiple genes with environmental factors that affect the embryonic development of the affected system. Examples of these include neural tube defects, congenital heart defects, congenital hip dysplasia, and cleft lip or palate. Research is adding information about factors that might cause congenital anomalies (Chuangsuwanich et al., 1998; Hoek, Brown, & Susser, 1998; Queisser-Luft et al., 1996; Schaefer et al., 1997; Yerkes et al., 1998).

A disease or disorder that is transmitted from generation to generation is termed *genetic* or *hereditary*. A **congenital** disorder is one that is present at birth and can be caused by genetic or environmental factors, or both. Some congenital disorders such as inborn errors of metabolism and mental retardation are not malformations.

Congenital anomalies are evident in 2% to 3% of all live births (Steele, 1997), but this number increases to about 6% by 5 years of age, when more anomalies are diagnosed. In addition, the incidence of congenital malformations in fetuses that are spontaneously aborted is higher than that in infants who are born alive, thus also adding to the overall incidence. Major congenital defects are the leading cause of death in infants younger than 1 year of age in the United States and account for 20% of neonatal deaths. Although there has been a decrease in the incidences of other causes of neonatal mortality, the death rate associated with most congenital anomalies has essentially remained stable since 1932.

The most common major congenital anomalies that cause serious problems in the neonate are congenital heart disease, neural tube defects, cleft lip or palate, clubfoot, and congenital hip dysplasia. These are thought to result from the interaction of multiple genetic and environmental factors. Minor anomalies are less apparent but are important to identify because they may be a part of a characteristic pattern of malformations. That is, they may point to the presence of a more serious major anomaly and aid in its diagnosis. For example, about 15% of newborns have a minor anomaly; of these, only 1.4% also have a major anomaly. In contrast, only 0.5% of newborns have three or more minor anomalies, but the probability of these infants also having a major anomaly is 90% (Fanaroff & Martin, 1997). Minor malformations are more common in areas of the body that have variable features, such as the face and distal extremities. Some of the most common malformations include the lack of a helical fold of the pinna, complete or incomplete simian creases, and a capillary hemangioma other than on the face or posterior aspect of the neck.

The seriousness of congenital anomalies in terms of their effect on society is reflected in the more than six million hospital days and $200 billion a year required for the care and treatment of these neonates. Ways of preventing and detecting these anomalies are being improved continuously, as are techniques for the care of the fetus with certain anomalies. Promoting the availability of these services to populations at risk challenges community health care systems. An interdisciplinary team approach is vital for providing holistic care: the surgical treatment, rehabilitation, and education of the child, as well as psychosocial and financial assistance for the parents. Parental disappointment and disillusion add to the complexity of the nursing care needed for these infants.

Cardiovascular System Anomalies

During fetal development there are periods when cell division and differentiation of the organs and tissues of a particular body system are occurring rapidly. During these various sensitive, or critical, periods, particular body systems are more susceptible to environmental influences *early gestat.* than they are later in gestation. For example, the critical period for the cardiovascular system is from week 3 of embryonic development to week 8, a time when many women may not be aware that they are pregnant.

Congenital heart defects (CHDs) are anatomic abnormalities in the heart that are present at birth, although they may not be diagnosed immediately. Some type of cardiologic problem is present in 1 of every 100 live births (Daberkow-Carson & Washington, 1998). Ventricular septal defects, constituting more than 20% of all CHDs, are the most common type of acyanotic lesion. Tetralogy of Fallot, constituting 10% of all CHDs, is the most common type resulting in cyanosis. After prematurity, CHDs are the next major cause of death in the first year of life.

The etiology of CHDs is unknown in more than 90% of the cases. This is an important fact for parents to know, because they often feel guilt that they have done something to cause the defect. Maternal factors that are associated with a higher incidence of CHD include:

• Viral infections such as rubella
• Ingestion of folic acid antagonists or anticonvulsants such as phenytoin, progesterone, estrogen, lithium, or warfarin (Coumadin)
• Use of the acne medication isotretinoin (Accutane)
• Alcoholism
• Poor nutrition
• Radiation exposure
• Complications of pregnancy such as age over 40 or antepartal bleeding
• Metabolic disorders such as diabetes mellitus and phenylketonuria

There is also an increased likelihood of cardiac disease in low-birth-weight infants, especially those small for gestational age, as well as in premature infants and those with congenital infections. In addition, CHDs may be associated with other extracardiac defects such as renal agenesis, tracheoesophageal fistula, and diaphragmatic hernias.

Genetic factors are implicated in the pathogenesis of CHD. As a general rule, these defects are thought to be multifactorial in origin, involving both genetic and environmental influences; however, a familial occurrence of virtually all forms of CHD has been noted. If a family has one affected child, the risk for having a second child with CHD has been thought to be 1% to 3%; the risk for the acquisition of some defects is greater than this. For example, the risk for left-sided lesions such as hypoplastic left heart syndrome and coarctation of the aorta is higher (Wong, 1999). If the father is affected, the risk of having a child with CHD is 1% to 3%; it is 2% to 10% if the mother is affected. This inherited risk will become more important as children with CHD live longer and reproduce; therefore continuing epidemiologic studies are needed in this area.

Chromosomal abnormalities may also be associated with CHDs. For example, 45% of children with trisomy 21, or Down syndrome, have a cardiac defect. All children who have trisomy 18, the second most common chromosomal abnormality, have cardiac anomalies. About 95% of trisomy 18 fetuses miscarry, and the survivors usually die within the first year of life.

Although traditionally CHD has been classified as either cyanotic or acyanotic, a classification that categorizes cardiac defects physiologically is now considered more de-

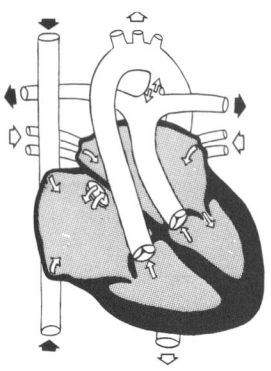

Complete transposition of great vessels

The anomaly is an embryologic defect caused by a straight division of the bulbar trunk without normal spiraling. As a result, the aorta originates from the right ventricle, and the pulmonary artery from the left ventricle. An abnormal communication between the two circulations must be present to sustain life.

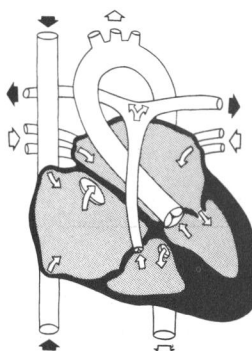

Tricuspid atresia

Tricuspid valvular atresia is characterized by a small right ventricle, large left ventricle, and usually a diminished pulmonary circulation. Blood from the right atrium passes through an atrial septal defect into the left atrium, mixes with oxygenated blood returning from the lungs, flows into the left ventricle, and is propelled into the systemic circulation. The lungs may receive blood through one of three routes: (1) a small ventricular septal defect, (2) patent ductus arteriosus, (3) bronchial vessels.

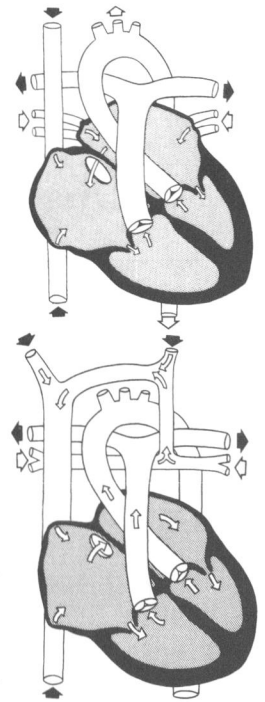

Atrial septal defects

An atrial septal defect is an abnormal opening between the right and left atria. Basically, three types of abnormalities result from incorrect development of the atrial septum. An incompetent foramen ovale is the most common defect. The high ostium secundum defect results from abnormal development of the septum secundum. Improper development of the septum primum produces a basal opening known as an ostium primum defect, frequently involving the atrioventricular valves. In general, left to right shunting of blood occurs in all atrial septal defects.

Anomalous venous return

Oxygenated blood returning from the lungs is carried abnormally to the right heart by one or more pulmonary veins emptying directly, or indirectly, through venous channels into the right atrium. Partial anomalous return of the pulmonary veins to the right atrium functions the same as an atrial septal defect. In complete anomalous return of the pulmonary veins, an interatrial communication is necessary for survival.

Fig. 40-1 Congenital heart abnormalities. *(Used with permission of Ross Products Division, Abbott Laboratories, Inc., Columbus, OH 43216. From Clinical Education Aid #7, Copyright 1976, Ross Products Division, Abbott Laboratories, Inc.)*

scriptive. The first of the four categories in this classification includes defects that result in increased pulmonary blood flow, often with congestive heart failure. Examples of the CHDs in this category are atrial and ventricular septal defects and patent ductus arteriosus (Fig. 40-1). The second category includes defects that involve decreased pulmonary blood flow and typically result in cyanosis. The most common example of this type of defect is tetralogy of Fallot; tricuspid atresia is a less common defect in this category. The third category includes those defects

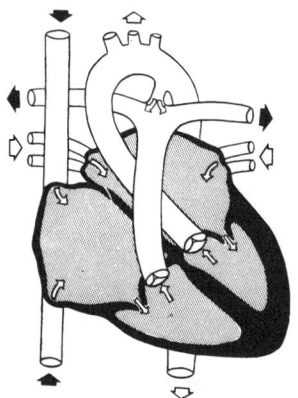

Patent ductus arteriosus

The patent ductus arteriosus is a vascular connection that, during fetal life, bypasses the pulmonary vascular bed and directs blood from the pulmonary artery to the aorta. Functional closure of the ductus normally occurs soon after birth. If the ductus remains patent after birth, the direction of blood flow in the ductus is reversed by the higher pressure in the aorta.

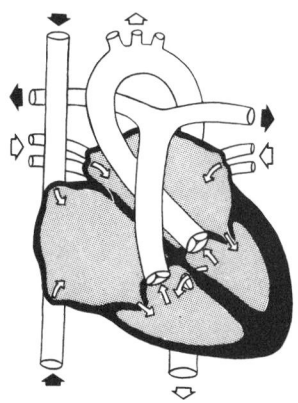

Ventricular septal defects

A ventricular septal defect is an abnormal opening between the right and left ventricle. Ventricular septal defects vary in size and may occur in either the membranous or muscular portion of the ventricular septum. Due to higher pressure in the left ventricle, a shunting of blood from the left to right ventricle occurs during systole. If pulmonary vascular resistance produces pulmonary hypertension, the shunt of blood is then reversed from the right to the left ventricle, with cyanosis resulting.

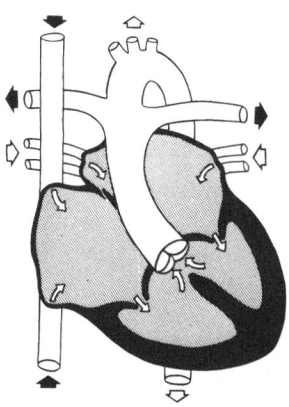

Truncus arteriosus

Truncus arteriosus is a retention of the embryologic bulbar trunk. It results from the failure of normal septation and division of this trunk into an aorta and pulmonary artery. This single arterial trunk overrides the ventricles and receives blood from them through a ventricular septal defect. The entire pulmonary and systemic circulation is supplied from this common arterial trunk.

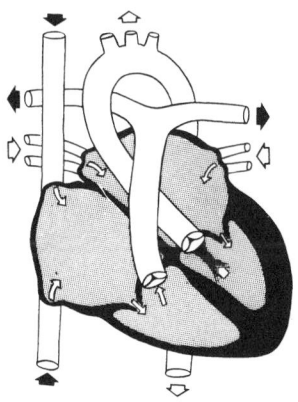

Subaortic stenosis

In many instances, the stenosis is valvular with thickening and fusion of the cusps. Subaortic stenosis is caused by a fibrous ring below the aortic valve in the outflow tract of the left ventricle. At times, both valvular and subaortic stenosis exist in combination. The obstruction presents an increased work load for the normal output of the left ventricular enlargement.

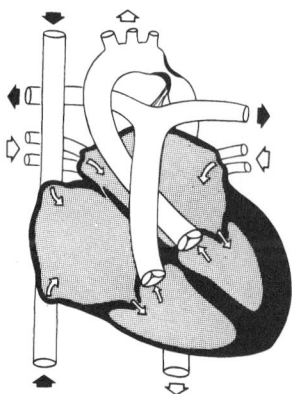

Coarctation of the aorta

Coarctation of the aorta is characterized by a narrowed aortic lumen. It exists as a preductal or postductal obstruction, depending on the position of the obstruction in relation to the ductus arteriosus. Coarctations exist with great variation in anatomic features. The lesion produces an obstruction to the flow of blood through the aorta causing an increased left ventricular pressure and work load.

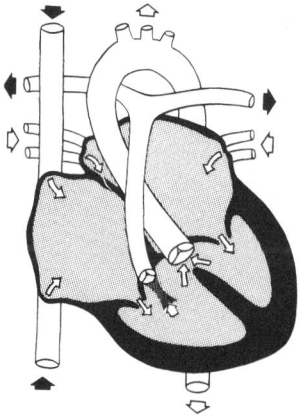

Tetralogy of Fallot

Tetralogy of Fallot is characterized by the combination of four defects: (1) pulmonary stenosis, (2) ventricular septal defect, (3) overriding aorta, (4) hypertrophy of right ventricle. It is the most common defect causing cyanosis in patients surviving beyond two years of age. The severity of symptoms depends on the degree of pulmonary stenosis, the size of the ventricular septal defect, and the degree to which the aorta overrides the septal defect.

Fig. 40-1, cont'd For legend see p. 1078

that cause obstruction to blood flow out of the heart. Pulmonary stenosis is an example of an obstruction to the flow of blood out of the right side of the heart that causes cyanosis. Coarctation of the aorta and subaortic stenosis are examples of obstructions to the flow of blood out of the left side of the heart that can result in congestive heart failure but not cyanosis. The fourth category comprises those complex cardiac anomalies that involve a flow of mixed saturated and desaturated blood in the heart or great vessels. These include such defects as transposition of the great vessels and total anomalous venous return.

Severe CHDs often are evident immediately after birth, especially defects that cause cyanosis such as transposition of the great vessels. Infants with these anomalies are transferred directly to special care nurseries or pediatric units. Even though the structural or functional anomalies are always present at birth, some affected newborns may be asymptomatic. Some of these CHDs, such as a small coarctation of the aorta, become apparent only as the infant or child is exposed to stresses such as growth demands or infection.

If symptoms are present at birth, they may be obvious with the first cry, which may be weak and muffled or loud and breathless. Affected newborns may be cyanotic and unrelieved by oxygen treatment, with the cyanosis increasing whenever the child is in the supine position or cries. The bluish-gray, dusky color of cyanotic infants may be mild, moderate, or severe. Other infants may be acyanotic and pale, with or without mottling on exertion, which includes crying, feeding, or stooling.

The affected newborn's activity level varies from restlessness to lethargy, and possibly unresponsiveness, except to pain. Persistent bradycardia (resting heart rate of less than 80 to 100 beats/min) or tachycardia (rate exceeding 160 to 180 beats/min) may be noted (Wong, 1999). The cardiac rhythm may be abnormal, and murmurs may be heard. Signs of congestive heart failure, diminished cardiac output, and decreased tissue perfusion may be evident.

Because the cardiac and respiratory systems function together, cardiac disease may be manifested by respiratory signs and symptoms. The respiratory rate should be determined when the newborn is in a resting state. Abnormal findings may include tachypnea, which is a rate of 60 breaths per minute or more; retractions with nasal flaring; grunting occurring with or without exertion; and dyspnea, which may worsen when the infant is supine or exerting itself.

A major role of the nurse is to assess infants for abnormal findings, which, if observed, must be reported immediately. Newborns exhibiting these symptoms require prompt diagnosis and appropriate therapy in a neonatal or pediatric intensive care unit. Interventions planned if a nursing diagnosis of decreased cardiac output is made include administering oxygen as ordered, as well as cardiotonic and other medications such as diuretics that rid the body of accumulated fluid, decreasing the workload of the heart by maintaining a thermoneutral environment, feeding using the gavage method if necessary, and preventing crying if this precipitates cyanosis. Various diagnostic tests such as echocardiography and cardiac catheterization are performed to obtain specific information about the defect and the need for surgical intervention.

Central Nervous System Anomalies

Most congenital anomalies of the central nervous system (CNS) result from defects in the closure of the neural tube during fetal development. Although the cause of **neural tube defects** is unknown, they are thought to stem from the interaction of many genes that is in turn influenced by factors in the fetal environment. Environmental influences such as treatment with valproic acid (an anticonvulsant), treatment with methotrexate (a chemotherapeutic medication), and alcohol consumption have been implicated. Excessive maternal body heat exposure during the early first trimester, such as from a significant febrile illness or extensive hot tub exposure, may also increase the risk of a neural tube defect (Elias & Hobbs, 1998). Studies have shown that a maternal folic acid deficit has a direct bearing on failure of the neural tube to close; therefore in 1993 the American Academy of Pediatrics issued recommendations that folic acid be taken by women of childbearing age (Morrow & Kelsey, 1998). Although a neural tube defect is usually an isolated defect, it can occur with some chromosomal abnormalities and syndromes and also with other defects such as cleft palate, ventricular septal defect, tracheoesophageal fistula, diaphragmatic hernia, imperforate anus, and renal anomalies. Some neural tube defects can be diagnosed prenatally with fetal ultrasonography and the finding of elevated levels of alpha-fetoprotein in the amniotic fluid and maternal serum.

Encephalocele and Anencephaly

Encephalocele and anencephaly are abnormalities resulting from failure of the anterior end of the neural tube to close. An encephalocele is a herniation of the brain and meninges through a skull defect. Treatment consists of surgical repair and shunting to relieve hydrocephalus, unless a major brain malformation is present. Most of these infants will have some degree of cognitive deficit. **Anencephaly** is the absence of both cerebral hemispheres and of the overlying skull. It is a condition that is incompatible with life; many of the infants are stillborn or die within a few days of birth. Comfort measures are provided until the infant eventually dies of respiratory failure.

Spina Bifida

Spina bifida, the most common defect of the CNS, results from failure of the neural tube to close at some point. There are two categories of spina bifida: spina bifida occulta and spina bifida cystica. Spina bifida occulta is a malformation in which the posterior portion of the laminas fails to close but the spinal cord or meninges do not herniate or protrude through the defect (Fig. 40-2). It is usually asymptomatic and may be not diagnosed unless there are associated problems. Spina bifida cystica includes meningocele and myelomeningocele. A meningocele is an external sac that contains meninges and cerebrospinal fluid (CSF) and that protrudes through a defect in the vertebral column. A **myelomeningocele** is similar, except that it also contains nerves; therefore the infant has motor and sensory deficits below the lesion. Myelomeningocele occurs in approximately 0.4 to 1 per 1000 live births in the United States each year, with this number varying by region of the country (Ball & Bindler, 1999).

A myelomeningocele, which is visible at birth and most often in the lumbosacral area, is usually covered with a very fragile, thin membrane (see Fig. 40-2). The sac can tear easily, allowing CSF to leak out, as well as providing an entry for infectious agents into the CNS. Myelomeningocele usually is associated with an Arnold-Chiari malformation, which results from the improper development and downward displacement of part of the brain into the cervical spinal canal. This in turn results in the development of hydrocephalus, which affects about 90% of children with myelomeningocele, although it may not be present at birth. The long-term prognosis in an affected infant can be determined to a large extent at birth, with the degree of neurologic dysfunction related to the level of the lesion, which determines the nerves involved. Although decisions regarding closure of the sac and treatment traditionally have been a matter of controversy, many physicians now recommend that treatment be instituted regardless of the level of the lesion, unless there is a severe CNS anomaly, advanced hydrocephalus at birth, severe anoxic brain damage, active CNS infection, or a congenital malformation or syndromes incompatible with long-term survival. Prenatal diagnosis of myelomeningocele has made possible a scheduled cesarean birth, allowing more careful delivery of the infant's back to try to prevent rupture of the meningeal sac.

A major preoperative nursing intervention for a neonate with a myelomeningocele is to protect the protruding sac from injury to prevent its rupture and resultant risk of CNS infection. Such infants should be positioned in a side-lying or prone position to prevent pressure on the sac until surgical repair is done. If the infant is allowed to be held, the nurse or parent must be careful to keep the defect from being injured. The sac should be covered with a sterile, moist, nonadherent dressing and sterile techniques used in its care. The skin around the defect must be cleansed and dried carefully to prevent breakdown, which would establish a portal of entry for infectious agents. Because a lack of normal innervation may prevent the bladder from emptying completely, the nurse should use Credé's method at regular intervals to express urine from the bladder.

Other nursing care involves an assessment of the infant's neurologic function that includes the status of the following: apparent paralysis of lower extremities; the flac-

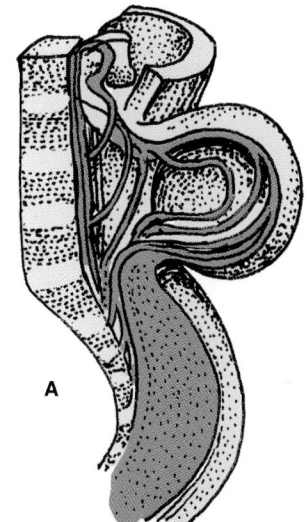

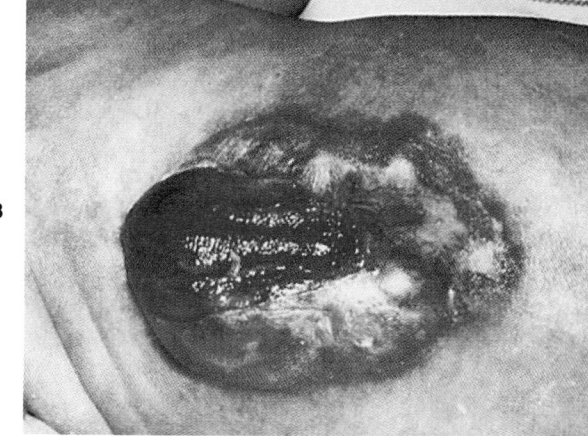

Fig. 40-2 A, Myelomeningocele. Note absence of vertebral arches. **B,** Myelomeningocele (spina bifida). *(From Zitelli, B., & Davis, H. [1997]. Atlas of pediatric physical diagnosis. [3rd ed.]. St. Louis: Mosby.)*

cidity and spasticity of muscles below the defect; and sphincter control, as evidenced by the number and character of voidings and stools, as well as the leakage of urine and stool. The infant's head circumference is measured and other neurologic assessments are performed to determine the presence and degree of hydrocephalus.

A major nursing intervention is providing support and needed information to parents as they begin to learn to cope with an infant who has immediate needs for intensive care and probably will have long-term needs as well. Surgical repair is often done in the neonatal period, preferably within the first 24 hours. Very early closure can prevent CNS infection and trauma to the exposed nerves. It can also prevent stretching of other nerve roots, which can occur as the sac continues to enlarge after birth. Surgical shunt procedures to prevent increasing hydrocephalus may be needed. Other problems, such as infection, are treated as they occur.

Hydrocephalus

Hydrocephalus refers to a condition in which the ventricles of the brain are enlarged as a result of an imbalance between the production and absorption of the CSF. It is almost always caused by interference with the circulation and absorption of CSF. Congenital hydrocephalus usually arises as a result of a malformation in the brain or an intrauterine infection. It occurs in approximately 3 to 4 per 1000 live births (Jackson & Harvey, 1996). About one third of all cases of congenital hydrocephalus result from stenosis of the aqueduct of Sylvius in the brain. Hydrocephalus frequently occurs in conjunction with a myelomeningocele, which blocks the flow of CSF.

An infant with congenital hydrocephalus will initially have a bulging anterior fontanel and a head circumference that increases at an abnormal rate, resulting from the increase in CSF pressure (Fig. 40-3). Enlargement of the forehead with depressed eyes that are rotated downward, causing a "setting sun" sign, occurs as the condition worsens. If the surgical shunting of excess CSF from the brain is not done soon after birth, the resulting increasing intracranial pressure will lead to irreversible neurologic damage, as evidenced by palpably widening sutures and fontanels, lethargy, poor feeding, vomiting, irritability, opisthotonos, and a high-pitched, shrill cry.

Nursing actions appropriate to the needs of a newborn with hydrocephalus include careful documentation of the ongoing observations. The occipitofrontal circumference of the head is measured daily at its largest point, and neurologic assessments are done frequently. If the infant's head is large, the placement of sheepskin or a flotation mattress under the infant and frequent position changes are necessary to prevent skin breakdown resulting from the pressure.

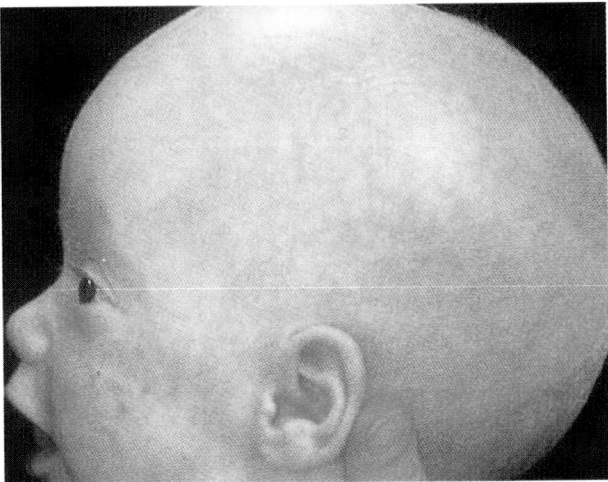

Fig. 40-3 Infantile hydrocephalus. The characteristic appearance is an enlarged head, thinning of the scalp, distended scalp veins, and a full fontanel. *(From Booth, I., & Wozniak, E. [1984]. Pediatrics. Baltimore: Williams & Wilkins.)*

The infant's heavy head should be supported carefully during holding or turning, and positioning in the crib should be done in such a way that a patent airway is maintained. The method, amount, and frequency of feeding are determined by the infant's tolerance and energy level. The nurse should be alert to the possibility of projectile vomiting, which is a frequent occurrence in the presence of increased intracranial pressure, and maintain aspiration precautions. Nonnutritive sucking, touching, and cuddling needs should be met.

Diagnosis is made by computed tomography (CT) and magnetic resonance imaging (MRI), and antenatal diagnosis can be made by fetal ultrasonography. The surgical correction of hydrocephalus involves the placement of a shunt that goes from the ventricles of the brain usually to the peritoneum to allow the drainage of excess CSF. Damaged or destroyed brain tissue cannot be restored; the long-term prognosis in affected infants depends on the presence and extent of such tissue damage, along with the cause of the hydrocephalus, the presence of concurrent neurologic problems, and the long-term success of the shunt procedure.

Microcephaly

Microcephaly refers to a small brain in a generally normally formed head. It can be an autosomal recessive disorder or caused by a chromosomal abnormality; exposure of the woman to x-rays; or rubella, cytomegalovirus, or other maternal infections. Microcephalic infants require supportive nursing care and medical observation to determine the extent of the psychomotor retardation that almost always accompanies this abnormality. There is no treatment. Parents need support to learn to care for a child with such cognitive impairment.

Respiratory System Anomalies

Screening for congenital anomalies of the respiratory system is necessary even in infants who are apparently normal at birth. Respiratory distress at birth or shortly thereafter may be the result of lung immaturity or anomalous development. Congenital laryngeal web and bilateral choanal atresia are readily apparent at birth. Respiratory distress caused by diaphragmatic hernia and tracheoesophageal fistula may appear immediately or be delayed, depending on the severity of the defect.

Laryngeal Web and Choanal Atresia

A laryngeal web, which is uncommon, results from the incomplete separation of the two sides of the larynx and is most often between the vocal cords. **Choanal atresia** (Fig. 40-4) is the most common congenital anomaly of the nose; it is a bony or membranous septum located between the nose and the pharynx. Inability to pass a suction catheter through the nose into the pharynx usually leads to its detection. Nearly half of the infants with choanal atresia have other anomalies. Infants with either a laryngeal web or choanal atresia require emergency surgery.

Diaphragmatic Hernia

Diaphragmatic hernia results from a defect in the formation of the diaphragm, allowing the abdominal organs to be displaced into the thoracic cavity. It occurs in approximately 1 in 3000 to 4000 live births (Finer et al., 1998); however, if stillbirths resulting from this defect are included, the incidence increases to 1 in 2000. Herniation of the abdominal viscera into the thoracic cavity may cause severe respiratory distress and represent a neonatal emergency (Fig. 40-5). The defect and herniation may be minimal and easily repaired, or the defect may be so extensive that the viscera present in the thoracic cavity during embryonic life have prevented the normal development of pulmonary tissue. The defect is usually on the left because that is the side of the diaphragm that fuses last.

Most congenital diaphragmatic hernias are discovered prenatally on ultrasound studies and in some research institutions may be repaired by fetal surgery. At birth most affected infants have severe respiratory distress, and respiratory assessment reveals worsening distress as the bowels fill with air. Typically the breath sounds are diminished and bowel sounds are heard in the chest. Heart sounds may be heard on the right side of the chest because the heart has been displaced there by the abdominal contents. Physical examination reveals a flat or scaphoid abdomen and a prominent ipsilateral chest. Diagnosis can be made on the basis of the x-ray study finding of loops of intestine in the thoracic cavity and the absence of intestine in the abdominal cavity.

Preoperative nursing interventions include participating in the stabilization of the infant's condition until surgical repair can be done. The infant should be positioned with the head and chest elevated and the affected side downward to allow the normal lung to expand. Gastric contents are aspirated and suction applied to decompress the gastrointestinal tract and prevent further cardiothoracic compromise. Oxygen therapy, mechanical ventilation, and the correction of acidosis are necessary in infants with large defects. Extracorporeal membrane oxygenation (ECMO) may be used in infants with severe circulatory and respiratory complications. The prognosis depends largely on the degree of pulmonary development and the success of diaphragmatic closure, but the prognosis in severe cases is poor. The Extracorporeal Life Support Organization (ELSO) registry, which is the largest registry of infants with congenital diaphragmatic hernia, reports on the outcome of infants treated with ECMO. There was a 59% survival rate of the 2627 infants who were registered by mid-1997. Of those survivors, a significant number had chronic lung disease with long-term oxygen dependency, feeding difficulties, and gastroesophageal reflux (Finer et al., 1998). There has been some success with fetal repair, but the mortality rate associated with it is higher than that associated with current conventional management, including ECMO.

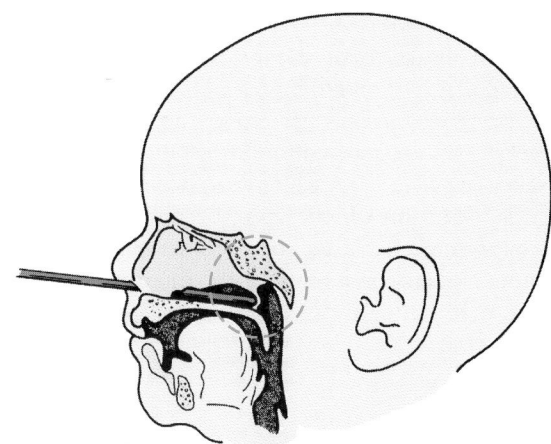

Fig. 40-4 Choanal atresia. Posterior nares are obstructed by membrane or bone either bilaterally or unilaterally. Infant becomes cyanotic at rest. With crying, newborn's color improves. Nasal discharge is present. Snorting respirations often are observed with increased respiratory effort. Newborn may be unable to breathe and eat at the same time. Diagnosis is made by noting inability to pass small feeding tube through one or both nares. *(Used with permission of Ross Products Division, Abbott Laboratories, Inc., Columbus, OH 43216. From Clinical Education Aid #6, Copyright 1963, Ross Products Division, Abbott Laboratories, Inc.)*

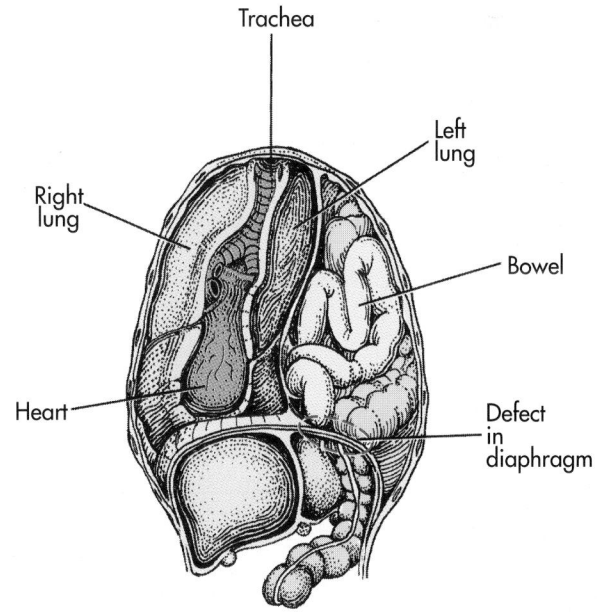

Fig. 40-5 Diaphragmatic hernia. *(Used with permission of Ross Products Division, Abbott Laboratories, Inc., Columbus, OH 43216. From Clinical Education Aid #6, Copyright 1963, Ross Products Division, Abbott Laboratories, Inc.)*

Gastrointestinal System Anomalies

Anomalies in the gastrointestinal system can occur anywhere along the gastrointestinal tract, from the mouth to the anus. Some anomalies, such as cleft lip, omphalocele, and gastroschisis, are apparent at birth. Others, including cleft palate, esophageal atresia, pyloric stenosis, intestinal obstructions, and imperforate anus, become apparent as the infant is further assessed or becomes symptomatic. These anomalies arise as a result of the interrupted development of that particular organ at a crucial point during organogenesis.

Cleft Lip and Palate

Cleft lip or palate is a commonly occurring congenital midline fissure, or opening, in the lip or palate resulting from failure of the primary palate to fuse (Fig. 40-6). One or both deformities may occur, and nasal deformity may also be present. Multiple genetic and, to a lesser extent, environmental factors, such as maternal infection, radiation exposure, alcohol ingestion, and treatment with medications such as corticosteroids, some tranquilizers, and anticonvulsants, appear to be involved in their development.

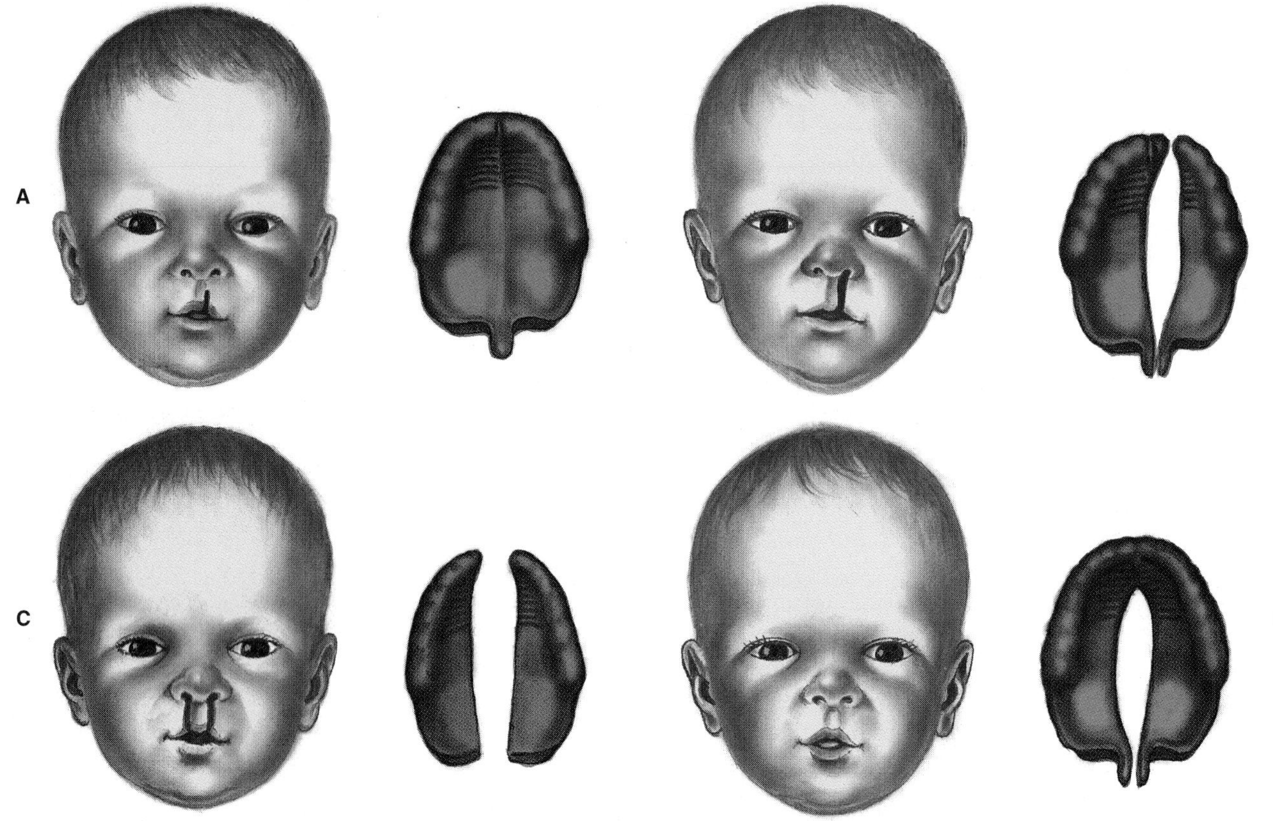

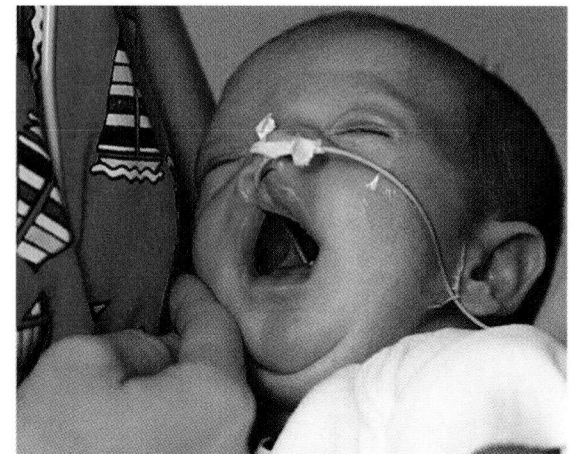

Fig. 40-6   Variations in clefts of lip and palate at birth. **A,** Notch in vermilion border. **B,** Unilateral cleft lip and cleft palate. **C,** Bilateral cleft lip and cleft palate. **D,** Cleft palate. **E,** Infant with complete unilateral cleft lip. Note the feeding tube. (*A-D,* From Wong, D. [1999]. Whaley and Wong's nursing care of infants and children [6th ed.]. St. Louis: Mosby. *E,* From Dickason, E., Silverman, B., & Kaplan J. [1998]. Maternal-infant nursing care [3rd ed.]. St. Louis: Mosby.)

Cleft lip with or without cleft palate occurs in approximately 1 in 800 live births (Balasubrahmanyam et al., 1998). It is more common in Native American and Asians and less common in African-Americans. It is more common in males. The defect can range from a simple notch in the lip to complete separation of the lip that extends to the floor of the nose. The treatment for a cleft lip is surgical repair, which usually is done between 6 and 12 weeks of age, if the infant is healthy and free of infection. Advances in surgical techniques have made it possible for some infants, particularly those with unilateral cleft lip, to have a near-normal appearance. The results of the repair depend on the severity of the defect, with more severe bilateral cleft lip requiring surgical repair done in stages.

Anomalies of the palate often occur in association with cleft lip. Cleft palate alone occurs in approximately 1 in 2000 live births (Balasubrahmanyam et al., 1998). It is more common in females and occurs more frequently as a constituent of certain syndromes. This defect can range from a cleft in the uvula to a complete cleft of the hard and soft palates that may be unilateral, bilateral, or midline. Feeding is difficult because the cleft lip renders the newborn unable to maintain a seal around a nipple, and the cleft palate renders the infant unable to form a vacuum to maintain suction when feeding. In addition, the inability to suck and swallow normally allows milk to pool in the nasopharynx, which increases the likelihood of aspiration. Furthermore, as the infant attempts to suck, milk often comes out through the cleft and out of the nares. Although the degree of difficulty depends on the size of the cleft, feeding problems are greater in infants with a cleft palate than in those with a cleft lip. Regardless of the extent and type of defect, feeding may become a very frustrating experience for parents. Breastfeeding can be successful in some infants (Darzi et al., 1996). There are special nipples, bottles, and appliances available to aid in feeding (Fig. 40-6, E). In general, parents of infants with these defects need a great deal of education and support as they learn to feed their baby, to prevent what should be a normal part of infant care from becoming a very frustrating experience.

The type of surgical repair done to close the cleft palate is based on the degree of the cleft and, as with a cleft lip, if severe, may necessitate repair done in stages. Repair is begun at 6 to 18 months, after some development of the affected area has occurred. Early repair helps avert some of the speech problems that may occur in people with palate defects. Long-term care is often necessary for children with a cleft palate and involves the combined efforts of a health care team comprising acute care and community nurses; social workers; ear, nose, and throat and plastic surgeons; speech therapists; and orthodontists.

Parents of infants with a cleft lip or palate need much support, particularly in the case of a cleft lip, because this is both a cosmetic and functional defect. Recognizing that this may interfere with normal parent-infant bonding in the neonatal period, the nurse must assess for this and intervene appropriately.

Esophageal Atresia and Tracheoesophageal Fistula

Esophageal atresia (EA) and tracheoesophageal fistula (TEF), the most life-threatening anomalies of the esophagus, often occur together, although they can also occur singly. **Esophageal atresia** is a congenital anomaly in which the esophagus ends in a blind pouch or narrows into a thin cord, thus failing to form a continuous passageway to the stomach. TEF is an abnormal connection between the esophagus and trachea.

Hydramnios is a common finding in pregnancy, particularly if the fetus has an EA without a TEF. More than half of the infants have associated anomalies, most often cardiac and gastrointestinal tract ones. Variations of the anomalies are possible, depending on the presence or absence of a TEF, the site of the fistula, and the location and degree of the esophageal obstruction. The most common variant is the combination of a proximal EA, in which the esophagus ends in a blind pouch, with a distal TEF, in which the lower esophagus exits the stomach and is connected to the trachea by a fistula, rather than forming a continuous tube to the upper esophagus (Fig. 40-7). This defect occurs in approximately 1 in 3000 live births (Stapleton, 1996).

Infants with the life-threatening anomaly EA with TEF show significant respiratory difficulty immediately after birth. EA with or without TEF results in excessive oral secretions, drooling, and feeding intolerance. When fed, the infant may swallow, but then cough and gag and return the fluid through the nose and mouth. Respiratory distress can result from aspiration or from the acute gastric distention produced by the TEF. Choking, coughing, and cyanosis occur after even a small amount of fluid is taken by mouth.

Nursing interventions are supportive until surgery is performed.

NURSE ALERT *Any infant with excessive oral secretions and respiratory distress should not be fed orally until a physician is consulted.*

The infant with EA and TEF is placed in a semi-Fowler's position, which facilitates respiratory efforts and diminishes the reflux of gastric contents into the trachea. A double-lumen catheter is placed in the proximal esophageal pouch and attached to continuous suction to remove secretions and decrease the possibility of aspiration. The infant requires close observation and intervention to maintain a patent airway. Other supportive measures include maintaining fluid and electrolyte balance intravenously, and thermoregulation. Surgical correction, done in one stage if possible, consists of ligating the fistula and anastomosing the two segments of the esophagus.

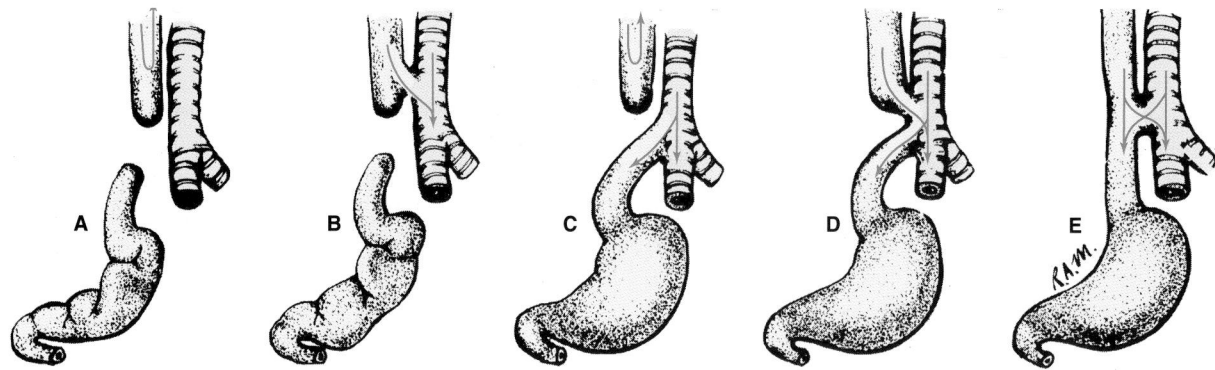

Fig. 40-7 Congenital atresia of esophagus and tracheoesophageal fistula. **A,** Upper and lower segments of esophagus end in blind sac, occurring in 5% to 8% of such infants. **B,** Upper segment of esophagus ends in atresia and connects to trachea by fistulous tract, occurring rarely. **C,** Upper segment of esophagus ends in blind pouch; lower segment connects with trachea by small fistulous tract, occurring in 80% to 95% of such infants. **D,** Both segments of esophagus connect by fistulous tracts to trachea, occurring in less than 1% of such infants. Infant may aspirate with first feeding. **E,** Esophagus is continuous but connects by fistulous tract to trachea; known as *H-type.* *(From Wong, D. [1999]. Whaley and Wong's nursing care of infants and children [6th ed.]. St. Louis: Mosby.)*

Prematurity increases the risk of poor outcome. In addition, major congenital cardiac and chromosomal anomalies have been found to be predictors of a poor outcome (Chondhury et al., 1999). The mortality rate for these infants is reported as high as 50%. The survival rate for infants in a good-risk category exceeds 95% (Ryckman, Flake, & Balisteri, 1997).

Omphalocele and Gastroschisis

Omphalocele and gastroschisis are two of the more common congenital defects that occur in the abdominal wall. They are rare, however, with omphalocele occurring in approximately 1 in 5000 live births. The incidence of gastroschisis is about 1 to 3 in 10,000 live births (Wong, 1999). An **omphalocele** is a covered defect of the umbilical ring into which varying amounts of the abdominal organs may herniate (Fig. 40-8). Although it is covered with a peritoneal sac, the sac may rupture during or after birth. Many infants born with an omphalocele are premature, and more than half have other serious syndromes or anomalies involving the gastrointestinal, cardiac, genitourinary, musculoskeletal, and nervous systems.

Gastroschisis is the herniation of the bowel through a defect in the abdominal wall to the right of the umbilical cord (Fig. 40-8, *B*). No membrane covers the contents, as occurs with an omphalocele. Unlike infants with omphalocele, these infants rarely have associated anomalies.

The preoperative nursing care for infants with either defect is similar. Exposure of the viscera causes problems with thermoregulation and fluid and electrolyte balance. Before closure is performed, the exposed viscera are covered with moistened saline gauze and plastic wrap. Antibiotics, fluid and electrolyte replacement, gastric decompression, and

thermoregulation are needed for physiologic support. If complete closure is impossible because of the small size of the defect and the large amount of viscera to be replaced, a Silastic (Dow Corning, Midland, MI) silo pouch is created and sewn to the fascia of the abdominal defect. This protects the contents as they are gradually placed back into the abdominal cavity. The defect is closed surgically after the reduction of the contents that have been exposed is completed, which usually takes 7 to 10 days. Gastric decompression is necessary preoperatively to prevent aspiration pneumonia and to allow as much bowel as possible to be placed into the abdomen during surgery. Surgery is usually performed soon after birth. With improved surgical treatment, nutritional support, and medical management, the prognosis has improved for infants born with an abdominal wall defect. It is estimated that more than 80% of infants born with an omphalocele survive, as do more than 90% of those born with gastroschisis (Wong, 1999).

Parental support is essential, because the infant has an obvious disfiguring anomaly that can be shocking and repulsive in appearance. Depending on the size of the defect, the infant may also be critically ill preoperatively. The nurse must be aware of the effect this may have on parental bonding and intervene appropriately as the parents cope with this crisis.

Gastrointestinal Obstruction

Congenital intestinal obstruction can occur anywhere in the gastrointestinal tract and occur in the form of atresia, which is a complete obliteration of the passage; partial obstruction, in which the symptoms may vary in severity and sometimes not be detected in the neonatal period; or malrotation of the intestine, which leads to twisting of the

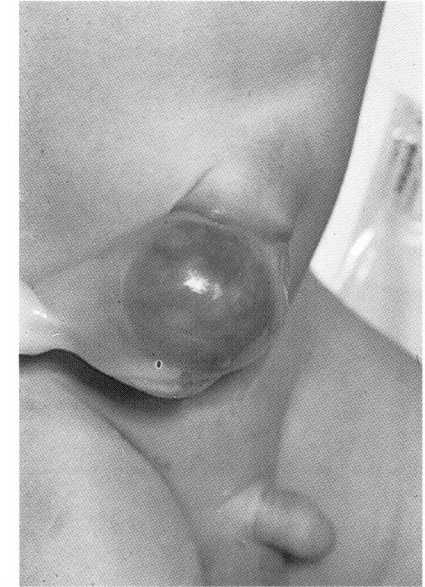

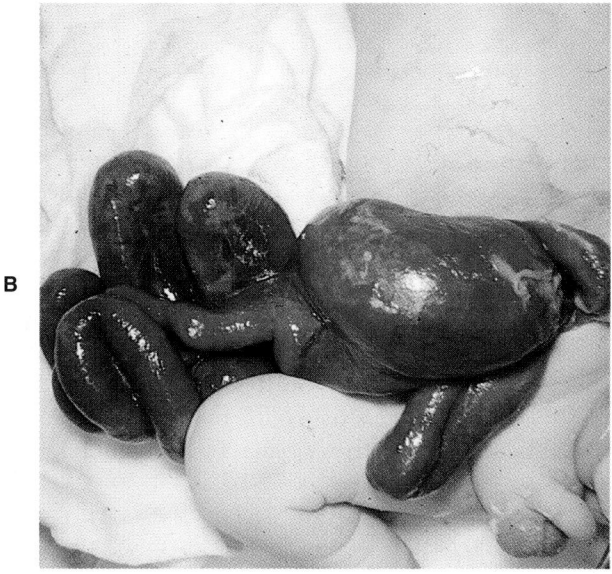

Fig. 40-8 **A,** Omphalocele. **B,** Gastroschisis of bowel and stomach. *(A, From O'Doherty, N. [1986]. Neonatology: Micro atlas of the newborn. Nutley, NJ: Hoffmann-La Roche. **B,** Courtesy Wyeth-Ayerst Laboratories, Philadelphia, PA.)*

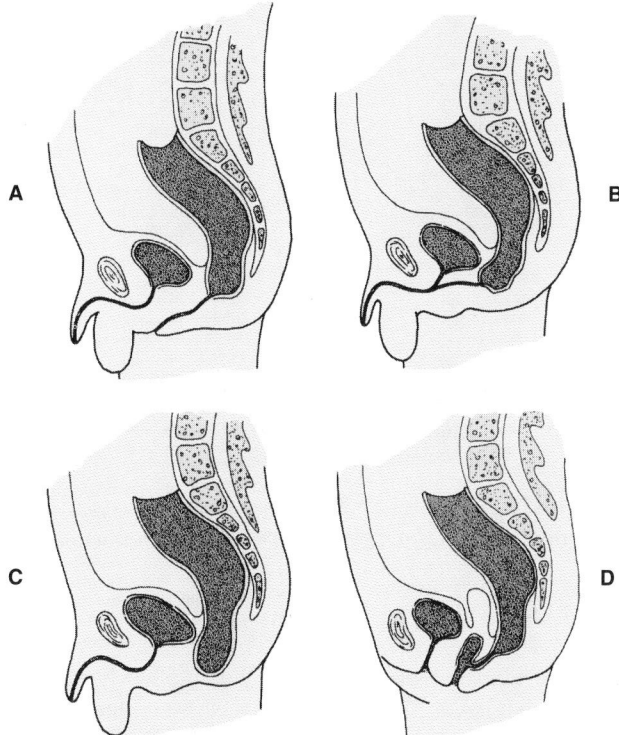

Fig. 40-9 Types of imperforate anus. Anal sphincter muscle may be present and intact. **A,** High lesion opening onto perineum through narrow fistulous tract. **B,** High lesion ending in fistulous tract to urinary tract. **C,** Low lesion in bowel passes through puborectal muscle. **D,** High lesion ending in fistulous tract to vagina.

intestine (volvulus) and obstruction. EA, discussed previously, is a type of gastrointestinal obstruction. Meconium ileus is an obstruction caused by impacted meconium and is the earliest symptom of cystic fibrosis, a life-threatening chronic illness. Infants with this type of obstruction should be tested for cystic fibrosis, because 95% of infants with meconium ileus have cystic fibrosis. Meconium ileus occurs in 7% to 25% of patients with cystic fibrosis (Holland, Price, & Bensard, 1998).

In addition to hydramnios in the pregnant woman, the infant shows the following cardinal signs and symptoms: bilious vomiting, abdominal distention, and failure to pass normal amounts of meconium in the first 24 hours. High intestinal obstruction is characterized by vomiting, even if the infant is not being fed orally. A low obstruction is characterized primarily by distention, with vomiting occurring later. Abdominal distention can elevate the diaphragm, which causes respiratory difficulties. Careful evaluation must be done to make a correct diagnosis.

Nursing care is aimed at supporting the infant until surgical intervention can be carried out to eliminate the obstruction. Oral feedings are discontinued, a nasogastric tube is placed for suction, and intravenous therapy is initiated to provide needed fluid and electrolytes. In infants with an intestinal obstruction, surgery consists of resecting the obstructed area of bowel and anastomosing the nonaffected bowel. In recent years the survival rate for these infants has risen to 85% to 90% as a result of better treatments, better neonatal intensive care, and a better understanding of the total problem.

Imperforate Anus

Imperforate anus is a term used to describe a wide range of congenital disorders involving the anus and rectum (Fig. 40-9). These anomalies are relatively common,

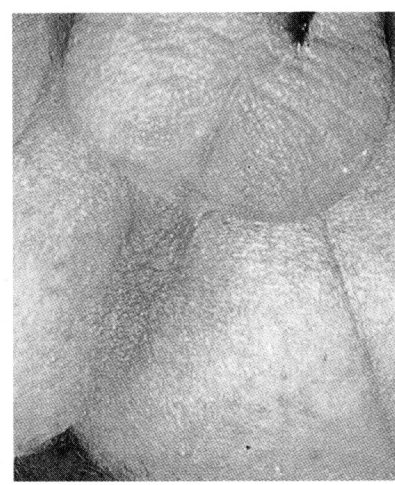

Fig. 40-10 Imperforate anus. *(From Chessell, G. et al. [1984]. Diagnostic picture tests in clinical medicine [vol. 2]. St. Louis: Mosby.)*

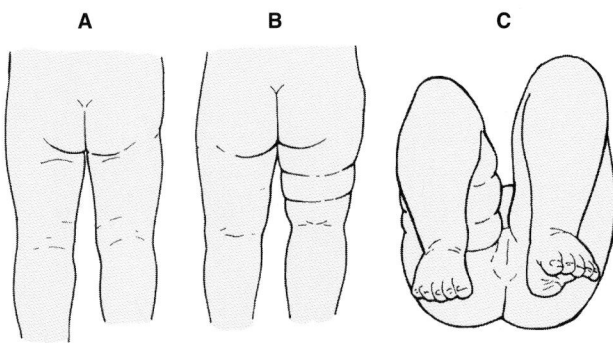

Fig. 40-11 Congenital dysplasia of hip. **A,** Normal gluteal and popliteal skin creases. **B,** Abnormal skin creases and asymmetry of skinfolds. **C,** Apparent shortening of femur. Femoral head is displaced. *(Used with permission of Ross Products Division, Abbott Laboratories, Inc., Columbus, OH 43216. From Clinical Education Aid #15, Copyright 1965, Ross Products Division, Abbott Laboratories.)*

with an incidence of approximately 1 in 5000 live births (Holland, Price, & Bensard, 1998). Occurring more in male than in female infants, they result from the failure of anorectal development in weeks 7 and 8 of gestational life. Such infants have no anal opening, and frequently there is also a fistula from the rectum to the peritoneum or genitourinary system (Fig. 40-10). They can be further classified according to the location of the defect into a "high" or "low" type, which determines the treatments necessary, as well as the prognosis. Infants with high anomalies, which occur primarily in males, require a colostomy in the neonatal period, with corrective surgery done in stages over time. Low anomalies may involve stenotic areas or there may be a thin translucent membrane covering the anal opening. Treatment for such a membrane is excision followed by daily dilation, which parents are taught to do. Other low lesions are surgically corrected by anoplasty. The preoperative nursing care is similar to that described for other gastrointestinal obstructions.

Musculoskeletal System Anomalies

The two most common musculoskeletal system anomalies seen in neonates are developmental dysplasia of the hip and congenital clubfoot. Both of these conditions must be detected and treated early for them to be successfully corrected.

Developmental Dysplasia of the Hip

Developmental dysplasia of the hip (DDH) consists of disorders that result from the abnormal development of one or all of the components of the hip joint, resulting in instability of the hip. This causes one or both of the femoral heads to be displaced from the hip socket, or acetabulum. The dislocated femoral head does not exert pressure on the acetabulum, causing delayed development of the femoral head and failure of the acetabulum to form normally. The etiology is considered to be multifactorial, with genetic factors involved, and females are more often affected than males. Risk factors for the defect include breech presentation, a positive family history, the birth order (firstborn), and prenatal maternal oligohydramnios with fetal compression and deformation. The effect of maternal hormones during pregnancy may foster hip joint capsule laxity, especially in the female. Although as many as 1 in 100 newborns will have an unstable hip that the examiner can dislocate, only 1 in 1000 will have a hip that is truly dislocated. Infants presenting in the breech position have a 20% chance of having DDH (Ballock & Richards, 1997; Novacheck, 1996).

The examiner tests for an unstable or actually dislocated femoral head by abducting the hips and feeling for a click when the femoral head passes back into the acetabulum (see Fig. 26-13). Other diagnostic clues include an asymmetric number of skinfolds, one knee higher than the other when the hips and knees are flexed to 90 degrees (Galeazzi sign), and limited hip abduction (Fig. 40-11).

Early detection, often by the nurse during a routine newborn assessment, allows for early treatment, which is more effective than later treatment and can prevent complications. Treatment involves the use of a Pavlik harness, a dynamic device that keeps the hips and knees flexed, the hips abducted, and the femoral head in the acetabulum (Fig. 40-12). Worn continuously for 3 to 6 months, it promotes the development of muscle and cartilage, resulting in a stable hip. If the infant is treated between 1 and 8 months of age, the harness is effective 80% to 90% of the time (Wong, 1999). If not effective, traction, casting, and even surgery may be necessary to stabilize the hip.

In addition to the major intervention of assessing and helping identify the disorder, another key nursing inter-

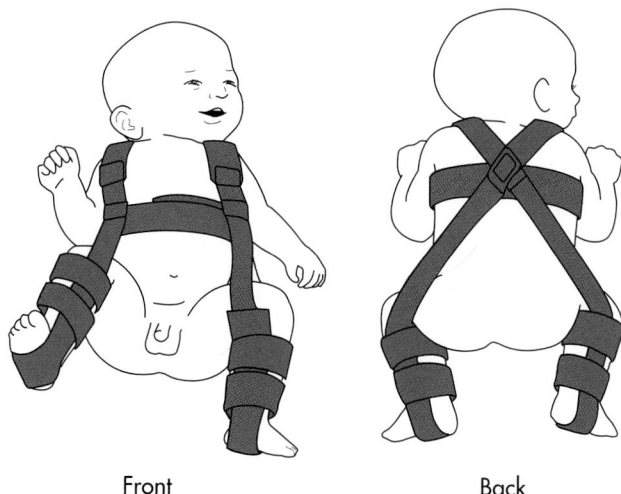

Front   Back

Fig. 40-12 Treatment for congenital hip dislocation by application of the Pavlik harness. *(From Ball, J. [1998]. Mosby's pediatric patient teaching guides. St. Louis: Mosby.)*

vention is teaching the parents about the care of the infant, who will remain in the harness continuously during the treatment. Because this occurs during a time of maximum growth, it will be necessary for them to adjust the infant's care to accommodate the infant's changing needs. Continuing thorough follow-up care is necessary, as well as psychosocial support for the family.

Clubfoot

Clubfoot is a congenital deformity in which portions of the foot and ankle are twisted out of a normal position. These can be of varying degrees of severity and assume a variety of combinations of abnormal positions. The most common, seen in approximately 95% of infants with clubfoot, is talipes equinovarus. In this abnormality, the foot appears C shaped, pointing downward and inward; the ankle is inverted; and the Achilles tendon is shortened. The foot appears small, wide, and stiff, and the lower leg appears small because of hypoplasia of the calf muscles. Unless treated, further stiffening occurs, and bony changes will result.

Clubfoot is one of the most common congenital anomalies, occurring in approximately 1 per 1000 live births, with two times more males than females affected (Grover, 1996). The condition is bilateral in approximately 50% of cases. The exact cause is unknown, but possibilities include a genetic predisposition, in utero compression, and abnormal embryonic development. Treatment begins soon after birth. This consists of manipulation and frequent serial casting, which is necessary because of the rapid growth of the infant. If this is ineffective, surgical correction is necessary. Although a controversial issue, the optimal age for surgery is generally acknowledged to be between 4 and 12 months. Treatment, which may continue into adolescence, often results in good function of the foot, although

the feet may differ in size. The deformity may recur, and repeat surgery may then be necessary.

Because these infants are often placed in a cast before they are discharged, the nurse must teach the parents the way to care for an infant in a cast, including protecting the cast and assessing the toes for neurovascular compromise. This is particularly important because of the growth of the child, which could cause the child to outgrow the cast. As is true with the birth of any child with any anomaly, the nurse should be supportive of the parents as they learn the ways in which to meet the infant's normal needs, as well as those brought about by the infant's physical problem.

Genitourinary System Anomalies

Anomalies involving the genitourinary system can be distressing to parents because they may be readily apparent and, in the case of some conditions, because of the concern about sexuality and reproductive functioning. These anomalies range from obvious anomalies of the external genitalia, such as hypospadias, to those involving internal organs that may not be detected but may cause damage to the urinary tract. An example of the latter is an obstruction in the urinary tract that can cause hydronephrosis, which is the abnormal collection of urine in the renal pelvis that can eventually destroy the kidney.

Hypospadias and Epispadias

Hypospadias constitutes a range of penile anomalies associated with an abnormally located urinary meatus. The meatus can open below the glans penis or anywhere along the ventral surface of the penis, the scrotum, or the perineum. One of the most common congenital anomalies, it is thought to affect approximately 1 in 250 male births, although the exact incidence is unknown (Paulozzi, Erickson, & Jackson, 1997). It is classified according to the location of the meatus and the presence or absence of chordee, which is a ventral curvature of the penis. The cause is unknown, although it is thought to be of multifactorial inheritance.

Mild cases of hypospadias are often repaired for cosmetic reasons and involve a single surgical procedure. In more severe cases, several operations are required to reconstruct the urethral opening and correct the chordee, thereby straightening the penis. The goals are to improve the appearance of the genitalia and make it possible for the child to be able to urinate in a standing position and have a sexually adequate organ. It is vital that these infants not be circumcised, because the foreskin may be needed during surgical repair. Repair is done early, often during or soon after the first year of life, so that the child's body image is not impaired.

Epispadias, a rare anomaly, results from failure of urethral canalization. About 55% of the affected infants are males who have a widened pubic symphysis and a broad spadelike penis with the urethra opened on its dorsal surface (Bellinger, 1997). In females there is a wide urethra and a bifid clitoris. Severity ranges from a mild to a severe anomaly that is associated with exstrophy of the bladder. Surgical correction is necessary, and affected male infants should not be circumcised.

Exstrophy of the Bladder

The most common bladder anomaly is exstrophy (Fig. 40-13), which often occurs in conjunction with epispadias. It is rare, occurring in approximately 1 in 40,000 live births (Bellinger, 1997). It results from the abnormal development of the bladder, abdominal wall, and pubic symphysis that causes the bladder, urethra, and ureteral orifices to all be exposed. The bladder is visible in the suprapubic area as a red mass with numerous folds, with urine draining from it onto the infant's skin. The bladder is covered with a sterile, nonadherent dressing to protect its delicate surface until closure can be performed. It is recommended that reconstructive surgery be started in the neonatal period, preferably with the bladder being closed during the first or second day of life. Parents will need much support as they deal with caring for an infant who has such an obvious defect. Repair is completed before school age, if possible, although some children never attain normal voiding patterns and later may be considered for surgery for urinary diversion.

Sexual Ambiguity

Sexual ambiguity in the newborn (Fig. 40-14) often is discovered by the nurse during a physical assessment. Erroneous or abnormal sexual differentiation may be a genetic aberration, such as congenital adrenal hypoplasia, which can be life threatening because of the deficiency of all adrenal cortical hormones involved. Other possible causes of sexual ambiguity include chromosomal abnor-

malities, defective sex hormone synthesis in males, and the placental transfer of masculinizing agents to female fetuses. Gender assignment should be based on data gathered from the following sources: maternal and family history, including the ingestion of steroids during pregnancy and relatives with ambiguous genitalia or who died during the neonatal period; physical examination; chromosomal analysis (results are available in 2 to 3 days); endoscopy, ultrasonography, and radiographic contrast studies; biochemical tests, such as analysis of urinary steroid excretion, which helps detect several of the adrenal cortical syndromes; and, in some instances, laparotomy or gonad biopsy.

Therapeutic intervention, including any surgery, should be started as soon as possible. Any child born with ambiguous genitalia should not receive a sex assignment until the appropriate sex of rearing may be properly assessed and assigned. An appropriate sex assignment should be based on the following: potential for mature sexual function, potential fertility, and the long-term psychologic and intellectual impact on the child and family (Finegold, 1997). Parents need much support as they learn to deal with this very challenging situation.

Teratoma

A **teratoma** is an embryonal tumor that may be solid, cystic, or mixed. It is composed of at least two and usually three types of embryonal tissue: ectoderm, mesoderm, and endoderm. This rare tumor in the neonate may occur in the skull, cervical area, mediastinum, abdomen, or sacral area, with more than half located in the sacrococcygeal

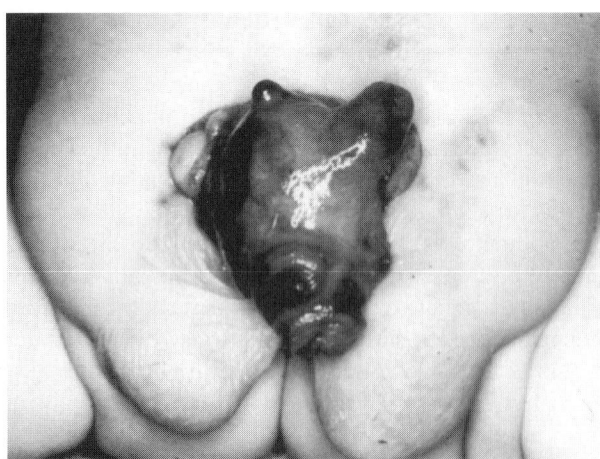

Fig. 40-13 Exstrophy of bladder. *(Courtesy Edward S. Tank, MD, Division of Urology, Oregon Health Science University, Portland, OR.)*

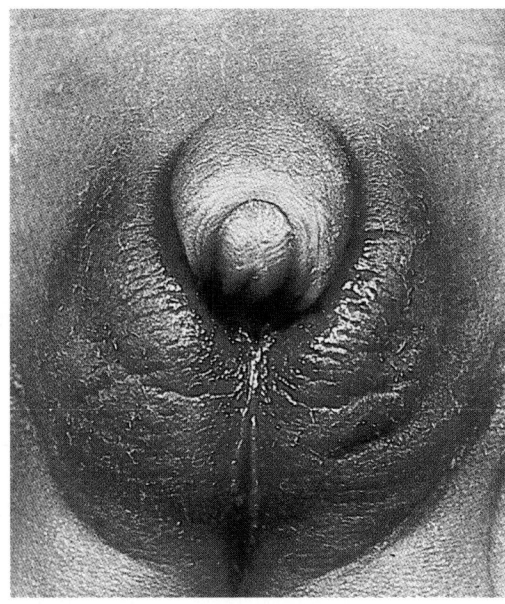

Fig. 40-14 Ambiguous external genitals (i.e., structure can be enlarged clitoral hood and clitoris or malformed penis). *(Courtesy Edward S. Tank, MD, Division of Urology, Oregon Health Science University, Portland, OR.)*

area. A cervical teratoma may compress the esophagus in utero and produce polyhydramnios. After birth, compression of the upper airway from the mass may create a surgical emergency (Nakayama, 1997). The treatment of choice is complete surgical resection. Approximately 80% of all teratomas are benign, and no additional therapy is needed after complete resection done in the neonatal period. If the tumor is not surgically resected before the infant is 1 to 2 months old, the likelihood of the teratoma becoming malignant increases rapidly.

CARE MANAGEMENT

Prenatal Diagnosis

Refined testing procedures are available to monitor fetal development. Prenatal diagnostic techniques such as amniocentesis, ultrasonography, alpha-fetoprotein measurements, chorionic villus sampling, percutaneous umbilical cord blood sampling, and gene probes contribute information to the database (see Chapter 29). Although they represent a valuable adjunct to prenatal care, these tests cannot identify all congenital disorders. Furthermore, there are ethical issues surrounding such testing, and the nurse must be prepared to support the family's decision regarding these tests. If a disorder is detected and the family decides to proceed with the pregnancy, the advantage is that appropriate care can be made available for the infant immediately at birth.

In addition to testing, the history and medical information in the prenatal record is reviewed for factors that are associated with congenital disorders. These factors include various medical, surgical, and social conditions and their treatments (see Chapter 33); maternal infection (see Chapter 8); maternal endocrine and metabolic disorders (see Chapter 32); and infection and drug dependence in the newborn (see Chapter 39).

Perinatal Diagnosis

Many congenital anomalies require intervention soon after birth. By careful observations in the birth room or nursery, the nurse can identify most of these conditions. An excessive amount of amniotic fluid, **hydramnios,** is commonly associated with congenital anomalies in the newborn, and such infants should be examined closely at the earliest possible time.

Oligohydramnios, which is an insufficient amount of amniotic fluid, is associated primarily with anomalies of the urinary tract that prevent normal micturition in utero. It is most often associated with renal agenesis or dysplasia and obstructive lesions in the lower urinary tract. Anomalies of the ears sometimes occur with renal abnormalities. Bilateral renal agenesis, resulting in oligohydramnios, commonly manifests as Potter syndrome, which is characterized by atypical facial appearance consisting of a flat nose, recessed chin, epicanthal folds, and low-set abnormal ears; limb abnormalities; pulmonary hypoplasia; and

fetal growth restriction. These conditions may be diagnosed prenatally.

Postnatal Diagnosis

Apgar scoring and a brief assessment are completed for all neonates after birth. Any deviations from normal are reported to the physician or midwife immediately. A thorough assessment of all body systems follows, with identification of both visible anomalies and those that might not be visible. Because the etiology and prevention of most congenital disorders remains unknown, it is still necessary to rely on immediate diagnosis and initiation of treatment to reduce the mortality rate of these children (Druschel, Hughes, & Olsen, 1996).

Some infants have multiple congenital anomalies. A recognized pattern of malformations is referred to as a *syndrome.* The most common is Down syndrome (Table 40-1, Fig. 40-15), with diagnosis confirmed early in the neonatal period.

Genetic diagnosis. Diagnostic procedures for the detection of genetic disorders are performed after birth at any time from the postnatal period through adulthood. There are many tests for various disorders; only the most frequently used ones are discussed here.

Biochemical tests. The most widespread use of postnatal testing for genetic disease is the routine screening of newborns for inborn errors of metabolism such as phenylketonuria (PKU), which is mandatory in most states in the United States. **Inborn errors of metabolism** is the term applied to a large group of disorders caused by a metabolic defect that results from the absence of or change in a protein, usually an enzyme, and mediated by the action of a certain gene. These defects can involve any substrate produced from protein, carbohydrate, or fat metabolism. Inborn errors of metabolism are recessive disorders, and, for this reason, for them to occur, a person must receive a defective gene from each parent. The parents usually are unaffected because their normal dominant gene directs the synthesis of sufficient protein to meet their metabolic needs under normal circumstances. With the advent of new biochemical techniques, it is now possible to detect the abnormal gene responsible for causing an increasing number of these disorders.

PKU results from a deficiency of the enzyme phenylalanine dehydrogenase (see Chapter 14). The test for PKU is not reliable, however, until the newborn has ingested an ample amount of the amino acid phenylalanine, a constituent of both human and cow milk.

NURSE ALERT *The nurse must document the initial ingestion of milk and perform the test at least 24 hours after that time.*

The current trend toward early infant discharge from the hospital has the potential to cause neonates with a disorder such as PKU not to be screened as frequently as in

TABLE 40-1 Common Autosomal Aberrations

SYNDROME	CHROMOSOMAL ABNORMALITY AND NOMENCLATURE	AVERAGE INCIDENCE* (LIVE BIRTHS)	MAJOR CLINICAL MANIFESTATIONS
Cri-du-chat	Deletion of short arm of no. 5 chromosome—46,XY,5p	1:50,000	Distinctive weak, high-pitched mewlike cry resembling the cry of a cat; small head; hypertelorism; failure to thrive; severe mental retardation
Trisomy 13 (Patau)	Trisomy of no. 13 chromosome—47,XY,+13	1:4000 to 1:15,000	Cleft lip and palate (frequently bilateral); ear malformations; microphthalmia; polydactyly; eye defects; cardiac defects; mental retardation; early death
Trisomy 18 (Edwards)	Trisomy of no. 18 chromosome—47,XY,+18	1:3500 to 1:8000	Deformed and low-set ears; micrognathia; rocker-bottom feet; overlapping (index over third) fingers; prominent occiput; hypertelorism; cardiac defects; failure to thrive and early death; mental retardation
Trisomy 21 (Down)	Trisomy of no. 21 chromosome—47,XY,+21 (trisomy); 46,XY,+(14;21) (translocation); 46,XY/47,XY,+21 (mosaic)	1:700†	Brachycephaly with flat occiput; inner epicanthal folds; small ears, nose, and mouth with protruding tongue; muscular hypotonia; broad, short hands with stubby fingers and simian palmar crease; broad, stubby feet with wide space between big and second toes; mental retardation; variable life expectancy

Modified from Wong, D. (1999). *Whaley and Wong's nursing care of infants and children* (6th ed.). St. Louis: Mosby.
*Data from Nora, J., & Fraser, F. (1989). *Medical genetics: Principles and practice* (3rd ed.). Philadelphia: Lea & Febiger.
†Risk related to maternal age: 30 years, 1/900; 35 years, 1/300; 40 years, 1/100; 45 years, 1/30.

the past. In response to this, the American Academy of Pediatrics (1996) has made the following recommendations:
- Obtain a subsequent sample before 2 weeks of age if the initial specimen is collected before the newborn is 24 hours old.
- Designate a primary care provider to all newborns before discharge for adequate newborn screening follow-up.
- Collect the initial specimen as close as possible to discharge or no later than 7 days after birth.

If the infant is found to have PKU, a diet low in phenylalanine is begun soon after birth. Breastfeeding or partial breastfeeding may be possible for some infants if the phenylalanine levels are monitored carefully and remain within acceptable limits (Kirby, 1999). Although severe mental retardation is seen less in affected children living in countries where there is neonatal screening for PKU, many affected children have some intellectual impairment.

Galactosemia, caused by a deficiency of the enzyme galactose 1-phosphate uridyltransferase, results in the inability to convert galactose to glucose. Galactosemia can be detected by measuring the blood levels of galactose in the urine of newborns suspected of having the disease who have ingested formula containing galactose. Early symptoms are vomiting, weight loss, and CNS symptoms, including poor feeding, drowsiness, and seizures. If the disorder goes untreated, the galactose levels will continue to increase and the affected infant will show failure to thrive, mental retardation, cataracts, jaundice, hepatomegaly, and cirrhosis of the liver, with death possibly occurring in the first month of life. Therapy consists of eliminating galactose from the diet.

Congenital hypothyroidism results from a deficiency of thyroid hormones and affects approximately 1 of every 3600 to 5000 newborns (American Academy of Pediatrics, 1996). All states in the United States routinely screen for hypothyroidism. This can be done by measuring thyroxine (T_4) in a drop of blood obtained from a heel stick at 2 to 5 days of age. At this time the normally expected increase in T_4 would be lacking in newborns with hypothyroidism. It is more often included as part of the newborn screen done in the first 24 to 48 hours or before discharge. Early screening may have false-positive results, but this is better than failure to detect infants with hypothyroidism. Treatment is thyroid hormone replacement. If untreated, symptoms usually appear after 6 weeks and include bradycardia; hypothermia; hypotension; hyporeflexia; abdominal distention; umbilical hernia; coarse, dry hair; thick, dry skin that feels cold; anemia; widely patent cranial sutures; and retarded bone age beginning at birth. The most disabling problem, however, is delayed development of the nervous system, leading to severe mental retardation (Wong, 1999).

Cytologic studies. Abnormalities can occur in either the autosomes or the sex chromosomes. Chromosomal disorders often can be diagnosed on the basis of the clinical manifestations alone. However, an infant may have a clinical appearance that is only suggestive of a problem. Cytologic studies must be done to confirm or rule out a suspected diagnosis.

Disorders in the number or structure of chromosomes can be diagnosed by a *karyotype* (see Fig. 14-2), which is a photographic enlargement of the chromosomes arranged by their numbered pairs.

Abnormalities of the sex chromosomes make up about half of all the chromosomal abnormalities occurring in the newborn. The most common test for sex chromosome abnormalities is the buccal smear, using cells scraped from the mucosa inside the mouth. When prepared and stained, these show the number of inactive X chromosomes, also known as an *X-chromatin mass* or a *Barr body*. Each cell, whether male or female, has one genetically active X chromosome. Therefore a normal female has one active X chromosome and one Barr body, which is on the inactive X chromosome. A normal male has no Barr bodies, because he has only one genetically active X chromosome.

Dermatoglyphics. Dermatoglyphics is the study of the patterns formed by the ridges in the skin on the digits, palms, and soles. Development of these ridges begins during the thirteenth week of gestation and is complete by the nineteenth week. Thus many genetic and chromosomal disorders will also affect the ridges. The addition or deletion of genetic material produces alterations in the loops, swirls, and arches of the finger and toe prints, in the palm lines, and in the flexion creases on the palms of the hands and soles of the feet. Characteristic dermatoglyphic patterns have been noted for almost all the chromosomal abnormalities, such as Down syndrome.

An infant with Down syndrome may have a single, palmar crease (see simian crease in Fig. 40-15), a single flexion crease of the fifth digit, and an open-field pattern on the ball of the foot (Subjansky & Matthews, 1998). The characteristic dermatoglyphic feature in a child with Turner syndrome is the large size of the dermal patterns on the fingers and toes. Certain fingerprint patterns may also be found in those people who have cardiac valvular problems later in life. Asymmetry of palmar ridges has been reported in congenital anomalies such as cleft lip and palate and congenital vertebral anomaly (Goldberg et al., 1997).

The nursing diagnoses formulated for an infant born with a congenital anomaly depend on the anomaly the infant has. For example, the diagnoses in an infant born with

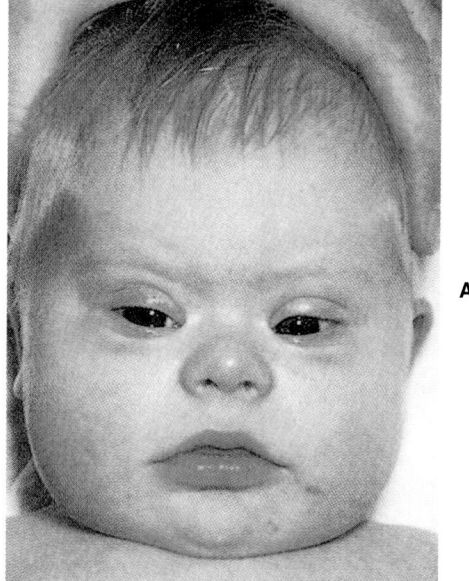

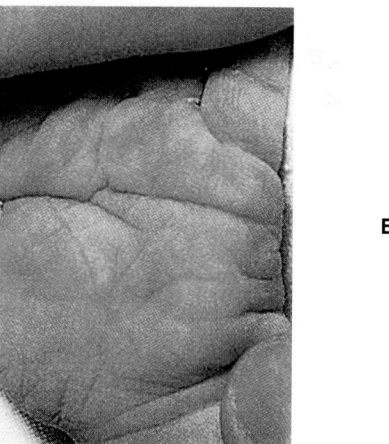

Fig. 40-15   A, Clinical features of Down syndrome. **B,** Simian crease. *(From Zitelli, B., & Davis, H. [1997]. Atlas of pediatric physical diagnosis [3rd ed.]. St. Louis: Mosby.)*

a CHD causing cyanosis will relate to inadequate oxygenation of body tissues, such as "activity intolerance related to imbalance between oxygen supply and demand." General nursing diagnoses pertaining to the care of neonates with congenital abnormalities include the following:

▮ Nursing Diagnoses _____

Newborn
- Risk for injury or death related to
  - presence of a congenital disorder
- Risk for infection related to
  - anomaly or its treatment
- Risk for impaired gas exchange, nutrition, or mobility related to
  - congenital anomaly

Continued

▮ Nursing Diagnoses—cont'd

- Risk for altered growth and development related to
  - inborn error of metabolism

Parents and Family

- Dysfunctional grieving or spiritual distress related to
  - birth of a child with a defect
- Risk for ineffective individual or family coping related to
  - birth of a child with a defect
- Knowledge deficit related to
  - cause of disorder, its management, alternative courses of action, community resources, prognosis, and the care needed by the child after discharge
- Anxiety related to
  - uncertainty regarding prognosis or ability to care for child
- Risk for altered parenting related to
  - birth of a child with a disorder or defect

Collaborative Care

Newborn

A collaborative health team approach that includes specialists (e.g., orthodontists, physical therapists, geneticists) and community service representatives is needed in the care of infants with some disorders. Surgical intervention in the neonatal period may be necessary for the infant requiring either immediate correction or a palliative procedure to relieve the symptoms of the anomaly until definitive correction can be done. However, the complications induced by the stress of surgery may upset the delicate metabolic balance in a neonate already attempting to adapt to its extrauterine environment. This is compounded by the fact that there is only a limited amount of nutrient reserves normally present in the neonate and these reserves are already being drawn on by the energy-expending processes involved in rapid growth. Any surgical procedures performed during this time of growth place additional demands on these reserves. There is also a higher morbidity and mortality rate in neonates than in older children or adults undergoing similar procedures. However, despite these problems unique to neonates, advances in surgical techniques, anesthesia, and the nursing care given in intensive care nurseries have together been responsible for lessening the risk of surgery in neonates.

The health care team must be highly skilled to meet the needs of these infants. These needs are similar to those of the compromised infant. In addition to stabilization of the infant's condition, other preoperative interventions, such as orogastric tube placement for abdominal decompression, the management of open lesions, and the maintenance of fluid and electrolyte balance, are implemented to manage specific anomalies.

Postoperatively the infant is returned to the intensive care nursery, where close monitoring is maintained. The infant's respiratory efforts are supported; this often requires suctioning and usually mechanical ventilation. Constant surveillance is necessary to detect any respiratory complications resulting from the anesthesia. A pulse oximeter is attached to measure the oxygen saturation in hemoglobin, which closely correlates with arterial oxygen saturation. Oxygen is provided as needed. An indwelling gastric catheter attached to intermittent suction is placed to remove gastric secretions, thereby preventing aspiration and the abdomen from becoming distended. The infant's fluid, electrolyte, and acid-base status are monitored and adjusted as needed. Urinary output is monitored and should equal 1 to 2 ml/kg/hr. Other nursing interventions are focused on caring for the surgical site, maintaining thermoregulation, and promoting comfort.

Parents and Family

While the infant is receiving optimal care, the parents, too, have needs that must be met as they deal with the crisis of having an infant with an abnormal condition. Their reactions are carefully assessed and are likely to be those typical of a grief response. Facilitating their understanding of the information given them about their infant's condition is a vital nursing intervention. A newly diagnosed disorder often implies the need for the implementation of a therapeutic regimen. For example, the disorder may be an inborn error of metabolism, such as PKU, which requires consistent and rigid adherence to a diet. The family of such an infant may need help with securing the required formula and receiving counseling from the clinical dietitian. The importance of maintaining the diet, keeping an adequate supply of special preparations, and avoiding the use of unauthorized substitutions must be impressed on the family.

Referral to appropriate agencies is another essential component of the follow-up management, and the nurse should make the parents aware of all possible sources of aid, including pertinent literature, parent groups, and national organizations. Many organizations and foundations, such as the Cystic Fibrosis Foundation and the Muscular Dystrophy Association, provide services and equipment for affected children. There are also numerous parent groups the family can join where they can share experiences and derive mutual support in coping with problems similar to those of other group members. Nurses should be familiar with the services available in their community that provide assistance and education to families with these special problems (see Appendix D).

A major nursing function is providing emotional support to the family during all aspects of the care of the child born with a defect or disorder. The feelings stemming from the real or imagined threat posed by a congenital anomaly are as varied as the people being counseled. Responses may include apathy, denial, anger, hostility, fear, embarrassment, grief, and loss of self-esteem (see Chapter 42).

Parents benefit from seeing before-and-after pictures of other babies born with the same defect. Coupled with other verbal and nonverbal supportive care, this visual reassurance may be effective in allaying their concerns.

Families need much information, guidance, and support as they make decisions regarding the care of their infant. Once they have been given the facts and possible consequences and all the assistance they need in problem solving, the final decision regarding a course of action must be their own. It is then incumbent on health care providers to support the decision of the family.

KEY POINTS

- Hyperbilirubinemia is caused by a variety of factors, including maternal-fetal Rh and ABO incompatibility.
- Erythroblastosis fetalis leads to anemia, edema, and the cytotoxic effects of unconjugated bilirubin.
- The injection of $Rh_0(D)$ immune globulin in Rh-negative and Coombs' test–negative women bestows passive immunity and also minimizes the possibility of isoimmunization.
- An Rh-negative woman may receive Rh-positive red blood cells (RBCs) from the fetus if the cellular layer separating fetal and maternal circulation is disrupted.
- Neonatal exchange transfusion with type O, Rh-negative RBCs serves to treat anemia and acidosis and to remove bilirubin, maternal antibodies, and fetal RBCs that are beginning to hemolyze.
- Perinatal events such as hypoxia and cold stress increase the infant's susceptibility to the neurotoxic effects of bilirubin.
- Major congenital defects are the leading cause of death in infants younger than 1 year of age in the United States and account for 20% of neonatal deaths.
- Hydramnios and oligohydramnios are associated with the occurrence of many congenital anomalies.
- Current technology permits the prenatal diagnosis of many congenital anomalies and disorders.
- The curative and rehabilitative problems of an infant with a congenital disorder are often complex and require a multidisciplinary approach to care.
- The supportive care given to the parents of infants with an abnormal condition must begin at birth or at the time of diagnosis and continue for years.

CRITICAL THINKING EXERCISES

1 You are caring for Donna, who is 21 years old, married, and has just given birth to her first child, Erik, who has been diagnosed as having a ventricular septal defect. Donna is in good health, and her pregnancy was uneventful, except for an upper respiratory infection the week before. You are talking with her as she is holding Erik.
  a. She asks, "What did I do wrong to cause Erik to have a heart defect? Was it because of the cold I had last week? Will he die? If I have more children, will they have heart defects, too?" How would you respond to these questions?
  b. Identify health care team members that you will include as you plan the care for Donna and Erik.
  c. You are assisting as Donna feeds Erik. She is anxious and states that she fears Erik will "turn blue." What is your response?
  d. What are your priority nursing diagnoses at this time? Describe your rationale for these diagnoses.
  e. What nursing actions would you select and implement?
  f. What are the criteria for evaluating the nursing care of Erik and his parents?

2 On the same day, you are also caring for Dianna, who is 30 years old and has just given birth to Ben, who has a cleft lip and palate.
  a. What are your priority nursing diagnoses at this time?
  b. Why might Ben and Erik have feeding problems? Describe the feeding-related interventions that would be most appropriate for each infant. Dianna wishes to breastfeed Ben. What is your response?
  c. How do you think Dianna might respond to her son's having a cleft lip and palate?
  d. How will this defect affect Ben's growth and development?

3 Shaquelle, an African-American, has given birth at term to Maya, who is now 48 hours old, and is about to be discharged from the hospital. Shaquelle is having some difficulty breastfeeding Maya, despite many suggestions from her mother-in-law, who lives next door. The nursery nurse assesses Maya, thinks she has jaundice, and arranges to have blood drawn for a bilirubin level. Her bilirubin level is 6 mg/dl, and all other labs are normal.
  a. Is it likely that the jaundice is pathologic?
  b. What do you think the treatment will be?
  c. What feeding recommendations should the nurse make?
  d. What assessments regarding Maya's hydration status can you teach Shaquelle to do at home?
  e. What follow-up care will be needed for Maya?

References

American Academy of Pediatrics Committee on Genetics. (1996). Newborn screening facts. *Pediatrics* 98, 473-481.

Augustine, M. (1999). Hyperbilirubinemia in the healthy term newborn. *Nurse Pract* 24, 24-41.

Balasubrahmanyam, G., Scherer, N., & Martin, J. (1998). Cleft lip and palate: Keys to successful management. *Contemp Pediatr* 15, 133-153.

Ball, J., & Bindler, R. (1999). *Pediatric nursing: Caring for children* (2nd ed.). Stamford, CT: Appleton & Lange.

Ballock, R., & Richards, B. (1997). Hip dysplasia: Early diagnosis makes a difference. *Contemp Pediatr* 14, 108-117.

Bellinger, M. (1997). Urologic disorders. In B. Zitelli & H. Davis (Eds.). *Atlas of pediatric physical diagnosis* (3rd ed.). St. Louis: Mosby.

Booth, I., & Wozniak, E. (1984). *Pediatrics*. Baltimore: Williams & Wilkins.

Bratlid, D. (1996). Criteria for treatment of neonatal jaundice. *J Perinatol* 16, 583-588.

Chessell, G. et al. (1984). *Diagnostic picture tests in clinical medicine* (vol. 2). St. Louis: Mosby.

Chondhury, S. et al. (1999). Survival of patients with esophageal atresia: Influence of birth weight, cardiac anomaly, and late respiratory complications. *J Pediatr Surg* 34, 70-74.

Chuangsuwanich, A. et al. (1998). Epidemiology of cleft lip and palate in Thailand. *Ann Plast Surg* 41, 7-10.

Daberkow-Carson, E., & Washington, R. (1998). Cardiovascular diseases and surgical interventions. In G. Merenstein & S. Gardner (Eds.). *Handbook of neonatal intensive care* (4th ed.). St. Louis: Mosby.

Darzi, M., Chowdri, N., & Bhat, A. (1996). Breastfeeding or spoon feeding after cleft lip repair: A prospective, randomized study. *Br J Plast Surg* 49, 24-26.

Dennery, P., & Rodgers, P. (1996). Ontogeny and developmental regulation of heme oxygenase. *J Perinatol* 16, 579-583.

Dickason, E., Silverman, B., & Kaplan, J. (1998). *Maternal-infant nursing care* (3rd ed.). St. Louis: Mosby.

Dixit, R., & Gartner, L. (1999). The jaundiced newborn: Minimizing the risks. *Contemp Pediatr* 16, 166-183.

Drummond, G., Valaes, T., & Kappas, A. (1996). Control of bilirubin production by synthetic heme analogs: Pharmacologic and toxicologic considerations. *J Perinatol* 16, 572-579.

Druschel, C., Hughes, J., & Olsen, C. (1996). Mortality among infants with congenital malformations. *Public Health Rep* 111, 359-365.

Elias, E., & Hobbs, N. (1998). Spina bifida: Sorting out the complexities of care. *Contemp Pediatr* 15, 156-171.

Fanaroff, A., & Martin, R. (1997). *Neonatal-perinatal medicine: Diseases of the fetus and infant* (6th ed.). St. Louis: Mosby.

Finegold, D. (1997). Endocrinology. In B. Zitelli & H. Davis (Eds.). *Atlas of pediatric physical diagnosis* (3rd ed.). St. Louis: Mosby.

Finer, N. et al. (1998). Congenital diaphragmatic hernia: Developing a protocolized approach. *J Pediatr Surg* 33, 31-37.

Frank, C., Cooper, S., & Merenstein, G. (1998). Jaundice. In G. Merenstein & S. Gardner (Eds.). *Handbook of neonatal intensive care* (4th ed.). St. Louis: Mosby.

Goldberg, C. et al. (1997). Fluctuating asymmetry and vertebral malformation: A study of dermatoglyphics in congenital spine deformities. *Spine* 22, 775-779.

Grover, G. (1996). Rotational problems of the lower extremity: In-toeing and out-toeing. In C. Berkowitz (Ed.). *Pediatrics: A primary care approach*. Philadelphia: W.B. Saunders.

Hoek, H., Brown, A., & Susser, E. (1998). The Dutch famine and schizophrenia spectrum disorders. *Soc Psychiatry Psychiatr Epidemiol* 33, 373-379.

Holland, R., Price, F., & Bensard D. (1998). Neonatal surgery. In G. Merenstein & S. Gardner (Eds.). *Handbook of neonatal intensive care* (4th ed.). St. Louis: Mosby.

Jackson, P., & Harvey, J. (1996). Hydrocephalus. In P. Jackson & J. Vessey (Eds.). *Primary care of the child with a chronic condition* (2nd ed.). St. Louis: Mosby.

Kirby, R. (1999). Maternal phenylketonuria: A new cause for concern. *J Obstet Gynecol Neonatal Nurs* 28(3), 227-234.

Morrow, J., & Kelsey, K. (1998). Folic acid for prevention of neural tube defects: Pediatric anticipatory guidance. *J Pediatr Health Care* 12, 55-59.

Nakayama, D. (1997). Surgery. In B. Zitelli & H. Davis (Eds.). *Atlas of pediatric physical diagnosis* (3rd ed.). St. Louis: Mosby.

Nora, J., & Fraser, F. (1989). *Medical genetics: Principles and practice* (3rd ed.). Philadelphia: Lea & Febiger.

Novacheck, T. (1996). Developmental dysplasia of the hip. *Pediatr Clin North Am* 43, 829-848.

O'Doherty, N. (1986). *Neonatology: Micro atlas of the newborn*. Nutley, NJ: Hoffmann-La Roche.

Paulozzi, L., Erickson, D., & Jackson, R. (1997). Hypospadias trends in two U.S. surveillance systems. *Pediatrics* 100, 831-834.

Queisser-Luft, A. et al. (1996). Serial examination of 20,248 newborn fetuses and infants: Correlations between drug exposure and major malformations. *Am J Med Genet* 70, 99-101.

Ryckman, F., Flake, A., & Balisteri, W. (1997). Upper gastrointestinal disorders. In A. Fanaroff & R. Martin (Eds.). *Neonatal-perinatal medicine: Diseases of the fetus and infant* (6th ed.). St. Louis: Mosby.

Schaefer, U. et al. (1997). Congenital malformations in offspring of women with hyperglycemia first detected during pregnancy. *Am J Obstet Gynecol* 177, 1165-1171.

Stapleton, S. (1996). The infant with tracheoesophageal fistula and esophageal atresia. *Mother Baby Journal* 1, 13-16.

Steele, M. (1997). Common chromosomal disorders. In B. Zitelli & H. Davis (Eds.). *Atlas of pediatric physical diagnosis* (3rd ed.). St. Louis: Mosby.

Subjansky, E., & Matthews, A. (1998). Genetic disorders, malformations, and inborn errors of metabolism. In G. Merenstein & S. Gardner (Eds.). *Handbook of neonatal intensive care* (4th ed.). St. Louis: Mosby.

Wandstrat, T. (1997). $Rh_o(D)$ immune globulin. *Mother Baby Journal* 2, 45-48.

Wong, D. (1999). *Whaley and Wong's nursing care of infants and children* (6th ed.). St. Louis: Mosby.

Wong, D., & Perry, S. (1998). *Maternal child nursing care*. St. Louis: Mosby.

Yerkes, E. et al. (1998). Role of angiotensin in the congenital anomalies of the kidney and urinary tract in the mouse and the human. *Kidney Int Suppl* 67, S75-77.

Zitelli, B., & Davis, H. (1997). *Atlas of pediatric physical diagnosis* (3rd ed.). St. Louis: Mosby.

41

Nursing Care of the High Risk Newborn

Shannon E. Perry

LEARNING OBJECTIVES

- Define the key terms.
- Compare and contrast the characteristics of preterm, term, postterm, and postmature neonates.
- Discuss respiratory distress syndrome and the approach to treatment.
- Compare methods of oxygen therapy.
- Describe nursing interventions for nutritional care of the preterm infant.
- Discuss the pathophysiology of retinopathy of prematurity and bronchopulmonary dysplasia, and identify risk factors that predispose preterm infants to these problems.

- List the signs and symptoms of perinatal asphyxia.
- Describe meconium aspiration syndrome.
- Plan developmentally appropriate care.
- Examine the needs of parents of high risk infants.
- Evaluate a neonatal transport plan.
- Identify appropriate responses and interventions the nurse can use in caring for families experiencing anticipatory grief or loss and grief in the neonatal period.
- Identify topics for nursing research related to high risk newborns.

KEY TERMS

anticipatory grief
bronchopulmonary dysplasia (BPD)
continuous positive airway pressure (CPAP)
corrected age
extracorporeal membrane oxygenation (ECMO)
extremely low birth weight (ELBW)

hypoglycemia
insensible water loss (IWL)
kangaroo care
mechanical ventilation
meconium aspiration syndrome (MAS)
necrotizing enterocolitis (NEC)
neutral thermal environment (NTE)

nonnutritive sucking
patent ductus arteriosus (PDA)
periventricular-intraventricular hemorrhage (PV-IVH)
respiratory distress syndrome (RDS)
retinopathy of prematurity (ROP)
total parenteral nutrition

 odern technology and expert nursing care have made important contributions to improving the health and overall survival of high risk infants. However, infants who are born considerably before term and survive are particularly susceptible to the development of sequelae related to their preterm birth. These conditions, which can also occur in term and near-term infants, but not as frequently, include necrotizing enterocolitis, bronchopulmonary dysplasia, intraventricular and periventricular hemorrhage, and retinopathy of prematurity. The focus of this chapter

BOX 41-1   Resuscitation of Extremely Premature Infants

There are many different opinions about the resuscitation of extremely preterm infants weighing between 500 and 750 g. Ethical issues that nurses caring for such infants are confronted with include:
- Whether to resuscitate?
- Who should decide?
- Is the cost of resuscitation justified?
- Do the benefits of technology outweigh the burdens in relation to the quality of life?

All people involved (health care providers and parents) should participate in the discussions in which these controversial issues are resolved.

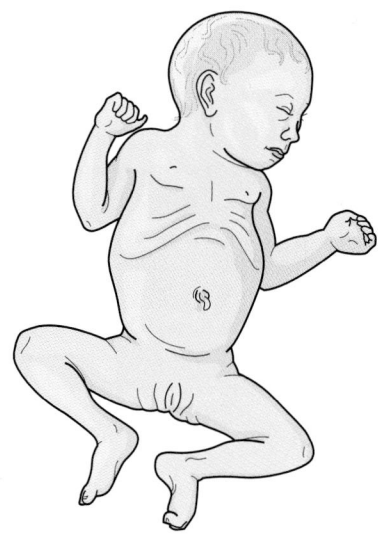

Fig. 41-1   Retractions: Substernal, subcostal, and intercostal retractions are evident. *(Courtesy Ross Laboratories, Columbus, OH.)*

is on care of the preterm infant. Care of other high risk infants with gestational age-related problems is also discussed.

PRETERM INFANTS

Preterm infants are at risk because their organ systems are immature and they lack adequate reserves of bodily nutrients. The potential problems and care needs of the preterm infant weighing 2000 g differ from those of the term, postterm, or postmature infant of equal weight. If these infants have physiologic disorders and anomalies as well, these affect the infant's response to treatment. In general, the closer infants are to term from the standpoint of both gestational age and birth weight, the easier their adjustment to the external environment. The cost of the care required by low birth weight (LBW) infants is estimated to be in the billions of dollars each year.

There are varying opinions about the practical and ethical dimensions of resuscitation of **extremely low birth weight** infants (those infants whose birth weight is 1000 g or less). Some of the ethical issues associated with resuscitation of these infants are in Box 41-1.

CARE MANAGEMENT

Assessment and Nursing Diagnoses

For the high risk infant, an accurate assessment of gestational age (see Chapter 27) is critical in helping the nurse identify the potential problems the newborn is likely to experience. The response of the preterm or postterm infant to extrauterine life is different from that of the term infant. By understanding the physiologic basis of these differences, the nurse can assess these infants, determine the response of the preterm or postterm infant, and discern which potential problems are most likely to occur.

Respiratory function. The preterm infant is likely to have difficulty making the pulmonary transition from intrauterine to extrauterine life. Numerous problems may af-

fect the respiratory systems of preterm infants and may include the following:
- Decreased number of functional alveoli
- Deficient surfactant levels
- Smaller lumen in the respiratory system
- Greater collapsibility or obstruction of respiratory passages
- Insufficient calcification of the bony thorax
- Weak or absent gag reflex
- Immature and friable capillaries in the lungs
- Greater distance between functional alveoli and the capillary bed

In combination, these deficits severely hinder the infant's respiratory efforts and can produce respiratory distress or apnea.

Respiratory difficulty often follows a progressive pattern. Infants normally breathe between 30 to 60 breaths/min, relying significantly on their abdominal muscles to accomplish this (Hagedorn, Gardner, & Abman, 1998). However, the respiratory rate may increase without a change in rhythm. Early signs of respiratory distress include flaring of the nares and an expiratory grunt. Depending on the cause, retractions may begin as subcostal, suprasternal, or clavicular retractions (Fig. 41-1). If the infant shows increasing respiratory effort, for example, seesaw breathing patterns, retraction, flaring of the nares, expiratory grunts, and apneic spells (Fig. 41-2), this indicates deepening distress. A compromised infant's color progresses from pink to circumoral cyanosis and then to generalized cyanosis. Acrocyanosis deepens. (Acrocyanosis is a normal finding in the neonate, but central cyanosis indicates the existence of an underlying problem.)

Periodic breathing is a respiratory pattern commonly seen in premature infants. Such infants exhibit 5- to 10-

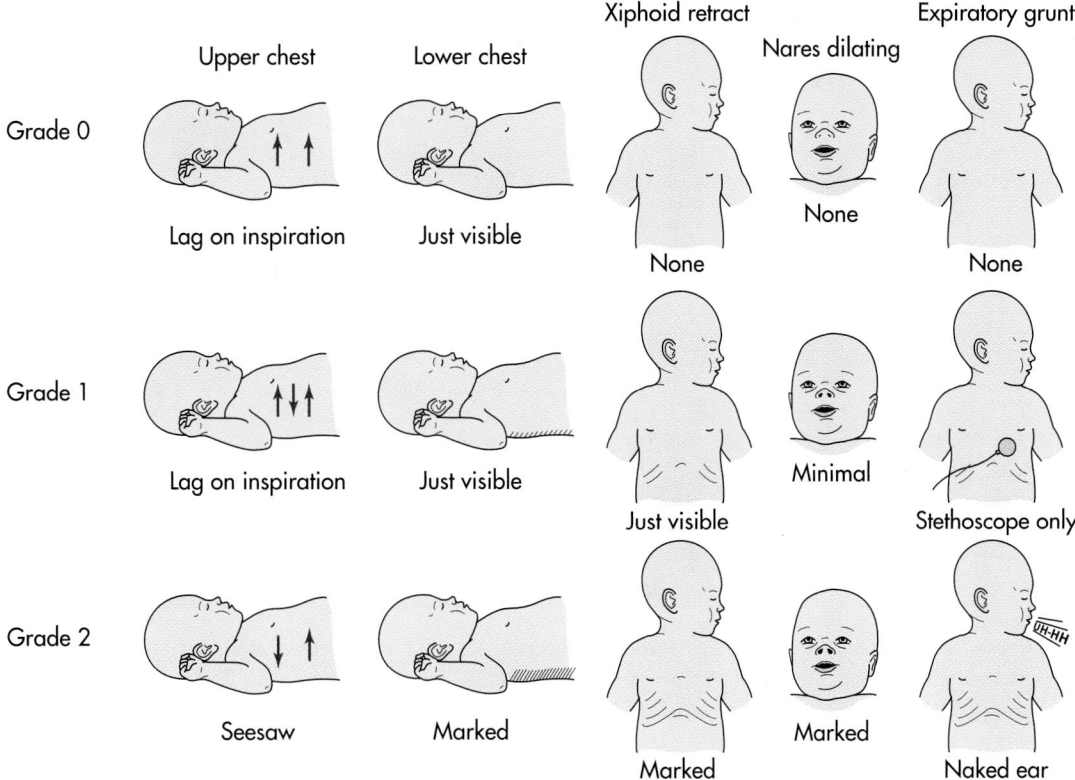

	Upper chest	Lower chest	Xiphoid retract	Nares dilating	Expiratory grunt
Grade 0	Lag on inspiration	Just visible	None	None	None
Grade 1	Lag on inspiration	Just visible	Just visible	Minimal	Stethoscope only
Grade 2	Seesaw	Marked	Marked	Marked	Naked ear

Fig. 41-2 Observation of retractions. Silverman-Anderson index of respiratory distress is determined by grading each of five arbitrary criteria: *grade 0,* no respiratory difficulty; *grade 1,* moderate difficulty; and *grade 2,* maximum difficulty. The retraction score is a sum of these values; a total score of 0 indicates no dyspnea, whereas a total score of 10 indicates maximum respiratory distress. *(Modified from Silverman, W., & Anderson, D. [1956]. A controlled clinical trial of effects of water mist on obstructive respiratory signs, death rate and necropsy findings among premature infants. Pediatrics 17, 1.)*

second respiratory pauses followed by 10 to 15 seconds of compensatory rapid respirations. Such periodic breathing should not be confused with apnea, which is a 15- to 20-second cessation of respiration. The nurse needs to be prepared to provide oxygen and ventilation as necessary (Cloherty & Stark, 1997).

Cardiovascular function. Evaluation of heart rate and rhythm, skin color, blood pressure, perfusion, pulses, oxygen saturation, and acid-base status provides information on the cardiovascular status. The nurse must be prepared to intervene if symptoms of hypovolemia, shock, or both, are found. These symptoms include hypotension, slow capillary refill (>3 seconds), and continued respiratory distress despite the provision of oxygen and ventilation.

An accurate and timely blood pressure reading can assist in making an early diagnosis of cardiorespiratory disease and in monitoring the effects of fluid therapy. Blood pressure readings can be obtained by the Doppler method or by an electronic monitor (Fig. 41-3).

Maintaining body temperature. Preterm infants are susceptible to temperature instability as a result of numerous factors. Preterm infants are at high risk for heat loss because of the large body surface area in relation to weight.

Other factors that place preterm infants at risk for temperature instability include the following:
- Minimal insulating subcutaneous fat
- Limited stores of brown fat (an internal source for the generation of heat present in normal term infants)
- Decreased or absent reflex control of skin capillaries (shiver response)
- Inadequate muscle mass activity (rendering the preterm infant unable to produce its own heat)
- Poor muscle tone resulting in more body surface area being exposed to the cooling effects of the environment
- Friable (easily damaged) capillaries
- An immature temperature regulation center in the brain

The goal of thermoregulation is to create a **neutral thermal environment (NTE),** which is the environmental temperature at which oxygen consumption is minimal but adequate to maintain the body temperature (Cloherty & Stark, 1997). Armed with the knowledge of the four mechanisms of heat transfer (convection, conduction, radiation, and evaporation), the nurse can then create an environment for the preterm infant that prevents temperature instability (see Chapter 26). The infant will be kept in a radiant warmer or isolette with control settings at a

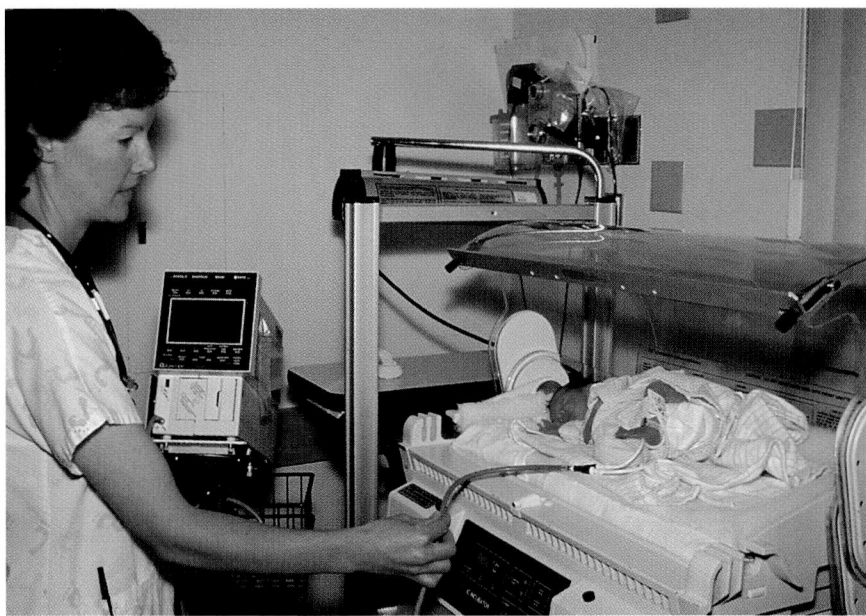

Fig. 41-3 Preparing to assess a newborn's blood pressure. Note stethoscopes for auscultation and electronic equipment. Blood pressure cuff should cover no more than 75% of the upper arm. *(Courtesy Michael S. Clement, MD, Mesa, AZ.)*

BOX 41-2 | **Signs of Cold Stress**

Skin temperature	Decreases before other signs.
Respiratory rate	Initially increases, then apneic spells occur.
Heart rate	Initially increases, then bradycardia occurs.
Skin color	Mottled with acrocyanosis increasing to cyanosis.
Physical activity	Increased in term infants without respiratory distress.
	Decreased in term infants with respiratory distress.
	Decreased in premature infants.
Thermoregulatory control	Unstable in premature infants.

---

temperature to maintain the NTE. Signs of cold stress are listed in Box 41-2.

Central nervous system function. The preterm infant's central nervous system (CNS) is susceptible to injury as a result of the following problems:

- Birth trauma that includes damage to immature structures
- Bleeding from fragile capillaries
- An impaired coagulation process, including prolonged prothrombin time
- Recurrent anoxic episodes
- Predisposition to hypoglycemia

Research data indicate that the developing nervous system has the ability to reorganize neural connection after injury, meaning that some injuries that would be permanent in adults are not so in infants. Certain neurologic signs appear to be predictive of later neurologic abnormalities. These signs include hypotonia, a decreased level of activity, weak cry for more than 24 hours, and an inability to coordinate suck and swallow (Fanaroff & Martin, 1997). Ongoing assessment and documentation of these neurologic signs is needed for the purpose of discharge teaching and making follow-up recommendations, as well as for their predictive value.

Maintaining adequate nutrition. The goal of neonatal nutrition is to promote normal growth and development (Cloherty & Stark, 1997). However, the maintenance of adequate nutrition in the preterm infant is complicated by problems with intake and metabolism. The preterm infant has the following disadvantages with regard to intake: weak or absent suck, swallow, and gag reflexes; a small stomach capacity; and weak abdominal muscles. The preterm infant's metabolic functions are compromised by a limited store of nutrients, a decreased ability to digest proteins or absorb nutrients, and immature enzyme systems.

The nurse must continuously assess the infant's ability to take in and digest nutrients. Some preterm infants require gavage or intravenous (IV) feedings instead of oral feedings.

Maintaining renal function. The preterm infant's immature renal system is unable to (1) adequately excrete metabolites and drugs; (2) concentrate urine; or (3) maintain acid-base, fluid, or electrolyte balance (Cloherty &

Stark, 1997). Therefore intake and output, as well as specific gravity, must be assessed. Laboratory tests must be done to assess acid-base and electrolyte balance. Medication levels are also monitored in preterm infants because certain medications can overwhelm the immature system's ability to excrete them.

Maintaining hematologic status. The preterm infant is also particularly predisposed to hematologic problems due to the following problems:

- Increased capillary friability
- Increased tendency to bleed (prolonged prothrombin time and partial thromboplastin time)
- Slowed production of red blood cells resulting from rapid decrease in erythropoiesis after birth
- Loss of blood due to frequent blood sampling for laboratory tests
- Decreased red blood cell survival related to the relatively larger size of the red blood cell and its increased permeability to sodium and potassium

The nurse assesses such infants for any evidence of bleeding from puncture sites and the gastrointestinal (GI) tract. Infants are also examined for signs of anemia (decreased hemoglobin and hematocrit levels, pale skin, increased apnea, lethargy, tachycardia, and poor weight gain) (Fanaroff & Martin, 1997).

Resisting infection. Preterm infants are at increased risk for infection because they have a shortage of stored maternal immunoglobulins, an impaired ability to make antibodies, and a compromised integumentary system (thin skin and fragile capillaries). Preterm infants exhibit various nonspecific signs and symptoms of infection (Box 41-3). Early identification and treatment of sepsis are essential (see Chapter 39). As with all aspects of care, strict handwashing is the single most important measure to prevent iatrogenic infections.

Growth and Development Potential

Although it is impossible to predict with complete accuracy the growth and development potential of each preterm infant, some findings support an anticipated favorable outcome in the absence of ongoing medical sequelae that can affect growth, such as bronchopulmonary dysplasia, necrotizing enterocolitis, and CNS problems. The lower the birth weight, the greater the likelihood of negative sequelae. The growth and development milestones (e.g., motor milestones, vocalization, growth) are corrected for gestational age until the child is approximately 2½ years of age (Avery, Fletcher, & MacDonald, 1994).

The age of a preterm newborn is corrected by adding the gestational age and the postnatal age. For example, an infant born at 32 weeks of gestation 4 weeks ago would now be considered 36 weeks of age. The infant's **corrected age** at 6 months after the birth date is then 4 months, and the infant's responses are accordingly evaluated against the norm expected for a 4-month-old infant.

BOX 41-3   Signs and Symptoms of Infection

- Temperature instability
  - Hypothermia
  - Hyperthermia
- CNS changes
  - Lethargy
  - Irritability
- Changes in color
  - Cyanosis, pallor
  - Jaundice
- Cardiovascular instability
  - Poor perfusion
  - Hypotension
  - Bradycardia/tachycardia
- Respiratory distress
  - Tachypnea
  - Apnea
  - Retractions, nasal flaring, grunting
- Gastrointestinal problems
  - Feeding intolerance
  - Vomiting
  - Diarrhea
  - Glucose instability
- Metabolic acidosis

There are certain measurable factors that predict normal growth and development. The preterm infant experiences catch-up body growth during the first 2 to 3 years of life, with maximum growth occurring between 36 and 40 weeks of postconceptional age (Fanaroff & Martin, 1997). The head is the first to experience catch-up growth, followed by a gain in weight and height (Cloherty & Stark, 1997). At the infant's discharge from the hospital, which usually occurs between 37 and 40 weeks of postconceptional age, the infant should exhibit the following characteristics:

- An ability to raise the head when prone and to hold the head parallel with the body when tested for the head lag response
- An ability to cry with vigor when hungry
- An appropriate amount and pattern of weight gain according to a growth grid
- Neurologic responses appropriate for corrected age

At 39 to 40 weeks of corrected age, the infant should be able to focus on the examiner's or parent's face and to follow with his or her eyes.

Of very low-birth-weight (VLBW) survivors, approximately 15% to 25% will have neurologic and/or cognitive disabilities in varying degrees of severity (Avery, Fletcher, & MacDonald, 1994).

Parental Adaptation to Preterm Infant

The experience of parents whose infant is born prematurely or is otherwise high risk is different from the experience of parents whose infant is born at term and is normal (Shields-Poe & Pinelli, 1997; Wereszczak, Miles, & Holditch-Davis, 1997). This may cause parental attachment and the adaptation to the parental role to differ as well.

Parental tasks. Parents of preterm infants must accomplish numerous psychologic tasks before effective relationships and parenting patterns can evolve. These tasks include the following:

- Experiencing **anticipatory grief** over the potential loss of an infant. The parent grieves in preparation for the infant's possible death, although the parent clings to the hope that the child will survive. This begins during labor and lasts until the infant dies or shows evidence of surviving. Anticipatory grief occurs when families have knowledge of an impending loss, such as when a baby is admitted to an NICU with problems or when a diagnosis of an anencephalic fetus is made by ultrasonography. The baby is still alive, but the prognosis is poor. Being able to anticipate the loss gives families an opportunity to plan, feel more in control of their situation, and say good-bye in a special way. However, some individuals or family members may distance or detach themselves from the experience or from their loved ones as a way of protecting themselves from the pain of loss and grief.
- The mother's acceptance of her failure to give birth to a healthy, full-term infant. Grief and depression typify this phase, which persists until the infant is out of danger and is expected to survive.
- Resuming the process of relating to the infant. As the baby's condition begins to improve and the baby gains weight, feeds by nipple, and is weaned from the isolette, the parent can begin the process of developing an attachment to the infant that was interrupted by the infant's critical condition at birth.

- Learning about the ways in which this baby differs in terms of his or her special needs and growth patterns and caregiving needs and growth and development expectations.
- Adjusting the home environment to accommodate the needs of the new infant. Parents are encouraged to limit the number of visitors to minimize exposure of the infant to pathogens. The environmental temperature may need to be altered to optimize conditions for the infant. Grandparents and siblings also react to the birth of the preterm infant. Parents must deal with the grief of grandparents and the bewilderment and anger of the infant's siblings at the seemingly disproportionate amount of parental time spent on the newborn.

Parental responses. Parents progress in interactions with their infants from maintaining an *en face* position, stroking, and touching their infant to assuming some child care activities, such as feeding, bathing, and changing the infant (Fig. 41-4). Parents go through numerous phases of adjustment as they learn to parent their infant. Nurses assist the transition to parenthood through their teaching and support of parental efforts.

Parenting disorders. The incidence of physical and emotional abuse has been found to be greater in infants who, because of preterm birth or illness, are separated from their parents for a time after birth (Fanaroff & Martin, 1997). Physical abuse includes varying degrees of poor nutrition, poor hygiene, and battering. Emotional abuse ranges from subtle disinterest to outright dislike of the infant to abandonment.

NURSE ALERT *Parents may also show preferential treatment toward the brothers and sisters of the infant, nag the infant, have extremely high expectations of the infant, or show other types of overt or covert negative parental responses.*

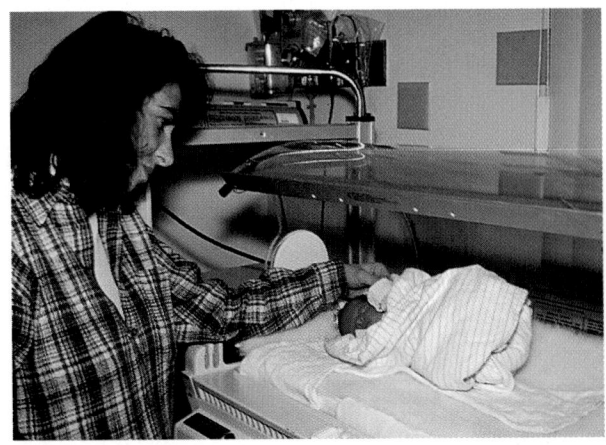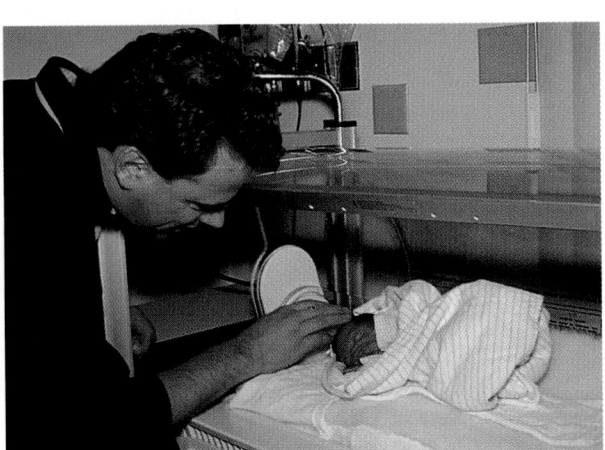

Fig. 41-4 **A,** Mother interacts with her premature infant by touch. **B,** Father interacts with his baby by stroking and touching baby with fingertip. *(Courtesy Michael S. Clement, MD, Mesa, AZ.)*

Factors surrounding the birth may predispose parents to treat their infant this way because subconsciously they have rejected the infant. These factors might include parental pain and anxiety, a heavy financial burden because of the cost of the infant's care, unresolved anticipatory grief, a threat to self-esteem, or the fact that the infant was the product of an unwanted pregnancy. The goal of health professionals is to identify abuse and neglect early so that further problems can be prevented and, in turn, the incidence of such abuse can be reduced.

Potential nursing diagnoses for high risk infants and their parents include the following:

▋ Nursing Diagnoses _____

- Impaired gas exchange related to
  - decreased number of functional alveoli
  - deficiency of surfactant
- Ineffective breathing pattern related to
  - inadequate chest expansion, secondary to infant position
- Ineffective thermoregulation related to
  - immature thermoregulation center
- Risk for infection related to
  - invasive procedures
  - decreased immune response
- Anxiety (parental) related to
  - lack of knowledge regarding infant condition
  - lack of knowledge regarding infant cues

Expected Outcomes of Care

The plan of nursing care for the preterm infant is directed by the physiologic needs of the infant's immature systems and often involves emergency treatments and procedures. Nursing care is a critical element in determining the infant's chances for survival, as well as normal development. In addition to meeting the infant's physical needs, nursing care is planned in conjunction with parents to promote parent-infant attachment and interaction. Expected outcomes are presented in client-centered terms and include that the infant will do the following:
- Maintain physiologic functioning.
- Maintain adequate nutrition.
- Experience no or minimal hematologic problems.
- Remain free of infection.
- Not develop retinal problems.
- Not suffer trauma to the immature musculoskeletal system.
- Experience attachment to parents.

Expected outcomes for the parents include that they will do the following:
- Perceive the infant as potentially normal (if this is medically substantiated).
- Provide care comfortably.
- Experience pride and satisfaction in the care of their infant.

- Organize their time and energies to meet the love, attention, and care needs of the other members of the family, as well as their own needs.

Plan of Care and Interventions

The best environment for fetal growth and development is the uterus of a healthy, well-nourished woman. The goal of care for the preterm infant is to provide an extrauterine environment that approximates the healthy intrauterine environment in order to promote normal growth and development. Physicians, nurses, and respiratory therapists work together as a team to provide the intensive care needed.

The admission of a preterm newborn to the intensive care nursery usually represents an emergency situation. Immediately after admission, a rapid initial evaluation is done to determine the infant's need for lifesaving treatment. Resuscitation is started in the birthing unit, and the newborn's need for warmth and oxygen is provided for during transfer to the nursery.

Nursing care is focused on the continuous assessment and analysis of the infant's physiologic status. Nurses fulfill many roles in providing the intensive and extended care that these infants require. In addition, they are the support persons and teachers during the first phase of the parents' adjustment to the birth of their preterm infant.

The nurse uses many technologic support systems to monitor the body responses and maintain the body functions of the infant. Technical skill needs to be combined with a gentle touch and concern about the traumatic effects of harsh lighting and the volume of machinery noise. The NICU environment may be a major contributing factor to learning and behavioral problems in preterm infants (Blackburn, 1998).

Physical Care

The environmental support measures for the preterm infant typically consist of the following equipment and procedures:
- An isolette or radiant warmer placed over the infant to control body temperature (NTE)
- Oxygen administration, depending on the infant's cardiopulmonary and circulatory status
- Electronic monitors as needed for the observation of respiratory and cardiac functions
- Assistive devices for positioning the infant in neutral flexion
- Clustering of care and minimization of stimulation

Various metabolic support measures that may be instituted consist of the following:
- Parenteral fluids to help support nutrition and maintain normal arterial blood gas (ABG) levels and acid-base balance
- IV access to facilitate the administration of antibiotic therapy if sepsis is a concern

- Blood work to monitor ABG levels, pH, blood glucose levels, electrolytes, and the status of blood cultures

Maintaining Body Temperature

The high risk infant is susceptible to heat loss and its complications. In addition, LBW infants may be unable to increase their metabolic rate because of impaired gas exchange, caloric intake restrictions, or poor thermoregulation. Transepidermal water loss is greater because of skin immaturity in very premature infants (those at less than 28 weeks of gestation) and can contribute to temperature instability.

High risk infants are cared for in the thermoneutral environment created by use of an external heat source. The infant is attached by a probe to an external heat source supplied by a radiant warmer or a servocontrolled incubator. This idealized environment maintains an infant's normal body temperature between 36.5° and 37.2° C. Maintaining a thermoneutral condition in the youngest, most immature infants decreases the need for them to generate additional heat. As a result, excessive oxygen consumption is prevented in such compromised infants (Blake & Murray, 1998).

Oxygen Therapy

Clinical criteria for identifying the need for oxygen administration include increased respiratory effort, respiratory distress with apnea, tachycardia, bradycardia, and central cyanosis with or without hypotonia. In addition, the need for oxygen should be substantiated by biochemical data (arterial oxygen pressure [PaO$_2$] of less than 60 mm Hg or an oxygen saturation of less than 92%). High risk infants often require saturations of more than 95% to maintain respiratory stability because their hemoglobin levels are frequently low. As the PaO$_2$ falls, less oxygen is released from the hemoglobin, which increases the risk for cellular hypoxia (Hagedorn, Gardner, & Abman, 1998).

Oxygen administered to an infant is warmed and humidified to prevent cold stress and drying of the respiratory mucosa. During the administration of oxygen, the concentration, volume, temperature, and humidity of the gas are carefully controlled. Delivery of oxygen for more than a few minutes requires the use of special equipment (hood, nasal cannula, positive-pressure mask, or endotracheal tube) because the concentration of free-flow oxygen cannot be monitored accurately (Hagedorn, Gardner, & Abman, 1998). Free-flow oxygen into an incubator should not be used because the concentration fluctuates dramatically every time the doors or portholes are opened. The indiscriminant use of oxygen may be hazardous. Possible complications of oxygen therapy include retinopathy of prematurity and bronchopulmonary dysplasia.

NURSE ALERT *Administration of a therapeutic level of oxygen for a severely depressed infant could cause significant physiologic harm if given to an infant with mild respiratory disease (Hagedorn, Gardner, & Abman, 1998).*

Infants who need oxygen should have their respiratory status assessed accurately every 1 to 2 hours; this includes a continuous pulse oximetry reading and at least one ABG measurement (Hagedorn, Gardner, & Abman, 1998). The interventions implemented are then determined on the basis of the findings yielded by the clinical assessment, including telemetry (pulse oximetry or tcPO$_2$ monitoring) and laboratory tests (Hagedorn, Gardner, & Abman, 1998). The interventions ordered are those that can directly manage the underlying disease process and range from hood oxygen administration to ventilator therapy.

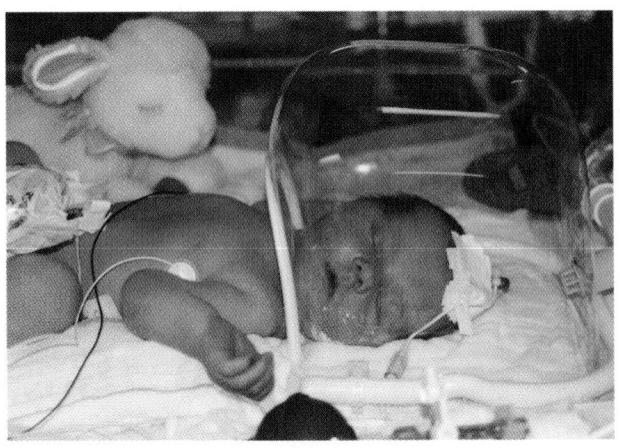 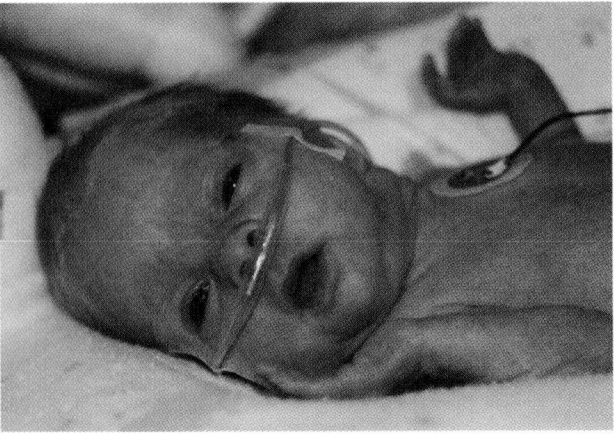

A **B**

Fig. 41-5 **A,** Infant under hood. **B,** Infant with nasal cannula. *(Courtesy Victoria Langer, RNC, MSN, NNP; from Dickason, E., Silverman, B., & Kaplan J. [1998]. Maternal-infant nursing care [3rd ed.]. St. Louis: Mosby.)*

Hood therapy. Oxygen can be administered by a hood to infants who do not require mechanical pressure support. The hood is a clear plastic cover that is sized to fit over the head and neck of the infant (Fig. 41-5, *A*). Inside the hood the infant receives the correct amount of oxygen. The nurse checks the oxygen level every 1 to 2 hours because the concentration must be adjusted in response to the infant's condition.

Nasal cannula. Infants requiring low-flow amounts of oxygen can benefit from the use of a nasal cannula (Fig. 41-5, *B*). These are of particular value for older infants who are recuperating but still require supplemental oxygen. They are the preferred method for home oxygen administration (Hagedorn, Gardner, & Abman, 1998). They permit the infant to receive an adequate, continuous flow of oxygen while allowing optimal vision, positioning, and parental holding. Infants can also breastfeed while receiving oxygen by this method. However, the nasal prongs must be inspected frequently to make sure they are not partially obstructed by milk or secretions (Hagedorn, Gardner, & Abman, 1998). Nasal cannulas allow easier feedings and psychosocial interactions (Ludington-Hoe et al., 1994).

Continuous positive airway pressure therapy. Infants who are unable to maintain an adequate PaO_2 despite the administration of oxygen by hood or nasal cannula may require the delivery of oxygen using **continuous positive airway pressure (CPAP).** CPAP infuses oxygen or air under a preset pressure (Fig. 41-6, *A*) by means of nasal prongs, a face mask, or an endotracheal tube. An orogastric tube should be used for decompression of the stomach during use of nasal prongs (Hagedorn, Gardner, & Abman, 1998). CPAP increases the functional residual capacity, improves the diffusion time of pulmonary gases, including oxygen, and can decrease pulmonary shunting. If implemented early enough, CPAP may preclude the need for mechanical ventilation (Hagedorn, Gardner, & Abman, 1998). CPAP can cause vascular shunting in the pulmonary beds, which can lead to persistent pulmonary hypertension and severe respiratory distress.

Mechanical ventilation. Mechanical ventilation must be implemented if other methods of therapy cannot correct abnormalities in oxygenation (Hagedorn, Gardner, & Abman, 1998). Its use is indicated whenever blood gas values reveal the existence of severe hypoxemia or severe hypercapnia (Fig. 41-6, *B*). The condition of the infant suffering from apnea with bradycardia, ineffective respiratory effort, shock, asphyxia, infection, meconium aspiration syndrome, respiratory distress syndrome, or congenital defects that affect ventilation may also deteriorate and require intubation to reverse the process (Hagedorn, Gardner, & Abman, 1998). Dexamethasone may be administered to prevent chronic lung disease (Garland et al., 1999).

The ventilator settings are determined by the infant's particular needs. The ventilator is set to provide a prede-

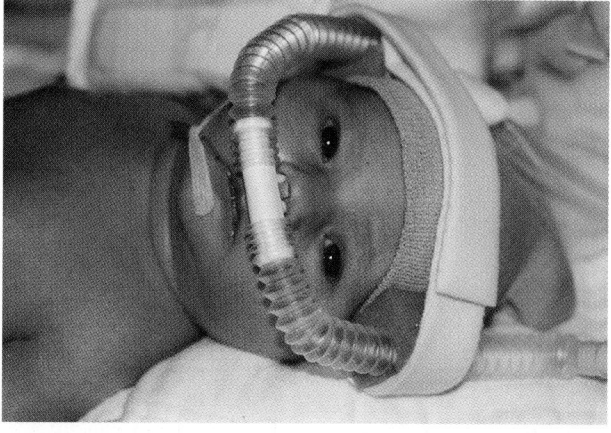

A

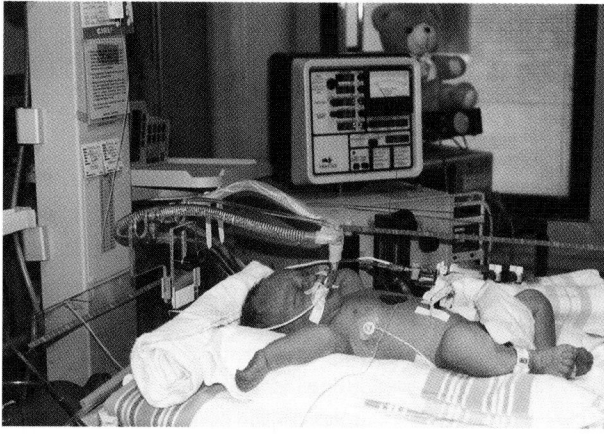

B

Fig. 41-6 A, Infant receiving ventilatory assistance with continuous positive airway pressure (CPAP). **B,** Infant intubated and on ventilator. *(Courtesy Victoria Langer, RNC, MSN, NNP; from Dickason, E., Silverman, B., & Kaplan J. [1998]. Maternal-infant nursing care [3rd ed.]. St. Louis: Mosby.)*

termined amount of oxygen to the infant during spontaneous respirations and also to provide mechanical ventilation in the absence of spontaneous respirations (Hagedorn, Gardner, & Abman, 1998). See Box 41-4 for explanation of ventilator terminology.

Surfactant administration. Surfactant can be administered as an adjunct to oxygen and ventilation therapy. Before 34 weeks of gestation, most infants do not produce enough surfactant to survive extrauterine life (American Academy of Pediatrics, 1999; Hagedorn, Gardner, & Abman, 1998). As a result, lung compliance is decreased, and not enough gas exchange occurs as the lungs become atelectatic and require greater pressures to expand. By administering artificial surfactant, respiratory compliance is improved until the infant can generate enough surfactant on his or her own. Exogenous surfactant is manufactured from human or bovine amniotic fluid and is given in several doses through an endotracheal tube (Hagedorn,

BOX 41-4 Definitions of Ventilator Terminology

Peak inspiratory pressure (PIP)	The peak level of pressure on inspiration. High pressures may cause overdistention, which can cause complications such as a pneumothorax.
Positive end-expiratory pressure (PEEP)	Creates mechanical continuous positive airway pressure (CPAP). The therapeutic range is 3 to 8 cm H_2O (Wong, 1999).
Rate	The frequency with which the ventilator delivers the specified volume of gases (oxygen and air) to the infant. This provides the minimal number of breaths per minute needed for adequate oxygenation.
Inspiration/ expiration ratio (I:E)	The amount of time during each breath spent on inspiration versus expiration.
Mean airway pressure (MAP)	The amount of pressure exerted on the airway throughout the respiratory cycle. The average pressure is constant on high-frequency ventilators but varies during inspiratory and expiratory cycles on the conventional mode of ventilation.

From Hagedorn, M., Gardner, S., & Abman, S. (1993). Respiratory distress. In G. Merenstein & S. Gardner (Eds.). *Handbook of neonatal intensive care* (3rd ed.). St. Louis: Mosby; and Wong, D. (1999). *Whaley and Wong's nursing care of infants and children* (6th ed). St. Louis: Mosby.

Gardner, & Abman, 1998). As with any drug therapy, the infant must be monitored for the occurrence of potential side effects such as a patent ductus arteriosus and pulmonary hemorrhage. Use of this drug has been associated with a significantly reduced length of time on ventilators and oxygen therapy, and an increased survival rate in premature infants (see Medication Guide) (Hagedorn, Gardner, & Abman, 1998).

Extracorporeal membrane oxygenation therapy. Infants with severe pulmonary dysfunction who are at more than 34 weeks of gestation may be candidates for **extracorporeal membrane oxygenation (ECMO)** therapy. ECMO makes use of cardiopulmonary bypass to oxygenate the infant's blood outside the body through a membrane oxygenator. The membrane oxygenator serves as an artificial lung while the infant's lungs heal. Because of the massive systemic anticoagulation therapy required in the pump tubing and the increased risk for hemorrhage, the criteria for its use are very strict, and the use of this therapy is therefore limited (Donovan, Schwartz, & Moles, 1998). The risk for intraventricular hemorrhages in prema-

MEDICATION GUIDE

Surfactant Replacement:
Bovine Lung Extract: Beractant (Survanta)
Artificial Surfactant: Colfosceril (Exosurf)

ACTION

These medications provide exogenous surfactant to correct deficiency in lung immaturity.

INDICATIONS

Surfactants are used in the prevention and treatment of respiratory distress syndrome in premature infants.
- For *prevention,* drug is administered within 15 minutes of birth to infants with clinical manifestations of surfactant deficiency or with a birth weight less than 1250 g.
- For *treatment,* drug is administered to infants with confirmed diagnosis of respiratory distress syndrome, preferably within 8 hours of birth.

DOSAGE

Dosage depends on drug used. Administer via endotracheal tube

ADVERSE REACTIONS

Adverse reactions include respiratory distress immediately after administration and bradycardia and oxygen desaturation.

NURSING CONSIDERATIONS

Observe infant's condition for changes. Diuresis may occur with improvement. Ventilator settings may need changing as the infant's ability to oxygenate increases.

ture infants is particularly high, and for this reason ECMO therapy cannot be used in them. ECMO has been successful in the treatment of various acute and chronic lung diseases, including meconium aspiration syndrome and persistent pulmonary hypertension (Hagedorn, Gardner, & Abman, 1998).

High-frequency ventilation. Other modes of ventilator therapies include high-frequency oscillator ventilation, jet ventilation, flow interruption ventilation, and liquid ventilation (Cools & Offringa, 1999; Donovan, Schwartz, & Moles, 1998; Plavka et al., 1999). These methods of high-frequency ventilation work by providing smaller volumes of oxygen at a significantly more rapid rate (more than 300 breaths/min) than traditional mechanical ventilators do. As a result, the intrathoracic pressure is decreased, and along with this, the risk of barotrauma. In liquid ventilation the surface tension is reduced while oxygenation is improved through the recreation of a fetal lung environment. Instead of air pressure, an experimental oxygenated lipid solution is pumped continuously through the lungs.

Nitric oxide therapy. Inhaled nitric oxide (NO), delivered as a gas, causes potent and sustained pulmonary vasodilation in the pulmonary circulation (Donovan, Schwartz, & Moles, 1998; Hagedorn, Gardner, & Abman, 1998). NO binds with hemoglobin in red blood cells and is inactivated after metabolism. In the few studies conducted using human infants, positive results were seen: oxygen saturation improved and no toxic effects from methemoglobin or increased levels of nitrogen oxide were documented. Currently, inhaled nitric oxygen therapy is not approved by the Food and Drug Administration. Several multicenter studies are currently being conducted (Donovan, Schwartz, & Moles, 1998; Hagedorn, Gardner, & Abman, 1998).

Weaning from Respiratory Assistance

Respiratory assistance is weaned slowly as the infant's status improves. The infant is ready to be weaned from respiratory assistance once the ABG and oxygen saturation levels are maintained within normal limits. A spontaneous, adequate respiratory effort must be present, and the infant must show improved muscle tone during increased activity. Weaning is done in a stepwise and gradual manner. This may consist of the infant being extubated, placed on continuous positive airway pressure, and then weaned to oxygen by means of a hood or nasal cannula. Throughout the weaning process the infant's oxygen levels are monitored by pulse oximetry, tcPO$_2$ monitoring, and blood gas levels.

The goal of weaning is the withdrawal of all oxygen support. However, some infants do not achieve this before discharge from the hospital and may require home oxygen therapy for several months. Throughout the weaning period, the infant is assessed for signs and symptoms indicating poor tolerance of the process. These include an increased pulse, respiratory distress, or cyanosis, or a combination of these. If these occur, the amount of oxygen being delivered is increased, and weaning proceeds more slowly while further assessments are done. Underlying causes of intolerance of weaning may be bronchopulmonary dysplasia, a patent ductus arteriosus, or CNS damage (Hagedorn, Gardner, & Abman, 1998).

Nutritional Care

It is not always possible to provide enteral (by the GI route) nourishment to a high risk infant. Such infants are often too ill or weak to breastfeed or bottle feed because of respiratory distress or sepsis (Townsend, Johnson, & Hay, 1998). Early enteral feeding of the asphyxiated neonate with a low Apgar score is also avoided to prevent bowel necrosis. In such cases, nutrition is provided parenterally. Those infants who require parenteral nutrition may have one or more of the following problems (Townsend, Johnson, & Hay, 1998):

- Lack of a coordinated suck-and-swallow reflex
- Inability to suck because of a congenital anomaly
- Respiratory distress requiring aggressive ventilator support
- Asphyxiation with a potential for necrotizing enterocolitis

Type of nourishment. The types of formulas used, the mode and volume of feeding, and the feeding schedule of the infant are determined on the basis of the findings yielded by assessment of the following variables:
- Initially, the birth weight, then the current weight of the preterm infant
- Pattern of weight gain or loss (infants weighing less than 1500 g require more energy for growth and thermoregulation and may gain weight poorly with either breastfeedings or bottle feedings)
- Presence or absence of suck-and-swallow reflex in all infants at less than 35 weeks of gestation
- Behavioral readiness to take oral feedings
- Physical condition, including presence or absence of bowel sounds, abdominal distention, or bloody stools, as well as presence and degree of respiratory distress or apneic episodes
- Residual from previous feeding, if being gavage fed
- Malformations (especially GI defects such as omphalocele or esophageal atresia), including the need for a gastrostomy feeding tube
- Renal function, including urinary output and laboratory values (nitrogen balance, electrolyte balance, glucose level); premature infants are especially susceptible to altered renal function

Weight and fluid loss or gain. For many reasons, the caloric, nutrient, and fluid requirements of high risk infants are greater than those of the term, normal newborn. One reason is that premature or dysmature (malnourished) newborns often have limited stores of nutrients and fluids. In addition, symptomatic or asymptomatic hypoglycemia, electrolyte imbalances, or other metabolic disturbances can develop in an infant whose nutritional intake is poor. Such hypoglycemia may cause serious damage to carbohydrate-dependent brain cells.

The infant's weight is measured and recorded daily, and the rate of weight loss or gain is calculated. Further depletion of weight and metabolic stores can occur as a result of one or a combination of the following factors:
- Birth asphyxia
- Increased respirations or respiratory effort
- Patent ductus arteriosus
- Hypothermic environment
- Insensible fluid loss caused by evaporation (with radiant heat or phototherapy)
- Vomiting, diarrhea, and dysfunctional absorption from the GI tract
- Growth demands (a premature infant's growth rate approximates that of fetal growth during the last trimester and is at least two times faster than a term infant's growth rate after birth)

- Inability of the renal system to concentrate urine and maintain an adequate rate of urea excretion, as well as infant's inadequate response to antidiuretic hormone

The high risk newborn is predisposed to have weight and fluid losses because of the greater amount of fluid needed to meet the demands of the increased cellular metabolic processes (resulting from stress, repair, or growth). The body weight of premature infants weighing less than 1500 g consists of 83% to 89% water, compared with the term infant's water content of 71% (Denne et al., 1998). Most of this water is in the extracellular fluid compartment. Even with the early institution of fluid and nutrition intake, the premature infant's weight and fluid losses seem exaggerated. Inadequate fluid intake, resulting from either delayed administration or insufficient volume, can further cause weight and fluid losses in the premature infant.

Insensible water loss (IWL) is an evaporative loss that occurs largely through the skin. Approximately 30% of this IWL comes from the respiratory tract. The total IWL in a normal infant ranges anywhere from 30 to 60 ml/kg/24 hr (Blake & Murray, 1998). The effects of radiant warmers, incubators, phototherapy, and other factors can augment the IWL. Some of this loss can be prevented by humidifying the respiratory gases administered.

During the first week of extrauterine life, the premature infant can lose up to 15% of his or her birth weight. In contrast, a weight loss of up to only 10% is acceptable in a term AGA infant (Adcock, Consolvo, & Berry, 1998). After the initial week, a premature infant's loss or gain during each 24-hour period should not exceed 2% of the previous day's weight. (To calculate a weight loss or gain, see Box 41-5.) Weight loss may be caused by increased stooling or voiding, increased evaporative losses, inadequate volume or incorrect fluid administration, and problems with malabsorption. Implementation of interventions and frequent reassessment of the infant and its environment are necessary to correct the problems (Townsend, Johnson, & Hay, 1998). Such interventions include adjusting the incubator temperature; monitoring and adjusting the volume and type of fluids being administered; assessing the urinary output, including the specific gravity; and assessing the blood glucose levels. The glucose determinations are used to assess urine osmolarity and hence renal function. High glucose levels (greater than 125 mg/dl) can stimulate an excessive osmotic diuresis (Wong, 1999). Weight gain may be due to overfeeding or fluid retention. The nurse reports and records the findings and continues to assess the infant's fluid status, urinary output, and blood glucose levels. The interventions implemented are determined by the infant's specific disorder and nutritional needs.

Elimination patterns. The infant's elimination patterns are also assessed. This includes the frequency of urination, as well as the amount, color, pH, and specific gravity of the urine. The assessment of the infant's bowel movements includes the frequency of stooling and the character of the stool, as well as whether there is constipation, diarrhea, or loss of fats (steatorrhea). All of these findings are documented. The nurse may request guaiac tests to assess for blood in the stool, tests to detect stool-reducing substances, and a pH determination to assess for malabsorption (Townsend, Johnson, & Hay, 1998). Infants with unexplained abdominal distention are assessed carefully to rule out the presence of hypomotility or obstructions of the GI tract.

Oral feeding. Nourishment by the oral route is preferred for the infant who has adequate strength and GI function. The best milk for an infant is that of its mother. Breast milk may be fed by breast or bottle. Formula may be fed by bottle or a supplementer (see Fig. 28-3). Throughout the feeding, the nurse assesses the newborn's tolerance of the procedure. When the infant breastfeeds, the nurse assists the mother by providing support and help, as necessary.

The needs of the high risk infant must be considered when determining the type and frequency of the feedings. Many high risk infants cannot suck well enough to breastfeed or bottle feed until they have recovered from their initial illness or matured physically (greater than 32 weeks of gestation). Mothers of high risk infants are encouraged to continue pumping breast milk, especially if theirs is a very premature infant who may not breastfeed for many weeks (Townsend, Johnson, & Hay, 1998). Because of the significant breastfeeding attrition rates among these mothers, they need support and encouragement every few days to continue pumping while their infant is not yet able to nurse. If there is no available breast milk (from the mother or a milk bank), commercial formula is used. The calories, protein, and mineral content of commercial formulas vary (see Chapter 28). The type of nipple selected ("preemie," regular, orthodontic) depends on the infant's ability to

---

■ BOX 41-5 | **Calculation of a Weight Loss or Gain**

EXAMPLE 1

Day 4	1,750 g
Day 5	1,730 g
	20 g loss

$$\frac{20}{1,750} = \frac{X\%}{100\%}$$

$$1,750X = 2,000$$

$$1,750\overline{)2,000.0}^{\;1.1}$$

$$X = 1.1\% \text{ weight loss}$$

EXAMPLE 2

Day 4	1,750 g
Day 5	1,790 g
	40 g gain

$$\frac{40}{1,750} = \frac{X\%}{100\%}$$

$$1,750X = 4,000$$

$$1,750\overline{)4,000.00}^{\;2.3}$$

$$X = 2.3\% \text{ weight gain}$$

suck from the specific type of nipple. The nurse also considers the energy the infant needs to expend in the process.

Overfeeding of the preterm infant should be avoided because this can lead to abdominal distention, with apnea, vomiting, and possibly aspiration of the feeding. The nurse monitors the infant's abdominal girth when distention is obvious.

Gavage feeding. Gavage feeding is a method of providing nourishment to the infant who is compromised by respiratory distress, the infant who is too immature to have a coordinated suck-and-swallow reflex, or the infant who is easily fatigued by sucking. In gavage feeding, breast milk or formula is given to the infant through a nasogastric or orogastric tube. This spares the infant the work of sucking.

Gavage feeding can be done either with an intermittently placed tube or continuously through an indwelling catheter. Infants who cannot tolerate large-bolus feedings (those on ventilators for more than a week) are given continuous feedings. Breast milk or formula can be supplied intermittently using a syringe with gravity-controlled flow or can be given continuously using an infusion pump. The type of fluid instilled is recorded with every syringe change. The volume of the continuous feedings is recorded hourly, and the residual gastric aspirate is measured every 4 hours. Residuals of less than a quarter of a feeding can be refed to the infant to prevent the loss of gastric electrolytes. Feeding is stopped if the residual is greater than a quarter of the feeding and is not resumed until the infant can be assessed for a possible feeding intolerance (Townsend, Johnson, & Hay, 1998).

The orogastric route for gavage feedings is preferred because most infants are preferential nose breathers. However, some infants do not tolerate oral tube placement. A small nasogastric feeding tube can be placed in older infants who would otherwise gag or vomit or in ones who are learning to suck (Townsend, Johnson, & Hay, 1998). To insert the tube, the nurse should follow the sequence given in the Procedure box.

To begin the feeding, the nurse connects the barrel of a syringe to the gavage tube. While crimping the feeding tube, the nurse pours the specified amount of breast milk or formula into the syringe. The nurse then releases the crimp in the tube and allows the feeding to flow down by gravity (Fig. 41-7). The infant usually tolerates the feeding better if the rate approximates that of an oral feeding (about 1 ml/min). The parent or nurse can swaddle or hold the infant to help the infant associate the feeding with positive interactions. The parents are encouraged to talk to their infant during the feedings.

Once the prescribed volume has been delivered, the nurse crimps or pinches the tube and removes the syringe. The gavage tube is capped (or the nurse continues to pinch it) while removing it in one steady motion. Capping the tube (or pinching it off) prevents breast milk or formula from leaking from the tube and being aspirated during removal of the tube.

PROCEDURE

Inserting a Gavage Feeding Tube

1. Measure the length of the gavage tube from the tip of the nose to the lobe of the ear to the midpoint between the xiphoid process and the umbilicus (Fig. 41-7, A). Mark the tube with a piece of tape.
2. Lubricate the tip of the tube with sterile water and insert gently through the nose or mouth (Fig. 41-7, B) until the predetermined mark is reached. Placement of the tube in the trachea will cause the infant to gag, cough, or become cyanotic.
3. Check correct placement of the tube by:
   a. Pulling back on the plunger to aspirate stomach contents. Lack of fluid is not necessarily evidence of improper placement. Aspiration of respiratory secretions may be mistaken for stomach contents; however, the pH of the stomach contents is much lower (more acidic) than the pH of respiratory secretions.
   b. Injecting a small amount of air (1 to 3 ml) into the tube while listening for gurgling or by using a stethoscope placed over the stomach. Ensure that the tube is inserted to the mark; it is possible to hear air entering the stomach even if the tube is positioned above the gastroesophageal (cardiac) sphincter.
4. Tape the tube in place and also tape it to the cheek to prevent accidental dislodgment and incorrect positioning (Fig. 41-7, C).
   a. Assess the infant's skin integrity before taping the tube.
   b. Edematous or very premature infants should have a pectin barrier placed under the tape to prevent abrasions (Lund & Durand, 1998).
5. Tube placement must be assessed before each feeding.

After the feeding, the infant is positioned to prevent aspiration. The documentation of the procedure includes the size of the feeding tube, the amount and quality of the residual from the previous feeding, the type and quantity of fluid instilled (sterile water, breast milk, or formula), and the infant's response to the procedure.

Gastrostomy feedings. Infants with certain congenital malformations require gastrostomy feedings. This involves the surgical placement of a tube through the skin of the abdomen into the stomach. The tube is then taped in an upright position to prevent trauma to the incision site. After the site heals, the nurse initiates small bolus feedings per the physician's orders. Feedings by gravity are done slowly over 20 to 30 minutes. Special care must be taken to prevent rapid bolusing of the fluid because this may

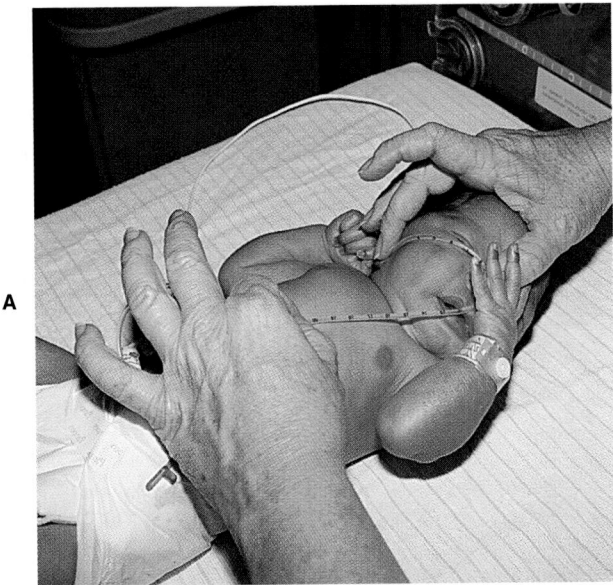

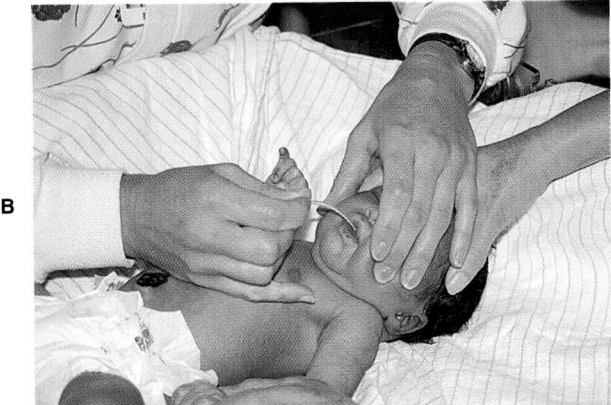

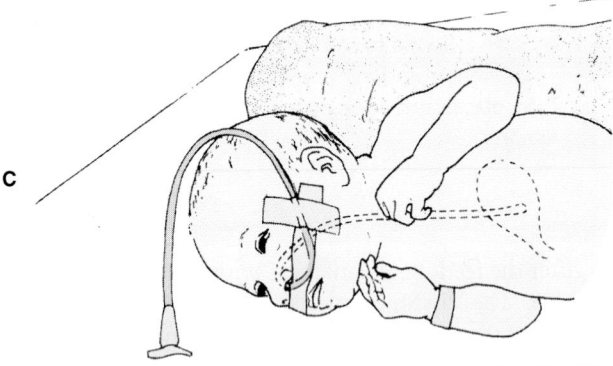

Fig. 41-7 Gavage feeding. **A,** Measurement of gavage feeding tube from tip of nose to earlobe and to midpoint between end of xyphoid process and umbilicus. Tape may be used to mark correct length on tube. **B,** Insertion of gavage tube using orogastric route. **C,** Indwelling gavage tube, nasogastric route. After feeding by orogastric or nasogastric tube, infant is propped on right side for 1 hour to facilitate emptying of stomach into small intestine. Note rolled towel for support. (**A** and **B** courtesy Marjorie Pyle, RNC, Lifecircle, Costa Mesa, CA.)

lead to abdominal distention, GI reflux into the esophagus, or respiratory compromise. Meticulous skin care at the tube insertion site is necessary to prevent skin breakdown or infections. In addition, intake and output are monitored scrupulously because these infants are prone to diarrhea until regular feedings are established.

Parenteral fluids. Feeding supplemental parenteral fluids is indicated for infants who are unable to obtain sufficient fluids or calories by enteral feeding (Fig. 41-8). Some of these infants are dependent on **total parenteral nutrition (TPN)** for extensive periods. The nurse assesses and documents the following in infants receiving parenteral fluids or TPN:

- Type and infusion rate of the solution
- Functional status of the infusion equipment, including the tubing and infusion pump
- Infusion site for possible complications (phlebitis, infiltration, dislodgment)
- Caloric intake
- Infant's responses to therapy

The physician orders TPN per the hospital protocol. These orders must specify the electrolytes and nutrients desired, as well as the volume and rate of infusion. The amounts of calories, protein, and fat are determined on the basis of the individual infant's energy needs (Lefrak & Dowling, 1998).

While caring for the infant receiving parenteral fluids or TPN, the nurse secures and protects the insertion site (Fig. 41-9). In addition to observing the principles of asepsis, the nurse must observe the principles of neonatal skin care (Lund & Durand, 1998). The nurse should also inspect the infusion site for signs of infiltration and reposition the infant frequently to maintain body alignment and protect the site. Parents of infants need to be given explanations about TPN and the way in which the IV equipment and solutions affect their infant.

Advancing infant feedings. Feedings are advanced as assessment data and the infant's ability to tolerate the feedings warrant it. Documentation of a premature infant's sucking patterns can also be used to determine its readiness to nipple feed. Feedings are advanced from passive (parenteral and gavage) to active (nipple and breastfeeding). At each step, the nurse must carefully assess the infant's response to prevent overstressing the infant.

The infant receiving nutrition parenterally is gradually weaned off of this type of nutrition. To do this, the nourishment given by continuous or intermittent gavage feedings is increased while the parenteral fluids are decreased.

Feedings are advanced slowly and cautiously because, if feedings are advanced too rapidly, the infant may experience vomiting (with an attendant risk of aspiration), diarrhea, abdominal distention, and apneic episodes. Rapid advancement of feedings may also cause fluid retention with cardiac compromise or a pronounced diuresis with hyponatremia.

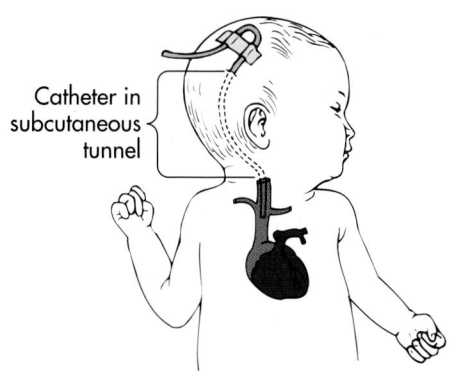

Catheter in subcutaneous tunnel

Fig. 41-8   Total parenteral nutrition (TPN). Close-up showing infusion site and internal placement of catheter into descending vena cava.

If the infant needs additional calories, a commercial human milk fortifier can be added to the gavaged breast milk, or the number of calories per 30 ml of commercial formula can be increased. Soy and elemental formulas are used only for infants with very special dietary needs, such as allergies to cow's milk or chronic malabsorption (Townsend, Johnson, & Hay, 1998). Calories in breast milk can be lost if the cream separates and adheres to the tubing during continuous infusion. This problem is decreased if microbore tubing is used for both continuous and intermittent gavage feedings.

The infant receiving gavage feedings progresses to bottle feeding or breast milk feedings. To do this, the gavage feedings are decreased as the infant's ability to suckle breast milk or formula improves. Often during this transition the infant is fed by both nipple and gavage feeding to ensure the intake of both the prescribed volume of food and nutrients. However, an increased respiratory effort is a documented problem in premature infants who have a gavage tube that is left in place during nipple feedings (Shiao, Youngblut, & Anderson, 1995), so nurses must watch for this. The parents need support during this transition because many families measure their parenting competence by how well they can feed their infant (Green, 1994).

As the time of discharge nears, the appropriate method of feeding, as well as the assessments pertaining to the method (e.g., tolerance of feedings, status of gavage tube placement), are reviewed with the parents. The parents should be encouraged to interact with the infant by talking and making eye contact with the infant during the feeding. This interaction is encouraged to stimulate the psychosocial development of the infant and to facilitate bonding and attachment.

Nonnutritive sucking.   If the infant is nourished by the gavage or the parenteral route, **nonnutritive sucking** is encouraged (Fig. 41-10) for several reasons. Allowing the infant to suck on a pacifier during gavage or between oral

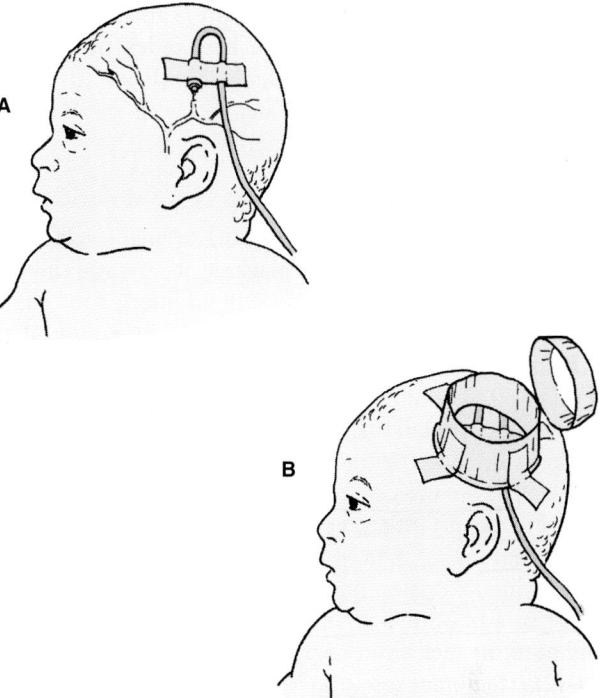

Fig. 41-9   **A,** Venipuncture of scalp vein. **B,** Paper cup protecting venipuncture site.

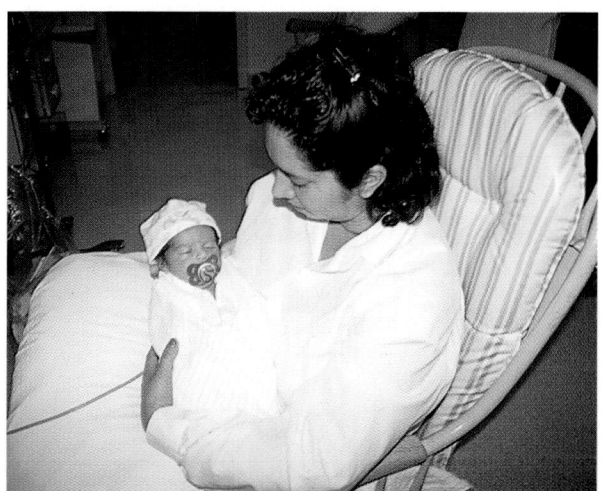

Fig. 41-10   Nonnutritive sucking by infant. *(Courtesy Marjorie Pyle, RNC, Lifecircle, Costa Mesa, CA.)*

feedings may improve oxygenation. In addition, such nonnutritive sucking may lead to a decreased energy expenditure with less restlessness and promote faster attachment to the nipple when oral feedings are initiated (Lefrak & Dowling, 1998).

Mothers of premature infants should be encouraged to let their premature infants start sucking at the breast during kangaroo care because some infant's suck-and-swallow reflexes may be coordinated as early as 32 weeks of gestation.

Infants with intrauterine growth restriction (IUGR) may have an age-appropriate sucking reflex but require thermoregulatory support, making it difficult to breast-feed. These infants may also benefit from nonnutritive sucking at the breast for short periods.

Environmental Concerns

Infants in NICUs are also exposed to high levels of auditory input from the various machine alarms, and this can have adverse effects (Fig. 41-11). In addition, continuous noise levels of 45 to 85 decibels (db) are common in NICUs. An incubator alone produces a constant noise level of 60 to 80 db (Haubrich, 1998), and each new piece of life-support equipment used adds another 20 db to the background noise (Strauch, Brandt, & Edwards-Beckett, 1993). The infant's hearing may be damaged if it is exposed to a constant decibel level of 90 db or frequent decibel swings higher than 110 db.

The infant's vision may be altered by respiratory equipment or a phototherapy mask, making it difficult for the infant to interact with caregivers and family members (Fig. 41-12). The infant may also be unable to establish diurnal and nocturnal rhythms because of the continuous exposure to overhead lighting. In addition, sedation or pain medications affect the way in which the infant perceives the environment.

An additional concern in the care of infants is that environmental hazards can be potentiated by some drugs used for infant therapy. Diuretics (especially furosemide [Lasix]), antibiotics (gentamicin), and anti-malarial agents can potentiate noise-induced hearing loss (Haubrich, 1998).

NURSE ALERT *Therefore routine hearing screening should be performed in all infants before discharge, with universal screening completed by no later than the third month of life.*

Nurses can modify the environment to provide a developmentally supportive milieu. In that way, the infant's neurobehavioral and physiologic needs can be met better, the infant's developing organization can be supported, and growth and development fostered (Blackburn, 1998).

Developmental Care

The goal of developmental care is to support each infant's efforts to become as well-organized, competent, and stable as possible. Developmental care includes all care procedures and the physical and social aspects of care in the NICU (Als, 1998). The caregiver uses the infant's own behavior and physiologic functioning as the basis for planning care and providing interventions. Through caregiver observation, the infant's strengths, thresholds for disorganization, and areas in which the infant is vulnerable can be identified (Als, 1998). The family is included in developmental care as the primary coregulators (Als, 1998). Working together, the family and other caregivers provide opportunities to enhance the strengths of the family and the infant and to reduce the stress that is associated with the birth and care of high risk infants.

Lowering light and noise levels by instituting "quiet hours" during each 8-hour shift and positioning are just two of the ways in which nurses can support infants in their development (Gray et al., 1998). Sleep interruptions are minimized and positioning and bundling the infant help promote self-regulation and prevent disorganization (Petryshen et al., 1997).

Positioning. The motor development of preterm infants permits less flexion than their full-term counterparts. Caregivers can provide a variety of positions for infants; sidelying and prone are preferred to supine. Body containment with use of blanket rolls, swaddling, holding the infant's arms in a crossed position, and secure holding provide boundaries and promote self-regulation during feed-

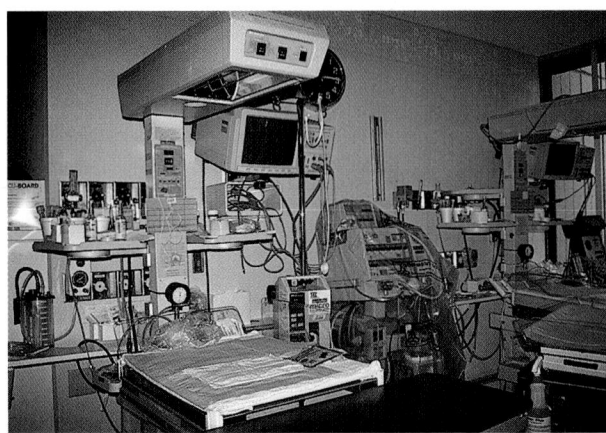

Fig. 41-11 Significant environmental stimulation. Note bed, wall oxygen attachments, monitor, ventilator, incubator, and pumps, all of which have alarm systems. *(Courtesy Marjorie Pyle, RNC, Lifecircle, Costa Mesa, CA.)*

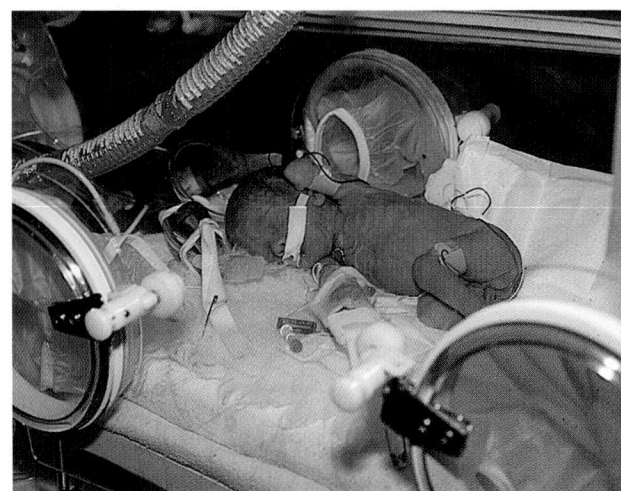

Fig. 41-12 Ventilator-dependent infant. *(Courtesy Marjorie Pyle, RNC, Lifecircle, Costa Mesa, CA.)*

ing, procedures, and other stressful interventions (Gardner & Lubchenco, 1998). The prone position encourages flexion of the extremities; a sling or hiproll assists in maintenance of flexion. Use of a sheepskin prevents abrasion of the knees (Gardner & Lubchenco, 1998). Holding the limbs close to the body when the infant is moved decreases stimulation that produces jerky, uncoordinated movements (Wong, 1999). Proper body alignment is necessary to prevent developmental problems that may affect the ability to walk as the child matures.

Reducing inappropriate stimuli. Staff can reduce unnecessary noise by closing doors or portholes on incubators quietly, placing gently only necessary objects on top of incubators, keeping radios at low volume, speaking quietly, and handling equipment noiselessly. Earmuffs may also reduce auditory input (Wong, 1999).

Infants can be protected from light by dimming the lights during the night, placing a blanket over the incubator (Fig. 41-13), or covering the infant's eyes with a mask. Sleep-wake cycles can be induced with such measures. Infants need periods when they are completely undisturbed (Wong, 1999).

Infant communication. Infants communicate their needs and ability to tolerate sensory stimulation through physiologic responses. The nurses and parents of high risk infants must therefore be alert to such cues. Although full-term infants may thrive on stimulation, this same stimulation in high risk infants can instead provoke physical symptoms of stress and anxiety (Blackburn, 1998; Gardner & Lubchenco, 1998).

Problems with noxious stimuli and barriers to normal contact may cause anxiety and tension. Clues to overstimulation include averting the gaze, hiccuping, gagging, or regurgitating food. Term infants exhibit a startle reflex, and premature infants move all of their limbs in an uncoordinated fashion in response to noxious stimuli. An irregular respiratory rate or an increased heart rate may develop in

severely distressed infants, and they may then be unable to regain a calm state.

A relaxed infant state is indicated by stabilization of vital signs, closed eyes, and a relaxed posture. Nonintubated infants may make soothing verbal sounds when they are relaxed. Infants requiring artificial ventilation cannot cry audibly and often show their distress through posturing; they then relax once their needs are met. As high risk infants heal and mature, they increasingly respond to stimuli in a self-regulated manner rather than with a dissociated response. Infants who do not show increased self-regulation should be evaluated for a neurologic problem.

Infant stimulation. A neonatal individualized developmental care and assessment program (NIDCAP) routinely integrates aspects of neurodevelopmental theory with caregivers' observations, environmental interventions, and parental support (Gardner & Lubchenco, 1998). Routine reassessment is built into the program's design. Developmental stimuli may consist of such simple measures as placing a waterbed on the top of the infant's mattress or kangaroo (skin-to-skin) holding. The simplest calming technique is to contain the infant's extremities close to the body using both hands. The care of the infant is organized to allow extended periods of undisturbed rest and sleep. Pain medications or sedatives should be administered consistently, per the unit's protocol.

Infants acquire a sense of trust as they learn the feel, sound, and smell of their parents (Gardner & Lubchenco, 1998). High risk infants must also learn to trust their caregivers to obtain comfort. However, caregivers in the nursery may also inflict pain as part of the care they must give. For this reason, it is important for both the parents and the caregivers of such infants to employ comforting interventions such as removing painful stimuli, stopping hunger, and changing wet or soiled clothing to foster trust (Green, 1994).

When the infant is ready for stimulation, the nurse has many options. All infants can tolerate being held, even if only for short periods. Additional ways for the nurse or parents to stimulate infants include cuddling, rocking, singing, and talking to the infant (Fig. 41-14). These activities are beneficial, increase weight gain, and decrease time to discharge (Standley, 1998). Stroking the infant's skin during medical therapy can provide tactile stimulation. The caregiver responds to the infant's cues by offering reassurance, providing for nonnutritive sucking, stroking the infant's back, and talking to the infant.

Mobiles and decals that can be changed frequently may also be placed within the infant's visual range to stimulate the infant visually. Wind-up musical toys provide rhythmic distractions as long as they are not too loud. If the infant is receiving phototherapy, the protective eye patches are removed periodically (e.g., during feeding) so that the infant can see the caregiver's face for short, comforting sessions.

Kangaroo care. Kangaroo care (skin-to-skin holding) helps infants to directly interact with their parents (Gale & VandenBerg, 1998). In this technique the infant, dressed

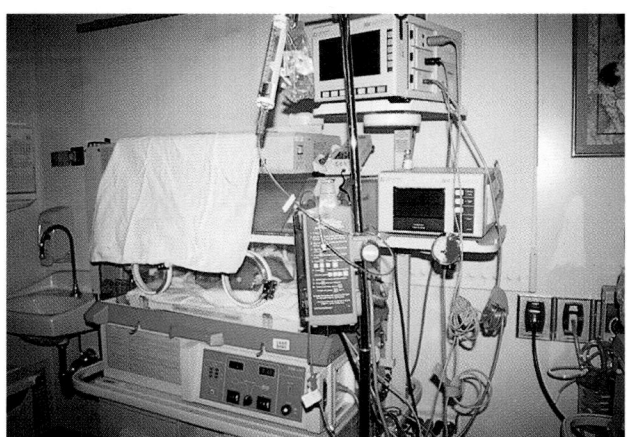

Fig. 41-13 Infant in double-walled incubator with a blanket for a light shield. *(Courtesy Marjorie Pyle, RNC, Lifecircle, Costa Mesa, CA.)*

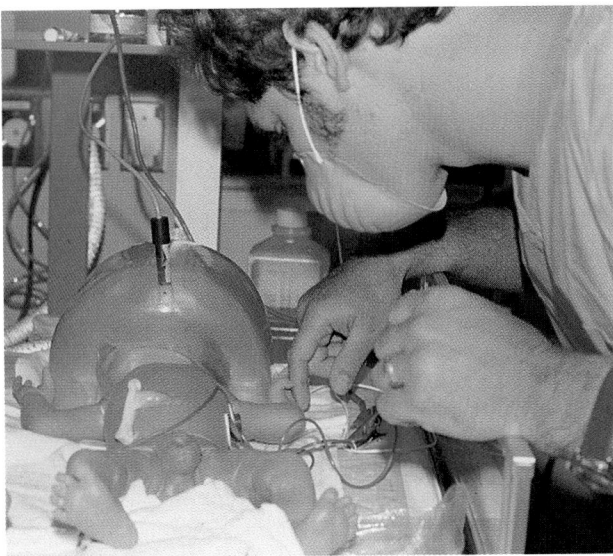

Fig. 41-14 A father caresses his tiny preterm infant in the NICU. *(Courtesy Marjorie Pyle, RNC, Lifecircle, Costa Mesa, CA.)*

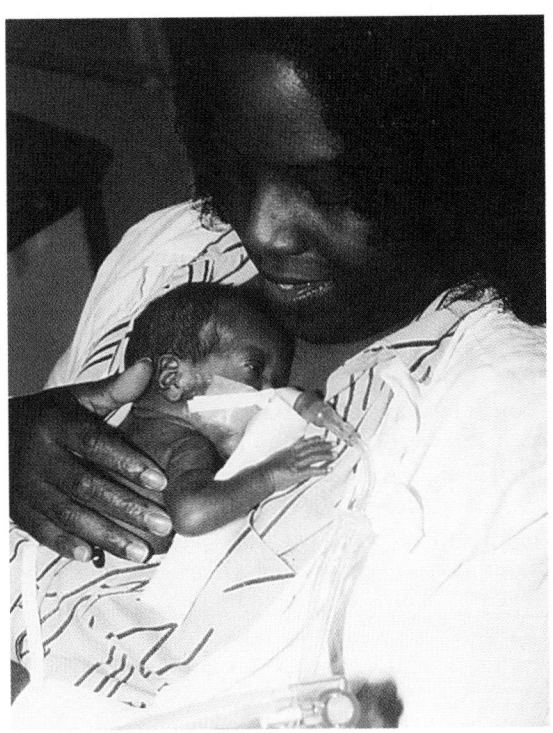

Fig. 41-15 Kangaroo care. Parent wraps her shirt around the infant. *(From Gale, G., Franck, L., & Lund, C. [1993]. Skin-to-skin holding of the intubated premature infant. Neonatal Netw 12[6], 51.)*

only in a diaper, is placed directly on the parent's bare chest and then covered with the parent's clothing or a warmed blanket (Fig. 41-15). In this way, the parent's body temperature also functions as an external heat source that enhances the infant's temperature regulation. Even ventilator-dependent infants weighing under 1 kg have been found to benefit from this measure, although they usually tolerate it for only 30 minutes or less at a time (see Research box).

Kangaroo holding was originally developed in Bogota, Colombia, where radiant warmers and incubators were in severely short supply. Although such care has its roots in severe economic hardships, it stems from a deep respect for natural processes. Infants and parents who participate in such kangaroo care have been observed to have dramatically better outcomes. The mothers report increased breast milk output and fewer feelings of helplessness related to their experiences in the NICU. The infants have been found to maintain their temperatures and oxygenation levels better and to experience fewer episodes of crying, apnea, and periodic respirations. They have also been observed to be alert and quiet longer and to have slightly higher heart rates. Kangaroo care also meets developmental needs by fostering neurobehavioral development (Ludington-Hoe et al., 1994).

Parental Support

The nurse as the support person and teacher is responsible for shaping the environment and making the caregiving responsive to the needs of the parents and infant. Nurses are instrumental in helping parents learn who their infant is and to recognize behavioral cues in his or her development (VandenBerg, 1999).

If a high risk birth has been anticipated, the family can be given a tour of the NICU or shown a video to prepare

them for the sights and activities of the unit. After the birth, the parents can be given a booklet, be shown a video, or have someone describe what they will see when they go to the unit to see their infant. As soon as possible, the parents should see and touch their infant so that they can begin to acknowledge the reality of the birth and the infant's true appearance and condition. They will need encouragement as they begin to accomplish the psychologic tasks imposed by the high risk birth. For the following reasons, a nurse or physician should be present during the parents' first visit to see the infant:

- To help them "see" the infant rather than focus on the equipment. The importance and purpose of the apparatus that surrounds their infant should also be explained to them.
- To explain the characteristics normal for an infant of their baby's gestational age; in this way parents do not compare their child with a full-term, healthy infant.
- To encourage the parents to express their feelings about the pregnancy, labor, and birth and the experience of having a high risk infant.
- To assess the parents' perceptions of the infant to determine the appropriate time for them to become actively involved in care (see Guidelines/Guías box).

As soon as possible after the birth, the parents are given the opportunity to meet the infant in the *en face* position, to touch the infant, and to see his or her favorable characteristics. As soon as possible, depending primarily on her physi-

RESEARCH

Parents' Perception of Skin-to-Skin Care with Their Preterm Infants Requiring Assisted Ventilation

Skin-to-skin care has been used in nurseries in the United States as well as with critically ill neonates. According to one survey, at least 34 intensive care nurseries in the United States provide skin-to-skin care to mothers and their infants who require assisted ventilation. However, little research has been published addressing the responses of seriously ill infants or the feelings of their parents during skin-to-skin care. The purpose of this study was to explore parents' perception of skin-to-skin care with their preterm infant who is on assisted ventilation, and to elucidate factors influencing the decision to continue or discontinue skin-to-skin care.

A naturalistic inquiry was used to obtain a detailed subjective description of the experience of parents (N = 9) who had participated in skin-to-skin care. This design incorporated two interviews, one conducted immediately after two skin-to-skin care sessions and a follow-up interview conducted several months later.

Three themes emerged: (a) ambivalence of parents toward skin-to-skin care, including subthemes of yearning to hold the infant and apprehension to do so; (b) need of a supportive environment; and (c) special quality of the parent-infant interaction, including subthemes of intense connectedness and active parenting. Perceptions of apprehension, need for a supportive environment, and active parenting differed between parents who continued skin-to-skin care

during their infants' hospitalization and parents who did not. Three of the four parents who discontinued skin-to-skin care in the hospital resumed when their infants were home.

The author concluded that differences in narratives of the parents emphasized the importance of individualizing the skin-to-skin experience to the needs of the parent and infant. Parents who resumed skin-to-skin care at home valued the experience while their infant was hospitalized but needed interventions to alleviate their apprehension, enhance their feeling of autonomy, and modify the environment.

CLINICAL APPLICATION

Nursing actions such as providing privacy, expressing a positive attitude toward skin-to-skin care, and offering to assist may alleviate anxiety and provide enough encouragement for a parent who values the skin-to-skin experience. Indicating to a parent when his/her nurturing actions are followed by improvement in physiologic or behavioral status of the infant may increase that parent's confidence in his or her ability to contribute to the infant's well-being during skin-to-skin holding. Exploration by nurse and parent of ways to provide a facilitative environment for skin-to-skin care will optimize the experience for both parent and infant.

Source: Neu, M. (1999). Parents perception of skin-to-skin care with their preterm infants requiring assisted ventilation. *J Obstet Gynecol Neonatal Nurs* 28(2), 157-164.

---

cal condition, the mother is encouraged to visit the nursery as desired and help with the infant's care. When the family cannot be present physically, staff members devise appropriate methods to keep them in almost constant touch with the newborn, such as with daily phone calls, notes written as if by the infant, or photographs of the infant.

Some hospitals have support groups for the parents of infants in NICUs. These groups help parents experiencing anxiety and grief by encouraging them to share their feelings. Hospitals also often arrange to have an experienced NICU parent make contact with a new group member to provide additional support. The volunteer parents provide support by making hospital visits, phone calls, and home visits.

Many NICUs use volunteers in varying capacities. After they have gone through the orientation program, volunteers can perform tasks such as holding the infants, stocking bedside cabinets, assembling parent packets, and, in some nurseries, feeding the infants.

Some high risk infants can be discharged earlier than the expected time (Gamblian, Hess, & Kenner, 1998). The

criteria showing an infant's readiness for early discharge are that the infant's physiologic condition is stable, the infant is receiving adequate nutrition, and the infant's body temperature is stable. The parents, or other caregivers, also need to exhibit a physical, emotional, and educational readiness to assume responsibility for the care of the infant. Ideally, the home environment is adequate for meeting the needs of the infant. The parents also need to show that they know the way to take the infant's temperature, know the signs and symptoms to report, and understand the dietary needs of the infant (Brooten, 1995).

Parent Education

Cardiopulmonary resuscitation. Sudden infant death syndrome (SIDS) is 8 to 10 times more likely to develop in preterm infants than in term infants. Furthermore, it has been found that infants discharged from an NICU are about twice as likely to die unexpectedly during the first year of life as infants in the general population. Instruction in cardiopulmonary resuscitation (CPR) is essential for parents of all infants but especially for those of infants at

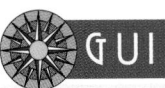

Intensive Care Nursery—Parent Teaching on First Visit

He/she is small but strong.
Él/ella es pequeño/pequeña pero fuerte.

This is a special bed that keeps the baby warm with radiant heat.
Esta es una cama especial que mantiene al bebé caliente con calor radiante.

The baby is breathing by himself on room air.
El bebé está respirando solo en el aire ambiente.

The baby has an IV so we can give him fluids.
El bebé tiene un cateter intrevenoso para administrarle líquidos.

The baby has an umbilical catheter so that we may administer fluids and nutrients and so we may draw blood for laboratory testing.
El bebé tiene un cateter umbilical que nos permite administrar líquidos y nutrimentos al bebé y nos permite obtener muestras de sangre para hacer pruebas.

This nasogastric tube allows us to feed the baby.
Este tubo nasogastrica nos permite alimentar a su bebé.

This endotracheal tube delivers air directly to the lungs.
Este tubo endotraqueal entrega aire directamente a los pulmones.

risk for life-threatening events (see Chapter 27). Infants considered at risk include those who are premature, have apnea or bradycardia spells, or have a tendency to choke. Before taking their infant home, parents must be able to administer CPR. All parents should be encouraged to obtain instruction in CPR at their local Red Cross or other community agency.

Evaluation

The nurse uses the previously stated expected outcomes of care to evaluate the effectiveness of the physical and psychosocial aspects of care (see Plan of Care).

COMPLICATIONS IN HIGH RISK INFANTS

Respiratory Distress Syndrome

Respiratory distress syndrome (RDS) refers to a lung disorder usually affecting premature infants. Maternal and fetal conditions associated with a decreased incidence and severity of RDS include female infant, African-American race, maternal pregnancy-induced hypertension, maternal drug abuse, maternal steroid therapy

(betamethasone), chronic retroplacental abruption, prolonged rupture of membranes, and IUGR (Hagedorn, Gardner, & Abman, 1998). The incidence and severity of RDS increase with a decrease in the gestational age. Perinatal asphyxia, hypovolemia, male infant, white race, maternal diabetes (types 1 and 2), second-born twin, familial predisposition, maternal hypotension, cesarean birth without labor, hydrops fetalis, and third-trimester bleeding are all factors that place an infant at increased risk for RDS (Hagedorn, Gardner, & Abman, 1998). The incidence of RDS in infants weighing less than 1500 g is 56% (Hack et al., 1995).

RDS is caused by a lack of pulmonary surfactant, which leads to progressive atelectasis, loss of functional residual capacity, and a ventilation-perfusion imbalance with an uneven distribution of ventilation. This surfactant deficiency may be caused by insufficient surfactant production, abnormal composition and function, disruption of surfactant production, or a combination of these factors. The sequence of events that occurs is further compromised by the weak respiratory muscles and an overly compliant chest wall common to premature infants. Lung capacity is further compromised by the presence of proteinaceous material and epithelial debris in the airways. The resulting decreased oxygenation, cyanosis, and metabolic or respiratory acidosis can cause the pulmonary vascular resistance (PVR) to be increased. This increased PVR can lead to right-to-left shunting and a reopening of the ductus arteriosus and foramen ovale (Merenstein & Gardner, 1998) (Fig. 41-16).

Clinical symptoms of RDS are listed in Box 41-6. These respiratory symptoms usually appear immediately after birth or within 6 hours of birth. Physical examination reveals crackles, poor air exchange, pallor, the use of accessory muscles (retractions), and occasionally apnea. Radiographic findings include a uniform reticulogranular appearance and air bronchograms (Fanaroff & Martin, 1997). The infant's clinical course typically is variable. There is usually an increased oxygen requirement and increased respiratory effort as atelectasis, a loss of functional residual capacity, and ventilation-perfusion imbalance worsen.

However, RDS is a self-limiting disease, with the respiratory symptoms abating after 72 hours. This disappearance of respiratory symptoms coincides with the production of surfactant in the type 2 cells of the alveoli.

The treatment for RDS is supportive. Adequate ventilation and oxygenation must be established and maintained in an attempt to prevent ventilation-perfusion mismatch and atelectasis. Exogenous surfactant may be administered at birth or shortly after birth, and this has the effect of altering the typical course of RDS. Positive-pressure ventilation, CPAP, and oxygen therapy may be needed during the respiratory illness. However, the prevention of complications associated with mechanical ventilation is also critical. These complications include pulmonary interstitial emphysema, pneumothorax, pneumomediastinum, and

NURSING DIAGNOSIS Ineffective breathing pattern related to pulmonary and neuromuscular immaturity, decreased energy, fatigue

Expected Outcome *Infant exhibits adequate oxygenation (i.e., ABGs and acid-base within normal limits [WNL], oxygen saturations 92% or greater, respiratory rate and pattern WNL, breath sounds clear, absence of grunting, nasal flaring, minimal retractions, skin color WNL).*

Nursing Interventions/*Rationales*

Position neonate prone or supine, avoiding neck hyperextension *to promote optimum air exchange.* Use a sidelying position after feeding or in cases of excessive mucous production *to avoid aspiration.* Avoid Trendelenburg's position *because it can cause increased intracranial pressure and reduce lung capacity.*

Suction nasopharynx, trachea, and endotracheal tube as indicated *to remove mucus.* Avoid oversuctioning *because it can cause bronchospasm, bradycardia, hypoxia, and predispose neonate to intraventricular hemorrhage.*

Administer percussion, vibration, and postural drainage as prescribed *to facilitate drainage of secretions.*

Administer oxygen and monitor neonatal response *to maintain oxygen saturation.*

Maintain a neutral thermal environment *to conserve oxygen use.*

Monitor arterial blood gases, acid-base balance, oxygen saturation, respiratory rate and pattern, breath sounds, and airway patency; observe for grunting, nasal flaring, retractions, and cyanosis *to detect signs of respiratory distress.*

NURSING DIAGNOSIS Ineffective thermoregulation related to immature temperature regulation and minimal subcutaneous fat stores

Expected Outcome *Infant exhibits maintenance of stable body temperature within normal range for postconceptional age (36.5° to 37.2° C).*

Nursing Interventions/*Rationales*

Place neonate in a prewarmed radiant warmer *to maintain stable temperature.*

Place temperature probe on neonatal abdomen *to control heat levels in radiant warmer.*

Take axillary temperature periodically *to monitor temperature and cross-check functioning of warmer unit.*

Avoid infant exposure to cool air and drafts, cold scales, cold stethoscopes, cold examination tables, and prolonged bathing *that predispose the infant to heat loss.*

Monitor probe frequently *as detachment can cause overheating or warmer-induced hyperthermia.*

Transfer infant to a servocontrolled open warmer bed or incubator *when temperature has stabilized.*

NURSING DIAGNOSIS Risk for infection related to immature immune system

Expected Outcome *Infant exhibits no evidence of nosocomial infection.*

Nursing Interventions/*Rationales*

Institute scrupulous handwashing techniques before and after handling neonate, ensure all supplies and/or equipment are clean before use, and ensure strict aseptic technique with invasive procedures *to minimize exposure to infective organisms.*

Prevent contact with persons who have communicable infections and instruct parents in infection control procedures *to minimize infection risk.*

Administer prescribed antibiotics *to provide coverage for infection during sepsis workup.*

Continuously monitor vital signs for stability *as instability, hypothermia, or prolonged temperature elevations serve as indicators for infection.*

NURSING DIAGNOSIS Risk for nutrition alteration less than body requirements related to inability to ingest nutrients secondary to immaturity

Expected Outcomes *Infant receives adequate amount of nutrients with sufficient caloric intake to maintain positive nitrogen balance; demonstrates steady weight gain.*

Nursing Interventions/*Rationales*

Administer parenteral fluid/total parenteral nutrition (TPN) as prescribed *to provide adequate nutrition and fluid intake.*

Monitor for signs of intolerance to TPN, *which can interfere with effective replenishment of nutrients.*

Periodically assess readiness to orally feed (i.e., strong suck, swallow, and gag reflexes) *to provide appropriate transition for TPN to oral feeding as soon as neonate is ready.*

Advance volume and concentration of formula when orally feeding per unit protocol *to avoid overfeeding and feeding intolerance.*

If mother desires to breastfeed when neonate is stable, demonstrate how to express milk *to establish and maintain lactation until infant can breastfeed.*

From Wong, D., & Perry, S. (1998). *Maternal child nursing care.* St. Louis: Mosby.

Continued

PLAN ᵒꜰ CARE | High Risk Premature Newborn—cont'd

NURSING DIAGNOSIS Risk for fluid volume deficit/excess related to immature physiology

Expected Outcome *Infant exhibits evidence of fluid homeostasis.*

Nursing Interventions/*Rationales*

Administer parenteral fluids as prescribed and regulate carefully *to maintain fluid balance.* Avoid hypertonic fluids such as undiluted medications, and concentrated glucose because *they can cause excess solute load on immature kidneys.*

Implement strategies (use of plastic covers and increase of ambient humidity) *that minimize insensible water loss.*

Monitor hydration status (i.e., skin turgor, blood pressure, edema, weight, mucous membranes, fontanels, urine specific gravity, electrolytes) and intake and output *to evaluate for evidence of dehydration or overhydration.*

NURSING DIAGNOSIS Risk for impaired skin integrity related to immature skin structure, immobility, or invasive procedures

Expected Outcome *Infant's skin remains intact with no evidence of irritation or injury.*

Nursing Interventions/*Rationales*

Cleanse skin as needed with plain warm water and apply moisturizing agents to skin *to prevent dryness and reduce friction across skin surface.*

When performing procedures: minimize use of tape and apply a skin barrier between tape and skin; use transparent elastic film for securing central and peripheral lines; use limb electrodes for monitoring or attach with hydrogel and rotate electrodes frequently; remove adhesives with soap and water rather than alcohol or acetone-based adhesive removers *to minimize skin damage.*

Monitor use of thermal devices such as warmers or heating pads carefully *to prevent burns.*

Monitor skin closely for evidence of redness, rash, irritation, bruising, breakdown, ischemia, and infiltration *to detect and treat potential complications early.*

NURSING DIAGNOSIS Risk for injury related to increased intracranial pressure and intraventricular hemorrhage secondary to immature central nervous system

Expected Outcome *Infant will exhibit normal intracranial pressure (ICP) with no evidence of intraventricular hemorrhage.*

Nursing Interventions/*Rationales*

Institute minimum stimulation protocol (i.e., minimal handling, clustering care techniques, avoidance of sudden head movements to one side, undisturbed sleep periods, light variations to simulate day and night, limiting personnel and equipment noise in environment) *to decrease stress responses, which can increase ICP.*

Institute ordered pharmacologic and nonpharmacologic pain control methods *to manage pain and reduce physical stress.*

Avoid hypertonic solutions and medications *as they increase cerebral blood flow.*

Elevate head of bed 15 to 20 degrees *to decrease ICP.*

Monitor vital signs *for evidence of ICP.*

Recognize signs of overstimulation (i.e., flaccidity, yawning, irritability, crying, staring, active averting) *so stimulation can be stopped to allow rest.*

NURSING DIAGNOSIS Altered parenting related to separation and interruption of parent/infant attachment secondary to premature birth

Expected Outcomes *Parents establish contact with neonate; demonstrate competent parenting skills and willingness to care for neonate.*

Nursing Interventions/*Rationales*

Before parents' first visit to the NICU, prepare them by explaining what the neonate will look like, what the equipment will look like and its function *to diminish fear and decrease sense of shock.*

Keep parents informed about infant's condition (improvements and setbacks) and important aspects of infant's care; encourage and answer parental questions; actively listen to parent concerns *to establish trust, open communication, and caring atmosphere to aid in coping.*

Encourage parents to visit the NICU often; to name infant; to touch, hold, or caress infant as physical condition permits; to be actively involved in infant's care; to bring personal items (i.e., clothing, stuffed animals, or pictures of family) *to allow for formation of emotional bond.*

Reinforce parent involvement and praise care endeavors to *increase self-confidence in their contribution.*

Encourage parents to bring other siblings to visit; explain to siblings what they are seeing; encourage siblings to draw pictures or write letters for infant and place in or near infant's crib *to promote family involvement, help ease sibling fears, and let them contribute to infant's care.*

Refer parents to social services as needed *to ensure comprehensive care.*

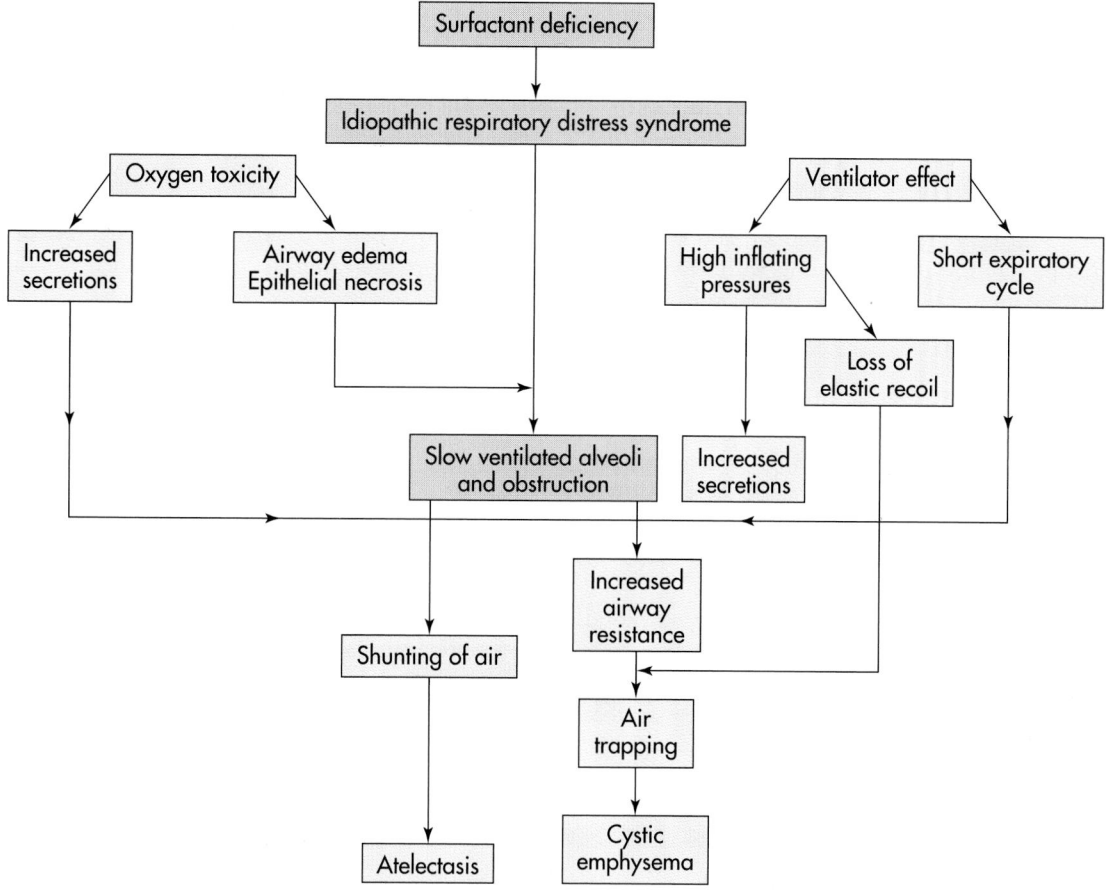

Fig. 41-16 Pathogenesis of respiratory distress syndrome (RDS). *(From Merenstein, G., & Gardner, S. [1998]. Handbook of neonatal intensive care [4th ed.]. St. Louis: Mosby.)*

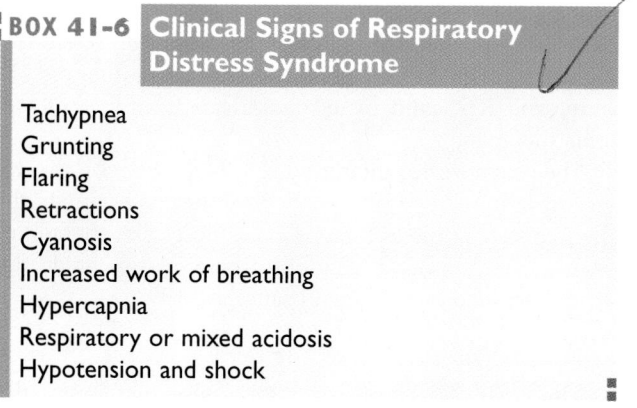

BOX 41-6 **Clinical Signs of Respiratory Distress Syndrome**

Tachypnea
Grunting
Flaring
Retractions
Cyanosis
Increased work of breathing
Hypercapnia
Respiratory or mixed acidosis
Hypotension and shock

TABLE 41-1 **Normal Arterial Blood Gas Values for Neonates**

VALUE	RANGE
pH	7.33-7.42
Arterial oxygen pressure (PaO_2)	50-80 mm Hg
Carbon dioxide pressure ($PaCO_2$)	38-48 mm Hg
Bicarbonate (HCO_3)	20-24 mEq/L
Oxygen saturation	>90%

From Dickason, E., Silverman, B., & Kaplan, J. (1998). *Maternal-infant nursing care* (3rd ed.). St Louis: Mosby.

pneumopericardium. The mortality and morbidity rates associated with RDS are attributed to the immature organ systems of the infant and the complications associated with the treatment of the disease (Fanaroff & Martin, 1997).

Acid-base balance is evaluated by monitoring the ABG values (Table 41-1). Frequent blood sampling requires arterial access accomplished either by umbilical artery catheterization or by a peripheral arterial line. Pulse oximetry and transcutaneous carbon dioxide and oxygen monitors document trends in ventilation and oxygenation. Capillary blood gas values indicate the pH and PCO_2 status in infants who are in a more stable condition (Cloherty & Stark, 1997).

The maintenance of an NTE continues to be of critical importance in infants with RDS because infants suffering from hypoxemia are unable to increase their metabolic rate when cold stressed (Fanaroff & Martin, 1997).

The clinical and radiographic presentation (radiodense lung fields and air bronchograms) of neonatal pneumonia may be similar to that of RDS. Fluid in the minor tissue may also be noted in infants with neonatal pneumonia. Therefore sepsis evaluation, including blood culture, complete blood count (CBC) with differential, and occasionally a lumbar puncture, is done in infants with RDS to rule out neonatal pneumonia. Broad-spectrum antibiotics are begun while the results of cultures are awaited (Cloherty & Stark, 1997).

Fluid and nutrition need to be maintained in the critically ill infant with RDS. Parenteral nutrition can be implemented to provide protein and fats to promote a positive nitrogen balance. Daily monitoring of the electrolyte values, urinary output, specific gravity, and weight help evaluate the infant's hydration status (Cloherty & Stark, 1997; Fanaroff & Martin, 1997).

The need for frequent blood sampling may make blood transfusions necessary. The critically ill infant usually needs to have a venous hematocrit level of more than 40% to maintain adequate oxygen-carrying capacity (Fanaroff & Martin, 1997).

> **NURSE ALERT** *Directed-donor blood has become more frequently requested. This is donor blood usually obtained from a family member or close friend of the family who has the same blood type as the infant or a compatible blood type. It may be necessary to notify the infant's family of the potential need for blood transfusion on admission to allow for the processing of directed-donor blood.*

Reassuring the family that stringent testing of all blood products is done may alleviate some of their anxiety about the transmission of blood-borne pathogens. Because some religions prohibit the use of blood transfusions, it is critical to obtain a complete history from the family, including their religious preference. Alternative strategies for maintaining the hematocrit may need to be employed in these instances.

Complications Associated with Oxygen Therapy

Retinopathy of Prematurity

Retinopathy of prematurity (ROP) is a complex multicausal disorder that affects the developing retinal vessels of premature infants. The normal retinal vessels begin to form in utero at approximately 16 weeks in response to an unknown stimulus. These vessels continue to develop until they reach maturity at approximately 42 to 43 weeks postconception. Once the retina is completely vascularized, the retinal vessels are not susceptible to ROP. The mechanism of injury in ROP is unclear. Oxygen tensions that are too high for the level of retinal maturity initially

result in vasoconstriction. After oxygen therapy is discontinued, neovascularization occurs in the retina and vitreous, with capillary hemorrhages, fibrotic resolution, and possible retinal detachment. Cicatricial (scar) tissue formation and consequent visual impairment may be mild or severe. The entire disease process in severe cases may take as long as 5 months to evolve. Examination by an ophthalmologist before discharge and a schedule for repeat examinations thereafter are recommended for the parents' guidance.

The key to the management of ROP is prevention and early detection of premature birth. Circumferential cryopexy, laser photocoagulation, vitamin E therapy, and decreasing the intensity of ambient light are used in the treatment of ROP, with varying results (Fanaroff & Martin, 1997).

Bronchopulmonary Dysplasia

Bronchopulmonary dysplasia (BPD) is a chronic pulmonary iatrogenic condition caused by barotrauma from pressure ventilation and oxygen toxicity (Hagedorn, Gardner, & Abman, 1998). The etiology of BDP is multifactorial and includes pulmonary immaturity, surfactant deficiency, lung injury and stretch, barotrauma, inflammation caused by oxygen exposure, fluid overload, ligation of a patent ductus arteriosus, and a familial predisposition (Hagedorn, Gardner, & Abman 1998).

Clinical symptoms of BPD include tachypnea, retractions, nasal flaring, increased work of breathing, exercise intolerance (to handling and feeding), and tachycardia (Hagedorn, Gardner, & Abman, 1998). Auscultation of the lung fields in affected infants typically reveals crackles, decreased air movement, and occasionally expiratory wheezing. The treatment for BPD includes oxygen therapy, nutrition, fluid restriction, and medications (diuretics, corticosteroids, bronchodilators). However, the key to the management of BPD is prevention by preventing prematurity and RDS and by using surfactant and other less toxic therapies.

The prognosis for infants with BPD depends on the degree of pulmonary dysfunction. Most deaths occur within the first year of life as a result of cardiorespiratory failure, sepsis, or respiratory infection; in some infants the deaths are sudden and unexplained (Bancalari, 1997).

Patent Ductus Arteriosus

The ductus arteriosus is a normal muscular contractile structure in the fetus connecting the left pulmonary artery and the dorsal aorta. The duct constricts after birth as oxygenation, the levels of circulating prostaglandins, and the muscle mass increase. Other factors that promote ductal closure include catecholamines, low pH, bradykinin, and acetylcholine (Zahka & Patel, 1997). When the fetal ductus arteriosus fails to close after birth, **patent ductus arteriosus (PDA)** occurs. The incidence of PDA in premature infants weighing less than 1500 g is 40% to 60%, with an increased percentage of cases occurring in premature infants weighing less than 1000 g (Gomella, Cunningham, & Eyal, 1994).

The clinical presentation in an infant with a PDA includes systolic murmur, active precordium, bounding peripheral pulses, tachycardia, tachypnea, crackles, and hepatomegaly. The systolic murmur is heard best at the second or third intercostal space at the upper left sternal border. An active precordium is caused by an increased left ventricular stroke volume. In addition, a widened pulse pressure may result in an increase in peripheral pulses (Daberkow-Carson & Washington, 1998; Zahka & Patel, 1997).

Radiographic studies in infants with PDA typically show cardiac enlargement and pulmonary edema. ABG findings reveal hypercapnia and metabolic acidosis. Echocardiography can demonstrate a PDA and can quantitate the amount of blood shunting across the PDA (Daberkow-Carson & Washington, 1998).

The PDA can be managed medically or surgically. Medical management consists of ventilatory support, fluid restriction, and the administration of diuretics and indomethacin. Indomethacin is a prostaglandin synthetase inhibitor that blocks the effect of the arachidonic acid products on the ductus and causes the PDA to constrict (Daberkow-Carson & Washington, 1998). Ventilatory support is adjusted based on the ABG values. Fluid restriction is implemented to decrease cardiovascular volume overload in association with the diuretic therapy. Surgical ligation is done when a PDA is clinically significant and medical management has failed (Daberkow-Carson & Washington, 1998).

The nursing care of the infant with PDA focuses on supportive care. The infant needs an NTE, adequate oxygenation, meticulous fluid balance, and parental support.

Periventricular-intraventricular hemorrhage. Periventricular-intraventricular hemorrhage (PV-IVH) is one of the most common types of brain injury that occurs in neonates and is among the most severe from the standpoint of both short- and long-term outcomes. The true incidence of PV-IVH is unknown, but approximately 50% of infants who die in the first few days of life experience hemorrhage (Moe & Paige, 1998). Use of prenatal corticosteroids can reduce the incidence to about 25% (Reed & Blumer, 1997). The general estimate is 20% to 30% in infants less than 32 weeks of gestation or under 1500 g (Moe & Paige, 1998).

The pathogenesis of PV-IVH includes intravascular factors (fluctuating or increasing cerebral blood flow, increases in cerebral venous pressures, and coagulopathy), vascular factors, extravascular factors, and nursery care. PV-IVH events typically occur within the first hours or days of life.

PV-IVH is classified according to a grading system of I to IV, with grade I being the least severe and grade IV the most severe (Moe & Paige, 1998) (Box 41-7).

BOX 41-7 Classification of Periventricular-Intraventricular Hemorrhage

GRADE I

Isolated germinal matrix hemorrhage

GRADE II

Intraventricular hemorrhage with normal ventricular size

GRADE III

Intraventricular hemorrhage with acute ventricular dilatation

GRADE IV

Intraventricular hemorrhage with parenchymal hemorrhage

From Moe, P., & Paige, P. (1998). Neurologic disorders. In G. Merenstein & S. Gardner (Eds.). *Handbook of neonatal intensive care* (4th ed.). St. Louis: Mosby.

The long-term neurodevelopmental outcome is determined by the severity of the PV-IVH. Infants with grade I or II usually have good outcomes; infants with grade III and IV often have long-term morbidity (Moe & Paige, 1998).

Nursing care focuses on recognition of factors that increase the risk of PV-IVH, interventions to decrease the risk of bleeding, and supportive care to infants who have bleeding episodes. The infant is positioned with the head in midline and the head of the bed elevated slightly to prevent or minimize fluctuations in intracranial blood pressure. NTE is maintained, as well as oxygenation. Rapid infusions of fluids should be avoided. Blood pressure is monitored closely for fluctuations. The infant is monitored for signs of pneumothorax because it often precedes PV-IVH.

Necrotizing Enterocolitis

Necrotizing enterocolitis (NEC) is an acute inflammatory disease of the GI mucosa, commonly complicated by perforation. This often fatal disease occurs in about 2% to 5% of newborns in NICUs. Although the cause is unknown, the factors listed in Box 41-8 are known to contribute to its development. Breastfeeding seems to lower the incidence of NEC.

Reversal of perinatal asphyxia within 30 minutes may prevent GI tract insult and thus prevent the pathophysiologic events that trigger NEC. After 30 minutes the distribution of cardiac output tends to be directed more toward the heart and brain and away from the abdominal organs. Therefore prompt birth of the intrauterine-asphyxiated fetus or ventilation of the asphyxiated newborn may be beneficial to the GI tract, as well as to other organs.

BOX 41-8 Proposed Risk Factors for Necrotizing Enterocolitis

Asphyxia
Respiratory distress syndrome
Umbilical artery catheter
Exchange transfusion
Early enteral feedings/hyperosmolar feedings
Patent ductus arteriosus
Congenital heart disease
Polycythemia
Anemia
Shock
Gastrointestinal infection

The onset of NEC in the full-term infant usually occurs between 4 and 10 days after birth. In the preterm infant the onset may be delayed for up to 30 days. The signs of developing NEC are nonspecific, which is characteristic of many neonatal diseases. Some generalized signs include decreased activity, hypotonia, pallor, recurrent apnea and bradycardia, decreased oxygen saturation values, respiratory distress, metabolic acidosis, oliguria, hypotension, decreased perfusion, temperature instability, and cyanosis. GI symptoms include abdominal distention, increasing or bile-stained residual gastric aspirates, vomiting (bile or blood), grossly bloody stools, abdominal tenderness, and erythema of the abdominal wall (Holland, Price, & Bensard, 1998).

A diagnosis of NEC is confirmed by a radiographic examination that reveals bowel loop distention, pneumatosis intestinalis, pneumoperitoneum, portal air, or a combination of these findings. The abnormal radiographic findings are caused by the bacterial colonization of the GI tract associated with NEC, resulting in ileus. Pneumatosis intestinalis, pneumoperitoneum, and portal air are caused by gas produced by the bacteria that invade the wall of the intestines and escape into the peritoneum and portal system when perforation occurs. The laboratory evaluation in such infants consists of a CBC with differential, coagulation studies, ABG analysis, measurement of serum electrolyte levels, and blood culture (Korones & Bada-Ellzey, 1993). The white blood cell count on the CBC may be either increased or decreased. The platelet count and coagulation study findings may be abnormal, showing thrombocytopenia and disseminated intravascular coagulation (DIC). Electrolyte levels may be abnormal with leaking capillary beds and fluid shifts with the infection.

Treatment in such infants is supportive. Oral or tube feedings are discontinued to rest the GI tract. An orogastric tube is placed and attached to low wall suction to provide gastric decompression. Parenteral therapy (often TPN) is begun. Because NEC is an infectious disease, control of the infection is imperative, with an emphasis on careful handwashing before and after infant contact. Antibiotic therapy may be instituted, and surgical resection is performed if perforation or clinical deterioration occurs. Therapy is usually prolonged, and recovery may be delayed by the formation of adhesions, the development of the complications associated with bowel resection, the occurrence of short gut syndrome (especially if the ileocecal valve is removed), or the development of intolerance to oral feedings.

A decrease in the incidence of NEC correlates with the use of nonnutritive sucking during gavage feedings (Pickler & Terrell, 1994). The authors hypothesize that nonnutritive sucking has this effect because it makes the GI tract less susceptible to the factors that precipitate NEC by promoting gastric motility and thus increasing the release of gastric enzymes. The improvement in the infant's behavioral organization brought about by nonnutritive sucking also appears to play a role in this.

INFANT PAIN RESPONSES

The physiology of pain and pain assessment in the newborn were discussed in Chapter 27. This discussion focuses on pain assessment and management in the preterm infant.

Pain Assessment

Assessment of pain in the neonate is difficult because evaluation must be based on physiologic changes and behavioral observations. Although behaviors such as vocalizations, facial expressions, body movements, and general state are common to all infants, they vary with different situations. Crying associated with pain is more intense and sustained. Facial expression is the most consistent and specific characteristic; scales are available to systematically evaluate facial features, such as eye squeeze, brow bulge, and open mouth and taut tongue (Grunau & Craig, 1987; Grunau, Johnston, & Craig, 1990; Hadjistavropoulos et al., 1997). Most infants respond with increased body movements but the infant may be experiencing pain even when lying quietly with eyes closed (Shapiro, 1989). The preterm infant's response to pain may be behaviorally blunted or absent. An infant who receives a muscle-paralyzing agent such as vecuronium will also be incapable of mounting a behavioral or visible pain response (Box 41-9).

NURSE ALERT *When in doubt about pain in infants, base your decision on the following rule: Whatever is painful to an adult or child is painful to an infant unless proved otherwise.*

Several pain assessment tools have been developed for the assessment of pain in the neonate. One pain assessment tool used by nurses in the neonatal intensive care setting is called the *CRIES* (Table 41-2). This tool was developed for use by nurses who work with premature and

BOX 41-9 Manifestations of Acute Pain in the Neonate

PHYSIOLOGIC RESPONSES
Vital Signs: Observe for Variations

Increased heart rate
Increased blood pressure
Rapid, shallow respirations

Oxygenation

Decreased transcutaneous O_2 saturation ($tcPO_2$)
Decreased arterial O_2 saturation (SaO_2)

Skin: Observe Color and Character

Pallor and flushing
Diaphoresis
Palmar sweating

Other Observations

Increased muscle tone
Dilated pupils
Decreased vagal nerve tone
Increased intracranial pressure
Laboratory evidence of metabolic or endocrine
  changes
  Hyperglycemia
  Lowered pH
  Elevated corticosteroids

BEHAVIORAL RESPONSES
**Vocalizations: Observe Quality, Timing,
and Duration**

Crying
Whimpering
Groaning

**Facial Expression: Observe Characteristics, Timing,
and Orientation of Eyes and Mouth (see Fig. 27-13)**

Grimaces
Brow furrowed
Chin quivering
Eyes tightly closed
Mouth open and squarish

**Body Movements and Posture: Observe Type,
Quality, and Amount of Movement or Lack of
Movement; Relationship to Other Factors**

Limb withdrawal
Thrashing
Rigidity
Flaccidity
Fist clenching

**Change in State: Observe Sleep, Appetite,
Activity Level**

Changes in sleep/wake cycles
Changes in feeding behavior
Changes in activity level
Fussiness, irritability
Listlessness

From Wong, D. (1999). *Whaley and Wong's nursing care of infants and children* (6th ed.). St. Louis: Mosby.

full-term infants. CRIES is an acronym for the physiologic and behavioral indicators of pain used in the tool. The indicators include crying, requiring increased oxygen, increased vital signs, expression, and sleeplessness. Each indicator is scored from 0 to 2—similar to the Apgar score for neonates. The total possible pain score, which represents the worst pain, is 10. A pain score greater than 4 should be considered significant. This tool has been tested for reliability and validity for postoperative pain in infants between the ages of 32 weeks of gestation and 20 weeks post-term (Bildner & Krechel, 1996; Krechel & Bildner, 1995).

Memory of Pain

Premature infants are subjected to a variety of repeated noxious stimuli, including multiple heel sticks, venipuncture, endotracheal intubation and suctioning, arterial sticks, chest tube placement, and lumbar puncture. The effects of pain caused by such procedures are not fully

known, but researchers have begun to investigate potential consequences.

Nurses' anecdotal reports suggest that infants show memory by exhibiting defensive behaviors when painful procedures are repeated. Nurses often describe infants who stiffen and withdraw when touched because human touch has repeatedly been associated with pain. Such infants often become hypervigilant and gaze intently at the hands rather than at the eyes of people who approach them (Penticuff, 1987).

These reports not only indicate that infants remember painful events but also show that continual exposure to pain affects development, especially in response to human contact.

Consequences of Untreated Pain in Infants

Despite current research on the neonate's experience of pain, infant pain remains inadequately managed. The

TABLE 41-2   CRIES Neonatal Postoperative Pain Scale

	0	1	2
Crying	No	High pitched	Inconsolable
Requires O$_2$ for Sat >95%	No	<30%	>30%
Increased vital signs	Heart rate and blood pressure equal or less than preoperative state	Heart rate and blood pressure <20% of preoperative state	Heart rate and blood pressure >20% of preoperative state
Expression	None	Grimace	Grimace/grunt
Sleepless	No	Wakes at frequent intervals	Constantly awake

CODING TIPS FOR USING CRIES

Crying	The characteristic cry of pain is *high pitched*.
	If no cry or cry that is not high pitched, score 0
	If cry high pitched but infant is easily consoled, score 1
	If cry is high pitched and infant is inconsolable, score 2
Requires O$_2$ for saturation >95%	Look for *changes* in oxygenation. Infants experiencing pain manifest decreases in oxygenation as measured by tCO$_2$ or oxygen saturation. (Consider other causes of changes in oxygenation, such as atelectasis, pneumothorax, oversedation.)
	If no oxygen is required, score 0.
	If <30% O$_2$ is required, score 1.
	If >30% O$_2$ is required, score 2.
Increased vital signs	Note: measure blood pressure last because this may wake child, causing difficulty with other assessments. Use baseline preoperative parameters from a nonstressed period.
	Multiply baseline HR × 0.2, then add this to baseline HR to determine the HR that is 20% over baseline. Do likewise for BP. Use mean BP.
	If HR and BP are both unchanged or less than baseline, score 0.
	If HR or BP is increased but increase is <20% of baseline, score 1.
	If either one is increased >20% over baseline, score 2.
Expression	The facial expression most often associated with pain is a grimace.
	This may be characterized by brow lowering, eyes squeezed shut, deepening of the nasolabial furrow, open lips and mouth.
	If no grimace is present, score 0.
	If grimace alone is present, score 1.
	If grimace and noncry vocalization grunt is present, score 2.
Sleepless	This parameter is scored based on the infant's state during the hour preceding this recorded score.
	If the child has been continuously asleep, score 0.
	If he/she has awakened at frequent intervals, score 1.
	If he/she has been awake constantly, score 2.

BP, Blood pressure; *HR,* heart rate.
Neonatal pain assessment tool developed at the University of Missouri-Columbia.
From Krechel, S., & Bildner, J., (1995) CRIES: A new neonatal postoperative pain measurement score: Initial testing of validity and reliability, *Pediatr Anaesth* 5, 53-61.

mismanagement of infant pain is partially due to misconceptions regarding the effects of pain on the neonate, as well as a lack of knowledge of immediate and long-term consequences of untreated pain. Infants respond to noxious stimuli through physiologic indicators (increased heart rate and blood pressure, variability in heart rate and intracranial pressure, and decreases in arterial oxygen saturations and skin blood flow) and behavioral indicators (muscle rigidity, facial expression, crying, withdrawal, and sleeplessness) (Anand, Grunau, & Oberlander, 1997;

Bildner & Krechel, 1996). The physiologic and behavioral indicators, as well as a variety of neurophysiologic responses to noxious stimulation, are responsible for acute and long-term consequences of pain.

Pain Management

Nonpharmacologic measures to alleviate pain include repositioning, swaddling, containment, cuddling, rocking, music, reducing environmental stimulation, tactile comfort measures, and nonnutritive sucking (Campos, 1989;

Franck, 1987a; Franck, 1987b; Shapiro, 1989). However, nonpharmacologic measures may not be sufficient to decrease physiologic distress, even if behavioral responses such as crying are lessened (Gunnar, Fisch, & Malone, 1984; Marchette et al., 1991). In premature infants, additional stimulation such as stroking may *increase* physiologic distress (Brown, 1987).

Morphine is the most widely used opioid analgesic for pharmacologic management of neonatal pain, with fentanyl as an effective alternative. Continuous or bolus epidural or IV infusion of opioids provides effective and safe pain control (Farrington et al., 1993; Haberkern et al., 1996). Other methods of relieving pain are epidural/intrathecal infusion, local and regional nerve blocks, and topical anesthetics (Choonara, 1992; Ochsenreither, 1997; Taddio et al., 1998; Yaster et al., 1994).

Parents are universally concerned that their infants are suffering pain during procedures. Nurses need to address these concerns and encourage the parents to speak with the health care professionals involved. Parents have the right to withhold consent for invasive procedures and are entitled to honest answers from those responsible for the infant's care. When appropriate, they can also help provide comfort measures for the infant. It is important that parents are aware that nurses are sensitive to the infant's pain and are reassured that the infant will not suffer unduly (Butler, 1988; Shapiro, 1989).

POSTMATURE INFANTS

A pregnancy that is prolonged beyond 42 weeks is a postterm pregnancy, and the infant who is born is called postmature. Postmaturity can be associated with placental insufficiency, resulting in a fetus who has a wasted appearance (dysmaturity) at birth due to loss of subcutaneous fat and muscle mass. There may be meconium staining of the fingernails, and the hair and nails may be long. The skin may peel off. Not all postmature infants will show signs of dysmaturity; some will continue to grow in utero and be large at birth.

The perinatal mortality rate is significantly higher in the postmature fetus and neonate. One reason for this is that during labor and birth the increased oxygen demands of the postmature fetus may not be met. Insufficient gas exchange in the postmature placenta also increases the likelihood of intrauterine hypoxia, which may result in the passage of meconium in utero, thereby increasing the risk for meconium aspiration syndrome. Of all the deaths that occur in postmature newborns, one half occur during labor and birth, about one third occur before the onset of labor, and one sixth occur during the postpartum period.

Meconium Aspiration Syndrome

Meconium staining of the amniotic fluid can be indicative of nonreassuring fetal status, especially in a vertex presentation. It appears in from 8% to 20% of all births. Many infants with meconium staining exhibit no signs of depression at birth; however, the presence of meconium in the amniotic fluid necessitates careful supervision of labor and close monitoring of fetal well-being. The presence of a team skilled at neonatal resuscitation is required at the birth of any infant with meconium-stained amniotic fluid. The mouth and nares of the infant should be suctioned on the perineum before the infant's first breath.

LEGAL TIP Standard of Care—Meconium Aspiration

When there are particles of meconium in the amniotic fluid, the standard of care is that the infant should be suctioned below the vocal cords immediately after birth. The nurse's responsibility is to notify the appropriate personnel to be at the birth and have suctioning equipment available.

If meconium is not removed from the airway at birth, it can migrate down to the terminal airways, causing mechanical obstruction leading to **meconium aspiration syndrome (MAS)**. It is also possible that the fetus aspirated meconium in utero. Such meconium aspiration can cause a chemical pneumonitis. These infants may develop persistent pulmonary hypertension of the newborn (PPHN), further complicating their management.

Persistent Pulmonary Hypertension of the Newborn

The term *persistent pulmonary hypertension of the newborn (PPHN)* is applied to the combined findings of pulmonary hypertension, right-to-left shunting, and a structurally normal heart. PPHN may present either as a single entity or as the main component of MAS, congenital diaphragmatic hernia, RDS, hyperviscosity syndrome, or neonatal pneumonia or sepsis. PPHN is also called *persistent fetal circulation* (PFC) because the syndrome includes a reversion to fetal pathways for blood flow.

A brief review of the characteristics of fetal blood flow can help in the visualization of the problems with PPHN (see Fig. 14-9). In utero, oxygen-rich blood leaves the placenta via the umbilical vein, goes through the ductus venosus, and enters the inferior vena cava. From there it empties into the right atrium and is mostly shunted across the foramen ovale to the left atrium, effectively bypassing the lungs. This blood enters the left ventricle, leaves via the aorta, and preferentially perfuses the carotid and coronary arteries. Thus the heart and brain receive the most oxygenated blood. Blood drains from the brain into the superior vena cava, reenters the right atrium, proceeds to the right ventricle, and exits via the main pulmonary artery. The lungs are a high-pressure circuit, needing only enough perfusion for growth and nutrition. The ductus arteriosus (connecting the main pulmonary artery and the aorta) is the path of least resistance for the blood leaving the right side of the fetal heart, shunting most of the cardiac output away from the lungs and toward the systemic system. This *right-to-left shunting* is the key to fetal circulation.

After birth, both the foramen ovale and the ductus arteriosus close in response to various biochemical processes, pressure changes within the heart, and dilation of the pulmonary vessels. This dilation allows virtually all of the cardiac output to enter the lungs, become oxygenated, and provide oxygen-rich blood to the tissues for normal metabolism. Any process that interferes with this transition from fetal to neonatal circulation may precipitate PPHN. PPHN characteristically proceeds into a downward spiral of exacerbating hypoxia and pulmonary vasoconstriction. Prompt recognition and aggressive intervention are required to reverse this process.

The infant with PPHN is typically born at term or postterm and presents with tachycardia and cyanosis. Management depends on the underlying cause of the persistent pulmonary hypertension. The use of ECMO has improved the chances of survival in these infants (see earlier discussion).

Another mode of treatment for PPHN and other respiratory disorders of the newborn is high-frequency ventilation, a group of assisted-ventilation methods that deliver small volumes of gas at high frequencies and limit the development of high airway pressure, thus reducing barotrauma (Fanaroff & Martin, 1997).

CARE MANAGEMENT

To ensure the safe birth of the fetus, it becomes important to determine whether the pregnancy is actually prolonged and also whether there is any evidence of fetal jeopardy as a result.

Most postmature infants are oversized but otherwise normal, with advanced development and bone age. A postmature infant will have some, but not necessarily all, of the following physical characteristics:

- Generally a normal skull, but the reduced dimensions of the rest of the body make the skull look inordinantly large
- Dry, cracked (desquamating), parchmentlike skin at birth
- Hard nails extending beyond the fingertips
- Profuse scalp hair
- Depleted subcutaneous fat layers, leaving the skin loose and giving the infant an "old person" appearance
- Long and thin body
- Absent vernix
- Often meconium staining (golden yellow to green) of skin, nails, and cord, indicative of a hypoxic episode in utero
- May have an alert, wide-eyed appearance symptomatic of chronic intrauterine hypoxia

Possible nursing diagnoses for the postmature infant include the following:

⁞ Nursing Diagnoses _____

- Impaired airway clearance related to
  - meconium aspiration syndrome
- Ineffective thermoregulation related to
  - immature thermoregulation center
- Risk for injury related to
  - birth trauma
- Risk for injury secondary to hypoglycemia related to
  - depleted glycogen stores

Immediate outcomes of care are that the postmature newborn will do the following:

- Initiate and maintain respirations.
- Experience no CNS trauma or infection.
- Have any birth trauma identified and treated promptly without sequelae.

The long-term expected outcome is that the infant will not experience adverse effects of postmaturity.

The immediate care rendered to postmature infants is similar to that given to preterm infants. Potential complications experienced by postmature infants include polycythemia, hypothermia, hypoglycemia, and meconium aspiration. See other sections for the management and care of these complications.

The nurse can be assured that care was effective when the short-term outcomes for care have been achieved. Long-term follow-up will be needed to evaluate whether there are any adverse effects as a result of postmaturity.

OTHER PROBLEMS RELATED TO GESTATION

Small for Gestational Age and Intrauterine Growth Restriction

Infants who are small for gestational age (e.g., weight falls below the 10th percentile expected at term) and infants who have IUGR (rate of growth does not meet expected growth pattern) are considered high risk, with the perinatal mortality rate 5 to 20 times greater than that for the normal term infant (Kliegman, 1997).

Common problems that affect small-for-gestational age (SGA) IUGR infants are perinatal asphyxia, meconium aspiration, hypoglycemia, and heat loss.

Perinatal Asphyxia

Commonly, IUGR infants have been exposed to chronic hypoxia for varying periods before labor and birth. Labor is a stressor to the normal fetus, but it is an even greater stressor for the growth-restricted fetus. The chronically hypoxic infant is severely compromised even by a normal labor and has difficulty compensating after birth. The alert, wide-eyed appearance of such newborns is attributed to the prolonged fetal hypoxia. Appropriate management and resuscitation are essential for these depressed infants.

The birth of SGA babies with perinatal asphyxia may be associated with a maternal history of heavy cigarette smoking; preeclampsia; low socioeconomic status; multifetal gestation; gestational infections such as rubella, cytomegalovirus, and toxoplasmosis; advanced diabetes mellitus; and cardiac problems. The nursing staff must be alert to and prepared for possible perinatal asphyxia during the birth of an infant in a woman with such a history. Sequelae to perinatal asphyxia include MAS and hypoglycemia.

Hypoglycemia

All stressed infants are at risk for the development of hypoglycemia. Such stress may include perinatal asphyxia and IUGR. The definition of **hypoglycemia** differs for the term and the preterm infant. Hypoglycemia occurring within the first 3 days of life in the term infant is defined as a blood glucose level of less than 40 mg/dl; that occurring in the preterm infant within the same time frame is defined as a blood glucose level of less than 25 mg/dl. Symptoms of hypoglycemia include poor feeding, hypothermia, and diaphoresis. CNS symptoms can include tremors and jitteriness, weak cry, lethargy, floppy posture, convulsions, or coma. Diagnosis is confirmed by blood glucose determinations performed by the laboratory when suspected or by unit visual methods using reagent strips such as Chemstrip-BG or Dextrostix (McGowan, Hagedorn, & Hay, 1998).

Heat Loss

For numerous reasons, SGA infants are particularly susceptible to temperature instability, and close attention must be paid to them to maintain thermoneutrality. These reasons include the fact that they have less muscle mass, less brown fat, less heat-preserving subcutaneous fat, and little ability to control skin capillaries. Nursing considerations in these infants focus on the maintenance of thermoneutrality to promote recovery from perinatal asphyxia, because cold stress jeopardizes such recovery (Blake & Murray, 1998).

⦂ CARE MANAGEMENT

Several physical findings are characteristic of the SGA neonate:
- Generally a normal skull, but the reduced dimensions of the rest of the body make the skull look inordinantly large
- Reduced subcutaneous fat stores
- Loose and dry skin
- Diminished muscle mass, especially over buttocks and cheeks
- Sunken abdomen (scaphoid) as opposed to the well-rounded abdomen seen in normal infants
- Thin, yellowish, dry, and dull umbilical cord (normal cord is gray, glistening, round, and moist)
- Sparse scalp hair
- Wide skull sutures (inadequate bone growth)

The nursing care given to the SGA infant is determined by the nature of the clinical problems and is the same as that given to the preterm infant with the same problems. Gas exchange is supported by maintaining a clear airway and preventing cold stress. Hypoglycemia is treated with oral feedings (e.g., breast milk, formula, dextrose solution) per the hospital protocol. Parenteral infusions may be necessary. An external heat source is used until the infant's temperature is stabilized (radiant warmer or isolette). The nursing support given to parents is also similar to that given to parents of preterm infants.

Large for Gestational Age

The large-for-gestational age (LGA), or oversized, infant traditionally has been regarded as one weighing 4000 g or more at birth. An infant is considered LGA despite gestation when the weight falls above the 90th percentile on growth charts or two standard deviations above the mean weight for gestational age. Certain fetal disorders can also result in LGA infants. These include transposition of the great vessels and Beckwith-Wiedemann syndrome (Korones, 1995).

Birth trauma, especially in infants with a breech or shoulder presentation, is a serious hazard for the oversized neonate. Asphyxia or CNS injury, or both, may occur. All pregnancies of more than 42 weeks of gestation need to be carefully evaluated. All large fetuses are monitored during a trial of labor, and preparation is made for cesarean birth if a nonreassuring fetal status or poor progress of labor occurs. LGA newborns may be preterm, term, or postterm; they may be the infants of diabetic (or prediabetic) mothers; and they may be postmature. Each of these problems carries special concerns. Regardless of any coexisting potential problems, the oversized infant is at risk just by virtue of its size.

⦂ CARE MANAGEMENT

The nurse assesses the LGA infant for gestational age, hypoglycemia, and trauma resulting from vaginal or cesarean birth. The blood glucose levels of LGA infants are monitored, and any hypoglycemia is corrected. Any specific birth injuries are identified and treated appropriately. Care depends on the LGA infant's condition.

DISCHARGE PLANNING

Discharge planning for the high risk infant begins at the time of admission. Throughout the infant's hospitalization, the discharge planning coordinator gathers information from all of the health care team members. This information is used to determine the infant's and family's readiness for discharge (Green, 1994). Nurses are very influential members of the planning team because as the direct caregivers throughout the infant's hospitalization they have a firsthand knowledge of the infant and the family.

As the home care needs of the infant's parents are assessed, steps are taken to eliminate any knowledge deficits.

Information is provided about infant care, especially as it pertains to the particular infant's home needs (e.g., the administration of oxygen, gastrostomy feedings). Parent education includes having them give return demonstrations of their infant care skills to show whether they are becoming increasingly independent in the provision of this care. Parents should also obtain an age-appropriate car seat before the discharge of their infant. Instruction in infant CPR should be offered to all parents before discharge.

As the home care of medically fragile clients is expanded to the pediatric population, early teaching and planning become a necessity. Goldberg, Gardner, and Gibson (1994) cite an example of a health care maintenance organization that saved more than a million dollars in hospital charges by having a ventilator-dependent client live at home. More facilities are investigating such home care options as one way to provide long-term care for the compromised infant.

Referrals for appropriate resources also need to be made. Social service involvement is especially important for young or psychosocially high risk parents (e.g., substance abusers or those with a mental illness). Social services can also provide parents with information about financial assistance (Aid to Families with Dependent Children, Medicaid, Crippled Children's Program, Social Security Disability). As our understanding of genetics increases, appropriate counseling, referral, and follow-up will become more important (Scanlon & Fibison, 1995).

Infants with developmental disabilities, or those infants who may be at risk for further problems (premature infants), are referred to appropriate community programs. Many community resources that give assistance with special educational and medical needs have been mandated by Federal Public Law #102-119 (Jenkins, Covington, & Plotnick, 1994). Such services range from family counseling to physical therapy. Some hospitals also offer infant stimulation and development programs for the parents of at-risk infants. Nursing is recognized by this law as one of the 10 qualified disciplines that can provide these services.

Referrals are made for home health assistance, as appropriate (some medical plans cover these services). These health care providers can perform actual nursing functions, as well as provide some relief from the emotional burden of caring for an infant with medical problems. Special attention should be given to parents' feelings of uncertainty, anxiety, and overwhelming frustration. Parents often experience these emotions during the planning for an infant's home care, especially if the infant has had a severe or prolonged illness (Catlett, Miles, & Holditch-Davis, 1994).

TRANSPORT TO A REGIONAL CENTER

If a hospital is not equipped to care for a high risk mother and fetus or a high risk infant, transfer to a specialized perinatal or tertiary care center is arranged. Maternal trans-

port ideally occurs with the fetus in utero because this has two distinct advantages:

1. The associated neonatal morbidity and mortality are decreased.
2. Infant-parent attachment is supported, thereby avoiding separation of the parents and infant.

For a variety of reasons, however, it is not always possible to transport the mother before the birth. These reasons include imminent birth and unanticipated problems. Therefore, physicians and nurses in level 1 and 2 facilities must have the skills and equipment necessary for making an accurate diagnosis and implementing emergency interventions to stabilize the infant's condition until transport can occur (Box 41-10) (Pettett, Sewell, & Merenstein, 1998). The goal of these interventions is to maintain the infant's condition within the normal physiologic range. Specific attention is given to the following areas:

- Vital signs
- Oxygen and ventilation
- Thermoregulation
- Acid-base balance
- Fluid and electrolyte levels
- Glucose level
- Developmental interventions

The transport team may consist of physicians, nurse-practitioners, nurses, and respiratory therapists. Commonly a nurse trained in neonatal intensive care and a respiratory therapist constitute the team. The team must have expertise in resuscitation, stabilization, and provision of critical care during the transport. In a neonatal transport, the team should provide information for the parents about the tertiary center (Box 41-11). Transport teams can integrate an individual developmental plan of care into their caregiving efforts, thereby initiating multidisciplinary interventions early in the infant's life (Little, Riddle, & Soule, 1994).

The birth of any high risk infant can cause profound parental stress. Such parents can grieve the loss of the ideal infant. They are fearful of the possible eventual outcomes for the infant. They must also deal with the technologic world surrounding their infant, and amid all the equipment, it is sometimes difficult for them to perceive the infant and respond to its needs. Parents of high risk infants who have been transported to regional centers therefore need special support. As one way to deal with this problem, many intensive care units provide the family with a handbook or pictures of the tertiary care unit to help them understand what is going on around them (Prukop, 1994).

TRANSPORT FROM A REGIONAL CENTER

Infants may need to be transferred back to the referring facility. Often premature infants who require thermoregulation and gavage feedings can be cared for in community hospitals closer to the parents' home. This allows parents to visit their infant more easily and to work with their per-

BOX 41-10 Neonatal Resuscitation Supplies and Equipment

SUCTION EQUIPMENT

Bulb syringe
Mechanical suction
5 (or 6), 8, 10 French suction catheters
8 French feeding tube and 20 ml syringe
Meconium aspirator

BAG-AND-MASK EQUIPMENT

Infant resuscitation bag with a pressure-release valve or pressure gauge; the bag must be capable of delivering 90% to 100% oxygen
Face masks—newborn and premature sizes (cushioned-rim masks preferred)
Oral airways—newborn and premature sizes
Oxygen source with intact flowmeter and tubing

INTUBATION EQUIPMENT

No. 0 (premature) and No. 1 (term newborn) laryngoscope with straight blades
Extra bulbs and batteries for laryngoscope
2.5, 3.0, 3.5, and 4.0 mm endotracheal tubes
Stylet
Scissors
Gloves

MEDICATIONS

1:10,000 epinephrine; 3 or 10 ml ampules
0.4 mg/ml naloxone hydrochloride in 1 ml ampules or 1.0 mg/ml in 2 ml ampules

Volume expander—one or more
Normal saline
Ringer's lactate
Albumin (5%)/saline solution
Sodium bicarbonate 4.2% (5 mEq/10 ml) in 10 ml ampules
250 ml of 10% dextrose
30 ml of sterile water
30 ml of normal saline

OTHER EQUIPMENT AND SUPPLIES

Radiant warmer
Stethoscope
$\frac{1}{2}$ or $\frac{3}{4}$ in wide adhesive tape
1, 3, 5, 10, 20, and 50 ml syringes
25, 21, and 18 gauge needles
Alcohol sponges
Umbilical artery catheterization tray
Umbilical tape
3 $\frac{1}{2}$, 5 French umbilical catheters
Three-way stopcocks
5 French feeding tube
Cardiotachometer with ECG oscilloscope (desirable)

Used with permission of the American Academy of Pediatrics. (1994). *Textbook of neonatal resuscitation.* Elk Grove Village, IL: American Academy of Pediatrics.

BOX 41-11 Information for Parents About the Tertiary Center

- Exact location of the unit—address, map
- Visiting hours and hospital rules
- Telephone numbers
- Names of individuals likely to be involved with the baby's care
- Information of the special care unit—what it is, what it does

- Location of parking facilities, nearby lodging, and rules regarding young children (siblings)
- Any particular rules or regulations regarding the special care unit

From Pettitt, G., Sewell, S., & Merenstein, G. (1998). Regionalization and transport in perinatal care. In G. Merenstein & S. Gardner (Eds.). *Handbook of neonatal intensive care* (4th ed.). St. Louis: Mosby.

sonal health care provider on the long-range expected outcomes for the infant. Specialized incubators make these trips possible (Fig. 41-17). However, parents may express mixed feelings about such return transports and may be reluctant to adapt to a different facility and group of caregivers. To minimize some of these concerns it is important to give the parents very clear information about return transports during the initial discharge planning.

Although at the time of discharge parents may not recognize the need for information on the various resources available to help them in the care of their infant, they can be given such lists of agencies and telephone numbers for

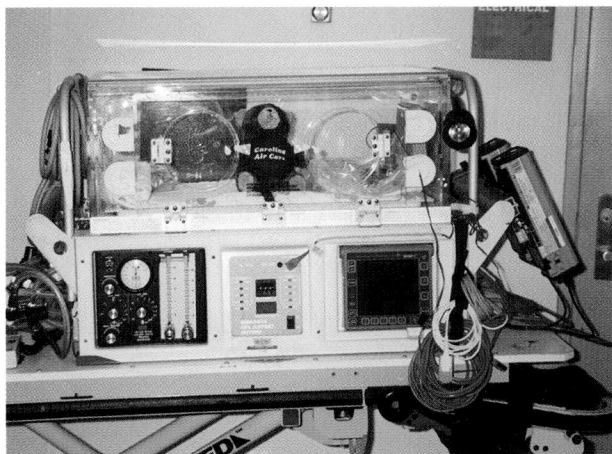

Fig. 41-17 Total life support system for transport of high risk newborns. *(Courtesy UNC Hospitals, Carolina Air Care, Chapel Hill, NC.)*

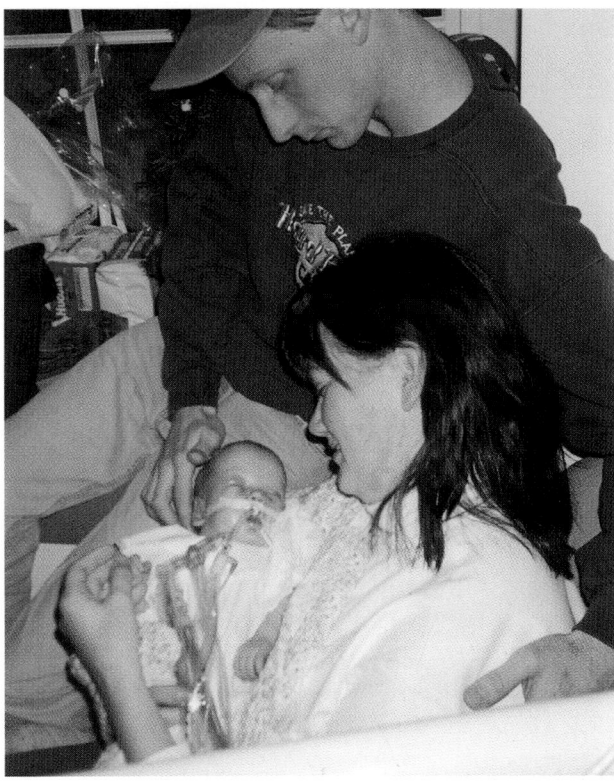

Fig. 41-18 Parents comfort their dying infant. *(Courtesy family of Laura Turner, Cary, NC.)*

later use. Providing them with a client-specific directory covering special programs, social support, community, and funding resources can help them make the transition to the home care of their infants. As the nurse continually reinforces the idea that the infant will go home, this will prompt the parents to plan for the days ahead and therefore be ready to take their infant home when the time comes.

Anticipatory Grief

Families experience anticipatory grief when they are told of the impending death of their infant (Gardner, Merenstein, & Castello, 1998). Anticipatory grief prepares and protects parents who are facing a loss. Parents who have an infant with a debilitating disease (with or without a congenital deformity), but one that may not necessarily threaten the life of the child, may also experience anticipatory grief. An alteration in relationships, a change in lifestyle, and a very real threat to their hopes and dreams for the future may affect the day-to-day interaction of the family with their infant and the staff. Nurses can help facilitate the family's grieving process. If the nurse observes that a family member's day-to-day interactions with the infant change, the nurse should assess the situation and request psychosocial support or intervention by a chaplain or social worker, if necessary.

Loss of an Infant

Parents who know their infant is going to die experience a very difficult time. Before the infant's death, the parents need to direct their attention, energy, and caregiving activities toward the dying infant (Fig. 41-18). However, some parents find it difficult to visit their infant even for short periods once a terminal diagnosis has been made. Grandparents also grieve but often are unsure how to comfort their own child (the infant's parent) during the period

of impending death. Health care professionals can help by involving the family in the infant's care, providing privacy, answering questions, and preparing them for the inevitability of the death (see Chapter 42).

The nursing staff also experiences grief (Gardner, Merenstein, & Costello, 1998). Many primary staff nurses find themselves grieving as if the infant were their own because they often have been the primary caregiver for weeks, or even months. Managers and other staff members must acknowledge this grief. Talking about the infant or attending the funeral may help the affected staff members resolve their feelings about the infant's death.

KEY POINTS

- Preterm infants are at risk for problems stemming from the immaturity of their organ systems.
- Nurses who work with preterm and other high risk infants observe them for respiratory distress and other early symptoms of physiologic disorders.
- The adaptation of parents to preterm or high risk infants differs from that of parents to normal full-term infants.

KEY POINTS—cont'd

- Nurses can facilitate the development of a positive parent-child relationship.

- Nurses' skills in interpreting data, making decisions, and initiating therapy in newborn intensive care units are crucial to ensuring infants' survival.

- Parents need special instruction (e.g., CPR, oxygen therapy, suctioning, developmental care) before they take a high risk infant home.

- SGA infants are considered at risk because of fetal growth restriction.

- The high incidence of nonreassuring fetal status among postmature infants is related to the progressive placental insufficiency that can occur in a postterm pregnancy.

- Specially trained nurses may transport high risk infants to and from special care units.

- Parents need assistance with coping with anticipated grief or loss and grief.

CRITICAL THINKING EXERCISES

1 A multiparous woman has a preterm infant who was born at 28 weeks of gestation and was transported to a special care nursery. The woman does not live in the city where the hospital was located, and she is to be discharged tomorrow. It is anticipated that the infant will require a stay in the hospital for at least 8 more weeks and will likely require oxygen therapy at home after discharge. What information should the transport team provide the parents? What kinds of assistance will this mother need now and after the infant goes home? Identify resources in the community that may have services she can use.

2 Identify an infant with intrauterine growth restriction (IUGR). Is the growth restriction symmetric or asymmetric? Review the prenatal and postnatal history. Identify reasons why an infant is growth restricted. Identify problems that might occur with this infant.

3 During a scheduled clinical experience in the NICU or a special care nursery, observe a transport team leaving to pick up an infant from a referring hospital or bringing in an infant to the special care nursery.
  a. Who are the transport team members?
  b. What equipment are they using?
  c. How was the referral made?
  d. What communication links are there between the special care nursery and the Level 1 and Level 2 hospitals in the surrounding area?

References

Adcock, E., Consolvo, C., & Berry, D. (1998). Fluid and electrolyte management. In G. Merenstein & S. Gardner (Eds.). *Handbook of neonatal intensive care* (3rd ed.). St. Louis: Mosby.

Als, H. (1998). Developmental care in the newborn intensive care unit. *Curr Opin Pediatr* 10(2), 138-142.

American Academy of Pediatrics Committee on Fetus and Newborn. (1999). Surfactant replacement therapy for respiratory distress syndrome. *Pediatrics* 103(3), 684-685.

American Heart Association/American Academy of Pediatrics. (1994). *Textbook of neonatal resuscitation.* Dallas: American Heart Association.

Anand, K., Grunau, R., & Oberlander, T. (1997). Developmental character and long-term consequences of pain in infants and children. *Child Adolesc Psychiatric Clin North Am* 6(4), 703-724.

Avery, G., Fletcher, M., & MacDonald, M. (1994). *Neonatology: Pathophysiology and management of the newborn* (4th ed.). Philadelphia: Lippincott.

Bancalari, E. (1997). The respiratory system: Neonatal chronic lung disease. In A. Fanaroff & R. Martin (Eds.). *Neonatal-perinatal medicine: Diseases of the fetus and infant.* St. Louis: Mosby.

Bildner, J., & Krechel, S. (1996). Increasing staff nurse awareness of postoperative pain management in the NICU. *Neonatal Netw* 15, 11-16.

Blackburn, S. (1998). Environmental impact of the NICU on developmental outcomes. *J Pediatr Nurs* 13(5), 279-289.

Blake, W., & Murray, J. (1998). Heat balance. In G. Merenstein & S. Gardner (Eds.). *Handbook of neonatal intensive care* (3rd ed.). St. Louis: Mosby.

Brooten, D. (1995). Perinatal care across the continuum: Early discharge and nursing home follow-up. *J Perinat Neonatal Nurs* 9(1), 38-44.

Brown, L. (1987). Physiologic responses to cutaneous pain in neonates. *Neonatal Netw* 6(3), 18-22.

Butler, N. (1988). How to raise professional awareness of the need for adequate pain relief for infants. *Birth* 15(1), 38-41.

Campos, R. (1989). Soothing pain-elicited distress in infants with swaddling and pacifiers. *Child Dev* 60, 781-792.

Catlett, A., Miles, M., & Holditch-Davis, D. (1994). Maternal perceptions of illness severity in premature infants. *Neonatal Netw* 13(2), 45-49.

Cloherty, J., & Stark, A. (1997). *Manual of neonatal care* (4th ed.). Boston: Little, Brown.

Choonara, I. (1992). Management of pain in newborn infants. *Semin Perinatol* 16(1), 32-40.

Cools, F., & Offringa, M. (1999). Meta-analysis of elective high frequency ventilation in preterm infants with respiratory distress syndrome. *Arch Dis Chld Fetal Neonatal Ed* 80(1), F15-20.

Daberkow-Carson, E. & Washington, R. (1998). Cardiovascular diseases and surgical interventions. In G. Merenstein & S. Gardner (Eds.). *Handbook of neonatal intensive care* (4th ed.). St. Louis: Mosby.

Denne, S. et al. (1998). Nutrition and metabolism in the high-risk neonate. In A. Fanaroff & R. Martin (Eds.). *Neonatal-perinatal medicine: Diseases of the fetus and infant.* St. Louis: Mosby.

Dickason, E., Silverman, B., & Kaplan, J. (1998). *Maternal-infant nursing care* (3rd ed.). St. Louis: Mosby.

Donovan, E., Schwartz, J., & Moles, L. (1998). New technologies applied to the management of respiratory dysfunction. In C. Kenner, J. Lott, & A. Flandermeyer (Eds.). *Comprehensive neonatal nursing. A physiologic perspective* (2nd ed.). Philadelphia: W.B. Saunders.

Fanaroff, A., & Martin, R. (1997). *Neonatal-perinatal medicine: Diseases of the fetus and infant* (6th ed.). St. Louis: Mosby.

Farrington, E. et al. (1993). Continuous intravenous morphine infusion in postoperative newborn infants. *Am J Perinatol* 10(1), 84-87.

Franck, L. (1987a). Comfort measures and analgesia. *Neonatal Netw* 16(4), 65.

Franck, L. (1987b). A national survey of the assessment and treatment of pain and agitation in the neonatal intensive care unit. *J Obstet Gynecol Neonatal Nurs* 16, 387-393.

Gale, G., Franck, L., & Lund, C. (1993). Skin to skin (kangaroo) holding of the intubated premature infant. *Neonatal Netw* 12(6), 49-57.

Gale, G., & VandenBerg, K. (1998). Kangaroo care. *Neonatal Netw* 17(5), 69-71.

Gamblian, V., Hess, D., & Kenner, C. (1998). Early discharge from the NICU. *J Pediatr Nurs* 13(5), 296-301.

Gardner, S., & Lubchenco, L. (1998). The neonate and the environment: Impact on development. In G. Merenstein & S. Gardner (Eds.). *Handbook of neonatal intensive care* (4th ed.). St. Louis: Mosby.

Gardner, S., Merenstein, G., & Costello, A. (1998). Grief and perinatal loss. In G. Merenstein & S. Gardner (Eds.). *Handbook of neonatal intensive care* (4th ed.). St. Louis: Mosby.

Garland, J. et al. (1999). A three-day course of dexamethasone therapy to prevent chronic lung disease in ventilated neonates: A randomized trial. *Pediatrics* 104 (1 pt 1), 91-99.

Goldberg, A., Gardner, G., & Gibson, L. (1994). Home care: The next frontier of pediatric practice. *J Pediatr* 125 (5 pt 1), 686-690.

Gomella, T., Cunningham, M., & Eyal, F. (1994). *Neonatology: Management, procedure, on-call problems, diseases and drugs* (3rd ed.). Norfolk, CT: Appleton & Lange.

Gray, K. et al. (1998). Developmentally supportive care in a neonatal intensive care unit: A research utilization project. *Neonatal Netw* 17(2), 33-38.

Green, M. (Ed.). (1994). *Bright futures, guidelines for health supervision of infants, children, and adolescents.* Arlington, VA: National Center for Education in Maternal and Child Health.

Grunau, R., & Craig, K. (1987). Pain expression in neonates: Facial action and cry. *Pain* 28, 395-410.

Grunau, R., Johnston, C., & Craig, K. (1990). Neonatal facial and cry responses to invasive and noninvasive procedures. *Pain* 42(3), 295-305.

Gunnar, M., Fisch, R., & Malone, S. (1984). The effects of a pacifying stimulus on behavioral and adrenocortical responses to circumcision in the newborn. *J Acad Child Psychiatry* 23(1), 34-38.

Haberkern, C. et al. (1996). Epidural and intravenous bolus morphine for postoperative analgesia in infants. *Can J Anaesth* 43(12), 1203-1210.

Hack, M. et al. (1995). Very-low-birth-weight outcomes of the National Institute of Child Health and Human Development Neonatal Network, November 1989 to October 1990. *Am J Obstet Gynecol* 172(2 pt 1), 457-464.

Hadjistavropoulos, H. et al. (1997). Judging pain in infants: Behavioural, contextual, and developmental determinants. *Pain* 73(3), 319-324.

Hagedorn, M., Gardner, S., & Abman, S. (1998). Respiratory diseases. In G. Merenstein & S. Gardner (Eds.). *Handbook of neonatal intensive care* (4th ed.). St. Louis: Mosby.

Haubrich, K. (1998). Assessment and management of auditory dysfunction. In C. Kenner, J. Lott, & A. Flandermeyer (Eds.). *Comprehensive neonatal nursing—A physiologic perspective* (2nd ed.). Philadelphia: W.B. Saunders.

Holland, R., Price, F., & Bensard, D. (1998). Neonatal surgery. In G. Merenstein & S. Gardner (Eds.). *Handbook of neonatal intensive care* (4th ed.). St. Louis: Mosby.

Jenkins, J., Covington, C., & Plotnick, J. (1994). Early childhood interventions: The law. *MCN Am J Matern Child Nurs* 19(3), 135-139, 142.

Kliegman, R. (1997). Intrauterine growth retardation. In A. Fanaroff & R. Martin (Eds.). *Neonatal-perinatal medicine. Diseases of the fetus and infant.* St. Louis: Mosby.

Korones, S. (1995). *High risk infants: The basis for intensive care* (5th ed.). St. Louis: Mosby.

Korones, S., & Bada-Ellzey, H. (1993). *Neonatal decision making.* St. Louis: Mosby.

Krechel, S., & Bildner, J. (1995). CRIES: A new neonatal postoperative pain measurement score: Initial testing of validity and reliability. *Pediatric Anaesthesia* 5, 53-61.

Lefrak, L., & Dowling, D. (1998). Nutrition: Physiologic basis of metabolism and management of enteral and parenteral nutrition. In C. Kenner, J. Lott, & A. Flandermeyer (Eds.). *Comprehensive neonatal nursing—A physiologic perspective* (2nd ed.). Philadelphia: W.B. Saunders.

Little, D., Riddle, B., & Soule, C. (1994). The power in our hands: Integrating developmental care into neonatal transport. *Neonatal Netw* 13(7), 19-22.

Korones, S. (1995). *High risk infants: The basis for intensive care* (5th ed.). St. Louis: Mosby.

Ludington-Hoe, S. et al. (1994). Kangaroo care: Research results, practice implications and guidelines. *Neonatal Netw* 13(1), 19-27.

Lund, C., & Durand, D. (1998). Skin and skin care. In G. Merenstein & S. Gardner (Eds.). *Handbook of neonatal intensive care* (4th ed.). St. Louis: Mosby.

Marchette, L. et al. (1991). Pain reduction interventions during neonatal circumcision. *Nurs Res* 40(4), 241-244.

McGowan, J., Hagedorn, M., & Hay, W. (1998). Glucose homeostasis. In G. Merenstein & S. Gardner (Eds.). *Handbook of neonatal intensive care* (4th ed.). St. Louis: Mosby.

Meis, P. et al. (1998). The preterm prediction study: Risk factors for indicated preterm births. Maternal-Fetal Medicine Units Network of the National Institute of Child Health and Human Development. *Am J Obstet Gynecol* 178(3), 562-567.

Merenstein, G., & Gardner, S. (1998). *Handbook of neonatal intensive care* (4th ed.). St. Louis: Mosby.

Moe, P., & Paige, P. (1998). Neurologic disorders. In G. Merenstein & S. Gardner (Eds.). *Handbook of neonatal intensive care* (4th ed.). St. Louis: Mosby.

Neu, M. (1999). Parents' perception of skin-to-skin care with their preterm infants requiring assisted ventilation. *J Obstet Gynecol Neonatal Nurs* 28(2), 157-164.

Ochsenreither, J. (1997). Epidural analgesia in infants. *Neonatal Netw* 16(6), 79-84.

Penticuff, J. (1987). Neonatal nursing ethics: Toward a consensus. *Neonatal Netw* 5, 7-16.

Petryshen, P. et al. (1997). Comparing nursing costs for preterm infants receiving conventional vs. developmental care. *Nurs Econ* 15(3), 138-145, 150.

Pettitt, G., Sewell, S., & Merenstein, G. (1998). Regionalization and transport in perinatal care. In G. Merenstein & S. Gardner (Eds.). *Handbook of neonatal intensive care* (4th ed.). St. Louis: Mosby.

Pickler, R., & Terrell, B. (1994). Nonnutritive sucking and necrotizing enterocolitis. *Neonatal Netw* 13(8), 15-18.

Plavka, R. et al. (1999). A prospective randomized comparison of conventional mechanical ventilation and very early high frequency oscillatory ventilation in extremely premature newborns with repiratory distress syndrome. *Intensive Care Med* 25(1), 68-75.

Prukop, S. (Ed.). (1994). *Lucile Salter Packard Children's Hospital at Stanford NICU parent handbook.* Palo Alto, CA: Mead Johnson Nutritionals.

Reed, M., & Blumer, J. (1997). Pharmacologic treatment of the fetus. In A. Fanaroff & R. Martin (Eds.). *Neonatal-perinatal medicine. Diseases of the fetus and infant.* St. Louis: Mosby.

Scanlon, C., & Fibison, W. (1995). *Managing genetic information: Implications for nursing practice.* Washington, DC: American Nurses Association.

Shapiro, C. (1989). Pain in the neonate: Assessment and intervention. *Neonatal Netw* 8(1), 7-21.

Shiao, S., Youngblut, J., & Anderson, G. (1995). Nasogastric tube placement: Effects on breathing and sucking in low birth weight infants. *Nurs Res* 44(2), 82-88.

Shields-Poe, D., & Pinelli, J. (1997). Variables associated with parental stress in neonatal intensive units. *Neonatal Netw* 16(1), 29-37.

Silverman, W., & Anderson. (1956). A controlled clinical trial of effects of water mist on obstructive respiratory signs, death rate, and necropsy findings among premature infants. *Pediatrics* 17(1), 1-10.

Standley, J. (1998). The effect of music and multimodal stimulation on responses of premature infants in neonatal intensive care. *Pediatr Nurs* 24(6), 532-538.

Strauch, C., Brandt, S., & Edwards-Beckett, J. (1993). Implementation of a quiet hour: Effect on noise level and infant sleep states. *Neonatal Netw* 12(2), 31-35.

Taddio, A. et al. (1998). A systematic review of lidocaine-prilocaine cream (EMLA) in the treatment of acute pain in neonates. *Pediatrics* 101(2), E1.

Townsend, S., Johnson, C., & Hay, W. (1998). Enteral nutrition. In G. Merenstein & S. Gardner (Eds.) *Handbook of neonatal intensive care* (4th ed.). St. Louis: Mosby.

VandenBerg, K. (1999) What to tell parents about the developmental needs of their baby at discharge. *Neonatal Netw* 18(1), 57-59.

Wereszczak, J., Miles, M., & Holditch-Davis, D. (1997). Maternal recall of the neonatal intensive care unit. *Neonatal Netw* 16(4), 33-40.

Wong, D. (1999). *Whaley and Wong's nursing care of infants and children* (6th ed.). St. Louis: Mosby.

Wong, D., & Perry, S. (1998). *Maternal child nursing care.* St. Louis: Mosby.

Yaster, M. et al. (1994). Local anesthetics in the management of acute pain in children. *J Pediatr* 124(2), 165-176.

Zahka, K., & Patel, C. (1997). The cardiovascular system: Congenital defects. In A. Fanaroff & R. Martin (Eds.). *Neonatal-perinatal medicine. Diseases of the fetus and infant.* St. Louis: Mosby.

Loss and Grief

Margaret Shandor Miles, and Esther Mergerman

LEARNING OBJECTIVES

- Define the key terms.
- Understand the personal and societal issues that may complicate responses to perinatal loss.
- Describe emotional, behavioral, cognitive, and physical responses commonly experienced during the grieving process associated with perinatal loss.
- Formulate appropriate nursing diagnoses for parents experiencing perinatal loss.
- Identify specific nursing interventions to meet the special needs of parents and their families related to perinatal loss and grief.

- Develop expected outcome criteria to evaluate nursing care for grieving families.
- Differentiate among helpful and nonhelpful responses in caring for parents experiencing loss and grief.
- Identify topics for nursing research related to perinatal loss and grief.

KEY TERMS

acute distress	disorganization	perinatal loss
bereavement	grief	reorganization
bittersweet grief	intense grief	search for meaning
complicated bereavement	miscarriage	

ecoming pregnant and giving birth are important developmental milestones that are anticipated by most men and women in our society. Becoming a parent gives one social status, expands one's capacity for caring and loving for another, and adds immense responsibility to one's life. However, loss can be associated with pregnancy and birth. During pregnancy parents plan for the birth, imagine what the birth will be like, and develop an image of the appearance of the baby. The reality of childbirth may not be what the parents have dreamed of or hoped for. In particular, the experience of premature labor and preterm birth or cesarean birth all involve a loss of the expected pregnancy and birth plans. Parents also may grieve over the sex or appearance of their child. For some parents, loss is associated with the birth of an infant who has a birth defect or chronic illness.

Although having children can be a strong desire and goal for women and men, not everyone is successful in achieving parenthood. For some couples infertility may thwart their plans and desires for parenthood and cause intense feelings of grief. When couples undergo infertility treatments, feelings of loss may intensify, especially when treatments fail and/or a pregnancy ends in a miscarriage (Lukse & Vacc, 1999). Women, in particular, experience high distress during this time (Mori et al., 1997).

Many women and their partners, whether infertile or not, experience miscarriage in the early months of pregnancy. Miscarriage affects the personal identity of the woman, and causes guilt, depression, and anxiety (Frost & Condon, 1996). Others may have an ectopic pregnancy or experience a fetal death. Women and their partners who experience a successful pregnancy may suddenly be confronted with stillbirth at time of birth. All of these experiences may be called **perinatal loss.** Others may experience intense grief following infant death (Kavanaugh, 1997). These others include women who give birth prematurely to an infant who survives only a few hours or who dies after days, weeks, or months in an intensive care unit. In addition, a woman may give birth to an infant with severe congenital anomalies or other serious health problems; these infants also may die after a few hours, days, weeks, or months in an intensive care unit.

The statistics on perinatal loss and death of an infant are grim. Approximately 19.7 of each 1000 of all pregnancies are ectopic pregnancies, taking place outside the uterus, usually in a uterine tube (Pisarska & Carson, 1999). Ectopic pregnancies accounted for 9% of maternal deaths in 1992 (Pisarska & Carson, 1999). A **miscarriage**—a pregnancy that ends before 20 weeks of gestation—is reported to account for 15% to 20% of all pregnancies (Zinaman et al., 1996). In addition, each year approximately 5 of every 1000 births end in stillbirth or fetal deaths (those occurring after 20 weeks of gestation). Newborn death, death of a baby born showing signs of life such as respiratory effort, heart rate, pulsating cord at birth and/or muscle irritability, regardless of gestational age, accounts for almost 27,000 deaths per year in the United States (Guyer et al., 1998). In addition, 18,000 infants die in the early postpartum period from prematurity, birth defects, and other acute illnesses (Guyer et al., 1998).

Thus parents can experience grief before or during the childbearing experience. Grief involves the painful feelings and related behavioral and physical responses to a major loss. Grief can be particularly difficult with perinatal losses for a number of reasons. There is the societal belief that there are no barriers to getting pregnant, and there is an expectation that once a woman is pregnant the result will be a healthy live infant. As a result, our society tends to minimize perinatal loss and to lack understanding of the associated pain. Women and men who undergo perinatal losses struggle with these issues themselves and, because of these societal attitudes, they may not receive the support they need. In addition, many perinatal losses are hidden or private, in that others may not know about the infertility or the early pregnancy that ended in miscarriage. Too, perinatal losses may be intensified for couples who delay pregnancy until the woman's career and the family's financial status is at the right point to take on the responsibilities of a child. Feelings of helplessness and loss of control can be very difficult when the couple experiences infertility or miscarriage. In many instances of perinatal loss, the lack of an identified cause for the loss can complicate grief. This is particularly difficult for women, who often feel personally responsible for infertility, miscarriage, and infant death. In addition, some couples endure repeated losses, which can be devastating. All of these issues can reduce the support to bereaved women and men who experience perinatal losses.

Nurses have an important role in helping parents who experience perinatal loss. Nurses encounter these parents in a variety of settings, including the antepartum, labor and delivery, postpartum, and gynecologic units of hospitals, and obstetric, gynecologic, and infertility outpatient clinics and offices. In these settings, nurses have opportunities to provide sensitive and caring interventions to parents. Indeed, parents have reported that their nurses were an important resource in helping them cope with their grief. Nurses in many inpatient settings have developed protocols that provide clear direction to all staff in how to help parents through this difficult process. In addition, many institutions now have follow-up programs involving telephone calls, home visits, and support groups that are effective in helping parents after discharge.

The focus of this chapter is to prepare the beginning nurse to provide sensitive, supportive, and therapeutic interventions to parents experiencing perinatal loss in a variety of settings. An overview of the grief process is presented as a guide for assessing and understanding the responses of bereaved women, men, and their families. Guidelines for intervention are given, and specific intervention approaches are discussed.

GRIEF RESPONSES

Grief or **bereavement** has been described as a cluster of painful responses experienced by individuals coping with the death of someone with whom they had a close relationship, generally a relative or close friend (Lindemann, 1944; Osterweis, Solomon, & Green, 1984; Parkes, 1972, 1983). Many authors believe there are overlapping phases in the grief process, but most do not believe that grief is experienced in "stages." There is an early period of acute distress and shock followed by a period of intense grief. Commonly, the manifestations of grief during the phase of intense grief include emotional, cognitive, behavioral, and physical responses. The phase of reorganization is reached when the individuals return to their usual level of functioning in society and have more good than bad days. However, this does not mean that the pain associated with the death is gone. The duration of grief varies with the individual, but there is general agreement that grief is a long-term process that can extend for months and years. With a very close relationship such as with one's baby, some aspects of grief never truly end. Another way of

BOX 42-1 Conceptual Model of Parental Grief

PHASE OF ACUTE DISTRESS

Shock
Numbness
Intense crying
Depression

PHASE OF INTENSE GRIEF

Loneliness, emptiness, and yearning
Guilt
Anger, resentment, bitterness, irritability
Fear and anxiety (especially about getting pregnant
  again)
Disorganization
Difficulties with cognitive processing
Sadness and depression
Physical symptoms

REORGANIZATION

Search for meaning
Reduction of distress
Reentering normal life activities with more enthusiasm
Can make future plans, including decision about
  another pregnancy

Adapted from Miles, M. (1980). *The grief of parents...when a child dies.* Oak Brook, IL: Compassionate Friends, Inc.; Miles, M. (1984). Helping adults mourn the death of a child. In H. Wass, & C. Corr (Eds.). *Childhood and death.* New York: Hemisphere.

conceptualizing the grief process is through the achievement of certain tasks of mourning. Worden (1991) identified four tasks: (1) Accepting the loss, (2) working through the pain, (3) adjusting to the environment, and (4) moving on. He proposes that these four "tasks of mourning" must be completed in order to resolve grief.

Miles (1984) and Miles and Demi (1986, 1997) proposed a conceptual model of parental grief, based on the work of Lindemann (1944), Parkes (1972, 1983), and Worden (1991). In addition, the model proposes that the grief responses of parents are closely linked to their self-image as a mother or father. Parental grief responses occur in three overlapping phases of grief—acute distress, intense grief, and reorganization (Box 42-1).

Acute Distress

The loss of a pregnancy or death of an infant is an acute and distressing experience for mothers and fathers who planned for and expected a normal healthy infant as the outcome. The loss encompasses a loss of their identity as a mother or father and the loss of their many dreams related to parenthood. The immediate reaction to news of a perinatal loss or infant death encompasses a period of **acute distress.** Parents generally are in a state of shock and

numbness. They may feel a sense of unreality and confusion, as though they were in a bad dream or in a fog or trancelike state. Disbelief and denial can occur. However, parents also feel very sad and depressed. Intense outbursts of emotion and crying are common. However, lack of affect, euphoria, and calmness may occur and may reflect numbness, denial, or a personal way of coping with stress.

It is during this time of acute distress that parents face the first task of grief, accepting the reality of the loss. The pregnancy has ended or the baby has died and their life has changed. While parents are often required to make many decisions, such as naming the infant or funeral arrangements, normal functioning is impeded and decisions are difficult to make. These decisions are especially painful and difficult for young couples who have limited or no previous experience with death. In these cases, their parents, friends, ministers, or other relatives may be available to help them cope. However, it is important that the mother and father ultimately make the decisions that are right for them.

Intense Grief

The phase of **intense grief** encompasses many difficult emotions, including loneliness, emptiness, and yearning; guilt, anger, and fear; disorganization and depression; and physical symptoms. During this time parents are working on two additional tasks of mourning: working through the pain and adjusting to life without the wished-for-child. Being able to adjust to the environment after the loss means learning how to accommodate the changes that the loss has brought. Issues such as deciding what to do about the nursery and baby clothes, how to handle comments of co-workers when returning to work, and how to cope with insensitive family members and friends are among the problems bereaved parents face during this phase of grief.

In the early months after the loss, parents often experience feelings of loneliness, emptiness, and yearning. The mother may report that her arms ache to hold or nurse her baby and that she wakes to the sound of a baby crying. When her milk comes in, it is particularly poignant when there is no baby to take to breast. Both mothers and fathers may be preoccupied with thoughts about the wished-for-child. Some women cope with these feelings by avoiding memories and by not talking about the baby, while others want to reminisce and discuss their loss over and over. Taking down the baby's room is particularly difficult during this period. Some women want the room taken down before they go home, whereas others want the room left intact until they have had time to grieve their loss.

During this phase of intense grief, guilt may emerge from the deep feelings of helplessness in not somehow preventing the pregnancy loss or the death of the infant. Mothers are particularly vulnerable to feel guilt because of their sense of responsibility for the well-being of the fetus and baby. With many perinatal losses, there is no clear cause of the event, leaving the woman to speculate about what she might have done or not done to cause the loss. Guilt also may be intense if a mother thinks she is being punished for some unrelated event such as having had a prior induced abortion.

Another common response during this phase of grief is anger, resentment, bitterness, or irritability. Anger is particularly poignant if the loss is perceived as senseless and there is a need to blame others. Anger may be focused on the health care team who failed to save the pregnancy or infant. For some parents, anger is vented toward a God who allowed the loss to occur. This can lead to a spiritual crisis. Anger also occurs toward family, friends, and peers when they do not provide the support bereaved parents need and want. Some parents focus their resentment on parents who do not appreciate their children or who neglect and abuse them. A sense of bitterness or generalized irritability, rather than frank anger, may be another response.

Fear and anxiety can occur during the grief process as a profound worry that something else bad might happen to another. Fear and anxiety are particularly poignant when the couple thinks about another pregnancy. At this time, they must come to grips with whether or not they can cope with another potential loss.

Deep sadness and depression occur when the parent is faced with the full awareness of the reality of the loss. This often occurs several months after a perinatal loss and can continue for some time. Sadness and depression are often accompanied by **disorganization** and problems with cognitive processing. This leads to behavioral changes such as difficulty in getting things done, an inability to concentrate, restlessness, confused thought processes, difficulty in solving problems, and poor decision making. Disorganization and depression often cause difficulties in keeping up with work and family expectations.

Physical symptoms of grief include fatigue, headaches, dizziness, or backaches. Parents are at risk for developing health problems, such as colds or hypertension. The grieving process makes it difficult for bereaved parents to sleep. Their appetites may be depressed or voracious. Lack of sleep and inadequate nutrition and fluids can complicate other grief responses.

Grief responses are very personal, ongoing, and difficult to cope with. Some parents may suppress or deny their feelings because of societal indifference toward pregnancy loss and infant death. Suppression of feelings may, on the surface, be more socially acceptable. However, denying the pain of grief may lead to eventual physical and emotional distress or illness. Sometimes parents begin to think they are the only individuals who have ever had such a rough time and that they may be going crazy. While bereaved parents have many ups and downs for many months and even years after a child's death, few parents actually become mentally ill or commit suicide. It is important to verbalize fears about one's mental health and to know that others have felt the same.

Reorganization

From the time of the pregnancy loss or infant death, parents attempt to understand "why?" This leads to a long and intense **search for meaning**. At first the "why" is focused on the cause of death. Finding few good answers, parents focus next on "why me, why mine?" These questions lead some parents into an existential search about the meaning of life and death. "What does my loss mean to my life?" "What is life all about?" "What do I do with the rest of my life?" This search continues into the phase of reorganization and may lead to profound changes in the parents' views about the fragility of life.

Time helps to slowly ease the painful feelings of grief. Over time, the pain becomes less frequent. **Reorganization** occurs when the parent is better able to function at home and work, experiences a return of self-esteem and confidence, can cope with new challenges, and has placed the loss in perspective. Reorganization begins to peak sometime after the first year as parents begin to achieve the task of moving on with their lives. Enjoying the simple pleasures of life without feeling guilty, nurturing self and others, developing new interests, and reestablishing relationships are all signs of moving on. For some women and families, another pregnancy and the birth of a subsequent child is an important step to be able to move on with their lives. However, we do not use the term "recovery" because the grief related to perinatal loss can continue in varying degrees for life. Parents have shared that they will never forget the baby who has died and they are not the same person as before the loss. The term **"bittersweet grief,"** coined by Kowalski (1984), refers to the grief response that occurs with reminders of the loss. This typically happens at special anniversary dates related to the loss. Grief feelings also can be triggered after a subsequent live birth (Box 42-2).

The Grief of Fathers

Much of the literature and research on grief following perinatal loss and infant death has focused on the mother. Less is known about the experiences of fathers. The response of fathers may be more variable and depend on the level of identification with the pregnancy. With early miscarriage or ectopic pregnancy, some fathers may not have a strong investment in the wished-for-child. However, many fathers do grieve deeply for a miscarriage (Puddifoot & Johnson, 1997; Schaap et al., 1997). Fathers are profoundly affected by a stillbirth or death of an infant. Fathers also are distressed by the grief of the mother and often feel helpless as to how to help her with the intense pain. Some fathers appear stoic and unemotional to maintain the societal expectation that he be "strong" for the mother and other family members. But it is important to realize that fathers may be experiencing deep pain beneath their calm and quiet appearance. Because fathers don't easily share feelings or ask for help, special efforts are needed to help them realize that they too have a right to support from others in their pain.

BOX 42-2   Bittersweet Grief

To Jessica Mayo—on her 11th Birthday
   Sunday, November 18, 1990
"The child born on the Sabbath day,
is bonny and blithe and good and gay."
   Sundays are special days.
   . . . a day of rest, a day to play.
   A day to reflect on days past.
   . . . a day to thank God for all that we bless.
   I bless your memory.
   I wish you were here.
On your eleventh birthday I still want to share.
   . . . Your dreams of the future.
   . . . Our memories past.
      My baby's first cry.
   My daughter's first laugh.
I was told you were an angel in heaven above.
   Eleven years later, I'm an expert . . .
   At long-distance love.
   On your third birthday I wrote my first poem
to you.
   Eight years later, it's still true
   ". . . no birthday cake,
   no presents unwrapped . . .
no pictures of you in your party hat.
   But the candles are lit,
      Never to go out
For they burn forever in my heart.
      Love, Mom"
Kathie Rataj Mayo
1990

Used with permission of Bereavement Services. Copyright Lutheran Hospital—La Crosse, Inc., a Gundersen Lutheran Affiliate, La Crosse, WI.

CARE MANAGEMENT

Nursing care of mothers and fathers experiencing a perinatal loss begins the first time they are faced with the potential loss of their pregnancy or death of their infant. Supportive interventions are important both at the time of the loss and after the parents have returned home.

Assessment and Nursing Diagnoses

An important step in the nursing process involves assessment. Several key areas to address include the following:
- The nature of the parental attachment with the pregnancy or infant, the meaning of the pregnancy and infant to the parent, and the related losses they are experiencing.

   Each pregnancy and birth has a special meaning to parents. Whether a woman has experienced a miscarriage or ectopic pregnancy, stillbirth, or death of an infant, it is important to gain some understanding of parents' perceptions of their unique loss.

Listening to parents tell their story and being sensitive to the language used to describe their experience can help one gain an understanding of the meaning of the loss. Open-ended questions are helpful: "Tell me about your labor and birth with Lucas." Or "When did you know you were miscarrying?" Mothers who have had a previous pregnancy loss may feel less attached, which can increase their feelings of guilt when a loss occurs (see Research box).
- The circumstances surrounding the loss, including the level of preparation for the loss and the parents' level of understanding about the cause of the loss or death, and any related unresolved issues are important.

   While listening to the parents' stories, it is important to uncover any special experiences that may make their losses even more poignant. A history of infertility, repeated pregnancy losses, a previous stillbirth, or infant death can make this loss even more painful. In addition, other life circumstances such as illness of another family member, loss of a job, or other family stresses can increase the distress of parents. It is also helpful to know whether the mother and father perceived the loss to be totally unexpected or whether they had some forewarning or preparation.
- The immediate response of the mother and father to the loss, whether their responses are complementary or problematic, and how their responses match with their past experiences, personalities, and behavioral and cultural backgrounds.

   An understanding of the usual responses to grief described earlier can be helpful in attempting to understand the unique grief responses of the mother and father and other family members. As nurses work with families, they may uncover information about how the individual or family responded to a previous loss, or a personality or behavioral trait that may interact in their responses to this grief. In particular, it is important to know about any history of infertility, previous pregnancy losses, or infant deaths and evaluate how that might affect parental responses (Armstrong & Hutti, 1998; Lukse & Vacc, 1999). It also is important to be sensitive to different expectations during grief for men and women from different cultural groups (see section on cultural and spiritual needs of parents later in this chapter).
- The social support network of the parent (e.g., extended family, friends, co-workers, church) and the extent to which it has been activated.

   Support during a perinatal loss is important to most couples. However, it is important to assess the amount of support and the type of support from others that a couple wants. Some prefer to handle the tragedy alone for a time. Others want assistance in calling other family members, friends, and clergy to be with them and to help them with decisions.

Nursing diagnoses may include physiologic and psychosocial problems experienced by the individual mother or father, or problems occurring within the couple or family because of the loss and subsequent grief. Examples of nursing diagnoses include the following:

Nursing Diagnoses

- Anxiety related to
  - lack of experience regarding how to manage the loss
  - worry about the partner
  - intense concern over not achieving a pregnancy
  - becoming pregnant again because of risk of another loss
- Ineffective family or individual coping related to
  - inability to make decisions as a family
  - difficulties in communication within the family
  - conflictual coping patterns between mother and father
- Powerlessness related to
  - high risk pregnancy and birth
  - unexpected cesarean birth
  - hospitalization
- Altered family processes related to
  - maternal depression leading to changes in role function
  - inadequate communication of feelings between the grieving mother and father
  - lack of attention and support to siblings
- Fatigue and sleep pattern disturbance related to
  - inability to fall asleep because of grief
  - waking in the night and thinking about the loss
  - fatigue related to loss of sleep
- Dysfunctional grieving related to
  - prolonged denial or avoidance of the loss
  - intense guilt related to the loss
  - continued anger about the loss
  - serious depressive symptoms and despair
  - loss of self-esteem
  - intense grieving patterns that continue for over a year
  - continued high anxiety about getting pregnant again
  - social isolation due to grief
- Self-esteem disturbance related to
  - prolonged feelings of poor self-worth because of the loss
  - feeling unworthy of having a child
- Spiritual distress related to
  - anger with God
  - confusion about why prayers were not answered
- Altered thought processes related to
  - difficulty making decisions
  - inability to get organized
  - poor work performance
  - confused thinking

RESEARCH

Pregnancy After Perinatal Loss: The Relationship Between Anxiety and Prenatal Attachment

Perinatal loss continues to be a complicated, shattering experience in the lives of parents and families at a time when the happiness of a birth is anticipated. Past clinical studies focused on grief responses after perinatal loss and interventions to facilitate adaptation for the parents at the time of loss. However, the research did not focus on the effects of grieving on the mother during a subsequent pregnancy nor on the relationship of anxiety to concerns about the current pregnancy and prenatal attachment with the fetus. The purpose of this study was to examine the relationships between anxiety-related concerns about the pregnancy and the development of prenatal attachment.

A convenience sample was comprised of 31 expectant mothers, 16 of whom had previously experienced a late pregnancy, stillbirth, or neonatal death (loss group), and 15 primiparas. Anxiety levels for all subjects were measured using the Pregnancy Outcome Questionnaire. Their prenatal attachment was measured using the Prenatal Attachment Inventory. Women who had experienced a previous pregnancy loss had a higher level of anxiety related to concerns about the pregnancy and decreased prenatal attachment with the child in the current pregnancy. Women in their first pregnancy had decreased anxiety compared to the loss group. Higher levels of prenatal attachment were also shown in the primiparous group.

CLINICAL APPLICATION

Nurses must be aware of the difficult emotions that can accompany grief after perinatal loss. The anxiety mothers often experience during a subsequent pregnancy may be overwhelming. Nurses must carefully counsel expectant mothers regarding their increased concerns about their current pregnancy. Actions to decrease the level of anxiety are needed. These could include a more thorough assessment of the mother's support system, increased information for parents regarding their concerns about the current pregnancy, and more frequent prenatal visits and testing, such as ultrasound examination. Allowing parents to share their previous experience and the uniqueness of the lost child can help them look forward to the new child as a separate infant and to the pregnancy as a separate event.

Source: Armstrong, D., & Hutti, M. (1998). Pregnancy after perinatal loss: The relationship between anxiety and prenatal attachment. *J Obstet Gynecol Neonatal Nurs* 27(2), 183-189.

Expected Outcomes of Care

Expected outcomes are set and prioritized in client-centered terms according to the mutual goals chosen by the client and the nurse. Nursing actions are then selected to meet the expected outcomes, which may include that the woman/family will do the following:

- Actualize the loss.
- Share experiences and verbalize feelings of grief.
- Understand the normal grief responses they may experience at the time of and following the loss.
- Demonstrate increasing independence in participating in and making decisions that meet their needs and reflect their religious and cultural beliefs.
- Identify family and community resources for support.
- Discuss problems or issues involving relationships with other family members.
- Verbalize satisfaction with their health care professionals.

Plan of Care and Interventions

Interventions and support for parents from the nursing and medical staff following a perinatal loss or infant death are extremely important in their healing. While parents often cannot recall details of their experiences at the time of death, they may recall vividly minor events that were perceived as particularly painful or particularly helpful. The interventions provided below are general ideas about what may be helpful to parents. However, care must be individualized to each parent and family. In a large longitudinal study of parents following a perinatal death, Rand and associates (1998) found that parents appreciated the opportunity to make choices about their needs. The authors suggested that providers should not bias parents nor make presumptions that would limit their choices or force them to make choices they do not want. Furthermore, the cultural and spiritual beliefs and practices of individual parents and families must be considered.

Help the Mother, Father, and Other Family Members Actualize the Loss

When a loss or death occurs, the nurse should be sure that parents have been honestly told about the situation by their physician or others on the health care team. It is important for their nurse to be with them during this time. With infant death, caregivers need to use the words "dead" and "died," rather than "lost" or "gone," to assist the bereaved in accepting this reality. Parents need opportunities to tell their story about the events, experiences, and feelings surrounding the loss. This can help them come to terms with the reality of their loss. Listening to their pain and allowing time for them to absorb the information are important.

One way of actualizing the loss is to tell the parents the sex of the baby and give them the option of naming the fetus or to help them to name an infant who has died. Choosing a name helps make the baby a member of their family so that the baby can be remembered in a special way. Once the baby is named, the nurse should use the name when referring to the baby. While naming can be helpful, it is important not to create the sense that the parents have to name the "baby," especially in the case of a miscarriage when the sex is not known.

> **NURSE ALERT** *A caution about naming is important. There are cultural taboos and rules in some religious faiths that prohibit the naming of an infant who has died. It is very important to be sensitive to this possibility and not impose naming on such parents.*

It is helpful to most mothers and fathers to have a choice about whether or not they want to see the fetus or baby. Many experts believe that seeing the fetus/baby helps parents face the reality of the loss and reduces painful fantasies about what the baby did or did not look like. Approach the subject with a question such as, "Some parents have found it helpful to see their baby, would you like time to consider this?" However, this need to see differs greatly between parents who experience a miscarriage or ectopic pregnancy and those who experience a stillbirth or newborn death. The need or willingness to see also may vary greatly among family members. It is extremely important to determine what each parent really wants to do. This should not be a joint decision made by one person or a decision made for the parents by grandparents or others. Parents may need to think about their answers when asked about seeing the baby. It is a good policy for the nurse to first tell them about this option and then give them time to think about it. Later the nurse can return and ask each parent what they decided. If they decided negatively, it is appropriate to check with them again before they leave the hospital.

In preparation for the visit with the baby, parents appreciate explanations about what to expect. Descriptions of how their baby looks is important. For example, babies may have red, peeling skin like a bad sunburn, dark discoloration similar to bruises, molding of the head that makes the head look soft and swollen, or birth defects. The nurse should make the baby look as normal as possible and remember that parents see their baby with different eyes than health care professionals. Bathing the baby, applying lotion to the baby's skin, combing hair, placing identification bracelets on the arm and leg, dressing the baby in a diaper and special outfit, sprinkling powder in the baby's blanket, and wrapping the baby in a pretty blanket conveys to the parents that their baby has been cared for in a special way (Fig. 42-1). The use of powder and lotion stimulates the parent's senses and provides pleasant memories of their baby.

It is more complicated if the fetus died several days or weeks before birth or if decapitation or dismemberment occurred. Consultation with a local funeral director can help the nurse prepare the baby to be seen by his or her

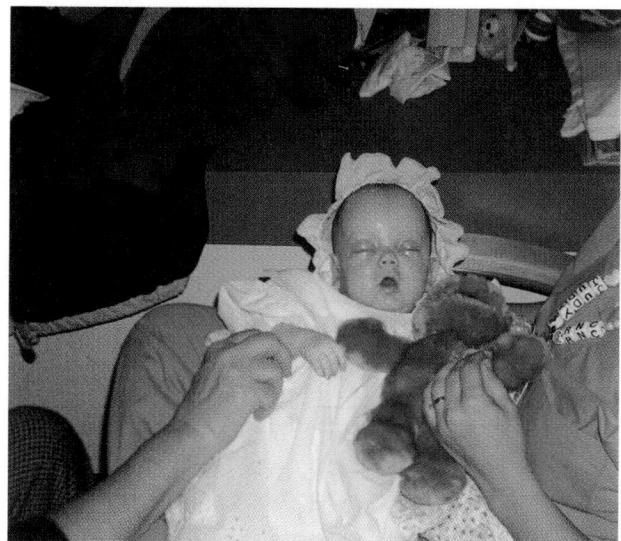

Fig. 42-1 Laura. *(Courtesy Amy and Ken Turner, Cary, NC)*

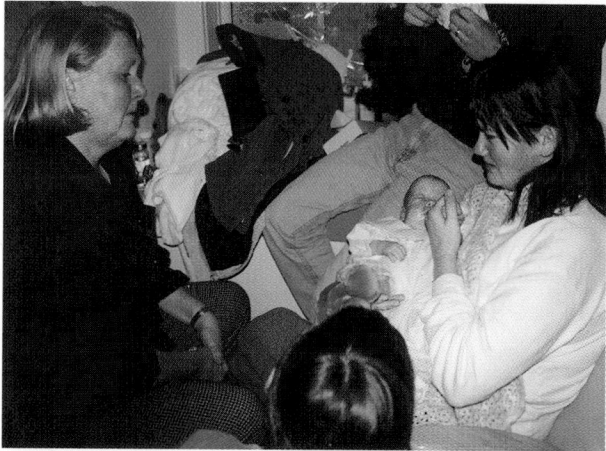

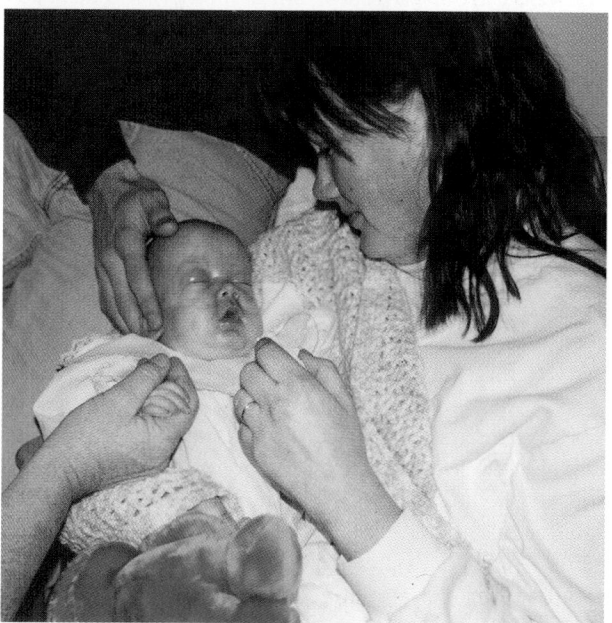

Fig. 42-2 Laura's family members say a special good-bye. *(Courtesy Amy and Ken Turner, Cary, NC)*

parents. If the baby has been in the morgue, he or she can be placed underneath a warmer for 20 to 30 minutes and wrapped in a warm blanket before being brought to the parents. Cold cream rubbed over stiffened joints can help in positioning the baby.

When bringing the baby to the parents, it is important to treat the baby as one would a live baby. Holding the baby close, touching a hand or cheek, using the baby's name, and talking with the parents about the special features of their child conveys that it is all right for them to do likewise. If a baby has a congenital anomaly, the nurse can desensitize the family by pointing out aspects of the baby that are normal. Nurses can help parents explore the baby's body as they desire. Parents often seek to identify family resemblances. A good question might be: "Who in your family does Angela resemble?"

When possible, families should be given the opportunity to bathe and dress their baby. This can be an important ritual for many families. Some babies' skins are fragile, and may crack or ooze when touched. Parents can still apply lotion with cotton balls, sprinkle powder, tie ribbons, fasten the diaper, and place amulets, medallions, rosaries, or special toys or mementos in their baby's hands or alongside their baby. They may want to perform other parenting activities, such as combing hair, wrapping the baby in a blanket, or placing the baby in a crib. They may have special clothes at home, or they may want to purchase a special outfit in which to dress their baby.

Parents need to be offered time alone with their baby if they wish. They also need to know when the nurse will return and how to call if they should need anything. If at all possible, the family should be placed in a private room, and when possible the room should have a rocking chair for the parents to sit in when holding their baby. This offers the mother and father special time together with their baby and

with other family members (Fig. 42-2). Marking the door to the room with a special card can be helpful in reminding the staff that this family has experienced a loss (Fig. 42-3).

It is difficult to predict how long and how often parents will need to spend time with their baby. These moments are the only ones they will have to parent their child while their child's physical presence is still with them. Some parents need only a few minutes, others need hours. It is extremely painful for some parents to say good-bye to their baby. They will tell the nurse when they are ready verbally and nonverbally. The nurse should watch for cues that the parents have had enough time with their baby, such as when parents are no longer holding their child close to them or have placed the baby back in the crib. Asking parents whether they have had enough time usually makes the parents feel that the nurse thinks they have had enough time, which may not be the case. When a baby is taken too

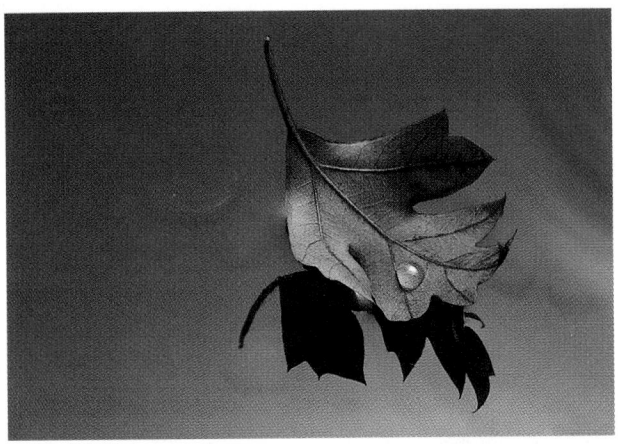

Fig. 42-3 Door card for room of mother who has had a perinatal loss. *(Used with permission of Bereavement Services. Copyright Lutheran Hospital—La Crosse, Inc., a Gundersen Lutheran Affiliate, La Crosse, WI.)*

soon from parents, it leaves them feeling as though the baby was "ripped from their arms too soon." Heiman, Yankowitz, and Wilkins (1997) found that 85% of parents in their study would have appreciated additional opportunities to see their baby and 44% felt they did not have adequate time with the baby. Thus sensitivity to parental needs in actualizing the loss and coping with the reality of the death is essential for their healing.

While it is important for parents to be given all of these options regarding their loss, nurses need to understand that anything they say or do can feel intrusive to the parents. Thus, one should never impose expectations on parents. Giving the parents information in writing can be a helpful way for parents to think about options until they are more capable of making a decision.

Help the Parents with Decision Making

At the time of a perinatal loss and especially if the loss was of an infant, parents have many decisions to make at a time when they are experiencing great distress. Mothers, fathers, and extended families look to the medical and nursing staff for guidance in knowing what decisions they must and can make, and in understanding the options related to those decisions. Thus, it is a primary responsibility of the nurse to help them because decisions made during the time of their loss will provide their memories for a lifetime.

One decision might be related to conducting an autopsy or donation of body parts or organs. An autopsy can be instrumental in determining the cause of death. For some families this information is helpful in understanding why their loss occurred, processing their grief, and perhaps preventing another loss. Other parents may feel that their baby has been through enough. They prefer not to have further information about the cause of death. Some religions prohibit autopsy or limit the choice to times when it may help prevent another loss. (Options for the type of autopsy, such as excluding the head, are available to parents.) Parents may need time to make this decision. There is no

need to rush them, unless there was evidence of contagious disease or maternal infection at the time of death.

Organ donation can be an aid to grieving and an opportunity for the family to see something positive associated with their experience. The physician is usually the first to offer this opportunity to the family. Organ donation of eyes from a baby can occur if the baby was born alive at 36 weeks of gestation or more.

Another important decision relates to spiritual rituals that may be helpful and important to parents. Support from the clergy is an option that should be offered to all parents. Parents may wish to have their own pastor, priest, rabbi, or spiritual leader contacted, or they may wish to see the hospital's chaplain. They may choose to do neither. Members from the clergy may offer the parents the opportunity for baptism when appropriate. Other rituals that may be important include a blessing, a naming ceremony, anointing, ritual of the sick, memorial service, or prayer.

One of the major decisions parents must make has to do with disposition of the body. Parents should be given information about the choices for the final disposition of their baby, regardless of gestational age. The nurses must be aware, however, of cultural and spiritual beliefs that may dictate the choices of parents. In the instance of a baby younger than 20 weeks of gestation, many hospitals will offer to make the final disposition arrangements. Babies under 20 weeks of gestation are considered to be products of conception. Embryos, uterine tubes removed with an ectopic pregnancy, and tissue from a pregnancy obtained during a dilation and curettage, are all considered tissue. Should parents want to know what arrangements the hospital makes for their babies, the nurse should know the hospital's policies and procedures and answer the parents' questions honestly. Many hospitals are currently reviewing and changing their policies regarding cremation and burial of fetuses younger than 20 weeks of gestational age. In most states, if a baby is at least 20 weeks and 1 day of gestational age or is born alive, it is the parents' responsibility to make the final arrangements for their baby.

LEGAL TIP

There are laws in all states governing what constitutes a live birth. In most states a live birth is considered to be any products of conception expelled from a woman that show any signs of life. Signs of life are considered to be any muscle irritability, respiratory effort, or heart rate, regardless of gestational age. All nurses should be knowledgeable about their state laws regarding what constitutes a live birth and what forms must be completed and filed in the case of fetal death, stillbirth, or newborn death.

Final disposition of all identifiable babies, regardless of gestational age, includes burial or cremation. Depending on the cemetery's policies, casketed babies or the ashes from cremated babies can be buried in a special place designated for babies, at the foot of an already deceased relative, in a separate plot, or in a mausoleum. Ashes may also be scattered in a designated area; many states have regulations regarding where ashes can be scattered. A local funeral director or a state's Vital Statistics Bureau should have information about the state's rules, codes, and regulations regarding live births, burial requirements, transportation of the deceased by parents, and cremation.

In making final arrangements for their baby, parents may want a special service. They may choose to have a service in the hospital chapel, visitation at a funeral home or their own home, a funeral service, or a graveside service. Parents can make any of these services as special, personal, and memorable as they like. They can choose special music, poetry, or prose written by others or themselves.

If the family has decided on a funeral and burial, they still have decisions about what funeral home to call and where to bury the baby. Many couples may be living in an area distant from their family homes and they may want to bury their child in their hometown or family cemetery. If the family desires cremation, they may want to have the option of obtaining the ashes. It is important to determine whether or not this will be done by the facility conducting the cremation.

Families may have many other decisions related to their needs but many do not know what they need at the time of loss. Their hopes, dreams, self-esteem, and role expectations have been shattered. However, all families can make a choice once it has been offered and they have some time to consider what their needs might be. It is rare for a mother or family to know exactly what is needed and to be willing to verbalize those needs. When a mother or family is able to verbalize needs, it is extremely important for the nurse to respond positively. The nurse should do everything in his or her power to see that the needs are met. Unmet needs can form the basis of "if only" that may plague a mother or family for a lifetime. Unmet needs can be the foundation for the development of complicated bereavement.

Families become unaware of time frames and do not care about the change of shifts or any needs the hospital system might have in "moving things along." When families are pushed or rushed into making decisions, in most cases they make a decision in response to the health care system's needs, not their own. Thus, the timing for actions such as naming the baby, seeing and holding the baby, disposition of the body, and funeral arrangements should never be rushed. In some cases, it is feasible that the mother may be discharged home before these decisions are made. Then the family can think about them in the comfort of their home and contact the hospital in the following days to give their answers.

Help the Bereaved to Acknowledge and Express Their Feelings

One of the most important goals of the nurse is to help parents express their grief. This involves allowing the parents to talk about their loss and the meaning it has for

---

BOX 42-3 What to Say and What Not to Say to Bereaved Parents

WHAT TO SAY

"I'm sad for you."
"How are you doing with all of this?"
"This must be hard for you."
"What can I do for you?"
"I'm sorry."
"I'm here, and I want to listen."

WHAT NOT TO SAY

"God had a purpose for her."
"Be thankful you have another child."
"The living must go on."
"I know how you feel."
"It's God's will."
"You have to keep on going for her sake."
"You're young, you can have others"
"We'll see you back here next year, and you'll be happier"
"Now you have an angel in heaven."
"This happened for the best."
"Better for this to happen now, before you knew the baby."
"There was something wrong with the baby anyway."

Used with permission of Bereavement Services. Copyright Lutheran Hospital—La Crosse, Inc., a Gundersen Lutheran Affiliate, La Crosse, WI.

---

their lives, and to share their emotional pain. The nurse should listen patiently during the story of loss or grief but listening is hard work and can be painful for the helper. The feelings and emotions of expressed grief can overwhelm health care professionals. Being with someone who is terribly sad and crying or sobbing can be extremely difficult. The initial impulse is to touch the person or to hand the person a tissue. Although such a response may seem supportive at the time, the expression of emotion may be stopped or stifled. The bereaved person will let you know when he or she is ready for a tissue by beginning to wipe the eyes or nose, raising the head, and looking around for or reaching for a tissue. Careful assessment is important before using touch as a therapeutic technique. If touch is used inappropriately, the bereaved person will stiffen, pull away, look at the spot that was touched, or stop the expression of feelings and emotions.

Another common response to reduce the sense of helplessness is to say something that you think will reduce the pain of the parents. Bereaved parents have identified many unhelpful responses made to them by well meaning health care professionals, family, and friends. The nurse should resist the temptation to give advice or to use clichés in offering support to the bereaved (Box 42-3).

Nurses need to be comfortable with their own feelings of grief and loss to effectively support and care for bereaved persons. The nurse should have a presence of self, the willingness to be alongside, quietly supporting the bereaved in whatever expressions of feelings or emotions are appropriate for them. This presence leaves parents feeling that they were cared for. Leaning forward, nodding the head, and saying "Uh-huh" or "Tell me more" is often encouragement enough for the bereaved person to tell his or her story. Sitting through the silence can be therapeutic; silence gives the bereaved person an opportunity to collect thoughts and to process what he or she is sharing.

Bereaved persons have many questions surrounding the event of their loss that can leave them feeling guilty. This is particularly true for mothers. Such questions include "What did I do?" "What caused this to happen?" "What do you think I should have, could have done?" Part of the grief process for bereaved parents is figuring out what happened, their role in the loss, why it happened to them, and why it happened to their baby. The nurse needs to recognize that the answers to these questions must be answered by the bereaved themselves; it is part of their healing. For example, a bereaved mother might ask, "Do you think that I shouldn't have painted the baby's room? Did that cause my baby to die?" An appropriate response to her might be, "I understand you need to find an answer for why your baby died, but we really don't know why she died. What are some of the other things you have been thinking about?" Trying to give bereaved parents answers when there are no clear answers or trying to squelch their guilt feelings by telling them they should not feel guilty does not help them process their grief. In reality, many times there are no definite answers to the question of why this terrible thing has happened to them. However, when there is factual information such as data about the frequency of miscarriages in pregnant women, or the fact that there usually is no clear cause of a stillbirth, can be helpful.

Feelings of anger, guilt, and sadness can occur immediately but often become more problematic in the early days and months after a loss. When a bereaved person expresses feelings of anger, it can be helpful to identify the feeling by simply saying, "You sound angry," or "You look angry." The nurse's willingness to sit down and listen to these feelings of anger can help the bereaved move past those surface feelings into the underlying feelings of powerlessness and helplessness in not being able to control the many aspects of the situation.

Normalize the Grief Process and Facilitate Positive Coping

While helping parents share their feelings of pain, it is critical to help them understand their grief responses and feel they are not alone in these painful responses. Most parents are not prepared for the raw feelings that they experience nor the fact that these painful, complex feelings and related behavioral reactions continue for many weeks or months. Thus, reassuring them of the normality of their responses and preparing them for the length of their grief is important. The nurse can help the parent be prepared for the emptiness, loneliness, and yearning; for the feelings of helplessness that can lead to anger, guilt, and fear; and for the cognitive processing problems, disorganization, difficulty making decisions; and sadness and depression that are part of the grief process. Books and pamphlets about grief, if short and sensitive, can be given to parents to take home. Many parents have reported feelings of fear that they were going crazy because of the many emotions and behavioral responses that leave them feeling totally out of control in the months following the loss. It is essential for the nurse to reassure and educate bereaved parents about the grief process, including the physical, social, and emotional responses of individuals and families. Offering health teaching on the bereavement process alone is not enough, however. In the initial days after a loss, other strategies include follow-up phone calls, referrals to a perinatal grief support group, or providing a list of publications or web sites intended for helping parents who have experienced a perinatal loss. As with any referral, however, the nurse should herself read the materials or check out the web sites first (Box 42-4; see also Appendix D).

It is particularly important to help couples understand that they may respond and grieve in very different ways (Wallerstedt & Higgins, 1996). Discongruent grieving can lead to serious marital problems and be a risk factor for complicated bereavement (Schaap et al., 1997). Thus, it is helpful to remind the couple to be understanding and patient with each other. Fathers may need to be encouraged to share their grief with their wives because of the desire to protect the woman from his pain

Nurses can reinforce positive coping efforts and attempt to prevent negative coping. They can remind the parents of the importance of being patient and being good to themselves during the grief process. Additional suggestions are to encourage attempts to resume normal activities; reinforce and encourage positive ways to hold onto memories of the pregnancy or baby, while letting go; and help the parent to organize a plan for daily activities, if needed. In particular, nurses should discourage overdependence on drugs and alcohol.

Meet the Physical Needs of the Postpartum Bereaved Mother

Coping with loss and grief after childbirth can be an overwhelming experience for the woman and her family. One particularly difficult aspect of the loss is the sound of crying babies and the happiness of other families on the unit who have given birth to healthy infants. The mother should be given the opportunity to decide if she wants to remain on the maternity unit or be moved to another hospital unit. She should also be helped to understand the pluses and minuses of each choice. Postpartum care may not be as good on another hospital unit. Thus, mothers may want to remain on the maternity unit where the staff nurses are better prepared to meet their physical and emo-

BOX 42-4 Web Sources for When a Baby Dies

AAPC
American Association of Pastoral Counselors
http://www.aapc.org
Growth House, Inc.
Page to grief related to pregnancy, including miscarriage, stillbirth, termination of pregnancy, and neonatal death
http://www.growthhouse.org
Griefnet
A collection of resources of value to those who are experiencing loss and grief
http://www.griefnet.org
HAND
Houston's Aid in Neonatal Death: Supporting grieving parents in the greater Houston area with the rest of the world via the Internet
http://www.hern.org/~hand
Hannah's Prayer
Christian support for fertility challenges
http://www.hannah.org
Hygeia™
An on-line journal for pregnancy and neonatal loss: Dr. Michael Berman
http://www.connix.com/~hygeia/
Miscarriage Support and Information Resources
Comprehensive resource list
http://www.pinelandpress.com/support/miscarriage.html

OBGYN.net
List of resources for loss and bereavement
http://www.obgyn.net/woman/loss/loss.htm
Pen-Parents, Inc.
An international nonprofit support network for bereaved parents
http://www.penparents.org
A Place to Remember
Uplifting resources for those who have been touched by a crisis in pregnancy or the birth of a baby
http://www.aplacetoremember.com
SHARE
Pregnancy and Infant Loss Support, Inc.
http://www.nationalshareoffice.com
SIDS NETWORK
Sudden infant death syndrome (SIDS) information web site
http://www.sids-network.org
The Compassionate Friends
A self-help organization for bereaved parents and siblings
http://www.compassionatefriends.org

---

tional needs. The physical needs of a bereaved mother are the same as those of any woman who has given birth. The cruel reality for many bereaved mothers is that their milk may come in and there is no baby to nurse, their afterpains remind them of their emptiness, and gas pains feel as though a baby is still moving inside. The nurse needs to assure that the mother receives appropriate medications to reduce these physical symptoms. Adequate rest, diet, and fluids must be offered to replenish her physical strength.

Mothers need postpartum care instructions upon discharge. They also need ideas about how to cope with problems with sleep such as decreasing food or fluids that contain caffeine, limiting alcohol and nicotine consumption, exercising regularly, using strategies for rest, taking a warm bath or drinking warm milk before bedtime, relaxation exercises, restful music, or a massage.

Assist the Bereaved in Communicating with, Supporting, and Getting Support from Family

Providing sensitive care to bereaved parents means including their families in the grief process. Grandparents and siblings are particularly important when a perinatal loss has occurred. However, it is up to the parents to decide to what extent they want family involved in their grief process. If it is the parents' desire, children, grandparents,

extended family members, and friends should be allowed to be involved in the rituals surrounding the death. This includes seeing and holding the baby. Such visits afford others the opportunity to become acquainted with the baby, to understand the parents' loss, to offer their support, and to say good-bye (see Fig. 42-2). This experience helps parents explain to their surviving children who their brother or sister was and what death means, offers the children answers to their questions in a concrete manner, and helps the children in expressing their grief. Involving extended family and friends enables the parents to mobilize their social support system of people who will support the family not only at the time of loss but also in the future.

Parents also need information about how grief affects a family. They may need help in understanding and coping with the potential differing responses of various family members. Frustrations may arise because of the insensitive or inadequate responses of other family members. Parents may need help in determining ways to let family members know how they feel and what they need.

Create Memories for Parents to Take Home

Parents may want tangible mementos of their baby to allow them to actualize the loss. Some may want to bring in a previously purchased baby book. Special memory

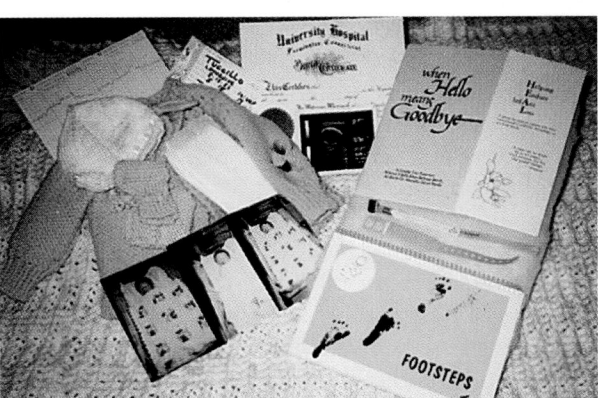

Fig. 42-4   A memory kit assembled at the University of Connecticut Health Center, Farmington, CT. It includes pictures of the infant, clothing, death certificate, footprints, ID bands, fetal monitor printout, and ultrasound picture. *(From Dickason, E., Silverman, B., & Kaplan, J. [1998]. Maternal-infant nursing care [3rd ed.]. St. Louis: Mosby.)*

books, cards, and information on grief and mourning are available for purchase by parents or hospitals or clinics through national perinatal bereavement organizations (Fig. 42-4).

The nurse can provide information about the baby's weight, length, and head circumference to the family. Footprints and handprints can be taken and placed with the other information on a special card or in a memory or baby book. Sometimes it is difficult to obtain good handprints or footprints. Application of alcohol or acetone on the palms or soles can help the ink adhere to make the prints clearer, especially for small babies. When making prints, have a hard surface underneath the paper to be printed. The baby's heel or palm is placed down first, the foot or hand is rolled forward, keeping the toes or fingers extended. It may be helpful to have a partner in doing this procedure. If the print does not turn out, tracing around the baby's hands and feet can be done, although this distorts the actual size. A form of plaster of paris can also be used to make an imprint of the baby's hand or foot.

Parents often appreciate articles that were in contact with or used in caring for the baby. This might include the tape measure used to measure the baby, baby lotions, combs, clothing, hats, blankets, crib cards, and identification bands. The identification band helps the parents remember the size of the baby and personalizes the mementos. The nurse should ask parents if they wish to have these articles before giving them to the parents. A lock of hair may be another important keepsake. Parents need to be asked for permission before cutting a lock of hair, which can be removed from the nape of the neck where it is not noticeable.

Pictures are the most important memento a parent can have. Photographs should be taken whenever there is an identifiable baby and when it is culturally acceptable to the family. It does not matter how tiny the baby is, what the baby looks like, or how long the baby has been dead. Pictures should be taken by an instant-print camera as well as a 35 mm camera. Pictures should include close-ups of the baby's face, hands, and feet. The baby should be clothed in some of the pictures, and wrapped in a blanket with a hat or gown. Pictures should also be taken of the unclothed baby. If there are any congenital anomalies, close-ups of the anomalies should also be taken. Flowers, blocks, stuffed animals, or toys can be placed in the background to make the picture more special. The parents or siblings may also want to have their pictures taken holding the baby. Keeping a camera nearby and taking pictures when parents are spending special time with their baby can provide wonderful memories. Some parents may have their own camera or video camera and would like the nurse to record them holding or parenting their baby as they bathe, dress, or diaper their baby.

Communicate Using a Caring Framework

Mothers, fathers, and extended families look to the nursing staff for support and understanding during the time of loss. Nurses have an important role in providing sensitive care to parents at the time of a perinatal loss. One model for conceptualizing intervention is that developed by Swanson-Kauffman based on her research with women experiencing perinatal loss (Swanson-Kauffman, 1986, 1988). The framework identifies five components in a caring concept:
1. Knowing
2. Being with
3. Doing for
4. Enabling
5. Maintaining belief

Knowing implies that the nurse has taken the time to understand the perception of the loss and its meaning to the woman and her family. *Being with* involves how the nurse conveys acceptance of the various feelings and perceptions of each family member. *Doing for* refers to the activities performed by the nurse that provide for the physical care, comfort, and safety for the woman and her family. This may include offering pain medication, sitz baths, maintaining the patency of the intravenous line, postpartum checks, and back rubs. *Enabling* occurs when the nurse offers the woman and her family options for care. Offers of information, anticipatory guidance, choices for decision making, and support during hospitalization and after discharge help the family feel more in control of a situation in which they feel very much out of control. Enabling raises their self-esteem and allows them to feel more comfortable in asking for options according to their needs for memories and closure, rather than to the nurse's perception of their needs. *Maintaining belief* involves encouraging the woman and her family to believe in their own ability to pick up the pieces and begin to heal. The nurse spends time with the family, learns their inner strengths and coping abilities, and points out these inner resources to the family by saying, "I know this is a difficult time for you, but I have seen some of your inner strength and know that you will be able to make it through all of this."

Be Concerned About Cultural and Spiritual Needs of Parents

Parents who experience perinatal loss can be from widely diverse cultural and ethnic groups. In addition, parents belong to many different religious groups. Many of the responses that were described and the interventions suggested in this chapter are based on Euro-American views of perinatal grief and loss. Although it is thought that there are no particular differences in the individual, intrapersonal experiences of grief based on culture, ethnicity, or religion, there are many differences in mourning rituals, traditions, and behavioral expressions of grief (Cowles, 1996). Thus, the practices suggested earlier may not be appropriate for parents from other cultural, ethnic, and religious groups, and the nurse must consider the potential unique responses and needs of parents from different groups (Hebert, 1998). This involves understanding the cultural orientation and beliefs of the individual parent, the partner, the extended family, and the larger community to which they belong.

Cultural and religious differences can affect the way parents respond to a perinatal loss. This includes their way of communicating with health care professionals, as well as their emotional and behavioral responses and family interaction patterns. Some groups, such as Orthodox Jews, may not support the notion of grieving perinatal loss because the fetus or stillborn infant is not considered a person. Mothers from some cultural groups may have intense somatic symptoms. In some cultures such as Muslims, decisions are communal (Hebert, 1998). Expressions of grief may range from quiet and stoic to dramatic and hysterical for different Native American groups. Native Americans from many tribes would not respond well to an "interviewing" or "questioning" approach (Lawson, 1990). Mexican-American mothers may be very demonstrative in their grief, while also struggling with the view that hardship is "God's will" (Lawson, 1990).

With perinatal loss, culture and religious beliefs can affect issues such as seeing the child, naming the child, and taking pictures. Some cultural and religious groups do not believe in naming an infant who dies younger than 30 days of age. Picture taking can conflict with beliefs of some cultures, such as some Native Americans, Eskimos, Amish, Hindu, and Muslim. Families from these cultures should be sensitively offered this opportunity but not pushed into having a picture taken.

There are many different taboos and expectations related to death for different religious groups. Autopsies are not allowed by some religions except under unusual circumstances. Cremation is forbidden by the Jewish religion, Baha'is, and the Greek Orthodox Church (Harakas, 1999). It is discouraged or allowed only under unusual circumstances in the Church of Jesus Christ of Latter-Day Saints. Embalming is not allowed for Jews, Baha'is, and Muslims.

Culture and religious beliefs also influence the customs surrounding death. Many religious groups have rituals, such as prayers, ritualistic washing and shrouding, or anointing with oil, that are performed at the time of death. Baptism is extremely important for Roman Catholics and some Protestant groups. Baptism can be performed by a lay person, such as a nurse, in an emergency situation where a priest cannot be there in a timely fashion (Box 42-5).

Many Protestant groups believe that baptism is conducted at the age of reason and parents from these religions would not want their baby baptized. When bereaved parents need a referral for grief counseling, cultural considerations are paramount. Native Americans, for example, are best referred to native healers and counselors rather than to Western biomedical therapists (Lawson, 1990).

Provide Sensitive Care at and Following Discharge

When leaving the hospital, it is customary for all mothers to be taken out in a wheelchair. This can be a devastating experience for the mother who has experienced a pregnancy loss. Leaving the hospital without a baby in her arms is a very empty and painful experience. It is especially difficult if others are seen leaving with babies. Thus, the discharge of mothers and fathers who have experienced a perinatal loss should be done with great sensitivity to their feelings. They should not be discharged at a time when other mothers with live babies are leaving. Giving the mother a special flower to carry in her arms can be a thoughtful gesture.

BOX 42-5 Infant Baptism

In an emergency, baptism may be performed by anyone by pouring water over the forehead (or products of conception) and saying "I baptize you in the name of the Father and of the Son and of the Holy Spirit." The person performing the baptism needs only to have the intention of baptizing and does not necessarily have to believe in infant baptism for the baptism to be valid. If the infant has no signs of life, the person performing the baptism can add "If you are alive, I baptize you..." In the Greek Orthodox tradition, baptism is only for the living; thus a miscarried or stillborn infant would not be baptized. If the infant is born alive and in serious danger of death, the infant can be lifted up while saying "The servant of God is baptized in the name of the Father and the Son and Holy Spirit" (Harakas, 1999)

The grief of the mother and her family does not end with discharge; rather it really begins once they return home, attend the funeral, and start to live their lives without their baby. Follow-up phone calls after a loss may be helpful to some parents. However, it needs to be determined when parents do not want a follow-up call, which often is the case following early loss. Follow-up calls let the parents know they are still thought of and cared about. The calls are made at predictably difficult times such as the first week at home, 1 month to 6 weeks later, 4 to 6 months after the loss, and at the anniversary of the death. Families who experienced a miscarriage, ectopic pregnancy, or death of a premature baby may appreciate a phone call on the due date. The calls provide an opportunity for parents to ask questions, share their feelings, seek advice, and receive information to help them in processing their grief.

A grief conference can be planned when parents return for an appointment with their doctor, nurses, and other health care providers. At the conference, the loss or death of the infant is discussed in detail, parents are given information about the baby's autopsy report and genetic studies, and they have opportunities to ask the questions that have arisen since their baby's death. Parents appreciate the opportunity to review the events of hospitalization, go over the baby's and/or mother's chart with their primary health care provider, and talk with those who cared for them during hospitalization. In addition, parents have opportunities to share their grief. This gives health care professionals the opportunity to assess how the family is coping with their loss and provide additional information and education on grief.

Some parents are very interested in finding a perinatal or parent grief support group. They appreciate the opportunity to talk with others who have been through similar experiences. A grief support group also can be helpful in sharing feelings and gaining an understanding of the normality of the grief process. Over time, it may be the only place where a bereaved parent can talk about their wished-for-child and their grief. However, not all parents find such groups helpful. When referring to a group, it is important to know something about the group and how it operates. For example, if a group has a religious base for their interventions, a nonreligious parent would likely find the group nonhelpful. If parents experiencing a perinatal loss are referred to a parental grief group, they might feel overwhelmed with the grief of parents whose older children have died of cancer, suicide, or homicide. In addition, their grief might be minimized by participants. Thus, the needs of the parents must be matched with the focus of the group.

Provide Postmortem Care

Preparation of the baby's body to be taken to the morgue depends on the procedures and protocols developed by individual hospitals. Transport to the morgue is also done according to the agency procedures. Postmortem care can be an emotional and sometimes difficult task for the nurse depending on the gestational age and condition of the baby's skin. However, nurses may find that doing postmortem care helps them find closure in their own grief related to a perinatal loss. This is particularly true for neonatal intensive care nurses who have cared for an infant for several hours, days, or weeks.

Evaluation

The evaluation of nursing care is made more difficult by the shock and numbness of the bereavement process and the varied grief responses of the parents and other family members during hospitalization. The achievement of expected outcomes is assured when the positive integration of the perinatal loss is expressed by the family (see Plan of Care).

One approach to evaluation is the use of checklists. Many hospitals have checklists that are used in providing care, mobilizing members of the multidisciplinary health care team, communicating options the family has chosen, and keeping track of all the details in meeting the needs of bereaved parents (Figs. 42-5 and 42-6). Such checklists may be a permanent part of the chart. Documentation in the nursing notes of primary concerns, grief responses, health teaching, health care advice, and any referrals of the mother or other family members is essential to ensure continuity and consistency of care.

SPECIAL LOSSES

Prenatal Diagnoses with Negative Outcome

Early prenatal diagnostic tests such as ultrasonography, chorionic villi sampling, and amniocentesis can determine the well-being of the embryo or fetus. Reasons for prenatal testing include history of chromosomal abnormality in the family; three or more miscarriages; older maternal age; lack of fetal growth, movement, or heartbeat; and diabetes mellitus or other chronic illnesses. If the health care provider is certain that the baby has a serious genetic defect that would lead to death in utero or after birth (congenital anomalies incompatible with life or genetic disorders with severe mental retardation) the choice of interruption of a pregnancy may be offered. Abortion is controversial, and this may prevent parents from sharing this decision with other family members or friends. This limits their support systems after their loss (Lorenzen & Holzgreve, 1995).

The decision to terminate a pregnancy paves the way for feelings such as guilt, despair, sadness, depression, and anger. The nurse's role is to be a good listener. It is important to assess how these families feel about the experience and to offer options for their memories as appropriate. Healing can take place when words can be given to feelings and needs can be met.

PLAN ᵒᶠ CARE | Fetal Death: 20 Weeks of Gestation

> **NURSING DIAGNOSIS** Dysfunctional grieving related to fetal death, as evidenced by intense expressions of grief for prolonged period of time

Expected Outcome: *Client will identify appropriate ways to deal with grief.*

Nursing Interventions/*Rationales*

Prepare family for viewing fetus by cleaning body and wrapping in clean blanket *to initiate and support the grieving process in a supportive setting.*

Allow family quiet time to hold and view fetus. Take pictures for family to keep *to provide reality to death and support the grieving process.*

Provide a certificate for the family with vital statistics, along with identification bands, lock of hair and footprints *to provide reality of situation and support the grieving process.*

Provide spiritual support as needed to assist with religious services, such as baptism and memorial services *to provide spiritual support and assist with religious practices.*

Refer to appropriate community support groups to facilitate grieving with group input and *to share experiences.*

> **NURSING DIAGNOSIS** Situational low self-esteem related to fetal death as evidenced by client's intense feelings of guilt

Expected Outcomes: *Client will exhibit positive self-comments and adapt to death of fetus in a timely manner.*

Nursing Interventions/*Rationales*

Provide private time for expressions of feelings through therapeutic communication and active listening *to validate feelings.*

Identify client's perception and feelings about fetal death *to correct any misconceptions and alleviate guilt.*

Assist client to identify positive coping mechanisms and support systems *to promote feelings of self-worth.*

Refer to appropriate health professionals for further evaluation and counseling, such as social service *to provide ongoing assistance as needed.*

The parent who decides to continue the pregnancy also requires emotional support. The time of labor and birth can be particularly difficult. The nurse should remember that parents may be grieving not only the loss of the perfect child but the loss of expectations for their child's future.

Loss of One in a Multiple Birth

The death of a twin or baby in a multifetal gestation during pregnancy, labor, or birth or after birth requires parents to parent and grieve at the same time. Such a death imposes a confusing and ambivalent induction into parenthood (Swanson-Kauffman, 1988). Parents feel that they cannot do anything right. They cannot parent their surviving child with all the joy and enthusiasm of new parents because their surviving child reminds them of what they have lost. They cannot give over completely and grieve in the manner they need to because their surviving child demands their attention. These parents are at risk for altered parenting and complicated bereavement.

It is important to help the parents acknowledge the birth of all their babies. Parents should be treated as bereaved families, and all the options previously discussed should be offered. Pictures should be taken of the babies and parents should be offered the opportunity to hold their babies in their arms and have time to say good-bye to the baby who has died.

Bereaved parents should be warned that well-meaning family members or friends may say, "Well at least you have the other baby," implying that there should be no grief because they are lucky to have one at all. Parents need to be able to anticipate insensitivity to their loss and be empowered to say to those people, "That is not how I feel." By simply setting a boundary on what their feelings are, they are able to acknowledge the baby who died and then have an opportunity to share more about their feelings if they so choose.

Bereaved parents of multiples have special problems in coping with life without their anticipated "extra special" family, telling their surviving child about his or her twin, dealing with the possibility of that child's feelings of survivor guilt, and deciding on how to celebrate birthdays, death days, or special holidays.

Adolescent Grief

Adolescent pregnancy accounts for many births in the United States. Each year, many adolescents experience perinatal loss particularly as elective abortion or miscarriage. Although adolescent participants have been included in the samples of research done in all areas of perinatal bereavement, their particular responses to perinatal loss have not been specifically identified. Adolescents grieve the loss

SAMPLE

RTS Bereavement Services
CHECKLIST FOR ASSISTING PARENT(S) EXPERIENCING MISCARRIAGE/ECTOPIC PREGNANCY

RTS Counselor _____ Date _____

Mother's name _____ Age _____ Due date _____

Date of beginning of miscarriage _____ Date of surgery _____

# of Miscarriages _____ # of Children _____ Religion _____

Address _____ Occupation _____

Phone number (   ) _____ Marital status _____

Father's name _____ Age _____ Occupation _____

Address _____ Phone number (   ) _____

Baby's name _____ Sex _____

Support people available _____ Children's names: _____

Problem areas _____ Physician _____

OK to send written material to home address ☐ Yes ☐ No

Date	Time	See Miscarriage Protocol RTS Manual	Comments	Initials
		Notify/Assign RTS counselor ☐ Yes ☐ No		
		Pastoral Care ☐ Yes ☐ No		
		Offered: ☐ Blessing ☐ Memorial Service ☐ Naming Ceremony ☐ Burial		
		Asked: "Would you like someone with you now?" ☐ Yes ☐ No		
		D&C/Surgical procedure discussed ☐ Yes ☐ No		
		Saw baby or tissue ☐ Mother ☐ Father		
		Touched and/or held baby ☐ Mother ☐ Father		
		If RH negative, RhoGAM given within 72 hrs ☐ Yes ☐ No		
		Patient's room flagged with door card ☐ Yes ☐ No		
		Photos taken: ☐ 35 mm ☐ Polaroid ☐ Given to parents ☐ On file		
		Footprints & handprints/weight & length: ☐ Given to parents ☐ On file		
		Grief process discussed ☐ Yes ☐ No		
		Incongruent grief discussed ☐ Yes ☐ No		
		Grief packet given ☐ Yes ☐ No		
		Info Brochure given to parents re: RTS PSG ☐ Yes ☐ No		
		Name/business card given ☐ Yes ☐ No		
		Regular OB/Midwife notified _____ ☐ Memo ☐ Verbally		
		Childbirth Educator notified _____ ☐ Yes ☐ No		
		Telephone number verified ☐ Yes ☐ No Optimal call time _____		
		Preg & Inf Loss Card sent to RTS Secretary ☐ Yes ☐ No		
		Given option to transfer from Maternity Unit ☐ Yes ☐ No		
		Genetic Studies ordered ☐ Yes ☐ No		
		Sex determination desired (tissue in NS only) ☐ Yes ☐ No		
		Would like another parent to call: ☐ Yes ☐ No ☐ Ask later		
		Parent contact: _____ Follow-up calls: eg. ☐ 1 wk, ☐ 3 wk, ☐ 4 mo, ☐ due date/anniv. date		

Forms for burial or cremation of:
  a) Products of conception - 2 copies of "Request for Return of Products of Conception to Patients" (1 copy-chart, 1 copy-lab). Obtain forms from histology.
  b) Identifiable baby less than 20 wk or less than 350 gm - 2 copies of "Request for Return of Products of Conception to Patients" (1-chart, 1-lab). "Notice of Removal" #DOH 5043 - Responsible party for burial signs this form (either parent or a funeral director). Pink copy goes to responsible party. "Final Disposition of a Human Corpse" #DOH 5045 is required for any age identifiable baby that goes across state lines.
Note: Some cemeteries may require a "Final Disposition of a Human Corpse" report for their own recordkeeping.

Fig. 42-5   Sample checklist for assisting parents experiencing miscarriage/ectopic pregnancy. *(Used with permission of Bereavement Services. Copyright Lutheran Hospital—La Crosse, Inc., a Gundersen Lutheran Affiliate, La Crosse, WI.)*

RTS Bereavement Services
CHECKLIST FOR ASSISTING PARENT(S) EXPERIENCING STILLBIRTH OR NEWBORN DEATH

SAMPLE

Mother's discharge date:_____

Mother's name:_____

Address: _____

Phone number: (   ) _____

Father's name: _____

Address: _____

Phone number: (   ) _____

Optimal call time:_____

RTS Counselor: _____

Unit:_____ Ext _____

Regular OB MD/Midwife:_____

Religion: _____

Age _____ Gr ___ Para ___ L.C. ___ Due date _____

Previous loss: _____

Date/Time delivered: _____

Date/Time death: _____

Baby's name: _____ Sex: _____

Children's name(s): _____ Age: _____

_____ Age: _____

_____ Age: _____

Support people

Attending MD &/or Pediatrician _____

Notify Peds Nurse Practitioner _____

Date	Time		Comments	Initials
		Notify/Assign RTS counselor ☐ Yes ☐ No		
		Pastoral Care notified ☐ Yes ☐ No		
		Funeral Home notified: ☐ Yes ☐ No Family Burial: ☐ Yes ☐ No		
		Saw baby when born and/or after delivery: ☐ Mother ☐ Father		
		Touched and/or held baby: ☐ Mother ☐ Father		
		☐ Siblings ☐ Grandparents ☐ Friends		
		Offered private time with their baby: ☐ Yes ☐ No		
		Baptism offered: (use seashell as vessel, give to parents) ☐ Yes ☐ No		
		Remembrance of Blessing offered: ☐ Yes ☐ No		
		(can offer for any perinatal loss) ☐ Given to parents		
		Given option to transfer off Maternity Unit: ☐ Yes ☐ No		
		Patient's room flagged with door card ☐ Yes ☐ No		
		Autopsy: ☐ Yes ☐ No Genetic studies: ☐ Yes ☐ No		
		Genetic Associate notified: ☐ Yes ☐ No		
		Regular Physician/Midwife notified of death: ☐ Yes ☐ No		
		Memo sent to Physician/Midwife: ☐ Yes ☐ No		
		Section of Fetal monitor strip: ☐ Given to parents ☐ On file		
		ID Bands/Crib cards/Tape measure: ☐ Given to parents ☐ On file		
		Footprints/Handprints/Weight/Length recorded on		
		"In Memory Of" sheet: ☐ Given to parents ☐ On file		
		Lock of hair offered: (ask permission) ☐ Yes ☐ No		
		☐ Given to parents ☐ On file		
		Mementos (clothing, hat , blanket, pacifier, crib cards, basin, baby ring,		
		bear, thermometer, silk flower) ☐ Given to parents ☐ On file		
		Complimentary birth keepsake ☐ Given to parents ☐ On file		
		RTS Photos taken:		
		(clothed, unclothed, w. props, family photo)		
		1) Polaroid - 3 or more ☐ Given to parents ☐ On file		
		2) 35 mm (6-12 pictures) ☐ Given to parents ☐ On file		
		3) Medical photos: ☐ Yes ☐ No		

Fig. 42-6 Sample checklist for assisting parents experiencing stillbirth or newborn death. *(Used with permission of Bereavement Services. Copyright Lutheran Hospital—La Crosse, Inc., a Gundersen Lutheran Affiliate, La Crosse, WI.)*

Date	Time		Comments	Initials
		Informed about postponing funeral until mother is able to attend: ☐ Yes ☐ No		
		Services/Funeral arrangements, options discussed: ☐ Self-transport ☐ Gravesite service ☐ Visitation ☐ Hospital chapel ☐ Cremation ☐ Funeral home ☐ Burial at foot or head of relative's grave ☐ Specific area for babies in cemetery ☐ Plan own service		
		Funeral arrangements made by: ☐ Mother ☐ Father Discussed: ☐ Seeing baby at funeral home ☐ Taking pictures there ☐ Providing outfit/toy for baby ☐ Dressing baby at funeral home		
		Grief information packet given to: ☐ Mother ☐ Father		
		Discussed grief process/incongruent grief with: ☐ Mother ☐ Father		
		Discussed grief conference: ☐ Yes ☐ No		
		RTS Parents Support Group brochure given to: ☐ Mother ☐ Father		
		RTS business card given to: ☐ Mother ☐ Father		
		Pregnancy & Infant Loss Card sent to RTS secretary: ☐ Yes ☐ No		
		Follow-up calls: 1 week: . . . . 3 weeks: . . . . Due date: . . . . 6-10 months: . . . . Anniversary date:		
		Grief conference planned with parents: Date _____ Time _____ Place _____ Letter of confirmation sent: ☐ Yes ☐ No		
		Parent Support Group, first meeting attended: Date: _____ Follow-up meetings attended: Dates _____		
		Would like another parent to call: ☐ Yes ☐ No ☐ Ask later Parent contact: _____		

Forms Needed: Report of fetal death (Photocopy and save for mother.)
                  Autopsy if ordered
                  Record of death
                  Genetics protocol (folder) if ordered
                  Notice of removal of a human corpse from an institution
                  Final disposition form
                  If funeral home involved - Final disposition will be completed by them.
                  Original certificate of death (for NB death only)

Note: <u>Family Burial</u> - Check with your funeral home.

** You may wish to list your hospital and state forms that are necessary, as required by your state laws and your institution.

Fig. 42-6, cont'd For legend see p. 1151

of their babies through miscarriage, stillbirth, or newborn death and need the emotional support from the nurses who care for them. However, nurses and other health care professionals, as well as family members, often believe that the adolescent's loss of her baby was for the best so that the adolescent can move on with her life. Adolescent girls, then, may not receive the support they need from staff and family. In addition, adolescent girls usually do not have the support from the father of the baby as compared to older women who have a perinatal loss. Thus, there is a great need to provide sensitive care to all adolescents who experience any type of perinatal loss.

The first step for the nurse in caring for a bereaved adolescent is to acknowledge the significance of giving birth, no matter what age the mother might be. Second, the nurse should make additional efforts to develop a trusting relationship in working with the adolescent. Third, the nurse should offer options for saying good-bye, anticipatory guidance, support, and information to meet the adolescent at the point of her need. It may take longer for adolescents to process their grief because of their level of cognitive and emotional maturation. Being patient, saving mementos, and giving the adolescent information on how to contact the nurse are interventions that can help the adolescent accept the reality of the loss and process her grief.

Maternal Death

It is extremely rare for a woman to die in childbirth, but it does happen. The occurrence of maternal deaths is 7.5 per 100,000 each year (Centers for Disease Control and Prevention, 1998). The father and extended family who is faced with not only mourning the death of a wife and mother but also the death of the baby have a particularly difficult time. On the other hand, the father may be faced with parenting a baby without a surviving mother. Death of a mother disrupts the family structure and leaves the father with the care of a baby at a time when he is greatly distressed. Thus the father and extended family, especially other children and grandparents, need supportive grief counseling at the time of death and following discharge for them to heal after such a devastating loss.

The nursing care of families at this time is similar to that already described. Options need to be offered, memories made, and mementos obtained and held for the family until they are ready for them. These families are at risk for complicated bereavement and altered parenting of the surviving baby and other children in the family. Referral to social services to help the family mobilize support systems and for counseling can help combat potential problems before they develop. Such a referral may be beneficial not only at the time of the loss but also in the future.

The emotional toll that a maternal death can take on the nursing and medical staff must also be addressed. Guilt, anger, fear, sadness, and depression are all common responses to a maternal death. The staff may want to review the situation surrounding the events, the chart, and their responses in the forum of a mortality-morbidity review and a critical incident debriefing to help in coping with the feelings and emotions that result after a maternal death. Attending memorial or funeral services may benefit staff and family.

COMPLICATED BEREAVEMENT

While most parents cope adequately with the pain of their grief and return to some level of normal functioning, some parents have extremely intense grief reactions that last for a very long time; this response is **complicated bereavement.** There are other parents whose grief from one loss is exaggerated or intensified by other past losses. A long preloss pregnancy, a more neurotic personality, more preexisting psychiatric symptoms, and not having other living children are important risk factors for stronger grief reactions (Janssen et al., 1997).

Evidence of complicated grief includes continued obsession with yearning and loneliness, intense and continued guilt or anger, relentless depression or anxiety that interferes with role functioning, abuse of drugs (including prescription medications) or alcohol, severe relationship difficulties, continued feelings of inadequacy and low self-esteem, and suicidal thoughts or threats (Hunfeld, Wladimiroff, & Passchier, 1997). Hunfeld and co-workers (1997) also found that feelings of inadequacy, in particular, were strongly and positively related to distress after 4 years. Such individuals should be referred for counseling. It is the responsibility of a qualified mental health professional to determine whether or not the parent is experiencing a normal, albeit intense grief response or whether they also are having a serious mental health problem such as depression. However, it is important to refer to a therapist or counselor who is experienced in grief counseling and knows how to help the bereaved, because there are therapists and counselors who do not have an understanding of the special needs related to grief.

Therapy is a big step. The highest number of cancellations and "no shows" in a therapist's practice are intakes, or first visits; therefore, anything the nurse can do for a family or individual to help with that major hurdle would be helpful. However, it is also important to remember that people may have symptoms but may not, for whatever reason, be ready to deal directly with these symptoms or may not have the energy to make the call. Enlisting a family member to encourage parents to seek such assistance may be helpful.

 EY POINTS

- Parental and infant attachment can begin before pregnancy with many hopes and dreams for the future.

- The gestational age of the baby influences neither the severity of the grief response nor the bereavement process.

- When a baby or a mother dies, all members of a family are affected, but no two family members grieve in the same way.

- When birth represents death, the role of the nurse is critical in caring for the woman and her family, regardless of the age of the woman or stage of gestation.

- An understanding of the grief process is fundamental in the implementation of the nursing process.

- Assessment of each family member's perception and experience of the loss is important.

- Therapeutic communication and counseling techniques can help families identify their feelings, feel comfortable in expressing their grief, and understand their bereavement process.

- Follow-up after discharge can be an important component in providing care to families who have experienced a loss.

- Nurses need to be aware of their own feelings of grief and loss to provide a nonjudgmental environment of care and support for bereaved families.

CRITICAL THINKING EXERCISES

1 *Identify community resources and support groups for parents who have experienced the following:*
   a. *Infertility*
   b. *Birth of a less than perfect child*
   c. *Death of a baby through miscarriage, stillbirth, or newborn death.*
   What services do each of these resources/groups provide?

2 *Attend a support group meeting. You should ask permission of the group leader before you attend the group.*
   a. *Discuss your reactions to the meeting.*
   b. *Describe the information you identified as useful in understanding the needs of bereaved families.*
   c. *Identify what you learned as useful in providing care to families at the time of their loss.*

3. *Role play a situation in which a family has experienced a newborn death and the nurse is bringing their baby to them.*
   a. *Discuss how it felt to be the nurse.*
   b. *Discuss how it felt to be the parents.*

4 *Prepare a presentation on caring for families experiencing perinatal loss and grief for one of the following groups:*
   a. *Labor and birth nurses*
   b. *Mother and baby nurses*
   c. *Nurses working in antepartum clinic settings*
   d. *Nurses working in home care*
       Give the presentation to your clinical group and ask for constructive criticism from your peers. Use the constructive comments to revise and improve the presentation.

References

Armstrong, D., & Hutti, M. (1998). Pregnancy after perinatal loss: The relationship between anxiety and prenatal attachment. *J Obstet Gynecol Neonatal Nurs* 27, 183-189.

Centers for Disease Control and Prevention. (1998). Maternal mortality–United States, 1982-1996. *MMWR* 47, 705-707.

Cowles, K. (1996). Cultural perspectives of grief: An expanded concept analysis. *J Adv Nurs* 23, 287-294.

Frost, M., & Condon, J. (1996). The psychological sequelae of miscarriage: A critical review of the literature. *Aust N Z J Psychiatry* 30(1), 54-62.

Guyer, B. et al. (1998). Annual summary of vital statistics–1997. *Pediatrics* 102(6), 1333-1347.

Harakas, S. (RHarakas@aol.com). (1999, May 17). E-mail to M. Miles. (mmiles@email.unc.edu).

Hebert, M. (1998). Perinatal bereavement in its cultural context. *Death Studies* 22, 61-78.

Heiman, J., Yankowitz, J., & Wilkins, J. (1997). Grief support programs: Patients' use of services following the loss of a desired pregnancy and degree of implementation in academic centers. *Am J Perinatol* 14, 587-591.

Hunfeld, J., Wladimiroff, J., & Passchier, J. (1997). Prediction and course of grief four years after perinatal loss due to congenital anomalies: A follow-up study. *Br J Med Psychol* 70, 85-91.

Janssen, H. et al. (1997). A prospective study of risk factors predicting grief intensity following pregnancy loss. *Arch Gen Psychiatry* 54, 56-61.

Kavanaugh, K. (1997). Parents' experience surrounding the death of a newborn whose birth is at the margin of viability. *J Obstet Gynecol Neonatal Nurs* 26, 43-51.

Kowalski, K. (1984). Perinatal death: An ethnomethodological study of factors influencing parental bereavement. Doctoral dissertation, University of Colorado.

Lawson, L. (1990). Culturally sensitive support for grieving parents. *MCN Am J Matern Child Nurs* 15, 76-79.

Lindemann, E. (1944). Symptomatology and management of acute grief. *Am J Psychiatry* 101, 141-148.

Lorenzen, J., & Holzgreve, W. (1995). Helping parents to grieve after second trimester termination of pregnancy for fetopathic reasons. *Fetal Diagn Ther* 10(3), 147-156.

Lukse, M., & Vacc, N. (1999). Grief, depression, and coping in women undergoing infertility treatment. *Obstet Gynecol* 93, 245-251.

Miles, M. (1980). *The grief of parents...when a child dies.* Compassionate Friends, Inc., P.O. Box 1347, Oak Brook, IL 60521.

Miles, M. (1984). Helping adults mourn the death of a child. In H. Wass & C. Corr. (Eds.). *Children and death.* Washington, D.C.: Hemisphere Publishing.

Miles, M., & Demi, A. (1986). Guilt in bereaved parents. In T. Rando (Ed.). *Parental loss of a child: Clinical and research considerations.* Champaign, IL: Research Press.

Miles, M., & Demi, A. (1997). Historical and contemporary theories of grief. In I. Corless, B. Germino, & M. Pittman-Lindeman (Eds.). *Dying, death and bereavement.* Boston, MA: Jones & Bartlett.

Mori, E. et al. (1997). Anxiety of infertile women undergoing IVF-ET: Relation to the grief process. *Gynecol Obstet Invest* 44, 157-162.

Osterweis, M., Solomon, F., & Green, M. (Eds.). (1984). *Bereavement: Reactions, consequences, and care.* Washington, D.C.: National Academy Press.

Parkes, C. (1972). *Bereavement: Studies of grief in adult life.* New York: International Universities Press.

Parkes, C. & Weiss, R. (1983). *Recovery from bereavement.* New York: Basic Books.

Pisarska, M., & Carson, S. (1999). Incidence and risk factors for ectopic pregnancy. *Clin Obstet Gynecol* 42(1), 2-8.

Puddifoot, J., & Johnson, M. (1997). The legitimacy of grieving: The partner's experience at miscarriage. *Soc Sci Med* 45, 837-845.

Rand, C. et al. (1998). Parental behavior after perinatal death: Twelve years of observations. *J Psychosomatic Obstet Gynecol* 19, 44-48.

Schaap, A. et al. (1997). Long-term impact of perinatal bereavement: Comparison of grief reactions after intrauterine versus neonatal death. *Eur J Obstet Gynecol Reprod Biol* 74, 161-167.

Swanson-Kauffman, K. (1986). Caring in the instance of unexpected early pregnancy loss. *Top Clin Nurs* 8, 37-46.

Swanson-Kauffman, K. (1988). There should have been two: Nursing care of parents experiencing perinatal death of a twin. *J Perinat Neonatal Nurs* 2, 78-85.

Wallerstedt, C., & Higgins, P. (1996). Facilitating perinatal grieving between the mother and the father. *J Obstet Gynecol Neonatal Nurs* 25, 389-394.

Worden, W. (1991). *Grief counseling and grief therapy: A handbook for the mental health practitioner.* New York: Springer.

Zinaman, M. et al. (1996). Estimates of human fertility and pregnancy loss. *Fertil Steril* 65 (3), 503-509.

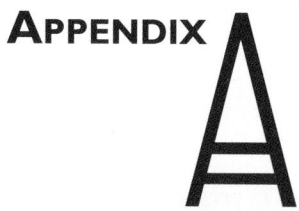
Standard Laboratory Values: Pregnant and Nonpregnant Women

	NONPREGNANT	PREGNANT
HEMATOLOGIC VALUES		
Complete Blood Count (CBC)		
Hemoglobin, g/dl	12 to 16*	>11*
Hematocrit, PCV, %	37 to 47	>33*
Red blood cell (RBC) volume, per ml	1600	1500 to 1900
Plasma volume, per ml	2400	3700
RBC count, million/mm³	4.2 to 5.4	5 to 6.25
White blood cells, total per mm³	5000 to 10,000	5000 to 15,000
Polymorphonuclear cells, %	55 to 70	60 to 85
Lymphocytes, %	20 to 40	15 to 40
Erythrocytes sedimentation rate, mm/hr	20/hr	Elevated second and third trimesters
MCHC, g/dl packed RBCs (mean corpuscular hemoglobin concentration)	32 to 36	No change
MCH (mean corpuscular hemoglobin) per picogram (less than a nanogram)	27 to 31	No change
MCV/μm³ (mean corpuscular volume) per cubic micrometer	80 to 95	No change
Blood Coagulation and Fibrinolytic Activity†		
Factors VII, VIII, IX, X		Increase in pregnancy, return to normal in early puerperium; factor VIII increases during and immediately after birth
Factors XI, XIII		Decrease in pregnancy
Prothrombin time (PT)	11 to 12.5 sec	Slight decrease in pregnancy
Partial thromboplastin time (PTT)	60 to 70 sec	Slight decrease in pregnancy and again decrease during second and third stage of labor (indicates clotting at placental site)
Bleeding time	1 to 9 min (Ivy)	No appreciable change
Coagulation time	6 to 10 min (Lee/White)	No appreciable change
Platelets	150,000 to 400,000/mm³	No significant change until 3 to 5 days after birth and then a rapid increase (may predispose woman to thrombosis) and gradual return to normal

	NONPREGNANT	PREGNANT
HEMATOLOGIC VALUES—cont'd		
Blood Coagulation and Fibrinolytic Activity†—cont'd		
Fibrinolytic activity		Decreases in pregnancy and then abrupt return to normal (protection against thromboembolism)
Fibrinogen	200 to 400 mg/dl	Increased levels late in pregnancy
Mineral/Vitamin Concentrations		
Vitamin B_{12}, folic acid, ascorbic acid	Normal	Moderate decrease
Serum proteins		
Total, g/dl	6.4 to 8.3	5.5 to 7.5
Albumin, g/dl	3.5 to 5.0	Slight increase
Globulin, total, g/dl	2.3 to 3.4	3 to 4
Blood glucose		
Fasting, mg/dl	70 to 105	Decreases
2-hour postprandial, mg/dl	<140	Under 140 after a 100 g carbohydrate meal is considered normal
HEPATIC VALUES		
Bilirubin total	Not more than 1 mg/dl	Unchanged
Serum cholesterol	120 to 200 mg/dl	Increases from 16 to 32 weeks of pregnancy; remains at this level until after birth
Serum alkaline phosphatase	42 to 128 U/L	Increases from week 12 of pregnancy to 6 weeks after birth
Serum globulin albumin	2.3 to 3.4 g/dl	Slight increase
RENAL VALUES		
Bladder capacity	1300 ml	1500 ml
Renal plasma flow (RPF), ml/min	490 to 700	Increases by 25%
Glomerular filtration rate (GFR), ml/min	88 to 128	Increases by 50%
Nonprotein nitrogen (NPN), mg/dl	25 to 40	Decreases
Blood urea nitrogen (BUN), mg/dl	10 to 20	Decreases
Serum creatinine, mg/dl	0.5 to 1.1	Decreases
Serum uric acid, mg/dl	2.0 to 6.6	Decreases
Urine glucose	Negative	Present in 20% of pregnant women
Intravenous pyelogram (IVP)	Normal	Slight-to-moderate hydroureter and hydronephrosis; right kidney larger than left kidney

From Pagana, K., & Pagana, T. (1997). *Mosby's diagnostic and laboratory test reference* (3rd ed.). St Louis: Mosby.
*At sea level. Permanent residents of higher levels (e.g., Denver) require higher levels of hemoglobin.
†Pregnancy represents a hypercoagulable state.

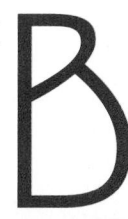
Standard Laboratory Values in the Neonatal Period

	NEONATAL
1. HEMATOLOGIC VALUES	
Clotting factors	
Activated clotting time (ACT)	2 min
Bleeding time (Ivy)	2 to 7 min
Clot retraction	Complete 1 to 4 hr
Fibrinogen	125 to 300 mg/dl*

	TERM	PRETERM
Hemoglobin (g/dl)	14.5 to 22.5	15 to 17
Hematocrit (%)	44 to 72	45 to 55
Reticulocytes (%)	0.4 to 6	Up to 10
Fetal hemoglobin (% of total)	40 to 70	80 to 90
Red blood cells (RBCs)/mm³	4.0^6 to 6.0^6	
Platelet count/mm³	84,000 to 478,000	120,000 to 180,000
White blood cells (WBCs)/mm³	9000 to 30,000	10,000 to 20,000
Neutrophils (%)	54 to 62	47
Eosinophils and basophils (%)	1 to 3	
Lymphocytes (%)	25 to 33	33
Monocytes (%)	3 to 7	4
Immature WBC (%)	10	16

*dl refers to deciliter (1 dl = 100 ml); this conforms to the SI system (standardized international measurements).

			NEONATAL
2. BIOCHEMICAL VALUES			
Bilirubin, direct			0 to 1 mg/dl
Bilirubin, total	Cord:		<2 mg/dl
	Peripheral blood:	0 to 1 day	6 mg/dl
		1 to 2 days	8 mg/dl
		3 to 5 days	12 mg/dl
Blood gases		Arterial:	pH 7.31 to 7.45
			Pco_2 33 to 48 mm Hg
			Po_2 50 to 70 mm Hg
		Venous:	pH 7.28 to 7.42
			Pco_2 38 to 52 mm Hg
			Po_2 20 to 49 mm Hg
α_1-Fetoprotein			0
Fibrinogen			150 to 300 mg/dl
Serum glucose			40 to 60 mg/dl

NEONATAL

3. URINALYSIS

Color	Clear, straw
Specific gravity	1.001 to 1.018
pH	5 to 7
Protein	Negative
Glucose	Negative
Ketones	Negative
RBCs	Rare
WBCs	0 to 4
Casts	Rare
17-Ketosteroids	Under 1
17-Hydroxycorticosteroids	Same
Urinary calcium	5 mg/kg of body weight
Urinary sodium	20% of adult values
Urinary vanillylmandelic acid (VMA)	<1.0 mg/24 hr

Volume: 20 to 40 ml excreted daily in the first few days; by week 1, 24-hr urine volume close to 200 ml
Protein: may be present in first 2 to 4 days
Osmolarity (mOsm/L): 100 to 600

4. URINE SCREENING TESTS FOR INBORN ERRORS OF METABOLISM

Benedict's test: for reducing substances in the urine—glucose, galactose, fructose, lactose; phenylketonuria (PKU), alkaptonuria, tyrosyluria, and tyrosinosis may give a positive Benedict's test result.
Ferric chloride test: an immediate green color for PKU, histidinemia, and tyrosinuria; a gray to green color for presence of phenothiazines, isoniazid; red to purple color for presence of salicylates or ketone bodies.
Dinitrophenylhydrazine test: for PKU, maple syrup urine disease, Lowe's syndrome.
Cetyltrimethylammonium bromide test: for mucopolysaccharides: immediate positive reaction in gargoylism (Hurler syndrome); delayed, moderately positive reaction for Marfan, Morquio-Ullrich, and Murdoch syndromes.
Metachromatic stain (or urine sediment): granules (free or as inclusion bodies in cells) are seen in metachromatic leukodystrophy; may also be seen rarely in Tay-Sachs and other lipid diseases of central nervous system.
Amino acid chromatography: aminoaciduria may be normal in newborns; chromatography may be helpful to detect hypophosphatasia and argininosuccinicaciduria.
Diaper test, Phenistix test, and Dinitrophenylhydrazine (DNPH) test: simple, inexpensive tests for PKU; used for screening; most useful when infant is at least 6 weeks of age.

5. BLOOD SERUM PHENYLALANINE TESTS

Guthrie inhibition assay methods: drops of blood placed on filter paper; laboratory uses bacterial growth inhibition test; phenylalanine level above 8 mg/dl blood: diagnostic of PKU. Effective in newborn period; used also to monitor PKU diet; blood easily obtained by heel or finger puncture; inexpensive; used for wide-scale screening.

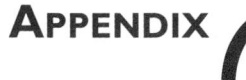

Relationship of Drugs to Breast Milk and Effect on Infant

The drugs listed in this appendix have been categorized by their major use. The ratings given are those published by the American Academy of Pediatrics (AAP) Committee on Drugs. These ratings label drugs that transfer into human milk. Drugs without a rating were not included in the AAP list. The ratings are described as follows:

1. Drugs that are contraindicated during breastfeeding
2. Drugs of abuse that are contraindicated during breastfeeding
3. Radioactive compounds that require temporary cessation of breastfeeding
4. Drugs with unknown effects on breastfeeding but may be of concern
5. Drugs that have been associated with significant effects on some breastfeeding infants and should be given to breastfeeding mothers with caution
6. Maternal medication usually compatible with breastfeeding
7. Food and environmental agents: effect on breastfeeding

DRUG	EXCRETED IN MILK	% ADULT DOSE IN MILK	AAP RATING	COMMENTS
ANALGESICS AND ANTIINFLAMMATORY DRUGS (NONNARCOTIC)				
Acetaminophen (Datril, Tylenol)	Yes	0.04 to 1.85	6	Detoxified in liver. Avoid in immediate postbirth period; otherwise no problems with therapeutic dose.
Aspirin (Bayer, Anacin, Bufferin, Excedrin, etc.)	Yes	10.55 ± 10.45	6	Long history of experience shows complications rare. Can cause interference with platelet aggregation and diminished factor XII (Hageman factor) at birth. When mother requires high, continuing level of medication for arthritis, aspirin is drug of choice. Observe infant for bruisability. Platelet aggregation can be evaluated. Salicylism seen only in maternal overdosing. Mother should increase vitamin C and vitamin K intake.
Ibuprofen (Advil, Nuprin, Motrin, etc.)	Yes	<0.8	6	No apparent effects in therapeutic doses.
Indomethacin (Indocin)	Yes	0.11 to 0.98	6	Convulsions in breastfed neonate (case report). Used to close patent ductus arteriosus. Insufficient data as to effect on other vessels. May be nephrotoxic.

DRUG	EXCRETED IN MILK	% ADULT DOSE IN MILK	AAP RATING	COMMENTS
ANALGESICS AND ANTIINFLAMMATORY DRUGS (NONNARCOTIC)—cont'd				
Mefenamic acid (Ponstel)	Yes	0.036 to 0.8	6	No apparent effect on infant at therapeutic doses; infant able to excrete via urine.
Naproxen (Naproxyn, Anaprox, Naprosyn, Aleve)	Yes	1.1		Less toxic in adults than some other organic derivatives.
Propoxyphene (Darvon)	Yes	Trace amounts	6	Only symptoms detectable would be failure to feed and drowsiness. On daily, around-the-clock dosage, infant could consume 1 mg/day.
ANTIINFECTIVES (May change intestinal flora of infant and sensitize for later allergic reaction)				
Acyclovir (Zovirax)	Yes	5.6 ±4.4	6	Minimal absorption through maternal skin.
Ampicillin (Polycillin, Amcill, Omnipen, Penbritin)	Yes	0.05 to 0.04		Sensitivity resulting from repeated exposure; diarrhea or secondary candidiasis.
Carbenicillin (Pyopen, Geopen)	Yes	0.001		Levels not significant. Drug is given to neonate. Not well absorbed from gastrointestinal (GI) tract.
Cefazolin (Ancef, Kefzol)	Yes	0.075	6	Probably not significant. Detected in milk if given intravenously (IV).
Cephalexin (Keflex)	Yes	0.86 ±0.35		Completely gone by 8 hours; absorption less in first few months.
Cephalothin (Keflin)	Yes	0.4		Negligible.
Chloramphenicol (Chloromycetin)	Yes	1.6	4	Gray syndrome. Infant does not excrete drug well, and small amounts may accumulate. Contraindicated. May be tolerated in older infant with mature glycuronide system.
Colistin (Colymycin)	Yes	0.07		Not absorbed orally.
Demeclocycline (Declomycin)	Yes	Trace		Not significant in therapeutic doses. Can be given to infants. Drug remains in milk 3 days after dose.
Erythromycin (Ilosone, E-Mycin, Erythrocin)	Yes	0.1 to 2.1	6	Higher concentrations have been reported in milk than in plasma. Should not be given under 1 month of age because of risk of jaundice. Dose in milk higher when given IV to mother.
Gentamicin	Yes			Not absorbed from GI tract, may change gut flora. Drug is given to newborns directly.
Isoniazid (Nydrazid)	Yes	2.3		Infant at risk for toxicity, but need for breast milk may outweigh risk.
Kanamycin (Kantrex)	Yes	0.95	6	Infant absorbs little from GI tract. Infants can be given drug.
Metronidazole (Flagyl)	Yes	0.13 to 36	4	Caution should be exercised because of its high milk concentrations. Contraindicated when infant under 6 months; may cause neurologic disorders and blood dyscrasia. AAP says to discard milk for 12 hours if mother takes 2-g dose.

ANTIINFECTIVES—cont'd

Nitrofurantoin (Furadantin, Macrodantin)	Yes	0.6	6	No significant effect in therapeutic doses except in infant with G6PD deficiency.
Novobiocin (Albamycin, Cathomycin)	Yes	0.15		Infant can be given drug directly.
Nystatin (Mycostatin)	No	Not absorbed orally		Can be given to infant directly.
Oxacillin (Prostaphlin)	No	Trace		
Penicillin G, benzathine (Bicillin)	Yes	0.8		Clinical need should supersede possible allergic responses.
Penicillin G, potassium	Yes	0.8		Infant can be given penicillin directly. Parents should be told to inform physician that infant has been exposed to penicillin because of potential sensitivity.
Streptomycin	Yes	0.5	6	Not to be given more than 2 weeks. Ototoxic and nephrotoxic with long use. Is given to infants directly.
Sulfisoxazole (Gantrisin)	Yes	0.45	6	To be avoided during first month after birth; may cause kernicterus.
Tetracycline HCl (Achromycin, Panmycin, Sumycin)	Yes	0.3 to 4.8	6	Not enough to treat an infection in an infant. May cause discoloration of the teeth in the infant; the antibiotic, however, may be largely bound to the milk calcium. Do not give longer than 10 days or repeatedly.

ANTICOAGULANTS

Coumarin derivatives Dicumarol (bishydroxy-coumarin), warfarin (Panwarfin)	Yes	6.5	6	Monitor prothrombin time. Give vitamin K to infant. Discontinue if surgery or trauma occurs. Drug of choice if mother to continue breastfeeding. May cause bleeding.
Heparin	No			Heparin ineffective orally.

ANTICONVULSANTS AND SEDATIVES (Barbiturates may pass into milk but do not sedate infant)

Magnesium sulfate	Yes	0.5	6	May produce sedation in infant.
Pentobarbital (Nembutal)	Yes	Traces		Depends on liver for detoxification so may accumulate in first week of life until infant is able to detoxify. No problem for older infant in usual doses.
Phenytoin (Dilantin)	Yes	1.4 to 7.2	6	No problem if mother's dose is in therapeutic range.
Phenobarbital (Luminal)	Yes	1.5		Sleepiness and decreased sucking possible. On usual analeptic doses, infants alert and feed well. On hypnotic doses, infants depressed and difficult to rouse.
Sodium bromide (Bromo-Seltzer and over-the-counter sleeping aids)	Yes	6, 7		Drowsy, decreased crying, rash, decreased feeding. No longer available in the United States.

ANTIHISTAMINES (May suppress lactation; administer after nursing; all pass into breast milk)

Brompheniramine (Dimetane)	Yes	Unknown		Drugs used in neonates. May cause sedation or decreased feeding, or may produce stimulation and tachycardia. Should avoid long-acting preparations, which may accumulate in infant.
Diphenhydramine (Benadryl)	Yes	Unknown		When combined with decongestants, may cause decrease in milk.
Promethazine (Phenergan)	Yes	Unknown	6	Passage into breast is expected; increases serum prolactin levels.

AUTONOMIC DRUGS

Atrophine sulfate*	Yes	Traces	6	Hyperthermia, atropine toxicity, infants especially sensitive; also inhibits lactation. Infant dose 0.01 mg/kg.
Ergotamine	Yes	Unknown	1	May inhibit lactation.
Neostigmine	No	No known harm to infant		
Propantheline bromide (Pro-Banthine)	No	Uncontrolled data indicate no measurable levels		Drug rapidly metabolized in maternal system to inactive metabolite. Mother should avoid long-acting preparations, however.

CARDIOVASCULAR DRUGS

Diazoxide (Hyperstat)				Arteriolar dilators and antihypertensive, given only IV, not active orally.
Digoxin	Yes	0.07 to 14	6	Not detected in infant's plasma.
Hydralazine (Apresoline)	Yes	0.8	6	Jaundice, thrombocytopenia, electrolyte disturbances possible.
Methyldopa (Aldomet)	Yes	0.02 to 0.09		Galactorrhea. No specific data except as affects mother's milk production.
Propranolol (Inderal)	Yes	Traces		Risk of effect almost nonexistent.
Quinidine	Yes	4.1	6	Arrhythmia may occur.

CATHARTICS

Cascara	Yes	Low	6	Causes colic and diarrhea in infant.
Milk of magnesia	No	None	6	No effect.
Mineral oil	No	None	6	No effect.
Phenolphthalein	Unknown	Unknown	6	Reported to cause symptoms in some.
Rhubarb	Unknown	None	6	None in syrup form. Fresh rhubarb may give symptoms of colic and diarrhea.
Saline cathartics	No	None	6	No effect.
Senna	No	None	6	None
Stool softeners and bulk-forming laxatives	No	None	6	No effect.
Suppositories (for constipation)	No	None	6	Not absorbed.

DIURETICS

Furosemide (sulfamoylan-thranilic acid) (Lasix)	Possible	Not found in all samples		Drug is given to children under medical management.
Spironolactone (Aldactone)	Yes	Canrenone, a metabolite, appears	6	Acts as antagonist of aldosterone; causes sodium excretion and potassium retention. The metabolite apparently has some activity.

*An ingredient in many prescription and nonprescription drugs.

DIURETICS—cont'd

Thiazides (Diuril, Enduron, Esidrix, HydroDiuril, Oretic, Thiuretic tablets)	Yes	0.25 to 0.43	6	Risk of dehydration and electrolyte imbalance, especially sodium loss, which would require monitoring. Watch weight and wet diapers and take an occasional specific gravity reading of urine and serum sodium to indicate status of infant. Risk, however, is extremely low. May suppress lactation because of dehydration in mother.

HORMONES AND CONTRACEPTIVES

Contraceptives (oral) Ethinyl estradiol, mestranol, 19-nortestosterone, norethindrone (Norlutin)	Yes	0.16 ±0.14	6	May diminish milk supply. May decrease vitamins, protein, and fat in milk. Most significant concern is long-range influence of hormone on young infant, which is not certain. Reports of feminization of infant.
Corticotropin	Yes	1.1	6	May decrease quantity and quality of milk.
Cortisone	Yes	Significant amounts		May affect infant in therapeutic doses.
Epinephrine (Adrenalin)	Yes			Destroyed in GI tract of infant.
Estrogen	Yes	0.1	6	Risks as with oral contraceptives. May alter quality and quantity of milk.
Insulin	No			Destroyed in intestinal tract.
Medroxyprogesterone acetate (Provera)	Yes	0.86 to 5	6	6-month injection may affect milk supply; 3-month injection should not decrease supply.
Prednisone	Yes	0.06 to 3.6	6	Minimum amount not likely to cause effect on infant in short course.
Tolbutamide (Orinase)	Yes	18	6	Watch for jaundice.

NARCOTICS

Cocaine	Yes	Significant levels in milk	1, 2	No metabolites or drug found in milk after 36 hours or in infant's urine after 60 hours.
Codeine	Yes	5 ±2	6	No effect in therapeutic level and transient use. Can accumulate. Individual variation. Watch for neonatal depression. Asians metabolize drug less than Caucasians do.
Heroin	Yes		2	Level in milk enough to cause addiction in infant.
Marijuana (Cannabis sativa L.)	Yes		2	Shown in laboratory animals to produce structural changes in nursling's brain cells; impairs DNA and RNA formation. Infant at risk of inhaling smoke during feeding or when held by person who is smoking.
Meperidine (Demerol)	Yes	Trace		Trace amounts may accumulate if drug taken around the clock when infant is neonate. Watch for drowsiness and poor feeding.

NARCOTICS—cont'd

Methadone	Yes	2.2	6	When dosage not excessive, infant can be breastfed if monitored for evidence of depression and failure to thrive. Suggest mother take daily dose after evening feeding and supplement formula at next feeding.
Morphine	Yes	0.8 to 1.2	6	Single doses have minimum effect. Potential for accumulation. May be addicting to neonate. Amounts in breast milk too variable to consider breastfeeding as means of treating withdrawal symptoms.
Percodan (oxycodone [derived from opiate thebaine], aspirin, phenacetin, caffeine)	Yes	Unknown		Consider for its component parts. In neonatal period, sleepiness and failure to feed, which increase maternal engorgement and neonatal weight loss, have been observed, probably caused by oxycodone.

PSYCHOTROPIC AND MOOD-CHANGING DRUGS

Alcohol (Ethanol)	Yes	1 to 19.5	6	Milk may smell like alcohol. Ethanol in doses of 1 to 2 g/kg to mother causes depression of milk-ejection reflex (dose dependent). No acetaldehyde found because infant cannot metabolize ethanol.
Amphetamine	Yes	6.1 ±0.1	2	Has caused stimulation in infants with jitteriness, irritability, sleeplessness. Long-acting preparations cumulative.
Benzodiazepines* Chlordiazepoxide (Librium)	Yes			Not sufficient to affect infant first week when glucuronyl system needed for detoxification. May accumulate. May cause jaundice. Older infant, no apparent problem.
Diazepam (Valium)	Yes	2 to 4.7	4	Detoxified in glucuronyl system. In first weeks of life may contribute to jaundice. Metabolite active. Effect on infant: hypoventilation, drowsiness, lethargy, weight loss. Single doses over 10 mg contraindicated during breastfeeding. Accumulation in infant possible.
Haloperidol (Haldol)	Yes	0.15 to 2	4	An antipsychotic: animal studies in nurslings show behavior abnormalities.
Lithium carbonate (Eskalith, Lithane, Lithonate)	Yes	1.8		Measurable lithium in infant's serum. Infant kidney can clear lithium; however, lithium inhibits adenosine 3′,5′-cyclic monophosphate, significant for brain growth. Also affects amine metabolism. Report of cyanosis and poor muscle tone and ECG changes in nursing infant.
Meprobamate (Miltown, Equanil)	Yes	2 to 4 times maternal plasma level		If therapy continued, infant should be followed closely.

*Alcohol enhances the effects of these drugs.

PSYCHOTROPIC AND MOOD-CHANGING DRUGS—cont'd

Drug	In milk	Ratio	Ref	Comments
Phencyclidine (PCP)	Yes		I	Animal studies show PCP in milk even after drug has been discontinued for 40 days.
Phenothiazines				
Chlorpromazine (Thorazine)	Yes	0.07 to 0.2		Drowsiness and lethargy in infants.
Thioridazine (Mellaril)	Yes	No information		Thioridazine is less potent in general than other phenothiazines. Probably safe.
Trifluoperazine (Stelazine)	Yes	Minimum		
Tricyclic antidepressants				Apparently no accumulation. No infants who have been observed showed symptoms.
Amitriptyline (Elavil)	Yes	0.8 ±0.2	4	Watch for depression or failure to feed; increases maternal prolactin secretion.
Desipramine (Norpramin, Pertofrane)		I	4	
Imipramine (Tofranil)	Yes	0.1	4	

STIMULANTS

Drug	In milk	Ratio	Ref	Comments
Caffeine	Yes	0.66 to 10	6	Accumulates when intake moderate and continual. Causes jitteriness, wakefulness, and irritability. Caffeine present in many hot and cold drinks. Consider if infant very wakeful.
Theobromine	Yes	20	7	No adverse symptoms observed in the infants. Chocolate the most common cause of exposure.
Theophylline	Yes	<I to 15	6	Irritability, fretfulness.

THYROID AND ANTITHYROID MEDICATIONS

Drug	In milk	Ratio	Ref	Comments
Thiouracil	Yes	0.3 to 2.6	6	Get baseline levels of T_3, T_4, and TSH before and 6 weeks after mother starts medication.
Thyroid and thyroxine	Yes	0.3 to 2.6	6	Does not produce adverse symptoms on long-range follow-up study. Noted to improve milk supply of hypothyroid mothers. No contraindication.

MISCELLANEOUS

Drug	In milk	Ratio	Ref	Comments
DPT	Yes	Minimum		Does not interfere with immunization schedule.
Methotrexate	Yes	0.93	I	Antimetabolite. Infant would receive 0.26 g/dl, which researchers consider nontoxic for infant.
Nicotine	Yes		2	Decreases milk production. Smoking may interfere with let-down reflex if smoking started before onset of a feeding. Smoke exposure may be a concern.
Poliovirus vaccine	No			Live vaccine taken orally. Not necessary to withhold breastfeeding 30 minutes before and after dose. Provide booster after infant no longer breastfeeding.

MISCELLANEOUS—cont'd

Rh antibodies	Yes		Destroyed in GI tract; not effective orally.
Rubella virus vaccine	Yes	Minimum	Will not confer passive immunity. Mother should not be given vaccine when at risk for pregnancy.
Tuberculin test	No		Tuberculin-sensitive mothers can adaptively immunize their infants through breast milk, and that immunity may last several years.
Chest x-rays			No effect.

Compiled from Lawrence, R. (1999). *Breastfeeding: A guide for the medical profession* (5th ed.). St. Louis: Mosby; The Committee on Drugs, American Academy of Pediatrics. (1994). The transfer of drugs and other chemicals into human breast milk. *Pediatrics* 93(1), 137-150.

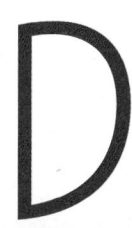
Resources

This appendix includes community and national resources, national clearinghouses, journals, and nursing organizations of interest to maternity and women's health nurses.

COMMUNITY AND NATIONAL RESOURCES

Academy for Guided Imagery
P.O. Box 2070
Mill Valley, CA 94942
(800) 726-2070
http://www.healthy.net/agi/

AIDS Network Hotline
(800) 342-2437 (AIDS)

AIDS Resource List
http://www.hivnet.org/aidsres.html

American Academy of Husband-Coached Childbirth
P.O. Box 5224
Sherman Oaks, CA 91413
(800) 422-4784

American Academy of Pediatrics
141 Northwest Point Blvd.
Elk Grove, IL 60007-1098
(847) 228-5005
http://www.aap.org

American Association of Acupuncturists and Oriental Medicine
4104 Lake Boone Trail, Suite 201
Raleigh, NC 27607-6518
(919) 787-5181

American Cancer Society
1599 Clifton Rd., NE
Atlanta, GA 30329
(800) ACS-2345
http://www.cancer.org

American Cleft Palate Association
1218 Grandview Ave.
Pittsburgh, PA 15211
(412) 681-1376
(800) 24-CLEFT

American College of Obstetricians and Gynecologists
409 12th St., SW
Washington, DC 20024
(800) 762-2264
http://www.acog.com

American Diabetes Association
Diabetes Information Service Center
1660 Duke St.
Alexandria, VA 22314
(800) 342-2383
http://www.diabetes.org

American Fertility Foundation
2131 Magnolia Ave., Suite 201
Birmingham, AL 35256
(205) 251-9764

American Heart Association
Women's heart information: 1-888-MYHEART
(1-888-694-3278)
(800) 242-8721
http://www.americanheart.org

American Red Cross
430 17th St., NW
Washington, DC 20006
(202) 737-8300
http://www.redcross.org

American Society for Reproductive Medicine
1209 Montgomery Hwy.
Birmingham, AL 35316
(205) 978-5000
http://www.asrm.com

Anorexia Nervosa and Related Eating Disorders Inc.
http://www.amred.com

Association for Childbirth at Home, International
P.O. Box 39498
Los Angeles, CA 90039
(213) 667-0839

Association of Maternal and Child Health Programs
1220 19th St., NW, Suite 801
Washington, DC 20036
(202) 775-0436
http://www.amchp.org

Baby Center
(Source for expectant parents)
http://www.babycenter.com

Bereavement Services/RTS
Lutheran Hospital–La Crosse
1910 South Ave.
La Crosse, WI 54601
(608) 791-4747
(800) 362-9567

Cancernet
http://www.cancernet.nei.nih.gov

CDC National Prevention Information Network
http://www.cdcnpin.org

Center for Sickle Cell Disease
2121 Georgia Ave., NW
Washington, DC 20059
(202) 636-7930

Centers for Disease Control and Prevention
1600 Clifton Rd., NE
Atlanta, GA 30333
(404) 329-1819
(404) 329-3286
http://www.cdc.gov

Childbirth Graphics
P.O. Box 21207
Waco, TX 76702
(800) 229-3366

Compassionate Friends
(Following death of an infant)
P.O. Box 1347
Oak Brook, IL 60521
(312) 990-0010

COPE (Coping with the Overall Pregnancy/Parenting Experience)
37 Clarendon St.
Boston, MA 02116
(617) 357-5588

C/SEC, Inc. (Cesarean/Support Education and Concern)
22 Forest Rd.
Framingham, MA 01701
(508) 877-8266

Doulas of North America (DONA)
1100 23rd Ave. East
Seattle, WA 98112
(206) 324-5440
http://www.dona.com

Endometriosis Association
8585 North 76th Place
Milwaukee, WI 53223
(414) 355-2200
(800) 992-3636
http://www.ivf.com/endohtml.html

Environmental Protection Agency (EPA)
Public Information Center
Room PM 211-B
401 M St., SW
Washington, DC 20460
(202) 382-7550
http://www.epa.gov

Gynecologic Cancer Foundation
http://www.sgo.org/gcf

Harvard Eating Disorders Center
356 Boylston St.
Boston, MA 02166
(888) 236-1188
http://www.hedc.org

Healing Touch International, Inc.
12477 W. Cedar Drive, Suite 202
Lakewood, CO 80228
(303) 989-7982
http://www.healingtouch.net

Health Web: Evidence Based Health Care
http://www.uic.edu/depts/lib/health/hw/ebhc

Healthy Mothers, Healthy Babies Coalition
409 12th St., SW
Washington, DC 20024
(202) 863-2458

Human Genome Project and ELSI (Ethical, Legal, and Social Implications in Genetics)
http://www.nhgri.nih.gov

Hysterectomy Educational Resource and Services (HERS)
422 Byrn Mawr Ave.
Bala Cynwyd, PA 19004
(215) 667-7757
http://www.ccon.com/hers

Institute for Women's Policy Research
1400 20th St., NW, Suite 104
Washington, DC 20036
(202) 785-5100
http://www.iwpr.org

International Association of Infant Massage
http://www.infantmassage.com

International Childbirth Education Association (ICEA)
P.O. Box 20048
Minneapolis, MN 55420
(612) 854-8660
http://www.icea.org

International Lactation Consultant Association
201 Brown Ave.
Evanston, IL 60202-3601
(708) 260-8874

Lact-Aid
(Provides information and services to promote breastfeeding)
P.O. Box 1066
Athens, TN 37303
(614) 744-9090

La Leche League
1400 N. Meacham Rd.
Schaumburg, IL 60173
(800) 525-3243 (24-hour line)
http://www.lalecheleague.org

Lamaze International
1200 19th St., NW, Suite 300
Washington, DC 20036-2422
(800) 368-4404
(202) 857-1128
http://www.lamaze-childbirth.com

March of Dimes Birth Defects Foundation
National Foundation/March of Dimes
1275 Mamaroneck Ave.
White Plains, NY 10605
(914) 428-7100
(888) 663-4637 (MODIMES)
http://www.modimes.org

Maternity Center Association, Inc.
281 Park Ave. South, 5th Floor
New York, NY 10010
(212) 777-5000

Mining Company Guide to Pregnancy and Birth
http://pregnancy/miningco.com

National Abortion Federation Consumer Hotline
1156 15th St., NW, Suite 700
Washington, DC 20005
(800) 772-9100

National Alliance of Breast Cancer Organizations
9 East 37th St., 10th Floor
New York, NY 10016
(800) 719-0154
http://www.nabco.org

National Association for Sickle Cell Disease
3345 Wilshire Blvd., Suite 1106
Los Angeles, CA 90010-1880
(213) 736-5455
(800) 421-8453

National Association of Childbearing Centers
3123 Gottschall Rd.
Perkiomenville, PA 18074
(215) 234-8068

National Association of Parents and Professionals for Safe Alternatives in Childbirth (NAPSAC)
P.O. Box 267
Marble Hill, MO 63764
(314) 238-2010

National Breast Cancer Coalition
P.O. Box 66373
Washington, DC 20035
(202) 296-7477
(800) 935-0434

National Cancer Institute Cancer Information Service
(800) 4-CANCER
http://www.nci.nih.gov

National Center for Complementary and Alternative Medicine (NCCAM)
P.O. Box 8218
Silver Spring, MD 20907-8218
(888) 644-6226
http://altmed.od.nih.gov/nccam/

National Cervical Cancer Coalition
http://www.nccc-online.org

National Coalition Against Sexual Assault
912 North 2nd St.
Harrisburg, PA 17102
(717) 232-6771

National Coalition of Feminist and Lesbian Cancer Projects
P.O. Box 90437
Washington, DC 20090
(202) 332-5536

National Coalition of Hispanic Health and Human Services Organizations (COSSMHO)
1030 15th St., NW, Suite 1053
Washington, DC 20005
(202) 387-5000
http://www.cossmho.org

National Council of Women's Organizations
Women's Health
1126 16th St., NW, Suite 411
Washington, DC 20036
(202) 331-7343
http://womensorganizations.org/healthtopic_toc.cfm

National Domestic Violence and Abuse Hotline
(800) 799-SAFE

National Down Syndrome Congress
1800 Dempster St.
Park Ridge, IL 60068-1146
(708) 823-7550
(800) 232-6372

National Down Syndrome Society Hotline
666 Broadway
New York, NY 10012
(800) 221-4602

National Foundation for Jewish Genetic Diseases, Inc.
250 Park Ave., Suite 1000
New York, NY 10177
(212) 371-1030

National Institute of Child Health and Human Development (NICHD)
National Institutes of Health
9000 Rockville Pike
Bldg. 31, Room 2A32
Bethesda, MD 20892
(301) 496-4000
http://www.nih.gov

National Institutes of Health Information Page
http://www.nih.gov/health

National Organization of Mothers of Twins Clubs, Inc.
P.O. Box 23188
Albuquerque, NM 87192
(505) 275-0955

National Organization on Adolescent Pregnancy, Parenting, and Prevention
2401 Pennsylvania Ave., Suite 350
Washington, DC 20037
(202) 293-8370
http://www.noappp.org

National Organization for Women (NOW) Legal Defense and Education Fund
99 Hudson St.
New York, NY 10013-2871
(212) 925-6635

National Osteoporosis Foundation
1150 17th St., NW, Suite 500
Washington, DC 20036
(800) 223-9994
http://www.nof.org

National Ovarian Cancer Coalition
2335 East Atlantic Blvd., #401
Pompano Beach, FL 33062
(888) 682-7426
http://ww.ovarian.org

National Perinatal Association
101½ South Union St.
Alexandria, VA 22314-3323
(703) 549-5523

National Resource Center for Domestic Violence
(800) 537-2238

National Right to Life Committee
419 7th St., NW, Suite 500
Washington, DC 20004
(202) 626-8800

National Sexually Transmitted Diseases Hotline
(800) 227-8922

National Sudden Infant Death Syndrome Foundation
10500 Little Patuxent Parkway, Suite 420
Columbia, MD 21044
(301) 964-8000
(800) 221-7437

National Women's Health Resource Center
120 Albany St., Suite 820
New Brunswick, NJ 08901
(877) 986-9472
http://www.healthywomen.org

New York Times on the Web Women's Health
http://www.nytimes.com/specials/women/whome/index.html

Office of Minority Health Resource Center
P.O. Box 37337
Washington, DC 20013-7337
(301) 587-1938

Parent Care, Inc.
(Neonatal intensive care unit family support)
101½ South Union
Alexandria, VA 22314-3323
(703) 836-4678

Parenthood After Thirty
451 Vermont
Berkeley, CA 94707
(415) 524-6635

Parents of Prematures
13613 NE 26th Place
Bellevue, WA 98005
(206) 883-6040

Parents Without Partners
8807 Colesville Rd.
Silver Spring, MD 20910
(301) 588-9354
(800) 637-7974

Planned Parenthood Federation of America, Inc.
810 Seventh Ave.
New York, NY 10019
(800) 230-PLAN
http://www.plannedparenthood.org

Pregnancy and Infant Loss
1421 East Wayzata Blvd., Suite 40
Wayzata, MN 55391
(614) 473-9372

Premenstrual Syndrome Action

P.O. Box 16292
Irving, CA 92713
(714) 854-4407

Reach to Recovery
(*see* American Cancer Society)
(breast cancer)

Read Natural Childbirth Foundation
P.O. Box 956
San Rafael, CA 94915
(415) 456-8462

Resolve, Inc.
(Impaired fertility)
1310 Broadway, Dept. GM
Summerville, MA 02144-1713
(617) 623-0744
(888) 299-1585
http://www.resolve.org

Sex Information and Education Council of the United States
(Provides publications [e.g., "Sexual relations in pregnancy and postpartum"] and teaching aids)
130 W. 42nd St., Suite 350
New York, NY 10036
http://www.siecus.org

Society for Women's Health Research
1828 L St., NW, Suite 625
Washington, DC 20036
(202) 223-8224
http://www.womens-health.org

Soy Protein Council
(202) 467-6610
http://spcouncil.com

Special Supplemental Nutrition Program for Women, Infants, and Children (WIC)
Food and Consumer Service
3101 Park Center Dr., Room 819
Alexandria, VA 22302
(703) 305-2286
http://www.usda.gov/fns/wic.html

Spina Bifida Association of America
4590 McArthur Blvd., NW, Suite 250
Washington, DC 20007-4226
(800) 621-3141

Susan G. Koman Breast Cancer Foundation
(800) 462-9273

The Touch Research Institute
http://www.miami.edu/touch-research/home.html

NATIONAL CLEARINGHOUSES

Breastfeeding Resources
http://www.parentsplace.com/expert/lactation/

Food and Drug Administration (FDA)
Office of Consumer Affairs
Public Inquiries
5600 Fishers Lane (HFE-88)
Rockville, MD 20857
(301) 443-3170
http://www.fda.gov

Infertility Resources
http://www.ihr.com/infertility/index.html

International Council on Infertility Information Dissemination
(703) 379-9178
http://www.inciid.org

National AIDS Information Clearinghouse
P.O. Box 6003
Rockville, MD 20849-6003
(800) 458-5231 (English and Spanish)

National Clearinghouse for Alcohol and Drug Abuse Information
P.O. Box 426
Dept DQ
Kensington, MD 20795
(800) 729-6686
http://www.health.org

National Clearinghouse for Family Planning Information
P.O. Box 10716
Rockville, MD 20850
(703) 558-4990

National Clearinghouse for Human Genetic Disease
(Provides information about inherited diseases)
National Center for Education in Maternal and Child Health
38th and R Sts., NW
Washington, DC 20057

Sudden Infant Death Syndrome Clearinghouse
8201 Greensboro Dr., Suite 600
McLean, VA 22102
(723) 821-8955

NURSING JOURNALS

Alternative Therapies in Health and Medicine
101 Columbia
Aliso Viejo, CA 92656
(800) 899-1712
http://www.alternative-therapies.com

AWHONN's Lifelines
2000 L St., NW, Suite 740
Washington, DC 20036
(202) 261-2400
http://www.awhonn.org

Birth: Issues in Prenatal Care and Education
(Formerly Birth and Family Journal)
Blackwell Scientific Publications, Inc.
3 Cambridge Center, Suite 208
Cambridge, MA 02142
(617) 876-7000

Bookmarks
(Complimentary annotated catalog of book reviews)
ICEA Supplies Center
P.O. Box 20048
Minneapolis, MN 55420

Canadian Nurse
The Canadian Nurses Association
50 The Driveway
Ottawa, Canada K2P1E2

The Female Patient
Division Excerpta Medica
301 Gibraltar Dr.
P.O. Box 528
Morris Plains, NJ 07950

Journal of Nurse-Midwifery
Elsevier Science, Inc.
655 Avenue of the Americas
New York, NY 10010
(212) 989-5800

Journal of Obstetric, Gynecologic, and Neonatal Nursing (JOGNN)
J.B. Lippincott Co.
12107 Insurance Way
Hagerstown, MD 21740

Journal of Perinatal and Neonatal Nursing
Aspen Publishers, Inc.
7201 McKinney Circle
Frederick, MD 21701
(800) 234-1660

Maternal/Newborn Advocate
The National Foundation/March of Dimes
P.O. Box 2000
White Plains, NY 10602

MCN The American Journal of Maternal Child Nursing
555 W. 57th St.
New York, NY 10019

Mother-Baby Journal/Neonatal Network
1410 Neotomas Ave., Suite 107
Santa Rosa, CA 95405
(707) 569-1415
www.neonatalnetwork.com

Nurse Practitioner: A Journal of Primary Nursing Care
3845 42nd Ave., NE
Seattle, WA 98105

Nursing Research
555 W. 57th St.
New York, NY 10019

Women's Health Issues
The Jacob's Institute for Women's Health
409 12th St., SW
Washington, DC 20024
(888) 4ES-INFO

NURSING ORGANIZATIONS

American College of Nurse Midwives
818 Connecticut Ave., NW, Suite 900
Washington, DC 20006
(202) 728-9860
http://www.midwife.org

American Holistic Nurses' Association
P.O. Box 2130
Flagstaff, AZ 86003
http://www.ahna.org

American Nurses Association
600 Maryland Ave., SW
Suite 100 W
Washington, DC 20024
(800) 274-4262
http://www.ana.org

The Association of Women's Health, Obstetric, and Neonatal Nurses (AWHONN)
2000 L St., NW, Suite 740
Washington, DC 20036
(800) 673-8499 (United States)
(800) 245-0231 (Canada)
http://www.awhonn.org

Canadian Nurses Association
50 The Driveway
Ottawa, Ontario K2P 1E2
(613) 237-2133
http://www.cna-nurses.ca

Midwives Alliance of North America
United States and Canada
c/o Concord Midwifery Service
30 South Main St.
Concord, NH 03301
(603) 225-9586

National Association of Neonatal Nurses (NAAN)
701 Lee St., Suite 450
Des Plaines, IL 60016
(800) 451-3795
http://www.nann.org

National League for Nursing (NLN)
61 Broadway
New York, NY 10006
(800) 669-9656
http://www.nln.org

National Perinatal Association
3500 E. Fletcher Ave., Suite 205
Tampa, FL 33613
(813) 971-1008

HUMAN MILK BANKING ASSOCIATION OF NORTH AMERICA (HMBANA) MEMBER BANKS

HMBANA Executive Office
P.O. Box 370464
West Hartford, CT 06137-0464
(860) 232-8809

Community Human Milk Bank
Georgetown University Hospital
Washington, DC 20007
(202) 784-2177

Lactation Support Service
British Columbia Children's Hospital
Vancouver, British Columbia, Canada V6H 3V4
(604) 875-2345, ext. 7607

Mothers' Milk Bank
Medical Center of Delaware
Wilmington, DE 19579
(302) 733-2340

Mothers' Milk Bank
Central Baptist Hospital
Lexington, KY 40503
(606) 275-6502

Mothers' Milk Bank
Presbyterian/St. Luke's Medical Center
Denver, CO 80218
(303) 869-1888

Mothers' Milk Bank
Valley Medical Center
San Jose, CA 95128
(408) 998-4550

Regional Milk Bank
The Medical Center of Central Massachusetts
Worcester, MA 01605
(508) 793-6005

Triangle Mothers' Milk Bank
Wake Medical Center
Raleigh, NC 27610
(919) 250-8599

Glossary

abdominal Belonging or relating to the abdomen and its functions and disorders.

a. birth Birth of a child through a surgical incision made into the abdominal wall and uterus; cesarean birth.

a. gestation Implantation of a fertilized ovum outside the uterus but inside the peritoneal cavity.

ABO incompatibility Hemolytic disease that occurs when the mother's blood type is O and the newborn's is A, B, or AB.

abortion Termination of pregnancy before the fetus is viable and capable of extrauterine existence, usually less than 20 weeks of gestation (or when the fetus weighs less than 500 g).

complete a. Abortion in which fetus and all related tissue have been expelled from the uterus.

elective a. Termination of pregnancy chosen by the woman that is not required for her physical safety.

habitual (recurrent) a. Loss of three or more successive pregnancies for no known cause.

incomplete a. Loss of pregnancy in which some but not all the products of conception have been expelled from the uterus.

induced a. Intentionally produced loss of pregnancy by woman or others.

inevitable a. Threatened loss of pregnancy that cannot be prevented or stopped and is imminent.

missed a. Loss of pregnancy in which the products of conception remain in the uterus after the fetus dies.

septic a. Loss of pregnancy in which there is an infection of the products of conception and the uterine endometrial lining, usually resulting from attempted termination of early pregnancy.

spontaneous a. Loss of pregnancy that occurs naturally without interference or known cause; preferred term is *miscarriage*.

therapeutic a. Pregnancy that has been intentionally terminated for medical reasons.

threatened a. Possible loss of a pregnancy; early symptoms are present (e.g., the cervix begins to dilate).

abruptio placentae Partial or complete premature separation of a normally implanted placenta.

abstinence Refraining from sexual intercourse periodically or permanently.

access to care Opportunity to receive health care services.

accreta, placenta See *placenta accreta*.

acid mantle Covering of skin formed by uppermost horny layer of epidermis, sweat, superficial fat, metabolic products, and external substances.

acidosis Increase in hydrogen ion concentration resulting in a lowering of blood pH below 7.35.

acini cells Milk-producing cells in the breast.

acme Highest point (e.g., of a contraction).

acoustic stimulation test Antepartum test to elicit fetal heart rate response to sound; performed by applying sound source (laryngeal stimulator) to maternal abdomen over the fetal head.

acquaintance Process used by parents to get to know or become familiar with their new infant; an important step in attachment.

acrocyanosis Peripheral cyanosis; blue color of hands and feet in most infants at birth that may persist for 7 to 10 days.

acromion Projection of the spine of the scapula (forming the point of the shoulder); used to explain the presentation of the fetus.

active phase Phase in first stage of labor from 4 to 7 cm dilation.

acupressure Massage technique applied to specific points along certain energy pathways of the body called *meridians*. A form of treatment based in the theories of traditional Chinese medicine.

acupuncture A form of treatment using slender needles to stimulate points along energy pathways to correct, enhance, and rebalance the flow of body energy.

adequate intakes (AIs) Recommended nutrient intakes estimated to meet the needs of almost all healthy people in the population. They are provided for nutrients or age-group categories where the available information is not sufficient to warrant establishing recommended dietary allowances.

adnexa Adjacent or accessory parts of a structure.
   uterine a. Ovaries and uterine (fallopian) tubes.

adolescence That period of an individual's transformation from a child to an adult.

adult respiratory distress syndrome (ARDS) Set of symptoms including decreased compliance of lung tissue, pulmonary edema, and acute hypoxemia. The condition is similar to respiratory distress syndrome of the newborn.

afibrinogenemia Absence or decrease of fibrinogen in the blood such that the blood will not coagulate. In obstetrics, this condition occurs from complications of abruptio placentae or retention of a dead fetus.

afterbirth Lay term for the placenta and membranes expelled after the birth of the child.

afterbirth pains (afterpains) Painful uterine cramps that occur intermittently for approximately 2 or 3 days after birth and that result from contractile efforts of the uterus to return to its normal involuted condition.

afterload Ventricular wall tension during systole, or the resistance the blood meets as blood is ejected from the ventricles.

AGA Appropriate (growth) for gestational age.

agenesis Failure of an organ to develop.

agonist-antagonist compounds An *agonist* is an agent that activates something; an *antagonist* is an agent that blocks something.

albuminuria Presence of readily detectable amounts of albumin in the urine.

alkalosis Abnormal condition of body fluids characterized by a tendency toward an increased pH, such as from an excess of alkaline bicarbonate or a deficiency of acid.

allopathic, standard, or Western medicine Interchangeable terms used to describe the current U.S. health care system. With foundations in germ theory and reductionism, standard medical practice often focuses on one body system or disease complex. Treatments are often pharmaceutical or surgical and produce effects that are different from those of the disease complex.

alpha-fetoprotein (AFP) Fetal antigen; elevated levels in amniotic fluid are associated with neural tube defects.

alternative and complementary therapies Nontraditional approaches to health care and healing, often philosophically different from Western medicine. Often involve interventions that are said to induce healing from within the client or improve the internal environment so that the body, mind, or spirit can heal. Often referred to as "natural healing." Might be used in place of or in conjunction with standard health care practices. Also defined as therapeutic modalities not commonly taught by U.S. medical schools or available in U.S. hospitals. *Alternative therapy* often refers to those modalities used in place of conventional (or other) health care. *Complementary therapy* refers to those modalities used in conjunction with conventional (or other) health care. Many therapies can be either alternative or complementary.

amenorrhea Absence or suppression of menstruation.

amniocentesis Procedure in which a needle is inserted through the abdominal and uterine walls into the amniotic fluid; used for assessment of fetal health and maturity.

amnioinfusion Infusion of normal saline warmed to body temperature through an intrauterine catheter into the uterine cavity in an attempt to increase the fluid around the umbilical cord and prevent compression during uterine contractions.

amnion Inner membrane of two fetal membranes that form the sac and contain the fetus and the fluid that surrounds it in utero.

amnionitis Inflammation of the amnion, occurring most frequently after early rupture of membranes.

amniotic Pertaining or relating to the amnion.
   a. fluid Fluid surrounding fetus derived primarily from maternal serum and fetal urine.
   a. fluid embolism Embolism resulting from amniotic fluid entering the maternal bloodstream during labor and birth after rupture of membranes; this is often fatal to the woman if it is a pulmonary embolism.
   a. fluid index (AFI) Estimation of amount of amniotic fluid by means of ultrasound to determine excess or decrease.
   a. sac Membrane "bag" that contains the fetus and fluid before birth.

amniotomy Artificial rupture of the fetal membranes (AROM), using a plastic Amnihook or surgical clamp.

analgesia Absence of pain without loss of consciousness.

analgesic Any medication or agent that relieves pain.

anaphylaxis Immediate hypersensitivity reaction characterized by local reactions such as urticaria or by systemic reactions; may be fatal.

android pelvis Male type of pelvis; heart-shaped inlet.

anencephaly Congenital deformity characterized by the absence of cerebrum, cerebellum, and flat bones of skull.

anesthesia Partial or complete absence of sensation with or without loss of consciousness.

aneuploidy Having an abnormal number of chromosomes.

announcement phase The first developmental task experienced by expectant fathers as identified by May. During this phase the expectant father accepts the biologic fact of pregnancy.

anomaly Organ or structure that is malformed or in some way abnormal with reference to form, structure, or position.

anovulatory Failure of the ovaries to produce, mature, or release eggs.

anoxia Absence of oxygen.

antenatal Occurring before or formed before birth (newborn).

> **a. glucocorticoids** Medications given 24 hours before a preterm birth between 24 and 34 weeks of gestation to accelerate fetal lung maturation.

antepartal Before labor (maternal).

anthropoid pelvis Pelvis in which the anteroposterior diameter is equal to or greater than the transverse diameter; oval inlet.

antibody Specific protein substance made by the body that exerts restrictive or destructive action on specific antigens, such as bacteria, toxins, or Rh factor.

anticipatory grief Grief that predates the loss of a beloved object.

antigen Protein foreign to the body that causes the body to develop antibodies (e.g., bacteria, dust, Rh factor).

Apgar score Numeric expression of the condition of a newborn obtained by rapid assessment at 1 and 5 minutes of age; developed by Dr. Virginia Apgar.

apnea Cessation of respirations for more than 15 seconds associated with generalized cyanosis.

Apt test Differentiation of maternal and fetal blood when there is vaginal bleeding. It is performed as follows: Add 0.5 ml of blood to 4.5 ml of distilled water. Shake. Add 1 ml of 0.25 N sodium hydroxide. Fetal and cord blood remain pink for 1 or 2 minutes. Maternal blood becomes brown in 30 seconds.

areola Pigmented ring of tissue surrounding the nipple.

> **secondary a.** During the fifth month of pregnancy, a second faint ring of pigmentation seen around the original areola.

arterial pressure catheter A Teflon intravenous catheter, usually 20 gauge, that is placed in an artery and connected to a hemodynamic monitor by means of a pressure line to provide continuous measurements of the systolic, diastolic, and mean arterial blood pressures.

arteriolar vasospasm Diameter of arteriolar vessels diminishes, impeding blood flow to all organs and raising blood pressure.

Asherman's syndrome Intrauterine adhesions after inflammation and infection; one cause of impaired fertility.

asphyxia Decreased oxygen with or without excess of carbon dioxide in the body.

> **perinatal a.** Condition occurring in utero with the following biochemical changes: hypoxemia (lowering of PO_2), hypercapnia (increase in PCO_2), and respiratory and metabolic acidosis (reduction of blood pH).

aspiration pneumonia Inflammatory condition of the lungs and bronchi caused by the inhalation of vomitus containing acid gastric contents.

assisted reproductive therapies (ARTs) Treatments for infertility, including in vitro fertilization procedures, embryo adoption, embryo hosting, and therapeutic insemination.

asynclitism Oblique presentation of the fetal head at the superior strait of the pelvis; the pelvic planes and those of the fetal head are not parallel.

ataractics Drugs capable of promoting tranquility; a tranquilizer.

atelectasis Pulmonary pathosis involving alveolar collapse.

atony Absence of muscle tone.

atresia Absence of a normally present passageway.

> **biliary a.** Absence of the bile duct.
>
> **choanal a.** Complete obstruction of the posterior nares, which open into the nasopharynx, with membranous or bony tissue.
>
> **esophageal a.** Congenital anomaly in which the esophagus ends in a blind pouch or narrows into a thin cord, thus failing to form a continuous passageway to the stomach.

attachment A specific and enduring affective tie to another person.

attitude Body posture or position.

> **fetal a.** Relation of fetal parts to each other in the uterus (e.g., all parts flexed, all parts flexed except neck is extended).

augmentation of labor Stimulation of ineffective uterine contractions after labor has started spontaneously but is not progressing satisfactorily.

autoimmune disorders Body produces antibodies against itself, causing tissue damage.

autoimmunization Development of antibodies against constituents of one's own tissues (e.g., a man may develop antibodies against his own sperm).

autolysis "Self-digestive" process by which the uterus returns to a nonpregnant state after childbirth. The decrease in estrogen and progesterone levels after childbirth results in this destruction of excess hypertrophied uterine tissue.

autosomal inheritance Characteristics transmitted by genes on the autosomes, not the sex chromosomes.

autosomes Any of the paired chromosomes other than the sex (X and Y) chromosomes.

azoospermia Absence of sperm in the semen.

bacteremic shock Shock that occurs in septicemia when endotoxins are released from certain bacteria into the bloodstream.

bag of waters Lay term for the sac containing amniotic fluid and fetus.

ballottement (1) Movability of a floating object, such as a fetus. (2) Diagnostic technique using palpation: a floating object, when tapped or pushed, moves away and then returns to touch the examiner's hand.

Bandl's ring Abnormally thickened ridge of uterine musculature between the upper and lower segments that occurs after a mechanically obstructed labor, with the lower segment thinning abnormally.

barotrauma Tissue damage caused by pressure, often applied to the lungs.

Bartholin's glands Two small glands situated on either side of the vaginal orifice that secrete small amounts of mucus during coitus and that are homologous to the bulbourethral glands in the male.

basal body temperature Lowest body temperature of a healthy person taken immediately after awakening and before getting out of bed.

basalis, decidua See *decidua basalis.*

bearing-down effort "Secondary powers"; energy exerted by the woman during contractions to push out the baby.

behavioral assessment Assessment of activity, feeding and sleeping patterns, and responsiveness.

behavioral repertoire A set of behaviors (actions and reactions) that both parent and infant use to facilitate interactions.

Bell's palsy See *palsy, Bell's.*

bereavement The feelings of loss, pain, desolation, and sadness that occur after the death of a loved one.

best practice A program or service that has been recognized for excellence.

bicornuate uterus Anomalous uterus that may be either a double or single organ with two horns.

biliary atresia See *atresia, biliary.*

bilirubin Yellow or orange pigment that is a breakdown product of hemoglobin. It is carried by the blood to the liver, where it is chemically changed and excreted into the bile or is conjugated and excreted by the kidneys.

Billings method See *ovulation method.*

bimanual Performed with both hands.

   b. palpation Examination of a woman's pelvic organs done by placement of one hand on the abdomen and one or two fingers of the other hand into the vagina.

biofeedback Technique that teaches the client to consciously control certain body functions usually thought of as unconscious (e.g., breathing, heart rate). Often involves electronic instrumentation that provides immediate visual and auditory feedback to assist the learning process.

biophysical profile (BPP) Noninvasive assessment of the fetus and its environment using ultrasonography and uterine fetal monitoring; includes fetal breathing movements, gross body movements, fetal tone, reactive fetal heart rate, and qualitative amniotic fluid volume.

biopsy Removal of a small piece of tissue for microscopic examination and diagnosis.

biorhythmicity Cyclic changes that occur with established regularity, such as sleeping and eating patterns.

biparietal diameter Largest transverse diameter of the fetal head; extends from one parietal bone to the other.

bipolar disorders Depression with previous or current manic episodes.

birth plan A tool by which parents can explore their childbirth options and choose those that are most important to them.

birth rate Number of live births per 1000 population per year. See also *fertility.*

Bishop score Rating system to evaluate inducibility of the cervix; a higher score increases the rate of successful induction of labor.

bittersweet grief The resurgence of feelings and emotions that occur on remembering a loved one after the bereavement process has lessened.

blastocyst Stage in the development of a mammalian embryo, occurring after the morula stage, that consists of an outer layer, or trophoblast, and a hollow sphere of cells enclosing a cavity.

blended family Family form that includes stepparents and stepchildren.

bloody show Vaginal discharge that originates in the cervix and consists of blood and mucus; increases as cervix dilates during labor.

body boundaries Boundaries that serve to separate the self from the nonself and provide a feeling of safety.

body image Person's subjective concept of his or her physical appearance.

bonding A process by which parents, over time, form an emotional relationship with their infant.

Bradley method Husband-coached childbirth using labor breathing techniques.

Braxton Hicks sign Mild, intermittent, painless uterine contractions that occur during pregnancy. These contractions occur more frequently as pregnancy advances but do not represent true labor.

Brazelton assessment Method for assessing the interactional behavior of a newborn.

breakthrough bleeding Escape of blood occurring between menstrual periods; may be noted by women using chemical contraception (birth control pills).

breast self-examination (BSE) Self-examination of the breasts.

breast shells Rigid plastic cups that are worn inside a bra to put pressure on the areola to help a nipple protrude or to protect sore nipples from the pressure of clothing.

breech presentation Presentation in which buttocks or feet are nearest the cervical opening and are born first; occurs in approximately 3% of all births.

   complete b.p. Simultaneous presentation of buttocks, legs, and feet.

   footling (incomplete) b.p. Presentation of one or both feet.

frank b.p. Presentation of buttocks, with hips flexed so that thighs are against abdomen.

bregma Point of junction of the coronal and sagittal sutures of the skull; the area of the anterior fontanel of the fetus.

brim Edge of the superior strait of the true pelvis; the inlet.

bronchopulmonary dysplasia (BPD) Pulmonary condition affecting preterm infants who have experienced respiratory failure and have been oxygen dependent for more than 28 days.

brown fat Source of heat unique to neonates that is capable of greater thermogenic activity than ordinary fat. Deposits are found around the adrenals, kidneys, and neck, between the scapulas, and behind the sternum for several weeks after birth.

bruit, uterine See *uterine bruit.*

calendar method See *rhythm method.*

***Candida* vaginitis** Vaginal, fungal infection; formerly called *moniliasis.*

candidiasis Infection of the skin or mucous membrane by a yeastlike fungus, *Candida albicans;* see *thrush.*

capacitation Enzymatic process resulting in removal of plasma protein over acrosome of sperm; prerequisite for sperm to fertilize an ovum.

capillary hydrostatic pressure Pressure in the arterial capillary system to promote the movement of fluid across the semipermeable membrane of the capillary wall from the vessel into the interstitial space. Measured as the pulmonary capillary wedge pressure (PCWP).

capsularis, decidua See *decidua capsularis.*

caput Occiput of fetal head appearing at the vaginal introitus preceding birth of the head.

c. succedaneum Swelling of the tissue over the presenting part of the fetal head caused by pressure during labor.

carcinoma Malignant, often metastatic epithelial neoplasm; cancer.

cardiac decompensation A condition of heart failure in which the heart is unable to maintain a sufficient cardiac output.

cardiac output (CO) Volume of blood ejected from the left ventricle in 1 minute, measured in liters per minute. Cardiac output is the product of stroke volume and heart rate (CO = HR × SV).

cardinal movements of labor The mechanism of labor in a vertex presentation; includes engagement, descent, flexion, internal rotation, extension, external rotation (restitution), and expulsion.

carpal tunnel syndrome Pressure on the median nerve at the point at which it goes through the carpal tunnel of the wrist. It causes soreness, tenderness, and weakness of the muscles of the thumb.

carrier Individual who carries a gene that does not exhibit itself in physical or chemical characteristics but that can be transmitted to children (e.g., a female carrying the trait for hemophilia, which is expressed in male offspring).

caul Hood of fetal membranes covering fetal head during birth.

cephalhematoma NOTE: This is spelled *cephalohematoma* in some sources. Extravasation of blood from ruptured vessels between a skull bone and its external covering, the periosteum. Swelling is limited by the margins of the cranial bone affected (usually parietals).

cephalic Pertaining to the head.

c. presentation Presentation of the fetal head.

cephalocaudal development Principle of maturation that development progresses from the head to tail (rump).

cephalopelvic disproportion (CPD) Condition in which the infant's head is of such a shape, size, or position that it cannot pass through the mother's pelvis.

cerclage Use of nonabsorbable suture to keep a premature dilating cervix closed; released when pregnancy is at term to allow labor to begin.

cervical cap Individually fitted contraceptive barrier for the cervix.

cervical cauterization Destruction (usually by heat or electric current) of the superficial tissue of the cervix.

cervical conization Excision of a cone-shaped section of tissue from the endocervix.

cervical funneling Effacement of the internal cervical os.

cervical intraepithelial neoplasm (CIN) Uncontrolled and progressive abnormal growth of cervical epithelial cells.

cervical mucus method See *ovulation method.*

cervical os "Mouth" or opening to the cervix.

cervical ripening Process of effecting physical softening and distensibility of the cervix in preparation for labor and birth

cervicitis Cervical infection.

cervix Lowest and narrow end of the uterus; the "neck." The cervix is situated between the external os and the body, or corpus, of the uterus, and its lower end extends into the vagina.

cesarean birth Birth of a fetus by an incision through the abdominal wall and uterus.

cesarean hysterectomy Removal of the uterus immediately after the cesarean birth of an infant.

Chadwick's sign Violet color of vaginal mucous membrane that is visible from about the fourth week of pregnancy; caused by increased vascularity.

chloasma Increased pigmentation over bridge of nose and cheeks of pregnant women and some women taking oral contraceptives; also known as *mask of pregnancy.*

choanal atresia See *atresia, choanal.*

cholecystitis Acute or chronic inflammation of the gallbladder.

cholelithiasis Presence of gallstones in the gallbladder.

choreoathetoid cerebral palsy Condition characterized by both choreiform (jerky, ticlike, twitching) and athetoid (slow, writhing) movements.

chorioamnionitis Inflammatory reaction in fetal membranes to bacteria or viruses in the amniotic fluid, which then become infiltrated with polymorphonuclear leukocytes.

chorion Fetal membrane closest to the intrauterine wall that gives rise to the placenta and continues as the outer membrane surrounding the amnion.

chorionic villus (villi) Tiny vascular protrusions on the chorionic surface that project into the maternal blood sinuses of the uterus and that help form the placenta and secrete human chorionic gonadotropin.

chorionic villus sampling (CVS) Removal of fetal tissue from placenta for genetic diagnostic studies.

chromosome Element within the cell nucleus carrying genes and composed of DNA and proteins.

circumcision

 female c. Religious or cultural removal of a portion of the clitoris and labia; practiced in some Third World countries but illegal in the United States. Mutilating procedure that can cause problems in childbirth.

 male c. Excision of the prepuce (foreskin) of the penis, exposing the glans; may be done for religious or cultural reasons.

claiming process Process by which the parents identify their new baby in terms of likeness to other family members, differences, and uniqueness.

cleft lip Incomplete closure of the lip. Lay term used is harelip.

cleft palate Incomplete closure of the palate or roof of mouth; a congenital fissure.

climacteric The period of a woman's life when she is passing from a reproductive to a nonreproductive state, with regression of ovarian function. The cycle of endocrine, physical, and psychosocial changes that occurs during the termination of the reproductive years. Also called *climacterium.*

clinical benchmark Process used to compare one's own performance against the performance of the best in an area of service.

clitoris Female organ analogous to male penis; a small, ovid body of erectile tissue situated at the anterior junction of the vulva.

clonus (ankle) Spasmodic alternation of muscular contraction and relaxation; counted in beats.

clubfoot Congenital deformity in which portions of the foot and ankle are twisted out of a normal position.

coitus Penile-vaginal intercourse.

 c. interruptus Intercourse during which penis is withdrawn from vagina before ejaculation.

cold stress Excessive loss of heat that results in increased respirations and nonshivering thermogenesis to maintain core body temperature.

colloid osmotic pressure (COP) Pressure in the arterial capillary system to prevent the movement of fluid across the semipermeable membrane of the capillary wall from the vessel into the interstitial space. The COP measures the "pulling" pressure of proteins in the plasma to retain fluid inside the vessel.

colostrum The fluid in the breast from pregnancy into the early postpartal period. It is rich in antibodies, which provide protection from many diseases; high in protein, which binds bilirubin; and laxative acting, which speeds the elimination of meconium and helps loosen mucus.

colporrhaphy Procedure of suturing the vagina for the purpose of narrowing the vagina, as in anterior or posterior vaginal repair surgery.

colposcopy Examination of vagina and cervix with a colposcope to identify neoplastic or other changes.

complement Naturally occurring blood component that is a factor in the destruction of bacteria.

complete abortion See *abortion, complete.*

complete breech presentation See *breech presentation, complete.*

complicated bereavement The persistent feelings of anger, guilt, loss, pain, and sadness over time that lead to feelings of hopelessness, helplessness, and diminishing self-worth. Signs and symptoms of clinical depression, which is different from the normal depression of bereavement.

conception Union of the sperm and ovum resulting in fertilization; formation of the one-celled zygote.

conceptional age In fetal development the number of completed weeks since the moment of conception. Because the moment of conception is almost impossible to determine, conceptional age is estimated at 2 weeks less than gestational age.

conceptus Embryo or fetus, fetal membranes, amniotic fluid, and the fetal portion of the placenta.

condom Mechanical barrier worn on the penis for contraception or to protect against STIs; a "rubber."

condyloma acuminatum (*plural* condylomata acuminata) Wartlike growth on the skin usually seen near the anus or external genitals caused by human papillomavirus (HPV); genital warts. (Must be differentiated from condyloma latum seen in secondary syphilis.)

congenital Present or existing before birth as a result of either hereditary or prenatal environmental factors.

congenital rubella syndrome Complex of problems, including hearing defects, cardiovascular abnormalities, and cataracts, caused by maternal rubella in the first trimester of pregnancy.

conjoined twins See *twins, conjoined.*

conjugate

 diagonal c. Radiographic measurement of distance from inferior border of symphysis pubis to sacral promontory; may be obtained by vaginal examination; 12.5 to 13 cm.

 true c. (conjugata vera) Radiographic measurement of distance from upper margin of symphysis pubis to sacral promontory; 1.5 to 2 cm less than diagonal conjugate.

conjunctivitis Inflammation of the mucous membrane that lines the eyelids and is reflected onto the eyeball.

conscious relaxation Technique used to release the mind and body from tension through conscious effort and practice.

contraception Prevention of impregnation or conception.

contractility Force and velocity of ventricular contractions when preload and afterload are held constant.

contraction ring See *Bandl's ring.*

contractions

  duration Period from the beginning of the contraction to the end.

  frequency How often the contractions occur–the period from the beginning of one contraction to the beginning of the next.

  intensity Strength of the contraction at its peak.

  interval Period between uterine contractions, timed from the end of one contraction to the beginning of the next.

  resting tone The tension in the uterine muscle between contractions.

contraction stress test (CST) Test to stimulate uterine contractions for the purpose of assessing fetal response; a healthy fetus does not react to contractions, whereas a compromised fetus demonstrates late decelerations in the fetal heart rate that are indicative of uteroplacental insufficiency.

Coombs' test Indirect: determination of Rh-positive antibodies in maternal blood; direct: determination of maternal Rh-positive antibodies in fetal cord blood. A positive test result indicates the presence of antibodies or titer.

coping mechanism Any effort directed at stress management. It can be task oriented and involve direct problem-solving efforts to cope with the threat itself or be intrapsychic or ego-defense oriented with the goal of regulating one's emotional distress.

copulation Coitus; sexual intercourse.

corpus luteum Yellow body. After rupture of the graafian follicle at ovulation, the follicle develops into a yellow structure that secretes progesterone and some estrogen in the second half of the menstrual cycle, atrophying about 3 days before sloughing of the endometrium in menstrual flow. If impregnation occurs, it continues to produce the hormones until the placenta can take over this function.

cotyledon One of the 15 to 28 visible segments of the placenta on the maternal surface, each made up of fetal vessels, chorionic villi, and an intervillous space.

counterpressure Pressure to sacral area of back during uterine contractions.

couplet care One nurse, educated in both mother and infant care, functions as the primary nurse for both mother and infant (also known as mother-baby care or single-room maternity care).

Couvade syndrome The phenomenon of expectant fathers' experiencing pregnancy-like symptoms

Couvelaire uterus See *uterus, Couvelaire.*

CPAP Continuous positive airway pressure.

cradle cap Common seborrheic dermatitis of infants consisting of thick, yellow, greasy scales on the scalp.

craniotabes Localized softening of cranial bones.

creatinine Substance found in blood and muscle; measurement of levels in maternal urine correlates with amount of fetal muscle mass and therefore fetal size.

crib death Unexpected and sudden death of an apparently normal and healthy infant that occurs during sleep and with no physical or autopsic evidence of disease. Also referred to as *sudden infant death syndrome (SIDS).*

cri-du-chat syndrome Rare congenital disorder recognized at birth by a kitten-like cry, which may prevail for weeks and then disappear. Other characteristics include low birth weight, microcephaly, "moon face," wide-set eyes, strabismus, and low-set misshapen ears. Infants are hypotonic; heart defects and mental and physical retardation are common. Also called *cat-cry syndrome.*

critical path The exact timing of all key incidents that must occur to achieve the standard outcomes within the diagnosis related group (DRG)–specific length of stay.

crowning Stage of birth when the top of the fetal head can be seen at the vaginal orifice as the widest part of the head distends the vulva.

cryosurgery Local freezing and removal of tissue without injury to adjacent tissue and with minimum blood loss, done with special equipment.

cryptorchidism Failure of one or both of the testicles to descend into the scrotum. Also called undescended testis.

cul-de-sac of Douglas Pouch formed by a fold of the peritoneum dipping down between the anterior wall of the rectum and the posterior wall of the uterus; also called *Douglas's cul-de-sac, pouch of Douglas,* and *rectouterine pouch.*

culdocentesis Puncture of cul-de-sac of Douglas through the vagina for aspiration of fluid.

Cullen's sign Faint, irregularly formed, hemorrhagic patches on the skin around the umbilicus. The discolored skin is blue-black and becomes greenish brown or yellow. Cullen's sign may appear 1 to 2 days after the onset of anorexia and the severe, poorly localized abdominal pains characteristic of acute pancreatitis. Cullen's sign is also present in massive upper gastrointestinal hemorrhage and ruptured ectopic pregnancy.

cultural context Setting in which one considers the individual's and the family's beliefs and practices (culture).

curettage Scraping of the endometrium lining of the uterus with a curet to remove the contents of the uterus (as is done after an incomplete miscarriage or induced abortion) or to obtain specimens for diagnostic purposes.

cycle of violence Pattern of three phases: period of increasing tension, the abusive episode, and a period of contrition and kindness.

cystocele Bladder hernia: injury to the vesicovaginal fascia during labor and birth may allow herniation of the bladder into the vagina.

cytology Study of cells, including their formation, origin, structure, function, biochemical activities, and pathology.

daily fetal movement counts (DFMCs) Maternal assessment of fetal activity; the number of fetal movements within a specific time are counted.

death Cessation of life.

> **fetal d.** Intrauterine death; death of a fetus weighing 500 g or more of 20 weeks of gestation or more.

> **infant d.** Death during the first year of life.

> **maternal d.** Death of a woman as a result of a pregnancy or birth-related problem.

> **neonatal d.** Death of a newborn within the first 28 days after birth.

> **perinatal d.** Death of a fetus of 20 weeks of gestation or older or death of a neonate 28 days old or younger.

decidua Mucous membrane, lining of uterus, or endometrium of pregnancy that is shed after giving birth.

> **d. basalis** Maternal aspect of the placenta made up of uterine blood vessels, endometrial stroma, and glands. It is shed in lochial discharge after delivery.

> **d. capsularis** That part of the decidual membranes surrounding the chorionic sac.

> **d. vera** Nonplacental decidual lining of the uterus.

decrement Decrease or stage of decline, as of a contraction.

deep tendon reflexes (DTRs) Reflex caused by stimulation of tendons, such as elbow, wrist, knee, triceps, and ankle jerk reflexes.

delivery (birth) Expulsion of the child with placenta and membranes by the mother or their extraction by the obstetric practitioner.

> **abdominal d.** See *abdominal birth*.

ΔOD$_{450}$ (delta OD$_{450}$) Delta optical density (or absorbance) at 450 nm, obtained by spectral analysis of amniotic fluid. This prenatal test is used to measure the degree of hemolytic activity in the fetus and to evaluate fetal status in women sensitized to the Rh factor.

demand feeding Feeding a newborn every third hour or when the baby cries to be fed, whichever comes first.

deoxyribonucleic acid (DNA) Intracellular complex protein that carries genetic information, consisting of two purines (adenine and guanine) and two pyrimidines (thymine and cytosine).

depression An intense and pervasive sadness with severe and labile mood swings.

depressive reactions Depression related to the postpartum period including postpartum blues, postpartum nonpsychotic depression, and postpartum psychosis.

DES Diethylstilbestrol; female fetus is predisposed to reproductive tract malformations and (later) dysplasia if her mother ingested this medication during pregnancy.

desquamation Shedding of epithelial cells of the skin and mucous membranes.

developmental crisis Severe, usually transient, stress that occurs when a person is unable to complete the tasks of a psychosocial stage of development and is therefore unable to move on to the next stage.

developmental task Physical or cognitive skill that a person must accomplish during a particular age period to continue developing, such as walking, which precedes the development of the sense of autonomy in the toddler period.

developmental theory Theoretic approach for viewing the family. The developmental perspective sees family members pass through phases of growth from dependence through active independence to interdependence.

diabetes mellitus Systemic disorder of carbohydrate, protein, and fat metabolism; caused by deficient insulin production or ineffective use of insulin at the cellular level.

diaphragmatic hernia Congenital malformation of diaphragm that allows displacement of the abdominal organs into the thoracic cavity.

diastasis recti abdominis Separation of the two rectus muscles along the median line of the abdominal wall. This is often seen in women with repeated childbirths or with a multiple gestation (e.g., triplets). In the newborn it is usually attributable to incomplete development.

Dick-Read method An approach to childbirth based on the premise that fear of pain produces muscular tension, producing pain and greater fear. The method includes teaching physiologic processes of labor, exercise to improve muscle tone, and techniques to assist in relaxation and prevent the fear-tension-pain mechanism.

dietary reference intakes (DRIs) New nutritional recommendations being prepared for the United States, consisting of the recommended dietary allowances, adequate intakes, and tolerable upper intake levels, the upper limit of intake associated with low risk in almost all members of a population.

dilation of cervix Stretching of the external os from an opening a few millimeters in size to an opening large enough to allow the passage of the infant.

dilation and curettage (D&C) Vaginal procedure in which the cervical canal is stretched enough to admit passage of an instrument called a *curet* (or *curette*). The endometrium of the uterus is scraped with the curet to empty the uterine contents or to obtain tissue for examination.

diploid number Having two sets of chromosomes; found normally in somatic (body) cells; 23 sets or 46 chromosomes.

discordance Discrepancy in size (or other indicator) between twins.

disorganization A dimension of bereavement characterized by depression, anorexia, difficulty in concentration, and a generalized feeling of not feeling good about oneself physically and emotionally.

disparate twins See *twins, disparate.*

disseminated intravascular coagulation (DIC) Pathologic form of coagulation in which clotting factors are consumed to such an extent that generalized bleeding can occur; associated with abruptio placentae, eclampsia, intrauterine fetal demise, amniotic fluid embolism, and hemorrhage.

dizygotic Related to or proceeding from two zygotes (fertilized ova).

dizygotic twins See *twins, dizygotic.*

Döderlein's bacillus Gram-positive bacterium occurring in normal vaginal secretions.

dominant trait Gene that is expressed whenever it is present in the heterozygous gene state (e.g., brown eyes are dominant over blue).

Doppler blood flow analysis Device for measuring blood flow noninvasively in the fetus and placenta to detect intrauterine growth restriction.

Douglas's cul-de-sac See *cul-de-sac of Douglas.*

doula Experienced assistant hired to give the woman support during labor and birth.

Down syndrome Abnormality involving the occurrence of a third chromosome, rather than the normal pair (trisomy 21), that characteristically results in a typical picture of mental retardation and altered physical appearance. This condition was formerly called mongolism.

drug dependence (addiction) Physical or psychologic dependence or both on a substance.

dry labor Lay term referring to labor in which amniotic fluid has already escaped. A "dry birth" does not exist.

Dubowitz assessment Estimation of gestational age of a newborn based on criteria developed for that purpose.

ductus arteriosus In fetal circulation an anatomic shunt between the pulmonary artery and arch of the aorta. It is obliterated after birth by a rising PO_2 and a change in intravascular pressures in the presence of normal pulmonary function. It normally becomes a ligament after birth but in some instances remains patent.

ductus venosus In fetal circulation, a blood vessel carrying oxygenated blood between the umbilical vein and the inferior vena cava, bypassing the liver. It is obliterated and becomes a ligament after birth.

Duncan's mechanism Delivery of placenta with the maternal surface presenting, rather than the shiny fetal surface.

dys- Prefix meaning abnormal, difficult, painful, faulty.

dysfunctional labor Abnormal uterine contractions that prevent normal progress of cervical dilation and effacement.

dysfunctional uterine bleeding (DUB) Abnormal bleeding from the uterus for reasons that are not readily established.

dysmaturity See *intrauterine growth restriction (IUGR).*

dysmenorrhea
>   **primary d.** Painful menstruation beginning 2 to 6 months after menarche, related to ovulation.
>   **secondary d.** Painful menstruation related to organic disease such as endometriosis, pelvic inflammatory disease, or uterine neoplasm.

dyspareunia Painful sexual intercourse, for either sex.

dysplasia Any abnormal development of tissues or organs.

dystocia Prolonged, painful, or otherwise difficult birth because of mechanical factors produced by the passenger (the fetus) or the passage (the pelvis and soft tissues of the birth canal of the mother), inadequate powers (uterine and other muscular activity), or maternal position.

ecchymosis Bruise; bleeding into tissue caused by direct trauma, serious infection, or bleeding diathesis.

eclampsia Severe complication of pregnancy of unknown cause and occurring more often in the primigravida; characterized by tonic and clonic convulsions, coma, high blood pressure, albuminuria, and oliguria occurring during pregnancy or shortly after birth.

ectoderm Outer layer of embryonic tissue giving rise to skin, nails, and hair.

ectopic Out of normal place.
>   **e. pregnancy** Implantation of the fertilized ovum outside of its normal place in the uterine cavity. Locations include the abdomen, uterine tubes, and ovaries.

edema Generalized accumulation of interstitial fluid.
>   **dependent e.** Edema of lower or most dependent parts of body where hydrostatic pressure is greater.
>   **pitting e.** Edema that leaves a small depression or pit when pressure is applied to a swollen area.

effacement Thinning and shortening or obliteration of the cervix that occurs during late pregnancy or labor or both.

effleurage Gentle stroking used in massage.

Eisenmenger syndrome Pulmonary hypertension characterized by elevated pulmonary vascular resistance and right-to-left (or bidirectional) shunting in either atria or ventricles.

ejaculation Sudden expulsion of semen from the male urethra.

elective abortion See *abortion, elective.*

electronic fetal monitoring (EFM) Electronic surveillance of fetal heart rate by external and internal methods.

embolus Any undissolved matter (solid, liquid, or gaseous) that is carried by the blood to another part of the body and obstructs a blood vessel.

embryo Conceptus from the second or third week of development until about the eighth week after conception, when mineralization (ossification) of the skeleton begins. This period is characterized by cellular differentiation and predominantly hyperplastic growth.

emotional lability Rapid mood changes from irritability to anger or sadness to joy and cheerfulness; often seen in the first trimester of pregnancy.

endocarditis Inflammation of the inner layer of the heart muscle (endocardium).

endocervical Pertaining to the interior of the canal of the cervix of the uterus.

endocrine glands Ductless glands that secrete hormones into the blood or lymph.

endometriosis Tissue closely resembling endometrial tissue but located outside the uterus in the pelvic cavity. Symptoms may include pelvic pain or pressure, dysmenorrhea, dyspareunia, abnormal bleeding from the uterus or rectum, and sterility.

endometritis Postpartum uterine infection, often beginning at the site of the placental implantation.

endometrium Inner lining of the uterus that undergoes changes caused by hormones during the menstrual cycle and pregnancy; decidua.

endorphins Endogenous opioids secreted by the pituitary gland that act on the central and peripheral nervous systems to reduce pain.

energy healing A variety of techniques and disciplines that are said to augment, modulate, stimulate, or remedy certain deficiencies or blocks in the human energy system.

en face Face-to-face position in which the parent's and infant's faces are approximately 20 cm apart and on the same plane.

engagement In obstetrics, the entrance of the fetal presenting part into the superior pelvic strait and the beginning of the descent through the pelvic canal.

engorgement Distention or vascular congestion. In obstetrics, the process of swelling of the breast tissue brought about by an increase in blood and lymph supply to the breast, which precedes true lactation. It lasts about 48 hours and usually reaches a peak between the third and fifth postbirth days.

engrossment A parent's absorption, preoccupation, and interest in his or her infant; term typically used to describe the father's intense involvement with his newborn.

enterocele Herniation of the peritoneum of the posterior cul-de-sac between the uterosacral ligaments into the rectovaginal septum.

entoderm Inner layer of embryonic tissue giving rise to internal organs such as the intestine.

entrainment Phenomenon observed in the microanalysis of sound films in which the speaker moves several parts of the body and the listener responds to the sounds by moving in ways that are coordinated with the rhythm of the sounds. Infants have been observed to move in time to the rhythms of adult speech but not to random noises or disconnected words or vowels. Entrainment is believed to be an essential factor in the process of maternal-infant bonding.

epicanthus Fold of skin covering the inner canthus and caruncle that extends from the root of the nose to the median end of the eyebrow; characteristically found in certain races but may occur as a congenital anomaly.

epidural block Type of regional anesthesia produced by injection of a local anesthetic into the epidural (peridural) space.

epidural blood patch A patch formed by a few millimeters of the mother's blood occluding a tear or hole in the dura mater around the spinal cord.

episiotomy Surgical incision of the perineum at the end of the second stage of labor to facilitate birth and to avoid laceration of the perineum.

epispadias Defect in which the urethral canal terminates on the dorsum of the penis or above the clitoris (rare).

Epstein's pearls Small, white blebs found along the gum margins and at the junction of the soft and hard palates. They are a normal manifestation and are typically seen in the newborn. Similar to Bohn's nodules.

epulis Tumorlike benign lesion of the gingiva seen in pregnant women.

equilibrium State of balance or rest resulting from the equal action of opposing forces, as with calcium and phosphorus in the body. In psychiatry, a state of mental or emotional balance.

Erb-Duchenne paralysis Paralysis caused by physical injury to the upper brachial plexus, occurring most often in childbirth from forcible traction during birth. The signs of Erb's paralysis include loss of sensation in the arm and paralysis and atrophy of the deltoid, the biceps, and the branchialis muscles. Also called *Erb's palsy.*

ergot Drug obtained from *Claviceps purpurea,* a fungus, which stimulates the smooth muscles of blood vessels and the uterus, causing vasoconstriction and uterine contractions.

erythema toxicum Innocuous pink papular neonatal rash of unknown cause, with superimposed vesicles appearing within 24 to 48 hours after birth and resolving spontaneously within a few days.

erythroblastosis fetalis Hemolytic disease of the newborn usually caused by isoimmunization resulting from Rh incompatibility or ABO incompatibility.

esophageal atresia See *atresia, esophageal.*

estimated date of birth (EDB) Approximate date of birth. Usually determined by calculation using Nägele's rule; "due date."

estradiol An estrogen.

estriol Major metabolite of estrogen that increases during the second half of pregnancy with an intact fetoplacental unit (normal placenta, normal fetal liver and adrenals) and normal maternal renal function.

estrogen Female sex hormone produced by the ovaries and placenta.

estrogen replacement therapy (ERT) Exogenous estrogen given to women during and after menopause to prevent hot flashes, mood changes, osteoporosis, and genitourinary symptoms.

ethics Systematic inquiry into the principles of right and wrong conduct, of virtue and vice, and of good and evil as they relate to conduct.

eutocia Normal or natural labor or birth.

evidence-based practice Practice based on analysis of research findings.

exchange transfusion Replacement of 75% to 85% of circulating blood by withdrawal of the recipient's blood and injection of a donor's blood in equal amounts, the purposes of which are to prevent an accumulation of bilirubin in the blood above a dangerous level, to prevent the accumulation of other by-products of hemolysis in hemolytic disease, and to correct anemia and acidosis.

expressive style Expectant father's strong emotional response to partner's pregnancy.

expulsive Having the tendency to drive out or expel.

> **e. contractions** Labor contractions that are characteristic of the second stage of labor.

extended family Family form that includes the nuclear family and other blood-related persons.

external cephalic version (ECV) Turning the fetus to a vertex position by exertion of pressure on the fetus externally through the maternal abdomen.

extracorporeal membrane oxygenation (ECMO) Oxygenation of blood external to body using cardiopulmonary bypass and a membrane oxygenator. Used primarily for newborns with refractory respiratory failure or meconium aspiration syndrome.

extrauterine Occurring outside the uterus.

> **e. pregnancy** Pregnancy in which the fertilized ovum implants itself outside the uterus.

extrusion reflex Infant automatically extends tongue when it is stimulated.

facies Pertaining to the appearance or expression of the face; certain congenital syndromes typically cause a specific facial appearance.

FAD Fetal activity determination; also called *fetal activity test (FAT)*.

failure to thrive Condition in which neonate's or infant's growth and development patterns are below the norms for age.

fallopian tubes Two canals or oviducts extending laterally from each side of the uterus through which the ovum travels, after ovulation, to the uterus; also called *uterine tubes*.

false labor Uterine contractions that do not result in cervical dilation, are irregular, are felt more in front, often do not last more than 20 seconds, and do not become longer or stronger.

false pelvis Part of the pelvis superior to a plane passing through the linea terminalis (brim or outlet).

family dynamics Process by which family members assume varying social roles.

family functions Activities carried out within families for the well-being of family members, including biologic, economic, educational, psychologic, and sociocultural aspects.

family stress theory Theory that explains how families react and adapt to stressors that they experience.

family systems theory Theory that conceptualizes the family as a unit and focuses on observing interactions among family members.

family violence Interpersonal violence, including child, elder, sibling, and spouse.

fantasy child The imagined dream child; the "ideal" unborn child.

fantasy mom A composite of the ideal mother ("super-mom") whom a woman envisions in her mind's eye but who may have enviable but totally unrealistic accomplishments to her credit.

feeding readiness cues Infant responses that indicate optimal times to begin a feeding. The baby may make mouthing motions, suck a fist, or awaken and cry.

Ferguson reflex Reflex contractions of the uterus after stimulation of the cervix.

ferning (arborization) test The appearance of a fern-like pattern found on slides of certain fluids.

> **ovulation f.t.** Test in which cervical mucus, placed on a slide, dries in a branching pattern in the presence of high estrogen levels at the time of ovulation.

fertile period Period before and after ovulation during which the human ovum can be fertilized; usually 3 days before and 4 days after ovulation.

fertility Quality of being able to reproduce; also number of births per 1000 women ages 15 through 44 years. See also *birth rate*.

fertilization Union of an ovum and a sperm.

fetal Pertaining or relating to the fetus.

> **f. alcohol effect (FAE)** Lesser set of the same symptoms that make up fetal alcohol syndrome.
>
> **f. alcohol syndrome (FAS)** Congenital abnormality or anomaly resulting from excessive maternal alcohol intake during pregnancy. It is characterized by typical craniofacial and limb defects, cardiovascular defects, intrauterine growth restriction, and developmental delay.
>
> **f. asphyxia** See *asphyxia, fetal*.
>
> **f. attitude** See *attitude, fetal*.
>
> **f. compromise** Evidence such as a nonreassuring fetal heart rate pattern that indicates the fetus may be in jeopardy.
>
> **f. death** See *death, fetal*.
>
> **f. lie** Relation of the fetal spine to the maternal spine; that is, in vertical lie, maternal and fetal spines are parallel and the fetal head or breech presents; in transverse lie, fetal spine is perpendicular to the maternal spine and the fetal shoulder presents.

f. membrane See *membrane.*

f. presentation The part of the fetus that enters the pelvic inlet first.

f. heart rate (FHR) Beats per minute of the fetal heart. Normal range is 110 to 160 beats per minute.

  acceleration Increase in fetal heart rate, usually seen as a reassuring sign.

  baseline Average fetal heart rate between uterine contractions.

  bradycardia Baseline fetal heart rate below 110 beats per minute.

  deceleration Slowing of fetal heart rate attributed to a parasympathetic response and described in relation to uterine contractions.

    early d. Onset corresponding to onset of uterine contraction, related to fetal head compression.

    late d. Onset after peak of contraction, continuing into interval after contraction; caused by uteroplacental insufficiency.

    prolonged d. Slowing of fetal heart rate lasting longer than 2 minutes.

    variable d. Onset at any time unrelated to contraction; caused by cord compression.

  tachycardia Baseline fetal heart rate above 160 beats per minue.

f. scalp spiral electrode Internal signal source for electronically monitoring the fetal heart rate.

f. tobacco syndrome Diagnostic term applicable to infants who fit the following criteria: mother who smoked more than 5 cigarettes a day during pregnancy and had no prenatal evidence of hypertension; infant has symmetric growth restriction, weighs less than 2500 g, and has no other cause of intrauterine growth restriction.

fetotoxic Poisonous or destructive to the fetus.

fetus Child in utero from approximately the eighth week after conception until birth.

fibroid Fibrous, encapsulated connective tissue tumor, especially of the uterus.

fimbria Structure resembling a fringe, particularly the fringelike end of the uterine tube.

first stage Stage of labor from the onset of regular uterine contractions to full dilation of the cervix.

fissure Groove or open crack in tissue.

fistula Abnormal tubelike passage that forms between two normal cavities, possibly congenital or caused by trauma, abscesses, or inflammatory processes.

flaccid Having relaxed, limp, or absent muscle tone.

flaring of nostrils Widening of nostrils (alae nasi) during inspiration in the presence of air hunger; sign of respiratory distress.

flexion Opposite of extension. In obstetrics, resistance to the descent of the baby down the birth canal causes the head to flex, or bend, so that the chin approaches the chest. Thus the smallest diameter (suboccipitobregmatic) of the vertex presents.

focusing phase Third developmental task experienced by expectant fathers as identified by May. This phase is characterized by the father's active involvement in both the pregnancy and his relationship with his infant.

follicle Small secretory cavity or sac.

  graafian f. Mature, fully developed ovarian cyst containing the ripe ovum. The follicle secretes estrogens, and after ovulation the corpus luteum develops within the ruptured graafian follicle and secretes estrogen and progesterone.

follicle-stimulating hormone (FSH) Hormone produced by the anterior pituitary during the first half of the menstrual cycle. Stimulates development of the graafian follicle.

fomites Nonliving material on which disease-producing organisms may be conveyed (e.g., bed linen).

fontanel Broad area, or soft spot, consisting of a strong band of connective tissue contiguous with cranial bones and located at the junctions of the bones.

  anterior f. Diamond-shaped area between the frontal and two parietal bones just above the baby's forehead at the junction of the coronal and sagittal sutures.

  mastoid f. Posterolateral fontanel, usually not palpable.

  posterior f. Small, triangular area between the occipital and parietal bones at the junction of the lambdoidal and sagittal sutures.

  sagittal f. Soft area located in the sagittal suture, halfway between the anterior and posterior fontanels; may be palpated in normal newborns and in some neonates with Down syndrome.

  sphenoid f. Anterolateral fontanel usually not palpable.

footling (incomplete) breech presentation See *breech presentation, footling.*

foramen ovale Septal opening between the atria of the fetal heart. The opening normally closes shortly after birth, but if it remains patent, surgical repair usually is necessary.

forceps Curved-bladed instruments used to protect head of fetus during birth and to apply traction to assist birth.

forceps-assisted birth Birth in which forceps are used to assist in delivery of the fetal head.

foreskin Prepuce, or loose fold of skin covering the glans penis.

fornix Any structure with an arched or vaultlike shape.

  f. of the vagina Anterior and posterior spaces, formed by the protrusion of the cervix into the vagina, into which the upper vagina is divided.

fourth stage of labor Initial period of recovery from childbirth. It is usually considered to last for the first 1 to 2 hours after the expulsion of the placenta.

fourth trimester Another term for the puerperium; the 3-month interval after the birth of the newborn that includes return of the reproductive organs to their nonpregnant state and psychologic adaptation to parenthood.

frank breech presentation See *breech presentation, frank.*

fraternal twins Nonidentical twins that come from two separate fertilized ova.

free-standing birth center A center that provides prenatal care, labor and birth, and postbirth care outside of a hospital setting.

frenulum Thin ridge of tissue in midline of undersurface of tongue extending from its base to varying distances from the tip of the tongue.

friability Easily broken. May refer to a fragile condition of the cervix, especially during pregnancy, that causes the cervix to bleed easily when touched.

Friedman's curve Labor curve; pattern of descent of presenting part and of dilation of cervix; partogram.

FSH See *follicle-stimulating hormone.*

fundus Dome-shaped upper portion of the uterus between the points of insertion of the uterine tubes.

funic souffle See *souffle, funic.*

funis Cordlike structure, especially the umbilical cord.

galactorrhea Lactation not associated with childbirth or breastfeeding; a symptom of a pituitary gland tumor.

galactosemia Inherited, autosomal recessive disorder of galactose metabolism, characterized by a deficiency of the enzyme galactose-1-phosphate uridyltransferase.

gamete Mature male or female germ cell; the mature sperm or ovum.

gastroschisis Abdominal wall defect at base of umbilical stalk.

gastrostomy Surgical creation of an artificial opening into the stomach through the abdominal wall, performed to feed a client when oral feeding is not possible.

gate control theory Proposed in 1965 by Melzack and Wall, this theory explains the neurophysical mechanism underlying the perception of pain: the capacity of nerve pathways to transmit pain is reduced or completely blocked by using distraction techniques.

gavage Feeding by means of a tube passed through the nose or mouth to the stomach.

gender identity Sense or awareness of knowing to which sex one belongs. The process begins in infancy, continues throughout childhood, and is reinforced during adolescence.

gene Factor on a chromosome responsible for hereditary characteristics of offspring.

genetic Dependent on the genes. A genetic disorder may or may not be apparent at birth.

genetic counseling Process of determining the occurrence or risk of occurrence of a genetic disorder within a family and of providing appropriate information and advice about the courses of action that are available, whether care of a child already affected, prenatal diagnosis, termination of a pregnancy, sterilization, or artificial insemination is involved.

genitalia Organs of reproduction.

genome Complete copy of genetic material in an organism.

genotype Hereditary combinations in an individual determining physical and chemical characteristics. Some genotypes are not expressed until later in life (e.g., Huntington's chorea); some hide recessive genes, which can be expressed in offspring; and others are expressed only under the proper environmental conditions (e.g., diabetes mellitus appearing under the stress of obesity or pregnancy).

gestation Period of intrauterine fetal development from conception through birth; the period of pregnancy.

gestational age In fetal development, the number of completed weeks counting from the first day of the last normal menstrual cycle.

gestational diabetes Glucose intolerance first recognized during pregnancy.

gestational trophoblastic neoplasia (GTN) Persistent trophoblastic tissue that is presumed to be malignant.

GIFT Gamete intrafallopian transfer of ova and washed sperm into uterine tubes.

gingivitis Inflammation of the gums characterized by redness, swelling, and tendency to bleed.

glans penis Smooth, round head of the penis, analogous to the female glans clitoris.

glomerulonephritis Noninfectious disease of the glomerulus of the kidney, characterized by proteinuria, hematuria, decreased urine production, and edema.

glucose tolerance test A test of the body's ability to use carbohydrates; used as a screening measure for gestational diabetes.

glycosuria Presence of glucose (a sugar) in the urine.

glycosylated hemoglobin (Ghb) Glycohemoglobin, a minor hemoglobin with glucose attached. Ghb A1c concentration represents the average blood glucose level over the previous several weeks and is a measurement for glycemic control in diabetic therapy.

gonad Gamete-producing, or sex, gland; the ovary or testis.

gonadotropic hormone Hormone that stimulates the gonads.

gonadotropin-releasing hormone (GnRH) Hormone released from hypothalamus that stimulates pituitary gland to produce FSH and LH.

Goodell's sign Softening of the cervix, a probable sign of pregnancy, occurring during the second month.

graafian follicle (vesicle) See *follicle, graafian.*

gravida Pregnant woman.

gravidity Number of times a woman has been pregnant.

grief responses The physical, emotional, social, and cognitive responses to the death of a loved one.

grieving process A complex of somatic and psychologic symptoms associated with some extreme sorrow or loss, specifically the death of a loved one.

growth spurts Times of increased neonatal growth that usually occur at approximately 6 to 10 days, 6 weeks, 3 months, and 4 to 5 months. The increased caloric needs necessitate more frequent feedings to increase the amount of milk needed.

grunt, expiratory Sign of respiratory distress (hyaline membrane disease [respiratory distress syndrome, or RDS] or advanced pneumonia) indicative of the body's attempt to hold air in the alveoli for better gaseous exchange.

guided imagery The use of imagination and thought processes in a purposeful way to change certain physiologic and emotional conditions.

gynecoid pelvis Pelvis in which the inlet is round instead of oval or blunt; typical female pelvis.

gynecology Study of the diseases of the female, especially of the genital, urinary, and rectal organs.

habitual (recurrent) abortion See *abortion, habitual.*

habituation An acquired tolerance from repeated exposure to a particular stimulus. Also called *negative adaptation;* a decline and eventual elimination of a conditioned response by repetition of the conditioned stimulus.

haploid number Having half the normal number of chromosomes found in somatic (body) cells; 23 chromosomes.

harlequin sign Rare color change of no pathologic significance occurring between the longitudinal halves of the neonate's body. When infant is placed on one side, the dependent half is noticeably pinker than the superior half.

healing The integrating and balancing of the body, mind, and spirit. May or may not affect physical healing from illness. Often perceived as improved sense of well-being, acceptance, and inner peace and harmony.

healing touch A combination of energetic healing techniques used by nurses and other health care professionals.

health promotion Motivation to increase well-being and actualize health potential.

Hegar's sign Softening of the lower uterine segment that is classified as a probable sign of pregnancy and that may be present during the second and third months of pregnancy and is palpated during bimanual examination.

HELLP syndrome Condition characterized by hemolysis, elevated liver enzymes, and low platelet count; a form of severe preeclampsia.

hematocrit Volume of red blood cells per deciliter (dl) of circulating blood; packed cell volume (PCV).

hematoma Collection of blood in a tissue; a bruise or blood tumor.

hematopoiesis Production of blood cells.

hemoconcentration Increase in the number of red blood cells in proportion to the volume, resulting from either a decrease in plasma volume or increased erythropoiesis.

hemodilution An increase in fluid content of blood, resulting in diminution of the proportion of formed elements.

hemoglobin Component of red blood cells consisting of globin, a protein, and hematin, an organic iron compound.

   h. electrophoresis Test to diagnose sickle cell disease in newborns. Cord blood is used.

hemolytic disease of the newborn Breakdown of fetal red blood cells by maternal antibodies, usually from an Rh-negative mother.

hemorrhagic disease of newborn Bleeding disorder during first few days of life based on a deficiency of vitamin K.

hemorrhagic shock Clinical condition in which the peripheral blood flow is inadequate to return sufficient blood to the heart for normal function, particularly oxygen transport to the organs or tissue.

hereditary Pertaining to a trait or characteristic transmitted from parent to offspring by way of the genes; used synonymously with the term *genetic.*

hermaphrodite Person having genital and sexual characteristics of both sexes.

heterozygous Having two dissimilar genes at the same site, or locus, on paired chromosomes (e.g., at the site for eye color, one chromosome carrying the gene for brown, the other for blue).

high risk Increased possibility of suffering harm, damage, loss, or death. See also *risk factor.*

hirsutism Condition characterized by the excessive growth of hair.

holism Philosophy that states that the whole is greater than the sum of its parts. In healing, refers to consideration and treatment of the whole client as a unified being. May include alternative and complementary modalities, but it is more a philosophical base than a modality in and of itself.

holistic medicine Health care treatment with techniques not commonly taught in U.S. medical schools or widely available in U.S. hospitals. May include a variety of disciplines involving diet, exercise, vitamin and nutritional supplements, bodywork, or alternative pharmacologic agents. Philosophy of medicine that encompasses holism.

holistic nursing Nursing practice that stems from the philosophy of holism, one that views the client as an integrated whole, and influenced by a variety of internal and external factors, including the biopsychosocial and spiritual dimensions of the person.

Homans' sign Early sign of phlebothrombosis of the deep veins of the calf in which there are complaints of pain when the leg is in extension and the foot is dorsiflexed.

home birth Planned birth of the child at home, usually done under the supervision of a midwife.

homologous Similar in structure or origin but not necessarily in function.

homologous insemination Insemination in which the semen specimen is provided by the husband. The procedure is used primarily in cases of impotence or when the husband is incapable of sexual intercourse because of some physical disability.

homosexual family Family in which parents form a homosexual union. Children may be the offspring of a previous heterosexual union, adopted, or conceived by one or both members of a homosexual couple through artificial insemination.

homozygous Having two similar genes at the same locus, or site, on paired chromosomes.

hormone Chemical substance produced in an organ or gland that is conveyed through the blood to another organ or part of the body, stimulating it to increased functional activity or secretion. See also specific hormones.

hormone replacement therapy (HRT) Progestin and estrogen given for menopausal symptoms. See *estrogen replacement therapy.*

hot flash (flush) Transient sensation of warmth experienced by some women during or after menopause, resulting from autonomic vasomotor disturbances that accompany changes in the neurohormonal activity of the ovaries, hypothalamus, and pituitary gland.

human chorionic gonadotropin (hCG) Hormone that is produced by chorionic villi; the biologic marker in pregnancy tests.

hyaline membrane disease (HMD) See *respiratory distress syndrome (RDS).*

hydatidiform mole (molar pregnancy) Gestational trophoblastic neoplasm usually resulting from fertilization of egg that has no nucleus or an inactivated nucleus.

hydramnios (polyhydramnios) Amniotic fluid in excess of 1.5 liters; often indicative of fetal anomaly and frequently seen in poorly controlled, insulin-dependent, diabetic pregnant women even if there is no coexisting fetal anomaly.

hydrocele Collection of fluid in a saclike cavity, especially in the sac that surrounds the testis, causing the scrotum to swell.

hydrocephalus Accumulation of fluid in the subdural or subarachnoid spaces.

hydrops fetalis Most severe expression of fetal hemolytic disorder, a possible sequela to maternal Rh isoimmunization; infants exhibit gross edema (anasarca), cardiac decompensation, and profound pallor from anemia, and seldom survive.

hymen Membranous fold that normally partially covers the entrance to the vagina.

hymenal tag Normally occurring redundant hymenal tissue protruding from the floor of the vagina of a newborn female that disappears spontaneously within a few weeks after birth.

hyperbilirubinemia Elevation of unconjugated serum bilirubin concentrations.

hyperemesis gravidarum Abnormal condition of pregnancy characterized by protracted vomiting, weight loss, and fluid and electrolyte imbalance.

hyperesthesia Unusual sensibility to sensory stimuli, such as pain or touch.

hyperglycemia Excess glucose in the blood.

hyperplasia Increase in number of cells; formation of new tissue.

hyperreflexia Increased action of the reflexes.

hyperthyroidism Excessive functional activity of the thyroid gland.

hypertonic uterine dysfunction Uncoordinated, painful, frequent uterine contractions that do not cause dilation and effacement; primary dysfunctional labor.

hypertrophic cardiomyopathy Enlargement and loss of elasticity of the heart muscle, that is, the septum and the left ventricle, causing impaired filling during diastole resulting in decreased cardiac output.

hypertrophy Enlargement, or increase in size, of existing cells.

hyperventilation Rapid, shallow (or prolonged, deep) respirations resulting in respiratory alkalosis: a decrease in H^+ concentration and Pco_2 and an increase in the blood pH and the ratio of $NaHCO_3$ to H_2CO_3. Symptoms may include faintness, palpitations, and carpopedal (hands and feet) muscular spasms.

hypocalcemia Deficiency in calcium often seen in preterm infants, in infants of diabetic mothers, or after long stressful labor in full-term infants.

hypofibrinogenemia Deficient level of a blood-clotting factor, fibrinogen, in the blood; in obstetrics, it occurs after complications of abruptio placentae or retention of a dead fetus.

hypogastric arteries Branches of the right and left iliac arteries carrying deoxygenated blood from the fetus through the umbilical cord, where they are known as umbilical arteries, to the placenta.

hypoglycemia Less than normal amount of glucose in the blood, usually caused by administration of too much insulin, excessive secretion of insulin by the islet cells of the pancreas, or dietary deficiency.

hypospadias Anomalous positioning of urinary meatus on undersurface of penis or close to or just inside the vagina.

hypothalamus Portion of the diencephalon of the brain forming the floor and part of the lateral wall of the third ventricle. It activates, controls, and integrates the peripheral autonomic nervous system, endocrine processes, and many somatic functions, such as body temperature, sleep, and appetite.

hypothermia Temperature that falls below normal range, that is, below 35° C, usually caused by exposure to cold.

hypothyroidism Deficiency of thyroid gland activity with underproduction of thyroxine.

hypotonic uterine dysfunction Weak, ineffective uterine contractions usually occurring in the active phase of labor; often related to cephalopelvic disproportion (CPD) or malposition of the fetus.

hypoxemia Reduction in arterial P_{O_2} resulting in metabolic acidosis by forcing anaerobic glycolysis, pulmonary vasoconstriction, and direct cellular damage.

hypoxia Insufficient availability of oxygen to meet the metabolic needs of body tissue.

hysterectomy Surgical removal of the uterus.

TAH-BSO Total abdominal hysterectomy and bilateral salpingo-oophorectomy; removal of uterus, both tubes, and both ovaries.

TVH Total vaginal hysterectomy.

hysterosalpingography Recording by x-rays of the uterus and uterine tubes after they are injected with radiopaque material.

hysterotomy Surgical incision into the uterus.

iatrogenic Caused by a health care provider's words, actions, or treatment.

icterus neonatorum Jaundice in the newborn.

idiopathic peripartum cardiomyopathy A primary disease of the heart muscle with no apparent cause, occurring during the peripartum period.

IDM Infant of a diabetic mother.

immunity

acquired i. Protection against microorganisms that develops in response to actual infection or transfer of antibody from an immune donor.

active i. Protection against specific microorganisms that develops in response to actual infection or vaccination.

natural i. Nonspecific protection against microorganisms. Natural immunity is the first line of defense and includes skin and phagocytic cells.

passive i. Protection against specific microorganisms that develops in response to the transfer of antibody or lymphocytes from an immune donor.

immunocompetent Ability of the immune system to respond appropriately to foreign antigens and to develop antigen-specific antibodies.

immunoglobin

IgA Primary immunoglobulin in colostrum.

IgG Transplacentally acquired immunoglobulin that confers passive immunity to the fetus against the infections to which the mother is immune.

IgM Immunoglobulin neonate can manufacture soon after birth. Fetus produces it in the presence of amnionitis.

immunology The study of the components essential to the recognition and disposal of foreign (nonself or antigenic) material and maintenance of body defenses.

impaired fertility Inability to conceive or to carry fetus to live birth at a time a couple chooses to do so.

implantation Embedding of the fertilized ovum in the uterine mucosa; nidation.

impotence Term designating a man's inability, partial or complete, to perform sexual intercourse or to achieve orgasm; erectile dysfunction.

inborn error of metabolism Hereditary deficiency of a specific enzyme needed for normal metabolism of specific chemicals (e.g., deficiency of phenylalanine hydroxylase results in phenylketonuria [PKU]; a deficiency of hexosaminidase results in Tay-Sachs disease).

incompetent cervix Cervix that is unable to remain closed until a pregnancy reaches term because of a mechanical defect in the cervix resulting in dilation and effacement usually during the second or early third trimester of pregnancy. *Premature dilation of the cervix* is the preferred term.

incomplete abortion See *abortion, incomplete.*

increment Increase, or buildup, as of a contraction.

induced abortion See *abortion, induced.*

induction Stimulation of uterine contractions before the spontaneous onset of labor.

inertia Sluggishness or inactivity; in obstetrics, refers to the absence or weakness of uterine contractions during labor.

inevitable abortion See *abortion, inevitable.*

infant Child who is under 1 year of age.

infective endocarditis Inflammation of the inner layer of the heart muscle (endocardium), caused by a bacterial infection.

infertility Decreased capacity to conceive.

informed consent Choice based on full comprehension of relevant information.

inhalation analgesia Reduction of pain by administration of anesthetic gas. Occasionally given during the second stage of labor. Consciousness is retained to allow the woman to follow instructions and to avoid the adverse effects of general anesthesia.

inlet Passage leading into a cavity.

pelvic i. Upper brim of the pelvic cavity.

insemination Introduction of semen into the vagina or uterus for impregnation.

therapeutic donor i. Introduction of donor semen by instrument injection into the vagina or uterus for impregnation.

instrumental style Characteristic style displayed by expectant fathers that emphasizes tasks to be accomplished.

insulin Hormone produced by the beta cells of the pancreatic islets of Langerhans; promotes glucose transport into the cells; aids in protein and lipid synthesis.

integrative health care Encompasses complementary and alternative therapies in combination with conventional Western modalities of treatment.

internal os Inside mouth or opening.

intertuberous diameter Distance between ischial tuberosities. Measured to determine dimension of pelvic outlet.

intervillous space Irregular space in the maternal portion of the placenta, filled with maternal blood and serving as the site of maternal-fetal gas, nutrient, and waste exchange.

intoxication Development of a reversible substance-specific syndrome caused by the recent ingestion of or exposure to a substance. The symptoms of intoxication are attributable to the direct physiologic effects of the substance on the central nervous system.

intrapartum During labor and birth.

intrathecal Within the subarachnoid space.

intrauterine device (IUD) Small plastic or metal form placed in the uterus to prevent implantation of a fertilized ovum.

intrauterine growth restriction (IUGR) Fetal undergrowth of any cause, such as deficient nutrient supply or intrauterine infection, or associated with congenital malformation; birth weight below population 10th percentile corrected for gestational age.

intrauterine pressure catheter (IUPC) Catheter inserted into uterine cavity to assess uterine activity and pressure by electronic means.

intrauterine resuscitation Interventions initiated when nonreassuring fetal heart rate patterns are noted and are directed at improving intrauterine blood flow.

introitus Entrance into a canal or cavity such as the vagina.

intussusception Prolapse of one segment of bowel into the lumen of the adjacent segment.

in utero Within or inside the uterus.

in vitro fertilization Fertilization in a culture dish or test tube.

inversion Turning end for end, upside down, or inside out.
  i. of uterus Condition in which the uterus is turned inside out so that the fundus intrudes into the cervix or vagina, caused by a too vigorous removal of the placenta before it is detached by the natural process of labor.

involution (1) Rolling or turning inward. (2) Reduction in size of the uterus after birth and its return to its non-pregnant condition.

isoimmune hemolytic disease Breakdown (hemolysis) of fetal/neonatal Rh-positive red blood cells because of Rh antibodies formed by an Rh-negative mother who had been previously exposed to Rh-positive red blood cells.

isoimmunization Development of antibodies in a species of animal with antigens from the same species (e.g., development of anti-Rh antibodies in an Rh-negative person).

ITP Idiopathic thrombocytopenic purpura.

IVF-ET In vitro fertilization and embryo transfer

jaundice Yellow discoloration of the body tissues caused by the deposit of bile pigments (unconjugated bilirubin); icterus.
  breast milk j. Term used by some clinicians to describe late-onset (after day 5) jaundice in the breastfed infant. A cause for this phenomenon has not been conclusively identified. See *physiologic j.*
  pathologic j. Jaundice usually first noticeable within 24 hours after birth; caused by some abnormal condition such as an Rh or ABO incompatibility and resulting in bilirubin toxicity (e.g., kernicterus).
  physiologic j. Yellow tinge to skin and mucous membranes in response to increased serum levels of unconjugated bilirubin; not usually apparent until after 24 hours; also called *neonatal jaundice, physiologic hyperbilirubinemia.*

kangaroo care Skin-to-skin infant care, especially for preterm infants, which provides warmth to infant. Infant is placed naked or diapered against mother's or father's bare chest and is covered with parent's shirt or a warm blanket.

karyotype Schematic arrangement of the chromosomes within a cell to demonstrate their numbers and morphology.

Kegel exercises Pelvic muscle exercises to strengthen the pubococcygeal muscles.

kernicterus Bilirubin encephalopathy involving the deposit of unconjugated bilirubin in brain cells, resulting in death or impaired intellectual, perceptive, or motor function and adaptive behavior.

ketoacidosis The accumulation of ketone bodies in the blood as a consequence of hyperglycemia; leads to metabolic acidosis.

Kleihauer-Betke test Laboratory test that detects the presence of fetal blood cells in the maternal circulation.

labia majora Two folds of skin containing fat and covered with hair that lie on either side of the vaginal opening and form each side of the vulva. (Singular, *labium majus.*)

labia minora Two thin folds of delicate, hairless skin inside the labia majora. (Singular, *labium minus.*)

labor Series of processes by which the fetus is expelled from the uterus; parturition; childbirth.
  active phase Phase in first stage of labor from 4 to 7 cm in dilation.
  first stage Stage of labor from the onset of regular uterine contractions to full dilation of the cervix.
  latent phase Phase in first stage of labor from none to 3 cm in dilation.
  second stage Stage of labor from full dilation of the cervix to the birth of the baby.
  third stage Stage of labor from the birth of the baby to the expulsion of the placenta.
  transition phase Phase in first stage of labor from 8 to 10 cm in dilation.

labor, delivery, recovery (LDR) A single room where all steps of the birth process occur. Avoids having to move the woman to different rooms for each phase of the birth process. The woman is moved to a postpartum room after recovery.

labor, delivery, recovery, postpartum (LDRP) A single room where all steps of the birth process and hospitalization occur. The woman stays in the same room throughout her hospitalization.

laceration Irregular tear of wound tissue; in obstetrics, it usually refers to a tear in the perineum, vagina, or cervix caused by childbirth.

lactase Enzyme necessary for the digestion of lactose.

lactation Function of secreting milk or period during which milk is secreted.

l. consultant A health care professional who has specialized training in breastfeeding.

l. suppression Stopping the production of breast milk through the use of medication (rare) or nonpharmacologic interventions.

lactogen Medication or other substance that enhances the production and secretion of milk.

lactogenesis stage I Initial synthesis of milk components (colostrum) that begins during pregnancy.

lactogenesis stage II Beginning of milk production 2 to 5 days postpartum.

lactose intolerance Inherited absence of the enzyme lactose.

lactosuria Presence of lactose in the urine during late pregnancy and during lactation. Must be differentiated from glycosuria.

Lamaze (psychoprophylaxis) method Method of preparation for childbirth developed in the 1950s by a French obstetrician, Fernand Lamaze, that gained popularity in the United States in the 1960s. It requires practice at home and coaching during labor and birth. The goals are to minimize fear and the perception of pain and to promote positive family relationships by using both mental and physical preparation.

lambdoid suture Suture line extending across the posterior third of the skull, separating the occipital bone from the two parietal bones, and forming the base of the triangular posterior fontanel.

Laminaria **tent** Cone of dried seaweed that swells as it absorbs moisture. Used to dilate the cervix nontraumatically in preparation for an induced abortion or in preparation for induction of labor.

lanugo Downy, fine hair characteristic of the fetus between 20 weeks of gestation and birth that is most noticeable over the shoulder, forehead, and cheeks but is found on nearly all parts of the body except the palms of the hands, soles of the feet, and the scalp.

laparoscopy Examination of the interior of the abdomen by insertion of a small telescope through the anterior abdominal wall.

large for gestational age (LGA) Exhibiting excessive growth for gestational age.

last menstrual period (LMP) Date of the first day of the last menstrual bleeding.

latch-on Attachment of the infant to the breast for feeding.

latent phase Phase in first stage of labor from none to 3 cm in dilation.

lecithin A phospholipid that decreases surface tension; surfactant.

lecithin/sphingomyelin ratio Ratio of lecithin to sphingomyelin in the amniotic fluid. It is used to assess maturity of the fetal lung.

leiomyoma Benign smooth muscle tumor.

Leopold's maneuvers Four maneuvers for diagnosing the fetal position by external palpation of the mother's abdomen.

letdown or letdown reflex See *milk ejection reflex.*

letting-go phase Interdependent phase after birth in which the mother and family move forward as a system with interacting members.

leukorrhea White or yellowish mucous discharge from the cervical canal or the vagina that may be normal physiologically or caused by pathologic states of the vagina and endocervix (e.g., *Trichomonas vaginalis* infections).

LH See *luteinizing hormone (LH).*

libido Sexual drive.

lie Relationship existing between the long axis of the fetus and the long axis of the mother. In a longitudinal lie, the fetus is lying lengthwise or vertically, whereas in a transverse lie, the fetus is lying crosswise or horizontally in the uterus.

lightening Sensation of decreased abdominal distention produced by uterine descent into the pelvic cavity as the fetal presenting part settles into the pelvis. It usually occurs 2 weeks before the onset of labor in nulliparas.

linea nigra Line of darker pigmentation seen in some women during the latter part of pregnancy that appears on the middle of the abdomen and extends from the symphysis pubis toward the umbilicus.

linea terminalis Line dividing the upper (false) pelvis from the lower (true) pelvis.

lithotomy position Position in which the woman lies on her back with her knees flexed and with abducted thighs drawn up toward her chest.

live birth Birth in which the neonate, regardless of gestational age, manifests any heartbeat, breathes, or displays voluntary movement.

living ligature Configuration of smooth muscle fibers of the uterus that gives them the capacity to ligate blood vessels and control blood loss after abortion, miscarriage, and childbirth.

local infiltration anesthesia Process by which a substance such as a local anesthetic drug is deposited within the tissue to anesthetize a limited region.

lochia Vaginal discharge during the puerperium consisting of blood, tissue, and mucus.

l. alba Thin, yellowish to white, vaginal discharge that follows lochia serosa on about the tenth day after birth and that may last from 2 to 6 weeks postpartum.

l. rubra Red, distinctly blood-tinged vaginal flow that follows birth and lasts 2 to 4 days.

l. serosa Serous, pinkish brown, watery vaginal discharge that follows lochia rubra until about the tenth day after birth.

low birth weight (LBW) An infant birth weight of less than 2500 g.

low spinal (saddle) block anesthesia Type of regional anesthesia produced by injection of a local anesthetic solution into the cerebrospinal fluid intrathecal (subarachnoid) space in the spinal canal.

L/S ratio See *lecithin/sphingomyelin ratio.*

lunar month Four weeks (28 days).

luteinizing hormone (LH) Hormone produced by the anterior pituitary that stimulates ovulation and the development of the corpus luteum.

luteotropin (LTH) Lactogenic hormone; prolactin; an adenohypophyseal hormone.

lysozyme Enzyme with antiseptic qualities that destroys foreign organisms and that is found in blood cells of the granulocytic and monocytic series and is also normally present in saliva, sweat, tears, and breast milk.

maceration (1) Process of softening a solid by soaking it in a fluid. (2) Softening and breaking down of fetal skin from prolonged exposure to amniotic fluid as seen in a postterm infant. Also seen in a dead fetus.

macroglossia Hypertrophy of tongue or tongue large for oral cavity; seen in some preterm neonates and in neonates with Down syndrome.

macrophage Any phagocytic cell of the reticuloendothelial system, including Kupffer cells in the liver, splenocytes in the spleen, and histocytes in the loose connective tissue.

macrosomia Large body size as seen in neonates of diabetic or prediabetic mothers.

magnetic resonance imaging (MRI) Noninvasive nuclear procedure for imaging tissues with high fat and water content; in obstetrics, uses include evaluation of fetal structures, placenta, and amniotic fluid volume.

malpractice Professional negligence that is the proximate cause of injury or harm to a client, resulting from a lack of professional knowledge, experience, or skill that can be expected in others in the profession or from a failure to exercise reasonable care or judgment in the application of professional knowledge, experience, or skill.

mammary gland Compound gland of the female breast that is made up of lobes and lobules that secrete milk for nourishment of the young. Rudimentary mammary glands exist in the male.

mammography X-ray examination technique used to screen for and evaluate breast lesions.

managed care System of guiding care to promote efficiency and cost-effectiveness.

Marfan syndrome An inherited disorder that is an autosomal dominant trait resulting in an abnormal condition characterized by elongation of the bones, causing significant musculoskeletal disturbances. Also usually associated with cardiovascular and eye abnormalities.

mask of pregnancy See *chloasma.*

mastectomy Excision, or removal, of the mammary gland.

> **modified radical m.** Removal of breast tissue, skin, and axillary nodes.

mastitis Infection in a breast, usually confined to a milk duct, characterized by influenza-like symptoms and redness and tenderness in the affected breast.

maternal adaptation Process that a woman goes through in adjusting to her version of the maternal role; includes three phases: taking in, taking hold, and letting go.

maternal mortality Death of a woman related to childbearing.

maturation (1) Process of attaining maximum development. (2) In biology, a process of cell division during which the number of chromosomes in the germ cells (sperm or ova) is reduced to one half the number (haploid) characteristic of the species.

maturational crisis Crisis that arises during normal growth and development, such as puberty.

McDonald's sign Easy flexion of the fundus on the cervix.

mean arterial pressure (MAP) Average of systolic and diastolic blood pressures. An MAP of greater than 90 mm Hg in the second trimester is associated with an increase in the incidence of pregnancy-induced hypertension in the third trimester.

meatus Opening from an internal structure to the outside (e.g., urethral meatus).

mechanical ventilation Technique used to provide predetermined amount of oxygen; requires intubation.

meconium First stools of infant: viscid, sticky; dark greenish brown, almost black; sterile; odorless.

> **m. aspiration syndrome (MAS)** Function of fetal hypoxia: with hypoxia, the anal sphincter relaxes and meconium is released; reflex gasping movements draw meconium and other particulate matter in the amniotic fluid into the infant's bronchial tree, obstructing the airflow after birth.

> **m. ileus** Lower intestinal obstruction by thick, putty-like, inspissated (dried) meconium that may be the result of deficiency of trypsin production in the newborn with cystic fibrosis.

> **m.-stained fluid** In response to hypoxia, fetal intestinal activity increases and anal sphincter relaxes, resulting in the passage of meconium, which imparts a greenish coloration.

meditation Any activity that focuses the attention in the present moment and quiets and relaxes the mind and body in the process.

meiosis Process by which germ cells divide and decrease their chromosomal number by one half.

membrane(s) Thin, pliable layer of tissue that lines a cavity or tube, separates structures, or covers an organ or structure; in obstetrics, the amnion and chorion surrounding the fetus.

artificial rupture of m. (AROM) Rupture of membranes using a plastic Amnihook or surgical clamp.

premature rupture of m. (PROM) Rupture of amniotic sac and leakage of amniotic fluid beginning at least 1 hour before onset of labor at any gestational age.

preterm premature rupture of m. (PPROM) PROM that occurs before 37 weeks of gestation.

spontaneous rupture of m. (SROM) Rupture of membranes by natural means.

menarche Onset, or beginning, of menstrual function.

meningomyelocele Saclike protrusion of the spinal cord through a congenital defect in the vertebral column.

menopausal hormone therapy (MHT) Hormonal therapy for menopausal symptoms, usually estrogen and progestin.

menopause From the Greek word *mēn* (month) and Greek word *pausis* (cessation), the actual permanent cessation of menstrual cycles; so diagnosed after 1 year without menses.

menorrhagia Abnormally profuse or excessive menstrual flow.

menses (menstruation) (Latin plural of *mensis* "month.") Periodic vaginal discharge of bloody fluid from the nonpregnant uterus that occurs from the age of puberty to menopause.

mentum Chin, a fetal reference point in designating position (e.g., "left mentoanterior" [LMA], meaning that the fetal chin is presenting in the left anterior quadrant of the maternal pelvis).

mesoderm Embryonic middle layer of germ cells giving rise to all types of muscles, connective tissue, bone marrow, blood, lymphoid tissue, and urogenital system.

metastasis Process by which tumor cells spread from site of origin to distant parts of the body.

metrorrhagia Abnormal bleeding from the uterus, particularly when it occurs at any time other than the menstrual period.

microcephaly Congenital anomaly characterized by abnormal smallness of the head in relation to the rest of the body and by underdevelopment of the brain, resulting in some degree of mental retardation.

midwife One who practices the art of helping and aiding a woman to give birth.

certified nurse m. Registered nurse with advanced education in midwifery.

lay m. Midwife who learned skills through practice; has no formal education in midwifery

milia Unopened sebaceous glands appearing as tiny, white, pinpoint papules on forehead, nose, cheeks, and chin of a neonate that disappear spontaneously in a few days or weeks.

milk ejection reflex (MER) Release of milk caused by the contraction of the myoepithelial cells within the milk glands in response to oxytocin; also called *letdown*.

milk-leg Thrombophlebitis of femoral vein resulting in edema of leg and pain; may occur after difficult vaginal birth.

milk transfer Infant's removal of milk from the breast, which is dependent on correct latch-on and the efficiency of the baby's suck, as well as the mother's milk ejection reflex.

miscarriage Spontaneous abortion; lay term usually referring to the loss of the fetus.

missed abortion See *abortion, missed.*

mitleiden "Suffering along," or the psychosomatic symptoms of fathers-to-be.

mitosis Process of somatic cell division in which a single cell divides, but both of the new cells have the same number of chromosomes as the first.

mitral valve prolapse (MVP) A disorder in which one or both of the cusp(s) of the mitral valve protrude backward into the left atrium during ventricular systole, resulting in incomplete closure of the valve. A midsystolic click or a late systolic murmur may be heard.

mitral valve stenosis Narrowing of the opening of the mitral valve caused by stiffening of valve leaflets, obstructing the blood flow from the atrium to the ventricle.

mittelschmerz Abdominal pain in the region of an ovary during ovulation that usually occurs midway through the menstrual cycle. Present in many women, mittelschmerz is useful for identifying ovulation, thus pinpointing the fertile period of the cycle.

molding Overlapping of cranial bones or shaping of the fetal head to accommodate and conform to the bony and soft parts of the mother's birth canal during labor.

mongolian spot Bluish gray or dark nonelevated pigmented area usually found over the lower back and buttocks present at birth in some infants, primarily nonwhite. The spot usually fades by school age.

mongolism See *Down syndrome.*

moniliasis See *candidiasis.*

monitrice One trained in psychoprophylactic methods and who supports women during labor.

monosomy Chromosomal aberration characterized by the absence of one chromosome from the normal diploid complement.

monozygotic Originating or coming from a single fertilized ovum, such as identical twins.

monozygotic twins See *twins, monozygotic.*

mons veneris Pad of fatty tissue and coarse skin that overlies the symphysis pubis in the woman and that, after puberty, is covered with hair.

Montgomery's glands (tubercles) Small, nodular prominences (sebaceous glands) on the areolas around the nipples of the breasts that enlarge during pregnancy and lactation.

mood disorders Disorders that have a disturbance in the prevailing emotional state as the dominant feature. Cause is unknown.

moratorium phase The second developmental task experienced by expectant fathers as identified by May. During this phase the expectant father adjusts to the reality of pregnancy.

morbidity (1) Condition of being diseased. (2) Number of cases of disease or of sick persons in relationship to a specific population; incidence.

morning sickness Nausea and vomiting that affect some women during the first few months of their pregnancy; may occur at any time of day.

Moro's reflex Normal, generalized reflex in a young infant elicited by a sudden loud noise or by striking the table next to the child, resulting in flexion of the legs, an embracing posture of the arms, and usually a brief cry. Also called startle reflex.

mortality (1) Quality or state of being subject to death. (2) Number of deaths in relation to a specific population; incidence.

  fetal m. Number of fetal deaths per 1000 births (or per live births). See also *death, fetal.*

  infant m. Number of deaths per 1000 children 1 year of age or younger.

  maternal m. Number of maternal deaths per 100,000 births.

  neonatal m. Number of neonatal deaths per 1000 births (or per live births). See also *neonatal mortality.*

  perinatal m. Combined fetal and neonatal mortality. See also *death, perinatal.*

morula Developmental stage of the fertilized ovum in which there is a solid mass of cells resembling a mulberry.

mosaicism Condition in which some somatic cells are normal, whereas others show chromosomal aberrations.

mourning The process of finding the answers to the questions surrounding the loss, coping with grief responses, and determining how to live again.

multifetal pregnancy Pregnancy in which there is more than one fetus in the uterus at the same time; multiple pregnancy.

multigravida Woman who has been pregnant two or more times.

multipara Woman who has carried two or more pregnancies to viability, whether they ended in live infants or stillbirths.

mutation Change in a gene or chromosome in gametes that may be transmitted to offspring.

mutuality Component of parent-infant attachment; infant behaviors and characteristics call forth corresponding parent behaviors and characteristics.

myelomeningocele External sac containing meninges, spinal fluid, and nerves that protrudes through defect in vertebral column.

Nägele's (or Naegele's) rule Method for calculating the estimated date of birth (EDB) or "due date."

narcotic antagonist A compound such as naloxone (Narcan) that promptly reverses the effects of narcotics such as meperidine (Demerol).

natal Relating or pertaining to birth.

navel Depression in the center of the abdomen, where the umbilical cord was attached to the fetus; umbilicus.

necrotizing enterocolitis (NEC) Acute inflammatory bowel disorder that occurs primarily in preterm or low-birth-weight neonates. It is characterized by ischemic necrosis (death) of the gastrointestinal mucosa, which may lead to perforation and peritonitis; formula-fed infants are at higher risk for this disease.

negligence Commission of an act that a prudent person would not have done or the omission of a duty that a prudent person would have fulfilled, resulting in injury or harm to another person. In particular, in a malpractice suit a professional person is negligent if harm to a client results from such an act or such a failure to act, but it must be proved that other prudent persons of the same profession would ordinarily have acted differently under the same circumstances.

neonatal abstinence syndrome Signs and symptoms associated with drug withdrawal in the neonate.

neonatal mortality Statistical rate of infant death during the first 28 days after live birth, expressed as the number of such deaths per 1000 live births in a specific geographic area or institution in a given period of time.

neonatal narcosis Central nervous system depression in the newborn caused by a narcotic; may be exhibited by respiratory depression, hypertonia, lethargy, and delay in temperature regulation.

neonatology Branch of medicine that studies care of the neonate.

neoplasia Growth of new tissue; tumor that serves no physiologic function; may be benign or malignant.

neural tube Tube formed from fusion of the neural folds from which develop the brain and spinal cord.

  n. t. defect Improper development of tube resulting in malformation of brain or spinal cord; see alpha-fetoprotein.

neutral thermal environment (NTE) Environment that enables the neonate to maintain a body temperature of at least 36.5° C with minimum use of oxygen and energy.

nevus Natural blemish or mark; a congenital circumscribed deposit of pigmentation in the skin; mole.

  n. flammeus Port-wine stain; reddish, usually flat, discoloration of the face or neck. Because of its large size and color, it is considered a serious deformity.

  n. vasculosus (strawberry hemangioma) Elevated lesion of immature capillaries and endothelial cells that regresses over a period of years.

nidation Implantation of the fertilized ovum in the endometrium, or lining, of the uterus.

nipple confusion Difficulty experienced by some infants in mastering breastfeeding after having been given a pacifier or bottle. This problem appears to be more related to tactile sensation than flow of liquid.

nipple cup A device used to make inverted nipples erectile.

nonmaleficence The principle in bioethics directing us to act so as to avoid causing harm.

nonnutritive sucking Use of a pacifier by infants.

nonreassuring fetal heart rate pattern Fetal heart rate pattern that indicates the fetus is not well oxygenated and requires intervention.

nonshivering thermogenesis Infant's method of producing heat from brown fat by increasing metabolic rate.

nonstress test (NST) Evaluation of fetal response (fetal heart rate) to natural contractile uterine activity or to an increase in fetal activity.

normoglycemia Blood glucose level within normal limits; glycemic control.

nosocomial Pertaining to a hospital.

nuchal cord Encircling of fetal neck by one or more loops of umbilical cord.

nuclear family Family form consisting of parents and their dependent children.

nulligravida Woman who has never been pregnant.

nullipara Woman who has not yet carried a pregnancy to viability.

nurse-practitioner Registered nurse who has additional education to practice nursing in an expanded role.

observer style Characteristic style described by May that is displayed by expectant fathers who show a detached approach to involvement in their partner's pregnancy.

occipitobregmatic Pertaining to the occiput (the back part of the skull) and the bregma (junction of the coronal and sagittal sutures) or anterior fontanel.

occiput Back part of the head or skull.

oligohydramnios Abnormally small amount or absence of amniotic fluid; often indicative of fetal urinary tract defect.

oliguria Urine output below 25 to 30 ml by the kidneys for 2 consecutive hours (in adults).

omphalitis Inflammation of the umbilical stump characterized by redness, edema, and purulent exudate in severe infections.

omphalocele Congenital defect resulting from failure of closure of the abdominal wall or muscles and leading to hernia of abdominal contents through the navel.

oocyte Primordial or incompletely developed ovum.

oogenesis Formation and development of the ovum.

operculum Plug of mucus that fills the cervical canal during pregnancy.

ophthalmia neonatorum Infection in the neonate's eyes usually resulting from gonorrheal or other infection contracted when the fetus passes through the birth canal (vagina).

opisthotonos Tetanic spasm resulting in an arched, hyperextended position of the body.

oral glucose tolerance test Test for blood glucose after oral ingestion of a concentrated sugar solution.

orchitis Inflammation of one or both of the testes, characterized by swelling and pain, often caused by mumps, syphilis, or tuberculosis.

orifice Normal mouth, entrance, or opening, to any aperture.

os Mouth, or opening.
  external o. (o. externum) External opening of the cervical canal.
  internal o. (o. internum) Internal opening of the cervical canal.
  o. uteri Mouth, or opening, of the uterus.

ossification Mineralization of fetal bones.

osteoporosis Deossification of bone tissue resulting in structural weakness; decreased bone mass increasing risk of fractures, especially after menopause.

outlet Opening by which something can leave.
  pelvic o. Lower aperture, or opening, of the true pelvis.

ovary One of two glands in the female situated on either side of the pelvic cavity that produces the female reproductive cell, the ovum, and two known hormones, estrogen and progesterone.

ovulation Periodic ripening and discharge of the ovum from the ovary, usually 14 days before the onset of menstrual flow.
  o. method Control of fertility using evaluation of cervical mucus throughout the menstrual cycle; ovulation occurs just after the appearance of the peak mucus sign; Billings method.

ovum Female germ, or reproductive cell, produced by the ovary; egg.

oxygen toxicity Oxygen overdosage that results in pathologic tissue changes (e.g., retinopathy of prematurity, bronchopulmonary dysplasia).

oxytocics Drugs that stimulate uterine contractions, thus accelerating childbirth and preventing postbirth hemorrhage. They may be used to increase the letdown reflex during lactation.

oxytocin Hormone produced by the posterior pituitary that stimulates uterine contractions and the release of milk in the mammary gland (letdown reflex).
  o. challenge test (OCT) Evaluation of fetal response (fetal heart rate) to contractile activity of the uterus stimulated by exogenous oxytocin (Pitocin).

Paco$_2$ Partial pressure of carbon dioxide in arterial blood.

palmar erythema Rash on the surface of the palms sometimes seen in pregnancy.

palsy Permanent or temporary loss of sensation or ability to move and control movement; paralysis.
  Bell's p. Peripheral facial paralysis of the facial nerve (cranial nerve VII), causing the muscles of the unaffected side of the face to pull the face into a distorted position.
  Erb's p. See *Erb-Duchenne paralysis.*

Pao₂ Partial pressure of oxygen in arterial blood.

Papanicolaou (Pap) smear Microscopic examination using scrapings from the cervix, endocervix, or other mucous membranes that will reveal, with a high degree of accuracy, the presence of premalignant or malignant cells.

para Usually expressed as a number that refers to parity. See *parity.*

paracervical block Type of regional anesthesia produced by injection of a local anesthetic into the lower uterine segment just beneath the mucosa adjacent to the outer rim of the cervix (3 and 9 o'clock positions).

parental adjustment Process that a person goes through in adapting to the parental role; includes three stages: expectations, reality, and transition to mastery.

parity Number of past pregnancies that have reached viability, regardless of whether the infant or infants were alive or stillborn. See *para.*

parturient Woman giving birth.

parturition Process or act of giving birth.

patent Open.

pathogen Substance or organism capable of producing disease.

pathologic jaundice See *jaundice, pathologic.*

peau d'orange Orange peel–like skin secondary to cancerous lesions and seen over edematous breasts.

pedigree Shorthand method of depicting family lines of individuals that is usually used for tracing manifestations of a physical or chemical disorder.

pelvic Pertaining or relating to the pelvis.

p. exenteration Surgical removal of all reproductive organs and adjacent tissues

p. inflammatory disease (PID) Infection of internal reproductive structures and adjacent tissues usually secondary to sexually transmitted infections.

p. inlet See *inlet, pelvic.*

p. outlet See *outlet, pelvic.*

p. relaxation Refers to the lengthening and weakening of the fascial supports of pelvic structures.

p. tilt (rock) Exercise used to help relieve low back discomfort during menstruation and pregnancy.

pelvimetry Measurement of dimensions and proportions of the pelvis to determine its capacity and ability to allow the passage of the fetus through the birth canal.

pelvis Bony structure formed by the sacrum, coccyx, innominate bones, and symphysis pubis and the ligaments that unite them.

android p. See *android pelvis.*

anthropoid p. See *anthropoid pelvis.*

gynecoid p. See *gynecoid pelvis.*

platypelloid p. See *platypelloid pelvis.*

true p. Pelvis below the linea terminalis.

penis Male organ used for urination and copulation.

percutaneous umbilical blood sampling (PUBS) Procedure during which the fetal umbilical vessel is accessed for blood sampling or for transfusions.

perimenopause Period of transition of changing ovarian activity before menopause and through first few years of amenorrhea.

perinatal Of or pertaining to the time and process of giving birth or being born.

perinatal period Period extending from the twentieth or twenty-eighth week of gestation through the end of the twenty-eighth day after birth.

perinatologist Physician who specializes in fetal and neonatal care.

perineum Area between the vagina and rectum in the female and between the scrotum and rectum in the male.

periodic breathing Sporadic episodes of cessation of respirations for periods of 10 seconds or less not associated with cyanosis typically noted in preterm infants.

periods of reactivity (newborn infant) First period (within 30 minutes after birth): brief cyanosis, flushing with crying; crackles, nasal flaring, grunting, retractions; heart sounds loud, forceful, irregular; alert; mucus; no bowel sounds; followed by period of sleep. Second period (4 to 8 hours after birth): swift color changes; irregular respiratory and heart rates; mucus with gagging; meconium passage; temperature stabilizing.

peripartum heart failure Inability of the heart to maintain an adequate cardiac output. Heart failure occurring during pregnancy.

periventricular Intraventricular hemorrhage, a common type of brain injury in preterm infants; prognosis depends on severity of hemorrhage.

pessary Device placed inside the vagina to function as a supportive structure for the uterus.

petechiae Pinpoint hemorrhagic areas caused by numerous disease states involving infection and thrombocytopenia and occasionally found over the face and trunk of the newborn because of increased intravascular pressure in the capillaries during birth.

pH Hydrogen ion concentration.

phenotype Expression of certain physical or chemical characteristics in an individual resulting from interaction between genotype and environmental factors.

phenylketonuria (PKU) Recessive hereditary disease that results in a defect in the metabolism of the amino acid phenylalanine caused by the lack of an enzyme, phenylalanine hydroxylase, that is necessary for the conversion of the amino acid phenylalanine into tyrosine. If PKU is not treated, brain damage may occur, causing severe mental retardation.

phimosis Tightness of the prepuce, or foreskin, of the penis.

phlebitis Inflammation of a vein with symptoms of pain and tenderness along the course of the vein, inflammatory swelling and acute edema below the obstruction, and discoloration of the skin because of injury or bruise to the vein, possibly occurring in acute or chronic infections or after procedures or childbirth.

phlebothrombosis Formation of a clot or thrombus in the vein; inflammation of the vein with secondary clotting.

phocomelia Developmental anomaly characterized by the absence of the upper portion of one or more limbs so that the feet or hands or both are attached to the trunk of the body by short, irregularly shaped stumps, resembling the fins of a seal.

phosphatidylglycerol A phospholipid, a component of pulmonary surfactant; its presence in amniotic fluid is considered a sign of fetal lung maturity when the pregnancy is complicated by maternal diabetes.

phototherapy Utilization of lights to reduce serum bilirubin levels by oxidation of bilirubin into water-soluble compounds that are then processed in the liver and excreted into bile and urine.

physiologic jaundice See *jaundice, physiologic.*

phytoestrogens Plant compounds that have a weak estrogenic effect in the human body; used in the management of menopause as an alternative or complement to conventional hormone replacement therapy.

pica Unusual craving during pregnancy (e.g., of laundry starch, dirt, red clay).

pinch test Determines if nipples are everted or inverted by placing thumb and forefinger on areola and pressing inward. The nipple will stand erect or invert.

placenta Latin, flat cake; afterbirth, specialized vascular disk-shaped organ for maternal-fetal gas and nutrient exchange. Normally it implants in the thick muscular wall of the upper uterine segment.

    abruptio p. See *abruptio placentae.*

    battledore p. Umbilical cord insertion into the margin of the placenta.

    circumvallate p. Placenta having a raised white ring at its edge.

    p. accreta Invasion of the uterine muscle by the placenta, thus making separation from the muscle difficult if not impossible.

    p. increta Deep penetration in myometrium by placenta.

    p. percreta Perforation of uterus by placenta.

    p. previa Placenta that is abnormally implanted in the thin, lower uterine segment and that is typed according to proximity to cervical os: total—completely occludes os; partial—does not occlude os completely; and marginal—placenta encroaches on margin of internal cervical os.

    p. succenturiata Accessory placenta.

placental Pertaining or relating to the placenta.

    p. infarct Localized, ischemic, hard area on the fetal or maternal side of the placenta.

    p. souffle See *souffle, placental.*

platypelloid pelvis Broad pelvis with a shortened anteroposterior diameter and a flattened, oval, transverse shape.

plethora Deep, beefy-red coloration of a newborn caused by an increased number of blood cells (polycythemia) per volume of blood.

plugged ducts Milk ducts blocked by small curds of dried milk.

podalic Concerning or pertaining to the feet.

    p. version Shifting of the position of the fetus so as to bring the feet to the outlet during labor.

polycythemia Increased number of erythrocytes per volume of blood, which may be caused by large placental transfusion, fetus transfusion, or maternal-fetal transfusion, or it may be attributable to hypovolemia resulting from movement of fluid out of vascular into interstitial compartment.

polydactyly Excessive number of digits (fingers or toes).

polyhydramnios See *hydramnios.*

polyp Small tumorlike growth that projects from a mucous membrane surface.

polyuria Excessive secretion and discharge of urine by the kidneys.

position Relationship of an arbitrarily chosen fetal reference point, such as the occiput, sacrum, chin, or scapula on the presenting part of the fetus to its location in the front, back, or sides of the maternal pelvis.

positive signs of pregnancy Definite indication of pregnancy (e.g., hearing the fetal heartbeat, visualization and palpation of fetal movement by the examiner, sonographic examination).

posterior Pertaining to the back.

    p. fontanel See *fontanel, posterior.*

postmature infant Infant born at or after the beginning of week 43 of gestation or later and exhibiting signs of dysmaturity.

postnatal Happening or occurring after birth (newborn).

postpartum Happening or occurring after birth (mother).

    p. blues A letdown feeling, accompanied by irritability and anxiety, which usually begins 2 to 3 days after giving birth and disappears within a week or two. Sometimes called the "baby blues."

    p. depression Depression occurring within 6 months of childbirth, lasting longer than postpartum blues and characterized by a variety of symptoms that interfere with activities of daily living and care of the baby.

    p. hemorrhage Excessive bleeding after childbirth; traditionally defined as a loss of 500 ml or more after a vaginal birth

    p. psychosis Symptoms begin as postpartum blues or depression but are characterized by a break with reality. Delusions, hallucinations, confusion, delirium, and panic can occur.

postterm pregnancy Pregnancy prolonged past 42 weeks of gestation (also called *postdate pregnancy*).

posttraumatic stress disorder An anxiety disorder characterized by an acute emotional response to a traumatic event or situation such as sexual abuse.

precipitous labor Rapid or sudden labor of less than 3 hours beginning from onset of cervical changes to completed birth of neonate.

preconception care Care designed for health maintenance before pregnancy.

preeclampsia Disease encountered after 20 weeks of gestation or early in the puerperium; a vasospastic disease process characterized by increasing hypertension, proteinuria, and hemoconcentration.

pregestational diabetes Diabetes mellitus type 1 or type 2 that exists before pregnancy.

pregnancy Period between conception through complete birth of the products of conception. The usual duration of pregnancy in the human is 280 days, 9 calendar months, or 10 lunar months.
> **abdominal p.** See *abdominal gestation.*
> **ectopic p.** See *ectopic pregnancy.*
> **extrauterine p.** See *extrauterine pregnancy.*

pregnancy-induced hypertension (PIH) Hypertensive disorders of pregnancy including preeclampsia, eclampsia, and transient hypertension.

preload The stretch of myocardial fiber at end-diastole. The ventricular end-diastole pressure and volume reflect this parameter.

premature dilation of the cervix See *incompetent cervix.*

premature infant Infant born before completing week 37 of gestation, irrespective of birth weight; preterm infant.

premature rupture of membranes (PROM) See *membrane(s).*

premenstrual syndrome Syndrome of nervous tension, irritability, weight gain, edema, headache, mastalgia, dysphoria, and lack of coordination occurring during the last few days of the menstrual cycle preceding the onset of menstruation.

premonitory Serving as an early symptom or warning.

prenatal Occurring or happening before birth.

prepartum Before birth; before giving birth.

prepuce Fold of skin, or foreskin, covering the glans penis of the male.
> **p. of the clitoris** Fold of the labia minora that covers the glans clitoris.

presentation That part of the fetus that first enters the pelvis and lies over the inlet: may be head, face, breech, or shoulder.
> **breech p.** See *breech presentation.*
> **cephalic p.** See *cephalic presentation.*

presenting part That part of the fetus that lies closest to the internal os of the cervix.

pressure edema Edema of the lower extremities caused by pressure of the heavy pregnant uterus against the large veins; edema of fetal scalp after cephalic presentation (caput succedaneum).

presumptive signs of pregnancy Manifestations that are suggestive of pregnancy but are not absolutely positive. These include the cessation of menses, Chadwick's sign, morning sickness, and quickening.

preterm birth Birth occurring before 37 weeks of gestation.

preterm premature rupture of membranes (PPROM) See *membrane(s).*

prevention Desire to avoid illness, detect it early, or maintain optimal functioning when illness is present.

previa, placenta See *placenta previa.*

primary survey The immediate response after trauma: the *ABC's* of resuscitation: establishment and maintenance of an airway, ensuring adequate breathing, and maintenance of an adequate circulatory volume.

primigravida Woman who is pregnant for the first time.

primipara Woman who has carried a pregnancy to viability whether the child is dead or alive at the time of birth.

primordial Existing first or existing in the simplest or most primitive form.

probable signs of pregnancy Manifestations or evidence that indicates that there is a definite likelihood of pregnancy. Among the probable signs are enlargement of abdomen, Goodell's sign, Hegar's sign, Braxton Hicks sign, and positive hormonal tests for pregnancy.

prodromal Serving as an early symptom or warning of the approach of a disease or condition (e.g., prodromal labor).

progesterone Hormone produced by the corpus luteum and placenta whose function is to prepare the endometrium of the uterus for implantation of the fertilized ovum, develop the mammary glands, and maintain the pregnancy.

prolactin A pituitary hormone that triggers milk production.

prolapsed cord Protrusion of the umbilical cord in advance of the presenting part.

proliferative phase of menstrual cycle Preovulatory, follicular, or estrogen phase of the menstrual cycle.

promontory of the sacrum Superior projecting portion of the sacrum at the junction of the sacrum and L5.

prophylactic (1) Pertaining to prevention or warding off of disease or certain conditions. (2) Condom, or "rubber."

proscription Forbidden; taboo.

prostaglandin (PG) Substance present in many body tissues; has a role in many reproductive tract functions; used to induce abortions, cervical ripening for labor induction.

proteinuria Presence of protein in urine.

pruritus Itching.

pseudocyesis Condition in which the woman has all the usual signs of pregnancy, such as enlargement of the abdomen, cessation of menses, weight gain, and morning sickness, but is not pregnant; phantom or false pregnancy.

pseudopregnancy See *pseudocyesis.*

psychoprophylaxis Mental and physical education of the parents in preparation for childbirth, with the goal of minimizing fear and pain and promoting positive family relationships.

ptyalism Excessive salivation.

puberty Period in life in which the reproductive organs mature and one becomes functionally capable of reproduction.

pubic Pertaining to the pubis.

pubis Pubic bone forming the front of the pelvis.

pudendal block Injection of a local anesthetizing drug at the pudendal nerve root to produce numbness of the genital and perianal region.

puerperal infection Infection of the pelvic organs during the postbirth period; childbed fever.

puerperium Period after the third stage of labor and lasting until involution of the uterus takes place, usually about 3 to 6 weeks.

pulmonary artery catheter (PAC) A flow-directed, balloon-tipped multilumen catheter made of polyvinyl chloride that is inserted into the pulmonary artery to provide continuous measurements of pulmonary artery pressure when the balloon is deflated and pulmonary capillary wedge pressures when the balloon is inflated. Sometimes called a Swan-Ganz catheter.

pulmonary artery pressure (PAP) Systolic and diastolic pressures of blood in the pulmonary artery; reflects right afterload.

pulmonary capillary wedge pressure (PCWP) Pressure when the balloon of the pulmonary artery catheter (PAC) is inflated to obstruct right-sided pressures and to reflect left-sided pressures. Value is obtained during diastole, with the mitral valve open; it reflects left preload.

pulmonary vascular resistance A measure for the tension required for the ejection of blood from the right ventricle into the circulation (afterload).

pulse oximetry Noninvasive method of monitoring oxygen levels by detecting the amount of light absorbed by oxygen-carrying hemoglobin.

pyrosis A burning sensation in the epigastric and sternal region from stomach acid (heartburn).

quickening Maternal perception of fetal movement; usually occurs between weeks 16 and 20 of gestation.

radioimmunoassay Pregnancy test that tests for the beta subunit of human chorionic gonadotropin using radioactively labeled markers.

rape-trauma syndrome Characteristic symptoms seen in victims of rape and consisting of several phases; similar to posttraumatic stress syndrome.

recessive trait Genetically determined characteristic that is expressed only when present in the homozygotic state.

reciprocity Type of body movement or behavior that provides the observer with cues, such as the behavioral cues infants provide to parents and parents' responses to cues.

recommended dietary allowances (RDAs) Recommended nutrient intakes estimated to meet the needs of almost all (97% to 98%) of the healthy people in the population.

reconstituted family See *blended family.*

rectocele Herniation or protrusion of the rectum into the posterior vaginal wall.

referred pain Discomfort originating in a local area such as cervix, vagina, or perineal tissues but felt in the back, flanks, or thighs.

reflection Looking within for solutions and answers to certain dilemmas, using intuition and inner wisdom as guides for attainment of healing.

reflex Automatic response built into the nervous system that does not need the intervention of conscious thought (e.g., in the newborn, rooting, gagging, grasp).

reflex bradycardia Slowing of the heart in response to a particular stimulus.

refractory oliguria Oliguria not corrected with fluid challenge.

regional anesthesia Anesthesia of an area of the body by injection of a local anesthetic to block a group of sensory nerve fibers.

regurgitate Vomiting or spitting up of solids or fluids.

relaxation The absence or alleviation of mental, physical, and emotional tension through purposeful activities that quiet the mind and body.

residual urine Urine that remains in the bladder after urination.

respiratory distress syndrome (RDS) Condition resulting from decreased pulmonary gas exchange, leading to retention of carbon dioxide (increase in arterial Pco_2). Most common neonatal causes are prematurity, perinatal asphyxia, and maternal diabetes mellitus; hyaline membrane disease (HMD).

restitution In obstetrics, the turning of the fetal head to the left or right after it has completely emerged from the introitus as it assumes a normal alignment with the infant's shoulders.

resuscitation Restoration of consciousness or life in one who is apparently dead or whose respirations or cardiac function or both have ceased.

retained placenta Retention of all or part of the placenta in the uterus after birth.

retinopathy of prematurity (ROP) Associated with hyperoxemia, resulting in eye injury and blindness in premature infants.

retraction (1) Drawing in or sucking in of soft tissues of chest, indicative of an obstruction at any level of the respiratory tract from the oropharynx to the alveoli. (2) Retraction of uterine muscle fiber. After contracting, the muscle fiber does not return to its original length but remains slightly shortened, a unique attribute of uterine muscle that aids in preventing postdelivery hemorrhage and results in involution.

retroflexion Bending backward.

r. of uterus Condition in which the body of the uterus is bent backward at an angle with the cervix, the position of which usually remains unchanged.

retrolental fibroplasia (RLF) See *retinopathy of prematurity.*

retroversion Turning or a state of being turned back.

r. of uterus Displacement of the uterus; the body of the uterus is tipped backward with the cervix pointing forward toward the symphysis pubis.

Rh factor Inherited antigen present on erythrocytes. The individual with the factor is known as positive for the factor.

Rh immune globulin (RhIG) Solution of gamma globulin that contains Rh antibodies. Intramuscular administration of Rh immune globulin (trade name RhoGAM) prevents sensitization in Rh-negative women who have been exposed to Rh-positive red blood cells.

rheumatic heart disease Permanent damage of the heart muscle and valves secondary to an autoimmune reaction in the heart tissue precipitated by rheumatic fever.

rhythm method Contraceptive method in which a woman abstains from sexual intercourse during the ovulatory phase of her menstrual cycle; calendar method.

ribonucleic acid (RNA) Element responsible for transferring genetic information within a cell; a template, or pattern.

ring of fire Burning sensation as vagina stretches and fetal head crowns.

risk factors Factors that cause a person or a group of people to be particularly vulnerable to an unwanted, unpleasant, or unhealthful event.

risk taking Intentional behaviors with uncertain outcomes.

rite of passage Significant life event indicating movement from one maturational level to another.

Ritgen maneuver Procedure used to control the birth of the head.

rooming-in unit Maternity unit designed so that the newborn's crib is at the mother's bedside or in a nursery adjacent to the mother's room.

rooting reflex Normal response of the newborn to move toward whatever touches the area around the mouth and to attempt to suck. This reflex usually disappears by 3 to 4 months of age.

rotation In obstetrics, the turning of the fetal head as it follows the curves of the birth canal downward.

rubella vaccine Live attenuated rubella virus given to clients who have not had rubella or who are serologically negative. Exposure to the rubella virus through vaccination causes the client to form antibodies, producing active immunity.

Rubin's test Transuterine insufflation of the uterine tubes with carbon dioxide to test their patency; infrequently used.

rugae Folds in the vaginal mucosa and scrotum.

sac, amniotic See *amniotic sac.*

sacroiliac Of or pertaining to the sacrum and ilium.

sacrum Triangular bone composed of five united vertebrae and situated between L5 and the coccyx; forms the posterior boundary of the true pelvis.

safe passage Normal uneventful birth process for mother and child.

safe period The days in the menstrual cycle that are not designated as fertile days, that is, before and after ovulation.

safer sex Use of protection whenever body fluids (semen, blood, vaginal secretions) are exchanged.

sagittal suture Band of connective tissue separating the parietal bones, extending from the anterior to the posterior fontanel.

salpingo-oophorectomy Removal of a uterine tube and an ovary.

Schultze's mechanism Delivery of the placenta with the fetal surfaces (shiny in appearance) presenting.

scrotum Pouch of skin containing the testes and parts of the spermatic cords.

second stage Stage of labor from full dilation of the cervix to the birth of the baby.

secondary areola See *areola, secondary.*

secondary survey A complete physical assessment of all body systems after immediate resuscitation and stabilization after trauma to mother and fetus.

secretory phase of menstrual cycle Postovulatory, luteal, progestational, premenstrual phase of menstrual cycle; 14 days in length.

secundines Fetal membranes and placenta expelled after childbirth; afterbirth.

self-care Client provides care for self as part of plan of care.

semen Thick, white, viscid secretion discharged from the urethra of the male at orgasm; the transporting medium of the sperm.

semen analysis Examination of semen specimen to determine liquefaction, volume, pH, sperm density, and normal morphology.

sensitization Development of antibodies to a specific antigen.

sensory behavior Responses of the five senses; indicate a readiness for social interaction.

sepsis Bacterial infections of the bloodstream.

septic abortion See *abortion, septic.*

sex chromosome Chromosome associated with determination of gender: the X (female) and Y (male) chromosomes. The normal female has two X chromosomes, and the normal male has one X and one Y chromosome.

sexual decision making Selection of choices concerned with intimate and sexual behavior.

sexual history Past and present health conditions, lifestyle behaviors, knowledge, and attitudes related to sex and sexuality.

sexual response cycle The phases of physical changes that occur in response to sexual stimulation and sexual tension release.

sexuality The part of life that has to do with being male or female.

sexually transmitted infections (STIs) Infections transmitted as a result of sexual activity with an infected individual; also called sexually transmitted diseases (STDs).

shake test "Foam" test for lung maturity of fetus; more rapid than determination of lecithin/sphingomyelin ratio.

Sheehan syndrome Postpartum necrosis of the pituitary gland resulting from hypovolemic shock and disseminated intravascular coagulation.

sibling rivalry Negative behaviors exhibited by siblings in response to the addition of a new baby in the family.

sickle cell hemoglobinopathy Abnormal crescent-shaped red blood corpuscles in the blood.

Sims' position Position in which the client lies on the left side with the right knee and thigh drawn upward toward the chest.

single-parent family Family form characterized by one parent (male or female) in the household. This may result from loss of spouse by death, divorce, separation, desertion, or birth of a child to a single woman.

single-room maternity care (SRMC) Variation of care sites where one nurse provides care to a mother and infant, that is, mother-baby units, LDRPs.

singleton A single fetus.

situational crisis Crisis that arises suddenly in response to an external event or a conflict concerning a specific circumstance. The symptoms are transient, and the episode is usually brief.

sitz bath Application of moist heat to the perineum by sitting in a tub or basin filled with warm water.

sleep-wake cycles Variations in states of newborn consciousness.

small for gestational age (SGA) Inadequate growth for gestational age.

smegma Whitish secretion around labia minora and under foreskin of penis.

somatic pain Perineal discomfort resulting from stretching of perineal tissues.

sonogram See *ultrasonography*.

souffle Soft, blowing sound or murmur heard by auscultation.

    funic s. Soft, muffled, blowing sound produced by blood rushing through the umbilical vessels and synchronous with the fetal heart sounds.

    placental s. Soft, blowing murmur caused by the blood current in the placenta and synchronous with the maternal pulse.

    uterine s. Soft, blowing sound made by the blood in the arteries of the pregnant uterus and synchronous with the maternal pulse.

sperm Male sex cell. Also called *spermatozoon, spermatozoa.*

spermatogenesis Process by which mature spermatozoa are formed, during which the diploid chromosome number (46) is reduced by half (haploid, 23).

spermicide Chemical substance that kills sperm by reducing their surface tension, causing the cell wall to break down by a bactericidal effect or by creating a highly acidic environment. Also called *spermatocide.*

spina bifida occulta Congenital malformation of the spine in which the posterior portion of laminas of the vertebrae fails to close but there is no herniation or protrusion of the spinal cord or meninges through the defect. The newborn may have a dimple in the skin or growth of hair over the malformed vertebrae.

spinnbarkeit Formation of a stretchable thread of cervical mucus under estrogen influence at time of ovulation.

spirituality The individual's connection to one's own values, purpose, and meaning of life. May encompass organized religion or belief in higher power or authority. Recognition of wisdom, imagination, spirit, intuition. A perception of the unity of nature and the interconnectedness of all beings. Inner strength.

splanchnic engorgement Excessive filling or pooling of blood within the visceral vasculature that occurs after the removal of pressure from the abdomen, such as birth of an infant, removal of an excess of urine from bladder, removal of large tumor.

spontaneous abortion See *abortion, spontaneous.*

spontaneous rupture of membranes (SROM) Rupture of membranes by natural means.

squamocolumnar junction Site in the endocervical canal where columnar epithelium and squamous epithelium meet; also called *transformation zone.*

squamous intraepithelial lesion (SIL) Term used to describe neoplastic changes of the cervix.

square window Angle of wrist between hypothenar prominence and forearm; one criterion for estimating gestational age of neonate.

standard body weight An appropriate weight for height; a body mass index (BMI) within the normal range.

state-related behavior Behavioral responses dependent on current state of infant.

station Relationship of the presenting fetal part to an imaginary line drawn between the ischial spines of the pelvis.

sterility (1) State of being free from living microorganisms. (2) Complete inability to reproduce offspring.

sterilization Process or act that renders a person unable to produce children.

stillbirth The birth of a baby after 20 weeks of gestation and 1 day or weighing 350 g (depending on the state code) that does not show any signs of life.

stress urinary incontinence (SUI) Loss of urine occurring with increased abdominal pressure (e.g., with coughing or sneezing).

striae gravidarum ("stretch marks") Shining reddish lines caused by stretching of the skin, often found on the abdomen, thighs, and breasts during pregnancy. These streaks turn to a fine pinkish white or silver tone in time in fair-skinned women and brownish in darker-skinned women.

stroke volume Volume of blood ejected from the left ventricle during one cardiac cycle.

subinvolution Failure of a part (e.g., the uterus) to reduce to its normal size and condition after enlargement from functional activity (e.g., pregnancy).

suboccipitobregmatic diameter Smallest diameter of the fetal head–follows a line drawn from the middle of the anterior fontanel to the undersurface of the occipital bone.

supine hypotension Shock; fall in blood pressure caused by impaired venous return when gravid uterus presses on ascending vena cava, when woman is lying flat on her back; vena cava syndrome.

supply meets demand Physiologic basis for determining milk production. The volume of milk produced equals the amount of milk removed from the breast.

support systems Network from which people receive help in times of crisis.

surfactant Phosphoprotein necessary for normal respiratory function that prevents the alveolar collapse (atelectasis). See also *lecithin* and *L/S ratio.*

suture (1) Junction of the adjoining bones of the skull. (2) Procedure uniting parts by their being sewn together.

Svo₂ monitoring Percentage of saturation of hemoglobin with oxygen in mixed venous and arterial blood monitored with a fiberoptic pulmonary artery catheter that is connected to a bedside microprocessor. The SvO₂ reflects the balance between oxygen delivery and oxygen use.

symphysis pubis Fibrocartilaginous union of the bodies of the pubic bones in the midline.

synchrony Fit between an infant's cues and the parent's response.

syndactyly Malformation of digits, often seen as a fusion of two or more toes to form one structure.

systemic analgesia Analgesics administered either intramuscularly or intravenously that cross the blood-brain barrier and provide central analgesic effects.

systemic lupus erythematosus (SLE) A chronic inflammatory connective tissue disease affecting many systems, that is, the integumentary, renal, and nervous systems.

systemic vascular resistance (SVR) A measure of the tension required for the ejection of blood from the left ventricle into the circulation (afterload) and is derived by calculation as follows: SVR = [(MAP − CVP)/CO] × 80.

taboo Proscribed (forbidden) by society as improper and unacceptable; a proscription.

tachypnea Excessively rapid respiratory rate (e.g., in neonates, respiratory rate of 60 breaths/min or more).

taking-hold phase Period after birth characterized by a woman becoming more independent and more interested in learning infant care skills; learning to be a competent mother is an important task.

taking-in phase Period after birth characterized by the woman's dependency; maternal needs are dominant, and talking about the birth is an important task.

talipes equinovarus Deformity in which the foot is extended and the person walks on the toes.

telangiectasia Permanent dilation of groups of superficial capillaries and venules.

telangiectatic nevi ("stork bites") Clusters of small, red, localized areas of capillary dilation frequently seen in neonates at the nape of the neck or lower occiput, upper eyelids, and nasal bridge that can be blanched with pressure of a finger.

teratogenic agent Any drug, virus, or irradiation, the exposure to which can cause malformation of the fetus.

teratogens Nongenetic factors that cause malformations and disorders in utero.

teratoma Tumor composed of different kinds of tissue, none of which normally occurs together or at the site of the tumor.

term infant Live infant born between weeks 38 and 42 of completed gestation.

term pregnancy Gestation that continues until at least 38 weeks.

testis One of the glands contained in the male scrotum that produces the male reproductive cell, or sperm, and the male hormone, testosterone; testicle.

tetany, uterine Extremely prolonged uterine contractions.

thalassemia An anemia affecting Mediterranean and Southeast Asian populations in which there is an insufficient amount of globin produced to fill the red blood cells.

therapeutic abortion See *abortion, therapeutic.*

therapeutic donor insemination See *insemination, therapeutic donor.*

therapeutic rest Administration of analgesics to decrease pain and induce rest for management of hypertonic uterine dysfunction.

therapeutic touch A modern interpretation of the laying-on-of-hands for healing, as interpreted by Dolores Krieger, PhD, RN, and Dora Kunz, a noted healer. Originally taught within nursing programs.

thermal shift Drop and subsequent rise in basal body temperature around the time of ovulation.

thermistor probe Automatic sensor used to monitor skin temperature of infant under radiant warmer.

thermogenesis Creation or production of heat, especially in the body.

thermoregulation Control of temperature.

third stage Stage of labor from the birth of the baby to the expulsion of the placenta.

threatened abortion See *abortion, threatened.*

thrombocytopenia Abnormal hematologic condition in which the number of platelets is reduced, usually by destruction of erythroid tissue in bone marrow because of certain neoplastic diseases or an immune response to a drug.

thrombocytopenic purpura Hematologic disorder characterized by prolonged bleeding time, decreased number of platelets, increased cell fragility, and purpura, which result in hemorrhages into the skin, mucous membranes, organs, and other tissue.

thromboembolism Obstruction of a blood vessel by a clot that has become detached from its site of formation.

thrombophlebitis Inflammation of a vein with secondary clot formation.

thrombus Blood clot obstructing a blood vessel that remains at the place it was formed.

thrush Fungal infection of the mouth or throat that is characterized by the formation of white patches on a red, moist, inflamed mucous membrane and is caused by *Candida albicans.*

toco- (toko-) Combining form that means childbirth or labor.

tocolysis See *tocolytic therapy.*

tocolytic therapy Medications used to relax the uterus, to suppress preterm labor, or for version.

tocotransducer Electronic device for measuring uterine contractions.

TORCH infections Infections caused by organisms that damage the embryo or fetus; acronym for *t*oxoplasmosis, *o*ther (e.g., syphilis), *r*ubella, *c*ytomegalovirus, and *h*erpes simplex.

toxemia Term previously used for hypertensive states of pregnancy.

toxicology screen Laboratory analysis of blood or urine to test for alcohol or drug content. Urine drug screening is the most common because it is noninvasive.

toxic shock syndrome A severe acute disease usually caused by *Staphylococcus aureus;* associated with high-absorbency tampon use during menstruation.

tracheoesophageal fistula Congenital malformation in which there is an abnormal tubelike passage between the trachea and esophagus.

traditional Chinese medicine Ancient methods of healing that combine herbs, energy healing, and movement as a pathway to health. Seeks to heal on deeper levels, rather than just treat symptoms.

transformation zone See *squamocolumnar junction.*

transition—labor See *transition phase.*

transition period—newborn Period from birth to 4 to 6 hours later; infant passes through period of reactivity, sleep, and second period of reactivity.

transition phase Phase in first stage of labor from a cervical dilation of 8 to 10 cm.

transition to parenthood Period of time from the preconception parenthood decision through the first months after birth of the baby during which parents define their parental roles and adjust to parenthood.

translocation Condition in which a chromosome breaks and all or part of that chromosome is transferred to a different part of the same chromosome or to another chromosome.

trial of labor (TOL) Period of observation to determine if a laboring woman is likely to be successful in progressing to a vaginal birth.

***Trichomonas* vaginitis** Inflammation of the vagina caused by *Trichomonas vaginalis,* a parasitic protozoon, and characterized by persistent burning and itching of the vulvar tissue and a profuse, frothy, white discharge.

trimester One of 3 periods of about 3 months each into which pregnancy is divided.

trisomy Condition whereby any given chromosome exists in triplicate instead of the normal duplicate pattern.

trophoblast Outer layer of cells of the developing blastodermic vesicle that develops the trophoderm or feeding layer, which will establish the nutrient relationships with the uterine endometrium.

trophoblastic disease A condition in which trophoblastic cells covering the chorionic villi proliferate and undergo cystic changes, which may be malignant.

tubal ligation Abdominal procedure in which the uterine tubes are tied off and a section is removed to interrupt tubal continuity and thus sterilize the woman.

tubercles of Montgomery Small papillae on surface of nipples and areolae that secrete a fatty substance that lubricates the nipples.

twins Two neonates from the same impregnation developed within the same uterus at the same time.

    conjoined t. Twins who are physically united; Siamese twins.

    disparate t. Twins who are different (e.g., in weight) and distinct from one another.

    dizygotic t. Twins developed from two separate ova fertilized by two separate sperm at the same time; fraternal twins.

    monozygotic t. Twins developed from a single fertilized ovum; identical twins.

ultrasonography Use of high-frequency sound waves for a variety of obstetric diagnoses and for fetal surveillance.

ultrasound transducer External signal source for monitoring fetal heart rate electronically.

umbilical cord (funis) Structure connecting the placenta and fetus and containing two arteries and one vein encased in a tissue called Wharton's jelly. The cord is ligated at birth and severed; the stump falls off in 4 to 10 days.

umbilicus Navel, or depressed point in the middle of the abdomen that marks the attachment of the umbilical cord during fetal life.

urethra Small tubular structure that drains urine from the bladder.

urinary frequency Need to void often or at close intervals.

urinary meatus Opening, or mouth, of the urethra.

uterine Referring or pertaining to the uterus.

   u. adnexa See *adnexa, uterine.*

   u. atony Relaxation of uterus; leads to postpartum hemorrhage.

   u. bruit Abnormal sound or murmur heard while auscultating the uterus.

   u. ischemia Decreased blood supply to the uterus.

   u. prolapse Falling, sinking, or sliding of the uterus from its normal location in the body.

   u. souffle See *souffle, uterine.*

uteroplacental insufficiency (UPI) Decline in placental function–exchange of gases, nutrients, and wastes–leading to fetal hypoxia and acidosis; evidenced by late fetal heart rate decelerations in response to uterine contractions.

uterus Hollow muscular organ in the female designed for the implantation, containment, and nourishment of the fetus during its development and expulsion of fetus during labor and birth; also organ of menstruation.

   Couvelaire u. Interstitial myometrial hemorrhage after premature separation (abruption) of placenta. A purplish-bluish discoloration of the uterus and board-like rigidity of the uterus are noted.

   inversion of u. See *inversion of uterus.*

   retroflexion of u. See *retroflexion of uterus.*

   retroversion of u. See *retroversion of uterus.*

vaccination Intentional injection of antigenic material given to stimulate antibody production in the recipient.

vacuum-assisted birth Birth involving attachment of vacuum cup to fetal head and using negative pressure to assist in birth of the fetus.

vacuum curettage Uterine aspiration method of early abortion.

vagina Normally collapsed musculomembranous tube that forms the passageway between the uterus and the entrance to the vagina.

vaginal birth after cesarean (VBAC) Giving birth vaginally after having had a previous cesarean birth.

vaginismus Intense, painful spasm of the muscles surrounding the vagina.

Valsalva maneuver Any forced expiratory effort against a closed airway such as holding one's breath and tightening the abdominal muscles (e.g., pushing during the second stage of labor).

variability Normal irregularity of fetal cardiac rhythm; short term–beat-to-beat changes; long term–rhythmic changes (waves) from the baseline value.

varicocele Enlargement of veins of the spermatic cord.

varicosity (varicose veins) Swollen, distended, and twisted veins that may develop in almost any part of the body but are most commonly seen in the legs, caused by pregnancy, obesity, congenital defective venous valves, and occupations requiring much standing.

vasectomy Ligation or removal of a segment of the vas deferens, usually done bilaterally to produce sterility in the male.

VDRL test Abbreviation for Venereal Disease Research Laboratories test, a serologic flocculation test for syphilis.

vernix caseosa Protective gray-white fatty substance of cheesy consistency covering the fetal skin.

version Act of turning the fetus in the uterus to change the presenting part and facilitate birth.

   external cephalic v. See *external cephalic version.*

   podalic v. Shifting of the fetus's position so as to bring the feet to the outlet during birth.

vertex Crown or top of the head.

   v. presentation Presentation in which the fetal head is nearest the cervical opening and is born first.

very low birth weight (VLBW) Refers to infant weighing 1500 g or less at birth.

viable, viability Capable, capability of living, as in a fetus that has reached a stage of development, usually 22 menstrual weeks (20 weeks of gestation), which will permit it to live outside the uterus.

visceral pain Discomfort from cervical changes and uterine ischemia located over the lower portion of the abdomen and radiating to the lumbar area of the back and down the thighs.

vulva External genitalia of the female that consist of the labia majora, labia minora, clitoris, urinary meatus, and vaginal introitus.

vulvar self-examination (VSE) Systematic examination of the vulva by the client.

vulvectomy Surgical removal of all or parts of the vulva.

warm line A help line, or consultation service, for families to access; most often for support of newborn care and postpartum care after hospital discharge.

weaning Process of changing from breastfeeding or bottle feeding to drinking from a cup.

Wharton's jelly White, gelatinous material surrounding the umbilical vessels within the cord.

witch's milk Secretion of a whitish fluid for about a week after birth from enlarged mammary tissue in the neonate, presumably resulting from maternal hormonal influences.

withdrawal (1) Physiologic or cognitive changes that occur after removal of the substance in the substance-dependent person; (2) removing penis from vagina before ejaculation (coitus interruptus).

womb See *uterus.*

X chromosome Sex chromosome in humans existing in duplicate in the normal female and singly in the normal male.

X linkage Genes located on the X chromosome.

Y chromosome Sex chromosome in the human male necessary for the development of the male gonads.

ZIFT Zygote intrafallopian transfer.

zona pellucida Inner, thick membranous envelope of the ovum.

zygote Cell formed by the union of two reproductive cells or gametes; the fertilized ovum resulting from the union of a sperm and an ovum.

Index

A

ABCX theory; *see* Family stress theory
Abdomen
  auscultation of, 709
  hernias, 908-909
  newborn assessments
    circumference, 696*t*, 706, *707*
    description of, 108
    initial assessment, 717
    parameters, 701-702*t*, 709
  postpartum appearance, 585
  trauma
    blunt, 932
    penetrating, 932-933
Abduction, of newborn, 603
ABO blood groups
  classification of, 1072
  incompatibility in, 1072-1073
Abortion
  care management approach, 201
  complications after, 203
  elective, 200
  epidemiologic data regarding, 200
  first trimester, 201-202
  incidence of, 4
  induced, 200-201
  methods of
    dilation and evacuation,
      202-203
    methotrexate, 202
    mifepristone, 196, 202
    prostaglandins, 203
    vacuum aspiration, 201-202
  nursing considerations, 203
  psychologic sequelae of, 201
  second trimester, 202-203
  spontaneous; *see* Miscarriage
  therapeutic, 200
Abortus, 4

Abruptio placentae
  classification of, 855
  clinical manifestations of, 855-856
  definition of, 855
  electronic fetal monitoring, 935
  etiology of, 855
  fetal mortality, 856
  home care for, 857
  hospital care for, 856-857
  illustration of, *855*
  incidence of, 855
  maternal hypertension and, 855
  maternal mortality, 856
  neonatal mortality, 856
  placenta previa and, differential diagnosis
    between, 851*t*
  risk factors, 855
  trauma and, 935
Abstinence
  neonatal syndrome, 1063, *1064*
  periodic, as contraceptive method,
    181-182
Abuse; *see also* Violence
  childhood, 227
  physical
    anatomic areas of, 105
    description of, 104-105
    indicators of, 106
    medical history questions regarding,
      102
    prenatal care assessments, 396
    screening for, 104-106, *105*
  sexual
    care management approach, 238-239
    definition of, 237
    labor in victims of, 518
    perpetuation of, 238
    psychopathologic consequences of,
      238
    resource information and
      organizations, 244
    types of, 237-238
  substance; *see* Substance abuse

Acculturation, 22
Acesulfame K, 361
Acetaminophen, 1159
Acid-base balance
  fetal assessments, 506
  pregnancy-induced changes, 345
Acid mantle, 752
Acinus, 92-93
Acoustic stimulation test, of fetal heart rate,
  810
Acquired immunity, 100
Acquired immunodeficiency syndrome; *see*
  also Human immunodeficiency virus
  description of, 163
  in neonates, 4
  opportunistic infections associated with,
    163
  resources for, 1167
Acquired resistance, 100
Acrocyanosis, 682, 706
Acroesthesia, 349
Acupressure
  for childbirth pain management, 440,
    470-471
  for cocaine abuse, 946
  definition of, 54
  history of, 59
  for pregnancy-related nausea and
    vomiting, 61-62,
    62
Acupuncture, 54, 61, 1167
Acute distress, 1136
Acyclovir
  breastfeeding and, 1160
  for herpes simplex virus, 152*t*, 160, 1056
Adaptations
  of grandparents
    to newborn, 652-654
    to pregnancy, 389
  to labor
    circulation, 460
    heart rate, 459-460
    respiration, 460

Page numbers in *italics* indicate illustrations;
t indicates tables.

GUIDELINES/GUÍAS

TEACHING guidelines

MEDICATION GUIDE

CULTURAL considerations

RESEARCH

continued

RESEARCH—CONT'D

PROCEDURE

EMERGENCY

SIGNS OF POTENTIAL COMPLICATIONS

THE CITY OF MIRRORS

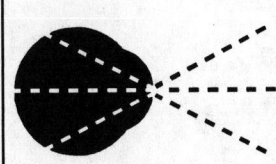

This Large Print Book carries the
Seal of Approval of N.A.V.H.

THE CITY OF MIRRORS

JUSTIN CRONIN

WHEELER PUBLISHING
A part of Gale, Cengage Learning

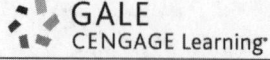

GALE
CENGAGE Learning·

Farmington Hills, Mich • San Francisco • New York • Waterville, Maine
Meriden, Conn • Mason, Ohio • Chicago

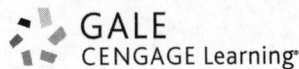

LIBRARY OF CONGRESS CATALOGING-IN-PUBLICATION DATA

Names: Cronin, Justin, author.
Title: The city of mirrors / Justin Cronin.
Description: Large print edition. | Waterville, Maine : Wheeler Publishing Large Print, 2016. | Series: The passage trilogy ; 3 | Series: Wheeler Publishing large print hardcover
Identifiers: LCCN 2016015321 | ISBN 9781410489968 (hardback) | ISBN 1410489965 (hardcover)
Subjects: LCSH: Survival—Fiction. | Large type books. | BISAC: FICTION / Horror. | GSAFD: Epic fiction. | Suspense fiction.
Classification: LCC PS3553.R542 C58 2016b | DDC 813/.54—dc23
LC record available at https://lccn.loc.gov/2016015321

Published in 2016 by arrangement with Ballantine Books, an imprint of Random House, a division of Penguin Random House LLC

For my family

And how am I to face the odds
Of man's bedevilment and God's?
I, a stranger and afraid
In a world I never made.
— A. E. HOUSMAN, *Last Poems*

CONTENTS

PROLOGUE

From the Writings of the First Recorder ("The Book of Twelves")

Presented at the Third Global Conference on the North American Quarantine Period

Center for the Study of Human Cultures and Conflicts

University of New South Wales, Indo-Australian Republic

April 16–21, 1003 A.V.

[Excerpt 2 begins.]

CHAPTER FIVE

1 Thus did it come to pass that Amy and her fellows returned to Kerrville, in the place of Texas.

2 And there they were to learn that three among them had been lost. And these were Theo and Mausami, his wife; and Sara, who was called Sara the Healer, wife of Hollis.

3 For in the place of Roswell, where they had taken shelter, a great army of virals had laid siege, killing every kind. And only two of their company survived. And these were

Hollis the Strong, husband of Sara, and Caleb, son of Theo and Mausami.

4 And a great sadness was upon them all, for the friends that they had lost.

5 And in the place of Kerrville, Amy went to live among the Sisters, who were women of GOD. And likewise did Caleb do the same, to be cared for by Amy.

6 And in that same period, Alicia, who was Alicia of Blades, and Peter, the Man of Days, took up arms with the Expeditionary, who were soldiers of Texas, to search for the Twelve. For they had learned that to kill one of the Twelve was to kill his Many also, sending their souls unto the LORD.

7 And many battles were joined; and many lives were lost. But neither could they slay the Twelve, nor find the places wherein they dwelled. For such was not the will of GOD at that time.

8 And in this manner did the years pass, five in sum.

9 And at the end of that time, Amy received a sign; and this sign was a dream. And in that dream Wolgast came to her, appearing as a man. And Wolgast said:

10 "My master is waiting; and the place of his waiting is a great ship in which he dwells. For a change is upon the land. Soon I will come for you, to show you the way."

11 And that man was Carter, Twelfth of Twelve, who was to be called Carter the Sorrowful; a man righteous in his generation, and beloved of GOD.

12 And thus did Amy wait for Wolgast's return.

1 But there was also in that time another city of mankind, in the place of Iowa. And this was known as the Homeland.

2 And in that place abided a race of men who had drunk the blood of a viral, so that they might live, ruling for many generations. And these were called Redeyes. And the greatest of these was Guilder the Director, a man of the Time Before.

3 And the viral from which they took their sustenance was Grey, called the Source. For in his blood was the seed of Zero, father of the Twelve. And Grey abided in chains, wherein he suffered greatly.

4 And in that place the people lived as captives to serve the Redeyes, doing all they wished. And one of these captives was Sara the Healer, taken at the place of Roswell, whose friends knew not that she lived.

5 And Sara had a daughter, Kate; but the child was taken away. And the Redeyes told Sara that her daughter had not survived, causing a great woe in her heart.

6 And it came to pass that the child was given to a woman of the Redeyes. And this was Lila, wife of Wolgast.

7 For Lila's daughter had died in the Time Before; and though many years had passed, the wound was still sharp in her mind. And she took comfort in Kate, imagining her to be the daughter she had lost.

8 And it came to pass that certain people of the Homeland rose up against their oppres-

sors; and these were the Insurgents. And Sara joined with them. And she was sent to Lila to serve her in the Dome, wherein the Redeyes dwelled, that she might learn more about their ways. And in this manner did she discover that her daughter yet lived.

9 And in that same time also, Alicia and Peter discovered the lair of Martínez, Tenth of Twelve, in the place of Carlsbad; and there they did battle with his Many. But they did not find Martínez, who had fled from that place.

10 For Zero had commanded Guilder the Director to build a mighty fortress, wherein the Twelve should reside, to feed upon the blood of beasts and the blood of the Homelanders also. For their Many had devoured nearly every living thing upon the earth, making it a wasteland, fit neither for man nor viral, nor any kind of animal.

11 And in accordance with this design, the Twelve told their Many to leave their places of darkness; and they died. And this was known as the Casting Off.

12 And the Twelve commenced their journeys to the Homeland, a distance of many miles, so that they might preside over the earth.

CHAPTER SEVEN

1 But there was one who did not heed Zero's words; and this was Carter the Sorrowful, Twelfth of Twelve. And he instructed Wolgast to guide Amy to the place wherein he dwelled, that they two might join against his fellows.

2 And Amy heeded this command and left the place of Kerrville for the place of Houston. And in her company was Lucius the Faithful, who was a helpmate to her, and a man righteous in the eyes of GOD.

3 And in the place of Houston, Amy found the ship, which was the *Chevron Mariner;* and in its belly Carter dwelled. And many things passed between them. And when Amy emerged, her body was no longer that of a child, but of a woman; and in the company of Lucius she set out for the Homeland, to do battle with the Twelve.

4 And in that time also, Peter, the Man of Days; and Michael, who was called Michael the Clever; and Hollis, husband of Sara, likewise journeyed to the Homeland, to learn what was there. For they had come to believe that Sara was held captive in that place and many others also.

5 And with them were two companions. And the first of these was Lore, who was Lore the Pilot. And the second was a criminal, called Tifty the Gangster.

6 And in that same period, Alicia likewise made her way to the place of Iowa, pursuing Martínez, Tenth of Twelve, whom she had vowed to slay. For Martínez was the most evil of these demons, a killer of many women, and a scourge upon the earth.

7 But Alicia was taken captive at the Homeland, and endured many tribulations at the hands of the Redeyes and their helpmates, who were called Cols. And the worst of the Cols was Sod. But Alicia was strong and did not yield.

8 And when one night Sod came to her cell, so that he might have his dark way with her again, Alicia said: "Loosen my chains, so that you may take your pleasure more easily." And she wrapped the chains around his neck, killing him in this manner. And she made her escape, slaying many others.

9 And in the wilderness beyond the walls of the Homeland, Amy appeared to her; and Alicia saw that she was now a woman in body as well as mind. And Amy comforted her; for they were sisters in blood.

10 But Alicia had a secret; and this was the blood-hunger. For the seed of the Twelve was growing strong within her, making her a viral. And this was a great heaviness in her heart, for she loved her fellows deeply, and did not wish to be apart from them.

11 And in that same time, Sara was discovered by the Redeyes; and she was made a captive, and suffered many violations. For Guilder the Director desired that all who had risen up against him should know his wrath in fullest measure.

12 But the hour of reckoning was at hand; for Amy and Alicia had joined with the Insurgents, to take arms against the Redeyes. And among them a plan was hatched to liberate the people of the Homeland and destroy the Twelve and rescue Sara also.

CHAPTER EIGHT

1 And it came to pass that Peter and his fellows arrived in the place of Iowa, so that all were in attendance, making a mighty force.

And the greatest of these was Amy.

2 For she had surrendered to the Redeyes, saying: "I am the leader of the Insurgents; do with me as you will." For it was her design that Guilder in his fury should unleash the Twelve to kill her.

3 And all did come to pass as Amy had foreseen; and the hour of her execution was established. And this would occur in the Stadium, a great amphitheater from the Time Before, so that the people of the Homeland might see.

4 And Alicia and the others concealed themselves in that place, so that when the Twelve were revealed, they could use their weapons upon them and upon the Redeyes also.

5 And Amy was brought before the crowd, and bound in chains; and upon an armature of metal she was made to hang. And Guilder took great delight in her suffering, exhorting the multitudes to do likewise.

6 But Amy would not give him satisfaction. And Guilder commanded the Twelve to devour her, so that all in attendance might know his power, bowing down before him.

7 But Amy saw that she was not alone; for among the Twelve was Wolgast, who had taken Carter's place, so that he might protect her. And Amy said to the Twelve:

8 "My brothers, hello. It is I, Amy, your sister." And no more words were spoken by her.

9 For she began to shake, and her body became as a bright light shattering the darkness; and with a furious roar Amy became as one of them, taking the form of

a viral, mighty to behold. And this was the Letting Go. And one to see was Peter, and another Alicia, and a third Lucius, and all the others also.

10 And the chains were broken, and a great battle joined; and a great victory was won. And many lives were lost. And one of these was Wolgast, who sacrificed himself to save Amy; for his love for her was like unto a father's for his child.

11 And in this manner the Twelve perished from off the face of the earth, freeing all its people.

12 But of Amy's fate, her friends knew nothing; for she was nowhere to be found.

■ ■ ■ ■

I
THE DAUGHTER

■ ■ ■ ■

98–101 A.V.

There is another world but it is this one.
— PAUL ÉLUARD

1

CENTRAL PENNSYLVANIA
August 98 A.V.
Eight months after the liberation of the Homeland

The ground yielded easily under her blade, unlocking a black smell of earth. The air was hot and moist; birds were singing in the trees. On her hands and knees, she stabbed the dirt, chopping it loose. One handful at a time, she scooped it away. Some of the weakness had abated but not all. Her body felt loose, disorganized, drained. There was pain, and the memory of pain. Three days had passed, or was it four? Perspiration beaded on her face; she licked her lips to taste the salt. She dug and dug. The sweat ran in rivulets, falling into the earth. That's where everything goes, Alicia thought, in the end. Everything goes into the earth.

The pile beside her swelled. How deep was enough? Three feet down, the soil began to change. It became colder, with the odor of clay. It seemed like a sign. She rocked back on her boots and took a long drink from her canteen. Her hands were raw; the flesh at the base of her thumb had peeled back in a sheet. She placed the web of her hand to her mouth and used her teeth to sever the flap of skin and spat it into the dirt.

Soldier was waiting for her at the edge of the clearing, his jaws loudly working on a stand of waist-high grass. The grace of his haunches, his rich mane and blue roan coat, the magnificence of his hooves and teeth and the great black marbles of his eyes: an aura of splendor surrounded him. He possessed, when he chose, an absolute calm, then, in the next moment, could perform remarkable deeds. His wise face lifted at the sound of her approach. *I see. We're ready.* He turned in a slow arc, his neck bent low, and followed her into the trees to the place where she had pitched her tarp. On the ground beside Alicia's bloody bedroll lay the small bundle, swaddled in a stained blanket. Her daughter had lived less than an hour, yet in that hour Alicia had become a mother.

Soldier watched as she emerged. The baby's face was covered; Alicia drew back the cloth. Soldier bent his face to the child's, his nostrils flaring, breathing in her scent. Tiny nose and eyes and rosebud mouth, startling in their humanness; her head was covered in a cap of soft red hair. But there was no life, no breath. Alicia had wondered if she would be capable of loving her — this child conceived in terror and pain, fathered by a monster. A man who had beaten her, raped her, cursed her. How foolish she'd been.

She returned to the clearing. The sun was directly overhead; insects buzzed in the grass, a rhythmic pulsing. Soldier stood beside her as she laid her daughter in the grave. When her labor had started, Alicia had begun to pray. *Let her be all right.* As the hours of agony dissolved into one another, she had felt death's cold presence inside her. The pain pounded through her, a wind of

steel; it echoed in her cells like thunder. Something was wrong. *Please, God, protect her, protect us.* But her prayers had fallen into the void.

The first handful of soil was the hardest. How did one do it? Alicia had buried many men. Some she'd known, and some she hadn't; only one she'd loved. The boy, Hightop. So funny, so alive, then gone. She let the dirt sift through her fingers. It struck the cloth with a pattering sound, like the first spits of rain upon leaves. Bit by bit her daughter disappeared. *Goodbye,* she thought, *goodbye, my darling, my one.*

She returned to her tent. Her soul felt shattered, like a million chips of glass inside her. Her bones were tubes of lead. She needed water, food; her stores were exhausted. But hunting was out of the question, and the creek, a five-minute walk down the hillside, felt like miles away. The needs of the body: what did they matter? Nothing mattered. She lay on her bedroll and closed her eyes, and soon she was asleep.

She dreamed of a river. A wide, dark river, and above it the moon was shining. It laid its light across the water like a golden road. What lay ahead Alicia did not know, only that she needed to cross this river. She took her first cautious step upon its glowing surface. Her mind felt divided: half marveled at this unlikely mode of travel; the other half did not. As the moon touched the far shore, she realized she had been deceived. The shining pathway was dissolving. She broke into a run, desperate to reach the other side before the river swallowed her. But the distance was too great; with every step she took, the horizon leapt farther away. The water sloshed around her ankles, her knees, her waist. She had no strength to fight

23

its pull. *Come to me, Alicia. Come to me, come to me, come to me.* She was sinking, the river was taking her, she was plunging into darkness . . .

She awoke to a muted orange light; the day had nearly passed. She lay motionless, assembling her thoughts. She had grown accustomed to these nightmares; the pieces changed but never the feeling of them — the futility, the fear. Yet this time something was different. An aspect of the dream had traveled into life; her shirt was sopping. She looked down to see the widening stains. Her milk had come in.

Staying was not a conscious decision; the will to move on was simply absent. Her strength returned. It approached with small steps; then, like a guest long awaited, it arrived all at once. She constructed a shelter of deadfall and vines, using the tarp as a roof. The woods abounded with life: squirrels and rabbits, quail and doves, deer. Some were too quick for her but not all. She set traps and waited to collect her kill or took them on her cross: one shot, a clean death, then dinner, raw and warm. At the end of each day when the light had faded, she bathed in the creek. The water was clear and shockingly cold. It was on such an excursion that she saw the bears. A rustling ten yards upstream, something heavy moving in the brush; then they appeared at the edge of the creek, a mother and a pair of cubs. Alicia had never seen such creatures in the flesh, only in books. They prowled the shallows together, pushing the mud with their snouts. There was something loose and half-formed about their anatomy, as if the muscles were not firmly stitched to the skin beneath their heavy, twig-tangled coats. A cloud of insects

24

sparkled around them, catching the last of the light. But the bears did not appear to notice her or, if they did, did not think she was important.

The summer faded. One day, a world of fat green leaves, dense with shadow; then the woods exploded with riotous color. In the morning, the floor of the forest crunched with frost. Winter's cold descended with a feeling of purity. Snow lay heavy on the land. The black lines of the trees, the small footprints of birds, the whitewashed sky, bleached of all tone: everything had been pared to its essence. What month was it? What day? As time wore on, food became a problem. For hours, whole days even, she barely moved, conserving her strength; she hadn't spoken to a living soul in nearly a year. Gradually it came to her that she was no longer thinking in words, as if she had become a creature of the forest. She wondered if she was losing her mind. She began to talk to Soldier, as if he were a person. *Soldier,* she would say, *what should we have for dinner? Soldier, do you think it's time to gather wood for the fire? Soldier, does the sky look like snow?*

One night she awoke in the shelter and realized that for some time she'd been hearing thunder. A wet spring wind was blowing in directionless gusts, hurling around in the treetops. With a feeling of detachment, Alicia listened to the storm's approach; then it was suddenly upon them. A blast of lightning forked the sky, freezing the scene in her eyes, followed by an earsplitting clap. She let Soldier inside as the heavens opened, ejecting raindrops heavy as bullets. The horse was shivering with terror. Alicia needed to calm him; just one panicked movement in the tiny space and his massive body would blow the shelter to pieces.

You're my good boy, she murmured, stroking his flank. With her free hand she slipped the rope around his neck. *My good, good boy. What do you say? Keep a girl company on a rainy night?* His body was tense with fear, a wall of coiled muscle, and yet when she applied slow force to draw him downward, he allowed it. Beyond the walls of the shelter, the lightning flashed, the heavens rolled. He dropped to his knees with a mighty sigh, turned onto his side beside her bedroll, and that was how the two of them slept as the rain poured down all night, washing winter away.

She abided in that place for two years. Leaving was not easy; the woods had become a solace. She had taken its rhythms as her own. But when Alicia's third summer began, a new feeling stirred: the time had come to move on. To finish what she'd started.

She passed the rest of the summer preparing. This involved the construction of a weapon. She left on foot for the river towns and returned three days later, hauling a clanking bag. She understood the basics of what she was attempting, having watched the process many times; the details would come through trial and error. A flat-topped boulder by the creek would serve as her anvil. At the water's edge, she stoked her fire and watched it burn down to coals. Maintaining the right temperature was the trick. When she felt she had it right, she removed the first piece from the sack: a bar of O1 steel, two inches wide, three feet long, three-eighths of an inch thick. From the sack she also withdrew a hammer, iron tongs, and thick leather gloves. She placed the end of the steel bar in the fire and watched its color change as the

metal heated. Then she got to work.

It took three more trips downriver for supplies, and the results were crude, but in the end she was satisfied. She used coarse, stringy vines to wrap the handle, giving her fist a solid purchase on the otherwise smooth metal. Its weight was pleasant in her grip. The polished tip shone in the sun. But the first cut would be the true test. On her final trip downriver, she had wandered upon a field of melons, the size of human heads. They grew in a dense patch, tangled with vines of grasping, hand-shaped leaves. She'd selected one and carried it home in the sack. Now she balanced it atop a fallen log, took aim, and brought the sword down in a vertical arc. The severed halves rocked lazily away from each other, as if stunned, and flopped to the ground.

Nothing remained to hold her in place. The night before her departure, Alicia visited her daughter's grave. She did not want to do this at the last second; her exit should be clean. For two years the place had gone unmarked. Nothing had seemed worthy. But leaving it unacknowledged felt wrong. With the last of her steel, she'd fashioned a cross. She used the hammer to tap it into the ground and knelt in the dirt. The body would be nothing now. Perhaps a few bones, or an impression of bones. Her daughter had passed into the soil, the trees, the rocks, even the sky and animals. She had gone into a place beyond knowing. Her untested voice was in the songs of birds, her cap of red hair in the flaming leaves of autumn. Alicia thought about these things, one hand touching the soft earth. But she had no more prayers inside her. The heart, once broken, stayed broken.

"I'm sorry," she said.

Morning dawned unremarkably — windless, gray, the air compacted with mist. The sword, sheathed in a deer-hide scabbard, lay across her back at an angle; her blades, tucked in their bandoliers, were cinched in an X over her chest. Dark, gogglelike glasses, with leather shields at the temples, concealed her eyes. She fixed the saddlebag in place and swung onto Soldier's back. For days he'd roamed restlessly, sensing their imminent departure. *Are we doing what I think we're doing? I rather like it here, you know.* Her plan was to ride east along the river, to follow its course through the mountains. With luck, she'd reach New York before the first leaves fell.

She closed her eyes, emptying her mind. Only when she had cleared this space would the voice emerge. It came from the same place dreams did, like wind from a cave, whispering into her ear.

Alicia, you are not alone. I know your sorrow, because it's my own. I'm waiting for you, Lish. Come to me. Come home.

She tapped Soldier's flanks with her heels.

2

The day was just ending when Peter returned to the house. Above him, the immense Utah sky was breaking open in long fingers of color against the deepening blue. An evening in early autumn: the nights were cold, the days still fair. He made his way homeward along the murmuring river, his pole over his shoulder, the dog ambling at his side. In his bag were two fat trout, wrapped in golden leaves.

As he approached the farmstead, he heard music

coming from the house. He removed his muddy boots on the porch, put down his bag, and eased inside. Amy was sitting at the old upright piano, her back facing the door. He moved in quietly behind her. So total was her concentration that she failed to notice his entry. He listened without moving, barely with breath. Amy's body was swaying slightly to the music. Her fingers moved nimbly up and down the keyboard, not so much playing the notes as calling them forth. The song was like a sonic embodiment of pure emotion. There was a deep heartache inside its phrases, but the feeling was expressed with such tenderness that it did not seem sad. It made him think of the way time felt, always falling into the past, becoming memory.

"You're home."

The song had ended without his noticing. As he placed his hands on her shoulders, she shifted on the bench and tilted her face upward.

"Come here," she said.

He bent to receive her kiss. Her beauty was astonishing, a fresh discovery every time he looked at her. He tipped his head at the keys. "I still don't know how you do that," he said.

"Did you like it?" She was smiling. "I've been practicing all day."

He told her he did; he loved it. It made him think of so many things, he said. It was hard to put into words.

"How was the river? You were gone a long while."

"Was I?" The day, like so many, had passed in a haze of contentment. "It's so beautiful this time of year, I guess I just lost track." He kissed the top of her head. Her hair was freshly washed,

29

smelling of the herbs she used to soften the harsh lye. "Just play. I'll get dinner going."

He moved through the kitchen to the back door and into the yard. The garden was fading; soon it would sleep beneath the snow, the last of its bounty put up for winter. The dog had gone off on his own. His orbits were wide, but Peter never worried; always he would find his way home before dark. At the pump Peter filled the basin, removed his shirt, splashed water on his face and chest, and wiped himself down. The last rays of sun, ricocheting off the hillsides, lay long shadows on the ground. It was the time of day he liked best, the feeling of things merged into one another, everything held in suspension. As the darkness deepened he watched the stars appear, first one and then another and another. The feeling of the hour was the same as Amy's song: memory and desire, happiness and sorrow, a beginning and an ending joined.

He started the fire, cleaned his catch, and set the soft white meat in the pan with a dollop of lard. Amy came outside and sat beside him while they watched their dinner cook. They ate in the kitchen by candlelight: the trout, sliced tomatoes, a potato roasted in the coals. Afterward they shared an apple. In the living room, they made a fire and settled on the couch beneath a blanket, the dog taking his customary place at their feet. They watched the flames without speaking; there was no need for words, all having been said between them, everything shared and known. When a certain time had passed, Amy rose and offered her hand.

"Come to bed with me."

Carrying candles, they ascended the stairs. In

30

the tiny bedroom under the eaves they undressed and huddled beneath the quilts, their bodies curled together for heat. At the foot of the bed, the dog exhaled a windy sigh and lowered himself to the floor. A good old dog, loyal as a lion: he would remain there until morning, watching over the two of them. The closeness and warmth of their bodies, the common rhythm of their breathing: it wasn't happiness Peter felt but something deeper, richer. All his life he had wanted to be known by just one person. That's what love was, he decided. Love was being known.

"Peter? What is it?"

Some time had passed. His mind, afloat in the dimensionless space between sleep and waking, had wandered to old memories.

"I was thinking about Theo and Maus. That night in the barn when the viral attacked." A thought drifted by, just out of reach. "My brother never could figure out what killed it."

For a moment, Amy was silent. "Well, that was you, Peter. You're the one who saved them. I've told you — don't you remember?"

Had she? And what could she mean by such a statement? At the time of the attack, he had been in Colorado, many miles and days away. How could he have been the one?

"I've explained how this works. The farmstead is special. Past and present and future are all the same. You were there in the barn because you needed to be."

"But I don't remember doing it."

"That's because it hasn't happened yet. Not for you. But the time will come when it does. You'll be there to save them. To save Caleb."

Caleb, his boy. He felt a sudden, overwhelming

31

sadness, an intense and yearning love. Tears rose to his throat. So many years. So many years gone by.

"But we're here now," he said. "You and me, in this bed. That's real."

"There's nothing more real in the world." She nestled against him. "Let's not worry about this now. You're tired, I can tell."

He was. So very, very tired. He felt the years in his bones. A memory touched down in his mind, of looking at his face in the river. When was that? Today? Yesterday? A week ago, a month, a year? The sun was high, making a sparkling mirror of the water's surface. His reflection wavered in the current. The deep creases and sagging jowls, the pockets of flesh beneath eyes dulled by time, and his hair, what little remained, gone white, like a cap of snow. It was an old man's face.

"Was I . . . dead?"

Amy gave no answer. Peter understood, then, what she was telling him. Not just that he would die, as everyone must, but that death was not the end. He would remain in this place, a watchful spirit, outside the walls of time. That was the key to everything; it opened a door beyond which lay the answer to all the mysteries of life. He thought of the day he'd first come to the farmstead, so very long ago. Everything inexplicably intact, the larder stocked, curtains on the windows and dishes on the table, as if it were waiting for them. That's what this place was. It was his one true home in the world.

Lying in the dark, he felt his chest swell with contentment. There were things he had lost, people who had gone. All things passed away. Even the earth itself, the sky and the river and the

32

stars he loved, would, one day, come to the end of their existence. But it was not a thing to be feared; such was the bittersweet beauty of life. He imagined the moment of his death. So forceful was this vision that it was as if he were not imagining but remembering. He would be lying in this very bed; it would be an afternoon in summer, and Amy would be holding him. She would look just as she did now, strong and beautiful and full of life. The bed faced the window, its curtains glowing with diffused light. There would be no pain, only a feeling of dissolution. *It's all right, Peter,* Amy was saying. *It's all right, I'll be there soon.* The light would grow larger and larger, filling first his sight and then his consciousness, and that was how he would make his departure: he would leave on waves of light.

"I do love you so," he said.

"And I love you."

"It was a wonderful day, wasn't it?"

She nodded against him. "And we'll have many more. An ocean of days."

He pulled her close. Outside, the night was cold and still. "It was a beautiful song," he said. "I'm glad we found that piano."

And with these words, curled together in their big, soft bed beneath the eaves, they floated off to sleep.

I'm glad we found that piano.
  That piano.
  That piano.
  That piano . . .

Peter ascended to consciousness to find himself naked, wrapped in sweat-dampened sheets. For a moment, he lay motionless. Hadn't he been . . . ?

33

And wasn't he . . . ? His mouth tasted like he'd been eating sand; his bladder was dense as a rock. Behind his eyes, the first stab of his hangover was making its presence felt.

"Happy birthday, Lieutenant."

Lore lay beside him. Not so much *beside* as coiled around, their bodies knotted together, slick with perspiration where they touched. The shack, just two rooms with a privy out back, was one they'd used before, though its ownership wasn't clear to him. Beyond the foot of the bed, the small window was a gray square of predawn summer light.

"You must be mistaking me for somebody else."

"Oh, believe me," she said, placing a finger against the center of his chest, "there's no mistaking you. So how does it feel to be thirty?"

"Like twenty-nine with a headache."

She smiled seductively. "Well, I hope you liked your present. Sorry I forgot the card."

She unwound herself, swiveled to the edge of the bed, and snatched her shirt from the floor. Her hair had grown long enough to need tying back; her shoulders were wide and strong. She wrenched herself into a pair of dirty gaps, shoved her feet into her boots, and turned her upper body to face him again.

"Sorry to run, *mi amigo,* but I've got tankers to move. I'd make you breakfast, only I seriously doubt there's anything here." She leaned forward to kiss him, quickly, on the mouth. "Give my love to Caleb, okay?"

The boy was spending the night with Sara and Hollis. Neither ever asked Peter where he was going, though certainly they had guessed the kind of thing it was. "I'll do that."

34

"And I'll see you the next time I'm in town?" When Peter said nothing, she cocked her head and looked at him. "Or . . . maybe not."

He didn't really have an answer. What passed between them wasn't love — the subject had never come up — but it was also more than physical attraction. It fell into the gray space between the two, neither one thing nor the other, and that was where the problem lay. Being with Lore reminded him of what he couldn't have.

Her face fell. "Well, shit. And I was so damn *fond* of you, Lieutenant."

"I don't know what to say."

She sighed, looking away. "I guess it's not like this could have lasted. I just wish I'd thought to dump you first."

"I'm sorry. I shouldn't have let things go so far."

"Believe me, it'll pass." She lifted her face toward the ceiling and took a long, steadying breath, then touched a tear away. "Fuck it all, Peter. See what you made me do?"

He felt awful. He hadn't planned this; up until a minute ago, he'd expected that the two of them would just drift in the current of whatever-this-was until they lost interest or new people came along.

Lore asked, "This isn't about Michael, is it? Because I told you, that's over."

"I don't know." He paused, shrugged. "Okay, maybe a little. He's going to find out if we keep this up."

"So he finds out — so what?"

"He's my friend."

She wiped her eyes and gave a quiet, bitter laugh. "Your loyalty is admirable, but trust me, I'm the last thing on Michael's mind. He'd prob-

35

ably thank you for taking me off his hands."

"That's not true."

She shrugged. "You're only saying that because you're being nice. Which is maybe why I like you so much. But you don't have to lie — we both know what we're doing. I keep telling myself I'll get him out of my system, but of course I never do. You know what kills me? He can't even tell me the truth. That goddamn redhead. What is it with her?"

For a moment Peter felt lost. "Are you talking about . . . Lish?"

Lore looked at him sharply. "Peter, don't be dense. What do you think he's doing out in that stupid boat of his? Three years since she's gone, and he still can't get her out of his head. Maybe if she were still around, I'd stand a chance. But you can't compete with a ghost."

It took Peter another moment to process this. A mere minute ago he wouldn't have said that Michael even *liked* Alicia; the two used to quarrel like a couple of cats over a clothesline. But underneath, Peter knew, they were not so unlike — the same cores of strength, the same resolve, the same stubborn refusal to be told no when an idea stuck in their teeth. And, of course, a long history was there. Was that what Michael's boat was all about? That it was his way of mourning the loss of her? They'd all done it in their own fashion. For a time, Peter had been angry with her. She had abandoned them without explanation, not even saying goodbye. But a lot had changed; the world had changed. Mostly what he felt was a pure ache of loneliness, a cold, empty place in his heart where Alicia had once stood.

"As for you," Lore said, rubbing her eyes with

the back of her wrist, "I don't know who she is, but she's a lucky girl."

There was no point in denying it. "I really am sorry."

"So you've said." With a pained smile, Lore clapped her palms on her knees. "Well, I've got my oil. A girl could hardly ask for more. Do me a favor and feel like shit, okay? You don't have to drag it out or anything. A week or two is fine."

"I feel like shit now."

"Good." She leaned forward and took his mouth with a deep kiss that tasted of tears, then pulled abruptly away. "One for the road. See you around, Lieutenant."

The sun was just rising as Peter made his way up the stairs to the top of the dam. His hangover had settled in for the long haul, and a day spent swinging a hammer on a blazing rooftop wasn't going to improve it any. He could have done with an extra hour of sleep, but after his conversation with Lore, he wanted to clear his head before reporting to the jobsite.

The breaking day met him when he reached the top, softened by a low-hanging stratum of clouds that would burn off within the hour. Since Peter's resignation from the Expeditionary, the dam had become a site of totemic importance in his mind. In the days leading up to his fateful departure for the Homeland, he had brought his nephew here. Nothing especially noteworthy had occurred. They had taken in the view and talked about Peter's journeys with the Expeditionary and about Caleb's parents, Theo and Maus, then gone down to the impoundment to swim, something Caleb had never done before. An ordinary outing, yet by the

end of that day, something had changed. A door had opened in Peter's heart. He had not understood it at the time, but on the far side of this door lay a new way of being, one in which he would assume the responsibilities of being the boy's father.

That was one life, the one that people knew about. Peter Jaxon, retired officer of the Expeditionary turned carpenter and father, citizen of Kerrville, Texas. It was a life like anybody else's, with its satisfactions and travails, and he was glad to live it. Caleb had just turned ten. Unlike Peter, who at that age was already serving as a runner of the Watch, the boy was experiencing a childhood. He went to school, he played with his friends, he did his chores without much prodding and only occasional complaint, and every night after Peter tucked him in, he drifted into dreams on the cushioning knowledge that the next day would be just like the last. He was tall for his age, like a Jaxon; the little-boy softness had begun to leave his face. Every day he looked a little bit more like his father, Theo, though the subject of his parents never came up anymore. Not that Peter was avoiding it; the boy just didn't ask. One evening, after Peter and Caleb had been living on their own for six months, the two of them were playing chess when the boy, hovering over his next move, said, simply, with no more weight than if he were inquiring about the weather, *Would it be okay if I called you Dad?* Peter was startled; he had failed to see this coming. *Is that what you want to do?* Peter asked, and the boy nodded. *Uh-huh,* he said. *I think that would be good.*

As for his other life: Peter could not say quite what it was, only that it existed, and that it hap-

38

pened at night. His dreams of the farmstead included a range of days and events, but the tone was always the same: a feeling of belonging, of home. So vivid were these dreams that he awoke with the sensation that he had actually traveled to another place and time, as if his hours of waking and sleeping were two sides of the same coin, neither one more real than the other.

What were these dreams? Where did they come from? Were they the product of his own mind, or was it possible that they derived from an outside source — even from Amy herself? Peter had told no one about the first night of the evacuation from Iowa when Amy had come to him. His reasons were many, but most of all he couldn't be sure the whole thing had actually happened. He had entered the moment from deep sleep, Sara and Hollis's daughter out cold on his lap, the two of them bundled up in the Iowa cold beneath a sky so drunk with stars he had felt himself to be float-ing among them, and there she was. They had not spoken, but they didn't need to. The touch of their hands was enough. The moment had lasted forever and was over in a flash; the next thing Pe-ter knew, Amy was gone.

Had he dreamed that, too? The evidence said so. Everyone believed that Amy had died in the stadium, killed in the blast that had killed the Twelve. No trace of her had been found. And yet the moment had felt so real. Sometimes he was convinced that Amy was still out there; then the doubts would creep in. In the end, he kept these questions to himself.

He stood awhile, watching the sun spread its light over the Texas hills. Below him, the face of the impoundment was as still and reflective as a

mirror. Peter would have liked a swim to shake off his hangover, but he needed to fetch Caleb and take him to school before reporting to the jobsite. He wasn't much of a carpenter — he'd really only ever learned to do one thing, which was be a soldier — but the work was regular and kept him close to home, and with so much construction going on, the Housing Authority needed all the warm bodies they could get.

Kerrville was busting at the seams; fifty thousand souls had made the journey from Iowa, more than doubling the population in just a couple of years. Absorbing so many hadn't been easy and still wasn't. Kerrville had been built on the principle of zero population growth; couples weren't allowed to have more than two children without paying a hefty fine. If one did not survive to adulthood, they could have a third, but only if the child died before the age of ten.

With the arrival of the Iowans, the whole concept had gone out the window. There had been food shortages, runs on fuel and medicine, sanitation problems — all the ills that went with too many people wedged into too little space, with more than enough resentment on both sides to go around. A hastily erected tent city had absorbed the first few waves, but as more arrived, this temporary encampment had quickly descended into squalor. While many of the Iowans, after a lifetime of enforced labor, had struggled to adjust to a life in which not every decision was made for them — a common expression was "lazy as a Homelander" — others had gone in the opposite direction: violating curfew, filling Dunk's whorehouses and gambling halls, drinking and stealing and fighting and generally running amok. The

only part of the population that seemed happy was the trade, which was making money hand over fist, operating a black market in everything from food to bandages to hammers.

People had begun to openly talk about moving outside the wall. Peter supposed this to be just a matter of time; without a single viral sighting in three years, drac or dopey, the pressure was mounting on the Civilian Authority to open the gate. Among the populace, the events in the stadium had become a thousand different legends, no two exactly the same, but even the most hard-core doubters had begun to accept the idea that the threat was really over. Peter, of all people, should have been the first to agree.

He turned to look out over the city. Nearly a hundred thousand souls: there was a time when this number would have knocked him flat. He had grown up in a town — a world — of fewer than a hundred people. At the gate, the transports had gathered to take workers down to the agricultural complex, chuffing diesel smoke into the morning air; from everywhere came the sounds and smells of life, the city rising, stretching its limbs. The problems were real but small when compared to the promise of the scene. The age of the viral was over; humankind was finally on the upswing. A continent stood for the taking, and Kerrville was the place where this new age would begin. So why did it seem so meager to him, so frail? Why, standing on the dam on an otherwise encouraging summer morning, did he feel this inward shiver of misgiving?

Well, thought Peter, so be it. If being a parent taught you one thing, it was that you could worry all you wanted, but it wouldn't change a thing.

He had a lunch to pack and "be good"s to say and a day of honest, simple work to wrestle to the ground, and twenty-four hours from now, he'd start it all over again. *Thirty*, he mused. *Today, I turn thirty years old.* If anyone had asked him a decade ago if he'd live to see it, let alone be raising a son, he would have thought they were crazy. So maybe that was all that really mattered. Maybe just being alive, and having someone to love who loved you back, was enough.

He had told Sara that he didn't want a party, but of course the woman would do something. *After all we've been through, thirty means something. Come by the house after work. It'll just be the five of us. I promise it won't be any big deal.* He picked up Caleb at school and went home to wash, and a little after 1800 they arrived at Sara and Hollis's apartment and stepped through the door and into the party that Peter had refused. Dozens of people were there, crammed into two tiny, airless rooms — neighbors and co-workers, parents of Caleb's friends, men he had served with in the Army, even Sister Peg, who, in her dour gray frock, was laughing and chatting away like everybody else. At the door Sara hugged him and wished him happy birthday, while Hollis put a drink in his hand and clapped him on the back. Caleb and Kate were giggling so fiercely they could barely contain themselves. "Did you know about this?" Peter asked Caleb. "And what about you, Kate?" "Of course we knew!" the boy exclaimed. "You should see your face, Dad!" "Well, you're in big trouble," Peter said, using his cross-dad voice, though he was laughing, too.

There was food, drink, cake, even some pres-

ents, things people could make or scrounge, some of them jokes: socks, soap, a pocketknife, a deck of cards, a huge straw hat, which Peter put on so everybody could enjoy a laugh. From Sara and Hollis, a pocket compass, a reminder of their journeys together, though Hollis also slipped him a small steel flask. "Dunk's latest, something special," he said with a wink, "and don't ask me how I got it. I still have friends in low places."

When the last presents had been opened, Sister Peg presented him with a large piece of paper rolled into a tube. *Happy Birthday to Our Hero,* it read, with the signatures — some legible, some not — of all the children in the orphanage. A lump rising in his throat, Peter put his arms around the old woman, surprising them both. "Thank you, everyone," he said. "Thank you one and all."

It was close to midnight when the party broke up. Caleb and Kate had fallen asleep on Sara and Hollis's bed, the two of them piled together like a couple of puppies. Peter and Sara sat at the table while Hollis cleaned up.

"Any word from Michael?" Peter asked her.

"Not a peep."

"Are you worried?"

She frowned sharply, then shrugged. "Michael's Michael. I don't get this thing with the boat, but he's going to do what he wants to do. I sort of thought Lore might settle him down, but I guess that's done."

Peter felt a stab of guilt; twelve hours ago he'd been in bed with the woman. "How are things at the hospital?" he asked, hoping to change the subject.

"It's a madhouse. They've got me delivering

43

babies. Lots and lots of babies. Jenny's my assistant."

Sara was speaking of Gunnar Apgar's sister, whom they'd found at the Homeland. Pregnant, Jenny had returned to Kerrville with the first batch of evacuees and arrived just in time to deliver. She'd gotten married a year ago to another Iowan, though Peter didn't know if the man was actually the father. A lot of the time, these things were improvised.

"She's sorry she couldn't make it," Sara continued. "You're sort of a big deal to her."

"I am?"

"To lots of people, actually. I can't tell you how many times people have asked me if I know you."

"You're kidding."

"I'm sorry, didn't you read that poster?"

He shrugged, embarrassed, though part of him was pleased. "I'm just a carpenter. Not too good at it, either, if you want to know the truth."

Sara laughed. "Whatever you say."

The hour was long past curfew, but Peter knew how to avoid the patrols. Caleb's eyes barely opened as he hoisted him onto his back and headed home. He had just tucked the boy into bed when he heard a knock on the door.

"Peter Jaxon?"

The man in the doorway was a military officer, with the epaulets of the Expeditionary on his shoulders.

"It's late. My boy's asleep. What can I do for you, Captain?"

He offered Peter a sealed piece of paper. "Have a good night, Mr. Jaxon."

Peter quietly closed the door, cut the wax with his new pocketknife, and opened the message.

44

Mr. Jaxon:

Might I ask you to pay me a call in my office on Wednesday at 0800? Arrangements have been made with your work supervisor to excuse your late arrival at the jobsite.

Sincerely,
Victoria Sanchez
President, Texas Republic

"Dad, why was there a soldier at the door?"

Caleb had wandered into the room, rubbing his eyes with his fists. Peter read the message again. What could Sanchez want with him?

"It's nothing," he said.

"Are you in the Army again?"

He looked at the boy. Ten years old. He was growing so fast.

"Of course not," he said, and put the note aside. "Let's get you back to bed."

3

RED ZONE
Ten Miles West of Kerrville, Texas
July 101 A.V.

Lucius Greer, the Man of Faith, took his position on the platform in the hour before dawn. His weapon: a bolt-action .308, meticulously restored, with a polished wooden stock and an optical sight, its glass clouded by time but still usable. He was down to four rounds; he'd have to return to Kerrville soon, to trade for more. But on this morning of the fifty-eighth day, this was no concern. A single shot was all he'd need.

A gentle mist had settled overnight in the glade. His trap — a bucket of crushed apples — was a

45

hundred yards upwind, nestled in the tall grass. Sitting motionless, his legs folded under him and his rifle resting on his lap, Lucius lay in wait. He had no doubt that his quarry would make an appearance; the smell of fresh apples was irresistible.

To pass the time, he offered a simple prayer: *My God, Lord of the Universe, be my guide and solace, give me the strength and wisdom to do Your will in the days ahead, to know what is required of me, to be worthy of the charge You have placed in my care. Amen.*

Because something was coming; Lucius could feel it. He knew it the same as he knew his own heartbeat, the wind of breath in his chest, the carriage of his bones. The long arc of human history was headed toward the hour of its final test. When this hour would come there was no knowing, but come it surely would, and it would be a time for warriors. For men like Lucius Greer.

Three years had passed since the liberation of the Homeland. The events of that night were still with him, indelible memories flashed upon his consciousness. The bedlam of the stadium, and the virals making their entrance; the insurgency's unleashing of their firepower upon the redeyes and Alicia and Peter advancing on the stage, guns drawn, firing again and again; Amy in chains, a meager figure, and then the roar that rose from her throat as she'd released the power within herself; her body transforming, shedding its human shape, and then the snap of the chains as she freed herself and her bold leap, quick as lightning, upon the monstrous enemies; the chaos and confusion of battle, and Amy trapped beneath Martínez, Tenth of Twelve; the bright flash of destruction, and the absolute quiet of aftermath,

46

the whole world arrested into stillness.

By the time Lucius had returned to Kerrville, the following spring, he knew he could no longer dwell among people. The meaning of that night was clear; he had been called to a solitary existence. Alone, he had constructed his modest hut along the river only to feel the pull of something deeper, summoning him into the wilderness. *Lucius, lay yourself bare. Put down your lendings; cast aside all worldly comforts that you may know me.* With nothing but a blade and the clothes on his back, he had ventured into the dry hills and beyond, no destination but the deepest solitude he could find so that his life might find its true shape. Days without food, his feet torn and bloody, tongue thick in his mouth from thirst: as the weeks went by, with only the rattlesnakes and cacti and scorching sun for company, he had begun to hallucinate. A stand of saguaros became rows of soldiers at attention; lakes of water appeared where there were none; a line of mountains took the form of a walled city in the distance. He experienced these apparitions uncritically, with no awareness of their falsehood; they were real because he believed them to be so. Likewise did the past and present blend in his mind. At times he was Lucius Greer, major of the Expeditionary; at others, a prisoner of the stockade; at still others, a young recruit, or even his boyhood self.

For weeks he wandered in this condition, a being of multiple worlds. Then one day he awoke to discover himself lying in a gully beneath an obliterating midday sun. His body was grotesquely emaciated, covered with scratches and sores; his fingers were bloody, some of the nails torn away. What had happened? Had he done this to himself?

He possessed no recollection, only a sudden, overwhelming awareness of the image that had come to him during the night.

Lucius had received a vision.

He had no sense of where he was, only that he needed to walk north. Six hours later, he found himself on the Kerrville Road. Mad with thirst and hunger, he continued to walk until just before nightfall, when he saw the sign with the red X. The hardbox was amply stocked: food, water, clothes, gas, weapons and ammo, even a generator. Most welcome of all to his eyes was the Humvee. He washed and cleaned his wounds and spent the night on a soft cot, and in the morning he fueled up the vehicle, charged the battery and filled the tires, and headed east, reaching Kerrville on the morning of the second day.

At the edge of the Orange Zone he abandoned the Humvee and made his way into the city on foot. There, in a dark room in H-town, among men he did not know and whose names were never offered, he sold three of the carbines from the hardbox to buy a horse and other supplies. By the time he arrived at his hut, night was falling. It stood modestly among the cottonwoods and swamp oaks at the edge of the river, just one room with a packed-dirt floor, yet the sight of it filled his heart with the warmth of return. How long had he been away? It seemed like years, whole decades of life, and yet it was just a matter of months. Time had come full circle; Lucius was home.

He unsaddled, tied up his horse, and entered the hut. A nest of fluff and twigs on the bed indicated where something had made its home in his absence, but the sparse interior was otherwise

unaltered. He lit the lantern and sat at the table. At his feet was the duffel bag of supplies: the Remington, a box of cartridges, fresh socks, soap, a straight razor, matches, a hand mirror, a half dozen quill pens, three bottles of dewberry ink, and sheets of thick, fibrous paper. At the river he filled his washbasin, then returned to the house. The image in the mirror was neither more nor less shocking than he expected: cheeks cratered, eyes sunk way back in his skull, skin scorched and blistered, a tangle of madman's hair. The lower half of his face was buried beneath a beard that a family of mice would gladly live in. He had just turned fifty-two; the man in the mirror was an easy sixty-five.

Well, he said to himself, if he was going to be a soldier again, even an old, broken-down one, he damn well ought to look the part. Lucius hacked away at the worst of his hair and beard, then used the straight razor and soap to shave himself clean. He tossed the soapy water out the door and returned to the table, where he'd laid out his paper and pens.

Lucius closed his eyes. The mental picture that had come to him that night in the gully wasn't like the hallucinations that had dogged him during his sojourn in the desert. It was more like a memory of something lived. He brought its details into focus, his mind's eye roaming its visual expanse. How could he ever hope to capture something so magnificent with his amateur's hand? But he would have to try.

Lucius began to draw.

A rustling in the brush: Lucius drew the rifle-scope to his eye. There were four of them, rooting

through the dirt, snuffling and grunting: three sows and a boar, reddish brown, with large, razor-sharp tusks. A hundred and fifty pounds of wild pig for the taking.

He fired.

While the sows scattered, the boar staggered forward, shuddered with a deep twitch, and went down on its front legs. Lucius held the image in his scope. Another twitch, deeper than the first, and the animal flopped on its side.

Lucius scrambled down the ladder and went to where the animal lay in the grass. He rolled the boar onto the tarp, dragged it to the tree line, looped the animal's hind legs together, set the hook, and began to hoist him up. When the boar's head reached the height of Lucius's chest, he tied off the rope, positioned the basin beneath the hog, drew his knife, and slashed the animal's throat.

A gush of hot blood splattered into the basin. The boar would produce as much as a gallon. When the boar had emptied out, Lucius funneled the blood into a plastic jug. With more time on his hands, he would have gutted and butchered the animal and smoked the meat for trade. But it was day fifty-eight, and Lucius needed to be on his way.

He lowered the corpse to the ground — at least the coyotes would get the benefit — and returned to the hut. He had to admit it: the place looked like a madman lived there. A little over two years since Lucius had first put pen to paper, and now the walls were covered with the fruits of his labor. He'd branched out from ink to charcoal, graphite pencil, even paint, which cost a bundle. Some were better than others — viewing them in chronological order, one could trace his slow, at

times frustratingly inept self-education as an artist. But the best ones satisfyingly captured the image Lucius carted around in his head all day like the notes of a song he couldn't shake except by singing.

Michael was the only person who'd seen the pictures. Lucius had kept his distance from everyone, but Michael had tracked him down through somebody on the trade, a friend of Lore's. One evening over a year ago Lucius had returned from setting his traps to find an old pickup parked in his yard and Michael sitting on the open tailgate. Over the years Greer had known him, he had grown from a rather meek-looking boy to a well-made specimen of manhood in its prime: hard and sleek, with strong features and a certain severity around the eyes. The sort of companion you could count on in a bar fight that began with a punch to the nose and ended with running like hell.

"Holy damn, Greer," he said, "you look like shit on a biscuit. What does a man have to do to get a little hospitality around this place?"

Lucius got the bottle. At first it wasn't quite clear what Michael wanted. He seemed changed to Lucius, a little at loose ends, a bit sunk down into himself. One thing Michael had never been was quiet. Ideas and theories and various campaigns, however cockeyed and half-baked, shot from the man like bullets. The intensity was still there — you could practically warm your hands on the man's skull — but it had a darker quality, the feel of something caged, as if Michael were chewing on something he didn't have words for.

Lucius had heard that Michael had quit the refinery, split from Lore, built some kind of boat

51

and spent most of his time on it, sailing out alone into the Gulf. What the man was looking for in all that empty ocean, he never got around to saying, and Lucius didn't press; how would he have explained his own hermitic existence? But over the course of the evening they passed together, getting drunker and drunker on a bottle of Dunk's Special Recipe No. 3 — Lucius wasn't much of a drinker these days, though the stuff came in handy as a solvent — he came to think that Michael didn't really *have* a reason for appearing at his doorstep beyond the basic human urge to be around another person. Both of them were doing their time in the wilderness, after all, and maybe what Michael really wanted, when you boiled away the bullshit, was a few hours in the company of someone who understood what he was going through — this profound impulse to be alone just when all of them should have been dancing for joy and having babies and generally celebrating a world where death didn't reach down from the trees and snatch you just for the hell of it.

For a while they caught up on news of the others: Sara's job at the hospital and her and Hollis's long-awaited move out of the refugee camps into permanent housing; Lore's promotion to crew chief at the refinery; Peter's resignation from the Expeditionary to stay home with Caleb; Eustace's decision, which surprised no one, to resign from the Expeditionary and return with Nina to Iowa. A tone of optimistic good cheer glazed the surface of the conversation, but it only went so deep, and Lucius wasn't fooled; always lurking beneath the surface were the names they weren't saying.

Lucius had told nobody about Amy — only he knew the truth. On the matter of Alicia's fate,

Lucius had nothing to offer. Nor, apparently, did anybody else; the woman had vanished into the great Iowa emptiness. At the time, Lucius had been unconcerned — Alicia was like a comet, given to long, unannounced absences and blazing, unanticipated returns — but as the days went by with no sign of her, Michael trapped in his bed with his casted leg in a sling, Lucius watched the fact of her disappearance burning in his friend's eyes like a long fuse looking for a bomb. *You don't get it,* he told Lucius, practically levitating off his bed with frustration. *This isn't like the other times.* Lucius didn't bother to contradict him — the woman needed absolutely nobody — nor did he try to stop Michael when, twelve hours after the cast came off, the man saddled up and rode into a snowstorm to look for her — a highly questionable move, considering how much time had passed, and the fact that he could barely walk. But Michael was Michael: you didn't tell the man no, and there was something oddly personal about the whole thing, as if Alicia's leaving was a message just for him. He returned five days later, half-frozen, having run a one-hundred-mile perimeter, and said no more about it, not that day or all the days after; he'd never even said her name.

They had all loved her, but there existed a kind of person, Lucius knew, whose heart was unknowable, who was born to stand apart. Alicia had stepped into the ether, and with three years gone by, the question in Lucius's mind wasn't what had become of her but if she'd really been there in the first place.

It was well past midnight, after the last glasses had been poured and tossed back, when Michael finally raised the subject that, in hindsight, had

been plaguing him all night.

"Do you really think they're gone? The dracs, I mean."

"Why would you ask that?"

Michael cocked an eyebrow. "Well, do you?"

Lucius framed his answer carefully. "You were there — you saw what happened. Kill the Twelve and you kill the rest. If I'm not mistaken, that was your idea. It's a little late to change your mind."

Michael glanced away and said nothing. Had the answer satisfied him?

"You should come sailing with me sometime," he said finally, brightening somewhat. "You'd really like it. It's a big wide world out there. Like nothing you've ever seen."

Lucius smiled. Whatever was eating the man, he wasn't ready to talk about it. "I'll give it some thought."

"Consider it a standing invitation." Michael got to his feet, one hand clutching the edge of the table for balance. "Well, I, for one, am completely hammered. If it's all right with you, I think it's time for me to go throw up and pass out in my truck."

Lucius gestured toward his narrow cot. "The bed's yours if you want it."

"That's sweet of you. Maybe when I get to know you better."

He stumbled to the door, where he turned to cast his bleary gaze around the tiny room.

"You're quite the artist, Major. Those are interesting pictures. You'll have to tell me about them sometime."

And that was all; when Lucius awoke in the morning, Michael was gone. He thought he might see the man again, but no more visits were

forthcoming; he supposed Michael had gotten what he was looking for, or else he'd decided that Lucius didn't have it. *Do you really think they're gone . . . ?* What would his friend have said if Lucius had actually answered his question?

Lucius put these disconcerting thoughts aside. Leaving the jug of boar's blood in the shade of the hut, he walked down the hillside to the river. The water of the Guadalupe was always cold, but here it was colder; where the river made a bend there was a deep hole — twenty feet to the bottom — fed by a natural spring. Tall banks of white limestone encircled the edge. Lucius stripped off his boots and trousers, grabbed the rope he'd left in place, took a deep breath, and dove in a clean arc into the water. With every foot of his descent the temperature dropped. The satchel, made of heavy canvas, was secured beneath an overhang, protected from the current. Lucius tied the rope to the satchel's handle, tugged it free of the overhang, blew the air from his lungs, and ascended.

He climbed out on the opposite shore, walked downstream to a shallow spot, crossed the river again, and followed a path to the top of the limestone wall. There he sat at the edge, took the rope in his hands, and hauled up the satchel.

He dressed again and carried the satchel back to the hut. There, at the table, he removed the contents: eight more jugs, for nine gallons total — the same amount of blood, more or less, that coursed through the circulatory systems of half a dozen human adults.

Once it was out of the river, his prize would quickly spoil. He strung the jugs together and gathered his supplies — three days' worth of food

and water, the rifle and ammo, a blade, a lantern, a length of sturdy rope — and carried them out to the paddock. Not even 0700, but already the sun was blazing. He saddled his horse, slid the rifle into its holder, and slung the rest over the horse's withers. He never bothered with a bedroll; he'd be riding through the night, arriving in Houston on the morning of the sixtieth day.

With a tap of his heels to the horse's flanks, he was off.

4

GULF OF MEXICO
Twenty-two Nautical Miles South-southeast of Galveston Island
0430: Michael Fisher awoke to the pattering of rain on his face.

He drew his back upright against the transom. No stars but, to the east, a narrow transect of ditchwater dawn light hovered between the horizon and the clouds. The air was dead calm, though this wouldn't last; Michael knew a storm when he smelled one.

He unfastened his shorts, jutted his pelvis over the stern, and released a urine stream of satisfying volume and duration into the waters of the Gulf. He wasn't especially hungry, hunger being something he'd taught his body to ignore, but he took a moment to go below and mix a batch of powdered protein and drink it down in six throat-pumping gulps. Unless he was mistaken, and he almost never was, the morning would bring its share of excitement; best to face it with a full belly.

He was back on deck when the first jag of lightning forked the horizon. Fifteen seconds later,

the thunder arrived in a long, rolling peal, like a grumpy god clearing its throat. The air had picked up, too, in the disorganized manner of an approaching squall. Michael unhooked the self-steerer and took the tiller in his fist as the rain arrived in earnest: a hot, needling, tropical rain that soaked him in a second. About the weather, Michael lacked any strong opinion. Like everything else, it was what it was, and if this was to be the storm that finally sent him to the bottom, well, it wasn't like he hadn't asked for it.

Really? Alone? In that thing? Are you crazy? Sometimes the questions were kindly meant, an expression of genuine concern; even total strangers tried to talk him out of it. But more often than not, the speaker was already writing him off. If the sea didn't kill him, the barrier would — that blockade of floating explosives said to encircle the continent. Who in his right mind would tempt fate like that? And especially now, when not a single viral had been seen for, what, going on thirty-six months? Wasn't a whole continent sufficient space for a restless soul to roam around in?

Fair enough, but not every choice came down to logic; a lot came from the gut. What Michael's gut was telling him was that the barrier didn't exist, that it had never existed. He was raising his middle finger to history, a hundred years of humanity saying, *Not me, no way, you go on ahead without me.* That or playing Russian roulette. Which, given his family history, wasn't necessarily out of the question.

His parents' suicide wasn't something he liked to think about, but of course he did. In some room in his brain, a movie of that morning's events was constantly running. Their gray, empty faces, and

57

the tautness of the ropes around their necks. The slight creaking sound they made. The elongated shapes of their bodies, the absolute, unoccupied looseness of them. The darkness of their toes, bloated with pooled blood. Michael's initial reaction had been complete incomprehension: he'd stared at the bodies for a good thirty seconds, trying to parse the data, which came to him in a series of free-floating words he couldn't stick together (*Mom, Dad, hanging, rope, barn, dead*), before an explosion of white-hot terror in his eleven-year-old brain sent him dashing forward to scoop their legs into his arms to push their bodies upward, all the while screaming Sara's name so she could come and help him. They'd been dead for many hours; his efforts were pointless. Yet one had to try. A lot of life, Michael had learned, came down to trying to fix things that weren't fixable.

So, the sea, and his solo wanderings upon it. It had become a home of a kind. His boat was the *Nautilus.* Michael had taken the name from a book he'd read years ago, when he was just a Little in the Sanctuary: *Twenty Thousand Leagues Under the Sea,* an old yellowed paperback, pages popping loose, and on its cover the image of a curious, armor-plated vehicle that seemed like a cross between a boat and an undersea tank, entwined in the suctioning tentacles of a sea monster with one huge eye. Long after the details of the story had fallen away from his mind, the image had stayed with him, seared into his retinas; when it came time to christen his craft, after two years of planning and execution and plain old guesswork, *Nautilus* had seemed a natural. It was as if he'd been storing the name in his brain for later use.

Thirty-six feet from stern to bowsprit with a six-

foot draft, one main and one headsail, masthead-rigged, with a small cabin (though he almost always slept on the deck). He'd found it in a boat-yard near San Luis Pass, tucked away in a ware-house, still standing on blocks. The hull, made of polyester resin, was sound, but the rest was a mess — deck rotted, sails disintegrated, anything metal fatigued beyond use. It was, in other words, perfect for Michael Fisher, first engineer of Light and Power and oiler first class, and within a month he'd quit the refinery and cashed in five years of unspent paychecks to buy the tools he needed and hire a crew to bring them down to San Luis. *Really? Alone? In that thing?* Yes, Michael told them, unfolding his drawing on the table. Really.

How ironic that after all those years of blowing on the embers of the old world, trying to relight civilization with its leftover machines, in the end it should be the most ancient form of human propulsion that seized him. The wind blew, it back-eddied along the edge of the sail, it created a vacuum that the boat forever tried to fill. With every voyage he took, he went a little longer, a little farther, a little more crazily *out there*. He'd traced the coasts at the start, getting the feel of things. North and east along the coast to oil-mucked New Orleans and its depressing plume of gooey, river-borne, chemical stink. South to Padre Island, with its long, wild stretches of sand as white as talc. As his confidence grew, his trajectories expanded. From time to time he came across the anachronistic leavings of mankind — clumps of rusted wreckage piled along the shoals, ersatz atolls of bobbing plastic, derelict oil rigs bestriding massive slicks of pumped-out sludge — but soon he left all of these behind, driving his craft

59

deeper into the heart of an oceanic wilderness. The water's color darkened; it contained incredible depths. He shot the sun with his sextant, plotting his course with a stub of pencil. One day it occurred to him that beneath him lay nearly a mile of water.

The morning of the storm, Michael had been at sea for forty-two days. His plan was to make Freeport by noon, restock, rest for a week or so — he really needed to put on some weight — and set out again. Of course, there would be Lore to contend with, always an uncomfortable business. Would she even speak to him? Just glare at him from a distance? Grab him by the belt and drag him into the barracks for an hour of angry sex that, against his better judgment, he couldn't make himself refuse? Michael never knew what it would be or which made him feel worse; he was either the asshole who had broken her heart or the hypocrite in her bed. Because the one thing he couldn't find the words to explain was that she had nothing to do with any of it: not the *Nautilus,* or his need to be alone, or the fact that, although she was in every way deserving, he could not love her in return.

His thoughts went, as they often did, to the last time he'd seen Alicia — the last time anyone had, as far as he knew. Why had she chosen him? She had come to him in the hospital, on the morning before Sara and the others had left the Homeland to return to Kerrville. Michael wasn't sure what time it was; he was asleep and awoke to see her sitting by his bed. She had this . . . *look* on her face. He sensed that she'd been sitting there for some time, watching him as he slept.

— Lish?

She smiled.

— Hey, Michael.

That was it, for at least another thirty seconds. No *How are you feeling?* or *You look kind of ridiculous in that cast, Circuit,* or any of the thousand little barbs that the two of them had fired at each other since they were little kids.

— Can you do something for me? A favor.

— Okay.

But the thought went unfinished. Alicia looked away, then back again.

— We've been friends a long time, haven't we?

— Sure, he said. Absolutely we have.

— You know, you were always so damn smart. Do you remember . . . now, when was this? I don't know, we were just a couple of kids. I think Peter might have been there, Sara, too. We all snuck up to the Wall one night, and you gave this speech, an actual speech, I swear to God, about how the lights worked, the turbines and the batteries and all the rest of it. You know, up until then, I thought that they just came on by themselves? Seriously. God, I felt so dumb.

He shrugged, embarrassed.

— I was kind of a showoff, I guess.

— Oh, don't apologize. I thought it right then: That kid's really got something. Someday, when we need him, he's going to save our sorry asses.

Michael hadn't known what to say. Never had he seen anyone who looked so lost, so weighed down by life.

— What did you want to ask me, Lish?

— Ask you?

— You said you needed a favor.

She frowned, as if the question didn't quite make sense to her.

— I guess I did, didn't I?

— Lish, are you okay?

She rose from her chair. Michael was about to say something else, he wasn't sure what, when she leaned forward, brushed his hair aside, and, amazing him utterly, kissed him on the forehead.

— Take care of yourself, Michael. Will you do that for me? They're going to need you around this place.

— Why? Are you going somewhere?

— Just promise me.

And there it was: the moment when he'd failed her. Three years later and still he was reliving it over and over, like a hiccup in time. The moment when she told him she was leaving for good, and the one thing he could have said to keep her there. *Somebody loves you, Lish. I love you. Me, Michael. I love you and I've never stopped and never ever will.* But the words got tangled up somewhere between his mouth and his brain, and the moment slipped away.

— Okay.

— Okay, she said. And then was gone.

But the storm, on the morning of his forty-second day at sea: lost in these thoughts, Michael had let his attention drift — had noted, but failed to fully process, the sea's growing hostility, the absolute blackness of the sky, the accumulating fury of the wind. Too quickly it arrived with an earsplitting blast of thunder and a massive, rain-saturated gust that slapped the boat like a giant hand, heeling it hard. *Whoa,* thought Michael, scrambling up the transom. *What the holy fuck.* The moment had passed to reef the sail; the only thing to do was take the squall head-on. He tightened the mainsheet and steered his boat close

to the wind. Water was pouring in — foaming over the bow, dumping from the heavens in sheets. The air was lit with voltage. He locked the main in his teeth, pulled it as tight as it could go, and snapped it down in the block.

All right, he thought. *At least you let me take a piss first. Let's see what you've got, you bastard.*

Into the storm he went.

Six hours later he emerged, his heart soaring with victory. The squall had blown through, carving a pocket of blue air behind it. He had no idea where he was; he had been thrown far off course. The only thing to do was head due west and see where he made landfall.

Two hours later, a long gray line of sand appeared. He approached it on a rising tide. Galveston Island: he could tell from the wreckage of the old seawall. The sun was high, the winds fair. Should he turn south for Freeport — home, dinner, a real bed, and all the rest — or something else? But the events of the morning made this prospect seem depressingly tame, a too-meager conclusion to the day.

He decided to scout the Houston Ship Channel. He could anchor for the night there, then proceed to Freeport in the morning. He examined his chart. A narrow wedge of water separated the north end of the island from the Bolivar Peninsula; on the far side lay Galveston Bay, a roughly circular basin, twenty miles wide, leading at its northeastern edge to a deep estuary, lined with the wreckage of shipyards and chemical plants.

Running before the wind, he made his way into the bay. Unlike the brown-tinged surf of the coastline, the water was clear, almost translucent,

with a greenish cast. Michael could even see fish, dark shapes running below the surface. In places the shoreline was clotted with huge masses of debris, but elsewhere it seemed scrubbed clean.

The afternoon had begun to fade as he approached the estuary's mouth. A large, dark shape stood in the channel. As he neared, the image came into focus: a massive ship, hundreds of feet long. It had come to rest midway between two stanchions of a suspension bridge that traversed the channel. He guided his craft closer. The ship was listing slightly to port, bow-down, the tops of its massive propellers just visible above the waterline. Was it aground? How had it gotten there? Probably the same way he had, pulled by the tides through Bolivar Pass. Across the stern, dripping with rust, was written the vessel's name and registry:

BERGENSFJORD
OSLO, NORWAY

He drew the *Nautilus* alongside the closest stanchion. Yes, a ladder. He tied off, dropped his sails, then went below to fetch a pry bar, a lantern, an assortment of tools, and two one-hundred-yard lengths of heavy rope. He put his supplies in a backpack, returned to the deck, took a steadying breath, and began to climb.

Michael didn't care for heights. Not much else got to him, except for that. At the refinery, circumstances often placed him somewhere far above the ground — swinging from a harness on the towers, chipping off the rust — and over time he'd become more brave about it, insofar as his crew could tell. But exposure went only so far in

64

its curative effects. The ladder, steel rungs set into the concrete of the stanchion, was not, on close inspection, anywhere near as sturdy as it had appeared from below. Some of the rungs seemed barely attached. By the time he reached the top, his heart felt like it was stuffed against the back of his throat. He lay on his back on the suspension bridge's roadway, just breathing, then peered over the edge. He guessed it was a hundred and fifty feet down to the ship's deck, maybe more. Jesus.

He tied the rope to the railing and watched it fall. The trick would be using his feet to control his descent. Taking the rope in his hands, he leaned backward over the edge, swallowed hard, and stepped off.

For half a second he believed he had made the biggest mistake of his life. What a stupid idea! He was going to plummet like a rock to the deck. But then his feet found the rope, wrapping it in a death grip. Hand over hand, he made his way down.

Michael guessed the boat had been some kind of freight vessel. He headed for the stern, where an open metal staircase led to the pilothouse. At the top of the stairs he came to a heavy door with a handle that refused to move. He popped the handle loose with the pry bar and inserted the tip of a screwdriver into the mechanism. A bit of jiggling, tumblers clacking, and with a second pop of the pry bar the door swung free.

An eye-watering ammoniac funk filled the air — air that nobody had breathed for a century. Beneath the broad windshield, with its view of the channel, was the ship's control panel: rows of switches and dials, flat-panel displays, computer keyboards. In one of the three high-backed chairs that faced the panel was a body. Time had turned

it into little more than a shrunken brown stain encased by the moldy tatters of its clothing. Military-style epaulets with three stripes decorated the shoulders of its shirt. An officer, Michael thought, perhaps the captain himself. The cause of death was apparent: a hole in his skull, no bigger than the tip of Michael's pinkie, marked the spot of the bullet's entry. On the floor, beneath the man's outstretched right hand, lay a revolver.

Michael found other bodies below decks. Nearly all were in their beds. He didn't linger, merely added them to the count, forty-two corpses in all. Had they killed themselves? The orderliness of the bodies said so, yet the method was not apparent. Michael had seen this sort of thing before, but never so many, all in one place.

Traveling downward into the ship, he came to a room that was different from the others, with not one or two beds but many — narrow bunks attached two high on the bulkheads, the space bisected by a slim corridor. The crew's quarters? Many of the cots were empty; he counted only eight bodies, including two that were naked, their limbs wound together in the cramped space of a lower bunk.

This space was more cluttered than the others. Rotted articles of clothing and miscellaneous objects covered much of the floor. Many of the walls beside the bunks were decorated: faded photographs, religious images, postcards. He gently freed one of the photographs and held it up to his lantern. A dark-haired woman, smiling for the camera, cradling an infant in her lap.

Something caught his eye.

A large sheet of paper, thin as tissue, taped to the bulkhead: at the top, in ornate lettering, were

the words INTERNATIONAL HERALD TRIBUNE.
Michael loosened the tape and laid the paper
across the bunk.

HUMANITY IN PERIL
Crisis Deepens as Death Toll Soars Worldwide
Virus extends its deadly reach to all continents
Ports and borders overrun as millions flee the spread of infection
Major cities in chaos as massive blackouts darken Europe

ROME (AP), May 13 — The world stood on the
edge of chaos Tuesday night as the disease
known as the Easter Virus continued its deadly
march across the globe.

Although the disease's rapid spread makes
estimates of the dead difficult, U.N. health officials say the toll numbers in the hundreds of
millions.

The virus, an airborne variant of the one that
decimated North America two years ago,
emerged in the Caucasus region of central Asia
just fifty-nine days ago. Health officials have
been at pains to identify either a source of the
virus or an effective treatment.

"What we can say at this point is that this
pathogen is unusually vigorous and highly lethal,"
said Madeline Duplessis, Chairman of the World
Health Organization's Executive Board, speaking
from its headquarters in Geneva. "Morbidity rates
are running very close to 100 percent."

Unlike the North American strain, the Easter
Virus does not require close physical contact to
pass from person to person and can travel great
distances attached to dust motes or respiratory
droplets, causing many health officials to liken it

to the Spanish influenza epidemic of 1918, which killed as many as 50 million people worldwide. Travel bans have done little to slow its spread, as have attempts by officials in many cities to prevent people from congregating in public places.

"I fear we are on the verge of losing control of the situation," said Italian Health Minister Vincenzo Monti in an extended press briefing, during which coughing could be heard throughout the room. "I cannot stress enough the importance that people stay indoors. Children, adults, the elderly — none has been spared the effects of this cruel epidemic. The only way to survive this disease is not to catch it."

Absorbed through the lungs, the Easter Virus acts swiftly to overwhelm the body's defenses, attacking the respiratory system and digestive tracts. Early symptoms include disorientation, fever, headache, coughing, and vomiting with little or no warning. As the pathogen takes hold, victims experience massive internal hemorrhaging, typically leading to death within 36 hours, though some cases have been reported in which healthy adults have succumbed within as little as two hours. In rare instances, victims of the illness have exhibited the transformative effects of the North American strain, including a marked increase in aggressiveness, but whether any of these individuals have survived past the 36-hour threshold is not known.

"This appears to be happening in a small percentage of cases," Duplessis told reporters. "Why these individuals are different, we simply don't know at this time."

WHO officials have speculated that the disease

may have traveled from North America via ship or aircraft, despite the international quarantine imposed by the United Nations in June two years ago. Other theories of the pathogen's origins include an avian source, connected to the massive die-off of several species of migrating songbirds in the southern Ural Mountains just prior to the disease's appearance.

"We're looking at everything," Duplessis said. "We're leaving no stone unturned."

A third theory is that the epidemic is the work of terrorists. Responding to continued speculation in the press, Interpol Secretary-General Javier Cabrera, the former United States Secretary of Homeland Security and a member of the U.S. government in exile in London, told reporters, "At this time, no group or individual has claimed responsibility that we are aware of, though our investigation continues." Cabrera went on to state that the international law enforcement organization, with 190 member states, possesses no evidence that any terrorist group or sponsoring country has the capability to create such a virus.

"Despite the many challenges, we continue to coordinate our efforts with law enforcement and intelligence agencies around the world," Cabrera said. "This is a global crisis warranting a global response. Should any credible evidence arise that the epidemic is man-made, rest assured that we will bring the perpetrators to justice."

With most of the globe now under some form of martial law, riots have engulfed hundreds of cities, with fierce fighting reported in Rio de Janeiro, Istanbul, Athens, Copenhagen, Prague, Johannesburg, and Bangkok, among many oth-

ers. Responding to the rising tide of violence, the United Nations, meeting in an emergency session at its headquarters in The Hague, urged the nations of the world to exercise restraint in the use of deadly force.

"Now is not the time for humankind to turn upon itself," said U.N. Secretary-General Ahn Yoon-dae in a printed statement. "Our common humanity must be a guiding light in these dark days."

Power outages throughout Europe continue to hamper relief efforts and add to the chaos. As of Tuesday night, darkness extended from as far north as Denmark to southern France and northern Italy. Similar failures have been reported throughout the Indian subcontinent, Japan, and Western Australia.

Landline and cellular communications networks have also been adversely affected, cutting many cities and towns off from the outside world. In Moscow, water shortages and high winds are being blamed for the unchecked fires that have left much of the city in ashes and killed thousands.

"The whole thing is gone," said one eyewitness. "Moscow is no more."

Also on the rise are reports of mass suicides and so-called "death cults." Early Monday in Zurich, police officers, responding to reports of a suspicious smell, discovered a warehouse containing more than 2,500 bodies, including children and infants. According to police, the group had used secobarbital, a powerful barbiturate, mixing it with a powdered fruit drink to make a lethal cocktail. Though the majority of victims appeared to have taken the drug voluntarily, some of the bodies had been bound at the ankles

and wrists.

Speaking to the press, Zurich Chief of Police Franz Schatz described the scene as one of "unspeakable horror."

"I cannot imagine the despair that led these people to end not only their own lives but those of their children," Schatz said.

Around the globe, huge crowds have flocked to houses of worship and important religious sites to seek spiritual comfort during the unprecedented crisis. In Mecca, Islam's holiest city, millions continue to gather despite food and water shortages that have added to the suffering. In Rome, Pope Cornelius II, whom many eyewitnesses claimed appeared ill, addressed the faithful Tuesday evening from the balcony of the papal residence, exhorting them to "place your lives in the hands of an almighty and merciful God."

As bells tolled throughout the city, the pontiff said, "If it is God's will that these should be the last days of humanity, let us meet our heavenly father with peace and acceptance in our hearts. Do not abandon yourselves to despair, for ours is a living and loving God, in whose hands of mercy his children have rested since time's beginning and will rest until its end."

As the death toll rises, health officials worry that the unburied remains of the deceased may be accelerating the spread of infection. Struggling to keep pace, officials in many European locales have employed open pit graves. Others have resorted to mass burials at sea, moving the bodies of the deceased by freight cars to coastal sites.

Yet despite the risks, many of the bereaved

are taking matters into their own hands, using any available patch of ground to bury their loved ones. In a scene typical of cities around the world, Paris's famed Bois de Boulogne, one of Europe's most storied urban parks, is now the site of thousands of graves.

"It is the last thing I could do for my family," said Gerard Bonnaire, 36, standing by the freshly dug grave of his wife and young son, who had succumbed within six hours of each other. After fruitless attempts to notify officials, Bonnaire, who identified himself as an executive with the World Bank, asked neighbors to help him move the bodies and dig a grave, which he had marked with family photographs and his son's stuffed parrot, a beloved toy.

"All I can hope is to join them as soon as possible," Bonnaire said. "What is left for any of us now? What can we do but die?"

It took Michael a moment to realize he had come to the end. His body felt numb, almost weightless. He raised his eyes from the paper and looked around the compartment, as if searching for someone to tell him that he was mistaken, that it was all a lie. But there was no one, only bodies, and the great, creaking weight of the *Bergensfjord.*

Good God, he thought.

We're alone.

5

The woman in bed 16 was making a ruckus. With each contraction, she released a volley of curses at her husband that would make an oiler blush. Worse, her cervix was barely dilated, just two

centimeters.

"Try to keep calm, Marie," Sara told her. "Yelling and screaming won't make it any better."

"Goddamnit," Marie screeched at her husband, "you did this to me, you son of a bitch!"

"Is there anything you can do?" her husband asked.

Sara wasn't sure if he meant to ease his wife's pain or to shut her up. From the cowed look on his face, she guessed that the verbal abuse was nothing new. He worked in the fields; Sara could tell by the crescents of dirt under his fingernails.

"Just tell her to breathe."

"What do you call *this?*" The woman puffed up her cheeks and blew out two sarcastic breaths.

I could hit her with a hammer, Sara thought. *That would do the trick.*

"For God's sake, tell that woman to zip it!" The voice came from the next bed, occupied by an old man with pneumonia. He finished his plea with a spasm of wet coughing.

"Marie, I really need you to work with me here," Sara said. "You're upsetting the other patients. And there's really nothing I can do at this point. We just have to let nature take its course."

"Sara?" Jenny had come up behind her. Her brown hair was askew, lacquered to her forehead with sweat. "A woman's come in. She's pretty far along."

"Just a second." Sara gave Marie a firm look: *No more nonsense.* "Are we clear on this?"

"Fine," the woman huffed. "Have it your way."

Sara followed Jenny to admissions, where the new woman lay on a gurney, her husband standing beside her, holding her hand. She was older than the patients Sara was used to seeing, maybe

forty, with a drawn, hard face and crowded teeth. Shocks of gray ran through her long, damp hair. Sara quickly read her chart.

"Mrs. Jiménez, I'm Dr. Wilson. You're thirty-six weeks along, is that correct?"

"I'm not sure. About that."

"How long have you been bleeding?"

"A few days. Just spotting, but then this morning it got worse and I started to hurt."

"I told her she should have come sooner," her husband explained. He was a large man in dark blue coveralls; his hands were big as bear paws. "I was at work."

Sara checked the woman's heart rate and blood pressure, then drew up the gown and placed her hands on her belly, gently pressing. The woman winced in pain. Sara moved her hands lower, touching here and there, searching for the site of the abruption. That was when she noticed the two boys, young teenagers, sitting off to the side. She exchanged a look with the man but said nothing.

"We have a birthright certificate," the man said nervously.

"Let's not worry about that now." From the pocket of her coat, Sara withdrew the fetoscope and pressed the silver disk against the woman's abdomen, holding up a hand for silence. A strong, swishing click filled her ears. She recorded the baby's heart rate on the chart, 118 bpm — a little low, but nothing too concerning yet.

"Okay, Jenny, let's get her into the OR." She turned to the woman's husband. "Mr. Jiménez —"

"Carlos. That's my first name."

"Carlos, everything's going to be fine. But you'll want your children to wait here."

The placenta had separated from the uterine wall; that's where the blood was coming from. The tear might clot on its own, but the fact that the baby was in a breech position complicated matters for a vaginal delivery, and at thirty-six weeks, Sara saw no reason to wait. In the hall outside the OR, she explained what she intended to do.

"We could hold off," she told the woman's husband, "but I don't think that's wise. The baby might not be getting enough oxygen."

"Can I stay with her?"

"Not for this." She took the man by the arm and looked him in the eye. "I'll take care of her. Trust me, there'll be lots for you to do later."

Sara called for the anesthetic and a warmer while she and Jenny washed up and put on their gowns. Jenny cleaned the woman's belly and pubic area with iodine and bound her to the table. Sara rolled lights into place, snapped on her gloves, and poured the anesthetic into a small dish. Using forceps, she dipped a sponge into the brown liquid, then placed this into the compartment of the breathing mask.

"Okay, Mrs. Jiménez," she said, "I'm going to put this on your face now. It will smell a little strange."

The woman looked at her with helpless terror. "Is this going to hurt?"

Sara smiled to reassure her. "Believe me, you won't care. And when you wake up, your baby will be here." She positioned the breather on the woman's face. "Just take slow, even breaths."

The woman was out like a light. Sara rolled the tray of instruments, still warm from the boiler, into place and drew up her mask. With a scalpel she cut a transverse incision at the top of the

woman's pubic bone, then a second to open the uterus. The baby appeared, coiled head-down in the amniotic sac, its fluid tinged pink with blood. Sara carefully punctured the sac and reached inside with forceps.

"Okay, get ready."

Jenny moved beside her with a towel and a basin. Sara drew the baby through the incision, sliding her hand beneath its head as it emerged and hooking her thumb and pinkie beneath its shoulders. *Her* arms; the baby was a girl. One more slow pull and she came free. Holding her in the towel, Jenny suctioned her mouth and nose, rolled her onto her stomach, and rubbed her back; with a wet hiccup, the child began to breathe. Sara clamped the umbilicus, snipped it with a pair of shears, drew out the placenta, and dropped it into the basin. While Jenny put the baby in the warmer and checked her vitals, Sara sutured the woman's incisions. Minimal blood, no complications, a healthy baby: not bad for ten minutes' work.

Sara drew the mask off the woman's face. "She's here," she whispered into her ear. "Everything's fine. She's a healthy baby girl."

Her husband and sons were waiting outside. Sara gave everyone a moment together. Carlos kissed his wife, who had begun to come around, then lifted the baby from the warmer to hold her. Each of the sons took a turn.

"Do you have a name for her?" Sara asked.

The man nodded, his eyes shining with tears. Sara liked him for this; not all the fathers were so sentimental. Some seemed barely to care.

"Grace," he said.

Mother and daughter were wheeled down the

hall. The man sent his boys away, then reached into the pocket of his jumpsuit and nervously handed Sara the piece of paper she was expecting. Couples who were going to have a third baby were allowed to purchase the right to do so from a couple who had had fewer than their legal allotment. Sara disliked the practice; it seemed wrong to her, buying and selling the rights to making a person, and half the certificates she saw were forgeries, purchased on the trade.

She examined Carlos's document. The paper was government-issue stock, but the ink wasn't even close to the correct color, and the seal had been embossed on the wrong side.

"Whoever sold you this, you should get your money back."

Carlos's face collapsed. "Please, I'm just a hydro. I don't have enough to pay the tax. It was totally my fault. She said it wasn't the right day."

"Good of you to admit, but I'm afraid that's not the issue."

"I'm begging you, Dr. Wilson. Don't make us give her to the sisters. My sons are good boys, you can see that."

Sara had no intention of sending baby Grace to the orphanage. On the other hand, the man's certificate was so palpably false that somebody in the census office was bound to flag it.

"Do us both a favor and get rid of this. I'll record the birth, and if the paperwork bounces back, I'll make something up — tell them I lost it or something. With any luck, it'll get misplaced in the shuffle."

Carlos made no move to accept the certificate; he seemed not to comprehend what Sara was telling him. She had no doubt that he had mentally

rehearsed this moment a thousand times. Not once, in all that time, had he imagined that somebody would simply make his problem go away.

"Go on, take it."

"You'd really do that? Won't you get in trouble?"

She pushed the paper toward him. "Tear it up, burn it, shove it in a trash can somewhere. Just forget we had this conversation."

The man returned the certificate to his pocket. For a second, he seemed about to hug her but stopped himself. "You'll be in our prayers, Dr. Wilson. We'll give her a good life, I swear."

"I'm counting on it. Just do me a favor."

"Anything."

"When your wife tells you it's not the right day, believe her, okay?"

At the checkpoint, Sara showed her pass and made her way home through darkened streets. Except for the hospital and other essential buildings, the electricity was shut off at 2200. Which was not to say that the city went to bed the minute the power was cut; in darkness, it acquired a different kind of life. Saloons, brothels, gaming halls — Hollis had told her plenty of stories, and after two years in the refugee camp, there wasn't much that Sara hadn't seen herself.

She let herself into the apartment. Kate had long since been put to bed, but Hollis was waiting up, reading a book by candlelight at the kitchen table.

"Anything good?" she asked.

With Sara working so many late hours at the hospital, Hollis had become quite a reader, checking out armfuls of books from the library and

78

reading them from a stack he kept by his side of the bed.

"It's a little heavy on the mumbo jumbo. Michael recommended it a while ago. It's about a submarine."

She hung her coat on the hook by the door. "What's a submarine?"

Hollis closed the book and removed his reading glasses — another new development. Little half-moon lenses, cloudy and scratched, set in a black plastic frame: Sara thought they made him look distinguished, though Hollis said they made him feel old.

"Apparently, it's a boat that goes underwater. Sounds like bullshit to me, but the story's not bad. Are you hungry? I can fix you something if you want."

She was, but eating felt like too much effort. "All I want to do is go to bed."

She checked on Kate, who was sound asleep, and washed up at the sink. She paused to examine herself in the mirror. No doubt about it, the years were starting to show. Fans of wrinkles had formed around her eyes; her blond hair, which she now wore shorter and pulled back, had thinned somewhat; her skin was beginning to lose its tightness. She'd always thought of herself as pretty and, in a certain light, still was. But sometime in the midst of life she had passed the apex. In the past, when she'd looked at her reflection, she had still seen the little girl she'd once been; the woman in the mirror had still been an extension of her girlhood self. Now it was the future she saw. The wrinkles would deepen; her skin would sag; the lights of her eyes would dim. Her youth was fading, easing into the past.

And yet this thought did not disturb her, or not very much. With age came authority, and with authority came the power to be useful — to heal and comfort and bring new people into the world. *You'll be in our prayers, Dr. Wilson.* Sara heard words like these nearly every day, but she had never become inured to them. Just that name, Dr. Wilson. It still amazed her to hear someone say it and know they were speaking to her. When Sara had arrived in Kerrville, three years ago, she'd reported to the hospital to see if her nurse's training could be of any use. In a little windowless room, a doctor by the name of Elacqua quizzed her at length — bodily systems, diagnostics, treatments for illness and injury. His face showed no emotion as he responded to her answers with marks on a clipboard. The grilling lasted over two hours; by its conclusion, Sara felt like she was stumbling blind in a windstorm. What use could her meager training be to a medical establishment that was so far ahead of the homespun remedies of the Colony? How could she have been so naïve? "Well, I guess that about covers it," Dr. Elacqua said. "Congratulations." Sara was knocked flat; was he being ironic? "Does this mean I can be a nurse?" she asked. "A nurse? No. We have plenty of nurses. Report back here tomorrow, Ms. Wilson. Your training starts at oh-seven-hundred sharp. My guess is twelve months should do it." "Training for what?" she asked, and Elacqua, whose lengthy inquisition was a mere shadow of things to come, said, with unconcealed impatience, "Perhaps I'm not being clear. I don't know where you learned it, but you know twice as much as you have any right to. You're going to be a doctor."

And then, of course, there was Kate. Their beautiful, amazing, miraculous Kate. Sara and Hollis would have liked to have had a second child, but the violence of Kate's birth had inflicted too much damage. A disappointment, and not without irony, as day by day new babies traveled into the world beneath her hands, but Sara was hardly entitled to complain. That she should have found her daughter at all, and that the two of them should have been reunited with Hollis and escaped the Homeland to travel back to Kerrville to be a family together — *miracle* was hardly the word. Sara was not religious in the churchgoing sense — the sisters all struck her as good people, if a bit extreme in their beliefs — but only an idiot would fail to feel the actions of providence. You couldn't wake up each day in a world like that and not spend a solid hour just thinking of ways to be grateful.

She thought rarely of the Homeland, or as rarely as she could. She still had dreams about it — though, strangely, these dreams did not focus on the worst things that had happened to her there. Mostly they were dreams of feeling hungry and cold and helpless, or the endlessly turning wheels of the grinder in the biodiesel plant. Sometimes she was simply looking at her hands with a feeling of perplexity, as if trying to remember something she was supposed to be holding; from time to time she dreamed about Jackie, the old woman who had befriended her, or else Lila, for whom Sara's complex feelings had distilled over time to a kind of sorrowful sympathy. Once in a while, her dreams were flat-out nightmares — she was carrying Kate in blinding snow, the two of them being chased by something terrible — but these had

81

abated. So that was one more thing to be thankful for: eventually, perhaps not soon but someday, the Homeland would become just one more memory in a life of memories, an unpleasant recollection that made the others all the sweeter.

Hollis was already out cold. The man slept like a fallen giant; his head hit the pillow, and soon he was snoring away. Sara extinguished the candle and slid beneath the covers. She wondered if Marie had delivered her baby yet, and if she was still yelling at her husband; she thought of the Jiménez family and the look on Carlos's face as he lifted baby Grace into his arms. Maybe *grace* was the word she was looking for. It was possible they'd still get flagged by the census office, but Sara didn't think so. Not with so many babies being born. Which was the thing. That was the heart of the matter. A new world was coming; a new world was already here. Maybe that was what getting older taught you, when you looked in the mirror and saw the passage of time in your face, when you looked at your sleeping daughter and saw the girl you once were and would never be again. The world was real and you were in it, a brief part but still a part, and if you were lucky, and maybe even if you weren't, the things you'd done for love would be remembered.

6

The sky over Houston released the night slowly, darkness easing to gray. Greer made his way into the city. Where the Katy Freeway met the 610 in a tangle of collapsed ramps and overpasses, he arced north, away from the bayous and swamps, with their sucking mud and impenetrable foliage,

bypassing the liquefied inner neighborhoods for higher ground, then followed a wide avenue of junked cars south to the downtown lagoon.

The rowboat was where he'd left it two months ago. Greer tied up his horse, dumped out the mosquito-infested rainwater, and dragged the craft to the water's edge. Across the lagoon, the *Chevron Mariner* lay at its improbable angle, a great temple of rust and rot lodged among the listing towers of the city's central core. He laid his supplies in the bottom of the boat, set it afloat, and rowed away from shore.

In the lobby of One Allen Center, he tied off at the base of the escalators and ascended, the duffel bag with its sloshing contents slung over his shoulder. The ten-story climb through mold-befouled air left him dizzy and short of breath. In the empty office, he pulled up the rope he'd left in place and lowered the bag to the deck of the *Mariner,* then climbed down behind it.

He always fed Carter first.

On the port side, just about amidships, a hatch lay flush with the deck. Greer knelt beside it and removed the jugs of blood from the bag. He tied three together by their handles with one of the ropes. The sun was angled behind him, raking the deck with light. With a heavy wrench he unscrewed the safety bolts, turned the handle, and opened the hatch.

A shaft of sunshine spilled into the space below. Carter lay curled in a fetal position near the forward bulkhead, his body in shadow, away from the light. Old jugs and coils of rope were piled in a heap on the floor. Hand over hand, Greer lowered the jugs. Only when they reached bottom did Carter stir. As he scuttled on all fours toward

83

the blood, Greer released the rope, closed the hatch, and replaced the safety bolts.

Now, Amy.

Greer moved to the second hatch. The trick was to move fast but not with panicked recklessness. The scent of blood: for Amy, it could not be contained by something as meager as the thin plastic membrane of the jugs; her hunger was too strong. Greer set his supplies within quick reach, unwrenched the bolts, and placed them to the side. A deep breath to calm his nerves; then he opened the hatch.

Blood.

She leapt. Lucius dropped the jugs, slammed the hatch, and shoved the first bolt into place as Amy's body made contact. The metal clanged as if hit by a giant hammer. He threw his body across it; another blow came, knocking the wind from his chest. The hinges were bending; unless he could get the remaining bolts in place, the hatch wouldn't hold. He'd managed to get two more into their holes when Amy struck again; Greer watched helplessly as one of the bolts jogged free and rolled across the deck. His hand stabbed outward and seized it at the very edge of his reach.

"Amy," he yelled, "it's me! It's Lucius!" He shoved the bolt into place and smacked it with the head of the wrench, driving it home. "The blood is there! Follow the scent of the blood!"

Three turns on the wrench and the bolt locked down, bringing the fourth hole back into alignment. He rammed its bolt into place. One last pound on the underside of the hatch, halfhearted; then it was over.

Lucius, I didn't mean it . . .

"It's all right," he said.

84

I'm sorry . . .

He picked up his tools and put them in the empty duffel. Below him, in the hold of the *Chevron Mariner,* Amy and Carter were drinking their fills. It always happened like this; Greer should have been used to it by now. Yet his heart was pounding, his mind and body flying with adrenaline.

"I'm yours, Amy," he said. "I always will be. Whatever comes, you know that."

And with these words, Lucius made his way across the deck of the *Mariner* and climbed back through the window.

7

Amy returned to awareness to find herself on all fours in the dirt. Her hands were gloved; a plastic flat of impatiens rested on the ground close by and, beside it, a rusty trowel.

"You all right there, Miss Amy?"

Carter was sitting on the patio, legs akimbo beneath the wrought-iron table, fanning his face with his big straw hat. On the table were two glasses of iced tea.

"That man takes good care of us," he said, and sighed with satisfaction. "Haven't eaten my fill like that since I don't remember when."

Amy rose unsteadily to her feet. A deep lassitude enveloped her, as if she had just awoken from a long nap.

"Come and sit a minute," Carter said. "Give the body a chance to digest. Feeding day like a day off round here. Them flowers can wait."

Which was true; there were always more flowers. As soon as Amy finished planting a flat, a new

85

one would appear by the gate. It was the same with the tea: one minute the table was bare; in the next, two sweating glasses awaited. By what unseen agency these things arrived, Amy did not know. It was all part of this place and its own particular logic. Every day a season, every season a year.

She removed her gloves and crossed the lawn to sit across from Carter. The greasy taste of blood lingered in her mouth. She sipped the tea to clear it away.

"It's good to keep your strength up, Miss Amy," Carter said. "Ain't no prize for starving yourself."

"I just don't . . . like it." She looked at Carter, who was still fanning himself with his hat. "I tried to kill him again."

"Lucius knows the situation well enough. I doubt he takes it personal."

"That's not the point, Anthony. I need to learn to control it the way you do."

Carter frowned. He was a man of compact expression, small gestures, thoughtful pauses. "Don't be so hard on yourself. You ain't had but three years to get used to things. You still just a baby in the way of being what we are."

"I don't feel like a baby."

"What you feel like then?"

"A monster."

She'd spoken too sharply; she glanced away, feeling ashamed. After feeding, she always passed through a period of doubt. How strange it all was: she was a body in a ship, but her mind lived here, with Carter, among the plants and flowers. Only when Lucius brought the blood did these two worlds touch each other, and the contrast was disorienting. Carter had explained that this place

was nothing particular to the two of them; the difference was that they could see it. There was one world, of flesh and blood and bone, but also another — a deeper reality that ordinary people could glimpse only fleetingly, if at all. A world of souls, both the living and the dead, in which time and space, memory and desire, existed in a purely fluid state, the way they did in dreams.

Amy knew this to be so. She felt as if she'd always known it — that even as a little girl, a purely *human* girl, she had sensed the existence of this other realm, this world-behind-the-world, as she had come to call it. She supposed that many children did the same. What was childhood if not a passage from light to dark, of the soul's slow drowning in an ocean of ordinary matter? During her time in the *Chevron Mariner,* a great deal of the past had become clear. Vivid recollections had inched their way back to her, approaching on memory's delicate feet, until things that had happened ages past felt like recent occurrences. She recalled a time, long ago, in the innocent period she thought of as "before" — before Lacey and Wolgast, before Project NOAH, before the Oregon mountaintop where they had made their home and then her long, solo wanderings in a people-less world with only the virals for company — when animals had spoken to her. Larger animals, like dogs, but also smaller ones that nobody paid attention to — birds and even insects. She'd thought nothing of this at the time; it was simply the way things were. Nor did it trouble her that nobody else seemed to hear them; it was part of the world's arrangement that the animals spoke only to her, always addressing her by name, as if they were old friends, telling her stories about

their lives, and it made her happy to be the recipient of the special gift of their attention when so much else in her life seemed to make no sense at all: her mother's lurching emotions and long absences, their drifting from place to place, the strangers that came and went with no apparent purpose.

All this had gone on without repercussion until the day Lacey had taken her to the zoo. At the time, Amy did not yet fully comprehend that her mother had deserted her — that she would never see the woman again — and she'd welcomed the invitation; she'd heard of zoos but had never been to one. She entered the grounds to an animal buzz of welcome. After the confusing events of the previous day — her mother's abrupt departure and the presence of the nuns, who were nice but in a slightly stilted way, as if they were reciting their kindnesses off a card of instructions — here was a familiar comfort. In a burst of energy, she broke away from Lacey and dashed to the polar bear tank. Three were basking in the sun; a fourth was swimming under the water. How magnificent they were, how amazing! Even now, so many years later, it gave her pleasure to remember them, their wonderful white fur and great muscular bodies and expressive faces, which seemed to contain all the wisdom of the universe. As Amy approached the glass, the one in the water paddled toward her. Though she knew that her communication with the creatures of the natural world was best conducted in private, her excitement could not be contained. She felt suddenly sorry that such a stately creature should be forced to live like a prisoner, sunning himself on phony rocks and being gawked at by people who did not appreciate

him. "What's your name?" she asked the bear. "I'm Amy."

His answer was a collision of incompatible consonants, as were the names of the other bears, which he courteously offered. Were these things real? Had she, a little girl, simply imagined them? But no; all of it had happened, she believed, precisely as she recalled. As she stood at the glass, Lacey came up beside her. She was wearing a look of deep concern. "There now, Amy," Lacey advised. "Not so close." To put her unease at bay, and because Amy had detected in this kindly woman with her melodious accent an openness to extraordinary phenomena — the zoo, after all, had been her idea — she explained the situation as simply as she knew how. "He has a bear name," she told Lacey. "It's something I can't pronounce."

Lacey frowned. "The bear has a name?"

"Of course he does," said Amy.

She returned her attention to her new friend, who was bumping his nose against the glass. Amy was about to ask him about his life, if he missed his Arctic home, when the water was rocked by a tremendous splash. A second bear had leapt into the tank. With paws big as hubcaps he swam toward her, taking his place beside the first bear, who was licking the glass with his immense pink tongue. A collective exhalation of oohs and aahs ascended from the crowd; people began to snap pictures. Amy placed her hand against the glass in greeting, but something felt wrong. Something was different, and it wasn't very good. The bears' great black eyes seemed to be looking not at her but *through* her, with a gaze of such intensity that she could not look away. She felt herself dissolving into it, as if she were melting, and with this

came a falling sensation, like putting her foot on a step that wasn't there.

Amy, the bears were saying. *You're Amy Amy Amy Amy Amy . . .*

Things were happening. Some sort of commotion. As Amy's awareness widened, she became conscious of other sounds, other voices, coming from all around — not human but animal. The hoots of monkeys. The shrieks of birds. The roars of jungle cats and the concussing hooves of elephants and rhinoceroses stamping the ground in panic. As the third and then the fourth bear leapt into the tank, displacing its contents with their white-furred tonnage, a wall of frigid water bulged over the lip. It crashed down upon the crowd, unleashing mayhem.

It's her, it's her, it's her, it's her . . .

She was kneeling by the glass, soaked to the bone, her head bowed to its slick surface. Her mind swirled with the voices, a chorus of black dread. She felt as if the universe were bending around her, swathing her in darkness. They would die, all these animals. That is what her presence meant to them. The bears and monkeys and birds and elephants: all of them. Some would starve in their cages; others would perish by more violent means. Death would take them all, and not just the animals. The people, too. The world would die around her, and she would be left standing at the center, alone.

It's coming, death is coming, you're Amy, Amy, Amy . . .

"You remembering, ain't you?"

Amy's mind returned to the patio. Carter was looking at her pointedly.

90

"I'm sorry," she said. "I didn't mean to snap at you."

" 'Sall right. I felt the same, there at the beginning. Took some getting used to."

The feeling of summer had faded; autumn would soon come. In the blue-green water of the pool, the body of Rachel Wood would rise. Sometimes, when Amy was tending flowers near the gate, she would see the woman's black Denali slowly cruising past. Through the tinted windows she could make out Rachel in her tennis clothes, staring at the house. But the car never stopped, and when Amy waved at her, the woman never waved back.

"How much longer do you think we have to wait?"

"That depends on Zero. Man got to show his hand sooner or later. So far as he knows, I'm gone with the rest of them."

It was the water, Carter had explained, that protected them. Its cold embrace was nothing Fanning's mind could penetrate. As long as they stayed where they were, Fanning couldn't find them.

"But he'll come," said Amy.

Carter nodded. "He's bided his time a good while, but the man wants this thing done. It's what he's wanted from the start. Everything over."

The wind was picking up — an autumn wind, damp and raw. Clouds had moved in, denuding the light. It was the time of day when a certain silence always fell.

"We're quite a pair, aren't we?"

"That we are, Miss Amy."

"I was wondering if maybe you could drop the 'miss.' I should have said that long ago."

91

"I just meant it respectful. But as long as you're asking, I'd like that."

The leaves were spinning down. They fluttered across the lawn, the patio, the pool deck, tossing in the wind like skeletal hands. Amy thought of Peter, how she missed him. Wherever he was now, she hoped that happiness would find him in his life. That was the price she'd paid; she had given him up.

She took a last sip of tea to clear the blood taste from her mouth and drew on her gloves. "Ready?"

"Right you are." Carter donned his hat. "We best get to work on them leaves."

8

"Michael!"

His sister took her last two steps at a jog and wrapped him in a hug that made his ribs crunch.

"Whoa. I'm glad to see you, too."

The nurse at the desk was staring at them, but Sara couldn't be contained. "I can't believe it," she said. "What are you doing here?" She stepped back and looked him over with a motherly eye. One part of him felt embarrassed; another part would have been disappointed if she hadn't. "God, you're thin. When did you get here? Kate will be thrilled." She glanced at the nurse, an older woman in a boiled smock. "Wendy, this is my brother, Michael."

"The one with the sailboat?"

He laughed. "That's me."

"Please tell me you're staying," Sara said.

"Just a couple of days."

She shook her head and sighed. "I guess I'll have to take what I can get." She was clutching his up-

92

per arm as if he might float away. "I'm off in an hour. Don't go *anywhere,* okay? I know you, Michael. I mean it."

He waited for her, and together they walked to the apartment. How odd it was to be back on dry land, with its disconcerting stillness underfoot. After three years mostly alone, the hum of so much packed humanity felt like something scraping his skin. He did his best to conceal his agitation, believing it would pass, though he also wondered if his time at sea had wrought a fundamental change in his temperament that would bar him from ever living among people again.

With a stab of guilt, he noted how much Kate had changed. The baby in her was gone; even her curls had straightened. The two of them played go-to with Hollis while Sara made supper; when dinner was over, Michael got into bed with her to tell her a story. Not a story from a book: Kate demanded something from real life, a tale of his adventures at sea.

He chose the story of the whale. This was something that had happened about six months before, far out in the Gulf. It was late at night, the water calm and gleaming beneath a full moon, when his boat began to lift, as if the sea were rising. A dark bulge emerged off his port side. At first he didn't know what it was. He had read about whales but never seen one, and his sense of such a creature's dimensions was vague, even disbelieving. How could something so big be alive? As the whale slowly breached the surface, a spout of water shot from its head; the creature rolled lazily onto its side, one massive flipper lifting clear. Its flanks, shiny and black, were encrusted with

93

barnacles. Michael was too amazed to be afraid; only later did it occur to him that with one slap of its tail, the whale could have shattered his boat to pieces.

Kate was staring at him, wide-eyed. "What happened?"

Well, Michael went on, that was the funny thing. He had expected the whale to move on, but it didn't. For nearly an hour it ran alongside the *Nautilus.* Occasionally it would duck its enormous head beneath the surface, only to reappear a few moments later with a spout from its blowhole, like a big wet sneeze. Then, as the moon was setting, the creature descended and did not reappear. Michael waited. Was it finally gone? Several minutes passed; he began to relax. Then, with an explosion of seawater, it reared upward off his starboard bow, hurling its massive body high into the air. It was, Michael said, like watching a city lift into the sky. *See what I can do? Don't mess with me, brother.* It crashed back down with a second detonation that blasted him broadside and left him drenched. He never saw it again.

Kate was smiling. "I get it. He was playing a joke on you."

Michael laughed. "I guess maybe he was."

He kissed her good night and returned to the main room, where Hollis and Sara were putting up the last of the dishes. The power had been cut for the night; a pair of candles flickered on the table, exuding greasy trails of smoke.

"She's quite a kid."

"Hollis gets the credit," Sara said. "I'm so busy at the hospital I sometimes feel like I barely see her."

Hollis grinned. "It's true."

94

"I hope a mat on the floor is all right," Sara said. "If I'd known you were coming, I could have gotten a proper cot from the hospital."

"Are you kidding? I usually sleep sitting up. I'm not even sure I actually sleep anymore."

Sara was wiping down the stove with a cloth. A little too aggressively — Michael could sense her frustration. It was an old conversation.

"Look," Michael said, "you don't have to worry about me. I'm fine."

Sara exhaled sharply. "Hollis, talk to him. I know I won't get anywhere."

The man shrugged helplessly. "What do you want me to say?"

"How about 'People love you, stop trying to get yourself killed.' "

"It's not like that," Michael said.

"What Sara is trying to say," Hollis interjected, "is we all hope you're being careful."

"No, that's not at all what I'm saying." She looked at Michael. "Is it Lore? Is that the reason?"

"Lore has nothing to do with it."

"Then tell me, because I'd really like to understand this, Michael."

How should he explain himself? His reasons were so tangled together that they weren't anything he could assemble into an argument. "It just feels right. That's all I can say."

She resumed her overzealous scrubbing. "So you *feel* like you should be scaring the hell out of me."

Michael reached for her, but she shook him away. "Sara —"

"Don't." She refused to look at him. "Don't tell me this is okay. Don't tell me any of this is okay. Goddamnit, I told myself I wouldn't do this. I have to get up early."

Hollis moved in behind her. He placed one hand on her shoulder, the other on the rag, bringing it to a halt and gently taking it from her hand. "We've talked about this. You've got to let him be."

"Oh, listen to you. You probably think it's just great."

Sara had begun to cry. Hollis turned her around and drew her into him. He looked past her shoulder at Michael, who was standing awkwardly by the table. "She's just worn out is all. Maybe you could give us a minute?"

"Sure, yeah."

"Thank you, Michael. The key's right by the door."

Michael let himself out of the apartment and exited the complex. With nowhere to go, he took a seat on the ground near the entrance where nobody would bother him. He hadn't felt this bad in a long time. Sara had always been a worrier, but he didn't like upsetting her; it was one of the reasons he came to the city so rarely. He would have liked to make her happy — find someone to marry, settle down with a job just like everybody else, have kids. His sister deserved some peace of mind after all she'd done, stepping in to look after him when their parents had died, though she'd just been a kid herself. Everything they did and said to each other contained this unspoken fact. If things had happened differently, they might have been just like any other brother and sister, their importance to one another fading over time as new connections took precedence. But not the two of them. New people would take the stage, but there would always be a room in their hearts in which only the two of them resided.

When he felt like he'd waited a suitable time, he returned to the apartment. The candles were doused; Sara had left a mat and pillow for him. He undressed in the dark and lay down. Only then did he notice the note that Sara had propped on his pack. He lit a candle and read.

I'm sorry. I love you. All eyes. — S

Just three sentences, but they were all he needed. They were the same three sentences that the two of them had been saying to each other every day of their lives.

He awoke to see Kate's face just inches from his own.

"Uncle Michael, *wake . . . up.*"

He drew himself up on his elbows. Hollis was standing by the door. "Sorry. I told her to leave you alone."

It took Michael a moment to gather himself. He wasn't used to sleeping so late. He wasn't used to sleeping at all. "Is Sara here?"

"Gone for hours." He beckoned to his daughter. "Let's go — we're going to be late."

Kate rolled her eyes. "Daddy's scared of the sisters."

"Your daddy's a smart man. Those ladies make my insides twist."

"Michael," said Hollis, "you're not helping."

"Right." He looked at the girl. "Do as your daddy says, sweetheart."

Kate surprised him with a sudden, forceful hug. "Will you be here when I get back?"

"Sure I will."

He listened to their footsteps descending the

stairs. You had to hand it to the kid. Pure emotional blackmail, but what could he do? He dressed and washed up at the sink. Sara had left rolls for breakfast, but he wasn't really hungry. He could find something later if he needed to, assuming he actually felt like eating.

He grabbed his pack and headed out.

Sara was finishing her morning rounds when one of the nurses fetched her. She made her way to the reception area to find Sister Peg standing at the desk.

"Sister, hello."

Sister Peg was one of those people who changed any room she entered, tightening every screw. Her age was anybody's guess — at least sixty, though it was said that she'd looked exactly the same for twenty years. A figure of legendary cantankerousness, though Sara knew better; beneath the stern exterior was a woman devoted completely to the children in her care.

"Might I have a word with you, Sara?"

Moments later, they were headed to the orphanage. As they drew near, Sara could hear the whoops and cries of children; morning recess was in full swing. They entered through the garden gate.

"Dr. Sara, Dr. Sara!"

Sara didn't make it five steps onto the playground before the children descended. They knew her well, but part of their excitement, she understood, was the presence of any visitor. She extricated herself with promises to stay longer next time and followed Sister Peg into the building.

The girl was sitting on the table in the little room Sara used for exams. Her eyes flicked up as

98

Sara entered. She could have been twelve or thirteen; it was difficult to tell through the layers of filth. She was wearing a grimy burlap frock, knotted over one shoulder; her feet, blackened with dirt and covered with scabs, were bare.

"Domestic Security brought her in late last night," Sister Peg said. "She hasn't spoken a word."

The girl had been caught trying to break into an ag storehouse. Sara could see why: she looked half-starved.

"Hello, I'm Dr. Sara. Can you tell me your name?"

The girl, peering intently at Sara from under the hood of her matted hair, gave no reply. Her eyes — the only part of her body that had moved since Sara entered the room — darted to Sister Peg, then back at Sara.

"We tried to find out who her parents are," Sister Peg said, "but there's no record of anybody looking for her."

Sara guessed there wouldn't be. She removed her stethoscope from her bag and showed the girl. "I'm going to listen to your heart — would that be okay?"

No words, yet the girl's eyes said she could. Sara slid the knotted side of the frock from her shoulder. She was thin as a reed, but her breasts had just begun to show. At the feel of the cold disk on her skin, the girl flinched slightly, but that was all.

"Sara, you should look at this."

Sister Peg was staring at the girl's back. It was covered with burns and lash marks. Some were old, others still weeping. Sara had seen it before, but never like this.

She looked at the girl. "Honey, can you tell me

who did this to you?"

"I don't think she can talk," Sister Peg said.

Sara had begun to grasp the situation. The girl allowed Sara to hold her chin. Sara moved her other hand beside the girl's right ear. She snapped her fingers three times; the girl did not react. She swapped hands to test the other ear. Nothing. Looking into the girl's eyes, Sara then pointed to her own ear and slowly shook her head, meaning no. The girl nodded.

"That's because she's deaf."

Then a surprising thing happened. The girl reached for Sara's hand. With her index finger, she began to draw a series of lines in Sara's upturned palm. Not lines, Sara realized. Letters. P. I. M.

"Pim," Sara said. She glanced at Sister Peg, then looked back at the girl. "Pim — is that your name?"

She nodded. Sara took the girl's palm. SARA, she wrote, and pointed at herself. "Sara." She looked up. "Sister, can you get me something to write with?"

Sister Peg departed the room, returning moments later with one of the handheld chalkboards the children used for their lessons.

WHERE ARE YOUR PARENTS? Sara wrote.

Pim took the board. She erased Sara's words with her palm, then gripped the chalk awkwardly in her fist.

— DED

— WHEN?

— MOM THEN DAD LONG TIM

— WHO HURT YOU?

— MAN

— WHAT MAN?

— DONT KNW GOT AWAY

The next question pained her, but it had to be asked.

— DID HE HURT YOU ANYWHERE ELSE?

The girl hesitated, then nodded. Sara's heart sank.

— WHERE?

Pim took the board.

— GIRLPLACE

Without taking her eyes off the girl, Sara said, "Sister, can you give us a minute?"

When Sister Peg was gone, Sara wrote, MORE THAN ONCE?

The girl nodded.

— NEED TO LOOK. WILL BE CAREFUL.

Pim's whole body clenched. She shook her head vigorously back and forth.

— PLEASE, wrote Sara. HAVE TO MAKE SURE YOU ARE OK.

Pim took the chalkboard and quickly scribbled, MY FALT PROMISST NOT TO TELL

— NO. NOT YOUR FAULT.

— PIM BAD

Sara didn't know if she wanted to cry or be sick. She'd seen some things in her life — terrible things — and not just at the Homeland. You couldn't walk the hospital halls without encountering the worst of human nature. A woman with a broken wrist and an excuse about falling down a flight of stairs, reciting how it had happened while her husband looked on, coaching her with his eyes. An old man with advanced malnutrition dumped at the door by relatives. One of Dunk's whores, her body ravaged with disease and misuse, clutching a fistful of Austins to rid herself of the baby she was carrying so she could get back on

101

the stool. You hardened your heart because there was no other way to get through the day, but the children were the worst. The children you couldn't look away from. In Pim's case, it wasn't hard to reconstruct the story. Her parents dead, somebody had offered to take the girl in, a family member or neighbor, everyone thinking how kind and generous that person was, to assume responsibility for this poor orphan who couldn't hear or talk, and after that nobody had bothered to check.

"No, honey, no." Sara took Pim's hands and looked into her eyes. There was a soul in there, tiny, terrified, discarded by the world. There wasn't anybody more alone on the face of the earth, and Sara understood what was being asked of her, just for being human.

Not even Hollis knew the story. It wasn't that Sara was afraid to tell him; she knew the kind of man he was. But silence was a decision she'd made long ago. At the Homeland, it was said, everybody had taken their turn, and Sara's had come in due course. She had endured it as best she knew how, and when it was over, she imagined a box, made of steel with a strong lock. Then she took the memory and put it in the box.

She took the board and wrote:
— SOMEBODY HURT ME THERE ONCE TOO.

The girl studied the board with the same guarded expression. Perhaps ten seconds passed. She took up the chalk again.
— SECRET?
— YOU ARE THE ONLY PERSON I EVER TOLD.

The girl's face was changing. Something was letting go.

Sara wrote: WE ARE THE SAME. SARA IS GOOD. PIM IS GOOD. NOT OUR FAULT.

A film of tears appeared in the surface of the girl's eyes. A single drop edged over the barrier and spilled down her cheek, cutting a river in the dirt. Her lips were closed; the muscles of her neck and jaw grew taut, then began to quiver. A strange new sound entered the room. It was a kind of growl, like an animal's. It felt like something fighting to get out.

And then it did. The girl opened her mouth and released a howl that seemed to shatter the very idea of human language, distilling it to a single sustained vowel of pain. Sara wrapped her in a tight embrace. Pim was wailing, shaking, fighting to break free, but Sara wouldn't let her. "It's all right," she said. "I won't let you go, I won't let you go." And she held her that way until the girl was quiet again, and for a long time after.

9

The capitol building, housed in what had once been Texas First Trust Bank — the name was still engraved in the building's limestone fascia — was just a short walk from the school. A directory in the lobby listed the various departments: Housing Authority, Public Health, Agriculture and Commerce, Printing and Engraving. Sanchez's office was located on the second floor. Peter ascended the stairs, which opened onto a second open area with a desk, behind which sat a Domestic Security officer in an unnaturally clean uniform. Peter felt suddenly embarrassed to be dressed in his ratty work clothes, carrying a bag full of rattling tools and nails.

"Help you?"

"I'm here to see President Sanchez. I have an appointment."

"Name?" His eyes had returned to his desk; he was filling out some kind of form.

"Peter Jaxon."

It was like a light going on in the man's face. "You're Jaxon?"

Peter dipped his head.

"Holy smokes." The man just sat there, awkwardly staring. It had been some time since Peter had gotten this kind of reaction. On the other hand, he rarely met anybody new these days. Never, in fact.

"Maybe you could let somebody know?" Peter said finally.

"Right." The officer popped from his chair. "Just a second. I'll tell them you're here."

Peter noted the word "them." Who else would be attending the meeting? For that matter, why was he here at all? In the hours of mulling over the president's note, he'd come up empty. Maybe it was just as Caleb had suggested and they really *did* want him back in the Army. If so, it was going to be a short conversation.

"You can come right back, Mr. Jaxon."

The officer took Peter's tool bag and led him down a long hallway. Sanchez's door was open. She rose from behind her desk as Peter entered: a small woman with mostly white hair, sharp features, and a strong gaze. A second person, a man with a tight, bristly beard, was seated across from her. He looked familiar, though Peter couldn't place him.

"Mr. Jaxon, it's good to see you." Sanchez stepped around her desk and extended her hand.

"Madam President. It's an honor."

"Please," she said, "it's Vicky. Let me introduce you to Ford Chase, my chief of staff."

"I believe we've met, Mr. Jaxon."

Now Peter remembered: Chase had attended the inquest after the destruction of the bridge on the Oil Road. The memory was unpleasant; he'd taken an instant disliking to the man. Compounding Peter's distrust, Chase was wearing a necktie, the most incomprehensible article of clothing in the history of the world.

"And of course you know General Apgar," Sanchez said.

Peter turned to see his former commanding officer rising from the couch. Gunnar had aged a little, his clipped hair gone gray, his brow more deeply furrowed. A bit of a paunch stretched the buttons of his uniform. The urge to salute was strong, but Peter held it in check, and the two men shook.

"Congratulations on the promotion, sir." To the surprise of no one who had served under the man, Apgar had been named general of the Army after Fleet had stepped down.

"I regret it every day. Tell me, how's your boy?"

"He's doing well, sir. Thanks for asking."

"If I wanted you to call me 'sir,' I wouldn't have accepted your resignation. Which is my second-biggest regret, by the way. I should have put up more of a fight."

Peter liked Gunnar; the man's presence put him at his ease. "It wouldn't have done you any good."

Sanchez led them to a small sitting area with a sofa and a couple of leather armchairs surrounding a low table with a stone top, on which rested a long tube of rolled paper. For the first time Peter

had a chance to look at his surroundings: a wall of books, a curtainless window, a chipped desk piled high with paper. A pole stood behind it bearing the Texas flag, the only ceremonial object in the room. Peter took one of the chairs, across from Sanchez. Apgar and Chase sat to the side.

"To begin, Mr. Jaxon," Sanchez said, "I'm sure you're wondering why I asked you to come see me. I'd like to request a favor. To put this in context, let me show you something. Ford?"

Chase unrolled the paper on the table and weighed down the corners. A surveyor's map: Kerrville stood at the center, its walls and perimeter lines clearly marked. To the west, along the Guadalupe, three large areas were blocked off with cross-hatching, each with a notation: SP1, SP2, SP3.

"At the risk of sounding grandiose, what you're looking at is the future of the Texas Republic," Sanchez said.

Chase explained, "SP stands for 'settlement parcel.' "

"These are the most logical areas for moving out the population, at least to start. There's water, arable soil in the bottoms, good land for grazing. We're going to proceed in stages, using a lottery system for people who want to leave."

"Which will be a lot of them," Chase added.

Peter looked up. Everyone was waiting for his reaction.

"You don't seem pleased," Sanchez said.

He searched for the words. "I guess . . . I never really thought this day would come."

"The war is over," Apgar said. "Three years without a single viral. It's what we've been fighting for, all these years."

Sanchez was leaning forward. There was something tremendously attractive about the woman, an undeniable force. Peter had heard this about her — she was said to have been a great beauty in her youth, with a list of suitors a mile long — but it was an entirely different matter to experience it.

"History will remember you, Peter, for all you've done."

"It was more than just me."

"I know that, too. There's more than enough congratulations to go around. And I'm sorry about your friends. Captain Donadio is a great loss. And Amy, well . . ." She paused. "I'll be honest with you. The stories about her — I was never quite sure what to believe. I'm not sure I completely understand them now. What I do know is that none of us would be having this conversation if not for Amy, and for you. You're the one who brought her to us. That's what the people know. And it makes you very important. You could say there's no one like you." Her eyes remained fixed on his face; she had a way of making it feel as if they were the only two people in the room. "Tell me, how do you like working for the Housing Authority?"

"It's all right."

"And it gives you the chance to raise your boy. To be around for him."

Peter sensed a strategy unfolding. He nodded.

"I never had children," Sanchez said, somewhat regretfully. "One of the costs of the office. But I understand your feelings. So let me say right off that I'm sensitive to your priorities, and nothing about what I'm proposing would get in the way of that. You'll be there for him, just as you are now."

Peter knew a half-truth when he heard one. On

107

the other hand, Sanchez's approach was so carefully laid he couldn't help but admire it.

"I'm listening."

"What would you say, Peter, to joining my staff?"

The notion was so ludicrous he almost laughed. "Forgive me, Madam President —"

"Please," the woman cut in with a smile, "it's Vicky."

He had to admit it, the woman was masterful. "There's so much wrong with the idea I don't even know where to begin. Just for starters, I'm not a politician."

"And I'm not asking you to be one. But you are a leader, and the people know it. You're too valuable a resource to sit on the sidelines. Opening the gate isn't just about making more room, though we absolutely need it. This represents a fundamental change in how we do just about everything. A lot of details have to be hammered out, but within the next ninety days I'm planning to suspend martial law. The Expeditionary is going to be recalled from the territories to assist with resettlement, and we'll be transitioning to a full civilian government. It's a big adjustment, giving everybody a place at the table, and it's going to be messy. But it absolutely has to happen, and this is the right moment."

"With all due respect, I don't see what this has to do with me."

"It has everything to do with you, actually. Or at least I hope so. Your position is unique. The military respects you. The people love you, especially the Iowans. But those are only two legs of the tripod. The third is the trade. They're going to have a field day with this. Tifty Lamont may be dead, but your previous relationship with him

gives you access to their chain of command. There's no question of shutting them down, we couldn't if we tried. Vice is a fact of life — an ugly fact, but a fact nonetheless. You know Dunk Withers, yes?"

Peter nodded. "We've met."

"More than met, if what my sources tell me is correct. I've heard about the cage. That was quite a stunt."

She was referring to Peter's first encounter with Tifty at his underground compound north of San Antonio. As a cathartic entertainment, members of the trade leadership would face off against virals in hand-to-hand combat, the others betting on the outcome. Dunk had gone into the cage first, dispatching a dopey with relative ease, followed by Peter, who had taken on a full-blown drac in order to secure Tifty's agreement to escort them to Iowa.

"It seemed like the thing to do at the time."

Sanchez smiled. "That's my point. You're a man who does what needs to be done. As for Dunk, the man's not half as smart as Lamont was, and I wish he were. Our agreement with Lamont was a simple one. The man was sitting on some of the best-preserved military hardware we'd seen in years. We couldn't have outfitted the Army without him. Keep the worst stuff in check, we told him, keep the guns and ammo coming, and you can go about your business. He understood the sense of it, but I doubt Dunk will. The man's a pure opportunist, and he has an ugly streak."

"So why not just put him in the stockade?"

Sanchez shrugged. "We could, and it may come to that. General Apgar thinks we should round up the lot of them, seize the bunker and the gambling

halls, and put an end to it. But somebody else would slide into his spot before the ink was dry, and we'd be back to square one. It's a case of supply and demand. The demand is there — who will supply the goods? The card tables, the lick, the prostitutes? I don't like it, but I'd rather deal with a known quantity, and for now that's Dunk."

"So you want me to talk to him."

"Yes, in time. Corralling the trade is important. So is keeping the military and the civilian population fully on board during the transition. You're the one man who has stock with all three. Hell, you could probably have my job if you asked for it, not that I'd wish it on my worst enemy."

Peter had the unsettling feeling that he had already agreed to something. He looked at Apgar, whose face said, *Believe me, I've been down this road.*

"What exactly are you asking?"

"For now, I'd like to name you as a special adviser. A go-between, if you like, between the stakeholders. We can come up with a more specific title later. But I want you out in front, where everyone can see you. Your voice should be the first one people hear. And I promise you that you'll be home for supper every day with your boy."

The temptation was real: no more sweltering days swinging a hammer. But he was also tired. Some essential energy had left him. He'd done enough, and what he wanted now was a quiet, simple life. To take his boy to school and do a day of honest labor, and put his boy to bed at night and spend eight sweet hours someplace else entirely — the only place where he had ever been truly happy.

"No."

Sanchez startled; she wasn't used to being denied so succinctly. "No?"

"That's it. That's my answer."

"Surely there's something I can say that will change your mind."

"I'm flattered, but this has to be somebody else's problem. I'm sorry."

Sanchez didn't seem angry, merely puzzled. "I see." The disarming smile returned. "Well, I had to ask."

She rose to her feet, everyone else following suit. Now it was Peter's turn to be surprised; he realized he'd expected her to put up more of a fight. At the door, she shook his hand in parting.

"Thank you for taking the time to meet with me, Peter. The offer stands, and I hope you'll reconsider. You could do a lot of good. Promise me you'll think about it?"

There seemed no harm in agreeing. "I'll do that."

"General Apgar can show you out."

So that was it. He felt a little amazed, and wondered, as one always did when a door closed, if he had made the right choice.

"Peter, one last thing," Sanchez said.

He turned at the threshold. The woman had returned to her desk.

"I was meaning to ask. How old is your boy?"

The question seemed harmless enough. "He's ten."

"And it's Caleb, yes?"

Peter nodded.

"It's a wonderful age. His whole life ahead of him. When you stop to think about it, it's the children we're really working for, isn't it? We'll be

111

long gone, but our decisions in the next few months will determine the kind of world they're going to live in." She smiled. "Well. Food for thought, Mr. Jaxon. Thank you again for coming."

He followed Gunnar out the door. Halfway down the hall, Peter heard the man chuckling under his breath.

"She's good, isn't she?"

"Yeah," said Peter. "She's good all right."

10

Michael had three things in his bag. The first was the newspaper. The second was a letter.

He had found it in the breast pocket of the captain's uniform. The envelope was unmarked; the man had never intended to send it. The letter, less than a page, was written in English.

My darling boy,

I know now that you and I are never to meet in this life. Our fuel is nearly exhausted; our last hope of reaching the refuge is gone. Last night, the crew and passengers took a vote. The result was unanimous. Death by dehydration is a fate none desires. Tonight will be the last we share on earth. Entombed in steel, we will drift in the currents until such time as almighty God chooses to take us to the bottom.

I obviously have no hope that these last words will reach you. I can only pray that you and your mother have been spared the devastation and somehow survived. What awaits me now? The Holy Quran says: "To Allah belongeth the Mystery of the heavens and the

earth. And the Decision of the Hour of Judgment is as the twinkling of an eye, or even quicker: for Allah hath power over all things." Surely we are His and to Him we shall return. In spite of all that has happened, I have faith that my immortal soul will pass into His hands, and that when at last we meet, it shall be in paradise.

My final thoughts in life are with you. Baraka Allahu fika.

Your loving father,
Nabil

Michael mused on these words as he made his way through the streets of H-town. He was accustomed to scenes of abandonment and devastation; he had crossed ruined cities that contained skeletons by the thousands. But never before had the dead spoken so directly to him. In the captain's quarters, he had found the man's passport. His full name was Nabil Haddad. He had been born in the Netherlands, in a city called Utrecht, in 1971. Michael found no further evidence of the boy in the cabin — no photographs or other letters — but the emergency contact named in his passport was a woman named Astrid Keeble, with a London address. Perhaps she was the boy's mother. Michael wondered what had happened between the three of them, that the captain never should have seen his son. Perhaps the boy's mother wouldn't allow it; perhaps for some reason the man did not feel worthy. Yet he had felt the need to write to him, knowing that in a few hours he would be dead and the letter would travel no farther than his own pocket.

But that wasn't all the letter told him. The *Ber-*

gensfjord had been going somewhere; it had had a destination. Not "a refuge," "*the* refuge." A safe haven where the virus could not reach them.

Hence the third thing in Michael's bag, and his need for the man they called the Maestro.

If the man had a real name, Michael didn't know it. The Maestro also had the habit of speaking in disconcertingly butchered sentences while always referring to himself in the third person; it took some getting used to. He was quite old, possessing a sinewy twitchiness that made him seem less like a man than some kind of overgrown rodent. He had once been an electrical engineer for the Civilian Authority; long retired, he had become Kerrville's go-to man for electronic antiquities. Crazy as a caged bird, and not a little paranoid, but the man knew how to make an old hard drive confess its secrets.

The Maestro's shed was unmissable; it was the only building in H-town with solar panels on the roof. Michael knocked loudly and stepped back for the camera; the Maestro wanted a good look at you first. A moment passed, and then a series of heavy locks opened.

"Michael." The Maestro stood in a narrow wedge of open door, wearing a work apron and a plastic visor with flip-down lenses.

"Hello, Maestro."

The man's eyes darted up and down the street. "Quickly," he said, waving Michael inside.

The shed's interior was like a museum. Old computers, office machines, oscilloscopes, flat-panels, huge bins of handhelds and cellphones: the sight of so much circuitry always gave Michael a tingly thrill.

"How can the Maestro be of assistance?"

114

"I've got an antique for you."

Michael removed the third thing from his bag. The old man took it in his hand and examined it quickly.

"Gensys 872HJS. Fourth generation, three terabytes. Late prewar." He looked up. "Where?"

"I found it on a derelict ship. I need to recover the files."

"A closer look, then."

Michael followed him to one of several workbenches, where he laid the drive on a cloth mat and flipped down the lenses of his visor. With a minuscule screwdriver he removed the case and perused the interior parts.

"Moisture damage. Not good."

"Can you fix it?"

"Difficult. Expensive."

Michael removed a wad of Austins from his pocket. The old man counted it on the bench.

"Not enough."

"It's what I've got."

"The Maestro doubts that. Oil man like yourself?"

"Not anymore."

He studied Michael's face. "Ah. The Maestro remembers. He has heard some crazy stories. True?"

"Depends on what you heard."

"Hunting for the barrier. Sailing out alone."

"More or less."

The old man pursed his rubbery lips, then slid the money into the pocket of his apron. "The Maestro will see what he can do. Come back tomorrow."

Michael returned to the apartment. In the mean-

time he'd been to the library, adding a heavy book to his satchel: *The Reader's Digest Great World Atlas.* It wasn't one that people were permitted to check out. He'd waited for the reference librarian to be distracted, concealed it in his bag, and slipped outside.

Once again, he was called upon for a bedtime story. This one was about the storm. Kate listened with tense excitement, as if the story might end with him drowned in the sea, despite the fact that he was sitting right in front of her. With Sara, the subject of the previous night did not come up. This was their way; a lot was said by saying nothing. She also seemed distracted. Michael assumed that something had happened at the hospital and let it go at that.

In the morning he left the apartment before anyone else was awake. The old man was waiting for him.

"The Maestro has done it," he declared.

He led Michael to a CRT. His hands scurried over the keyboard; a glowing map appeared on the screen. "The ship. Where?"

"I found it in Galveston Bay, at the mouth of the ship channel."

"Long way from home."

The Maestro walked Michael through the data. Departing from Hong Kong in mid-March, the *Bergensfjord* had sailed to Hawaii, then passed through the Panama Canal into the Atlantic. According to the time line Michael had established from the newspaper, that much would have occurred before the outbreak of the Easter Virus. They had made port in the Canary Islands, perhaps to refuel, then continued north.

At this point, the data changed. The ship had

traveled in circles up and down the coast of northern Europe. A brief foray to the Strait of Gibraltar, then it reversed course without entering the Mediterranean and returned to Tenerife. Several weeks elapsed, and they set sail again. The epidemic would have been widespread by this time. They passed through the Strait of Magellan and headed north toward the equator.

In midocean, the ship appeared to stop. After two motionless weeks, the data ended.

"Can we tell where they were headed?" Michael asked.

Another screen of data appeared: these were course plottings, the Maestro explained. He scrolled down the page and directed Michael's attention to the last one.

"Can you back that up for me?" Michael asked.

"Already done." The old man produced a flash drive from his apron; Michael put it in his pocket. "The Maestro is curious. Why so important?"

"I was thinking of taking a vacation."

"The Maestro has already checked. Empty ocean. Nothing there." His pale eyebrows lifted. "But something, perhaps?"

The man was no fool. "Perhaps," said Michael.

He left Sara a note. *Sorry to run. Visiting an old friend. Hope to be back in a few days.*

The second transport to the Orange Zone left at 0900. Michael rode it to the end of the line, got off, and waited as the bus drove away. The posted sign read:

YOU ARE ENTERING THE RED ZONE.
PROCEED AT OWN RISK.
WHEN IN DOUBT, RUN.

117

If you only knew, he thought. Then he began to walk.

11

Sara returned to the orphanage before the start of her morning shift. Sister Peg greeted her at the door.

"How is she doing?" Sara asked.

The woman looked more harried than usual; it had been a long night for her. "Not very well, I'm afraid."

Pim had woken up screaming. Her howls were so loud that they had awakened the entire dormitory. For the time being, they had put her in Sister Peg's quarters.

"We've had abused children before, but nothing so extreme. Another night like that . . ."

Sister Peg led Sara to her room, a monastic space with just the bare-bones necessities. The only decoration was a large cross on the wall. Pim was awake and sitting on the bed with her knees tight to her chest. But as Sara entered, some of the tension released from her face. *Here is an ally, someone who knows.*

"I'll be outside if you need me," Sister Peg said.

Sara sat on the bed. The grime was gone, the mats in her hair teased straight or cut away. The sisters had dressed her in a plain wool tunic.

— HOW ARE YOU FEELING TODAY? Sara wrote on the chalkboard.

— OK

— SISTER SAID YOU COULDN'T SLEEP.

Pim shook her head.

Sara explained to Pim that she needed to change her dressings. The girl flinched as Sara eased away

118

the bandages but made no sound. Sara applied antibiotic salve and a cream of cooling aloe and rewrapped her.

— I'M SORRY IF THAT HURT.

Pim shrugged.

Sara looked her in the eye. IT WILL BE OK, she wrote. Then, when the girl did nothing: IT GETS BETTER.

— NO MOR NITEMERES?

Sara shook her head. "No."

— HOW?

There was, of course, the easy thing to say: *Give it time*. But that wasn't the truth, or at least not the whole truth. What took the pain away, Sara knew, was other people — Hollis, and Kate, and being a family.

— IT JUST DOES, she wrote.

It was nearly 0800; Sara had to leave, though she didn't want to. She packed up her kit and wrote:

— I HAVE TO GO NOW. TRY TO REST. THE SISTERS WILL TAKE CARE OF YOU.

— COME BACK? Pim wrote.

Sara nodded.

— DO YU SWEAR?

Pim was looking at her intently. People had been throwing her away her entire life; why should Sara be different?

"Yes," she said, and crossed her heart. "I swear."

Sister Peg was waiting for Sara in the hall. "How is she?"

The day had only just started, yet Sara felt completely drained. "The wounds on her back aren't the real problem. I wouldn't be surprised if she has more nights like that."

"Is there any chance of finding a relative?

119

Somebody who can take her in?"

"I think that would be the worst thing for her."

Sister Peg nodded. "Yes, of course. That was stupid of me."

Sara gave the woman a roll of gauze, boiled cloth pads, and a jar of ointment. "Change her dressings every twelve hours. There's no sign of infection, but if anything starts to look worse, or she gets a fever, send for me right away."

Sister Peg was frowning at the objects in her hand. Then, brightening a little, she looked up. "I meant to thank you for the other night. It was nice to get out. I should do it more often."

"Peter was happy to have you there."

"Caleb has grown so much. Kate, too. Sometimes it's easy to forget how lucky we are. Then you see something like this . . ." She let the thought pass. "I'd better get back to the children. Where would they be without mean old Sister Peg?"

"It's a good act, if you don't mind my saying so."

"Does it show? I'm really just an old softie at heart."

She walked Sara out. At the doorway, Sara paused. "Let me ask you something. In the course of a year, say, how many children get adopted?"

"In a year?" The woman seemed startled by the question. "Zero."

"None at *all*?"

"It happens, but very rarely. And it's never the older children, if that's what you're asking. Sometimes a baby will be left here and a relative will come and claim it within a few days. But once a child has been here awhile, the odds are good they'll stay."

"I didn't know."

Her eyes searched Sara's face. "The two of us aren't so very different, you know. Ten times a day our jobs give us good reason to cry. And yet we can't. We wouldn't be any use to anyone if we did."

It was true; but it didn't make Sara's heart feel any less heavy. "Thank you, Sister."

She headed for the hospital. Her mood was bleak. As she entered the building, Wendy urgently waved her over to the desk.

"There's somebody waiting for you."

"A patient?"

The woman looked around to make sure she wasn't overheard. She lowered her voice to a whisper. "He says he's from the *census office.*"

Uh-oh, thought Sara. *That was fast.* "Where is he?"

"I told him to wait, but he went to look for you on the ward. Jenny's with him."

"You let *Jenny* talk to him? Are you nuts?"

"There wasn't anything I could do! She was standing right there when he asked for you!" Wendy lowered her voice again. "It's about that woman with the abruption, isn't it?"

"Let's hope not."

At the door to the ward, Sara took a clean smock from the shelf. Two things worked in her favor. The first was her rank. She was a doctor, and although she didn't like to do it, she could throw her weight around if she had to. A certain peremptory tone; veiled or not-so-veiled references to unnamed persons of substantial influence; the mantle of the higher calling, busy day, lives to save: Sara had learned the tricks. Second, she hadn't done anything illegal. Failing to file the

proper paperwork was not a crime — more like an error. She was safe, more or less, but this wouldn't help Carlos or his family. Once the fraud was discovered, Grace would be taken away.

She stepped into the ward. Jenny was standing with a man who possessed the unmistakable look of a bureaucrat: soft, balding, and flat-footed, with pasty skin that rarely saw sunshine. Jenny's glance met hers with a look of barely concealed panic: *Help!*

"Sara," she began, "this is —"

She didn't let the girl finish. "Jenny, could you please check the laundry for blankets? I think we're running low."

"We are?"

"Now, please."

She scurried away.

"I'm Dr. Wilson," Sara said to the man. "What is this about?"

The man cleared his throat. He seemed a little nervous. Good. "There was a woman who delivered a girl here four nights ago." He fumbled through the papers he was holding. "Sally Jiménez? I believe you were the doctor on duty."

"And you are?"

"Joe English. I'm from the census office."

"I have a lot of patients, Mr. English." She pretended to think. "Oh, yes, I remember. A healthy girl. Is there an issue?"

"No birthright certificate was filed with the census form. The woman has two sons."

"I'm sure I took care of it. You'll have to check again."

"I spent all yesterday looking for it. It definitely wasn't sent to my office."

122

"Your office never makes mistakes? Loses paper-work?"

"We're very thorough, Dr. Wilson. According to the nurse at the desk, Mrs. Jiménez was released three days ago. We always talk to the family first, but they don't seem to be home. Her husband hasn't been to work since the birth."

Dumb move, Carlos, Sara thought. "I can't be responsible for people once they leave here."

"But you *are* responsible for filing the proper documentation. Without a valid birthright, I'm going to have to move her case up the line."

"Well, I'm sure there was one. You're mistaken. Is that all? I'm very busy here."

He regarded her for an uncomfortably long moment. "For now, Dr. Wilson."

Wherever the Jiménez family had gone, Sara knew it wouldn't take long for the census office to track them down. There were only so many places to hide.

She tried to put them out of her mind. She'd done her best to help, and the situation was out of her hands. Sister Peg was right; she had a job to do. It was important, and she was good at it. That was what mattered most.

In the middle of the night, she awoke with the feeling that a powerful dream had ejected her from sleep. She rose and checked on Kate. She felt certain that her daughter had been in this dream, if peripherally; she had not been the focus — rather, a witness, almost a judge. Sara sat on the edge of her daughter's cot and watched the night pass through her. The girl was deeply asleep, her lips slightly parted, her chest expanding and contracting with long, even breaths, filling the air

123

with her unmistakable scent. At the Homeland, in the time before Sara had found her again, it was Kate's smell that had given her the strength to go on. She'd kept a baby curl in an envelope, hidden away in her bunk, and each night she had taken it out and pressed it to her face. This act was, Sara knew, a form of prayer — not that Kate was still alive, because she'd believed absolutely that her daughter was dead, but that wherever she was, wherever her spirit had gone, it felt like home.

"Is everything okay?"

Hollis was standing behind her. Kate stirred, rolled over, and then was quiet again.

"Come back to bed," he whispered.

"I can sleep in. I'm on second shift."

Hollis said nothing.

"All right," she said.

When dawn came, Sara was wide awake. Hollis told her to stay in bed, but she got up anyway; she wouldn't return from the hospital until after dinner and wanted to take Kate to school. She was half-drunk with exhaustion, although this fact did not seem like a compromising influence on her judgment but a source of clarity. At the door of the school, she hugged her daughter tightly. It did not seem so long ago that Sara had needed to kneel to do this; now the crown of Kate's head reached Sara's chest.

"Mom?"

The hug had gone on for some time. "Sorry." Sara released her. The other children were streaming past. She realized what she was feeling. She was happy; a weight had lifted from her heart. "Go on, kiddo," she said. "I'll see you later."

The records office opened at nine o'clock. Sara waited on the steps in the dappled shade of a live

oak. It was a pleasant summer morning; people were striding past. How quickly life could change, she thought.

When the clerk unlocked the door, Sara rose and followed the woman inside. She was older, with a pleasant, weathered face and a row of bright false teeth. She took her time situating herself behind the counter before looking Sara's way, pretending to notice her for the first time.

"Can I help you?"

"I need to transfer a birthright."

The clerk licked her fingers and removed a form from a slotted shelf, then placed it on the counter and dipped her quill in a bottle of ink. "Whose?"

"Mine."

The woman's pen halted over the paper. She raised her face with an expression of concern. "You seem young, honey. Are you sure?"

"Please, can we just do this?"

Sara sent the form to the census office with a note attached — *Sorry! Found it after all!* — and went to the hospital. The day passed quickly; Hollis was still awake when she got home. She waited until they were in bed to make her announcement.

"I want to have another child."

He rose on his elbows and turned toward her. "Sara, we've been through this. You know we can't."

She kissed him, long and tenderly, then drew back to meet his eyes. "Actually," she said, "that's not exactly true."

12

Ten moves, and Caleb had Peter completely boxed

in. A feint with a rook, a knight cruelly sacrificed, and the enemy forces swarmed over him.

"How the heck did you do that?"

Peter didn't really mind, though it would be nice to win once in a while. The last time he'd beaten Caleb, the boy had had a nasty cold and had dozed off midway through the game. Even then, Peter had barely eked out the victory.

"It's easy. You think I'm on defense, but I'm not."

"Laying a trap."

The boy shrugged. "It's like a trap in your head. I make you see the game the way I need you to." He was setting up the pieces again; one victory was not enough for the night. "What did the soldier want?"

Caleb had a way of changing the subject so abruptly that sometimes Peter struggled to keep up. "It was about a job, actually."

"What kind?"

"To tell you the truth, I'm not really sure." He shrugged and looked at the board. "It's not important. Don't worry about it — I'm not going anywhere."

They were listlessly moving pawns.

"I still want to be a soldier, you know," the boy said, "like you were."

From time to time, the boy brought this up. Peter's feelings were mixed. On the one hand, he had a parent's intense desire to keep Caleb away from any danger. But he also felt flattered. The boy was, after all, expressing interest in the same life he had chosen.

"Well, you'd be good at it."

"Do you miss it?"

"Sometimes. I liked my men, I had good friends.

126

But I'd rather be here with you. Plus, it looks like those days are over. Not much need for an army when there's nobody to fight."

"Everything else seems like it would be boring."

"Boredom is underrated, believe me."

They played in silence.

"Somebody asked me about you," Caleb said. "A kid at school."

"What was the question?"

Caleb squinted at the board, reached toward his bishop, stopped, and moved his queen one space forward. "Just, what it's like, you being my dad. He knew a lot about you."

"Which kid was this?"

"His name is Julio."

He wasn't one of Caleb's usual friends. "What did you tell him?"

"I told him you worked on roofs all day."

For once, Peter held Caleb to a draw. He put the boy to bed and poured himself a drink from Hollis's flask. Caleb's words had stung a little. Peter wasn't truly tempted by Sanchez's offer, but the whole thing had left a bad taste in his mouth. The woman's manipulation was transparent, as it was meant to be — that was the genius of it. She had simultaneously aroused his natural sense of duty and made it clear that she was not a woman to be messed with. *I'll have you in the end, Mr. Jaxon.*

Just you try, he thought. I'll be right here, reminding my kid to brush his teeth.

They were reroofing an old mission close to the center of town. Empty for decades, it was now being converted to apartments. Peter's crew had spent two weeks dismantling the rotted belfry and

127

had begun to strip off the old slates. The roof was steeply pitched; they worked on twelve-inch-wide horizontal boards, called cleats, anchored by metal brackets nailed into the sheeting and spaced at six-foot intervals. A pair of ladders, lying flush with the roof at the ends of the cleats, acted as staircases connecting them.

All morning they worked shirtless in the heat. Peter was on the uppermost cleat with two others, Jock Alvado and Sam Foutopolis, who went by the name Foto. Foto had worked construction for years, but Jock had been there just a couple of months. He was young, seventeen or so, with a narrow, acned face and long greasy hair he wore in a ponytail. Nobody liked him; his movements were too sudden, and he talked too much. It was an unwritten rule of the roofing crews not to remark on the danger. It was a form of respect. Looking down, Jock liked to say stupid things like "Wow, that would hurt" and "That would most definitely fuck a person *up*."

At noon they broke for lunch. Climbing down was too much trouble, so they ate where they were. Jock was talking about a girl he had seen in the market, but Peter was barely listening. The sounds of the city drifted upward in an aural haze; from time to time a bird floated past.

"Let's get back to it," Foto said.

They were using pry bars and mallets to chip out the old tiles. Peter and Foto moved to the third cleat; Jock was working below them to the right. He was still talking about the woman — her hair, a certain way she walked, a look that passed between them.

"Will he ever shut up?" Foto said. He was a thick, muscular man, his black beard sprinkled

with gray.

"I think he just likes the sound of his own voice."

"I'm going to throw his ass off this roof, I swear." Foto glanced up, squinting into the sun. "Looks like we missed a couple."

Several tiles remained along the ridgeline. Peter slid his bar and mallet into his tool belt. "I'll go."

"Forget it, lover boy can do it." He yelled down, "Jock, get up there."

"I'm not the one who missed those. That was Jaxon's section."

"It's yours now."

"Fine," the boy huffed. "Whatever you say."

Jock unclipped his harness, scrambled up the ladder to the uppermost cleat, and wedged his pry bar under one of the tiles. As he lifted the mallet to strike, Peter realized he was straight above them.

"Wait a sec—"

The tile popped free. It sang past, narrowly missing Foto's head.

"You idiot!"

"Sorry, I didn't see you there."

"Where did you *think* we were?" Foto said. "You did that on purpose. And clip in, for Christ's sake."

"It was an accident," Jock said. "Calm down. You'll have to move."

They shifted to the side. Jock finished up and had begun to climb down when Peter heard a pop. Jock let out a yelp. A second pop, and with a loud clatter the ladder rocketed down the roof with Jock still attached. At the last second he lunged clear and began to slide down the roof on his belly. After his first cry, he hadn't made a sound. His hands were madly searching for something to grab

hold of, his toes digging into the tiles to slow his descent. Nobody had ever fallen that Peter knew of. Suddenly this seemed not possible but inevitable; Jock was the one chosen.

Ten feet from the edge his body halted. His hand had found something: a rusty spike.

"Help!"

Peter unclipped and scrambled down to the lowest cleat. Gripping a bracket, he leaned out. "Take my hand."

The boy was frozen with terror. His right hand was clutching the spike, his left gripping the edge of a tile. Every inch of him was pressed to the surface.

"If I move I'll fall."

"No, you won't."

Far below, people had stopped on the street to look.

"Foto, toss me my safety line," Peter said.

"It won't reach. I'll have to reset the anchor."

The spike was bending under Jock's weight. "Oh God, I'm slipping!"

"Stop squirming. Foto, hurry up with that rope."

Down it came. Peter had no time to clip in; the boy was about to fall. As Foto pulled the line taut through the block, Peter wrapped it around his forearm and lunged toward Jock. The spike broke loose; Jock began to slide.

"I've got you!" Peter yelled. "Hold on!"

Peter had him by the wrist. Jock's feet were inches from the edge.

"Find something to grip," Peter said.

"There's nothing!"

Peter didn't know how much longer he could hold him. "Foto, can you pull us up?"

"You're too heavy!"

"Tie it off and get down here with some brackets."

A small crowd had gathered on the street. Many were pointing upward. The distance to the ground had enlarged, becoming an infinite space that would swallow them whole. A few seconds passed; then Foto was moving across the cleat above them.

"What do you want me to do?"

Peter said, "Jock, there's a small lip at the edge just below you. Try to find it with your feet."

"It's not there!"

"Yes, it is — I'm looking right at it."

A moment later, Jock said, "Okay, got it."

"Take a deep breath, okay? I'm going to have to let you go for a second."

Jock tightened his grip on Peter's wrist. "Are you kidding me?"

"I can't get you up unless I do. Just lie still. I guarantee, the lip will hold you if you don't move."

The man had no choice. Slowly he released his grip.

"Foto, toss me a bracket."

Peter caught it with his free hand, wedged it under a seam in the tiles, removed a nail from his tool belt, and pressed it into the gap until it bit. Three strokes of the mallet drove it home. He set the second nail, then lowered himself a few feet.

"Toss me another."

"Please," Jock moaned, "hurry."

"Deep breaths. This will all be over in a minute."

Peter set three more brackets in place. "Okay, carefully reach up and to your left. Got it?"

Jock's hand gripped the bracket. "Yeah. Jesus."

"Now pull yourself up to the next one. Take your time — there's no hurry."

Bracket by bracket, Jock ascended. Peter fol-

131

lowed him up. Jock was sitting on the cleat, gulping water from a canteen. Peter crouched beside him.

"Okay?"

Jock nodded vaguely. His face was pale, his hands trembling.

"Just take a minute," Peter said.

"Hell, take the whole day," said Foto. "Take the rest of your life."

Jock was staring into space. Though he wasn't really seeing anything, Peter guessed.

"Try to relax," Peter said.

Jock glanced down at Peter's harness. "You weren't clipped in?"

"There wasn't time."

"So you just . . . did all that. Holding the rope."

"It worked, didn't it?"

Jock looked away. "I thought I was dead for sure."

"You know what gets me?" Foto said. "That little shit didn't even thank you."

They'd knocked off early; the two of them were sitting on the front steps, passing a flask. They'd seen the last of Jock; he'd turned in his tool belt and walked off.

"That was smart, with the brackets," Foto continued. "I wouldn't have thought of that."

"You might have. I just got there first."

"That kid is fucking lucky, is all I have to say. And look at you, not even rattled."

It was true: he'd felt invincible, his mind perfectly focused, his thoughts clear as ice. In fact, there was no lip at the edge of the roof; the surface was perfectly smooth. *I make you see the game the way I need you to.*

132

Foto capped the flask and got to his feet. "So I guess I'll see you tomorrow."

"Actually, I think that's it for me," Peter said.

Foto stared at him, then gave a quiet chuckle. "Anybody else, I'd figure they were worried about getting killed. You'd probably like it if somebody fell every day so you could catch them. What will you do instead?"

"Somebody's offered me a job. I thought I wasn't interested, but maybe I am."

The man nodded evenly. "Whatever it is, it's got to be more interesting than this. It's true what they say about you." They shook hands. "Good luck to you, Jaxon."

Peter watched him go, then walked to the capitol. As he entered Sanchez's office, she glanced up from her papers.

"Mr. Jaxon. That was fast. I thought I was going to have to work a little harder."

"Two conditions. Actually, three."

"The first is your son, of course. I've given you my word. What else?"

"I want direct access to you. No middlemen."

"What about Chase? The man's my chief of staff."

"Just you."

She thought only a moment. "If that's what it takes. What's the third?"

"Don't make me wear a necktie."

The sun had just set when Michael knocked on the door of Greer's cabin. There was no light inside, no sound. *Well, I've walked too long to wait out here,* he thought. *I'm sure Lucius won't mind.*

He put his bag on the floor and lit the lamp. He looked around. Greer's pictures: How many were

133

there? Fifty? A hundred? He stepped closer. Yes, his memory had not betrayed him. Some were hasty sketches; others had obviously required hours of focused labor. Michael selected one of the paintings, untacked it from the wall, and laid it on the table: a mountainous island, bathed in green, seen from the bow of a ship, which was just visible at the bottom edge. The sky above and behind the island was a deep twilight blue; at its center, at forty-five degrees to the horizon, was a constellation of five stars.

The door flew open. Greer stood at the threshold, pointing a rifle at Michael's head.

"Flyers, put that *down*," Michael said.

Greer lowered the gun. "It's not loaded anyway."

"Good to know." Michael tapped the paper with his finger. "Remember when I said you should tell me about these?"

Greer nodded.

"Now would be the time."

The constellation was the Southern Cross — the most distinctive feature of the night sky south of the equator.

Michael showed Greer the newspaper, which the man read without reaction, as if its contents came as no surprise to him; he described the *Bergensfjord* and the bodies he'd found; he read the captain's letter aloud, the first time he had done this. It felt very different to speak the words, as if he were not overhearing a conversation but enacting it. For the first time, he glimpsed what the man had intended by writing a letter that could never be sent; it imparted a kind of permanence to the words and the emotions they contained. Not a letter but an epitaph.

134

Michael saved the data from the *Bergensfjord*'s navigational computer for last. The ship's destination had been a region of the South Pacific roughly halfway between northern New Zealand and the Cook Islands; Michael used the atlas to show Greer. When the ship's engines had failed, they had been fifteen hundred miles north-northeast of their goal, traveling in the equatorial currents.

"So how did it end up in Galveston?" Greer asked.

"It shouldn't have. It should have sunk, just like the captain said."

"Yet it didn't."

Michael frowned. "It's possible the currents could have pushed it here. I don't really know much about it. I'll tell you one thing it means. There's no barrier and never was."

Lucius looked at the newspaper again. He pointed midway down the page. "This here, about the virus having an avian source —"

"Birds."

"I'm familiar with the word, Michael. Does it mean the virus could still be out there?"

"If they're carriers, it might be. Sounds like the people in charge never figured it out, though."

" 'In rare instances,' " Greer read aloud, " 'victims of the illness have exhibited the transformative effects of the North American strain, including a marked increase in aggressiveness, but whether any of these individuals have survived past the thirty-six-hour threshold is not known.' "

"That got my attention, too."

"Are they talking about virals?"

"If so, they're a different strain."

"Meaning they could still be alive. Killing the

135

Twelve wouldn't have affected them."

Michael didn't say anything.

"Good God."

"You want to know what's funny?" Michael said. "Maybe *funny*'s not the right word. The world quarantined us and left us to die. In the end, it's the only reason we're still here."

Greer rose from the table and fetched a whiskey bottle from the shelf. He poured two glasses, handed one to Michael, and sipped. Michael did the same.

"Think about it, Lucius. That ship traveled halfway around the world, never bumping into anything, never running aground, never down-flooding in a storm. Somehow it manages to make its way perfectly intact, into Galveston Bay, right under our noses. What are the odds?"

"Not good, I'd say."

"So you tell me what it's doing here. You're the one who drew those pictures."

Greer poured more into his glass but didn't drink it. He was silent for a moment, then said, "It's what I saw."

"What do you mean, 'saw'?"

"It's difficult to explain."

"None of this is easy, Lucius."

Greer was staring into his glass, turning it around on the tabletop. "I was in the desert. Don't ask me what I was doing there — it's a long story. I hadn't had anything to eat or drink for days. Something happened to me in the night. I'm not really sure what to call it. I guess it was a dream, though it was stronger than that, more real."

"This image, you mean. The island, the five stars."

Lucius nodded. "I was on a ship. I could feel it

136

moving under me. I could hear the waves, smell the salt."

"Was it the *Bergensfjord*?"

He shook his head. "All I know is, it was big."

"Were you alone?"

"There may have been other people there, but I couldn't see them. I couldn't turn around." Greer looked at him pointedly. "Michael, are you thinking what I think you're thinking?"

"That depends."

"That the ship is meant for us. That we're supposed to go to the island."

"How else can you explain it?"

"I can't." He frowned skeptically. "This isn't at all like you. To put so much faith in a picture drawn by a crazy man."

For a moment, neither man spoke. Michael sipped his whiskey.

"This ship," Greer said. "Will it float?"

"I don't know how much damage there is below the waterline. The lower decks are flooded, but the engine compartment's dry."

"Can you fix it?"

"Maybe, but it'd take an army. And lots of money, which we don't have."

Greer drummed his fingers on the table. "There are ways around that. Assuming we had the manpower, how long would we need?"

"Years. Hell, maybe decades. We'd have to drain her, build a drydock, float her in. And that's just for starters. The damn thing's six hundred feet long."

"But it could be done."

"In theory."

Michael studied his friend's face. They had yet to touch on the missing piece, the one question

from which all the rest descended.

"So how much time do you think we have?" Michael asked.

"Until what?"

"Until the virals come back."

Greer didn't answer right away. "I'm not sure."

"But they *are* coming."

Greer looked up. Michael saw relief in the man's eyes; he had been alone with this for too long. "Tell me, how did you figure it out?"

"It's the only thing that makes sense. The question is, how did *you?*"

Greer drained his whiskey, poured another, and drank that, too. Michael waited.

"I'm going to tell you something, Michael, and you can never tell anybody what you know. Not Sara, not Hollis, not Peter. *Especially* not Peter."

"Why him?"

"I don't make the rules, I'm sorry. I need your word on this."

"You have it."

Greer drew a long breath and let the air out slowly. "I know the virals are coming back, Michael," he said, "because Amy told me."

13

Rain was falling as Alicia approached the city. Seen from above in the soft morning light, the river was as she'd imagined it: wide, dark, ceaselessly flowing. Beyond it rose the spires of the city, dense as a forest. Ruined piers jutted from the banks; wrecks of ships were washed against the shoals. In a century, the sea had risen. Parts of the island's southern tip looked submerged, water lapping against the sides of the buildings.

She picked her way north, hopscotching through the detritus, searching for a way across. The rain stopped, started, stopped again. It was late afternoon when she reached the bridge: two massive struts, like giant twins, holding the decks aloft with cables slung over their shoulders. The thought of crossing it filled Alicia with a profound anxiety she dared not show, but Soldier sensed it anyway. The smallest notch of reluctance in his gait: *This again?*

Yes, she thought. This.

She veered inland and located the ramp. Barricades, gun emplacements, military vehicles stripped bare by a century of weather, some overturned or lying on their sides: there had been a battle here. The upper deck was choked with the carcasses of automobiles, painted white by the droppings of birds. Alicia dismounted and led Soldier through the wreckage. With every step her apprehension increased. The feeling was automatic, like an allergy, a sneeze barely held in abeyance. She kept her eyes forward, putting one foot in front of the next.

About mid-span they came to a place where the roadway had collapsed. Cars lay in a twisted heap on the deck below. A narrow ledge along the guardrail, four feet wide at the most, presented the only viable pathway.

"No big deal," Alicia said to Soldier. "Nothing to it."

The height was irrelevant; it was the water she feared. Beyond the edge lay a swallowing maw of death. Step by step, gelid with dread, she led Soldier across. How strange, she thought, to fear nothing but this.

The sun was behind them when they reached

the far side. A second ramp guided them to street level, into an area of warehouses and factories. She remounted Soldier and headed south, along the backbone of the island. The numbered streets ticked down. Eventually the factories gave way to blocks of apartments and brownstones, interspersed with vacant lots, some barren, others like miniature jungles. In some places the streets were flooded, dirty river water bubbling up through the manholes. Never had Alicia been in such a place; the island's sheer density astounded her. She was aware of the tiniest sounds and movements: pigeons cooing, rats scurrying, water dripping down the walls of the buildings' interiors. The acrid spore-smell of mold. The funk of rot. The stench of the city itself, death's temple.

Evening came on. Bats flittered in the sky. She was on Lenox Avenue, in the 110s, when a wall of vegetation rose in her path. At the heart of the abandoned city, a woodland had taken root, flowering to massive dimensions. At its edge she brought Soldier to a halt and tuned her thoughts to the trees; when the virals came, they came from above. It wasn't her they'd want, of course; Alicia was one of them. But there was Soldier to consider. She allowed a few minutes to go by, and when she was satisfied that they would pass in safety, tapped her heels to his flanks.

"Let's go."

Just like that, the city vanished. They could have been in the mightiest of ancient forests. Night had fallen in full, lit by a waning rind of moon. They came to a wide field of feathered grass tall enough to swish against her thighs; then the trees again staked their claim upon the land.

They emerged up a flight of stone steps onto

Fifty-ninth Street. Here the buildings had names. Helmsley Park Lane. Essex House. The Ritz-Carlton. The Plaza. She jogged east to Madison Avenue and headed south again. The buildings grew taller, towering above the roadway; the street numbers continued their relentless decline. Fifty-sixth. Fifty-first. Forty-eighth. Forty-third.

Forty-second.

She dismounted. The building was like a fortress, smaller than the great towers that surrounded it but with a royal aspect. A castle, fit for a king. High, arched windows gazed darkly upon the street; along the roofline, at the center of the facade, a stone figure stood with his arms outstretched in welcome. Beneath this, etched into the building's face, chiseled in moonlight, were the words GRAND CENTRAL TERMINAL.

Alicia, I'm here. Lish, I'm so glad that you have come.

She could feel her brothers and sisters plainly now. They were everywhere beneath her, a vast repository curled in slumber in the bowels of the city. Did they sense her presence also? There was, Alicia realized, a single hour that all the days since your birth pointed you toward. What you thought was a maze of choices, all the possibilities of what your life might become, was, in fact, a series of steps you took along a road, and when you reached your destination and looked back, only one path — the one chosen for you — was visible.

She clipped a rope to Soldier's bridle. Two nights before, camped on the outskirts of Newark, she'd prepared a pine-knot torch. Now, crouched on the sidewalk, she shaved a pile of tinder, ignited it with her firesteel, and dipped the end of the torch in the flames until the pitch began to burn.

She rose, holding it aloft. The torch, which would burn for hours, gave off a smoky orange light. She cinched her bandoliers tight to her chest, then reached her right hand over the opposite shoulder to withdraw her sword from its sheath. Bright-edged, hard-tipped, the cords at the handle worn from hours of practice, the object had no symbolic meaning for her; it was simply a tool. She swooped it slowly back and forth, feeling its power meld with her own. Soldier was watching her. When the moment felt right, Alicia resheathed her weapon and opened the door to the terminal.

"It's time."

She led him inside. Broken glass crunched underfoot; she heard the squeaks of rats. Ten feet past the door, two options: straight ahead, down a sloping hallway to the station's lower level, or left, through an arched portal.

She went left.

Space expanded around her. She was in the main room of the station, but it did not seem like a station — more like a church. A place where vast crowds gathered to commune with one another in the company of some higher presence. Shafts of moonlight pulsed from the high windows onto the floor, spreading like a pale yellow liquid. The silence was intense; she could hear the blood swishing in her ears. Looking up, she saw what she thought was the sky until she realized it was a painting. Stars were strewn across the ceiling, and in their midst were figures — a bull, a ram, a man pouring water from a pitcher.

"Alicia. Hello."

She startled. It was his voice. An audible, distinctly human-sounding voice.

"I'm over here."

The sound came from the far end of the room. Alicia moved toward it, guiding Soldier beside her. Ahead she saw a structure. It looked like a small house. Positioned on top, like a crown, was a large, four-faced clock. As she approached, the clock was the first thing to capture the glow of her torch, not so much reflecting the light as absorbing it, causing its faces to shine with an orange luster.

"Up here, Lish."

A broad flight of stairs ascended to a balcony. She released the rope and placed her hand against Soldier's neck. His coat was damp with sweat. She pressed her palm against it with a calming gesture: *Wait here.*

"Don't worry, your friend will be safe. He's a magnificent companion, Lish. More than I even imagined. Every inch a soldier, like you. Like my Lish."

She ascended the stairs, making no effort to conceal herself — there was no point. What form of creature awaited her? The voice was human, meager in a way, but the body surely wouldn't be. He would be a giant, a monster of gargantuan dimensions, a titan of his race.

She reached the top. To her right was a bar with stools, straight ahead an area of tables, some overturned, others still set with china and silverware.

Sitting at one of the tables was a man.

Was it a trick? Had he done something to her mind? He was sitting at ease, his hands folded on his lap, wearing a dark suit, a white shirt, collar undone at his throat. Sandy hair, almost red, with a sharp widow's peak; a slight sag around the jowls; eyes with a certain indefinable intensity.

143

Suddenly nothing around her seemed real. It was all a gigantic joke. He was like any man, a figure in a crowd, no one a person would notice.

"Does my appearance surprise you?" he asked. "Perhaps I should have warned you."

His voice aroused her to action. She dropped the torch and the sword came out as she strode toward him; she swung it away from her body, cocked her hip, transferring energy to the large muscle groups — shoulders, pelvis, legs — and brought it around, halting its flight just inches from his neck.

"What the hell are you?"

Not a muscle had flinched. Even his face was relaxed. "What do I look like?"

"You're not human. You can't be."

"You might ask yourself the same thing. What it means, to be human." He tipped his head toward her blade. "If you're going to use that, I suggest you get on with it."

"Is that what you want?"

He angled his face toward the ceiling. At the corners of his mouth, dagger-like incisors revealed themselves. They were the teeth of a predator, and yet the face before her was mild. "I've been waiting here rather a long time, you know. In a hundred years, you get around to thinking about pretty much everything. All the things you did, the people you knew, the mistakes you made. The books you read, the music you listened to, how the sun felt, the rain. It's all still there inside you. But it's not enough, is it? That's the thing. The past is never enough."

The sword was still poised at his neck. How simple he was making this, how easy. He was looking at her with an expression of perfect calm. One

144

swift blow, and she would be free.

"We're two of a kind, you see." His voice was placid, almost teacherly. "So much regret. So many things lost."

Why hadn't she done it? Why had she failed to strike? A strange immobility had taken hold — not a physical paralysis; more a dimming of her will.

"I have no doubt you're more than capable." He touched a spot on his neck. "Right about here, I think. That should do the trick."

Something was wrong. Something was terribly wrong. All she had to do was pull back the sword and let fly, yet she could not make herself do it.

"You can't, can you?" He frowned; his tone was almost regretful. "Patricide goes against the grain after all."

"I killed Martínez. I watched him die."

"Yes, but you did not belong to him, Lish. You belong to me. The viral that bit you was one of mine. Amy is but one part of you; I am the other. You could no more use that sword on me than you could on her. I'm surprised you hadn't figured that out."

She felt the truth of his words. The sword, the sword; she could not move the sword.

"But I don't think you came to kill me. I don't think that's why you're here at all. I can see it. You have questions. There are things you want to know."

She answered through gritted teeth: "I don't want anything from you."

"No? Then I'll ask you something instead. Tell me, Alicia, what did being human ever get you?"

She felt disoriented; none of this made sense.

"It's a simple question, really. Most things are,

145

in the end."

"I had friends," she said, and heard the shakiness in her voice. "People who loved me."

"Did they? Is that why you left them?"

"You don't know what you're talking about."

"I think I do. Your mind is an open book to me. Peter, Michael, Sara, Hollis, Greer. And Amy. The great and powerful Amy. I know all about them. Even the boy, Hightop, who died in your arms. You promised him you would keep him safe. But in the end you could not save him."

Her being was dissolving; the sword was like an anvil in her hand, incomparably dense.

"What would your friends say to you now? I'll answer for you. They would call you a monster. They would hound you from their midst, if they didn't kill you first."

"Shut up, goddamnit."

"You're not one of them. You never have been, not since the day the Colonel took you outside the walls and left you there. You sat there under the trees and cried all night. Isn't that so?"

How could he know these things?

"Did he comfort you, Alicia? Did he tell you he was sorry? You were just a little girl, and he left you all alone. You have always been . . . alone."

The last of her resolve was failing; it was all she could do to hold the sword aloft.

"I know, because I know *you,* Alicia Donadio. I know your secret heart. Don't you see? That's why you've come to me. I'm the only one who does."

"Please," she begged. "Please stop talking."

"Tell me. What did you name her?"

She was undone; she had nothing left. Whoever she'd been, or wanted to be, she felt that person leaving her.

146

"Tell me, Lish. Tell me your daughter's name."

"Rose." The word came out with a choking sound. "I named her Rose."

She had begun to sob. At some uncharted distance, the sword fell clattering to the floor. The man had risen and put his arms around her, drawing her into a warm embrace. She made no resistance, having none to offer. She cried and cried. Her little girl. Her Rose.

"That's why you came here, isn't it?" His voice was soft, close to her ear. "That's what this place is for. You came to speak your daughter's name."

She nodded against him. She heard herself say, "Yes."

"Oh, my Alicia. My Lish. Do you know where you are? All your journeys are ended. What is home but a place where you are truly known? Say it with me. 'I've come home.' "

A flicker of resistance; then she let it go. "I've come home."

" 'And I am never leaving here.' "

How easy it suddenly was. "And I am never leaving here."

A moment passed; he stepped away. Through her tears, she looked at his kind face, so full of understanding. He pulled a chair from the table.

"Now, sit with me," he said. "We have all the time in the world. Sit with me, and I will tell you everything."

■ ■ ■ ■

II
THE LOVER

■ ■ ■ ■

28–3 B.V.
(1989–2014)

from Morn
To Noon he fell, from Noon to dewy Eve,
A Summers day; and with the setting Sun
Dropped from the Zenith like a falling Star.
— MILTON, *Paradise Lost*

14

Behind every great hatred is a love story.

For I am a man who has known and tasted love. I say "a man" because that is how I know myself. Look at me, and what do you see? Do I not take the form of a man? Do I not feel as you do, suffer as you do, love as you do, mourn as you do? What is the essence of a man, if not these things? In life I was a scientist, called Fanning. Fanning, Timothy J., holder of the Eloise Armstrong Distinguished Chair in Biochemical Sciences, Columbia University. I was known and respected, a figure of my times. My opinions were sought on many subjects; I walked the hallways of my profession with my head held high. I was a man of connections. I shook hands, kissed cheeks, made friends, took lovers. Fortune and treasure flowed my way; I supped at the flower of the modern world. City apartments, country houses, sleek automobiles, good wine: all of these were things I had. I dined in fine restaurants, slept in upscale hotels; my passport was fat with visas. Thrice I wooed and thrice I wed, and although these unions came to naught, each was, in its final measure, no matter of regret. I worked and rested, danced and wept, hoped and remembered — even, from time to

time, prayed. I lived, in sum, a life.

Then, in a jungle in Bolivia, I died.

You will know me as Zero. Such is the name that history has bestowed upon me. Zero the Destroyer, Great Devourer of the World. That this history shall never be written is a circumstance of ontological debate. What becomes of the past when there is no man to record it? I died and then was brought to life, the oldest tale there is. I arose from the dead, and what did I behold? I was in a room of the bluest light — pure blue, cerulean blue, the blue the sky would be if it were married to the sea. My arms, legs, even my head were bound; I was a captive in that place. Scattered images lit my mind, flashes of light and color that refused to gather into meaning. My body was humming. That is the only word. I was to learn that I had just emerged from the final stages of my transformation. I had yet to see my body, being inside it.

Tim, can you hear me?

A voice, coming from everywhere and nowhere. Was I dead? Was this the voice of God, addressing me? Perhaps the life I'd lived had been not so worthy, and things had gone the other way.

Tim, if you can hear me, lift a hand.

This did not seem too much for God, any god, to ask.

That's it. Now the other one. Excellent. Well done, Tim.

You know this voice, I said to myself. You are not dead; it is the voice of a human being, like you. A man who calls you by name, who says "well done."

That's it. Just breathe. You're doing fine.

The nature of the situation was becoming clear.

152

I had been ill in some manner. Perhaps I had suffered seizures; that would explain the restraints. I could not yet recall the circumstances, how I had come to be in this place. The voice was the key. If I could identify its owner, all would be revealed.

I'm going to undo the straps now, okay?

I felt a release of pressure; triggered by some remote mechanism, my bindings had surrendered their hold.

Can you sit up, Tim? Can you do that for me?

It was also true that, whatever my ailment was, the worst had passed. I did not feel ill — quite the contrary. The humming sensation, which originated in my chest, had enlarged to an orchestral, whole-body vibrato, as if all the molecules of my anatomy were playing a single note. The sensation was deeply, almost sexually pleasurable. My loins, the tips of my toes, even the roots of my hair — never had I experienced anything so exquisite.

A second voice, deeper than the first: *Dr. Fanning, I'm Colonel Sykes.*

Sykes. Did I know a man named Sykes?

Can you hear us? Do you know where you are?

A hole had opened inside me. Not a hole: a maw. I was hungry. Deeply, madly hungry. Mine was the appetite not of a human being but of an animal. A hunger of claws and teeth, of burrowing in, of soft flesh beneath the jaws and hot juices exploding upon the palate.

Tim, you've got us pretty worried in here. Talk to me, buddy.

And just like that the gates of memory opened, releasing a flood. The rain forest, with its steamy air and dense green canopy full of hooting animals; the stickiness of my skin and the omnipresent swarm of insects around my face; the soldiers,

153

scanning the trees with their rifles as we walked, their faces streaked with jungle paint; the statues, manlike figures of monstrous form, warning us away even as they called us forward, summoning us deeper into the heart of this vile place; the bats.

They'd come at night, swarming our encampment. Bats by the hundreds, the thousands, the ten thousands, a flapping multitude. They blotted out the heavens. They took the sky by storm. The gates of hell had opened and this was its disgorgement, its black vomitus. They seemed not to fly but to swim, moving in organized waves, like a school of airborne fish. They fell upon us, all wings and teeth and vicious little squeaks of joy. I remembered the shots, the screams. I was in a place of blue light and a voice that knew my name but in my mind I was running for the river. I saw a woman, writhing on the banks. Her name was Claudia; she was one of us. The bats had covered her like a cloak. Imagine it, the horror. Almost no part of her was visible. She twitched in a demonic dance of agony. In truth, my first instinct was to do nothing. I did not possess the heart of a hero. Yet sometimes we discover things about ourselves we never knew. I took two great leaps and tackled her, sending the two of us plunging into the fetid jungle water. I felt the hot stab of the bats' teeth in the flesh of my arms and neck. The water boiled with blood. Such was their fury that even the water did not deter them; they would feed upon us even as they drowned. I locked Claudia's neck in my elbow and dove down, though I knew this would come to nothing; the woman was already dead.

I remembered all these things, and then one more. I remembered a man's face. It hovered

above me, framed by jungle sky. I was insensate, burning with fever. The air around me throbbed with the din of the helicopter's blades. The man was yelling something. I tried to focus on his mouth. *It was alive,* he was saying — my friend, Jonas Lear, was saying — *it was alive, it was alive, it was alive . . .*

I lifted my head and looked. The room was barren, like a cell. On the wall across from me, a wide, dark window showed my reflection.

I saw what I'd become.

I did not rise. I launched. I rocketed across the room and hit the window with a thud. Behind the glass, the two men lurched backward. Jonas and the second one, Sykes. Their eyes were wide with fear. I pounded. I roared. I opened my jaws to display my teeth so they would know the measure of my rage. I wanted to kill them. No, not kill. "Kill" is too dull a word for that which I desired. I wanted to annihilate them. I wanted to tear them limb from limb. I wanted to crack their bones and bury my face in the wet remains. I wanted to reach inside their chests and yank out their hearts and devour the bloody meat as the last stray current twitched the muscle and watch their faces as they died. They were yelling, screaming. I was not what they'd bargained for. The glass was bowing, shuddering beneath my blows.

A blast of white-hot brightness engulfed the room. I felt as if I'd been shot by a hundred arrows. I stumbled backward and fell curling to the floor. A clattering of gears above, and with a bang the bars fell, sealing me away.

Tim, I'm sorry. This was never my intention. Forgive me . . .

Perhaps he was. It made no difference. Even

155

then, huddled in agony, I knew that their advantage was temporary; it held no weight. The walls of my prison could not help but eventually yield to my power. I was the dark flower of mankind, ordained since time's beginning to destroy a world that had no God to love it.

From one, we became Twelve. That, too, is a matter of record. From my blood the ancient seed was taken and passed into others. I came to know these men. At first, they alarmed me. Their human lives had been very different from my own. They possessed no conscience, no pity, no philosophy. They were like brute animals, their bestial hearts full of the blackest of deeds. That such men existed I had long understood, but evil, to be truly comprehended, must be felt, experienced. One must enter into it, as into a lightless cave. One by one they came into my mind, and I into theirs. Babcock was the first. What terrible dreams he possessed — though they were, in truth, no worse than my own. The others followed in due course, each added to the fold. Morrison and Chávez. Baffes and Turrell. Winston and Sosa, Echols and Lambright, Reinhardt and Martínez, vilest of all. Even Carter, whose memories of suffering blew upon the dying embers of compassion in my heart. Over time, in the company of these troubled souls, I underwent an expanding sense of mission. They were my heirs, my acolytes; alone among them, I possessed the capacity to lead. They did not despise the world, as I did; to such men, the world is nothing, as everything is nothing. Their appetites knew no moderation; unguided, they would bring down swift and total destruction upon us all. They were mine to command, but

how to make them follow?

What they needed was a god.

Nine and one, I commanded them, in my best god voice. *Nine are yours but one is mine, as you are mine. Into the tenth shall be planted the seed so that we will be Many, millions-fold.*

A reasonable person might ask, Why did you do it? If I possessed the power to lead them, surely I could have put a stop to everything. The rage was part of it, yes. All that I loved had been taken from me, and that which I did not love as well, which was my human life. So, too, did the biological imperatives of my remanufactured self; could you ask a hungry lion to ignore the bounty of the veldt? I do not note these things to seek the pardon of any person, because my actions are unpardonable, nor to say I'm sorry, although I am. (Does that surprise you to hear? That Timothy Fanning, called Zero, is sorry? It's true: I'm sorry about everything.) I merely wish to set the stage, to place my mental contours in their proper context. What did I desire? To make the world a wasteland; to bring upon it the mirrored image of my wretched self; to punish Lear, my friend, my enemy, who believed he could save a world that was not savable, that never deserved saving in the first place.

Such was my wrath in those early days. Yet I could not ignore the metaphysical aspects of my condition indefinitely. As I boy, I spoke often to the Almighty. My prayers were shallow and childish, as if I were speaking to Santa Claus: spaghetti for dinner, a new bike at my birthday, a day of snow and no school. "If, Lord, in your infinite mercy, it would not be too much trouble . . ." How ironic! We are born faithful and afraid, when

it should be the opposite; it is life that teaches us how much we stand to lose. As a grown man, I mislaid the impulse, like many people. I would not say I was a nonbeliever; rather, that I gave little if any thought to celestial concerns. It did not seem to me that God, whoever he was, would be the sort of god to take an interest in the minutiae of human affairs, or that this fact released us from the duty to go about our lives in a spirit of decency to others. It is true that the events of my life brought me into a state of nihilistic despair, yet even in the darkest hours of my human life — the hours that, to this day, I dwell in — I blamed no one but myself.

But as love turns to grief, and grief becomes anger, so must anger yield to thought, in order to know itself. My symbolic properties were inarguable. Made by science, I was a perfect industrial product, the very embodiment of mankind's indefatigable faith in itself. Since our first, furry ancestor scraped flint on stone and banished night with fire, we have climbed heavenward on a ladder made of our own arrogance. But was that all? Was I the final proof that humanity dwelled in an unwatched cosmos of no purpose, or was I something more?

Thus did I contemplate my existence. In due course, these ruminations led me to but one conclusion. I had been made for a purpose. I was not the author of destruction; I was its instrument, forged in heaven's workshop by a god of horrors.

What could I do but play the part?

As to my present, more human-seeming incarnation: all I can say is that Jonas was right about one

thing after all, though the bastard never knew it. The events I am about to describe occurred just a few days after my emancipation, in a certain benighted prairie hamlet by the name (I was later to learn) of Sewanee, Kansas. To this day my recollections of that early period are drowned in joy. What soaring liberty! What bountiful slaking of my appetites! The world of night seemed a glorious banquet to my senses, an infinite buffet. Yet I moved with a certain caution. No roadhouse-tavern massacres. No families slaughtered whole in their beds. No fast-food emporia painted red, patrons strewn willy-nilly in bloody dismemberment. These things would come eventually; but for the time being, I sought to leave a lighter footprint. Each night, as I made my way east, I dined upon only a handful, and only in situations in which I could do so at my ease, and swiftly dispose of the remains.

Thus my heart sang an aria of delight at the sight of the truck.

The vehicle, a preposterously bloated and over-appointed quad cab pickup — smokestacks, dual-lies, lights on the roll bar, Confederate-flag decal on the bumper — was parked nose-in at the lip of a flooded quarry. Its isolation was ideal, as was the distracted state of its occupants: a man and a woman in full passionate flagrante, enjoying each other as much as I was about to enjoy them. For a time, I merely watched. My gaze was not carnal; rather, I observed with the curiosity of the scientist. Why this crummy place to do the deed? Why the awkward confines of a pickup (the man was practically crushing his beloved against the dashboard) to unleash their animal splendor? Surely there were enough beds in the world to go

159

around. They were not young, far from it — he bald and rather portly, she scrawny and loose-skinned, the two of them a spectacle of aging flesh. What about this place had called out to them? Was it nostalgia? Had they come here when they were young? Was I witnessing a reenacted glory of youth? Then it came to me. They were married. They just weren't married to each other.

I took the woman first. Astride her companion on the wide bench seat, so wildly was she pumping upon his anatomy — fists gripping the head-rest, skirt bunched around her waist and under-pants swinging from a bony ankle, her face angled toward the ceiling like a supplicant — that as I yanked open the door she seemed more irritated than alarmed, as if I had interrupted her in the midst of a particularly important train of thought. This, of course, did not last long, no more than a couple of seconds. It is an interesting truth that the human body, liberated from its head, is in essence a bag of blood with a built-in straw. Holding her headless torso upright, I positioned my mouth around this jetting orifice and gave it a long, muscular suck. I wasn't expecting anything much. It seemed likely that her small-town diet, rich in preservatives, would give her blood a chemical taste. But this turned out not to be the case. The woman was, in fact, delicious. Her blood was a veritable bouquet of complex flavors, like a well-aged wine.

Two more robust sucks and I cast her aside. By this time her associate, pants puddled around his ankles, gleaming penis in rapid deflation, had gathered the wherewithal to shimmy toward the driver's side of the cab, where he was frantically attempting to isolate the truck's key from a ring

of them. The ring was enormous. It was positively janitorial. Fingers trembling, he jammed one key into the slot and then another, all to no avail, muttering a chain of "oh God"s and "holy fuck"s that were only a lightly retooled rendition of the ecstatic sounds and filthy encouragements he'd been breathing into his companion's ear mere seconds ago.

The comedy was exquisite. Speaking frankly, I couldn't get enough of it.

Which was my grand mistake. Had I killed him more quickly, not pausing to savor this risible display, the world we know would be a different place. As it was, my delay gave him time to locate the correct key, shove it into the ignition, turn the engine over, and reach for the gearshift before I shot into the cab, grabbed his head, tipped it to the side, and crushed his windpipe under my jaws with a gristly crunch. So enraptured was I with the bloody feast of my hapless victim that I failed to notice what was happening — that he had put the truck in gear.

Our species' aversion to water is well known; water is death to us. We sink like stones, our bodies lacking the buoyancy of adipose tissue. Of my plunge into the quarry I possess only a fractured recollection. The truck's slow progress to the lip of the abyss; the snatch of gravity and the inevitable plunge; water all around me, a cocoon of cold death, engulfing my eyes and nose and lungs. From small mistakes come great catastrophes; invincible in most other aspects, I had found the quickest way to die. As the truck touched down with a soft thump upon the quarry's watery floor, I extricated myself from the cab and began to crawl along the bottom. Even in

161

my panicked state, the irony was not lost on me. Subject Zero, World Destroyer, scuttling like a crab! My only hope was to feel my way to the edge of the pit and scale my way to freedom. Time was my enemy; I had but one bottled breath with which to save myself. A wall of rock met my desperate grasp; I began to climb. Hand over hand I made my ascent. My vision swirled with darkness, the end was closing in . . .

How I came in due course to find myself on hands and knees — pink-fleshed, inarguably human-looking hands and knees — whilst gagging out great volumes of boggy vomitus is a question I shall leave to the theologians. For die I surely did; the body remembers these things. Having freed myself from the quarry's waters, I had yet succumbed and for some period of time lain as a drowned corpse upon the rocks, only to be shot back into existence.

Death's doorway, it seemed, was not marked EXIT ONLY after all.

The last of the quarry's waters expelled, I managed, in a state of dazed astonishment, to rise. Where was I? When was I? *What* was I? Such was my disorientation that it seemed that I might have dreamed it all — then, conversely, that I was dreaming *this*. I held up a hand before the moon. It was, in every visible aspect, the hand of a human being — the hand of Timothy Fanning, holder of the Eloise Armstrong Chair, et cetera. I looked down upon the rest of me; with tremulous digits I probed my face, my chest and stomach, my pale legs; naked by moonlight, I investigated each feature of my physical person like a blind man reading braille.

I'll be goddamned, I thought.

I had come to rest on a rocky shelf jutting from the quarry wall; a narrow switchback led me to the top, where I emerged into an area of rusted machinery half-buried by weeds. The hour was unknown to me. Save for the moon, no lights burned anywhere. The landscape was one of such uninhabited desolation the world might have ended already.

The quarry's waters would conceal my second victim, but there was the woman to consider; the last thing I wanted was a police manhunt to complicate matters. I circled the quarry to the parking area. The sight of her aroused no remorse, just the sort of perfunctory, quickly dispatched pity one might feel reading a newspaper account of some distant catastrophe over one's second slice of morning toast. Two distant splashes — body, head — and into the watery deep she went.

None of which did anything to solve the problem of being a naked, full-grown man at large in an unknown countryside. I needed clothes, shelter, a story. Also, a certain mental agitation, like an inaudible siren in my brain, told me that, should daybreak find me in the open, nothing happy would ensue.

The main highway was too risky. I headed for the woods, hoping that I might eventually come to some lesser-traveled thoroughfare. At length I emerged into a landscape of freshly planted fields bisected by a dirt road. In the distance I saw a light and headed toward it. A small, rather dilapidated one-story house of nondescript design, little more than a box in which to store a human life: the light I'd seen was a lamp in one of the two front windows. There was no car in the driveway, suggesting that the house was unoc-

cupied, the light left burning in anticipation of its owner's return.

The door obediently opened onto a living room of particleboard furniture, country-themed bric-a-brac, and a television the size of a Jumbotron. A quick survey of the interior — four rooms and a kitchen — confirmed my impression that no one was home. My inspection further revealed that the occupant was a woman, had attended nursing school at Wichita State, was in her late forties, possessed a soft, moonlike face and gray hair she didn't do much with, wore a size twenty, was frequently photographed in a state of rosy-cheeked inebriation in ethnic-themed restaurants (wearing a plastic lei, flirting shamelessly with the mariachis, holding up a flaming fondue spike), and that she lived alone. From her wardrobe I selected the most neutral things I could find — a pair of sweatpants, voluminous on my midsized masculine frame, a hooded sweatshirt, likewise huge, and a pair of flip-flops — and entered the bathroom.

The sight that greeted me in the mirror was not wholly unexpected. By this time it had become apparent to me that the physical act of drowning had not wholly restored me to my human state but wrought upon my person something more like costumery. The virus remained; my death had merely excited it into some new interaction with its host. Many attributes had been preserved. Vision, hearing, smell: all had retained their super-charged acuteness. Though I had yet to put them to a proper test, my limbs — indeed, my entire physical carriage, bones to blood — hummed with bestial strength.

Yet these things hardly prepared me for what I

saw. My complexion was unnaturally pale, almost cadaverous. My hair, which had miraculously grown back, triangulated at my forehead to a comically perfect widow's peak. My eyes possessed the alien rosiness of an albino's. But the final detail was the one that stopped me flat. At first I thought it was a joke. Behind the corners of my upper lip, amidst otherwise ordinary dentition, two white points dripped like icicles — or, more precisely, fangs.

Dracula. Nosferatu. Vampyre. I can barely utter the names without a roll of the eyes. Yet here I was, Jonas Lear's fantasy incarnate, a legend come to life.

The crunch of tires on gravel aroused me; as I emerged from the lavatory, a pair of headlights raked the room. I ducked behind a coat tree just in time for the door to fling open with a gust of spring air. The woman, whose name was Janet Duff — I'd gotten this from the framed diploma hung above the bill-cluttered desk in her bedroom — lumbered inside, wearing the flowered smock, white polyester trousers, and sensible shoes of a nurse coming off the late-night shift. Without missing a beat she deposited her ring of keys on the table by the door, kicked off her shoes, flung her overstuffed purse onto a chair, and made her way back to the kitchen, from whence ensued the sound of an opening refrigerator and the splash and glug of a tumbler being filled. A moment in which to down a soul-soothing quantity of wine (I could smell it: cheap Chablis, from a box, probably), and Nurse Duff returned to the living room bearing a glass the approximate size of a paint can, turned on the giant TV, and plopped down on the sofa, settling into its cushions like a

punctured parade float.

How she had failed to notice me behind the coat tree I couldn't guess, except to say that my new condition had afforded me the ability to stand with a stillness that functioned as a kind of camouflage, rendering me nearly invisible to the casual, world-weary eye. I watched her flick through various programs — a cop drama, the Weather Channel, a prison documentary — until she settled on a reality show about, what else, competitive cupcake making. Her back was to me. Sip by sip, the wine went down. I guessed it wouldn't be long before the alcohol-anesthetized Nurse Duff began to snore. But with dawn's blade sliding toward me, and my various needs pressing down — cash, an automobile, a safe place to wait out the daylight hours — I saw no reason for delay. I emerged from my concealment and stepped behind her.

"Ahem."

I did not kill her immediately. Again, I seek not pardon but patience with my tale. There was data to collect, and for that, Nurse Duff needed to be alive.

A taste and the deed was done. At once, the woman fell into a swoon — eyes rolled back, breath expelled, every inch gone flabbily slack. Like an eager groom I picked her up and carried her to the bedroom, where I lay her on the comforter, then retreated to the bathroom and filled the tub. By the time I returned, the change had commenced. A white froth bubbled from her lips. Her fingers began to twitch, her hands. She began to moan, then grunt, then fell silent as a series of hard spasms shook her frame so violently

166

I thought dear Nurse Duff would snap like a cracker.

Then it happened. The closest visual approximation I can offer is a time-accelerated video of a flower breaking into blossom. With a cartilaginous crunch, her fingers commenced their elongation. Her hair suddenly detached from her skull and fell fanlike onto the pillow. As if doused by acid, her facial features blandified until no trace of personality remained. By this time her convulsions had ceased; her eyes were closed, her face almost peaceful. I sat on the bed beside her, murmuring gentle encouragements. A green light had begun to emanate from her, bathing the room in a nursery-soft glow. Her jaw unhinged; with something like a dog's sneeze, her teeth shot from her mouth like a handful of corn kernels, making way for the barricade of lances that ascended bloodily from her gums.

It was ghastly. It was beautiful.

She opened her eyes. For a long moment, she stared at me. What pathos in that gaze! We are, each of us, a character in our own story; that is how we make sense of our lives. But the woman who had been Nurse Duff — help maid to the sick and suffering, collector of quilts and butter churns, drinker of mai tais, margaritas, and Bahama Mamas; daughter, sister, dreamer, healer, spinster — had become unknown to herself. She was a part of me now, an extension of my will; had I desired, I could have made her hop on one foot while playing an invisible ukulele.

"You don't have to be afraid," I said, taking her hand in mine. "It's all for the best, you'll see."

Once again, I lifted her into my arms. My strength was such that her considerable bulk

seemed toylike. A memory came to me — I had carried a woman like this once. Though the circumstances were very different, she, too, had seemed to weigh almost nothing. The recollection aroused a feeling of tenderness so overwhelming that for a moment I doubted my actions. But there were things to learn, and the duty I was about to perform was, in its backhanded way, a kindness.

I carted Nurse Duff to the bathroom and suspended her body above the tub. Through some lingering womanly instinct, she had looped her arms around my neck; she had yet to notice the water, as was my hope. I was gazing deep into her eyes, beaming thoughts of reassurance. Her trust in me was absolute. What was I to her? Father? Lover? Deliverer? God?

The spell was broken the moment her body touched the water. She began to thrash wildly, fighting to free herself. But her strength was far outmatched by mine. Pressing her by the shoulders, I forced her gargoyle's face below the surface. Her panic and confusion rippled through me. What betrayal! What incomprehensible deceit! Others would have been moved to mercy, yet these feelings only strengthened my resolve. I felt her take the first breath of water. It ricocheted through her like a hiccup. She took a second, then a third, filling her lungs. A last agonal spasm and she was gone.

I stepped back. The first test had been passed; here was the second. Waiting for the restoration of her human form, I counted off the seconds; when nothing happened, I hoisted her from the water and arranged her facedown on the floor, thinking this might encourage the process. But more minutes ticked away, and I was forced to concede

168

that no change was forthcoming; Nurse Duff had permanently departed from this life.

I retreated from the room and sat on the woman's bed to ponder the situation. The only conclusion I could draw was that the transformative effect of death by water was for me alone — that my descendants possessed no such gift of resurrection. Yet why this should be so — why I should be sitting there, looking altogether like the man I'd once been, while she should be lying dead on the bathroom floor like a beached sea monster — was beyond my power to explain. Was I simply a more robust version of our species, being the alpha, the original, the Zero? Or could the difference be one not of body but of mind? That I had wanted to live, while she had not? I considered my emotions. I didn't really have any. I had drowned an innocent woman in a bathtub, yet my feelings were utterly colorless. From the moment I'd sunk my incisors into the soft meat of her neck and taken the first, candy-sweet sip, she had ceased to exist as an entity distinct from myself; rather, she'd been a kind of appendage. Killing her had seemed no more morally noteworthy than trimming a fingernail. So perhaps that was where the difference lay. In the only way that really mattered, Nurse Duff was already dead when I'd shoved her in the water.

Simultaneously, alarm bells were ringing inside me. The light in the room was changing; daybreak, my nemesis, was at hand. I moved hastily through the house, drawing every drape and shade, locking doors both front and back. For the next twelve hours, I was going nowhere.

I awoke in delicious darkness, having discovered

the most refreshing dream-free sleep I had ever known. No knock on the door had aroused me; Nurse Duff's departure from the world had yet to be noticed, though surely this would come. I made my preparations quickly. On America's byways, even a vampire, especially one who wishes to fly beneath the radar, needs money to get by. In a cat-shaped cookie jar, I discovered twenty-three hundred dollars in soft bills, more than enough, and a .38 revolver, which no person in the history of the planet needed less than I.

My plan was to zigzag my way east, avoiding major highways. The journey would take five, perhaps six nights. Nurse Duff's well-worn Corolla, with its detritus of candy wrappers, pop cans, and worthless scratch-offs, would suffice for the time being but would have to be discarded soon; somebody was bound to catch wind of the dead demon in the bathroom and note her missing automobile. I also felt — and looked — ridiculous in the woman's oversized sweat suit and shower shoes; a more suitable costume was in the offing.

Eight hours later I was in southern Missouri, where I commenced the pattern that would organize my life for the duration. Each new daybreak found me safely ensconced in an off-brand motel behind closed drapes, duct-taped cardboard panels, and a Do Not Disturb sign; once night fell, I would set out again and drive without stopping until an hour or two before dawn. In Carbondale, Illinois, I decided to ditch the Corolla. I was also very hungry. I lingered at my hotel past dark, sitting in my parked car, so that I might observe the comings and goings of my fellow travelers and identify an appropriate

provider of nutrition, clothes, and transport. The man I selected was my approximate height and weight; he also seemed, conveniently, inebriated. As he entered his room I pushed in behind him, killed him tidily before he could utter more than a drunken whimper — he tasted rancidly of nicotine and bar-pour whiskey — wrapped his body in the shower curtain to conceal the stench of putrefaction, shoved him in the closet, helped myself to the contents of his wallet and suitcase (Dockers, no-iron sport shirts of obnoxious plaid, six sets of underpants and a pair of "novelty" boxers with the words KISS ME, I'M IRISH stenciled on the crotch), and skedaddled in his plushly appointed, thoroughly American sedan. The business cards in his wallet identified him as a regional sales manager for a manufacturer of industrial air-circulation equipment. I might as well have been him.

In this manner I hunt-and-pecked my way across the great featureless slab of the American Middle West. As the nights and miles slithered by, road hypnosis cast my mind into the past. I thought of my parents, long dead, and the town where I was raised — a doppelgänger to the many anonymous hamlets that I, King of Destruction, passed through unremarkably, just a pair of headlights drifting downstream in the dark. I thought of people I'd known, friends I'd made, women I'd bedded. I thought of a table with flowers and crystal and a view of the sea, and a night — a sad and beautiful night — when in falling snow I had carried my beloved home. I thought of all these things, and many more besides, but most of all, I thought of Liz.

The lights of New York rose from wretched New

Jersey on the evening of the sixth day. Eight million souls: my senses were singing like a soprano. I entered Manhattan via the Lincoln Tunnel, abandoned the car on Eighth Avenue, and set out on foot. I stopped in the first tavern I came to, an Irish pub with a heavily lacquered bar and sawdust on the floor. Among the patrons, nothing seemed out of the ordinary; such is the insularity of New Yorkers that what was happening in the middle of the country had yet to coalesce into a feeling of general crisis. Seated alone at the bar, I ordered a Scotch, not intending to drink it, but discovered that I wanted to and, more interestingly, that it caused no ill effects. It was delicious, its most subtle flavors dancing upon my palate. I was on my third when I realized two other things: I was not the least drunk, and I badly needed to piss. In the men's room my body released a stream so powerfully percussive it made the porcelain chime. This, too, was immensely satisfying; it seemed there was no bodily pleasure that had not been amplified a hundred-fold.

But the real object of my attention was the television above the bar. A Yankees game was on. I waited until the last pitch was thrown and asked the bartender if he would switch to CNN.

I did not have to wait long: "Colorado Killing Spree," read the chyron at the bottom of the screen. The madness was spreading. Reports were coming in from locales throughout the state: whole families obliterated in their beds, towns without a man or woman left alive, a roadside restaurant of patrons gutted like trout. But there were also survivors — bitten, but alive. *It just looked at me. It wasn't human. It gave off this kind of glow.* The ravings of the traumatized or some-

thing more? No one had done the math yet, but I did. Per my instructions, for every nine killed, one had been called into the fold. The hospitals were filling with the sick and injured. Nausea, fever, spasms, then . . .

"That's some creepy shit."

I turned to the man sitting next to me. When had the adjacent stool become occupied? A certain urban type, manufactured by the thousands: balding and lawyerish, with an intelligent, slightly pugnacious face, a speckling of day-old beard, and a little paunch he kept meaning to do something about. Wingtips and a blue suit and starched white shirt, necktie loose around his throat. Somebody was waiting for him at home, but he couldn't quite bring himself to face them yet, not after the day he'd just had.

"Don't I know it."

On the bar before him sat a glass of wine. Our eyes met for what seemed an unusually long time. I noted the overwhelming odor of nervous perspiration he'd attempted to cloak with cologne. His eyes traveled the length of my torso, pausing at my mouth on the upswing. "Haven't I seen you in here before?"

Ah, I thought. I darted my eyes around the room. There were no women at all. "I don't think so. I'm new."

"Are you meeting anyone?"

"Not until now."

He smiled and put out his hand — the one without the wedding ring. "I'm Scott. Let me buy you a drink."

Thirty minutes later, wearing his suit, I left him in an alleyway, twitching and frothing.

I thought of visiting my old apartment but discarded the idea; it was not, had never been, home. What is home to a monster? To anyone? There exists for each of us a geographical fulcrum, a place so saturated with memory that within its precinct the past is always present. It was late, after two A.M., when I entered the main hall at Grand Central Terminal. The restaurants and shops had long since closed, sealed behind their grates; the board above the ticket windows listed only morning trains. Just a few souls lingered: the ubiquitous transit police in their Kevlar vests and creaking leather accoutrements, a couple in evening wear racing for a train that had long since departed, an old black man pushing a dust mop, earphones stuffed in his head. At the center of the marbled hall stood the information booth with its legendary timepiece. *Meet me at the kiosk, the one with the four-faced clock . . .* It was New York's most celebrated rendezvous point, perhaps the most famous in the world. How many fateful encounters had occurred in this place? How many assignations had commenced, what nights of love? How many generations walked the earth because a man and a woman had arranged to meet here, beneath this storied timepiece of gleaming brass and opalescent glass? I tilted my face toward the barrel-vaulted ceiling, 125 feet overhead. In my young adulthood, its beauty had been muted by layers of coal soot and nicotine, but that was the old New York; a thorough cleaning in the late nineties had restored its gold-leaf astrological images to their original luster. Taurus, the bull;

Gemini, the twins; Aquarius, bearing his water; a milky smear of galactic arm, as one sees only on the clearest of nights. A little-known fact, though not unacknowledged by my scientist's eye, is that the ceiling of Grand Central is actually backward. It is a mirror image of the night sky; lore holds that the artist was working from a medieval manuscript that showed the heavens not from within but from without — not mankind's view but God's.

I took a seat at the top of the west balcony steps. One of the transit cops gave me a quick eyeball, but as I was now dressed for the part of respectable white-collar professional and was neither asleep nor visibly drunk, he left me alone. I took logistical stock of my surroundings. Grand Central was more than a train station; it was a principal nexus of the city's substrata, its vast underground world of tunnels and chambers. People by the hundreds of thousands flowed through this place each and every day, most never looking beyond the tips of their own shoes. It was perfect, in other words, for my purpose.

I waited. The hours moved by, and then the days. No one seemed to notice me or, if they did, to care. Too much else was going on.

And then after some unknown interval of time had passed, I heard a sound I had not heard before. It was the sound that silence makes when there is no one left to listen. Night had fallen. I rose from my place on the steps and walked outside. There were no lights burning anywhere; the blackness was so complete I might have been at sea, miles from any shore. I looked up and beheld the most curious of sights. Stars by the hundreds, the thousands, the millions, locked in

their slow turning above the empty world, as they had done since time's beginning. Their pins of light fell upon my face like pattering drops of rain, streaming out of the past. I did not know what I was feeling, only that I felt it; and I began, at last, to weep.

15

And thus to my woeful tale.

Observe him, a capable young man of passable looks, slender and shaggy-haired, tan from a summer of honest outdoor work, good with math and things mechanical, not without ambition and bright hopes and possessing a solitary, inward-looking personality, alone in his bedroom beneath the eaves as he packs his suitcase of folded shirts and socks and underwear and not much else. The year is 1989; our setting is a provincial town named Mercy, Ohio — famous, briefly, for its precision brassworks, said to produce the finest shell casings in the history of modern warfare, though that, like much else of the town, is long faded. The room, which is to be unoccupied within the hour, is a shrine to the young man's youth. Here is the display of trophies. Here are the soldier bedside lamp and matching martial-themed curtains; here the shelves of serial novels featuring intrepid trios of underappreciated teenagers whose youthful intellects enable them to solve crimes their elders cannot. Here, tacked to the neutral plaster walls, are the pennants of sports teams and the conundrumous M. C. Escher etching of hands drawing each other and, opposite the sagging single bed, the era-appropriate poster of the erect-nippled *Sports Illustrated*

swimsuit model, beneath whose lubricious limbs and come-hither gaze and barely concealed pudenda the boy has furiously masturbated night after adolescent night.

But the boy: he undertakes his packing with the puzzled solemnity of a mourner at a child's funeral, which is the scene's appropriate analogue. The problem is not that he cannot make his belongings fit — he can — but the opposite: the meagerness of the bag's contents seems mismatched with the grandeur of his destination. Tacked above his cramped little-boy's desk, a letter gives the clue. *Dear Timothy Fanning,* it reads on elaborately decorated letterhead with a crimson, shield-shaped emblem and the ominous word VERITAS bespeaking ancient wisdoms. *Congratulations, and welcome to the Harvard class of 1993!*

It is early September. Outside, an earthbound, misting rain, tinged by summer's green, hugs the little hamlet of houses and yards and storefront commercial concerns, one of which belongs to the boy's father, the town's lone optometrist. This places the boy's family in the upper reaches of the town's constricted economics; they are, by the standards of that time and place, well-off. His father is known and appreciated; he walks the streets of Mercy to a chorus of amiable hellos, because who is more admirable and worthy of gratitude than the man who has placed the spectacles upon your nose that enable you to see the things and people of your life? As a child, the boy loved to visit his father's office and try on all the eyeglasses that decorated the racks and display cases, longing for the day when he would need a pair of his own, though he never did: his eyes were perfect.

177

"Time to go, son."

His father has appeared in the door: a short, barrel-chested man whose gray flannel trousers, by gravitational necessity, are held aloft by clip-on suspenders. His thinning hair is wet from the shower, his cheeks freshly scraped by the old-fashioned safety razor he favors despite modern innovations in shaving technology. The air around him sings with the smell of Old Spice.

"If you forget anything, we can always send it to you."

"Like what?"

His father shrugs amiably; he is trying to be helpful. "I don't know. Clothes? Shoes? Did you take your certificate? I'm sure you'll want that."

He is speaking of the boy's second-place award in the Western Reserve District 5 Science Day competition. "The Spark of Life: Gibbs-Donnan Equilibrium and Nernst Potential at the Critical Origin of Cell Viability." The certificate, in a plain black frame, hangs on the wall above his desk. The truth is, it embarrasses him. Don't all Harvard students win first prize? Nevertheless, he makes a show of gratitude for being reminded and places it atop the pile of clothing in the open suitcase. Once in Cambridge, it will never make it out of his bureau drawer; three years later, he will discover it beneath a pile of miscellaneous papers, regard it with a quick, bitter feeling, and pitch it into the trash.

"That's the spirit," his father says. "Show those Harvard smarties who they're dealing with."

From the base of the stairs, his mother's voice ascends in an insistent song: "Tim-o-thy! Are you ready yet?"

She never calls him "Tim"; always it is "Tim-

178

othy." The name embarrasses him — it feels both courtly and diminutive at the same time, as if he were a little English lord on a velvet cushion — though he also secretly likes it. That his mother vastly prefers him to her husband is no secret; the reverse is also true. The boy loves her far more easily than he loves his father, whose emotional vocabulary is limited to manly pats on the back and the occasional boys-only camping trip. Like many only children, the boy is aware of his value in the household economy, and nowhere is this value more lofty than in his mother's eyes. *My Timothy,* she likes to say, as if there are others not hers; he is her only one. *You are my special Timothy.*

"Haaa-rold! What are you doing up there? He's going to miss the bus!"

"For Pete's sake, just a minute!" He returns his eyes to the boy. "Honestly, I don't know what she's going to do without you to worry about. That woman's going to drive me crazy."

A joke, the boy understands, but in his father's voice he detects an undertone of seriousness. For the first time he considers the full emotional dimensions of the day. His life is changing, but his parents' lives are changing, too. Like a habitat abruptly deprived of a major species, the household will be wrenched into realignment by his departure. Like all young people, he has no idea who his parents really are; for eighteen years he has experienced their existence only insofar as it has related to his own needs. Suddenly his mind is full of questions. What do they talk about when he's not around? What secrets do they hold from each other, what aspirations have been left to languish? What private grievances, held in check

by the shared project of child rearing, will now, in his absence, lurch into the light? They love him, but do they love each other? Not as parents or even husband and wife but simply as people — as surely they must have loved each other at one time? He hasn't the foggiest; he can no more grasp these matters than he can imagine the world before he was alive.

Compounding the difficulty is the fact that the boy has never been in love himself. Though the social patterns of Mercy, Ohio, are such that even a modestly attractive person can find opportunities in the sexual marketplace, and the boy, although a virgin, has been from time to time its beneficiary, what he has experienced is merely love's painless presage, the expression without the soul. He wonders if this is a lack within himself. Is there a part of the brain from which love comes that in his case has drastically malfunctioned? The world is awash in love — on the radio, in movies, in the pages of novels. Romantic love is the common cultural narrative, yet he seems immune to it. Thus, though he has yet to taste the pain that comes with love, he has experienced pain of a different, related sort: the fear of facing a life without it.

They meet the boy's mother in the kitchen. He expects to find her dressed and ready to go, but she is wearing her flowered housecoat and terrycloth slippers. Through some unspoken agreement it has been determined that his father alone will accompany him to the station.

"I packed you a lunch," she declares.

She thrusts a paper sack into his hands. The boy unfolds the crinkled top: a peanut butter sandwich in waxed paper, cut carrots in a baggie, a pint of

milk, a box of Barnum's Animal Crackers. He is eighteen: he could devour the contents of ten such bags and still be hungry. It's a meal for a child, yet he finds himself absurdly grateful for this small present. Who knows when his mother will make him lunch again?

"Do you have enough money? Harold, did you give him any cash?"

"I'm fine, Mom. I have plenty from the summer."

His mother's eyes have begun to pool with tears. "Oh, I said I wouldn't do this." She waves her hands in front of her face. "Lorraine, I said, don't you dare cry."

He steps into her warm embrace. She is a substantial woman, good to hug. He breathes in the smell of her — a dusty, fruit-sweet aroma, tinged with the chemical scent of hairspray and the off-gassing nicotine of her breakfast cigarette.

"You can let him go now, Lori. We're going to be late."

"Harvard. My Timothy is going to Harvard. I just can't believe it."

The ride to the bus station, in a neighboring town, takes thirty minutes along rural highways. The car, a late-model Buick LeSabre with a soft suspension and seats of crushed velour, makes the roadway beneath them seem vague, as if they are levitating. It is his father's one self-indulgence: every two years a new LeSabre appears in the driveway, all but indistinguishable from the last. They pass the last houses and ease into the countryside. The fields are fat with corn; birds wheel over the windbreaks. Here and there a farmhouse, some pristinely kept, others in disrepair — paint flaking, foundations tipping, uphol-

stered furniture on the porches and abandoned toys in the yards. Everything the boy sees touches his heart with fondness.

"Listen," his father says, as they are approaching the station, "there's something I wanted to say to you."

Here it comes, the boy thinks. This impending announcement, whatever it is, is the reason they've left his mother behind. What will it be? Not girls or sex; apart from one awkward conversation when he was thirteen, the subject has never been raised. Study hard? Keep your nose to the grindstone? But these things, too, have already been said.

His father clears his throat. "I didn't want to say this before. Well, maybe I did. I probably should have. What I'm trying to say is that you're destined for big things, son. *Great* things. I've always known that about you."

"I'll do my best, I promise."

"I know you will. That's not really what I'm saying." His father hasn't looked at the boy once. "What I'm saying is, this isn't the place for you anymore."

The remark is deeply unsettling. What can his father intend?

"It doesn't mean we don't love you," the man continues. "Far from it. We only want what's best."

"I don't understand."

"The holidays, okay. It wouldn't make sense for you not to be here for Christmas. You know how your mother is. But otherwise . . ."

"You're telling me you don't want me to come home?"

His father is speaking rapidly, his words not so much spoken as unleashed. "You can call, of

182

course. Or we can call you. Every couple of weeks, say. Or even once a month."

The boy has no idea what to make of any of this. He also detects a note of falsehood in his father's words, a manufactured rigidity. It is as if he's reading them off a card.

"I don't believe what you're saying."

"I know this is probably hard to hear. But it really can't be helped."

"What do you mean, it can't be helped? Why can't it be?"

His father draws a breath. "Listen, you'll thank me later. Trust me on that, okay? You might not think so now, but you've got your whole life ahead of you. That's the point."

"That's not the goddamned point!"

"Hey, let's watch the language. There's no reason for that kind of talk."

Suddenly the boy is on the verge of tears. His departure has become a banishment. His father says nothing more, and the boy understands that a border has been reached; he'll get nothing more from the man. *We only want what's best. You've got your whole life.* Whatever his father is actually feeling lies hidden behind this barricade of clichés.

"Dry your tears, son. There's no reason to make a mountain out of a molehill."

"What about Mom? Is this her idea, too?"

His father hesitates; the boy detects a flash of pain on the man's face. A hint of something genuine, a deeper truth, but in the next instant it's gone.

"You don't have to worry about her. She understands."

The car has come to a halt; the boy looks up, amazed to discover that they've arrived at the sta-

tion. Three bays, one with a bus awaiting; passengers are filing aboard.

"You've got your ticket?"

Speechless, the boy nods; his father extends his hand. He feels like he's being fired from a job. When they shake, his father squeezes before he does, mashing his fingers together. The handshake is awkward and embarrassing; they're both relieved when it's over.

"Go on now," his father urges with false cheer. "You don't want to miss your bus."

There is no rescuing the moment. The boy gets out, still clutching his paper sack of lunch. It feels totemic, the last vestige of a childhood not so much departed as obliterated. He hoists his suitcase from the trunk and pauses to see if his father will emerge from the Buick. Perhaps in a gesture of last-minute conciliation the man will carry his bag to the bus, even send him away with a hug. But no such thing happens. The boy advances to the bus, places his bag in one of the open bays, and takes his place in line.

"Cleveland!" the driver bellows. "All aboard for Cleveland!"

There is some confusion at the head of the line. A man has lost his ticket and is attempting to explain. While everyone waits for the matter to be sorted out, the woman just ahead of the boy turns toward him. She is maybe sixty, with neatly pinned hair, shimmering blue eyes, and a bearing that strikes him as grand, even aristocratic — someone who should be boarding an ocean liner, not a dirty motor coach.

"Now, I bet a young man like you is off somewhere interesting," she says merrily.

He doesn't feel like talking — far from it. "Col-

184

lege," he explains, the word thick in his throat. When the woman doesn't respond, he adds, "I'm going to Harvard."

She reveals a smile of absurdly false teeth. "How *marvelous*. A Harvard man. Your parents must be very proud."

His turn comes; he hands his ticket to the driver, moves down the aisle, and selects a seat at the rear because it is as far away from the woman as possible. In Cleveland he will change buses for New York; after a night sleeping on a hard bench in the Port Authority station, his suitcase tucked under his legs, he will catch the first bus to Boston, departing at five A.M. As the big diesel rumbles to life, he finally turns his face toward the window. The rain has returned, dotting the glass. The spot where his father parked is empty.

As the bus backs away, he opens the bag in his lap. It's surprising, how hungry he is. He tears into the sandwich; six bites and it's gone. He downs the milk without removing the carton from his lips. The carrots are next, devoured in an instant. He barely tastes any of it; the point is simply to eat, to fill an empty space. When all else is done, he opens the little box of cookies, pausing to regard its colorful illustrations of caged circus creatures: the polar bear, the lion, the elephant, the gorilla. Barnum's Animal Crackers have been a staple of his childhood, yet it is only now that he notices that the animals are not alone in their cages; each is a mother with her baby.

He places a cookie on his tongue and lets it melt, coating the walls of his mouth with its vanilla sweetness, then another and another, until the box is empty, then closes his eyes, waiting for sleep to come.

Why do I relate this scene in the third person? I suppose because it's easier. I know my father meant well, but it took me many years to process the pain of his decree. I have forgiven him, of course, but absolution is not the same as understanding. His unreadable face, his casually declarative tone: all these years later, I still puzzle over the apparent ease with which he dispatched me from his life. It seems to me that one of the great rewards of raising a son would be the simple enjoyment of his company as he moves into the real business of adulthood. But having no son of my own, I can neither confirm nor deny this.

So it was that I arrived at Harvard University in September 1989 — the Soviet Union on the brink of collapse, the economy in a state of general decline, the national mood one of weary boredom with a decade of drift — friendless, orphaned in all but name, with few possessions and no idea what would become of me. I had never set foot on the campus or, for that matter, traveled east of Pittsburgh, and after the past twenty-four hours in transit, my mind was in such a state that everything around me possessed an almost hallucinatory quality. From South Station I took the T to Cambridge (my first ride on a subway) and ascended from the cigarette-strewn platform into the hubbub of Harvard Square. It appeared that the season had changed during my journey; muggy summer had yielded to tart New England autumn, the sky so shockingly blue it was practically audible. In my jeans and slept-in T-shirt, I shivered as a dry breeze moved over me. The hour

was just shy of noon, the square thick with people, all of them young, all apparently at perfect ease with their surroundings, moving purposefully in pairs or packs, the talk and laughter passing between them with the crisp assuredness of batons in a relay race. I had entered an alien realm, but this was home to them. My destination was a dormitory named Wigglesworth Hall, though, reluctant to ask anyone for directions — I doubted they'd even stop to talk to me — and discovering that I was famished, I made my way up the block away from the square, looking for someplace inexpensive to eat.

I was to learn later that the restaurant I chose, Mr. and Mrs. Bartley's Burger Cottage, was a beloved Cambridge landmark. I stepped inside to an eye-watering assault of weaponized onion smoke and the roar of a crowd. Half the city appeared to have shoved itself into the cramped space, filling the long tables, everyone trying to talk over everybody else, including the cooks, who were shouting out their orders like quarterbacks calling signals. On the wall above the grill was an enormous blackboard bearing elaborate descriptions in colored chalk of the most off-puttingly garnished burgers I had ever heard of: pineapple, blue cheese, fried egg.

"Just you?"

The man addressing me looked more like a wrestler than a waiter — a huge, bearded fellow wearing an apron as stained as a butcher's. I nodded dumbly.

"Singles at the counter only," he commanded. "Grab a stool."

A place had just come free. As the waitress behind the counter whisked away the previous oc-

cupant's dirty plate, I slid my suitcase against the base of the counter and took a seat. It wasn't very comfortable, but at least my luggage was hidden from view. I took my map out of my pocket and began to look it over.

"What'll you have, hon?"

The waitress, a harried-looking older woman with sweat stains at the armpits of her Burger Cottage T-shirt, stood before me, pad and pencil poised.

"A cheeseburger?"

"Lettuce, tomato, onion, pickle, ketchup, mayo, mustard, Swiss, cheddar, provolone, American, what kind of bun, toasted or plain?"

It was like trying to catch bullets from a machine gun. "Everything, I guess."

"You want four different kinds of cheese?" She had yet to lift her eyes from her pad. "I'll have to charge you extra."

"I didn't mean that. Sorry. Just the cheddar. Cheddar is fine."

"Toasted or plain?"

"I'm sorry?"

Her eyes, weary with boredom, rose at last. "Do . . . you . . . want . . . your bun . . . toasted . . . or . . . plain?"

"Jesus, Margo, take it easy on the guy, will you?"

The voice had come from the man sitting to my right. I had studiously kept my eyes forward, but now I turned to look. He was tall, broad-shouldered but not overtly muscular, with the sort of well-proportioned face that gives the impression of having been made more carefully than most people's. He was dressed in a rumpled oxford shirt tucked into faded Levi's; a pair of sunglasses was perched on his head, held in place

by the folds of his wavy brown hair. One ankle, his right, was propped on the opposite knee, showing a scuffed penny loafer without a sock. In the periphery of my vision he had registered as a full-fledged adult, but I now saw that he couldn't have been more than a year or two older than I was. The difference was one not of age but of bearing. Everything about him radiated an aura of belonging, that he was a scion of the tribe and fluent in its customs.

He closed his book, placed it on the counter next to his empty coffee cup, and gave me a disarming smile that said, *Don't worry, I've got this.*

"The man wants a cheeseburger with the works. Toasted bun. Cheddar cheese. Fries with that, I think. How about a drink?" he asked me.

"Um, milk?"

"And a milk. No," he said, correcting himself, "a shake. Chocolate, no whip. Trust me."

The waitress looked at me doubtfully. "Okay with you?"

The whole exchange had left me baffled. On the other hand, a shake did sound good, and I was in no mood to turn away a kindness. "Sure."

"Attaboy." My neighbor climbed down from his stool and tucked his book under his arm in a way that suggested all books should be carried in precisely this manner. I saw but did not understand the title: *Principles of Existential Phenomenology.* "Margo here will take good care of you. The two of us go way back. She's been feeding me since I was in short pants."

"I liked you better then," Margo said.

"And you wouldn't be the first to say so. Now, chop-chop. Our friend looks hungry."

The waitress left without another word. Their

repartee suddenly became clear to me. Not the banter of friends but something rather like a precocious nephew and his aunt. "Thanks," I said to my companion.

"*De nada.* Sometimes this place is like a big rudeness contest, but it's worth the hassle. So where did they put you?"

"I'm sorry?"

"What dorm. You're an incoming freshman, aren't you?"

I was amazed. "How did you know that?"

"The powers of my mind." He tapped his temple, then laughed. "That and the suitcase. So, which is it? I hope they didn't put you in one of the Union dorms. You want to be in the Yard."

The distinction meant nothing to me. "Someplace called Wigglesworth."

My answer obviously pleased him. "You're in luck, friend. You'll be right in the middle of the action. Of course, what qualifies as action around this place can be a little staid. It's usually people tearing their hair out at four A.M. over a problem set." He gave my shoulder a manly clap. "Don't worry. Everybody feels a little lost at first."

"I kind of get the feeling you didn't."

"I'm what you'd call a special case. Harvard brat from birth. My father teaches in the philosophy department. I'd tell you who he is, but then you might feel you should take one of his courses out of gratitude, which would be, pardon me, a huge fucking mistake. The man's lectures are like a bullet to the brain." For the second time in as many days, I was to receive a handshake from a man who seemed to know more about my life than I did. "Anyway, good luck. Out the door, take a left, go down a block to the gate. Wigglesworth is

on your right."

With that, he was gone. Only then did I realize that I had neglected to get his name. I hoped I might see him again, though not too soon, and that when I did, I could report that I had ably inserted myself into my new life. I also made a note that at the earliest opportunity I would go shopping for a white oxford shirt and loafers; at least I could look the part. My cheeseburger and fries arrived, shimmering deliciously with grease, and beside it the promised chocolate shake, standing tall in an elegant, fifties-era glass. It was more than a meal; it was an omen. I was so thankful that I might have said grace, and nearly did.

College days, Harvard days: the feeling of time itself changed in those early months, everything rushing past at a frenetic pace. My roommate was named Lucessi. His first name was Frank, though neither I nor anyone I knew ever used it. We were friends of a sort, thrust together by circumstances. I had expected everyone at the college to be some version of the fellow I'd met at the Burger Cottage, with a quick-talking social intelligence and an aristocrat's knowledge of local practices, but, in fact, Lucessi was more typical: weirdly smart, a graduate of the Bronx High School of Science, hardly the winner of any prizes for physical attractiveness or personal hygiene, his personality laden with tics. He had a big, soft body, like a poorly filled stuffed animal's, large damp hands he had no idea what to do with, and the roving, wide-eyed gaze of a paranoiac, which I thought he might be. His wardrobe was a combination of a junior accountant's and a middle schooler's: he favored high-waisted pleated pants, heavy brown

191

dress shoes, and T-shirts emblazoned with the emblem of the New York Yankees. Within five minutes of our meeting he had explained to me that he had scored a perfect 1600 on his SATs, intended to double major in math and physics, could speak both Latin and ancient Greek (not just read: actually *speak*), and had once caught a home run launched from the bat of the great Reggie Jackson. I might have viewed his companionship as a burden, but I soon saw the advantages; Lucessi made me appear well-adjusted by comparison, more confident and attractive than I actually was, and I won not a few sympathy points among my dormitory neighbors for putting up with him, as one might have for tending to a farty dog. The first night we got drunk together — just a week after our arrival, at one of the countless freshman keg parties that the administration seemed content to overlook — he vomited so helplessly and at such extended duration that I spent the night making sure he didn't die.

My goal was to be a biochemist, and I wasted no time. My course load was crushing, my only relief a distribution course in art history that required little more than sitting in the dark and looking at slides of Mary and the baby Jesus in various beatific poses. (The class, a legendary refuge for science majors meeting their humanities requirement, bore the nickname "Darkness at Noon.") My scholarship was generous, but I was used to working and wanted pocket money; for ten hours a week, at a wage just above minimum, I shelved books at Widener Library, pushing a wobbly cart through a maze of stacks so isolated and byzantine that women were warned against visiting them alone. I thought the job would kill

me with boredom, and for a while it nearly did, but over time I came to like it: the smell of old paper and the taste of dust; the deep hush of the place, a sanctuary of silence broken only by the squeaking wheels of my cart; the pleasant shock of pulling a book from the shelves, removing the card, and discovering that nobody had checked it out since 1936. A twinge of anthropomorphic sympathy for these underappreciated volumes often inspired me to read a page or two, so that they might feel wanted.

Was I happy? Who wouldn't be? I had friends, my studies to occupy me. I had my quiet hours in the library in which to woolgather to my heart's content. In late October, I lost my virginity to a girl I met at a party. We were both very intoxicated, didn't know each other at all, and though she didn't say as much — we barely spoke, beyond the usual preliminary blather and a brief negotiation over the mechanically baffling mechanism of her brassiere — I suspected she was a virgin, too, and that her intention was simply to get the thing done as expeditiously as possible so that she could move on to other, more satisfying encounters. I suppose I felt the same. When it was over, I left her room quickly, as if from the scene of a crime, and in four years I laid eyes on her only twice more, both times at a distance.

Yes, I was happy. My father was right: I had found my life. I dutifully telephoned every two weeks, reversing the charges, but my parents — indeed, my whole small-town Ohio childhood — began to fade from my mind, the way dreams do in the light of day. Always these calls were the same. First I would speak with my mother, who usually answered — the suggestion being that she

193

had spent two weeks waiting by the phone — and then my father, whose jovial tone seemed contrived to remind me of his parting edict, and finally both together. I could easily imagine the scene: their faces angled close together with the receiver between them as they called out their valedictory "I love you"s and "I'm proud of you"s and "be good"s, my father's eyes locked in an optic death grip on the clock above the kitchen sink, watching his money drain away at thirty cents a minute. Their voices aroused great feelings of tenderness in me, almost of pity, as if I were the abandoner and they the abandoned, yet I was always relieved when these calls ended, the click of the receiver releasing me back into my true existence.

Before I knew it, the leaves had turned, then fallen, their desiccated carcasses everywhere underfoot, suffusing the air with a sweet smell of decay; the week before Thanksgiving the first snow fell, my inaugural New England winter, damp and raw. It felt like one more baptism in a year of them. There had been no discussion of my returning home for the Thanksgiving break, and Ohio was too far in any case — I'd have wasted half the time on the bus — so I accepted an invitation to spend the holiday with Lucessi in the Bronx. Stupidly, I had expected a scene of Italian life straight out of Hollywood: a cramped apartment above a pizza parlor, everyone yelling and screaming at one another, his father leaking armpitty garlic sweat through his undershirt and his mustached mother, in a housecoat and slippers, throwing up her hands and wailing *"Mamma mia"* every thirty seconds.

What I found couldn't have been more differ-

ent. They lived in Riverdale, which, though technically the Bronx, was as tony as any neighborhood I'd ever seen, in a huge stone Tudor that looked as if it had been hijacked from the English countryside. No spaghetti and meatballs here, no household shrines to the Madonna, no arm-waving drama of any sort; the house was as stultifying as a tomb. Thanksgiving dinner was served by a Guatemalan housemaid in an aproned uniform, and afterward, everybody repaired to a room they actually called "the study," to listen to a radio broadcast of Wagner's interminable *Ring* cycle. Lucessi had told me that his family was in "the restaurant business" (thus the pizza parlor of my imagination), but in fact his father was chief financial officer of the restaurant division of Goldman Sachs, to whose Wall Street offices he commuted every day in a Lincoln Continental the size of a tank. I'd known that Lucessi had a younger sister; he had failed to mention that she was a bona fide Mediterranean goddess, quite possibly the most beautiful girl I'd ever laid eyes on — regally tall, with lustrous black hair, a complexion so creamy I wanted to drink it, and a habit of traipsing into a room wearing nothing more than a slip. Her name was Arianna. She was home from boarding school, someplace in Virginia where they rode horses all day, and when she wasn't lounging around in her underwear, reading magazines and eating buttered toast and talking loudly on the phone, she was striding through the house in tall riding boots and clanking spurs and tight breeches, a costume no less powerful than the slip in its ability to send the blood dumping to my loins. Arianna was completely out of my league, in other words, a fact as obvious as the

weather, yet she went out of her way to remind me of it, calling me "Tom" no matter how many times her brother corrected her and nailing me with looks of such dismissive contempt it was like being doused by cold water.

My final night in Riverdale, I awoke sometime after midnight to discover that I was hungry. I had been instructed to treat the house "as if it were my own" — laughably impossible — yet I knew I would not sleep unless I put something in my stomach. I slipped on a pair of sweatpants and crept downstairs to the kitchen, where I discovered Arianna at the table in a flannel bathrobe, paging through *Cosmopolitan* with her elegant hands and spooning cereal into her flawlessly formed, generously lipped mouth. A box of Cheerios and a gallon of milk sat on the counter. My first instinct was to retreat, but she had already noticed me, standing like an idiot in the doorway.

"Do you mind?" I asked. "I thought I'd get a snack."

Her attention had already returned to her magazine. She took a bite of cereal and gave a backhanded wave. "Do what you want."

I helped myself to a bowl. There was no place else to sit, so I joined her at the table. Even in the flannel bathrobe, her face without makeup and her hair uncombed, she was magnificent. I had no idea what to say to such a creature.

"You're looking at me," she said, turning a page.

I felt the blood rushing to my cheeks. "No, I wasn't."

She said nothing more. I had no place to put my eyes, so I looked at my cereal. The crunch of my chewing seemed intensely loud.

"What are you reading?" I asked finally.

She sighed irritably, closed her magazine, and looked up. "Okay, fine. Here I am."

"I was just trying to make conversation."

"Can we not? Please? I've seen you watching me, Tim."

"So you know my name."

"Tim, Tom, whatever." She rolled her eyes. "Oh, all right. Let's get this over with."

She parted the top of her robe. Beneath it she was wearing only a bra of shimmering pink silk. The sight aroused me indescribably.

"Go on," she urged.

"Go on what?"

She was looking at me with an expression of bored mockery. "Don't be dense, Harvard boy. Here, let me help you."

She took my hand and placed it, rather mechanically, against her left breast. A magnificent breast it was! I had never touched a goddess before. Its spherical softness, sheathed in high-dollar silk with a scallop of delicate lace at the edges, filled my palm like a peach. I sensed she was making fun of me, but I hardly cared. What would happen now? Would I be permitted to kiss her?

Apparently not. As I was constructing a complete sexual narrative in my head, the wonderful things we might do together, culminating in breathy intercourse upon the kitchen floor, she abruptly pulled my hand away and let it fall on the table with the same contemptuous gesture one might use for dropping trash into a bin.

"So," she said, reopening her magazine, "did you get what you wanted? Did that satisfy you?"

I was utterly flummoxed. She turned a page, then another. What the hell had just happened?

"I don't understand you at all," I said.

"Of course you don't." She looked up again, wrinkling her nose in distaste. "Tell me something. Why are you even friends with him? I mean, all things considered, you seem sort of normal."

This was, I supposed, what passed for a compliment. It also aroused in me a fiercely protective instinct toward her brother. Who was she to talk about him like that? Who did she think she was, teasing me this way?

"You're awful," I said.

She gave a nasty little laugh. "Sticks and stones, Harvard boy. Now, if you'll excuse me, I'm trying to read."

And that was the end of it. I returned to bed, so sexually charged I barely slept, and in the morning, before anybody else in the house was awake, Lucessi's father drove us to the train station in his monstrous Lincoln. As we disembarked, in an awkward reversal of customary courtesy, he thanked me for coming in a manner that suggested that he, too, felt a little baffled by my friendship with his son. A picture was emerging: Lucessi was the runt of the litter, an object of family-wide pity and embarrassment. I felt profoundly sorry for him, even as I recognized his situation's similarity to my own. We were a couple of castaways, the two of us.

We boarded the train. I was exhausted and didn't feel like talking. For a while we bumped along in silence. Lucessi was the first to speak.

"Sorry about all that." He was drawing meaningless shapes on the window with his index finger. "I'm sure you were hoping for something more exciting."

I hadn't told him what had happened and, of course, never would. It was also true that my anger

198

had softened, replaced by a budding curiosity. Something altogether unexpected about the world had been glimpsed. This life his family led; I had known that such wealth existed, but that is not the same as sleeping under its roof. I felt like an explorer who'd stumbled upon a golden city in the jungle.

"Don't worry about it," I said. "I had a great time."

Lucessi sighed, settled back, and closed his eyes. "They can be the stupidest people on earth," he said.

What fascinated me, of course, was money. Not just because of the things it could buy, though these were appealing (Lucessi's sister being Exhibit A). The deeper attraction lay in something more atmospheric. I had never been around wealthy people but had not felt this as a lack; I had never been around Martians, either. There were plenty of rich kids at Harvard, of course, the ones who'd gone to exclusive prep schools and addressed each other with preposterous nicknames like "Trip" and "Beemer" and "Duck." But in day-to-day existence, their affluence was easily overlooked. We lived in the same crappy dormitories, sweated through the same papers and tests, ate the same atrocious food in the dining hall, like co-residents of a kibbutz. Or so it seemed. Visiting Lucessi's house had opened my eyes to a hidden world that lay beneath the egalitarian surface of our lives, like a system of caves under my feet. Except for Lucessi, I actually knew very little about my friends and classmates. It seems improbable to say so now, but the thought had never occurred to me that there could be something so

fundamentally different about them.

In the weeks after Thanksgiving, I took clearer stock of my surroundings. There was a boy who lived down the hall whose father was the mayor of San Francisco; a girl I knew slightly, who spoke with a heavy Spanish accent, was said to be the daughter of a South American dictator; one of my lab partners had confided to me, apropos of nothing, that his family owned a summer house in France. All this information coalesced into a whole new awareness of where I was, and the thought made me incredibly self-conscious, even as I longed to learn more about it, to penetrate its social codes and see where I might fit.

Equally fascinating to me was the fact that Lucessi himself wanted nothing to do with any of it. Throughout the weekend, he had made no secret of his contempt for his sister, his parents, even the house, which he called, in typical Lucessian fashion, "an idiotic pile of rock." I attempted to draw him out on this subject but got nowhere; my overtures actually made him angry and snappish. What I had begun to discern in my roommate was the price of being too smart. He possessed an intellect capable of calculating reams of data without taking pleasure in any of it. To Lucessi, the world was a collection of interlocking systems divorced from all meaning, a surface reality governed only by itself. He could, for instance, recite the batting averages of every player on the New York Yankees, but when I asked him who his favorite was, he had no answer. The only emotion he seemed capable of was disdain for other people, though even that possessed a quality of childish bewilderment, as if he were a bored toddler in a man's body, forced to sit at the grown-

ups' table and listen to incomprehensible conversations about the price of real estate and who was divorcing whom. I believe this pained him — he wasn't aware what the problem was, only that it existed — resulting in a kind of nihilistic loneliness: he both despised and envied everybody else, except for me, to whom he attributed a similar vision of the world, simply because I was always around and didn't make fun of him.

As for his unhappy fate: perhaps I didn't value him enough as a friend. Sometimes I think I might have been the only friend he ever had. And it is strange, after so many years, that from time to time my thoughts still turn to him, even though he was, after all, but a minor actor in my life. Probably it is the idleness of my circumstances that draws me to the recollection. With so many years to fill, one inevitably gets around to everything, opens each drawer of the mind to rustle around inside it. I did not know Lucessi well; no man could. Yet the failure to know a person does not rule out his importance in our lives. I wonder: how would Lucessi regard me now? Were he to wander, miraculously alive, into this prison of my own making, this becalmed memorial to things lost, ascend the marble staircase with his graceless Lucessian gait and stand before me in his clunky shoes and ill-fitting trousers and Yankees' jersey stinking of unwashed Lucessian sweat, what would he tell me? *See?* he might say. *Now you get it, Fanning. Now you really get it, after all.*

I returned to Ohio for Christmas. I was glad to be home, but mine was the exile's gladness; none of it seemed to pertain to me anymore, as if I'd been gone for years, not months. Harvard was not my

201

home, at least not yet, but neither was Mercy, Ohio. The very idea of home, of one true place, had become odd to me.

My mother did not appear well. She had lost a great deal of weight, and her smoker's cough had worsened. A glaze of sweat appeared on her brow at the smallest exertion. I paid this little mind, accepting at face value my father's explanation that she had overdone it making ready for the holidays. I dutifully went through the sentimental motions: tree trimming and pie baking, a trip to Midnight Mass (we never attended church otherwise), opening my presents while my parents looked on — an awkward ceremony that is the bane of all only children — but my heart was nowhere in this, and I departed two days early, explaining that with exams still ahead of me, I needed to get back to my studies. (I did, but that wasn't the reason.) Just as he'd done in September, my father drove me to the station. The rains of summer had been replaced by snow and biting cold, the warm wind through open windows by a blast of desiccated air from the dashboard vents. It would have been the perfect time to say something meaningful, if either of us could have imagined what such a thing might be. When the bus pulled away, I did not look back.

About the remainder of that first year, there is not much else to say. My grades were good — better than good. Though I knew I had done well, I was still astonished to see my first-semester report with its barricade of A's, each emphatically embossed into the paper by the old-fashioned dot matrix printer. I did not use this as an opportunity to slack off but redoubled my efforts. I also, for a brief time, acquired a girlfriend, the daughter of

the South American dictator. (He was actually the Argentine minister of finance.) What she saw in me I have no idea, but I wasn't going to interrogate the point. Carmen possessed a good deal more sexual experience than I did — a *great* deal. She was the kind of woman who used the word "lover," as in "I have taken you as my," and she applied herself to pleasure's project with greedy abandon. She was blessed with a single room, rare for a freshman, and in that hallowed precinct of draped scarves and female aromas she introduced me to what might have passed for actual, grown-up eroticism, working her way through the full menu of bodily delights, appetizers to dessert. We did not love each other — that sainted emotion still eluded me, and Carmen had little use for it — nor was she what I would call conventionally attractive. (I can say this because I wasn't, either.) She was a little heavy, and her face possessed a slightly masculine bulk around the jawline, which looked like a boxer's. But unclothed, and in the heat of passion, crying out naughty things in her Argentine-inflected Spanish, she was the most sensual creature who ever walked the earth, a fact magnified a hundred-fold by her own awareness of it.

Between these carnal escapades — Carmen and I would often race back to her room between classes for an hour of furious copulation — and my voluminous classwork and, of course, my hours at the library — time well spent replenishing myself for our next encounter — I saw less and less of Lucessi. He'd always kept odd hours, studying through the night and living on naps, but as the semester wore on, his comings and goings became more erratic. When I slept over at

Carmen's, I might not see him for several days in a row. By this time I had widened my society beyond the walls of Wigglesworth to include a number of Carmen's friends, all of them far more cosmopolitan than I was. Lucessi obviously resented this, but any effort to pull him into the circle was sternly rebuffed. His hygiene took another dip; our room stank of socks and the trays of moldy food he brought back from the cafeteria and never removed. Many times I entered to find him sitting on his bed, barely dressed, muttering to himself and making odd, twitchy hand gestures, as if involved in earnest conversation with some unseen party. At bedtime — whenever he decided that was, even if it was the middle of the day — he would smear his face with a layer of acne cream as thick as a mime's makeup; he began to sleep with a scuba diver's knife in a rubber sheath strapped to his leg. (This should have disturbed me more than it did.)

I worried about him, but not very much; I was simply too busy. Despite my new, more interesting circle of friends, I had always assumed that the two of us would continue to room together. At the end of the year, all freshmen entered a lottery to determine which of the Harvard houses they would live in for the next three years. This was regarded as a rite of passage as socially determinant as whom one married, and it possessed two aspects. The first was which house one sought to live in. There were twelve, each with its own reputation: the preppy house, the artsy house, the jock house, and so forth. The most desirable were the ones located along the Charles River — extremely fancy real estate for the price of an undergraduate tuition. The least were the ones in

the old Radcliffe Quad, far up Garden Street. To be "quadded" was tantamount to exile, one's life forever chained to a schedule of shuttle buses that, inconveniently, stopped running long before the party had ended.

The second aspect was, of course, who would room with whom. This made for an uncomfortable few weeks as people sorted out their allegiances and prioritized their friendships. Rejecting one's freshman roommate in favor of other parties was common but no less awkward than a divorce. I considered having this very conversation with Lucessi, then found that I didn't have the heart. Who else would be willing to room with him? Who else would tolerate his quirks, his doleful personality, his unhealthful aromas? On top of which, come to think of it, nobody else had asked me. Lucessi, it seemed, was mine.

As the day of the lottery approached, I sought him out to see what he wanted to do. I told him I thought we might go in for Winthrop House, or else Lowell. Quincy, maybe, as a backup. They were river houses but without the distinct social slant of some of the others. This conversation occurred in the middle of the afternoon of a warm spring day that Lucessi had apparently slept through. He was sitting at his desk, wearing only briefs and an undershirt, fussing with a calculator as I spoke, punching in meaningless digits with the eraser end of a pencil. A white crust of dried toothpaste ringed his mouth.

"So what do you think?"

Lucessi shrugged. "I already entered."

His words made no sense. "What are you talking about?"

"I asked for a single in the quad."

Psycho singles, they were called. Housing for the maladjusted; rooms for people who couldn't handle roommates.

"It's pretty nice up there, actually," Lucessi went on. "Quieter. You know. Anyway, it's done."

I was dumbfounded. "Lucessi, what the hell? The lottery's next week. I thought we were going to go together."

"I just kind of assumed you didn't want to. You have lots of friends. I thought you'd be happy."

"*You're* supposed to be my friend." I strode furiously around the room. "Is that what this is about? I can't believe you're doing this. Look at this place. Look at *you.* Who else do you have? And you're doing this to *me?*"

These awful, unrecallable words: Lucessi's face crumpled like a wad of paper.

"Christ, I'm sorry. I didn't mean —"

He didn't let me finish. "No, you're right. I really am pretty pathetic. Believe me, it's nothing I haven't heard before."

"Don't talk about yourself like that." My guilt was excruciating. I sat on his bed, trying to get him to look at me. "I shouldn't have said what I did. I was just upset."

"That's okay. Forget it." A moment went by, Lucessi frowning at the calculator. "Did I ever tell you I was adopted? I'm not even related to her. Not technically, anyway."

The comment came from so far out of left field it took me a moment to realize that he was talking about Arianna.

"Everybody always thinks it's the other way around," he continued. "I mean, God, just look at her. But no. My parents got me out of some orphanage. They didn't think they could have kids.

206

Eleven months later, wouldn't you know, along comes Miss Perfect."

I had never heard a confession of such absolute misery. What was there to say? And why was he telling me this now?

"She really hates me, you know. I mean *hates*. You should hear the things she calls me."

"I'm sure that's not true."

Lucessi shrugged hopelessly. "They all do it. They think I don't know, but I do. Okay, I'm king of the dorks. It's not like I haven't figured that out. But Arianna. You've seen her — you know what I'm talking about. Jesus, it just kills me."

"Your sister is a total bitch. She probably treats everybody like that. Just forget about her."

"Yeah, well. That's not really the issue." He lifted his gaze from the calculator and looked me dead in the eye. "You've been really nice to me, Tim, and I appreciate it. I mean that. Promise me we'll stay friends, okay?"

I realized what Lucessi was doing. What I'd thought was jealousy or self-pity was actually a kind of backhanded generosity. Just as my father had done, Lucessi was severing his ties to me because he thought I'd be better off. The worst part was, I knew he was right.

"Sure," I said. "Of course we will."

He held out his hand. "Shake on it? So I know you're not too mad."

We shook, neither of us believing it meant a thing.

"So that's it?" I said.

"I guess so, yeah."

He was in love with her, of course. Though he'd told me as much, this was the part of the story

that took me a long time — too long — to figure out. He loved the thing he also hated, and it was destroying him. The other thing Lucessi had told me, without actually saying it, was that he was in the process of flunking all his courses. His living arrangements were moot, because he wouldn't be returning.

In the meantime, this left me with the problem of finding a place to live. I felt betrayed, and angry with myself for having so badly misunderstood the situation, but also resigned to my fate, which seemed somehow deserved. It was as if I'd lost some cosmic game of musical chairs; the song had stopped, I was left standing, and there was simply nothing to be done about it. I called around to see if anybody I knew was looking for a third or a fourth to round out a suite, but no one was, and rather than dig deeper into my list of acquaintances and embarrass myself further, I stopped asking. There were no singles in any of the River Houses, but it was still possible to enter the lottery as a "floater"; I'd be placed on a waiting list for each of the three houses I chose, and if a student dropped out over the summer, the university would give me his slot. I put in for Lowell, Winthrop, and Quincy, no longer caring which one I got, and waited to hear.

The year came to an end. Carmen and I went our separate ways. One of my professors had offered me a job working in his lab. The pay was negligible, but it was an honor to be asked, and it would keep me in Cambridge for the summer. I rented a room in Allston from a woman in her eighties who favored Harvard students; except for her collection of cats, which was voluminous — I was never quite sure how many there were — and

the overwhelming stink of the litter boxes, the situation was close to ideal. I left early and returned late, usually taking my meals at one of the many cheap eateries on the fringes of Cambridge, and the two of us rarely saw each other. All my friends were gone for the summer, and I expected to be lonely, but it didn't turn out that way. The year had left me enervated and overstuffed, as if by a too-rich meal, and I was glad for the quiet. My job, which involved collating reams of data on the structural biology of plasma cells in mice, could be conducted virtually without interaction with another human being. Sometimes I barely spoke for days.

It shames me to say this, but during that silent summer, I forgot all about my parents. I do not mean that I ignored them. I mean that I forgot that they existed at all. I had told them in a letter where I would be staying and why but hadn't given them the phone number, because I didn't know it at the time — an omission I never got around to correcting. I did not call them and they could not call me, and as the summer wore on, this casual oversight became a psychological buffer that eradicated them from my thoughts. Doubtless, in some pocket of my mind I knew what I was doing, and I would need to contact them before the fall to file the proper paperwork for my scholarship; but at the level of conscious awareness, they simply ceased to matter.

Then my mother died.

My father informed me of this in a letter. Suddenly, a great deal was made clear to me. A month before I'd left for Harvard, my mother had been diagnosed with uterine cancer. She had delayed surgery — a total abdominal hysterectomy — until

after my departure, not wanting to cast a shadow over this occasion. Postoperative biopsies had revealed that the cancer was an aggressive and rare adenosarcoma that left her with no hope of recovery. By winter, she had metastases in her lungs and bones. There was simply nothing to be done. It was, my father said, her dying desire that the son she loved so much should suffer no interruption in his progress toward the fulfillment of all her proud hopes: in other words, that I should go about my life and know nothing. She had died two weeks previously, her ashes buried without funereal pageant, in accordance with her wishes. She had not suffered much, my father wrote, rather coldly, and it was on loving thoughts of me that she had traveled into the life to come.

He wrote in closing, *Probably you're angry with me, with both of us, for keeping this secret from you. If it's any consolation, I wanted you to know, but your mother wouldn't hear of it. When I told you that day at the bus to leave us behind, those were her words, not mine, though she eventually made me see the wisdom of them. Your mother and I were happy together, I believe, but never for a moment did I doubt that you were the great love of her life. She wanted only what was best for you, her Timothy. You may wish to return home, but I encourage you to wait. I am doing reasonably well, under the circumstances, and can see no reason for you to interrupt your studies for what would be, in the end, a painful distraction that would serve no purpose. I love you, son. I hope you know that, and that you can forgive me — forgive us both — and that when we next meet, it will be not to mourn your mother's passing but to celebrate your triumphs.*

I read this letter standing in the front hallway of

the house of a woman I barely knew, cats nosing around my feet, at ten o'clock on a warm night in early August when I was nineteen years old. What I experienced is nothing I have words for, and I will not make the attempt. The urge to telephone him was strong; I wanted to scream at him until my throat ripped open, until my words were blood. So was the urge to get on a bus to Ohio, go straight to the house, and strangle him in his bed — the bed he had shared with my mother for nearly thirty years and where, no doubt, I had been conceived. But I did neither. I realized I was hungry. The body wants what it wants — a useful lesson — and I availed myself of the old woman's larder to make myself a cheese sandwich on stale bread with a glass of the same milk she left in saucers all around the house. The milk had turned, but I drank it anyway, and that is what I remember most vividly of all: the taste of sour milk.

16

The remainder of the summer passed in an emotionless haze. At some point I received a letter informing me that I had been placed in Winthrop House with an as-yet-unnamed roommate who was returning from a year abroad. That I cared nothing about this news is a gross understatement. As far as I was concerned, I could have gone on living with the old woman and her dirty litter boxes. About my mother, I told no one. I worked at the lab right up until the first day of the new semester, leaving no transitional interval in which I might find myself with nothing to distract me. My professor asked me if I wanted to

continue working with him during the academic year, but I turned him down. Perhaps this was unwise, and he seemed shocked that I should decline such a privilege, but it would leave no time for the library, whose consoling silence I missed.

I come now to the part of the story in which my situation changed so radically that I recall it as a kind of plunge, as if I had been merely floating on the surface of my life until then. This commenced the day I moved into Winthrop House. Lucessi and I had sold off our Salvation Army furniture, and I arrived with little more than the same suitcase I'd brought to Harvard a year ago, a desk lamp, a box of books, and the impression that I had once again slipped into an anonymity so pure that I could have changed my name if I wanted to with nobody the wiser. My quarters, two rooms arranged railroad-apartment-style with a bathroom at the rear, was on the fourth floor facing the Winthrop quadrangle, with a view of Boston's modest skyline behind it. There was no sign of my roommate, whose name I was yet to learn. I spent some time mulling over which space to choose as my own — the interior room was smaller but more private; on the other hand, I would have to endure my roommate trooping through at all hours to the toilet — before deciding that, to get things off on the right foot, I would await his arrival, so that we might decide together.

I had finished carting the last of my belongings up the stairs when a figure appeared in the doorway, his face obscured by the stack of cardboard boxes in his arms. He advanced into the room, groaning with effort, and lowered them to the floor.

"You," I said.

It was the man I'd met at the Burger Cottage. He was wearing frayed khaki pants and a gray T-shirt that said HARVARD SQUASH, with crescents of sweat under the arms.

"Wait," he said, peering at me. "I know you. How do I know you?"

I explained our meeting. At first he professed no recollection; then a look of recognition dawned.

"Of course. The guy with the suitcase. I'm guessing this means you found Wigglesworth." A thought occurred to him. "No offense, but wouldn't that make you a sophomore?"

It was a fair question, with a complicated answer. Though I'd been admitted as a freshman, I had enough AP credits to graduate in three years. I'd given this matter little thought, always expecting to hang around for the full four. But in the weeks since receiving my father's letter, the option to bang out my education at a quickstep and skedaddle had grown more appealing. Evidently the Harvard higher-ups had thought so, too, since they'd housed me with an upperclassman.

"I guess that makes you a real smarty-pants, doesn't it?" he said. "So, let's have it."

He had a way of speaking that was both elusively sarcastic and somehow complimentary at the same time. "Have what?"

"You know. Name, rank, serial number. Your major, place of origin, that sort of thing. The history of yourself, in other words. Keep it simple — my memory is for shit in this heat."

"Tim Fanning. Biochemistry. Ohio."

"Nicely done. Though if you ask me tomorrow I probably won't remember, so don't be offended."

He stepped forward, hand extended. "Jonas Lear, by the way."

I did my best to respond with a manly grip. "Lear," I repeated. "Like the jet?"

"Alas, no. More like Shakespeare's mad king." He glanced around. "So, which of these luxury compartments have you selected as your own?"

"I thought it would be fair to wait."

"Lesson number one: Never wait. Law of the jungle and so forth. But since you're determined to be a nice guy, we can flip for it." He pulled a coin from his pocket. "Call it."

Up the coin went before I could respond. He snatched it from the air and slapped it to his wrist

"I guess . . . heads?"

"Why does everybody call heads? Someone should do a study." He lifted his hand. "Well, what do you know, it's heads."

"I guess I was thinking of the smaller one."

He smiled. "See? How hard was that. I would have gone the same way."

"You never told me what you were studying."

"Right you are. That was rude of me." He tossed a pair of finger quotes into the air. "Organismic and Evolutionary Biology."

I'd never heard of it. "That's an actual major?"

He'd bent to open one of the boxes. "So my transcript tells me. Plus, it's fun to say. It sounds a little dirty." He glanced up and smiled. "What? Not what you expected?"

"I would have said — I don't know — something more lively. History, maybe. Or English."

He removed an armload of textbooks and began loading them onto the shelves. "Let me ask you something. Of all the possible subjects in the world, why did you choose biochemistry?"

214

"I suppose because I'm good at it."

He turned, hands on his hips. "Well, there you have it. The truth is, I'm just crazy about amino acids. I put them in my martini."

"What's a martini?"

His face drew back. "James Bond? Shaken, not stirred? They don't have these movies in Ohio?"

"I know who James Bond is. I mean, I don't know what's in one."

His mouth curved into a mischievous grin. "Ah," he said.

We were on our third drink when we heard a girl's voice calling his name and the sound of footsteps coming up the stairs.

"In here!" Lear yelled.

The two of us were seated on the floor with the tools of Lear's enterprise spread before us. I have never met anyone else who traveled with not only a fifth of gin and a bottle of vermouth but the sort of bartending gizmos — jiggers, shakers, tiny, delicate knives — one sees only in old movies. A bag of ice swooned in a puddle of meltwater beside an open jar of olives from the market up the street. Ten-thirty in the morning, and I was completely hammered.

"Jesus, look at you."

I hauled my addled eyes into focus on the figure in the doorway. A girl, wearing a summer dress of pale blue linen. I note the dress first because it is the easiest thing to describe about her. I do not mean to say that she was beautiful, although she was; rather, I wish to make a case that there was about her something distinctive and therefore unclassifiable (unlike Lucessi's sister, whose ice-pick perfection was a dime a dozen and had left

215

no lasting mark on me). I could note the particulars — her figure, slender and small-breasted, almost boyish; the petite formation of her sandaled toes, darkened by street grime; her heart-shaped face and damp blue eyes; her hair, pale blond, unmanaged by clips or barrettes, cut to her shining, sun-touched shoulders — but the whole, as they say, was greater than the sum of its parts.

"Liz!" Lear made a big show of getting to his feet, trying not to spill his drink. He threw his arms around her in a clumsy hug, which she pushed back from with a look of exaggerated distaste. She was wearing small, wire-framed eyeglasses, perfectly round, that on another woman might have seemed mannish but in her case didn't at all.

"You're drunk."

"Not in the least. More like in the most. Not as bad as my new roomie here." He propped his free hand against the side of his mouth and spoke in an exaggerated whisper: "Don't tell him, but a minute ago he appeared to be melting." He lifted his glass. "Have one?"

"I have to meet my adviser in half an hour."

"I'll take that as a yes. Tim, this is Liz Macomb, my girlfriend. Liz, Tim. Don't recall his last name, but I'm sure it'll come to me. Say your hellos while I fix this girl a cocktail."

The polite thing to do would have been to stand, but somehow this seemed too formal, and I decided against it. Also, I wasn't sure I could actually accomplish this.

"Hi," I said.

She sat on the bed, folded her slender legs beneath herself, and drew the hem of her dress over her knees. "How do you do, Tim? So you're

216

the lucky winner."

Lear was sloppily pouring gin. "Tim here is from Ohio. That's about all I remember."

"Ohio!" She spoke this word with the same delight she might have used for Pago Pago or Rangoon. "I've always wanted to go there. What's it like?"

"You're kidding."

She laughed. "Okay, a little. But it's your home. Your *patria.* Your *pays natal.* Tell me anything."

Her directness was totally disarming. I struggled to come up with something worthy of it. What was there to say about the home I'd left behind?

"It's pretty flat, I guess." I winced inwardly at the lameness of the remark. "The people are nice."

Lear handed her a glass, which she accepted without looking at him. She took a tiny sip, then said, "Nice is good. I like nice. What else?"

She had yet to avert her eyes from my face. The intensity of her gaze was unsettling, though not unwelcome — far from it. I saw that she had a faint swirl of peach fuzz, dewy with sweat, above her upper lip.

"There really isn't very much to tell."

"And your people? What do they do?"

"My father's an optometrist."

"An honorable profession. I can't see past my nose without these things."

"Liz is from Connecticut," Lear added.

She took a second, deeper sip, wincing pleasurably. "If it's all right with you, Jonas, I'll speak for myself."

"What part?" I said, as if I knew the first thing about Connecticut.

"Little town called Greenwich, dah-ling. Which I'm supposed to hate, there's probably no place

217

more hateable, but I can't seem to manage it. My parents are angels, and I adore them. Jonas," she said, gazing into her glass, "this is really *good.*"

Lear dragged a desk chair to the center of the room and lowered himself onto it backward. I made a mental note that this would be how I sat from now on.

"I'm sure you can describe it better than that," he said, grinning.

"This again. I'm not some dancing monkey, you know."

"Come on, pumpkin. We're totally wasted."

" 'Pumpkin.' Listen to you." She sighed, puffing out her cheeks. "Fine, just this once. But to be clear, I'm only doing this because we have company."

I had no idea what to make of this exchange. Liz sipped again. For an unnervingly long interval, perhaps twenty seconds, silence gripped the room. Liz had closed her eyes, like a medium at a séance attempting to conjure the spirits of the dead.

"It tastes like —" She frowned the thought away. "No, that's not right."

"For God's sake," Lear moaned, "don't be such a tease."

"Quiet." Another moment slipped by; then she brightened. "Like . . . the air of the coldest day."

I was amazed. She was exactly right. *More* than right: her words, rather than functioning as a mere decoration of the experience, actually deepened its reality. It was the first time that I felt the power of language to intensify life. The phrase was also, coming from her lips, deeply sexy.

Lear gave an admiring whistle through his teeth. "That's a good one."

I was frankly staring at her. "How did you do that?"

"Oh, just a talent I have. That and twenty-five cents will get you a gumball."

"Are you some kind of writer?"

She laughed. "God, no. Have you met those people? Total drunks, every one."

"Liz here is one of those English majors we were talking about," Lear said. "A burden on society, totally unemployable."

"Spare me your crass opinions." She directed her next words to me: "What he's not telling you is that he's not quite the self-involved bon vivant he makes himself out to be."

"Yes, I am!"

"Then why don't you tell him where you were for the last twelve months?"

In my state of information overload, and under the influence of three strong drinks, I had over-looked the most obvious question in the room. Why had Jonas Lear, of all people, needed a floater for a roommate?

"Okay, I'll do it," Liz said. "He was in Uganda."

I looked at him. "What were you doing in Uganda?"

"Oh, a little of this, a little of that. As it turns out, they've got quite a civil war going on. Not what the brochure promised."

"He was working in a refugee camp for the U.N.," Liz explained.

"So I dug latrines, handed out bags of rice. It doesn't make me a saint."

"Compared to the rest of us, it does. What your new roommate hasn't told you, Tim, is that he has serious designs on saving the world. I'm talk-

ing major savior complex. His ego is the size of a house."

"Actually, I'm thinking of giving it up," Lear said. "It's not worth the dysentery. I've never shat like that in my life."

"Shit, not 'shat,' " Liz corrected. " 'Shat' is not a word."

These two: I could barely keep up, and the problem wasn't merely that I was smashed, or already half in love with my new roommate's girlfriend. I felt like I had stepped straight from Harvard, circa 1990, into a movie from the 1940s, Spencer Tracy and Katharine Hepburn duking it out.

"Well, I think English is a great major," I remarked.

"Thank you. See, Jonas? Not everyone is a total philistine."

"I warn you," he told her, wagging a finger my direction, "you're talking to another dreary scientist."

She made a face of exasperation. "Suddenly in my life it's raining scientists. Tell me, Tim, what kind of science do you do?"

"Biochemistry."

"Which is . . . ? I've always wondered."

I found myself strangely happy to be asked this question. Perhaps it was just a matter of who was asking it.

"The building blocks of life, basically. What makes things live, what makes them work, what makes them die. That's about all there is to it."

She nodded approvingly. "Well, that's nicely said. I'd say there's a bit of the poet in you after all. I'm beginning to like you, Tim from Ohio." She polished off her drink and set it aside. "As for

220

me, I'm really here to form a philosophy of life. An expensive way to do it, but it seemed like a good idea at the time, and I've decided to go with it."

This luxurious ambition — four years of college at twenty-three grand a pop to amass a personality — struck me as another alien aspect of her that I was hoping to learn more about. I say alien, but what I mean is angelic. By this point, I was utterly convinced that she was a creature of the spheres.

"You don't approve?"

Something in my face must have said so. I felt my cheeks grow warm. "I didn't say that."

"You didn't say anything. Piece of advice. 'That man that hath a tongue, I say, is no man, if with his tongue he cannot win a woman.' "

"I'm sorry?"

"Shakespeare, *Two Gentlemen of Verona*. In plain English, when a woman asks you a question, you better answer."

"If you want to get her into bed," Lear added. He looked at me. "You'll have to excuse her. She's like the Shakespeare channel. I don't understand half the things she says."

I knew almost nothing about Shakespeare. My experience of the bard was limited, like many people's, to a dutiful slog through *Julius Caesar* (violent, occasionally exciting) and *Romeo and Juliet* (which, until that moment, I'd found patently ridiculous).

"I just meant I've never met anybody who thinks that way."

She laughed. "Well, if you want to hang around with me, bub, better bone up. And with that," she said, rising from the bed, "and speaking of which,

221

I must be off."

"But you're not *half* as drunk as we are," Lear protested. "I was hoping to have my way with you."

"Weren't you just." At the doorway, she looked back at me. "I forgot to ask. Which are you?"

One more question I had no answer for. "Come again?"

"Fly? Owl? A.D.? Tell me you're not Porcellian."

Lear answered in my stead: "Actually, our boy here, though technically a junior, has yet to experience this aspect of Harvard life. It's a complicated story I'm much too drunk to explain."

"So, you're not in a club?" she said to me.

"There are clubs?"

"*Final* clubs. Somebody pinch me. You really don't know what they are?"

I had heard the term, but that was all. "Are they some kind of fraternity?"

"Um, not exactly," Lear said.

"What they are," Liz explained, "are anachronistic dinosaurs, elitist to the core. Which also happen to throw the best parties. Jonas is in the Spee Club. Like his daddy and his daddy's daddy and all the Lear daddies since fish grew legs. He's also the whattayacallit. Jonas, what *do* you call it?"

"The punchmaster."

She rolled her eyes. "And what a title that is. Basically, it means he's in charge of who gets in. Honeybunch, do something."

"I only just met the guy. Maybe he's not interested."

"Sure I am," I said, though I wasn't sure at all. What was I letting myself in for? And what did something like that cost? But if it meant spending more time in Liz's company, I would have walked

through fire. "Absolutely. I'd definitely be interested in something like that."

"Good." She smiled victoriously. "Saturday night. Black tie. See, Jonas? It's settled."

I had no doubt that it was.

The first problem: I didn't own a tuxedo.

I had worn one once in my life, a powder-blue rental with navy velvet accents, paired with a ruffled shirt that only a pirate could have loved and a clip-on bow tie fat as a fist. Perfect for the island-themed senior prom at Mercy Regional High School ("A Night in Paradise!") but not the rarefied chambers of the Spee Club.

I intended to rent one, but Jonas convinced me otherwise. "Your tuxedo life," he explained, "has only just begun. What you need, my friend, is a *battle tux.*" The shop he took me to was called Keezer's, which specialized in recycled formal wear cheap enough to vomit on without compunction. A vast room, unfancy as a bus station, with moth-eaten animal heads on the walls and air so choked with naphthalene it made my sinuses sting: from its voluminous racks I selected a plain black tux, a pleated shirt with yellow stains under the arms, a box of cheap studs and cuff links, and patent leather dress shoes that hurt only when I walked or stood. In the days leading up to the party, Jonas had adopted a persona that was somewhere between a wise young uncle and a guide dog for the blind. The selection of the tux was mine, but he insisted on choosing my tie and cummerbund, examining dozens before settling on pink silk with a pattern of tiny green diamonds.

"Pink?" Needless to say, it wasn't anything that would have flown in Mercy, Ohio. A powder-blue

tux, yes. A pink tie, no. "Are you sure about this?"

"Trust me," he said. "It's the kind of thing we do."

The party, as I understood it, would be a sort of elaborate first date. Members would have the chance to look over fresh prospects, called "punchees." I was worried that I didn't have anyone to bring, but Jonas assured me that I was better off alone. That way, he explained, I would have the opportunity to impress the flotilla of un-escorted women imported for the occasion from other colleges.

"Get two of them into bed, and you're definitely in."

I laughed at the absurdity. "Why only two?"

"I mean at the same time," he said.

I had not seen Liz since my first day in Win-throp House. This did not seem strange to me, as she lived in Mather, far down the river, and moved in an artsier crowd. I had, however, through discreet, well-spaced questioning, managed to learn more about her connection to Jonas. They were not, in fact, a strictly Harvard couple but had known each other since childhood. Their fathers had been prep school roommates, and the two families had vacationed together for years. This made sense to me; in hindsight, their verbal jousting had sounded as much like an exchange between two precocious siblings as a romantic twosome's. Jonas claimed that for many years, they actually couldn't stand each other; it wasn't until they were fifteen, and forced to endure two foggy weeks with their parents on a remote island off the coast of Maine, that their mutual antipathy had boiled over into what it really was. They'd kept this from their families — even Jonas con-

fessed that there was something vaguely incestuous about the whole thing — confining their passions to secret, summertime trysts in barns and
boathouses while their parents got drunk on the
patio, not really thinking of themselves as
boyfriend-girlfriend until they'd both wound up
at Harvard and discovered that they actually liked
each other after all.

This account also explained, at least partly, the
oddness of their relationship. What else but shared
history could bond two people who possessed
such fundamentally incompatible temperaments,
such divergent visions of life? The more I grew to
know them both, the more I came to understand
how truly different they were. That they had traveled in the same social circles as children, attended virtually interchangeable country day and
boarding schools, and been able to navigate the
New York subway system, the Paris Métro, and
the London tube by the time they were twelve
said nothing about who they really were as people.
It is possible for the same circumstances that draw
two souls together to keep them forever at arm's
length. Herein lies the truth of love, and the essence of all tragedy. I was not yet wise enough to
understand this, nor would I be, until many years
had passed. Yet I believe that from the start I
sensed this, and that it was the source of my affinity, the force that pulled me to her.

The day of the party arrived. The daylight hours
were all desultory preamble; I got nothing done.
Was I nervous? How does the bull feel when he is
marched into the ring and notices the cheering
crowds and the man with his cape and sword?
Jonas had gone off for the day — I didn't know
where — and as the clock neared eight, the ap-

pointed hour, he had yet to show himself. The midwesterner in me was forever disturbed by the regional differences in what was and was not considered late, and by nine-thirty, when I decided to dress (I had entertained the girlish fantasy that Jonas and I would do this together), my anxiety was such that it verged on anger. It seemed likely that his promise had been forgotten and I would spend the evening like a jilted groom, watching TV in a tuxedo.

The other difficulty lay in the fact that I did not know how to tie a bow tie. Probably I couldn't have accomplished this in any event; my hands were actually shaking. Managing the studs and cuff links felt like trying to thread a needle with a hammer. It took me ten full minutes of cursing like a longshoreman to lodge them in their proper holes, and by the time I was done, my face was damp with sweat. I mopped it away with a bad-smelling towel and examined myself in the full-length mirror on the bathroom door, hoping for some encouragement. I was an unremarkable-looking sort of boy, neither one thing nor the other; although naturally slender, and without significant blemishes, I had always felt my nose was too big for my face, my arms too long for my body, my hair too bulky for the head it sat atop. Yet the face and figure I beheld in the mirror did not look so unpromising to me. The sleek black suit and shiny shoes and starch-hardened shirt — even, against my expectations, the pink cummerbund — did not appear unnatural on me. Instantly I regretted the powder-blue getup I'd worn to prom; who knew that something as simple as a black suit could gentrify one's appearance so thoroughly? For the first time, I dared to think

that I, this plain boy from the provinces, might pass through the doors of the Spee Club without an alarm going off.

The door sailed open; Jonas charged into the outer room. "Fuck, what time is it?" He marched straight past me to the bathroom and turned on the shower. I followed him to the door.

"Where have you been?" I said, realizing too late how peevish this sounded. "No big deal, but it's almost ten."

"I had a lab due." He was peeling off his shirt. "This thing doesn't really get going until eleven. Didn't I tell you?"

"No."

"Oh. Well, sorry."

"How do you tie a bow tie?"

He had stripped to his boxers. "Hell if I know. Mine's a clip-on."

I retreated to the outer room. Jonas called out over the water, "Has Liz been here?"

"Nobody's been here."

"She was supposed to meet us."

My anxiety had now focused entirely on the matter of my tie. I returned to the mirror and withdrew it from my pocket. The gist, I'd heard, was to tie it like a pair of shoes. How much harder could it be? I'd been tying my own shoes since I was two.

The answer was: a lot harder. Nothing I did made the ends come out even close to the same length. It was as if the silk were possessed.

"Now, don't you look spiffy."

Liz had come in through the open door. Or, rather, a woman who *resembled* Liz; in her place stood a creature of pure understated glamour. She was wearing a slender black cocktail dress

227

scooped low at the neck and high-heeled shoes of shiny red leather; she had added something to her hair, making it full and rich, and exchanged her glasses for contacts. A long string of pearls, no doubt real, dangled deep into her décolletage.

"Wow," I said.

"And *that*," she said, tossing her clutch on the sofa, "is the very syllable that every woman longs to hear." A cloud of complex scent had followed her into the room. "Having some troubles with your neckwear, I see?"

I held out the villainous article. "I have no idea what I'm doing."

"Let's have a look." She stepped toward me and took it from my hand. "Ah," she said, examining it, "here's the problem."

"What?"

"It's a bow tie!" She laughed. "As it so happens, you've come to the right person. I do this for my father all the time. Hold still."

She draped the tie around my neck and positioned it under the collar. In her heels, she was nearly as tall as I was; our faces were inches apart. With her eyes intently focused on the base of my throat, she engaged in her mysterious business. I had never been so close to a woman I was not about to kiss. My gaze instinctively went to her lips, which looked soft and warm, then downward, following the path of the pearls. The effect was like a low-voltage current passing through each cell of my body.

"Eyes up here, buster."

I knew I was blushing. I looked away. "Sorry."

"You're a man, what can you do? You're like pull toys. It must be awful." A final adjustment; then she stepped back. That heat in her cheeks:

was she blushing, too? "There you go. Have a look."

She retrieved a compact from her clutch and gave it to me. It was made of a material that was smooth to the touch, like polished bone; it felt warm in my hand, as if it were radiating a pure, womanly energy. I opened it, revealing its bay of flesh-toned powder and small round mirror, in which my face looked back at me, floating above the flawlessly knotted pink bow tie.

"Perfect," I said.

The shower shut off with a groan, widening my awareness. I had forgotten all about my roommate.

"Jonas," Liz called, "we're late!"

He bounded into the room, clutching a towel around his waist. I had the feeling of being caught doing something I shouldn't have.

"So, are you two going to stand around and watch me dress? Unless —" Looking at Liz, he gave his towel a suggestive jostle, like an exotic dancer teasing an audience. *"Ça te donne du plaisir, mademoiselle?"*

"Just hurry it up. We're late."

"But I asked in French!"

"You'll want to work on your accent. We'll meet you outside, thank you very much." She gripped me by the arm, steering me toward the door. "Come on, Tim."

We took the stairs to the courtyard. A college campus on a Saturday night follows principles of its own: it awakens just as the rest of the world is readying for slumber. Music came from everywhere, pouring out of the windows; laughing figures moved through the darkness; voices lit the night from all directions. As we stepped through

229

the breezeway, a girl hurried past, holding the hem of her dress with one hand, a bottle of champagne in the other.

"You'll do fine," Liz assured me.

We were standing just beyond the gate. "Do I look worried?" Though, of course, I was.

"All you have to do is act like you belong. That's really the whole point. Of most things, actually."

Away from Jonas, she had become somebody slightly different: more philosophical, even a little world-weary. I sensed that this was closer to the truth of her.

"I forgot to mention," Liz said, "I've got somebody I'd like you to meet. She'll be at the party."

I wasn't sure what I thought of this.

"We're cousins," she went on. "Well, second cousins. She goes to B.U."

The offer was disorienting. I had to remind myself that what had transpired upstairs had been an innocent flirtation, nothing more — that she was somebody else's girlfriend.

"Okay."

"Try not to sound too excited."

"What makes you think we'd hit it off?"

The remark came off too blunt, even a little resentful. But if she took offense, she didn't show it. "Just don't let her drink too much."

"Is that a problem?"

She shrugged. "Steph can be a bit of a party girl, if you know what I mean. That's her name, Stephanie."

Jonas caught up with us, all grins and apologies. We made our way to the party, which was just three blocks away. Previously, he had pointed out the Spee Club building to me, a brick townhouse with a walled side garden I had passed a thousand

230

times. A college party is usually a loud affair, belching out a wide perimeter of sound, but not this one. There was no evidence that anything was going on inside, and for a second I thought Jonas might have gotten the night wrong. He stepped up to the door and withdrew a single key on a fob from the pocket of his tux. I had seen this key before, lying on his bureau, but had not connected it to anything until now. The fob was in the form of a bear's head, the symbol of the Spee.

We followed him inside. We were in an empty foyer, the floor painted in alternating black and white squares, like a chessboard. I did not feel as if I were going to a party — parachuting at night into an alien country was more like it. The spaces I could see were dark and masculine and, for a building inhabited by college students, remarkably neat. A clack of ivory: nearby, someone was playing pool. On a pedestal in the corner stood a large stuffed bear — not a teddy bear, an actual bear. It was rearing up on its hind legs, clawed hands reaching forward as if it were going to maul some invisible attacker. (That, or play the piano.) From overhead came a swell of liquor-loosened voices.

"Come on," Jonas said.

He led us back to a flight of stairs. Seen from the street, the building had appeared deceptively modest in its dimensions, but not inside. We ascended toward the noise and heat of the crowd, which had spilled from two large rooms onto the landing.

"Jo-man!"

As we made our entry, Jonas's neck was clamped in the elbow of a large, red-haired man in a white dinner jacket. He had the florid complexion and

231

thickened waist of an athlete gone to seed.

"Jo-man, Jo-Jo, the big Jo-ster." Unaccountably, he gave Jonas a big smooch on the cheek. "And Liz, may I say you are looking *especially* tasty tonight."

She rolled her eyes. "So noted."

"Does she love me? I'm asking, does this girl just love me?" With his arm still draped around Jonas, he looked at me with an expression of startled concern: "Sweet Jesus, Jonas, tell me this isn't the guy."

"Tim, meet Alcott Spence. He's our president."

"And roaring drunk, too. So tell me, Tim, you're not gay, are you? Because, no offense, you look a little gay in that tie."

I was caught totally off guard. "Um —"

"Kidding!" He roared with laughter. We were being pressed on all sides now, as more party-goers ascended the stairs behind us. "Seriously, I'm just messing with you. Half the guys in here are *huge* fags. I myself am what you call a sexual omnivore. Isn't that right, Jonas?"

He grinned, playing along. "It's true."

"Jonas here is one of my most special friends. *Very* special. So you just go ahead and be as gay as you feel you need to be."

"Thanks," I said. "But I'm not gay."

"Which is also totally fine! That's what I'm saying! Listen to this guy. We're not the Porcellian, you know. Seriously, those guys can*not* stop fucking each other."

How much did I want a drink at that moment? Very, very much.

"Well, I've enjoyed our little chat," Alcott merrily continued, "but I must be off. Hot date in the sauna with a certain sophomore from the Univer-

232

sity of Loose Morals and some *cocaina más excelente.* You kids run along and have fun."

He faded into the throng. I turned to Jonas. "Is everybody here like that?"

"Actually, no. A lot of them can come on pretty strong."

I looked at Liz. "Don't you dare leave me."

She laughed wryly. "Are you kidding?"

We fought our way to the bar. No lukewarm keg beer here: behind a long table, a white-shirted bartender was frantically mixing drinks and passing out bottles of Heineken. As he shoveled ice into my vodka tonic — I'd learned my freshman year to stick to clear liquor when I could — I had the urge to send him some clandestine message of Marxist-inspired fellowship. "I'm actually from Ohio," I might have told him. "I shelve books at the library. I don't belong here any more than you do." ("P.S. Stand ready! The Glorious Workers' Revolution commences at the stroke of midnight!")

Yet as he placed the drink in my hand, a new feeling came upon me. Perhaps it was the way he did it — automatically, like a high-speed robot, his attention already focused to the next partygoer in line — but the thought occurred to me that I'd done it. I'd passed. I had successfully snuck into the other world, the hidden world. This was where I had been headed, all along. I gave myself a moment to soak in the sensation. Joining the Spee: what I had believed utterly impossible just moments before suddenly seemed like a fait accompli, a thing of destiny. I would take my place among its membership, because Jonas Lear would pave the way. How else to explain the extraordinary coincidence of our second meeting? Fate had

put him in my path for a reason, and here it was, in the rich atmosphere of privilege that radiated from everywhere around me. It was like some new form of oxygen, one I'd been waiting all my life to breathe, and it made me feel weirdly alive.

So caught up was I in this new line of thought that I failed to notice Liz standing right in front of me. With her was a new person, a girl.

"Tim!" she yelled over the music that had erupted in the room behind us. "This is Steph!"

"Pleased to meet you!"

"Likewise!" She was short, hazel-eyed, with a spray of freckles and glossy brown hair. Unremarkable compared to Liz, but pretty in her own way — *cute* would be the word — and smiling at me in a manner that told me Liz had laid the groundwork. She was holding a nearly empty glass of something clear. Mine was empty, too. Was it my first or my second?

"Liz says you go to B.U.!"

"Yeah!" Because the music was so loud, we were standing very close. She smelled like roses and gin.

"Do you like it?"

"It's okay! You're a biochem major, right?"

I nodded. The most banal conversation in history, but it had to be done. "What about you?"

"Poli-sci! Hey, do you want to dance?"

I was an awful dancer, but who wasn't? We made our way to the light-confettied ballroom and began our awkward attempt to perform this intimate act, pretending we hadn't met each other thirty seconds ago. The dance floor was already full, the music having been strategically withheld until everybody was adequately liquored; I glanced around for Liz but didn't find her. I supposed she

was too cool to make a fool of herself in this way and hoped she didn't see me. Stephanie, not to my surprise, was an enthusiastic dancer; what I hadn't banked on was that she'd be so good at it. Whereas my moves were an ungainly mimicry of actual dancing, wholly unrelated to this song or any other, hers possessed a lithe expressiveness that verged on actual grace. She spun, twirled, gyrated. She did things with her hips that elsewise might have looked indecent but under the circumstances seemed ordained by a different, less constricted morality. She also managed to keep her attention on me the whole time, wearing a warmly seductive smile, her eyes focused like lasers. What had Liz called her? A "party girl"? I was beginning to see the advantages.

We broke after the third song for yet another drink, slung them back like sailors on leave, and returned to the floor. I'd eaten no dinner, and the booze was doing its work. The evening dissolved into a haze. At some point I found myself talking to Jonas, who was introducing me to other members of the club, and then playing pool with Alcott, who was not such a bad fellow after all. Everything I did and said seemed charmed. More time passed, and then Stephanie, whom I'd briefly lost track of, was pulling me by the hand back toward the music, which pumped without ceasing like the night's own heartbeat. I had no idea what time it was and didn't care. More fast dancing, the song downshifted, and she wrapped her arms around my neck. We'd barely spoken, but now this warm, good-smelling girl was in my arms, her body pressed against mine, the tips of her fingers stroking the hairs at the back of my neck. Never had I received such an undeserved present. What

was happening to my anatomy was nothing she could have missed; nor did I want her to. When the song ended, she placed her lips against my ear, her breath a sweet exhalation that made me shudder.

"I have coke."

I found myself, then, sitting beside her on a deep leather couch in a room that looked like something in a hunting lodge. From her purse she produced a small packet made of notebook paper, sealed by complex folding. She used my Harvard ID to arrange the coke in two fat lines on the coffee table and rolled a dollar bill into a tube. Cocaine was an aspect of college life that I had not experienced but did not see the harm of. She bent to the table, sucked the powder deep into her sinuses with a delicate, girlish snort, and passed me the bill so that I might do the same.

It wasn't bad at all. It was, in fact, very good. Within seconds of the powder's purchase, I experienced a Roman-candle rush of well-being that seemed not a departure from reality but a deeper entry into truth. The world was a fine place full of wonderful people, an enchanted existence worthy of the utmost enthusiasm. I looked at Stephanie, who was quite beautiful now that I had eyes to see, and sought the words to explain this revelation on a night of many.

"You're a really good dancer," I said.

She leaned forward and took my mouth with hers. It was not a schoolgirl's kiss; it was a kiss that said there were no rules if I didn't want there to be. It did not take long before our bodies were a confusion of tongues and hands and skin. Things were being slid aside, unlatched, unzipped. I felt like I had plummeted into a vortex of pure

sensuality. It was different than it had been with Carmen. It had no edges, no roughness. It felt like being melted. Stephanie was astride my lap and drawing her panties aside and down she went, enveloping me; she began to move in a wondrous, aquatic fashion, like an anemone undulating on the tides, rocking and rising and plunging, each variation accompanied by the creak of leather upholstery. Mere hours since I'd been pacing my room, consigned to a night of humiliated loneliness, and here I was, fucking a girl in a cocktail dress.

"Whoa. Sorry, bud."

It was Jonas. Stephanie was off me like a shot. A moment of frantic activity as the pants were yanked upward, the dress downward, various articles of underclothing rammed into adjustment. Standing in the doorway, my roommate was in a state of barely contained hilarity.

"Jesus," I said. I was pulling up my fly, or trying to. My shirttail was stuck in the zipper. More comedy. "You could have knocked."

"And you could have locked the door."

"Jonas, did you find her?" Liz appeared behind him. As she stepped into the room, her eyes widened. "Oh," she said.

"They were getting better acquainted," Jonas offered, laughing.

Stephanie was smoothing down her hair; her lips were swollen, her face flushed with blood. I had no doubt mine was the same.

"I can see that," Liz said. Her mouth was set in a prim line; she didn't look at me. "Steph, your friends are waiting for you outside. Unless you want me to tell them something else."

This was clearly impossible; the balloon of pas-

sion had been punctured. "No, I guess I should go." She fetched her shoes from the floor and turned to me. I was, ridiculously, still sitting on the sofa. "Well, thanks," she said. "It was really nice to meet you."

Should we kiss? Shake hands? What was I supposed to say? "You're welcome" didn't seem like it would cut it. In the end, the gap between us was too wide; we didn't even touch.

"You, too," I said.

She followed Liz from the room. I felt miserable — not only because of my painfully blockaded loins, but also because of Liz's unmistakable disappointment in me. I had revealed myself to be just like every other guy: a pure opportunist. It wasn't until that moment that I fully realized how important her opinion of me had become.

"Where is everybody?" I asked Jonas. The building was remarkably quiet.

"It's four o'clock in the morning. Everybody's gone. Except for Alcott. He's passed out in the pool room."

I looked at my watch. So it was. Whether from the adrenaline or the coke counteracting the booze, my thoughts had cleared. Cringe-inducing snippets of the night came back to me: knocking a drink onto a member's date, attempting a Cossack dance to the B-52's "Love Shack," laughing too loudly at a joke that was actually somebody's sad story about his disabled brother. What had I been thinking, getting so drunk?

"Are you okay? You want us to wait?"

I'd never wanted anything less in my life. I was already calculating which park bench I could sleep on. Did people do that anymore? "You guys go ahead. I'll be along."

"Don't worry about Liz, if that's what you're thinking. This was totally her idea."

"It was?"

Jonas shrugged. "Well, maybe not that you'd actually bone her cousin on the couch. But she wanted you to feel . . . I don't know. Included."

This made me feel even worse. Stupidly, I had assumed that Liz was doing her cousin a favor, when it was the other way around.

"Listen, Tim, I'm sorry —"

"Forget it," I said, and waved my roommate away. "I'm fine, really. Go home."

I waited ten minutes, gathered myself together, and left the building. Jonas hadn't said where he and Liz were going; back to her place, probably, but I couldn't chance it. I made my way down to the river and began to walk. I had no destination in mind; I suppose I was performing a kind of penance, though for what, precisely, I could not say. I had, after all, done exactly what was expected of me by the standards of that time and place.

Gray dawn found me, a pathetic figure in his tuxedo, five miles away on the Longfellow Bridge, overlooking the Charles River Basin. The first rowers were out, carving the waters with their long, elegant oars. It is at such moments that revelations are said to come, but none did. I had wanted too much and embarrassed myself; there wasn't anything more to say than that. I was badly hungover; blisters had formed on both feet from my too-tight shoes. The thought occurred to me that I hadn't spoken to my father in a very long time, and I was sorry about that, though I knew I would not call him.

By the time I got back to Winthrop, it was nearly

nine o'clock. I keyed the lock and found Jonas freshly shaved and sitting on his bed, shoving his legs into a pair of jeans.

"Jesus, look at you," he said. "Did you get mugged or something?"

"I went for a walk." Everything about him radiated cheerful urgency. "What's going on?"

"We're leaving, is what's going on." He got to his feet, shoving his shirt into the waistband of his jeans. "You better change."

"I'm exhausted. I'm not going anywhere."

"Better rethink that. Alcott just phoned. We're driving down to Newport."

I had no idea what to make of this ridiculous claim. Newport was at least two hours away. All I wanted to do was climb into my bed and sleep. "What are you talking about?"

Jonas snapped on his watch and stepped to the mirror to brush his hair, still damp from the shower. "The after-party. Just members and punchees this time. The ones who, you know, passed. Which would include you, my friend."

"You're joking."

"Why would I joke about a thing like that?"

"Gee, I don't know. Maybe because I made a total jackass of myself?"

He laughed. "Don't be so hard on yourself. You got a little wasted, so what? Everybody really liked you, especially Alcott. Apparently, your escapade in the library made quite an impression."

My stomach dropped. "He knows?"

"Are you serious? Everybody knows. It's Alcott's house we're going to, by the way. You should see this place. It's like something in a magazine." He turned from the mirror. "Earth to Fanning. Am I talking to myself here?"

240

"Um, I guess not."

"Then for fucksake, get dressed."

17

The fall was a marathon of parties, each more extravagant than the last. Nights at restaurants I could never afford, strip clubs, a harbor cruise on a sixty-foot boat owned by an alumnus who never came out of his cabin. Bit by bit, the candidates dropped away, until only a dozen remained. Just after the Thanksgiving holiday, an envelope appeared under my door. I was to report to the club at midnight. Alcott met me in the entryway, instructed me not to speak, and handed me a pewter cup of powerful rum, which he told me to down. The building seemed empty; all the lights were out. He led me to the library, blindfolded me, and told me to wait. Some minutes passed. I was feeling quite drunk and having trouble maintaining my balance.

Then I heard, from behind me, an alarming sound — a low, animal growling, like a dog about to attack. I spun, stumbling, and whipped off the blindfold as the bear reared up before me. It seized me bodily, hurled me to the ground, and pounced on top of me, pushing the wind from my chest. In the dark room all I could make out was its great black bulk and gleaming teeth, poised above my neck. I screamed, utterly convinced that I was about to die — a prank, intended to be harmless, had obviously gone terribly wrong — until I realized that the bear, rather than tearing my throat open, had begun to hump me.

The lights came on. It was Alcott, wearing a bear suit. All the members were there, including

Jonas. An explosion of general hilarity, and then the champagne came out. I had been accepted.

The dues were a hundred and ten dollars a month — more than I had to spare, less than I could do without. I signed on for extra hours at the library and found I could make up the difference easily enough. I had spent Thanksgiving at Jonas's house in Beverly, but Christmas was a problem. I had told him nothing about my situation, and did not want to be the object of his pity. A semester of nonstop parties had also put me badly behind in my studies. I was at a loss as to what to do until I hit upon the idea of calling Mrs. Chodorow, the woman whose house I had lived in for the summer. She agreed to let me stay, even offered to let me have my room for free — it would be nice, she said, to have a young person around for the holidays. On Christmas Eve, she invited me downstairs, and the two of us passed the afternoon together, baking cookies for her church and watching the Yule log on TV. She'd even bought me a present, a pair of leather gloves. I had thought I was immune to holiday sentiment, but I was so touched that my eyes actually welled with tears.

It wasn't until February that I decided to call Stephanie. I felt bad about what had happened and had meant to apologize sooner, but the longer I'd waited, the more difficult this had become. I assumed that she'd just hang up on me, but she didn't. She seemed genuinely happy to hear from me. I asked her if she wanted to meet for coffee, and the two of us discovered that, even sober, we liked each other. We kissed under an awning in the falling snow — a much different kind of kiss, shy, almost courtly — and then I put her in a cab

to Back Bay, and when I returned to my room, the phone was already ringing.

Thus were the terms established for the next two years of my life. Somehow, the universe had forgiven me my trespasses, my vain ambitions, my casual, self-interested cruelties. I should have been happy and for the most part was. The four of us — Liz and Jonas, Stephanie and I — became a quartet: parties, movies, weekend ski trips to Vermont, and lusty, drunken outings to Cape Cod, where Liz's family had a house left conveniently unoccupied during the off-season. I did not see Stephanie during the week, nor did Jonas see much of Liz, whose life did not seem otherwise to intersect with his own, and the rhythms appeared to work. From Monday to Friday, I worked my tail off; come Friday night, the fun began.

My grades were excellent, and my professors took notice. I was encouraged to begin thinking about where I would pursue my doctoral work. Harvard was at the top of my list, but there were other considerations. My adviser was lobbying for Columbia, the chairman of the department for Rice, where he had taken his PhD and still had close professional connections. I felt like a racehorse up for auction but hardly minded. I was in the gate; soon the bell would ring, and I would commence my mad dash down the track.

Then Lucessi killed himself.

This was in the summer. I'd remained in Cambridge, staying at Mrs. Chodorow's, and had resumed working at the lab. I hadn't spoken to Lucessi since the last day of our freshman year — indeed, had barely thought of him beyond a mild curiosity, never acted on, as to his fate. It was his sister, Arianna, who telephoned me. How she'd

tracked me down, I didn't think to ask. She was clearly in shock; her voice was flat and emotionless, laying out the facts. Lucessi had been working in a video store. He appeared, at first, to have taken his expulsion more or less in stride. The experience had chastened but not broken him. There were vague plans about his attending the local community college, perhaps reapplying to Harvard in a year or two. But across the winter and spring, his tics had gotten worse. He became sullen and uncommunicative, refusing to talk to anyone for days. The low-grade muttering became more or less continual, as if he were engaged in conversation with imaginary persons. A number of disturbing obsessions took hold. He would spend hours reading the daily newspaper, underlining random sentences in wholly unrelated articles, and claimed that the CIA was watching him.

Gradually it became apparent that he was in the throes of a psychotic episode, perhaps even full-blown schizophrenia. His parents made arrangements to have him admitted to a psychiatric hospital, but the night before he was to leave, he disappeared. Apparently he had taken the train to Manhattan. With him, in a canvas bag, was a length of sturdy rope. In Central Park, he had selected a tree with a large rock beneath its boughs, flung the rope over one of the branches, put the noose in place, and stepped off. The distance was not enough to break his neck; he could have regained a foothold on the boulder at any time. But such was his determination that he hadn't done this, and death had been caused by slow strangulation — a horrendous detail I wished Arianna had not shared with me. In his pocket

was a note: *Call Fanning.*

The funeral was scheduled for the following Saturday. Under the circumstances, the family wanted to proceed quietly, with a brief service confined to close family and friends. That I was to be among them was ordained by his note, although I told Arianna that I didn't know what to make of it, which was true. We'd been friends, but not great friends. Our bond had hardly gone deep enough to earn my inclusion in his final thoughts. I wondered if he intended this note as a punishment of some kind, though I could not think what sin I had committed to warrant it. The other possibility was that he was sending me a message of an altogether different nature — that his death was, in a way only he could understand, a demonstration for my benefit. But what it could mean, I hadn't the foggiest.

Jonas was spending the summer on an archaeological dig in Tanzania; Stephanie had won a coveted internship in Washington, working on Capitol Hill, but at the time of Lucessi's death was traveling with her parents in France and could not be reached. I did not think that Lucessi's death had shaken me all that badly, but of course it had — my emotions, like Arianna's, were blunted by shock — yet I showed the good sense to call the one person I trusted whom I could actually get on the phone. Liz's family was on the Cape, but she was working at a bookshop in Connecticut. I'm sorry about your friend, she said. You shouldn't be alone. Meet me at Grand Central at the main kiosk, the one with the four-faced clock.

My train got into Penn Station early Friday morning. I took the 1 train uptown to Forty-

245

second Street, changed to the 7, and arrived at Grand Central at the height of the rush. Except to change buses at Port Authority in the middle of the night, I had never been to New York City, and as I ascended the ramp into the terminal's main concourse, I was, like many a traveler through the ages, bowled over by the majesty of its dimensions. I felt as though I'd entered the grandest of cathedrals, not some mere way station but a destination in its own right, worthy of pilgrimage. Even the tiniest sound seemed magnified by the sheer size of the place. The smoke-stained ceiling, with its images of constellated stars, soared so majestically overhead it seemed to rewrite the dimensions of the world. Liz was waiting for me at the kiosk, wearing a light summer dress and carrying an overnight bag. She hugged me far longer and more tightly than I was prepared for, and it was in the shelter of her embrace that I suddenly felt the weight of Lucessi's death, like a cold stone at the center of my chest.

"We're staying at my parents' apartment in Chelsea," she said. "I won't take no for an answer."

We took a cab downtown, through streets clogged with traffic and great walls of pedestrians that surged forward at every intersection. This was early 1990s New York, a time when the city seemed on the verge of unmanageable chaos, and although I was, later in life, to live in a very different Manhattan — safe, tidy, and affluent — my first impression of the city was so indelible, so charged with heat and light, that it remains my truest vision of the place. The apartment was on the second floor of a brownstone just off Eighth Avenue — two small rooms, compactly furnished, with a view across Twenty-eighth Street of a small

theater known for incomprehensible avant-garde productions and a men's haberdashery called World of Shirts and Socks. Liz had explained that her parents only used the place when they came into the city to shop or take in a show. Probably nobody had been there in months.

The funeral was at ten the next morning. I called Arianna to tell her where I was staying, and she said that she'd arrange for a car to meet us in the morning and drive us to Riverdale. There was no food in the apartment, so Liz and I went up the street to a small café with tables on the sidewalk. She told me what she knew of Jonas, which wasn't very much. She'd received only three letters, none very long. I'd never quite understood what he was doing there — he was a biologist, or wanted to be, not an archaeologist — though I knew it had to do with extracting fossilized pathogens from the bones of early hominids.

"Basically," she said, "he's squatting in the dirt all day long, dusting rocks with a paintbrush."

"Sounds like fun."

"Oh, to him it is."

I knew this to be so. Sharing a room with the man had taught me that, despite his fun-loving exterior, Jonas was deeply serious about his studies, sometimes verging toward obsession. The core of his passion lay in the idea that the human animal was a truly unique organism, evolutionarily distinct. Our powers of reason, of language, of abstract thought — none of these was matched anywhere else in the animal kingdom. Yet despite these gifts, we remained chained to the same physical limitations as every other creature on the earth. We were born, we aged, we died, all of it in a relatively short span of time. From an evolution-

ary point of view, he said, this simply made no sense. Nature craved balance, yet our brains were completely out of sync with the short shelf life of the bodies that housed them.

Think about it, he said: What would the world be like if human beings could live two hundred years? Five hundred? How about a thousand? What leaps of genius would a man be capable of, with a millennium of accumulated wisdom on which to draw? The great mistake of modern biological science, he believed, was to assume that death was natural, when it was anything but, and to view it in terms of isolated failures of the body. Cancer. Heart disease. Alzheimer's. Diabetes. Trying to cure them one by one, he said, was as pointless as swatting at a swarm of bees. You might get a couple, but the swarm would kill you in the end. The key, he said, lay in confronting the whole *question* of death, to turn it on its head. Why should we have to die at all? Could it be that somewhere within the deep molecular coding of our species lay the road map to a next evolutionary step — one in which our physical attributes would be brought into equilibrium with our powers of thought? And wouldn't it make sense that nature, in its genius, intended for us to discover this for ourselves, employing the unique endowments it had afforded us?

He was, in short, making a case for immortality as the apotheosis of the human state. This sounded like mad science to me. The only things missing from his argument were a slab of reassembled body parts and a lightning rod, and I'd told him as much. For me, science wasn't about the big picture but the small one — the same modestly ambitious, hunt-and-peck investigations that Jonas

248

decried as a waste of time. And yet his passion was attractive — even, in its own crackpot way, inspiring. Who wouldn't want to live forever?

"The thing I don't get is why he thinks the way he does," I said. "He seems so sensible otherwise."

My tone was light, but I could tell I'd hit on something. Liz called the waiter over and asked for another glass of wine.

"Well, there's an answer for that," she said. "I thought you knew."

"Knew what?"

"About me."

This was how I came to learn the story. When Liz was eleven, she had been diagnosed with Hodgkin's disease. The cancer had originated in the lymph nodes surrounding her trachea. Surgery, radiation, chemotherapy — she'd had it all. Twice she'd gone into remission, only to have the disease return. Her current remission had lasted four years.

"Maybe I'm cured, or so they tell me. I guess you never know."

I had no idea how to respond. The news was deeply distressing, but anything I might have offered would have been an empty platitude. Yet in a way I could not put my finger on, the information did not seem entirely new to me. I had felt it from the day we'd met: there was a shadow over her life.

"I'm Jonas's pet project, you see," she continued. "I'm the problem he wants to solve. It's pretty noble, when you think about it."

"I don't believe that," I said. "He worships you. It's totally obvious."

She sipped her wine and returned it to the table. "Let me ask you something, Tim. Name one thing

about Jonas Lear that isn't perfect. I'm not talking about the fact that he's always late or picks his nose at traffic lights. Something important."

I searched my thoughts. She was right. I couldn't.

"This is what I'm saying. Handsome, smart, charming, destined for great things. That's our Jonas. Since the day he was born, everybody's loved him. And it makes him feel guilty. *I* make him feel guilty. Did I tell you he wants to marry me? He tells me all the time. *Say the word, Liz, and I'll buy the ring.* Which is ridiculous. Me, who might not live past twenty-five, or whatever the statistics say. And even if the cancer doesn't come back, I can't have children. The radiation took care of that."

It was getting late; I could feel the city changing around me, its energies shifting. Down the block, people were stepping from the theater, hailing cabs, going in search of drinks or food. I was tired and overloaded by the emotions of the last few days. I signaled the waiter for the bill.

"I'll tell you something else," Liz said as we were paying the tab. "He really admires you."

This was, in some ways, the strangest news of all. "Why would he admire *me*?"

"Oh, a lot of reasons. But I think it comes down to the fact that you're something he can't ever be. Authentic, maybe? I'm not talking about being modest, although you are. Too modest, if you ask me. You underestimate yourself. But there's something . . . I don't know, pure about you. A resilience. I saw it the moment I met you. I don't mean to put you on the spot, but the one good thing about cancer, and I mean the *only* thing, is it teaches you to be honest."

250

I felt embarrassed. "I'm just a kid from Ohio who did well on his SATs. There's nothing interesting about me at all."

She paused, gazing into her glass, then said, "I've never asked you about your family, Tim, and I don't mean to pry. All I know is what Jonas has told me. You never mention them, they never call, you spend all your breaks in Cambridge with this woman and her cats."

I shrugged. "She's not so bad."

"I'm sure she isn't. I'm sure she's a saint. And I like cats as much as the next person, in the right quantity."

"There's not really much to tell."

"I doubt that very much."

A silence followed. I discovered that swallowing took a great deal of effort; my windpipe felt as if it had constricted. When at last I spoke, the words seemed to come from another place entirely.

"She died."

Behind her glasses, Liz's eyes were intently fixed on my face. "Who died, Tim?"

I swallowed. "My mother. My mother died."

"When was this?"

It would all come out now; there was simply no stopping it. "Last summer. It was just before I met you. I didn't even know she was sick. My father wrote me a letter."

"And where were you?"

"With the woman and her cats."

Something was happening. Something was coming undammed. I knew that if I didn't move immediately — stand up, walk around, feel the beating of my heart and the action of air in my lungs — I would fall apart.

"Tim, why didn't you tell us?"

I shook my head. I felt suddenly ashamed. "I don't know."

Liz reached across the table and gently took my hand. Despite my best efforts, I had begun to cry. For my mother, for myself, for my dead friend Lucessi, whom I knew I had failed. Surely I could have done something, said something. It wasn't the note in his pocket that told me so. It was the fact that I was alive and he was dead, and I of all people should have understood the pain of living in a world that didn't seem to want him. I did not want to take my hand away — it felt like the only thing anchoring me to the earth. I was in a dream in which I was flying and could not make myself land were it not for this woman who would save me.

"It's all right," Liz was saying, "it's all right, it's all right . . ."

Time moved then; we were walking, I didn't know where. Liz was still holding my hand. I sensed the presence of water, and then the Hudson emerged. Decrepit piers jutted long fingers into the water. Across the river's broad expanse, the lights of Hoboken made a diorama of the city and its lives. The air tasted of salt and stone. There was a kind of park along the water's edge, filthy and abandoned-looking; it did not seem safe, so we headed north along Twelfth Avenue, neither of us speaking, before turning east again. I had given no thought at all to what would happen next but now began to. In the last hour, Liz had spoken of things that I felt certain she had told no other person, just as I had done with her. There was Jonas to think of, but we were also a man and a woman who had shared the most intimate truths, things that, once said, could never

be unsaid.

We arrived at the apartment. No words of consequence had passed between us for many minutes. The tension was palpable — surely she could feel it, too. I couldn't say for certain what I wanted, only that I didn't want to be away from her, not for a minute. I was standing dumbly in the middle of the tiny room, searching my mind for the words to capture how I felt. Something needed to be said. And yet I could say nothing.

It was Liz who broke the silence. "Well, I'm going to turn in. The sofa folds out. There are sheets and blankets in the closet. Let me know if you need anything else."

"Okay."

I could not make myself move toward her, though I wanted to, very badly. On the one hand there was Liz, and all we had shared, and the fact that, in every way, I loved her and probably had since the day we'd met; on the other, there was Jonas, the man who'd given me a life.

"Your friend Lucessi. What was his first name?"

I actually had to think. "Frank. But I never called him that."

"Why do you think he did it?"

"He was in love with somebody. She didn't love him back."

Not until that moment had this chain of thought, in all its starkness, come clear to me. *Call Fanning,* my friend had written. *Call Fanning to tell him that love is all there is, and love is pain, and love is taken away.*

"What time is the car?" she asked.

"Eight o'clock."

"I'm going with you, you know."

"I'm glad you are."

A frozen moment passed.

"Well," Liz said, "I guess that's it." She retreated to the bedroom door, where she paused and turned to face me again. "Stephanie is a lucky girl, you know. I'm just saying that in case you haven't figured it out."

Then she was gone. I stripped to my boxers and lay on the couch. Under different circumstances, I might have felt foolish, daring to think that such a woman would take me into her bed. But I actually felt relieved; Liz had chosen the honorable route, making the decision for both of us. It occurred to me that not once, neither at the restaurant nor as we'd walked, had I thought of Stephanie in the context of any betrayal I might have contemplated. The day felt like a year; through the windows, I heard the wash of the city, an oceanic sound. It seemed to creep into my chest, where it matched itself to the rhythm of my breathing. Exhaustion poured through my bones, and soon I drifted off.

Sometime later, I awoke. I had the unmistakable sense of being watched. A sensation, vaguely electrical, lingered on my forehead, as if I had been kissed. I rose onto my elbows, expecting to see someone standing over me. But the room was empty, and I thought I must have dreamed this.

About the funeral, there is little to say. To describe it in detail would be a violation of its confidential grief, its closed circuit of pain. During the service, I kept my eyes on Arianna, wondering what she was feeling. Did she know? I wanted her to know, but I also didn't; she was just a girl. No good could come of it.

I declined the family's invitation to lunch; Liz

254

and I returned to the apartment to retrieve my luggage. On the platform at Penn Station she hugged me, then, revising her thoughts, kissed me quickly on the cheek.

"So, okay?"

I didn't know if she meant me or the two of us. "Sure," I said. "Never better."

"Call me if you get too blue."

I stepped aboard. Liz was watching me through the windows as I made my way down the car to find an empty seat. I remembered boarding the bus to Cleveland, that long-ago September day — the drops of rain on the window, my mother's crinkled bag in my lap, looking to see if my father had stayed to watch my departure, finding him gone. I took a seat beside the window. Liz had yet to move. She saw me, smiled, waved; I waved back. A deep mechanical shudder; the train began to move. She was still standing there, following my carriage with her gaze, as we entered the tunnel and disappeared.

18

May 1992: The last of my coursework had been completed. I was to graduate summa cum laude; offers of generous graduate fellowships had come my way. MIT, Columbia, Princeton, Rice. Harvard, which had decided it had not seen the last of me if I cared to stay on. It was the obvious choice, one I felt bound to make in the end, though I had not committed, preferring to savor the possibilities for as long as I could. Jonas would be going back to Tanzania for the summer, then heading to the University of Chicago to start his doctoral work; Liz would be going to Berkeley for

255

her master's in Renaissance literature; Stephanie was returning to Washington to work for a political consulting firm. The graduation ceremony itself would not happen until the first week of June. We had entered a nether time, a caesura between what our lives had been and what they would become.

In the meanwhile, there were parties — lots of them. Roiling keggers, black-tie balls, a garden fete where everyone drank mint juleps and all the girls wore hats. In my trusty battle tux and pink tie — wearing it had become a trademark — I danced the Lindy, the Electric Slide, the Hokey Pokey, and the Bump; at any given hour of the day, I was either drunk or hungover. An hour of triumph, but it came at a cost. For the first time in my life, I felt the pain of missing people I had not yet left.

The week before graduation, Jonas, Liz, Stephanie, and I drove down to the Cape, to Liz's house. No one was talking about it, but it seemed unlikely that the four of us would be together again for some time. Liz's parents were there, having just opened the house for the season. I had met them before, in Connecticut. Her mother, Patty, came across as a bit of a society doyenne, with a brisk, somewhat phony graciousness and a lock-jawed accent, but her father was one of the most likable and easygoing people I'd ever met. A tall, bespectacled man (Liz had gotten his vision) with an earnest face, Oscar Macomb had been a banker, retired early, and now, in his words, spent his days "noodling around with money." He worshipped his daughter — that was plain to anyone with eyes; less apparent, though undeniable, was that he vastly preferred her to his wife,

whom he regarded with the bemused affection one might give to an overbred poodle. With Liz, the man was all smiles — the two of them would frequently chatter away in French — and his warmth extended to anybody in her circle, including me, whom he had nicknamed "Ohio Tim."

The house, in a town called Osterville, stood on a bluff overlooking Nantucket Sound. It was enormous, room upon room, with a wide back lawn and rickety stairs to the beach. No doubt it was worth many millions of dollars, just for the land alone, though in those days I had no ability to calculate such things. Despite its size, it had a homey, unfussy feel. Most of the furniture looked like you could pick it up for pennies at a yard sale; in the afternoons, when the wind swung around, it tore through the house like the offensive line of the New York Giants. The ocean was still too cold for swimming, and because it was so early in the season, the town was mostly deserted. We spent our days lying on the beach, pretending not to be freezing, or lazing around on the porch, playing cards and reading, until evening arrived and the drinks came out. My father might have had a beer before dinner while he watched the news on television, but that was the extent of it; my mother never drank at all. In the Macomb household, cocktail hour was religion. At six o'clock everyone would gather in the living room or, if the evening was pleasant, on the porch, whereupon Liz's father would present us with a silver tray of the evening's concoction — whiskey old-fashioneds, Tom Collinses, vodka martinis in chilled glasses with olives on sticks — accompanied by dainty porcelain cups of nuts warmed in the oven. This was followed by ample quantities of wine with

dinner and sometimes whiskey or port afterward. I had hoped our days on the Cape would give my liver a chance to recuperate; there was no chance of that.

Jonas and I were sharing a bedroom, the girls another, located at opposite ends of the house with Liz's parents in between. When we'd come here during the academic term, we'd had the place, and our choice of sleeping arrangements, to ourselves. But not this time. I'd expected that the situation would lead to a certain amount of creeping around in the wee hours, but Liz forbade it. "Please do not shock the grown-ups," she said. "We'll all be shocking them soon enough."

Which was just as well. By this time, I had begun to tire of Stephanie. She was a wonderful girl, but I did not love her. There was nothing about her that made this so; she was in every way deserving. My heart was simply elsewhere, and it made me feel like a hypocrite. Since the funeral in New York, Liz and I had not spoken of my mother, or her cancer, or the night when we had walked the city streets together but in the end had chosen to step back from the abyss and keep our allegiances intact. Yet it was clear that the night had left its mark on both of us. Our friendship, until that time, had flowed through Jonas. A new circuit had been opened — not through him but around him — and along this pathway pulsed a private current of intimacy. We knew what had happened; we had been there. I had felt it, and I was sure she'd felt it too, and the fact that we'd done nothing only deepened this connection, even more than if we'd fallen into bed together. We would be sitting on the porch, each of us reading one of the mildew-smelling paperbacks left behind by other

258

guests; we would look up at just the same moment, our eyes would meet, an ironic smile would flash at the corners of her mouth, which I'd return in kind. *Look at us,* we were saying to each other, *aren't we the trusty twosome. If only they knew how loyal we are. We should get a prize.*

I intended to do nothing about this, of course. I owed Jonas that much and more. Nor did I think Liz would have welcomed the attempt. The connection she shared with Jonas, one of long history, ran deeper than ours ever could. The house, with its endless warren of rooms and ocean views and shabbily genteel furnishings, reminded me how true this was. I was a visitor to this world, welcomed and even, as Liz had told me, admired. But a tourist nonetheless. Our night together, though indelible, had been just that: a night. Still, it thrilled me just being around her. The way she held her drink to her lips. Her habit of pushing her glasses to her forehead to read the smallest print. How she smelled, which I will not attempt to name, because it wasn't like anything else. Pain or pleasure? It was both. I wanted to bathe in her existence. Was she dying? I tried not to think about it. I was happy to be near her at all and accepted the situation as it stood.

Two days before our departure, Liz's father announced that we would be eating lobsters for dinner. (He did all the cooking; I'd never seen Patty so much as fry an egg.) This was for my benefit; he had learned, to his alarm, that I had never eaten one. He returned from the fish market in the late afternoon bearing a sack of squirming red-black monsters, removed one with a carnivore's grin, and made me hold it. No doubt I looked horrified; everyone had a good laugh, but I

didn't mind. I loved her father a little for it, in fact. A lazy rain had been falling all day, sapping our energy; now we had a purpose. As if in acknowledgment of this fact, the sun emerged in time for the festivities; Jonas and I carried the dining table out to the back porch. I had noticed something about him. In the last couple of days, he had adopted a manner I could only describe as secretive. Something was afoot. At the cocktail hour, we drank bottles of dark beer (the only proper accompaniment, Oscar explained); then on to the main event. With great solemnity, Oscar presented me with a lobster bib. I had never understood this infantile practice; no one else was wearing one, and I felt a bit resentful until I cracked a claw and sprayed lobster juice all over myself, to an explosion of table-wide hilarity.

Imagine the perfection of the scene. The table with its red-checkered cloth; the ridiculous bounty of the feast; the golden sunset streaming toward us across the sound, then sinking into the sea with a final flash like an elegant gentleman tipping his hat in farewell. The candles came out, polishing our faces with their flickering glow. How had my life led me to such a place, among such people? I wondered what my parents would have said. My mother would have been pleased for me; wherever she was, I hoped its rules included the power to observe the living. As for my father, I didn't know. I had severed all ties completely. I saw now how unfair I'd been and vowed to get in touch. Perhaps it was not too late for him to make my graduation.

When we'd finished dessert — a strawberry-rhubarb pie — Jonas clinked his glass with his fork.

"Everybody, if I could have your attention."

He rose and moved around the table so that he was standing next to Liz. With a little grunt of effort, he turned her chair so she was facing him.

"Jonas," she said with a laugh, "what the hell are you doing?"

His hand fumbled in his pocket, and I knew. My stomach plunged, then the rest of me. As he bent to one knee, my friend withdrew the small velvet box. He opened the lid and held it before her. A huge, nervous grin was on his face. I saw the stone. It was enormous, made for a queen.

"Liz, I know we've talked about it. But I wanted to make it official. I feel like I've loved you all my life."

"Jonas, I don't know what to say." She looked up and laughed uneasily. Her cheeks were flushed with embarrassment. "This is so corny!"

"Say yes. That's all you have to do. I promise to give you everything you want in life."

I wanted to be ill.

"C'mon," Stephanie said. "What are you waiting for?"

Liz looked at her father. "At least tell me he asked you first."

The man was smiling, a conspirator. "That he did."

"And what did you tell him, O wise man?"

"Honey, it's really your decision. It's a big step. But I'll say I'm not opposed."

"Mom?"

Ever so slightly, the woman was crying. She nodded ardently, speechless.

"God," Stephanie moaned, "I can't stand the suspense! If you don't marry him, I will."

As Liz looked back at Jonas, did her eyes pause

261

at my face? My memory says she did, though perhaps I imagined this.

"Well, I, um —"

Jonas removed the ring from the box. "Put it on. That's all you have to do. Make me the happiest man alive."

She stared at it, expressionless. The damn thing was fat as a tooth.

"Please," said Jonas.

She looked up. "Yes," she said, and nodded. "My answer is yes."

"You really mean it?"

"Don't be dense, Jonas. Of course I mean it." At last she smiled. "Get over here."

They embraced, then kissed; Jonas slid the ring onto her finger. I looked out over the water, unable to bear the scene. But even its broad blue expanse seemed to mock me.

"Oh!" Liz's mother cried. "I'm so happy!"

"Now, no sneaking around tonight, you two," her father laughed. "You're in separate rooms for the duration. Save it for the wedding night."

"Daddy, don't be gross!"

Jonas turned to her father and extended his hand. "Thank you, sir. Thank you from the bottom of my heart. I'll do everything in my power to make her happy."

They shook. "I know you will, son."

Out came the champagne, which Liz's father had kept in the wings. Glasses were filled, then raised.

"To the happy couple," Oscar said. "Long lives, happiness, a house full of love."

The champagne was delicious. It must have cost a bundle. I could barely swallow it down.

■ ■ ■ ■

I couldn't sleep. I didn't want to.

As soon as I was sure Jonas was out cold, I snuck from the house. It was well after midnight; the moon, fat and white, had risen over the sound. I had no plan, only the desire to be alone with my feelings of desolation. I removed my shoes and took the stairs to the beach. Not a breath of wind blew; the world felt stuck. The tiniest of waves lapped upon the shore. I began to walk. The sand beneath my feet was still damp from the day of rain. The houses above me were all dark, some still boarded up, like tombs.

At a distance I saw someone sitting in the sand. It was Liz. I halted, uncertain what to do. She was holding a champagne bottle. She lifted it to her mouth and took a long drink. She noticed me, then looked away, but the damage was done; I couldn't turn back now.

I sat on the sand beside her. "Hey."

"Of course it would be you," she said, slurring her words.

"Why 'of course'?"

She took another swig. The ring was on her finger. "I noticed you didn't say anything tonight. It's considered polite, you know, to congratulate the bride-to-be."

"Okay, congratulations."

"You say that with such conviction." She sighed mournfully. "Jesus, am I drunk. Get this away from me."

She passed me the bottle. Just the dregs remained; I wished there were more. There were times to be sober, and this wasn't one of them. I

polished it off and tossed it away.

"If you didn't want to, why did you say yes?"

"With everyone staring at me? You try it."

"So back out. He'll understand."

"No, he won't. He'll ask and ask, and I'll eventually give in and be the luckiest woman on earth, to be married to Jonas Lear."

We were quiet for a time.

"Can I ask you something?" I said.

She laughed sarcastically. Her gaze was cast over the sea. "Why not? Everybody's doing it."

"That night in New York. I was asleep, and something happened. I felt something."

"Did you now."

"Yes, I did." I waited. Liz said nothing. "Did you . . . kiss me?"

"Now, why would I do a thing like that?"

She was looking right at me. "Liz —"

"Shhh." A frozen moment followed. Our faces were just a foot apart. Then she did something puzzling. She took off her glasses and put them in my hand.

"You know, without these, I can't see anything. What's funny is that it's like nobody can see me, either. Isn't that strange? I kind of feel invisible."

I absolutely could have done it. *Should* have done it, long before. Why hadn't I? Why hadn't I taken her in my arms and pressed my mouth to hers and told her how I felt, consequences be damned? Who's to say I couldn't give her just as good a life? *Marry me*, I thought. *Marry me instead. Or don't marry anyone at all. Stay just as you are, and I will love you forever, as I do now, because you are the other half of me.*

"Oh, God," she said. "I think I'm going to throw up."

Then she did; she turned her face away and retched onto the sand. I held her hair back as all the lobster and champagne came up and out of her.

"I'm sorry, Tim." She was crying a little. "I'm so sorry."

I lifted her to her feet. She was mumbling more apologies as I draped her arm over my shoulders. She was close to dead weight now. Somehow I managed to haul her up the stairs and prop her in a chair on the divan on the porch. I was at a total loss; how would this look? I couldn't take her up to her room, not with Stephanie there. I doubted I could have gotten her up the stairs anyway without waking the entire house. I drew her upright again and carried her to the living room. The sofa would have to do; she could always say she'd had trouble sleeping and come downstairs to read. A crocheted blanket lay across the back of the sofa; I pulled it over her. She was fast asleep now. I got a glass of water from the kitchen and put it on the coffee table where she could find it, then took a chair to watch her. Her breathing became deep and even, her face slack. I allowed some more time to pass to be certain she would not be sick again, and got to my feet. There was something I needed to do. I bent over her and kissed her on the forehead.

"Good night," I whispered. "Good night, good-bye."

I crept up the stairs. Dawn wasn't far off; through the open windows, I could hear the birds beginning to sing. I made my way down the hall to the room I shared with Jonas. I gently turned the handle and stepped inside, but not before I heard, behind me, the snap of a closing door.

■ ■ ■ ■

The cab rolled up the drive at six A.M. I was waiting on the porch with my bag.

"Where to?" the driver asked.

"The bus station."

He glanced up through the windshield. "You really live in this place?"

"No chance of that."

I was putting my bag in the trunk when the door of the house opened. Stephanie came striding down the walk, wearing one of the long T-shirts she slept in. It was actually one of mine.

"Sneaking off, are you? I saw the whole thing, you know."

"It wasn't what you thought."

"Sure it wasn't. You're a total asshole, you know that?"

"I'm aware of that, yes."

She rocked her face upward, hands on her hips. "God. How could I be so blind? It was totally obvious."

"Do me a favor, will you?"

"Are you kidding me?"

"Jonas can't ever know."

She laughed bitterly. "Oh, believe me, the last thing I want is to get mixed up with this mess. It's your problem."

"Feel free to think of it that way."

"What do you want me to tell them? As long as I'm being such a fucking liar."

I thought for a moment. "I don't care. A sick relative. It doesn't really matter."

"Just tell me: did you ever think about *me* in any of this? Did I even once cross your mind?"

266

I didn't know what to say.

"Fuck you," she said, and strode away.

I lowered myself into the cab. The driver was filling out a slip of paper on a clipboard. He glanced at me through the rearview. "Kinda rough, pal," he said. "Trust me, I've been there."

"I'm not really in the mood to talk, thanks."

He tossed his clipboard onto the dash. "I was only trying to be nice."

"Well, don't," I said, and with that we drove away.

19

I left them all behind.

I did not attend graduation. Back in Cambridge, I packed my belongings — three years later, there still wasn't much — and telephoned the biochemistry department at Rice. Of all the programs I had been accepted to, it possessed the virtue of being the farthest away, in a city I knew nothing about. It was a Saturday, so I had to leave a message, but yes, I told them, I'd be coming. I thought about abandoning my tuxedo; perhaps the next occupant would get some use out of it. But this seemed peevish and overly symbolic, and I could always throw it out later. Waiting outside, double-parked, was a rental car. As I closed my suitcase, the phone began to ring, and I ignored it. I carried my things downstairs, dropped off my key at the Winthrop House office, and drove away.

I arrived in Mercy in the middle of the night. I felt as if I'd been gone for a century. I slept in my car outside the house and awoke to the sound of tapping on the window. My father.

"What are you doing here?"

He was wearing a bathrobe; he had come out of the house to get the Sunday paper and noticed the car. He had aged a great deal, in the manner of someone who no longer cared much about his appearance. He had not shaved; his breath was bad. I followed him into the house, which seemed eerily the same, though it was very dusty and smelled like old food.

"Are you hungry?" he asked me. "I was going to have cereal, but I think I have some eggs."

"That's all right," I said. "I wasn't really planning on staying. I just wanted to say hello."

"Let me put some coffee on."

I waited in the living room. I had expected to be nervous, but I wasn't. I wasn't really feeling much of anything. My father returned from the kitchen with two mugs and sat across from me.

"You look taller," he said.

"I'm actually the same height. You must remember me wrong."

We drank our coffee.

"So, how was college? I know you just graduated. They sent me a form."

"It was fine, thank you."

"That's all you've got to say about it?" The question wasn't peevish; he merely seemed interested.

"Mostly." I shrugged. "I fell in love. It didn't really work out, though."

He thought for a moment. "I suppose you'll want to visit your mother."

"That would be nice."

I asked him to stop at a grocery store so I could pick up some flowers. They didn't have much, just daisies and carnations, but I did not think my mother would mind, and I told the girl behind the counter to wrap them with some greens to make

them nice. We drove out of town. The interior of my father's Buick was full of fast-food trash. I held up a bag from McDonald's. A few dried-out fries rattled inside it.

"You shouldn't eat this stuff," I said.

We arrived at the cemetery, parked, and walked the rest of the way. It was a pleasant morning. We were passing through a sea of graves. My mother's headstone was located in the area for cremations: smaller headstones, spaced close together. Hers had just her name, Lorraine Fanning, and the dates. She had been fifty-seven.

I put the flowers down and stepped back. I thought about certain days, things we'd done together, about being her son.

"It's not bad to be here," I said. "I thought it might be."

"I don't come all that much. I guess I should." My father took a long breath. "I really screwed this up. I know that."

"It's all right. It's all over now."

"I'm kind of falling apart. I have diabetes, my blood pressure's through the roof. I'm forgetting things, too. Like yesterday, I had to sew a button on my shirt, and I couldn't find the scissors."

"So go to a doctor."

"It seems like a lot of trouble." He paused. "The girl you're in love with. What's she like?"

I thought for a moment. "Smart. Beautiful. Kind of sarcastic, but in a funny way. There wasn't one thing that did it, though."

"I think that's how it's supposed to be. That's how it was with your mother."

I looked up, into the spring day. Seven hundred miles away, in Cambridge, the graduation ceremony would be just getting rolling. I wondered

269

what my friends were thinking about me.

"She loved you very much."

"I loved her, too." I looked at him and smiled. "It's nice here," I said. "Thanks for bringing me."

We returned to the house.

"If you want I can make up your room," my father said. "I left it just as it was. It's probably not very clean, though."

"Actually, I need to get going. I have a long drive."

He seemed a little sad. "Well. All right then." He walked me to my car. "Where are you off to?"

"Texas."

"What's there?"

"Texans, I guess." I shrugged. "More school."

"Do you need any money?"

"They're giving me a stipend. I should be all right."

"Well, let me know if you need more. You're welcome to it."

We shook hands and then, somewhat awkwardly, embraced. If I'd had to guess, I would have said my father wasn't going to live much longer. This turned out to be true; we would see each other only four more times before the heart attack that killed him. He was alone in the house when it happened. Because it was a weekend, several days would pass before anybody noticed he was missing and thought to look.

I got into the car. My father was standing above me. He motioned with his hand for me to roll down the window. "Call me when you get there, okay?"

I told him I would, and I did.

In Houston, I rented the first apartment I looked

270

at, a garage studio with a view of the back of a Mexican restaurant, and got a job shelving books at the Rice library to tide myself over for the summer. The city was strange-looking and hotter than the mouth of hell, but it suited me. We search for ourselves in our surroundings, and everything I saw was either brand-new or falling apart. Most of the city was quite ugly — a sea of low-rise retail, shabby apartment complexes, and enormous, overcrowded freeways piloted by maniacs — but the area around the university was rather posh, with large, well-kept houses and wide boulevards flanked by live oaks so perfectly manicured they looked less like trees than sculptures of trees. For six hundred dollars, I bought my first car, a snot-yellow 1983 Chevy Citation with bald tires, 230,000 miles on the odometer, and a sagging vinyl ceiling I used a staple gun to reattach. I'd heard nothing from Liz or Jonas, but of course they had no idea where I was. There was a time in America when it was still possible to disappear by going left when everybody expected you to go right. With a little digging, they probably could have found me — a few well-placed calls to a few department chairs — but this presupposed that they would want to. I had no idea what they would want. I didn't think I ever had.

Classes began. About my studies, there is not much to say except that they occupied me utterly. I made friends with the department secretary, a black woman in her fifties who basically ran the place; she confided to me that nobody in the department had actually expected me to come. I was, in her words, "a prize thoroughbred they had bought for pennies on the dollar." To describe my fellow graduate students as antisocial would be

271

the understatement of the century; no lawn parties here. Their minds were utterly unfettered by thoughts of fun. They also despised me for the naked favoritism shown me by my professors. I kept my head down, my nose to the stone. I adopted the practice of taking long drives in the Texas countryside. It was windblown, flat, without meaningful demarcation, every square of dirt the same as every other. I liked to pull the car to the side of the road someplace completely arbitrary and just look at it.

The one eastern habit I retained was reading *The New York Times,* and in this manner I learned that Liz and Jonas had made it official. This was in the fall of '93; a year had passed. "Mr. and Mrs. Oscar Macomb, of Greenwich, Connecticut, and Osterville, Massachusetts, are pleased to announce the marriage of their daughter, Elizabeth Christina, to Jonas Abbott Lear of Beverly, Massachusetts. The bride, a graduate of Harvard, recently completed a master's degree in literature at the University of California, Berkeley, and is currently a doctoral student in Renaissance studies at the University of Chicago, where the groom, also a Harvard graduate, is pursuing a PhD in microbiology."

Two days later, I received a large manila envelope from my father. Inside was another envelope, to which he'd affixed a sticky note, apologizing for taking so long to forward it. It was an invitation, of course, postmarked the previous June. I put it aside for a day, then, the next night, in the company of a bottle of bourbon, sat at the kitchen table and peeled back the flap. Ceremony to be held September 4, 1993, St. Andrew's-by-the-Sea, Hyannis Port. Reception to follow at the home of

Oscar and Patricia Macomb, 41 Sea View Avenue, Osterville, Massachusetts. In the margin was a message:

Please please please come. Jonas says so too. We miss you terribly.

Love, L

I looked at this for some time. I was sitting in the window of my apartment, facing the alley behind the restaurant, with its reeking Dumpsters. As I watched, a kitchen worker, a small, round-bellied Hispanic man in a stained apron, came through the door. He was carrying a garbage bag; he opened one of the Dumpsters, tossed the bag inside, and closed the lid with a clang. I expected him to go back inside, but instead he lit a cigarette and stood there, inhaling the smoke with long, hungry drags.

I rose from the table. I kept them in my bureau, wrapped in a sock: Liz's glasses. I had put them in my pocket that night on the beach and forgotten all about them until I was in the cab, by which time it was too late to return them. Now I put them on; they were a little small for my face, the lenses quite strong. I sat back down at the window and watched the man smoke in the alleyway, the image distorted and far away, as if I were looking through the wrong end of a telescope or sitting at the bottom of the sea, gazing upward through miles of water.

20

Here I must leap ahead in time, because that is what time did. I finished my degree at a quickstep;

273

this was followed by a postdoc at Stanford, then a faculty appointment at Columbia, where I was tenured in due course. Within professional circles, I became well known. My reputation increased; the world came calling. I traveled widely, speaking for lucrative fees. Grants flowed my way without difficulty; such was my reputation, I barely had to fill out the forms. I became the holder of multiple patents, two purchased by pharmaceutical concerns for outrageous sums that set me up for life. I refereed important journals. I sat on elite boards. I testified before Congress and was, at various times, a member of the Senate Special Commission on Bioethics, the President's Council on Science and Technology, the NASA advisory board, and the U.N. Task Force on Biological Diversity.

Along the way, I married. The first time, when I was thirty, lasted four years, the second half that. Each woman had, at one time, been my student, a matter of some awkwardness — chummy glances from male colleagues, raised eyebrows from the higher-ups, frosty exchanges with my female co-workers and the wives of friends. Timothy Fanning, that lothario, that dirty old man (though I had not turned forty). My third wife, Julianna, was just twenty-three the day we married. Our union was impulsive, forged in the furnace of sex; two hours after she graduated, we attacked each other like dogs. Though I was very fond of her, I found her bewildering. Her tastes in music and movies, the books she read, her friends, the things she thought important: none made a lick of sense to me.

I was not, like many a man of a certain age, trying to prop up my self-esteem with a young woman's body. I did not mourn the years' unravel-

ing, or fear death unduly, or grieve my waning youth. To the contrary, I liked the many things my success had brought me. Wealth, esteem, authority, good tables at restaurants and hot towels on planes — the whole kit and caboodle that history awards the conquerors: for all of these, I had time's passage to thank. Yet what I was doing was obvious, even to me. I was trying to recapture the one thing I had lost, that life had denied me. Each of my wives, and the many women in between — all far younger than I was, the age gap widening with every one I took into my bed — was a facsimile of Liz. I speak neither of their appearances, though all belonged to a recognizable physical type (pale, slender, myopic), nor of their temperaments, which possessed a similar brainy combativeness. I mean that I wanted them to *be* her, so I could feel alive.

That Jonas and I should cross paths was inevitable; we belonged to the same world. Our first reunion occurred at a conference in Toronto in 2002. Enough time had gone by that we both managed to make no reference to my abrupt severing of the relationship. We were all "how the hell are you" and "you haven't changed a bit" and vowed to keep in better touch, as if we'd been in touch at all. He had returned to Harvard, of course — it ran in the family. He felt himself to be on the verge of some kind of breakthrough, though he was secretive about this, and I didn't press. Of Liz, he offered only the bare-bones professional data. She was teaching at Boston College; she liked it, her students worshipped her, she was working on a book. I told him to say hello for me and let it go at that.

The following year, I received a Christmas card.

It was one of those photograph cards that people use to parade their beautiful children, though the image showed only the two of them. The shot had been taken in some arid locale; they were dressed head to foot in khaki and wearing honest-to-God pith helmets. A note from Liz was written on the back, penned in a hurried script, as if added at the last second: *Jonas said he ran into you. Glad you're doing well!*

Year by year, the cards kept coming. Each showed them in a different exotic setting: atop elephants in India, posing before the Great Wall of China, standing at the bow of a ship in heavy parkas with a glacial coastline in the background. All very cheery, yet there was something depressing about these photos, a mood of compensation. *What a great life we're having! Really! Swear to God!* I began to notice other things. Jonas was the same hale specimen he'd always been, but Liz was aging precipitously, and not just physically. In previous pictures, her eyes had been distracted in a manner that made the photo seem incidental to the moment. Now she looked at the camera dead-on, like a hostage made to pose with a newspaper. Her smile felt manufactured, a product of her will. Was I imagining this? Furthermore, was it fancy on my part that her darkening gaze was a message meant for me? And what of their bodies? In the first photograph, taken in the desert, Lear was standing behind her, wrapping her with his arms. Year by year, they separated. The last one I received, in 2010, had been taken at a café beside a river that was unmistakably the Seine. They were sitting across from each other, far out of arm's reach. Glasses of wine stood on the table. My old roommate's was nearly empty. Liz had touched

hers not at all.

At the same time, rumors began to swirl about Jonas. I had always known him to be a man of ardent if somewhat outlandish passions, but the stories I heard were disturbing. Jonas Lear, it was said, had gone off the deep end. His research had drifted into fantasy. His last paper, published in *Nature,* had danced around the subject, but people had begun to use the V-word in connection to him. He hadn't published anything since, or appeared at the usual conferences, where a good deal of barroom hilarity transpired at his expense. Some of his colleagues even went so far as to conjecture that his tenure was in jeopardy. A certain amount of schadenfreude was built into our profession, the theory being that one man's fall was another man's rise. But I became genuinely worried for him.

It was not long after Julianna tossed in the towel on our ersatz marriage that I received a call from a man named Paul Kiernan. I had met him once or twice; he was a cell biologist at Harvard, a junior colleague of Jonas's, with an excellent reputation. I could tell that the conversation made him uncomfortable. He had learned of our long association; the gist of his call was his concern that his tenure case might be adversely affected by his connection to Jonas. Might I write a letter on his behalf? My initial instinct was to tell him to grow up, that he was lucky to even know such a man, gossip be damned. But given the ignominious workings of tenure committees, I knew he had a point.

"A lot of it has to do with his wife, actually," Paul said. "You've got to feel for the guy."

I practically dropped the phone. "What are you

talking about?"

"I'm sorry, I thought you knew, being such good friends and all. She's very sick, it doesn't look good. I guess I shouldn't have said anything."

"I'll write your letter," I said, and hung up.

I was completely at a loss. I looked up Liz's number at Boston College and began to dial, then put the phone back in its cradle. What would I say, after so many years? What right did I have at this late date to reinsert myself into her life? Liz was dying; I'd never stopped loving her, not for a second, but she was another man's wife. At a time like this, their bond was paramount; if I had learned anything from my parents, it was that the journey of death was one that spouses took together. Maybe it was just the old cowardice returning, but I did not pick up the phone again.

I waited for news. Every day I checked the *Times'* obituary page, in a grim death watch. I was short with colleagues, avoided my friends. I had turned the apartment over to Julianna and sublet a one-bedroom in the West Village, making it easy to disappear, to recede into the fringes of life. What would I do when my Liz was gone? I realized that in some drawer of my brain I had kept the idea that someday, somehow, we would be together. Perhaps they would divorce. Perhaps Jonas would die. Now I had no hope.

Then one night, close to Christmas, the phone rang. It was nearly midnight; I had just settled into bed.

"Tim?"

"Yes, this is Tim Fanning." I was annoyed by the lateness of the call and did not recognize the voice.

"It's Liz."

My heart crashed into my ribs. I could not form words.

"Hello?"

"I'm here," I managed to say. "It's good to hear your voice. Where are you?"

"I'm in Greenwich, at my mother's."

I noted that she did not say "my parents'." Oscar was no more.

"I need to see you," she said.

"Of course. Of course you can." I was madly fumbling in the drawer for a pencil. "I'll drop everything. Just tell me where and when."

She would be taking the train into the city the next day. She had something to do first, and we planned to meet at Grand Central at five o'clock, before she returned to Greenwich.

I left my office well ahead of time, wanting to arrive first. It had rained all day, but as the early winter darkness fell, the rain changed to snow. The subway was jammed; everything felt like it was moving in slow motion. I arrived at the station and took my position beneath the clock with minutes to spare. The heedless crowds streamed by — commuters in raincoats with umbrellas tucked under the arms, the women wearing running shoes over their stockings, snow clinging to everyone's hair. Many were carrying shopping bags brightly decorated for the season. Macy's. Nordstrom. Bergdorf Goodman. Just the thought of these happy, hopeful people irritated me more than I can say. How could they think about Christmas at a time like this? How could they think about anything at all? Didn't they know what was about to happen in this place?

Then she appeared. The sight of her nearly

undid me; I felt as if I were awakening from a long sleep. She was wearing a dark trench coat; a silk scarf covered her hair. She threaded her way toward me through the hurrying mobs. It was absurd, but I was afraid that she would never make it, that the crowds would swallow her, as in a dream. She caught my eye, smiled, and made a "move along" gesture behind the back of a man who was blocking her path. I pushed my way to her.

"And there you are," she said.

What followed was the warmest, most deeply felt hug of my life. Just the smell of her drowned my senses in joy. Yet happiness was not the only thing I felt. Every bone, every edge of her pressed against me; it was as if I were holding a bird.

She pulled away. "You look great," she said.

"So do you."

She gave a little laugh. "You're such a liar, but I do appreciate the sentiment." She removed her scarf, revealing a scrim of pale hair, the kind that grows back after chemo. "What do you think of my new holiday 'do? I'm guessing you know the story."

I nodded. "I got a call from a colleague of Jonas's. He told me."

"That would be Paul Kiernan, that little weasel. You scientists are such gossips."

"Are you hungry?"

"Never. But I could use a drink."

We climbed the stairs to the bar on the west balcony. Even this small effort seemed to enervate her. We took a table near the edge with a view of the grand hall. I ordered a Scotch, Liz a martini and a glass of water.

"Do you remember when you met me here the

first time?" I asked.

"You had a friend, wasn't it? Something awful had happened."

"That's right. Lucessi." I hadn't said the name in years. "It meant a lot to me, you know. You really took care of me."

"Comes with the service. But if I remember correctly, it was at least half the other way around. Maybe more than half." She paused, then said, "You really do look good, Tim. Success suits you, but I always knew it would. I've kind of kept tabs. Tell me one thing. Are you happy?"

"I'm happy now."

She smiled. Her lips were thin and white. "An excellent dodge, Dr. Fanning."

I reached across the table and took her hand. It was cold as ice. "Tell me what's going to happen."

"I'm going to die, that's what."

"I can't accept that. There has to be something they can do. Let me make some calls."

She shook her head. "They've all been made. Believe me, I'm not going down without a fight. But it's time to raise the white flag."

"How long?"

"Four months. Six if I'm lucky. That's where I was today. I've been seeing a doc at Sloan Kettering. It's all over the place. His words."

Six months: it was nothing. How had I let all the years go by? "Jesus, Liz —"

"Don't say it. Don't say you're sorry, because I'm not." She squeezed my hand. "I need a favor, Tim."

"Anything."

"I need you to help Jonas. I'm sure you've heard the stories. They're all true. He's in South America right now, on his great goose chase. He can't ac-

cept any of this. He still thinks he can save me."

"What can *I* do?"

"Just talk to him. He trusts you. Not just as a scientist but as his friend. Do you know how much he still talks about you? He follows your every move. He probably knows what you ate for breakfast this morning."

"That makes no sense. He should hate me."

"Why would he hate you?"

Even then, I couldn't say the words. She was dying, and I couldn't tell her.

"Leaving the way I did. Never telling him why."

"Oh, he knows why. Or thinks he does."

I was shocked. "What did you tell him?"

"The truth. That you finally figured out you were too good for us."

"That's insane. And it wasn't the reason."

"I know it wasn't, Tim."

A silence passed. I sipped my drink. Announcements were being made; people were hurrying to their trains, riding into the winter dark.

"We were a couple of good soldiers, you and I," Liz said. She gave a brittle smile. "Loyal to a fault."

"So he never figured out that part."

"Are we talking about the same Jonas here? He couldn't even imagine such a thing."

"How has it been with him? I don't just mean now."

"I can't complain."

"But you'd like to."

She shrugged. "Sometimes. Everyone does. He loves me, he thinks he's helping. What else could a girl ask for?"

"Somebody who understood you."

"That's a tall order. I don't think I even under-

stand myself."

I felt suddenly angry. "You're not some high school science project, damnit. He just wants to feel noble. He should be here with you, not trooping around, where was it? South America?"

"It's the only way he has of dealing with this."

"It's not fair."

"What's fair? I have cancer. That isn't fair."

I understood, then, what she was saying to me. She was afraid, and Jonas had left her alone. Maybe she wanted me to bring him home; maybe what she really needed was for me to tell him how he'd failed her. Maybe it was both. What I knew was that I'd do absolutely anything she asked.

I became aware that neither of us had spoken for a while. I looked at Liz; something was wrong. She'd begun to perspire, though the room was quite cold. She took a shuddering breath and reached weakly for her glass of water.

"Liz, are you all right?"

She sipped. Her hand was shaking. She returned the glass to the table, nearly spilling it, dropped her elbow, and braced her forehead against her palm.

"I don't think I am, actually. I think I'm going to faint."

I rose quickly from my chair. "We need to get you to a hospital. I'll get a cab."

She shook her head emphatically. "No more hospitals."

Where then? "Can you walk?"

"I'm not sure."

I threw some cash onto the table and helped her to her feet. She was on the verge of collapse, giving me nearly all of her weight.

"You're always carrying me, aren't you?" she

283

murmured.

I got her into a cab and gave the driver my address. The snow was falling heavily now. Liz leaned back against the seat and closed her eyes.

"The lady okay?" the driver asked. He was wearing a turban and had a heavy black beard. I knew he meant, Is she drunk? "The lady looks sick. No puking in my cab."

I handed him a hundred-dollar bill. "Does this help?"

The traffic was like glue. It took us nearly thirty minutes to get downtown. New York was softening under the snow. A white Christmas: how happy everyone was going to be. My apartment was on the second floor; I would have to carry her. I waited for a neighbor to come through the door and asked him to hold it open, guided Liz out of the cab, and lifted her into my arms.

"Wow," my neighbor said. "She doesn't look too good."

He followed us to my apartment door, took the key from my pocket, and opened that as well. "Do you want me to call 911?" he asked.

"It's okay, I've got this. She had a little too much to drink is all."

He winked despicably. "Don't do anything I wouldn't do."

I got her out of her coat and carried her into the bedroom. As I lay her on my bed, she opened her eyes and turned her face toward the window.

"It's snowing," she said, as if this were the most amazing thing in the world.

She closed them again. I removed her glasses and shoes, draped a blanket over her, and doused the lights. There was an overstuffed chair close to the window where I liked to read. I sat down and

waited in the dark to see what would happen next.

Sometime later, I awoke. I looked at my watch: it was nearly two A.M. I went to Liz and placed my palm to her forehead. She felt cool, and I believed that the worst had passed.

Her eyes opened. She looked around cautiously, as if she wasn't quite sure where she was.

"How are you feeling?" I asked.

She didn't answer right away. Her voice was very soft. "Better, I think. Sorry to scare you."

"That's perfectly all right."

"It happens sometimes like that, but it goes away. Until sometime when it doesn't, I guess."

I had nothing to say to that. "Let me get you some water."

I filled a glass in the bathroom and brought it to her. She lifted her head off the pillow and sipped. "I was having the strangest dream," she said. "The chemo is what does it. The stuff's like LSD. I thought that was over, though."

A thought occurred to me. "I have a present for you."

"You do?"

"Wait here."

I kept her glasses in my desk. I returned to the bedroom and placed them in her hand. She studied them for a long moment.

"I was wondering when you'd get around to giving these back."

"I like to put them on sometimes."

"And here I didn't get you anything. I'm just appalling." She was crying, just a little. She looked up, meeting my eye. "You're not the only one who blew it you know."

"Liz?"

She reached out her hand and touched my cheek. "It's funny. You can live your whole life and then suddenly know that you didn't do it right at all."

I wrapped her fingers with my own. Outside, the snow fell upon the sleeping city.

"You should kiss me," she said.

"Do you want me to?"

"I think that's the dumbest thing you've ever said."

I did. I brought my mouth to hers. It was a soft, quiet kiss — *peaceful* would be the word — the kind that obliterates the world and makes all time turn around it. Infinity in a moment, the hem of creation brushing the face of the waters.

"I should stop," I said.

"No, you shouldn't." She began to unbutton her blouse. "Just please be careful with me. I'm kind of breakable, you know."

21

We became lovers. I don't think I'd ever truly understood the word. I don't mean just sex, though there was that — unhurried, meticulous, a form of passion I had never known existed. I mean that we lived as richly as two people ever could, with a feeling of absolute rightness. We left the apartment only to walk. A deep cold had followed the snow, sealing the city in whiteness. Jonas's name was never mentioned. It wasn't a subject we were avoiding. It had simply ceased to matter.

We both knew she would have to return eventually; she could not simply step out of her life. Nor could I imagine the two of us being apart for one minute of the time she had left. I believed she felt

the same. I wanted to be there when it happened. I wanted to be touching her, holding her hand, telling her how much I loved her as she faded away.

One morning the week after Christmas, I awoke in bed alone. I found her in the kitchen, sipping tea, and knew what she was about to tell me.

"I have to go back."

"I know," I said. "Where?"

"Greenwich first. My mother must be worried. Then Boston, I suppose." She didn't have to say more; her meaning was plain. Jonas would be home soon.

"I understand," I said.

We took a cab to Grand Central. Few words had been spoken since her announcement. I felt like I was being taken to face a firing squad. Be brave, I told myself. Be the sort of man who stands tall with his eyes open, waiting for the guns' report.

Her train was called. We walked to the platform where it awaited. She put her arms around me and began to cry. "I don't want to do this," she said.

"Then don't. Don't get on the train."

I felt her hesitancy. Not just the words; I felt it in her body. She couldn't make herself let go.

"I have to."

"Why?"

"I don't know."

People were hurrying past. The customary announcement crackled overhead: *All aboard for New Haven, Bridgeport, Westport, New Canaan, Greenwich . . .* A door was closing; soon it would be sealed.

"Then come back. Do what you have to do, and

then come back. We can go someplace."

"Where?"

"Italy, Greece. An island in the Pacific. It doesn't matter. Somewhere nobody can find us."

"I want to."

"Say yes."

A frozen moment; then she nodded against me. "Yes."

My heart soared. "How long do you need to tie things up?"

"A week. No, two."

"Make it ten days. Meet me here, under the clock. I'll have everything ready."

"I love you," she said. "I think I did from the start."

"I loved you even before that."

A last kiss, she stepped toward the train, then turned and embraced me again.

"Ten days," she said.

I made ready. There were things I needed to do. I composed a hasty email to my dean, requesting a leave of absence. I wouldn't be around to know if it had been accepted, but I hardly cared. I could imagine no life beyond the next six months.

I called a friend who was an oncologist. I explained the situation, and he told me what would happen. Yes, there would be pain, but mostly a slow receding.

"It's not something you should manage on your own," he said. When I didn't reply, he sighed. "I'll phone in a prescription."

"For what?"

"Morphine. It will help." He paused. "At the end, you know, a lot of people take more than they should, strictly speaking."

I said I understood and thanked him. Where should we go? I had read an article in the *Times* about an island in the Aegean where half the population lived to be a hundred. There was no valid scientific explanation; the residents, most of whom were goat herders, took it as a fact of life. A man was quoted in the article as saying, "Time is different here." I bought two first-class tickets to Athens and found a ferry schedule online. A boat traveled to the island only once a week. We would have to wait two days in Athens, but there were worse places. We would visit the temples, the great, indestructible monuments of a lost world, then vanish.

The day arrived. I packed my bags; we would be going straight from the station to the airport for a ten P.M. flight. I could barely think straight; my emotions were an indescribable jumble. Joy and sadness had fused together in my heart. Foolishly, I had planned nothing else for the day and was forced to sit idly in my apartment until late afternoon. I had no food on hand, having cleaned out the refrigerator, but doubted I could have eaten anyway.

I took a cab to the station. Five o'clock was, once again, the appointed hour. Liz would be taking an Amtrak train to Stamford, to see her mother, in Greenwich, one last time, then a local to Grand Central. With each passing block my feelings annealed into a pure sense of purpose. I knew, as few men did, why I had been born in the first place; everything in my life had called me forward to this moment. I paid the cabbie and went inside to wait. It was a Saturday, the crowds light. The opalescent clock faces read 4:36. Liz's train was due in twenty minutes.

My pulse quickened as the announcement came over the speakers: *Now arriving at track 16 . . .* I considered going to the platform to head her off, but we might lose each other in the crowd. Passengers surged into the main hall. Soon it became clear that Liz was not among them. Perhaps she had taken a later train; the New Haven line ran every thirty minutes. I checked my phone, but there were no messages. The next train came, and still no Liz. I began to worry that something had happened. It did not occur to me yet that she had changed her mind, though the idea was waiting in the wings. At six o'clock I called her cell, but it went straight to voicemail. Had she shut it off?

Train by train, my panic grew. It was now obvious that Liz would not be coming, and yet I continued to wait, to hope. I was hanging by my fingertips over an abyss. Time and again I tried her cell, with the same result. *This is Elizabeth Lear. I'm not available to take your call.* The clocks' hands mocked me with their turning. It was nine, then ten. I had waited five hours. What a fool I'd been.

I left the station and began to walk. The air was cruel; the city seemed like a huge dead thing, some monstrous joke. I did not button my coat or put on my gloves, preferring to feel the pain of the wind. Sometime later I looked up to find I was on Broadway, near the Flatiron. I realized I had left my suitcase at the station. I thought to go back and retrieve it — surely somebody would have turned it in — but the flame of this impulse quickly extinguished itself. A suitcase — who cared? Of course there was the morphine to consider. Perhaps whoever found it would enjoy themselves.

Drinking myself blind seemed like the next logical step. I entered the first restaurant I came to, in the lobby of an office building — sleek and upscale, full of chrome and stone. A few couples were still eating, though it was after midnight. I took a place at the bar, ordered a Scotch, finished it before the bartender had returned the bottle to the rack, and requested a refill.

"Excuse me. You're Professor Fanning, aren't you?"

I turned to the woman sitting a few stools away. She was young, a little heavy but quite striking, Indian or Middle Eastern, with raven-black hair, full cheeks, and a bow-shaped mouth. Above her generically sexy black skirt she wore a filmy top the color of cream. A glass of something with fruit in it sat on the bar in front of her, its rim stained with crescents of rust-colored lipstick.

"I'm sorry?"

She smiled. "I guess you don't remember me." When I didn't reply, she added, "Molecular Biology 100? Spring 2002?"

"You were my student."

She laughed. "Not much of one. You gave me a C minus."

"Oh. Sorry about that."

"Trust me, no offense taken. The human race has a lot to thank you for, actually. Many people are alive today because I didn't go to med school."

I had no recollection of her; hundreds of young women like her came and went from my classes. It is also not the same thing to see someone from the distance of a podium at eight o'clock in the morning, wearing sweatpants and furiously tapping a laptop, as to find them sitting three stools away in a bar, dressed for a night of adventure.

291

"So, where did you end up?" A dull remark; I was simply looking for something to say, since conversation was now inevitable.

"Publishing, where else?" She leveled her gaze at me. "You know, I had the biggest crush on you. I'm talking *major*. A lot of the girls did."

I realized she was drunk, making such a confession without even telling me her name.

"Miss — ?"

She moved to the stool next to mine and extended her hand. Her nails were perfectly manicured, painted to match her lips. "Nicole."

"It's been a long night for me, Nicole."

"I could sort of tell, the way you put away that Scotch." She touched her hair for no reason. "What do you say, Professor? Buy a girl a drink? It's your chance to make up for that C."

She was plainly amusing herself, a woman who knew what she had, what it could do. I glanced past her; just a handful of other people were in the room. "Aren't you — ?"

"With anyone?" She gave a little laugh. "Like, did my date step out for a smoke?"

I felt suddenly flustered; I hadn't meant the question as a come-on. "I mean, a pretty girl like you. I just assumed."

"Well, you assumed wrong." With the tips of her fingers she picked a cherry from her glass and raised it slowly to her lips. Her eyes locked onto my face; she placed it on her tongue, balancing it there for a half second before popping the stem and curling the red meat into her mouth. It was the hokiest thing I'd ever seen.

"Don't you know, Professor? Tonight I'm all yours."

■ ■ ■ ■

We were in a taxi. I was very drunk. The cab was bouncing through narrow streets and we were kissing like teenagers, drinking each other's mouths in furious gulps. I appeared to have lost all volition; things were simply happening of their own accord. There was something I wanted, I didn't know what. One of my hands had found its way up her skirt, lost in a feminine country of skin and lace; the other was lifting her buttocks toward me, pulling our hips together. She unlatched my trousers and eased me free, then dropped her head to my lap. The cabbie glanced back, said nothing. Up and down she went, my fingers entwined in the lush mane of her hair. My head was spinning, I could hardly breathe.

The taxi halted. "Twenty-seven fifty," the driver said.

It was like being splashed by cold water. I hurriedly rearranged myself and paid. When I exited the car, the girl — Natalie? Nadine? — was already waiting on the steps to her building, smoothing down the front of her skirt. Something loud and large was rattling overhead; I thought we might be in Brooklyn, near the Manhattan Bridge overpass. More grappling at the door and she pushed me away.

"Wait here." Her face was flushed; she was breathing very fast. "I have something to take care of. I'll buzz you in."

She was gone before I could object. Standing on the sidewalk, I tried to reassemble the order of the night's events. Grand Central, the hours of hopeless waiting. My desolate walk through the

icy streets. The warm oasis of the bar, and the girl — Nicole, that was it — smiling and moving closer and putting her hand on my knee and the two of us making our hasty, inevitable exit. I could remember these things, yet none of them seemed completely real. Abandoned in the cold, I felt a rush of panic. I did not want to be alone with my thoughts. How could she have done it? How could Liz have left me standing there, train after train? If the door didn't buzz soon, I knew, I would literally detonate.

A few agonizing minutes passed. I heard the door open and turned in time to see a woman emerge from the building. She was older, heavyset, perhaps Hispanic. Her body, buried in a bunchy down coat, was hunched against the wind. She had failed to notice me standing in the shadows; I slid behind her and grabbed the door just before it closed.

The lobby encased me with its sudden warmth. I scanned the mailboxes. Nicole Forood, apartment zero. I descended the stairs to the basement, where a single door awaited. I knocked with my knuckles, then, when no one responded, with my fist. My frustration was indescribable. My feelings had annealed to a pure desperation, almost like anger. My fist was raised again when I heard footsteps inside. The complicated unlocking of a New York apartment door commenced; then it opened just enough for me to see the girl's face on the other side of the chain. She had taken off her makeup, revealing an otherwise plain face, flawed by traces of acne. Another man would have understood the meaning, but my agitation was such that my brain could not compute the data.

"Why did you leave me?"

"I don't think this is a good idea. You should go."

"I don't understand."

Her face was as rigid as a blind man's. "Something's come up. I'm sorry."

How could this be the same girl who had laid siege to me in the bar? Was this some kind of game? I wanted to blow the chain off its anchors and burst through the door. Maybe that was what she wanted me to do. She sort of seemed the type.

"It's late. I shouldn't have left you out there, but I'm going to shut the door now."

"Please, just let me warm up for a minute. I promise I'll go after that."

"I'm sorry, Tim. I had a good time. Maybe we can do it again sometime. But I really have to go."

I'll admit it: part of my mind was computing the strength of the chain that held the door. "You don't trust me, is that the reason?"

"No, that's not it. It's just —" She didn't finish.

"I swear I'll behave. Whatever you want." I offered a sheepish smile. "The truth is, I'm still a little drunk. I really need to sober up."

I could see the indecision in her face. My appeal was doing its work.

"Please," I said. "It's freezing out there."

A moment passed; her face relaxed. "Just a few minutes, okay? I have to be up early."

I held up three fingers. "Scout's honor."

She closed the door, undid the chain, and opened it again. Disappointingly, the skirt and filmy top had been replaced by a robe and a shapeless flannel nightgown. She stepped aside to let me enter.

"I'll put on some coffee."

The apartment had a dingy look: a small living

area with high-set windows facing the street, a galley kitchen with dishes teetering in the sink, a narrow hallway that led, presumably, to the bedroom. The couch, which faced an old tube-style television, was heaped with laundry. There were few books in sight, nothing on the walls except a couple of cheap museum posters of water lilies and ballerinas.

"Sorry it's such a mess," she said, and waved at the sofa. "Just shove that stuff aside if you want."

Nicole's back was to me. She filled a pot at the tap and began to pour the water into a stained coffee machine. Something peculiar was happening to me. I can only describe it as a kind of astral projection. It was as if I were a character in a movie, observing myself from a distance. In this divided state, I watched myself approach her from behind. She was sifting ground beans into the machine. I was about to put my arms around her when she sensed my presence and spun toward me.

"What are you doing?"

My body was pressing her against the counter. I began to kiss her neck. "What do you think I'm doing?"

"Tim, stop. I mean it."

I was burning from within. My senses were swarming. "God, you smell so good." I was licking, tasting. I wanted to drink her.

"You're scaring me. I need you to leave."

"Say you're her." Where were these words coming from? Who was talking? Was it me? "Say it. Tell me how sorry you are."

"Goddamnit, stop!"

With surprising strength, she shoved me away. I fell against the counter, barely staying on my feet.

When I looked up, she was pulling a long knife from a drawer. She aimed it at me like a pistol.

"Get out."

Darkness was spreading inside me. "How could you do it? How could you leave me standing there?"

"I'll scream."

"You bitch. You fucking bitch."

I lurched toward her. What were my intentions? Who was she to me, this woman with the knife? Was she Liz? Was she even a person, or merely a mirror in which I beheld the image of my wretched self? To this day, I do not know; the moment seems the property of another man entirely. I do not say this to exonerate myself, which is impossible, only to describe events as accurately as I can. With one hand I reached to cover her mouth; with the other I grabbed her arm, jerking the knife downward. Our bodies collided in a soft crash, and then we were falling to the floor, my body on top of hers, the knife between us.

The knife. The knife.

As we hit the floor, I felt it. There was no mistaking the sensation, or the sound it made.

The events that followed are no less strange to my memory, benighted by horror. I was in a nightmare in which the great, unrecallable act had been committed. I rose from her body. A pool of blood, rich and dark, almost black, was spreading beneath it; more was on my shirt, a crimson splash. The blade had entered just below the girl's sternum, driven deep into her thoracic cavity by my falling weight. She was looking at the ceiling; she let out a little gasp, no louder than a person would make who had suffered a mild surprise. *Is my life over?*

Is that all? This stupid little thing and that's the end? Bit by bit, her eyes lost focus; an unnatural stillness eased across her face.

I turned to the sink and vomited.

The decision to hide my tracks was not one I recall making. I did not have a plan; I merely enacted one. I did not yet think of myself as a killer; rather, I was a man who had been involved in a serious accident that would be misunderstood. I stripped to my undershirt; the girl's blood had not seeped through. I cast my eyes around for the things I might have touched. The knife of course; that would have to be disposed of. The front door? Had I touched the knob, the frame? I had seen the shows on television, the ones with the good-looking detectives combing crime scenes for the minutest evidence. I knew their prowess to be wildly overstated for dramatic purposes, but they were my only reference. What invisible traces of me were, even now, touching down upon the surfaces of the woman's apartment, awaiting collection and study, pointing to my guilt?

I rinsed my mouth and washed the knobs and sink with a sponge. The knife I cleaned as well, then wrapped it in my shirt and deposited it carefully in the pocket of my coat. I did not look at the body again; to do so would have been unbearable. I scrubbed the counters and turned to appraise the rest of the apartment. Something seemed different. What was I seeing?

I heard a sound, coming from down the hall.

What is the worst thing? The deaths of millions? A whole world lost? No: the worst thing is the sound I heard.

Details I had failed to notice emerged in my vision. The pile of laundry, full of tiny pink gar-

ments. The bright toys of plush and plastic strewn across the floor. The distinctive, fecal aroma masked by sweet powder. I remembered the woman I had seen coming from the building. The timing of her departure had been no accident.

The sound came again; I wanted to flee but could not. That I had to follow it was my penance; it was the stone I would carry for life. Slowly I moved down the hall, terror accompanying my every step. A pale, vigilant light shone through the partly open door. The odor grew stronger, coating my mouth with its taste. At the threshold I paused, petrified, yet knowing what was required of me.

The little girl was awake and looking about. Six months, a year — I was not a good judge of these things. A mobile of cardboard-cutout animals dangled above her crib. She was waving her arms and kicking her legs against the mattress, causing the animals to jostle on their strings; she made the sound again, a joyful little squeal. *See what I can do? Mama, come look.* But in the other room her mother lay in a pool of blood, her eyes staring into time's abyss.

What did I do? Did I fall before her and beg her forgiveness? Did I pick her up with my unclean hands, the hands of a killer, and tell her I was sorry for her motherless life? Did I call the police and take my shameful vigil beside her crib to wait for them?

None of these. Coward that I was, I ran.

And yet the night does not end there. You could say it never has.

A flight of stairs led from Old Fulton Street to the Brooklyn Bridge walkway. At the midpoint of the bridge, I removed the knife and bloody shirt

and dropped them into the water. The hour was approaching five A.M.; soon the city would arise. Already the traffic was thickening — early commuters, taxis, delivery trucks, even a few bicyclists, their faces masked against the cold, whizzing past me like wheeled demons. There is no being who feels more anonymous, more forgotten, more alone than a New York pedestrian, if he so chooses, but this is an illusion: our comings and goings are tracked to a fault. In Washington Square I bought a cheap baseball cap from a street vendor to hide my face and found a pay phone. Calling 911 was out of the question, as the call would be instantly traced. From information I got the number for the *New York Post,* dialed it, and asked for the city desk.

"Metro."

"I'd like to report a murder. A woman's been stabbed."

"Hang on a second. Who am I speaking to?"

I gave the address. "The police don't know yet. The door's unlocked. Just go look," I said and hung up.

I made two more calls, to the *Daily News* and the *Times,* from different pay phones, one on Bleecker Street, the other on Prince. By this time, the morning was in full swing. It seemed to me I should return to my apartment. It was the natural place for me to be and, more to the point, I had no place else to go.

Then I remembered my abandoned suitcase. How this might connect me to the girl's death I could not foresee, but it was, at the very least, a thread best cut quickly. I took the subway uptown to Grand Central. At once I became aware of the station's heavy police presence; I was now a

murderer, sentenced to a preternatural awareness of my surroundings, a life of constant fear. At the kiosk, I was directed to the lost and found, located on the lower level. I showed my driver's license to the woman behind the counter and described the bag.

"I think I left it in the main concourse," I said, attempting to sound like one more flustered traveler. "We just had so much luggage, I think that's how I forgot it."

My story didn't interest her even vaguely. She disappeared into the racks of luggage and returned a minute later with my suitcase and a piece of paper.

"You'll need to fill this out and sign at the bottom."

Name, rank, serial number. It felt like a confession; my hands were shaking so badly I could barely hold the pen. How absurd I was being: one more filled-out form in a city that generated a felled forest of paper every day.

"I need to photocopy your license," the woman said.

"Is that really necessary? I'm in a bit of a hurry."

"Honey, I don't make the rules. You want your bag or don't you?"

I handed it over. She ran it through the machine, gave it back, and stapled the copy to the form, which she shoved into a drawer under the counter.

"I bet you get a lot of bags," I remarked, thinking I should say something.

The woman rolled her eyes. "Baby, you should see the stuff that comes in here."

I took a cab to my apartment. Along the way, I inventoried my situation. The girl's apartment, as far as I could tell, was clean; I'd washed every

surface I'd touched. No one had seen me enter or leave, except the cabbie; that could be a problem. There was the bartender to consider, as well. *Excuse me. You're Professor Fanning, aren't you?* I couldn't recall if he'd been within earshot, though he'd certainly had a good look at both of us. Had I paid with cash or a credit card? Cash, I thought, but I couldn't be sure. The trail was there, but could anyone follow it?

Upstairs, I opened the suitcase on my bed. No surprise, the morphine was gone, but everything else was there. I emptied my pockets — wallet, keys, cellphone. The battery had died in the night. I plugged it into the charger on the nightstand and lay down, though I knew I would not sleep. I didn't think I would ever sleep again.

My phone chirped as the battery awoke. Four new messages, all from the same number, with a 401 area code. Rhode Island? Who did I know in Rhode Island? Then, as I was holding it, the phone rang.

"Is this Timothy Fanning?"

I didn't recognize the voice. "Yes, this is Dr. Fanning."

"Oh, you're a doctor. That explains it. My name is Lois Swan. I'm a nurse in the ICU at Westerly Hospital. A patient was brought here yesterday afternoon, a woman named Elizabeth Lear. Do you know her?"

My heart lurched into my throat. "Where is she? What happened?"

"She was taken off an Amtrak train from Boston and brought here by ambulance. I've been trying to reach you. Are you her physician?"

The nature of the call was becoming clear to me. "That's right," I lied. "What's her condition?"

"I'm afraid that Mrs. Lear has passed away."

I didn't say anything. The room was dissolving. Not just the room, the world.

"Hello?"

I made an effort to swallow. "Yes, I'm here."

"She was unconscious when they brought her in. I was alone with her when she woke up. She gave me your name and number."

"Was there a message?"

"I'm sorry, no. She was very weak. I wasn't even sure I heard the number right. She died just a few minutes later. We tried to reach her husband, but apparently he's overseas. Is there anybody else we should notify?"

I hung up. I placed a pillow over my face. Then I began to scream.

22

The story of the girl's death was plastered on the front pages of the tabloids for several days, and in this manner I learned more about her. She was twenty-nine, from College Park, Maryland, the daughter of Iranian immigrants. Her father was an engineer, her mother a school librarian; she had three siblings. For six years she had worked at Beckworth and Grimes, ascending to the rank of associate editor; she and the baby's father, an actor, were recently divorced. Everything about her was ordinary and admirable. A hard worker. A devoted friend. A beloved daughter and doting mother. For a time, she had wanted to be a dancer. There were many photos of her. In one, she was just a child herself, wearing a leotard and performing a little-girl plié.

Two days later I received a call from Jonas, relay-

ing the news of Liz's death. I did my best to act surprised and discovered that I actually was a little, as if, hearing his broken voice, I were experiencing the loss of her for the first time all over again. We talked awhile, sharing stories of the past. From time to time we laughed over something funny she had done or said; at others, the phone went silent for long intervals in which I heard him crying. I listened to the spaces in the conversation for any indication that he'd known, or suspected, about the two of us. But I detected nothing. It was just as Liz had said: his blindness was total. He couldn't even imagine such a thing.

I was still slightly amazed that nothing had happened to me: no knock on the door, no dark men in suits standing beyond the chain, displaying their badges. *Dr. Fanning, mind if we have a word with you?* None of the stories mentioned the bartender or the cabbie, which I took to be a good sign, though eventually, I believed, the law would come calling. My penance would be extracted; I would fall to my knees and confess. The universe could simply make no sense otherwise.

I took a shuttle to Boston for the funeral. The ceremony was held in Cambridge, within sight of Harvard Yard. The church was packed. Family, friends, colleagues, former students; in her too-short years, Liz had been much loved. I took a pew in back, wanting to be invisible. I knew many, recognized others, felt the weight of all. Among the mourners was a man whom, beneath his puffy alcoholic's face, I knew to be Alcott Spence. Our eyes met briefly as we followed Liz's casket outside, though I do not think he remembered who I was.

After the burial, the inner circle repaired to the

Spee Club for a catered lunch. I had told Jonas that I needed to return early and couldn't make it, but he insisted so ardently that I had little choice. There were toasts, remembrances, a great deal of drinking. Every second was torture. As people were leaving, Jonas pulled me aside.

"Let's go out to the garden. There's something I need to talk to you about."

So here it was, I thought. The whole mess was about to come out. We exited through the library and sat on the steps that led down to the courtyard. The day was unusually warm, a mocking foretaste of spring — a spring I believed I would not see. Surely I would be living in a cell by then.

He reached into the inside pocket of his jacket and removed a flask. He took a long pull and passed it to me.

"Old times," he said.

I didn't know how to respond. The conversation was his to steer.

"You don't have to say it. I know I fucked up. I should have been there. That may be the worst thing."

"I'm sure she understood."

"How could she?" He drank again and wiped his mouth. "The truth is, I think she was leaving me. Probably I deserved it."

I felt my stomach drop. On the other hand, if he'd known it was me, he would have already said so. "Don't be ridiculous. She was probably just going to see her mother."

He gave a fatalistic shrug. "Yeah, well, last time I checked, you don't need a passport to go to Connecticut."

I had failed to consider this. There was nothing to say.

"That's not the reason I asked you out here, though," he went on. "I'm sure you've heard the stories about me."

"A little."

"Everybody thinks I'm a big joke. Well, they're wrong."

"Maybe this isn't the day for this, Jonas."

"Actually, it's the perfect day. I'm close, Tim. Very, very close. There's a site in Bolivia. A temple, at least a thousand years old. The legends say there's a grave there, the body of a man infected with the virus I've been searching for. It's nothing new — there are lots of stories like that. Too many for all this to be nothing, in my opinion, but that's another argument. The thing is, I've got hard evidence now. A friend at the CDC came to me a few months back. He'd heard about my work, and he'd happened across something he thought would interest me. Five years ago, a group of four American tourists showed up at a hospital in La Paz. All of them had what looked like hantavirus. They'd been on some kind of ecotour in the jungle. But here's the thing. They all had terminal cancer. The tour was one of those last-wish things. You know, do the stuff you always wanted to do before you check out."

I had no idea where he was headed. "And?"

"Here's where it gets interesting. All of them recovered, and not just from the hanta. From the cancer. Stage four ovarian, inoperable glioblastoma, leukemia with full lymphatic involvement — not a trace of it was left. And they weren't just cured. They were *better* than cured. It was as if the aging process had been reversed. The youngest one was fifty-six, the oldest seventy. They looked like twenty-year-olds."

"That's quite a story."

"Are you kidding? It's *the* story. If this pans out, it will be the most important medical discovery in history."

I was still skeptical. "So why haven't I heard about it? It isn't in any of the literature."

"Good question. My friend at the CDC suspects the military got involved. The whole thing went over to USAMRIID."

"Why would they want it?"

"Who knows? Maybe they just want the credit, though that's the optimistic view. One day you have Einstein, puzzling over the theory of relativity, the next you've got the Manhattan Project and a big hole in the ground. It's not like it hasn't happened before."

He had a point. "Have you examined them? The four patients."

Jonas took another pull of the whiskey. "Well, that's a bit of a wrinkle. They're all dead."

"But I thought you said —"

"Oh, it wasn't the cancer. They all seemed to kind of . . . well, speed up, like their bodies couldn't handle it. Somebody took a video. They were practically bouncing off the walls. The longest any of them lasted was eighty-six days."

"That's a mighty big wrinkle."

He gave me a hard look. "Think about it, Tim. Something's out there. I couldn't find it in time to save Liz, and that'll haunt me the rest of my days. But I can't stop now. Not just in spite of her; *because* of her. A hundred and fifty-five thousand human beings die every day. How long have we been sitting here? Ten minutes? That's over a thousand people just like Liz. People with lives, families who love them. I need you, Tim.

307

And not just because you're my oldest friend, and the smartest guy I know. I'll be honest: I'm having a hard time with the money. Nobody wants to back this anymore. Maybe your credibility could, you know, grease the gears a bit."

My credibility. If he only knew how little that was worth. "I don't know, Jonas."

"If you can't do it for me, do it for Liz."

I'll admit, the scientist in me was intrigued. It was also true that I wanted nothing to do with this project, or with Jonas, ever again. In the slender ten minutes in which a thousand human beings had perished, I had come, very profoundly, to despise him. Perhaps I always had. I despised his obliviousness, his monstrous ego, his self-aggrandizing pomp. I despised his naked manipulation of my loyalties and his unwavering faith that the answer to everything lay within his grasp. I despised the fact that he didn't know one god-damn thing about anything at all, but most of all, I despised him for letting Liz die alone.

"Can I give it some thought?" An easy dodge; I had no such intentions.

He began to say something, then stopped himself. "Got it. You have your reputation to consider. Believe me, I know how it goes."

"It's not that. It's just a big commitment. I have a lot on my plate these days."

"I'm not going to let you off easy, you know."

"I was pretty sure you wouldn't."

We were silent for a time. Jonas was looking at the garden, though I knew he wasn't seeing it.

"It's funny — I always knew this day would come. Now I can't believe it. It's like it's not even happening, you know? I feel like I'll go back to the house and there she'll be, grading papers at

her desk or stirring something in the kitchen." He blew out a breath and looked at me. "I should have been a better friend to you, all these years. I shouldn't have let so much time pass."

"Forget it," I said. "It was my fault, too."

The conversation ended there. "Well," Jonas said, "thank you for being here, Tim. I know you'd come anyway, just for her. But it means a lot to me. Let me know what you decide."

I sat awhile after he'd gone. The building was quiet; the mourners had left, returning to their lives. How lucky they were, I thought.

I heard nothing more from Jonas. Winter yielded to spring, then summer, and I began to believe that the dots hadn't been connected after all and I would remain a free man. Bit by bit, the girl's death ceased to hang over my every thought and action. It was still there, of course; the memory touched down often and without warning, paralyzing me with guilt so deep I could hardly draw a breath. But the mind is nimble; it seeks to preserve itself. One particularly clement summer day, cool and dry with a sky so crisp it looked like a great blue dome snapped down over the city, I was walking to the subway from my office when I realized that for a full ten minutes I hadn't felt utterly ruined. Perhaps life could go on, after all.

I returned to teaching in the fall. A bevy of new graduate assistants awaited me; as if the administration took delight in torturing me, most were female. But to say that those days were over for me would be the understatement of the century. Mine was a monk's existence, as it would be henceforth. I did my work, I taught my classes, I sought the company of no one, man or woman. I

309

heard, secondhand, that Jonas had found funding for his expedition after all and was gearing up for Bolivia. Good riddance, I thought.

On a day in late January, I was grading labs in my office when there was a knock on the door.

"Come."

Two people, a man and a woman: I instantly knew who, and what, they were. My face probably betrayed my guilt in a heartbeat.

"Got a minute, Professor Fanning?" the woman said. "I'm Detective Reynaldo, this is Detective Phelps. We'd like to ask you a few questions, if you don't mind."

"Of course." I feigned surprise. "Sit down, Detectives."

"We'll stand, if that's all right."

The conversation lasted barely fifteen minutes, but it was enough to let me know that the noose was tightening. A woman had come forward — the babysitter. She was an illegal, which explained the long delay. Though she had glimpsed me quickly, the description she provided matched the bartender's. He did not recall my name but had overheard the part of our conversation in which she confessed her crush on me, using the phrase "a lot of the girls did." This led them to Nicole's college transcript and eventually to me, who bore a remarkable resemblance to the sitter's description of the suspect. A *very* remarkable resemblance.

I made the customary denials. No, I had never been to the bar in question. No, I did not recall the girl from my classes; I had seen the story in the papers but had made no connection. No, I could not recall my whereabouts that night. When, exactly? Probably I was in bed.

310

"Interesting. In bed, you say?"

"Perhaps I was reading. I'm a bit of an insomniac. I really don't recall."

"That's strange. Because according to the TSA, you were scheduled to be on a flight to Athens. Any thoughts on that you'd care to share at this point, Dr. Fanning?"

The cold sweat of the criminal dampened my palms. Of course they would know this. How could I have been so dumb?

"Very well," I said, doing my best to seem annoyed. "I wish this hadn't had to come out, but since you insist on prying into my personal life, I was going away with a friend. A *married* friend."

A single eyebrow lasciviously lifted. "Care to tell us her name?"

My mind was racing. Could they connect us? I'd paid for the tickets in cash and bought them separately to cover our tracks. Our seats weren't even next to each other's; I'd planned to sort it out before we boarded.

"I'm sorry, I can't do that. It's not my place."

"A gentleman doesn't kiss and tell, huh?"

"Something like that."

Detective Reynaldo smiled imperiously, enjoying herself. "A gentleman who runs off with another man's wife. Doubt you'll win any prizes for that."

"I don't claim to, Detective."

"So why didn't you go?"

I gave my most innocent shrug. "She changed her mind. Her husband is a colleague of mine. It was a stupid idea to begin with. That's really all there is to it."

For ten full seconds neither of us spoke — a gap I was obviously meant to fill, incriminating myself.

311

"Well, that's all for now, Dr. Fanning. Thank you for taking time out of your busy day." She gave me her card. "You think of anything else, you call me, all right?"

"I'll do that, Detective."

"And I do mean anything."

I waited thirty minutes to make sure they were well clear of the building, then took the subway home. How long did I have? Days? Hours? How much paperwork did they need to get me into a lineup?

I could think of only one option. I called Jonas's office, then his cell, but got no answer. I would have to risk an email.

Jonas — I've given some thought to your proposal. Sorry it took me so long. Not sure how much I can offer at this late date, but I'd like to sign on. When do you leave? — TF

I waited at my computer, hitting the Refresh button over and over. Thirty minutes later his reply came.

Delighted. We leave in three days. Have already cleared your visa with State. Don't ever say I'm not a man with connections. How many more do you need for your team? Knowing you, you'll bring a flotilla of attractive female grad assistants, which we could sure use to brighten up the place.

Move your ass, buddy. We're going to change the world. — JL

23

There is not much more to say. I went. I was infected. Of those infected, I alone survived. And thus was built a race to establish dominion over the earth.

There was a night when Jonas came to see me in my chamber. This was long after my transformation, by which time I had adjusted to my circumstances. I could not know what the hour was, such things having lost all meaning in my captive state. My plans were well under way. I and my co-conspirators had identified the avenue of our escape. The weak-minded men who watched over us: day by day we had infiltrated their thoughts, filling their minds with our black dreams, bringing them into the fold. Their flabby souls were collapsing; soon they would be ours.

His voice came over the speaker: "Tim, it's Jonas."

This was not his first visit. Many was the time I had seen his face behind the glass. Yet he had not addressed me directly since the day of my awakening. The last years had wrought startling changes to his appearance. Long-haired, wild-bearded, crazed-eyed, he had become the very image of the mad scientist I had always thought him to be.

"I know you can't talk. Hell, I'm not even sure you can understand me."

I felt a confession coming. I was, I admit, only vaguely interested in what he had to say. His disturbed conscience — what did I care? His visit had also interrupted my feeding schedule. Though in life I had not much cared for the taste of wild game, I had come to enjoy raw rabbit very much.

"Something bad is happening. I'm really losing

control of this thing."

Indeed, I thought.

"God, I miss her, Tim. I should have listened to her. I should have listened to *you.* If only you could talk to me."

You will hear from me soon enough, I thought.

"I've got one more chance, Tim. I still believe this can work. Maybe if I pull it off, I can get the military to back away. I can still turn everything around."

Hope springs eternal, does it not?

"The thing is, it has to be a child." He was silent for a moment. "I can't believe I'm saying this. They just brought her in. I don't even want to know what they did to get her here. Jesus, Tim, she's just a little kid."

A child, I thought. Here was an intriguing wrinkle; no wonder Jonas despised himself. I delighted in his misery. I had learned how low a man could sink; why shouldn't he?

"They're calling her Amy NLN. No last name. They got her from some orphanage. God almighty, she doesn't even have a proper name. She's just some girl from nowhere."

I felt my heart go out to this unlucky child, plucked from her life to become the last pitiable hope of a crazy man. Yet even as I considered this, a new thought was bearing fruit inside me. A little girl, bathed in the innocence of youth: of course. The symmetry was undeniable; it was a message, meant for me. To face her, that would be the test. I heard the rumble of distant armies joining. This girl from nowhere. This Amy NLN. Who was alpha, who omega? Who the beginning and who the end?

"Did you love her, Tim? You can tell me."

Yes, I thought. Yes and yes and yes. She was the only thing that ever mattered. I loved her more than any man could. I loved her enough to watch her die.

"The police came to me, you see. They knew the two of you were supposed to be on the same plane. You know what's funny? I was actually happy for her. She deserved someone who could love her the way she needed. The way I never could. I guess what I'm saying is, I'm glad it was you."

Was it possible? Had my eyes — the eyes of a beast, a demon — begun to shed tears?

"Well." Jonas cleared his throat. "I guess that's what I came to say. I'm sorry about all this, Tim. I hope you know that. You were the best friend I ever had."

Now it is dark. Stars soar above the vacant city, heaven's diadem. A century since the last person walked here, and still one cannot travel its streets, as I do, without seeing one's face reflected a thousand-fold. Shop windows. Bodegas and brownstones. The mirrored flanks of skyscrapers, great vertical tombs of glass. I look, and what do I see? Man? Monster? Devil? A freak of cold nature or heaven's cruel utensil? The first is intolerable to think, the second no less so. Who is the monster now?

I walk. Listen closely, and one still hears the footfalls of a throng, engraved in stone. At the center has grown a forest. A forest in New York! A great green eruption, alive with animal sounds and smells. There are rats everywhere, of course. They grow to fantastic dimensions. Once I saw one that I thought might be a dog, or a wild pig,

or something brand-new to the world. The pigeons wheel, the rain falls, the seasons turn without us; in winter, all is dressed with snow.

City of memories, city of mirrors. Am I alone? Yes and no. I am a man of many descendants. They lie hidden away. Some are here, those who once called this island home; they slumber beneath the streets of the forgotten metropolis. Others lie elsewhere, my ambassadors, awaiting final use. In slumber they become themselves again; in dreams, they relive their human lives. Which world is the real one? Only when they're aroused does the hunger obliterate them, taking them over, their souls spilling into mine, and so I leave them as they are. It is the only mercy I can offer.

Oh, my brothers, Twelve in sum, you were sorely used by this world! I spoke to you like the god you thought I was, though in the end I could not save you. I would not say I failed to see this coming. From the start, your fates were written; you could not help being what you were, which was the truth of us. Consider the species known as man. We lie, we cheat, we want what others have and take it; we make war upon each other and the earth; we harvest lives in multitudes. We have mortgaged the planet and spent the cash on trifles. We may have loved, but never well enough. We never truly knew ourselves. We forgot the world; now it has forgotten us. How many years will pass before jealous nature reclaims this place? Before it is as if we never existed at all? Buildings will crumble. Skyscrapers will come crashing to the ground. Trees will sprout and spread their canopies. The oceans will rise, rinsing the rest away. It is said that one day all will be water again; a vast

ocean will blanket the world. *In the beginning, God created the heaven and the earth. And the earth was without form, and void; and darkness was upon the face of the deep. And the Spirit of God moved upon the face of the waters.* How will God, if there is a God, remember us? Will he even know our names? All stories end when they have returned to their beginnings. What can we do but remember in his stead?

I go abroad, into the streets of the empty city, always returning. I take my place upon the steps, beneath the inverted heavens. I watch the clock; its mournful faces stay the same. Time frozen at the moment of man's departure, the last train exiting the station.

■ ■ ■ ■

III
THE SON

■ ■ ■ ■

TEXAS REPUBLIC
POP. 204,876
MARCH 122 A.V.
TWENTY-ONE YEARS AFTER
THE DISCOVERY OF THE *BERGENSFJORD*

All the world's a stage,
And all the men and women merely players:
They have their exits and their entrances,
And one man in his time plays many parts.
— SHAKESPEARE, *As You Like It*

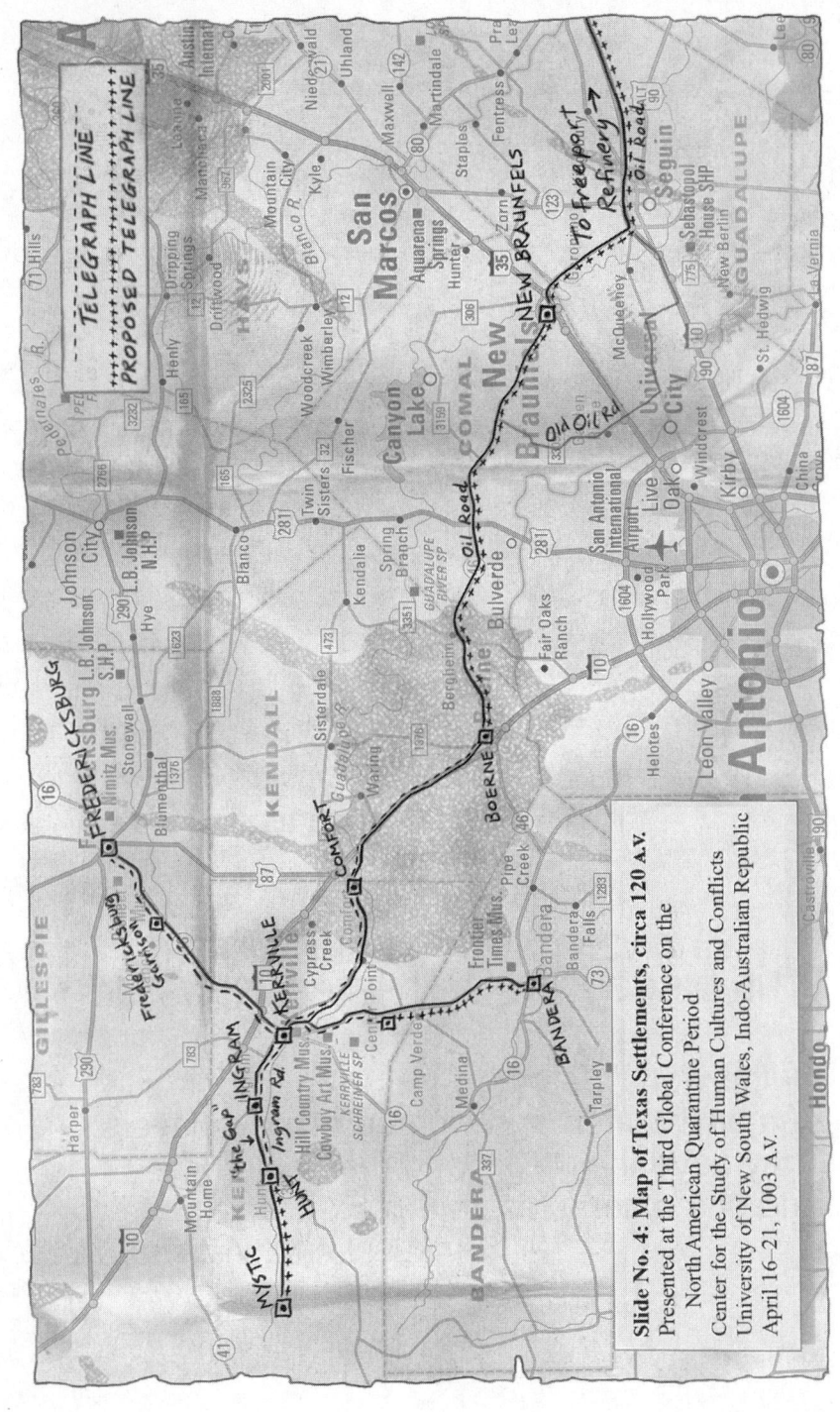

Slide No. 4: Map of Texas Settlements, circa 120 A.V.
Presented at the Third Global Conference on the
North American Quarantine Period
Center for the Study of Human Cultures and Conflicts
University of New South Wales, Indo-Australian Republic
April 16–21, 1003 A.V.

24

Peter Jaxon, age fifty-one, president of the Texas Republic, stood at the Kerrville gate in the pale dawn light, waiting to say goodbye to his son.

Sara and Hollis had just arrived; Kate was working at the hospital but had promised that her husband, Bill, would bring the girls. Caleb was loading the last of their gear into the wagon while Pim, in a loose cotton dress, stood nearby, holding baby Theo. Two strong horses, fit for plowing, idled in their harnesses.

"I guess that's it," Caleb said, as he finished lashing the final crate. He was wearing a long-sleeved work shirt and overalls; he'd let his hair grow long. He checked the load on his rifle, a lever-action .30-06, and put it up on the seat. "We really should get moving if we're going to make Hunt by dark."

They were headed to one of the outer settlements, a two-day ride on the buckboard. The land had only just been incorporated, though people had been homesteading there for years. Caleb had spent most of two years preparing the place — framing the house, digging the well, laying out fences — before returning for Pim and the baby. Good soil, the clear water of the river, woods

heavy with game: there were worse places, Peter thought, to start a life.

"You can't go yet," Sara said. "The girls will be heartbroken if you leave without seeing them."

Sara had, simultaneously, signed these words for Pim, who now turned to her husband with a stern look.

You know how Bill is, Caleb signed. *We could be here all day.*

No. We wait.

There was no point in arguing when Pim had made up her mind. Caleb always said it was the woman's stubbornness that had kept them together while he was stationed with the Army on the Oil Road, and Peter didn't doubt it. The two of them had married the day after Caleb had finally capitulated and resigned his commission — not, as he often pointed out, that there was much of an Army remaining to resign from. Like nearly everything else in Kerrville, the Army had scattered to the winds; barely anyone remembered the Expeditionary, disbanded twenty years ago, when the Texas Code had been suspended. It had been one of the great disappointments of Caleb's life that there was nobody left to fight anymore. He'd spent his years in the service as a glorified ditch digger, assigned to the construction of the telegraph line between Kerrville and Boerne. It was a different world than the one Peter had known. The city walls went unmanned; the perimeter lights had gone out one by one and never been repaired; the gate hadn't been shut in a decade. A whole generation had grown to adulthood thinking the virals were little more than exaggerated boogeymen in scary stories told by their elders,

who, in the fashion of all old people since the dawn of time, believed theirs had been the vastly harder and more consequential life.

But it was like Kate's husband, Bill, to be late. The man had his positive qualities — he was far more easy-going than Kate, counterbalancing her often humorless maturity — and there was no question that he adored their daughters. But he was scattered and disorganized, liked the lick and cards, and lacked anything approximating a work ethic. Peter had tried to bring him into the administration as a favor to Sara and Hollis, offering him a low-level job with the Bureau of Taxation that required little more than the ability to use a stamp. But as with Bill's brief forays into carpentry, farriering, and driving a transport, it wasn't long before he drifted away. Mostly he seemed content to look after his daughters, make Kate the occasional meal, and sneak out to the tables at night — both winning and losing but, according to Kate, always winning just a little more.

Baby Theo had begun to fuss. Caleb used the delay to pick the horses' hooves while Sara took Theo from Pim to change his diaper. Just when it had begun to seem that Bill wouldn't show, Kate appeared with the girls, Bill bringing up the rear with a sheepish look on his face.

"How did you get away?" Sara asked her daughter.

"Don't worry, Madam Director — Jenny's got it covered. Plus, you love me too much to fire me."

"You know, I really hate it when you call me that."

Elle and her younger sister, Merry, who everybody called Bug, dashed to Pim, who knelt and hugged them together. The girls' signing abilities

were limited to simple phrases, and all exchanged *I love you,* circling their hearts with a flat palm.

Visit me, Pim signed, then glanced up at Kate, who explained what she was asking.

"Can we?" Bug asked eagerly. "When?"

"We'll see," Kate said. "Maybe after the baby is born."

This was a sore subject; Sara had wanted Pim to delay their departure until after the birth of their second child. But that wouldn't be until nearly the end of the summer, far too late to plant. Nor did Pim, in her obstinate way, plan to return alone for the birth. *I've done it before,* she said. *How hard can it be?*

"Please, Mom?" Elle begged.

"I said, we'll see."

Hugs all around. Peter glanced at Sara; she was feeling it, too. Their children were leaving for good. It was what you were supposed to want, the thing you worked for, yet facing it was a different matter.

Caleb shook Peter's hand, then pulled him into a masculine embrace. "So I guess this is it. Mind if I say some stupid things? Like, I love you. You're still a terrible chess player, though."

"I promise to practice. Who knows? Maybe you'll find me out there before too long."

Caleb grinned. "See? That's what I've been telling you. No more politics. It's time to find a nice girl and settle down."

If you only knew, Peter thought. *Every night I close my eyes and do just that.*

He lowered his voice slightly. "Did you do like I asked?"

Caleb sighed indulgently.

"Humor your old man."

"Yeah, yeah, I dug it."

"And you used the steel framing I sent out? It's important."

"I did it just like you said, I promise. At least I've got someplace to sleep when Pim kicks me out."

Peter looked up at his daughter-in-law, who had climbed onto the bench. Baby Theo, worn out by all the attention, had passed out in her arms.

Look after him for me, Peter signed.

I will.

The babies, too.

She smiled at him. *The babies, too.*

Caleb lifted himself onto the buckboard.

"Be safe," Peter said. "Good luck."

The indelible moment of departure: everyone stepped back as the wagon moved through the gate. Bill and the girls were the first to leave, followed by Kate and Hollis. Peter had a full schedule ahead of him, but he couldn't quite bring himself to start his day.

Nor, apparently, could Sara. They stood together without speaking, watching the wagon bearing their children away.

"Why do I feel sometimes like they're parenting us?" Sara said.

"They will be, soon enough."

Sara snorted. "Now *there's* something to look forward to."

The wagon was still in sight. It was crossing the old fence line to the Orange Zone. Beyond it, only a fraction of the fields had been plowed for planting; there simply wasn't enough manpower. Nor were there that many mouths remaining to feed; the population of Kerrville itself had shrunk to

just about five thousand. Make that 4,997, thought Peter.

"Bill's a mess," Peter said.

Sara sighed. "And yet Kate loves him. What's a mother to do?"

"I could try again with a job."

"I'm afraid he's a lost cause." She glanced at him. "Speaking of which, what's this about you not running for reelection?"

"Where did you hear that?"

She shrugged coyly. "Oh, just around the halls."

"Meaning Chase."

"Who else? The man is chomping at the bit. So, is it true?"

"I haven't decided. Maybe ten years is enough, though."

"People will miss you."

"I doubt they'll even notice."

Peter thought she might ask him about Michael. What had he heard? Was her brother okay at least? They avoided the details, a painful reality. Michael on the trade, rumors of some crazy project, Greer in cahoots with Dunk, an armed compound on the ship channel with trucks full of lick and God knew what else leaving every day.

But she didn't. Instead Sara asked, "What does Vicky think?"

The question pierced him with guilt. He'd been meaning to visit the woman for weeks, months even.

"I need to go see her," he said. "How is she doing?"

The two of them were still standing shoulder to shoulder as their eyes traced the course of the wagon. It was little more than a speck now. It crested a small rise, began to sink, then was gone.

326

Sara turned toward him.

"I wouldn't wait," she said.

His day dissolved into the customary duties. A meeting with the collector of taxes to decide what to do about homesteaders who refused to pay; a new judicial appointment to make; an agenda to set for the upcoming meeting of the territorial legislature; various papers to sign, which Chase placed in front of him with only cursory description. At three o'clock, Apgar appeared in Peter's door. Did the president have a minute? Everybody else on the staff simply called him by his first name, as he preferred, but Gunnar, a stickler for protocol, refused. Always he was "Mr. President."

The subject was guns — specifically, a lack of them. The Army had always run on a combination of reconditioned civilian and military weaponry. A lot had come from Fort Hood; plus, the old Texas had been a well-armed place. Virtually every house, it seemed, had a gun cabinet in it, and there were weapon-manufacturing facilities throughout the state, offering a bountiful supply of parts for repair and reloading. But a lot of time had passed, and certain guns lasted longer than others. Metal-framed pistols, like the old Browning 1911, SIG Sauer semiautos, and army-issue Beretta M9s, were close to indestructible with adequate maintenance. So were most revolvers, shotguns, and bolt-action rifles. But polymer-framed pistols, like Glocks, as well as M4 and AR-15 rifles, the bread and butter of the military, did not enjoy the same indefinite shelf life. As their plastic casings cracked with fatigue, more and more were retired; others had leaked via the

trade into civilian hands; some had simply vanished.

But that was only part of the problem. The more pressing issue was a dwindling supply of ammunition. Decades had passed since a prewar cartridge had been fired; except for the stockpiles in Tifty's bunker, which were vacuum-sealed, the primer and cordite didn't last more than twenty years. All of the Army's rounds had been either reloaded from spent brass or manufactured with empty casings taken from two munitions plants, one near Waco and a second in Victoria. Casting lead for bullets was easy; far trickier was engineering a propellant. Weapons-grade cordite required a complicated cocktail of highly volatile chemicals, including large quantities of nitroglycerine. It could be done, but it wasn't easy, and it necessitated both manpower and expertise, both of which were in very short supply. The Army was down to just a couple thousand soldiers — fifteen hundred spread throughout the townships, and a garrison of five hundred in Kerrville. They had no chemists at all.

"I think we both know what we're talking about here," Peter said.

Apgar, seated across the paper-stacked expanse of Peter's desk, was looking at his nails. "I didn't say I liked it. But the trade has the manufacturing capacity, and it's not like we haven't dealt with them before."

"Dunk's not Tifty."

"What about Michael?"

Peter frowned. "Sore subject."

"The guy was an OFC. He knows how to cook oil — he can do this."

"What about this boat of his?" Peter asked.

"He's *your* friend. You tell me what it's all about."

Peter took a long breath. "I wish I could. I haven't seen the guy in over twenty years. On top of which, we tell the trade we're out of ammo, we've tipped our hand. Dunk will be sitting in this chair in a weekend."

"So threaten him. He comes through for us or that's it, the deal's off, we storm the isthmus and put him out of business."

"Across that causeway? It'd be a bloodbath. He'll smell a bluff before I stop talking."

Peter leaned back in his chair. He imagined himself laying out Apgar's terms to Dunk. What could the man do but laugh in his face?

"This is all stick. There's no way it's going to work. What can we offer him?"

Gunnar scowled. "What, besides money, guns, and whores? Last time I checked, Dunk had all of those in plentiful supply. Plus, the guy's practically a folk hero. You know what happened last Sunday? Out of the blue, a five-ton full of women shows up at the encampment in Bandera where they're housing the road crews. The driver has a note. 'Compliments of your good friend Dunk Withers.' On a fucking *Sunday*."

"Did they send them away?"

Gunnar snorted through his nose. "No, they took them to church. What do you think?"

"Well, there has to be something."

"You could ask him yourself."

A joke, but not entirely. There was also Michael to consider. Despite everything, Peter liked to think that the man would at least agree to talk to him.

"Maybe I'll do that."

329

As Gunnar rose, Chase appeared in the doorway.

"What is it, Ford?" Peter asked.

"We've got another sinkhole. A big one. Two houses this time."

This had been happening all spring. A rumbling in the earth; then, within moments, the ground would collapse. The largest hole had been over fifty feet wide. *This place really is falling apart,* Peter thought.

"Anybody hurt?" he asked.

"Not this time. Both houses were empty."

"Well, that's lucky." Ford was still looking at him expectantly. "Is there something else?"

"I'm thinking we should make a statement. People are going to want to know what you're doing about it."

"Such as what? Telling the ground to behave itself?" When Ford said nothing, Peter sighed. "Fine, write something up, and I'll sign it. Engineering on the case, situation in hand, et cetera." He raised an eyebrow at Ford. "Okay?"

Apgar looked like he was about to laugh. *Jesus,* Peter thought, *it never ends.* He got to his feet.

"Come on, Gunnar. Let's get some air."

He had become president not because he desired the job particularly but as a favor to Vicky. Right after her election to a third term, she had developed a tremor in her right hand. This was followed by a series of accidents, including a fall on the capitol steps that had broken her ankle. Her handwriting, always precise, decayed to a scrawl; her speech adopted a weirdly monotonic quality, lacking all inflection; the tremors spread to her other hand, and she began to make involuntary rocking motions with her neck. Peter and Chase

had managed to hide the situation by keeping her public schedule to a minimum, but halfway into her second year, it became clear that she could no longer continue. The Texas Constitution, which had superseded the Code of Modified Martial Law, allowed her to name a president pro tem.

At the time, Peter was serving as secretary of territorial affairs, a position he had taken on midway through her second term. It was one of the most visible jobs in the cabinet, and Vicky made no secret of the fact that she was grooming him for something more. Still, he had assumed that Chase would be the one to step in; the man had been with her for years. When Vicky called Peter to her office, he wholly expected a meeting to discuss the transition to Chase's administration; what he found was a judge with a Bible. Two minutes later, he was president of the Texas Republic.

This was, he came to understand, what the woman had intended from the start: to create her successor from the ground up. Peter had stood for election two years later, won easily, and ran unopposed for his second term. Some of this was his personal popularity as a chief executive; as Vicky had predicted, his stock was very high. But it was also true that he had assumed the office at a time when it was easy to make people happy.

Kerrville itself was on its way to becoming irrelevant. How long before it was just one more provincial town? The farther out people settled, the less the idea of centralized authority held sway. The legislature had relocated to Boerne and almost never met. Financial capital had followed human capital to the townships; people were opening businesses, trading commodities at

market-established prices, negotiating life on their own terms. In Fredericksburg, a group of private investors had pooled their money to open a bank, the first of its kind. There were still problems, and only the federal administration possessed the resources for major infrastructure projects: roads, dams, telegraph lines. But even this wouldn't last indefinitely. When Peter was being honest with himself, he understood that he was not so much running the place as guiding it into port. Let Chase have his chance, he thought. Two decades in public life, with its endless closed-door bickering, was plenty for any man. Peter had never farmed; he'd never so much as planted a tomato. But he could learn, and best of all, a plow had no opinions.

Vicky had retired to a small, wood-frame house on the east side of town. A lot of the neighborhood was empty, folks having cleared out long ago. It was getting dark when he stepped onto the porch. A single light was burning in the front parlor. He heard footsteps; then the door opened to reveal Meredith, Vicky's partner, wiping her hands on a cloth.

"Peter." About sixty, she was a petite woman with sharp blue eyes. She and Vicky had been together for years. "I didn't know you were coming."

"I'm sorry, I should have sent word."

"No, come in, of course." She stepped back. "She's awake — I was just about to feed her some supper. I know she'll be happy to see you."

Vicky's bed was in the parlor. As Peter entered, she glanced in his direction, her head jerking side to side against the elevated pillows.

"Ssss . . . bout tahm . . . Misss . . . ter . . . P . . .

p . . . reeee . . . sa . . . dent."

It was as if she were swallowing the words, then spitting them out again. He drew a chair to the side of her bed. "How are you feeling?"

"Toooo . . . day . . . n . . . not ssso . . . b . . . b . . . a-duh."

"I'm sorry I've been away."

Her hands were moving about restlessly on the blanket. She gave a crooked smile. "Thasss . . . oh . . . k . . . *kay*. Aaas you . . . caaan see . . . I . . . fff . . . been . . . bizzz . . . ee."

Meredith appeared in the door with a tray, which she placed on the bedside table. On the tray were a bowl of clear broth and a glass of water with a straw. She cupped the back of Vicky's head to lift it forward from the pillow and tied a cotton bib around her neck. Night had fallen, making mirrors of the windows.

"Do you want me to do it?" Peter asked Meredith.

"Vicky, do you want Peter to help you with dinner?"

"W . . . w . . . why . . . n . . . n . . . not."

"Small sips," Meredith told him, and patted him on the arm. She gave him the faintest of smiles; her face was heavy with fatigue. The woman probably hadn't slept a solid night in months and was simply grateful for the help. "If you need me, I'll be in the kitchen."

Peter began with the water, holding the straw to Vicky's lips, which were flaked with dryness, then moved on to the broth. He could see the tremendous effort it required for her to swallow even the tiniest amount. Most of it dribbled from the corners of her mouth; he used the bib to wipe her chin.

"Sss . . . sss . . . fun . . . neee."

"What's that?"

"You . . . ffff . . . fff . . . eed . . . ing . . . me. Like . . . a . . . bay . . . beeee."

He gave her more of the broth. "The least I could do. You spoon-fed me more than once."

Her neck made a sinewy pumping motion as she tried to swallow. It exhausted him, just watching it.

"How . . . ssss . . . the . . . cam . . . p . . . p . . . aign?"

"Not really gotten started yet. Been a bit tied up."

"Yyyyy . . . you're . . . f . . . full of . . . sh . . . sh . . . shit."

She had him dead to rights, but of course she always did. He fed her another spoonful, without much luck. "Caleb and Pim left for the townships today."

"You're . . . j . . . j . . . ust . . . blue. It . . . will . . . lll . . . passss."

"What? You don't think I can farm?"

"I . . . I kn . . . know . . . you . . . P . . . eter. You'lllll . . . go . . . c . . . c . . . craze . . . ee."

She said nothing else. Peter put the bowl aside; she'd consumed only a fraction. When he looked up again, Vicky's eyes were closed. He doused the lamp and watched her. Only in sleep did the restless turmoil of her body cease. A few minutes passed; he heard a sound behind him and saw Meredith standing in the kitchen doorway.

"It happens like that," the woman said quietly. "One minute she's there, the next . . ." She left the thought unfinished.

"Is there anything I can do?"

Meredith placed one hand on his arm and met

334

his eye. "She was so proud of you, Peter. It made her so happy, watching all you've done."

"Will you call me if you need me? Anything at all."

"I think this was a perfect visit, don't you? Let's let it be the last one."

He returned to Vicky's bedside and lifted one of her hands from the blanket. The woman didn't stir. He held it for a minute, thinking about her, then leaned down and kissed her on the cheek, something he had never done before.

"Thank you," he whispered.

He followed Meredith to the porch. "She loved you, you know," the woman said. "It wasn't the kind of thing she said very often, not even to me. That's just how she was. But she did."

"I loved her, too."

"She knows you did." They embraced. "Good-bye, Peter."

The street was silent, no lights burning. He touched a finger to his eye; it came away wet. Well, he was the president, he could cry if he wanted to. His son was gone; others would follow. He had entered the era of his life when things would drop away. Peter tipped his face to the sky. It was true, what they said about the stars. The more you looked, the more you saw. They were a comfort, their watchful presence a force of reassurance; yet this had not always been so. He stood and looked at them, remembering a time when the sight of so many stars had meant something else entirely.

25

They spent the night in Hunt, sleeping on the ground by the wagon, and arrived in Mystic Town-

ship on the second afternoon. The town was a threadbare outpost: a small main street with just a few houses, a general store, and a government building that acted as everything from the post office to the jail. They passed through and followed the river road west through a tunnel of thickening foliage. Pim had never been to the townships before; everything she saw seemed to fascinate her. *Look at the trees,* she signed to the baby. *Look at the river. Look at the world.*

The day had begun to fade when they reached the homestead. The house stood on a rise looking down toward the Guadalupe, with a paddock for the horses, fields of black soil between, and a privy in the rear. Caleb stepped down from the buckboard and reached up for Theo, who was sleeping in a basket.

"What do you think?"

Since Theo's birth, Caleb had made it his habit to speak and sign simultaneously whenever the boy was present. With nobody else around, he would grow up thinking that talking and signing were really no different from each other.

You did all this?

"Well, I had help."

Show me the rest.

He led her inside. There were two rooms on the main floor, with real glass windows and a kitchen with a stove and a pump, and a flight of stairs that led to a loft where the three of them would sleep. The floor, of sawn oak planks, felt solid underfoot.

"It'll be too hot to sleep inside in the summer, but I can build a sleeping porch out back."

Pim was smiling; she looked as if she couldn't believe her eyes. *When will you have time for that?*

"I'll do it, don't worry."

They unloaded a night's worth of gear. In a few days, Caleb would have to return to town, an eight-mile ride, to begin the process of securing stock: a milk cow, a goat or two, chickens. His seeds were ready to plant; the soil had been turned. They would be growing corn and beans in alternating rows, with a kitchen garden out back. The first year would be a race against time. After that, he hoped, things would settle into a more predictable rhythm, though life would never be easy, by any means.

They ate a simple dinner and lay down on the mattress he had moved inside from the wagon to the floor of the main room. He'd wondered if Pim would be afraid or at least anxious, being out here, just the three of them. She'd never spent a night beyond the city walls. But the opposite seemed true; she appeared completely at ease, eager to see how their situation unfolded. Of course, there was a reason. The things that had happened to her when she was a young girl had become for her a source of strength.

Pim had crept up on his life slowly. At the beginning, when Sara had brought her home from the orphanage, she had hardly seemed like a person to him. Her blunt gestures and guttural groans unnerved him. Extending even the simplest kindness was met with incomprehension, even anger. The situation had started to change when Sara taught Pim sign language. They moved through this improvisationally, beginning by spelling out every word, then advancing to whole phrases and ideas that could be captured with a single swoop of the hand. A book from the library had been involved, but later, when Kate gave it to Caleb to study, he realized that many of the gestures Pim

used were made up: a bubble of private language that only she and her mother — and, to a degree, Kate and her father — shared. Caleb was, by this point, fourteen or fifteen. He was a clever boy, unused to problems he could not solve. Also, Pim had begun to seem interesting to him. What sort of person was she? The fact that he could not communicate with her as he could with everybody else was both frustrating and attractive. He made a point of carefully observing Pim's interactions with members of her family to encode these gestures into memory. Alone in his room, he practiced in front of a mirror for hours, signing both sides of dialogues on arbitrary topics. *How are you today? I am very well, thank you. What do you think of the weather? I enjoy the rain but am looking forward to warmer days.*

It became important that he delay the unveiling of his new abilities until he had acquired the confidence to engage her on a range of subjects. The opportunity presented itself on an afternoon outing their families had taken together to the spillway. While everyone else was enjoying their picnic by the water, he had climbed to the top of the dam. There he saw Pim, sitting on the concrete, writing in her journal. She was always writing; Caleb had wondered about this. She glanced up as he made his approach, her dark eyes narrowing on him in their intense way, then looked away dismissively. Her brown hair, long and glossy and tucked behind her ears, flared with captured sunshine. He stood for a moment, observing her. She was three years older than he was, basically an adult in his eyes. She had also become very pretty, though in a no-nonsense way that came across as condescending, even a little icy.

338

His presence was obviously unwelcome, but it was too late to back out. Caleb walked up to her. She regarded him with her head slightly cocked to the side, wearing an expression of bored mirth.

Hello, he signed.

She closed her book around her pencil. *You want to kiss me, don't you?*

The question was so unexpectedly direct that he actually startled. Did he? Was that what this was all about? Now she really *was* laughing at him — laughing with her eyes.

I know you know what I'm saying, she signed.

He found the answer with his hands: *I learned.*

For me or for yourself?

He felt caught. *Both.*

Have you kissed anyone before?

He hadn't. It was something he had been meaning to get around to. He knew he was blushing.

A few times.

No, you haven't. Hands don't lie.

He recognized the truth of this. All his study and practice, yet he'd failed to notice the obvious fact, which Pim had laid bare to him in mere seconds: signing was a language of complete forthrightness. Within its compact rhetoric, little space remained for evasion, for the self-protecting half-truths that were most of what people said to one another.

Do you want to?

She stood and faced him. *Okay.*

So they did. He closed his eyes, thinking this was something he should do, tilted his head slightly, and leaned forward. Their noses bumped, then passed each other, their lips meeting in a soft collision. It was over before he knew it.

Did you like it?

339

He barely believed this was actually happening. He spelled out his answer: *Lots.*

Open your mouth this time.

That was even better. A soft pressure entered his mouth that he realized was her tongue. He followed her lead; now they were kissing for real. He had always imagined the act to be a simple grazing of surfaces, lips upon lips, but kissing was, he now understood, far more complex. It was more a mingling than a touching. They did this for a while, exploring one another's mouths, then she backed away in a manner that indicated that the kissing was over. Caleb wished it weren't; he could have done it for a long while more. Then he understood the nature of the interruption. Sara was calling to them from the bottom of the dam.

Pim smiled at him. *You're a good kisser.*

And that was all, at least for a time. In due course, they had kissed again, and done different things as well, but it hadn't amounted to much, and other girls had come along. Yet always those slender minutes on the dam remained in his mind as a singular point in his life. When he joined the Army, at eighteen, his CO said he should find someone back home to write to. He chose Pim. His letters were all cheerful nonsense, complaints about the food and lighthearted stories of his friends, but hers were unlike anything he'd ever read, richly observant and full of life. At times they read like poetry. A single phrase, even describing something trivial — how the sun looked on leaves, a passing remark by an acquaintance, the smell of cooking food — would catch his mind and linger for days. Unlike sign language, with its unequivocal compactness, Pim's words on the page seemed to overflow with feeling — a

richer kind of truth, closer to the heart of her. He wrote to Pim as often as he could, hungering for more of her. It was her voice he was hearing — hearing at last — and it wasn't long before he began to fall in love with her. When he told her, not in a letter but in person when he returned to Kerrville on a three-day pass, she laughed with her eyes, then signed, *When did you finally figure it out?*

To these memories, Caleb drifted into sleep. Sometime later he awoke to find her gone. He didn't worry; Pim was something of a night owl. Theo was still asleep. Caleb slid into his trousers, lit the lantern, got his rifle from its place by the door, and stepped outside. Pim was sitting with her back against the stump he used for splitting.

Everything okay?

Douse the light, she signed. *Come sit.*

She was wearing only her nightgown, though it was actually quite chilly; her feet were bare. He took his place beside her and extinguished the lantern. In the dark, they had a system. She took his hand and in his palm signed in miniature: *Look.*

At what?

Everything.

He understood what she was saying, between the lines. This is ours.

I like it here.

I'm glad.

Caleb detected movement in the brush. The sound came again, a grassy rustling to their left. Not a raccoon or possum — something larger.

Pim sensed his sudden alertness. *What?*

Wait.

He relit the lantern, casting a pool of light on the ground. The rustling was coming from several

341

places now, though generally in the same direction. He positioned the rifle under his arm and clenched it to his side with his elbow. Holding the lantern in one hand, the rifle in the other, he crept forward, toward the heart of the sounds.

The light caught something: a flash of eyes.

It was a young deer. It froze in the light, staring at him. He saw the others, six in all. For a moment nothing moved, man and deer regarding one another with mutual astonishment. Then, as if guided by a common mind, the herd turned as one and burst away.

What could he do? What else could Caleb Jaxon do but laugh?

26

"Okay, Rand, try it now."

Michael was lying on his back, wedged into the slender gap between the floor and the base of the compressor. He heard the valve opening; gas began to move through the line.

"What's it say?"

"Looks like it's holding."

Don't you dare leak, Michael thought. *I've given you half my morning.*

"Nope. Pressure's dropping."

"God*damn*it." He'd checked every seal he could think of. Where the hell was the gas coming from? "The hell with it. Shut it off."

Michael wriggled free. They were on the lower engineering level. From the catwalk above came the sounds of metal striking metal, the crackling hiss of arc welders, men calling to one another, all of it amplified by the acoustics of the engine compartment. Michael hadn't seen sunshine for

forty-eight hours.

"Any ideas?" he asked Rand.

The man was standing with his hands in the pockets of his trousers. There was something equine about him. He had small eyes, delicate-seeming in his strong face, and black wavy hair that, despite his age — somewhere north of forty-five — failed to show more than scattered threads of gray. Calm, reliable Rand. He had never spoken of a wife or girlfriend; he never visited Dunk's whores. Michael had never pressed, the matter being one of supreme unimportance.

"It could be someplace in the charger," Rand suggested. "Tight fit, though."

Michael looked up at the catwalk and yelled, to whomever might hear him, "Where's Patch?"

Patch's real name was Byron Szumanski. The nickname came from the anomalous square of white in his otherwise coal-black stubble. Like many of Michael's men, he had been raised in the orphanage; he'd done a stint in the military, learning a thing or two about engines along the way, then worked for the civilian authority as a mechanic. He had no relatives, had never married and professed no desire to do so, possessed no bad habits Michael knew of, didn't mind the isolation, wasn't a talker, took orders without complaint, and liked to work — perfect, in other words, for Michael's purposes. A wiry five foot three, he spent whole days in pockets of the ship so cramped that another man wouldn't have been able to draw a breath. Michael paid him accordingly, though nobody could complain about the wages. Every cent Michael made from the stills went straight to the *Bergensfjord*.

A face appeared above: Weir's. He drew his

343

welder's mask up to his forehead. "I think he's on the bridge."

"Send somebody to get him."

As Michael bent for his tool bag, Rand rapped him on the arm. "We've got company."

Michael looked up; Dunk was coming down the stairs. Michael needed the man, just as Dunk needed him, but their relationship was not an easy one. Needless to say, Dunk knew nothing of Michael's true purpose; he regarded the *Bergensfjord* as an eccentric distraction, an elaborate pastime on which Michael wasted his time — time better spent putting more money in Dunk's pockets. That the man had never bothered to wonder just why Michael needed to refloat a six-hundred-foot freighter was just more evidence of his limited intelligence.

"Great," Michael said.

"You want me to get some guys together? He looks pissed."

"How can you tell?"

Rand moved away. At the base of the stairs Dunk halted, propped his hands on his hips, and surveyed the room with an expression of weary irritation. The tattoos on his face ended abruptly at his former hairline. A lifetime of hard living had done him few favors in the aging department, but he was still built like a tank. For entertainment, he liked to lift a truck by its bumper.

"What can I do for you, Dunk?"

He had a way of smiling that made Michael think of a cork in a bottle. "I really should get down here more often. I don't know what half this stuff is. Take those things over there." He wagged a meaty finger, thick as a sausage.

"Water jacket pumps."

"What do they do?"

The day was getting away without much to show for it; now he had to deal with this. "It's kind of technical. Not really your thing."

"Why am I here, Michael?"

Guessing games, as if they were five years old. "A sudden interest in marine repair?"

Dunk's eyes hardened on Michael's face. "I'm here, Michael, because you're not meeting your obligation to me. Mystic's open for settlement. That means demand. I need the new boiler up and running. Not later. Today."

Michael aimed his voice at the catwalk. "Has anybody found Patch yet?"

"We're looking!"

He turned toward Dunk again. What an ox the man was. He should've been strapped to a plow. "I'm kind of busy at the moment."

"Allow me to remind you of the terms. You do your magic with the stills, I give you ten percent of the profits. It's not hard to remember."

Michael yelled up to the catwalk again. "Sometime today would be nice!"

The next thing Michael knew, he was rammed up against the bulkhead, Dunk's forearm pressing against his throat.

"Do I have your attention now?"

The man's broad, pitted nose was inches from Michael's; his breath was sour as old wine.

"Easy, amigo. We don't have to do this in front of the kids."

"You work for *me,* goddamnit."

"If I could point something out. Breaking my neck might feel good in the moment, but it won't get you any more lick."

"Everything okay, Michael?"

Rand was standing behind Dunk with two others, Fastau and Weir. Rand was clutching a long wrench; the other two had lengths of pipe. They were holding these implements in an offhand manner, as if they'd merely picked them up in the course of a day's work.

"Just a little misunderstanding," Michael replied. "How about it, Dunk? We don't need to have a problem here. You've got my attention, I promise."

Dunk's arm pressed tighter against his throat. "Fuck you."

Michael glanced over Dunk's shoulder at Weir and Fastau. "You two, go check on the stills, see what the situation is, then report back to me. Got it?" He returned his attention to Dunk. "Got this covered. I'm hearing you loud and clear."

"Twenty years. I've had it with your bullshit. This . . . hobby of yours."

"Totally understand your feelings. I spoke out of turn. New boilers up and running, no problem."

Dunk kept glowering at him. It was hard to say how things were going to go. Finally, giving Michael a last hard shove against the bunker, Dunk backed away. He turned toward Michael's men and nailed them with a hard look.

"You three should be more careful."

Michael withheld his coughing until Dunk was out of sight.

"Jesus, Michael." Rand was staring at him.

"Oh, he's just having a bad day. He'll cool off. You two, back to work. Rand, you're with me."

Weir frowned. "You don't want us to go to the stills?"

"No, I don't. I'll look in on them later."

They walked away.

"You shouldn't goad him like that," Rand said.

Michael paused to cough again. He felt a little foolish, though on the other hand, the whole thing had been strangely gratifying. It was nice when people were themselves. "Have you seen Greer anywhere?"

"He took a launch up the channel this morning."

So, feeding day. Michael always worried — Amy still tried to kill Greer every time — but the man took it in stride. Except for Rand, who'd been with them from the beginning, none of Michael's men knew about that part of things: Amy, Carter, the *Chevron Mariner,* the jugs of blood that Greer dutifully delivered every sixty days.

Rand glanced around. "How long do you think we have before the virals come back?" he asked quietly. "It's got to be close by now."

Michael shrugged.

"It's not that I'm not grateful. We all are. But people want to be ready."

"If they do their damn jobs, we'll be long gone before it happens." Michael hitched his tool bag onto his shoulder. "And for fucksake, will somebody *please* go find Patch. I don't want to wait around all morning."

It was evening when Michael finally emerged from the bowels of the ship. His knees were killing him; he'd done something to his neck, too. He'd never found the leak, either.

But he would; he always did. He would find it, and every other leak and rusty rivet and frayed wire in the *Bergensfjord*'s miles of cables and wires and pipes, and soon, in a matter of months, they would charge the batteries and test-fire the

347

engines, and if all went as it should, they'd be ready. Michael liked to imagine that day. The pumps engaging, water pouring into the dock, the retaining wall opening, and the *Bergensfjord,* all twenty thousand tons of her, sliding gracefully from her braces into the sea.

For two decades, Michael had thought of little else. The trade had been Greer's idea — a stroke of genius, really. They needed money, a lot of it. What did they have to sell? A month after he'd shown Lucius the newspaper from the *Bergensfjord,* Michael had found himself in the back room of the gambling hall known as Cousin's Place, sitting across a table from Dunk Withers. Michael knew him to be a man of extraordinary temper, lacking all conscience, driven by only the most utilitarian concerns; Michael's life meant nothing to him, because no one's did. But Michael's reputation had preceded him, and he'd done his homework. The gates were about to open; people would be flooding into the townships. The opportunities were many, Michael pointed out, but did the trade possess the capacity to meet a rapidly growing demand? What would Dunk say if Michael told him that he could triple — no, *quadruple* — his output? That he could also guarantee an uninterrupted flow of ammunition? And furthermore, what if Michael knew about a place where the trade could operate in complete safety, beyond the reach of the military or the domestic authority but with quick access to Kerrville and the townships? That, in sum, he could make Dunk Withers richer than he could imagine?

Thus was the isthmus born.

A great deal of time was wasted at the start. Before Michael could so much as tighten a single

bolt on the *Bergensfjord,* he had to win the man's confidence. For three years he had overseen the construction of the massive stills that would make Dunk Withers a legend. Michael was not unaware of the costs. How many fistfights would leave a man bloodied and toothless, how many bodies would be dumped into alleyways, how many wives and children would be beaten or even killed, all because of the mental poison he provided? He tried not to think about it. The *Bergensfjord* was all that mattered; it was a price she demanded, paid in blood.

Along the way, he laid the groundwork for his true enterprise. He began with the refinery. Cautious inquiries: Who seemed bored? Dissatisfied? Restless? Rand Horgan was the first; he and Michael had worked the cookers together for years. Others followed, recruited from every corner. Greer would leave for a few days, then return with a man in a jeep with nothing but a duffel bag and his promise to stay on the isthmus for five years in exchange for wages so outrageous they would set him up for life. The numbers accumulated; soon they had fifty-four stout souls with nothing to lose. Michael noticed a pattern. The money was an inducement, but what these men really sought was something intangible. A great many people drifted through their lives without a feeling of purpose. Each day felt indistinguishable from the last, devoid of meaning. When he unveiled the *Bergensfjord* to each new recruit, Michael could see a change in the man's eyes. Here was something beyond the scope of ordinary days, something from before the time of mankind's diminishment. It was the past Michael was giving these men and, with it, the future. *We're actually going*

to fix it? they always asked. *Not "it,"* Michael corrected. *"Her." And no, we're not going to fix her. We're going to wake her up.*

It didn't always take. Michael's rule was this: At the three-year mark, once Michael was certain of a man's loyalty, he took him to an isolated hut, sat him in a chair, and gave him the bad news. Most took it well: a moment of disbelief, a brief period of bargaining with the cosmos, requests for evidence Michael declined to provide, resistance eventually yielding to acceptance and, finally, a melancholy gratitude. They would be among the living, after all. As for those who didn't last three years, or failed the test of the hut, well, that was unfortunate. Greer was the one to take care of this; Michael kept his distance. They were surrounded by water, into which a man could quietly vanish. Afterward, his name was never mentioned.

It took two years to repair the dock, another two to pump and refloat the hull, a fifth to back her in. The day they set her hull in the braces, sealed the doors, and drained the water from the dock was the most anxious of Michael's life. The braces would hold, or not; the hull would crack, or it wouldn't. A thousand things could go wrong, and there would be no second chances. As a layer of daylight appeared between the receding water and the bottom of the hull, his men erupted in cheers, but Michael's emotions were different. He felt not elation but a sense of fate. Alone, he took the stairs to the bottom of the dock. The cheers had quieted; everyone was watching him. With water pooling around his ankles, he stepped toward her cautiously, as if approaching some great, holy relic. Clear of the water, she had become something new. The sheer size of her, her indomitable

bulk — it staggered the mind. The curvature of her hull below the waterline possessed an almost feminine softness; from her bow jutted a bulbous shape, like a nose or the front of a bullet. He moved under her; all her weight was above him now, a mountain suspended over his head. He reached up and placed a hand against her hull. She was cold; a humming sensation met the tips of his fingers. It was as if she were breathing, a living thing. A deep certainty flowed into his veins: here was his mission. All other possibilities for his life dropped away; until the day he died, he would have no purpose but this.

Except to sail the *Nautilus,* Michael had not left the isthmus since. A show of solidarity, politically wise, but in his heart he knew the real reason. He belonged nowhere else.

He walked to the bow to look for Greer. A damp March wind was blowing. The isthmus, part of an old shipyard complex, jutted into the channel a quarter mile south of the Channel Bridge. A hundred yards offshore, the *Nautilus* lay at anchor. Her hull was still tight, her canvas crisp. The sight made him feel disloyal; he had not sailed her in months. She was the forerunner; if the *Bergens-fjord* was his wife, then the *Nautilus* was the girl who had taught him to love.

He heard the launch before he saw it, churning under the Channel Bridge in the silvery light. Michael descended to the service dock as Greer guided the boat in. He tossed Michael a line.

"How did it go?"

Greer tied off the stern, passed Michael his rifle, and climbed onto the pier. Just past seventy, he had aged the way bulls did: one minute they'd be

huffing and snorting, looking to gore you; the next you'd find them lying in a field, covered in flies.

"Well," Michael offered, "she didn't kill you — that's a plus."

Greer didn't answer. Michael sensed that the man was troubled; the visit had not gone well.

"Lucius, did she say something?"

"Say? You know how this works."

"Actually, I've never really known."

He shrugged. "It's a feeling I have. *She* has. Probably it's nothing."

Michael decided not to press. "There was something else I wanted to bring up with you. I had a little run-in with Dunk today."

Greer was coiling rope. "You know how he gets. This time tomorrow he'll have forgotten all about it."

"I don't think he's going to let this one go. It was bad."

Greer looked up.

"It was my fault. I was egging him on."

"What happened?"

"He came down to the engine room. The usual bullshit about the stills. Rand and a couple of guys practically had to pull him off me."

Greer's brow furrowed. "There's been too much of this."

"I know. He's getting to be a problem." Michael paused, then said, "It may be time."

Greer was silent, taking this in.

"We've talked about it."

Greer thought for a moment, then nodded. "Under the circumstances, you may be right."

They went over the names: who they could count on, who they couldn't, who was somewhere

352

in between and would have to be carefully handled.

"You should lie low for now," Greer said. "Rand and I will make the arrangements."

"If you think that's best."

The spotlights had come on, drenching the dock with light. Michael would be working most of the night.

"Just get that ship ready," said Greer.

Sara glanced up from her desk; Jenny was standing in the doorway.

"Sara, you need to see something."

Sara followed her downstairs to the wards. Jenny pulled back the curtain to show her. "The DS found him in an alley."

It took Sara a moment to recognize her own son-in-law. His face had been beaten to a pulp. Both of his arms were in casts. They moved back outside.

Jenny said, "I only just saw the chart and realized who it was."

"Where's Kate?"

"She's on the evening shift."

It was nearly four o'clock. Kate would be walking in the door any second.

"Head her off."

"What do you want me to say?"

Sara took a moment to think. "Send her to the orphanage. Aren't they due for a visit?"

"I don't know."

"Figure it out. Go."

Sara entered the ward. As she approached, Bill looked up with the eyes of a man who knew his day was about to get worse.

"Okay, what happened?" she asked.

353

He turned his face away.

"I'm disappointed in you, Bill."

He spoke through split lips: "I kinda figured."

"How much do you owe them?"

He told her. Sara dropped into a chair by the bed. "How could you be so goddamned stupid?"

"It wasn't like I planned this."

"You know they'll kill you. Probably I should just let them."

He surprised her by starting to cry.

"Cripes, don't do that," she said.

"I can't help it." Snot was running from his thickened nose. "I love Kate, I love the girls. I'm really, really sorry."

"Sorry doesn't help. How much time have they given you to come up with the money?"

"I can earn it all back. Just stake me for one night. I won't need much, just enough to get started."

"Does Kate fall for stuff like this?"

"She doesn't have to know."

"It was a rhetorical question, Bill. How much time?"

"The usual. Three days."

"What's usual about it? On second thought, don't tell me." She got to her feet.

"You can't tell Hollis. He'll kill me."

"He might."

"I'm sorry, Sara. I screwed up, I know that."

Jenny appeared, a little breathless. "Okay, looks like she bought it."

Sara glanced at her watch. "That gives you about an hour, Bill, before your wife shows up. I suggest you come clean and beg for mercy."

The man looked terrified. "What are you going to do?"

"Nothing you deserve."

27

Caleb was building a chicken coop when he saw a figure walking up the dusty road. It was late in the afternoon; Pim and Theo were resting in the house.

"Saw your smoke." The man who stood before him had a pleasant, weathered face and a thick, woolly beard. He was wearing a wide straw hat and suspenders. "Since we're going to be neighbors, thought I'd come by to say hello. Phil Tatum's the name."

"Caleb Jaxon." They shook.

"We're just on the other side of that ridge. Been there a bit, before most folks. There's me and my wife, Dorien. We got a grown boy just started his own place up toward Bandera. Did you say Jaxon?"

"That's right. He's my father."

"I'll be damned. What are you doing way out here?"

"Same as everyone, I guess. Making do." Caleb removed his gloves. "Come in and meet my family."

Pim was sitting in a chair by the cold hearth with Theo on her lap, showing him a picture book.

"Pim," Caleb said, signing along, "this is our neighbor, Mr. Tatum."

"How do you do, Mrs. Jaxon?" He was holding his hat against his chest. "Please, don't get up on my account."

I'm very pleased to meet you.

Caleb realized his error. "I should have explained. My wife is deaf. She says she's pleased to meet you."

The man nodded evenly. "Got a cousin like that, passed a while back. She learned to read lips a little, but the poor thing just lived in her own world." He raised his voice, the way a lot of people did. "That's a fine-looking boy you have, Mrs. Jaxon."

What's he saying?

You're beautiful and he wants to go to bed with you. He turned to their guest, who was still fingering the brim of his hat. "She says thank you, Mr. Tatum."

Don't be rude. Ask him if he wants something to drink.

Caleb repeated the question.

"Have to be home before supper, but I reckon I could sit for a bit, thank you."

Pim filled a pitcher with water, added slices of lemon, and placed it on the table, where the two men sat. They talked about little things: the weather, other homesteads in the area, where Caleb should get his livestock and at what price. Pim had gone off with Theo; she liked to take him down to the river, where the two of them would just sit quietly. It became clear to Caleb that the man and his wife were a little lonely. Their son had gone off with a woman he'd met at a dance in Hunt, barely saying goodbye.

"Couldn't help notice your wife is expecting," Tatum said. They had finished the water; now they were just talking.

"Yes, she's due in September."

"There's a doc in Mystic when the time comes." He gave Caleb the information.

"That's very kind. Thank you." Caleb sensed the presence of a sad history in the man's offer. The Tatums had had another child, perhaps more than one, who had failed to survive. This was all far in the past, but not really.

"Much obliged to you both," Tatum said at the door. "It's nice to have some young people around."

That night, Caleb replayed the conversation for Pim. She was bathing Theo in the sink. He had fussed at the start but now seemed to be enjoying himself, batting the water around with his fists.

I should call on his wife, Pim signed.

Do you want me to go with you? He meant to translate for her.

She looked at him like he had lost his mind. *Don't be ridiculous.*

This conversation stayed with him for several days. Somehow, in all his planning, Caleb had failed to consider that they would need other people in their lives. Some of this was the fact that with Pim he shared a private richness that made other relationships seem trivial. Also, he was not innately social; he preferred his own thoughts to most human interaction.

It was true, as well, that Pim's world was more limited than most people's. Beyond her family, it was confined to a small group of those who, if they could not sign, were able to intuit her meanings. She was often alone, which did not seem to trouble her, and she filled much of this time by writing. Caleb had peeked at her journals a few times over the years, unable to resist this small crime; like her letters, her entries were wonderfully written. While they sometimes expressed

357

doubts or concern over various matters, generally they communicated an optimistic view of life. They also contained a number of sketches, though he had never seen her draw. Most depicted familiar scenes. There were a great many drawings of birds and animals, as well as the faces of people she knew, although none of him. He wondered why she had never let him see them, why she had drawn them in secret. The best ones were the seascapes — remarkable, because Pim had never seen the ocean.

Still, she would want friends. Two days after Phil had stopped by, Pim asked Caleb if he would mind looking after Theo for a few hours; she wanted to visit the Tatums and planned to bring a johnnycake. Caleb spent the afternoon working in the garden while Theo napped in a basket. He began to worry as the day drew to a close, but just before dark Pim returned in high spirits. When Caleb asked her how they had been able to carry on a conversation for close to five hours, Pim smiled. *It doesn't matter with women,* she signed. *We always understand each other just fine.*

The next morning, Caleb took the buckboard into town for supplies and to reshoe one of the horses, the big black gelding they called Handsome. Pim had also written a letter to Kate and asked him to post it. Besides these errands, he wanted to establish contact with more people from the area. He could ask the men he met about their wives, with the hope of expanding Pim's circle, so that she would not feel lonely.

The town was not encouraging. Just a few weeks had passed since he and Pim had passed through on their way to the farmstead; at the time there

had been people about, but now the place seemed lifeless. The town office was closed, as was the farrier. But he had better luck at the mercantile. The owner was a widower named George Pettibrew. Like many men on the frontier, he had a taciturn manner, slow to warm up, and Caleb had never managed to learn much about him. George followed him as he moved through the cluttered space, placing his order — a sack of flour, beet sugar, a length of heavy chain, sewing thread, thirty yards of chicken wire, a sack of nails, lard, cornmeal, salt, oil for the lanterns, and fifty pounds of feed.

"I'd also like to buy some ammo," Caleb said, as George was tallying the bill at the counter. "Thirty-aught-six."

The man made a certain expression: *You and everybody else.* He continued jotting figures with a stub of pencil. "I can give you six."

"How many in a box?"

"Not boxes. Rounds."

It seemed like a joke. "That's all? Since when?"

George poked his thumb over his shoulder. Tacked to the wall behind the counter was a sign.

$100 BOUNTY
MOUNTAIN LION
PRESENT CARCASS AT HUNT TOWNSHIP OFFICE TO COLLECT.

"Folks cleaned me out, not that I had much to begin with. Ammo's scarce these days. I'll give 'em to you for a buck apiece."

"That's ridiculous."

George shrugged. Business was business; it was all the same to him. Caleb wanted to tell him to

359

stick it, but on the other hand, a mountain lion was nothing to mess with. He rolled off the bills.

"Think of it as an investment," George said, depositing the money in his lockbox. "You bag that cat, this won't seem so much, will it?"

Everything went into the wagon. Caleb surveyed the empty street. It really *was* awfully damn quiet for the middle of the day. He found it a little unnerving, though mostly he felt disappointed that he would return with so little to show for his visit.

He was about to drive out of town when he remembered the doctor Tatum had told him about. It would be good to introduce himself. The doctor's name was Elacqua. According to Tatum, he had once worked at the hospital in Kerrville and retired to the townships. There weren't many houses, and the doctor's was easy to find: a small frame structure, painted a cheerful yellow, with a sign that read, BRIAN ELACQUA, M.D. hanging off the porch. A pickup truck with rusted fenders was parked in the yard. Caleb tied up the horses and knocked. A single eye peeked through the curtain on the door's window.

"What do you want?" The voice was loud, almost hostile.

"Are you Dr. Elacqua?"

"Who's asking?"

Caleb regretted coming; there was obviously something wrong with the man. He thought he might be drunk. "My name is Caleb Jaxon. Phil Tatum is my neighbor, he said you were the doctor in town."

"Are you sick?"

"I just wanted to say hello. We're new out here. My wife is expecting. It's all right — I can come back later."

But as Caleb stepped off the porch, the door opened. "Jaxon?"

"That's right."

The doctor had the look of a derelict, thick at the waist, with a wild mane of snow-white hair and a beard to match. "You might as well come in."

His wife, a nervous woman in a shapeless housedress, served them some kind of bad-tasting tea in the parlor. No explanation was offered for Elacqua's curt behavior at the door. Maybe that was just how things were done out here, Caleb thought.

"How far along is your wife?" Elacqua asked, after they'd gotten past the formalities. He had, Caleb noted, put a little something in his tea from a pocket flask.

"About four months." Caleb saw an opening. "My mother-in-law is Sara Wilson. Maybe you know her."

"Know her? I trained her. I thought her daughter worked at the hospital, though."

"That's Kate. My wife is Pim."

He thought for a moment. "I don't remember a Pim. Oh, the mute." He shook his head sadly. "The poor thing. Nice of you, to marry her."

Caleb had heard statements like this before. "I'm sure she thinks it's the other way around."

"On the other hand, who wouldn't want a wife who couldn't talk? I can barely put two thoughts together around here."

Caleb just looked at him.

"Well," Elacqua said, and cleared his throat, "I can pay a call if she'd like, just to see how things are going."

At the door, Caleb remembered Pim's letter. He

361

asked Elacqua if he would mind posting it for him when the office opened.

"I can try. Those people are never there."

"I was wondering about that," Caleb said. "The town seems kind of empty."

"I didn't notice." He frowned doubtfully. "Could be the mountain lion, I guess. That happens out here."

"Has anyone been attacked?"

"Not that I've heard, just livestock. With the bounty, a lot of folks are out looking. Stupid, if you ask me. Those things are nasty."

Caleb rode out of town. At least he'd tried to post the letter. As for Elacqua, he seriously doubted Pim would want anything to do with the man. The mountain lion didn't concern him unduly. It was simply the price one paid for life on the frontier. Still, he would tell Pim not to take Theo to the river for a while. The two of them should stay near the house until the matter was resolved.

They ate their supper and went to bed. Rain was falling, making a peaceful pattering on the roof. In the middle of the night, Caleb awoke to a sharp cry. For a terrifying second he thought something had happened to Theo, but then the sound came again, from outside. It was fear he was hearing — fear and mortal pain. An animal was dying.

In the morning he searched the brush behind the house. He came to an area of broken branches; tufts of short, stiff hair, tacky with blood, were spread over the ground. He thought it might have been a raccoon. He scanned the area for tracks, but the rain had washed them away.

The next day he walked over the ridge to the Tatums'. Their operation was much larger than his own, with a good-sized barn and a house with a standing-seam metal roof. Boxes of bluebonnets hung beneath the front windows. Dorien Tatum greeted him at the door, a plump-cheeked woman with gray hair in a bun; she directed him to the far edge of the property, where her husband was clearing brush.

"A mountain lion, you say?" Phil removed his hat to mop his brow in the heat.

"That's the word in town."

"We've had 'em before. Long gone by now, I'd guess. They're restless sons of bitches."

"I thought so, too. Probably it's nothing."

"I'll keep a lookout, though. Thank your wife for the johnnycake, won't you? Dory really enjoyed her visit. Those two were writing messages to each other for hours."

Caleb made to leave, then stopped. "What's it usually like in town?"

Tatum was drinking from a canteen. "What you mean?"

"Well, it was pretty quiet. It seemed odd, in the middle of the day." Now that he'd said it, he felt a little silly. "The town office was shut, the farrier, too. I was hoping to get one of the horses reshod."

"Folks are usually around. Maybe Juno's taken sick." Juno Brand was the farrier.

"Maybe that's it."

Phil smiled through his beard. "Go round in a day or two. I bet you'll find him. But you get hard up for something, you let us know."

Caleb had decided not to tell Pim about what he'd found in the woods; there seemed no good

363

reason to alarm her, and a dead raccoon meant nothing. But that night as they were cleaning up the dishes, he repeated his request that she and Theo stay close to the house.

You worry too much, she signed.

Sorry.

Don't be. She turned at the sink to surprise him with a lingering kiss. *It's one of the reasons I love you.*

He wagged his eyebrows cornily. *Does this mean what I think it does?*

Let me get Theo down first.

But there was no need. The boy was already asleep.

28

She began the night, as she began all nights, atop the partially constructed office tower at the corner of Forty-third and Fifth Avenue. The air was blustery, with a hint of warmth; stars bedecked the heavens, thick as dust. The shapes of great buildings crenellated the sky in silhouettes of perfect blackness. The Empire State. Rockefeller Center. The magnificent Chrysler Building, Fanning's favorite, soaring above everything around it with its graceful art deco crown. The hours after midnight were the ones Alicia liked best. The quiet was richer somehow, the air purer. She felt closer to the core of things, the world's rich chroma of sound and scent and texture. The night flowed through her, a coursing in the blood. She breathed it in and out. A darkness indomitable, supreme.

She crossed the roof to the construction crane and began to climb. Attached to the exposed gird-ers of the building's upper floors, it soared another

hundred feet above the roof. There were stairs, but Alicia never bothered, stairs being a thing of the past, a quaint feature of a life she barely recalled. The boom, hundreds of feet long, was positioned parallel with the building's west face. She made her way down the catwalk to the boom's tip, from which a long hooked chain dangled in the darkness. Alicia winched it up, released the brake, and drew the hook backward along the boom. Where the boom met the mast was a small platform. She laid the hook there, returned to the tip, and reset the chain's brake. Then, back to the platform. A keen anticipation filled her, like a hunger about to be slaked. Standing erect, head held high, she gripped the hook in her fists.

And stepped off.

She plunged down and away. The trick was to release the hook at just the right moment, when her speed and upward momentum existed in perfect balance. This would occur roughly two-thirds up the back side of the hook's arc. She swung through the bottom, still accelerating. Her body, her senses, her thoughts — all were attuned, at one with speed and space.

She released the hook. Her body inverted; she tucked her knees to her chest. Three aerial rolls and she uncoiled. The flat-topped roof across the street: that was the target. It rose in greeting. *Welcome, Alicia.*

Touchdown.

Her powers had expanded. It was as if, in the presence of her creator, some powerful mechanism within her had been fully unleashed. The aerial spaces of the city were trivial; she could vault vast distances, alight on the narrowest ledges, cling to the tiniest cracks. Gravity was a toy to her; she

ranged above Manhattan like a bird. In the glass faces of skyscrapers her reflected image dove and darted, plunged and swooped.

She found herself, sometime later, above Third Avenue, near the demarcation between land and sea; a few blocks south of Astor Place, the encroaching waters began, bubbling up from the island's flooded underworld. She descended, ping-ponging between buildings, to the street. Broken shells lay everywhere among the dried husks of ocean weeds swept inward by storm surges. She knelt and pressed her ear to the pavement.

They were definitely moving.

The grate pulled away easily; she dropped into the tunnel, lit her torch, and began to walk south. A ribbon of dark water sloshed at her feet. Fanning's Many had been eating. Their droppings were everywhere, rank, ureic, as were the skeletal remains of their feeding — mice, rats, the small creatures of the city's clammy substratum. Some of the droppings were fresh, a few days old at the most.

She passed through the Astor Place station. Now she could feel it: the sea. The great bulge of it, always pressing, seeking to enlarge its domain, to drown the world with its cold blue weight. Her heart had quickened; the hairs stood up along her arms. *It's only water,* she told herself. *Only water* . . .

The bulkhead appeared. A thin spray of water, almost a mist, shot from its edges. She stepped toward it. A moment's hesitation; then she extended a hand to touch its frigid face. On the other side, untold tons of pressure lay in stasis, stalemated for a century by the weight of the door. Fanning had explained the history. The entire Manhattan subway system lay below sea level; it

366

had been a disaster waiting to happen. After Hurricane Wilma had flooded the tunnels, the city fathers had constructed a series of heavy doors to hold the water in check. In the throes of the epidemic, when the electricity had failed, a fail-safe mechanism had sealed them. There they had rested for over a century, holding the encroaching ocean at bay.

Don't be afraid, don't be afraid . . .

She heard a skittering behind her. She spun, raising her torch. At the edge of the darkness, a pair of orange eyes flared. A large male but skinny, the bumps of his ribs showing; he squatted, frog-like, between the tracks, a rat gripped in his mouth with the very tips of his teeth. The rat squirmed and squeaked, its bald tail whipping.

"What are you looking at?" Alicia said. "Get out of here."

The jaws clamped shut. An arcing pop of blood and a sucking sound and the viral spat the empty bag of bones and fur to the ground. Alicia's stomach tumbled, not with nausea but hunger; she hadn't eaten for a week. The viral extended its claws, petting the air like a cat. It cocked his head: *What sort of being is this?*

"Go on." She waved the torch like a pike. "Shoo. Scat."

A last look, almost fond. It darted away.

Fanning had already prepared for daybreak by drawing the shades. He was sitting at his usual table on the balcony above the main hall, reading a book by candlelight. His eyes lifted as she approached.

"Good hunting?"

Alicia took a chair. "I wasn't hungry."

"You should eat."

"So should you."

His attention returned to his book. Alicia glanced at the title: *The Tragedy of Hamlet, Prince of Denmark.*

"I went to the library."

"So I see."

"It's a very sad play. No, not sad. Angry." Fanning shrugged. "I haven't read it for years. It seems different to me now." He found a certain page, looked at her, and raised a professorial finger. "Have a listen."

The spirit I have seen
May be the devil, and the devil hath power
T' assume a pleasing shape; yea, and perhaps
Out of my weakness and my melancholy,
As he is very potent with such spirits,
Abuses me to damn me. I'll have grounds
More relative than this. The play's the thing
Wherein I'll catch the conscience of the king.

When Alicia said nothing, he raised an eyebrow at her. "You're not a fan?"

Fanning's moods were like this. He could go silent for days, brooding incessantly, then, without warning, would emerge. Lately he had adopted a tone of dry cheerfulness, almost smug.

"I can see why you like it."

" 'Like' may not be the word."

"The end doesn't make sense, though. Who's the king?"

"Precisely."

Wedges of sunlight peeked through the drapes, making pale stripes on the floor. Fanning seemed unperturbed by them, though his sensitivity was

far greater than her own. For Fanning, the sun's touch was deeply painful.

"They're waking up, Tim. Hunting. Moving through the tunnels."

Fanning continued reading.

"Are you listening?"

He looked up with a frown. "Well, what of it?"

"That's not our agreement."

His attentions had returned to his book, though he was only pretending to read. She got to her feet. "I'm going to see Soldier."

He yawned, showing his fangs, and gave her a pale-lipped smile. "I'll be here."

Alicia cinched on her goggles, exited onto Forty-third, and headed north on Madison Avenue. Spring had come on sluggishly; only a few trees were budding out, and pockets of snow still lay in the shadows. The stable was located on the east side of the park at Sixty-third, just south of the zoo. She removed Soldier's blanket and led him out of his stall. The park felt static, as if caught between the seasons. Alicia sat on a boulder at the edge of the pond and watched the horse graze. He had taken on the years with dignity; he tired more easily, but only a little, and was still strong, his gait firm. Strands of white had appeared in his tail and whiskers, more on the feathers at his feet. She watched him eat his fill, then saddled him and climbed aboard.

"A little exercise, boy, what do you say?"

She guided him across the meadow, into the shade of the trees. A memory came to her of the day she'd first seen him, all that coiled wildness inside him, standing alone outside the wreckage of the Kearney garrison, waiting for her like a message. *I am yours as you are mine. For each of*

us there will always be one. Past the trees she brought him to a trot, then a canter. To their left lay the reservoir, a billion gallons, lifeblood of the city's green heart. At the Ninety-seventh Street Transverse, she dismounted.

"Back in a jiff."

She made her way into the woods, removed her boots, and scaled a suitable tree at the edge of the glade. There, balanced on her haunches, she waited.

Eventually her wish was granted: a young doe tiptoed into view, ears flicking, neck bent low. Alicia watched the animal approach. Closer. Closer.

Fanning hadn't moved from the table. He looked up from his book, smiled. "What's this I see?"

Alicia heaved the doe off her shoulders, onto the bar top. Its head hung with the looseness of death, the pink tongue unspooling from its mouth like a ribbon.

"I told you," she said. "You really need to eat."

29

The first gunshots rang out on schedule, a series of distant pops from the end of the causeway. It was one A.M. Michael was concealed with Rand and the others outside the Quonset hut. The door swung open with a blaze of light and laughter; a man stumbled out, his arm draped over the shoulders of one of the whores.

He died with a gurgle. They left him where he fell, blood darkening the earth from the wire's incision around his neck. Michael stepped up to the woman. She wasn't one he knew. Rand's hand

was covering her mouth, dampening her terrified shrieks. She couldn't have been a day over eighteen.

"Nothing's going to happen to you, if you keep quiet. Understand?"

She was a well-fed girl with short, red hair. Her eyes, heavily made up, were open very wide. She nodded.

"My friend is going to uncover your mouth, and you're going to tell me what room he's in."

Cautiously, Rand drew his hand away.

"The last one, at the end of the hall."

"You're certain?"

She nodded vigorously. Michael gave her a list of names. Four were playing cards in the front room; two more were back in the stalls.

"Okay, get out of here."

She dashed away. Michael looked at the others. "We go in in two groups. Rand with me; the rest of you hover in the outer room until everybody's ready."

Eyes flicked up from the tables as they entered, but that was all. They were comrades, no doubt stopping by the hut for the same reasons everyone did: a drink, some cards, a few minutes of bliss in the stalls. The second group spread out across the room while Michael and the others faded to the hallway and took their positions outside the doors. The signal was passed, the doors were flung open.

Dunk was on his back, naked, a woman busily rocking astride his hips. "Michael, what the fuck?" But when he saw Rand and the others, his expression changed. "Oh, give me a break."

Michael looked at the whore. "Why don't you take a walk?"

She snatched her dress from the floor and ran

371

out the door. From elsewhere in the building came an assortment of screams and shouts, the sound of glass breaking, a single gunshot.

"It was going to happen sooner or later," Michael said to Dunk. "Might as well make the best of it."

"You think you're so fucking smart? You'll be dead the minute you walk out of here."

"We've pretty much cleaned house, Dunk. I was saving you for last."

Dunk's face lit with a phony smile; beneath the bluster, the man knew he was looking into an abyss. "I get it. You want a bigger share. Well, you've certainly earned it. I can make that happen for you."

"Rand?"

The man moved forward, gripping the wire in his fists. Three others grabbed Dunk as he attempted to rise and shoved him hard onto the mattress.

"For fucksake, Michael!" He was squirming like a fish. "I treated you like a son!"

"You have no idea how funny that is."

As the wire slipped around Dunk's neck, Michael stepped from the room. The last of Dunk's lieutenants was putting up a bit of a struggle in the second stall, but then Michael heard a final grunt and the thump of something heavy striking the floor. Greer met him in the front room, where bodies lay strewn amid overturned card tables. One of them was Fastau; he'd been shot through the eye.

"Are we done?" Michael asked.

"McLean and Dybek got away in one of the trucks."

"They'll stop them at the causeway. They aren't

going anywhere." Michael looked at Fastau, lying dead on the floor. "We lose anyone else?"

"Not that I've heard."

They loaded the bodies into the five-ton that waited outside. Thirty-six corpses in all, Dunk's inner circle of murderers, pimps, thieves: they'd be carted to the dock, loaded onto a launch, and dumped in the channel.

"What about the women?" Greer asked.

Michael was thinking of Fastau — the man had been one of his best welders. Any loss at this point was a concern.

"Have Patch put them under guard in one of the machine sheds. Once we're ready to move, get them on a transport out of here."

"They'll talk."

"Well, consider the source."

"I see your point."

The truck with the bodies drove away.

"I don't mean to press," Greer said, "but have you decided about Lore?"

The question had preoccupied Michael for weeks. Always he came back to the same answer. "I think she's the only one I trust enough to do this."

"I agree."

Michael turned toward Greer. "Are you sure you don't want to be the one to run things around here? I think you'd be good at it."

"That's not my role. The *Bergensfjord* is yours. Don't worry, I'll keep the troops in line."

They were quiet for a time. The only lights burning were the big spots on the dock. Michael's men would be working through the night.

"There's something I've been meaning to bring up," Michael said.

Greer cocked his head.

"In your vision, I know you couldn't see who else was on the ship —"

"Just the island, the five stars."

"I understand that." He hesitated. "I'm not sure how to put this. Did it . . . *feel* like I was there?"

Greer seemed perplexed by the question. "I really couldn't say. That wasn't part of it."

"You can be honest with me."

"I know I can."

The sound of gunfire from the causeway: five shots, a pause, then two more, deliberate, final. Dybek and McLean.

"I guess that's that," said Greer.

Rand walked up to them. "Everybody's assembled at the dock."

Suddenly Michael felt the weight of it. Not ordering the deaths of so many; that had been easier than expected. He was in charge now — the isthmus was his. He checked the magazine on his sidearm, decocked the hammer, and slid the pistol back into its holster. From now on, he would never be apart from it.

"All right, that oil ships in thirty-six days. Let's get this show on the road."

30

IOWA FREESTATE
(Formerly the Homeland)
Pop. 12,139

Sheriff Gordon Eustace began the morning of March 24 — as he did every March 24 — by hanging his holstered revolver on the bedpost.

Because carrying a weapon wouldn't be right. It wouldn't be respectful. For the next few hours,

he'd be just a man, like any man, standing in the cold on aching joints to think about the way things might have been.

He kept a room at the back of the jail. For ten years, since the night he couldn't make himself return to the house, that was where he'd slept. He'd always considered himself the sort of man who could pick himself up and get on with things, and it wasn't as if he was the first person whose luck had turned bad. But something had gone out of him and never come back, and so this was where he lived, in a cinder-block box with nothing but a bed and a sink and a chair to sit in and a toilet down the hall, nobody but drunks sleeping it off for company.

Outside the sun was rising in a halfhearted, March-in-Iowa way. He heated a kettle on the stove and carried it to the basin with his straight razor and soap. His face looked back in the old cracked mirror. Well, wasn't that a pretty sight. Half his front teeth gone, left ear shot off to a pink nub, one eye clouded and useless: he looked like something in a children's story, the mean old ogre under the bridge. He shaved, splashed water on his face and under his arms, and dried himself off. All he had on hand for breakfast were some leftover biscuits, hard as rocks. Sitting at the table, he worked them over with his back teeth and washed them down with a shot of corn liquor from the jug beneath the sink. He wasn't much of a drinker, but he liked one in the morning, especially this morning of all mornings, the morning of March 24.

He put on his hat and coat and stepped outside. The last of the snow had melted, turning the earth to mud. The jailhouse was one of the few build-

ings in the old downtown that anybody still used; most had been empty for years. Blowing on his hands, he made his way past the ruins of the Dome — nothing left of it now but a pile of rocks and a few charred timbers — and down the hill into the area that everybody still called the Flatland, though the old workers' lodges had long since been dismantled and used as firewood. Some folks still lived down here, but not many; the memories were too bad. The ones who did were generally younger, born after the days of the red-eyes, or else very old and unable to break the psychological chains of the old regime. It was a squalid dump of shacks without running water, miasmatic rivers of sewage running in the streets, and a roughly equivalent number of dirty children and skinny dogs picking through the trash. Eustace's heart broke every time he saw it.

It wasn't supposed to be this way. He'd had plans, hopes. Sure, a lot of people had accepted the offer to evacuate to Texas in those first years; Eustace had expected that. *Fine,* he'd thought, *let them go.* The ones who remained would be the hearty souls, the true believers who viewed the end of the redeyes not merely as a liberation from bondage but something more: the chance to right a wrong, start over, build a new life from the bottom up.

But as he'd watched the population drain away, he'd begun to worry. The people who stayed behind weren't the builders, the dreamers. Many were simply too weak to travel; some were too afraid; others so accustomed to having everything decided for them that they were incapable of doing much of anything at all. Eustace had made a run at it, but nobody had the slightest idea how to

make a city work. They had no engineers, no plumbers, no electricians, no doctors. They could operate the machines the redeyes left behind, but nobody knew how to fix them when they broke. The power plant had failed within three years, water and sanitation within five; a decade later, almost nothing functioned. Schooling the children proved impossible. Few of the adults could read, and most didn't see the sense of it. The winters were brutal — people froze to death in their own houses — and the summers were almost as bad, drought one year and drenching rains the next. The river was foul, but people filled their buckets anyway; the disease that everyone called "river fever" killed scores. Half the cattle had died, most of the horses and sheep, and all of the pigs.

The redeyes had left behind all the tools to build a functioning society but one: the will to actually do it.

The road through the Flatland joined the river and took him east to the stadium. Just beyond it was the cemetery. Eustace made his way through the rows of headstones. A number were decorated — guttered candles, children's toys, the long-desiccated sprigs of wildflowers exposed by the retreating snow. The arrangement was orderly; the one thing people were good at was digging graves. He came to the one he was looking for and crouched beside it.

NINA VORHEES EUSTACE
SIMON TIFTY EUSTACE
BELOVED WIFE, BELOVED SON

They had perished within a few hours of each other. Eustace was not told of this until two days

377

later; he was roiling with fever, his mind adrift in psychotic dreams he was glad to have no memory of. The epidemic had cut through the city like a scythe. Who lived and who died seemed random; a healthy adult was as likely to succumb as an infant or someone in their seventies. The illness came on quickly: fever, chills, a cough from deep in the lungs. Often it would seem to run its course only to come roaring back, overwhelming the victim within minutes. Simon had been three years old — a watchful boy with intelligent eyes and a joyful laugh. Never had Eustace felt a love so deep for anyone, not even for Nina. The two of them joked about it — how, by comparison, their affection for each other seemed minor, though of course that wasn't quite true. Loving their boy was just another way of loving each other.

He spent a few minutes by the grave. He liked to focus on little things. Meals they'd shared, snippets of conversation, quick touches traded for no reason, just to do it. He hardly ever thought about the insurgency; it seemed to have no bearing anymore, and Nina's ferocity as a fighter made up but one small part of the woman she was. Her true self was something she had shown only to him.

A feeling of fullness told him it was time to go. So, another year. He touched the stone, letting his hand linger there as he said goodbye, and made his way back through the maze of headstones.

"Hey, mister!"

Eustace spun around as a chunk of ice the size of a fist sailed past his head. Three boys, teenagers, stood fifty feet away among the headstones, guffawing like idiots. But when they got a look at him, the laughter abruptly ceased.

"Shit! It's the sheriff!"

They dashed away before Eustace could say a word. It was too bad, really; there was something he wanted to tell them. *It's okay,* he would have said. *I don't mind. He would have been about your age.*

When he returned to the jail, Fry Robinson, his deputy, was sitting at the desk with his boots up, snoring into his collar. He was just a kid, really, not even twenty-five, with a wide, optimistic face and a soft round jaw he barely had to shave. Not the smartest but not the dumbest either; he'd stayed on with Eustace longer than most men did, which counted for something. Eustace let the door bang behind himself, sending Fry jolting upright.

"Jesus, Gordo. What the hell did you do that for?"

Eustace strapped on his gun. It was mostly for show; he kept it loaded, but the ammunition the redeyes had left behind was nearly gone, and what remained was unreliable. On more than one occasion, the hammer had fallen on a dud.

"Did you feed Rudy yet?"

"I was just about to before you woke me up. Where'd you go? I thought you were still back there."

"Went to visit Nina and Simon."

Fry gave him a blank stare; then he understood. "Shit, it's the twenty-fourth, isn't it?"

Eustace shrugged. What was there to say?

"I can look after things here if you want," Fry offered. "Why don't you take the rest of the day off?"

"And do what?"

"Sleep or something. Get drunk."

"Believe me, I've thought about it."

Eustace carried Rudy's breakfast back to his cell: a couple of stale biscuits and a raw potato cut into slices.

"Rise and shine, partner."

Rudy lifted his emaciated frame off his bunk. Thieving, fighting, being a general, all-around pain in the ass: the man was in jail so often he actually had a favorite cell. This time the charge was drunk and disorderly. With a lurid snort he excavated a wad of phlegm, hawked it into the bucket that served as a toilet, and shuffled to the bars, beltless pants hoisted in his fist. Maybe I should let him keep his belt next time, Eustace thought. The man might do us all a favor and hang himself. Eustace slid the plate through the slot.

"That's it? Biscuits and a potato?"

"What do you want? It's March."

"The service isn't what it used to be around this place."

"So stay out of trouble for once."

Rudy sat on the bunk and took a bite of one of the biscuits. The man's teeth were disgusting, brown and wobbly-looking, though Eustace was hardly one to talk. Crumbs spurted from his mouth as he spoke. "When's Abel coming?"

Abel was the judge. "How should I know?"

"I need a clean bucket, too."

Eustace was halfway down the hall.

"I'm serious!" Rudy yelled. "It stinks in here!"

Eustace returned to the front and sat behind his desk. Fry was wiping down his revolver, something he did about ten times a day. The thing was like his pet. "What's his problem?"

"Didn't care much for the cuisine."

Fry frowned with contempt. "He should be

380

grateful. I didn't get much more than that myself." He stopped and sniffed the air. "Jesus, what's that smell?"

"Hey, assholes," Rudy yelled from the back, "got a present for you!"

Rudy was standing in his cell holding the now-empty bucket with a triumphant look on his face. Shit and piss were running down the hallway in a brown river.

"This is what I think of your fucking potato."

"Goddamnit," Fry yelled, "you're cleaning this up!"

Eustace turned to his deputy. "Hand me the key."

Fry unhooked the ring from his belt and passed it to Eustace. "I mean it, Rudy." He jabbed a finger in the air. "You're in a heap of trouble, my friend."

Eustace unlocked the door, stepped into the cell, closed the door behind himself, reached with the keys back through the bars, and locked the door again. Then he deposited the ring deep in his pocket.

"What the hell is this?" Rudy asked.

"Gordon?" Fry looked at him cautiously. "What are you doing?"

"Just give me a sec."

Eustace drew his revolver, spun it around in his hand, and slapped the butt across Rudy's face. The man stumbled backward and toppled to the floor.

"Are you out of your mind?" Rudy scrabbled backward until he was against the wall of the cell. He worked his tongue around and spat a bloodied tooth into his palm. He held it up by its long, rot-

ten root. "Look at this! How am I supposed to eat now?"

"I doubt you'll miss it much."

"You had that coming, you piece of shit," Fry said. "Come on, Gordo, let's get this asshole a mop. I think he's learned his lesson."

Eustace didn't think so. *Teach the man a lesson* — what did that actually mean? He wasn't sure what he was feeling, but it was coming to him. Rudy was holding out his tooth with a look of righteous indignation on his face. The sight of it was thoroughly disgusting; it seemed to encapsulate everything wrong with Eustace's life. He reholstered his gun, letting Rudy think the worst was over, then hauled him to his feet and slammed his face against the wall. A damp crunch, like a fat cockroach popping underfoot: Rudy released a howl of pain.

"Gordon, seriously," Fry said. "Time to open that door."

Eustace wasn't angry. Anger had left him, years ago. What he felt was relief. He hurled the man across the cell and got to work: his fists, the butt of the revolver, the points of his boots. Fry's pleas for him to stop barely registered in his consciousness. Something had come uncorked inside him, and it was elating, like riding a horse at full gallop. Rudy was lying on the floor, his face protectively buried in his arms. *You pathetic excuse for a human being. You worthless waste of skin. You are everything that's wrong with this place, and I am going to make you know it.*

He was in the process of lifting Rudy by his collar to slam his head against the edge of the bunk — what a satisfying crack that was going to make — when a key turned in the lock and Fry grabbed

him from behind. Eustace connected with an elbow to Fry's midriff, knocking him away, and wrapped Rudy's neck in the crook of his arm. The man was like a big rag doll, a fleshy sack of loosely organized parts. He tightened his biceps against Rudy's windpipe and shoved his knee into his back for leverage. One hard yank and that would be the end of him.

Then: snowflakes. Fry was standing over him, heaving for breath, holding the fire poker he'd just used on Eustace's head.

"Jesus, Gordo. What the hell was *that*?"

Eustace blinked his eyes; the snowflakes winked out one by one. His head felt like a split log; he was a little sick to his stomach, too.

"Got a little carried away, I guess."

"It wasn't like the guy didn't deserve it, but what the fuck."

Eustace turned his head to get a look at the situation. Rudy was curled into a fetal ball with his hands jammed between his legs. His face looked like raw meat.

"I really did a number on him, didn't I?"

"The man never traded on his looks anyway." Fry directed his voice at Rudy. "You hear me? You breathe one word of this, they're going to find you in a ditch, you asshole." Fry looked at Eustace. "Sorry, I didn't mean to hit you so hard."

"That's okay."

"Don't mean to rush you, but it's probably best if you vacate the premises for the time being. Think you can stand?"

"What about Abel?"

"I'll handle it. Let's get you on your feet."

Fry helped him up. Eustace had to hold on to the bars for a second to make the floor feel solid.

The knuckles of his right hand were bloody and swollen, skin split along the bone. He tried to close it into a fist, but the joints wouldn't go that far.

"Okay?" Fry was looking at him.

"I think so, yeah."

"Just go clear your head. You might want to take care of that hand, too."

At the door of the cell, Eustace stopped. Fry was easing Rudy into a seated position. His shirt was a bib of blood.

"You know, you were right," Eustace said.

Fry glanced up. "How's that?"

Eustace didn't feel sorry about what he'd done, though he supposed he might later on. A lot of things were like that; the reaction you were supposed to have took its time getting there.

"Maybe I should have taken the day off after all."

31

Alicia began to spend her nights in the stable.

Fanning took little notice of her absence. *That horse of yours,* he might comment, barely lifting his eyes from one of the books that now completely occupied his waking hours. *I don't see why you feel the need, but it's really none of my business.* His mind seemed distant, his thoughts veiled. Yes, he was different; something had shifted. The change felt tectonic, a rumbling from deep in the earth. He wasn't sleeping, there was that — if indeed their kind could be said to sleep. In the past, the daylight hours had brought forth in him a kind of melancholy exhaustion. He would fade into a trancelike state — eyes closed, hands

384

folded in his lap with his fingers tidily meshed. Alicia knew his dreams. The clocks' hands remorseless turning. The anonymous crowds streaming past. His was a nightmare of infinite waiting in a universe barren of pity — without hope, without love, without the purpose that only hope and love could bear upon it.

She had a dream like that of her own. Her baby. Her Rose.

She sometimes thought about the past. "New York," Fanning liked to say, "has always been a place of memory." She missed her friends as the dead might miss the living, citizens of a realm she had permanently departed. What did Alicia remember? The Colonel. Being a little girl in the dark. Her years on the Watch, how true they felt. There was a night that came back to her often; it seemed to define something. She had taken Peter up to the roof of the power station to show him the stars. Side by side they had lain on the concrete, still warm with the day's crushing heat, the two of them just talking, beneath a night sky made more remarkable by the fact that Peter had never seen it before. It brought them out of themselves. *Have you ever thought about it?* Alicia had asked him. *Thought about what?* he'd asked; and she'd said, nervously — she couldn't seem to stop herself — *You're going to make me say it? Pairing, Peter. Having Littles.* She understood, much later, what she was really asking of him: to save her, to lead her into life. But it was too late; it had always been too late. Since the night the Colonel had abandoned her, Alicia hadn't really been a person anymore; she had given it up.

So, the years. Fanning said time was different for their kind, and it was. The days' ceaselessly

melding, season into season, year into year. What were they to each other? He was kind. He understood her. *We have traveled the same road,* he said. *Stay with me, Lish. Stay with me, and all of it is ended.* Did she believe him? There were times when he seemed to know the deepest truths of her. What to say, what to ask, when to listen and for how long. *Tell me about her.* How soft his voice was, how gentle. It was like no voice she had ever heard; it felt like floating in a bath of tears. *Tell me about your Rose.*

Yet there was another part of him, veiled, impenetrable. His long, brooding silences disturbed her, as did instances of a slightly off-key cheerfulness that seemed wholly manufactured. He began to venture out at night, something he had not done in years. He made no announcement; he would simply be gone. Alicia decided to follow him. For three nights he wandered without apparent destination, a forlorn figure haunting the streets; then, on the fourth night, he surprised her. With deliberate strides he made his way downtown, into the West Village, and halted before a nondescript residential building, five stories tall, with a flight of steps connecting the front door to the street. Alicia concealed herself behind a rooftop parapet at the top of the block. Several minutes passed, Fanning studying the building's face. Suddenly it came to her: Fanning had lived here once. Something seemed to click inside him, and he marched up to the door, forced it with his shoulder, and disappeared inside.

He was gone for a long while. An hour, then two. Alicia began to be concerned. Unless Fanning appeared soon, there would not be time for him to return to the station before sunrise. Finally

he emerged. At the bottom of the steps, he stopped. As if sensing her presence, he cast his eyes around the street, then looked straight toward her. Alicia ducked below the parapet and pressed her body to the rooftop.

"I know you're there, Alicia. But it's all right."

When she looked again, the street was empty.

He made no mention of the night's events, and Alicia did not press. She had glimpsed something, a clue, but its meaning eluded her. Why, after all this time, would he make such a pilgrimage?

He never left again.

What was going to happen next, Fanning must have anticipated; Alicia was obviously meant to do it. The building was a wreck on the inside. Black spatters of mold scaled the walls, and the floors were soft underfoot. In the stairwell, water dripped from a leak in the ceiling, high above. She ascended to the second floor, where a door stood open in invitation. The interior of the apartment had been largely spared the destruction. The furniture, though caked with dust, was all neatly arranged; books and magazines and various decorative objects still occupied their places, just as, Alicia supposed, they had been in the final hours of Fanning's human life. As she moved through the fastidious rooms she became aware of what she was feeling. Fanning wanted her to know the man he'd been. A new, deeper intimacy had been offered her.

She entered the bedroom. It seemed different from the other spaces of the apartment, possessing an intangible sense of more recent occupation. The furniture was simple: a desk, a dresser, an upholstered chair by the window, a bed, neatly

made. Bisecting the center of the mattress was a depression of distinctly human dimensions. A similar divot marked the pillow.

A pair of eyeglasses rested on the bedside table. Alicia knew whom they'd belonged to; they were part of the story. She gently picked them up. They were petite, with wire frames. The cratered bed, the linens, the glasses within reach. Fanning had lain here. And he had left all of this for her to see.

To see, she thought. What did he want her to see?

She lay on the bed. The mattress was formless beneath her, its internal structure long collapsed. Then she put on the glasses.

She could never explain it; the moment she had looked through the lenses, it was as if she had *become* him. The past poured through her, the pain. The truth hit her heart like voltage. Of course. Of course.

Daybreak found her at the bridge. Her fear of the churning waters, though strong, seemed trivial; she pushed it aside. The sun cast its long, golden rays behind her. Upon Soldier's back she made her way across, following her shadow.

32

They found Bill in the retaining pool at the bottom of the spillway. The night before, he'd slipped out of the hospital, taking his clothes and shoes. After that, the trail went cold. Someone said they had seen him at the tables, although the man demurred; he could be thinking of a different night, he said. Bill was always at the tables. It would have been more remarkable if he weren't.

It was the fall that had killed him: a hundred feet from the top of the dam, then the long slide to the pool, where his body had wedged against a drain. His legs were shattered, his chest caved in; otherwise, he looked the same. Had he jumped or was he pushed? His life was not what they had thought it to be; Sara wondered how much Kate had kept from her. But it was not a question to ask.

The matter of his debts remained. Pooling their savings with Kate's, Sara and Hollis could assemble less than half the amount owed. Three days after the burial, Hollis took the money to the building in H-town that everyone still called Cousin's Place, though Cousin himself had been dead for years. Hollis hoped that this token of good faith, combined with his old connections, would square the matter. He returned, shaking his head dispiritedly. The players had changed; he had no clout. "This is going to be a problem," he said.

Kate and the girls were bedding down at Sara and Hollis's house. Kate seemed benumbed, a woman who had accepted a fate she had long seen coming, but the girls' grief was shattering to witness. In their young eyes, Bill was simply their father. Their love for him was uncolored by the knowledge that he had, in a sense, shunned them, choosing a path that would take him away from them forever. As they grew, the wound would morph into a different kind of injury — one not of loss but of rejection. Sara would have done anything in her power to spare them this pain. But there was nothing.

The only thing to do was hope that the situation would blow over. Two more days passed, and Sara

came home to find Hollis sitting at the table in the kitchen, looking grim. Kate was on the floor playing cards with the girls, but Sara could see this was intended as a distraction; something serious had happened. Hollis showed her the note that had been slid under the door. In blocky handwriting, like a child's, two words: "Adorable girls."

Hollis kept a revolver in a lockbox under the bed. He loaded it and gave it to Sara.

"Anybody comes through that door," he instructed, "shoot them."

He didn't tell her what he'd done, though that was the night Cousin's Place burned to the ground. In the morning, Sara went with Kate to the post office to mail the letter that would, in all likelihood, arrive in Mystic Township many days after she did. *Coming for a visit,* Kate wrote to Pim. *The girls can't wait to see you.*

33

Yes, I am tired. Tired of waiting, tired of thinking. I am tired of myself.

My Alicia: how good you have been to me. *Solamen miseris socios habuisse doloris:* "It is a comfort to the wretched to have companions in misery." When I think of you, Alicia, and what we are to each other, I am reminded of my first trip to a barbershop as a boy. Indulge me — memory is my method in all things, and the story has more bearing than you think. In my boyhood town, there was only one. It was a kind of clubhouse. On a Saturday afternoon, escorted by my father, I entered this sacred masculine space. The details were intoxicating. The odors of tonic, leather, talc.

The combs lounging in their disinfecting aquamarine bath. The hiss and crackle of AM radio, broadcasting manly contests upon green fields. My father beside me, I waited on a chair of cracked red vinyl. Men were being barbered, lathered, whisked. The owner of the shop had been a World War II bomber pilot of some renown. Upon the wall behind the cash register hung a photograph of his young warrior self. Beneath his snipping shears and buzzing razor, each small-town cranium emerged a perfect simulacrum of his own, on the day he'd donned his goggles, wrapped a scarf around his neck, and crossed the eaves of heaven to blast the samurai to smithereens.

My turn arrived; I was summoned forth. Many smiles and winks were exchanged among the witnesses. I took my seat — a board balanced upon the chair's chrome arms — as the barber, like a toreador flashing his cape, shook out the curtain with which he meant to dress me, wrapped toilet paper around my neck, and draped my body in decapitating plastic. That was when I noticed the mirrors. One on the wall before me, one behind, and my likeness — a reflection of a reflection of a reflection — caroming down the corridor of cold eternity. The sight brought forth an existential nausea. Infinity: I knew the term, yes, but the world of boyhood is finite and firm. To gaze into the heart of it, and to see my likeness stamped a million-fold upon its face, disconcerted me profoundly. The barber, meanwhile, had set blithely about his task, simultaneously engaged in lighthearted conversation with my father on various adult subjects. I thought that focusing my eyes solely upon the first image might somehow

banish the others, but the effect was the opposite: I was made even more aware of the innumerable shadow selves lurking behind him, ad infinitum, infinitum, infinitum.

But then something else happened. My discomfort waned. The lush sensory package of the place, combined with the delicate tickling of the barber's shears upon my neck, eased me into a state of trancelike fascination. The idea came to me: I was not just one small thing. I was, in fact, a multitude. Looking farther, I believed I detected among my infinite fellows certain subtle differences. This one's eyes were a bit closer together, a second's ears were positioned a fraction higher on his head, a third sat just a little lower in his chair. To test my theory, I commenced to make small adjustments — angling my gaze, wrinkling my nose, winking one eye and then the other. Each version of me responded in kind, and yet I discerned the tiniest lag, the barest hitch of time, between my action and its manifold duplication. The barber warned me that if I did not hold still he might accidently cut my ear off — more virile laughter — but his words made no impact, so thoroughly was I enjoying my new discovery. It became a kind of game. Fanning says: Stick out your tongue. Fanning says: Raise one finger. What delicious power I possessed! "Come on, son," my father commanded, "quit your fussing," but I wasn't fussing — far from it. Never had I felt so alive.

Life wrests that feeling from us. Day by day, the sublime glimpses of childhood pass away. It is love, of course, and only love, that restores us to ourselves, or so we hope, but that is taken away. What is left when there is no love? A rope and rock.

I have been dying forever. That is what I mean to say. I have been dying as you are dying, my Alicia. It was you I saw in the mirror, that long-ago morning of boyhood; it is you I see now, as I walk these streets of glass. There is one love, made of hope, and another, made of grief.

I have, my Alicia, loved you.

Now you are gone; I knew this day would come. The look on your face as you strode into the hall: there was wrath in it, yes. How angry you were with me, how your eyes flashed with feelings of betrayal, how the words spat with righteous fury from your lips. *This isn't our deal,* you said. *You said you would leave them alone.* But you know as well as I that we cannot; our purpose is ordained. Hope is none but vapid sweetness to the tongue, without the taste of blood. What are we, Alicia, but the gauntlet through which humanity must pass? We are the knife of the world, clamped between God's teeth.

Forgive me, Alicia, my modest deceit. You made it rather easy. In my defense, I did not lie. I would have told you, had you asked; you believed because you wanted to. You might ask yourself, Who, my dear, was following whom? Who the watcher and who the watched? Night after night you prowled the tunnels like a schoolmarm counting heads. Honestly, your gullibility was a little disappointing. Did you truly believe that all my children are here? That I could have been so careless? That I would be content to bide a meaningless eternity? I am a scientist, methodical in all things; my eyes are everywhere, seeing all. My descendants, my Many: I walk with them, I haunt the night, I see as they see, and what do I behold?

The great city defenseless, all but abandoned. The small towns and farms, staking their claim. Humanity bursting with ripeness, flowing over the land. They have forgotten us; their minds have returned to the ordinary concerns of life. How will the weather be? What will I wear to the dance? Whom should I marry? Shall I have a child? What will I name it?

What would you tell them, Alicia?

The heavens toy with me; I will have satisfaction. I have waited long enough for this savior, this Girl from Nowhere, this Amy NLN. She taunts me with her silence, her limitless, tactical calm. To flush me out, that is her aspiration, and so she shall have it. I know what you are thinking, Alicia. Surely I must despise her, for the deaths of my ignoble fellows, my Twelve. Far from it! The day she faced them was one of the happiest of my long, unhappy exile. Her sacrifice was supreme. It was positively God-kissed. It gave me — dare I use the word? — hope. Without alpha, there can be no omega; without beginning, no end.

Bring her to me, I told you. *My quarrel is not with humankind; it is but ransom to the nobler purpose. Bring her to me, my darling, my Lish, and I will spare the rest.*

Oh, I have no illusions. I know what you will do. Always I have known, and I have loved you no less for it — to the contrary. You are the better part of me; each of us must play his role.

Thus the long-awaited day. You asked, Who is the king, whose conscience we must catch? Is it I, or is there another? Shall the creator be moved to pity his creation? Soon we will know. The stage is set, the lights go down, the actors take their marks.

Let it begin.

■ ■ ■ ■

IV
THE HEIST

■ ■ ■ ■

MAY 122 A.V.

The jury, passing on the prisoner's life,
May in the sworn twelve have a thief or two
Guiltier than him they try.

— SHAKESPEARE,
Measure for Measure

34

"Everybody, kill your engines."

0440 hours: in darkness they rowed the final fifty yards to shore and dragged the launches onto the sand. A few hundred yards south, the glow of burning butane flickered in the sky. Michael checked his rifle, racked his sidearm, and returned it to its holster. Everyone else did the same.

They broke into three groups and scuttled up the dunes. Rand's squad would take the workers' quarters, Weir's the radio and control rooms. Michael's team, the largest, would rendezvous with Greer's to secure the Army barracks and armory. That's where the shooting would be.

Michael pressed the radio to his mouth. "Lucius, are you in position?"

"Roger that. Waiting on your signal."

The refinery was protected by a two-tiered fence line with guard towers; the remainder of the perimeter was a gauntlet of trip-wire mines. The only access from the north was straight through the gate. Greer would lead the frontal assault using a tanker truck equipped with a plow. A pair of trucks full of men would follow. A pickup at the rear, armed with a fifty-caliber and a grenade launcher, would dispense with the towers if need

be. Michael's orders were to avoid casualties if possible, but if it came to that . . .

The teams dispersed at a quick step. Michael and his men took up positions around the barracks, a long Quonset hut with doors front and rear. They were expecting fifty well-armed men inside, perhaps more.

"Team one."

"Good to go."

"Team two."

"Roger that."

Michael checked his watch: 0450. He looked at Patch, who nodded.

Michael raised his flare gun and fired. A popping flash and the compound appeared around them in blocks of light and shadow. A second later, Patch launched the gas canister from its tube. Shouts and gunfire from the gate, and then a crash as the semi plowed through the fence. Gas had begun to sift under the door of the barracks. As it flew open, Michael's men released a barrage of grazing fire into the dirt. The fleeing soldiers lurched backward in confusion. More men were careening into them from behind, choking and coughing and sputtering.

"On your knees! Drop your weapons! Hands on your heads!"

The soldiers had nowhere to run; onto their knees they went.

"Everyone, report."

"Team two, secure."

"Lucius?"

"No casualties. Headed your way."

"Team one?"

Michael's men had moved forward to wrap the soldiers' wrists and ankles with heavy cord. Most

were still coughing, a few vomiting helplessly.

"Team one, report."

A grainy crackle of static; then, a voice, not Rand's: "Secure."

"Where's Rand?"

A pause, followed by laughter. "You'll have to give him a minute. That woman sure packs a wallop."

It had been too easy. Michael had expected more of a fight — *any* kind of fight.

"These guns are practically empty."

Greer showed him; none of the soldiers' magazines had more than two rounds.

"What about the armory?"

"Clean as a whistle."

"That's actually not so good."

From Greer, a tight nod. "I know. We'll have to do something about that."

It was Rand who brought Lore to him. Her wrists were bound. At the sight of him she startled, then quickly composed herself.

"I guess you missed me, Michael?"

"Hello, Lore." Then, to Rand: "Take those off."

Rand cut her loose. Lore had nailed him with a hard right cross. His left eye was half-shut, his cheek marked with the imprint of her fist. Michael felt almost proud.

"Let's go someplace and talk," he said.

He led Lore into the station chief's office. *Her* office: for fifteen years, the refinery had been Lore's to run. Michael sat behind the desk to make a point; Lore sat across from him. The day had broken, warming the room with its light. She looked older, of course, aged by sun and work, but the raw physicality was still there, the strength.

399

"So how's your pal Dunk?"

Michael smiled at her. "It's good to see you. You haven't changed a bit."

"Are you trying to be funny?"

"I mean it."

She glanced away, a furious look on her face. "Michael, what do you want?"

"I need fuel. Heavy diesel, the dirty stuff."

"Going into the oil business? It's a hard life — I don't recommend it."

He took a long breath. "I know this doesn't make you happy. But there's a reason."

"Is that right?"

"How much do you have?"

"You know what I always liked best about you, Michael?"

"No, what?"

"I don't remember either."

It was true: she was just the same. Michael felt a frisson of attraction. Her power had not abated.

He leaned back in his chair, balanced the tips of his fingers together, and said, "You have a major delivery to the Kerrville depot scheduled in five days. Add that to what's in the storage tanks, I'm figuring you've got somewhere in the neighborhood of eighty thousand gallons."

Lore shrugged indifferently.

"So I should take that as a yes?"

"You should take it up your ass, actually."

"I'm going to find out anyway."

She sighed. "Okay, fine. Yes, eighty thousand, more or less. Does that satisfy you?"

"Good. I'm going to need it all."

Lore cocked her head. "I beg your pardon?"

"With twenty tanker trucks, I'm thinking we can move it all in just under six days. After that, we'll

400

release your people. No harm, no foul. You've got my word."

Lore was staring at him. "Move it *where?* What the hell do you need eighty thousand gallons for?"

Ah.

The tanker trucks were being loaded; the first convoy would be ready to move by 0900. For Michael, five days of looking at his watch, yelling at everyone: *Hurry the hell up.*

One wrinkle, maybe small, maybe not. When Weir's men had stormed the communications hut, the radio operator had been in the midst of sending a message. There was no way to know what it was, because the man was dead — the morning's only fatality.

"How the hell did that happen?"

Weir shrugged. "Lombardi thought he had a weapon. It looked like he was drawing on us."

The weapon was a stapler.

"Have any messages come in since?" Michael asked, thinking, *Lombardi, of course it would be you, you trigger-happy asshole.*

"Nothing so far."

Michael cursed himself. The man's death was regrettable, but that wasn't the true source of his anger. They should have taken out the radio first. A stupid mistake, probably not the first.

"Get on the horn," he said, then thought the better of it. "No, wait until twelve hundred. That's when they expect the refinery to check in."

"What should I tell them?"

" 'Sorry, we shot the radio operator. He was waving office supplies at us.' "

Weir just looked at him.

"I don't know, something *normal.* 'Everything's

401

peachy, how are you, isn't it a nice day?' "

The man hurried away. Michael walked to the Humvee, where Lore was waiting in the backseat. Rand was handcuffing her to the safety rail.

"You should take somebody else with you," Rand said.

Michael accepted the key to the cuffs and got in the cab. He glanced at Lore through the mirror. "You promise to be good or do you need a babysitter?"

"The man you shot. His name was Cooley. The guy wouldn't squash a bug."

Michael looked at Rand. "I'll be fine. Just get that diesel moving."

The drive to the channel took three hours. Lore barely uttered a word, and Michael made no effort to draw her out. It had been a hard morning for her — the end of a career, the death of a friend, a public humiliation — all at the hands of a man she had every reason to despise. She needed time to adjust, especially considering the things Michael was about to tell her.

They passed through the wires and made their way down the causeway. He brought the truck to a halt behind the machine shed at the edge of the quay. From here, the *Bergensfjord* wasn't visible. He wanted a grand unveiling.

"So why am I here?"

Michael opened Lore's door and unlocked her wrists. As she climbed out of the Humvee, he withdrew his sidearm and held it out to her.

"What's this?"

"A gun, obviously."

"And you're giving it to me?"

"You get to pick. Shoot me, take the truck, you'll

402

be back in Kerrville by nightfall. Stay, and you'll know what this is all about. But there are rules."

Lore said nothing, merely raised an eyebrow.

"Rule one is you can't leave unless I allow it. You're not a prisoner, you're one of us. Once I tell you what's happening, you'll see the necessity. Rule two is I'm in charge. Speak your mind, but never question me in front of my men."

She was looking at him as if he'd lost all sense. Still, the offer had to be made; the woman had to choose.

"Why in hell would I want to join you?"

"Because I'm going to show you something that will change everything you thought you knew about your life. And because, deep down, you trust me."

She stared at him, then laughed. "The comedy never stops, does it?"

"I wasn't fair to you, Lore. I'm not proud of what I did — you deserved better than that. But there *was* a reason. I said you haven't changed, which is true. That's why I brought you here. I need your help. I can see why you'd say no, but I hope you won't."

She eyed him suspiciously. "Where exactly *is* Dunk?"

"This was never about the trade. I needed money and manpower. More than that, I needed secrecy. Five weeks ago, Dunk and all his lieutenants went into the channel. There is no trade anymore. Only me, and those loyal to me." He nudged the gun toward her. "The mag is full, and there's one in the pipe. What you do with it is up to you."

Lore accepted the pistol. For a long moment she looked at it, until, with a heavy sigh, she slid it

403

into the waistband of her jeans at the base of her spine.

"If it's all right with you, I'm keeping this."

"That's fine. It's yours now."

"I must be out of my mind."

"You made the right choice."

"I regret it already. I'm only going to say this one time, but you really broke my heart, you know that?"

"I do. And I apologize."

A brief silence. Then she nodded, just once: case closed. "So?"

"Brace yourself."

He wanted Lore to see the *Bergensfjord* from below. That was the best way. Not just to see her but to *experience* her; only then could her meaning be grasped. They took the stairs to the floor of the drydock. Michael waited as Lore approached the hull. The ship's flanks were smooth and gracefully curved, every rivet tight. Beneath the *Bergensfjord's* massive propellers, Lore came to a halt, gazing upward. Michael would let her speak first. Above them, the clang of footfalls, men calling to one another, the whine of a pneumatic drill, the ship's vast square footage of metal amplifying every sound like a giant tuning fork.

"I knew there was a boat . . ."

Michael was standing beside her. She turned to face him. In her eyes a struggle was being waged.

"She's called the *Bergensfjord*," Michael said.

Lore spread her hands and looked around. "All this?"

"Yes. For her."

Lore moved forward, extended her right hand over her head, and pressed it against the hull —

just as Michael had done on the morning they'd drained the water from the dock, revealing the *Bergensfjord* in all her rusted, invincible glory. Lore held it there, then, as if startled, broke away.

"You're scaring me," she said.

"I know."

"Please tell me you were just keeping your hands busy. That I'm not seeing what I think I'm seeing."

"What do you think you're seeing?"

"A lifeboat."

Some color had drained from her face; she seemed uncertain where to direct her eyes.

"I'm afraid it is," Michael said.

"You're lying. You're making this up."

"It's not good news — I'm sorry."

"How could you possibly *know*?"

"There's a lot to explain. But it's going to happen. The virals are coming back, Lore. They were never really gone."

"This is crazy." Her confusion turned to anger. "*You're* crazy. Do you know what you're saying?"

"I'm afraid I do."

"I don't want anything to do with this." She was backing away. "This can't be true. Why don't people know? They would *know*, Michael."

"That's because we haven't told them."

"Who the hell is 'we'?"

"Me and Greer. A handful of others. There's no other way to say this, so I just will. Anybody who's not on this boat is going to die, and we're running out of time. There's an island in the South Pacific. We believe it's safe there — maybe the only safe place. We have food and fuel for seven hundred passengers, maybe a few more."

He hadn't expected this to be easy. Under ideal

circumstances, he would have softened the blow. But Lore would cope, because that was her nature, the meat and marrow of Lore DeVeer. What had passed between them years ago was, for her, a painful memory perhaps, a quick jolt of anger and regret that touched her from time to time, but not for Michael. She was part of his life, and a good part, because she was one of the few people who had ever understood him. There were people who simply made existence more bearable; Lore was one.

"That's why I brought you here. We have a long voyage ahead of us. I need the diesel, but that's not all. The men who work for me, well, you've met them. They're hard workers, and they're loyal, but that only goes so far. I need *you*."

Her struggle was not over. There was more talking to be done. Nevertheless, Michael saw his words taking hold.

"Even if what you say is true," Lore said, "what can *I* possibly do?"

The *Bergensfjord:* he had given her everything. Now he would give her this.

"I need you to learn how to drive her."

35

The funeral was held in the early morning. A simple gravesite service: Meredith had requested that no general announcement of Vicky's death be made until the following day. Despite her high profile, Vicky had been a guarded person, sharing her private life with just a handful of people. *Let it just be us.* Peter offered a few words, followed by Sister Peg. The last to speak was Meredith. She appeared composed; she'd had years to prepare.

Still, she said, with a hitch in her voice, one was never really ready. She then went on to tell a series of hilarious stories that left them all weeping with laughter. At the end, everyone was saying the same thing. *Vicky would have been so pleased.*

They adjourned to the house that was now Meredith's alone. The bed in the parlor was gone. Peter moved among the mourners — government officials, military, a few friends — then, as he was preparing to leave, Chase took him aside.

"Peter, if you have a second, there's something I'd like to discuss with you."

Here it comes, he thought. The timing made sense; now that Vicky was gone, the man felt that the path had been cleared for him. They stepped into the kitchen. Chase appeared uncharacteristically anxious, fiddling with his beard. "This is a little awkward for me," he admitted.

"You can stop right there, Ford. It's okay — I've decided not to run again." It surprised Peter a little, how easily the words had come. He felt a burden lifting. "I'll give you my full endorsement. You should have no problems."

Chase looked perplexed, then laughed. "I'm afraid you've got it wrong. I want to resign."

Peter was dumbstruck.

"I was waiting until Vicky . . . well. I knew she'd be disappointed in me."

"But I thought you always wanted it."

Chase shrugged. "Oh, there was a time when I did. When she picked you, I was pretty sore, I won't deny it. But not anymore. We've had our differences along the way, but the woman was right, you were the man for the job."

How could Peter have so badly misjudged? "I don't know what to say."

"Say, 'Good luck, Ford.' "

He did just that. "What will you do?"

"Olivia and I are thinking Bandera. It's good cattle land out there. The telegraphs are in, the town's first on the drawing board for the rail line. I figure fifty years from now, I'll make my grandkids rich."

Peter nodded. "It's a sound plan."

"You know, if you're really not running again, I'd be willing to talk about a partnership."

"You're serious?"

"It was actually Olivia's idea. The woman knows me; I'm all about the details. You want to fix the sewers on time, I'm your guy. But a cattle operation takes more than that. It takes nerve, and it takes capital. Just your name on the operation will open a lot of doors."

"I really don't know anything about cows, Ford."

"And I do? We'll learn. That's what everybody's doing these days, isn't it? We'd be a good team. We have so far."

Peter had to admit it: the notion was intriguing. Somehow, through the years, he had failed to notice that he and Chase had become, of all things, friends.

"But who's going to run if you don't?"

"Does it matter? We're half a government now. Another ten years, this place will be empty, a relic. People will be making their own ways. My guess is, the next guy to sit in that chair will be the one to turn the lights off. Personally, I'm glad it won't be you. I'm your adviser, so let this be my last piece of advice: go out strong, get rich, leave a fortune behind. Have a *life*, Peter. You've earned it. The rest will take care of itself."

Peter couldn't argue the point. "How soon do

you need my answer?"

"I'm not Vicky. Take time to think it over. It's a big step, I know that."

"Thank you," Peter said.

"What for?"

"All of it."

From Chase, a grin. "You're welcome. The letter's on your desk, by the way."

After Chase had gone, Peter lingered in the kitchen; he emerged a few minutes later to find that nearly everyone had left. He said goodbye to Meredith and stepped onto the porch, where Apgar was waiting with his hands in his pockets.

"Chase bowed out."

An eyebrow went up. "Did he now?"

"You wouldn't by any chance feel like running for president?"

"Ha!"

A young officer jogged up the path. He was out of breath and sweating hard, evidently having run a great distance.

"What is it, son?" Peter said.

"Sirs," he said between gulps of air, "you need to see something."

The truck was parked in front of the capitol. Four soldiers were standing guard. Peter unlatched the tailgate and drew the canvas aside. Military crates filled the space, packed to the ceiling. Two of the soldiers extricated a crate from the first row and lowered it to the ground.

"I haven't seen one of these in years," Apgar said.

The crates had come from Dunk's bunker. Inside, vacuum-sealed in plastic strips, lay ammunition: .223, 5.56, 9mm, .45 ACP.

Apgar broke the seal on a round, held it up to the light, and whistled admiringly. "This is the good stuff. Original Army." He rose and turned to one of the soldiers. "Corporal, how many rounds do you have in your sidearm?"

"One and one, sir."

"Give it here."

The soldier handed it over. Apgar dropped the magazine, cleared the chamber, and topped the magazine off with a fresh cartridge. He racked the slide and held out the gun to Peter. "You want the honors?"

"Be my guest."

Apgar aimed the pistol at a square of earth ten feet away and pulled the trigger. There was a satisfying boom as dirt leapt up.

"Let's see what else we've got," Peter said.

They removed a second crate. This one contained a dozen M16s with extra thirty-round magazines, similarly sealed, looking fresh as the day they were made.

"Did anybody see the driver?" Peter asked.

Nobody had; the truck had simply appeared.

"So why would Dunk be sending us this?" Apgar asked. "Unless you brokered some kind of deal you didn't tell me about."

Peter shrugged. "I didn't."

"Then how do you explain it?"

Peter couldn't.

36

She crossed into Texas on old Highway 20. The morning of the forty-third day; Alicia had traveled half the breadth of a continent. The going had been slow at the start — cutting her way through

the detritus of the coast, working inland across the rocky folds of the Appalachians, then the way had loosened and she'd begun to make good time. The days grew warmer, the trees burst into flower, springtime spread over the land. Whole days passed in heavy rain; then the sun exploded over the earth. Unbelievable nights, wide and starlit, the moon rolling through its cycle as she rode.

But now they stopped to rest. In the shade of a gas station awning Alicia lay on the ground while Soldier grazed nearby. Just a few hours and they'd press on. Her bones grew heavy; she felt herself plummeting into sleep. Throughout her journey, this had been the pattern. Days of wakefulness, her mind so alert it was almost painful, then she'd fall like a bird shot from the sky.

She dreamed of a city. Not New York; it was no city she had ever seen or known. The vision was majestic. In the darkness, it floated like an isle of light. Mighty ramparts surrounded it, protecting it from all danger. From within came noises of life: voices, laughter, music, the delighted shrieks of children at play. The sounds fell upon her like a shimmering rain. How Alicia longed to be among the inhabitants of that happy city! She made her way toward it and walked its perimeter, searching for a way in. There seemed to be none, but then she found a door. It was tiny, fit for a child. She knelt and turned the handle, but the door wouldn't budge. She became aware that the voices had faded. Above her, the city wall soared into blackness. *Let me in!* She began to pound the door with her fists; panic was consuming her. *Somebody, please! I'm all alone out here!* Still the door refused her. Her cries became howls, and then she saw: there was no door. The wall was perfectly

411

smooth. *Don't leave me!* On the far side, the city
had fallen silent: the people, the children, all gone.
She pounded till she could pound no more and
collapsed to the ground, sobbing into her hands.
Why did you leave me, why did you leave me . . .

She awoke in twilight. Lying motionless, she
blinked the dream away, then rose on her elbows
to see Soldier standing at the edge of the shelter.
He angled one dark eye at her.

"All right already. I'm coming."

Kerrville was four days away.

37

Kate and the girls had been with them a little
more than a month. At the start, Caleb hadn't
minded. It was good for Pim to have family
around, and the girls adored Theo. But as the
weeks passed, Kate's mood only seemed to
darken. It filled the house like a gas. She did few
chores and spent long hours sleeping, or else sitting on the front steps, staring into space.

How long is she going to mope around like that?

Pim was cleaning up the breakfast dishes. She
dried her hands on a towel and looked at him
squarely. *She's my sister. She just lost her husband.*

She's better off, Caleb thought, but didn't say
so; he didn't have to.

Give her time, Caleb.

Caleb left the house. In the dooryard, Elle and
Bug were playing with Theo, who had learned to
crawl. The boy was capable of astonishing speed;
Caleb reminded the girls to keep an eye on their
cousin and not wander far from the house.

He was hitching the horses to the plow when he
heard a cry of shock and pain. He dashed back to

412

the yard as Kate and Pim came running from the house.

"Get them off! Get them off!"

Elle's bare legs were swarming with ants — hundreds of them. Caleb scooped her up and ran to the trough, the little girl writhing and shrieking in his arms. He plunged her into the water and began frantically stripping the ants from her legs, running his hands up and down her skin. The ants were on him too; he felt the electrical sting of their teeth boring into his arms, his hands, inside the collar of his shirt.

At last Elle quieted, her screams yielding to hic-cupy sobs. A dark scrim of ant corpses had floated to the surface of the trough. Caleb lifted her out and handed her to Kate, who wrapped her in a towel. Her legs were covered with welts.

There's ointment inside, Pim signed.

Kate carried Elle away. Caleb drew his shirt over his head and shook it out, sending ants scattering. He had plenty of bites too, but nothing like his niece.

Where are Theo and Bug? he asked.

In the house.

It had been a hard spring for ants. People were saying it was the weather — the wet winter, the dry spring, the early summer, shockingly warm. The woods were bursting with their mounds, some reaching gigantic proportions.

Pim gave him a look of concern. *Is there anything we can do?*

This can't last forever. We should keep the kids inside until it passes.

But it didn't pass. The next morning, the ground around the house was swarming. Caleb decided to burn the mounds. From the shed he retrieved a

413

can of fuel and carried it to the edge of the woods. He chose the largest pile, a yard wide and half as high, splashed it with kerosene, tossed a match, and stepped back to watch.

As black smoke roiled upward, ants exploded from the mound in a massive horde. Simultaneously, the hardened earth of the mound's surface began to bulge volcanically, then split open like a piece of rotten fruit. Soil cascaded down the sides. Caleb lurched back. What the hell was down there? It must have been a gigantic colony, millions of the little bastards, driven to mad panic by the smoke and flames.

The mound collapsed.

Caleb stepped gingerly forward. The last of the flames were sputtering out. All that remained was a shallow indentation in the earth.

Pim came up beside him. *What happened?*

Not sure.

From where he stood, he counted five other mounds.

I'm taking the wagon. Stay inside.

Where are you going? Pim signed.

I need to get more gas.

38

The Possum Man was missing.

The Possum Man, but also dogs — lots of dogs. The city was usually crawling with them, especially in the flatland. You couldn't walk ten paces down there without seeing one of the damn things, all skinny legs and matted fur and gooey eyes, snuffling through a garbage pile or crouched to take a wormy shit in the mud.

But suddenly, no dogs.

The Possum Man lived on the river near the old perimeter. He looked like what he did: pale and pointy-nosed, with dark, slightly bulging eyes and ears that stuck out from the sides of his face. He kept a woman half his age, though not the sort that anyone would want. According to her, they'd heard noise in the yard late at night. They figured it might be foxes, which had gotten into the hutches before. The Possum Man had grabbed his rifle and gone out to look. One shot, then nothing.

Eustace was kneeling by what was left of the hutches, which looked like they'd been hit by a tornado. If there were tracks, Eustace couldn't find any; the earth in the yard was packed too hard. Possum corpses were strewn around, torn to bloody chunks, although a few yards away a pair of them fidgeted in the dirt, staring at him woefully, like traumatized witnesses. They were actually kind of cute. As the closest one loped toward him, Eustace extended his hand.

"Don't want to do that," the woman warned. "They're nasty fuckers. Bite your finger off."

Eustace yanked his hand away. "Right."

He stood and looked at the woman. Her name was Rena, Renee, something like that, as scragglylooking a thing as he'd ever laid eyes on. It was entirely possible that her parents had given her to the Possum Man in exchange for food. Such bargains were common.

"You said you found the rifle."

She retrieved it from the house. Eustace worked the bolt, kicking out an empty cartridge. He asked her where she'd found it. Her eyes didn't look in quite the same direction; it made her a little hard to talk to.

"Just about where you're standing."

"And you didn't hear anything else. Only the one shot."

"Happened like I said."

He was beginning to wonder if maybe she'd done it — shot the Possum Man, dragged his body to the river, busted up the hutches to cover her tracks. Well, if she had, she probably had a good enough reason, and Eustace sure as hell wasn't going to do anything about it.

"I'll put the word out. He turns up, you let us know."

"You sure you don't want to come inside, Sheriff?"

She was giving him a look. It took Eustace a second to figure out what it was. Her off-kilter gaze traveled the length of his body, then lingered pointedly. The gesture was supposed to be seductive but was more like livestock trying to sell itself.

"Folks say you ain't got a woman."

Eustace wasn't perturbed. Well, maybe a little. But the woman had been treated like property all her life; she had no other way of doing things.

"Don't believe everything you hear."

"But what'll I do he's dead?"

"You've got two possums, don't you? Make more."

"Them there? Them's both boys."

Eustace handed back the rifle. "I'm sure you'll think of something."

He returned to the jail. Fry, at his desk with his boots up, was paging through a picture book.

"She try to poke you?" Fry asked, not looking up.

Eustace sat behind his desk. "How'd you know?"

"They say she does that." He turned a page.

416

"Think she killed him?"

"She mighta." Eustace gestured at the book. "What you got there?"

Fry held it up to show him. *Where the Wild Things Are.*

"That's a good one," Eustace said.

The door swung open and a man entered, banging dust from his hat. Eustace recognized him; he and his wife farmed a patch of ground on the other side of the river.

"Sheriff. Deputy." He nodded at each of them in turn.

"Help you, Bart?"

He cleared his throat nervously. "It's my wife. I can't find her anywhere."

It was nine A.M. By noon, Eustace had heard the same story fourteen times.

39

It was midafternoon by the time Caleb reached town on the buckboard. The place seemed totally dead — no people anywhere. In two hours on the road, he hadn't seen a single soul.

The door of the mercantile was locked. Caleb cupped his eyes to the glass. Nothing, no movement inside. He stilled his body, listening to the quiet. Where the hell was everybody? Why would George close up in the middle of the day? He walked around to the alley. The back door stood ajar. The frame was splintered; the door had been forced.

He returned to the buckboard for his rifle.

He nudged the door open with the tip of the barrel and moved inside. He was in the storeroom. The space was tightly packed — sacks of feed

piled high, coils of fencing, spools of chain and rope — leaving only a narrow corridor through which to pass.

"George?" he called. "George, are you in here?"

He felt and heard crunching underfoot. One of the bags of feed had been torn open. As he knelt to look, he heard a high-pitched clicking above his head. He lurched back, swinging the barrel of the rifle upward.

It was a raccoon. The animal was sitting on top of the pile. It lifted onto its hind legs, rubbing its two front paws together, and gave him a look of absolute innocence. *That mess on the floor? Nothing to do with me, pal.*

"Go on, beat it." Caleb poked the barrel of the rifle forward. "Get your ass out of here before I make you into a hat."

The raccoon scampered down the pile and out the door. Caleb took a breath to calm his heart and passed through the beaded curtain into the store. The lockbox where George kept the day's receipts sat beneath the counter in its usual spot. He moved through the aisles, finding nothing amiss. A flight of stairs behind the counter led to the second floor — presumably, George's living quarters.

"George, if you're there, it's Caleb Jaxon. I'm coming up."

He found himself in a single large room with upholstered furniture and curtains on the windows. The homeyness of it surprised him — he had expected a scene of bachelor squalor. But George had been married once. The room was divided into two areas, one for living, the other for sleeping. A kitchen table; a couch and chairs with lace doilies on the headrests; a cast-iron bed

with a sagging mattress; an ornately carved wardrobe of a type that usually stayed within a family, traveling the road of several generations. All seemed orderly enough, but as Caleb surveyed the space, he began to notice certain things. A dining chair had been knocked over; books and other objects — a kitchen pot, a ball of yarn, a lantern — were tossed about the floor; a large, free-standing mirror had shattered in its frame, the glass cracked in concentric circles, like a reflective spider's web.

As he moved toward the bed, the odor hit him: the rancid, biological reek of old vomitus. George's chamber pot sat on the floor near the headboard; that was where the smell was coming from. Blankets were bunched at the foot of the mattress as if kicked aside by a restless sleeper. On the bedside table lay George's gun, a long-barreled .357 revolver. Caleb opened the cylinder and pushed the ejection rod. Six cartridges fell into his palm; one had been fired. He turned around and swept the pistol over the room, then lowered the gun and stepped toward the fractured mirror. At the epicenter of the cracks was a single bullet hole.

Something had happened here. George had obviously been ill, but there was more to it. A robbery? But the lockbox hadn't been touched. And the bullet hole was strange. A stray shot, perhaps, though something about it seemed deliberate — as if, lying in bed, George had shot his own reflection.

In the alley, he filled his jugs from the tank and loaded them onto the buckboard. It wouldn't do to leave without paying; he made his best guess and left the bills under the counter with a note:

"Nobody here, door unlocked. Took fifteen gallons of kerosene. If the money isn't enough, I'll be back in a week and can pay you then. Sincerely, Caleb Jaxon."

On the way out of town, he stopped at the town office to report what he'd found. At least someone should fix the door of the mercantile and lock the place up until they knew what had happened to George. But nobody was there, either.

Dusk was settling down when he returned to the house. He unloaded the kerosene, put the horses in the paddock, and entered the house. Pim was sitting with Kate by the cold woodstove, writing in her journal.

Did you get what you needed?

He nodded. Strange how Kate was now the silent one. The woman had barely glanced up from her knitting.

How was town?

Caleb hesitated, then signed: *Very quiet.*

They ate corn cakes for supper, played a few hands of go-to, and went to bed. Pim was out like a light, but Caleb slept badly; he barely slept at all. All night his mind seemed to skip over the surface of sleep like a stone upon water, never quite breaking the skin. As dawn approached, he gave up trying and crept from the house. The ground was moist with dew, the last stars receding into a slowly paling sky. Birds were singing everywhere, but this wouldn't last; to the south, where the weather came from, a wall of flickering clouds roiled at the horizon. So: a spring storm. Caleb guessed he had maybe twenty minutes before it arrived. He gave himself another minute to watch it, then retrieved the first jug of kerosene

420

from the shed and lugged it to the edge of the woods.

He didn't know what he was seeing. It simply made no sense. Perhaps it was the light. But no.

The mounds were gone.

40

0600 hours: Michael Fisher, Boss of the Trade, stood on the quay to watch the morning light come on. A thick, cloudy dawn; the waters of the channel, caught between tides, were absolutely motionless. How long since he'd slept? He was not so much tired — he was well past that — as running on some reserve of energy that felt vaguely lethal, as if he were burning himself up. Once it was gone, that would be the end of him; he would vanish in a puff of smoke.

He'd emerged from the bowels of the *Bergensfjord* with some vague intention he couldn't recall; the moment he'd hit fresh air, the plan had fled from his mind. He'd drifted down to the edge of the wharf and found himself just standing there. Twenty-one years: amazing how so much time could slip by. Events grabbed hold of you and in the blink of an eye there you were, with sore knees and a sour stomach and a face in the mirror your barely recognized, wondering how all of it had happened. If that was really your life.

The *Bergensfjord* was nearly ready. Propulsion, hydraulics, navigation. Electronics, stabilizers, helm. The stores were loaded, the desalinators up and running. They'd stripped the ship to the simplest configuration; the *Bergensfjord* was basically a floating gas tank. But a lot had been left to chance. For instance: Would she actually float?

421

Computations on paper were one thing; reality was another. And if she did, could her hull, cobbled together from a thousand different plates of salvaged steel, a million screws and rivets and patch welds, withstand a journey of such duration? Did they have enough fuel? What about the weather, especially when they attempted to round Cape Horn? Michael had read everything he could find about the waters he intended to cross. The news was not good. Legendary storms, crosscurrents of such violence that they could snap your rudder off, waves of towering dimensions that could downflood you in a second.

He sensed someone coming up behind him: Lore.

"Nice morning," she said.

"Looks like rain."

She shrugged, looking over the water. "Still nice, though."

She meant, How many more mornings will we have? How many dawns to watch? Let's enjoy it while we can.

"How are things in the pilothouse?" Michael asked.

She blew out a breath.

"Don't worry," he said. "You'll get it."

A bit of pink was in the clouds now. Gulls swooped low over the water. It really was a fine morning, Michael thought. He felt suddenly proud. Proud of his ship, his *Bergensfjord*. She had traveled halfway around the world to test his worthiness. She had given them a chance and said, *Take it if you can.*

A glow of light appeared on the causeway.

"There's Greer," he said. "I better go."

Michael made his way up the quay and met the

first tanker truck just as Greer stepped down from the cab.

"That's the last of it," Greer said. "We tapped out at nineteen tankers, so we left the last one behind."

"Any problems?"

"A patrol eyeballed us south of the barracks at Rosenberg. I guess they just assumed we were on the way to Kerrville. I thought they'd be onto us by now, but apparently they're not."

Michael glanced over Greer's shoulder and signaled to Rand. "You got this one?"

Men were swarming over the tankers. Rand gave him a thumbs-up.

Michael looked at Greer again. The man was obviously worn out. His face had thinned to skull-like proportions: cheekbones ridged like knives, eyes red-rimmed and sunk into their pockets, skin waxy and damp. A frost of white stubble covered his cheeks and throat; his breath was sour.

"Let's get something to eat," Michael said.

"I could go for some shut-eye."

"Have breakfast with me first."

They'd erected a tent on the quay with a commissary and cots for resting. Michael and Greer filled their bowls with watery porridge and sat at a table. A few other men were hunched over their breakfasts, robotically shoveling the gruel into their mouths, faces slack with exhaustion. Nobody was talking.

"Everything else good to go?" Greer asked.

Michael shrugged. *More or less.*

"When do you want us to flood the dock?"

Michael took a spoon of the porridge. "She should be ready in a day or two. Lore wants to inspect the hull herself."

"Careful woman, our Lore."

Patch appeared on the far side of the tent. Eyes unfocused, he shambled across the space, lifted the lid on the pot, decided against it, and took one of the cots instead, not so much lying down as succumbing, like a man felled by a bullet.

"You should catch a few winks yourself," Greer said.

Michael gave a painful laugh. "Wouldn't that be nice?"

They finished breakfast and walked to the loading area, where Michael's pickup was parked. Two of the tankers were already drained and standing off to the side. An idea took shape in Michael's mind.

"Let's leave one tanker full and move it to the end of the causeway. Do we have any of those sulfur igniters left?"

"We should."

No further explanation was necessary. "I'll let you see to it."

Michael got in the pickup and placed his Beretta in the bracket under the steering wheel; a short-barreled shotgun with a pistol grip and a sidesaddle of extra shells was clamped between the seats. His rucksack rested on the passenger seat: more rounds, a change of clothes, matches, a first-aid kit, a pry bar, a bottle of ether and a rag, and a cardboard folder sealed with twine.

Michael started the engine. "You know, I've never been in jail before. What's it like?"

Greer grinned through the open window. "The food's better than it is here. The naps are sensational."

"So, something to look forward to."

Greer's expression sobered. "He can't know

424

about her, Michael. Or about Carter."

"You're not making my job any easier, you know."

"It's how she wants it."

Michael regarded his friend for another few seconds. The man really did look terrible. "Go sleep," he said.

"I'll add it to my to-do list."

The two men shook. Michael put the truck in gear.

41

"Everybody, settle down!"

The auditorium was packed, all the seats taken, with more people crowded into the back and along the aisles. The room stank of fear and unwashed skin. At the front of the room, the mayor, red-faced and sweating, pointlessly banged his gavel on the podium, yelling for silence, while behind him, the members of the Freestate Council — as ineffective a group of individuals as Eustace had ever laid eyes on — found papers to shuffle and buttons to adjust, guiltily averting their gazes like a group of students caught cheating on a test.

"My wife's missing!"

"My husband! Has anybody seen him?"

"My kids! Two of them!"

"What happened to all the dogs? Did anybody else notice that? No dogs anywhere!"

More banging of the gavel. "Goddamnit, people, please!"

And so on. Eustace glanced at Fry, who was standing on the other side of the room and sending him a look that said, *Oh boy, ain't this going to be fun.*

425

Finally the room quieted enough for the mayor to be heard. "Okay, that's better. We know everybody's worried and wants answers. I'm going to bring up the sheriff, who can maybe shed some light. Gordon?"

Eustace took the podium and got to it. "Well, we don't know much more at this point than everybody else. About seventy folks have gone missing over the last couple of nights. Mind, these are the ones we know about. Deputy Fry and I haven't gotten out to all the farms yet."

"So why aren't you out looking for them?" a voice yelled.

Eustace parsed the man's face from the crowd. "Because I'm standing here talking to you, Gar. Now just button it so I can get through this."

A voice barked from the other side of the room: "Yeah, shut your mouth and let the man talk!"

More yelling, anxious voices volleying back and forth. Eustace let it run its course.

"Like I was saying," he continued, "we don't know where these folks have gone off to. What seemed to have happened is that, for whatever reason, these individuals got up in the middle of the night, went outside, and didn't come back."

"Maybe somebody's taking them!" Gar yelled. "Maybe that person is right here in this room!"

The effect was instantaneous; everybody started looking at everybody else. A low murmuring rippled through the room. *Could it be . . . ?*

"We're not ruling anything out at this point," Eustace said, aware of how weak this sounded, "but that doesn't seem so likely. We're talking about a lot of people."

"Maybe it's more than one person doing this!"

"Gar, you want to come up here and run this

426

meeting?"

"I'm just saying —"

"What you're doing is scaring people. I'm not having you start a panic, people looking sideways at each other. For all we know, these folks have gone off on their own. Now, pipe down before I lock you up."

A woman in the front row rose to her feet. "Are you saying my boys ran away? They're six and seven!"

"No, I'm not saying that, Lena. We just don't have any more information than what I'm telling you. The best thing people can do is stay in their homes till we sort this out."

"And what about my wife?" Eustace couldn't see who was talking. "Are you saying she just up and left me?"

The mayor, stepping forward to retake the podium, held up both hands. "I think what the sheriff is trying to express —"

"He's not 'expressing' anything! You heard him! He doesn't know!"

Everybody started shouting again. There was no taking this thing back; it was spiraling out of control. Eustace glanced across the stage at Fry, who tipped his head toward the wings. As the mayor resumed banging his gavel, Eustace slipped backstage and met Fry at the door. The two men stepped outside.

"Well, that was sure productive," Fry said. "Glad to get out before the shooting started."

"I wouldn't joke about that. We're going to be on the top of everybody's list if we don't figure this thing out."

"Think they're still alive?"

"Not really."

427

"What do you want to do?"

The day was bright and warm, the sun midpoint in a cloudless sky. Eustace remembered a day like this one: spring on the cusp of summer, the earth unclenching its fist, thick green leaves, rich with fragrance, fattening the trees. A walk by the river, Simon balanced on his shoulders, Nina beside him; the day like a marvelous gift, and then the moment, unmistakable, when the boy had had his fill; returning to the house and putting him down for his nap, Nina beckoning to him from the doorway with her special smile, the one only for him, and the two of them tiptoeing to their room to make quiet, lazy love on a sunny afternoon. Always the joke: *How can you kiss this damn ugly face of mine?* But she could; she did. The last such day; for Eustace, there would never come another.

"Let's find those missing people."

42

Apgar found Peter where he always was: at his desk, wading through a mass of paperwork. Just two days without Chase's organizing presence, and Peter felt completely swamped.

"Got a minute?"

"Make it fast."

Apgar took the chair across from him. "Chase really sandbagged you. You shouldn't have let him off the hook so easily."

"What can I say? I'm too nice."

Apgar cleared his throat. "We've got a problem."

He was filling out a form. "Are you quitting, too?"

"Probably not the moment for that. I got a message from Rosenberg this morning. A lot of tank-

ers moving through there in the last few days, but none of it is showing up here."

Peter raised his head.

"You heard me."

"What does the refinery say?"

"Everything on schedule, blah blah blah. Then, as of this morning, not a peep, and we can't raise them."

Peter leaned back in his chair. *Good God.*

"I've got men on the way to the refinery to check it out," Apgar continued, "but I think I know what we'll find. You've got to hand it to the guy for balls, anyway."

"What the hell would Dunk need our oil for?"

"My bet is, he doesn't. It's a play. He wants something."

"Such as?"

"You've got me there. It isn't going to be small, though. Light and Power says we have enough gas on hand for ten days, a few more if we ration. Even if we can secure the refinery, no way we can get enough slick back into the system to keep the lights burning. In less than two weeks, this city goes dark."

Dunk had them in a vise. Peter had to admit, begrudgingly, that it was sort of brilliant. But one piece didn't fit.

"So he sends us a truck full of guns and ammo, then hijacks all our oil? It seems contradictory."

"Maybe the guns came from somebody else."

"That was bunker ammo. Only the trade has that stuff."

Apgar shifted in his chair. "Well, here's another piece to consider. First you've got Cousin's Place going up in smoke, then there's a rumor going around that one of Dunk's women showed up in

the city saying that something happened out there. A lot of shooting."

"A power play by one of his guys, you mean."

"Could be just gossip. And I don't see how it fits, but it's something to consider."

"Where is she now?"

"The woman?" Apgar almost laughed. "Who the hell knows?"

The guns and the oil were connected, but how? It didn't feel like Dunk; holding a city hostage was out of his league, and the Army now had enough weaponry to take the isthmus and put him out of business. It would be a slaughter on both sides — the causeway was a kill box — but once the dust settled, Dunk Withers would find himself either lying dead in a ditch with fifty holes in him or swinging from a rope.

So suppose, Peter thought, the oil wasn't just a play. Suppose it was actually *for* something.

"What do we know about this boat of his?" he asked.

Apgar frowned. "Not a lot. Nobody from the outside has laid eyes on the damn thing in years."

"But it's big."

"So folks say. You think that's got something to do with it?"

"I don't know what to think. But there's something we're missing. Have we spread that ammo around?"

"Not yet. It's still in the armory."

"Get it done. And let's send a patrol to scout the isthmus. How long till we hear from Freeport?"

"A couple of hours."

It was a little after three P.M. "Let's get men on the perimeter. Tell them it's a training exercise.

And get some engineers on the gate. The thing hasn't been closed in a decade."

Apgar gave him a look of caution. "Folks will notice that."

"Better safe than sorry. None of this makes sense to us, but it does to someone."

"What about the isthmus? We don't want to wait too long to get a plan in place."

"I won't. Write it up."

Apgar rose. "I'll get it on your desk within the hour."

"That quick?"

"There's only one way in. Not a lot to say." He turned at the door. "This is completely fucked, I know, but maybe it's the opportunity we've been waiting for."

"That's a way of looking at it."

"I'm just glad it isn't Chase sitting in that chair."

He left Peter alone. Just five minutes, and the piles of paper on his desk now seemed completely trivial. He swiveled his chair to face the window. The day had begun with clear skies, but now the weather was turning. Low clouds hovered over the city, a heavy gray mass. A gust of wind tossed the treetops, followed by a flash, whitening the sky. As thunder rolled behind it, the first drops of rain, heavy and slow, tapped the glass.

Michael, he thought, *what the hell are you up to?*

43

Anthony Carter, Twelfth of Twelve, had just shut off the mower when he looked toward the patio and noticed that the tea had arrived.

So soon? Could it be noon again already? He angled his chin to the sky — an oppressive sum-

431

mer Houston sky, pale like something bleached. He removed his hankie and then his hat to mop the sweat from his forehead. A glass of tea would surely hit the spot.

Mrs. Wood, she knew that. Though of course it wasn't Mrs. Wood who brought it. Carter couldn't say just who it was. The same someone who delivered the flats of flowers and bags of mulch to the gate, who fixed his tools when they broke, who made time turn how it did in this place, every day a season, every season a year.

He pushed his mower to the shed, wiped it clean, and made his way to the patio. Amy was working in the dirt on the far side of the lawn. There was some ginger there, it grew like crazy, always needing cutting back, bordered by the beds where Mrs. Wood liked to put some summer color. Today it was three flats of cosmos, the pink ones that Miss Haley loved, picking them and putting them in her hair.

"Tea's here," Carter said.

Amy looked up. She was wearing a kerchief around her neck; there was dirt on her hands and face where she'd wiped the sweat away.

"You go ahead." She batted a gnat from her face. "I want to get these in first."

Carter sat and sipped the tea. Perfect as always, sweet but not too sweet, and the ice made a pleasant tinkling against the sides of the glass. From behind him, in the house, came the bright drifting notes of the girls' playing. Sometimes it was Barbies or dress-ups. Sometimes they watched TV. Carter heard the same movies playing over and over — *Shrek* was one, and *The Princess Bride* — and he felt sorry for the two of them, Miss Haley and her sister, all alone and stuck inside the house,

waiting for their mama to come home. But when Carter peeked in the windows, there was never anybody there; the inside and the outside were two different places, and the rooms were empty, not even any furniture to tell that people lived there.

He'd had some time to think on that. He'd thought about a lot of things. Such as, what this place exactly *was*. The best he could come up with was that it was a kind of waiting room, like at a doctor's office. You bided your time, maybe flipping through a magazine, and then when your turn came, a voice would call your name and you'd go on to the next place, whatever that was. Amy called the garden "the world behind the world," and that seemed right to Carter.

How the day got on, he thought. He'd have to get back to work soon; there was a sprinkler head needed replacing, and the pool to skim, and all that edging to do. He liked to keep the yard just so for the day when Mrs. Wood would return. *Mr. Carter, what a beautiful job you've done taking care of the place. You're a godsend. I don't know what I ever did without you.* He liked to think of the things they'd say to each other when that day came. The two of them would have a good talk, just like they used to, sitting on the patio the way any two friends would do.

But for the moment, Carter was content to settle in a spell while the edge came off the heat. He unlaced his boots and closed his eyes. The garden was a place for thinking your thoughts, and that was what he did now. He remembered Wolgast coming to him in Terrell, which was the death house, and then a ride in a van with deep cold and snowy mountains all around, and then the

433

doctors giving him a shot. It made him sick something awful, but that wasn't the worst of it. The worst was the voices in his head. *I am Babcock. I am Morrison. I am Chávez Baffes Turrell Winston Sosa Echols Lambright Martínez Reinhardt . . .* He saw pictures too, horrible things, people dying and such, like he was dreaming someone else's dreams. He'd been to school for a bit, and they'd read a book by Mr. William Shakespeare. Carter hadn't actually read much of it himself. The words in the book were like something chopped up in a blender, that's how confusing it was. But the teacher, Mrs. Coe, a pretty white lady who decorated the walls of her classroom with posters of animals and mountain climbers and sayings like "Reach for the stars" and "Be a friend to make a friend," had showed the class a video. Carter liked it, how everybody was always getting in swordfights and dressed like a pirate, and Mrs. Coe explained that the main guy, who was named Hamlet, and was also a prince, was going crazy because somebody had killed his daddy by pouring poison in his ear. There was more to the story, but Carter remembered that part, because that's what the voices reminded him of. Like poison poured in his ear.

Things had gone on like that for a while, Carter wasn't sure how long. The others were whispering away, saying various things, ugly things, but mostly what they said was their names, over and over, like they couldn't get enough of themselves. Then they fell quiet like the air before a storm and that was when Carter heard him: Zero. "Heard" wasn't exactly the word. Zero could make you think with his own mind. Zero came into his head and it was like taking a step that wasn't there and tumbling

434

down a lightless hole and at the bottom of the hole was a train station. Folks were hurrying in winter coats, and the voice over the loudspeaker was calling out the numbers of the tracks and what was going where. New Haven. Larchmont. Katonah. New Rochelle. Carter didn't know those places. It was cold. The floor was slick with melted snow. He was standing at the kiosk, the one with the four-faced clock. He was waiting for someone, someone important. One train arrived and then another. Where was she? Had something happened? Why hadn't she called, why did she fail to answer? Train after train, the anticipation intense, then, as the last passengers hurried by, the cruelest dashing of his hopes. His heart was shattering, yet he couldn't make himself move. The hands of the clock mocked him with their turning. *She said she would be here, where was she, how he longed to hold her in his arms, Liz you are the only thing that ever mattered, let me be the one to hold you as you slip away . . .*

After that, Carter had gone plain crazy. It was like one long bad dream in which he was watching himself do the worst kinds of things and couldn't stop. Eating folks. Tearing them to bits. Some he didn't kill but only tasted, no rhyme or reason to it, it was just a thing he did because that's what Zero wanted. He remembered a couple in a car. They were driving somewhere in a hurry and Carter had come down on them from the trees. *Leave those people be,* he was telling himself, *what they ever done to you,* but the hungry part of him paid this no mind, it did what it liked, and what it liked was killing folks. He landed hard on the hood and gave them a good long look at him, his teeth and claws and what he was about

435

to do. The two of them were young. There was the man at the wheel and the woman beside him who Carter guessed was his wife. She had short blond hair and eyes that were wide and staring. The car began to fishtail. They were sliding all over the place. The man was yelling *Holy shit!* and *What the fuck!* but the woman barely reacted. Her eyes slid right through Carter, her face as blank as paper, like the sight of a monster on the hood was nothing her brain knew what to do with, and it stopped Carter flat, that's how weird it was, and that was when he noticed the gun — a big shiny pistol with a barrel you could fit your finger in, which the man was trying to aim over the steering wheel. *Now, don't be pointing that,* the one part of him, the still-Carter part, was thinking; *you don't ever point a gun at no one, Anthony;* and maybe it was the memory of his mama's voice or else the way the car was swerving in long looping arcs like a kid on a swing pumping higher and higher and faster and faster, but for a second Carter froze, and as the car began to roll the gun went off in a blast of noise and light and Carter felt a sharp little sting in his shoulder, not much more than a bee might do, and the next thing Carter knew, he was rolling on the pavement.

He came up in time to see the car banging down on its side. It spun in a 360 and crashed down onto its roof with an explosion of glass and a shriek of tearing metal. It began to roll down the asphalt like a log, over and over, bright bits of things hurling away, until it flopped one last time onto its roof and came, at last, to rest.

Everything was very still; they were deep in the country, miles from any town. Debris littered the roadway in a wide, glittering plume. He smelled

gasoline, and something hot and sharp, like melted plastic. He knew he should feel something but didn't know what. His thoughts were all mixed up inside him like single frames from a movie he couldn't put in order. He scuttled his way to the car and crouched to look. The two of them were hanging upside down from their seatbelts, the dashboard crunched up against their waists. The man was dead, on account of the big piece of metal in his head, but the woman was alive. She was staring forward, wide-eyed, blood all over her — her face and shirt, her hands and hair, her lips and tongue and teeth. Black smoke was coiling from under the dash. A piece of glass crunched under Carter's foot and her face swiveled toward him, slowly, no other part of her moving, tracing the source of the sound.

"Is somebody there?" Bubbles of blood formed at her lips as they curved around the words. "Please. Is . . . any . . . body . . . there?"

She was looking right at him. That was when Carter realized she couldn't see. The woman was blind. With a soft *whump* the first flames appeared, licking under the dash.

"Oh, God," she moaned. "I can hear you breathing. For the love of God, please answer me."

Something was happening to him, something strange. Like the woman's sightless eyes were a mirror, and what he saw in them was himself — not the monster they'd made him into but the man he used to be. As if he were waking up and remembering who he was. He tried to answer. *I'm here,* he wanted to say. *You're not alone. I'm sorry about what I done.* But his mouth would not make words. The flames were spreading, the cabin filling with smoke.

"Oh God, I'm burning, please, oh God, oh God . . ."

The woman was reaching for him. Not *for* him, he realized. *To* him. Something was clutched in her hand. A hard spasm shook her; she had begun to choke on the blood that was pouring from her mouth. Her fingers opened and the object fell to the ground.

It was a pacifier.

The baby was in the backseat, still strapped in its carrier upside down. Any second the car was going to blow. Carter dropped to the ground and slithered through the back window. The baby was awake and crying now. The carrier would never fit — he'd have to take the baby out of it. He released the buckle, guided the child's shoulders through the straps, and just like that the soft crying weight of a baby filled his arms. A little girl, wearing pink pajamas. Holding her tight to his chest, Carter wriggled free of the car and began to run.

But that was all he remembered. The story ended there. He never did know what became of that baby girl. For Anthony Carter, Twelfth of Twelve, made it all of three steps before the flames found what they were looking for, the gas in the tank ignited, and that car was blown to smithereens.

He never took another one.

Oh, he ate. Rats, possums, raccoons. Now and again a dog, which he always felt sorry about. But it wasn't long before the world went quiet, and there weren't so many people around to tempt him, and then one day after more time had passed, he realized there weren't any people at all.

He'd closed himself to Zero, too — closed it to

all of them. Carter wanted no part in what they were about. He built a wall in his mind, Zero and the others on one side and him on the other; and though the wall was thin and Carter could hear them if he chose to, he never sent anything back.

It was a lonely time.

He watched his city drown. He'd made a place for himself in that building, One Allen Center, on account of it was high and at night he could stand on the rooftop, among the stars, and feel close to them for company. Year by year the waters rose around the bases of the buildings, and then one night a great wind came barreling down. Carter had been through a hurricane or two in his day, but this wasn't like any storm he'd ever seen. It set the skyscraper swaying like a drunk. Walls were cracking, windows popping from their frames, everything was in an uproar. He wondered if the end of the world was coming, if God had just grown sick and tired of it all. As the waters rose and the building rocked and the heavens howled, he took to praying, telling God to take him if that's what he wanted, saying he was sorry over and over about the things he'd done, and if there was a better place to go to, he knew he didn't deserve it any but hoped he'd get a chance to see it, assuming God could forgive him, which Carter didn't think he could.

Then he heard a sound. A terrifying, heart-rending, inhuman sound, as if the gates of hell had opened and released a million screaming souls into the whirlwind. From out of the blackness a great dark shape emerged. It grew and grew and then the lightning flashed and Carter saw what it was, though he could not believe it. A ship. In downtown Houston. She was headed straight for

him, her great keel dragging along the street, bearing down upon the towers of the Allen Center like God's own bowling ball and the buildings were the pins.

Carter dropped to the floor and covered his head, bracing for the impact.

Nothing happened. Suddenly, everything went quiet; even the wind had stopped. He wondered how this could be so, the sky so furious one minute and still the next. He rose and peered out the window. Above him, the clouds had opened like a porthole. The eye, Carter thought, that's what this was; he was in the eye of the storm. He looked down. The ship had come to rest against the side of the tower, parked like a cab at the curb.

He climbed down the face of the building. How much time he had before the storm returned, Carter couldn't say. All he knew was that the ship being there felt like a message. At length he found himself in the bowels of the vessel, its maze of passages and pipes. Yet he did not feel lost; it was as if an unseen influence was guiding his every action. Oily seawater sloshed around his feet. He chose a direction, then another, drawn by this mysterious presence. A door appeared at the end of the corridor — heavy steel, like the door of a bank vault. T1, it was marked: Tank No. 1.

The water will protect you, Anthony.

He started. Who was speaking to him? The voice seemed to come from everywhere: from the air he breathed, the water sloshing at his feet, the metal of the ship. It enfolded him like a blanket of perfect softness.

He cannot find you here. Abide here in safety, and she will come to you.

That was when he felt her: Amy. Not dark, like

440

the others; her soul was made of light. A great sob racked his body. His loneliness was leaving him. It lifted from his spirit like a veil, and what lay behind it was a sorrow of a different kind — a beautiful, holy kind of sorrow for the world and all its woes. He was holding the wheel. Slowly it turned under his hands. Outside, beyond the walls of the ship, the wind was howling again. The rain lashed, the sky rolled, the seas tore through the streets of the drowned city.

Come inside, Anthony.

The door opened; Carter stepped through. His body was in the ship, the *Chevron Mariner,* but Carter was in that place no more. He was falling and falling and falling, and when the falling stopped he knew just where he was, even before he opened his eyes, because he could smell the flowers.

Carter realized he'd finished his tea. Amy was done with the cosmos and was tidying up the beds. Carter thought to tell her to rest a spell, he'd get to the weeds directly, but he knew that she'd refuse; when there was work to do, she did it.

The waiting was hard for her. Not just because of the things she'd have to face, but for what she'd given up. She never said a word about it, that wasn't Amy's way, but Carter could tell. He knew what it was like to love a person and lose them in this life.

Because Zero would come calling. That was a fact. Carter knew that man, knew he wouldn't rest until the whole world was a mirror to his grief. Thing was, Carter couldn't help but feel a little sorry for him. Carter had been in that sta-

tion himself. Weren't the question the man had wrong, it was his way of asking it.

Carter got up from his chair, put on his hat, and went to where Amy was kneeling in the dirt.

"Have a good nap?" she asked, looking up.

"Was I sleeping?"

She tossed a weed onto the pile. "You should have heard yourself snoring."

Now, that was news to Carter. Although, come to think of it, he might have rested his eyes there for a second.

Amy rocked back on her heels and held her arms wide over the newly planted beds. "What do you think?"

He stepped back to look. Everything was neat as a pin. "Those cosmos is pretty. Mrs. Wood will like 'em. Miss Haley, too."

"They'll need water."

"I'll see to it. You should get out of the sun for a bit. Tea's still there you want it."

He was hooking the hose to the spigot near the gate when he heard the soft pressure of tires on asphalt and saw the Denali coming down the street. It halted at the corner, then crept forward. Carter could just make out the shape of Mrs. Wood's face through the darkly tinted windows. The car cruised slowly by the house, barely moving but never stopping either, the way a ghost might do, then accelerated and sped away.

Amy appeared beside him. "I heard the girls playing earlier." She, too, was looking down the street, though the Denali was long gone. "I brought you this."

Amy was holding a wand. For a second Carter was unable to connect the idea of it to anything else. But it was for the cosmos, of course.

442

"Are you okay?" she asked.

Carter responded with a shrug. He threaded the wand to the end of the hose and opened the spigot. Amy returned to the patio while Carter dragged the hose to the beds and began to water them down. It hardly mattered, he knew; autumn would be here soon. The leaves would pale and fall, the garden fade, the wind grow raw. Frost would wick the tips of the grass, and the body of Mrs. Wood would rise. All things found their ends. But still Carter went on with it, passing his wand over the flowers, back and forth, back and forth, his heart always believing that even the smallest things could make a difference.

44

All day long the rain poured down. Everyone was antsy, trapped in the house. Caleb could tell that Pim's patience with her sister was wearing thin, and he felt a row coming. A few days ago, he might have welcomed such a development, if only to get it over with.

Dusk was near when the clouds broke. A radiant sun streamed low across the fields, everything sopping and glinting in the light. Caleb scanned the ground around the house for ants; finding none, he declared that they could go out to enjoy the last of the day. All that remained of the mounds were ovals of depressed mud barely distinguishable from the surrounding earth. Relax, he told himself. You're letting the isolation get to you, that's all.

Kate and Pim supervised the children making mud pies while Caleb went to check on the horses. He'd built an open-sided shelter on the far side of

the paddock to give them cover from the weather, and that was where he found them now. Handsome seemed none the worse for wear, but Jeb was breathing hard and showing the whites of his eyes. He was also holding his left rear hoof off the ground. The horse let him bend the joint long enough for Caleb to see a small puncture wound in the raised central structure of the hoof. Something long and sharp was stuck in there. He walked to the shed and returned with a halter, needle-nosed pliers, and a rope. He was fixing Jeb's halter when he saw Kate coming his way.

"He doesn't look so happy."

"Got a pricker in his hoof."

"Could you use an extra set of hands?"

He was fine on his own, but the woman's sudden interest in helping out wasn't anything he was going to say no to. "The ropes should hold him. Just keep a hand on his halter."

Kate gripped the leather near the horse's mouth. "He looks sick. Should he be breathing like that?"

Caleb was crouched at the rear of the animal. "You're the doctor — you tell me."

He lifted the horse's foot. With his other hand, he angled the pliers to the wound. There wasn't much to grab hold of. As the tips made contact, the animal shoved his weight backward, whinnying and tossing his head.

"Keep him still, damn it!"

"I'm trying!"

"He's a horse, Kate. Show him who's boss."

"What do you want me to do, slug him?"

Jeb was having none of it. Caleb left the shelter and returned with a length of three-quarter-inch chain, which he ran through the halter, up and over the horse's nose. He tightened the chain

against Jeb's jaw and gave the ends to Kate.

"Hold this," he said. "And don't be nice."

Jeb didn't like it, but the chain worked. Caught in the tips of the pliers, the offending article slowly emerged. Caleb held it up in the light. About two inches long, it was made of a rigid, nearly translucent material, like the bone of a bird.

"Some kind of thorn, I guess," he said.

The horse had relaxed somewhat but was still breathing rapidly. Flecks of spittle hung from the corners of his mouth; his neck and flanks were glossed with sweat. Caleb washed the hoof with water from a bucket and poured iodine into the wound. Handsome was lingering near the shelter, watching them cautiously. While Kate held the halter, Caleb sheathed the hoof in a leather sock and secured it with twine. There wasn't much else he could do at this point. He'd leave the animal tied up for the night and see how he was in the morning.

"Thanks for your help."

The two of them were standing at the door of the shed; the light was just about gone.

"Look," Kate said finally, "I know I haven't been especially good company these days."

"It's fine, forget it. Everybody understands."

"You don't need to be nice about it, Caleb. We've known each other too long."

Caleb said nothing.

"Bill was an asshole. Okay, I get that."

"Kate, we don't have to do this."

She didn't seem angry, merely resigned. "I'm just saying I know what everybody thinks. And they're not wrong. People don't even know the half of it, actually."

"So why did you marry him?" Caleb was sur-

prised at himself; the question had just popped out. "Sorry, that was a little direct."

"No, it's a fair question. Believe me, I've asked it myself." A moment passed; then she brightened a little. "Did you know that when Pim and I were kids we used to have fights over who would get to marry you? I'm talking physical fights — slapping, hair pulling, the whole thing."

"You're kidding."

"Don't look so happy, I'm surprised one of us didn't end up in the hospital. One time, I stole her diary? I think I was thirteen. God, I was such a little shit. There was all this stuff in there about you. How *good-looking* you were, how *smart* you were. Both your names with a big fat heart drawn around them. It was just disgusting."

Caleb found the thought hilarious. "What happened?"

"What do you think? She was older, the fights weren't exactly fair." Kate shook her head and laughed. "Look at you. You love this."

It was true, he did. "It's a funny story. I never knew about any of it."

"And don't flatter yourself, bub — I'm not about to throw myself at your feet."

He smiled. "That's a relief."

"Plus, it would seem a little incestuous." She shuddered. "Seriously, gross."

Night had fallen over the fields. Caleb realized what he'd been missing: the feeling of Kate's friendship. As kids, they'd been as close as any two siblings. But then life had happened — the Army, Kate's medical training, Bill and Pim, Theo and the girls and all their plans — and they'd mislaid each other in the shuffle. Years had passed

since they'd really spoken, the way they were do-ing now.

"But I didn't answer your question, did I? Why I married Bill. The answer is pretty simple. I married him because I loved him. I can't think of a single good reason *why* I did, but a person doesn't get to pick. He was a sweet, happy, worthless man, and he was mine." She stopped, then said, "I didn't come out here to help you with the horses, you know."

"You didn't?"

"I came to ask you what's making you so nervous. I don't think Pim has noticed, but she's going to."

Caleb felt caught. "It's probably nothing."

"I know you, Caleb. It's not nothing. And I have my girls to think about. Are we in trouble?"

He didn't want to answer, but Kate had him dead to rights.

"I'm not sure. We might be."

A loud whinny in the paddock broke his thoughts. They heard a crash, then a series of hard, rhythmic bangs.

"What the hell is *that?*" Kate said.

Caleb grabbed a lantern from the shed and raced across the paddock. Jeb lay on his side, his head tossing violently. His hind hooves were knocking against the wall of the shelter in spas-modic jerks.

"What's wrong with him?" Kate said.

The animal was dying. His bowels released, then his bladder. A trio of convulsions barreled through his body, followed by a final, violent tremor, every part of him stiffening. He held this position for several seconds, as if stretched on wires. Then the air went out of him and he was still.

Caleb crouched beside the carcass, lifting the lantern over the animal's face. A bubbly froth, tinged with blood, was running from his mouth. One dark eye stared upward, shining with reflected light.

"Caleb, why are you holding a gun?"

He looked down; so he was. It was George's revolver, the big .357, which he'd hidden in the shed. He must have grabbed it when he'd retrieved the lantern — an action so automatic as to escape his conscious awareness. He'd cocked the hammer, too.

"You need to tell me what's going on," Kate said.

Caleb released the hammer and swiveled on his heels toward the house. The windows shimmered with candlelight. Pim would be making supper, the girls playing on the floor or looking at books, Baby Theo fussing in his high chair. Maybe not; maybe the boy was already asleep. He sometimes did that, passing out cold at dinnertime only to awaken hours later, howling with hunger.

"Answer me, Caleb."

He rose, slipped the pistol into the waistband of his trousers, and drew his shirt over the butt to conceal it. Handsome was standing at the edge of the light, his head bent low like a mourner's. The poor guy, Caleb thought. It was as if he knew that the job would fall to him to drag the carcass of his only friend across the field to a patch of useless ground where, come morning, Caleb would use the rest of his fuel to burn it.

45

By late afternoon, Eustace and Fry had canvassed

most of the outermost farms. Overturned furniture, beds disturbed, pistols and rifles lying where they'd fallen, a round or two fired, if that.

And not a living soul.

It was after six o'clock when they finished checking the last one, a dump of a place four miles downriver, near the old ADM ethanol plant. The house was tiny, just one room, the structure hammered together from scrap lumber and decaying asphalt shingles. Eustace didn't know who'd lived out here. He guessed he never would.

Eustace's bad leg was aching hard; they'd have just enough time to make it back to town before dark. They mounted their horses and turned north, but a hundred yards later Eustace held up.

"Let's have a peek at that factory."

Fry was leaning over the pommel. "We ain't got but two hands of light, Gordo."

"You want to go back without something to show for it? You heard those folks."

Fry thought for a moment. "Let's be quick on it."

They rode into the compound. The plant comprised three long, two-story buildings arranged in a U, with a fourth, much larger than the others, closing the square — a windowless concrete bulk connected to the grain bins by a maze of pipes and chutes. The skeletal husks of rusted vehicles and other machinery filled the spaces between the weeds. The air had stilled and cooled; birds were flitting through the glassless windows of the buildings. The three small structures were just shells, their roofs long collapsed, but the fourth was mostly tight. This was the one Eustace was interested in. If you were going to hide a couple hundred people, that would be a place to do it.

"You got a windup in your saddlebag, don'tcha?" Eustace asked.

Fry retrieved the lantern. Eustace turned the crank until the bulb began to glow.

"Thing won't last more than about three minutes," Fry warned. "You think they're in there?"

Eustace was checking his gun. He closed the cylinder and reholstered the weapon but left the strap off. Fry did the same.

"Guess we're going to find out."

One of the loading dock doors stood partially open; they dropped and rolled through. The smell hit them like a slap.

"I guess that answers that," Eustace said.

"Fuck *me,* that's nasty." Fry was pinching his nose. "Do we really need to look?"

"Get ahold of yourself."

"Seriously, I think I'm gonna puke."

Eustace gave the lantern a few more cranks. A hallway lined with lockers ran to the main work space of the building. The smell grew more intense with every step. Eustace had seen some bad things in his day, but he was pretty sure this was going to be the worst. They came to the end of the hallway, and a pair of swinging doors.

"I'm thinking this might be the time to ask about a raise," Fry whispered.

Eustace drew his pistol. "Ready?"

"Are you fucking kidding me?"

They pushed through. Several things hit Eustace's senses in close order. The first thing was the stench — a miasma of rot so gaggingly awful that Eustace would have lost his lunch on the spot if he'd actually bothered to eat. To this was added a sound, a dense vibrato that stroked the air like the humming of an engine. In the center of the

room was a large, dark mass. Its edges appeared to be moving. As Eustace stepped forward, flies exploded from the corpses.

They were dogs.

As he raised his pistol he heard Fry yell, but that was as far as he got before a heavy weight crashed into him from above and knocked him to the floor. All those people gone; he should have seen this coming. He tried to crawl away, but something awful was occurring inside him. A kind of . . . swirling. So this was how it was going to be. He reached for his gun to shoot himself but his holster was empty of course, and then his hands went numb and watery, followed by the rest of him. Eustace was plunging. The swirling was a whirlpool in his head and he was being sucked down into it, down and down and down. *Nina, Simon. My beloveds, I promise I will never forget you.*

But that was exactly what happened.

■ ■ ■ ■

V
THE MANIFEST

■ ■ ■ ■

We must take the current when it serves,
Or lose our ventures.
— SHAKESPEARE, *Julius Caesar*

46

It was nearly nine o'clock when Sister Peg walked Sara out.

"Thank you for coming," the old woman said. "It always means so much."

A hundred and sixteen children, from the tiniest babies to young adolescents; it had taken Sara two full days to examine them all. The orphanage was a duty she could have let go of long ago. Certainly Sister Peg would have understood. Yet Sara had never been able to bring herself to do this. When a child got sick in the night, or was down with a fever, or had leapt from a swing and landed wrong, it was Sara who answered the call. Sister Peg always greeted her with a smile that said she hadn't doubted for a second who would be gracing her door. *How would the world get on without us?*

Sara figured that Sister Peg had to be eighty by now. How the old woman continued to manage the place, its barely contained chaos, was a miracle. She had softened somewhat with the years. She spoke sentimentally of the children, both those in her care and the ones who had moved on; she kept track of their lives, how they made their ways in the world, and whom they

married and their children if they had them, the way any mother would do. Though Sara knew the woman would never say as much, they were her family, no less than Hollis and Kate and Pim were Sara's; they belonged to Sister Peg, and she to them.

"It's no trouble, Sister. I'm glad to do it."

"What do you hear from Kate?"

Sister Peg was one of the few people who knew the story.

"Nothing so far, but I didn't expect to. The mail is so slow."

"That was a hard thing, with Bill. But Kate will know what to do."

"She always seems to."

"Would it be all right if I worried about you?"

"I'll be fine, really."

"I know you will. But I'm going to worry anyway."

They said their goodbyes. Sara made her way home through darkened streets; no lights burned anywhere. It had something to do with the supply of fuel for the generators — a minor hiccup at the refinery, that was the official word.

She found Hollis dozing in his reading chair, a kerosene lantern burning on the table and a book of intimidating thickness resting on his belly. The house, where they had lived for the past ten years, had been abandoned in the first wave of settlement — a small wooden bungalow, practically falling down. Hollis had spent two years restoring it, in his off hours from the library, which he was now in charge of. Who would have thought it, this bear of a man passing his days pushing a cart through the dusty shelves and reading to children? Yet that was what he loved.

She hung her jacket in the closet and went to the kitchen to warm some water for tea. The stove was still hot — Hollis always left it that way for her. She waited for the kettle to boil, then poured the water through the strainer filled with herbs she'd taken from the canisters that stood in a neat line on the shelf above the sink, each one marked in Hollis's hand: "lemon balm," "spearmint," "rosehips," and so on. It was a librarian's habit, Hollis said, to fetishize the smallest details. Left to herself, Sara would have had to spend thirty minutes looking for everything.

Hollis stirred as she entered the living room. He rubbed his eyes and smiled groggily. "What time is it?"

Sara was sitting at the table. "I don't know. Ten?"

"Guess I fell asleep there."

"The water's hot. I can make you some tea." They always drank tea together at the end of the day.

"No, I'll get it."

He lumbered into the kitchen and returned with a steaming mug, which he placed on the table. Rather than sit, he moved behind her, took her shoulders in his hands, and began, with gathering pressure, to work his thumbs into the muscles. Sara let her head slump forward.

"Oh, that's good," she moaned.

He kneaded her neck for another minute, then cupped her shoulders and moved them in a circular motion, unleashing a series of pops and cracks.

"Ouch."

"Just relax," Hollis said. "God, you're tight."

"You would be too, if you just gave physicals to a hundred kids."

"So tell me. How is the old witch?"

"Hollis, don't be nasty. The woman's a saint. I hope I've got half her energy at her age. Oh, right there."

He continued his pleasurable business; bit by bit, the tensions of the day drained away.

"I can do you next if you want," Sara said.

"Now you're talking."

She felt suddenly guilty. She tipped her face backward to look at him. "I have been ignoring you a little, haven't I?"

"Comes with the territory."

"Getting old, you mean."

"You look pretty good to me."

"Hollis, we're *grandparents*. My hair's practically white; my hands look like beef jerky. I won't lie — it depresses me."

"You talk too much. Lean forward again."

She dropped her head to the table and nestled it into her arms. "Sara and Hollis," she sighed, "that old married couple. Who knew we'd be those people someday?"

They drank their tea, undressed, and got into bed. Usually there were noises at night — people talking in the street, a barking dog, the various small sounds of life — but with the power out, everything was very quiet. It was true: it had been a while. A month, or was it two? But the old rhythm, the muscle memory of marriage, was still there, waiting.

"I've been thinking," Sara said after.

Hollis was nestled behind her, wrapping her in his arms. Two spoons in a drawer, they called it. "I thought you might be."

"I miss them. I'm sorry. It's just not the same. I thought I'd be okay with it, but I'm just not."

458

"I miss them, too."

She rolled to face him. "Would you really mind so much? Be honest."

"That depends. Do you think they need a librarian in the townships?"

"We can find out. But they need doctors, and I need you."

"What about the hospital?"

"Let Jenny run it. She's ready."

"Sara, you do nothing but *complain* about Jenny."

Sara was taken aback. "I do?"

"Nonstop."

She wondered if this was true. "Well, *somebody* can take over. We can just go for a visit to start, to see how it feels. Get the lay of the land."

"They may not actually want us out there, you know," Hollis said.

"Maybe not. But if it seems right, and everyone's agreed, we can put in for a homestead. Or build something in town. I could open an office there. Hell, you've got enough books right here to start a library of your own."

Hollis frowned dubiously. "All of us crammed into that tiny house."

"So we'll sleep outside. I don't care. They're our *kids*."

He took a long breath. Sara knew what Hollis was going to say; it was just a matter of hearing him say it.

"So when do you want to leave?"

"That's the thing," she said, and kissed him. "I was thinking tomorrow."

Lucius Greer was standing under the spotlights at the base of the drydock, watching a distant figure

459

swinging over the side of the ship in a bosun's chair.

"For godsakes," Lore yelled. "Who did this fucking weld?"

Greer sighed. In six hours, Lore had seen very little that she actually approved of. She lowered the chair to the dock and stepped free.

"I need half a dozen guys down here now. Not the same jokers who did these welds, either." She angled her face upward. "Weir! Are you up there?"

The man's face appeared at the rail.

"String up three more chairs. And go get Rand. I want these seams redone by sunrise." Lore looked at Greer from the corner of her eye. "Don't say it. I ran that refinery for fifteen years. I know what I'm doing."

"You won't hear any complaints from me. That's why Michael wanted you here."

"Because I'm a hard-ass."

"Your words, not mine."

She stood back, hands resting on her hips, eyes distractedly scanning the hull. "So tell me something," she said.

"All right."

"Did you ever think it was all bullshit?"

He liked Lore, her directness. "Never."

"Not once?"

"I wouldn't say the thought never crossed my mind. Doubt is human nature. It's what we do with it that matters. I'm an old man. I don't have time to second-guess things."

"That's an interesting philosophy."

A pair of ropes drifted down the flank of the *Bergensfjord,* then two more.

"You know," Lore said, "all these years, I wondered if Michael would ever find the right

woman and settle down. Never in my wildest dreams did I imagine my competition was twenty thousand tons of steel."

Rand appeared at the gunwale. He and Weir began to hitch up the bosun's chairs.

"Do you still need me here?" Greer asked.

"No, go sleep." She waved up at Rand. "Hang on, I'm coming up!"

Greer left the dock, got in his truck, and drove down the causeway. The pain had gotten bad; he wouldn't be able to hide it much longer. Sometimes it was cold, like being stabbed by a sword of ice; other times it was hot, like glowing embers tossing around inside him. He could hardly keep anything down; when he actually managed to take a piss, it looked like an arterial bleed. There was always a bad taste in his mouth, sour and ureic. He'd told himself a lot of stories over the last few months, but there was really only one ending he could see.

Near the end of the causeway the road narrowed, hemmed in on either side by the sea. A dozen men armed with rifles were stationed at this bottleneck. As Greer drew alongside, Patch stepped from the cab of the tanker and came over.

"Anything going on out there?" Greer asked.

The man was sucking at something in his teeth. "Looks like the Army sent a patrol. We saw lights to the west just after sundown, but nothing since."

"You want more men out here?"

Patch shrugged. "I think we're okay for tonight. They're just sniffing us out at this point." He focused on Greer's face. "You okay? You don't look too good."

"Just need to get off my feet."

"Well, the cab of the tanker is yours if you want

it. Catch a few winks. Like I said, there's nothing going on out here."

"I've got some other things to see to. Maybe I'll come back later."

"We'll be here."

Greer turned the truck around and drove away. Once he was out of sight, he pulled to the side of the causeway, got out, placed a hand against the fender for balance, and threw up onto the gravel. There wasn't much to come up, just water and some yolky-looking blobs. For a couple of minutes he remained in that position; when he decided there was nothing more, he retrieved his canteen from the cab, rinsed his mouth, poured some water into his palm, and splashed his face. The aloneness of it — that was the worst part. Not so much the pain as carrying the pain. He wondered what would happen. Would the world dissolve around him, receding like a dream, until he had no memory of it, or would it be the opposite — all the things and people of his life rising up before him in vivid benediction until, like a man gazing into the sun on a too-bright day, he was forced to look away?

He tipped his face to the sky. The stars were subdued, veiled by a moist sea air that made them seem to waver. He brought his thoughts to bear upon a single star, as he had learned to do, and closed his eyes. *Amy, can you hear me?*

Silence. Then: *Yes, Lucius.*

Amy, I'm sorry. But I think that I am dying.

47

A spring afternoon: Peter was working in the garden. Rain had worked through in the night,

but now the sky was clear. Stripped to his shirt-sleeves, he jabbed his hoe into the soft dirt. Months of eating from the canning jars while they watched the snow fall; how good it would be, he thought, to have fresh vegetables again.

"I brought you something."

Amy had snuck up behind him. Smiling, she held out a glass of water. Peter took it and sipped. It was ice cold against his teeth.

"Why don't you come inside? It's getting late."

So it was. The house lay long in shadow, the last rays of light peeking over the ridge.

"There's a lot to be done," he said.

"There always is. You can get back to work tomorrow."

They ate their supper on the sofa, the old dog nosing around their feet. While Amy washed up, Peter set a fire. The wood caught with crackling quickness. The rich contentment of a certain hour: beneath a heavy blanket, they watched the flames leap up.

"Would you like me to read to you?"

Peter said he thought that would be nice. Amy left him briefly and returned with a thick, brittle volume. Settling back on the sofa, she opened the book, cleared her throat, and began.

"*David Copperfield,* by Charles Dickens. Chapter One. I Am Born."

Whether I shall turn out to be the hero of my own life, or whether that station will be held by anybody else, these pages must show. To begin my life with the beginning of my life, I record that I was born (as I have been informed and believe) on a Friday, at twelve o'clock at night. It was remarked that the clock began to strike, and I

began to cry, simultaneously.

How wonderful, to be read to. To be carried from this world and into another, borne away on words. And Amy's voice, as she told the story: that was the loveliest part. It flowed through him like a benign electric current. He could have listened to her forever, their bodies close together, his mind in two places simultaneously, both within the world of the story, with its wonderful rain of sensations, and here, with Amy, in the house in which they lived and always had, as if sleep and wakefulness were not adjacent states with firm boundaries but part of a continuum.

At length he realized that the story had stopped. Had he dozed off? Nor was he on the sofa any longer; in some manner, unaware, he had made his way upstairs. The room was dark, the air cold above his face. Amy was sleeping beside him. What was the hour? And what was this feeling he had — the sense that something was not right? He drew the blankets aside and went to the window. A lazy half-moon had risen, partially lighting the landscape. Was that movement, there, at the edge of the garden?

It was a man. He was dressed in a dark suit; gazing upward at the window, he stood with his hands behind his back, in a posture of patient observation. Moonlight slanted across him, sharpening the angles of his face. Peter experienced not alarm but a feeling of recognition, as if he had been waiting for this nighttime visitor. Perhaps a minute passed, Peter watching the man in the yard, the man in the yard watching him. Then, with a courteous tip of his chin, the stranger turned away and walked off into the darkness.

"Peter, what is it?"

He turned from the window. Amy was sitting up in bed.

"There was somebody out there," he said.

"Somebody? Who?"

"Just a man. He was looking at the house. But he's gone now."

Amy said nothing for a moment. Then: "That would be Fanning. I was wondering when he'd show up."

The name meant nothing to Peter. Did he know a Fanning?

"It's all right." She drew the blanket aside for him. "Come back to bed."

He climbed under the covers; at once, the memory of the man receded into unimportance. The warm pressure of the blankets, and Amy beside him; these were all he needed.

"What do you think he wanted?" Peter asked.

"What does Fanning ever want?" Amy sighed wearily, almost with boredom. "He wants to kill us."

Peter awoke with a start. He'd heard something. He drew a breath and held it. The sound came again: the creak of a floorboard underfoot.

He rolled, reached his right hand to the floor, and took the weight of the pistol in his grip. The creak had come from the front hallway; it sounded like one person; they were trying to keep quiet; they didn't know he was awake; surprise was therefore on his side. He rose and crossed the room to the front window; his security detail, two soldiers stationed on the porch, were gone.

He thumbed off the safety. The bedroom door was closed; the hinges, he knew, were loud. The

moment the door opened, the intruder would be alerted to his presence.

He pulled the door open and moved at a quick-step down the hall. The kitchen was empty. Without missing a stride, he turned the corner into the living room, extending the pistol.

A man was seated in the old wooden rocker by the fireplace. His face was turned partially away, his eyes focused on the last embers glowing in the grate. He appeared to take no notice of Peter at all.

Peter stepped behind him, leveling the gun. Not a tall man but solidly built, his broad shoulders filling the chair. "Show me your hands."

"Good. You're awake." The man's voice was calm, almost casual.

"Your hands, damnit."

"All right, all right." He held his hands away from his body, fingers spread.

"Get up. Slowly."

He lifted himself from his chair. Peter tightened the grip on his pistol. "Now face me."

The man turned around.

Holy shit, thought Peter. *Holy, holy shit.*

"You think maybe you could stop pointing that thing at me?"

Michael had aged, but of course they all had. The difference was that the Michael he knew — his mental image of the man — had leapt forward two decades in an instant. It was, in a way, like looking in a mirror; the changes you didn't notice in yourself were laid bare in the face of another.

"What happened to the security detail?"

"Not to worry. Their headaches will be historic, though."

"The shift changes at two, in case you were wondering."

Michael looked at his watch. "Ninety minutes. Plenty of time, I'd say."

"What for?"

"A conversation."

"What did you do with our oil?"

Michael frowned at the gun. "I mean it, Peter. You're making me nervous."

Peter lowered the weapon.

"Speaking of which, I brought you a present." Michael gestured toward his pack on the floor. "Do you mind — ?"

"Oh, please, make yourself at home."

Michael removed a bottle, wrapped in stained oilcloth. He uncovered it and held it up for Peter to see.

"My latest recipe. Should strip the lining right off your brainpan."

Peter retrieved a pair of shot glasses from the kitchen. By the time he returned, Michael had moved the rocking chair to the small table in front of the sofa; Peter sat across from him. On the table was a large cardboard folder. Michael cut the wax on the bottle, poured two shots, and raised his glass.

"Compadres," he said.

The taste exploded into Peter's sinuses; it was like drinking straight alcohol.

Michael smacked his lips appreciatively. "Not bad, if I do say so myself."

Peter stifled a cough, his eyes brimming. "So, did Dunk send you?"

"Dunk?" Michael made a sour face. "No. Our old friend Dunk is taking a very long swim with his cronies."

"I suspected as much."

"No need to thank me. Did you get the guns?"

"You left out the part about what they're for."

Michael picked up the folder and untied the cords. He withdrew three documents: a painting of some kind; a single sheet of paper, covered in handwriting; and a newspaper. The masthead said INTERNATIONAL HERALD TRIBUNE.

Michael poured a second shot into Peter's glass and pushed it toward him. "Drink this."

"I don't want another."

"Believe me, you do."

Michael was waiting for Peter to say something. His friend was standing at the window, looking out into the night, though Michael doubted he was seeing much of anything.

"I'm sorry, Peter. I know it's not good news."

"How can you be so damn *sure*?"

"You're going to have to trust me."

"That's all you've got? *Trust* you? I'm committing about five felonies just *talking* to you."

"It's going to happen. The virals are coming back. They were never really gone to begin with."

"This is . . . insane."

"I wish it were."

Michael had never felt so sorry for anyone since the day he'd sat on the porch with Theo, a lifetime ago, and told him the batteries were failing.

"This other viral —" Peter began.

"Fanning. The Zero."

"Why do you call him that?"

"It's how he knows himself. Subject Zero, the first one infected. The documents Lacey gave us in Colorado described thirteen test subjects, the Twelve plus Amy. But the virus had to come from

somewhere. Fanning was the host."

"So what's he waiting for? Why didn't he attack us years ago?"

"All I know is, I'm glad he didn't. It's bought us the time we needed."

"And Greer knows this because of some . . . vision."

Michael waited. Sometimes, he knew, that was what you had to do. The mind refused certain things; you had to let resistance run its course.

"Twenty-one years since we opened the gate. Now you waltz in here and tell me it was all a big mistake."

"I know this is hard, but you couldn't know. No one could. Life had to go on."

"Just what would you have me tell people? Some old man had a bad dream, and I guess we're all dead after all?"

"You're not going to tell them anything. Half of them won't believe you; the other half will lose their minds. It'll be pandemonium — everything will fall apart. People will do the math. We only have room for seven hundred on the ship."

"To go to this island." Peter gestured dismissively at Greer's painting. "This picture in his head."

"It's more than a picture, Peter. It's a map. Who really knows where it comes from? That's Greer's department, not mine. But he saw it for a reason, I know that much."

"You always seemed so goddamned *sensible*."

Michael shrugged. "I admit, the whole thing took some getting used to. But the pieces fit. You read that letter. The *Bergensfjord* was headed there."

"And just who decides who goes? You?"

"You're the president — that's ultimately your call. But I think you'll agree —"

"I'm not *agreeing* to anything."

Michael took a breath. "I think you'll agree that we need certain skills. Doctors, engineers, farmers, carpenters. We need leadership, obviously, so that includes you."

"Don't be absurd. Even if what you say is right, which is ridiculous, there's no way I'd go."

"I'd rethink that. We'll need a government, and the transition should be as smooth as possible. But that's a subject for later." Michael removed a small, leather-wrapped notebook from his pack. "I've drafted a manifest. There are some names, people I know who fit the bill, and we've included their immediate families. Age is a factor, too. Most are under forty. Otherwise there are job descriptions grouped by category."

Peter accepted the notebook, opened it to the first page, and began to read.

"Sara and Hollis," he said. "That's good of you."

"You don't have to be sarcastic. Caleb's in there, too, in case you were wondering."

"What about Apgar? I don't see him anywhere."

"The man is what? Sixty-five?"

Peter shook his head with a look of disgust.

"I know he's your friend, but we're talking about rebuilding the human race."

"He's also general of the Army."

"As I said, these are just recommendations. But take them seriously. I've given the matter a lot of thought."

Peter read the rest without comment, then looked up. "What's this last category, these fifty-six spots?"

"Those are my men. I've promised them places

on the ship. I won't go back on that."

Peter tossed the notebook onto the table "You've lost your mind."

Michael leaned forward. "This is going to *happen,* Peter. You need to accept it. And we don't have a lot of time."

"Twenty years, and now this is a big emergency."

"Rebuilding the *Bergensfjord* took what it took. If I could have finished faster, I would have. We'd be long gone."

"And just how do you propose we get people to this boat of yours without starting a panic?"

"Probably we can't. That's what the guns are for."

Peter just stared at him.

"There are three options that I can see," Michael continued. "The first is a public lottery for the available slots. I'm opposed to that, obviously. Option two is we make our selections, tell the people on the manifest what's happening, give them the choice of either staying or going, and do our best to keep order while we get them out of here. Personally, I think that would be a disaster. No way we could keep a lid on things, and the Army might not back us. Option three is we tell the passengers nothing, apart from a few key individuals we know we can trust. We round up the rest and get them out in the dead of night. Once they're at the isthmus, we give them the good news that they're the lucky ones."

"*Lucky?* I can't believe we're even talking like this."

"Make no mistake, that's what they are. They'll get to live their lives. More than that. They'll be starting over, someplace that's truly safe."

"And this boat of yours can actually get them

there? This derelict?"

"I hope she can. I *believe* she can."

"You don't sound convinced."

"We've done our best. But there aren't any guarantees."

"So those seven hundred lucky people might be going straight to the bottom of the ocean."

Michael nodded. "That might be exactly what happens. I've never lied to you, and I'm not going to start now. But she managed to cross the world once. She'll do it again."

The conversation was broken by a burst of voices outside and three hard bangs on the door.

"Well," Michael said, and clapped his knees. "It looks like our time is over. Think about what I've told you. In the meanwhile, we need to make this look right." He reached into his pack and withdrew the Beretta.

"Michael, what are you doing?"

He pointed the gun halfheartedly at Peter. "Do your best to act like a hostage."

Two soldiers burst into the room; Michael rose to his feet, raising his hands. "I surrender," he said, just in time for the closest one to take two long strides toward him, raise the butt of his rifle, and send it crashing into Michael's skull.

48

Rudy was hungry. *Really* fucking hungry.

"Hello!" he called, pressing his face to the bars to aim his voice down the lightless corridor. "Did you forget about me? Hey, assholes, I'm starving in here!"

Yelling was pointless; nobody had been in the office since early afternoon — not Fry and not

Eustace, either. Rudy plopped down on his bunk, trying not to think about his empty stomach. What he would have given for one of those stupid potatoes now.

He rocked back on the cot and tried to get comfortable. There were lots of spots that still hurt; every position Rudy tried made him ache in a different way. Okay, he'd pretty much asked for a beating. He wouldn't say he hadn't. But what would have happened if Fry hadn't gotten the door open? Dead Rudy, that's what.

For a while he drifted. Little squirts of liquid burbled in his gut. He wasn't sure what time it was; late, probably, though without Fry coming back to bring him his meals, the day had lost its rhythm. He wouldn't have minded a book to occupy himself, if there were any light to see by or if he could actually read, which he couldn't, having never understood the point of it.

Fucking Gordon Eustace.

More time slipped by. His mind was floating on the crest of sleep when a jolt of dread aroused him.

Somewhere outside, a woman was screaming.

The window was positioned high on the wall; Rudy had to stand on his tiptoes and grip the bars to keep his nose above the sill. There were lots of sounds now — shots, shouts, screams. A darkened figure tore past the window, then two more.

"Hey!" Rudy yelled after them. "Hey, I'm in here!"

Something was happening, and it was nothing good. He yelled some more, but nobody stopped or even answered. The screaming died down and then picked up again, louder than before, a lot of

people at once. Maybe it wasn't such a good idea to be telling everybody where he was, Rudy thought. He released his grip and backed away from the window. Whatever was going on out there, he was trapped like a rat in a can. Better to just shut up.

The world went quiet again. Maybe a minute passed before Rudy heard the front door of the building open. He dropped to the floor and scrambled beneath the cot. The squeak of a chair, a shuffling sound, a drawer being opened: somebody was searching for something. Then Rudy heard it: the jingling of keys.

"Sheriff?"

No answer.

"Deputy Fry? That you?"

A soft green light filled the corridor.

Simultaneously, at the farthest outskirts of Mystic Township, Texas, three virals were emerging from the earth.

Like pupae struggling free of their protective coverings, the members of the pod appeared in stages: first the pearlescent tips of their claws, then the long bony fingers, followed by a busting of soil that laid bare their sleek, inhuman faces to the stars. They rose, shaking off the dirt with a doglike motion, and stretched their slumberous limbs. A moment was required to ascertain their situation. It was night. They were in a field. The field was freshly turned. The first to emerge, the dominant member of the pod, was the widowed shopkeeper, George Pettibrew; the second was the town farrier, Juno Brand; the third was a fourteen-year-old girl from Hunt Township who had been taken up four nights ago when she'd made a

midnight run to the outhouse of her family's farm. These identities lay beyond their powers of recollection, for they had none; all they had was a mission.

They saw the farmhouse.

A lazy curlicue of smoke chuffed from its chimney pipe. They circled the structure, taking stock. It possessed two doors, front and rear. Though it was not in their natures to bother with a door, nor with the dainty human custom of turning a handle, such was their task that this was what they did.

They entered. Their senses roamed the space. A sound from above.

Somebody was snoring.

The first viral, the alpha, crept up the stairs. So fine were his movements that not even a floorboard creaked; he barely parted air. The faint glow of a lantern issued from the room at the top, carelessly left burning after the house's inhabitants had retired for the night. In the big bed, two were sleeping, a man and a woman.

The viral bent to the woman. She was on her left side, one arm crooked beneath the pillows, the second exposed upon the blankets. Under the subdued light of the lantern, her skin shimmered deliciously. The viral unlocked his jaws and lowered his face toward her. The barest prick, his teeth delicately sliding into the microscopic spaces of her flesh, and it was done.

She stirred, moaned, rolled over. Perhaps she dreamed that she was pruning roses and got punctured by a thorn.

The viral moved to the other side of the bed. Only the man's head and neck were exposed. The viral sensed as well that the man, whose snores

rattled with a phlegmy texture, was not as deeply asleep as the woman. Leaning forward, the viral tilted his head to one side, as if to aim a kiss.

The man's eyes flew open. "Holy fucking shit!"

He shoved the palm of one hand against the viral's forehead to hold him at bay while reaching the other hand beneath the pillow. "Dory!" he bellowed, "Dory, wake up!" The viral was stunned into inaction: this was not how things were supposed to be. And that name, Dory. It jostled his mind. Did he know a Dory? Did he know the man as well? Had the two of them, at one time, been people in his life? And what was the man reaching for beneath his pillow?

It was a gun. With a howl, the man shoved the barrel into the viral's mouth, pressing the muzzle up against his palate, and fired.

A thunder clap, a parabola of blood, the viral's brain matter caroming through the crown of his skull to splatter on the ceiling. The body rocked forward, dead weight. The woman was awake now, immobilized with terror and screaming to beat the band. The other virals vaulted up the stairs. Shoving the corpse aside, the man fired at the first one as it burst through the door. He wasn't really aiming anymore. He was simply squeezing the trigger. The third shot connected in a general way, but that was the extent of it. Two more shots and the hammer fell on an empty chamber. As one of the virals leapt toward him, the man grabbed the only thing he could think of — the kerosene lantern — and hurled it at his attackers.

His aim was true. The viral exploded in flames.

And then everything was on fire.

The feeling hit Amy like a punch to the gut. She

doubled over, the trowel falling from her hand, and dropped to her hands and knees in the dirt.

"Amy, are you all right?"

Carter was kneeling beside her. She tried to answer but couldn't; her breath stopped in her chest.

"You hurting somewhere? Tell me what's wrong."

At the same moment, Caleb Jaxon awoke to the disconcerting smell of smoke. He had spent the night in a chair by the door, George's pistol on the table, his rifle cradled in his lap. His first thought was that his own house was burning; he jerked upright, panic pounding through him. But, no, the room was all in order; the smell came from someplace else. He grabbed the pistol and stepped outside. To the west, beyond the ridgeline, the sky was lit with fire.

"Please, Miss Amy," Carter said. "You scaring me."

She was shaking; she could not speak. Such pain they felt, such terror. So many, all at once. Her breath unlocked; air flowed back into her lungs.

"It's started."

■ ■ ■ ■ ■

VI
ZERO HOUR

■ ■ ■ ■ ■

The fire which seems extinguished often
slumbers beneath the ashes.
— PIERRE CORNEILLE, *Rodogune*

49

Just after daybreak, Caleb shook Pim by the shoulder.

Something's happened at the Tatums'.

She sat upright, instantly awake. *What?*

Caleb opened the fingers of both hands and moved them in a rotating motion in front of his chest: *Fire.*

Pim shoved the blankets aside. *I'm coming with you.*

Stay here. I'll look.

She's my friend.

Pim was referring to Dory, of course.

Okay, he signed.

The children were still out cold. While Pim dressed, Caleb awakened Kate to tell her what was happening.

"What do you think it means?" Her voice was groggy, but her eyes were clear.

"I don't know." He pulled the revolver from his waistband and held it out. "Keep this handy."

"Any idea what I'm supposed to be shooting at?"

"If I knew, I'd tell you. Stay inside — we won't be long."

Caleb met Pim in the yard. She was gazing

481

toward the ridgeline, hands on her hips. A thick column of white smoke, the color of a summer cloud, billowed at a distance. The color meant the fire was out.

Jeb? she signed.

The horse was lying where he had fallen. Handsome had wandered to the far end of the paddock, keeping his distance.

He died last night.

Pim's face was all business. *How?*

Maybe colic. I didn't want to upset you.

I'm your wife. She signed these words with brisk anger. *I saw you give Kate a gun. Tell me what's happening.*

Caleb had no answer.

All that remained of the farmhouse was a pile of charred timbers and glowing ash. The heat had been so intense that the glass in the windows had melted. It would be several hours, perhaps a day, before Caleb could look for bodies, though he doubted there'd be anything left but bones and teeth.

Do you think they got out? Pim asked.

Caleb could only shake his head. How had it happened? A loose ember from the stove? A lantern knocked aside? Something small, and now they were gone.

He noticed something else. The paddock was empty. The gate stood open; the ground around it looked scraped, as if someone had killed the horses and dragged the carcasses away. What did it mean?

Let's check the barn, he signed.

Caleb entered first. It took his eyes a moment to

adjust to the darkness. At the rear, in deep shadow, was a hump on the floor.

It was Dory. She was lying in a fetal position. Her hair was burned away, brows and lashes gone, her face swollen and scorched. Her nightdress was charred in places, in others fused to her flesh. Her right arm and both legs were blackened to a crisp; elsewhere the skin had bubbled, as if boiled from within.

He knelt beside her. "Dory, it's Caleb and Pim."

Her right eye opened the thinnest crack; the other seemed welded shut. She flicked her gaze toward him. From her throat came a sound, half moan, half gurgle. Caleb couldn't imagine such agony. He wanted to be ill.

Pim brought a bucket and ladle. She knelt beside Dory, cupped the woman's head to lift it slightly, and held the ladle to her lips. Dory managed a small sip, then sputtered the rest from her mouth.

We have to get her back, Pim signed. *Kate will know what to do.*

That the woman was still alive was a miracle; surely she would not survive long. Still, they had to try. A wheelbarrow stood propped against the wall. Caleb rolled it over and fetched a pair of saddle pads from the tack bin and laid them in the bottom.

Take her legs.

Caleb positioned himself behind Dory and hooked his elbows under her shoulders. The woman began to shriek and buck at the waist. After the longest five seconds of his life, they managed to get her into the wheelbarrow. A tacky substance came away on Caleb's bare forearms: pieces of Dory's skin.

Her cries subsided. She was breathing in shallow, rapid jerks. The trip would be unbearable for her; each jostle would bring fresh waves of torture. As Caleb hoisted the bars of the wheelbarrow, he saw another problem. Dory was not a small woman. Keeping the whole thing balanced would take every ounce of his strength.

Give me a side, Pim signed.

Caleb shook his head firmly. *The baby.*

I'll stop if I'm tired.

Caleb didn't want to, but Pim wouldn't be deterred. They rolled Dory to the door. As sunlight fell across her, her whole body recoiled, sending the wheelbarrow tipping dangerously to the side.

It's her eyes, Pim signed. *They must be burned.*

She returned to the barn and came back with a cloth, which she moistened in the bucket and then draped over the upper half of the woman's face. Her body began to relax.

Let's go, Pim signed.

It took almost an hour to get Dory back to the house, by which time the woman had lapsed into a merciful unconsciousness. Kate rushed out to meet them. When she saw Dory, she turned back toward the door, where Elle and Bug were standing watchfully, curious about all the excitement. Theo was nosing through Bug's legs like a puppy.

"Get back in the house," she ordered. "And take your cousin with you."

"We want to look!" Elle whined.

"Now."

They faded inside. Kate crouched next to Dory. "Dear God."

"We found her in the barn," Caleb explained.

484

"Her husband?"

"No sign of him."

Kate looked toward Pim. *The girls shouldn't see.*

Pim nodded. *I'll take them out back.*

"We need a tarp or strong blanket," Kate said to Caleb. "We can put her in the back room, away from the children."

"Will she survive?"

"She's a mess, Caleb. There's not a lot I can do."

Caleb retrieved one of the heavy wool blankets he used for the horses. They spread it on the ground next to the wheelbarrow, then lifted Dory from the cart and lowered her onto the blanket, tied the corners together, and ran a length of two-by-four through the ends to fashion a makeshift sling. As they hoisted her off the ground, she made a noise from back in her throat that sounded like a strangled scream. Caleb shuddered; he could barely listen to this anymore. That Dory hadn't died seemed a cruelty of immense proportions. They carried her into the house, to the small storage room where the girls had been sleeping, and laid her on the pallet. Caleb nailed a saddle pad to the tiny window as a shade.

"I need to get that nightgown off." Kate gave Caleb a grave look. "This will be . . . bad."

He swallowed. He could barely bring himself to look at the woman, at her charred and bubbled flesh.

"I'm not good with things like this," he admitted.

"Nobody is, Caleb."

He realized something else. He'd waited too long; now they were stranded, waiting for the woman to die. With only one horse, they couldn't

485

use the buckboard to take Dory to Mystic. And Pim would never leave her.

"I'll need clean cloths, a bottle of alcohol, scissors," Kate commanded. "Boil the scissors, and don't touch them afterward, just lay them in a cloth. Then go look after the children. Pim can help me here. You'll want to keep them away from the house for a while."

Caleb didn't feel insulted, only grateful. He retrieved the things she'd asked for, brought them to the room, and traded places with Pim. By the kitchen garden, the girls were playing with their dolls, making beds for them out of leaves and sticks, while Theo toddled around.

"Come on, children, let's go for a walk to the river."

He lodged Theo on his hip and took Elle by the hand. She, in turn, took her sister's, as they had learned to do, making a chain. They were halfway to the river when a scream severed the air. The sound shot through Caleb like a bullet.

Lucius, it's started. I need you now.

Greer had been driving since before dawn. "Just get this boat ready," he'd told Lore. He swung past Rosenberg in the dark, jogged northwest, and hit Highway 10 as the sun was rising behind him.

He would reach Kerrville by four o'clock, five at the latest. What would the darkness bring?

Amy, I am coming.

50

Michael came to consciousness in darkness. Lying on his bunk, he fingered the wound on his head. His hair was rigid with dried blood; he was lucky

they hadn't broken his skull. But he supposed an armed criminal in the president's house warranted at least one good blow to the melon. Not an ideal way to get a night's rest, though, on the whole, not entirely unwelcome.

He slept some more; when he awoke, soft daylight was coming through the window. A clunk of tumblers, and a pair of DS officers appeared. One was holding a tray. While the other stood guard, the first placed the tray on the floor.

"Much obliged, guys."

The two walked off. Probably they'd been instructed not to talk to him. Michael lifted the tray and put it on the bunk. A bowl of boiled oats, scrambled eggs, a peach — a better meal than he'd had in days. They'd given him only a spoon — no fork, of course — so he ate the eggs with that, followed by the porridge. He saved the peach for last. Juice exploded over his chin. Fresh fruit! He'd forgotten what it was like.

More time passed. At last he heard footsteps and voices in the hall. Peter, most likely, with someone else in tow. Apgar? Sooner or later, the conversation was going to have to widen.

But it wasn't Peter.

Sara stood in the doorway. She'd changed less than he would have thought. Older, of course, but she'd aged gracefully, the way some women could, the ones who didn't fight it, who accepted the passage of time.

"I don't believe my eyes."

"Hello, Sara."

Michael sat up on his bunk as his sister stepped inside. She was carrying a small leather bag. A guard moved in behind her, holding a baton.

"Goddamnit, Michael." She was standing apart

from him.

"I know." An absurd remark: What did it mean? I know I hurt you? I know how this must look? I know I'm the worst brother in the world?

"I am so . . . angry at you."

"You have a right."

An eyebrow lifted. "That's all you have to say?"

"How about, I'm sorry."

"Are you kidding me? You're *sorry*?"

"You look well, Sara. I've missed you."

"Don't even try. And you look like hell."

"Oh, this is one of my better days."

"Michael, what are you *doing* here? I thought I'd never see you again."

He searched her face. Did she know? "What did Peter tell you?"

"Just that you'd been arrested and you had a gash in your head." She lifted the bag a little. "I'm here to sew you up."

"So he didn't say anything else."

She made a face of disbelief. "Like what, Michael? That they'll probably hang you? He didn't have to."

"Don't worry. Nobody's getting hanged."

"Twenty-one years, Michael." Her right hand, the one not holding the bag, was clenched into a fist, as if she might strike him. "Twenty-one years without a message, a letter, nothing. Help me understand this."

"I can't explain right now. But you have to know there *was* a reason."

"Do you know what I had to do? Do you? Ten years ago, I said, That's it, he's never coming back. He might as well be dead. I *buried* you, Michael. I put you in the ground and forgot about you."

"I did some awful things, Sara."

At last the tears came. "I took *care* of you. I *raised* you. Did you ever think of that?"

He rose from the bunk. Sara let the bag drop to the floor, raised her fists, and began to pummel his chest. She was crying in earnest now.

"You *asshole,*" she said.

He pulled her into a tight embrace. She struggled in his arms, then let him hold her. The guard was watching them warily; Michael shot him a look: *Back off.*

"How could you do this to me?" she sobbed.

"I never wanted to hurt you, Sara."

"You left me, just like they did. You're no better than they were."

"I know."

"Damn you, Michael, *damn* you."

He held her that way for a long time.

"That's quite a story."

It was late morning; Peter had cleared the office. He and Apgar were seated at the conference table, waiting for Chase. A short retirement for the man, thought Peter.

"I know it is," Peter answered.

"Do you believe him?"

"Do *you?*"

"You're the one who knows the man."

"That was twenty years ago."

Chase appeared in the door. "Peter, what's going on? Where is everybody? This place is a tomb." He was dressed in the jeans, work shirt, and heavy boots of the cattleman he had announced his intention to become.

"Have a seat, Ford," Peter said.

"Will this take long? Olivia's waiting for me. We're meeting some people at the bank."

489

Peter wondered how many of these conversations he was going to have to have. It was like leading people to the edge of a cliff, showing them the view, and then shoving them off.

"I'm afraid so," he said.

Alicia saw the first mounds just outside of Fredericksburg — three domes of earth, each the length of a man, bulging from the ground in the shade of a pecan tree. Riding on, she came to the outermost farmstead. She dismounted in the packed-dirt yard. No sounds of life reached her from the house. She stepped inside. Furniture overturned, objects strewn about, a rifle on the floor, beds unmade. The inhabitants had been infected as they'd slept; now they slept in the earth, beneath the pecan tree.

She watered Soldier at the trough and continued on her way. The rocky hills rose and fell. Soon she saw more houses — some nestled discreetly in the folds of the land, others exposed on the flats, surrounded by hard-won fields of newly tilled soil. There was no need to look more closely; the stillness told Alicia all she needed to know. The sky seemed to hang above her with an infinite weariness. She had expected it to happen like this, at the outer edges first. The first ones taken up, then more and more, an army swelling its ranks, metastasizing as it moved toward the city.

The town itself was abandoned. Alicia rode the length of the dusty main street, past the small stores and houses, some new, others reclaimed from the past. Just a few days ago, people had gone about their daily lives here: raised families, conducted business and trade, talked of small things, gotten drunk, cheated at cards, argued,

fought with their fists, made love, stood on the porches to greet their fellow citizens as they passed. Had they known what was happening? Did the fact creep upon them slowly — first one person missing, a curiosity barely remarked on, then another and another, until the meaning dawned — or had the virals swooped down in a rush, a single night of horror? At the southern edge of town, Alicia came to a field. She began to count. Twenty mounds. Fifty. Seventy-five.

At one hundred, she gave up counting.

51

The day moved on. Still Dory did not die.

From the room where the woman lay, Caleb heard only small sounds — moans, murmurs, a chair shifting on the floor. Kate or Pim might appear briefly, to fetch some small implement or boil more cloths. Caleb sat in the yard with the children, though he had no energy to amuse them. His mind drifted to undone chores, but then another voice would speak to him, saying it was for naught; they would soon be leaving this place, all his proud hopes dashed.

Kate came out and sat beside him on the stoop. The children had gone down for a nap in the house.

"So?" he asked.

Kate squinted into the afternoon light. A strand of hair, golden blond, was plastered to her forehead; she tucked it away. "She's still breathing, anyway."

"How long will this take?"

"She should be dead already." Kate looked at him. "If she's still alive in the morning, you should

491

take Pim and the kids and get out of here."

"If anybody's staying, it's me. Just tell me what to do."

"Caleb, I can handle it."

"I know you can, but I'm the one who got us into this mess."

"What were you going to do? A horse gets sick, some people go missing, a house burns down. Who's to say any of it's related?"

"I'm still not leaving you here."

"And, believe me, I appreciate the gesture. I never was much of a country gal, and this place gives me the creeps. But it's my *job*, Caleb. Let me do it, and we'll get along fine."

For a while they sat without talking. Then Caleb said, "I could use your help with something."

Jeb's body had swollen and stiffened in the heat. They lashed his hind legs together, set Handsome into his plow harness, and began the slow process of dragging the body to the far edge of the field. When Caleb felt they were far enough away from the house, they led Handsome back to the shelter and brought out one of the jugs of fuel. Caleb dragged some deadfall from the woods and placed it over the corpse, building a pyre; he splashed kerosene over it, recapped the can, and stepped back.

Kate asked, "Why did you call him Jeb?"

Caleb shrugged. "Just the name he came with."

Nothing remained to be said. Caleb struck a match and tossed it forward. With a whoosh, flames enveloped the pile. There was no wind to speak of; the thick smoke rose straight skyward, full of popping sparks. For a while it smelled like mesquite; then it became something else.

"That's that, I guess," he said.

They walked back toward the house. As they approached, Pim appeared in the doorway. Her eyes were very wide.

Something is happening, she signed.

The room was cool and dark. Only Dory's face was showing; the rest was covered by boiled clothes.

"Mrs. Tatum," Kate said, "can you hear me? Do you know where you are?"

Staring at the ceiling, the woman seemed completely unaware of them. A remarkable change had occurred. Remarkable, but also disturbing. The harsh appearance of the burns on her face had softened. Their color was now pinkish, almost dewy; in other patches, her skin was white as talc. Dory shifted slightly in her bed, exposing her left hand and forearm from under the cloths. Before, it had been a gruesome claw of cooked flesh. In its stead was a recognizable human hand — blisters gone, charred bits flaked off to reveal skin of rosy newness beneath.

Kate looked up at Pim. *How long has she been awake?*

She wasn't. That just happened.

"Mrs. Tatum," Kate said, more commandingly, "I'm a doctor. You've been in a fire. You're at the Jaxons' farm; Caleb and Pim are with me. Do you remember what happened?"

Her gaze, wandering the room in a desultory fashion, located Kate's face.

"Fire?" she murmured.

"That's right, there was a fire at your house."

"Ask her if she knows what started it," Caleb said.

"Fire," Dory repeated. "Fire."

"Yes, what do you remember about the fire?"

Pim stepped forward and knelt by the bed. She gently lifted Dory's exposed hand, placed the tip of her index finger in the woman's palm, and began to form letters.

"Pim," Dory said.

But that was all; the light in her eyes faded. She closed them again.

"Caleb, I'm going to examine her," Kate said. Then, to Pim: *Stay and help.*

Caleb waited in the kitchen. The children, mercifully, were still asleep. A few minutes passed, and the women appeared.

Kate gestured to the back door. *Let's talk outside.*

The light had shifted toward evening. "What's happening to her?" Caleb asked, signing simultaneously.

"She's getting better, that's what."

"How is that possible?"

"If I knew, I'd bottle it. The burns are still bad — she's not out of the woods yet. But I've never seen anybody heal so fast. I thought the shock alone would kill her."

"What about her waking up like that?"

"It's a good sign, her recognizing Pim. I don't think she understood much else, though. She may never."

"You mean she'll stay like this?"

"I've seen it happen." Kate addressed her sister directly: *You should stay with her. If she wakes up again, try to get her talking.*

What about?

Easy stuff. Keep her mind off the fire for now.

Pim returned to the house.

"This changes things," Caleb said.

"I agree. We may be able to move her sooner

than I thought. Do you think you can find a vehicle in Mystic?"

He recalled the pickup he'd seen in Elacqua's yard.

Kate seemed surprised. "*Brian* Elacqua?"

"That's him."

"That drunken old cuss. I'd wondered what had become of him."

"That was pretty much my experience of the man."

"Still, I'm sure he'd help us."

Caleb nodded. "I'll ride in in the morning."

Sara was waiting on the porch with their bags when Hollis appeared, sitting atop a sorry-looking mare. With him was a man Sara didn't know, riding a second horse, a black gelding with a back as bowed as a hammock and ancient, runny eyes.

"What's this I see?" Sara said. "Oh, two of the worst horses I ever laid eyes on."

The two men dismounted. Hollis's companion was a squat-looking man wearing overalls but no shirt. His hair was long and white; there was something cunning in his face. Hollis and the man exchanged a few words, shook hands, and the man walked off.

"Who's your friend?" Sara asked.

Hollis was tying the horses to the porch rail. "Just somebody I knew in the old days."

"Husband, I thought we talked about a truck."

"Yeah, about that. Turns out a truck costs actual money. Also, there's no gas to be had. On the upside, Dominic threw in the tack for free, so we are not, technically, one hundred percent penniless at the moment."

"Dominic. Your shirtless friend."

495

"He kind of owed me a favor."

"Should I ask?"

"Probably best if you don't."

They returned to the house, lightened their gear, loaded the remains into saddlebags, and secured them to the horses. Hollis took the mare, Sara the gelding. She was getting the best of the deal, though not by much. Years had passed since she'd even been on a horse, but the feeling was automatic, touching a deep chord of physical memory. Bending forward in the saddle, Sara gave three firm pats to the side of the horse's neck. "You're not such a bad old guy, are you? Maybe I'm being too hard on you."

Hollis looked up. "I'm sorry, were you addressing me?"

"Now, now," Sara said.

They made their way to the gate and descended the hill. Scattered workers were toiling in the fields beneath a late afternoon sun. Here and there a pennant still hung limply from its pole, marking the location of a hardbox; the watchtowers with their warning horns and sharpshooter platforms jutted from the valley floor, unmanned for years.

At the outer edge of the Orange Zone, the road forked: west toward the river townships, east toward Comfort and the Oil Road. Hollis drew up and took his canteen from his belt. He drank and passed it to Sara. "How's the old boy doing?"

"A perfect gentleman." She wiped her mouth with the back of her hand and gestured eastward with the canteen. "Looks like somebody's in a hurry."

Hollis saw it too: the boiling dust plume of a vehicle, driving fast toward the city.

"Maybe we could see if he'd trade for the

horses," Hollis said, not seriously.

Sara examined him for a moment, flicking her eyes up and down. "I have to say, you look rather dashing up there. Takes me back a bit."

Hollis was leaning forward, bracing his weight with both hands on the pommel. "I used to like to watch you ride, you know. If I was on the day shift on the Watch, I'd sometimes wait on the Wall until you came back with the herd."

"Really? I was not aware."

"It was a little creepy of me, I admit that."

She felt suddenly happy. A smile came to her face, the first in days. "Oh, what could you do?"

"I wasn't the only one. Sometimes you drew quite a crowd."

"Then lucky you, things working out like they did." She capped the canteen and handed it back. "Now let's go see our babies."

52

"Hey, good afternoon, everybody."

Two DS officers manned the stockade's outer room — one sitting at his desk, a second, much older, standing behind the counter. Greer recognized the second one immediately; years ago, the man had been one of his jailors. Winthrop? No, Winfield. He'd been just a kid then. As their gazes locked, Lucius could see a series of rapid calculations unfolding behind the man's eyes.

"I'll be damned," Winfield said.

His hand dropped to his sidearm, but the movement was startled and clumsy, giving Greer ample time to raise the shotgun from beneath his coat and level it at the man's chest. With a loud clack, he chambered a shell. "Tut tut."

Winfield froze. The younger one was still sitting behind his desk, staring wide-eyed. Greer nudged the shotgun toward him. "You, weapon on the floor. You too, Winfield. Let's be quick now."

They placed their pistols on the ground. "Who is this guy?" the younger one said.

"Been a while, Sixty-two," Winfield said, using Greer's old inmate number. He seemed more amused than angry, as if he'd run into an old friend of dubious reputation who'd lived up to expectations. "Heard you've been keeping yourself busy. How's Dunk?"

"Michael Fisher," Greer said. "Is he here?"

"Oh, he's here, all right."

"Any more DS in the building? We keep the nonsense to a minimum, this doesn't have to be a problem."

"Are you serious? I don't give a shit one way or the other. Ramsey, toss me the keys."

Winfield opened the door to the cellblock. Greer followed a few paces behind the two men, keeping the shotgun trained on their backs. Michael, lying on his bunk, rose on his elbows as the door to his cell opened.

"This is sudden," he remarked.

Greer ordered Winfield and the other one into the cell, then looked at Michael. "Shall we?"

"Nice seeing you, Sixty-two," Winfield called after them. "You haven't changed a bit, you fucker."

Greer shut the door, turned the lock, and pocketed the key. "Keep it down in there," he barked through the slot. "I don't want to have to come back here." He turned to look at Michael. "What happened to your head? That looks like it hurt."

"Not to sound ungrateful, but I'm thinking your being here is not good news."

"We're moving to Plan B."

"I didn't know we had one of those."

Greer handed him Winfield's pistol. "I'll explain on the way."

Peter, Apgar, and Chase were looking over Michael's passenger manifest when shouts erupted in the hall: "Put it down! Put it down!"

A crash; a gunshot.

Peter reached into his desk for the pistol he kept there. "Gunnar, what have you got?"

"Nothing."

"Ford?"

The man shook his head.

"Get behind my desk."

The handle of the door jiggled. Peter and Apgar took positions against the wall on either side. The wood shuddered: somebody was kicking it.

The door blew open.

As the first man entered, Apgar tackled him from behind. A shotgun skittered away. Apgar pinned him with his knees, one hand on his throat, the other lifted, ready to strike. He stopped.

"Greer?"

"Hello, General."

"Michael," Peter said, lowering his gun, "what the *fuck*."

Three soldiers charged into the room, rifles drawn.

"Hold your fire!" Peter yelled.

With visible uncertainty, the soldiers complied.

"What was that gunshot outside, Michael?"

The man waved casually. "Oh, he missed. We're fine."

499

Peter was shaking with anger. "You three," he said to the soldiers, "clear the room."

They made their departure. Apgar climbed off Greer. Chase, meanwhile, had come out from behind Peter's desk.

Michael gestured in Chase's direction. "Is he okay?"

"In what sense?"

"I mean does he *know*?"

"Yeah," Chase said tersely, "I know."

Peter was still furious. "The two of you, what do you think you're doing?"

"Under the circumstances, we thought a direct approach was best," Greer replied. "We have a vehicle outside. We need you to come with us, Peter, and we need to leave right now."

Peter's patience was at its end. "I'm not going anywhere. You don't start talking sense, I'll toss your asses in the stockade myself and throw away the key."

"I'm afraid the situation has changed."

"So the virals aren't coming back after all? This is all some kind of joke?"

"I'm afraid it's the opposite," Greer said. "They're already here."

53

Amy was going to miss this place.

They had decided to leave the rest of their chores undone for the day. There seemed no point in finishing them now. *Sometimes,* Carter told her, *you got to let a garden tend itself.*

She felt sick, almost feverish. Could she control it? Would she kill him? And what of the water?

You got to do it the way Zero done, Carter had

told her. *Ain't no other way to go back to the way you were.*

The girls were watching a movie in the house. It was one Amy remembered, from being just a girl herself: *The Wizard of Oz.* The movie had terrified her — the tornado, the field of poppies, the wicked witch with her sickly green skin and battalion of airborne monkeys in bellman's hats — but she had also loved it. Amy had watched it in the motel where she and her mother had lived. Her mother would put on her little skirt and stretchy top to go out to the highway, and before she left she'd sit Amy down in front of the television with something to eat, something greasy in a bag, and tell her: *You sit tight now. Mama will be back soon. Don't you open that door for nobody.* Amy could see the guilt in her mother's eyes — she understood that leaving a child by herself wasn't something her mother was supposed to do — and Amy's heart always went out to her, because she loved her, and the woman was so remorseful and sad all the time, as if life was a series of disappointments she could do nothing to stop. Sometimes her mother could barely get out of bed all day, and then night would fall, and the skirt and the top and the television would go on, and she'd leave Amy alone again.

The night of *The Wizard of Oz* had been their last in the motel, or so Amy recalled. She'd watched cartoons for a while and, when these were over, a game show, and then she flipped around the dial until the movie caught her eye. The colors were odd, too vivid. That was the first thing she noticed. Lying on the bed, which smelled like her mother — a mélange of sweat, and perfume, and something distinctly her own — Amy settled in to

501

watch. She entered the story when Dorothy, having rescued her dog from the clutches of the evil Miss Gulch, was racing from the storm. The tornado whisked her away; she found herself in the land of the Munchkins, who sang about their happy lives. But, of course, there was the problem of the feet — the feet of the Wicked Witch of the East, sticking out from beneath Dorothy's tornado-driven house.

It went on from there. Her attention was complete. She understood Dorothy's desire to go home. That was the heart of the story, and it made sense to Amy. She hadn't been home in a long time; she barely remembered it, just a shadowy sense of certain rooms. As the movie drew to a close, and Dorothy clicked her heels together and awoke in the bosom of her family, Amy decided to try this. She had no ruby slippers, but her mother had a pair of boots, very tall, with pointed heels. Amy slid them on. They rose up her skinny, little-girl legs nearly to her crotch; the heels were very high, making it difficult to walk. She took tender steps around the room to get the hang of it, and when she felt comfortable she closed her eyes and tapped the heels together, three times. *There's no place like home, there's no place like home, there's no place like home . . .*

So convinced was she of the magical power of this gesture that when she opened her eyes she was shocked to discover that nothing had happened. She was still in the motel, with its dirty carpet and dull immovable furniture. She yanked off the boots, hurled them across the room, threw herself down on the bed, and began to cry. She must have fallen asleep, because the next thing she saw was her mother's frightened face, loom-

ing over her. She was shaking Amy roughly by the shoulder; her top was stained and torn. *Come on now, honey,* her mother said. *Wake up now, baby. We got to go, right now.*

Carter was skimming the pool. The first leaves were falling, crisp and brown.

"I thought we were taking the day off," Amy said.

"We are. Just got to get these here. Bothers me seeing them."

She was sitting on the patio. Inside, the girls had reached the part of the movie where Dorothy and her companions entered the Emerald City.

"They should turn it down a bit," Carter remarked. He was dragging the skimmer along the edges, trying to work some small bit of debris into the net. "Girls are going to wreck their ears."

Yes, she would miss it here. The softness of the place, its cool feeling of green. The small tasks that filled their days of waiting. Carter lay the skimmer on the pool deck and took a chair across from her. They listened to the movie for a while. When the Wicked Witch melted, the girls erupted in happy shrieks.

"How many times they watch that?" Carter asked.

"Oh, quite a few."

"When I was a boy, seemed like it was on TV about half the time. Scared the wits out of me." Carter paused. "I always did like that movie, though."

They loaded the Humvee with cans of fuel. Sitting in the cargo compartment were plastic bins of supplies Greer had brought with him — rope and tackle, a spinner net, a pair of wrenches,

503

blankets, a simple cotton frock.

"I'd be happier if we could bring Sara along," Peter said. "She'd know better than any of us what to do."

Greer heaved a jug over the tailgate. "Not a good idea at this point. We need to keep the number of people to a minimum."

"We have to get word out to the townships," Peter told Apgar. "People need to take shelter. Basements, interior rooms, whatever they've got. In the morning, we can send out vehicles to bring as many back as we can."

"I'll see to it."

Peter glanced at Chase. "Ford? You've got the chair."

"Understood."

Peter addressed Apgar again: "My son and his family —"

The general didn't let him finish. "I'll radio the detachment in Luckenbach. We'll get some men out there."

"Caleb's got a hardbox on the property."

"I'll pass that along."

Greer was waiting at the wheel, Michael riding shotgun. Peter climbed in back.

"Let's go," he said.

It was 1830. The sun would set in two hours.

54

Sara and Hollis were making good time. They had entered the zone everybody called the Gap — a stretch of empty road between Ingram and Hunt Township. They were hugging the Guadalupe now, which gurgled pleasantly in the shallows. Fat live oaks stretched their canopies over the road-

way; then they came to an open stretch, the low sun in their faces, then more trees and shade.

"I think this guy needs a break," Sara said.

They dismounted and led the horses to the edge of the river. Standing on the bank, Hollis's mare dipped her long face to the water without hesitation, but the gelding seemed uncertain. Sara removed her boots, rolled up her pants, and led him into the shallows to drink. The water was wonderfully cold, the river bottom made of smooth limestone, firm underfoot.

After the horses had drunk their fill, Sara and Hollis took a moment to let the animals wander. The two of them sat on a rocky outcrop that jutted over the edge of the water. The vegetation on the banks was thick — willows, pecans, oaks, a scrub of mesquites and prickly pears. Evening insects were hatching from the water in ascending motes of light. A hundred yards upstream, the river paused in a wide, deep pool.

"It's so peaceful out here," Sara said.

Hollis nodded, his face full of contentment.

"I think I could get used to this."

She was thinking of a certain place in the past. It was many years ago, when she and Hollis and all the others had traveled east with Amy to Colorado. Theo and Maus were gone by this time, left behind at the farmstead so Maus could have her baby. They'd crossed the La Sal Range and descended to a wide valley of tall grass and blue skies and stopped to rest. In the distance, snow-capped, the peaks of the Rockies loomed, though the air was still mild. Sitting in the shade of a maple tree, Sara had experienced a feeling she'd never really had before — a sense of the world's beauty. Because it really *was* beautiful. The trees,

the light, the way the grass moved in the breeze, the mountains' glinting faces of ice: how had she failed to notice these things before? And if she had, why had they seemed different, more ordinary, less charged with life? She had fallen in love with Hollis, and she understood, sitting under the maple tree with her friends around her — Michael had, in fact, fallen asleep, hugging his shotgun over his chest like a child's stuffed animal — that Hollis was the reason. It was love, and only love, that opened your eyes.

"We better go," Hollis said. "It'll be dark soon."

They gathered the horses and rode on.

General Gunnar Apgar, standing at the top of the wall, watched the shadows stretching over the valley.

He glanced at his watch: 2015 hours. Sunset was minutes away. The last transports bringing workers in from the fields were churning up the hill. All of his men had taken up positions along the top of the wall. They had new guns and fresh ammunition, but their numbers were small — far too few to watch every inch of a six-mile perimeter, let alone defend it.

Apgar wasn't a religious man. Many years had passed since a prayer had found his lips. Though it made him feel a little foolish, he decided to say one now. *God,* he thought, *if you're listening, sorry about the language, but if it's not too much trouble, please let this all be bullshit.*

Footsteps banged down the catwalk toward him.

"What is it, Corporal?"

The soldier's name was Ratcliffe — a radio operator. He was badly winded from his run up the stairs. He bent at the waist and put his hands

506

on his knees, taking in great gulps of air between words. "General, sir, we got the message out like you said."

"How about Luckenbach?"

Ratcliffe nodded quickly, still looking at the ground. "Yeah, they're sending a squad." He paused and coughed. "But that's the thing. They were the only ones who answered."

"Catch your breath, Corporal."

"Yes, sir. Sorry, sir."

"Now tell me what you're talking about."

The soldier drew himself erect. "It's just like I said. Hunt, Comfort, Boerne, Rosenberg — we're not getting anything back. No acknowledgment, nothing. Every station except Luckenbach is off-line."

The last bus was passing through the gate. Below, in the staging area, workers were filing off. Some were talking, telling jokes and laughing; others separated themselves quickly from the group and marched away, headed home for the night.

"Thanks for passing that along, Corporal."

Apgar watched him totter away before turning to look over the valley again. A curtain of darkness was sweeping over the fields. *Well,* he thought, *I guess that's that. It would have been nice if it could have lasted longer.* He descended the stairs and walked to the base of the gate. Two soldiers were waiting with a civilian, a man of about forty, dressed in stained coveralls and holding a wrench the size of a sledgehammer.

The man spat a wad of something onto the ground. "Gate should be working fine now, General. I got everything well greased, too. The thing will be quiet as a cat."

507

Apgar looked at one of the soldiers. "Are all the transports in?"

"As far as we know."

He tipped his face to the sky; the first stars had appeared, winking from the darkness.

"Okay, gentlemen," he said. "Let's lock it up."

Caleb was sitting on the front stoop, watching the night come on.

That afternoon, he'd inspected the hardbox, which he hadn't looked at in months. He'd built it only to please his father; it had seemed silly at the time. Tornadoes happened, yes, some people had even been killed, but what were the chances? Caleb had cleared the hatch of leaves and other debris and descended the ladder. The interior was cool and dark. A kerosene lantern and jugs of fuel stood along one wall; the hatch sealed from the inside with a pair of steel crossbars. When Caleb had shown the shelter to Pim, their second night at the farm, he'd felt a little embarrassed by the thing, which seemed like an expensive and unwarranted indulgence, completely out of step with the optimism of their enterprise. But Pim had taken it in stride. *Your father knows a thing or two,* she signed. *Stop apologizing. I'm glad you took the time.*

Now, looking west, Caleb took measure of the sun. Its bottom edge was just kissing the top of the ridgeline. In its final moments, it appeared to accelerate, as it always did.

Going, going, gone.

He felt the air change. Everything around him seemed to stop. But in the next instant, something caught his eye — a rustling, high in a pecan tree at the edge of the woods. What was he seeing? Not birds; the motion was too heavy. He got to

508

his feet. A second tree shuddered, then a third.

He recalled a phrase from the past. *When they come, they come from above.*

He had levered a round into the chamber of his rifle when, behind him, in the house, a voice cried out his name.

"Hold up a second," Hollis said.

An Army truck was tipped on its side in the roadway; one of its back wheels was still spinning with a creaking sound.

Sara quickly dismounted. "Somebody might be hurt."

Hollis followed her to the truck. The cab was empty.

"Maybe they walked out of here," Hollis said.

"No, this just happened." She looked down the road then pointed. "There."

The soldier was lying on his back. He was breathing in quick bursts, eyes open, staring at the sky. Sara dropped to her knees beside him. "Soldier, look at me. Can you speak?" He was acting like a man who was badly injured, yet there was no blood, no obvious sign of anything broken. The sleeves of his uniform bore the two stripes of a corporal. He rolled his face toward her, exposing a small wound, bright with blood, at the base of his throat.

"Run," he croaked.

Caleb burst into the house. Pim was holding Theo, backing away from the door to Dory's room; Bug and Elle were clustered at her legs.

Kate's voice: "Caleb, come quick!"

Dory was thrashing on the bed, spittle spewing from her lips. With a sound like a sneeze, her teeth

509

flew from her mouth. Kate was standing by the bed, holding the revolver.

"Shoot her!" Caleb yelled.

Kate seemed not to hear him. With a sickening crunch, Dory's fingers elongated, gleaming claws extending from their tips. Her body had begun to glow. Her jaw unlocked; her mouth opened wide, revealing the picketed teeth.

"Shoot her now!"

Kate was frozen in place. As Caleb raised the rifle, Dory jolted upright, rolled into a crouch, and sprang toward the two of them. A confusion of bodies, Dory crashing into Kate, Kate crashing into Caleb; the rifle spat from his hand and skittered across the floor. On his hands and knees, Caleb scrambled toward it. He was yelling for Pim to run, though of course the woman couldn't hear him. His hand found the weapon, and he rolled onto his back. Kate was pushing herself backward toward the opposite wall; Dory stood above her, jaws flexing, fingers extended, strumming the air. Caleb lifted his back off the floor, widened his knees, and leveled the rifle at her with both hands.

"Dory Tatum!"

At the sound of her name, she stiffened, as if struck by a curious thought.

"You're Dory Tatum! Phil is your husband! Look at me!"

She turned toward him, exposing her upper body. *One shot,* thought Caleb, taking the center of her chest into his sights, and then he squeezed the trigger.

The soldier began to shake. The motion began at his fingers, which bent into clawlike shapes, like the talons of a hawk. A groan poured from deep

in his throat. The shaking hardened into a whole-body convulsion, his spine arcing, spittle boiling to his lips. Sara was on her feet and backing away. She knew what she was seeing. It seemed impossible, and yet it was happening before her eyes. She sensed movement above her, yet she could not tear her eyes away from the soldier, whose transformation was occurring with unheard-of speed.

"Sara, come on! We have to get out of here!"

One of the horses whinnied and tore past her. It made it all of fifty feet down the road before a glowing shape swooped down and knocked it off its feet. Jaws tore into the horse's neck with a ripping sound.

Sara's mind snapped back into a wider awareness. Hollis was pulling her by the wrist. *The river!* he yelled. *We have to get to the river!* With a hard yank, he hauled her into the cover of the trees; they began to run. Shapes bounded above them, limb to limb. Branches whipped her face and arms. Where was the river, their salvation? Sara could hear it but could not locate it in the dark.

"Jump!"

In midair, she realized what was happening. They had leapt from a cliff. As she hit the surface, a new, deeper darkness, the darkness of water, enveloped her. It seemed she would never stop descending, but at last her feet touched the bottom. She pushed off and shot to the surface.

"Hollis!" She twisted in the water, blindly searching. "Hollis, where are you?"

"Over here. Keep your voice down."

She was spinning frantically, trying to locate the source of the voice. "I can't find you."

"Stay where you are."

Hollis appeared, treading water beside her. "Are you hurt?"

Was she? She took stock of her body. She didn't think she was.

"What's happening? Where did they come from?"

"I don't know."

"Don't leave me."

"Breathe, Sara."

She fought to calm herself. In, out, in, out.

"It looks like there are pockets at the base of the cliff," Hollis said. "We're going to swim there. Can you do it?"

She nodded. The water was freezing; her teeth had begun to chatter.

"Stay close."

With a smooth breaststroke he glided away, Sara following. The cliff took form above her. It wasn't as tall as she'd thought, perhaps twenty feet, and irregularly shaped, with blocky protrusions of pale limestone cantilevered over the pool. The water became shallower; Sara realized she could stand. Hollis guided her beneath an outcrop. A flat-topped boulder rose above the surface of the water. Hollis helped her up.

"We should be safe here for the night," he said.

Shivering, Sara leaned against him; Hollis put his arm around her and drew her close. She thought of her children, out there in the dark. She buried her face in Hollis's chest and began to cry.

Dory melted to the ground like a puppet cut from its strings. Caleb stepped over the body. Kate was still propped against the wall, her body inert, numbed by shock and fear.

"There's more out there," Caleb said. "We have

to get to the shelter."

She looked at him with an unfocused gaze.

"Kate, snap out of it."

He couldn't wait. He grabbed her by the wrist and shoved her out the door. Pim was huddled by the hearth with the children. She hadn't heard the shot, but he knew she had felt it, shuddering through the frame of the house.

Caleb signed a single word: *Go.*

He dropped the rifle and scooped Elle and Bug into his arms, balancing them on the points of his hips; Pim was carrying Theo. They raced out the back door into the yard. Pim was ahead of him, Kate behind. The darkness was coming alive. The crowns of the trees tossed as if by the wind of an approaching storm. Pim and Theo reached the shelter first. Caleb dropped the girls to their feet and hauled the door of the hardbox open. Pim scrambled down the ladder and raised her arms to take Theo and then the girls, Caleb following.

At the top of the ladder, he stopped. Kate was standing thirty feet away.

"Kate, come on!"

She drew her collar aside. At the base of her throat, a wound had bloomed with blood. Caleb's stomach dropped; all sensation left him.

"Shut the door," she said.

She was holding the revolver. He couldn't move.

"Caleb, please!" She collapsed to her knees. A deep tremor shook her body. She was cradling the gun in her lap, attempting to lift it. She rocked her head skyward as a second jolt moved through her. "I'm begging you!" she sobbed. "If you love me, shut the door!"

His windpipe clamped; he could barely breathe. Behind her, shapes were dropping from the trees.

Caleb reached above his head, taking the handle in his grip.

"I'm sorry," he whispered.

He drew down the door, sealing them in blackness, and shoved the crossbars into place. The children were crying. He felt for the lantern, took a box of matches from his pocket. His hands were trembling as he lit the wick. Pim was huddled with the children against the wall.

Her eyes grew very wide. *Where's Kate?*

From outside, a shot.

■ ■ ■ ■

VII
THE AWAKENING

■ ■ ■ ■

At the round earth's imagin'd corners, blow
Your trumpets, angels, and arise, arise
From death, you numberless infinities
Of souls.

— JOHN DONNE, *Holy Sonnets*

55

Peter awoke to a clattering of branches dragging against the side of the Humvee. He shook off his sluggishness and sat up.

"Where are we?"

"Houston," Greer said. Michael was asleep in the passenger seat. "Not long now."

A few minutes later, Greer brought the vehicle to a halt. To the east, the darkness had begun to soften.

"Let's be quick now," Greer said.

Peter and Michael unloaded their gear. They were at the edge of the lagoon; to the east, skyscrapers of incredible height cut black rectangles against the diminishing stars. Greer dragged a rowboat into the shallows. Michael sat in the bow, Peter the stern; Greer climbed into the middle, facing backward. The boat sank nearly to the gunwale but remained afloat.

"I was a little worried about that," Greer confessed.

With broad strokes he propelled them across the lagoon. Peter watched the city's core harden into its full dimensions. The *Mariner* soared into view, its great wide stern riding high above the water. Inside One Allen Center they tied off,

gathered their supplies, and began to climb.

From a window on the tenth floor, they dropped to the deck. Dawn was a few minutes away. Greer had refurbished a small crane of a type once used to lower cargo over the side of the ship. He spread the net beneath it, tightened the spring on the spinner joint, and attached it to the rope that ran through the block at the end of the boom. A second rope would be used to swing the boom over the water. Greer would manage the first rope, Michael the second. Peter's job was to act as bait — Greer's theory being that Peter was the person Amy was least likely to kill.

Greer handed him the wrench. "Remember, she's not the Amy we know."

They took up their positions. Peter fit the tip of the wrench around the first bolt.

"They're here," said Amy.

Carter was sitting across the table from her. "Feel it, too."

Her heart was racing; she felt a little dizzy. It always came on like this, with a sensation of physical acceleration that culminated in an abrupt expulsion from one world to the next, as if she were a rock hurled from a sling.

"I wish you were coming with me," she said.

"Long as I'm here, they're safe. You know that."

She did. If Carter died, the dopeys, his Many, would die with him. Without them, Amy and Carter stood no chance.

She looked around the garden one last time, saying goodbye. She closed her eyes.

Two bolts to go, one on each side. Peter loosened the first, leaving it in place. As he fit the head of

the wrench around the second bolt, a massive force, like a giant fist, struck the hatch from the opposite side. The deck beneath his knees shuddered from the impact.

"Amy, it's me! It's Peter!"

Another *wang;* the loosened bolt popped from the hole and bounced across the deck. He had seconds to spare. With a final yank, he freed the last bolt and began to run.

The hatch blew skyward.

Amy alighted on the deck, compressing to a reptilian crouch. Her body was glossy and compact, annealed with hard muscle beneath the crystalline sheath of skin. Peter was standing just beyond the net. For a moment she seemed puzzled by her surroundings; then her head slanted with a darting motion, taking him into her sights. She scuttled forward. Peter saw no recognition in her eyes.

"Amy." He lifted a hand toward her and spread his fingers. "It's me."

She halted, inches from the net.

"It's Peter."

Rising, Amy stepped forward. Greer pulled the rope; the net engulfed her and shot upward, her weight freeing the spinner from its brake. The net began to twirl, faster and faster. Amy was screaming and thrashing in its grasp. Michael yanked the second rope, swinging the boom over the side of the ship.

Greer let go. The rope holding the net shrieked through the block. Peter ran to the rail. He had just enough time to see the splash before Amy vanished into the oily water.

Darkness.

She was spinning and twisting and falling. Her senses swarmed with the awful, chemical-tasting water. It filled her mouth. It filled her nose and eyes and ears, a grip of pure death. She touched down upon the mucky bottom. The net held her body fast in its tangle. She needed to breathe. To breathe! She was thrashing, clawing, but there was no escaping its grasp. The first bubble of air rose from her mouth. *No,* she thought, *don't breathe!* This simple thing, to open one's lungs and take in the air: the body demanded it. A second bubble and her throat opened and the water slammed into her. She began to choke. The world was dissolving. No, it was she who was dissolving. Her body felt untethered to her thoughts, a thing apart, no longer hers. Her heart began to slow. A new darkness came upon her. It spread from within. *This is what it's like,* she thought. Panic, and pain, and then the letting go. *This is what it's like to die.*

Then she was somewhere else.

She was playing a piano. This was strange, because she'd never learned. Yet here she was, playing not just well but expertly, fingers prancing across the keys. There was no sheet music before her; the song came from her head. A sad and beautiful song, full of tenderness and the sweet sorrows of life. Why did it seem entirely new to her but also remembered, like something from a dream? As she played, she began to discern patterns in the notes. Their relationship was not

arbitrary; they moved through discernible cycles. Each cycle carried a slight variation of the song's emotional core, a melodic line that never wholly departed but supported the rest like laundry on a string. How astonishing! She felt as if she were speaking an entirely new language, far more subtle and expressive than ordinary speech, capable of communicating the deepest truths. It made her happy, very happy, and she went on playing, her fingers dexterously moving, her spirit soaring with delight.

The song turned a corner; she could sense its end approaching. The final notes descended. They hung like dust motes in the air, then were gone.

"That was wonderful."

Peter was standing behind her. Amy leaned the back of her head against his chest.

"I didn't hear you come in," she said.

"I didn't want to disturb you. I know how much you like to play. Will you play me another?" he asked.

"Would you like that?"

"Oh, yes," he said. "Very much."

"Pull her up!" Peter yelled.

Greer was looking at his watch. "Not yet."

"Goddamnit, she's drowning!"

Greer continued looking at his watch with infuriating patience. At last he looked up.

"Now," he said.

She played for a long while, song after song. The first was light, with a humorous energy; it made her feel as if she were at a gathering of friends, everyone talking and laughing, darkness thickening outside the windows as the party went on and

on into the small hours of the night. The next one was more serious. It began with a deep, sonorous chord at the bass end of the keyboard, with a slightly sour tone. A song of regret, of acts that could not be recalled, mistakes that could never be undone.

There were others. One was like looking at a fire. Another like falling snow. A third was horses galloping through tall grass beneath a blue autumn sky. She played and played. There was so much feeling in the world. So much sadness. So much longing. So much joy. Everything had a soul. The petals of flowers. The mice of the field. The clouds and rain and the bare limbs of trees. All these things and many others were in the songs she played. Peter was still behind her. The music was for him, an offering of love. She felt at peace.

They swung the net over the side and lowered it to the deck. Greer drew a knife and began to slash at the filaments.

In the net was the body of a woman.

"Hurry," Peter said.

Greer hacked away. He was fashioning a hole. "Take her feet."

Michael and Peter drew Amy free and laid her faceup on the deck. The sun was rising. Her body was limp, with a bluish cast. On her head, a scrim of black hair.

She wasn't breathing.

Peter dropped to his knees; Michael straddled her at the waist, stacked his palms, and positioned them on Amy's sternum. Peter slid his left hand beneath her neck, lifting it slightly to open the airway; with his other hand he pinched her nose. He fit his mouth over hers and blew.

"Amy."

Her fingers stilled, bringing a sudden silence to the room. She lifted her hands above the keyboard, palms flat, fingers extended.

"I need you to do something for me," Peter said.

She reached over her shoulder, took his left hand, and placed it against her cheek. His skin was cold and smelled of the river, where he liked to spend his days. How wonderful everything was. "Tell me."

"Don't leave me, Amy."

"What makes you think I'm going someplace?"

"It's not time yet."

"I don't understand."

"Do you know where you are?"

She wanted to turn around to see his face and yet could not. "I do. I think I do. We're at the farmstead."

"Then you know why you can't stay."

She was suddenly cold. "But I want to."

"It's too soon. I'm sorry."

She began to cough.

"I need you with me," Peter said. "There are things we have to do."

The coughing became more intense. Her whole body shook with it. Her limbs were like ice. What was happening to her?

"Come back to me, Amy."

She was choking. She was going to vomit. The room began to fade. Something else was taking its place. A sharp pain struck her chest, like the blow of a fist. She doubled over, her body curling around the impact. Foul-tasting water poured

from her mouth.

"Come back to me, Amy. Come back to me . . ."

"Come back to me."

Amy's face was slack, her body still. Michael was counting out the compressions. Fifteen. Twenty. Twenty-five.

"Goddamnit, Greer!" Peter yelled. "She's dying!"

"Don't stop."

"It's not working!"

Peter bent his face to hers once more, pinched her nose, and blew.

Something clicked inside her. Peter pulled away as her mouth opened wide in a throttled gasp. He rolled her over, slipped an arm beneath her torso to lift her slightly, and pounded her on the back. With a retching sound, water jetted from her mouth onto the deck.

There was a face. That was the first thing she became aware of. A face, its features vague, and behind it only sky. Where was she? What had occurred? Who was this person who was looking at her, floating in the heavens? She blinked, trying to focus her eyes. Slowly the image resolved. A nose. The curving shape of ears. A broad, smiling mouth and, above it, eyes that glittered with tears. Pure happiness filled her like a bursting star.

"Oh, Peter," she said, raising a hand to his cheek. "It is so good to see you."

■ ■ ■ ■

VIII
THE SIEGE

■ ■ ■ ■

Thick as autumnal leaves or driving sand,
The moving squadrons blacken all the strand.
— HOMER, *The Iliad*

56

All night long, the virals pounded.

It happened in bursts. Five minutes, ten, their fists and bodies slamming against the door — a period of silence, then they would begin again.

Eventually the intervals between the attacks grew longer. The girls gave up their crying and slept, their heads buried in Pim's lap. More time passed with no sounds outside; finally, the virals did not return.

Caleb waited. When would dawn come? When would it be safe to open the door? Pim, too, had fallen asleep; the terrors of the night had exhausted all of them. He leaned his head against the wall and closed his eyes.

He awoke to muffled voices outside; help had arrived. Whoever it was had begun to knock.

Pim awoke. The girls were still asleep. She signed a simple question mark.

It's people, he replied.

Still, it was with some anxiety that he unbarred the door. He pushed it just a little; a crack of daylight blasted his eyes. He shoved the door open the rest of the way, blinking in the light.

Standing before him, Sara dropped to her knees.

"Oh, thank God," she said.

Hollis was with her; the two were barefoot, soaked to the bone.

"We were coming to see you when they attacked," Hollis explained. "We hid in the river."

Pim lifted the children out and climbed up behind them. Sara embraced her, weeping. "Thank God, thank God." She knelt and drew the girls into her arms. "You're safe. My babies are safe."

Caleb's relief melted away. He realized what was about to happen.

"Kate," Sara yelled. "Come out now!"

Nobody said anything.

"Kate?"

Hollis looked at Caleb. The younger man shook his head. Hollis stiffened, wavering on his feet, the blood draining from his face. For a moment Caleb thought his father-in-law might collapse.

"Sara, come here," Hollis said.

"Kate?" Her voice was frantic. "Kate, come out!"

Hollis grabbed her around the waist.

"Kate! You answer me!"

"She's not in the hardbox, Sara."

Sara thrashed in his arms, trying to break free. "Hollis, let me go. Kate!"

"She's gone, Sara. Our Kate is gone."

"Don't say that! Kate, I'm your mother, you come out here right now!"

Her strength left her; she dropped to her knees, Hollis still holding her around the waist. "Oh, God," she moaned.

Hollis's eyes were closed in anguish. "She's gone. She's gone."

"Please, no. Not her."

"Our little girl is gone."

Sara lifted her face to the heavens. Then she

began to howl.

The light was soft and featureless; low, wet clouds blotted the sun. Peter lifted Amy into the vehicle's cargo bay and put a blanket over her. A bit of color had flowed back into her face; her eyes were closed, though it seemed she was not asleep but, rather, in a kind of twilight, as if her mind were floating in a current, the banks of the world flowing past.

Greer's voice was tight: "We better get moving."

Peter rode in the back with Amy. The going was slow, the dirt track crowded by brush. In the dark, Peter had absorbed almost nothing of the landscape. Now he saw it for what it was: an inhospitable swamp of lagoons, ruined structures clawed by vines, the earth vague, like something melted. Sometimes standing water obscured the roadway, its depth unknown; Greer plowed through.

The foliage began to thin; a cyclonic tangle of highway overpasses appeared. Greer threaded through the detritus beneath the freeway, located a ramp, and ascended.

For a time they followed the highway; then Greer veered away. Despite the violent jostling of the Humvee, Amy had yet to stir. They skirted a second region of collapsed overpasses, then climbed up the bank, back onto the highway.

Michael turned in his seat. "Easier going from here."

Rain began to fall, pattering the windshield; then the clouds broke, revealing a strong Texas sun. Amy gave a sigh of wakefulness; Peter looked to find that her eyes had opened. She blinked at him, then, squinting fiercely, covered her eyes with her arms.

"It's bright," she said.

"What was that?" Greer said from the front.

"She says it's bright."

"She's been in the dark for twenty years — the light may bother her awhile." Greer bent forward to reach under his seat. "Give her these."

Over his shoulder, he passed Peter a pair of dark glasses. The lenses were scratched and pitted, the frames made from soldered wire. He slipped the glasses over her face, wrapping the wires gently behind her ears.

"Better?"

She nodded. Her eyes closed once more. "I'm so tired," she murmured.

Peter leaned forward. "How much farther?"

"We should make it before sundown, but it will be close. We're going to need fuel, too. There should be some in the hardbox west of Sealy."

They continued in silence. Despite the tension, Peter felt himself drifting off. He slept for two hours, awakening to find that the truck had stopped. Greer and Michael were toting two heavy plastic jugs of fuel from the hardbox. His thoughts were fuzzy; his limbs, heavy and slow, moved like pooled liquid. Everywhere in his body, he felt his age.

Michael glanced his way as he stepped out. "How's she doing?"

"Still asleep."

Greer was pouring gas through a funnel into the truck's tank. "She'll be okay. Sleep is what she needs."

"Let me take the wheel for a while," Peter offered. "I know the way from here."

Greer bent to cap the can and wiped his hands on his shirt. "Better if Michael does for now.

530

There's a few tricky spots ahead."

They found Kate at the edge of the woods. The gun was still in her hand, her finger curled inside the trigger guard. One shot, through the sweet spot: Kate, thorough to the last, had wanted to be sure.

They had no time to bury her. They decided to take her into the house and lay her in the bed Caleb and Pim had shared, since they would never be coming back here. Hollis and Caleb carried her inside. It did not seem right to leave her in her blood-stained clothes; Pim and Sara undressed her, washed her body, and put her in one of Pim's nightgowns, made of soft blue cotton. They placed a pillow beneath her head and tucked a blanket tightly around her; Pim, weeping silently, brushed her sister's hair. A final question: Should they let the girls see her? Yes, Sara said. Kate was their mother. They needed to say goodbye.

Caleb waited outside. It was midmorning, cruelly bright. Nature mocked him with its disregard. The birds sang, the breeze blew, the clouds scudded overhead, the sun moved in its lazy, fateful arc. Handsome lay dead in the field; a crowd of buzzards jabbed at the banquet of his flesh, flapping their enormous wings. All was a ruin, yet the world did not seem to know or care. In the bedroom, Caleb had told Kate he loved her and kissed her on the forehead. Her skin was shockingly cold, but that was not the most disturbing thing. He realized he was expecting her to say something. *It didn't hurt too much.* Or *It's okay, Caleb, I don't blame you. You did the best you could.* Maybe she would say something sarcastic, such as *Seriously? You're going to tuck me into bed?*

531

I'm not a child, you know. I bet this is a lot of fun for you, Caleb. Yet there was nothing. Her body existed, but all that had made her distinct as a person was absent. Her voice was gone; never would it be heard again.

Pim came out first, with the girls. Elle was crying softly; Bug looked merely confused. A few minutes passed before Sara and Hollis emerged.

"If you're ready, we should get moving," Caleb said.

Hollis nodded. Sara, standing apart, was gazing toward the trees. Her eyes were glassy, her face unnaturally still, as if some essential element of life had left it. She cleared her throat and spoke:

"Husband, will you do something for me?"

"All right."

She looked him in the eye. "Kill every last fucking one of them."

The going was slow. Soon all three children were being carried — Bug on Caleb's shoulders, Elle on her grandfather's back, Theo in his sling, Pim and Sara taking turns. They were deep into the afternoon by the time they reached town. The streets were devoid of life. In Elacqua's yard, they found the truck, still parked where Caleb had seen it. Caleb got in the driver's seat. He'd hoped the key would be in the ignition, but it wasn't. He searched the cab to no avail and climbed back out.

"Do you know how to hot-wire a truck?" he asked Hollis.

"Not really."

Caleb looked toward the house. A window on the top floor was broken, smashed from its frame. Glass and splintered wood littered the ground

beneath it.

"Somebody's going to have to go inside to look."

"I'll do it," said Hollis.

"This is my responsibility. Stay here."

Caleb left the rifle with Hollis and took the revolver. The air in the house was so still it felt unbreathed. He crept from room to room, opening drawers and cabinets. Finding no keys, he climbed the stairs. There were two rooms with closed doors on either side of a narrow hall. He opened the first door. Here was where Elacqua and his wife had slept. The bed was unmade; beside it, lace curtains shifted slightly in the breeze coming through the broken window. He searched all the drawers, then stepped to the window and waved down. Hollis gazed up with a questioning look. Caleb shook his head.

One room to go. What if they couldn't find the keys? He'd seen no other vehicles in town. That didn't mean there weren't any, but they were running out of time.

Caleb took a breath and pushed the door with his foot.

Elacqua was lying on the bed fully clothed. The room reeked of piss and rancid breath. At first Caleb thought the man was dead, but then he gave a wet snort and rolled onto his side. An empty whiskey bottle stood on the floor beside the bed. The man wasn't dead, just dead drunk.

Caleb shook him roughly by the shoulders. "Wake up."

Elacqua, eyes still closed, batted clumsily at Caleb's hand. "Leave me alone," he mumbled.

"Dr. Elacqua, it's Caleb Jaxon. Pull yourself together."

His tongue moved heavily in his mouth. "You . . . bitch."

Caleb had a sense of what had occurred. Cast out from his marital bed, the man had anesthetized himself into oblivion and missed the whole thing. Perhaps he'd been drunk to begin with and that was why his wife had sent him packing. In either case, Caleb practically envied him; the disaster had passed him by. How had the virals missed him? Maybe he just smelled too bad; maybe that was the solution. Maybe they should all get drunk and stay that way.

He shook Elacqua again. The man's eyes fluttered open. They roamed blearily, finally landing on Caleb's face.

"Who the hell are you?"

There was no point in attempting to explain the situation; the man was too far gone. "Dr. Elacqua, look at me. I need the keys to your truck."

Caleb might have been asking him the most incomprehensible question in the world. "Keys?"

"Yes, the keys. Where are they?"

His eyes lost focus; he closed them again, his head, with its wild mane of hair, relaxing into the pillow. Caleb realized there was one place he hadn't looked. The man's trousers were soaked with urine, but there was nothing to be done about that. Caleb patted him down. At the base of the man's left front pocket, Caleb felt something sharp. He slid his hand in and pulled it out: a single key, tarnished with age, on a small metal ring.

"Gotcha."

His thoughts were broken by the roar of engines coming down the street. Caleb went to the window. Sara and the others were waving franti-

cally toward the source of the sound, yelling, "Hey! Over here!"

Caleb stepped onto the porch as the trucks, three Army five-tons, halted in front of the house. A broad-chested man in uniform stepped from the cab of the first truck: Gunnar Apgar.

"Caleb. Thank God."

They shook. Hollis and Sara had joined them. Apgar looked the group over. "Is this all of you?"

"There's one more in the house, but we'll need some help getting him out. He's pretty drunk."

"You're kidding." When Caleb said nothing, Apgar addressed a pair of soldiers who had disembarked from the second vehicle: "Haul him out here, on the double."

They trotted up the steps.

"We've been working our way west, looking for folks," Apgar said.

"How many survivors have you found?"

"You're it. We're not even finding any *bodies.* The virals either dragged them off or they've been turned."

Hollis asked, "What about Kerrville?"

"No sign of them yet. Whatever's going on, it's happening out here first." He paused, his expression suddenly uncertain. "There's something else you ought to know, Caleb. It's about your father."

Peter took the wheel east of Seguin. Amy had awakened briefly in midafternoon, asking for water. Her fever was down, and her eyes seemed to be bothering her less, though she complained of a headache and was still very weak. Squinting out a side window, she asked how much farther they had to go. She was wearing the blanket like a shawl over her head and shoulders. Three hours,

Greer said, maybe four. Amy considered this answer, then said, very softly, "We should hurry."

They crossed the Guadalupe and turned north. The first township they'd come to was just east of the old city of Boerne. It wasn't much, but there was a telegraph station. Only two hands of daylight remained when they pulled into the small central square.

"Awfully quiet around here," Michael said.

The streets were empty. Odd for this hour, Peter thought. They disembarked into ghostly silence. The town comprised just a few buildings: a general store, a township office, a chapel, and a handful of shoddily erected houses, some half-constructed, as if their builders had lost interest.

"Anybody here?" Michael yelled. "Hello?"

"Feels strange," Greer said.

Michael reached into the Humvee and released the shotgun from the holder. Peter and Greer checked their pistols.

"I'll stay with Amy," Greer said. "You two go find the telegraph station."

Peter and Michael crossed the square to the township office. The door stood open, another oddity. Everything appeared normal inside, but still there were no signs of life.

"So where the hell did everybody go?" Peter said.

The telegraph was in a small room in the rear of the building. Michael sat at the operator's desk and examined the log, a large, leather-bound ledger.

"The last message from here was sent Friday, five-twenty P.M., to Bandera station. The intended recipient was Mrs. Nills Grath."

"What was the message?"

" 'Happy birthday, Aunt Lottie.' " Michael looked up. "Nothing after that, at least that anybody bothered to record."

Today was Sunday. Whatever had happened here, Peter thought, it had happened sometime in the last forty-eight hours.

"Send a message to Kerrville," Peter instructed. "Let Apgar know we're coming."

"My Morse is a little rusty. I'll probably tell him to make me a sandwich."

Michael threw a switch on the panel and began tapping the key. A few seconds later, he stopped.

"What's wrong?"

Michael pointed to the panel. "See this meter? The needle should move when the plates touch."

"So?"

"So I'm talking to myself here. The circuit won't close."

Peter knew nothing about it. "Is that something you can fix?"

"Not a chance. There's a break in the line, could be anywhere between here and Kerrville. The storm might have knocked down a pole. A lightning strike could do it, too. It doesn't take much."

They exited through the back door. An old gas generator was crouched like a monster in the weeds, beside a rusted pickup and a buckboard with a broken axle and tall grass poking through the floorboards. Trash of all kinds — construction debris, busted packing crates, barrels with their seams split open — littered the yard. The wreckage of the frontier, flung out the door the moment it had outlived its usefulness.

"Let's check some of the other buildings," Peter said.

They entered the nearest house. It was one

537

story, with two rooms. Dirty dishes were stacked on a table; flies twisted above them in the air. In the back room was a washbasin on a stand, a wardrobe, and large feather bed covered by a quilt. The bed was sturdy and carefully made, with a tableau of interlocking flowers, quite detailed, carved into the headboard; somebody had taken their time with it. A marriage bed, thought Peter.

But where were the people? What had happened that the inhabitants should vanish before they had a chance to clear the dirty dishes from the table? Peter and Michael returned to the main room as Greer came through the door.

"What's the holdup?"

"The telegraph's not working," Michael said.

"What's wrong with it?"

"Break in the line someplace."

Greer leveled his eyes at Peter. "We really have to get moving."

What weren't they seeing? What was this haunted place trying to tell him? Peter's eyes fell upon something on the floor.

"Peter, did you hear me?" Greer pressed. "If we're going to make it back before dark, we need to leave right now."

Peter crouched to get a closer look, simultaneously gesturing toward the table. "Hand me that dishrag."

Using a corner of the cloth, he took hold of the object. The virals' teeth had a way of catching the light, almost prismatic, with a pearlescent, milky luster. The tip was so sharp it seemed to fade into invisibility, too small for the naked eye to discern.

"I don't think Zero's sending an army," Peter said.

"Then what's he doing?" Michael asked.

Peter looked at Greer; the older man's expression said he thought the same.

"I think he's growing one."

57

By the time the convoy reached Kerrville, it was nearly seven o'clock. The group disembarked into a state of siege. Along the top of the wall, soldiers were scurrying back and forth, handing out magazines and other gear. Fifty-caliber machine guns were positioned on either side of the gate. Apgar had exited the cab and was standing with Ford Chase, pointing at one of the spotlights. As Chase moved away, Caleb stepped up.

"General, I'd like my commission back."

Apgar frowned. "I have to say, that's a first. Nobody ever asks to get back in the Army."

"You can bust me to private — I don't care."

The general looked past Caleb's shoulder toward Pim, who was standing with Sara and the children.

"You clear this with your CO?"

"I'd be lying if I said she was happy about it. But she gets it. She lost her sister last night."

Apgar beckoned to a noncom manning the gates. "Sergeant, take this man to the armory and get him suited up. One brass bar."

"Thank you, General," said Caleb.

"You may rethink that later. And your old man's going to have my ass for this."

"Have we heard anything?"

Apgar shook his head. "Try not to worry, son. He's been through worse than this. Report to Colonel Henneman on the platform. He'll tell you where to go."

Caleb went to Pim and hugged her. He placed his palm against the curve of her belly, then kissed Theo on the forehead.

Be careful, she signed.

"We're going to the hospital," Sara said. "There's a hardbox in the basement. We're moving the patients down there."

The sergeant shifted impatiently on his feet. "Sir, we'd better go."

Caleb looked at his family a final time. He felt a gap widening, as if he were viewing them from the end of a lengthening tunnel.

I love you, Pim signed.

I love you, too.

He jogged away.

From Boerne, Greer took the wheel. They were driving into the sun now. Michael was in the passenger seat, Peter in the back with Amy.

They saw no other vehicles, no signs of life at all. The world seemed dead, an alien landscape. The shadows of the hills were lengthening; evening was coming on. Greer, squinting into the harsh light, wore a look of great intensity — his arms and back rigid as wood, his fingers clenching the wheel. Peter saw the muscles of his jaw bunching; the man was grinding his teeth.

They passed through Comfort. The ruins of ancient buildings — restaurants, gas stations, hotels — lined the highway, sand-scoured and scavenged to the bones. They came to the settlement on the west side of the city, away from the wreckage of the old world. Like Boerne, the town was abandoned; they didn't stop.

Fifteen miles to go.

■ ■ ■ ■

Sara and the others met Jenny at the door to the hospital. The woman was on the verge of wild-eyed panic.

"What's going on? There are soldiers everywhere. A Humvee just rolled by with a bullhorn, telling everybody to take shelter."

"There's an attack coming. We have to get these people to the basement. How many patients are on the wards?"

"What do you mean, an attack?"

"I mean *virals,* Jenny."

The woman blanched but said nothing.

"Listen to me." Sara took Jenny's hands and made the woman look at her. "We don't have a lot of time here. How many?"

Jenny gave her head a little shake, as if trying to focus her thoughts. "Fifteen?"

"Any children?"

"Just a couple. One boy has pneumonia, the other a broken wrist we just set. We've got one woman in labor, but she's early."

"Where's Hannah?"

Hannah was Jenny's daughter, a girl of thirteen; her son was grown and gone. Jenny and her husband had long since parted ways.

"Home, I think?"

"Run and get her. I can handle the situation until you're back."

"God, Sara."

"Just be quick."

Jenny darted from the building. Pim, holding Theo, was standing with the girls. Sara crouched before them. "I need you to go with your Auntie

Pim now."

Elle looked fearful and lost; snot was running from her nose. Sara wiped it with the bottom edge of her shirt.

"Where are we going?" the girl asked woefully.

People were scurrying past — nurses, doctors, orderlies with stretchers. Sara glanced up at Pim, then looked at her granddaughter again. "Downstairs to the basement," Sara answered. "You'll be safe there."

"I want to go home."

"It's just for a little while."

She hugged Elle, then her sister; Pim led the girls to the stairs. As they descended, Sara turned to her husband. She recognized the look on his face. It was the same one he'd worn the night after Bill had been killed, when he'd shown her the note.

"It's okay," she said.

"You're sure?"

"I've got things in hand here. Go before I change my mind."

No more words were necessary. Hollis kissed her and strode out the door.

They turned off Highway 10. From here, it was a straight shot south on a gravel road to the city. The truck shook fiercely as they pounded through the potholes. Wind whipped through the open windows; the sun, coming across their right shoulders, was low and bright.

"Michael, take the wheel and keep it steady." Greer reached below his seat. "Peter, give her this."

Peter leaned forward to receive the pistol. A round was already chambered.

"You won't have time to aim," he said to Amy. "Just point and shoot, like you're pointing your finger."

She took the gun from him. Her expression was uncertain, yet her grip seemed firm.

"You have fifteen rounds. You'll have to be close — don't try to shoot them from a distance."

"Unlock the shotgun," Greer said.

Michael freed the weapon. An extended magazine tube ran below the barrel, holding eight shells. "What's in here?" he asked Greer.

"Slugs, big ones. No room for slop, but it'll put one down fast."

The shape of the city emerged in the distance. Standing on the hill, it looked as small as a toy.

"This is going to be tight," Greer said.

The last patients were being brought down from the main floor. Jenny stood at the door of the hardbox with a clipboard, checking names off a list, while Sara and the nursing staff moved among the cots, doing their best to make sure everyone was comfortable.

Sara came to the cot that held the pregnant woman Jenny had spoken of. She was young, with thick, dark hair. While Sara took her pulse, she looked quickly at the girl's chart. A nurse had checked her an hour ago; her cervix had been barely dilated. Her name was Grace Alvado.

"Grace, I'm Dr. Wilson. Is this your first baby?"

"I was pregnant one other time, but it didn't take."

"And how old are you?"

"Twenty-one."

Sara stopped; the age was right. If this was the same Grace, Sara had last seen her when she was

just a day old.

"Are your parents Carlos and Sally Jiménez?"

"You knew my folks?"

Sara almost smiled; she might have, on a different day. "This might surprise you, Grace, but I was there the day you were born." She looked toward the girl's companion, who was sitting on a packing crate on the other side of the cot. He was older, maybe forty, with a rough look to him, though like many new fathers he seemed a little overwhelmed by the sudden urgency of events after months of waiting.

"Are you Mr. Alvado?"

"Call me Jock. Everybody does."

"I need you to keep her relaxed, Jock. Deep breaths, and no pushing for now. Can you do that for me?"

"I'll try."

Jenny came up behind Sara. "Everybody's in," she said.

Sara put her hand on Grace's arm. "Just focus on having your baby, okay?"

The basement door was made of heavy steel, set into walls of thick concrete. Sara was about to close it when the room plunged into darkness. An anxious murmuring, and then people began to shout.

"Everybody, settle down, please!" Sara said.

"What happened to the lights?" a voice cried from the darkness.

"The Army's just diverting current to the spots, that's all."

"That means the virals are coming!"

"We don't know that. Everyone, just try to keep calm."

Jenny was standing beside her. "Is that really

what they're doing?" she asked quietly.

"Do I know? Go check the storage room for lanterns and candles."

The woman returned a couple of minutes later. Lamps were lit and distributed around the space. The yells had fallen to whispers and, then, in the gloom, a tense silence.

"Jenny, give me a hand."

The door weighed four hundred pounds. Sara and Jenny pulled it closed and turned the wheel to engage the bolts.

A quarter of Apgar's men had taken up positions within five hundred yards of the gate; the rest were spread at regular intervals along the walls and connected by radio. Caleb was in charge of a squad of twelve men. Six of them had been stationed at Luckenbach — part of a small contingent who'd made it to a hardbox as the garrison was overrun. No officers had survived, orphaning them in the chain of command. Now they were Caleb's.

A man came banging down the catwalk toward him. Hollis wore no uniform, but a standard-issue chest pack was cinched to his frame, holding half a dozen spare magazines and a long, sheathed knife. An M4 dangled from its sling across his broad frame, the muzzle pointed downward; a pistol was holstered to his thigh.

He gave a crisp salute. "Private Wilson, sir."

It was absurd, Hollis speaking to him this way. He almost seemed like he was play-acting. "You're kidding me."

"The women and children are secure. I was told to report to you."

His face was set in a way that Caleb had never

seen before. This large, gentle man, collector of books and reader to children, had become a warrior.

"I made a promise, Lieutenant," Hollis reminded him. "I believe you were there at the time."

The spots came on, spilling a defensive perimeter of stark white light at the base of the wall. Radios began to crackle; a tremor of energy moved up and down the catwalk.

A call went out: "Eyes up!"

The *clack* of chambering rounds. Caleb pointed his rifle over the wall and flicked off the safety. He glanced to his right, where Hollis stood at the ready: feet wide, stock set, eyes trained down the barrel in perfect alignment. His body was somehow both tense and relaxed, purposeful and at ease with itself. It had the look of an old feeling stitched to the bones, summoned effortlessly to the surface when called upon.

Where would the virals come from? How many would there be? His chest was opening and closing arrhythmically; his vision seemed unnaturally confined. He forced himself to take a long, deep breath. *Don't think,* he told himself. *There are times for thinking, but this isn't one of them.*

A glowing point appeared in the distance, straight north. Adrenaline hit his heart; he hardened the stock against his shoulder. The light began to bob, then to separate like a dividing cell. Not virals: headlights.

"Contact!" a voice yelled. "Thirty degrees right! Two hundred yards!"

"Contact! Twenty left!"

For the first time in over two decades, the horn began to wail.

■ ■ ■ ■

Greer shoved the accelerator to the floor. The speedometer leapt, the fields flying past in a blur, the engine roaring, the frame of the truck shuddering.

"They're dead behind us!" Michael yelled.

Peter swiveled in his seat. Points of light were rising from the fields.

"Look out!" Greer yelled.

Peter turned around in time to see three virals leap into the headlights. Greer took aim and sliced through the pod. As bodies barreled over the hood, Peter slammed forward and bounced back into his seat. When he looked again, a single viral was clinging to the hood of the truck.

Michael pointed the shotgun over the dash and fired.

The glass exploded. Greer swerved to the left; Peter was thrown against the door, Amy on top of him. They were barreling through a bean field, moving laterally to the gate. Greer swerved the opposite way; the chassis tipped to the left, threatened to roll; then the wheels slammed down. Greer crested a rise and the truck went briefly airborne before spinning back onto the road. An ominous *clunk* from below; they began to decelerate.

Peter yelled to Greer, "What's wrong?"

Smoke was pouring from the grille; the engine roared pointlessly. "We must have hit something — the transmission's blown. On your right!"

Peter turned, took the viral in his sights, and squeezed the trigger, missing cleanly. Again and again he fired. He had no idea if he was hitting

anything. The slide locked back; the magazine was empty. The lighted perimeter was still a hundred yards away.

"I'm out!" Michael yelled.

As the truck floated to a halt, flares arced from the catwalk, dragging contrails of light and smoke above their heads. Peter turned to Amy. She was slumped against the door, the pistol, unfired, dangling in her hand.

"Greer," Peter said, "help me."

He pulled her from the cab. Her motions were as heavy and loose as a sleepwalker's. The flares began their lazy, flickering descents. As Amy's legs unfolded from the truck, Greer stepped around the front of the vehicle, shoving fresh shells into the shotgun's magazine. He slapped the gun into Peter's hand and slid his right shoulder under Amy's arm to take her weight.

"Cover us," he said.

Caleb helplessly watched the truck's approach. The virals were still well out of reach for even the luckiest shot. Up and down the wall, voices were yelling to hold fire, to wait until they were in range.

He saw the truck stop. Four figures emerged. At the rear of the group, one man turned and fired a shotgun into the heart of an approaching pod. One shot, two shots, three, flames blooming from the gun's muzzle in the darkness.

Caleb knew that man to be his father.

He had stepped into the harness and clipped in before he was even aware he was doing it. The action was automatic; he had no plan, only instinct.

"Caleb, what the hell are you doing?"

Hollis was staring at him. Caleb hopped to the top of the rampart and turned his back toward

the fields.

"Tell Apgar we'll need a squad at the pedestrian portal. Go."

Before Hollis could say anything else, Caleb pushed off. A long arc away from the wall and his boots touched concrete; he shoved himself away again. Two more pushes and he landed in the dirt. He unclipped and swung his rifle around.

His father was running with the others up the hill, just inside the lighted perimeter. Virals were massing at the edges. Some were covering their eyes; others had crouched into low, ball-like shapes. A moment's hesitation, their instincts warring inside them. Would the lights be enough to hold them back?

The virals charged.

The machine guns opened up; Caleb ducked reflexively as bullets whizzed over his head, slicing into the creatures with a wet, slapping sound. Blood splashed; flesh was cleaved from bone; whole pieces of the virals' bodies winged away. They seemed not merely to die but to disintegrate. The machine guns pounded, round after round. A slaughter, yet always there were more, surging into the lights.

"The portal!" Caleb called. He was running forward at a forty-five-degree angle to the wall, waving above his head. "Head for the portal!"

Caleb dropped to one knee and began to fire. Did his father see him? Did he know who he was? The bolt locked back; thirty rounds, gone in a heartbeat. He dropped the magazine, reached into his chest pack for a fresh one, and shoved it into the receiver.

Something crashed into him from behind. Breath, sight, thought: all left him. He felt himself

549

sailing, almost hovering. This seemed extraordinary. In the midst of his flight, he had just enough time to marvel at the lightness of his body compared to other things. Then his body grew heavy again and he slammed into the ground. He was rolling down the incline, his rifle whipping around on its sling. He tried to control his body, its wild tumble down the hill. His hand found the lower unit of the rifle, but his index finger got tangled in the trigger guard. He rolled again, onto his chest, the rifle wedged between his body and the ground, and there was no stopping it; the gun went off.

Pain! He came to rest on his back, the rifle lying over his chest. Had he shot himself? The ground was spinning under him; it refused to be still. He blinked into the spotlights. He didn't feel the way he imagined a shot person would. The pain was in two places: his chest, which had received the explosive force of the rifle's firing, and a spot on his forehead, near the outer edge of his right eyebrow. He reached up, expecting blood; his fingers came away dry. He understood what had happened. The ejecting cartridge, ricocheting off the ground, had pinged upward into his face, narrowly missing his eye. *You are fucking lucky, Caleb Jaxon,* he thought. *I really hope nobody saw that.*

A shadow fell across him.

Caleb raised the rifle, but as his left hand reached forward to balance the barrel he realized the mag well was empty; the magazine had been stripped away. He had, at various times of his life, imagined the moment of his own death. These imaginings had not included lying on his back with an empty rifle while a viral tore him to pieces. Perhaps, he considered, that's the way it was for

everybody: *Bet you didn't think of this.* Caleb dropped the rifle. His only hope was his sidearm. Had he racked it? Had he remembered to free the safety? Would the gun even be there, or had it, like the rifle's magazine, been stripped from his person? The shadow had taken the form of a human silhouette, but it wasn't human, not at all. The head cocked. The claws extended. The lips retreated, revealing a dark cave dripping with teeth. The pistol was in Caleb's hand and rising.

A burst of blood; the creature curled around the hole at the center of its chest. With an almost tender gesture, it reached up with one clawed hand and touched the wound. It raised its face with a bland expression. *Am I dead? Did you do that?* But Caleb hadn't; he hadn't even pulled the trigger. The shot had come from over Caleb's shoulder. For a second they studied one another, Caleb and this dying thing; then a second figure stepped from Caleb's right, shoved the muzzle of a shotgun into the viral's face, and fired.

It was his father. With him was a woman, barefoot, in a plain frock, the kind the sisters wore. Her hair was the barest patina of darkness on her skull. In her outstretched hand, she held the pistol she had used to fire the first, fatal shot.

Amy.

"Peter . . ." she said. And melted to her knees.

Then they were running.

No words were passed that Caleb would later recall. His father was carrying Amy over his shoulder; two other men were with them; one of them had the shotgun his father had cast aside. The portal was open; a squad of six soldiers had formed a firing line in front of it.

551

"Get down!"

The voice was Hollis's. All of them hit the dirt. Shots screamed past them, then ceased abruptly. Caleb lifted his face. Over the barrel of his rifle, Hollis was waving them on.

"Run your asses off!"

His father and Amy entered first, Caleb following. A barrage of gunfire erupted behind them. The soldiers were shouting to one another — *On your left! On your right! Go, go!* — firing their rifles as, one by one, they backed through the narrow doorway. Hollis was the last to enter. He dropped his rifle, swung the door around, and began to close it, clutching the wheel that, once turned, would set the bolts. Just as the lip of the door was about to make contact with the frame, it stopped.

"Need some help here!"

Hollis was bracing the door with his shoulder. Caleb sprang forward and pushed; others did the same. Still, the gap began to widen. An inch, then two more. Half a dozen men were piled against the door. Caleb swiveled his body so his back was braced against it and dug the heels of his boots into the earth. But the end was ordained; even if they could hold the door a few minutes longer, the virals' strength would outlast them.

He saw a way.

Caleb dropped his hand to his belt. He hated grenades; he could not put aside the irrational fear that they would detonate of their own accord. Thus it was with some psychological effort that he freed one from his belt and pulled the pin. Holding the striker lever in place, he angled his face to the edge of the door. He needed more space; the gap between the door and its frame was too narrow. Nobody was going to like what he

was about to do, but he had no time to explain. He stepped back; the door lurched inward six inches. A hand appeared at the edge, clawed fingers curling with a searching gesture around the lip. A chorus of yells erupted. *What are you doing? Push the goddamn door!* Caleb relaxed his grip on the grenade, freeing the striker lever.

"Catch," he said, and shoved it through the opening.

He thrust his shoulder against the door. Eyes closed, he counted off the seconds, like a prayer. *One Mississippi, two Mississippi, three Mississippi . . .*

A boom.

The ping of shrapnel.

Dust falling.

58

"We need a corpsman over here right now!"

Peter lowered Amy to the ground. Her lips moved haltingly; then she asked, very softly, "Are we inside?"

"Everyone's safe."

Her skin was pale, her eyes heavy-lidded. "I'm sorry, I thought I could make it on my own."

Peter looked up. "Where's my son? Caleb!"

"Right here, Dad."

His boy was standing behind him. Peter rose and drew him into a fierce hug. "What the hell were you doing out there?"

"Coming to get you." There were scratches on his arms and face; one of his elbows was bleeding.

"What about Pim and Theo?" Peter couldn't help it; he was talking in bursts.

"They're safe. We got here a few hours ago."

Peter was suddenly overcome. Thoughts crowded his mind from all directions. He was exhausted, he needed water, the city was under attack, his son and his family were safe. Two medics appeared with a stretcher; Greer and Michael lifted Amy onto it.

"I'll go with her to the aid station," Greer said.

"No, I'll do it."

Greer took his arm above the elbow and looked at him squarely. "She'll be fine, Peter — we did it. Just go do your job."

They bore her away. Peter looked up to see Apgar and Chase striding toward him. Above them, the gunfire had fallen to random spattering.

"Mr. President," said Apgar, "I would appreciate it if in the future you did not cut it quite so close."

"What's our status?"

"The attack appears to have come only from the north. We've got no sightings elsewhere on the wall."

"What do we hear from the townships?"

Apgar hesitated. "Nothing."

"What do you mean *nothing?*"

"Everybody's off the air. We ran patrols this morning as far west as Hunt, south to Bandera and as far north as Fredericksburg. No survivors, and almost no bodies. At this point, we have to assume they've all been overrun."

Peter had no words. Over two hundred thousand people, gone.

"Mr. President?"

Apgar was looking at him. Peter swallowed and said, "How many people do we have inside the wall?"

"Including military, four, maybe five thousand,

554

tops. Not a lot to fight with."

"What about the isthmus?" Michael asked the general.

"As a matter of fact, we got a call on the radio from them a couple of hours ago. Someone named Lore, wondering where you were. They didn't know anything about last night's attack, so I guess the dracs missed them. That or they were too smart to try to cross that causeway."

Above them, the guns fell silent.

"Maybe that's it for tonight," Chase said. He scanned their faces hopefully. "Maybe we scared them off."

Peter didn't think so; he could tell that Apgar didn't think so, either.

"We need to make some decisions, Peter," Michael cut in. "The window's closing fast. We should be talking about getting people out of here."

The idea suddenly seemed absurd. "I'm not leaving these people undefended, Michael. This thing has started. Right now, I need everybody who can hold a pitchfork on that wall."

"You're making a mistake."

From the catwalk: "Contact! Two thousand yards!"

The first thing they saw was a line of light in the distance.

"Soldier, give me your binoculars."

The spotter handed them over; Peter brought the lenses to his eyes. Standing beside him on the platform, Apgar and Michael were also scanning north.

"Can you tell how many there are?" Peter asked the general.

"They're too far out to tell." Apgar unclipped the walkie on his belt and brought it to his mouth. "All stations, what are you seeing?"

A crackle of static, then: "Station one, negative."

"Station two, no contact."

"Station three, same here. We're not seeing anything."

And so on, around the perimeter. The line of light began to stretch, though it appeared to come no closer.

"What the hell are they doing?" Apgar said. "They're just waiting out there."

"Hang on." Michael pointed. "Thirty degrees left."

Peter followed his aim. A second line was forming.

"There's another," Apgar said. "Forty right, near the tree line. Looks like a large pod. More coming in from the north, too."

The main line was now several hundred yards long. Virals were streaming in from all directions, moving toward the central mass.

"This is no scouting party," Peter said.

Apgar bellowed, "Runners, get ready to move!" He turned to Peter. "Mr. President, we need to get you to safety."

Peter addressed one of the spotters: "Corporal, hand me that M16."

"Peter, please, this is not a good idea."

The soldier passed Peter the weapon. He freed the magazine, blew on the top round to clear any dust, reseated it in the well, and pulled the charging handle. "You know, Gunnar, I think that's the first time in ten years you've called me by my first name."

The conversation ended there. A low, rumbling

sound rolled toward them. With each second, it increased in intensity.

"What am I hearing?" Michael said.

It was the sound of feet striking the earth. The mass continued to thicken, its great, heaving volume barreled toward them. In its wake, a cloud of dust boiled high in the air.

"Holy God," Peter said. "It's everyone."

Apgar lifted his voice over the din: "Hold fire till they reach the perimeter!"

The horde was three hundred yards out and closing fast. It seemed less like an army than some great spectacle of nature — an avalanche, a hurricane, a flood. The platform began to hum, its bolts and rivets vibrating in rhythm to the seismic impact of the virals' charge.

"Will that gate hold?" Peter asked Apgar. He, too, had given up his binoculars for a rifle.

"Against this?"

Two hundred yards. Peter pressed the stock of the weapon against his clavicle.

"Ready!" Apgar bellowed.

One hundred yards.

"Aim!"

Everything stopped.

The virals had halted just beyond the edge of the lights. Not just halted — they were frozen in place, as if a switch had been thrown.

"What the *hell* . . . ?"

The mass began to divide into halves, creating a corridor. Starting at the rear, it flowed down the middle with a rippling on either side. The motion seemed somehow reverential, as if the virals were making way for a great king to pass among them, bowing as he passed. A dark shape was pushing forward through the heart of the horde. It ap-

peared to be some sort of animal. It approached the city with painstaking slowness, the corridor unfurling before it. All guns were trained on the spot where it would emerge. A hundred feet, fifty, twenty. The front wall of virals separated, opening like a doorway to reveal the shockingly ordinary figure of a person on horseback.

"Is that him?" Apgar said. "Is that Zero?"

The rider moved forward into the lights. Halfway to the gate, he brought his horse to a halt and dismounted. Not "he," Peter realized. *She.* The glare of the spotlights ricocheted off the lenses of the dark glasses that obscured the upper half of her face. A scabbard containing some kind of weapon, a sword or long gun, lay slantwise across her back; crisscrossing her upper body, she wore a pair of bandoliers.

Bandoliers.

"Holy goddamn," Michael breathed.

Peter's mind was tumbling down a hole in time. "Hold your fire!" He raised his arms high and wide above his head. "Everyone stand down!"

Her back erect, the woman angled her face toward the top of the wall. "I am Alicia Donadio, captain of the Expeditionary! Where is Peter Jaxon?"

59

Thirty minutes had passed; everyone was in position. Standing back from the portal, Peter nodded at Henneman.

"Open it, Colonel."

Henneman turned the wheel and backed away. From inside the tunnel came a slow clop of hooves. A frisson of energy rippled through the

line of soldiers facing the portal; all guns were raised, all eyes arrowed over the barrels. A shadow elongated across the wall of the tunnel; then Alicia emerged. One hand held a short rope attached to the horse's bridle; the second lay easily at her side. Her hair, that distinctive red crown, was pulled tight to her scalp, its length corralled into a densely woven braid that fell midway down her back. On her upper body she wore a T-shirt without sleeves, revealing the muscularity of her arms and shoulders; below, loose trousers, cinched at the waist, and a pair of leather boots. A quick scan of the crowd, the lights of the staging area rebounding off the lenses of her goggles like search beams, another step forward, and there she paused, awaiting instructions.

"Move forward," Peter said. "Slowly."

She advanced another twenty feet; Peter ordered her to stop.

"Blades first. Toss them forward."

"That's all you have to say?"

He had a sudden feeling of unreality; it was as if he were talking to a ghost. "The blades, Lish."

She glanced to Peter's right. "Michael. I didn't notice you standing there."

"Hello, Lish."

"And Colonel Apgar." Alicia gave a quick nod from the chin. "It's nice to see you, sir."

"It's 'General' to you, Donadio." The man's arms were folded over his chest; his face was a hard scowl. "Mr. President, say the word and this is done."

" 'Mr. President'?" From Alicia, a wry frown. "You've come up in the world, Peter."

The old banter, the jokey tone: was it a trick? "I said, take them off."

In a manner that struck him as leisurely, Alicia unbuckled the straps and tossed her bandoliers to the ground.

"Now the sword," Peter said.

"I'm here to talk, that's all."

Peter lifted his voice toward the top of the wall. "Snipers! Target the horse!" Then, to Alicia: "Soldier, isn't it?"

If he'd rattled her, she didn't show it. Nevertheless, she drew the scabbard over her head and lobbed it forward.

"Now the goggles," Peter said.

"I'm no threat, Peter. I'm just the messenger."

He waited.

"As you like."

Off they came, revealing her eyes. Their orange color had grown stronger, more piercing. Time had not moved for her; she hadn't aged a day. Yet something was different, a quality not so much seen as felt, like the prickling of a storm's approach long before the clouds arrived. Her gaze did not wander but held him straight. A look of challenge, though now that her face was unconcealed, there was something naked about her, almost vulnerable. Her confidence was a ruse; feelings of uncertainty lay beneath.

"Hit the lights."

Three portable banks of sodium vapor lamps were positioned behind him. They went off like a gun, blasting Alicia in the face. As her hands flew upward, half a dozen soldiers charged forward and shoved her face-first to the ground. With a loud whinny, Soldier reared up on his hind legs and pawed violently at the air. One of the soldiers jammed the barrel of a pistol against the base of Alicia's skull while the others covered her body.

"Somebody control that animal," Peter barked. "If it makes any trouble, shoot it."

"Leave him alone!"

"Colonel Henneman, shackle the prisoner."

As two soldiers led the horse away, Henneman holstered his pistol, stepped forward, and chained Alicia's wrists and ankles. A third chain connected the shackles behind her back.

"Rise and face me," Peter said.

Alicia rocked upright into a kneeling position. Her eyes were clamped shut, her face angled down and away from the harsh glare of the lights, like someone dodging a blow.

"I'm trying to save your lives, Peter."

"You have an interesting way of showing it."

"You need to hear what I have to say."

"So talk."

A moment passed; then she began: "There's a man — more than a man, a kind of viral, but he looks like us. His name is Fanning. He's in New York City, in a building called Grand Central. He's the one who sent me."

"So that's where you've been all this time?"

Alicia nodded. "There are things I never told you, Peter. Things I *couldn't* tell you. The viral part of me was always stronger than I let on. The feeling got worse and worse — I knew I couldn't control it for long. Right after Iowa, I began to hear Fanning in my head. That's why I went to New York. I intended to kill him. Or he could kill me. I didn't really care which. I just wanted it all to be over."

"So why didn't you?"

"Believe me, I wanted to. I wanted to slice his damn head off. But I couldn't. The viral that bit me in Colorado wasn't Babcock's. It was Fan-

ning's. It's his virus I carry. I belong to him, Peter."

I belong to him. The phrase was chilling. Peter glanced at Apgar to see if the full meaning had registered. It had.

"Fanning and I had a deal. If I stayed with him, he'd leave you alone."

"Looks like he changed his mind."

She shook her head emphatically. "I didn't have any part in that. By the time I figured out what he was doing, it was too late to stop it. All along he was waiting for you to spread out, your defenses to drop. It's Amy he wants. If I bring her to him, he'll call it off."

So there it was. "What does he want with her?"

"I don't know."

"Don't you lie to me."

"Where is she, Peter?"

"I have no idea. Nobody's seen Amy in over twenty years."

Alicia's tone had shifted; all her bluster was gone. "Listen to me, *please.* There's no stopping this. You've seen what he can do. He's not like the others. The others were *nothing.*"

"We have walls. We have lights. We've fought them before. Go back and tell him that."

"Peter, you don't get it. He doesn't have to *do* anything. You have, what, just a few thousand soldiers? And how much food? How much gas? Give him what he wants. It's your only chance."

"Private Wilson, step forward please."

Hollis moved into the lights.

"You remember Hollis, don't you, Lish? Why don't you say hello."

Her head was bowed. "Why do you even ask me that?"

562

"How about his daughter, Kate? She would have been a little girl the last time you saw her."

Alicia nodded.

"*Say* it. Say you remember Kate."

"Yes, I remember her."

"I'm glad you do. She grew up to be a doctor, just like her mother. Two little girls of her own. Then one of your friends bit her last night. Want to know what happened next?"

Alicia was silent.

"*Do* you?"

"Just get on with it, Peter."

"All right, I will. That little girl you remember? She shot herself."

Her silence infuriated him. What had happened to her? What had she become?

"You don't have anything to say for yourself?"

"What do you want me to say? That I'm sorry? You can do what you want with me, but that won't stop a thing."

Peter's pulse was pounding; his hands were clenched. He jabbed a finger at her. "*Look at him.* I'll get Sara out here, Kate's daughters, too. You can tell all of them how fucking sorry you are."

Alicia said nothing.

"Two hundred thousand people, Lish. And you come here and talk about surrender? Like he's your *friend?*"

Her shoulders shook. Was she crying?

"I'll ask you again. What does Fanning want with Amy?"

Her head rocked from side to side. "I don't know."

"Gunnar, give me your sidearm."

Apgar drew his pistol, spun it in his hand, and passed it to Peter. Peter released the magazine,

checked it, and shoved it back into the well, making a loud show of it.

Michael said, "Peter, what the hell are you doing?"

"This woman is a viral. She's in league with the enemy."

"It's Alicia! She's one of us!"

Peter strode forward and leveled the barrel at Alicia's temple. "Tell me, goddamnit."

"I know she's here," Alicia murmured. "I can hear it in your voice."

He thumbed back the hammer and spoke through gritted teeth. He was running on instinct now, a blind white fury, obliterating all thought. "Answer the question or I am going to put a bullet through your head."

"Wait."

He turned. Amy, clutching Greer's arm for balance, was standing at the edge of the circle.

"Lucius, get her the hell out of here."

Two soldiers moved to block their path. One pressed a hand against Greer's chest. The man tensed, then, apparently changing his mind, permitted this.

"Let me talk to her," Amy said.

The idea was ludicrous. The woman could barely stand; a puff of wind would have knocked her to her knees.

"I mean it, Greer."

"I understand you're angry," Amy said, "but there's more to this than you know."

She spoke to him as one might address a dangerous animal or a man poised at the lip of an abyss. Peter was suddenly conscious of the pistol's slick weight in his hand.

"Lucius can stay where he is," Amy said, "but if

you want answers, you need to let me through."

Peter looked back at Alicia. The woman's head hung in submission; she seemed small, frail, broken. Had he really been about to shoot her? This seemed impossible, yet in the moment, something had taken him over, beyond his control.

"Please, Peter."

The moment stretched; everyone was staring.

"All right," he said. "Let her pass."

The soldiers stepped back. Amy's shadow lay long on the ground as she approached Alicia's cowed figure. Using her body to shield Alicia's face from the light, Amy crouched before her.

"Hello, sister. It's good to see you."

"I'm sorry, Amy." Her shoulders shook. "I'm so sorry."

"Don't be." Tenderly, Amy lifted Alicia's chin with the tips of her fingers. "Do you know how proud I am of you? You've been so very strong."

Tears were coursing down Alicia's cheeks, cutting bright streaks in the dirt. "How can you say that to me?"

Amy smiled into her face. "Because we're sisters, isn't that so? Sisters in blood. My thoughts have never been far from you, you know."

Alicia said nothing.

"He comforted you, didn't he?"

Her lips were wet, tears rolling off her chin. "Yes."

"He took you in, cared for you. He made you feel that you were not alone."

Alicia's voice was barely more than a whisper. "Yes."

"Do you see? That's why I'm so proud of you. Because you didn't give in, not in your heart."

"But I did."

"No, sister. I know what it's like to be alone. To be outside the walls. But that's over now." Without breaking Alicia's gaze, Amy lifted her voice to the assembly. "Everyone, are you listening? You can put your guns down. This woman is a friend."

"Hold your positions," Peter commanded.

Amy swiveled her face toward him. "Peter, didn't you hear me? She's with us."

"I need you to step away from the prisoner."

In confusion, Amy looked back at Alicia, then at Peter once more.

"It's okay," Alicia said. "Do as he says."

"Lish —"

"He's only doing what he has to. You really need to back away now."

An uncertain moment passed; Amy got to her feet. Another pause, her expression tentative, and she backed away. Alicia dropped her head.

Peter said, "Colonel, go ahead."

Henneman approached Alicia from behind. He had donned a pair of heavy rubber gloves; in his hands was a metal rod wrapped with copper wire, one end connected by a long cord to the generator powering the lights. As the tip of the rod made contact with the base of Alicia's neck, she jerked upright, her shoulders pulled back and her chest thrust forward, as if she'd been impaled. She made no sound at all. For a few seconds she stayed that way, every muscle taut as wire. Then the air let out of her and she toppled face-first into the dirt.

"Is she out?"

Henneman nudged Alicia's ribs with the toe of his boot. "Looks like it."

"Peter, *why?*"

"I'm sorry, Amy. But I can't trust her."

A truck was backing toward them. Two men

jumped down from the cargo bay and dropped the tailgate.

"All right, gentlemen," Peter said. "Let's haul this woman to the stockade. And watch yourselves. You don't want to forget what she is."

60

0530: Peter stood with Apgar on the catwalk, watching the day come on. An hour before dawn, the horde had departed — a vast, silent retreat, like a wave beating back from shore to enfold itself in the dark bulk of the sea. All that remained was a wide swath of trampled earth and, beyond, fields of broken corn.

"I guess that's it for the night," Apgar said.

His voice was heavy, resigned. They waited, not talking, each man alone in his thoughts. A few minutes went by, and then the horn blasted — an expansion of sound like a great intake of breath, followed by the inevitable exhalation, sighing over the valley, then gone. Across the city, frightened people would be emerging from basements and shelters, out of closets and from under their beds. Old people, neighbors, families with children. They would look at each other wide-eyed and weary: Is it over? Are we safe?

"You should get some sleep," Apgar said.

"So should you."

Yet neither man moved. Peter's stomach was sour and empty — he couldn't remember when he'd eaten last — while the rest of him seemed numb, almost weightless. His face felt tight, like paper. The body's demands: the world could end, yet you'd still have to take a piss.

"You know," Apgar said, and yawned into his

567

fist, "I think Chase was onto something. Maybe we should leave this to the kids to sort out."

"It's an interesting idea."

"So, would you have actually shot her?"

The question had plagued him all night. "I don't know."

"Well, don't beat yourself up. I wouldn't have had a problem with it." A pause, then: "Donadio was right about one thing. Even if we manage to hold them back, we don't have the gas to keep the lights burning for more than a few nights."

Peter stepped to the rampart. A gray morning, the light indifferent and worn: it seemed suitable. "I let this happen."

"We all did."

"No, this is on me. We never should have opened those gates."

"What were you going to do? You can't keep people locked up forever."

"You're not letting me off the hook here."

"I'm just pointing out the reality. You want to blame someone, blame Vicky. Hell, blame *me*. The decision to open the townships was made long before you came along."

"I'm the one in that chair, Gunnar. I could have stopped it."

"And had a revolution on your hands. Once the dracs disappeared, this was a done deal. I'm surprised we kept this place running as long as we did."

No matter what Gunnar said, Peter knew the truth. He'd let down his guard, allowing himself to believe that it was all in the past — the war, the virals, the old way of doing things — and now two hundred thousand people were gone.

Henneman and Chase came clomping down the

catwalk. Chase looked like he'd slept under a bridge somewhere, but Henneman, always a stickler for appearance, had somehow managed to get through the night with barely a hair out of place.

"Orders, General?" the colonel asked.

It was not the time to drop their defenses, but the men needed rest. Apgar put them on a four-hour rotation: one-third on the wall, one-third patrolling the perimeter, one-third in their racks.

"So what now?" Chase asked, as Henneman moved away.

But Peter had ceased listening; an idea was forming at the back of his mind. Something old; something from the past.

"Mr. President?"

Peter turned to face the two men. "Gunnar, what are our weak points? Besides the gate."

Apgar thought for a moment. "The walls are sound. The dam's basically impregnable."

"So it's the gate that's the problem."

"I'd say so."

Would it work? It just might.

"My office," said Peter. "Two hours."

"Open the door."

The officer keyed the lock; Peter stepped inside. Alicia was sitting on the floor of the cell. Her arms and legs were shackled in front; a third chain connected her hands to a heavy iron ring in the wall. Thick fabric had been used to cover the window, muting the light.

"About time," she said drolly. "I was beginning to think you'd forgotten me."

"I'll knock when I'm done," Peter told the guard.

He left them alone. Peter sat on the cot facing

Alicia. A silent moment, the two regarding each other across a distance that felt far vaster than it was.

"How are you feeling?" he asked.

"Oh, you know." A shrug, dismissive. "Beats a bullet to the brain. You had me going for a second there."

"I was angry. I still am."

"Yeah, I sensed that." Her eyes took slow measure of his face. "Now that I have a chance to really look at you, I've got to say, you're holding up nicely. That snow on the roof suits you."

He smiled, just a little. "And you look the same."

She glanced around the tiny box of a room. "And you're really running the show here? President and all that."

"That seems to be the case."

"Like it?"

"The last couple of days haven't been so hot."

These wry exchanges, like a dance to a song that only the two of them could hear: he couldn't help himself; he'd missed them.

"You've put me in a bind, Lish. That was a pretty big splash you made last night."

"My timing wasn't the best."

"As far as this government is concerned, you're a traitor."

She looked up. "And what does Peter Jaxon think?"

"You've been gone a long time. Amy seems to believe you're on our side, but she's not the one calling the shots."

"I am on your side, Peter. But that doesn't change the situation. In the end, you're going to have to give her up. You can't beat him."

"See, this is where I have a problem. I've never

heard you talk that way, not about anything."

"This is different. *Fanning* is different. He's been controlling everything from the start. The only reason we were able to kill the Twelve was because he *let* us. We're all pieces on a board to him."

"So why would you trust him now?"

"Maybe I'm not being clear. I don't."

" 'He comforted you.' 'He took care of you.' Am I remembering this correctly?"

"He did, Peter. But that's not the same thing."

"You're going to have to do better than that."

"Why? So you'll believe me? The way I see it, you don't have a choice."

"Who am I talking to here? You or Fanning?"

Her eyes sharpened with anger; his words had hit the mark. "I took an oath, Peter. Same as you, same as Apgar, same as every man on that wall last night. I stayed with Fanning because I believed he'd leave Kerrville alone. Yes, he was good to me. I never said he wasn't. Believe it or not, I actually feel sorry for the guy, until I remember what he is."

"And what's that?"

"The enemy."

Was she lying? For the moment, it didn't matter; that she *wanted* him to believe her was leverage he could use.

"Tell me what we're up against, how many dracs are out there."

"I think what you saw last night."

"The rest of Fanning's forces are in New York, in other words. He's holding them in reserve."

Alicia nodded. "I wasn't followed, if that's what you mean. The rest are in the tunnels under the city."

"And you don't know what he wants with Amy?"

"If I knew, I'd tell you. Trying to understand Fanning is a fool's errand. He's a complicated man, Peter. I was with him for twenty years, and I never figured him out completely. Mostly, he just seems sad. He doesn't like what he is, but he sees a kind of justice in it. Or, at least, he wants to."

Peter frowned. "I'm not following."

Alicia took a moment to form her thoughts. "In the station, there's a clock. Long ago, Fanning was supposed to meet a woman there." She looked up. "It's a long story. I can give you all of it, but it'd take hours."

"Give me the short version."

"The woman's name was Liz. She was Jonas Lear's wife."

Peter was caught short.

"Yeah, it surprised me, too. They all knew each other. Fanning loved her since they were young. When she married Lear, he pretty much gave up on the whole thing, but not really. Then she got sick. She was dying, some kind of cancer. Turns out she loved him, too; she had all along. She and Fanning were going to run away, spend her last days together. You should hear him tell the story, Peter. It'd just about rip your heart out. The clock was where they were going to meet, but Liz never showed. She'd died on the way, but Fanning didn't know that; he thought she'd changed her mind. That night he got drunk in a bar and went home with a woman. She was a stranger, nobody he knew. He killed her."

"So he's a murderer, in other words."

Alicia made an expression of demurral. "Well, it was sort of an accident, the way he tells it. He was half out of his mind; he thought his life was basically over. She pulled a knife on him, they

struggled, she fell on it."

"Putting him on death row, like the Twelve."

"No, he got away with it. He actually felt awful about the whole thing. He was plenty mixed up, but he was no hardened killer, at least not yet. It was later that he went to South America with Lear, which is where the virus comes from. Lear had been looking for it for years; he thought he could use it to save his wife, though that was a moot point by then. Fanning describes the guy as totally obsessed."

"Was that how Fanning caught the virus?"

Alicia nodded. "As far as I can tell from Fanning's story, it happened by chance, though in his head Lear was responsible. After Fanning got infected, Lear brought him back to Colorado. He was still hoping to use the virus as a kind of cure-all, but the military got involved. They wanted to use it as a weapon, make some kind of super-soldier out of it. That was when they brought in the twelve inmates."

Peter thought for a moment. Then, his thoughts crystallizing: "What about Amy? Why did the Army make her?"

"They didn't; that was Lear. He used a different virus, not descended from the one Fanning carried. That's why she's not the same as the others. That, plus she was so young. I think he maybe knew that the whole thing had gone bad and was trying to make it right."

"It's a strange way of doing it."

"Like I said, Fanning is pretty much of the opinion that the man was off his rocker. Either way, in Fanning's mind, Amy is the fish that got away. Killing the Twelve was a test — not of us, since we never stood a chance against them. Fan-

ning was testing *her.* I don't know why I didn't think of it at the time, his positioning them all in one place like that. He was never particularly fond of them, to put it mildly. A bunch of psychotics, is how he puts it."

"And he's not?"

Alicia shrugged. "Depends on your definition. If you mean he doesn't know right from wrong, I'd have to say no. He's pretty well versed on the subject, actually. Which is the strangest thing about him, the part I could never really get. Your ordinary drac doesn't care one way or another — it's just an eating machine. Fanning thinks about *everything.* Maybe Michael could keep up with him, but I never could. Talking to him was like being dragged by a horse."

"So why test her? What was he trying to find out?"

Alicia glanced away, then said, "I think he wanted to know if she really was different from the rest of them. I don't think he wants to kill her. That'd be too obvious. If I had to guess, I'd say it all comes down to his feelings about Lear. Fanning hated the guy. Really *hated.* And not just because of what Lear did to him. It goes deeper than that. Lear made Amy as a way to set things straight. Maybe Fanning just can't sit with that. Like I said, he mostly seems miserable. He sits in that station staring at the clock as if time stopped for him when Liz didn't show."

Peter waited for more, but Alicia seemed to end there. "Last night you called him a man."

She nodded. "At least that's how he looks, though there are a few differences. He's sensitive to light, much more than I am. He never sleeps, or almost never. Likes his dinner warm. And" —

she used her thumb and forefinger to indicate her incisors — "he's got these."

Peter frowned. "Fangs?"

She nodded. "Just these two."

"Was he always that way?"

"Actually, no. At the start, he was exactly like the rest of them. But something happened, an accident. He fell into a flooded quarry. This was early on, just a few days after he broke out of the NOAH lab. None of us can swim; Fanning went straight to the bottom. When he woke up, he was lying on the shore, looking like he does now." She paused, eyes narrowing on his face, as if struck by a sudden thought. "Is that what happened to Amy?"

"Something like that."

"But you're not going to tell me."

Peter left it there. "Could water change back his Many?"

"Fanning says no, just him."

Peter rose from the cot. A wave of lightheadedness passed through him: he really needed to lie down, even for just a few minutes. But it seemed important not to show her how exhausted he was — an old habit, from the days when the two of them had stood the Watch together, each always trying to best the other. *I can do this, can you?*

"Sorry about those chains."

Alicia lifted her wrists, examining them with a neutral expression — as if they were not her hands but someone else's. She shrugged and let them fall to her lap again. "Forget it. It's not like I'm making this easy for you."

"Do you need anything? Food, water?"

"My diet is a little peculiar these days."

Peter understood. "I'll see what I can do."

A silent moment, each of them acknowledging the awkwardness of the situation.

"I know you don't want to believe me," Alicia said. "Hell, I wouldn't. But I'm telling you the truth."

Peter said nothing.

"We were *friends,* Peter. All those years, you were the one person I could always rely on. We stood for each other."

"Yes, we did."

"Just tell me that still counts for something."

As he looked at her, his mind went back to the night when they had said goodbye to each other at the Colorado garrison, so many years ago — the night before he had ridden up the mountain with Amy. How young they'd been. Standing outside the soldiers' barracks, the cold wind lancing through them, he had loved Alicia fiercely, as he had never loved anyone in his life — not his parents or Auntie or even his brother Theo: no one. It was not the love of a man for a woman, or a brother for a sister, but something leaner, pared to its essence: a binding, subatomic energy that had no words to name it. Peter could no longer recall what they'd said to one another; only the impression remained, like footprints in snow. It was one of those moments when it had still seemed possible to understand life and what was meant by living one — he had been young enough to still believe that such a thing was possible — and the recollection carried a striking vividness of emotion, as if three decades had not passed since that cold and distant hour in which he had stood in the sheltering light of Alicia's courage. But then he blinked the memory away, his mind returned to the present, and what remained was only a

great weight of sadness at the center of his chest. Two hundred thousand souls gone, and Alicia at the center of it all.

"Yes," he said. "It counts. But I'm afraid it doesn't change a thing."

He gave three hard bangs on the door. Tumblers turned and the guard appeared.

"Don't be dumb, Peter. Fanning's everything I say he is. I don't know what you're planning, but don't."

"Thank you," he said to the guard. "I'm finished here."

The chain attaching Alicia to the wall rattled as she yanked on it. "Listen to me, goddamnit! It's no good, fighting him!"

But these words barely reached his ears; Peter was already striding down the hall.

61

And now, my Alicia, you reside among them.

How do I know this? I know it as I know everything; I am a million minds, a million histories, a million roving pairs of eyes. I am everywhere, my Alicia, watching you. I have watched you since the beginning, taking measure and stock. Would it be too much to say that I felt your arrival on the day you were born into this world — a wet, squealing nugget, the hot blood of protest already pouring through your veins? Impossible, of course; yet it seems so. Such is the bewitching way of providence: all seems ordained, all known, both in forward and reverse.

What an entrance you made! With what bold declaration, what showmanship, what authoritative poise did you step into the city's lights and

stake your claim! How could the occupants of the besieged metropolis fail to swoon under your spell, enchanted by the drama of your arrival? *I am Alicia Donadio, captain of the Expeditionary!* Forgive, Alicia, these windy flights; my mood is grandiose. Not since the great Achilles stood without the battlements of mighty Troy has our pocket of creation seen the likes of you. Within those walls, no doubt, a great parliament commences. Debates, edicts, threats and counter-threats — the customary swordplay of a city under siege. Do we fight? Do we run? Earnest and admirable, yet — and you must pardon the analogy — these discussions are to the outcome what splashing is to drowning: they only make the whole thing go faster.

In your absence, Alicia, I have, so to speak, taken a page from your book. Night after night the dark beckons me; my feet cast me wandering anew into the streets of mighty Gotham. Summer has come at last upon this isle of exile. In the branches the songbirds twitter; the trees and flowers clutter the breeze with their airborne sexual excreta; newborn creatures of every ilk undertake their first uncertain adventures in the grass. (Last night, recalling your concerns for my strength, I devoured a litter of six young bunnies in your honor.) What is this new restlessness inside me? Adrift among Manhattan's maze of glass and steel and stone, I feel closer to you, yes, but something else as well: a sense of the past so glowingly intense it is practically hallucinatory. It was in summer, after all, when I traveled to New York for my friend Lucessi's funeral, when this city first laid its hand of love upon me. I close my eyes and there I am, with her, my Liz, the woman and the place indel-

ible, one and the same. The appointed hour at the clock, and then our exit into the moist human heat of the season's early rush; the abrupt encapsulation of the taxi, with its cracked vinyl bench and feeling of a million prior occupants; the parade of heaving humanity clogging the streets and sidewalks; the impatiently perfunctory honking of horns and the catlike mating shrieks of sirens; the majestic towers of midtown, glazed and shining with the hour's exhausted light; my bright, almost painful awareness of everything, a rush of undifferentiated data to my brain, all of it permanently inseparable from the beloved and eternal *her.* Her shining, sun-blessed shoulders. The faint, womanly aroma of her perspiration in the sealed space of the taxi. Her wan, expressive face, with its touch of mortality, and her myopic gaze, always peering deeper into things. The perfection of her hand in my own as we wandered the dark streets together, alone among millions. It has been said that in ancient times there was only one gender; in that blissful state, humankind existed until, as punishment, the gods divided each of us in two, a cruel mitosis that sent each half forever spinning across the earth in search of its mate, so that it could be whole again.

That was how her hand felt in my own, Alicia: as if, of all men upon the earth, I had found that one.

Did she kiss me that night as I was sleeping? Was it a dream? Is there a difference? That is my New York, as it was once so many's: the kiss one dreams of.

All lost, all gone — as is the city of your love, Alicia, the city of your Rose. *Call Fanning,* my friend Lucessi wrote. *Call Fanning to tell him that*

love is all there is, and love is pain, and love is taken away. How many hours did he hang there? How many days and nights did my mother linger, floating in a sea of agony? And where was I? What fools we are. What fools we mortals be.

Thus does the hour of reckoning approach. Unto God I issue my just complaint; 'twas he who cruelly dangled love before our eyes, like a brightly colored toy above a baby's crib. From nothing he made this world of woe; to nothing it shall return.

I know she's here, you said. *I can hear it in your voice.*

And I in yours, my Alicia. I in yours.

62

Two soldiers, rifles dangling, stood at the end of the walkway. As Peter approached, they stiffened, popping quick salutes.

"All quiet here?" Peter asked.

"Dr. Wilson went in a while ago."

"Anyone else?" He wondered if Gunnar had visited, or maybe Greer.

"Not since we came on duty."

The door opened as he mounted the porch: Sara, carrying her small leather satchel of instruments. Their eyes met in a way that Peter understood. He embraced her and backed away.

"I don't know what to say," Peter began. Her hair was damp and pressed to her forehead, her eyes swollen and bloodshot. "We all loved her."

"Thank you, Peter." Her words were flat, without emotion. "Is it true about Alicia?"

He nodded.

"What are you going to do with her?"

"I don't know at this point. She's in the stockade."

Sara didn't say anything; she didn't have to. Her face said it all. *We trusted her; now look.*

"How's Amy?" Peter asked.

Sara heaved a sigh. "You can see for yourself. I'm a little out of my depth here, but as far as I can tell, she's fine. Fine as in *human.* A little malnourished, and she's very weak, but the fever's gone. If you brought her in here and didn't tell me who she was, I'd say she was a perfectly healthy woman in her mid-twenties who'd just come off a bad bout of the flu. Somebody please explain this to me."

As compactly as he could, Peter related the story: the *Bergensfjord,* Greer's vision, Amy's transformation.

"What are you going to do?" Sara said.

"I'm working on it."

Sara seemed dazed; the information had begun to sink in. "I guess maybe I owe Michael an apology. Funny to think about that at a time like this."

"There's a meeting in my office at oh-seven-thirty. I need you there."

"Why me?"

There were lots of reasons; he went with the simplest. "Because you've been part of this from the beginning."

"And now part of the end," Sara said grimly.

"Let's hope not."

She fell silent, then said, "A woman came into the hospital yesterday in labor. Early stages, we might have just sent her home, but she and her husband were there when the horn went off. Along about three A.M. she decides to have her baby. A baby, in the middle of all this." Sara

looked at Peter squarely. "Know what I wanted to tell her?"

He shook his head.

"Don't."

The bedroom door was ajar; Peter paused at the threshold. The drapes were shut, bathing the room in a thin, yellowish light. Amy was turned on her side — eyes closed, face relaxed, one arm tucked beneath the pillow. He was about to retreat when her eyes fluttered open.

"Hey." Her voice was very soft.

"It's okay, go back to sleep. I just wanted to check on you."

"No, stay." She cast her eyes groggily around the room. "What time is it?"

"I'm not sure. Early."

"Sara was here."

"I know. I saw her leave. How are you feeling?"

She frowned pensively. "I don't . . . know." Then, eyes widening as if the idea surprised her: "Hungry?"

Such an ordinary want; Peter nodded. "I'll see what I can do."

In the kitchen he lit the kerosene stove — he hadn't used it in months — then went outside to tell the soldiers what he needed. While he waited, he washed up; by the time they returned, carrying a small basket, the fire was ready to go. Buttermilk, eggs, a potato, a loaf of dense, dark bread, and mixed-berry jam in a jar sealed with wax. He set to work, happy to have this small chore to take his mind from other things. In a cast-iron pan he fried the potatoes and then the eggs; the bread he cut into thick slices and smeared with jam. How long since he'd cooked a meal for another person?

Probably for Caleb, as a boy. Years ago.

He arranged Amy's breakfast on a tray, added a glass of buttermilk, and carried it all to the bedroom. He'd wondered if she'd fall asleep again in his absence; instead he found her alert and sitting up. She had pulled the drapes aside; evidently the light had ceased to trouble her. A smile blossomed at the sight of him, standing in the doorway like a waiter with his tray.

"Wow," she said.

Peter placed the tray on her lap. "I'm not much of a cook."

Amy was staring at the food as if she were a prisoner released from years in jail. "I don't even know where to start. The potatoes? The bread?" She smiled decisively. "No, the milk."

She drained the glass and set to work on the rest, jabbing the food with her fork like a field hand.

Peter dragged a chair to the bedside. "Maybe you should slow down."

She glanced up, speaking around a mouthful of eggs. "Aren't you going to eat?"

He was famished but enjoyed watching her. "I'll get something later."

Peter went to the kitchen to refill her glass; by the time he returned, her plate was empty. He handed her the buttermilk and watched her polish it off. A healthy color had flowed back into her cheeks.

"Come sit by me," she said.

Peter cleared her tray and perched on the edge of the bed. Amy slipped her hand into his. "I've missed you," she said.

It felt so unreal, to be sitting here, talking to her. "I'm sorry I got old."

583

"Oh, I think I've got you beat there."

He almost laughed. There was so much he wanted to say, to tell her. She looked just as she did in his dreams; the short hair was the only difference. Her eyes, the warmth of her smile, the sound of her voice — all were the same.

"What was it like, in the ship?"

She dropped her face; her thumb moved gently over the top of his hand. "Lonely. Strange. But Lucius took care of me." She looked at him again. "I'm sorry, Peter. You couldn't know."

"Why?"

"Because I wanted you to live your life. To be . . . happy. I heard Caleb call you 'Dad.' I'm glad, for both of you."

"He's married, you know. His wife is Pim."

"Pim," Amy repeated, and smiled.

"They have a son, too. They named him Theo."

She gently squeezed his hand. "So there's a life, right there. What else made you happy? I want to know."

You did, he thought. *You made me happy. I've been with you every night since you were gone. I've lived a whole life with you, Amy.* But he could not find the words to say this.

"That night in Iowa," he began. "That was real, wasn't it?"

"I'm not sure I even know what real is anymore."

"I mean, it happened. It wasn't a dream."

Amy nodded. "Yes."

"Why did you come to me?"

Amy's eyes darted away, as if the memory pained her. "I'm not sure I know. I was confused, the change had happened so fast. Probably I shouldn't have done it. I was so ashamed of what I was."

584

"Why would you think that?"

"I was a monster, Peter."

"Not to me."

Their eyes met and held; her hand was warm, though not with fever; it was the warmth of life. A thousand times he'd held it, and yet this was also the first.

"Is Alicia all right?" Amy asked.

"Oh, she's tougher than that. What do you want me to do with her?"

"I don't think that's my decision."

"It's not. But I still need to know what you think."

"This isn't simple for her. She's been with him a long time. I think there's a lot she's not telling us."

"Like what?"

Amy thought for a moment, then shook her head. "I can't tell. She's very sad. But it's like there's a locked box inside her. I can't get past it." Their eyes met again. "She needs you to trust her, Peter. I'm one side of her; Fanning's the other. Between us, there's you. It's you she's really here to see. She needs to know who she is. Not just who she is: *what* she is."

"So what is she?"

"What she always was. Part of this, part of *us*. You're her family, Peter. You have been from the start. She needs to know that you still are."

Peter felt the truth of her words. But knowing something was not the same thing as believing it. That was the hell of it, he thought.

"You're not going with her," he said. "I can't allow it."

"You may not have a choice about that. Alicia's right, the city can't stand indefinitely. Sooner or

585

later, I'll have to face him."

"I don't care. I lost you once. I'm not doing it again."

Footsteps in the hall: Peter turned as Caleb appeared in the doorway, Pim behind him. For a moment, Peter's son appeared dumbstruck. A warm light switched on in his eyes.

"It's really you," he said.

Amy smiled. "Caleb, I believe I would like to hug you."

Peter stepped back; Amy rose on her elbows as Caleb leaned over the bed and the two embraced. When at last they parted, they still held one another by the elbows, each beaming into the other's happy face. Peter understood what he was seeing: the deep bond that Amy and his son shared, forged in the days before Iowa, when Amy had looked after him in the orphanage.

"You look so grown-up," Caleb said, laughing.

Amy laughed, too. "So do you."

Caleb turned to his wife, speaking and signing simultaneously. "Amy, this is Pim, my wife. Pim, Amy."

How do you do, Pim? Amy signed.

Very well, thank you, Pim replied.

Amy's hands were moving with expert speed. *It's a beautiful name. You're just as I pictured you.*

You, too.

Caleb stared at the two women; only then did it occur to Peter that the exchange he had just witnessed was, technically, impossible.

"Amy," Caleb said, "how did you *do* that?"

She frowned at her splayed fingers. "Now, I don't think I know. I suppose the sisters must have taught me."

"None of them can sign."

She dropped her hands to her lap and looked up. "Well, somebody must have. How else could I have done it?"

More footsteps; an atmosphere of official briskness accompanied Apgar into the bedroom.

"Mr. President, I'm sorry for the interruption, but I thought I might find you here." His chin lifted toward the bed. "Pardon me, ma'am. How are you feeling?"

Amy was sitting up now, hands folded in her lap. "Much better, thank you, General."

He narrowed his attention on Caleb. "Lieutenant, aren't you supposed to be in your rack?"

"I wasn't tired, sir."

"That wasn't what I asked. And don't look at your father — he's not interested."

Caleb took Amy's hand and gave it a final squeeze. "Get better, okay?"

"Now, Mr. Jaxon."

Caleb exchanged a hasty, unreadable sign with Pim and exited the room. "If you're done here," Apgar said, "it's time. People will be waiting."

Peter turned to Amy. "I better go."

Amy appeared not to have heard him; her eyes were fixed on Pim's. The seconds stretched as the two women regarded each other with a crackling intensity, as if engaged in a private, inaudible conversation.

"Amy?"

She startled, breaking the circuit. It seemed to take her a moment to assemble her sense of her surroundings. Then she said, very calmly, "Of course."

"And you'll be all right here?" Peter said.

Another smile, but not the same — more of reassurance than something genuine. There was

something hollow about it, even forced.

"Perfectly."

63

"Mirrors," Chase repeated.

Around the conference table, clockwise from Peter's left, sat the players, Peter's war cabinet: Apgar, Henneman, Sara, Michael, Greer.

"It doesn't have to be a mirror specifically. Anything reflective will work, just as long as they can see themselves."

Chase took a long breath and folded his hands on the table. "This is the craziest thing I've ever heard."

"It's not crazy at all. Thirty years ago, in Las Vegas, Lish and I were running from a pod of three and got cornered in a kitchen. We were out of ammunition, pretty much defenseless. A bunch of pots and pans were hanging from the ceiling. I grabbed one to use as a club, but when I held it out at the first viral, it stopped the bastard cold, like it was hypnotized. And this was just a copper pot. Michael, back me up here."

"He's right. I've seen it, too."

Apgar asked Michael, "So what does it do to them? Why does it slow them down?"

"Hard to say. My guess would be some kind of residual memory."

"Meaning what?"

"Meaning, they don't like what they see, because it doesn't conform to some other aspect of their self-image." He turned toward Peter. "Do you remember the viral you fought in Tifty's cage?"

Peter nodded.

"After you killed her, you said something to

Tifty. 'Her name was Emily. Her last memory was kissing a boy.' How did you know that?"

"It was a long time ago, Michael. I can't really explain it. She was looking at me, and it just happened."

"Not just looking. She was *staring.* You both were. People don't look a viral in the eye when it's about to rip them in half. The natural impulse is to look away. You didn't. And just like the mirror, it stopped her flat." Michael paused, then said, with deeper certainty, "The more I think about this, the more sense it makes. It explains a lot of things. When a person gets taken up, their first impulse is to go home. Dying people feel the same way. Sara, am I right about that?"

She nodded. "It's true. Sometimes it's even the last thing people say. 'I want to go home.' I can't tell you how often I've heard it."

"So a viral is a person infected with a virus, strong, superaggressive. But somewhere deep down, they remember who they were. During the transitional phase, let's say, that memory gets buried, but it doesn't go away, not completely. It's just a kernel, but it's there. Eyes are reflective, just like mirrors. When they see themselves, the memory rises to the surface, and it confuses them. That's what stops them, a sort of nostalgia. It's the pain of remembering their human lives and seeing what they've become."

"That's quite . . . a theory," Henneman said.

Michael shrugged. "Maybe. Maybe I'm just talking out of my exhaust pipe, and it wouldn't be the first time. But let me ask you something, Colonel. How old are you?"

"I'm sorry?"

"Sixty? Sixty-three?"

589

He scowled a little. "I'm fifty-eight, thank you."

"My mistake. Ever look in a mirror?"

"I try to avoid it."

"Precisely my point. In your mind, you're the same person you always were. Hell, between my ears I'm still just a seventeen-year-old kid. But the reality is different, and it's depressing to look at. I don't see any twenty-year-olds around this table, so I'm guessing I'm not alone."

Peter turned toward his chief of staff. "Ford, what do we have that reflects? We'd need to cover the whole gate, and it's best if we have at least a hundred yards on either side, more if we can do it."

He thought for a moment. "Galvanized roofing metal could work, I suppose. It's pretty shiny."

"How much do we have?"

"A lot of that stuff has moved out to the townships, but we should have enough. We can strip some houses if we come up short."

"Get engineering on it. We also need to reinforce that gate. Tell them to weld the damn thing shut if they have to. The portal, too."

Chase frowned. "How will people get out?"

" 'Out' is not the issue right now. For the time being, they won't."

"Mr. President, if I may," Henneman cut in. "Assuming this all works — a big *if,* in my opinion — we still have a couple hundred thousand virals running loose out there. We can't stay inside the walls forever."

"I hate to contradict you, Colonel, but that's exactly what we did in California. First Colony stood for almost a century, with a fraction of the resources. We're down to just a few thousand people, a sustainable population if we manage it

right. Within these walls we have enough arable land for planting and livestock. The river gives us a good continuous source for drinking water and irrigation. With some modification, we can still run oil up from Freeport in smaller loads, and the refinery itself is defensible. With careful rationing, using all of our refined petroleum for the lights, we should be fine for a very long time."

"And weaponry?"

"Tifty's bunker can supply us for a while, and probably we can remanufacture more, at least to last for a few more years. After that, we use crossbows, longbows, and incendiaries. We made it work at First Colony. We'll do it here."

Silence from around the table; everybody was thinking the same thing, Peter knew. *It comes to this.*

"All due respect," Michael said, "but this is bullshit, and you know it."

Peter turned toward him.

"So maybe the mirrors slow them down. Fanning is still out there. If what Alicia said is true, the virals we saw last night are just the tip of the spear. He's holding an entire army in reserve."

"Let me worry about that."

"Don't patronize me. I've been thinking about this for twenty years."

Apgar scowled. "Mr. Fisher, I suggest you stop talking."

"Why? So he can get us all killed?"

"Michael, I want you to listen to me very carefully." Peter wasn't angry; he had expected the man to object. What mattered now was making sure everyone stayed on board. "I know your feelings. You've made them very clear. But the situation has evolved."

"The time line has moved up, that's all. We're pissing away our chance sitting around like this. We should be loading buses right now."

"Maybe it would have worked before. But we start moving people out of here now, there'll be a riot. This place will come apart. And there's no way we can move seven hundred people to the isthmus in daylight. Those buses would be caught in the open. They wouldn't stand a chance."

"We don't stand a chance anyway. The *Bergensfjord* is all we have. Lucius, don't just sit there."

Greer's face was calm. "This isn't our decision. Peter is in charge."

"I don't believe what I'm hearing." Michael looked around the room, then back at Peter. "You're just too goddamn obstinate to admit you're beaten."

"Fisher, that's enough," Apgar warned.

Michael turned toward his sister. "Sara, you can't be buying this. Think about the girls."

"I am thinking about them. I'm thinking about everybody. I'm with Peter. He's never steered us wrong."

"Michael, I need to know you're with us," Peter said. "It's that simple. Yes or no."

"Okay, no."

"Then you're dismissed. The door is that way."

Peter wasn't quite sure what was going to happen next. For several seconds, Michael looked him dead in the eye. Then, with an angry sigh, he rose from the table.

"Fine. You make it through the night, you let me know. Lucius, are you coming?"

Greer glanced at Peter, eyebrows raised.

"It's all right," said Peter. "Somebody needs to look after him."

The two men departed. Peter cleared his throat and continued: "The important thing is that we get through tonight. I expect every able-bodied person to man those walls, but we'll need shelters for the rest. Ford?"

Chase rose, crossed to Peter's desk, and returned with a rolled tube of paper, which he unfurled on the table and weighed down at the corners.

"This is one of the builders' original schematics. Hardboxes were constructed here" — he pointed — "here, and here. All three date to the early days of the city, and none has been used in decades, not since the Easter Incursion. I don't imagine they're in very good shape, but with some reinforcement, we can use them in a pinch."

"How many people can we fit?" Peter asked.

"Not many, at most a few hundred. Now, over here," he continued, "you've got the hospital, which can fit, oh, maybe another hundred. Another, smaller box is underneath this building, the old bank vault. Full of files and other junk, but basically in good shape."

"What about basements?"

"There aren't a lot. A few beneath commercial buildings, some of the old apartment complexes, and we can safely assume there are a few in private hands. But the way the city was built, almost everything is on slab or pier. The soil by the river is mostly clay, so no basements at all. That extends from H-town all the way to the southern wall."

Not good, Peter thought. So far, they had accounted for fewer than a thousand people.

"Now, here's the granddaddy." Chase directed everyone's attention to the orphanage, which was marked "HB1." "When they moved the government from Austin, one of the reasons they chose

Kerrville is because of this. While the walls were being constructed, they needed a safe place to overnight the workers and the rest of the government. This end of the city sits on top of a large formation of limestone, and it's full of pockets. The largest one is underneath the orphanage, and it's deep, at least thirty feet below the surface. According to the old records, it was originally used by the sisters as part of the Underground Railroad, a place to hide runaway slaves before the Civil War."

"How do we get down there?" Apgar asked.

"I went and looked this morning. The hatch is under the floorboards in the dining area. There's a flight of wooden stairs, pretty rickety but usable, that leads down to the cave. Dank as a tomb, but it's big. If we pack folks in, it can hold another five hundred at least." Chase looked up. "Now, before anybody asks, I went through the census data last night. It's just an estimate, but here's how things break down. Inside the walls, we have about eleven hundred children under the age of thirteen. Not counting military, the remainder divvies up about pretty evenly in terms of gender, but the population skews old. We've got a lot of people over sixty. Some of them will want to fight, but I don't see that they'll be much help, frankly."

"So what about the rest?" Peter asked.

"Of the remainder, we're looking at roughly thirteen hundred men of fighting age. About the same number of women, maybe slightly less. It's safe to assume some of the women will choose to defend the wall, and there's no reason they shouldn't. The problem is armament. We have weapons for only about five hundred civilians. There are probably plenty of guns floating around

out there, but there's no way to know how many. We'll just have to wait and see what appears when the time comes."

Peter looked at Apgar. "What about ammunition?"

From the general, a frown. "Not too good. Last night cost us badly. We've got maybe twenty thousand rounds on hand in a mix of calibers, mostly nine-millimeter, forty-five, and five fifty-six. Plenty of shot shells, but they're only good for close quarters. For the big guns, we're down to about ten thousand rounds in fifty-cal. If the dracs charge that gate, our ammo won't last long."

The situation boiled down disconcertingly: maybe a thousand defenders on the wall, enough ammunition to last a few minutes at most, hardboxes for a thousand, and two thousand unarmed civilians with nowhere to hide.

"There's got to be someplace we can put people," Peter said. "Somebody, give me something."

"As a matter of fact," Chase said, "I've got an idea about that." He rolled out another map: a schematic of the dam. "We use the drainage tubes. There are six, each a hundred feet long, so maybe a hundred and fifty people apiece. The downstream openings are barred; no viral has ever gotten through. The only access on the upstream side is through the waterworks, and there are three heavy doors between the tubes and the outside. The beauty of it is, even if the dracs breach the walls, there's no reason they'd think to look there. The people inside would be completely hidden."

It made sense. "Ford, I think you just earned your pay for the month. Gunnar?"

Apgar, lips pursed, nodded. "It's a hell of an

idea, actually."

"Everybody else?"

From the room, a murmur of agreement.

"Good, it's settled. Chase, you're in control of the civilian side. We need to start moving people to shelter as soon as possible, no last-minute rushes. Children under thirteen to the orphanage, starting with the youngest. Sara, how many patients do you have in the hospital?"

"Not many. Twenty or so."

"We can use the basement hardbox for some of the overflow, plus the hardboxes on the west side of town. Gunnar, I'll need a security detachment on all of these. Children only, plus mothers with young kids. But no men. If they can walk, they can fight."

"And if they won't?"

"Martial law is martial law. If they don't take your advice, I'll back your decision, but we don't want to stir things up."

Apgar received his meaning with a tight nod.

"The rest who don't want to fight go in the tubes. I want all sheltered civilians in place by eighteen hundred hours, but let's make this orderly to keep panic to a minimum. Colonel, you oversee assembling the civilian force. Send out a couple of squads to go house to house and put out a call for any additional weaponry. People can keep one rifle or pistol of their own, but any extras go into the armory for redistribution. As of this moment, any working firearm is property of the Texas military."

"I'll get it done," Henneman said.

Peter addressed the group: "We don't know how long we'll have to hold them off, people. It might be minutes, it might be hours, it might be all

night. They might not attack at all, just wait us out. But if the dracs get in, the orphanage is our fallback position. We protect the children. Is that clear?"

Silent nods passed around the table.

"Then we're adjourned. I'll want everybody back here at fifteen hundred. Gunnar, stay behind a minute. I need a word."

They waited as the room emptied. Apgar, elbows resting on the table, eyed Peter over his meshed fingers. "So?"

Peter rose and stepped to the window. The square was quiet, with no one about, everything becalmed in the summer heat. Where was everybody? Probably hiding in their houses, Peter thought, afraid to come out.

"Fanning will have to be dealt with," he said. "This will never end otherwise."

"This would be the part of the conversation when you tell me you're going to New York."

Peter turned around. "I'll need a small contingent — say, two dozen men. We can use the portables as far north as Texarkana, maybe a little farther before we run out of fuel. On foot, we should reach New York by winter."

"That's suicide."

"I've done it before."

Apgar looked at him pointedly. "And you were fucking lucky, if you'll excuse my saying so. Never mind that you're thirty years older and New York is two thousand miles away. According to Donadio, it's crawling with dracs."

"I'll take Alicia with me. She knows the territory, and the virals won't attack her."

"After last night's performance? Be serious."

"The city won't stand unless we kill him. Sooner

597

or later, that gate will fail."

"I don't disagree. But taking on Fanning with two dozen soldiers doesn't seem like much of a plan to me."

"What do you suggest? That we hand Amy over?"

"You should know me better than that. On top of which, once we give her to Donadio, we've got nothing. No cards to play."

"So what, then?"

"Well, have you given any more thought to Fisher's boat?"

Peter was speechless.

"Don't get me wrong," Apgar continued. "I don't trust the man any farther than I can throw him, and I'm glad you tossed his ass out of here. I don't tolerate division in the ranks, and he was way out of line. Also, I have no idea if that thing will even float."

"I don't believe what I'm hearing."

Apgar let a moment pass. "Mr. President. Peter. I'm your military adviser. I'm also your friend. I know you, how you think. It's served you well, but the situation is different. If it were up to me I'd say sure, go down swinging. The gesture might be symbolic, but symbolism matters to old war-horses like us. I hate these things, and I always have. But by any measure, this isn't going to end well. Like it or not, you're the last president of the Texas Republic. That pretty much leaves you in charge of the fate of the human race. Maybe Fisher's full of shit. You know the man, so that's your call. But seven hundred is better than nothing."

"This place will come apart. There's no way we'll be able to mount a coherent defense."

"No, probably we won't."

Peter turned back to the window. It really was awfully damn quiet out there. He had the unsettled sense of observing the city from some distant future time: buildings empty and abandoned, dead leaves rolling in the streets, every surface being slowly reclaimed by wind and dust and years — the permanent silence of lives stopped, all the voices gone.

"Not that I'm objecting," he said, "but is this first-name thing going to be a habit?"

"When I need it, yeah."

Below him in the square, a group of boys appeared. The oldest of them couldn't have been more than ten. What were they doing out there? Then Peter grasped the situation: one of the boys had a ball. At the center of the square, he dropped it on the ground and kicked it, sending the rest scurrying after it. A pair of five-tons pulled into the square; soldiers disembarked and began to set up a line of tables. More were hauling out crates of weaponry and ammunition to be distributed among the civilian inductees. The boys took only cursory notice, lost in their game, which appeared to have nothing in the way of formal structure: no rules or boundaries, no objectives or way to keep score. Whoever possessed the ball tried to keep it away from the others, until he was bested by one of his companions, thus starting the mad chase all over again. Peter's thoughts took him back many years, first to the formless contests that had diverted Caleb and his friends for hours and their contagious youthful energy — *just five more minutes, Dad, there's still plenty of light, please just one more game* — and then to his own boyhood: that brief, innocent span in which he had existed

in total obliviousness, outside the flow of history and the accumulated weight of life.

He turned from the window. "Do you remember the day Vicky summoned me to her office to offer me a job?"

"Not really, no."

"As I was leaving, she called me back. Asked about Caleb, how old he was. She said — and I think I have this right — 'It's the children we're doing this for. We'll be long gone, but our decisions will determine the kind of world they're going to live in.' "

Apgar gave a slow nod. "Come to think of it, maybe I do remember. She was a cunning old broad, I'll give her that. It was a masterpiece of manipulation."

"No chance I could turn her down. It was just a matter of time before I surrendered."

"So what's your point?"

"The point is, this patch of ground doesn't just belong to us, Gunnar. It belongs to *them*. First Colony was dying. Everyone had given up. But not here. That's why Kerrville has survived as long as it has. Because the people here have refused to go quietly."

"We're talking about the survival of our species."

"I know we are. But we need to earn the right, and abandoning three thousand people to save seven hundred isn't an equation I can sit with. So maybe it all ends here. Tonight, even. But this city is ours. This *continent* is ours. We run, Fanning wins, no matter what. And Vicky would say the same thing."

A moment of stalemate passed, the two men looking at each other. Then:

600

"That's a nice speech," Apgar said.

"Yeah, I bet you didn't know I was such a deep thinker."

"So that's it?"

"That's it," said Peter. "That's my final word. We stay and fight."

64

Sara descended the stairs to the basement. Grace was at the end of the second row of cots, sitting up, her baby resting in her lap. The woman looked tired but also relieved. She offered a small smile as Sara approached.

"He's fussing a little," she said.

Sara took the baby from her, laid him on the adjacent cot, and unwound the blanket to examine him. A big, healthy boy with curly black hair. His heart was loud and strong.

"We're calling him Carlos, after my father," Grace said.

During the night, Grace had told Sara the story. Fifteen years ago, her parents had moved out to the townships, settling in Boerne. But her father had had little luck as a farmer and had been forced to take a job with the telegraph crews, leaving the family alone for months at a time. After he'd been killed in a fall from a pole, Grace and her mother — her two older brothers had long since moved on — had returned to Kerrville to live with relatives. But it had been a hard life, and her mother, too, had passed, though Grace shared no details. At seventeen, Grace had gone to work in an illegal saloon — she was vague about her duties, which Sara didn't want to know — and this was how she'd met Jock. Not an auspicious

beginning, although the two were, Grace asserted, very much in love, and when she'd turned up pregnant, Jock had done the honorable thing.

Sara rewrapped the baby and returned him to his mother, assuring her that everything was fine. "He'll complain a bit until your milk comes in. Don't worry — it doesn't mean anything."

"What's going to happen to us, Dr. Wilson?"

The question seemed too large. "You're going to take care of your son, that's what."

"I heard about that woman. They say she's some kind of viral. How could that be?"

Sara was caught off guard — but of course people would be talking. "Maybe she is — I don't know." She put a hand on Grace's shoulder. "Try to rest. The Army knows what it's doing."

She found Jenny in the storage room, taking inventory of their supplies: bandages, candles, blankets, water. More boxes had been brought down from the first floor and stacked against the wall. Her daughter, Hannah, was helping her — a freckled, disarmingly green-eyed girl of thirteen, with long, coltish legs.

"Sweetheart, could your mom and I have a minute? Go see if they need anything upstairs."

The girl left them alone. Quickly, Sara reviewed the plan. "How many people do you think we can fit in here?" she asked.

"A hundred, anyway. More if we really stuff them in, I guess."

"Let's set up a desk at the front door to count heads. No men get in, only women and children."

"What if they try?"

"Not our problem. The military will handle it."

Sara examined four more patients — the boy with pneumonia; a woman in her forties who had

rushed in with breathing trouble that she feared was a heart attack but was nothing more than panic; two little girls, twins, who had come down with acute diarrhea and fever in the night — then returned to the first floor in time to see a pair of five-tons roar up to the entrance. She stepped outside to meet them.

"Sara Wilson?"

"That's right."

The soldier turned back to the first truck in line. "Okay, start unloading."

Moving in pairs, the soldiers began carting sandbags to the entrance. Simultaneously, a pair of Humvees with .50-caliber machine guns attached to their roofs backed up to the building and took flanking positions on both sides of the door. Sara watched this numbly; the strangeness of all of it was catching up with her.

"Can you show me the other entrances?" the sergeant asked.

Sara led him around to the back and side doors. Soldiers arrived with sheets of plywood and began hammering them into the molding.

"Those won't keep a drac out," Sara said. They were standing at the front of the building, where more sheets of plywood were being used to cover the windows.

"They're not for the dracs."

Sweet Jesus, she thought.

"Do you have a weapon, ma'am?"

"This is a hospital, Sergeant. We don't just leave guns lying around."

He walked to the first truck and returned with a rifle and pistol. He held them out. "Take your pick."

Everything about his offer went against the

grain; a hospital still meant something. Then she thought of Kate.

"All right, the pistol." She tucked it into her waistband.

"You've used one before?" the sergeant said. "I can give you the basics if you want."

"That won't be necessary."

In the stockade, Alicia was gauging the strength of the chains.

The bolt on the wall was negligible — one hard yank should do it — but the shackles were a problem. They were constructed of a hardened alloy of some sort. Probably they had come from Tifty's bunker; the man had made a science of viral containment. So even if she freed herself from the wall, she'd still be as trussed up as a hog for slaughter.

The thought of sleep enticed her. Not merely to obliterate time but to carry her thoughts away. But her dreams, always the same, were nothing she cared to revisit: the brilliantly lit city dissolving to darkness; the happy cries of life within waning, then gone; the pitiless, disappearing door.

And then there was the other issue: Alicia wasn't alone.

The feeling was subtle, but she could tell Fanning was still there: a sort of low-grade hum in her brain, more tactile than aural, like a breeze pushing over the surface of her mind. It made her feel angry and sick and tired of everything, ready to be done with it all.

Get out of my head, goddamnit. Haven't I done what you asked? Leave me the hell alone.

The promised food did not appear. Peter had forgotten, or else he'd decided that a hungry Alicia

was safer than a full one. It could be a tactic to make her pliable: *Food is on the way; wait, no, it isn't.* In either event, she was perversely glad; part of her still hated it. The moment her jaws sank into flesh, hot blood squirting upon her palate, a chorus of revulsion erupted in her head: *What the hell are you doing?* Yet always she drank her fill until, thoroughly disgusted with herself, she sank back on her heels and let the lassitude engulf her.

The hours moved sluggishly. At last the door opened.

"Surprise."

Michael stepped into the room. A small metal cage was pressed against his chest.

"Five minutes, Fisher," the guard said, and slammed the door behind him.

Michael put the cage on the floor and took a seat on the cot, facing her squarely. In the cage was a brown rabbit.

"How'd you get in?" Alicia asked.

"Oh, they know me pretty well around here."

"You bribed them."

Michael seemed pleased. "As it happens, a little money changed hands, yes. Even in these troubled times, a man has to think about his family. That, plus nobody else had the stomach to bring you breakfast." He nodded toward the cage. "Apparently, the little bundle of fur is somebody's pet. Goes by Otis."

Alicia allowed herself a good, long look at Michael. The boy she'd known was gone, replaced by a middle-aged man of sinewy hardness, compact and capable. His face had a chiseled look, nothing wasted. Though his eyes still possessed their twinkling, busy alertness, a darker aspect lay within them, more knowing: the eyes of experi-

ence, of a man who had seen things in his life.

"You've changed, Michael."

He shrugged carelessly. "This is something I hear a lot."

"How've you been keeping yourself?"

"Oh, you know me." A cockeyed smile. "Just keeping the lights burning."

"And Lore?"

"Can't say that worked out."

"Sorry to hear it."

"You know how it goes. I got the potted plants, she took the house. For the best, really." He angled his head at the floor again, where the caged rabbit was anxiously working its cheeks. "Aren't you going to eat?"

She wanted to, very badly. The intoxicating scent of warm meat, warm life; the swish and throb of the animal's blood surging through its veins, as if she'd cupped a seashell to her ear: her anticipation was intense.

"It's not a pretty sight," she said. "Probably best if I wait."

For several seconds, they just looked at each other.

"Thanks for standing up for me last night," Alicia said.

"No thanks necessary. Peter was way out of line."

She searched his face. "Why don't you hate me, Michael?"

"Why would I do that?"

"Everybody else seems to."

"I guess I'm not everybody else then. You could say I don't have a lot of fans in these parts myself."

"I hardly believe that."

"Oh, trust me. I'm lucky I'm not living down

606

the hall."

A smile, unbidden, rose to her lips; it was good to talk to a friend. "Sounds interesting."

"That would be one word for it." He placed the tips of his fingers together, a man making a point. "I always knew you were out there, Lish. Maybe the others gave up on you. But I never did."

"Thanks, Circuit. That means something. That means a lot."

He grinned. "Now, seeing as it's you, I'll let that nickname slide."

"Talk to him, Michael."

"I've made my opinion known."

"What's he going to do?"

He shrugged. "What Peter always does. Hurl himself at the problem until he bashes his way through it. I love the guy, but he's a bit of an ox."

"It won't work this time."

"No, it won't."

He was watching her intently — though, unlike Peter's, his gaze held no suspicion. She was a confidante, a co-conspirator, a trusted part of his world. His eyes, his tone of voice, the manner in which his body occupied space: all radiated an undeniable force.

"I've thought a lot about you, Lish. For a long time, I believed I was in love with you. Who knows? Maybe I still am. I hope that doesn't embarrass you."

Alicia was dumbstruck.

"I see from your expression that this comes as a surprise. Just take it as a compliment, which is how it's meant. What I'm saying is that you matter a great deal to me, and you always have. When you appeared last night, I realized something. Do you want to know what that was?"

Alicia nodded, still at a loss for words.

"I realized I'd been waiting for you all along. Not just waiting. Expecting." He paused. "Do you remember the last time we saw each other? It was the day you came to visit me in the hospital."

"Of course I do."

"For the longest time I wondered: Why me? Why did Alicia pick me, of all people, at just that moment? I would have guessed Peter would be the one. The answer came to me when I thought about something you said. 'Someday, that boy's going to save our sorry asses.' "

"We were talking about when we were kids."

"That's right. But we were talking about a lot more than that." He leaned forward. "Even then, you knew, Lish. Maybe not knew. But you felt it, the shape of things, just as I did. Just as I do now, sitting here twenty years later talking to you in a jail cell. Now, 'why' is another question. I don't have an answer to that one and I've stopped asking. And as for how this is all going to play out, your guess is as good as mine. Given the general direction of the last twenty-four hours, I'm not especially optimistic. But either way, I can't do this without you."

The sound of tumblers; the guard appeared in the doorway. "Fisher, I said five minutes. You need to get the hell out of here."

Michael reached into his shirt pocket and waved a wad of bills over his shoulder, not even bothering to look as the guard snatched it and skulked away.

"God, they're idiots," he sighed. "Do they actually think money's going to be worth anything this time tomorrow?" He reached into his pocket again

and removed a folded sheet of paper. "Here, take this."

Alicia opened it: a map, hastily sketched in Michael's hand.

"When the time comes, follow the Rosenberg road south. Just beyond the garrison, you'll come to an old farm with a water tank on your left. Take the road after it and follow it straight east, fifty-two miles."

Alicia looked up from the paper. Something new was in his eyes: a kind of wildness, almost manic. Beneath Michael's controlled exterior, his aura of self-possessing strength, was a man aflame with belief.

"Michael, what's at the end of that road?"

Alone again, Alicia drifted. So, there had been a woman for Michael, after all. His ship, his *Bergensfjord.*

We are the exiles, he had told her in parting. *We are the ones who understand the truth and always have; that is our pain in life.* How well he knew her.

The rabbit was watching her guardedly. His black eyes, unblinking, shone like drops of ink; in their curved surfaces Alicia could see the ghost of her face reflected, a shadow self. She realized her cheeks were wet; why could she not stop crying? She scooted forward to the cage, undid the latch, and reached inside. Soft fur filled her hand. The rabbit made no attempt to escape; he was either tame, a pet as Michael claimed, or too frightened to react. She lifted the animal free and placed him on her lap.

"It's all right, Otis," she said. "I'm a friend." And she stayed that way, stroking the soft fur, for a very long time.

65

Footsteps, and the creak of the opening door: Amy opened her eyes.

Hello, Pim.

The woman halted in the entryway. She was tall, with an oval face and expressive eyes, and wearing a simple cotton dress of blue fabric. Beneath its soft drape, her belly arced with the bulge of her pregnancy.

I'm glad that you've come back to see me, Amy signed.

A look of deep uncertainty, and Pim stepped to her bedside.

May I? Amy asked.

Pim nodded. Amy cupped her palm against the curving cloth. The force within, being so new, exuded a pure feeling of life — if it were a color, it would be the white of summer clouds — but was also full of questions. Who am I? What am I? Is this the world? Am I everything, or just a part?

Show me the rest, Amy signed.

Pim sat on the bed, facing away. Amy unfastened the buttons of her dress and drew the fabric aside. The stripes on her back, the burns — they were faded, though not erased. Time had given them a ridged and burrowed quality, like roots running under soil. Amy ran the tips of her fingers along their lengths. In the untouched places Pim's skin was soft, with a pulsing warmth, but the muscles were hard beneath, as if forged with remembered pain.

Amy buttoned the dress; Pim swiveled on the mattress to face her.

I've dreamed about you, Pim signed. *I feel like I've known you all my life.*

And I you.

Pim's eyes were full of inexpressible emotion. *Even when . . .*

Amy took her hands to quiet them. *Yes,* she replied. *Even then.*

From the pocket of her dress, Pim withdrew a notebook. It was small but possessed the thickness of stiff parchment paper stitched together. *I brought you this.*

Amy accepted it and opened the covers, which were wrapped in soft hide. Here it was, page after page. The drawings. The words. The island with its five stars.

Who else has seen this? she signed.

Only you.

Not even Caleb?

Pim shook her head. A film of tears coated the surface of her eyes; she appeared completely overcome, beyond words. *How do I know these things?*

Amy closed the notebook. *I cannot say.*

What does it mean?

I think it means you will live; your baby will live. A pause, then: *Will you help me?*

In the living room, she found paper and a pen. She wrote the note, folded it into thirds, and gave it to Pim, who hurried away. Alone again, Amy went to the bathroom off the hall. Above the washbasin was a small round mirror. The changes that had occurred to her person had been felt rather than observed; she had yet to see herself. She stepped to the mirror. The face she beheld did not seem to be her own, and yet it was also the person she had long felt herself to be: a woman with dark hair, a well-sculpted though not overtly angular face, pale unblemished skin, and

deep-set eyes. Her hair was as short as a boy's, showing the curves of her skull, and bristly to the touch, like the end of a broom. The reflection possessed a disquieting ordinariness; she might have been anyone, just another woman in the crowd, yet it was within this face, this body, that all her thoughts and perceptions — her sense of self — resided. The urge to reach out and touch the mirror was strong, and she allowed herself to do so. As her finger made contact with the glass, her reflection responding in kind, a shift occurred. *This is you,* her mind told her. *This is the one true Amy.*

It was time.

To quiet one's mind, to bring it to a condition of absolute motionlessness — that was the trick. Amy liked to use a lake. This body of water was not imaginary; it was the lake in Oregon where Wolgast, in their first days together at the camp, had taught her to swim. She closed her eyes and willed herself to go there; gradually the scene arose in her thoughts. The cusp of night, and the first stars punching through a blue-black sky. The wall of shadow where tall pines, rich with fragrance, stood regally along the rocky shore. The water itself, cold and clear and sharp-tasting, and the downy duff of needles carpeting the bottom. In this mental construct, Amy was both the lake and the swimmer in the lake; ripples moved outward along its surface in accordance with her motions. She took a breath and dove down, into an unseen world; when the bottom appeared, she began to move along it with a smooth, gliding motion. Far above her, the ripples of her entry dispersed concentrically across the surface. When the last of these disturbances touched their fingers

612

to the shore, and the lake's surface returned to perfect balance, the state she required would be achieved.

The ripples touched. The lake stilled.

Can you hear me?

Silence. Then:

Yes, Amy.

I think that I am ready, Anthony. I think I am ready at last.

Michael had been waiting at the gate for nearly an hour. Where the hell was Lucius? It was nearly 1030; they were cutting it close as it was. Men were welding heavy brackets in place to lay iron beams across the gate. More were hammering sheets of galvanized roofing metal to the outside face. If Greer didn't show up soon, they'd be locked inside like everybody else.

At last Greer appeared, striding briskly through the portal from outside. He climbed into the truck and nodded toward the windshield. "Let's go."

"She's fooling herself."

Greer gave him a look: don't go there.

Michael turned the engine over, angled his head out the window, and yelled to the foreman of the work crew: "Coming through!" When the man failed to turn around, he leaned on the horn. "Hey! We need to get out!"

That got the foreman's attention; he strode up to the driver's window. "The hell you honking at me for?"

"Tell those guys to get out of the way."

He spat onto the ground. "Nobody's supposed to go outside. We're working here."

"Yeah, well, we're different. Tell them to move or get run over. How would that be?"

The man looked like he was about to say something but stopped himself. He turned back toward the gate. "Okay, clear a path for this guy."

"Much obliged," Michael said.

The foreman spat again. "It's your funeral, asshole."

Yours, too, thought Michael.

66

1630 hours: the last of the evacuees were being moved into the dam; the hardboxes were full; the few remaining civilian inductees were awaiting their assignments. There had been a few incidents — some arrests, even a few shots fired. Yet most people saw the sense of what they were being asked to do; their own lives were on the line.

But processing the inductees was taking longer than expected. Long lines, confusion about weapons and who reported to whom, the distribution of equipment and delegation of duties: Peter and Apgar were trying to assemble an army in half a day. Some barely knew how to hold a gun, much less load and fire it. Ammo was at a premium, but a target range had been set up in the square, using sandbags as a backstop. A crash course for the uninitiated — three shots, good or bad — and off they went to the wall.

Just a few weapons remained, pistols only; the rifles were gone, except for a few that would be held in reserve. Tempers were short; everyone had been standing in the hot sun for hours. Peter was positioned to the side of the processing desk with Apgar, watching the last few men come through. Hollis was checking off names.

A man approached the desk — forties, lean in

614

the manner of someone to whom life had not been kind, with a high, domed forehead and old acne scars on his cheeks. A hunting rifle hung from his shoulder. It took Peter a moment to recognize him.

"Jock, isn't it?"

The man nodded — somewhat sheepishly, Peter thought. Twenty years gone by, yet Peter could tell that the memory of that day on the roof still affected him. "I don't think I ever really thanked you, Mr. President."

Apgar glanced at Peter. "What'd you do?"

Jock said, "He saved my life, is what he did." Then, to Peter: "I've never forgotten it. Voted for you both times."

"What became of you? No more roofs, I'll bet."

Jock shrugged; his regular life, like everyone's, was receding into the past. "Worked as a mechanic, mostly. Just got married, too. My wife had a baby last night."

Peter remembered Sara's story. He gestured toward Jock's rifle, a lever-action .30-30. "Let's see your weapon."

Jock handed it over. The action was jerky, the trigger like mush, the glass of the scope gouged and pitted.

"When was the last time you fired this?"

"Never. Got it from my dad years ago."

Hollis looked up. "We don't have any thirty-thirty."

"How many rounds do you have for this?" Peter asked Jock.

The man held out his open palm, showing four cartridges, old as the hills.

"This thing is worthless. Hollis, get this man a proper rifle."

The gun was produced: one of Tifty's M16s, fresh and gleaming.

"A wedding present," Peter said, passing it off to Jock. "Report to the range. They'll get you ammo and show you how to use it."

The man looked up, blindsided. His face was full of gratitude; no one had ever given him such a present. "Thank you, sir." A crisp nod and he moved away.

"Okay, what was that about?" Apgar asked.

Peter's eyes followed Jock as he made his way to the range. "For luck," he said.

In the orphanage, the last of the women and children were descending into the shelter. It had been decided that only women with children under five would be allowed to accompany their offspring; there had been many tearful scenes of separation, agonizing and awful. Quite a few mothers claimed their children were younger than they obviously were; in those instances that seemed close, or close enough, Caleb let them through. He simply didn't have the heart to say no.

Caleb worried about Pim; the shelter was rapidly filling. At last she arrived, explaining that the children had spent the morning at Kate and Bill's house. For Pim a painful pilgrimage, Kate's ghost everywhere, but a helpful distraction for the girls: a few hours in familiar rooms, playing with familiar toys. They'd bounced on their old beds for half an hour, Pim said.

And yet something was off; Caleb sensed the presence of words unsaid. They were standing by the open hatch. One of the sisters, positioned on the platform below, reached up to assist the

616

children, first Theo, then the girls. As Pim's turn came, Caleb took her by the elbow.

What is it?

She hesitated. Yes, something was there.

Pim?

A flicker of uncertainty in her eyes; then she composed herself. *I love you. Be careful.*

Caleb let the matter rest. Now was not the time, the hatch standing open, everyone waiting. Sister Peg was observing from the side. Caleb had already broached the question of whether or not Sister Peg would be joining the children underground. "Lieutenant," she'd said with a reproachful look, "I'm eighty-one years old."

Caleb hugged his wife and helped her down. As her hands gripped the top rung, she raised her eyes, for a last look. A cold weight dropped inside him. She was his life.

Keep our babies safe, he signed.

More children came through; then, suddenly, the shelter was full. From outside the building a cry went up, followed by a voice from a megaphone, ordering the crowd to disperse.

Colonel Henneman strode into the hall. "Jaxon, I'm putting you in charge here."

It was the last thing Caleb wanted. "I'd be more use on the wall, sir."

"This isn't a debate."

Caleb felt the presence of an unseen hand. "Does my father have something to do with this?"

Henneman ignored the question. "We'll need men on the roof and the perimeter and two squads inside. Are we clear? Nobody else gets inside. How you accomplish that is up to you."

Dire words. Also inevitable. People would do anything to survive.

Michael and Greer picked up the first survivors north of Rosenberg, a group of three soldiers — stunned, starving, their carbines and pistols drained. The virals had attacked the barracks two nights ago, they said, tearing through the place like a tornado, destroying everything, vehicles and equipment, the generator and radio, ripping the roofs off the Quonsets like they were opening tins of meat.

There were others. A woman, one of Dunk's girls, with black hair streaked white, walking barefoot along the roadway with her tippy shoes dangling from her fingertips and a story about hiding in a pump house. A pair of men from one of the telegraph crews. An oiler named Winch — Michael recalled him from the old days — sitting cross-legged by the side of the road, carving meaningless shapes in the ground with a six-inch knife and babbling incoherently. His face was chalky with dust, his coveralls black with dried blood, though it was not his own. All took their places in the back of the truck in stunned silence, not even asking where they were going.

"These are the luckiest people on the planet," Michael said, "and they don't even know it."

Greer watched the landscape flow past, dry scrub yielding to the dense tangle of the coastal shelf. The intensity of the last twenty-four hours had kept the pain at bay, but now, in the unstructured silence of his thoughts, it roared back. An omnipresent, low-grade urge to vomit tossed his gut; his saliva was thick and brassy-tasting; his bladder pulsed with unexpressed fullness, febrile and enormous. When they'd stopped to pick up

the woman, Greer had stepped into the scrub with the hope of passing water, but all he'd managed to produce was a pathetic crimson-tinted trickle.

South of Rosenberg, they swung east toward the ship channel. Muddy water sprayed up behind them; each bang of the truck's carriage on the gullied roadway threw fresh punches of pain. Greer wanted a drink of water very badly, if only to clear the taste in his mouth, but when Michael drew his canteen from under his seat, took a long pull, and offered it to him, all the while staring out the windshield, Greer waved it off. From Michael, a sideways glance — *You're sure?* — and for that moment the man seemed to know something, or at least suspect. But when Greer said nothing, Michael wedged the canteen between his knees and capped it with a shrug.

The air in the truck changed, and then the sky; they were approaching the channel.

"For fucksakes, I only just came from here," said the woman.

Five more miles and the causeway appeared. Patch and his men were waiting at the bottleneck. Barriers of razor wire had been laid across it. As the truck drew to a halt, Patch stepped up to the driver's window.

"Didn't expect you back so soon."

"What has Lore told you?" Michael asked.

"Just the bad parts. No sign of them here, though." Then, glancing into the back of the vehicle, "I see you've brought some friends."

"Where is she?"

"The ship, I guess. Rand says she's driving everybody crazy down there."

Michael turned toward their passengers. "You three," he said to the soldiers, "get out."

They were looking around with bewilderment. "What do you want us to do?" one asked — the highest-ranking among them, a corporal with eyes empty as a cow's and the soft, baby-fatted face of a fifteen-year-old.

"I don't know," Michael said dryly, "be soldiers? Shoot at things?"

"I told you, we haven't got any ammo."

"Patch?"

The man nodded. "I'll fix them up."

"This is Patch," Michael said to the three. "He's your new CO."

They looked blankly at one another. "Aren't you guys, like, criminals?" the one said.

"Right now, do you honestly give a damn?"

"Come on now," Patch cut in, "be good fellows and do like the man says."

Looking askance at one another, the soldiers disembarked. Once Patch and the others had pulled the barrier aside, Michael gunned the engine and roared down the causeway. Rand met them at the shed, shirtless and sweating, a greasy rag knotted around his head.

"What's our status?" Michael asked, stepping down. "Have you flooded the dock?"

"There's a problem. Lore found another bad section. There are soft spots all through it."

"Where?"

"Starboard bow."

Fuck." Michael gestured toward their remaining passengers, who were standing in a group, staring with befuddlement. "Figure out what to do with these people."

"Where'd you get them?"

"Found them on the way."

"Isn't that Winch?" Rand asked. The man was

muttering into his collar. "What the hell happened to him?"

"Whatever it was, it wasn't nice," Michael answered.

Rand's eyes darkened. "Is it true about the townships? That they're all gone?"

Michael nodded. "Yeah, looks like we're it."

Greer interrupted: "Michael, I think we need to take extra men up to the causeway. It'll be dark in a few hours."

"Rand, how about it?"

"I guess we can spare a few. Lombardi and those other guys."

"You two," Rand said to the telegraph men, "come with me. And you," he said to the woman, "what can you do?"

She arched her eyebrows.

"Besides that, I mean."

She thought for a moment. "Cook a little?"

"A little's better than what we've got. You're hired."

Michael strode down the ramp to the ship. A crane with a sling had been moved into place on the dock, near the bow, where six men in bosun's chairs hung over the side. At the far end of the weir, men in welding masks and heavy gloves were using circular saws to cut the replacement from a larger plate, sparks jetting from their blades.

Lore, standing at the rail, saw him and came down. "Sorry, Michael." She was practically yelling to make herself heard over the whine of the saws. "The timing isn't great, I know."

"What the hell, Lore?"

"Did you want her to sink? Because she would have. I'm not the one who missed it. You should be thanking me."

This was more than a delay; it was a catastrophe. Until the hull was tight, they couldn't flood the dock; until they flooded the dock, they couldn't fire the engines. Just flooding the dock would take an additional six hours. "How long do you figure to replace it?" he asked.

"To cut the plates, pull out the old ones, lower them into place, rivet, and weld, I'd say sixteen hours, minimum."

There was no reason to question her; it wasn't something that could be rushed. He turned on his heels and headed down the dock.

"Where are you going?" Lore called after him.

"To cut some fucking steel."

68

The time was 1730; the sun would set in three hours. For the moment, Peter had done all he could. He was well past the need to sleep but wanted a moment to collect himself. He thought of Jock as he walked to the house. He had no particular allegiance to the man; he had been a callow and obnoxious kid who had nearly gotten Peter killed. The rifle was probably wasted on him. But Peter recognized that day on the roof as a turning point, and he believed in second chances.

The security detail was gone.

Peter darted up the stairs and raced into the house. "Amy?" he called.

A silence, then: "In here."

She was sitting on the bed, facing the door, hands folded neatly in her lap.

"Are you all right?" he asked.

She looked up. Her face changed; she gave him a melancholy smile. A peculiar quiet took the

room — not merely an absence of sound but something deeper, more fraught. "Yes. I'm fine." She patted the mattress. "Come sit with me."

He took a place beside her. "What is it? What's wrong?"

She took his hand, not looking at him. He sensed she was on the verge of some announcement.

"When I was in the water, I went someplace," she said. "At least, my mind did. I'm not sure I can explain this right. I was so happy there."

He realized what she was saying. "The farmstead."

Her eyes found his.

"I've been there, too." Strangely, he felt no surprise; the words had been waiting to be said.

"I was playing the piano."

"Yes."

"And we were together."

"Yes. We were. Just the two of us."

How good to say it, to speak the words. To know that he was not alone with his dreams after all, that there was some reality to it, though he could not know what that reality was, only that it existed. He existed. Amy existed. The farmstead, and their happiness in that place, existed.

"You asked me this morning why I came to you in Iowa," Amy said. "I didn't tell you the truth. Or, at least, not all of it."

Peter waited.

"When you change, you get to keep one thing, one memory. Whatever was closest to your heart. From all your life, just the one." She looked up. "What I wanted to keep was you."

She was crying, just a little: small, jeweled tears that hung suspended on the tips of her lashes, like

drops of dew upon leaves. "Peter, will you do something for me?"

He nodded.

"Please kiss me."

He did. He did not so much kiss her as fall into the world of her. Time slowed, stopped, moved in an unhurried circle around them, like waves around a pier. He felt at peace. His senses were soaring. His mind was in two places, this world and also the other: the world of the farmstead, a place beyond space, beyond time, where only the two of them resided.

They parted. Their faces were inches apart. Amy cupped his cheek, her eyes locked on his.

"I'm sorry, Peter."

The remark was strange. Her gaze deepened.

"I know what you're planning to do," she said. "You wouldn't survive it."

Something came undone inside him. All strength drained from his body. He tried to speak but couldn't.

"You're tired," Amy said.

She caught him as he fell.

Amy laid him on the bed. In the outer room, she pulled her frock over her head and replaced it with the clothing that Greer had fetched for her: heavy canvas pants with pockets, leather boots, a tan shirt, the sleeves torn away, with the insignia of the Expeditionary on the shoulders. They possessed a warm, human odor — a smell of work, of life. Whoever had owned these articles was small; the fit was nearly perfect. On the back porch the soldiers slept soundly, like babies, hands tucked under their cheeks, lost to all cares. Amy gently relieved one of his pistol and tucked it into her

trousers, against her spine.

A deep quiet held the street, everyone in hiding, bracing for the storm. As Amy made her way toward the center of town, soldiers began to take notice, yet none spoke to her; their minds were elsewhere, what did one woman matter? The exterior of the stockade was unguarded. Amy strode purposefully to the door and stepped inside.

She counted three men. Behind the counter, the officer in charge glanced up.

"Help you, soldier?"

The sound of tumblers: Alicia raised her eyes. Amy?

"Hello, sister."

Alicia looked past her but saw no one; Amy was alone.

"What are you doing here?" she asked.

Amy was unlocking the shackles. She handed Alicia her goggles. "I'll explain on the way."

In the outer room, the guards lay asleep on the floor. Following Greer's directions, Amy and Alicia made their way via backstreets and trash-strewn alleys into H-town. Soon the southern wall rose into view. Amy entered a small house, little more than a hut. There was no furniture at all. In the main room, she drew a threadbare rug aside to reveal a hatch with a ladder. One of the trade's stash houses, Amy explained, though Alicia had already figured that out. They descended into a cool, damp space that smelled of rotten fruit.

"There," Amy said, pointing.

The shelves, stocked with liquor, pulled away to reveal a tunnel. At the far end they came to another ladder and, ten feet up, a metal hatch set

into concrete. Amy turned the ring and pushed.

They were outside the city, a hundred yards outside the wall in a copse of trees. Soldier and a second horse were tied up, obliviously grazing. As Alicia climbed free of the hatch, Soldier raised his head: *Ah. There you are. I was beginning to wonder.*

Her sword and bandoliers were hanging from the saddle. Alicia strapped on her blades while Amy covered the hatch with brush.

"You should be the one to ride him," Alicia said. She was also holding out the sword.

Amy considered this. "All right," she said.

She angled the sword over her shoulders and swung up onto Soldier's back. Alicia mounted the second horse, a dark bay stallion, quite young but with a fierce look to him. It was late afternoon, the sun harsh and white.

They rode away.

The dream of the farmstead was different. Peter was lying in bed. The room was full of moonlight, making the walls seem to glow. The sheets were cold; it was this coldness that had aroused him. He had a sense of having slept a long time.

Amy's side of the bed was empty.

He called her name. His voice sounded weak in the darkness, barely a presence. He rose and went to the window. Amy was standing in the yard, facing away from the house. Her posture meant something; panic surged in his heart. She began to walk — away from the house, away from him and the life they had known, her figure silhouetted by the moonlight, growing smaller. Peter could neither move nor cry out. He felt as if his soul were being wrenched from his body. *Don't leave me, Amy . . .*

626

He awoke with a start; his heart was pounding, his body glazed with sweat. Apgar's face swam into focus.

"Mr. President, something has happened."

He didn't have to say the rest. Peter knew at once. Amy was gone.

■ ■ ■ ■

IX
THE TRAP

■ ■ ■ ■

Blood ran in torrents, drenched was all the
    earth,
As Trojans and their alien helpers died.
Here were men lying quelled by bitter death
All up and down the city in their blood.

— QUINTUS SMYRNAEUS,
The Fall of Troy

69

The saws had silenced; the steel had been cut. On the ship's starboard flank, a gaping hole revealed the hidden decks and passageways within. The sun was receding, sparkling over the channel's waters; the spotlights had been lit.

Rand was operating the crane. From the floor of the dock, Michael watched the first plate descending in its cradle. Voices volleyed through the dock, more from up on deck, where Lore commanded.

The required height was achieved. Men scurried over the surface, hammers and pneumatic guns swaying from their belts; others guided the plate from inside. With a clang, the huge steel sheet made contact. Michael ascended the stairs and crossed the gangway to the deck.

"So far so good," Lore said.

They were, improbably, on schedule. The passing hours were like a funnel, drawing them down to a single moment. Every decision was binding; there would be no second chances.

Lore went to the rail and yelled down a barrage of orders, trying to make her voice heard over the roar of the generators and the whine of the guns; Michael moved beside her. The first plate lay flush against the side. They had six more to go.

"Want to know how they did it?"

Lore looked at him strangely.

"How the passengers killed themselves."

He had not meant to raise the subject. It seemed to have arisen of its own accord, one more secret he wanted to be rid of.

"Okay."

"They'd saved some fuel. Not much but enough. They sealed the doors and rerouted the engine's exhaust back into the ship's ventilation. It would have been like falling asleep."

Lore's face showed no expression. Then, with a small nod: "I'm glad you said something."

"Maybe I shouldn't have."

"Don't apologize."

He realized why he had told her. If it came to that, they could do the same thing.

70

The light was leaving them.

Runners had begun to move; from the command post on the catwalk, Peter felt, with cold clarity, the thinness of their defense. A six-mile perimeter, men without training, an enemy like no other, lacking all fear.

Though Apgar said nothing on the subject, Peter could read the man's thoughts. Maybe Amy had gone with Alicia to give herself up; maybe the dracs wouldn't come, after all. Maybe they would anyway; maybe that was the point. He remembered his dream: the image of Amy in the moonlight, walking away, not looking back. All that kept him going was the certainty of what lay ahead in the next few hours. He had a role to play, and he would play it.

Chase arrived on the platform. Peter almost didn't recognize his chief of staff. The man was dressed in an officer's uniform, though the insignia had been removed, cut away roughly as if in a hurry, perhaps out of respect; he was toting a rifle, trying to seem a certain way with it. The gun looked like it had been hanging over a fireplace for years. Peter was about to say something, then stopped himself. Apgar raised a skeptical eyebrow, but that was the extent of it.

"Where's Olivia?" Peter asked finally.

"In the president's hardbox." Chase seemed uncertain. "I hope that's all right."

The three men listened as the stations called in. All stood ready, braced for attack. The shadows lengthened over the valley. It was a beautiful evening in summer, the clouds ripening with color.

71

Amy did not have to know the place. The place, she knew, would come to her.

They galloped away from the sun, the ground flying beneath them. Dust rose in a gritty cloud; clods of dirt flew up from the horses' hooves. A certain feeling built within her. It magnified with every mile, like a radio signal growing stronger, calling them forward. Soldier's gait was powerful and smooth. *You have taken wonderful care of our friend,* Amy told him. *How brave you are, how strong. You will always be remembered. Green fields await you; you will spend a noble eternity among your kind.*

Soldier's gallop faded to a walk. They brought their horses to a halt and dismounted. The rich foam of his efforts boiled from Soldier's mouth;

633

his dark flanks flashed with sweat.

"Here," Amy said.

Alicia nodded but said nothing; Amy detected within her friend an edge of fear. She stepped away and stood in silence, waiting. The wind moved by her ears, through her hair, then faded to nothing. All seemed frozen, sealed in a great calm. The day's last minutes ticked away. On the ground before her, her shadow stretched — longer, longer. She felt the moment of the sun's union with the earth, its first touch upon the line of hills, audible, like a sigh. She closed her eyes and sent her mind diving into darkness; the ripples widened on the lake's tranquil surface high above.

Anthony, I'm here.

First, silence. Then:

Yes, Amy. They are ready. They are yours.

Night was falling.

Come to me, she thought.

Night fell.

72

They were called dopeys. But in their lives, they had been many things.

They hailed from every quarter of the continent, every state and city. Seattle, Washington. Albuquerque, New Mexico. Mobile, Alabama. The toxic chemical swamp of New Orleans and the windswept flatlands of Kansas City and the icebound canyons of Chicago. As a body, they were a statistician's dream, a perfect representative sampling of the inhabitants of the Great North American Empire. They came from farms and small towns, faceless suburbs and sprawling metropolises; they were every color and creed;

they had lived in trailers, houses, apartments, mansions with views of the sea. In their human states, each had occupied a discrete and private self. They had hoped, hated, loved, suffered, sung, and wept. They had known loss. They had surrounded and comforted themselves with objects. They had driven automobiles. They had walked dogs and pushed children on swing sets and waited in line at the grocery store. They had said stupid things. They had kept secrets, nurtured grudges, blown upon the embers of regret. They had worshipped a variety of gods or no god at all. They had awakened in the night to the sound of rain. They had apologized. They had attended various ceremonies. They had explained the history of themselves to psychologists, priests, lovers, and strangers in bars. They had, at unexpected moments, experienced bolts of joy so unalloyed, so untethered to events, that they seemed to come from above; they had longed to be known and, sometimes, almost were.

Heirs to the viral lineage of Anthony Carter, Twelfth of Twelve, they were intrinsically less bloodthirsty than their counterparts; it had been remarked many times by human observers that the dopeys satisfied their appetites with an attitude of joyless obligation, and that it was this characteristic, singular among virals, that made them easier to kill. *Dumb as a dopey* was the phrase. This was true, while also concealing a deeper truth. Indeed they did not like it; the butchery of innocents disturbed them. Yet within them lay an unexpressed ferocity, unwitnessed by humankind. For more than a century they had waited, anticipating the day when the call would come to release this hidden power.

In their lives, they had been many things. Then they were another. Now they were an army.

First in twilight, then in blackness, beneath the Texas stars, they roared west, a wall of noise and dust. At the head of the pod, like the point of a spear, a pair of riders led the way. For Alicia, the sensation was one of pure momentum; she was leading as much as she was being led, joined to a primal force. For Amy, the feeling was one of expansion, an internal amassing of souls. The moment Carter had surrendered his forces to her command, they had ceased to be external entities. They had become extensions of her awareness and her will: her Many.

Come with me. Come with me come with me come with me . . .

Ahead, like lights upon a distant shore, the besieged city appeared.

"Weapons up!"

All along the catwalk, the snap of magazines, the clack of bolts, rounds hammering into chambers. The last shadows were gone, drowned in the gloom.

It didn't take long.

A glowing line appeared to the east. Second by second it thickened, spreading over the land. A feeling of fate, of destiny: it hung like a fog. The city seemed meager in its face.

"Here they come!"

The horde rumbled toward them. Its speed was tremendous. Random shots split the air — men adrenalized with terror who could not restrain the urge to fire their weapons.

Peter pressed the radio to his mouth. "Hold your fire! Wait till they're in range!"

The stars were disappearing, blotted out by the great dust cloud that ascended in the virals' wake. The pod had taken the form of an arrowlike wedge.

"Looks like the negotiation phase is over," Apgar said.

More panicked shots; the pod kept coming. They would drive straight through the gate, splitting it like a bull's-eye.

"Hang on a second," Apgar said. He was watching through binoculars. "Something's off."

"What are you seeing?"

He hesitated, then said, "They're moving differently. Short leaps, long strides in between, like the older ones do." He pulled the lenses away. "I think these are dopeys."

Something was happening. The pod was decelerating.

From the spotting platform, a cry went up: "Riders! Two hundred yards!"

Prepare yourselves.

Amy slowed Soldier to a canter, then a trot.

We will defend this city. We will hold this gate, my brothers and sisters of blood.

Flowing like a liquid, her forces spread. Amy moved among them. She dared not show fear; her courage would be theirs. She rode with her back erect, Soldier's reins held lightly in one hand, the other extended in a gesture of blessing, like a priest.

They were people once, like you. But they follow another, the Zero.

A thousand long, three hundred deep, Amy's forces formed a protective barrier along the northern wall and turned to face the field. To the

east, the first edge of moon was peeking above the hills.

Do not hesitate, for they will not. Kill them, my brothers and sisters, but always with a blessing of mercy in your heart.

She felt the eyes of the soldiers upon her, the posts and crosshairs of their guns. The great dust cloud was settling. A taste of grit was in her mouth.

Stand tall. Have courage. Show him who and what you are.

They brought their horses to a halt at the front of the line. Amy removed the pistol from her belt, passed it to Alicia, and drew the sword from over her back. The grip possessed a satisfying thickness, comfortable in the hand. She rocked her wrist to turn its blade in the air.

"This is a fine weapon, sister."

"I was sort of guessing when I made it."

Her mind was composed, her thoughts ordered and calm. There was fear, but also relief and, on top of this, curiosity about what would come.

"I've never gone into battle," she said. "What is it like?"

"It's very . . . busy."

Amy considered this.

"Things happen fast. You won't even be aware of them until later. Most will seem like they happened to somebody else."

"I suppose that makes a lot of sense." Then: "Alicia, if I don't survive —"

"One other thing."

"What's that?"

Alicia met her eye. "You're not allowed to say things like that."

■ ■ ■ ■

On the rampart, chaos reigned. Runners were dashing, fingers were twitching on triggers, nobody knew what to do. *Hold fire? They're virals! And why are they facing the wrong direction?*

"I mean it," Peter barked into the radio, "all stations, stand down now!" He tossed Apgar the radio and turned to the closest runner. "Private, get me a harness."

"Peter, you are *not* going out there," Apgar said.

"Amy can protect me. You can see it for yourself. They're here to defend us."

"I don't care if they're here to fix the plumbing — you've lost your goddamn mind. Do not make me tackle you, because I will absolutely do that."

The soldier darted his eyes to Peter, then the general, then back again. "Sir, should I get the harness or not?"

"Private, you take one step and I'm going to pitch you over that wall," Apgar said.

Another cry from the spotter: "We have movement! The riders are moving away!"

Peter looked up. "What do you mean *away?*"

A face floated over the rail. A quick conferral with someone behind him, then the man pointed due north. "Across the field, sir!"

Peter stepped back to the edge of the rampart and raised his binoculars. "Gunnar, are you seeing this?"

"What are they doing?" Apgar said. "Are they surrendering?"

With a puff of dust, Amy and Alicia brought their horses to a halt. Amy drew and raised the

sword. It was not a gesture of capitulation but defiance.

They were setting themselves as bait.

"Fanning, do you hear me?!"

Amy's words dwindled into the gloom.

"If you want me, come and get me!"

"Should we go further out?" Alicia asked.

"If we do, we might not make it back." Then, raising her voice again: "Are you listening? I'm right here, you bastard!"

Alicia waited. Still nothing. Then:

You have done well, Alicia.

She pressed her hands over her ears, a pointless reflex; Fanning's voice was inside her.

Everything I could have wished for, you have accomplished. Her army is nothing, I can whisk it away. You have given me that, and so much more.

"Shut up! Leave me alone!"

Amy was staring at her. "Lish, what is it? Is it Fanning?"

Do you feel it, Alicia? Fanning's voice was smooth, taunting. It was like an oily liquid spreading through her brain. *Of course you do. You always could. Haunting the streets, counting heads. They are a part of you as I am a part of you.*

Alicia heard the sound then. No, not heard: sensed. A kind of . . . scratching. Where was it coming from?

She must come to me in ruins. That will be the truest test. To feel what I feel. What we feel, my Alicia. To know despair. A world without hope, without purpose, everything lost.

"Alicia, tell me what's happening."

I know your dreams, Alicia. The great walled city and its sounds of life within. The music and the

640

happy cries of children. Your longing to be among them, and the door you cannot enter. Did you know even then, Alicia? Did you know what lay in store?

The sound grew more intense. The blood was throbbing in her neck; she thought she might be ill.

My Alicia, it is already done. Can you feel it? Can you feel . . . them?

Her mind slammed back to awareness. She turned in her saddle. Beyond the barrier of Amy's army, the lights of the city shone.

Outside, she thought. I'm outside, just like in the dream.

"Oh, God, no."

Sara was trying to make herself breathe.

A hundred and twenty souls were crammed in the basement. Candles and lanterns, spread throughout the space, cast odd, animated shadows. Sara's pistol lay in her lap, her hand upon it, loose but ready.

Jenny and Hannah had organized a game of duck, duck, goose to distract some of the children. Others were occupying themselves with smuggled toys. A few were crying, though probably they did not know why; they were channeling the anxiety of the adults.

Sara was sitting on the floor with her back against the door. Its metal face was cool against her skin. Would it hold? Various scenes unfolded in her mind: pounding on the door, the metal bulging, everyone screaming, backing away, then the final crack and death pouring in, engulfing them all.

She was watching Jenny and Hannah. Jenny was terrified — the woman wore her emotions like a

coat — but Hannah had a steady streak in her. It was she who had initiated the game. There were people, Sara knew, who were like this, the ones who could not be ruffled or else didn't show it, who possessed great internal reservoirs of calm. Hannah was racing around the circle on her long legs, grinning with conspiracy, pursued by a little boy. Hannah was going to let him catch her, of course; she made a stagy show of her surrender that sent the boy into a fit of happy giggles, which, for a moment, put Sara at ease. She remembered such games, how much fun they were, their object so simple and pure. She had played duck, duck, goose as a girl, then, later, with Kate and her friends. But in the next instant, this thought was replaced by another. Kate, she thought, Kate, where are you, where have you gone? Your body lies in a bed far from home; your spirit has flown. I am lost without you. Lost.

"Dr. Wilson, are you okay?"

Holding Carlos, Grace was standing above her. Sara touched her tears away. "How's he doing?"

"He's a baby — he doesn't know anything."

Sara made a place beside her; Grace lowered herself to the floor.

"Are we going to be safe here?" Grace asked.

"Sure."

A silence; then Grace shrugged. "You're lying, but that's okay. I just wanted to hear you say it." She turned her face toward Sara. "You were the one who transferred your birthright to my parents, weren't you?"

"I guess they told you."

"Just that it was the doctor. I don't see any other women doctors around the place, though, so I figured it had to be you. Why did you do it?"

There was probably an answer, but Sara couldn't think of it. "It just felt like the thing to do."

"My folks were good to me. Things weren't easy, but they loved me as well as anyone could. We always said a prayer for you at supper. I thought you should know."

From baby Carlos, a yawn; sleep was near. For a minute or so, Sara and Grace watched the game together. Suddenly Grace looked up.

"What's that noise?"

"Station six. We have movement."

Peter grabbed the radio. "Say again."

"Not sure." A pause. "Looks like it's gone now."

Station 6 was at the south end of the dam.

"Everyone, maintain readiness!" Apgar yelled. "Hold your positions!"

Peter barked into the mike: "What are you seeing?"

A crackle, and then the voice said, "Forget it, I was wrong."

Peter looked at Chase. "What's below station six?"

"Just scrub."

"Enough for cover?"

"Some."

Peter took up the radio again. "Station six, report. What did you see?"

"I'm telling you, it's nothing," the voice repeated. "Looks like just another sinkhole opening up."

From his post on the roof of the orphanage, Caleb Jaxon did not hear the sound so much as feel it: a disturbance lacking a discernible source, as if the air were bristling with a swarm of invisible

bees. He scanned the city with his binoculars. All seemed ordinary, unchanged, yet as his mind stilled, he became aware of other sounds, coming from several directions. The crack of wood splintering. The crash and tinkle of fracturing glass. A rumble, lasting perhaps five seconds, of an unknown type. Around him, and on the ground below, some of his men had begun to sense these things as well; their conversations halted, one man or the other saying, *Do you hear that? What* is *that?* Eyes burning from lack of sleep, Caleb peered into the darkness. From the roof, he had a clear view of the capitol building and the city's central square. The hospital was four blocks east.

He unhitched his radio from his belt. "Hollis, are you there?" His father-in-law was stationed at the entrance to the hospital.

"Yeah."

Another crash. It came from deep within the streets of the city. "Are you hearing this?"

A gap, then Hollis said: "Roger that."

"What are you seeing? Any movement?"

"Negative."

Caleb brought his binoculars to bear on the capitol. A pair of trucks and a long table remained in the square, left behind when the inductions were complete. He took up the radio again. "Sister, can you hear me?"

Sister Peg was waiting by the hatch. "Yes, Lieutenant."

"I'm not sure, but I think something's going on out here."

A pause. "Thank you for telling me, Lieutenant Jaxon."

He clipped the radio to his belt. His grip on his rifle tightened reflexively. Though he knew a

644

round was seated in the chamber, he gently drew back the charging handle to double-check. Through the tiny window, the brass casing gleamed.

The radio crackled: Hollis. "Caleb, come back."

"What have you got?"

"Something's out there."

Caleb's heart accelerated. "Where?"

"Headed for the square, northwest corner."

Caleb pressed the binoculars to his brow again. With vexing slowness, the square came into focus. "I'm not seeing anything."

"It was there a second ago."

Still scanning, Caleb lifted the radio to his mouth to call the command platform.

"Station one, this is station nine . . ."

He stopped in mid-sentence; his vision had grazed something. He swept the lenses back the way they'd come.

The table in the square had been overturned; behind it, the nose of one of the trucks was pointed upward at a forty-five degree angle, its rear wheels sunk deep into the earth.

A sinkhole. A big one, opening up.

Peter turned away from the battlefield. The buildings of the city were shapes against the dark, lit by angled moonlight.

Chase was beside him. "What is it?"

The feeling prickled his skin like static electricity: all eyes. "There's something we're not seeing." He held up a hand. "Hang on. Did you hear that?"

"Hear what?" Apgar's eyes narrowed as he cocked his head "Wait. Yeah."

"Like . . . rats inside walls."

"I hear it, too," Chase said.

Peter grabbed the mike. "Station six, anything out there?"

Nothing.

"Station six, report."

Sister Peg stepped into the kitchen pantry. The rifle was stashed on the top shelf, wrapped in oilcloth. It had belonged to her brother, rest his soul; he had served with the Expeditionary, years ago. She remembered the day the soldier had arrived at the orphanage with the news of his death. He had brought her brother's locker of effects. Nobody had checked the contents, or else the rifle would have been taken back into inventory. Or so Sister Peg had supposed at the time. Most of the belongings in her brother's locker contained no trace of him and did not seem worth keeping. But not his gun. Her brother had held it, used it, fought with it; it stood for what he was. It was more than a remembrance; it was a gift, as if he'd left it behind so that someday she would have it when she needed it.

She moved the ladder into place and, with gingerly steps, brought the gun down and placed it on the table where the sisters kneaded bread. Sister Peg had cared for the weapon meticulously; the action was tight and well lubed. She liked the way it fired, with a decisive trigger and a good, clean snap. Once a year, in May — the month of her brother's death — Sister Peg would remove her frock, don the clothes of an ordinary worker, and take the transport out to the Orange Zone. The rifle rode beside her, concealed in a duffel bag. Beyond the windbreak she would set up a target of cans, sometimes apples or a melon, or

sheets of marked paper nailed to a tree.

She carried the rifle, now loaded, to the dining hall. Over the years the gun had grown heavier in her arms, but she could still manage it, including the recoil, which was dampened by a buffer tube with a spring connected to the pad. This was very important for follow-up shots. She chose a position by the hatch with a clear view of the hallway and the windows on either side of the room.

She thought she should take a moment to pray. But, as she was holding a loaded rifle, conventional prayer did not seem entirely suitable. Sister Peg hoped that God would help her, but it was her belief that He much preferred for people to attend to themselves. Life was a test; it was up to you to pass it or not. She raised the gun to her clavicle and angled one eye down the length of the barrel.

"Not my children," she said and pulled the charging handle, snapping the first round into the chamber. "Not tonight."

"Rider inbound!"

A tense new energy shivered along the rampart. Something was shifting. The viral barrier parted, forming a corridor like the one the previous night. Down this hallway a single rider galloped toward them. All along the catwalk, eyes took purchase upon the posts and slots of gunsights; gathering pressure flowed from shoulders to forearms to the padded tips of index fingers. The order to hold fire was clear, yet the urge to do otherwise was strong. Still the rider kept on coming. Raised in the saddle, this person — the gender was as yet unknowable — was yelling incomprehensible words. While one hand clutched the reins, the

other swayed in the air over the rider's head, a gesture of ambiguous meaning. Was it a threat? A plea for forbearance?

On the command platform, Peter understood what was about to happen. The inductees had no experience; they lacked the mental muscle memory of military training; they existed in only the most general way within a chain of command. The second Alicia reached the lighted perimeter, he would lose control of the situation. "Hold your fire!" he was yelling. "Don't shoot!" But words went only so far.

Alicia hit the lighted perimeter at a full gallop. "It's a trap!"

Her words made no sense to him.

She pulled up, skidding to a halt. "It's a trap! They're inside!"

A shout came from Peter's left: "It's that woman from last night!"

"She's a viral!"

"Shoot her!"

The first bullet speared Alicia's right thigh, shattering her femur; the second caught her in the left lung. The horse's front legs folded, sending her pitching forward over its neck. The first pops became a full-throated barrage. Dust kicked up around her as she crawled behind the fallen animal, which now lay riddled and dead. Shots were connecting. Bullets were finding their mark. Alicia experienced them like a fusillade of punches. Her left palm, speared like an apple. The ilium of her right pelvis, shrapnelized like an exploding grenade. Two more to the chest, the second of which ricocheted off her fourth rib, plunged diagonally through her thoracic cavity, and cracked her second lumbar vertebrae. She did

648

her best to shove herself beneath the fallen horse. Blood splashed from its flesh as the bullets pounded.

Lost, she thought, as a curtain of darkness fell. *Everything is lost.*

The majority of virals emerged inside the city at four points: the central square, the southeast corner of the impoundment, a large sinkhole in H-town, and the staging area inside the main gate. Others had piloted their way through the pocketed earth to emerge in smaller pods throughout the city. The floors of houses; abandoned lots, weedy and untended, where children had once played; the streets of densely packed neighborhoods. They dug and crawled. They traced the sewage and water lines. They were clever; they sought the weakest points. For months they had moved through the geological and man-made fissures beneath the city like an infestation of ants.

Go now, their master ordered. *Fulfill your purpose. Do that which I've commanded.*

On the catwalk, Peter did not have long to consider Alicia's words of warning. Amid the roar of guns — many of the soldiers, gripped by the frenzy of a mob, were firing upon the dopeys as well — the structure lurched under him. It was as if the metal grate beneath his feet were a carpet that had been lifted and shaken at one end. The sensation shot to his stomach, a swirl of nausea, like seasickness. He looked side to side, searching for the source of this motion, simultaneously becoming aware that he was hearing screams. A second lurch and the structure jolted downward. His balance failed; knocked backward, he fell to the floor of the catwalk. Guns were blasting, voices

yelling. Bullets whizzed over his face. *The gate,* someone cried, *they're opening the gate! Shoot them! Shoot those fuckers!* A groan of bending metal, and the catwalk began to tip away from the wall.

He was rolling toward the edge.

He had no way to stop himself; his hands found nothing to grab. Bodies tumbled past, launching into the dark. As he rolled over the lip, one hand seized slick metal: a support strut. His body swung around it like a pendulum. He would not be able to hold on; he had merely paused. Beneath him, the city spun, lit with screams and gunfire.

"Take my hand!"

It was Jock. He had lodged himself under the rail, one arm dangling over the edge. The catwalk had paused at a forty-five-degree angle to the ground.

"Grab on!"

A series of pops: the last bolts were yanking free of the wall. Jock's fingertips, inches from Peter's, could have been a mile away. Time was moving in two streams. There was one, of noise and haste and violent action, and a second, coincidental with the first, in which Peter and everything around him seemed caught in a lazy current. His grip was failing. His other hand flailed uselessly, trying to grasp Jock's.

"Pull yourself up!"

Peter tore away.

"I've got you!"

Jock was gripping him by the wrist. A second face appeared under the rail: Apgar. As the man reached down, Jock heaved Peter upward; Apgar caught him by the belt. Together they hauled him the rest of the way.

The catwalk began to fall.

The slaughter had commenced.

Freed from hiding, the virals poured over the city. They swarmed the ramparts, flinging men into space. They launched from the ground and rooftops like a glowing fireworks display. They burst through the floors of hardboxes to butcher the occupants and exploded through the floors of buildings to haul the hiding inhabitants from closets and out from under their beds. They stormed the gate, which, although formidable, was not designed to repel an attack from within; all that was required to open the city to invasion was to tear the crossbars from their braces, free the brake, and push.

The pod that emerged near the impoundment was likewise charged with a specific mission. Throughout the day, their delicate sensorium had detected the footfalls of a great number of people, all headed in the same direction. They had heard the roar of vehicles and the barks of bullhorns. They had heard the word "dam." They had heard the word "shelter." They had heard the word "tubes." Those that sought a direct entry to the dam were confounded. As Chase had predicted, there was no way in. Others, like an elite assault force, homed in on a compact building nearby. This was guarded by a small contingent of soldiers, who died swiftly and badly. Jaws snapping, fingers trilling, eyes restlessly roaming, the virals took measure of the interior. The room was full of pipes. Pipes meant water; water meant the dam. A flight of stairs descended.

They arrived in a hallway with walls of sweating stone. A ladder took them deeper underground, a

second deeper still. A dense humanity lay near. They were coming closer. They were homing in.

They reached a metal door with a heavy ring. The first viral, the alpha, opened the door and slid inside, the others following.

The room was ripe with the odor of men. A row of lockers, a bench, a table bearing the remains of a hastily abandoned meal. Connected to a complex assembly of pipes and gears was a panel with six steel wheels the size of manhole covers.

Yes, said Zero. *Those.*

The alpha gripped the first wheel. INLET NO. 1 it was marked.

Turn it.

Six wheels. Six tubes.

Eight hundred dying cries.

Pistol extended, Sara approached the storage room and gently dislodged the door with her foot.

"Maybe it was just mice," Jenny whispered.

The scratching sounded again. It was coming from behind a stack of crates. Sara placed the lantern on the floor and pushed the pistol out with both hands. The crates were piled four high. One on the bottom began to move, jostling those above it.

"Sara —"

The crates went tumbling. Sara fell back as the viral burst through the floor, twisting in midair to attach itself to the ceiling like a roach. She fired the pistol blindly. The viral seemed not to care at all about the gun or else knew that Sara was too startled to aim. The pistol's slide locked back; the magazine was spent. Sara turned, shoved Jenny from the room, and began to run.

■ ■ ■ ■

At the base of the wall, Alicia, immobilized, broken, lay alone. Her breathing was labored and damp, punctuated by small, exquisitely painful hitches. Blood was in her mouth. Her vision seemed skewed; images refused to resolve. She had no sense of time at all. She might have been shot thirty seconds ago. It might have been an hour.

A dark shape materialized above her: Soldier, bowing his head to hers. *Oh, see what you've done to yourself,* he said. *I leave you for a minute and look what happens.* His warm breath kissed her face; he dipped closer, nuzzling her, exhaling softly through his nostrils.

My good boy. She raised one bloody hand to his cheek. *My great, my magnificent Soldier, I am sorry.*

"Sister, what have they done to you?"

Amy was kneeling beside her. The woman's shoulders shook with a sob; she buried her face in her hands. "Oh no," she moaned. "Oh no."

The spotlights had gone out. Alicia heard gunshots and cries, but these were distant, dimming. A merciful darkness enveloped her. Amy was holding her hand. It seemed that all that had gone before was a journey, that the road had brought her here and ended. The night slid into silence. She felt suddenly cold. She drifted away.

Wait.

Her eyes flew open. A breeze was pushing over her — dense, gritty — and with it a rumble, like thunder, though the sound did not stop. It rolled and rolled, its volume accumulating, the air swirling with windblown matter. The ground beneath

653

them began to shake; with a whinny, Soldier reared up, his hooves slashing the air.

Her army is nothing. I can whisk it away.

Alicia raised her head just in time to see them coming.

Peter, Apgar, and Jock were racing down the falling catwalk. Its failure proceeded in sections, like dominoes falling in a line. Peter's orders to fall back to the orphanage, the city's last line of defense, went unheeded; a state of panic reigned. The problem was not merely the serial collapse of the catwalk, from which soldiers were falling a hundred feet to their deaths. The virals had also stormed its length. Some men were hurled, others devoured, twitching and screaming as the virals' jaws sank home. Yet a third group were bitten and subsequently left to their own devices. As had been witnessed in the townships, Fanning's virus did its work with unprecedented swiftness; in short order, a growing percentage of Kerrville's defenders were turning on their former comrades.

A hundred yards downstream from the vanished command post, Peter, Apgar, and Jock found themselves boxed in. Behind them, the catwalk's failure continued, span by span; ahead, the virals were coming toward them. No flight of stairs lay within reach.

"Oh, hell," said Apgar. "I always hated doing this."

They unfurled the ropes over the side. Jock was no fan of heights, either; the incident on the mission roof had scarred him for life. Yet it was also true that in the last twenty-four hours a change had occurred. He had always believed himself to be a flimsy man, a chip in the current of life. But

654

since the birth of his son, and the burst of love this had produced, he had discovered within himself a solidity of character he had never thought possible, an expanding sense of life's importance and his place within its web. He wanted to be a man of whom it could be said that he had put others before himself and died in their defense. Thus the newly inducted and personally transformed Private Jock Alvado shoved his terror aside, stepped over the rail, and turned his back on the maw of space below him; Peter and Apgar did the same.

They jumped.

A hundred feet with only the friction of their hands and feet to slow them: they landed hard on the packed dirt. Peter and Apgar came up quickly, but Jock did not. He had sprained, perhaps broken, his ankle. Peter pulled him upright and threw the man's arm over his shoulder.

"Christ, you're heavy."

They ran.

The basement was a death trap.

As Sara ran for the door, a scream volleyed behind her, sharp, like metal being cut, then the room erupted in cries. She was carrying a little girl; she had scooped her up without thinking. She would have carried more if she could; she would have carried them all.

Jenny reached the door first. People were surging behind her. Suddenly the woman couldn't move; the weight of panicked bodies had immobilized her, pressing her against the metal. She was yelling for people to back away but could scarcely be heard. The shrieks of the children were like the highest notes of a scale, impossibly shrill.

The door burst open; a hundred people attempted to cram through at once. Blind instinct had taken hold — to flee, to survive whatever the cost. People were falling, children being trampled underfoot. Virals ricocheted around the room, flinging themselves from wall to wall, victim to victim. Their enjoyment was obscene. One was carrying a child in its mouth and shaking it like a dog with a rag doll. As Sara wedged through the door, a faceless woman wrenched the little girl from her arms and shoved ahead, knocking her to the floor at the base of the stairs. People were thundering past. A familiar face emerged from the chaos: Grace, holding her baby. She was huddled against the wall of the stairwell. Upstairs, guns were popping. Sara gripped the woman by the sleeve to make her look at her. *Stay with me, hold my hand.*

Jenny and Hannah were waving to her from the top of the stairs. Sara half-pulled, half-dragged Grace to the lobby. Beyond the doors, a fierce battle raged. Children were screaming, mothers were huddled with their children, no one knew where to go. A few were running blindly out the door, into the heart of it. The virals were behind them and coming up the stairs.

A huge crash: the front of the building detonated inward. Bricks, shards of glass, splintered plywood went flying. Suddenly an Army five-ton was standing in the lobby. Hollis was at the wheel.

"Everybody, get in!"

Amy covered Alicia's body with her own. Her army was dying; she felt them leaving her, souls draining into the ether. *You did not fail me,* she thought. *It was I who erred. Go peacefully — at last*

you are free.

Fanning's virals broke through. Amy buried her face against Alicia's neck, holding her close. It would happen quickly, faster than light. She thought of Peter, then of nothing at all.

It felt as if they were inside a flock of birds; as if the air around them had turned into a million flapping wings.

From the roof of the orphanage, Caleb watched the city die.

He had heard the catwalk collapse, a terrific crash. The scene before him possessed an odd quality of disconnection. It was as if he were observing events that did not wholly pertain to him, unfolding at a great remove. Though when the shooting started, he knew, he would feel differently. Twenty-five men: how long could they last?

The gunshots faded, the flash of fired rounds, the pitiable, anguished screams. The city was sliding into silence, a place of ghosts. A moment of stunning quiet; then a new sound accumulated. Caleb pressed his eyes to the binoculars. An Army five-ton, draped in canvas, was roaring toward them from the square, flanked by a pair of Humvees. The men on the turrets were firing wildly, others shooting through the windows of the cab. Simultaneously Caleb became aware of a second, more compact movement to his right. He swung his lenses around. Impenetrable darkness; then two figures appeared. A third man was being carried.

Apgar.

His father.

They would intersect with the truck near the

front of the building. Caleb's feet barely touched the ladder as he descended. One of the Humvees veered away from the other vehicles; virals were clinging to it. It crashed onto its side and began to roll, like an animal trying to shake off a swarm of hornets. The five-ton was moving too quickly; it was going to crash into the building. At the last second, the driver cut the wheel to the left and screeched to a stop.

Hollis leapt from the cab, Sara from the bed. Everyone was grabbing children and hauling them through the door. Caleb vaulted over the sandbags and raced toward his father and the general.

"Take him," his father said.

Caleb threaded an arm around the injured man's back. The situation took shape in Caleb's mind: the orphanage would be their final stand. In the dining room, Sister Peg waited by the open hatch. The woman was holding a rifle. The sight was so odd that Caleb's mind simply rejected it. "Hurry!" Sister Peg yelled. His father and Apgar were ordering men to take positions at the windows. Hands reached up through the opening in the floor to help the children, who funneled into the hatch with a slowness painfully out of sync with everything else that was occurring. People were pushing and shoving, women screaming, babies crying. Caleb smelled gasoline. An empty fuel can lay on its side on the floor, a second by the pantry door. Their presence made no sense — it was in the same category of unaccountable details as Sister Peg's rifle. Men were hurling dining chairs through the windows. Others were upending tables to act as barricades. All the things of the world were colliding. Caleb took a position at the closest window, pointed his rifle into the

darkness, and began to fire.

For Peter Jaxon, last president of the Texas Republic, the final seconds of the night were nothing he had anticipated. Once the catwalk had begun its collapse, and the nature of the situation had become clear to him, he wholly intended to die. This was the only honorable outcome he could foresee. Amy was gone, his friends were gone, the city was gone, and he had only himself to blame. Surviving Kerrville's destruction would be an unthinkable disgrace.

The last of the civilians had descended through the hatch, but would the door hold? Judging from the events of the last ten minutes, Peter could only conclude that, like everything else, it was bound to fail. Fanning, however he'd done it, knew everything.

Still, one had to try. Symbolism counted for something, as Apgar had said. The virals were amassing outside; they would storm the building as a horde. Still firing from the window, Peter ordered the men to fall back to the shelter; they had nothing left to defend except themselves. Many were out of ammo, anyway. A final shot from Peter's rifle and the charger locked back. He cast the gun aside and drew his pistol.

"Mr. President, time to go."

Apgar was standing behind him.

"I thought you were calling me Peter now."

"I mean it. You need to get down that hole right now."

Peter squeezed off a round. Maybe he connected, maybe not. "I'm not going anywhere."

Peter would never be sure what Apgar had hit him with. The butt of his pistol? The leg of a

broken chair? A thud at the back of his skull and his legs melted, followed by the rest of him.

"Caleb," he heard Apgar say, "help me get your father out of here."

His body lacked all volition; his thoughts were like slick ice, impossible to hold. He was being dragged, then lifted, then lowered once again. He felt, oddly, like a child, and this feeling morphed into a memory — an impossible memory, in which he was a little boy again, not merely a boy but an infant, being passed from hand to hand. He saw faces above him. They floated enormously, their features bloated and vague. He was being laid upon a wooden platform. A single face came into focus: his son's. But Caleb wasn't a boy anymore, he was a man, and the situation had reversed. Caleb was the father and he the son, or so it seemed. It was a pleasant inversion, inevitable in its way, and Peter felt happy that he had lived long enough to see this.

"It's all right, Dad," Caleb said, "you're safe now."

And then the light went out.

Apgar slammed the hatch and listened as the bolts sealed from inside.

"You could have gone," said Sister Peg.

"So could you." He rose and looked at her. Everything felt suddenly calm. "The gas was a good idea."

"I thought so, too."

"Ready?"

Sounds above: the virals were tearing through the roof. Apgar lifted a rifle from the floor, checked the magazine, and shoved it back into the well. Sister Peg withdrew the box of matches from

the pocket of her tunic. She struck one, tossed it. A river of blue flame snaked along the floor, then separated, running in several directions.

"Shall we?" Apgar said.

They walked briskly down the hall. Thick smoke was boiling up. At the door they halted.

"You know," said Sister Peg, "I think I'll stay after all."

His eyes searched her face.

"I think it's best this way," she explained. "To be . . . with them."

Of course that's what she would want. To affirm his understanding, Apgar cupped her chin, leaned his face forward, and kissed her lightly on the lips.

"Well," she managed. Tears rose to her throat. She had never been kissed by a grown man before. "I didn't expect that."

"I hope you didn't mind."

"You always were a lovely boy."

"That's nice of you to say."

She took his hands and held them. "God bless and keep you, Gunnar."

"And you as well, Sister."

Then he was gone.

She faded back into the hall. In the dining room, flames were leaping up the walls; the smoke was dense and swirling. Sister Peg began to cough. She lay down on the hatch. Her time in the physical world was ending. She had no fear of what would come, the hand of love into which her spirit would pass. Fire took the building in its grip. The flames shot up, consuming all. As the smoke snaked inside her, Sister Peg's mind filled up with faces. Faces by the hundreds, the thousands. Her children. She would be with them again.

All around the building, the virals were watch-

ing. They stood in abeyance, the glow of the flames glazing their denuded faces. They had been vanquished; fire was a barrier they could not cross. Still they waited, ever hopeful. The hours passed. The building burned and burned and burned some more. The embers were still glowing when dawn came, a blade of light sweeping over the silent city.

■ ■ ■ ■

X
THE EXODUS

■ ■ ■ ■

To war and arms I fly.

— RICHARD LOVELACE,
To Lucasta, Going to the Wars

"Greer."

He was dead to the world. In a different one, a voice was calling his name.

"Lucius, wake up."

He jerked to consciousness. He was sitting in the cab of the tanker. Patch was standing on the running board by the open door. Through the windshield, a foggy dawn.

"What time is it?" His mouth was dry.

"Oh-six-thirty."

"You should have woken me up."

"What do you think I just did?"

Greer stepped down. The water was still, birds swooping low over its glassy surface. "Anything happen while I was asleep?"

Patch shrugged in his wiry way. "Nothing major. Just before sunrise, we saw a small pod working its way down the shore."

"Where?"

"Base of the channel bridge."

Greer frowned. "And this didn't strike you as important?"

"They never came all that close. It didn't seem worth the trouble to wake you."

Greer got in his truck and drove down the

isthmus. Lore was standing on the dock, hands perched on her hips, studying the hull. The repair was nearing completion.

"How long till we fill?" he asked.

"Three, maybe four hours." She raised her voice. "Rand! Watch that chain!"

"Where is he?" Greer asked.

"Quonset hut, I think."

He found Michael sitting at the shortwave.

"Kerrville, come back, please. This is Isthmus station." A momentary pause and he repeated the call.

"Anything?" Greer asked.

Michael shook his head. His expression was blank, his mind far away in worry.

"I have some other news. A viral pod was sighted near the bridge a while ago."

Michael turned sharply. "Did they approach?"

"Patch says no."

Michael sat back. He rubbed his face with a heavy hand. "So they know we're here."

"It would seem so."

The bolts were still too hot to touch. Peter was standing on the platform just below the hatch. His mind had cleared, but his headache felt like an ice pick buried in the back of his skull.

"It's got to be light out," Sara said. "What should we do?"

Caleb and Hollis were there as well. Peter scanned their faces; both wore the same expression: of weariness and defeat, the power of decision beyond them. None had slept a wink.

"Wait, I guess."

An hour or so passed. Peter was dozing on the platform when he heard knocking on the hatch.

He reached up to touch the surface; the metal had cooled somewhat. He removed his jersey and wrapped it around his hands; beside him, Caleb did the same. They each took a lever and turned. Cracks of daylight appeared at the edges and, with them, a strong smell of smoke. Water dripped through. They pushed the hatch open the rest of the way.

Chase was standing over them, holding a bucket. His face was black with soot. Peter climbed the ladder, the others following. They emerged into a scene of ruin. The orphanage was gone, reduced to a smoldering wreckage of ashes and collapsed beams. The heat was still intense. Behind Peter's chief of staff stood a group of seven: three soldiers of diverse ranks and four civilians, including a teenage girl and a man who had to be at least seventy. All were holding buckets, their clothes sodden, arms and faces black as coal. They had wetted down a path through the ashes, clearing a way out of the destruction. The fire had leapt to several adjacent buildings, which were burning to various degrees.

"It's good to see you, Mr. President."

As with everyone who had survived the night, Chase's survival was a story of luck and timing. When the catwalk had begun to fail, he had just stepped away from the command deck in search of more ammunition. This placed him near the stairs on the west side of the gate. He had made it to the bottom just in time to see the whole thing come crashing to the ground. Two soldiers had recognized him; they'd hustled him into a truck to get him to the president's hardbox, but they hadn't made it very far before they were attacked,

the driver yanked through the windshield. As the vehicle rolled, Chase was thrown clear. His rifle empty and the hardbox far out of reach, he had run for the closest building, a small wood-framed house that the tax office used for storage. Among the boxes of meaningless paperwork, he was joined over the next two hours by the seven survivors with whom he now stood. For the rest of the night they had remained there, trying not to attract attention to themselves, waiting for an end that never came.

Since daybreak, more survivors had emerged, but not very many. The sight of so many bodies was jarring, sickening. The vultures had begun to alight, pecking at the meat. It was nothing for the children to see. During the night, Sara had counted heads. The shelter contained 654 souls, mostly women and children. Sara descended the ladder to help Jenny organize their removal.

"What about the other hardboxes?" Peter asked.

Chase's face was grim. "They got in through the floors."

"Olivia?"

Chase shook his head.

"I'm sorry, Ford."

He shook his head faintly. None of this was registering completely yet.

"What about the tubes?"

"Flooded. I don't know how they did it, but they did."

Peter's stomach dropped; a wave of cold dizziness passed through him.

"Peter?" Chase was gripping his arm; suddenly, he was the strong one.

"No survivors?" Peter asked.

Chase shook his head. "There's something else

you need to see."

It was Apgar. The man was alive, though barely. He lay on the ground beside an overturned Humvee. His legs were crushed beneath the frame, though that was not the worst of it; on his left hand, which lay across his chest, was a semicircular imprint of teeth. He was still in the shade, but the sun would soon find him.

Peter knelt beside him. "Gunnar, can you hear me?"

The man's awareness seemed divided. Then, with a faint start, his eyes alighted on Peter's face.

"Peter, hello." His voice was bland, lacking emotion except, perhaps, for a touch of mild surprise.

"Just lie still."

"Oh, I'm not going anywhere." His legs had been crushed to a pulp, yet he seemed to be experiencing no pain at all. He lifted his wounded hand with a vague gesture. "Can you believe this shit?"

"Does anybody have any water?"

Caleb produced a canteen; just an inch or two sloshed in the bottom. Peter cupped the man's neck to lift his head and held the spout to his lips. Peter wondered why Apgar had not yet turned. Of course, there was a range; it varied person to person. A few weak sips, water dribbling from the corners of his mouth, and Apgar leaned back.

"It's true what they say. You can feel it inside you." He took a long, shuddering breath. "How many survivors?"

Peter shook his head. "Not many."

"Don't blame yourself."

"Gunnar —"

"Take this as my last piece of official advice. You've done all you could. It's time to get these

669

people out of here." The general licked his lips and lifted the bloody hand again. "But let's not let this go on too long. I don't want people to see me like this."

Peter turned his face and scanned the group: Chase, Hollis, Caleb, a few of the soldiers. All were staring. He felt benumbed; none of it seemed real yet.

"Somebody give me something."

Hollis produced a knife. Peter accepted its cold weight into his hand. For a moment he doubted he could find the strength to do what was required of him. He crouched beside Apgar again, holding the blade a little behind himself to keep it from view.

"It's been an honor to serve under you, Mr. President."

Through a throat thickened with tears, Peter raised his voice, speaking words no one had said in over twenty years. "This man is a soldier of the Expeditionary! It is time for him to take the trip! All hail, General Gunnar Apgar! Hip hip —"

"Hooray!"

"Hip hip —"

"Hooray!"

"Hip hip —"

"Hooray!"

Apgar took a long breath and let it out slowly. His face became peaceful.

"Thank you, Peter. I'm ready now."

Peter tightened his grip on the knife.

There were two more.

Peter was looking at Apgar's body. The man had died quickly, almost inaudibly. A grunt as the knife

went in, his eyes opening wide, death easing into them.

"Somebody get me a blanket."

No one spoke.

"Goddamnit, what's the matter with you people? You —" He jabbed a finger at one of the soldiers. "What's your name, Private?"

The man seemed a little dazed. "Sir?"

"What, you don't know your own name? Are you that stupid?"

He swallowed nervously. "It's Verone, sir."

"Organize a burial detail. I want everyone gathered at the parade ground in thirty. Full military honors, do you read me?"

He glanced at the others.

"Is there a problem, soldier?"

"Dad —" Caleb gripped him by an arm and made his father look at him. "I know this is painful. We all understand how you felt about him. I'll get a blanket, all right?"

The tears had begun to flow; his jaw trembled with confined fury. "We're not just leaving him here for the birds, goddamnit."

"There are a lot of bodies out here. We really don't have time."

Peter shook him off. "This man was a hero. He's the reason any of us are still alive."

Caleb spoke in measured tones: "I know that, Dad. Everyone does. But the general was right. We really have to think about what comes next."

"I'll tell you what comes next. We bury this man."

"Mr. President —"

Peter turned: Jock. Someone had wrapped his ankle and found him a pair of crutches. He was sweating and a little out of breath.

671

"What the hell is it now?"

The man seemed uncertain.

"For God's sake, just say it."

"It looks like . . . somebody's alive outside."

The gate was gone: one of the doors had been knocked askew and was hanging from a single hinge; the other lay on the ground a hundred feet inside the wall. As they moved through the opening, Peter's first, impossible impression was that it had snowed in the night. A fine, pale dust coated every surface. A moment passed before he grasped the meaning. Carter's army lay dead; their bones, now in sunlight, had begun their dissolution.

Amy was sitting near the base of the wall, arms wrapping her knees, gazing across the field. Covered in ash, she looked like a ghost, a specter from a children's story. A few feet beyond her, beside Soldier's body, lay Alicia. The horse's throat was torn open, among other things. Flies were buzzing around him, dipping in and out of his wounds.

Peter strode forward with gathering speed. Amy turned her face toward him.

"He didn't kill us," she said. She spoke as if in a daze. "Why didn't he kill us?"

Her presence barely registered in Peter's mind; it was Alicia he wanted. "You knew!" He barreled past Amy, seized Alicia by the arm, and rolled her faceup. "You fucking knew all along!"

Amy cried, "Peter, stop!"

He dropped to his knees and straddled Alicia's waist; his fingers wrapped her throat. His eyes and mind filled with the loathsome sight of her. "He was my friend!"

More voices, not just Amy's, were yelling at him,

but this was a matter of no importance. They might just as well have been calling to him from the moon. Alicia was making a gurgling sound; her lips were paling to a bluish color. She was squinting into the morning light. Through these narrow slits, their gazes met. In her eyes, Peter saw not fear but fatalistic acceptance. *Go ahead,* her eyes said. *We've done everything else together, why not this?* Beneath the pads of his thumbs, he felt the stringy gristle of her trachea. He shifted them downward, positioning them in the spoon-like depression at the base of her throat. Hands had grabbed him. Some were tugging at his shoulders, others attempting to pry his fingers from her neck. "He was my friend and you killed him! You killed all of them!" One hard push to crush her larynx and that would be the end of her. "Say it, you traitor! Say you knew!"

A tremendous force yanked him away. He crashed onto his back in the dust. Hollis.

"Take a breath, Peter."

The man had positioned himself between Peter and Alicia, who had begun to cough. Amy was kneeling beside her, cradling her head.

"We all heard her," Hollis said. "She was trying to warn us."

Peter's face was burning; his hands, clenched into fists, shook with adrenaline. "She lied to us."

"I understand your anger. We all do. But she didn't know."

Peter's awareness expanded. The others were watching him in mute incomprehension. Caleb. Chase. Jock, leaning on his crutches. The old man, who was, for some reason, still carrying his bucket.

"Now, do I have your agreement to leave her be — yes or no?" Hollis said.

673

Peter swallowed. The fog of fury had begun to dissipate. Another moment and he nodded.

"All right, then," said Hollis.

He extended a hand and pulled Peter to his feet. Alicia's coughing had eased somewhat. Amy looked up. "Caleb, run and get Sara."

Amy waited by Alicia until Sara arrived. At the sight of Alicia, she startled.

"You're kidding me." Her voice was dispassionate, lacking all pity.

"Please, Sara," said Amy. There were tears in her eyes.

"You think I'm helping *her*?" Sara scanned the others. "She can go to hell."

Hollis took her by the shoulders to make her look at him. "She's not our enemy, Sara. Please believe me. And we're going to need her."

"What for?"

"To help us get out of here. Not just you and me. Pim. Theo. The girls."

A moment passed; Sara sighed and broke away. She crouched beside Alicia, passing her eyes quickly over her without expression, then looked up. "I'm not doing this with an audience. Amy, you stay. The rest of you, a little space, please."

The group backed away. Caleb took Peter aside.

"Dad? Okay?"

He wasn't sure what to say. His anger had faded, but not his doubt. He glanced past his son's shoulder. Sara was moving her hands over Alicia's chest and stomach, pressing with her fingertips.

"Yeah."

"Everybody understands."

Caleb said nothing more; neither did anyone else. A few more minutes went by before Sara rose and went to them.

"She's broken up pretty badly." Her tone was indifferent; she was doing a job, that was all. "I can't really tell the full extent. And in her case, things will probably happen differently. A couple of the gunshot wounds have closed up already, but I don't know what's happening inside. She's got a broken back, and about six other fractures I can detect."

"Will she live?" Amy asked.

"If she were anyone else, she'd be dead already. I can sew her up and set her leg. She needs to be immobilized. As for the rest . . ." She shrugged without feeling. "Your guess is as good as mine."

Caleb and Chase returned with a stretcher; they carried Alicia inside. All the survivors had been brought out of the shelter and had gathered in the staging area. Jenny and Hannah were moving through the group with buckets of water and ladles. Here and there, a person was sobbing; others were talking quietly or just gazing into space.

"So what now?" Chase asked.

Peter felt unattached to everything, almost floating. Particles of ash, bitter-smelling, drifted down. The fires had begun to spread. Leaping from building to building, they would sweep down to the river, consuming everything in their path. Other parts of the city, spared from the flames, would take longer — years, decades. Rain, wind, the devouring teeth of time — all would do their work. Peter could see it in his mind. Kerrville would become one more ruin in a world of them. He was suddenly crushed by the simplicity of it all. The city had fallen; the city was gone. He felt it keenly: the stab of defeat.

"Caleb?"

"Here, Dad."

Peter turned. His son was waiting; everyone was. "We need vehicles. Buses, trucks, whatever you can find. Fuel, too. Hollis, you go with him. Ford, what do we have for power?"

"Everything's out."

"The barracks have a backup generator. See if we can get it running. We need to get a message to Michael, tell him we're coming. Sara, you'll be in charge here. People will need food and water, enough for the day. But everybody needs to stay put. No wandering off, no looking for family or retrieving belongings."

"What about a search party?" Amy asked. "There could still be people out there."

"Take two men and a vehicle. Start on the other side of the river and work your way back. Stay clear of shaded areas, and keep out of the buildings."

"I'd like to help," Jock said.

"Fine, do your best but be quick about it. You've got one hour. No passengers unless they're injured. Anyone who can walk can make it here on their own."

"What if we find more infected who haven't turned yet?" Caleb asked.

"That's up to them. Make the offer. If they don't take it, leave them where they are. It won't make any difference." He paused. "Is everyone clear?"

Nods and murmurs passed around the group.

"Then that's it," Peter said. "We're done here. Sixty minutes, people, and we're gone."

74

They were 764 souls.

They were dirty, exhausted, terrified, confused.

They rode in six buses, three to a seat; four five-tons, crammed with people; eight smaller trucks, both military and civilian, their cargo beds full of supplies — water, food, fuel. They had only a few weapons, and barely any ammunition. Among their numbers, they counted 532 children under the age of thirteen, 309 of these below the age of six. They included 122 mothers of children three and younger, including 19 women who were still nursing infants. Of the remaining 110, there were 68 men and 42 women of various ages and backgrounds. Thirty-two were, or had been, soldiers. Nine were over the age of sixty; the oldest, a widow who had sat in her house through the night, muttering to herself that all the noise outside was just a bunch of goddamn nonsense, was eighty-two. They included mechanics, electricians, nurses, weavers, shopkeepers, bootleggers, farmers, farriers, a gunsmith, and a cobbler.

One of the passengers was the drunken doctor, Brian Elacqua. Too inebriated to comprehend the orders to relocate to the dam, he had found himself, as night had fallen, wondering where everyone had gone. He had passed the twenty-four hours since his return to Kerrville drinking himself into oblivion in the abandoned house that had once been his — a miracle he had managed to find it — and awakened to a silence and darkness that disturbed him. Departing his house in search of more liquor, he reached the square just as gunfire erupted along the wall. He was profoundly disoriented and still quite drunk. Dimly he wondered, Why were people shooting? He decided to head for the hospital. It was a place he knew, a touchstone. Also, maybe someone could tell him what in the hell was going on. As he made

his way there, his apprehension mounted. The gunfire had continued, and he was hearing certain other sounds as well: vehicles racing, cries of distress. As the hospital came into sight, a shout went up, followed by a barrage of shooting. Elacqua hit the dirt. He had no idea what to make of any of this; it seemed entirely unconnected to him. Also, he wondered, with sudden concern, what had become of his wife? It was true that she despised him, yet he was accustomed to her presence. Why was she not here?

These questions were shoved aside by the sound and shock of a tremendous impact. Elacqua peeled his face off the ground. A truck had crashed into the front of the building. Not just into: it had rammed straight through the wall. He got to his feet and stumbled toward it. Perhaps someone was injured, he thought. Perhaps they needed help. "Get in!" a man yelled from the cab. "Everybody in the truck!" Elacqua wobbled his way up the steps and beheld a scene of such disorder that his addled brain could not compute it. The room was full of screaming women and children. Soldiers were shoving and tossing them into the cargo bed while simultaneously shooting over their heads in the direction of the stairwell. Elacqua was caught in the crush. From the chaos, his mind distilled the image of a familiar face. Was that Sara Wilson? He had a sense that he'd seen her rather recently, though he could not pull the memory into shape. Either way, getting into the truck seemed like a good idea. He fought his way through the melee. Children were scrambling all around and underfoot. The driver of the vehicle was racing the engine. By this time, Elacqua had reached the tailgate. The truck was packed with

people, barely any room at all. Also, there was the problem of getting one foot onto the bumper to hoist himself into the cargo compartment, an act requiring a degree of physical coordination he didn't think he could muster.

"Help me," he moaned.

A hand, heaven-sent, reached down. Up and into the truck he went, tumbling over bodies as the vehicle shot forward. A syncopation of bone-jarring bangs followed as the truck sailed out of the building and down the steps. Through the fog of terror and confusion, Brian Elacqua experienced a revelation: his life had been unworthy. It might not have begun that way — he'd meant to be a good and decent man — but over the years he had strayed far from the path. If I get out of this, he thought, I won't ever touch a drink again.

Which was how, sixteen hours later, Brian Elacqua came to find himself on a school bus of 87 women and children, deep in the physical and existential sorrows of acute alcohol withdrawal. It was still early morning, the light soft, with a golden color. He had, with many others, watched from the window as the city faded, then disappeared from sight. He wasn't completely sure where they were going. There was talk of a ship that would take them to safety, though he found this difficult to fathom. Why had he, of all people, a man who had squandered his life, the most worthless of worthless drunks, survived? Seated on the bench beside him was a little girl with strawberry-blond hair, tied in back with a ribbon. He supposed she was four or five. She was wearing a loose dress of thick woven fiber; her feet were dirty and bare, covered with numerous scratches and scabs. At her waist she clutched a

ratty stuffed toy, some kind of animal, a bear or maybe a dog. She had yet to acknowledge him in any manner, her eyes staring forward. "Where are your parents, honey?" Elacqua asked. "Why are you alone?" "Because they're dead," the little girl stated. She did not look at him as she spoke. "They're all dead."

And with that, Brian Elacqua dropped his face to his hands, his body shaking with tears.

At the wheel of the first bus, Caleb was watching the clock. The hour was approaching noon; they had been on the road a little more than four hours. Pim and Theo sat behind him with the girls. He was down to half a tank; they planned to stop in Rosenberg, where a tanker from the isthmus would meet them to refuel. The bus was quiet; no one was talking. Lulled by the rocking of the chassis, most of the children had fallen asleep.

They had passed through the last of the outer townships when the radio crackled: "Pull over, everyone. Looks like we've lost one."

Caleb brought the bus to a halt and stepped down as his father, Chase, and Amy emerged from the lead Humvee. One of the buses, the fourth in line, was parked with its hood open. Steam and liquid were pouring from its radiator.

Hollis was standing on the bumper, slapping at the engine with a rag. "I think it's the water pump."

"Can you do anything about it?" Caleb's father said. "It'd have to be fast."

Hollis jumped down. "No chance. These old things aren't built for this. I'm surprised it's taken this long for one to conk out."

"As long as we're stopped," Sara suggested, "probably the children need to go."

"Go where?"

"To the bathroom, Peter."

Caleb's father sighed impatiently. Any minute of delay was a minute they'd be driving in darkness at the other end. "Just watch for snakes. That's all we need right now."

The children filed off and were led into the weeds, girls on one side of the buses, boys on the other. By the time the convoy was ready to move again, they had been stopped for twenty minutes. A hot Texas wind was blowing. It was 0130 hours, the sun poised above them like the head of a hammer in the sky.

The patch was complete, the dock ready to fill. Michael, Lore, and Rand, in one of six pump houses along the weir, were preparing to open the vents to the sea. Greer was gone, headed with Patch to Rosenberg in the last tanker truck.

"Shouldn't we say something?" Lore asked Michael.

"How about 'Please open, you bastard'?"

The wheel had not been turned in seventeen years.

"That'll have to do," said Lore.

Michael wedged a pry bar between the spokes; Lore was holding a mallet. Michael and Rand gripped the bar and leaned in.

"Hit it now."

Lore, positioned to the side, swung the mallet. It glanced off the top of the rim.

"For God's sake." Michael's jaws were clenched, his face reddened with effort. "Hit the bastard."

Blow after blow: still the wheel refused to turn.

681

"This isn't great," Rand said.

"Let me try," said Lore.

"How's that going to help?" Then, when Lore just stared at him, he stepped aside. "Suit yourself."

Lore left the pry bar where it was, gripping the wheel instead.

"You've got no leverage," Rand said. "That'll never work."

Lore ignored him. She planted her feet wide. The muscles in her arms tightened, thick ropes stretched over bone.

"This is pointless," Michael said. "We have to think of something else."

Then, miraculously, the wheel began to turn. An inch, then two. They all heard it: water had begun to move. A fine spray shot through the vent on the floor of the dock. With a jolt, the wheel released. Below them, the seas began to pour in. Lore backed away, flexing her fingers.

"We must have loosened it," Rand said lamely.

She gave them a droll smile.

The time was fast approaching.

His army was gone. Carter had felt the dopeys leaving him: a scream of terror, and a blast of pain, and then the letting go. Their souls had passed through him like wind, a whorl of memories, waning, then gone.

He did the last of his chores for the day with a solemn feeling. A deck of low clouds moved over the sky as he rolled his mower to the shed, padlocked the door, and turned to face the yard so that he might survey his handiwork. The crisp lawn, every blade just so. The tailored edges along the walkways with their bit of monkey grass to

682

mark them. The trees all limbed up and the flowers, banks of them, like a carpet of color beneath the hedges. That morning, a dwarf Japanese cutleaf maple had appeared by the gate. Mrs. Wood had always wanted one. Carter had rolled it in its plastic pot to the corner of the yard and set it in the ground. Cut-leafs had an elegant feel to them, like the hands of a beautiful woman. It felt like an act of completion to plant it there, a final gift to the yard he'd tended for so long.

He wiped his brow. The sprinklers came on, scattering a fine mist over the lawn. Inside the house, the little girls were laughing. Carter wished he could see them, talk to them. He imagined himself sitting on the patio while watching them play in the yard, tossing a ball or chasing each other. Little girls needed time in the sunshine.

He hoped he didn't stink too bad. He sniffed his armpits and supposed he'd pass all right. At the kitchen window, he inspected his reflection. It was a long time since he'd bothered to do that. He supposed he looked like he always had, which wasn't really one thing or the other, just a face like most people's.

For the first time in over a century, Carter opened the gate and stepped through.

The air wasn't any different here; he wondered why he'd thought it might be. The busy city made a whooshing sound in the background but the street was otherwise quiet, all the big houses staring back at him with no particular interest. He walked to the end of the drive to wait, fanning himself with his hat.

It was the hour when everything changes. The birds, the insects, the worms in the grass — all know this. Cicadas were buzzing in the trees.

1700: Greer and Patch had been waiting in the tanker truck for two hours. Patch was reading a magazine — reading or perhaps just looking at it. It was called *National Geographic Kids;* the pages were brittle and popped out when he turned them. He nudged Greer on the shoulder and held it out to show him a picture.

"Think it'll be like that?"

A jungle scene: fat green leaves, brightly colored birds, everything wreathed in vines. Greer was too preoccupied to look very closely.

"I don't know. Maybe."

Patch took it back. "I wonder if there's people out there."

Greer used binoculars to scan the horizon to the north. "I doubt it."

"Because if there is, I hope they're friendly. Seems like a lot to go through if they're not."

Another fifteen minutes passed.

"Maybe we should go look for them," Patch suggested.

"Hang on. I think this is them."

A cloud of dust had formed in the distance. Greer watched through the binoculars as the image of the convoy took shape. The two men climbed down from the cab as the first vehicle drew up.

"What kept you?" Greer asked Peter.

"We lost two buses. A busted radiator and a broken axle."

All of the vehicles took diesel except the smaller pickups, which carried their own extra fuel. Greer organized a team to pour the diesel off into jugs; they began moving down the line to refill the

buses. The children were allowed off but told not to wander far.

"How long is this going to take?" Chase asked Greer.

It took almost an hour. The shadows had begun to stretch. They had fifty more miles to go, but these would be the hardest. None of the buses would be able to travel more than twenty miles per hour over the rough terrain.

The convoy began to move again.

The dock had been filling for seven hours. Everything was ready — batteries charged, bilge pumps on, engines ready to fire. Chains had been fixed to hold the *Bergensfjord* in place. Michael was in the pilothouse with Lore. The sea had risen a yard past the waterline — within a reasonable margin of error but disturbing nonetheless.

"I can't stand this," Lore said.

She was pacing around the tiny space, all her energy suddenly having nowhere to go. Michael picked up the microphone from the panel. "Rand, what are you seeing down there?"

He was moving through the corridors below-decks, checking seams. "All good so far, no leaks. She seems tight."

Higher and higher the water rose, wrapping the hull in its cold embrace. Still the ship refused to budge.

"Flyers, this is killing me," groaned Lore.

"That's not an expression I've ever heard you use," Michael said.

"Well, I kind of see the sense of it now."

Michael held up a hand; he'd felt something. He willed all his senses to focus. The sensation came again: the tiniest shudder, rippling through

685

the hull. His eyes met Lore's; she'd detected it, too. The great creature was coming to life. The deck shifted beneath him with a deep moan.

"Here we go!" Lore cried.

The *Bergensfjord* began to lift from her braces.

At the end of the block, the Denali appeared, turning the corner with painstaking care. Carter stepped into the road and positioned himself in its path. He did not hold up his hand or in any way indicate his wish that it should stop. He stepped aside as the car came to a halt in front of him. With a hushed, mechanical purr, the driver's window drew down. Crisp air and a smell of leather flowed out onto his face.

"Mr. Carter?"

"It's good to see you, Mrs. Wood."

She was wearing her tennis clothes. The silver packages in back, the baby seat with its mobile of plush toys, the sunglasses perched on her head: all the same as the morning they'd met.

"You're looking well," he said.

Her eyes narrowed on his face, as if she were attempting to read small print. "You stopped me."

"Yes, ma'am."

"I don't understand. Why did you do that?"

"Why don't you pull into the driveway? We can have us a talk."

She glanced around in confusion.

"You go on now," he assured her.

Rather reluctantly, she turned the Denali into the driveway and shut off the engine. Carter stepped to the driver's-side window again. The motor was making a quiet ticking sound. Hands locked on the steering wheel, Rachel stared

straight out the windshield, as if afraid to look at him.

"I don't think I'm supposed to be doing this," she said.

"It's all right," Carter said.

Her voice sharpened with panic. "But it's *not* all right. It's not all right at all."

Carter opened her door. "Why don't you come and see the yard, Mrs. Wood? Kept it nice for you."

"I'm *supposed* to drive the car. That's what I *do.* That's my *job.*"

"Just this morning planted one of those cut-leaf maples you like. You should see how pretty it is."

For a moment she was silent. Then: "A cut-leaf maple, you say?"

"Yes, ma'am."

She nodded pensively to herself. "I always thought it would be just the right thing for that corner. You know the one I mean?"

"Absolutely I do."

She turned to look at him. For a moment she studied his face, her blue eyes slightly squinted. "You're always thinking of me, aren't you, Mr. Carter? You always know just the thing to say. I don't think I've ever had a friend like you."

"Oh, I expect you have."

"Oh, please. I have people, sure. Lots of people in Rachel Wood's life. But never anyone who understands me the way you do." She looked at him kindly. "But you and me. We're quite a pair, aren't we?"

"I'd say we are, Mrs. Wood."

"Now, if I've said it once, I've said it a thousand times. It's Rachel."

He nodded. "Anthony, then."

Her face opened as if she'd discovered some-

thing. "Rachel and Anthony! We're like two characters in a movie."

He held out a hand. "Why don't you come on now, Rachel? It'll all be fine, you'll see."

Accepting his hand for balance, she exited the car. By the open door she paused with great deliberateness and filled her lungs with air.

"Now, that's a wonderful smell," she said. "What is that?"

"Cut the lawn just now. I suspect that's it."

"Of course. Now I remember." She smiled with satisfaction. "How long has it been since I smelled new-mown grass? Smelled anything, for that matter."

"Garden's waiting on you. Lots of good smells there."

He made a circle with his arm; Rachel let him lead the way. The shadows were stretching over the ground; evening was about to fall. He steered her to the gate, where she came to a stop.

"Do you know how you make me feel, Anthony? I've been trying to think how to say it."

"How's that?"

"You make me feel *seen*. Like I was invisible until you came along. Does that sound crazy? Probably it does."

"Not to me," said Carter.

"I think I sensed it right away, that morning under the overpass. Do you remember?" A feeling of distance came into her eyes. "It was all so upsetting. Everyone honking and yelling and you there with your sign. 'HUNGRY, ANYTHING WILL HELP. GOD BLESS YOU.' I thought, that man means something. He's not just there by accident. That man's come into my life for a purpose."

Carter opened the latch; they stepped through.

688

She was still clutching his arm, the two of them like a couple walking down the aisle. Her steps were solemn and measured; it was as if each one required a separate act of will.

"Now, Anthony, this really *is* lovely."

They were standing by the pool. The water was perfectly still and very blue. Around them, the yard made an effulgent display of color and life.

"Honestly, I can hardly believe my eyes. After all this time. You must have worked so hard."

"Wasn't any trouble. I had some help, too."

Rachel looked at him. "Really? Who was that?"

"Woman I know. Named Amy."

Rachel pondered this. "Now," she declared, raising a finger to her lips, "I believe I met an Amy not too long ago. I believe I gave her a lift. About so tall, with dark hair?"

Carter nodded.

"A very sweet girl. And what skin. Absolutely *glorious* skin." She smiled suddenly. "And what have we here?"

Her eyes had fallen on the cosmos. She separated from him and walked across the lawn to the beds, Carter following.

"These are just beautiful, Anthony."

She knelt before the flowers. Carter had planted two shades of pink: the first a deep solid, the second softer with green flares, on long, tippy stems.

"May I, Anthony?"

"You go on and do as you like. Planted them for you."

She selected one of the deeper pink and pinched off the stem. Holding it between thumb and forefinger, she rotated it slowly, breathing softly through her nose.

"Do you know what the name means?" she asked.

"Can't say I do."

"It's from the Greek. It means 'balanced universe.' " She rocked back onto her heels. "It's funny, I have no idea how I know that. Probably I learned it in school."

A quiet passed.

"Haley loves these." Rachel was looking at the flower, gazing at it as if it were a talisman or the key to a door she couldn't quite unlock.

"That she does," Carter answered.

"Always putting them in her hair. Her sister's, too."

"Miss Riley. Cute as a bug, that one."

A soft night was coming on between the branches of the trees. Rachel pointed her face to the sky.

"I have so many memories, Anthony. Sometimes it's all so hard to sort out."

"Things will come to you," he assured her.

"I remember the pool."

It was happening. Carter crouched beside her.

"That morning, how terrible everything was. The air so raw." She took a long, mournful breath. "I was so sad. So incredibly sad. Like a great black ocean and there you are, floating in it, drifting, no land anywhere, nothing to want or hope for. It's just you and the water and the darkness and you know it will always be like that, forever and ever."

She fell silent, lost in these old, troubled thoughts. The air had cooled; the lights of the city, coming on, reflected off the cloud deck, making a pale glow. Then:

"That was when I saw you. You were in the yard with Haley. Just . . ." She shrugged. "Showing her

690

something. A toad, maybe. A flower. You were always doing that, showing her little things to make her happy." She shook her head slowly. "But that was the thing. I *knew* it was you, I *believed* it was you. But that wasn't who I saw."

She was staring at the ground, dry-eyed, beyond feeling. It would all pour forth now, the memories, the pain, the horrors of that day.

"It was Death, Anthony."

Carter waited.

"I know that's an old idea. A *crazy* idea. And you so sweet to me, to all of us. But I saw you standing there with Haley and I thought, Death has come. He's here, he's outside right now with my little girl. It's all a mistake, a horrible mistake, I'm the one he wants. *I'm* the one who needs to die."

The day was fading, colors draining, the sky releasing the last of its light. She raised her face; her eyes were beseeching, moist and wide.

"That's why I did what I did, Anthony. It wasn't fair. It wasn't right, I know that. There are things that can never be forgiven. But that is why."

Rachel had begun to cry. Carter put his arms around her as she collapsed into his weight. Her skin was warm and sweet-smelling, just a hint of her perfume lingering. How small she was, and he not a big man in the slightest. She might have been a bird there, just a little bit of a thing cupped in his hand.

The girls were laughing in the house.

"Oh God, I left them," Rachel sobbed. She was clutching his shirt in her fists. "How could I leave them? My babies. My beautiful baby girls."

"Hush now," he said. "Time to let go of all the old things."

They stayed like that for a time, holding each other. Night had descended in full; the air was still and moist with dew. The little girls were singing. The song was sweet and wordless, like the songs of birds.

"They waitin' on you," said Carter.

She shook her head against his chest. "I can't face them. I can't."

"You be strong, Rachel. Be strong for your babies."

She let him slowly draw her to her feet and took his arm, gripping it tightly with both hands, just above the elbow. With small steps, Carter led her around the pool toward the back door. The house was dark. Carter had expected it to be this way but could not say why that should be so. It was simply a part, another part, of the way things were in this place.

They stopped before the door. From deep in the house, more laughter and the creaking of springs: the girls were jumping on the beds.

"Aren't you going to open it?" Rachel asked.

Carter didn't answer. Rachel looked at him closely; something shifted in her face. She understood that he would not be going with her.

"Have to be this way," he explained. "You go on, now. Tell them hello for me, won't you? Tell them I've been thinking on them, every day."

She regarded the knob with a deep tentativeness. Inside, the girls were laughing with wild delight.

"Mr. Carter —"

"Anthony."

She placed a palm upon his cheek. She was crying again; come to think of it, Carter was crying a little himself. When she kissed him, he tasted not

just the softness of her mouth and the warmth of her breath but also the saltiness of their tears conjoining — not a taste of sorrow, strictly speaking, though there was sorrow in it.

"God bless you, too, Anthony."

And before he knew it — before the feel of her kiss had faded from his lips — the door had opened and she was gone.

76

2030 hours: the light was almost gone, the convoy moving at a creep.

They were in a coastal tableland of tangled scrub, the road pocked with potholes in places, in others rippled like a washboard. Chase was driving, his gaze intent as he fought the wheel. Amy was riding in back.

Peter radioed Greer, who was driving the tanker at the rear of the column. "How much farther?"

"Six miles."

Six miles at twenty miles per hour. Behind them, the sun had been subsumed into a flat horizon, erasing all shadows.

"We should see the channel bridge soon," Greer added. "The isthmus is just south of there."

"Everyone, we need to push it," Peter said.

They accelerated to thirty-five. Peter swiveled in his seat to make sure the convoy was keeping pace. A gap opened, then narrowed. The cab of the Humvee flared as the first bus in line turned on its headlights.

"How much faster should we go?" Chase asked.

"Keep it there for now."

There was a hard bang as they rocketed through a deep hole.

"Those buses are going to blow apart," Chase said.

A scrim of light appeared ahead: the moon. It lifted swiftly from the eastern horizon, plump and fiery. Simultaneously, the channel bridge rose up before them in distant silhouette — a stately, vaguely organic figure with its long scoops of wire slung from tall trestles. Peter took up the radio again.

"Drivers, anybody seeing anything out there?"

Negative. Negative. Negative.

Through the windscreen of the pilothouse, Michael and Lore were watching the drydock doors. The portside door had opened without complaint; the starboard was the problem. At a 150-degree angle to the dock, the door had stopped cold. They'd been trying to open it the rest of the way for nearly two hours.

"I'm out of ideas here," Rand radioed from the quay. "I think that's all we're going to get."

"Will we clear it?" Lore asked. The door weighed forty tons.

Michael didn't know. "Rand, get down to engineering. I need you there."

"I'm sorry, Michael."

"You did your best. We'll have to manage." He hung the microphone back on the panel. *Fuck.*

The lights on the panel went dead.

Twenty-eight miles west, the same summer moon had risen over the *Chevron Mariner.* Its blazing orange light shone down upon the deck; it shimmered over the oily waters of the lagoon like a skin of flame.

With a bang like a small explosion, the hatch

694

detonated skyward. It seemed not so much to fly as to leap, soaring into the nighttime sky of its own volition. Up and up it sailed, spinning on its horizontal axis with a whizzing sound; then, like a man who's lost his train of thought, it appeared to pause in mid-flight. For the thinnest moment, it neither rose nor fell; one might easily have been forgiven for thinking it was charged with some magical power, capable of thwarting gravity. But, not so: down it plunged, into the befouled waters.

Then: Carter.

He landed on the foredeck with a *clang,* absorbing the impact through his legs and simultaneously compressing his body to a squat: hips wide, head erect, one splayed hand touching the deck for balance, like an offensive tackle preparing for the snap. His nostrils flared to taste the air, which was imbued with the freshness of freedom. A breeze licked at his body with a tickling sensation. Sights and sounds bombarded his senses from all directions. He regarded the moon. His vision was such that he could detect the smallest features of its face — the cracks and crevices, craters and canyons — with an almost lurid quality of three dimensions. He felt the moon's roundness, its great rocky weight, as if he were holding it in his arms.

Time to be on his way.

He ascended to the top of One Allen Center. High above the drowned city, Carter took measure of the buildings: their heights and handholds, the fjord-like gulfs between them. A route materialized in his mind; it had the force, the clarity of a premonition, or something absolutely known. A hundred yards to the first rooftop, perhaps another fifty to the second, a long two hundred to

the third but with a drop of fifty feet that would expand his reach . . .

He backed to the far edge of the platform. The key was, first, to create an accumulation of velocity, then to spring at precisely the right moment. He lowered to a runner's crouch.

Ten long strides and he was up. He soared through the moonlit heavens like a comet, a star unlocked. He made the first rooftop with room to spare. He landed, tucked, rolled; he came up running and launched again.

He'd been saving up.

In the cargo bay of the third vehicle in the convoy, among the other injured, Alicia lay immobilized. Thick rubber cords strapped her to her stretcher at the shoulders, waist, and knees; a fourth lay across her forehead. Her right leg was splinted from ankle to hip; one arm, her right, was pinned across her chest. Various other parts of her were bandaged, stitched, bound.

Inside her body, the rapid cellular repair of her kind was under way. But this was an imperfect process, and complicated by the vastness and complexity of her wounds. This was especially true of the winglike flange of her right hip, which had been pulverized. The viral part of her could accomplish many things, but it could not reassemble a jigsaw puzzle. It might have been said that the only thing keeping Alicia Donadio alive was habit — her predisposition to see things through, just as she had always done. But she no longer had the heart for any of it. As the bone-banging hours passed, that she had failed to die seemed more and more like a punishment, and proof enough of Peter's words. *You traitor. You knew. You killed*

them. You killed them all.

Sara was sitting on the bench above her. Alicia undestood that the woman hated her; she could see it in her eyes, in the way she looked at her — or, rather, didn't — as she went about attending to Alicia's injuries: checking the bandages, measuring her temperature and pulse, dribbling the horrible-tasting elixir into her mouth that kept her in a pain-numbed twilight. Alicia wished she could say something to the woman, whose hatred she deserved. *I'm sorry about Kate.* Or *It's all right, I hate myself enough as it is.* But this would only make things worse. Better Alicia should accept what was offered and say nothing.

Besides, none of this mattered now; Alicia was asleep, and dreaming. In this dream, she was in a boat, and all around was water. The seas were calm, covered in mist, without a visible horizon. She was rowing. The creak of the oars in their locks, the swish of water moving under their blades: these were the only sounds. The water was dense, with a slightly viscous texture. Where was she going? Why had the water ceased to terrify her? Because it didn't; Alicia felt perfectly at home. Her back and arms were strong, her strokes compact, nothing wasted. Rowing a boat was something she did not recall ever doing, yet it felt completely natural, as if the knowledge had been inscribed into her muscles for later use.

On she rowed, her blades elegantly slicing through the inky murk. She became aware that something was moving in the water — a shadowy bulk gliding just beneath the surface. It appeared to be following her, maintaining a watchful distance. Her mind did not register its presence as menacing; rather, it merely seemed to be a natural

feature of the environment, one she might have anticipated if she'd thought about it in advance.

"Your boat is very small," said Amy.

She was sitting in the stern. Water was running from her face and hair.

"You know we can't go," Amy stated.

The remark was puzzling. Alicia continued to row. "Go where?"

"The virus is in us." Amy's voice was dispassionate, without any perceptible tone. "We can't ever leave."

"I don't understand what you're talking about."

The shape had begun to circle them. Great bulges of water began to rock the boat from side to side.

"Oh, I think you do. We're sisters, aren't we? Sisters in blood."

The motion increased in intensity. Alicia drew the oars into the boat and clutched the gunwales for balance. Her heart turned to lead; bile bubbled in her throat. Why had she failed to foresee the danger? So much water all around them, and her little boat, so small as to be nothing. The hull began to rise; suddenly they were no longer in contact with the water. A great blue bulk emerged under them, water streaming from its encrusted flanks.

"You know who that is," Amy said impassively.

It was a whale. They were balanced like a pea atop its immense, horrible head. Higher and higher it lifted them into the air. One flick of its monstrous tail and it would send them soaring; it would crash down upon them and smash their boat to pieces. A hopeless terror, that of fate, took her in its grasp. From the stern, Amy issued a bored sigh.

698

"I'm so . . . tired of him," she said.

Alicia tried to scream, but the sound stopped in her throat. They were rising, the sea was falling away, the whale was looming up . . .

She awoke with a slam. She blinked her eyes and tried to focus. It was night. She was in the back of the truck, and the truck was bouncing hard. Sara's face floated into view.

"Lish? What is it?"

Her lips moved slowly around the words: "They're . . . coming."

From the rear of the convoy, the sound of guns.

Shit. Shit shit shit.

Michael took the stairs from the pilothouse three at a time; he raced across the deck, his feet barely touching steel, and down the hatch. He was yelling into his radio, "Rand, get down here right now!"

He hit the engineering catwalk at a sprint, grabbed the poles of the ladder, and slid the rest of the way. The engines were quiet, everything stopped. Rand appeared above him.

"What happened?"

"Something tripped the main!"

Lore, on the radio: "Michael, we're hearing shots up here."

"Say again?"

"*Gunshots,* Michael. I'm looking down the isthmus now. We've got lights coming this way from the mainland."

"Headlights or virals?"

"I'm not sure."

He needed current to trace the problem. At the electrical panel, he switched diagnostics over to the auxiliary generator. The meters jumped to life.

"Rand!" Michael bellowed. "What are you seeing?"

Rand was positioned at the engine-control array on the far side of the room, checking dials. "Looks like its something in the water jacket pumps."

"That wouldn't trip the main! Look farther up the line!"

A brief silence; then Rand said, "Got it." He tapped a dial. "Pressure's flatlined on the starboard-side charger. Must have shut down the system."

Lore again: "Michael, what's going on down there?"

He was strapping on his tool belt. "Here," he said, tossing Rand the radio, "you talk to her."

Rand looked lost. "What should I say?"

"Tell her to get ready to engage the props straight from the pilothouse."

"Shouldn't she wait for the system to repressurize? We could blow a header."

"Just get on the electrical panel. When I tell you, switch the system back over to the main bus."

"Michael, talk to me," Lore said. "Things are looking very fucking serious up here."

"Go," Michael told Rand.

He raced aft, plugged in his lantern, dropped to his back, and wedged himself under the charger.

This goddamn leak, he thought. It's going to be the death of me.

The convoy hit the isthmus doing sixty miles an hour. Buses were bounding; buses were going airborne. The tanker, last in the line, had failed to keep up. The virals were close behind and massing. The barrier of razor wire appeared in the headlights.

Peter yelled into the radio, "Everyone keep going! Don't stop!"

They careened straight through the barrier. Chase stamped the brakes and pulled to the side as the convoy roared past with inches to spare, pushing a wall of wind that buffeted the vehicle like a howling gale. Peter, Chase, and Amy leapt from the cab.

Where was the tanker?

It lumbered into view at the base of the causeway — lamps blazing, engine roaring, traveling toward them like a well-lit rocket in slow motion. Past the turn it began to accelerate. Two virals were crouched on the roof of the cab. Chase raised his rifle and squinted through the scope.

"Ford, don't," Peter warned. "You hit that tank, it could blow."

"Quiet. I can do this."

A bullet split the air. One of the virals tumbled away. Ford was taking aim at the second when it dropped to the hood: no shot.

"Shit!"

From the cab, a pair of shotgun blasts came in rapid succession; the windshield shattered outward into the moonlight. There was a hissing groan of brakes. The viral flopped backward into the conical glare of the truck's headlights and disappeared beneath the front wheels with a wet burst.

Suddenly the cab was at a right angle to the causeway; the tanker was jackknifing. The whole thing began to swing crosswise. As its back wheels touched the water, the rear of the truck abruptly decelerated, swinging the cab in the opposite direction like a weight on a string. The truck was less than a hundred yards away now. Peter could see Greer fighting the wheel for control, but his

efforts were now pointless; the vehicle's angular momentum had assumed command.

It flopped onto its side. The cab separated from its cargo, which rammed it from behind in a second crunch of glass and metal. A long, screeching skid, and the whole thing came to rest, lying driver side up at a forty-five-degree angle to the roadway.

Peter dashed toward it, Chase and Amy close behind. Fuel was gushing everywhere; black smoke billowed from the undercarriage. The virals were funneling onto the isthmus; they would arrive within seconds. Patch was dead, his head crushed from behind; what was left of him was spread-eagled over the dashboard. Greer was lying on top of him, soaked in blood. Was it Patch's or his own? He was staring upward.

"Lucius, cover your eyes."

Peter and Chase began to kick what was left of the windshield. Three hard blows and the glass caved inward. Amy climbed inside and took the man by the shoulders while Peter took his legs. "I'm okay," Greer muttered, as if to apologize. As they hauled him out, the first fingers of flame appeared.

Chase and Peter each took a side. They ran.

Passengers had massed at the narrow gangway, attempting to shove their way through the bottleneck. Cries of panic stabbed the air. Men were scrambling over the deck of the ship to free the chains that held it in place. Many of the children seemed dazed and uncertain, drifting on the dock like a herd of sheep in the rain.

Pim and the girls were already on the ship. At the top of the gangway, Sara was lifting the small-

est children aboard, pulling others by the hand to hasten them; Hollis and Caleb were shepherding the children from the rear. A man charged from behind, nearly knocking Hollis over. Caleb grabbed him, threw him to the pavement, and shoved a finger into his face.

"You wait your goddamn turn!"

They weren't going to make it, Caleb thought. People had resorted to using the chains, attempting to drag themselves hand over hand to the ship. A woman lost her grip; with a cry, she plunged into the water. She came up, her face visible for only a moment, arms waving over her head: she didn't know how to swim. She sank back down.

Where were his father and the others? Why hadn't they come?

From the causeway, an explosion; all faces turned. A ball of fire was rising in the sky.

Wedged under the charger, Michael was trying to trace the faint hiss of leaking gas. Keep cool, he told himself. Do this by the numbers, joint by joint.

"Anything?" Rand was standing at the base of the charger.

"You're not helping."

It was no use. The leak was too small; it must have bled for hours.

"Get me some soapy water," he called. "I need a paintbrush, too."

"Where the hell am I going to get that?"

"I don't care! Figure it out!"

Rand darted away.

The blast hit them like a slap, hurling them forward, off their feet. Debris whizzed past: tires,

engine parts, shards of metal sharp as knives. As a wall of heat soared over him, Peter heard a scream and a great crunch of metal and splintering glass.

He was lying facedown in the mud. His thoughts were disordered; none seemed related to any of the others. A raglike bundle lay to his left. It was Chase. The man's clothes and hair were smoking. Peter crawled to him; his friend's eyes stared sightlessly. Cradling the back of the man's head, he felt something soft and damp. He turned Chase onto his side.

The back of the man's skull was gone.

The Humvee was totaled, crushed and burning. Greasy smoke clotted the air. It coated the insides of Peter's mouth and nose with its rancid taste. With every breath it drilled into his lungs, deeper and deeper.

"Amy, where are you?" He staggered toward the Humvee. "Amy, answer me!"

"I'm here!"

She was pulling Greer clear of the water. The two of them emerged covered in gooey mud and collapsed to the ground.

"Where's Chase?" She had pink burns on her face and hands.

"Dead." Crouched, he asked Greer, "Can you walk?"

The man was holding his head in his hands. Then, glancing up: "Where's Patch?"

The burning truck would hold the virals at bay, but once the fires died, the horde would come streaming down the isthmus. The three of them had nothing to fight with except Amy's sword, which still lay in its scabbard over her back.

A harsh white light raked their faces; a pickup was racing down the roadway toward them. Peter

hooded his eyes against the glare. The driver skidded to a stop.

"Get in," Caleb said.

Alicia saw only the sky. The sky and the back of a man's head. She sensed the presence of a crowd. Her stretcher jostled beneath her, there were voices, people crying, everything rushing around her.

Don't take me. Her body was broken; she lay loose as a doll. *I'm one of them. I don't belong.*

Clanging footsteps: they were crossing the gangway. "Put her over there," someone said. The stretcher-bearers lowered her to the deck and hurried away. A woman was sitting beside her, her body curled around a blanketed bundle. She was murmuring into the bundle, some kind of repeated phrase that Alicia could not make out, though it possessed the rote rhythm of prayer.

"You," Alicia said.

One syllable; it felt like lifting a piano. The woman failed to notice her.

"You," she repeated.

The woman looked up. The bundle was a baby. The woman's grip on it was almost ruthless, as if she feared someone might snatch it away at any moment.

"I need you . . . to help me."

The woman's face crumpled. "Why aren't we moving?" She bent her face to the baby again, burying it in the cloth. "Oh, God, why are we still here?"

"Please . . . listen."

"Why are you talking to me? I don't even know you. I don't know who you are."

"I'm . . . Alicia."

705

"Have you seen my husband? He was here a second ago. *Has anybody seen my husband?*"

Alicia was losing her. In another moment, she'd be gone. "Tell me . . . her name."

"What?"

"Your baby. Her . . . name."

It was as if nobody had ever asked her such a question.

"Say it," Alicia said. "Say . . . her name."

She shook with a sob. "He's a boy," she moaned. "His name is Carlos."

A moment passed, the woman weeping, Alicia waiting. There was chaos all around, and yet it felt as if they were alone, she and this woman she did not know, who could have been anyone. *Rose, my Rose,* Alicia thought, *how I have failed you. I could not give you life.*

"Will you . . . help me?"

The woman wiped her nose with the back of a wrist. "What can *I* do?" Her voice was utterly hopeless. "I can't *do* anything."

Alicia licked her lips; her tongue was heavy and dry. There would be pain, a lot of it; she would need every ounce of strength.

"I need you . . . to untie . . . my straps."

Soaring leap after soaring leap, Carter made his way down the channel toward the isthmus. The mushroom shapes of chemical tanks. The rooftops of buildings. The great, forgotten debris fields of industrial America. He moved swiftly, his power inexhaustible, like a huge heaving engine.

A great backlit shape rose before him: the channel bridge. He unleashed his body skyward; up he flew, seizing a handhold just below the bridge's shattered surface. A moment of calibra-

tion and he hurled himself upward again, grabbed a guy wire with one hand, and somersaulted to the deck.

Below, the unfolding battle was laid out before him like a model. The ship and the mob of people funneling aboard; the truck roaring down the causeway; the barricade of flames and the viral horde amassed behind it. Carter cocked his head to calculate his arc; he needed more height.

Using one of the support wires, he climbed to the top of the tower. The water shone below him still as glass, like a great smooth mirror to the moon. He felt some uncertainty, even a bit of fear; he pushed it aside. The tiniest fleck of doubt and he would fail, he would plummet into the abyss. To traverse such a distance — to master its breadth — one needed to enter an abstract realm. To become not the jumper but the jump, not an object in space but space itself.

He compressed to a crouch. Energy expanded outward from his core and gushed into his limbs.
Amy, I am coming.

From the pilothouse, Lore was watching the viral horde through binoculars. Blockaded by the flaming wreckage, it appeared as a column of thrumming light that stretched far back onto the mainland and beyond, widening to encompass virtually all of the far shore.

She raised the radio to her mouth. "I don't want to rush you, Michael, but whatever's wrong, you have got to fix it *right the fuck now.*"

"I'm trying here!"

Something was happening to the horde, a kind of . . . rippling. A rippling but also a compacting, like the gathering action of a spring. Beginning at

the rear, the motion slithered forward, gathering speed as it proceeded down the causeway toward the flames. The truck was lying lengthwise across the roadway. What was she seeing?

The head of the column crashed into the burning tanker like a battering ram. Gouts of smoke and fire shot into the sky. The tanker began to creep forward, scraping along the roadway. Burning virals peeled off into the water as more were propelled from behind into the destruction.

Lore looked down from the rail. The chains connecting the hull to the dock had been released; dozens of people were splashing helplessly in the water. At least a hundred, including some children, remained on the dock. Panicked cries knifed the air. *"Get out of my way!" "Take my daughter!" "Please, I'm begging you!"*

"Hollis!" she cried.

The man looked up. Lore pointed toward the isthmus. She realized her mistake: others on the dock had seen her. The mob surged forward, everyone attempting to wedge themselves onto the narrow gangway simultaneously. Blows were thrown, bodies hurled; people were trampled in the crush. From the center of the melee came the crack of a gunshot. Hollis rushed forward, arms swinging like a swimmer's, carving a path through the chaos. More shots; the crowd scattered, revealing a lone man with a pistol and two bodies on the ground. For a second the man just stood there, as if amazed by what he'd done, before he turned and charged up the gangway. Too late for him: he made it all of five steps before Hollis grabbed him by the collar, pulled him backward, placed his other hand under the man's buttocks, hoisted him over his head — the man flailing his arms and

legs like an overturned turtle — and hurled him over the rail.

Lore grabbed the radio: "Michael, it's getting ugly up here!"

A froth of bobbles appeared. Rand passed Michael a three-foot length of pipe and a tub of grease. Michael wrenched the old pipe free, greased the threads of its replacement, and fitted it into place. Rand had returned to the panel.

"Switch it over!" Michael yelled.

The lights flickered; the mixers began to spin. Pressure flowed into the lines.

"Here we go!" Rand cried.

Michael wriggled free. Rand tossed him the radio.

"Lore —"

Everything died again.

She had failed; her army was gone, scattered to dust. With all her heart Amy wanted to be on that ship, to depart this place and never come back. But she could never leave, not on this boat or any other. She would stand on the dock as it sailed away.

How I wanted to have that life with you, Peter, she thought. *I'm sorry, I'm sorry, I'm sorry.*

The truck was racing east, Caleb at the wheel, Peter, Amy, and Greer in the cargo bed. Ahead the lights of the dock loomed; behind them, across the widening distance, Amy saw the burning tanker pivoting. The first virals appeared through the breach. Their bodies were burning. They staggered forward, man-sized wicks of flame. The gap continued to widen, opening like a door.

Amy turned to the window of the cab. "Caleb—"

He was looking through the mirror. "I see them!"

Caleb floored it; the truck shot forward, sending Amy tumbling. Her head impacted the metal floor with a *clang* and a burst of disorienting pain. Lying on her back, her face to the sky, Amy saw the stars. Stars by the hundreds, the thousands, and one of them was falling. It grew and grew, and she knew what this star was.

"Anthony."

Carter's aim was true; as the truck zoomed past, he landed behind it on the causeway, rolled, and came up on his feet. The virals were careening toward him. He drew himself erect.

Brothers, sisters.

He sensed their confusion. Who was this strange being who had dropped into their path?

I am Carter, Twelfth of Twelve. Kill me if you can.

"What the hell happened?"

"I don't know!"

The radio squawked: Lore. "Michael, we have *got* to go *right now.*"

Rand was madly checking gauges. "It's not the charger — it has to be electrical."

Michael stood before the panel in utter desolation. It was hopeless; he was beaten. His ship, his *Bergensfjord,* had denied him. His paralysis became anger; his anger turned to rage. He slammed a fist against the metal. "You bitch!" He reared back, struck again. "You heartless bitch! You do this to me?" With tears of frustration brimming, he grabbed a wrench from the deck and

710

began to slam it against the metal, again and again. "I've . . . given . . . you . . . *everything!*"

A sudden rumble, like the roar of a great caged beast. Lights came on; all the gauges leapt.

"Michael," said Rand, "what the hell did you do?"

"That's got it!" Lore cried.

The sound increased in intensity, humming through the ship's plating. Rand yelled over the din: "Pressure's holding! Two thousand rpm! Four! Five! Six thousand!"

Michael snatched the radio from the floor. "Engage the screws!"

A groan. A shudder, deep in the bones.

The *Bergensfjord* began to move.

They skidded into the loading area. Amy leapt from the back of the truck before it stopped moving.

"Amy, stop!"

But the woman was already gone, racing toward the causeway. "Caleb, take Lucius and get on that boat."

Standing by the cargo bed, his son seemed stunned.

"Do it!" Peter ordered. "Don't wait!"

He took off after her. With every step he willed himself to go faster. His breath was heaving in his chest, the ground flying beneath him. The gap between them began to narrow. Twenty feet, fifteen, ten. A final burst of speed and he grabbed her around the waist, sending both of them rolling on the ground.

"Let me go!" Amy was on her knees, fighting to break free.

"We have to leave *right now.*"

There were tears in her voice. "They'll kill him!"

Carter coiled. He flexed his fingers, claws glinting. He flexed his toes, feeling the taut wires of ligaments. Blueing moonlight doused him like a benediction.

Reaching one hand forward, Amy released a wail of pain. "Anthony!"

He charged.

They had to clear eight hundred feet.

At the rear of the vessel, a wall of foam churned up. Shouts rose from the dock: *"They're leaving without us!"* The last of the passengers rushed forward, shoving themselves onto the ramp, which had begun to scrape along the pier as the *Bergensfjord* pulled away.

Standing at the rail, Pim watched the scene unfold in silence. The bottom lip of the gangway was inching toward the edge; soon it would fall. Where was her husband? Then she saw him. Supporting Lucius, he was racing at a quick-step down the pier. She began to sign emphatically to any who might see: *That's my husband!* And: *Stop this ship!* But, of course, no one could make sense of her.

The gangway was clotted with people. Crammed between the guardrails, they squeezed forward onto the deck of the ship only one or two at a time, ejected from the squirming mass. Pim began to moan. She was not aware that she was doing this at first. The sound had emerged of its own volition, an expression of violent feeling that could not be contained — just as, twenty-one years ago, in Sara's arms, she had wailed with such ferocity that she might have been mistaken for a dying animal. As the volume increased, the sound began

to form a distinctive shape altogether new in the life of Pim Jaxon: she was about to make words.

"Caaay . . . leb! Ruuuuunnnn!"

The lip of the gangway halted. It had lodged against a cleat at the edge of the pier. Under the pressure of the ship's accelerating mass, it began to twist on its axis. Rivets were popping, metal buckling. Caleb and Greer were steps away. Pim was waving, shouting words she couldn't hear but felt — felt with every atom of her body.

The gangway began to fall.

Still chained to the ship, it cantilevered into the side of the hull. Bodies plunged into the water, some wordlessly, their fate accepted, others with pitiful cries. At the bottom of the ramp, Caleb had hooked an elbow through the rail while simultaneously holding on to Greer, whose feet were balanced on the lowest rung. The *Bergensfjord* was gathering speed, dragging a roiling whirlpool. As the stern passed by, the ones in the water were dragged under, into the propeller's froth. Perhaps a cry, a hand reaching up in vain, and they were gone.

In the bowels of the *Bergensfjord,* Michael was running. Deck by deck he ascended, legs flying, arms swinging, heart pumping in his mouth. With a burst he flung himself into open air. The point of the bow was passing the end of the drydock door.

They weren't going to clear it. No goddamn way.

He took the stairs to the pilothouse three at a time and charged through the door. "Lore —"

She was staring out the windscreen. "I know!"

"Give it more rudder!"

"You don't think I did that?"

The gap between the door and the ship's right

flank was narrowing. Twenty yards. Ten. Five.

"Oh, shit," Lore breathed.

Peter and Amy were racing down the dock.

The ship was departing; she was gliding away. Gunfire spattered from the fantail, bullets whizzing over their heads; the virals had broken through.

A crash.

The side of the hull had collided with the end of the drydock door. A long scraping sound followed, the irresistible force of the ship's momentum meeting the immovable object of the door's weight. The hull trembled even as it failed to decelerate, thrusting forward.

The great wall of steel slid heartlessly by. In another few seconds, the *Bergensfjord* would be gone. There was no way to board. Peter saw something hanging off the side of the ship: the fallen gangway, still attached at the top. Two people were clinging to it.

Caleb. Greer.

With one arm crooked around the gangway rail, his son was calling to them while pointing at the end of the pier. The drydock door had been nudged away from the ship; it now stood at an acute angle to the moving hull. When the gangway passed the end of the door, the gap between them would narrow to a jumpable distance.

But Amy was no longer beside him; Peter was alone. He spun and saw her, standing a hundred feet behind him, facing away.

"Amy, come on!"

"Get ready to jump!" Caleb yelled.

The virals had reached the far end of the pier. Amy drew her sword and called to Peter over her

shoulder, "Get on that ship!"

"What are you doing? We can make it!"

"Don't make me explain! Just go!"

Suddenly he understood: Amy did not intend to leave. Perhaps she never had.

Then he saw the girl.

Far out of his reach, she was crouched behind a giant spool of cable. Strawberry hair tied with a ribbon, scratches on her face, a stuffed animal gripped tightly to her chest with arms thin as twigs.

Amy saw her, too.

She sheathed her sword and dashed forward. The virals were charging down the dock. The little girl was frozen with terror. Amy swung her onto her hip and began to run. With her free hand she waved Peter forward. "Don't wait! I'll need you to catch us!"

He raced down the drydock door. The bottom of the gangway was thirty feet away and closing fast. Caleb yelled, "Do it now!"

Peter leapt.

For an instant it seemed he had jumped too soon; he would plunge into the roiling water. But then his hands caught the rail of the gangway. He pulled himself up, found his footing, and turned around. Amy, still holding the girl, was running down the top of the wall. The gangway was passing them by; she was never going to make it. Peter reached out as Amy took five bounding strides, each longer than the last, and flung herself over the abyss.

Peter could not remember the moment when he grabbed her hand. Only that he'd done it.

They had cleared the dock. Michael ran down

715

from the pilothouse and dashed to the rail. He saw a deep dent, fifty feet long at least, though the wound was high above the waterline. He looked toward shore. A hundred yards aft, at the end of the dock, a mass of virals was watching the departing ship like a crowd of mourners.

"Help!"

The voice came from the stern.

"Someone's fallen!"

He raced aft. A woman, clutching an infant, was pointing over the rail.

"I didn't know she was going to jump!"

"Who? Who was it?"

"She was on a stretcher, she could barely walk. She said her name was Alicia."

A coiled rope lay on the deck. Michael pushed the button on the radio. "Lore, kill the props!"

"What?"

"Do it! Full stop!"

He was already wrapping the rope around his waist, having shoved the radio into the hand of the woman, who stared at him in confusion.

"Where are you going?" the woman asked.

He stepped over the rail. Far below, the waters swirled in a maelstrom. *Kill them,* he thought. *Dear God, Lore, kill those screws now.*

He jumped.

Toes pointed, arms outstretched, he pierced the surface like a spike; instantly the current grabbed him, shoving him down. He slammed into the mucky bottom and began to roll along it. His eyes stung with salt; he could see nothing at all, not even his hands.

He fell straight into her.

A confusion of limbs: they were both tumbling,

spiraling along the bottom. He grabbed her belt and drew her body into his and wrapped his arms around her waist.

The slack ran out.

A hard yank; Michael felt as if he were being sliced in two. Still holding Alicia, he vaulted upward at a forty-five-degree angle. Michael had already been in the water for thirty seconds; his brain was screaming for air. The screws had stopped turning, but this no longer mattered. They were being pulled along by the boat's momentum. Unless they broke the surface soon, they'd drown.

Suddenly, a whining sound: the screws had reengaged. *No!* Then Michael realized what had happened: Lore had reversed the engines. The tension on the rope began to soften, then was gone. A new force gripped them. They were being sucked forward, toward the spiraling props.

They were going to be chopped to bits.

Michael looked up. High above, the surface shimmered. What was the source of this mysterious, beckoning light? The sound of the screws abruptly ceased; now he understood Lore's intentions. She was creating enough slack in the line for them to ascend. Michael began to kick. *Alicia, don't give up. Help me do this. Unless you do, we're dead.* But it was no use; they were sinking like stones. The light receded pitilessly.

The rope went taut again. They were being pulled.

As they broke the surface, Michael opened his mouth wide, sucking in a vast gulp of air. They were beneath the stern, a mountain of steel soaring above them; the light he'd seen was the moon. It shone down upon them, fat and full, spilling

717

across the surface of the water.

"It's all right, I've got you," Michael said. Alicia was coughing and sputtering in his arms; from high above, a lifeboat floated down. "I've got you, I've got you, I've got you."

77

Carter's eyes were full of stars.

He lay on the causeway, bloodied and broken. Some parts of him felt as if they were absent, no longer attached. There was no pain; rather, his body felt distant, beyond his command.

Brothers, sisters.

They stood around him in a circle. Toward them, he felt only love. The ship was gone; it was streaming away. He felt a great love for everything; he would have wrapped the world with his heart if he could. At the edge of the causeway, moonlight skittered across the water, making a glowing road for him to travel.

Let me do this. Let me feel it coming out of me. Let me be a man again, before I die.

Carter began to crawl. The virals stepped back, allowing him to pass. There was in their comportment a feeling of respect, as if they were pupils, or soldiers accepting the sword of their enemy. Across the roadway, Carter made his passage. His left hand, reaching out, was the first part of him to touch the sea. The water was cool and welcoming, rich with salt and earth. A billion living things coursed through it; to them he would be joined.

Brothers, sisters, I thank you.

He slipped beneath the surface of the water.

■ ■ ■ ■

XI
THE CITY OF MIRRORS

■ ■ ■ ■

I wear the chain I forged in life. . . .
I made it link by link, and yard by yard;
I girded it on of my own free will,
and of my own free will I wore it.
— CHARLES DICKENS, *A Christmas Carol*

78

Dawn at sea.

The *Bergensfjord* lay at anchor, her great engines at rest. The sky was low, the water blank as stone; far away, a screen of rain fell into the Gulf. Most of the passengers were sleeping on the deck. Their bodies lay in disorder, as if felled all at once. They were a hundred miles from land.

Amy stood at the bow, Peter beside her. Her mind was drifting, refusing to attach to any thought but one. Anthony was gone. She was all that remained.

The little girl's name was Rebecca. Her mother had died in the attack, her father years ago. Amy's feeling of her — her body's weight and heat, the desperate force with which she'd clung to her as they had soared through space — was still palpable. Amy did not think it would ever depart; the sensation had become a part of her, stitched to her bones. It had defined the moment, making the choice for her. It was not only Rebecca that Amy had seen on the pier but her own little-girl self, who had, after all, been just as alone, abandoned by the great heaving engine of the world and in need of saving.

For some time, perhaps ten minutes, neither she

nor Peter spoke. Like her, Peter was only half present, staring into space — the pale dawn sky, the sea, limitlessly calm.

It was Amy who broke the silence. "You better go talk to her."

In the small hours of the night, a decision had been reached. Amy could not go; neither could Alicia. If the survivors were going to make a new life for themselves, all traces of the old terrors needed to be left behind. What mattered now was for others to accept it.

"She didn't do this, Peter."

He glanced at her but said nothing.

"Neither did you," she added.

Another silence. With all her heart she wanted him to believe this, yet she knew it was impossible for him to think otherwise.

"You need to make peace with her, Peter. For both your sakes."

The sun was rising unremarkably behind the clouds; the sky was devoid of color, its edges blended imperceptibly into the horizon. The rain kept its distance. Michael had assured them that the weather wouldn't be a problem; he knew how to read these things.

"Well," Peter said with a sigh, "I suppose I better do this."

He left her and descended to the crew's quarters. The air belowdecks was cooler, smelling of wet metal and rust. Most of Michael's men were snoring in their racks, using this brief hiatus to rest and prepare themselves for what lay ahead.

Alicia lay on a lower bunk at the far end of the corridor. Peter pulled up a stool and cleared his throat. "So."

Staring upward, she had yet to look at him. "Say

what's on your mind."

He wasn't entirely sure what that was. *I'm sorry I tried to strangle you?* Or *What were you thinking?* Perhaps he meant *Go to hell.*

"I'm here to offer a truce."

"A truce," Alicia repeated. "Sounds like Amy's idea."

"You tried to kill yourself, Lish."

"And it would have worked, too, if Michael hadn't decided to be the hero. I've got a bit of a bone to pick with the guy."

"Did you think the water would change you back?"

"Would it make you feel better if I did?" She blew out a breath. "I'm afraid that's not an option for me. Fanning was pretty clear on that score. No, I'd have to say that drowning was pretty much the goal."

"I can't believe that."

"Peter, what do you want? If you're here to pity me, I'm not interested."

"I'm aware of that."

"What you mean to say is that you need me."

He nodded. "That would be fair."

"And, under the circumstances, it's best if we bury the hatchet. Comrades, brothers-in-arms, no division within the ranks."

"More or less, yes."

With painful slowness, she turned her face toward him. "Want to know what I was thinking? While your hands were around my throat, I mean."

"If you want to tell me."

"I was thinking, Well, if anybody's going to strangle me, I'm glad it's my old friend Peter."

She'd spoken these words without bitterness; she was merely stating a fact.

723

"I was wrong," he said. "You didn't deserve it. I don't know what's between you and Fanning. I doubt I'll ever get it, frankly. But I sold you short."

She weighed his words, then shrugged. "So, you screwed up. Short of an outright apology, I guess I'll have to take that."

"I guess you will."

She gave him a look of warning. "I said I can get you in there, and I can. But you're throwing your life away."

"I'd say it's the opposite."

Alicia made a sound that began as a laugh but turned into a cough — deep, hacking. Her eyes clamped shut with pain. Peter waited for it to subside.

"Lish, are you all right?"

Her cheeks were flushed; spittle flecked her lips. "Do I look all right?"

"On the whole, you've seemed better."

She shook her head indulgently, the way a mother might with a hopeless child. "You never change, Peter. Fifty years I've known you, and you're still the same guy. Maybe that's why I can't stay mad at you."

"And I'll take that." He stood. "Need anything before we leave?"

"A new body would be nice. This one seems to have run its course."

"Short of that."

Alicia thought for a moment, then smiled. "I don't know — how about another rabbit?"

He found his son on deck, sitting on a wooden crate and watching Michael making his preparations on the fantail.

"You mind?" he asked.

724

Caleb scooted over.

"Where's Pim?"

"Asleep." His son turned and gave him a hard look. "Help me understand this."

"I'm not sure I can."

"Then why? What difference could it possibly make now?"

"People will come back someday. If Fanning's still alive, it starts all over again."

"You're going because of her."

Peter was speechless.

"Oh, don't look so surprised," Caleb went on. "I've known about it for years."

Peter didn't know how to respond. In the end, he could only admit the truth. "Well, you're right."

"Of course I'm *right.*"

"Let me finish. Amy does have something to do with this, but she's not the only reason." He brought his thoughts into focus. "Here's the best way I have to explain it. It's a story about your father. At the Colony, we had a tradition. We called it standing the Mercy. When a person was taken up, a relative would wait for them each night on the city wall. We'd set out a cage with a lamb inside as bait. Seven nights, waiting for them to come home, and if they did, it was that person's job to kill them. It was usually the responsibility of the closest male relative, so when your father disappeared, I had to stand for him."

Caleb was watching his face closely. "How old were you?"

"Twenty, twenty-one? Just a kid."

"But he didn't come back. He'd been taken to the Haven."

"Yes, but I didn't know that. Seven nights, Caleb. That's a lot of time to think about killing a

725

person, especially my own brother. At the start, I wondered if I actually could. Our parents had died, Theo was the only person I had left in the world. But as the nights passed, I came to understand something. There was something worse than killing him, and that would be letting somebody else do it. If the situation were reversed, if I had been the one taken up, I wouldn't have wanted it any other way. I didn't want to do it, believe me, but I owed him that much. The responsibility was mine and no one else's." Peter gave his words a moment to sink in. "That's what this is like, son. I don't know why it has to be me. That's a question I can't answer. But it doesn't matter. Pim and the kids — those are your responsibilities. You were put on earth to protect them till your last breath. That's your job. This is mine. You need to let me do it."

Aboard the *Nautilus,* Michael was issuing instructions to the crewmen who would assist in launching her. The hull had been wrapped in thick rope webbing; a steel boom and a system of blocks would be used to lift her from her cradle and lower her over the side. Once she was in the water, they would cut her free, raise the mast, and set sail for New York.

"He'll kill you," Caleb said.

Peter said nothing.

"And if you succeed? Amy can't leave. You said so yourself."

"No, she can't."

"So what then?"

"Then I live my life. Just like you're going to live yours."

Peter waited for his son to say more; when he didn't, he put his hand on Caleb's shoulder. "You

have to accept this, son."

"It's not easy."

"I know it's not."

Caleb tipped his face upward. He swallowed, hard, and said, "When I was a kid, my friends always talked about you. Some of what they said was true, a lot of it was total bullshit. The funny thing was, I felt bad for you. I won't say I didn't like the attention, but I also knew you didn't want people to think of you like that. It kind of stumped me. Who wouldn't want to be a big deal, some kind of hero? Then one day it hit me. You felt that way because of me. I was the choice you'd made, and the rest didn't matter to you anymore. You would have been perfectly happy if the world just forgot about you."

"It's true. That's how I saw it."

"I felt so goddamn *lucky*. When you started working for Sanchez, I thought things might change, but they never did." He looked at Peter again. "So now you ask me if I can just let you go. Well, I can't. I don't have that in me. But I do understand."

They sat without speaking for a time. Around them, the ship was waking up, passengers rising, stretching their limbs. *Did that really happen?* they thought, their eyes blinking against an unfamiliar, oceanic light. *Am I really on a ship? Is that the sun, the sea?* How stunned they must be, thought Peter, by the infinite calm of it all. Voices accumulated — mostly the children, for whom a night of terror, abruptly and in a manner completely unforeseen, had opened a door to an entirely new existence. They had gone to sleep in one world and awakened in another, so dissimilar as to seem, perhaps, an altogether different ver-

sion of reality. As the minutes passed, many of the passengers were drawn magnetically to the rail — pointing, whispering, chattering among themselves. As he listened, memories poured through him, as well as a sense of all the things he would never see.

Michael walked toward them. The man's eyes darted toward Caleb, quickly sizing up the situation, then back to Peter. Shuffling his hands in his pockets, he said, gently, almost as if he were apologizing, "The supplies are all aboard. I think we're about ready here."

Peter nodded. "Okay." But he made no move to do anything about this.

"Do you . . . want me to tell the others?"

"I think that would be good."

Michael walked away. Peter turned to his son. "Caleb —"

"I'm all right." He rose from the crate, holding himself stiffly, like a man with a wound. "I'll get Pim and the children."

Everyone gathered at the *Nautilus*. Lore and Rand operated the winch that hoisted Alicia, still strapped to her stretcher, to the cockpit. Michael and Peter carried her down to the boat's small cabin, then descended the ladder to join the others: Caleb and his family; Sara and Hollis; Greer, who had rebounded well enough from the crash to join them on deck, though his head was bandaged and he stood unsteadily, one hand braced against the hull of the *Nautilus*. Everywhere on the ship, people were watching; the story had spread. It was 0830 hours.

The final goodbyes: no one knew where to start. It was Amy who broke the stalemate. She em-

braced Lucius, the two of them exchanging quiet words that no one else could hear, then Sara and then Hollis, who, of everyone, more so even than Sara, seemed undone by the weight of it all, hugging Amy tightly against his chest.

But, of course, Sara was steeling herself. Her composure was a ruse. She would not go to Michael; she simply could not bear to. Finally, as the various farewells proceeded around them, it was he who went to her.

"Oh, damn you, Michael," she said miserably. "Why are you always doing this to me?"

"I guess it's my talent."

She wrapped her arms around him. Tears squeezed from the corners of her eyes. "I lied to you, Michael. I never gave you up. Not for a day."

They parted; Michael turned to Lore. "I guess this is it."

"You always knew that you wouldn't be going, didn't you?"

Michael didn't answer.

"Oh, hell," Lore said. "I guess I kind of knew it, too."

"Take care of my ship," Michael said. "I'm counting on you."

Lore took his cheeks in her hands and kissed him, long and tenderly. "Stay safe, Michael."

He climbed aboard the *Nautilus*. At the base of the ladder, Peter shook Greer's hand, then Hollis's; he hugged Sara long and hard. He had already said goodbye to Pim and the children. His son would be the last. Caleb was standing to the side. His eyes were tight, withholding tears; he would not cry. Peter felt, suddenly, as if he were marching to his death. Likewise was he struck, as never before, by a sense of pride. This strong man

before him. Caleb. His son, his boy. Peter pulled him into a firm embrace. He would not hold on long; if he did, he might not let go. It's children, he thought, that give us our lives; without them we are nothing, we are here and then gone, like the dust. A few seconds, recording all he could, and he stepped back.

"I love you, son. You make me very proud."

He climbed the ladder to join the others on the deck. Rand and Lore began to crank the winch. The *Nautilus* rose from her cradle and swung over the side. With a soft splash, the boat settled into the water.

"Okay, hold us there!" Michael called up.

They used their knives to cut the net. It passed beneath their stern, half-floating, then was dragged under the surface by its weight. Peter and Amy attached the guy wires while Michael set the lines that would pull the mast erect. They had begun to drift away from the *Bergensfjord.* When everything was ready, Michael commenced turning the winch. The mast rose into position; he locked it in place and unstrapped the sail from the boom. The distance to the *Bergensfjord* had increased to fifty yards. The air was warming, with a gentle breeze. The great ship's engines had come on. A new sound emerged, one of chains. Beneath the *Bergensfjord*'s bow, the anchor appeared, water streaming as it ascended. The ship's rail was lined with faces; people were watching them. Some began to wave.

"Okay, we're ready," Michael said.

They raised the mainsail. It flapped emptily, but then Michael pulled the tiller to one side and the bow veered slowly off the wind. With a pop, the canvas filled.

"We'll raise the jib once we're clear," said Michael.

Their velocity was, to Peter, quite startling. The boat, heeling slightly, possessed a stable feel, the point of its bow slicing cleanly through the water. The *Bergensfjord* receded behind them. The sky seemed infinitely deep.

It happened gradually, then all at once: they were alone.

79

Log of the *Nautilus*
Day 4: 27°95'N, 83°99'W. Wind SSE 10–15, gusts to 20.
Skies clear, seas running 3–4 feet.
After three days of light air, we are finally making decent headway, running at 6–8 knots. I expect we will reach Florida's west coast by nightfall, just north of Tampa. Peter seems to be finally getting his sea legs. After three days vomiting over the side, he announced today that he was hungry. From Lish, not very much; she sleeps most of the time and has said virtually nothing. Everyone is worried about her.

Day 6: 26°15'N, 79°43'W. Wind SSE 5–10, shifting.
Partly cloudy. Seas running 1–2 feet.
We have rounded the Florida peninsula and turned north. From here we will leave the coast behind and make a straight shot for the Outer Banks of North Carolina. Heavy clouds all night but no rain. Lish is still very weak. Amy finally talked her into eating, and Peter and I drew straws. He was the winner, though I guess it

731

depends on how you look at it. I was a little nervous about Sara's instructions and I'm no good with needles, so Amy took over. One pint. We'll see if it helps.

Day 9: 31°87'N, 75°25'W. Winds SSE 15–20, gusts to 30.
Skies clear. Seas running 5–7 feet.
A horrible night. The storm hit just before sunset — huge seas, high winds, driving rain. Everyone was up all night working the bailers. Blown way off course, and the self-steerer is shot. We've taken on water, but the hull seems tight. Running reefed in heavy air, no jib.

Day 12: 36°75'N, 74°33'W. Winds NNE 5–10.
Patchy clouds. Seas running 2–3 feet.
We have decided to head west for the coast. Everyone is exhausted and needs to rest. On the bright side, Lish seems to have turned a corner. Her back is the issue; she's still in a lot of pain and can barely bend at all. My turn with the needle. Lish seemed to have a little fun with that. "Oh, buck up, Circuit," she said. "A girl's got to eat. Maybe your blood will make me smarter."

Day 13: 36°56'N, 76°27'W. Winds NNE 3–5.
Seas running 1–2 feet.
Lying at anchor at the mouth of the James River. Fantastic wreckage everywhere — huge naval vessels, tankers, even a submarine. Lish's mood has improved. At sunset she asked us to bring her up on deck.

A beautiful starlit night.

Day 15: 38°03'N, 74°50'W. Winds light and

variable. Seas 2–3 feet.
Under way again with fair winds. Running at 6 knots. Everyone feels it — we are getting closer.

Day 17: 39°63'N, 75°52'W. Winds SSE 5–10. Seas 3–5 feet.
Tomorrow we reach New York.

80

The four of them sat in the cockpit in the gathering dusk. They were lying at anchor; off the port bow, a long sandy line. The southern edge of Staten Island, once populated by a dense humanity, now exposed, swept clean, a wilderness.

"So, we're all in agreement?" Peter said, scanning the group. "Michael?"

Seated by the tiller, he was fingering a pocketknife, opening and closing the blade. His face had been crisped by salt and wind; through his beard, the color of sand, his teeth shone white. "I told you before. If you say that's the plan, then that's the plan."

Peter turned to Alicia. "Last chance to weigh in here."

"Even if I said no, you wouldn't listen."

"I'm sorry, that's not good enough."

She looked at him guardedly. "He's not going to just surrender, you know. 'I'm sorry, I guess I was wrong after all.' Not really the man's style."

"That's why I need you in the tunnel with Michael."

"I belong in the station with you."

Peter looked at her pointedly. "You can't kill him — you said so yourself. You can barely walk. I know you're angry and you don't want to hear

this. But you need to put your feelings aside and leave that part to me and Amy. You'd only slow us down, and I need you to protect Michael. Fanning's virals won't attack you. You can give him cover."

Peter could see that his words had stung. Alicia glanced away, then back, her eyes narrowed with warning. "You realize that he knows we're coming. I seriously doubt any of this has escaped his attention. Waltzing into the station plays straight into his hands."

"That's the idea."

"And if this doesn't work?"

"Then we all die and Fanning wins. I'm willing to hear a better idea. You're the expert on the man. Tell me I'm wrong and I'll listen."

"That's not fair."

"I know it's not."

A brief silence passed. Alicia sighed in surrender. "Fine, I can't. You win."

Peter looked toward Amy. After two weeks at sea, her hair had grown out somewhat, softening her features while also making them seem clearer somehow, sturdier and more defined. "I think it all depends on what Fanning wants," she said.

"From you, you mean."

"Maybe he just intends to kill me, and if so, there's not a lot to stop him. But he's gone to a lot of trouble to get me here if that's all he has in mind."

"What do *you* think he wants?"

The light was nearly gone; from the shore, the long shushing of waves.

"I don't know," she said. "I agree with Lish, though. The man has something to prove. Beyond that . . ." She trailed off, then continued: "The

important thing is to make sure he's in that station. Get him there and keep him there. We shouldn't wait for Michael. We need to be there when the water hits. That's our moment."

"So you agree with the plan."

She nodded. "Yes. I think it's our best chance."

"Let's look at that drawing."

Alicia had sketched a simple map: streets and buildings, but also what lay beneath them and points of access. To this she added verbal descriptions: how things looked and felt, certain landmarks, places where their passage would be obstructed by forest growth or collapsed structures, the sea's margins where it lapped over the southern tier of the island.

"Tell me about the streets around the station," Peter said. "How much shade is there for the virals to move in?"

Alicia thought for a moment. "Well, a lot. Midday you'd get more sun, but the buildings are all very tall. I'm talking sixty, seventy stories. It's like nothing you've ever seen in your life, and it can get pretty dark at street level any time of day." She drew their attention to the drawing again. "I'd say your best bet would be here, at the station's west exit."

"Why there?"

"Two blocks west, there's a construction site. The building's fifty-two stories tall, not huge by the standards of what's around it, but the top thirty stories are only framed in. There's good sun around the base, even late in the day. You can see it from the station — there's an external elevator and a crane up the side of the building. I used to spend a lot of time up there."

"On the crane, you mean?"

Alicia shrugged. "Yeah, well. It was kind of a thing with me."

She offered no more explanation; Peter decided not to press. He pointed to another spot on the map, a block east of the station. "What's this?"

"The Chrysler Building. It's the tallest thing around there, almost eighty stories. The top is made of this kind of shiny metal, like a crown. It's highly reflective. Depending on where the sun is, it can throw a lot of light."

The day was over; the temperature had dropped, drawing dew from the air. As a silence settled, Peter realized they had come to the end of the conversation. In a little under eight hours they would raise the sails, the *Nautilus* would make the final leg to Manhattan, and whatever was bound to happen there would happen. It was unlikely that all of them would survive, or even that any of them would.

"I'll take the watch," said Michael.

Peter looked at him. "We seem well protected here. Is that necessary?"

"The bottom's pretty sandy. The last thing we need is a dragging anchor right now."

"I'll stay, too," Lish said.

Michael smiled. "Can't say I'd mind the company." Then, to Peter: "It's fine, I've done it a million times. Go sleep. You two are going to need it."

Night spread her hands over the sea.

All was still: only the sounds of the ocean, deep and calm, and the lap of waves against the hull. Peter and Amy lay curled together on the cabin's only bunk, her head resting on his chest. The night was warm, but belowdecks the air felt cool, almost

736

cold, chilled by the water encircling the bulkhead.

"Tell me about the farmstead," Amy said.

Peter needed a moment to gather his answer; lulled by the boat's motion and the feeling of closeness, he had, in fact, been skating on the edge of sleep.

"I'm not sure how to describe it. They weren't like ordinary dreams — they were far more real than that. Like every night I went someplace else, another life."

"Like . . . a different world. Real, but not the same."

He nodded, then said, "I didn't always remember them, not in detail. It was mostly the feeling that lasted. But some things. The house, the river. Ordinary days. The music you played. Such beautiful songs. I could have listened to them forever. They seemed so full of life." He stopped, then said, "Was it the same for you?"

"I think so, yes."

"But you're not sure."

She hesitated. "It only happened the one time, when I was in the water. I was playing for you. The music came so easily. As if the songs had been inside me and I was finally letting them out."

"What happened then?" Peter asked.

"I don't remember. The next thing I knew I woke up on the deck, and there you were."

"What do you think it means?"

She paused before answering. "I don't know. All I know is that for the first time in my life, I was truly happy."

For a while they listened to the quiet creaking of the boat.

"I love you," Peter said. "I think I always have."

"And I love you."

She drew herself closer against him; Peter replied in kind. He took her left hand, slipped her fingers through his, pulled it to his chest, and held it there.

"Michael's right," she said. "We should sleep."

"All right."

Soon she felt his breathing slow. It eased into a deep, long rhythm, like waves upon the shore. Amy closed her eyes, although she knew it was no use. She would lie awake for hours.

On the deck of the *Nautilus,* Michael was watching the stars.

Because a person could never grow tired of them. All his many nights at sea, the stars had been his most loyal companions. He preferred them to the moon, which seemed to him too frank, always begging to be noticed; the stars maintained a certain cagey distance, permitting the mystery of their hidden selves to breathe. Michael knew what the stars were — exploding balls of hydrogen and helium — as well as many of their names and the arrangements they made in the night sky: useful information for a man alone at sea in a small boat. But he also understood that these things were an imposed ordering that the stars themselves possessed no knowledge of.

Their vast display should have made him feel tiny and alone, but the effect was exactly the opposite; it was in daylight that he felt his solitude most keenly. There were days when his soul ached with it, the feeling that he had moved so far away from the world of people that he could never go back. But then night would fall, revealing the sky's hidden treasure — the stars, after all, weren't gone during the day, merely obscured — and his loneli-

738

ness would recede, supplanted by the sense that the universe, for all its inscrutable vastness, was not a hard, indifferent place in which some things were alive and others not and all that happened was a kind of accident, governed by the cold hand of physical law, but a web of invisible threads in which everything was connected to everything else, including him. It was along these threads that both the questions and the answers to life pulsed like an alternating current, all the pains and regrets but also happiness and even joy, and though the source of this current was unknown and always would be, a person could feel it if he gave himself a chance; and the time when Michael Fisher — Michael the Circuit, First Engineer of Light and Power, Boss of the Trade and builder of the *Bergensfjord* — felt it most was when he was looking at the stars.

He thought of many things. Days in the Sanctuary. Elton's blind, rigid face and the hot, cramped quarters of the battery hut. The gassy stink of the refinery, where he had left boyhood behind and found his course in life. He thought of Sara, whom he loved, and Lore, whom he also loved, and Kate and the last time he had seen her, her compact youthful energy and easy affection for him on the night when he had told her the story of the whale. All so long ago, the past forever retreating to become the great internal accumulation of days. Probably his time on earth was reaching its end. Maybe something came after, beyond one's physical existence as a person; on this subject, the heavens were obscure. Greer certainly thought so.

Michael knew that his friend was dying. Greer had tried to conceal it, and nearly had, but Michael had figured it out. No one thing in particular

had told him this; it was simply his sense of the man. Time was outstripping him — as, sooner or later, it did everyone.

And, of course, he thought about his ship, his *Bergensfjord.* She would be far away now, somewhere off the coast of Brazil, churning south beneath the selfsame starry sky.

"It's beautiful out here," Alicia said.

She was sitting across from him, reclining lengthwise on the bench, a blanket covering her legs. Her head, like his, was tipped upward, her eyes glazed by starlight.

"I remember the first time I saw them," she continued. "It was the night the Colonel left me outside the Wall. They absolutely terrified me." She pointed toward the southern horizon. "Why is that one so bright?"

He followed her finger. "Well, that's not a star, actually. It's the planet Mars."

"How can you tell?"

"You'll see it most of the summer. If you look closely, you can see that it has a slight red tint. It's basically a big, rusty rock."

"And that one?" Directly overhead this time.

"Arcturus."

In the dark, her expression was hidden from his view, though he imagined her frowning with interest. "How far away is it?"

"Not very, as these things go. About thirty-seven light-years. That's how long it takes the light to get here. When the light you're seeing left Arcturus, we were both a couple of kids. So when you look at the sky, what you're actually seeing is the past. But not just *one* past. Every star is different."

She laughed lightly. "That kind of messes with

my head when you put it that way. I remember you telling me about this stuff when we were kids. Or trying to."

"I was pretty obnoxious. Probably I was just trying to impress you."

"Show me more," she said.

He did just that; Michael traced the sky. Polaris and the Big Dipper. Bright Antares and blue-tinted Vega and her neighbors, the small cluster known as Delphinius the Dolphin. The broad galactic band of the Milky Way, running horizon to horizon, north to south, bisecting the eastern sky like a cloud of light. He told her all he could think of, her interest never wavering, and when he was done, she said, "I'm cold."

Alicia scooted forward from the transom; Michael crossed over and wedged himself behind her, his legs positioned on either side of her waist. He pulled the blanket up, wrapping the two of them, drawing her in for warmth.

"We haven't talked about what happened on the ship," Alicia said.

"We don't have to if you don't want."

"I feel like I owe you an explanation."

"You don't."

"Why did you come in after me, Michael?"

"I didn't really give it a lot of thought. It was a heat-of-the-moment thing."

"That's not an answer."

He shrugged, then said, "I guess you could say I don't much like it when people I care about try to kill themselves. I've been down that road before. I take it kind of personally."

His words stopped her flat. "I'm sorry. I should have thought —"

"And there's absolutely no reason you would

741

have. Just don't do it again, okay? I'm not such a great swimmer."

A silence fell. It was not uncomfortable but the opposite: the silence of shared history, of those who can speak without talking. The night was full of small sounds that, paradoxically, seemed to magnify the quiet: each shifting touch of water against the hull; the pinging of the lines against the spars; the creak of the anchor line in its cleat.

"Why did you name her *Nautilus*?" Alicia asked. The back of her head was resting against his chest.

"It was something from a book I read when I was a kid. It just seemed to fit."

"Well, it does. I think it's nice." Then, quietly: "What you said, in the cell."

"That I loved you." He felt no embarrassment, only the calm of truth. "I just thought you should know. It seemed like a big waste otherwise. I've kind of had it with secrets. It's okay — you don't have to say anything about it."

"But I want to."

"Well, a thank-you would be nice."

"It's not that simple."

"Actually, it's exactly that simple."

She fit the fingers of one hand into his, pressing their palms together. "Thank you, Michael."

"And you are most welcome."

The air was damp, mist falling, beads clinging to every surface. At an indeterminate distance, waves were hissing on the sand.

"God, the two of us," she said. "We've been fighting our whole lives."

"That we have."

"I'm so . . . tired of it." She drew his arm tighter around her waist. "I thought about you, you know. When I was in New York."

"Did you now?"

"I thought: What is Michael doing today? What is he doing to save the world?"

He laughed lightly. "I'm honored."

"As you should be." A pause; then she spoke again. "Do you ever think about them? Your parents."

The question, though unexpected, did not seem strange. "Once in a while. It was a long time ago, though."

"I don't really remember mine. They died when I was so young. Just little things, I guess. My mother had a silver hairbrush she liked. It was very old; I think it belonged to my grandmother. She used to visit me in the Sanctuary and brush my hair with it."

Michael considered this. "Now, that sounds right to me. I think I recall something like that happening."

"You do?"

"She'd put you on a stool in the dormitory, by the big window. I remember her humming — not a song exactly, more like just notes."

"Huh," Alicia said after a moment. "I didn't know anyone was paying attention."

They were quiet for a time. Even before she said the words, Michael sensed their approach. He did not know what she was about to tell him, only that she was.

"Something . . . happened to me in Iowa. A man raped me there, one of the guards. He got me pregnant."

Michael waited.

"She was a girl. I don't know if it was what I am or something else, but she didn't survive."

When Alicia fell silent, Michael said, "Tell me

about her."

"She was Rose. That's what I named her. She had such beautiful red hair. After I buried her, I stayed with her awhile. Two years. I thought it would help, make things easier somehow. But it never did."

He felt, suddenly, closer to Alicia than he had to anyone in his life. Painful as this story was, telling him was a gift she had given him, the heart of who she was, the stone she carried and how love had happened in her life.

"I hope it's okay I told you."

"I'm very glad you did."

Another silence, then: "You're not really worried about the anchor, are you?"

"Not really, no."

"That was nice, what you did for them." Alicia tipped her head upward. "It's such a beautiful night."

"Yes, it is."

"No, more than beautiful," she said and squeezed his hand, nestling against him. "It's perfect."

81

So, at the last, a story.

A child is born into this world. She is lost, alone, in due course both befriended and betrayed. She is the carrier of a special burden, a singular vocation that is only hers to bear. She wanders in a wasteland, a ruin of grief and tormented dreams. She has no past, only a long, blank future; she is like a convict with an unknown sentence, never visited in the cell of her interminable imprisonment. Any other soul would be broken by this

fate, and yet the child abides; she dares to hope that she is not alone. That is her mission, the role for which she has been cast at heaven's cruel audition. She is hope's last vessel on the earth.

Then, a miracle: a city appears to her, a bright walled city on a hill. Her prayers have been answered! Shining like a beacon, it has the aspect of a prophecy fulfilled. The key turns in the lock; the door swings open. Ensconced within its walls she discovers a wondrous race of men and women who have, like her, endured. They become hers, after a fashion. In the eyes of this wordless child, the most prescient among them perceive an answer to their most persistent questions; as they have relieved her loneliness, so has she relieved theirs.

A journey commences. The world's dark arrangement is revealed. The child grows; she leads her companion to a glorious victory. By her hand, seeds of hope are scattered over the land, promise bubbles forth from every spring and stream. And yet she knows this flowering is an illusion, the merest respite. There can be no safety; her triumphs have but scratched the crust. Below lies the dark core, that great iron ball beneath all things. Its compressed weight is fantastic; it is older than time itself. It is a vestige of the blackness that predates all existence, when a formless universe existed in a state of chaotic un-creation, lacking awareness even of itself.

She falters. She has doubts. She becomes indecisive, even fearful. Hers is the greatest of all errors; she has grown attached to life. She has dared, unwisely, to love. In her mind a contest rages, that of one who questions fate. Is she merely a lunatic's puppet? Is she destiny's slave or its

author? Must she turn away from all the things and people she has grown to love? And is this love a reflection of some grand design, a taste of an ordered and divine creation? Is it truth or a departure from the truth? Romantic love, fraternal love, the love of a parent for a child and the love returned in kind — are they a mirror to God's face or the bitterest gall in a cosmos of sound and fury, signifying nothing?

As for me: there was a time in my life when I put aside all doubt and supped at the flower of heaven. What sweet juice was there! What balm to all suffering, the soul's holy ache! That my Liz was dying did not countermand my joy; she had come to me like a messenger, in the hours when all is laid bare, to reveal my purpose on the earth. All my days, I had scrutinized the tiniest workings of life. I had gone about this task blandly, never fathoming my true motive. I gazed upon the smallest shapes and processes of nature, seeking divinity's fingerprints. Now the evidence had come to me not at the end of a microscope but in the face of this slender, dying woman and the touch of her hand across a café table. My long, lonely hours — like yours, Amy — seemed not an exile or imprisonment but a test that I had passed. I was loved! Me, Timothy Fanning of Mercy, Ohio! Loved by a woman, loved by a god — a great, fatherly god, who, measuring my trials, had found me worthy. I had not been made for nothing! And not just loved; I had been charged as heaven's escort. The blue Aegean, where ancient gods and heroes were said to dwell; the whitewashed house one climbed a flight of stairs to reach; the humble bed and homespun furnishings; the workaday sounds of village life, and a

746

terrace with a view of olive groves and the wild sea beyond; the soft white light of eternal mornings, growing brighter and brighter and brighter still. In my mind's eye I saw it, saw it all. In my arms she would pass from this life to the next, which surely existed after all, love having come to me — to both of us — at last.

Not an hour would have gone by, her body grown cold in my embrace, before I would have followed her from this world. That, too, was part of my design. I would take the last pills, the ones I'd saved for myself, and slip away in silence, so that together we would be bound eternally to each other and to an invincible universe. My resolve was implacable, my thoughts lucid as ice. I possessed not an iota of doubt. Thus at the anointed hour of our rendezvous I took my position at the kiosk, waiting for my angel to appear. In my suitcase, the instruments of our mortal deliverance slept like stones. Little did I know that this was but a foretaste of the wider ruin — that the hurrying travelers flowing around me possessed no inkling that death's prince stood among them.

Thrice have I been fathered; thrice betrayed. I will have satisfaction.

You, Amy, have dared to love, as once I did. You are hope's deluded champion, as I am sworn to be its enemy. I am the voice, the hand, the pitiless agent of truth, which is the truth of nothing. We were, each of us, made by a madman; from his design we forked like roads in a dark wood. It has ever been thus, since the materials of life assembled and crawled from nature's muck.

Your band approaches; the time grows sweeter by the hour. I know that he is with you, Amy. How could he fail to stand at your side, the man who

made you human?

Come to me, Amy. Come to me, Peter.

Come to me, come to me, come to me.

82

It emerged like a vision, the great city, soaring from the sea like a castle or some vast holy relic. A ruin of staggering dimensions: it boggled the senses, its scope too massive to hold in the mind. The morning sun, low, slanting, blazed off the faces of the towers, ricocheting from the glass like bullets.

Peter joined Amy at the bow. She seemed almost preternaturally calm; a profound intensity radiated off her like heat from a stove. Minute by minute the metropolis loomed higher.

"Good God, it's enormous," Peter said.

She nodded, though this was only half the truth. Fanning's presence saturated the city. It was as if a background hum she'd been hearing all her life, so omnipresent as to be barely noticeable, were increasing in volume. She felt a heaviness. That was the only word. A terrible exhausted heaviness with everything.

They had decided to come in from the west. On tepid air they sailed up the Hudson, searching for a place to dock. Daylight was everything; they needed to move quickly. The tide was strong, pushing against them like an invisible hand.

"Michael . . ."

He was working the lines and tiller, seeking to harness any breath of wind. "I know."

The river was dark as ink; its force was immense. The day turned toward afternoon. At times they seemed stopped cold.

"This is impossible," said Michael.

By the time they found a place to tie off, it was four o'clock. Clouds had moved in from the south; the air was sultry, smelling of decay. Four, perhaps five hours of daylight remained. From the cabin, Michael retrieved the backpack of explosives, as well as a long spool of cable and the detonator, a wooden box with a plunger. It seemed primitive, but that was the point, he explained. The simple things were always the most reliable, and there would be no second chances to get this right. In the cockpit, they armed themselves and reviewed the plan a final time.

"Make no mistake," Alicia said, "this island is a deathtrap. It gets dark, we're done."

They disembarked. They were in the West Twenties. The roadway was choked with the skeletons of cars; glassless windows stared at them like the mouths of caves. Here they would diverge, Michael and Lish south to Astor Place, Peter and Amy across midtown to Grand Central. Michael had fashioned a crude crutch for Alicia from a boat oar.

"Sixty minutes," Peter said. "Good luck."

They parted cleanly, no goodbyes.

Peter and Amy walked north along Fifth Avenue. Block by block, the vertical core of the city rose, fashioning narrow fjords between the buildings. In places the pavement was buckled with the roots of trees, in others collapsed into craters that varied in size from a few yards to the width of the street, forcing them to creep along the edge. As they moved up the island, Peter took note of the landmarks: the Empire State, dizzyingly tall, like a single imperious finger pointing to the sky; the

749

Chrysler Building, with its curved crown of burnished metal; the library, sheathed in a feathery cloak of vines, its broad front steps guarded by a pair of pedestaled lions. At the corner of Forty-second and Fifth, the half-constructed tower Alicia had described came into view. The exposed girders of its upper floors possessed a reddish appearance — the product of decades of slow oxidation. An exterior elevator ascended to the top of the structure; from there, the crane rose another ten or fifteen stories, its horizontal boom parallel to the building's west flank, high above Fifth Avenue.

So far, they had seen no trace of Fanning's virals — no scat or animal carcasses, no sounds of movement from the buildings. Except for pigeons, the city seemed dead. Each of them had a semi-automatic rifle and a pistol; Amy also carried the sword. She had offered it to Alicia, but the woman had refused. "Peter's right," Alicia said. "I've got no use for it. Just do me a favor and cut the bastard's head off."

They approached from the west, via Forty-third to Vanderbilt; between the buildings, a view of Grand Central emerged. Compared to what was around it, the structure seemed modest in its dimensions, nestled like a heart in the bosom of the city. The streets around it were open to the sun, though an elevated roadway encircled the perimeter at balcony level, creating a zone of darkness beneath.

Amy checked her watch: twenty minutes to go. "We need to scout that door," she said.

A risk, but Peter agreed. If they moved cautiously and kept low, maintaining an upward line of sight, they would be able to detect any virals

beneath the overpass before they got too close.

Which was, Peter later realized, precisely what Fanning had intended them to do: to look *up*. Never mind Alicia's warnings not to under-estimate their adversary. Never mind that the street was suspiciously carpeted in vines, or that with each step forward the air thickened with the damp, septic odor of an open sewer. Never mind the faint sound of rustling, which might have been caused by rats but wasn't. One careless moment was all it took. They crept beneath the overpass, every ounce of their attention focused on the empty ceiling.

Peter and Amy never even saw them coming.

Michael watched the numbers of the streets decline. A few were impassable, choked with vegetation or debris, others empty, as if forgotten by time. In some of the buildings, trees were grow-ing; flocks of startled pigeons burst forth in their path, wheeling upward in huge, flapping clouds.

At the corner of Eighteenth and Broadway, they paused to rest. Alicia was breathing hard, her face glazed with sweat. "How much farther?" Michael asked.

She coughed and cleared her throat. "Eleven blocks."

"I can do this on my own, you know."

"Not a chance."

The crutch was too unstable; they left it behind and went on, Michael supporting Alicia from one side. A rifle dangled over her shoulder. Her steps were labored, more hobble than walk. From time to time, she issued a tiny gasp he knew she was trying to hide. The minutes dripped away. They came to a small shelter of elaborate iron scroll-

work, painted white with pigeon guano. The smell of the sea had grown strong.

"This is it," she said.

From his pack, Michael removed a lantern and lit the wick. As they descended the stairs, he detected small movements along the floor. He paused and raised the lantern. Rats were scurrying everywhere, long brown ropes of them hugging the edges of the walls.

"Yuck," he said.

They reached the bottom. Arched brick columns supported the roof above the tracks. On the tiled wall, a sign in gold lettering read ASTOR PLACE.

"Which direction?" Michael felt turned around in the dark.

"This way. South."

He dropped onto the rail bed. Alicia handed him her rifle, and he helped her down. As they passed into the tunnel, the air became colder. Water sloshed at their feet. He counted their steps. At one hundred, the light of his lantern caught a frisson of movement: the hissing spray of water that shot from the edges of the bulkhead. He stepped forward and pressed his hand against the thick metal. Behind it lay untold tons of pressure, the weight of the sea, like an unfired cannon.

"How much time?" Alicia asked. She was leaning against the wall, scanning the tunnel with the rifle.

They had used forty-five minutes. He stripped off his pack and removed his supplies. Alicia was keeping watch on the far end of the tunnel. He twisted the wires of the blasting caps together, then clipped the end to the cable from the spool. Keeping everything dry would be a challenge; he had to prevent water from contacting the fuses.

He returned the dynamite to his pack and searched the door for something to hang it on. Its surface was absolutely smooth.

"There," Alicia said.

Beside the bulkhead, a long rusty screw jutted from the wall. Michael hung his pack on it, handed Alicia the detonator, and began to pull out the cable from the spool.

"Let's go."

They emerged into the Astor Place station and scrambled onto the platform. Unspooling the cable behind them, they headed for the stairs and ascended to the first landing. A particle-filled daylight filtered down from street level. Kneeling, Michael placed the plunger on the floor, split the cable with his teeth, and threaded one wire into each of the two slotted screws on the top of the box. Alicia was sitting on the step below him, goggles pushed up onto her forehead, her rifle pointed into the blackness below. Circles of sweat drenched her shirt at the throat and armpits; her jaw was tight with pain. As he tightened the wing nuts, their eyes met.

"That ought to do it," Michael said.

Ten minutes to go.

Amy in darkness: First came the pain, a sharp-edged thudding at the back of her skull. This was followed by the sensation of being dragged. Her thoughts refused to organize. Where was she? What had occurred? What force was pulling her along? Solitary pictures drifted by, pushed by mental winds: a television screen of spitting static; fat, feathered snowflakes descending from an inky sky; Carter's garden, a carpet of living color; the tossing, blue-black sea. There was the floor —

dirty, scuffed. Her tongue was dense and heavy in her mouth. She tried to make a sound, but none would come. The floor passed by in aortal jerks, timed to the rhythm of the tugging pressure on her wrists. The idea of resistance took hold, but when she attempted to move her limbs, she found she had no power to act; her body had been sundered from her will.

She sensed, then saw, a light, a kind of filtered glowing, and in the next instant everything changed: how the air moved on her skin, the way sound behaved, her intuitive sense of the physical parameters around her. Noises expanded and leapt away; the air smelled different, less confined, with a biological tang.

"Leave her there, please."

The voice — nonchalant, even a little bored — came from someplace ahead. The pressure on her wrists released; her face slammed into the floor. A hot, glowing ball ricocheted around the interior of her skull like an ember spat from a fire.

"*Gently,* for God's sake."

Consciousness ebbed, then, like a dark wave returning to shore, broke upon her again. She tasted blood in her mouth; she had bitten her tongue. The floor was cool against her cheek. The light, what was it? And the sound? A low-grade murmuring, not made by voices per se but by a volume of breathing bodies. She sensed the presence of faces. Faces and also hands, lurking in a fog. Her brain told her: *Look harder, Amy. Focus your eyes and look.*

It wasn't good. It wasn't good at all.

She was surrounded by virals. The first layer was crouched around her at a distance of just a yard or two — jaws clicking, throats amphibiously

bobbing, hooked fingers caressing the air with small, syncopated movements, as if tapping the keys of invisible pianos. This was bad, but not the worst of it. The room writhed and throbbed, a population of hundreds. They carpeted the walls. They gazed down from the balconies like spectators at a contest. They filled each nook and corner and perched atop every ledge. The space was squirming like a pit of snakes.

"That all went rather smoothly," the voice drolly continued. "I'm a little bit amazed, actually. I was worried that their enthusiasm might get the better of them. They do that."

She was still having difficulty bringing her mind and her body into alignment, to forge the proper chain of command. Everything seemed delayed and out of sync. The voice seemed to emanate from everywhere around her, as if the air were speaking. It flowed over and into her like slick oil, lodging with cloying, buttery sweetness at the back of her throat.

"Would it be too obvious to say how long I've waited to meet you? But I have. Since the day Jonas told me of your existence, I've wondered, When will we meet? When will my Amy come to me?"

"My Amy." Why was the voice calling her that? She discovered the sky. No, not the sky: the ceiling, far above, and on it the image of the stars with gilded figures floating among them.

"Oh, you should have heard the man. How *guilty* he felt. How *sorry* he was. 'Jesus, Tim, you should see her. She's just a little kid. She doesn't even have a proper last name. She's just some girl from nowhere.' "

The backward stars, thought Amy. As if the

heavens were being viewed from without, or were reflected in a mirror. She felt her thoughts attaching to this notion, and as they did, new ideas began to form. As if stumbling from a dream, her mind began to open to her circumstances; memories were rising to the surface. An image entered her mind: Peter, his body airborne, crashing through a plate-glass window.

A dark chuckle. "Not really funny, I suppose, when you put it in the context of a few billion corpses. Still, the whole thing was quite a performance. Jonas missed his true calling. He should have been an actor."

Fanning, she thought.

The voice was Fanning.

And everything came slamming back.

"I waited so long, Amy." A heavy sigh. "Always hoping that my Liz would be on the next train. Do you know what that's like? But how could you. How could anyone?"

She struggled onto all fours. She was in the west end of the hall. To her right, the ticket windows, barred like cells in a jail; to her left, the shadowy recesses of train platforms. Shrouded windows, both behind her and to her right, pulsed with a febrile glow. Ahead, at a distance of perhaps a hundred feet, stood the kiosk, topped by its pearlescent clocks. A man was standing there. An altogether unremarkable-looking man, wearing a dark suit. He was positioned in profile, back erect and chin tipped slightly upward, left hand tucked casually in the pocket of his suit coat, his attention aimed at the dark maws of the tunnels.

"How alone she must have felt at the end, how afraid. No words of comfort. Not the touch of a hand for company."

Still he did not look at her. All around her, the virals trilled and stroked, flexed and snapped. She had the sense that they were kept at bay only by the thinnest of invisible barriers.

" 'I have known the evenings, mornings, afternoons, I have measured out my life with coffee spoons.' That's T. S. Eliot, in case you were wondering. An oldie but a goodie. When it came to existential exhaustion, the man was one smart cookie."

Where was Peter? Had the virals killed him? What of Michael and Alicia? She thought: Water. She thought: Time. How much had passed? But the answer to this question was like an empty drawer in her brain. Moving just her eyes, she scanned for something to use as a weapon. But there was nothing, only the virals and the inverted heavens and her heart beating in her throat.

"Oh, I had my books, my thoughts. I had my memories. But those things only take a man so far." Fanning paused, then said, with more directness, "Consider this place, Amy. Imagine it as it once was. Everyone hurrying, rushing here, rushing there. The appointments. The assignations. The dinners with friends. How gloriously alive it was. All our lives, the one thing we never seem to have enough of is time. Time to work. Time to eat. Time to sleep. Time to love and be loved before it's time to die." He shrugged. "But I digress. You came to kill me, wasn't it?"

He turned to face her. His right hand, now revealed, held the sword.

"Just to clear the decks, let me say that I don't hold it against you in the least. *Au contraire, mon amie.* That's French, by the way. Liz always said it was the mark of a truly cultured person. I never

757

had much of a knack for languages, but with a century to kill, you get around to trying new things. Any preference? Italian, Russian, German, Dutch, Greek? How about Latin? We could do this whole thing in Norwegian if you'd like."

Close your mouth, Amy's brain commanded her. *Use the silence, because it's all you have.*

Fanning's face soured. "Well, your choice. I was only trying to make a little small talk." He gave a backhanded wave. "Let's have a look at you."

More hands upon her: a large, smooth male and a slightly smaller female, with a wispy diadem of white hair on her otherwise featureless skull. They seized her by the upper arms and whisked her forward, her feet skimming the tile, and dumped her unceremoniously to the floor.

"I said gently, for fucksake!"

Looming like a thundercloud, Fanning stood above her, his aura of merry confidence replaced by jaw-clenched rage.

"You." He pointed the sword at the large male. "Get over here."

A spark of hesitation in the creature's eyes — or did she imagine this? The viral scuttled forward. It dropped to its knees at Fanning's feet and bowed its head submissively, like a subdued dog.

Fanning raised his voice to the room. "Everyone, are you listening? Are you hearing my words, goddamnit? This woman is our guest! She is not a piece of luggage for you to toss around as you please! I expect you to treat her with respect!"

As he raised the sword, Amy covered her head. A crack, followed by a grinding sound and then the thump of something heavy hitting the floor. A wet stickiness splashed the side of her face and, with it, a rotten smell, as if a door had blown open

onto a room of corpses.

"Oh, for the love of God."

The viral was still on its knees, its headless torso folded forward to the floor. Dark, rhythmic spurts were convulsing from its severed neck, forming a glossy pool on the floor. Fanning was staring at the front of his pants with revulsion. His suit, Amy realized, was rotten and threadbare. It hung on his body with the unstructured looseness of rags.

"Look at this," he moaned. "This is never going to come out. They're like pets, the mess they make. And the stink. Just god-awful."

It was absurd, all of it. What had she expected? Not this. Not this whirlwind of instantly changeable moods and thoughts. This man before her: there was something almost pathetic about him.

"Well, now," he said, and smiled nonsensically. "Let's get you to your feet, shall we?"

She was hauled upright. Fanning stepped forward; from his pocket he produced a handkerchief, flapped it open with a flourish, and dabbed the blood from her face. His eyes seemed both close and far away, peculiarly magnified, as if she were observing them through a telescope. On his cheeks and chin was a dusting of whitish beard; his teeth were gray, dead-looking. He hummed tunelessly as he went about this chore, then took a step back, lips pursed, brow furrowed, examining his handiwork with a slow nod.

"Much better." He regarded her at uncomfortable length, then declared, "I have to say, there's something very appealing about you. A certain innocence. Though I'm guessing there's more there than meets the eye."

"Where's Peter?"

His eyes widened. "She speaks! I was beginning

to wonder." Then, dismissively: "Not to worry about your friend. Delayed in traffic, I expect. As for me, I'm glad the two of us can have this chance to talk amongst ourselves. I hope this doesn't seem too forward, but I feel a certain kinship with you, Amy. Our journeys are not so very different when you think about it. But first: where, pray tell, is my friend Alicia? This specimen of overgrown table cutlery tells me she's around here some-place."

Amy didn't answer.

"Nothing to share on the subject? Have it your way. Do you know what you are, Amy? I've given it a lot of thought."

Let him talk, she told herself. Time was what she needed. Let him use the minutes.

"You're . . . an apology."

Fanning said nothing further. The virals held her fast. He stepped away toward the train tun-nels, where he resumed his original position, gaz-ing forlornly into the blackness.

"For a long time, I wanted to kill you. Well, perhaps not 'wanted.' You can't help being what you are, any more than I can. It wasn't anything personal. You were merely a symbol, a stand-in for the thing I hated most." He turned the sword in his hand, studying the blade. "Imagine it, Amy. Imagine the folly of the man. He actually *believed* he could make everything all right, that he could atone for his crimes. But he couldn't. Not after what he did to Liz. To me, to you." He looked up. "She was nothing to me, the other one. Just some woman in a bar, looking for a night of fun, a bit of company in her lonely little life. I regret that intensely."

Amy waited.

"I thought I could forget about it. But that was the night. I see that now. It was the night the truth of the world opened to me. It wasn't the woman that did it. No, it was the child. The little girl in the crib. Do you know that I can still smell her, Amy? That sweet soft odor that all babies have. It's practically holy. Her little fingers and toes, the smoothness of her skin. Her whole life was in her eyes. All of us begin that way. You, me, everyone. Full of love, full of hope. I could see it: she trusted me. Her mother lay dead on the kitchen floor, but here was this man, come to answer her cries. Would I give her a bottle? Change her diaper? Perhaps I would pick her up, take her on my lap and read her a story. She had no idea what I'd done, what I *was*. I felt so sorry for her. But that wasn't the reason. I felt sorry because she'd had to be born in the first place. I should have killed her right then. It would have been a mercy."

A silence caught and held. Then:

"I see from your expression that I appall you. Believe me, I appall myself sometimes. But the truth is the truth. There's no one watching over us. That's the cold heart of it, the grand delusion. Or if there is, he's the cruelest kind of bastard, letting us believe he cares. I'm nothing, compared to him. What kind of God would allow her mother to die like that? What God would let Liz be all alone at the end, not the touch of a hand or a single word of kindness to help her leave her life? I'll tell you what kind, Amy. The same one who made me." He turned toward her again. "Your friends on the boat will be back, you know. Don't be surprised — I know all about it. I practically watched them sail away from the pier. Oh, maybe not soon. But eventually. Their curiosity will get

761

the better of them. It's simple human nature. All of this will be dust by then, but here I'll be, waiting."

Do it, Alicia, she thought. *Do it, Michael. Do it now.*

"What do I want, Amy? The answer is quite simple: I want to save you. More than that. I want to teach you. To make you see the truth." His expression darkened. "Hold her tightly, please."

The clock had run down. Michael glanced at Alicia. "Ready?"

She nodded.

"You might want to cover your ears."

He shoved down the plunger.

"What the hell, Circuit?"

He drew up the bar and tried again. Nothing. He pulled the positive wire, touched it lightly to the contact, and pressed the plunger a third time. A spark leapt.

He had current; the problem was at the other end.

"Stay here."

He unscrewed the second wire, grabbed the plunger box and lantern, and tore down the stairs.

The strength of the virals' grip increased with a hot jab. The pain was eye-watering; bits of confettied light danced in her vision.

"Bring him in, please."

Peter.

Two virals dragged him from the direction of the tunnels. His body hung floppily, facedown, the tips of his boots skimming the floor.

"It's the only way, Amy. I wish there were another, but there simply isn't."

762

Amy could barely think. The slightest movement ignited shrieks of agony. It felt as if the bones of her upper arms were about to shatter under the pressure of the virals' hands, to crumble into dust.

"Ah, here we are."

The virals halted, still holding Peter by the shoulders. Blood was dripping from his hair, flowing down the creases of his face. Fanning stepped toward him, sword extended. Amy's breath stopped in her throat. He positioned the flat of the blade beneath Peter's chin and, with cruel slowness, tilted his face upward.

"You care about this man, do you not?"

Peter found Amy with his eyes but seemed unable to focus. His mouth was moving soundlessly, with what might have been a sigh or groan.

"Answer the question."

"Yes," she said.

"So much that you would do anything to save him, in fact."

Her vision swam. To be undone so easily; that was the cruelest thing.

"Say it, Amy. Let me hear the words."

Her answer came out with a choking sound: "Yes, I'd do anything to save him." Her head rolled forward in defeat; she had nothing left. "Please, just let him go."

One flick of the wrist and his throat would open like paper. Peter's eyes were closed, preparing for death. That or he had slipped back into a merciful unconsciousness.

"Let me show you something," Fanning said. "It's a little talent I've discovered. Jonas would get a real kick out of this."

He did something strange: he began to undress. First the suit coat, which he folded in half and lay

neatly on the floor with the sword, then his shirt, unbuttoning it to reveal a fan of downy white chest hair and a smooth, leanly muscled trunk.

"I have to say, it's good to finally get out of these clothes." He had knelt to untie his shoes. "To put aside these *trappings*."

Shoes, socks, pants. The air around him had begun to change. It fluttered like waves of heat above a desert road. He rocked his head toward the ceiling; a sheen of oily sweat appeared on his skin. He licked his lips with a slow tongue and began to roll his shoulders and neck, his eyes half-lidded, lost in sensation.

"God, that's good," he said.

With a bony pop, Fanning arced his back and moaned with pleasure. His hair was ejecting in clumps; fat, throbbing veins pulsed beneath the skin of his face and chest, tatting a bluish web. He rocked his jaw, showing his fangs. His fingers, from which long, yellowish nails now protruded, flexed restlessly.

"Isn't it . . . wonderful?"

Michael hit the tunnel, Alicia shouting his name behind him. Rats were suddenly everywhere, an undulating wave of them, flowing toward the bulkhead.

The screw had torn loose; the pack lay in the water. The fuses were soaked and useless.

"Fuck!"

His eyes fell on a small electrical panel, at eye level, just to the right of the bulkhead. The ground was boiling with rats. They were swarming around his ankles, brushing against his legs with their soft, nauseating weight. With the tip of a screwdriver, he popped the door and waved the lantern

over the interior.

"Get back!"

Alicia was standing a few yards behind him. Thirty feet away, a viral was crouched on the floor of the tunnel; a second clung to the ceiling, its inverted head rocking side to side. The long, bald tail of a rat was whipping from its mouth.

"Go on, beat it!" The virals merely looked at her. "Get out of here!"

The inside of the panel was a tangled mess of wires connected to a breaker board. Give me an hour, Michael thought, and I can do something with this, no problem.

"These guys look hungry, Circuit. Tell me you've figured this out."

God, how he hated that name. He was pulling wires free, attempting to separate them into some kind of coherence, to trace them back to their source.

"More coming!"

He glanced over his shoulder. The walls of the tunnel had begun to glow green. There was a skittering sound, like dry leaves rolling on pavement. "I thought these guys were your friends!"

Alicia fired at the viral on the ceiling. Her aim was unsteady; sparks flew up. The viral skittered backward, dropped, and came up on all fours. "I don't think it's me they're interested in!"

He sliced off a length of cable, stripped the ends, and screwed them to the plunger. Holding the wire, he gave a final look into the panel. He would have to take a wild guess. This one? No, that.

A barrage of fire behind him. "I'm not kidding, Michael, we've got about ten seconds!"

With four quick turns, he spliced the ends of the wires together. Alicia was backing toward him,

firing in short bursts. The sound reverberated off the walls of the tunnel, hammering his eardrums. Good God, he was tired of this sort of thing. Tired of guesswork and laboring in the dark, tired of leaking valves and bad circuits and busted relays — tired of things not working, things that refused to bend to his will.

"Need some help here!" Alicia yelled.

Her rifle drained, Alicia tossed it aside and drew a pair of blades from her belt, one for each fist. Michael grabbed her around the waist and pulled her into him.

The tunnel was a squirming mass.

They fell backward as the first viral careened forward. Michael drew his sidearm and fired two shots, the first sparking off its shoulder, the second catching it in the left eye. A splash of blood and with a shriek it skidded to the floor. They were scooting backward toward the bulkhead, Michael firing his pistol, shoving his heels against the concrete, one arm encircling Alicia's waist to drag her with him through the fetid water. He had fifteen rounds in the gun, another two magazines stashed in a pocket, useless and out of reach.

The slide locked back.

"Oh, shit, Michael."

So: the end of the line. How slow its approach, how sudden its arrival. We never truly believe it's coming, he thought, and then before we know it, it's here. All the things we've done in our lives, and the undone things as well, extinguished in an instant. He dropped the gun and pulled Alicia tight against him. His hand was on the plunger.

"Close your eyes," he said.

The change was complete.

Fanning's face was still tipped upward, lips parted, eyes shut. A sigh of satisfaction heaved from deep in his chest. The being before her was not one Amy had ever seen or imagined — still recognizable as himself but neither wholly man nor wholly viral. An amalgam, half one and half the other, as if a new version of the species had been born into the world. There was something of the rodent about him, the nose snoutlike and full-nostriled, the ears triangulated at the top and swept back from the curve of his skull. His hair was gone, replaced by pinkish natal fuzz. His teeth were the same, though the mouth itself had enlarged into a kind of windblown grin, giving a full view of his fangs, which dripped from the corners. His limbs possessed a thin-boned delicacy; the index fingers of both hands had elongated to curve-tipped points.

Amy thought of a giant wingless bat.

He stepped toward her. His eyes locked on hers; she dared not look away, no matter how much she wanted to. Fear had paralyzed her limbs. They felt far away and useless, loose as liquid. As Fanning neared, his right hand rose. The digits were webbed with a translucent membrane. The daggered index finger, jointed in the middle, unfurled toward her face. Her eyes clamped shut instinctively. A prick of pressure on her cheek, not quite hard enough to break the skin: every molecule in her body shuddered. With lascivious slowness the nail traced downward, following the curve of her face. As if he were tasting her flesh through his finger.

"How good it is to let the truth come out."

His voice, too, had altered, possessing a high, hidden note with a squeaking sound. The air

767

around him smelled of animals. The small, burrowing things of the world.

"Open your eyes, Amy."

Fanning was standing beside Peter. The virals
had hauled him upright.

"This man, he is your curse, as Liz was mine.
It's love that enslaves us, Amy. It is the play within
the play, the stage on which the tragic drama of
our human lives unfolds. That is the lesson I have
to teach you."

And with these words, Fanning opened his jaws
wide, tipped Peter's face upward on the end of
one long, webbed digit — tenderly, like a mother
with her child — and clamped his jaws around
Peter's neck.

The squeak of current from the plunger was not
enough to open the bulkhead all the way; but it
was enough to get things started. As the door's
counterweights jolted downward, creating a gap
between the door and the floor of the tunnel, Michael and Alicia were blasted by a jet of water. In
less than a second, the tunnel became a roaring
river. Michael attempted to rise, but the force was
too great, he could find no traction, and then they
were tumbling, hurtled downstream in the roiling
water.

They plunged into the station, going like a shot.
There was no real light, only a vague glow from
the stairway, glimpsed fleetingly as they passed.
Water filled his nose and mouth, foul-tasting —
he imagined this to be the taste of rats — and
threatening to choke him. They were riding just
beneath the platform. Gripping Alicia by the wrist,
Michael reached out with his free hand and made
a desperate lunge for the edge. His fingers touched

but tore away.

They passed through the station. The water was rising fast; soon it would be over their heads. The next station would come at Fourteenth Street — much too far. Ahead, a faint glow appeared. As they neared, the light congealed into a discrete shaft — an opening in the roof of the tunnel.

"There's a ladder!" Alicia cried. Her head went under again.

"What?"

Her face reemerged; she was fighting for breath. She pointed. "A ladder on the wall!"

They were sailing straight for it. Alicia grabbed hold first. Michael spun around her body, then, using his left hand, reached out, seized a rung, and hooked an elbow through it. At the top of the ladder was a metal grate, daylight beyond it.

"Can you make it?" Michael said.

They were being pummeled by the current. Lish shook her head.

"Try, damn it!"

Her strength was gone; she had nothing left. "I can't."

He would have to pull her up. Michael reached above her head and drew himself free of the water. The grate presented a different problem; unless he could find a way to open it, they were going to drown anyway. At the top of the ladder, he raised one hand and pushed. Nothing, not the slightest tremor. He reared back and shoved the heel of his palm into the slatted metal. He punched the grate again, and again. On the fourth blow, it burst open.

He shoved it aside, climbed out, and pressed his body to the pavement. The rising water had lifted Alicia halfway up the ladder. The light seemed to

make a kind of halo around her face.

He reached down. "Take my hand —"

But that was all he said, his words cut short as a wall of water slammed into her — into both of them — bursting like a geyser through the open grate and blowing Michael halfway across the street.

The collapse of the bulkhead just south of the Astor Place station — one of eight retention dams protecting the subway lines of Manhattan from the greedy Atlantic — was the first in a series of events that no person, Michael included, could have anticipated. Freed from incarceration, the water shot through the tunnel with the hammering power of a hundred locomotives. It ripped and tore. It blasted to bits. It detonated and crushed and destroyed, plowing through the structural underpinnings of lower Manhattan like a scythe through wheat. Eight blocks north of Astor Place, at Fourteenth Street, the water jumped the tracks. While the main body churned straight north beneath Lexington Avenue, toward Grand Central, the rest veered west on the Broadway line, roaring toward the bulkhead at Times Square, which would subsequently fail as well, flooding everything beneath the pavement south of Forty-second Street between Broadway and Eighth Avenue and opening the whole West Side to the sea.

And it was only just getting started.

In its thundering wake, the water left a trail of destruction. Manhole covers blew sky-high. Sewers exploded. Streets buckled and collapsed. Beneath the ground, a chain reaction had commenced. Like the ocean of which it was a part,

the raging water sought only the expansion of its domain; the prize was the island itself, which, after a century of sodden neglect, was rotten to the core.

On the corner of Tenth Street and Fourth Avenue, Michael returned to consciousness with the unsettled sense that the world's relationship to gravity had altered. It was as if every object were moving away from every other in a state of general repulsion. He blinked his eyes and waited for this feeling to stop, but it did not. A great font of water was jetting from the grate, high into the air, dissolving at the top into a sparkling mist that cast a rainbow above the flooded street. In his mentally fogged state, Michael stared at it in astonishment, not yet connecting the sight to anything else, while also noting, rather blandly, that other things were occurring: loud things, concussive things, things that warranted further consideration if only he could marshal his thoughts. The street seemed to be sinking — either that or everything else was getting taller — and bits of material were sailing off the faces of the buildings.

Wait a second.

The structure he was looking at — a nondescript, mid-rise office building of dark tinted glass — was doing something peculiar. It appeared to be . . . breathing. A deep respiratory flexing, like a baby's first breaths of life. It was as if this anonymous structure, one of thousands like it on the island, had awakened after decades of abandoned slumber. Spidering cracks materialized in its reflective face. Michael sat upright, balancing on his palms. The pavement had begun to undulate disturbingly beneath him.

The glass exploded.

Michael rolled and flattened himself to the ground, covering his head as a million shards rained down. Whole plates detonated on the pavement. He was yelling at the top of his lungs. Nonsensical words, vile curses, an aural vomitus of terror. He was about to be diced to ribbons. There wouldn't be enough of him left to bury, not that there would be anybody around to do that. The seconds passed, glass cascading all around him, Michael waiting, for the second time that day, to die.

He didn't.

He lifted his face from the pavement. The sun was gone, the air grown dim. Tiny, twinkling shards covered his body, clinging to his arms and hands and hair and the fabric of his clothing. A gritty wind swirled the air. The sky, it seemed, had begun to issue snow. No, not snow. Paper. A single page dropped lazily into his hands. "Memo," it read at the top. And, beneath that, "From: HR Department. To: All employees. Re: Benefits enrollment period." Michael was momentarily transfixed by the strangeness of these words. They felt like a code. Within their mysterious phrasing lay an entire reality, a world lost in time.

Suddenly the paper was gone; a gust of air had stripped it from his hand. The street was darkening. A roaring sound came from his left. Second by second it increased, as did the wind. He turned his head to look uptown, toward the source of the noise.

A great gray monster was roaring toward him.

He scrambled to his feet. His head was swimming; his legs felt like wet sand.

He ran, nonetheless, like hell.

■ ■ ■ ■

The first building to fall was not the one Michael saw. By this time, the collapse of midtown Manhattan was several minutes old. From the south edge of Central Park to Washington Square, edifices large and small were in the process of acute structural liquefaction, melting and toppling into the gobbling sinkhole that the island's central core was on its way to becoming. Some fell independently, crumpling vertically into their foundations like prisoners felled by a firing squad. Others were encouraged by their neighbors, as building after building teetered and toppled into others. A few, such as the great glass tower on the east side of the trapezoidal city block at Fifty-fifth and Broadway, appeared to succumb entirely through the power of suggestion: *My fellows are giving up the ghost — why don't I do that also?* The process might have been likened to a swiftly moving metastasis; it leapt across the boulevards as if from organ to organ, it churned through the avenues of blood, it wrapped its lethal fingers around the bones of steel. Dust clouds roared in a great carcinogenic regurgitation, blackening the skies.

An ersatz night fell over Manhattan.

Beneath Grand Central Station, the water arrived from two directions: first via the Lexington Avenue subway line from Astor Place, then, a few seconds later, through the Forty-second Street shuttle line from Times Square. The currents converged; like a tsunami compressing as it approached the shore, the water's power magnified a thousand-fold as it tore up the stairs.

"You ungrateful bitch!" Fanning cried. "What have you done?"

He said no more; the water arrived, a pounding wall, blasting them off their feet. In a blink, the main hall was subsumed. Amy went under. She was rolling, tossing, her sense of direction obliterated. The water was six feet deep and rising. Glass was shattering, things were falling, everything was in a tumult. She broke the surface in time to see the hall's high windows burst inward; the current grabbed her, sending her under again. She flailed helplessly, searching for something to grasp. The body of a viral careened into her. It was the female with the hair. Through the roaring murk, Amy glimpsed her eyes, full of terrified incomprehension. She sank and was gone.

Amy was being swept toward the balcony stairs. She impacted hard — more bells, more pain — but she managed to grab hold of the rail with her right hand. Her lungs cried out for air; bubbles rose from her mouth. The urge to breathe could not be forestalled much longer. The only thing to do was let the current take her, in the hope that she would be carried to safety.

She let go of the rail.

She smashed into the stairs again, but at least she was moving in the right direction. If she'd been carried into the tunnels, she would have drowned. A second shock wave hit her, squirting her upward.

She landed on the balcony, clear of the water at last. On her hands and knees, she coughed and retched, foul-tasting water spewing from her mouth.

Peter.

Hurled up the stairs by the same current, he

was lying just a few feet behind her. Where was Fanning? Had he been pulled under like the other virals, carried to the bottom by his weight? As she thought this, the floor lurched. The air cracked. She looked up to see a large chunk of the ceiling detach and tumble to the water.

The building was coming down.

Peter's chest was moving rapidly. The change had yet to begin. She shook him by the shoulders, called his name; his eyes fluttered open, then squinted at her face. She saw no recognition in them, only vague puzzlement, as if he could not quite place her.

"I'm going to get you out of here."

She drew him up by his arms and folded his body over her right shoulder. Her balance wavered, but she managed to hold on. The floor was sliding and undulating like the deck of a boat. Hunks of ceiling continued to break away as the building's structural underpinnings failed.

She looked around. To her right, a door.

Run, she thought. *Run and keep on running.*

Then they were outside, though it hardly seemed so. The sky was dark as night, the sun eclipsed by dust, the great city unrecognizable. A vast immolation, everything rushing to ruin. The noise hammered her ears, roaring from all directions. She was on the elevated roadway on the west side of the station. It was tipped at a precarious angle; cracks were spreading, whole sections collapsing. Amy picked a direction; under Peter's weight, the best she could manage was a jog. Instinct was her only guide. To run. To survive. To carry Peter away.

The road sloped down to street level. She could go no farther; her legs were giving way. At the base of the ramp, she eased Peter to the ground.

He was trembling — shaking with small, sharp spasms, like the chills of a fever, but growing stronger, more defined. Amy knew what he would want. He would want to die while still a man. The mortal instruments lay everywhere among the wreckage: segments of rebar sharp as knives, hunks of twisted metal, shards of glass. Suddenly she knew: this was what Fanning had intended, all along. That she should be the one. *It's love that enslaves us, Amy.* She was beaten; it was all for nothing in the end. She would be alone again.

As she knelt beside him, a great sob shook her, the pain of her too-long life, forestalled for a century, unleashed. The glimpse of life she'd been given: how fleeting it was. Better, perhaps, never to have had it. Peter had begun to moan. The virus churned inside him; it bore him away.

She made her choice: a three-foot length of steel with a triangulated tip. What function had it served? Part of a signpost? The frame of a window that had once gazed out upon the busy world? The underpinnings of a mighty tower soaring to the sky? She knelt again by Peter's body. The man inside was leaving. She bent and touched his cheek. His skin was damp and feverish. The blinking had commenced. Blink. Blink, blink.

A voice from behind: "Goddamn you!"

She went hurling through the air.

Michael sprinted down Fourth Avenue, the debris cloud roaring behind him. There would be no outrunning it. He turned right onto Eighth Street. At the ends of the block, both in front and behind, the cloud roared past with a tornadic whoosh, then, as if suddenly recalling his presence — *Oh, Michael, sorry I forgot you* — turned the corners,

barreling toward him from two directions.

He dove through the nearest door and slammed it behind him. Some kind of clothing shop, coats and dresses and shirts hanging disembodied on the racks. A wide window with mannequins propped upon an elevated platform faced the street.

The cloud arrived.

The window burst inward; Michael's hands shot up to protect his eyes. Dust engulfed the room, blasting him backward. Pricks of pain announced themselves all over his body — his arms and hands, the base of his throat, the parts of his face that had been exposed — as if he'd been attacked by a swarm of bees. He tried to rise; only then did he discover the long shard of glass embedded in his right thigh. It seemed strange that it didn't hurt more — it should have hurt like hell — but then the pain arrived, annihilating his thoughts. He was coughing, choking, drowning in the dust. He scrambled back from the window and crashed into a clothing rack. He yanked a shirt from its hanger. It was made of some kind of gauzy material. He wadded it in his fist and pressed it to his mouth and nose. Breath by hungry breath, oxygen flowed back into his lungs.

He tied the shirt around the lower half of his face. With stinging eyes, he looked out upon the dark street. He was inside the cloud. Everything was silent except for a faint pattering: the sound of airborne particles falling upon the pavement and the roofs of abandoned cars. His hands and arms were slick with blood; his leg, where the long piece of glass was buried, screamed with the slightest motion. He drew his blade and cut, then tore, the leg of his trousers away. The glass, a long,

narrow splinter, irregularly edged and slightly curved, had entered at an angle; the wound was roughly halfway between his groin and his knee on the inside flank of his leg. *Good Christ,* he thought. *Another few inches higher and that thing would have sliced my nuts off.*

He reached over his head to yank another shirt from the rack and used it to wrap the exposed end of the shard. He supposed it was possible that removing the glass would open the wound wider, but the pain was unendurable. Unless he removed it, he wouldn't be going anywhere. To do it quickly: that was the best way.

He took the wrapped shard in his fist. He counted to three. He pulled.

All up and down the block, man-sized figures, moving in the dust, halted in their tracks and swiveled their faces toward the sound of Michael's scream.

"This was a temple!"

Fanning's hand caught her across the cheek. The blow sent her careening backward.

"You do this to *me?* To *my* city?"

She raised her hands to protect her face. Instead Fanning yanked her by the collar, hauled her up until her feet left the pavement, and tossed her away.

"I am going to take my time with you. You're going to *want* me to kill you. You are going to *beg.*"

He came at her again, and again. Tosses, slaps, kicks. She discovered herself lying facedown. She felt detached from everything. Her thoughts possessed a lazy, unmoored quality. They seemed on the verge of some permanent and final severing, as if with the next blow they would sail up and

away from her body, swallowed into the sky like a balloon cut from its string.

Yet, to yield, to accept death: the mind forbade it. The mind demanded, against all sense, to go on. Fanning was somewhere behind her. Amy's awareness of him was less as a physical presence than an abstract force, like gravity, a well of darkness into which she was being relentlessly sucked. She began to crawl. Why wouldn't Fanning just kill her? But he'd said so himself: he wanted her to feel it. To feel life leaking out of her, drip by drip.

"Look at me!"

A crack to her midriff lifted her off the ground; Fanning had kicked her. The wind sailed from her chest.

"I said, look at me!"

He kicked her again, burying his foot below her sternum and flipping her onto her back.

He was holding the sword over his head.

"We were supposed to meet at the kiosk!"

We?

"You said you would be there! You said we would be together!"

What was he seeing? Who was she to him? The transformation: it had done something to his mind.

"I never should have loved you!"

She rolled away as the sword came down. It struck the pavement with a single-noted clang. Fanning howled like a wounded animal.

"I wanted to die with you!"

She was on her back again. Fanning had raised the sword above his head, ready to swing. She raised her arms in forbearance. One chance was all she had.

"Tim, don't."

Fanning froze.

"I wanted to be there. To be with you. That was all I ever wanted."

His arms tensed. At any second, the blade would fall. "I waited all night! How could you do that to me? Why didn't you come, why?"

"Because . . . I died, Tim."

For a moment nothing happened. *Please,* she thought.

"You . . . died."

"Yes. I'm sorry. I didn't mean to."

His voice was numb. "On the train."

Amy spoke cautiously, keeping her voice even. "Yes. I was coming to see you. They carried me off. I couldn't stop them."

Fanning's eyes floated away from her face. He glanced around uncertainly.

"But I'm here now, Tim. That's what matters. I'm sorry it took me so long."

How long could she sustain the lie? The sword was everything. If she could convince Fanning to give it to her . . .

"We can still do it," she said. "There's a way we can always be together, just like we planned."

He looked back at her.

"Come with me, Tim. There's a place we can go. I've seen it."

Fanning said nothing. She sensed her words gaining traction in his mind.

"Where?" he asked.

"It's the place where we can start over. We can do it right this time. All you have to do is give me the sword." She extended her hand. "Come with me, Tim."

Fanning's eyes were locked on hers. Everything

was inside them, the whole history of the man he'd been. The pain. The loneliness. The interminable hours of his life. Then:

"You."

She was losing him. "Give me the sword, Tim. That's all you have to do."

"You're not her."

She felt it all collapsing. "Tim, it's me. It's Liz."

"You're . . . Amy."

Fifty yards away, lying faceup on the ground, the man known as Peter Jaxon had begun to disappear.

His mind straddled two worlds. In the first, one of darkness and commotion, Fanning was hurling Amy through the air. Peter sensed this rather dimly; he could not recall why it should be so. Nor could he intervene, his powers to act, even to move at all, having abandoned him.

In the other was a window.

A shade, drawn over it, glowed with summer light. The image felt familiar, like déjà vu. *The window,* Peter thought. *It means I must be dying.* As he fought to focus his eyes, to bring himself back to reality, the light began to change. It was becoming something else: not a window in his mind but something physical. Through the dust-filled darkness was an opening, like a corridor ascending to a higher world, and through this tunnel a shining shape appeared. It teased at his memory; he knew what it was, if only he could summon the image forth. The picture sharpened. It resembled a crown, multilayered, each layer arched as it narrowed to a spiked peak. Sunlight flared upon its mirrored face, shooting a bright beam down the corridor, which was a hole in the

clouds, into his eyes.

The Chrysler Building.

The corridor collapsed; darkness folded over him again. But now he knew: the night in which he dwelled was false. The sun was still up there. Above the cloud of dust it shone, bright as day. If he could get to the sun, if he could somehow lead Fanning into its light . . .

But this thought was lost as a great force gripped him, like a vortex. Its power was colossal. He felt himself being pulled, down and down and down. What lay at the bottom he did not know, only that when he reached it, he would be forever lost. Somewhere distant, his body was changing. Racked with convulsions, it hammered on the pavement of the broken city. Bones elongated. Teeth showered from his gums. He was sinking into a sea of everlasting darkness in which no trace of himself would remain. *No! Not yet!* He searched for something, anything, to hold on to. In his mind's eye, Amy's face appeared. The picture was not imagined but taken from life. They were sitting on his bed. Their faces were close, their hands entwined. Teardrops hung upon her eyelashes like beads of light. *You get to keep one thing,* she told him. *What I wanted to keep was you.*

Was you, thought Peter.

You.

He fell.

The pain in Michael's leg exploded. Removing the glass had peeled the skin back like the rind of an orange, exposing the fibrous, subtly pulsating muscle beneath. Another backward reach above his head produced a long, silk scarf. He twirled it into a thick rope and tied it tightly around the

wound. The fabric was instantly saturated. Was he doing this right? He wished Sara were here. Sara would know what to do. The things that came into your mind at a time like this: the brain was not kind, it had no sense of fairness, it taunted you with thoughts of the things you did not have or couldn't do.

The noise outside had subsided as the destruction marched north. The air had an unnatural chemical smell, bitter and burnt. For the first time since he'd awakened on the street, his mind went to Alicia, the look on her face as the water crashed into her and swept her away. She was gone. Alicia was gone.

From the street, a crunch of glass.

Michael froze. The noise came again.

Footsteps.

Pushing with her heels, Amy scrambled backward. "Tim, don't! It's me!"

"Don't call me that!"

She had lost him; the spell was broken. In his eyes, the look of white-hot fury had returned. Suddenly Fanning raised his head. A new emotion came into his face, one of unanticipated pleasure.

"And what have we here?"

It was Peter. The transformation was complete; his body, sleek, powerful, had joined the anonymous horde.

"There's a good fellow." Fanning's lips pulled back into a smile, showing his fangs. "Why don't you join us?"

Peter moved toward them through the rubble, legs bent, arms held away from his body. His steps seemed uncertain; his back and shoulders rippled with an undulating motion, like a man stretching

after a long night of sleep or adjusting himself inside a new suit of clothes.

"Allow me, Amy, to make a point."

With a flick of his wrist Fanning tossed the sword, handle first, to Peter, who snatched it robotically from the air.

"Let's see who's in there, shall we?" Fanning strode toward him, straightened his back and tapped the center of his chest. "Right about here, I should think."

Peter was staring at the sword, as if puzzling over its function. What was this alien object in his hand?

"Come on, now. I promise I won't move a muscle."

Peter took another step forward. His movements were jerky, as if the parts of his body could not completely coordinate. The muscles of his arms and shoulders tightened as he attempted to lift the blade.

"Getting heavier, I see."

Another step and Peter stopped. He was within striking distance now. Fanning made no effort to defend himself; his batlike face radiated confidence, almost amusement. The sword, at a forty-five-degree angle to the ground, refused to rise.

"Here, let me help you."

With the long-nailed tip of his index finger, Fanning guided the blade to a horizontal position. He moved slightly forward until the point made contact with his chest, just below the sternum.

"One good thrust should do it."

A growl of effort rose from deep in Peter's throat. The seconds stretched, every part of his body drawn taut. A pop of air expelled from his lungs; he melted to his knees, the sword clanging

on the pavement.

"You see, Amy? It is simply not possible. This man belongs to me now."

Like the viral in the hall, Peter had bowed his head in abject surrender. Fanning placed a hand on his shoulder. It was as if he were patting an especially obedient dog. "Do me a favor, won't you?" Fanning asked him.

Peter raised his head.

"Would you please kill her?"

Michael pushed backward from the window on his palms, leaving a wide trail of blood on the floor. There was more than one viral out there, he could sense it; they were like wraiths, there and not there, shadowy figures gliding and shifting in the dust.

Searching. Hunting.

Once they found him, he wouldn't make it two steps. He scooted to the rear of the room, where there was a long counter and, behind it, a doorway half-hidden by a curtain. As he slipped behind the counter, the floor began to shake again. The feeling gathered in intensity like a revving engine. Clothes racks toppled. Mirrors shattered and burst outward. Chunks of plaster severed from the ceiling and detonated on the floor. Curled into a ball, arms wrapped around his head, Michael thought, *God, whoever you are, I am sick of your shit. I am not your plaything. If you're going to kill me, please stop screwing around and get it over with.*

The shaking subsided. From all up and down the street, Michael heard the crack of windows popping free of their frames and crashing on the pavement. The virals still lurked out there, but

maybe the commotion had put them off his trail. Maybe they were cowering in some dark corner, as he was. Maybe they were dead.

He peeked around the counter. The place looked like a wrecking ball had hit it, nothing left intact except for a free-standing, full-length mirror, which stood anomalously on the right side of the room like a bewildered survivor surveying the wreckage of some terrible catastrophe. Angled slightly toward the front of the store, the mirror's face gave him a partial view of the street.

A pod of three emerged in the murk. They seemed to be drifting aimlessly, looking around as if lost. Michael willed his body into absolute stillness. If they couldn't hear him, maybe they'd pass him by. For several seconds they continued their confused wandering, until one of them stopped abruptly. Standing in profile, the viral rotated its face from side to side, as if attempting to triangulate the source of a sound. Michael held his breath. The creature paused and angled its chin upward, holding this position for another several seconds before swiveling toward the storefront. Its nose was twitching like a rat's.

Peter stepped toward her. There was no point in trying to get away; the outcome would be the same. Time had given up its customary course. Everything seemed to happen in a manner both rushed and strangely sluggish; her vision had narrowed, the city around her fading to a collection of shadows.

She was crying, though not for herself. She couldn't have said what she was crying for; her tears possessed an abstract quality of sadness, though something else as well. Her trials were

ended. In a way, she was glad. How strange, to put down life like a heavy load she had been too long forced to carry. She hoped she would go to the farmstead. How happy she had been there. She remembered the piano, the music flowing forth, Peter's hands resting on her shoulders, the joy of his touch. How happy they had been, together.

"It's all right," she murmured. Her voice felt distant, not quite her own. It spilled from her lips on shallow, rapid breaths. "It's all right, it's all right."

Peter positioned the sword so that the tip was pointed at the base of her throat. The gap narrowed, then stopped, flesh mere inches from steel. His head cocked to the side; in another second he would strike.

"Well?" Fanning said.

Their gazes met and held. To know and be known: that was the final desire, the heart of love. It was the one thing she could give him. A huge force was bursting open inside her. It was a kind of light. She would have beamed it straight into his heart if she could.

"You're Peter," Amy whispered, and went on whispering, so that he would be hearing these words. "You're Peter, you're Peter, you're Peter . . ."

The blood, thought Michael.

They can smell my blood.

He wasn't sure he could stand, let alone run. He had painted a road of red on the floor, leading them straight to him. He pressed his back against the counter and drew his knees to his chest. The virals had entered the store. He heard a kind of

787

wet snuffling, like the noise of hogs rooting in mud; they were sucking the blood off the floor. Michael felt a weird surge of protectiveness. *Hey, leave my blood alone!* On and on went their lascivious slurping. So intense was their focus that Michael began to think about the curtained door. What lay beyond it? Was it a dead end or was there, perhaps, a hallway that led deeper into the building — to the street, even? The doorway was only partially concealed by the counter. For some interval of time, depending on how fast he was able to go, he would be exposed.

He peeked around the corner, using the angled mirror to survey the room. The virals, on their hands and knees, were busily pressing their mouths to the floor, their tongues swirling like mopheads. Michael scooted down the length of the counter so he was as close as possible to the door, which was positioned ten feet behind him and to his right. If he could move the virals to the opposite corner of the room, the counter would obscure him completely.

Michael unwound the scarf from his leg. The fabric was bloated with blood. He formed it into a ball, tied off the ends to hold the shape, and rose on his knees, keeping the top of his head just below the lip of the counter. Pulling back his arm, he counted to three. Then he lobbed the scarf across the room.

It impacted the far wall with a splat. Michael dropped to his stomach and began to crawl. From behind him, he heard scurrying, then a series of clicks and snarls. It was better than he'd hoped; the virals were fighting over the rag. He slipped beneath the curtain and kept going. Now he couldn't see a goddamn thing. He crawled another

few feet, until he was away from the door, and attempted to rise. The instant the foot of his injured leg touched the ground was one he was pretty sure he would always remember. The pain was simply spectacular. He reached into his shirt pocket for a box of matches. Fumbling in the dark, he managed to remove one without dumping out the rest, and scraped it on the striker.

He was in a narrow hallway of high brick walls that led deeper into the building. Metal racks of empty hangers lined the walls. The air was clearer here, less dust-choked. He pulled the kerchief down from his face. An opening to his left dead-ended in a small room of curtained booths. He looked down; drops of blood had followed him like a trail of crumbs. More blood sloshed in his boot. The match burned down; he flicked it away, lit another, and went on.

Eight matches later, Michael concluded that there was no way out. Branching hallways always led him back to the central corridor. Who designed a building like this? How long before the virals' interest in the rag exhausted itself and they followed the blood?

He came to a final room. It appeared to be a kitchen, with a stove and sink and cabinets lining two of the four walls; in the center was a small square table covered with open cans and plastic bottles. Two brown-boned skeletons lay on a cratered mattress, curled together. In all of New York, these were the first human remains Michael had encountered. He crouched beside them. One of them was much smaller than the other, who appeared to be a grown woman, with a desiccated tangle of long hair. A mother and her child? Probably they had holed up together during the crisis.

For a century they had lain here, their last loving moment captured for all time. It made him feel like an interloper, as if he had violated the sanctity of a tomb.

A window.

It was covered by a cage, hinged shutters of crisscrossing wire, held in place by metal bars bolted to the wall. The two halves were joined with a padlock. The match burned down, scorching his fingertips; he flung it away. As his eyes adjusted he realized a faint glow was coming through the window, just enough to see by. He looked around the room for something to use as a lever. *Think, Michael.* On the table was a butter knife. The floor lurched again with a single, horizontal bang. Plaster dust rained down. He wedged the knife into the curved arm of the lock. His hands felt cold and slightly numb, at the edge of his ability to command them; the loss of blood was catching up to him. He tightened his arms and shoulders and twisted the blade, hard.

It snapped in two.

That was it; enough already. Michael was done. He sank to the floor and braced his back against the wall so that he could see them coming.

Peter was standing in a field of knee-high grass. The color of everything was peculiar, possessing an unnatural, off-kilter vividness that accentuated the smallest movements in the landscape. A breeze was blowing. The land was perfectly flat, though in the far distance mountains jostled the horizon. It was neither day nor night but something in between, the light soft and shadowless. What was this curious place? How had he come to be here? He searched his memory; only then did he realize

that he did not, in fact, know who he was. He felt vaguely alarmed. He was alive, he existed, yet he seemed to have no history he could recall.

He heard the sound of running water and walked toward it. The action was automatic, as if an invisible intelligence were piloting his body. After some time had passed, he came upon a river. The water moved lazily, murmuring around scattered rocks. Leaves spiraled in its current like upturned hands. He followed the river downstream to a bend where it gathered in a pool. The surface of the water was still, almost solid-looking. He felt a peculiar agitation. It seemed that within the pool's depths lay an answer, though the question eluded him. It was on the tip of his tongue, yet when he tried to focus on it, it darted up and away from his thoughts like a bird. He knelt at the edge of the pool and looked down. An image appeared: a man's face. It was disturbing to look at. The face was his, yet it might as well have been a stranger's. He reached out and with his index finger broke the surface. Concentric rings bloomed outward from the point of contact; then the image reassembled. With this came the sense, distant at first, but growing stronger, of recognition. He knew who he was, if only he could manage to recall. *You're* . . . It was as if he were attempting to lift a boulder with his mind. *You're* . . . *you're* . . .

Peter.

He lurched backward. A dam was bursting in his mind. Images, faces, days, names — they poured forth in a torrent, almost painful. The scene around him — the field and the river and the flat light of the sky — began to disperse. It was washing away. Behind it lay a wholly different

791

reality, of objects and people and events and ordered time. *I am Peter Jaxon,* he thought, and then he said it:

"I am Peter Jaxon."

Peter stumbled backward; the sword fell from his hand.

"What do you think you're doing?" Fanning barked. "I said, kill her."

Peter's head swiveled; his eyes narrowed on Fanning's face. It was happening, thought Amy. He was remembering. The muscles of his legs compressed.

He sprang.

He rammed Fanning headlong. Surprise was on his side: Fanning went sailing. He crashed back down and rolled end over end, coming to rest against a concrete pylon. He rose onto all fours but his movements were sluggish. He gave his head a horsey shake and spat on the ground.

"Well, *this* is unexpected."

Then Amy was being lifted; Peter had gathered her into his arms. Together they raced down Forty-third Street on soaring strides. Where was he taking her? Then she understood: the partially constructed office tower. She tipped her face skyward, but the dust was too thick to see if the building's upper floors rose above the cloud deck. Peter halted at the base of the elevator shaft. He swung her onto his back, scrambled ten feet up the shaft's outer structure, guided Amy back around his waist, lowered her through the bars to the elevator's roof, and followed her down. His purpose in all this was unknown to her. He hoisted her onto his back again, using his elbows to compress her legs around his waist to tell her

to hold on to him as tightly as possible. All of this had transpired in just a matter of seconds. The elevator's cables, three of them, were set into a steel plate affixed to a crossbar on the elevator's roof. Peter gathered the cables into his fists and set his feet wide. Amy, her arms hooked around his shoulders and her legs squeezing his waist like a vise, felt a gathering pressure in his body. Peter began to groan through his teeth. Only then did she grasp his intentions. She closed her eyes.

The plate tore free; Amy and Peter launched skyward, Peter gripping the cables, Amy riding his back like the shell of a turtle. Five stories, ten, fifteen. The elevator's counterweight plunged past. What would happen when they reached the top? Would they shoot through the roof into space?

Suddenly the whole cage shuddered; the counterweight had reached the bottom. The tension on the cable was instantly gone. Hurled upward, Amy found herself looking down at the base of the shaft. She was alone in the air, unattached to anything. Her body slowed as she approached the apogee of her ascent and for a second seemed to hover. *I am going to fall,* she thought. How far away the ground was. She would hit it going a hundred miles an hour, maybe more. *I am falling.*

A jolt: Peter, still gripping the cable, had seized her by the wrist. He pumped his legs, shifting his center of gravity to swing Amy in progressively wider arcs. Amy saw his target, an opening in the wall of the shaft not far below them.

He flung her away.

She landed on the floor and rolled to a halt. They were still inside the dust cloud. The adrenaline of their ascent had sharpened her thoughts. Everything was coming into a fine, almost granular

focus. She scrambled to the edge and looked down into a dizzying maw of space.

Fanning was climbing up the side of the building.

The air concussed with a titanic roar. The building on the opposite side of Forty-third Street began to melt straight down into itself like a man felled at the knees. The floor under Amy began to shake. The vibration deepened; sounds of buckling metal rippled through the structure as the floor tipped abruptly toward the street. Loose materials — rusted tools, sawhorses, moisture-swollen pieces of drywall, a bucket of nails — slid past her and sailed into the abyss. She was on her stomach, pressing herself to the floor. The angle was increasing. She was slipping, her hands and feet could gain no traction, gravity was taking hold . . .

"Peter, help!"

The sweet pressure of his hand on her arm halted her slide; he was lying on his stomach, the crowns of their heads just touching. The floor gave another downward lurch, yet he held on, his toes digging into the concrete. With gathering force, he drew her back from the edge.

"Ah," said Fanning. His face had appeared above the lip of the floor. "*There* you are."

Michael heard a faint metallic ringing from the hallway — the sound of hangers jostling on racks. A short silence ensued; the trail of his blood, crisscrossing the various hallways and doubling back, had momentarily perplexed them. The delay was excruciating. If only he would just pass out. If anything, he felt more alert than ever.

Maybe he should make a noise. Call out to them, to get the whole thing over with. *Hey, I'm in*

here, idiots! Come and fucking get it!

Such a stupid, arbitrary place to die. He'd never thought he'd die in bed; it wasn't that sort of world, and he wasn't that sort of person. But some damn kitchen?

A kitchen.

Standing up was out of the question. But the top of the stove lay within his reach. Vertigo sloshed through his brain as he rocked onto his knees; straining forward, he grabbed hold of the skillet. He spat on the underside and wiped the metal with the hem of his shirt. His reflection was vague and undetailed, more a general outline of a human face than any particular person, but it was what he had.

The sounds were coming closer.

They raced up the stairs. Two flights brought them to the roof. The dust was as thick as ever, though in the western sky a paler region, weak but discernible, showed the sun's location.

They had to get higher. They had to get above the cloud.

Amy looked up. The boom of the crane was rocking like the neck of a pecking bird. A long, hooked cable swayed from its tip. A stairway inside the crane's mast ascended to the top.

They began to climb. Where was Fanning? Watching them, no doubt — enjoying himself, choosing his moment.

They clanged the rest of the way to the top. The swaying was getting worse. The whole thing felt unstable, as if at any moment the crane might peel away from the side of the building. They were still inside the cloud. The skyline of midtown Manhattan was a smoldering wreckage, the

795

destruction continuing to extend outward from its epicenter. A rumble, a cloud, and another building toppled. Broad gaps existed where whole blocks had once stood.

"Hello up there!"

Fanning was halfway up the mast. Gripping a bar with one hand, he leaned out and waved to them with merry confidence. "Not to worry, I'll be there soon!"

A narrow catwalk led to the end of the boom. Amy crawled along it, Peter following. The boom was slamming up and down. She kept her eyes aimed forward; she didn't dare look down into the void. Even a glimpse would paralyze her.

They reached the end; there was no place else to go.

"God*damn* I like a view."

Fanning had reached the top of the mast and was now standing fifty feet behind them. Back arched, chest puffed out, he let his gaze travel over the ruined city.

"You've really made a mess of things, haven't you? Speaking as a New Yorker, I have to say, this brings back some very unpleasant memories."

A sudden warmth touched Amy's cheek. She looked to her left, across Fifth Avenue. The glass facade of the building on the far side shone with a faint orange color. Which made no sense; the building faced east, away from the sun. The light, she realized, was a reflection.

Fanning huffed a sigh. "Well. Looks to me like we've reached the end of the line. I'd ask you to stand aside, Peter, but you don't seem to be a very good listener."

The violence of the crane's movement intensified. Far below, the hooked chain was swaying like

a pendulum. The glow of the glass was growing brighter. Where was the light coming from?

"What do you say? Perhaps the two of you could hold hands and throw yourselves off. I'll be glad to wait."

There was a flash. A ray of intense sunlight, angling off the steel crown of the Chrysler Building, had broken through the murk.

It shot Fanning directly in the face.

Suddenly the crane tipped away from the side of the building. The bolts attaching the mast to the structure's outer girders were breaking away. With a groan, the boom began to arc over Fifth Avenue, slowly at first, then with gathering velocity. The mast was tipping from its base. They were moving both down and away, the boom falling like a hammer toward the glass tower across the street. It would spear the building at a forty-five-degree angle, going like a shot.

Oh please, thought Amy. She was hugging the edges of the catwalk. *Make it stop.*

Glass exploded around them.

The virals did not so much enter as pop into the room. The first one, the alpha, bounded straight over the table, landing in front of him. Michael thrust the pan out toward its face.

It froze.

The other two seemed confused, unable to decide what to do. It was as Michael had hoped; he had disrupted their chain of command. He moved the pan a little to the side; the viral's gaze tracked it unerringly. This discovery would have intrigued him if he weren't so terrified. Hardly daring to breathe, Michael slowly drew the pan toward himself. The viral obediently followed; it

seemed utterly entranced. Inch by inch, the gap between them closed. Michael shifted the pan to the left, making the viral turn its face.

A broken butter knife, thought Michael. *I better get this right.*

He struck.

The end of the crane's boom speared the glass tower at the northwest corner of Forty-third and Fifth at the thirty-second floor. Such was the force of impact that it continued its downward course through two more floors, while also embedding itself deeper within the structure. Here it came to rest in precarious balance, mast and boom forming the upper legs of an isosceles triangle suspended three hundred feet above the street.

Amy returned to consciousness with only partial recollection of these events: a sensation of wild descent, culminating in a chaos so total that her mind could not sort its components. She was lying on the floor, her body twisted and her knees drawn up, her left arm extended past her head. Ahead lay a region of light and wind and swirling dust, which, after a moment, showed itself to be a gaping hole in the side of the building. To her left, the end of the boom sloped downward into the floor, swaying from side to side with a soporific creaking sound. The air was otherwise weirdly still. Something rough and bulky lay beneath her: the chain. It was still attached to the tip of the boom. She felt profound puzzlement at having survived, at the mere fact of being alive. That was her only emotion. As she rolled onto her stomach, her center of gravity, distorted by her long plunge through space, swayed nauseatingly inside her. Nevertheless, she managed to push herself onto

her hands and knees and crawled toward the end of the boom.

Peter was lying facedown on the catwalk. He did not, at first, appear to be living. There was blood everywhere, and his neck was bent away from her at an unnatural angle. One arm dangled over the edge. But as Amy inched forward, calling his name, she detected a faint respiratory stirring, followed by a twitch of his exposed hand. I'm coming, she cried, I'm coming to get you. Just hang on.

She didn't have much time; the crane's tenuous state of balance would not last long. At any moment the whole thing would wrench free and topple to the street below. Kneeling on the catwalk, Amy slid her hands beneath Peter's shoulders. She was panting for air; perspiration dripped into her mouth and eyes. In a series of jerks, she drew him to the end of the boom and slid him onto the floor.

She rolled him onto his back. His body seemed completely inert, yet his eyes were open. Amy cupped his chin to make him look at her. His tongue swished behind his teeth with a gurgling sound; he was attempting to speak.

"You're hurt," she said. "Don't try to talk."

The muscles of his face compressed. His eyes were open very wide. She realized he wasn't looking at her. He was looking *behind* her.

A single word, the last one of his life, burst from Peter's lips: *"Fanning."*

The fractured end of the butter knife sank into the creature's eye with a spurt of clear fluid. Michael tried to hold on, but the metal slipped from his fingers as the creature emitted a high-pitched

799

squeal and staggered backward, the blade still embedded. Now Michael had nothing but the pan to work with. As one of the others shot forward, he swung it as hard as he could, connecting with the side of the creature's skull. He fell onto his side, still pressed to the wall. He raised the pan before his face.

The viral batted it away.

Michael rolled onto his stomach and buried his head in his arms.

Roaring with rage, Fanning blasted into her. A second of confusion and she was on her back, Fanning straddling her waist, claws coiled around her neck. The skin of his face was blackened and charred, the flesh separated in long, puckered slits that exposed the musculature beneath; his lips were gone, transforming his mouth into a skeleton's grin of naked teeth. Bits of damp, stringy material dangled from his eye sockets; the orbs within had burst. She tried to breathe, but no air passed the knot of pressure on her throat. Jets of spittle flew from Fanning's mouth into her eyes. Her hands batted at his arms and face, but her efforts were weak and vague. The floor began to shake; the crane was breaking loose. The walls of her vision were compacting around her like a narrowing tunnel. She abandoned her flailing and swept her hands along the floor. *He's blind,* she told herself. *He can't see what you're doing.* The shaking deepened; with a shriek of torquing metal, the boom jerked upward.

There it was, in her hand. The chain.

As she wound it around Fanning's neck, his face and body startled; Amy felt a momentary easing of the pressure on her windpipe. The boom had

begun to back out the side of the building. She quickly formed a second loop and tossed it over his head.

Fanning released her and sat upright. He raised a searching hand to his throat. The slack was running out.

"Look for her," said Amy.

He made no cry. He exited the world in a blink. He was there one second and gone the next, plucked into the whirling dust, his body thus to join the ashes of the vanished city.

And then it was over.

For a long time Michael waited. The silence seemed like a trick. But as the seconds passed and nothing happened, he realized something had changed. There was, all around him, a deep stillness, as if he were alone in the room.

He uncovered his eyes and looked.

The virals were dead. The one that had knocked the pan away lay at his feet, curled in a fetal position. The other two were on the far side of the room in a similar posture — even the one with the blade in its eye, from which still issued a trail of blood-tinged fluid. There was something tender about their postures. It was as if, overcome by a sudden exhaustion, they had lain on the floor and gone to sleep.

He used the stove to pull himself upright and limped down the hall, following the trail of his own blood. He took a scarf from one of the racks, rebandaged his leg, and ventured outside. A low evening sun, punching through the dust, flared the clouds with color. He made his way east to Lafayette Street and turned north. It wasn't until he'd traveled another block that he knew for

certain what had happened.

The virals lay everywhere. On the sidewalks. On the street. On the roofs of old cars. All in the same fetal posture, curled like children in their beds, worn out by a too-long day. A sight less of death than of a vast, collective repose. Their bodies, like the city of which they had so long been a part, were crumbling to dust. It was a scene of wonder. A great, sad, and joyous wonder, too heavy for one mind to bear. He stumbled forward. Uptown, the rumbling of destruction persisted. For months, years, centuries even, the immolation would continue, the great metropolis finally folding itself into the sea. But now, as Michael moved among the bodies, an infinite quiet prevailed, the world pausing in acknowledgment, history held in time's cupped hand.

And Michael Fisher did the only thing he could. He fell to his knees and wept.

Peter had begun to die.

Amy felt his spirit fade; Fanning was leaving him. His eyes were open, yet the light inside was dimming. Soon it would be gone.

Don't leave me. She lifted his hand and pressed it to her cheek; his flesh was growing cold. The muscles of his face relaxed toward death. *Please,* she said, and shuddered with a sob, *don't leave me alone.*

The time had come to let him go, to say goodbye, yet the prospect was unendurable; it could not be accepted. There was a way, perhaps. The gravest act — a betrayal, even. She momentarily had the sensation of being outside her body, watching herself, as she took the shard of glass from off the floor and slashed the edge across her

palm. Blood rose from the wound and swiftly gathered in a rich, crimson puddle. She took Peter's hand and did the same. A last flicker of doubt, then she placed his palm against her own and meshed their fingers together. She felt a tiny twitch; with accumulating pressure, Peter folded his fingers over the back of her hand.

She closed her eyes.

■ ■ ■ ■

XII
THE WILD BEYOND

■ ■ ■ ■

Though my soul may set in darkness,
it will rise in perfect light;
I have loved the stars too fondly
to be fearful of the night.

— SARAH WILLIAMS,
"The Old Astronomer to His Pupil"

83

At the top of Central Park, away from the destruction, Amy and Michael pitched their camp. It had taken them nearly a week to find each other; the center of the island was blocked by impenetrable mountains of debris. It was on the morning of the sixth day that Amy had heard him calling. Michael emerged from the rubble, a ghostly figure, covered with ash. By this time, Amy knew Alicia was gone; her presence, her spirit, these were nowhere in the world. Still, when Michael told her what had happened, the reality undid her. She sat on the ground and wept.

— And Peter? Michael asked tentatively.

Not looking up, Amy shook her head. No.

They remained there for three weeks to rest and gather supplies. Michael slowly regained his strength. Together they constructed a simple smokehouse and set snares to catch small game. Elsewhere in the park they found a variety of edible plants, even some apple trees, fat with glossy fruit. Michael worried that the water in the reservoir would be tainted by seawater, but it wasn't; they retrieved the water filter from the *Nautilus* to clean it of debris. From time to time they would hear the rumble of another building's

collapse, followed by a silence that seemed somehow deeper in the aftermath. At first this unnerved them, but eventually the noise became commonplace, nothing even to acknowledge.

The days were long, the sun hot. One early morning they awoke to a blast of thunder. Storm after storm crashed through the city. When at last the sun returned, the air was different. A sparkling freshness lay upon the park, dust washed from the leaves of the trees.

It was on their final night that Michael produced the bottle of whiskey. He had found it in an apartment building when he'd gone to scavenge tools and clothes. The cap was sealed, the glass caked with dust so thick it was like a layer of soil. Sitting by the fire, Michael was the first to try it. "Absent friends," he said, raising the bottle, and took a long swallow. As his throat bobbed, he began to cough while also, somehow, wearing an expression of triumph.

"Oh, you're going to like this," he wheezed, and handed it to her.

Amy took a small sip, to get the feel, then, as Michael had done, tipped her head back and let the whiskey fill her mouth. A rich, smoky taste bloomed on her tongue, filling her sinuses with tingling warmth.

Michael looked at her inquisitively, eyebrows raised. "You might want to go easy," he warned. "That's a hundred-and-twenty-year-old Scotch you're drinking."

She took a second pull, savoring the flavor more deeply.

"It tastes . . . like the past," she said.

In the morning they broke camp and headed south, through the park and down Eighth Avenue.

At the water's edge they loaded the last of Michael's supplies into the *Nautilus.* He would head first for Florida, where he would restock, then make the long jump to the coast of Brazil, hugging the land until he reached the Strait of Magellan. Once through, a final stop to rest and re-supply and he would set sail for the South Pacific.

"Are you sure you can find them?" Amy asked.

He shrugged carelessly, though they both understood the danger of what he was attempting. "After all this, how hard can it be?" He stopped, looked at her, then said with a note of caution, "I know you don't think you can come with me —"

"I can't, Michael."

He hunted for words. "It's just . . . how will you get along? All alone."

Amy did not have an answer, at least not one she believed would make sense to him. "I'll have to manage." She looked at his sad face. "I'll be all right, Michael."

They had agreed that a clean break would be best. Yet as the moment of separation arrived, this seemed not just foolish but impossible. They embraced, holding each other for a long time.

"She loved you, you know," Amy said.

He was crying a little; they both were. He shook his head. "I don't know that she did."

"Perhaps not the way you wanted. But it was the way she knew how." Amy drew back a little and placed a hand to his cheek. "Hold on to that, Michael."

They parted. Michael stepped down into the cockpit; Amy cast off the lines. A snap of the sail and the boat streamed away. Michael waved once over the transom; Amy waved in reply. *God bless*

and keep you, Michael Fisher. She watched the image recede into the vastness.

She put on her pack and hiked north. By the time she reached the bridge, it was early afternoon. A strong summer sun gleamed upon the surface of the water, far below. She made her way across and on the opposite side stopped to drink and rest, then donned her pack once more and continued on her journey.

Utah was four months away.

From the observation deck of the Empire State Building — one of the last intact structures between Grand Central and the sea — Alicia watched the *Nautilus* sail down the Hudson.

It had taken her most of two days to make the climb. Two hundred and four flights of stairs, most in total darkness, an agonizing ascent on her makeshift crutch and, when the pain became too great, her hands and knees. For hours she had lain on various landings, perspiring and breathing hard, wondering if she could go on. Her body was broken; her body was done. In those places where there was no pain, she felt only a creeping numbness. One by one, the lights of life were winking out inside her.

But her mind, her thoughts: these were her own. No Fanning, no Amy. How she'd escaped the subway tunnel she possessed no memory of; somehow she had been ejected onto dry land. The rest was fragments, flashes. She remembered Michael's face, backlit by sunshine, and his hand reaching down; the water slamming into her, its power immeasurable, large as a planet's; all volition gone, her body plunging and tumbling; the first involuntary gulp, making her choke, her

throat opening instinctively to take a second breath, pulling the water deeper into her lungs; pain, and then a merciful lessening of pain; a feeling of dispersal, her body and her thoughts losing their distinctiveness, like a radio signal fading from range; and then nothing at all.

She'd awakened to find herself in the most perplexing circumstance. She was sitting on a bench; around her, a small park of overgrown trees and a playground deep in tall, feathered grass. Slowly her awareness expanded. Vast crags of debris surrounded the perimeter although the park itself was miraculously untouched. The sun was out; birds twittered in the trees, a peaceful sound. Her clothing was soaked and her mouth tasted of salt. She sensed a gap in time between remembered events and her present situation, the calm of which seemed wholly anachronistic, like nothing she had ever known. She wondered, somewhat dully, if she was dead — if she was, in fact, a ghost. But when she attempted to stand, and the pain volleyed through her body, she knew this wasn't so; surely death would bring an absence of bodily sensation.

That was when she realized it. The virus was gone.

Not transmuted into some new state, as it had been in Fanning and Amy, restoring their human appearance while leaving other traits intact. The virus was nowhere inside her at all. Somehow the water had killed it, and then returned her to life.

How was this possible? Had Fanning lied to her? But when she searched her memory she realized he had never told her, in so many words, that the water would kill her, she who was neither wholly viral nor wholly human but poised between the

two. Perhaps he had sensed the truth; perhaps he simply hadn't known. What irony! She had hurled herself off the fantail of the *Bergensfjord* intending to die, yet it was the water that had been her salvation in the end.

But to be alive. To smell and hear and taste the world in proper proportion. To be alone in one's mind at last. She inhaled the sensation like the purest air. How amazing, how wondrous and unexpected. To be purely and simply *a person* again.

Fanning was dead. The wreckage of the city told her so first, then the bodies, curled and crumbling to ash. She took shelter in a ruined bodega. Perhaps the others were searching for her; perhaps they weren't, believing her dead. On the morning of the second day she heard someone calling. It was Michael. "Hello!" His voice ricocheted through the becalmed streets. "Hello! Is anybody there?" *Michael!* she answered. *Find me! I'm here!* But then she realized that she had not, in fact, spoken these words aloud.

It was very puzzling. Why would she not call out to him? What was this impulse to be silent? Why could she not tell him where she was? His calls faded, then were gone.

She waited for the meaning of this to become clear, so that a plan might emerge. The days moved by. When it rained, she set pots outside the store to catch the drops, and in that manner she slaked her thirst, though she had neither food nor the means to locate it, a fact that seemed oddly unimportant; she wasn't hungry at all. She slept a great deal: whole nights, many days as well. Long, deep states of unconsciousness in which she dreamed with fascinating emotional and sensory

vividness. Sometimes she was a little girl, sitting outside the wall of the Colony. At others, a young woman, standing the Watch with cross and blades. She dreamed of Peter. She dreamed of Amy. She dreamed of Michael. She dreamed of Sara and Hollis and Greer and, quite often, of her magnificent Soldier. Whole days, whole episodes of her life replayed before her eyes.

But the greatest of these dreams was the dream of Rose.

It began in a forest — misty, dark, like something from a childhood tale. She was hunting. On cautious, nearly floating steps she progressed beneath the trees' dense canopy, bow at the ready. From all around came the small noises and movements of game in the brush, yet her targets remained elusive. No sooner would she identify the location of a particular sound — a cracking twig, the rustle of dry leaves — than it would swing behind her or shift to the side, as if the woodland's inhabitants were toying with her.

She emerged into an area of rolling fields of open grassland. The sun had set, but darkness was yet to fall. As she walked, the grass grew taller. It rose to her waist, then to her chest. The light — soft, faintly glowing — remained uniform and appeared to have no source. From somewhere ahead she heard a new sound. It was laughter. A bright, bubbly, little-girl laughter. *Rose!* she cried, for she knew instinctively that the voice was her daughter's. *Rose, where are you!* She tore forward. The grass whipped her face and eyes. Desperation gripped her heart. *Rose, I can't see you! Help me find you!*

— Here I am, Mama!

— Where?

Alicia caught a flicker of movement, ahead and to the right. A flash of red hair.

— Over here! the girl teased. She was laughing, playing a game. Can't you see me? I'm right here!

Alicia plunged toward her. But like the animals in the forest, her daughter seemed to be everywhere and nowhere, her calls coming from all directions.

— Here I am! Rose sang. Try to find me!

— Wait for me!

— Come find me, Mama!

Suddenly the grass was gone. She found herself standing on a dusty road sloping upward toward the crest of a small hill.

— Rose!

No answer.

— Rose!

The road beckoned her forward. As she walked, she began to have a sense of her environment, or at least the kind of place it was. It was beyond the world she knew while also a part of it, a hidden reality that could be glimpsed as if from the corner of the eye but never wholly entered into in this life. With each step, her anxiety softened. It was as if an invisible power, purely benevolent, was guiding her. As she mounted the hill, she heard, once again, the bright, distant music of her daughter's laughter.

— Come to me, Mama, she sang. Come to me.

She reached the top of the rise.

And there Alicia awakened. What waited in the valley beyond the hilltop was not yet hers to see, though she believed she knew what it was, as she also knew the meaning of the other dreams, of Peter and Amy and Michael and all those whom she had loved and been loved by in return.

She was saying goodbye.

A night came when Alicia dreamed no more. She awoke with a feeling of fullness. All she had meant to do had been accomplished; the work of her life was complete.

On the crutch she had fashioned from scrap wood she made her way through the debris, three blocks north and one block west. Even this short distance left her gasping with pain. It was mid-morning when she began her ascent; by nightfall she had reached the fifty-seventh floor. Her water was nearly gone. She slept on the floor of a windowed office, so that the sun would wake her, and at dawn she resumed her climb.

Was it coincidence that this was the very same morning that Michael set sail? Alicia preferred to think it wasn't. That the sight of the *Nautilus*, pulling away on the wind, was a sign, and meant for her. Could Michael feel her? Did he, in some manner, sense that she was observing him from above? Impossible, and yet it pleased Alicia to think so — that he might suddenly look up, startled, as if touched by a sudden breeze. The *Nautilus* was departing the inner harbor, headed for open sea. Sunlight glimmered dazzlingly upon the water. Clutching the balustrade, Alicia watched as the tiny shape became smaller and smaller, fading into nonexistence. *Of all people, Michael,* she thought. And yet he had been the one. He had been the one to save her.

A tall fence, curved inward at the top, fixed into the top of the balustrade, had once formed a barricade around the perimeter of the platform; many sections remained, but not all. Alicia had saved a little water. She drank it now. How sweet it was,

the scavenged rain. She experienced a profound sense of the interconnectedness of all things, the eternal rising and falling of life — how the water, which had begun as the sea, had ascended, gathered into clouds, and descended from the sky as rain, to be gathered in the pots she'd laid. Now it had become a part of her.

Alicia sat on the balustrade. Below, on the outer side, was a small ledge. She rotated her body, using her hands to assist her disobedient legs over the rail. Faced away from the building, she scooted a few inches forward on the concrete until her feet touched the ledge. How did one do it? How did one say farewell to the world? She took a long breath and let the air out slowly. She realized she was crying. Not with sadness — no, not that — although her tears did not seem unrelated to sadness. They were tears of sadness and happiness conjoined, everything over and done.

My darling, my Rose.

Pushing with her palms, she drew herself erect. Space jumped away beneath her; she pointed her eyes to the sky.

Rose, I am coming. I will be with you soon.

Some might have said she fell. Others, that she flew. Both were true. Alicia Donadio — Alicia of Blades, the New Thing, Captain of the Watch and Soldier of the Expeditionary — would die as she had lived.

Always soaring.

Night came on.

Amy was somewhere in New Jersey. She had left the main thoroughfares behind, moving into the wild backcountry. Her arms and legs were heavy, full of a deep, almost pleasurable exhaustion. As

darkness fell, she made her camp in a field of winking fireflies, ate her simple supper, and lay down beneath the stars.

Come to me, she thought.

All around her, and all above, the small lights of heaven danced. A stout full moon rose from the trees, sharpening the shadows.

I'm waiting for you. I'll always wait. Come to me.

A pure silence; not even the air was moving. Time passed in its languid course. Then, like the brush of a feather inside her:

Amy.

At the far edge of the field, in the boughs of the trees, she saw and heard a rustling; Peter dropped down. He had just eaten, a squirrel or mouse perhaps, or some small bird; she could feel his contentment, the rich satisfaction he had taken in the act, like waves of warmth washing through her blood. Amy rose as he moved toward her, passing among the fireflies. There were so many, it was as if he — as if the two of them — were swimming together in a sea of stars. *Amy.* His voice like a soft wind of longing, breathing her name. *Amy, Amy, Amy.*

She raised her hand; Peter did the same. The gap between them closed. Their fingers meshed and fell together, the soft pressure of Peter's palm against her own.

Am I . . . ?

She nodded. — Yes.

And . . . I'm yours? I belong to you?

She sensed his confusion. The trauma was still fresh, the disorientation. She tightened her fingers, pressing their palms together, and held his eyes with hers.

— You are mine, and I am yours. We belong to

each other, you and I.

A pause, then: *We are each other's. You are mine and I am yours.*

— Yes, Peter.

Peter. He held the thought for a moment. *I am Peter.*

She cupped his cheek.

— Yes.

I am Peter Jaxon.

Her vision swam with tears. The moonlit night was fantastically still, everything held in abeyance, the two of them like actors on a stage of dark wings with a single spotlight falling upon them.

— Yes, that is who you are. You are my Peter.

And you are my Amy.

As she made her way west — and then for many years after — he was to come to her each night in this manner. The conversation would be repeated countless times, like a chant or prayer. Each visit was as if it were the first; at the start he retained no memory, either of the previous nights or of the events that had preceded them, as if he were a wholly novel creature in the world, born anew each night. But slowly, as the years became decades, the man inside the body — the essential spirit — reasserted itself. Never would he speak again, though they would talk of many things, words flowing through the touch of their hands, the two of them alone among the stars.

But that came later. Now, standing in the field of fireflies, beneath the summer moon, he asked her:

Where are we going?

She smiled through her tears.

— Home, said Amy. My Peter, my love. We are going home.

■ ■ ■ ■

Michael had cleared the harbor. Over the transom, the image of the city grew faint. The moment of decision was upon him. South, as he'd told Amy, or a new direction entirely?

It wasn't even a question.

He tacked the *Nautilus,* turning in a northeasterly direction. The wind was fair, the seas light, with a gentle green color. The following afternoon he rounded the tip of Long Island and leapt into open sea. Three days after leaving New York, he made landfall at Nantucket. The island was arrestingly beautiful, with long beaches of pure white sand and crashing surf. There appeared to be no buildings at all, or none he could see; all traces of civilization had been swept away by the ocean's hand. Anchored in a sheltered cove, he made his final calculations, and at dawn, he set sail again.

Soon the ocean changed. It grew darker, with a solemn look. He had passed into a wild zone, far from any land. He felt not fear but excitement and, beneath this, a thrilling rightness. His boat, his *Nautilus,* was sound; he had the wind and sea and stars to guide him. He hoped to reach the English coast in twenty-three days, though perhaps that wouldn't happen. There were many variables. Maybe it would take a month, or longer; maybe he'd end up in France, or even Spain. It didn't matter.

Michael Fisher was going to find what was out there.

Fanning came to awareness of his surroundings slowly, and in parts. First there was a sensation of cold sand on his feet; this was followed by the sound of waves, gently pushing upon a tranquil shore. After an unknown interval of time had passed, other facts emerged. It was night. Stars thick as powder lay across a sky of velvety blackness, immeasurably deep. The air was cool and still, as after a daylong rain. Above and behind him, atop a steep bluff of eelgrass and beach plum, were houses; their white faces shone faintly with the reflected light of the moon, which was ascending from the sea.

He began to walk. The hems of his trousers were damp; he seemed to have mislaid his shoes, or else he had arrived in this place without them. He had no destination in mind, merely a sense that walking was something the situation called for. The unanticipated nature of his circumstances, its feeling of elastic reality, aroused in him no anxiety. Quite the contrary: everything felt inevitable, reassuringly so. When he tried to recall anything that might have happened prior to his being in this place, he could think of nothing. He knew who he was, yet his personal history seemed devoid of narrative coherence. There was a time, he knew, when he had been a child. And yet that period of his life, like all others, registered only as a collection of emotional and sensory impressions with a metaphoric aspect. His mother and his father, for example, resided in his memory not as individuated beings but as a feeling of warmth and safety, like being cradled in a bath. The town where he'd grown up, whose name he did not

recall, was not a discrete civic unit of buildings and streets but a view through a window screen of rain pattering upon summer leaves. It was all very peculiar, not unsettling but simply unexpected, especially the fact that his adult life seemed almost completely unknown to him. He knew that in his life he had been happy, also sad; for a long time he had been very, very lonely. Yet when he tried to reconstruct the circumstances, all he remembered was a clock.

For a great while, in this unforeseen and generally pleasant state of unremembering, he made his way down the broad boulevard of sand at the water's edge. The moon, having cleared the horizon, had ceased its upward arc. The tide was high, boastfully so, the sky immense. At length he became aware of a figure in the distance. For a time the figure grew no closer; then, with a telescoping quality, the gap began to narrow.

Liz was sitting on the sand with her arms wrapped around her shins, gazing over the water. She was wearing a white dress of some diaphanous material, light as a nightgown; her feet, like his, were bare. He vaguely recalled that something had happened to her, very unfortunate, though he couldn't say what that thing might have been; she had gone away, that was all, and now she had returned. He was happy, very happy to see her, and although she indicated no awareness of his presence, he felt very much as if she were expecting him.

"Liz, hello."

She looked up; her eyes twinkled with starlight. "Well, there you are," she said, smiling. "I was wondering when you'd get here. Do you have something for me?"

In fact, he did. He was holding her glasses. How curious this fact was.

"May I have them, please?"

She accepted the glasses, turned her face once again toward the water, and put them on. "There," she remarked, with a nod of satisfaction, "that's much better. I can't see a damn thing without them. All of this beauty was practically wasted on me, if you want to know the truth. But now I can see everything just fine."

"Where are we?" he asked.

"Why don't you sit?"

He lowered himself onto the sand beside her.

"That is an excellent question," Liz said. "The beach, would be the answer. This is the beach."

"How long have you been here?"

She touched a finger to her lips. "Now, isn't that funny. Even just a few minutes ago, I think I would have said for quite some time. But now that you're here, it doesn't seem like very much at all."

"Are we alone?"

"Alone? Yes, I should think so." She paused; a look of mischief came into her face. "You don't recognize any of this, do you? That's all right; it takes a little while to adjust. Believe me, when I first got here, I didn't have a clue what was going on."

He looked around. It was true; he had been in this place.

"I always wondered," Liz continued. "What would have happened if you had kissed me that night? How would our lives have been different? Of course, you might well have, if I hadn't gotten so drunk. What a self-pitying fool I made of myself. The whole thing was totally my fault from

the get-go."

At once he remembered. The beach below her parents' house on Cape Cod: that's where they were. The place where, long ago, he had let life pass by, failing to say what his heart knew.

"How are we . . . here?"

"Oh, I think 'how' is not the question."

"What's the question, then?"

"The question, Tim, is 'why.' "

She was looking at him absorbedly. It was a gaze meant to comfort, as if he were ill. She had taken his hand in hers without his quite being aware of it. It felt warm as a cup of tea.

"It's all right," she said softly. "You can let it out now."

Suddenly his mind seemed to plunge. He remembered everything. The past reared up inside him, complete. He saw faces; he inhabited days; he lived the hour of his birth and each that followed. He felt as if he were choking; his lungs could find no air.

"That's all you have to do, is let it out."

She had put her arms around him. He was trembling, weeping, such tears as he had never wept in his life. All his sorrows, all his pain, the terrible things he'd done.

"Everything is forgiven, my darling, my love. All is forgiven, nothing is lost. Everything you have loved will come back to you. That is why you have come."

He moaned and shook. He cast his cries upward to the heavens. The waves moved in and out in their ancient rhythm; the stars poured down their primordial light upon him.

I'm here, Liz, his Liz, was saying. *It's over now, everything will be all right. Oh, beloved, I am here.*

823

It took some time. It took days, weeks, years. But this was unimportant. It would pass in a blink, not even. All things fell into the past but one; and what that was, was love.

■ ■ ■ ■

XIII
THE MOUNTAIN AND THE STARS

■ ■ ■ ■

And thence we came forth, to see again
the stars.
— DANTE ALIGHIERI, *Inferno*

85

"Shut it off," Lore said.

Rand stared at her, expressionless. They were on the engineering deck — heat stifling, air throbbing with the engines' rhythmic roar. Rand's broad, bare chest shone with sweat.

"You're sure about this?"

They were down to their last ten thousand pounds of fuel.

"Please," Lore said, "don't argue with me. It's not like we have a choice."

Rand raised the radio to his mouth. "That's it, gents. We're powering down. Weir, switch the generator to the auxiliary bus — bilges, lights, and desalinators only."

A crackle, then Weir's voice came through: "Lore said that?"

"Yeah, she said it. I'm looking right at her."

A moment passed; the thrumming ceased, replaced by a low electrical hum. Above them caged bulbs flickered, failed, then, as if with reluctance, sparked back to life.

"So that's it?" Rand asked. "We're dead in the water?"

Lore had no answer to that.

"I'm sorry, I shouldn't have said it that way."

She made some vague gesture. "Forget it."

"I know you did your best. Everyone does."

She had nothing to say. They were twenty thousand tons of steel, drifting in the ocean.

"Maybe something will still work out," Rand offered.

Lore ascended through the ship to the deck and climbed the stairs to the pilothouse. It was the morning of their thirty-ninth day at sea, the equatorial sun already blazing like a furnace. Not a breath of wind moved the air; the sea was absolutely flat. Many of the passengers were camped on deck, huddled in the shade of canvas shelters. On the charting table were the sheets of thick, fibrous paper on which Lore had run her final computations. The currents when they'd rounded the Horn had nearly stopped them cold; running at full throttle, they had barely powered through, huge waves blasting over the deck, everybody vomiting helplessly. They had made it eventually, but day by day, as Lore watched the fuel gauges drop, the cost grew painfully evident. They had stripped everything they could and jettisoned it into the sea: pieces of bulkhead, doors, the loading crane. Anything to reduce weight, to buy one more mile with the fuel they had. It wasn't enough. They had come up five hundred miles short.

Caleb entered the pilothouse. Like Rand, he was shirtless, the skin of his shoulders and cheeks flaking with sunburn. "What's going on? Why did we stop?"

From the helm, Lore shook her head.

"Jesus." For a second he seemed dazed, then looked up. "How long?"

"We can keep the desalinators running about a week."

"And then?"

"I really don't know, Caleb."

He had the look of a man who needed to sit down. He took a place on the bench by the chart table. "People are going to figure it out, Lore. We can't just turn off the engines and not tell them anything."

"What do you want me to say?"

"We could lie, I guess."

"There's an idea. Why don't you come up with something?"

Her sense of failure was overwhelming; she had spoken too curtly. "Sorry, you didn't deserve that."

Caleb took a long breath. "It's all right, I get it."

"Tell everyone it's just a minor repair, nothing to worry about," Lore said. "That should buy us a day or two."

Caleb stood and put one hand on her shoulder. "It's not your fault."

"Who else is there?"

"I mean it, Lore. It's just bad luck." He tightened his grip, giving her a sharp squeeze that offered no comfort at all. "I'll put the word out."

After he'd gone, she sat alone for a time. She was exhausted, filthy, beaten. Without its engines, the ship felt soulless, inert as stone.

I'm sorry, Michael, she thought, *I did everything I could, but it wasn't enough.*

She dropped her face to her hands.

It was late in the day when she descended into the hull. She met Sara as the woman was closing the door to Greer's cabin.

"How is he?"

Sara shook her head tersely: not well. "I don't see how things can go on much longer." She paused, then said, "Caleb told me about the engines."

Lore nodded halfheartedly.

"Well, let me know if I can do anything to help. Maybe it just wasn't meant to be."

"You're not the first to say that."

When Lore said nothing else, Sara sighed. "See if you can get him to eat. I left a tray by his cot."

She watched the woman move down the passageway, then quietly turned the handle and stepped inside. The air had an unwashed smell of sweat and urine and sour breath and something else, like fermenting fruit. Greer was lying faceup on his bunk with a sheet pulled to his chin, his arms lying at his sides. At first Lore thought he was dozing — he slept most of the time now — but at the sound of her entry, he rotated his face toward her.

"I wondered when I'd see you."

Lore drew a stool to the edge of the cot. The man was a shadow of a shadow, a shell of bones. His flesh, a sickly yellow, possessed a damp, translucent appearance, like the inner layers of an onion.

"I guess you noticed," she said.

"Hard not to."

"Don't try to cheer me up, okay? A lot of people are doing that, and it's already getting old. Now, what's this I hear about you not eating?"

"Hardly seems worth the bother."

"Nonsense. Let's scoot you up."

He was too weak to rise off the mattress on his own; Lore drew him to a sitting position and

wedged a pillow between his back and the bulk-head.

"All right?"

He offered a faint, courageous smile. "Never better."

On the tray were a cup of water and a bowl of porridge, also a spoon and cloth. She draped the cloth over Greer's chest and began to spoon the porridge into his mouth. He worked his lips and tongue hesitatingly, as if these simple actions required tremendous concentration. Still, he managed a good amount before waving her off. She wiped his chin and held the cup of water to his lips. He took a small sip; she could tell he was humoring her. She had noticed, while feeding him, a basin at the foot of the bed, stained with blood.

"Happy now?" he asked, as she put the cup aside.

She almost laughed. "What a question."

"Michael picked you for a reason. That's no less true now than it was thirty-nine days ago."

Suddenly the tears came. "Oh, goddamnit, Lucius. What am I going to tell people?"

"You're not going to tell them anything yet."

"They're going to figure it out. Probably a lot of them already have."

Greer gestured to the bedside table. "Open that drawer," he said. "The top one."

Inside she found a single sheet of heavy paper, folded into thirds and sealed with wax. For several seconds she just looked at it, dumbfounded.

"It's from Michael," Greer said.

She took it in her hand. It weighed almost nothing — it was only paper — but it felt like far more; it felt like a letter from the grave. She wiped her

face with the back of her wrist. "What does it say?"

"That's between the two of you. All he told me was that you weren't supposed to open it until we arrived at the island. His orders."

"So why are you giving it to me now?"

"Because I think you need it. He believed in you. He believed in the *Bergensfjord.* The situation is what it is; I won't tell you different. But things may work out yet."

She hesitated, then said, "He told me how the passengers died. How they killed themselves, sealing the ship and channeling back the engines' exhaust."

"Don't get ahead of yourself, Lore."

"I'm only saying he knew it was a possibility. He wanted me to be ready."

"We're not there yet. A lot of things can happen between now and then."

"I wish I had your faith."

"Feel free to use mine. Or Michael's. God knows I borrowed his lots of times. We all did. None of us would be here if we hadn't."

A brief silence passed.

"Tired?" Lore asked.

His eyes were heavy-lidded. "A little, yeah."

She put her hand on his arm. "You just rest, all right? I'll come check on you later."

She rose and went to the door.

"Lore?"

She turned at the threshold; Greer was looking at the ceiling.

"A thousand years," he said. "That's how long."

Lore waited for more but there was none. Finally she said, "I don't understand."

Greer swallowed. "In case Amy and the others fail. That's how long before anybody can go back."

He took a deep breath and let the air out slowly, closing his eyes. "I'm only saying this because I might not be around to tell you later."

She let herself into the passageway and returned to the pilothouse, where she sat at the chart table. The sky beyond the windscreen showed evening coming on. A mass of clouds, as thick and textured as wads of unspun cotton, had moved in from the south; perhaps they'd be lucky and get some rain. She watched as the sun dipped to the horizon, flaring the sky with its final light. A sudden weariness enfolded her. Poor Lucius, she thought. Poor everyone. The world could do without her for a while, she decided, and she laid her head on the table, cradling it with her arms, and soon was fast asleep.

She dreamed of many things. In one dream, she was a girl again, lost in a forest; in another, she was stuck inside a closet; in a third, she was carrying a heavy object of unknown type and could not put it down. These dreams were not pleasant, but neither were they nightmares. Each unfolded seamlessly into the next, depriving them of their full power — no climax was reached, no mortal moment of terror — and as sometimes occurred, she was also aware that she was dreaming, that the landscape she inhabited was harmlessly symbolic.

The final dream of Lore's thirty-ninth night at sea was hardly a dream at all. She was standing in a field. All was quiet, yet she knew a danger was approaching. The color of the air began to change, first to yellow, then to green. The hair on her arms and the back of her neck rose, as if with a static charge; simultaneously, a great wind swirled up

around her. She tilted her face to the sky. Clouds of black and silver had begun to form a whirlpool overhead. With a crackling explosion and a biting smell of ozone, a bolt of lightning jagged the ground in front of her, blinding her utterly.

She began to run. Sheets of rain commenced to fall as, above her, the furious, whirlpooling clouds congealed into a single, fingerlike cone. The ground was shaking, thunder crashing; trees were bursting into flames. The storm was pursuing her. It would sweep her into oblivion. As the finger touched down behind her, the air was rent by a deafening, animal roar. Its power seized her like a fist; suddenly the ground was gone. A voice, far away, was calling her name. She was lifting into the air, she was soaring higher and higher, she was being hurled off the face of the earth . . .

"Lore, wake up!"

Her head jerked from the table. Rand was staring at her. Why was he so wet? And why was everything moving?

"What the hell are you doing?" Rand barked. Rain and seawater were pelting against the windscreen. "We're in real trouble here."

As she attempted to rise from the bench, the deck heaved sideways. The door flew open with a bang, rain and wind blasting into the pilothouse. Another groan from deep within the hull and the deck began to heel in the opposite direction. Lore went tumbling, sliding down the deck and smacking into the bulkhead. For a moment it seemed that they would just keep going, but then the motion reversed. Gripping the edge of the table for balance, she fought her way upright.

"When the hell did this start?"

Rand was clutching the edge of the pilot's seat.

"About thirty minutes ago. It just whipped up from nowhere."

They were taking the sea broadside. The lightning flashed, the heavens shook; huge waves were crashing over the rails.

"Get below and fire the engines," she ordered.

"That'll use the rest of our fuel."

"No choice." She strapped herself into the pilot seat; water was sloshing over the floor. "Without helm control, this is going to pound us to pieces. I just hope we have enough left to get through this. We'll need all the thrust you've got."

As Rand exited, Caleb appeared out of the storm. The man's face was white as a ghost's, whether with terror or seasickness, Lore couldn't tell.

"Is everyone below?" she asked.

"Are you kidding me? It's like a screaming contest down there."

She yanked the straps tight. "This is going to be rough, Caleb. We need every hatch sealed. Tell people to tie themselves down however they can."

He nodded grimly, turned to go.

"And shut that fucking door!"

The ship heeled into the next trough, listing at a perilous angle before rolling up the other side. With nearly all of their fuel gone, they had no ballast; it wouldn't take much to capsize them. She looked at her watch; it was 0530. Dawn would soon be breaking.

"Goddamnit, Rand," she muttered. "Come on, come on . . ."

The pressure gauges leapt; power flowed through the panel. Lore set the rudder, gripped the throttle control, and opened it wide. The compass was spinning like a top. With excruciating slowness,

the bow began to turn into the wind.

"Come on, girl!"

The bow bit and held, plummeting into the next trough as if down a mountainside. Spray blasted over the deck. For a second, the front of the ship was almost fully submerged; then it ascended, the hull rearing upward like a great rising beast.

"That's the way!" Lore shouted. "Do it for Mama!"

She drove into the howling darkness.

For twelve full hours, the storm raged. Many times, as giant waves crashed over the bow, Lore believed the end had come. Each time, the foredeck plunged into the abyss; each time, it rose again.

The storm did not so much fade as simply stop. One second the wind was howling, the rain lashing; in the next it was all over. It was as if they had simply passed from one room into the next, one of violence, the other of almost perfect calm. With cramped hands, Lore unfastened her straps. She had no idea what was going on belowdecks, nor did this question, at that moment, concern her very much. She was tired and thirsty and badly needed to pee. She squatted over the pot she kept in the pilothouse and stepped outside to toss the contents over the side.

The clouds had begun to break apart. She stood at the rail for a moment and watched the evening sky. She had no idea where they were; she hadn't been able to read the compass since the storm had begun. They had survived, but at what cost? Their fuel was nearly exhausted. Beneath the stern of the *Bergensfjord,* the screws were softly churning, pushing them through the motionless sea.

Rand emerged from the main hatch and ascended the stairs toward her. He took a place beside her at the rail.

"I've got to admit, it sure is pretty out here," he said. "Funny how it's like that after a storm."

"What's the situation belowdecks?"

His shoulders were slumped, his eyes rimmed with dark circles of fatigue; a bit of something, vomit perhaps, was caught in his beard. "We've got the bilges working — we should be dry pretty soon. You have to hand it to Michael, the guy knew how to build a boat."

"Any injuries?"

Rand shrugged. "Few broken bones, I heard. Some cuts and scrapes. Sara's taking care of it. Lucky thing no one's going to want to eat for a week, seeing as how we're so low on food. The smell is pretty bad down there." He looked at her for a moment, then said, carefully, "Want me to shut down the engines? It's your call."

She considered this question. "In a minute," she said.

For a while they stood together without talking, watching the sun descend over the starboard side. The last of the clouds were separating, lit from within by a purpling light. An area of water near the port bow had begun to boil with fish, feeding near the surface. As Lore watched, a large bird with black-tipped wings and a yellowish head swooped low over the surface, reached down with its bill — a quick, sharp jab — hauled a fish free, tossed it backward into its gullet, and began to climb away.

"Rand. That's a bird."

"I know it's a bird. I've seen birds before."

"Not in the middle of the ocean you haven't."

She darted into the pilothouse and returned with the binoculars. Her pulse was racing, her heart was in her mouth. She pressed the lenses to her eyes and scanned the horizon.

"Anything?"

She held up a hand. "Quiet."

She made a slow circle. Facing due south, she stopped.

"Lore, what are you seeing?"

She held the image in the lenses for an extra few seconds to be sure. Holy damn, she thought. She lowered the binoculars.

"Get Greer up here," she said.

By the time they were able to bring him up on deck, darkness was falling. Lucius did not appear to be in pain; that part had passed. His eyes were closed; he did not seem to know where he was or what was happening. With Sara supervising, Caleb and Hollis served as stretcher-bearers. Others had gathered around; word had spread throughout the ship. Pim was there, with Theo and the girls; Jenny and Hannah; Jock and Grace, holding their infant son; the men of the crew, weary after the long battle of the storm. All stood aside as the stretcher passed.

They carried him to the bow and lowered the gurney. Lore crouched beside him and wrapped one hand with her fingers. His skin was cold and dry, loose on the bones.

"Lucius, it's Lore."

From deep in his throat, a soft moan.

"I have something to show you. Something wonderful."

She slipped the palm of her left hand beneath his neck and gently tipped his face forward,

toward the bow.

"Open your eyes," she said.

His lids separated to make the thinnest slits, then a little more. It was if he were using the last of his strength to perform this tiny act. All stood silent, waiting. The island was well within sight now, directly ahead: a single mountain, lushly green, soaring from the sea, and, above it, a cross of five bright stars, punching through the twilight.

"Do you see?" she whispered.

The breath in his chest was barely a presence; death was in his face. A long moment passed as he struggled to focus. At last the faintest of smiles curled his lips.

"It's . . . beautiful," Greer said.

86

Lucius Greer lived three more days, thus earning the distinction of being the first settler on the island, as yet unnamed, to die upon its soil. He spoke no more words; it could not have been said that he regained full consciousness. Yet from time to time, as Sara or one of the others attended to him, the smile would reappear, as if rising from a happy dream.

They buried him in a clearing surrounded by tall palms with a view of the sea. Apart from the men who had worked on the boat, few of the ship's complement knew the man or even who he was, least of all the children, who had heard only vague rumors of a dying man in a cabin, and whose shouts of play could be heard throughout the ceremony. Nobody minded; it seemed suitable. Lore was the first to speak, followed by Rand and Sara. They had decided in advance that each

would tell a story. Lore spoke of his friendship with Michael; Rand, the tales Greer had told him about his life in the Expeditionary; Sara, the day she and Greer had met, so many years ago, in Colorado, and all that had happened there. When this was done, they formed a line so each could place a stone upon the grave, which bore a simple marker Lore had fashioned from pieces of drift-wood:

LUCIUS GREER
SEER, SOLDIER, FRIEND

It was the next morning that a small group used two of the dinghies to return to the *Bergensfjord,* which waited at anchor a thousand yards offshore. There had been some disagreement on the matter — the ship contained all manner of usable materials — but Lore was firm and, as captain, had final say. We let her rest, she told them. It's what Michael wanted.

She had not, in fact, opened Michael's letter until their second day on the island, by which time she had begun to suspect what it said. She could not say why this should be so; perhaps it was merely her sense of the man. Thus it was without undo surprise, only a pleasant sense of hearing his voice, that she read the three simple sentences the letter contained.

Look in aft storage locker #16.
Scuttle the ship.
Start over.

Love, M

The storage locker contained a crate of explosives, as well as spools of cable and a radio detona-

tor. Michael had left instructions for their proper distribution. Caleb and Hollis ran the cables through the passageways while Lore and Rand distributed the explosives throughout the hull. The fuel tanks, now nearly empty, were full of highly combustible diesel fumes. Lore turned on the mixers, opened the valves, and set the final charge.

There was no further discussion about what would happen next; the job was Lore's. The men returned to the dinghies. Lore took a final tour through the ship, its silent rooms and passageways. She thought of Michael as she walked, for the two, Michael and the *Bergensfjord,* were one and the same in her mind. She was sad but also full of gratitude, for all he had given her.

She ascended to the deck and headed aft. The detonator was a small metal box operated by a key. She removed the key, which she wore on a chain around her neck, and carefully inserted it into the slot. Rand and the others were waiting below in their boats.

"Goodbye, Michael."

She turned the key and dashed for the stern. Beneath her, explosions were ripping through the hull, headed toward the fuel tanks. She hit the fantail at a dead sprint, took three long steps, and launched.

Lore DeVeer, captain of the *Bergensfjord,* airborne.

She entered the water cleanly, with barely a splash. All around her, a beautiful blue world appeared. She rolled onto her back and gazed upward. A few seconds passed; then a flash of light lit the surface. The water shook with a muffled boom.

She emerged just a few yards from the boats. Behind her, the *Bergensfjord* was in flames, a huge cloud of black smoke soaring skyward. Caleb helped her in.

"That was a nice dive," he said.

She sat on the bench. The *Bergensfjord* was sinking from the stern. As its bow lifted clear of the water, exposing its massive, bulbous nose, shouts went up from the beach; the children, thrilled by the marvelous display, were cheering. When the hull reached a forty-five-degree angle, the ship began to slide backward, accelerating with astonishing speed. Lore closed her eyes; she did not want to witness the final moment. When she opened them, the *Bergensfjord* was gone.

They rowed back toward shore. As they approached the beach, Sara came jogging down the sand to meet them.

"Caleb, I think you'd better come," she said.

Pim's membranes had ruptured. Caleb found her underneath a tarp hung between trees on one of the thin mattresses they'd stripped from the *Bergensfjord*. Her face was calm, though damp in the tropical heat. During the last few weeks, her hair had grown incomparably thick, its color deepening to a rich chestnut that flared with red in the sun.

Hey, he signed.

Hey yourself. Then, with a smile: *You should see your expression. Don't worry, I'll be done in no time.*

He looked at Sara. "How is she really?" He was signing simultaneously; no secrets, not now.

"I don't see any problems. She's only a little short of her due date. And she's right: for a second birth, things tend to go faster."

Theo's birth had taken forever, nearly twenty hours from the first contraction to the last. It had just about crushed Caleb with worry, though less than a minute after Theo hit the air, Pim was all smiles, demanding to hold him.

"Just hang around," Sara told him. "Hollis can look after Theo and the girls."

Caleb could tell that there was something the woman wasn't saying. He moved away, Sara following.

"Out with it," he said.

"Well. The thing is, I'm hearing two heartbeats."

"Two," he repeated.

"Twins, Caleb."

He stared at her. "And you didn't know this until now?"

"Sometimes it happens." She reached out and took him by the upper arm. "She's strong — she's done this before."

"Not with two."

"It's not so very different until the end."

"Good God. How am I going to tell them apart?" A foolish concern, and yet it was the first thought to enter his mind.

"You'll figure it out. Plus, they might not be identical."

"Really? How does *that* work?"

She laughed lightly. "You don't know the first thing about this, do you?"

His stomach churned with anxiety. "I guess not."

"Just stay with her. The contractions are still far apart, there's really nothing for me to do at this point. Hollis will keep the kids amused." She gave him a parental look. "Okay?"

Caleb nodded. He felt completely overwhelmed.

"Attaboy," she said.

He watched her head down the beach and returned to the shelter. Pim was jotting in her notebook. It was one he hadn't seen before, handsomely bound with leather. A bottle of ink sat on the sand beside her, as well as a pile of books from Hollis's stash. Pim looked up, closing the diary with a muffled clap as Caleb sat on the sand.

She told you.

Yes.

Pim, too, was grinning at him in a manner that verged on laughter. He felt like he'd wandered into the wrong room at a party, one in which everybody knew everybody else and he knew exactly no one.

Relax, she signed. *It's no big deal.*

How do you know?

Because women know. She drew a sharp breath, her face scrunching with pain. Caleb saw it in her eyes: her lighthearted attitude was a cover. His wife was steeling herself for what would come. Hour by hour, she would go further away from him, into the place where all her strength came from.

Pim? Okay?

A few seconds went by; her face relaxed as she expelled a long breath. She tipped her head at the pile of books. *Read to me?*

He lifted the first volume from the pile. Caleb had never been much for reading; he found it tedious, no matter how much his father-in-law had attempted to persuade him otherwise. At least the title made sense to him: *War and Peace.* Perhaps, contrary to all his expectations, it would actually be interesting. The book was enormous; it felt like it weighed ten pounds. He opened the cover and turned to the first page, which was

covered in dispiritingly minuscule print, like a wall of ink.

You're sure about this? he signed.

Pim's eyes were bright, her hands folded together over her belly. *Yes, please. It's one of my father's favorites. I've been meaning to read it for ages.*

Full of dread, yet anxious to please her, Caleb sat on the sand, balanced the book on his lap, and began to sign:

" *'Well, prince, Genoa and Lucca are now no more than private estates of the Bonaparte family. No, I warn you, that if you do not tell me we are at war, if you again allow yourself to palliate all the infamies and atrocities of this Antichrist (upon my word, I believe he is), I don't know you in future, you are no longer my friend, no longer my faithful slave, as you say.'* "

And so on. Caleb was totally baffled; nothing seemed to be happening, just obscure conversations that went nowhere, full of references to places and characters he couldn't keep track of, even a little. The signing was laborious; many words he did not know and had to spell out. Yet Pim seemed to be enjoying herself. At unforeseen moments, she would issue small sighs of pleasure, or her eyes would widen with anticipation, or she would smile at what Caleb supposed was the book's equivalent of a joke. It wasn't long before his hands were exhausted. Pim's contractions continued, the gaps between them shortening over time while their durations increased. When this happened, Caleb would pause in his reading, waiting for the pain to end; Pim would nod to tell him it was over, and he would begin reading again.

The hours moved by. Sara visited at regular

intervals, taking Pim's pulse, touching her belly here and there, reporting that all was well, things were moving normally. Of *War and Peace,* she only remarked, eyebrows raised, "Good luck."

Others came by: Lore and Rand, Jenny and Hannah, as well as several people Pim had befriended on the ship. In midafternoon, Hollis brought Theo and the girls. The boy could have cared less, sitting on the ground beside his mother and attempting to fill his mouth with sand, but for the girls, the birth of a cousin — not just one but, magically, a pair of them — was a long-anticipated excitement, like a present waiting to be unwrapped. During their weeks on the ship with little to amuse them, Elle's signing had improved. No longer was she limited to the most elementary phrases. With Pim she chattered away, oblivious to the woman's discomfort, though Pim didn't seem to mind or, if she did, managed not to show it.

"All right," Hollis said finally, clapping his hands together, "your aunt needs her rest. Let's go look for shells, shall we?"

The girls complained, but off they went, Theo riding his grandfather's hip. Pim's eyes followed them. *She looks so much like Kate,* she signed.

Which one?

She paused. *Both of them.*

The afternoon faded. Caleb had become aware of a certain energy being directed at the tent from multiple directions. Word had gone around: a baby was being born. Eventually Pim told him to stop reading. *Let's save the rest for later,* she said, by which she meant: nothing besides having these babies is going to happen for a while. The contractions intensified, long and deep. Caleb called for

846

Sara. A quick exam, then she looked at him pointedly.

"Go wash your hands. We'll need a couple of clean towels, too."

Jenny had heated a pot of water. Caleb did as Sara instructed and returned to the tent. Pim had begun to make a great deal of noise. The sounds she made were different than other people's. There was something more raw about them, almost animalistic. Sara hiked up Pim's skirt and laid one of the towels beneath her pelvis.

Ready to push?

Pim nodded.

"Caleb, sit next to her. I need you to translate what I say."

The next contraction seized her. Pim clamped her eyes tight, raising her knees and bending her chin to her chest.

"That's the way," Sara said. "Keep going."

Another few seconds, torturous to Caleb, and then Pim relaxed, gasping for breath, her head falling back onto the sand. Caleb hoped for some respite, but virtually no time passed before the next contraction. The long, listless afternoon had become a battle. Caleb took one of her hands and began to write in her palm. *I love you. You can do this.*

"Here we go," said Sara.

Pim coiled and bore down. Sara had placed her hands beneath Pim's pelvis with her palms open, as if to catch a ball. A dark, round cap of hair appeared, slithered back inside, then emerged once more. Pim was puffing rapidly through pursed lips.

"One more time," Sara said.

Caleb signed the words, though Pim took no

notice. It hardly mattered; her body was in control now — she was merely following its commands. She gripped Caleb's arm for balance, rose up, and buried her fingers into his flesh as every part of her compressed.

The head appeared again, and then the shoulders; with a slippery sound the baby slid free, into Sara's hands. A girl. The baby was a girl. Sara passed her to Jenny, who was kneeling beside her. Jenny quickly snipped the cord and balanced the baby along her forearm; cupping the baby's face with her palm, she began to rub her tiny, blue-skinned back with a tender, circular motion. The air of the shelter had a smoky smell, as well as a note of something sweet, almost floral.

The baby made a small, wet sound, like a sneeze.

"Piece of cake," Jenny said with a smile.

"We're not done here, Caleb," Sara said. "The next one's yours."

"You're kidding."

"You have to earn your keep around this place. Just follow Jenny's lead."

Pim rocked forward again. Her last push seemed less effortful; the path had been cleared. A single sustained straining and the second child arrived.

A boy.

Sara passed him to Caleb. The cord, a glistening rope of veins, was still attached. The boy was warm against Caleb's skin, his color dull, almost gray. He placed his son along his arm as Jenny had done and began to rub. The lightness of his body was stupendous; how astounding that a person could grow from this small thing, that not just people but every living creature upon the earth had begun this way. Caleb felt swept into a miracle. Something soft and wet filled his palm;

the baby's chest expanded with a gulp of air.

One life had left them; now two had entered. Pim, her face glazed with relief, was already holding their daughter. Sara cut the cord, washed the little boy with a damp cloth, wrapped him in a blanket, and gave him back to Caleb. An unanticipated longing washed over him; how he wished his father were here. For weeks he had kept this feeling at bay. Holding his son in his arms, he could no longer.

Tears poured from his eyes.

87

They named the girl Kate; the boy was Peter.

Two months had passed. Quickly the joy of the settlers' arrival had been put aside as everyone turned to the concerns of making the island a home. Hunting parties were organized, food gathered, fishing nets laid, vines harvested and trees felled for the construction of shelters. The island seemed eager to fulfill their needs. Many things were new. Bananas. Coconuts. Huge tusked boars, nasty as hell and not to be messed with but which, when taken, provided bountiful meat. In the jungle, less than a hundred yards from the beach, a mountain stream, descending in a dazzling waterfall, filled a rocky grotto with water so cold and fresh it made their heads pound.

It was Hollis who suggested that the first civic structure should be a school. This seemed sensible; without something to organize their days, the children would run wild as mice. He selected a site, organized a party, and got to work. When Caleb happened to mention that they had very few books, the big man laughed. "Seems to me

we're starting over in more ways than one," he said. "I guess we'll just have to write some."

It did not take long for the memories of their old life to recede. That was, perhaps, the most amazing thing. Everything was new: the food they ate, the air they breathed, the sound of the wind in the palm fronds, the rhythm of days. It was as if a blade had fallen onto their lives, carving it into a time before and a time after. Ghosts were always with them, the people they had lost. Yet everywhere, on the beach and in the jungle, was always the sound of children.

The mantle of leadership had naturally fallen to Lore. At first she'd demurred: *What do I know about running a town?* Yet the precedent had been set; that she'd been captain was hard to put aside in people's minds, and she commanded the respect not only of the crew, who had served under her, but of the people she had brought safely to shore. A vote was held; over her objections, which had come to seem only halfhearted, she was elected by acclaim. Some discussion followed as to what her title should be; she opted for "mayor." She organized a cabinet of sorts: Sara would be in charge of all medical matters; Jenny and Hollis would oversee the school; Rand and Caleb would supervise construction of all the residential structures; Jock, who'd turned out to be a fine shot with a bow, would organize the hunting parties; and so on.

They had yet to investigate much of the island, which was far bigger than it had originally appeared. It was decided that two scouting parties would set out, circling the mountain in opposite directions. Rand led one party, Caleb the other. They returned a week later, reporting that the

island, rather than standing alone, was the south-ernmost of what appeared to be a chain. Two more were visible from the high cliffs of the island's northern side, with a third, perhaps, lurking in the far distance. They had also found no traces of prior inhabitation. That did not mean it wasn't there; perhaps one day they would discover evidence that people had been here before. But for now, the island's unspoiled quality, its wild-ness and beneficence, spoke in tones of solitude.

It was a hopeful time. Not without cares; there was much to do. But they had begun.

For many weeks, Pim had been considering what to do with her book. The work was complete, the words polished. Of course, the story it told went only so far; the end was unknown to her. But she had done all she could.

The decision to bury it, or in some similar man-ner conceal it, had come upon her slowly, and with some surprise. She had long supposed that eventually she would show it to other people. Yet day by day the idea grew that these writings were not, in fact, for anyone still living but served a grander purpose. She attributed this intuition to the same mysterious influence that had led her to write these pages in the first place, and to write them as she had. One early morning, not long after Caleb's return from scouting the island, she awoke to a feeling of great calm. Caleb and the children were still asleep. Pim rose quietly, gathered her journal and shoes, and stepped out-side.

The first rays of dawn were crawling upward from the horizon. Soon the settlement would awaken, but for now, Pim had the beach to herself.

The world had a way of speaking to you if you let it; the trick was learning to hear. She stood for a moment, savoring the quiet, listening for what the world was telling her this morning.

She turned away from the water and headed into the jungle.

She had no destination; she would let her feet carry her where they chose. She found herself walking beneath thick foliage roughly parallel with the beach, perhaps two hundred yards inland. All of this had been explored, of course. Dew was dripping from the leaves; the rising sun saturated the jungle canopy with a warm green light. The ground became uneven, folded into rocky ridges. At times she was forced to crawl on her hands and knees. At the top of a ridge she saw, below her, a gentle depression, guarded on three sides by rock walls roped with vines. Jeweled beads of water trickled down the face of the farthest wall, collecting at the base in a pool. She carefully descended. Something about this place felt new and undiscovered; it possessed a feeling of sanctuary. Crouched by the pool, she filled her cupped hands and drank. The water was clean and tasted like stone.

She rose and surveyed her surroundings. Something was here; she could sense it. Something she was meant to find.

As she scanned the rocky perimeter, her eyes fell upon a zone of shadow within the dense vegetation. She made her way toward it. It was a cave, the opening curtained by vines. She drew them aside. Here was a likely place — indeed, an ideal place — in which to conceal her journal. She reached down into the pocket of her dress; yes, a box of matches, one of the last. She scraped

a match on the striker and extended it into the cave's mouth. The space was not especially large, more like the room of a house. The match burned down to her fingertips. She extinguished it with a flick of her wrist, struck a second, and followed its light inside.

At once Pim became aware that she had entered not merely a natural formation but somebody's home. The space was furnished with a table, a large bed, and two chairs, all fashioned from rough-cut logs roped together with vines. Other objects, similarly primitive in their manufacture, littered the floor: simple stone tools, baskets of dried fronds woven together, plates and cups of unfired clay. She lit another match and approached the bed. Shadows stretched before her, revealing a human form beneath the brittle blanket. She drew it aside. The body, what persisted of it — dried bones the color of wood, a whorl of hair — lay curled on its side, its arms tucked protectively against its chest. Whether male or female, Pim could not discern. Carved into the wall beside the bed were a series of marks, small slashes cut into the stone. Pim counted thirty-two. Did they represent days? Months? Years? The bed was unnecessarily large for one person; there were two chairs, not one. Somewhere, probably not far, would be the grave of the cave's other inhabitant.

Pim stepped outside. That she was meant to conceal her journal in this place was apparent; the cave was a repository of the past. Still, she longed to know more. Who were these people? Where had they come from? How had they died? Standing at the edge of the pool, she could feel the presence of these silenced lives. She made her way around

the walls. Gradually, as if a veil had lifted from her eyes, other artifacts emerged. Shards of pottery. A wooden spoon. A circle of stones where a fire had once been laid. On the far side of the pool, she came to a tangle of bushes with thick, waxy leaves. Something lurked behind it — a curved shape, bulging from the ground.

It was a boat — more precisely, a lifeboat. The fiberglass hull, about twenty feet long, was settled deeply into the soil. Vines entwined it, rendering it nearly invisible; a thick duff of organic matter carpeted the bottom, small plants growing from it. How long had it rested here, slowly sinking into the jungle floor? Years, decades, even more. She circled the hull, hunting for clues. It yielded nothing until she reached the stern. Affixed to the transom, partially obscured by vegetation, was a wooden plaque — faded, brittle, riven with rot. Spectral letters were etched into its surface. She crouched and pulled the vines aside.

For a time she did not move, so profound was her astonishment. How could it be so? But as the minutes passed, a new feeling rose within her. She remembered the storm, the great wind howling down, carrying them to shore when all seemed lost. Destiny was too small a word; there was a force at work that ran far deeper, a thread woven into the fabric of all things. When more time had elapsed she rose and returned to the clearing. She had no intentions; she was acting by instinct. At the edge of the pool she knelt once more. There, in the water's placid surface, she beheld the image of her face: a young face, smooth and unlined, though this, she knew, would change. Time would have its way, as it did for everyone. Her babies would grow; she, and all the people she loved,

would recede, becoming memories, then memories of memories, and finally nothing at all. It was a sad thought, but it also made her happy in a way that felt new. This island of refuge: It was meant to be theirs. It had waited for them all along, so that history could begin again. That's what the words on the plaque had told her.

Perhaps a time would come when it would feel right to share this with the others. On that day, she would lead them to the boat and show them what she had discovered. But not just yet. For now — like her journals and the story they told — it would be her secret, this message from the past, engraved upon the transom of a derelict lifeboat.

BERGENSFJORD
OSLO, NORWAY

88

Carter held his breath as long as he could. Bubbles rose around his face; his lungs were screaming for air. The world above seemed miles away, though in fact it was only a few feet. Finally he could endure it no longer. He pushed off and zoomed to the surface, exploding into the summer sunshine.

"Do it again, Anthony!"

Haley was clinging to his back. She was wearing a pink two-piece suit and cobalt-blue goggles that made her look like an enormous bug.

"All right," he laughed, "just give me a second. Besides, it's Riley's turn."

Haley's sister was sitting on the pool deck, dangling her feet in the water. Her bathing suit

was one piece, green, with a flouncy skirt and a single plastic daisy appliquéd onto one shoulder strap; she was wearing orange water wings. Carter could toss her into the water for hours without her getting bored.

"Again! Again!" demanded Haley.

Rachel walked toward them from the garden. She was dressed in shorts and a white T-shirt streaked with dirt; on her head, a broad straw hat. In one gloved hand she held a pair of shears, in the other a basket of freshly cut flowers of various types and colors.

"Girls, let Anthony catch his breath."

"I don't mind," Carter said. He was clinging to the side. "It's no bother."

"See?" said Haley. "He says he doesn't mind."

"That's because he's being polite." Rachel removed her gloves and dropped them into the basket. Her face shone with sweat and sun. "How about some lunch?"

"What do we have?" Haley asked.

"Let me think." Her mother frowned theatrically. "Hot dogs?"

"Yay! Hot dogs!"

Rachel broke into a smile. "I guess that decides it. Hot dogs it shall be. Do you want one, Anthony?"

He nodded. "I can always take a hot dog."

She returned to the house. Carter climbed from the pool and got towels for himself and the girls.

"Can we swim more?" Haley asked, as he was rubbing her hair. It was blond, with flecks of a copper color. Riley's was a soft, heathery brown, quite long. She liked to wear it in pigtails when she swam.

"Depends on what your mama says. Maybe after lunch."

She made her eyes grow wide. That was the kind of girl she was, always putting on a show to get what she wanted. It was the funniest thing. "If you say yes, she'll have to say it, too."

"Don't work that way, you know that. We'll just have to see."

He squeezed the last of the water from her hair, sent the two of them off to play, and sat at the wrought-iron table to catch his breath and watch. There were toys all over the yard — Barbies, stuffed animals, a brightly colored plastic play set Haley was too big for but still liked to fool with, the two of them pretending it was other things, such as the counter at a store. Haley had gone off in one direction, her sister in another.

"Look!" Riley yelled. "I found a toad!"

She was crouched over the path by the garden gate.

"Is that right?" Carter said. "You go on and bring that over here and let me have a look."

She walked to the patio with cupped palms extended before her, her big sister following.

"Now, that there is one handsome toad," Carter declared. The creature, a mottled tan color, was breathing rapidly, loose skin flapping along its sides.

"I think it's disgusting," Haley said with a sour face.

"Can I keep him?" Riley asked. "I want to name him Pedro."

"Pedro," Carter repeated with a slow nod. "Sounds like a fine name. Now, of course," he went on, "he may already got one. That's something to consider. Something he goes by with the

other toads."

The little girl's face pinched with a frown. "But toads don't have names."

"Now, how you know? Do you speak toad?"

"That's silly," the older girl stated. She was tugging at the bottom of her suit. "Don't listen to him, Riley."

Carter leaned forward in his chair and raised a finger, drawing their attention to his face. "I'm going to tell you something true now, both of you," he said. "And that is this: everything got a name. It's got a way to know itself. That's an important lesson in life."

The smaller girl stared at him. "Trees?"

"Sure," he replied.

"Flowers?"

"Trees, flowers, animals. Everything living."

Haley looked at him askance. "You're making this up."

Carter smiled. "Not in the least. Grown folks know things, you'll see."

"I still want to keep him," Riley insisted.

"Maybe so. And I'm sure Mr. Toad would like that just fine. But a toad belongs in the grass, with the other toads who know him. Plus, your mama would pitch a fit she knew I let you keep him."

"I *told* you," Haley moaned.

Carter sat back. "You two go on now. You can play with him a bit if you like, but leave him be after that."

They scampered away. Carter rose to put on his shirt and sat back down. The sun was mild on his face in the dappled shade of the live oaks; from far away, he heard a quiet wash of traffic. A few minutes passed before Rachel came out the back

door, bearing a tray of the promised hot dogs. Riley's had ketchup and cheese, Haley's mustard; Carter's had all three. For herself, Rachel had made a salad. She returned to the kitchen and came back out with paper plates and a bag of chips, then once more with drinks: milk for the girls, a pitcher of tea for the grown-ups.

"Riley found a toad," Carter remarked. "Wanted to keep it as a pet."

Rachel put the hot dogs onto plates and laid out napkins. "Of course she did. I'm assuming you said no." She looked up and raised her voice. "Girls, come for lunch!"

They ate their hot dogs and chips and drank their tea and milk. Afterward, cherry popsicles for dessert. By the time they finished, the girls were starting to fade. Usually Riley took a nap after lunch; Haley would put up a fuss but wasn't too old for one, especially after the morning they'd had, hours and hours of playing in the pool in the hot sun. With promises of more swimming later, they ushered the girls into the house, Carter carrying Riley, who was already half asleep. In the girls' bedroom, he passed her off to Rachel, who removed Riley's damp suit, replaced it with a T-shirt and underpants, and tucked her into bed. Haley was already under the covers.

"Now, I want you two to sleep," Rachel said from the door. "No fooling around." She closed the door with a quiet click. "Come to think of it," she said, "I could go for a nap myself."

Carter nodded. "I was thinking the same thing. Girls just about wore me out."

In the bedroom, he traded his bathing suit for an old pair of shorts he liked, soft from laundering, and lay down on top of the comforter. Rachel

moved in beside him. He put his arm around her and pulled her close. Her hair had a clean, sweet smell he loved. It was just about the nicest thing there was.

"You know," she said softly, "I was thinking."

"What's that now?"

She shrugged against his chest. "Just how wonderful this morning was. The garden was so beautiful."

Carter pulled her tighter against him to say he thought the same.

"I could do this forever," she said.

Forever was what they had. Soon her breathing steadied, long and low, like waves upon a placid shore. Its rhythm moved into him in a soft current, taking him with her.

What happiness, thought Carter, and closed his eyes. What happiness at last.

■ ■ ■ ■ ■

XIV
THE GARDEN
BY THE SEA

■ ■ ■ ■

343 A.V.

This bud of love, by summer's ripening breath,
May prove a beauteous flower when next we
meet.

— SHAKESPEARE,
Romeo and Juliet

89

She had chosen a spot in sight of the river. The earth was softer here, but that was not the only reason. As dawn broke over the ridgeline, Amy began to dig. The river was low, as it always was in summer; mist floated atop the water like smoke. She dug first to the calls of birds, then, as the heat built, to the stillness spreading over the land.

Stopping now and then to rest, she finished at midday. At the river's edge she splashed her face and cupped her palms to drink. She was sweating profusely in the heat. For a time she sat on a rock to gather herself, her shovel resting above her on the bank. In the shallows she detected the shapes of trout, tucked behind rocks. Protected from the current, they held themselves in place with small flicks of their tails, lying in wait for the insects that washed downstream to their open mouths.

The body was swathed in a sheet. Amy used a wooden bier and ropes, tackled to a sturdy tree limb, to lower it. Her thoughts were ordered and calm; she'd had years to prepare for this moment. But at the first pattering of soil upon the shroud, she experienced a rush of emotion, an upwelling of feeling she had no name for. It seemed like many things at once; it came not from her mind

but from a deeper place, almost physical. Tears mixed with the perspiration streaming down her face. One shovelful at a time, the body disappeared, becoming one with the earth.

She tamped the surface and knelt by the grave. She would erect no marker; the proper memorial would be made in due course. Perhaps an hour passed; she possessed no sense of time, nor had the need to. Her heart felt heavy and full. As the sun touched the line of the hills, she pressed one palm to the freshly turned earth.

"Goodbye, my love," she said.

Peter had died, as he had long believed he would, on a summer afternoon. Four nights ago, he had failed to return to the house. This had happened before, when his wanderings took him too far to make it back before first light. But when he didn't appear the next night, Amy went to look for him. She found him curled beneath an overhang on the east side of the mesa, his body wedged tightly against the rocks. He was only partially conscious. His breathing was quick and thin, his skin pallid, his hands dry and cold. She wrapped him in a blanket and lifted him into her arms; the lightness of his body shocked her. She carried him back to the house and upstairs to the bedroom. She had already closed the shutters. She laid him in the bed and got in next to him, holding him as he slept, and the next morning she sensed something, a presence. Death had entered the house. He seemed to experience no pain, just a kind of fading. He did not regain awareness of his surroundings, or did not seem to. The hours passed. She would not leave him, not for a moment. At midday, his breathing slowed until it was barely

perceptible. Amy waited. A moment came when she realized he had slipped away.

Now, her task complete, she returned to the house and made a simple dinner for herself. She tidied the kitchen and put her dishes away. The quiet of eternity had settled over the rooms. Darkness came on. The stars wheeled above the silent land. She had preparations to make, but these could wait until morning. She did not want to go upstairs — those days were over. She bedded down on the sofa, curled beneath a blanket, and soon was fast asleep.

Dawn's soft glow in the windows awakened her. Standing on the porch, she took measure of the day, then returned to the house to prepare her supplies. She had fashioned a simple pack with a wooden frame she could carry on her back. Into this went the things for her journey: a blanket, some simple tools, extra clothing, food for a couple of days, a plate and cup, a tarp, a coil of rope, a sharp knife, bottles of water. That which she lacked or had failed to anticipate, she could find along the way. Upstairs, she washed and dressed. In the mirror above the stand, she saw her face. She, too, had aged. She might have been a woman of forty, perhaps forty-five. Ribbons of gray, almost white, threaded through her long hair. Crinkles fanned from the corners of her eyes; her lips had thinned and paled, becoming almost colorless. How much time would go by before this face, her face, was observed by another living soul? Would this even happen, or would she pass from the world unseen?

In the living room, Amy sat at the piano. Its existence was nothing she'd ever been able to account for; when she and Peter had arrived at the farm-

stead, all those years ago, the piano was waiting, a gift from beyond. Every night, Amy played it; the music was the force that summoned Peter home. Now, placing her hands above the keys, she waited for something to come to her; with a quiet chord she began, letting her hands tell her where to go. Bright notes filled the house. Within the song's phrases lay all that she felt. It passed through her in waves, rising and falling, circling and returning, a language of pure emotion. *I never grow tired of it,* Peter always told her. He would stand behind her, placing his hands on her shoulders with the gentlest touch to feel the music as she did, as a force that flowed from within. *I could listen to you play forever, Amy.*

Every song is a love song, she thought. Every song is for you.

She came to the end. Her hands stilled above the keys; the last notes hovered, faded, and were gone. So, the moment of parting. A lump had lodged in her throat. She cast her eyes a final time about the room. It was just a room, like any other — simple furnishings, a hearth blackened with long use, candles on the tables, books — but it meant vastly more. It meant everything. Here they had lived.

She rose, put on her pack, and strode out the door, not looking back.

She reached California in the fall. First the deserts, scorched by the sun, then mountains emerged from the haze, their great blue backs surging above the arid valley. Two more days in sight of them and she began to climb. The temperature declined; cool green woodlands waited at the top. Beneath her, the valleys and mountains of

the high Mojave undulated in the haze. The wind was fierce and dry on her face.

At length, the Colony Wall appeared. It was still towering in places, in others crumbled to ruin, barriers of vegetation poking through the rubble. Amy scrambled over the detritus and made her way to the center of town. Great trees stood where none had grown before; most of the buildings were gone, collapsed into their foundations. Yet a handful of the larger ones remained. She came to the structure that had been known as the Sanctuary. The roof had caved in; the building was a shell. She mounted the steps to look through a window that had, miraculously, remained unbroken. It was caked with grime; she used a dampened cloth to make a small porthole and cupped her eyes to the glass. Open to the sky, the interior had become a forest.

It took her some time to get her bearings, but eventually she located the stone. It had settled into the earth somewhat; many of the names inscribed into its face had washed away to mere depressions, scarcely legible. Still, she was able to discern certain surnames. Fisher. Wilson. Donadio. Jaxon.

Evening was approaching. She removed her pack and withdrew her tools: chisels and gouges of various sizes, picks, and two hammers, one large, one small. For a time she sat on the ground, surveying the stone. Her eyes traveled over the stoic surface as she planned her attack. She could have waited until morning, but the moment seemed right. She selected a spot, took up her chisel and hammer, and began.

She finished on the morning of the third day. Her

hands were bloody and raw. The sun was high in the sky as she stood back to examine her handiwork. The quality of the inscription was unpracticed but, on the whole, better than she'd hoped. She slept that day and all the next night and, in the morning, refreshed, packed her camp and descended the mountain. She headed west, first away from the sun and then toward it. The land was empty, without history, devoid of life. The days passed in windswept silence, until, one morning, Amy heard the sea. On the air was the scent of flowers. The sound, a low roaring, expanded; suddenly the Pacific appeared. Its blue expanse seemed infinite; she felt as if she were beholding an entire planet. White-tipped waves crashed upon the shore. She made her way through banks of wild roses and eelgrass down to the wide beach at the water's edge. She felt uneasy but also consumed by a sudden urge. She stripped off her pack and then her clothes and sandals. As the first wave broke across her body, its power nearly knocked her off her feet; a second claimed her, and rather than resist, she dove down into the surging water. She could no longer touch the bottom — it had happened that fast. She experienced no fear, only a wild, startled joy. It was as if she had rediscovered a wholly natural condition in which she was connected to the forces of creation. The water was wonderfully cold and salty. With the barest motions of her arms and legs, she could keep herself afloat. She allowed herself to bob freely in the swells, then dove down again. Beneath the surface she opened her eyes but could see virtually nothing, just vague shapes; she rolled her body to look up. Brilliant sunshine ricocheted off the face of the water, making a kind of halo. Gazing at this

heavenly light, she held her breath as long as she could, hidden in this unseen world beneath the waves.

She decided to remain awhile. Every morning she swam, each time moving farther out. She was not testing her resolve; rather, she was waiting for a new impulse to emerge. Her body felt clean and strong, her mind rinsed of all care. She was entering a new phase of life. She spent her days just sitting and watching the waves or taking long walks up and down the sandy expanse. Her needs were simple and few; she discovered a grove of oranges and, near that, great banks of blackberries, and these were what she ate. She missed Peter, but the feeling was not the same as missing something she had lost. He was gone but would always be a part of her.

Content as she was, she realized over the months that her journey had not ended. The beach was a way station, a place of preparation for the final leg. When spring came, she broke camp and made her way north. She had no destination in mind; she would let the land speak to her. The terrain grew more rugged: rocky promontories, the heart-stopping beauty of the California coast, towering trees blasted by the salted winds into strange, grasping shapes that cantilevered over the sea. She passed her days walking, the sun's hands pressing on her shoulders, the ocean beside her, curling and falling; at night she bedded down beneath the stars or, if it was raining, a tarp suspended on a cord between the limbs of a tree. She saw animals of every type: the small ones, squirrels and rabbits and groundhogs, but also larger, statelier creatures, antelope and bobcats and even bears, great dark shapes shambling

through the brush. She was alone on a continent that man had conquered and then left. Soon no trace of his long habitation would remain; it would all be new again.

Spring became summer, summer fall. The days were crisp and cool, and at night she built a fire for warmth. She was north of San Francisco, she didn't know quite where. One morning she awoke under her tarp and knew at once that something had changed. She emerged into a world of soft white light and silence; snow had fallen in the night. Fat flakes floated soundlessly down from the sky. She tipped her face upward, receiving them. Flakes clung to her lashes and hair; she opened her mouth to taste them on her tongue. A flood of memories engulfed her. It was as if she were a girl again. She lay on her back and extended her legs and arms, moving them back and forth to carve a shape in the snow: a snow angel.

She understood, then, the nature of the force that was drawing her north. She did not arrive until spring and even then was caught by surprise. It was early morning, the forest air thick with mist. The sea, far below, at the base of a tall cliff, was heavy and dark. In the dense shade of trees, she was cresting a rise when all of a sudden a feeling of completeness overwhelmed her, so arresting that it froze her in her tracks. She ascended the rest of the way and emerged into a clearing with a view of the ocean, and there her heart seemed to stop.

The field was carpeted with the most lustrous show of wildflowers she had ever seen — flowers by the hundreds, the thousands, the millions. Purple irises. White lilies. Pink daisies. Yellow buttercups and red columbines and many others she

knew no names for. A breeze had arisen; the sun had broken through the clouds. She shrugged off her pack and walked slowly forward. It was as if she were wading into a sea of pure color. The tips of her fingers brushed the petals of the flowers as she passed. They seemed to bow their heads in salutation, welcoming her into their embrace. In a trance of beauty, Amy moved among them. Corridors of golden sunshine fell over the field; far away, across the sea, a new age had begun.

Here she would make her garden. She would make her garden, and wait.

■ ■ ■ ■

EPILOGUE:
THE MILLENNIALIST

■ ■ ■ ■

INDO-AUSTRALIAN REPUBLIC
POP. 186 MILLION
1003 A.V.

The past is never dead. It's not even past.
— WILLIAM FAULKNER,
Requiem for a Nun

90

Third Global Conference on the North American
   Quarantine Period
Center for the Study of Human Cultures and
   Conflicts
University of New South Wales, Indo-Australian
   Republic
April 16–21, 1003 A.V.
Transcript: Plenary Session 1

Welcoming Address by Dr. Logan Miles
**Professor and Chair of Millennial Studies,
   University of New South Wales, and Direc-
   tor of the Chancellor's Task Force on North
   American Research and Reclamation**

Good morning and welcome, everyone. I'm happy
to see so many esteemed colleagues and valued
friends in the audience today. We have a busy
schedule, and I know everyone is eager to get
started with the presentations, so I will keep these
opening remarks brief.

This gathering, our third, brings together
researchers from every settled territory, in virtually every field of study. Among our numbers, we
count scholars in disciplines as various as human

anthropology, systems theory, biostatistics, environmental engineering, epidemiology, mathematics, economics, folklore, religious studies, philosophy — and on and on. We are a diverse group, with a range of methodologies and interests. But we are united by a common purpose, one that runs far deeper than any specific field of study. It is my hope that this conference will serve not only as a springboard for innovative scholarly collaboration but also as an occasion for reflection — the opportunity for all of us, individually and collectively, to consider the broader, humanistic questions that lie at the heart of the North American Quarantine and its history. This is especially important now, as we pass the millennial mark and the project of North American reclamation, under the authority of the Trans-Pacific Council and the Brisbane Accord, moves into its second phase.

A millennium ago, human history very nearly came to an end. The viral pandemic we know as the Great Catastrophe killed over seven billion people and brought humanity to the edge of extinction. Some among us would assert that this event was an arbitrary occurrence — nature's way of shuffling the deck. Every species, no matter how successful, eventually encounters a force greater than itself, and it was simply our turn. Others have postulated that the wound was self-inflicted, the consequence of mankind's rapacious assault upon the very biological systems that sustained our existence. We made war on the planet, and the planet fought back.

Yet there are many — and I count myself among them — who look at the history of the Great Catastrophe and see not merely a tale of suffering

and loss, arrogance and death, but also one of hope and rebirth. How and where the virus originated is a door that science has yet to unlock. Where did it come from? Why did it vanish from the earth? Is it still out there, waiting? We may never know the answers, and in the last instance, I pray we never do. What *is* known is that our species, against the greatest odds, endured. On an isolated island in the South Pacific, a pocket of humanity survived, eventually to spread the seeds of a reborn civilization across the Southern Hemisphere and establish a second age of humankind. It has been a long struggle, fraught with peril, and we have far to go. History teaches us that there are no guarantees, and we ignore the lessons of the Great Catastrophe at our peril. But the example of our forebears is no less instructive. Our instinct for survival is indomitable; we are a species of unconquerable will and the capacity for hope. And should that day come again when the forces of nature rise up against us, humanity will not go quietly.

Until very recently, very little of substance was known about our ancestors. Scripture tells us that they made their passage to the South Pacific from North America, and that they carried with them a warning. North America, it was said, was a land of monsters; to return was to bring death and ruin down upon the world once more. Until a thousand years had passed, no man or woman should set foot there. This injunction has been a central tenet of our civilization, encoded as law by virtually every civic and religious institution since the foundation of the republic. No scientific evidence has heretofore existed to support this claim or, even, its source. We have, so to speak, taken the

matter on faith. But it lies at the core of who we are.

Much has changed in the last few years. With the discovery of the ancient writings we know as "The Book of Twelves," new light has been shed on the past. Concealed in a cave on the southernmost of the Holy Isles, this text, of unknown authorship, has for the first time lent historical credence to our common lore, even as it has deepened the mysteries of our origins. Dating from the second century A.V., "The Book of Twelves" recounts an epic contest on the North American continent between a small band of survivors and a race of beings called virals. At the center of this struggle is the young girl Amy — the Girl from Nowhere. Possessing unique powers of body and spirit, she leads her fellows — Peter, the Man of Days; Alicia of Blades; Michael the Clever; Sara the Healer; Lucius the Faithful; et al. — in the fight to save humanity. The tale and its cast of characters are familiar to all, of course. No document in our history has been the subject of as much study, speculation, and, in many cases, outright skepticism as this manuscript. Certainly elements of the narrative are far-fetched, more the province of religion than science. Yet from the moment of its discovery, nearly everyone has agreed that it is a document of extraordinary importance. That it should be found in the Holy Isles, the cradle of our civilization, forges the first tangible link between North America and the lore that has shaped and guided us for nearly a millennium.

I am a historian. I deal in facts, in evidence. My professional creed dictates that only through the prisms of doubt and patient scholarship can the

truth of the past be revealed. But one thing my various travels in the past have taught me, ladies and gentlemen, is that behind every legend lies an element of truth.

May I have the first slide please?

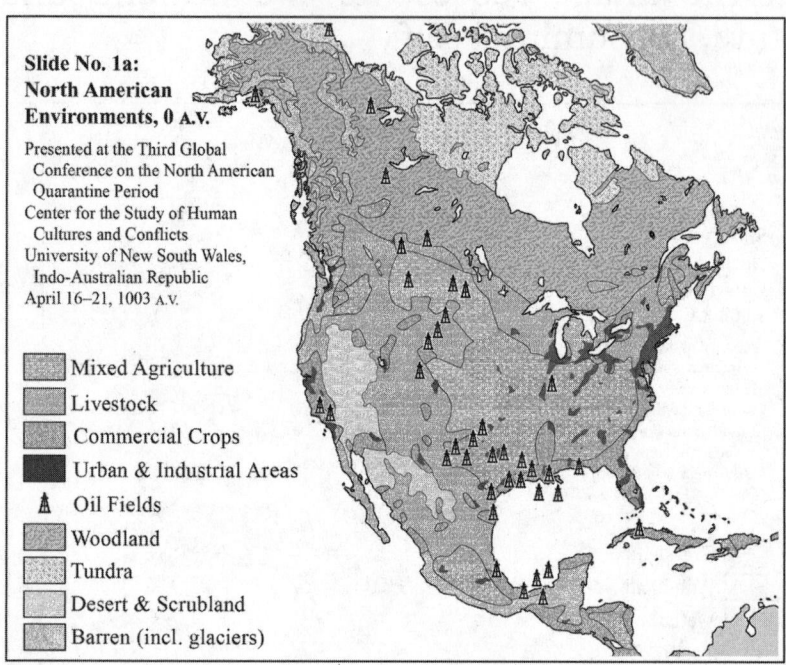

Slide No. 1a:
North American
Environments, 0 A.V.

Presented at the Third Global
 Conference on the North American
 Quarantine Period
Center for the Study of Human
 Cultures and Conflicts
University of New South Wales,
 Indo-Australian Republic
April 16–21, 1003 A.V.

Mixed Agriculture
Livestock
Commercial Crops
Urban & Industrial Areas
Oil Fields
Woodland
Tundra
Desert & Scrubland
Barren (incl. glaciers)

Since our return to North America, thirty-six months ago, a great deal has been learned about the state of the continent both before and during the Quarantine Period. These two images represent two very different North Americas. The contrast could not be more vivid. On the top we see a reconstruction of the continent as it stood in the final years of the American Imperial Period. Cities of millions dominated both coasts. Unsustainable agricultural practices had decimated virtually all of the continent's interior plains. Heavy industry, powered by fossil fuels, had rendered vast swaths of land virtually uninhabit-

able, the soil and water fouled by heavy metals and chemical by-products. Though some wilderness remained, primarily in the alpine regions of the Appalachian uplift, the northern Pacific coast, and the Intermountain West, there is little doubt that the image represents a continent, and a culture, consuming itself.

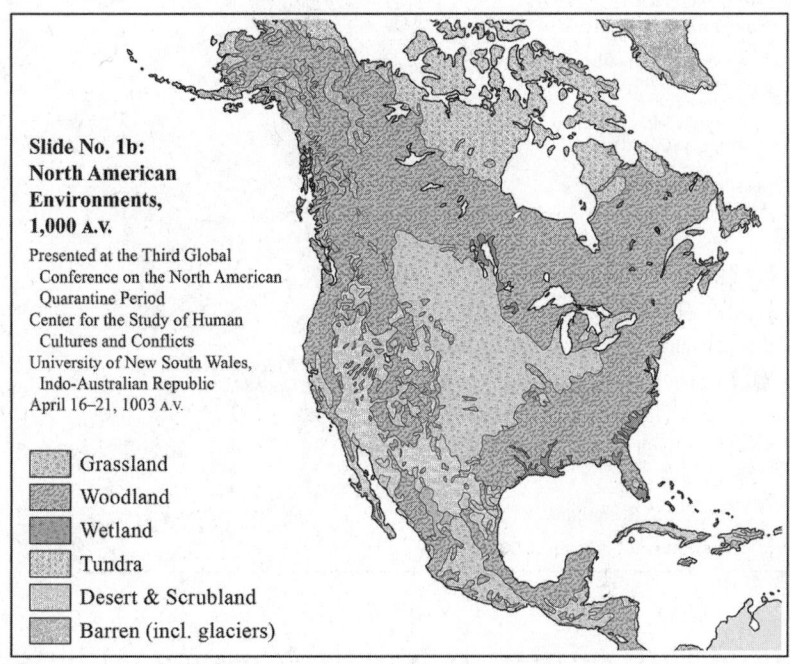

Slide No. 1b:
North American Environments, 1,000 A.V.

Presented at the Third Global
Conference on the North American
Quarantine Period
Center for the Study of Human
Cultures and Conflicts
University of New South Wales,
Indo-Australian Republic
April 16–21, 1003 A.V.

Grassland
Woodland
Wetland
Tundra
Desert & Scrubland
Barren (incl. glaciers)

On the bottom we see North America as it now stands. Airship reconnaissance, conducted from floating platforms situated beyond the two-hundred-mile quarantine line, has revealed a pristine wilderness stunning in its organic diversity. Virgin forests now rise where once stood huge cities and poisonous industrial complexes. Gone are the tamed fields of the continent's interior plains, replaced by grasslands of incomparable biological richness. Most significantly, a majority of the great coastal metropolises, including New

York, Philadelphia, Boston, Baltimore, Washington, D.C., Miami, New Orleans, and Houston, have all but disappeared, subsumed by rising sea levels. Nature, as is its wont, has reclaimed the land, wiping away the leavings of the imperialistic power that once radiated from its shores.

Powerful images, indeed — but hardly unexpected. It is at ground level that our most startling findings have occurred.

Next slide?

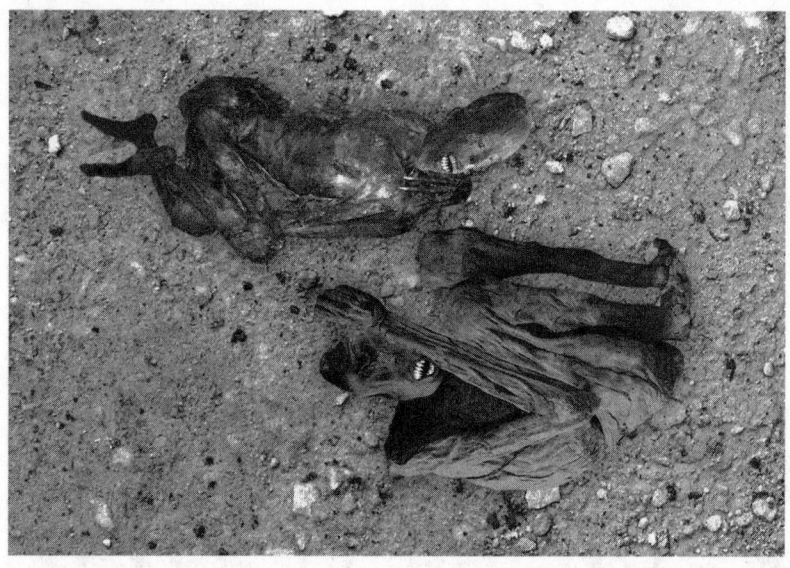

These mummified remains, one male, one female, were recovered twenty-three months ago in an arid basin at the foot of Southern California's San Jacinto Mountains. Their monstrous appearance is inarguable. Note the elongation of the bones, particularly those of the hands and feet, which have taken on a clawlike aspect; the softening of the facial support structure, creating an almost fetal blandness, devoid of personality; the massive jaws and radically altered dentition. Yet,

surprisingly, genetic testing indicates that they are, in fact, human beings — a paramutational counterpart of our species, endowed with the physiological attributes of nature's most fearsome predators. Excavated at a depth of just under two meters, these remains were found in the midst of many others, suggesting a mass die-off of some kind, probably occurring at or near the end of the first century A.V. — the same time frame to which carbon dating has attributed the writing of "The Book of Twelves."

Are these the "virals" that our forebears warned us of? And if they are, how did these dramatic changes come about? To this there appears to be an answer.

Next slide?

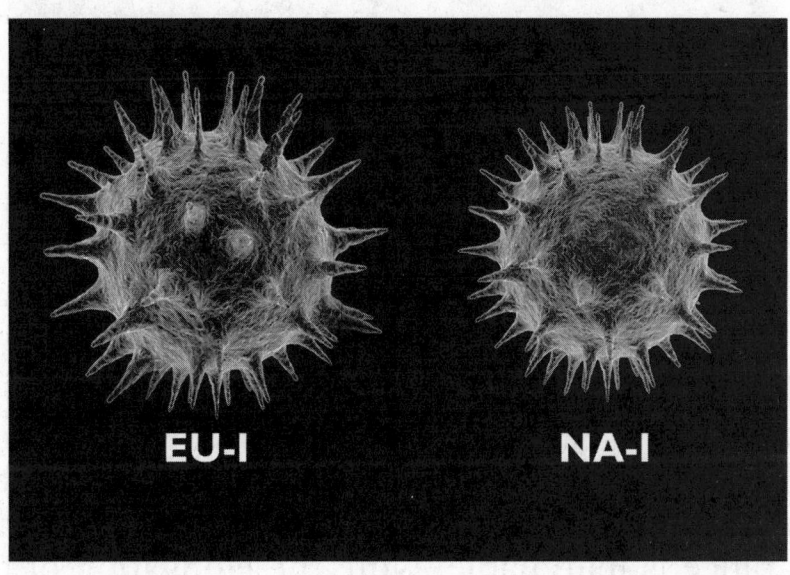

On the left we see the EU-1 strain of the GC virus, taken from the body of the so-called "frozen man," a polar researcher who succumbed to the infection a millennium ago. This virus, we believe,

was the primary biological agent of the Great Catastrophe, a microorganism of such robustness and lethality that it was able to kill its human host within hours and virtually wiped out the world's population in fewer than eighteen months.

I draw your attention now to the virus on the right, which was extracted from thymus tissue of one of the two corpses found in the Los Angeles basin. We now believe this to be a precursor to the EU-1 strain. Whereas the virus on the left contains a considerable quantity of genetic material from an avian source — more specifically, *Corvus corax,* known as the common raven — the one on the right does not. In its stead we find genetic material linking it to an altogether different species. Though our teams have yet to identify this organism's genetic author, it bears some resemblance to *Rhinolophus philippinnensis,* or the large-eared horsehoe bat. We are calling this virus NA-1, or North America–1.

In other words, the Great Catastrophe was caused not by a single virus but by two: one in North America and a second, descendant strain that subsequently appeared elsewhere in the world. From this fact, researchers have built a tentative chronology of the epidemic. The virus first emerged in North America, infiltrating the human population from an unknown vector, though in all likelihood a species of bat; at some later point, the NA-1 virus changed, acquiring avian DNA; this new, second strain, far more aggressive and lethal, subsequently made its way from North America to the rest of the world. Why the EU-1 strain failed to bring about the physical changes caused by NA-1 we can only speculate. Perhaps in some instances it did. But by and large,

the consensus of opinion is that it simply killed its victims too quickly.

What does this mean for us? Put succinctly, the "virals" of "The Book of Twelves" are not fiction. They are not, as some have claimed, a mere literary device, a metaphor for the predatory rapaciousness of North American culture in the B.V. period. They existed. They were real. "The Book of Twelves" describes these beings as a manifestation of an almighty deity's displeasure with mankind. That is a matter for each of us to weigh in the privacy of his or her own conscience. So, too, is the story of the man known as Zero and the twelve criminals who acted as the original vectors of infection. Speaking for myself, the jury is still out. But in the meantime, we know who and what the virals were: ordinary men and women, infected with a disease.

But what of humanity? What of the story of Amy and her followers? I turn now to the matter of survivors.

Next slide?

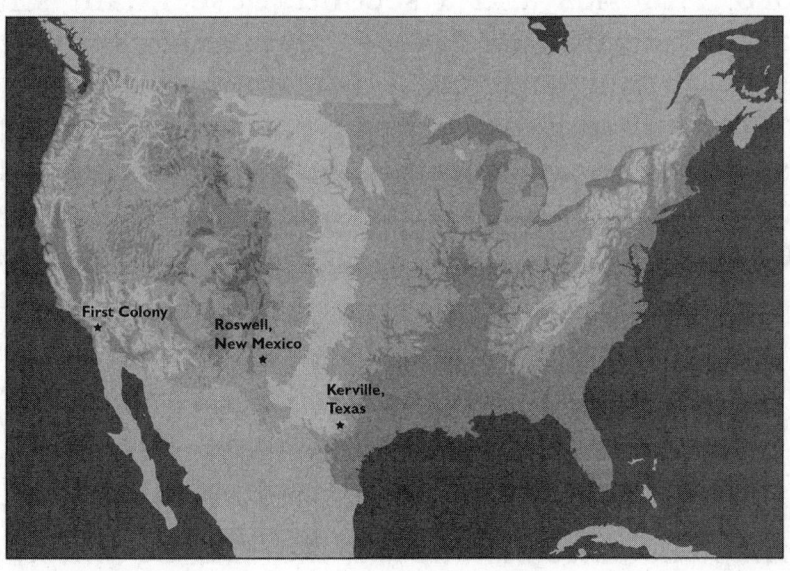

As everyone here certainly knows, it has been an exciting year in the field — very exciting, indeed. Excavations of several newly discovered human settlements in the North American West, dating from the first century of the Quarantine Period, have begun to bear fruit. Much of this work is still in its infancy. Yet I think it's no overstatement to say that what we've uncovered in the last twelve months alone has signaled a truly radical reconceptualizing of the period.

Our understanding of the early Quarantine Period has long presupposed that no human inhabitants remained in North America between the Equatorial Isthmus and the Hudson Frontier Line following the year zero. The disruption to the continent's biological and social infrastructures was believed to have been so complete as to render the continent incapable of supporting human life, let alone any kind of organized culture.

We now know — and once again, the last year has been extraordinary — that this view of the Quarantine Period is incomplete. Indeed, there were survivors. Just how many, we may never know. But based on the findings of the last year, we now think it possible, indeed very likely, that they numbered in the tens of thousands, living in a number of communities throughout the Intermountain West and the Southern Plains.

The size and configuration of these settlements varied considerably, from a mountaintop village housing just a few hundred inhabitants to a city-sized compound in the hills of central Texas. But all give evidence of human habitation well after the continent was thought to have been depopulated. These communities also share a number of distinctive traits, most significantly a culture that

was both classically survivalist and, paradoxically, deeply attentive to the social practice of being *human.* Within these protected enclaves, the men and women who survived the Great Catastrophe, and generations of their descendants, went about their lives, as men and women do. They married and had children. They formed governments and engaged in trade. They built schools and places of worship. They kept records of their experience — I am speaking, of course, about the documents known to everyone in this room, indeed to people throughout the settled territories, as "The Book of Sara" and "The Book of Auntie" — and, perhaps, even sought contact with others like themselves, beyond the walls of these isolated islands of humanity.

Using "The Book of Twelves" as a road map, research teams on the ground have identified three such settlements, all named within those writings. These include Kerrville, Texas; Roswell, New Mexico, the site of what has been called the "Roswell Massacre"; and the community we know as First Colony, in the San Jacinto Mountains of Southern California.

May I have the next image, please?

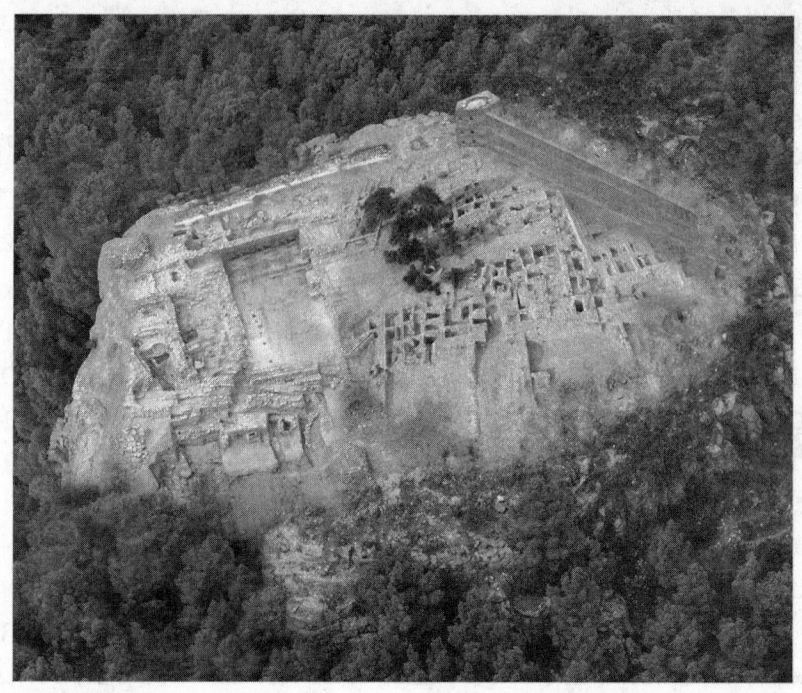

The photograph we see here provides an aerial view of the layout of the First Colony site, which might, for our purposes today, be considered a "typical" human settlement of the Quarantine Period. Situated on an arid plateau two thousand meters above the Los Angeles coastal formation, and guarded to the west by a granite ridge rising an additional fifteen hundred meters, the settlement presents itself very like a walled medieval city — roughly five square kilometers, irregularly shaped, with high ramparts defining the outer perimeter. These steel-and-concrete fortifications, which stood twenty meters high, appear to have been constructed right around the time of the Great Catastrophe. This conforms to "The Book of Twelves," which asserts that First Colony was constructed to house children evacuated from the eastern coastal city of Philadelphia. Beyond these

fortifications, the terrain now presents a mixture of alpine forest and high desert chaparral, but soil samples taken both within and outside the walls indicate that the mountainside was decimated by fire as recently as fifty years ago, and during the first century of the Quarantine Period, the terrain was almost entirely denuded.

The entire settlement seems to have been surrounded by banks of high-pressure sodium vapor lamps. These were powered, we believe, by a stack of proton exchange membrane fuel cells, connected by a buried cable to an array of wind-powered turbines, also dating from the pre-Q period, located forty-two kilometers to the north, in the San Gorgonio Pass. Seismic activity has substantially altered the northern slope of the mountain, and we have yet to locate the power trunk connecting First Colony to its primary energy source. But we hope this will happen in due course.

Inside the walls, we find several discrete zones of human activity, arranged in a ringlike formation and leading to a central core. The outer ring, which has received the most extensive excavation, seems to have served as a staging platform for defense. From these areas we have recovered a range of artifacts, including, at the lowest levels, a variety of conventional firearms of the pre-Q period, yielding at the upper levels to more homemade weaponry, such as knives, longbows, and crossbows. Though more primitive, these armaments were surprisingly sophisticated in their design and manufacture, with arrow points honed to a width of just fifty microns — sufficient, we believe, to pierce the crystalline-silicate breastplate of an infected human.

Moving farther in, we find discrete regions for sanitation, agriculture, livestock, commerce, and housing. Structures in the eastern and northern quadrants of the interior appear also to have served as domiciles, perhaps for married couples or families. The exposed foundation we see near the center seems to have been some kind of school dating from the pre-Q period but converted by the citizens of First Colony to perform a variety of civic functions. We believe that this building, the most substantial structure on the site, could have been employed as a final refuge in the event that the colony's outer defenses were penetrated. But in daily life, it seems to have served as a kind of communal nursery or hospital.

On their own, these findings are remarkable enough. But there is more. "The Book of Twelves" speaks of First Colony as the place from which Amy and her fellows traveled east, eventually coming into contact with other survivors, including an armed force from Texas, known as the Expeditionary. Is there any archaeological record to support these claims?

I draw your attention now to the large, open area at the center, and in particular to the object located on the northwest corner.

May I have the next image?

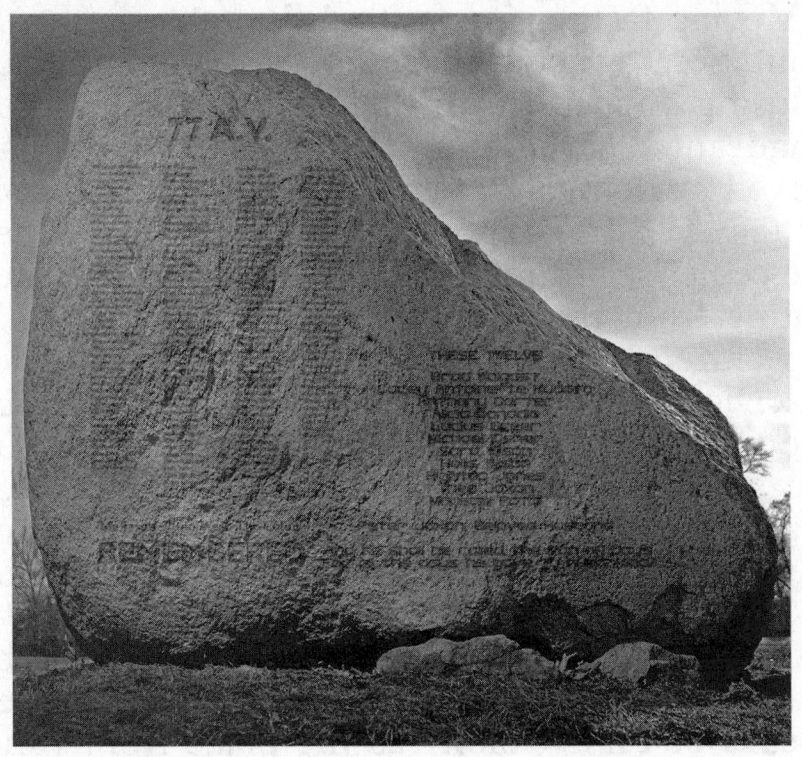

This object, which we are calling the First Colony Stone, sits adjacent to the settlement's central public space. The stone itself is an ordinary granitic boulder of the type found throughout the San Jacinto uplift, standing three meters high, with a basal radius of about four meters. Etched into its surface we find three distinct groups of writings. The first group, by far the most extensive, begins with a date, 77 A.V., followed by a list of what appears to be 206 names in four columns. As we can see, they are presented in family groups and include seventeen different surnames. Though there is some debate on this point, the arrangement suggests that these individuals may have perished in a single event, perhaps one associated with the massive earthquake that struck California at about that time.

Below this we see a second group of three names, also legible: Ida Jaxon, Elton West, and a person named as "The Colonel," evidently a military leader of some stature. Beneath these markings we see the single word "Remembered." Our best guess is that these individuals may have perished in some kind of battle, perhaps one in which the fate of the Colony itself was determined.

It is the third grouping, however, that is the most provocative. As we can see, the etching is much less sophisticated, and exposure to the elements has rendered the names unreadable to the naked eye. Significantly, wear-pattern analysis indicates that these markings date to about 350 A.V., well after the settlement was abandoned. Again, there's some disagreement on this point, but prevailing opinion holds that these markings are, like the others, a memorial of some kind. Digital enhancement reveals names well known to all.

May I have the final slide?

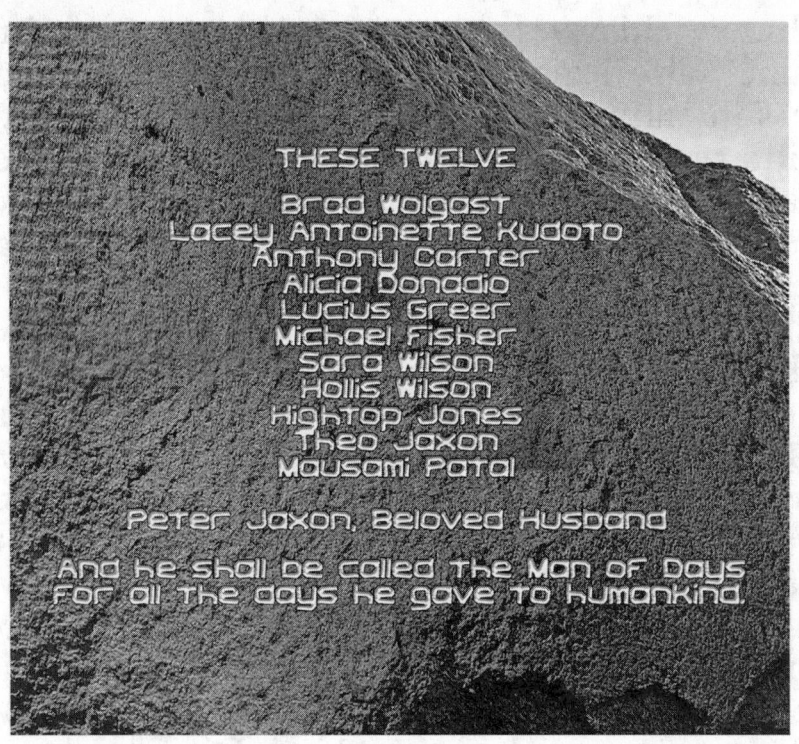

THESE TWELVE

Brad Wolgast
Lacey Antoinette Kudoto
Anthony Carter
Alicia Donadio
Lucius Greer
Michael Fisher
Sara Wilson
Hollis Wilson
Hightop Jones
Theo Jaxon
Mausami Patal

Peter Jaxon, Beloved Husband

And he shall be called The Man of Days
For all the days he gave to humankind.

Of Amy, the Girl from Nowhere, there is no mention. Perhaps we shall never learn who she was, if she existed at all.

There is much we do not understand. We don't know who these people were. We don't know what role they may have played, if any, in the extinction of the paramutational race known as virals. And we don't know what became of them, how they died. This gathering, I hope, will open the door to addressing some of these mysteries. But even more, what I wish is for all of us to come away with a deeper appreciation of the most fundamental questions that define us. History is more than data, more than facts, more than science and scholarship. These things are merely the means to a greater end. History is a *story* — the story of ourselves. Where do we come from? How have we

survived? How can we avoid the mistakes of the past? Do we matter, and if we do, what is our proper place upon the earth?

I shall put the question another way: Who are we?

In a very real and pressing sense, the study of the North American Quarantine Period is far more than an academic investigation of the past. It is — and I think everyone in the room would echo this notion — a crucial step toward safeguarding the long-term health and survival of our species. This is all the more pressing now, as we contemplate humanity's long-awaited return to that feared and vacant continent.

91

For Logan Miles, age fifty-six, professor of millennial studies and director of the Chancellor's Task Force on North American Research and Reclamation, it has been a good morning. A very good morning, indeed.

The conference is off to a roaring start. Hundreds of scholars are in attendance; press interest is intense. Before he reaches the door of the ballroom, a wall of reporters surrounds him. What does it all mean, they want to know, these names on the stone? Were the twelve disciples of Amy real people? What will be the effect on North American reclamation? Are the first settlements going to be delayed?

"Patience, everyone," Logan says. Flashbulbs fire into his face. "You know what I do, neither more nor less."

Free of the crowd, he departs the building via a rear exit off the kitchens. It is a pleasant autumn

morning, dry and blue-skied, with an easterly breeze coming off the harbor; high above, a pair of airships float serenely, accompanied by the vibrato buzzing of their massive propellers. The sight always brings his son to mind; Race, a pilot in the air service, has just been promoted to captain, with a ship of his own — a great achievement, especially for a man so young. Logan pauses to take in the air before making his way around the corner of the building toward the campus's central quadrangle. The usual protestors linger by the steps, forty or fifty of them, holding their signs: "NORTH AMERICA = DEATH," "SCRIPTURE IS LAW," "THE QUARANTINE MUST STAND." Most are older — country people, adherents to the old ways. Among them are perhaps a dozen Ammalite clergy, as well as a scattering of Disciples, women dressed in plain gray robes tied with a simple cord at the waist, their heads shorn in the manner of the Savior. They have been there for months, always showing up at precisely eight A.M., as if clocking in for a job. At the start, Logan found them irritating, even a little disturbing, but as time went by, their presence acquired a quality of doomed listlessness, easily ignored.

The walk to his office takes ten minutes, and he is both pleased and surprised to find the building practically empty. Even the department secretary has flown the coop. He makes his way to his office, on the second floor. In the past three years, he has become an infrequent visitor; most of his work is now in the capitol, and he sometimes doesn't set foot on campus for weeks at a stretch, not counting his visits to North America, which have devoured whole months. With its walls of bookshelves, enormous teakwood desk — a

splurge to mark his promotion to department chair, fifteen years ago — and overall atmosphere of professorial seclusion, the room always reminds him of both how far he's come and the unlikely role that has been thrust upon him. He has reached a kind of pinnacle; yet it is still true that from time to time he misses his old life, its quiet and routine.

He is sorting through a file of papers — a tenure committee report, graduation forms requiring his signature, a caterer's bill — when he hears a knock and looks up to see a woman standing in the doorway: thirty or perhaps thirty-five and quite striking, with auburn hair, an intelligent face, and energetic hazel eyes. She wears a tailored suit of dark navy and high, somewhat tippy heels; a well-used leather satchel hangs from her shoulder. Logan senses that he has seen her before.

"Professor Miles?" She does not wait for permission to enter but insinuates herself into the room.

"I'm sorry, Miss . . ."

"Nessa Tripp, *Territorial News and Record*." As she steps to his desk, she extends her hand. "I was hoping I might have a minute of your time."

A reporter, of course; Logan recalls her from the press conference. Her grip is firm — not masculine but meant to convey a message of professional seriousness. Logan catches the high note of her perfume, subtly floral.

"I'm afraid I'm going to have to disappoint you. This is quite a busy day for me. I've really said all I have to say for one morning. Perhaps you could call my secretary to schedule an appointment."

She ignores the suggestion, knowing full well that it's a dodge; nobody would schedule anything. She offers a smile, rather coquettish, meant to

895

charm. "I promise, it won't take long. I have only a few questions."

Logan doesn't want to. He dislikes dealing with the press, even under the most scripted of circumstances. Many times he has opened the morning paper to find himself misquoted or his words taken entirely out of context. Yet he can tell that this woman can't be brushed off so easily. Better to face the music now, quickly, and move on.

"Well, I suppose . . ."

Her face beams. "Wonderful."

She takes a chair across from him and digs into her bag for a notebook, followed by a small recorder, which she places on the desk. "To start, I was wondering if I could get a little bit of personal information, just for background. There's very little about you that I could find, and the university press office wasn't much help."

"There's a reason. I'm a very private person."

"And I can respect that. But people want to know about the man behind the discovery, wouldn't you agree? The world is watching, Professor."

"I'm really not very interesting, Miss Tripp. I think you'll find me rather boring."

"I hardly believe that. You're just being modest." She flips quickly through her notebook. "Now, from what I can gather, you were born in . . . Headly?"

A softball question, to get things started. "Yes, my parents raised horses."

"And you were an only child."

"That's correct."

"Sounds like you didn't much care for it."

His tone, evidently, has betrayed him. "It was a childhood like any other. There were some good

896

points, some bad."

"Too isolated?"

Logan shrugs. "When you're my age, these sorts of feelings soften a great deal, though at the time I probably saw it that way. In the end, it wasn't the life for me — that's really all there is to say."

"Still, Headly is a very traditional place. Some would even say backward."

"I don't think the people there would see it that way."

A quick smile. "Perhaps I misspoke. What I mean is, it's a long way from a horse farm in Headly to heading the chancellor's task force on resettlement. Would that be fair to say?"

"I suppose. But I never had any doubts that I would go to university. My parents were country people, but they let me chart my own course."

She looks at him warmly. "So, a bookish boy, then."

"If you like."

This is followed, once again, by a brief trip to her notes. "Now," she says, "I have here that you're married."

"I'm afraid your information is a little out of date. I'm divorced."

"Oh? When was that?"

The question makes him uncomfortable. Still, it is a matter of public record; he has no reason not to answer. "Six years ago. All very amicable. We're still good friends."

"And your ex-wife, she's a judge, yes?"

"She was, with the Sixth Family Court. But she's left that now."

"And you have a son, Race. What does he do?"

"He's a pilot in the air service."

Her face brightens. "How marvelous."

Logan nods. Obviously she knows all of this.

"And what does he have to say about your discoveries?"

"We haven't really talked about it, not recently."

"But he must be proud of you," she says. "His own father, in charge of an entire continent."

"I think that's a bit of an overstatement, don't you?"

"I'll rephrase. Going back to North America — you'd have to concede it's pretty controversial."

Ah, thinks Logan. *Here we go.* "Not to most people. Not according to the polls."

"But certainly to some. The church, for instance. What do you make of their opposition, Professor?"

"I don't make anything."

"But surely you've thought about it."

"It's not my place to hold one voice above any other. North America — not just the place but the *idea* of the place — has sat at the center of humankind's sense of itself for a millennium. The story of Amy, whatever the truth is, belongs to everyone, not just the politicians or the clergy. My job is simply to take us there."

"And what do *you* think the truth is?"

"It doesn't matter what I think. People will have to judge the evidence for themselves."

"That sounds very . . . dispassionate. Detached, even."

"I wouldn't say that. I care a great deal, Miss Tripp. But I don't leap to conclusions. Take these names on the stone. Who were they? All I can tell you is that they were people, that they lived and died a very long time ago, and that somebody thought well enough of them to make a memorial. That's what the *evidence* says. Maybe we'll

learn more, maybe we won't. People can fill in the blanks however they like, but that's faith, not science."

For a moment she appears nonplussed; he is not being a cooperative subject. Then, reviewing her notes again: "I'd like to go back to your childhood for a moment. Would you say you come from a religious family, Professor?"

"Not especially."

"But somewhat." Her tone is leading.

"We went to church," Logan concedes, "if that's what you're asking. It's hardly unusual in that part of the world. My mother was Ammalite. My father wasn't really anything."

"So she was a follower of Amy," Nessa says, nodding along. "Your mother."

"It's just the way she was raised. There are beliefs, and there are habits. In her case, I'd say it was mostly a habit."

"What about you? Would you say you're a religious man, Professor?"

So, the heart of the matter. He feels a growing caution. "I'm a historian. It seems like more than enough to occupy myself."

"But history could be said to be a kind of faith. The past isn't something you can actually *know*, after all."

"I wouldn't say that."

"No?"

He settles back to gather his thoughts. Then: "Let me ask you something. What did you have for breakfast, Miss Tripp?"

"I beg your pardon?"

"It's a straightforward question. Eggs? Toast? A yogurt, perhaps?"

She shrugs, playing along. "I had oatmeal."

"And you're quite certain? No doubts in your mind."

"None."

"How about last Tuesday? Was it oatmeal or something else?"

"Why this curiosity about my breakfast?"

"Indulge me. Last Tuesday. It wasn't very long ago, surely you ate something."

"I haven't the foggiest."

"Why not?"

"Because it's not important."

"Not worth remembering, in other words."

She shrugs again. "I suppose not."

"Now, how about that scar on your hand?" He gestures toward the one holding the poised pen. The mark, a series of pale, semicircular depressions, runs from the base of her index finger to the top of her wrist. "How did you get that? It looks to be quite old."

"You're very observant."

"I don't mean to be impertinent. Merely demonstrating a point."

She shifts uncomfortably in her chair. "If you must know, I was bitten by a dog. I was eight years old."

"So you *do* remember that. Not what you ate last week, but something that happened long ago."

"Yes, of course. It scared the hell out of me."

"I'm sure it did. Was it your dog or a neighbor's? A stray, perhaps?"

Her expression grows irritated. Not irritated: exposed. As he watches, she reaches with her other hand to the scar and covers it with her palm. The gesture is involuntary; she isn't aware that she is doing it, or is only partly cognizant.

"Professor, I fail to see the point in all this."

"So it was *your* dog."

She startles.

"Forgive me, Miss Tripp, but if it wasn't, you wouldn't be so defensive. The way you covered your hand just now? It tells me something else."

She moves her hand away deliberately. "And what's that?"

"Two things. One, you believe it was your fault. Perhaps you were playing too roughly. Perhaps you teased him, not meaning to, or maybe a little. Either way, you were part of it. You did something, and the dog responded by biting you."

She shows no reaction. "And what's the other?"

"That you never told anyone the truth."

The look on her face tells Logan that he has hit the mark. There is a third thing, of course, that has gone unstated: the dog was put down, perhaps unjustly. Nevertheless, after a moment passes, she breaks into a grin. *Two can play at this game.*

"That's quite a trick, Professor. I'll bet your students love it."

Now he's the one who smiles. "Touché. But it's not a trick, Miss Tripp, not entirely. The point is a meaningful one. History isn't what you had for breakfast. That's meaningless data, gone with the wind. History is that scar on your hand. It's the stories that leave a mark, the past that refuses to stay past."

She hesitates. "You mean . . . like Amy."

"Exactly. Like Amy."

Their eyes meet. Over the course of the interview, a subtle shift has occured. A barrier has unexpectedly fallen, or so it feels. Logan notes yet again how attractive she is — the word he thinks of, somewhat old-fashioned, is "lovely" — and that she wears no ring. It has been a while for

him. Since his divorce, Logan has dated only occasionally and never for long. He does not still love his ex-wife; that isn't the problem. The marriage, he has come to understand, was really a kind of elaborate friendship. He isn't sure quite what the problem is, though he has begun to suspect that he is simply one of those people who is destined to be alone, a creature of work and duty and not much else. Is his interlocutor's flirtatious manner merely a tactic, or is there more to it? He knows that he is, for his age, passably appealing. He swims fifty laps each morning, is still blessed with a full head of hair, favors pricey, well-tailored suits and somewhat splashy ties. He is aware of women and maintains a certain courtly style — holding doors, offering his umbrella, rising when a female companion excuses herself from the table. But age is age. Nessa calls him "Professor," the appropriate mode of address, yet the word also carries a reminder that he is at least twenty years older than she is: old enough, technically, to be her father.

"Well," he says, rising from his chair. "If you'll excuse me, Miss Tripp, I'm afraid I'll have to stop there. I'm running late for a lunch engagement."

She seems caught off guard by this announcement — jarred from some complex mental state by this ordinary detail of a day. "Yes, of course. I shouldn't have kept you so long."

"May I show you out?"

They make their way through the silent building. "I'd like to talk more," she says, as they are standing on the front steps. "Perhaps once the conference is over?"

She retrieves a card from her bag and hands it to him. Logan glances at it quickly — "Nessa

Tripp, Features, *Territorial News and Record,*" with both home and office numbers — and slips it into the pocket of his suit coat. Another silence; to fill it, he offers his hand. Students flow by, singly and in groups, those on bicycles weaving through the stream like waves around a pier. The air is alive with the buzz of youthful voices. Nessa lets her hand linger an extra second in his, though perhaps it is he who does this.

"Well. Thank you for your time, Professor."

Her watches her walk down the steps. At the bottom, she turns.

"One last thing. Just for the record, the dog wasn't mine."

"No?"

"He was my brother's. His name was Thunder."

"I see." When she says nothing else, he asks, "If you don't mind my asking, what became of him?"

"Oh, you know." Her tone is casual, even a little cruel. She raises her index fingers to make air quotes. "My father took him to 'a farm.' "

"I'm sorry to hear it."

She laughs. "Are you kidding? Couldn't have happened to a nastier son of a bitch. I was lucky he didn't bite my hand off." She hikes her bag higher on her shoulder. "Call me when you're ready, okay?"

She smiles as she says this.

Logan takes a streetcar to the harbor. By the time he arrives at the restaurant, it is nearly one o'clock, and the hostess directs him to the table where his son is waiting. Tall and rangy, with pale blond hair, he takes after his mother. He is wearing his pilot's uniform — black slacks, a starched white shirt with epaulets on the shoulders, and a

dark, narrow tie clipped to the front of his shirt. At his feet rests the fat briefcase he always carries when he flies, emblazoned with the insignia of the air service. When he catches sight of Logan, he puts down his menu and rises, smiling warmly.

"Sorry I'm late," Logan says.

They embrace — a quick, manly hug — and settle in. It is a restaurant they have been coming to for years. The view from their table embraces the busy waterfront. Pleasure boats and larger commercial craft ply the water, which sparkles in the bright autumn sunshine; offshore, wind turbines stand in echelon, propellers spinning in the ocean breeze.

Race orders a chicken sandwich and tea, Logan a salad and sparkling water. He apologizes once again for his lateness and the short time they will have together, their first visit in months. Their talk is light and easy — his son's twin boys, his travels, the travails of the conference and Logan's next trip to North America, scheduled for late winter. It is all familiar and comfortable, and Logan relaxes into it. He has been away too long, depriving himself of the enjoyment of his son's company. He has certain regrets about Race's childhood. Logan was too absent, too distracted by work, and much was left to the boy's mother. This capable, handsome man in uniform: what has Logan done to deserve such a prize?

As the waitress takes their plates, Race clears his throat and says, "There's something I've been meaning to talk to you about."

Logan detects a note of anxiety in his son's voice. His first impulse, born of his own experience, is that there is trouble in the marriage. "Of course. Say what's on your mind."

His son folds his hands on the table. Now Logan is certain: something is wrong. "The thing is, Dad, I've decided to leave the air service."

Logan is stunned beyond words.

"You're surprised," his son tenders.

Logan searches frantically for a response. "But you love it. You've wanted to fly since you were young."

"I still do."

"Then why?"

"Kaye and I have been talking. All this travel is hard on us, hard on the boys. I'm gone all the time. I'm missing too much."

"But you were just promoted. An airship captain. Think what that means."

"I have thought about it. This isn't easy, believe me."

"Is this Kaye's idea?"

Logan is aware that his words sound somewhat accusing. He is fond of his son's wife, an elementary school art teacher, but has always found her a bit too fanciful — the effect, he supposes, of her spending so much time around children.

"It was, at first," Race answers. "But the more we discussed it, the more it made sense. Our life is just too chaotic. We need things to be simpler."

"Things will get easier, son. It's always hard, with young children. You're just tired, that's all."

"My mind's made up, Dad. There really isn't anything you can say to change it."

"But what will you do instead?"

Race hesitates; Logan realizes the core of his announcement is coming. "I was thinking of the ranch. Kaye and I would like to buy it from you."

He is speaking of Logan's parents' horse farm. After his father died, Logan sold off a quarter sec-

tion to pay the estate taxes; for reasons he cannot quite name, he kept the rest, though he hasn't visited it for years. The last time he saw it, the house and outbuildings were a wreck, falling down and full of mice. Weeds were growing in the roof gutters.

"We've saved the money," Race says. "We'll give you a fair price."

"You can have it for a dollar, as far as I'm concerned. That's not the issue." He regards his son for a moment, utterly nonplussed. The request makes no sense to him at all. "Really? This is what the two of you want?"

"It's not just me and Kaye. The boys love the idea."

"Race, they're four years old."

"That's not what I meant. They spend half their time in daycare. I see them two weeks out of four if I'm lucky. Boys like that — they need fresh air, room to roam."

"Trust me, son, country life is much more appealing in the abstract."

"You turned out fine. Take it as a compliment."

He feels a growing frustration. "But what will you do out there? You don't know anything about horses. Even less than I do."

"We've thought about that. We're planning on starting a vineyard."

It is a pie-in-the-sky plan if ever he heard one; it has dreamy Kaye written all over it.

"We had the land checked out," Race continues, "and it's close to ideal — dry summers, damp winters, the right kind of soil. I have some investors, too. It won't happen overnight, but in the meantime, Kaye can teach at the township school. She already has an offer. If we're careful with

906

money, that should tide us over until we're up and running."

Gone unspoken, of course, is the underlying criticism: Race wants to be around for his boys, a deep part of their lives, as Logan failed to do for him.

"You're really *certain* about this?"

"We are, Dad."

A brief silence passes as Logan searches for something to say that might dissuade his only child from this ludicrous plan. But Race is a grown man; the land is just sitting there; he has expressed the desire to sacrifice something important on behalf of his family. What can Logan do but agree?

"I guess I can call the lawyer to get the ball rolling," he concedes.

His son seems surprised; for the first time, it occurs to Logan that Race expected he might say no. "You mean it?"

"You've made your case. It's your life. I can't argue with it."

His son looks at him earnestly. "I meant what I said. I want to pay you what it's worth."

Logan wonders: What is something like that worth? Nothing. Everything.

"Don't worry about the money," he insists. "We'll figure that out when the time comes."

The waitress arrives with the bill, which Race, in jocular spirits, insists on paying. Outside, a car is waiting to take him to the airfield. Race thanks his father again, then says, "So I'll see you Sunday at Mom's?"

Logan is momentarily confused. He has no idea what his son is talking about. Race senses this.

"The party? For the boys?"

Now Logan remembers: a birthday party for the twins, who are turning five. "Of course," he says, embarrassed by the lapse.

Race waves this away with a laugh. "It's fine, Dad. Don't worry about it."

The driver is standing by the door. "Captain Miles, I'm afraid we really have to be going."

Logan and his son shake hands. "Just don't be late, okay?" Race admonishes him. "The boys are excited to see you."

The next morning, back from his morning swim, Logan sees Nessa's article in the paper. Page 1, below the fold; it is neutral, as these things go. The conference and his opening address, mention of the protestors and "the ongoing controversy," snippets of their conversation in his office. Curiously, this disappoints him. His words seem wooden and performed. The article contains a perfunctory stiffness; Nessa has described him as "professorial" and "reserved," both of which are true enough but feel reductive. Is that all he is? Is that what he's become?

For two days the conference occupies him utterly. There are panels and meetings, lunches and, in the evenings, gatherings for drinks and dinner. His moment of triumph, and yet he feels a growing depression. Some of this is Race's announcement; Logan does not like to think of his son abandoning his accomplishments to eke out a living in the middle of nowhere. Headly cannot even be said to be a proper town. There is a mercantile, a post office, a hotel, a farm supply store. The school, which includes all grades, is housed in a single, ugly building made of concrete and possesses neither playing fields nor a library. He

thinks of Race wearing a broad-brimmed hat, a sweat-sodden kerchief encircling his neck and insects buzzing around his face, shoving a spade into the unforgiving earth while his wife and children, bored beyond measure, fidget in the house. Scenes of provincial life: Logan should have sold the place years ago. It is all a terrible mistake he is powerless to correct.

On Thursday night, his conference duties concluded, he returns to the courtyard apartment where he has lived since his divorce. It was, like many things in life, meant to be temporary, but six years later, here he is. It is compact, tidy, without much character; most of the furniture was purchased in haste during the confusing early days of separation. He makes a simple dinner of pasta and greens, sits down to eat in front of the television, and the first thing he sees is his own face. The footage was taken immediately after the conference's closing ceremonies. There he is, microphones hovering around his head, his face washed to corpselike whiteness by the harsh glare of the television crew's lights. "STUNNING REVELATIONS," the banner at the bottom of the screen reads. He turns it off.

He decides to call Olla, his ex-wife. Perhaps she can shed some light on their son's perplexing plans. Olla lives at the edge of the city in a small house, a cottage really, that she shares with her partner, Bettina, a horticulturalist. Olla insisted that the relationship did not overlap with the marriage, that it began later, though Logan suspects otherwise. It makes no difference; in a way, he is glad. That Olla should take up with a woman — he had always known her to be bisexual — has made things easier for him. It would be more dif-

ficult for him if she were married to a man, if a man were in her bed.

Bettina is the one who answers. Their relationship is wary but cordial, and she fetches Olla to the phone. In the background Logan can hear the chirps and squawks of Bettina's collection of caged birds, which is voluminous — finches, parrots, parakeets.

"We just saw you on TV," Olla starts off.

"Really? How did I look?"

"Quite dashing, actually. Confidence-inspiring. A man at the top of his game. Bette, wouldn't you agree? She's nodding."

"I'm glad to hear it."

This light, easy banter. Very little has changed, in a way. They were always friends who could talk.

"How does it feel?" Olla asks.

"How does what feel?"

"Logan, don't be modest. You've made quite a splash. You're *famous.*"

He changes the subject. "By any chance, have you talked to Race lately?"

"Oh, that," Olla sighs. "I wasn't really surprised. He's been hinting at it for a while, actually. I'm surprised you didn't see it coming."

Just one more thing he has missed. "What do you make of it?" he says, then adds, jumping the gun, "I think it's a huge mistake."

"Maybe. But he knows his own mind — Kaye, too. It's what they want. Are you going to sell it to them?"

"I didn't really have a choice."

"There's always a choice, Logan. But if you're asking my opinion, you did the right thing. The place has been sitting there too long. I always wondered why you didn't let it go. Maybe this

910

was the reason."

"So that my son could toss his career away?"

"Now you're being cynical. It's a nice thing, what you're doing. Why not let yourself just look at it that way?"

Her voice is even, careful. Her words, not rehearsed exactly, are nonetheless things that have been imagined in advance. Logan has the unsettling sense, yet again, that he is a step behind everyone, a quantity to be managed by those who know better than he does.

"Your feelings are complicated, I know that," Olla goes on, "but a lot of time has passed. In a way, it's not just a new start for Race. It's a new start for you."

"I wasn't aware I needed one."

A pause at the other end of the line; then Olla says, "I apologize. That didn't come out right. What I mean to say is that I worry about you."

"Why would you worry about *me*?"

"I know you, Logan. You don't let go of things."

"I'm just afraid that our son is about to make the worst error of his life. That this is all some romantic whim."

In the silence that follows, Logan thinks of Olla standing in her kitchen, telephone receiver pressed to her ear. The room is cozy, low-ceilinged; copper pots and dried herbs, tied into bunches with twine, hang from the beams. She will be twirling the phone cord around her index finger, a lifelong habit. Other images, other memories: the way she pushes her eyeglasses up to her forehead to read small print; the reddish spot that flares on her forehead whenever she is angry; her habit of salting her food without tasting it. Divorced, but still the keepers of shared history, the inventory of

911

each other's lives.

"Let me ask you something," Olla says.

"All right."

"You're all over the news. You've been working toward this your whole life. The way I see it, you're getting more than you ever could have asked for. Are you enjoying *any* of this? Because it doesn't sound as if you are."

The question is peculiar. Enjoying it? Is that what one is supposed to do? "I haven't thought about it that way."

"Then maybe it's time you should. Put aside the big questions for a while and just live your life."

"I thought I was."

"Everyone does. I miss you, Logan, and I liked being married to you. I know you don't believe that, but it's true. We had a wonderful family, and I'm very proud of all you've accomplished. But Bettina makes me happy. This *life* makes me happy. In the end, it isn't very complicated. I want you to have that, too."

He has nothing to say; she has him dead to rights. Does he feel hurt? Why should he? It is only the truth. It occurs to him suddenly that this is precisely what Race is asking from him. His son wants to be happy.

"So we'll see you Sunday?" Olla asks, steering the conversation back to firmer ground. "Four o'clock — don't be late."

"Race told me the same thing."

"That's because he knows you the same as I do. Don't be insulted — we're all used to it by now." She pauses. "Come to think of it, why don't you bring someone?"

He's not sure what to make of this curious sug-

912

gestion. "That isn't the province of ex-wives, generally speaking."

"I'm serious, Logan; you have to start somewhere. You're a celebrity. Surely there's someone you can invite."

"There isn't. Not really."

"What about what's-her-name, the biochemist."

"Olla, that was two years ago."

Olla sighs — a wifely sound, a sound of marriage. "I'm only trying to help. I don't like to see you like this. It's your big moment. You shouldn't do it alone. Just think about it, all right?"

The call over, Logan broods. The sun has set, darkening the room. "Like this"? What is he like? And "celebrity": the word is strange. He is not a celebrity. He is a man with a job who lives alone, who comes home to an apartment that looks like a suite at a hotel.

He pours himself a glass of wine and walks to the bedroom. In the closet he finds his suit coat and, in an outer pocket, Nessa's card. She answers on the third ring, slightly breathless.

"Miss Tripp, it's Logan Miles. Am I disturbing you?"

She seems unsurprised by the call. "I just came back from a run. Give me a moment, will you? I need to get a glass of water."

She puts down the phone. Logan listens to her footsteps, then hears a tap running. Is he hearing anything — anyone — else? He doesn't think so. Thirty seconds and she returns.

"I'm glad you called, Professor. Did you see the article? I suppose you must have."

"I thought it was very good."

She laughs lightly. "You're lying, but that's all right. You didn't give me very much to work with.

913

You're a secretive man. I wish we could have spoken longer."

"Yes, well, that's the reason I called, you see. I was wondering, Miss Tripp —"

"Please," she interrupts, "call me Nessa."

He feels suddenly flustered. "Nessa, of course." He swallows and wades in. "I know it's short notice, but I was wondering if, perhaps, you'd like to join me for a party this Sunday at four o'clock."

"Why, Professor." She sounds coyly amused. "Are you asking me on a date?"

Logan knows it at once: he is making a fool of himself. He has no idea if she is even available. The invitation is preposterous.

"I have to warn you," he says, backing away, "it's a birthday party for a couple of five-year-olds. My grandsons, actually." How smooth of you, he thinks, telling her you're a grandfather. With every word, he feels like he is digging his own grave. "Twins," he adds, rather pointlessly.

"Will there be a magician?"

"I'm sorry?"

"Because I'm very fond of magicians."

Is she making fun of him? This was a terrible idea. "Of course, I understand if you're not free. Perhaps another time —"

"I'd love to," she says.

Sunday arrives, sunny and bright. Logan passes the morning buying presents for the boys — a hop-a-long for Noa; for his brother, Cam, the more cerebral of the duo, a construction set — takes a swim to settle his nerves and waits for the hour to come. At three o'clock he retrieves his car from the garage — undriven for many weeks, it is, to his dismay, rather dusty — and drives to the

address Nessa has provided. He finds himself in front of a large, modern apartment complex three blocks from the harbor; Nessa is waiting by the entrance. She is dressed in white slacks, a peach-colored top, and low-heeled, open-toed sandals. Her hair is loose and freshly washed. She is holding a large package wrapped in silver paper. Logan disembarks to open her door.

"That's very thoughtful of you," he says of the parcel, "but you didn't need to bring a present."

"It's a tether ball," she says, pleased. She places the box on the backseat with the others. "You don't think they're too young? My nephews play with theirs for hours."

This is the first mention of her family, which is, Logan learns, quite large. Raised in a northern suburb, where her parents still live — her father is a postmaster — she is the fourth of six children. Three of them, her older sisters and a younger brother, are married with families of their own. So, Logan thinks, she is alone but not unacquainted with the life he has led, that customary life of children and duty and never enough time. Logan has already explained that the party will be held at his ex-wife's house, a fact on which Nessa has made no comment. He wonders if this is a reportorial habit, withholding her thoughts so that others will reveal more of themselves, then chastises himself for being suspicious; maybe it makes no difference to someone of her generation, raised in a more ethically malleable world of constantly changing partners.

The drive to Olla's takes thirty minutes. Their talk comes easily. Little mention is made of the conference. He questions her about her work, if she enjoys it, which she says she does. She likes

915

the travel, meeting new people, learning about the world and trying to shape it into stories. "I was always like that, even as a kid," she explains. "I'd sit in my room and write for hours. Silly stuff mostly, elves and castles and dragons, but as I got older, I got more interested in real things."

"Do you still write fiction?"

"Oh, once in a while, just for fun. Every reporter I know has a half-written novel in their desk somewhere, usually pretty awful. It's like a disease we all have, this wish to get below the surface somehow, to find some kind of larger pattern."

"Do you think that's possible?"

She considers the question, looking out the windshield. "I think there is one. Life *means* something. It's not just going to work and making dinner and taking your car to the repair shop. Wouldn't you agree?"

They are passing through an outer neighborhood: tidy houses set far back from the road, mailboxes standing at attention at the curb, dogs barking from the yards as they drive by.

"I think most people would," Logan says. "At least, we hope so. It can be very hard to see, though."

She seems pleased with his answer. "So you have your way, and I have mine. Some people go to church. I write stories. You study history. They're not really so very different." She glances over at him, then returns her gaze to the passing world. "I have a friend who's a novelist. He's rather famous — maybe you've heard of him. The man's a total mess, drinks a liter a day, barely bothers to change his clothes, the whole cliché of the tortured artist. I asked him once, Why do you do it if it makes you feel so awful? Because seriously, the

man's not going to make it to forty the way he lives. His books are thoroughly depressing, too."

"What did he say?"

" 'Because I can't stand not knowing.' "

They arrive. The door stands open in welcome; the road in front of the house is lined with cars. Parents and children of various ages are making their way up the path, the youngest ones dashing ahead, bearing the presents they cannot wait to see opened, their magical contents revealed. Logan hadn't realized the party would be so large; who are all these people? Companions of the boys from play school, neighbors, colleagues of Race and Kaye and their families, Olla's sisters and their husbands, a few old friends Logan recognizes but in some cases hasn't seen for years.

Olla greets them as they enter. She is wearing a willowy dress, a large, somewhat clumsy necklace, neither shoes nor makeup. Her hair, gray since her early forties, falls unmanaged to her shoulders. Gone forever is the barrister in a polished suit and heels, replaced by a woman of simpler, more relaxed habits and tastes. She kisses Logan on both cheeks and turns to Nessa to shake hands, her eyes bright with barely concealed surprise; never did his ex-wife imagine that her dare would be accepted. Nessa goes to the kitchen to fetch drinks while Logan and Olla carry their presents to the spare room off the hall, where a huge pile of gifts rests on the bed.

"Who is she, Logan?" Olla says enthusiastically. "She's lovely."

"You mean young."

"That's entirely your business. How did you meet her?"

He tells her about the interview. "It was kind of

a shot in the dark," he admits. "I was surprised she said yes, an old codger like me."

Olla smiles. "Well, I'm glad you asked her. And she certainly seems to like you."

In the living room he moves among the adults, greeting those he knows, introducing himself to those he doesn't. Nessa is nowhere to be found. Logan exits through the patio doors onto the ample, sloped lawn, which is flanked by elaborate gardens, Bettina's handiwork. The children are madly dashing around according to some secret code of play. He spies Nessa seated with Kaye at the edge of the patio, the two of them locked in animated talk, but before he can go over, Race grips him by the arm.

"Dad, you should have told me," he says with mischievous delight. "Holy moly."

"Blame your mother. It was her idea, me bringing a date."

"Well, good for her. Good for you. Boys," he calls, "come say hello to your grandfather."

They break away from their game and trot toward him. Logan kneels to gather their small, warm bodies in his arms.

"Did you bring us presents?" Cam asks, beaming.

"Of course I did."

"Come play with us," Noa begs, tugging at his hand.

Race rolls his eyes. "Boys, let your grandfather catch his breath."

Logan glances past his grandsons and sees that Nessa has already joined the children. "What, do I look too old?" He smiles at the boys. He is full of memories of other parties, when Race was small. "What are the rules?"

"You freeze when you get tagged," Noa explains, wide-eyed. It is as if he is announcing a discovery that will change the fate of mankind. "When everybody freezes, you win."

"Show me the way," he says.

The party roars forward, riding the children's energy, which seems inexhaustible, an engine that can't run down. Logan allows himself to be tagged as quickly as possible, though Nessa does not, dodging and weaving until, with a shriek, she succumbs. A pair of ponies arrive by trailer, sway-backed and balding, like moth-eaten clothes. They are so docile they seem drugged; the man in charge looks like he slept under a bridge. Never mind: the children are thrilled. Cam and Noa take the first rides, while the rest form a line to wait their turns.

"Having a good time?" Logan, approaching Nessa from the side, hands her a glass of wine. Her brow is damp with perspiration. Parents are snapping pictures, hoisting their children onto the backs of the mangy ponies.

"Loads," she says with a smile.

"Fun comes so naturally to them. Children, I mean."

Nessa sips the wine. "Your daughter-in-law is adorable. She told me about their plans."

"You approve?"

"Approve? I think it's marvelous. You must be thrilled for them."

Is it simply the mood of the afternoon that he suddenly feels this way? Not thrilled, perhaps, but certainly more comfortable with the notion. Yes, why not, he thinks. A vineyard in the country. Open spaces, cool, moist dawns, a night sky exploding with stars. Who wouldn't want that?

"*And* you can keep the land in the family," Nessa goes on. She lifts her glass in a little toast. "A bit of history, no? Sounds to me like that would be right up your alley."

The great ceremony comes: the presents are unwrapped. The boys barely acknowledge each one before tearing into the next. Hamburgers and hot dogs, chips, strawberries and slices of melon, cake. Among the children, heads begin to droop, minor disagreements flare, eyes grow heavy-lidded. As evening comes on, they make their departures while some of the adults linger, drinking on the patio. Everyone seems to acknowledge Nessa as an important new presence, especially Bettina, who in the gathering dusk gives Nessa a tour of her gardens.

By the time they leave, there are almost no cars out front. Nessa, exhausted and perhaps a little drunk, leans back in her seat as they pull away.

"You have a wonderful family," she says sleepily.

It's true, Logan thinks; he does. Even his ex-wife, who, despite their difficulties, has emerged at this late stage of life as an advocate for his happiness. Under the influence of the day he feels something long-clenched relaxing inside him. Life is not so bad, so purely dutiful, as he has thought. As they drive, his mind travels to the ranch. He has already spoken to his lawyer to set the paperwork in motion. Soon his son and his family will be there, infusing it with fresh life, fresh memories.

"I was thinking," Logan begins, "perhaps I should drive out and have a look at the old place. I haven't been there for years."

Nessa nods dreamily. "I think that's a good idea."

"Would you like to come? It would only be for a couple of days. Next weekend, say."

Nessa's eyes are closed. Another mistake; he has gotten ahead of himself. She is drunk; he is taking advantage of this moment of warm feeling. Perhaps she has fallen asleep.

"It could be useful to you," he offers quickly. "Another article, perhaps."

"An article," Nessa repeats neutrally. Another moment lapses. "So, just to be clear, you're asking me to go away with you for the weekend to help me write an article."

"Yes, I suppose. If that's what you want."

"Pull over."

"Are you feeling ill?" The worst is upon him. The night is ruined.

"Please, just do it."

He draws the car to the side of the road. He expects her to burst from the door, but instead she turns to face him.

"Nessa, are you all right?"

She seems about to laugh. Before he can utter another word, she takes his cheeks in her hands and draws him toward her, crushing his mouth with a kiss.

They have lunch together on Tuesday, see a film the following night, and on Saturday depart in the early morning. The city falls away as they drive deep into the heart of the country. The day is cool, with fat white clouds, though the temperature begins to rise as they make their way west, away from the sea.

It is just noon when they arrive in Headly. The town has improved somewhat. More commercial concerns now line the dusty main street, and the

921

school has expanded. A new municipal hall stands at the top of the square. They check in to the inn — Logan has booked separate rooms, not wanting to assume too much — and, with a picnic lunch, drive on to the ranch.

The sight is dispiriting. The land, untended for years, is weedy and wild; the barn has caved in, as well as many of the outbuildings. The house is only a little better — paint peeling, porch tipping to one side, gutters languishing off the eaves. Logan stands in silence for a moment, taking it in. The house was never large, but like all revisited places it seems a lesser version of the one held in memory. Its degraded condition disturbs him. Yet he also feels the upwelling of an emotion he hasn't experienced in years: a sense of homecoming, of home.

"Logan? All right?"

He turns to Nessa. She is standing slightly apart from him. "Strange to be back," he says and shrugs diffidently, though the word "strange" hardly does the situation justice.

"It's really not so bad, you know. I'm sure they can fix it up."

He does not want to enter the house yet. They put their blanket on the ground and lay out their picnic: bread and cheese, fruit, smoked meat, lemonade. The site they have selected has a view of the parched hills; the sun is hot but clouds scud past, creating brief intervals of shade. As they eat, Logan points out the sites, explaining the history: the barns, the paddocks, the fields where horses once grazed, the thickets where he spent idle hours as a boy, lost in worlds of his own imagining. He begins to relax; the tension between what he remembers and what he now sees softens; the

past flows forth, wanting to be told — though there is, of course, more to the story.

The moment comes when the house can no longer be avoided. Logan takes the key from his pocket — it has lain in his desk drawer, untouched, for years — and lets them in. The door opens directly onto the front parlor. The air is stale. Some of the furnishings remain: a couple of armchairs, shelves, the desk where his father did his accounts. A thick layer of dust coats every surface. They move deeper into the house. All the kitchen cabinets stand open, as if explored by hungry ghosts. Despite the staleness, smells assault him, tinged with the past.

They press on to the back room. Logan is drawn to it as if by a magnetic force. There, covered by a tarp, is the unmistakable shape of the piano. He pulls the cloth aside and raises the fallboard, exposing the keys, which are as yellow as old teeth.

"Do you play?" Nessa asks.

They are the first words either of them has spoken since entering the house. Logan depresses a key, expelling a sour note. "Me? No." The sound hovers in the air, then is gone. "I'm afraid I haven't been completely honest with you," he says, looking up. "You asked me if I came from a religious family. My mother was what used to be known as an 'Amy dreamer.' Are you familiar with the term?"

Nessa frowns. "Isn't that a myth?"

"You mean, hasn't modern science rebranded the phenomenon? In conventional terms, I suppose you could say she was crazy. Schizophrenic with a tendency toward grandiosity. That's more or less what the doctors told us."

"But you don't think so."

Logan shrugs. "It's not really a yes-or-no question. Sometimes I do, sometimes I don't. At least she came by it honestly. Her maiden name was Jaxon."

Nessa is visibly taken aback. "You're First Family?"

Logan nods. "It's not something I like to talk about. People make assumptions."

"I hardly think these days anyone would make much of it."

"Oh, you'd be surprised. Out here, folks put stock in a thing like that."

Nessa pauses, then asks, "What about your father?"

"My father was a simple man. *Straightforward* would be the term. If he had a religion, it was horses. That, and my mother. He loved her a great deal, even when things got bad. When they married, according to him, she was just like anybody else. Perhaps a little more devout than most, but that wasn't so unusual in these parts. It wasn't until later that she started having spells. Visions, episodes, waking dreams, whatever you like to call them."

"Was the piano hers?"

Nessa has correctly intuited this. "My mother was a country girl, but she came from a musical family. From an early age she was quite good. Some people said she was a prodigy, even. She could have gone on to a real career, but then she met my father, and that was that. They were very traditional in that way. She still played sometimes, though I think she had mixed feelings about it."

Logan takes a steadying breath before continuing: "Then one night I woke up and heard her playing. I was very young, six, maybe seven. The

924

music wasn't like anything I'd heard before. Incredibly beautiful, hypnotic almost. I can't even describe it. It swept me up completely. After a while, I went downstairs. My mother was still playing, though she wasn't alone. My father was there, too. He was sitting in a chair with his face in his hands. My mother's eyes were wide open, but she wasn't looking at the keys or anything else. Her face had a kind of erased blankness to it. It was as if some outside force was borrowing her body for its own intentions. It's hard to explain — maybe I'm not telling it right — but I knew instinctively that the person playing the piano wasn't my mother. She'd become someone else. 'Penny, stop,' my father was saying — pleading, really. 'It's not real, it's not real.' "

"It must have been terrifying."

"It was. There he was, this proud man, strong as a bull, completely helpless, shaking with tears. It rocked me to the core. I wanted to get the hell out of there and pretend the whole thing had never happened, but then my mother stopped playing." Logan snaps his fingers for emphasis. "Just like that, right in the middle of a phrase, as if somebody had thrown a switch. She stood up from the piano and marched right past me like I wasn't even there. 'What's happening,' I asked my father, 'what's wrong with her?' But he didn't answer me. We followed her outside. I didn't know what time it was, though it was late, the middle of the night. She stopped at the edge of the porch, looking out over the fields. For a little while nothing happened — she just stood there, the same empty look on her face. Then she began to mutter something. At first I couldn't tell what she was saying. One phrase, over and over. 'Come to me,'

925

she was saying. 'Come to me, come to me, come to me.' I'll never forget it."

Nessa is watching his face intently. "Who do you think she was talking to?"

Logan shrugs. "Who knows? I don't remember what happened after that. I suppose I went to bed. A few days later, the same thing happened. Over time it became a kind of nightly ritual. *Oh, Mom's playing the piano again at four A.M.* During the day she seemed fine, but then that changed, too. She became harried, obsessive, or else wandered around the house in a kind of daze. That's when the painting started."

" 'Painting'?" Nessa repeats. "You mean, pictures?"

"Come on, I'll show you."

He escorts her upstairs. Three tiny bedrooms, tucked under the eaves; in the ceiling of the hallway is a hatch with a cord. Logan pulls it down and unfolds the rickety wooden stairs that lead to the attic.

They ascend into the cramped, low-ceilinged space. Standing a dozen deep, his mother's paintings line nearly a whole wall. Logan kneels and draws the protective cloth aside.

It is like opening a door onto a garden. The paintings, of various sizes, depict a landscape of wildflowers, the colors burning with an almost supernatural brightness. Some show a background of mountains; others, the sea.

"Logan, these are beautiful."

They are. Bound up in pain, they are, nevertheless, creations of stunning beauty. He takes the first one and brings it to Nessa, who holds it in her hands.

"It's . . ." she begins, then stops. "I'm not even

sure how to say it."

"Unearthly?"

"I was going to say haunting." She looks up. "And they're all the same?"

"Different viewpoints, and her style improved over time. But the subjects are identical. The fields, the flowers, the ocean in the background."

"There are hundreds."

"Three hundred and seventy-two."

"What do you think this place is? Was it some-place she'd been?"

"If it is, I never saw it. Neither did my father. No, I think the image came from inside her head someplace. Like the music."

Nessa considers this. "A vision."

"Perhaps that's the word."

She examines the painting again. A long silence follows.

"What became of her, Logan?"

He takes a long breath to steady himself. "It eventually got to be too much. The spells, the craziness. I was sixteen when my father had her committed. He visited every week, sometimes more, but he wouldn't let me see her; I gather her state was rather bad. My junior year in college, she killed herself."

For a moment, Nessa says nothing. And, really, what is there to say? Logan has never known. One minute there, in another one gone. All of it far in the past, nearly forty years ago.

"I'm sorry, Logan. That must have been very hard."

"She left a note," he adds. "It wasn't very long."

"What did it say?"

The rope, the chair, the silent building after everyone had gone to bed: this is where his

imagination ends. He has never permitted it to go further, to envision the mortal moment.

" 'Let her rest.' "

They return to the inn. There, for the first time, in Nessa's room, they make love. The act is unhurried; they conduct it without words. Her body, firm and smooth, is extraordinary to him, as wondrous a present as he has ever received. In the aftermath, they sleep.

Night is falling when Logan awakens to the sound of running water. The shower shuts off with a groan and Nessa emerges from the bathroom in a soft robe, a towel wrapping her hair. She sits on the edge of the bed.

"Hungry?" she asks, smiling.

"There aren't a lot of choices. I thought we'd go to the restaurant downstairs."

She kisses him on the mouth. The kiss is brisk, but she allows her face to linger close to his. "Go dress."

She returns to the bathroom to finish her preparations. How swiftly life can change, Logan thinks. There was no one, now there is someone; he is not alone. Telling the story of his mother was, he realizes, his intention from the start; he has no other way of explaining who he is. That is what two people must give to each other, he thinks: the history of themselves. How else can we hope to be known?

He puts on his trousers and shirt to go next door to change for dinner, but as he enters the hallway he hears his name being called.

"Dr. Miles, Dr. Miles!"

The voice belongs to the hotel proprietor, a small, deeply tanned man with jet black hair and

a nervously formal manner, who bounds up the stairs. "There is a phone call for you," he says with excitement. He pauses to catch his breath, waving air into his face. "Someone has been trying to reach you all day."

"Really? Who?" As far as Logan is aware, nobody knows he's here.

The proprietor glances at the door to Nessa's room, then back again. "Yes, well," he says, and clears his throat self-consciously, "they are on the phone now. They say it is quite urgent. Please, I will show you the way."

Logan follows him downstairs, through the lobby, to a small room behind the check-in desk, where a large black telephone rests on an otherwise empty table.

"I will leave you to it," the proprietor says with a curt bow.

Alone, Logan picks up the receiver. "This is Professor Miles."

A woman's voice, unknown to him, says, "Dr. Miles, please hold while I patch you through to Dr. Wilcox."

Melville Wilcox is the on-site supervisor at First Colony. Such calls happen only rarely, and always with considerable advance planning; only by positioning a chain of airships across the Pacific, a tenuous and expensive arrangement, can a signal be relayed. Whatever Wilcox wants, it's bound to be important. For a full minute, the line crackles with empty static; Logan has begun to think the call's been lost when Wilcox comes on the line.

"Logan, can you hear me all right?"

"Yes, I can hear you fine."

"Good, I've been trying to set this up for days.

Are you sitting down? Because you might want to."

"Mel, what's happening there?"

His voice grows excited. "Six days ago, an unmanned reconnaissance airship surveying the coast of the Pacific Northwest took a photo. A *very* interesting photo. Do you have access to an imager?"

Logan scans the room. To his surprise, there is one.

"Give me the number," Wilcox says. "I'll have Lucinda send it over."

Logan fetches the proprietor, who enthusiastically provides the information and offers to man the machine.

"Okay, they're sending it," Wilcox says.

The imager emits a shriek. "The connection has been made, I believe," the proprietor declares.

"Why don't you just tell me what it is?" Logan asks Wilcox.

"Oh, believe me, it's better if you see this for yourself."

A series of mechanical clunks and the machine draws a piece of paper from the tray. As the print head moves noisily back and forth, Logan becomes aware of a second sound, coming from outside — a kind of rhythmic beating. He has only just realized what he is hearing when Nessa enters the room, dressed for dinner. She looks animated, even a little alarmed.

"Logan, there's a lifter out there. It looks like it's about to land on the front lawn."

"And here we are," the proprietor announces.

With a triumphant smile, he places the transmitted picture onto the desk. It is the image of a house, seen from above. Not a ruin — an actual

house. It is encircled by a fence; within this perimeter are a second, smaller structure, a privy perhaps, and the neatly planted rows of a vegetable garden.

"Well?" Wilcox says. "Did you get it?"

There is more. In the field adjacent to the house, rocks have been arranged on the ground to make letters, large enough to be read from the air.

"What is it, Logan?" Nessa asks.

Logan looks up; Nessa is staring at him. The world, he knows, is about to change. Not just for him. For everyone. Outside the walls of the inn, the racket reaches a crescendo as the lifter touches down.

"It's a message," he says, showing Nessa the paper.

Three words: COME TO ME.

92

Six days have passed. Logan and Nessa, in the observation lounge, sit in silence.

On an airship, time moves differently. The excitement of travel quickly wanes, replaced by a kind of mental and physical hibernation; the days seem shapeless, the ship itself barely to move at all. Logan and Nessa, the only passengers, the objects of obscene fussing by a staff that far outnumbers them, have passed the time sleeping, reading, playing cards. In the evening, after eating by themselves in the too-large dining room, they have their pick of movies from the ship's collection and watch alone or with members of the crew.

But now, with their destination in view, time snaps back into line. The ship is headed north, tracing the northern California coastline at an

altitude of two thousand feet. Towering cliffs wreathed by morning fog, mighty forests of ancient trees, the indomitable greatness of the sea where it collides with the land: Logan's heart stirs, as it always does, at the sight of this wild, untouched place.

"Is it what you thought it would be?" he asks Nessa.

Looking raptly out the window, she has barely spoken a word since breakfast.

"I'm not sure what I thought." She turns her face toward him, lips pressed together and eyes slightly squinted, like someone puzzling out a problem. "It's beautiful, but there's something else to it. A different feeling."

Not much later, the platform appears. Standing a hundred meters above the ocean's surface, it has the appearance of a rigid structure, though it is, in fact, floating at anchor. The airship moves gracefully into place and attaches at the nose to the docking tower; ropes and chains are lowered; the vessel is drawn slowly downward to the deck. As Logan and Nessa disembark, Wilcox strides toward them with a rolling gait: a heavyset man with an untidy beard peppered with gray, his face and arms bronzed by sun and wind.

"Welcome back," Wilcox says as they shake. "And you," he says, turning, "must be Nessa."

Wilcox is aware of Nessa's role, although he is, Logan knows, not entirely comfortable with it, believing it is too soon to involve the press. But that is part of Logan's design. Security is never as tight as it should be; word will get out, and once it does, they will lose control of the narrative. He'd rather get ahead of the situation by giving the story to one person, someone they can trust.

"Do you need to eat, clean up?" Wilcox asks. "The bird's fueled and ready whenever you want."

"How long will it take to get to the site?" Logan asks.

"Ninety minutes, about."

Logan looks at Nessa, who nods. "I see no reason to delay," he says.

The lifter waits on a second, slightly elevated platform, its props pointed upward. As they walk to it, Wilcox brings Logan up to speed. Per Logan's instructions, no one has approached the house, although the building's inhabitant, a woman, has been sighted several times, working in the yard. Wilcox's team has moved equipment to the camp in order to bag the house, if that's what Logan wants to do.

"Does she know she's being watched?" Logan asks.

"She'd have to, with all those lifters going in and out, but she doesn't act like it." They take their seats in the bird. From the portfolio under his arm, Wilcox removes a photo and hands it to Logan. The image, taken from a great distance, is grainy and flattened; it shows a woman with a nimbus of white hair, hunched before a vegetable patch. She is wearing what appears to be a kind of thickly woven sack, almost shapeless; her face, angled downward, is obscured.

"So who is she?" Wilcox says.

Logan just looks at him.

"I know what you're thinking," Wilcox says, holding up a hand in forbearance, "and pardon me, but no fucking way."

"She's the sole human inhabitant of a continent that's been depopulated for nine hundred years. Give me another theory and I'll listen."

"Maybe people came back without our knowing it."

"Possible. But why just her? Why haven't we found anybody else in thirty-six months?"

"Maybe they don't want to be found."

"She has no problem with it. 'Come to me' sounds like an engraved invitation."

The conversation is drowned out by the roar of the lifter's engines; a lurch and they are airborne again, rising vertically. When a sufficient altitude is achieved, the nose tips upward as the rotors move to a horizontal position. The lifter accelerates, coming in low over the water and then the coast. The ocean vanishes. All below them is trees, a carpet of green. The noise is tremendous, each of them encased in a bubble of their own thoughts; there will be no more talking until they land.

Logan is drifting at the edge of sleep when he feels the lifter slowing. He sits up and looks out the window.

Color.

That is the first thing he sees. Reds, blues, oranges, greens, violets: extending from the forested base of the mountains to the sea, flowers paint the earth in an array of hues so richly prismatic it is as if light itself has shattered. The rotors tilt; the aircraft begins to descend. Logan breaks his gaze from the window to find Nessa staring at him. Her eyes are full of a mute wonder that is, he knows, a mirror to his own.

"My God," she mouths.

The camp is situated in a narrow depression separated from the wildflower field by a stand of trees. In the main tent, Wilcox presents his team, about a dozen researchers, some of whom Logan is acquainted with from previous trips. In turn, he

introduces Nessa to the group, explaining only that she has come as "a special adviser." The house's resident, he is told, has been working in the garden since morning.

Logan issues instructions. Everybody is to wait here, he says; under no circumstances should anyone approach the house until he and Nessa report back. In Wilcox's tent, they strip to their underclothes and don their yellow biosuits. The afternoon is bright and hot; the suits will be sweltering. Wilcox tapes the joints of their gloves and checks their air supplies.

"Good luck," he says.

They make their way through the trees, into the field. The house stands about two hundred meters distant.

"Logan . . ." Nessa says.

"I know."

Everything is perfect. Everything is just the same, without the slightest deviation. The flowers. The mountains. The sea. The way the wind moves and the light falls. Logan keeps his eyes forward, lest he be consumed by the powerful emotions roiling inside him. Slowly, in their bulky suits, he and Nessa make their way across the field. The house, one story, is homey and neat: wide-planked siding weathered to gray, a simple porch, a sod roof, from which a haze of green grass grows.

As promised, the woman is working in the dooryard, which is planted in rosebushes of several colors. Logan and Nessa halt just outside the picket fence. Kneeling in the dirt, the woman doesn't notice them, or appears not to. She is profoundly old. With gnarled hands — fingers bent and stiffened, skin puckered in folds, knuckles fat as walnuts — she is plucking weeds and

935

placing them in a bucket.

"Hello," Logan says.

She offers no reply, just continues her work. Her movements are patient and focused. Perhaps she has not heard him. Perhaps she is hard of hearing or deaf.

Logan tries again: "Good afternoon, ma'am."

She stops in the manner of someone alerted by a distant sound; slowly she raises her face. Her eyes are rheumy, damp and faintly yellow. She squints at him for perhaps ten seconds, fighting to focus. Some of her teeth are gone, giving her mouth a pursed appearance.

"So, you've decided to come up, then," she says. Her voice is a coarse rasp. "I was wondering when that would happen."

"My name is Logan Miles. This is my friend Nessa Tripp. I was hoping we could talk with you. Would that be all right?"

The woman has resumed her weeding. She has also begun, faintly, to mutter to herself. Logan glances at Nessa, whose face, behind her plastic mask, drips with sweat, as does his own.

"Would you like some help?" Nessa asks the woman.

The question appears to puzzle her. The woman shifts backward onto her haunches. "Help?"

"Yes. With the weeding."

Her mouth puckers. "Do I know you, young lady?"

"I don't believe so," Nessa replies. "We've only just arrived."

"From where?"

"Far away," says Nessa. "*Very* far away. We've come a great distance to see you." She points toward the field of rocks. "We got your message."

The woman's yellowed eyes follow Nessa's gesture. "Oh, that," she says after a moment. "Set that up a long time ago. Can't really remember the reason for it. You say you want to help with the weeding, though — that's fine. Come on through the gate."

They enter the yard. Nessa, taking the lead, kneels before the rose beds and begins to work, scooping the dirt aside with her thick gloves; Logan does the same. Best, he thinks, to let the woman get used to their presence before pressing her further.

"The roses are lovely," Nessa says. "What kind are they?"

The woman doesn't answer. She is scraping the ground with a metal claw. She appears to take no interest in them whatsoever.

"So, how long have you been here?" Logan asks.

The woman's hands stop, then, after a beat, resume working. "Started work early this morning. Garden doesn't rest."

"No, I meant in this place. How long have you lived here?"

"Oh, a long time." She plucks another weed and, unaccountably, places the green tip between her front teeth and nibbles on it, her jaws working like a rabbit's. With a sound of dissatisfaction, she shakes her head and tosses it in the bucket.

"Those suits you're wearing," she says. "I think I've seen those before."

Logan is perturbed. Has someone else been here? "When was that, do you think?"

"Don't remember." She purses her lips. "I doubt they're very comfortable. You can wear what you like, though. It's not really my business."

More time passes. The pail is nearly full.

"Now, I don't believe we got your name," Logan says to the woman.

"My name?"

"Yes. What are you called?"

It is as if the question makes no sense to her. The woman lifts her head and angles her gaze toward the sea. Her eyes narrow in the bright oceanic light. "No one around here to call me anything."

Logan glances at Nessa, who nods cautiously. "But surely you have a name," he presses.

The woman doesn't answer. The murmuring has returned. Not murmuring, Logan realizes: humming. Mysterious notes, almost tuneless but not quite.

"Did Anthony send you?" she asks.

Once again, Logan looks at Nessa. Her face says that she, too, has made the connection: Anthony Carter, the third name on the stone.

"I don't believe I know Anthony," Logan tenders. "Is he around here?"

The woman frowns at the absurdity of this question, or so it seems. "He went home a long time ago."

"Is he a friend of yours?"

Logan waits for more, but there is none. The woman takes a single rose between her thumb and forefinger. The petals are fading, brittle and brown. From the pocket of her dress she removes a small blade and clips the stem at the first tier of leaves and drops the wilted bloom in the pail.

"Amy," Logan says.

She stops.

"Is that you? Are you . . . Amy?"

With painstaking, almost mechanical slowness, she swivels her face. She regards him for a mo-

ment, expressionless, then frowns as if puzzled. "You're still here."

Where would they have gone? "Yes," says Nessa. "We came to see you."

She shifts her eyes to Nessa, then back to Logan. "Why are you still here?"

Logan senses a deepening presence in her gaze. Her thoughts are taking clearer form.

"Are you . . . real?"

The question stops him. But of course it makes sense that she would ask this. It is the most natural question in the world, when one has been alone so long. *Are you real?*

"As real as you are, Amy."

"Amy," she repeats. It is as if she is tasting the word. "I think my name was Amy."

More time goes by. Logan and Nessa wait.

"Those suits," she says. "They're because of me, aren't they?"

It surprises him, the thing he does next. Yet he experiences not the slightest hesitation; the act feels ordained. He removes his gloves and reaches up to the clasp that holds his helmet in place.

"Logan —" Nessa warns.

He pulls the helmet over his head and places it on the ground. The taste of fresh air swarms his senses. He breathes deeply, enriching his lungs with the scents of flowers and the sea.

"I think this is much better, don't you?" he asks.

Tears have risen at the corners of the woman's eyes. A look of wonder comes. "You're really here."

Logan nods.

"You've come back."

Logan takes her hand. It is nearly weightless, and alarmingly cold. "I'm sorry it took us so long. I'm sorry you have been alone."

A tear spills down her weathered cheek. "After all this time, you've come back."

She is dying. Logan wonders how he knows this, but then the answer comes: his mother's note. "Let her rest." He has always assumed she was speaking of herself. But now he understands that the message was for him, for this day.

"Nessa," he says, not breaking his gaze from Amy, "go back to camp and tell Wilcox to gather his team and call for a second lifter."

"Why?"

He turns his face to look at her. "I need them to leave. All their gear, everything except a radio. Deliver the message and then come back. I would be very grateful if you could do that for me, please."

She pauses, then nods.

"Thank you, Nessa."

Logan watches as she passes through the flowers, into the trees, and out of sight. So much color, he thinks. So much life everywhere. He feels tremendously happy. A weight has lifted from his life.

"My mother dreamed of you, you know."

Amy's head is bowed. Tears fall down her cheeks in glistening rivers. Is she happy? Is she sad? There is a joy so powerful it is like sadness, Logan knows, just as the opposite is also true.

"Many people have. This place, Amy. The flowers, the sea. My mother painted pictures of it, hundreds of them. She was telling me to find you." He pauses, then says, "You were the one who wrote the names on the stone, weren't you?"

She gives the barest nod, grief flowing, rising out of the past.

"Brad. Lacey. Anthony. Alicia. Michael. Sara.

Lucius. All of them, your family, your Twelve."

Her answer comes in a whisper. "Yes."

"And Peter. Peter most of all. 'Peter Jaxon, Beloved Husband.' "

"Yes."

Logan cups her chin and gently raises her face. "It was a world you gave us, Amy. Do you see? We are your children. Your children, come home."

A quiet moment passes — a holy moment, Logan thinks, for within it he experiences an emotion entirely new to him. It is the feeling of a world, a reality, expanding beyond its visible borders, into a vast unknown; and likewise does he believe that he — that everyone, the living and the dead and those yet to come — belong to this greater existence, one that outstrips time. That is why he has come: to be an agent of this knowledge.

"Will you do something for me?" he asks.

She nods. Their time together will be brief; Logan knows this. A day, a night, perhaps no more.

"Tell me the story, Amy."

DRAMATIS PERSONAE

(In chronological order)

B.V., Ohio, Cambridge, and New York

Timothy Fanning, a student
Harold and Lorraine Fanning, his parents
Jonas Lear, a student
Frank Lucessi, a student
Arianna Lucessi, his sister
Elizabeth Macomb, a student
Alcott Spence, a ne'er-do-well
Stephanie Healey, a student
Oscar and Patty Macomb, parents of Elizabeth
  Macomb
Nicole Forood, an editor
Reynaldo and Phelps, police detectives

A.V., Texas Republic

Alicia Donadio, a soldier
Peter Jaxon, a laborer
Amy Bellafonte Harper, the Girl from Nowhere
Lore DeVeer, an oiler
Caleb Jaxon, adopted son of Peter Jaxon
Sara Wilson, a physician
Hollis Wilson, her husband; a librarian
Kate Wilson, their daughter

943

Sister Peg, a nun
Lucius Greer, a mystic
Michael Fisher, an explorer
Jenny Apgar, a nurse
Carlos and Sally Jiménez, expectant parents
Grace Jiménez, their daughter
Anthony Carter, a gardener
Pim, a foundling
Victoria Sanchez, president of the Texas Republic
Gunnar Apgar, general of the Army
Ford Chase, president's chief of staff
The Maestro, an antiquarian
Foto, a laborer
Jock Alvado, a laborer
Theo Jaxon, infant son of Caleb and Pim Jaxon
Bill Speer, a gambler
Elle and Merry ("Bug") Speer, daughters of Kate
  Wilson Speer and Bill Speer
Meredith, partner of Victoria Sanchez
Rand Horgan, a mechanic
Byron "Patch" Szumanski, a mechanic
Weir, a mechanic
Fastau, a mechanic
Dunk Withers, a criminal
Phil and Dorien Tatum, farmers
Brian Elacqua, a physician
George Pettibrew, a shopkeeper
Gordon Eustace, a lawman
Fry Robinson, his deputy
Rudy, an Iowan
The Possum Man's wife, an Iowan
Rachel Wood, a suicide
Haley and Riley Wood, her daughters
Alexander Henneman, an officer
Hannah, a teenage girl, daughter of Jenny Apgar

A.V., INDO-AUSTRALIAN REPUBLIC

Logan Miles, a scholar

Nessa Tripp, a reporter

Race Miles, a pilot, son of Logan and Olla Miles

Kaye Miles, a teacher, wife of Race Miles

Olla Miles, ex-wife of Logan Miles

Bettina, a horticulturalist, partner of Olla Miles

Noa and Cam Miles, twin sons of Race and Kaye Miles

Melville Wilcox, an archaeologist

ACKNOWLEDGMENTS

Thanks and yet more ponies to the usual suspects: Mark Tavani, Libby McGuire, Gina Centrello, Bill Massey, and the spectacular editing, marketing, production, sales, and publicity teams at Ballantine, Orion, and my many publishers around the world. Y'all are going to need a bigger barn.

To Ellen Levine, my agent and friend of twenty years: you are a true treasure in my life.

In the course of writing the Passage trilogy, I've called upon the expertise of many individuals on subjects ranging from epidemiology to military strategy. My gratitude to all. A special shout-out to Dr. Annette O'Connor of La Salle University, who has advised me on scientific questions since the beginning.

Although I generally adhere to a policy of strict realism in matters of geography and landscape, this is not always possible. Respectful apologies to the fine citizens of Kerrville, Texas, for liberties taken with the area's topography. Similar adjustments have been made to the Houston Ship Channel and environs.

To Leslie, I say again: Without you, nothing.

Finally, special thanks to my daughter, Iris, who challenged me ten years ago to write a story about

"a girl who saves the world."
Darlin', here it is.

ABOUT THE AUTHOR

Justin Cronin is the *New York Times* bestselling author of *The Passage, The Twelve, The City of Mirrors, Mary and O'Neil* (which won the PEN/ Hemingway Award and the Stephen Crane Prize), and *The Summer Guest.* Other honors for his writing include a fellowship from the National Endowment for the Arts and a Whiting Writers' Award. A Distinguished Faculty Fellow at Rice University, he divides his time between Houston, Texas, and Cape Cod, Massachusetts.

enterthepassage.com
Facebook.com/justincroninauthor
@jccronin

ПРЕДИСЛОВИЕ

В соответствии с этим авторы словаря поставили себе целью отобрать и включить в словарь наиболее употребительные слова, составляющие основу словарного состава английского языка. Узкоспециальная терминология, малоупотребительные слова и вышедшие из употребления значения слов в словарь не вошли.

При подготовке данного издания словаря его словник был тщательно пересмотрен. В словарь включены слова и словосочетания, связанные с полетами в космос, исследованиями космического пространства и новой техникой. Многие из таких слов, еще не зафиксированных английскими словарями, взяты непосредственно из прессы.

Стремясь наиболее полно показать многозначность слов, которые по своей важности и общенародности должны быть отнесены к числу наиболее употребительных, авторы особенно тщательно разработали значения и фразеологию корневых слов, напр.: man, hand, good, to come, to get, to see и др. Особенное внимание было обращено на разработку предлогов, поскольку они многозначны и, как правило, не совпадают в своих значениях и употреблении с предлогами в русском языке.

В словаре принято следующее расположение значений в словарной статье: значения слов располагаются по степени их употребительности в языке и сочетаемости с другими словами, чтобы читатель, работающий со словарем, мог всегда найти самое употребительное значение неизвестного ему слова в начале словарной статьи. Это, по мнению авторов словаря, должно облегчить читателю нахождение нужного значения слова.

Особое внимание уделяется в словаре фразеологическим единицам, как представляющим наибольшие трудности для глубокого понимания читаемого текста. В связи с этим в расположении названных сочетаний принят такой порядок:

а) устойчивые сочетания нефразеологического типа, напр.: to take seats, to catch fire, тесно связанные с данным значением слова, приводятся непосредственно при значении;

б) пословицы, поговорки и фразеологические единицы, не связанные непосредственно с данными значениями слова, помещаются в конце словарной статьи и отделяются от остальной части статьи знаком ромб (◇);

в) фразеологические единицы, построенные по типу: подлежащее (имя существительное), сказуемое, прямое дополнение (имя существительное) — помещаются в словаре один раз под словом, выполняющим в данном выражении функцию подлежащего, напр.: the early bird catches to worm следует искать под bird;

г) фразеологические единицы, построенные по типу: неопределенная форма глагола или повелительное наклонение, прямое дополнение (имя существительное) — помещаются в словаре один раз под словом, выполняющим функцию прямого дополнения, напр.: to wear one's heart on one's sleeve следует искать под heart;

д) фразеологические единицы, не содержащие сказуемого и начинающиеся с прилагательного, помещаются только под этим прилагательным, напр.: slow but steady следует искать под slow;

е) фразеологические единицы, не содержащие ни имени существительного, ни имени прилагательного, но содержащие сказуемое, выраженное непереходным глаголом, помещаются под словом, обозначающим данное сказуемое, напр.: don't halloo till you are out of the wood следует искать под halloo;

ж) фразеологические единицы, построенные по типу: определение, определяемое (имя существительное), как правило, даются под соответствующим определяемым (существительным), а под определением дается лишь перевод данного значения с указанием в скобках случаев его употребления;

з) фразеологические единицы, состоящие из глагола с последующим предлогом или наречием, помещаются под соответствующим глаголом, напр.: cheer up следует искать под cheer;

и) фразеологические единицы, состоящие из глагола-связки и прилагательного или наречия, помещаются под соответствующим знаменательным словом, напр.: to fly open следует искать под open.

В связи с тем, что существительные в английском языке часто выступают в атрибутивной функции, что создает значительные трудности для понимания текста, в данном словаре при существительных указывается их атрибутивное употребление.

Стремясь к тому, чтобы словарь в возможно большей степени соответствовал научным положениям, принятым при преподавании специальных языковедческих дисциплин на факультетах и отделениях английского языка педагогических институтов, составители словаря подробнее разработали в словаре проблему омонимии, имеющую в английском языке особо важное значение. Так, было признано целесообразным и соответствующим научным положениям современной лексикологии рассматривать слова, образовавшиеся путем корневого (бессуффиксального) словообразования, как отдельные слова, обладающие собственной системой морфологических признаков, выражающих грамматическую категорию данной части речи. Это позволило принять следующий порядок их подачи в словаре:

1. Слова-омонимы, возникшие как вследствие исторического схождения различавшихся в древнем периоде слов, напр.: work — работа (из др.-англ. weorc) и to work — работать (из др.-англ. wyrcan), так и в результате корневого (бессуффиксального) способа словообразования, столь характерного для системы словообразования английского языка нового периода, и относящиеся к различным частям речи (так называемые лексико-грамматические омонимы), напр.: green — зеленый, green — зеленый цвет, молодость, сила и т. д., to green — зеленеть, красить в зеленый цвет и т. д., выделяются в отдельные словарные статьи, обозначенные светлыми римскими цифрами, напр.:

work I [wə:k] *n* 1) работа *и т. д.*
work II *v* 1) работать *и т. д.*

Слова-омонимы располагаются в словаре в порядке частей речи, общепринятом в наших лингвистических трудах — имена существительные, имена прилагательные, имена числительные, местоимения, глаголы, наречия, частицы, предлоги, союзы [1].

От этого принципа, однако, допускаются отступления в том случае, если то или иное слово-омоним оказывается явно более употребительным, чем то слово-омоним или те слова-омонимы, которые должны ему предшествовать согласно приведенному выше порядку расположения частей речи. Так, напр., среди слов-омонимов green порядок следования будет таким:

green I [griːn] *a* 1) зелёный *и т. д.*
green II *n* 1) зелёный цвет *и т. д.*
green III *v* 1) зеленеть *и т. д.*

2. Слова-омонимы, возникшие из этимологически разных источников (так называемые л е к с и- ч е с к и е о м о н и м ы) и относящиеся как к одной и той же части речи, так и к различным частям речи, располагаются в порядке частей речи данного этимологического гнезда и обозначаются надстрочной светлой арабской цифрой, помещенной справа от слова. Напр., слова-омонимы этимологи- ческих гнезд rest (из др.-англ. ræst — отдых) и rest (из фр. rester) располагаются следующим образом:

rest[1] I [rest] *n* 1) отдых, покой *и т. д.*
rest[1] II *v* 1) отдыхать; лежать (спокойно) *и т. д.*
rest[2] I *n* остаток *и т. д.*
rest[2] II *v* оставаться.

3. В словаре выделены о м о г р а ф ы, т. е. слова, имеющие одно и то же написание, но различный звуковой состав. Вследствие этого они рассматриваются как разные слова. Они обозначаются в словаре строчными светлыми буквами, набранными курсивом и помещенными вверху справа от слова. Напр., слова-омографы salve, произносимое [saːv], salve, произносимое [sælv], и salve, произносимое [ˈsælvɪ], даются следующим образом:

salve[a] I [saːv] *n* 1) целебная мазь *и т. д.*
salve[u] II *v* 1) смазывать мазью *и т. д.*
salve[b] [sælv] *v* спасать имущество *(на море, от огня)*.
salve[c] [ˈsælvɪ] *int* здорово! *(приветствие при встрече)*.

В целях удобства пользования приложенными к словарю фонетическими таблицами они помещены перед текстом словаря.

При подготовке восьмого издания были приняты во внимание критические замечания, сделанные в рецензиях, полученных Издательством.

Составители словаря считают своим долгом выразить благодарность рецензентам и всем лицам, которые взяли на себя нелегкий труд внимательно ознакомиться с предыдущими изданиями словаря и сообщить в Издательство свои критические замечания.

Авторы выражают большую признательность доценту Н. К. Матвееву за предоставление в их распоряжение своих лексических разработок по газетно-политическому тексту.

Составители словаря надеются, что лица, пользующиеся данным словарем будут и в дальнейшем сообщать свои замечания об этой книге, что несомненно приведет к улучшению ее качества.

При работе над словарем были использованы следующие лексикографические пособия:
The Concise Oxford Dictionary, 1956.
The Pocket Oxford Dictionary, 1942.
The American College Dictionary, 1947.
H o r n b y A. S., G a t e n b y E. V., W a k e f i e l d H. The Advanced Learner's Dictionary of Current English, London, 1957.
W y l d H. C. The Universal Dictionary of the English Language, London, 1956.
W e b s t e r's New International Dictionary of the English Language, Springfield, Mass., 1957.
W e b s t e r's Third New International Dictionary of the English Language, Springfield, Mass., 1964.
W e b s t e r's New World Dictionary of the American Language, New York, 1962.
B r e w e r's Dictionary of Phrase and Fable, revised ed., Cassel, London, 1965.
D a n i e l J o n e s. An English Pronouncing Dictionary, 11th ed., London, 1957.
The Shorter Oxford English Dictionary, 3d ed., Oxford, 1962.
К у н и н А. В. Англо-русский фразеологический словарь, 3-е изд., М., 1967.
М ю л л е р В. К. Англо-русский словарь, 12-е изд., М., 1965.
С л о в а р ь р у с с к о г о я з ы к а, тт. I—IV, Академия наук СССР — Институт русского языка, Государственное издательство иностранных и национальных словарей, М., 1957—1961.
Отраслевые словари, вышедшие в СССР за последние 10 лет.

Обо всех замеченных в словаре недочетах и желательных изменениях просьба сообщить в издательство «Русский язык», 103012, Москва, Старопанский пер., д. 1/5.

1970 г.

---

[1] Грамматика русского языка, т. I, Фонетика и морфология, с. 21—41, Институт языкознания АН СССР, М., 1953.

О ПОЛЬЗОВАНИИ СЛОВАРЕМ

Заглавные английские слова расположены в алфавитном порядке. Каждое такое слово, а также сложное слово, пишущееся через дефис, образует отдельную словарную статью.

Следует, однако, отметить, что многие сложные слова, напр.: liberty-man, doorbell, chest-of-drawers, lily-of-the-valley, зафиксированные в данном словаре в дефисном или слитном написании, могут встретиться в различных текстах в трех написаниях: дефисном, раздельном или слитном.

Отдельные з н а ч е н и я внутри словарной статьи отмечаются светлой арабской цифрой со скобкой. В данном издании порядок подачи значений несколько видоизменен в соответствии с подачей значений в словаре А. Хорнби (A. S. Hornby).

Л е к с и ч е с к и е о м о н и м ы даются как отдельные заглавные слова и обозначаются светлыми арабскими надстрочными цифрами.

Л е к с и к о - г р а м м а т и ч е с к и е о м о н и м ы даются как отдельные заглавные слова и обозначаются светлыми римскими цифрами.

О м о г р а ф ы даются как отдельные заглавные слова и обозначаются надстрочными светлыми латинскими буквами курсивом.

Если ф р а з е о л о г и ч е с к и е е д и н и ц ы, а также сочетания глагола с послелогом имеют несколько значений, то переводы их отмечаются русскими буквами со скобкой: а), б) и т. д.

Каждое заглавное слово снабжено ф о н е т и ч е с к о й т р а н с к р и п ц и е й, данной в квадратных скобках непосредственно за этим словом.

В омонимах фонетическая транскрипция приводится при первом слове. Сложные слова транскрибируются полностью.

Фонетическая транскрипция проверена по словарю Д. Джоунза (D. Jones), введен нейтральный гласный [ə] перед слоговыми [l], [m] и т. д., набранный курсивом. Он означает, что слово имеет два варианта произношения.

При каждом заглавном слове указывается его г р а м м а т и ч е с к а я к а т е г о р и я (светлым курсивом).

Специальные т е р м и н ы, когда это необходимо, снабжаются условными пометами: *бот., тех.* и т. п.

Разговорные выражения, американизмы и т. п. также отмечаются соответствующими пометами: *разг., амер.* и т. п.

Заглавное слово в примерах и фразеологии заменяется тильдой (~).

Если слово в одном из значений пишется с прописной буквы, то после цифры указывается в скобках начальная прописная буква с точкой, напр.: **eminence** [´eminəns] *n* 1) ...3) (E.) преосвяще́нство.

При ссылке на другое слово в случае тождества дается помета *см.*

Если в словаре приводится с о к р а щ е н н а я (стяженная) ф о р м а, то рядом указывается полная форма, напр.: **can't** *разг.*=cannot; **wasn't** *разг.*=was not; **we're** *разг.*=we are.

Если слово или значение слова употребляется только в известном с о ч е т а н и и, то после указания на часть речи или за цифрой, выделяющей соответствующее значение, ставится двоеточие, а затем приводится данное сочетание.

Атрибутивное употребление имени существительного дается после всех значений за арабской цифрой со скобкой с пометой *attr.*

Множественное число имен существительных, отклоняющееся от обычной формы, приводится в скобках непосредственно за указанием грамматической категории, напр.: **foot** [fut] *n* (*pl* feet) нога́...

Эти же формы приводятся на своем алфавитном месте со ссылкой на форму единственного числа. Если формы единственного и множественного числа совпадают, то слово снабжается указанием (*pl без измен.*).

В данном издании в глагольных статьях более строго проведено разграничение между глаголами с предложным управлением и глаголами с наречиями и предлогами (послелогами).

С о ч е т а н и я г л а г о л а с п о с л е л о г а м и приводятся отдельно после всех значений за знаком прямоугольник (□) в алфавитном порядке послелогов, выделенных жирным шрифтом.

У п р а в л е н и е при глаголе дается после перевода в скобках курсивом. В трудных случаях показывается также и русское управление.

Формы прошедшего времени и причастия прошедшего времени глаголов с чередованием гласного приводятся при неопределенной форме. Кроме того, они даются на своем алфавитном месте как самостоятельные вокабулы со ссылкой на неопределенную форму. Так же подаются и супплетивные глаголы. Напр.:

sing II *v* (*past* sang; *p. p.* sung)...
sang [sæŋ] *past см.* sing II.
sung [sʌŋ] *p. p. см.* sing II.
go [gou] *v* (*past* went; *p. p.* gone)...
went [went] *past см.* go.
gone [gɔn] *p. p. см.* go.

С т е п е н и с р а в н е н и я прилагательных и наречий, отклоняющиеся от обычной формы, указываются при прилагательном и даются на своем месте по алфавиту.

Имена прилагательные, употребляющиеся предикативно, снабжаются пометой *predic.*

После всех значений и относящейся к ним фразеологии за знаком ромб (◇) даются пословицы, поговорки и фразеология, не имеющая прямой связи с приведенными значениями.

Перед текстом словаря помещены «Фонетико-орфографические замечания».

После текста словаря даны географические названия, наиболее употребительные сокращения, принятые в Англии и США, и список имен.

ФОНЕТИКО-ОРФОГРАФИЧЕСКИЕ ЗАМЕЧАНИЯ
NOTES ON PRONUNCIATION AND SPELLING

Ниже даются основные сведения о звуках английского языка и их буквенном изображении. Произношение указано по международной фонетической системе.

I
Гласные
Vowels

i: — долгий **и**
ɪ — краткий, открытый **и**
e — **э** в словах **эти, экий**
æ — более открытый, чем **э**
ɑ: — долгий, глубокий **а**
ɔ — краткий, открытый **о**
ɔ: — долгий **о** со слабым округлением губ
u — краткий **у** со слабым округлением губ
u: — долгий **у** без сильного округления губ
ʌ — краткий гласный, приближающийся к русскому **а** в словах: **варить, бранить.** Английский гласный почти всегда стоит под ударением
ə: — долгий гласный, несколько напоминающий немецкий ö в слове hören, но со слабым округлением губ
ə,ə — безударный гласный, напоминающий русский гласный в словах: **нужен, водяной, молоток, комната**

Двугласные
Dipthongs

eɪ — э́й	ɔɪ — о́ɪ
ou — о́у	ɪə — и́ᵃ
aɪ — а́й	ɛə — э́ᵃ
au — а́у	uə — у́ᵃ

От звука к букве
Sounds represented by more than one letter

Далее рассматриваются случаи, когда один и тот же звук имеет несколько способов буквенного выражения:

[i:]

e	ee	ea	ie	ei
he	green	read	field	receive
she	tree	speak	chief	perceive
we	keep	teach	thief	conceive

[ɑ]

a+r	a+ss	a+st	a+sk	a+sp	a+lf	a+lm	a+nt	ea
car	class	past	ask	grasp	half	calm	plant	heart
farm	pass	cast	bask	clasp	calf	palm	can't	hearth
dark	grass	mast	task					

[ɔ]

o+r	a+ll	au	aw	augh	ough	wa+r
short	all	sauce	draw	taught	thought	war
horse	call	autumn	claw	caught	brought	warm
	fall			daughter	fought	

[uː]		
o	oo	ou
do	spoon	soup
who	too	group
move	fool	rouble

[ɜː]			
i+r	e+r	u+r	ea+r
shirt	berth	fur	learn
dirt	her	turn	earn
birth		burn	year

[ʌ]			
u	o	ou	oo
but	son	young	blood
gun	love	trouble	flood
must	some	country	

[au]	
ou	ow
found	how
round	now
count	down

[ou]			
o	oa	ow	o+ll, ld
phone	boat	know	roll
tone	moan	slow	bold
stone	road	flow	cold

[ɔɪ]	
oi	oy
boil	boy
coin	toy

[aɪ]					
i	y	igh	i+gn	i+ld	i+nd
nice	sky	high	sign	child	mind
write	fly	light		wild	kind
kite	my	right		mild	bind

[eɪ]				
a	ai	ay	ey	eigh
take	rain	day	they	eight
sake	plain	say	grey	freight
lame	pain	may		neighbour

[ɪə]		[ɛə]		[uə]	
e+re	ea+r	a+re	e+re	oo+r	our
here	ear	care	there	poor	tour
mere	hear	dare	where		
	fear	fare			

От буквы к звуку

Letter represented by more than one vowel sound

Ниже рассматриваются случаи, когда данная буква выражает несколько звуков:

Aa

[eɪ]	[æ]	[ɑː]	[ɔː]	[ɔ]	[ə]
make	cat	farm	tall	watch	about
plate	bag	past	salt	wash	around
same	catch	grass	walk	what	
		ask			

[iː]	[e]	[ɪ]	[əː]	[ɪə]	[ɑː]
he	men	begin	her	mere	clerk
meet	pen	behind	berth	here	sergeant
	best		serve		

Ii					Oo				

[aɪ]	[ɪ]	[iː]	[əː]	[a(ɪ)ə]	[ou]	[ɔ]	[uː]	[ʌ]	[ɔː]
fine	is	machine	fir	fire	bone	not	do	son	more
bind	pick	ravine	bird	hire	home	got	who	come	for
sign	ink			wire		long	move	above	floor

Yy			Uu			

[aɪ]	[ɪ]	[j]	[juː]	[ʌ]	[u]	[əː]
sky	shaky	yes	tune	cut	put	lur
my	fully	yacht	fume	fuss	pull	hurt
by	kitty	yawn	mute	plum	full	turn

II

Согласные

Consonants

p — п
b — б
m — м
w — звук, образующийся с положением губ, как при **б**, но с маленьким отверстием между губами, как при свисте
f — ф
v — в
θ — *(без голоса)* ⎫ оба звука образуются при помощи языка, кончик которого помещается между
ð — *(с голосом)* ⎬ передними зубами
s — с
z — з
t — т, произнесенное не у зубов, а у десен
d — д　　　»　　　　　»　　　　　»
n — н　　　»　　　　　»　　　　　»
l — л　　　»　　　　　»　　　　　»
r — звук, несколько похожий на очень твердый русский **ж**; произносится без вибрации кончика языка в отличие от русского **р**
ʃ — мягкий русский **ш**

АНГЛИЙСКИЙ АЛФАВИТ
ENGLISH ALPHABET

Aa	[eɪ]	Jj	[dʒeɪ]	Ss	[es]
Bb	[biː]	Kk	[keɪ]	Tt	[tiː]
Cc	[siː]	Ll	[el]	Uu	[juː]
Dd	[diː]	Mm	[em]	Vv	[viː]
Ee	[iː]	Nn	[en]	Ww	[ˈdʌbljuː]
Ff	[ef]	Oo	[ou]	Xx	[eks]
Gg	[dʒiː]	Pp	[piː]	Yy	[waɪ]
Hh	[eɪtʃ]	Qq	[kjuː]	Zz	[zed]
Ii	[aɪ]	Rr	[ɑː]		

ABBREVIATIONS USED IN THE DICTIONARY

ав.—авиация
австрал.—уротребительно в Австралии
авто—автомобильное дело
амер.—американизм
анат.—анатомия
англ.—английский
археол.—археология
архит.—архитектура
астр.—астрономия
бакт.—бактериология
без измен.—без измения
безл.—безличная форма
библ.—библиское выражение
биол.—биология
бирж.—биржевое выражение
бот.—ботаника
бухг.—бухгалтерия
вет.—ветеринария
вин.—винительный (падеж)
воен.—военное дело
вопр.—вопросительный
вспом.—вспомогательный
г.—город; год
геогр.—география
геол.—геология
гидр.—гидротехника
гл.—глагол
горн.—горное дело
грам.—грамматика; грамматический термин
груб.—грубое выражение
дет.—детское выражение
диал.—диалект
дип.—дипломатия
др.—другой, другие
ед. ч.—единственное число
ж. -д.—железнодорожное дело
жив.—живопись
ж.р.—женский род
зоол.—зоология
изъяв. накл.—изъявительное наклонение
инд.—употребительно в Индии
ирл.—употребительно в Ирландии
ирон.—ироническое выражение
иск.—искусство
ист.—исторический
карт.—карточная игра
кино—кинематография
ком.—коммерческий термин
косв. п.—косвенный падеж
косм.—космонавтика
кто-л.—кто-ливо
кул—кулинария
л.—лицо
ласк.—ласкательная форма
лингв.—лингвистика
лит.—литературоведение, литературный
лог.—логика
.мат.—математика

aeron.—aeronautics
Austral.—Australian
auto—automotive
Amer.—Americanism
anat.—anatomy
Eng.—English
archaeol.—archaeology
archit.—architecture
astron.—astronomy
bacteriol.—bacteriology
—— —does not change[*]
impers.—impersonal form
bibl.—biblical
biol.—biology
St. Ex.—stock exchange
bot.—botany
bkg.—bookkeeping
vet.—veterinary medicine
acc.—accusative (case)
mil.—military
interrog.—interrogative
aux.—auxiliary [verb]
C.—city; *y./yr.*—year
geog.—geography; geographical
geol.—geology; geologic
hydral. engin.—hydraulic engineering
vb.—verb
min.—mining
gram.—grammar; grammatical term
vulg.—vulgar(ism)
juv.—juvenile
dial.—dialect(al)
dipl.—diplomacy
—— —other, others[*]
sing.—singular
rail.—railroad; railway
paint.—painting
fem.—feminine
zool.—zoology
indic.—indicative mood
Ind.—Indian
Ir.—Irish
iron.—ironic(al)
—— —art[*]
hist.—historical
—— —card game[*]
cine.—cinema(tography)
comm.—commerce; commercial
obl. csc.—oblique case
cosmonaut.—cosmonautics
s.o.—someone
cul.—culinary
pers.—person
affec. fm.—affectionate form
ling.—linguistics
liter.—literary
log.—logic
math.—mathematics

*The notation "——" indicates no conventional equivalent English abbreviation.

мед.—медицина	*med.*—medical; medicine
мест.—местонмение	*pron.*—pronoun
метео.—метеорология	*meteor.*—meteorology
мин.—минералогия	*mineral*—mineralogy
миф.—мифология	*myth.*—mythology
мн. ч.—множественное чиесло	*pl.*—plural
мор.—морское дело	*naut.*—nautical
муз.—музыка, музыкальный	*mus.*—music(al)
напр.—например	*e.g.*—for example
наст. вр.—настоящее время	*pres.*—present tense
обыкн.—обыкновенно	*usu.*—usually
о-в(а)—остров(а)	*Is.*—island(s)
особ.—особенно	*esp.*—especially
отрщ.—отрицательный	*neg.*—negative
охот.—охота	—— —hunting*
парл.—парламентское выражение	*parl.*—parliamentary
перен.—переносное значение	*fig.*—figurative
повел. накл.—повелительное наклонение	*imper.*—imperative mood
погов.—поговорка	—— —saying, adage*
полигр.—полиграфия	*prntg.*—printing
полит.—политика	*pol.*—political
полит. эк.—политическая экономия	*pol. econ.*—political economics
посл.—пословица	*prov.*—proverb
поэт.—поэтическое выражение	*poet.*—poetic(al)
превосх. ст.—превосходная степень	*superl.*—superlative degree
презр.—презрительно	—— —contemptuous*
преим.—преимущественно	—— —largely*
пренебр.—пренебрежительно	—— —disdainful*
прил.—прилагательное	*adj.*—adjective
прич.—причастие	*part.*—participle
прош. вр.—прошедшее время	*past*—past tense
р.—река	*r.*—river
радио.—радиотехника	*rad.*—radio
разг.—разговорное слово, выражение	*coll.*—colloquial
рел.—религия	*relig.*—religion
ритор.—риторическое выражение	*rhet.*—rhetorical
род.—родительный (падеж)	*gen.*—genitive (case)
с.м.—смотри	*see*—see
собир.—собирательно	*collect.*—collective(ly)
сокр.—сокращение, сокращенно	*abbr.*—abbreviation; abbreviated
спорт.—физкультура и спорт	—— —sport(s)*
ср.—сравни	*cf.*—compare
сравн. ст.—сравнительная степень	*comp.*—comparative degree
стил.—стилистика; стилистический термин	*styl.*—stylistics
стр.—строительное дело	*constr.*—construction
сущ.—существительное	*n.*—noun
с. -х.—сельское хозяйство	*agric.*—agriculture
тв.—творительный (падеж)	*instr.*—instrumental (case)
театр.—театральное выражение	*theatr.*—theatrical
текст.—текстильное дело	*text.*—textiles
тех.—техника	*tech.*—technical
тж.—также	—— —also*
тлв.—телевидение	*tele. (TV)*—television
унив.—университетский	*univ.*—university
употр.—употребляется	—— —in use*
уст.—устаревшее слово или выражение	*obs.*—obsolete
фарм.—фармакология	*pharm.*—pharmaceutical
физ.—физика	*phys.*—physics
физиол.—физиология	*physiol.*—physiology
филос.—филослфия	*philos.*—philosophy
фин.—финансы	*fin.*—finance
фольк.—фольклор	*folkl.*—folklore
фон.—фонетика	*phon.*—phonetics
хим.—хнмия	*chem.*—chemistry
церк.—церковное выражение	*eccl.*—ecclesiastical
ч.—число	*num.*—number
что-л.—что-либо	*sth.*—something
шахм.—шахматы	—— —chess*
шк.—школьное выражение	*sch. sl.*—school slang
шотл.—употребительно в Шотландии	*Scot.*—Scottish
шутл.—шутливо	*joc.*—jocular
эвф.—эвфемизм	*euph.*—euphemism
эк.—экономика	*econ.*—economics
эл.—элекротехника	*E.E.*—electrical engineering
юр.—юридический термин	*leg.*—legal (term)

A

A, a[1] [eɪ, ə] *n* 1-я *буква англ. алфавита*; ◇ from A to Z от нача́ла до конца́; по́лностью; A 1 *разг.* первокла́ссный, превосхо́дный.

a[2] [eɪ (*сильная форма*), ə (*слабая форма*)] 1) *грам. неопределённый член, артикль — служебное слово, с помощью которого говорящий выделяет в своей речи возникшее в его созна́нии общее понятие, отграничивая его от других общих понятий*: a book кни́га (*а не тетра́дь*); a town го́род (*а не дере́вня*); 2) оди́н; it costs a rouble сто́ит (оди́н) рубль; 3): a few не́сколько; a great (*или* a good) many о́чень мно́го.

aback [ə'bæk] *adv* наза́д, сза́ди; ◇ taken ~ смущённый, засти́гнутый враспло́х; поражённый.

abaft [ə'bɑːft] *adv мор.* 1) на корме́, в сто́рону кормы́; 2) сза́ди, позади́.

abandon I [ə'bændən] *v* 1) оставля́ть, покида́ть; 2) отка́зываться от; броса́ть (*привы́чку*); 3) : to ~ oneself to предава́ться чему́-л.; to ~ oneself to the idea склоня́ться к мы́сли.

abandon II *n* непринуждённость.

abandoned [ə'bændənd] *a* 1) забро́шенный, поки́нутый; 2) распу́щенный, распу́тный.

abandonment [ə'bændənmənt] *n* 1) оставле́ние; 2) отка́з от; 3) забро́шенность; 4) непринуждённость.

abase [ə'beɪs] *v* 1) снижа́ть; понижа́ть (*в чи́не и т. п.*); 2) унижа́ть.

abasement [ə'beɪsmənt] *n* 1) сниже́ние; пониже́ние (*в чи́не и т. п.*); 2) униже́ние.

abash [ə'bæʃ] *v* смуща́ть; приводи́ть в замеша́тельство.

abashment [ə'bæʃmənt] *n* смуще́ние; замеша́тельство.

abate [ə'beɪt] *v* 1) уменьша́ть, ослабля́ть; смягча́ть; 2) снижа́ть (*це́ну и т. п.*); 3) уменьша́ться; ослабева́ть; затиха́ть (*о буре, эпидемии и т. д.*); 4) устраня́ть, прекраща́ть; 5) притупля́ть (*остриё*); 6) аннули́ровать, отменя́ть.

abatement [ə'beɪtmənt] *n* 1) уменьше́ние, смягче́ние; 2) сниже́ние (*цен и т. п.*); 3) аннули́рование, отме́на.

abbacy ['æbəsɪ] *n* до́лжность *или* зва́ние абба́та.

abbess ['æbɪs] *n* настоя́тельница монастыря́, аббати́са.

abbey ['æbɪ] *n* абба́тство; монасты́рь.

abbot ['æbət] *n* абба́т.

abbreviate [ə'briːvɪeɪt] *v* сокраща́ть.

abbreviation [ə,briːvɪ'eɪʃən] *n* 1) сокраще́ние; 2) аббревиату́ра.

ABC ['eɪ'biː'siː] *n* 1) алфави́т, а́збука; 2) осно́вы; нача́тки; ABC of chemistry осно́вы хи́мии; 3) железнодоро́жный алфави́тный указа́тель; 4) *attr* просто́й, просте́йший.

ABC-book ['eɪ'biː'siːbuk] *n* буква́рь.

abdicate ['æbdɪkeɪt] *v* отка́зываться (*от права и т. п.*); слага́ть полномо́чия; отрека́ться (*от престо́ла*).

abdication [,æbdɪ'keɪʃən] *n* отрече́ние (*от престо́ла*).

abdomen ['æbdəmen] *n* 1) *анат.* брюшна́я по́лость; 2) брюшко́ (*насекомого*).

abdominal [æb'dɔmɪnl] *a* брюшно́й.

abdominous [æb'dɔmɪnəs] *a* то́лстый, пуза́тый.

abduct [æb'dʌkt] *v* похища́ть, наси́льно увози́ть (*особ. женщину, ребёнка*).

abduction [æb'dʌkʃən] *n* похище́ние (*особ. женщины, ребёнка*).

abductor [æb'dʌktə] *n* 1) похити́тель; 2) *анат.* отводя́щая мы́шца.

abecedarian I [,eɪbiːsiː'dɛərɪən] *a* 1) располо́женный в алфави́тном поря́дке; 2) а́збучный, элемента́рный; 3) неве́жественный, малогра́мотный.

abecedarian II *n амер.* обуча́ющий(ся) гра́моте.

abed [ə'bed] *adv* в посте́ли.

aberration [,æbə'reɪʃən] *n* 1) заблужде́ние; уклоне́ние от пра́вильного пути́; 2) слабоу́мие; 3) *биол.* отклоне́ние от норма́льного ти́па; 4) *физ., астр.* аберра́ция.

abet [ə'bet] *v* поощря́ть, подде́рживать (*что-л. дурное*).

abeyance [ə'beɪəns] *n* 1) вре́менное безде́йствие; 2) вре́менная отме́на (*закона и т. п.*).

abhor [əb'hɔː] *v* испы́тывать отвраще́ние.

abhorrence [əb'hɔrəns] *n* 1) у́жас; отвраще́ние; 2) предме́т, вызыва́ющий у́жас *или* отвраще́ние.

abhorrent [əb'hɔrənt] *a* 1) отврати́тельный; ненави́стный; 2) несовмести́мый.

abidance [ə'baɪdəns] *n* 1) соблюде́ние; ~ by rules соблюде́ние пра́вил; 2) пребыва́ние.

abide [ə'baɪd] *v* (*past, p. p.* abode, *редко* abided) 1) ждать; 2) *разг.* (*в отрицательных и вопросительных предложениях*) терпе́ть; мири́ться с кем-л., чем-л.; I cannot (who can) ~ it я не могу́ (кто мо́жет) мири́ться с э́тим; 3) *уст.* пребыва́ть; жить; □ to ~ by оставаться ве́рным кому́-л., чему́-л.; приде́рживаться чего́-л.; to ~ by one's promises исполня́ть свои обеща́ния; to ~ by the law соблюда́ть зако́ны.

abiding [ə'baɪdɪŋ] *a* постоя́нный.

ability [ə'bɪlɪtɪ] *n* 1) спосо́бность; уме́ние; to the best of one's abilities в ме́ру свои́х сил; 2) *pl* дарова́ния, тала́нты; 3) *юр.* компете́нция, правомо́чность; 4) *фин.* платёжеспосо́бность.

15

abject ['æbdʒekt] *a* 1) ни́зкий, жа́лкий, презре́нный; 2) уни́женный.

abjection [æb'dʒekʃən] *n* униже́ние; прини́женность.

abjuration [ˌæbdʒuə'reɪʃən] *n* отрече́ние.

abjure [əb'dʒuə] *v* 1) отрека́ться; 2) отка́зываться.

ablation [æb'leɪʃən] *n* 1) *мед.* удале́ние; 2) *геол.* разруше́ние *(пород)*.

ablaze I [ə'bleɪz] *a predic* 1) в огне́, в пла́мени; to be ~ пыла́ть; 2) сверка́ющий; 3) возбуждённый.

ablaze II *adv* в огне́.

able ['eɪbl] *a* 1) спосо́бный; тала́нтливый; 2) уме́лый; to be ~ мочь, быть в состоя́нии; уме́ть.

able-bodied ['eɪbl'bɔdɪd] *a* кре́пкий, здоро́вый.

abloom [ə'bluːm] *adv* в цвету́.

ablush [ə'blʌʃ] *a predic* покрасне́в, в смуще́нии.

ablution [ə'bluːʃən] *n* 1) обыкн. pl омове́ние; 2) *тех.* промы́вка.

ably ['eɪblɪ] *adv* уме́ло, ло́вко.

abnegate ['æbnɪgeɪt] *v* 1) отка́зывать себе́ *(в чём-л.)*; 2) отка́зываться *(от прав и т. п.)*; 3) отрица́ть.

abnegation [ˌæbnɪ'geɪʃən] *n* 1) отка́з *(от чего-л.)*; отрече́ние; 2) отрица́ние.

abnormal [æb'nɔːməl] *a* 1) ненорма́льный; *мед.* патологи́ческий; 2) непра́вильный.

abnormality [ˌæbnɔː'mælɪtɪ] *n* 1) ненорма́льность; 2) уро́дство; 3) непра́вильность; 4) анома́лия.

abnormity [æb'nɔːmɪtɪ] *см.* abnormality.

aboard I [ə'bɔːd] *adv* 1) *см.* aboard II; 2) вдоль.

aboard II *prep* на корабле́, на борту́; на кора́бль, на борт; to go ~ a ship сесть на кора́бль.

abode I [ə'boud] *n* местопребыва́ние; жили́ще; to take up *(или* to make) one's ~ посели́ться.

abode II *past, p. p. см.* abide.

aboil [ə'bɔɪl] *a predic:* ~ with indignation в си́льном негодова́нии.

abolish [ə'bɔlɪʃ] *v* отменя́ть, уничтожа́ть, упраздня́ть *(обычаи, учреждения)*.

abolition [ˌæbə'lɪʃən] *n* отме́на, уничтоже́ние, упраздне́ние.

abolitionism [ˌæbə'lɪʃənɪzəm] *n ист.* аболиционизм *(движение за освобождение негров в США)*.

A-bomb ['eɪ'bɔm] *n* а́томная бо́мба.

abominable [ə'bɔmɪnəbl] *a* отврати́тельный, отта́лкивающий; проти́вный.

abominate [ə'bɔmɪneɪt] *v* испы́тывать отвраще́ние.

abomination [əˌbɔmɪ'neɪʃən] *n* 1) отвраще́ние; 2) что-л. отврати́тельное.

aboriginal I [ˌæbə'rɪdʒənl] *n* тузе́мец.

aboriginal II *a* тузе́мный, коренно́й; исконный.

aborigines [ˌæbə'rɪdʒɪniːz] *n pl* тузе́мцы; коренны́е жи́тели.

abort [ə'bɔːt] *v* 1) преждевре́менно разреша́ться от бре́мени; 2) потерпе́ть неуда́чу.

abortion [ə'bɔːʃən] *n* 1) вы́кидыш; або́рт; 2) неуда́ча.

abortive [ə'bɔːtɪv] *a* 1) преждевре́менный *(о родах)*; 2) неуда́вшийся, беспло́дный; 3) недора́звитый.

abound [ə'baund] *v* 1) име́ться в большо́м коли́честве; 2) изоби́ловать, кише́ть *(чем-л.— in, with)*.

about I [ə'baut] *adv* 1) приблизи́тельно, о́коло; ~ fifty miles о́коло пяти́десяти миль; 2) неподалёку, недалеко́; he is somewhere ~ он где́-то недалеко́; 3) почти́; ~ ready почти́ гото́в; 4) вокру́г, круго́м; look ~ посмотри́те круго́м.

about II *prep* 1) *в пространственном значении служит для выражения:* а) *местонахождения данного предмета* круго́м, вокру́г; there are large factories ~ the town вокру́г го́рода нахо́дятся больши́е заво́ды; б) *нахождения где-то в пределах данного ограниченного пространства* где́-то в, где́-то на, в преде́лах; he is ~ the house (the garden, the factory, the town) он где́-то в до́ме (в саду́, на заво́де, в го́роде); 2) *во временном значении выражает близость к определённому моменту* о́коло; he left ~ five o'clock он ушёл *(или* уе́хал) о́коло пяти́ часо́в; 3) *указывает .на наличие чего-л. у кого-л.* при, с; have you any money (a watch, a document) ~ you? у вас с собо́й есть де́ньги (часы́, докуме́нт)?; 4) *указывает на предмет, на который направлена речь, мысль* о, относи́тельно; yesterday we were talking ~ you вчера́ мы говори́ли о вас.

above I [ə'bʌv] *adv* 1) наверху́, наве́рх; the blue sky ~ голубо́е не́бо над голово́й; 2) вы́ше; from what has been said ~ из того́, что бы́ло ска́зано вы́ше.

above II *prep* 1) *в пространственном значении указывает на местонахождение над чем-л.* над; high ~ the city высоко́ над го́родом; 2) *во временном значении указывает на что-л., происшедшее до определённого времени, периода и т. п.* не да́лее чем, до; not traced ~ the fifth century просле́живается до V ве́ка; 3) *указывает на численное превышение* бо́лее, свы́ше; the weight of this load is ~ 3 tons вес э́того гру́за бо́лее 3 тонн; 4) *указывает на превосходство над чем-л.—* вы́ше, свы́ше; this is ~ me э́то вы́ше моего́ понима́ния.

above-board I [ə'bʌv'bɔːd] *a predic* откры́тый, че́стный.

above-board II *adv* откры́то, че́стно. •

above-mentioned [ə'bʌv'menʃənd] *a* вышеупомя́нутый.

abrade [ə'breɪd] *v* 1) стира́ть; сдира́ть *(кожу)*; 2) *тех.* шлифова́ть.

abrasion [ə'breɪʒən] *n* 1) (и)стира́ние; изно́с; 2) сса́дина; 3) *геол.* абра́зия, истира́ние пород; 4) шлифо́вка.

abrasive I [ə'breɪzɪv] *n тех.* абрази́в.

abrasive II *a* шлифова́льный.

abreast [ə'brest] *adv* 1) на одно́й ли́нии, в ряд; 2) на у́ровне, в у́ровень; ~ with the times в но́гу с ве́ком; 3) *мор.* на тра́верзе.

abridge [ə'brɪdʒ] *v* 1) сокраща́ть; 2) ограни́чивать *(свободу, права)*; 3) лиша́ть *(чего-л.— of)*.

abridg(e)ment [ə'brɪdʒmənt] *n* 1) сокраще́ние; 2) ограниче́ние *(свободы, прав)*; 3) сокращённое изложе́ние, конспе́кт.

abroach [əˈbroutʃ] *a predic* откупоренный.

abroad [əˈbrɔːd] *adv* 1) за границей, за границу; from ~ из-за границы; 2) широко, повсюду; 3) вне дома, снаружи; 4) в заблуждении.

abrogate [ˈæbrougeit] *v* отменять (*закон, обычай*).

abrogation [ˌæbrouˈgeiʃən] *n* отмена, уничтожение.

abrupt [əˈbrʌpt] *a* 1) внезапный; 2) резкий, грубый (*о манерах, речи*); 3) обрывистый, крутой; 4) отрывистый.

abruption [əˈbrʌpʃən] *n* разрыв, отрыв; отделение.

abruptness [əˈbrʌptnis] *n* 1) внезапность; 2) резкость, грубость (*речи и т. п.*); 3) обрывистость, крутизна; 4) отрывистость.

abscess [ˈæbsis] *n* нарыв, гнойник.

abscond [æbˈskɔnd] *v* 1) скрыться, уйти украдкой; 2) скрываться (*от суда, преследования*).

absconder [əbˈskɔndə] *n* скрывающийся (*от правосудия*).

absence [ˈæbsəns] *n* 1) отсутствие; неявка; отлучка; ~ without leave самовольная отлучка; 2) неимение, недостаток; 3) рассеянность, невнимание (*тж.* ~ of mind).

absent[a] [ˈæbsənt] *a* 1) отсутствующий; 2) рассеянный.

absent[b] [æbˈsent] *v*: to ~ oneself отсутствовать, отлучаться; to ~ oneself from smth. уклоняться от чего-л.

absentee [ˌæbsənˈtiː] *n* 1) отсутствующий; 2) живущий вне дома; 3) уклоняющийся от чего-л.

absenteeism [ˌæbsənˈtiːizəm] *n* длительное отсутствие; непосещение.

absently [ˈæbsəntli] *adv* рассеянно.

absent-minded [ˈæbsəntˈmaindid] *a* рассеянный, невнимательный.

absent-mindedness [ˈæbsəntˈmaindidnis] *n* рассеянность.

absolute [ˈæbsəluːt] *a* 1) полный, совершенный, абсолютный; безусловный; nominative ~ *грам.* номинативный оборот, *напр.:* she being away... когда она уехала...; 2) абсолютный; неограниченный (*о власти*); 3) чистый, без примеси.

absolutely [ˈæbsəluːtli] *adv* 1) совершенно, абсолютно; безусловно; 2) независимо, самостоятельно.

absolution [ˌæbsəˈluːʃən] *n* 1) освобождение от наказания, оправдание по суду; 2) прощение; 3) *церк.* отпущение грехов.

absolutism [ˈæbsəluːtizəm] *n* *полит.* абсолютизм.

absolve [əbˈzɔlv] *v* 1) освобождать (*от обязательства и т. п.*); 2) прощать, оправдывать; 3) *церк.* отпускать (*грехи*).

absorb [əbˈsɔːb] *v* 1) поглощать; впитывать, всасывать; ~ed in thoughts погружённый в мысли; 2) *тех.* амортизировать.

absorbable [əbˈsɔːbəbl] *a* легко поглощаемый, всасываемый.

absorbedly [əbˈsɔːbidli] *adv* с большим вниманием.

absorbent I [əbˈsɔːbənt] *n* поглотитель, всасывающее вещество.

absorbent II *a* всасывающий, впитывающий.

absorber [əbˈsɔːbə] *n* *тех.* 1) поглотитель, всасывающее вещество; 2) амортизатор.

absorbing I [əbˈsɔːbiŋ] *n* поглощение, всасывание.

absorbing II *a* 1) поглощающий; всасывающий; 2) увлекательный, захватывающий.

absorption [əbˈsɔːpʃən] *n* 1) поглощение; впитывание, всасывание; 2) погружённость (*в мысли и т. п.*).

absorptive [əbˈsɔːptiv] *a* поглощающий; всасывающий.

abstain [əbˈstein] *v* воздерживаться (*от* — from); не употреблять (*спиртных напитков и т. п.*; from).

abstainer [əbˈsteinə] *n* непьющий, трезвенник.

abstemious [æbˈstiːmjəs] *a* воздержанный, умеренный.

abstention [æbˈstenʃən] *n* 1) воздержание; 2) уклонение (*особ. от подачи голоса на выборах*).

abstinence [ˈæbstinəns] *n* воздержание.

abstinency [ˈæbstinənsi] *n* умеренность, воздержанность (*особ. в пище*).

abstinent [ˈæbstinənt] *a* 1) умеренный, воздержанный; 2) непьющий.

abstract[a] I [ˈæbstrækt] *n* 1) краткое изложение, резюме; 2) абстракция; отвлечённое понятие; in the ~ отвлечённо, абстрактно.

abstract[a] II *a* отвлечённый, абстрактный.

abstract[b] [æbˈstrækt] *v* 1) извлекать, отделять (from); 2) рассматривать отвлечённо (from); 3) суммировать, резюмировать; 4) *эвф.* унести, утащить.

abstracted [æbˈstræktid] *a* задумчивый; рассеянный.

abstractedly [æbˈstræktidli] *adv* 1) абстрактно, отвлечённо; отдельно (from); 2) рассеянно.

abstractedness [æbˈstræktidnis] *n* 1) отвлечённость; 2) рассеянность.

abstraction [æbˈstrækʃən] *n* 1) отвлечение; отвлечённость, абстракция; 2) рассеянность.

abstruse [æbˈstruːs] *a* 1) трудный для понимания; неясный; 2) глубокий (*о мысли и т. п.*).

absurd [əbˈsəːd] *a* 1) нелепый, абсурдный; 2) смешной, глупый.

absurdity [əbˈsəːditi] *n* 1) нелепость, абсурдность; глупость; 2) нелепый поступок.

abundance [əˈbʌndəns] *n* 1) изобилие, богатство; 2) множество; there are ~ who... многие...; ◇ ~ of the heart избыток (*или* наплыв) чувств.

abundant [əˈbʌndənt] *a* обильный; изобилующий, богатый (*чем-л.* — in).

abuse[a] [əˈbjuːs] *n* 1) брань, оскорбление; 2) плохое обращение, порча; 3) злоупотребление; 4) неправильное употребление; извращение.

abuse[b] [əˈbjuːz] *v* 1) бранить; оскорблять; 2) плохо обращаться, портить; 3) злоупотреблять; 4) неправильно употреблять.

abusive [əˈbjuːsiv] *a* бранный; оскорбительный.

abut [əˈbʌt] *v* 1) граничить, примыкать (on, upon); 2) упираться (*во что-л.* — on, against).

abutment [əˈbʌtmənt] *n* 1) общая граница, межа; 2) *стр.* опора арки *или* свода.

abysm [əˈbizəm] *n* *поэт.* бездна, пучина.

abysmal [əˈbizməl] *a* 1) бездонный, глубокий; 2) полный, крайний (*о невежестве и т. п.*).

abyss [ə'bɪs] *n* 1) бе́здна, пучи́на; про́пасть; 2) первозда́нный ха́ос; 3) не́дра земли́.

abyssal [ə'bɪsəl] *a* глуби́нный; глубоково́дный.

acacia [ə'keɪʃə] *n* ака́ция.

academic I [ˌækə'demɪk] *n* 1) учёный; 2) *pl* чи́сто теорети́ческие аргуме́нты, до́воды; 3) *pl* университе́тское одея́ние.

academic II *a* 1) академи́ческий; университе́тский; 2) академи́чный, отвлечённый.

academical I [ˌækə'demɪkəl] *n* *pl* университе́тское одея́ние.

academical II *a* академи́ческий, университе́тский.

academically [ˌækə'demɪkəlɪ] *adv* теорети́чески; отвлечённо.

academician [əˌkædə'mɪʃən] *n* акаде́мик.

academy [ə'kædəmɪ] *n* 1) (A.) акаде́мия; Academy of Sciences of the USSR Акаде́мия нау́к СССР; 2) вы́сшее уче́бное заведе́ние; *тж.* сре́днее (ча́стное) уче́бное заведе́ние; 3) специа́льная шко́ла; military ~ вое́нное учи́лище; ~ of music музыка́льная шко́ла.

accede [æk'siːd] *v* 1) соглаша́ться (*с мне́нием и т. п.*); 2) вступа́ть (*в до́лжность и т. п.*); 3) присоединя́ться (*к организа́ции и т. п.*).

accelerate [æk'seləreɪt] *v* ускоря́ть(ся).

accelerated [æk'seləreɪtɪd] *a физ.* уско́ренный.

acceleration [ækˌselə'reɪʃən] *n* ускоре́ние.

accelerative [æk'selərətɪv] *a* ускори́тельный.

accelerator [æk'seləreɪtə] *n* 1) ускори́тель; 2) *хим.* катализа́тор.

accent[a] ['æksənt] *n* 1) ударе́ние; знак ударе́ния; primary ~ *фон.* гла́вное ударе́ние; 2) акце́нт, произноше́ние; 3) *pl поэт.* речь.

accent[b] [æk'sent] *v* 1) де́лать ударе́ние; ста́вить знак ударе́ния; *перен.* подчёркивать, акценти́ровать; 2) произноси́ть.

accentual [æk'sentʃuəl] *a* 1) относя́щийся к ударе́нию; 2) тони́ческий.

accentuate [æk'sentʃueɪt] *v* де́лать ударе́ние; *перен.* подчёркивать.

accentuation [ækˌsentʃu'eɪʃən] *n* 1) ударе́ние; *перен.* подчёркивание; 2) произноше́ние, вы́говор.

accept [ək'sept] *v* 1) принима́ть; 2) соглаша́ться; признава́ть пра́вильным; допуска́ть; 3) относи́ться *или* принима́ть благоскло́нно; 4) *ком.* акцептова́ть.

acceptability [əkˌseptə'bɪlɪtɪ] *n* прие́млемость, допусти́мость.

acceptable [ək'septəbl] *a* 1) прие́млемый, допусти́мый; 2) прия́тный.

acceptance [ək'septəns] *n* 1) приня́тие, приём; 2) согла́сие; одобре́ние; благоскло́нное отноше́ние; ~ of persons лицеприя́тное отноше́ние, лицеприя́тие; 3) *ком.* акце́пт.

acceptation [ˌæksep'teɪʃən] *n* при́нятое значе́ние сло́ва *или* выраже́ния.

accepted [ək'septɪd] *a* общепри́нятый; общепри́знанный.

access ['ækses] *n* 1) до́ступ; досту́пность; easy of ~ досту́пный; 2) по́дступ, подхо́д; прохо́д; 3) при́ступ (*боле́зни, гне́ва*); 4) приближе́ние.

accessary I [æk'sesərɪ] *n* 1) помо́щник; соуча́стник; 2) сопровожде́ние; дополне́ние.

accessary II *a predic* 1) (со)уча́ствующий; 2) *см.* accessory II 1).

accessible [æk'sesəbl] *a* 1) досту́пный; достижи́мый; 2) поддаю́щийся (*чему-л.* — to); пода́тливый.

accession [æk'seʃən] *n* 1) прибавле́ние; приро́ст; 2) ‛до́ступ; 3) вступле́ние (*в до́лжность и т. п.*); 4) согла́сие; 5) припа́док; при́ступ (*боле́зни*).

accessory I [æk'sesərɪ] *n* 1) *pl* принадле́жности; 2) соуча́стник, сообщник.

accessory II *a* 1) дополни́тельный; второстепе́нный; 2) случа́йный, побо́чный.

accidence ['æksɪdəns] *n* 1) *грам.* морфоло́гия; 2) осно́вы како́го-л. предме́та; 3) авари́йность.

accident ['æksɪdənt] *n* 1) слу́чай; случа́йность; by ~ случа́йно; pure ~ чи́стая случа́йность; 2) несча́стный слу́чай; ава́рия; fatal ~ несча́стный слу́чай со смерте́льным исхо́дом; industrial ~ несча́стный слу́чай на произво́дстве; without ~ безопа́сно; благополу́чно; 3) обстоя́тельство; 4) осо́бенность; сво́йство; 5) *геол.*: ~ of the ground скла́дка *или* неро́вность ме́стности.

accidental [ˌæksɪ'dentl] *a* 1) случа́йный; неча́янный; 2) вспомога́тельный; второстепе́нный.

accidentally [ˌæksɪ'dentəlɪ] *adv* случа́йно; неча́янно.

acclaim I [ə'kleɪm] *n* бу́рные аплодисме́нты; *перен.* одобре́ние.

acclaim II *v* 1) бу́рно аплоди́ровать; приве́тствовать; 2) провозглаша́ть.

acclamation [ˌæklə'meɪʃən] *n* 1) шу́мное, дру́жное одобре́ние; voted (*или* carried) by ~ при́нято единогла́сно; 2) *обыкн. pl.* ова́ция.

acclimate [ə'klaɪmeɪt] *см.* acclimatize.

acclimation [ˌæklaɪ'meɪʃən] *см.* acclimatization.

acclimatization [əˌklaɪmətaɪ'zeɪʃən] *n* акклиматиза́ция.

acclimatize [ə'klaɪmətaɪz] *v* акклиматизи́ровать(ся).

acclivity [ə'klɪvɪtɪ] *n* подъём (*холма́, горы́*).

acclivous [ə'klaɪvəs] *a* поднима́ющийся вверх (*о доро́ге*).

accolade [ˌækə'leɪd] *n ист.* обря́д посвяще́ния в ры́цари.

accommodate [ə'kɔmədeɪt] *v* 1) предоставля́ть жильё, помеще́ние; 2) ока́зывать услу́гу; 3) снабжа́ть (*with*); 4) согласо́вывать; ула́живать; примиря́ть; 5) приспоса́бливать.

accommodating [ə'kɔmədeɪtɪŋ] *a* 1) любе́зный, услу́жливый; 2) усту́пчивый, сгово́рчивый; 3) приспособля́ющийся; 4) вмеща́ющий.

accommodation [əˌkɔmə'deɪʃən] *n* 1) жильё; помеще́ние; 2) *pl* удо́бства (*в кварти́ре и т. п.*); 3) ссу́да; 4) соглаше́ние, компроми́сс; 5) приспособле́ние.

accompaniment [ə'kʌmpənɪmənt] *n* 1) сопровожде́ние; 2) *муз.* аккомпанеме́нт.

accompanist [ə'kʌmpənɪst] *n* аккомпаниа́тор.

accompany [ə'kʌmpənɪ] *v* 1) сопровожда́ть; 2) *муз.* аккомпани́ровать.

accomplice [ə'kɔmplɪs] *n* соуча́стник (преступле́ния).

accomplish [ə'kɔmplɪʃ] *v* 1) исполня́ть, выполня́ть; заверша́ть; 2) соверше́нствовать; достига́ть соверше́нства.

accomplished [ə'kɔmplɪʃt] *a* 1) зако́нченный, заверше́нный; соверши́вшийся (*о собы́тии, фа́кте*); 2) образо́ванный; хорошо́ воспи́танный.

accomplishment [ə'kɔmplɪʃmənt] *n* 1) выполне́ние; заверше́ние; 2) достиже́ние; 3) образова́ние; хоро́шее воспита́ние; 4) благоустро́йство.

accord I [ə'kɔːd] *n* 1) согла́сие; with one ~ единоду́шно; of one's own ~ доброво́льно; 2) соглаше́ние; 3) соотве́тствие, гармо́ния; 4) *муз.* акко́рд.

accord II [ə'kɔːd] *v* 1) соотве́тствовать, гармони́ровать (*with*); 2) приходи́ть к соглаше́нию; 3) ока́зывать (*приём, честь*); жа́ловать.

accordance [ə'kɔːdəns] *n* согла́сие, соотве́тствие; in ~ with согла́сно, в соотве́тствии с.

accordant [ə'kɔːdənt] *a* 1) согла́сный, созву́чный; 2) соотве́тственный.

according [ə'kɔːdɪŋ] *adv:* ~ as соотве́тственно; ~ to согла́сно; по утвержде́нию, по слова́м.

accordingly [ə'kɔːdɪŋlɪ] *adv* 1) соотве́тственно; 2) поэ́тому, таки́м о́бразом.

accordion [ə'kɔːdjən] *n* аккордео́н; гармо́ника.

accost I [ə'kɔst] *n* приве́тствие; обраще́ние (*к кому́-л.*).

accost II *v* 1) приве́тствовать; обраща́ться к кому́-л.; заговори́ть с кем-л.; 2) пристава́ть (*обыкн. о проститу́тке*); 3) *мор.* прича́ливать.

accouchement [ə'kuːʃmɑːŋ] *n* ро́ды.

accoucheur [ˌækuː'ʃəː] *n* акуше́р.

account I [ə'kaunt] *n* 1) счёт; расчёт; подсчёт; to keep ~s вести́ счета́; for ~ of за счёт (*кого́-л.*); on ~ в счёт; ~ current (*сокр.* a/c) теку́щий счёт; to square (*или* to settle) ~s with smb. а) рассчита́ться с кем-л.; б) своди́ть счёты с кем-л.; to take (of) принима́ть в расчёт, учи́тывать; 2) отчёт; бала́нс; to give an ~ of smth. дава́ть отчёт в чём-л.; 3) докла́д, сообще́ние; отчёт; to render an ~ of a) описа́ть (подро́бно); б) объясни́ть (*свои́ посту́пки, своё поведе́ние*); 4) оце́нка, мне́ние; by all ~s по о́бщему мне́нию; 5) причи́на, основа́ние; on ~ of по причи́не, из-за; on no ~ ни в ко́ем слу́чае; 6) вы́года; по́льза; to turn to ~ испо́льзовать; 7) ва́жность, значе́ние; of no ~, of small ~ не име́ющий значе́ния; to make little ~ of не придава́ть значе́ния, не обраща́ть внима́ния; ◇ on one's own ~ на свой страх и риск; to call to ~ призва́ть к отве́ту; to take into ~ принима́ть во внима́ние.

account II [ə'kaunt] *v* счита́ть за; рассма́тривать как; to ~ him a hero счита́ть его́ геро́ем; □ to ~ for объясня́ть, быть причи́ной.

accountability [əˌkauntə'bɪlɪtɪ] *n* отве́тственность; подотчётность.

accountable [ə'kauntəbl] *a* 1) отве́тственный (*за что-л.— for; пе́ред кем-л.— to*); 2) объясни́мый.

accountancy [ə'kauntənsɪ] *n* счетово́дство; бухгалте́рия.

accountant [ə'kauntənt] *n* 1) бухга́лтер; 2) *юр.* отве́тчик.

accountant-general [ə'kauntənt,dʒenərəl] *n* гла́вный бухга́лтер.

accounting [ə'kauntɪŋ] *n* учёт; отчётность; cost ~ калькуля́ция сто́имости.

accredit [ə'kredɪt] *v* 1) уполномо́чивать; аккредитова́ть (*посла́ и т. п.*); 2) доверя́ть (*что-л. кому́-л.*); 3) припи́сывать (*что-л. кому́-л.*); наделя́ть (*кого́-л. чем-л.*).

accredited [ə'kredɪtɪd] *a* 1) официа́льно при́знанный; аккредито́ванный; 2) общепри́нятый.

accretion [æ'kriːʃən] *n* 1) разраста́ние; 2) сраста́ние, сраще́ние; 3) прираще́ние, нараще́ние.

accrue [ə'kruː] *v* 1) прибавля́ться; нараста́ть (*осо́б. о проце́нтах*); 2) достава́ться, выпада́ть на до́лю (*кому́-л.— to*); 3) происходи́ть (*от чего́-л.— from*).

accumulate [ə'kjuːmjuleɪt] *v* 1) нака́пливать, аккумули́ровать; 2) скопля́ться.

accumulation [əˌkjuːmju'leɪʃən] *n* 1) накопле́ние, собира́ние, аккумуля́ция; primitive ~ *полит. эк.* первонача́льное накопле́ние; 2) скопле́ние; ма́сса.

accumulative [ə'kjuːmjulətɪv] *a* 1) накопи́вшийся; 2) скло́нный к стяжа́тельству.

accumulator [ə'kjuːmjuleɪtə] *n* 1) собира́тель; 2) стяжа́тель; 3) *эл.* аккумуля́тор; 4) *тех.* колле́ктор.

accuracy ['ækjurəsɪ] *n* то́чность; аккура́тность, тща́тельность; with pinpoint ~ с преде́льной то́чностью.

accurate ['ækjurɪt] *a* то́чный; аккура́тный, тща́тельный; пра́вильный.

accursed [ə'kəːsɪd] *a* 1) прокля́тый; злополу́чный; 2) отврати́тельный.

accurst [ə'kəːst] *см.* accursed.

accusal [ə'kjuːzəl] *ре́дко см.* accusation.

accusation [ˌækju'zeɪʃən] *n* обвине́ние; *юр. тж.* обвини́тельный акт; to bring an ~ against smb. обвиня́ть кого́-л.; to be under an ~ of smth. обвиня́ться в чём-л.

accusative I [ə'kjuːzətɪv] *n грам.* вини́тельный паде́ж.

accusative II *a грам.* вини́тельный.

accuse [ə'kjuːz] *v* обвиня́ть (*в чём-л.— of*).

accused [ə'kjuːzd] *n* (the ~) обвиня́емый.

accuser [ə'kjuːzə] *n* обвини́тель.

accustom [ə'kʌstəm] *v* приуча́ть; to ~ oneself приуча́ться, привыка́ть.

accustomed [ə'kʌstəmd] *a* 1) привы́кший, приу́ченный (*к чему́-л.— to*); 2) обы́чный; привы́чный.

ace [eɪs] *n* 1) очко́; 2) туз (*в ка́ртах*); кость в одно́ очко́ (*в домино́*); 3) о́чень ма́ленькое коли́чество; чу́точка; within an ~ of на волосо́к от; 4) ас, первокла́ссный лётчик; 5) изве́стный спортсме́н.

acerbity [ə'səːbɪtɪ] *n* 1) те́рпкость; 2) ре́зкость (*то́на и т. п.*).

acetic [ə'siːtɪk] *a* у́ксусный.

acetous ['æsɪtəs] *a* у́ксусный; ки́слый.

acetylene [ə'setɪliːn] *n* 1) ацетиле́н; 2) *attr* ацетиле́новый.

ache I [eɪk] *n* (тупа́я) боль.

ache II *v* 1) боле́ть; 2) жа́ждать чего́-л.

acheless ['eɪklɪs] *a* безболе́зненный.

achievable [ə'tʃiːvəbl] *a* достижи́мый.

achieve [ə'tʃiːv] *v* 1) достига́ть; 2) соверша́ть; 3) доводи́ть до конца́.

achievement [ə'tʃiːvmənt] *n* 1) достиже́ние; 2) выполне́ние, заверше́ние.

achromatic [ˌækrou'mætɪk] *a* ахроматический, бесцветный.

acid I ['æsɪd] *n* кислота; nitric ~ азотная кислота; prussic ~ синильная кислота.

acid II *a* 1) кислый; 2) *хим.* кислотный.

asidify [ə'sɪdɪfaɪ] *v* окислять(ся).

asidity [ə'sɪdɪtɪ] *n* кислотность.

acid-proof ['æsɪd'pruːf] *a* кислотоупорный.

acidulated [ə'sɪdjuleɪtɪd] *a* 1) кисловатый; подкислённый; 2) недовольный.

acidulous [ə'sɪdjuləs] *a* кисловатый.

acknowledge [ək'nɔlɪdʒ] *v* 1) признавать; допускать; 2) подтверждать получение (*письма и т. п.*); 3) вознаграждать (*за услугу и т. п.*).

acknowledgement [ək'nɔlɪdʒmənt] *n* 1) признание; 2) подтверждение; расписка в получении; 3) вознаграждение; благодарность; in ~ of в благодарность за, в знак признательности; 4) указание *или* ссылка на источник.

aclinic [ə'klɪnɪk] *a:* ~ line магнитный экватор.

acme ['ækmɪ] *n* высшая точка; кульминационный пункт.

acne ['æknɪ] *n* угорь, прыщ.

acock [ə'kɔk] *adv* набекрень.

acolyte ['ækəlaɪt] *n* служитель; помощник.

acorn ['eɪkɔːn] *n* жёлудь.

acoustic [ə'kuːstɪk] *a* 1) акустический, звуковой; 2) *анат.* слуховой.

acoustics [ə'kuːstɪks] *n* акустика; учение о звуке.

acquaint [ə'kweɪnt] *v* 1) знакомить (*с кем-л., с чем-л.*); осведомлять; to ~ oneself with знакомиться с чем-л.; to be ~ed with быть знакомым с; 2) извещать, сообщать.

acquaintance [ə'kweɪntəns] *n* 1) знакомство; nodding ~ шапочное знакомство; speaking ~ знакомство, позволяющее заговорить при встрече; to make the ~ of smb. познакомиться с кем-л.; to cultivate the ~ поддерживать знакомство (*c — of*); 2) знакомый.

acquest [æ'kwest] *n* 1) приобретение; 2) *юр.* благоприобретённое имущество.

acquiesce [ˌækwɪ'es] *v* молча соглашаться; □ to ~ in принимать.

acquiescence [ˌækwɪ'esns] *n* молчаливое согласие; покорность.

acquiescent [ˌækwɪ'esnt] *a* податливый; покорный.

acquire [ə'kwaɪə] *v* 1) приобретать; получать; 2) снискать; 3) овладевать (*навыком и т. п.*).

acquirement [ə'kwaɪəmənt] *n* 1) приобретение; 2) овладение; 3) *pl* познания; навыки.

acquisition [ˌækwɪ'zɪʃən] *n* приобретение.

acquisitive [æ'kwɪzɪtɪv] *a* 1) стяжательный; 2) восприимчивый.

acquit [ə'kwɪt] *v* 1) выплачивать (*долг*); выполнять (*обязанность и т. п.*); to ~ oneself of promise выполнить обещание; 2) освобождать(ся) от чего-л.; 3) оправдывать.

acquittal [ə'kwɪtl] *n* 1) выполнение (*обязанности*); 2) освобождение (*от долга и т. п.*); 3) оправдание.

acquittance [ə'kwɪtns] *n* 1) уплата долга; освобождение от долга; 2) расписка об уплате.

acre ['eɪkə] *n* акр (*около 0,4 га*).

acreage ['eɪkərɪdʒ] *n* количество акров; площадь земли в акрах.

acrid ['ækrɪd] *a* 1) острый, едкий (*на вкус; о запахе*); раздражающий; 2) резкий; колкий, язвительный.

acridity [æ'krɪdɪtɪ] *n* 1) едкость; 2) резкость; язвительность.

acrimonious [ˌækrɪ'mounjəs] *a* 1) язвительный; жёлчный; 2) *уст.* едкий.

acrimony ['ækrɪmənɪ] *n* 1) язвительность; жёлчность; 2) *уст.* едкость.

acrobacy ['ækrəbəsɪ] *n* *ав.* высший пилотаж.

acrobat ['ækrəbæt] *n* акробат.

acrobatic [ˌækrə'bætɪk] *a* акробатический.

acrobatics [ˌækrə'bætɪks] *n* акробатика; aerial ~ фигурные полёты.

acronym ['ækrənɪm] *n* *лингв.* акроним.

acropolis [ə'krɔpəlɪs] *n* акрополь.

across I [ə'krɔs] *adv* 1) поперёк; a line drawn ~ линия, линия поперёк; 2) на ту сторону, на той стороне (*реки, канала, дороги*); by this time he is ~ к этому времени он уже прибыл на ту сторону; 3) крест-накрест; with arms ~ сложив руки крест-накрест.

across II *prep* в пространственном значении указывает на: а) *движение с одной стороны реки, канала, улицы и т. п.* на другую черрез; we sailed ~ the bay мы переплыли через залив; б) *местонахождение по другую сторону реки, канала и т. п.* через, на той стороне, по ту сторону; this man lives ~ the street (the road) этот человек живёт через улицу (дорогу); в) *пересечение (на любых средствах транспорта) территории или водного пространства* через, сквозь; the motor-car went ~ the field машина проехала через поле (*или* полем).

acrostic [ə'krɔstɪk] *n* акростих.

act I [ækt] *n* 1) дело, поступок; действие; акт; 2) постановление, указ; Act of grace амнистия; 3) документ, акт; 4) акт, действие (*пьесы*); ◊ to play (*или* to plead) the baby ~ ссылаться на неопытность; to sue an ~ against smb. подавать в суд на кого-л.

act II *v* 1) поступать, действовать; вести себя; 2) играть (*роль*); 3) действовать, влиять (*на — on*).

acting I ['æktɪŋ] *n* *театр.* игра.

acting II *a* 1) действующий; 2) исполняющий обязанности; ~ in charge по поручению.

action ['ækʃən] *n* 1) действие; поступок; joint ~ совместные действия; to take ~ начать действовать; принять меры; to put in ~ приводить в действие; 2) деятельность, работа; 3) действие механизма, механизм; 4) судебный процесс; иск; 5) сражение, бой; in ~ в бою; to bring into ~ вводить в бой; to go into ~ начать сражение; to come out of ~ выйти из боя; б) выходить из строя; to be killed (*или* to fall) in ~ пасть на поле боя.

activated ['æktɪveɪtɪd] *a* активированный.

active ['æktɪv] *a* 1) активный; деятельный, энергичный; 2) действующий; 3) *грам.* действительный.

activity [æk'tɪvɪtɪ] *n* 1) деятельность; 2) активность; энергия.

actor ['æktə] *n* актёр.

actress ['æktrɪs] *n* актри́са.

actual ['æktʃuəl] *a* 1) действи́тельный; реа́льный; настоя́щий; 2) теку́щий, совреме́нный.

actuality [ˌæktʃu'ælɪtɪ] *n* 1) действи́тельность; реа́льность; 2) реали́зм (*в искусстве*).

actualize ['æktʃuəlaɪz] *v* 1) осуществля́ть; реализова́ть; 2) изобража́ть реалисти́чески.

actually ['æktʃuəlɪ] *adv* 1) факти́чески, в действи́тельности, на са́мом де́ле; 2) в да́нный моме́нт, в настоя́щее вре́мя; 3) да́же, как ни стра́нно.

actuate ['æktʃueɪt] *v* 1) приводи́ть в де́йствие *или* в движе́ние; 2) побужда́ть, стимули́ровать.

actuation [ˌæktʃu'eɪʃən] *n* 1) приведе́ние в де́йствие; 2) побужде́ние, стимули́рование.

acuity [ə'kjuːɪtɪ] *n* острота́ (*восприятия, вкуса*).

acumen [ə'kjuːmen] *n* проница́тельность.

acuminate [ə'kjuːmɪneɪt] *v* 1) заостря́ть; 2) придава́ть остроту́.

acute [ə'kjuːt] *a* 1) о́стрый; 2) проница́тельный (*об уме*); 3) высо́кий, ре́зкий, пронзи́тельный (*о звуке*).

acuteness [ə'kjuːtnɪs] *n* 1) острота́; 2) проница́тельность (*ума*); 3) ре́зкость, пронзи́тельность (*звука*).

ad [æd] *сокр. разг. см.* advertisement.

adage ['ædɪdʒ] *n* изрече́ние, посло́вица.

adamant ['ædəmənt] *n* 1) алма́з; 2) *attr* твёрдый; непреклóнный.

adamantine [ˌædə'mæntaɪn] *a* 1) твёрдый (как алма́з); 2) несокруши́мый.

adapt [ə'dæpt] *v* 1) приспоса́бливать, пригоня́ть (*to, for*); to ~ oneself приспоса́бливаться; 2) адапти́ровать (*текст*); переде́лывать (*лит. произведение*).

adaptability [əˌdæptə'bɪlɪtɪ] *n* 1) приспособля́емость; 2) приго́дность, примени́мость.

adaptable [ə'dæptəbl] *a* легко́ приспоса́бливаемый.

adaptation [ˌædæp'teɪʃən] *n* 1) приспособле́ние, адапта́ция; light ~ адапта́ция гла́за к све́ту; 2) переде́лка (*лит. произведения*).

adapter [ə'dæptə] *n* 1) тот, кто приспоса́бливает, де́лает приго́дным; 2) тот, кто переде́лывает литерату́рное произведе́ние; 3) *тех.* ада́птер; держа́тель; наконе́чник.

add [æd] *v* прибавля́ть, присоединя́ть; дополня́ть; □ to ~ **in** включа́ть; to ~ **to** добавля́ть; увели́чивать; to ~ **together**, to ~ **up** скла́дывать, подсчи́тывать; сумми́ровать.

addenda [ə'dendə] *pl см.* addendum.

addendum [ə'dendəm] *n* (*pl* addenda) приложе́ние, дополне́ние.

adder ['ædə] *n* 1) гадю́ка; 2) *амер.* уж; ◊ flying ~ стрекоза́.

addict[a] ['ædɪkt] *n* наркома́н.

addict[b] [ə'dɪkt] *v* пристрасти́ться (*к чему-л.— to*); предава́ться (*чему-л.— to; обыкн.* to ~ oneself).

addiction [ə'dɪkʃən] *n* скло́нность к чему́-л., па́губная привы́чка.

addition [ə'dɪʃən] *n* 1) прибавле́ние, увеличе́ние; дополне́ние; in ~ to в дополне́ние; к тому́ же; a useful ~ це́нное доба́вление; 2) *мат.* сложе́ние; 3) *хим.* при́месь.

additional [ə'dɪʃənl] *a* дополни́тельный, доба́вочный; накладно́й (*о расходах*).

addle I ['ædl] *a* 1) ту́хлый; без заро́дыша (*о яйце*); 2) пусто́й, взба́лмошный; пу́таный.

addle II *v* 1) ту́хнуть, по́ртиться (*о яйце*); 2) пу́тать.

addle-brained ['ædlbreɪnd] *см.* addle-headed.

addle-headed ['ædlˌhedɪd] *a* пустоголо́вый, безмо́зглый.

address I [ə'dres] *n* 1) а́дрес; 2) обраще́ние; речь; election ~ предвы́борное обраще́ние к избира́телям; 3) ло́вкость, нахо́дчивость; уме́ние держа́ться; 4) *pl* уха́живание; to pay one's ~es уха́живать.

address II *v* 1) адресова́ть; надпи́сывать а́дрес; 2) обраща́ться к кому́-л. (*с речью, письмом*); 3) : to ~ oneself to принима́ться, бра́ться за что-л.

addressee [ˌædre'siː] *n* адреса́т.

adduce [ə'djuːs] *v* представля́ть, приводи́ть (*в качестве доказательства, примера*).

adduction [ə'dʌkʃən] *n* приведе́ние (*доказа́тельств, примеров*).

adept I ['ædept] *n* 1) знато́к; 2) приве́рженец, после́дователь; 3) алхи́мик.

adept II *a* о́пытный, све́дущий; иску́сный.

adequacy ['ædɪkwəsɪ] *n* 1) соотве́тствие, адеква́тность; 2) доста́точность.

adequate ['ædɪkwɪt] *a* 1) соотве́тствующий, адеква́тный; 2) доста́точный; 3) отвеча́ющий тре́бованиям.

adequation [ˌædɪ'kweɪʃən] *n* 1) выра́внивание; 2) эквивале́нт.

adhere [əd'hɪə] *v* 1) (про́чно) прикле́иваться, пристава́ть, прилипа́ть; 2) приде́рживаться (*чего-л.— to*); остава́ться ве́рным (*чему-л.— to*).

adherence [əd'hɪərəns] *n* 1) привя́занность; ве́рность, приве́рженность; 2) пло́тное соедине́ние; 3) *тех.* сцепле́ние.

adherent I [əd'hɪərənt] *n* приве́рженец; после́дователь.

adherent II *a* 1) пло́тно соединённый, прилега́ющий; 2) кле́йкий, ли́пкий.

adhesion [əd'hiːʒən] *n* 1) прилипа́ние; 2) *тех.* сцепле́ние; притяже́ние; тре́ние; 3) ве́рность чему́-л., приве́рженность к чему́-л.

adhesive I [əd'hiːsɪv] *n* кле́йкое вещество́.

adhesive II *a* ли́пкий, кле́йкий; свя́зывающий.

adieu I [ə'djuː] *n* проща́ние; to take (*или* to make) one's ~ проща́ться.

adieu II *int* проща́й(те)!

adiposity [ˌædɪ'pɔsɪtɪ] *n* ожире́ние, ту́чность.

adit ['ædɪt] *n* 1) вход; прохо́д; 2) по́дступ; 3) приближе́ние; 4) *горн.* што́льня, галере́я.

adjacency [ə'dʒeɪsənsɪ] *n* 1) бли́зость, сосе́дство; сме́жность; 2) *pl* окре́стности.

adjacent [ə'dʒeɪsənt] *a* сосе́дний, бли́зкий; сме́жный, примыка́ющий.

adjectival [ˌædʒek'taɪvəl] *a* *грам.* в ка́честве прилага́тельного.

adjective I ['ædʒɪktɪv] *n* *грам.* и́мя прилага́тельное.

adjective II *a* дополни́тельный; несамостоя́тельный, зави́симый.

adjoin [ə'dʒɔɪn] *v* 1) примыка́ть, прилега́ть, быть сме́жным; 2) присоединя́ть, соединя́ть.

adjourn [ə'dʒəːn] *v* 1) откла́дывать, отсро́чивать; 2) объявля́ть переры́в (*заседания и т. п.*); 3) переноси́ть заседа́ние в друго́е помеще́ние; *разг.* переходи́ть в друго́е ме́сто; 4) закрыва́ть заседа́ние, расходи́ться.

adjournment [ə'dʒəːnmənt] *n* 1) отсро́чка; 2) переры́в (*в заседании*).

adjudge [ə'dʒʌdʒ] *v* 1) выноси́ть пригово́р, осужда́ть; 2) присужда́ть (*что-л. кому-л.*).

adjudg(e)ment [ə'dʒʌdʒmənt] *n* 1) вынесе́ние пригово́ра, осужде́ние; 2) присужде́ние.

adjudicate [ə'dʒuːdıkeıt] *v* юр. суди́ть; выноси́ть реше́ние; пригова́ривать.

adjunct ['ædʒʌŋkt] *n* 1) помо́щник; адъю́нкт; 2) дополне́ние, прида́ток; 3) *грам.* определе́ние.

adjuration [ˌædʒuə'reıʃən] *n* 1) заклина́ние, мольба́; 2) кля́тва.

adjure [ə'dʒuə] *v* 1) заклина́ть; умоля́ть; 2) *уст.* приводи́ть к прися́ге.

adjust [ə'dʒʌst] *v* 1) приспоса́бливать; прила́живать, пригоня́ть, устра́ивать; 2) приводи́ть в поря́док; 3) ула́живать (*спор и т. п.*); 4) регули́ровать, устана́вливать, выверя́ть.

adjustable [ə'dʒʌstəbl] *a* регули́руемый; передвижно́й.

adjuster [ə'dʒʌstə] *n* монтёр, устано́вщик, сбо́рщик.

adjusting [ə'dʒʌstıŋ] *a* 1) устано́вочный, регули́рующий; 2) сбо́рочный (*о цехе*).

adjustment [ə'dʒʌstmənt] *n* 1) регули́рование; приспособле́ние; 2) *тех.* устано́вка, сбо́рка; вы́верка; 3) *воен.* корректиро́вка.

adjuvant I ['ædʒuvənt] *n* помо́щник.

adjuvant II *a* поле́зный, спосо́бствующий.

admeasure [æd'meʒə] *v* 1) отмеря́ть; устана́вливать преде́лы, грани́цы; 2) размеря́ть; распределя́ть.

admeasurement [æd'meʒəmənt] *n* 1) отме́ривание; 2) разме́р; 3) распределе́ние, разде́л.

administer [əd'mınıstə] *v* 1) вести́ дела́; управля́ть; 2) соверша́ть; отправля́ть (*правосудие*); 3) прописа́ть, дава́ть (*лекарство*); 4) спосо́бствовать, соде́йствовать.

administrate [əd'mınıstreıt] *v* управля́ть.

administration [ədˌmınıs'treıʃən] *n* 1) управле́ние дела́ми; администра́ция; 2) министе́рство; прави́тельство; 3) отправле́ние (*правосудия*); 4) назначе́ние *или* примене́ние (*лекарств*).

administrative [əd'mınıstrətıv] *a* 1) администрати́вный; администрати́вно-хозя́йственный; 2) исполни́тельный (*о власти*).

administrator [əd'mınıstreıtə] *n* 1) администра́тор; управля́ющий; 2) чино́вник; 3) *юр.* опеку́н.

admirable ['ædmərəbl] *a* восхити́тельный, замеча́тельный.

admiral ['ædmərəl] *n* 1) адмира́л; 2) фла́гманский кора́бль.

admiralty ['ædmərəltı] *n* 1) адмиралте́йство; 2) (A.) вое́нно-морско́е министе́рство (*Англии*).

admiration [ˌædmə'reıʃən] *n* 1) восхище́ние; 2) предме́т восхище́ния.

admire [əd'maıə] *v* 1) восхища́ться; любова́ться; 2) *амер.* си́льно хоте́ть (*сделать что-л.*).

admirer [əd'maıərə] *n* покло́нник, обожа́тель.

admiringly [əd'maıərıŋlı] *adv* восхищённо, с восхище́нием.

admissible [əd'mısəbl] *a* допусти́мый; прие́млемый.

admission [əd'mıʃən] *n* 1) допуще́ние; приня́тие; 2) призна́ние (*правильным, верным*); 3) до́ступ; вход; 4) *тех.* впуск; подво́д (*воды, воздуха*); 5) *attr* вступи́тельный (*о взносе и т. п.*); входно́й (*о плате, билете*).

admissive [əd'mısıv] *a* досту́пный.

admit [əd'mıt] *v* 1) впуска́ть, допуска́ть; 2) позволя́ть; разреша́ть; it doesn't ~ of doubt здесь нет ме́ста сомне́нию; 3) принима́ть; признава́ть (*правильным, действительным*); 4) допуска́ть, соглаша́ться; 5) вмеща́ть (*о помеще́нии*).

admittance [əd'mıtəns] *n* до́ступ; вход; по ~ ! вход воспрещён!

admittedly [əd'mıtıdlı] *adv* предположи́тельно.

admix [əd'mıks] *v* 1) преме́шивать; 2) сме́шивать(ся).

admixture [əd'mıkstʃə] *n* 1) при́месь; 2) смесь.

admonish [əd'mɒnıʃ] *v* 1) убежда́ть, увещева́ть; сове́товать; 2) предупрежда́ть, предостерега́ть (*о чём-л. — of*); 3) извеща́ть, напомина́ть (*о чём-л. — of*).

admonishment [əd'mɒnıʃmənt] *n* 1) увеща́ние; 2) предупрежде́ние, предостереже́ние; 3) напомина́ние, указа́ние.

admonition [ˌædmə'nıʃən] *n* 1) *см.* admonishment; 2) замеча́ние; вы́говор.

admonitory [əd'mɒnıtərı] *a* увещева́ющий; предостерега́ющий.

ado [ə'duː] *n* 1) шум, суета́, хло́поты; much ~ about nothing мно́го шу́му из ничего́; 2) затрудне́ние.

adobe [ə'doubı] *n* 1) необожжённый кирпи́ч; сама́н; 2) сама́нная постро́йка.

adolescence [ˌædou'lesns] *n* ю́ность.

adolescent I [ˌædou'lesnt] *n* ю́ноша; де́вушка; подро́сток.

adolescent II *a* ю́ношеский; ю́ный.

adopt [ə'dɒpt] *v* 1) усыновля́ть; 2) принима́ть; усва́ивать; 3) заи́мствовать (*слово из другого языка*); 4) выбира́ть, брать по своему́ вы́бору.

adoptee [ˌædɒp'tiː] *n* усыновлённый; приёмыш.

adoption [ə'dɒpʃən] *n* 1) усыновле́ние; 2) приня́тие; усвое́ние; 3) заи́мствование (*из другого языка*); 4) вы́бор.

adoptive [ə'dɒptıv] *a* 1) приёмный, усыновлённый; 2) восприи́мчивый.

adorable [ə'dɔːrəbl] *a* восхити́тельный.

adoration [ˌædɔː'reıʃən] *n* обожа́ние; поклоне́ние.

adore [ə'dɔː] *v* обожа́ть; поклоня́ться.

adorer [ə'dɔːrə] *n* покло́нник, обожа́тель.

adorn [ə'dɔːn] *v* украша́ть.

adornment [ə'dɔːnmənt] *n* украше́ние.

adown [ə'daun] *adv* *уст., поэт.* внизу́, вниз.

adrenal I [æd'riːnəl] *n* *анат.* надпо́чечная железа́.

adrenal II *a* *анат.* надпо́чечный.

adrift [ə'drıft] *adv* по тече́нию; по во́ле волн; по во́ле слу́чая; to cut ~ пусти́ть по тече́нию; to go ~ дрейфова́ть; to turn ~ вы́гнать и́з дому; бро́сить на произво́л судьбы́.

adroit [ə'drɔıt] *a* ло́вкий, прово́рный; нахо́дчивый.

adulate ['ædjuleıt] *v* льстить, низкопокло́нничать.

adulation [ˌædjuˈleɪʃən] *n* низкая лесть, низкопоклонство.

adulatory [ˈædjuleɪtərɪ] *a* льстивый, угодливый.

adult I [ˈædʌlt] *n* взрослый человек.

adult II *a* взрослый, зрелый.

adulterant [əˈdʌltərənt] *n* примесь.

adulterate I [əˈdʌltəreɪt] *a* 1) поддельный, фальсифицированный; 2) виновный в прелюбодеянии; 3) внебрачный, незаконнорождённый.

adulterate II *v* фальсифицировать (*продукты*); *перен.* подтасовывать (*факты и т. п.*).

adulteration [əˌdʌltəˈreɪʃən] *n* фальсификация, подделка.

adulterer [əˈdʌltərə] *n* виновный в прелюбодеянии.

adultery [əˈdʌltərɪ] *n* адюльтер, нарушение супружеской верности.

adumbrate [ˈædʌmbreɪt] *v* 1) описывать в общих чертах; делать набросок; 2) предвещать; 3) омрачать.

adumbration [ˌædʌmˈbreɪʃən] *n* 1) набросок; общее представление; 2) омрачение.

adust [əˈdʌst] *a* 1) опалённый; выжженный; высохший; 2) загорелый; 3) жёлчный, угрюмый.

advance I [ədˈvɑːns] *n* 1) продвижение; *воен.* наступление; 3) успех; прогресс; 4) аванс; ссуда; 5) повышение (*в должности, в цене*); 6) *обыкн.* *pl* первый шаг к чему-л., предложение; to make ~s делать авансы; 7) предварение, опережение; in ~ раньше, заранее; вперёд; in ~ of а) впереди; б) раньше; to be in ~ а) опередить; б) идти вперёд, спешить (*о часах*).

advance II *v* 1) двигать(ся) вперёд; продвигать(ся); 2) *воен.* наступать; 3) выдвигать; 4) делать успехи; развивать(ся); 5) платить авансом; давать ссуду; 6) повышать(ся) (*в должности, в цене*).

advanced [ədˈvɑːnst] *a* 1) выдвинутый вперёд; 2) продвинутый; повышенного типа; 3) успевающий (*об ученике*); 4) передовой; ◊ ~ in years престарелый.

advance-guard [ədˈvɑːnsɡɑːd] *n* авангард.

advancement [ədˈvɑːnsmənt] *n* 1) продвижение; 2) успех; прогресс; 3) повышение.

advantage I [ədˈvɑːntɪdʒ] *n* преимущество; благоприятное положение; mutual ~ взаимная выгода; to take (*или* to make) ~ of smth. воспользоваться чем-л.; to take ~ of smb. перехитрить кого-л.; to score an ~ получить преимущество; to ~ выгодно; to show smth. to the best ~ представить что-л. в самом выгодном свете.

advantage II [ədˈvɑːntɪdʒ] *v* благоприятствовать; давать преимущество; способствовать; продвигать.

advantageous [ˌædvənˈteɪdʒəs] *a* выгодный, благоприятный.

advent [ˈædvənt] *n* 1) приход, прибытие; вступление; появление; 2) (A.) *рел.* пришествие.

adventitious [ˌædvenˈtɪʃəs] *a* 1) добавочный; 2) побочный, случайный.

adventure I [ədˈventʃə] *n* 1) приключение; 2) рискованное предприятие; авантюра; 3) событие; 4) переживание.

adventure II *v* 1) рисковать; 2) осмеливаться (*сделать что-л.*).

adventurer [ədˈventʃərə] *n* искатель приключений; авантюрист.

adventuress [ədˈventʃərɪs] *n* искательница приключений; авантюристка.

adventurous [ədˈventʃərəs] *a* 1) смелый; 2) рискованный; 3) предприимчивый.

adverb [ˈædvəb] *n* *грам.* наречие.

adverbial [ədˈvəːbjəl] *a* *грам.* наречный.

adversary [ˈædvəsərɪ] *n* противник, соперник.

adversative [ədˈvəːsətɪv] *a* 1) выражающий противоположность; 2) *грам.* противительный.

adverse [ˈædvəːs] *a* 1) неблагоприятный; враждебный; вредный; 2) противный (*о ветре*); 3) расположенный напротив.

adversity [ədˈvəːsɪtɪ] *n* 1) неблагоприятная обстановка; 2) невзгоды, несчастья.

advert [ədˈvəːt] *v* 1) ссылаться; упоминать; 2) обращать *или* привлекать внимание.

advertence [ədˈvəːtəns] *n* внимательное отношение; внимание.

advertency [ədˈvəːtənsɪ] *см.* advertence.

advertise [ˈædvətaɪz] *v* помещать объявление; рекламировать; to ~ for smth. искать что-л. по объявлению.

advertisement [ədˈvəːtɪsmənt] *n* объявление; реклама.

advertiser [ˈædvətaɪzə] *n* 1) лицо, помещающее объявление; 2) газета с объявлениями.

advertize [ˈædvətaɪz] *см.* advertise.

advice [ədˈvaɪs] *n* 1) совет; консультация (*врача, юриста и т. п.*); 2) извещение; *pl* сообщение.

advisable [ədˈvaɪzəbl] *a* 1) целесообразный; желательный; 2) рекомендуемый.

advise [ədˈvaɪz] *v* 1) советовать; 2) давать совет, консультировать; 3) извещать, уведомлять; 4) советоваться (*с кем-л.— with*); консультироваться (*у кого-л., с кем-л.— with*).

advised [ədˈvaɪzd] *a* 1) осведомлённый; 2) обдуманный; 3) рассудительный.

advisedly [ədˈvaɪzɪdlɪ] *adv* обдуманно; сознательно.

adviser [ədˈvaɪzə] *n* советник; консультант; советчик.

advisory [ədˈvaɪzərɪ] *a* совещательный; консультативный.

advocacy [ˈædvəkəsɪ] *n* 1) защита; 2) пропаганда (*взглядов и т. п.*); 3) адвокатура.

advocateᵃ [ˈædvəkɪt] *n* 1) защитник; сторонник; 2) адвокат.

advocateᵇ [ˈædvəkeɪt] *v* защищать, выступать в защиту; поддерживать; отстаивать.

aegis [ˈiːdʒɪs] *n* защита; under the ~ of под эгидой (*кого-л.*).

aerate [ˈeɪəreɪt] *v* 1) проветривать; 2) газировать.

aeration [ˌeɪəˈreɪʃən] *n* 1) проветривание, вентиляция; 2) газирование.

aerial I [ˈɛərɪəl] *n* антенна.

aerial II *a* 1) воздушный; эфирный; *перен.* нереальный; 2) надземный.

aerie [ˈɛərɪ] *n* 1) орлиное гнездо; 2) дом высоко в горах; 3) выводок (*хищной птицы*).

aeriform [ˈɛərɪfɔːm] *a* газообразный, воздушный; *перен.* нереальный.

aerify [ˈɛərɪfaɪ] v 1) превращáть в газообрáзное состоя́ние; 2) газировать.

aerobatics [ˌɛərəˈbætɪks] n вы́сший пилотáж, фигу́рные полёты.

aerocarrier [ˈɛərəˌkærɪə] n авианóсец.

aerodrome [ˈɛərədroum] n аэродрóм.

aerodynamics [ˈɛəroudaɪˈnæmɪks] n аэродинáмика.

aerolite [ˈɛərəlaɪt] n аэроли́т, кáменный метеори́т.

aeronaut [ˈɛərənɔːt] n аэронáвт.

aeronautics [ˌɛərəˈnɔːtɪks] n аэронáвтика.

aeronavigation [ˌɛərəˌnævɪˈgeɪʃən] n аэронавигáция.

aerophone [ˈɛərəfoun] n радиотелефóн.

aeroplane [ˈɛərəpleɪn] n самолёт, аэроплáн.

aeroport [ˈɛərəpɔːt] n аэропóрт.

aerostat [ˈɛərəstæt] n аэростáт; воздýшный шар.

aerostatics [ˌɛərouˈstætɪks] n 1) аэростáтика; 2) воздухоплáвание.

aerostation [ˌɛərouˈsteɪʃən] n воздухоплáвание.

aerotechnics [ˌɛərouˈtekniks] n авиатéхника.

aery [ˈɛərɪ] см. aerie.

aesthete [ˈiːsθiːt] n эстéт.

aesthetic [iːsˈθetɪk] a эстети́ческий.

aesthetics [iːsˈθetɪks] n эстéтика.

afar [əˈfɑː] adv далекó, вдалекé, вдали́ (тж. ~ off); издалекá, и́здали (тж. from ~).

affability [ˌæfəˈbɪlɪtɪ] n приветливость; любéзность, вéжливость.

affable [ˈæfəbl] a привéтливый; любéзный, вéжливый.

affair [əˈfɛə] n 1) дéло; that is my ~ это моё дéло; mind your own ~s не вмéшивайтесь в чужи́е делá; domestic ~s внýтренние делá (госудáрства); an ~ of honour a) дéло чéсти; б) дуэ́ль; a poor ~ разг. ги́блое дéло; 2) pl дея́тельность, заня́тия; 3) воен. дéло, сты́чка.

affect¹ [əˈfekt] v 1) воздéйствовать, влия́ть (на когó-л.); 2) трóгать, волновáть; 3) затрáгивать, задевáть (интерéсы); 4) поражáть (о болéзни).

affect² [əˈfekt] v 1) притворя́ться, дéлать вид; 2) чáсто употребля́ть, люби́ть (что-л.).

affectation [ˌæfekˈteɪʃən] n 1) показнáя любóвь; притвóрство; 2) жемáнство; аффектáция; 3) искýсственность (языкá, сти́ля).

affected¹ [əˈfektɪd] a 1) трóнутый; задéтый; 2) поражённый (болéзнью); 3) повреждённый.

affected² a 1) искýсственный; 2) показнóй; притвóрный.

affection [əˈfekʃən] n 1) привя́занность, любóвь (к чему-л., кому-л.— for, towards); 2) волнéние; 3) болéзнь.

affectionate [əˈfekʃnɪt] a любя́щий; нéжный.

affective [əˈfektɪv] a эмоционáльный.

afferent [ˈæfərənt] a центростреми́тельный (о нéрве).

affiance I [əˈfaɪəns] n 1) довéрие (к — in); 2) обручéние.

affiance II v давáть обещáние при обручéнии.

affidavit [ˌæfɪˈdeɪvɪt] n юр. пи́сьменное показáние под прися́гой; to swear (или to make) an ~ давáть показáния под прися́гой; to take an ~ снимáть показáния.

affiliate [əˈfɪlɪeɪt] v 1) присоединя́ть(ся) в кá-

честве филиáла (with, to); 2) принимáть в члéны; 3) юр. усыновля́ть; 4) юр. устанáвливать отцóвство; перен. устанáвливать áвторство.

affiliation [əˌfɪlɪˈeɪʃən] n 1) присоединéние; 2) приня́тие в члéны; члéнство; 3) юр. усыновлéние; 4) юр. установлéние отцóвства; перен. установлéние áвторства.

affinage [əˈfɪnɪdʒ] n тех. рафини́рование, очи́стка.

affined [əˈfaɪnd] a срóдный.

affinity [əˈfɪnɪtɪ] n 1) свóйство; 2) рóдственность, бли́зость, схóдство, (с)родствó; linguistic ~ языковóе родствó; 3) привлекáтельность; 4) влечéние.

affirm [əˈfəːm] v 1) утверждáть; 2) подтверждáть.

affirmation [ˌæfəːˈmeɪʃən] n 1) утверждéние; 2) подтверждéние.

affirmative I [əˈfəːmətɪv] n: to answer in the ~ отвéтить утверди́тельно.

affirmative II a утверди́тельный, положи́тельный.

affixᵃ [ˈæfɪks] n 1) прибавлéние, придáток; 2) грам. áффикс.

affixᵇ [əˈfɪks] v 1) прикрепля́ть (to, on); приклéивать (мáрку); 2) приклáдывать (пéчать); стáвить (пóдпись); 3) дéлать припи́ску; 4) придавáть (смысл и т. п.).

afflict [əˈflɪkt] v причиня́ть страдáние; огорчáть, опечáливать.

affliction [əˈflɪkʃən] n 1) огорчéние; печáль; 2) несчáстье.

affluence [ˈæfluəns] n 1) наплы́в, притóк; 2) изоби́лие; богáтство.

affluent I [ˈæfluənt] n притóк (реки́).

affluent II a 1) прилива́ющий, притекáющий; 2) оби́льный; богáтый.

afflux [ˈæflʌks] n 1) прили́в, притóк, скоплéние; 2) мед. прили́в крóви.

afford [əˈfɔːd] v 1) позволя́ть себé, имéть срéдства; I can ~ buying this book я могý позвóлить себé купи́ть эту кни́гу; 2) предоставля́ть (возмóжность); 3) давáть, приноси́ть (урожáй и т. п.); доставля́ть (удовóльствие и т. п.).

afforest [æˈfɔrɪst] v засади́ть лéсом, облеси́ть.

afforestation [æˌfɔrɪsˈteɪʃən] n лесонасаждéние, облесéние.

affranchise [əˈfræntʃaɪz] v освобождáть (от рáбства, обязáтельства и т. п.).

affray [əˈfreɪ] n нарушéние обществéнного спокóйствия, скандáл, дрáка.

affricate [ˈæfrɪkɪt] n фон. аффрикáта.

affront I [əˈfrʌnt] n оскорблéние (публи́чное); to put an ~ upon, to offer an ~ to нанести́ оскорблéние (кому-л.).

affront II v 1) оскорбля́ть; 2) смéло встречáть или смотрéть в лицó (опáсности и т. п.).

Afghan I [ˈæfgæn] n 1) афгáнец; афгáнка; the ~s афгáнцы; 2) афгáнский язы́к; пуштý.

Afghan II a афгáнский.

afield [əˈfiːld] adv в пóле; на пóле; far ~ далекó; вдалекé.

afire [əˈfaɪə] adv в огнé; to set ~ поджигáть.

aflame [əˈfleɪm] adv в плáмени, в огнé; to set ~ поджигáть.

aflat [əˈflæt] adv в ýровень; наравнé; плóско.

afloat [əˈflout] adv 1) на водé, на плавý; в движёнии; to bring ~ снять с мéли; 2) в мóре; на корабле; во флóте; 3) в ходý; в разгáре (*деятельности и т. п.*).

afoot [ə'fut] *adv* 1) пешкóм; 2) на ходý; в движéнии, в дéйствии.

afore I [ə'fɔː] *adv* 1) *мор.* впередú; 2) *уст.* рáньше, прéжде.

afore II *prep* пéред.

afore- [ə'fɔː-] *pref* выше-; aforenamed вышенáзванный; aforesaid вышескáзанный, вышеупомя́нутый.

aforecited [ə'fɔːˌsaɪtɪd] *a* вышеприведённый, вышеукáзанный.

aforenamed [ə'fɔːneɪmd] *a* вышенáзванный, вышеупомя́нутый.

aforethought [ə'fɔːθɔːt] *a* преднамéренный, умы́шленный.

aforetime [ə'fɔːtaɪm] *adv* нéкогда, прéжде, в былóе врéмя.

afraid [ə'freɪd] *a predic* испýганный; to be ~ of боя́ться; to make ~ пугáть.

afresh [ə'freʃ] *adv* снóва, опя́ть, сы́знова.

African I ['æfrɪkən] *n* африкáнец; африкáнка; the ~s африкáнцы.

African II *a* африкáнский.

Africander [ˌæfrɪ'kændə] *n* африкáндер (*уроженец Южной Африки европейского происхождения, особ. голландец*).

Afrikaans [ˌæfrɪ'kɑːns] *n* африкáанс (*бурский язык*).

aft [ɑːft] *adv мор.* на кормé, к кормé.

after I ['ɑːftə] *prep* 1) *в пространственном значении выражает:* а) *местонахождение позади или после данного предмета* за; the boys were placed in a line one ~ another мáльчики бы́ли вы́строены в шерéнгу одúн за другúм; б) *движение одного человека, животного за другим, вдогонку* за; the dog ran ~ him собáка побежáла за ним; 2) *во временном значении указывает на:* а) *последовательную смену явлений, событий, фактов* пóсле; ~ dinner sit a while, ~ supper walk a mile пóсле обéда отдохнú немнóго, пóсле ýжина погуля́й побóльше; б) *промежуток времени, после которого действие произошло или произойдет* спустя́, пóсле, чéрез; ~ ten years чéрез дéсять лет; 3) *выражает сходство с оригиналом или подражание чему-л.* по, с; this picture is ~ Riepin а) э́то кóпия с Рéпина; б) э́та картúна вы́полнена в манéре Рéпина; this text is ~ Dickens э́тот текст состáвлен по произведéниям Дúккенса; ~ the latest fashion по послéдней мóде; 4) *выражает внимание, заботу о ком-л.* о, за; to inquire (ask) ~ smb. справля́ться (спрáшивать) о ком-л.

after II *a* 1) послéдующий; 2) *мор.* зáдний, кормовóй.

after III *adv* 1) сзáди, позадú; 2) затéм, потóм, пóзднее, спустя́.

after IV *conj* пóсле тогó как.

afterbirth ['ɑːftəbəːθ] *n анат.* послéд, дéтское мéсто.

afterbody ['ɑːftəˌbɔdɪ] *n* послéдняя ступéнь ракéты-носúтеля.

aftercrop ['ɑːftəkrɔp] *n с.-х.* вторóй урожáй.

after-effect ['ɑːftərɪˌfekt] *n* 1) послéдствие, результáт; 2) *мед.* послéдствие.

afterglow ['ɑːftəglou] *n* вечéрняя заря́.

after-grass ['ɑːftəgrɑːs] *n* отáва.

aftermath ['ɑːftəmæθ] *n* 1) *см.* after-grass; 2) послéдствия.

afternoon ['ɑːftə'nuːn] *n* врéмя пóсле полýдня, послеобéденное врéмя; in the ~ днём, пóсле полýдня, пополýдни; in the ~ of life на склóне лет; good ~! дóбрый день!; здрáвствуйте! (*при встрече во второй половине дня*); до свидáния! (*при расставании во второй половине дня*).

afterpiece ['ɑːftəpiːs] *n* дивертисмéнт.

aftertaste ['ɑːftəteɪst] *n* остаю́щийся прúвкус; осáдок.

'afterthought ['ɑːftəθɔːt] *n* 1) запоздáлая мысль; I had an ~ мне э́то тóлько потóм пришлó в гóлову; 2) раздýмье о прóшлом.

after-treatment ['ɑːftəˌtriːtmənt] *n* послéдующая обрабóтка.

afterwards ['ɑːftəwədz] *adv* впослéдствии, потóм, в бýдущем.

again [ə'gen, ə'geɪn] *adv* 1) снóва, опя́ть, ещё раз; ~ and ~ снóва и снóва, то и дéло; as much ~ ещё стóлько же, вдвóе; as far ~ вдвóе дáльше; 2) крóме тогó, к томý же; 3) с другóй стороны́.

against [ə'genst, ə'geɪnst] *prep* 1) *выражает действие, направленное в противоположную сторону* прóтив, в; he rode ~ the wind он скакáл прóтив вéтра; 2) *указывает на опору, фон* о, обо, на, к; the sick man leaned ~ the wall больнóй прислонúлся к стенé; the pictures stand out ~ the dark wall картúны выделя́ются на фóне тёмной стены́; the rain beat ~ the windows дождь барабáнил в óкна; 3) *указывает на столкновение двух предметов* на, с; the ship ran ~ a crag корáбль наскочúл на скалý; I ran ~ my friend я столкнýлся со своúм дрýгом; 4) *выражает противодействие чему-л., несогласие с чем-л.* прóтив; he did it ~ my will он сдéлал э́то прóтив моéй вóли; 5) *указывает на ожидание чего-л.* на, про; ~ a rainy day на чёрный день; 6) *указывает на определенный срок* к, на; ~ the end of the week к концý недéли.

agape [ə'geɪp] *a predic* разúнув рот, с разúнутым ртом.

agaric ['ægərɪk] *n бот.* пластúнчатый гриб.

agate ['ægət] *n* агáт.

agave [ə'geɪvɪ] *n бот.* агáва; столéтник.

age I [eɪdʒ] *n* 1) вóзраст; great ~ преклóнный вóзраст; to bear one's ~ well казáться молóже своúх лет; to be (*или* to act) one's ~ *разг.* вестú себя́ соотвéтственно вóзрасту; 2) совершеннолéтие (*тж.* full ~); to come of ~ достúгнуть совершеннолéтия; to be of ~ быть совершеннолéтним; to be under ~ быть несовершеннолéтним; lawful ~ граждáнское совершеннолéтие; 3) век, эпóха, перúод; Middle Ages срéдние векá; 4) поколéние; 5) *разг.* дóлгий срок, вéчность; we have not seen you for ~s мы не вúдели вас цéлую вéчность; 6) стáрость.

age II *v* 1) старéть, стáриться; 2) стáрить.

aged[a] ['eɪdʒɪd] *a* пожилóй, стáрый.

aged[b] [eɪdʒd] *a* в вóзрасте ...

ageless ['eɪdʒlɪs] *a* нестарéющий.

agency ['eɪdʒənsɪ] *n* 1) агéнтство; óрган (*учреждение, организация*); tourist ~ бюрó путешéствий; 2) деятельность; действие; 3) средство; содействие; 4) посредничество; by (*или* through) the ~ of посредством; при помощи; 5) фактор, сила.

agenda [ə'dʒendə] *n pl* 1) повестка дня; 2) памятная книжка.

agent ['eidʒənt] *n* 1) агент; представитель; constituency ~ доверенное лицо в избирательном округе; publicity ~ агент по рекламе; 2) деятель; исполнитель; ticket ~ кассир билетной кассы; 3) действующая сила; причина; фактор; colouring ~ красящее вещество; physical ~ физическое тело.

age-old ['eidʒould] *a* вековой, очень давний.

agglomerate [ə'glɔməreit] *v* собирать(ся), скоплять(ся).

agglomeration [ə‚glɔmə'reiʃən] *n* 1) накопление; скопление; 2) *тех.* агломерация.

agglutinate[a] [ə'gluːtinit] *a* 1) склеенный; 2) *лингв.* агглютинативный.

agglutinate[b] [ə'gluːtineit] *v* склеивать.

agglutination [ə‚gluːti'neiʃən] *n* 1) склеивание; 2) *лингв.* агглютинация.

agglutinative [ə'gluːtinətiv] *a* 1) склеивающий; 2) *лингв.* агглютинативный.

aggrandize [ə'grændaiz] *v* 1) увеличивать, усиливать; повышать; 2) преувеличивать; приукрашивать; возвеличивать.

aggravate ['ægrəveit] *v* 1) отягощать; усугублять; 2) *разг.* раздражать.

aggravating ['ægrəveitiŋ] *a* отягчающий; усугубляющий.

aggravation [‚ægrə'veiʃən] *n* усугубление, ухудшение.

aggregate[a] I ['ægrigit] *n* 1) совокупность; собрание, скопление; in the ~ как целое, в целом; 2) агрегат.

aggregate[a] II *a* совокупный; собранный вместе, общий.

aggregate[b] ['ægrigeit] *v* 1) объединять; соединять; 2) собираться вместе; 3) *разг.* равняться, составлять (*сумму*).

aggregation [‚ægri'geiʃən] *n* 1) собирание; 2) агрегат; 3) масса, смесь.

aggression [ə'greʃən] *n* нападение, агрессия.

aggressive [ə'gresiv] *a* 1) нападающий, агрессивный; наступательный; 2) *амер.* энергичный, настойчивый.

aggressor [ə'gresə] *n* 1) агрессор; 2) зачинщик.

aggrieve [ə'griːv] *v* огорчать, обижать.

aghast [ə'gɑːst] *a predic* поражённый ужасом, в ужасе; ошеломлённый.

agile ['ædʒail] *a* подвижной, проворный; живой (*об уме*).

agility [ə'dʒiliti] *n* подвижность, проворство, ловкость.

agio ['ædʒou] *n* 1) *фин.* лаж; 2) биржевая игра.

agiotage ['ædʒətidʒ] *n* 1) биржевая игра; 2) ажиотаж.

agitate[1] ['ædʒiteit] *v* 1) волновать, возбуждать; to ~ oneself волноваться, беспокоиться; 2) мешать, взбалтывать, встряхивать; 3) обсуждать, рассматривать (*планы и т. п.*).

agitate[2] *v* агитировать (*for*).

agitation[1] [‚ædʒi'teiʃən] *n* 1) волнение, смятение; 2) размешивание, взбалтывание; 3) дискуссия, обсуждение.

agitation[2] *n* агитация.

agitator[1] ['ædʒiteitə] *n тех.* мешалка.

agitator[2] *n* агитатор.

aglet ['æglit] *n* 1) аксельбант; 2) металлический наконечник шнурка; 3) серёжка (*орешника, берёзы*).

aglow I [ə'glou] *a predic* раскалённый, пылающий, ярко горящий; *перен.* возбуждённый; the cheeks are ~ with health щёки пышут здоровьем.

aglow II *adv* в пламени.

agnail ['ægneil] *n* заусеница.

agnate I ['ægneit] *n* родственник по мужской линии.

agnate II *a* родственный.

agnomen [æg'noumen] *n* прозвище.

agnostic [æg'nɔstik] *n филос.* агностик.

agnosticism [æg'nɔstisizəm] *n филос.* агностицизм.

ago [ə'gou] *adv* тому назад; long ~ давно.

agog [ə'gɔg] *a predic* в возбуждении, в нетерпении.

a-going [ə'gouiŋ] *a predic* в движении, на ходу; to set ~ пустить в ход.

agonize ['ægənaiz] *v* 1) мучить; 2) быть в агонии; сильно мучиться; 3) отчаянно бороться.

agony ['ægəni] *n* 1) мучение, страдание; 2) сильная боль; 3) агония.

agrarian [ə'grɛəriən] *a* аграрный.

agree [ə'griː] *v* 1) соглашаться (*с чем-л. — to; с кем-л. — with*); принимать (*предложение и т. п.*); условливаться (*о чём-л. — on, upon*); 2) уживаться, ладить; 3) соответствовать, гармонировать; 4) *грам.* согласовываться; 5) быть подходящим (*о климате, пище и т. п.; with*); 6) согласовывать, приводить в порядок (*счета и т. п.*).

agreeable [ə'griəbl] *a* 1) приятный, милый; 2) согласный; 3) соответствующий.

agreeably [ə'griəbli] *adv* 1) приятно; 2) согласно; 3) соответственно.

agreement [ə'griːmənt] *n* 1) (взаимное) согласие; to be in ~ with а) соглашаться, быть согласным с, разделять чьё-л. мнение; б) соответствовать, не противоречить чему-л.; 2) соглашение, договор; collective ~ коллективный договор; to break an ~ нарушить соглашение; 3) *грам.* согласование.

agricultural [‚ægri'kʌltʃurəl] *a* сельскохозяйственный, земледельческий.

agriculture ['ægrikʌltʃə] *n* сельское хозяйство, земледелие.

agriculturist [‚ægri'kʌltʃərist] *n* агроном.

agrimony ['ægriməni] *n* репейник.

agronomic(al) [‚ægrə'nɔmik(əl)] *a* агрономический.

agronomics [‚ægrə'nɔmiks] *n* агрономия.

agronomist [əg'rɔnəmist] *n* агроном.

agronomy [əg'rɔnəmi] *n* 1) сельское хозяйство, земледелие; 2) агрономия.

aground I [ə'graund] *a predic мор.* сидящий на мели; *перен.* находящийся в затруднительном положении.

aground II *adv мор.* на мели; *перен.* в затруднении; без средств; to be ~ сидеть на мели; to run ~ сесть на мель.

ague [ˈeɪgjuː] *n* малярия; озноб.

aguish [ˈeɪgjuːʃ] *a* 1) малярийный; 2) подверженный малярии; 3) перемежающийся.

ah [ɑː] *int* ax!, a!

aha [ɑːˈhɑː] *int* ага!

ahead I [əˈhed] *a predic*: to get (*или* to be) ~ of опередить.

ahead II *adv* вперёд; впереди; ~ of time раньше времени.

aheap [əˈhiːp] *adv* в куче.

ahem [mˈmm] *int* гм!

ahorse(back) [əˈhɔːs(bæk)] *adv* верхом (на лошади).

aid I [eɪd] *n* 1) помощь; 2) помощник; *разг.* адъютант; 3) *ист.* налог; 4) *обыкн. pl.* вспомогательные средства; пособия; training ~s учебные пособия; visual ~s наглядные пособия.

aid II *v* помогать.

aide-de-camp [ˈeɪddəˈkɑːŋ] *n* (*pl* aides-de-camp [ˈeɪdzdəˈkɑːŋ]) адъютант.

aiglet [ˈeɪglɪt] *см.* aglet.

aigrette [ˈeɪgret] *n* 1) султан, плюмаж; эгрет; 2) *тех.* пучок *или* сноп лучей.

aiguille [ˈeɪgwiːl] *n* 1) остроконечная вершина; пик; 2) игла.

ail [eɪl] *v* беспокоить; причинять боль, страдание; болеть.

aileron [ˈeɪlərɔːn] *n обыкн. pl. ав.* элерон.

ailing I [ˈeɪlɪŋ] *n* нездоровье.

ailing II *a* нездоровый, больной.

ailment [ˈeɪlmənt] *n* нездоровье, недомогание.

aim I [eɪm] *n* 1) цель; намерение; 2) прицел; to take ~ прицелиться; 3) прицеливание.

aim II *v* 1) целиться, прицеливаться (*at*); 2) метить, целить (*at*); 3) стремиться; намереваться.

aimless [ˈeɪmlɪs] *a* бесцельный.

ain't [eɪnt] *разг.* = am not; are not.

air I [ɛə] *n* 1) воздух; атмосфера; stale ~ затхлый, спёртый воздух; to take the ~ прогуливаться, дышать воздухом; 2) ветерок; 3) (внешний) вид; наружность; 4) *обыкн. pl.* важный вид; жеманничанье; to put on (*или* to give oneself, to assume) ~s важничать; ~s and graces жеманство, манерность; 5) *муз.* мелодия; ария; ◇ by ~ самолётом; to be in the ~ а) быть в неопределённом положении, висеть в воздухе; б) носиться (*о слухах и т. п.*); to be on the ~ передаваться (*или* выступать) по радио; to beat the ~ ≅ толочь воду в ступе; to clear the ~ разрядить атмосферу; to saw the ~ сильно жестикулировать, размахивать руками; hot ~ *разг.* болтовня; похвальба.

air II *a* 1) воздушный; 2) авиационный.

air III *v* 1) проветривать; 2) сушить (*бельё и т. п.*); 3) выставлять напоказ.

air-balloon [ˈɛəbəˌluːn] *n* воздушный шар; аэростат.

air-barrage [ˈɛəˈbærɑːʒ] *n* воздушное заграждение (*аэростатами*).

air-base [ˈɛəbeɪs] *n* авиабаза.

air-bladder [ˈɛəˌblædə] *n* плавательный пузырь.

air-blast [ˈɛəblɑːst] *n* 1) дутьё; 2) воздуходувка.

airborne [ˈɛəbɔːn] *a* 1) перевозимый по воздуху; *воен.* авиадесантный; 2) *predic* находящийся в воздухе; to become ~ оторваться от земли.

air-brake [ˈɛəbreɪk] *n* пневматический тормоз.

air-bridge [ˈɛəbrɪdʒ] *n* «воздушный мост».

air-built [ˈɛəbɪlt] *a* несбыточный; призрачный, химерический.

air-chamber [ˈɛəˌtʃeɪmbə] *n* воздушная камера.

air-conditioning [ˈɛəkənˈdɪʃənɪŋ] *n* кондиционирование воздуха.

air-cooled [ˈɛəkuːld] *a тех.* с воздушным охлаждением.

aircraft [ˈɛəkrɑːft] *n* 1) самолёт; *собир.* самолёты; авиация; robot ~ управляемый самолёт-снаряд; manned ~ пилотируемый воздушный корабль; 2) *attr* авиационный; ~ carrier авианосец.

air-crew [ˈɛəkruː] *n* экипаж самолёта.

air-cushion [ˈɛəˌkuʃɪn] *n* 1) надувная подушка; 2) *тех.* пневматическая подушка.

airdrome [ˈɛədroum] *n амер.* аэродром.

air-exhauster [ˈɛərɪgˌzɔːstə] *n* вытяжной вентилятор.

airfield [ˈɛəfiːld] *n* аэродром.

air-freighter [ˈɛəˌfreɪtə] *n* грузовой самолёт.

air-ga(u)ge [ˈɛəgeɪdʒ] *n* манометр.

air-gun [ˈɛəgʌn] *n* 1) духовое ружьё; 2) *тех.* пульверизатор.

air-hammer [ˈɛəˌhæmə] *n* пневматический молот.

air-highway [ˈɛəˌhaɪweɪ] *n* воздушная трасса.

air-hole [ˈɛəhoul] *n* 1) *ав.* воздушная яма; 2) отдушина; 3) полынья (*на реке*).

air-hostess [ˈɛəˌhoustɪs] *n* бортпроводница, стюардесса.

airily [ˈɛərɪlɪ] *adv* 1) воздушно, легко; 2) легкомысленно; беззаботно.

airing [ˈɛərɪŋ] *n* 1) проветривание, вентиляция; to give an ~ to проветрить и просушить (*что-л.*); 2) прогулка; to take (*или* to do for) an ~ пойти погулять.

air-jacket [ˈɛəˌdʒækɪt] *n* (надувной) спасательный пояс.

airless [ˈɛəlɪs] *a* 1) безвоздушный; 2) безветренный; душный.

air-lift [ˈɛəlɪft] *n ав.* «воздушный мост»; воздушная перевозка.

air-line [ˈɛəlaɪn] *n* авиалиния.

air-liner [ˈɛəˌlaɪnə] *n* воздушный лайнер; рейсовый пассажирский самолёт.

air-lock [ˈɛəlɔk] *n* 1) тамбур газоубежища; 2) *тех.* воздушная пробка.

air-mail [ˈɛəmeɪl] *n* воздушная почта, авиапочта.

airman [ˈɛəmən] *n* лётчик.

air-mechanic [ˈɛəmɪˌkænɪk] *n* бортмеханик.

air-monger [ˈɛəˌmʌŋgə] *n* фантазёр; прожектёр.

airplane [ˈɛəpleɪn] *n* самолёт, аэроплан; ambulance ~ санитарный самолёт.

air-pocket [ˈɛəˌpɔkɪt] *n* (*ав.* воздушная яма; 2) *тех.* воздушный мешок.

airport [ˈɛəpɔːt] *n* аэропорт.

air-proof [ˈɛəpruːf] *см.* air-tight.

air-raid [ˈɛəreɪd] *n* воздушный налёт.

air-route [ˈɛəruːt] *n* воздушная трасса.

airscrew [ˈɛəskruː] *n* пропеллер, воздушный винт.

air-shaft [ˈɛəʃɑːft] n вентиляционная шахта.

airshed [ˈɛəʃed] n ангар.

airship [ˈɛəʃɪp] n дирижабль.

airsickness [ˈɛəˌsɪknɪs] n воздушная болезнь.

air-strip [ˈɛəstrɪp] n лётная полоса; посадочная площадка.

air-tight [ˈɛətaɪt] a воздухонепроницаемый, герметический.

air-unit [ˈɛəˌjuːnɪt] n авиачасть.

airway [ˈɛəweɪ] n 1) воздушная трасса; 2) гор. вентиляционная выработка.

airwoman [ˈɛəˌwumən] n лётчица.

airworthy [ˈɛəˌwəːðɪ] a годный к полёту (о самолёте).

airy [ˈɛərɪ] a 1) воздушный, лёгкий; грациозный; 2) весёлый; 3) легкомысленный, ветреный.

aisle [aɪl] n 1) крыло здания; боковой придел (храма); 2) проход (между рядами).

ait [eɪt] n островок.

aitch-bone [ˈeɪtʃboun] n 1) крестцовая кость; 2) огузок.

ajar¹ [əˈdʒɑː] a predic полуоткрытый, приоткрытый.

ajar² adv в разладе.

ajog [əˈdʒɔg] adv мелкой рысью.

a-kimbo [əˈkɪmbou] adv подбоченясь, руки в боки.

akin [əˈkɪn] a predic родственный; сродни.

alabaster [ˈæləbɑːstə] n алебастр, гипс.

alack [əˈlæk] int уст. увы!

alacrity [əˈlækrɪtɪ] n живость, готовность.

alarm I [əˈlɑːm] n 1) тревога; сигнал тревоги; air-raid ~ воздушная тревога; to give (или to sound) the ~ бить тревогу; to ring the ~ ударить в набат; false ~ ложная тревога; 2) тревога, страх.

alarm II v 1) поднять тревогу; 2) встревожить, взволновать.

alarm-clock [əˈlɑːmˈklɔk] n будильник.

alarming [əˈlɑːmɪŋ] a тревожный.

alarmist [əˈlɑːmɪst] n паникёр.

alarm-post [əˈlɑːmpoust] n место сбора войск при тревоге.

alarum [əˈlɛərəm] n будильник.

alas [əˈlɑːs] int увы!

Albanian I [ælˈbeɪnjən] n 1) албанец; албанка; the ~s албанцы; 2) албанский язык.

Albanian II a албанский.

albatross [ˈælbətrɔs] n альбатрос.

albescent [ælˈbesənt] a белеющий; беловатый.

albino [ælˈbiːnou] n альбинос.

Albion [ˈælbjən] n поэт. Альбион, Англия.

album [ˈælbəm] n альбом.

albumen [ˈælbjumɪn] n 1) (яичный) белок; 2) биол., хим. белок.

albumin [ˈælbjumɪn] n хим. альбумин.

alchemist [ˈælkɪmɪst] n алхимик.

alchemy [ˈælkɪmɪ] n алхимия.

alcohol [ˈælkəhɔl] n алкоголь, спирт.

alcoholic I [ˌælkəˈhɔlɪk] n алкоголик.

alcoholic II a алкогольный.

Alcoran [ˌælkɔˈrɑːn] n коран.

alcove [ˈælkouv] n 1) ниша; альков; 2) беседка.

alder [ˈɔːldə] n ольха.

alderman [ˈɔːldəmən] n ольдермен, член городского управления.

ale [eɪl] n пиво, эль; ginger ~ имбирное пиво; Adam's ~ шутл. вода.

alee [əˈliː] adv с подветренной стороны; в подветренную сторону.

ale-house [ˈeɪlhaus] n пивная.

alembic [əˈlembɪk] n: through the ~ of fancy сквозь призму воображения.

alert I [əˈləːt] n тревога; сигнал тревоги; ◊ on the ~ настороже.

alert II a 1) бдительный; to keep ~ быть бдительным; 2) живой, проворный.

alert III v 1) насторожить; сделать бдительным; 2) воен. поднимать по тревоге.

alertness [əˈləːtnɪs] n 1) бдительность; 2) проворство.

Alexandrine I [ˌælɪgˈzændraɪn] n александрийский стих.

Alexandrine II a александрийский.

alexandrite [ˌælɪgˈzændraɪt] n мин. александрит.

alfalfa [ælˈfælfə] n бот. люцерна.

alfresco [ælˈfreskou] adv на открытом воздухе.

alga [ˈælgə] n (pl algae [ˈældʒiː]) морская водоросль.

algebra [ˈældʒɪbrə] n алгебра.

algebraic(al) [ˌældʒɪˈbreɪk(əl)] a алгебраический.

Algerian I, II [ælˈdʒɪərɪən] см. Algerine I, II.

Algerine I [ˌældʒəˈriːn] n алжирец; алжирка; the ~s алжирцы.

Algerine II a алжирский.

alias I [ˈeɪlɪæs] n вымышленное имя.

alias II adv иначе (называемый).

alibi [ˈælɪbaɪ] n юр. алиби.

alien I [ˈeɪljən] n чужестранец, иностранец.

alien II a 1) чужой; чуждый; далёкий (от — to, from); 2) иностранный.

alien III v 1) поэт. отдалять; 2) юр. отчуждать.

alienable [ˈeɪljənəbl] a отчуждаемый.

alienate [ˈeɪljəneɪt] v 1) отчуждать; отдалять; 2) отвращать (from).

alienation [ˌeɪljəˈneɪʃən] n 1) отчуждение; отдаление; 2) умопомешательство (обыкн. mental ~).

alienist [ˈeɪljənɪst] n психиатр.

alight¹ [əˈlaɪt] v 1) слезать, сходить; спешиваться; выходить (из вагона, экипажа); 2) спускаться, садиться (о птицах и т. п.); 3) ав. приземляться.

alight² a predic 1) зажжённый; в огне; 2) освещённый.

align [əˈlaɪn] v 1) ставить, выстраивать в ряд; выравнивать; 2) выравниваться; строиться; равняться.

alignment [əˈlaɪnmənt] n 1) выравнивание; 2) воен. равнение, линия строя.

alike I [əˈlaɪk] a predic похожий, подобный.

alike II adv подобно; точно так же.

aliment [ˈælɪmənt] n 1) пища; 2) содержание (кого-л.); поддержка.

alimentary [ˌælɪˈmentərɪ] a 1) пищевой; 2) питательный; 3) пищеварительный (о канале, тракте).

alimentation [ˌælɪmenˈteɪʃən] n 1) питание; кормление; 2) содержание (кого-л.).

alimony ['ælɪmənɪ] *n* 1) алименты; 2) содержание; 3) питание.

aline [ə'laɪn] *см.* align.

aliquant ['ælɪkwənt] *a мат.* некратный.

aliquot ['ælɪkwɔt] *a мат.* кратный.

alive [ə'laɪv] *a predic* 1) живой, в живых; 2) бодрый, живой; 3) живо воспринимающий *(to)*; to be ~ to smth. ясно понимать; сознавать что-л.; 4) кишащий *(with)*; 5) *тех.* действующий, работающий; 6) *эл.* под током *или* напряжением; ◇ to keep ~ поддерживать *(жизнь, интерес)*; look ~! живо!; no man ~ никто; any man ~ кто-нибудь.

alkali ['ælkəlaɪ] *n (pl тж.* alkalies ['ælkəlaɪz]) *хим.* 1) щёлочь; 2) *attr* щелочной; содовый.

alkaline ['ælkəlaɪn] *a хим.* щелочной.

all I [ɔːl] *n* 1) всё; все; целое *(of)*; ~ is well всё хорошо; ~ of it всё это (в целом); ~ of you все (без исключения); after ~ после всего, в конце концов; at ~ вообще; in ~ всё вместе; ~ but почти; кроме; чуть не; ~ but impossible всё возможное; for ~ I know насколько я знаю; not at ~ совсем не, отнюдь не, вовсе нет; 2) всё имущество; he lost his ~ он потерял всё, что имел.

all II *a* 1) весь; ~ day весь день; ~ his life вся его жизнь; ~ this всё это; and ~ that и всё такое; for ~ that несмотря на ~ всё то, при всём том; ~ the others все остальные; we ~ agree мы все согласны; 2) всякий; to renounce ~ attempt отказаться от всякой попытки.

all III *adv* полностью, целиком; совершенно; ~ the better тем лучше; ~ one безразлично; ~ the same a) тем не менее, всё же; б) безразлично; ~ at once совершенно внезапно, вдруг; ~ alone a) совершенно самостоятельно, без всякой помощи; б) в полном одиночестве; ~ over a) повсюду; б) полностью, совершенно; that is he ~ over! это так на него похоже!; ~ over with кончено, покончено *(с кем-л., чем-л.)*.

Allah ['ælə] *n* аллах.

allay [ə'leɪ] *v* 1) уменьшать, ослаблять; 2) успокаивать *(боль)*; сдерживать *(волнение)*.

all-clear [ɔːl'klɪə] *n* сигнал отбоя воздушной тревоги.

allegation [ˌæleˈgeɪʃən] *n* заявление; (голословное) утверждение.

allege [ə'ledʒ] *v* 1) утверждать, заявлять; 2) ссылаться на что-л., объяснять чем-л.

allegiance [ə'liːdʒəns] *n* верность, преданность; лояльность.

allegoric(al) [ˌæleˈgɔrɪk(əl)] *a* аллегорический, иносказательный.

allegory ['ælɪgərɪ] *n* 1) аллегория; 2) эмблема.

all-embracing ['ɔːlɪm'breɪsɪŋ] *a* всеобъемлющий.

allergy ['ælədʒɪ] *n* аллергия.

alleviate [ə'liːvɪeɪt] *v* облегчать, смягчать *(боль и т. п.)*.

alleviation [əˌliːvɪ'eɪʃən] *n* облегчение.

alley ['ælɪ] *n* 1) узкая улица, переулок; узкий проход между домами; blind ~ тупик; 2) аллея; 3) кегельбан *(тж.* skittle-~).

alleyway ['ælɪˌweɪ] *амер. см.* alley 2).

alliance [ə'laɪəns] *n* 1) союз; 2) брачный союз; 3) родство; общность.

allied [ə'laɪd] *a* 1) союзный; 2) родственный, близкий.

alligation [ˌælɪ'geɪʃən] *n* сплав; смешение.

alligator ['ælɪgeɪtə] *n* 1) *зоол.* аллигатор; 2) *тех.* камнедробилка.

all-in ['ɔːlɪn] *a* 1) включающий всё, всеобъемлющий; 2) *разг.* переутомлённый, выдохшийся.

all-in-all I ['ɔːlɪn'ɔːl] *n* предмет любви, всё *(для кого-л.)*.

all-in-all II *a* 1) чрезвычайно важный, решающий; 2) очень дорогой *(кому-л.)*.

all-in-all III *adv* 1) в целом, в общем; 2) целиком, полностью.

alliteration [əˌlɪtə'reɪʃən] *n* аллитерация.

all-metal ['ɔːl'metl] *a* цельнометаллический.

allocate ['æləkeɪt] *v* 1) распределять, назначать; 2) локализовать.

allocation [ˌæləˈkeɪʃən] *n* 1) распределение, назначение; 2) локализация.

allocution [ˌæləuˈkjuːʃən] *n* речь, обращение.

allopathy [ə'lɔpəθɪ] *n* аллопатия.

allot [ə'lɔt] *v* 1) распределять (по жребию); раздавать; 2) назначать; предназначать.

allotment [ə'lɔtmənt] *n* 1) распределение; назначение; 2) доля, часть; *перен.* участь, удел; 3) участок земли, надел.

all-out I ['ɔːl'aut] *a* 1) полный; тотальный; 2) решительный *(о наступлении и т. п.)*.

all-out II *adv* изо всех сил; полностью; to go ~ бороться изо всех сил; из кожи вон лезть.

allow [ə'lau] *v* 1) позволять, разрешать; 2) допускать, соглашаться *(that)*; 3) выдавать, выплачивать *(периодически)*; 4) *амер.* высказываться, утверждать *(that)*; 5) принимать во внимание, учитывать *(что-л.— for)*; делать скидку *или* поправку *(на что-л.— for)*.

allowance I [ə'lauəns] *n* 1) позволение, разрешение; 2) допущение; 3) принятие во внимание; скидка, поправка на что-л.; to make ~s for принимать во внимание; 4) *тех.* допуск; 5) (периодическая) выдача; содержание; паёк; house ~ *воен.* квартирные деньги.

allowance II *v* 1) разрешать, позволять; 2) выдавать содержание, паёк.

allowedly [ə'laudlɪ] *adv* по общему признанию.

alloy[a] ['ælɔɪ] *n* 1) сплав; 2) проба *(золота, серебра)*.

alloy[b] I [ə'lɔɪ] *n* примесь.

alloy[b] II *v* 1) сплавлять *(металлы)*; 2) подмешивать.

all-powerful ['ɔːl'pauəful] *a* всемогущий.

all right ['ɔːl'raɪt] *adv разг.* хорошо, ладно; ничего.

all-round ['ɔːl'raund] *a* всесторонний, многосторонний.

All-Russian ['ɔːl'rʌʃən] *a* всероссийский.

allseed ['ɔːlˌsiːd] *n бот.* многосемянное растение.

all-sufficient ['ɔːlsə'fɪʃənt] *a* способный обходиться без импорта *(о стране и т. п.)*.

allude [ə'luːd] *v* намекать; упоминать; ссылаться; подразумевать.

All-Union ['ɔːl'juːnjən] *a* всесоюзный.

allure [ə'ljuə] *v* 1) завлекать, заманивать; 2) пленять, очаровывать.

allurement [ə'ljuəmənt] *n* 1) обольще́ние; 2) привлека́тельность.

alluring [ə'ljuərɪŋ] *a* 1) соблазни́тельный, зама́нчивый; 2) привлека́тельный.

allusion [ə'luːʒən] *n* намёк; упомина́ние.

allusive [ə'luːsɪv] *a* содержа́щий намёк (*на —to*); иносказа́тельный.

alluvia [ə'luːvjə] *pl см.* alluvium.

alluvial [ə'luːvjəl] *a геол.* аллювиа́льный; нано́сный.

alluvium [ə'luːvjəm] *n* (*pl* alluvia) *геол.* аллю́вий; нано́сные образова́ния.

ally[a] ['ælaɪ] *n* сою́зник.

ally[b] [ə'laɪ] *v* соединя́ть; to ~ oneself соединя́ться, вступа́ть в сою́з; to be allied to быть свя́занным, быть бли́зким.

ally[c] ['ælɪ] *n* мра́морный ша́рик (*для игры*).

almanac ['ɔːlmənæk] *n* альмана́х, календа́рь.

almighty I [ɔːl'maɪtɪ] *a* 1) всемогу́щий; the Almighty бог; 2) *разг.* ужа́сный.

almighty II *adv разг.* чрезвыча́йно, ужа́сно.

almond ['ɑːmənd] *n* 1) минда́ль; 2) *анат.* миндалеви́дная железа́, минда́лина.

almost ['ɔːlmoust] *adv* почти́.

alms [ɑːmz] *n* ми́лостыня.

alms-house ['ɑːmzhaus] *n* богаде́льня.

aloe ['ælou] *n* 1) *бот.* ало́э; 2) *pl* сабу́р (*слабительное*).

aloft [ə'lɔft] *adv* наверху́; наве́рх.

alone I [ə'loun] *a predic* оди́н; одино́кий; he can do it ~ он мо́жет сде́лать э́то сам (*или* оди́н); to let (*или* to leave) ~ оста́вить в поко́е.

alone II *adv* то́лько, исключи́тельно; he ~ can do it то́лько он мо́жет сде́лать э́то.

along I [ə'lɔŋ] *adv* 1) вдоль; из конца́ в коне́ц; 2) вперёд; ◊ ~ with вме́сте; с собо́й; all ~ всё вре́мя; (all) ~ of *разг.* всле́дствие, из-за.

along II *prep* вдоль, по.

along-shore [ə'lɔŋ'ʃɔː] *adv* вдоль бе́рега.

alongside [ə'lɔŋ'saɪd] 1) вдоль; ~ with наряду́ с; 2) *мор.* борт о́ борт, у бо́рта; ~ of бок о́ бок.

aloof I [ə'luːf] *a predic* 1) отчуждённый; 2) холо́дный, равноду́шный.

aloof II *adv* пода́ль, вдали́, в стороне́; to hold (*или* to keep, to stand) ~ стоя́ть *или* держа́ться в стороне́.

aloofness [ə'luːfnɪs] *n* отчуждённость.

aloud [ə'laud] *adv* 1) гро́мко; вслух; 2) *разг.* си́льно, я́вно.

alp [ælp] *n* 1) го́рная верши́на; 2) го́рное па́стбище (в Швейца́рии).

alpha ['ælfə] *n* а́льфа; ◊ Alpha and Omega а́льфа и оме́га, нача́ло и коне́ц; са́мое гла́вное; ~ plus *разг.* превосхо́дный.

alphabet ['ælfəbɪt] *n* алфави́т; а́збука.

alphabetic(al) [ˌælfə'betɪk(əl)] *a* алфави́тный; а́збучный.

alphabetically [ˌælfə'betɪkəlɪ] *adv* в алфави́тном поря́дке.

Alpine ['ælpaɪn] *a* альпи́йский.

Alpinist ['ælpɪnɪst] *n* альпини́ст.

already [ɔːl'redɪ] *adv* уже́.

also ['ɔːlsou] *adv* та́кже, то́же; ◊ ~ ran *разг.* а) неуда́чливый уча́стник состяза́ния; б) посре́дственность (*о челове́ке*).

alt [ælt] *n муз.* альт.

altar ['ɔːltə] *n* алта́рь.

alter ['ɔːltə] *v* 1) изменя́ть(ся); 2) переде́лывать.

alteration [ˌɔːltə'reɪʃən] *n* переме́на; измене́ние; переде́лка.

altercate ['ɔːltəkeɪt] *v* препира́ться, ссо́риться.

altercation [ˌɔːltə'keɪʃən] *n* перебра́нка, ссо́ра.

alternate[a] [ɔːl'təːnɪt] *a* череду́ющийся, перемежа́ющийся.

alternate[b] ['ɔːltəːneɪt] *v* чередова́ть(ся).

alternating ['ɔːltəːneɪtɪŋ] *a* перемежа́ющийся; переме́нный (*тж. о то́ке*).

alternation [ˌɔːltəː'neɪʃən] *n* чередова́ние.

alternative I [ɔːl'təːnətɪv] *n* вы́бор; альтернати́ва; I had no (other) ~ у меня́ не́ было вы́бора.

alternative II *a* 1) взаи́мно исключа́ющий; альтернати́вный; 2) *тех.* переме́нный.

although [ɔːl'ðou] *conj* хотя́; несмотря́ на.

altimeter ['æltɪmɪːtə] *n* высотоме́р, альтиме́тр.

altitude ['æltɪtjuːd] *n* 1) высота́; высота́ над у́ровнем мо́ря; to grab for ~ а) *ав.* стара́ться набра́ть высоту́; б) *разг.* разозли́ться; 2) глубина́; 3) *обыкн. pl* возвы́шенность; *перен.* высо́кое положе́ние; знамени́тость; 4) *attr ав.* высо́тный.

alto ['æltou] *n муз.* 1) альт; 2) контра́льто.

altogether I [ˌɔːltə'geðə] *n:* an ~, the ~ це́лое; (in) the ~ *разг.* обнажённый (*о моде́ли худо́жника*).

altogether II *adv* в о́бщем, в це́лом; всего́; for ~ навсегда́.

altruism ['æltruɪzəm] *n* альтруи́зм.

altruistic [ˌæltru'ɪstɪk] *a* альтруисти́ческий.

alum ['æləm] *n* квасцы́.

alumina [ə'ljuːmɪnə] *n* о́кись алюми́ния, глинозём.

aluminium [ˌæljuˈmɪnjəm] *n* алюми́ний.

aluminum [ə'ljuːmɪnəm] *амер. см.* aluminium.

alumnus [ə'lʌmnəs] *n* (*pl* alumni [ə'lʌmnaɪ]) (бы́вший) пито́мец, воспи́танник (*шко́лы или университета*).

alveolar [æl'vɪələ] *a анат., фон.* альвеоля́рный.

alveolus [æl'vɪələs] *n* (*pl* alveoli [æl'vɪəlaɪ]) *анат.* альвео́ла.

always ['ɔːlwəz] *adv* всегда́; not ~ иногда́, не всегда́.

am [æm (*си́льная фо́рма*), əm, m (*слабые фо́рмы*)] 1-е л. ед. ч. наст. вр. гл. to be.

amadou ['æməduː] *n* трут.

amalgam [ə'mælgəm] *n* 1) амальга́ма; 2) смесь.

amalgamate I [ə'mælgəmeɪt] *a* соединённый, объединённый; сме́шанный (*обыкн. о языке́*).

amalgamate II *v* 1) сме́шивать(ся); соединя́ть(ся), объединя́ть(ся); 2) амальгами́ровать; соединя́ть(ся) с рту́тью.

amalgamation [əˌmælgə'meɪʃən] *n* 1) соедине́ние, слия́ние; 2) амальгама́ция; смеше́ние.

amass [ə'mæs] *v* 1) собира́ть; 2) накопля́ть.

amassment [ə'mæsmənt] *n* 1) ку́ча, гру́да; скопле́ние; 2) накопле́ние.

amateur ['æmətəː] *n* 1) люби́тель; дилета́нт; 2) *attr* люби́тельский.

amateurish [ˌæmə'təːrɪʃ] *a* люби́тельский; дилета́нтский.

amaze I [ə'meɪz] *n поэт.* изумле́ние.

amaze II *v* изумля́ть.

amazement [ə'meızmənt] *n* изумле́ние, удивле́ние.

amazing [ə'meızıŋ] *a* удиви́тельный, порази́тельный.

Amazon ['æməzən] *n* амазо́нка.

ambassador [æm'bæsədə] *n* 1) посо́л; Ambassador Extraordinary and Plenipotentiary чрезвыча́йный и полномо́чный посо́л; 2) посла́нец, ве́стник.

ambassadorial [æm,bæsə'dɔːrıəl] *a* посо́льский.

ambassadress [æm'bæsədrıs] *n* 1) жена́ посла́; 2) же́нщина-посо́л; 3) посла́нница, ве́стница.

amber ['æmbə] *n* 1) янта́рь; 2) *attr* янта́рный.

ambergris ['æmbəgriːs] *n* (се́рая) а́мбра.

ambidexter ['æmbı'dekstə] *a* 1) владе́ющий одина́ково обе́ими рука́ми; 2) двули́чный.

ambidexterity ['æmbıdeks'terıtı] *n* 1) одина́ковое владе́ние обе́ими рука́ми; 2) двули́чность, двуру́шничество.

ambient ['æmbıənt] *a* окружа́ющий.

ambiguity [,æmbı'gjuːıtı] *n* двусмы́сленность.

ambiguous [æm'bıgjuəs] *a* 1) двусмы́сленный; 2) нея́сный; сомни́тельный.

ambit ['æmbıt] *n* преде́лы, грани́цы; *перен.* сфе́ра.

ambition [æm'bıʃən] *n* 1) честолю́бие, амби́ция; 2) стремле́ние, цель, предме́т жела́ний.

ambitious [æm'bıʃəs] *a* честолюби́вый.

amble I ['æmbl] *n* 1) и́ноходь; 2) лёгкая похо́дка.

amble II *v* 1) идти́ и́ноходью (*о лошади*); 2) е́хать на иноходце; 3) идти́ лёгкой похо́дкой.

ambler ['æmblə] *n* иноходец.

ambrosia [æm'brouzjə] *n* 1) *миф.* амбро́зия, пи́ща бого́в (*тж. перен.*); 2) перга́.

ambulance ['æmbjuləns] *n* 1) полево́й го́спиталь; 2) санита́рная пово́зка; каре́та ско́рой по́мощи; 3) *attr* санита́рный.

ambulatory ['æmbjulətərı] *a* 1) передвижно́й; вре́менный; 2) амбулато́рный (*о больном*).

ambuscade I [,æmbəs'keıd] *n* заса́да.

ambuscade II *v* 1) скрыва́ться, находи́ться в заса́де; 2) устра́ивать заса́ду.

ambush I ['æmbuʃ] *n* заса́да; to make (*или* to lay) an ~ устра́ивать заса́ду; to lie in ~ находи́ться в заса́де.

ambush II *v* 1) находи́ться в заса́де; 2) напада́ть из заса́ды.

ameer [ə'mıə] *n* эми́р.

ameliorate [ə'miːljəreıt] *v* улучша́ть(ся).

amelioration [ə,miːljə'reıʃən] *n* улучше́ние.

ameliorative [ə'miːljərətıv] *a* улучша́ющий (-ся).

amen I ['ɑː'men] *int* ами́нь.

amen II *n* ами́нь; to say ~ to соглаша́ться с чем-л.

amenability [ə,miːnə'bılıtı] *n* 1) отве́тственность; подсу́дность; 2) досту́пность; податливость.

amenable [ə'miːnəbl] *a* 1) отве́тственный; подсу́дный; 2) сгово́рчивый; (легко́) поддаю́щийся.

amend [ə'mend] *v* 1) исправля́ть(ся); улучша́ть(ся); 2) поправля́ть; вноси́ть попра́вки (*в законопроект и т. п.*); 3) *уст.* чини́ть.

amendable [ə'mendəbl] *a* исправи́мый, поправи́мый.

amendment [ə'mendmənt] *n* 1) исправле́ние (*недоста́тков*); улучше́ние; 2) попра́вка (*к законопроекту и т. п.*).

amends [ə'mendz] *n pl* компенса́ция, возмеще́ние; to make ~ компенси́ровать, возмеща́ть.

amenity [ə'miːnıtı] *n* 1) прия́тность; любе́зность; 2) *pl* удово́льствия; 3) *pl* удо́бства.

amerce [ə'məːs] *v* 1) штрафова́ть; 2) нака́зывать.

amercement [ə'məːsmənt] *n* 1) наложе́ние штра́фа; 2) штраф; 3) наказа́ние.

American I [ə'merıkən] *n* америка́нец; америка́нка; the ~s америка́нцы.

American II *a* америка́нский. -

americanism [ə'merıkənızəm] *n* американи́зм.

americanize [ə'merıkənaız] *v* 1) американизи́ровать(ся); 2) употребля́ть американи́змы.

americium [,æmə'rısıəm] *n хим.* аме́риций.

amethyst ['æmıθıst] *n* амети́ст.

amiability [,eımjə'bılıtı] *n* 1) любе́зность; дружелю́бие; 2) привлека́тельность.

amiable ['eımjəbl] *a* 1) любе́зный; дружелю́бный; 2) привлека́тельный.

amicability [,æmıkə'bılıtı] *n* дружелю́бие.

amicable ['æmıkəbl] *a* дру́жеский; дру́жественный.

amid [ə'mıd] *prep* среди́, посреди́, ме́жду.

amidships [ə'mıdʃıps] *adv* в середи́не корабля́.

amidst [ə'mıdst] *см.* amid.

amir [ə'mıə] *см.* ameer.

amiss [ə'mıs] *adv* 1) оши́бочно; не в поря́дке; нела́дно, пло́хо; not ~ недурно; 2) неуда́чно, некста́ти; to come ~ приходи́ть некста́ти, не во́время; ◊ to take ~ обижа́ться; what's ~ ? в чём де́ло?; to draw ~ вводи́ть в заблужде́ние.

amity ['æmıtı] *n* дру́жба.

ammeter ['æmıtə] *n эл.* ампермétр.

ammonia [ə'mounjə] *n хим.* аммиа́к; 2) *разг.* нашаты́рный спирт (*тж.* liquid ~).

ammoniac [ə'mounıæk] *a хим.* аммиа́чный.

ammunition [,æmju'nıʃən] *n* боеприпа́сы; сна́ряды, патро́ны.

amnesty I ['æmnestı] *n* 1) амни́стия; 2) созна́тельное попусти́тельство.

amnesty II *v* амнисти́ровать.

amoeba [ə'miːbə] *n* (*pl тж.* amoebae [ə'miːbiː] *зоол.* амёба.

amok [ə'mɔk] *см.* amuck.

among [ə'mʌŋ] *prep* 1) среди́, ме́жду; 2) из, из числа́, из среды́.

amongst [ə'mʌŋst] *см.* among.

amoral [æ'mɔrəl] *a* амора́льный.

amorous ['æmərəs] *a* 1) влюблённый; 2) влю́бчивый; 3) любо́вный.

amorousness ['æmərəsnıs] *n* 1) влюблённость; 2) влю́бчивость.

amorphous [ə'mɔːfəs] *a* бесфо́рменный; амо́рфный; некристалли́ческий.

amortisation [ə,mɔːtı'zeıʃən] *n* амортиза́ция; погаше́ние до́лга.

amortise [ə'mɔːtaız] *v* 1) амортизи́ровать; погаша́ть долг; 2) отчужда́ть иму́щество.

amount I [ə'maunt] *n* 1) су́мма, ито́г; 2) коли́чество; a considerable ~ of значи́тельное коли́чество чего-л.; in ~ по коли́честву; 3) значе́ние, ва́жность.

amount II *v* 1) составля́ть; достига́ть; равня́ться (*чему-л.* — *to*); 2) быть равноси́льным, равнозна́чным.

amour [ə'muə] *n* любо́вь; любо́вная интри́га.

ampere ['æmpɛə] *n эл.* ампе́р.

ampersand ['æmpəsænd] *n* знак & (= and).

Amphibia [æm'fɪbɪə] *n pl зоол.* земново́дные, амфи́бии.

amphibian I [æm'fɪbɪən] *n* 1) *зоол.* амфи́бия; 2) *ав.* самолёт-амфи́бия.

amphibian II *a* земново́дный.

amphibious [æm'fɪbɪəs] *a* земново́дный.

amphitheatre ['æmfɪˌθɪətə] *n* амфитеа́тр.

ample ['æmpl] *a* 1) вполне́ доста́точный; обма́льный; 2) просто́рный; обши́рный; 3) простра́нный.

amplification [ˌæmplɪfɪ'keɪʃən] *n* 1) расшире́ние, увеличе́ние; 2) преувеличе́ние; 3) *радио* усиле́ние.

amplifier ['æmplɪfaɪə] *n радио* усили́тель.

amplify ['æmplɪfaɪ] *v* 1) расширя́ть(ся), увели́чивать(ся); 2) преувели́чивать; 3) *радио* уси́ливать.

amplitude ['æmplɪtjuːd] *n* 1) *физ., астр.* амплиту́да; 2) полнота́; оби́лие; 3) широта́, разма́х.

amply ['æmplɪ] *adv* 1) доста́точно; оби́льно; 2) простра́нно.

ampoule ['æmpuːl] *n* а́мпула.

amputate ['æmpjuteɪt] *v* отнима́ть, ампути́ровать.

amputation [ˌæmpju'teɪʃən] *n* ампута́ция.

amuck [ə'mʌk] *adv*: to run ~ а) в я́рости набра́сываться на всех; б) обезу́меть, быть вне себя́.

amulet ['æmjulɪt] *n* амуле́т, талисма́н.

amuse [ə'mjuːz] *v* забавля́ть; развлека́ть; you ~ me вы меня́ смеши́те.

amusement [ə'mjuːzmənt] *n* развлече́ние, заба́ва.

amusing [ə'mjuːzɪŋ] *a* заба́вный, занима́тельный.

an [æn (*сильная форма*), эп (*слабая форма*)] *см.* a II; *употребляется перед словами, начинающимися с гласного или немого* h (heir, hour, honour, honest *и их производными*): an apple я́блоко; an hour час; an honest man че́стный челове́к.

ana ['ɑːnə] *n* 1) сбо́рник изрече́ний, выска́зываний; 2) *pl* анекдо́ты; воспомина́ния (*о каком-л. лице́*).

anachronism [ə'nækrənɪzəm] *n* анахрони́зм.

anaemia [ə'niːmjə] *n мед.* малокро́вие, анеми́я.

anaemic [ə'niːmɪk] *a мед.* малокро́вный, анеми́чный.

anaesthesia [ˌænɪs'θiːzjə] *n* обезбо́ливание, анестезия.

anaesthetic I [ˌænɪs'θetɪk] *n* обезбо́ливающее, анестези́рующее сре́дство.

anaesthetic II *a* обезбо́ливающий, анестези́рующий.

anaesthetize [æ'niːsθɪtaɪz] *v* обезбо́ливать, анестези́ровать.

analogical [ˌænə'lɔdʒɪkəl] *a* осно́ванный на анало́гии, аналоги́ческий.

analogous [ə'næləgəs] *a* аналоги́чный, схо́дный.

analogy [ə'nælədʒɪ] *n* анало́гия; схо́дство; by ~ with, on the ~ of по анало́гии с.

analyse ['ænəlaɪz] *v* 1) анализи́ровать; 2) *хим., физ.* разлага́ть; 3) *грам.* разбира́ть (*предложе́ние*).

analysis [ə'næləsɪs] *n* (*pl* analyses [ə'næləsiːz]) 1) ана́лиз; 2) *хим., физ.* разложе́ние; 3) *грам.* разбо́р; sentence ~ синтакси́ческий разбо́р.

analyst ['ænəlɪst] *n* 1) анали́тик; 2) лабора́нт-хи́мик.

analytic(al) [ˌænə'lɪtɪk(əl)] *a* аналити́ческий.

anamnesis [ˌænæm'niːsɪs] *n* 1) воспомина́ние; 2) *мед.* ана́мнез.

anapaest ['ænəpiːst] *n лит.* ана́пест.

anarchic(al) [æ'nɑːkɪk(əl)] *a* анархи́ческий.

anarchist ['ænəkɪst] *n* анархи́ст.

anarchy ['ænəkɪ] *n* ана́рхия.

anathema [ə'næθɪmə] *n* 1) ана́фема, отлуче́ние от це́ркви; 2) прокля́тие.

anatomical [ˌænə'tɔmɪkəl] *a* анатоми́ческий.

anatomize [ə'nætəmaɪz] *v* 1) анатоми́ровать; 2) анализи́ровать, разбира́ть крити́чески.

anatomy [ə'nætəmɪ] *n* 1) анато́мия; 2) анатоми́рование; 3) *разг.* скеле́т, о́чень худо́й челове́к.

ancestor ['ænsɪstə] *n* пре́док.

ancestral [æn'sestrəl] *a* насле́дственный, родово́й.

ancestry ['ænsɪstrɪ] *n* 1) пре́дки; 2) происхожде́ние.

anchor I ['æŋkə] *n* 1) я́корь; to be (*или* to lie, to ride) at ~ стоя́ть на я́коре; to cast (*или* to drop) ~ броса́ть я́корь; to weigh (*или* to raise) ~ снима́ться с я́коря; to come to ~ стать на я́корь, бро́сить я́корь; 2) я́корь спасе́ния; си́мвол наде́жды; 3) *тех.* а́нкер.

anchor II *v* 1) ста́вить *или* стать на я́корь; 2) укрепи́ть(ся); установи́ться; 3) остепени́ться; 4) скрепля́ть, закрепля́ть.

anchorage ['æŋkərɪdʒ] *n* 1) я́корная стоя́нка; 2) стоя́нка на я́коре; 3) я́корный сбор; 4) закрепле́ние; укрепле́ние; анкера́ж; 5) опо́ра, я́корь спасе́ния.

anchoret ['æŋkəret] *n* отше́льник, анахоре́т.

anchorite ['æŋkəraɪt] *см.* anchoret.

anchovy ['æntʃəvɪ] *n* анчо́ус.

ancient I ['eɪnʃənt] *n*: the ~s а) дре́вние наро́ды; б) анти́чные писа́тели.

ancient II *a* 1) дре́вний, ста́рый; 2) анти́чный.

ancle ['æŋkl] *см.* ankle.

and [ænd (*сильная форма*), ənd, ən, n (*слабые формы*)] *conj* 1) *соедини́тельный союз* и; Jack ~ Jill Джек и Джил; 2) *противи́тельный союз* a; I live in London and he lives in Moscow я живу́ в Ло́ндоне, а он в Москве́; 3) *разг. между глаголами вместо* to: try ~ do it постара́йтесь сде́лать э́то.

andiron ['ændaɪən] *n* подста́вка для дров в ками́не.

anecdote ['ænɪkdout] *n* анекдо́т, заба́вный слу́чай; коро́ткий расска́з.

anecdotic(al) [ˌænek'dɔtɪk(əl)] *a* анекдоти́чный, анекдоти́ческий.

anemone [ə'nemənɪ] *n бот.* анемо́н.

anew [ə'njuː] *adv* 1) сно́ва; 2) за́ново; по-но́вому.

anfractuous [æn'fræktʃuəs] *a* 1) изви́листый; 2) сло́жный, запу́танный.

angel ['eɪndʒəl] *n* 1) áнгел; guardian ~ áнгел-хранúтель, дóбрый гéний; lost ~ пáдший áнгел; 2) *разг.* лицó, окáзывающее финáнсовую поддéржку; 3) *ист.* золотáя монéта.

angelic [æn'dʒelɪk] *a* áнгельский.

anger I ['æŋgə] *n* гнев.

anger II *v* сердúть, раздражáть.

angina [æn'dʒaɪnə] *n* ангúна.

angle[1] ['æŋgl] *n* 1) ýгол; right ~ прямóй ýгол; oblique ~ косóй ýгол; 2) угóльник; 3) тóчка зрéния; to get (*или* to use) a new ~ on smth. посмотрéть на что-л. с инóй тóчки зрéния.

angle[2] I *n* рыболóвный крючóк.

angle[2] II *v* удúть рыбý; *перен.* закúдывать ýдочку.

angler ['æŋglə] *n* 1) рыболóв; 2) *зоол.* морскóй чёрт.

Anglican I ['æŋglɪkən] *n* член англикáнской цéркви.

Anglican II *a* 1) англикáнский; 3) *амер.* англúйский.

Anglo-Saxon I ['æŋglou'sæksən] *n* 1) англосáкс; 2) древнеанглúйский язык.

Anglo-Saxon II *a* англосаксóнский.

angrily ['æŋgrɪlɪ] *adv* сердúто, гнéвно.

angry ['æŋgrɪ] *a* 1) сердúтый, гнéвный; раздражённый; to get ~ at рассердúться на что-л.; to grow ~ with рассердúться на когó-л.; to make ~ рассердúть, разгнéвать; to be ~ with smb. сердúться на когó-л.; 2) воспалённый (*о ра-не и т. п.*).

anguish ['æŋgwɪʃ] *n* сúльное страдáние, жестóкая боль, мучéние.

angular ['æŋgjulə] *a* 1) угловóй, угóльный; с углáми; 2) угловáтый, невлóвкий; 3) худóй.

angularity [,æŋgju'lærɪtɪ] *n* угловáтость.

anhydride [æn'haɪdraɪd] *n хим.* ангидрúд.

anhydrite [æn'haɪdraɪt] *n мин.* ангидрúт, безвóдный гипс.

anhydrous [æn'haɪdrəs] *a хим.* безвóдный.

anil ['ænɪl] *n* индúго.

aniline ['ænɪliːn] *n хим.* 1) анилúн; 2) *attr* анилúновый.

animadvert [,ænɪmæd'vəːt] *v* критиковáть, осуждáть (on).

animal I ['ænɪməl] *n* живóтное.

animal II *a* живóтный; скóтский.

animate[a] ['ænɪmɪt] *a* живóй; оживлённый; (во)одушевлённый.

animate[b] ['ænɪmeɪt] *v* оживлять; вдохновлять; воодушевлять; ободрять.

animated ['ænɪmeɪtɪd] *a* оживлённый.

animation [,ænɪ'meɪʃən] *n* оживлéние; воодушевлéние; жúвость.

animosity [,ænɪ'mɔsɪtɪ] *a* 1) враждéбность, злóба; 2) враждá.

animus ['ænɪməs] *n* 1) неприязнь; предубеждéние; 2) враждéбность.

ankle ['æŋkl] *n* лодыжка.

anklet ['æŋklɪt] *n* ножнóй браслéт.

anna ['ænə] *n* áнна (*индийская монета*).

annalist ['ænəlɪst] *n* летопúсец; историóграф.

annals ['ænlz] *n pl* аннáлы, лéтопись.

anneal [ə'niːl] *v* 1) *тех.* отжигáть (*стекло*); прокáливать, отпускáть (*сталь*); 2) закалять (*характер, волю*).

annex[a] ['æneks] *n* 1) дополнéние, приложéние (*к документу и т. п.*); 2) пристрóйка, флúгель.

annex[b] [ə'neks] *v* 1) присоединять, аннексúровать; 2) прилагáть; дéлать приложéние (*к книге и т. п.*).

annexation [,ænek'seɪʃən] *n* присоединéние, аннéксия.

annihilate [ə'naɪəleɪt] *v* 1) уничтожáть; истреблять; 2) *уст.* упразднять, аннулúровать.

annihilation [ə,naɪə'leɪʃən] *n* 1) уничтожéние; истреблéние; 2) *уст.* упразднéние, отмéна.

anniversary I [,ænɪ'vəːsərɪ] *n* годовщúна.

anniversary II *a* ежегóдный, годовóй.

Anno Domini I ['ænou'dɔmɪnaɪ] *adv* нóвой эры.

Anno Domini II *n разг.* стáрость.

annotate ['ænouteɪt] *v* 1) аннотúровать; 2) снабжáть примечáниями.

annotation [,ænou'teɪʃən] *n* 1) аннотáция; 2) примечáние.

announce [ə'nauns] *v* 1) объявлять; заявлять; извещáть; сообщáть; 2) доклáдывать (*о чьём-л. прихóде и т. п.*).

announcement [ə'naunsmənt] *n* объявлéние; извещéние; сообщéние; spot ~ *разг.* объявлéние (*после обычной радиопередачи*).

announcer [ə'naunsə] *n* дúктор.

annoy I [ə'nɔɪ] *n уст., поэт.* досáда; неприятность.

annoy II *v* 1) досаждáть, раздражáть; 2) надоедáть; беспокóить.

annoyance [ə'nɔɪəns] *n* 1) досáда; раздражéние; 2) надоедáние.

annoying [ə'nɔɪɪŋ] *a* досáдный; раздражáющий; надоéдливый; how ~ ! какáя досáда!

annual I ['ænjuəl] *n* 1) однолéтнее растéние; 2) ежегóдник (*книга*).

annual II *a* ежегóдный; годовóй.

annually ['ænjuəlɪ] *adv* ежегóдно.

annuity [ə'njuːɪtɪ] *n* ежегóдная рéнта; life ~ пожúзненная рéнта.

annul [ə'nʌl] *v* аннулúровать; отменять; уничтожáть.

annular ['ænjulə] *a* кольцеобрáзный; кольцевóй.

annulet ['ænjulet] *n* 1) колéчко; 2) *архит.* поясóк колóнны, завитóк.

annulment [ə'nʌlmənt] *n* аннулúрование; отмéна; уничтожéние.

annunciate [ə'nʌnʃeɪt] *v* объявлять; возвещáть.

annunciation [ə,nʌnsɪ'eɪʃən] *n* 1) объявлéние; возвещéние; 2) (A.) *рел.* благовéщение.

anode ['ænoud] *n эл.* анóд.

anodyne I ['ænoudaɪn] *n* болеутоляющее срéдство.

anodyne II *a* болеутоляющий, успокáивающий.

anointment [ə'nɔɪntmənt] *n* 1) смáзывание; 2) *рел.* помáзание.

anomalous [ə'nɔmələs] *a* непрáвильный, ненормáльный.

anomaly [ə'nɔməlɪ] *n* аномáлия.

anon [ə'nɔn] *adv уст.* сейчáс, тóтчас; ever and ~ то и дéло.

anonym ['ænənɪm] *n* 1) анонúм; 2) псевдонúм.

anonymity [,ænə'nɪmɪtɪ] *n* анонúмность.

anonymous [ə'nɔnɪməs] *a* анонúмный.

anorak ['ænəræk] *n* спортúвная кýртка с капюшóном.

another [ə'nʌðə] *pron* другой; ещё один; one ∼ друг друга; one with ∼ вместе; в среднем.

anoxia [ə'nɒksɪə] *n мед.* кислородное голодание.

answer I ['ɑːnsə] *n* 1) ответ; in ∼ to в ответ на; confused ∼ туманный ответ; 2) *мат.* решение; ответ (*задачи*); 3) *юр.* письменное объяснение ответчика по делу.

answer II *v* 1) отвечать; откликаться; 2) открыть (*дверь — на звонок, стук и т. п.*); ответить (*по телефону*); 3) отвечать (*требованиям и т. п.*); удовлетворять; соответствовать; 4) быть ответственным; ручаться (*за — for*); 5) удаваться, иметь успех; □ to ∼ back *груб.* дерзить, огрызаться.

answerable ['ɑːnsərəbl] *a* ответственный (*перед — to, за — for*).

answerless ['ɑːnsəlɪs] *a* безответный.

an't [ɑːnt] *разг.* = am not, are not.

ant [ænt] *n* муравей; white ∼ термит.

antagonism [æn'tægənɪzəm] *n* 1) антагонизм; вражда; 2) сопротивление, противодействие (*to, against*).

antagonist [æn'tægənɪst] *n* антагонист, соперник, противник.

antagonistic [æn,tægə'nɪstɪk] *a* 1) антогонистический, враждебный; 2) противодействующий.

antagonize [æn'tægənaɪz] *v* 1) противодействовать; 2) вызывать вражду, антагонизм; 3) *амер.* сопротивляться.

Antarctic [ænt'ɑːktɪk] *n* (the ∼) Антарктика.

antarctic *a* антарктический, южнополярный.

ant-bear ['ænt'bɛə] *n зоол.* муравьед.

ant-eater ['ænt,iːtə] *см.* ant-bear.

antecedence [,æntɪ'siːdəns] *n* 1) предшествование; 2) первенство, приоритет.

antecedent I [,æntɪ'siːdənt] *n* 1) предшествующее, предыдущее; 2) *pl* прошлая жизнь, прошлое; 3) *мат.* предыдущий член отношения.

antecedent II *a* 1) предшествующий, предыдущий (*to*); 2) априорный, предполагаемый.

antechamber ['æntɪ,tʃeɪmbə] *n* прихожая, передняя.

antedate I ['æntɪ'deɪt] *n* дата, поставленная задним числом (*особ. в письме*).

antedate II *v* 1) датировать задним числом; 2) предшествовать; 3) предвосхищать.

antediluvian I ['æntɪdɪ'luːvjən] *n* 1) старомодный человек; 2) глубокий старик.

antediluvian II *a* допотопный.

antelope ['æntɪloup] *n* антилопа.

antemeridian ['æntɪmə'rɪdɪən] *a* утренний, дополуденный.

ante meridiem ['æntɪmə'rɪdɪəm] *adv* до полудня (*сокр.* a. m.).

antenna [æn'tenə] *n* (*pl* antennae [æn'teniː]) 1) *радио* антенна; 2) *зоол.* щупальце, усик.

anterior [æn'tɪərɪə] *a* 1) передний; 2) предшествующий (*to*).

anteriority [,æntɪərɪ'ɒrɪtɪ] *n* первенство.

anteriorly [æn'tɪərɪəlɪ] *adv* раньше, прежде.

ante-room ['æntɪrum] *n* передняя.

ant-fly ['æntflaɪ] *n* крылатый муравей.

anthem I ['ænθəm] *n* 1) гимн; national ∼ государственный *или* национальный гимн; 2) церковный хорал.

anthem II *v поэт.* петь гимны.

anther ['ænθə] *n бот.* пыльник.

ant-hill ['ænthɪl] *n* муравейник.

anthology [æn'θɒlədʒɪ] *n* антология.

anthracite ['ænθrəsaɪt] *n* антрацит.

anthrax ['ænθræks] *n мед.* 1) карбункул; 2) сибирская язва.

anthropoid I ['ænθrəpɔɪd] *n* человекообразная обезьяна, антропоид.

anthropoid II *a* человекообразный.

anthropology [,ænθrə'pɒlədʒɪ] *n* антропология.

anthropophagy [,ænθrə'pɒfədʒɪ] *n* людоедство.

anti- ['æntɪ-] *pref* противо-, анти-; antibiotic антибиотик.

anti-aircraft ['æntɪ'ɛəkrɑːft] *a* противовоздушный; зенитный.

antibiotic ['æntɪbaɪ'ɒtɪk] *n* антибиотик.

antic I ['æntɪk] *n* 1) *обыкн. pl* гримасы, ужимки; 2) *уст.* гротеск; 3) *уст.* шут, фигляр.

antic II *a уст.* шутовской.

antichrist ['æntɪkraɪst] *n* антихрист.

anticipant [æn'tɪsɪpənt] *a* ожидающий; предчувствующий, предвидящий.

anticipate [æn'tɪsɪpeɪt] *v* 1) предвидеть, предчувствовать, ожидать; 2) предупреждать, предвосхищать; 3) делать что-л. раньше времени.

anticipation [æn,tɪsɪ'peɪʃən] *n* ожидание, предчувствие; by ∼ заранее; in ∼ of в ожидании чего-л.

anticipatory [æn'tɪsɪpeɪtərɪ] *a* 1) предупреждающий, предварительный; 2) преждевременный.

anticlerical ['æntɪ'klerɪkl] *a* актиклерикальный.

anticyclone ['æntɪ'saɪkloun] *n* антициклон.

antidote ['æntɪdout] *n* противоядие (*against, for, to*).

anti-fascist I ['æntɪ'fæʃɪst] *n* антифашист.

anti-fascist II *a* антифашистский.

antifreeze ['æntɪ'friːz] *n авто* антифриз.

anti-imperialistic ['æntɪɪm,pɪərɪə'lɪstɪk] *a* антиимпериалистический.

antimech(anized) ['æntɪ'mek(ənaɪzd)] *a амер.* противотанковый.

anti-missile ['æntɪ'mɪsaɪl] *a* противоракетный.

antimony ['æntɪmənɪ] *n хим.* сурьма.

antipathetic [æn,tɪpə'θetɪk] *a* антипатичный.

antipathy [æn'tɪpəθɪ] *n* антипатия, отвращение.

antipodal [æn'tɪpədl] *a* диаметрально противоположный.

antipodes [æn'tɪpədiːz] *n pl* 1) *геогр.* антиподы; 2) антиподы, противоположности.

antiquarian I [,æntɪ'kwɛərɪən] *n* собиратель, любитель древностей; антиквар.

antiquarian II *a* антикварный.

antiquary ['æntɪkwərɪ] *n* собиратель древностей; антиквар.

antiquated ['æntɪkweɪtɪd] *a* 1) устаревший; 2) старомодный.

antique I [æn'tiːk] *n* 1) антикварная вещь; 2) произведение античного искусства; the ∼ античный стиль, античное искусство; 3) *полигр.* антиква (*шрифт*).

antique II *a* 1) древний; старинный; 2) античный; 3) старомодный.

antiquity [æn'tɪkwɪtɪ] *n* 1) древность; старина; high ∼ глубокая древность; 2) античность; 3) *pl* древности.

antirrhinum [ˌæntɪ'raɪnəm] *n* бот. льви́ный зев.

antiscorbutic I ['æntɪskɔ:'bjuːtɪk] *n* противоцинго́тное сре́дство.

antiscorbutic II *a* противоцинго́тный.

anti-Semite [ˌænti'siːmaɪt] *n* антисеми́т.

anti-Semitism [ˌænti'siːmɪtɪzəm] *n* антисемити́зм.

antiseptic I [ˌæntɪ'septɪk] *n* дезинфици́рующее сре́дство.

antiseptic II *a* антисепти́ческий.

antisocial [ˌæntɪ'souʃəl] *a* 1) антиобще́ственный; 2) неприве́тливый, необщи́тельный.

antitank [ˌæntɪ'tæŋk] *a* противота́нковый.

antithesis [æn'tɪθɪsɪs] *n* (*pl* antitheses [æn'tɪθɪsiːz]) 1) противоположе́ние; антите́за; 2) контра́ст (*of, between*); пряма́я противоположность (*of, to*).

antitoxic ['æntɪ'tɔksɪk] *a* противоя́дный.

antitoxin ['æntɪ'tɔksɪn] *n* противоя́дие, антитокси́н.

anti-trade ['æntɪ'treɪd] *n* антипасса́т (*ветер*).

antler ['æntlə] *n* оле́ний рог.

antonym ['æntənɪm] *n* анто́ним.

anus ['eɪnəs] *n* анат. за́дний прохо́д.

anvil ['ænvɪl] *n* накова́льня.

anxiety [æŋ'zaɪətɪ] *n* 1) беспоко́йство, трево́га; 2) стра́стное жела́ние (*чего-л.* — *for, to* + *Inf*).

anxious ['æŋkʃəs] *a* 1) озабо́ченный, обеспоко́енный, встрево́женный (*about*); 2) стра́стно жела́ющий (*чего-л.* — *for, to* + *Inf*); 3) беспоко́йный, трево́жный, тру́дный (*о времени*).

any I ['enɪ] *a* 1) *в отрицательных и вопросительных предложениях* како́й-либо, како́й-нибудь; have you ~ English books? у вас есть каки́е-нибудь англи́йские кни́ги?; 2) *в отрицательных и вопросительных предложениях как показатель части от целого; по-русски не переводится:* have you ~ butter? у вас есть ма́сло?; 3) *в утверди́тельных предложе́ниях* любо́й; ~ schoolboy would know it любо́й шко́льник зна́ет это.

any II *pron* 1) *в отрицательных и вопросительных предложениях* кто́-нибудь, кто́-либо; does ~ of you know it? зна́ет ли кто́-нибудь из вас об э́том?; 2) ско́лько-нибудь.

any III *adv* не́сколько, в како́й-то ме́ре; do you feel ~ better? вам немно́го лу́чше?; ◊ it ins't ~ good э́то никуда́ не годи́тся.

anybody ['enɪˌbɒdɪ] *pron* кто́-нибудь; вся́кий; ◊ to be ~ представля́ть собо́й что́-нибудь.

anyhow ['enɪhau] *adv* 1) ка́к-нибудь; так и́ли ина́че; 2) во вся́ком слу́чае; во что́ бы то ни ста́ло; 3) ко́е-ка́к; he does his work ~ он рабо́тает ко́е-ка́к; things are all ~ дела́ нева́жны.

anyone ['enɪwʌn] *pron* кто́-нибудь; вся́кий; любо́й; ~ could do it вся́кий мог бы сде́лать это.

anything ['enɪθɪŋ] *pron* 1) *в вопросительных и отрицательных предложениях* что́-нибудь; do you see ~? вы что́-нибудь ви́дите?; one can't say ~ more бо́льше ничего́ нельзя́ сказа́ть; 2) *в утвердительных предложениях* всё; что уго́дно; you can do ~ you like мо́жете де́лать всё, что хоти́те; ◊ ~ but далеко́ не, совсе́м не; if ~ пожа́луй, е́сли хоти́те.

anyway ['enɪweɪ] *adv* во вся́ком слу́чае; как бы то ни́ было.

anywhere ['enɪwɛə] *adv* 1) *в вопросительных*

и отрицательных предложениях где́-нибудь, куда́-нибудь; 2) *в утвердительных предложениях* где уго́дно, куда́ уго́дно, везде́.

anywise ['enɪwaɪs] *adv* каки́м-нибудь о́бразом.

aorta [eɪ'ɔːtə] *n* ао́рта.

apace [ə'peɪs] *adv* бы́стро.

apanage ['æpənɪdʒ] *см.* appanage.

apart [ə'pɑːt] *adv* 1) в стороне́; отде́льно; в сто́рону; to set ~ отложи́ть, отдели́ть; to stand ~ стоя́ть, держа́ться в стороне́; 2) по́рознь, в отде́льности; to take ~ разбира́ть на ча́сти; to know ~ (уме́ть) различа́ть, понима́ть ра́зницу; 3) кро́ме; незави́симо; jesting (*или* joking) ~ шу́тки в сто́рону, кро́ме шу́ток; 4): ~ from... не говоря́ о...

apartheid [ə'pɑːthaɪd] *n* апартеи́д.

apartment [ə'pɑːtmənt] *n* 1) ко́мната; *pl* кварти́ра; 2) *амер.* кварти́ра; 3) *attr* многокварти́рный.

apartness [ə'pɑːtnɪs] *n* обосо́бленность.

apathetic [ˌæpə'θetɪk] *a* безразли́чный, равноду́шный, апати́чный.

apathy ['æpəθɪ] *n* безразли́чие, апа́тия.

apatite ['æpətaɪt] *n* *мин.* апати́т.

ape I [eɪp] *n* обезья́на; *перен. тж.* подража́тель; to act (*или* to play) the ~ обезья́нничать, передра́знивать; ◊ to lead ~s in hell умере́ть ста́рой де́вой.

ape II *v* обезья́нничать, подража́ть; передра́знивать.

aperient I [ə'pɪərɪənt] *n* *мед.* слаби́тельное.

aperient II *a* *мед.* слаби́тельный.

aperture ['æpətʃuə] *n* 1) отве́рстие; 2) *стр.* проём; пролёт.

apery ['eɪrɪ] *n* 1) обезья́нничанье, подража́ние; 2) обезья́ний пито́мник.

apex ['eɪpeks] *n* (*pl тж.* apices) 1) верши́на, верху́шка; 2) *стр.* конёк кры́ши.

aphis ['eɪfɪs] *n* (*pl* aphides ['eɪfɪdiːz]) тля.

aphorism ['æfərɪzəm] *n* афори́зм, кра́ткое изрече́ние.

aphoristic [ˌæfə'rɪstɪk] *a* афористи́чный.

aphtha ['æfθə] *n* (*pl* aphthae ['æfθiː]) 1) моло́чница (*болезнь*); 2) *pl* а́фты, я́звы во рту; 3) *вет.* я́щур.

apiarist ['eɪpjərɪst] *n* пчелово́д.

apiary ['eɪpjərɪ] *n* па́сека.

apical ['æpɪkəl] *a* верху́шечный, верши́нный.

apices ['eɪpɪsiːz] *pl см.* apex.

apiculture ['eɪpɪkʌltʃə] *n* пчелово́дство.

apiece [ə'piːs] *adv* за шту́ку; за *или* на ка́ждого; с головы́.

apish ['eɪpɪʃ] *a* 1) обезья́ний; 2) обезья́нничающий; глу́пый.

a-plenty [ə'plentɪ] *adv* *амер.* в изоби́лии, в избы́тке.

apocope [ə'pɔkəpɪ] *n* *лингв.* апоко́па.

apocryphal [ə'pɔkrɪfəl] *a* 1) апокрифи́ческий; 2) недостове́рный.

apogee ['æpoudʒiː] *n* апоге́й.

apologetic(al) [əˌpɔlə'dʒetɪk(əl)] *a* 1) извиня́ющийся; 2) защити́тельный, апологети́ческий.

apologetics [əˌpɔlə'dʒetɪks] *n* апологе́тика.

apologist [ə'pɔlədʒɪst] *n* сторо́нник, защи́тник, апологе́т.

apologize [ə'pɔlədʒaɪz] *v* извиня́ться (*в чём-л.* — *for, перед кем-л.* — *to*); опра́вдываться.

apology [ə'pɔlədʒɪ] *n* 1) извине́ние; to make

(*или* to offer) an ~ извиняться; 2) оправдание, объяснение, защита; 3) *разг.*: an ~ for с позволения сказать.

apoplectic [ˌæpəˈplektɪk] *a* апоплексический.

apoplexy [ˈæpəpleksɪ] *n* паралич, удар.

apostasy [əˈpɒstəsɪ] *n* отступничество; измена (*делу, партии*).

apostate I [əˈpɒstɪt] *n* отступник; изменник.

apostate II *a* отступнический.

apostatize [əˈpɒstətaɪz] *v* отступаться (*from*).

apostle [əˈpɒsl] *n* апостол.

apostrophe[1] [əˈpɒstrəfɪ] *n ритор.* апострофа.

apostrophe[2] *n* апостроф (*знак* ').

apotheosis [əˌpɒθɪˈousɪs] *n* (*pl* apotheoses [əˌpɒθɪˈousiːz]) прославление; апофеоз.

appal [əˈpɔːl] *v* пугать; ужасать.

appalling [əˈpɔːlɪŋ] *a* ужасный.

appallingly [əˈpɔːlɪŋlɪ] *adv* ужасно, чрезвычайно.

appanage [ˈæpənɪdʒ] *n* 1) удел; 2) цивильный лист; 3) свойство, атрибут.

apparatus [ˌæpəˈreɪtəs] *n* (*pl тж. без измен.*) 1) прибор, аппарат, инструмент; docking ~ *косм.* стыковочное устройство; 2) орган; digestive ~ органы пищеварения; 3) гимнастический снаряд.

apparel I [əˈpærəl] *n* 1) *церк.* украшение на облачении; 2) *уст.* одежда; платье.

apparel II *v* одевать, наряжать.

apparent [əˈpærənt] *a* 1) видимый; очевидный, явный; to become ~ обнаруживаться, выявляться; 2) кажущийся; 3) *юр.* бесспорный.

apparently [əˈpærəntlɪ] *adv* по-видимому; очевидно.

apparition [ˌæpəˈrɪʃən] *n* 1) появление; 2) видение; призрак, привидение; 3) *астр.* видимость.

apparitor [əˈpærɪtɔː] *n* 1) судебный исполнитель; 2) служитель, педель (*в университете*).

appeal I [əˈpiːl] *n* 1) призыв, обращение (*к кому-л.*— to); World Peace Council's Appeal Обращение Всемирного Совета Мира; 2) просьба (*о чём-л.*— for); 3) привлекательность; to make an ~ to smb. привлекать кого-л. к себе; 4) влечение; 5) *юр.* апелляция; право апелляции.

appeal II *v* 1) апеллировать; обращаться; взывать; to ~ to reason апеллировать к здравому смыслу; to ~ to the country назначить новые выборы; 2) привлекать; 3) *юр.* подавать апелляционную жалобу.

appear [əˈpɪə] *v* 1) показываться, появляться; 2) выступать (публично); 3) выходить из печати; появляться; 4) казаться; it ~s кажется; 5) *личная форма глагола* to appear + *Inf другого глагола переводится по-русски сложноподчинённым предложением с формой* кажется *в главном предложении и личной формой другого глагола в придаточном предложении*: he ~s to think... он, по-видимому, думает...; 6) явствовать; it will ~ by what follows из последующего будет ясно.

appearance [əˈpɪərəns] *n* 1) появление; to put in (*или* to make) an ~ появляться; показываться; 2) вид, наружность; видимость; at first ~ с первого взгляда; to (*или* in) all ~ по всей видимости; судя по всему; 3) явление; призрак; ◊ to save (*или* to keep up) ~s соблюдать приличия.

appeasable [əˈpiːzəbl] *a* сговорчивый, покладистый.

appease [əˈpiːz] *v* 1) успокаивать; умиротворять;

ублажать; 2) облегчать, смягчать (*боль и т. п.*); 3) утолять.

appeasement [əˈpiːzmənt] *n* 1) успокоение; умиротворение; 2) смягчение; 3) удовлетворение, утоление.

appellant I [əˈpelənt] *n* апеллянт.

appellant II *a* 1) апеллирующий; 2) *юр.* апелляционный.

appellate [əˈpelɪt] *a* апелляционный.

appellation [ˌæpeˈleɪʃən] *n* 1) имя, название; 2) номенклатура.

appellative I [əˈpelətɪv] *n* 1) имя, название; 2) *грам.* имя существительное нарицательное.

appellative II *a грам.* нарицательный.

appellee [ˌæpeˈliː] *n* ответчик, обвиняемый.

append [əˈpend] *v* 1) привешивать; присоединять; 2) прибавлять, прилагать (*к письму, книге*).

appendage [əˈpendɪdʒ] *n* 1) привесок; придаток; 2) приложение.

appendant I [əˈpendənt] *n* придаток.

appendant II *a* 1) привешенный, присоединённый; 2) принадлежащий; зависимый.

appendices [əˈpendɪsiːz] *pl см.* appendix.

appendicitis [əˌpendɪˈsaɪtɪs] *n мед.* аппендицит.

appendix [əˈpendɪks] *n* (*pl тж.* appendices) 1) дополнение; приложение (*к книге и т. п.*); 2) *анат.* червеобразный отросток, аппендикс.

appertain [ˌæpəˈteɪn] *v* принадлежать (*to*); относиться (*к* — to).

appetence [ˈæpɪtəns] *n* 1) желание (*of, for, after*); 2) влечение (*for*).

appetency [ˈæpɪtənsɪ] *см.* appetence.

appetite [ˈæpɪtaɪt] *n* 1) аппетит; 2) склонность, вкус, охота.

appetizer [ˈæpɪtaɪzə] *n* что-л., возбуждающее аппетит, придающее вкус; закуска перед обедом.

appetizing [ˈæpɪtaɪzɪŋ] *a* аппетитный; привлекательный.

applaud [əˈplɔːd] *v* 1) аплодировать; 2) одобрять; приветствовать (*решение и т. п.*).

applause [əˈplɔːz] *n* 1) аплодисменты; 2) одобрение.

apple [ˈæpl] *n* 1) яблоко; 2) яблоня; ◊ Adam's ~ кадык; ~ of the eye а) зрачок; б) зеница ока; ~ of discord яблоко раздора.

apple-cart [ˈæplˈkɑːt] *n*: to upset one's ~ расстраивать чьи-л. планы.

apple-pie [ˈæplˈpaɪ] *n* яблочный пирог.

apple-tree [ˈæplˈtriː] *n* яблоня.

appliance [əˈplaɪəns] *n* 1) принадлежность; приспособление; 2) электроприбор (*тж.* electric ~); 3) применение.

applicable [ˈæplɪkəbl] *a* применимый, пригодный, подходящий (*to*).

applicant [ˈæplɪkənt] *n* 1) проситель; 2) претендент, кандидат.

application [ˌæplɪˈkeɪʃən] *n* 1) обращение, просьба; заявление; 2) применение, употребление; 3) прикладывание (*пластыря и т. п.*); 4) прилежание.

applied [əˈplaɪd] *a* прикладной.

apply [əˈplaɪ] *v* 1) обращаться (*к кому-л.*— to; *за чем-л.*— for); 2) применять; прилагать; прикладывать; 3) касаться, относиться (*to*); 4): to ~ oneself to усердно заниматься чем-л., отдавать все силы чему-л.

appoint [ə'pɔɪnt] v 1) назначать, определять; 2) предписывать; 3) снаряжать, оборудовать.

appointee [əpɔɪn'tiː] n назначенный.

appointive [ə'pɔɪntɪv] a амер. замещаемый по назначению (о должности).

appointment [ə'pɔɪntmənt] n 1) назначение; 2) предписание; 3) условленная встреча, свидание; to keep an ~ явиться в назначенное время; прийти на свидание; 4) должность; to hold an ~ занимать должность, состоять в должности; 5) обыкн. pl оборудование; мебель; снаряжение.

apportion [ə'pɔːʃən] v 1) распределять, делить (пропорционально, соразмерно); 2) назначать (часть, долю; кому-л.— to); наделять.

apportionment [ə'pɔːʃənmənt] n пропорциональное распределение.

apposite ['æpəzɪt] a удачный; подходящий (to).

apposition [ˌæpə'zɪʃən] n 1) прикладывание; ~ of seal приложение печати; 2) грам. приложение.

appraisal [ə'preɪzəl] n оценка.

appraise [ə'preɪz] v оценивать.

appraisement [ə'preɪzmənt] n оценка.

appraiser [ə'preɪzə] n оценщик, таксатор.

appreciable [ə'priːʃəbl] a 1) заметный, ощутимый; 2) поддающийся определению, оценке.

appreciate [ə'priːʃɪeɪt] v 1) оценивать; 2) (высоко) ценить; отдавать должное; 3) повышать(ся) (о ценности чего-л.); 4) воспринимать, различать; 5) понимать; признавать.

appreciation [əˌpriːʃɪ'eɪʃən] n 1) определение, различение; 2) признание; понимание; (высокая) оценка; 3) признательность, благодарность; 4) повышение ценности.

apprehend [ˌæprɪ'hend] v 1) понимать, постигать; схватывать; 2) задерживать, арестовывать; 3) опасаться; предчувствовать (что-л. дурное).

apprehensible [ˌæprɪ'hensəbl] a постижимый.

apprehension [ˌæprɪ'henʃən] n 1) способность схватывать; схватывание, понимание; 2) представление, понятие, мнение; 3) захват; арест; 4) опасение; предчувствие (дурного).

apprehensive [ˌæprɪ'hensɪv] a 1) сообразительный, понятливый; восприимчивый (к — of); 2) полный страха, предчувствий.

apprentice I [ə'prentɪs] n 1) ученик, подмастерье; to go ~ стать подмастерьем; to bind ~ to отдавать в учение (ремеслу); 2) новичок.

apprentice II v отдавать в учение.

apprenticeship [ə'prentɪʃɪp] n учение; ученичество; to serve one's ~ работать учеником (у мастера).

apprise [ə'praɪz] v извещать.

apprize [ə'praɪz] v уст. оценивать; (высоко) ценить.

approach I [ə'proutʃ] n 1) приближение; перен. подход; easy of ~ легкодоступный; difficult of ~ труднодоступный; 2) подступ, подход.

approach II v 1) приближаться; подходить; 2) обращаться к кому-л.; делать предложение.

approachable [ə'proutʃəbl] a доступный.

approbate ['æproubeɪt] v 1) одобрять; 2) санкционировать.

approbation [ˌæprə'beɪʃən] n 1) одобрение; 2) санкция.

approbatory [ə'proubətrɪ] a одобрительный.

appropriate[a] [ə'prouprɪɪt] a 1) свойственный, присущий; 2) подходящий.

appropriate[b] [ə'prouprɪeɪt] v 1) присваивать; 2) предназначать; ассигновать.

appropriation [əˌprouprɪ'eɪʃən] n 1) присвоение (обыкн. незаконное); 2) назначение; ассигнование.

approval [ə'pruːvəl] n одобрение; утверждение; on ~ по одобрении, по утверждении.

approve [ə'pruːv] v 1) одобрять; 2) санкционировать; 3) проявлять, показывать.

approvingly [ə'pruːvɪŋlɪ] adv одобрительно.

approximate[a] [ə'prɔksɪmɪt] a приблизительный; близкий (к — to).

approximate[b] [ə'prɔksɪmeɪt] v 1) приближаться, почти равняться; 2) приближать.

approximately [əˌprɔksɪmɪtlɪ] adv приблизительно.

approximation [əˌprɔksɪ'meɪʃən] n приближение; приближённое значение.

approximative [ə'prɔksɪmətɪv] a приблизительный; приближённый.

appurtenance [ə'pəːtɪnəns] n принадлежность, придаток.

appurtenant · [ə'pəːtɪnənt] a принадлежащий; относящийся к.

apricot ['eɪprɪkɔt] n абрикос.

April ['eɪprəl] n 1) апрель; 2) attr апрельский.

April-fool-day ['eɪprəl'fuːldeɪ] n день весёлых обманов, первое апреля.

apron ['eɪprən] n 1) передник; фартук; 2) полость (в экипаже); 3) театр. авансцена; 4) ав. площадка перед ангаром; 5) гидр. порог.

apron-string ['eɪprən'strɪŋ] n завязка передника; ◇ to be tied to one's wife's ~s ≅ быть под башмаком у жены.

apropos I ['æprəpou] a своевременный, уместный.

apropos II adv 1) кстати; 2) относительно, по поводу.

apt [æpt] a 1) способный (к чему-л.— at); 2) склонный (к чему-л.— to); 3) подходящий.

aptitude ['æptɪtjuːd] n 1) способность; 2) склонность (к чему-л.— for); готовность.

aqualung ['ækwəlʌŋ] n акваланг.

aquamarine [ˌækwəmə'riːn] n аквамарин.

aquarelle [ˌækwə'rel] n акварель.

aquarium [ə'kwɛərɪəm] n (pl тж. aquaria [ə'kwɛərɪə]) аквариум.

aquatic [ə'kwætɪk] a 1) водяной; 2) водный.

aquatics [ə'kwætɪks] n водный спорт.

aqueduct ['ækwɪdʌkt] n 1) акведук; 2) анат. канал, проход.

aqueous ['eɪkwɪəs] a 1) водяной; водянистый; 2) геол. осадочный.

aquiline ['ækwɪlaɪn] a орлиный.

Arab I ['ærəb] n 1) араб; арабка; the ~s арабы; 2) арабская лошадь; ◇ street (или city) arab беспризорный ребёнок.

Arab II a арабский.

arabesque I [ˌærə'besk] n арабеска.

arabesque II a фантастический, причудливый.

Arabian I [ə'reɪbjən] n см. Arab I 1).

Arabian II a арабский.

Arabic I ['ærəbɪk] n арабский язык.

Arabic II *a* ара́бский; арави́йский.
arable I ['ærəbl] *n* па́шня, па́хотная земля́.
arable II *a* па́хотный.
arbalest ['ɑːbəlest] *n* арбале́т, самостре́л.
arbiter ['ɑːbɪtə] *n* арби́тр, третейский судья́.
arbitrage ['ɑːbɪtrɪdʒ] *n* арбитра́ж, третейский суд.
arbitrament [ɑːˈbɪtrəmənt] *n* 1) реше́ние арби́тра; 2) арбитра́ж.
arbitrary ['ɑːbɪtrərɪ] *a* 1) произво́льный, необосно́ванный; 2) капри́зный; невы́держанный; 3) деспоти́чный.
arbitrate ['ɑːbɪtreɪt] *v* 1) реша́ть третейским судо́м; 2) передава́ть (вопро́с) в арбитра́ж; 3) быть третейским судьёй.
arbitration [ˌɑːbɪˈtreɪʃən] *n* третейский суд, арбитра́ж; ~ of exchange эк. валю́тный арбитра́ж.
arbitrator ['ɑːbɪtreɪtə] *n* арби́тр, третейский судья́.
arbor ['ɑːbə] *n* тех. вал, ось, шпи́ндель.
arboreal [ɑːˈbɔːrɪəl] *a* древе́сный.
arboreous [ɑːˈbɔːrɪəs] *a* 1) леси́стый; 2) древе́сный; 3) древови́дный.
arboriculture ['ɑːbərɪkʌltʃə] *n* разведе́ние дере́вьев и куста́рников; лесово́дство.
arbour ['ɑːbə] *n* бесе́дка (*из зеле́ни*).
arc [ɑːk] *n* 1) *мат.* дуга́; 2) ра́дуга; 3) электри́ческая дуга́; 4) *attr* дугово́й.
arcade [ɑːˈkeɪd] *n* 1) пасса́ж (*с магази́нами*); 2) *архит.* арка́да; сво́дчатая галере́я.
Arcadian [ɑːˈkeɪdjən] *a* идилли́ческий; се́льский.
arch[1] I [ɑːtʃ] *n* 1) а́рка, свод; 2) дуга́.
arch[1] II *v* 1) перекрыва́ть а́ркой; 2) изгиба́ть дуго́й.
arch[2] *a* хи́трый, лука́вый.
arch- [ɑːtʃ-] *pref* архи-; ~-liar архилгу́н.
archaeological [ˌɑːkɪəˈlɔdʒɪkəl] *a* археологи́ческий.
archaeologist [ˌɑːkɪˈɔlədʒɪst] *n* архео́лог.
archaeology [ˌɑːkɪˈɔlədʒɪ] *n* археоло́гия.
archaic [ɑːˈkeɪɪk] *a* архаи́ческий, устаре́лый.
archaism ['ɑːkeɪɪzəm] *n* архаи́зм; устаре́вшее сло́во *или* выраже́ние.
archangel ['ɑːkˌeɪndʒəl] *n* арха́нгел.
archbishop ['ɑːtʃˈbɪʃəp] *n* архиепи́скоп.
archduke ['ɑːtʃˈdjuːk] *n* ист. эрцге́рцог.
arched [ɑːtʃt] *a* а́рочный, сво́дчатый; изо́гнутый.
arch-enemy ['ɑːtʃˈenɪmɪ] *n* 1) закля́тый враг; 2) сатана́.
archer ['ɑːtʃə] *n* 1) стрело́к из лу́ка; 2) (A.) Стреле́ц (*созве́здие*).
archery ['ɑːtʃərɪ] *n* стрельба́ из лу́ка.
archetype ['ɑːkɪtaɪp] *n* прототи́п; моде́ль.
archipelago [ˌɑːkɪˈpelɪgou] *n* (*pl тж.* archipelagoes [ˌɑːkɪˈpelɪgouz]) архипела́г; гру́ппа острово́в.
architect ['ɑːkɪtekt] *n* архите́ктор; зо́дчий; *перен.* творе́ц; ~ of his own fortunes кузне́ц своего́ сча́стья.
architectonic [ˌɑːkɪtekˈtɔnɪk] *a* архитекту́рный; структу́рный.
architectonics [ˌɑːkɪtekˈtɔnɪks] *n* архитекто́ника.
architectural ['ɑːkɪˈtektʃərəl] *a* архитекту́рный.
architecture ['ɑːkɪtektʃə] *n* 1) архитекту́ра; зо́дчество; 2) структу́ра; the ~ of a speech построе́ние ре́чи.
archival [ɑːˈkaɪvəl] *a* архи́вный.

archive ['ɑːkaɪv] *n обыкн. pl* архи́в.
archivist ['ɑːkɪvɪst] *n* архива́риус.
archly ['ɑːtʃlɪ] *adv* лука́во.
archway ['ɑːtʃweɪ] *n* сво́дчатый прохо́д, прохо́д под а́ркой.
archwise ['ɑːtʃwaɪz] *adv* в фо́рме а́рки, дугообра́зно.
arctic I ['ɑːktɪk] *n* 1) (the A.) А́рктика; 2) *pl амер. разг.* тёплые бо́ты.
arctic II *a* поля́рный, се́верный.
ardency ['ɑːdənsɪ] *n* жар, пыл; рве́ние.
ardent ['ɑːdənt] *a* 1) горя́чий; пы́лкий; ре́вностный; 2) пыла́ющий.
ardently ['ɑːdəntlɪ] *adv* горячо́, пы́лко.
ardour ['ɑːdə] *n* жар, пыл; рве́ние.
arduous ['ɑːdjuəs] *a* 1) тру́дный; 2) круто́й (*о подъёме и т. п.*); недосту́пный; 3) энерги́чный; напряжённый.
are [ɑː (*сильная форма*), ə, ə (*слабые формы*)] *мн. ч. наст. вр. изъяв. накл. ел.* to be.
area ['ɛərɪə] *n* 1) пло́щадь; простра́нство; 2) зо́на; о́бласть, райо́н; *перен.* сфе́ра; охва́т; 3) вну́тренний дво́рик (*ниже у́ровня у́лицы*).
arena [əˈriːnə] *n* аре́на; ме́сто де́йствия.
aren't [ɑːnt] *разг.* = are not.
arête [æˈreɪt] *n* о́стрый гре́бень горы́.
argent ['ɑːdʒənt] *a* сере́бряный, серебри́стый (*о цве́те*).
argil ['ɑːdʒɪl] *n* гонча́рная гли́на.
Argonaut ['ɑːgənɔːt] *n* 1) *миф.* аргона́вт; 2) *амер. уст.* золотоиска́тель; 3) (a). *зоол.* кора́блик (*моллю́ск*).
argot ['ɑːgou] *n* жарго́н; арго́.
arguable ['ɑːgjuəbl] *a* спо́рный, тре́бующий доказа́тельства.
argue ['ɑːgjuː] *v* 1) спо́рить (*с кем-л. — with, against; о чём-л. — for, about, against*); аргументи́ровать; to ~ against (in favour of) smth. приводи́ть до́воды про́тив (в по́льзу) чего́-л.; 2) дока́зывать; утвержда́ть; 3) обсужда́ть; 4) убежда́ть (*into*); разубежда́ть (*out of*); □ to ~ away отде́латься (*доказа́в несостоя́тельность чего-л.*).
argument ['ɑːgjumənt] *n* спор; диску́ссия; 2) до́вод, аргуме́нт, доказа́тельство; to put aside an ~ отводи́ть до́вод; 3) кра́ткое содержа́ние.
argumentation [ˌɑːgjumenˈteɪʃən] *n* 1) аргумента́ция; 2) спор.
argumentative [ˌɑːgjuˈmentətɪv] *a* 1) спо́рный, дискуссио́нный; 2) лю́бящий спо́рить; 3) логи́чный; доказа́тельный.
argus-eyed ['ɑːgəsˌaɪd] *a* зо́ркий; бди́тельный.
argute ['ɑːgjuːt] *a* 1) о́стрый; проница́тельный; 2) ре́зкий, пронзи́тельный (*о зву́ке*).
arid ['ærɪd] *a* сухо́й, засу́шливый; беспло́дный (*о по́чве*); *перен.* сухо́й, ску́чный.
aridity [æˈrɪdɪtɪ] *n* су́хость, засу́шливость; беспло́дность (*по́чвы*).
Aries ['ɛəriːz] *n* Ове́н (*созве́здие*).
aright [əˈraɪt] *adv* пра́вильно.
arise [əˈraɪz] *v* (*past* arose; *p. p.* arisen) 1) возника́ть, появля́ться; 2) происходи́ть; проистека́ть (*from*); 3) *уст., амер.* поднима́ться; встава́ть; *поэт.* воскреса́ть; 4) *уст.* доноси́ться (*о зву́ках*).
arisen [əˈrɪzn] *p. p. см.* arise.

aristocracy [ˌærɪsˈtɔkrəsɪ] *n* аристокра́тия.

aristocrat [ˈærɪstəkræt] *n* аристокра́т.

aristocratic [ˌærɪstəˈkrætɪk] *a* аристократи́ческий.

arithmetic [əˈrɪθmətɪk] *n* арифме́тика.

arithmetical [ˌærɪθˈmetɪkəl] *a* арифмети́ческий.

arithmometer [ˌærɪθˈmɔmɪtə] *n* арифмо́метр.

ark [ɑːk] *n* я́щик; ковче́г; Noah's ∼ Но́ев ковче́г.

arm[1] [ɑːm] *n* 1) рука́ (*от кисти до плеча*); with open ∼s с распростёртыми объя́тиями; 2) пере́дняя ла́па (*животного*); 3) рука́в; 4) ру́чка (*кресла*); 5) ветвь (*дерева*); 6) *тех.* плечо́ (*рычага*); рукоя́тка; ∼ of a balance коро́мысло весо́в; ◊ the long ∼ of the law си́ла зако́на.

arm[2] **I** *n* обыкн. *pl.* 1) ору́жие; in ∼s вооружённый; to ∼s! к ору́жию!; under ∼s под ружьём; up in ∼s а) гото́вый к борьбе́; б) охва́ченный восста́нием; to bear ∼s носи́ть ору́жие; служи́ть в а́рмии; to lay down ∼s сложи́ть ору́жие; сда́ться; to take up ∼s бра́ться за ору́жие; to present ∼s *воен.* брать на карау́л; 2) род войск; 3) вое́нная профе́ссия; 4) герб.

arm[2] **II** *v* 1) вооружа́ть(ся); 2) бра́ться за ору́жие.

armada [ɑːˈmɑːdə] *n* арма́да; the Invincible Armada *ист.* «Непобеди́мая арма́да».

armament [ˈɑːməmənt] *n* 1) вооруже́ние; bloated ∼s чрезме́рные вооруже́ния; 2) *обыкн. pl* вооружённые си́лы.

armature [ˈɑːmətʃʊə] *n* 1) вооруже́ние; броня́; 2) *зоол., бот.* па́нцирь; 3) *тех.* армату́ра; 4) *эл.* я́корь.

arm-chair [ˈɑːmˈtʃɛə] *n* кре́сло.

armed [ɑːmd] *a* вооружённый; укреплённый.

Armenian I [ɑːˈmiːnjən] *n* 1) армяни́н; армя́нка; the ∼s армя́не; 2) армя́нский язы́к.

Armenian II *a* армя́нский.

armful [ˈɑːmful] *n* оха́пка (*чего-л.*).

arm-hole [ˈɑːmhoul] *n* про́йма.

arm-in-arm [ˈɑːmɪnˈɑːm] *adv* под руку.

arming [ˈɑːmɪŋ] *n* вооруже́ние.

armistice [ˈɑːmɪstɪs] *n* прекраще́ние вое́нных де́йствий, кратковре́менное переми́рие.

armless[1] [ˈɑːmlɪs] *a* 1) безру́кий; 2) не име́ющий ветве́й.

armless[2] *a* безору́жный.

armlet [ˈɑːmlɪt] *n* 1) нарука́вник; 2) брасле́т; 3) небольшо́й зали́в (*реки*).

armor I, II [ˈɑːmə] *амер. см.* armour I, II.

armored [ˈɑːməd] *амер. см.* armoured.

armour I [ˈɑːmə] *n* 1) броня́ (*корабля, танка*); 2) бронета́нковые войска́; 3) вооруже́ние; доспе́хи; па́нцирь; 4) скафа́ндр; 5) *зоол., бот.* па́нцирь; 6) *attr* бронирова́нный.

armour II *v* покрыва́ть бронёй.

armour-bearer [ˈɑːməˌbɛərə] *n* *ист.* оруженосец.

armour-clad I [ˈɑːməˌklæd] *n* бронено́сец.

armour-clad II *a* бронено́сный; бронирова́нный, оде́тый в броню́.

armoured [ˈɑːməd] *a* бронирова́нный.

armourer [ˈɑːmərə] *n* 1) владе́лец оружейного заво́да; *уст.* оруже́йный ма́стер; 2) *воен.* каптена́рмус.

armour-piercing [ˈɑːməˈpɪəsɪŋ] *a* бронебо́йный.

armour-plated [ˈɑːməpleɪtɪd] *a* брониро́ванный.

armoury [ˈɑːmərɪ] *n* 1) склад ору́жия, арсена́л; 2) *амер.* оруже́йный заво́д; 3) *амер.* уче́бный мане́ж; 4) (A.) Оруже́йная пала́та (*Кремля*).

arm-pits [ˈɑːmpɪts] *n pl* подмы́шки.

arm-saw [ˈɑːmsɔː] *n* ручна́я пила́.

army [ˈɑːmɪ] *n* 1) а́рмия; the Soviet Army Сове́тская А́рмия; the Army in the Field де́йствующая а́рмия; standing ∼ постоя́нная а́рмия; to enter (*или* to go into, to join) the ∼ поступи́ть на вое́нную слу́жбу; 2) мно́жество; 3) *attr* арме́йский, относя́щийся к а́рмии.

army-beef [ˈɑːmɪbiːf] *n* *воен. разг.* мясны́е консе́рвы.

aroma [əˈroumə] *n* арома́т.

aromatic [ˌærouˈmætɪk] *a* арома́тный, аромати́чный.

arose [əˈrouz] *past см.* arise.

around I [əˈraund] *adv* 1) круго́м; вокру́г, повсю́ду; 2) *амер.* побли́зости; о́коло.

around II *prep* 1) вокру́г; 2) по; за; о́коло; to wander ∼ the town броди́ть по го́роду; ∼ the corner за угло́м; 3) *амер.* приблизи́тельно; ∼ a thousand о́коло ты́сячи.

arouse [əˈrauz] *v* 1) буди́ть; 2) пробужда́ть (*силы, спосо́бности*); возбужда́ть (*чу́вство, жела́ние*).

arraign [əˈreɪn] *v* 1) привлека́ть к суду́; предъявля́ть обвине́ние; обвиня́ть; 2) придира́ться, находи́ть недоста́тки.

arraignment [əˈreɪnmənt] *n* привлече́ние к суду́; обвине́ние.

arrange [əˈreɪndʒ] *v* 1) устра́ивать; подготовля́ть; 2) приводи́ть в поря́док; 3) усло́вливаться, сгова́риваться, догова́риваться; 4) ула́живать (*спор и т. п.*); приходи́ть к соглаше́нию; 5) приспоса́бливать, переде́лывать; 6) *муз.* аранжи́ровать.

arrangement [əˈreɪndʒmənt] *n* 1) приведе́ние в поря́док; 2) подгото́вка; *pl* приготовле́ния; 3) распоряже́ние; 4) соглаше́ние, договорённость; to make ∼s усло́вливаться; 5) приспособле́ние, переде́лка; 6) *муз.* аранжиро́вка.

arrant [ˈærənt] *a* 1) су́щий, отъя́вленный; отпе́тый; 2) *уст.* стра́нствующий.

array I [əˈreɪ] *n* 1) *поэт.* наря́д, облаче́ние, одея́ние; 2) (боево́й) поря́док; строй; 3) войска́; 4) це́лый ряд, большо́е коли́чество; ма́сса, мно́жество.

array II *v* 1) наряжа́ть, облача́ть; украша́ть; to ∼ oneself in all one's finery разоде́ться в пух и прах; 2) выстра́ивать (*войска́ и т. п.*).

arrear [əˈrɪə] *n* 1) *pl* долги́, задо́лженность; to be in ∼s име́ть задо́лженность; отстава́ть (*в чём-л.*); 2) *уст.* за́дняя сторона́, часть; in ∼ of позади́.

arrearage [əˈrɪərɪdʒ] *n* 1) отстава́ние, отста́лость; 2) оста́ток; 3) *pl* долги́, недои́мки.

arrest I [əˈrest] *n* 1) аре́ст, задержа́ние; under ∼ под аре́стом; под запре́том; 2) заде́ржка, остано́вка.

arrest II *v* 1) заде́рживать, остана́вливать; приостанови́ть (*реше́ние суда́*); 2) аресто́вывать; 3) прико́вывать (*внима́ние*); 4) *тех.* тормози́ть; выключа́ть (*маши́ну*).

arrester [ə'restə] *n* 1) *тех.* задерживающее приспособление; 2) *эл.* разрядник; lightning ~ молниеотвод; 3) предохранитель.

arresting [ə'restɪŋ] *a* 1) задерживающий, останавливающий; 2) привлекающий внимание; поражающий.

arrival [ə'raɪvəl] *n* 1) прибытие, приезд; 2) вновь прибывший; 3) *разг.* новорождённый.

arrive [ə'raɪv] *v* 1) прибывать, приезжать; to ~ at a conclusion приходить к заключению; to ~ at a decision принимать решение; 2) наступать (*о времени, событии*); 3) добиться успеха, признания.

arrogance ['ærəgəns] *n* высокомерие, надменность.

arrogant ['ærəgənt] *a* 1) высокомерный, надменный; 2) самонадеянный, нахальный.

arrogate ['ærougeɪt] *v* 1) самонадеянно претендовать, требовать без основания; 2) без основания приписывать (*что-л. кому-л.*).

arrogation [,ærou'geɪʃən] *n* самонадеянность; неоснова́тельные претензии.

arrow ['ærou] *n* 1) стрела; 2): broad ~ британское правительственное клеймо (*тж.* broad arrow-head); 3) стрелка (*на чертежах и т. п.*); ◇ an ~ left in one's quiver неиспользованное средство.

arrow-head ['æroʊhed] *n* 1) наконечник, остриё стрелы; 2) *воен.* строй «клин».

arrow-headed ['ærou,hedɪd] *a* заострённый; клинообра́зный.

arrowy ['ærouɪ] *a* 1) стреловидный; остроконечный; 2) язвительный.

arsenal ['ɑːsɪnl] *n* арсена́л.

arsenic[a] ['ɑːsnɪk] *n хим.* мышьяк.

arsenic[b] [ɑː'senɪk] *a хим.* мышьяко́вый.

arsenical [ɑː'senɪkəl] *см.* arsenic[b].

arson ['ɑːsn] *n* поджог.

art[1] [ɑːt] *n* 1) искусство; the Fine Arts изящные искусства; 2) ремесло́; 3) ловкость; умение, знание; 4) хитрость, коварство; 5) *attr* искусный; 6) *attr* художественный; ◇ to be ~ and part in быть причастным к чему-л.; black ~ чёрная ма́гия.

art[2] *уст.* 2-е л. ед. ч. наст. вр. изъяв. накл. гл. to be.

arterial [ɑː'tɪərɪəl] *a* 1) артериа́льный; 2) разветвля́ющийся.

arteriosclerosis [ɑː'tɪərɪouskliə'rousɪs] *n мед.* артериосклероз.

artery ['ɑːtərɪ] *n* арте́рия.

artesian [ɑː'tiːzjən] *a* артезиа́нский.

artful ['ɑːtful] *a* хитрый; ло́вкий.

artichoke ['ɑːtɪtʃouk] *n* артишо́к; ◇ Jerusalem ~ земляна́я гру́ша.

article I ['ɑːtɪkl] *n* 1) статья; leading ~ передова́я статья; 2) пара́граф, разде́л, пункт; 3) (отде́льный) предме́т; ~s of general consumption предме́ты широ́кого потребле́ния; 4) *грам.* член, арти́кль; definite ~ определённый член (the); indefinite ~ неопределённый член (a, an); ◇ in the ~ of death в момент смерти.

article II *v* 1) излага́ть по пу́нктам; 2) предъявля́ть обвине́ние (*кому-л.* — against; *в чём-л.* — for); 3) отдава́ть в уче́ние (по контра́кту).

articular [ɑː'tɪkjulə] *a* суставно́й.

articulate[a] [ɑː'tɪkjulɪt] *a* 1) членоразде́льный; я́сный; 2) чле́нистый; коле́нчатый; 3) *тех.* шарни́рный.

articulate[b] [ɑː'tɪkjuleɪt] *v* 1) произноси́ть отчётливо, я́сно; 2) соединя́ть, свя́зывать (*обыкн. в pass*).

articulation [ɑː,tɪkju'leɪʃən] *n* 1) членоразде́льное произноше́ние; 2) *лингв.* артикуля́ция; 3) сочлене́ние.

artifice ['ɑːtɪfɪs] *n* 1) ло́вкость; иску́сство; 2) хи́трость; 3) изобрете́ние; вы́думка, зате́я.

artificer [ɑː'tɪfɪsə] *n* 1) реме́сленник; те́хник; 2) изобрета́тель (*of*).

artificial [,ɑːtɪ'fɪʃəl] *a* иску́сственный; неесте́ственный.

artillerist [ɑː'tɪlərɪst] *n* артиллери́ст.

artillery [ɑː'tɪlərɪ] *n* 1) артилле́рия; 2) *attr* артиллери́йский.

artilleryman [ɑː'tɪlərɪmən] *n* артиллери́ст.

artisan [,ɑːtɪ'zæn] *n* реме́сленник; мастерово́й.

artist ['ɑːtɪst] *n* худо́жник; ма́стер; арти́ст.

artiste [ɑː'tiːst] *n* арти́ст эстра́ды.

artistic(al) [ɑː'tɪstɪk(əl)] *a* артисти́ческий, худо́жественный.

artistry ['ɑːtɪstrɪ] *n* мастерство́; артисти́чность.

artless ['ɑːtlɪs] *a* 1) безыску́сственный; простоду́шный; просто́й; 2) неиску́сный; нело́вкий.

arty ['ɑːtɪ] *a разг.* с прете́нзией на худо́жественность.

Aryan I ['eərɪən] *n* арие́ц.

Aryan II *a* арийский.

as I [æz (*сильная форма*), əz (*слабая форма*)] *adv* 1) как; do as you like де́лайте, как хоти́те; 2) так; as... as так же... как; he is as tall as I am он так же высо́к, как и я; as well as в тако́й же ме́ре, так же; as well та́кже (*обычно в конце предложения*); 3) в ка́честве; *тж. переводится тв. падежом*; to work as a ᛫ teacher рабо́тать учи́телем.

as II *pron* кото́рый, како́й, что; I had the same books as you had у меня́ бы́ли таки́е же кни́ги, как и у вас.

as III *conj* 1) когда́, в то вре́мя как; as I was walking in the street I met doctor B. когда́ я шёл по у́лице, я встре́тил до́ктора Б.; 2) так как, поско́льку; as it was getting dark I took the tram так как темне́ло (станови́лось темно́), я сел в трамва́й; 3) как ни, хотя́; clever as he is... как он ни умён...; as if, as though как бу́дто бы; as to, as for что каса́ется; as it were а) так сказа́ть; б) как бы то ни было.

asbestine [æz'bestɪn] *a* асбе́стовый; несгора́емый.

asbestos [æz'bestɔs] *n мин.* асбе́ст, го́рный лён.

ascend [ə'send] *v* 1) поднима́ться; всходи́ть; 2) восходи́ть; 3) возноси́ться.

ascendancy [ə'sendənsɪ] *n* власть, доминиру́ющее влия́ние (*over*).

ascendant I [ə'sendənt] *n* 1) влия́ние, преоблада́ние, власть; 2) гороско́п; ◇ in the ~ на подъёме.

ascendant II *a* 1) восходя́щий; 2) преоблада́ющий, госпо́дствующий.

ascendency [ə'sendənsɪ] *см.* ascendancy.

ascendent I, II [ə'sendənt] *см.* ascendant I, II.

ascension [ə'senʃən] *n* 1) восхождéние, подъём; 2) *амер.* прихóд; ~ to power прихóд к влáсти.

ascensional [ə'senʃənl] *a* 1) восходя́щий; 2) подъёмный.

ascent [ə'sent] *n* 1) восхождéние, подъём; 2) крутизнá, крутóй склон, подъём.

ascertain [,æsə'teɪn] *v* устанáвливать, выясня́ть, убеждáться.

ascetic I [ə'setɪk] *n* аскéт.

ascetic II *a* аскети́ческий.

asceticism [ə'setɪsɪzəm] *n* аскети́зм.

ascribe [əs'kraɪb] *v* припи́сывать (*качества, авторство, причину; to*).

ascription [əs'krɪpʃən] *n* припи́сывание.

aseptic I [æ'septɪk] *n* асепти́ческое срéдство.

aseptic II *a* асепти́ческий, стери́льный.

ash¹ [æʃ] *n* я́сень; mountain (*или* wild) ~ ряби́на.

ash² *n* 1) *обыкн. pl* золá, пéпел; to burn to ~es, to lay in ~es сжечь дотлá; 2) *pl* прах, остáнки.

ashamed [ə'ʃeɪmd] *a predic* пристыжённый; to be (*или* to feel) ~ of smth. стыди́ться чего-л; to feel ~ for smb. стыди́ться за кого-л.

ash-bin ['æʃbɪn] *n* 1) ýрна, я́щик для мýсора; 2) *тех.* зóльник.

ash-box ['æʃbɔks] *n тех.* зóльник.

ash-can ['æʃkæn] *амер. см.* ash-bin 1).

ashen¹ ['æʃn] *a* я́сеневый.

ashen² *a* 1) пéпельный, из пéпла; 2) пéпельного цвéта; 3) мéртвенно-блéдный.

ashet ['æʃɪt] *n* большóе блю́до.

ashore [ə'ʃɔː] *adv* к бéрегу, на бéрег, на берегý; to go ~ сходи́ть на бéрег; to run ~ наскочи́ть на бéрег, на мель.

ash-pan ['æʃpæn] *см.* ash-box.

ash-pit ['æʃpɪt] *см* ash-box.

ash-pot ['æʃpɔt] *n* пéпельница.

ash-tray ['æʃtreɪ] *n* 1) пéпельница; 2) *тех.* зóльник.

ashy ['æʃɪ] *a* 1) пéпельный; 2) покры́тый пéплом, золóй; 3) пéпельного цвéта; блéдный.

Asian I ['eɪʃən] *n* азиáт.

Asian II *a* азиáтский.

Asiatic I, II [,eɪʃɪ'ætɪk] *см.* Asian I, II.

aside I [ə'saɪd] *adv* в стóрону; в сторонé; отдéльно; ~ from за исключéнием; to put ~ отложи́ть; to set ~ аннули́ровать, отменя́ть; to speak ~ говори́ть в стóрону; to take ~ отвести́ в стóрону; to lay the book ~ отложи́ть кни́гу (*перестать читать*).

aside II *n* словá, произноси́мые (актёром) в стóрону.

ask [ɑːsk] *v* 1) спрáшивать; 2) проси́ть; 3) приглашáть; 4) трéбовать; it ~s (for) attention э́то трéбует внимáния; 5) осведомля́ться (*o — after, about, for*); ◊ to ~ for trouble, to ~ for it *сленг* напрáшиваться на неприя́тность; to ~ (out) in church оглашáть (*имена вступающих в брак*).

askance [əs'kæns] *adv* 1) и́скоса, кóсо; 2) с подозрéнием; to look ~ at smb. смотрéть на когó-л. подозри́тельно.

askant [əs'kænt] *см.* askance.

askew [əs'kjuː] *adv* кóсо, кри́во; и́скоса.

aslant I [ə'slɑːnt] *adv* кóсо, нáискось.

aslant II *prep* поперёк.

asleep I [ə'sliːp] *a predic* 1) спя́щий; сóнный; to be ~ спать; to fall ~ заснýть; 2) онемéвший, затёкший.

asleep II *adv* во снé.

aslope [ə'sloup] *adv* кóсо, покáто.

a-smoke [ə'smouk] *adv* в дымý.

asp¹ [æsp] *n* оси́на.

asp² *n* 1) *зоол.* áспид; гадю́ка; 2) *поэт.* ядови́тая змея́.

asparagus [əs'pærəgəs] *n* спáржа.

aspect ['æspekt] *n* 1) вид; 2) тóчка зрéния; аспéкт; 3) нарýжность; выражéние (*лица, глаз*); 4) *грам.* вид.

aspen I ['æspən] *n* оси́на.

aspen II *a* оси́новый.

asperity [æs'perɪtɪ] *n* 1) шерохóватость, нерóвность; 2) сурóвость (*климата и т. п.*); 3) рéзкость, жёсткость (*характера*); 4) *pl* трýдности.

asperse [əs'pəːs] *v* 1) обры́згивать, кропи́ть (*with*); 2) позóрить; клеветáть.

aspersion [əs'pəːʃən] *n* 1) обры́згивание (*with*); 2) клеветá; to cast ~s on smb. клеветáть на когó-л.

asphalt I ['æsfælt] *n* асфáльт; битýм.

asphalt II *v* асфальти́ровать.

asphyxiant [æs'fɪksɪənt] *n* удушáющее отравля́ющее вещество.

asphyxiate [æs'fɪksɪeɪt] *v* вызывáть удýшье.

aspic¹ ['æspɪk] *n см.* asp² 2).

aspic² *n* заливнóе (из мя́са).

aspirant I [əs'paɪərənt] *n* претендéнт, кандидáт (*to, after, for*).

aspirant II *a* стремя́щийся; добивáющийся.

aspirateᵃ ['æspərɪt] *n фон.* придыхáтельный соглáсный, аспирáт.

aspirateᵇ ['æspəreɪt] *v* 1) произноси́ть с придыхáнием; 2) *тех.* всáсывать.

aspiration [,æspə'reɪʃən] *n* 1) стремлéние, желáние, чáяние (*after, for*); 2) *фон.* придыхáние; 3) *тех.* всáсывание.

aspire [əs'paɪə] *n* стреми́ться, домогáться (*to, after, at*).

asquint [ə'skwɪnt] *adv* кóсо, и́скоса.

ass [æs] *n* осёл; ◊ to make an ~ of oneself а) стáвить себя́ в глýпое положéние; б) валя́ть дуракá, дурáчиться; to act (*или* to play) the ~ валя́ть дуракá; sell your ~ перестáньте дéлать (*или* говори́ть) глýпости.

assail [ə'seɪl] *v* 1) нападáть, атаковáть; 2) энерги́чно брáться за что-л.; набрáсываться (*на работу и т. п.*); 3) забрáсывать (*вопросами и т. п.; with*).

assailable [ə'seɪləbl] *a* уязви́мый.

assailant [ə'seɪlənt] *n* нападáющая сторонá; проти́вник.

assassin [ə'sæsɪn] *n* (наёмный) уби́йца.

assassinate [ə'sæsɪneɪt] *v* убивáть.

assassination [ə,sæsɪ'neɪʃən] *n* уби́йство.

assault I [ə'sɔːlt] *n* 1) атáка, штурм; нападéние; *перен.* напáдки; 2) *юр.* словéсное оскорблéние и угрóза физи́ческим наси́лием; ~ and battery оскорблéние дéйствием; 3) *attr воен.* штурмовóй.

assault II *v* атаковáть, штурмовáть; нападáть.

assaulter [ə'sɔːltə] *n* *юр.* нападающая сторона.

assay I [ə'seɪ] *n* испытание; анализ; проба (*металлов*).

assay II *v* проводить испытание, анализ; определять пробу (*металлов*).

assemblage [ə'semblɪdʒ] *n* 1) собирание; сбор; 2) скопление; собрание; коллекция; 3) *тех.* сборка, монтаж.

assemble [ə'sembl] *v* 1) собирать(ся); 2) созывать; 3) *тех.* монтировать.

assembly [ə'semblɪ] *n* 1) собрание; ассамблея; constituent ~ учредительное собрание; General Assembly Генеральная Ассамблея; 2) (A.) законодательное собрание; 3) *тех.* сборка; 4) агрегат; 5) *воен.* сигнал сбора; 6) *attr* сборочный; ~ line сборочный конвейер; ~ hall сборочный цех.

assembly-room [ə'semblɪrum] *n* зал для балов, концертов, собраний *и т. п.*

assent I [ə'sent] *n* 1) согласие; уступка; to nod ~ кивнуть в знак согласия; 2) санкция.

assent II *v* 1) соглашаться, давать согласие; уступать (*чьему-л. желанию*); 2) санкционировать.

assert [ə'sɜːt] *v* 1) утверждать; заявлять; 2) отстаивать; защищать; to ~ oneself а) отстаивать свои права; б) предъявлять чрезмерные претензии; в) важничать.

assertion [ə'sɜːʃən] *n* 1) утверждение; заявление; a mere ~ голословное утверждение; 2) защита, отстаивание (*своих прав и т. п.*).

assertive [ə'sɜːtɪv] *a* 1) утвердительный, положительный; 2) настойчивый; напористый.

assess [ə'ses] *v* 1) определять сумму налога, штрафа; 2) облагать налогом; штрафовать; 3) оценивать имущество для обложения налогом.

assessable [ə'sesəbl] *a* подлежащий обложению.

assessment [ə'sesmənt] *n* 1) обложение; 2) сумма обложения; 3) оценка имущества для обложения налогом.

assessor [ə'sesə] *n* 1) консультант (*при судье и т. п.*); 2) податной инспектор.

asset [ˈæset] *n* 1) *pl* *фин.* актив; ~s and liabilities актив и пассив; 2) *pl* *юр.* имущество несостоятельного должника; 3) положительное качество, достоинство.

asseverate [ə'sevəreɪt] *v* 1) торжественно заявлять; 2) утверждать.

asseveration [ə‚sevə'reɪʃən] *n* 1) торжественное заявление; 2) утверждение.

assiduity [‚æsɪ'djuːɪtɪ] *n* 1) прилежание, усердие; 2) *pl* ухаживание.

assiduous [ə'sɪdjuəs] *a* прилежный, усердный.

assign I [ə'saɪn] *v* 1) назначать; определять (*срок, границы*); 2) ассигновать; предназначать; 3) передавать (*имущество и т. п.*); 4) приписывать.

assign II *n* *юр.* правопреемник.

assignation [‚æsɪg'neɪʃən] *n* 1) назначение; 2) ассигнование, выделение; 3) передача (*прав, имущества*); 4) условленная встреча; 5) ассигнация.

assignee [‚æsɪ'niː] *n* 1) уполномоченный; представитель; 2) *юр.* правопреемник.

assignment [ə'saɪnmənt] *n* 1) назначение; выделение, распределение; ассигнование; 2) переда-

ча (*прав, имущества*); документ о передаче; 3) приписывание.

assimilate [ə'sɪmɪleɪt] *v* 1) уподоблять(ся), ассимилировать(ся) (*to, with*); 2) сравнивать (*to, with*); 3) ассимилировать(ся), усваивать(ся).

assimilation [ə‚sɪmɪ'leɪʃən] *n* 1) уподобление; 2) ассимиляция, усвоение; 3) сравнение.

assist [ə'sɪst] *v* 1) помогать; содействовать; 2) принимать участие (*in*); 3) присутствовать (*at*).

assistance [ə'sɪstəns] *n* помощь, содействие.

assistant [ə'sɪstənt] *n* помощник; ассистент.

assize [ə'saɪz] *n* 1) судебное разбирательство (с присяжными); 2) *pl* выездная сессия суда; 3) *ист.* твёрдо установленная цена; такса.

associate[a] I [ə'souʃiɪt] *n* 1) товарищ, коллега; участник; компаньон; 2) младший член корпорации; член-корреспондент (*научного общества*).

associate[a] II *a* объединённый; связанный; союзный.

associate[b] [ə'souʃieɪt] *v* 1) соединять(ся); объединять(ся); 2) ассоциировать(ся); 3) присоединяться; вступать (*в общество и т. п.*); 4) общаться (*with*).

association [ə‚sousɪ'eɪʃən] *n* 1) соединение; 2) общество, ассоциация; 3) ассоциация; связь представлений, идей; 4) общение, близость.

assonance [ˈæsənəns] *n* созвучие; ассонанс.

assonant [ˈæsənənt] *a* созвучный.

assort [ə'sɔːt] *v* 1) сортировать; группировать; 2) снабжать ассортиментом (*товаров*); 3) согласовываться, гармонировать (*with*).

assortment [ə'sɔːtmənt] *n* 1) сортировка; 2) ассортимент, подбор.

assuage [ə'sweɪdʒ] *v* 1) успокаивать, облегчать (*боль и т. п.*); смягчать (*вину и т. п.*); 2) утолять (*голод*).

assuagement [ə'sweɪdʒmənt] *n* 1) успокоение, облегчение (*боли и т. п.*); смягчение (*вины и т. п.*); 2) болеутоляющее средство.

assume [ə'sjuːm] *v* 1) брать на себя (*ответственность и т. п.*); 2) присваивать; 3) принимать (*вид, форму*); 4) напускать на себя (*важность и т. п.*); 5) симулировать; 6) допускать, предполагать.

assuming [ə'sjuːmɪŋ] *a* самонадеянный.

assumption [ə'sʌmpʃən] *n* 1) принятие на себя; присвоение; 2) предположение, допущение; 3) притворство; 4) самонадеянность; высокомерие.

assumptive [ə'sʌmptɪv] *a* 1) предполагаемый, допускаемый; 2) самонадеянный; высокомерный.

assurance [ə'ʃuərəns] *n* 1) уверение, заверение; гарантия; 2) уверенность; 3) уверенность в себе; самоуверенность; самонадеянность; 4) страхование (*обыкн.* life ~, fire ~).

assure [ə'ʃuə] *v* 1) уверять; заверять (*кого-л.*); to ~ oneself убеждаться; 2) гарантировать, обеспечивать; 3) страховать.

assured [ə'ʃuəd] *a* 1) уверенный; 2) гарантированный, обеспеченный; 3) самоуверенный; 4) застрахованный.

assuredly [ə'ʃuərɪdlɪ] *adv* конечно, несомненно.

assuredness [ə'ʃuədnɪs] *n* 1) уверенность; 2) самоуверенность.

aster [ˈæstə] *n* астра.

asterisk I [ˈæstərɪsk] *n полигр.* звёздочка (знак*).

asterisk II *v полигр.* отмечать звёздочкой.

astern [əsˈtəːn] *adv мор.* 1) на корме, за кормой; 2) назад.

asteroid I [ˈæstərɔɪd] *n* 1) *астр.* малая планета, астероид; 2) *зоол.* морская звезда.

asteroid II *a* звездообразный.

asthma [ˈæsmə] *n* астма; одышка.

asthmatic I [æsˈmætɪk] *n* астматик.

asthmatic II *a* астматический; страдающий астмой.

astir [əsˈtəː] *a predic* 1) в движении; 2) на ногах; вставши с постели; 3) в волнении, в возбуждении.

astonish [əsˈtɔnɪʃ] *v* удивлять, изумлять.

astonishing [əsˈtɔnɪʃɪŋ] *a* удивительный, изумительный.

astonishment [əsˈtɔnɪʃmənt] *n* удивление, изумление.

astound [əsˈtaund] *v* поражать.

astounding [əsˈtaundɪŋ] *a* поразительный.

astraddle [əsˈtrædl] *adv* широко расставив ноги; верхом.

astrakhan [ˌæstrəˈkæn] *n* 1) каракуль; 2) *attr* каракулевый.

astray [əsˈtreɪ] *adv*: to go (*или* to run) ~ сбиться с пути; to lead ~ ввести в заблуждение.

astride [əsˈtraɪd] *adv* верхом (на — of); to get ~ «оседлать».

astringent I [əsˈtrɪndʒənt] *n* вяжущее средство.

astringent II *a* вяжущий.

astrolabe [ˈæstrouleɪb] *n геод.* астролябия.

astrologer [əsˈtrɔlədʒə] *n* астролог, звездочёт.

astrology [əsˈtrɔlədʒɪ] *n* астрология.

astronaut [ˌæstrəˈnɔːt] *n* астронавт, космонавт.

astronautics [ˌæstrəˈnɔːtɪks] *n* астронавтика, космонавтика.

astronomer [əsˈtrɔnəmə] *n* астроном.

astronomic(al) [ˌæstrəˈnɔmɪk(əl)] *a* астрономический.

astronomy [əsˈtrɔnəmɪ] *n* астрономия.

astute [əsˈtjuːt] *a* 1) проницательный; 2) хитрый.

asunder [əsˈʌndə] *adv* порознь, отдельно друг от друга; to rush ~ броситься в разные стороны; to tear ~ разорвать на куски, на части.

asylum [əsˈaɪləm] *n* 1) убежище, приют; 2) психиатрическая больница; lunatic ~ сумасшедший дом.

asymmetric [ˌæsɪˈmetrɪk] *a* несимметричный, асимметричный.

at [æt (*сильная форма*), ət (*слабая форма*)] *prep* 1) *в пространственном значении указывает на:* а) *нахождение в непосредственной близости от другого предмета* у, около; at the window у окна; at the door у двери, у подъезда; б) *присутствие или участие в процессе, совершающемся в определённом месте* в, на; at the lesson (lecture, meeting, factory, market, concert, theatre) на уроке (лекции, собрании, фабрике *или* заводе, рынке, в концерте, в театре); at school в школе; at war на войне; в) *местонахождение в пределах небольшого населённого пункта, города* в; he lives at a small town on живёт в маленьком городке; at Yarmouth в Ярмуте; г) *присутствие во время еды* за; at breakfast (lunch,

dinner, supper, tea, table) за завтраком (вторым завтраком, обедом, ужином, чаем, столом); 2) *во временном значении указывает на момент, время действия в, на или переводится наречием;* at ten o'clock в десять часов; at noon (midnight) в полдень (полночь); at dawn (day-break, sunrise, sunset) на заре (рассвете, восходе солнца, закате); at first (last, the outset, present) сначала (наконец, в начале, в настоящее время); 3) *выражает:* а) *характер протекания действия; переводится обстоятельством образа действия:* the flowers are at their best цветы совсем распустились; the sport was at its height, the sliding was at the quickest, the laughter was at the loudest, when a sharp smart crack was heard веселье было в самом разгаре, катание на коньках достигло предельной скорости, смех звучал громче всего, когда послышался негромкий, но резкий треск; б) *состояние субъекта; переводится наречием или описательным оборотом:* I am at a loss (at my wit's end, at leisure, at ease) я не знаю, что делать (потерял голову, имею свободное время, чувствую себя свободно, не стесняюсь); they are at daggers drawn (at war, at peace) они живут как кошка с собакой (в состоянии войны, в мире); в) *темп действия:* at a quick rate быстрым темпом; at full gallop (full speed, a trot, a foot's pace, a snail's pace) галопом (полным ходом, рысью, шагом, черепашьим шагом); 4) *указывает на вознаграждение, цену* по, за; at a good price (a high rate, a high salary, high remuneration) за большую цену (по высокой ставке, за высокую зарплату, за большое вознаграждение); 5) *с глаголами* aim, fire, fly, hit, rush, throw *и др., а также* look, jeer, sneer, laugh, smile, hint *и др. выражает целеустремлённость действия* в, над, на; he aimed at me он прицелился в меня; he rushed at me он бросился ко мне; he laughed at me он смеялся надо мной; he smiled at me он улыбнулся мне.

at-a-boy [ˈætəˌbɔɪ] *int амер. сленг* молодец!

ate [et] *past см.* eat.

atheism [ˈeɪθɪɪzəm] *n* безбожие, атеизм.

atheist [ˈeɪθɪɪst] *n* безбожник, атеист.

atheistic [ˌeɪθɪˈɪstɪk] *a* атеистический.

athenaeum [ˌæθɪˈniːəm] *n* 1) литературный *или* научный клуб; the Athenaeum «Атенеум», литературный клуб в Лондоне; 2) библиотека.

Athenian I [əˈθiːnjən] *n* афинянин.

Athenian II *a* афинский.

athirst [əˈθəːst] *a predic* 1) испытывающий жажду; 2) жаждущий; стремящийся (к чему-л. — for).

athlete [ˈæθliːt] *n* 1) атлет; 2) силач.

athletic [æθˈletɪk] *a* атлетический.

athletics [æθˈletɪks] *n* атлетика.

at-home [ətˈhoum] *n разг.* приём гостей.

athwart I [əˈθwɔːt] *adv* 1) поперёк; наискось; перпендикулярно; 2) *мор.* на траверзе; на пересечку курса; to run ~ врезаться в борт судна.

athwart II *prep* 1) поперёк; через; 2) вопреки, против.

a-tilt [əˈtɪlt] *adv* наперевес.

Atlantic I [ətˈlæntɪk] *n* Атлантический океан (*тж.* ~ Ocean).

Atlantic II *a* атлантический.

atlas[1] [ˈætləs] *n* 1) (географический) атлас; 2) *анат.* атлант.

atlas² *n* атла́с (*материя*).

atmosphere ['ætməsfɪə] *n* 1) атмосфе́ра; во́здух; 2) атмосфе́ра, окружа́ющая обстано́вка.

atmospheric [,ætməs'ferɪk] *a* атмосфе́рный, атмосфери́ческий.

atmospherics [,ætməs'feriks] *n pl* *радио* атмосфе́рные поме́хи.

atoll [ə'tɔl] *n* кора́лловый о́стров, ато́лл.

atom ['ætəm] *n* 1) а́том; 2) мельча́йшая части́ца; to break to ~s разби́ть вдре́безги; not an ~ of ни ка́пли, ни те́ни (*чего-л.*); 3) *attr* а́томный.

atomaniac I ['ætə,meɪnɪæk] *n* проповедник а́томной войны́.

atomaniac II *a* проповедующий а́томную войну́.

atomic [ə'tɔmɪk] *a* а́томный.

atomicity [,ætə'mɪsɪtɪ] *n* а́томность; вале́нтность.

atomize ['ætəmaɪz] *v* распыля́ть.

atomizer ['ætəmaɪzə] *n* 1) пульвериза́тор; 2) *тех.* форсу́нка.

atom-monger ['ætəm,mʌŋgə] *n* *разг.* поджига́тель войны́.

atom-smasher ['ætəm,smæʃə] *n* *физ.* ускори́тель я́дерных части́ц.

atom-smashing ['ætəm,smæʃɪŋ] *n* *физ.* расщепле́ние а́томного ядра́.

atone [ə'toun] *v* 1) загла́живать, искупа́ть (*вину*); 2) возмеща́ть, компенси́ровать; 3) примиря́ть; ула́живать (*ссору*).

atonement [ə'tounmənt] *n* 1) искупле́ние; распла́та; 2) возмеще́ние, компенса́ция; 3) примире́ние.

atonic [æ'tɔnɪk] *a* 1) *грам.* безуда́рный; 2) *мед.* ослабленный; с пони́женным то́нусом.

atop [ə'tɔp] *adv* наверху́, на верши́не.

atrocious [ə'trouʃəs] *a* 1) жесто́кий; ужа́сный; 2) скве́рный.

atrocity [ə'trɔsɪtɪ] *n* 1) жесто́кость; *pl* зве́рства; 3) гру́бая оши́бка, про́мах.

atrophied ['ætrəfɪd] *a* 1) атрофи́рованный; 2) истощенный.

atrophy I ['ætrəfɪ] *n* 1) атрофи́я; 2) ослабле́ние, истоще́ние.

atrophy II *v* 1) атрофи́роваться; 2) истоща́ть(ся).

attaboy ['ætə,bɔɪ] *см.* at-a-boy.

attach [ə'tætʃ] *v* 1) прикрепля́ть, присоединя́ть; свя́зывать; to ~ oneself to the party вступи́ть в па́ртию; 2) привя́зывать, привлека́ть к себе́; to be ~ed to привяза́ться к кому́-л.; 3) припи́сывать; придава́ть (*значение и т. п.; to*); 4) *юр.* налага́ть аре́ст, аресто́вывать; 5) *воен.* придава́ть.

attaché [ə'tæʃeɪ] *n* атташе́ (*посольства*).

attaché-case [ə'tæʃɪkeɪs] *n* пло́ский ко́жаный чемода́нчик (*для бумаг*).

attached [ə'tætʃt] *a* 1) привя́занный, пре́данный; 2) прикрепленный.

attachment [ə'tætʃmənt] *n* 1) привя́занность, пре́данность; 2) прикрепле́ние; 3) *юр.* наложе́ние аре́ста; 4) *тех.* приспособле́ние; принадле́жность.

attack I [ə'tæk] *n* 1) ата́ка, наступле́ние; нападе́ние; *перен.* напа́дки; 2) при́ступ боле́зни, припа́док.

attack II *v* 1) атакова́ть, напада́ть; 2) поража́ть (*о болезни*); 3) разруша́ть.

attackable [ə'tækəbl] *a* уязви́мый.

attain [ə'teɪn] *v* 1) дости́гнуть, доби́ться; 2) получи́ть.

attainability [ə,teɪnə'bɪlɪtɪ] *n* достижи́мость.

attainable [ə'teɪnəbl] *a* достижи́мый.

attainment [ə'teɪnmənt] *n* 1) достиже́ние, приобрете́ние; 2) *pl* зна́ния, на́выки.

attaint I [ə'teɪnt] *n* пятно́, позо́р.

attaint II *v* 1) пригова́ривать к сме́рти *или* изгна́нию с лише́нием прав; 2) поража́ть (*о болезни*); зараżáть; 3) позо́рить, бесче́стить.

attar ['ætə] *n* ро́зовое ма́сло.

attemper [ə'tempə] *v* 1) умеря́ть, смягча́ть; 2) регули́ровать; приспоса́бливать (*to*); настра́ивать (*to*); 3) сме́шивать в соотве́тствующих пропо́рциях.

attempt I [ə'tempt] *n* 1) попы́тка; про́ба; 2) покуше́ние; an ~ upon the life покуше́ние на жизнь.

attempt II *v* 1) пыта́ться, про́бовать; предпринима́ть; 2) покуша́ться.

attend [ə'tend] *v* 1) посеща́ть (*лекции, собра́ния*); прису́тствовать (*at*); 2) быть внима́тельным; 3) уха́живать (*за больны́м и т. п.*); забо́титься; следи́ть; обслу́живать (*on, upon*); 4) сопровожда́ть; провожа́ть.

attendance [ə'tendəns] *n* 1) прису́тствие; посеще́ние; 2) посеща́емость; to take ~ прове́рить прису́тствующих (*на заня́тиях*); 3) ухо́д, обслу́живание; medical ~ медици́нское обслу́живание; 4) аудито́рия, пу́блика; ◊ to dance ~ (up)on прислу́живаться, ходи́ть на за́дних ла́пках.

attendant I [ə'tendənt] *n* сопровожда́ющее, обслу́живающее *или* прису́тствующее лицо́; провожа́тый; слуга́.

attendant II *a* 1) сопровожда́ющий, сопу́тствующий; 2) обслу́живающий; 3) прису́тствующий.

attention [ə'tenʃən] *n* 1) внима́ние; внима́тельность; to attract ~ to привлека́ть внима́ние к; to call (*или* to pay) ~ to обраща́ть внима́ние на; to compel ~ прико́вывать внима́ние; with due ~ с до́лжным внима́нием; to be all ~ сосредото́чить всё внима́ние; to slip one's ~ ускользну́ть от чего́-л. внима́ния; 2) забо́тливость; забо́та; 3) ухо́д (*за больны́м и т. п.*); обслу́живание; 4) *pl* уха́живание; to pay ~s to a lady уха́живать за да́мой; 5): ~! *воен.* сми́рно!

attentive [ə'tentɪv] *a* 1) внима́тельный; 2) забо́тливый; 3) ве́жливый, предупреди́тельный.

attenuateᵃ [ə'tenjuɪt] *a* 1) худо́й; стро́йный; 2) разжиженный.

attenuateᵇ [ə'tenjueɪt] *v* 1) истоща́ть, ослабля́ть; 2) разжижа́ть.

attenuation [ə,tenju'eɪʃən] *n* 1) истоще́ние; ослабле́ние; 2) разжиже́ние; 3) *тех., радио* затуха́ние.

attest [ə'test] *v* 1) удостоверя́ть; свиде́тельствовать; 2) приводи́ть к прися́ге; 3) *юр.* дава́ть свиде́тельские показа́ния (*to*); 4) зачисля́ть *или* поступа́ть на вое́нную слу́жбу.

attestation [,ætes'teɪʃən] *n* 1) удостовере́ние (*подписи, документа*); 2) свиде́тельское показа́ние; 3) приведе́ние к прися́ге.

Attic ['ætɪk] *a* атти́ческий; класси́ческий.

attic ['ætɪk] *n* манса́рда; черда́к; ве́рхний эта́ж.

attic-stor(e)y ['ætɪk'stɔːrɪ] *n* черда́чный эта́ж.

attire I [ə'taɪə] *n* наря́д; украше́ние.

attire II *v* наряжа́ть, одева́ть.

attitude ['ætɪtjuːd] *n* 1) пози́ция; отноше́ние (*к чему-л.— to*): ~ of mind склад ума́; a devil-may-care ~ наплева́тельское отноше́ние; 2) по́за; оса́нка; to strike an ~ приня́ть по́зу.

attitudinize [ˌætɪˈtjuːdɪnaɪz] *v* принима́ть театра́льные по́зы.

attorney [əˈtəːnɪ] *n* пове́ренный, адвока́т; Attorney General генера́льный атто́рней; мини́стр юсти́ции (*в США*); letter (*или* warrant) of ~ дове́ренность; power of ~ полномо́чие; дове́ренность; by ~ по дове́ренности.

attract [əˈtrækt] *v* 1) притя́гивать, привлека́ть; 2) пленя́ть, прельща́ть.

attraction [əˈtrækʃən] *n* 1) притяже́ние, тяготе́ние; 2) привлека́тельность; 3) аттракцио́н.

attractive [əˈtræktɪv] *a* привлека́тельный, зама́нчивый.

attribute[a] [ˈætrɪbjuːt] *n* 1) сво́йство, характе́рный при́знак, характе́рная черта́, атрибу́т; 2) *грам.* определе́ние.

attribute[b] [əˈtrɪbjuːt] *v* припи́сывать, относи́ть (*к — to*).

attribution [ˌætrɪˈbjuːʃən] *n* 1) припи́сывание, отнесе́ние (*к — to*); 2) власть, компете́нция.

attributive I [əˈtrɪbjutɪv] *n* 1) атрибу́т; 2) *грам.* определе́ние.

attributive II *а грам.* определи́тельный, атрибути́вный.

attrition [əˈtrɪʃən] *n* 1) изна́шивание, истира́ние; 2) истоще́ние, изнуре́ние.

attune [əˈtjuːn] *v* настра́ивать (*муз. инструмент*).

auburn [ˈɔːbən] *a* золоти́сто-кашта́новый, рыжева́тый.

auction I [ˈɔːkʃən] *n* аукцио́н; to put up to ~, to sell by ~ продава́ть с аукцио́на; Dutch ~ «голла́ндский аукцио́н» (*распрода́жа, на кото́рой цена́ снижа́ется, пока́ не найдётся покупа́тель*).

auction II *v* продава́ть с аукцио́на (*обыкн.* to ~ off).

auctioneer I [ˌɔːkʃəˈnɪə] *n* аукциони́ст.

auctioneer II *v* производи́ть аукцио́нную прода́жу.

audacious [ɔːˈdeɪʃəs] *a* 1) сме́лый; де́рзкий; 2) на́глый.

audacity [ɔːˈdæsɪtɪ] *n* 1) сме́лость, де́рзость; 2) на́глость.

audibility [ˌɔːdɪˈbɪlɪtɪ] *n* слы́шимость.

audible [ˈɔːdəbl] *a* слы́шный, вня́тный; слы́шимый.

audibly [ˈɔːdəblɪ] *adv* вслух, гро́мко, вня́тно; *перен.* я́вно.

audience [ˈɔːdjəns] *n* 1) аудито́рия; пу́блика; зри́тели; a numerous ~ многочи́сленная аудито́рия; 2) (ра́дио)слу́шатели; 3) аудие́нция (*у кого́-л. — of, with*); to give ~ назна́чить аудие́нцию; вы́слушать; 4) слу́шание (*де́ла в суде́*).

audit I [ˈɔːdɪt] *n* прове́рка счето́в; реви́зия отчётности.

audit II *v* проверя́ть счета́; ревизова́ть отчётность.

audition [ɔːˈdɪʃən] *n* 1) слух; 2) слу́шание, выслу́шивание; про́ба голосо́в.

auditor [ˈɔːdɪtə] *n* 1) ревизо́р, контролёр; 2) слу́шатель.

auditorial [ˌɔːdɪˈtɔːrɪəl] *a* ревизио́нный, контро́льный.

auditorium [ˌɔːdɪˈtɔːrɪəm] *n* аудито́рия; зри́тельный зал.

auditory I [ˈɔːdɪtərɪ] *n* аудито́рия; слу́шатели.

auditory II *a* слухово́й.

Augean [ɔːˈdʒiːən] *a:* ~ stables а́вгиевы коню́шни.

auger [ˈɔːgə] *n* сверло́, бура́в.

aught [ɔːt] *n* что́-нибудь, что́-то; не́что; for ~ I know наско́лько я зна́ю.

augment[a] [ˈɔːgmənt] *n грам.* прираще́ние.

augment[b] [ɔːgˈment] *v* 1) увели́чивать(ся); 2) *грам.* присоединя́ть (*приста́вку и т. п.*).

augmentation [ˌɔːgmenˈteɪʃən] *n* 1) увеличе́ние, повыше́ние; 2) прираще́ние.

augmentative [ɔːgˈmentətɪv] *a* 1) увели́чивающий(ся); 2) *грам.* увеличи́тельный (*о су́ффиксе*).

augur I [ˈɔːgə] *n* авгу́р, прорица́тель.

augur II *v* предвеща́ть; предска́зывать.

augural [ˈɔːgjurəl] *a* предвеща́ющий.

augury [ˈɔːgjurɪ] *n* 1) гада́ние; предска́зание; 2) предзнаменова́ние; 3) предчу́вствие.

August [ˈɔːgəst] *n* 1) а́вгуст; 2) *attr* а́вгустовский.

august [ɔːˈgʌst] *a* вели́чественный; благоро́дный.

Augustinian [ˌɔːgəsˈtɪnɪən] *n* августи́нец (*мона́х*).

aunt [ɑːnt] *n* тётя, тётка.

auntie [ˈɑːntɪ] *n* тётушка.

aura [ˈɔːrə] *n* лёгкое дунове́ние.

aural [ˈɔːrəl] *a* 1) ушно́й; 2) слухово́й (*о восприя́тии*).

aurally [ˈɔːrəlɪ] *adv* на слух, у́стно.

aureate [ˈɔːrɪɪt] *a* золоти́стый; позоло́ченный.

aureola [ɔːˈrɪələ] *n* орео́л, сия́ние, ве́нчик.

aureole [ˈɔːrɪoul] *см.* aureola.

auricle [ˈɔːrɪkl] *n* 1) нару́жное у́хо (*живо́тных*); 2) *анат.* предсе́рдие.

auricular [ɔːˈrɪkjulə] *a* 1) ушно́й, слухово́й; 2) ска́занный на́ ухо, по секре́ту.

auriferous [ɔːˈrɪfərəs] *a* золотоно́сный.

aurist [ˈɔːrɪst] *n* врач по ушны́м боле́зням.

aurochs [ˈɔːrɔks] *n зоол.* зубр.

aurora [ɔːˈrɔːrə] *n поэт.* авро́ра, у́тренняя заря́; ~ australis ю́жное сия́ние; ~ borealis се́верное сия́ние.

auroral [ɔːˈrɔːrəl] *a* 1) у́тренний; сия́ющий, румя́ный как заря́; 2) свя́занный с се́верным *или* ю́жным сия́нием.

auscultation [ˌɔːskəlˈteɪʃən] *n мед.* выслу́шивание.

auspice [ˈɔːspɪs] *n* 1) предзнаменова́ние; 2) *pl* покрови́тельство; under the ~s of под покрови́тельством, при соде́йствии.

auspicious [ɔːsˈpɪʃəs] *a* благоприя́тный.

Aussie [ˈɔːsɪ] *n сленг* австрали́ец; dinkum ~ настоя́щий австрали́ец.

austere [ɔːsˈtɪə] *a* 1) суро́вый, стро́гий; аскети́ческий; 2) просто́й (*о сти́ле*); 3) те́рпкий.

austerity [ɔːsˈterɪtɪ] *n* 1) стро́гость, суро́вость; аскети́зм; 2) простота́ (*сти́ля*); 3) те́рпкость.

austral [ˈɔːstrəl] *a* ю́жный.

Australian I [ɔːsˈtreɪljən] *n* австрали́ец; австрали́йка; the ~s австрали́йцы.

Australian II *a* австрали́йский.

Austrian I [ˈɔːstrɪən] *n* австри́ец; австри́йка; the ~s австри́йцы.

Austrian II *a* австри́йский.

autarchy [ˈɔːtɑːkɪ] *n* 1) абсолю́тная мона́рхия; 2) *эк.* авта́ркия.

authentic [ɔːˈθentɪk] *a* по́длинный, достове́рный; аутенти́чный.

authentically [ɔ:'θentɪkəlɪ] *adv* по́длинно, достове́рно.

authenticate [ɔ:'θentɪkeɪt] *v* устана́вливать по́длинность; удостоверя́ть.

authenticity [,ɔ:θen'tɪsɪtɪ] *n* по́длинность, достове́рность; аутенти́чность.

author ['ɔ:θə] *n* 1) а́втор, писа́тель; joint ~s соа́вторы; 2) созда́тель; творе́ц; 3) инициа́тор; вино́вник.

authoress ['ɔ:θərɪs] *n* писа́тельница.

authoritarian I [ɔ:,θɔrɪ'tɛərɪən] *n* сторо́нник авторита́рной вла́сти.

authoritarian II *a* авторита́рный.

authoritative [ɔ:'θɔrɪtətɪv] *a* 1) авторите́тный; 2) вла́стный; повели́тельный.

authority [ɔ:'θɔrɪtɪ] *n* 1) власть; полномо́чие (to+Inf, for); 2) *обыкн. pl* вла́сти, нача́льство; 3) авторите́т; влия́ние; вес; to cary ~ име́ть влия́ние; 4) авторите́т, авторите́тный специали́ст; 5) авторите́тный исто́чник (*книга и т. п.*); 6) доказа́тельство, основа́ние, до́вод.

authorization [,ɔ:θəraɪ'zeɪʃən] *n* 1) разреше́ние, са́нкция; 2) полномо́чие.

authorize ['ɔ:θəraɪz] *v* 1) разреша́ть, санкциони́ровать; 2) поруча́ть, уполномо́чивать; 3) опра́вдывать, объясня́ть.

authorized ['ɔ:θəraɪzd] *a* 1) санкциони́рованный; 2) авторизо́ванный (*о переводе*).

authorless ['ɔ:θəlɪs] *a* анони́мный.

authorship ['ɔ:θəʃɪp] *n* а́вторство.

auto ['ɔ:tou] *n разг.* автомоби́ль.

auto- ['ɔ:tou-] *pref* авто-, само-.

autobiographic ['ɔ:tou,baɪou'græfɪk] *a* автобиографи́ческий.

autobiography [,ɔ:toubaɪ'ɔgrəfɪ] *n* автобиогра́фия.

auto-camp ['ɔ:tou,kæmp] *n* автопансиона́т.

autocar ['ɔ:toukɑ:] *n* автомоби́ль.

auto-court ['ɔ:tou,kɔ:t] *n амер.* моте́ль.

autocracy [ɔ:'tɔkrəsɪ] *n* самодержа́вие, автокра́тия.

autocrat ['ɔ:təkræt] *n* самоде́ржец.

autocratic(al) [,ɔ:tə'krætɪk(əl)] *a* 1) самодержа́вный; 2) деспоти́ческий, самовла́стный.

autogenesis [,ɔ:tou'dʒenɪsɪs] *n биол.* автогене́з, самозарожде́ние.

autogenous [ɔ:'tɔdʒɪnəs] *a* автоге́нный.

autogiro [,ɔ:tou'dʒaɪərou] *n* автожи́р, вертолёт.

autograph ['ɔ:təgrɑ:f] *n* 1) авто́граф; 2) оригина́л ру́кописи.

autographic [,ɔ:tə'græfɪk] *a* собственнору́чно напи́санный.

automat ['ɔ:təmæt] *n амер.* рестора́н-автома́т.

automata [ɔ:'tɔmətə] *pl см.* automaton.

automatic I [,ɔ:tə'mætɪk] *n* 1) автомати́ческий аппара́т; автома́т; 2) автомати́ческое ору́жие; 3) пистоле́т.

automatic II *a* 1) автомати́ческий; 2) машина́льный, непроизво́льный.

automatical [,ɔ:tə'mætɪkəl] *см.* automatic II.

automation [,ɔ:tə'meɪʃən] *n* автоматиза́ция.

automatism [ɔ:'tɔmətɪzəm] *n* автомати́зм; непроизво́льное движе́ние, де́йствие.

automaton [ɔ:'tɔmətən] *n* (*pl тж.* automata) автома́т.

automobile I ['ɔ:təməbi:l] *n* автомоби́ль.

automobile II *a* автомоби́льный.

automotive [,ɔ:tə'moutɪv] *a* 1) самодви́жущийся; 2) автомоби́льный.

autonomist [ɔ:'tɔnəmɪst] *n* сторо́нник автоно́мии.

autonomous [ɔ:'tɔnəməs] *a* автоно́мный.

autonomy [ɔ:'tɔnəmɪ] *n* 1) автоно́мия; самоуправле́ние; 2) пра́во на самоуправле́ние; 3) автоно́мное госуда́рство; автоно́мная о́бласть.

autopsy ['ɔ:təpsɪ] *n мед.* вскры́тие (*трупа*).

autorifle ['ɔ:təraɪfl] *n амер.* ручно́й пулемёт.

auto-road ['ɔ:təroud] *n* автостра́да.

autostrada ['ɔ:tou,streɪdə] *см.* auto-road.

autosuggestion ['ɔ:tousə'dʒestʃən] *n* самовнуше́ние.

autotruck ['ɔ:tətrʌk] *n амер.* грузови́к.

autotype I ['ɔ:tətaɪp] *n* автоти́пия.

autotype II *v* де́лать автоти́пный сни́мок.

autumn ['ɔ:təm] *n* 1) о́сень; deep ~ по́здняя о́сень; 2) *attr* осе́нний.

autumnal [ɔ:'tʌmnəl] *a* осе́нний.

auxiliary I [ɔ:g'zɪljərɪ] *n* 1) помо́щник; 2) *грам.* вспомога́тельный глаго́л; 3) *pl* вспомога́тельные сою́зные войска́.

auxiliary II *a* вспомога́тельный; дополни́тельный.

avail I [ə'veɪl] *n* по́льза, вы́года; of ~ поле́зный, приго́дный; of no ~, without ~ бесполе́зный; to little ~ малополе́зный.

avail II *v* быть поле́зным, приго́дным; to ~ (oneself) of испо́льзовать (*что-л.*), воспо́льзоваться (*чем-л.*).

availability [ə,veɪlə'bɪlɪtɪ] *n* 1) приго́дность; поле́зность; 2) нали́чие; 3) ассортиме́нт.

available [ə'veɪləbl] *a* 1) нали́чный, име́ющийся (*в распоряже́нии*); досту́пный; 2) (при)го́дный; поле́зный; 3) действи́тельный (*о биле́те и т. п.*).

avalanche ['ævəlɑ:nʃ] *n* лави́на, снежный обва́л.

avarice ['ævərɪs] *n* ску́пость; жа́дность.

avaricious [,ævə'rɪʃəs] *a* скупо́й; жа́дный.

avast [ə'vɑ:st] *int мор.* стой!, стоп!

ave I ['ɑ:vɪ] *n* проща́ние.

ave II *int* приве́т! (*особ. как проща́ние*).

avenge [ə'vendʒ] *v* мстить; to ~ oneself отомсти́ть за себя́.

avengeful [ə'vendʒful] *a* мсти́тельный.

avenger [ə'vendʒə] *n* мсти́тель.

avenue ['ævɪnju:] *n* 1) алле́я, доро́га (*к до́му и т. п.*); 2) путь; сре́дство; 3) *амер.* широ́кая у́лица; проспе́кт.

aver [ə'və:] *v* утвержда́ть.

average I ['ævərɪdʒ] *n* 1) сре́днее число́, сре́дняя величина́; at (*или* on, upon) the ~ в сре́днем; below (above) the ~ ни́же (вы́ше) сре́днего; 2) убы́ток от ава́рии су́дна; 3) распределе́ние убы́тка ме́жду владе́льцами.

average II *a* 1) сре́дний; 2) обы́чный, норма́льный.

average III *v* 1) выводи́ть сре́днее число́; 2) составля́ть в сре́днем.

averment [ə'və:mənt] *n* 1) утвержде́ние; 2) доказа́тельство.

averse [ə'və:s] *a* нераспо́ложенный, нескло́нный; пита́ющий отвраще́ние (*к—to, from*).

aversely [ə'və:slɪ] *adv* неохо́тно.

aversion [ə'və:ʃən] *n* 1) неприя́знь, антипа́тия (to, from, for); 2) неохо́та (to+Inf); 3) предме́т антипа́тии.

avert [ə'vəːt] *v* 1) отводить (*глаза, руку*); отвлекать (*мысли*); 2) отвращать (*опасность, беду*).

avertible [ə'vəːtəbl] *a* предотвратимый.

aviary ['eɪvjərɪ] *n* вольер для птиц.

aviate ['eɪvɪeɪt] *v* летать на самолёте; управлять самолётом.

aviation [,eɪvɪ'eɪʃən] *n* 1) авиация; liaison ~ авиация связи; 2) *attr* авиационный.

aviator ['eɪvɪeɪtə] *n* лётчик, пилот.

aviculture ['eɪvɪkʌltʃə] *n* птицеводство.

avid ['ævɪd] *a* жадный, алчный (*of, for*).

avidity [ə'vɪdɪtɪ] *n* жадность, алчность.

aviette [,eɪvɪ'et] *n* авиетка, небольшой самолёт.

avigation [,ævɪ'geɪʃən] *n* амер. аэронавигация.

aviso [ə'vaɪzou] *n* 1) фин. авизо; 2) мор. посыльное судно.

avocation [,ævou'keɪʃən] *n* 1) любимое занятие (*в свободное время*); 2) (основная) профессия; призвание, склонность.

avoid [ə'vɔɪd] *v* 1) избегать; уклоняться; 2) юр. аннулировать.

avoidable [ə'vɔɪdəbl] *a* которого можно избежать.

avoidance [ə'vɔɪdəns] *n* 1) избежание; 2) отмена, аннулирование; 3) вакансия.

avouch [ə'vautʃ] *v* 1) подтверждать; утверждать, уверять; 2) ручаться, гарантировать; 3) признаваться.

avow [ə'vau] *v* признавать; to ~ oneself признаваться, признать себя.

avowal [ə'vauəl] *n* (открытое) признание.

avowed [ə'vaud] *a* открыто признанный.

avowedly [ə'vauɪdlɪ] *adv* открыто, гласно.

avulsion [ə'vʌlʃən] *n* отрыв.

await [ə'weɪt] *v* ждать, ожидать.

awake I [ə'weɪk] *a predic* бодрствующий; проснувшийся; *перен.* бдительный; to be ~ а) проснуться; б) бодрствовать; to be ~ to ясно сознавать что-л.

awake II *v* (*past* awoke; *p. p.* awoke, awaked) 1) будить; *перен.* пробуждать; 2) просыпаться; *перен.* пробуждаться; to ~ to осознать.

awaken [ə'weɪkən] *v* 1) пробуждать (*чувство, стремление*); 2) просыпаться.

award I [ə'wɔːd] *n* 1) решение (*суда, жюри*); 2) присуждение (*премии, награды*); 3) награда; 4) наказание.

award II *v* присуждать что-л.; награждать чем-л.

aware [ə'wɛə] *a predic* сознающий, знающий (*of*); to be ~ of (*или* that) сознавать, отдавать себе отчёт в чём-л.

awash [ə'wɔʃ] *a predic* 1) на поверхности воды, на волнах; 2) смытый водой.

away I [ə'weɪ] *a predic* 1) отсутствующий; he is ~ from home его нет дома; 2) находящийся на расстоянии (*стольких-то километров и т. п.*); six miles ~ на расстоянии шести миль.

away II *adv* 1) *выражает удаление, движение от данного предмета* прочь; *переводится также гл. совершенного вида с префиксами* у-, от-; to go ~ уходить; go ~ please! уходите, пожалуйста!; ~ with you! убирайтесь вон!; ~ with it! уберите это прочь!; 2) *выражает отдалённость, расстояние от данного предмета* вдали; from home he felt lonely вдали от дома он скучал; far ~ далеко; 3) *выражает передачу в собственность другому лицу, пре-*

кращение использования, существования, исчезновение; *передаётся гл. с префиксами* у-, от-, раз-, рас-; I have given the money ~ я отдал деньги; to waste ~ растрачивать; 4) *выражает непрерывно продолжающееся действие; переводится гл.* продолжать *с инфинитивом основного глагола*: the soldiers fired ~ солдаты продолжали стрелять.

awe I [ɔː] *n* благоговейный страх; to keep (*или* to hold) in ~ внушать страх, благоговение; to stand in ~ бояться (*кого-л.— of*); испытывать трепет (*перед кем-л.— of*).

awe II *v* внушать страх, благоговение.

awesome ['ɔːsəm] *a* страшный, внушающий страх.

awestruck ['ɔːstrʌk] *a* поражённый, проникнутый благоговейным страхом.

awful ['ɔːful] *a* 1) *разг.* ужасный; 2) внушающий страх, благоговение *или* почтение.

awfully[a] ['ɔːfulɪ] *adv* ужасно.

awfully[b] ['ɔːflɪ] *adv разг.* чрезвычайно, крайне.

awhile [ə'waɪl] *adv* (на) некоторое время; wait ~ подождите немного.

awkward ['ɔːkwəd] *a* 1) неуклюжий, неловкий (*о человеке, движении*); 2) неудобный; неловкий, затруднительный (*о положении и т. п.*); 3) опасный.

awkwardness ['ɔːkwədnɪs] *n* 1) неуклюжесть; 2) неловкость.

awl [ɔːl] *n* шило.

awn [ɔːn] *n* ость (*колоса*).

awning ['ɔːnɪŋ] *n* тент, навес.

awoke [ə'wouk] *past, p. p. см.* awake II.

awry I [ə'raɪ] *a predic* 1) кривой, косой; 2) искажённый; 3) неправильный.

awry II *adv* 1) косо, вкось; to look ~ смотреть косо, коситься; 2) неправильно, плохо; to take ~ толковать неправильно *или* в дурную сторону.

ax(e) I [æks] *n* 1) топор; секира; to get the ~ *разг.* быть казнённым; 2) (the ~) *разг.* резкое сокращение бюджета; ◊ to put the ~ in the helve разрешить трудный вопрос, преодолеть затруднение.

ax(e) II *v* 1) рубить топором; 2) сокращать (*бюджет, штаты*), проводить жёсткий режим экономии.

axes[1] ['æksɪz] *pl см.* ax(e) I.

axes[2] ['æksiːz] *pl см.* axis.

axial ['æksɪəl] *a* осевой.

axiom ['æksɪəm] *n* аксиома.

axiomatic(al) [,æksɪə'mætɪk(əl)] *a* не требующий доказательства, самоочевидный.

axis ['æksɪs] *n* (*pl* axes) ось.

axle ['æksl] *n тех.* ось, вал.

axle-box ['ækslbɔks] *n тех.* букса, подшипниковая коробка.

axled ['æksld] *a тех.* осевой.

axle-pin ['ækslpɪn] *n тех.* чека.

axle-tree ['æksltriː] *n* колёсный вал, ось.

ay I [aɪ] *n* (*pl* ayes [aɪz]) положительный ответ; голос «за» (*при голосовании*); the ayes have it большинство за (*при голосовании*).

ay II *int* да.

ayah ['aɪə] *n инд.* няня-туземка.

aye [eɪ] *adv уст.* всегда; for ~ навсегда.

Azerbaijanian I [ɑː,zəːbaɪ'dʒɑːnɪən] *n* 1) азербайджанец; азербайджанка; the ~s азербайджанцы; 2) азербайджанский язык.

Azerbaijanian II *a* азербайджа́нский.
azimuth [ˈæzɪməθ] *n* а́зимут.
azote [əˈzout] *n* азо́т.
azotic [əˈzɔtɪk] *a* азо́тный; азо́тистый.
azure I [ˈæʒə] *n* лазу́рь; небе́сная лазу́рь.
azure II *a* голубо́й, лазу́рный.

B

B, b [biː] *n* 1) 2-я бу́ква англ. алфави́та; 2) *муз.* но́та си.
babble I [ˈbæbl] *n* 1) ле́пет; бормота́ние; гул (*голосо́в, толпы́*); 2) болтовня́; 3) журча́ние.
babble II *v* 1) лепета́ть; бормота́ть; 2) болта́ть; вы́болтать, проболта́ться; 3) журча́ть.
babbler [ˈbæblə] *n* болту́н.
babe [beɪb] *n поэт.* младе́нец, ребёнок; ◊ ~s and sucklings, ~s in the wood простаки́, дове́рчивые, нео́пытные лю́ди.
baboo [ˈbɑːbuː] *n* 1) господи́н (*обраще́ние*); 2) *ист.* чино́вник-инди́ец, пи́шущий по-англи́йски.
baboon [bəˈbuːn] *n* бабуи́н (*обезья́на*).
baby [ˈbeɪbɪ] *n* 1) младе́нец, ребёнок; 2) *attr* ма́лый, небольшо́й; ◊ to hold the ~ а) не име́ть свобо́ды де́йствий; б) нести́ неприя́тную отве́тственность.
babyhood [ˈbeɪbɪhud] *n* младе́нчество.
babyish [ˈbeɪbɪʃ] *a* де́тский, ребя́ческий.
Bacchanal [ˈbækənl] *a* вакхи́ческий; разгу́льный.
baccy [ˈbækɪ] *n разг.* табачо́к.
bachelor[1] [ˈbætʃələ] *n* холостя́к.
bachelor[2] *n* бакала́вр.
bacillus [bəˈsɪləs] *n* (*pl* bacilli [bəˈsɪlaɪ]) баци́лла.
back I [bæk] *n* 1) спина́; to be (*или* to lie) on one's ~ а) быть побеждённым; б) лежа́ть больны́м; to give smb. the ~ игнори́ровать кого́-л., пренебрега́ть кем-л.; he is glad to see the ~ of он сча́стлив, что отде́лался от (*кого́-л.*); to turn one's ~ upon smb. поки́нуть кого́-л., отверну́ться от кого́-л.; with one's ~ to the wall прижа́тый к стене́; to crouch one's ~ before гнуть спи́ну пе́ред (*кем-л.*); 2) за́дняя часть *или* оборо́тная сторона́ чего́-л.: спи́нка (*сту́ла, пла́тья*); изна́нка; корешо́к (*кни́ги*); ~ of the hand ты́льная пове́рхность руки́; at the ~ of one's mind подсозна́тельно; to be at the ~ of быть та́йной причи́ной чего́-л.; 3) гре́бень (*волны́, холма́*); ~ of the ship киль су́дна; 4) *спорт.* защи́тник; ◊ an edge cell целико́м, по́лностью; to break the ~ of а) преодоле́ть препя́тствие *или* са́мую тру́дную часть чего́-л.; отде́латься от; б) разори́ть кого́-л.; в) сокруши́ть, сломи́ть сопротивле́ние; it breaks the camel's ~ ≅ э́то после́дняя ка́пля; to get (*или* to put, to set) one's ~ up рассерди́ть(ся), разозли́ть(ся); on the ~ of в дополне́ние к; to put one's ~ into мно́го рабо́тать над чем-л.; the ~ of beyond край све́та.
back II *a* 1) за́дний; отдалённый; 2) запозда́лый; устаре́вший; ста́рый (*о но́мере журна́ла, газе́ты*); просро́ченный (*о платеже́*).

back III *adv* 1) наза́д, обра́тно; I am glad to see you ~ я рад, что вы верну́лись; ~ and forth взад и вперёд; туда́ и сюда́; there and ~ туда́ и обра́тно; 2) в стороне́ (*от чего́-л.*), вдали́; 3) тому́ наза́д; as far ~ as... ещё в..., уже́ в... (*о да́те*); 4): ~ of, ~ from *амер.* позади́; ◊ to go ~ from (*или* upon) one's word отступа́ться от своего́ сло́ва; не сдержа́ть сло́ва; to go ~ on smb. преда́ть кого́-л.
back IV *v* 1) подде́рживать, подкрепля́ть; 2) помога́ть; субсиди́ровать; 3) служи́ть спи́нкой, фо́ном, подкла́дкой; 4) класть на подкла́дку; 5) грани́чить, соприкаса́ться (*с — on, upon*); 6) оса́живать (*ло́шадь, экипа́ж*); дава́ть за́дний ход; 7) отступа́ть, пя́тить(ся); to ~ and fill *мор.* лави́ровать; *перен.* колеба́ться, быть в нереши́тельности; 8) держа́ть пари́ за кого́-л.; ста́вить (*на ло́шадь*); 9) индосси́ровать (*ве́ксель*); 10) е́здить верхо́м; сади́ться в седло́; 11) приуча́ть (*ло́шадь*) к седлу́; □ to ~ **down** отступа́ться от чего́-л.; to ~ **out** уклоня́ться, отступа́ть от чего́-л. (*of*); to ~ **up** подде́рживать.
backache [ˈbækeɪk] *n* боль в спине́ *или* пояснице.
back-bencher [ˈbækˈbentʃə] *n* заднескаме́ечник, рядово́й депута́т парла́мента, не занима́ющий официа́льного поста́.
backbit [ˈbækbɪt] *past см.* backbite.
backbite [ˈbækbaɪt] *v* (*past* backbit; *p. p.* backbitten) злосло́вить; клевета́ть.
backbiter [ˈbækˌbaɪtə] *n* клеветни́к.
backbitten [ˈbækˌbɪtn] *p. p. см.* backbite.
backbone [ˈbækboun] *n* 1) спинно́й хребе́т, позвоно́чник; to the ~ до мо́зга косте́й; 2) осно́ва, суть; 3) твёрдость хара́ктера.
back-breaking [ˈbækˌbreɪkɪŋ] *a* изнури́тельный.
back-chat [ˈbæktʃæt] *n разг.* 1) нахо́дчивый, ко́лкий отве́т; 2) перебра́нка.
back-cloth [ˈbækklɔθ] *n* 1) *театр.* за́дник; 2) *кино* экра́н.
back-country [ˈbækˌkʌntrɪ] *n* 1) вну́тренние райо́ны страны́; 2) *воен.* глубо́кий тыл.
backdoor I [ˈbækdɔː] *n* чёрный ход, за́дний ход.
backdoor II *a* закули́сный, та́йный.
backer [ˈbækə] *n* 1) подде́рживающий кого́-л.; покрови́тель; 2) держа́щий пари́; ста́вящий на ло́шадь.
backfire [ˈbækˈfaɪə] *n* 1) *тех.* обра́тная вспы́шка; 2) встре́чный ого́нь (*как сре́дство борьбы́ с лесны́м пожа́ром*).
backgammon [bækˈgæmən] *n* игра́ в трикта́к.
background [ˈbækgraund] *n* 1) за́дний план; фон; to stay in the ~ остава́ться в тени́, на за́днем пла́не; 2) подоплёка.
backhand I [ˈbækhænd] *n* 1) по́черк с накло́ном букв вле́во; 2) уда́р сле́ва (*в те́ннисе*).
backhand II *a* 1) нанесённый ты́льной стороно́й руки́ (*об уда́ре*); 2) неи́скренний; двусмы́сленный.
backhanded [ˈbækˈhændɪd] *a* 1) *см.* backhand II 1); 2) косо́й, с накло́ном вле́во (*о по́черке*); 3) сомни́тельный, двусмы́сленный (*о комплиме́нте*).
backing [ˈbækɪŋ] *n* 1) подде́ржка; 2) подкла́дка; 3) осно́ва; 4) за́дний ход; враще́ние про́тив

часово́й стре́лки; ◊ ~ and filling колеба́ние, нереши́тельность.

backlog ['bæklɔg] n накопи́вшиеся невы́полненные дела́, зава́л рабо́ты.

backmost ['bækmoust] a са́мый за́дний.

backside ['bæk'saɪd] n за́дняя сторона́; зад.

back-sight ['bæk,saɪt] n прице́л.

backslide ['bæk'slaɪd] v отступа́ть(ся).

backslider ['bæk'slaɪdə] n отсту́пник.

backstairs I ['bæk'steəz] n чёрная, за́дняя ле́стница.

backstairs II a закули́сный, та́йный.

backstitch ['bækstɪtʃ] n стро́чка (в шитье́).

back-talk ['bæktɔk] n разг. де́рзкий, ре́зкий отве́т.

backward I ['bækwəd] a 1) обра́тный (о движе́нии); 2) отста́лый; запозда́лый; 3) отстаю́щий; 4) ме́длящий; 5) ро́бкий, засте́нчивый.

backward II adv 1) наза́д, обра́тно; 2) за́дом; 3) наоборо́т, за́дом наперёд; 4) к ху́дшему.

backwards ['bækwədz] см. backward II.

backwash ['bækwɔʃ] n 1) вода́, отбра́сываемая винто́м парохо́да; волна́ от парохо́да; 2) ав. завихре́ние.

backwater ['bæk,wɔtə] n запру́женная вода́; за́водь; перен. засто́й.

backwoods ['bækwudz] n pl лесна́я глушь.

bacon ['beɪkən] n копчёная свина́я груди́нка, беко́н; ◊ to save one's ~ разг. спаса́ть свою́ шку́ру.

bacteria [bæk'tɪərɪə] pl см. bacterium.

bacteriological [bæk,tɪərɪə'lɔdʒɪkəl] a бактериологи́ческий.

bacteriologist [bæk,tɪərɪ'ɔlədʒɪst] n бактерио́лог.

bacteriology [bæk,tɪərɪ'ɔlədʒɪ] n бактериоло́гия.

bacterium [bæk'tɪərɪəm] n (pl bacteria) бакте́рия.

bad I [bæd] a (compar worse I; superl worst I) 1) плохо́й, дурно́й; 2) испо́рченный; to go ~ сгнить, испо́ртиться; 3) развращённый; поро́чный; 4) больно́й; to feel ~ чу́вствовать себя́ пло́хо; to look ~ пло́хо вы́глядеть; име́ть больно́й вид; to be taken ~ заболе́ть; 5) нездоро́вый, вре́дный; 6) си́льный (о бо́ли, хо́лоде); серьёзный (о боле́зни); гру́бый (об оши́бке); 7) фальши́вый (о деньга́х); 8) безнадёжный (о до́лге).

bad II n неуда́ча; убы́ток; £ 500 to the ~ пятьсо́т фу́нтов сте́рлингов убы́тку; ◊ to go to the ~ поги́бнуть, мора́льно опусти́ться; from ~ to worse всё ху́же и ху́же; ≅ из огня́ да в по́лымя; to go from ~ to worse ухудша́ться.

bade [beɪd] past см. bid I.

badge [bædʒ] n 1) знак, значо́к; 2) эмбле́ма, си́мвол.

badger I ['bædʒə] n барсу́к.

badger II v 1) трави́ть; 2) раздража́ть, изводи́ть.

badly ['bædlɪ] adv (compar worse II; superl worst II) пло́хо, ду́рно; 2) си́льно, о́чень; ~ wounded тяжело́ ра́нен; I want it ~ мне э́то о́чень ну́жно; to be ~ off си́льно нужда́ться (в чём-л. — for).

badminton ['bædmɪntən] n бадминто́н.

bad-tempered ['bæd'tempəd] a раздражи́тельный.

baffle ['bæfl] v 1) сбива́ть с то́лку; ста́вить в тупи́к; 2) расстра́ивать пла́ны; препя́тствовать, меша́ть.

bag I [bæg] n 1) мешо́к; 2) портфе́ль; 3) су́мка; shopping ~ хозя́йственная су́мка; 4) ягдта́ш; добы́ча (охо́тника); 5) pl мешки́ (под глаза́ми); 6) вы́мя; 7) pl бога́тство; 8) pl сленг штаны́ (тж. pair of ~s); ◊ to empty the ~ рассказа́ть, ничего́ не скрыва́я, вы́ложить начистоту́; ~ and baggage со все́ми пожи́тками; ~ of bones истощённый челове́к; ≅ ко́жа да ко́сти.

bag II v 1) класть в мешо́к; 2) охот. уби́ть, подстрели́ть; 3) собира́ть, коллекциони́ровать; 4) разг., шутл. стащи́ть, взять; I have ~ged some of your cigarettes я стащи́л у вас не́сколько папиро́с; 5) наполня́ть(ся) во́здухом, надува́ть(ся); 7) висе́ть мешко́м (об оде́жде); 7) ав. сбить самолёт; ◊ ~s I!, ~s! шк. чур-чура́!

bagatelle [,bægə'tel] n пустя́к, безде́лица.

bagful ['bægful] n мешо́к (как ме́ра).

baggage ['bægɪdʒ] n 1) бага́ж; 2) воен. обо́з; 3): impudent ~ наха́лка; silly ~ ду́ра; sly (или saucy) ~ плуто́вка, озорни́ца; 4) attr бага́жный; 5) attr вью́чный (о живо́тном).

bagger ['bægə] n землечерпа́лка; черпа́к.

baggy ['bægɪ] a мешкова́тый.

bagman ['bægmən] n разг. коммивояжёр.

bagpipe ['bægpaɪp] n муз. волы́нка.

bail[1] I [beɪl] n 1) поручи́тельство, зало́г; 2) поручи́тель; to go ~ for поручи́ться (за кого́-л.).

bail[1] II v руча́ться; брать на пору́ки (тж. to ~ out).

bail[2] I n ру́чка (ведра́ или ча́йника).

bail[2] II v вычёрпывать во́ду (из ло́дки); ◊ to ~ out a) вы́броситься с парашю́том; б) (в спе́шке) поки́нуть подби́тый танк.

bailee [beɪ'liː] n лицо́, кото́рому дове́рены това́ры на хране́ние.

bailey ['beɪlɪ] n 1) ист. двор, стена́ за́мка; 2): Old Bailey Центра́льный уголо́вный суд (в Ло́ндоне).

bailie ['beɪlɪ] n шотл. член городско́го управле́ния, ба́льи.

bailiff ['beɪlɪf] n 1) суде́бный при́став; 2) управля́ющий име́нием.

bailment ['beɪlmənt] n 1) освобожде́ние на пору́ки; 2) юр. переда́ча иму́щества на хране́ние.

bairn [bɛən] n шотл. ребёнок.

bait[1] I [beɪt] n 1) прима́нка; нажи́вка; to jump at the ~, to swallow the ~ попа́сться на у́дочку (тж. перен.); 2) искуше́ние; 3) остано́вка в пути́ (для еды́ и о́тдыха).

bait[1] II v 1) наса́живать нажи́вку, класть прима́нку; 2) остана́вливаться в пути́ (для еды́ и о́тдыха); 3) корми́ть ло́шадь (в пути́); получа́ть корм (о ло́шади).

bait[2] I n я́рость, гнев.

bait[2] II v 1) трави́ть соба́ками; 2) дразни́ть, изводи́ть.

baize [beɪz] n 1) ба́йка; 2) attr ба́йковый.

bake [beɪk] v 1) печь(ся); запека́ть(ся); to be ~d with heat запе́чься, растре́скаться от жары́ (о губа́х); 2) затвердева́ть; 3) загора́ть на со́лнце; 4) обжига́ть (кирпичи́).

bakehouse ['beɪkhaus] n пека́рня.

bakelite ['beɪkəlaɪt] n тех. бакели́т.

baker ['beɪkə] *n* пе́карь; бу́лочник.
baker-legged ['beɪkəlegd] *a* кривоно́гий.
bakery ['beɪkərɪ] *n* 1) пека́рня; 2) бу́лочная.
baksheesh ['bækʃiːʃ] *n* 1) взя́тка, бакши́ш; 2) чаевы́е.
balance I ['bæləns] *n* 1) весы́; Danish ~ безме́н; spring ~ пружи́нные весы, безме́н; 2) равнове́сие; ~ of power полити́ческое равнове́сие; to strike a ~ восстанови́ть равнове́сие, примири́ть; to keep ~ сохраня́ть равнове́сие, споко́йствие; 3) ма́ятник; 4) противове́с; 5) эк. бала́нс; оста́ток; ~ of trade акти́вный бала́нс (вне́шней торго́вли); 6) *разг.* оста́ток, оста́вшаяся часть; ~ of the day коне́ц дня.
balance II *v* 1) уравнове́шивать; 2) взве́шивать, сопоставля́ть (*with, by, against*); 3) баланси́ровать; сохраня́ть равнове́сие; *перен.* колеба́ться (*between*); 4) эк. подводи́ть бала́нс.
balance-bridge ['bælənsbrɪdʒ] *n* подъёмный мост.
balanced ['bælənst] *a* уравнове́шенный; гармони́чный.
balancer ['bælənsə] *n* эквилибри́ст.
balance-sheet ['bælənsʃiːt] *n* бала́нс.
balconied ['bælkənɪd] *a* с балко́ном, с балко́нами.
balcony ['bælkənɪ] *n* балко́н.
bald [bɔːld] *a* 1) лы́сый; плеши́вый; 2) оголённый; лишённый расти́тельности, пе́рьев, ме́ха; 3) просто́й, бесцве́тный (*о стиле и т. п.*); 4) неприкра́шенный; непр́икрытый (*о недоста́тках*); 5) с бе́лым пятно́м на лбу (*о живо́тном*).
baldachin ['bɔːldəkɪn] *n* балдахи́н.
balderdash ['bɔːldədæʃ] *n* вздор.
bald-headed I ['bɔːld'hedɪd] *a* лы́сый; плеши́вый.
bald-headed II *adv:* to go ~ *сленг* а) идти́ напроло́м; де́йствовать безрассу́дно; б) с жа́ром принима́ться за что-л.
baldly ['bɔːldlɪ] *adv* откры́то, пря́мо; напрями́к; ску́дно, убо́го.
baldric ['bɔːldrɪk] *n* пе́ревязь (*для меча́, ро́га*): портупе́я.
bale[1] I [beɪl] *n* 1) ки́па, тюк; 2) *pl* това́р.
bale[1] II *v* укла́дывать в ки́пы, тюки́.
bale[2] *v см.* bail[2] II.
bale[3] *n поэт., уст.* бе́дствие.
baleen [bə'liːn] *n* кито́вый ус.
balefire ['beɪlˌfaɪə] *n* сигна́льный ого́нь, костёр.
baleful ['beɪlful] *a поэт.* 1) па́губный, ги́бельный; 2) мра́чный.
balk I [bɔːk] *n* 1) ба́лка, брус; *мор.* бимс; the ~s черда́чное помеще́ние; 2) невспа́ханная полоса́ земли́; межа́; 3) препя́тствие, поме́ха, заде́ржка; 4) про́мах, оши́бка; неуда́ча.
balk II *v* 1) препя́тствовать, меша́ть; заде́рживать; 2) пропуска́ть; игнори́ровать; 3) не опра́вдывать наде́жд; 4) отка́зываться; уклоня́ться; 5) арта́читься, упира́ться (*о ло́шади*).
Balkan ['bɔːlkən] *a* балка́нский.
ball[1] I [bɔːl] *n* 1) шар; мяч; клубо́к; 2) баллотиро́вочный шар; 3) пу́ля; *ист.* ядро́; ◇ ~ of the eye глазно́е я́блоко; ~ of the knee коле́нная ча́шка; ~ of fortune игру́шка судьбы́; the ~ is with you ва́ша о́чередь, о́чередь за ва́ми; to have

the ~ at one's feet быть господи́ном положе́ния; име́ть ша́нсы на успе́х; to keep up the ~, to keep the ~ rolling подде́рживать, продолжа́ть разгово́р; three ~s вы́веска ростовщика́.
ball[1] II *v* собира́ть(ся), свива́ть(ся) в клубо́к.
ball[2] *n* бал, танцева́льный ве́чер; to open the ~ откры́ть бал; *перен.* взять на себя́ инициати́ву.
ballad ['bæləd] *n* балла́да (*лирико-эпи́ческая поэ́ма наро́дного хара́ктера*).
ballade [bæ'lɑːd] *n* балла́да (*лири́ческая песнь*).
ballad-monger ['bæləd,mʌŋgə] *n* пренебр. рифмоплёт.
ballast I ['bæləst] *n* 1) балла́ст; 2) о́пыт(ность); убежде́ния, усто́и.
ballast II *v* 1) грузи́ть, снабжа́ть балла́стом; придава́ть усто́йчивость (*тж. перен.*); 2) *ж.-д.* засыпа́ть балла́стом.
ball-bearing ['bɔːl'bɛərɪŋ] *n* шарикоподши́пник.
ballet ['bæleɪ] *n* бале́т.
ballet-dancer ['bæleɪ,dɑːnsə] *n* арти́ст, арти́стка бале́та; балери́на.
ballet-master ['bæleɪ,mɑːstə] *n* балетме́йстер.
ballistics [bə'lɪstɪks] *n* балли́стика.
balloon I [bə'luːn] *n* 1) возду́шный шар; неуправля́емый аэроста́т; barrage ~ аэроста́т загражде́ния; captive ~ привязно́й аэроста́т; 2): trial ~ про́бный шар.
balloon II *v* 1) поднима́ться на аэроста́те; 2) раздува́ться как шар.
ballot I ['bælət] *n* 1) избира́тельный бюллете́нь; баллотиро́вочный шар; to mark one's ~ запо́лнить свой избира́тельный бюллете́нь; 2) голосова́ние (*особ. та́йное*); баллотиро́вка; second ~ повто́рное голосова́ние, баллоти́рование; successive ~s многоступе́нчатые вы́боры; to take a ~ голосова́ть; 3) жеребьёвка.
ballot II *v* 1) голосова́ть, баллоти́ровать; 2) тяну́ть жре́бий.
ballot-box ['bælətbɔks] *n* избира́тельная у́рна; баллотиро́вочный я́щик.
ballot-paper ['bælət,peɪpə] *n* избира́тельный бюллете́нь.
ball-room ['bɔːlruːm] *n* танцева́льный зал.
ballyhoo ['bælɪ'huː] *n амер.* крича́щая рекла́ма; шуми́ха.
ballyrag ['bælɪræg] *v сленг* гру́бо шути́ть, издева́ться.
balm [bɑːm] *n* бальза́м.
balmy ['bɑːmɪ] *a* 1) души́стый; 2) мя́гкий, не́жный; 3) успока́ивающий; цели́тельный.
baloney [bə'lounɪ] *см.* boloney.
balsam ['bɔːlsəm] *n* 1) бальза́м; 2) *бот.* бальзами́н.
baluster ['bæləstə] *n* 1) баля́сина; 2) *pl* балюстра́да.
balustrade [,bæləs'treɪd] *n* балюстра́да.
bamboo [bæm'buː] *n* 1) бамбу́к; 2) *attr* бамбу́ковый.
bamboozle [bæm'buːzl] *v сленг* обма́нывать, мистифици́ровать.
ban [bæn] *n* 1) запреще́ние; 2) объявле́ние вне зако́на; пригово́р об изгна́нии; 3) *церк.* ана́фема, прокля́тие.

ban II *v* 1) запреща́ть, налага́ть запре́т; 2) *уст.* проклина́ть.

banal [bə'nɑːl] *a* бана́льный, изби́тый.

banality [bæ'nælɪtɪ] *n* бана́льность.

banana [bə'nɑːnə] *n* 1) бана́н; 2) *attr* бана́новый.

band[1] I [bænd] *n* 1) отря́д, гру́ппа (*рабочих и т. п.*); 2) орке́стр; brass ~ духово́й орке́стр; jazz ~ джаз-ба́нд; string ~ стру́нный орке́стр.

band[1] II *v* объединя́ть(ся) (*часто* to ~ together).

band[2] *n* ба́нда; ◊ it beats the ~ *амер.* э́то превосхо́дит всё, э́то невероя́тно.

band[3] I *n* 1) обод, о́бруч; 2) тесьма́, завя́зка; ле́нта; 3) *уст.* связь, у́зы.

band[3] II *v* 1) свя́зывать; обвя́зывать; 2) окружа́ть, обрамля́ть.

bandage I ['bændɪdʒ] *n* повя́зка, бинт.

bandage II *v* перевя́зывать, бинтова́ть; де́лать перевя́зку.

bandbox ['bændbɔks] *n* карто́нка (*для шляп, лент и т. п.*); ◊ to look as if one came out of a ~ быть оде́тым с иго́лочки.

bandit ['bændɪt] *n* (*pl тж.* banditti) банди́т.

banditti [bæn'dɪtiː] *n* 1) *pl см.* bandit; 2): a ~ ша́йка разбо́йников, ша́йка банди́тов.

bandmaster ['bænd,mɑːstə] *n* капельме́йстер, дирижёр.

bandoleer [,bændə'lɪə] *n* патронта́ш.

bandolier [,bændə'lɪə] *см.* bandoleer.

band-saw ['bændsɔː] *n* ле́нточная пила́.

bandsman ['bændzmən] *n* оркестра́нт.

bandstand ['bændstænd] *n* эстра́да для орке́стра.

bandwag(g)on ['bænd,wægən] *n*: to climb on the ~, to be (*или* to get) into the ~ а) примкну́ть к стороне́, име́ющей ша́нсы на успе́х (*на выборах и т. п.*); б) заня́ть ви́дное, вы́годное положе́ние.

band-wheel ['bændwiːl] *n* приводно́е колесо́.

bandy[1] ['bændɪ] *v* 1) перебра́сываться (*мячом*); обме́ниваться (*ударами, бра́нными слова́ми*); 2) распространя́ть (*слухи*).

bandy[2] *n спорт.* 1) хокке́й; 2) клю́шка.

bandy[3] *a* криво́й (*о ногах*).

bandy-legged ['bændɪlegd] *a* кривоно́гий.

bane [beɪn] *n поэт.* ги́бель, несча́стье; прокля́тие; the ~ of my life несча́стье, прокля́тие мое́й жи́зни.

baneful ['beɪnful] *a* ги́бельный, губи́тельный.

bang[1] I [bæŋ] *n* уда́р; стук; звук уда́ра, взры́ва; with a ~ с шу́мом, с гро́хотом.

bang[1] II *v* 1) уда́рить(ся); сту́кнуть(ся); 2) хло́пнуть (*дверью и т. п.*); гро́хнуть; с шу́мом захло́пнуть(ся); 3) бить, тузи́ть; 4) *сленг* превзойти́; □ to ~ **away** загрохота́ть (*об орудиях*).

bang[1] III *adv* вдруг, как раз; to go ~ взорва́ться, си́льно хло́пнуть; вы́стрелить (*о ружье*).

bang[1] IV *int* бац!

bang[2] I *n* чёлка.

bang[2] II *v* подстрига́ть во́лосы чёлкой.

bangle ['bæŋgl] *n* брасле́т.

bang-up ['bæŋ'ʌp] *a сленг* первокла́ссный, превосхо́дный.

banish ['bænɪʃ] *v* 1) изгоня́ть, высыла́ть; 2) отгоня́ть мы́сли, изгоня́ть из па́мяти.

banishment ['bænɪʃmənt] *n* изгна́ние, вы́сылка.

banister ['bænɪstə] *n обыкн. pl* балюстра́да, пери́ла ле́стницы.

banjo ['bændʒou] *n* ба́нджо (*муз. инструмент*).

bank[1] I [bæŋk] *n* 1) бе́рег реки́; 2) вал, на́сыпь; 3) нано́с, зано́с; ~ of snow снежный сугро́б; ~ of clouds гряда́ облако́в; 4) о́тмель, ба́нка; 5) *ав.* крен.

bank[1] II *v* 1) де́лать на́сыпь; окружа́ть ва́лом; образова́ть нано́сы; 2) *ав., авто* накреня́ться.

bank[2] I *n* 1) банк; The Bank Англи́йский банк; 2) *карт.* банк; to break the ~ сорва́ть банк; 3) *attr* ба́нковый, ба́нковский.

bank[2] II *v* 1) класть де́ньги в банк; держа́ть де́ньги в ба́нке; 2) быть банки́ром; 3) *карт.* держа́ть банк; 4) наде́яться, рассчи́тывать (*on, upon*).

bankable ['bæŋkəbl] *a фин.* учи́тываемый.

bank-bill ['bæŋkbɪl] *n* 1) ве́ксель; 2) *амер. см.* bank-note.

bank-book ['bæŋkbuk] *n* лицево́й счёт (*в ба́нке*).

banker[1] ['bæŋkə] *n* 1) банки́р; 2) *карт.* банкомёт.

banker[2] *n* землеко́п.

banking[1] ['bæŋkɪŋ] *n* ба́нковое де́ло.

banking[2] *n ав.* крен, вира́ж.

bank-note ['bæŋknout] *n* ба́нковый биле́т, банкно́т.

bank-rate ['bæŋkreɪt] *n* учётная ста́вка ба́нка.

bankrupt I ['bæŋkrəpt] *n* банкро́т; несостоя́тельный должни́к.

bankrupt II *a* несостоя́тельный, обанкро́тившийся; to go ~ обанкро́титься.

bankrupt III *v* привести́ к банкро́тству; разори́ть.

bankruptcy ['bæŋkrəpsɪ] *n* банкро́тство.

banksman ['bæŋksmən] *n горн.* рукоя́тчик, рабо́чий у у́стья ша́хты.

banner ['bænə] *n* 1) зна́мя; флаг; стяг; to join (*или* to follow) the ~ (of) стать под знамёна; *перен.* после́довать (за); 2) *амер.* заголо́вок в газе́те кру́пным шри́фтом, «ша́пка»; 3) *attr* наилу́чший, образцо́вый; гла́вный.

banner-bearer ['bænə,beərə] *n* знамено́сец.

banner-cry ['bænəkraɪ] *n* боево́й клич.

banns [bænz] *n pl* оглаше́ние в це́ркви имён вступа́ющих в брак.

banquet I ['bæŋkwɪt] *n* банке́т, (зва́ный) обе́д; пир; funeral ~ поми́нки; a regular ~ о́чень хоро́ший обе́д.

banquet II *v* дава́ть банке́т в честь кого́-л.; пирова́ть.

bantam ['bæntəm] *n* 1) банта́мка (*порода кур*); *перен.* ма́ленький, но сме́лый и энерги́чный челове́к; 2) боксёр легча́йшего ве́са; 3) *attr* ма́ленький, ка́рликовый.

bantam-weight ['bæntəm,weɪt] *n спорт.* легча́йший вес, «вес петуха́».

banter I ['bæntə] *n* добро́душное поддра́знивание.

banter II *v* добро́душно поддра́знивать.

bantling ['bæntlɪŋ] *n* 1) ребёнок; 2) *презр.* отро́дье.

baptism ['bæptɪzəm] *n* креще́ние; ~ of fire боево́е креще́ние.

baptist [ˈbæptɪst] *n* 1) крести́тель; 2) бапти́ст.

baptize [bæpˈtaɪz] *v* 1) крести́ть; *перен.* очища́ть(ся); 2) дава́ть и́мя, про́звище; окрести́ть.

bar[1] I [bɑː] *n* 1) брусо́к (*металла, дерева, мыла и т. п.*); ~ of chocolate пли́тка шокола́да; 2) засо́в; 3) прегра́да, препя́тствие; 4) заста́ва; 5) *pl* решётка; 6) о́тмель, бар; 7) полоса́ (*света*); 8) *муз.* та́ктовая черта́.

bar[1] II *v* 1) запира́ть на засо́в; 2) прегражда́ть; 3) запреща́ть; исключа́ть; □ to ~ in не выпуска́ть, запира́ть; to ~ out не впуска́ть.

bar[1] III *prep* исключа́я, за исключе́нием.

bar[2] *n* 1) (the ~) адвокату́ра; to be at the ~ быть адвока́том; to be called to the ~ получи́ть пра́во адвока́тской пра́ктики; to go to the ~ стать адвока́том; 2) барье́р в суде́, отделя́ющий скамью́ подсуди́мых; ◇ ~ of conscience суд со́вести; ~ of public opinion суд обще́ственного мне́ния.

bar[3] *n* 1) сто́йка, прила́вок; 2) бар, небольшо́й рестора́н.

barb [bɑːb] *n* 1) ость (*колоса*); 2) боро́дка (*птичьего пера*); 3) колю́чка; *перен.* жа́ло; 4) зазу́брина, зубе́ц.

barbarian I [bɑːˈbɛərɪən] *n* ва́рвар.

barbarian II *a* ва́рварский.

barbaric [bɑːˈbærɪk] *a* ва́рварский.

barbarism [ˈbɑːbərɪzəm] *n* 1) ва́рварство; 2) *лингв.* варвари́зм.

barbarity [bɑːˈbærɪtɪ] *n* 1) ва́рварство, жесто́кость; 2) гру́бость (*вкуса и т. п.*).

barbarous [ˈbɑːbərəs] *a* 1) ва́рварский, ди́кий; 2) гру́бый, жесто́кий.

barbecue I [ˈbɑːbɪkjuː] *n* 1) ту́ша, зажа́ренная целико́м; 2) *амер.* пра́зднество на откры́том во́здухе, во вре́мя кото́рого ту́ши жа́рятся целико́м.

barbecue II *v* жа́рить ту́шу целико́м.

barbed [bɑːbd] *a* колю́чий, с колю́чками; *перен.* ядови́тый, ко́лкий.

bar-bell [ˈbɑːbel] *n* *спорт.* шта́нга.

barber[1] [ˈbɑːbə] *n* парикма́хер, цирю́льник.

barber[2] *n* 1) пар над водо́й в моро́зный день; 2) си́льный моро́зный ве́тер.

barber(r)y [ˈbɑːbərɪ] *n* *бот.* барбари́с.

bard[1] [bɑːd] *n* *поэт.* бард, поэ́т; the Bard of Avon Шекспи́р; the Bard of Ayrshire Ро́берт Бернс.

bard[2] *n* *ист.* ко́нский доспе́х.

bare I [bɛə] *a* 1) го́лый, обнажённый; to lay ~ обнару́жить; разоблачи́ть; 2) пусто́й; лишённый чего́-л.; 3) бе́дный, ску́дный; неприкра́шенный; 4) потёртый; поно́шенный; 5) мале́йший, незначи́тельный; едва́ доста́точный; a ~ hundred pounds каки́е-то (незначи́тельные) сто фу́нтов сте́рлингов; ◇ to be ~ of credit a) име́ть плоху́ю репута́цию; б) быть неизве́стным.

bare II *v* обнажа́ть; раскрыва́ть.

bareback I [ˈbɛəbæk] *a* неосёдланный.

bareback II *adv* без седла́.

barebacked [ˈbɛəbækt] *см.* bareback I.

barefaced [ˈbɛəfeɪst] *a* 1) безборо́дый; безу́сый; 2) бессты́дный, на́глый, бессо́вестный.

barefoot I [ˈbɛəfut] *a* босо́й.

barefoot II *adv* босико́м.

barefooted [ˈbɛəˈfutɪd] *a* босо́й, босоно́гий.

bare-headed [ˈbɛəˈhedɪd] *a* с непокры́той голово́й.

barely [ˈbɛəlɪ] *adv* 1) про́сто, то́лько; 2) едва́, лишь; 3) откры́то, я́сно.

bareness [ˈbɛənɪs] *n* неприкры́тость, нагота́.

bargain I [ˈbɑːgɪn] *n* 1) сде́лка; a hard ~ невы́годная сде́лка; to close (*или* to make, to strike) a ~ заключи́ть сде́лку; прийти́ к соглаше́нию; 2) дёшево ку́пленная вещь; ◇ Dutch ~, wet ~ сде́лка, зако́нченная вы́пивкой; that's a ~! по рука́м!, де́ло решённое!; into the ~ в прида́чу, прито́м; to make the best of a bad ~ не уныва́ть, не па́дать ду́хом в беде́.

bargain II *v* 1) торгова́ться; 2) ста́вить усло́вием, догова́риваться; □ to ~ for быть гото́вым к, рассчи́тывать, ожида́ть; it is more than I ~ed for э́того я не ожида́л.

bargainer [ˈbɑːgɪnə] *n* 1) торго́вец; 2) торгу́ющийся.

bargain-sale [ˈbɑːgɪnseɪl] *n* дешёвая распрода́жа.

barge I [bɑːdʒ] *n* 1) ба́ржа́, ба́рка; 2) адмира́льский ка́тер; 3) экскурсио́нный туристи́ческий парохо́д.

barge II *v* 1) перевози́ть, плыть на ба́рже́; 2) пошату́ываться, идти́ шата́ясь; неуклю́же дви́гаться (*тж.* to ~ about, to ~ along); □ to ~ against натолкну́ться на; to ~ in вторга́ться; to ~ into *см.* to ~ against.

bargee [bɑːˈdʒiː] *n* ло́дочник с баржи́; ◇ lucky ~ *разг.* счастли́вчик.

bargeman [ˈbɑːdʒmən] *см.* bargee.

baritone [ˈbærɪtoun] *см.* barytone.

barium [ˈbɛərɪəm] *n* *хим.* ба́рий.

bark[1] I [bɑːk] *n* 1) кора́ (*дерева*); 2) *сленг* ко́жа; 3) хини́н (*тж.* Peruvian ~, Jesuits' ~); ◇ with the ~ on *амер.* неотёсанный (*о челове́ке*).

bark[1] II *v* 1) сдира́ть кору́, окоря́ть; 2) сдира́ть ко́жу; 3) покрыва́ться ко́ркой; 4) дуби́ть.

bark[2] I *n* 1) лай; 2) звук вы́стрела; 3) *разг.* ка́шель; ~ his ~ is worse than his bite ≅ не бо́йся соба́ки, кото́рая ла́ет.

bark[2] II *v* 1) ла́ять; 2) *разг.* ка́шлять; 3) говори́ть повели́тельно; ря́вкать; ◇ to ~ up the wrong tree а) непра́вильно обвини́ть кого́-л.; б) *амер.* напа́сть на ло́жный след.

bark[3] *n* барк (*трёхма́чтовое су́дно*).

barkeeper[1] [ˈbɑːˌkiːpə] *n* сто́рож при заста́ве.

barkeeper[2] *n* буфе́тчик.

barker [ˈbɑːkə] *n* 1) крику́н; 2) *амер.* аукциони́ст; 3) зазыва́ла; глаша́тай; 4) револьве́р.

barkery [ˈbɑːkərɪ] *n* дуби́льный заво́д.

barking[1] [ˈbɑːkɪŋ] *n* 1) око́рка; 2) дубле́ние коро́й.

barking[2] I *n* лай.

barking[2] II *a* ла́ющий.

barley [ˈbɑːlɪ] *n* 1) ячме́нь; 2) *attr* ячме́нный; ◇ to cry ~ проси́ть поща́ды.

barleycorn [ˈbɑːlɪkɔːn] *n* ячме́нное зерно́; ◇ John Barleycorn Джон Ячме́нное Зерно́ (*олицетворе́ние спиртны́х и со́лодовых напи́тков*).

barm [bɑːm] *n* (пивны́е) дро́жжи; заква́ска.

barmaid [ˈbɑːmeɪd] *n* буфе́тчица.

barman [ˈbɑːmən] *n* буфе́тчик; ба́рмен.

barmy ['bɑːmɪ] *a* 1) пенистый, бродильный; 2) *разг.* свихнувшийся, спятивший (*тж.* ~ on the crumpet).

barn [bɑːn] *n* 1) амбар; 2) *презр.* сарай (*о большом неуютном помещении*); 3) *амер.* конюшня, коровник; 4) *амер.* трамвайный парк.

barnacle ['bɑːnəkl] *n* 1) *зоол.* морская уточка (*моллюск*); 2) надоедливый, неотвязный человек.

barn-door I ['bɑːn'dɔː] *n* ворота амбара; ◇ not to be able to hit a ~ быть плохим стрелком.

barn-door II *a*: ~ fowl домашняя птица.

barometer [bə'rɔmɪtə] *n* барометр.

baron ['bærən] *n* барон; ◇ ~ of beef толстый филей.

baronage ['bærənɪdʒ] *n* 1) бароны, сословие баронов *или* пэров; 2) титул барона.

baroness ['bærənɪs] *n* баронесса.

baronet ['bærənɪt] *n* баронет.

baronetcy ['bærənɪtsɪ] *n* титул баронета.

baronial [bə'rounjəl] *a* баронский.

barony ['bærənɪ] *n* 1) владения барона; 2) титул барона.

baroque I [bə'rouk] *n* барокко.

baroque II *a* в стиле барокко; *перен.* причудливый.

barque [bɑːk] *см.* bark[3].

barrack I ['bærək] *n* барак; *pl* казармы.

barrack II *v* 1) размещать в бараках, казармах; 2) громко высмеивать (*участников спортивного состязания*); улюлюкать.

barrage ['bærɑːʒ] *n* 1) преграда; заграждение; 2) плотина, запруда; 3) заградительный огонь; 4) *attr* заградительный.

barrel I ['bærəl] *n* 1) бочка, бочонок; 2) баррель (*мера жидкости и сыпучих тел*); 3) *амер.* деньги для финансирования политической кампании; 4) *тех.* цилиндр, вал, барабан; 5) *воен.* ствол (*ружья, орудия*).

barrel II *v* наливать в бочку, в бочки.

barrel-organ ['bærəl,ɔːgən] *n* шарманка.

barren ['bærən] *a* 1) бесплодный; неплодородный; 2) бессодержательный, скучный.

barrenness ['bærənnɪs] *n* 1) бесплодие; неплодородность; 2) бедность, бессодержательность.

barret ['bærət] *n* берет.

barricade I [,bærɪ'keɪd] *n* 1) баррикада; 2) *attr* баррикадный.

barricade II *v* баррикадировать.

barrier ['bærɪə] *n* 1) барьер; заграждение; 2) застава; шлагбаум; 3) препятствие, помеха.

barring ['bɑːrɪŋ] *prep* исключая, за исключением.

barrister ['bærɪstə] *n* адвокат.

barrow[1] ['bærou] *n* 1) холм; 2) *археол.* могильник, курган.

barrow[2] *n* 1) ручная тележка; 2) тачка (*тж.* wheel-barrow); 3) носилки (*тж.* hand-barrow).

bartender ['bɑː,tendə] *n* *амер.* буфетчик; содержатель бара.

barter I ['bɑːtə] *n* товарообмен; меновая торговля.

barter II *v* 1) менять, обменивать (*на — for*); вести меновую торговлю; 2) променять (*тж.* to ~ away).

barytone ['bærɪtoun] *n* баритон.

basalt ['bæsɔːlt] *n* *мин.* базальт.

bascule-bridge ['bæskjuːl'brɪdʒ] *n* подъёмный мост.

base[1] I [beɪs] *n* 1) основа, основание; 2) база, опорный пункт; 3) подножие (*горы*); 4) *архит.* пьедестал, цоколь; 5) *спорт.* место старта; 6) *attr* основной, базовый.

base[1] II *v* 1) основывать, базировать (*на — on, upon*); to ~ oneself on основываться на; 2) закладывать основание.

base[2] *a* 1) низменный, низкий, подлый; 2) неблагородный (*о металлах*).

baseball ['beɪsbɔːl] *n* *спорт.* бейсбол.

base-court ['beɪskɔːt] *n* задний двор.

baseless ['beɪslɪs] *a* необоснованный.

basement ['beɪsmənt] *n* 1) фундамент; 2) (полу)подвальный этаж.

bases ['beɪsiːz] *pl см.* basis.

bash I ['bæʃ] *n* *разг.* сильный удар.

bash II *v* *разг.* сильно ударять.

bashful ['bæʃful] *a* застенчивый, робкий.

basic ['beɪsɪk] *a* основной.

basically ['beɪsɪkəlɪ] *adv* в основе, по существу.

basin ['beɪsn] *n* 1) таз, миска; 2) бассейн; водоём; 3) бухта; 4) бассейн (*реки*).

basis ['beɪsɪs] *n* (*pl* bases) 1) основание, базис; 2) исходный пункт; 3) *амер. воен.* база.

bask [bɑːsk] *v* 1) греться (*на солнце, у огня; in*); 2) наслаждаться (*in*); блаженствовать.

basket ['bɑːskɪt] *n* 1) корзина; 2) *attr* плетёный.

basket-ball ['bɑːskɪtbɔːl] *n* *спорт.* баскетбол.

basketful ['bɑːskɪtful] *n* полная корзина (*чего-л.*).

basketry ['bɑːskɪtrɪ] *n* плетёные изделия.

basket-work ['bɑːskɪtwəːk] *см.* basketry.

basque [bæsk] *n* баска (*род лифа*).

bas-relief ['bæsrɪ,liːf] *n* барельеф.

bass[a1] [bæs] *n* окунь.

bass[a2] *n см.* bast.

bass[b] I [beɪs] *n* бас.

bass[b] II *a* басовый, низкий.

bassoon [bə'suːn] *n* *муз.* фагот.

bass-relief ['bæsrɪ,liːf] *см.* bas-relief.

bass-wood ['bæswud] *n* американская липа.

bast [bæst] *n* лыко, луб, мочало.

bastard I ['bæstəd] *n* 1) внебрачный ребёнок; 2) *груб.* ублюдок; 3) помесь, гибрид.

bastard II *a* 1) внебрачный; 2) поддельный; притворный; 3) необычный (*о форме или размере*).

baste[1] [beɪst] *v* смётывать, шить на живую нитку.

baste[2] *v* поливать жаркое соком (*во время жаренья*).

baste[3] *v* 1) бить, колотить; 2) прерывать (*вопросами*); забрасывать (*словами*).

bastion ['bæstɪən] *n* *воен. ист.* бастион; *перен.* крепость.

bat[1] [bæt] *n* летучая мышь; ◇ to have ~s in the belfry *разг.* быть ненормальным *или* эксцентричным; as blind as a ~ совершенно слепой.

bat[2] [bæt] *n* 1) бита (*для крикета, бейсбола*); (теннисная) ракетка; 2) игрок (*в крикет, бейсбол*); a good ~ хороший игрок (*в крикет, бейсбол*);

3) *разг.* си́льный уда́р; ◊ off one's own ~ самостоя́тельно, без посторо́нней по́мощи.

bat[2] II *v* ударя́ть бито́й.

bat[3] *n разг.* шаг; to go full ~ идти́ бы́стрым ша́гом.

bat[4] *v амер.* мига́ть, морга́ть.

bat[5] *n сленг* 1) беззабо́тное весе́лье; 2) *амер.* гуля́нка, кутёж.

batata [bɑ'tɑːtə] *n бот.* бата́т.

batch [bætʃ] *n* 1) вы́печка, коли́чество вы́печенного хле́ба; 2) па́ртия, гру́ппа; ~ of workmen па́ртия рабо́чих; 3) ку́ча; па́чка; ◊ of the same ~ того́ же со́рта.

bate[1] [beɪt] *v* 1) убавля́ть, уменьша́ть, ослабля́ть; 2) сде́рживать; зата́ить (*дыха́ние и т. п.*); 3) слабе́ть, притупля́ться.

bate[2] *n* я́рость, гнев.

Bath [bɑːθ] *n*: go to ~! убира́йся к чёрту!

bath I [bɑːθ, *pl* bɑːðz] *n* 1) ва́нна; купа́ние в ва́нне; to have (*или* to take) a ~ приня́ть ва́нну (*ср.* bathe I); 2) ва́нная ко́мната (*тж.* bath-room); 3) ба́ня; купа́льное заведе́ние; ◊ ~ of blood резня́, крова́вая ба́ня.

bath II *v* мы́ть(ся), купа́ть(ся).

bathe I [beɪð] *n* купа́ние; to have a ~ вы́купаться (*ср.* bath I 1).

bathe II *v* 1) окуна́ть(ся), погружа́ть(ся); купа́ть(ся), обмыва́ть(ся); 2) омыва́ть (*берега́*); 3) залива́ть (*о све́те*).

bather ['beɪðə] *n* 1) купа́ющийся; 2) купа́льщик, -ица.

bathing ['beɪðɪŋ] *n* 1) купа́ние; 2) *attr* купа́льный.

bathing-box ['beɪðɪŋbɔks] *n* раздева́льня (для купа́ющихся).

bathing-place ['beɪðɪŋpleɪs] *n* морско́й куро́рт.

bat-horse ['bæthɔːs] *n* вью́чная ло́шадь.

bathrobe ['bɑːθroub] *n* (купа́льный) хала́т.

bath-room ['bɑːθrum] *n* ва́нная ко́мната.

bath-tub ['bɑːθtʌb] *n* ва́нна.

bathyscaphe ['bæθɪskeɪf] *n* батиска́ф.

bathysphere ['bæθɪsfɪə] *n* батисфе́ра.

bating ['beɪtɪŋ] *prep* за исключе́нием.

batiste [bæ'tiːst] *n* бати́ст.

batman ['bætmən] *n* денщи́к, вестово́й, ордина́рец.

baton ['bætən] *n* 1) полице́йская дуби́нка; 2) дирижёрская па́лочка; 3) жезл.

batsman ['bætsmən] *n* отбива́ющий, бью́щий (*в бейсбо́ле или кри́кете*).

battalion [bə'tæljən] *n* батальо́н; *амер. тж.* артиллери́йский дивизио́н.

batten[1] I ['bætn] *n* доска́; ре́йка; пла́нка, дра́нка.

batten[1] II *v* зола́чивать, скрепля́ть доска́ми; □ to ~ **down** *мор.* задра́ивать (*лю́ки*).

batten[2] *v* 1) объеда́ться, жире́ть; 2) процвета́ть за счёт други́х; 3) отка́рмливать; 4) станови́ться плодоро́дной, тучне́ть (*о по́чве*).

batter[1] I ['bætə] *v* 1) си́льно бить, колоти́ть; долби́ть; 2) мять, расплю́щивать; 3) ре́зко критикова́ть, громи́ть; 4) разбива́ть артиллери́йским огнём.

batter[2] *n см.* batsman.

batter[3] I *n архит.* усту́п, укло́н (*стены́*).

batter[3] II *v архит.* отклоня́ться, име́ть укло́н.

battered ['bætəd] *a* 1) изби́тый, разби́тый; 2) изно́шенный; потрёпанный; 3) мя́тый.

battery ['bætərɪ] *n* 1) *воен.* батаре́я; to mask one's batteries а) замаскирова́ть свои́ ору́дия; б) скрыва́ть свои́ наме́рения; 2) *эл.* батаре́я; solar batteries со́лнечные батаре́и; 3) *юр.* побо́и, оскорбле́ние де́йствием.

batting ['bætɪŋ] *n* вати́н.

battle I ['bætl] *n* 1) би́тва, бой, сраже́ние; to join ~ вступа́ть в бой; to commit to ~ вводи́ть в бой; to deliver a ~ дать бой; pitched ~ реши́тельный бой; 2) побе́да, успе́х сраже́ния; 3) борьба́.

battle II *v* би́ться, боро́ться (*с — with, against, за — for*).

battle-cruiser ['bætl,kruːzə] *n* лине́йный кре́йсер.

battle-cry ['bætlkraɪ] *n* 1) боево́й клич; 2) призы́в, ло́зунг.

battledore ['bætldɔː] *n* 1) валёк, ска́лка; 2) раке́тка (*для игры́ в вола́н*); ~ and shuttlecock игра́ в вола́н.

battle-field ['bætlfiːld] *n* по́ле сраже́ния, би́твы.

battle-fleet ['bætlfliːt] *n* лине́йный флот.

battle-ground ['bætlgraund] *n* 1) райо́н сраже́ния; теа́тр вое́нных де́йствий; 2) предме́т спо́ра.

battlement ['bætlmənt] *n обыкн. pl* зубча́тые сте́ны; зубцы́ (*сте́ны, ба́шни*).

battle-piece ['bætlpiːs] *n жив., лит.* бата́льная сце́на, карти́на.

battle-plane ['bætlpleɪn] *n* штурмово́й самолёт.

battle-ship ['bætlʃɪp] *n* лине́йный кора́бль, линко́р.

battle-tried ['bætltraɪd] *a* с боевы́м о́пытом; обстре́лянный.

bauble ['bɔːbl] *n* 1) безделу́шка; 2) безде́лица, пустя́к.

baubling ['bɔːblɪŋ] *a* пустя́чный.

baulk I, II [bɔːk] *см.* balk I, II.

bauxite ['bɔːksaɪt] *n* бокси́т.

bawbee [bɔː'biː] *n шотл.* полпе́нни.

bawdy I ['bɔːdɪ] *n* непристо́йность.

bawdy II *a* непристо́йный.

bawl [bɔːl] *v* крича́ть, ора́ть, накрича́ть (*на — at*); □ to ~ **out** а) выкри́кивать; б): to ~ smb. out накрича́ть на кого́-л.

bay[1] [beɪ] *n* 1) зали́в, бу́хта; 2) уще́лье.

bay[2] *n* 1) ла́вр(овое де́рево); 2) *pl* лавро́вый вено́к, ла́вры.

bay[3] *n* 1) *стр.* пролёт (*моста́, между коло́ннами и т. п.*); 2) вы́ступ с окно́м (*в ко́мнате*); «фона́рь».

bay[4] I *n* лай; ◊ at ~ в безвы́ходном положе́нии; to be (*или* to stand) at ~, to turn to ~ отча́янно, из после́дних сил защища́ться; to bring to ~ а) загна́ть (*зве́ря*); б) припере́ть к стене́; to keep at ~ не подпуска́ть бли́зко, держа́ть на почти́тельном расстоя́нии.

bay[4] II *v* 1) ла́ять; 2) гнать, пресле́довать.

bay[5] I *n* гнедо́й конь.

bay[5] II *a* гнедо́й.

bayonet I ['beɪənɪt] *n* 1) штык; 2) *attr* штыково́й.

bayonet II *v* коло́ть штыко́м.

bazaar [bə'zɑː] *n* 1) (восточный) база́р; 2) благотвори́тельный база́р.

bazooka [bə'zuːkə] *n* воен. (реакти́вный) противота́нковый гранатомёт «базу́ка».

be [biː] *v* (*past: sg* was, *pl* were; *p. p.* been) 1) быть; существова́ть, жить; I think, therefore, I am я мы́слю, сле́довательно, я существу́ю; 2) быва́ть, находи́ться; прису́тствовать; he is in the garden он нахо́дится в саду́; has anyone been? кто́-нибудь заходи́л?, кто́-нибудь был?; 3) чу́вствовать себя́; how are you? как вы пожива́ете?, как вы себя́ чу́вствуете?; 4) сто́ить; how much is it? ско́лько э́то сто́ит?; 5) *является глаголом-связкой и в настоящем времени по-русски не переводится*: he is my father он мой оте́ц; he is thirty years old ему́ три́дцать лет; I am cold мне хо́лодно; I am hungry я го́лоден; it is bad weather today сего́дня плоха́я пого́да; it is all over всё ко́нчено; here he is вот он; 6) *является вспомогательным глаголом*: а) *в сочетании с прич. прош. вр.* (*past participle*) *переходных глаголов образует страдательный залог* (*passive voice*): the lesson was explained by the teacher уро́к был объяснён учи́телем; б) *в сочетании с прич. прош. вр.* (*past participle*) *некоторых непереходных глаголов образует формы перфекта* (*perfect tenses*) *со значением невозвратности*: the sun is set со́лнце се́ло; the train is gone по́езд ушёл; в) *в сочетании с прич. наст. вр.* (*present participle*) *образует конкретные формы* (*continuous tenses*): he is swimming он плывёт; г) *в сочетании с прич. наст. вр.* (*present participle*) *глаголов движения принимает значение ближайшего будущего*: he is leaving next week он уе́дет на сле́дующей неде́ле; I am coming home tomorrow я верну́сь домо́й за́втра; I am going to write to him at once я сейча́с же ему́ напишу́; 7) *в сочетании с инфинитивом означает намерение, возможность, долженствование*: I am to go on Monday я до́лжен отпра́виться в понеде́льник; this book is to come э́та кни́га должна́ появи́ться; I am to inform you изве́щаю вас, я до́лжен вас извести́ть; the book was not to be found кни́гу нельзя́ бы́ло найти́; can you tell me where the book is to be had? скажи́те мне, где мо́жно доста́ть э́ту кни́гу?; □ to be **about** а) *в сочетании с инфинитивом соответствует русскому* собира́ться, намерева́ться; б) быть за́нятым чем-л.; в) быть на нога́х (*не в постели → о больном*); to be **abroad** распространя́ться (*о слухах*); to be **away** быть в отсу́тствии; уе́хать; to be **back** верну́ться; to be **down** быть больны́м, лежа́ть (*в лихорадке и т. п.; with*); to be **for** а) быть, стоя́ть за кого́-л., что́-л.; б) отправля́ться в; to be **in** а) прийти́, быть на рабо́те; б) прибы́ть (*о пароходе, поезде и т. п.*); прийти́ (*домой, на работу и т. п.*); в) наступи́ть (*о сезоне*); поспе́ть (*о фруктах, ягодах*); г) прийти́ к вла́сти (*о политических партиях*); д) to be in for име́ть в перспекти́ве; to be **off** уходи́ть, уезжа́ть; to be **on** происходи́ть (*о выборах и т. п.*); идти́ (*о войне, битве*); to be **out** *в сочетании с инфинитивом соответствует русскому* быть гото́вым (*сделать что-л.*); to be **up** а) зако́нчиться; all is up with him

с ним всё ко́нчено; the Parliament is up се́ссия парла́мента закры́лась; б) встать, подня́ться; быть на нога́х; to be up all night не спать всю ночь; в) повы́ситься (*в цене, количестве и т. п.*); the corn is up хлеб вздорожа́л; г) случи́ться, произойти́; something is up что́-то случи́лось, что́-то происхо́дит; what's up? что случи́лось?; в чём де́ло?; what are you up to? что вы заду́мали?, что вы замышля́ете?; it is up to you to decide вам реша́ть, реша́ть бу́дете вы; ◊ to let be оста́вить в поко́е; as it were е́сли бы не; как бу́дто; так сказа́ть.

be- [bɪ-] *pref* 1) *со значением* круго́м, вокру́г *служит для усиления глагола*: besiege, becloud; 2) *служит для образования переходных глаголов от непереходных, а также от существительных и прилагательных, напр.*: belabour, befriend, belittle.

beach I [biːtʃ] *n* морско́й бе́рег, пляж, о́тмель; взмо́рье; ◊ to be on the ~ а) разори́ться, быть в тру́дном положе́нии; «быть на мели́»; б) *мор. сленг* быть в отста́вке.

beach II *v* 1) наскочи́ть, сесть на мель; 2) вытя́гивать (*лодку*) на бе́рег.

beacon I ['biːkən] *n* 1) сигна́льный ого́нь; ма́як; radio ~ радиома́як; 2) ба́кен, буй; 3) фона́рь, ука́зывающий ме́сто перехо́да че́рез у́лицу; flashing ~ светофо́р; 4) предостереже́ние.

beacon II *v* 1) свети́ть, ука́зывать путь; 2) снабжа́ть буя́ми, ба́кенами.

bead I [biːd] *n* 1) бу́сина; *pl* бу́сы, би́сер; 2) *pl* чётки; to tell one's ~s чита́ть моли́твы, перебира́ть чётки; 3) ка́пля; 4) пузырёк (*воздуха*); 5) му́шка (*ружья*); to draw a ~ on прице́ливаться, наводи́ть на.

bead II *v* 1) нани́зывать бу́сы; 2) украша́ть бу́сами, би́сером.

beadle ['biːdl] *n* 1) педе́ль при университе́те; 2) церко́вный сторож.

beadledom ['biːdldəm] *n* формали́зм, канцеля́рщина.

beady ['biːdɪ] *a* 1) ма́ленький и блестя́щий (*о глазах*); 2) покры́тый бу́синками *или* ка́плями.

beagle ['biːgl] *n* 1) коротконо́гая го́нчая, бигль; 2) сы́щик; шпио́н.

beak ['biːk] *n* 1) клюв; 2) крючкова́тый нос; 3) но́сик (*чайника и т. п.*); 4) *ист.* вы́ступ на носу́ боево́го корабля́.

beaker ['biːkə] *n* 1) лаборато́рный стака́н; 2) ку́бок, ча́ша.

beam I [biːm] *n* 1) луч, пучо́к луче́й; 2) сия́ние; улы́бка; 3) ба́лка, брус; перекла́дина; 4) *мор.* бимс; ширина́ су́дна; 5) коромы́сло весо́в; ◊ to be on the ~ быть на пра́вильном пути́.

beam II *v* сия́ть (*тж. перен.*); излуча́ть (*свет, тепло*).

beam-end ['biːm'end] *n*: to be on one's ~s а) *мор.* опроки́нуться, быть на боку́; б) быть в опа́сности; быть в безвы́ходном положе́нии.

bean [biːn] *n* боб; French ~, kidney ~ фасо́ль; ◊ full of ~s горя́чий; живо́й, энерги́чный; в припо́днятом настрое́нии; to have too much ~s быть горя́чим (*о лошади*); he knows how many ~s make five ≅ он себе́ на уме́; to give smb. ~s вздуть, наказа́ть кого́-л.; руга́ть кого́-л.; стро́го обойти́сь с кем-л.; it gave me ~s э́то причини́ло мне боль, доста́вило мно́го страда́ний; not to have a ~ не име́ть ни гроша́; old ~ дружи́ще, старина́; to spill the ~s a) вы́дать секре́т, проболта́ться; б) расстро́ить пла́ны.

bean-pod ['biːnpɔd] *n* стручо́к.

bear¹ I [bɛə] *n* 1) медве́дь; polar ~, white ~ бе́лый медве́дь; 2) *астр.* Great (Little) Bear Больша́я (Ма́лая) Медве́дица; 3) спекуля́нт, игра́ющий на пониже́ние (*на бирже*).

bear¹ II *v* игра́ть на пониже́ние (*на бирже*).

bear² *v* (*past* bore; *p. p.* born, borne) 1) нести́; to ~ in mind, to ~ in view име́ть в виду́; по́мнить; учи́тывать; 2) выде́рживать груз *или* тя́жесть; 3) рожда́ть, производи́ть; плодоноси́ть; 4) терпе́ть, выноси́ть, переноси́ть; 5) опира́ться (*на — on*); 6): to ~ oneself держа́ться, вести́ себя́; □ to ~ **away** а) ~ away the prize завоева́ть, вы́играть приз; to ~ **down** а) преодолева́ть; б) *мор.* подходи́ть с наве́тренной стороны́; в) устремля́ться (*к — upon*); г) влия́ть (*на — upon*); to ~ **off** отклоня́ться; to ~ **on** каса́ться, име́ть отноше́ние к; to ~ **out** подтвержда́ть, совпада́ть; to ~ **up** а) подде́рживать; держа́ться; б) *мор.* держа́ться по ве́тру; to ~ **upon** *см.* to ~ **on**; to ~ **with** мири́ться с, относи́ться терпи́мо к.

bearable ['bɛərəbl] *a* терпи́мый; сно́сный.

beard¹ [biəd] *n* 1) борода́; 2) ость (*колоса*).

beard² *v* откры́то выступа́ть про́тив.

bearded ['biədid] *a* борода́тый.

beardless ['biədlis] *a* безборо́дый.

bearer ['bɛərə] *n* 1) несу́щий, принося́щий *или* подде́рживающий что-л.; 2) носи́льщик; 3) пода́тель; предъяви́тель; 4) плодонося́щее расте́ние; a good (bad) ~ расте́ние, принося́щее хоро́ший (плохо́й) урожа́й; 5) *тех.* опо́ра.

beargarden ['bɛəˈgɑːdn] *n* шу́мное ме́сто, «база́р».

bearing ['bɛəriŋ] *n* 1) отноше́ние; in all its ~s со всех сторо́н, во всех отноше́ниях; to have a ~ on, upon smth. име́ть отноше́ние к чему́-л., име́ть влия́ние на что-л.; 2) *pl* положе́ние, направле́ние; координа́ты; пе́ленг, а́зимут; to lose one's ~s заблуди́ться; *перен.* растеря́ться; to find (*или* to get, to take) one's ~s сориенти́роваться, осмотре́ться; 3) поведе́ние, мане́ра держа́ться; military ~ вое́нная вы́правка; 4) плодоноше́ние; 5) *тех.* подши́пник; roller ~ ро́ликовый подши́пник; 6) *pl* деви́з (*на гербе*); ◊ beyond (*или* past) all ~s нестерпи́мо.

bearish ['bɛəriʃ] *a* медве́жий; гру́бый.

bearleader ['bɛəˌliːdə] *n* 1) вожа́к (*медведя*); 2) *шутл.* гуверне́р, сопровожда́ющий молоды́х люде́й.

bearskin ['bɛəskin] *n* 1) медве́жья шку́ра; 2) высо́кая мехова́я ша́пка (*английских гвардейцев*).

beast [biːst] *n* зверь, живо́тное; скоти́на, скот (*тж. перен.*); ~ of prey хи́щный зверь; ~ of burden вью́чное живо́тное.

beastly I ['biːstli] *a* 1) живо́тный; гру́бый; 2) *разг.* отврати́тельный, ужа́сный.

beastly II *adv разг.* ужа́сно, стра́шно; отврати́тельно.

beat I [biːt] *n* 1) бой (*барабана*); 2) бие́ние (*сердца*); такт; ритм; отбива́ние та́кта; колеба́-

ние (*маятника*); 3) дозо́р, обхо́д; to be on the ~ обходи́ть дозо́ром; 4) привы́чная де́ятельность; 5) *амер. сленг* газе́тная сенса́ция; 6) *амер. сленг* безде́льник.

beat II *v* (*past* beat; *p. p.* beat, beaten) 1) бить, колоти́ть; 2) ударя́ть, стуча́ть; 3) би́ться, разбива́ться (*о волнах*; against); 4) выбива́ть; 5) отбива́ть (*такт*); би́ться (*о сердце*); 6) побива́ть, побежда́ть; 7) превосходи́ть; 8) кова́ть (*металл*; *тж.* to ~ out); 9) *мор.* лави́ровать; □ to ~ **away** отбива́ть, отража́ть; to ~ **back** отбива́ть, отража́ть; to ~ **down** а) подави́ть, сломи́ть (*сопротивление и т. п.*); б) сбить, сни́зить (*цену*), вы́торговать; to ~ **into** вбива́ть; to ~ **off** отбива́ть, отража́ть; to ~ **out** а) выбива́ть, кова́ть; б) разъясня́ть; в) *амер.* изнуря́ть, доводи́ть до кра́йней уста́лости; to ~ **up** а) взбива́ть (*яйца, сливки*); б) избива́ть; в) *мор.* продвига́ться про́тив тече́ния, про́тив ве́тра; г) набира́ть (*рекрутов*); ◊ to ~ it *амер.* удира́ть; ~ it! прочь!, убира́йся!; that ~s me! я поражён, не могу́ э́того пости́чь.

beatax(e) ['biːtæks] *n* моты́га, оку́чник.

beaten I ['biːtn] *p. p. см.* beat II.

beaten II *a* 1) би́тый, побеждённый; разби́тый; 2) изби́тый, бана́льный; 3) утомлённый, изму́ченный; 4) проторённый; 5) ко́ваный.

beater ['biːtə] *n* 1) бью́щий, колотя́щий; 2) *охот.* заго́нщик; 3) колоту́шка, выбива́лка; би́ло, трепа́ло.

beatific [ˌbiːəˈtifik] *a* блаже́нный, счастли́вый.

beatify [biːˈætifai] *v* 1) осчастли́вить; 2) *церк.* канонизи́ровать.

beating ['biːtiŋ] *n* 1) битьё, (теле́сное) наказа́ние; 2) бие́ние (*сердца, крыльев*); 3) пораже́ние.

beatitude [biːˈætitjuːd] *n* блаже́нство.

beau [bou] *n* (*pl* beaux) 1) щёголь; 2) кавале́р, покло́нник.

beautician [bjuːˈtiʃən] *n* космети́чка.

beautiful ['bjuːtəful] *a* прекра́сный; краси́вый.

beautify ['bjuːtifai] *v* украша́ть; де́лать прекра́сным.

beauty ['bjuːti] *n* 1) красота́; пре́лесть; that's the ~ of it вот в чём пре́лесть; you are a ~! *ирон.* хоро́ш ты, не́чего сказа́ть!; 2) краса́вица; ◊ ~ is but skin deep ≅ нельзя́ суди́ть по нару́жности.

beauty-sleep ['bjuːtisliːp] *n* ра́нний сон (*до полуночи*).

beauty-spot ['bjuːtispɔt] *n* му́шка (*на лице*).

beaux [bouz] *pl см.* beau.

beaver¹ ['biːvə] *n* 1) бобр; 2) бобро́вый мех; 3) касто́ровая шля́па; 4) *сленг* борода́ч; polar ~ седоборо́дый челове́к; 5) *attr* бобро́вый.

beaver² *n ист.* забра́ло.

becalmed [biˈkɑːmd] *a мор.* 1) сти́хший (*о ветре*); успоко́ившийся (*о море*); 2) попа́вший в штиль (*о судне*).

became [biˈkeim] *past см.* become.

because [biˈkɔz] *conj* потому́ что, так как; ~ of из-за, всле́дствие.

beck¹ [bek] *n* киво́к, приве́тствие; ◊ to have at one's ~ име́ть в своём распоряже́нии; to be at smb.'s ~ and call быть всеце́ло в чьём-л. распоряже́нии.

beck² *v см.* beckon.

beckon ['bekən] *v* кива́ть, подзыва́ть кивко́м.

becloud [bɪˈklaud] v заволакивать тучами; *перен.* затемнять, затуманивать.

become [bɪˈkʌm] v (*past* became; *p. p.* become) 1) делаться, становиться; 2) случаться; what has ~ of him? что с ним случилось?; 3) годиться; 4) быть к лицу.

becoming [bɪˈkʌmɪŋ] a 1) подобающий, приличествующий; 2) (идущий) к лицу.

bed I [bed] n 1) кровать; постель; hospital ~ больничная койка; feather ~ перина; spring ~ пружинный матрац; to go to ~ ложиться спать; to take to one's ~ заболеть, слечь в постель; to keep one's ~ быть больным, лежать в постели; to leave one's ~ встать с постели, выздороветь; to make the ~ стлать постель; to get up on the wrong side of the ~ *перен.* встать с левой ноги; 2) клумба; гряда, грядка; 3) *поэт.* смертное ложе, могила (*тж.* narrow ~); 4) *ж.-д.* полотно (*тж.* railway ~); 5) дно (*моря, реки*); 6) *геол.* пласт, залегание; 7) *тех.* основание; станина; ◊ ~ of down, ~ of roses лёгкая, приятная жизнь; it's not all a ~ of roses *посл.* ≅ жизнь прожить — не поле перейти; ~ of thorns неприятное, трудное положение; to be brought to ~ (of a boy, girl) разрешиться от бремени (мальчиком, девочкой).

bed II v 1) сажать, высаживать в грядки (*обыкн.* to ~ out); 2) класть подстилку (*скоту*); 3) класть на основание; настилать.

bedabble [bɪˈdæbl] v замочить, забрызгать (*грязной водой и т. п.*).

bedaub [bɪˈdɔːb] v запачкать краской; замазать.

bed-clothes [ˈbedklouðz] n pl постельное бельё.

bedding [ˈbedɪŋ] n 1) постель, постельные принадлежности; 2) подстилка (*для скота*); 3) основание; ложе; 4) *геол.* напластование, залегание.

bedeck [bɪˈdek] v украшать.

bedevil [bɪˈdevl] v 1) терзать, мучить; 2) сбивать с толку.

bedew [bɪˈdjuː] v обрызгивать; покрывать росой; орошать (*слезами*).

bedfellow [ˈbedˌfelou] n 1) сосед по койке, по постели; 2) *уст.* супруг(а).

bedgown [ˈbedgaun] n женская ночная сорочка.

bed-head [ˈbedhed] n изголовье (постели).

bedim [bɪˈdɪm] v затемнять, затуманивать (*рассудок, глаза*).

bedlam [ˈbedləm] n дом для умалишённых; *перен.* бедлам, сумасшедший дом.

bedlamite [ˈbedləmaɪt] n сумасшедший.

bedouin [ˈbeduɪn] n (*pl тж. без измен.*) бедуин.

bedpost [ˈbedpoust] n столбик кровати; ◊ between you and me and the ~ между нами (говоря).

bedrabbled [bɪˈdræbld] a промокший и забрызганный грязью.

bedraggle [bɪˈdrægl] v запачкать, замочить.

bedrid(den) [ˈbedˌrɪd(n)] a прикованный к постели болезнью.

bed-rock [ˈbedˈrɔk] n 1) *геол.* коренная порода, бедрок; 2) суть; основной принцип; to get down to (*или* to reach) ~ выяснить истину, добраться до сути дела.

bedroom [ˈbedrum] n спальня.

bed-side [ˈbedsaɪd] n: to sit at a person's ~ ухаживать за больным, сидеть у постели больного.

bed-sitting-room [ˈbedˈsɪtɪŋrum] n жилая комната (*спальня и гостиная вместе*).

bedsore [ˈbedsɔː] n пролежень.

bedspread [ˈbedspred] n покрывало (на постель).

bedstead [ˈbedsted] n кровать.

bedtime [ˈbedtaɪm] n время ложиться спать.

bee [biː] n 1) пчела; *перен.* трудолюбивый человек; worker ~ рабочая пчела; as brisk as a ~ проворный, быстрый; as busy as a ~ очень занятый; 2) *амер.* компания, собравшаяся для прогулки, развлечений *или* для совместной работы; ◊ to have a ~ in one's bonnet быть с причудой, иметь «пунктик» помешательства.

bee-bread [ˈbiːˌbred] n перга.

beech I [biːtʃ] n бук(овое дерево).

beech II a буковый.

beechen [ˈbiːtʃən] *см.* beech II.

beef [biːf] n (*pl* beeves) 1) говядина; horse ~ конина; corned ~ солонина; 2) туша; 3) мускулы (*человека*).

beefateria [ˌbiːfəˈtɪərɪə] n *амер.* ресторан, специализирующийся на приготовлении мясных блюд.

beefeater [ˈbiːfˌiːtə] n 1) лейб-гвардеец (*при англ. дворе*); 2) *ист.* страж в Тауэре.

beefsteak [ˈbiːfˈsteɪk] n бифштекс.

beef-witted [ˈbiːfˈwɪtɪd] a глупый.

beefy [ˈbiːfɪ] a крепкий, мускулистый; мясистый.

bee-garden [ˈbiːˌgɑːdn] n пасека.

beehive [ˈbiːhaɪv] n улей.

bee-line [ˈbiːlaɪn] n прямая (воздушная) линия.

bee-master [ˈbiːˌmɑːstə] n пчеловод, пасечник.

been [biːn] *p. p. см.* be.

beer [bɪə] n пиво; small ~ слабое пиво; *перен.* пустяки; ◊ to chronicle small ~ заниматься пустяками; to think no small ~ of oneself быть о себе высокого мнения.

beerhouse [ˈbɪəhaus] n пивная.

beeswax [ˈbiːzwæks] n воск.

beet [biːt] n свёкла; red ~ красная свёкла; white ~ сахарная свёкла.

beetle[1] [ˈbiːtl] n жук; ◊ blind as a ~ совершенно слепой.

beetle[2] I n *тех.* баба, кувалда, трамбовка.

beetle[2] II v *тех.* 1) трамбовать; 2) дробить камни.

beetle[3] I a нависший.

beetle[3] II v нависать.

beetle-browed [ˈbiːtlˌbraud] a с нависшими бровями; нахмуренный.

beetroot [ˈbiːtruːt] n свекловица; свёкла.

beeves [biːvz] pl *см.* beef.

befall [bɪˈfɔːl] v (*past* befell; *p. p.* befallen) происходить, случаться.

befallen [bɪˈfɔːlən] *p. p. см.* befall.

befell [bɪˈfel] *past. см.* befall.

befit [bɪˈfɪt] v подходить, приличествовать.

befog [bɪˈfɔg] v затуманивать.

befool [bɪˈfuːl] v одурачивать.

before I [bɪˈfɔː] adv 1) вперёд, впереди; 2) раньше, прежде; уже; ~ long вскоре; long ~ задолго до; shortly ~ незадолго до.

before II *prep* 1) пе́ред; 2) впереди́; to be ~ others быть впереди́ други́х (*в чём-л.* — *in*); 3) до.

before III *conj* 1) пре́жде чем; 2) скоре́е чем; he would die ~ lying он скоре́е умрёт, чем солжёт.

beforehand [bɪˈfɔːhænd] *adv* зара́нее; заблаговре́менно; to be ~ with опереди́ть кого́-л. в чём-л.

befoul [bɪˈfaul] *v* па́чкать, оскверня́ть.

befriend [bɪˈfrend] *v* помога́ть, подде́рживать.

beg [beg] *v* 1) проси́ть, умоля́ть (*кого́-л.* — *of, from, о чём-л.* — *for*); 2) ни́щенствовать; to go (a) begging а) ни́щенствовать; б) не име́ть спро́са; быть вака́нтным (*о до́лжности*); 3): I ~ to differ позво́лю себе́ не согласи́ться; we ~ to enclose при сём прилага́ем.

began [bɪˈgæn] *past см.* begin.

beget [bɪˈget] *v* (*past* begot; *p. p.* begotten) 1) рожда́ть, производи́ть; 2) порожда́ть.

beggar I [ˈbegə] *n* 1) ни́щий, попроша́йка; 2): insolent ~ наха́л; poor ~ бедня́га; little ~s малыши́; ◇ ~ on horseback вы́скочка; ≅ воро́на в павли́ньих пе́рьях.

beggar II *v* 1) доводи́ть до нищеты́; разоря́ть; 2) не поддава́ться (*описа́нию*).

begin [bɪˈgɪn] *v* (*past* began; *p. p.* begun) начина́ть(ся); ◇ to ~ with во-пе́рвых, пре́жде всего́.

beginner [bɪˈgɪnə] *n* 1) начина́ющий; 2) новичо́к.

beginning [bɪˈgɪnɪŋ] *n* 1) нача́ло; 2) исто́чник.

begone [bɪˈgɔn] *int* убира́йся!

begot [bɪˈgɔt] *past см.* beget.

begotten [bɪˈgɔtn] *p. p. см.* beget.

begrudge [bɪˈgrʌdʒ] *v* 1) испы́тывать разочарова́ние, неудовлетворённость; 2) зави́довать; 3) жале́ть, неохо́тно дава́ть (*что-л. кому́-л.*).

beguile [bɪˈgaɪl] *v* 1) занима́ть внима́ние, вре́мя; корота́ть вре́мя; 2) обма́нывать, вводи́ть в заблужде́ние; обма́ном вовлека́ть (*into*).

beguilement [bɪˈgaɪlmənt] *n* 1) развлече́ние; 2) обма́н.

begum [ˈbeɪgəm] *n* бегу́ма (*зна́тная да́ма в Индии*).

begun [bɪˈgʌn] *p. p. см.* begin.

behalf [bɪˈhɑːf] *n*: in ~ of, in smb.'s ~ в по́льзу, ра́ди, для кого́-л., on ~ of, on smb.'s ~ от и́мени кого́-л.

behave [bɪˈheɪv] *v* 1) вести́ себя́, поступа́ть; 2) вести́ себя́ хорошо́ (*тж.* to ~ oneself); 3) рабо́тать (*о маши́не, механи́зме и т. п.*).

behaviour [bɪˈheɪvjə] *n* 1) поведе́ние; обраще́ние, мане́ры; proper ~ хоро́шее поведе́ние; 2) *тех.* режи́м (рабо́ты).

behead [bɪˈhed] *v* отруби́ть го́лову, обезгла́вить.

beheld [bɪˈheld] *past, p. p. см.* behold.

behind I [bɪˈhaɪnd] *adv* сза́ди, позади́, за, по́сле; to leave ~ оста́вить (позади́, по́сле себя́); to fall ~ отстава́ть; to be ~ запа́здывать.

behind II *prep* позади́, за, по́сле.

behind III *n разг.* зад.

behindhand I [bɪˈhaɪndhænd] *a predic* 1) отста́лый, запозда́вший; 2) задолжа́вший, в долгу́.

behindhand II *adv*: wise ~ ≅ за́дним умо́м кре́пок.

behold [bɪˈhould] *v* (*past, p. p.* beheld) уви́деть; заме́тить; ~! смотри́!

beholden [bɪˈhouldən] *a predic* обя́занный (*кому́-л.* — *to*).

beholder [bɪˈhouldə] *n* зри́тель, очеви́дец.

behoof [bɪˈhuːf] *n*: in (*или* on, for, to) smb.'s ~, in (*или* on, for, to) the ~ of в по́льзу, в интере́сах кого́-л.

behoove [bɪˈhuːv] *v* надлежа́ть.

behove [bɪˈhouv] *см.* behoove.

being I [ˈbiːɪŋ] *n* 1) созда́ние, челове́к, существо́; human ~s лю́ди; 2) бытие́, существова́ние, жизнь; ~ determines consciousness бытие́ определя́ет созна́ние; to call into ~ вы́звать к жи́зни.

being II *a* существу́ющий, настоя́щий; for the time ~ а) в настоя́щее вре́мя; б) на не́которое вре́мя.

being III *pres. p.* бу́дучи.

belabour [bɪˈleɪbə] *v* бить, колоти́ть; трепа́ть.

belated [bɪˈleɪtɪd] *a* засти́гнутый темното́й; запозда́лый.

belaud [bɪˈlɔːd] *v* восхваля́ть.

belch I [beltʃ] *n* 1) отры́жка; 2) столб огня́; 3) гул изверже́ния; гро́хот ору́дий.

belch II *v* 1) рыга́ть; 2) изверга́ть (*ого́нь, ла́ву и т. п.*); 3) изрыга́ть (*руга́тельства*).

belcher [ˈbeltʃə] *n* пёстрое кашне́.

beleaguer [bɪˈliːgə] *v* осажда́ть.

belfry [ˈbelfrɪ] *n* колоко́льня.

Belgian I [ˈbeldʒən] *n* бельги́ец; бельги́йка; the ~s бельги́йцы.

Belgian II *a* бельги́йский.

belie [bɪˈlaɪ] *v* 1) оболга́ть, оклевета́ть; 2) дава́ть неве́рное представле́ние о чём-л., противоре́чить; 3) не опра́вдывать (*наде́жд, дове́рия и т. п.*).

belief [bɪˈliːf] *n* 1) ве́ра, дове́рие (*in*); 2) убежде́ние, мне́ние; to the best of my ~ наско́лько я понима́ю, наско́лько мне изве́стно; beyond ~ невероя́тно; 3) ве́рование, рели́гия.

believable [bɪˈliːvəbl] *a* вероя́тный, правдоподо́бный.

believe [bɪˈliːv] *v* 1) ве́рить (*in*); 2) доверя́ть; 3) полага́ть; I ~ so ка́жется, так; я так полага́ю; I ~ not едва́ ли; полага́ю, что нет.

believer [bɪˈliːvə] *n* ве́рующий; true ~ правове́рный.

belittle [bɪˈlɪtl] *v* преуменьша́ть; умаля́ть, принижа́ть.

bell¹ [bel] *n* 1) ко́локол, колоко́льчик; alarm ~ наба́т(ный ко́локол); to sound a ~ звони́ть в ко́локол; 2) звоно́к; to pull the ~ позвони́ть; дёрнуть звоно́к; to answer the ~ пойти́ откры́ть дверь (*на звоно́к*); there goes the ~! звоно́к!; 3) *бот.* ча́шечка цветка́; 4) *pl мор.* скля́нки; ◇ to bear (*или* to carry) away the ~ быть пе́рвым, получи́ть приз, победи́ть (*на состяза́нии*); to ring the ~ име́ть успе́х.

bell² I *n* крик, рёв (*оле́ня*).

bell² II *v* крича́ть, реве́ть, мыча́ть.

bell-boy [ˈbelbɔɪ] *n* коридо́рный (*в гости́нице*).

belle [bel] *n* краса́вица; цари́ца (*ба́ла и т. п.*).

belles-lettres [ˈbelˈletr] *n pl* беллетри́стика.

bell-flower [ˈbelˌflauə] *n бот.* колоко́льчик.

bell-hop [ˈbelhɔp] *амер. сленг см.* bell-boy.

bellicose ['belɪkous] *a* войнственный.

bellicosity [,belɪ'kɔsɪtɪ] *n* войнственность.

belligerency [bɪ'lɪdʒərənsɪ] *n* состояние войны́.

belligerent I [bɪ'lɪdʒərənt] *n* воюющая сторона́.

belligerent II *a* воюющий; находящийся в состоянии войны́.

bellow I ['belou] *n* мыча́ние; рёв (*тж. перен.*).

bellow II *v* 1) мыча́ть; реве́ть (*тж. перен.*); 2) греме́ть, громыха́ть.

bellows ['belouz] *n pl* воздуходу́вные мехи́; a pair of ~ ручны́е мехи́.

bell-wether ['bel,weðə] *n* бара́н-вожа́к (*с колокольчиком*).

belly I ['belɪ] *n* 1) живо́т, брю́хо; желу́док; *перен.* аппети́т; обжо́рство; 2) *мор.* «пу́зо» па́руса.

belly II *v* надува́ться (*обыкн.* to ~ out).

belly-ache[1] ['belieɪk] *n* боль в животе́.

belly-ache[2] *v сленг* ворча́ть; хны́кать.

belly-band ['belɪbænd] *n* подпру́га.

belly-pinched ['belɪpɪntʃt] *a* голода́ющий; изголода́вшийся.

belong [bɪ'lɔŋ] *v* 1) принадлежа́ть (*to*); 2) относи́ться (*к — to, амер. with, among*); 3) происходи́ть, быть ро́дом.

belongings [bɪ'lɔŋɪŋz] *n pl* 1) принадле́жности; ве́щи, пожи́тки; 2) пристро́йки, слу́жбы.

beloved I [bɪ'lʌvd] *n* возлю́бленный, люби́мый.

beloved II *a* возлю́бленный, люби́мый.

below I [bɪ'lou] *adv* внизу́; ни́же.

below II *prep* ни́же; под.

belt I [belt] *n* 1) по́яс, ре́мень; портупе́я; to hit below the ~ а) нанести́ уда́р ни́же по́яса; б) нанести́ преда́тельский уда́р; to tighten one's ~ подтяну́ть по́яс потуже; 2) по́яс, зо́на; 3) *тех.* приводно́й ре́мень; ◇ to hold the ~ быть победи́телем (*в состяза́нии*).

belt II *v* 1) опоя́сывать; 2) подпоя́сывать; 3) поро́ть ремнём.

belting ['beltɪŋ] *n* приводны́е ремни́; ремённая переда́ча.

belt-saw ['beltsɔː] *n* ле́нточная пила́.

bemire [bɪ'maɪə] *v* грязни́ть, покрыва́ть гря́зью.

bemoan [bɪ'moun] *v* опла́кивать.

bench I [bentʃ] *n* 1) скамья́; 2) верста́к; 3) ме́сто (*в парла́менте*); cross ~ скамья́ для беспарти́йных чле́нов парла́мента; front ~ ме́сто в пе́рвых ряда́х парла́мента (*см.* frontbencher); 4) ме́сто судьи́; суд; *собир.* су́дьи; to be raised to the ~ стать судьёй; 5) вы́ставка (*собак; тж.* ~ show).

bench II *v* выставля́ть на вы́ставке (*собак*).

bench-warmer ['bentʃ,wɔːmə] *n сленг* бездо́мный, безрабо́тный.

bend I [bend] *n* 1) сгиб; изги́б; 2) излу́чина (*реки*); 3) *мор.* у́зел; 4) *тех.* коле́но.

bend II *v* (*past, p. p.* bent) 1) гну́ть(ся), сгиба́ть(ся), склоня́ть(ся); 2) изгиба́ть(ся); повора́чивать (*о реке́, доро́ге и т. п.*); 3) сосредото́чивать (*мы́сли, внима́ние*); направля́ть (*шаги́, взо́ры*).

beneath I [bɪ'niːθ] *adv* внизу́.

beneath II *prep* под, ни́же; ~ one ни́же чьего́-л. досто́инства.

Benedictine [,benɪ'dɪktɪn] *n* бенедикти́нец (*мона́х*).

benediction [,benɪ'dɪkʃən] *n* благослове́ние.

benefaction [,benɪ'fækʃən] *n* 1) благодея́ние; 2) поже́ртвование.

benefactor ['benɪfæktə] *n* 1) благоде́тель; 2) же́ртвователь.

benefice ['benɪfɪs] *n* бенефи́ция, прихо́д.

beneficence [bɪ'nefɪsəns] *n* благодея́ние, до́брое де́ло.

beneficent [bɪ'nefɪsənt] *a* благоде́тельный.

beneficial [,benɪ'fɪʃəl] *a* благотво́рный; поле́зный.

beneficiary [,benɪ'fɪʃərɪ] *n* 1) *ист.* владе́лец фео́да *или* бенефи́ции; 2) *юр.* бенефициа́рий.

benefit I ['benɪfɪt] *n* 1) по́льза, вы́года; for the ~ of для, ра́ди, в по́льзу (*чего́-л.*); for your ~ ра́ди вас; to the ~ of с вы́годой для; to give smb. the ~ of one's experience подели́ться с кем-л. свои́м о́пытом; 2) содержа́ние, пе́нсия; страхово́е посо́бие; unemployment ~ посо́бие по безрабо́тице; 3) *театр.* бенефи́с; 4) *attr* благотвори́тельный.

benefit II *v* 1) извлека́ть по́льзу, вы́году (*из — by*); 2) помога́ть, приноси́ть по́льзу.

benefit-night ['benɪfɪtnaɪt] *см.* benefit I 3).

benevolence [bɪ'nevələns] *n* 1) доброжела́тельность; доброта́; 2) ще́дрость, благотвори́тельность; 3) милосе́рдие.

benevolent [bɪ'nevələnt] *a* 1) доброжела́тельный; 2) ще́дрый; благотвори́тельный; 3) милосе́рдный.

Bengalee I [beŋ'gɔːlɪ] *n* 1) бенга́лец; бенга́лка; 2) бенга́льский язы́к.

Bengalee II *a* бенга́льский.

Bengali I, II [beŋ'gɔːlɪ] *см.* Bengalee I, II.

benighted [bɪ'naɪtɪd] *a* 1) засти́гнутый но́чью, темното́й; 2) тёмный, неве́жественный.

benign [bɪ'naɪn] *a* 1) до́брый, мя́гкий; 2) благотво́рный, поле́зный (*о кли́мате, во́здухе*); 3) плодоно́сный (*о по́чве*); 4) *мед.* доброка́чественный.

benignant [bɪ'nɪgnənt] *см.* benign.

benignity [bɪ'nɪgnɪtɪ] *n* доброта́.

bent[1] I [bent] *n* скло́нность, накло́нность, влече́ние; to the top of one's ~ вдо́воль.

bent[1] II *past, p. p. см.* bend II.

bent[2] *n* по́ле, боло́тистая лугови́на; to go (*или* to flee) to the ~ вы́браться на ло́но приро́ды.

benumb [bɪ'nʌm] *v* приводи́ть в оцепене́ние; 2) парализова́ть (*чу́вства, де́йствия*).

benzene ['benziːn] *n* бензо́л.

benzine ['benziːn] *n* бензи́н.

benzyl ['benzɪl] *n хим.* бензи́л.

bequeath [bɪ'kwiːð] *v* завеща́ть.

bequest [bɪ'kwest] *n* насле́дство, посме́ртный дар.

berate [bɪ'reɪt] *v амер.* брани́ть, руга́ть.

berberry ['bɜːbərɪ] *см.* barber(r)y.

bereave [bɪ'riːv] *v* (*past, p. p.* bereaved, bereft) лиша́ть, отнима́ть (*жизнь, наде́жды и т. п.; of*).

bereaved [bɪ'riːvd] *a* лиши́вшийся бли́зких, осироте́вший.

bereavement [bɪ'riːvmənt] *n* тяжёлая утра́та.

bereft [bɪ'reft] *past, p. p. см.* bereave; ~ of reason умалишённый.

beret ['bereɪ] *n* бере́т.

berg [bɜːg] *n* а́йсберг.

berry I ['berı] *n* 1) я́года; 2) икри́нка; 3) *амер. сленг* до́ллар.

berry II *v* 1) приноси́ть я́годы; 2) собира́ть я́годы.

berth [bə:θ] *n* 1) ко́йка; каю́та; спа́льное ме́сто; 2) я́корная стоя́нка; 3) положе́ние; до́лжность; ◊ to give a wide ~ to держа́ться на расстоя́нии, избега́ть.

beryl ['berıl] *n* бери́лл.

beseech [bı'si:tʃ] *v* (*past, p. p.* besought) проси́ть, умоля́ть, упра́шивать.

beseem [bı'si:m] *v* подоба́ть, прили́чествовать.

beset [bı'set] *v* (*past, p. p.* beset) 1) окружа́ть; осажда́ть (*вопросами и т. п.*); 2) прегражда́ть (*путь*).

beside [bı'saıd] *prep* 1) ря́дом, близ, о́коло; 2) по сравне́нию с; 3) ми́мо; ◊ ~ oneself вне себя́.

besides [bı'saıdz] *adv* кро́ме того́; поми́мо; сверх того́.

besiege [bı'si:dʒ] *v* осажда́ть.

besieger [bı'si:dʒə] *n* осажда́ющий; осажда́ющая сторона́.

beslaver [bı'slævə] *v* 1) замусо́лить; 2) чрезме́рно льсти́ть.

beslubber [bı'slʌbə] *v* па́чкать, мара́ть.

besmear [bı'smıə] *v* запа́чкать, заса́лить.

besmirch [bı'smə:tʃ] *v* 1) запа́чкать (*ли́пким*); 2) замара́ть (*репута́цию*).

besom I ['bi:zəm] *n* метла́.

besom II *v* мести́, вымета́ть.

besought [bı'sɔ:t] *past, p. p. см.* beseech.

bespangle [bı'spæŋgl] *v* осыпа́ть блёстками.

bespatter [bı'spætə] *v* забры́згивать, обры́згивать; ~ with abuse осыпа́ть руга́тельствами; ~ with flattery осыпа́ть ле́стью.

bespeak [bı'spi:k] *v* (*past* bespoke; *p. p.* bespoke, bespoken) 1) зара́нее догова́риваться; зака́зывать (*това́ры*); 2) обнару́живать; пока́зывать, говори́ть о.

bespoke [bı'spouk] *past, p. p. см.* bespeak.

bespoken [bı'spoukən] *p. p. см.* bespeak.

besprent [bı'sprent] *a поэт.* 1) обры́зганный; 2) усы́панный.

besprinkle [bı'sprıŋkl] *v* обры́згивать, окропля́ть.

best I [best] *a* (*superl см.* good I, well² II) 1) лу́чший; 2) бо́льший; the ~ part of бо́льшая часть чего́-л.; 3) *употребля́ется для усиле́ния значе́ния сущ.*: ~ liar отъя́вленный лжец; ~ thrashing си́льная по́рка.

best II *adv* (*superl см.* well² I) 1) лу́чше всего́; you had ~ to... лу́чше бы вы (*сде́лали что-л.*); 2) бо́льше всего́; the ~ hated man са́мый ненави́стный челове́к.

best III *n означа́ет что-л. са́мое лу́чшее:* at (the very) ~ в лу́чшем слу́чае; to be at one's ~ быть в уда́ре; быть на высоте́; to make the ~ of things быть дово́льным, не уныва́ть; to make the ~ of one's way идти́ бы́стро, спеши́ть; to the ~ of one's power по ме́ре сил; to the ~ of one's knowledge наско́лько изве́стно; he did it for the ~ он сде́лал э́то с лу́чшими наме́рениями; to do one's ~ (с)де́лать всё возмо́жное; to try one's ~ сде́лать всё от тебя́ зави́сящее; one's (Sunday) ~ пра́здничное пла́тье; ◊ to

have (*или* to get) the ~ of it победи́ть, взять верх.

best² *v разг.* обману́ть, перехитри́ть; взять верх.

bestead [bı'sted] *v* (*past* besteaded; *p. p.* bested, bestead) помога́ть.

bested [bı'sted] *p. p. см.* bestead.

bestial ['bestjəl] *a* 1) ско́тский, живо́тный; 2) жесто́кий, гру́бый.

bestir [bı'stə:] *v* де́лать уси́лия, стара́ться; ~ yourself! пошеве́ливайся!

bestow [bı'stou] *v* 1) дава́ть, дари́ть; награжда́ть; 2) помеща́ть; размеща́ть; can you ~ us somewhere for the night? мо́жете ли вы устро́ить нас где́-нибудь на ночь?

bestowal [bı'stouəl] *n* дар; награ́да.

bestrew [bı'stru:] *v* (*past* bestrewed; *p. p.* bestrewed, bestrewn) 1) усыпа́ть, обсыпа́ть (*with*); 2) разбра́сывать.

bestrewn [bı'stru:n] *p. p. см.* bestrew.

bestridden [bı'strıdn] *p. p. см.* bestride.

bestride [bı'straıd] *v* (*past* bestrode; *p. p.* bestridden) 1) сиде́ть *или* сади́ться верхо́м; 2) стоя́ть расста́вив но́ги; 3) переки́нуться (*о ра́дуге, мо́сте и т. д.*).

bestrode [bı'stroud] *past см.* bestride.

bet I [bet] *n* 1) пари́; 2) ста́вка.

bet II *v* (*past, p. p.* bet, betted) держа́ть пари́ (*за — on; про́тив — against*); you ~! *разг.* бу́дьте уве́рены!, мо́жете быть уве́рены!; коне́чно!

betake [bı'teık] *v* (*past* betook; *p. p.* betaken): to ~ oneself to a) прибе́гнуть к чему́-л.; б) отпра́виться к кому́-л. *или* куда́-л.; to ~ oneself to one's heels удира́ть.

betaken [bı'teıkən] *p. p. см.* betake.

bethink [bı'θıŋk] *v* (*past, p. p.* bethought): to ~ oneself вспо́мнить, поду́мать (*of*).

bethought [bı'θɔ:t] *past, p. p. см.* bethink.

betimes [bı'taımz] *adv* 1) своевре́менно; 2) ра́но.

betook [bı'tuk] *past см.* betake.

betray [bı'treı] *v* 1) предава́ть; изменя́ть; выдава́ть; 2) обма́нывать, соблазня́ть (*же́нщину*).

betrayal [bı'treıəl] *n* преда́тельство; изме́на.

betrayer [bı'treıə] *n* преда́тель; изме́нник.

betroth [bı'trouð] *v* обручи́ть, помо́лвить.

betrothal [bı'trouðəl] *n* помо́лвка, обруче́ние.

better I ['betə] *a* (*compar см.* good I, well² II) лу́чший; to be (*или* to get) ~ чу́вствовать себя́ лу́чше; no ~ than a fool про́сто глуп, про́сто дура́к; twice as long and ~ длинне́е бо́лее чем в два ра́за; ◊ ~ off бога́че; for ~ for worse что бы ни случи́лось; to be ~ than one's word сде́лать бо́льше, чем обеща́л.

better II *adv* (*compar см.* well² I) лу́чше; he had ~ go ему́ лу́чше бы́ло бы пойти́; he is ~ loved than ever он бо́лее люби́м, чем когда́-либо; to think ~ of переду́мать; перемени́ть мне́ние о; ◊ all the ~, so much the ~ тем лу́чше.

better III *n:* one's ~ бо́лее иску́сный челове́к; one's ~s вышестоя́щие ли́ца; to get the ~ of a) взять верх над кем-л., победи́ть; б) испо́льзовать что-л. наилу́чшим о́бразом; to think (all) the ~ of smb. быть лу́чшего мне́ния о ком-л.

better IV *v* исправля́ть(ся), улучша́ть(ся); to ~ oneself получи́ть повыше́ние (*по слу́жбе*); получи́ть приба́вку (*к жа́лованью*).

better[2] *n* держащий пари.

betting ['betɪŋ] *n* пари.

bettor ['betə] *см.* better[2].

between [bɪ'twiːn] *prep* между; ~ ourselves между нами, конфиденциально; ◇ betwixt and ~ ни то ни сё.

betwixt [bɪ'twɪkst] *поэт., уст. см.* between.

bevel I ['bevəl] *n тех.* скос, уклон, наклон.

bevel II *v* 1) скашивать; стёсывать острые края; 2) кривиться, коситься.

beverage ['bevərɪdʒ] *n* напиток.

bevy ['bevɪ] *n* 1) общество (*обыкн. женщин*); стая (*птиц*); стадо (*косуль*).

bewail [bɪ'weɪl] *v* оплакивать, скорбеть.

beware [bɪ'wɛə] *v* беречься, остерегаться.

bewilder [bɪ'wɪldə] *v* смущать; ставить в тупик, сбивать с толку.

bewilderment [bɪ'wɪldəmənt] *n* 1) смущение, замешательство; 2) путаница.

bewitch [bɪ'wɪtʃ] *v* 1) заколдовывать; зачаровывать; 2) очаровывать.

bewray [bɪ'reɪ] *v* (невольно) выдавать (*тайну и т. п.*).

beyond I [bɪ'jɔnd] *prep* 1) по ту сторону, за; вне; 2) позже; 3) сверх, выше; it is ~ me это выше моего понимания.

beyond II *adv* вдали, на расстоянии.

beyond III *n* (the ~) загробная жизнь.

bi- [baɪ-] *pref со значением* дву-; bilateral двусторонний; bicarbonate *хим.* двууглекислый.

bias I ['baɪəs] *n* 1) склон, уклон, покатость; 2) косая линия, диагональ; to cut on the ~ резать, кроить по косой линии; 3) склонность, пристрастие (*towards*); предубеждение (*against*); влияние; 4) *радио* смещение.

bias II *v* оказывать влияние (*обыкн. плохое*); склонять (*к чему-л.*); внушать предубеждение (*против кого-л.— against*).

bias III *adv* косо; по диагонали.

bib[1] [bɪb] *n* 1) детский нагрудник, «слюнявчик»; 2) верхняя часть, грудь фартука; ◇ one's best ~ and tucker лучшее платье.

bib[2] *v* много, часто пить.

bibber ['bɪbə] *n* пьяница.

Bible ['baɪbl] *n* библия.

biblical ['bɪblɪkəl] *a* библейский.

bibliography [ˌbɪblɪ'ɔgrəfɪ] *n* библиография.

bibliophile ['bɪblɪoufaɪl] *n* библиофил.

bicameral [baɪ'kæmərəl] *a полит.* двухпалатный.

bicarbonate [baɪ'kɑːbənɪt] *n хим.* двууглекислая соль; ~ of soda *разг.* сода (*питьевая*).

bicentenary I [ˌbaɪsen'tiːnərɪ] *n* двухсотлетие.

bicentenary II *a* двухсотлетний.

bicentennial [ˌbaɪsen'tenjəl] *a* двухсотлетний; повторяющийся каждые двести лет.

biceps ['baɪseps] *n анат.* бицепс, двуглавая мышца.

bichloride [baɪ'klɔːraɪd] *n хим.* двухлористый состав; ~ of mercury сулема.

bicker I ['bɪkə] *n* перебранка; потасовка.

bicker II *v* 1) ссориться; журчать (*о ручье*); стучать (*о дожде*); 3) колыхаться, мерцать (*о свете, пламени*).

bickering ['bɪkərɪŋ] *n* 1) перебранка, потасовка; стычка; 2) перестрелка.

biconcave [baɪ'kɔnkeɪv] *a* двояковогнутый.

biconvex [baɪ'kɔnveks] *a* двояковыпуклый.

bicycle I ['baɪsɪkl] *n* велосипед; to ride a ~ ездить на велосипеде.

bicycle II *v* ездить на велосипеде.

bicyclist ['baɪsɪklɪst] *n* велосипедист.

bid I [bɪd] *v* (*past* bade, bid; *p. p.* bidden, bid) 1) предлагать (цену) (*for*); to ~ fair сулить, обещать; 2) приказывать; do as you are ~ (den) делайте, как приказано; 3) приглашать (*гостей*); 4) *уст.* просить; □ to ~ against, to ~ up набавлять цену.

bid II *n* 1) предложение (цены); заявка (*на торгах*); 2) предлагаемая цена; 3) *амер.* приглашение.

bidden ['bɪdn] *p. p. см.* bid I.

bidder ['bɪdə] *n* покупщик (*на торгах*).

bidding ['bɪdɪŋ] *n* 1) предложение цены; 2) приказание.

biennial I [baɪ'enɪəl] *n бот.* двухлетнее растение.

biennial II *a* двухлетний, двухгодичный; повторяющийся каждые два года.

bier [bɪə] *n* 1) похоронные носилки, дроги; 2) гроб.

biff I [bɪf] *n амер. сленг* сильный удар.

biff II *v амер. сленг* ударять.

bifurcate[a] ['baɪfəkɪt] *a* раздвоённый.

bifurcate[b] ['baɪfəkeɪt] *v* раздваивать(ся), разветвляться.

bifurcation [ˌbaɪfəː'keɪʃən] *n* раздвоение, разветвление.

big [bɪg] *a* 1) большой, крупный; высокий; 2) взрослый; 3) важный, значительный; to look ~ иметь важный вид; to go ~ *амер. разг.* иметь успех; 4) благородный, великодушный; 5) беременная (*тж.* ~ with child); ~ with news *перен.* полный новостей; 6) хвастливый; to talk ~ хвастаться; ◇ to grow (*или* to get) too ~ for one's boots *разг.* стать самонадеянным, самодовольным.

bigamy ['bɪgəmɪ] *n* двоебрачие, бигамия.

Big Ben ['bɪg'ben] *n* Большой Бен (*часы на здании англ. парламента*).

bight [baɪt] *n* 1) излучина (*реки*); бухта; 2) *мор.* бухта (*троса*).

bigot ['bɪgət] *n* 1) фанатик; изувер; 2) человек, не терпящий возражений.

bigoted ['bɪgətɪd] *a* нетерпимый, фанатичный.

bigotry ['bɪgətrɪ] *n* фанатизм; слепая приверженность к чему-л.

bigwig ['bɪgwɪg] *n сленг* важная персона, «шишка».

bijou ['biːʒuː] *n* (*pl* bijoux ['biːʒuːz]) безделушка, драгоценность.

bijou II *a* маленький и изящный.

bike I, II [baɪk] *сокр. разг. см.* bicycle I, II.

bikini [bɪ'kiːnɪ] *n* бикини (*купальный костюм*).

bilateral [baɪ'lætərəl] *a* двусторонний.

bilberry ['bɪlbərɪ] *n* черника; red ~ брусника.

bile [baɪl] *n* 1) жёлчь; 2) раздражительность, брюзгливость.

bilge I [bɪldʒ] *n* 1) подводная часть судна; 2) трюмная вода; 3) наиболее широкая часть бочки; 4) *разг.* чепуха, ерунда.

bilge II *v* 1) получить пробоину в подводной части; дать течь; 2) раздуться, распухнуть.

biliary ['bɪljərɪ] *a* жёлчный.

bilingual [baɪ'lɪŋgwəl] *a линг.* двуязы́чный.

bilious ['bɪljəs] *a* 1) страда́ющий разли́тием жёлчи; жёлчный; 2) раздражи́тельный.

bilk [bɪlk] *v* уклоня́ться от упла́ты (*по счета́м и т. п.*); ускольза́ть (*от креди́тора и т. п.*); обма́нывать.

bill[1] I [bɪl] *n* 1) счёт; to foot the ~ нести́ расхо́ды; 2) ве́ксель, тра́тта (*тж.* ~ of exchange); 3) *амер.* банкно́т; a five-dollar ~ бума́жка в 5 до́лларов; 4) спи́сок; докуме́нт; ~ of fare меню́; ~ of lading накладна́я; коносаме́нт; ~ of parcels факту́ра, накладна́я; ~ of health каранти́нное свиде́тельство; ~ of sale закладна́я; 5) плака́т, афи́ша; програ́мма (*спекта́кля, конце́рта*); ◊ to fill the ~ *амер.* выполня́ть все тре́бования, де́лать всё, что ну́жно; соотве́тствовать назначе́нию.

bill[1] II *v* 1) раскле́ивать плака́ты, афи́ши; объявля́ть в афи́шах; 2) *амер.* обеща́ть.

bill[2] *n* 1) законопрое́кт, билль; to pass the ~ приня́ть законопрое́кт; to throw out the ~ отклони́ть законопрое́кт; 2) *юр.* иск; to find a true ~ переда́ть де́ло в суд; to ignore the ~ прекрати́ть де́ло.

bill[3] I *n* 1) клюв; 2) у́зкий мыс; 3) носо́к я́коря.

bill[3] II *v* ласка́ться (*тж.* to ~ and coo).

bill[4] *n* 1) *уст.* алеба́рда; 2) садо́вые но́жницы, сека́тор (ы).

billboard ['bɪlbɔːd] *n* доска́ для объявле́ний, афи́ш.

billet[1] I ['bɪlɪt] *n* 1) о́рдер на посто́й солда́т; 2) ме́сто расквартирова́ния; *pl* кварти́ры; to go into ~s располага́ться на кварти́рах (*о во́йсках*); 3) назначе́ние, положе́ние, до́лжность.

billet[1] II *v* расквартиро́вывать (*войска́*).

billet[2] *n* 1) поле́но, чурба́н; 2) *метал.* болва́нка, загото́вка.

billet-doux ['bɪleɪ'duː] *n шутл.* любо́вная запи́сочка.

billiard-marker ['bɪljəd‚mɑːkə] *n* маркёр.

billiards ['bɪljədz] *n pl* билья́рд.

billion ['bɪljən] *n* биллио́н; *амер.* миллиа́рд.

billow I ['bɪlou] *n* 1) больша́я волна́; вал; *перен.* лави́на; 2) *поэт.* мо́ре.

billow II *v* вздыма́ться, волнова́ться.

billowy ['bɪlouɪ] *a* 1) волну́ющийся (*о мо́ре*); 2) неро́вный, волни́стый (*о ме́стности*).

bill-poster ['bɪl‚poustə] *n* раскле́йщик афи́ш.

bill-sticker ['bɪl‚stɪkə] *см.* bill-poster.

billy-goat ['bɪlɪgout] *n* козёл.

bi-monthly I ['baɪ'mʌnθlɪ] *a* двухме́сячный.

bi-monthly II *adv* ка́ждые два ме́сяца.

bin [bɪn] *n* 1) деревя́нный ларь, за́кром; бу́нкер; 2) му́сорный я́щик; 3) мешо́к для сбо́ра хме́ля.

bin- [baɪn-, bɪn-] *pref* со значе́нием дву- (*перед гла́сными*); binocular бинокуля́рный.

binary ['baɪnərɪ] *a* двойно́й, сдво́енный.

bind [baɪnd] *v* (*past, p. p.* bound) 1) вяза́ть, свя́зывать; завя́зывать; привя́зывать; закрепля́ть; 2) обя́зывать; to ~ oneself обяза́ться, взять на себя́ обяза́тельство; to be bound быть вы́нужденным; bound to win уве́ренный в побе́де; 3) свя́зывать, скрепля́ть (*бето́ном и т. п.*); 4) затвердева́ть (*о гли́не и т. п.*); 5) перепле-

та́ть (*кни́гу*); ▢ to ~ up а) перевя́зывать (*ра́ну*); б) переплета́ть в о́бщий переплёт; в): bound up with (те́сно) свя́занный с кем-л., чем-л.

binder ['baɪndə] *n* 1) тот, кто свя́зывает, завя́зывает; 2) переплётчик; 3) свя́зующее вещество́ (*клей, цеме́нт и т. п.*); 4) сноповяза́лка.

binding I ['baɪndɪŋ] *n* 1) переплёт (*кни́ги*); 2) обши́вка, око́вка.

binding II *a* 1) связу́ющий; 2) обя́зывающий.

bindweed ['baɪndwiːd] *n бот.* вьюно́к.

bine [baɪn] *n бот.* 1) побе́г; 2) сте́бель ползу́чего расте́ния.

binocular [baɪ'nɔkjulə] *a* бинокуля́рный.

binoculars [bɪ'nɔkjuləz] *n pl* бино́кль.

binomial [baɪ'noumjəl] *n мат.* бино́м, двучле́н.

biochemistry [baɪou'kemɪstrɪ] *n* биохи́мия.

biographer [baɪ'ɔgrəfə] *n* био́граф.

biographic(al) [‚baɪou'græfɪk(əl)] *a* биографи́ческий.

biography [baɪ'ɔgrəfɪ] *n* биогра́фия; campaign ~ биогра́фия кандида́та, публику́емая пе́ред вы́борами.

biologic(al) [‚baɪə'lɔdʒɪk(əl)] *a* биологи́ческий.

biologist [baɪ'ɔlədʒɪst] *n* био́лог.

biology [baɪ'ɔlədʒɪ] *n* биоло́гия.

bionics [baɪ'ɔnɪks] *n* био́ника.

bipartisan [baɪ'pɑːtɪzən] *a* двупарти́йный.

biped I ['baɪped] *n* двуно́гое живо́тное.

biped II *a* двуно́гий.

bipedal ['baɪ‚pedl] *см.* biped II.

biplane ['baɪpleɪn] *n* бипла́н.

biquadratic [‚baɪkwɔ'drætɪk] *n мат.* биквадра́тное уравне́ние (*тж.* ~ equation).

birch I [bəːtʃ] *n* 1) берёза; 2) ро́зга; 3) *attr* берёзовый.

birch II *v* сечь ро́згой.

birchen ['bəːtʃən] *a* берёзовый, сде́ланный из берёзы.

bird [bəːd] *n* 1) пти́ца; ~ of passage перелётная пти́ца; ~ of prey хи́щная пти́ца; 2): gay ~ весельча́к; queer ~ чуда́к; ◊ a ~ in the hand is worth two in the bush *посл.* ≅ не сули́ журавля́ в не́бе, а дай сини́цу в ру́ки; old ~ ≅ стре́ляный воробе́й; an old ~ is not caught with chaff *посл.* ста́рого воробья́ на мяки́не не проведёшь; the early ~ ра́нняя пта́шка; the early ~ catches the worm ≅ кто ра́но встаёт, тому́ бог даёт; ~s of a feather пти́цы одного́ полёта; to give smb. the ~ а) освиста́ть кого́-л.; б) уво́лить, вы́ставить кого́-л.; to get the ~ а) быть освиста́нным; б) быть уво́ленным.

bird-cage ['bəːdkeɪdʒ] *n* 1) кле́тка (*для птиц*); 2) *сленг* ночле́жка.

birdie ['bəːdɪ] *n* пти́чка, пта́шка.

bird's-eye ['bəːdzaɪ] *a*: ~ view вид с пти́чьего полёта; *перен.* о́бщая перспекти́ва.

birth [bəːθ] *n* 1) рожде́ние; artist by ~ худо́жник по призва́нию; to give ~ to а) роди́ть, произвести́ на свет; б) дава́ть нача́ло чему́-л.; 2) нача́ло, исто́чник; 3) ро́ды; two at a ~ дво́йня; 4) происхожде́ние.

birthday ['bəːθdeɪ] *n* день рожде́ния.

birth-mark ['bəːθmɑːk] *n* ро́динка, роди́мое пятно́.

birth-place ['bəːθpleɪs] *n* ме́сто рожде́ния, ро́дина.

birth-rate ['bə:θreɪt] *n* процéнт рождáемости.

biscuit ['bɪskɪt] *n* 1) сухóе печéнье; ship's ~ сухáрь; 2) неглазирóванный фарфóр, бисквѝт; 3) *attr* свéтло-корѝчневый.

bisect [baɪ'sekt] *v* разрезáть, делѝть пополáм.

bisector [baɪ'sektə] *n мат.* биссектрѝса.

bisexual ['baɪ'seksjuəl] *a* двуполый.

bishop ['bɪʃəp] *n* 1) епѝскоп; 2) *шахм.* слон; 3) «бѝшоп» (*напиток*).

bishopric ['bɪʃəprɪk] *n* 1) сан епѝскопа; 2) епáрхия.

bismuth ['bɪzməθ] *n хим.* вѝсмут.

bison ['baɪsn] *n* бизóн.

bissextile I [bɪ'sekstaɪl] *n* високóсный год.

bissextile II *a* високóсный.

bit¹ [bɪt] *n* 1) кусóчек; небольшóе количество; dainty ~ лáкомый кусóчек; every ~ as совершéнно как, в тóчности; a ~ немнóго; a ~ of a fool, a coward *etc* немнóго глуповáт, трусовáт *и т. п.*; ~ by ~ понемнóгу, постепéнно; not a ~ нискóлько, ничýть; 2) мéлкая монéта; three-penny ~ монéта в 3 пéнса; short ~ *амер.* монéта в 10 цéнтов; ◊ to do one's ~ испóлнить свой долг, внестѝ свою лéпту; to give a ~ of one's mind говорѝть откровéнно, напрямѝк.

bit² I *n* 1) удилá; мундштýк; *перен.* уздá; to draw ~ сдéрживать лóшадь; 2) лéзвие; 3) бур; сверлó; 4) бородка (*ключа*).

bit² II *v* взнуздывать; *перен.* сдéрживать, обуздывать.

bit³ *past, p. p. см.* bite II.

bitch [bɪtʃ] *n* сýка; сáмка.

bite I [baɪt] *n* 1) укýс; 2) клёв (*рыбы*); 3) едá, кусóк; 4) схвáтывание, зажáтие.

bite II *v* (*past* bit; *p. p.* bit, bitten) 1) кусáть(ся); жáлить; щипáть (*о морозе*); *перен.* задевáть, колóть; 2) клевáть (*о рыбе; тж. перен.*); 3) пронзáть, колóть (*об оружии*); 4) побивáть (*о морозе*); 5) разъедáть (*о кислоте, ржавчине*); 6) зацеплять, схвáтывать; the wheels will not ~ колёса скользят; 7) поддавáться (*обману*); 8): bitten with захвáченный (*идеей*) (*энтузиазмом и т. п.*); □ to ~ off откýсывать; ◊ once bitten twice shy *посл.* ≅ обжёгшись на молокé, бýдешь дуть и нá воду.

biter ['baɪtə] *n* кусáющееся живóтное; ◊ the ~ bit ≅ попáлся, котóрый кусáлся.

biting ['baɪtɪŋ] *a* 1) éдкий; язвѝтельный, кóлкий; 2) рéзкий (*о ветре, морозе*).

bitten ['bɪtn] *p. p. см.* bite II.

bitter I ['bɪtə] *n* 1) гóречь; 2) *обыкн. pl* гóрькое пѝво.

bitter II *a* 1) гóрький; *перен. тж.* мучѝтельный; 2) рéзкий; ожесточённый; жгýчий (*о ненависти*); 3) éдкий (*о сатире*); 4) злéйший (*о враге*).

bitter III *adv* гóрько; рéзко, жестóко; it was ~ cold было óчень хóлодно, был сѝльный морóз.

bitumen ['bɪtjumɪn] *n* битýм; асфáльт.

bivouac I ['bɪvuæk] *n* бивáк.

bivouac II *v* располагáться на бивáк.

bizarre [bɪ'zɑ:] *a* стрáнный, причýдливый; эксцентрѝчный.

blab I ['blæb] *n* болтýн.

blab II *v* (раз)болтáть.

blabber ['blæbə] *n* болтýн; сплéтник.

---

black I [blæk] *a* 1) чёрный; 2) тёмный; мрáчный; to look ~ казáться, быть мрáчным, подáвленным; имéть недовóльный, сердѝтый вид; хмýриться; 3) зловéщий; 4) безрáдостный, унылый; ◊ ~ and blue в синякáх; ~ and tan чёрный с корѝчневыми пятнами; (in) ~ and white чёрным по бéлому; ~ in the face a) побагровéвший (*от раздражения*); б) сѝльно рассéрженный.

black II *n* 1) черногá; чёрный цвет; 2) чёрная крáска; carbon ~ лáмповая кóпоть (*краска*); 3) чернокóжий; 4) чёрное *или* трáурное плáтье.

black III *v* 1) чернѝть; 2) чѝстить вáксой; □ to ~ out а) затемнять; выключáть свет; б) вычёркивать, вымáрывать; в) засекрéчивать.

black-ball ['blækbɔ:l] *v* забаллотѝровать.

black-beetle ['blæk'bi:tl] *n* чёрный таракáн.

blackberry ['blækbərɪ] *n* ежевѝка.

blackbird ['blækbə:d] *n* чёрный дрозд.

black-board ['blækbɔ:d] *n* клáссная доскá.

black-cock ['blækkɔk] *n* тéтерев.

black-earth ['blækə:θ] *n* чернозём.

blacken ['blækən] *v* 1) чернéть; 2) чернѝть; пáчкать.

blackguard I ['blægɑ:d] *n* негодяй; подлéц.

blackguard II *a* мéрзкий.

black-head ['blækhed] *n* ýгорь (*на лице*).

blacking ['blækɪŋ] *n* вáкса.

blacking-out ['blækɪŋaut] *n* 1) затемнéние; выключéние свéта; 2) провáл пáмяти; 3) вымáривание (*текста цензором*); 4) засекрéчивание.

blackish ['blækɪʃ] *a* черновáтый.

black-jack I ['blæk'dʒæk] *n амер. сленг* дубѝнка.

black-jack II *v амер. сленг* бить, избивáть дубѝнкой.

black-lead ['blæk'led] *n* графѝт.

blackleg I ['blækleg] *n* 1) мошéнник, жýлик; 2) штрейкбрéхер.

blackleg II *v* 1) мошéнничать; 2) быть штрейкбрéхером.

black-list ['blæklɪst] *v* вносѝть в чёрный спѝсок.

blackmail I ['blækmeɪl] *n* шантáж, вымогáтельство.

blackmail II *v* шантажѝровать, вымогáть дéньги.

blackmailer ['blæk,meɪlə] *n* шантажѝст, вымогáтель.

blackness ['blæknɪs] *n* 1) черногá; темнотá; 2) мрáчность.

black-out ['blækaut] *n* 1) затемнéние; отсýтствие электрѝческого свéта; 2) затмéние, провáл пáмяти; 3) *ав., косм.* чёрная пеленá (*при перегрузке*); 4) *attr* затемнённый; 5) *attr* засекрéченный.

blacksmith ['blæksmɪθ] *n* кузнéц.

black-soil ['blæksɔɪl] *см.* black-earth.

blackthorn ['blækθɔ:n] *n* тёрн, тернóвник.

blacky ['blækɪ] *a* черновáтый.

bladder ['blædə] *n* 1) пузырь; 2) кáмера; football ~ кáмера футбóльного мячá; 3) мочевóй пузырь; 4) болтýн, пустомéля.

blade [bleɪd] *n* 1) лéзвие (*ножа, бритвы*); 2) лóпасть (*весла, винта*); 3) *бот.* ýзкий лист; 4) *разг.* пáрень; a jolly old ~ весельчáк, жизнерáдостный пáрень.

blaeberry ['bleɪbərɪ] *см.* bilberry.

blah [blɑ] *n амер. разг.* преувеличение, вздор.

blain [bleɪn] *n* нарыв, чирей.

blame I [bleɪm] *n* 1) обвинение, порицание; упрёк; 2) ответственность; вина; to shift the ~ on smb. свалить вину на кого-л.; to cast (*или* to lay, to put) the ~ on smb. взвалить, возложить ответственность, вину на кого-л.; to bear the ~ нести ответственность; принять на себя вину.

blame II *v* порицать; обвинять, винить; to be to ~ заслуживать порицания; быть виновным.

blameful ['bleɪmful] *a* заслуживающий порицания, осуждения.

blameless ['bleɪmlɪs] *a* безупречный.

blameworthy ['bleɪm,wɜːðɪ] *a* заслуживающий порицания.

blanch [blɑntʃ] *v* 1) белить; 2) белеть, бледнеть; 3) чистить (*миндаль*); 4) лудить; чистить, полировать (*металл*); □ to ~ **over** обелять, оправдывать.

bland [blænd] *a* 1) мягкий; нежный; вежливый; 2) иронический; 3) умеренный, мягкий (*о климате*).

blandish ['blændɪʃ] *v* 1) льстить; 2) улещивать.

blank I [blæŋk] *n* 1) пустое, свободное место; пробел; пустота; 2) пустой лотерейный билет; to draw a ~ вынуть пустой номер; *перен.* потерпеть неудачу; 3) тире (*заменяющее нецензурное слово*); 4) *амер.* бланк; 5) холостой патрон; 6) *тех.* болванка.

blank II *a* 1) чистый, неисписанный; 2) незаполненный, пустой (*о бланке и т. п.*); 3) холостой (*о патроне*); 4) пустой, бессодержательный; невыразительный; to look ~ быть в замешательстве, быть озадаченным; 5) абсолютный, полный; 6) *амер.* Н-ский, N (*о не подлежащем оглашению*); the Blank Pursuit Squadron Н-ская истребительная эскадрилья; General Blank генерал N.

blank III *v амер.* наносить крупное поражение.

blanket I ['blæŋkɪt] *n* 1) шерстяное одеяло; 2) попона; 3) *геол.* (поверхностный) слой; покров; нанос; 4) *attr* общий, полный, всеобъемлющий; ◊ a wet ~ а) человек, расхолаживающий других; б) что-л., действующее расхолаживающе; to throw a wet ~ over охладить пыл.

blanket II *v* 1) покрывать одеялом; 2) заглушить, замять (*скандал, вопрос и т. п.*).

blankly ['blæŋklɪ] *adv* 1) безучастно; 2) прямо, решительно; 3) крайне.

blankness ['blæŋknɪs] *n* 1) пустота; 2) смущение.

blare I [blɛə] *n* трубный звук.

blare II *v* трубить.

blarney I ['blɑnɪ] *n* лесть.

blarney II *v* льстить.

blaspheme [blæs'fiːm] *v* богохульствовать; оскорблять, поносить.

blasphemous ['blæsfɪməs] *a* богохульный.

blasphemy ['blæsfɪmɪ] *n* богохульство.

blast I [blɑst] *n* 1) сильный порыв ветра; струя воздуха; тяга; in (out of) ~ работающая полным ходом (нератотающая) (*о доменной печи*); in full ~ *перен.* полным ходом, вовсю; 2) взрывная волна; 3) звук духового инструмен-

та; 4) подрывной заряд; 5) *тех.* воздуходувка, вентилятор; 6) пагубное влияние; 7) вредитель (*растений*).

blast II *v* 1) взрывать; 2) портить; вредить; 3) *разг.* проклинать.

blast-down ['blɑst'daun] *n* посадка (на другую планету).

blast-furnace ['blɑst,fɜːnɪs] *n* доменная печь.

blast-off ['blɑstɔːf] *n* старт (космического корабля); пуск ракеты.

blatant ['bleɪtənt] *a* 1) крикливый; 2) явный, несомненный (*о лжи*); вопиющий (*о несправедливости*).

blather I, II ['blæðə] *см.* blether I, II.

blatherskite ['blæðəskaɪt] *см.* bletherskate.

blaze[1] I [bleɪz] *n* 1) яркое пламя; in a ~ в огне, в пламени; 2) вспышка (*огня, страсти*); 3) яркий свет *или* цвет; *перен.* блеск, великолепие; ~ of publicity огласка; 4): go to ~s! убирайся к чёрту!; what the ~s! что за чёрт!; like ~s изо всех сил; неистово.

blaze[1] II *v* 1) гореть, пылать; 2) сверкать, сиять; □ to ~ **away** а) *воен.* вести непрерывный огонь; б) делать что-л. с увлечением; to ~ **up** вспыхнуть.

blaze[2] I *n* 1) белое пятно (*на лбу животного*); 2) зарубка (*на дереве*).

blaze[2] II *v* делать зарубки (*на деревьях*); указывать путь зарубками.

blaze[3] разглашать (*тж.* to ~ abroad).

blazer ['bleɪzə] *n* 1) спортивная куртка; 2) *сленг* наглая ложь.

blazing ['bleɪzɪŋ] *a* 1) горящий, пылающий; палящий; 2) явный; горячий (*о следе*).

blazon I ['bleɪzn] *n* 1) герб; 2) прославление.

blazon II *v* 1) украшать гербами, геральдическими знаками; 2) прославлять; □ to ~ **abroad** разглашать, распространять (*новости и т. п.*).

blazonry ['bleɪznrɪ] *n* 1) геральдика; 2) гербы, геральдические знаки.

bleach [bliːtʃ] *v* 1) белить; отбеливать(ся); 2) побелеть; 3) обесцвечивать.

bleak[1] [bliːk] *n* уклейка (*рыба*).

bleak[2] *a* 1) голый, открытый, незащищённый от ветра; 2) холодный; 3) мрачный; 4) бесцветный.

blear I [blɪə] *a* затуманенный; неясный.

blear II *v* затуманивать; делать неясным.

blear-eyed ['blɪəraɪd] *a* 1) с затуманенными глазами; 2) непредусмотрительный.

bleat I [bliːt] *n* 1) блеяние; 2) мычание (*телёнка*).

bleat II *v* 1) блеять; 2) мычать (*о телёнке*); 3) говорить невнятно *или* неразумительно (*тж.* to ~ out).

bleb [bleb] *n* 1) волдырь; 2) пузырёк воздуха (*в воде, стекле*).

bled [bled] *past, p. p. см.* bleed.

bleed [bliːd] *v* (*past, p. p.* bled) 1) кровоточить; истекать кровью; 2) проливать кровь (*за for*); 3) давать сок, сочиться (*о растениях*); 4) *мед.* пускать кровь; 5) подвергаться вымогательству; 6) вымогать деньги; to ~ white выманить последние деньги, обобрать до нитки.

bleeding I ['bliːdɪŋ] *n* 1) кровотечение; 2) кровопускание.

bleeding II *a* истекающий кровью; кровоточащий.

blemish I ['blemɪʃ] *n* недостаток; пятно, порок.

blemish II *v* портить; пятнать, порочить.

blench[1] [blentʃ] *v* 1) отступать от чего-л.; уклоняться; 2) закрывать глаза на что-л.

blench[2] *v* 1) белить; отбеливать; 2) обесцвечивать; 3) выцветать.

blend I [blend] *n* смесь.

blend II *v* (*past, p. p.* blended, blent) 1) смешивать; делать смесь; 2) соединять, сочетать; 3) смешиваться; соединяться, сочетаться; 4) стираться (*об оттенках, различиях*); незаметно переходить в другой оттенок (*о краске*).

blent [blent] *past, p. p. см.* blend II.

bless [bles] *v* (*past, p. p.* blessed, blest) 1) освящать; благословлять; 2) осчастливливать; 3) *уст.* славословить; 4) *эвф.* проклинать; I'm ~ed!, ~ me!, ~ my soul! чёрт возьми!, будь я проклят!

blessed ['blesɪd] *a* 1) счастливый; блаженный, благословенный; 2) *эвф.* проклятый.

blessedness ['blesɪdnɪs] *n* блаженство, счастье; single ~ *шутл.* холостая жизнь.

blessing ['blesɪŋ] *n* 1) благословение; 2) молитва до *или* после еды; 3) дар природы; благо, благодеяние; ◊ a ~ in disguise неприятность, оказавшаяся благодетельной.

blest I [blest] *past, p. p. см.* bless.

blest II *a см.* blessed.

blether I ['bleðə] *n* болтовня, вздор.

blether II *v* болтать вздор.

bletherskate ['bleðəskeɪt] *n разг.* болтун.

blew[1] [bluː] *past см.* blow[2] II.

blew[2] *past см.* blow[3] II.

blight I [blaɪt] *n* 1) болезнь растений; 2) насекомые-паразиты на растениях; 3) душный воздух; 4) то, что портит удовольствие, разрушает планы *и т. д.*

blight II *v* 1) приносить вред (*растениям*); 2) вредить, портить.

blighter ['blaɪtə] *n сленг* нудный, надоедливый человек.

blind[1] I [blaɪnd] *a* 1) слепой; to go ~ ослепнуть; to be ~ to не быть в состоянии оценить что-л.; to go it ~ действовать вслепую, наобум; 2) нечёткий; неясный; 3) безрассудный; 4) *сленг* (вдребезги) пьяный (*тж.* ~ drunk, ~ to the world).

blind[1] II *n*: the ~ (*употр. как pl*) слепые.

blind[1] III *v* 1) ослеплять; слепить; 2) затемнять, затмевать.

blind[2] *n* 1) штора, занавеска; маркиза; Venetian ~ жалюзи; 2) предлог, отговорка.

blindage ['blaɪndɪdʒ] *n* блиндаж.

blind-alley ['blaɪnd'ælɪ] *a* бесперспективный, безвыходный (*см. тж.* alley 2).

blinders ['blaɪndəz] *n pl* шоры.

blindfold I ['blaɪndfould] *a* с завязанными глазами.

blindfold II *v* завязывать глаза.

blindfold III *adv* вслепую, слепо.

blindly ['blaɪndlɪ] *adv* 1) не видя, ощупью; 2) безрассудно, слепо.

blind-man's-buff ['blaɪndmænz'bʌf] *n* жмурки (*игра*).

blindness ['blaɪndnɪs] *n* слепота; *перен. тж.* ослепление.

blink I [blɪŋk] *n* 1) мерцание; мигание; in a ~ в один миг; 2) отблеск полярных льдов (*на горизонте; тж.* iceblink); ◊ on the ~ *амер. разг.* в плохом состоянии, не в порядке.

blink II *v* 1) мигать, моргать; щуриться; 2) мерцать; блеснуть; 3) игнорировать (*факт*); закрывать глаза (*на что-л.*).

blinkers ['blɪŋkəz] *см.* blinders.

blirt [blɜːt] *v диал.* зарыдать; разрыдаться.

bliss [blɪs] *n* блаженство.

blissful ['blɪsful] *a* блаженный.

blister I ['blɪstə] *n* 1) волдырь; 2) *мед.* вытяжной пластырь.

blister II *v* 1) покрываться волдырями; 2) вызывать волдыри; 3) *разг.* надоедать.

blithe [blaɪð] *a* весёлый, жизнерадостный.

blithesome ['blaɪðsəm] *см.* blithe.

blitz I [blɪts] *n* 1) молниеносная война; 2) воздушное нападение; бомбёжка.

blitz II *v* (раз)бомбить; to be ~ed подвергнуться воздушному нападению.

blizzard ['blɪzəd] *n* буран, сильная метель.

bloat I [blout] *n см.* bloater.

bloat[1] II *v* коптить сельдь.

bloat[2] *v* распухать, раздуваться.

bloated ['bloutɪd] *a* 1) распухший; разжиревший; *перен.* раздутый, чрезмерный; 2) надутый, напыщенный.

bloater ['bloutə] *n* копчёная сельдь.

blob [blɔb] *n* 1) капля; 2) комочек; 3) *сленг* ноль (*при счёте в крикете*).

blobber-lipped ['blɔbəlɪpt] *a* толстогубый.

bloc [blɔk] *n полит.* блок; the communist and non-party ~ блок коммунистов и беспартийных.

block I [blɔk] *n* 1) бревно; чурбан; 2) кубик (*игрушка*); 3) плаха; 4) глыба; 5) квартал (*города*); жилой массив; 6) затор (*движения*); 7) *тех.* блок; 8) болван (*для шляп*); 9) группа соединённых предметов; in ~ гуртом, массой.

block II *v* 1) преграждать (*путь*); задерживать, препятствовать; блокировать (*обыкн.* to ~ up); 2) *парл.* задерживать прохождение законопроекта; □ to ~ in, to ~ out набрасывать вчерне.

blockade I [blɔ'keɪd] *n* блокада; to raise (to run) the ~ снять (прорвать) блокаду.

blockade II *v* блокировать.

block-buster ['blɔk,bʌstə] *n разг.* тяжёлая фугасная бомба.

blockhead ['blɔkhed] *n* болван.

blockhouse ['blɔkhaus] *n* 1) блокгауз; 2) бревенчатый дом, сруб.

bloke [blouk] *n разг.* парень.

blond(e) I [blɔnd] *n* блондин(ка).

blond(e) II *a* белокурый, светлый.

blood [blʌd] *n* 1) кровь; *перен.* жизнь; to let one's ~ пустить кровь; to spit ~ харкать кровью; to shed the ~ of пролить чью-л. кровь, убить; to shed one's ~ проливать кровь (*за что-л. — for*); 2) темперамент; пыл; bad ~ враждебность; to make one's ~ boil приводить в бешенство; to stir ~ возбуждать энтузиазм; in cold ~ хладнокро́вно; it made his ~ run cold у него́ кровь в жи́лах засты́ла; his ~ is up он в раздражённом состоя́нии; his ~ is warm (*или* hot) он вспы́льчив; 3) род, происхожде́ние; full ~ чистокро́вная ло́шадь; half ~ полукро́вная ло́шадь; blue ~ «голуба́я кровь», аристокра́т; it runs in his ~ э́то у него́ в крови́, в роду́; 4) сок (*виногра́дный и т. п.*); 5) *attr* кровяно́й; 6) *attr* (чи́сто)кро́вный.

blooded ['blʌdɪd] *a* 1) окрова́вленный; 2) чистокро́вный; 3) *воен.* понёсший поте́ри, обескро́вленный.

blood-guilty ['blʌd,gɪltɪ] *a* вино́вный в уби́йстве *или* сме́рти.

blood-horse ['blʌdhɔːs] *n* чистокро́вная ло́шадь.

bloodhound ['blʌdhaund] *n* ище́йка; *перен.* сы́щик.

bloodiness ['blʌdɪnɪs] *n* кровожа́дность.

bloodless ['blʌdlɪs] *a* 1) бескро́вный; 2) бле́дный; 3) вя́лый.

blood-letting ['blʌd,letɪŋ] *n* кровопуска́ние.

blood-poisoning ['blʌd,pɔɪznɪŋ] *n* зараже́ние кро́ви.

bloodshed(ding) ['blʌdʃed(ɪŋ)] *n* кровопроли́тие.

bloodshot ['blʌdʃɔt] *a* нали́тый кро́вью (*о глаза́х*).

blood-stained ['blʌdsteɪnd] *a* запа́чканный кро́вью; *перен.* запя́тнанный кро́вью.

blood-sucker ['blʌd,sʌkə] *n* пия́вка; *перен.* кровопи́йца.

blood-thirsty ['blʌd,θəːstɪ] *a* кровожа́дный.

blood-vessel ['blʌd,vesl] *n* кровено́сный сосу́д.

bloodworm ['blʌdwəːm] *n* дождево́й червь.

bloody I ['blʌdɪ] *a* 1) окрова́вленный; 2) крова́вый; 3) кровожа́дный; 4) *груб.* прокля́тый (*пи́шется тж.* b—y).

bloody II *v* окрова́вить, запа́чкать кро́вью.

bloody III *adv груб.* черто́вски, о́чень.

bloom I [bluːm] *n* 1) цвете́ние; цвето́к; in ~ в цвету́; 2) расцве́т; 3) румя́нец; 4) пушо́к (*на плода́х*).

bloom II *v* цвести́, быть в цвету́; *перен.* расцвета́ть.

bloomer ['bluːmə] *n разг.* гру́бая оши́бка.

bloomers ['bluːməz] *n pl* же́нские спорти́вные шарова́ры.

blooming[1] ['bluːmɪŋ] *a* цвету́щий.

blooming[2] *n тех.* блю́минг.

bloomy ['bluːmɪ] *a* цвету́щий.

blossom I ['blɔsəm] *n* 1) цвето́к (*на фрукто́вых дере́вьях*); in ~ в цвету́; 2) расцве́т.

blossom II *v* цвести́; распуска́ться, расцвета́ть.

blot I [blɔt] *n* 1) пятно́; 2) кля́кса; 3) пятно́ позо́ра, бесче́стье.

blot II *v* 1) па́чкать; 2) покрыва́ть кля́ксами; 3) промока́ть (*черни́ла; тж.* to ~ out); 4) бесче́стить; □ to ~ out а) вычёркивать, стира́ть; б) уничтожа́ть; в) закрыва́ть, затемня́ть.

blotch I [blɔtʃ] *n* 1) прыщ; у́горь; 2) пятно́, кля́кса; 3) *шк. сленг* промока́шка.

blotch II *v* покрыва́ть пя́тнами, кля́ксами.

blotter ['blɔtə] *n* 1) промока́шка; 2) писа́ка; 3) *амер.* мемориа́л; торго́вая кни́га.

blotting-paper ['blɔtɪŋ,peɪpə] *n* промока́тельная бума́га.

blouse [blauz] *n* 1) блу́зка; ко́фточка; 2) (рабо́чая) блу́за.

blow[1] [blou] *n* уда́р; at a ~, at one ~ одни́м уда́ром; сра́зу, за оди́н раз; to come to ~s дойти́ до рукопа́шной; to exchange ~s дра́ться; to fetch (*или* to strike) a ~ ударя́ть, наноси́ть уда́р; to strike a ~ for выступа́ть в защи́ту, помога́ть; to strike a ~ against противоде́йствовать.

blow[1] I *n* 1) дунове́ние; to have (*или* to go for) a ~ подыша́ть све́жим во́здухом; 2) *мор.* бу́ря; 3) хвастовство́; 4) *тех.* проду́вка; одна́ пла́вка.

blow[2] II *v* (*past* blew; *p. p.* blown) 1) дуть; раздува́ть; выдува́ть; продува́ть; 2) развева́ть; 3) уноси́ть, гнать, сдува́ть ве́тром; 4) труби́ть; 5) тяжело́ дыша́ть, пыхте́ть; 6) сморка́ть (*нос*); 7) *разг.* транжи́рить де́ньги; □ to ~ about, to ~ abroad распространя́ть (*слух, изве́стие*); «раззвони́ть», to ~ in а) *сленг* внеза́пно появи́ться, влете́ть; б) *тех.* заду́ть до́менную печь; to ~ off: ~ off steam а) *тех.* выпустить пар; б) дать вы́ход избы́тку эне́ргии; to ~ out а) гаси́ть, туши́ть; б) *тех.* вы́дуть до́менную печь; to ~ over проходи́ть, минова́ть; to ~ up а) надува́ть, раздува́ть; б) взрыва́ть; в) рассерди́ться, вспыли́ть; отчита́ть (*кого́-л.*); дать взбу́чку; to ~ upon дискредити́ровать, оговори́ть; ◇ ~ high, ~ low во что бы то ни ста́ло; to ~ hot and cold колеба́ться; (постоя́нно) меня́ть свою́ пози́цию.

blow[3] I *n* цвет, цвете́ние: in full ~ в по́лном цвету́.

blow[3] II *v* (*past* blew; *p. p.* blown) 1) цвести́; 2) расцвета́ть.

blowing ['blouɪŋ] *n* 1) дутьё; 2) уте́чка (*га́за, па́ра*).

blowing-up ['blouɪŋ'ʌp] *n* 1) взрыв; 2) *сленг* взбу́чка, нагоня́й.

blowlamp ['bloulæmp] *n* пая́льная ла́мпа.

blown[1] [bloun] *p. p. см.* blow[2] II.

blown[2] *p. p. см.* blow[3] II.

blown[3] *a* запыха́вшийся.

blow-off ['blouɔf] *n* отделе́ние (*ступе́ней раке́ты*).

blow-out ['blouaut] *n* 1) разры́в (*ши́ны*); проры́в (*плоти́ны и т. п.*); (внеза́пная) уте́чка (*га́за, па́ра и т. п.*); 2) *разг.* шу́мное весе́лье; кутёж; 3) вспы́шка гне́ва; ссо́ра; 4) *амер.* волне́ния; беспоря́дки.

blowtorch ['bloutɔtʃ] *см.* blowlamp.

blow-up ['blou'ʌp] *n* 1) взрыв; 2) взбу́чка, нагоня́й; 3) *см.* blow-out 2), 3) *и* 4).

blowy ['blouɪ] *a* ве́треный.

blowzy ['blauzɪ] *a* 1) краснощёкий; 2) грубова́тый на вид; 3) неря́шливый, растрёпанный.

blub [blʌb] *сокр. шк. сленг см.* blubber[1] II.

blubber[1] I ['blʌbə] *n* рёв, плач.

blubber[1] II *v* реве́ть, гро́мко пла́кать.

blubber[2] *a* то́лстый (*о губа́х*).

blubber[3] *n* 1) во́рвань; 2) *зоол.* меду́за.

bludgeon I ['blʌdʒən] *n* дуби́нка.

bludgeon II *v* бить дуби́н(к)ой.

blue I [bluː] *a* 1) голубо́й, си́ний; dark ~, deep ~ (тёмно-)си́ний; 2) принадлежа́щий к па́ртии то́ри; 3) непристо́йный; to make the air ~ скверносло́вить; ◇ to look ~ вы́глядеть пода́вленным, уны́лым; things look ~ дела́ пло́хи; to feel ~ хандри́ть; to drink till all's ~ о́чень си́льно напи́ться.

blue II *n* 1) си́ний, голубо́й цвет; лазу́рь; си́няя, голуба́я кра́ска; Cambridge ~ све́тло-си́ний цвет; Oxford ~ тёмно-си́ний цвет; Berlin ~, Prussian ~ берли́нская лазу́рь; 2) си́нька; 3) синева́ (*моря, неба*); *поэт.* не́бо, небеса́; мо́ре; 4) оде́жда си́него цве́та; 5) *pl* хандра́; in the ~s в мра́чном настрое́нии.

blue III *v* 1) окра́шивать в си́ний цвет; 2) сини́ть (*бельё*); 3) *сленг* прома́тывать де́ньги.

Bluebeard ['blu:biəd] *n* Си́няя Борода́; *перен. тж.* женоуби́йца.

bluebell ['blu:bel] *n бот.* 1) ди́кий гиаци́нт; 2) колоко́льчик.

bluebottle ['blu:,bɔtl] *n* 1) василёк; 2) мясна́я му́ха.

blueing ['blu:iŋ] *n амер.* си́нька.

bluejacket ['blu:,dʒækit] *n разг.* матро́с англи́йского вое́нного фло́та.

blueprint ['blu:print] *n* светоко́пия, си́нька.

bluestocking ['blu:,stɔkiŋ] *n* «си́ний чуло́к»; педа́нтка.

bluff[1] I [blʌf] *n* отве́сный бе́рег; утёс.

bluff[1] II a 1) отве́сный, круто́й; 2) прямо́й; грубова́то-доброду́шный.

bluff[2] I *n* обма́н, блеф.

bluff[2] II *v* обма́нывать, вводи́ть в заблужде́ние.

bluish ['blu:iʃ] *a* голубова́тый; синева́тый.

blunder I ['blʌndə] *n* гру́бая оши́бка (*тж.* gross ~).

blunder II *v* 1) идти́ спотыка́ясь (*on, along*); 2) сде́лать гру́бую оши́бку; 3) испо́ртить (*дело*); не спра́виться (*с делом*); □ to ~ **away** пропусти́ть, упусти́ть (*по недосмотру*); to ~ **out** сболтну́ть; to ~ **upon** случа́йно найти́, натолкну́ться на что-л.

blunt I [blʌnt] *n* 1) то́лстая коро́ткая игла́; 2) *сленг* нали́чные де́ньги.

blunt II *a* 1) тупо́й; 2) прямо́й, ре́зкий.

blunt III *v* тупи́ть; притупля́ть.

bluntly ['blʌntli] *adv* пря́мо, ре́зко.

blur I [blə:] *n* 1) нея́сные очерта́ния; 2) кля́кса; 3) пятно́.

blur II *v* 1) де́лать нея́сным; затума́нивать; затемня́ть (*сознание и т. п.*); 2) па́чкать, мара́ть.

blurb [blə:b] *n* рекла́мное объявле́ние о кни́ге; изда́тельская анноти́ция.

blurt [blə:t] *v* вы́палить; сболтну́ть не поду́мав (*тж.* to ~ out).

blush I [blʌʃ] *n* 1) кра́ска стыда́, смуще́ния; to put to the ~ пристыди́ть, заста́вить покрасне́ть; 2) взгляд; at the first ~ на пе́рвый взгляд.

blush II *v* 1) красне́ть, вспы́хивать (*от смуще́ния, стыда́; at, for, with*); she ~ed deeply она́ гу́сто покрасне́ла; 2) стыди́ться, красне́ть (*за — for*).

bluster I ['blʌstə] *n* 1) вой бу́ри; 2) шу́мное хвастовство́, самохва́льство; пусты́е угро́зы.

bluster II *v* 1) бушева́ть; 2) угрожа́ть, шуме́ть.

boa ['bouə] *n* 1) уда́в; 2) боа́, горже́тка.

boar [bɔ:] *n* 1) бо́ров; 2) ди́кий каба́н (*тж.* wild ~).

board[1] I [bɔ:d] *n* 1) доска́; junction ~ комму́татор; 2) борт (*судна*); on ~ на корабле́, на

пароходе; *амер.* в ваго́не; to go on ~ сесть на кора́бль, парохо́д; to go by the ~ упа́сть за́ борт; *перен.* быть вы́брошенным за́ борт; 3) кры́шка переплёта; 4) *pl* сце́на, подмо́стки; to be on the ~s, to tread (*или* to walk) the ~s быть актёром; 5) *мор.* галс; ◇ above ~ че́стно, откры́то.

board[1] II *v* 1) обшива́ть доска́ми; настила́ть до́ски; 2) сесть на кора́бль, парохо́д, по́езд, самолёт; 3) *мор.* лави́ровать.

board[2] I *n* 1) накры́тый стол; 2) стол, пита́ние; ◇ to sweep the ~ а) *карт.* забра́ть все ста́вки; б) завладе́ть всем.

board[2] II *v* 1) столова́ться (*у кого-л. — with*); 2) корми́ть (*столующихся*).

board[3] *n* правле́ние; сове́т; колле́гия; министе́рство; school ~ шко́льный сове́т, педагоги́ческий сове́т; the Board of Education министе́рство просвеще́ния (*в Англии*); the Board of Trade министе́рство торго́вли (*в Англии*); торго́вая пала́та (*в США*).

boarder ['bɔ:də] *n* пансионе́р.

boarding-house ['bɔ:diŋhaus] *n* пансио́н, меблиро́ванные ко́мнаты со столо́м.

boarding-school ['bɔ:diŋsku:l] *n* закры́тое уче́бное заведе́ние; *перен.* тюрьма́.

boast I [boust] *n* 1) хвастовство́, бахва́льство; 2) предме́т го́рдости; the ~ of one's family го́рдость семьи́; to make ~ of хвали́ться чем-л.

boast II *v* 1) хва́стать(ся) (*of, about, that*); 2) горди́ться.

boaster ['boustə] *n* хвасту́н.

boastful ['boustful] *a* хвастли́вый.

boat I [bout] *n* 1) су́дно; ло́дка; шлю́пка; flying ~ *ав.* лета́ющая ло́дка; to take ~ сесть на кора́бль, парохо́д; in the same ~ *перен.* в одина́ковых усло́виях; 2) со́усник.

boat II *v* ката́ть(ся) на ло́дке; перевози́ть в ло́дке.

boat-hook ['bouthuk] *n* баго́р.

boating ['boutiŋ] *n* 1) ката́ние на ло́дке; to go ~ ката́ться на ло́дке; 2) ло́дочный спорт.

boatman ['boutmən] *n* ло́дочник.

boat-race ['boutreis] *n спорт.* состяза́ние по гре́бле, гребны́е го́нки.

boatswain ['bousn] *n* бо́цман.

bob[1] I [bɔb] *n* 1) ко́ротко подстри́женные во́лосы; 2) подре́занный хвост; 3) ги́ря ма́ятника; отве́с; грузи́ло; 4) *мор.* лот.

bob[1] II *v* 1) кача́ться; подска́кивать; ста́лкиваться; 2) приседа́ть; 3) ко́ротко стричь во́лосы.

bob[2] *n* (*pl* без измен.) *разг.* ши́ллинг.

bobber ['bɔbə] *n* поплаво́к.

bobbery ['bɔbəri] *n* 1) шум, гам; 2) *attr* шу́мный, беспоко́йный.

bobbin ['bɔbin] *n* кату́шка; шпу́лька.

bobbish ['bɔbiʃ] *a сленг* весёлый, оживлённый.

bobby ['bɔbi] *n разг.* полисме́н.

bobby-soxer ['bɔbi,sɔksə] *n амер. разг.* де́вочка-подро́сток.

bob-sled ['bɔbsled] *см.* bob-sleigh.

bob-sleigh ['bɔbslei] *n спорт.* бо́бслей.

bobtail ['bɔbteil] *n* 1) подре́занный хвост; 2) ло́шадь *или* соба́ка с подре́занным хвосто́м.

bode [boud] *v* 1) предвеща́ть, предска́зывать; сули́ть; 2) предчу́вствовать.

bodeful ['boudful] *a* зловещий.

bodice ['bɔdɪs] *n* 1) лиф; корсаж; 2) лифчик, бюстгальтер.

bodily I ['bɔdɪlɪ] *a* физический, телесный.

bodily II *adv* 1) лично; 2) целиком.

body I ['bɔdɪ] *n* 1) туловище; тело; to keep ~ and soul together поддерживать существование; heavenly ~ небесное тело, небесное светило; 2) труп; 3) *разг.* человек; 4) основная часть (*чего-л.*); корпус, кузов; фюзеляж; ствол дерева; 5) группа людей, корпорация; ~ of electors, elective ~ избиратели; corporate ~ корпоративная организация; diplomatic ~ дипломатический корпус; legislative ~ законодательный орган; in a ~ в полном составе; 6) масса; 7) *воен. разг.* соединение, часть; the main ~ главные силы.

body II *v* придавать форму, воплощать (*тж.* to ~ forth).

body-cloth ['bɔdɪklɔθ] *n* попона.

body-guard ['bɔdɪgɑːd] *n* 1) телохранитель; 2) личная охрана.

Boer ['bouə] *n* бур (*потомок голландских поселенцев в Южной Африке*).

boffin ['bɔfɪn] *n шутл.* учёный, разрабатывающий научные методы ведения войны (*тж.* backroom boy).

bog I [bɔg] *n* болото.

bog II *v*: to be ~ged, to ~ down увязнуть.

bog-berry ['bɔgˌberɪ] *n* клюква.

bogey ['bougɪ] *см.* bogy.

boggle ['bɔgl] *v* 1) пугаться; 2) сомневаться, колебаться (*at, about*); 3) лицемерить; 4) портить, неумело обращаться с чем-л.

boggy ['bɔgɪ] *a* болотистый.

bogie ['bougɪ] *n* тележка.

bogle ['bougl] *n* привидение; 2) пугало.

bogus ['bougəs] *a* поддельный, фиктивный.

bogy ['bougɪ] *n* 1) дьявол; домовой; 2) пугало; *дет.* бука.

Bohemian[1] I [bou'hiːmjən] *n* богемец.

Bohemian[1] II *a* богемский.

Bohemian[2] I *n* 1) человек богемы; 2) цыган.

Bohemian[2] II *a* богемный.

boil I [bɔɪl] *n* кипение; точка кипения.

boil[1] II *v* 1) кипеть; 2) кипятить(ся), варить(ся); 3) сердиться, кипятиться; □ to ~ away a) (продолжать) кипеть; б) выкипать; ~ down a) уваривать, выпаривать; б) сокращать; to ~ over перекипать, убегать (*о кипящем*).

boil[2] *n* фурункул, нарыв.

boiled [bɔɪld] *a* варёный; кипячёный.

boiler ['bɔɪlə] *n* 1) (паровой) котёл; 2) кипятильник; бак для кипячения; 3) овощи, годные для варки.

boiler-house ['bɔɪləhaus] *n* котельная.

boiler-room ['bɔɪlərum] *n* котельное отделение.

boiling I ['bɔɪlɪŋ] *n* 1) кипение; 2) кипячение; ◊ the whole ~ *сленг* все, вся компания.

boiling II *a* кипящий.

boiling-point ['bɔɪlɪŋpɔɪnt] *n* точка кипения; ◊ to be at ~ быть очень рассерженным.

boisterous ['bɔɪstərəs] *a* бурный; шумливый.

bold [bould] *a* 1) смелый, предприимчивый; 2) самоуверенный; дерзкий, наглый, бесстыдный (*тж.* ~ as brass); 3) отчётливый; чёткий; 4) крутой, обрывистый (*о береге*).

bold-faced ['bouldfeist] *a* наглый.

boldly ['bouldlɪ] *adv* 1) смело; 2) дерзко, нагло.

bole [boul] *n* ствол, пень.

boletus [bou'liːtəs] *n* моховик (*гриб*); edible ~ белый гриб.

boll [boul] *n* семенная коробочка.

boloney [bə'lounɪ] *n сленг* вздор, ерунда; абсурд.

Bolshevik I ['bɔlʃɪvɪk] *n* большевик.

Bolshevik II *a* большевистский.

Bolshevism ['bɔlʃɪvɪzəm] *n* большевизм.

Bolshevist I, II ['bɔlʃɪvɪst] *см.* Bolshevik I, II.

bolster I ['boulstə] *n* 1) валик (под подушку); 2) *тех.* подушка.

bolster II *v* 1) подкладывать валик под подушку; 2) поддерживать (*тж.* to ~ up); 3) *шк.* бросаться подушками.

bolt[1] I [boult] *n* 1) засов, задвижка; 2) болт; 3) стрела; 4) молния; удар грома; a ~ from the blue гром среди ясного неба; 5) кусок (*холста*); вязанка (*хвороста и т. п.*).

bolt[1] II *v* 1) запирать на засов; 2) скреплять болтами; □ to ~ in запереть (*кого-л.*) внутри; to ~ out a) захлопнуть дверь (*перед или за кем-л.*), выставить за дверь; б) выболтать, разболтать.

bolt[1] III *adv*: ~ upright прямо; как стрела.

bolt[2] I *n* 1) бегство; to make a ~ броситься (*бежать*); 2) *амер.* измена (*убеждениям, партии и т. п.*).

bolt[2] II *v* 1) броситься (*бежать*); понести (*о лошади*); 2) глотать, не прожёвывая; 3) *амер.* изменить своей партии; не поддерживать кандидата своей партии.

bolt[3] *v* 1) просеивать, отсеивать; 2) расследовать, рассматривать.

bolter[1] ['boultə] *n* 1) горячая лошадь; 2) *амер.* отколовшийся от *или* изменивший своей партии.

bolter[2] *n* сито, решето.

bomb I [bɔm] *n* бомба; (миномётная) мина; ручная граната; incendiary (atomic, hydrogene, napalm, nuclear) ~ зажигательная (атомная, водородная, напалмовая, ядерная) бомба; buzz (*или* flying winged) ~ самолёт-снаряд; delayed--action (*или* time) ~ бомба замедленного действия; demolition (*или* high-explosive) ~ фугасная бомба.

bomb II *v* бомбардировать; *разг.* бомбить; □ to ~ out a) разбомбить район; б) бомбардировками принудить к уходу; ~ed out families семьи, оставшиеся без крова вследствие бомбардировки.

bombard [bɔm'bɑːd] *v* бомбардировать (*тж. перен.*).

bombardment [bɔm'bɑːdmənt] *n* бомбардировка.

bombast I ['bɔmbæst] *n* напыщенность.

bombast II *a см.* bombastic.

bombastic [bɔm'bæstɪk] *a* напыщенный.

bomber ['bɔmə] *n* 1) *ав.* бомбардировщик; 2) гранатомётчик.

bombing ['bɔmɪŋ] *n* 1) бомбардировка, бомбёжка; 2) бомбометание; метание ручных гранат.

bomb-proof ['bɔmpruːf] *a* не пробиваемый бомбами.

bomb-shell ['bɔmʃel] *n* 1) неожи́данность; 2) *attr* внеза́пный.

bombshelter ['bɔm,ʃeltə] *n* бомбоубе́жище.

bonbon ['bɔnbɔn] *n* конфе́та.

bond I [bɔnd] *n* 1) у́зы; *pl* око́вы; *перен.* тюре́мное заключе́ние; in ~s в тюрьме́; 2) сде́рживающая си́ла; 3) *pl* облига́ции; бо́ны; 4) долгово́е обяза́тельство.

bond II *v* 1) закла́дывать иму́щество; 2) подпи́сывать обяза́тельство.

bond III *a уст.* крепостно́й.

bondage ['bɔndɪdʒ] *n* ра́бство; *перен.* зави́симость, ярмо́.

bondholder ['bɔnd,houldə] *n* держа́тель облига́ций.

bondman ['bɔndmən] *n* крепостно́й; вилла́н; раб.

bondsman ['bɔndzmən] *n* 1) *см.* bondman; 2) поручи́тель.

bone I [boun] *n* 1) кость; *pl* скеле́т; to set a ~ вправля́ть кость (*при вы́вихе*); to the ~ наскво́зь, до косте́й, целико́м; 2) те́ло, оста́нки; ◊ a ~ of contention предме́т спо́ра; ≅ я́блоко раздо́ра; to cut to the ~ сни́зить (*це́ны и т. п.*) до ми́нимума; to feel in one's ~s *разг.* быть соверше́нно уве́ренным; to make no ~s of the matter не колеба́ться; не стесня́ться; сме́ло и откры́то обсужда́ть; to make old ~s дожи́ть до ста́рости; to have a ~ to pick with smb. име́ть, своди́ть счёты с кем-л.; to give smb. a ~ to pick «бро́сить кость» кому́-л., задо́брить.

bone II *v* 1) снима́ть мя́со с косте́й; 2) *сленг* красть; ▢ to ~ **up** *амер.* зубри́ть; поду́чивать, повторя́ть.

bone-dry ['boun'draɪ] *a* 1) иссо́хший, вы́сохший; 2) *амер.* сухо́й (*о зако́не*).

bonedust ['boundʌst] *n* костяна́я мука́.

boner ['bounə] *n амер. сленг* 1) си́льный уда́р в спи́ну; 2) неуда́ча, про́мах, оши́бка.

bone-setter ['boun,setə] *n* костопра́в.

bonfire ['bɔn,faɪə] *n* костёр.

bonnet ['bɔnɪt] *n* 1) да́мская шля́па; ка́пор, че́пчик; Gipsy ~ широкопо́лая шля́па; 2) шотла́ндская ша́почка; 3) *тех.* капо́т; колпа́к; кожу́х; 4) *разг.* сообщник.

bonny ['bɔnɪ] *a* 1) краси́вый, здоро́вый; 2) хоро́ший.

bonus ['bounəs] *n* пре́мия.

bony ['bounɪ] *a* 1) кости́стый; 2) костля́вый.

booby ['bu:bɪ] *n* болва́н, дура́к.

boodle ['bu:dl] *n* 1) толпа́; ку́ча; 2) *амер.* взя́тка.

book I [buk] *n* 1) кни́га; juvenile ~s кни́ги для ю́ношества; correspondence ~ журна́л входя́щих и исходя́щих бума́г; ~ of reference, reference ~ спра́вочник; to produce a ~ напеча́тать, изда́ть кни́гу; 2) (the B.) би́блия; 3) либре́тто; 4) *attr* кни́жный; ◊ to be ~ то́чно, то́чно по the ~s быть в спи́сках, быть чле́ном; to be in smb.'s good (bad, black) ~s быть у кого́-л. на хоро́шем (плохо́м) счету́; to be deep in smb.'s black ~s быть у кого́-л. в неми́лости; to be out of smb.'s ~s перестать по́льзоваться расположе́нием кого́-л.; to bring to ~ призва́ть к отве́ту; to suit smb.'s ~ совпада́ть с чьи́ми-л. пла́нами, наме́рениями.

book II *v* 1) регистри́ровать, заноси́ть в кни́гу; 2) зака́зывать, брать, выдава́ть (*биле́т*); 3) приглаша́ть; ◊ I'm ~ed! я попа́лся!

bookbinder ['buk,baɪndə] *n* переплётчик.

bookbinding ['buk,baɪndɪŋ] *n* переплётное де́ло.

bookcase ['bukkeɪs] *n* кни́жный шкаф.

booking-clerk ['bukɪŋklɑːk] *n* касси́р биле́тной ка́ссы.

booking-office ['bukɪŋ,ɔfɪs] *n* 1) биле́тная ка́сса; 2) конто́ра гости́ницы.

bookish ['bukɪʃ] *a* кни́жный; педанти́чный.

book-keeper ['buk,ki:pə] *n* бухга́лтер.

book-keeping ['buk,ki:pɪŋ] *n* бухгалте́рия, счетово́дство.

booklet ['buklɪt] *n* 1) брошю́ра; 2) кни́жечка.

book-maker ['buk,meɪkə] *n* 1) букме́кер (*на ска́чках*); 2) компиля́тор.

bookmark ['bukmɑːk] *n* закла́дка (*в кни́ге*).

bookseller ['buk,selə] *n* книготорго́вец; second--hand ~ букини́ст.

bookselling ['buk,selɪŋ] *n* кни́жная торго́вля.

book-shelf ['bukʃelf] *n* кни́жная по́лка.

book-shop ['bukʃɔp] *n* кни́жный магази́н.

bookstall ['bukstɔːl] *n* кни́жный кио́ск.

bookstand ['bukstænd] *n* кни́жный шкаф.

bookstore ['bukstɔː] *n амер.* кни́жный магази́н.

bookworm ['bukwə:m] *n* кни́жный червь.

boom[1] [bu:m] *n* 1) *мор.* утле́гарь; 2) *мор.* загражде́ние (*из брёвен, це́пи*); 3) *тех.* стрела́ (*кра́на*).

boom[2] I *n* 1) гул; 2) бум (*в торго́вле*); 3) шуми́ха; сенса́ция.

boom[2] II *v* 1) гуде́ть; 2) производи́ть сенса́цию; реклами́ровать, создава́ть шуми́ху; 3) бы́стро расти́ (*о це́нах и т. п.*).

boomerang ['bu:məræŋ] *n* бумера́нг.

boomster ['bu:mstə] *n амер. сленг* спекуля́нт.

boon I [bu:n] *n* 1) бла́го; благодея́ние; 2) преиму́щество.

boon II *a* 1) весёлый; прия́тный; 2) *поэт.* ще́дрый; 3) *поэт.* благотво́рный (*о кли́мате, приро́де и т. п.*).

boor [buə] *n* гру́бый, невоспи́танный челове́к.

boorish ['buərɪʃ] *a* гру́бый, невоспи́танный; неуклю́жий.

boost I [bu:st] *n амер. разг.* 1) подде́ржка, по́мощь; 2) повыше́ние.

boost II *v* 1) поднима́ть, подта́лкивать (*сни́зу или сза́ди*); to ~ a plane into the air подня́ть самолёт в во́здух (*о раке́тном или реакти́вном дви́гателе*); 2) повыша́ть, всеме́рно развива́ть, расширя́ть; 3) подде́рживать; прота́скивать (*кандида́та и т. п.*); 4) создава́ть шуми́ху, реклами́ровать; 5) *эл.* повыша́ть напряже́ние.

booster ['bu:stə] *n* 1) раке́та-носи́тель (*тж.* booster-vehicle); 2) пе́рвая ступе́нь раке́ты-носи́теля (*тж.* booster-rocket).

boot[1] I [bu:t] *n* 1) боти́нок; high ~, riding ~ сапо́г; lace ~s боти́нки на шнурка́х; 2) *амер. разг.* новичо́к, новобра́нец; ◊ to get the ~ быть уво́ленным; to give the ~ уво́лить; the ~ is on the other leg обстоя́тельства измени́лись; to die in one's ~s а) умере́ть скоропости́жной *или* наси́льственной сме́ртью; б) умере́ть на своём посту́.

boot[1] II *v разг.* увольня́ть, выгоня́ть со слу́жбы (*тж.* to ~ out, to ~ round).

boot² I *n*: to ~ в прида́чу, вдоба́вок.

boot² II *v*: what ~s (it) to? кака́я по́льза от э́того?; it little ~s, it ~s not бесполе́зно.

bootblack ['bu:tblæk] *n* чи́стильщик сапо́г.

booth [bu:ð] *n* 1) бу́дка; пала́тка, кио́ск; 2) каби́на.

bootlace ['bu:tleɪs] *n* шнуро́к для боти́нок.

bootlegger ['bu:t,legə] *n* *амер.* торго́вец контраба́ндными *или* самого́нными спиртны́ми напи́тками.

bootless ['bu:tlɪs] *a* бесполе́зный.

bootmaker ['bu:t,meɪkə] *n* сапо́жник.

boots [bu:ts] *n* коридо́рный (*в гости́нице*).

boot-top ['bu:ttɔp] *n* голени́ще.

boot-tree ['bu:ttri:] *n* сапо́жная коло́дка.

booty ['bu:tɪ] *n* добы́ча; награ́бленное добро́; ◇ to play ~ прои́грывать, завлека́я нео́пытного игрока́; спосо́бствовать вы́игрышу партнёра.

booze I [bu:z] *n* *разг.* попо́йка, пья́нка.

booze II *v* *разг.* пья́нствовать.

boracic [bə'ræsɪk] *a* бо́рный.

borax ['bɔ:ræks] *n* *хим.* бура́.

border I ['bɔ:də] *n* 1) грани́ца; 2) край; 3) кайма́, кро́мка; бордю́р.

border II *v* 1) грани́чить (*с — on, upon*); 2) окаймля́ть.

borderland ['bɔ:dəlænd] *n* пограни́чная о́бласть, пограни́чная полоса́; *перен.* грань, грани́ца.

border-line ['bɔ:dəlaɪn] *a* демаркацио́нный; пограни́чный; *перен.* грани́чащий (*с чем-л.*); находя́щийся на гра́ни (*чего́-л.*).

bore¹ I [bɔ:] *n* 1) ску́чный челове́к; 2) что-л. ску́чное; ску́ка.

bore¹ II *v* надоеда́ть; докуча́ть; I am ~d мне надое́ло.

bore² I *n* 1) вы́сверленное отве́рстие; 2) *воен.* кана́л ствола́ ору́жия; кали́бр ору́жия; 3) бурова́я сква́жина (*тж.* ~ hole).

bore² II *v* сверли́ть; бура́вить; *перен.* (с трудо́м) пробива́ться.

bore³ *n* высо́кий прили́в (*в у́зких у́стьях рек*).

bore⁴ *past см.* bear¹.

boreal ['bɔ:rɪəl] *a* се́верный.

boredom ['bɔ:dəm] *n* ску́ка, тоска́.

borer ['bɔ:rə] *n* 1) бура́в, бур; сверло́; 2) бури́льщик.

boric ['bɔ:rɪk] *a* бо́рный.

boring¹ I ['bɔ:rɪŋ] *n* 1) буре́ние; 2) бурова́я сква́жина.

boring¹ II *a* сверля́щий.

boring² I *n* надоеда́ние.

boring² II *a* надое́дливый; ску́чный.

born I [bɔ:n] *p. p. см.* bear²; to be ~ роди́ться; ~ in 1919 роди́лся в 1919 г.

born II *a* рождённый; прирождённый; in all my ~ days за всю мою́ жизнь.

borne [bɔ:n] *p. p. см.* bear².

borough ['bʌrə] *n* 1) небольшо́й го́род с самоуправле́нием (*тж.* county ~); 2) го́род, име́ющий депута́та в парла́менте.

borrow ['bɔrou] *v* 1) брать взаймы́, занима́ть (*у кого́-л. — of, from*); 2) заи́мствовать.

bosh I [bɔʃ] *n* *сленг* глу́пости.

bosh II *v* *шк. сленг* дразни́ть.

bosh III *int сленг* глу́пости!

bosom ['buzəm] *n* 1) грудь; the wide ~ of пе-

рен. ширь (*мо́ря, равни́ны и т. п.*); 2) па́зуха; 3) ло́но, не́дра.

bosom-friend ['buzəmfrend] *n* закады́чный друг.

boss¹ [bɔs] *a* 1) вы́ступ, вы́пуклость, ши́шка; 2) сту́пица колеса́.

boss² I *n* *разг.* 1) хозя́ин, предпринима́тель; вороти́ла; 2) надсмо́трщик; ста́рший рабо́чий, ма́стер; 3) *горн.* штейгер.

boss² II *v* управля́ть, хозя́йничать.

botanical [bə'tænɪkəl] *a* ботани́ческий.

botanist ['bɔtənɪst] *n* бота́ник.

botany ['bɔtənɪ] *n* бота́ника.

botch I [bɔtʃ] *n* 1) гру́бая запла́та; 2) плоха́я рабо́та.

botch II *v* 1) де́лать гру́бые запла́ты; 2) по́ртить рабо́ту.

botcher ['bɔtʃə] *n* плохо́й рабо́тник.

both I [bouθ] *pron* о́ба; и тот и друго́й.

both II *a* о́ба.

both III *adv*: ~ ... and ... как... так и...; ~ brother and sister go in for sports как брат, так и сестра́ увлека́ются спо́ртом.

bother I ['bɔðə] *n* 1) беспоко́йство, хло́поты; 2) исто́чник беспоко́йства.

bother II *v* 1) надоеда́ть; беспоко́ить; 2) беспоко́иться; волнова́ться; ◇ oh, ~ it! *разг.* прокля́тие!, чёрт возьми́!

bothersome ['bɔðəsəm] *a* надое́дливый; беспоко́йный.

bothy ['bɔθɪ] *n* *шотл.* хи́жина.

bottle I ['bɔtl] *n* 1) буты́лка; to bring up on the ~ иску́сственно вска́рмливать; a ~ за буты́лкой (вина́); to crack (*или* to crush) a ~ (of wine) распи́ть буты́лку (вина́); 2) пузырёк, флако́н.

bottle II *v* 1) разлива́ть по буты́лкам; 2) *сленг* пойма́ть, схвати́ть; □ to ~ **up** скрыва́ть, сде́рживать (*негодова́ние и т. п.*).

bottle-green ['bɔtlgri:n] *a* буты́лочного цве́та, тёмно-зелёный.

bottle-neck ['bɔtlnek] *n* 1) го́рлышко буты́лки; 2) у́зкий прохо́д, прое́зд; *перен.* у́зкое ме́сто.

bottle-screw ['bɔtlskru:] *n* што́пор.

bottom I ['bɔtəm] *n* 1) дно; to go to the ~ пойти́ ко дну; to send to the ~ потопи́ть; 2) ни́жняя часть, низ; основа́ние, фунда́мент; 3) осно́ва; суть; причи́на; to be at the ~ of быть причи́ной чего́-л.; at the ~ в осно́ве; to get (down) to the ~ of, to touch the ~ a) добра́ться до су́ти де́ла; б) испи́ть ча́шу до дна; 4) сиде́нье (*сту́ла*); 5) *разг.* зад; ◇ to knock the ~ out of вы́бить по́чву из-под ног; from the ~ of the heart от всей души́; to stand on one's own ~ быть незави́симым.

bottom II *a* ни́жний; кра́йний, после́дний.

bottom III *v* 1) приде́лывать дно, дни́ще; 2) стро́ить, осно́вывать (*на — on, upon*); 3) косну́ться дна; измеря́ть глубину́; 4) добра́ться до су́ти, вполне́ поня́ть.

bottom-land ['bɔtəmlænd] *n* по́йма; доли́на.

bottomless ['bɔtəmlɪs] *a* 1) бездо́нный; *перен.* неизмери́мый, непостижи́мый; 2) не име́ющий сиде́нья (*о сту́ле*).

bottommost ['bɔtəmmoust] *a* са́мый ни́жний.

bough [bau] *n* сук.

bought [bɔ:t] *past, p. p. см.* buy I.

boulder ['bouldə] *n* 1) валу́н; 2) га́лька, голы́ш.

boulevard ['bu:lvɑ:] *n* 1) бульва́р; 2) *амер.* широ́кая у́лица, обса́женная дере́вьями.

bounce I [bauns] *n* 1) прыжо́к, скачо́к; отско́к; 2) хвастовство́; на́глая ложь; 3) си́льный, внеза́пный уда́р; 4) *амер. сленг* увольне́ние.

bounce II *v* 1) подпры́гивать; отска́кивать; 2) влета́ть, врыва́ться (*into*); вылета́ть, ри́нуться вон (*из — out of*); 3) хва́стать(ся); 4) *амер. сленг* увольня́ть.

bounce III *adv* вдруг, внеза́пно.

bouncer ['baunsə] *n* 1) хвасту́н; 2) хвастовство́; на́глая ложь; 3) о́чень высо́кий челове́к; о́чень больша́я вещь.

bound¹ I [baund] *n* 1) грани́цы; 2) *обыкн. pl* грани́цы, преде́л; to set ∼s to ограни́чивать; to go beyond the ∼s of reason поступа́ть безрассу́дно.

bound¹ II *v* 1) грани́чить; 2) ограни́чивать, сде́рживать.

bound² I *n* прыжо́к, скачо́к; at a ∼ одни́м прыжко́м; by leaps and ∼s с большо́й быстрото́й.

bound² II *v* 1) отска́кивать; 2) пры́гать, скака́ть; 3) набега́ть (*о волне*).

bound³ *past, p. p. см.* bind.

bound⁴ *a* гото́вый к отправле́нию; направля́ющийся (*в, к — for*); homeward ∼ возвраща́ющийся на ро́дину; направля́ющийся домо́й; outward ∼ гото́вый к вы́ходу в мо́ре; направля́ющийся за грани́цу.

boundary ['baundərı] *n* грани́ца.

boundless ['baundlıs] *a* безграни́чный, беспреде́льный.

bounteous ['bauntıəs] *a* ще́дрый; оби́льный.

bountiful ['bauntıful] *см.* bounteous.

bounty ['bauntı] *n* 1) ще́дрость; 2) пода́рок; 3) поощри́тельная пре́мия (*в торго́вле, се́льском хозя́йстве и т. п.*).

bouquet ['bukeı] *n* буке́т.

bourgeois I ['buəʒwɑ] *n* буржуа́.

bourgeois II *a* буржуа́зный.

bourgeoisie [ˌbuəʒwɑ'zi:] *n* буржуази́я; petty ∼ ме́лкая буржуази́я.

bout [baut] *n* 1) черёд, круг; раз; this ∼ на э́тот раз; at one ∼ ра́зом; 2) припа́док, при́ступ; drinking ∼ запо́й; 3) схва́тка, борьба́.

bovine ['bouvaın] *a* 1) быча́чий; бы́чий; 2) медли́тельный; тупо́й.

bowᵃˡ [bau] *n* покло́н; to make one's ∼ откла́няться; to take a ∼ выходи́ть, раскла́ниваться на аплодисме́нты; *амер. разг.* заслужи́ть призна́ние, похвалу́.

bowᵃˡ II *v* 1) склоня́ться, сгиба́ться (*to, before*); 2) кла́няться; 3) сгиба́ть, гнуть.

bowᵃ² *n* нос (*корабля́*)

bowᵇ [bou] *n* 1) лук (*ору́жие*); 2) смычо́к; 3) дуга́; ра́дуга; 4) бант; 5) *стр.* а́рка; ◊ to draw a ∼ at a venture а) сде́лать что-л. наугáд, наудáчу; б) случáйно сдéлать мéткое замечáние; to draw a long ∼ преувели́чивать.

bowels ['bauəlz] *n pl* 1) кишки́; вну́тренности; 2) не́дра; 3) сострада́ние, жа́лость.

bower ['bauə] *n* бесе́дка.

bowery I ['bauərı] *a* обса́женный дере́вьями; тени́стый.

bowery II *n амер.* ху́тор, фе́рма.

bowie-knife ['bouı'naıf] *n амер.* дли́нный охо́тничий нож.

bow-knot ['bounɔt] *n* бант.

bowl¹ [boul] *n* 1) ку́бок, ча́ша; the ∼ пи́ршество; 2) ва́за (*для цвето́в*).

bowl² I *n* 1) шар; 2) *pl* игра́ в шары́.

bowl² II *v* игра́ть в шары́; □ to ∼ along бы́стро идти́, кати́ться; to ∼ over сбить с ног; *перен.* привести́ в замеша́тельство.

bow-legged ['boulegd] *a* кривоно́гий.

bowler ['boulə] *n* котело́к (*мужска́я шля́па* тж. ∼ hat); battle ∼ *воен. сленг* стально́й шлем.

bowling-alley ['boulıŋ'ælı] *n* 1) лужа́йка для игры́ в шары́; 2) кегельба́н.

bowling-green ['boulıŋgri:n] *см.* bowling-alley 1).

bowman ['boumən] *n* стрело́к (*из лу́ка*), лу́чник.

bow-pot ['boupɔt] *n* 1) ва́за, горшо́к для цвето́в; 2) буке́т.

bowsprit ['bousprıt] *n мор.* бушпри́т.

bow-string ['boustrıŋ] *n* тетива́.

box¹ I [bɔks] *n* 1) коро́бка; 2) я́щик; сунду́к; 3) бу́дка (*часово́го, сто́рожа и т. п.*); 4) *теа́тр.* ло́жа; 5) ко́злы (*экипа́жа*); 6) сто́йло; ◊ in the wrong ∼ в нело́вком положе́нии; to be in the same ∼ быть в одина́ковом положе́нии (*с кем-л.*).

box¹ II *v* 1) класть в я́щик, коро́бку; 2) подава́ть (*докуме́нты*) в суд; 3) отделя́ть перего́родкой; □ to ∼ up вти́скивать.

box² I *n* 1) уда́р; ∼ on the ear(s) пощёчина; 2) бокс.

box² II *v* 1) бить кулака́ми; 2) бокси́ровать.

box³ *n бот.* самши́т.

boxcalf ['bɔks'kɑf] *n* хро́мовая ко́жа.

boxer ['bɔksə] *n* боксёр.

boxing ['bɔksıŋ] *n спорт.* бокс.

boxing-glove ['bɔksıŋglʌv] *n* боксёрская перча́тка.

box-keeper ['bɔks,ki:pə] *n теа́тр.* капельди́нер.

box-office ['bɔks'ɔfıs] *n* театра́льная ка́сса.

box-up ['bɔks'ʌp] *n сленг* пу́таница.

boxwood ['bɔkswud] *см.* box³.

boy [bɔı] *n* 1) ма́льчик, ю́ноша; old ∼ старина́, дружи́ще; 2) *мор.* ю́нга; 3) бой (*слуга́-тузе́мец*).

boycott I ['bɔıkət] *n* бойко́т.

boycott II *v* бойкоти́ровать.

boyhood ['bɔıhud] *n* о́трочество.

boyish ['bɔıʃ] *a* о́троческий; мальчи́шеский.

boyishness ['bɔıʃnıs] *n* ребя́чество, ребя́чливость.

brace I [breıs] *n* 1) связь; скре́па; подпо́рка; 2) па́ра; 3) *полигр.* фигу́рная ско́бка; 4) *тех.* коловоро́т; 5) *мор.* брас.

brace II *v* 1) свя́зывать; скрепля́ть; подпира́ть; 2) бодри́ть, укрепля́ть; to ∼ oneself up подбодри́ться, взять себя́ в ру́ки; 3) заключа́ть в фигу́рные ско́бки.

bracelet ['breıslıt] *n* 1) брасле́т; 2) *pl* нару́чники.

braces ['breısız] *n pl* подтя́жки.

bracing I ['breısıŋ] *n* связь, крепле́ние.

bracing II *a* бодря́щий, живи́тельный.

bracket I ['brækıt] *n* 1) ско́бка; square ∼ пря-

ма́я ско́бка; to put in ~s заключа́ть в ско́б-
ки; 2) кронште́йн, консо́ль; бра.

bracket II *v* заключа́ть в ско́бки; *перен.* ста́-
вить на одну́ до́ску с кем-л.

brackish ['brækɪʃ] *a* солонова́тый (*о воде*).

bradawl ['brædɔːl] *n* ши́ло.

brag I [bræg] *n* хвастовство́.

brag II *a амер.* первокла́ссный.

brag III *v* хва́статься.

braggart I ['brægət] *n* хвасту́н.

braggart II *a* хвастли́вый.

braggery ['brægərɪ] *n* хвастовство́.

brahmin ['brɑːmɪn] *n* брами́н.

braid I [breɪd] *n* 1) коса́ (*волос*); 2) шнуро́к,
тесьма́.

braid II *v* 1) плести́; заплета́ть; 2) *тех.* оплета́ть; 3) обшива́ть шнурко́м, тесьмо́й.

brain I [breɪn] *n* 1) мозг; to blow out one's ~s
пусти́ть пу́лю в лоб; 2) *pl* мозги́ (*кушанье; тж.*
dish of ~s); 3) *обыкн. pl* ум; у́мственные спо-
со́бности; to beat (*или* to cudgel, to rack) one's
~s лома́ть го́лову (*над чем-л.*—*about, with*); to
get smth. on the ~ мно́го ду́мать о чём-л.; to
turn smb.'s ~ вскружи́ть кому́-л. го́лову; сбива́ть
кого́-л. с то́лку; 4) электро́нная вычисли́тельная
маши́на (*тж.* electronic ~).

brain II *v* размозжи́ть го́лову.

brainless ['breɪnlɪs] *a* безмо́зглый.

brain-sick ['breɪnsɪk] *a* психи́чески больно́й;
сумасше́дший.

brain-storm ['breɪnstɔːm] *n* душе́вное потрясе́-
ние.

brainy ['breɪnɪ] *a* у́мный, мозгови́тый.

braird I [breəd] *n* пе́рвые ростки́; всхо́ды.

braird II *v* всходи́ть (*о посевах*).

braise [breɪz] *v* туши́ть (*мясо*).

brake[1] I [breɪk] *n* то́рмоз; emergency ~ тормоз экстренного торможе́ния; запасно́й то́рмоз.

brake[1] II *v* тормози́ть.

brake[2] *n* па́поротник.

brake[3] *n* ча́ща, за́росли; куста́рник.

brakesman ['breɪksmən] *n* 1) тормозно́й кон-
ду́ктор; 2) машини́ст ша́хтной подъёмной маши́ны.

brake-van ['breɪkvæn] *n* тормозно́й ваго́н.

braky ['breɪkɪ] *a* поро́сший куста́рником.

bramble ['bræmbl] *n бот.* кумани́ка.

bran [bræn] *n* о́труби; вы́севки.

branch I [brɑːntʃ] *n* 1) ветвь, ве́тка; 2) фи-
лиа́л, отделе́ние; 3) о́трасль (*науки, знания*);
4) рука́в (*реки*); отро́г (*горной цепи*); ответвле́ние
(*дороги*); 5) ли́ния родства́.

branch II *v* 1) раски́дывать ве́тви; 2) развет-
вля́ться, расходи́ться (*тж.* to ~ away, to ~ off);
□ to ~ **out** нача́ть но́вое де́ло; расши́рить пред-
прия́тие.

branchia(e) ['bræŋkɪə, -kiː] *n pl* жа́бры.

branchy ['brɑːntʃɪ] *a* ветви́стый.

brand I [brænd] *n* 1) клеймо́; тавро́; *перен.*
пятно́; 2) (фабри́чная) ма́рка; сорт, ка́чество;
3) головёшка.

brand II *v* 1) клейми́ть; выжига́ть, прижига́ть
калёным желе́зом; *перен.* оставля́ть отпеча́ток (*в
памяти*); 2) клейми́ть, позо́рить, облича́ть.

brandish ['brændɪʃ] *v* разма́хивать (*оружием и т. п.*); угрожа́ть.

brand-new ['brænd'njuː] *a* но́вый, с иго́лочки.

brandy ['brændɪ] *n* конья́к; во́дка, бре́нди;
cherry ~ вишнёвка.

bran-new ['bræn'njuː] *см.* brand-new.

brash I [bræʃ] *n* обло́мки.

brash II *a* хру́пкий.

brass I [brɑːs] *n* 1) лату́нь, жёлтая медь;
2) (the ~) *муз.* духовы́е инструме́нты, «медь»;
3) *сленг* де́ньги; 4) *сленг* бессты́дство.

brass II *a* лату́нный.

brassard ['bræsɑːd] *n* нарука́вная повя́зка.

brassière ['bræsɪə] *n* бюстга́льтер.

brassy ['brɑːsɪ] *a* 1) ме́дный (*о цвете*);
2) металли́ческий (*о звуке, привкусе*); 3) на-
ха́льный, на́глый.

brat [bræt] *n пренебр.* отро́дье.

bravado [brə'vɑːdou] *n* (*pl тж.* bravadoes)
брава́да; бесце́льно де́рзкая вы́ходка.

brave I [breɪv] *a* 1) хра́брый, сме́лый; 2) *уст.*
превосхо́дный, прекра́сный; 3) *уст.* наря́дный.

brave II *v* 1) сме́ло встреча́ть (*опасность*);
2) брави́ровать; to ~ it out держа́ться вызы-
ва́юще.

bravery ['breɪvərɪ] *n* 1) хра́брость, сме́лость;
2) великоле́пие; пы́шность.

bravo ['brɑː'vou] *int* бра́во!

brawl I [brɔːl] *n* 1) ссо́ра, перебра́нка; 2) жур-
ча́ние (*ручья*).

brawl II *v* 1) ссо́риться, гро́мко перебра́ни-
ваться; 2) журча́ть.

brawler ['brɔːlə] *n* сканда́ли́ст, крику́н.

brawn [brɔːn] *n* 1) му́скулы; му́скульная си́ла;
2) засо́ленная свини́на.

brawny ['brɔːnɪ] *a* си́льный, му́скулистый.

bray[1] [breɪ] *v* толо́чь.

bray[2] I *n* 1) крик осла́; 2) си́льный шум,
ре́зкие зву́ки.

bray[2] II *v* 1) крича́ть (*об осле*); 2) шуме́ть;
издава́ть ре́зкие зву́ки.

braze [breɪz] *v* спа́ивать, сва́ривать; пая́ть
твёрдым припо́ем.

brazen I ['breɪzn] *a* 1) ме́дный, бро́нзовый;
2) пронзи́тельный, ре́зкий (*о звуке*); 3) бессты́д-
ный, на́глый (*тж.* ~-faced).

brazen II *v*: to ~ out на́гло вести́ себя́;
брать бессты́дством.

brazen-faced ['breɪznfeɪst] *см.* brazen I, 3).

brazier[1] ['breɪzjə] *n* ме́дник.

brazier[2] *n* жаро́вня.

Brazilian I [brə'zɪljən] *n* брази́лец; бразилиа́н-
ка; the ~s брази́льцы.

Brazilian II *a* брази́льский.

breach I [briːtʃ] *n* 1) наруше́ние (*правил, долга и т. п.*); ~ of faith изме́на; ~ of justice не-
справедли́вость; ~ of privilege наруше́ние прав
парла́мента; 2) разры́в (*отношений*); 3) проло́м,
проры́в, брешь; 4) интерва́л; ◊ to stand in the ~
приня́ть на себя́ гла́вный уда́р.

breach II *v* прола́мывать; де́лать брешь.

bread [bred] *n* хлеб; *перен.* сре́дства к су-
ществова́нию; daily ~ насу́щный хлеб; stale ~
чёрствый хлеб; ~ and cheese а) ску́дная еда́;
б) сре́дства к существова́нию; to make one's ~
зараба́тывать на хлеб; ◊ to know on which side
one's ~ is buttered *погов.* не забыва́ть свои́х ин-
тере́сов; знать что к чему́; быть себе́ на уме́.

bread-and-butter ['bredənd'bʌtə] *a*: ~ miss

школьница; де́вочка шко́льного во́зраста; ~ letter письмо́ с выраже́нием благода́рности.

bread-stuffs ['bredstʌfs] *n pl* 1) зерно́; 2) мука́.

breadth [bredθ] *n* 1) ширина́; 2) поло́тнище; 3) широта́ (*взгля́дов*); ◊ to a hair's ~ то́чь-в-то́чь.

breadthways ['bredθweiz] *adv* в ширину́.

breadthwise ['bredθwaiz] *см.* breadthways.

bread-winner ['bred,winə] *n* 1) корми́лец (семьи́); 2) исто́чник существова́ния (семьи́).

break I [breik] *n* 1) проло́м, проры́в; просве́т; щель, брешь; 2) наступле́ние чего́-л.; ~ of day рассве́т; 3) перело́м, измене́ние (*в пого́де, в настрое́нии*); 4) интерва́л, переры́в; *шк.* переме́на; 5) *разг.* случай, возмо́жность; to get a ~ (*неожи́данно*) доби́ться успе́ха; to give smb. a ~ предоста́вить кому́-л. возмо́жность (*попра́вить оши́бку и т. п.*); 6) *амер. полит.* раско́л; 7) *амер.* обмо́лвка, оши́бка; to make a bad ~ сде́лать ло́жный шаг; соверши́ть оши́бку; 8) *амер.* паде́ние цен.

break II *v* (*past* broke; *p. p.* broken) 1) лома́ть(ся); разбива́ть(ся); рвать(ся); разруша́ть(ся); 2) взла́мывать; 3) порыва́ть (*отноше́ния; c — with*); 4) рассе́иваться; 5) света́ть; the day ~s света́ет; 6) наруша́ть (*обеща́ние, зако́н и т. п.*); прерыва́ть (*сон, путеше́ствие и т. п.*); 7) разме́нивать (*де́ньги*); 8) сломи́ть; подорва́ть; осла́бе́ть (*от боле́зни*); 9) тренирова́ть, воспи́тывать; 10) избавля́ть(ся); отуча́ть(ся) (*of*); 11) вспа́хивать, поднима́ть (*целину́*); 12) поби́вать (*реко́рд*); 13) разори́ть(ся); □ to ~ **away** а) вы́рваться (*из тюрьмы́ и т. п.*); б) рассе́яться (*о ту́чах и т. п.*); в) отдели́ться, отпа́сть; to ~ **down** а) полома́ть(ся), слома́ть(ся); б) разби́ть(ся); в) подава́ться, ослабева́ть; г) сломи́ть; д) не вы́держать, потеря́ть самооблада́ние; to ~ **forth** разрази́ться; to ~ forth into tears распла́каться; to ~ **in** а) объезжа́ть (*ло́шадь*); б) вла́мываться; в) прерыва́ть (*разгово́р*); to ~ **into** а) вла́мываться; б) разрази́ться; to ~ **off** а) отла́мывать; б) внеза́пно прекраща́ть; прерыва́ть; обрыва́ть; to ~ **out** а) выла́мывать; б) разрази́ться, вспы́хнуть (*о войне́, пожа́ре и т. п.*); to ~ **through** прорыва́ться; to ~ **up** а) разбива́ть; б) прекраща́ть; в) расходи́ться (*о собра́нии*); г) закрыва́ться на кани́кулы; г) меня́ться (*о пого́де*).

breakable ['breikəbl] *a* ло́мкий, хру́пкий.

breakage ['breikidʒ] *n* 1) поло́мка; поврежде́ние; ава́рия; 2) *обыкн. pl* лом, бой, поло́манные предме́ты; 3) *обыкн. pl* убы́ток, причинённый поло́мкой.

break-down ['breikdaun] *n* 1) поло́мка, ава́рия; 2) упа́док (*сил, здоро́вья*); 3) разва́л, разру́ха, круше́ние; 4) *воен.* переры́в (*в снабже́нии*).

breaker¹ ['breikə] *n* 1) тот, кто лома́ет, разруша́ет; 2) наруши́тель (*зако́на и т. п.*); 3) буру́н; 4) ледоре́з; бык (*моста́*); 5) *эл.* выключа́тель; 6) *тех.* дроби́лка; 7) *горн.* отбо́йщик.

breaker² *n* небольшо́й бочо́нок.

breakfast I ['brekfəst] *n* за́втрак; to have (*или* to take) ~ за́втракать.

breakfast II *v* за́втракать.

breaking ['breikiŋ] *n* 1) ло́мка; 2) дробле́ние;

3) наступле́ние, нача́ло; перело́м; 4) *амер.* распа́ханная, по́днятая целина́; 5) проры́в (*плоти́ны*).

breakneck ['breiknek] *a* опа́сный.

breakstone ['breikstoun] *n* ще́бень.

break-up ['breikʌp] *n* 1) разва́л, распа́д, разру́ха; 2) перело́м (*пого́ды*); нача́ло, наступле́ние; the spring ~ наступле́ние весны́; 3) переры́в (*на кани́кулы*).

breakwater ['breik,wɔːtə] *n* волноло́м, волноре́з; мол.

bream [briːm] *n* лещ.

breast I [brest] *n* 1) грудь; 2) со́весть, душа́, се́рдце; ◊ to make a clean ~ of чистосерде́чно призна́ться.

breast II *v* стать гру́дью про́тив чего́-л.

breast-stroke ['breststrouk] *n спорт.* брасс (*стиль пла́вания*).

breath [breθ] *n* 1) дыха́ние; вздох; to bate (*или* to catch, to hold) one's ~ затаи́ть дыха́ние; to save one's ~ молча́ть; to be out of ~ запыха́ться; зады́ха́ться; to draw ~ дыша́ть; жить; to draw a deep ~ глубоко́ вздохну́ть, вздохну́ть с облегче́нием; to draw (*или* to breathe) one's last ~ умере́ть; to fetch (*или* to take) ~ перевести́ дух, передохну́ть; to gather ~ собира́ться с ду́хом; 2) дунове́ние; ◊ below (*или* under) one's ~ шёпотом; all in a ~, in one ~, in the same ~ одни́м ду́хом, в одно́ мгнове́ние; to give ~ to промо́лвить сло́во; to spend ~, to waste ~ напра́сно тра́тить слова́, говори́ть на ве́тер.

breathe [briːð] *v* 1) дыша́ть; 2) жить; 3) вздохну́ть, передохну́ть; to ~ again (*или* freely) свобо́дно вздохну́ть; 4) ти́хо говори́ть; not to ~ a word не пророни́ть ни сло́ва; 5) слегка́ дуть (*о ве́тре*); 6) вдохну́ть (*что-л. в кого́-л. — into*); 7) испуска́ть (*за́пах*); ◊ to ~ upon smb. очерни́ть кого́-л.

breather ['briːðə] *n разг.* коро́ткая переды́шка.

breathing ['briːðiŋ] *n* 1) дыха́ние; 2) дунове́ние; 3) *фон.* придыха́ние.

breathless ['breθlis] *a* 1) безды́ха́нный; 2) запыха́вшийся; задыха́ющийся; сде́рживающий дыха́ние; 3) безве́тренный; неподви́жный (*о воде́, во́здухе*).

breath-taking ['breθ,teikiŋ] *a* порази́тельный, захва́тывающий.

bred [bred] *past, p. p. см.* breed II.

breeches ['britʃiz] *n pl* бри́джи; ◊ to wear the ~ держа́ть му́жа под башмако́м.

breed I [briːd] *n* поро́да; поколе́ние; of the same ~ одного́ скла́да, ти́па.

breed II *v* (*past, p. p.* bred) 1) выводи́ть, разводи́ть; 2) порожда́ть, вызыва́ть; 3) выси́живать (*птенцо́в*); вска́рмливать; воспи́тывать; 4) размножа́ться; ◊ bred in bone врождённый.

breeder ['briːdə] *n* 1) производи́тель; 2) *с.-х.* селекционе́р; cattle ~ ското́во́д.

breeding ['briːdiŋ] *n* 1) разведе́ние, выведе́ние; 2) воспи́танность; ill ~ невоспи́танность, плохи́е мане́ры.

breeze¹ ['briːz] *n* о́вод (*тж.* ~-fly).

breeze² *n* 1) лёгкий ветеро́к, бриз; 2) слух, но́вость; 3) *разг.* ссо́ра, перебра́нка.

breezy ['briːzi] *a* 1) прохла́дный, све́жий; 2) откры́тый (*ве́тру*); 3) живо́й, весёлый.

brethren ['breðrɪn] *n pl* бра́тья, собра́тья.

breviary ['briːvjərɪ] *n церк.* тре́бник.

brevity ['brevɪtɪ] *n* кра́ткость, сжа́тость.

brew [bruː] *v* 1) вари́ть (*пиво*); 2) зава́ривать (*чай*); сме́шивать, приготовля́ть (*пунш*); 3) затева́ть; замышля́ть; 4) назрева́ть, надвига́ться; □ to ~ **up** *воен. разг.* подже́чь (*танк*); ◊ drink as you have ~ed ≅ завари́л ка́шу, сам и расхлёбывай.

brewer ['bruːə] *n* пивова́р.

brewery ['bruərɪ] *n* пивова́ренный заво́д.

briar ['braɪə] *см.* brier.

briary ['braɪərɪ] *см.* briery.

bribable ['braɪbəbl] *a* подку́пный, прода́жный.

bribe I [braɪb] *n* взя́тка, по́дкуп.

bribe II *v* дава́ть взя́тку, подкупа́ть.

briber ['braɪbə] *n* взяткода́тель.

bribery ['braɪbərɪ] *n* взя́точничество.

bribetaker ['braɪb,teɪkə] *n* взя́точник.

bric-à-brac ['brɪkəbræk] *n* 1) стари́нные ве́щи, ре́дкости; 2) ста́рый хлам.

brick I [brɪk] *n* 1) кирпи́ч; 2) брусо́к (*чего-л.*); 3) *разг.* сла́вный па́рень (*тж.* a regular ~); ◊ gold ~ *амер.* обма́н, надува́тельство; to sell a gold ~ наду́ть, обману́ть; to drop a ~ допусти́ть беста́ктность; сде́лать про́мах; to make ~s without straw а) рабо́тать, не име́я ну́жного материа́ла; б) приступи́ть к де́лу с него́дными сре́дствами; затева́ть безнадёжное де́ло.

brick II *a* кирпи́чный.

brick III *v* класть кирпичи́; □ to ~ **in**, to ~ **up** закла́дывать кирпичо́м; замуро́вывать.

brick-field ['brɪkfiːld] *n* кирпи́чный заво́д.

bricklayer ['brɪk,leɪə] *n* ка́менщик.

brickwork ['brɪkwəːk] *n* кирпи́чная кла́дка.

bridal I ['braɪdl] *n* сва́дьба.

bridal II *a* сва́дебный.

bride [braɪd] *n* неве́ста; новобра́чная; ~ elect наречённая (неве́ста).

bridecake ['braɪdkeɪk] *n* сва́дебный пиро́г.

bridegroom ['braɪdgrum] *n* жени́х; новобра́чный

bridesmaid ['braɪdzmeɪd] *n* подру́жка неве́сты.

bridesman ['braɪdzmən] *n* ша́фер, дру́жка.

bridge¹ I [brɪdʒ] *n* 1) мост; мо́стик; floating ~ наплавно́й мост; паро́м; 2) *мор.* (капита́нский) мо́стик; 3) перено́сица.

bridge¹ II *v* стро́ить мост; соединя́ть мосто́м.

bridge² n карт. бридж.

bridle I ['braɪdl] *n* узда́; to give a horse the ~ отпусти́ть пово́дья; *перен.* дать во́лю.

bridle II *v* 1) взну́здывать; 2) обу́здывать, сде́рживать; 3) вски́нуть го́лову (*в гневе; в знак презре́ния и т. п.*); □ to ~ **up** задра́ть нос.

brief I [briːf] *n* 1) сво́дка, резюме́; 2) *см.* briefing; 3) *юр.* кра́ткое изложе́ние де́ла; to hold ~ for вести́ де́ло в суде́ (*об адвока́те*); *перен.* защища́ть, быть сторо́нником; 4) па́пское бре́ве.

brief II *a* кра́ткий, сжа́тый; in ~ вкра́тце, ко́ротко.

brief III *v* 1) резюми́ровать, кра́тко излага́ть; 2) *ав.* инструкти́ровать (лётчиков) пе́ред боевы́м вы́летом; 3) поруча́ть адвока́ту веде́ние де́ла в суде́.

brief-case ['briːfkeɪs] *n* ручно́й чемода́нчик.

briefing ['briːfɪŋ] *n ав.* кра́ткий инструкта́ж лётчиков пе́ред вы́летом.

briefly ['briːflɪ] *adv* кра́тко, сжа́то.

brier¹ ['braɪə] *n* шипо́вник.

brier² *n* 1) ве́реск; 2) кури́тельная тру́бка (*из ко́рня ве́реска*).

briery ['braɪərɪ] *a* колю́чий.

brig [brɪg] *n мор.* бриг.

brigade [brɪ'geɪd] *n* 1) брига́да; shock ~ уда́рная брига́да; 2) отря́д, кома́нда.

brigadier [,brɪgə'dɪə] *n* 1) бригади́р; 2) брига́дный генера́л.

brigand ['brɪgənd] *n* разбо́йник, банди́т.

brigandage ['brɪgəndɪdʒ] *n* разбо́й, бандити́зм.

bright I [braɪt] *a* 1) я́ркий; 2) блестя́щий; 3) сия́ющий; 4) прозра́чный; я́сный; 5) смышлёный; расторо́пный; 6) живо́й, весёлый.

bright II *adv* я́рко, блестя́ще.

brighten ['braɪtn] *v* 1) освеща́ть(ся); озаря́ть(ся); проясня́ться; 2) очища́ть, придава́ть блеск; 3) оживля́ться (*тж.* to ~ up).

brilliance ['brɪljəns] *n* я́ркость; блеск; великоле́пие.

brilliancy ['brɪljənsɪ] *см.* brilliance.

brilliant I ['brɪljənt] *n* бриллиа́нт.

brilliant II *a* блестя́щий; сверка́ющий.

brim I [brɪm] *n* 1) край; 2) по́ле (*шля́пы*).

brim II *v* наполня́ть(ся), быть по́лным до краёв; □ to ~ **over** перелива́ться че́рез край.

brimful ['brɪm'ful] *a* по́лный до краёв.

brimstone ['brɪmstən] *n* се́ра.

brindle(d) ['brɪndl(d)] *a* полоса́тый; пёстрый.

brine I [braɪn] *n* 1) рассо́л, соляно́й раство́р; 2) солёная вода́; мо́ре; 3) *поэт.* слёзы.

brine II *v* соли́ть, заса́ливать.

bring [brɪŋ] *v* (*past, p. p.* brought) 1) приноси́ть; привози́ть; приводи́ть; 2) причиня́ть; доводи́ть (*до — to*); 3) убежда́ть; □ to ~ **about** а) вызыва́ть; приводи́ть к (*чему-л.*); б) повора́чивать круго́м (*кора́бль и т. п.*); to ~ **back** вспомина́ть; to ~ **down** а) уби́ть, подстрели́ть; повали́ть; сбить (*самолёт*); б) снижа́ть (*це́ны*); в) унижа́ть; to ~ **forth** производи́ть, (по)рожда́ть; to ~ **forward** а) представля́ть, выдвига́ть (*до́вод, предложе́ние*); б) привлека́ть внима́ние к; в) перенести́ на бо́лее ра́нний срок (*о собра́нии и т. п.*); to ~ **in** а) вводи́ть; б) приноси́ть (*дохо́д*); в) вноси́ть (*предложе́ние*); г) выноси́ть (*пригово́р*); to ~ **into** вводи́ть; to ~ **into** play, to ~ **into** action приводи́ть в де́йствие; осуществля́ть; to ~ **into** world рожда́ть; to ~ **off** а) спаса́ть; б) *разг.* доби́ться успе́ха; заверши́ть; to ~ **on** навлека́ть, вызыва́ть; вести́ к; to ~ **out** а) выводи́ть; выявля́ть; б) публикова́ть, выпуска́ть в свет; ста́вить (*пье́су*); в) вывози́ть (*де́вушку в свет*); to ~ **over** переубеди́ть, обрати́ть; to ~ **round** приводи́ть в себя́; to ~ **through** а) вы́лечить; б) вы́вести (*из затрудне́ния*); to ~ **to** а) останови́ть(ся); б) приводи́ть в созна́ние; to ~ **under** подавля́ть, покоря́ть; подчиня́ть; to ~ **up** а) воспи́тывать, вска́рмливать; б) поднима́ть (*вопро́с*); в) останови́ться; *мор.* стать *или* ста́вить на я́корь; ◊ to ~ to bear ока́зывать давле́ние; (по)влия́ть на; to ~ to pass соверша́ть, осуществля́ть.

brink [brɪŋk] *n* край (*обрыва, крутого берега*); *перен.* грань.

brinkmanship ['brɪŋkmənʃɪp] *n*: policy of ~ политика балансирования на грани войны.

briny I ['braɪnɪ] *a* солёный.

briny II *n сленг* море.

brisk I [brɪsk] *a* 1) живой, оживлённый; проворный; 2) бодрящий, свежий (*о ветре*); 3) игристый (*о напитках*).

brisk II *v* оживлять(ся) (*тж.* to ~ up).

brisket ['brɪskɪt] *n* грудинка.

bristle I ['brɪsl] *n* щетина; to set up one's ~s ощетиниться.

bristle II *v* 1) ощетиниться; *перен.* рассердиться; 2) подняться дыбом; 3) изобиловать (*with*).

bristly ['brɪslɪ] *a* щетинистый; колючий.

British I ['brɪtɪʃ] *n*: the ~ (*употр. как pl*) англичане, британцы.

British II *a* (велико)британский.

Britisher ['brɪtɪʃə] *n амер. разг.* англичанин, британец.

Briton ['brɪtn] *n* 1) *ист.* бритт; 2) англичанин, британец; North ~ шотландец.

brittle ['brɪtl] *a* ломкий, хрупкий.

broach I [broutʃ] *n* 1) вертел; 2) шпиль (*церкви*); 3) сверло.

broach II *v* 1) пробуравить *или* початьь (*бочку вина*); 2) открыть, вскрыть (*ящик и т. п.*); 3) начать обсуждение (*вопроса*).

broad I [brɔːd] *a* 1) широкий; 2) обширный; 3) полный, ясный; явный; яркий; резко выраженный (*об акценте*); 4) общий, в общих чертах; 5) терпимый; 6) грубый, непристойный.

broad II *adv* 1) широко; открыто; 2) вполне.

broadcast I ['brɔːdkɑːst] *n см.* broadcasting I.

broadcast II *a* 1) радиовещательный; 2) рассеянный, разбросанный.

broadcast III *v* (*past* broadcasted; *p. p.* broadcast) 1) передавать по радио; 2) распространять; 3) разбрасывать семена.

broadcaster ['brɔːd,kɑːstə] *n* диктор.

broadcasting I ['brɔːd,kɑːstɪŋ] *n* радиовещание, радиопередача.

broadcasting II *a* радиовещательный.

broaden ['brɔːdn] *v* расширять(ся); распространять(ся).

broad-gauge ['brɔːdgeɪdʒ] *a* 1) ширококолейный; 2) широкий, широких взглядов.

broadly ['brɔːdlɪ] *adv* широко; вполне; ~ speaking вообще говоря, в общем.

broad-minded ['brɔːd'maɪndɪd] *a* широких взглядов.

broadness ['brɔːdnɪs] *n* грубость, вольность, нескромность (*в разговоре*).

broadsheet ['brɔːdʃiːt] *n* 1) лист бумаги с текстом на одной стороне; 2) плакат.

broadside ['brɔːdsaɪd] *n* 1) борт корабля; 2) орудия одного борта; 3) бортовой залп; 4) поток брани, упрёков; 5) *см.* broadsheet.

broadsword ['brɔːdsɔːd] *n* палаш.

broadways ['brɔːdweɪz] *adv* вширь, в ширину, поперёк.

broadwise ['brɔːdwaɪz] *см.* broadways.

brocade [brə'keɪd] *n* парча.

brock [brɔk] *n* барсук.

brogue[1] [broug] *n* грубый башмак.

brogue[2] *n* провинциальный акцент (*особ. ирландский*).

broil[1] [broɪl] *n* ссора, шум.

broil[2] I *n* жареное мясо.

broil[2] *v* 1) жарить(ся) на огне; 2) палить, жарить (*о солнце*); 3) жариться на солнце.

broke I [brouk] *past см.* break II.

broke II *a* разорённый; в стеснённых обстоятельствах, без денег.

broken I ['broukən] *p. p. см.* break II.

broken II *a* 1) разбитый; разрушенный; 2) нарушенный; 3) разорившийся; 4) неровный, пересечённый (*о местности*); 5) прерывистый (*о голосе*); 6) ломаный (*о языке*); 7) неустойчивый (*о погоде*); 8) выезженный (*о лошади*).

broken-down ['broukən'daun] *a* 1) надломленный (*о здоровье*); 2) сломленный; 3) не годный к работе (*о лошади*); 4) разорившийся.

broken-hearted ['broukən'hɑːtɪd] *a* убитый горем.

brokenly ['broukənlɪ] *adv* урывками; отрывисто, судорожно.

broken-winded ['broukən'wɪndɪd] *a* запалённый (*о лошади*).

broker ['broukə] *n* 1) маклер; 2) комиссионёр, посредник.

bromide ['broumaɪd] *n* 1) *хим.* соль бромистоводородной кислоты, бромид; 2) снотворное; 3) *разг.* заурядный человек; 4) *разг.* избитая фраза, банальность.

bromine ['broumiːn] *n хим.* бром.

bronchi ['brɔŋkaɪ] *n pl анат.* бронхи.

bronchia ['brɔŋkɪə] *см.* bronchi.

bronchial ['brɔŋkjəl] *a* бронхиальный.

bronchitis [brɔŋ'kaɪtɪs] *n* бронхит.

broncho ['brɔŋkou] *см.* bronco.

bronco ['brɔŋkou] *n амер.* дикая *или* малообъезженная лошадь.

broncobuster ['brɔŋkou'bʌstə] *n амер.* ковбой, объезжающий лошадь.

bronze I [brɔnz] *n* 1) бронза; 2) изделия из бронзы.

bronze II *a* бронзовый.

brooch [broutʃ] *n* брошь.

brood I [bruːd] *n* 1) выводок; 2) куча, стая.

brood II *v* 1) высиживать (*птенцов*); 2) размышлять (*о чём-л. — on, over*); вынашивать (*мысль*); 3) нависать (*о тучах и т. п.; on, over*).

brood-hen ['bruːdhen] *n* наседка.

broody ['bruːdɪ] *a* наседка, клуша (*тж.* ~ hen).

brook[1] [bruk] *n* ручей.

brook[2] *v* терпеть, выносить.

brooklet ['bruklɪt] *n* ручеёк.

broom I [bruːm] *n* метла, веник.

broom II *v* мести.

broth [brɔθ] *n* бульон, отвар; жидкий суп; Scotch ~ перловый суп.

brother ['brʌðə] *n* 1) брат; ~ german, full ~ родной брат; 2) собрат; коллега; 3) земляк.

brotherhood ['brʌðəhud] *n* 1) братские отношения; 2) братство.

brother-in-law ['brʌðərɪnlɔː] *n* (*pl* brothers-in-law) зять, шурин, деверь, свояк.

brotherly I ['brʌðəlɪ] *a* братский.

brotherly II *adv* по-братски.

brought [brɔːt] *past, p. p. см.* bring.

brow[1] [brau] *n* 1) бровь; to bend (*или* to

contract, to knit) one's ~s хму́риться; 2) *поэт.* лоб, чело́; 3) вы́ступ (*скалы*); верши́на (*холма*).

brow² *n мор.* мо́стки, схо́дни.

brow-ague ['brau͵eɪgjuː] *n* мигре́нь.

browbeat ['braubiːt] *v* (*past* browbeat; *p. p.* browbeaten) запу́гивать (*надменностью*).

brown I [braun] *a* 1) кори́чневый; бу́рый; 2) сму́глый, загоре́лый; 3) ка́рий (*о глазах*); 4) суро́вый, небелёный (*о полотне*).

brown II *n* 1) кори́чневый цвет; кори́чневая кра́ска; 2) *сленг* медя́к, пе́нни.

brown III *v* 1) подрумя́ниваться; 2) загора́ть; 3) вороні́ть (*сталь*); ◊ to be ~ed off быть сы́тым по го́рло.

brownie ['brauni] *n* 1) домово́й; 2) шокола́дное пиро́жное.

browse I [brauz] *n* ве́тки, молоды́е побе́ги (*как корм*).

browse II *v* 1) корми́ть (*скот*) ве́тками, молоды́ми побе́гами (*on*); 2) объеда́ть, ощи́пывать (*листья, ветки; on*); 3) пасти́сь; 4) чита́ть (*беспорядочно*).

Bruin ['bruːɪn] *n* Ми́шка, медве́дь (*в сказках*).

bruise I [bruːz] *n* синя́к, кровоподтёк.

bruise II *v* 1) ста́вить синяки́; 2) уда́ром сде́лать вмя́тину, впа́дину; 3) толо́чь; 4) скака́ть сломя́ го́лову.

brumous ['bruːməs] *a* холо́дный, тума́нный.

brunch [brʌntʃ] *n разг.* по́здний за́втрак.

brunette [bruːˈnet] *n* брюне́тка.

brunt [brʌnt] *n* гла́вный уда́р.

brush¹ I [brʌʃ] *n* 1) щётка; 2) кисть; 3) (ли́сий *или* бе́личий) хвост; 4) чи́стка щёткой; to have a ~ почи́стить щёткой; 5) куста́рник, ча́ща, за́росль.

brush¹ II *v* 1) чи́стить щёткой; 2) причёсывать; 3) (слегка́) заде́ть (*тж.* to ~ against); □ to ~ aside отмета́ть, отстраня́ть от себя́; to ~ away, to ~ off а) смахну́ть; б) отмахну́ться, отде́латься; to ~ over а) тро́нуть ки́стью; б) слегка́ заде́ть; в) счи́стить пыль; to ~ up а) чи́стить(ся); приводи́ть (себя́) в поря́док; б) освежа́ть в па́мяти.

brush² I *n* 1) сты́чка, схва́тка; 2) цара́пина; сса́дина.

brush² II *v* ри́нуться (*тж.* to ~ off); □ to ~ by проскользну́ть ми́мо.

brushwood ['brʌʃwud] *n* 1) куста́рник, ча́ща; 2) хво́рост.

brushy ['brʌʃɪ] *a* 1) косма́тый; лохма́тый; 2) щети́нистый; 3) покры́тый куста́рником.

brusque [brusk] *a* гру́бый, ре́зкий.

brutal ['bruːtl] *a* гру́бый; зве́рский, жесто́кий.

brutality [bruːˈtælɪtɪ] *n* гру́бость; зве́рство, жесто́кость.

brute I [bruːt] *n* живо́тное, зверь, скоти́на (*о человеке*).

brute II *a* живо́тный, гру́бый.

brutish ['bruːtɪʃ] *a* 1) жесто́кий, зве́рский; 2) тупо́й, живо́тный; чу́вственный.

bubble I ['bʌbl] *n* 1) пузы́рь, пузырёк (*воздуха*); 2) кипе́ние, бурле́ние; бу́льканье; 3) ду́тое предприя́тие, «мы́льный пузы́рь»; ◊ to prick the ~ показа́ть ничто́жество, развенча́ть.

bubble II *v* пузы́риться, кипе́ть, бурли́ть, бу́лькать (*тж.* to ~ over, to ~ up).

buccaneer I [͵bʌkəˈnɪə] *n* пира́т.

buccaneer II *v* занима́ться морски́м разбо́ем.

buck¹ I [bʌk] *n* 1) саме́ц (*об олене, зайце, кролике*); 2) де́нди, франт; ◊ to pass the ~ to smb. *амер.* свали́ть отве́тственность на кого́-л.

buck¹ II *v* станови́ться на дыбы́; брыка́ться; □ to ~ against *амер.* проти́виться, выступа́ть про́тив; to ~ off сбра́сывать с седла́; to ~ up *разг.* а) спеши́ть; б) оживля́ться, проявля́ть эне́ргию; ~ up! встряхни́сь, (под)бодри́сь!

buck² *v* распи́ливать на брёвна.

buck³ I *n* болтовня́, хвастовство́.

buck³ II *v* болта́ть; хва́статься.

buck⁴ *n амер. сленг* до́ллар.

buck-basket ['bʌk͵bɑːskɪt] *n* бельева́я корзи́на.

bucket¹ I ['bʌkɪt] *n* 1) ведро́; 2) черпа́к, ковш (*землечерпалки и т. п.*); ◊ to give (to get) the ~ уво́лить (уво́литься) со слу́жбы; to kick the ~ умере́ть.

bucket¹ II *v* че́рпать.

bucket² *v* 1) скака́ть сломя́ го́лову; 2) си́льно грести́.

buckish ['bʌkɪʃ] *a* щеголева́тый.

buckle I ['bʌkl] *n* пря́жка.

buckle II *v* 1) застёгивать пря́жкой (*тж.* to ~ up, to ~ on); 2) сгиба́ть; гнуть, выгиба́ть; 3) сгиба́ться, подава́ться; □ to ~ to принима́ться за де́ло.

buckram I ['bʌkrəm] *n* 1) клеёный холст, клеёнка; 2) чо́порность; 3) ви́димость си́лы, кре́пости.

buckram II *a* 1) чо́порный; 2) си́льный *или* кре́пкий то́лько на вид.

buck-shot ['bʌkʃɔt] *n* кру́пная дробь.

buckskin ['bʌkskɪn] *n* 1) оле́нья ко́жа; 2) *pl* штаны́ из оле́ньей ко́жи.

buckstick ['bʌkstɪk] *n* хвасту́н.

buckwheat ['bʌkwiːt] *n* 1) гречи́ха; 2) *attr* гре́чневый.

bucolic [bjuːˈkɔlɪk] *a* 1) буколи́ческий, пастора́льный; 2) *шутл.* се́льский.

bud I [bʌd] *n* 1) *бот.* по́чка; 2) буто́н; ◊ to nip in the ~ подави́ть в заро́дыше, пресе́чь в ко́рне.

bud II *v* 1) дава́ть по́чки; пуска́ть ростки́; 2) *зоол.* размножа́ться почкова́нием; 3) развива́ться.

buddhism ['budɪzəm] *n* будди́зм.

buddhist ['budɪst] *n* будди́ст.

budge [bʌdʒ] *v* шевели́ть(ся); (по)шевельну́ть(ся).

budget I ['bʌdʒɪt] *n* бюдже́т; ◊ ~ of news ку́ча новосте́й.

budget II *v* предусма́тривать в бюдже́те (*for*).

budgetary ['bʌdʒɪtərɪ] *a* бюдже́тный.

buff [bʌf] *n* 1) то́лстая бу́йволовая *или* быча́чья ко́жа; 2) ко́жа челове́ка; in ~ го́лый, на-гишо́м; 3) ту́скло-жёлтый цвет.

buffalo ['bʌfəlou] *n* бу́йвол; бизо́н.

buffer¹ ['bʌfə] *n* 1) бу́фер; 2) *attr* бу́ферный.

buffer² *n сленг:* old ~ ста́рый хрыч, стари-ка́шка.

buffetᵃ¹ I ['bʌfɪt] *n* уда́р.

buffetᵃ¹ II *v* 1) наноси́ть уда́р; 2) боро́ться.

buffetᵃ² *n* буфе́т, го́рка.

buffet[b] ['bufeɪ] *n* буфе́т, заку́сочная.
buffoon I [bʌ'fuːn] *n* шут.
buffoon II *a* шутовско́й.
buffoon III *v* изобража́ть шута́, фигля́рничать.
buffoonery [bʌ'fuːnərɪ] *n* шутовство́.
bug [bʌg] *n* 1) клоп; *разг.* насеко́мое; жук; 2) *сленг* «пу́нктик», помеша́тельство; to go ~s сойти́ с ума́; 3) *амер.* техни́ческий дефе́кт; ◊ big ~ *сленг* ва́жная персо́на, «ши́шка».
bugaboo ['bʌgəbuː] *n* пу́гало; бу́ка.
bugbear ['bʌgbeə] *см.* bugaboo.
buggy[1] ['bʌgɪ] *n* 1) лёгкая одноме́стная *или* двухме́стная коля́ска; 2) ма́ленькая вагоне́тка.
buggy[2] *a* киша́щий клопа́ми.
bughouse ['bʌghaus] *n* *амер. сленг* сумасше́дший дом.
bugle I ['bjuːgl] *n* рожо́к, горн.
bugle II *v* труби́ть в рог, игра́ть на го́рне.
bugler ['bjuːglə] *n* 1) горни́ст; 2) *воен.* сигнали́ст.
build I [bɪld] *n* 1) фо́рма; констру́кция; стиль; 2) телосложе́ние.
build II *v* (*past, p. p.* built) 1) стро́ить, сооружа́ть; создава́ть; 2) вить (*гнёзда*); 3) осно́вывать(ся), полага́ться (*на — on*) □ to ~ **into** вде́лывать в сте́ну; to ~ **up** а) воздвига́ть; создава́ть; стро́ить; to be built up быть застро́енным дома́ми; б) укрепля́ть (*здоро́вье*); в) закла́дывать кирпичо́м; to ~ **upon** осно́вывать на; рассчи́тывать на.
builder ['bɪldə] *n* строи́тель.
building ['bɪldɪŋ] *n* 1) зда́ние; строе́ние, сооруже́ние; 2) строи́тельство.
building-up ['bɪldɪŋ'ʌp] *n* строи́тельство, постро́ение.
built [bɪlt] *past, p. p. см.* build II.
bulb [bʌlb] *n* 1) лу́ковица; 2) электри́ческая ла́мпочка.
bulbaceous [bʌl'beɪʃəs] *a* 1) лу́ковичный; 2) вы́пуклый.
bulbous ['bʌlbəs] *см.* bulbaceous.
Bulgarian I [bʌl'gɛərɪən] *n* 1) болга́рин; болга́рка; the ~s болга́ры; 2) болга́рский язы́к.
Bulgarian II *a* болга́рский.
bulge I [bʌldʒ] *n* 1) вы́пуклость; 2) *разг.* вздутие цен; 3) (*обыкн.* the ~) *сленг* преиму́щество; to have (to get) the ~ on smb. име́ть (получи́ть) преиму́щество над кем-л.
bulge II *v* 1) выпя́чиваться, выдава́ться; 2) вздува́ться, распуха́ть; увели́чиваться (*в объёме, коли́честве*); 3) набива́ть (*мешо́к, кошелёк и т. п.*).
bulging ['bʌldʒɪŋ] *a* 1) вы́пуклый; навы́кате (*о глаза́х*); 2) оттопы́ривающийся.
bulgy ['bʌldʒɪ] *см.* bulging.
bulk I [bʌlk] *n* 1) объём; вмести́мость; 2) бо́льшая часть чего-л.; 3) основна́я ма́сса; большо́е коли́чество; to sell (to buy) in ~ продава́ть (покупа́ть) о́птом, гурто́м; 4) величина́, больши́е разме́ры; 5) груз (*су́дна*); to break ~ начина́ть разгру́зку; ◊ in ~ без упако́вки.
bulk II *v* 1) каза́ться больши́м, ва́жным (*тж.* to ~ large); 2) ссыпа́ть в ку́чу, нагроможда́ть; □ to ~ **up** соста́вить значи́тельную су́мму, коли́чество *и т. п.*
bulkhead ['bʌlkhed] *n* *мор.* перебо́рка.

bulky ['bʌlkɪ] *a* большо́й; громо́здкий; гру́зный.
Bull [bul] *n* Теле́ц (*созве́здие*).
bull[1] I [bul] *n* 1) бык; 2) саме́ц (*о слоне́, ките́ и др. кру́пных живо́тных*); 3) *бирж.* спекуля́нт, игра́ющий на повыше́ние; ◊ to take the ~ by the horns де́йствовать реши́тельно, напрями́к, взять быка́ за рога́.
bull[1] II *v* 1) *бирж.* игра́ть на повыше́ние; 2) повыша́ть це́ну; повыша́ться в цене́.
bull[2] *n* противоре́чие, неле́пость.
bull[3] *n* *сленг* моне́та в пять ши́ллингов; half a ~ полкро́ны.
bull[4] *n* (па́пская) бу́лла.
bulldog ['buldɒg] *n* бульдо́г; *перен.* упо́рный челове́к.
bulldoze ['buldouz] *v* *амер. сленг* запу́гивать, шантажи́ровать; принужда́ть.
bulldozer ['bul,douzə] *n* бульдо́зер.
bullet ['bulɪt] *n* пу́ля; percussion ~ разрывна́я пу́ля; stray ~ шальна́я пу́ля.
bulletin ['bulɪtɪn] *n* бюллете́нь, сво́дка; news ~ переда́ча после́дних изве́стий (*по ра́дио и т. п.*).
bullfight ['bulfaɪt] *n* бой быко́в.
bullfighter ['bul,faɪtə] *n* тореадо́р, матадо́р.
bullfighting ['bul,faɪtɪŋ] *см.* bullfight.
bullfinch ['bulfɪntʃ] *n* снеги́рь.
bullhead ['bulhed] *n* болва́н.
bullheaded ['bul'hedɪd] *a* упря́мый, упо́рный; насто́йчивый.
bullion ['buljən] *n* сли́ток зо́лота *или* серебра́.
bullock ['bulək] *n* вол.
bull's-eye ['bulzaɪ] *n* 1) *мор.* иллюмина́тор; 2) слухово́е окно́; 3) центр, я́блоко мише́ни.
bully[1] I ['bulɪ] *n* 1) зади́ра; хвасту́н; 2) хулига́н.
bully[1] II *v* 1) задира́ть; запу́гивать, трети́ровать.
bully[2] I *a* *амер.* первокла́ссный, великоле́пный.
bully[2] II *int амер.*: ~ for you! бра́во!
bully[3] *n* мясны́е консе́рвы (*тж.* ~ beef).
bullyrag ['bulɪræg] *см.* ballyrag.
bulrush ['bulrʌʃ] *n* камы́ш, тростни́к.
bulwark ['bulwək] *n* 1) (крепостно́й) вал, бастио́н; 2) опло́т; 3) мол.
bumble-bee ['bʌmblbiː] *n* шмель; ◊ it's plain as a ~ on a fried egg *погов.* ≅ э́то я́сно как день.
bumbledom ['bʌmbldəm] *n* *разг.* бюрократи́зм; мелкочино́вное чва́нство.
bumbo ['bʌmbou] *n* холо́дный пунш.
bump I [bʌmp] *n* 1) глухо́й уда́р; столкнове́ние; 2) ши́шка, о́пухоль; 3) вы́гиб, вы́пуклость; 4) *ав.* возду́шная я́ма.
bump II *v* 1) уда́рять(ся), ушиба́ть(ся); 2) наска́кивать, налета́ть (*тж.* to ~ into); □ to ~ **off** *амер. сленг* устрани́ть кого́-л., уби́ть.
bump III *adv* внеза́пно, вдруг.
bumper ['bʌmpə] *n* 1) стака́н (вина́), по́лный до краёв; 2) *тех.* ба́мпер; амортиза́тор; 3) *attr* небыва́лого большо́й, оби́льный.
bumpkin ['bʌmpkɪn] *n* неотёсанный па́рень; нело́вкий, засте́нчивый челове́к.
bumptious ['bʌmpʃəs] *a* самоуве́ренный.
bumpy ['bʌmpɪ] *a* уха́бистый.
bun[1] [bʌn] *n* сла́дкая бу́лочка с изю́мом.
bun[2] *n* 1) (коро́ткий) хво́стик; 2) кро́лик.
bunch I [bʌntʃ] *n* 1) свя́зка, пучо́к; буке́т (*цвето́в*); ~ of fives *сленг* пятерня́, кула́к, ру-

ка; 2) *разг.* компа́ния; the best of the ~ лу́чший из всех.

bunch II *v* собира́ться *или* держа́ться вме́сте.

buncombe ['bʌŋkəm] *см.* bunkum.

bundle I ['bʌndl] *n* свя́зка, узело́к; вяза́нка.

bundle II *v* 1) свя́зывать в у́зел (*тж.* to ~ up); на́спех упако́вывать ве́щи (*тж.* to ~ in); 2) бы́стро уйти́, убра́ться (*тж.* to ~ out, off, away); 3) выпрова́живать (*тж.* to ~ out, off, away).

bung I [bʌŋ] *n* 1) заты́чка, втулка; 2) *сленг* ложь.

bung II *v* 1) затыка́ть, заку́поривать; *перен.* закрыва́ть; ~ed up заплы́вший (*о глазах*); 2) *сленг* швыря́ть (*камни*).

bungalow ['bʌŋgəlou] *n* бу́нгало, одноэта́жный ле́тний дом.

bungle I ['bʌŋgl] *n* 1) плоха́я, гру́бая рабо́та; 2) пу́таница; ошибка.

bungle II *v* 1) пло́хо рабо́тать; 2) напу́тать.

bungler ['bʌŋglə] *n* плохо́й рабо́тник.

bunk[1] I [bʌŋk] *n* ко́йка.

bunk[1] II *v* *амер.* *разг.*: to ~ it спать (на ко́йке).

bunk[2] I *n* *сленг* бе́гство.

bunk[2] II *v* *сленг* исче́знуть, убра́ться.

bunk[3] *n* *амер.* *сокр.* *см.* bunkum.

bunker ['bʌŋkə] *n* 1) *мор.* у́гольная я́ма, бу́нкер; 2) *воен.* дот.

bunkum ['bʌŋkəm] *n* вздор, болтовня́, пусты́е фра́зы.

bunny ['bʌnɪ] *n* *дет.* кро́лик.

bunt I [bʌnt] *n* уда́р; пино́к, толчо́к.

bunt II *v* 1) ударя́ть; пиха́ть; 2) бода́ть(ся).

bunting[1] ['bʌntɪŋ] *n* овся́нка (*птица*).

bunting[2] *n* 1) мате́рия для фла́гов; 2) *собир.* фла́ги.

buoy I [bɔɪ] *n* ба́кен, буй.

buoy II *v* 1) (*обыкн.* to ~ up) подде́рживать на пове́рхности; *перен.* подде́рживать, поднима́ть (*настроение и т. п.*); 2) ста́вить ба́кены.

buoyancy ['bɔɪənsɪ] *n* 1) плаву́честь, спосо́бность держа́ться на пове́рхности; 2) бо́дрость, эне́ргия; жизнера́достность; 3) повыша́тельная тенде́нция (*на бирже*).

buoyant ['bɔɪənt] *a* 1) плаву́чий, спосо́бный держа́ться на пове́рхности; 2) бо́дрый, энерги́чный; жизнера́достный.

bur [bəː] *n* 1) репе́й(ник); 2) назо́йливый челове́к.

Burberry ['bəːbərɪ] *n* непромока́емое пальто́.

burden[1] I ['bəːdn] *n* 1) тя́жесть; но́ша; груз; 2) бре́мя; гнёт; 3) накладны́е расхо́ды; 4) *мор.* тонна́ж; грузоподъёмность.

burden[1] II *v* 1) нагружа́ть; 2) обременя́ть, отягоща́ть.

burden[2] *n* 1) припе́в, рефре́н; 2) те́ма; основна́я мысль; суть; лейтмоти́в.

burdensome ['bəːdnsəm] *a* обремени́тельный, тяжёлый.

burdock ['bəːdɔk] *n* лопу́х, репе́йник.

bureau [bjuə'rou] *n* (*pl* bureaux, bureaus [bjuə'rouz]) 1) бюро́; пи́сьменный стол; конто́рка; 2) *амер.* комо́д с зе́ркалом; 3) бюро́; конто́ра; комите́т.

bureaucracy [bjuə'rɔkrəsɪ] *n* 1) бюрокра́тия; 2) бюрократи́зм.

bureaucrat ['bjuəroukræt] *n* бюрокра́т.

bureaucratic [,bjuərou'krætɪk] *a* бюрократи́ческий.

burgess ['bəːdʒɪs] *n* 1) горожа́нин, граждани́н (*муниципального города*); 2) *ист.* член парла́мента от самоуправля́ющегося го́рода *или* от университе́та.

burgh ['bʌrə] *шотл.* *см.* borough.

burglar ['bəːglə] *n* (ночно́й) вор-взло́мщик.

burglary ['bəːglərɪ] *n* (ночна́я) кра́жа со взло́мом.

burgle ['bəːgl] *v* 1) соверша́ть кра́жу со взло́мом; 2) обворо́вывать.

burgundy ['bəːgəndɪ] *n* бургу́ндское (кра́сное) вино́.

burial ['berɪəl] *n* по́хороны.

burial-ground ['berɪəlgraund] *n* кла́дбище.

burial-service ['berɪəl,səːvɪs] *n* заупоко́йная слу́жба.

burke [bəːk] *v* 1) подави́ть в заро́дыше; запрети́ть (*книгу, журнал*); 2) замя́ть (*дело*); обойти́ молча́нием.

burlap ['bəːlæp] *n* (джу́товый) холст; дерю́га, мешкови́на.

burlesque I [bəː'lesk] *n* 1) бурле́ск, паро́дия; карикату́ра; 2) *амер.* фарс.

burlesque II *a* пароди́йный.

burlesque III *v* пароди́ровать.

burly ['bəːlɪ] *a* здоро́вый, пло́тный, доро́дный.

Burmese I [bəː'miːz] *n* 1) бирма́нец; бирма́нка; the ~ (*употр. как pl*) бирма́нцы; 2) бирма́нский язы́к.

Burmese II *a* бирма́нский.

burn[1] [bəːn] *шотл.* ручей.

burn[2] I *v* (*past, p. p.* burnt) 1) горе́ть; пыла́ть; сгора́ть; to ~ with anger пыла́ть зло́бой; 2) жечь; сжига́ть; выжига́ть; прожига́ть; зажига́ть; 3) обжига́ть; 4) *мед.* прижига́ть; 5) загора́ть; 6) подгора́ть; □ to ~ **away** а) сгора́ть; б) сжига́ть; to ~ **down** а) сжига́ть дотла́; б) догора́ть; to ~ **into** вреза́ться (*в память*), запа́сть (*в душу*); to ~ **out** выжига́ть; выгора́ть; to ~ **up** а) зажига́ть; б) сжига́ть; to ~ up the road *амер.* е́хать с большо́й ско́ростью; ◊ to ~ с избы́тком.

burn[2] II *n* 1) ожо́г; 2) клеймо́; 3) выжига́ние (*травы, кустарника*).

burner ['bəːnə] *n* горе́лка.

burning I ['bəːnɪŋ] *n* 1) горе́ние; 2) о́бжиг, обжига́ние, прока́ливание.

burning II *a* горя́щий; *перен.* жгу́чий; горя́чий; животрепе́щущий.

burnish I ['bəːnɪʃ] *n* полиро́вка; блеск.

burnish II *v* полирова́ть.

burnt [bəːnt] *past, p. p.* *см.* burn[2] I.

burr[1] I [bəː] *n* 1) заднеязы́чное произноше́ние зву́ка r; карта́вость; 2) шум, гро́хот (*колёс*).

burr[1] II *v* карта́вить.

burr[2] *n* *см.* bur.

burr[3] *n* вене́ц (*вокруг светила*).

burr[4] *n* рва́ный край (*бумаги*); заусе́нец (*на металле*).

burr[5] *n* 1) точи́льный ка́мень; 2) известня́к.

burro ['burou] *n* *разг.* осёл.

burrow I ['bʌrou] *n* норá.

burrow II *v* рыть норý, ход; прятаться; *перен.* дойскиваться до чего-л., «раскáпывать».

burst [bə:st] *n* 1) взрыв; вспышка; 2) разрыв (снаряда); пулемётная очередь; 3) внезáпное проявлéние; порыв; 4) запóй.

burst II *v* (*past, p. p.* burst) 1) лóпаться; взрывáться; разрывáться; 2) взрывáть; 3) прорвáться (*о пламени, плотине и т. п.*); ворвáться; □ to ~ **in** a) разразиться, вспыхнуть; б) внезáпно появиться, ворвáться; to ~ **into**: to ~ into blossom распуститься, расцвести: to ~ into applause разразиться аплодисмéнтами; to ~ into (a storm of) tears залиться слезáми; to ~ into laughter разразиться смéхом; to ~ into flame вспыхнуть, загорéться; to ~ **out** a) воскликнуть; б) разразиться; вспыхнуть (*о войне, эпидемии*); to ~ out laughing (crying) разразиться смéхом (слезáми); to ~ **up** a) взрывáть(ся); б) *разг.* потерпéть неудáчу; to ~ **with**: to ~ with envy лóпнуть от зáвисти; to ~ with joy сиять от удовóльствия, светиться рáдостью; to ~ with pride сиять гóрдостью.

burthen ['bə:ðən] *поэт. см.* burden.

bury ['berı] *v* 1) хоронить; зарывáть (в зéмлю); 2) прятать; to ~ one's face in one's hands закрыть лицó рукáми; to ~ one's hands in one's pockets засýнуть, спрятать рýки в кармáны.

burying-ground ['berıŋgraund] *n* клáдбище.

burying-place ['berıŋpleıs] *см.* burying-ground.

bus, 'bus [bʌs] *n* 1) автóбус; 2) *сленг* пассажирский самолёт; ◊ to miss the ~ *сленг* потерпéть неудáчу, упустить слýчай.

bus, 'bus II *v* éхать в автóбусе.

bush I [buʃ] *n* 1) куст; кустáрник; 2) обширные малонаселённые прострáнства, покрытые кустáрником, буш (*в Африке и в Австралии*); 3) густые вóлосы; ~ of hair копнá волóс; ◊ to take to the ~ стать бродягой; to beat about the ~ ходить вокрýг да óколо, подходить к дéлу осторóжно.

bush II *v* обсáживать кустáрником.

bushel ['buʃl] *n* бýшель (*мера объёма=* =36,3 *л.*); ◊ under a ~ тáйно, секрéтно.

bushing ['buʃıŋ] *n тех.* втýлка.

Bushman ['buʃmən] *n* бушмéн; the Bushman бушмéны.

bush-ranger ['buʃ,reındʒə] *n австрал.* бродяга, бéглый престýпник.

bushwhacker ['buʃ,wækə] *n* 1) *австрал.* живýщий в леснóй глуши; 2) *амер. ист.* партизáн (*в гражданской войне*); 3) *амер. ист.* дезертир (*в гражданской войне*).

bushy ['buʃı] *a* 1) зарóсший кустáрником; 2) густóй, пушистый.

business[a] ['bıznıs] *n* 1) дéло; занятие; профéссия; on ~ по дéлу; the ~ of the day (*или* of the meeting) повéстка дня; to mean ~ поступáть серьёзно, дéльно; go about your ~! mind your own ~! не вмéшивайтесь не в своё дéло!; what is your ~? что вам нáдо?; to send smb. about his ~ прогнáть, увóлить когó-л.; good ~! хорóшее дéло!; здóрово!; a pretty ~! *ирон.* хорóшенькое дéло!; 2) обязанность; to make it one's ~ считáть своéй обязанностью; to stick to one's ~ быть усéрдным, исполнительным;

3) коммéрческая дéятельность; slack ~ вялая торгóвля; 4) коммéрческое, торгóвое предприятие, фирма; big ~ крýпный капитáл; to set up in ~ начáть торгóвое дéло; 5) (выгодная) сдéлка; ◊ to have no ~ to не имéть прáва, основáний (*сделать что-л.*); to do the ~ for smb. a) погубить, разорить когó-л.; б) убить когó-л.

business[b] ['bıznıs] *n см.* busyness.

business-like ['bıznıslaık] *a* 1) делóвой, практичный; 2) тóчный, чёткий.

bust[1] [bʌst] *n* бюст.

bust[2] *n см.* burst I, 4).

bust[3] *v сленг* 1) обанкрóтиться; потерпéть неудáчу (*тж.* to ~ up); 2) запить; 3) *см.* burst II.

bustle I ['bʌsl] *n* суматóха, суетá.

bustle II *v* 1) торопиться; суетиться; 2) торопить.

busy I ['bızı] *a* 1) занятый, дéятельный; прилéжный; 2) беспокóйный, суетливый.

busy II *v* давáть рабóту, занимáть чем-л.; to ~ oneself занимáться.

busy III *n сленг* сыщик.

busy-body ['bızı,bɔdı] *n* хлопотýн; человéк, сýющий нос в чужие делá.

busyness ['bızınıs] *n* занятость; деловитость.

but I [bʌt (*сильная форма*), bət (*слабая форма*)] *conj* 1) но, а, тем не мéнее, однáко; I should like to come ~ I haven't time я бы пришёл, но у меня нет врéмени, 2) éсли бы не; как не; ~ for éсли бы не; ~ then но затó, но с другóй сторóны; cannot ~... не могý не..., не мóжет не...; she would have fallen ~ that he caught her онá упáла бы, éсли бы он не удержáл её; 3) во всяком слýчае; you can ~ try во всяком слýчае вы мóжете попрóбовать.

but II *adv* тóлько; ~ just тóлько что; he was ~ a child он был ещё ребёнком; he left ~ an hour since он ушёл тóлько час томý назáд; he spoke ~ in jest он говорил тóлько в шýтку.

but III *prep* крóме, за исключéнием; anything ~ всё, что угóдно, тóлько не...; they are all wrong ~ him они все ошибáются, крóме негó; no one ~ me никтó за исключéнием, крóме меня; the last ~ one предпослéдний.

but IV *pron* кто бы, котóрый бы.

but V *n, v* только в выражении: ~ me no ~s прошý без возражéний, пожáлуйста без «но».

butcher I ['butʃə] *n* 1) мясник; 2) убийца, палáч.

butcher II *v* 1) забивáть (*скот*); 2) убивáть с бессмысленной жестóкостью; 3) искажáть (*текст*).

butchery ['butʃərı] *n* бóйня.

butler ['bʌtlə] *n* дворéцкий.

butt[1] [bʌt] *n* большáя бóчка (*вместимостью* 490,96 *л.*).

butt[2] *n* 1) тóлстый конéц чегó-л.; кóмель (*дерева*); 2) приклáд (*винтовки*); 3) *разг.* окýрок; 4) кáмбала.

butt[3] *n* 1) цель, мишéнь; 2) *pl* стрéльбище, полигóн.

butt[4] I *n* 1) удáр (*головой, рогами*); 2) *тех.* стык, тóрец.

butt[4] II *v* 1) удáрять(ся) головóй; натыкáться; 2) бодáться; 3) располагáть впритык; □ to ~ **in** *разг.* вмéшиваться.

butte [bjuːt] *n амер.* одинокая возвышенность; одинокий холм.

butt-end [ˈbʌtˈend] *n* остаток, отрезок; толстый конец.

butter [ˈbʌtə] *n* 1) масло; artificial ~ маргарин; 2) лесть.

butter II *v* 1) намазывать маслом; маслить *(еду)*; 2) льстить *(тж.* to ~ up).

buttercup [ˈbʌtəkʌp] *n* лютик.

butter-fingers [ˈbʌtəˌfiŋgəz] *n (pl без измен.)* растяпа.

butterfly [ˈbʌtəflaɪ] *n* бабочка.

buttermilk [ˈbʌtəmɪlk] *n* 1) пахтанье; 2) *амер.* кефир.

butter-nut [ˈbʌtənʌt] *n* орех серый калифорнийский.

buttocks [ˈbʌtəks] *n pl* ягодицы.

button I [ˈbʌtn] *n* 1) пуговица; 2) кнопка; to press the ~ *перен.* нажать все кнопки; пустить в ход связи; 2) бутон; ◊ he is a ~ short, he has not all his ~s он не совсем нормален, у него винтика не хватает.

button II *v* 1) пришивать пуговицы; 2) застёгивать(ся) на пуговицы *(обыкн.* to ~ up).

buttonhole I [ˈbʌtnhoul] *n* 1) петля; 2) цветок в петлице; бутоньерка.

buttonhole II *v* 1) метать петли; 2) держать за пуговицу (разговаривая); *перен.* осаждать *(вопросами).*

buttons [ˈbʌtnz] *n* мальчик-посыльный.

buttress I [ˈbʌtrɪs] *n стр.* подпора, устой, бык; опора *(тж. перен.).*

buttress II *v* поддерживать, служить опорой.

buxom [ˈbʌksəm] *a* миловидный; полный *(обыкн. о женщине).*

buy I [baɪ] *v (past, p. p.* bought) 1) купить, покупать; 2) подкупать; □ to ~ in а) закупать; б) выкупать *(на аукционе)*; to ~ off откупаться; to ~ out выкупать; to ~ over подкупать; to ~ up скупать; ◊ I'll ~ it *сленг* я не знаю, сдаюсь *(в ответ на загадку и т. п.).*

buy II *n* покупка.

buyer [ˈbaɪə] *n* покупатель.

buzz I [bʌz] *n* жужжание; гул.

buzz II *v* 1) жужжать; гудеть; 2) распространять *(слухи)*; 3) бросать, швырять; 4) проноситься *(тж.* to ~ along); □ to ~ about увиваться, надоедать; to ~ off удаляться.

by I [baɪ] *adv* 1) рядом, поблизости; he lives close by он живёт поблизости; it's near by это совсем рядом; 2) мимо; he passed by он проходил мимо; in times gone by в прошлые времена; 3) в сторону; про запас; he put the newspaper by for the moment он на некоторое время отложил газету; he is laying by money for a new radioset он откладывает деньги на новый радиоприёмник; ◊ by and by вскоре; by and large в целом, в общем.

by II *prep* 1) *в пространственном значении указывает на:* а) *местонахождение неподалёку от другого предмета* у, около; by the fireside у камина; б) *движение мимо предмета* мимо; we went by the old tower, by the gate мы прошли мимо старой башни, калитки; в) *движение через определённый пункт, место и т. п.* через; we travelled by the town N мы ехали через город N; 2) *во временном значении выражает:* а) *приближение к*

определённой точке во времени к; I shall be here by 7 o'clock я буду здесь к семи часам; б) *действие в пределах отрезка времени больше часа — переводится наречиями:* by day днём; by night ночью; 3) *указывает на средство, способ передвижения* на, по; *иногда переводится наречием:* by tram (train, rail, boat, bicycle, land, water, sea, air) на трамвае (поездом, по железной дороге, пароходом, на велосипеде, сухим путём, водным путём, морем, по воздуху); 4) *указывает на автора — переводится род. или тв. падежом:* have you read "The Young Guard" by Fadeyev? вы читали «Молодую гвардию» Фадеева?; do you like the 6th symphony by Tchaikovsky? вам нравится 6-я симфония Чайковского?; 5) *указывает на субъект действия в предложении, сказуемое которого стоит в пассивной форме — переводится тв. падежом:* Moscow was founded by Yury Dolgoroocky in 1147 Москва была основана Юрием Долгоруким в 1147 г.; 6) *указывает на характер действия — переводится наречием:* by chance (degrees) случайно (постепенно); by retail в розницу; 7) *указывает на меры веса, длины и т. п. в применении к торговле — переводится наречием:* by the pound (the yard) на фунты (ярдами); 8) *указывает на множитель или делитель* на; five by six is thirty пять, умноженное на шесть, равно тридцати; 9) *указывает на различие между сравниваемыми величинами* на; bread is cheaper now by 5 kopecks хлеб теперь подешевел на 5 копеек; ◊ by the by кстати.

by- [baɪ-] *pref со значениями:* 1) вторичный; by-product побочный продукт; 2) отдалённый, лежащий в стороне; by-road малопроезжая дорога; 3) находящийся поблизости; bystander свидетель, очевидец.

bye-bye[a] [ˈbaɪbaɪ] *n дет.* бай-бай.

bye-bye[b] [ˈbaɪˈbaɪ] *int разг. см.* good-bye[b].

bye-law [ˈbaɪlɔː] *см.* by-law.

by-election [ˈbaɪˌlekʃən] *n* дополнительные выборы.

Byelorussian I [ˌbjeləˈrʌʃən] *n* 1) белорус; белоруска; the ~s белорусы; 2) белорусский язык.

Byelorussian II *a* белорусский.

by-end [ˈbaɪend] *n* побочная *или* скрытая цель.

bygone I [ˈbaɪgɔn] *n обыкн. pl* прошлое; прошлые обиды; ◊ to let ~s be ~s *посл.* забыть прошлое; ≅ что было, то прошло.

bygone II *a* прошлый.

by-law [ˈbaɪlɔː] *n* 1) устав; 2) постановление местных властей *или* организаций.

by-name [ˈbaɪneɪm] *n* прозвище, кличка.

by-no-means [ˈbaɪnouˈmiːnz] *adv* отнюдь не; никоим образом, ни в коем случае.

bypass I [ˈbaɪpɑːs] *n* 1) обход; 2) обводный канал; 3) обходная дорога.

bypass II *v* 1) обходить *(тж. перен.)*; 2) окружать, окаймлять.

bypath [ˈbaɪpɑːθ] *n* уединённая дорога; окольный путь.

by-place [ˈbaɪpleɪs] *n* уединённое место, забытый уголок.

byplay [ˈbaɪpleɪ] *n театр.* немая сцена; эпизод.

by-product [ˈbaɪˌprɔdəkt] *n* побочный продукт.

by-road ['baɪroud] *n* малопроéзжая дорóга.

bystander ['baɪ,stændə] *n* зри́тель, свидéтель, очеви́дец.

bystreet ['baɪstriːt] *n* глухáя ýлица; боковáя ýлица.

by-way ['baɪweɪ] *n* 1) второстепéнная, малопроéзжая дорóга; просёлочная дорóга; 2) второстепéнные *или* малоизýченные óбласти (*знáния*).

by-word ['baɪwəːd] *n* 1) поговóрка; 2) олицетворéние (*обыкн. чего-л. плохóго*); «при́тча во язы́цех».

by-work ['baɪwəːk] *n* побóчная рабóта.

Byzantine I [bɪ'zæntaɪn] *n* византи́ец.

Byzantine II *a* византи́йский.

C

C, c [siː] *n* 1) 3-я бýква *англ.* алфави́та; 2) *муз.* нóта до.

cab¹ I [kæb] *n* 1) экипáж, кеб; извóзчик; такси́ (*тж.* motor-~); 2) бýдка (*на паровóзе*); 3) каби́на (*води́теля, пилóта*).

cab¹ II *v разг.* éхать на извóзчике (*тж.* to ~ it).

cab² I *n сленг* подстрóчный перевóд; шпаргáлка.

cab² II *v сленг* пóльзоваться подстрóчным перевóдом, шпаргáлкой.

cabal I [kə'bæl] *n* 1) интри́га; 2) кли́ка.

cabal II *v* интриговáть; занимáться интри́гами; составля́ть зáговор.

cabana [kə'bɑːnə] *n* 1) мáленький дóмик (*деревéнского ти́па*); 2) *амер.* купáльня.

cabaret ['kæbəreɪ] *n* кабарé.

cabbage ['kæbɪdʒ] *n* 1) капýста; 2) *attr* капýстный.

cabbage-head ['kæbɪdʒ,hed] *n* 1) кочáн (капýсты); 2) *разг.* тупи́ца.

cabby ['kæbɪ] *n разг.* извóзчик; такси́ст.

cabin ['kæbɪn] *n* 1) хи́жина; лачýга; 2) каю́та; second ~ каю́та 2-го клáсса; 3) каби́на, бýдка; pressurized (*или* sealed) ~ *ав., косм.* гермети́ческая каби́на.

cabin-boy ['kæbɪnbɔɪ] *n мор.* ю́нга.

cabinet I ['kæbɪnɪt] *n* 1) кабинéт; 2) кабинéт мини́стров, прави́тельство; inner ~ англи́йский кабинéт мини́стров в ýзком состáве; 3) шкатýлка; 4) гóрка; бюрó; 5) я́щик (*радиоприёмника*).

cabinet II *a* 1) кабинéтный; 2) прави́тельственный.

cabinet-maker ['kæbɪnɪt,meɪkə] *n* 1) столя́р-краснодерéвец; 2) *шутл.* премьéр-мини́стр (*формирýющий нóвое прави́тельство*).

cable I ['keɪbl] *n* 1) кáбель; канáт, трос; 3) телегрáмма.

cable II *v* 1) телеграфи́ровать; 2) закрепля́ть (*канáтом, трóсом*).

cablegram ['keɪblgræm] *разг. см.* cable I, 3).

cabman ['kæbmən] *n* 1) извóзчик; 2) шофёр такси́.

caboose [kə'buːs] *n* 1) *мор.* кáмбуз; 2) *амер.* служéбный вагóн в товáрном пóезде.

cabotage ['kæbətɑːʒ] *n мор.* каботáж.

cab-stand ['kæbstænd] *n* стоя́нка (*извóзчиков, такси́*).

cacao [kə'kɑːou] *n* 1) какáовое дéрево (*тж.* ~-tree); 2) какáо (*боб и напи́ток*).

cachalot ['kæʃəlɔt] *n* кашалóт.

cache [kæʃ] *n* тáйный запáс (*провиáнта и т. п.*), тайни́к; arms ~ тáйный склад орýжия.

cackle I ['kækl] *n* 1) кудáхтанье; готóтанье; 2) болтовня́, хвастовствó; 3) хихи́канье.

cackle II *v* 1) кудáхтать; готóтать; 2) болтáть; 3) хихи́кать.

cacophony [kæ'kɔfənɪ] *n* неблагозвýчие, какофóния.

cactus ['kæktəs] *n* кáктус.

cad [kæd] *n* хам.

cadastral [kə'dæstrəl] *a юр.* кадáстровый.

cadaverous [kə'dævərəs] *a* 1) трýпный; 2) блéдный как мертвéц.

caddie ['kædɪ] *n* мáльчик (*прислýживающий при игрé в гольф или тéннис*).

caddish ['kædɪʃ] *a* грýбый, вульгáрный.

caddy¹ ['kædɪ] *n* чáйница.

caddy² ['kædɪ] *n см.* caddie.

cadence ['keɪdəns] *n* 1) ритм; *муз.* кадéнция; 2) интонáция; повышéние *или* понижéние гóлоса.

cadet [kə'det] *n* 1) млáдший сын; 2) курсáнт воéнного учи́лища; кадéт.

cadge [kædʒ] *v* 1) попрошáйничать; 2) торговáть вразнóс; набивáться со свои́м товáром (*об ýличном разнóсчике*).

cadger ['kædʒə] *n* 1) попрошáйка; тунея́дец; 2) разнóсчик; ýличный торгóвец.

cadmium ['kædmɪəm] *n хим.* кáдмий.

cadre [kɑːdr] *n* 1) рáмка, óстов; схéма; 2) *воен.* кáдровый состáв.

cadres ['kɑːdəz] *n pl* кáдры, штат.

caesura [sɪ'zjuərə] *n* (*pl тж.* caesurae [sɪ'zjuəriː]) цезýра.

cafe ['kæfeɪ] *n* кафé.

cafeteria [,kæfɪ'tɪərɪə] *n* кафетéрий.

cage I [keɪdʒ] *n* 1) клéтка; *перен.* тюрьмá; 2) лифт, каби́на; 3) *горн.* клеть (*в шáхтах*).

cage II *v* сажáть в клéтку; *перен.* заключáть в тюрьмý.

Cain [keɪn] *n* Кáин; братоуби́йца; ◊ to raise ~ *амер.* шумéть, буя́нить.

caisson [kə'suːn] *n* 1) *тех.* кессóн; 2) *воен.* заря́дный я́щик.

cajole [kə'dʒoul] *v* умáслить, упроси́ть; склони́ть к чемý-л. (*into*); вы́манить (*out of, from*).

cajolement [kə'dʒoulmənt] *n* умáсливание, упрáшивание, улéщивание.

cajolery [kə'dʒoulərɪ] *см.* cajolement.

cake [keɪk] *n* 1) торт, кекс, пирóжное; лепёшка (*овся́ная*); *pl* олáдьи; 2) кусóк (*мы́ла и т. п.*); пли́тка (*табакá, прессóванного чáя и т. п.*), брусóк; 3) лепёшка гря́зи, гли́ны (*на одéжде*); ◊ ~s and ale весéлье; to go like hot ~s раскупáться нарасхвáт (*о товáре*); to take the ~ оказáться победи́телем; you cannot eat your ~ and have it too *посл.* ≅ нельзя́ сдéлать так, чтóбы и вóлки бы́ли сы́ты и óвцы цéлы.

caky ['keɪkɪ] *a* ли́пкий, клéйкий.

calabar [,kælə'bɑː] *n* сéрая бéлка (*мех*).

calabash ['kæləbæʃ] *n* 1) ты́ква-горля́нка; 2) бутýлка *или* кури́тельная трýбка (*из ты́квы-горля́нки*).

calaber ['kæləbə] *см.* calabar.

calaboose ['kæləˌbuːs] *n амер. разг.* тюрьма́.

calamitous [kə'læmɪtəs] *a* 1) па́губный; вредоно́сный; 2) бе́дственный.

calamity [kə'læmɪtɪ] *n* (стихи́йное) бе́дствие; большо́е несча́стье.

calash [kə'læʃ] *n* 1) коля́ска; 2) верх коля́ски.

calcareous [kæl'kɛərɪəs] *a* известко́вый.

calcification [ˌkælsɪfɪ'keɪʃn] *n* обызвествле́ние.

calcify ['kælsɪfaɪ] *v* обызвествля́ть(ся).

calcination [ˌkælsɪ'neɪʃn] *n тех.* прока́ливание, кальцини́рование.

calcine ['kælsaɪn] *v* 1) *тех.* прока́ливать, кальцини́ровать; 2) сжига́ть дотла́.

calcium ['kælsɪəm] *n хим.* ка́льций.

calculability [ˌkælkjulə'bɪlɪtɪ] *n* исчисли́мость, измеря́емость.

calculable ['kælkjuləbl] *a* 1) поддаю́щийся счёту, измере́нию; 2) надёжный.

calculate ['kælkjuleɪt] *v* 1) вычисля́ть; подсчи́тывать; калькули́ровать; 2) рассчи́тывать (*на что-л.— on*); 3) *амер.* предполага́ть.

calculating-machine ['kælkjuleɪtɪŋmə'ʃiːn] *n* арифмо́метр.

calculation [ˌkælkju'leɪʃn] *n* 1) расчёт; 2) вычисле́ние, калькуля́ция; 3) *амер.* предположе́ние.

calculator ['kælkjuleɪtə] *n* 1) вычисли́тель, калькуля́тор; 2) арифмо́метр, счётчик (*прибор*); 3) расчётные табли́цы.

calculus ['kælkjuləs] *n* (*pl тж.* calculi ['kælkjulaɪ]) 1) *мед.* ка́мень (*напр., в почках*); 2) *мат.* исчисле́ние; differential ~ дифференциа́льное исчисле́ние; integral ~ интегра́льное исчисле́ние.

caldron ['kɔːldrən] *см.* cauldron.

Caledonia [ˌkælɪ'dounjə] *n поэт.* Шотла́ндия, Каледо́ния.

Caledonian I [ˌkælɪ'dounjən] *n поэт.* шотла́ндец.

Caledonian II *a поэт.* шотла́ндский.

calendar I ['kælɪndə] *n* 1) календа́рь; loose-leaf (tear-off) ~ насто́льный (отрывно́й) календа́рь; 2) *амер.* пове́стка дня; 3) *юр.* спи́сок дел (*назна́ченных к слу́шанию*); 4) о́пись (*докуме́нтов, бума́г*); 5) свя́тцы.

calendar II *v* 1) заноси́ть в спи́сок, о́пись; регистри́ровать; 2) составля́ть и́ндекс.

calf[1] [kɑːf] *n* (*pl* calves) 1) телёнок; in ~, with ~ сте́льная (*о коро́ве*); 2) детёныш (*оленёнок, слонёнок и т. п.*); 3) простофи́ля, телёнок; 4) теля́чья ко́жа (*тж.* calf-skin); bound in ~ переплетённый в теля́чью ко́жу; ◊ golden ~ золото́й теле́ц.

calf[2] *n* (*pl* calves) икра́ (*ноги́*).

calf-bound ['kɑːfbaund] *a* переплетённый в теля́чью ко́жу.

calf-love ['kɑːflʌv] *n* ю́ношеское увлече́ние, де́тская любо́вь.

calf-skin ['kɑːfskɪn] *n* теля́чья ко́жа, опо́ек.

calibrate ['kælɪbreɪt] *v* калиброва́ть; градуи́ровать; выверя́ть.

calibration [ˌkælɪ'breɪʃn] *n* калиброва́ние; градуиро́вка; вы́верка.

calibre ['kælɪbə] *n* 1) кали́бр; 2) досто́инство; уде́льный вес (*челове́ка*).

calico I [ˌkælɪkou] *n* (*pl тж.* calicoes ['kælɪkouz]) 1) коленко́р; 2) *амер.* си́тец.

calico II *a* 1) коленко́ровый; 2) *амер.* си́тцевый.

Californian I [ˌkælɪ'fɔːnjən] *n* калифорни́ец.

Californian II *a* калифорни́йский.

calk[1] I [kɔːk] *n* 1) шип (*в подко́ве или башмаке́*); 2) *амер.* подко́вка (*на каблуке́*).

calk[1] II *v* 1) подко́вывать на шипа́х; 2) *амер.* набива́ть подко́вки (*на каблуки́*).

calk[2] *v* кальки́ровать.

call I [kɔːl] *n* 1) крик; вы́крик; о́клик; зов; a ~ for help крик о по́мощи; within ~ поблизости, неподалёку; the ~ of the cuckoo крик куку́шки; the ~ of the nightingale пе́ние соловья́; 2) призы́в, зов; 3) вы́зов (*в суд и т. п.*); 4) сигна́л; свисто́к; 5) вы́зов, звоно́к (*по телефо́ну*); long-distance ~ междугоро́дный телефо́нный разгово́р; 6) визи́т, посеще́ние; to pay a ~ сде́лать визи́т; morning ~ у́тренний визи́т; 7) захо́д (*парохо́да в порт*); остано́вка (*по́езда на ста́нции*); 8) тре́бование (*упла́ты де́нег*); 9) нужда́, необходи́мость; there's no ~ to worry нет основа́ний трево́житься.

call II *v* 1) (по)зва́ть; оклика́ть; 2) называ́ть(ся); 3) созыва́ть; 4) вызыва́ть, выклика́ть; 5) заходи́ть (*за кем-л.— for; в учрежде́ние, порт и т. п.— at, к знако́мым и т. п.— on*); навеща́ть (*кого́-л.— on*); приходи́ть в го́сти (*к кому́-л.— on*); быть в гостя́х; 6) призыва́ть (*кого́-л.— on*), апелли́ровать (*к кому́-л.— on*); 7) (раз)буди́ть; 8) счита́ть; 9) радирова́ть, посыла́ть позывны́е (*по ра́дио*); ☐ to ~ **away** отзыва́ть; to ~ **back** a) звать обра́тно; б) брать наза́д (*слова́ и т. п.*); to ~ **down** a) крича́ть (*стоя́щему внизу́*); б) призыва́ть (*прокля́тия и т. п.*); упрека́ть; в) руга́ть; обзыва́ть; to ~ **for** a) тре́бовать; б) предусма́тривать; зака́зывать; to be ~ed for до востре́бования; to ~ **forth** вызыва́ть, возбужда́ть; to ~ **in** a) вызыва́ть (*врача́*); б) тре́бовать возвраще́ния (*до́лга*); в) изъя́ть из обраще́ния (*де́ньги*); to ~ **off** a) отменя́ть (*собра́ние и т. п.*); to be ~ed off не состоя́ться; б) отзыва́ть (*посла́*); в) отвлека́ть (*внима́ние*); to ~ **out** a) закрича́ть, кри́кнуть; гро́мко окли́кнуть (*of*); б) выкри́кивать; в) вызыва́ть (*на дуэ́ль*); г) производи́ть набо́р (*в а́рмию*); to ~ **over** вызыва́ть по спи́ску; де́лать перекли́чку; to ~ **up** a) призыва́ть (*в а́рмию*); б) (по)звони́ть по телефо́ну; в) вы́полнить; г) вызыва́ть *или* воскреша́ть в па́мяти; д) (по)зва́ть наве́рх.

call-boy ['kɔːlbɔɪ] *n* 1) ма́льчик-коридо́рный (*в гости́нице, на парохо́де*); 2) *театр.* помо́щник режиссёра.

call-down ['kɔːl'daun] *n амер.* нагоня́й.

caller ['kɔːlə] *n* посети́тель, визитёр.

calling ['kɔːlɪŋ] *n* 1) призва́ние; 2) профе́ссия.

callipers ['kælɪpəz] *n pl* кронци́ркуль.

call-loan ['kɔːlloun] *n ком.* заём с вы́платой до́лга по пе́рвому тре́бованию.

callosity [kæ'lɔsɪtɪ] *n* 1) затверде́ние; мозо́ль; 2) гру́бость (*чувств*).

callous ['kæləs] *a* 1) огрубе́лый, мозо́листый; 2) бессерде́чный, чёрствый.

call-over ['kɔːlˌouvə] *n* перекли́чка.

callow ['kælou] *a* 1) неопери́вшийся; 2) нео́пытный (*о челове́ке*); 3) *ирл.* заливно́й (*о лу́ге*).

call-up [ˈkɔːlˈʌp] *n* призы́в (на вое́нную слу́жбу).

callus [ˈkæləs] *n* мозо́ль; затвердѐние.

calm I [kɑːm] *n* 1) споко́йствие; тишина́; 2) зати́шье; 3) штиль, безвѐтрие; 4) *разг.* дѐрзость.

calm II *a* 1) споко́йный; ти́хий; ми́рный; 2) безвѐтренный; 3) *разг.* наха́льный, на́глый.

calm III *v* успока́ивать; умиротворя́ть; ▢ to ~ **down** успока́ивать(ся); улѐчься; сти́хнуть.

caloric I [kəˈlɔrɪk] *n* теплота́.

caloric II *a* теплово́й.

calorie [ˈkælərɪ] *n физ.* кало́рия.

calorimeter [ˌkæləˈrɪmɪtə] *n физ.* калори́метр.

calumet [ˈkæljumet] *n* тру́бка ми́ра (*у инде́йцев*).

calumniate [kəˈlʌmnɪeɪt] *v* клевета́ть, поро́чить.

calumniator [kəˈlʌmnɪeɪtə] *n* клеветни́к.

calumniatory [kəˈlʌmnɪeɪtərɪ] *a* клеветни́ческий.

calumny [ˈkæləmnɪ] *n* клевета́.

calve [kɑːv] *v* 1) (о)тели́ться (*тж. о слона́х, кита́х и т. п.*); 2) отрыва́ться от ледников́ (*об айсбергах*).

calves [kɑːvz] *pl см.* calf.

calvish [ˈkɑːvɪʃ] *a* 1) теля́чий; 2) глу́пый.

calx [kælks] *n* 1) ока́лина; 2) зола́; 3) и́звесть.

calyx [ˈkeɪlɪks] *n* (*pl тж.* calyces [ˈkeɪlɪsiːz]) *бот.* ча́шечка.

cam [kæm] *n тех.* па́лец, кула́к, эксцѐнтрик.

Cambria [ˈkæmbrɪə] *n поэт.* Уэ́льс.

Cambrian I [ˈkæmbrɪən] *n* уроже́нец, жи́тель Уэ́льса.

Cambrian II *a* уэ́льский.

cambric [ˈkeɪmbrɪk] *n* бати́ст.

came [keɪm] *past см.* come.

camel [ˈkæməl] *n* верблю́д; Arabian ~ одного́рбый верблю́д; Bactrian ~ двуго́рбый верблю́д.

cameleer [ˌkæmɪˈlɪə] *n* пого́нщик верблю́дов.

camellia [kəˈmiːljə] *n* каме́лия.

cameo [ˈkæmɪou] *n* каме́я.

camera [ˈkæmərə] *n* 1) фотоаппара́т; 2) *стр.* сво́дчатое покры́тие *или* помеще́ние; 3) *юр.* кабине́т судьи́.

camera-man [ˈkæmərəmæn] *n* фоторепортёр; кинооперáтор.

cami-knickers [ˈkæmɪˌnɪkəz] *n pl* да́мская комбина́ция (*с панталонами*).

camion [ˌkæmɪˈjɔːŋ] *n* грузови́к; подво́да.

camomile [ˈkæməmaɪl] *n* рома́шка.

camouflage I [ˈkæmuflɑːʒ] *n* маскиро́вка, камуфля́ж.

camouflage II *v* маскирова́ть; применя́ть маскиро́вку.

camp I [kæmp] *n* 1) ла́герь; internment ~ ла́герь для интерни́рованных *или* военнопле́нных; pioneer ~ пионе́рский ла́герь; summer ~ ле́тний ла́герь; prison ~ ла́герь для заключённых; inter-racial ~ ла́герь, где прово́дят ле́тние кани́кулы бе́лые и не́гры; 2) бива́к; стоя́нка; 3) *амер.* до́мик (*в лесу*).

camp II *v* 1) располага́ться ла́герем; 2) жить по-бива́чному; to go ~ing выезжа́ть на све́жий во́здух, проводи́ть о́тпуск на све́жем во́здухе (*в палатке*); ▢ to ~ **out** жить в пала́тках *или* на откры́том во́здухе.

campaign I [kæmˈpeɪn] *n* кампа́ния (*тж. поли-*

тическая); похо́д; press ~ кампа́ния в печа́ти; to launch a ~ нача́ть кампа́нию (*в печати и т. п.*).

campaign II *v* уча́ствовать в кампа́нии, похо́де.

camp-bed [ˈkæmpˈbed] *n* похо́дная *или* складна́я крова́ть.

camp-chair [ˈkæmpˈtʃɛə] *n* складно́й стул.

camp-fever [ˈkæmpˌfiːvə] *n* сыпно́й тиф.

camp-fire [ˈkæmpˌfaɪə] *n* ла́герный костёр.

camp-follower [ˈkæmpˌfɔlouə] *n* гражда́нское лицо́, сопровожда́ющее во́инскую часть.

camphor [ˈkæmfə] *n* 1) камфара́; 2) *attr* камфа́рный.

camp-stool [ˈkæmpstuːl] *n см.* camp-chair.

campus [ˈkæmpəs] *n амер.* террито́рия университе́та, колле́джа *и т. п.* (*включая парк, цветники и т. п.*); университе́тский двор.

cam-shaft [ˈkæmʃɑːft] *n тех.* распределительный вал.

can[1] [kæn (*сильная форма*), kən, kn (*слабые формы*)] *v* (*past* could) модáльный глаго́л, входя́щий в соста́в сло́жного модáльного сказу́емого мочь; уме́ть; *последующий смыслово́й глаго́л употребля́ется без части́цы* to: I ~ speak English я уме́ю говори́ть по-англи́йски; *отрица́тельные и вопроси́тельные фо́рмы употребля́ются без глаго́ла* to do: ~ you translate this article? мо́жете ли вы перевести́ э́ту статью́?; No, I cannot (*разг.* can't) нет, я не могу́; I can't help it я не могу́ ничего́ поде́лать.

can[2] **I** [kæn] *n* 1) бидо́н; 2) жестяна́я коро́бка *или* ба́нка (*для консерви́рования*); ба́нка консе́рвов; garbage ~ а) я́щик для му́сора; б) *сленг* жилье́ в рабо́чем посёлке.

can[2] **II** *v* консерви́ровать (*проду́кты*).

Canadian I [kəˈneɪdjən] *n* кана́дец; кана́дка; the ~s кана́дцы.

Canadian II *a* кана́дский.

canal [kəˈnæl] *n* 1) (ороси́тельный) кана́л; 2) *анат.* прото́к, прохо́д; alimentary ~ пищевари́тельный кана́л, тракт.

canalization [ˌkænəlaɪˈzeɪʃən] *n* 1) канализа́ция; 2) проведе́ние кана́лов.

canal-lock [kəˈnællɔk] *n* шлюз.

canard [kæˈnɑːd] *n* ло́жный слух, «у́тка».

canary I [kəˈnɛərɪ] *n* канаре́йка.

canary II *a* све́тло-жёлтый, канаре́ечного цве́та.

cancel [ˈkænsəl] *v* 1) отменя́ть, аннули́ровать; 2) вычёркивать; 3) погаша́ть (*марки*); 4) *мат.* сокраща́ть (*тж.* to ~ out).

cancellation [ˌkænsəˈleɪʃən] *n* 1) отме́на; аннули́рование; 2) вычёркивание; 3) погаше́ние (*марки*); 4) *мат.* сокраще́ние.

cancer [ˈkænsə] *n* 1) *мед.* рак; 2) зло, бе́дствие; 3) (C.) созве́здие Ра́ка.

cancroid I [ˈkæŋkrɔɪd] *n мед.* ракообра́зная о́пухоль.

cancroid II *a зоол., мед.* ракообра́зный.

candid [ˈkændɪd] *a* 1) и́скренний; прямо́й (*ответ и т. п.*); чистосерде́чный; 2) беспристра́стный.

candidacy [ˈkændɪdəsɪ] *n* кандидату́ра; to nominate (to withdraw) a ~ предложи́ть (снять) кандидату́ру.

candidate [ˈkændɪdɪt] *n* кандида́т; presidential ~, ~ for the presidency кандида́т на пост президе́нта; to challenge (*или* to execute) ~s отводи́ть кандида́тов.

candidature ['kændɪdɪtʃə] *n* кандидату́ра; to put up ~s выставля́ть кандида́тов (*на вы́борах*).

candied ['kændɪd] *a* 1) заса́харенный, в са́харе; 2) заса́харившийся; 3) *уст.* льсти́вый.

candle ['kændl] *n* свеча́, све́чка; ◊ to burn the ~ at both ends *погов.* жечь свечу́ с двух концо́в; прожига́ть жизнь; is not fit to hold a ~ to *погов.* ≅ в подмётки не годи́тся.

candle-end ['kændlend] *n* ога́рок.

candlelight ['kændllaɪt] *n* 1) свет свечи́; 2) иску́сственное освеще́ние; 3) су́мерки.

candlestick ['kændlstɪk] *n* подсве́чник.

candour ['kændə] *n* 1) и́скренность; прямота́; чистосерде́чие; 2) беспристра́стность.

candy I ['kændɪ] *n* 1) ледене́ц; 2) *pl амер.* конфе́ты; сла́дости.

candy II *v* 1) вари́ть в са́харе; 2) заса́харивать(ся).

cane I [keɪn] *n* 1) камы́ш, тростни́к; 2) тросто́чка; трость; па́лка; 3) са́харный тростни́к; 4) па́лочка (*сургуча́ и т. п.*).

cane II *v* 1) бить тро́стью, па́лкой; 2) вда́лбливать уро́к (*обыкн.* to ~ into); 3) плести́ из тростника́.

canful ['kænful] *n* бидо́н (*объём жи́дкости, ра́вный бидо́ну*).

canicular [kə'nɪkjulə] *a:* ~ days зно́йные дни (*коне́ц ию́ля — нача́ло а́вгуста*).

canine ['keɪnaɪn] *a* соба́чий.

canister ['kænɪstə] *n* 1) металли́ческая ча́йница; 2) коро́бка противога́за.

canker ['kæŋkə] *n* 1) я́зва; червото́чина; 2) *с.-х.* вреди́тель; 3) боле́знь плодо́вых дере́вьев.

cankered ['kæŋkəd] *a* разъеда́емый я́звой.

cankerous ['kæŋkərəs] *a* 1) поражённый я́звой; 2) разъеда́ющий.

canned [kænd] *a* консерви́рованный.

cannery ['kænərɪ] *n* консе́рвный заво́д.

cannibal ['kænɪbəl] *n* людое́д.

cannibalism ['kænɪbəlɪzəm] *n* людое́дство.

cannon ['kænən] *n* (*pl без изме́н.*) ору́дие; пу́шка.

cannonade I [ˌkænə'neɪd] *n* канона́да; оруди́йный ого́нь.

cannonade II *v* обстре́ливать оруди́йным огнём.

cannon-ball ['kænənbɔ:l] *n* 1) *уст.* пу́шечное ядро́; 2) *амер.* по́езд-экспре́сс.

cannon-bit ['kænənbɪt] *n* мундшту́к (*удила́*).

cannoneer [ˌkænə'nɪə] *n* канони́р, артиллери́ст.

cannon-shot ['kænənʃɔt] *n* пу́шечный вы́стрел.

cannot ['kænɔt]: I ~ я не могу́ (*см.* can¹).

canny ['kænɪ] *a* 1) ло́вкий, хи́трый; себе́ на уме́; 2) осторо́жный.

canoe I [kə'nu:] *n* челно́к; байда́рка (*тж.* Indian ~); ◊ to paddle one's own ~ де́йствовать самостоя́тельно.

canoe II *v* плыть в челноке́, на байда́рке.

canon ['kænən] *n* 1) пра́вило, крите́рий; 2) *церк.* кано́н.

cañon ['kænjən] *см.* canyon.

canonical [kə'nɔnɪkəl] *a* канони́ческий.

canoodle [kə'nu:dl] *v амер. сленг* ласка́ть, не́жить.

canopy ['kænəpɪ] *n* балдахи́н; наве́с; по́лог;

the ~ of heaven *поэт.* не́бо, небеса́; the ~ of leaves *поэт.* сень дере́вьев.

can't [kɑ:nt] *разг.* = cannot.

cant¹ I [kænt] *n* 1) кося́к; 2) накло́н; накло́нное положе́ние; 3) отклоне́ние от прямо́й; 4) *амер.* обтёсанное бревно́, брус; 5) толчо́к, уда́р.

cant¹ II *v* 1) отклоня́ться от прямо́й; 2) принима́ть, придава́ть накло́нное положе́ние; наклоня́ть; 3) перевёртывать.

cant² I *n* 1) жарго́н (*воровско́й и т. п.*); 2) ходя́чее словцо́; 3) лицеме́рие, ха́нжество.

cant² II *v* 1) говори́ть на жарго́не; 2) говори́ть лицеме́рно; 3) спле́тничать; руга́ть.

Cantabrigian [ˌkæntə'brɪdʒɪən] *n* студе́нт (*тж.* бы́вший) Ке́мбриджского университе́та.

cantankerous [kən'tæŋkərəs] *a* сварли́вый; вздо́рный.

cantata [kæn'tɑ:tə] *n* канта́та.

canteen [kæn'ti:n] *n* 1) продукто́вый магази́н (*в во́инской ча́сти*); 2) фля́га; 3) похо́дный я́щик со столо́выми принадле́жностями; 4) буфе́т; столо́вая.

canter¹ I ['kæntə] *n* лёгкий гало́п; ◊ to win at (*или* in) а ~ легко́ дости́гнуть побе́ды; вы́играть с лёгкостью.

canter¹ II *v* идти́ *или* пусти́ть ло́шадь лёгким гало́пом.

canter² *n* 1) говоря́щий на жарго́не; 2) лицеме́р, ханжа́.

Canterbury ['kæntəbərɪ] *a:* ~ bell *бот.* колоко́льчик сре́дний; ~ tales Кентербери́йские расска́зы Чо́сера.

canterbury ['kæntəbərɪ] *n* шка́фчик, этаже́рка (*с отделе́ниями для нот, бума́г и т. п.*).

canticle ['kæntɪkl] *n рел.* песнь, гимн.

cantilever ['kæntɪli:və] *n стр.* консо́ль (*моста́*), кронште́йн.

canting ['kæntɪŋ] *a* лицеме́рный, неи́скренний; ха́нжеский.

canto ['kæntou] *n* песнь (*часть поэ́мы*).

cantonᵃ ['kæntɔn] *n* канто́н; о́круг.

cantonᵇ [kən'tu:n] *v* расквартиро́вывать (*войска́*).

cantonmentᵃ [kən'tu:nmənt] *n* 1) *воен.* бара́ки; winter ~ зи́мние кварти́ры; 2) вое́нное поселе́ние (*в Индии*).

cantonmentᵇ [kæn'tɔnmənt] *n амер.* постоя́нный ла́герь.

Canuck [kə'nʌk] *n сленг* 1) кана́дец францу́зского происхожде́ния; 2) *амер.* кана́дец.

canvas ['kænvəs] *n* 1) холст, паруси́на; брезе́нт; 2) канва́; 3) карти́на, полотно́; 4) паруса́; ◊ under ~ а) в пала́тках; б) под паруса́ми.

canvass I ['kænvəs] *n* 1) собира́ние голосо́в (*пе́ред вы́борами*); предвы́борная агита́ция; 2) обсужде́ние, дебати́рование; 3) *амер.* официа́льный подсчёт голосо́в.

canvass II *v* 1) собира́ть голоса́ (*пе́ред вы́борами*); быть агита́тором; 2) обсужда́ть; дебати́ровать; 3) домога́ться зака́зов; собира́ть подпи́ску (*на изда́ния*).

canyon ['kænjən] *n* уще́лье, кань́он.

caoutchouc ['kautʃuk] *n* каучу́к.

cap I [kæp] *n* 1) ке́пка; ша́пка; фура́жка; fore-and-aft ~ пило́тка; 2) че́пец; 3) шля́пка (*гриба́*); 4) верху́шка, кры́шка; 5) *тех.* колпачо́к; голо́вка; 6) писто́н, ка́псюль (*тж.* percussion ~); 7) коленная ча́шка; ◊ ~ and bells шутовско́й колпа́к; ~ and gown бере́т и плащ (форма англ. студентов и профессоров); the ~ fits погов. ≅ не в бровь, а в глаз; to set one's ~ at smb. завлека́ть кого́-л., стара́ться жени́ть кого́-л. на себе́.

cap II v 1) надева́ть (кепку, шапку); 2) наса́живать (колпачок); вставля́ть (капсюль); 3) присужда́ть учёную сте́пень (в шотл. университете); 4) перещеголя́ть; превзойти́.

capability [ˌkeɪpəˈbɪlɪtɪ] n 1) спосо́бность; 2) pl возмо́жности.

capable [ˈkeɪpəbl] a 1) спосо́бный (на что-л. — of); ода́рённый; 2) поддаю́щийся; восприи́мчивый (of).

capacious [kəˈpeɪʃəs] a просто́рный, вмести́тельный.

capacitor [kəˈpæsɪtə] n радио конденса́тор.

capacity [kəˈpæsɪtɪ] n 1) спосо́бность; ода́рённость; 2) ёмкость, вмести́мость (тж. holding ~); 3): in the ~ of в ка́честве; 4) компете́нция; 5) тех. мо́щность, производи́тельность; idle ~ резе́рвная мо́щность; labour ~ производи́тельность труда́.

cap-à-pie [ˌkæpəˈpiː] adv с головы́ до ног; armed ~ вооружённый до зубо́в.

cape¹ I [keɪp] n мыс.

cape¹ II a южноафрика́нский.

cape² I n плащ; наки́дка.

caper I [ˈkeɪpə] n 1) прыжо́к; 2) обыкн. pl проде́лки; to cut ~s выде́лывать антраша́, дура́читься.

caper II v 1) пры́гать; 2) дура́читься, шали́ть.

capful [ˈkæpful] n по́лная ша́пка (чего-л.).

capillarity [ˌkæpɪˈlærɪtɪ] n капилля́рность.

capillary I [kəˈpɪlərɪ] n капилля́р.

capillary II a капилля́рный; то́нкий (как волос).

capital¹ [ˈkæpɪtl] n капита́л; fixed ~ основно́й капита́л; floating ~, circulating ~ оборо́тный капита́л; industrial ~ промы́шленный капита́л.

capital² I (n 1) столи́ца; 2) прописна́я, загла́вная, больша́я бу́ква; in ~s загла́вными бу́квами.

capital² II a 1) капита́льный; основно́й; 2) гла́вный; 3) разг. превосхо́дный; 4) загла́вный (о букве); 5) юр. уголо́вный (о преступлении); 6) сме́ртный (о приговоре, казни).

capital³ n архит. капите́ль.

capitalism [ˈkæpɪtəlɪzəm] n капитали́зм.

capitalist I [ˈkæpɪtəlɪst] n капитали́ст.

capitalist II a капиталисти́ческий.

capitalistic [ˌkæpɪtəˈlɪstɪk] a капиталисти́ческий.

capitalize [ˈkæpɪtəlaɪz] v капитализи́ровать, превраща́ть в капита́л.

capitally [ˈkæpɪtlɪ] adv 1) превосхо́дно, замеча́тельно; 2) чрезвыча́йно; основа́тельно.

capitation [ˌkæpɪˈteɪʃən] n 1) обложе́ние нало́гом «с головы́»; 2) attr поду́шный (о налоге).

Capitol [ˈkæpɪtl] n 1) Капито́лий (в дре́внем Ри́ме); 2) зда́ние конгре́сса США; 3) амер. зда́ние, в кото́ром помеща́ются о́рганы госуда́рственной вла́сти шта́та.

capitulate [kəˈpɪtjuleɪt] v сдава́ться, капитули́ровать.

capitulation [kəˌpɪtjuˈleɪʃən] n сда́ча, капитуля́ция.

cap-paper [ˈkæpˌpeɪpə] n обёрточная бума́га.

cap-peak [ˈkæpiːk] n козырёк фура́жки.

caprice [kəˈpriːs] n капри́з, причу́да.

capricious [kəˈprɪʃəs] a капри́зный; непостоя́нный.

Capricorn [ˈkæprɪkɔːn] n Козеро́г (созвездие).

capsize [kæpˈsaɪz] v опроки́дывать(ся) (о корабле, лодке, телеге и т. п.).

capsule [ˈkæpsjuːl] n 1) ка́псюль; 2) мембра́на.

captain I [ˈkæptɪn] n 1) капита́н; sea ~ флотово́дец; поэт. вели́кий морепла́ватель; 2) капита́н спорти́вной кома́нды; 3) амер. команди́р ро́ты, эскадро́на, батаре́и; 4) полково́дец; 5) руководи́тель; 6) нача́льник пожа́рной кома́нды; 7) мор. капита́н I ра́нга.

captain II v руководи́ть (чем-л.).

caption [ˈkæpʃən] n 1) загла́вие; заголо́вок (статьи, главы); 2) кино титр, на́дпись на экра́не; 3) юр. аре́ст.

captious [ˈkæpʃəs] a приди́рчивый.

captivate [ˈkæptɪveɪt] v пленя́ть, очаро́вывать; увлека́ть.

captivating [ˈkæptɪveɪtɪŋ] a увлека́тельный; чару́ющий.

captive I [ˈkæptɪv] n пле́нник, пле́нный; заключённый.

captive II a взя́тый в плен; to hold ~ держа́ть в плену́.

captivity [kæpˈtɪvɪtɪ] n плен.

captor [ˈkæptə] n захва́тывающий в плен.

capture I [ˈkæptʃə] n 1) захва́т; плене́ние; пои́мка; 2) добы́ча, трофе́й.

capture II v 1) захвати́ть, взять (город); 2) пойма́ть; взять в плен; 3) захвати́ть, увле́чь.

car [kɑː] n 1) ваго́н (трамвая, амер. тж. железнодоро́жный); coach ~ пассажи́рский ваго́н; lounge ~, soft-seated ~ мя́гкий ваго́н; platform ~ амер. ж.-д. платфо́рма (вагон); sleeping ~ см. sleeping-car; smoking ~ амер. ваго́н для куря́щих; observation ~ ваго́н с больши́ми о́кнами; parlor ~ амер. сало́н-ваго́н; through ~ ваго́н прямо́го сообще́ния; 2) автомоби́ль; goods ~ грузови́к, грузово́й автомоби́ль; ambulance ~ маши́на ско́рой по́мощи; armoured ~ бронемаши́на; bubble ~ ма́ленький автомоби́ль; pleasure ~ автомоби́ль для экску́рсий, прогу́лок; to come by ~ прие́хать на (авто)маши́не; to get into a ~ сади́ться в (авто)маши́ну; to get out of a ~ выходи́ть из (авто)маши́ны; 3) гондо́ла дирижа́бля; 4) амер. каби́на ли́фта; 5) поэт. колесни́ца, экипа́ж.

carafe [kəˈrɑːf] n графи́н.

caramel [ˈkærəmel] n 1) караме́ль; 2) жжёный са́хар.

carat [ˈkærət] n кара́т (единица веса драгоценных камней = 0,2053 г.)

caravan [ˌkærəˈvæn] n 1) карава́н; 2) киби́тка, фурго́н.

caraway [ˈkærəweɪ] n тмин.

carbide [ˈkɑːbaɪd] n хим. карби́д.

carbine [ˈkɑːbaɪn] n караби́н.

carbo-hydrate [ˈkɑːbouˈhaɪdreɪt] n хим. углево́д.

carbolic I [kɑːˈbɒlɪk] n карбо́ловая кислота́ (тж. ~ acid).

carbolic II a карбо́ловый.

carbon [ˈkɑːbən] n 1) хим. углеро́д; 2) эл. у́гольный электро́д; 3) хими́чески чи́стый у́голь; absorbent ~ активи́рованный у́голь; 4) attr у́гольный.

carbonate [ˈkɑːbənɪt] n хим. карбона́т.

carbonic [kɑːˈbɔnɪk] a хим. у́гольный, углеро́дный; углеро́дистый.

carbonite [ˈkɑːbənaɪt] n 1) кокс; 2) карбони́т (взрывчатка).

carbonize [ˈkɑːbənaɪz] v обу́гливать; карбонизи́ровать; обжига́ть; коксова́ть.

carbon-paper [ˈkɑːbənˌpeɪpə] n копирова́льная бума́га.

carbuncle [ˈkɑːbʌŋkl] n мед., мин. карбу́нкул.

carburettor [ˈkɑːbjuretə] n карбюра́тор.

carcass [ˈkɑːkəs] n 1) пренебр. труп, те́ло; 2) ту́ша; 3) карка́с, о́стов; 4) разва́лины, обло́мки; 5) воен. ист. зажига́тельный снаря́д.

card [kɑːd] n 1) ка́рта (игра́льная); plain ~ нефигу́рная ка́рта; to shuffle the ~s тасова́ть ка́рты; 2) pl ка́рты; игра́ в ка́рты; 3) ка́рточка; откры́тка; birthday ~ поздрави́тельная ка́рточка (с днём рожде́ния); calling ~, visiting ~ визи́тная ка́рточка; coach ~ поса́дочный тало́н (на авто́бус); food ~ продово́льственная ка́рточка; New Year ~ нового́дняя поздрави́тельная откры́тка; 4) биле́т (чле́нский, пригласи́тельный); Party ~ парти́йный биле́т; ~ of admission про́пуск; 5) карту́шка (ко́мпаса); 6) разг. челове́к; «тип»; a queer ~ чуда́к; 7) амер. объявле́ние в газе́те, публика́ция; ◊ one's best ~ са́мый гла́вный аргуме́нт; to have a ~ up one's sleeve име́ть ко́зырь про запа́с; замы́слить что-л.; to play one's ~s well (badly) хорошо́ (пло́хо) испо́льзовать обстоя́тельства; to put one's ~s on the table, to show one's ~s раскры́ть свои́ ка́рты, пла́ны; to throw up one's ~s (с)пасова́ть; при́знать возмо́жно, вероя́тно.

cardan [kɑːˈdæn] n тех. карда́н.

cardboard [ˈkɑːdbɔːd] n карто́н.

carder [ˈkɑːdə] n текст. 1) ка́рдная маши́на; 2) чеса́льщик, -ица; ворси́льщик, -ица.

cardiac I [ˈkɑːdɪæk] n сре́дство, возбужда́ющее серде́чную де́ятельность.

cardiac II a анат. серде́чный.

cardigan [ˈkɑːdɪɡən] n шерстяно́й дже́мпер.

cardinal I [ˈkɑːdɪnl] n кардина́л.

cardinal II a 1) основно́й, гла́вный, кардина́льный; 2) я́рко-кра́сный, пунцо́вый.

care I [kɛə] n 1) забо́та, попече́ние; in ~ of smb., in smb.'s ~ на чьём-л. попече́нии; c/o (чита́ется care of) для переда́чи (на пи́сьмах); under the ~ of под присмо́тром, под наблюде́нием (кого́-л.); возглавля́ется (кем-л.); to take ~ а) забо́титься (о — of, about); б) взять на воспита́ние (кого́-л.— of); в) смотре́ть (за кем-л.— for); take ~! осторо́жно!, береги́тесь!; 2) наблюде́ние (врача́); the best of ~ идеа́льный ухо́д; 3) внима́ние, тща́тельность.

care II v 1) забо́титься, проявля́ть забо́ту (о — about); уха́живать (за детьми́, больны́ми); 2) интересова́ться (чем-л.— for); люби́ть (кого́-л.— for); 3) име́ть жела́ние, хоте́ть (с после́дующим гл. в Inf); ◊ I don't ~! мне всё равно́!

career I [kəˈrɪə] n 1) заня́тие, профе́ссия; 2) амер. профе́ссия диплома́та; 3) карье́ра, успе́х; 4) карье́р; in full ~ во весь опо́р.

career II v мча́ться (тж. to ~ about, along, over, through).

careerist [kəˈrɪərɪst] n карьери́ст.

careful [ˈkɛəful] a 1) забо́тливый (for, of); 2) стара́тельный; тща́тельный; аккура́тный; 3) вни-

ма́тельный; 4) то́чный (о подсчёте и т. п.); 5) осторо́жный.

carefully [ˈkɛəfulɪ] adv осторо́жно, с большо́й осторо́жностью.

carefulness [ˈkɛəfulnɪs] n 1) забо́тливость; 2) стара́тельность; тща́тельность; аккура́тность; 3) внима́тельность; 4) осторо́жность.

care-laden [ˈkɛəleɪdn] a обременённый забо́тами.

careless [ˈkɛəlɪs] a 1) беззабо́тный; беспе́чный; 2) легкомы́сленный; 3) невнима́тельный; 4) неаккура́тный.

carelessness [ˈkɛəlɪsnɪs] n 1) беззабо́тность; 2) легкомы́слие; a piece of ~ легкомы́сленный посту́пок; 3) невнима́тельность; 4) неаккура́тность.

caress I [kəˈres] n ла́ска.

caress II v ласка́ть.

caressing [kəˈresɪŋ] n ла́сковый, láска́ющий.

care-taker [ˈkɛəˌteɪkə] n 1) сто́рож (в до́ме, кварти́ре и т. п.); 2) храни́тель, смотри́тель (зда́ния).

care-worn [ˈkɛəwɔːn] a изму́ченный забо́тами.

cargo [ˈkɑːɡou] n груз корабля́.

cariboo [ˈkærɪbuː] см. caribou.

caribou [ˈkærɪbuː] n кана́дский оле́нь.

caricature I [ˌkærɪkəˈtʃuə] n карикату́ра.

caricature II v изобража́ть в карикату́рном ви́де.

carious [ˈkɛərɪəs] a гнило́й, карио́зный.

carload [ˈkɑːloud] n ваго́н (как ме́ра груза).

carman [ˈkɑːmən] n 1) во́зчик; 2) вагоновожа́тый.

Carmelite [ˈkɑːmɪlaɪt] n кармели́т (монах).

carmine [ˈkɑːmaɪn] n карми́н.

carnage [ˈkɑːnɪdʒ] n избие́ние, резня́.

carnal [ˈkɑːnl] a 1) теле́сный, пло́тский; 2) чу́вственный.

carnation [kɑːˈneɪʃən] n 1) кра́сная гвозди́ка; 2) кра́сный, а́лый цвет.

carnival [ˈkɑːnɪvəl] n 1) карнава́л; 2) бу́рное весе́лье; 3) ма́сленица.

carnivore [ˈkɑːnɪvɔː] n плотоя́дное живо́тное.

carnivorous [kɑːˈnɪvərəs] a плотоя́дный.

carol I [ˈkærəl] n 1) весёлая песнь (особ. рожде́ственский гимн); 2) ра́достное щебета́ние (птиц).

carol II v воспева́ть, сла́вить.

carotid [kəˈrɔtɪd] n анат. со́нная арте́рия.

carousal [kəˈrauzəl] n 1) кутёж; попо́йка; 2) амер. карусе́ль.

carp[1] [kɑːp] n карп; саза́н.

carp[2] v придира́ться (at); находи́ть недоста́тки.

carpenter I [ˈkɑːpɪntə] n пло́тник.

carpenter II v пло́тничать.

carpentry [ˈkɑːpɪntrɪ] n пло́тничное де́ло; пло́тничные рабо́ты.

carpet I [ˈkɑːpɪt] n ковёр (тж. травы́, цвето́в); runner ~ ковро́вая доро́жка; ◊ on the ~ на обсужде́нии (о вопро́се); to have smb. on the ~ сде́лать вы́говор кому́-л.

carpet II v 1) устила́ть ковра́ми, цвета́ми; 2) вызыва́ть для вы́говора, замеча́ния.

carpet-bag [ˈkɑːpɪtbæɡ] n саквоя́ж.

carpet-bagger [ˈkɑːpɪtˌbæɡə] n 1) полити́ческий де́ятель, живу́щий вне своего́ избира́тельного о́круга; 2) разг. полити́ческий авантюри́ст; 3) амер. сленг северя́нин, доби́вшийся влия́ния и бога́тства на ю́ге (в эпо́ху гражда́нской войны́ 1861—1865 гг.).

carpet-knight [ˈkɑːpɪtnaɪt] n 1) солда́т, отси́живающийся в тылу́; 2) сало́нный шарку́н.

carpet-sweeper ['kɑːpɪt,swiːpə] *n* пылесо́с.

carriage ['kærɪdʒ] *n* 1) экипа́ж; ~ and pair (four) экипа́ж, запряжённый па́рой (четвёркой); 2) *ж.-д.* ваго́н; composite ~ комбини́рованный ваго́н; corridor ~ пу́льмановский ваго́н; the first--class ~ ваго́н пе́рвого кла́сса; saloon ~ сало́н--ваго́н; 3) перево́зка; сто́имость перево́зки; 4) мане́ра держа́ть себя́; оса́нка; 5) *тех.* каре́тка; ра́ма; 6) *воен.* лафе́т, стано́к (*орудия*); 7) *ав.* шасси́; 8) выполне́ние; проведе́ние (*законопроекта в парламенте*).

carriage-free ['kærɪdʒ'friː] *n* пересы́лка беспла́тно.

carrier ['kærɪə] *n* 1) во́зчик; носи́льщик; посы́льный; 2) бага́жник (*на велосипеде, мотоцикле*); 3) транспортёр; 4) *мор.* авиано́сец (*тж.* aircraft ~); cruiser ~ кре́йсер-авиано́сец; 5) *амер.* почтальо́н (*тж.* letter ~); 6) *мед.* бациллоноси́тель; 7) *тех.* держа́тель; кронште́йн.

carrier-pigeon ['kærɪə,pɪdʒɪn] *n* почто́вый го́лубь.

carrier-rocket ['kærɪə,rɔkɪt] *n* раке́та-носи́тель.

carrion I ['kærɪən] *n* па́даль.

carrion II *a* гни́лостный; отврати́тельный.

carrot ['kærət] *n* морко́вь.

carry ['kærɪ] *v* 1) нести́; носи́ть; 2) везти́; (пере-)вози́ть; 3) подде́рживать, нести́ на себе́ тя́жесть (*о колоннах и т. п.*); 4) держа́ться, вести́ себя́; to ~ oneself well хорошо́ держа́ться; 5) проводи́ть (*звук и т. п.*); 6) доводи́ть; 7) убира́ть (*сено*); 8) передава́ть, разноси́ть (*новости*); 9) доноси́ться, долета́ть; 10) проводи́ть (*кандидата*); принима́ть (*решение*); 11) содержа́ть в себе́, име́ть; 12) *воен.* захва́тывать, брать при́ступом; 13) приноси́ть (*доход, проценты*); 14) увле́чь за собо́й; 15) *амер.* продава́ть, торгова́ть; □ to ~ away а) уноси́ть, увози́ть; б) сноси́ть (*ветром*); в) увлека́ть, охва́тывать (*о чувстве*); to ~ back: to ~ smb. back напомина́ть кому́-л. про́шлое; to ~ forward а) продвига́ть (*дело*); б) *см.* to ~ over б); to ~ off а) уноси́ть, похища́ть; своди́ть в моги́лу; б) выи́грывать (*приз*); в) it off well не пока́зывать ви́да; to ~ on а) продолжа́ть; ~ on! продолжа́ть рабо́ту!; б) соверша́ть; в) *разг.* флиртова́ть (*with*); to ~ out а) выполня́ть, осуществля́ть; б) выноси́ть (*покойника*); to ~ over а) перевози́ть; б) *бухг.* переноси́ть на другу́ю страни́цу; to ~ through доводи́ть до конца́; заверша́ть; ◊ to ~ all before one преодолева́ть препя́тствия; to ~ too far а) заходи́ть сли́шком далеко́; б) заводи́ть сли́шком далеко́.

carry-all ['kærɪ,ɔːl] *n* 1) больша́я су́мка; вещево́й мешо́к; 2) *амер.* кры́тый экипа́ж.

cart I [kɑːt] *n* теле́га; пово́зка; двуко́лка; to put the ~ before the horse а) де́лать что-л. ши́ворот--навы́ворот; б) опережа́ть собы́тия; ◊ in the ~ *разг.* в затрудни́тельном положе́нии.

cart II *v* 1) везти́ в теле́ге; 2) е́хать в теле́ге; 3) *разг.* легко́ побежда́ть, наноси́ть пораже́ние (*в игре, состязании*).

cartel [kɑː'tel] *n* 1) *эк.* карте́ль; 2) соглаше́ние об обме́не пле́нными.

carter ['kɑːtə] *n* во́зчик.

cartful ['kɑːtful] *n* воз (*как мера груза*); a ~ of hey воз се́на.

cart-horse ['kɑːthɔːs] *n* ломова́я ло́шадь.

cartilage ['kɑːtɪlɪdʒ] *n* хрящ.

cartilaginous [,kɑːtɪ'lædʒɪnəs] *a* хрящево́й.

cart-load ['kɑːtloud] *см.* cartful.

cartographer [kɑː'tɔgrəfə] *n* карто́граф.

cartography [kɑː'tɔgrəfɪ] *n* картогра́фия.

cartoon I [kɑː'tuːn] *n* 1) карикату́ра (*преим. политическая*); 2) карто́н (*этюд для фрески*).

cartoon II *v* рисова́ть карикату́ры.

cartoonist [kɑː'tuːnɪst] *n* карикатури́ст.

cartridge ['kɑːtrɪdʒ] *n* 1) патро́н; blank ~ холосто́й патро́н; ink ~ сте́ржень, штифт с па́стой (*в шариковой ручке*); 2) кату́шка (*с фотографическими плёнками*); 3) *attr* патро́нный.

cartridge-belt ['kɑːtrɪdʒ,belt] *n* 1) пулемётная ле́нта; 2) патронта́ш.

cartridge-paper ['kɑːtrɪdʒ,peɪpə] *n* пло́тная бума́га (*для черчения, рисования*).

cart-road ['kɑːtroud] *n* просёлочная доро́га.

cart-track ['kɑːttræk] *см.* cart-road.

carve [kɑːv] *v* 1) выреза́ть, ре́зать (*по дереву, кости*); 2) гравирова́ть; 3) ре́зать (*мясо за столом*); □ to ~ out отреза́ть; to ~ up разделя́ть (*наследство, территорию*).

carver ['kɑːvə] *n* 1) ре́зчик (*по дереву*); 2) гравёр; 3) нож (*для нарезания мяса*).

carving ['kɑːvɪŋ] *n* 1) резна́я рабо́та; 2) резьба́ по де́реву.

cascade [kæs'keɪd] *n* 1) небольшо́й водопа́д; 2) *эл.* каска́д.

case[1] [keɪs] *n* 1) слу́чай; in ~ (of) в слу́чае; in any ~ во вся́ком слу́чае; is it the ~ that..? пра́вда, что..?, ве́рно, что..?; it is not the ~ э́то не так; to put (the) ~ that... предположи́м, что...; this is especially the ~ э́то осо́бенно ве́рно; gone ~ *разг.* безнадёжный слу́чай; 2) состоя́ние, положе́ние; as the ~ stands при да́нном положе́нии дел; to clinch the ~ *разг.* реши́ть исхо́д де́ла; 3) *юр.* де́ло, ка́зус; фа́кты, доказа́тельства, до́воды; to try a ~ вести́ суде́бный проце́сс; to have a good ~ располага́ть фа́ктами, подтвержда́ющими правоту́; to make out one's ~ доказа́ть свою́ правоту́; to state one's ~ изложи́ть своё де́ло; 4) *грам.* паде́ж; common ~ о́бщий паде́ж; subjective ~ имени́тельный паде́ж; possessive ~ притяжа́тельный паде́ж; objective ~ объе́ктный паде́ж; 5) *мед.* больно́й, пацие́нт; ра́неный; cot ~ лежа́чий больно́й; walking ~ ходя́чий больно́й.

case[2] I [keɪs] *n* 1) я́щик, коро́бка; vanity ~ да́мская су́мочка; cigar(ette) ~ портсига́р; 2) (доро́жный) несессе́р (*тж.* dressing-case); 3) футля́р, чехо́л; кры́шка (*переплёта*); 4) *тех.* кожу́х; 5) *полигр.* набо́рная ка́сса; 6) витри́на; 7) *воен.* ги́льза.

case[2] II *v* 1) класть (*в ящик, футляр и т. п.*); 2) вставля́ть в опра́ву; обкла́дывать, покрыва́ть.

case-hardened ['keɪs,hɑːdnd] *a* 1) закалённый; 2) нечувстви́тельный, загрубе́лый.

casein ['keɪsɪɪn] *n* *хим.* казеи́н.

casemate ['keɪsmeɪt] *n* *воен.* казема́т.

casement ['keɪsmənt] *n* 1) ство́рчатый око́нный переплёт; 2) *поэт.* окно́.

cash I [kæʃ] *n* 1) *разг.* де́ньги; in ~ при деньга́х; out of ~ не при деньга́х; без де́нег; short of ~ ма́ло де́нег; 2) зво́нкая моне́та; ~ down нали́чными деньга́ми; ~ on delivery (*сокр.* C.O.D.) нало́женным платежо́м; hard ~ нали́чные, зво́нкая моне́та; net ~, spot ~ нали́чные де́ньги; нали́чный расчёт; spare ~ свобо́дные де́ньги; to pay ~ плати́ть нали́чными деньга́ми; to roll in ~ располага́ть деньга́ми; 3) *attr* нали́чный (*о деньгах, расчёте*).

cash II *v* получа́ть де́ньги по че́ку.

cashier[a] [kæˈʃɪə] *n* касси́р.

cashier[b] [kəˈʃɪə] *v* 1) увольня́ть; 2) *воен.* разжа́ловать.

cashless [ˈkæʃlɪs] *a* 1) не име́ющий нали́чных де́нег; 2) безнали́чный.

cashmere [kæʃˈmɪə] *n* кашеми́р.

casing [ˈkeɪsɪŋ] *n* 1) обши́вка; опа́лубка; 2) *авто* покры́шка; 3) кожу́х; футля́р.

cask [kɑːsk] *n* бо́чка, бочо́нок.

casket [ˈkɑːskɪt] *n* 1) шкату́лка; 2) у́рна с пра́хом; *амер.* гроб.

casque [kæsk] *n* *ист., поэт.* шлем.

cassation [kæˈseɪʃən] *n* касса́ция.

cassock [ˈkæsək] *n* ря́са, сута́на.

cassowary [ˈkæsəweərɪ] *n* *зоол.* казуа́р.

cast I [kɑːst] *n* 1) броса́ние, мета́ние; забра́сывание (*сети, удочки и т. п.*); 2) бросо́к; 3) число́ очко́в (*на кости*); 4) риск (*или* to set, to stake) on a ~ поста́вить на ка́рту; 5) *театр.* соста́в исполни́телей (*в данном спектакле*); распределе́ние роле́й; 6) склад (*ума, характера*); тип; 7) выраже́ние (*лица*); 8) подсчёт; вычисле́ние; 9) отте́нок; 10) поворо́т, отклоне́ние; a ~ in the eye лёгкое косогла́зие; 11) ме́сто (*в телеге, повозке*); 12) образе́ц, обра́зчик; 13) фо́рма (*для отливки*); изло́жница.

cast II *v* (*past, p. p.* cast) 1) броса́ть; 2) кида́ть, швыря́ть; 3) отбра́сывать (*тень*); 4) сбра́сывать (*кожу*); меня́ть (*рога*); теря́ть (*зубы*); роня́ть (*листья*); 5) подсчи́тывать (*часто* to ~ up); 6) распределя́ть (*роли*); подбира́ть (*актёров*) на роль (*в фильме*); 7) опуска́ть (*избирательный бюллетень*); 8) *тех.* отлива́ть, формова́ть; □ to ~ **about** а) обду́мывать, раски́дывать умо́м (*for*); б) подыска́ть (*тему разговора и т. п.; for*); to ~ **aside** отверга́ть, отбра́сывать; to ~ **away** отбра́сывать; to be ~ away потерпе́ть кораблекруше́ние; to ~ **back** возвраща́ть(ся) (*в прежнее состояние*); to ~ **down** а) поверга́ть в уны́ние; б) опуска́ть (*глаза*); сверга́ть; to ~ **off** а) броса́ть, покида́ть; б) зака́нчивать рабо́ту; в) сбра́сывать око́вы; г) *мор.* отдава́ть (*канат*); отва́ливать (*на шлюпке*); to ~ **out** а) изверга́ть (*пищу*); б) выгоня́ть; to ~ **up** а) вски́дывать (*глаза*); б) подсчи́тывать, вычисля́ть.

castanets [ˌkæstəˈnets] *n pl* кастанье́ты.

castaway I [ˈkɑːstəˌweɪ] *n* 1) потерпе́вший кораблекруше́ние; 2) отве́рженный; па́рия.

castaway II *a* отве́рженный.

caste [kɑːst] *n* ка́ста; привилегиро́ванный класс; to lose ~ опусти́ться.

castigate [ˈkæstɪgeɪt] *v* 1) нака́зывать; поро́ть; 2) бичева́ть (*словами*); 3) подверга́ть суро́вой кри́тике; 4) исправля́ть (*лит. произведение*).

castigation [ˌkæstɪˈgeɪʃən] *n* 1) наказа́ние; по́рка; 2) бичева́ние (*словами*); 3) суро́вая кри́тика; 4) исправле́ние (*лит. произведения*).

casting [ˈkɑːstɪŋ] *n* *тех.* литьё, отли́вка.

casting-vote [ˈkɑːstɪŋˈvout] *n* реша́ющий го́лос (*при равенстве голосов*).

cast iron [ˈkɑːstˈaɪən] *n* чугу́н.

cast-iron [ˈkɑːstˌaɪən] *a* 1) чугу́нный; твёрдый; 2) непрекло́нный; желе́зный.

castle I [ˈkɑːsl] *n* 1) за́мок; дворе́ц; 2) *шахм.*

ладья́, тура́; 3) тверды́ня, убе́жище; ◊ to build ~s in the air (*или* in Spain) стро́ить возду́шные за́мки; фантази́ровать.

castle II *v* *шахм.* рокирова́ть(ся).

castle-builder [ˈkɑːslˌbɪldə] *n* фантазёр.

castor[1] [ˈkɑːstə] *n* 1) *мед.* бобро́вая струя́; 2) *сленг* касто́ровая шля́па.

castor[2] *n* 1) пе́речница; 2) *pl* судо́к; 3) колёсико (*на ножках мебели*).

castrate [kæsˈtreɪt] *v* кастри́ровать, холости́ть.

castration [kæsˈtreɪʃən] *n* кастра́ция.

casual [ˈkæʒjuəl] *a* 1) случа́йный; 2) непостоя́нный; нерегуля́рный; 3) непреднаме́ренный; 4) небре́жный.

casuals [ˈkæʒjuəlz] *n pl* вое́нные, ожида́ющие назначе́ния.

casualty [ˈkæʒjuəltɪ] *n* 1) несча́стный слу́чай; 2) ра́неный; уби́тый; to extricate casualties выноси́ть ра́неных; 3) *pl воен.* поте́ри уби́тыми и ра́неными; to inflict casualties наноси́ть уро́н; to sustain casualties понести́ поте́ри.

cat [kæt] *n* 1) кот; ко́шка; 2) *разг.* скло́чная же́нщина; 3) *разг.* ко́шка (*плеть*); 4) двойно́й трено́жник; 5) *мор.* кат; ◊ it rains ~s and dogs дождь льёт как из ведра́; to bell the ~ рискова́ть чем-л. ра́ди други́х; to fight like Kilkenny ~s ожесточённо дра́ться; to let the ~ out of the bag *погов.* вы́дать секре́т; like a ~ on hot bricks *погов.* ≅ как на горя́чих у́гольях; no room to swing a ~ *погов.* ≅ я́блоку не́где упа́сть; we shall see how the ~ jumps поживём — уви́дим; to see which way the ~ jumps, to wait for the ~ to jump *погов.* ≅ выжида́ть, куда́ поду́ет ве́тер; it's enough to make a ~ laugh о́чень смешно́.

cataclysm [ˈkætəklɪzəm] *n* 1) пото́п; 2) переворо́т (*социальный, политический*); катакли́зм.

catacomb [ˈkætəkoum] *n* 1) подземе́лье; 2) *обыкн. pl* катако́мбы.

catafalque [ˈkætəfælk] *n* катафа́лк.

catalog [ˈkætələg] *амер. см.* catalogue.

catalogue I [ˈkætələg] *n* 1) катало́г; subject ~ предме́тный катало́г; 2) прейскура́нт; priced ~ катало́г с це́нами; 3) *амер.* уче́бный план, програ́мма.

catalogue II *v* каталогизи́ровать, вноси́ть в катало́г.

cataloguer [ˈkætələgə] *n* каталогиза́тор.

catamaran [ˌkætəməˈræn] *n* 1) катамара́н; 2) *разг.* сварли́вая же́нщина.

cat-and-dog [ˈkætəndˈdɔg] *a:* ~ life семе́йные дря́зги; постоя́нные скло́ки.

catapult I [ˈkætəpʌlt] *n* 1) катапу́льта; 2) рога́тка.

catapult II *v* 1) катапульти́ровать; 2) стреля́ть из рога́тки.

cataract [ˈkætərækt] *n* 1) водопа́д; 2) ли́вень; 3) *мед.* катара́кта.

catastrophe [kəˈtæstrəfɪ] *n* 1) катастро́фа; несча́стье; 2) развя́зка (*в драме*).

catastrophic [ˌkætəˈstrɔfɪk] *a* катастрофи́ческий.

catcall I [ˈkætkɔːl] *n* свист, освИ́стывание.

catcall II *v* освИ́стывать.

catch I [kætʃ] *n* 1) пои́мка; 2) уло́в; добы́ча; 3) вы́годное приобрете́ние; вы́года; 4) кова́рный вопро́с; лову́шка; 5) щеко́лда; защёлка; 6) то́рмоз; 7) заде́ржка (*дыхания*); поте́ря на мгнове́ние (*голоса*).

catch II *v* (*past, p. p.* caught) 1) лови́ть; пойма́ть; 2) заста́ть (*за чем-л.— in, at*); 3) схвати́ть; 4) заста́ть (*о буре, дожде и т. п.*); to be caught попа́сть (*под дождь и т. п.*); быть засти́гнутым (*дождём, снегом, грозой*); 5) попа́сть, ра́нить; 6) зацепи́ть; 7) поспе́ть (*на поезд*); 8) запу́таться (*в проволоке и т. п.*); 9) зарази́ться, схвати́ть (*болезнь*); 10) привле́чь, порази́ть, увле́чь; 11) понима́ть, схва́тывать (*смысл*); 12) прищеми́ть (*палец и т. п.*); 13) стать, замёрзнуть (*о реке, пруде*); ▢ to ~ at a) пыта́ться схвати́ть что-л. *или* ухвати́ться за что-л.; б) обра́доваться чему́-л.; to ~ away утащи́ть; to ~ off *амер. сленг* засну́ть; to ~ on приви́ться, сде́латься мо́дным; to ~ out обнару́жить; to ~ up a) догна́ть, нагна́ть; б) прерва́ть (*оратора*); в) бы́стро схвати́ть (*словечко*); г) подхвати́ть (*словечко*); ◊ you will ~ it! бу́дет тебе́ на оре́хи!

catching ['kætʃɪŋ] *a* 1) зара́зный, прили́пчивый; 2) привлека́тельный.

catchpenny ['kætʃˌpenɪ] *a* рассчи́танный на дешё́вый успе́х и привлече́ние покупа́телей (*особ. об изда́ниях*).

catchpole ['kætʃpoul] *n* суде́бный при́став, суде́бный исполни́тель.

catchword ['kætʃwəːd] *n* 1) ходово́е выраже́ние, сло́во; 2) ло́зунг, призы́в; 3) *полигр.* колонти́тул; 4) *театр.* ре́плика.

catchy ['kætʃɪ] *a* 1) легко́ запомина́ющийся (*о мело́дии*); 2) привлека́тельный.

categorical [ˌkætɪˈgɔrɪkəl] *a* 1) категори́ческий; реши́тельный; 2) безусло́вный; я́сный.

category ['kætɪgərɪ] *n* катего́рия; разря́д; класс.

catenation [ˌkætɪˈneɪʃən] *n* сцепле́ние.

cater[1] ['keɪtə] *v* 1) поставля́ть проду́кты (*for*); 2) развлека́ть, доставля́ть удово́льствие (*to*).

cater[2] *n* четвёрка (*в ка́ртах*); четы́ре очка́ (*в костя́х*).

caterer ['keɪtərə] *n* поставщи́к (*проду́ктов*).

caterpillar ['kætəpɪlə] *n* 1) гу́сеница; 2) *attr* гу́сеничный.

caterwaul I ['kætəwɔːl] *n* мяу́канье; *разг.* коша́чий конце́рт.

caterwaul II *v* мяу́кать; *разг.* устра́ивать конце́рт (*о ко́шках*).

catgut ['kætgʌt] *n* 1) струна́; 2) стру́нные инструме́нты.

cathedral [kəˈθiːdrəl] *n* собо́р (*кафедра́льный*).

cathode ['kæθoud] *n* *эл.* като́д.

catholic I ['kæθəlɪk] *n* като́лик.

catholic II *a* 1) католи́ческий; 2) всеохва́тывающий; 3) *церк.* вселе́нский.

catholicism [kəˈθɔlɪsɪzəm] *n* католи́чество, католици́зм.

catkin ['kætkɪn] *n* серёжка (*на и́ве, берёзе и т. п.*).

cat-like ['kætlaɪk] *a* коша́чий; мя́гкий, неслы́шный.

cat-o'-nine-tails ['kætəˈnaɪnteɪlz] *n* плеть, ко́шка-девятихво́стка.

cat's-meat ['kætsmiːt] *n* кони́на, покупа́емая для ко́шек.

cat's-paw ['kætspɔː] *n* 1) рябь на воде́; 2) ору́дие в рука́х кого́-л.

catsup ['kætsəp] *см.* ketchup.

cattle ['kætl] *n* (*pl без изме́н.*) 1) кру́пный рога́тый скот; horned (dairy, pedigree, prize) ~ рога́тый (моло́чный, племенно́й, премиро́ванный) скот;

store ~ скот, предназна́ченный на убо́й; 2) *сленг* ло́шади, живо́тные (*о лю́дях*).

cattle-box ['kætlbɔks] *n ж.-д.* ваго́н для скота́.

cattle-dealer ['kætlˌdiːlə] *n* торго́вец ското́м.

cattle-leader ['kætlˌliːdə] *n* ноздрево́е кольцо́.

cattleman ['kætlmən] *n* 1) пасту́х; 2) ско́тник.

cattle-pen ['kætlpen] *n* заго́н для скота́.

cattle-plague ['kætlpleɪg] *n* чума́ рога́того скота́.

cattle-ranch ['kætlrɑːntʃ] *n* животново́дческая фе́рма, животново́дческое хозя́йство.

Caucasian I [kɔːˈkeɪʒən] *n* кавка́зец.

Caucasian II *a* кавка́зский.

caucus ['kɔːkəs] *n* 1) *амер.* предвы́борное закры́тое собра́ние парти́йных ли́деров; 2) поли́тика подтасо́вки вы́боров.

caught [kɔːt] *past, p. p. см.* catch II.

caul [kɔːl] *n* 1) че́пчик; 2) *анат.* околопло́дный пузы́рь; ◊ to be born with a ~ ≅ роди́ться в соро́чке.

cauldron ['kɔːldrən] *n* котёл.

cauliflower ['kɔlɪflauə] *n* цветна́я капу́ста.

caulk [kɔːk] *v* конопа́тить; смоли́ть (*су́дно*).

causal ['kɔːzəl] *a* причи́нный; кауза́льный.

causality [kɔːˈzælɪtɪ] *n* причи́нность; причи́нная связь.

causative ['kɔːzətɪv] *a* 1) причи́нный; 2) *грам.* каузати́вный.

cause I [kɔːz] *n* 1) причи́на; prime ~ первопричи́на; to spot the ~ of the trouble вы́яснить причи́ну непола́док; 2) основа́ние, по́вод; there's no ~ нет никаки́х основа́ний (*для чего́-л.— for*); 3) де́ло; to support the ~ of the working class стоя́ть за де́ло рабо́чего кла́сса; the ~ of peace де́ло ми́ра; 4) *юр.* де́ло, проце́сс; lost ~ про́игранное де́ло; to plead a ~ защища́ть де́ло в суде́; 5) заинтересо́ванная сторона́.

cause II *v* 1) вызыва́ть, производи́ть; влия́ть (*быть причи́ной*); 2) заставля́ть, веле́ть (*с после́дующим гл. в Inf*).

'**cause** [kɔːz] *разг. см.* because.

causeless ['kɔːzlɪs] *a* беспричи́нный, необосно́ванный; беспричи́нный.

causeway I ['kɔːzweɪ] *n* 1) насыпна́я доро́га; да́мба; 2) мостки́.

causeway II *v* 1) стро́ить доро́гу; 2) настила́ть мостки́.

causey ['kɔːzeɪ] *см.* causeway.

caustic I ['kɔːstɪk] *n* 1) е́дкое вещество́; lunar ~ ля́пис; 2) язви́тельность, сарка́зм.

caustic II *a* 1) *хим.* е́дкий; каусти́ческий; 2) язви́тельный, саркасти́ческий.

cauterize ['kɔːtəraɪz] *v* 1) прижига́ть; *перен.* клейми́ть; 2) де́лать нечувстви́тельным.

cautery ['kɔːtərɪ] *n* прижига́ние.

caution I ['kɔːʃən] *n* 1) (пред)осторо́жность; осмотри́тельность; 2) предостереже́ние; ~ ! *воен.* пригото́вься!

caution II *v* предостерега́ть (*against*).

cautionary ['kɔːʃnərɪ] *a* предупрежда́ющий, предостерега́ющий.

cautious ['kɔːʃəs] *a* осторо́жный; осмотри́тельный.

cavalcade [ˌkævəlˈkeɪd] *n* гру́ппа вса́дников, кавалька́да.

cavalier I [ˌkævəˈlɪə] *n* 1) вса́дник; 2) кавалёр; 3) *ист.* рыцарь; 4) *ист.* роялист *(в Англии XVII в.)*.

cavalier II *a* 1) бесцеремонный; 2) надменный; 3) *ист.* роялистский.

cavalry ['kævəlrı] *n* 1) конница, кавалерия; 2) *attr* кавалерийский.

cavalryman ['kævəlrımən] *n* кавалерист.

cave I [keɪv] *n* 1) пещера; 2) впадина; полость; 3) *полит.* фракция.

cave II *v* 1) выдалбливать; 2) создавать фракцию; □ to ~ in *a*) *(о почве, части здания)* вдавливать(ся); *б*) уступать, поддаваться.

cave-dweller ['keɪv‚dwelə] *n* пещерный человек.

cavendish ['kævəndɪʃ] *n* подслащённый плиточный табак.

cavern ['kævən] *n* 1) пещера; 2) полость; 3) *мед.* каверна.

caviar(e) ['kævɪɑ:] *n* икра *(рыбная)*.

cavil I ['kævɪl] *n* придирка.

cavil II *v* придираться *(к — at, about)*.

cavity ['kævɪtɪ] *n* полость; впадина; abdominal ~ брюшная полость.

caw I [kɔ:] *n* карканье.

caw II *v* каркать; *перен.* накликать беду.

cay [keɪ] *n* 1) коралловый риф; 2) песчаная отмель.

cayenne [keɪ'en] *n* красный стручковый перец.

cease [si:s] *v* прекращать(ся); переставать; ~ fire! *воен.* прекратить огонь!

cease-fire ['si:s‚faɪə] *n воен.* прекращение огня.

ceaseless ['si:slɪs] *a* непрерывный, беспрестанный.

cedar ['si:də] *n* 1) кедр; 2) *attr* кедровый.

cede [si:d] *v* уступать *(территорию; в споре)*.

ceiling ['si:lɪŋ] *n* 1) потолок *(тж. ав.)*; emergency ~ *ав.* максимальный потолок; 2) верхний предел зарплаты; 3) перекрытие, обшивка; 4) *attr* предельно высокий *(о цене и т. п.)*.

celebrate ['selɪbreɪt] *v* 1) праздновать; 2) прославлять; 3) совершать *(богослужение)*.

celebrated ['selɪbreɪtɪd] *a* знаменитый; прославленный.

celebration [‚selɪ'breɪʃən] *n* 1) празднование; 2) *pl* торжества; 3) прославление; 4) церковная служба.

celebrity [sɪ'lebrɪtɪ] *n* 1) известность; 2) знаменитость.

celerity [sɪ'lerɪtɪ] *n* быстрота.

celery ['selərɪ] *n* сельдерей.

celestial [sɪ'lestjəl] *a* 1) небесный; 2) прекрасный; божественный.

celibacy ['selɪbəsɪ] *n* безбрачие.

celibate I ['selɪbɪt] *n* 1) холостяк; 2) холостяцкая жизнь; безбрачие.

celibate II *a* 1) холостой; 2) холостяцкий; 3) *церк.* давший обет безбрачия.

cell [sel] *n* 1) камера *(тюремная)*; condemned ~ камера смертников; 2) *биол.* клетка; 3) ячейка; 4) келья; 5) *поэт.* могила; 6) *эл.* элемент; voltaic ~ гальванический элемент.

cellar ['selə] *n* 1) подвал *(особ. для провизии)*; 2) погреб *(особ. винный)*; 3) запас вин.

'cellist ['tʃelɪst] *сокр. разг. см.* violoncellist.

'cello ['tʃelou] *сокр. разг. см.* violoncello.

cellophane ['seləfeɪn] *n* 1) целлофан; 2) *attr* целлофановый.

cellular ['seljulə] *a* клеточный.

cellulate ['seljuleɪt] *a* состоящий из клеток, ячеистый.

cellule ['selju:l] *n биол.* клетка.

celluloid ['seljulɔɪd] *n* целлулоид.

cellulose I ['seljulous] *n* целлюлоза; клетчатка.

cellulose II *a* целлюлозный.

Celt [kelt] *n* кельт.

Celtic I ['keltɪk] *n* кельтский язык.

Celtic II *a* кельтский.

cement I [sɪ'ment] *n* 1) цемент; 2) замазка; 3) строительный раствор; 4) вяжущее вещество.

cement II *v* цементировать; скреплять *(тж. перен.)*.

cementation [‚si:men'teɪʃən] *n* цементирование; цементация.

cemetery ['semɪtrɪ] *n* кладбище.

censer ['sensə] *n* кадило.

censor I ['sensə] *n* цензор.

censor II *v* подвергать цензуре; просматривать *(с целью цензуры)*; проверять.

censorial [sen'sɔ:rɪəl] *a* цензурный.

censorious [sen'sɔ:rɪəs] *a* критический; осуждающий.

censorship ['sensəʃɪp] *n* 1) цензура; 2) должность цензора.

censure I ['senʃə] *n* осуждение; порицание.

censure II *v* порицать, осуждать; делать выговор.

census ['sensəs] *n* перепись.

census-paper ['sensəs‚peɪpə] *n* анкета переписи.

cent [sent] *n* цент *(= 0,01 доллара)*; ◊ I don't care a ~ мне наплевать; per ~ процент *(%)*.

centenarian I [‚sentɪ'nɛərɪən] *n* столетний человек.

centenarian II *a* столетний.

centenary I [sen'ti:nərɪ] *n* 1) столетняя годовщина; столетие; 2) празднование столетней годовщины.

centenary II *a* столетний.

center I ['sentə] *n амер.* 1) *см.* centre I; 2) станция, пункт *(обслуживания)*; boat ~ пункт проката лодок *или* яхт; service ~ станция обслуживания автомашин.

center II *v амер. см.* centre II.

centigrade ['sentɪgreɪd] *a* стоградусный *(о термометре)*.

centimeter ['sentɪ‚mi:tə] *амер. см.* centimetre.

centimetre ['sentɪ‚mi:tə] *n* сантиметр.

centner ['sentnə] *n* английский центнер *(= 45,36 кг)*.

central ['sentrəl] *a* 1) центральный; 2) основной; главный; ведущий.

centralization [‚sentrəlaɪ'zeɪʃən] *n* сосредоточение, централизация.

centralize ['sentrəlaɪz] *v* сосредоточивать, централизовать.

centre I ['sentə] *n* центр; середина; средоточие; dead ~ *тех.* мёртвая, нулевая точка; неподвижный центр; polling ~ избирательный участок.

centre II *v* 1) помещать(ся) в центре; 2) концентрировать(ся); сосредоточивать(ся); 3) *тех.* центрировать.

centric(al) ['sentrɪk(əl)] *a* центральный.

centrifugal [sen'trıfjugəl] *a* центробежный.

centrifuge ['sentrıfjuːdʒ] *n* центрифуга.

centripetal [sen'trıpıtl] *a* центростремительный.

century ['sentʃurı] *n* 1) столетие; век; 2) сотня *(чего-л.)*; 3) *амер. разг.* сто долларов.

cephalic [ke'fælık, se'fælık] *a анат.* головной.

cephalitis [ˌsefə'laıtıs] *n мед.* энцефалит.

ceramic [sı'ræmık] *a* гончарный; керамический.

ceramics [sı'ræmıks] *n* керамика; гончарное дело.

ceramist ['serəmıst] *n* гончар.

cereal I ['sıərıəl] *n* 1) *обыкн. pl* хлебные злаки, хлеба; 2) *амер.* кушанье *(из круп)*.

cereal II *a* зерновой; относящийся к хлебным злакам.

cerebellum [ˌserı'beləm] *n анат.* мозжечок.

cerebra ['serıbrə] *pl см.* cerebrum.

cerebral I ['serıbrəl] *a* 1) мозговой; 2) *фон.* церебральный.

cerebral II *n фон.* церебральный звук.

cerebrum ['serıbrəm] *n (pl тж.* cerebra) *анат.* головной мозг.

cerecloth ['sıəklɔθ] *n* навощённая холстина.

ceremonial I [ˌserı'mounjəl] *n* церемониал, обряд.

ceremonial II *a* 1) формальный; 2) церемониальный, обрядовый.

ceremonious [ˌserı'mounjəs] *a* 1) церемонный; манерный; 2) педантичный.

ceremony ['serımənı] *n* 1) церемония; обряд; 2) церемонность; формальность; to stand (up)on ~ церемониться; don't stand on ~! не церемоньтесь!, не стесняйтесь!

certain ['səːtn] *a* 1) определённый; 2) надёжный, верный; несомненный; he is ~ to come он обязательно придёт; 3) уверенный; to feel ~ быть уверенным; to make ~ of удостовериться *(в чём-л.)*; for ~ наверняка; 4) некий, какой-то; 5) некоторый, известный.

certainly ['səːtnlı] *adv* конечно; несомненно.

certainty ['səːtntı] *n* 1) несомненный факт; to bet on a ~ держать пари на определённую ставку; 2) уверенность; for a ~ наверняка; несомненно; with ~ уверенно, определённо.

certificate[a] [sə'tıfıkıt] *n* 1) удостоверение; свидетельство; ~ of birth, a birth ~ метрика; a health ~ справка о состоянии здоровья; a marriage ~ свидетельство о браке; 2) *амер.* аттестат.

certificate[b] [sə'tıfıkeıt] *v* удостоверять; выдавать удостоверение, свидетельство.

certification [ˌsəːtıfı'keıʃən] *n* 1) выдача удостоверения, свидетельства; 2) удостоверение.

certify ['səːtıfaı] *v* 1) удостоверять, заверять; 2) ручаться; 3) *мед.* выдавать свидетельство о психическом заболевании.

certitude ['səːtıtjuːd] *n* уверенность; убеждённость, определённость.

cessation [se'seıʃən] *n* 1) прекращение; ~ of hostilities прекращение военных действий; перемирие; 2) перерыв.

cession ['seʃən] *n* уступка, передача *(прав и т. п.)*.

cesspool ['sespuːl] *n* выгребная яма.

chafe I [tʃeıf] *n* 1) ссадина; 2) раздражение.

chafe II *v* 1) растирать; 2) тереть, натирать; 3) раздражаться, нервничать.

chafer ['tʃeıfə] *n* майский жук.

chaff I [tʃɑːf] *n* 1) мякина; 2) сечка *(из соломы, сена)*; 3) отбросы; 4) подтрунивание, подшучивание; 5) *attr* соломенный.

chaff II *v* 1) рубить, резать *(солому и т. п.)*; 2) подшучивать, поддразнивать.

chaffer ['tʃæfə] *v* торговаться.

chaffinch ['tʃæfıntʃ] *n* зяблик.

chaffy ['tʃɑːfı] *a* пустой, негодный.

chagrin I ['ʃægrın] *n* досада, большое огорчение.

chagrin II *v* огорчать.

chain I [tʃeın] *n* 1) цепь; цепочка; a ~ of mountains горная цепь, горный хребет; a ~ of events цепь, серия событий; 2) *pl* узы, оковы; 3) мерная цепь (= *19,8 м*); 4) *attr* цепной.

chain II *v* 1) сковывать; приковывать; 2) сажать на цепь *(обыкн.* to ~ up); *перен.* привязывать.

chain-mail ['tʃeınmeıl] *n* кольчуга.

chair I [tʃeə] *n* 1) стул; cane ~ плетёное кресло *(из камыша)*; easy ~ кресло; hammock ~ шезлонг; Bath ~ кресло на колёсах для больных; take a ~!, won't you take a ~? садитесь!; 2) кафедра; 3) профессура; 4) председательское место; to be in the ~ председательствовать; to leave the ~ закрыть собрание; to take the ~ а) занять председательское место; б) открыть собрание; ~!, ~! к порядку!; 5) председатель *(собрания)*; to elect the ~ выбирать председателя *(собрания)*; 6) *амер.* электрический стул.

chair II *v* поднимать и нести *(победителя)*.

chair-car ['tʃeəkɑː] *n амер. ж.-д.* пассажирский вагон с мягкими креслами; салон-вагон.

chairman ['tʃeəmən] *n* председатель.

chairwoman ['tʃeəˌwumən] *n* женщина-председатель.

chaise [ʃeız] *n* 1) фаэтон; 2) почтовая карета.

chalet ['ʃæleı] *n* 1) шале *(дом в швейцарском стиле)*; 2) *эвф.* уличная уборная.

chalk I [tʃɔːk] *n* 1) мел; 2) мелок *(для рисования, записи)*; ◊ by long ~s намного, значительно.

chalk II *v* писать, рисовать мелом; □ to ~ **out** намечать *(план)*; ◊ to ~ on the barn-door производить приблизительные подсчёты.

chalk-stone ['tʃɔːkstoun] *n* 1) известняк; 2) *мед.* подагрические отложения.

chalky ['tʃɔːkı] *a* 1) меловой; известковый; 2) *мед.* подагрический.

challenge I ['tʃælındʒ] *n* 1) оклик; 2) вызов *(на соревнование, на дуэль)*; 3) сомнение, возникшая проблема; to bring smth. into ~ поставить что-л. под сомнение; 4) *юр.* отвод *(присяжного заседателя)*; 5) *мор.* опознавательные *(сигналы)*.

challenge II *v* 1) окликать; спрашивать пропуск; 2) вызывать *(на соревнование, на дуэль)*; 3) сомневаться; оспаривать; 4) *юр.* отводить *(присяжного заседателя)*; 5) претендовать *(на внимание)*.

chamber ['tʃeımbə] *n* 1) палата; Gilded Chamber палата лордов; Lower Chamber нижняя палата; Second *(или* Upper) Chamber верхняя палата; Star Chamber *ист.* Звёздная палата *(тайный граж-*

данский и уголовный суд в Англии XVI — XVII вв.); Chamber of Commerce Торговая пала́та; 2) поэт. ко́мната, го́рница; 3) pl апарта́ме́нты; 4) pl конто́ра адвока́та; 5) тех. ка́мера; pressure ~, altitude ~ косм. бароска́мера; blast ~ косм. ка́мера сгора́ния; 6) attr ка́мерный.

chamberlain ['tʃeɪmbəlɪn] n 1) гофме́йстер; камерге́р; 2) казначе́й.

chambermaid ['tʃeɪmbəmeɪd] n го́рничная (в гости́нице и т. п.).

chameleon [kə'miːljən] n хамелео́н.

chamfer I ['tʃæmfə] n 1) жёлоб, вы́емка; 2) ско́шенная кро́мка; фа́ска.

chamfer II v 1) выда́лбливать; 2) стёсывать, ска́шивать.

chamois[a] ['ʃæmwɑ] n зоол. се́рна.

chamois[b] ['ʃæmɪ] n 1) за́мша; 2) attr за́мшевый.

champ I [tʃæmp] n ча́вканье.

champ II v 1) ча́вкать; 2) грызть удила́.

champagne [ʃæm'peɪn] n шампа́нское.

champaign ['tʃæmpeɪn] n равни́на.

champion I ['tʃæmpjən] n 1) чемпио́н; 2) победи́тель, пе́рвый призёр; 3) боре́ц, защи́тник, побо́рник; ~s of peace борцы́ за мир; сторо́нники ми́ра.

champion II a разг. первокла́ссный.

champion III v защища́ть; боро́ться за что-л.

championship ['tʃæmpjənʃɪp] n 1) пе́рвенство (в спорте); 2) зва́ние чемпио́на.

chance I [tʃɑːns] n 1) слу́чай; by ~ случа́йно; on the ~ в слу́чае; 2) случа́йность; неожи́данность; 3) удо́бный слу́чай; возмо́жность; a fair ~ удо́бный, подходя́щий случай; to have no ~ не име́ть возмо́жности; there is just a ~ вполне́ возмо́жно; give me a ~! a) да́йте мне возмо́жность!; б) прости́те меня на э́тот раз!; 4) сча́стье, уда́ча, шанс; let ~ decide пусть судьба́ реша́ет; the main ~ возмо́жность зарабо́тать де́ньги; to stand a good ~ име́ть все ша́нсы; to take one's ~ of рискну́ть, реши́ться (на что-л.).

chance II a случа́йный.

chance III v 1) случи́ться; if I ~ to be если мне случи́ться быть; 2) разг. рискну́ть (особ. to ~ it); □ to ~ upon случа́йно найти́, наткну́ться.

chancellery ['tʃɑːnsələrɪ] n канцеля́рия (посо́льства).

chancellor ['tʃɑːnsələ] n 1) ка́нцлер; Lord Chancellor a) лорд-ка́нцлер; председа́тель пала́ты ло́рдов (в Англии); б) верхо́вный судья́ (в Англии); Chancellor of the Exchequer мини́стр фина́нсов (в Англии); 2) пе́рвый секрета́рь посо́льства; 3) ре́ктор университе́та (в Англии).

chancery ['tʃɑːnsərɪ] n 1) (C.) суд ло́рда-ка́нцлера; 2) амер. «суд справедли́вости», «ка́нцлерский суд»; 3) архи́в; ◊ in ~ в тиска́х, в безвы́ходном положе́нии.

chancy ['tʃɑːnsɪ] a риско́ванный; ненадёжный.

chandelier [ˌʃændɪ'lɪə] n лю́стра.

chandler ['tʃɑːndlə] n продаве́ц москате́льных това́ров.

change I [tʃeɪndʒ] n 1) измене́ние; переме́на; for a ~ для разнообра́зия; you need a ~ вам нужна́ переме́на обстано́вки; 2) заме́на; 3) сме́-

на (белья́, пла́тья); 4) обме́н (де́нег); 5) сда́ча, ме́лкие де́ньги; small ~ a) ме́лочь; б) бана́льности; 6) переса́дка (на железной дороге, трамвае); 7) но́вая фа́за луны́, новолу́ние; 8) pl перезво́н (колоколов).

change II v 1) меня́ть(ся), изменя́ть(ся); 2) сменя́ть, заменя́ть; 3) переодева́ть(ся); 4) де́лать переса́дку (на железной дороге, трамвае); 5) переезжа́ть (на другую квартиру); 6) обме́ниваться (чем-л.); 7) меня́ть, разме́нивать (деньги).

changeability [ˌtʃeɪndʒə'bɪlɪtɪ] n изме́нчивость, неусто́йчивость; непостоя́нство.

changeable ['tʃeɪndʒəbl] a изме́нчивый, неусто́йчивый; непостоя́нный.

channel I ['tʃænl] n 1) кана́л; перен. путь; исто́чник (получения сведений и т. п.); 2) проли́в; the English Channel Ла-Ма́нш; 3) ру́сло; 4) сток, сто́чная кана́ва; 5) тех. желобо́к, вы́емка.

channel II v 1) рыть кана́л; 2) стр. де́лать вы́емки, пазы́.

chant I [tʃɑːnt] n 1) церк. песнопе́ние; 2) поэт. песнь.

chant II v 1) петь, распева́ть; 2) воспева́ть; 3) говори́ть нараспе́в.

chanty ['tʃɑːntɪ] n хорова́я матро́сская пе́сня (которую поют при подъёме тяжестей).

chaos ['keɪɔs] n ха́ос; беспоря́док.

chaotic [keɪ'ɔtɪk] a хаоти́ческий; беспоря́дочный.

chap[1] [tʃæp] n разг. па́рень, ма́лый; old ~ стари́на, прия́тель; merry ~ весельча́к; a funny little ~ чуда́к, смешно́й челове́к.

chap[2] n обыкн. pl 1) че́люсть (чаще животных, шутл. человека); 2) щека́.

chap[3] v растре́скиваться (о коже на руках, о земле).

chapel ['tʃæpəl] n 1) часо́вня; 2) це́рковь (тюре́мная, домовая и т. п.); 3) капе́лла (тж. певческая); 4) типогра́фия; рабо́тники типогра́фии.

chaperon I ['ʃæpəroun] n компаньо́нка (сопровождающая молодую девушку).

chaperon II v сопровожда́ть (молодую девушку).

chapiter ['tʃæpɪtə] n архит. капите́ль коло́нны.

chaplain ['tʃæplɪn] n капелла́н; свяще́нник.

chaplet ['tʃæplɪt] n 1) вено́к, ле́нта (на голове); 2) чётки; бу́сы.

chapman ['tʃæpmən] n коробе́йник.

chapter ['tʃæptə] n 1) глава́ (в книге); to the end of the ~ до са́мого конца́; 2) те́ма, сюже́т; ◊ a ~ of accidents непредви́денное стече́ние обстоя́тельств.

char [tʃɑː] v 1) обу́гливать(ся); 2) обжига́ть.

character I ['kærɪktə] n 1) хара́ктер; a man of fine (noble, strong, weak) ~ челове́к с хоро́шим (благоро́дным, си́льным, сла́бым) хара́ктером; 2) хара́ктерная осо́бенность; сво́йство, ка́чество; биол. при́знак; 3) репута́ция; 4) характери́стика; пи́сьменная рекоменда́ция; 5) фигу́ра, ли́чность; де́ятель; 6) роль; 7) тип; персона́ж (в литературном произведении); 8) чуда́к; 9) pl бу́квы, алфави́т; Chinese ~s кита́йские иеро́глифы.

character II ['kærɪktə] v уст., поэт. 1) запечатлева́ть; 2) характеризова́ть.

characteristic I [ˌkærɪktə'rɪstɪk] n 1) хара́ктерная черта; особенность; 2) *мат.* характери́стика (*логари́фма*).

characteristic II *a* характе́рный; типи́чный (*для кого-л.* — *of*).

characterization [ˌkærɪktəraɪˈzeɪʃən] *n* характери́стика.

characterize [ˈkærɪktəraɪz] *v* 1) характеризова́ть; 2) быть характе́рным.

charade [ʃəˈrɑːd] *n* шара́да.

charcoal [ˈtʃɑːkoul] *n* 1) древе́сный у́голь; 2) ра́шкуль, у́гольный каранда́ш; 3) рису́нок у́глем.

charge I [tʃɑːdʒ] *n* 1) обвине́ние; to bring the ~ home to smb. обвини́ть кого́-л.; 2) нагру́зка; *перен.* бре́мя; 3) руково́дство; отве́тственность (*по до́лжности*); обя́занности; 4) забо́та; попече́ние, надзо́р; to be in ~ of a) смотре́ть, присма́тривать (*за кем-л.*); б) заве́довать (*чем-л.*); to take ~ присма́тривать (*за кем-л.* — *of*); to give in ~ сдать под надзо́р (*кого́-л.*); 5) лицо́, находя́щееся на попече́нии; подопе́чный; 6) цена́, сто́имость; *pl* изде́ржки; расхо́ды; at his own ~ за его́ со́бственный счёт; additional ~s накладны́е расхо́ды; 7) заря́д (*электри́ческий, огнестре́льный*); 8) посла́ние (*епи́скопа*); *юр.* речь (*судьи́*); 10) *тех.* загру́зка; ши́хта; 11) *воен.* ата́ка; сигна́л к ата́ке; 12) *церк.* па́ства.

charge II *v* 1) обвиня́ть, предъявля́ть обвине́ние (*with*); 2) поруча́ть, вменя́ть в обя́занность (*что-л.* — *with*); 3) возлага́ть отве́тственность (*на кого́-л.; за* — *with*); 4) обременя́ть (*па́мять*); 5) насыща́ть (*чем-л.*); 6) запи́сывать на (*чей-л.*) счёт; 7) назнача́ть це́ну, проси́ть (*за что-л.* — *for*); how much (*или* what) do you ~ for? ско́лько сто́ит?; 8) заряжа́ть (*ору́жие, аккумуля́тор*); 9) *тех.* загружа́ть; засыпа́ть; 10) *воен.* атакова́ть (*особ. в ко́нном строю́*).

chargeable [ˈtʃɑːdʒəbl] *a* 1) подлежа́щий опла́те, обложе́нию; 2) заслу́живающий обвине́ния.

chargé d'affaires [ˈʃɑːʒeɪdæˈfɛə] *n* (*pl* chargés d'affaires) пове́ренный в дела́х.

charger [ˈtʃɑːdʒə] *n* 1) боево́й конь; 2) патро́нная обо́йма.

chariot [ˈtʃærɪət] *n* поэт., ист. колесни́ца.

charitable [ˈtʃærɪtəbl] *a* 1) благотвори́тельный; 2) ще́дрый; сострада́тельный.

charity [ˈtʃærɪtɪ] *n* 1) милосе́рдие; отзы́вчивость; 2) благотвори́тельность; ми́лостыня; 3) благотвори́тельное о́бщество.

charity-school [ˈtʃærɪtɪˌskuːl] *n* шко́ла для бе́дных дете́й (*организо́ванная благотвори́тельным о́бществом*).

charivari [ˌʃɑːrɪˈvɑːrɪ] *n* шум и гам.

charlatan I [ˈʃɑːlətən] *n* шарлата́н; зна́харь.

charlatan II *a* шарлата́нский.

charlotte [ˈʃɑːlət] *n* шарло́тка (*сла́дкое блю́до*).

charm I [tʃɑːm] *n* 1) обая́ние; очарова́ние; 2) *pl* ча́ры; 3) амуле́т; 4) брело́к.

charm II *v* 1) очаро́вывать, прельща́ть; околдо́вывать; 2) заколдо́вывать; 3) заклина́ть; прируча́ть (*змей*); 4) успока́ивать (*боль*).

charmer [ˈtʃɑːmə] *n* 1) *шутл.* чароде́йка, обая́тельная же́нщина; 2) заклина́тель (*змей*).

charming [ˈtʃɑːmɪŋ] *a* преле́стный, очарова́тельный; обая́тельный.

charnel-house [ˈtʃɑːnlhaus] *n* склеп.

chart I [tʃɑːt] *n* 1) морска́я ка́рта; temperature ~ ка́рта температу́р; weather ~ синопти́ческая ка́рта; 2) диагра́мма; табли́ца; схе́ма; чертёж.

chart II *v* наноси́ть на ка́рту; черти́ть ка́рту.

charter I [ˈtʃɑːtə] *n* 1) ха́ртия, гра́мота; The Great Charter *ист.* Вели́кая ха́ртия во́льностей (*1215 г.*); The People's Charter програ́мма чарти́стов (*1838 г.*); Universal Charter of Human Rights Всеми́рная ха́ртия прав челове́ка; 2) уста́в; 3) привиле́гия.

charter II *v* 1) дарова́ть (*ха́ртию, гра́моту*); 2) (за)фрахтова́ть (*су́дно*).

Charterhouse [ˈtʃɑːtəhaus] *n* дом для престаре́лых пенсионе́ров (*в Ло́ндоне*).

chartism [ˈtʃɑːtɪzəm] *n ист.* чарти́зм.

chartist [ˈtʃɑːtɪst] *n ист.* чарти́ст.

charwoman [ˈtʃɑːˌwumən] *n* подёнщица, убо́рщица.

chary [ˈtʃɛərɪ] *a* 1) осторо́жный; 2) сде́ржанный, скупо́й (*на слова́ и т. п.; of*).

chase[1] I [tʃeɪs] *n* 1) пого́ня, пресле́дование; to give ~ гна́ться, пресле́довать; 2) охо́та; 3) неогоро́женная террито́рия па́рка; 4) дичь; пресле́дуемый зверь; 5) пресле́дуемый кора́бль; ◊ a wild-goose ~ сумасбро́дная зате́я; пого́ня за неосуществи́мым.

chase[1] II *v* 1) гоня́ться (*за кем-л.*); охо́титься; 2) гна́ться, пресле́довать; 3) выгоня́ть, изгоня́ть (*из чего́-л.* — *from, out of*); *перен.* рассе́ивать, разгоня́ть.

chase[2] *v* гравирова́ть (*на мета́лле, ка́мне*).

chaser [ˈtʃeɪsə] *n* 1) пресле́дователь; 2) самолёт-истреби́тель; 3) морско́й охо́тник (*су́дно*).

chasing [ˈtʃeɪsɪŋ] *n* пресле́дование, пого́ня.

chasm [ˈkæzəm] *n* 1) про́пасть (*тж. перен.*); 2) пучи́на, бе́здна; 3) глубо́кая рассе́лина.

chassis [ˈʃæsɪ] *n* (*pl тж.* chassis [ˈʃæsɪz]) *ав.* ра́ма, шасси́.

chaste [tʃeɪst] *a* 1) целому́дренный; 2) стро́гий (*о сти́ле*); просто́й.

chasten [ˈtʃeɪsn] *v* 1) кара́ть; 2) очища́ть (*стиль*).

chastise [tʃæsˈtaɪz] *v* 1) нака́зывать, бить; 2) де́лать стро́гий вы́говор.

chastisement [ˈtʃæstɪzmənt] *n* дисциплина́рное взыска́ние; наказа́ние.

chastity [ˈtʃæstɪtɪ] *n* 1) целому́дрие; де́вственность; 2) чистота́, стро́гость (*сти́ля*).

chasuble [ˈtʃæzjubl] *n церк.* ри́за, облаче́ние.

chat I [tʃæt] *n* разгово́р, бесе́да; болтовня́; to have a ~ поговори́ть, побесе́довать; to have a nice ~ наговори́ться до́сыта.

chat II *v* бесе́довать, болта́ть.

chattels [ˈtʃætlz] *n pl* пожи́тки.

chatter I [ˈtʃætə] *n* 1) болтовня́; 2) щебета́ние; 3) дребезжа́ние.

chatter II *v* 1) треща́ть, болта́ть без у́молку; 2) щебета́ть; 3) стуча́ть (*зуба́ми*); 4) дребезжа́ть.

chatterbox [ˈtʃætəbɔks] *n* 1) болту́н, -нья; 2) *амер. воен. сленг* пулемёт.

chatterer [ˈtʃætərə] *n* болту́н, -нья.

chatty [ˈtʃætɪ] *a* болтли́вый.

chauffeur [ˈʃoufə] *n* шофёр, води́тель (*маши́ны*).

chauvinism ['ʃouvɪnɪzəm] *n* шовини́зм.

chauvinist ['ʃouvɪnɪst] *n* шовини́ст.

chaw [tʃɔ:] *v груб.* жева́ть; ча́вкать; □ to ~ **up** *амер.* разби́ть на́голову.

cheap I [tʃi:p] *a* дешёвый; ~ and nasty дёшево, да гни́ло.

cheap II *adv* дёшево; to hold ~ не дорожи́ть; to go ~ идти́ по дешёвой цене́; to get off ~ дёшево отде́латься; to feel ~ *сленг* чу́вствовать себя́ нело́вко, «не в свое́й таре́лке».

cheapen ['tʃi:pən] *v* 1) дешеве́ть; 2) снижа́ть це́ну.

cheat I [tʃi:t] *n* 1) обма́н; жу́льничество; 2) обма́нщик; жу́лик, плут; ◊ topping ~ *сленг* ви́селица.

cheat II *v* обма́нывать; обжу́ливать, надува́ть.

check[1] I [tʃek] *n* 1) остано́вка; заде́ржка; препя́тствие; 2) прове́рка, контро́ль; *перен.* узда́; loyalty ~ прове́рка лоя́льности (*в США*); to keep (*или* to hold) in ~ сде́рживать; to keep a ~ on проверя́ть; 3) га́лочка, пти́чка (*на поля́х*); 4) номеро́к (*в гардеро́бе*); бага́жная квита́нция; контрама́рка; 5) кле́тчатая ткань; кле́тка (*на тка́ни*); 6) *шахм.* шах; 7) *воен.* приостано́вка наступле́ния; ◊ to hand in one's ~s *разг.* умере́ть.

check[1] II *a* 1) контро́льный; 2) кле́тчатый.

check[1] III *v* 1) сде́рживать, приостана́вливать, остана́вливать; 2) *шахм.* объявля́ть шах; 3) проверя́ть, контроли́ровать; сверя́ть; □ to ~ **out** *амер.* а) уйти́ в отста́вку; б) освободи́ть но́мер (*в гости́нице*); to ~ **up** проверя́ть, ревизова́ть.

check[2] *n амер. см.* cheque.

checkerboard ['tʃekəbɔ:d] *n* ша́хматная доска́.

checkered ['tʃekəd] *a* 1) кле́тчатый; 2) пёстрый; 3) разнообра́зный.

checkmate I ['tʃek'meɪt] *n* 1) *шахм.* шах и мат; 2) круше́ние, по́лное пораже́ние.

checkmate II *v* 1) *шахм.* сде́лать мат; 2) расстро́ить (*пла́ны*); нанести́ пораже́ние.

check-off ['tʃek'ɔ:f] *n амер.* удержа́ние профсою́зных чле́нских взно́сов непосре́дственно из за́работной пла́ты.

check-room ['tʃekrum] *n амер.* 1) гардеро́бная; 2) ка́мера хране́ния.

check-up ['tʃek'ʌp] *n амер.* 1) прове́рка; реви́зия; 2) *attr* ревизио́нный.

cheek[1] [tʃi:k] *n* щека́; ◊ ~ by jowl *a)* бли́зкий, инти́мный; б) ря́дом, бок о́ бок; to one's own ~ *разг.* всё для себя́ одного́.

cheek[2] I *n* 1) *разг.* на́глость, наха́льство; де́рзость; to have the ~ to име́ть наха́льство; ~ brings success наха́льством всего́ добьёшься; 2) самоуве́ренность.

cheek[2] II *v разг.* наха́льничать, дерзи́ть.

cheek-bone ['tʃi:kboun] *n* скула́; with high ~s широкоску́лый.

cheeky ['tʃi:kɪ] *a разг.* на́глый, наха́льный; де́рзкий.

cheep I [tʃi:p] *n* писк.

cheep II *v* пища́ть.

cheer I [tʃɪə] *n* 1) одобри́тельное восклица́ние; three ~s for our captain! да здра́вствует капита́н!; 2) *pl* аплодисме́нты; 3) настрое́ние; to be of good (of bad) ~ быть в хоро́шем (в плохо́м) настрое́нии; 4) угоще́ние.

cheer II *v* 1) одобря́ть; 2) (об)ра́довать; 3) аплоди́ровать; 4) подба́дривать; 5) приве́тствовать (*гро́мкими во́згласами*); □ to ~ **on** подба́дривать кри́ками (*о боле́льщиках*); to ~ **up** утеша́ть, ободря́ть; ра́довать; ~ up! не уныва́й(те)!, держи́(те)сь!

cheerful ['tʃɪəful] *a* 1) весёлый; жизнера́достный; 2) в хоро́шем настрое́нии; 3) я́ркий (*о дне, цве́те и т. п.*).

cheerfulness ['tʃɪəfulnɪs] *n* жизнера́достность; бо́дрость.

cheerily ['tʃɪərɪlɪ] *adv* ра́достно, ве́село.

cheerio(h) ['tʃɪərɪ'ou] *int разг.* 1) приве́т! (*при встре́че*); 2) пока́! (*при расстава́нии*); 3) (за) ва́ше здоро́вье!

cheerless ['tʃɪəlɪs] *a* уны́лый, безра́достный, угрю́мый.

cheery ['tʃɪərɪ] *a разг.* живо́й, ра́достный, весёлый.

cheese[1] [tʃi:z] *n* сыр; a ~ голо́вка сы́ра; cottage ~ творо́г; green ~ молодо́й сыр; ripe ~ о́стрый (вы́держанный) сыр; ◊ to make ~s де́лать ревера́нсы.

cheese[2] *n сленг*: big ~ *амер.* ва́жная персо́на, «ши́шка».

cheese-cake ['tʃi:zkeɪk] *n* ватру́шка.

cheesemonger ['tʃi:z,mʌŋgə] *n* торго́вец моло́чными проду́ктами.

chef [ʃef] *n* шеф-по́вар.

chef-d'oeuvre [ʃeɪ'də:vr] *n* (*pl* chefs-d'oeuvre) шеде́вр.

chemical ['kemɪkəl] *a* хими́ческий.

chemicals ['kemɪkəlz] *n pl* химика́лии.

chemise [ʃɪ'mi:z] *n* же́нская соро́чка.

chemisette [,ʃemi:'zet] *n* вста́вка, мани́шка.

chemist ['kemɪst] *n* 1) хи́мик; 2) апте́карь.

chemistry ['kemɪstrɪ] *n* 1) хи́мия; organic (inorganic, industrial) ~ органи́ческая (неоргани́ческая, техни́ческая) хи́мия; agricultural ~ агрохи́мия; tracer ~ хи́мия ме́ченых а́томов; 2) *разг.* та́ктика; приёмы, фо́кусы.

cheque [tʃek] *n* чек; to cash a ~ получи́ть де́ньги по че́ку; to draw a ~ вы́дать чек.

cheque-book ['tʃekbuk] *n* че́ковая кни́жка.

chequer I ['tʃekə] *n* 1) *pl* ша́хматная доска́ (*вы́веска гости́ницы*); 2) *pl амер.* ша́шки; 3) *обыкн.* *pl* кле́тчатая мате́рия.

chequer II *v* 1) графи́ть в кле́тку; 2) располага́ть в ша́хматном поря́дке; 3) разнообра́зить.

chequer-wise ['tʃekəwaɪz] *adv* в ша́хматном поря́дке.

cherish ['tʃerɪʃ] *v* 1) леле́ять; 2) забо́тливо выра́щивать.

cherry I ['tʃerɪ] *n* ви́шня (*плод и де́рево*).

cherry II *a* вишнёвый; вишнёвого цве́та, я́рко-кра́сный.

cherry-pie ['tʃerɪ'paɪ] *n* 1) гелиотро́п; 2) пиро́г с ви́шнями.

cherry-stone ['tʃerɪstoun] *n* вишнёвая ко́сточка.

cherub ['tʃerəb] *n* (*pl тж.* cherubim ['tʃerəbɪm]) херуви́м.

chess [tʃes] *n* ша́хматы; to play ~ игра́ть в ша́хматы.

chess-board ['tʃesbɔ:d] *n* ша́хматная доска́.

chess-man ['tʃesmæn] *n* ша́хматная фигу́ра.

chess-player ['tʃes,pleɪə] *n* шахмати́ст.

chest [tʃest] *n* 1) большо́й я́щик; сунду́к;

carpenter's ~ я́щик с пло́тничьими инструме́нтами; a ~ of tea я́щик ча́я (около 108 англ. фунтов = около 49 кг); medicine ~ дома́шняя апте́чка; 2) казна́; military ~ войскова́я казна́; 3) грудна́я кле́тка.

chesterfield ['tʃestəfiːld] n 1) дли́нное одно-бо́ртное пальто́; 2) куше́тка.

chestnut I ['tʃesnʌt] n 1) кашта́н (тж. Spanish ~, sweet ~); 2) разг. каўрая, гнеда́я ло́шадь; 3) сленг изби́тый анекдо́т; 4) pl сленг пу́ли; ◊ to pull smb's ~ out of the fire ≅ чужи́ми рука́ми жар загреба́ть; таска́ть кашта́ны из огня́ для кого́-л.

chestnut II a 1) кашта́новый, кашта́нового цве́та; 2) разг. каўрый, гнедо́й.

chest-of-drawers ['tʃestəv,drɔːz] n комо́д.

chest-trouble ['tʃest,trʌbl] n хрони́ческая боле́знь лёгких.

chest-voice ['tʃestvɔis] n грудно́й го́лос.

chevalier [,ʃevə'liə] n 1) (благоро́дный) ры́царь; 2) кавале́р (о́рдена); ◊ ~ of industry (или of fortune) авантюри́ст.

cheviot ['tʃeviət] n шевио́т.

chevron ['ʃevrən] n наши́вка, шевро́н.

chevy I ['tʃevi] n охо́та, пого́ня.

chevy II v гна́ться.

chew I [tʃuː] n жва́чка.

chew II v 1) жева́ть; 2) размышля́ть, обду́мывать (upon, over).

chewing-gum ['tʃuːiŋgʌm] n жева́тельная рези́нка.

chicane [ʃi'kein] v 1) придира́ться; 2) занима́ться крючкотво́рством.

chicanery [ʃi'keinəri] n 1) приди́рка; 2) крючкотво́рство; 3) софи́стика.

chick [tʃik] n птене́ц; the ~s ребя́та, малыши́, мелюзга́.

chicken ['tʃikin] n 1) цыплёнок; птене́ц; перен. тж. малы́ш; 2) куря́тина; ◊ don't count one's ~s before they are hatched посл. ≅ цыпля́т по о́сени счита́ют; Mother Cary's ~ мор. буреве́стник.

chicken-hearted ['tʃikin,hɑːtid] a трусли́вый; малоду́шный.

chicken-liver ['tʃikin,livə] n трус.

chicken-pox ['tʃikinpɔks] n ветряна́я о́спа.

chicory ['tʃikəri] n цико́рий.

chid [tʃid] past. p. p. см. chide.

chidden ['tʃidn] p. p. см. chide.

chide [tʃaid] v (past chid; p. p. chid, chidden) 1) брани́ть, ворча́ть; 2) выть, реве́ть (о ветре).

chief I [tʃiːf] n 1) ли́дер; глава́, руководи́тель; нача́льник; прави́тель; вождь (племени, клана).

chief II a 1) гла́вный; основно́й; 2) руководя́щий.

chiefly ['tʃiːfli] adv гла́вным о́бразом; осо́бенно.

chieftain ['tʃiːftən] n 1) вождь (племени, клана); 2) атама́н (ша́йки); 3) поэт. военача́льник, полково́дец.

chiff-chaff ['tʃiftʃæf] n пе́ночка (птица).

chilblain ['tʃilblein] n отморо́женное ме́сто.

chilblained ['tʃilbleind] a отморо́женный.

child [tʃaild] n (pl children) 1) ребёнок; дитя́; from a ~ с де́тства; with ~ бере́менная; natural ~ внебра́чный ребёнок; to spoil the ~ балова́ть ре-

бёнка; 2) сын, дочь; 3) пото́мок, о́тпрыск; перен. дети́ще; ◊ a burnt ~ dreads the fire посл. ≅ пу́ганая воро́на куста́ бои́тся.

childbirth ['tʃaildbəːθ] n 1) ро́ды; she died in ~ она́ умерла́ от ро́дов; 2) рожда́емость.

childhood ['tʃaildhud] n де́тство.

childish ['tʃaildiʃ] a 1) де́тский; 2) инфанти́льный; 3) ребя́ческий; глу́пый.

childlike ['tʃaildlaik] a по-де́тски неви́нный, и́скренний.

children ['tʃildrən] pl см. child.

Chilean I ['tʃiliən] n чили́ец.

Chilean II a чили́йский.

chill I [tʃil] n 1) прохла́да; перен. хо́лодность, холодо́к (в обраще́нии); to take the ~ off немно́го согре́ться; 2) озно́б; to catch a ~ просту́диться; 3) тех. зака́лка.

chill II a холо́дный; перен. тж. расхола́живающий.

chill III v 1) охлажда́ть(ся); 2) чу́вствовать озно́б; 3) приводи́ть в уны́ние; удруча́ть; 4) тех. зака́ливать.

chilly I ['tʃili] a 1) прохла́дный (о пого́де); 2) зя́бкий; 3) холо́дный (об обраще́нии, приёме).

chilly II adv 1) хо́лодно; 2) неприве́тливо, су́хо.

chime I [tʃaim] n 1) набо́р колоколо́в; 2) pl колоко́льный звон; бой ба́шенных часо́в; 3) мело́дия; ритм; 4) гармо́ния; согла́сие.

chime II v 1) звони́ть (в колокола́); 2) проби́ть (о часа́х); выбива́ть мело́дию; 3) соотве́тствовать, гармони́ровать (in, with); □ to ~ in а) присоединя́ться к разгово́ру, пе́нию и т. п.; б) вто́рить; в) совпада́ть (с чем-л. — with).

chimera [kai'miərə] n химе́ра.

chimerical [kai'merikəl] a химери́ческий, фантасти́ческий; несбы́точный.

chimney ['tʃimni] n 1) ками́н; 2) труба́ (дымова́я, парохо́дная); дымохо́д; 3) ла́мповое стекло́; 4) рассе́лина (в скале́); 5) кра́тер (вулка́на).

chimney-corner ['tʃimni,kɔːnə] n ме́сто у каме́лька, ками́на; перен. ую́тный уголо́к.

chimney-piece ['tʃimnipiːs] n по́лка над ками́ном.

chimney-pot ['tʃimnipɔt] n дымова́я труба́ (нару́жная).

chimney-stack ['tʃimnistæk] n о́бщий дымохо́д.

chimney-stalk ['tʃimnistɔːk] n заводска́я труба́.

chimney-sweep(er) ['tʃimni,swiːp(ə)] n трубочи́ст.

chimpanzee [,tʃimpən'ziː] n шимпанзе́.

chin [tʃin] n подборо́док; to scrape one's ~ бри́ться; up to the ~ ≅ по́ уши, по го́рло.

China ['tʃainə] a кита́йский.

china I ['tʃainə] n фарфо́р; a piece of ~ фарфо́ровая ча́шка, статуэ́тка и т. п.

china II a фарфо́ровый.

china-clay ['tʃainə'klei] n каоли́н.

Chinaman ['tʃainəmən] n 1) пренебр. кита́ец; 2) (с.) торго́вец фарфо́ром; 3) кита́йское су́дно.

china-ware ['tʃainəwɛə] n фарфо́ровые изде́лия.

Chinawoman ['tʃainə,wumən] n пренебр. китая́нка.

Chinese I ['tʃai'niːz] n 1) кита́ец; китая́нка;

the ~ (*употр. как pl*) китайцы; 2) китайский язык.

Chinese II *a* китайский.

chink¹ [tʃɪŋk] *n* трещина, щель; скважина.

chink² I *n* 1) звон, звяканье (*стаканов, монет*); 2) *разг.* наличные деньги.

chink² II *v* звенеть, звякать (*о посуде, монетах*).

chink³ *n* приступ кашля *или* смеха.

chintz [tʃɪnts] *n* (вощёный) ситец.

chintz II *a* ситцевый.

chip I [tʃɪp] *n* 1) щепка; стружка; 2) обломок; осколок; 3) *pl разг.* чипсы, хрустящий картофель; ◊ a ~ of the old block вылитый отец (*о ребёнке*); as dry as a ~ совершенно сухой.

chip II *v* 1) отщипывать (*лучину*); стругать; 2) откалывать; отбивать; 3) ломаться, биться (*о посуде*); 4) пробивать яичную скорлупу (*о цыплятах*); 5) жарить картофель стружкой; □ to ~ in *разг.* вмешиваться, ввязываться (*в разговор, драку*).

chippy [tʃɪpɪ] *a* 1) зазубренный (*о ноже*); щербатый (*о посуде*); 2) *сленг* раздражительный (*с похмелья*); «не в своей тарелке».

chiropody [kɪˈɡɔrədɪ] *n* маникюр; педикюр.

chirp I [tʃəːp] *n* чириканье; щебетание.

chirp II *v* 1) чирикать; щебетать; 2) весело болтать.

chirpy [ˈtʃəːpɪ] *a* жизнерадостный, оживлённый; весёлый.

chirr I [tʃəː] *n* 1) стрекотание (*кузнечиков, сверчков*); 2) шуршание (*тростника*).

chirr II *v* 1) стрекотать (*о кузнечиках, сверчках*); 2) шуршать (*о тростнике*).

chirrup I [ˈtʃɪrəp] *n* щебет, щебетание.

chirrup II *v* щебетать.

chisel I [ˈtʃɪzl] *n* 1) резец; 2) *тех.* зубило, долото; boring ~ долото; cold ~ слесарное зубило; pointed ~ гравёрный резец; wood ~ стамеска; 3) (the ~) искусство скульптора, ваяние; 4) *разг.* надувательство.

chisel II *v* 1) ваять, высекать; 2) работать зубилом, долотом; 3) отделывать (*стиль произведения*); 4) *разг.* надувать.

chiselled [ˈtʃɪzld] *a* отделанный, точёный.

chit¹ [tʃɪt] *n* ребёнок; крошка; a ~ of a girl *пренебр.* девчонка.

chit² *n инд.* 1) донесение; 2) письменная характеристика; рекомендация; 3) письмо; записка.

chit-chat [ˈtʃɪttʃæt] *n* 1) болтовня; 2) сплетни, пересуды.

chivalric [ˈʃɪvəlrɪk] *см.* chivalrous.

chivalrous [ˈʃɪvəlrəs] *a* рыцарский; благородный.

chivalry [ˈʃɪvəlrɪ] *n* 1) рыцарство; 2) рыцари.

chloride I [ˈklɔːraɪd] *n хим.* хлорид; cuprous ~ хлористая медь.

chloride II *a хим.* хлористоводородный; хлористый.

chlorine [ˈklɔːriːn] *n хим.* хлор.

chloroform I [ˈklɔrəfɔːm] *n* хлороформ.

chloroform II *v* усыплять.

chlorophyll [ˈklɔrəfɪl] *n бот.* хлорофилл.

chlorous [ˈklɔːrəs] *a хим.* хлористый.

chock I [tʃɔk] *n* 1) клин; 2) подставка; 3) *тех.* тормозная колодка, башмак.

chock II *v* 1) подкладывать (*подстилку, подставку*); 2) *тех.* заклинивать; □ to ~ up а) заклинить; забить; б) заставить (*мебелью*).

chock-full [ˈtʃɔkful] *a* битком набитый.

chocolate I [ˈtʃɔkəlɪt] *n* 1) шоколад; 2) *pl* шоколадные конфеты; 3) шоколадный цвет.

chocolate II *a* шоколадного цвета, тёмно-коричневый.

choice I [tʃɔɪs] *n* 1) выбор; отбор; to make ~ of выбирать; отбирать; to make (*или* to take) one's ~ сделать для себя выбор, решить; I have no ~ but to... мне ничего другого не остаётся, как...; 3) выбранный предмет; 4) избранник, -ица; ◊ Hobson's ~ отсутствие выбора; наличие только одного предложения.

choice II *a* отборный, лучший.

choir I [ˈkwaɪə] *n* 1) хор; 2) хоры; клирос.

choir II *v поэт.* петь хором.

choke I [tʃouk] *n* 1) припадок удушья; 2) суженная часть (*трубы*); 3) *тех.* воздушная заслонка, дроссель.

choke II *v* 1) душить; 2) задыхаться (*от волнения и т. п.*); 3) поперхнуться; подавиться; давиться (*от кашля*); 4) заглушать (*растение*); □ to ~ down а) с трудом глотать (*пищу*); б) подавлять (*слёзы*); to ~ in *амер. разг.* держать язык за зубами; to ~ off принудить к отказу (*от намерения*); to ~ up засорять, заносить (*песком*); забивать (*проезд, проход*), загромождать.

choke-damp [ˈtʃoukdæmp] *n* рудничный газ.

choker [ˈtʃoukə] *n* 1) стоячий крахмальный воротник; 2) *сленг* галстук (*тж.* white ~).

cholera [ˈkɔlərə] *n* холера; summer ~ дизентерия.

choleric [ˈkɔlərɪk] *a* раздражительный, жёлчный.

choose [tʃuːz] *v* (*past* chose; *p. p.* chosen) 1) выбирать; cannot ~ but должен; 2) избирать; 3) предпочитать.

choos(e)y [ˈtʃuːzɪ] *a разг.* разборчивый, привередливый.

chop¹ I [tʃɔp] *n* 1) удар (*топором*); 2) отбивная котлета.

chop¹ II *v* 1) рубить (*топором*); 2) резать, крошить; 3) отчеканивать (*слова*); □ to ~ about обрубать, рубить; to ~ up крошить.

chop² *n обыкн. pl* челюсть.

chop² I *n* .1) перемена, колебание; 2) зыбь, лёгкое волнение (*на море*).

chop³ II *v* 1) обменивать, менять; 2) меняться, колебаться; □ to ~ about резко менять направление (*о ветре*); to ~ in ввязаться в разговор.

chop⁴ *n* клеймо, фабричная марка; first (second) ~ первый (второй) сорт.

chop-house [ˈtʃɔphaus] *n* дешёвый ресторан.

chopper [ˈtʃɔpə] *n* 1) косарь, колун; нож (*мясника*); 2) *амер.* контролёр, билетёр.

choppy [ˈtʃɔpɪ] *a* порывистый (*о ветре*).

chopsticks [ˈtʃɔpstɪks] *n pl* палочки для еды (*в Китае и т. п.*).

choral [ˈkɔrəl] *a* хоровой.

chorale [kɔˈrɑːl] *n* хорал.

chord¹ [kɔːd] *n* 1) *поэт.* струна; to touch the right ~ задеть за живое; 2) *мат.* хорда;

3) *анат.* связка; vocal ~s голосовы́е свя́зки; spinal ~ спинно́й мозг.

chord² *n* 1) *муз.* акко́рд; 2) га́мма (*красок*).

chorister ['kɔrɪstə] *n* хори́ст, пе́вчий.

chorus I ['kɔːrəs] *n* 1) хор; in ~ хо́ром; 2) музыка́льное произведе́ние для хорово́го исполне́ния; 3) припе́в.

chorus II *v* говори́ть *или* петь хо́ром.

chose [tʃouz] *past см.* choose.

chosen ['tʃouzn] *p. p. см.* choose.

chouse I [tʃaus] *n разг.* моше́нничество.

chouse II *v разг.* обма́нывать; выма́нивать.

chow [tʃau] *n разг.* еда́.

chowder ['tʃaudə] *n* густа́я похлёбка из ры́бы *или* моллю́сков (*со свини́ной, сухаря́ми, овоща́ми и т. п.*).

Christ [kraɪst] *n* Христо́с.

christen ['krɪsn] *v* 1) крести́ть; дава́ть и́мя при креще́нии; 2) называ́ть, дава́ть и́мя (*кораблю́ и т. п.*); 3) *разг.* по́льзоваться в пе́рвый раз, «обновля́ть».

Christian I ['krɪstʃən] *n* христиани́н; христиа́нка.

Christian II *a* христиа́нский.

Christianity [ˌkrɪstɪˈænɪtɪ] *n* христиа́нство.

christianize ['krɪstjənaɪz] *v* обраща́ть в христиа́нство.

Christmas ['krɪsməs] *n* 1) рождество́ (*сокр. тж.* Xmas); 2) *attr* рожде́ственский.

Christmas-box ['krɪsməsbɔks] *n* рожде́ственский пода́рок.

Christmas-tide ['krɪsməsˌtaɪd] *n* свя́тки.

Christmas-tree ['krɪsməstriː] *n* рожде́ственская ёлка.

chromatic [krəˈmætɪk] *a* 1) цветно́й; 2) *муз.* хромати́ческий.

chrome [kroum] *n хим.* хром.

chromic ['kroumɪk] *a хим.* хро́мовый.

chromium ['kroumjəm] *см.* chrome.

chromo ['kroumou] *n* хромолитогра́фия.

chromolithograph ['kroumouˈlɪθəɡrɑːf] *n* хромолитогра́фия.

chronic ['krɔnɪk] *a* 1) застаре́лый, хрони́ческий (*о боле́зни*); 2) постоя́нный, привы́чный.

chronicle I ['krɔnɪkl] *n* хро́ника; ле́топись.

chronicle II *v* 1) заноси́ть, запи́сывать (*в ле́топись, дневни́к*); 2) вести́ хро́нику (*в газе́те*); отмеча́ть в пре́ссе.

chronicler ['krɔnɪklə] *n* летопи́сец; хроникёр.

chronologic(al) [ˌkrɔnəˈlɔdʒɪk(əl)] *a* хронологи́ческий.

chronology [krəˈnɔlədʒɪ] *n* 1) хроноло́гия; 2) хронологи́ческая табли́ца.

chronometer [krəˈnɔmɪtə] *n* 1) хроно́метр; 2) *муз.* метроно́м.

chrysanthemum [krɪˈsænθəməm] *n* хризанте́ма.

chubby ['tʃʌbɪ] *a* пу́хлый (*о щека́х*); круглоли́цый.

chuck¹ [tʃʌk] *n* чурба́н.

chuck² I *n разг.* 1) швыря́ние; 2) (the ~) увольне́ние.

chuck² II *v разг.* 1) швыря́ть; 2): to ~ under the chin трепа́ть за подборо́док; □ to ~ **away** а) упуска́ть слу́чай; б) сори́ть (*деньга́ми*); to ~ **out** выгоня́ть, выводи́ть, выставля́ть (*посети́теля*); to ~ **up** бро́сить (*рабо́ту, до́лжность*); ◇ ~ it! замолчи́(те).

chuck³ I *n* 1) цыплёнок; *ласк.* цы́почка; 2) куда́хтанье; 3) понука́ние (*ло́шади*).

chuck³ II *v* 1) склика́ть дома́шнюю пти́цу; 2) понука́ть ло́шадь.

chuck³ III *int*: ~!, ~! цып, цып!

chuck⁴ *n сленг* еда́, пи́ща.

chuckle I ['tʃʌkl] *n* 1) дово́льный смешо́к, хихи́канье; 2) усме́шка; 3) ра́дость; 4) куда́хтанье.

chuckle II *v* 1) хихи́кать; 2) усмеха́ться; ра́доваться (*чему́-л.— over*); 3) куда́хтать.

chuckle-head ['tʃʌklhed] *n* болва́н.

chuff [tʃʌf] *n* 1) грубия́н; 2) скря́га.

chug [tʃʌɡ] *n* пыхте́нье.

chug *v* пыхте́ть.

chum I [tʃʌm] *n разг.* 1) прия́тель, това́рищ; new ~ переселе́нец, новосёл (*в Австра́лии*); 2) това́рищ по ко́мнате (*в общежи́тии*).

chum II *v разг.* 1) жить в одно́й ко́мнате (*с кем-л.— with; тж.* to ~ together); 2) дружи́ть (*с кем-л.— with*); □ to ~ **in**, to ~ **up** *разг.* сбли́зиться (*с кем-л.— with*).

chummy ['tʃʌmɪ] *a разг.* общи́тельный.

chump [tʃʌmp] *n* 1) чурба́н; 2) *разг.* голова́, башка́; he is off his ~ он тро́нулся, у него́ не все до́ма; 3) *разг.* болва́н, дура́к; 4) филе́йная часть (*мясно́й ту́ши*).

chunk [tʃʌŋk] *n* 1) кусо́к, ломо́ть; 2) корена́стый челове́к.

church [tʃəːtʃ] *n* це́рковь; the Church of England англика́нская це́рковь; to go into the Church принима́ть духо́вный сан; Free Church незави́симая це́рковь (*в Шотла́ндии*).

churchwarden ['tʃəːtʃˈwɔːdn] *n* 1) церко́вный ста́роста; 2) дли́нная кури́тельная тру́бка (*из гли́ны*).

churchy ['tʃəːtʃɪ] *a разг.* еле́йный.

churchyard ['tʃəːtʃˈjɑːd] *n* кла́дбище.

churl [tʃəːl] *n* 1) гру́бый, невоспи́танный челове́к; 2) скря́га.

churlish ['tʃəːlɪʃ] *a* 1) гру́бый, невоспи́танный; 2) скупо́й.

churn I [tʃəːn] *n* 1) маслобо́йка; 2) меша́лка.

churn II *v* 1) сбива́ть ма́сло; 2) взба́лтывать; вспе́нивать.

chut [tʃʌt] *int* ну! (*выража́ет нетерпе́ние*).

chute [ʃuːt] *n* 1) стремни́на, 2) круто́й скат.

'chute [ʃuːt] *n воен. разг.* парашю́т.

'chutist [ʃuːtɪst] *n воен. разг.* парашюти́ст.

cicada [sɪˈkɑːdə] *n* цика́да.

cicatrice ['sɪkətrɪs] *n* рубе́ц, шрам.

cicatrize ['sɪkətraɪz] *v* 1) заживля́ть; 2) зажива́ть.

cider ['saɪdə] *n* сидр.

cigar [sɪˈɡɑː] *n* сига́ра.

cigarette [ˌsɪɡəˈret] *n* папиро́са, сигаре́та.

cigarette-case [ˌsɪɡəˈretkeɪs] *n* портсига́р.

cigar-holder [sɪˈɡɑːˌhouldə] *n* мундшту́к.

cigar-store [sɪˈɡɑːstɔː] *n амер.* таба́чный магази́н.

ciliated ['sɪlɪeɪtɪd] *a* опушённый ресни́цами.

cinchona [sɪŋˈkounə] *n* 1) хи́нное де́рево; 2) хи́нная кора́; хини́н.

cinder ['sɪndə] *n* 1) шлак; 2) *обыкн. pl* тле́ющие у́гли; 3) *pl* пе́пел, зола́.

Cinderella [ˌsɪndəˈrelə] *n* Зо́лушка.

cinder-path ['sɪndəpɑːθ] *n* беговая (гаревая) дорожка.

cinema ['sɪnɪmə] *n* 1) кинотеатр; 2) (the ~) (кино)фильм.

cinematograph [,sɪnɪ'mætəgrɑːf] *n* 1) киноаппарат; 2) кинематограф, кинотеатр.

cinematographic [,sɪnɪ,mætə'græfɪk] *a* кинематографический.

cinematography [,sɪnɪmə'tɔgrəfɪ] *n* кинематография.

cinereous [sɪ'nɪərɪəs] *a* пепельный, пепельного цвета.

cinnamon ['sɪnəmən] *n* корица.

cinq(ue) [sɪŋk] *n* пятёрка (*в картах, домино и т. п.*).

cipher I ['saɪfə] *n* 1) нуль (*тж. перен.*); 2) арабская цифра; 3) шифр; in ~ зашифрованный; 4) ключ к шифру; 5) монограмма.

cipher II *v* 1) высчитывать (*обыкн.* to ~ out); вычислять; 2) шифровать, зашифровывать.

circa ['səːkə] *prep* около, приблизительно (*с датами*).

Circassian I [səː'kæʃən] *n* 1) черкес; черкешенка; the ~s черкесы; 2) черкесский язык.

Circassian II *a* черкесский.

circle I ['səːkl] *n* 1) круг (*тж. геогр.*); окружность; to complete the ~ замыкать круг; Arctic Circle Северный полярный круг; Antarctic Circle Южный полярный круг; 2) *астр.* орбита; 3) *театр.* ярус; *амер.* балкон; parquet ~ задние ряды партера, амфитеатр; upper ~ галёрка; 4) цикл, круговорот; 5) круг (*знакомых, друзей*); family ~ семейный круг; 6) область, сфера (*деятельности*); 7) кружок (*по учебной дисциплине*); 8) *pl* круги (*общественные*); business ~s деловые, финансовые круги; ◊ to square the ~ строить квадратуру круга; добиваться невозможного.

circle II *v* 1) вращаться; двигаться по кругу; 2) кружиться; 3) совершать кругосветное плавание.

circlet ['səːklɪt] *n* 1) кружок; 2) диадема; 3) браслет.

circuit ['səːkɪt] *n* 1) кругооборот; 2) длина окружности; 3) круговая поездка; объезд; to make a ~ of обходить, объезжать; 4) судебный округ; 5) члены выездной сессии суда; 6) *эл.* цепь; short ~ короткое замыкание; 7) цикл.

circuitous [səː'kjuːɪtəs] *a* окольный (*о пути*).

circular I ['səːkjulə] *n* 1) циркуляр; реклама, проспект.

circular II *a* 1) круглый; 2) круговой (*о движении*), вращательный; 3) циркулярный; 4) *мат.* дуговой; 5) винтовой (*о лестнице*).

circulate ['səːkjuleɪt] *v* 1) циркулировать (*о слухах, крови и т. п.*); 2) обращаться, находиться в обращении (*о деньгах*); 3) передавать(ся); 4) повторяться (*о периодической дроби*).

circulation [,səːkju'leɪʃən] *n* 1) кругооборот; повторяющийся цикл; 2) циркуляция (*крови и т. п.*); кровообращение; poor ~ плохое кровообращение; 3) обращение (*тж. денежное*); in ~ в обращении; to withdraw from ~ изымать из обращения; to put in ~ пускать в обращение (*о деньгах, банкнотах*); 4) тираж; распространение (*газет, журналов*); 5) распространение (*слухов и т. п.*).

circulator ['səːkjuleɪtə] *n* 1) носитель (*заразы*); 2) распространитель (*слухов и т. п.*).

circulatory ['səːkjuleɪtərɪ] *a* циркулирующий.

circum- ['səːkəm-] *pref* в сложных словах означает вокруг, кругом.

circumambulate [,səːkəm'æmbjuleɪt] *v* обходить; ходить вокруг; *перен.* ходить вокруг да около.

circumference [sə'kʌmfərəns] *n* 1) окружность (*круга*); 2) периферия.

circumferential [sə,kʌmfə'renʃəl] *a* периферический.

circumfluent [sə'kʌmfluənt] *a* обтекающий.

circumfluous [sə'kʌmfluəs] *a* 1) омываемый; окружённый водой; 2) *см.* circumfluent.

circumlocution [,səːkəmlə'kjuːʃən] *n* 1) уклончивый разговор; 2) многоречивость.

circumlocutory [,səːkəm'lɔkjutərɪ] *a* 1) уклончивый; 2) многоречивый.

circumnavigate [,səːkəm'nævɪgeɪt] *v* совершать кругосветное плавание.

circumnavigation ['səːkəm,nævɪ'geɪʃən] *n* кругосветное плавание.

circumnavigator [,səːkəm'nævɪgeɪtə] *n* мореплаватель (*совершающий кругосветные путешествия*).

circumscribe ['səːkəmskraɪb] *v* 1) ограничивать; 2) *мат.* описывать (*окружность*).

circumscription [,səːkəm'skrɪpʃən] *n* 1) ограничение; граница, предел; 2) надпись (*по краю монеты и т. п.*).

circumspect ['səːkəmspekt] *a* осмотрительный; осторожный.

circumspection [,səːkəm'spekʃən] *n* осмотрительность.

circumstance ['səːkəmstəns] *n* 1) обстоятельство, случай; 2) *pl* обстоятельства; under no ~s ни при каких обстоятельствах; 3) *pl* материальное положение; narrow ~s стеснённые обстоятельства; in bad (*или* straitened, poor, reduced) ~s в стеснённом материальном положении; in easy (*или* good, flourishing) ~s в хорошем материальном положении; 4) *pl* подробности, детали; 5) церемония.

circumstantial [,səːkəm'stænʃəl] *a* 1) подробный, обстоятельный; 2) случайный; косвенный.

circumvent [,səːkəm'vent] *v* 1) обмануть; перехитрить; 2) расстроить (*планы*).

circus ['səːkəs] *n* 1) цирк; 2) амфитеатр; 3) арена; 4) круглая площадь (*с радиально расходящимися улицами*).

cirri ['sɪraɪ] *pl см.* cirrus.

cirro-cumulus ['sɪrou'kjuːmjuləs] *n* перисто-кучевые облака.

cirro-stratus ['sɪrou'streɪtəs] *n* перисто-слоистые облака.

cirrus ['sɪrəs] *n* (*pl* cirri) 1) перистые облака; 2) *бот., зоол.* усик.

cistern ['sɪstən] *n* 1) цистерна; резервуар; 2) водоём.

citadel ['sɪtədl] *n* 1) цитадель, крепость; 2) твердыня; 3) убежище, прибежище.

citation [saɪ'teɪʃən] *n* 1) ссылка, цитата; 2) перечисление; 3) вызов (*в суд*); 4) *амер.* объявление благодарности в приказе.

cite [saɪt] *v* 1) ссылаться на; цитировать; 2) вызывать (*в суд*).

cither(n) ['sɪθə(n)] *n* *ист., поэт.* лира; кифара, цитра.

citizen ['sɪtɪzn] *n* 1) гражданин; гражданка; 2) горожанин; горожанка.

citizenship ['sɪtɪznʃɪp] *n* гражданство.

citron ['sɪtrən] *n* 1) сладкий лимон, цитрон; 2) цукат.

citrus ['sɪtrəs] *n* *бот.* *собир.* цитрусовые.

cits [sɪts] *n* *pl* *амер.* *воен.* *разг.* штатское платье.

city ['sɪtɪ] *n* 1) большой город; the City a) Сити (*торговая и деловая часть Лондона*); б) финансовые и коммерческие круги Лондона; 2) *амер.* станция (обслуживания); auto ~ центр по продаже автомобилей; discount ~ универсальный магазин по продаже товаров по сниженным ценам; 3) *attr* городской; муниципальный; ◊ the Holy City Иерусалим; the Empire City Нью-Йорк.

civic ['sɪvɪk] *a* гражданский.

civics ['sɪvɪks] *n* основы гражданственности.

civil ['sɪvl] *a* 1) гражданский; 2) штатский; 3) вежливый, учтивый.

civilian I [sɪ'vɪljən] *n* штатский (человек).

civilian II *a* штатский, гражданский.

civility [sɪ'vɪlɪtɪ] *n* учтивость; любезность.

civilization [,sɪvɪlaɪ'zeɪʃən] *n* цивилизация.

civilize ['sɪvɪlaɪz] *v* цивилизовать.

civilized ['sɪvɪlaɪzd] *a* цивилизованный, культурный.

civ(v)y ['sɪvɪ] *n* *сленг* 1) штатский (человек); 2) *pl* *воен.* штатское платье.

clack I [klæk] *n* 1) треск; 2) болтовня.

clack II *v* 1) трещать; 2) громко болтать.

clad [klæd] *past, p. p.* *см.* clothe.

claim I [kleɪm] *n* 1) требование; to push one's ~ выставлять свои требования; 2) *юр.* иск, претензия; to lay ~ to предъявлять права (*на*); to prosecute a ~ for damages возбудить иск о возмещении убытков; 3) утверждение; 4) *горн.* участок, отведённый под разработку ископаемых; заявка на отвод участка.

claim II *v* 1) требовать; 2) претендовать на что-л.; предъявлять претензии; 3) утверждать; 4) *юр.* возбуждать иск (*о возмещении убытков*).

claimant ['kleɪmənt] *n* 1) *юр.* истец; 2) претендент.

clairvoyance [klɛə'vɔɪəns] *n* 1) проницательность; 2) ясновидение.

clairvoyant [klɛə'vɔɪənt] *a* 1) проницательный; 2) ясновидящий.

clam [klæm] *n* (съедобный) моллюск.

clamant ['kleɪmənt] *a* 1) шумливый; 2) настойчивый; 3) вопиющий (*о несправедливости*).

clamber I ['klæmbə] *n* карабканье.

clamber II *v* 1) карабкаться; 2) виться (*о растении*).

clammy ['klæmɪ] *a* клейкий, липкий.

clamorous ['klæmərəs] *a* шумный, крикливый.

clamour I ['klæmə] *n* 1) шум, крики; 2) шумный протест.

clamour II *v* 1) шуметь, кричать; 2) шумно требовать (*чего-л.— for*); шумно протестовать (*against*); □ to ~ **down** заставить замолчать (*криками*); to ~ **out** шумным протестом заставить сделать что-л.

clamp I [klæmp] *n* 1) скоба, скрепа, клемма; 2) клетка (*кирпича*); штабель (*торфа*).

clamp II *v* 1) скреплять; 2) складывать (*в кучу*).

clan [klæn] *n* 1) клан; 2) клика.

clandestine [klæn'destɪn] *a* тайный.

clang I [klæŋ] *n* звон, лязг.

clang II *v* звенеть, лязгать.

clangour ['klæŋgə] *n* резкий звон; лязг.

clank I [klæŋk] *n* звон (*цепей*); бряцание.

clank II *v* греметь (*цепью*); бряцать.

clanship ['klænʃɪp] *n* 1) деление на кланы; 2) деление на враждебные партии.

clap I [klæp] *n* 1) удар (*грома; тж.* a ~ of thunder); 2) хлопанье (*в ладоши*).

clap II *v* 1) хлопать в ладоши; аплодировать; 2) хлопать (*крыльями, руками*); 3) похлопывать (*по плечу*); 4) упрятать, упечь (*в тюрьму; in*); 5) захлопнуть (*крышку*); 6) нахлобучить (*шапку*); □ to ~ **on** a) поднять (*паруса*); б) облагать (*налогом*); to ~ **up** спешно заключить, состряпать (*сделку и т. п.*).

clap-net ['klæp,net] *n* силок для птиц.

clapper ['klæpə] *n* 1) язык (*колокола*); 2) трещотка.

claptrap I ['klæptræp] *n* трескучая фраза; что-л. показное.

claptrap II *a* показной.

clarence ['klærəns] *n* четырёхместная карета.

clarendon ['klærəndən] *n* *полигр.* жирный шрифт.

claret I ['klærət] *n* 1) кларет (*сорт вина*); 2) цвет бордо; 3) *сленг:* to tap one's ~ разбить (*кому-л.*) нос в кровь, расквасить нос (*кому-л.*).

claret II *a* цвета бордо.

clarification [,klærɪfɪ'keɪʃən] *n* 1) очистка, очищение; 2) прояснение; уяснение.

clarify ['klærɪfaɪ] *v* 1) очищать, делать прозрачным; 2) прояснять(ся); 3) уяснять; 4) *амер.* освещать.

clarinet [,klærɪ'net] *n* *муз.* кларнет.

clarion I ['klærɪən] *n* 1) *поэт.* рожок; горн; 2) звук рожка.

clarion II *a* звонкий, громкий.

clarity ['klærɪtɪ] *n* 1) ясность; 2) прозрачность.

clash I [klæʃ] *n* 1) столкновение; 2) конфликт; 3) лязг (*оружия*); 4) гул, шум.

clash II *v* 1) сталкиваться; приходить в столкновение; to ~ into smb. столкнуться с кем-л.; 2) совпадать во времени (*о лекциях и т. п.*); 3) расходиться (*о мнениях*); 4) звонить (*во все колокола*); 5) производить шум, лязг; лязгать (*оружием*).

clasp I [klɑːsp] *n* 1) пряжка; застёжка; 2) рукопожатие; 3) объятия.

clasp II *v* 1) обнимать; 2) сжимать, пожимать (*руки*); 3) застёгивать, пристёгивать.

clasp-knife ['klɑːsp'naɪf] *n* складной нож.

class¹ I [klɑːs] *n* класс (*общественный*; the working ~ рабочий класс; the middle ~ средняя буржуазия; the upper ~ крупная буржуазия; аристократия; the proprietory ~ имущий класс; landed ~es помещики, землевладельцы.

class¹ II *a* классовый.

class² I *n* 1) *биол.* класс; 2) разряд, кате-

гория, сорт; 3) класс (*группа учащихся*); to take
a ~ взять класс (*для обучения*); to take ~es
брать уроки, учиться (*чему-л.— in*); 4) год при-
зыва (*в армию*); 5) класс (*на железной дороге, пароходе*); 6) *амер.* выпуск (*студентов одного года*); 7) *мор.* тип (*корабля*).

class² II *a* классный (*о занятиях*).

class² III *v* классифицировать; *перен.* ставить
в один ряд (*c — with*).

class-book ['klɑːsbuk] *n* учебник.

class-conscious ['klɑːs'kɔnʃəs] *a* сознательный;
имеющий классовое сознание.

class-consciousness ['klɑːs'kɔnʃəsnɪs] *n* классовое сознание.

class-fellow ['klɑːs'felou] *n* однокласник.

classic I ['klæsɪk] *n* 1) классик (*писатель, художник и т. п.*); 2) специалист по класси-
ческой филологии; 3) *pl* классические языки и
литература.

classic II *a* 1) классический; 2) образцовый.

classical ['klæsɪkəl] *a* классический.

classicism ['klæsɪsɪzəm] *n* 1) классицизм;
2) *лингв.* латинская *или* греческая идиома.

classification [‚klæsɪfɪ'keɪʃən] *n* классифика-
ция.

classify ['klæsɪfaɪ] *v* классифицировать.

classless ['klɑːslɪs] *a* бесклассовый.

class-list ['klɑːslɪst] *n* экзаменационная ведомость.

class-mate ['klɑːsmeɪt] *n* однокласник.

clatter I ['klætə] *n* 1) треск, стук, грохот;
звон (*посуды и т. п.*); 2) трескотня; шум (*голосов*).

clatter II *v* 1) греметь (*посудой и т. п.*);
2) шуметь; □ to ~ **along** двигаться с грохотом;
грохотать; to ~ **down** «загреметь» (*вниз по
лестнице*).

clause [klɔːz] *n* 1) *грам.* предложение; principal (subordinate) ~ главное (придаточное)
предложение; 2) статья; пункт (*в договоре и т. п.*);
saving ~ статья, содержащая оговорку; ◇ escalator ~ условие «скользящей шкалы».

clave [kleɪv] *past см.* cleave².

clavichord ['klævɪkɔːd] *n муз.* клавикорды.

clavicle ['klævɪkl] *n анат.* ключица.

claw I [klɔː] *n* 1) коготь; to cut (*или* to
pare) smb.'s ~s пообломать когти кому-л.;
2) лапа (*с когтями*); 3) клешня; 4) *презр.* рука; 5) *тех.* клещи.

claw II *v* 1) скрести, царапать, рвать (*когтями*); 2) загребать (*деньги и т. п.*).

clay [kleɪ] *n* 1) глина; plastic ~ глина для
лепки; 2) земля; 3) *поэт.* прах; 4) глиняная
трубка; ◇ to moisten one's ~ промочить горло.

clayey ['kleɪɪ] *a* глинистый.

claymore ['kleɪmɔː] *n* палаш (*шотл. горцев*).

clean I [kliːn] *n*: to give it a ~ вычистить.

clean II *a* 1) чистый; 2) чистоплотный, опрят-
ный; 3) хорошо сложённый (*о человеке*); 4) ловкий, меткий.

clean III *v* 1) чистить, очищать; 2) убирать
(*комнату*); мыть (*посуду*); □ to ~ **down**
а) сметать (*пыль*); б) чистить (*лошадь*); to ~
out *разг.* обчистить, обворовать; to be ~ed out
остаться без копейки; to ~ **up** прибирать; убирать (*со стола*).

clean IV *adv* 1) совершенно, начисто; 2) прямо, как раз.

clean-cut ['kliːn'kʌt] *a* 1) резко очерченный;
2) определённый, точный.

cleaner ['kliːnə] *n*: vacuum ~ пылесос.

clean-fingered ['kliːn'fɪŋgəd] *a* неподкупный.

clean-handed ['kliːn'hændɪd] *a* честный; невинный.

cleaning ['kliːnɪŋ] *n* чистка, уборка.

cleanliness ['klenlɪnɪs] *n* чистоплотность.

cleanlyᵃ ['klenlɪ] *a* чистоплотный.

cleanlyᵇ ['kliːnlɪ] *adv* чисто.

cleanse [klenz] *v* 1) чистить; 2) очищать;
3) дезинфицировать.

clean-shaven ['kliːnʃeɪvn] *a* чисто выбритый.

clean-up ['kliːnʌp] *n разг.* чистка, уборка.

clear I [klɪə] *a* 1) ясный (*тж. об уме*);
безоблачный; 2) прозрачный; 3) чистый (*тж. о весе, совести*); 4) чёткий, отчётливый; 5) понятный;
6) свободный (*о пути*); all ~ а) путь свободен; б) отбой (*после тревоги*); 7) целый, полный.

clear II *v* 1) очищать; 2) становиться ясным,
прозрачным; 3) рассеивать (*сомнения, подозрения*); 4) оправдывать (*обвиняемого*); 5) устранять (*препятствия*); 6) рассеиваться (*о тучах*);
7) расходиться (*о людях*); 8) миновать, пройти
мимо; 9) выполнить все таможенные формаль-
ности; 10) *спорт.* брать барьер, высоту; 11) уплатить, расплатиться; □ to ~ **away** а) убирать
(*со стола*); б) рассеиваться (*о тумане, облаках*); to ~ **off** *разг.* избавиться (*от чего-л.*);
удрать; сбежать; ~ off! убирайтесь!; to ~ **out**
разг. а) очищать, опорожнять; to be ~ed out
остаться без единой копейки; б) удаляться; to ~
up а) выяснять (*дело*); б) прибирать, убирать;
в) проясниться (*о погоде*).

clear III *adv* 1) ясно; ~ as noonday ясно как
день; 2) совсем, целиком; ◇ to get ~ away отделаться; to come ~ off выйти сухим из воды;
keep ~ of pickpockets! остерегайтесь воров!

clearance ['klɪərəns] *n* 1) очистка (*тж. ком.—
от пошлины*); 2) расчистка (*под пашню*); выруб-
ка (*леса*); 3) устранение препятствий; 4) разрешение (*на уход с государственной должности*);
5) *тех.* зазор, просвет.

clear-cut ['klɪə'kʌt] *a* 1) резко очерченный;
2) чёткий.

clearing ['klɪərɪŋ] *n* 1) прояснение; 2) выяснение; 3) поляна (*в лесу*); 4) расчищенный участок в лесу (*под пашню*); 5) *ком.* клиринг; 6) вскрытие (*реки*).

clearing-house ['klɪərɪŋhaus] *n* расчётная палата.

clearly ['klɪəlɪ] *adv* ясно, определённо.

clear-sighted ['klɪə'saɪtɪd] *a* проницательный,
обладающий даром предвидения.

cleavage ['kliːvɪdʒ] *n* 1) расщепление; 2) *геол.*
слоистость; 3) расхождение.

cleave¹ [kliːv] *v* (*past* clove, cleft; *p. p.* cloven,
cleft) 1) раскалывать(ся); 2) рассекать (*воду,
воздух*); 3) разрезать.

cleave² *v* (*past* cleaved, clave; *p. p.* cleaved)
оставаться верным (*кому-л., чему-л.— to*).

cleaver ['kliːvə] *n* большой нож мясника.

clef [klef] *n муз.* ключ.

cleft[1] I [kleft] *n* ущелье, теснина; рас- щелина.

cleft[1] II *a* расколотый, расщеплённый.

cleft[2] *past, p. p. см.* cleave[1].

cleg [kleg] *n* овод, слепень.

clemency ['klemənsı] *n* 1) мягкость (*характера, погоды*); 2) милосердие.

clement ['klemənt] *a* 1) мягкий (*о характере, погоде*); 2) милосердный.

clench I [klentʃ] *n* 1) сжимание (*кулаков*); стискивание (*зубов*); 2) *тех.* заклёпывание.

clench II *v* 1) захватывать, зажимать; 2) сжи- мать (*кулаки*); стискивать (*зубы*); 3) догова- риваться (*о сделке*); решать, улаживать (*спор*); 4) *тех.* клепать.

clencher ['klentʃə] *n* убедительный аргумент.

clergy ['kləːdʒı] *n* духовенство.

clergyman ['kləːdʒımən] *n* священник.

clerical I ['klerıkəl] *n* клерикал.

clerical II *a* 1) духовный; клерикальный; 2) канцелярский.

clerk [klɑːk, *амер.* kləːk] *n* 1) чиновник, канце- лярский работник; клерк; 2) секретарь; corres- pondence ~ письмоводитель; town ~ секретарь городского совета; 3) *амер.* приказчик; 4) *воен.* писарь; 5) *уст.* причётник; a parish ~ приходский псаломщик.

clever ['klevə] *a* 1) умный; 2) способный, одарён- ный; 3) ловкий; 4) искусный, умелый; 5) добро- душный.

cleverness ['klevənıs] *n* 1) одарённость; 2) лов- кость; 3) искусность, умение.

clew I [kluː] *n* 1) клубок; 2) путеводная нить; ключ к разгадке.

clew II *v* сматывать в клубок (*обыкн.* to ~ up).

cliché ['kliːʃeı] *n* 1) *полигр.* клише; 2) избитая фраза, штамп.

click I [klık] *n* 1) щёлканье (*затвора и т. п.*); 2) *тех.* защёлка, собачка.

click II *v* 1) щёлкать; 2) защёлкнуть (*дверь*); 3) прищёлкивать (*языком*).

client ['klaıənt] *n* 1) клиент; 2) покупатель; заказчик.

clientèle [ˌkliːɑːnˈteıl] *n* клиентура.

cliff [klıf] *n* утёс, скала.

cliffsman ['klıfsmən] *n* альпинист.

climate ['klaımıt] *n* климат.

climatic [klaıˈmætık] *a* климатический.

climatology [ˌklaıməˈtɔlədʒı] *n* климатология.

climax I ['klaımæks] *n* высшая точка; кульмина- ционный пункт.

climax II *v* дойти *или* довести до кульминации.

climb I [klaım] *n* подъём, восхождение; easy (difficult, hard) ~ лёгкий (трудный) подъём; to be on the ~ идти в гору, делать карьеру.

climb II *v* 1) взбираться; влезать, карабкаться; 2) подниматься; 3) виться (*о растении*); 4) *ав.* на- бирать высоту; 5) делать карьеру; ◻ to ~ **down** а) слезать; спускаться; б) уступать (*в споре*); to ~ **up** а) взбираться, карабкаться; б) виться кверху (*о растении*).

climber ['klaımə] *n* 1) альпинист; 2) вьющееся растение; 3) карьерист.

climbing-irons ['klaımıŋˈaıənz] *n pl* 1) мон- тёрские когти; 2) шипы (*на ботинках альпини- стов*).

clime [klaım] *n поэт.* 1) район, страна; 2) кли- мат.

clinch I, II [klıntʃ] *см.* clench I, II.

cling [klıŋ] *v* (*past, p. p.* clung) 1) цепляться; крепко держаться (*за —to*); 2) оставаться верным (*взглядам, обычаям, друзьям*); 3) липнуть, прили- пать; 4) льнуть; 5) облегать (*о платье*); 6) дер- жаться (*берега, улицы и т. п.*).

clingy ['klıŋı] *a* цепкий, прилипчивый.

clinic ['klınık] *n* 1) клиника; 2) *амер.* мастер- ская по ремонту (*телевизоров, авторучек и т. п.*).

clinical ['klınıkəl] *a* клинический.

clink[1] I [klıŋk] *n* звон (*стекла, металла*).

clink[1] II *v* звенеть.

clink[2] *n сленг* 1) тюрьма; 2) *воен.* «губа».

clinker ['klıŋkə] *n* 1) *стр.* клинкер; 2) шлак.

clip[1] I [klıp] *n* 1) стрижка; 2) настриженная шерсть; 3) *разг.* сильный удар; 4) *разг.* быстрый шаг.

clip[1] II *v* 1) стричь; 2) обрезать, отрезать; подре- зать (*деревья*); 3) глотать (*буквы или слоги*); 4) *разг.* дать тумака; 5) *разг.* быстро бежать; 6) *разг.* обманывать.

clip[2] I *n* 1) скрепка; 2) зажим, захват; 3) скоба; 4) щипцы; 5) патронная обойма; 6) *pl* клипсы.

clip[2] II *v* 1) скреплять; 2) зажимать.

clipper ['klıpə] *n мор.* клиппер.

clippers ['klıpəz] *n pl* ножницы *или* машинка (*для стрижки*).

clipping ['klıpıŋ] *n* газетная вырезка.

clique [kliːk] *n* клика.

cloak I ['klouk] *n* 1) плащ; 2) покров; 3) пред- лог; under the ~ of под маской, под предлогом.

cloak II *v* 1) накидывать плащ; 2) скрывать, окутывать.

cloak-room ['kloukrum] *n* 1) гардероб, разде- вальня; 2) камера хранения (*багажа*).

clock[1] *n* часы (*стенные, настольные, ба- шенные*); alarm ~ будильник; Dutch ~ часы (*с фигурками, выскакивающими при бое*); grand- father's ~ (старинные) стоячие часы, to set a ~ ставить часы (*на определённое время*); to get the ~ going again починить часы; the ~ gains (loses) часы спешат (отстают).

clock[2] *n* стрелка (*украшение на чулке*).

clock-face ['klɔkfeıs] *n* циферблат.

clockwise ['klɔkwaız] *adv* по часовой стрелке.

clock-work ['klɔkwəːk] *n* 1) часовой механизм; everything went like ~ всё шло как по часам; 2) *attr* точный; 3) *attr* заводной (*об игрушках*).

clod [klɔd] *n* 1) ком, глыба (*земли, глины и т. п.*); 2) мёртвое тело, прах; 3) увалень.

cloddish ['klɔdıʃ] *a* 1) глупый; 2) флегматичный.

clod-hopper ['klɔdˌhɔpə] *n* увалень.

clog I [klɔg] *n* 1) путы; *ист.* колодка; 2) башмак (*на деревянной подошве*); 3) препятствие; 4) засо- рение.

clog II *v* 1) спутывать (*лошадь*); 2) мешать; препятствовать; 3) забивать(ся), засорять(ся).

cloggy ['klɔgı] *a* 1) комковатый; 2) липкий, вязкий.

cloister I ['klɔıstə] *n* 1) монастырь; 2) *архит.* крытая аркада.

cloister II *v* заточать в монастырь.

cloistral ['klɔıstrəl] *a* 1) монастырский; 2) мона- шеский.

close^a I [klouz] *n* конéц; завершéние, окончáние; to bring to a ~ завершúть; довестú до концá; to draw to a ~ приближáться к концý.

close^a II *v* 1) закрывáть; 2) закáнчивать (*заня́тия и т. п.*); заключáть (*речь*); 3) *воен.* сомкнýть (*ряды́*); 4) сходúться, сближáться (*о войскáх*); 5) *эл.* замыкáть (*цепь*); □ to ~ **about** окýтывать; to ~ **down** а) применя́ть репрéссии; б) закрывáть, ликвидúровать (*учреждéние*); to ~ **in** а) наступáть; б) сокращáться (*о дня́х*); to ~ **on** приходúть к соглашéнию; to ~ **up** а) запечáтывать (*письма́*); б) сходúться; затя́гиваться, закрывáться (*о ра́не*); to ~ **upon** а) схватúть, сжать; б) брóсить послéдний взгляд; to ~ **with** вступáть в борьбý.

close^{b1} [klous] *n* 1) шкóльная площáдка; 2) огорóженное мéсто.

close^{b2} I *a* 1) блúзкий; 2) дýшный, спёртый; 3) подрóбный; тщáтельный; прúстальный; 4) тóчный (*о ко́пии, перево́де*); 5) закры́тый; скры́тый; keep oneself ~ сторонúться, держáться особняко́м; 6) стрóгий (*об аре́сте, изоля́ции*); 7) плóтный (*о тка́ни*); хорошó прúгнанный; облегáющий (*об оде́жде*); убóристый (*о по́черке*); густóй (*о ле́се и т. п.*); 8) сдéржанный, скры́тный; 9) огранúченный, тéсный; 10) *воен.* сóмкнутый (*о стро́е*); 11) скупóй, скáредный; 12) *фон.* закры́тый, ýзкий (*о гла́сном*).

close^{b2} II *adv* 1) блúзко; ~ **by** ря́дом, поблúзости; ~ **to** óколо; ~ **upon** почтú, приблизúтельно; 2) плóтно.

close-cropped ['klouskrɔpt] *a* кóротко острúженный.

closed [klouzd] *a* 1) закры́тый; закóнченный; 2) зáмкнутый.

close-down ['klous'daun] *n* прекращéние рабóты (*в связи́ с закры́тием предприя́тия*).

close-fisted ['klous'fistid] *a* скупóй, скáредный.

close-fitting ['klous'fitiŋ] *a* облегáющий (*о пла́тье*); хорошó прúгнанный.

closely ['klouslı] *adv* 1) блúзко, тéсно; 2) внимáтельно, подрóбно.

closeness ['klousnıs] *n* 1) блúзость; 2) духотá; 3) плóтность.

closet ['klɔzıt] *n* 1) *чаще амер.* чулáн; стеннóй шкаф; 2) *уст.* кабинéт; 3) убóрная.

close-up ['klousʌp] *n* 1) *кино, тлв.* крýпный план; 2) *амер.* тщáтельный осмóтр.

closing ['klouzıŋ] *a* заключúтельный.

closing-time ['klouzıŋtaım] *n* врéмя закры́тия (*магази́нов, учрежде́ний и т. п.*).

closure I ['klouʒə] *n* 1) закры́тие; 2) перегорóдка; 3) прекращéние прéний (*в парла́менте*).

closure II *v* прекращáть прéния.

clot I [klɔt] *n* 1) комóк; сгýсток; *мед.* тромб.

clot II *v* свёртываться; запекáться (*о кро́ви*).

cloth [klɔθ] *n* 1) ткань; сукнó; холст, полотнó; bound in ~ *полигр.* в цельнотканевом переплёте; 2) *pl* (cloths [klɔðz]) куски́ матéрии; 3) скáтерть; to draw the ~ убирáть со столá; to lay the ~ накрывáть на стол; 4) духóвный сан; the ~ духовéнство; ◊ of the same ~ той же профéссии.

clothe [klouð] *v* (*past, p. p.* clothed, clad) 1) одевáть; *перен.* облекáть; 2) покрывáть.

clothes [klouðz] *n pl* одéжда; плáтье; бельё (*тж. посте́льное*); fatigue ~ *разг.* рабóчее плáтье; спецодéжда; plain ~ штáтское плáтье; store ~

амер. готóвое плáтье; ◊ to make ~ for fishes *погов.* ≅ решетóм вóду носúть.

clothes-basket ['klouðz‚ba:skıt] *n* бельевáя корзúна.

clothes-line ['klouðzlaın] *n* бельевáя верёвка.

clothes-peg ['klouðzpeg] *n* зажúмка, защúпка (*для белья́*).

clothes-pin ['klouðzpın] *см.* clothes-peg.

clothes-press ['klouðzpres] *n* шкаф, комóд для белья́.

clothier ['klouðıə] *n* сукóнщик.

clothing ['klouðıŋ] *n* одéжда; обмундировáние.

cloud I [klaud] *n* 1) тýча; óблако; 2) клуб (*ды́ма, пы́ли*); 3) мнóжество, тýча (*птиц, насеко́мых и т. п.*); 4) что-л. омрачáющее; a ~ of grief óблако грýсти; 5) жúлка, помутнéние (*в камне*); 6) покрóв (*ночи, темноты́*); 7) недовóльство, грусть; ◊ under a ~ в немúлости; a ~ on one's brow хмýрый вид; to be in the ~s витáть в облакáх; every ~ has a silver lining ≅ нет хýда без добрá.

cloud II *v* 1) покрывáть(ся) тýчами, облакáми; 2) омрачáть(ся); 3) затемня́ть; 4) запя́тнать (*репута́цию*); □ to ~ **over**, to ~ **up** заволáкиваться.

cloudberry ['klaud‚berı] *n* морóшка.

cloud-burst ['klaudbə:st] *n* *амер.* лúвень.

cloud-capped ['klaudkæpt] *a* окýтанный облакáми (*о го́рных верши́нах*).

cloud-drift ['klauddrıft] *n* плывýщие облакá.

cloudiness ['klaudınıs] *n* óблачность.

cloud-kissing ['klaud‚kısıŋ] *a* *разг.* уходя́щий в поднебéсье (*о гора́х*).

cloudland ['klaudlænd] *n* скáзочная странá.

cloudless ['klaudlıs] *a* безóблачный.

cloudlet ['klaudlıt] *n* облачкó.

cloudy ['klaudı] *a* 1) óблачный; 2) тумáнный, нея́сный; 3) мýтный (*о жи́дкости*); 4) затумáненный (*о взгля́де*).

clough [klʌf] *n* ущéлье; лощúна.

clout I [klaut] *n* 1) лоскýт; тря́пка; 2) *разг.* затрéщина; 3) *тех.* шáйба.

clout II *v* 1) латáть, чинúть (*оде́жду*); 2) *разг.* дать затрéщину.

clove^1 [klouv] *n* 1) гвоздúка (*пря́ность*).

clove^2 *n* зубóк (*чеснока́*).

clove^3 *past см.* cleave^1.

cloven ['klouvn] *p. p. см.* cleave^1.

clover ['klouvə] *n* клéвер; ◊ to be (*или* to live) in ~ жить в рóскоши, в достáтке.

clown [klaun] *n* 1) клóун; шут; 2) грýбый, неотёсанный человéк.

clownish ['klaunıʃ] *a* 1) шутовскóй; 2) грýбый, неотёсанный.

cloy [klɔı] *v* пресыщáть.

club^1 I [klʌb] *n* клуб.

club^1 II *v* 1) устрáивать склáдчину (*with, together*); 2) собирáться вмéсте.

club^2 I *n* 1) дубúнка; 2) *спорт.* клю́шка; битá; булавá; Indian ~s булавы́; 3) *pl карт.* трéфы.

club^2 II *v* бить дубúнкой; лупúть.

clubman ['klʌbmən] *n* 1) член клýба; 2) *амер.* свéтский человéк.

clubwoman ['klʌb‚wumən] *n* член клýба (*о же́нщине*).

cluck I [klʌk] *n* кудáхтанье.

cluck II *v* кудáхтать.

clue [kluː] *n* 1) ключ (к разгадке); 2) нить (*рассказа, мысли*).

clump I [klʌmp] *n* 1) группа (*деревьев, кустов*); 2) глыба; 3) двойная подмётка.

clump II *v* 1) сажать отдельными группами; 2) тяжело ступать; 3) ставить двойную подмётку.

clumsy ['klʌmzı] *a* 1) неуклюжий; нескладный; 2) грубый, топорный; 3) бестактный.

clung [klʌŋ] *past, p. p. см.* cling.

cluster I ['klʌstə] *n* 1) пучок (*цветов*); кисть, гроздь; 2) купа (*деревьев*); 3) группа, скопление (*однородных предметов*); 4) пчелиный рой; 5) кучка (*людей*).

cluster II *v* 1) расти пучками, гроздьями; 2) тесниться.

clutch[1] I [klʌtʃ] *n* 1) хватка; 2) *pl* когти; лапы (*тж. перен.*); 3) *тех.* сцепление; 4) *тех.* зажим; защёлка.

clutch[1] II *v* 1) стиснуть, зажать; 2) схватить, ухватиться.

clutch[2] *n* выводок (*цыплят*).

clutter I ['klʌtə] *n* 1) суматоха; паника; 2) шум, гам.

clutter II *v* 1) создавать суматоху; суетиться; 2) шуметь.

co- [kou-] *pref в сложных словах указывает на совместность действий, усилий и т. п.*

coach[1] I [koutʃ] *n* 1) пассажирский вагон; 2) (туристский) автобус (*междугородного сообщения*); 3) карета; дилижанс.

coach[1] II *v* ехать в поезде, в карете.

coach[2] I *n* 1) репетитор; 2) инструктор; тренер.

coach[2] II *v* 1) натаскивать к экзаменам; 2) тренировать.

coach-box ['koutʃbɔks] *n* козлы.

coach-house ['koutʃhaus] *n* каретный сарай.

coachman ['koutʃmən] *n* кучер; возничий.

coadjutor [kou'ædʒutə] *n* помощник.

coagulate [kou'ægjuleıt] *v* 1) свёртывать(ся); створаживать(ся); 2) *хим.* коагулировать.

coagulation [kou,ægju'leıʃən] *n* 1) свёртывание; 2) *хим.* коагуляция.

coal I [koul] *n* (каменный) уголь; hard (*или* anthracite) ~ антрацит; brown ~ бурый уголь; coking ~ коксующийся уголь; to get ~ добывать уголь; to blow the ~s раздувать огонь (*тж. перен.*); ◊ to carry ~s to Newcastle *погов.* возить уголь в Ньюкасл; to call (*или* to haul) smb. over the ~s давать нагоняй, взбучку кому-л.

coal II *v* 1) грузить уголь; грузиться углем; 2) обугливаться.

coal-bed ['koulbed] *n* угольный пласт.

coal-black ['koul'blæk] *a* чёрный как смоль.

coal-box ['koulbɔks] *n* ящик для угля.

coal-dust ['kouldʌst] *n* угольная пыль.

coaler ['koulə] *n* 1) угольщик (*пароход*); 2) грузчик угля.

coalesce [,kouə'les] *v* 1) срастаться; 2) сходиться; объединяться (*в группы*); 3) создавать коалицию.

coalescence [,kouə'lesns] *n* сращение; соединение.

coal-field ['koulfiːld] *n* каменноугольный бассейн, район.

coal-gas ['koul'gæs] *n* светильный газ.

coal-heaver ['koul,hiːvə] *n* возчик угля.

coal-hole ['koulhoul] *n* подвал для угля.

coaling ['koulıŋ] *n* бункеровка, загрузка угля.

coaling-station ['koulıŋ,steıʃən] *n* угольная станция, база.

coalition [,kouə'lıʃən] *n* коалиция.

coalman ['koulmæn] *n* углекоп.

coal-master ['koul,mɑːstə] *n* угольный магнат.

coal-mine ['koulmaın] *n* каменноугольная шахта.

coal-pit ['koulpıt] *см.* coal-mine.

coal-scuttle ['koul,skʌtl] *n* ведёрко для угля.

coal-tar ['koul'tɑː] *n* каменноугольный дёготь, смола.

coaly ['koulı] *a* 1) содержащий уголь; 2) чумазый.

coarse [kɔːs] *a* 1) грубый; 2) крупный, простой (*о выделке и т. п.*); 3) сырой, необработанный (*о материале*); 4) невежливый; 5) непристойный; вульгарный.

coarsen ['kɔːsn] *v* грубеть.

coarseness ['kɔːsnıs] *n* грубость; непристойность.

coast I [koust] *n* 1) побережье; морской берег; the ~ is clear *перен.* путь свободен; 2) *амер.* снежные горы для катания на салазках.

coast II *v* 1) плавать вдоль побережья; 2) *амер.* кататься с гор на салазках.

coastal ['koustəl] *a* береговой, прибрежный.

coaster ['koustə] *n* 1) каботажное судно; 2) серебряный поднос (*для графина*).

coast-guard ['koustgɑːd] *n* береговая охрана.

coasting ['koustıŋ] *a* каботажное судоходство.

coast-line ['koustlaın] *n* береговая линия.

coastwise I ['koustwaız] *a* каботажный.

coastwise II *adv* вдоль побережья.

coat I [kout] *n* 1) пиджак; clawhammer ~, tail ~ фрак; morning ~ визитка; Eton ~ куртка; sack ~ простой пиджак; 2) мундир; френч; to wear the king's (*или* the queen's) ~ служить в английской армии; 3) верхнее платье; пальто; ~ and skirt дамский костюм; 4) шерсть, шкура (*животного*); мех; 5) слой (*краски*); 6) *анат.* оболочка, плева; 7) *тех.* облицовка; ◊ ~ of arms герб; you must cut your ~ according to your cloth *погов.* по одёжке протягивай ножки.

coat II *v* 1) красить, окрашивать; 2) покрывать слоем (*пыли, краски и т. п.*); 3) облицовывать.

coatee ['koutiː] *n* куртка; тужурка.

coat-hanger ['kout,hæŋgə] *n* вешалка, плечики (*для одежды*).

coating ['koutıŋ] *n.* 1) слой (*краски и т. п.*); 2) материал для пальто.

co-author [kou'ɔːθə] *n* соавтор.

coax [kouks] *v* 1) уговаривать; задабривать; 2) льстить; to ~ smth. out of smb. добиться чего-л. с помощью лести; □ to ~ **away** соблазнять.

coaxing ['kouksıŋ] *n* задабривание; упрашивание.

cobalt [kə'bɔːlt] *n* 1) *хим.* кобальт; 2) синяя краска.

cobble[1] I ['kɔbl] *n* 1) булыжник; 2) *pl* булыжная мостовая; 3) *pl* крупный уголь.

cobble[1] II *v* мостить булыжником.

cobble[2] *v* чинить (*обувь*).

cobbler ['kɔblə] *n* 1) уличный сапожник; 2) *пренебр.* плохой мастер; 3) *амер.* прохладительный напиток (*из вина с сахаром и лимоном*).

cobble-stone ['kɔblstoun] *n* булыжник.

cobby ['kɔbɪ] *a* коренастый.

coble ['koubl] *n* рыбачья лодка-плоскодонка.

cob-nut ['kɔbnʌt] *n* фундук (*орех*).

cobra ['koubrə] *n* кобра.

cobweb ['kɔbweb] *n* 1) паутина; *перен.* западня; 2) лёгкая ткань, вуаль; 3) *pl* тонкости; ◇ to blow (away) the ~s проветриться.

cobwebby ['kɔbwebɪ] *a* затянутый паутиной.

cocaine [kə'keɪn] *n* кокаин.

cock[1] I [kɔk] *n* 1) петух; fighting ~ бойцовый петух; ~ of the wood глухарь; 2) кран; 3) курок; at full ~ на полном взводе; 4) *ав.* сиденье лётчика; 5) вожак, коновод; ◇ the ~ of the walk главная персона; «шишка»; that ~ won't fight этот номер не пройдёт; to live like a fighting ~ жить припеваючи.

cock[1] II [kɔk] *v* 1) задирать (*нос*); 2) навострить уши (*тж.* to ~ up); 3) заламывать (*шляпу*); 4) взводить курок.

cock[2] I *n* копна.

cock[2] II *v* складывать сено в копны.

cockade [kɔ'keɪd] *n* кокарда.

cock-a-doodle-doo ['kɔkədu:dl'du:] *n* 1) кукареку; 2) *дет.* петух, петушок.

cock-a-hoop ['kɔkə'hu:p] *a* самодовольный.

cock-and-bull ['kɔkən'bul] *a:* ~ story небылицы.

cockatoo [,kɔkə'tu:] *n* какаду (*попугай*).

cockboat ['kɔkbout] *n* судовая шлюпка.

cockchafer ['kɔk,tʃeɪfə] *n* майский жук.

cocker ['kɔkə] *v* баловать (*ребёнка*); □ to ~ up потворствовать (*в чём-л.—in*).

cockerel ['kɔkərəl] *n* молодой петушок.

cock-eyed ['kɔkaɪd] *a* 1) косоглазый, косой; 2) *сленг* пьяный.

cock-fight(ing) ['kɔkfaɪt(ɪŋ)] *n* петушиный бой.

cockle[1] I ['kɔkl] *n* морщина, изъян (*в бумаге, стекле и т. п.*).

cockle[1] II *v* 1) морщиться; 2) покрываться барашками (*о море*); 3) завертывать(ся) винтом или спиралью.

cockle[2] *n* сердцевидка (*съедобный моллюск*); ◇ to warm the ~s of one's heart радовать сердце.

cock-loft ['kɔklɔft] *n* мансарда, чердак.

cockney ['kɔknɪ] *n* 1) уроженец Лондона, *особ.* восточной части; 2) кокни.

cockpit ['kɔkpɪt] *n* 1) кабина пилота; 2) *мор.* кубрик; 3) место петушиных боёв; *перен.* арена борьбы.

cockroach ['kɔkroutʃ] *n* таракан.

cockscomb ['kɔkskoum] *n* 1) петушиный гребень; 2) самодовольный хлыщ, фат.

cock-shot ['kɔkʃɔt] *n* мишень.

cock-sure ['kɔk'ʃuə] *a* 1) вполне уверенный (*в — of, about*); 2) самоуверенный; 3) несомненный; неизбежный (*о событии и т. п.*).

cocktail ['kɔkteɪl] *n* 1) коктейль; 2) выскочка; 3) лошадь с подрезанным хвостом.

cocky ['kɔkɪ] *a* самоуверенный, нахальный.

coco ['koukou] *n* кокосовая пальма.

cocoa ['koukou] *n* какао.

coco(a)-nut ['koukənʌt] *n* 1) кокосовый орех, кокос; 2) *сленг* башка; 3) *attr* кокосовый.

coco-nut-tree ['koukənʌt,tri:] *n* кокосовая пальма.

cocoon [kə'ku:n] *n* кокон.

cod I [kɔd] *n* треска.

cod II *v* *разг.* надувать, обманывать.

coddle I ['kɔdl] *n* неженка.

coddle II *v* нянчиться; изнеживать.

code I [koud] *n* 1) кодекс, свод законов; penal ~ уголовный кодекс; labour ~ кодекс законов о труде; 2) код, шифр; Morse ~ азбука Морзе; 3) свод сигналов.

code II *a* 1) шифрованный; 2) шифровальный.

code III *v* шифровать по коду; кодировать.

codex ['koudeks] *n* (*pl* codices) старинная рукопись, свиток.

cod-fish ['kɔdfɪʃ] *см.* cod I.

codger ['kɔdʒə] *n* *разг.* чудак.

codices ['koudɪsi:z] *pl см.* codex.

codicil ['kɔdɪsɪl] *n* приписка к завещанию.

codify ['kɔdɪfaɪ] *v* 1) кодифицировать; составлять свод законов; 2) шифровать.

codling ['kɔdlɪŋ] *n* мелкая треска.

co-education ['kou,edju:'keɪʃən] *n* совместное обучение.

coefficient I [,kouɪ'fɪʃənt] *n* 1) коэффициент; 2) содействующий фактор.

coefficient II *a* содействующий.

coerce [kou'ə:s] *v* принуждать, заставлять.

coercion [kou'ə:ʃən] *n* принуждение, насилие.

coercive [kou'ə:sɪv] *a* принудительный.

coeval I [kou'i:vəl] *n* сверстник; современник.

coeval II *a* одного возраста, времени.

coexist ['kouɪg'zɪst] *v* сосуществовать.

coexistence ['kouɪg'zɪstəns] *n* сосуществование.

coexistent ['kouɪg'zɪstənt] *a* сосуществующий.

coffee ['kɔfɪ] *n* кофе; instant ~ растворимый кофе.

coffee-bean ['kɔfɪ'bi:n] *n* кофейный боб.

coffee-cup ['kɔfɪkʌp] *n* маленькая (кофейная) чашка.

coffee-grinder ['kɔfɪ,graɪndə] *n* 1) кофейная мельница; 2) *воен. сленг* пулемёт.

coffee-grounds ['kɔfɪgraundz] *n pl* кофейная гуща.

coffee-mill ['kɔfɪmɪl] *n* кофейная мельница.

coffee-pot ['kɔfɪpɔt] *n* кофейник.

coffee-room ['kɔfɪrum] *n* столовая в гостинице.

coffer ['kɔfə] *n* 1) сундук; ящик; 2) *pl* казна; 3) *архит.* кессон (*потолка*); 4) *гидр.* кессон; шлюз.

coffin I ['kɔfɪn] *n* 1) гроб; 2) *мор. разг.* «старая калоша» (*о негодном к плаванию судне*); 3) фунтик, бумажный пакет; 4) лошадиное копыто.

coffin II *v* класть в гроб.

cog[1] [kɔg] *n* зубец, выступ.

cog[2] *v* жульничать.

cogency ['koudʒənsɪ] *n* убедительность, неоспоримость.

cogent ['koudʒənt] *a* убедительный, неоспоримый.

cogged [kɔgd] *a* зубчатый.

cogitate ['kɔdʒɪteɪt] *v* обдумывать, размышлять.

cogitation [,kɔdʒɪ'teɪʃən] *n* обдумывание, размышление.

cognac ['kounjæk] *n* коньяк.

cognate I ['kɔgneɪt] *n* 1) родственник; 2) *pl лингв.* родственные языки, слова.

cognate II *a* родственный; близкий, сходный.

cognition [kɔg'nɪʃən] *n* 1) познание, знание; 2) познавательная способность.

cognitive ['kɔgnɪtɪv] *a* познавательный.

cognizable [ˈkɔgnɪzəbl] *a* 1) познаваемый; 2) *юр.* подсудный.

cognizance [ˈkɔgnɪzəns] *n* 1) знание; to take ~ of заметить; 2) компетенция; 3) подсудность; 4) знак отличия; эмблема, герб.

cognizant [ˈkɔgnɪzənt] *a* знающий, осведомлённый (*о чём-л.—of*); познавший, осознавший.

cognomen [kɔgˈnoumen] *n* прозвище; фамилия.

cog-wheel [ˈkɔgwiːl] *n тех.* зубчатое колесо.

cohabit [kouˈhæbɪt] *v* сожительствовать.

cohabitation [ˌkouhæbɪˈteɪʃən] *n* сожительство.

coheir [ˈkouˈɛə] *n* сонаследник.

cohere [kouˈhɪə] *v* 1) согласовываться; 2) быть связанным, сцепленным.

coherence [kouˈhɪərəns] *n* 1) согласованность; связность, последовательность; 2) сцепление.

coherent [kouˈhɪərənt] *a* 1) согласованный, последовательный; связный (*о речи*); 2) сцепленный.

cohesion [kouˈhiːʒən] *n* 1) сцепление; сила сцепления; 2) спайка, сплочённость.

cohesive [kouˈhiːsɪv] *a* связующий.

coiffeur [kwɑˈfəː] *n* парикмахер.

coiffure [kwɑˈfjuə] *n* причёска.

coign [kɔɪn] *n архит.* внешний угол (*здания*); ◊ ~ of vantage выгодная позиция для наблюдения.

coil I [kɔɪl] *n* 1) верёвка, сложенная витками; кольцо (*о верёвке, змее и т. п.*); 2) *эл.* катушка; 3) *мор.* бухта (*троса*); 4) *тех.* змеевик.

coil II *v* 1) свёртывать кольцом, спиралью (*верёвку, проволоку*); 2) свернуться в кольцо (*о змее*); 3) извиваться; 4) *мор.* укладывать в бухту (*трос*).

coin I [kɔɪn] *n* монета; *разг.* деньги; bad ~ неполноценная монета; base (*или* false) ~ фальшивая монета; to spin a ~ подбрасывать монету; to pay one in his own ~ отплатить той же монетой кому-л.

coin II *v* 1) чеканить (*монету*); выбивать (*медаль*); 2) фабриковать (*измышления*); 3) создавать новые слова, выражения.

coinage [ˈkɔɪnɪdʒ] *n* 1) чеканка (*монет*); 2) металлические деньги; 3) монетная система; 4) вымысел, измышление; 5) создание новых слов, выражений.

coincide [ˌkouɪnˈsaɪd] *v* совпадать; соответствовать.

coincidence [kouˈɪnsɪdəns] *n* 1) совпадение; соответствие; 2) случайное стечение обстоятельств.

coincident [kouˈɪnsɪdənt] *a* совпадающий, соответствующий.

coiner [ˈkɔɪnə] *n* фальшивомонетчик.

coke I [kouk] *n* кокс.

coke II *v* коксовать.

coker(nut) [ˈkoukə(nʌt)] *n* кокосовый орех.

col [kɔl] *n* седловина (*горы*).

col- [kɔl-] *см.* com-.

colander [ˈkʌləndə] *n* дуршлаг.

cold I [kould] *n* 1) холод; to be left out in the ~ *перен.* почувствовать пренебрежение; to keep the ~ out содержать в тепле; 2) простуда; to catch (*или* to take) ~ простудиться; получить насморк; a ~ in the head насморк.

cold II *a* 1) холодный; 2) озябший, застывший; I am ~, I feel ~ мне холодно; 3) безучастный, равнодушный; 4) спокойный (*о цвете*); холодный (*о тоне, краске*).

cold-blooded [ˈkouldˈblʌdɪd] *a* 1) хладнокровный, невозмутимый; 2) зябкий; 3) *зоол.* холоднокровный.

cold-bloodedness [ˈkouldˈblʌdɪdnɪs] *n* хладнокровие.

cold-hearted [ˈkouldˈhɑːtɪd] *a* сухой, чёрствый, бессердечный.

coldish [ˈkouldɪʃ] *a* холодноватый.

cold-livered [ˈkouldˈlɪvəd] *a* бесстрастный.

coldness [ˈkouldnɪs] *n* 1) холод; 2) холодность.

cold-pig [ˈkouldˈpɪg] *v* обливать холодной водой (*чтобы разбудить*).

cold-shoulder [ˈkouldˈʃouldə] *v* принять холодно, неприветливо (*см. тж.* shoulder I, ◊).

cold-storage [ˈkouldˌstɔːrɪdʒ] *n* 1) холодильник; 2) хранение в холодильнике.

colic [ˈkɔlɪk] *n* колика.

collaborate [kəˈlæbəreɪt] *v* сотрудничать.

collaboration [kəˌlæbəˈreɪʃən] *n* сотрудничество.

collaborator [kəˈlæbəreɪtə] *n* сотрудник.

collapsable [kəˈlæpsəbl] *a* складной.

collapse I [kəˈlæps] *n* 1) обвал, разрушение (*здания*); 2) падение; крушение, гибель; 3) упадок жизнедеятельности (*организма*).

collapse II *v* 1) обваливаться, рушиться (*о здании*); 2) обессилеть; упасть духом; 3) потерпеть крах.

collar I [ˈkɔlə] *n* 1) воротник; воротничок; stand-up ~ стоячий воротничок; Eton ~ широкий отложной воротник; to turn up the ~ поднять воротник; 2) ожерелье; 3) ошейник; 4) хомут (*тж. перен.*); 5) *тех.* втулка; шайба; ◊ to work up to the ~ работать не покладая рук.

collar II *v* 1) схватить за воротник; 2) поймать, задержать.

collar-bone [ˈkɔləboun] *n* ключица.

collate [kɔˈleɪt] *v* сличать, тщательно сравнивать.

collateral [kɔˈlætərəl] *a* 1) второстепенный; 2) косвенный; 3) параллельный.

collation [kɔˈleɪʃən] *n* 1) сличение, сравнивание; 2) закуска; лёгкий завтрак *или* ужин.

colleague [ˈkɔliːg] *n* сослуживец, коллега.

collect [kəˈlekt] *v* 1) собирать; коллекционировать; 2) собираться (*о толпе*); 3) овладевать собой; сосредоточиваться.

collection [kəˈlekʃən] *n* 1) коллекция, собрание (*трудов*); 2) сбор, собирание; 3) скопление; 4) *pl* экзамены в конце триместра (*в Оксфордском университете*).

collective I [kəˈlektɪv] *n* 1) коллектив; 2) *грам.* собирательное имя существительное.

collective II *a* 1) коллективный; 2) соединённый, совокупный; 3) *грам.* собирательный.

collectively [kəˈlektɪvlɪ] *adv* сообща, все вместе.

collectivism [kəˈlektɪvɪzəm] *n* коллективизм.

collectivization [kəˌlektɪvaɪˈzeɪʃən] *n* коллективизация.

collector [kəˈlektə] *n* 1) коллекционер; 2) сборщик (*податей и т. п.*); 3) контролёр (*в поезде и т. п.*); 4) *тех.* коллектор; 5) *эл.* токосниматель; щётки.

college [ˈkɔlɪdʒ] *n* 1) колледж; 2) среднее учебное заведение; 3) специальное учебное заведение (*военное и т. п.*); Military College военная академия; 4) *амер.* университет; 5) коллегия; корпорация; electoral ~ *амер.* коллегия выборщиков (*избираемых в отдельных штатах для выборов президента и вице-президента*); 6) *сленг* тюрьма.

collegian [kə'liːdʒən] *n* 1) профессор *или* студент колледжа; 2) окончивший колледж; человек с университетским образованием.

collegiate I [kə'liːdʒiːt] *n* студент колледжа.

collegiate II *a* 1) университетский; 2) коллегиальный.

collide [kə'laid] *v* сталкиваться.

collie ['kɔli] *n* колли, шотландская овчарка.

collier ['kɔliə] *n* 1) углекоп; 2) угольщик (*корабль*); 3) матрос на угольщике.

colliery ['kɔljəri] *n* каменноугольная копь.

collision [kə'liʒən] *n* 1) столкновение (*поездов, пароходов и т. п.*); to come into ~ with столкнуться (*см. тж.* 2); 2) противоречие (*интересов*); стычка; to come into ~ (with) вступать в противоречие (*см. тж.* 1).

collocate ['kɔləkeit] *v* располагать; расставлять.

collocation [,kɔlə'keiʃən] *n* взаиморасположение; расстановка.

collodion [kə'loudjən] *n* коллодий.

collogue [kə'loug] *v* беседовать с глазу на глаз.

colloid I ['kɔlɔid] *n хим.* коллоид.

colloid II *a хим.* коллоидный.

colloquial [kə'loukwiəl] *a* разговорный (*о выражении, слове, стиле*).

colloquialism [kə'loukwiəlizəm] *n* разговорный оборот, разговорное выражение; просторечие.

colloquy ['kɔləkwi] *n* разговор; беседа.

collusion [kə'luːʒən] *n* сговор; тайная договорённость.

colon[1] ['koulən] *n* двоеточие.

colon[2] *n анат.* толстая кишка.

colonel ['kəːnl] *n* полковник.

colonelcy ['kəːnlsi] *n* звание полковника.

colonial I [kə'lounjəl] *n* 1) житель колонии; 2) *амер. ист.* солдат армии периода существования 13 колоний.

colonial II *a* 1) колониальный; относящийся к колониям; 2) *амер. ист.* относящийся к периоду существования 13 колоний.

colonialism [kə'lounjəlizəm] *n* колониализм.

colonialist [kə'lounjəlist] *n* сторонник колониальной системы.

colonist ['kɔlənist] *n* колонист; переселенец.

colonization [,kɔlənai'zeiʃən] *n* колонизация; заселение (*чужой территории*).

colonize ['kɔlənaiz] *v* 1) колонизировать; заселять (*чужую территорию*); 2) поселять(ся).

colonizer ['kɔlənaizə] *n* колонизатор.

colonnade [,kɔlə'neid] *n* 1) колоннада; 2) двойной ряд деревьев.

colony ['kɔləni] *n* колония; Crown Colony британская колония, не имеющая самоуправления.

colophony [kə'lɔfəni] *n* канифоль.

color ['kʌlə] *амер. см.* colour.

coloration [,kʌlə'reiʃən] *n* 1) расцветка, раскраска; 2) окрашивание.

colorific [,kɔlə'rifik] *a* 1) красящий; 2) красочный; 3) цветистый (*о стиле*).

colossal [kə'lɔsl] *a* 1) колоссальный; 2) *разг.* замечательный.

colossus [kə'lɔsəs] *n* колосс.

colour I ['kʌlə] *n* 1) цвет; оттенок; primary (secondary) ~s основные (составные) цвета; out of ~ выцветший, выгоревший; 2) тон, краска; water ~ акварель; airy (*или* light, transparent) ~s прозрачные краски; bright (*или* festive) ~s яркие краски; soft (cold) ~ мягкие (холодные) тона; 3) освещение (*чего-л.*); to give (*или* to lend) ~ правильно освещать (*что-л.— to*); to paint in glaring ~s описывать в ярких красках; to give a false ~ неправильно освещать (*что-л.— to*), давать неверное освещение (*чему-л.— to*); to put a false ~ on искажать (*факты и т. п.*); 4) румянец; to change ~ перемениться в лице; to lose ~ побледнеть, поблёкнуть; high ~, ~ in one's cheeks румянец; 5) окраска; колорит; local ~ местный колорит; 6) предлог; under ~ of под предлогом; 7) *pl* цветные платья; 8) *pl* флаг, национальные цвета; national ~s государственный флаг; to join the ~s поступить на военную службу; with the ~s на действительной военной службе; 9) *муз.* тембр; ◊ off ~ *разг.* не в духе; to come off with flying ~s добиться успеха, выйти победителем; to lower one's ~s отказаться от своих требований, уступить; to nail one's ~s to the mast настаивать на своём, упорствовать; to show one's true ~s показать, проявить свою сущность.

colour II *v* 1) красить, раскрашивать; 2) окрашивать; придавать оттенок; 3) краснеть (*о лице, плодах*); покрываться румянцем; 4) окрашиваться; принимать окраску.

colourable ['kʌlərəbl] *a* 1) поддающийся окраске; 2) благовидный; правдоподобный.

colouration [,kʌlə'reiʃən] *см.* coloration.

colour-blind ['kʌləblaind] *a* страдающий дальтонизмом.

colour-blindness ['kʌlə,blaindnis] *n* дальтонизм.

colour-box ['kʌləbɔks] *n* ящик с красками.

coloured ['kʌləd] *a* 1) окрашенный, раскрашенный; 2) цветной.

colouring ['kʌləriŋ] *n* 1) раскраска, расцветка; окраска; protective ~ *зоол., бот.* покровительственная, защитная окраска; 2) колорит, краски; 3) цвет лица, волос; 4) чувство красок, цвета (*у художника*).

colourless ['kʌlələs] *a* 1) бесцветный; бледный; 2) обесцвеченный; 3) ничем не примечательный.

colour-printing ['kʌlə,printiŋ] *n полигр.* (многокрасочная) цветная печать.

colour-process ['kʌlə,prouses] *см.* colour-printing.

colt [koult] *n* 1) жеребёнок; 2) *разг.* новичок.

column ['kɔləm] *n* 1) *архит., воен.* колонна; close ~ сомкнутая колонна; 2) столб(ик); vertebral ~, spinal ~ позвоночный столб; спинной хребет; a ~ of smoke столб дыма; 3) столбец (*в газете*); раздел, отдел (*объявлений в газете*); 4) *pl разг.* газета, журнал; 5) графа.

columnist ['kɔləmnist] *n амер.* фельетонист; обозреватель.

com- [kɔm-, kəm-] *pref* придающий значение совместного или взаимного действия; *перед словами, начинающимися с* l, n, r, *принимает соответственно формы* col-, con-, cor-.

comb I [koum] *n* 1) гребень; 2) гребёнка, гребешо́к; 3) скребни́ца; 4) со́ты; 5) конёк (*крыши*); 6) *текст.* чеса́льная маши́на; ◇ to set up one's ~ хорохо́риться, задава́ться; to cut the ~ of сбить спесь.

comb II *v* 1) чеса́ть, расчёсывать; 2) мять, трепа́ть (*лён и т. п.*); 3) чи́стить скребни́цей; 4) *воен.* «прочёсывать» (*разведкой, огнём*); □ to ~ out а) вычёсывать; б) *воен.* переосвиде́тельствовать (*солдат*).

combat I ['kɔmbət] *n* 1) бой; single ~ единобо́рство, поеди́нок; 2) *attr* боево́й; строево́й.

combat II *v* сража́ться, би́ться, боро́ться (*за — for, против — against, with*).

combatant I ['kɔmbətənt] *n* 1) солда́т; бое́ц; 2) бо́рющаяся сторона́; 3) побо́рник.

combatant II *a* боево́й, строево́й.

combative ['kɔmbətɪv] *a* 1) вои́нственный; 2) драчли́вый.

combination [,kɔmbɪ'neɪʃən] *n* 1) сочета́ние; комбина́ция; ~ of circumstances стече́ние обсто́ятельств; 2) соедине́ние; 3) *pl* комбина́ция (*дамское бельё*).

combinative ['kɔmbɪnətɪv] *a* комбинацио́нный; скло́нный к комбина́циям.

combinatorial [kəm,baɪnə'tourɪəl] *a* комбинато́рный.

combineᵃ [kəm'baɪn] *v* 1) соединя́ть(ся), объединя́ть(ся); 2) комбини́ровать; сме́шивать.

combineᵇ ['kɔmbaɪn] *n* 1) *с.-х.* комба́йн; 2) комбина́т, синдика́т; 3) *полит.* объедине́ние.

combings ['koumɪŋz] *n pl* очёски.

comb-out ['koum,aut] *n* 1) вычёсывание; 2) чи́стка (*служащих, членов союза и т. п.*).

combustibility [kəm,bʌstə'bɪlɪtɪ] *n* воспламеня́емость.

combustible [kəm'bʌstəbl] *a* горю́чий.

combustibles [kəm'bʌstəblz] *n pl* горю́чее, то́пливо.

combustion [kəm'bʌstʃən] *n* 1) горе́ние, сгора́ние; spontaneous ~ самовозгора́ние; 2) *хим.* окисле́ние (*органических веществ*).

come [kʌm] *v* (*past* came; *p. p.* come) 1) приходи́ть, подходи́ть; приезжа́ть; прибыва́ть; I'll ~ and see you tomorrow я зайду́ к вам за́втра; 2): to ~ into a fortune получи́ть насле́дство; to ~ into one's own получи́ть то, что полага́ется; to ~ into effect (*или* force) входи́ть в си́лу (*о законе, постановлении*); to ~ into bud дать по́чки; to ~ into blossom (*или* flower) распусти́ться (*о цветах, кустах, деревьях*); to ~ to oneself а) приходи́ть в себя́; б) образу́миться; 3) случа́ться, происходи́ть, быва́ть; how did you ~ to hear of it? как случи́лось, что вы услы́шали об э́том?; 4) получа́ться, выходи́ть; 5) доходи́ть, достига́ть: to ~ of age дости́гнуть совершенноле́тия; to ~ right прийти́ в поря́док; 6) обходи́ться; 7) происходи́ть, быть ро́дом (*из какого-л. места; of*); 8): ~!, ~! ну!, ну!; успоко́йтесь!; □ to ~ about случа́ться; происходи́ть; to ~ across случа́йно встре́титься, наткну́ться; to ~ after а) сле́довать (за); б) прийти́ по́зже друго́го; в) насле́довать; to ~ again возвраща́ться; *амер. сленг* повтори́ть ска́занное; to ~ along идти́ вме́сте; сопровожда́ть; ~ along! пойдём!, идём!; to ~ asunder распада́ться на ча́сти; to ~ at а) добира́ться; б) дока́пываться (*до истины*); в) набра́сываться;

to ~ away а) уходи́ть; ~ away! отойди́те!; б) отла́мываться; отска́кивать; to ~ back а) возвраща́ться; б) всплыва́ть (*о воспоминаниях*); to ~ before а) предше́ствовать; б) превосходи́ть; в) предста́ть (*перед судом*); to ~ by а) проходи́ть ми́мо; б) достава́ть, добыва́ть; в) *амер.* заходи́ть; to ~ down а) па́дать (*о снеге, дожде*); б) спуска́ться, опуска́ться; в) переходи́ть по тради́ции; г) па́дать, снижа́ться (*о ценах*); д) брани́ться; набра́сываться (*на — upon*); е) уплати́ть, расщедри́ться (*with*); to ~ forward а) отве́тить на призы́в, откли́кнуться; б) предлага́ть свои́ услу́ги (*for*); to ~ in а) войти́; ~ in, please! войди́те!; б) вступа́ть (*в должность*); в) сде́латься мо́дным, войти́ в мо́ду; г) *спорт.* прийти́ пе́рвым к фи́нишу; д) созрева́ть, поспева́ть; е) получи́ть свою́ до́лю (*for*); to ~ off а) удаля́ться; б) отрыва́ться (*о пуговицах и т. п.*); в) име́ть ме́сто; состоя́ться; г) отде́латься (*небольшим наказа́нием*); to ~ on а) наступа́ть; напада́ть; бро́ситься (*в атаку*); б) расти́; преуспева́ть, де́лать успе́хи; в) разрази́ться (*о буре*), налете́ть (*о шква́ле, ветре*); г) возника́ть (*о вопросе*); д) пора́жать (*о болезни*); е): ~ on! живе́й!; продолжа́йте!; to ~ out а) выходи́ть (*тж. перен. о кни́ге, журнале и т. п.*); б) появля́ться; обнару́живаться; вскрыва́ться (*о фактах*); в) забасто́вать; г) распуска́ться (*о листьях, цвета́х*); д) проявля́ться (*о фотопласти́нке*); е) вы́палить; вы́ступить (*с заявле́нием; with*); to ~ over а) приезжа́ть, переезжа́ть; перебра́ться; б) переходи́ть (*на чью-л. сто́рону*); в) овладева́ть, захва́тывать (*о чу́встве*); приходи́ть в го́лову; to ~ round а) заходи́ть (*в гости*); б) поправля́ться (*после боле́зни*); приходи́ть в себя́; в) обойти́, обману́ть; to ~ to приходи́ть в себя́, приходи́ть в созна́ние; to ~ under а) подходи́ть (*под рубрику, классифика́цию*); б) подпада́ть под влия́ние; to ~ up а) поднима́ться; б) выраста́ть; возника́ть; в) взойти́ (*о растении*), дава́ть ростки́; г) войти́ в мо́ду; д) поступи́ть в университе́т; е) приезжа́ть (*из небольшо́го в более кру́пный город*); ж) подходи́ть к, сравня́ться с (*to*); з) догна́ть, нагна́ть (*кого-л.— with*); и): ~ up! но, пошла́! (*к лошади*); to ~ upon а) набрести́ на; б) *воен.* произвести́ внеза́пную ата́ку; ◇ to ~ back as wise as one went ≅ верну́ться несо́лоно хлеба́вши.

come-and-go ['kʌmənd'gou] *n* 1) движе́ние взад и вперёд; 2) *attr* случа́йный (*о людях*).

come-at-able [kʌm'ætəbl] *a* досту́пный.

comedian [kə'mi:djən] *n* 1) а́втор коме́дий; 2) актёр-ко́мик.

comedienne [kə,medɪ'en] *n* коми́ческая актри́са.

come-down ['kʌmdaun] *n* паде́ние; упа́док.

comedy ['kɔmɪdɪ] *n* коме́дия.

comely ['kʌmlɪ] *a* хоро́шенький, милови́дный.

comer ['kʌmə] *n* приходя́щий, пришле́ц; the first ~ пе́рвый прише́дший; all ~s все, кто пришёл.

comestibles [kə'mestɪblz] *n pl* съестны́е припа́сы.

comet ['kɔmɪt] *n* коме́та.

comfort I ['kʌmfət] *n* 1) утеше́ние; успоко́ение; подде́ржка (*мора́льная*); 2) поко́й; 3) комфо́рт; 4) *pl* удо́бства; creature ~s ме́лкие предме́ты ли́чного потребле́ния (*папиросы и т. д.*); ◊ cold ~, Dutch ~ сла́бое утеше́ние.

comfort II *v* утеша́ть; успока́ивать.

comfortable ['kʌmfətəbl] *a* 1) удо́бный; комфорта́бельный; 2) утеши́тельный; 3) споко́йный, дово́льный.

comforter ['kʌmfətə] *n* 1) утеши́тель; а Job's ~ плохо́й утеши́тель; 2) шерстяно́й шарф, тёплое ка́шне; 3) *амер.* стёганое ва́тное одея́ло; 4) *амер. сленг* газе́та (*кото́рой накрыва́ются бездо́мные, ночу́я под откры́тым не́бом*).

comfortless ['kʌmfətlıs] *a* 1) неудо́бный, неую́тный; 2) печа́льный, безуте́шный.

comfy ['kʌmfı] *разг. см.* comfortable.

comic I ['kɔmık] *n* 1) кинокоме́дия; 2) *разг.* актёр-ко́мик.

comic II *a* коми́ческий, юмористи́ческий.

comical ['kɔmıkəl] *a* коми́чный; чудно́й, поте́шный.

comics ['kɔmıks] *n pl амер.* ко́микс; бульва́рный журна́л.

coming I ['kʌmıŋ] *n* прие́зд, прибы́тие; прихо́д.

coming II *a* 1) бу́дущий; наступа́ющий; ожида́емый; 2) многообеща́ющий (*о писа́теле*).

coming-in ['kʌmıŋ'ın] *n* ввоз (*това́ров*).

coming-out ['kʌmıŋ'aut] *n* вы́воз (*това́ров*).

comity ['kɔmıtı] *n* ве́жливость.

comma ['kɔmə] *n* запята́я; inverted ~s ка́вычки.

command I [kə'mɑːnd] *n* 1) кома́нда; прика́з; 2) кома́ндование, боево́е управле́ние; under ~ под кома́ндованием; to be in ~ кома́ндовать (*чем-л.— of*); at ~ в распоряже́нии; 3) вое́нный о́круг (*в А́нглии*); 4) госпо́дство, власть; 5) владе́ние (*собо́й, языко́м и т. п.*); to have a good ~ of a language хорошо́ (о)владе́ть языко́м.

command II *v* 1) кома́ндовать; 2) прика́зывать; yours to ~ к Ва́шим услу́гам; 3) госпо́дствовать (*над чем-л.*); 4) владе́ть (*собо́й, языко́м и т. п.*); to ~ oneself владе́ть собо́й; 5) распоряжа́ться (*су́ммами и т. п.*); 6) *воен.* держа́ть под обстре́лом.

commandant [,kɔmən'dænt] *n* 1) коменда́нт; 2) нача́льник вое́нной акаде́мии *или* вое́нного учи́лища.

commandeer [,kɔmən'dıə] *v* 1) реквизи́ровать; 2) привлека́ть в принуди́тельном поря́дке.

commander [kə'mɑːndə] *n* 1) команди́р; нача́льник; кома́ндующий; 2) *мор.* капита́н 3 ра́нга.

Commander-in-Chief [kə'mɑːndərın'tʃiːf] *n* 1) главнокома́ндующий; 2) *мор.* кома́ндующий фло́том *или* отде́льной эска́дрой.

command-in-chief [kə'mɑːndın'tʃiːf] *n* гла́вное кома́ндование.

commanding [kə'mɑːndıŋ] *a* 1) кома́ндующий; 2) домини́рующий; 3) внуши́тельный.

commandment [kə'mɑːndmənt] *n* за́поведь.

commando [kə'mɑːndou] *n воен.* 1) диверси́онно-деса́нтный отря́д; 2) бое́ц-деса́нтник.

commemorate [kə'meməreıt] *v* 1) пра́здновать (*годовщи́ну*); отмеча́ть (*собы́тие*); 2) служи́ть напомина́нием.

commemoration [kə,memə'reıʃən] *n* 1) пра́зднование (*годовщи́ны*); in ~ of в ознаменова́ние; 2) (С.) годово́й акт (*в Оксфо́рдском университе́те*).

commemorative [kə'memərətıv] *a* мемориа́льный, па́мятный.

commence [kə'mens] *v* начина́ть(ся).

commencement [kə'mensmənt] *n* 1) нача́ло; 2) день присужде́ния университе́тских степене́й (*в Ке́мбридже, Ду́блине и др.*); 3) *амер.* акт; а́ктовый день (*в амер. уче́бных заведе́ниях*).

commend [kə'mend] *v* 1) хвали́ть; рекомендова́ть; 2) *уст.* вверя́ть; поруча́ть; 3) *уст.* передава́ть приве́т, покло́н.

commendable [kə'mendəbl] *a* похва́льный.

commendation [,kɔmən'deıʃən] *n* похвала́.

commensurable [kə'menʃərəbl] *a* соизмери́мый (*с чем-л.— with, to*); пропорциона́льный (*to*).

commensurate [kə'menʃərıt] *a* соразме́рный (*with*); пропорциона́льный (*чему-л.— with, to*)

comment I ['kɔment] *n* 1) толкова́ние; коммента́рий; поясне́ние; 2) замеча́ние.

comment II *v* 1) комменти́ровать (*что-л.— upon*); 2) де́лать крити́ческие замеча́ния (*о чём-л.— upon*).

commentary ['kɔməntərı] *n* коммента́рий; running ~ радиорепорта́ж; to keep up a running ~ вести́ радиорепорта́ж.

commentation [,kɔmen'teıʃən] *n* 1) комменти́рование; толкова́ние (*те́кста*); 2) аннота́ция.

commentator ['kɔmenteıtə] *n* коммента́тор.

commerce ['kɔməːs] *n* 1) торго́вля; комме́рция; 2) обще́ние.

commercial I [kə'məːʃəl] *n разг.* 1) коммивояжёр (*тж.* ~ traveller); 2) *ра́дио, тлв.* рекла́ма и объявле́ния; рекла́мная переда́ча.

commercial II *a* торго́вый, комме́рческий.

commercialism [kə'məːʃəlızəm] *n* торга́шеский дух.

commingle [kɔ'mıŋgl] *v* сме́шивать(ся).

commiserate [kə'mızəreıt] *v* сочу́вствовать, выража́ть соболе́знование.

commiseration [kə,mızə'reıʃən] *n* соболе́знование.

commissar [,kɔmı'sɑː] *n* комисса́р.

commissariat [,kɔmı'seərıət] *n* 1) комиссариа́т; 2) *воен.* интенда́нтство.

commissary ['kɔmısərı] *n* 1) комисса́р; 2) *воен.* интенда́нт.

commission I [kə'mıʃən] *n* 1) комите́т, коми́ссия; interim ~ вре́менный комите́т (*или* коми́ссия); 2) полномо́чия, дове́ренность; компете́нция; to resign one's ~ а) сложи́ть свои́ полномо́чия; б) *воен.* вы́йти в отста́вку; 3) поруче́ние, зада́ние; 4) соверше́ние; ~ of murder соверше́ние уби́йства; 5) командиро́вка; 6) пате́нт на офице́рский чин (*в А́нглии*); 7) комиссио́нная прода́жа; 8) комиссио́нное вознагражде́ние; ◊ in ~ гото́в к пла́ванию (*о корабле́*); to come (to put) into ~ *мор.* вступа́ть (вводи́ть) в строй (*о корабле́*); out of ~ в неиспра́вности.

commission II *v* 1) назнача́ть на до́лжность; 2) уполномо́чивать; 3) поруча́ть; 4) *мор.* назнача́ть команди́ра корабля́; укомплекто́вывать ли́чным соста́вом (*корабля́*).

commissionaire [kə,mıʃə'nɛə] *n* 1) посы́льный; швейца́р; 2) аге́нт по подыска́нию рабо́ты (*для бы́вших военнослу́жащих в А́нглии*).

commissioner [kə'mıʃnə] *n* 1) член парла́мент-ской комиссии; 2) уполномоченный; High Commissioner Верховный комиссар (*в колонии*).

commit [kəˈmɪt] *v* 1) поручать, вверять; 2): to ~ oneself принимать на себя обязательства; 3) заключать (*в тюрьму*); 4) предавать (*огню, суду и т. п.*); 5) передавать (*законопроект в комиссию*); 6) совершать (*ошибку, преступление*); 7) *воен.* вводить в дело.

commitment [kəˈmɪtmənt] *n* 1) заключение под стражу; 2) предание суду; 3) совершение (*преступления и т. п.*); 4) обязательство.

committal [kəˈmɪtl] *n* 1) заключение в тюрьму; 2) передача (*законопроекта в комиссию*).

committeeᵃ [kəˈmɪtɪ] *n* 1) комитет; Central Committee Центральный Комитет; Executive Committee исполнительный комитет; Standing Committee постоянный комитет; ad hoc ~ специальный комитет; local ~ профком; strike (steering) ~ стачечный (организационный) комитет; 2) комиссия; credentials ~ мандатная комиссия; Joint Committee междуведомственная комиссия; Un-American Activities ~ комиссия по расследованию антиамериканской деятельности; to go into ~ передать вопрос на рассмотрение комиссии (*в англ. парламенте*); a check-up ~ *амер.* ревизионная комиссия.

committeeᵇ [ˌkɔmɪˈtiː] *n юр.* опекун (*при душевнобольном*).

commixture [kɔˈmɪkstʃə] *n* смешение; смесь.

commode [kəˈmoud] *n* комод.

commodious [kəˈmoudjəs] *a* просторный.

commodity [kəˈmɔdɪtɪ] *n* 1) товар; предмет широкого потребления; 2) *attr* товарный.

commodore [ˈkɔmədɔː] *n* 1) *мор.* коммодор (*звание между капитаном I ранга и контр-адмиралом*); 2) президент яхт-клуба.

common I [ˈkɔmən] *n* 1) общее, обычное; in ~ совместно; сообща; out of the ~ незаурядный; to have smth. in ~ with иметь что-л. сходное с (*кем-л.*); 2) общинная земля; 3) пустырь; 4) право на пользование общественным выгоном, землёй; ◇ on short ~s впроголодь.

common II *a* 1) общий; 2) общественный; 3) обыкновенный; обычный; 4) простой; 5) грубый; вульгарный; 6) *грам.* нарицательный.

commonage [ˈkɔmənɪdʒ] *n* право на общественный выгон.

commoner [ˈkɔmənə] *n* 1) человек из народа; 2) член палаты общин; First Commoner спикер; 3) студент, не получающий стипендии; 4) имеющий общинные права.

commonly [ˈkɔmənlɪ] *adv* 1) обычно, обыкновенно, заурядно; 2) дёшево, плохо.

commonplace I [ˈkɔmənpleɪs] *n* банальность, избитое выражение.

commonplace II *a* банальный, избитый, плоский.

commonplace-book [ˈkɔmənpleɪsˌbuk] *n* общая тетрадь (*для записи цитат, заметок и т. п.*).

common-room [ˈkɔmənrum] *n* профессорская (*тж.* senior ~); учительская (*в англ. университетах*).

commons [ˈkɔmənz] *n pl* 1) (the C.) палата общин (*тж.* House of Commons); 2) *ист.* третье сословие; 3) простой народ (*в отличие от высших классов*); 4) порция.

commonwealth [ˈkɔmənwelθ] *n* 1) государство;

республика; the Commonwealth (of England) Английская республика (1649—1660 гг.); 2) федерация; содружество; the (British) Commonwealth (of Nations) (Британское) Содружество (Наций).

commotion [kəˈmouʃən] *n* 1) волнение; 2) смятение; потрясение; 3) суматоха.

communal [ˈkɔmjunl] *a* 1) коммунальный, общественный; 2) общинный.

communeᵃ [ˈkɔmjuːn] *n* 1) коммуна; the (Paris) Commune Парижская Коммуна; 2) община.

communeᵇ [kəˈmjuːn] *v* беседовать, общаться (*с — with*).

communicable [kəˈmjuːnɪkəbl] *a* 1) сообщаемый; 2) сообщающийся; 3) приветливый; любезный; 4) заразный (*о болезни*).

communicate [kəˈmjuːnɪkeɪt] *v* 1) передавать, сообщать (*кому-л.— to*); 2) сообщаться (*с — with*); сноситься; 3) *церк.* причащаться.

communication [kəˌmjuːnɪˈkeɪʃən] *n* 1) сообщение; связь; коммуникация; vocal ~ устное сообщение; 2) средство сообщения, связи (*железная дорога, телеграф и т. п.*); 3) *pl воен.* коммуникационные линии, коммуникации.

communicative [kəˈmjuːnɪkətɪv] *a* разговорчивый, общительный.

communion [kəˈmjuːnjən] *n* 1) общение; 2) *церк.* причастие.

communiqué [kəˈmjuːnɪkeɪ] *n* официальное сообщение; коммюнике.

communism [ˈkɔmjunɪzəm] *n* коммунизм.

communist I [ˈkɔmjunɪst] *n* коммунист.

communist II *a* коммунистический; the Communist Party of the Soviet Union Коммунистическая партия Советского Союза; Leninist Young Communist League of the Soviet Union Всесоюзный Ленинский Коммунистический Союз Молодёжи; the Young Communist League Комсомол.

communistic [ˌkɔmjuˈnɪstɪk] *a* коммунистический.

community [kəˈmjuːnɪtɪ] *n* 1) община; the ~ общество, публика; 2) общность; ~ of interest общность интересов.

commutation [ˌkɔmjuːˈteɪʃən] *n* 1) замена; 2) смягчение (*наказания*); 3) *воен.* деньги, выдаваемые взамен натурального довольствия; 4) *эл.* переключение тока.

commutative [kəˈmjuːtətɪv] *a* заменяющий.

commutator [ˈkɔmjuːteɪtə] *n эл.* переключатель тока, коммутатор.

commute [kəˈmjuːt] *v* 1) обменивать (*одну вещь на другую*); заменять; 2) смягчать (*наказание*); 3) *эл.* переключать (*ток*); 4) *амер.* совершать регулярные поездки (*на поезде, пароходе и т. п.*).

commuter [kəˈmjuːtə] *n амер.* пассажир, имеющий сезонный билет.

compactᵃ¹ [ˈkɔmpækt] *n* соглашение, договор.

compactᵃ² *n* прессованная пудра.

compactᵇ I [kəmˈpækt] *a* 1) плотный; компактный; 2) сжатый (*о стиле*).

compactᵇ II *v* уплотнять.

companion I [kəmˈpænjən] *n* 1) товарищ; 2) спутник, попутчик; 3) компаньон; 4) компаньон(ка); соучастник; ~ in crime соучастник преступления; 5) справочник; Gardener's ~ спутник садовода; 6) один из парных предметов; 7) кавалер ордена (*низшей степени*).

companion II *v* сопровождать, быть компаньоном.

companionable [kəm'pænjənəbl] *a* общительный.

companion-in-arms [kəm'pænjənin,ɑːmz] *n* товарищ по оружию.

companionship [kəm'pænjənʃip] *n* компания; товарищество, товарищеские отношения.

company ['kʌmpəni] *n* 1) компания, общество; for ~ за компанию; in ~ with вместе с; to keep ~ with водить дружбу, водить компанию; to keep ~ *разг.* ухаживать (*за женщиной*); to keep (*или* to bear) smb.'s ~ сопровождать кого-л.; составлять компанию кому-л.; to part ~ а) разойтись в разные стороны, расстаться, распрощаться (*с — with*); б) порвать с кем-л.; present ~ always excepted о присутствующих не говорят; 2) общество, товарищество; insurance ~ страховое общество; railway ~ железнодорожная акционерная компания; 3) гости; to see a great deal of ~ принимать много гостей; 4) собеседник; to be good (bad) ~ быть приятным (скучным) собеседником; 5) труппа; 6) экипаж (*судна; тж.* the ship's ~); 7) *воен.* рота; 8) *attr* ротный.

comparable ['kɔmpərəbl] *a* сравнимый.

comparative I [kəm'pærətiv] *n грам.* сравнительная степень.

comparative II *a* сравнительный (*тж. грам.*); относительный.

compare I [kəm'pɛə] *v* 1) сравнивать; 2) сличать, сопоставлять; 3) уподоблять.

compare II *n уст.* сравнение; beyond ~, past ~ вне всякого сравнения.

comparison [kəm'pærisn] *n* 1) сравнение; in ~ with по сравнению с; to bear (*или* to stand) ~ with выдерживать сравнение с; 2) сходство.

compartment [kəm'pɑːtmənt] *n* 1) отделение; купе; 2) *мор., тех.* отсек.

compass I ['kʌmpəs] *n* 1) компас; буссоль; 2) *pl.* циркуль; 3) окружность, круг; 4) диапазон; границы; beyond my ~ за пределами моего понимания, моих возможностей.

compass II *v* 1) осуществлять (*намерение*); 2) замышлять (*что-л. скверное*); 3) *уст.* окружать, обносить (*стеной и т. п.*).

compassion [kəm'pæʃən] *n* сострадание, жалость; to have (*или* to take) ~ испытывать жалость, сострадание (*к кому-л. — on*).

compassionate[a] [kəm'pæʃənit] *a* сострадательный.

compassionate[b] [kəm'pæʃəneit] *v* относиться с жалостью, состраданием.

compatibility [kəm,pætə'biliti] *n* совместимость, согласованность.

compatible [kəm'pætəbl] *a* совместимый, согласующийся.

compatriot [kəm'pætriət] *n* соотечественник.

compeer [kɔm'piə] *n* ровня; товарищ.

compel [kəm'pel] *v* 1) заставлять; принуждать, вынуждать; 2) подчинять.

compelling [kəm'peliŋ] *a* неотразимый, непреодолимый.

compendia [kəm'pendiə] *pl см.* compendium.

compendious [kəm'pendiəs] *a* краткий, сокращённый.

compendium [kəm'pendiəm] *n* (*pl тж.* compendia) 1) конспект, краткая запись; 2) резюме.

compensate ['kɔmpenseit] *v* 1) возмещать, компенсировать; 2) вознаграждать; 3) *амер.* оплачивать (*услуги*); 4) *тех.* уравновешивать.

compensation [,kɔmpen'seiʃən] *n* 1) возмещение; компенсация; 2) вознаграждение; 3) *амер.* жалованье; 4) *тех.* уравновешивание.

compete [kəm'piːt] *v* 1) соревноваться, состязаться; 2) конкурировать.

competence ['kɔmpitəns] *n* 1) способность; 2) компетентность; 3) достаток; 4) *юр.* компетенция; полномочие.

competency ['kɔmpitənsi] *см.* competence.

competent ['kɔmpitənt] *a* 1) компетентный; 2) *юр.* правомочный; 3) имеющий достаточную власть.

competition [,kɔmpi'tiʃən] *n* 1) соревнование; socialist ~ социалистическое соревнование; to be in ~ with состязаться, соревноваться с (*кем-л.*); 2) состязание, матч; boxing (skiing, swimming) ~ соревнование по боксу (по лыжам, по плаванию); chess ~ шахматный турнир; 3) конкурс; конкурсный экзамен; 4) конкуренция; cut-throat (*или* severe) ~ жестокая конкуренция.

competitive [kəm'petitiv] *a* 1) конкурсный; 2) соревнующийся; 3) соперничающий, конкурирующий.

competitor [kəm'petitə] *n* конкурент, соперник.

compilation [,kɔmpi'leiʃən] *n* 1) компиляция; 2) компилирование.

compile [kəm'pail] *v* 1) составлять, компилировать; 2) собирать (*факты, данные*); 3) накапливать (*имущество*).

compiler [kəm'pailə] *n* составитель, компилятор.

complacence [kəm'pleisns] *см.* complacency.

complacency [kəm'pleisnsi] *n* 1) самодовольство; 2) благодушие.

complacent [kəm'pleisnt] *a* 1) самодовольный; 2) благодушный.

complain [kəm'plein] *v* 1) жаловаться (*тж. на боль*); подавать жалобу; 2) выражать недовольство; 3) *поэт.* испускать жалобный крик.

complaint [kəm'pleint] *n* 1) жалоба; недовольство; to lodge (*или* to make) а ~ подать жалобу (*на кого-л. — against*); 2) недомогание.

complaisance [kəm'pleizəns] *n* 1) услужливость; вежливость; 2) уступчивость.

complaisant [kəm'pleizənt] *a* 1) услужливый, любезный; вежливый; 2) уступчивый.

complement[a] ['kɔmplimənt] *n* 1) дополнение (*тж. грам.*); ~ of an angle *мат.* дополнение до прямого угла; 2) комплект; 3) штатный состав (*воинской части, корабля*).

complement[b] ['kɔmpliment] *v* 1) дополнять; служить дополнением; 2) укомплектовывать.

complementary [,kɔmpli'mentəri] *a* дополнительный, добавочный.

complete I [kəm'pliːt] *a* 1) полный; 2) цельный; законченный; 3) совершённый.

complete II *v* 1) заканчивать, завершать; 2) пополнять; комплектовать.

completely [kəm'pliːtlɪ] *adv* совершённо, полностью.

completeness [kəm'pliːtnɪs] *n* 1) полнота; 2) закóнченность.

completion [kəm'pliːʃən] *n* 1) завершéние, окончáние; 2) комплéкт.

complex I ['kɔmpleks] *n* кóмплекс.

complex II *a* 1) слóжный; запутанный; 2) кóмплексный, составнóй.

complexion [kəm'plekʃən] *n* 1) цвет лицá; 2) вид; оттéнок, аспéкт.

complexity [kəm'pleksɪtɪ] *n* 1) слóжность; запутанность; 2) кóмплексность.

compliance [kəm'plaɪəns] *n* 1) угóдливость, 2) подáтливость, устýпчивость; 3) соглáсие; in ~ with в соотвéтствии с, соглáсно.

compliant [kəm'plaɪənt] *a* 1) угóдливый; 2) подáтливый, устýпчивый.

complicacy ['kɔmplɪkəsɪ] *n* 1) слóжность, запутанность; 2) усложнéние.

complicate I ['kɔmplɪkeɪt] *a* запутанный.

complicate II *v* 1) усложнять; 2) *мед.* осложняться.

complicated ['kɔmplɪkeɪtɪd] *a* слóжный; запутанный.

complication [,kɔmplɪ'keɪʃən] *n* 1) слóжность; запутанность; слóжное положéние; 2) *мед.* осложнéние.

complicity [kəm'plɪsɪtɪ] *n* соучáстие (*в преступлении и т. п.*).

compliment[a] ['kɔmplɪmənt] *n* 1) комплимéнт; left-handed ~ сомнительный комплимéнт; to pay a ~ сказáть комплимéнт; 2) любéзность, одолжéние; 3) *pl* поклóн, привéт; *pl* please, present my ~s to... пожáлуйста, передáйте мой привéт...; with ~s с привéтом (*в письмах*). ~ **compliment**[b] ['kɔmplɪmənt] *v* 1) привéтствовать; поздравлять; 2) подарить (*что-л.— with*).

complimentary [,kɔmplɪ'mentərɪ] *a* 1) похвáльный; лéстный; 2) поздравительный; 3) пригласительный (*о билете*).

comply [kəm'plaɪ] *v* 1) исполнять (*прóсьбу, трéбование и т. п.*); 2) подчиняться (*прáвилам*); уступáть, соглашáться.

component I [kəm'pounənt] *n* компонéнт, составнáя часть.

component II *a* составнóй; составляющий.

comport [kəm'pɔːt] *v* 1): to ~ oneself вести себя; 2) соотвéтствовать (*with*).

compose [kəm'pouz] *v* 1) составлять; 2) сочинять (*стихи, мýзыку*); 3) компоновáть; 4) успокáивать; to ~ oneself успокáиваться; 5) улáживать (*ссóру, неприятность*); 6) *полигр.* набирáть.

composed [kəm'pouzd] *a* спокóйный, сдéржанный.

composer [kəm'pouzə] *n* композитор.

composing-machine [kəm'pouzɪŋmə,ʃiːn] *n* по *лигр.* набóрная машина.

composing-stick [kəm'pouzɪŋstɪk] *n* *полигр.* верстáтка.

composite I ['kɔmpəzɪt] *n* смесь.

composite II *a* 1) слóжный; составнóй; 2) *бот.* сложноцвéтный.

composition [,kɔmpə'zɪʃən] *n* 1) произведéние (*литератýрное, музыкáльное*); 2) компози·

ция, компонóвка (*в искусстве*); 3) составлéние; 4) сочинéние (*шкóльное*); 5) *хим.* состáв, соединéние; смесь, сплав; 6) уговóр, соглашéние (*о перéмирии, о выплате дóлга и т. п.*); 7) склад умá; харáктер; 8) *полигр.* набóр.

compositor [kəm'pɔzɪtə] *n* набóрщик.

compost ['kɔmpɔst] *n* *с.-х.* составнóе удобрéние, компóст.

composure [kəm'pouʒə] *n* спокóйствие, самообладáние.

compote ['kɔmpout] *n* компóт.

compound[a] I ['kɔmpaund] *n* 1) смесь, соединéние; 2) составнóе слóво; 3) *тех.* компáунд.

compound[a] II *a* 1) составнóй; слóжный; 2) *грам.* сложносочинённый (*о предложéнии*).

compound[b] [kəm'paund] *v* 1) смéшивать, соединять; составлять; 2) улáживать, примирять (*интерéсы*); 3) прощáть (*оскорблéние*).

comprehend [,kɔmprɪ'hend] *v* 1) понимáть, постигáть; 2) включáть, охвáтывать.

comprehensible [,kɔmprɪ'hensəbl] *a* понятный, постижимый.

comprehension [,kɔmprɪ'henʃən] *n* 1) понимáние; понятливость; it passes my ~ это выше моегó понимáния; 2) охвáт, включéние.

comprehensive [,kɔmprɪ'hensɪv] *a* 1) понятливый; 2) всесторóнний; подрóбный; исчéрпывающий, глубóкий.

compress[a] ['kɔmpres] *n* компрéсс.

compress[b] [kəm'pres] *v* сжимáть; сдáвливать.

compressed [kəm'prest] *a* сжáтый.

compression [kəm'preʃən] *n* 1) сжáтие; сдáвливание; 2) *тех.* компрéссия; уплотнéние.

comprise [kəm'praɪz] *v* 1) включáть; заключáть в себé; 2) содержáть, вмещáть.

compromise I ['kɔmprəmaɪz] *n* компромисс.

compromise II *v* 1) пойти на компромисс; 2) (с)компрометировать (*себя, кого-л.*).

compromiser ['kɔmprəmaɪzə] *n* соглашáтель, примирéнец.

compulsion [kəm'pʌlʃən] *n* принуждéние.

compulsive [kəm'pʌlsɪv] *a* принудительный; обязáтельный.

compulsory [kəm'pʌlsərɪ] *a* принудительный.

compunction [kəm'pʌŋkʃən] *n* угрызéния сóвести; раскáяние.

computable [kəm'pjuːtəbl] *a* исчислимый.

computation [,kɔmpjuː'teɪʃən] *n* подсчёт; вычислéние, расчёт.

compute [kəm'pjuːt] *v* подсчитывать; вычислять.

computer [kəm'pjuːtə] *n* 1) счётно-решáющее устрóйство; (электрóнно-)вычислительная машина; 2) вычислитель.

comrade ['kɔmrɪd] *n* товáрищ.

comrade-in-arms ['kɔmrɪdɪn,ɑːmz] *n* сорáтник.

comradeship ['kɔmrɪdʃɪp] *n* товáрищеские отношéния.

con[1] [kɔn] *v* зубрить, долбить.

con[2] *v* вести сýдно.

con- [kɔn-] *см.* com-.

concave I ['kɔn'keɪv] *a* вóгнутый.

concave II *n* *поэт.* небéсный свод.

concavity [kɔn'kævɪtɪ] *n* вóгнутая повéрхность.

concavo-concave [kɔn'keɪvou'kɔnkeɪv] *a* двояковóгнутый (*о линзе*).

concavo-convex [kɔn'keɪvou'kɔnveks] *a* двояко-выпуклый (*о линзе*).

conceal [kən'siːl] *v* 1) скрывать, утаивать; укрывать; прятать; 2) маскировать.

concealer [kən'siːlə] *n* укрыватель.

concealment [kən'siːlmənt] *n* 1) сокрытие, утаивание; укрывательство; 2) тайное убежище; тайник; 3) маскировка.

concede [kən'siːd] *v* 1) допускать, соглашаться; 2) уступать (*право*).

conceit [kən'siːt] *n* 1) самомнение; тщеславие; full of ~ высокого мнения о себе; самодовольный; out of ~ with разочарованный в; 2) причуда, фантазия.

conceited [kən'siːtɪd] *a* тщеславный; самодовольный.

conceivable [kən'siːvəbl] *a* постижимый, понятный, вразумительный.

conceive [kən'siːv] *v* 1) задумывать; 2) представлять себе; понимать; 3) формулировать, выражать; 4) почувствовать; 5) зачать.

concentrate I ['kɔnsentreɪt] *n* концентрат.

concentrate II *v* 1) концентрировать(ся); сосредоточивать(ся); 2) *хим.* сгущать, выпаривать; 3) *горн.* обогащать руду.

concentration [,kɔnsen'treɪʃən] *n* 1) концентрация; сосредоточение; 2) сгущение; 3) *горн.* обогащение руды; 4) *attr* концентрированный; 5) *attr* концентрационный (*о лагере*).

concentric [kɔn'sentrɪk] *a* 1) концентрический; 2) *воен.* сосредоточенный (*об огне*).

concept ['kɔnsept] *n* понятие, общее представление.

conception [kən'sepʃən] *n* 1) понимание; понятие; 2) концепция, мысль; 3) замысел (*художественный и т. п.*).

concern I [kən'səːn] *n* 1) дело, отношение, касательство; to have no ~ with не иметь отношения (*к чему-л.*); no ~ of mine это не моё дело; mind your own ~s! занимайтесь своим делом!; 2) интерес, участие; доля, пай; 3) забота; беспокойство; 4) значение, важность; 5) концерн, фирма; предприятие; 6) *pl* дела.

concern II *v* 1) касаться, иметь отношение к; his life is ~ed речь идёт о его жизни; 2) интересовать; to ~ oneself интересоваться; 3) заниматься (*вопросом, делом*); to be ~ed in быть заинтересованным (*или* замешанным) в чём-л.; 4) заботиться, беспокоиться; to be ~ed at (*или* for, about) быть огорчённым чем-л. (*или* за кого-л.).

concerned [kən'səːnd] *a* 1) имеющий отношение к чему-л.; 2) озабоченный; расстроенный.

concerning [kən'səːnɪŋ] *prep* относительно, в отношении.

concert[a] ['kɔnsət] *n* 1) концерт; 2) согласие; уговор; in ~ with совместно, по уговору.

concert[b] [kən'səːt] *v* сговариваться; договариваться.

concerto [kən'tʃəːtou] *n* концерт (*муз. форма*).

concession [kən'seʃən] *n* 1) уступка; 2) концессия.

concession(n)aire [kən,seʃə'nɛə] *n* концессионер.

concessive [kən'sesɪv] *a* 1) уступчивый; 2) *грам.* уступительный.

conch [kɔŋk] *n* раковина, ракушка.

conciliate [kən'sɪlɪeɪt] *v* 1) примирять; 2) снискать доверие.

conciliation [kən,sɪlɪ'eɪʃən] *n* примирение; умиротворение; замирение.

conciliator [kən'sɪlɪeɪtə] *n* 1) мировой посредник; примиритель; 2) *полит.* примиренец.

conciliatory [kən'sɪlɪətərɪ] *a* 1) примирительный; 2) примиренческий.

concise [kən'saɪs] *a* краткий, сокращённый; сжатый.

conciseness [kən'saɪsnɪs] *n* краткость.

conclave ['kɔnkleɪv] *n* 1) тайное совещание; 2) *церк.* конклав.

conclude [kən'kluːd] *v* 1) заключать; заканчивать (-ся); 2) делать вывод; 3) решать.

conclusion [kən'kluːʒən] *n* 1) заключение; a ~ of a treaty заключение договора; 2) окончание; to bring to a ~ заканчивать; in ~ в заключение; 3) вывод, заключение; to draw a ~ делать вывод; выводить заключение; to jump at (*или* to) a ~ делать поспешный вывод.

conclusive [kən'kluːsɪv] *a* 1) заключительный; 2) убедительный; 3) решающий.

concoct [kən'kɔkt] *v* 1) стряпать; 2) выдумывать (*небылицы*); измышлять.

concoction [kən'kɔkʃən] *n* 1) стряпня; 2) вымысел.

concomitant [kən'kɔmɪtənt] *a* сопутствующий.

concord ['kɔŋkɔːd] *n* 1) согласие; 2) конвенция, договор; 3) *грам.* согласование; 4) *муз.* гармония.

concordance [kən'kɔːdəns] *n* 1) согласие; соответствие; 2) алфавитный указатель слов *или* изречений (*встречающихся у данного автора*).

concordant [kən'kɔːdənt] *a* 1) согласующийся; 2) гармоничный.

concourse ['kɔŋkɔːs] *n* 1) стечение народа; 2) скопление (*чего-л.*); 3) *амер.* главный зал вокзала.

concrete[a] I ['kɔnkriːt] *n* 1) бетон; armoured (*или* reinforced) ~ железобетон; 2): in the ~ в действительности, реально.

concrete[a] II *a* 1) конкретный; реальный; 2) бетонный.

concrete[a] III *v* бетонировать; заливать бетоном.

concrete[b] [kən'kriːt] *v* сгущаться; затвердевать; твердеть.

concretion [kən'kriːʃən] *n* 1) сращение; 2) сгущение; коагуляция; 3) твёрдая сросшаяся масса; 4) *мед.* камень.

concubine ['kɔŋkjubaɪn] *n* 1) любовница; 2) наложница.

concur [kən'kəː] *v* 1) совпадать; 2) соглашаться, сходиться во мнениях; 3) способствовать, содействовать.

concurrence [kən'kʌrəns] *n* 1) совпадение; 2) стечение (*обстоятельств*); 3) содействие.

concurrent I [kən'kʌrənt] *n* конкурент.

concurrent II *a* 1) совпадающий; 2) параллельный; совместный, действующий совместно.

concussion [kən'kʌʃən] *n* 1) сотрясение (*обыкн. мозга*); 2) контузия.

condemn [kən'dem] *v* 1) осуждать; 2) приговаривать, выносить приговор; 3) выдавать, уличать; his looks ~ him его вид выдаёт его; 4) браковать, признавать негодным.

condemnation [,kɔndem'neɪʃən] *n* 1) осуждение; 2) приговор (*судебный*).

condemnatory [kən'demnətərɪ] *a* обвинительный.

condensation [ˌkɔnden'seɪʃən] *n* 1) сгущение; конденсация; to produce by ~ вываривать (*соль и т. п.*); 2) конденсированная масса; 3) краткость (*изложения*).

condense [kən'dens] *v* 1) сгущать(ся); 2) конденсировать; 3) сокращать (*изложение*); сжато выражать (*мысль*).

condenser [kən'densə] *n* 1) конденсатор; 2) холодильник; газоохладитель; 3) *эл.* лейденская банка.

condescend [ˌkɔndɪ'send] *v* снизойти; удостоить.

condescension [ˌkɔndɪ'senʃən] *n* 1) снисхождение; 2) снисходительность.

condiment ['kɔndɪmənt] *n* приправа.

condition I [kən'dɪʃən] *n* 1) условие; on ~ that при условии, что; если; to make it a ~ поставить условием; 2) *pl* обстоятельства; favourable ~s благоприятные обстоятельства; under existing ~s при данных обстоятельствах; в настоящих условиях; under such ~s при таких условиях; 3) состояние, положение; in good (bad) ~ в хорошем (плохом) состоянии; out of ~ в плохом состоянии; to be in no ~ не быть в состоянии; to change one's ~ жениться, выйти замуж; 4) *амер.* переэкзаменовка; «хвост».

condition II *v* 1) обусловливать; 2) приводить в надлежащее состояние.

conditional I [kən'dɪʃənl] *n грам.* условный союз; условное предложение; условное наклонение.

conditional II *a* условный (*тж. грам.*); обусловленный.

conditioned [kən'dɪʃənd] *a* 1) обусловленный; 2) условный (*о рефлексах*); 3) кондиционированный.

condolatory [kən'doulətrɪ] *a* выражающий соболезнование; сочувствующий.

condole [kən'doul] *v* выражать соболезнование; сочувствовать.

condolence [kən'douləns] *n* соболезнование; сочувствие; please, accept my ~ примите моё соболезнование.

condone [kən'doun] *v* 1) забывать, прощать; 2) *церк.* отпускать (*грехи*).

conduce [kən'djuːs] *v* способствовать (*чему-л. — to*), вести к.

conducive [kən'djuːsɪv] *a* способствующий.

conduct ['kɔndəkt] *n* 1) поведение; 2) ведение (*дел*); руководство.

conduct [kən'dʌkt] *v* 1) вести; to ~ oneself вести себя; he ~s himself well он хорошо себя ведёт; 2) сопровождать; 3) руководить, управлять; 4) командовать (*армией*); 5) *муз.* дирижировать; 6) *физ.* проводить (*тепло, электричество*).

conduction [kən'dʌkʃən] *n физ.* проводимость.

conductivity [ˌkɔndʌk'tɪvɪtɪ] *n физ.* проводимость; теплопроводность; электропроводность.

conductor [kən'dʌktə] *n* 1) (художественный) руководитель; дирижёр, капельмейстер; 2) кондуктор (*трамвая, автобуса*); вожатый (*трамвая*); *амер. ж.-д.* проводник; 4) *физ.* проводник.

conduit ['kɔndjuɪt] *n* 1) трубопровод; 2) водопроводная труба; 3) *эл.* изоляционная трубка.

cone [koun] *n* 1) конус; 2) шишка (*еловая, сосновая*).

coney ['kounɪ] *см.* cony.

confabulate [kən'fæbjuleɪt] *v* разговаривать.

confection [kən'fekʃən] *n* 1) сласти; 2) готовое женское платье, конфекцион.

confectioner [kən'fekʃnə] *n* кондитер.

confectionery [kən'fekʃnərɪ] *n* кондитерская.

confederacy [kən'fedərəsɪ] *n* 1) конфедерация, лига; 2) заговор.

confederate I [kən'fedərɪt] *n* 1) сообщник, соучастник (*преступления*); 2) член конфедерации, союзник; 3) конфедерат, сторонник южных штатов (*в гражданской войне 1861—1865 гг. в Америке*).

confederate II *a* союзный, федеральный.

confederate [kən'fedəreɪt] *v* объединять(ся) в союз, конфедерацию.

confederation [kənˌfedə'reɪʃən] *n* конфедерация, союз.

confer [kən'fəː] *v* 1) присваивать (*звание*); присуждать (*степень*); 2) совещаться, беседовать (*с кем-л. — together, with*).

confer[2] *imp* сопоставь, сравни.

conference ['kɔnfərəns] *n* 1) конференция; совещание; Cabinet Conference заседание министров; a round-table ~ конференция «круглого стола»; a summit ~ конференция, совещание на высшем уровне; 2) съезд.

conferment [kən'fəːmənt] *n* присвоение (*звания*); присуждение (*степени*).

confess [kən'fes] *v* 1) признаваться, признавать (*вину*); сознаваться; 2) исповедовать(ся).

confession [kən'feʃən] *n* 1) признание (*вины и т. п.*); 2) исповедь; 3) вероисповедание.

confessor [kən'fesə] *n* исповедник, духовник.

confidant [ˌkɔnfɪ'dænt] *n* (*ж. р.* confidante) доверенное лицо.

confide [kən'faɪd] *v* 1) доверять, полагаться на (*in*); 2) поверять (*секреты; кому-л. — to*); 3) поручать (*кому-л. — to*).

confidence ['kɔnfɪdəns] 1) доверие; to enjoy one's ~ пользоваться чьим-л. доверием; to give one's ~ to доверять; to place ~ in верить, доверять; 2) уверенность; 3) смелость, самонадеянность; 4) конфиденциальное сообщение; told in ~ конфиденциально, по секрету; in strict ~ под строжайшим секретом; to exchange ~s секретничать.

confident I ['kɔnfɪdənt] *n* доверенное лицо.

confident II *a* 1) уверенный (*в успехе и т. п.*); 2) смелый, самонадеянный.

confidential [ˌkɔnfɪ'denʃəl] *a* 1) конфиденциальный; секретный; 2) доверительный; 3) пользующийся доверием, надёжный.

configuration [kənˌfɪgju'reɪʃən] *n* очертания, форма; конфигурация.

confine ['kɔnfaɪn] *n обыкн. pl* пределы, рубеж; границы.

confine [kən'faɪn] *v* 1) ограничивать; 2) ограничиваться, держаться в пределах; 3) заключать в тюрьму; 4): to be ~d рожать; to be ~d to bed быть прикованным к постели.

confinement [kən'faɪnmənt] *n* 1) ограничение; 2) тюремное заключение; 3) роды.

confirm [kən'fəːm] *v* 1) подтверждать; 2) подкреплять, поддерживать (*мнение и т. п.*); 3) утверждать (*во владении, в должности, звании и т. п.*); 4) ратифицировать (*договор*); 5) *церк.* конфирмовать.

confirmation [ˌkɔnfə'meɪʃən] *n* 1) подтверждение; 2) подкрепление; 3) утверждение (*во владении, в должности, звании и т. п.*); 4) *церк.* конфирмация.

confirmed [kənˈfəːmd] *a* 1) хрони́ческий; 2) закоренéлый.

confiscate [ˈkɔnfɪskeɪt] *v* конфискова́ть; реквизи́ровать.

confiscation [ˌkɔnfɪsˈkeɪʃən] *n* конфиска́ция; реквизи́ция.

conflagration [ˈkɔnfləˈgreɪʃən] *n* большо́й пожа́р.

conflict[a] [ˈkɔnflɪkt] *n* 1) конфли́кт, столкновéние; 2) противорéчие; борьба́.

conflict[b] [kənˈflɪkt] *v* 1) противорéчить (кому́-л., чему́-л. — with); 2) быть в конфли́кте; боро́ться.

confluence [ˈkɔnfluəns] *n* 1) слия́ние (рек); пересечéние (дорог); мéсто слия́ния; 2) стечéние (наро́да).

confluent I [ˈkɔnfluənt] *n* прито́к (реки́).

confluent II *a* слива́ющийся.

conflux [ˈkɔnflʌks] *n* стечéние наро́да, толпа́.

conform [kənˈfɔːm] *v* 1) соотвéтствовать; сообразова́ться, согласо́вываться (с чем-л. — to); 2) приспоса́бливать(ся), принора́вливать(ся); 3) подчиня́ться пра́вилам (to).

conformation [ˌkɔnfɔːˈmeɪʃən] *n* 1) устро́йство; фо́рма; 2) рельéф мéстности; 3) подчинéние (пра́вилам).

conformist [kənˈfɔːmɪst] *n* конформи́ст.

conformity [kənˈfɔːmɪtɪ] *n* соотвéтствие, согласо́ванность.

confound [kənˈfaund] *n* 1) поража́ть, ста́вить в тупи́к, смуща́ть; 2) смéшивать, пу́тать; 3) разруша́ть (планы); ◊ ~ it! к чёрту!

confounded [kənˈfaundɪd] *a* 1) смущённый, поста́вленный в тупи́к; сби́тый с то́лку; 2) разг. прокля́тый; перен. а́дский, тяжёлый.

confoundedly [kənˈfaundɪdlɪ] *adv разг.* ужа́сно, стра́шно, чрезвыча́йно.

confront [kənˈfrʌnt] *v* 1) стоя́ть лицо́м к лицу́; столкну́ться; 2) смотрéть в лицо́ (опасности, смерти); 3) противостоя́ть (трудностям); 4) предъявля́ть (требования); 5) устро́ить о́чную ста́вку (with); 6) сличáть, сопоставля́ть.

confrontation [ˌkɔnfrʌnˈteɪʃən] *n* 1) о́чная ста́вка; 2) сопоставлéние, сличéние.

confuse [kənˈfjuːz] *v* 1) производи́ть беспоря́док; приводи́ть в беспоря́док; 2) спу́тывать, перепу́тывать; 3) приводи́ть в замеша́тельство, смуща́ть (обыкн. в pass); 4) помрача́ть созна́ние.

confused [kənˈfjuːzd] *a* 1) спу́танный, перепу́танный; 2) бессвя́зный; беспоря́дочный, тума́нный; 3) смущённый; в замеша́тельстве, сби́тый с то́лку.

confusion [kənˈfjuːʒən] *n* 1) беспоря́док, неразбери́ха; 2) пу́таница; 3) смущéние, замеша́тельство.

confutable [kənˈfjuːtəbl] *a* опровержи́мый.

confutation [ˌkɔnfjuːˈteɪʃən] *n* опровержéние.

confute [kənˈfjuːt] *v* опроверга́ть.

congeal [kənˈdʒiːl] *v* 1) замерза́ть, застыва́ть; 2) свёртываться, сгуща́ться; 3) замора́живать.

congelation [ˌkɔndʒɪˈleɪʃən] *n* 1) замерза́ние, застыва́ние; 2) свёртывание, сгущéние, затвердéние; 3) замора́живание.

congenial [kənˈdʒiːnjəl] *a* 1) ро́дственный, бли́зкий; (по духу, взглядам; with, to); конгениа́льный; 2) подходя́щий (к — to).

congeniality [kənˌdʒiːnɪˈælɪtɪ] *n* сродство́; бли́зость (по духу, взглядам); конгениа́льность.

congenital [kɔnˈdʒenɪtl] *a* прирождённый; врождённый.

congeries [kɔnˈdʒɪəriːz] *n* (pl без измен.) скоплéние; ма́сса; ку́ча.

congest [kənˈdʒest] *v* переполня́ть(ся).

congested [kənˈdʒestɪd] *a* 1) мед. перепо́лненный (кро́вью); 2) перенаселённый; тéсный.

congestion [kənˈdʒestʃən] *n* 1) мед. переполнéние (кро́вью); 2) перенаселённость, теснота́; 3) скоплéние; 4) перегру́женность, зато́р (в у́личном движéнии).

conglomerate[a] [kɔnˈglɔmərɪt] *n* 1) конгломера́т; 2) геол. обло́мочная го́рная поро́да.

conglomerate[b] [kɔnˈglɔməreɪt] *v* 1) собира́ть(ся); скопля́ть(ся); 2) превраща́ться в сли́тную ма́ссу.

conglomeration [kɔnˌglɔməˈreɪʃən] *n* 1) скоплéние; сгу́сток; 2) конгломера́ция, превращéние в сли́тную ма́ссу.

Congolese I [ˌkɔŋgəˈliːz] *n* конголéзец; конголéзка; the ~ (употр. как pl) конголéзцы.

Congolese II *a* конголéзский.

congratulate [kənˈgrætjuleɪt] *v* поздравля́ть (с — on, upon).

congratulation [kənˌgrætjuˈleɪʃən] *n* обыкн. pl поздравлéние.

congratulatory [kənˈgrætjulətərɪ] *a* поздрави́тельный.

congregate [ˈkɔŋgrɪgeɪt] *v* собира́ть(ся), ска́пливать(ся).

congregation [ˌkɔŋgrɪˈgeɪʃən] *n* 1) скоплéние, схо́дка; 2) собра́ние профессо́ров (в Кéмбриджском и О́ксфордском университéтах); 3) церк. прихожа́не; 4) общи́на.

congress [ˈkɔŋgres] *n* 1) съезд; конгрéсс; a medical ~ съезд враче́й; The World Peace Congress Всеми́рный конгрéсс сторо́нников ми́ра; 2) (the C.) конгрéсс США.

congressional [kɔŋˈgreʃənl] *a* 1) относя́щийся к конгрéссу; 2) избира́тельный (см. тж. district I).

Congressman [ˈkɔŋgresmən] *n* амер. конгрессмéн, член конгрéсса.

congruence [ˈkɔŋgruəns] *n* 1) соотвéтствие; 2) согласова́ние.

congruent [ˈkɔŋgruənt] *см.* congruous.

congruous [ˈkɔŋgruəs] *a* 1) соотвéтствующий; гармони́рующий; 2) мат. конгруэ́нтный, сравни́мый.

conic [ˈkɔnɪk] *a* кони́ческий.

conical [ˈkɔnɪkəl] *a* конусообра́зный; кони́ческий.

conifer [ˈkɔunɪfə] *n* хво́йное дéрево.

coniferous [kouˈnɪfərəs] *a* хво́йный.

conjectural [kənˈdʒektʃərəl] *a* предположи́тельный.

conjecture I [kənˈdʒektʃə] *n* предположéние; дога́дка.

conjecture II *v* предполага́ть, дéлать предположéние; предуга́дывать.

conjee [ˈkɔndʒiː] *n* ри́совый отва́р.

conjoin [kənˈdʒɔɪn] *v* соединя́ть(ся); сочета́ть(ся).

conjoint [ˈkɔndʒɔɪnt] *a* соединённый; объединённый.

conjugal [ˈkɔndʒugəl] *a* супру́жеский, бра́чный.

conjugality [ˌkɔndʒuˈgælɪtɪ] *n* супру́жество.

conjugate[a] ['kɔndʒugeɪt] v 1) спрягать (глагол); 2) соединяться; спариваться.

conjugate[b] ['kɔndʒugɪt] a 1) соединённый; спаренный; 2) мат. сопряжённый; 3) бот. парный; 4) лингв. родственный (о слове).

conjugation [,kɔndʒu'geɪʃən] n 1) спряжение (глагола); periphrastic ~ спряжение с помощью вспомогательного глагола; 2) соединение.

conjunct [kən'dʒʌŋkt] a соединённый; объединённый.

conjunction [kən'dʒʌŋkʃən] n 1) соединение, связь; in ~ with вместе, в связи с; 2) стечение (обстоятельств); 3) грам. союз.

conjunctional [kən'dʒʌŋkʃənəl] a грам. относящийся к союзу.

conjunctive I [kən'dʒʌŋktɪv] n грам. сослагательное наклонение.

conjunctive II a 1) связывающий; 2) анат. соединительный (о ткани).

conjuncture [kən'dʒʌŋktʃə] n 1) стечение обстоятельств; положение дел; 2) конъюнктура.

conjure[a] [kən'dʒuə] v умолять, заклинать.

conjure[b] ['kʌndʒə] v 1) показывать фокусы; 2) колдовать; заклинать; 3) изгонять духов (тж. to ~ away); 4) воскрешать в памяти, вызывать в воображении (тж. to ~ up).

conjurer ['kʌndʒərə] n 1) фокусник; 2) волшебник, колдун, заклинатель; ◊ he is no ~ ≅ он пороха не выдумает.

conjuror ['kʌndʒərə] см. conjurer.

conk I [kɔŋk] n сленг 1) нос; 2) перебои в моторе.

conk II v испортиться, сломаться (о машине; тж. to ~ out).

conky ['kɔŋkɪ] a сленг носатый.

connate ['kɔneɪt] a 1) врождённый; 2) рождённый или возникший одновременно.

connatural [kə'nætʃrəl] a 1) врождённый; 2) подобный, сходный.

connect [kə'nekt] v 1) соединять(ся), связывать (-ся); 2) ассоциировать.

connected [kə'nektɪd] a 1) связанный; соединённый; well ~ имеющий большие связи; 2) связный (о рассказе, речи).

connection [kə'nekʃən] n 1) связь; in this ~ в этой связи; in ~ with в связи с; 2) обыкн. pl связи, знакомства; to have a ~ иметь связи (among); 3) (при)соединение; 4) сочленение; 5) согласованность расписания (поездов, пароходов); 6) клиентура, покупатели; 7) родство; свойство; 8) родственник; свойственник; 9) половая связь; to form a ~ вступить в связь.

connective I [kə'nektɪv] n грам. соединительное слово.

connective II a 1) связующий; 2) анат. соединительный (о ткани).

connexion [kə'nekʃən] см. connection.

connivance [kə'naɪvəns] n потворство, попустительство.

connive [kə'naɪv] v потворствовать.

connoisseur [,kɔnɪ'sə:] n знаток.

connotation [,kɔnou'teɪʃən] n вторичное, дополнительное значение.

connote [kɔ'nout] v 1) иметь дополнительное значение (о слове); 2) иметь дополнительное следствие (о фактах).

connubial [kə'nju:bjəl] a брачный, супружеский.

conquer ['kɔŋkə] v 1) завоёвывать, покорять; побеждать; 2) преодолевать (затруднения, препятствия и т. п.); превозмогать; 3) отделаться (от привычки); 4) обуздывать, подавлять (чувства, страсти); 4) добиваться (своей цели).

conqueror ['kɔŋkərə] n 1) завоеватель; победитель; the Conqueror ист. Вильгельм Завоеватель; 2) спорт. решающая партия.

conquest ['kɔŋkwest] n 1) завоевание, покорение; победа; the (Norman) Conquest ист. завоевание Англии норманнами (в 1066 г.); 2) завоёванная территория.

consanguineous [,kɔnsæŋ'gwɪnɪəs] a единокровный.

consanguinity [,kɔnsæŋ'gwɪnɪtɪ] n кровное родство.

conscience ['kɔnʃəns] n совесть; good ~, clear ~ чистая совесть; bad ~, guilty ~ нечистая совесть, in (all) ~ разг. конечно, поистине; to have on one's ~ иметь на совести, чувствовать за собой вину; to have the ~ to иметь наглость, совести хватает (сказать, сделать что-л.); to make a matter of ~ поступать по совести.

conscientious [,kɔnʃɪ'enʃəs] a 1) добросовестный; 2) совестливый.

conscious ['kɔnʃəs] a 1) сознающий, чувствующий, ощущающий; to be ~ of знать, сознавать, чувствовать; to be ~ to the last быть в сознании до последней минуты; 2) сознательный, здравый.

consciousness ['kɔnʃəsnɪs] n 1) сознание; to recover ~, to regain ~ прийти в себя; очнуться; to lose ~ потерять сознание; 2) сознательность.

conscript I ['kɔnskrɪpt] n новобранец.

conscript II v призывать на военную службу.

conscription [kən'skrɪpʃən] n воинская повинность; набор; ~ of wealth обложение налогом лиц, не мобилизованных в армию.

consecrate I ['kɔnsɪkreɪt] v 1) посвящать; 2) освящать.

consecrate II a см. consecrated.

consecrated ['kɔnsɪkreɪtɪd] a 1) посвящённый; 2) освящённый.

consecration [,kɔnsɪ'kreɪʃən] n 1) посвящение; 2) освящение.

consecution [,kɔnsɪ'kju:ʃən] n 1) последовательность; течение, ход (событий); 2) грам. последовательность (времён); порядок (слов).

consecutive [kən'sekjutɪv] a последовательный.

consensus [kən'sensəs] n согласие, согласованность.

consent I [kən'sent] n 1) согласие; a half-hearted ~ вынужденное согласие; 2) разрешение.

consent II v 1) соглашаться; уступать; 2) разрешать.

consentient [kən'senʃənt] a согласный, согласующийся (с — with); совпадающий (с — to).

consequence ['kɔnsɪkwəns] n 1) (по) следствие; in ~ of вследствие, в результате; to take the ~s отвечать, нести ответственность за последствия; 2) значение, важность; of ~ важный, существенный; of no ~ неважный, несущественный; 3) влияние, влиятельное положение.

consequent I ['kɔnsɪkwənt] n 1) результат, последствие; 2) мат. последующий член (пропорции).

consequent II a 1) последовательный; следующий

(*за — on*); 2) вытека́ющий, явля́ющийся результа́том чего́-л.

consequential [͵kɔnsɪ'kwenʃəl] *a* 1) вытека́ющий, явля́ющийся сле́дствием; 2) самоуве́ренный, по́лный самомне́ния.

consequently ['kɔnsɪkwentlɪ] *adv* сле́довательно; поэ́тому; в результа́те.

conservancy [kən'səːvənsɪ] *n* 1) комите́т по регули́рованию судохо́дства и ры́бных про́мыслов; 2) охра́на приро́ды.

conservation [͵kɔnsəː'veɪʃən] *n* 1) (со)хране́ние; 2) спосо́бность по́мнить; 3) консерви́рование; 4) *см.* conservancy 2).

conservative I [kən'səːvətɪv] *n* 1) консерва́тор; реакционе́р; to go ~ стать консерва́тором; 2) (С.) *полит.* консерва́тор; член консервати́вной па́ртии.

conservative II *a* 1) консервати́вный; реакцио́нный; 2) охрани́тельный; охра́нный; 3) *разг.* скро́мный (*о подсчёте и т. п.*).

conservatoire [kən'səːvətwɑː] *n* консервато́рия.

conservator[a] ['kɔnsəːveɪtə] *n* 1) храни́тель (*музея и т. п.*); 2) член организа́ции по охра́не приро́ды.

conservator[b] [kən'səːvətə] *n* опеку́н.

conservatory [kən'səːvətrɪ] *n* 1) оранжере́я, тепли́ца; 2) *амер.* консервато́рия.

conserve I [kən'səːv] *n обыкн. pl* консерви́рованные фру́кты в са́харе; варе́нье.

conserve II *v* 1) сохраня́ть; храни́ть, бере́чь; 2) консерви́ровать.

consider [kən'sɪdə] *v* 1) рассма́тривать, обсужда́ть; 2) обду́мывать; размышля́ть; 3) полага́ть; счита́ть; 4) учи́тывать, принима́ть во внима́ние; взве́шивать (*за и против*); 5) проявля́ть уваже́ние к; счита́ться с.

considerable [kən'sɪdərəbl] *a* 1) значи́тельный; 2) ва́жный, ви́дный (*о положении человека*); 3) большо́й.

considerate [kən'sɪdərɪt] *a* внима́тельный; такти́чный, делика́тный.

consideration [kən͵sɪdə'reɪʃən] *n* 1) рассмотре́ние; обсужде́ние; under ~ рассма́триваемый; обсужда́емый; на рассмотре́нии; 2) *обыкн. pl* соображе́ние, мне́ние; 3) внима́ние; расчёт; leave out of ~ оставля́ть без внима́ния; to take into ~ принима́ть во внима́ние; in ~ of принима́я во внима́ние, учи́тывая; to pay serious ~ to обраща́ть серьёзное внима́ние на; on no ~ ни под каки́м ви́дом; 4) уваже́ние, предупреди́тельность; внима́тельность; 5) вознагражде́ние, мзда; 6) ва́жность, значи́тельность; of ~ по́льзующийся уваже́нием; выдаю́щийся (*о поэте, общественном деятеле и т. п.*); it's of no ~ э́то соверше́нно нева́жно; э́то не име́ет ро́вно никако́го значе́ния.

considering [kən'sɪdərɪŋ] *prep* учи́тывая, принима́я во внима́ние.

consign [kən'saɪn] *n* 1) передава́ть, препоруча́ть; 2) предава́ть (*земле*); 3) *ком.* отправля́ть груз, това́ры; 4) депони́ровать (*деньги*).

consignee [͵kɔnsaɪ'niː] *n* грузополуча́тель.

consignment [kən'saɪnmənt] *n* 1) груз, па́ртия това́ров; 2) отпра́вка това́ров; 3) *ком.* накладна́я, коносаме́нт.

consignor [kən'saɪnə] *n* грузоотправи́тель.

consist [kən'sɪst] *v* 1) состоя́ть (*из чего́-л. —*

of); 2) скла́дываться из, заключа́ться в, выража́ться в (*in*); 3) совмеща́ться, совпада́ть (*с — with*).

consistence [kən'sɪstəns] *n* консисте́нция.

consistency [kən'sɪstənsɪ] *n* 1) после́довательность; постоя́нство; сто́йкость; 2) консисте́нция.

consistent [kən'sɪstənt] *a* 1) совмести́мый, согласу́ющийся; 2) после́довательный; сто́йкий; 3) пло́тный.

consolation [͵kɔnsə'leɪʃən] *n* утеше́ние.

consolatory [kən'sɔlətərɪ] *a* утеши́тельный.

console[a] [kən'soul] *v* утеша́ть.

console[b] ['kɔnsoul] *n архит.* консо́ль.

console-mirror ['kɔnsoul͵mɪrə] *n* трюмо́.

consolidate [kən'sɔlɪdeɪt] *v* 1) укрепля́ть(ся); 2) объединя́ть (*территорию, общества и т. п.*); 3) *воен.* закрепля́ть (*захва́ченную пози́цию*); 4) *фин.* консолиди́ровать (*за́ймы*); 5) отвердева́ть, тверде́ть.

consolidated [kən'sɔlɪdeɪtɪd] *a* 1) консолиди́рованный; ~ annuities консолиди́рованная ре́нта (*в Англии*); 2) сво́дный (*о донесениях, сведениях и т. п.*); 3) затверде́вший.

consolidation [kən͵sɔlɪ'deɪʃən] *n* 1) укрепле́ние; 2) консолида́ция; 3) объедине́ние; 4) сво́дка; 5) *воен.* закрепле́ние (*захва́ченной пози́ции*); 6) отвердение, затвердева́ние.

consols [kən'sɔlz] *n pl фин.* консо́ли, консолиди́рованная ре́нта (*в Англии*).

consonance ['kɔnsənəns] *n* 1) созву́чие, гармо́ния; 2) согла́сие, еди́нство (*в мыслях, мне́ниях и т. п.*); in ~ with в согла́сии с; 3) *муз.* консона́нс.

consonant I ['kɔnsənənt] *n* 1) согла́сный звук; 2) бу́ква, изобража́ющая согла́сный звук.

consonant II *a* 1) согла́сный (*с — to*), совмести́мый (*с — with*); 2) созву́чный; гармони́чный.

consonantal [͵kɔnsə'næntl] *a грам.* согла́сный; оканчивающийся на согла́сный (*об основе*).

consort[a] ['kɔnsɔːt] *n* 1) супру́г; супру́га; prince ~ принц-консо́рт, супру́г ца́рствующей короле́вы; 2) *мор.* кора́бль сопровожде́ния; 3) спу́тник.

consort[b] [kən'sɔːt] *v* 1) обща́ться (*with*); 2) гармони́ровать; соотве́тствовать; 3) сопровожда́ть.

conspectus [kən'spektəs] *n* конспе́кт.

conspicuous [kən'spɪkjuəs] *a* 1) заме́тный, броса́ющийся в глаза́; обраща́ющий на себя́ внима́ние; 2) выдаю́щийся; ви́дный; находя́щийся на виду́.

conspiracy [kən'spɪrəsɪ] *n* 1) за́говор, та́йный сго́вор; 2) конспира́ция.

conspirator [kən'spɪrətə] *n* загово́рщик.

conspiratress [kən'spɪrətrɪs] *n* загово́рщица.

conspire [kən'spaɪə] *v* устра́ивать за́говор; та́йно сгова́риваться, замышля́ть.

constable ['kʌnstəbl] *n* консте́бль, полице́йский; Chief Constable нача́льник поли́ции (*в го́роде, гра́фстве*); ◊ to outrun the ~ жить не по сре́дствам, влеза́ть в долги́.

constabulary I [kən'stæbjulərɪ] *n* поли́ция, полице́йские си́лы.

constabulary II *a* полице́йский.

constancy ['kɔnstənsɪ] *n* 1) постоя́нство; 2) ве́рность (*принципам*); 3) твёрдость (*убежде́ний*).

constant I ['kɔnstənt] *n* 1) *мат.* постоя́нная величина́, конста́нта; 2) коэффицие́нт.

constant II *a* 1) постоя́нный; неизме́нный; 2) ве́рный (*принципам*); 3) твёрдый (*в убежде́ниях*).

constantly ['kɔnstəntlɪ] *adv* 1) постоя́нно; всегда́; 2) ча́сто, то и де́ло.

constellation [ˌkɔnstə'leɪʃən] *n* 1) созве́здие; 2) плея́да.

consternation [ˌkɔnstə'neɪʃən] *n* у́жас, испу́г.

constipate ['kɔnstɪpeɪt] *v мед.* вызыва́ть запо́р.

constipation [ˌkɔnstɪ'peɪʃən] *n мед.* запо́р.

constituency [kən'stɪtjuənsɪ] *n* 1) избира́тели; 2) избира́тельный о́круг; 3) покупа́тели, клиенту́ра; 4) подпи́счики (*на газету и т. п.*); ◊ to sweep a ~ получи́ть большинство́.

constituent I [kən'stɪtjuənt] *n* 1) избира́тель; 2) составна́я часть.

constituent II *a* 1) избира́тельный; 2) законода́тельный; учреди́тельный; 3) составно́й, составля́ющий.

constitute ['kɔnstɪtjuːt] *v* 1) назнача́ть; 2) образо́вывать, учрежда́ть, осно́вывать; 3) издава́ть *или* вводи́ть в си́лу зако́н; 4) составля́ть, быть составно́й ча́стью.

constitution[1] [ˌkɔnstɪ'tjuːʃən] *n* 1) конститу́ция, основно́й зако́н; 2) уста́в; 3) учрежде́ние, устро́йство; 4) *ист.* ука́з, уложе́ние.

constitution[2] *n* 1) телосложе́ние, склад; 2) соста́в, физи́ческое строе́ние.

constitutional[1] [ˌkɔnstɪ'tjuːʃənl] *a* конституцио́нный.

constitutional[2] I *n* моцио́н, прогу́лка.

constitutional[2] II *a* 1) *мед.* органи́ческий; 2) *хим.* структу́рный.

constitutive ['kɔnstɪtjuːtɪv] *a* 1) учреди́тельный; 2) составля́ющий, составно́й.

constitutor ['kɔnstɪtjuːtə] *n* учреди́тель, основа́тель.

constrain [kən'streɪn] *v* 1) вынужда́ть, принужда́ть; 2) сде́рживать; стесня́ть; 3) сажа́ть в тюрьму́.

constrained [kən'streɪnd] *a* 1) вы́нужденный, навя́занный; 2) напряжённый; сда́вленный (*о голосе*); смущённый (*об улыбке*); 3) неесте́ственный, натя́нутый (*о манерах*).

constrainedly [kən'streɪnɪdlɪ] *adv* 1) с напряже́нием, с уси́лием; 2) вы́нужденно, поневоле.

constraint [kən'streɪnt] *n* 1) принужде́ние; давле́ние; under ~ по принужде́нию; под давле́нием; 2) ско́ванность; стесне́ние; to feel ~ чу́вствовать себя́ нело́вко; 3) тюре́мное заключе́ние.

constrict [kən'strɪkt] *v* сжима́ть, стя́гивать; сда́вливать.

constriction [kən'strɪkʃən] *n* сжа́тие, сда́вливание.

constrictor [kən'strɪktə] *n* 1) *зоол.* уда́в, боа́; 2) *анат.* сокраща́тельная мы́шца.

construct [kən'strʌkt] *v* 1) стро́ить, сооружа́ть; конструи́ровать; 2) создава́ть, приду́мывать, сочиня́ть; 3) *грам.* составля́ть (*предложение*).

construction [kən'strʌkʃən] *n* 1) строи́тельство, стро́йка; under ~ находя́щийся в постро́йке, стро́ящийся; 2) зда́ние, постро́йка, сооруже́ние; 3) *грам.* констру́кция, структу́ра (*предложения*); 4) *мат.* построе́ние.

constructional [kən'strʌkʃənl] *a* структу́рный; конструкти́вный.

constructive [kən'strʌktɪv] *a* 1) строи́тельный; 2) конструкти́вный (*тж. о критике*); творче́ский, созида́тельный.

constructor [kən'strʌktə] *n* 1) строи́тель; 2) констру́ктор; 3) инжене́р-кораблестрои́тель.

construe [kən'struː] *v* 1) толкова́ть, истолко́вывать (*слова, действия*); понима́ть в осо́бом смы́сле; 2) де́лать синтакси́ческий разбо́р; 3) управля́ть; тре́бовать (*падежа и т. п.*).

consul ['kɔnsəl] *n* ко́нсул.

consular ['kɔnsjulə] *a* ко́нсульский.

consulate ['kɔnsjulɪt] *n* 1) ко́нсульство; 2) зва́ние ко́нсула.

consul-general ['kɔnsəl,dʒenərəl] *n* генера́льный ко́нсул.

consult [kən'sʌlt] *v* 1) сове́товаться (*c — with*); консульти́роваться; 2) справля́ться (*по книгам, словарям, у специалистов*); 3) посмотре́ть (*на часы*); 4) принима́ть во внима́ние, счита́ться (*с интересами и т. п.*).

consultant [kən'sʌltənt] *n* консульта́нт.

consultation [ˌkɔnsəl'teɪʃən] *n* 1) консульта́ция; 2) совеща́ние; обсужде́ние; 3) конси́лиум.

consultative [kən'sʌltətɪv] *a* совеща́тельный.

consulting [kən'sʌltɪŋ] *a* 1) консульти́рующий, даю́щий консульта́ции; 2) ле́чащий (*о враче*); 3) приёмный (*о часах врача*).

consume [kən'sjuːm] *v* 1) потребля́ть; расхо́довать; 2) пожира́ть (*тж. об огне, зависти и т. п.*); истребля́ть; 3) расточа́ть, прома́тывать (*средства и т. п.*); 4) истоща́ть, ча́хнуть.

consumer [kən'sjuːmə] *n* 1) потреби́тель; 2) *attr* широ́кого потребле́ния (*о товарах*).

consummate[a] [kən'sʌmɪt] *a* соверше́нный (*по качеству*); по́лный, зако́нченный.

consummate[b] ['kɔnsʌmeɪt] *v* 1) соверше́нствовать; 2) заверша́ть, доводи́ть до конца́.

consummation [ˌkɔnsʌ'meɪʃən] *n* 1) заверше́ние (*дела и т. п.*); 2) осуществле́ние; 3) жела́емый коне́ц, цель.

consumption [kən'sʌmpʃən] *n* 1) потребле́ние; расхо́дование; 2) туберкулёз лёгких; galloping ~ скороте́чная чахо́тка.

consumptive [kən'sʌmptɪv] *a* 1) туберкулёзный; 2) разруши́тельный.

contact ['kɔntækt] *n* 1) соприкоснове́ние; конта́кт; to come into ~ with прийти́ в соприкоснове́ние с; to make ~ а) установи́ть конта́кт; б) *эл.* включа́ть ток; to break ~ *эл.* выключа́ть ток; 2) *pl амер.* знако́мства, свя́зи; 3) *мат.* каса́ние; 4) *attr* конта́ктный.

contagion [kən'teɪdʒən] *n* 1) зара́за, инфе́кция; 2) инфекцио́нная боле́знь; 3) вре́дное влия́ние.

contagious [kən'teɪdʒəs] *a* 1) зара́зный, инфекцио́нный; 2) зарази́тельный (*о смехе*).

contain [kən'teɪn] *v* 1) содержа́ть (в себе́); вмеща́ть; 2) сде́рживать (*неприятеля, страсти*); to ~ oneself сде́рживаться; 3) *мат.* дели́ться без оста́тка.

container [kən'teɪnə] *n* 1) сосу́д, вмести́лище; 2) резервуа́р; конте́йнер; 3) *воен.* газобалло́н.

contaminate [kən'tæmɪneɪt] *v* 1) оскверня́ть; 2) заража́ть; 3) загрязня́ть, по́ртить.

contamination [kən,tæmɪ'neɪʃən] *n* 1) зараже́ние; 2) загрязне́ние; 3) разложе́ние, по́рча; 4) *лингв.* контамина́ция.

contemn [kən'tem] *v* презира́ть.

contemplate ['kɔntempleɪt] *v* 1) рассма́тривать; созерца́ть; 2) размышля́ть; обду́мывать; 3) предполага́ть, намерева́ться; 4) ожида́ть (*чего-л.*).

contemplation [ˌkɔntem'pleɪʃən] *n* 1) рассмотре́ние; 2) созерца́ние; 3) размышле́ние; разду́мье; 4) предположе́ние; is in ~ предполага́ется, намеча́ется; 5) ожида́ние (*чего-л.*).

contemplative ['kɔntempleɪtɪv] *a* созерца́тельный.

contemporaneity [kənˌtempərə'niːɪtɪ] *n* 1) совреме́нность; 2) одновреме́нность, совпаде́ние (*во времени*).

contemporaneous [kənˌtempə'reɪnjəs] *a* 1) совреме́нный; 2) одновреме́нный, совпада́ющий во вре́мени.

contemporary I [kən'tempərərɪ] *n* 1) совреме́нник; 2) све́рстник.

contemporary II *a* 1) совреме́нный; 2) одновре́менный.

contempt [kən'tempt] *n* 1) презре́ние (*к — for*); презри́тельное отноше́ние; пренебреже́ние; to hold in ~ презира́ть; to fall into ~ вызыва́ть к себе́ презри́тельное отноше́ние; *юр.* неуваже́ние к вла́сти; ~ of court неуваже́ние к суду́; ◇ in ~ of вопреки́, невзира́я на.

contemptible [kən'temptəbl] *a* презре́нный.

contemptuous [kən'temptʃuəs] *a* презри́тельный, пренебрежи́тельный.

contend [kən'tend] *v* 1) боро́ться; 2) состяза́ться; 3) спо́рить, оспа́ривать; 4) утвержда́ть, наста́ивать (*that*).

content[a1] ['kɔntent] *n* 1) *обыкн. pl* содержи́мое; содержа́ние (*книги, письма и т. п.*); 2) суть; основно́е содержа́ние; 3) вмести́мость, ёмкость, объём.

content[a2] *n* 1) дово́льство; чу́вство удовлетворе́ния; to one's heart's ~ до по́лного удовлетворе́ния; вво́лю; 2) член пала́ты ло́рдов, голосу́ющий за предложе́ние.

content[b] I [kən'tent] *a predic* 1) дово́льный, удовлетворённый (*with*); 2) согла́сный; 3) голосу́ющий за предложе́ние (*в палате лордов*).

content[b] II *v* удовлетворя́ть; to ~ oneself with удовлетворя́ться; дово́льствоваться чем-л.

contented [kən'tentɪd] *a* дово́льный; удовлетворённый (*чем-л. — with*).

contention [kən'tenʃən] *n* 1) спор, ссо́ра; 2) предме́т спо́ра, ссо́ры; 3) соревнова́ние.

contentious [kən'tenʃəs] *a* 1) спо́рный; 2) вздо́рный, приди́рчивый; 3) задо́рный.

contentment [kən'tentmənt] *n* удовлетворе́ние, удовлетворённость; дово́льство.

conterminous [kɔn'təːmɪnəs] *a* 1) сме́жный, име́ющий о́бщую грани́цу (*with, to*); 2) совпада́ющий.

contest[a] ['kɔntest] *n* 1) спор; 2) соревнова́ние, состяза́ние; beauty ~ ко́нкурс красоты́; close ~ *амер.* упо́рная борьба́ на вы́борах; three-cornered ~ предвы́борная борьба́ ме́жду представи́телями трёх полити́ческих па́ртий.

contest[b] [kən'test] *v* 1) спо́рить; 2) боро́ться (*за — for*); 3) отста́ивать и́стину; оспа́ривать чьё-л. утвержде́ние; 4) состяза́ться, выступа́ть в ка́честве конкуре́нта.

contestant [kən'testənt] *n* 1) проти́вник, со-

пе́рник; 2) уча́стник соревнова́ния; 3) кандида́т, претенде́нт; ~ for the presidency кандида́т в президе́нты.

contestee [kɔntes'tiː] *n* 1) кандида́т, баллоти́рующийся по тому́ же о́кругу; 2) уча́стник соревнова́ния.

context ['kɔntekst] *n* конте́кст.

contexture [kən'tekstʃə] *n* 1) компози́ция (*лит. произведения*); 2) структу́ра, ткань.

contiguity [ˌkɔntɪ'gjuːɪtɪ] *n* 1) соприкоснове́ние; 2) ассоциа́ция иде́й.

contiguous [kən'tɪgjuəs] *a* соприкаса́ющийся, прилега́ющий, сме́жный.

continence ['kɔntɪnəns] *n* 1) сде́ржанность; 2) воздержа́ние; целому́дрие.

continent[1] ['kɔntɪnənt] *n* 1) матери́к; контине́нт; 2) (the C.) Европе́йский контине́нт (*в противоположность Британским о-вам*); 3) (the C.) *амер. ист.* гру́ппа (пе́рвых) коло́ний.

continent[2] *a* 1) сде́ржанный; 2) возде́ржанный; целому́дренный.

continental I [ˌkɔntɪ'nentl] *n* жи́тель европе́йского контине́нта.

continental II *a* материко́вый; континента́льный.

contingency [kən'tɪndʒənsɪ] *n* случа́йность, непредви́денное обстоя́тельство.

contingent I [kən'tɪndʒənt] *n* континге́нт (*тж. вооружённых сил*).

contingent II *a* 1) случа́йный; непредви́денный; возмо́жный; 2) усло́вный.

continual [kən'tɪnjuəl] *a* постоя́нный, непреры́вный; беспреста́нный.

continually [kən'tɪnjuəlɪ] *adv* постоя́нно, непреры́вно.

continuance [kən'tɪnjuəns] *n* 1) продолжи́тельность, дли́тельность; of long ~ дли́тельный; 2) дли́тельное пребыва́ние (*в должности и т. п.*).

continuation [kənˌtɪnju'eɪʃən] *n* 1) продолже́ние; возобновле́ние; 2) *pl сленг* брю́ки.

continue [kən'tɪnjuː] *v* 1) продолжа́ть(ся); 2) остава́ться, пребыва́ть; 3) быть, служи́ть продолже́нием; 4) тяну́ться, простира́ться.

continued [kən'tɪnjuːd] *a* 1) продо́лженный, продолжа́ющийся; to be ~ продолже́ние сле́дует; 2) непреры́вный.

continuity [ˌkɔntɪ'njuːɪtɪ] *n* 1) непреры́вность; 2) после́довательная сме́на (*явлений, фактов и т. п.*).

continuous [kən'tɪnjuəs] *a* 1) непреры́вный; 2) сплошно́й; 3) постоя́нный; 4) *грам.* дли́тельный; 5) *радио* незатуха́ющий.

contort [kən'tɔːt] *v* 1) искривля́ть; 2) искажа́ть.

contortion [kən'tɔːʃən] *n* 1) искривле́ние; 2) искаже́ние.

contortionist [kən'tɔːʃnɪst] *n* 1) акроба́т, «челове́к-змея́»; 2) *театр.* мим.

contour I ['kɔntuə] *n* 1) очерта́ние. ко́нтур; 2) горизонта́ль; 3) *амер.* положе́ние дел; разви́тие собы́тий; 4) *attr* ко́нтурный.

contour II *v* 1) наноси́ть ко́нтур; 2) вычёрчивать горизонта́ли; 3) обходи́ть, огиба́ть.

contra- ['kɔntrə-] *pref в сложных словах обозначает* противо-.

contraband I ['kɔntrəbænd] *n* контраба́нда.

contraband II *a* контрабандный.

contrabandist ['kɔntrəbændɪst] *n* контрабандист.

contract[a] ['kɔntrækt] *n* 1) до́говор, контра́кт; соглаше́ние; labour ~ трудово́й до́говор; to enter into (*или* to make) a ~ with smb. заключи́ть до́говор с кем-л.; the ~ will not stand соглаше́ние не бу́дет име́ть си́лы; 2) *attr* сде́льный; догово́рный.

contract[b1] [kən'trækt] *v* 1) заключа́ть до́говор, соглаше́ние; 2) взять, приня́ть на себя́ обяза́тельства; 3) вступа́ть (*в брак, в союз*); 4) заводи́ть (*знакомство, дружбу*); 5) приобрета́ть (*привычку*); 6) влеза́ть (*в долги*); 7) схвати́ть (*болезнь*).

contract[b2] *v* 1) сокраща́ть(ся), сжима́ть(ся); су́живать(ся); 2) хму́рить (*брови*).

contracted[1] [kən'træktɪd] *a* 1) обусло́вленный до́говором; 2) *уст.* помо́лвленный.

contracted[2] *a* 1) нахму́ренный, смо́рщенный; 2) у́зкий, ограни́ченный (*о взглядах*); 3) *лингв.* сокращённый, стяжённый.

contractile [kən'træktaɪl] *a* сжима́ющий(ся), сокраща́ющий(ся).

contraction [kən'trækʃən] *n* 1) сжа́тие, сокраще́ние; уменьше́ние; 2) приобрете́ние (*привычки и т. п.*); 3) влеза́ние (*в долги*); 4) вступле́ние (*в брак*); 5) *лингв.* стяже́ние.

contractive [kən'træktɪv] *a* спосо́бный сокраща́ться, сжима́ться; сжима́ющийся, сокраща́ющийся.

contractor [kən'træktə] *n* 1) подря́дчик; 2) лицо́, подписа́вшее контра́кт; 3) *анат.* стя́гивающая мы́шца.

contradict [ˌkɔntrə'dɪkt] *v* 1) противоре́чить; 2) отрица́ть; опроверга́ть.

contradiction [ˌkɔntrə'dɪkʃən] *n* 1) противоре́чие; 2) опроверже́ние; 3) противополо́жность.

contradictious [ˌkɔntrə'dɪkʃəs] *a* противоречи́вый.

contradictor [ˌkɔntrə'dɪktə] *n* 1) оппоне́нт; проти́вник; 2) спо́рщик.

contradictory [ˌkɔntrə'dɪktərɪ] *a* 1) противоречи́вый; 2) противоре́чащий.

contradistinction [ˌkɔntrədɪs'tɪŋkʃən] *n* противопоставле́ние, различе́ние; in ~ to в отли́чие от.

contradistinguish [ˌkɔntrədɪs'tɪŋgwɪʃ] *v* противопоставля́ть, различа́ть.

contraposition [ˌkɔntrəpə'zɪʃən] *n* противополо́жение.

contrariety [ˌkɔntrə'raɪətɪ] *n* противоре́чие; разногла́сие.

contrariness ['kɔntrərɪnɪs] *n* упря́мство, своево́лие.

contrariwise ['kɔntrərɪwaɪz] *adv* 1) с друго́й стороны́; 2) наоборо́т; 3) в противополо́жном направле́нии.

contrary[a] I ['kɔntrərɪ] *n* противополо́жность; on the ~ наоборо́т; напро́тив; to the ~ ина́че, в обра́тном смы́сле.

contrary[a] II *a* 1) противополо́жный, обра́тный; to be ~ to противоре́чить; идти́ вразре́з с; 2) неблагоприя́тный; проти́вный (*о ветре*).

contrary[a] III *adv* вопреки́, несмотря́ на.

contrary[b] [kən'treərɪ] *a разг.* упря́мый, де́йствующий вопреки́ чему́-л.; своево́льный.

contrast[a] ['kɔntræst] *n* 1) противоположе́ние, противопоставле́ние; in ~ with по сравне́нию с; 2) противополо́жность; контра́ст; 3) отте́нок.

contrast[b] [kən'træst] *v* 1) противополага́ть, противопоставля́ть; 2) сопоставля́ть; 3) отлича́ться (*друг от друга*); контрасти́ровать.

contravene [ˌkɔntrə'viːn] *v* 1) наруша́ть (*правило, закон*); 2) идти́ вразре́з с; противоре́чить (*закону, правилу и т. п.*); 3) возража́ть, оспа́ривать.

contravention [ˌkɔntrə'venʃən] *n* наруше́ние (*правила, закона*).

contribute [kən'trɪbjuːt] *v* 1) соде́йствовать; способствовать; 2) же́ртвовать (*деньги*); 3) де́лать вклад (*в науку*); 4) писа́ть статьи́ (*для газеты, журнала*).

contribution [ˌkɔntrɪ'bjuːʃən] *n* 1) соде́йствие; 2) вклад (*вещественный, научный и т. п.*); 3) взнос; поже́ртвование; 4) статья́ (*газетная*); 5) сотру́дничество (*в журнале, газете*); 6) контрибу́ция; to lay under ~ облага́ть контрибу́цией.

contributor [kən'trɪbjutə] *n* 1) соде́йствующий; помо́щник; 2) а́втор стате́й, сотру́дник (*журнала, газеты*); 3) же́ртвователь.

contributory [kən'trɪbjutərɪ] *a* 1) соде́йствующий, способствующий; 2) де́лающий взно́сы; 3) сотру́дничающий.

contrite ['kɔntraɪt] *a* ка́ющийся, раска́ивающийся.

contrition [kən'trɪʃən] *n* раска́яние.

contrivance [kən'traɪvəns] *n* 1) изобрета́тельство; 2) изобрете́ние; 3) вы́думка, измышле́ние; 4) приспособле́ние (*механическое*).

contrive [kən'traɪv] *v* 1) изобрета́ть; выду́мывать; 2) замышля́ть, затева́ть; 3) ухитря́ться, умудря́ться; суме́ть; 4) устра́ивать (*свои дела*).

control I [kən'troul] *n* 1) управле́ние, руково́дство; remote ~ управле́ние на расстоя́нии; телеуправле́ние; mission ~ *косм.* кома́ндный пункт; to be in ~ of управля́ть, руководи́ть; to gain ~ получи́ть большинство́ (*при голосовании*); to lose ~ over (*или* of) потеря́ть управле́ние; 2) власть; to be beyond ~ вы́йти из-под влия́ния; 3) самооблада́ние; самоконтро́ль; 4) контро́ль, прове́рка; social ~ обще́ственный контро́ль; 5) регулиро́вка; 6) *pl* прибо́ры, рычаги́ управле́ния; 7) *attr* контро́льный.

control II *v* 1) управля́ть, руководи́ть; госпо́дствовать над кем-л.; 2) владе́ть (*тж. собой*); сде́рживать (*свои чувства*); 3) контроли́ровать; проверя́ть; 4) регули́ровать.

controllable [kən'trouləbl] *a* 1) управля́емый, регули́руемый; поддаю́щийся управле́нию, прове́рке, контро́лю; 2) послу́шный (*о механизме, животном и т. п.*).

controller [kən'troulə] *n* 1) контролёр, ревизо́р; 2) *тех.* контро́ллер.

controversial [ˌkɔntrə'vəːʃəl] *a* 1) спо́рный, дискуссио́нный; 2) лю́бящий спо́ры, поле́мику.

controversy ['kɔntrəvəːsɪ] *n* 1) спор, диску́ссия, поле́мика; without ~, beyond ~ беспо́рно; 2) спор, ссо́ра.

controvert ['kɔntrəvəːt] *v* 1) оспа́ривать, полемизи́ровать; 2) возража́ть, отрица́ть.

contumacious [ˌkɔntjuː'meɪʃəs] *a* неповину́ющийся, неподчиня́ющийся; непоко́рный.

contumacy ['kɔntjuməsı] *n* неповиновение, неподчинение.

contuse [kən'tjuːz] *v* контузить.

contusion [kən'tjuːʒən] *n* контузия.

convalesce [ˌkɔnvə'les] *v* выздоравливать.

convalescence [ˌkɔnvə'lesns] *n* выздоровление.

convalescent [ˌkɔnvə'lesnt] *a* выздоравливающий.

convene [kən'viːn] *v* 1) созывать (*собрание и т. п.*); 2) собираться, сходиться; 3) вызывать (*в суд*).

convener [kən'viːnə] *n* лицо, созывающее собрание; уполномоченный.

convenience [kən'viːnjəns] *n* 1) удобство; at your (early) ~ как вам будет угодно, удобно; 2) *pl* удобства, комфорт; 3) уборная; 4) пригодность; 5) (материальная) выгода, интерес; for the ~ of в интересах.

convenient [kən'viːnjənt] *a* удобный, пригодный, подходящий.

convent ['kɔnvənt] *n* монастырь (*обыкн. женский*).

convention [kən'venʃən] *n* 1) собрание; съезд; *ист.* конвент; 2) конвенция, соглашение, договор; 3) общее согласие; 4) обычай, условность.

conventional [kən'venʃənl] *a* 1) условный; 2) общепринятый; 3) конвенционный, условный.

conventionality [kənˌvenʃə'nælıtı] *n* условность.

converge [kən'vəːdʒ] *v* 1) сходиться (*о дорогах, линиях*); 2) сводить в одну точку, совмещать; 3) *мат.* приближаться (*к пределу*).

convergence [kən'vəːdʒəns] *n* 1) схождение (*дорог, линий*); 2) совпадение, совмещение; 3) *мат.* приближение (*к пределу*).

convergent [kən'vəːdʒənt] *a* сходящийся в одной точке.

converging [kən'vəːdʒıŋ] *a* 1) сходящийся, концентрический; 2) сосредоточенный (*об артиллерийском огне*).

conversable [kən'vəːsəbl] *a* 1) разговорчивый, общительный; 2) приятный (*о собеседнике*).

conversant ['kɔnvəsənt] *a* 1) знакомый (*с — with*); сведущий (*в — with*); to keep ~ держать в курсе; 2) относящийся к чему-л.

conversation [ˌkɔnvə'seıʃən] *n* разговор, беседа; речь; to carry on a ~ вести разговор, разговаривать, беседовать (*с кем-л. — with*).

conversational [ˌkɔnvə'seıʃənl] *a* 1) разговорный; 2) разговорчивый.

converse[a] [kən'vəːs] *v* беседовать, разговаривать.

converse[b] I ['kɔnvəːs] *n* 1) обратное положение, утверждение *или* отношение; 2) *мат.* обратная теорема.

converse[b] II *a* обратный; перевёрнутый.

conversely ['kɔnvəːslı] *adv* обратно; наоборот.

conversion [kən'vəːʃən] *n* 1) превращение; 2) переход (*из одного состояния в другое*), изменение; 3) перемена фронта; переход (*из одной партии в другую*); 4) обращение (*в другую веру*); 5) перевод (*мер, весов и т. п.*); 6) *лингв.* конверсия; 7) *фин.* конверсия (*ценных бумаг*); перерасчёт; 8) *юр.* присвоение (*денег, имущества*); 9) перестройка, переоборудование; 10) *тех.* переработка.

convert[a] ['kɔnvəːt] *n* 1) перешедший в другую партию; 2) *рел.* новообращённый.

convert[b] [kən'vəːt] *v* 1) превращать; 2) обращать (*в другую веру, на путь истины*); 3) *фин.* конвертировать (*ценные бумаги и т. п.*); 4) *юр.* присваивать (*деньги, имущество*).

convertible [kən'vəːtəbl] *a* 1) обратимый; 2) подлежащий конверсии.

convex ['kɔn'veks] *a* выпуклый, выгнутый.

convexity [kɔn'veksıtı] *n* выпуклость, выгнутость.

convey [kən'veı] *v* 1) перевозить, переправлять (*груз, пассажиров*); 2) проводить (*звук, электричество и т. п.*); доносить, передавать (*запах*); 3) сообщать (*известия*); 4) выражать, передавать (*мысль, идею и т. п.*); 5) *юр.* передавать в собственность (*имущество*).

conveyance [kən'veıəns] *n* 1) перевозка, транспортировка (*груза, пассажиров*); 2) экипаж (*обычно наёмный*); перевозочное средство; 3) сообщение (*идей и т. п.*); 4) *юр.* передача (*имущества*); акт передачи (*имущества*).

conveyer [kən'veıə] *n* *тех.* конвейер, транспортёр.

convict[a] ['kɔnvıkt] *n* осуждённый; каторжник.

convict[b] [kən'vıkt] *v* 1) доказать виновность; 2) признать виновным; осудить; 3) заставить осознать свою вину.

conviction [kən'vıkʃən] *n* 1) осуждение, приговор; признание кого-л. виновным; summary ~ приговор, вынесенный без участия присяжных заседателей; to have no previous ~ не иметь судимостей; 2) убеждение; to carry ~ убеждать; действовать убедительно; быть убедительным; 3) уверенность; убеждённость.

convince [kən'vıns] *v* 1) убедить, уверить; 2) заставить осознать (*ошибку, проступок и т. п.; of*).

convinced [kən'vınst] *a* убеждённый (*в чём-л. — of*).

convincible [kən'vınsəbl] *a* поддающийся убеждению.

convincing [kən'vınsıŋ] *a* убедительный.

convivial [kən'vıvıəl] *a* 1) праздничный; весёлый, радостный; 2) общительный, компанейский.

conviviality [kənˌvıvı'ælıtı] *n* весёлое, праздничное настроение.

convocation [ˌkɔnvə'keıʃən] *n* 1) созыв (*съезда, парламента и т. п.*); 2) *церк.* собор (*духовенства*).

convocational [ˌkɔnvə'keıʃənl] *a* относящийся к созыву (*съезда, парламента и т. п.*), собору (*духовенства*).

convoke [kən'vouk] *v* созывать (*съезд, парламент и т. п.*).

convoluted ['kɔnvəluːtıd] *a* 1) свёрнутый спиралью; 2) завитой, изогнутый.

convolution [ˌkɔnvə'luːʃən] *n* 1) виток, оборот (*спирали*); 2) извилина (*мозга*).

convolvulus [kən'vɔlvjuləs] *n* *бот.* вьюнок.

convoy I ['kɔnvɔı] *n* 1) сопровождение; конвой; 2) *воен.* транспортная колонна с конвоем; *мор.* караван судов (*сопровождаемый военными кораблями*); 3) *attr* сопровождающий, конвойный.

convoy II *v* сопровождать, конвоировать.

convulse [kən'vʌls] *v* 1) сотряса́ть, потряса́ть; 2) вызыва́ть су́дороги, конву́льсии; to be ~d ко́рчиться в конву́льсиях; *перен.* ко́рчиться от сме́ха.

convulsion [kən'vʌlʃən] *n* 1) су́дорога, конву́льсия; 2) *pl* су́дорожный смех; 3) потрясе́ние; 4) сотрясе́ние, колеба́ние (*почвы*).

convulsive [kən'vʌlsɪv] *a* су́дорожный, конвульси́вный.

cony ['koʊnɪ] *n* кро́личья шку́рка; кро́лик.

coo I [kuː] *n* воркова́ние.

coo II *v* воркова́ть.

cook I [kuk] *n* по́вар; повари́ха, куха́рка; *мор.* кок; ◇ too many ~s spoil the broth *посл.* ≅ у семи́ ня́нек дитя́ без гла́зу.

cook II *v* 1) гото́вить (*кушанья*); вари́ть (*пищу*); стря́пать; 2) вари́ться; жа́риться; to be ~ed *сленг* свари́ться, изму́читься (*от жары*); 3) *разг.* подде́лывать (*документы, счета*); 4) состря́пать (*извинение*); приду́мать (*небылицу; тж.* to ~ up).

cooker ['kukə] *n* 1) плита́, печь; 2) *воен.* похо́дная ку́хня; 3) кастрю́ля; pressure ~ кастрю́ля-скорова́рка; 4) фру́кты, иду́щие на ва́рку; 5) вы́думщик; 6) подде́лыватель (*счетов, документов*).

cookery ['kukərɪ] *n* кулина́рия; стряпня́.

cookery-book ['kukərɪbuk] *n* кулина́рная кни́га.

cook-house ['kukhaus] *n* 1) ку́хня (*вне дома*); 2) похо́дная ку́хня.

cookie ['kukɪ] *n* 1) *шотл.* бу́лочка; 2) *амер.* (дома́шнее) пече́нье.

cooking ['kukɪŋ] *n* приготовле́ние пи́щи, готовка; to do the ~ гото́вить (*обед, ужин и т. п.*).

cookout ['kukaut] *n амер.* 1) приготовле́ние пи́щи на откры́том во́здухе; 2) пикни́к.

cook-room ['kukrum] *n мор.* ка́мбуз.

cool I ['kuːl] *n* прохла́да.

cool II *a* 1) прохла́дный, све́жий; to get ~ осты́ть; 2) споко́йный; невозмути́мый; to keep ~ сохраня́ть споко́йствие, хладнокро́вие; 3) холо́дный, неприве́тливый; 4) на́глый, беззасте́нчивый; 5) *разг.* кру́гленький (*о сумме денег*); ◇ as ~ as a cucumber невозмути́мый, споко́йный.

cool III *v* 1) охлажда́ться, остыва́ть (*тж.* to ~ down); 2) охлажда́ть, студи́ть.

cooler ['kuːlə] *n* 1) холоди́льник; 2) *воен. сленг* гауптва́хта, «губа́»; 3) *сленг* ка́рцер.

cool-headed ['kuːl'hedɪd] *a* хладнокро́вный, рассуди́тельный.

coolie ['kuːlɪ] *n* ку́ли.

cooling ['kuːlɪŋ] *n* охлажде́ние.

coolness ['kuːlnɪs] *n* 1) прохла́да; 2) хладнокро́вие; 3) холодо́к, охлажде́ние (*в отношениях*).

coomb [kuːm] *n* ложби́на; овра́г.

coon [kuːn] *n амер.* 1) ено́т; 2) *разг.* хи́трый ма́лый; a gone ~ пропа́щий челове́к.

coop I [kuːp] *n* 1) кле́тка (*для птицы*); 2) ве́рша (*для ловли рыбы*).

coop II *v* 1) сажа́ть в кле́тку; 2) держа́ть взаперти́ (*тж.* to ~ in, to ~ up).

cooper I ['kuːpə] *n* 1) бо́ндарь; 2) кре́пкий спиртно́й напи́ток.

cooper II *v* де́лать *или* чини́ть бо́чки, бонда́рить.

co-operate [kou'ɔpəreɪt] *v* 1) сотру́дничать (*с кем-л. — with*); рабо́тать вме́сте в одно́й о́бласти (*in*); 2) соде́йствовать; 3) коопери́ровать(ся),

объединя́ть(ся); 4) *воен.* взаимоде́йствовать, де́йствовать совме́стно.

co-operation [kou,ɔpə'reɪʃən] *n* 1) коопера́ция; 2) сотру́дничество; international ~ междунаро́дное сотру́дничество; 3) коопери́рование, объедине́ние; 4) *воен.* взаимоде́йствие, совме́стные де́йствия; hair-line ~ чёткое взаимоде́йствие.

co-operative [kou'ɔpərətɪv] *a* 1) кооперати́вный; 2) совме́стный; 3) (охо́тно) сотру́дничающий.

co-operator [kou'ɔpəreɪtə] *n* коопера́тор.

co-opt [kou'ɔpt] *v* коопти́ровать.

co-optation [,kouɔp'teɪʃən] *n* коопта́ция, коопти́рование.

co-ordinateᵃ I [kou'ɔːdnɪt] *n мат.* координа́та.

co-ordinateᵃ II *a* 1) ра́вный по положе́нию, ра́нгу, пра́ву; 2) координи́рованный, согласо́ванный; 3) *мат.* той же сте́пени; 4) *грам.* сочинённый (*о предложении*); 5) координа́тный.

co-ordinateᵇ [kou'ɔːdɪneɪt] *v* 1) координи́ровать, согласо́вывать; приводи́ть в соотве́тствие; 2) устана́вливать пра́вильное соотноше́ние.

co-ordination [kou,ɔːdɪ'neɪʃən] *n* координа́ция, координи́рование, согласова́ние.

coot [kuːt] *n* 1) лысу́ха (*птица*); 2) *разг.* проста́к, шля́па.

cop¹ [kɔp] *n разг.* полице́йский.

cop² *v разг.* пойма́ть, заста́ть (*на месте преступления*); to ~ it *сленг* пойма́ть; сца́пать; you will ~ it *шк.* тебе́ попадёт.

copartner ['kou'pɑːtnə] *n* член това́рищества (*обыкн. торгового*).

copartnership ['kou'pɑːtnəʃɪp] *n* това́рищество на пая́х.

cope¹ [koup] *v* справля́ться (*с чем-л. — with*); боро́ться (*с кем-л., чем-л. — with*).

cope² *n* 1) *церк.* ма́нтия; 2): the ~ of heaven небе́сный свод; the ~ of night покро́в но́чи.

copeck ['koupek] *n* копе́йка.

coping ['koupɪŋ] *n* гре́бень кры́ши, стены́.

coping-stone ['koupɪŋstoun] *n* 1) карни́зный ка́мень; 2) коне́ц (*дела*); после́дний штрих; после́дняя ка́пля.

copious ['koupjəs] *a* 1) оби́льный; 2) многово́дный (*о потоке*); 3) многосло́вный (*об ораторе*); 4) бога́тый (*о словаре, стиле*); 5) плодови́тый (*о писателе*).

copper¹ I ['kɔpə] *n* 1) медь; 2) ме́дная *или* бро́нзовая моне́та; 3) ме́дный котёл; 4) *attr* ме́дный; ◇ to cool one's ~s опохмеля́ться.

copper¹ II *v* покрыва́ть ме́дью.

copper² *n разг.* полице́йский.

copperas ['kɔpərəs] *n хим.* (желе́зный) купоро́с.

copperhead ['kɔpəhed] *n* мокаси́новая змея́.

copperplate I ['kɔpəpleɪt] *n* ме́дная гравирова́льная доска́.

copperplate II *a* каллиграфи́ческий (*о по́черке*).

copper-smith ['kɔpəsmɪθ] *n* ме́дник.

coppery ['kɔpərɪ] *a* цве́та ме́ди.

coppice ['kɔpɪs] *n* небольша́я ро́ща; молода́я по́росль, подле́сок.

copse [kɔps] *см.* coppice.

copsewood ['kɔpswud] *n* подле́сок.

copula ['kɔpjulə] *n грам.* свя́зка.

copulate ['kɔpjuleɪt] *v зоол.* спа́риваться.

copulation [,kɔpju'leɪʃən] *n* 1) *зоол.* спа́ривание, слу́чка; 2) *грам.* связь, соедине́ние.

copulative I ['kɔpjulətɪv] *n грам.* соедини́тельный сою́з.

copulative II *a грам.* соедини́тельный, свя́зывающий.

copy I ['kɔpɪ] *n* 1) экземпля́р (*книги, журнала и т. п.*); 2) ру́копись; fair ~, clean ~ чистови́к, белови́к; foul ~, rough ~ чернови́к; 3) ко́пия (*документа и т. п.*); репроду́кция (*картины*); 4) материа́л для печа́ти (*особ. для газеты*); 5) образе́ц.

copy II *v* 1) спи́сывать (*тж. у соседа на экзамене*); перепи́сывать; 2) подража́ть; копи́ровать (*кого-л.*); 3) снима́ть ко́пию.

copy-book ['kɔpɪbuk] *n* тетра́дь.

copyholder ['kɔpɪhouldə] *n ист.* копиго́льдер.

copyist ['kɔpɪɪst] *n* 1) перепи́счик; 2) копиро́вщик.

copyright I ['kɔpɪraɪt] *n* а́вторское пра́во.

copyright II *a* обеспе́ченный, гаранти́рованный а́вторским пра́вом.

copyright III *v* осуществля́ть а́вторское пра́во.

coquet [kou'ket] *v* коке́тничать; флиртова́ть.

coquetry ['koukɪtrɪ] *n* коке́тство.

coquette [kou'ket] *n* коке́тка.

coquettish [kou'ketɪʃ] *a* коке́тливый, игри́вый.

cor- [kɔ-] *см.* com-.

coracle ['kɔrəkl] *n* рыба́чья ло́дка (*в Ирландии и Уэльсе*).

coral I ['kɔrəl] *n* кора́лл.

coral II *a* 1) кора́лловый; 2) кора́ллового цве́та.

coral-island ['kɔrəl,aɪlənd] *n* ато́лл.

cord I [kɔ:d] *n* 1) верёвка, бечёвка; 2) струна́; 3) *анат.* свя́зка; vocal ~s голосовы́е свя́зки; spinal ~ спинно́й мозг; 4) ру́бчик (*на материи*); 5) *pl* пли́совые брю́ки; 6) корд (*мера дров*).

cord II *v* перевя́зывать верёвкой (*тж.* to ~ up).

cordage ['kɔ:dɪdʒ] *n мор.* сна́сти; такела́ж.

corded ['kɔ:dɪd] *a* 1) перевя́занный верёвкой; 2) ру́бчатый, в ру́бчик (*о материи*).

cordial I ['kɔ:djəl] *n* 1) серде́чное сре́дство, лека́рство; 2) ликёр.

cordial II *a* 1) раду́шный, приве́тливый, тёплый; 2) серде́чный (*тж. перен.*).

cordiality [,kɔ:dɪ'ælɪtɪ] *n* раду́шие, приве́тливость, серде́чность.

cordon ['kɔ:dn] *n* 1) кордо́н (*военный, санитарный и т. п.*); 2) о́рденская ле́нта; аксельба́нты.

corduroy I ['kɔ:dərɔɪ] *n* 1) ру́бчатый плис; вельве́т; 2) *pl* пли́совые штаны́; 3) *амер.* бреве́нчатая гать (*тж.* ~ road).

corduroy II *v амер.* стро́ить бреве́нчатую мостову́ю, гать.

core I [kɔ:] *n* 1) сердцеви́на; вну́тренность; ядро́; to the ~ наскво́зь; rotten to the ~ наскво́зь прогни́вший; испо́рченный до мо́зга косте́й; 2) су́щность, суть; 3) *тех.* серде́чник.

core II *v* удаля́ть сердцеви́ну.

cored [kɔ:d] *a* по́лый.

coriander [,kɔrɪ'ændə] *n* гвозди́ка (*пряность*).

cork I [kɔ:k] *n* 1) про́бка; 2) поплаво́к; like a ~ плаву́чий; держа́щийся на воде́; 3) *бот.* луб; 4) *attr* про́бковый; 5) *attr* спаса́тельный; 6) *attr* лубяно́й.

cork II *v* 1) заку́поривать; затыка́ть про́бкой

(*тж.* to ~ up); 2) зата́ивать, сде́рживать (*чувства*).

corkage ['kɔ:kɪdʒ] *n* заку́поривание, отку́поривание (*бутылок*).

corker ['kɔ:kə] *n разг.* преде́л, верх (*лжи, наглости и т. п.*).

cork-screw I ['kɔ:kskru:] *n* што́пор.

cork-screw II *a* спира́льный, винтообра́зный.

cork-screw III *v* 1) дви́гаться по спира́ли; 2) проти́скиваться, пролеза́ть (*сквозь толпу*).

cork-tree ['kɔ:ktri:] *n* про́бковый дуб.

corky ['kɔ:kɪ] *a* 1) про́бковый; 2) *разг.* жизнера́достный, бо́дрый.

cormorant ['kɔ:mərənt] *n* 1) *зоол.* большо́й бакла́н; 2) прожо́рливый челове́к.

corn[1] I [kɔ:n] *n* 1) зерно́; 2) *собир.* хлеба́; часто пшени́ца; standing ~ хлеб на корню́; to cut the ~ жать рожь *и т. п.*; 3) *амер.* кукуру́за, ма́ис (*тж.* Indian ~); 4) *амер. разг.* ма́исовая во́дка; ◇ to measure others' ~ by one's own bushel ≅ ме́рить на свой арши́н.

corn[1] II *v тех.* гранули́ровать; зерни́ть.

corn[2] *v* соли́ть мя́со.

corn[3] *n* мозо́ль; pet ~ *шутл.* люби́мая мозо́ль; ◇ to tread on smb.'s ~s наступи́ть на люби́мую мозо́ль.

corn-chandler ['kɔ:n,tʃɑ:ndlə] *n* (ро́зничный) торго́вец зерно́м.

corn-cob ['kɔ:nkɔb] *n* сте́ржень кукуру́зного поча́тка.

cornel ['kɔ:nəl] *n* 1) *бот.* кизи́л; 2) *attr* кизи́ловый.

corner I ['kɔ:nə] *n* 1) у́гол; *перен.* тру́дное положе́ние (*тж.* a tight ~); to cut off a ~ пойти́ напрями́к; to drive into a ~ загна́ть в у́гол; *перен.* припере́ть к сте́нке; поста́вить в безвы́ходное положе́ние; to turn the ~ a) заверну́ть за́ угол; б) вы́йти из (опа́сного) положе́ния; 2) край, сторона́ (*света*); 3) (потайно́й) уголо́к, месте́чко; done in a ~ сде́ланный та́йно; warm ~ жа́ркий уча́сток бо́я, опа́сное ме́сто; 4) ску́пка това́ра (*в спекулятивных целях*); 5) *спорт.* углово́й уда́р; 6) *attr* углово́й.

corner II *v* 1) загоня́ть в у́гол, в тупи́к; ста́вить в безвы́ходное положе́ние; 2) скупа́ть това́ры (*со спекулятивными целями*).

corner-stone ['kɔ:nəstoun] *n* краеуго́льный ка́мень.

cornet ['kɔ:nɪt] *n* 1) *муз.* корне́т; 2) *воен. уст.* корне́т; 3) фу́нтик (*из бумаги*); 4) моро́женое в ва́фельных стака́нчиках.

cornet-à-piston(s) ['kɔ:nɪtə'pɪstən(z)] *n муз.* корне́т-а-писто́н.

corn-exchange ['kɔ:nɪks'tʃeɪndʒ] *n* хле́бная би́ржа.

corn-factor ['kɔ:n,fæktə] *n* торго́вец зерно́м.

corn-flour ['kɔ:n,flauə] *n* кукуру́зная, ри́совая мука́.

corn-flower ['kɔ:n,flauə] *n* василёк.

cornice ['kɔ:nɪs] *n* 1) *архит.* карни́з; 2) нави́сшая над про́пастью сне́жная глы́ба.

Cornish I ['kɔ:nɪʃ] *n ист.* ко́рнский язы́к.

Cornish II *a* корнуо́ллский.

corn-stalk ['kɔ:nstɔ:k] *n разг.* ды́лда, каланча́.

corny[1] ['kɔ:nɪ] *a* 1) хле́бный, зерново́й; 2) *разг.* бана́льный, изби́тый.

corny[2] *a* мозо́листый.

corolla [kə'rɔlə] *n бот.* ве́нчик.

corona [kə'rounə] *n* (*pl* coronae [kə'rouni:])
1) со́лнечная коро́на; кольцо́ (*вокруг солнца или
луны*); 2) коро́нка (*зуба*); 3) *амер.* поду́шка под
вьючное седло́.

coronal[a] I ['kɔrənl] *n* 1) коро́на, вене́ц; ве́н-
чик; 2) вено́к.

coronal[a] II *a* 1) вене́чный, корона́рный; 2) лоб-
ный.

coronal[b] [kə'rounl] *a* относя́щийся к (со́лнеч-
ной) коро́не.

coronate ['kɔrəneɪt] *v* короно́ва́ть.

coronation [,kɔrə'neɪʃən] *n* корона́ция.

coroner ['kɔrənə] *n* ко́ронер (*следователь, ведущий дела о насильственной или скоропостижной смерти*).

coronet ['kɔrənɪt] *n* 1) диаде́ма; 2) коро́на
(*пэров*); 3) *поэт.* вено́к.

corpora ['kɔːpərə] *pl см.* corpus.

corporal[1] ['kɔːpərəl] *n* капра́л.

corporal[2] *a* теле́сный; физи́ческий (*о недо-
статке*).

corporate ['kɔːpərɪt] *a* корпорати́вный; о́бщий.

corporation [,kɔːpə'reɪʃən] *n* 1) корпора́ция; municipal ~, the Corporation муниципалите́т;
2) *амер.* акционе́рное о́бщество; 3) *разг.* большо́й
живо́т.

corporator ['kɔːpəreɪtə] *n* член корпора́ции.

corporeal [kɔː'pɔːrɪəl] *a* теле́сный; физи́ческий;
веще́ственный, материа́льный.

corps [kɔː] *n* (*pl* corps [kɔːz]) 1) *воен.*
ко́рпус; provost ~ вое́нная поли́ция, полева́я
жандарме́рия; 2) *attr.* ко́рпусный.

corps-de-ballet [,kɔːdəbæ'leɪ] *n* кордебале́т.

corpse [kɔːps] *n* труп; the senseless ~ без-
дыха́нное те́ло.

corpulence ['kɔːpjuləns] *n* доро́дность, ту́чность.

corpulent ['kɔːpjulənt] *a* 1) доро́дный, пло́тный,
ту́чный; 2) мяси́стый (*о носе*).

corpus ['kɔːpəs] *n* (*pl* corpora) ко́декс, свод;
~ juris свод зако́нов; ~ delicti *юр.* соста́в пре-
ступле́ния.

corpuscle ['kɔːpʌsl] *n* 1) мельча́йшая части́ца;
red (white) ~s *физиол.* кра́сные (бе́лые) кро-
вяны́е тельца́; 2) *физ.* а́том; электро́н.

corpuscular [kɔː'pʌskjulə] *a* а́томный; мельча́й-
ший.

corral I [kɔ'rɑːl] *n* 1) *амер.* кора́ль, заго́н
(*для скота*); 2) ла́герь, окружённый повозка́-
ми.

corral II *v* загоня́ть, сгоня́ть.

correct I [kə'rekt] *a* 1) пра́вильный, ве́рный;
то́чный; 2) хоро́ший (*о вкусе*); 3) корре́ктный.

correct II *v* 1) исправля́ть, поправля́ть; 2) пра́-
вить (*корректуру*); 3) вноси́ть попра́вки (*в показания инструмента*); 4) корректи́ровать (*огонь артиллерии*); 5) нака́зывать; 6) нейтрализова́ть
(*вредное действие*).

correction [kə'rekʃən] *n* 1) исправле́ние, по-
пра́вка; to speak under ~ говори́ть, допуска́я
возмо́жность оши́бок; 2) испра́вленный вариа́нт.

corrective I [kə'rektɪv] *n* 1) корректи́в; 2) *мед.*
нейтрализу́ющее сре́дство.

corrective II *a* 1) исправля́ющий; 2) испра́ви-
тельный; 3) *мед.* нейтрализу́ющий.

correctness [kə'rektnɪs] *n* 1) пра́вильность,
то́чность; 2) корре́ктность, благопристо́йность.

corrector [kə'rektə] *n* исправля́ющий; ~ of the
press корре́ктор.

correlate I ['kɔrɪleɪt] *n* корреля́т; соотноси́-
тельное поня́тие.

correlate II *v* 1) находи́ться в соотве́тствии
(*c — with, to*); 2) приводи́ть в соотве́тствие
(*c — with, to*).

correlation [,kɔrɪ'leɪʃən] *n* соотноше́ние, кор-
реля́ция.

correlative I [kɔ'relətɪv] *n* корреля́т.

correlative II *a* соотноси́тельный, соотве́тствен-
ный.

correspond [,kɔrɪs'pɔnd] *v* 1) соотве́тствовать
(*чему-л.— with, to*); 2) быть аналоги́чным; сов-
пада́ть (*c — with, to*); 3) перепи́сываться (*c —
with*).

correspondence [,kɔrɪs'pɔndəns] *n* 1) соотве́т-
ствие (*между — between; одного... другому — of...
with или to; в чём-л.— in*); анало́гия; 2) пе-
репи́ска; пи́сьма, корреспонде́нция; 3) *attr.* заоч-
ный (*о курсах*).

correspondent I [,kɔrɪs'pɔndənt] *n* корреспон-
де́нт.

correspondent II *a* соотве́тствующий (*чему-л.—
to, with*).

corresponding [,kɔrɪs'pɔndɪŋ] *a* соотве́тствую-
щий, соотве́тственный.

corridor ['kɔrɪdɔː] *n* коридо́р.

corrigenda [,kɔrɪ'dʒendə] *n pl* спи́сок опеча́ток.

corrigible ['kɔrɪdʒəbl] *a* исправи́мый, по-
прави́мый.

corroborant [kə'rɔbərənt] *n мед.* тони́ческое,
укрепля́ющее сре́дство.

corroborate [kə'rɔbəreɪt] *v* подтвержда́ть, под-
крепля́ть фа́ктами (*теорию и т. п.*).

corroboration [kə,rɔbə'reɪʃən] *n* подтвержде́ние,
подкрепле́ние фа́ктами (*теории и т. п.*).

corrode [kə'roud] *v* 1) ржа́веть, подверга́ться
де́йствию корро́зии; 2) разъеда́ть; трави́ть (*кислотой*).

corrodible [kə'roudəbl] *a* подве́рженный корро́-
зии.

corrosion [kə'rouʒən] *n* 1) ржа́вление, корро́-
зия; 2) ржа́вчина.

corrosive I [kə'rousɪv] *n* е́дкое, разъеда́ющее
вещество́.

corrosive II *a* е́дкий, разъеда́ющий.

corrugate ['kɔrugeɪt] *v* 1) мо́рщить(ся); 2) *тех.*
гофрирова́ть.

corrugated ['kɔrugeɪtɪd] *a* волни́стый, гофри-
ро́ванный, рифлёный (*о железе*).

corrugation [,kɔru'geɪʃən] *n* 1) скла́дка, мор-
щи́на (*на лбу*); 2) *тех.* гофрирова́ние, рифле́-
ние (*железа*); 3) вы́боина (*на дороге*).

corrupt I [kə'rʌpt] *a* 1) испо́рченный; развращённый; 2) прода́жный, подкупно́й; 3) искажённый (*о тексте*).

corrupt II *v* 1) по́ртить(ся); развраща́ть(ся);
2) подкупа́ть; 3) гнить, разлага́ться; 4) искажа́ть
(*текст*).

corruptibility [kə,rʌptə'bɪlɪtɪ] *n* прода́жность,
подку́пность.

corruptible [kə'rʌptəbl] *a* поддаю́щийся по́рче,
развра́ту, по́дкупу.

corruption [kəˈrʌpʃən] *n* 1) пóрча, гниéние; 2) разложéние, разврáт; 3) продáжность, коррýпция; 4) искажéние (*текста*).

corsage [kɔːˈsɑːʒ] *n* корсáж.

corsair [ˈkɔːsɛə] *n ист.* 1) корсáр, морскóй разбóйник; 2) кáпер (*судно*).

corselet [ˈkɔːslɪt] *см.* corslet.

corslet [ˈkɔːslɪt] *n ист.* лáты.

cortège [kɔːˈteɪʒ] *n* кортéж, процéссия.

cortex [ˈkɔːteks] *n* (*pl* cortices [ˈkɔːtɪsiːz]) 1) корá головнóго мóзга; 2) корá (*дерева*).

corvée [ˈkɔːveɪ] *n* 1) *ист.* бáрщина; 2) тяжёлая рабóта.

corvette [kɔːˈvet] *n мор.* корвéт.

cosecant [ˈkouˈsiːkənt] *n мат.* косéканс.

cosher [ˈkɔʃə] *v* баловáть, нéжить.

co-signatory [ˈkouˈsɪgnətərɪ] *n* лицó *или* госудáрство, подписáвшее соглашéние совмéстно с другими.

cosily [ˈkouzɪlɪ] *adv* уютно; удóбно.

cosine [ˈkousaɪn] *n мат.* кóсинус.

cosiness [ˈkouzɪnɪs] *n* уют.

cosmetic I [kɔzˈmetɪk] косметическое срéдство.

cosmetic II *a* косметический.

cosmic [ˈkɔzmɪk] *a* 1) космический; 2) áтомный (*о бомбе*).

cosmonaut [ˈkɔzmənɔːt] *n* космонáвт.

cosmonautics [ˌkɔzməˈnɔːtɪks] *n* космонáвтика.

cosmonette [ˌkɔzməˈnet] *n* жéнщина-космонáвт.

cosmopolitan I [ˌkɔzməˈpɔlɪtən] *n* космополит.

cosmopolitan II *a* космополитический.

cosmopolit(an)ism [ˌkɔzməˈpɔlɪt(ən)ɪzəm] *n* космополитизм.

cosmos [ˈkɔzmɔs] *n* мир, кóсмос, вселéнная.

Cossack [ˈkɔsæk] *n* 1) казáк; 2) *attr* казáцкий.

cost I [kɔst] *n* 1) стóимость; ценá (*тж. перен.*); first ~ себестóимость; prime ~ фабричная себестóимость; initial ~ а) первоначáльная стóимость; основнáя стóимость; б) капитáльные затрáты; to count the ~ а) произвести предварительный расчёт; б) учéсть все обстоятельства; at the ~ of ценóй чегó-л.; at all ~s во что бы то ни стáло; 2) счёт; расхóды; издéржки; ~s of production издéржки произвóдства; at my ~ за мой счёт; 3) *pl* судéбные издéржки; ◊ to know (*или* to learn) to one's own ~ знать по сóбственному óпыту; испытáть на себé.

cost II *v* (*past, p. p.* cost) 1) стóить; 2) обходиться (*дорого, дёшево*); 3) расцéнивать (*товар*); калькулировать (*стоимость товара*).

costal [ˈkɔstl] *a* рёберный.

coster(monger) [ˈkɔstə(ˌmʌŋgə)] *n* уличный торгóвец (*фруктами, рыбой и т. п.*).

costless [ˈkɔstlɪs] *a* даровóй.

costly [ˈkɔstlɪ] *a* 1) дорогóй; цéнный; 2) роскóшный, пышный.

costume [ˈkɔstjuːm] *n* костюм.

costumier [kɔsˈtjuːmɪə] *n* костюмéр.

cosy I [ˈkouzɪ] *n* 1) стёганая покрышка, «бáба» (*на чайник, кофейник и т. п.*); 2) козéтка.

cosy II *a* удóбный, уютный.

cot[1] [kɔt] *n* 1) хлев, овчáрня; 2) *поэт.* деревéнский дóмик.

cot[2] *n* 1) дéтская кровáтка; 2) кóйка (*на корабле*); 3) *инд.* лёгкая похóдная кровáть.

cotangent [ˈkouˈtændʒənt] *n мат.* котáнгенс.

cote [ˈkout] *n* загóн, хлев, овчáрня.

co-tenant [ˈkouˈtenənt] *n* соарендáтор.

coterie [ˈkoutərɪ] *n* круг лиц, имéющих óбщие интерéсы; своя компáния.

cottage [ˈkɔtɪdʒ] *n* 1) избá; хижина; 2) коттéдж; зáгородный дом; 3) *амер.* дáча.

cottage-cheese [ˈkɔtɪdʒˈtʃiːz] *амер. см.* cream-cheese.

cottager [ˈkɔtɪdʒə] *n* 1) батрáк; 2) сéльский житель; 3) *амер.* дáчник.

cottar [ˈkɔtə] *n шотл.* батрáк (*живущий при ферме*).

cotter[1] [ˈkɔtə] *n см.* cottar.

cotter[2] *n тех.* клин, костыль; чекá.

cotton I [ˈkɔtn] *n* 1) хлóпок; хлопчáтник; 2) хлопчáтая бумáга; spun ~ бумáжная пряжа; 3) нитка; 4) вáта; absorbent ~ гигроскопическая вáта.

cotton II *a* 1) хлóпковый; 2) хлопчатобумáжный.

cotton III *v* 1) согласóвываться; уживáться (*с кем-л.— together, with*); 2) привязáться (*к — to*); □ to ~ up сблизиться, завязáть дружеские отношéния.

cotton-gin [ˈkɔtndʒɪn] *n* хлопкоочистительная машина.

cotton-lord [ˈkɔtnlɔːd] *n* текстильный магнáт.

cotton-mill [ˈkɔtnmɪl] *n* текстильная фáбрика.

cotton-planter [ˈkɔtnplɑːntə] *n* хлопковóд.

cotton-spinner [ˈkɔtnˌspɪnə] *n* 1) рабóчий-прядильщик; 2) владéлец текстильной фáбрики.

cotton-wool [ˈkɔtnˈwul] *n* 1) хлóпок-сырéц; 2) вáта.

couch I [kautʃ] *n* 1) кушéтка; 2) *поэт.* лóже; 3) лóговище, берлóга.

couch II *v* 1) лежáть (*о зверях*); 2) притаиться; 3) снимáть катарáкту (*с глаз*); 4) формулировать, выражáть.

cougar [ˈkuːgə] *n зоол.* пýма.

cough I [kɔf] *n* кáшель; to give a (slight) ~ кáшлянуть.

cough II *v* кáшлять; □ to ~ down кáшлем застáвить орáтора замолчáть; to ~ out, to ~ up а) выпалить; б) отхáркивать.

could [kud] *past см.* can[1].

coulee [ˈkuːlɪ] *n амер.* оврáг; пересóхшее рýсло.

coulisse [kuːˈliːs] *n* 1) *театр.* кулиса; 2) *тех.* желобóк.

coulomb [ˈkuːlɔm] *n эл.* кулóн.

council [ˈkaunsl] *n* 1) совéт (*организация*); World Peace Council Всемирный Совéт Мира; Security Council Совéт Безопáсности; city ~, town ~ муниципалитéт, городскóй совéт; common ~ муниципáльный совéт; the (King's Privy) Council государственный совéт; *ист.* тáйный совéт короля (*в Англии*); in Council королéвский, от имени короля (*закон, приказ и т. п.*); County Council совéт грáфства (*в Англии*); Council of Action комитéт дéйствия; Council of War воéнный совéт; 2) совещáние; консилиум (*врачей*); family ~ семéйный совéт; 3) церкóвный собóр.

councillor [ˈkaunsɪlə] *n* член совéта.

counsel I [ˈkaunsəl] *n* 1) обсуждéние, совещáние; to hold (*или* to take) ~ совеща́ться, обсужда́ть (*c — with*); 2) сове́т (*указание*); 3) наме́рение; to keep one's own ~ держа́ть свои́ наме́рения в секре́те; 4) адвока́т; ~ to the Crown адвока́т коро́ны; ~ for the defence адвока́т отве́тчика; ~ for the prosecution обвини́тель; the King's (the Queen's) Counsel короле́вский адвока́т; ◊ to take ~ of one's pillow ≅ у́тро ве́чера мудрене́е.

counsel II *v* сове́товать, дава́ть сове́т.

counsellor ['kaunslə] *n* 1) сове́тник, консульта́нт; 2) *амер., ирл.* адвока́т.

counsellor-at-law ['kaunslərət'lɔː] *n* адвока́т-консульта́нт (*в Ирландии*).

count¹ I [kaunt] *n* 1) (под)счёт; blood ~s ана́лиз кро́ви; to keep ~ вести́ (под)счёт; to lose ~ потеря́ть счёт; 2) *уст.* ито́г; ◊ on both ~s в том и друго́м отноше́нии.

count¹ II *v* 1) счита́ть, подсчи́тывать; 2) пересчи́тывать; 3) полага́ть, счита́ть; 4) идти́ в расчёт, име́ть значе́ние; this ~s for nothing э́то не име́ет никако́го значе́ния; this does not ~ э́то не счита́ется, э́то не идёт в расчёт; 5) рассчи́тывать (*на кого-л., что-л. — on, upon*); □ to ~ in включа́ть в счёт, подсчёт; to ~ off! *воен.* рассчита́йсь!; to ~ out а) не счита́ть, не учи́тывать; не принима́ть во внима́ние; б) *парл.* отложи́ть заседа́ние пала́ты за отсу́тствием кво́рума; в) *спорт.* счита́ть вы́бывшим из игры́; to ~ up подсчита́ть.

count² *n* граф (*не английского происхождения*).

countenance I ['kauntɪnəns] *n* 1) выраже́ние лица́; лицо́; to change one's ~ измени́ться в лице́; to keep one's ~ не пока́зывать ви́да; сохраня́ть серьёзный вид; to lose ~ потеря́ть самооблада́ние; to put out of ~ смуща́ть, приводи́ть в замеша́тельство; 2) соде́йствие, подде́ржка (*моральная*); одобри́тельный взгляд; to keep one in ~ ока́зывать подде́ржку; to give (*или* to lend) one's ~ to ока́зывать мора́льную подде́ржку; he finds no ~ он не нахо́дит подде́ржки (*в ком-л.— in*).

countenance II *v* ока́зывать подде́ржку; поощря́ть, относи́ться сочу́вственно.

counter¹ ['kauntə] *n* 1) прила́вок; lunch ~ буфе́т (*для прода́жи заку́сок и напи́тков*); 2) фи́шка (*в играх*); 3) пе́шка (*в ша́шках*).

counter² *n* счётчик, член счётной коми́ссии.

counter³ I *n* 1) за́дник (*сапога́*); 2) *спорт.* отраже́ние уда́ра рапи́рой; 3) вы́крюк (*конькобе́жная фигу́ра*).

counter³ II *a* противополо́жный.

counter³ III *adv* в обра́тном направле́нии; про́тив; to run ~ противоре́чить (*друг другу*).

counter³ IV *v* 1) (от)пари́ровать (*удар*); 2) противоде́йствовать, возража́ть.

counter- ['kauntə-] *pref сло́жным слова́м придаёт значе́ние* противо-, контр-.

counteract [,kauntə'rækt] *v* 1) противоде́йствовать; 2) нейтрализова́ть.

counteraction [,kauntə'rækʃən] *n* противоде́йствие, отве́тные де́йствия.

counter-attack I ['kauntərə,tæk] *n* контрата́ка, контрнаступле́ние.

counter-attack II *v* контратакова́ть, вести́ контрнаступле́ние.

counter-attraction ['kauntərə,trækʃən] *n* обра́тное притяже́ние.

counterbalance*a* ['kauntə,bæləns] *n* 1) противове́с; 2) *тех.* уравнове́шивающий механи́зм.

counterbalance*b* [,kauntə'bæləns] *v* уравнове́шивать.

counterblast ['kauntəblɑːst] *n* энерги́чный проте́ст, вы́пад.

counterblow ['kauntəblou] *n* контруда́р.

countercharge I ['kauntətʃɑːdʒ] *n* встре́чное обвине́ние.

countercharge II *v* 1) предъявля́ть встре́чное обвине́ние; 2) контратакова́ть.

counter-claim ['kauntəkleim] *n* встре́чный иск.

counter-clockwise ['kauntə'klɔkwaiz] *adv* про́тив часово́й стре́лки.

counterdeed ['kauntədiːd] *n* секре́тный до́говор (*аннули́рующий официа́льный до́говор*).

counter-espionage ['kauntərespɪə,nɑːʒ] *n* контрразве́дка.

counterfeit I ['kauntəfit] *n* 1) подде́лка, подло́г; 2) подставно́е лицо́; 3) притво́рщик.

counterfeit II *a* 1) подде́льный, подло́жный; 2) фальши́вый, неи́скренний.

counterfeit III *v* 1) подде́лывать (*де́ньги, по́дпись*); соверша́ть подло́г (*документов*); 2) подража́ть, имити́ровать; 3) притворя́ться, обма́нывать.

counterfeiter ['kauntəfitə] *n* 1) притво́рщик, обма́нщик; 2) фальшивомоне́тчик.

counterfoil ['kauntəfɔil] *n* корешо́к тало́на, че́ка *и т. п.*

countermand I [,kauntə'mɑːnd] *n* контрприка́з.

countermand II *v* 1) отда́ть контрприка́з; 2) отменя́ть прика́з, зака́з; 3) отзыва́ть (*челове́ка, во́инскую часть*).

countermark I ['kauntə,mɑːk] *n* про́бирное клеймо́.

countermark II *v* ста́вить клеймо́.

counter-measure ['kauntə,meʒə] *n* контрме́ра.

countermine*a* ['kauntə,main] *n* контрми́на.

countermine*b* [,kauntə'main] *v* 1) закла́дывать контрми́ны; 2) разруша́ть чьи-л. пла́ны.

counterpane ['kauntəpein] *n* покрыва́ло (*на крова́ти*).

counterpart ['kauntəpɑːt] *n* 1) двойни́к; 2) ко́пия; дублика́т.

counterpoise I ['kauntəpɔiz] *n* 1) противове́с; 2) *радио* противове́с анте́нны; 3) равнове́сие.

counterpoise II *v* уравнове́шивать.

counter-revolution ['kauntərevə,luːʃən] *n* контрреволю́ция.

counter-revolutionary I ['kauntərevə,luːʃnəri] *n* контрреволюционе́р.

counter-revolutionary II *a* контрреволюцио́нный.

countersign I ['kauntəsain] *n* 1) паро́ль; о́тзыв (*на о́клик часово́го*); 2) контрассигна́ция.

countersign II *v* ратифици́ровать; скрепля́ть (*подписью*).

countersignature [,kauntə'signɪtʃə] *n* скрепле́ние по́дписью (*документа*).

counterwork*a* ['kauntə,wəːk] *n* 1) противоде́йствие; 2) *pl воен.* противооса́дные рабо́ты.

counterwork*b* ['kauntə'wəːk] *v* 1) противоде́йствовать; расстра́ивать (*планы*); 2) вести́ подрывну́ю рабо́ту.

countess ['kauntıs] *n* графи́ня.

counting-house ['kauntıŋhaus] *n* 1) конто́ра; 2) бухгалте́рия.

countless ['kauntlıs] *a* бесчи́сленный, неисчисли́мый.

count-out [kaunt'aut] *n* 1) *парл.* перено́с заседа́ния пала́ты за отсу́тствием кво́рума; 2) отсчи́тывание 10 секу́нд (*даваемых упавшему боксёру, чтобы подняться*).

country ['kʌntrı] *n* 1) страна́; край; launching ~ страна́, запуска́ющая раке́ты и спу́тники; conscript ~ страна́, име́ющая во́инскую пови́нность; to forbid the ~ запрети́ть въезд в страну́; to plunge a ~ into war вве́ргнуть страну́ в войну́; 2) ро́дина; mother ~ ро́дина, оте́чество; 3) наро́д, населе́ние; to appeal (*или* to go) to the ~ распусти́ть парла́мент и назна́чить но́вые вы́боры; 4) террито́рия, ме́стность; Black ~ каменноуго́льный райо́н (*Стаффордшира и др.*); 5) дере́вня (*в противоположность городу*); се́льская ме́стность; in the ~ в дере́вне, за́ городом, на да́че; to the ~ в дере́вню, за́ город, на да́чу; 6) перифери́я, прови́нция; 7) *attr* се́льский, дереве́нский; за́городный; провинциа́льный.

country-house ['kʌntrı'haus] *n* 1) за́городный дом, да́ча; 2) поме́щичий особня́к.

countryman ['kʌntrımən] *n* 1) земля́к, сооте́чественник; 2) крестья́нин; се́льский жи́тель.

country-seat ['kʌntrı'si:t] *n* уса́дьба; поме́стье.

country-side ['kʌntrı'saıd] *n* 1) се́льская ме́стность; дере́вня (*в противоположность городу*); 2) перифери́я; 3) се́льское населе́ние.

countrywoman ['kʌntrı‚wumən] *n* 1) земля́чка, соотéчественница; 2) крестья́нка; се́льская жи́тельница.

county ['kauntı] *n* 1) гра́фство (*административная единица Англии*); 2) (the ~) населе́ние гра́фства; 3) *амер.* о́круг; 4) *attr* относя́щийся к гра́фству; *амер.* окружно́й.

coup [ku:] *n* успе́х; уда́чный ход.

coup d'état ['ku:deı'ta:] *n* госуда́рственный переворо́т; дворцо́вый переворо́т.

couple I ['kʌpl] *n* 1) па́ра; in ~s па́рами; a courting ~ жени́х и неве́ста; a married ~ муж и жена́, супру́ги; 2) *mex.* па́ра сил; 3) *эл.* термопа́ра, термоэлеме́нт.

couple II *v* 1) соединя́ть(ся); своди́ть в па́ры; 2) *ж.-д.* сцепля́ть (*вагоны*); 3) выбира́ть па́ру; 4) ассоции́ровать, свя́зывать (*тж.* to ~ together); 5) спа́риваться.

coupled ['kʌpld] *a* 1) в соедине́нии (*с кем-л.*— with); 2) па́рный.

coupler ['kʌplə] *n* 1) *ж.-д.* сце́пщик (*вагонов*); 2) *mex.* соедини́тельный прибо́р, му́фта.

couplet ['kʌplıt] *n* двусти́шие.

coupling ['kʌplıŋ] *n* 1) соедине́ние; rendezvous ~ *косм.* стыко́вка; 2) *ж.-д.* сце́пка (*вагонов*); 3) совокупле́ние, спа́ривание; 4) *mex.* соедини́тельная му́фта.

coupon ['ku:pɔn] *n* 1) купо́н; 2) тало́н (*продуктовой карточки*); 3) рекоменда́ция кандида́ту на вы́борах (*даваемая лидером партии*).

courage ['kʌrıdʒ] *n* хра́брость, отва́га, му́жество, сме́лость; бо́дрость ду́ха; to have the ~ of one's

opinions проявля́ть гражда́нское му́жество; to muster (*или* to pluck) up ~ набра́ться сме́лости, отва́житься; to pick up (*или* to summon) ~ собра́ться с ду́хом; to screw up one's ~ подбодри́ться, набра́ться хра́брости; ◊ Dutch ~ хра́брость во хмелю́; to take one's ~ in both hands осме́литься, пойти́ на риск.

courageous [kə'reıdʒəs] *a* хра́брый, отва́жный, сме́лый.

courier ['kurıə] *n* 1) курье́р (*тж. как название целого ряда газет*); посы́льный; 2) аге́нт.

course I [kɔ:s] *n* 1) ход, тече́ние (*событий*); in ~ of в проце́ссе (*совершения действия*); in due ~ в до́лжное вре́мя; до́лжным о́бразом; in the ~ of в тече́ние; to run its ~ продолжа́ться без переры́ва; идти́ свои́м чередо́м; to stay the ~ доводи́ть де́ло до конца́; to take its (*или* their) ~ брать своё; 2) курс (*следования корабля, самолёта*); маршру́т; направле́ние; ру́сло; 3) ли́ния поведе́ния; a ~ of action о́браз де́йствий; 4) курс; ~ of exchange (валю́тный) курс; 5) *pl* ку́рсы; correspondence ~s зао́чные ку́рсы; 6) блю́до (*за обедом*), ку́шанье; ◊ of ~ коне́чно.

course II *v* 1) пресле́довать; гна́ться (*за дичью*); 2) гоня́ться (*друг за другом*); 3) пуска́ть вскачь (*коня*); 4) течь, протека́ть.

courser ['kɔ:sə] *n* *поэт.* скаку́н, быстроно́гий конь.

court[1] [kɔ:t] *n* 1) (the ~) суд (*тж.* ~ of justice); *амер. тж.* су́дьи, чле́ны суда́; Supreme Court Верхо́вный суд; Court of Appeal апелляцио́нный суд; Supreme Court of Judicature верхо́вный суд А́нглии; circuit ~ выездна́я се́ссия суда́; prize ~ призово́й суд; spiritual ~ церко́вный суд; out of ~ не име́ющий пра́ва на слу́шание де́ла; to put out of ~ лиши́ть пра́ва на слу́шание де́ла в суде́; kangaroo ~ *амер. сленг* а) самосу́д; б) суде́бная распра́ва; 2) зда́ние суда́; 3) *attr* суде́бный; ~ martial вое́нный суд; drum-head ~ martial вое́нно-полево́й суд.

court[2] I *n* 1) двор; 2) площа́дка для игр; *спорт.* корт; hard (grass) ~ бетони́рованный (земляно́й) корт; 3) двор (*коронованной особы*); at ~ при дворе́; to hold a ~ устра́ивать приём при дворе́; 4) уха́живание; to pay one's ~ to smb. уха́живать за кем-л.; 5) *attr* придво́рный.

court[2] II *v* 1) уха́живать; 2) соблазня́ть (*into, to, from*); 3) льстить; добива́ться популя́рности.

court-card ['kɔ:tka:d] *n* фигу́рная ка́рта в коло́де.

courteous ['kə:tjəs] *a* ве́жливый, учти́вый.

courtesan [‚kɔ:tı'zæn] *n* куртиза́нка.

courtesy ['kə:tısı] *n* ве́жливость, учти́вость; by the ~ благодаря́ любе́зности; he did me the ~ он оказа́л мне честь; with scant ~ нелюбе́зно.

courtezan [‚kɔ:tı'zæn] *см.* courtesan.

courtier ['kɔ:tjə] *n* придво́рный; царедво́рец.

courtly ['kɔ:tlı] *a* изы́сканный, утончённый; церемо́нный.

court-martial ['kɔ:t'ma:ʃəl] *v* суди́ть вое́нным судо́м.

courtship ['kɔ:tʃıp] *n* уха́живание.

courtyard ['kɔ:t'ja:d] *n* вну́тренний двор (*замка и т. д.*).

cousin ['kʌzn] *n* 1) двою́родный брат, двою́родная сестра́ (*тж.* ~ german, first ~); second ~

троюродный брат, троюродная сестра: 2) родственник; to call ~s with smb. считать кого-л. родственником; country ~ деревенский житель, провинциал.

cove[1] [kouv] *n* 1) небольшая бухта; 2) укромный уголок; 3) *архит.* свод.

cove[2] *n разг.* парень; topping ~ палач.

covenant I ['kʌvɪnənt] *n* соглашение; *юр.* договор.

covenant II *v* заключать соглашение, договор.

coventrate ['kɔvəntreit] *v разг.* разбомбить.

Coventry ['kɔvəntrɪ] *n:* to send smb. to ~ прекратить знакомство, общение с кем-л.

cover I ['kʌvə] *n* 1) покрышка, обёртка; чехол; покрывало; 2) конверт; under the same ~ в том же конверте; 3) переплёт, крышка переплёта; to read a book from ~ to ~ прочесть книгу от корки до корки; 4) крышка; 5) прикрытие; укрытие, убежище; to take ~ укрыться; under ~ в укрытии, под защитой; 6) покров; 7) обшивка; 8) ширма, предлог; 9) прибор (*столовый*).

cover II *v* 1) покрывать, закрывать, прикрывать (*чем-л.— with*); to be (to remain) ~ed быть (остаться) в головном уборе; 2) скрывать (*чувства и т. п.*); 3) окутывать, охватывать, включать; 4) превосходить (*количеством*); 5) проходить, покрывать (*расстояние*); 6) простираться; 7) ограждать, защищать; 8) *амер. разг.* давать в прессу материал; 9) *воен.* становиться в затылок; 10) *воен.* прикрывать (*огнём*); 11) покрывать (*кобылу*); □ to ~ in забрасывать, закидывать землёй (*могилу*); to ~ over закрывать, покрывать; to ~ up спрятать, прикрыть.

coverage ['kʌvərɪdʒ] *n* охват.

coverall(s) ['kʌvərɔːl(z)] *n* комбинезон, спецодежда.

covering ['kʌvərɪŋ] *n* 1) покрышка, чехол, 2) оболочка.

coverlet ['kʌvəlɪt] *n* покрывало.

covert[a] [kʌvət] *a* скрытый, тайный.

covert[b] ['kʌvə] *n* 1) лесная чаща (*как убежище для дичи*); 2) коверкот.

covet ['kʌvɪt] *v* сильно желать; жаждать, мечтать.

covetous ['kʌvɪtəs] *a* жадный, алчный (*of*).

covey ['kʌvɪ] *n* 1) выводок (*куропаток*); *pl* куропатки; to spring a ~ спугнуть куропаток; 2) семья; группа (*обычно детей, женщин*).

cow[1] [kau] *n* 1) корова; dry ~ яловая корова; grunting ~ як; 2) *pl* молочный скот; to keep ~s держать, разводить скот; 3) самка (*слона, носорога, кита, моржа и т. п.*).

cow[2] *v* запугивать, терроризировать; заставлять слушаться (*запугиванием*).

coward I ['kauəd] *n* трус; a sad ~ отъявленный, отчаянный трус.

coward II *a поэт.* трусливый; боязливый.

cowardice ['kauədɪs] *n* трусость, малодушие.

cowardly I ['kauədlɪ] *a* малодушный, трусливый, подлый.

cowardly II *adv* трусливо.

cow-boy ['kaubɔɪ] *n* 1) пастух; 2) *амер.* ковбой.

cow-catcher ['kau͵kætʃə] *n амер. ж.-д.* скотосбрасыватель.

cower ['kauə] *v* сжиматься, съёживаться (*от страха или холода*).

cowherd ['kauhəːd] *n* пастух.

cowl [kaul] *n* 1) мантия с капюшоном; 2) капюшон; 3) *разг.* монах; 4) колпак (*над дымовой трубой*).

cowlick ['kaulɪk] *n* чуб, хохолок.

cowman ['kaumən] *n* 1) рабочий на ферме; 2) *амер.* скотопромышленник.

cow-pox ['kaupɔks] *n* телячья оспа.

cox [kɔks] *см.* coxswain.

coxcomb ['kɔkskoum] *n* 1) фат, хлыщ; 2) *уст.* шутовской колпак.

coxswain ['kɔksweɪn, *мор.* 'kɔksn] *n* рулевой; старшина (*на шлюпке*).

coy [kɔɪ] *a* застенчивый.

coyote ['kɔɪout] *n* степной волк, койот.

cozen ['kʌzn] *v* морочить, обманывать.

crab[1] I [kræb] *n* 1) краб; hermit ~ рак-отшельник; 2) *тех.* лебёдка; ворот; ◊ to catch a ~ «завязить» весло.

crab[1] II *v* придираться, подвергать критике.

crab[2] *n* 1) дикое яблоко; 2) дикая яблоня (*тж.* crab-tree).

crabby ['kræbɪ] *a* 1) несговорчивый, упрямый; 2) раздражительный.

crabcake ['kræbkeɪk] *n* котлета из крабов.

crack I [kræk] *n* 1) треск; щёлканье (*хлыста*); 2) трещина, щель; 3) удар, затрещина; 4) *сленг* кража со взломом; 5) *сленг* вор-взломщик; ◊ in a ~ в одно мгновение.

crack II *a разг.* знаменитый; искусный; первоклассный; отборный.

crack III *v* 1) производить треск, трещать; 2) щёлкать хлыстом; 3) трескаться, давать трещину; 4) ломаться (*о голосе*); 5) отпускать (*шутки*); 6) щёлкать, колоть (*орехи*); 7) *сленг* совершить кражу со взломом; 8) распить бутылку (*вина*); 9) вывести из строя (*лошадь, борца*); □ to ~ up а) превозносить; б) грохнуться, разбиться (*вдребезги*).

crack IV *adv* 1) прямо; 2) с треском.

crack-brained ['krækbreɪnd] *a* помешанный, ненормальный.

cracked [krækt] *a* ненормальный, помешанный.

cracker ['krækə] *n* 1) фейерверк; 2) хлопушка; 3) *pl* щипцы для орехов (*тж.* nut-crackers); 4) печенье; крекер; 5) *сленг* ложь; ◊ to be ~s *сленг* рехнуться.

crackle I ['krækl] *n* треск (*выстрелов*); потрескивание (*горящих дров*); хруст.

crackle II *v* трещать, потрескивать, хрустеть.

crackling ['kræklɪŋ] *n* хрустящая корочка.

cracknel ['kræknl] *n* рассыпчатое печенье.

cracksman ['kræksmən] *n* вор-взломщик.

cracky ['krækɪ] *a* 1) потрескавшийся; 2) легко трескающийся; 3) *разг.* помешанный, ненормальный.

cradle I ['kreɪdl] *n* 1) колыбель; from the ~ с младенчества; 2) истоки (*искусства и т. п.*); 3) *тех.* рама; 4) *горн.* лоток (*для промывки золотоносного песка*); 5) рычаг (*телефона*).

cradle II *v* убаюкивать.

cradling ['kreɪdlɪŋ] *n* 1) качание, убаюкивание; 2) *стр.* кружало, рама.

craft [krɑːft] *n* 1) ремесло; умение; potter's ~

кера́мика; 2) ло́вкость, иску́сство, сноро́вка; 3) хи́трость, обма́н; 4) цех (*ремесленный*); 5) *собир.* суда́, самолёты; small ~ ло́дки; 6) кора́бль, ло́дка, челно́к; landing ~ самохо́дная деса́нтная ба́ржа; 7) *attr* цехово́й.

craftsman ['krɑːftsmən] *n* 1) реме́сленник; 2) специали́ст, ма́стер (*своего дела*).

craftsmanship ['krɑːftsmənʃɪp] *n* мастерство́.

crafty ['krɑːftɪ] *a* 1) ло́вкий, иску́сный; 2) хи́трый, кова́рный.

crag¹ [kræg] *n* скала́, утёс.

craggy ['krægɪ] *a* скали́стый.

cragsman ['krægzmən] *n* альпини́ст.

crake [kreɪk] *n зоол.* коросте́ль.

cram [kræm] *v* 1) набива́ть, наполня́ть (*до отказа*); переполня́ть; 2) впи́хивать, вти́скивать (*во что-л.*— into, down); запи́хивать; 3) зака́рмливать, пи́чкать; 4) ната́скивать (*к экзаменам*); 5) зубри́ть, зау́чивать (*тж.* to ~ up).

crammer ['kræmə] *n* 1) репети́тор; 2) *сленг* ложь, враньё.

cramp¹ I [kræmp] *n* су́дорога, спа́зма.

cramp¹ II *v* 1) свя́зывать, стесня́ть (*движения*); 2) своди́ть (*судорогой*).

cramp² I *n тех.* скоба́.

cramp² II *v тех.* скрепля́ть скобо́й.

cramped [kræmpt] *a* 1) стеснённый, сти́снутый; 2) сведённый (*судорогой*); парализо́ванный; 3) неразбо́рчивый (*о почерке*); 4) ограни́ченный (*о человеке*); 5) сжа́тый (*о стиле*).

crampons ['kræmpənz] *n pl* шипы́ на подо́швах (*спортивной обуви*).

cranberry ['krænbərɪ] *n* клю́ква.

crane I [kreɪn] *n* 1) жура́вль (*птица*); 2) *тех.* подъёмный кран.

crane II *v* 1) вытя́гивать ше́ю; 2) поднима́ть кра́ном (*тяжести*); 3) колеба́ться, остана́вливаться пе́ред тру́дностями (at).

cranium ['kreɪnjəm] *n* (*pl* crania ['kreɪnjə]) че́реп.

crank¹ I [kræŋk] *n тех.* кривоши́п, коле́но; коле́нчатый рыча́г; рукоя́тка.

crank¹ II *a* расша́танный.

crank¹ III *v* 1) сгиба́ть; 2) заводи́ть маши́ну (*рукояткой*).

crank² *n* 1) при́хоть, причу́да; 2) челове́к с причу́дами.

cranked [kræŋkt] *a* коле́нчатый, изо́гнутый.

crankshaft ['kræŋkʃɑːft] *n* коле́нчатый вал.

cranky¹ ['kræŋkɪ] *a* 1) ша́ткий; расша́танный; 2) изви́листый, изгиба́ющийся.

cranky² *a* 1) капри́зный; име́ющий причу́ды; прихотли́вый; 2) эксцентри́чный.

crannied ['krænɪd] *a* потре́скавшийся.

cranny ['krænɪ] *n* сква́жина; щель; тре́щина.

crape [kreɪp] *n* креп; *перен.* тра́ур.

crapulence ['kræpjuləns] *n* похме́лье.

crash¹ I [kræʃ] *n* 1) гро́хот, треск; 2) ава́рия, круше́ние; 3) крах, банкро́тство.

crash¹ II *v* 1) упа́сть с гро́хотом; ру́хнуть (*часто* to ~ down); 2) уда́риться с гро́хотом (*обо что-л.*— against); столкну́ться (*тж.* to ~ together); наскочи́ть с тре́ском (*на что-л.*— into); 3) грохота́ть (*о громе; тж.* to ~ out); 4) потерпе́ть ава́рию, круше́ние.

.**crash¹** III *adv* с гро́хотом, с тре́ском.

crash² *n* холст.

crash-helmet ['kræʃˌhelmɪt] *n* защи́тный шлем (*мотоциклиста и т. п.*).

crash-land ['kræʃlænd] *v ав.* 1) соверши́ть вы́нужденную поса́дку; 2) разби́ться при поса́дке.

crass [kræs] *a* 1) кра́йний, полне́йший (*о глупости, невежестве*); 2) гру́бый.

crater ['kreɪtə] *n* 1) кра́тер (*вулкана*); 2) воро́нка от снаря́да.

cravat [krə'væt] *n* ше́йный плато́к; га́лстук; ◊ hempen ~ «пенько́вый га́лстук», верёвка пала́ча.

crave [kreɪv] *v* 1) стра́стно жела́ть, жа́ждать чего́-л. (for); 2) проси́ть, умоля́ть; 3) тре́бовать, вынужда́ть (*об обстоятельствах*).

craven I ['kreɪvən] *n* трус.

craven II *a* трусли́вый.

craving ['kreɪvɪŋ] *n* стра́стное жела́ние, жа́жда чего́-л. (for).

craw [krɔː] *n* зоб (*у птиц*).

crawfish ['krɔːfɪʃ] *см.* crayfish.

crawl I [krɔːl] *n* 1) по́лзание; at a ~ ме́дленно, по-черепа́шьи; 2) ме́дленное движе́ние; to go at a ~ ме́дленно прогу́ливаться; 3) (the ~) *спорт.* кроль (*стиль плавания*).

crawl II *v* 1) ползти́, по́лзти; 2) дви́гаться о́чень ме́дленно; тащи́ться; 3) пресмыка́ться; 4) кише́ть (*насекомыми*); 5) чу́вствовать мура́шки (*по телу*).

crawler ['krɔːlə] *n* 1) пресмыка́ющееся (живо́тное); 2) ползу́чее расте́ние; 3) вошь; 4) *разг.* такси́ст, ме́дленно е́дущий в ожида́нии пассажи́ра; 5) низкопокло́нник; 6) *pl* ползунки́.

crayfish ['kreɪfɪʃ] *n* рак.

crayon ['kreɪən] *n* 1) цветно́й мело́к, каранда́ш; 2) рису́нок цветны́м мелко́м, карандашо́м; 3) у́голь для рисова́ния; 4) каранда́ш для брове́й; 5) *эл.* у́голь в дугово́й ла́мпе.

craze I [kreɪz] *n* 1) ма́ния; 2) помеша́тельство, мо́да (*на что-л.*— for); to be the ~ быть в мо́де.

craze II *v* своди́ть с ума́.

crazed [kreɪzd] *a* 1) сумасше́дший; 2) увлечённый (about).

crazy ['kreɪzɪ] *a* 1) сумасше́дший; безу́мный; 2) стра́стно увлечённый чем-л.; поме́шанный на чём-л.; 3) разва́ливающийся, распада́ющийся; ша́ткий.

creak I [kriːk] *n* скрип.

creak II *v* скрипе́ть.

creaky ['kriːkɪ] *a* скрипу́чий.

cream I [kriːm] *n* 1) сли́вки; крем; sour ~ смета́на; to skim the ~ off снима́ть сли́вки (*тж. перен.*); 2) космети́ческий крем; cold ~ кольдкре́м; 3) «сли́вки», лу́чшая часть (*чего-л.*); соль (*рассказа*); 4) *attr* кре́мовый (*о цвете*); 5) *attr* сли́вочный (*о сырке и т. д.*).

cream II *v* 1) отста́иваться; 2) снима́ть сли́вки.

cream-cheese ['kriːm'tʃiːz] *n* сли́вочный сыр(о́к).

creamery ['kriːmərɪ] *n* 1) маслобо́йня; сырова́рня; 2) моло́чный магази́н.

creamy ['kriːmɪ] *a* жи́рный.

crease I [kriːs] *n* скла́дка.

crease II *v* 1) де́лать скла́дки; утю́жить (*брюки*); 2) мя́ться.

creasy ['kriːsɪ] *a* мя́тый; в скла́дках.

create [kriː'eɪt] *v* 1) твори́ть, создава́ть;

2) возводи́ть в зва́ние; to be ~d получи́ть зва́ние; 3) *разг.* сути́ться, поднима́ть шум.

creation [kri:'eɪʃən] *n* 1) созда́ние, творе́ние; созида́ние; 2) произведе́ние (*науки, искусства*); 3) мирозда́ние; 4) возведе́ние в зва́ние (*пэра и т. п.*).

creative [kri:'eɪtɪv] *a* тво́рческий; созида́тельный.

creator [kri:'eɪtə] *n* 1) творе́ц, созда́тель; 2) а́втор.

creature ['kri:tʃə] *n* 1) созда́ние, творе́ние; 2) челове́к (*обыкн. с эпитетом*); 3) живо́тное, живо́е существо́; 4) ста́вленник, креату́ра; 5) *презр.* тварь.

crèche [kreɪʃ] *n* де́тские я́сли.

credence ['kri:dəns] *n* ве́ра, дове́рие; to give ~ to оказа́ть дове́рие; to find ~ по́льзоваться дове́рием; to refuse ~ отказа́ть в дове́рии.

credentials [krɪ'denʃəlz] *n pl* 1) вери́тельные гра́моты (*посла*); 2) полномо́чия, манда́т.

credibility [,kredɪ'bɪlɪtɪ] *n* вероя́тность.

credible ['kredəbl] *a* 1) заслу́живающий дове́рия; 2) вероя́тный.

credit I ['kredɪt] *n* 1) дове́рие, ве́ра; to give ~ to доверя́ть; to place (*или* to put) ~ in доверя́ть (*кому-л.*); полага́ться (*на что-л.*); 2) хоро́шая репута́ция, честь; to add to one's ~ укрепля́ть репута́цию; to do smb. ~, to be to smb.'s ~ де́лать честь кому́-л.; 3) значе́ние, влия́ние; заслу́г; заслу́га; to have the ~ of име́ть заслу́ги; 5) *ком.* креди́т; on ~ в креди́т; 6) *бухг.* кре́дит.

credit II *v* 1) доверя́ть, ве́рить; 2) припи́сывать что́-л. кому́-л., наделя́ть кого́-л. чем-л. (*with*); 3) *бухг.* кредитова́ть (*счёт*).

creditable ['kredɪtəbl] *a* похва́льный, досто́йный награ́ды, заслу́живающий уваже́ния.

creditor ['kredɪtə] *n* 1) кредито́р, заимода́вец; 2) *бухг.* кре́дит, пра́вая сторона́ бухга́лтерской кни́ги.

credo ['kri:dou] *n* ве́рование, убежде́ния, кре́до.

credulity [krɪ'dju:lɪtɪ] *n* дове́рчивость.

credulous ['kredjuləs] *a* дове́рчивый.

creed [kri:d] *n* 1) ве́ра, вероуче́ние; 2) убежде́ния, кре́до.

creek [kri:k] *n* 1) небольшо́й зали́в, бу́хта; 2) рука́в (*реки*); 3) *амер.* ручёй; ре́чка; 4) овра́г.

creel [kri:l] *n* плетёная корзи́на для ры́бы.

creep [kri:p] *v* (*past, p. p.* crept) 1) по́лзать, ползти́; 2) стели́ться, ви́ться (*о растениях*); 3) кра́сться, подкра́дываться; 4) е́ле дви́гаться (*о старых и больных*); 5) чу́вствовать мура́шки по те́лу; this makes me ~ all over у меня́ от э́того пошли́ мура́шки по всему́ те́лу; □ to ~ **away** уполза́ть; to ~ **in** вполза́ть; to ~ **out** выполза́ть.

creeper ['kri:pə] *n* 1) ползу́чее расте́ние; 2) пресмыка́ющееся живо́тное.

creeps [kri:ps] *n pl разг.* мура́шки; this gave him the ~ у него́ мура́шки пошли́ по те́лу от э́того.

creepy ['kri:pɪ] *a* 1) вызыва́ющий ощуще́ние мура́шек; 2) пресмыка́ющийся.

creepy-crawly ['kri:pɪ'krɔːlɪ] *см.* creepy 1).

cremate [krɪ'meɪt] *v* кремирова́ть.

cremation [krɪ'meɪʃən] *n* креми́рование, крема́ция.

crematorium [,kremə'tɔːrɪəm] *n* (*pl тж.* crematoria [,kremə'tɔːrɪə]) кремато́рий.

crenellation [,krenɪ'leɪʃən] *n* зубцы́ (*на крепостно́й стене́*).

Creole ['kri:oul] *n* крео́л(ка).

creosote ['kri:əsout] *n хим.* креозо́т.

crêpe [kreɪp] *n* креп.

crepitate ['krepɪteɪt] *n* 1) хрусте́ть; 2) хрипе́ть.

crepitation [,krepɪ'teɪʃən] *n* 1) хруст; 2) хри́пы (*при воспале́нии лёгких*).

crept [krept] *past, p. p. см.* creep.

crepuscular [krɪ'pʌskjulə] *a* су́меречный, ту́склый; нея́сный.

crescent I ['kresnt] *n* 1) лу́нный серп, полуме́сяц; 2) полукру́г; 3) герб Ту́рции; *перен.* магомета́нство.

crescent II *a* 1) име́ющий фо́рму полуме́сяца, серпови́дный; 2) *поэт.* расту́щий, нараста́ющий.

cress [kres] *n* кресс-сала́т.

cresset ['kresɪt] *n* фа́кел.

crest I [krest] *n* 1) гребешо́к, хохоло́к (*птицы*); 2) гри́ва, хо́лка; 3) гре́бень шле́ма; 4) рису́нок, украша́ющий гербо́вый щит све́рху; family ~ фами́льный герб; 5) гре́бень (*горы, волны*); 6) конёк (*крыши*).

crest I *v* 1) украша́ть гре́бнем; уве́нчивать; 2) достига́ть верши́ны (*холма, волны*); 3) поднима́ться (*о волна́х*).

crested ['krestɪd] *a* 1) укра́шенный гре́бнем; 2) остроконе́чный.

crest-fallen ['krest,fɔːlən] *a* удручённый, упа́вший ду́хом.

cretin ['kretɪn] *n* крети́н, идио́т.

cretinous ['kretɪnəs] *a* слабоу́мный.

crevasse [krɪ'væs] *n* рассе́лина в леднике́.

crevice ['krevɪs] *n* щель, тре́щина; расще́лина.

crew¹ [kru:] *n* 1) экипа́ж корабля́; air ~ экипа́ж самолёта; 2) *обыкн. пренебр.* компа́ния, ша́йка; the whole ~ все; 3) *ж.-д.* парово́зная *или* конду́кторская брига́да; 4) *воен.* оруди́йный *или* пулемётный расчёт.

crew² *past см.* crow² II.

crewman ['kru:mən] *n* член экипа́жа (*самолёта*); space crewmen экипа́ж косми́ческого корабля́.

crib I [krɪb] *n* 1) де́тская крова́тка (*с боковы́ми се́тками*); 2) я́сли, кормушка; 3) хи́жина, лачу́га; 4) *разг.* подстро́чник; *шк.* шпарга́лка; 5) *разг.* плагиа́т.

crib II *v* 1) заключа́ть, запира́ть в те́сное помеще́ние; 2) *шк.* спи́сывать; 3) *разг.* соверша́ть плагиа́т.

cribbage ['krɪbɪdʒ] *n карт.* кри́бидж.

crick [krɪk] *n* растяже́ние мышц.

cricket¹ ['krɪkɪt] *n* сверчо́к ◊ as lively (*или* merry) as a ~ живо́й, жизнера́достный.

cricket² I *n спорт.* крике́т; ◊ not ~ *разг.* не по пра́вилам; нече́стно.

cricket² II *v* игра́ть в крике́т.

crier ['kraɪə] *n* 1) глаша́тай; 2) крику́н.

crime I [kraɪm] *n* 1) преступле́ние; to confess of the ~ созна́ться в преступле́нии; ~s against humanity преступле́ния про́тив челове́чности; 2) злоде́йние.

crime II *v воен.* кара́ть за наруше́ние уста́ва.

crime-sheet ['kraɪmʃi:t] *n воен.* штрафно́й спи́сок.

criminal I ['krɪmɪnl] *n* престу́пник.

criminal II *a* 1) престу́пный; 2) уголо́вный.

criminality [͵krɪmɪˈnælɪtɪ] *n* престу́пность.

criminate [ˈkrɪmɪneɪt] *v* 1) обвиня́ть в преступле́нии; инкримини́ровать; 2) осужда́ть, порица́ть.

criminology [͵krɪmɪˈnɔlədʒɪ] *n* кримналистика.

crimp[1] [krɪmp] *v* завива́ть (*волосы*); гофрирова́ть (*ткань*).

crimp[2] I *n* аге́нт, вербу́ющий солда́т и матро́сов обма́нным путём.

crimp[2] II *v* вербова́ть обма́нным путём.

crimson I [ˈkrɪmzn] *n* 1) тёмно-кра́сный цвет; 2) румя́нец.

crimson II *a* тёмно-кра́сный.

crimson III *v* гу́сто красне́ть.

cringe I [krɪndʒ] *n* раболе́пие, низкопокло́нство.

cringe II *v* 1) раболе́пствовать, низкопокло́нничать; подли́зываться; 2) съёживаться (*от страха*).

crinkle I [ˈkrɪŋkl] *n* изви́лина; скла́дка.

crinkle II *v* извива́ться, изгиба́ться.

crinkum-crankum [ˈkrɪŋkəmˈkræŋkəm] *n разг.* 1) запу́танное де́ло; 2) причу́да.

crinoline [ˈkrɪnəliːn] *n* 1) кринолин; 2) *мор. сленг* противоторпе́дная сеть.

cripple I [ˈkrɪpl] *n* кале́ка, инвали́д.

cripple II *v* кале́чить; лиша́ть трудоспосо́бности.

crisis [ˈkraɪsɪs] *n* (*pl* crises [ˈkraɪsiːz]) кри́зис; cabinet ~ прави́тельственный кри́зис; to bring to a ~ довести́ до кри́зиса.

crisis-ridden [ˈkraɪsɪs͵rɪdn] *a* поражённый кри́зисом.

crisp I [krɪsp] *a* 1) рассы́пчатый, хрустя́щий; ло́мкий; 2) бодря́щий, свёжий (*о воздухе*); 3) ре́зко очёрченный (*о чертах лица*); 4) чёткий, чека́нный (*о речи*); живо́й (*о стиле*); 5) вью́щийся, кудря́вый.

crisp II *v* 1) де́лать(ся) рассы́пчатым, ло́мким; 2) хрусте́ть; 3) завива́ть(ся).

criss-cross I [ˈkrɪskrɔs] *n* 1) крест (*вместо подписи*); 2) кре́стики (*детская игра*).

criss-cross II *a* перекрёстный, перекре́щивающийся.

criss-cross III *v* перекре́щивать(ся).

criss-cross IV *adv* крест-на́крест.

criterion [kraɪˈtɪərɪən] *n* (*pl* criteria [kraɪˈtɪərɪə]) крите́рий.

critic [ˈkrɪtɪk] *n* кри́тик.

critical [ˈkrɪtɪkəl] *a* 1) крити́ческий; 2) придирчивый, крити́чески настро́енный; 3) переломный, реша́ющий; 4) опа́сный (*о положении, состоянии*).

criticism [ˈkrɪtɪsɪzəm] *n* 1) кри́тика; scathing (slashing) ~ жесто́кая (уничтожа́ющая) кри́тика; 2) крити́ческая статья́; крити́ческое замеча́ние.

criticize [ˈkrɪtɪsaɪz] *v* 1) критикова́ть; 2) осужда́ть.

critique [krɪˈtiːk] *n* 1) кри́тика; 2) крити́ческая статья́.

croak I [krouk] *n* 1) ка́рканье; 2) ква́канье.

croak II *v* 1) ка́ркать (*тж. перен.*); 2) ква́кать; 3) брюзжа́ть.

Croat [ˈkrouət] *n* хорва́т; хорва́тка; the ~s хорва́ты.

Croatian [krouˈeɪʃjən] *a* хорва́тский.

crochet I [ˈkrouʃeɪ] *n* та́мбурная вы́шивка.

crochet II *v* вышива́ть та́мбуром.

croci [ˈkrousɪ] *pl см.* crocus.

crock[1] [krɔk] *n* 1) гли́няный кувши́н; 2) черепо́к.

crock[2] I *n* 1) заёзженная кля́ча; 2) *разг.* измо́танный челове́к.

crock[2] II *v* заёздить, измота́ть (*тж.* to ~ up).

crockery [ˈkrɔkərɪ] *n* фая́нсовая посу́да.

crocodile [ˈkrɔkədaɪl] *n* 1) крокоди́л; 2) *разг.* гуля́нье па́рами (*о школьницах*); 3) *attr* крокоди́ловый.

crocus [ˈkroukəs] *n* (*pl тж.* croci) *бот., тех.* кро́кус.

Croesus [ˈkriːsəs] *n* Крез; *перен.* бога́ч, фина́нсовый коро́ль.

croft [krɔft] *n* 1) приуса́дебный уча́сток (*пахотной земли*); 2) часть фе́рмы.

crofter [ˈkrɔftə] *n* ме́лкий аренда́тор.

cromlech [ˈkrɔmlek] *n археол.* кро́млех.

crone [kroun] *n* ста́рая карга́, стару́ха.

crony [ˈkrounɪ] *n* ста́рый друг.

crook I [kruk] *n* 1) крюк, крючо́к; 2) за́гнутый коне́ц; 3) изги́б (*реки, дороги*); поворо́т; 4) *разг.* жу́лик, плут; on the ~ обма́нным путём; 5) клюка́.

crook II *a см.* crooked.

crook III *v* 1) скрю́чивать(ся); сгиба́ть(ся); 2) изгиба́ть(ся), искривля́ть(ся); 3) лови́ть на крючо́к.

crook-back(ed) [ˈkrukbæk(t)] *a* горба́тый.

crooked [ˈkrukɪd] *a* 1) криво́й, изо́гнутый; 2) искривлённый; сго́рбленный; 3) нече́стный, непрямо́й.

croon I [kruːn] *n* ти́хое пе́ние, мурлы́канье.

croon II *v* напева́ть е́ле слы́шно; мурлы́кать (*песню*).

crop I [krɔp] *n* 1) урожа́й; heavy (poor) ~ бога́тый (плохо́й) урожа́й; 2) хлеб на корню́ (*тж.* growing ~, standing ~); in ~ под се́вом; out of ~ незасе́янный; под па́ром; under ~ засе́янный; 3) *с.-х.* культу́ра; technical ~s техни́ческие культу́ры; 4) мно́жество, ма́сса; 5) зоб (*у птицы*); 6) кнутови́ще; 7) ко́ротко подстри́женные во́лосы; Eton ~ же́нская стри́жка «под ма́льчика»; to have a ~ ко́ротко подстрига́ть во́лосы.

crop II *v* 1) дава́ть, приноси́ть урожа́й; роди́ть (*о земле*); 2) собира́ть урожа́й; 3) подстрига́ть, обреза́ть; 4) ощи́пывать, объеда́ть (*траву и т. п.*); □ to ~ out *геол.* выходи́ть на пове́рхность (*о пласте*); to ~ up а) неожи́данно возника́ть (*о вопросе и т. п.*); б) *см.* to ~ out.

crop-eared [ˈkrɔpɪəd] *a* 1) с обре́занными уша́ми; 2) ко́ротко подстри́женный (*ист. тж. о пуританах*).

cropper [ˈkrɔpə] *n* 1) жнец; 2) *амер.* издо́льщик; 3) коси́лка, жне́йка; 4) *с.-х.:* good ~ плодоно́сное расте́ние; 5) *разг.* тяжёлое паде́ние; to come a ~ гро́хнуться; *перен.* потерпе́ть крах.

croquet I [ˈkroukeɪ] *n* кроке́т.

croquet II *v* крокирова́ть.

cross I [krɔs] *n* 1) крест; Red Cross Кра́сный Крест; the Victoria Cross Крест короле́вы Викто́рии; to make one's ~ поста́вить крест (*вместо подписи*); 2) распя́тие; 3) испыта́ния, страда́ния; 4) *биол.* скре́щивание (*пород*), гибридиза́ция; 5) *биол.* гибри́д.

cross II *a* 1) попере́чный, пересека́ющийся; 2) проти́вный (*о ветре*); неблагоприя́тный; 3) противополо́жный; обра́тный (*о действии*); 4) перекрёстный; 5) *разг.* серди́тый, злой;

◊ as ~ as two sticks о́чень раздражённый.

cross III *v* 1) пересека́ть; переходи́ть (*у́лицу*); переправля́ться, переезжа́ть (*мо́ре, океа́н*); 2) скре́щивать (*ру́ки, шпа́ги и т. п.*); 3) крести́ться; 4) размину́ться, разойти́сь (*о лю́дях, пи́сьмах*); 5) противоде́йствовать, препя́тствовать (*пла́нам, во́ле и т. п.*); 6) *биол.* скре́щивать(ся); □ to ~ off, to ~ out вычёркивать; to ~ over переходи́ть, пересека́ть, переезжа́ть; переправля́ться.

cross-bar ['krɔsbɑː] *n тех.* попере́чина.

cross-beam ['krɔsbiːm] *n тех.* попере́чная ба́лка, крестови́на.

cross-bow ['krɔsbou] *n ист.* самостре́л, арбале́т.

cross-bred ['krɔsbred] *a* скрещённый, гибри́дный.

cross-breed ['krɔsbriːd] *n* по́месь, гибри́д.

cross-country I ['krɔs'kʌntrɪ] *n* пересечённая ме́стность.

cross-country II *a* вездехо́дный.

cross-cut ['krɔskʌt] *n* 1) кратча́йшее расстоя́ние; 2) попере́чный разре́з; 3) попере́чная пила́.

cross-examination ['krɔsɪɡˌzæmɪ'neɪʃən] *n* перекрёстный допро́с.

cross-examine ['krɔsɪɡ'zæmɪn] *v* подверга́ть перекрёстному допро́су.

cross-fire ['krɔsˌfaɪə] *n воен.* перекрёстный ого́нь.

cross-grained ['krɔsɡreɪnd] *a* упря́мый, своенра́вный.

crossing ['krɔsɪŋ] *n* 1) пересече́ние; скре́щивание; скреще́ние; 2) перекрёсток; 3) перехо́д (*че́рез у́лицу*); zebra ~ перехо́д для пешехо́дов, отме́ченный поло́сами; 4) *ж.-д.* перее́зд (*амер.* grade ~); пересече́ние двух железнодоро́жных ли́ний; high (*или* level) ~ перее́зд; 5) перепра́ва; 6) морско́й рейс; a rough ~ морско́й рейс в неспоко́йную пого́ду.

cross-legged ['krɔsleɡd] *a* скрести́в но́ги.

crossly ['krɔslɪ] *adv* серди́то; сварли́во.

cross-patch ['krɔspætʃ] *n* сварли́вый челове́к.

cross-question ['krɔs'kwestʃən] *см.* cross-examine.

cross-road ['krɔsroud] *n* перекрёсток; at the ~s на распу́тье.

cross-stitch ['krɔsstɪtʃ] *n* вы́шивка кресто́м.

crosswise ['krɔswaɪz] *adv* крест-на́крест.

cross-word ['krɔswəːd] *n* кроссво́рд.

crotchet ['krɔtʃɪt] *n* 1) причу́да, фанта́зия, конёк; 2) *муз.* четвертна́я но́та; 3) крючо́к.

crotcheteer [ˌkrɔtʃə'tɪə] *n* челове́к с причу́дами.

crotchety ['krɔtʃɪtɪ] *a* капри́зный, своенра́вный.

crouch [krautʃ] *v* 1) сгиба́ться; 2) притаи́ться; 3) раболе́пствовать, пресмыка́ться.

croup[1] [kruːp] *n* круп (*боле́знь*).

croup[2] *n* круп (*ло́шади*).

croupe [kruːp] *см.* croup[2].

croupier ['kruːpɪə] *n* 1) банкомёт, крупье́; 2) замести́тель председа́теля на банке́те.

crow[1] [krou] *n* воро́на; ◊ as the ~ flies ≅ по прямо́й ли́нии; to have a ~ to pick (*или* to pluck) with smb. име́ть счёты с кем-л.; white ~ «бе́лая воро́на».

crow[2] I *n* 1) пе́ние петуха́; 2) гу́канье, ра́достный крик младе́нца.

crow[2] II *v* (*past* crowed, crew; *p. p.* crowed) 1) петь (*о петухе́*); 2) выража́ть ра́дость кри́ком, гу́кать (*о младе́нце*); 3) ликова́ть; □ to ~ over восторжествова́ть.

crow-bar ['kroubɑː] *n* лом (*инструме́нт*).

crowd I [kraud] *n* 1) толпа́; in ~s ма́ссами; the ~ *пренебр.* «толпа́», просты́е обыва́тели; he might pass in a ~ он не ху́же други́х; 2) *разг.* компа́ния, гру́ппа люде́й; 3) толкотня́; 4) мно́жество, ма́сса (*чего́-л.*).

crowd II *v* 1) толпи́ться; 2) набива́ть(ся) битко́м; заполня́ть до преде́ла; 3) тесни́ть(ся); □ to ~ into проти́скиваться; to ~ out вытесня́ть.

crowded ['kraudɪd] *a* 1) перепо́лненный, битко́м наби́тый; 2) по́лный, напо́лненный.

crown I [kraun] *n* 1) коро́на; вене́ц; the Crown а) коро́ль, короле́ва; б) короле́вская власть, престо́л; 2) вено́к (*из цвето́в*); 3): the ~ of one's labours заверше́ние трудо́в; the ~ of the year коне́ц го́да; 4) маку́шка (*головы́*); голова́; 5) кро́на, верху́шка (*де́рева*); 6) тулья́ (*шля́пы*); 7) коро́нка (*зу́ба*); 8) кро́на (*моне́та=5 шиллингам*); 9) *attr* коро́нный.

crown II *v* 1) коронова́ть; венча́ть; 2) вознагражда́ть; 3) заверша́ть, зака́нчивать; увенчивать; 4) поста́вить коро́нку (*на зуб*).

crowned [kraund] *a* 1) уве́нчанный (*with*); 2): high (low) ~ с высо́кой (с ни́зкой) тулье́й (*о шля́пе*).

crow's-foot ['krouzfut] *n* 1) *pl* морщи́ны у угла́ гла́за; 2) *воен.* про́волочные си́лки.

crow's-nest ['krouznest] *n* 1) воро́нье гнездо́; 2) *мор.* наблюда́тельная вы́шка.

crucial ['kruːʃəl] *a* 1) реша́ющий (*об о́пыте, эксперименте*); крити́ческий (*о пери́оде*); 2) *анат.* крестови́дный.

crucible ['kruːsɪbl] *n* 1) рето́рта, ти́гель; 2) тяжёлое испыта́ние; in the ~ «в переде́лке».

cruciferous [kruː'sɪfərəs] *a бот.* крестоцве́тный.

crucifix ['kruːsɪfɪks] *n* распя́тие.

crucifixion [ˌkruːsɪ'fɪkʃən] *n* 1) распя́тие на кресте́; 2) тяжёлые страда́ния.

cruciform ['kruːsɪfɔːm] *a* крестообра́зный.

crucify ['kruːsɪfaɪ] *v* 1) распина́ть; 2) умерщвля́ть (*плоть*).

crude [kruːd] *a* 1) сыро́й, недозре́лый; 2) неперева́ренный (*о пи́ще*); 3) недоде́ланный; неочи́щенный; недорабо́танный (*о пла́не, прое́кте и т. п.*); 4) незре́лый; 5) гру́бый (*о мане́рах*).

crudity ['kruːdɪtɪ] *n* 1) незре́лость; 2) недорабо́танность (*пла́на, прое́кта*); 3) гру́бость (*манер*).

cruel [kruəl] *a* 1) жесто́кий; бессерде́чный; безжа́лостный; 2) тяжёлый, мучи́тельный, тя́жкий.

cruelly ['kruəlɪ] *adv* жесто́ко; безжа́лостно.

cruelty ['kruəltɪ] *n* жесто́кость; бессерде́чие, безжа́лостность.

cruet-stand ['kruːɪtstænd] *n* столо́вый судо́к.

cruise I [kruːz] *n* морско́е путеше́ствие, круи́з; рейс; a round-the-world ~ кругосве́тное пла́вание.

cruise II *v* пла́вать, соверша́ть рейсы; крейси́ровать; □ to ~ round кружи́ть (*над — over*).

cruiser ['kruːzə] *n* крейсер; armoured ~ броненосный крейсер.

crumb I [krʌm] *n* 1) крошка (*хлеба*); 2) мякиш (*хлеба*); 3) крупица, частица; ~s of information обрывки сведений.

crumb II *v* 1) крошить; 2) убирать крошки; 3) обсыпать крошками.

crumble ['krʌmbl] *v* 1) крошиться, осыпаться; 2) разрушаться; рушиться (*тж.* to ~ away); 3) померкнуть (*о славе*).

crumbly ['krʌmblɪ] *a* хрупкий, ломкий; непрочный.

crumby ['krʌmɪ] *a* 1) усыпанный крошками; 2) *амер.* дешёвый.

crummy ['krʌmɪ] *a разг.* 1) полный, упитанный; 2) обеспеченный, зажиточный; 3) *см.* crumby 2).

crump I [krʌmp] *n* 1) сильный удар; 2) *воен. сленг* фугасная бомба; фугаска.

crump II *v* 1) наносить сильный удар; 2) *воен. сленг* стрелять, обстреливать.

crumpet ['krʌmpɪt] *n* 1) слойка, пышка; 2) *сленг* голова, башка.

crumple ['krʌmpl] *v* 1) мять(ся); комкать(ся); морщиться; съёживаться; 2) падать духом; □ to ~ up а) смять в руке (*бумагу*); б) раздавить, смять (*противника*); в) рухнуть, свалиться.

crumpled ['krʌmpld] *a* мятый; скомканный.

crunch I [krʌntʃ] *n* 1) хруст; 2) скрип.

crunch II *v* 1) грызть, хрустеть; 2) скрипеть под ногами.

crunchy ['krʌntʃɪ] *a* хрустящий, шуршащий.

crusade I [kruːˈseɪd] *n* 1) *ист.* крестовый поход; 2) поход, кампания (*против чего-л.*).

crusade II *v* выступить походом; начать кампанию.

crusader [kruːˈseɪdə] *n* крестоносец.

crush I [krʌʃ] *n* 1) дробление, размельчение; 2) толкотня, давка; 3) *разг.* толпа, сборище; 4) сокрушительный удар; *воен.* разгром; 5) *сленг* сильное увлечение (*кем-л. — on*); 6) фруктовый сок.

crush II *v* 1) давить; дробить; размельчать (*в порошок*); 2) выжимать (*виноград*); 3) мять; 4) уничтожать, подавлять, сокрушать; *воен.* разгромить; □ to ~ down а) дробить, мельчить; б) подавлять (*восстание, оппозицию*); to ~ out подавлять (*восстание*); to ~ up толочь, дробить.

crushing ['krʌʃɪŋ] *a* 1) сокрушительный; сокрушающий; 2) ударный (*о силе*); 3) тяжкий (*о горе*).

crush-room ['krʌʃrum] *n театр.* фойе.

crust I [krʌst] *n* 1) корка (*хлеба*); to earn one's ~ *перен.* зарабатывать себе на кусок хлеба; 2) *геол.* земная кора; 3) наст (*на снегу*); корка (*льда*); 4) налёт, осадок (*вина на стенках бутылки*).

crust II *v* покрываться коркой; образовывать кору, наст.

crusted ['krʌstɪd] *a* 1) покрытый коркой, корой; налётом; настом; 2) закоренелый (*о привычках, предрассудках*); застарелый.

crusty ['krʌstɪ] *a* 1) покрытый коркой, корой; 2) сварливый, придирчивый.

crutch [krʌtʃ] *n* 1) *обыкн. pl* костыль; *перен.*

опора, поддержка; 2) вилка (*костыля*); поперечина (*костыля*); 2) стойка (*мотоцикла*).

crutched [krʌtʃt] *a* 1) пользующийся костылями; 2) имеющий поперечину.

crux [krʌks] *n* 1) затруднение; тупик, недоумение; 2) (the C.) созвездие Южного Креста.

cry I [kraɪ] *n* 1) крик; to give a ~ крикнуть; 2) плач; to have a good ~ выплакаться; 3) мольба; призыв (*о помощи*); 4) боевой клич; лозунг; 5) общественное одобрение (*for*); общественный протест (*against*); 6) слухи (*обычно тревожные*), молва; 7) крики разносчиков; 8) собачий лай; ◇ much ~ and little wool ≅ много шуму из ничего; it is a far ~ а) далёкое расстояние; б) большая разница; in full ~ в бешеной погоне.

cry II *v* 1) кричать, вопить; орать; 2) воскликнуть, вскрикнуть; 3) плакать; 4) умолять, взывать (*о помощи*); 5) оглашать, объявлять; □ to ~ down а) сбивать цену (*товара*); б) раскритиковать; в) заглушать криками; to ~ for настойчиво требовать, добиваться чего-л.; ~ off отказываться от (*сделки, предложения*); идти на попятный; to ~ out а) выкрикивать, вопить; б) жаловаться вслух; to ~ out (against) осуждать; высказывать осуждение, порицание; to ~ up расхваливать.

cry-baby ['kraɪˌbeɪbɪ] *n* плакса.

crying ['kraɪɪŋ] *a* 1) кричащий, плачущий; 2) вопиющий, возмутительный.

crypt ['krɪpt] *n* склеп.

cryptic ['krɪptɪk] *a* загадочный, сокровенный.

crystal I ['krɪstl] *n* 1) хрусталь; хрустальная посуда; 2) кристалл; 3) *поэт.* лёд, вода; глаз, слеза; 4) *амер.* стекло для карманных и ручных часов; 5) *радио* детекторный кристалл.

crystal II *a* 1) хрустальный; 2) прозрачный, чистый; кристальный; 3) кристаллический.

crystalline ['krɪstəlaɪn] *a* кристальный; прозрачный.

crystallization [ˌkrɪstəlaɪˈzeɪʃən] *n* образование кристаллов, кристаллизация.

crystallize ['krɪstəlaɪz] *v* 1) кристаллизовать (-ся); 2) принимать определённую форму; 3) засахаривать(ся) (*о фруктах*).

cub I [kʌb] *n* 1) детёныш, щенок (*хищного зверя*); 2) юнец; *пренебр.* молокосос.

cub II *v* щениться.

Cuban I ['kjuːbən] *n* кубинец; кубинка; the ~s кубинцы.

Cuban II *a* кубинский.

cubbing ['kʌbɪŋ] *n* охота на лисят.

cubbish ['kʌbɪʃ] *a* невоспитанный.

cube I [kjuːb] *n* куб.

cube II *v мат.* возводить в куб.

cubed [kjuːbd] *a мат.* в кубе; в третьей степени.

cub-hunting ['kʌbˌhʌntɪŋ] *см.* cubbing.

cubic(al) ['kjuːbɪk(əl)] *a* кубический.

cubicle ['kjuːbɪkl] *n* маленькая отдельная спальня в общежитии.

cuboid I ['kjuːbɔɪd] *n* 1) *анат.* кубовидная кость; 2) *мат.* кубоид.

cuboid II *a* имеющий форму куба.

cuckold I ['kʌkəld] *n* муж-рогоносец.

cuckold II *v* изменять своему мужу.

cuckoo[a] ['kuku] *n* 1) кукушка; the ~ calls кукушка кукует; 2) *разг.* разиня.

cuckoo[b] [ˈkuˈkuː] *int* ку-ку!

cucumber [ˈkjuːkəmbə] *n* огурец.

cud [kʌd] *n* жвачка; to chew the ~ жевать жвачку; *перен.* нудно повторять одно и то же.

cudbear [ˈkʌdbɛə] *n* 1) лакмус; 2) лакмусовый ягель (*краситель*).

cuddle I [ˈkʌdl] *n* объятия.

cuddle II *v* 1) сжимать в объятиях; прижимать к себе (*ребёнка*); 2) свернуться калачиком; 3) прижиматься (*друг к другу — together*).

cuddy[1] [ˈkʌdɪ] *n* 1) каюта (*небольшого корабля*); 2) будка (*на барже*); 3) чулан.

cuddy[2] *n* 1) осёл, простак.

cudgel I [ˈkʌdʒəl] *n* дубина; to take up the ~s for заступаться за кого-л.; отстаивать что-л. (*в споре*).

cudgel II *v* бить палкой.

cue[1] [kjuː] *n* 1) кий (*бильярдный*); 2) очередь, хвост.

cue[2] *n* 1) *театр.* реплика; 2) намёк; to give the ~ подсказать; to take one's ~ from smb. воспользоваться чьим-л. указанием.

cuff[1] [kʌf] *n* манжета; обшлаг.

cuff[2] I *n* удар кулаком; ~s and kicks пинки и удары.

cuff[2] II *v* бить кулаком, тузить.

cuff-links [ˈkʌflɪŋks] *n pl* запонки.

cuirass [kwɪˈræs] *n* кираса, панцирь.

cuirassier [ˌkwɪrəˈsɪə] *n ист.* кирасир.

cuisine [kwiːˈziːn] *n* подбор кушаний, кухня; стол (*питание*).

cul-de-sac [ˈkuldəˈsæk] *n* тупик (*тж. перен.*).

culinary [ˈkʌlɪnərɪ] *a* кулинарный.

cullender [ˈkʌlɪndə] *см.* colander.

culminate [ˈkʌlmɪneɪt] *v* 1) достигать высшей точки, апогея; 2) *астр.* кульминировать.

culmination [ˌkʌlmɪˈneɪʃən] *n* 1) высшая точка; кульминационный пункт; 2) *астр.* кульминация.

culpability [ˌkʌlpəˈbɪlɪtɪ] *n* виновность.

culpable [ˈkʌlpəbl] *a* преступный, виновный.

culprit [ˈkʌlprɪt] *n* 1) преступник; 2) обвиняемый.

cult [kʌlt] *n* культ.

cultivate [ˈkʌltɪveɪt] *v* 1) возделывать, обрабатывать; 2) культивировать (*растения*); улучшать сорт; 3) развивать (*способности, привычки и т. п.*).

cultivation [ˌkʌltɪˈveɪʃən] *n* 1) возделывание (*земли*); 2) выращивание *или* улучшение сортов (*с.-х. культур*); 3) культура (*растений, бактерий*); 4) развитие (*способностей и тому подобное*).

cultivator [ˈkʌltɪveɪtə] *n* 1) земледелец; агроном; 2) *с.-х.* культиватор.

cultural [ˈkʌltʃərəl] *a* культурный.

culture [ˈkʌltʃə] *n* 1) культура; socialist ~ социалистическая культура; Soviet ~ советская культура; 2) сельскохозяйственная культура; 3) разведение (*пчёл, рыб и т. п.*); 4) выращивание (*бактерий*).

cultured [ˈkʌltʃəd] *a* культурный, образованный.

culvert [ˈkʌlvət] *n* трубопровод; дренажная труба.

cumber I [ˈkʌmbə] *n* затруднение.

cumber II *v* 1) затруднять, стеснять, препятствовать; 2) блокировать (*дорогу*), мешать (*движению*).

cumbersome [ˈkʌmbəsəm] *a* 1) громоздкий; 2) затруднительный.

Cumbrian I. [ˈkʌmbrɪən] *n* житель Камберленда.

Cumbrian II *a* камберлендский.

cumbrous [ˈkʌmbrəs] *см.* cumbersome.

cum(m)in [ˈkʌmɪn] *n* тмин.

cumulative [ˈkjuːmjulətɪv] *a* 1) совокупный, общий; 2) сводный (*о каталоге, указателе*).

cumulus [ˈkjuːmjuləs] *n* (*pl* cumuli [ˈkjuːmjulaɪ]) кучевые облака.

cuneiform I [ˈkjuːnɪfɔːm] *n* клинописный знак.

cuneiform II *a* клинописный.

cunning I [ˈkʌnɪŋ] *n* 1) хитрость, коварство; 2) умение, ловкость.

cunning II *a* 1) изобретательный; хитрый, коварный; 2) *амер. разг.* прелестный; привлекательный.

cup I [kʌp] *n* 1) чашка; a ~ of tea чашка чаю; 2) кубок, чарка; чаша; to crush a ~ of wine распить бутылку вина; 3) доля, судьба; чаша жизни; to drain the ~ испить чашу жизни; to fill up the ~ а) переполнить чашу (терпения); б) переливаться через край; the ~ is full чаша (терпения) переполнилась; 4) вино; крюшон; to be in one's ~s быть навеселе; he is too fond of the ~ он любит выпить; 5) *спорт.* кубок; 6) *мед.* банка; 7) *бот.* чашечка (*цветка*); ◊ to be a ~ too low быть в подавленном настроении.

cup II *v мед.* ставить банки.

cup-bearer [ˈkʌpˌbɛərə] *n ист.* виночерпий.

cupboard [ˈkʌbəd] *n* буфет (*для посуды*).

cupful [ˈkʌpful] *n* (полная) чашка (*чего-либо*).

cupidity [kjuːˈpɪdɪtɪ] *n* алчность, жадность.

cupola [ˈkjuːpələ] *n* купол.

cupping-glass [ˈkʌpɪŋglɑːs] *n мед.* банка.

cuprous [ˈkjuːprəs] *a хим.* медный.

cur [kəː] *n* 1) *презр.* шавка; 2) грубый, невоспитанный человек.

curable [ˈkjuərəbl] *a* излечимый.

curacy [ˈkjuərəsɪ] *n* 1) сан священника; 2) приход (*церковный*).

curate [ˈkjuərɪt] *n* помощник приходского священника.

curative I [ˈkjuərətɪv] *n* целебное средство.

curative II *a* целебный.

curator [kjuəˈreɪtə] *n* 1) хранитель (*музея, библиотеки*); 2) член правления (*в англ. университетах*).

curb I [kəːb] *n* 1) узда, уздечка; 2) обуздание; узда.

curb II *v* обуздывать, усмирять.

curbstone [ˈkəːbstoun] *n* тумба.

curd I [kəːd] *n обыкн. pl* творог.

curd II *v* свёртываться (*о молоке, крови*); створаживаться.

curdle [ˈkəːdl] *v* 1) свёртываться (*о молоке, крови*); 2) застыть (*от ужаса*); оцепенеть.

cure I [kjuə] *n* 1) лекарство; средство (*против, от — for*); 2) лечение, курс лечения.

cure II *v* 1) лечить; вылечивать; 2) исправлять (*зло*); 3) консервировать (*продукты питания*).

cure-all ['kjuər,ɔːl] *n* панацея; средство от всех болезней.

cureless ['kjuəlɪs] *a* неизлечимый.

curfew ['kəːfjuː] *n* 1) *ист.* вечерний звон (*сигнал для гашения огней*); 2) комендантский час; сигнал о начале комендантского часа.

curio ['kjuərɪou] *n* антикварная вещь.

curiosity [,kjuərɪ'ɔsɪtɪ] *n* 1) любознательность; 2) любопытство; 3) странность; 4) антикварная вещь.

curious ['kjuərɪəs] *a* 1) любознательный; 2) любопытный; 3) возбуждающий любопытство, чудной, удивительный; 4) тщательный.

curl I [kəːl] *n* 1) локон, завиток; *pl* вьющиеся волосы; 2) завивка; 3) кольцо (*дыма*); 4) спираль.

curl II *v* 1) завивать(ся); виться (*о волосах*); 2) виться (*о дороге, тропинке*); 3) свёртываться в клубок; 4) клубиться (*о дыме, облаках*); □ to ~ **up** а) свёртываться, скручиваться (*от мороза, жары*); б) испытать потрясение.

curlicue ['kəːlɪkjuː] *n* завиток.

curling ['kəːlɪŋ] *a* вьющийся.

curling-irons ['kəːlɪŋ,aɪənz] *n pl* щипцы для завивки.

curling-tongs ['kəːlɪŋtɔŋz] *см.* curling-irons.

curl-paper ['kəːl,peɪpə] *n* папильотка.

curly ['kəːlɪ] *a* 1) вьющийся, кудрявый, курчавый; 2) волнистый; изогнутый.

curr [kəː] *v* ворковать; мурлыкать.

currant ['kʌrənt] *n* 1) смородина; black (red, white) ~s чёрная (красная, белая) смородина; 2) коринка (*тж.* dried ~s).

currency ['kʌrənsɪ] *n* 1) система денежных знаков; денежное обращение; to give ~ to пустить в обращение; 2) валюта, деньги; paper ~ бумажные деньги; 3) употребительность, распространённость (*слов, мнения и т. п.*); to gain ~ получить распространение.

current I ['kʌrənt] *n* 1) течение; струя; поток; 2) ход, течение (*событий*); 3) *эл.* ток; alternating ~, commuted ~ переменный ток; direct (primary) ~ постоянный (первичный) ток.

current II *a* 1) текущий (*о периоде времени, о событиях*); 2) общераспространённый (*о мнениях, словах и т. п.*); ходячий, находящийся в обращении (*о денежных знаках*); to pass (*или* to go, to run) ~ иметь обращение везде, быть общепринятым; 3) гладкий (*о стиле*).

curriculum [kə'rɪkjuləm] *n* (*pl* curricula [kə'rɪkjulə]) учебный план, программа (*института, университета*).

currier ['kʌrɪə] *n* кожевник.

currish ['kəːrɪʃ] *a* невоспитанный, грубый.

curry[1] ['kʌrɪ] *n* кэрри (*род острого мясного или яичного соуса*).

curry[2] *v* 1) чистить скребницей (*лошадь*); 2) выделывать кожу.

curry-comb ['kʌrɪ,koum] *n* скребница.

curse I [kəːs] *n* 1) проклятие; to pronounce a ~ upon проклинать (*кого-л.*); 2) ругательство; брань; 3) бич, бедствие; ◇ ~s come home to roost *посл.* ≅ как аукнется, так и откликнется; I don't care (*или* give) a ~ (for) мне до этого нет никакого дела; not worth a ~ ≅ гроша ломаного не стоит.

curse II *v* 1) проклинать; 2) ругаться; 3) мучиться, страдать от чего-л.

cursed ['kəːsɪd] *a* 1) проклятый; 2) отвратительный.

cursive ['kəːsɪv] *a* рукописный.

cursory ['kəːsərɪ] *a* 1) беглый, поверхностный; 2) достаточно свободный (*о чтении, письме*).

curt [kəːt] *a* 1) краткий, сжатый (*о стиле*); 2) грубый, отрывистый (*об ответе и т. п.*); 3) короткий.

curtail [kəː'teɪl] *v* 1) сокращать, уменьшать; 2) урезывать; укорачивать.

curtailment [kəː'teɪlment] *n* 1) сокращение, уменьшение; 2) урезывание; укорачивание.

curtain I ['kəːtn] *n* 1) занавеска; to draw the ~s задёрнуть занавески; 2) занавес; behind the ~ за кулисами; to ring the ~ down (up) дать звонок к спуску (поднятию) занавеса; the ~ rises, the ~ is raised занавес поднимается; the ~ falls, the ~ drops занавес падает, опускается; to draw the ~ а) приподнять завесу над чем-л.; б) скрыть, укрыть что-л.; 3) *воен.* завеса; ◇ iron ~ железный занавес.

curtain II *v* занавешивать.

curtain-fire ['kəːtn,faɪə] *n воен.* огневая завеса.

curtain-raiser ['kəːtn,reɪzə] *n* одноактная пьеса (*исполняемая до начала спектакля*).

curtsey I ['kəːtsɪ] *n* реверанс; to drop a ~ сделать реверанс.

curtsey II *v* делать реверанс.

curtsy I, II ['kəːtsɪ] *см.* curtsey I, II.

curvature ['kəːvətʃə] *n* кривизна, изгиб.

curve I [kəːv] *n* 1) кривая линия; 2) изгиб, кривизна; 3) график; диаграмма; 4) лекало; 5) *мат.* кривая.

curve II *v* 1) изгибать(ся); 2) гнуть(ся), сгибать(ся).

curvet I [kəː'vet] *n* курбет (*прыжок верховой лошади*).

curvet II *v* делать курбет.

curvilinear [,kəːvɪ'lɪnɪə] *a* криволинейный.

cushion I ['kuʃən] *n* 1) подушка (*диванная, кислородная*); 2) борт (*бильярдного стола*); 3) *тех.* прокладка.

cushion II *v* 1) подкладывать подушку; 2) успокоить, утихомирить; 3) ставить шар (*к борту бильярда*).

cushy ['kuʃɪ] *a сленг* лёгкий; выгодный (*о работе*).

cusp [kʌsp] *n* 1) рог месяца; 2) остриё копья; 3) пик (*горы*).

cuspidor ['kʌspɪdɔː] *n амер.* плевательница.

custard ['kʌstəd] *n* заварной крем.

custodian [kʌs'toudjən] *n* 1) хранитель (*музея, библиотеки*); 2) опекун.

custody ['kʌstədɪ] *n* 1) охрана; опёка, попечение; to have the ~ of охранять; to be in the ~ of находиться под охраной, опекой; 2) арест, заключение; заточение; in ~ в заключении, в тюрьме; military ~ гауптвахта; to take into ~ взять под стражу, арестовать; to give into ~ заключить под стражу.

custom ['kʌstəm] *n* 1) обычай; native ~s местные, туземные обычаи; 2) привычка; 3) клиенту́ра; 4) заку́пки; 5) *pl* тамо́женные по́шлины; 6) *attr амер.* изгото́вленный на зака́з.

customary ['kʌstəmərɪ] *a* обы́чный; привы́чный.

customer ['kʌstəmə] *n* 1) покупа́тель; клие́нт; *перен.* завсегда́тай; 2) *разг.* тип, субъе́кт; awkward (ugly, tough) ~ нескла́дный (опа́сный, непокла́дистый) челове́к; rum ~ стра́нный, подозри́тельный челове́к.

custom-house ['kʌstəmhaus] *n* тамо́жня.

cut I [kʌt] *n* 1) поре́з, разре́з; ра́на (*ножева́я, са́бельная*); 2) уда́р (*хлысто́м, па́лкой*); 3) покро́й (*пла́тья*); фасо́н (*стри́жки*); 4) вы́резка (*из кни́ги, журна́ла*); 5) филе́й; 6) сниже́ние (*цен, зарпла́ты*); сокраще́ние (*шта́тов*); 7) прекраще́ние знако́мства; to give smb. the ~ direct разнакоми́ться с кем-л.; 8) оскорбле́ние, вы́пад; 9) ре́заная пода́ча мяча́ (*в те́ннисе*); 10) отре́зок; a short ~ коро́ткий, кратча́йший путь; ◇ a ~ above *разг.* сто очко́в вперёд даст (*о челове́ке*); a ~ and thrust оживлённый спор.

cut II *v* (*past, p. p.* cut) 1) ре́зать, разреза́ть; среза́ть, отреза́ть; it ~s him to the heart (*или* to the quick) э́то задева́ет его́ за живо́е; 2) ра́нить (*ножо́м, са́блей*); наноси́ть ре́заную ра́ну (*кому́-л. — at*); 3) причиня́ть ре́жущую боль; 4) жать, коси́ть; убира́ть урожа́й; среза́ть (*цветы*); 5) стричь (*во́лосы, но́гти*); 6) кройть; 7) руби́ть, вали́ть (*лес*); 8) высека́ть (*из ка́мня*); выреза́ть, ре́зать (*по де́реву*); шлифова́ть, грани́ть (*драгоце́нные ка́мни*); 9) снижа́ть (*це́ны, нало́ги*); сокраща́ть (*шта́ты*); 10) пересека́ться (*о ли́ниях, доро́гах*); 11) снима́ть (*ка́рты*); 12) разнакоми́ться с кем-л., де́лать вид, что не замеча́ешь кого́-л.; to ~ smb. dead игнори́ровать кого́-л.; 13) *разг.* смота́ться, удра́ть; to ~ and run бы́стро удира́ть; □ to ~ across пересека́ть (*у́лицу и т. п.*); to ~ away а) среза́ть; обреза́ть; б) *разг.* удира́ть; to ~ down а) сокраща́ть (*расхо́ды*); б) руби́ть (*дере́вья*); to ~ in а) вме́шиваться (*в разгово́р, дела́*); вступа́ть в игру́ (*карто́чную*); вкли́ниваться (*между двумя́ маши́нами на у́лице*); б) *эл.* включа́ть; to ~ off а) отреза́ть; б) свести́ в моги́лу; в) перере́зать, разъедини́ть; прерва́ть (*связь*); to be ~ off *воен.* быть отре́занным; г): to ~ off with a shilling лиши́ть насле́дства; to ~ out а) выреза́ть; кройть; to be ~ out for the job быть сло́вно со́зданным для да́нной рабо́ты; б) отреза́ть су́дно от бе́рега; в) *карт.* вы́йти из игры́; to ~ over *разг.* бы́стро пройти́, пробежа́ть (*како́е-л. простра́нство*); to ~ under продава́ть деше́вле (*других фирм*); to ~ up разруба́ть, разреза́ть; ◇ to ~ and come again есть мно́го и с аппети́том; to ~ up rough *разг.* возмуща́ться.

cut-away ['kʌtəweɪ] *n* визи́тка.

cute [kjuːt] *a разг.* 1) у́мный; остроу́мный; нахо́дчивый; 2) *амер.* ми́лый, прия́тный.

cutlet ['kʌtlɪt] *n* отбивна́я котле́та; veal ~ теля́чья отбивна́я.

cut-out ['kʌtaut] *n* 1) *эл.* автомати́ческий выключа́тель; предохрани́тель; 2) очерта́ние, ко́нтур.

cutpurse ['kʌtpəːs] *n* вор-карма́нник.

cutter[1] ['kʌtə] *n* ка́тер.

cutter[2] *n* 1) ре́зчик (*по де́реву, ка́мню*); 2) закро́йщик; 3) фре́зер; 4) забо́йщик; 5) вру́бовая маши́на.

cut-throat ['kʌtθrout] *n* 1) уби́йца, головоре́з; 2) *attr* ожесточённый.

cutting I ['kʌtɪŋ] *n* 1) вы́резка (*из газе́ты, журна́ла*); press ~ газе́тная вы́резка; 2) вы́емка, транше́я; 3) *pl* обре́зки; опи́лки; 4) сниже́ние, уменьше́ние (*цен и т. п.*); 5) *бот.* черено́к.

cutting II *a* 1) ре́зкий, о́стрый; 2) прони́зывающий (*о ве́тре*).

cuttle-fish ['kʌtlfɪʃ] *n зоол.* карака́тица.

cutty ['kʌtɪ] *n* пе́нковая тру́бка.

cutwater ['kʌtˌwɔːtə] *n мор.* волноре́з.

cyanic [saɪ'ænɪk] *a* 1) голубо́й; 2) *хим.* циа́новый.

cyanide ['saɪənaɪd] *n хим.* соль циа́нистой кислоты́, циани́д.

cyanogen [saɪ'ænədʒɪn] *n хим.* 1) циа́н; 2) *attr* циа́новый.

cybernetics [ˌsaɪbəˈnetɪks] *n* киберне́тика.

cyclamen ['sɪkləmən] *n бот.* цикламе́н, альпи́йская фиа́лка.

cycle I ['saɪkl] *n* 1) цикл; зако́нченный круг разви́тия; пери́од; 2) *разг.* велосипе́д.

cycle II *v* 1) соверша́ть цикл разви́тия; повторя́ться цикли́чески; 2) е́здить на велосипе́де.

cycler ['saɪklə] *амер. см.* cyclist.

cyclic ['saɪklɪk] *a* 1) цикли́ческий; 2) *хим.* цикли́чный.

cyclical ['saɪklɪkəl] *см.* cyclic.

cyclist ['saɪklɪst] *n* велосипеди́ст.

cyclone ['saɪkloun] *n* цикло́н.

cyclopaedia [ˌsaɪkləˈpiːdjə] *n* энциклопе́дия.

cyclopaedic [ˌsaɪkləˈpiːdɪk] *a* энциклопеди́ческий.

cyclotron ['saɪklətrɔn] *n физ.* циклотро́н.

cygnet ['sɪgnɪt] *n* молодо́й ле́бедь.

cylinder ['sɪlɪndə] *n* 1) *мат., тех.* цили́ндр; 2) *тех.* вал, бараба́н; 3) газобалло́н.

cylindrical [sɪ'lɪndrɪkəl] *a* цилиндри́ческий.

cymbals ['sɪmbəlz] *n pl муз.* таре́лки.

Cymric ['kɪmrɪk] *a* уэ́льский, ки́мрский.

cynic ['sɪnɪk] *n* ци́ник.

cynical ['sɪnɪkəl] *a* цини́чный; непристо́йный.

cynicism ['sɪnɪsɪzəm] *n* цини́зм.

cynosure ['sɪnəzjuə] *n* 1) созве́здие Ма́лой Медве́дицы; 2) Поля́рная звезда́; *перен.* путево́дная звезда́.

cypher I, II ['saɪfə] *см.* cipher I, II.

cypress ['saɪprɪs] *n бот.* кипари́с.

Cyprian I ['sɪprɪən] *n* уроже́нец Ки́пра, киприо́т.

Cyprian II *a* ки́прский.

Cypriote ['sɪprɪout] *n* киприо́т.

Cyrillic [sɪ'rɪlɪk] *a*: ~ alphabet кири́ллица (*древнеславя́нский алфави́т*).

czar [zɑː] *n* царь.

Czech I [tʃek] *n* 1) чех; че́шка; the ~s че́хи; 2) че́шский язы́к.

Czech II *a* че́шский.

Czechoslovak I [ˌtʃekouˈslouvæk] *n* жи́тель Чехослова́кии.

Czechoslovak II *a* чехослова́цкий.

Czechoslovakian [ˌtʃekouslouˈvækjən] *см.* Czechoslovak II.

D

D, d [diː] *n* 1) 4-я буква англ. алфавита; 2) *муз.* нота ре.

'd [-d] *разг. сокр. от* had, should, would *после* I, you, he *и т. д.*

da [dɑ] *см.* dad.

dab¹ I [dæb] *n* 1) лёгкое прикосновение, лёгкий удар; 2) мазок; пятно.

dab¹ II *v* 1) слегка прикасаться; прикладывать что-л.; ударять, тыкать (*at*); клевать; 2) намазывать; 3) покрывать краской, делать лёгкие мазки.

dab² *n* камбала (*рыба*).

dab³ *n разг.* знаток, дока.

dabble ['dæbl] *v* 1) смачивать; 2) брызгать(ся), плескать(ся); 3) *разг.* заниматься чем-л. поверхностно, по-любительски.

dabbler ['dæblə] *n* любитель, дилетант.

dabby ['dæbɪ] *a* влажный, сырой.

dabster ['dæbstə] *n* знаток, специалист.

dace [deɪs] *n* елец (*рыба*).

dachshund ['dækshund] *n* такса (*собака*).

dactyl ['dæktɪl] *n лит.* дактиль.

dactylic I [dæk'tɪlɪk] *n обыкн. pl* дактилический стих.

dactylic II *a* дактилический.

dactylogram [dæk'tɪləgræm] *n* отпечаток пальца.

dactylography [,dæktɪ'lɔgrəfɪ] *n* дактилоскопия.

dad [dæd] *n разг.* папа, отец.

daddy ['dædɪ] *см.* dad.

dado ['deɪdou] *n* 1) *архит.* пьедестал; 2) панель.

daemon ['diːmən] *см.* demon.

daemonic [diː'mɔnɪk] *см.* demonic.

daffodil ['dæfədɪl] *n* 1) бледно-жёлтый нарцисс; 2) бледно-жёлтый цвет.

daft [dɑːft] *a* безумный; безрассудный; to go ~ потерять рассудок.

dag [dæg] *n* клок свалявшейся шерсти.

dagger I ['dægə] *n* 1) кинжал; at ~s drawn на ножах; 2) *полигр.* крестик; ◊ to look ~s бросать злобные взгляды; to speak ~s говорить озлобленно.

dagger II *v* 1) пронзать кинжалом; 2) *полигр.* отмечать крестиком.

daggle ['dægl] *v* волочить, тащить.

dago ['deɪgou] *n амер. презр.* даго (*прозвище итальянца, испанца, португальца*).

dahlia ['deɪljə] *n* георгин.

Dail Eireann [daɪl'ɛərən] *n* нижняя палата парламента Ирландской республики.

daily I ['deɪlɪ] *n* 1) ежедневная газета; 2) *разг.* приходящая работница.

daily II *a* ежедневный; суточный.

daily III *adv* ежедневно.

daintiness ['deɪntɪnɪs] *n* изысканность, утончённость.

dainty I ['deɪntɪ] *n* лакомство, деликатес.

dainty II *a* 1) лакомый; 2) изысканный; утончённый; 3) разборчивый.

dairy ['dɛərɪ] *n* 1) маслобойня; сыроварня; 2) молочная; 3) *см.* dairy-farm.

dairy-farm ['dɛərɪfɑːm] *n* молочная ферма.

dairying ['dɛərɪŋ] *n* молочное хозяйство.

dairymaid ['dɛərɪmeɪd] *n* 1) работница молочной фермы; 2) молочница.

dairyman ['dɛərɪmən] *n* 1) продавец молочных продуктов; 2) владелец или работник молочной фермы.

dais ['deɪɪs] *n* возвышение; помост; кафедра.

daisy ['deɪzɪ] *n* 1) маргаритка; 2) *сленг* что-л. первосортное.

dale [deɪl] *n поэт.* дол, долина; up hill and down ~ по горам и долам; ◊ to curse up hill and down ~ ≅ ругать на чём свет стоит.

dalesman ['deɪlzmən] *n* житель долин (*на севере Англии*).

dalliance ['dælɪəns] *n* 1) развлечение; шалость; 2) флирт; 3) безделье; 4) несерьёзное отношение к чему-л.

dally ['dælɪ] *v* 1) заниматься пустяками; болтаться без дела; 2) развлекаться; 3) кокетничать; флиртовать; □ to ~ away терять время; упускать возможность; to ~ off уклоняться от.

dam I [dæm] *n* дамба, плотина, запруда.

dam II *v* 1) запруживать воду (*часто* to ~ up); 2) препятствовать; сдерживать (*чувства и т. п.*); □ to ~ out отвести воду плотиной.

damage I ['dæmɪdʒ] *n* 1) вред, повреждение; 2) убыток, ущерб; 3) *pl юр.* компенсация за убытки; 4) *сленг* стоимость; what's the ~? сколько это стоит?

damage II *v* 1) вредить, портить; повреждать; 2) наносить ущерб, убыток; 3) дискредитировать; 4) ушибить.

damageable ['dæmɪdʒəbl] *a* легко портящийся.

damask I ['dæməsk] *n* 1) камчатная *или* дамастная ткань; 2) дамасская сталь; булат; 3) алый цвет.

damask II *a* 1) камчатный, дамастный; 2) из дамасской стали; 3) алый.

damask III *v* 1) ткать с узорами; 2) насекать сталь.

dame [deɪm] *n* дама; *шутл.* пожилая женщина.

damn I [dæm] *n* 1) проклятие; 2) ругательство; 3): not to care a ~ совершенно не интересоваться, «наплевать»; not worth a ~ ничего не стоит.

damn II *v* 1) проклинать; I'll be ~ed if будь я проклят, если; ~ it all! чёрт побери!; тьфу, пропасть!; 2) ругаться; 3) осуждать; 4) *разг.* провалить (*пьесу*).

damnable ['dæmnəbl] *a* 1) заслуживающий осуждения; 2) *разг.* отвратительный; ужасный.

damnably ['dæmnəblɪ] *adv* 1) отвратительно; 2) *разг.* ужасно, чертовски.

damnation I [dæm'neɪʃən] *n* 1) проклятие; may ~ take it! будь проклято!; 2) осуждение; 3) *разг.* освистание (*пьесы*).

damnation II *int* проклятие!

damnatory ['dæmnətərɪ] *a* осуждающий.

damned I [dæmd] *a* 1) проклятый; 2) ужасный, адский, дьявольский.

damned II *adv* ужасно, чертовски; it is ~ hot чертовски жарко.

damning I ['dæmɪŋ] *n* ругательство.

damning II *a* вызывающий осуждение.

damp I [dæmp] *n* 1) сырость, влажность; 2) уныние, подавленность; to cast a ~ over омрачить; 3) рудничный газ; 4) *сленг* выпивка.

damp II *a* сырой, влажный.

damp III *v* 1) смачивать, увлажнять; 2) обескураживать; угнетать, подавлять; 3) заглушать; ослаблять, тушить; 4) *тех.* тормозить, демпфировать.

dampen ['dæmpən] *v* 1) *см.* damp III; 2) отсыревать.

damper ['dæmpə] *n* 1) кто-л. *или* что-л., действующее угнетающе; 2) *тех.* глушитель; регулятор тяги; вьюшка (*в печи*); 3) *тех.* увлажнитель.

damping ['dæmpɪŋ] *n* 1) увлажнение; 2) *тех.* заглушение; торможение; 3) *радио* затухание.

dampish ['dæmpɪʃ] *a* сыроватый.

damp-proof ['dæmppru:f] *a* влагонепроницаемый.

dampy ['dæmpɪ] *a* сырой, влажный.

damsel ['dæmzəl] *n уст.* девица.

damson ['dæmzən] *n* тернослив, мелкая чёрная слива.

dance I [dɑ:ns] *n* танец; country ~ народный танец; 2) тур (*танца*); 3) танцы, танцевальный вечер; to give a ~ приглашать на танцевальный вечер; ◇ to lead smb. a pretty ~ *разг.* водить кого-л. за нос, заставить помучиться.

dance II *v* 1) танцевать, плясать; 2) прыгать, скакать; кружиться (*о листьях*); скользить (*о лучах*); ◇ to ~ to smb.'s tune (*или* pipe) плясать под чью-л. дудку; to ~ upon nothing быть повешенным.

dancer ['dɑ:nsə] *n* 1) танцующий; 2) танцор; танцовщица; танцовщик; ◇ merry ~s северное сияние.

dancing I ['dɑ:nsɪŋ] *n* танцы; пляска.

dancing II *a* танцевальный.

dandelion ['dændɪlaɪən] *n* одуванчик; Russian ~ кок-сагыз.

dander ['dændə] *n разг.* гнев, раздражение, негодование; to get one's ~ up рассердить(ся); выйти *или* вывести из терпения.

dandle ['dændl] *v* 1) качать (ребёнка) на руках *или* на коленях; 2) ласкать, баловать.

dandruff ['dændrəf] *v* перхоть.

dandy I ['dændɪ] *n* 1) щёголь, денди; 2) *мор.* шлюп с выносной бизанью; 3) двухколёсная телёжка.

dandy II *a* 1) щегольской, нарядный; 2) *разг.* великолепный.

dandy-brush ['dændɪbrʌʃ] *n* скребница.

dandyism ['dændɪɪzəm] *n* щегольство, дендизм.

Dane[1] [deɪn] *n* датчанин; датчанка; the ~s датчане.

Dane[2] *n* датский дог.

danger ['deɪndʒə] *n* 1) опасность; in ~ of one's life с опасностью для жизни; out of ~ вне опасности; to stand in ~ of one's life подвергать свою жизнь опасности; 2) угроза; a ~ to peace угроза миру.

dangerous ['deɪndʒrəs] *a* опасный; угрожающий; рискованный.

danger-signal ['deɪndʒə,sɪgnl] *n* 1) сигнал опасности; 2) *ж.-д.* сигнал «путь закрыт».

dangle ['dæŋgl] *v* 1) свисать, болтаться; 2) подвешивать; 3) соблазнять, дразнить; □ to ~ about, to ~ after, to ~ round волочиться за кем-л.

dangler ['dæŋglə] *n* 1) бездельник; 2) волокита.

Danish I ['deɪnɪʃ] *n* 1) датский язык; 2): the ~ (*употр. как pl*) датчане.

Danish II *a* датский.

dank [dæŋk] *a* сырой, влажный.

dap I [dæp] *n* 1) подпрыгивание мяча; 2) зазубрина.

dap II *v* 1) удить рыбу; 2) (слегка) погружать; 3) ударять(ся) о землю; подпрыгивать (*о мяче*).

dapper ['dæpə] *a* 1) нарядно одетый; 2) подвижной, живой.

dapple I ['dæpl] *a* пёстрый, пятнистый; в яблоках (*о лошади*).

dapple II *v* покрывать(ся) пятнами.

dapple-grey ['dæpl'greɪ] *a* серый в яблоках (*о коне*).

dare [deə] *v* (*past* dared, durst; *p. p.* dared; *3-е л. ед. ч. наст. вр. тж.* dare) 1) сметь; осмеливаться, отваживаться; I ~ say смею сказать, полагаю; пожалуй; 2) рисковать; 3) вызывать (*на — to*); бросать вызов.

dare-devil I ['deə,devl] *n* сорвиголова.

dare-devil II *a* безрассудный, отчаянный.

daring I ['deərɪŋ] *n* смелость; отвага.

daring II *a* смелый, отважный; дерзкий.

dark I [dɑ:k] *n* 1) тьма, темнота; at ~ в темноте, ночью; in the ~ в темноте; before (after) ~ до (после) наступления темноты; 2) неизвестность, неведение; to keep smb. in the ~ держать кого-л. в неведении; to be in the ~ about smth. а) не знать о чём-л.; б) не совсем понимать что-л.; 3) невежество; 4) *жив.* тень; the lights and ~s of a picture свет и тени в картине.

dark II *a* 1) тёмный; to get (*или* to grow) ~ темнеть; 2) смуглый; темноволосый; 3) непонятный, неясный; 4) тайный, секретный; to keep smth. ~ держать что-л. в секрете; to keep ~ скрываться; 5) невежественный, некультурный; 6) печальный; мрачный; 7) дурной, нечистый.

darken ['dɑ:kən] *v* 1) затемнять; делать тёмным; 2) становиться тёмным; мрачнеть; темнеть, меркнуть; 3) омрачать; 4) ослеплять.

darkish ['dɑ:kɪʃ] *a* темноватый.

darkle ['dɑ:kl] *v* 1) скрываться; темнеть, меркнуть; 2) хмуриться.

darkling I ['dɑ:klɪŋ] *a* темнеющий.

darkling II *adv* во тьме, в темноте.

darkly ['dɑ:klɪ] *adv* 1) мрачно; 2) непонятно, неясно; смутно.

darkness ['dɑ:knɪs] *n* тьма, темнота, мрак.

darkroom ['dɑ:k'rum] *n фото* камера-обскура, тёмная комната.

darksome ['dɑ:ksəm] *a поэт.* тёмный, мрачный; хмурый.

darling I ['dɑ:lɪŋ] *n* 1) любимый, -ая; my ~! дорогой мой!, дорогая моя!; голубчик!; 2) любимец; the ~ of fortune баловень судьбы.

darling II *a* любимый, дорогой; милый.

darn[1] I [dɑ:n] *n* 1) штопка; 2) заштопанное место.

darn[1] II *v* штопать.

darn[2] *v эвф.* проклинать, ругать.

darnel ['dɑ:nl] *n* плевел, сорная трава.

darning ['dɑ:nɪŋ] *n* штопанье.

dart I [dɑ:t] *n* 1) метательное копьё, дротик; стрела; 2) метание (*копья и т. п.*); 3) стремительное движение; 4) жало.

dart II *v* 1) метать (*стрелы, взгляды*); 2) устремля́ться, лете́ть стрело́й; □ to ~ **down** ри́нуться вниз; *ав.* пики́ровать.

darting ['dɑːtɪŋ] *a* бы́стрый, стреми́тельный.

dartingly ['dɑːtɪŋlɪ] *adv* бы́стро, стрело́й.

Darwinism ['dɑːwɪnɪzəm] *n* дарвини́зм.

dash I [dæʃ] *n* 1) стреми́тельный на́тиск, напо́р; *спорт.* рыво́к, бросо́к; to make a ~ бро́ситься, рвану́ться; 2) уда́р, взмах; at one ~ с одного́ ра́за; 3) мазо́к; штрих; ро́счерк; 4) тире́; 5) (вс)плеск; 6) при́месь чего́-л.; a ~ of purple пурпу́рный отте́нок; 7) эне́ргия; 8) рисо́вка; to cut a ~ рисова́ться, ва́жничать.

dash II *v* 1) отбро́сить, оттолкну́ть, швырну́ть; 2) разбива́ть(ся), разруша́ть(ся) (*тж.* *перен.*); 3) устреми́ться, ри́нуться; to ~ against (*или* upon) smth. наскочи́ть, натолкну́ться на что-л.; 4) бры́згать, плеска́ть; 5) наброса́ть, бы́стро написа́ть (*тж.* to ~ off); 6) подме́шивать; 7) подчёркивать; 8) смуща́ть, обескура́живать; 9) *сленг* проклина́ть.

dash-board ['dæʃbɔːd] *n* 1) крыло́ (*экипа́жа*); 2) *ав., авто* прибо́рная доска́, щито́к.

dasher ['dæʃə] *n* 1) челове́к, лю́бящий порисова́ться, пова́жничать; 2) *амер.* крыло́ (*экипа́жа*).

dashing ['dæʃɪŋ] *a* 1) стреми́тельный; 2) сме́лый, лихо́й; 3) франтова́тый.

dastard ['dæstəd] *n* трус, трусли́вый негодя́й.

dastardly ['dæstədlɪ] *a* трусли́вый; по́длый.

data ['deɪtə] *n pl* 1) *см.* datum; 2) да́нные; све́дения; фа́кты; *амер.* но́вости.

datable ['deɪtəbl] *a* поддаю́щийся дати́рованию.

date[1] I [deɪt] *n* 1) да́та; 2) пери́од, срок; out of ~ устаре́лый; up to ~ (вполне́) совреме́нный, нове́йший; 3) *амер. разг.* свида́ние.

date[1] II *v* 1) дати́ровать; 2) относи́ть(ся) к (*сро́ку, эпо́хе и т. п.*); 3) вести́ исчисле́ние (*от како́й-л. да́ты*).

date[2] *n* 1) фи́ник; 2) фи́никовая па́льма.

dateless ['deɪtlɪs] *a* 1) недати́рованный; 2) незапа́мятный; 3) *амер. разг.* неприглашённый.

date-palm ['deɪtpɑːm] *n* фи́никовая па́льма.

dative I ['deɪtɪv] *n грам.* да́тельный паде́ж.

dative II *a грам* да́тельный.

datum ['deɪtəm] *n* (*pl* data) да́нная величина́.

daub I [dɔːb] *n* 1) штукату́рка, обма́зка; 2) пачкотня́; 3) мазня́, неуме́лый рису́нок.

daub II *v* 1) обма́зывать, ма́зать (*гли́ной и т. п.*); 2) па́чкать; 3) малева́ть; пло́хо рисова́ть.

dauber ['dɔːbə] *n* плохо́й, неуме́лый худо́жник, мази́лка.

daubster ['dɔːbstə] *см.* dauber.

dauby ['dɔːbɪ] *a* 1) пло́хо, неуме́ло напи́санный (*о карти́не, рису́нке*); 2) кле́йкий, ли́пкий.

daughter ['dɔːtə] *n* 1) дочь; 2) *attr.* доче́рний.

daughter-in-law ['dɔːtərɪnlɔː] *n* (*pl* daughters-in-law) жена́ сы́на, неве́стка.

daughterly ['dɔːtəlɪ] *a* доче́рний.

daunt [dɔːnt] *v* запу́гивать; обескура́живать; nothing ~ed ничу́ть не смуща́ясь.

dauntless ['dɔːntlɪs] *a* неустраши́мый; сто́йкий.

dauphin ['dɔːfɪn] *n ист.* дофи́н.

davenport ['dævnpɔːt] *n* 1) небольшо́й пи́сьменный стол со мно́жеством я́щиков; 2) *амер.* софа́; дива́н-крова́ть.

davit ['dævɪt] *n мор.* шлюпба́лка.

davy ['deɪvɪ] *n сленг:* to take one's ~ кля́сться в том, что.

daw [dɔː] *n* га́лка.

dawdle I ['dɔːdl] *n* безде́льник.

dawdle II *v* безде́льничать; да́ром теря́ть вре́мя (*ча́сто* to ~ away).

dawdler ['dɔːdlə] *n* безде́льник, ло́дырь.

dawn I [dɔːn] *n* 1) рассве́т, у́тренняя заря́; about ~ пе́ред рассве́том, в предрассве́тных су́мерках; at ~ на рассве́те, на заре́; 2) нача́ло, зарожде́ние.

dawn II *v* 1) (рас)света́ть; 2) пока́зываться, появля́ться; наступа́ть; 3) станови́ться я́сным; it has ~ed upon him его́ осени́ло.

day [deɪ] *n* 1) день; су́тки; at ~ на рассве́те; before ~ до рассве́та; by ~ днём; every ~ ка́ждый день; all (the) ~ long весь день напролёт; by the ~ подённо; ~ about, every other ~ че́рез день; the ~ after tomorrow послеза́втра; the ~ before накану́не; the ~ before yesterday позавчера́; good ~ ! здра́вствуйте!; до свида́ния!; ~ in, ~ out изо дня в день; ~ off выходно́й день; polling ~ день вы́боров; first ~ воскресе́нье; one's natal ~ день рожде́ния; red-letter ~ пра́здничный, па́мятный день; banner ~, high ~ пра́здничный день; one ~ одна́жды; the other ~ неда́вно, на дня́х; some ~ когда́-нибудь; one fine ~ в оди́н прекра́сный день; from ~ to ~ со дня на́ день; to a ~ день в день; by ~, ~ after ~ день за днём; one of these ~s в ближа́йшие дни, на дня́х; this many a ~ мно́го дней тому́ наза́д, давно́; this ~ fortnight (week) че́рез две неде́ли (неде́лю); to name the ~ назна́чить день сва́дьбы; 2) вре́мя, пери́од; in these latter ~s, at the present ~ в на́ше вре́мя, тепе́рь; in the ~s of old в былы́е дни, времена́; in ~s to come в бу́дущем; one's palmy ~s пери́од расцве́та, крупне́йшего успе́ха; to close (*или* to end) one's ~s сконча́ться; 3) реша́ющий день; Victory Day День Побе́ды; to carry (*или* to win) the ~ одержа́ть побе́ду; to lose the ~ проигра́ть сраже́ние; Independence Day День незави́симости США; Inauguration Day день вступле́ния в до́лжность но́вого президе́нта США; 4) *геол.* ближа́йший к земно́й пове́рхности пласт; 5) *attr* дневно́й; ◊ the ~ after (before) the fair сли́шком по́здно (ра́но); to call it a ~ счита́ть де́ло сде́ланным; on one's ~ в уда́ре.

day-boarder ['deɪˌbɔːdə] *n шк.* полупансионе́р.

day-boy ['deɪbɔɪ] *n шк.* приходя́щий учени́к.

daybreak ['deɪbreɪk] *n* рассве́т; at ~ на рассве́те.

day-dream I ['deɪdriːm] *n* 1) грёзы, мечты́; 2) мечта́тельность.

day-dream II *v* грези́ть (наяву́).

day-dreamer ['deɪˌdriːmə] *n* мечта́тель, фантазёр.

day-girl ['deɪgɜːl] *n шк.* приходя́щая учени́ца.

day-labour ['deɪˌleɪbə] *n* подённая рабо́та.

day-labourer ['deɪˌleɪbərə] *n* подёнщик.

daylight ['deɪlaɪt] *n* 1) дневно́й свет; есте́ственное освеще́ние; to burn ~ а) зажига́ть свет днём; б) зря тра́тить вре́мя, си́лы; 2) рассве́т; 3) гла́сность, публи́чность; to let ~ into а) преда́ть гла́сности; б) *сленг* уби́ть, застрели́ть.

daylight-saving ['deɪlaɪtˌseɪvɪŋ] *n* перево́д ле́том часово́й стре́лки на час вперёд.

day-long I ['deɪlɔŋ] *a* для́щийся це́лый день.

day-long II *adv* весь день, день-деньско́й.

day-nursery ['deɪˌnɜːsrɪ] *n* дневны́е де́тские я́сли.

day-school ['deɪskuːl] *n* 1) шко́ла без пансио́на; 2) шко́ла с дневны́ми часа́ми заня́тий.

day-spring ['deɪsprɪŋ] *n поэт.* рассве́т, заря́.

day-star ['deɪstɑː] *n* у́тренняя звезда́.

day-time ['deɪtaɪm] *n* день, дневно́е вре́мя; in the ~ днём.

day-to-day ['deɪtə'deɪ] *a* повседне́вный, ежедне́вный, каждодне́вный.

daywork ['deɪwɜːk] *n* 1) подённая рабо́та; 2) *горн.* рабо́та на пове́рхности земли́.

daze I [deɪz] *n* изумле́ние; in a ~ изумлённо, с изумле́нием.

daze II *v* изумля́ть, ошеломля́ть.

dazzle I ['dæzl] *n* ослепи́тельный блеск.

dazzle II *v* ослепля́ть; поража́ть.

d — d I, II, [dæmd] *эвф. сокр. см.* damned I, II.

de- [dɪ-, de-] *pref* указывает на: 1) *лишение кого-л. чего-л. или отделение одного предмета от другого:* to dethrone лиши́ть тро́на, све́ргнуть; 2) *значение, обратное данному в простом слове:* merit заслу́га, demerit недоста́ток, дефе́кт; 3) *снижение качества, уменьшение количества:* to degrade дегради́ровать; to deduct вычита́ть.

deacon I ['diːkən] *n* дья́кон.

deacon II *v амер.* чита́ть псалмы́.

dead I [ded] *a* 1) мёртвый; 2) глухо́й; загло́хший; поту́хший; 3) неодушевлённый, неживо́й; 4) сухо́й, увя́дший (*о листьях, цветах и т. п.*); 5) безжи́зненный, вя́лый; 6) онеме́вший (*о руке, ноге, пальцах*); 7) по́лный, соверше́нный; ~ certainty по́лная уве́ренность; in ~ earnest соверше́нно серьёзно; 8) недоста́вленный (*о письме, открытке*); 9) *горн.* пусто́й; ◊ ~ as a doornail (вне вся́кого сомне́ния) мёртвый; ~ above the ears, ~ from the neck up *амер. сленг* глу́пый, тупо́й; ~ and gone давно́ проше́дший; to be ~ with hunger умира́ть с го́лоду.

dead II *n* 1): the ~ (*употр. как pl*) уме́ршие, поко́йники; 2): the ~ of night глуха́я ночь, глубо́кая ночь; ◊ on the ~ *амер. сленг* реши́тельно.

dead III *adv* соверше́нно, по́лностью; ~ broke соверше́нно разорённый; ~ against a) реши́тельно про́тив; б) пря́мо в лицо́ (*о ветре*); ~ drunk мертве́цки пья́ный; ~ tired сме́ртельно уста́лый.

dead-alive ['dedə'laɪv] *a* 1) безжи́зненный; 2) ску́чный, уны́лый, моното́нный.

dead-beat ['ded'biːt] *a* 1) разби́тый, сме́ртельно уста́лый; 2) *тех.* апериоди́ческий (*об измери́тельном прибо́ре*); успоко́енный (*о магни́тной стре́лке*).

deaden ['dedn] *v* 1) лиша́ть(ся) жи́вости, сил, эне́ргии, бле́ска; 2) де́лать(ся) нечувстви́тельным; 3) заглуша́ть, ослабля́ть.

deadfall ['dedfɔːl] *n амер.* западня́, капка́н.

deadhead ['dedhed] *n* беспла́тный посети́тель теа́тра; безбиле́тный пассажи́р, за́яц.

dead-house ['dedhaus] *n* мертве́цкая, морг.

dead-light ['dedlaɪt] *n* глухо́й иллюмина́тор, глухо́е окно́ в кры́ше.

dead-line ['dedlaɪn] *n* 1) черта́, кото́рую нельзя́ переступи́ть; 2) кра́йний срок (*чего-л.*).

deadlock ['dedlɔk] *n* мёртвая то́чка; тупи́к, безвы́ходное положе́ние.

deadly I ['dedlɪ] *a* 1) смерте́льный; смерто-

но́сный; 2) сме́ртный; 3) неумоли́мый, беспоща́дный; 4) *разг.* ужа́сный, стра́шный.

deadly II *adv* 1) смерте́льно; 2) чрезвыча́йно, ужа́сно.

deadman ['dedmæn] *n стр.* (а́нкерный) столб, сва́я (*врытые в землю*).

dead-nettle ['ded'netl] *n* глуха́я крапи́ва.

dead-office ['ded,ɔfɪs] *n* панихи́да.

dead-pan ['ded'pæn] *n* 1) невозмути́мый вид; невозмути́мость; бесстра́стное лицо́; 2) *attr* невозмути́мый.

dead-water ['ded,wɔːtə] *n* 1) стоя́чая вода́; 2) *мор.* кильва́тер.

dead-wind ['ded'wɪnd] *n* встре́чный ве́тер.

deaf I [def] *a* глухо́й; *перен. тж.* не жела́ющий слу́шать; ~ of an ear глухо́й на одно́ у́хо; ◊ ~ as an adder; ~ as a post ≅ глуха́я тете́ря.

deaf II *n*: the ~ (*употр. как pl*) глухи́е.

deaf-and-dumb ['defən'dʌm] *a* глухонемо́й.

deafen ['defn] *v* 1) оглуша́ть; 2) заглуша́ть (*звук*); 3) де́лать звуконепроница́емым.

deafening ['defnɪŋ] *a* 1) оглуши́тельный; 2) заглуша́ющий.

deaf-mute ['def'mjuːt] *n* глухонемо́й.

deafness ['defnɪs] *n* глухота́.

deal[1] I [diːl] *n* 1) коли́чество; до́ля; a great (*или* a good) ~ of мно́го, значи́тельное коли́чество; a great ~ *со сравн. ст. наречий означает* значи́тельно, гора́здо: a great ~ better гора́здо лу́чше; 2) *карт.* сда́ча.

deal[1] II *v* (*past, p. p.* dealt) 1) раздава́ть, распределя́ть (*тж.* to ~ out); 2) *карт.* сдава́ть.

deal[2] I *n разг.* 1) сде́лка; square ~ че́стная сде́лка; 2) сго́вор; a criminal ~ престу́пный сго́вор; ◊ New Deal «но́вый курс» (*система экономи́ческих мероприя́тий президе́нта Ф. Д. Ру́звельта*).

deal[2] II *v* (*past, p. p.* dealt) 1) торгова́ть (*чем-л.—in; с кем-л.—with*); име́ть де́ло (*с кем-л.—with*); 2) боро́ться с чем-л., стара́ться преодоле́ть что-л. (*with*); 3) рассма́тривать, реша́ть (*вопрос, проблему; with*); 4) поступа́ть, вести́ себя́; to ~ smb. cruelly поступи́ть, обойти́сь с кем-л. жесто́ко.

deal[3] I *n* ело́вая *или* сосно́вая доска́.

deal[3] II *a* сосно́вый.

dealer ['diːlə] *n* 1) торго́вец; retail ~ ро́зничный торго́вец; ~ in old clothes старьёвщик; 2) сдаю́щий ка́рты; 3): ~ in politics челове́к, занима́ющийся поли́тикой; ◊ a plain ~ прямо́й, открове́нный челове́к.

dealing ['diːlɪŋ] *n* 1) поведе́ние; 2) *pl* обще́ние, прия́тельские отноше́ния; 3) *pl* торго́вые дела́.

dealt[1] [delt] *past, p. p. см.* deal[1] II.

dealt[2] *past, p. p. см.* deal[2] II.

dean[1] [diːn] *n* 1) дека́н (*факультета*); 2) старшина́ дипломати́ческого ко́рпуса; 3) ста́рший свяще́нник; настоя́тель собо́ра.

dean[2] *n* доли́на.

deanery ['diːnərɪ] *n* 1) декана́т; 2) дека́нство; 3) дом свяще́нника; 4) церко́вный о́круг.

dear I [dɪə] *n* 1) возлю́бленный, -ая; ми́лый, -ая; 2) *разг.* пре́лесть.

dear II *a* 1) дорого́й, ми́лый; (*в обраще́нии тж.*) любе́зный, любе́знейший; Dear Sir ми́лостивый госуда́рь; 2) дорого́й, дорогосто́ящий.

dear III *adv* до́рого.

dear IV *int*: ~, ~!, oh ~!, ~ me! *выражает удивле́ние, сожале́ние, сочу́вствие, нетерпе́ние и т. п.*

. **dearly** ['dɪəlɪ] *adv* 1) о́чень; he would ~ love to он бы о́чень хоте́л *(сде́лать что-л.)*; 2) до́рого; *перен. тж.* дорого́й цено́й; 3) не́жно; to love ~ не́жно люби́ть.

dearness ['dɪənɪs] *n* дороговизна́.

dearth [dɜ:θ] *n* недоста́ток, ску́дость; недоста́ток пищевы́х проду́ктов; ~ of labour недоста́ток рабо́чей си́лы.

deary ['dɪərɪ] *n* дорого́й, дорога́я, ми́лочка *(обыкн. как обраще́ние)*.

death [deθ] *n* 1) смерть; *перен.* ги́бель, прекраще́ние, коне́ц; civil ~ гражда́нская смерть; natural (violent) ~ есте́ственная (наси́льственная) смерть; to be the ~ of smb. быть вино́вником чье́й-л. сме́рти, ги́бели; *разг.* умори́ть кого́-л.; at ~'s door при́ сме́рти, на поро́ге сме́рти; to ~ на́смерть, сме́ртельно; tired to ~ сме́ртельно уста́вший; to put to ~ казни́ть; 2) *attr* сме́ртный; ◊ to be ~ on *сленг* быть иску́сным в чём-л.

death-bed ['deθbed] *n* сме́ртное ло́же.

deathbell ['deθbel] *n* похоро́нный звон.

death-blow ['deθblou] *n* сме́ртельный уда́р, роково́й уда́р.

death-cup ['deθkʌp] *n* бле́дная пога́нка.

death-duties ['deθ,dju:tɪz] *n pl* нало́г на насле́дство.

death-feud ['deθfju:d] *n* сме́ртельная вражда́.

death-hunter ['deθ,hʌntə] *n* мародёр.

deathless ['deθlɪs] *a* бессме́ртный.

deathlike ['deθlaɪk] *a* подо́бный сме́рти; a ~ silence гробово́е молча́ние.

deathly I ['deθlɪ] *a* сме́ртельный, роково́й.

deathly II *adv* сме́ртельно.

death-rate ['deθreɪt] *n* сме́ртность, проце́нт сме́ртности.

death-rattle ['deθ,rætl] *n* предсме́ртный хрип.

death-roll ['deθroul] *n* спи́сок уби́тых.

death's-head ['deθshed] *n* че́реп *(как эмбле́ма сме́рти)*.

death-struggle ['deθstrʌgl] *n* аго́ния.

death-trap ['deθtræp] *n* опа́сное ме́сто, опа́сность.

death-warrant ['deθ,wɔrənt] *n* 1) о́рдер на приведе́ние в исполне́ние сме́ртного пригово́ра; 2) сме́ртный пригово́р.

deb [deb] *n разг.* дебюта́нтка.

débâcle [deɪ'bɑ:kl] *n* 1) вскры́тие реки́; 2) стихи́йный проры́в вод; 3) пани́ческое бе́гство; 4) разгро́м.

debar [dɪ'bɑ:] *v* 1) воспреща́ть; лиша́ть *(пра́ва на что-л)*; 2) исключа́ть; отстраня́ть.

debark [dɪ'bɑ:k] *v* выса́живать(ся); выгружа́ть(ся) *(с су́дна)*.

debarkation [,di:bɑ:'keɪʃən] *n* вы́садка; вы́грузка *(с су́дна)*.

debase [dɪ'beɪs] *v* 1) унижа́ть; 2) ухудша́ть *(ка́чество и т. п.)*; 3) подде́лывать *(де́ньги)*.

debasement ['dɪ'beɪsmənt] *n* 1) униже́ние; 2) ухудше́ние *(ка́чества и т. п.)*; 3) подде́лка.

debatable [dɪ'beɪtəbl] *a* 1) спо́рный; 2) оспа́риваемый.

dabate I [dɪ'beɪt] *n* 1) деба́ты, диску́ссия,

обсужде́ние; to open the ~ вы́ступить пе́рвым; 2) поле́мика; спор; beyond ~ бесспо́рно; 3) (the ~s) *pl* официа́льный отчёт о парла́ментских заседа́ниях.

debate II *v* 1) обсужда́ть, дебати́ровать, спо́рить; 2) оспа́ривать, добива́ться; 3) размышля́ть, обду́мывать.

debater [dɪ'beɪtə] *n* 1) спо́рящий, уча́стник диску́ссии; 2) спо́рщик.

debauch I [dɪ'bɔːtʃ] *n* 1) дебо́ш; .попо́йка; 2) разгра́т.

debauch II *v* 1) развраща́ть; соблазня́ть *(же́нщину)*; 2) по́ртить *(вкус и т. п.)*.

debauchee [,debɔ:'tʃi:] *n* 1) развра́тник; 2) гуля́ка.

debauchery [dɪ'bɔːtʃərɪ] *n* 1) разврат, распу́щенность; 2) пья́нство, невоздержа́нность.

debenture [dɪ'bentʃə] *n* долгово́е обяза́тельство, долгова́я распи́ска.

debilitate [dɪ'bɪlɪteɪt] *v* ослабля́ть.

debility [dɪ'bɪlɪtɪ] *n* сла́бость *(здоро́вья и т. п.)*.

debit I ['debɪt] *n бухг.* дебет; to put to the ~ записа́ть в дебет.

debit II *v бухг.* заноси́ть в дебет.

debonair [,debə'nɛə] *a* 1) жизнера́достный, весёлый; 2) доброду́шный, любе́зный.

debouch [dɪ'bautʃ] *v* выходи́ть на откры́тую ме́стность *(из уще́лья, ле́са)*.

debouchment [dɪ'bautʃmənt] *n* 1) вы́ход из уще́лья *или* укры́тия; 2) у́стье реки́.

debris ['debri:] *n* 1) оско́лки, обло́мки; 2) *геол.* обло́мки поро́д; 3) разва́лины.

debt [det] *n* долг; задо́лженность; ~ of honour долг че́сти; a bad ~ безнадёжный долг; National Debt госуда́рственный долг; in ~ в долгу́; to get *(или* to run) into ~ влезть в долги́; to get out of ~ заплати́ть все долги́, не име́ть долго́в; to contract ~s де́лать долги́; ◊ to pay the ~ of *(или* to) nature сконча́ться.

debtor ['detə] *n* должни́к; *бухг.* дебито́р.

debunk [di:'bʌŋk] *v разг.* развенча́ть; разоблача́ть.

debus [di:'bʌs] *v воен.* выса́живать(ся), выгружа́ть(ся) из автомаши́н.

début ['deɪbu:] *n* дебю́т; to make one's ~ дебюти́ровать.

débutant ['debju:tɑ:ŋ] *n* дебюта́нт.

débutante ['debju:tɑ:nt] *n* дебюта́нтка.

deca- ['dekə-] *pref* дека-, десяти-.

decade ['dekeɪd] *n* 1) десятиле́тие; 2) деся́ток.

decadence ['dekədəns] *n* 1) упа́док, ухудше́ние; 2) декаде́нтство, упа́дочничество *(в иску́сстве)*.

decadency ['dekədənsɪ] *см.* decadence.

decadent I ['dekədənt] *n* декаде́нт.

decadent II *a* декаде́нтский, упа́дочный.

decahedral [,dekə'hi:drəl] *a* десятигра́нный.

decalcify [di:'kælsɪfaɪ] *v* удаля́ть известко́вое вещество́.

decamp [dɪ'kæmp] *v* 1) снима́ться с ла́геря, выступа́ть из ла́геря; 2) удира́ть.

decampment [dɪ'kæmpmənt] *n* 1) выступле́ние из ла́геря; 2) внеза́пный ухо́д.

decant [dɪ'kænt] *v* 1) сце́живать, слива́ть; фильтрова́ть; 2) перелива́ть (вино́) из буты́лки в графи́н.

decanter [dɪ'kæntə] *n* графи́н.

decapitate [dɪ'kæpɪteɪt] *v* обезгла́вить.

decapitation [dɪ,kæpɪ'teɪʃən] *n* обезгла́вливание.

decarbonize [di:'ka:bənaɪz] *v* обезуглеро́живать.

decay I [dɪ'keɪ] *n* 1) гние́ние; *перен.* упа́док; разложе́ние; to fall into ~ разруша́ться, приходи́ть в упа́док; 2) расстро́йство (*здоровья*); 3) разруше́ние (*здания*).

decay II *v* 1) гнить, разлага́ться; по́ртиться; *перен.* приходи́ть в упа́док; 2) ухудша́ться (*о здоровье*).

decayed [dɪ'keɪd] *a* гнило́й.

decease I [dɪ'si:s] *n* смерть, кончи́на.

decease II *v* умере́ть, сконча́ться.

deceased I [dɪ'si:st] *n* (the ~) поко́йник.

deceased II *a* поко́йное, уме́рший.

decedent [dɪ'si:dənt] *n* *юр.* поко́йник.

deceit [dɪ'si:t] *n* обма́н; хи́трость.

deceitful [dɪ'si:tful] *a* 1) лжи́вый; лука́вый; 2) обма́нчивый.

deceive [dɪ'si:v] *v* обма́нывать; to ~ oneself обману́ться.

deceiver [dɪ'si:və] *n* обма́нщик.

decelerate [di:'seləreɪt] *v* уменьша́ть скорость; замедля́ть.

December [dɪ'sembə] *n* 1) дека́брь; 2) *attr* дека́брьский.

Decembrist [dɪ'sembrɪst] *n* *ист.* декабри́ст.

decency ['di:snsɪ] *n* прили́чие, благопристо́йность; *разг.* ве́жливость; by ~, in (common) ~ из прили́чия; human ~ (добро)поря́дочность, мора́ль.

decennary I [dɪ'senərɪ] *n* десятиле́тие.

decennary II *a* десятиле́тний (*о периоде, сроке*).

decennial [dɪ'senjəl] *a* десятиле́тний; происходя́щий ка́ждые де́сять лет.

decent ['di:snt] *a* 1) прили́чный; поря́дочный; 2) скро́мный; 3) *разг.* сла́вный, ми́лый.

decently ['di:sntlɪ] *adv* 1) прили́чно; поря́дочно; 2) скро́мно; 3) любе́зно, ми́ло.

decentralize [di:'sentrəlaɪz] *v* децентрализова́ть.

deception [dɪ'sepʃən] *n* 1) обма́н; притво́рство; 2) лука́вство, хи́трость.

deceptive [dɪ'septɪv] *a* обма́нчивый.

deci- ['desɪ-] *pref* деци- (*обозначает деся́тую часть*).

decide [dɪ'saɪd] *v* реша́ть(ся); принима́ть реше́ние; to ~ in favour of (against) smb. выноси́ть реше́ние в пользу (про́тив) кого́-л.; to ~ between сде́лать вы́бор, вы́брать.

decided [dɪ'saɪdɪd] *a* 1) реши́тельный (*о челове́ке, хара́ктере*); 2) определённый; бесспо́рный.

decidedly [dɪ'saɪdɪdlɪ] *adv* 1) реши́тельно; 2) определённо; несомне́нно.

deciduous [dɪ'sɪdjuəs] *a* 1) роня́ющий (*листья, опере́ние*); 2) опада́ющий; выпада́ющий; 3) прехо́дящий.

decigram(me) ['desɪgræm] *n* децигра́мм.

decilitre ['desɪ,li:tə] *n* децили́тр.

decimal I ['desɪməl] *n* десяти́чная дробь; recurring ~ периоди́ческая десяти́чная дробь.

decimal II *a* десяти́чный.

decimalize ['desɪməlaɪz] *v* 1) обраща́ть в десяти́чную дробь; 2) переводи́ть на десяти́чную систе́му.

decimate ['desɪmeɪt] *v* 1) казни́ть ка́ждого деся́того; *перен.* уничтожа́ть ма́ссами, коси́ть (*об эпиде́мии и т. п.*); 2) *ист.* взима́ть десяти́ну.

decimation [,desɪ'meɪʃən] *n* 1) казнь ка́ждого

десятого; *перен.* ма́ссовая ги́бель, опустоше́ние; 2) *ист.* взима́ние десяти́ны.

decimetre ['desɪ,mi:tə] *n* дециме́тр.

decipher I [dɪ'saɪfə] *n* расшифро́вка.

decipher II *v* 1) расшифро́вывать; 2) разбира́ть (*почерк и т. п.*).

decipherable [dɪ'saɪfərəbl] *a* поддаю́щийся расшифро́вке.

decision [dɪ'sɪʒən] *n* 1) реше́ние; заключе́ние; to arrive at a ~, to come to a ~ приня́ть реше́ние; 2) реши́мость; реши́тельность; a man of ~ реши́тельный челове́к; to lack ~ быть нереши́тельным.

decisive [dɪ'saɪsɪv] *a* 1) реша́ющий, име́ющий реша́ющее значе́ние; 2) реши́тельный; убеди́тельный (*о фа́ктах, ули́ках*).

decivilize [di:'sɪvɪlaɪz] *v* приводи́ть к одича́нию.

deck I [dek] *n* 1) па́луба; protective ~ *мор.* бронева́я па́луба; poor ~ *мор.* полуют; on ~ на па́лубе; to tread the ~ быть моряко́м; to clear the ~s (for action) а) *мор.* пригото́виться к бою; б) пригото́виться к де́йствиям; 2) коло́да (*карт*); cold ~ краплёные ка́рты.

deck II *v* 1) наряжа́ть, украша́ть; 2) настила́ть па́лубу.

deck-cabin ['dek,kæbɪn] *n* каю́та на па́лубе.

deck-chair ['dek,tʃeə] *n* шезло́нг.

-decker [-'dekə] *n*: one-~ (two-~) одинопа́лубное (двухпа́лубное) су́дно.

deck-hand ['dekhænd] *n* матро́с.

deck-house ['dekhaus] *n* *мор.* ру́бка.

decking ['dekɪŋ] *n* 1) опа́лубка; насти́л па́лубы; 2) па́лубный материа́л; 3) украше́ние.

deck-light ['deklaɪt] *n* *мор.* па́лубный иллюмина́тор.

deck-passenger ['dek,pæsɪndʒə] *n* па́лубный пассажи́р.

deck-roof ['dekru:f] *n* пло́ская кры́ша (*без парапе́та*).

declaim [dɪ'kleɪm] *v* 1) деклами́ровать; 2) говори́ть напы́щенно, торже́ственно; □ to ~ against выступа́ть про́тив кого́-л.

declamation [,deklə'meɪʃən] *n* 1) деклама́ция; 2) напы́щенная, торже́ственная речь.

declamatory [dɪ'klæmətərɪ] *a* 1) деклама́цио́нный; 2) напы́щенный.

declaration [,deklə'reɪʃən] *n* 1) деклара́ция; заявле́ние; 2) объявле́ние; ~ of war объявле́ние войны́; ~ of the poll объявле́ние результа́тов голосова́ния.

declarative [dɪ'klærətɪv] *a* декларати́вный.

declaratory [dɪ'klærətərɪ] *a* 1) декларати́вный; 2) объясни́тельный.

declare [dɪ'kleə] *v* 1) объявля́ть; провозглаша́ть; 2) заявля́ть; to ~ oneself призна́ться, откры́ться; I am surprised, I ~ призна́ться, я удивлён; 3) выска́зываться (*за — for, против — against*); □ to ~ off отка́зываться (*от сде́лки и т. п.*).

declared [dɪ'kleəd] *a* 1) объя́вленный; зая́вленный; 2) при́знанный.

déclassé [,deɪkla:'seɪ] *см.* declassed.

declassed [di:'kla:st] *a* деклассированный.

declension [dɪ'klenʃən] *n* 1) паде́ние; упа́док; 2) отклоне́ние; ухудше́ние; *грам.* склоне́ние; ◊ in the ~ of years на скло́не лет.

declensional [dɪ'klenʃənl] *a* *грам.* паде́жный.

declinable [dɪ'klaɪnəbl] *a* *грам.* склоня́емый.

declination [,deklı'neıʃən] *n* 1) наклóн; отклонéние; 2) *грам.* склонéние; 3) магнúтное склонéние; 4) *уст.* упáдок, падéние.

decline I [dı'klaın] *n* 1) упáдок; ухудшéние; to fall into a ~ ослабевáть (*особ. от болéзни*); 2) снижéние, падéние (*цен*); 3) склон, закáт (*жúзни, дня*); on the ~ на склóне, на закáте; the ~ of the moon лунá на ущéрбе.

decline II *v* 1) откáзываться; отклонять (*предложéние и т. п.*); уклоняться; 2) уменьшáться; спадáть (*о температýре*); идтú на ýбыль; 3) приходúть в упáдок, ухудшáться; 4) наклонять(ся); клонúть (-ся); 5) *грам.* склонять.

declivity [dı'klıvıtı] *n* склон, покáтость; уклóн (*пути*).

declivous [dı'klaıvəs] *a* покáтый; отлóгий.

declutch ['diː'klʌtʃ] *v тех.* разъединять; расцеплять.

decode ['diː'koud] *v* расшифрóвывать.

decolo(u)r [diː'kʌlə] *v* обесцвéчивать.

decolo(u)rant [diː'kʌlərənt] *n* обесцвéчивающее веществó.

decolo(u)ration [diː,kʌlə'reıʃən] *n* обесцвéчивание.

decolo(u)rize [diː'kʌləraız] *см.* decolo(u)r.

decompose [,diːkəm'pouz] *v* 1) разлагáть на составнýе чáсти; 2) разлагáться, гнить; 3) анализúровать; 4) *грам.* разбирáть (*предложéние*).

decomposite I [diː'kɔmpəzıt] *n* 1) веществó, состáвленное из слóжных частéй; 2) слóжное слóво.

decomposite II *a* состáвленный из слóжных частéй.

decomposition [,diːkɔmpə'zıʃən] *n* 1) разложéние; 2) распáд, гниéние.

decompound I [,diːkəm'paund] *см.* decomposite II.

decompound II *см.* decompose 1).

deconsecrate [diː'kɔnsıkreıt] *v* секуляризúровать (*церкóвное имýщество*).

decontaminate ['diːkən'tæmıneıt] *v* обеззарáживать; дегазúровать.

decontamination ['diːkən,tæmı'neıʃən] *n* обеззарáживание; дегазáция.

decorate ['dekəreıt] *v* 1) украшáть, декорúровать; 2) отдéлывать (*дом*); 3) награждáть óрденом, медáлью *и т. п.*

decorated ['dekəreıtıd] *a* 1) укрáшенный, декорúрованный; 2) награждённый óрденом, медáлью *и т. п.*

decoration [,dekə'reıʃən] *n* 1) украшéние; 2) *pl* прáздничное убрáнство (*флáги, гирлянды и т. п.*); 3) óрден, медáль *и т. п.*

decorative ['dekərətıv] *a* декоратúвный.

decorator ['dekəreıtə] *n* 1) декорáтор; 2) маляр, обóйщик.

decorous ['dekərəs] *a* прилúчный, пристóйный.

decorum [dı'kɔːrəm] *n* прилúчие, декóрум; этикéт.

decoy I [dı'kɔı] *n* 1) манóк; примáнка; 2) ловýшка, западня; 3) искушéние, соблáзн.

decoy II *v* замáнивать; завлекáть.

decoy-duck [dı'kɔıdʌk] *n* манóк; *перен.* примáнка.

decrease[a] ['diːkriːs] *n* уменьшéние, понижéние; убавлéние; to be on the ~ идтú на ýбыль, уменьшáться.

decrease[b] [diː'kriːs] *v* уменьшáть(ся); убывáть.

decree I [dı'kriː] *n* 1) декрéт, укáз; 2) решéние, постановлéние (*судá*).

decree II *v* издавáть укáз, декрéт; декретúровать.

decrement ['dekrımənt] *n* 1) уменьшéние, стéпень ýбыли; 2) *тех.* затухáние; 3) *радио* декремéнт.

decrepit [dı'krepıt] *a* 1) вéтхий; 2) дряхлый (*о людях*).

decrepitate [dı'krepıteıt] *v* 1) *тех.* обжигáть до растрéскивания; 2) потрéскивать на огнé.

decrepitation [dı,krepı'teıʃən] *n* 1) *тех.* обжигáние; 2) потрéскивание.

decrepitude [dı'krepıtjuːd] *n* 1) вéтхость; 2) дряхлость.

decrescent [dı'kresnt] *a* убывáющий (*обыкн. о лунé*).

decretive [dı'kriːtıv] *a* декрéтный.

decretory [dı'kriːtərı] *см.* decretive.

decry [dı'kraı] *v* осуждáть, порицáть, хулúть.

decumbent [dı'kʌmbənt] *a* 1) лежáщий, прилегáющий; 2) *бот.* стéлющийся по землé.

decuple I ['dekjupl] *n* удесятерённое колúчество.

decuple II *a* удесятерённый.

decuple III *v* удесятерять.

dedicate ['dedıkeıt] *v* 1) посвящáть; 2) надпúсывать (*кнúгу и т. п.*); 3) *разг.* открывáть, объявлять (*торжéственно*).

dedicated ['dedıkeıtıd] *a* прéданный; посвятúвший себя (*дóлгу, дéлу*).

dedication [,dedı'keıʃən] *n* посвящéние.

deduce [dı'djuːs] *v* 1) выводúть (*заключéние и т. п.; from*); 2) устанáвливать происхождéние (*от — from*).

deduct [dı'dʌkt] *v* вычитáть, отнимáть.

deduction [dı'dʌkʃən] *n* 1) вычитáние; 2) вычитáемое; 3) вывод, заключéние; 4) *лог.* дедýкция.

deductive [dı'dʌktıv] *a лог.* дедуктúвный.

deed I [diːd] *n* 1) постýпок, дéйствие; 2) дéло, факт; in ~ and not in name не на словáх, а на дéле; in (very) ~ на сáмом дéле, в действúтельности; 3) пóдвиг; 4) *юр.* докумéнт; акт.

deed II *v амер. юр.* передавáть по áкту.

deem [diːm] *v* полагáть, дýмать; считáть; ~ highly of smb. быть высóкого мнéния о ком-л.

deep I [diːp] *n* 1) глубóкое мéсто; глубинá; бéздна; 2) (the ~) *поэт.* мóре, океáн.

deep II *a* 1) глубóкий; ~ in love влюблённый пó уши; in debt пó уши в долгý; 2) поглощённый (*чем-л.*); ~ in his pursuit погружённый в свой занятия; to be ~ in thought глубокó задýматься; 3) тёмный, густóй (*о цвéте, крáске*); 4) нúзкий, глубóкий (*о звýке, гóлосе*); ◊ a ~ one *сленг* тóнкая бéстия.

deep III *adv* глубокó; сúльно; to go ~ into углубляться; to drink ~ сúльно пить; ~ into the night до глубóкой нóчи.

deep-drawn ['diːp'drɔːn] *a* вырвавшийся из глубины, глубóкий (*о вздóхе*).

deepen ['diːpən] *v* 1) углублять(ся); усúливать (-ся); 2) становúться темнéе, гýще (*о цвéте, крáсках*); 3) понижáть(ся) (*о звýке, гóлосе*).

deep-felt ['diːp'felt] *a* глубокó прочýвствованный.

deep-laid ['diːp'leıd] *a* тщáтельно разрабóтанный и секрéтный (*о плáне*).

deeply ['diːplı] *adv* глубокó.

deep-rooted [ˈdiːpˈruːtɪd] *a* глубоко́ укорени́вшийся.

deep-sea [ˈdiːpˈsiː] *a* глубоково́дный.

deep-seated [ˈdiːpˈsiːtɪd] *a* 1) вкорени́вшийся; 2) затаённый (*о чувстве*); 3) скры́тый (*о болезни*); глубо́кий (*о нарыве*).

deer [dɪə] *n* (*pl без измен.*) оле́нь; лань; *собир.* кра́сный зверь.

deer-forest [ˈdɪəˌfɔrɪst] *n* оле́ний запове́дник.

deer-hound [ˈdɪəhaund] *n* шотла́ндская борза́я.

deerskin [ˈdɪəskɪn] *n* оле́нья ко́жа, за́мша.

deface [dɪˈfeɪs] *v* 1) искажа́ть; уро́довать, обезобра́живать; 2) стира́ть, де́лать неразбо́рчивым, нечётким; 3) дискредити́ровать.

defacement [dɪˈfeɪsmənt] *n* 1) искаже́ние; уро́дование, обезобра́живание; 2) стира́ние.

de facto [diːˈfæktou] *adv* факти́чески, де-фа́кто.

defalcate [ˈdiːfælkeɪt] *v* присва́ивать (*чужое иму́щество*); соверша́ть растра́ту.

defalcation [ˌdiːfælˈkeɪʃən] *n* присвое́ние чужи́х де́нег; растра́та.

defalcator [ˈdiːfælkeɪtə] *n* растра́тчик.

defamation [ˌdefəˈmeɪʃən] *n* клевета́, бесче́стье.

defamatory [dɪˈfæmətərɪ] *a* клеветни́ческий, бесчестя́щий; позо́рящий.

defame [dɪˈfeɪm] *v* клевета́ть; поноси́ть; поро́чить, позо́рить.

default I [dɪˈfɔːlt] *n* 1) невыполне́ние обяза́тельств; 2) неявка (*в суд*); to go by ~ проходи́ть в отсу́тствии отве́тчика (*о судебном деле*); 3) недоста́ток чего-л.; отсу́тствие; in ~ of за неиме́нием; за отсу́тствием; 4) *спорт.* вы́ход из состяза́ния.

default II *v* 1) не вы́полнить (*обязательств и т. п.*); 2) не яви́ться в суд; 3) вы́нести зао́чное реше́ние; 4) *спорт.* вы́йти из состяза́ния.

defaulter [dɪˈfɔːltə] *n* 1) челове́к, не выполня́ющий обяза́тельств, уклоня́ющийся от я́вки в суд и т. п.; 2) банкро́т.

defeasance [dɪˈfiːzəns] *n* аннули́рование, отме́на.

defeasible [dɪˈfiːzəbl] *a* могу́щий быть аннули́рованным, отменённым.

defeat I [dɪˈfiːt] *n* 1) пораже́ние; to suffer a ~ потерпе́ть пораже́ние; 2) неуда́ча; расстро́йство (*планов*); круше́ние (*надежд*); 3) *юр.* аннули́рование.

defeat II *v* 1) наноси́ть пораже́ние; разбива́ть (*в бою*); одержа́ть побе́ду; 2) расстра́ивать (*планы и т. п.*); разруша́ть (*надежды*); 3) *юр.* аннули́ровать.

defeatism [dɪˈfiːtɪzəm] *n полит.* пораже́нчество.

defeatist [dɪˈfiːtɪst] *n полит.* пораже́нец.

defecate [ˈdefɪkeɪt] *v* 1) очища́ть(ся) (*от приме́сей и т. п.*); отста́ивать (*жидкость*); 2) испражня́ться.

defecation [ˌdefɪˈkeɪʃən] *n* 1) очище́ние; 2) испражне́ние.

defect [dɪˈfekt] *n* 1) недоста́ток, недочёт; поро́к; изъя́н; corporal ~ физи́ческий недоста́ток; 2) несоверше́нство; 3) поврежде́ние.

defection [dɪˈfekʃən] *n* отсту́пничество; дезерти́рство.

defective [dɪˈfektɪv] *a* 1) недоста́точный (*тж. грам. о глаголе*); несоверше́нный; 2) неиспра́вный; 3) дефекти́вный, у́мственно отста́лый.

defence [dɪˈfens] *n* 1) оборо́на; защи́та (*тж. юр. и спорт.*); anti-aircraft ~ противовозду́шная обо

ро́на; 2) *pl воен.* оборони́тельные сооруже́ния; 3) запреще́ние (*охоты, рыбной ловли и т. п.*).

defenceless [dɪˈfenslɪs] *a* беззащи́тный.

defencist [dɪˈfensɪst] *n полит.* оборо́нец.

defend [dɪˈfend] *v* 1) защища́ть(ся); оборо́нять (-ся); 2) отста́ивать (*мнение и т. п.*); поддерживать; 3) *юр.* выступа́ть защи́тником.

defendant [dɪˈfendənt] *n юр.* отве́тчик; подсуди́мый, обвиня́емый.

defender [dɪˈfendə] *n* защи́тник; the ~s of peace сторо́нники ми́ра.

defense [dɪˈfens] *амер. см.* defence.

defensible [dɪˈfensəbl] *a* 1) *воен.* удо́бный для оборо́ны; допуска́ющий оборо́ну; 2) опра́вдываемый.

defensive I [dɪˈfensɪv] *n* 1) оборо́на; 2) оборони́тельная пози́ция; to act (*или* to be, to stand) on the ~ обороня́ться, защища́ться.

defensive II *a* оборони́тельный.

defer[1] [dɪˈfəː] *v* 1) откла́дывать; отсро́чивать; 2) ме́длить, ме́шкать.

defer[2] *v* уважа́ть, счита́ться с чьим-л. мне́нием, уступа́ть (*to*).

deference [ˈdefərəns] *n* уваже́ние, почти́тельное отноше́ние; in (*или* out of) ~ to из уваже́ния к; with all due ~ при всём уваже́нии; to show ~ to относи́ться почти́тельно к.

deferent [ˈdefərənt] *a* 1) отводя́щий, выводя́щий (*о канале, протоке*); 2) *редко* почти́тельный.

deferential [ˌdefəˈrenʃəl] *a* почти́тельный.

deferment [dɪˈfəːmənt] *n* отсро́чка.

defiance [dɪˈfaɪəns] *n* 1) вы́зов (*на борьбу́ и т. п.*); 2) откры́тое неповинове́ние; пренебреже́ние; in ~ of а) вопреки́; б) с я́вным пренебреже́нием; to set at ~, to bid ~ to пренебрега́ть; проявля́ть неповинове́ние; не счита́ться, не обраща́ть внима́ния.

defiant [dɪˈfaɪənt] *a* вызыва́ющий.

defiantly [dɪˈfaɪəntlɪ] *adv* с вы́зовом, вызыва́юще.

deficiency [dɪˈfɪʃənsɪ] *n* 1) недоста́ток, нехва́тка; дефици́т; 2) *мед.* недоста́точность; oxygen ~ кислоро́дное голода́ние.

deficient [dɪˈfɪʃənt] *a.*1) недоста́точный, недостаю́щий, непо́лный, лишённый чего-либо (*in*); 2) несоверше́нный; 3) слабоу́мный (*тж.* mentally ~).

deficit [ˈdefɪsɪt] *n* дефици́т.

defilade I [ˌdefɪˈleɪd] *n воен.* есте́ственное укры́тие.

defilade II *v воен.* укрыва́ть.

defile[a1] [dɪˈfaɪl] *v* 1) грязни́ть, па́чкать; 2) оскверня́ть; 3) развраща́ть, по́ртить.

defile[a2] *v* дефили́ровать, проходи́ть у́зкой коло́нной (*о войсках*).

defile[b] [ˈdiːfaɪl] *n* дефиле́, тесни́на.

defilement [dɪˈfaɪlmənt] *n* 1) загрязне́ние; 2) оскверне́ние; 3) развраще́ние.

definable [dɪˈfaɪnəbl] *a* определи́мый.

define [dɪˈfaɪn] *v* 1) определя́ть; дава́ть определе́ние; 2) оче́рчивать, устана́вливать (*границы, формы*).

definite [ˈdefɪnɪt] *a* определённый; то́чный, я́сный.

definition [ˌdefɪˈnɪʃən] *n* 1) определе́ние; 2) определённость; то́чность, я́сность, чёткость.

definitive [dɪˈfɪnɪtɪv] *a* оконча́тельный; реши́тельный.

deflagrate ['defləgreɪt] *v* быстро сжигать *или* сгорать.

deflagration [ˌdeflə'greɪʃən] *n* (мгновенное) сгорание.

deflate [diː'fleɪt] *v* 1) выкачивать (*воздух, газ*); 2) *эк.* сокращать количество денежных знаков в обращении; 3) *амер.* снижать цены.

deflation [diː'fleɪʃən] *n* 1) выкачивание (*воздуха, газа*); 2) *эк.* дефляция.

deflect [dɪ'flekt] *v* 1) отклонять(ся) (*от — from*); 2) преломлять(ся).

deflection [dɪ'flekʃən] *n* 1) отклонение; изгиб; склонение магнитной стрелки; 2) преломление.

deflexion [dɪ'flekʃən] *см.* deflection.

deflower [diː'flauə] *v* 1) лишать невинности; 2) обрывать цветы; 3) портить.

defoliate^{*a*} [diː'foulɪt] *a* лишённый листьев.

defoliate^{*b*} [dɪ'foulieɪt] *v* лишать листвы.

defoliation [dɪˌfoulɪ'eɪʃən] *n* листопад.

deforest [dɪ'fɔrɪst] *v* обезлесить, вырубить леса.

deform [dɪ'fɔːm] *v* 1) уродовать; искажать; 2) *тех.* деформировать.

deformation [ˌdiːfɔː'meɪʃən] *n* 1) уродование; искажение; 2) *тех.* деформация.

deformity [dɪ'fɔːmɪtɪ] *n* уродство; уродливость.

defraud [dɪ'frɔːd] *v* 1) выманивать; 2) обманывать.

defray [dɪ'freɪ] *n* оплачивать.

defrayal [dɪ'freɪəl] *n* оплата, покрытие расходов.

defrayment [dɪ'freɪmənt] *см.* defrayal.

defrock ['diː'frɔk] *v* лишать духовного сана.

defrost [diː'frɔst] *v* размораживать.

deft [deft] *a* ловкий; проворный; искусный.

defunct I [dɪ'fʌŋkt] *n* (the ~) покойник, покойный.

defunct II *a* умерший.

defy [dɪ'faɪ] *v* 1) вызывать (*на состязание и т. п.*); бросать вызов; 2) проявлять неповиновение; игнорировать (*закон*); пренебрегать (*мнением и т. п.*); 3) не поддаваться (*описанию, определению*).

degas [diː'gæs] *v* дегазировать.

degeneracy [dɪ'dʒenərəsɪ] *n* вырождение.

degenerate^{*a*} I [dɪ'dʒenərɪt] *n* дегенерат; выродок.

degenerate^{*a*} II *a* выродившийся.

degenerate^{*b*} [dɪ'dʒenəreɪt] *v* вырождаться.

degeneration [dɪˌdʒenə'reɪʃən] *n* 1) вырождение; 2) *мед.* перерождение.

degenerative [dɪ'dʒenərətɪv] *a* вырождающийся, дегенеративный.

deglutition [ˌdiːglu'tɪʃən] *n* глотание, проглатывание.

degradation [ˌdegrə'deɪʃən] *n* 1) понижение; разжалование; 2) унижение; 3) упадок; деградация; 4) *биол.* вырождение; 5) *геол.* разрушение (*пород*).

degrade [dɪ'greɪd] *v* 1) унижать; 2) ухудшаться; вырождаться; деградировать; понижать; 3) снижать, уменьшать (*ценность и т. п.*); 4) понижать (*в чине, звании*); разжаловать; 5) *геол.* разрушать (*породу*).

degree [dɪ'griː] *n* 1) степень; ступень; by ~s постепенно; in some ~, to a certain ~ до известной степени; not in the least ~ ничуть, нисколько; to the last ~ до последней степени; 2) положение (*общественное*); ранг; 3) учёная степень, учёное

звание; honorary ~ почётное звание; to go up for a ~ быть кандидатом на присуждение учёной степени; to take one's ~ получить степень; 4) градус; 5) *грам.* степень сравнения; Comparative Degree сравнительная степень; Superlative Degree превосходная степень; 6) степень родства, колено; ◊ third ~ *амер.* допрос с применением пыток.

degressive [dɪ'gresɪv] *a* нисходящий; уменьшающийся.

dehydrate [diː'haɪdreɪt] *a* обезвоживать; сушить (*картофель и т. п.*).

dehydration [ˌdiːhaɪ'dreɪʃən] *n* *хим.* обезвоживание.

de-ice ['diː'aɪs] *v* *ав.* устранять обледенение.

deification [ˌdiːɪfɪ'keɪʃən] *n* 1) обожествление; 2) обоготворение.

deify ['diːɪfaɪ] *v* 1) обожествлять; 2) обоготворять; боготворить.

deign [deɪn] *v* удостаивать; снисходить; соблаговолить.

deism ['diːɪzəm] *n* деизм.

deist ['diːɪst] *n* деист.

deity ['diːɪtɪ] *n* 1) божественность; 2) божество.

deject [dɪ'dʒekt] *v* удручать, приводить в уныние, угнетать.

dejected [dɪ'dʒektɪd] *a* унылый, подавленный, печальный.

dejection [dɪ'dʒekʃən] *n* 1) уныние; подавленность; 2) *мед.* дефекация; 3) *геол.* лава, пепел.

déjeuner ['deɪʒəneɪ] *n* завтрак.

de jure [diː'dʒuərɪ] *adv* юридически, де-юре.

delate [dɪ'leɪt] *v* доносить.

delation [dɪ'leɪʃən] *n* донос.

delator [dɪ'leɪtə] *n* доносчик.

delay I [dɪ'leɪ] *n* 1) задержка; препятствие; 2) отсрочка, отлагательство; without ~ безотлагательно; 3) замедление; промедление, проволочка; опоздание; 4) *attr* замедленный; ~ action замедленного действия.

delay II *v* 1) задерживать; 2) откладывать; 3) медлить; опаздывать.

delectable [dɪ'lektəbl] *a* обыкн. ирон. приятный, доставляющий удовольствие.

delectation [ˌdiːlek'teɪʃən] *n* удовольствие, наслаждение.

delegacy ['delɪgəsɪ] *n* 1) делегация; 2) делегирование; 3) полномочия делегата.

delegate^{*a*} ['delɪgɪt] *n* делегат; депутат.

delegate^{*b*} ['delɪgeɪt] *v* 1) делегировать; уполномочивать; 2) поручать; передавать (*права и т. п.*).

delegation [ˌdelɪ'geɪʃən] *n* 1) делегация; 2) делегирование, посылка делегации.

delete [dɪ'liːt] *v* вычёркивать (*букву, слово и т. п.*); уничтожать (*тж. перен.*).

deleterious [ˌdelɪ'tɪərɪəs] *a* вредный.

deletion [dɪ'liːʃən] *n* вычёркивание; уничтожение (*тж. перен.*).

deliberate^{*a*} [dɪ'lɪbərɪt] *a* 1) намеренный, заранее обдуманный; умышленный, нарочитый; 2) осторожный; нерешительный; 3) неторопливый (*о движениях и т. п.*).

deliberate^{*b*} [dɪ'lɪbəreɪt] *v* 1) обдумывать; 2) обсуждать.

deliberately [dɪ'lɪbərɪtlɪ] *adv* 1) умышленно, намеренно; 2) осторожно; нерешительно; 3) медленно.

deliberation [dɪ,lɪbə'reɪʃən] n 1) размышле́ние; after long ~ по зре́лом размышле́нии; 2) осмотри́тельность, осторо́жность; 3) обсужде́ние; совеща́ние.

deliberative [dɪ'lɪbərətɪv] a совеща́тельный.

delicacy ['delɪkəsɪ] n 1) то́нкость; не́жность (красок, тонов и т. п.); утончённость; 2) сла́бость, хру́пкость; 3) делика́тность, щепети́льность; 4) ла́комство; деликате́с.

delicate ['delɪkɪt] a 1) то́нкий; не́жный; изя́щный; 2) сла́бый, хру́пкий; 3) делика́тный, щепети́льный; 4) щекотли́вый (о вопросе, положении); 5) чувстви́тельный (тж. о приборе).

delicatessen [,delɪkə'tesn] n pl делика́тесы.

delicious [dɪ'lɪʃəs] a 1) преле́стный; очарова́тельный; 2) вку́сный.

delict ['diːlɪkt] n юр. наруше́ние зако́на, правонаруше́ние.

delight I [dɪ'laɪt] n 1) наслажде́ние, удово́льствие; to the ~ к вели́кому удово́льствию; to take ~ in smth. получа́ть удово́льствие от чего-л., наслажда́ться чем-л.; 2) восхище́ние.

delight II v 1) доставля́ть удово́льствие; 2) восхища́ть(ся); 3) наслажда́ться.

delighted [dɪ'laɪtɪd] a дово́льный, сия́ющий.

delightful [dɪ'laɪtful] a восхити́тельный, очарова́тельный.

delimit [diː'lɪmɪt] v определя́ть грани́цы; размежёвывать.

delimitate [dɪ'lɪmɪteɪt] см. delimit.

delimitation [dɪ,lɪmɪ'teɪʃən] n определе́ние грани́ц; размежева́ние.

delineate [dɪ'lɪnɪeɪt] v 1) оче́рчивать, обрисо́вывать; 2) опи́сывать, изобража́ть.

delineation [dɪ,lɪnɪ'eɪʃən] n 1) очерта́ние, а́брис; 2) описа́ние, изображе́ние; о́черк.

delinquency [dɪ'lɪŋkwənsɪ] n 1) упуще́ние; 2) оши́бка; просту́пок; 3) правонаруше́ние; престу́пность.

delinquent I [dɪ'lɪŋkwənt] n престу́пник, правонаруши́тель.

delinquent II a 1) вино́вный; 2) амер. неупла́ченный.

delirious [dɪ'lɪrɪəs] a 1) находя́щийся в бреду́; to grow ~ впада́ть в бред; 2) бредово́й.

delirium [dɪ'lɪrɪəm] n 1) бред, бредово́е состоя́ние; 2) исступле́ние.

deliver [dɪ'lɪvə] v 1) передава́ть; вруча́ть; 2) доставля́ть (почту, товары); 3) представля́ть (отчёт и т. п.); 4) произноси́ть (речь); чита́ть (доклад, лекцию); 5) избавля́ть (from); 6) мед. принима́ть (роды); be ~ed of разреши́ться (от бремени; тж. перен. чем-л.); 7) наноси́ть (удар, пораже́ние); 8) выраба́тывать, производи́ть; □ to ~ **over** выдава́ть, предава́ть; to ~ **up** сдава́ть (крепость); to ~ oneself up сдава́ться.

deliverance [dɪ'lɪvərəns] n 1) избавле́ние, освобожде́ние; 2) вы́сказанное мне́ние, заявле́ние.

delivery [dɪ'lɪvərɪ] n 1) переда́ча; вруче́ние; 2) доста́вка; the early ~, the first ~ пе́рвая, у́тренняя доста́вка корреспонде́нции; special ~ а) спе́шная по́чта; б) сро́чная доста́вка; on ~ по доставле́нии; 3) мане́ра произнесе́ния ре́чи; театр. мане́ра исполне́ния; 4) ро́ды; 5) сда́ча, вы́дача; 6) тех. пита́ние, снабже́ние (водой, током); пода́ча (угля и т. п.).

delivery-boy [dɪ'lɪvərɪbɔɪ] n ма́льчик-посы́льный.

dell [del] n (леси́стая) доли́на.

delta ['deltə] n 1) де́льта (греческая бу́ква); 2) де́льта (реки́).

delude [dɪ'ljuːd] v вводи́ть в заблужде́ние, обма́нывать; to ~ oneself обма́нывать себя́, заблужда́ться.

deluge I ['deljuːdʒ] n 1) наводне́ние; пото́п; 2) ли́вень; перен. пото́к (слов и т. п.).

deluge II v затопля́ть; наводня́ть (тж. перен.).

delusion [dɪ'luːʒən] n 1) обма́н; 2) заблужде́ние; иллю́зия; to be (или to labour) under the ~ (жесто́ко) заблужда́ться; 3) мед. ма́ния.

delusive [dɪ'luːsɪv] a обма́нчивый, при́зрачный.

delve I [delv] n впа́дина; ры́твина.

delve II v 1) уст. копа́ть, рыть; 2) ры́ться (в кни́гах, архи́вах).

demagogic [,demə'gɔgɪk] a демагоги́ческий.

demagogue ['deməgɔg] n демаго́г.

demagogy ['deməgɔgɪ] n демаго́гия.

demand I [dɪ'mɑːnd] n 1) тре́бование, про́сьба; запро́с; payable on ~ опла́чиваемый по тре́бованию, по предъявле́нии; to have many ~s on one's time име́ть мно́го обя́занностей, дел; 2) потре́бность, спрос; in ~ име́ющий спрос.

demand II v 1) тре́бовать; 2) нужда́ться; this work ~s great patience э́та рабо́та тре́бует огро́много терпе́ния; 3) спра́шивать.

demarcate ['diːmɑːkeɪt] v разграни́чивать; проводи́ть демаркацио́нную ли́нию.

demarcation [,diːmɑː'keɪʃən] n разграниче́ние; демарка́ция.

démarche ['deɪmɑːʃ] n дема́рш, дипломати́ческий шаг.

demean[1] [dɪ'miːn] v уст.: to ~ oneself вести́ себя́.

demean[2] v унижа́ть; to ~ oneself унижа́ться, роня́ть своё досто́инство.

demeanour [dɪ'miːnə] n поведе́ние; мане́ра (держа́ться).

demented [dɪ'mentɪd] a сумасше́дший.

démenti [,deɪmɑː'tiː] n официа́льное опроверже́ние.

demerit [diː'merɪt] n недоста́ток, дефе́кт; дурна́я черта́.

demesne [dɪ'meɪn] n 1) владе́ние (землёй, недвижимостью); to hold in ~ владе́ть; 2) поме́стье, име́ние (не сдаваемое в аренду); владе́ние (земли, имущество); Royal ~, State ~ госуда́рственные зе́мли; 4) о́бласть, сфе́ра.

demi- ['demɪ-] pref полу-.

demigod ['demɪgɔd] n полубо́г.

demilitarize ['diː'mɪlɪtəraɪz] v демилитаризи́ровать, разоружа́ть.

demi-monde ['demɪ'mɔːnd] n полусве́т.

demise I [dɪ'maɪz] n 1) сда́ча в аре́нду; 2) переда́ча по насле́дству; 3) перехо́д коро́ны к насле́днику; отрече́ние от престо́ла; 4) смерть, кончи́на.

demise II v 1) сдава́ть в аре́нду; 2) передава́ть по насле́дству; оставля́ть по завеща́нию; 3) отрека́ться от престо́ла.

demission [dɪ'mɪʃən] n отка́з, отрече́ние; ухо́д в отста́вку; сложе́ние зва́ния.

demob ['diː'mɔb] сокр. разг. см. demobilize.

demobee [,dɪmə'biː] n разг. демобилизо́ванный.

demobilization [ˌdiːˌmoubɪlaɪˈzeɪʃən] *n* демобилизация.

demobilize [diːˈmoubɪlaɪz] *v* демобилизовать.

democracy [dɪˈmɔkrəsɪ] *n* 1) демократия; 2) демократизм; 3) (D.) *амер.* демократическая партия.

democrat [ˈdeməkræt] *n* 1) демократ; 2) (D.) *амер.* член демократической партии.

democratic [ˌdeməˈkrætɪk] *a* демократический; демократичный.

democratize [dɪˈmɔkrətaɪz] *v* демократизировать.

demolish [dɪˈmɔlɪʃ] *v* 1) сносить (*здание*), разрушать; 2) разбивать, опровергать (*теорию и т. п.*); 3) *разг.* уничтожить, съесть.

demolition [ˌdeməˈlɪʃən] *n* 1) разрушение, снос; 2) уничтожение.

demon [ˈdiːmən] *n* демон, дьявол, злой дух.

demoniac [dɪˈmouniæk] *a* 1) одержимый; 2) дьявольский.

demonic [diːˈmɔnɪk] *a* демонический.

demonstrable [ˈdemənstrəbl] *a* доказуемый.

demonstrate [ˈdemənstreɪt] *v* 1) доказывать; 2) показывать, демонстрировать; 3) проявлять (*чувства и т. п.*); 4) участвовать в демонстрации; 5) *воен.* производить демонстрацию.

demonstration [ˌdemənsˈtreɪʃən] *n* 1) показ, демонстрирование; 2) проявление (*чувств и т. п.*); 3) доказательство; 4) демонстрация; 5) *воен.* демонстрация сил.

demonstrationist [ˌdemənsˈtreɪʃənɪst] *см.* demonstrator 1).

demonstrative I [dɪˈmɔnstrətɪv] *n* *грам.* указательное местоимение.

demonstrative II *a* 1) наглядный, доказательный, убедительный; 2) демонстративный; 3) экспансивный; несдержанный; 4) *грам.* указательный.

demonstrator [ˈdemənstreɪtə] *n* 1) участник демонстрации, демонстрант; 2) демонстратор; ассистент профессора.

demoralization [dɪˌmɔrəlaɪˈzeɪʃən] *n* моральное разложение, деморализация.

demoralize [dɪˈmɔrəlaɪz] *v* 1) деморализовать; 2) подрывать дисциплину.

demos [ˈdiːmɔs] *n* демос, народ.

demote [dɪˈmout] *v* снижать (*в должности, звании и т. п.*).

demountable [dɪˈmauntəbl] *a* разборный, съёмный.

demur I [dɪˈməː] *n* 1) возражение; without ~ без возражений; 2) колебание.

demur II *v* 1) возражать; протестовать; 2) колебаться, сомневаться.

demure [dɪˈmjuə] *a* 1) серьёзный; степенный; 2) притворно-застенчивый, скромный.

den [den] *n* 1) логовище, берлога; 2) притон; 3) небольшой уютный кабинет; 4) каморка.

denary [ˈdiːnərɪ] *a* десятичный.

denationalize [diːˈnæʃnəlaɪz] *v* 1) лишать национальных прав, национального характера; 2) денационализировать.

denaturalize [diːˈnætʃrəlaɪz] *v* 1) лишать подданства, прав гражданства; 2) лишать природных свойств.

denature [diːˈneɪtʃə] *v* 1) изменять природные свойства; 2) денатурировать (*спирт*).

denazification [dɪˌnɑːzɪfɪˈkeɪʃən] *n* денацификация.

dendriform [ˈdendrɪfɔːm] *a* древовидный.

dene[1] [diːn] *n* долина.

dene[2] *n* дюна.

dengue [ˈdeŋgɪ] *n* тропическая лихорадка.

denial [dɪˈnaɪəl] *n* 1) отказ; flat ~ категорический отказ; 2) отречение; 3) отрицание; опровержение.

denigrate [ˈdenɪgreɪt] *v* чернить, порочить, клеветать.

denizen I [ˈdenɪzn] *n* 1) житель, обитатель; 2) иностранец, получивший права гражданства; 3) акклиматизировавшееся животное *или* растение; 4) заимствованное слово.

denizen II *v* 1) принимать в число граждан; натурализовать; 2) акклиматизировать (*животных и растения*); 3) вводить в употребление иностранное слово.

denominate I [dɪˈnɔmɪneɪt] *a* именованный (*о числе*).

denominate II *v* называть, именовать.

denomination [dɪˌnɔmɪˈneɪʃən] *n* 1) название, наименование; 2) достоинство (*монеты*); 3) вероисповедание; секта.

denominational [dɪˌnɔmɪˈneɪʃənl] *a* сектантский.

denominative [dɪˈnɔmɪnətɪv] *a* нарицательный.

denominator [dɪˈnɔmɪneɪtə] *n* *мат.* знаменатель.

denotation [ˌdiːnouˈteɪʃən] *n* 1) обозначение; 2) знак; 3) значение.

denotative [dɪˈnoutətɪv] *a* 1) указывающий (*на — of*); 2) означающий.

denote [dɪˈnout] *v* 1) означать, значить; 2) показывать, указывать на что-л.

denotement [dɪˈnoutmənt] *n* обозначение; знак.

denounce [dɪˈnauns] *v* 1) осуждать; обличать; 2) *дип.* денонсировать; 3) доносить.

denouncement [dɪˈnaunsmənt] *см.* denunciation.

dense [dens] *a* 1) густой; частый (*о лесе и т. п.*); 2) плотный (*о населении, ткани*); 3) крайний (*о невежестве и т. п.*); 4) тупой, глупый, несообразительный.

density [ˈdensɪtɪ] *n* 1) густота; 2) плотность; 3) *физ.* удельный вес; 4) глупость, тупость.

dent I [dent] *n* углубление, впадина.

dent II *v* вдавливать, оставлять след, выбоину.

dental I [ˈdentl] *n* *фон.* зубной звук.

dental II *a* 1) зубной; 2) зубоврачебный.

denticle [ˈdentɪkl] *n* зубчик.

denticulate(d) [denˈtɪkjuˌleɪt(ɪd)] *a* зубчатый; зазубренный.

dentifrice [ˈdentɪfrɪs] *n* зубной порошок, зубная паста.

dentist [ˈdentɪst] *n* зубной врач.

dentistry [ˈdentɪstrɪ] *n* лечение зубов.

dentition [denˈtɪʃən] *n* 1) прорезывание зубов; 2) расположение зубов.

denture [ˈdentʃə] *n* ряд зубов (*особ. искусственных*).

denudation [ˌdiːnjuːˈdeɪʃən] *n* обнажение, оголение.

denude [dɪˈnjuːd] *v* 1) обнажать, оголять; 2) лишать чего-л.; *разг.* обирать.

denunciation [dɪ,nʌnsɪ'eɪʃən] *n* 1) осуждение, обличение; обвинение; 2) денонсирование (*договора*).

denunciator [dɪ'nʌnsɪeɪtə] *n* 1) обвинитель; 2) доносчик.

deny [dɪ'naɪ] *v* 1) отрицать; не соглашаться; 2) отказывать(ся); to ~ oneself отказывать себе в чём-л.; 3) отрекаться; отпираться.

depart [dɪ'pɑːt] *v* 1) отправляться, отбывать; уезжать; уходить; 2) *уст.* умирать; 3) отступать, отклоняться (*от правила, обычая и т. п.*); to ~ from one's word (one's promise) нарушить своё слово (обещание).

departed I [dɪ'pɑːtɪd] *n* (the ~) покойник(и).

departed II *a* 1) былой, прошлый; 2) умерший.

department [dɪ'pɑːtmənt] *n* 1) отдел; отделение; цех; 2) область, отрасль (*науки, знания*); 3) ведомство; департамент; 4) *амер.* министерство; State Department государственный департамент (*министерство иностранных дел США*); Navy Department военно-морское министерство.

departmental [,diːpɑːt'mentl] *a* относящийся к определённому отделу, ведомству; ведомственный.

departure [dɪ'pɑːtʃə] *n* 1) отправление; отъезд; уход; to take one's ~ уходить; уезжать; 2) *уст.* кончина, смерть; 3) отступление, отклонение (*от правила, обычая*); 4) отправная точка; а new ~ новая линия поведения; новое направление.

depasture [diː'pɑːstʃə] *v* пасти(сь).

depend [dɪ'pend] *v* 1) зависеть (*от — on, upon*); it ~s now upon himself это зависит теперь от него самого; that ~s смотря по тому, в зависимости от; it depends! как сказать!; 2) полагаться (*на — on, upon*); ~ upon it будьте уверены; 3) быть на иждивении; 4) *уст.* висеть.

dependable [dɪ'pendəbl] *a* надёжный.

dependant I, II [dɪ'pendənt] *см.* dependent I, II.

dependence [dɪ'pendəns] *n* 1) зависимость (*upon*); 2) доверие, надежда; to put (*или* to place) one's ~ in (*или* on) полагаться, надеяться на; 3) зависимое, подчинённое положение; to live in ~ жить на иждивении; быть в зависимости (*от кого-л.*).

dependency [dɪ'pendənsɪ] *n* 1) зависимость, подчинённое положение; 2) зависимая страна, колония.

dependent I [dɪ'pendənt] *n* 1) иждивенец; 2) подчинённый; 3) *ист.* вассал.

dependent II *a* 1) зависимый; зависящий от, находящийся на иждивении; 2) подчинённый (*тж. грам. о предложении*).

depict [dɪ'pɪkt] *v* 1) изображать, рисовать; 2) описывать.

depicture [dɪ'pɪktʃə] *v* 1) *см.* depict; 2) представлять себе.

deplete [dɪ'pliːt] *v* 1) опорожнять; исчерпывать; истощать (*силы, запасы*); 2) очищать кишечник.

depletion [dɪ'pliːʃən] *n* 1) истощение (*запасов, средств*); 2) очищение кишечника.

depletive I [dɪ'pliːtɪv] *n* слабительное средство.

depletive II *a* слабительный.

deplorable [dɪ'plɔːrəbl] *a* плачевный; прискорбный.

deplore [dɪ'plɔː] *n* 1) оплакивать, сожалеть; 2) быть шокированным.

deploy I [dɪ'plɔɪ] *n* *воен.* развёртывание (*строя*).

deploy II *v* *воен.* развёртывать (*строй*).

deployment [dɪ'plɔɪmənt] *см.* deploy I.

depolarize [diː'pouləraɪz] *v* 1) *физ.* деполяризовать; 2) разрушать, подрывать (*убеждения и т. п.*).

depopulate [diː'pɔpjuleɪt] *v* 1) уменьшать *или* истреблять население; обезлюдить; 2) уменьшаться (*о населении*); обезлюдеть.

depopulation ['diː,pɔpjuː'leɪʃən] *n* 1) уменьшение *или* истребление населения; 2) безлюдье, отсутствие населения.

deport[1] [dɪ'pɔːt] *v* высылать, ссылать.

deport[2] *v*: to ~ oneself вести себя.

deportation [,diːpɔː'teɪʃən] *n* высылка; ссылка, изгнание.

deportee [,diːpɔː'tiː] *n* сосланный; высланный.

deportment [dɪ'pɔːtmənt] *n* манеры; поведение.

depose [dɪ'pouz] *v* 1) смещать (*с должности*); свергать (*с престола*); 2) *юр.* давать показания под присягой.

deposit I [dɪ'pɔzɪt] *n* 1) вклад (*в банк*), депозит; 2) осадок, отложение; 3) задаток; залог; 4) *горн.* залежь.

deposit II *v* 1) класть (*в банк*); сдавать на хранение; 2) класть (*тж. о яйцах*); 3) отлагать; давать осадок; 4) давать задаток; оставлять залог.

depositary [dɪ'pɔzɪtərɪ] *n* лицо, которому вверены вклады.

deposition[1] [,depə'zɪʃən] *n* 1) смещение (*с должности*); свержение (*с престола*); лишение (*власти*); 2) *юр.* показание под присягой.

deposition[2] *n* отложение, осадок.

depositor [dɪ'pɔzɪtə] *n* вкладчик.

depository [dɪ'pɔzɪtərɪ] *n* 1) хранилище, склад; *перен.* сокровищница; кладезь; 2) *см.* depositary.

depot[a] ['depou] *n* 1) склад; 2) *ж.-д.* депо; 3) *воен.* сборный пункт; 4) *attr* запасной, запасный.

depot[b] ['diːpou] *n* *амер.* железнодорожная станция.

deprave [dɪ'preɪv] *v* портить, развращать, разлагать.

depraved [dɪ'preɪvd] *a* испорченный, безнравственный.

depravity [dɪ'prævɪtɪ] *n* развращённость, безнравственность.

deprecate ['deprɪkeɪt] *v* 1) осуждать; не одобрять; возражать, протестовать; 2) *уст.* умолять; стараться отвратить (*что-л.*).

deprecation [,deprɪ'keɪʃən] *n* 1) осуждение; неодобрение; возражение, протест; 2) *уст.* мольба.

deprecative ['deprɪkeɪtɪv] *a* 1) неодобрительный, осуждающий; возражающий, протестующий; 2) *уст.* молящий об отвращении беды *и т. п.*

deprecatory ['deprɪkətərɪ] *a* старающийся умилостивить, задабривающий; просительный.

depreciate [dɪ'priːʃɪeɪt] *v* 1) обесценивать; 2) падать в цене, терять стоимость; 3) недооценивать, умалять; относиться с пренебрежением.

depreciatingly [dɪ'priːʃɪeɪtɪŋlɪ] *adv* пренебрежительно.

depreciation [dɪ,priːʃɪ'eɪʃən] *n* 1) обесценение;

2) амортизация; изнашивание; 3) умаление, пренебрежение.

depreciatory [dɪ'priːʃjətərɪ] *a* 1) обесценивающий; 2) умаляющий.

depredation [ˌdeprɪ'deɪʃən] *n обыкн. pl* грабёж; опустошение, разорение (*страны*).

depredator ['deprɪdeɪtə] *n* грабитель, мародёр.

depress [dɪ'pres] *v* 1) угнетать, подавлять; удручать; 2) ослаблять (*деятельность, активность*); 3) опускать; понижать (*голос и т. п.*).

depressing [dɪ'presɪŋ] *a* гнетущий, тягостный.

depression [dɪ'preʃən] *n* 1) угнетённое состояние, уныние; 2) *эк.* депрессия, застой; 3) падение, снижение (*давления и т. п.*); 4) впадина, углубление.

deprivation [ˌdeprɪ'veɪʃən] *n* 1) лишение; потеря; 2) отстранение (*от должности*).

deprive [dɪ'praɪv] *v* лишать (*чего-л. — of*).

depth [depθ] *n* 1) глубина; *pl* глубины; пучина; 2) середина; in the ~ of night глубокой ночью; in the ~ of winter среди зимы; 3) густота (*цвета*); ◊ to get (*или* to go) out of one's ~ потерять почву под ногами, растеряться.

deputation [ˌdepjuː'teɪʃən] *n* 1) депутация, делегация; 2) делегирование.

depute [dɪ'pjuːt] *v* 1) передавать полномочия (*заместителю*); 2) назначать заместителем; 3) делегировать.

deputize ['depjutaɪz] *v* 1) назначать депутатом, делегировать; 2) представлять кого-л.; 3) замещать, заменять; дублировать (*об актёре*).

deputy ['depjutɪ] *n* 1) депутат; делегат; представитель; 2) заместитель, помощник.

deracinate [dɪ'ræsɪneɪt] *v* вырывать с корнем; искоренять.

derail [dɪ'reɪl] *v* 1) устраивать крушение (*поезда*); 2) сходить с рельсов.

derailment [dɪ'reɪlmənt] *n* крушение (*поезда*).

derange [dɪ'reɪndʒ] *v* 1) приводить в беспорядок; расстраивать; 2) доводить до сумасшествия.

derangement [dɪ'reɪndʒment] *n* 1) приведение в беспорядок; 2) психическое расстройство.

Derby ['dɑːbɪ] *n* дерби (*скачки*).

derby ['dɑːbɪ] *n амер.* котелок (*мужская шляпа*).

derelict ['derɪlɪkt] *a* покинутый, брошенный, оставленный.

dereliction [ˌderɪ'lɪkʃən] *n* 1) оставление; 2) заброшенность; 3) упущение; нарушение долга; 4) отступление моря от берега.

deride [dɪ'raɪd] *v* высмеивать, осмеивать.

derision [dɪ'rɪʒən] *n* 1) высмеивание, осмеяние; насмешка; to have (*или* to hold) in ~ насмехаться; to be in ~ быть посмешищем; ~ посмешище.

derisive [dɪ'raɪsɪv] *a* 1) насмешливый, иронический; 2) смехотворный.

derisory [dɪ'raɪsərɪ] *см.* derisive.

derivation [ˌderɪ'veɪʃən] *n* 1) происхождение; начало, источник; 2) установление происхождения; этимология (*слова*); 3) отвод (*воды*); 4) *эл.* ответвление; 5) отклонение (*стрелки и т. п.*).

derivative I [dɪ'rɪvətɪv] *n* 1) *грам.* производное слово; 2) *мат.* производная (*функция*).

derivative II *a* производный.

derive [dɪ'raɪv] *v* 1) происходить от; 2) устанавливать происхождение; производить (*слово и т. п.*); 3) получать; извлекать; 4) наследовать (*черту характера, признак*); 5) отводить (*воду*); 6) *эл.* ответвлять.

derogate ['derəgeɪt] *v* 1) умалять (*заслуги и т. п.*); 2) унижаться, ронять своё достоинство.

derogation [ˌderə'geɪʃən] *n* 1) умаление (*заслуг, прав*); 2) унижение.

derogatory [dɪ'rɔgətərɪ] *a* 1) умаляющий; унижающий; 2) унизительный.

derrick ['derɪk] *n* 1) *тех.* деррик-кран, подъёмная машина; 2) буровая вышка.

derring-do ['derɪŋ'duː] *n* отчаянная храбрость.

dervish ['dɜːvɪʃ] *n* дервиш.

descant[a] ['deskænt] *n* 1) мелодия, напев; песня; 2) *муз.* дискант; 3) длинное рассуждение.

descant[b] [dɪs'kænt] *v* 1) напевать; 2) распространяться (*о чём-л. — ирон.*).

descend [dɪ'send] *v* 1) спускаться, сходить; 2) опускаться; снижаться; 3) происходить (*from*); 4) переходить, передаваться по наследству; 5) обрушиваться, нападать (*upon*).

descendant [dɪ'sendənt] *n* потомок; direct ~ потомок по прямой линии.

descent [dɪ'sent] *n* 1) спуск; снижение; controlled ~ *косм.* управляемый спуск; 2) склон, скат; 3) понижение (*температуры*); 4) передача по наследству; 5) происхождение; 6) поколение; 7) внезапное нападение (*особ. с моря*); десант.

describe [dɪs'kraɪb] *v* 1) описывать, изображать; характеризовать (*as*); 2) описывать (*круг, кривую*); чертить.

description [dɪs'krɪpʃən] *n* 1) описание; изображение; to baffle (*или* to beggar, to defy) all ~ не поддаваться описанию; to answer to the ~ соответствовать описанию; 2) вид, род, сорт.

descriptive [dɪs'krɪptɪv] *a* описательный; изобразительный; наглядный.

descry [dɪs'kraɪ] *v* разглядеть, заметить, увидеть.

desecrate ['desɪkreɪt] *v* осквернять (*святыню*).

desecration [ˌdesɪ'kreɪʃən] *n* осквернение; профанация.

desert[a] I ['dezət] *n* 1) пустыня; 2) *разг.* скучная тема, скучное занятие и т. п.

desert[a] II *a* пустынный; необитаемый.

desert[b1] [dɪ'zɜːt] *n* заслуга; to get (*или* to obtain, to meet with) one's ~s получить по заслугам.

desert[b2] *v* 1) покидать, оставлять; 2) *воен.* дезертировать.

deserter [dɪ'zɜːtə] *n* дезертир.

desertion [dɪ'zɜːʃən] *n* 1) оставление (*семьи и т. п.*); 2) дезертирство; 3) заброшенность.

deserve [dɪ'zɜːv] *v* заслуживать, быть достойным; to ~ well of one's country иметь большие заслуги перед родиной.

deservedly [dɪ'zɜːvɪdlɪ] *adv* заслуженно, по заслугам, по достоинству.

deserving [dɪ'zɜːvɪŋ] *a* достойный, заслуживающий (*внимания и т. п.*).

desiccate ['desɪkeɪt] *v* 1) высушивать, обезвоживать; 2) высыхать.

desiderata [dɪ,zɪdə'reɪtə] *pl см.* desideratum.

desiderate [dɪ'zɪdəreɪt] *v* чувствовать отсутствие чего-л.; желать чего-л.

desiderative [dɪ'zɪdərətɪv] *a* выражающий желание.

desideratum [dɪ,zɪdə'reɪtəm] *n* (*pl* desiderata) что-л. недостающее, желаемое.

design I [dɪ'zaɪn] *n* 1) замысел, намерение; by ~, with a ~ намеренно; 2) (злой) умысел; ~s upon smb. (дурные) замыслы против кого-л.; 3) проект, план; набросок; чертёж; 4) конструкция; 5) эскиз; рисунок; узор.

design II *v* 1) замышлять; намереваться; 2) предназначать; 3) составлять план; планировать, проектировать; 4) конструировать; 5) рисовать; делать наброски, эскизы.

designateᵃ ['dezɪgnɪt] *a* назначенный.

designateᵇ ['dezɪgneɪt] *v* 1) определять; обозначать; указывать; 2) назначать на должность (*as, to, for*); 3) предназначать.

designation [,dezɪg'neɪʃən] *n* 1) обозначение; указание; 2) назначение (на должность).

designedly [dɪ'zaɪnɪdlɪ] *adv* намеренно, умышленно.

designer [dɪ'zaɪnə] *n* 1) проектировщик, конструктор; 2) художник, модельер; 3) чертёжник; 4) интриган.

designing I [dɪ'zaɪnɪŋ] *n* 1) проектирование, конструирование; 2) интриганство.

designing II *a* 1) планирующий, проектирующий; 2) коварный.

desirability [dɪ,zaɪərə'bɪlɪtɪ] *n* желательность.

desirable [dɪ'zaɪərəbl] *a* желательный; желанный.

desire I [dɪ'zaɪə] *n* 1) (сильное) желание; страсть; 2) предмет желания; 3) просьба, требование.

desire II *v* 1) желать; хотеть; 2) просить, требовать.

desirous [dɪ'zaɪərəs] *a* жаждущий чего-л.; (сильно) желающий.

desist [dɪ'zɪst] *v* прекращать, переставать.

desk [desk] *n* 1) письменный стол; 2) конторка; 3) парта; 4) пюпитр.

desolateᵃ ['desəlɪt] *a* 1) необитаемый; покинутый; 2) запущенный; разрушенный; 3) унылый; несчастный, неутешный.

desolateᵇ ['desəleɪt] *v* 1) разрушать; опустошать; обезлюдить (*страну*); 2) покидать; делать несчастным.

desolation [,desə'leɪʃən] *n* 1) опустошение, разорение; запустение; 2) заброшенность, одиночество; уныние.

despair I [dɪs'pɛə] *n* 1) отчаяние; безнадёжность; to fall into ~ приходить в отчаяние; 2) источник огорчения.

despair II *v* отчаиваться; терять надежду (*на — of*).

despairingly [dɪs'pɛərɪŋlɪ] *adv* безнадёжно; с отчаянием; в отчаянии.

despatch [dɪs'pætʃ] *см.* dispatch.

desperado [,despə'rɑːdou] *n* отчаянный человек; сорвиголова.

desperate ['despərɪt] *a* 1) отчаявшийся, потерявший надежду; безрассудный; 2) отчаянный, безнадёжный; 3) ужасный, отъявленный.

desperation [,despə'reɪʃən] *n* 1) отчаяние, безнадёжность; 2) безрассудство; to drive to ~ *разг.* довести до крайности, до бешенства.

despicable ['despɪkəbl] *a* презренный.

despise [dɪs'paɪz] *v* презирать, не выносить.

despite I [dɪs'paɪt] *prep* несмотря на.

despite II *n*: in one's ~ назло кому-л.; in ~ of вопреки.

despiteful [dɪs'paɪtful] *a* злобный.

despoil [dɪs'pɔɪl] *v* грабить.

despoilment [dɪs'pɔɪlmənt] *n* грабёж, расхищение.

despoliation [dɪs,poulɪ'eɪʃən] *см.* despoilment.

despond [dɪs'pɔnd] *v* терять надежду, падать духом.

despondency [dɪs'pɔndənsɪ] *n* уныние, подавленность.

despondent [dɪs'pɔndənt] *a* унылый, подавленный.

despot ['despɔt] *n* деспот, тиран.

despotic [des'pɔtɪk] *a* деспотический.

despotism ['despətɪzəm] *n* 1) деспотизм; 2) деспотия.

dessert [dɪ'zɜːt] *n* 1) десерт, сладкое (блюдо); 2) *attr* десертный.

destination [,destɪ'neɪʃən] *n* назначение; место назначения.

destine ['destɪn] *v* предназначать; предопределять.

destined ['destɪnd] *a* предназначенный.

destiny ['destɪnɪ] *n* судьба.

destitute ['destɪtjuːt] *a* 1) сильно нуждающийся, бедный; 2) лишённый (*чего-л. — of*).

destitution [,destɪ'tjuːʃən] *n* лишения; нужда, бедность.

destroy [dɪs'trɔɪ] *v* разрушать; уничтожать, истреблять.

destroyer [dɪs'trɔɪə] *n* 1) разрушитель; 2) *мор.* эскадренный миноносец.

destruction [dɪs'trʌkʃən] *n* 1) разрушение; 2) разорение; 3) причина гибели *или* разорения.

destructive [dɪs'trʌktɪv] *a* 1) разрушительный; 2) вредный; пагубный, гибельный.

desuetude [dɪ'sjuːɪtjuːd] *n* неупотребительность; to fall into ~ выходить из употребления.

desultory ['desəltərɪ] *a* несвязный, отрывочный; беспорядочный.

detach [dɪ'tætʃ] *v* 1) отвязывать, откреплять, отделять; 2) *воен., мор.* выделять, отряжать, откомандировывать.

detachable [dɪ'tætʃəbl] *a* 1) отделимый; 2) отрывной.

detached [dɪ'tætʃt] *a* 1) отдельный, обособленный; одиночный; 2) независимый (*об уме и т. п.*); беспристрастный; 3) *воен., мор.* выделенный, откомандированный.

detachment [dɪ'tætʃmənt] *n* 1) отделение, разъединение; выделение; 2) обособленность, отчуждённость; 3) *воен., мор.* отряд, выделенное подразделение.

detail I ['diːteɪl] *n* 1) подробность, деталь; частность; in ~ подробно; to go (*или* to enter) into ~s вдаваться в подробности; 2) *pl* детали, части, элементы; 3) *воен.* наряд, команда.

detail II *v* 1) подробно рассказывать, перечисля́ть все дета́ли; 2) *воен.* откомандиро́вывать, выделя́ть, наряжа́ть.

detain [dɪ'teɪn] *v* 1) заде́рживать; заставля́ть ждать; 2) замедля́ть; меша́ть (*движению*); 3) уде́рживать (*деньги и т. п.*); 4) держа́ть под стра́жей.

detect [dɪ'tekt] *v* 1) обнару́живать, выявля́ть, открыва́ть; 2) *радио* детекти́ровать, выпрямля́ть.

detection [dɪ'tekʃən] *n* 1) откры́тие, обнаруже́ние; 2) *радио* детекти́рование.

detective I [dɪ'tektɪv] *n* сы́щик.

detective II *a* сыскно́й; детекти́вный.

detector [dɪ'tektə] *n* 1) *радио* дете́ктор; 2) *тех.* указа́тель, индика́тор.

détente [de'tɑːt, deɪ'tɔnt] *n полит.* разря́дка (междунаро́дной напряжённости).

detention [dɪ'tenʃən] *n* 1) задержа́ние; содержа́ние под стра́жей; 2) вы́нужденная заде́ржка; 3) *шк.* оставле́ние по́сле уро́ков (*наказание*).

deter [dɪ'təː]- *v* уде́рживать, отгова́ривать (*от чего-л.— from*).

detergent I [dɪ'təːdʒənt] *n* дезинфици́рующее сре́дство.

detergent II *a* очища́ющий.

deteriorate [dɪ'tɪərɪəreɪt] *v* ухудша́ть(ся); по́ртить(ся).

deterioration [dɪ,tɪərɪə'reɪʃən] *n* ухудше́ние; по́рча; изна́шивание.

deteriorative [dɪ'tɪərɪə,reɪtɪv] *a* ухудша́ющий(ся).

determinant I [dɪ'təːmɪnənt] *n* 1) реша́ющий, определя́ющий фа́ктор; 2) *мат.* детермина́нт, определи́тель.

determinant II *a* реша́ющий, определя́ющий.

determinate [dɪ'təːmɪnɪt] *a* 1) определённый; 2) оконча́тельный; 3) реши́тельный.

determination [dɪ,təːmɪ'neɪʃən] *n* 1) реши́тельность, реши́мость; 2) определе́ние; 3) реше́ние.

determinative I [dɪ'təːmɪnətɪv] *n* 1) реша́ющий фа́ктор; 2) *грам.* определя́ющее сло́во.

determinative II *a* определя́ющий, реша́ющий.

determine [dɪ'təːmɪn] *v* 1) определя́ть, устана́вливать; ограни́чивать; реша́ть(ся); 3) назнача́ть (*дату и т. п.*); 4) заставля́ть, побужда́ть (*to*); направля́ть (*внимание и т. п.*); 5) конча́ть; 6) конча́ться; истека́ть (*о сроке*).

determined [dɪ'təːmɪnd] *a* реши́тельный, твёрдый.

deterrent [dɪ'terənt] *a* сде́рживающий, препя́тствующий.

detest [dɪ'test] *v* пита́ть отвраще́ние; ненави́деть.

detestable [dɪ'testəbl] *a* отврати́тельный; ненави́стный.

detestation [,diːtes'teɪʃən] *n* 1) отвраще́ние; не́нависть; to hold (*или* to have) in ~ ненави́деть; 2) предме́т не́нависти, отвраще́ния.

dethrone [dɪ'θroun] *v* сверга́ть с престо́ла; *перен.* развенча́ивать.

dethronement [dɪ'θrounmənt] *n* сверже́ние с престо́ла; *перен.* развенча́ние.

detonate ['detouneɪt] *v* взрыва́ть(ся); детони́ровать.

detonation [,detou'neɪʃən] *n* взрыв; детона́ция.

detonator ['detouneɪtə] *n* детона́тор.

detour ['deɪtuə] *n* отклоне́ние (от прямо́го

пути́); око́льный путь; to make a ~ сде́лать крюк.

detract [dɪ'trækt] *v* 1) принижа́ть, умаля́ть; 2) уменьша́ть.

detraction [dɪ'trækʃən] *n* 1) приниже́ние, умале́ние; 2) злосло́вие.

detractive [dɪ'træktɪv] *a* 1) умаля́ющий; унижа́ющий; 2) поро́чащий.

detrain [diː'treɪn] *v* 1) выса́живать(ся) из по́езда; 2) выгружа́ть (ваго́ны).

detriment ['detrɪmənt] *n* уще́рб, вред; without ~ to без уще́рба для.

detrimental [,detrɪ'mentl] *a* 1) убы́точный; 2) вре́дный.

detrition [dɪ'trɪʃən] *n* стира́ние, изна́шивание от тре́ния.

detruncate [diː'trʌŋkeɪt] *v* укора́чивать, обруба́ть, среза́ть.

detune [diː'tjuːn] *v радио* расстра́ивать.

deuce[1] [djuːs] *n* 1) дво́йка, два очка́; 2) ра́вный счёт (*в те́ннисе*).

deuce[2] *n* чёрт (*в восклица́ниях*); ~ take it! чёрт возьми́!; what the ~ како́го чёрта; to play the ~ with по́ртить, губи́ть; ~ a bit ничу́ть.

deuced I [djuːst] *a* черто́вский; ужа́сный.

deuced II *adv* черто́вски, ужа́сно.

devaluation [,diːvælju'eɪʃən] *n* обесце́нение.

devastate ['devəsteɪt] *v* опустоша́ть, разоря́ть.

devastation [,devəs'teɪʃən] *n* опустоше́ние, разоре́ние.

develop [dɪ'veləp] *v* 1) развива́ть(ся); 2) соверше́нствовать; 3) обнару́живать(ся), проявля́ть(ся); 4) *фото* проявля́ть.

developer [dɪ'veləpə] *n фото* прояви́тель.

development [dɪ'veləpmənt] *n* 1) разви́тие; рост; расшире́ние; 2) усоверше́нствование; улучше́ние; 3) раскры́тие; обнаруже́ние; 4) положе́ние дел, обстоя́тельства; 5) *фото* проявле́ние.

deviate ['diːvɪeɪt] *v* отклоня́ться.

deviation [,diːvɪ'eɪʃən] *n* 1) отклоне́ние; девиа́ция (*компаса*); 2) *полит.* укло́н.

device [dɪ'vaɪs] *n* 1) приспособле́ние; устро́йство; механи́зм; 2) план, схе́ма; прое́кт; 3) сре́дство, спо́соб; 4) зате́я, изобрете́ние; 5) эмбле́ма; деви́з; ◊ left to one's own ~s предоста́вленный самому́ себе́.

devil I ['devl] *n* 1) дья́вол, чёрт; the ~ a bit чёрта с два; what the ~ како́го чёрта; a ~ to work рабо́тает как чёрт; 2) помо́щник, челове́к, рабо́тающий за друго́го; printer's ~ ма́льчик на посы́лках в типогра́фии; 3) (ло́вкий, хи́трый) па́рень; 4): poor ~ бедня́га; ◊ ~ among the tailors сумато́ха, сва́лка; blue ~s хандра́; between the ~ and the deep sea в безвы́ходном положе́нии; ≅ ме́жду двух огне́й; to raise the ~ шуме́ть, буя́нить; ~ take the hindmost! к чёрту отста́ющих!; to give the ~ his due отдава́ть до́лжное проти́внику; talk of the ~ and he will appear ≅ лёгок на поми́не; to play the ~ with причини́ть вред, испо́ртить.

devil II *v* рабо́тать на, за кого́-л. (*for*).

devildom ['devldəm] *n* дья́вольщина, чертовщи́на.

devil-fish ['devlfɪʃ] *n зоол.* 1) скат; 2) осьмино́г; 3) карака́тица.

devilish I ['devlɪʃ] *a* дья́вольский; а́дский.

devilish II *adv* дья́вольски, черто́вски, ужа́сно.

devil-may-care ['devlmeı'kɛə] *a* беспе́чный, безрассу́дный, бесшаба́шный.

devilry ['devlrı] *n* 1) дья́вольщина, чёрная ма́гия; 2) (дья́вольская) зло́ба; 3) прока́зы.

deviltry ['devltrı] *см.* devilry.

devious ['di:vjəs] *a* 1) отклоня́ющийся от прямо́го пути́; блужда́ющий; 2) око́льный, кру́жный; изви́листый; 3) отдалённый; уединённый; 4) нейскренний; нече́стный.

devise [dı'vaız] *v* 1) приду́мывать, изобрета́ть; плани́ровать; 2) *юр.* завеща́ть (*недвижимость*); 3) предназнача́ть.

devisee [,devı'zi:] *n юр.* насле́дник.

deviser [dı'vaızə] *n* 1) изобрета́тель; 2) *юр.* завеща́тель.

devisor [devı'zɔ:] *см.* deviser 2).

devoid [dı'vɔıd] *a* лишённый (*чего-л.— of*); не име́ющий (*чего-л.— of*); ~ of fear бесстра́шный.

devoir ['devwɑ:] *n* долг, обя́занность; *pl* акт ве́жливости; to pay one's ~s to smb. засвиде́тельствовать почте́ние кому́-л.

devolution [,di:və'lu:ʃən] *n* 1) переда́ча (*власти, полномо́чий и т. п.*); 2) *биол.* вырожде́ние, регре́сс.

devolve [dı'vɔlv] *v* 1) переходи́ть к кому́-л. (*о должности, обязанности*); 2) передава́ть (*обязанности, полномочия*); 3) переходи́ть по насле́дству.

Devonian I [de'vounjən] *n* 1) уроже́нец Де́воншира; 2) *геол.* дево́нский пери́од.

Devonian II *a* 1) девонши́рский; 2) *геол.* дево́нский.

devote [dı'vout] *v* посвяща́ть (себя́), отдава́ться (*чему-л. — to*).

devoted [dı'voutıd] *a* 1) пре́данный; 2) посвящённый (*чему-л., кому-л.*); 3) обречённый; 4) увлека́ющийся.

devotedly [dı'voutıdlı] *adv* пре́данно, не́жно.

devotee [,devou'ti:] *n* 1) энтузиа́ст (*чего-л. — of*); 2) фана́тик; свято́ша.

devotion [dı'vouʃən] *n* 1) пре́данность; привя́занность; 2) на́божность.

devotional [dı'vouʃənl] *a* благочести́вый; на́божный.

devour [dı'vauə] *v* пожира́ть; жа́дно есть; *перен.* поглоща́ть; уничтожа́ть; ~ed by anxiety снеда́емый беспоко́йством.

devouringly [dı'vauərıŋlı] *adv* жа́дно.

devout [dı'vaut] *a* 1) благочести́вый; благогове́йный; 2) ́искренний (*о положении и т. п.*).

dew I [dju:] *n* 1) роса́; 2) ка́пля, роси́нка, слеза́; 3) све́жесть.

dew II *v* 1) ороша́ть, сма́чивать; 2) *обыкн. безл.* покрыва́ть росо́й; it is beginning to ~ выпада́ет роса́.

dewberry ['dju:berı] *n* ежеви́ка.

dew-drop ['dju:drɔp] *n* ка́пля́ росы́, роси́нка.

dew-fall ['dju:fɔ:l] *n* вре́мя появле́ния росы́, ве́чер.

dew-point ['dju:pɔınt] *n физ.* то́чка росы́; температу́ра конденса́ции.

dewy ['dju:ı] *a* 1) роси́стый; покры́тый росо́й; 2) вла́жный; 3) све́жий, освежа́ющий.

dexter ['dekstə] *a* пра́вый.

dexterity [deks'terıtı] *n* ло́вкость, сноро́вка; прово́рство.

dexterous ['dekstərəs] *a* 1) ло́вкий; прово́рный; 2) иску́сный, уме́лый.

dextrose ['dekstrous] *n хим.* виногра́дный са́хар, глюко́за.

dextrous ['dekstrəs] *см.* dexterous.

di- [dı-, daı-] *pref* 1) дву-, двух-; dichromatic двухцве́тный; 2) см. dia-.

dia- ['daıə-] *pref означает* че́рез, сквозь.

diabetes [daıə'bi:ti:z] *n мед.* са́харная боле́знь, диабе́т.

diabetic I [,daıə'betık] *n* больно́й диабе́том, диабе́тик.

diabetic II *a* диабети́ческий.

diabolic(al) [,daıə'bɔlık(əl)] *a* 1) дья́вольский; 2) (о́чень) злой, жесто́кий.

diabolism [daı'æbəlızəm] *n* 1) колдовство́, волшебство́; 2) дья́вольская зло́ба, жесто́кость.

diacritic I [,daıə'krıtık] *n лингв.* диакрити́ческий знак.

diacritic II *a лингв.* диакрити́ческий.

diacritical [,daıə'krıtıkəl] *см.* diacritic II.

diadem I ['daıədem] *n* диаде́ма; вене́ц, коро́на.

diadem II *v* венча́ть коро́ной.

diagnose ['daıəgnouz] *n* ста́вить диа́гноз.

diagnosis [,daıəg'nousıs] *n* (*pl* diagnoses [,daıəg'nousi:z]) диа́гноз.

diagnostic I [,daıəg'nɔstık] *n* 1) симпто́м; 2) *pl* диагно́стика.

diagnostic II *a* диагности́ческий.

diagonal I [daı'ægənl] *n* диагона́ль.

diagonal II *a* диагона́льный, иду́щий на́искось.

diagram I ['daıəgræm] *n* диагра́мма; схе́ма.

diagram II *v* 1) составля́ть диагра́мму, схе́му; 2) представля́ть в ви́де диагра́ммы, схе́мы.

diagrammatic [,daıəgrə'mætık] *a* схемати́ческий.

dial I ['daıəl] *n* 1) цифербла́т; кру́глая шкала́; номерно́й диск (*автоматического телефона*); 2) *сленг* кру́глое лицо́, «луна́».

dial II *v* набира́ть но́мер (*по автоматическому телефо́ну*).

dialect ['daıəlekt] *n лингв.* диале́кт, наре́чие, го́вор.

dialectal [,daıə'lektl] *a лингв.* диалекта́льный.

dialectical [,daıə'lektıkəl] *a* диалекти́ческий.

dialectician [,daıəlek'tıʃən] *n* диале́ктик.

dialectics [,daıə'lektıks] *n* диале́ктика; Marxist ~ маркси́стская диале́ктика; natural ~ диале́ктика приро́ды.

dialectology [,daıəlek'tɔlədʒı] *n* диалектоло́гия.

dialogue ['daıəlɔg] *n* разгово́р; диало́г.

diameter [daı'æmıtə] *n* диа́метр.

diametral [daı'æmıtrəl] *a* диаметра́льный, попере́чный.

diametrical [,daıə'metrıkəl] *a* диаметра́льный.

diametrically [,daıə'metrıkəlı] *adv* диаметра́льно; ~ opposed диаметра́льно противополо́жный.

diamond I ['daıəmənd] *n* 1) алма́з; бриллиа́нт; black ~ чёрный алма́з; карбона́т; sham ~ фальши́вый бриллиа́нт; rough ~ нешлифо́ванный алма́з; *перен.* грубова́тый, но хоро́ший, че́стный челове́к; 2) алма́з для ре́зки стекла́; 3) ромб; 4) *pl карт.* бу́бны; 5) *амер.* площа́дка для игры́ в бейсбо́л; ◊ ~ cut ~ *погов.* ≅ нашла́ коса́ на ка́мень.

diamond II *a* 1) алма́зный; бриллиа́нтовый; 2) ромбови́дный.

diamond III *v* украша́ть бриллиа́нтами.

diamond-field ['daɪəməndfiːld] *n* алма́зная копь.

diapason [,daɪə'peɪsn] *n* 1) диапазо́н; 2) основно́й реги́стр орга́на.

diaper I ['daɪəpə] *n* 1) узо́рчатое полотно́; 2) пелёнка; 3) ромбови́дный узо́р.

diaper II *v* 1) украша́ть узо́ром; 2) *амер.* пелена́ть.

diaphanous [daɪ'æfənəs] *a* прозра́чный.

diaphragm ['daɪəfræm] *n* 1) диафра́гма; 2) перегоро́дка; 3) мембра́на; 4) *бот., зоол.* перепо́нка.

diarrhoea [,daɪə'rɪə] *n мед.* поно́с.

diary ['daɪərɪ] *n* 1) дневни́к; to keep a ~ вести́ дневни́к; 2) записна́я кни́жка-календа́рь.

diathermic [,daɪə'θəːmɪk] *a физ.* теплопрово́дный.

diathermy ['daɪə,θəːmɪ] *n мед.* диатерми́я.

diatribe ['daɪətraɪb] *n* диатри́ба, ре́зкая кри́тика.

dibble ['dɪbl] *v с.-х.* сажа́ть под кол.

dibs [dɪbz] *n pl* 1) ба́бки (*игра́*); 2) фи́шки; 3) *сленг* де́ньги.

dice I [daɪs] *n* 1) *pl см.* die¹; 2) игра́ в ко́сти.

dice II *v* 1) игра́ть в ко́сти; 2) наре́зать в фо́рме ку́биков; 3) графи́ть в кле́тку.

dicer ['daɪsə] *n* игро́к в ко́сти.

dichromatic [,daɪkrou'mætɪk] *a* двухцве́тный.

dick¹ [dɪk] *n сленг:* to take one's ~ кля́сться, утвержда́ть.

dick² *n амер. сленг* сы́щик.

dickens ['dɪkɪnz] *n разг.* чёрт.

dicker¹ ['dɪkə] *n* деся́ток, дю́жина (*кож, шкур и т. п.*).

dicker² I *n амер.* ме́лкая сде́лка.

dicker² II *v* торгова́ться по мелоча́м; заключа́ть ме́лкие сде́лки.

dickey ['dɪkɪ] *n* 1) (пристёгиваемая) мани́шка; 2) де́тский нагру́дник; 3) пта́шка; 4) осёл; 5) сиде́нье для ку́чера.

dicky¹ ['dɪkɪ] *n см.* dickey.

dicky² *a* 1) *сленг* сла́бый; неусто́йчивый; 2) ненадёжный.

dicta ['dɪktə] *pl см.* dictum.

dictaphone [,dɪktəfoun] *n* диктофо́н.

dictateᵃ ['dɪkteɪt] *n* 1) *обыкн. pl* предписа́ние; наставле́ние; веле́ние; 2) *полит.* дикта́т.

dictateᵇ [dɪk'teɪt] *n* 1) диктова́ть; 2) предпи́сывать; диктова́ть (*усло́вия и т. п.*).

dictation [dɪk'teɪʃən] *n* 1) дикто́вка; дикта́нт; 2) предписа́ние.

dictator [dɪk'teɪtə] *n* дикта́тор.

dictatorial [,dɪktə'tɔːrɪəl] *a* 1) дикта́торский (*о вла́сти*); 2) вла́стный, повели́тельный.

dictatorship [dɪk'teɪtəʃɪp] *n* диктату́ра; ~ of the proletariat диктату́ра пролетариа́та.

diction ['dɪkʃən] *n* 1) стиль, мане́ра выраже́ния мы́слей; 2) ди́кция.

dictionary ['dɪkʃənrɪ] *n* слова́рь; a pronouncing ~ фонети́ческий слова́рь.

dictum ['dɪktəm] *n* (*pl тж.* dicta) 1) изрече́ние; погово́рка; 2) (авторите́тное) заявле́ние.

did [dɪd] *past см.* doᵃ I.

didactic [dɪ'dæktɪk] *a* дидакти́ческий, поучи́тельный.

didactics [dɪ'dæktɪks] *n* дида́ктика.

diddle ['dɪdl] *v сленг* 1) обма́нывать, надува́ть; подшу́чивать (*над кем-л.*); 2) зря тра́тить вре́мя, болта́ться.

dido ['daɪdou] *n амер. разг.* ша́лость, прока́за, шу́тка; to cut up ~es дура́читься, шали́ть.

die¹ [daɪ] *n* (*pl* dice) игра́льная кость; фи́шка; *перен.* слу́чай; уда́ча; the ~ is cast жре́бий бро́шен; to be upon the ~ быть поста́вленным на ка́рту.

die² I *n* (*pl* dies) штамп; ма́трица.

die² II *v* штампова́ть, чека́нить.

die³ *v* 1) умира́ть (*от чего-л. — of, from; за что-л. — for*); 2) конча́ться; исчеза́ть; 3) ослабева́ть; замира́ть (*о зву́ках*); затиха́ть (*о ве́тре*); 4) *разг.* си́льно хоте́ть (*обыкн.* to be dying for); □ to ~ **away** a) увяда́ть; ча́хнуть; б) замира́ть, затиха́ть (*о зву́ке, ве́тре*); в) па́дать в о́бморок; to ~ off a) отмира́ть; б) умира́ть оди́н за други́м; to ~ **out** a) вымира́ть; б) прекраща́ться; ◇ to ~ in the last ditch стоя́ть на́смерть; to ~ in harness умере́ть на посту́; to ~ in one's boots умере́ть наси́льственной сме́ртью; never say ~! никогда́ не уныва́й(те), не отча́ивайтесь!

die-hard ['daɪhɑːd] *n полит.* твердоло́бый, консерва́тор.

diesis ['daɪɪsɪs] *n* (*pl* dieses ['daɪɪsiːz]) 1) *муз.* дие́з; 2) *полигр.* знак сно́ски в ви́де двойно́го кре́стика.

diet¹ I ['daɪət] *n* 1) пи́ща, стол; 2) дие́та.

diet¹ II *v* быть на дие́те; держа́ть кого́-л. на дие́те; to ~ oneself соблюда́ть дие́ту.

diet² *n* 1) парла́мент (*не англи́йский*); 2) (междунаро́дная) конфере́нция.

dietary I ['daɪətərɪ] *n* 1) дие́та; 2) паёк.

dietary II *a* диети́ческий.

dietetic [,daɪɪ'tetɪk] *a* дие(те)ти́ческий.

differ ['dɪfə] *v* 1) отлича́ться, различа́ться, ра́зниться (*from*); 2) не соглаша́ться, расходи́ться (*во мне́ниях и т. п.; from, with*); to agree to ~ отказа́ться от попы́ток убеди́ть друг дру́га.

difference I ['dɪfrəns] *n* 1) ра́зница, разли́чие; to split the ~ соглаша́ться, идти́ на компроми́сс; it makes a great ~ э́то больша́я ра́зница, э́то о́чень ва́жно; 2) отличи́тельный при́знак; specific ~ *биол.* видово́е разли́чие; 3) разногла́сие; ссо́ра; 4) *мат.* ра́зность.

difference II *v* 1) отлича́ть; 2) *мат.* вычисля́ть ра́зность.

different ['dɪfrənt] *a* 1) друго́й, непохо́жий; несхо́дный; that is quite ~ э́то совсе́м друго́е де́ло; 2) ра́зный; разли́чный.

differential I [,dɪfə'renʃəl] *n мат.* дифференциа́л.

differential II *a* 1) *мат.* дифференциа́льный; 2) различа́ющийся; 3) отличи́тельный.

differentiate [,dɪfə'renʃɪeɪt] *v* 1) различа́ть(ся); отлича́ть(ся); 2) дифференци́ровать(ся); 3) видоизменя́ться.

differentiation [,dɪfərenʃɪ'eɪʃən] *n* 1) различе́ние; 2) дифференциа́ция; 3) видоизмене́ние.

differently ['dɪfrəntlɪ] *adv* разли́чно; по-друго́му, ина́че.

difficult ['dɪfɪkəlt] *a* 1) тру́дный; 2) тяжёлый (*о хара́ктере и т. п.*); 3) затрудни́тельный.

difficulty ['dɪfɪkəltɪ] *n* 1) тру́дность; to stem

difficulties боро́ться с тру́дностями; 2) затрудне́ние; препя́тствие.

diffidence [ˈdɪfɪdəns] *n* скро́мность; ро́бость, неуве́ренность в себе́.

diffident [ˈdɪfɪdənt] *a* скро́мный; ро́бкий, неуве́ренный в себе́.

diffluent [ˈdɪfluənt] *a* 1) растека́ющийся, расплыва́ющийся; 2) переходя́щий в жи́дкое состоя́ние; 3) раствори́мый.

diffract [dɪˈfrækt] *v* преломля́ть, отклоня́ть (*лучи*).

diffuse[a] [dɪˈfjuːs] *a* 1) разбро́санный; рассе́янный (*о свете*); 2) многосло́вный.

diffuse[b] [dɪˈfjuːz] *v* 1) распространя́ть; рассе́ивать; 2) распыля́ть; рассыпа́ть, разбра́сывать.

diffusion [dɪˈfjuːʒən] *n* 1) распростране́ние; рассе́ивание; 2) *физ.* диффу́зия; 3) многосло́вие.

diffusive [dɪˈfjuːsɪv] *a* 1) распространя́ющийся; рассе́ивающийся; 2) *физ.* диффу́зный; 3) многосло́вный.

dig I [dɪg] *n разг.* 1) толчо́к, тычо́к; to give smb. a ~ in the ribs ткнуть кого́-л. в бок; 2) язви́тельное замеча́ние, насме́шка; to have a ~ at, to give one a ~ уязви́ть, заде́ть (*замеча́нием*); 3) *амер.* зубри́ла; 4) *pl* (снима́емая) ко́мната.

dig II *v* (*past, p. p.* dug) 1) копа́ть, рыть; 2) отка́пывать, выи́скивать; 3) *разг.* ты́кать, толка́ть; to ~ in the ribs, to ~ in the side ткнуть в бок; 4) *амер. разг.* усе́рдно рабо́тать; зубри́ть; □ to ~ down подка́пывать, подрыва́ть; to ~ for дока́пываться, иска́ть, выи́скивать; to ~ from выка́пывать; to ~ in, to ~ into a) зака́пывать, зарыва́ть; to ~ oneself in ока́пываться; б) вонза́ть (*шпоры и т. п.*); to ~ out a) выка́пывать, выи́скивать; б) *амер. разг.* поспе́шно уходи́ть, исчеза́ть; to ~ through прокопа́ть, проры́ть; to ~ up a) подка́пывать, подрыва́ть; б) поднима́ть целину́; в) *амер. разг.* добыва́ть, разы́скивать.

digest[a] [ˈdaɪdʒest] *n* кра́ткое изложе́ние, сво́дка; сбо́рник (*постановле́ний, анноте́ций и т. п.*); спра́вочник.

digest[b] [dɪˈdʒest] *v* 1) перева́ривать(ся) (*о пи́ще*); *перен.* усва́ивать; 2) осва́ивать (*террито́рию*); 3) систематизи́ровать; классифици́ровать; 4) переноси́ть, терпе́ть.

digestible [dɪˈdʒestəbl] *a* 1) удобовари́мый; 2) легко́ усва́иваемый.

digestion [dɪˈdʒestʃən] *n* 1) пищеваре́ние; 2) усвое́ние (*зна́ний и т. п.*).

digestive I [dɪˈdʒestɪv] *n* сре́дство, спосо́бствующее пищеваре́нию.

digestive II *a* 1) пищевари́тельный; 2) спосо́бствующий пищеваре́нию.

digger [ˈdɪgə] *n* 1) землеко́п; 2) горнорабо́чий; золотоиска́тель; 3) *сленг* австрали́ец; 4) приспособле́ние для копа́ния.

digging [ˈdɪgɪŋ] *n* 1) ко́пка, рытьё; земляны́е рабо́ты; 2) рудни́к; золоты́е при́иски; 3) *pl разг.* жили́ще; жильё.

digit [ˈdɪdʒɪt] *n* 1) па́лец; 2) ци́фра (*от 0 до 9*).

dignified [ˈdɪgnɪfaɪd] *a* 1) с чу́вством со́бственного досто́инства; 2) велича́вый; вели́чественный; 3) досто́йный (*о челове́ке*).

dignify [ˈdɪgnɪfaɪ] *v* 1) придава́ть досто́инство; облагора́живать; 2) удоста́ивать; 3) велича́ть.

dignitary [ˈdɪgnɪtərɪ] *n* сано́вник; высо́кое до́лжностно́е лицо́.

dignity [ˈdɪgnɪtɪ] *n* 1) досто́инство; благоро́дство; beneath one's ~ ни́же чьего́-л. досто́инства; to stand (up)on one's ~ держа́ться с больши́м досто́инством; 2) высо́кое зва́ние, сан, ти́тул; 3) *собир.* ли́ца высо́кого зва́ния; знать.

digraph [ˈdaɪgrɑːf] *n линг.* дигра́ф.

digress [daɪˈgres] *v* отступа́ть, отклоня́ться.

digression [daɪˈgreʃən] *n* отступле́ние, отклоне́ние.

dike I [daɪk] *n* 1) кана́ва, ров; 2) да́мба, плоти́на; 3) прегра́да, препя́тствие.

dike II *v* 1) ока́пывать рвом, кана́вой; 2) окружа́ть, защища́ть да́мбой; 3) осуша́ть, дрени́ровать ме́стность.

dilapidate [dɪˈlæpɪdeɪt] *v* 1) разруша́ть; 2) разва́ливаться; приходи́ть в упа́док; 3) расточа́ть.

dilapidated [dɪˈlæpɪdeɪtɪd] *a* 1) полуразру́шенный, ве́тхий; 2) разорённый.

dilapidation [dɪˌlæpɪˈdeɪʃən] *n* 1) обветша́ние; упа́док; 2) разоре́ние.

dilatation [ˌdaɪleɪˈteɪʃən] *n* 1) расшире́ние; 2) распростране́ние.

dilate [daɪˈleɪt] *v* 1) расширя́ть(ся); 2) распространя́ться, пуска́ться в подро́бности.

dilation [daɪˈleɪʃən] *см.* dilatation.

dilatory [ˈdɪlətərɪ] *a* 1) медли́тельный; 2) затяжно́й; 3) запозда́лый.

dilemma [dɪˈlemə] *n* диле́мма; затрудни́тельное положе́ние.

dilettante I [ˌdɪlɪˈtæntɪ] *n* (*pl* dilettanti [ˌdɪlɪˈtæntiː] дилета́нт, люби́тель.

dilettante II *a* дилета́нтский, люби́тельский.

diligence[a] [ˈdɪlɪdʒəns] *n* прилежа́ние, усе́рдие; трудолю́бие.

diligence[b] [ˈdɪlɪʒɑːns] *n* дилижа́нс.

diligent [ˈdɪlɪdʒənt] *a* приле́жный, усе́рдный; трудолюби́вый.

dill [dɪl] *n* укро́п.

dilly-dally [ˈdɪlɪdælɪ] *v разг.* колеба́ться; ме́шкать.

dilute I [daɪˈljuːt] *a* разба́вленный, разведённый.

dilute II *v* 1) разбавля́ть, разводи́ть, разжижа́ть; 2) выхола́щивать (*тео́рию и т. п.*).

dilution [daɪˈluːʃən] *n* 1) разбавле́ние, разжиже́ние; 2) ослабле́ние; 3) сла́бая концентра́ция.

dim I [dɪm] *a* 1) ту́склый, му́тный; 2) нея́сный; тума́нный (*о предме́тах, представле́ниях*); сму́тный (*о воспомина́ниях*); 3) тёмный, мра́чный (*о помеще́нии*); 4) сла́бый (*о зре́нии, восприя́тии*).

dim II *v* 1) де́лать ту́склым, тума́нным; 2) тускне́ть; затума́ниваться; □ to ~ out затемня́ть.

dime [daɪm] *n амер.* 1) моне́та в 10 це́нтов; 2) *attr* дешёвый (*о рома́не*).

dimension I [dɪˈmenʃən] *n* 1) измере́ние; 2) *pl* разме́ры, величина́.

dimension II *v* 1) проставля́ть разме́ры (*на чертеже́ и т. п.*); 2) придава́ть определённые разме́ры.

dimensional [dɪˈmenʃənl] *a* простра́нственный.

diminish [dɪˈmɪnɪʃ] *v* 1) уменьша́ть(ся); убавля́ть(ся); 2) унижа́ть.

diminished [dɪˈmɪnɪʃt] *a* 1) уме́ньшенный; осла́бленный; 2) уни́женный.

diminution [ˌdɪmɪˈnjuːʃən] *n* уменьшéние; сокращéние; ослаблéние.

diminutival [dɪˌmɪnjuˈtaɪvəl] *a грам.* уменьши́тельный.

diminutive I [dɪˈmɪnjutɪv] *n грам.* уменьши́тельное слóво; уменьши́тельный сýффикс.

diminutive II *a* 1) малюсенький; миниатю́рный; 2) *грам.* уменьши́тельный.

dimity [ˈdɪmɪtɪ] *n* 1) тóнкая бумáжная ткань; 2) ткань для занавéсок, портьéр.

dimness [ˈdɪmnɪs] *n* 1) тýсклость; 2) тумáнность.

dim-out [ˈdɪmaut] *n* затемнéние, светомаскирóвка.

dimple I [ˈdɪmpl] *n* 1) я́мочка (*на щеке, подбородке*); 2) небольшáя впáдина; 3) рябь (*на воде*).

dimple II *v* 1) ряби́ть (*воду*); 2) покрывáться я́мочками.

dimply [ˈdɪmplɪ] *a* 1) с я́мочками; 2) подёрнутый ря́бью (*о воде*).

din I [dɪn] *n* шум, грóхот.

din II *v* 1) шумéть; 2) долби́ть, повторя́ть однó и то же.

dine [daɪn] *v* 1) обéдать; to ~ out обéдать вне дóма; 2) угощáть обéдом; давáть обéд; ◊ to ~ with Duke Humphrey *шутл.* остáться без обéда.

diner [ˈdaɪnə] *n* 1) обéдающий; 2) вагóн-ресторáн.

diner-out [ˈdaɪnərˈaut] *n* человéк, чáсто обéдающий вне дóма, в гостя́х.

ding I [dɪŋ] *n* звон (кóлокола).

ding II *v* (*past, p. p.* dinged, dung) 1) звенéть; 2) *разг.* назóйливо повторя́ть, долби́ть.

ding-dong I [ˈdɪŋˈdɔŋ] *n* динь-дóн.

ding-dong II *a* череду́ющийся.

ding-dong III *adv разг.* настóйчиво, упóрно, серьёзно.

dingey [ˈdɪŋgɪ] *n* шлю́пка; я́лик.

dinghy [ˈdɪŋgɪ] *см.* dingey.

dingle [ˈdɪŋgl] *n* глубóкая лощи́на.

dingo [ˈdɪŋgou] *n* ди́нго (*дикая собака*).

dingy [ˈdɪndʒɪ] *a* тýсклый, тёмный; гря́зный.

dining-car [ˈdaɪnɪŋkɑː] *n* вагóн-ресторáн.

dining-room [ˈdaɪnɪŋrum] *n* столóвая.

dinkey [ˈdɪŋkɪ] *n амер. разг.* небольшóй паровóз; «куку́шка».

dinkum [ˈdɪŋkəm] *a австрал.* 1) настоя́щий, и́стинный; 2) чéстный, и́скренний.

dinky [ˈdɪŋkɪ] *a разг.* изя́щный; наря́дный.

dinner [ˈdɪnə] *n* обéд; to have (*или* to take) ~ обéдать; to give a ~ устрáивать звáный обéд; давáть обéд в честь когó-л.; basket ~ *амер.* пикни́к.

dinner-jacket [ˈdɪnəˌdʒækɪt] *n* смóкинг.

dinner-party [ˈdɪnəˌpɑːtɪ] *n* звáный обéд.

dinosaur [ˈdaɪnəsɔː] *n* динозáвр.

dint I [dɪnt] *n* 1) впáдина, след от удáра; 2): by ~ of посрéдством; путём.

dint II *v* оставля́ть след, впáдину.

diocese [ˈdaɪəsɪs] *n* епáрхия.

dioxide [daɪˈɔksaɪd] *n хим.* двуóкись.

dip I [dɪp] *n* 1) погружéние (*в воду и т. п.*); ныря́ние; to have (*или* to take, to go for) a ~ пойти́ вы́купаться, окуну́ться; 2) жи́дкость, раствóр (*для купания овец*); 3) уклóн, откóс; 4) склонé-

ние (магни́тной стрéлки); 5): at the ~ приспу́щен (*о флаге*); 6) мáканая свечá; 7) *сленг* вор-кармáнник.

dip II *v* (*past, p. p.* dipped, dipt) 1) погружáть, окунáть; 2) погружáться, окунáться; ныря́ть; 3) чéрпать, зачéрпывать; 4) спускáть (*флаг, парус*); 5) наклоня́ть (*голову при приветствии*); 6) спускáться, опускáться; □ to ~ out, to ~ up вычéрпывать.

diphtheria [dɪfˈθɪərɪə] *n мед.* дифтери́я, дифтери́т.

diphthong [ˈdɪfθɔŋ] *n фон.* дифтóнг.

diploma [dɪˈploumə] *n* диплóм; свидéтельство.

diplomacy [dɪˈplouməsɪ] *n* дипломáтия.

diplomaed [dɪˈplouməd] *a* имéющий, получи́вший диплóм.

diplomat [ˈdɪpləmæt] *n* дипломáт.

diplomatic [ˌdɪpləˈmætɪk] *a* 1) дипломати́ческий; 2) дипломати́чный, лóвкий, такти́чный.

diplomatics [ˌdɪpləˈmætɪks] *n* дипломати́ческое иску́сство.

diplomatist [dɪˈploumətɪst] *n* дипломáт.

dipper [ˈdɪpə] *n* 1) черпáк; ковш; 2) *амер.*: the (Big) Dipper Большáя Медвéдица; the Little Dipper Мáлая Медвéдица.

dipping [ˈdɪpɪŋ] *n* погружéние.

dipt [dɪpt] *past, p. p. см.* dip II.

dire [ˈdaɪə] *a* ужáсный, стрáшный; крáйний.

direct I [dɪˈrekt] *a* 1) прямóй; 2) непосрéдственный, прямóй; 3) откры́тый; я́сный, правди́вый (*об ответе и т. п.*); 4) диаметрáльный; ~ opposite диаметрáльно противополóжный.

direct II *v* 1) направля́ть (*тж. внимание, усилия*); 2) руководи́ть; управля́ть; 3) адресовáть; 4) нацéливать(ся); 5) укáзывать дорóгу; 6) прикáзывать.

direct III *adv* пря́мо; непосрéдственно.

direction [dɪˈrekʃən] *n* 1) направлéние; in the ~ of по направлéнию к; 2) руковóдство, управлéние; collective ~ коллекти́вное руковóдство; under the ~ of под руковóдством; 3) указáние, наставлéние; распоряжéние; *pl* директи́вы; 4) *обыкн. pl* áдрес (*на письме, посылке*); 5) дирéкция, правлéние; 6) *кино* режиссу́ра.

directive I [dɪˈrektɪv] *n* директи́ва.

directive II *a* 1) направля́ющий; 2) директи́вный.

directly I [dɪˈrektlɪ] *adv* 1) пря́мо; непосрéдственно; 2) немéдленно, тóтчас.

directly II *conj разг.* как тóлько.

directness [dɪˈrektnɪs] *n* прямотá; непосрéдственность.

director [dɪˈrektə] *n* 1) руководи́тель; дирéктор; 2) режиссёр; дирижёр.

directorate [dɪˈrektərɪt] *n* дирéкция; правлéние.

directorship [dɪˈrektəʃɪp] *n* дирéкторство.

directory I [dɪˈrektərɪ] *n* спрáвочник; указáтель; áдресная кни́га; telephone ~ телефóнная кни́га.

directory II *a* директи́вный; инструкти́вный.

directress [dɪˈrektrɪs] *n* директри́са.

direful [ˈdaɪəful] *a поэт.* ужáсный, стрáшный.

dirge [dəːdʒ] *n* 1) панихи́да; 2) погребáльная песнь.

dirigible I [ˈdɪrɪdʒəbl] *n* дирижáбль.

dirigible II *a* управля́емый.

dirk [dəːk] *n* 1) кинжа́л; 2) ко́ртик.

dirt [dəːt] *n* 1) грязь; му́сор; что́-л. гря́зное; 2) земля́, по́чва; грунт; 3) га́дость; непоря́дочность; to do smb. ~ сде́лать кому́-л. га́дость; 4) брань; to fling (*или* to cast, to throw) ~ at осыпа́ть бра́нью; to eat ~ проглоти́ть оскорбле́ние, терпе́ть униже́ние; 5) *attr* земляно́й, грунтово́й; ◇ as cheap as ~ *разг.* ≅ деше́вле па́реной ре́пы.

dirt-cheap ['dəːt'tʃiːp] *a разг.* о́чень дешёвый.

dirtily ['dəːtɪlɪ] *adv* гря́зно; *перен. тж.* ни́зко, по́дло.

dirtiness ['dəːtɪnɪs] *n* 1) грязь, неопря́тность; 2) га́дость, ни́зость.

dirty I ['dəːtɪ] *a* 1) гря́зный; 2) неприли́чный; скабрёзный; 3) ни́зкий; нече́стный (*об игроке́*); 4) бу́рный; нена́стный (*о пого́де*).

dirty II *v* па́чкать, загрязня́ть.

dis-[1] [dɪs-] *pref со значе́нием:* 1) *отрица́ния или противоположе́ния ка́честву, сво́йству, де́йствию, вы́раженному в сло́ве без пре́фикса* dis-: to please нра́виться, to displease не нра́виться; to agree соглаша́ться, to disagree не соглаша́ться; honest че́стный, dishonest нече́стный; 2) *разделе́ния, распаде́ния на составны́е ча́сти:* to dismember расчленя́ть; to disband распусти́ть (*войска́, а́рмию*); 3) *лише́ния прав, иму́щества и т. п.:* to disarm разоружи́ть; to disinherit лиши́ть насле́дства; 4) *усиле́ния де́йствия, вы́раженного просты́м глаго́лом:* to disannul аннули́ровать.

dis-[2] *pref со значе́нием* двойно́й; dissyllable двусло́жный.

disability [,dɪsə'bɪlɪtɪ] *n* 1) неспосо́бность; бесси́лие; 2) *юр.* неправоспосо́бность.

disable [dɪs'eɪbl] *v* 1) де́лать неспосо́бным, непри́го́дным; кале́чить; лиша́ть трудоспосо́бности; 2) *воен.* выводи́ть из стро́я; 3) *юр.* де́лать неправоспосо́бным, лиша́ть пра́ва.

disabled [dɪs'eɪbld] *a* нетрудоспосо́бный; искале́ченный.

disabuse [,dɪsə'bjuːz] *v* выводи́ть из заблужде́ния.

disaccord I [,dɪsə'kɔːd] *n* расхожде́ние, разногла́сие.

disaccord II *v* расходи́ться во взгля́дах; не соглаша́ться.

disadvantage [,dɪsəd'vɑːntɪdʒ] *n* 1) невы́годное положе́ние; taken at ~ захва́ченный враспло́х; 2) убы́ток, уще́рб, вред.

disadvantageous [,dɪsædvɑːn'teɪdʒəs] *a* невы́годный, неблагоприя́тный.

disaffected [,dɪsə'fektɪd] *a* 1) недово́льный; 2) нелоя́льный.

disaffection [,dɪsə'fekʃən] *n* 1) недово́льство; 2) нелоя́льность.

disaffirm [,dɪsə'fəːm] *v* 1) отрица́ть, отверга́ть; 2) *юр.* отменя́ть (*реше́ние*); аннули́ровать.

disafforest [,dɪsə'fɔrɪst] *v* выруба́ть леса́.

disagree [,dɪsə'griː] *v* 1) расходи́ться, не совпада́ть, противоре́чить друг дру́гу; 2) не соглаша́ться, расходи́ться во мне́ниях; ссо́риться; 3) быть неподходя́щим, вре́дным (*о пи́ще, кли́мате; with*).

disagreeable I [,dɪsə'grɪəbl] *n обыкн. pl* неприя́тности.

disagreeable II *a* 1) неприя́тный; 2) неприветливый.

disagreement [,dɪsə'griːmənt] *n* расхожде́ние во мне́ниях, разногла́сие; разла́д, ссо́ра.

disallow ['dɪsə'lau] *v* 1) отка́зывать; отверга́ть, отклоня́ть (*про́сьбу и т. п.*); 2) не разреша́ть, запреща́ть.

disappear [,dɪsə'pɪə] *v* исчеза́ть, пропада́ть, скрыва́ться.

disappearance [,dɪsə'pɪərəns] *n* исчезнове́ние.

disappoint [,dɪsə'pɔɪnt] *v* 1) разочаро́вывать; 2) обма́нывать, разруша́ть (*наде́жды и т. п.; of*).

disappointed [,dɪsə'pɔɪntɪd] *a* разочаро́ванный, расстро́енный.

disappointing [,dɪsə'pɔɪntɪŋ] *a* печа́льный, гру́стный, неутеши́тельный.

disappointment [,dɪsə'pɔɪntmənt] *n* 1) разочарова́ние; обма́нутая наде́жда; 2) доса́да, неприя́тность, огорче́ние.

disapprobation [,dɪsæprou'beɪʃən] *n* неодобре́ние.

disapproval [,dɪsə'pruːvəl] *n* неодобре́ние; осужде́ние.

disapprove ['dɪsə'pruːv] *v* не одобря́ть, порица́ть; осужда́ть; выража́ть неодобре́ние (*of*).

disapprovingly ['dɪsə'pruːvɪŋlɪ] *adv* неодобри́тельно.

disarm [dɪs'ɑːm] *v* 1) разоружа́ть(ся); 2) обезору́живать.

disarmament [dɪs'ɑːməmənt] *n* разоруже́ние.

disarrange ['dɪsə'reɪndʒ] *v* приводи́ть в беспоря́док, расстра́ивать, дезорганизова́ть.

disarrangement [,dɪsə'reɪndʒmənt] *n* беспоря́док, расстро́йство, дезорганиза́ция.

disarray I ['dɪsə'reɪ] *n* 1) беспоря́док; замеша́тельство; 2) беспоря́док, небре́жность в оде́жде.

disarray II *v* 1) приводи́ть в беспоря́док, в замеша́тельство; 2) *поэт.* снима́ть наря́д, оде́жду.

disaster [dɪ'zɑːstə] *n* бе́дствие, несча́стье; катастро́фа.

disastrous [dɪ'zɑːstrəs] *a* бе́дственный; катастрофи́ческий.

disavow ['dɪsə'vau] *v* 1) отрица́ть; отрека́ться; снима́ть с себя́ отве́тственность; 2) *полит.* дезавуи́ровать.

disavowal ['dɪsə'vauəl] *n* 1) отрица́ние; отрече́ние; отка́з (*от чего́-л.*); 2) *полит.* дезавуи́рование.

disband [dɪs'bænd] *v* 1) распуска́ть (*по дома́м*); *воен.* расформиро́вывать; 2) расходи́ться, рассе́иваться.

disbar [dɪs'bɑː] *v юр.* лиша́ть зва́ния адвока́та, лиша́ть пра́ва адвока́тской пра́ктики.

disbark [dɪs'bɑːk] *v* сдира́ть кору́.

disbelief ['dɪsbɪ'liːf] *n* неве́рие.

disbelieve ['dɪsbɪ'liːv] *v* не ве́рить; не доверя́ть.

disbeliever ['dɪsbɪ'liːvə] *n* неве́рующий.

disburden [dɪs'bəːdn] *v* освобожда́ть(ся) от тя́жести, от бре́мени.

disburse [dɪs'bəːs] *v* 1) раскоше́ливаться; 2) распла́чиваться; 3) расхо́довать.

disbursement [dɪs'bəːsmənt] *n* 1) расхо́д, тра́та; 2) вы́плата.

disc [dɪsk] *см.* disk.

discard [dɪs'kɑːd] *v* 1) сбра́сывать (*ка́рты*); 2) выбра́сывать (*за нена́добностью*); 3) отка́зываться (*от прежних взглядов*); отрека́ться (*от друзей*); 4) увольня́ть.

discern [dɪ'səːn] *v* 1) различа́ть, замеча́ть, я́сно ви́деть; 2) отлича́ть, понима́ть ра́зницу.

discernible [dɪ'səːnəbl] *a* различи́мый, заме́тный, ви́димый.

discerning [dɪ'səːnɪŋ] *a* 1) уме́ющий различа́ть, разбира́ющийся; 2) проница́тельный.

discernment [dɪ'səːnmənt] *n* 1) различе́ние; 2) проница́тельность.

discharge I [dɪs'tʃɑːdʒ] *n* 1) разгру́зка; 2) вы́стрел; залп; 3) *эл.* разря́д; 4) освобожде́ние (*заключённого*); 5) увольне́ние; 6) выделе́ние (*гно́я и т. п.*); 7) вытека́ние, сток; 8) вы́плата (*долга*); выполне́ние (*обязанностей*); 9) *тех.* выпускно́е отве́рстие, вы́ход, вы́пуск; 10) *текст., хим.* обесцве́чение тка́ней.

discharge II *v* 1) разгружа́ть(ся); 2) выпуска́ть заря́д, производи́ть вы́стрел; 3) *эл.* разряжа́ть; 4) освобожда́ть (*заключённого*); выпи́сывать (*из больни́цы*); 5) увольня́ть; распуска́ть (*коми́ссию*); 6) выпуска́ть (*дым*); выделя́ть (*гной*); вылива́ть(ся) (*о жи́дкости*); 7) упла́чивать (*долг*); выполня́ть (*обя́занности*); 8) *текст., хим.* обесцве́чивать.

dischargee [,dɪstʃɑː'dʒiː] *n амер.* демобилизо́ванный.

disci ['dɪskaɪ] *pl см.* discus.

disciple [dɪ'saɪpl] *n* 1) учени́к, после́дователь; 2) *церк.* апо́стол.

disciplinary ['dɪsɪplɪnərɪ] *a* 1) дисциплина́рный, исправи́тельный; 2) дисциплини́рующий.

discipline I ['dɪsɪplɪn] *n* 1) дисципли́на, поря́док; 2) дисциплини́рованность; 3) наказа́ние; 4) дисципли́на (*о́трасль нау́ки*).

discipline II *v* 1) дисциплини́ровать; 2) нака́зывать.

disclaim [dɪs'kleɪm] *v* 1) отка́зываться (*от свои́х прав*); 2) отрека́ться; не признава́ть.

disclaimer [dɪs'kleɪmə] *n* 1) отка́з (*от свои́х прав*); 2) отрече́ние; отрица́ние.

disclose [dɪs'klouz] *v* обнару́живать, раскрыва́ть, разоблача́ть.

disclosure [dɪs'klouʒə] *n* обнаруже́ние, раскры́тие, разоблаче́ние.

discolo(u)r [dɪs'kʌlə] *v* изменя́ть цвет, окра́ску; обесцве́чивать(ся).

discolo(u)ration [dɪs,kʌlə'reɪʃən] *n* измене́ние цве́та, окра́ски; обесцве́чивание.

discomfit [dɪs'kʌmfɪt] *v* 1) расстра́ивать (*пла́ны и т. п.*); 2) смуща́ть; раздража́ть; 3) *уст.* наноси́ть пораже́ние.

descomfiture [dɪs'kʌmfɪtʃə] *n* 1) расстро́йство пла́нов; 2) смуще́ние, замеша́тельство; 3) пораже́ние.

discomfort I [dɪs'kʌmfət] *n* 1) неудо́бство; нело́вкость; 2) беспоко́йство.

discomfort II *v* причиня́ть беспоко́йство.

discommode [,dɪskə'moud] *v* беспоко́ить, меша́ть.

discompose [,dɪskəm'pouz] *v* расстра́ивать, смуща́ть, волнова́ть, трево́жить.

discomposedly [,dɪskəm'pouzɪdlɪ] *adv* беспоко́йно, трево́жно.

discomposure [,dɪskəm'pouʒə] *n* беспоко́йство; замеша́тельство.

disconcert [,dɪskən'səːt] *v* 1) смуща́ть; приводи́ть в замеша́тельство; дезориенти́ровать; 2) расстра́ивать (*пла́ны*).

disconnect ['dɪskə'nekt] *v* 1) разъединя́ть, разделя́ть, разобща́ть; 2) *эл., тех.* выключа́ть.

disconnectedly ['dɪskə'nektɪdlɪ] *adv* бессвя́зно, отры́висто.

disconnection [,dɪskə'nekʃən] *n* разъедине́ние, разобще́ние.

disconsolate [dɪs'kɔnsəlɪt] *a* неуте́шный, печа́льный; несча́стный.

discontent I ['dɪskən'tent] *n* недово́льство; неудовлетворённость.

discontent II *a* недово́льный; неудовлетворённый.

discontent III *v* вызыва́ть недово́льство.

discontented ['dɪskən'tentɪd] *a* недово́льный; неудовлетворённый.

discontentedly ['dɪskən'tentɪdlɪ] *adv* недово́льно; с неудово́льствием.

discontentment ['dɪskən'tentmənt] *n* недово́льство, неудовлетворённость.

discontinuance [,dɪskən'tɪnjuəns] *n* прекраще́ние, переры́в.

discontinue ['dɪskən'tɪnjuː] *v* прерыва́ть(ся), прекраща́ть(ся); переставáть.

discontinuous ['dɪskən'tɪnjuəs] *a* преры́вистый, прерыва́ющийся.

discord[a] ['dɪskɔːd] *n* 1) разногла́сие, разла́д, раздо́ры; 2) *муз.* диссона́нс.

discord[b] [dɪs'kɔːd] *v* 1) расходи́ться во взгля́дах, мне́ниях (*with, from*); 2) *муз.* звуча́ть диссона́нсом; 3) дисгармони́ровать.

discordance [dɪs'kɔːdəns] *n* 1) разногла́сие; 2) *муз.* диссона́нс.

discordant [dɪs'kɔːdənt] *a* 1) несогла́сный, несхо́дный, противоречи́вый; 2) нестро́йный; диссони́рующий.

discount I ['dɪskaunt] *n* 1) ски́дка; *перен.* попра́вка на преувеличе́ние; at a ~ со ски́дкой, ни́же цены́; 2) *фин.* учёт векселе́й; проце́нт, ста́вка учёта.

discount II *v* 1) убавля́ть (*це́ну*); уменьша́ть (*дохо́д*); *перен.* де́лать попра́вку на преувеличе́ние; не доверя́ть; 2) *фин.* учи́тывать векселя́; 3) не принима́ть во внима́ние, в расчёт.

discountenance [dɪs'kauntɪnəns] *v* 1) не одобря́ть; обескура́живать; отка́зывать в подде́ржке; 2) смуща́ть; стыди́ть.

discourage [dɪs'kʌrɪdʒ] *v* 1) обескура́живать, расхола́живать; 2) отгова́ривать, отсове́товать (*from*).

discouragement [dɪs'kʌrɪdʒmənt] *n* 1) обескура́живание; 2) обескура́женность; уны́ние.

discourse I [dɪs'kɔːs] *n* 1) рассужде́ние (*у́стное и́ли пи́сьменное*); речь, ле́кция; 2) *уст.* бесе́да, разгово́р.

discourse II *v* 1) излага́ть, рассужда́ть; орато́рствовать; 2) бесе́довать.

discourteous [dɪs'kəːtjəs] *a* неве́жливый, неучти́вый; гру́бый.

discourtesy [dɪs'kəːtɪsɪ] *n* неве́жливость, неучти́вость; гру́бость.

discover [dɪs'kʌvə] *v* 1) де́лать откры́тие; открыва́ть; 2) обнару́живать, находи́ть; раскрыва́ть; узнава́ть.

discoverer [dıs′kʌvərə] *n* (перво)открыва́тель; а́втор откры́тия.

discovery [dıs′kʌvərı] *n* 1) откры́тие; revolutionary discoveries откры́тия, производя́щие переворо́т; 2) раскры́тие, обнаруже́ние; 3) развёртывание (*сюжета*).

discredit I [dıs′kredıt] *n* 1) недове́рие, сомне́ние; to throw ~ on подверга́ть сомне́нию; 2) дискредита́ция; поте́ря авторите́та; 2) лише́ние креди́та.

discredit II *v* 1) не доверя́ть, подверга́ть сомне́нию; 2) дискредити́ровать; подрыва́ть авторите́т, дове́рие.

discreditable [dıs′kredıtəbl] *a* 1) дискредити́рующий; позо́рящий; 2) позо́рный.

discreet [dıs′kri:t] *a* осторо́жный; сде́ржанный; благоразу́мный.

discrepancy [dıs′krepənsı] *n* 1) разногла́сие, противоре́чие; расхожде́ние; 2) разли́чие, несхо́дство.

discrepant [dıs′krepənt] *a* 1) разноречи́вый, противоречи́вый; 2) несхо́дный.

discrete [dıs′kri:t] *a* 1) отде́льный; разде́льный; 2) *филос.* абстра́ктный.

discretion [dıs′kreʃən] *n* 1) благоразу́мие, осторо́жность; свобо́да де́йствий; усмотре́ние; at the ~ of на усмотре́ние кого́-л.; to surrender at ~ сда́ться на ми́лость, на во́лю победи́теля; the years, the age of ~ во́зраст (*14 лет*), с кото́рого челове́к счита́ется отве́тственным за свои́ посту́пки; it′s just a matter of ~ э́то зави́сит от того́, как посмотре́ть на де́ло.

discriminate [dıs′krımıneıt] *v* 1) различа́ть, распознава́ть (*between*); отлича́ть (*from*); 2) дискримини́ровать; 3) относи́ться по-ра́зному.

discriminating [dıs′krımıneıtıŋ] *a* 1) уме́ющий (то́нко) различа́ть; разбира́ющийся, проница́тельный; 2) отличи́тельный (*о признаке и т. п.*); 3) дифференциа́льный (*о тарифе и т. п.*).

discrimination [dıs,krımı′neıʃən] *n* 1) дискримина́ция; race ~ ра́совая дискримина́ция; 2) уме́ние (то́нко) различа́ть; проница́тельность.

discriminative [dıs′krımınətıv] *см.* discriminating 1), 2).

discursive [dıs′kə:sıv] *a* 1) перескакивающий с одного́ предме́та на друго́й; 2) логи́ческий, после́довательный.

discus [′dıskəs] *n* (*pl* disci) диск.

discuss [dıs′kʌs] *v* 1) обсужда́ть, дискути́ровать; 2) *шутл.* есть, пить с удово́льствием, смакова́ть.

discussion [dıs′kʌʃən] *n* 1) обсужде́ние; диску́ссия; 2) перегово́ры.

disdain I [dıs′deın] *n* надме́нность; пренебреже́ние, презре́ние.

disdain II *v* 1) презира́ть; 2) смотре́ть свысока́; счита́ть ни́же своего́ досто́инства.

disdainful [dıs′deınful] *a* надме́нный; презри́тельный.

disease [dı′zi:z] *n* боле́знь; заболева́ние; catching ~ зара́зная боле́знь.

diseased [dı′zi:zd] *a* больно́й, заболе́вший.

disembark [′dısım′bɑ:k] *v* 1) сходи́ть на бе́рег (*с судна*); выса́живать(ся); 2) выгружа́ть (*с судна*).

disembarkation [,dısembɑ:′keıʃən] *n* вы́садка, вы́грузка на бе́рег.

disembarrass [′dısım′bærəs] *v* 1) выводи́ть из замеша́тельства, из затрудне́ния; 2) освобожда́ть (*от тру́дностей, хлопот; of*); 3) распу́тывать (*сло́жное положе́ние*); выпу́тываться (*из чего́-л.— from*).

disembody [′dısım′bɔdı] *v* 1) расформиро́вывать, распуска́ть (*войска*); 2) *рел.* освобожда́ть от теле́сной оболо́чки.

disembogue [,dısım′boug] *v* 1) впада́ть (*о реке; into*); 2) излива́ться, выска́зываться.

disembosom [,dısım′buzəm] *v* поверя́ть (*та́йну, заве́тную мысль*); открыва́ть ду́шу.

disembowel [,dısım′bauəl] *v* потроши́ть.

disembroil [,dısım′brɔıl] *v* распу́тывать.

disenchant [′dısın′tʃɑ:nt] *v* освобожда́ть от чар, от иллю́зий; разочаро́вывать.

disencumber [′dısın′kʌmbə] *v* освобожда́ть от бре́мени, от затрудне́ний.

disengage [′dısın′geıdʒ] *v* 1) освобожда́ть(ся); отвя́зывать(ся); 2) разъединя́ть(ся); выключа́ть (-ся); 3) *воен.* выходи́ть из бо́я.

disengaged [′dısın′geıdʒd] *a* 1) свобо́дный; неза́нятый; 2) несвя́занный, освобождённый; 3) разобщённый.

disengagement [,dısın′geıdʒmənt] *n* 1) освобожде́ние (*от чего́-л.*); свобо́да, несвя́занность; 2) есте́ственность (*ма́нер*), непринуждённость; 3) расторже́ние помо́лвки; 4) *воен.* вы́ход из бо́я; 5) *хим.* выделе́ние.

disentangle [′dısın′tæŋgl] *v* 1) распу́тывать(ся); 2) выпу́тываться из затрудне́ний.

disenthral(l) [,dısın′θrɔ:l] *v* освобожда́ть от ра́бства, отпуска́ть на во́лю.

disentitle [,dısın′taıtl] *v* 1) лиша́ть пра́ва на что-л.; 2) лиша́ть ти́тула.

disestablish [′dısıs′tæblıʃ] *v* 1) отменя́ть (*устано́вленное*); 2) отделя́ть це́рковь от госуда́рства.

disestablishment [,dısıs′tæblıʃmənt] *n* отделе́ние це́ркви от госуда́рства.

disfavour I [′dıs′feıvə] *n* 1) неми́лость; to fall into ~ впасть в неми́лость; to be in ~ быть в неми́лости; 2) неодобре́ние.

disfavour II *v* не одобря́ть.

disfiguration [dıs,fıgjuə′reıʃən] *см.* disfigurement.

disfigure [dıs′fıgə] *v* 1) обезобра́живать, уро́довать; 2) искажа́ть.

disfigurement [dıs′fıgəmənt] *n* 1) уро́дство; 2) искаже́ние.

disforest [dıs′fɔrıst] *v* выруба́ть леса́.

disfranchise [′dıs′fræntʃaız] *v* лиша́ть гражда́нских (*особ. избира́тельных*) прав.

disfrock [dıs′frɔk] *v* лиша́ть духо́вного са́на.

disgorge [dıs′gɔ:dʒ] *v* 1) изверга́ть (*ла́ву*); изрыга́ть (*пи́щу*); выбра́сывать (*клу́бы ды́ма и т. п.*); 2) впада́ть, влива́ться (*о реке*); 3) возвраща́ть присво́енное, захва́ченное.

disgrace [dıs′greıs] *n* 1) позо́р, бесче́стие; indelible ~ несмыва́емый позо́р; to bring a ~ upon smb. навле́чь позо́р на кого́-л.; 2) неми́лость, опа́ла; to be in ~ быть в неми́лости, в опа́ле.

disgrace II *v* 1) лишать милости, расположения; 2) позорить, бесчестить; унижать.

disgraceful [dɪs'greɪsful] *a* позорный, бесчестный.

disgruntled [dɪs'grʌntld] *a* недовольный, рассерженный.

disguise I [dɪs'gaɪz] *n* 1) переодевание, маскировка; in ~ переодетый; 2) личина, маска.

disguise II *v* 1) переодевать, маскировать; делать неузнаваемым; 2) скрывать под видом, под личиной.

disgust I [dɪs'gʌst] *n* отвращение.

disgust II *v* вызывать, внушать отвращение; to be ~ed чувствовать отвращение.

disgustful [dɪs'gʌstful] *a* отвратительный.

disgusting [dɪs'gʌstɪŋ] *см.* disgustful.

dish I [dɪʃ] *n* 1) блюдо, тарелка, миска; *pl* посуда; 2) блюдо, кушанье; standing ~ неизменное блюдо; *перен.* постоянная тема.

dish II *v* 1) накладывать на блюдо; 2) *разг.* обмануть, обойти (кого-л.); 3) *разг.* расстроить (чьи-л. планы); □ to ~ out разливать, раскладывать (кушанье); to ~ up а) подавать к столу; б) уметь преподнести (факты и т. п.).

dishabille [,dɪsæ'biːl] *n* небрежная домашняя одежда, дезабилье.

dishabituate [,dɪshə'bɪtʃueɪt] *v* отучать от привычки.

disharmonious [,dɪshɑː'mounjəs] *a* несогласный; дисгармоничный.

disharmony ['dɪs'hɑːmənɪ] *n* разногласие, расхождение; дисгармония.

dish-cloth ['dɪʃklɔθ] *n* кухонное полотенце.

dishearten [dɪs'hɑːtn] *v* приводить в уныние, обескураживать; don't be ~ed не унывайте.

dishevelled [dɪ'ʃevəld] *a* растрёпанный, взъерошенный.

dishonest [dɪs'ɔnɪst] *a* 1) нечестный; мошеннический; 2) недобросовестный.

dishonesty [dɪs'ɔnɪstɪ] *n* 1) нечестность; мошенничество; обман; 2) недобросовестность.

dishonour I [dɪs'ɔnə] *n* 1) бесчестье, позор; 2) неуплата по векселю.

dishonour II *v* 1) бесчестить, позорить; 2) *ком.* отказываться в уплате по векселю.

dishonourable [dɪs'ɔnərəbl] *a* 1) бесчестный, позорный; 2) позорящий, низкий.

dishouse [dɪs'haus] *v* лишать крова.

dish-washer ['dɪʃ,wɔʃə] *n* 1) судомойка; 2) *зоол.* трясогузка.

dish-water ['dɪʃ,wɔːtə] *n* помои.

disillusion I [,dɪsɪ'luːʒən] *n* разочарование.

disillusion II *v* разрушать иллюзии; разочаровывать.

disinclination [,dɪsɪnklɪ'neɪʃən] *n* 1) несклонность, нерасположение; 2) неохота, нежелание.

disincline ['dɪsɪn'klaɪn] *v* 1) быть не склонным, не расположенным (к чему-либо); 2) отбивать охоту.

disinfect [,dɪsɪn'fekt] *v* дезинфицировать.

disinfectant I [,dɪsɪn'fektənt] *n* дезинфицирующее средство.

disinfectant II *a* дезинфицирующий.

disinfection [,dɪsɪn'fekʃən] *n* дезинфекция.

disingenuous [,dɪsɪn'dʒenjuəs] *a* 1) неискренний; 2) нечестный; непорядочный.

disinherit ['dɪsɪn'herɪt] *v* лишать наследства.

disinheritance [,dɪsɪn'herɪtəns] *n* лишение наследства.

disintegrate [dɪs'ɪntɪgreɪt] *v* 1) разделять на составные части, раздроблять; 2) распадаться, разрушаться; раздробляться.

disintegration [dɪs,ɪntɪ'greɪʃən] *n* 1) разделение на составные части; раздробление; 2) распадение, разрушение.

disinter ['dɪsɪn'təː] *v* 1) выкапывать из могилы; 2) раскапывать, откапывать (что-л.).

disinterested [dɪs'ɪntrɪstɪd] *a* 1) бескорыстный, незаинтересованный; беспристрастный; 2) равнодушный, безучастный.

disinterestedness [dɪs'ɪntrɪstɪdnɪs] *n* бескорыстие.

disject [dɪs'dʒekt] *v* разбрасывать.

disjoin [dɪs'dʒɔɪn] *v* разъединять, разделять; разобщать.

disjoint [dɪs'dʒɔɪnt] *v* 1) разбирать, разрезать на части; расчленять; 2) вывихнуть.

disjointed [dɪs'dʒɔɪntɪd] *a* 1) расчленённый; 2) бессвязный (о речи); 3) вывихнутый.

disjunction [dɪs'dʒʌŋkʃən] *n* 1) разъединение; разобщение; 2) *эл.* размыкание (цепи).

disjunctive I [dɪs'dʒʌŋktɪv] *n* *грам.* разделительный союз.

disjunctive II *a* разъединяющий, разделительный.

disk [dɪsk] *n* 1) диск; круг; 2) *attr* дисковый.

dislike I [dɪs'laɪk] *n* нелюбовь, нерасположение, неприязнь; отвращение.

dislike II *v* не любить, чувствовать неприязнь, нерасположение, отвращение.

dislocate ['dɪsləkeɪt] *v* 1) вывихнуть; 2) нарушать, расстраивать; 3) смещать, сдвигать.

dislocation [,dɪslə'keɪʃən] *n* 1) вывих; 2) нарушение (движения и т. п.); 3) смещение, сдвиг.

dislodge [dɪs'lɔdʒ] *v* 1) удалять; выгонять (зверя из берлоги); 2) вытеснять, выбивать (неприятеля).

disloyal ['dɪs'lɔɪəl] *a* 1) нелояльный; 2) неверный, предательский.

disloyalty ['dɪs'lɔɪəltɪ] *n* 1) нелояльность; 2) неверность, предательство.

dismal ['dɪzməl] *a* мрачный, унылый; печальный; гнетущий; угрюмый.

dismals ['dɪzməlz] *n* (the ~) угнетённое, мрачное настроение.

dismantle [dɪs'mæntl] *v* 1) разбирать; демонтировать; снимать оборудование; 2) разоружать, расснащивать (судно).

dismay I [dɪs'meɪ] *n* 1) ужас, страх (перед чем-л.); 2) уныние.

dismay II *v* 1) ужасать, пугать; 2) смущать, обескураживать.

dismember [dɪs'membə] *v* 1) расчленять; разделять, разрывать на части; 2) *уст.* лишать членства.

dismemberment [dɪs'membəmənt] *n* расчленение.

dismiss [dɪs'mɪs] *v* 1) отпускать; распускать; 2) увольнять; 3) прогонять; гнать от себя (мысли, страхи); 4) отвергать, отклонять (обвинение и т. п.); 5) закрывать (собрание и т. п.).

dismissal [dɪs'mɪsəl] *n* 1) роспуск; 2) увольнéние; отстáвка; 3) удалéние; отстранéние от себя (*неприятной мысли и т. п.*); 4) закры́тие (*собрания и т. п.*).

dismission [dɪs'mɪʃən] *см.* dismissal.

dismount ['dɪs'maunt] *v* 1) слезáть с лóшади; спéшиваться; 2) выбивáть из седлá; сбрáсывать ездокá (*о лошади*); 3) снимáть (*с подстáвки, пьедестáла*).

disobedience [ˌdɪsə'biːdjəns] *n* непослушáние, неповиновéние.

disobedient [ˌdɪsə'biːdjənt] *a* непослýшный, непокóрный.

disobey ['dɪsə'beɪ] *v* не слýшаться, не повиновáться.

disoblige ['dɪsə'blaɪdʒ] *v* не считáться (*с кем-л., чем-л.*); быть нелюбéзным.

disobligingly ['dɪsə'blaɪdʒɪŋlɪ] *adv* нелюбéзно.

disorder I [dɪs'ɔːdə] *n* 1) беспорядок; 2) беспоря́дки (*массовые волнения*); 3) расстрóйство; нездорóвье.

disorder II *v* 1) приводи́ть в беспоря́док; 2) расстрáивать (*здорóвье*).

disorderly I [dɪs'ɔːdəlɪ] *a* 1) беспоря́дочный; неаккурáтный, неопря́тный; 2) беспокóйный, необýзданный; бýйный; 3) распýщенный.

disorderly II *adv* беспоря́дочно.

disorganization [dɪsˌɔːgənaɪ'zeɪʃən] *n* беспоря́док; дезорганизáция.

disorganize [dɪs'ɔːgənaɪz] *v* расстрáивать, дезорганизовáть.

disorientate [dɪs'ɔːrɪenteɪt] *v* вводи́ть в заблуждéние, дезориенти́ровать.

disown [dɪs'oun] *v* не признавáть свои́м, отрекáться.

disparage [dɪs'pærɪdʒ] *v* 1) унижáть; умаля́ть чьё-л. достóинство; 2) говори́ть пренебрежи́тельно; относи́ться с пренебрежéнием.

disparagement [dɪs'pærɪdʒmənt] *n* 1) унижéние, умалéние (*достоинства и т. п.*); 2) пренебрежéние.

disparagingly [dɪs'pærɪdʒɪŋlɪ] *adv* пренебрежи́тельно, с пренебрежéнием.

disparity [dɪs'pærɪtɪ] *n* нерáвенство, несоотвéтствие.

dispart [dɪs'pɑːt] *v* разделя́ть(ся).

dispassionate [dɪs'pæʃnɪt] *a* 1) спокóйный, бесстрáстный; 2) беспристрáстный.

dispatch I [dɪs'pætʃ] *n* 1) отпрáвка, отправлéние (*курьера, почты*); 2) сообщéние, донесéние; депéша (*дипломатическая*); 3) быстротá (*исполнения, работы*); 4) *разг.* уби́йство; **happy ~ a**) харáкири; **б**) мгновéнная смерть при кáзни.

dispatch II *v* 1) отправля́ть, посылáть (*курьера, почту*); 2) бы́стро справля́ться (*с чем-л.*); бы́стро есть; 3) *разг.* отправля́ть на тот свет.

dispatch-bearer [dɪs'pætʃˌbeərə] *n* дипломати́ческий курьéр.

dispatcher [dɪs'pætʃə] *n* диспéтчер; экспеди́тор.

dispatch-station [dɪs'pætʃ'steɪʃən] *n ж.-д.* стáнция отправлéния.

dispel [dɪs'pel] *v* разгоня́ть, рассéивать.

dispensable [dɪs'pensəbl] *a* необязáтельный.

dispensary [dɪs'pensərɪ] *n* аптéка (*обыкн. благотворительная*); *амер. тж.* амбулатóрия.

dispensation [ˌdɪspen'seɪʃən] *n* 1) раздáча,

распределéние; 2) освобождéние (*от обязательства, обета; with, from*); 3) отправлéние (*правосудия*).

dispense [dɪs'pens] *v* 1) раздавáть, распределя́ть, выдавáть; 2) приготовля́ть и раздавáть (*лекарства*); 3) освобождáть (*от обязанности и т. п.; from*); 4) отправля́ть (*правосудие*); □ **to ~ with** обходи́ться без чего-л.

dispenser [dɪs'pensə] *n* фармацéвт.

dispeople ['dɪs'piːpl] *v* обезлю́дить.

dispersal [dɪs'pəːsəl] *n* 1) рассéивание; 2) рассыпáние.

disperse [dɪs'pəːs] *v* 1) разбрáсывать; рассыпáть; 2) разгоня́ть; рассéивать(ся); 3) распространя́ть; 4) расходи́ться (*о толпе*).

dispersion [dɪs'pəːʃən] *n* 1) рассéивание; разбрáсывание; 2) разбрóсанность; 3) *физ., хим.* диспéрсия.

dispersive [dɪs'pəːsɪv] *a* рассéивающий.

dispirit [dɪ'spɪrɪt] *v* приводи́ть в уны́ние, удручáть.

dispirited [dɪ'spɪrɪtɪd] *a* уны́лый, удручённый.

displace [dɪs'pleɪs] *v* 1) перемещáть; переставля́ть; 2) замещáть, заменя́ть; вытесня́ть; 3) увольня́ть, смещáть; 4) имéть водоизмещéние (*о судне*).

displaced [dɪs'pleɪst] *a*: **~ persons** *полит.* перемещённые лица.

displacement [dɪs'pleɪsmənt] *n* 1) перемещéние; перестанóвка; 2) замещéние, замéна; 3) увольнéние, смещéние; 4) водоизмещéние; 5) *геол.* сдвиг (*пластов*).

display I [dɪs'pleɪ] *n* 1) покáз; вы́ставка; 2) проявлéние, выкáзывание (*какого-л. чувства, свойства*); 3) выставлéние напокáз, хвастовствó; **to make great ~ of smth.** выставля́ть что-л. напокáз; хвáстаться чем-л.; **this is mere ~** всё это тóлько показнóе.

display II *v* 1) покáзывать; выставля́ть (*напокáз*); 2) проявля́ть, выкáзывать; 3) хвáстать(ся) чем-л.; 4) выделя́ть осóбым шри́фтом.

displease [dɪs'pliːz] *v* 1) не нрáвиться, быть неприя́тным (*кому-л.*); 2) серди́ть, раздражáть.

displeased [dɪs'pliːzd] *a* недовóльный (*кем-л., чем-л. — at, by, with*).

displeasing [dɪs'pliːzɪŋ] *a* неприя́тный.

displeasure [dɪs'pleʒə] *n* неудовóльствие, недовóльство; досáда; **to be in ~ with** быть в неми́лости у кого-л.

disport [dɪs'pɔːt] *v refl* развлекáться; забавля́ться.

disposable [dɪs'pouzəbl] *a* такóй, котóрым мóжно распоряжáться, свобóдный.

disposal [dɪs'pouzəl] *n* 1) расположéние, размещéние; 2) передáча, продáжа; 3) распоряжéние; **at one's ~** в чьём-л. распоряжéнии; **к услýгам кого-л.**; избавлéние (*от чего-л. ненужного, неприятного*).

dispose [dɪs'pouz] *v* 1) располагáть (*в каком-л. порядке*); 2) располагáть (*к кому-л., чему-л.*); **to be ~d** быть располóженным, быть склóнным; □ **to ~ of a**) распоряди́ться чем-л. (*путём продажи, передачи*); **б**) избáвиться, освобóдиться от чего-л., кого-л.

disposition [ˌdɪspə'zɪʃən] *n* 1) склóнность к чему-л.; 2) расположéние дýха; нрав, харáктер;

social ~ общительный характер; -3) расположение; порядок; *воен.* диспозиция; дислокация; 4) *обыкн.* pl приготовления, планы; 5) распоряжение; to have in one's ~ иметь в своём распоряжении; to make a ~ of· распорядиться чем-л.

dispossess ['dɪspə'zes] *v* 1) лишать (права) собственности (*of*); отчуждать; 2) выселять.

dispossession [,dɪspə'zeʃən] *n* 1) лишение (права) собственности; отчуждение; 2) выселение.

dispraise I [dɪs'preɪz] *n* порицание, неодобрение.

dispraise II *v* порицать, не одобрять.

disproof ['dɪs'pruːf] *n* опровержение.

disproportion I [,dɪsprə'pɔːʃən] *n* непропорциональность, несоразмерность, диспропорция.

disproportion II *v* делать непропорциональным, несоразмерным.

disproportionate [,dɪsprə'pɔːʃnɪt] *a* непропорциональный, несоразмерный.

disprove ['dɪs'pruːv] *v* опровергать.

disputable [dɪs'pjuːtəbl] *a* спорный; сомнительный.

disputant [dɪs'pjuːtənt] *n* спорщик; участник диспута.

disputation [,dɪspjuː'teɪʃən] *n* спор; диспут.

dispute I [dɪs'pjuːt] *n* 1) диспут, дебаты; спор, полемика; beyond ~ бесспорно; 2) ссора, препирательство.

dispute II *v* 1) спорить (*с кем-л.* — *with, against; о чём-л.* — *on, about*); пререкаться; 2) обсуждать; дискутировать; 3) оспаривать (*первенство в состязании*); добиваться (*победы*); 4) противиться, противостоять; to arms отстаивать с оружием в руках; 5) подвергать сомнению (*правильность, достоверность*).

disqualification [dɪs,kwɔlɪfɪ'keɪʃən] *n* 1) дисквалификация; 2) негодность к чему-л. (*for*); неподготовленность.

disqualify [dɪs'kwɔlɪfaɪ] *v* 1) дисквалифицировать; 2) признавать негодным, неспособным к чему-л.; 3) делать негодным, неспособным к чему-л.

disquiet I [dɪs'kwaɪət] *n* беспокойство, тревога.

disquiet II *a* беспокойный, тревожный.

disquiet III *v* беспокоить, тревожить.

disquietude [dɪs'kwaɪtjuːd] *n* беспокойство, встревоженность.

disquisition [,dɪskwɪ'zɪʃən] *n* исследование, изыскание.

disrank [dɪs'ræŋk] *v*- разжаловать.

disregard I [dɪsrɪ'gɑːd] *n* невнимание; пренебрежение; игнорирование.

disregard II *v* не обращать внимания; игнорировать; пренебрегать.

disrepair ['dɪsrɪ'peə] *n* плохое состояние, неисправность; in ~ в неисправном состоянии.

disreputable [dɪs'repjutəbl] *a* 1) пользующийся дурной репутацией; 2) позорный, неприличный.

disrepute ['dɪsrɪ'pjuːt] *n* дурная слава, репутация.

disrespect I ['dɪsrɪs'pekt] *n* неуважение; непочтительность; грубость.

disrespect II *v* относиться непочтительно; грубо обращаться.

disrespectful [,dɪsrɪs'pektful] *a* непочтительный, невежливый.

disrobe ['dɪs'roub] *v* 1) раздевать; разоблачать (*тж. перен.*); 2) раздеваться.

disroot [dɪs'ruːt] *v* искоренять, вырывать с корнем.

disrupt [dɪs'rʌpt] *v* разрывать; разрушать; *перен.* подрывать (*здоровье, силы*).

disruption [dɪs'rʌpʃən] *n* разрыв, раскол; разрушение.

disruptive [dɪs'rʌptɪv] *a* разрушительный.

dissatisfaction ['dɪs,sætɪs'fækʃən] *n* неудовлетворённость, недовольство, досада.

dissatisfy ['dɪs'sætɪsfaɪ] *v* не удовлетворять.

dissect [dɪ'sekt] *v* 1) рассекать; 2) вскрывать, анатомировать; 3) анализировать.

dissection [dɪ'sekʃən] *n* 1) рассечение; 2) анатомирование, вскрытие (*трупа*); 3) анализ, разбор.

dissemble [dɪ'sembl] *v* 1) скрывать (*мысли, чувства*); 2) притворяться, лицемерить.

dissembler [dɪ'semblə] *n* лицемер, притворщик.

disseminate [dɪ'semɪneɪt] *v* 1) рассеивать, разбрасывать (*семена*); 2) распространять (*взгляды, учение*); 3) сеять (*недовольство*).

dissemination [dɪ,semɪ'neɪʃən] *n* 1) рассеивание, разбрасывание; 2) распространение.

dissension [dɪ'senʃən] *n* 1) разногласие; 2) раздоры, распри.

dissent I [dɪ'sent] *n* 1) несогласие; расхождение во взглядах, мнениях; 2) сектантство.

dissent II *v* 1) не соглашаться, расходиться во взглядах, мнениях (*from*); 2) *церк.* принадлежать к секте.

dissenter [dɪ'sentə] *n* 1) сектант; раскольник; 2) *амер.* оппозиционер.

dissentient [dɪ'senʃɪənt] *a* не соглашающийся, инакомыслящий; раскольнический.

dissertation [,dɪsəː'teɪʃən] *n* диссертация.

disserve ['dɪs'səːv] *v* оказать плохую услугу, навредить.

disservice ['dɪs'səːvɪs] *n* плохая услуга, вред.

dissever [dɪs'sevə] *v* разъединять(ся), разделять(ся), отделять(ся).

dissidence ['dɪsɪdəns] *n* разногласия; раскол.

dissident I ['dɪsɪdənt] *n* раскольник.

dissident II *a* инакомыслящий.

dissimilar ['dɪ'sɪmɪlə] *a* непохожий; отличный, несходный.

dissimilarity [,dɪsɪmɪ'lærɪtɪ] *n* несходство, различие.

dessimilation ['dɪsɪmɪ'leɪʃən] *n* *лингв.* диссимиляция.

dissimulate [dɪ'sɪmjuleɪt] *v* скрывать; притворяться; симулировать.

dissimulation [dɪ,sɪmju'leɪʃən] *n* притворство, лицемерие; симуляция.

dissipate ['dɪsɪpeɪt] *v* 1) рассеивать(ся); разгонять (*облака, мрак и т. п.*); 2) растрачивать, расточать (*время, силы, деньги*); 3) *разг.* кутить, вести беспутный образ жизни.

dissipated ['dɪsɪpeɪtɪd] *a* 1) рассеянный; 2) растраченный зря; 3) беспутный; распущенный.

dissipation [,dɪsɪ'peɪʃən] *n* 1) рассеяние; рассеивание; 2) расточение (*of*); 3) легкомысленные развлечения; беспутный образ жизни.

dissociable [dɪ'souʃəbl] *a* необщительный.

dissociate [dɪ'souʃɪeɪt] *v* 1) разъединять, разобщать; to ~ oneself from отмежёвываться от; прекращать общение; 2) *хим.* диссоциировать.

dissociation [dɪ,sousɪ'eɪʃən] *n* 1) разъединение, разобщение; отмежевание; 2) *хим.* разложение, распад.

dissoluble [dɪ'sɔljubl] *a* 1) растворимый; 2) расторжимый (*о договоре, союзе*).

dissolute ['dɪsəluːt] *a* беспутный.

dissolution [,dɪsə'luːʃən] *n* 1) растворение; разложение, распад (*на составные части*); 2) расторжение (*брака, договора*); 3) прекращение; закрытие; роспуск (*парламента и т. п.*); 4) смерть, конец; исчезновение.

dissolvable [dɪ'zɔlvəbl] *a* 1) растворимый; 2) разложимый; 3) расторжимый.

dissolve [dɪ'zɔlv] *v* 1) растворять(ся); разлагать(ся); разжижать(ся); таять; ~d in tears заливаясь слезами; 2) расторгать, аннулировать; 3) прекращать; распускать (*парламент и т. п.*); 4) постепенно исчезать.

dissolvent I [dɪ'zɔlvənt] *n* растворитель.

dissolvent II *a* растворяющий.

dissonance ['dɪsənəns] *n* 1) *муз.* диссонанс; 2) разлад.

dissonant ['dɪsənənt] *a муз.* 1) нестройный, диссонирующий; 2) вносящий разлад.

dissuade [dɪ'sweɪd] *v* 1) отговаривать (*от чего-л.* — from); отсоветовать (*что-л.* — from); 2) разубеждать (*кого-л.*).

dissuasion [dɪ'sweɪʒən] *n* разубеждение.

dissyllabic ['dɪsɪ'læbɪk] *a* двусложный.

dissyllable [dɪ'sɪləbl] *n* двусложное слово.

distaff ['dɪstɑːf] *n* 1) прялка; 2) женская работа; ◊ on the ~ side по женской линии (*семьи*).

distance I ['dɪstəns] *n* 1) расстояние; дистанция; at a ~ на известном расстоянии; 2) отдалённость; дальность; даль; in the ~ вдали; from a ~ издали; striking ~ досягаемость; beyond (within) striking ~ вне пределов (в пределах) досягаемости; 3) сдержанность (*в обращении*), холодность; at a respectful ~ на почтительном расстоянии; to keep one's ~ from smb. избегать кого-л.; to keep smb. at a ~ держать кого-л. на почтительном расстоянии; 4) промежуток, отрезок времени.

distance II *v* 1) оставлять далеко позади (*в состязании и т. п.*); 2) помещать на расстоянии.

distant ['dɪstənt] *a* 1) далёкий; дальний; отдалённый; three miles ~ на расстоянии трёх миль; 2) сдержанный, холодный.

distantly ['dɪstəntlɪ] *adv*: ~ related состоящий в дальнем родстве.

distaste I ['dɪsteɪst] *n* отвращение.

distaste II *v* питать отвращение.

distasteful [dɪs'teɪstful] *a* неприятный, противный (*to*).

distemper[1] [dɪs'tempə] *n* 1) нездоровье; душевное расстройство; 2) собачья чума.

distemper[2] **I** *n* 1) *жив.* темпера; 2) клеевая краска.

distemper[2] **II** *v* 1) *жив.* писать темперой; 2) красить клеевой краской (*стены*).

distempered [dɪs'tempəd] *a* 1) расстроенный (*о воображении*); 2) раздражённый.

distend [dɪs'tend] *v* раздувать(ся), надувать(ся).

distensible [dɪs'tensəbl] *a* растяжимый, эластичный.

distension [dɪs'tenʃən] *n* растяжение.

distil [dɪs'tɪl] *v* 1) очищать перегонкой (*жидкость*); дистиллировать; 2) гнать (*спирт и т. п.*); 3) извлекать эссенцию (*из растений*); *перен.* извлекать самое существенное; 4) сочиться; капать, стекать.

distillation [,dɪstɪ'leɪʃən] *n* дистилляция; перегонка; dry ~ сухая перегонка; возгонка.

distiller [dɪs'tɪlə] *n* 1) винокур; 2) аппарат для перегонки.

distillery [dɪs'tɪlərɪ] *n* винокуренный завод.

distinct [dɪs'tɪŋkt] *a* 1) ясный; отчётливый; 2) отдельный; особый; отличный (*от других*); 3) определённый; явный.

distinction [dɪs'tɪŋkʃən] *n* 1) различение, распознавание; 2) различие; отличие, разница; ~ without a difference (только) кажущееся различие; without any ~ без всякого различия; без исключения; to draw a ~ провести различие; 3) отличительная особенность; 4) индивидуальность, оригинальность; 5) знак отличия; 6) высокие качества; известность.

distinctive [dɪs'tɪŋktɪv] *a* особый; отличительный; характерный.

distinctly [dɪs'tɪŋktlɪ] *adv* 1) ясно, отчётливо; 2) заметно; определённо.

distinctness [dɪs'tɪŋktnɪs] *n* 1) ясность, отчётливость; 2) определённость.

distinguish [dɪs'tɪŋgwɪʃ] *v* 1) различать(ся); отличать(ся); 2) распознать, разглядеть; 3) отличать, выделять; характеризовать; to ~ oneself (by) отличиться, прославиться.

distinguishable [dɪs'tɪŋgwɪʃəbl] *a* различимый, отличимый.

distinguished [dɪs'tɪŋgwɪʃt] *a* 1) выдающийся, знаменитый; 2) характерный.

distort [dɪs'tɔːt] *v* 1) искажать, искривлять; 2) извращать (*факты*).

distortion [dɪs'tɔːʃən] *n* 1) искажение; искривление; 2) извращение.

distortionist [dɪs'tɔːʃənɪst] *см.* contortionist.

distract [dɪs'trækt] *v* 1) отвлекать (*внимание*); 2) смущать, расстраивать; сбивать с толку.

distracted [dɪs'træktɪd] *a* 1) рассеянный; 2) обезумевший, безумный.

distraction [dɪs'trækʃən] *n* 1) отвлечение внимания; 2) рассеянность; 3) развлечение; 4) смятение, отчаяние; 5) безумие; to love to ~ любить до безумия; to drive smb. to ~ довести кого-л. до отчаяния, до безумия.

distrain [dɪs'treɪn] *v юр.* накладывать арест на имущество в обеспечение долга.

distraught [dɪs'trɔːt] *a* обезумевший.

distress I [dɪs'tres] *n* 1) горе, страдание; 2) нужда, тяжёлое положение; 3) беда; бедствие; несчастье; in ~ в беде; терпящий бедствие (*о судне и т. п.*); 4) истощение, крайнее утомление.

distress II *v* 1) причинять горе, страдания; 2) истощать; утомлять.

distressful [dɪs'tresful] *a* 1) прискорбный, горестный; 2) многострадальный, скорбный.

distress-gun [dɪs'tresgʌn] *n* вы́стрел с корабля́ как сигна́л бе́дствия.

distressingly [dɪs'tresɪŋlɪ] *adv* прискорбно, грустно.

distributable [dɪs'trɪbjutəbl] *a* подлежа́щий распределе́нию, разда́че.

distribute [dɪs'trɪbjuːt] *v* 1) распределя́ть, раздава́ть; 2) (равноме́рно) разбра́сывать; (ро́вно) разма́зывать (*краску*); 3) распространя́ть; widely ~d широко́ распространённый; 4) размеща́ть, располага́ть.

distribution [ˌdɪstrɪ'bjuːʃən] *n* 1) распределе́ние; разда́ча; 2) распростране́ние; 3) размеще́ние, расположе́ние; 4) *лингв.* дистрибу́ция.

distributive I [dɪs'trɪbjutɪv] *n грам.* раздели́тельное сло́во.

distributive II *a* 1) распредели́тельный; 2) *грам.* раздели́тельный.

distributor [dɪs'trɪbjuːtə] *n* распредели́тель.

district I ['dɪstrɪkt] *n* райо́н, о́круг; о́бласть; congressional ~ *амер.* избира́тельный о́круг.

district II *v* дели́ть на райо́ны, округа́, райони́ровать.

distrust I [dɪs'trʌst] *n* недове́рие, сомне́ние; подозре́ние.

distrust II *v* не доверя́ть, сомнева́ться.

distrustful [dɪs'trʌstful] *a* недове́рчивый; подозри́тельный.

disturb [dɪs'təːb] *v* 1) беспоко́ить, меша́ть; 2) приводи́ть в беспоря́док; 3) наруша́ть (*поко́й, тишину́, душе́вное равнове́сие*); волнова́ть; 4) расстра́ивать (*пла́ны*); подрыва́ть (*дове́рие*); разруша́ть (*наде́жды*).

disturbance [dɪs'təːbəns] *n* 1) беспоко́йство; наруше́ние (*тишины́, поря́дка*); 2) волне́ние, трево́га.

disturber [dɪs'təːbə] *n* наруши́тель (*тишины́, поря́дка*).

disunion ['dɪs'juːnjən] *n* 1) разъедине́ние, разобще́ние; разделе́ние; 2) разногла́сие, разла́д.

disunite ['dɪsjuː'naɪt] *v* разъединя́ть(ся), разобща́ть(ся); разделя́ть(ся).

disuse[a] ['dɪs'juːs] *n* неупотребле́ние; to fall into ~ вы́йти из употребле́ния.

disuse[b] ['dɪs'juːz] *v* переста́ть употребля́ть.

disused ['dɪs'juːzd] *a* 1) неупотреби́тельный; 2) забро́шенный.

ditch I [dɪtʃ] *n* кана́ва, ров.

ditch II *v* 1) копа́ть кана́вы; ока́пывать рвом; 2) чи́стить кана́ву, ров; 3) попа́сть в кана́ву; сбра́сывать в кюве́т (*автомоби́ль*); 4) *ав.* соверша́ть вы́нужденную поса́дку на́ воду.

ditcher ['dɪtʃə] *n* 1) землеко́п; 2) канавокопа́тель (*маши́на*).

ditch-water ['dɪtʃˌwɔːtə] *n* стоя́чая вода́ (*в кана́вах*); ◊ dull as ~ ску́чный, ну́дный.

dithyramb ['dɪθɪræm(b)] *n* дифира́мб.

ditto ['dɪtou] *n* то же (*са́мое*), тот же, тако́й же, сто́лько же (*вме́сто повторе́ния*); to say ~ to smb. *разг.* подда́кивать кому́-л.

ditty ['dɪtɪ] *n* пе́сенка.

ditty-bag ['dɪtɪbæg] *n* мешо́чек солда́та, матро́са для иго́лок, ни́ток и др. мелоче́й.

ditty-box ['dɪtɪbɔks] *см.* ditty-bag.

diurnal [daɪ'əːnl] *a* 1) дневно́й (*в тече́ние дня*); 2) *астр.* су́точный; 3) *уст.* ежедне́вный.

divan [dɪ'væn] *n* 1) дива́н, куше́тка; 2) дива́н (*госуда́рственный сове́т в Ту́рции*).

dive I [daɪv] *n* 1) ныря́ние; погруже́ние; 2) *ав.* пики́рование; 3) *амер.* рестора́н-погребо́к.

dive II *v* 1) ныря́ть; погружа́ть(ся) (в во́ду); 2) су́нуть ру́ку (*в карма́н, в во́ду*); 3) *ав.* пики́ровать; 4) внеза́пно скрыва́ться, юркну́ть; 5) погружа́ться, углубля́ться (*в изуче́ние чего́-л.— into*).

diver ['daɪvə] *n* 1) водола́з; 2) ныря́льщик; 3) иска́тель же́мчуга; лове́ц гу́бок; 4) *pl* ныря́ющая пти́ца (*ныро́к, гага́ра и т. п.*); 5) *разг.* вор-карма́нник.

diverge [daɪ'vəːdʒ] *v* 1) расходи́ться; 2) отклоня́ться; уклоня́ться.

divergence [daɪ'vəːdʒəns] *n* 1) расхожде́ние, разногла́сие; 2) отклоне́ние.

divergency [daɪ'vəːdʒənsɪ] *см.* divergence.

divergent [daɪ'vəːdʒənt] *a* расходя́щийся; отклоня́ющийся.

divers ['daɪvəːz] *a уст.* ра́зный.

diverse [daɪ'vəːs] *a* 1) ино́й, отли́чный (*от чего́-л.*); 2) разнообра́зный, ра́зный.

diversiform [daɪ'vəːsɪfɔːm] *a* разнообра́зный, ра́зной фо́рмы.

diversify [daɪ'vəːsɪfaɪ] *v* разнообра́зить.

diversion [daɪ'vəːʃən] *n* 1) отклоне́ние; отво́д; 2) отвлече́ние внима́ния; 3) развлече́ние; 4) *воен.* отвлека́ющий уда́р.

diversity [daɪ'vəːsɪtɪ] *n* 1) несхо́дство; 2) разнообра́зие.

divert [daɪ'vəːt] *v* 1) отклоня́ть; отводи́ть (*во́ду*); 2) отвлека́ть (*внима́ние*); 3) развлека́ть, забавля́ть.

diverting [daɪ'vəːtɪŋ] *a* занима́тельный.

divest [daɪ'vest] *v* 1) раздева́ть; снима́ть оде́жду (*of*); 2) лиша́ть (*of*); to ~ oneself of изба́виться, отде́латься от чего́-л.

divide I [dɪ'vaɪd] *n* водоразде́л.

divide II *v* 1) дели́ть(ся); разделя́ть(ся); 2) разъединя́ть(ся); отделя́ть(ся); 3) *мат.* дели́ться без оста́тка; 4) расходи́ться (*о мне́ниях*); 5) градуи́ровать, наноси́ть деле́ния; 6) *парл.* голосова́ть.

divided [dɪ'vaɪdɪd] *a* 1) разделённый; 2) разде́льный; разъёмный; составно́й; 3) *фон.* пла́вный; 4) градуи́рованный.

dividend ['dɪvɪdend] *n* 1) *мат.* дели́мое; 2) *фин.* дивиде́нд.

dividers [dɪ'vaɪdəz] *n pl* ци́ркуль.

divination [ˌdɪvɪ'neɪʃən] *n* 1) предсказа́ние; 2) гада́ние, ворожба́.

divine I [dɪ'vaɪn] *n* духо́вное лицо́; богосло́в.

divine II *a* боже́ственный.

divine III *v* 1) предска́зывать, проро́чить; 2) (пред)уга́дывать.

diviner [dɪ'vaɪnə] *n* прорица́тель, проро́к.

diving ['daɪvɪŋ] *n* 1) ныря́ние; 2) водола́зное де́ло; 3) *ав.* пики́рование.

diving-bell ['daɪvɪŋbel] *n* водола́зный ко́локол.

diving-dress ['daɪvɪŋdres] *n* скафа́ндр.

divinity [dɪ'vɪnɪtɪ] *n* 1) боже́ственность, 2) божество́; 3) богосло́вие.

divisibility [dɪˌvɪzɪ'bɪlɪtɪ] *n* дели́мость.

divisible [dɪ'vɪzəbl] *a* дели́мый.

division [dɪ'vɪʒən] *n* 1) деле́ние; разделе́ние;

~ of labour разделе́ние труда́; 2) отделе́ние, отде́л; разде́л; 3) перегоро́дка; грани́ца; межа́; 4) разногла́сие, раздо́ры; 5) *воен.* диви́зия.

divisor [dɪ'vaɪzə] *n мат.* дели́тель.

divorce I [dɪ'vɔːs] *n* 1) разво́д; 2) отделе́ние, разделе́ние, разры́в.

divorce II *v* 1) разводи́ться; расторга́ть брак; to get ~d развести́сь; 2) отделя́ть, разъединя́ть.

divorcee [dɪˌvɔː'siː] *n* разведённый, -ая.

divulge [daɪ'vʌldʒ] *v* разглаша́ть.

Dixie .['dɪksɪ] *n* Ю́жные шта́ты США (*тж.* ~ Land).

dixie ['dɪksɪ] *n воен. разг.* похо́дный котело́к.

dixy ['dɪksɪ] *см.* dixie.

dizziness ['dɪzɪnɪs] *n* головокруже́ние.

dizzy I ['dɪzɪ] *a* 1) испы́тывающий головокруже́ние; I am ~, I feel ~ у меня́ голова́ кру́жится; 2) головокружи́тельный.

dizzy II *v* 1) вызыва́ть головокруже́ние; 2) ошеломля́ть.

doᵃ I [duː (*сильная форма*), du, də, d (*слабые формы*)] *v* (*past* did; *p. p.* done) 1) де́лать; 2) выполня́ть; 3) причиня́ть (*боль, неприятность и т. п.*); 4) исполня́ть роль; де́йствовать в ка́честве кого́-л.; 5) поступа́ть, вести́ себя́; 6) годи́ться, подходи́ть; быть доста́точным; that will do! a) хва́тит!; б) идёт!; 7) поко́нчить (*с — with*); have done! переста́ньте!, бро́сьте!; 8) пожива́ть; быть здоро́вым; поправля́ться; 9) гото́вить (*еду*); 10) *разг.* осма́тривать (*достопримеча́тельности*); 11) *разг.* обма́нывать (*тж.* to do brown); you have been done вас наду́ли; 12) *употребля́ется как вспомога́тельный гл. в отриц. и вопр. формах Present и Past Indefinite:* I do not know him я не зна́ю его́; I did not see him я не ви́дел его́; do you like it? нра́вится ли вам э́то?; did you know it? зна́ли ли вы э́то?; 13) *употребля́ется:* а) *для усиле́ния про́сьбы:* do tell ну, пожа́луйста, скажи́ (прошу́ тебя́); б) *для подчёркивания и усиле́ния:* I did see him я-то (действи́тельно) ви́дел его́; I do want to go я о́чень хочу́ пойти́; 14) *употребля́ется для заме́ны како́го-л. глаго́ла (вместо повторе́ния):* my dog goes where I do моя́ соба́ка идёт туда́ же, куда́ и (иду́); did you see him? — I did ви́дели ли вы его́? —Ви́дел; ▢ to do **again** переде́лывать; to do **away** a) устраня́ть; б) снима́ть, счища́ть; в) уничтожа́ть, искореня́ть (*with*); to do **by** обраща́ться (*с кем-л.*); to do **down** *разг.* взять верх, перехитри́ть; to do **for** *разг.* губи́ть, убива́ть; he is done for он поги́б; to do **in** *сленг* а) погуби́ть, уби́ть; б) обману́ть; to do **into** переводи́ть (*на другой язык*); to do **off** снима́ть; отвя́зывать; to do **on** надева́ть; to do **out** убира́ть, прибира́ть; to do **over** покрыва́ть, обкла́дывать, обма́зывать; to do **to** *см.* to do by; to do **up** a) приводи́ть в поря́док; ремонти́ровать; б) завёртывать (*пакет*); в) *обыкн. p. p.* утомля́ть, изма́тывать; to do **with** a) терпе́ть, выноси́ть; б) ла́дить с кем-л.; в) обходи́ться чем-л.; to do **without** обходи́ться без чего́-л.; ◇ how do you do? здра́вствуйте!; to do smb. good приноси́ть кому́-л. по́льзу.

doᵃ II *n сленг* 1) обма́н; мистифика́ция; 2) вечери́нка.

doᵇ [dou] *n муз.* но́та до.

do-all ['duːˌɔːl] *n* ма́стер на все ру́ки.

doat [dout] *см.* dote.

dobbin ['dɔbɪn] *n* ло́шадь (*обыкн. споко́йная, сми́рная*).

doc [dɔk] *n амер. разг.* до́ктор.

docile ['dousaɪl] *a* 1) послу́шный; 2) поня́тливый.

docility [dou'sɪlɪtɪ] *n* 1) послуша́ние; 2) поня́тливость.

dock¹ [dɔk] *n* щаве́ль.

dock² I *n* 1) док; dry ~, graving ~ сухо́й док; in dry ~ *разг.* безрабо́тный; wet ~ мо́крый, наливно́й док; 2) *амер.* при́стань; 3) *ж.-д.* тупи́к.

dock² II *v* 1) ста́вить су́дно в док; входи́ть в док (*о судне*); 2) стро́ить до́ки; 3) производи́ть стыко́вку, стыкова́ться (*о космических корабля́х*).

dock³ *n* ме́сто подсуди́мого в суде́, скамья́ подсуди́мых; in the ~ на скамье́ подсуди́мых.

dock⁴ I *n* обру́бленный хвост.

dock⁴ II *v* 1) обруба́ть (*хвост*); 2) ко́ротко стричь (*волосы*); 3) сокраща́ть, уреза́ть.

dockage¹ ['dɔkɪdʒ] *n* 1) стоя́нка судо́в в до́ках; 2) сбор за по́льзование до́ком.

dockage² *n разг.* сокраще́ние, уре́зывание.

docker ['dɔkə] *n* до́кер.

docket ['dɔkɪt] *n* 1) на́дпись на докуме́нте с кра́тким изложе́нием его́ содержа́ния; 2) этике́тка, ярлы́к; 3) квита́нция об упла́те по́шлины; 4) *юр.* спи́сок суде́бных дел.

docking ['dɔkɪŋ] *n* стыко́вка (*космических корабле́й*).

dock-master ['dɔkˌmɑːstə] *n* нача́льник до́ка, ве́рфи.

dockyard ['dɔkjɑːd] *n* 1) верфь; 2) адмиралте́йство.

doctor I ['dɔktə] *n* 1) до́ктор, врач; 2) до́ктор (*учёная сте́пень*); 3) вспомога́тельный механи́зм.

doctor II *v* 1) лечи́ть; 2) присужда́ть до́кторскую сте́пень; 3) нала́живать (*машину*); 4) подде́лывать; фальсифици́ровать (*продукты*).

doctorate ['dɔktərɪt] *n* до́кторская сте́пень.

doctrinaire I [ˌdɔktrɪ'nɛə] *n* доктринёр.

doctrinaire II *a* доктринёрский. .

doctrinal [dɔk'traɪnl] *a* догмати́ческий.

doctrine ['dɔktrɪn] *n* 1) уче́ние, доктри́на; 2) ве́ра, до́гма.

documentᵃ ['dɔkjumənt] *n* докуме́нт.

documentᵇ ['dɔkjument] *v* 1) подтвержда́ть докуме́нтами; 2) снабжа́ть докуме́нтами.

documentary I [ˌdɔkju'mentərɪ] *n* документа́льный фильм.

documentary II *a* документа́льный.

documentation [ˌdɔkjumen'teɪʃən] *n* подтвержде́ние докуме́нтами, документа́ция.

dodder¹ ['dɔdə] *n бот.* повили́ка.

dodder² *v* 1) дрожа́ть, трясти́сь (*от старости, слабости*); 2) мя́млить; ▢ to ~ **about**, to ~ **along** ковыля́ть.

doddery ['dɔdərɪ] *a* 1) дрожа́щий, трясу́щийся; 2) слабоу́мный, глу́пый.

dodge I [dɔdʒ] *n* 1) уклоне́ние, уве́ртка; 2) уло́вка, хи́трость; проде́лка; 3) *разг.* хи́трое устро́йство.

dodge II *v* 1) избега́ть, увёртываться, уклоня́ться; 2) хитри́ть, ло́вко извора́чиваться.

dodger ['dɔdʒə] *n* 1) хитре́ц; ловка́ч; 2) *амер.* рекла́ма, объявле́ние.

dodgy ['dɔdʒɪ] *a* 1) хи́трый, ло́вкий, изворо́тливый; 2) остроу́мный (*о приспособле́нии*).

doe ['dou] *n* сáмка олéня, крóлика, зáйца.

doer ['du:ə] *n* дéятель, исполнúтель, рабóтник.

doeskin ['douskɪn] *n* 1) олéнья кóжа; зáмша; 2) мя́гкая шерстяна́я ткань под зáмшу.

doesn't ['dʌznt] *разг.* = does not.

doff [dɔf] *v* снима́ть (*шля́пу, пальтó*).

dog I [dɔg] *n* 1) собáка; пёс; Eskimo ~ лáйка; 2) кобéль; самéц (*о волке, лисе*); 3) *разг.* пáрень; a jolly ~ весельчáк; a lazy ~ лентя́й; a lucky ~ счастлúвчик; a dirty ~ дрянь, свинья́; 4) *тех.* собáчка; защёлка; ◊ ~s of war ýжасы войны́; a ~ in the manger *погов.* ≅ не тронь лúхо, покá спит тúхо; to go to the ~s *разг.* погúбнуть, разорúться; пойтú прáхом; top ~ *разг.* хозя́ин положéния, победúтель; hot ~ бутербрóд с горя́чей сосúской; every ~ has his day *погов.* ≅ бýдет и на нáшей ýлице прáздник; to help a lame ~ over a stile помóчь в бедé; to be under ~ быть вы́нужденным повиновáться; not even a ~'s chance никакúх шáнсов.

dog II *v* 1) слéдовать по пятáм; выслéживать; 2) преслéдовать.

dog-cart ['dɔgkɑːt] *n* двухколёсный экипáж с мéстом для собáк под сидéньями.

dog-cheap I ['dɔgtʃiːp] *a* óчень дешёвый; ≅ дешéвле пáреной рéпы.

dog-cheap II *adv* óчень дёшево.

dog-collar ['dɔg,kɔlə] *n* 1) ошéйник; 2) высóкий воротнúк.

dog-days ['dɔgdeɪz] *n pl* сáмые жáркие дни лéта.

doge [doudʒ] *n ист.* дож.

dog-ear I, II ['dɔgɪə] *см.* dog's-ear I, II.

dog-eared ['dɔgɪəd] *a* с зáгнутыми углáми (*о страницах*).

dogged ['dɔgɪd] *a* упря́мый, упóрный, настóйчивый.

doggerel I ['dɔgərəl] *n* плохúе стихú.

doggerel II *a* плохóй, неумéлый (*о стихах*).

doggie ['dɔgɪ] *см.* doggy I.

doggish ['dɔgɪʃ] *a* 1) собáчий; 2) *разг.* криклúво-мóдный.

doggo ['dɔgou] *adv сленг* притаúвшись; to lie ~ притаúться.

doggy I ['dɔgɪ] *n* собáчка.

doggy II *a* 1) собáчий; 2) любя́щий собáк.

dog-hole ['dɔghoul] *n* собáчья конурá (*тж. перен.*).

dog-in-a-blanket ['dɔgɪnə'blæŋkɪt] *n* пýдинг с варéньем.

dog-lead ['dɔgliːd] *n* поводóк (*для собáк*).

dogma ['dɔgmə] *n* (*pl тж.* dogmata ['dɔgmətə]) 1) дóгма; учéние; 2) дóгмат.

dogmatic [dɔg'mætɪk] *a* 1) догматúческий; 2) категорúческий, не допускáющий возражéний.

dogmatically [dɔg'mætɪkəlɪ] *adv* 1) догматúчески; 2) категорúческим тóном.

dog-rose ['dɔgrouz] *n* дúкая рóза, шипóвник.

dog's-ear I ['dɔgzɪə] *n* зáгнутый уголóк странúцы.

dog's-ear II *v* загибáть уголкú странúц.

dogskin ['dɔgskɪn] *n* лáйка (*кожа*).

dog-sleep ['dɔgsliːp] *n* чýткий сон; сон уры́вками.

dog's-meat ['dɔgzmiːt] *n* 1) мя́со для собáк; *особ.* конúна; 2) пáдаль.

dog-tired ['dɔg'taɪəd] *a* устáлый как собáка.

dog-tooth ['dɔgtuːθ] *n* клык.

dogtrot ['dɔgtrɔt] *n* рысцá.

dog-violet ['dɔg,vaɪəlɪt] *n бот.* фиáлка собáчья.

doily ['dɔɪlɪ] *n* салфéточка.

doing ['duːɪŋ] *n обыкн. pl* делá, постýпки, поведéние.

doit [dɔɪt] *n* мéлкая монéта; *перен.* пустя́к, мéлочь; not worth a ~ грошá лóманого не стóит; don't care a ~ наплевáть.

doldrums ['dɔldrəmz] *n pl* 1) плохóе настроéние, уны́ние; 2) *мор.* штилевáя полосá.

dole[1] I [doul] *n* 1) небольшóе посóбие, вспомоществовáние; 2) (the ~) посóбие по безрабóтице; to be (*или* to go) on the ~ получáть (еженедéльное) посóбие по безрабóтице; 3) *уст.* небольшáя дóля, часть.

dole II *v* 1) выдавáть небольшóе посóбие; 2) неохóтно, скýпо выдавáть.

dole[2] *n поэт.* гóре, скорбь.

doleful ['doulful] *a* скóрбный, печáльный; меланхолúческий.

doll I [dɔl] *n* кýкла.

doll II *v амер. разг.* наряжáть; ~ed up разря́женный.

dollar ['dɔlə] *n* 1) дóллар; 2) *attr* дóлларовый.

dollish ['dɔlɪʃ] *a* кýкольный.

dollop ['dɔləp] *n разг.* большóй кусóк.

dolly I ['dɔlɪ] *n* 1) кýколка; 2) бельевóй валёк.

dolly II *v* бить бельё вальком.

dolor ['doulə] *амер. см.* dolour.

dolorous ['dɔlərəs] *a поэт.* печáльный, грýстный.

dolour ['doulə] *n поэт.* печáль, грусть; гóре.

dolphin ['dɔlfɪn] *n зоол.* дельфúн.

dolt [doult] *n* болвáн, дурáк.

doltish ['doultɪʃ] *a* тупóй, придуркóватый.

domain [də'meɪn] *n* 1) владéние; имéние; 2) óбласть, сфéра (*деятельности, науки*).

dome I [doum] *n* 1) кýпол; свод; 2) *поэт.* велúчественное здáние.

dome II *v* 1) крыть кýполом; 2) возвышáться в вúде кýпола.

domed [doumd] *a* куполообрáзный.

domestic I [də'mestɪk] *n* 1) прислýга; 2) *pl* товáры отéчественного произвóдства.

domestic II *a* 1) домáшний; семéйный; 2) домосéдливый; 3) внýтренний; отéчественный; 4) домáшний, ручнóй (*о животных*).

domesticate [də'mestɪkeɪt] *v* 1) привя́зывать к дóму, к семéйной жúзни; 2) приручáть (*животных*); культивúровать (*растения*); акклиматизúровать; 3) обучáть домовóдству.

domestication [də,mestɪ'keɪʃən] *n* 1) приручéние (*животных*); 2) привы́чка, любóвь к дóму, к семéйной жúзни.

domesticity [,doumes'tɪsɪtɪ] *n* домáшняя жизнь; домáшний уют.

domicile I ['dɔmɪsaɪl] *n* 1) (постоя́нное) местожúтельство; 2) дом, жилúще.

domicile II *v* поселúться на постоя́нное жúтельство.

dominance ['dɔmɪnəns] *n* госпóдство; влия́ние; преобладáние.

dominant ['dɔmɪnənt] *a* госпóдствующий; преоблада́ющий.

dominate ['dɔmɪneɪt] v 1) госпо́дствовать, вла́ствовать; владе́ть (*чу́вствами и т. п.*); 2) име́ть влия́ние на кого́-л.; 3) возвыша́ться; домини́ровать; преоблада́ть.

domination [,dɔmɪ'neɪʃən] n госпо́дство, преоблада́ние; власть.

domineer [,dɔmɪ'nɪə] v 1) вла́ствовать; повелева́ть; тира́нить; 2) вести́ себя́ высокоме́рно.

domineering [,dɔmɪ'nɪərɪŋ] a 1) деспоти́ческий, вла́стный; 2) высокоме́рный; 3) госпо́дствующий над, возвыша́ющийся над (*ме́стностью и т. п.*).

Dominican [də'mɪnɪkən] n доминика́нец (*мона́х*).

dominie ['dɔmɪnɪ] n *шотл.* шко́льный учи́тель.

dominion [də'mɪnjən] n 1) власть, влады́чество; 2) владе́ния; 3) доминио́н.

domino ['dɔmɪnou] n 1) *pl* домино́ (*игра́*); 2) домино́ (*маскара́дный костю́м*).

don¹ [dɔn] n 1) преподава́тель, глава́ колле́джа; 2) (D) дон (*испа́нский ти́тул*); 3) испа́нец; 4) *разг.* знато́к.

don² v надева́ть.

donate [dou'neɪt] v *амер.* дари́ть; же́ртвовать.

donation [dou'neɪʃən] n дар; пожертвова́ние.

donative I ['dounətɪv] n дар, пода́рок.

donative II a да́рственный.

donatory ['dounətərɪ] n получа́ющий пода́рок.

done I [dʌn] a 1) зако́нченный; 2) гото́вый, прожа́ренный; 3) уста́лый, изму́ченный (*тж.* ~ up); 4) обма́нутый (*тж.* ~ brown); ◊ ~ for а) разорённый; б) поги́бший, ко́нченный; в) уби́тый.

done II *p. p. см.* do¹¹ I.

donkey ['dɔŋkɪ] n осёл.

donnish ['dɔnɪʃ] a 1) педанти́чный; 2) ва́жный, наду́тый.

donor ['dounə] n 1) дари́тель, же́ртвователь; 2) *мед.* до́нор.

do-nothing ['duː,nʌθɪŋ] n безде́льник.

don't [dount] *разг.* = do not.

doodle-bomb ['duːdl,bɔm] n *воен. разг.* самолёт-снаря́д.

doom I [duːm] n 1) судьба́, рок; 2) ги́бель, смерть; 3) *уст.* пригово́р; 4) *ист.* зако́н; постановле́ние.

doom II v осужда́ть; обрека́ть (*на — to*); ~ed to failure обречённый на прова́л.

doomsday ['duːmzdeɪ] n *рел.* день стра́шного суда́; to wait till ~ ждать до второ́го прише́ствия (*т. е. бесконе́чно*); from now till ~ навсегда́.

door [dɔː] n 1) дверь; две́рца; front ~ пара́дный вход; emergency ~ запа́сный вы́ход; back ~ чёрный ход; jib ~ потайна́я дверь; next ~ ря́дом, по сосе́дству; to live next ~ жить в сосе́днем до́ме; next ~ to *перен.* о́чень бли́зко, почти́, на волосо́к от; at death's ~ на поро́ге сме́рти; to show smb. the ~ указа́ть на дверь кому́-л., вы́проводить, вы́ставить кого́-л.; to open a ~ to сде́лать возмо́жным; to close the ~ upon сде́лать невозмо́жным; to force an open ~ ломи́ться в откры́тую дверь; out of ~s на (откры́том) во́здухе; he is out of ~s его́ нет до́ма; within ~s в помеще́нии, до́ма; to turn out of ~ вы́гнать, вы́проводить; 2) *attr* дверно́й; ◊ to lay at smb.'s ~ обвиня́ть кого́-л.

doorbell ['dɔːbel] n дверно́й звоно́к.

door-handle ['dɔː,hændl] n дверна́я ру́чка.

door-keeper ['dɔː,kiːpə] n швейца́р.

doormat ['dɔːmæt] n полови́к у две́ри.

door-plate ['dɔːpleɪt] n дощёчка, табли́чка на дверя́х (*с фами́лией жильца́*).

door-post ['dɔːpoust] n дверно́й коса́к.

doorstep ['dɔːstep] n поро́г.

door-stone ['dɔːstoun] n ка́менная плита́ (*у вхо́да*).

doorway ['dɔːweɪ] n дверно́й проём, дверь, вход; *перен.* путь; in the ~ в дверя́х.

dope I [doup] n 1) густа́я сма́зка; 2) *разг.* нарко́тик; дурма́н (*тж. перен.*); 3) *амер. разг.* секре́тная информа́ция.

dope II v *разг.* 1) дава́ть *или* употребля́ть нарко́тики; *перен.* одурма́нивать; 2) предска́зывать на основа́нии секре́тной информа́ции.

dop(e)y ['doupɪ] a *сленг* 1) одурма́ненный; 2) одурма́нивающий.

Doric ['dɔrɪk] a *архит.* дори́ческий.

dormancy ['dɔːmənsɪ] n дремо́та; состоя́ние безде́йствия.

dormant ['dɔːmənt] a 1) дре́млющий; спя́щий, безде́йствующий; скры́тый (*о си́лах, спосо́бностях*); to lie ~ бездействовать; 2) находя́щийся в спя́чке (*о живо́тном*).

dormer ['dɔːmə] n слухово́е окно́ (*тж.* ~-window).

dormitory ['dɔːmɪtrɪ] n 1 о́бщая спа́льня; 2) общежи́тие.

dorp [dɔːp] n дереву́шка.

dorsal ['dɔːsəl] a *анат., зоол.* спинно́й.

dory ['dɔːrɪ] n *амер.* рыба́чья плоскодо́нная ло́дка.

dosage ['dousɪdʒ] n 1) дозиро́вка; 2) до́за.

dose I [dous] n 1) до́за, приём; lethal ~ смерте́льная до́за; 2) до́ля, по́рция; regular ~ *разг.* изря́дная по́рция; 3) ингредие́нт, прибавля́емый к вину́.

dose II v 1) дава́ть лека́рство до́зами; дози́ровать; 2) прибавля́ть спирт и т. п. к вину́.

doss I [dɔs] n *сленг* крова́ть, ко́йка (*в ночле́жном до́ме*).

doss II v *сленг* ночева́ть (*в ночле́жном до́ме*).

doss-house ['dɔshaus] n ночле́жный дом; ночле́жка.

dossier ['dɔsɪeɪ] n досье́.

dot¹ I [dɔt] n 1) то́чка; 2) кро́шка, малю́тка; кро́шечная вещь; ◊ off one's ~ *сленг* рехну́вшийся, помеша́вшийся; not a ~ or comma ро́вно ничего́.

dot¹ II v 1) ста́вить то́чки; 2) отмеча́ть пункти́ром; 3) усе́ивать; ◊ to ~ smb. one *разг.* уда́рить кого́-л., сту́кнуть.

dot² n прида́ное.

dotage ['doutɪdʒ] n ста́рческое слабоу́мие; to be in one's ~ впасть в де́тство.

dot-and-dash ['dɔtən'dæʃ] a пункти́рный (*о ли́нии*); ~ code а́збука Мо́рзе.

dot-and-go-one ['dɔtən'gouwʌn] n хромота́, прихра́мывание.

dotard ['doutəd] n вы́живший из ума́ стари́к.

dote [dout] v 1) впасть в де́тство; 2) безрассу́дно люби́ть (*on, upon*).

doting ['doutɪŋ] a лю́бящий, пре́данный.

dotted ['dɔtɪd] a пункти́рный.

dotty ['dɔtɪ] *a* 1) тóчечный; в тóчках; 2) *разг.* неустóйчивый; ~ on one's legs нетвёрдо стоя́щий на нога́х; 3) *разг.* рехну́вшийся.

double I ['dʌbl] *n* 1) двойнóе коли́чество; 2) двойни́к; 3) *воен.* бéглый шаг; at the ~ бегóм; 4) *театр.* дублёр; актёр, исполня́ющий две рóли в пьéсе; 5) изги́б (*реки*); крутóй поворóт, пéтля (*преслéдуемого звéря*); 6) увёртка, хи́трость; 7) *pl* па́рная игра́ в тéннис.

double II *a* 1) двойнóй, удвóенный, сдвóенный; па́рный; he is ~ her age он вдвóе ста́рше её; 2) двоя́кий; 3) двóйственный; двули́чный; двусмы́сленный; 4) *бот.* махрóвый.

double III *v* 1) удва́ивать; сдва́ивать; 2) удва́иваться; быть вдвóе бóльше; 3) скла́дывать вдвóе; 4) сжима́ть (*кулаки*); 5) дéлать изги́б (*о рекé*); *мор.* огиба́ть (*мыс*); 6) дéлать поворóты, пéтли (*о преслéдуемом звéре*); 7) *театр.*: to ~ a part дубли́ровать роль; to ~ the parts of исполня́ть две рóли в пьéсе; 8) *воен.* идти́ бéглым ша́гом; □ to ~ **back** повора́чивать обра́тно; запу́тывать след, дéлать пéтли; to ~ **forward** выбега́ть вперёд; to ~ **in** подгиба́ть, загиба́ть внутрь; to ~ **over** перебега́ть; to ~ **up** сгиба́ть(ся); скрю́чивать (-ся); to ~ **upon** *мор.* обойти́, окружи́ть (*неприя́тельский флот*).

double IV *adv* вдвóе; вдвойнé; вдвоём; двоя́ко; ~ as bright вдвóе светлéе; to ride ~ éхать вдвоём на однóй лóшади; to see ~ двои́ться в глаза́х (*у пья́ного*); to play ~ двуру́шничать, лицемéрить.

double-acting ['dʌbl,æktɪŋ] *a* двойнóго дéйствия.

double-barrelled ['dʌbl,bærəld] *a* 1) двуствóльный; 2) двусмы́сленный.

double-bass ['dʌbl'beɪs] *n муз* контраба́с.

double-bedded ['dʌbl,bedɪd] *a* с двумя́ крова́тями, с двуспа́льной крова́тью (*о кóмнате*).

double-breasted ['dʌbl'brestɪd] *a* двубóртный (*о пиджакé и т. п.*).

double-cross ['dʌbl'krɔːs] *v разг.* надува́ть, обма́нывать (*друг дру́га*).

double-dealer ['dʌbl'diːlə] *n* обма́нщик; двуру́шник.

double-dealing I ['dʌbl'diːlɪŋ] *n* двуру́шничество.

double-dealing II *a* двуру́шнический.

double-decker ['dʌbl'dekə] *n* 1) двухпа́лубное су́дно; 2) *разг.* двухэта́жный трамва́й *или* автóбус; 3) *ав. разг.* бипла́н.

double-dyed ['dʌbl'daɪd] *a* закоренéлый; отъя́вленный.

double-edged ['dʌbl'edʒd] *a* обоюдоóстрый.

double-faced ['dʌblfeɪst] *a* 1) двули́чный, лицемéрный; 2) двусторóнний (*о матéрии*).

double-lock ['dʌbl'lɔk] *v* запира́ть на два оборóта.

double-natured ['dʌbl'neɪtʃəd] *a* двóйственный.

double-quick I ['dʌbl'kwɪk] *a* óчень бы́стрый.

double-quick II *v амер.* идти́ ускóренным ша́гом.

double-quick III *adv* óчень бы́стро.

doublet ['dʌblɪt] *n* 1) дублéт; дублика́т; 2) дуплéт (*в билья́рде*); 3) *ист.* корóткий камзóл XV—XVII вв.; 4) *радио* двойна́я анте́нна; 5) *лингв.* дублéт.

double-tongued ['dʌbl'tʌŋd] *a* лжи́вый, нейскренний.

doubling ['dʌblɪŋ] *n* 1) удвоéние; сдва́ивание; 2) повторéние, дубли́рование; 3) внеза́пный поворóт (*напр., убега́ющего за́йца*); 4) улóвка, увёртка; уклóнчивость.

doubly ['dʌblɪ] *adv* вдвóе, вдвойнé.

doubt I [daut] *n* сомнéние; to make ~ сомнева́ться; to make no ~ быть увéренным; to settle smb.'s ~s разреши́ть чьи-л. сомнéния; beyond (a) ~ вне (вся́кого) сомнéния; no ~, without ~ несомнéнно.

doubt II *v* 1) сомнева́ться; 2) не доверя́ть, подозрева́ть.

doubtful ['dautful] *a* 1) пóлный сомнéний; сомнева́ющийся, колéблющийся; 2) нея́сный; сомни́тельный, подозри́тельный.

doubtless ['dautlɪs] *adv* 1) несомнéнно; 2) *разг.* (весьма́) вероя́тно.

douche I [duːʃ] *n* 1) душ; облива́ние; to throw a cold ~ upon smb. *перен.* вы́лить уша́т холóдной воды́ на когó-л.; 2) промыва́ние.

douche II *v* принима́ть душ, облива́ть(ся) водóй.

dough [dou] *n* 1) тéсто; 2) густа́я ма́сса, па́ста; 3) *амер. сленг* дéньги.

dough-boy ['dou,bɔɪ] *n* 1) пóнчик; 2) *амер. сленг* солда́т, пехоти́нец.

doughfaced ['doufeɪst] *a* 1) блéдный (*о цвéте лица́*); 2) слабохара́ктерный, пода́тливый.

doughnut ['dounʌt] *n* пирожóк, пóнчик.

doughtily ['dautɪlɪ] *adv* дóблестно, отва́жно.

doughtiness ['dautɪnɪs] *n* дóблесть, отва́га, му́жество.

doughty ['dautɪ] *a уст.* дóблестный, удалóй (*часто ирон.*).

- **doughy** ['douɪ] *a* 1) тестообра́зный; плóхо пропечённый; 2) блéдный (*о цвéте лица́*).

dour [duə] *a* сурóвый, стрóгий.

douse ['daus] *v* 1) погружа́ть(ся) в вóду, окуна́ть(ся); 2) *мор.* спуска́ть па́рус; 3) облива́ть, обры́згивать водóй; 4) туши́ть, гаси́ть.

dove [dʌv] *n* 1) гóлубь; Dove of Peace гóлубь ми́ра; 2) голу́бчик, голу́бушка (*обыкн. my ~*).

dove-colour ['dʌv,kʌlə] *n* си́зый цвет.

dove-cot, dove-cote ['dʌvkɔt, 'dʌvkout] *n* голубя́тня; to flutter the dove-cotes произвести́ переполóх, переполоши́ть.

dove-eyed ['dʌv'aɪd] *a* с неви́нным ви́дом.

dovelike ['dʌvlaɪk] *a* крóткий (как гóлубь).

doveling ['dʌvlɪŋ] *n* птенéц гóлубя, голубёнок.

dovetail I ['dʌvteɪl] *n тех., стр.* ла́сточкин хвост, ла́па, шип.

dovetail II *v* 1) *стр.* вяза́ть в ла́пу; 2) плóтно подгоня́ть; 3) тóчно подходи́ть (*друг к дру́гу*); соотвéтствовать; совпада́ть (*о показа́ниях и т. п.*).

dowager ['dauədʒə] *n* 1) вдова́ (*титулóванная*); the Queen ~ вдóвствующая королéва; 2) *разг.* величественная жéнщина.

dowdy I ['daudɪ] *n* плóхо, безвку́сно одéтая жéнщина.

dowdy II *a* 1) плóхо, безвку́сно одéтая (*о жéнщине*); 2) плохóй, безвку́сный (*о пла́тье*).

dower I ['dauə] *n* 1) вдóвья часть наслéдства; 2) прида́ное; 3) приро́дный дар; тала́нт.

dower II *v* 1) оставля́ть насле́дство вдове́; 2) наделя́ть тала́нтом (*with*).

down¹ [daun] *n* пух, пушо́к.

down² *n* холми́стая ме́стность.

down³ I *adv* 1) вниз; внизу́; the guests are ~ in the sitting-room го́сти внизу́ в гости́ной; 2) на зе́млю, на земле́; he fell ~ он упа́л на зе́млю; 3) *указывает на движение от центра к периферии, из столицы в провинцию, с севера на юг;* обы́чно не перево́дится: to go ~ to the country е́хать в дере́вню; to go ~ south е́хать на юг; 4) *придаёт глаголам значение совершенного вида; передаётся приглагольными префиксами* вы-, за-, с-; to write ~ записа́ть; to climb ~ слезть; to pay ~ вы́платить; 5) *указывает на ухудшение, уменьшение количества, размера, ослабление силы и т. п.; передаётся приглагольными префиксами* у-, вы-; to boil ~ вы́кипеть; to calm ~ успоко́ить(ся); 6) *указывает на связь более раннего периода времени с более поздним* вплоть до; ~ to our days вплоть до на́ших дней; ◊ to be ~ and out а) потерпе́ть по́лный крах; разори́ться; б) быть пода́вленным; ~ on one's luck в несча́стье; в тяжёлом положе́нии; ~ with! доло́й!

down³ II *prep* 1) по; ~ the road по доро́ге; 2) вниз по, вдоль по; ~ the river вниз по тече́нию реки́.

down³ III *n* спуск; ◊ to have a ~ on smb. име́ть зуб на кого́-л.

down³ IV *a* 1) напра́вленный кни́зу; 2) иду́щий из столи́цы, из большо́го го́рода (*о поезде*).

down³ V *v разг.* 1) спуска́ть, опуска́ть; 2) сбива́ть (*самолёт*); 3) подчиня́ть, покоря́ть; 4) опроки́нуть (*рюмочку*); ◊ to ~ tools забастова́ть, прекрати́ть рабо́ту.

down-and-outs ['daunənd'auts] *n pl* беднота́, голь.

downcast ['daunkɑːst] *a* 1) удручённый; пода́вленный, уны́лый; 2) опу́щенный вниз; 3) поту́пленный (*о взгляде*).

downfall ['daunfɔːl] *n* 1) паде́ние; *перен. тж.* ги́бель; 2) ли́вень; си́льный снегопа́д.

down-hearted ['daun'hɑːtɪd] *a* упа́вший ду́хом, уны́лый.

downhill I ['daun'hɪl] *n* склон.

downhill II *a* пока́тый.

downhill III *adv* вниз (по склону); под го́ру; to go ~ а) ухудша́ться (*о здоровье, состоянии и т. п.*); б) кати́ться по накло́нной пло́скости.

Downing Street ['daunɪŋ'striːt] *n* Да́унинг-стрит (*улица в Лондоне, на которой помещается министерство иностранных дел и резиденция премьер-министра; перен.* англи́йское прави́тельство).

downpour ['daunpɔː] *n* пото́к; ли́вень.

downright I ['daunrait] *a* 1) че́стный; прямо́й, открове́нный, я́сный; 2) я́вный (*о лжи и т. п.*); 3) отъя́вленный; соверше́нный.

downright II *adv* соверше́нно, о́чень.

downstair ['daun'stɛə] *см.* downstairs I.

downstairs I ['daun'stɛəz] *a* располо́женный в ни́жнем этаже́.

downstairs II *adv* 1) вниз; 2) внизу́; в ни́жнем этаже́.

downstream ['daun'striːm] *adv* (вниз) по тече́нию.

downtown I ['dauntaun] *a амер.* располо́женный в делово́й ча́сти го́рода.

downtown II *adv амер.* в делову́ю часть, в делово́й ча́сти го́рода.

downtrodden ['daun‚trɔdn] *a* угнетённый.

downward I ['daunwəd] *a* 1) спуска́ющийся; снижа́ющийся; 2) уны́лый, пода́вленный.

downward II *adv* вниз, кни́зу.

downwards ['daunwədz] *см.* downward II.

downy¹ ['daunɪ] *a* 1) пуши́стый, мя́гкий как пух; 2) *сленг* хи́трый, себе́ на уме́.

downy² *a* холми́стый.

dowry ['dauərɪ] *n* 1) прида́ное; 2) приро́дный дар; тала́нт.

doxy ['dɔksɪ] *n сленг* 1) ни́щенка; 2) потаску́шка.

doze I [douz] *n* дремо́та.

doze II *v* дрема́ть; □ to ~ off вздремну́ть.

dozen ['dʌzn] *n* 1) дю́жина; to pack in ~s пакова́ть, скла́дывать дю́жинами; long (*или* great, baker's, devil's) ~ чёртова дю́жина, трина́дцать; 2) *pl* мно́жество.

dozy ['douzɪ] *a* со́нный; дре́млющий.

drab¹ I [dræb] *n* 1) ту́скло-кори́чневый цвет; 2) се́рость, однообра́зие.

drab¹ II *a* 1) ту́скло-кори́чневый; 2) се́рый, однообра́зный, ску́чный.

drab² *n* 1) неря́ха; 2) *уст.* проститу́тка.

drabble ['dræbl] *v* забры́згать(ся), запа́чкать(-ся), замочи́ть(ся).

drachm ['dræm] *см.* dram 1).

draff [dræf] *n* помо́и; подо́нки; отбро́сы.

draft I [drɑːft] *n* 1) чертёж, план; эски́з; 2) прое́кт, набро́сок; 3) чек; получе́ние де́нег по че́ку; 4) отбо́р (*людей для определённой цели*); гру́ппа, отря́д; 5) тя́га.

draft II *v* 1) де́лать чертёж, набро́сок; составля́ть план, черновико́к; 2) отбира́ть (*людей*), производи́ть отбо́р.

draftee [‚drɑːf'tiː] *n амер.* призывни́к.

draftsman ['drɑːftsmən] *n* 1) чертёжник; 2) состави́тель законопрое́ктов, докуме́нтов.

drag I [dræg] *n* 1) дра́га, землечерпа́лка; 2) тяжёлая борона́; 3) то́рмоз; 4) торможе́ние; заде́ржка; 5) обу́за.

drag II *v* 1) тащи́ть, тяну́ть; волочи́ть; 2) (ме́дленно) тяну́ться; тащи́ться; 3) борони́ть; 4) чи́стить дно дра́гой; 5) букси́ровать; □ to ~ in а) вта́скивать; б) вовлека́ть; в) *разг.* притяну́ть за́ уши; to ~ on ску́чно тяну́ться; бесконе́чно дли́ться; to ~ out выта́скивать; to ~ up *разг.* воспи́тывать кое-ка́к.

draggle ['drægl] *v* 1) волочи́ться, тащи́ться (*по земле*); 2) па́чкать(ся) (*волочась по земле*).

drag-net ['drægnet] *n* 1) бре́день, нево́д; 2) сеть для ло́вли птиц.

dragon ['drægən] *n* драко́н.

dragon-fly ['drægənflaɪ] *n* стреко́за.

dragoon I [drə'guːn] *n воен.* драгу́н.

dragoon II *v* 1) посыла́ть кара́тельную экспеди́цию; 2) принужда́ть си́лой.

dragsman ['drægzmən] *n горн.* отка́тчик.

drain I [dreɪn] *n* 1) дрена́жная кана́ва, труба́; 2) водоото́к, водосто́к; канализацио́нная труба́; 3) *мед.* дрена́жная тру́бка; 4) расхо́дование, истоще́ние; уте́чка; a ~ on one's money

(strength) истоще́ние чьих-л. средств (сил);
5) *сленг* глото́к.

drain II *v* 1) дрени́ровать, осуша́ть; 2) спус-
ка́ть во́ду; 3) *мед.* дрени́ровать (*ра́ну*); 4) опо-
ро́жнить; пить до дна (*тж.* to ~ dry, to ~ the
dregs); 5) истоща́ть (*сре́дства, си́лы*).

drainage ['dreɪnɪdʒ] *n* 1) дрена́ж; осуше́ние;
2) канализа́ция; 3) сто́чные во́ды, нечисто́ты.

drainage-basin ['dreɪnɪdʒ‚beɪsɪn] *n* бассе́йн реки́.

drake [dreɪk] *n* се́лезень.

dram [dræm] *n* 1) дра́хма (*едини́ца ве́са*);
2) *разг.* глото́к спиртно́го.

drama ['drɑːmə] *n* дра́ма.

dramatic [drə'mætɪk] *a* 1) драмати́ческий;
2) драмати́чный; 3) театра́льный, де́ланный.

dramatics [drə'mætɪks] *n* драмати́ческое ис-
ку́сство.

dramatist ['dræmətɪst] *n* драмату́рг.

dramatize ['dræmətaɪz] *v* 1) драматизи́ровать,
инсцени́ровать (*лит. произведе́ние*); 2) поддава́ть-
ся переде́лке.

dramaturge ['dræmətəːdʒ] *n* драмату́рг.

dramaturgy ['dræmə‚təːdʒɪ] *n* драматурги́я.

drank [dræŋk] *past см.* drink II.

drape [dreɪp] *v* драпирова́ть(ся).

draper ['dreɪpə] *n* торго́вец тка́нями.

drapery ['dreɪpərɪ] *n* 1) драпиро́вка; 2) тка́-
ни; 3) магази́н тка́ней.

drastic ['dræstɪk] *a* 1) круто́й, реши́тельный
(*о ме́рах и т. п.*); ре́зкий; 2) сильноде́йствую-
щий (*о лека́рстве*).

draught[1] [drɑːft] *n* 1) тя́га; сквозня́к; 2) гло-
то́к; to drink at a ~ вы́пить за́лпом; 3) до́за
жи́дкого лека́рства; 4) *мор.* оса́дка; водоизме-
ще́ние; 5) *pl* ша́шки (*игра́*); 6) *см.* draft I 2),
4); 7) заки́дывание не́вода; уло́в (*тж.* a ~ of
fish).

draught[2] *см.* draft II.

draughtboard ['drɑːftbɔːd] *n* 1) ша́шечная дос-
ка́; 2) черте́жная доска́.

draughtsman ['drɑːftsmən] *n* 1) *см.* draftsman;
2) ша́шка (*в игре́*).

draw[1] I [drɔː] *n* 1) тя́га; натяже́ние; вытя́-
гивание; 2) жеребьёвка; лотере́я; 3) ничья́, игра́
вничью́; ниче́йный результа́т; 4) прима́нка; что-л.
привлека́тельное; to be a great ~ име́ть боль-
шо́й успе́х; 5) наводя́щий вопро́с; 6) *стр.* разво-
дна́я часть моста́.

draw[1] II *v* (*past* drew; *p. p.* drawn) 1) тащи́ть,
тяну́ть; волочи́ть; 2) натя́гивать; надвига́ть (*шапку*); 3) выта́скивать, вынима́ть, вырыва́ть (*тж.*
to ~ out); 4) извлека́ть, достава́ть; че́рпать;
5) получа́ть (*де́ньги, информа́цию*); 6) выводи́ть
(*заключе́ние*); 7) проводи́ть (*разли́чие*); 8) при-
влека́ть (*внима́ние и т. п.*); притя́гивать; 9) задёргивать, отдёргивать (*за́навес*); 10) име́ть тя́гу
(*хоро́шую, плоху́ю*); 11) приближа́ться, придви-
га́ться, подходи́ть(ся) (*о ча́се*); 12) наста́ивать (*о
ча́е*); 13) вызыва́ть (*слёзы, аплодисме́нты и т. п.*);
14) вызыва́ть (*кого́-л. на открове́нность, на раз-
гово́р и т. п.*); 15) конча́ть(ся) вничью́; 16) *мор.*
име́ть (*таку́ю-то*) оса́дку; □ to ~ **aside** отводи́ть
в сто́рону; to ~ **back** отступа́ть; to ~ **down**
а) спуска́ть (*што́ру и т. п.*); б) навлека́ть (*гнев
и т. п.*); to ~ **forth** вы́звать, породи́ть, яви́ться
причи́ной; to ~ **in** а) вовлека́ть; б) втя́гивать;

в) станови́ться коро́че (*о днях*); бли́зиться к
концу́ (*о дне*); г) сокраща́ть (*расхо́ды*); to ~ **off**
отводи́ть (*войска́*); to ~ **on** а) надева́ть, натя́-
гивать (*перча́тки и т. п.*); б) навлека́ть; в) при-
ближа́ться, наступа́ть; to ~ **out** а) затя́гиваться,
продолжа́ться; б) станови́ться длинне́е (*о днях*);
в) вызыва́ть (на открове́нность); to ~ **up** а) *refl*
подтяну́ться (*вну́тренне*); б) выстра́иваться (*о
войска́х*); to ~ **upon** че́рпать, брать (*из фо́ндов,
средств*); ◊ it mild! бу́дьте осторо́жнее!, сдер-
жи́тесь!, не преувели́чивайте!

draw[2] *v* (*past* drew; *p. p.* drawn) 1) чер-
ти́ть; рисова́ть; 2) составля́ть (*докуме́нт*); выпи́-
сывать (*чек*); □ to ~ **up** составля́ть, набра́сы-
вать (*докуме́нт, план и т. п.*).

drawback ['drɔːbæk] *n* 1) поме́ха, препя́тствие;
2) невы́годное положе́ние; 3) недоста́ток, отрица́-
тельная сторона́; 4) усту́пка (*в цене́*); 5) возвра́т-
ная по́шлина.

drawbridge ['drɔːbrɪdʒ] *n* разводно́й *или* подъёмный мост.

drawer[a] ['drɔːə] *n* черте́жник.

drawer[b] [drɔː] *n* выдвижно́й я́щик (*стола́ и т. п.*).

drawers [drɔːz] *n pl* кальсо́ны.

drawing ['drɔːɪŋ] *n* 1) рисова́ние; черче́ние;
out of ~ нарисо́ванный с наруше́нием перспек-
ти́вы; 2) рису́нок, чертёж.

drawing-block ['drɔːɪŋblɔk] *n* тетра́дь, блокно́т
для рисова́ния.

drawing-board ['drɔːɪŋbɔːd] *n* черте́жная доска́.

drawing-paper ['drɔːɪŋ‚peɪpə] *n* бума́га для ри-
сова́ния; черте́жная бума́га.

drawing-pen ['drɔːɪŋpen] *n* рейсфе́дер.

drawing-pin ['drɔːɪŋpɪn] *n* канцеля́рская кно́п-
ка.

drawing-room ['drɔːɪŋrum] *n* гости́ная.

drawl I [drɔːl] *n* протя́жное произноше́ние;
медли́тельность ре́чи.

drawl II *v* растя́гивать слова́; говори́ть ме́д-
ленно.

drawn[1] [drɔːn] *a* 1) нерешённый, с нея́сным
исхо́дом (*о сраже́нии*); зако́нчившийся вничью́
(*об игре́*); 2) искажённый, вы́тянувшийся (*о
лице́*).

drawn[2] *p. p. см.* draw[1] II.

drawn[3] *p. p. см.* draw[2].

dray [dreɪ] *n* подво́да.

dray-horse ['dreɪhɔːs] *n* ломова́я ло́шадь.

drayman ['dreɪmən] *n* ломово́й изво́зчик.

dread I [dred] *n* страх, боя́знь; to be (*или*
to live) in ~ of быть в постоя́нном стра́хе
пе́ред чем-л.

dread II *v* боя́ться, страши́ться.

dreadful ['dredful] *a* 1) стра́шный, ужа́сный;
2) *разг.* проти́вный, неприя́тный; ску́чный.

dreadnought ['drednɔːt] *n* 1) *мор.* дредно́ут;
2) то́лстое сукно́.

dream I [driːm] *n* 1) сон, сновиде́ние; 2) мечта́,
грёза.

dream II *v* (*past, p. p.* dreamt, dreamed)
1) ви́деть сон; сни́ться; 2) мечта́ть, вообража́ть;
3) помышля́ть (*обыкн. в отриц. предложе́ниях*);
□ to ~ **away** промечта́ть; to ~ **up** выду́мывать,
фантази́ровать.

dreamer ['driːmə] *n* мечта́тель; фантазёр.

dreamily ['driːmɪlɪ] *adv* мечта́тельно.

dream-land ['driːmlænd] *n* сказочная страна; мир грёз.

dreamless ['driːmlɪs] *a* без сновидений; без грёз.

dreamlike ['driːmlaɪk] *a* 1) сказочный; 2) призрачный.

dreamliner ['driːmˌlaɪnə] *n амер. разг.* поезд из спальных вагонов.

dreamt [dremt] *past, p. p. см.* dream II.

dreamy ['driːmɪ] *a* 1) мечтательный; непрактичный; 2) призрачный; неясный; смутный; 3) *поэт.* полный сновидений.

dreary ['drɪərɪ] *a* мрачный, унылый; скучный.

dredge¹ I [dredʒ] *n тех.* землечерпалка, экскаватор; драга.

dredge¹ II *v* производить землечерпательные работы.

dredge² *v* обсыпать (*мукой, сахаром*).

dredger ['dredʒə] *n* землечерпалка, экскаватор.

dreg [dreg] *n* 1) *pl* подонки, осадок; отбросы; to drink (*или* to drain) to the ~s пить до дна; 2) небольшой остаток; not a ~ ни капельки.

drench I [drentʃ] *n* 1) промокание; 2) ливень; 3) доза лекарства (*для животного*).

drench II *v* 1) (про)мочить (насквозь); 2) вливать лекарство (*животному*).

drencher ['drentʃə] *n разг.* проливной дождь.

dress I [dres] *n* 1) платье, одежда; evening ~ фрак; вечернее платье; fancy ~ маскарадный костюм; full ~ парадная форма; low ~ платье с низким вырезом, декольте; morning ~ а) домашнее платье; б) визитка; to dip a ~ красить платье; 2) одеяние, внешний покров.

dress II *v* 1) одевать(ся); наряжать(ся); украшать(ся); 2) причёсывать; делать причёску; 3) перевязывать (*рану*); 4) приготовлять; приправлять (*кушанье*); разделывать (*тушу*); 5) убирать, украшать; 6) чистить (*лошадь*); 7) выделывать (*кожу*); 8) подрезать (*растения*); 9) *воен.* равняться; ~! равняйсь!; □ to ~ **down** *разг.* давать нагоняй, разносить; to ~ **out** вырядиться; to ~ **up** одевать(ся), наряжать(ся).

dress-circle ['dresˈsəːkl] *n театр.* бельэтаж.

dress-coat ['dresˈkout] *n* фрак.

dresser¹ ['dresə] *n* 1) *разг.* наряжающийся; 2) *театр.* костюмёр; 3) хирургическая сестра; 4) кожевник.

dresser² *n* 1) кухонный буфет; 2) *амер. разг.* туалетный столик.

dressing ['dresɪŋ] *n* 1) одевание; 2) отделка; 3) перевязочные средства; field ~ *воен.* индивидуальный пакет; 4) приправа (*к кушанью*); 5) удобрение; 6) *воен.* равнение; 7) *разг.* нагоняй, головомойка; to give a good ~ down задать хорошую головомойку.

dressing-case ['dresɪŋkeɪs] *n* 1) (дорожный) несессер; 2) санитарная сумка.

dressing-gown ['dresɪŋgaun] *n* халат (*домашний*).

dressing-room ['dresɪŋrum] *n* актёрская уборная.

dressing-table ['dresɪŋˌteɪbl] *n* туалетный столик.

dressmaker ['dresˌmeɪkə] *n* портниха.

dress-preserver ['drespriˈzəːvə] *n* подмышник.

dress-shield ['dresʃiːld] *см.* dress-preserver.

dressy ['dresɪ] *a* 1) любящий, умеющий нарядно одеваться; 2) нарядный; изящный.

drew¹ [druː] *past см.* draw¹ II.

drew² *past см.* draw².

dribble I ['drɪbl] *n* 1) капанье; просачивание; 2) тонкая струйка.

dribble II *v* 1) капать; течь; 2) пускать слюни; 3) вести мяч (*в футболе*); 4) гнать шар в лузу (*в бильярде*).

drib(b)let ['drɪblɪt] *n* 1) небольшое количество; капелька; by ~s по капельке; in ~s понемногу; 2) незначительная сумма.

drier ['draɪə] *см.* dryer.

drift I [drɪft] *n* 1) (медленное) течение; снос (*ветром или водой*); 2) *мор.* дрейф; *ав.* снос; 3) направление, тенденция; 4) смысл (слов); 5) нанос; сугроб (*снега*); куча (*песка*); 6) *горн.* штрек.

drift II *v* 1) сносить(ся) течением, ветром; дрейфовать; 2) наносить, наметать (*в кучу — о снеге, песке*); 3) быть пассивным, предоставлять всё судьбе; □ to ~ **apart** разойтись.

driftage ['drɪftɪdʒ] *n* 1) снос, дрейф (*судна*); 2) предметы, выброшенные на берег моря.

drifter ['drɪftə] *n* 1) дрифтер (*судно для лова рыбы или траления мин*); 2) рыбак, плавающий на дрифтере; 3) *разг.* бродяга.

drift-ice ['drɪftaɪs] *n* дрейфующий лёд.

drift-wood ['drɪftwud] *n* 1) сплавной лесоматериал; 2) лес, прибитый к берегу моря.

drill¹ I [drɪl] *n* сверло; бур; сверлильный станок.

drill¹ II *v* сверлить; бурить.

drill² I *n* 1) (строевое) учение; муштра; 2) тренировка; физическое упражнение; 3) *attr* учебный.

drill² II *v* 1) обучать, тренировать; 2) проходить (строевое) обучение; тренироваться.

drill³ I *n с.-х.* 1) борозда; 2) рядовая сеялка.

drill³ II *v с.-х.* сеять рядами.

drill⁴ *n* тик (*ткань*).

driller¹ ['drɪlə] *n* 1) сверлильный станок; 2) сверловщик; 3) бурильщик.

driller² *n* инструктор.

drillhole ['drɪlhoul] *n* буровая скважина.

drilling¹ ['drɪlɪŋ] *n* сверление; бурение.

drilling² *n* (строевое) учение; муштровка.

drilling³ *n* посев рядовой сеялкой.

drink I [drɪŋk] *n* 1) питьё, напиток; to have a ~ попить, напиться; give him a ~ дайте ему попить; soft ~s *разг.* безалкогольные напитки; 2) спиртной напиток (*тж.* strong ~); small ~ пиво; in ~ пьяный; 3) глоток, стакан, порция (*вина и т. п.*).

drink II *v* (*past* drank; *p. p.* drunk) 1) пить; 2) пьянствовать, пить; to ~ hard, to ~ like a fish сильно пьянствовать; 3) впитывать; всасывать влагу (*о растениях*); □ to ~ **down** выпить залпом; to ~ **in** жадно впитывать; упиваться; to ~ **off** *см.* to ~ down; to ~ **to** пить за здоровье, поднимать бокал за; to ~ **up** *см.* to ~ down.

drinkable ['drɪŋkəbl] *a* годный для питья.

drinker ['drɪŋkə] *n* 1) пьющий; 2) пьяница.

drinking-bout ['drɪŋkɪŋbaut] *n* попойка.

drinking-fountain ['drɪŋkɪŋ,fauntɪn] *n* питьевой фонтанчик.

drinking-song ['drɪŋkɪŋsɔŋ] *n* застольная песня.

drinking-water ['drɪŋkɪŋ,wɔːtə] *n* питьевая вода.

drip I [drɪp] *n* капанье; шум падающих капель.

drip II *v* капать; падать каплями.

dripping I ['drɪpɪŋ] *n* 1) капанье; 2) *pl* падающие капли.

dripping II *a* 1) каплющий; 2) мокрый, промокший.

dripping-pan ['drɪpɪŋpæn] *n* сковорода, противень.

drive I [draɪv] *n* 1) поездка, прогулка (*в автомобиле, экипаже*); 2) дорога, подъездная аллея (*к дому*); 3) побуждение, стимул; 4) преследование (*зверя, неприятеля*); облава; 5) энергичные усилия; 6) принуждение; подстёгивание (*в работе*); 7) гонка, спешка; armaments ~ гонка вооружений; 8) *амер.* кампания (*общественная*); to put on a ~ начать кампанию; 9) *воен.* наступление, атака; 10) *спорт.* удар; 11) сплав, гонка (*леса*); 12) *тех.* привод, передача.

drive II *v* (*past* drove; *p. p.* driven) 1) везти, ехать (*в автомобиле, экипаже и т. п.*); 2) управлять (*автомобилем*); править (*лошадьми*); 3) приводить в движение; 4) гнать; преследовать; 5) вбивать, вколачивать (*гвоздь*); 6) доводить, приводить; to ~ out of one's senses сводить с ума; to ~ to despair доводить до отчаяния; 7) мчаться, нестись; 8) вести (*торговлю*); заключать (*сделку и т. п.*); заниматься (*чем-л.*); 9) переутомлять, перегружать работой; 10) заставлять, принуждать, побуждать; 11) прокладывать (*туннель, дорогу*); □ to ~ at *разг.* метить; клонить к чему-л., добиваться чего-л.; to ~ away прогонять; разгонять, рассеивать; to ~ in загонять; to ~ into вбивать; *перен.* втолковывать; to ~ out а) выбивать; вытеснять; б) проехаться, прокатиться (*в автомобиле, экипаже*); to ~ up подъехать, подкатить.

drive-in ['draɪv'ɪn] *n* 1) кино на открытом воздухе, которое смотрят, не выходя из (авто)машины; 2) ресторан, закусочная, где можно поесть, не выходя из (авто)машины (*тж.* drive-in restaurant, drive-in lunch-room).

drivel I ['drɪvl] *n* 1) слюни; сопли; 2) глупая, бессмысленная болтовня.

drivel II *v* 1) распустить слюни, сопли; 2) болтать ерунду.

driveller ['drɪvlə] *n* 1) слюнявый ребёнок; 2) дурень, идиот.

driven ['drɪvn] *p. p. см.* drive II; ~ ashore выброшенный на берег.

driver ['draɪvə] *n* 1) водитель, шофёр; кучер; машинист; 2) погонщик скота; 3) *разг.* надсмотрщик; 4) *тех.* ведущее колесо; 5) *спорт.* клюшка.

driving ['draɪvɪŋ] *n* 1) езда, катание; 2) *тех.* передача, привод; 3) вождение (*автомобиля и т. п.*); 4) *мор.* дрейф.

driving-belt ['draɪvɪŋbelt] *n* приводной ремень.

driving-wheel ['draɪvɪŋwiːl] *n* ведущее колесо.

drizzle I ['drɪzl] *n* мелкий дождь, изморось.

drizzle II *v* моросить.

drogue [droug] *n* 1) плавучий якорь; 2) *ав.* привязной аэростат, «колбаса».

droll [droul] *a* забавный; смешной; чудной.

drollery ['droulərɪ] *n* шутка; юмор.

dromedary ['drʌmədərɪ] *n* одногорбый верблюд, дромадер.

drone I [droun] *n* 1) трутень; *перен.* бездельник, тунеядец; 2) жужжание.

drone II *v* 1) жужжать, гудеть; 2) *шутл.* говорить, читать монотонно; 3) бездельничать.

droningly ['drounɪŋlɪ] *adv* монотонно.

droop I [druːp] *n* 1) свисание, опускание; 2) уныние; 3) увядание; 4) *муз.* понижение тона.

droop II *v* 1) свисать, склоняться, поникать; 2) повесить, понурить (*голову*); потупить (*глаза, взор*); 3) увядать; 4) *поэт.* клониться к закату; 5) падать духом, унывать.

drop I [drɔp] *n* 1) капля; ~ by ~, by ~s капля за каплей; in ~s очень медленно, по капле; 2) *pl* капли (*лекарство*); 3) глоток; to take a ~ too much глотнуть лишнего; 4) леденец, драже; 5) (внезапное) падение (*цен, температуры и т. д.*); снижение; 6) расстояние (*сверху вниз*); ◇ a ~ in the bucket, a ~ in the ocean ≅ капля в море; to have a ~ in one's eye быть навеселе.

drop II *v* 1) капать, литься каплями; 2) проливать (*слёзы*); 3) ронять; бросать; терять; 4) проронить (*слово*); обронить (*намёк*); 5) опускать (*письмо в ящик*); 6) сбрасывать (*с самолёта*); 7) покидать; бросать (*семью*); 8) прекращать (*разговор, переписку*); бросать (*привычку*); ~ it! брось(те)!, оставь(те)!; 9) падать, спадать; опускаться; снижаться; 10) довозить; оставлять; высаживать; 11) понижать (*голос*); потупить (*глаза*); 12) *амер. разг.* увольнять; □ to ~ across *разг.* случайно встретить, наскочить; to ~ away расходиться, уходить один за другим; to ~ behind отставать; to ~ in а) зайти, заглянуть (*к кому-л.*); б) входить один за другим; to ~ into заглянуть, зайти (*куда-л.*); to ~ off а) расходиться; б) засыпать; в) умирать; г) опадать (*о листьях*); д) уменьшаться; to ~ out а) выпадать, исчезать; б) пропускать, не включать; to ~ through провалиться (*о плане и т. п.*); ◇ to ~ from sight исчезнуть из поля зрения; to ~ from the clouds (*или* from the skies) ≅ свалиться как снег на голову.

drop-curtain ['drɔp,kəːtn] *n* падающий занавес.

droplet ['drɔplɪt] *n* капелька.

dropper ['drɔpə] *n* пипетка.

droppings ['drɔpɪŋz] *n pl* 1) капли (*дождя, стекающего жира, воска со свечей*); 2) помёт животных (*экскременты*).

drop-scene ['drɔpsiːn] *n* 1) *см.* drop-curtain; 2) заключительная сцена, финал.

dropsical ['drɔpsɪkəl] *a* 1) страдающий водянкой; 2) отёчный; опухший.

dropsy ['drɔpsɪ] *n* водянка.

dross [drɔs] *n* 1) отбросы, остатки; угольная пыль; 2) *тех.* окалина, шлак.

drossy ['drɔsɪ] *a* 1) нечистый; сорный; 2) *тех.* шлаковый; 3) никчёмный, негодный.

drought [draut] *n* 1) засуха; 2) сухость воздуха.

droughty ['drautɪ] *a* 1) сухой; засушливый; 2) *уст.* испытывающий жажду.

drouth [drauθ] *поэт. см.* drought.

drove¹ [drouv] *past см.* drive II.

drove² *n* гурт, ста́до; *перен.* толпа́; to stand in ~s толпи́ться.

drover ['drouvə] *n* 1) гуртовщи́к, 2) скотопромы́шленник.

drown [draun] *v* 1) тону́ть; to be ~ed утону́ть; 2) топи́ть(ся); 3) затопля́ть, залива́ть (*тж. перен.*); ~ed in tears залива́ясь слеза́ми; ~ed in sleep погружённый в сон; 4) заглуша́ть (*звук, голос*).

drowse I [drauz] *n* дремо́та, полусо́н.

drowse II *v* 1) дрема́ть; быть вя́лым, со́нным; 2) усыпля́ть, наводи́ть сон; 3) безде́йствовать.

drowsiness ['drauzɪnɪs] *n* сонли́вость; вя́лость.

drowsy ['drauzɪ] *a* 1) со́нный, дре́млющий; сонли́вый; 2) снотво́рный, усыпля́ющий; 3) вя́лый.

drowsy-head ['drauzɪhed] *n* со́ня.

drub [drʌb] *v* 1) (по)би́ть, (по)колоти́ть; 2) вбива́ть в го́лову (*кому-л.* — into); 3) вы́бить из головы́ (out of); 4) стуча́ть; ударя́ть.

drubbing ['drʌbɪŋ] *n* побо́и.

drudge I [drʌdʒ] *n* 1) исполня́ющий тяжёлую, ну́дную рабо́ту; 2) раб.

drudge II *v* исполня́ть тяжёлую, ну́дную рабо́ту.

drudgery ['drʌdʒərɪ] *n* тяжёлая, ну́дная рабо́та.

drudgingly ['drʌdʒɪŋlɪ] *adv* 1) с трудо́м; 2) стара́тельно.

drug I [drʌg] *n* 1) лека́рство; 2) нарко́тик; 3) нехо́дкий това́р.

drug II *v* 1) подме́шивать яд, нарко́тики; 2) дава́ть, употребля́ть лека́рство *или* нарко́тики.

druggist ['drʌgɪst] *n* апте́карь.

drugstore ['drʌgstɔ:] *n амер.* апте́ка, апте́карский магази́н; апте́ка-заку́сочная.

drum [drʌm] *n* 1) бараба́н; 2) бараба́нный бой; шум; 3) *тех.* бараба́н, цили́ндр; 4) *анат.* бараба́нная перепо́нка; 5) *attr* бараба́нный.

drum II *v* 1) бить в бараба́н; 2) бараба́нить, стуча́ть; 3) хло́пать кры́льями; 4) вда́лбливать; □ to ~ up созыва́ть; зазыва́ть.

drumfire ['drʌmˌfaɪə] *n воен.* урага́нный ого́нь (*тж. перен.*).

drumhead ['drʌmhed] *n* 1) ко́жа на бараба́не; 2) *анат.* бараба́нная перепо́нка.

drummer ['drʌmə] *n* 1) бараба́нщик; 2) *амер. разг.* коммивояжёр.

drumstick ['drʌmstɪk] *n* 1) бараба́нная па́лочка; 2) но́жка варёной ку́рицы, гуся́ *и т. п.*

drunk I [drʌŋk] *n* 1) пья́ный, пья́ница; 2) *сленг* попо́йка; дебо́ш.

drunk II *a predic* пья́ный; *перен.* опьянённый; blind ~, dead ~ мертве́цки пьян; to get ~ напи́ться пья́ным; ◇ ~ as a fiddler, ~ as a lord ≅ пьян в сте́льку.

drunk III *p. p. см.* drink II.

drunkard ['drʌŋkəd] *n* пья́ница; алкого́лик; a sad ~ го́рький пья́ница.

drunken ['drʌŋkən] *a* пья́ный.

drunkenness ['drʌŋkənnɪs] *n* 1) опьяне́ние, хмель; 2) пья́нство.

dry I [draɪ] *a* 1) сухо́й; to suck ~ вы́сосать, истощи́ть; 2) ску́чный; безразли́чный; бесстра́стный; 3) вы́сохший (*о колодце и т. п.*); 4) испы́тывающий жа́жду (*о человеке*); 5) сухо́й, несла́дкий (*о вине*); 6) *амер.* сухо́й (*о зако́не*); to go ~ запреща́ть прода́жу *или* не употребля́ть спиртны́х напи́тков.

dry II *v* суши́ть(ся); со́хнуть, высыха́ть; *перен.* иссяка́ть; □ to ~ up a) высу́шивать; б) высыха́ть, иссяка́ть; в) прекраща́ться (*о бесе́де, обсужде́нии*); ~ up! *разг.* замолчи́(те)!; переста́нь(те)!

dryad ['draɪəd] *n миф.* лесна́я ни́мфа, дриа́да.

Dryasdust ['draɪəzdʌst] *n* педа́нт, «суха́рь».

dryasdust ['draɪəzdʌst] *a* сухо́й, ску́чный.

dryer ['draɪə] *n* 1) суши́льщик; 2) суши́льный прибо́р, суши́лка; 3) сиккати́в.

dryish ['draɪɪʃ] *a* сухова́тый.

dryly ['draɪlɪ] *adv* су́хо, сухи́м то́ном.

dry-nurse I ['draɪnə:s] *n* ня́ня, ня́нька.

dry-nurse II *v* ня́нчить.

dry-rot ['draɪ'rɔt] *n* 1) суха́я гниль (*древеси́ны*); 2) мора́льное разложе́ние.

dry-shod ['draɪ'ʃɔd] *adv* не замочи́в ног.

dual I ['djuːəl] *n грам.* дво́йственное число́.

dual II *a* двойно́й, дво́йственный.

dualism ['djuːəlɪzəm] *n* дуали́зм.

duality [djuː'ælɪtɪ] *n* дво́йственность.

dub¹ [dʌb] *v* 1) посвяща́ть в ры́цари; 2) дава́ть ти́тул; *шутл.* дава́ть про́звище; 3) сма́зывать жи́ром (*ко́жу*).

dub² *v* дубли́ровать (*фильм*); озву́чивать (*нсмо́й фильм*).

dubiety [djuː'baɪətɪ] *n* 1) сомне́ние, колеба́ние; 2) сомни́тельное де́ло.

dubious ['djuːbjəs] *a* 1) сомни́тельный; подозри́тельный; 2) сомнева́ющийся, коле́блющийся.

dubitative ['djuːbɪtətɪv] *a* сомнева́ющийся; нереши́тельный.

ducal ['djuːkəl] *a* ге́рцогский.

ducat ['dʌkət] *n* 1) дука́т (*золота́я моне́та*); 2) моне́та; *pl* де́ньги.

duchess ['dʌtʃɪs] *n* герцоги́ня.

duchy ['dʌtʃɪ] *n* ге́рцогство.

duck¹ [dʌk] *n* 1) у́тка; 2) ути́ное мя́со; 3) *ласк.* голу́бка, голу́бушка; ◇ to make ~s and drakes of, to play ~s and drakes with расточа́ть, прома́тывать; like water off a ~'s back ≅ как с гу́ся вода́; a fine day for young ~s *шутл.* дождли́вая пого́да; lame ~ а) кале́ка; неуда́чник; б) *сленг* банкро́т; в) *ав. сленг* повреждённый самолёт; like a ~ in a thunderstorm с расте́рянным ви́дом.

duck² I *n* 1) ныря́ние; 2) бы́стрый накло́н головы́ *или* сгиба́ние ту́ловища (*чтобы уклони́ться от уда́ра*).

duck² II *v* 1) ныря́ть; бы́стро окуна́ть(ся); 2) бы́стро наклоня́ть го́лову *или* сгиба́ть ту́ловище; 3) *разг.* приседа́ть, де́лать reveráns.

duck³ *n* 1) паруси́на; 2) *pl* паруси́новые брю́ки.

ducking ['dʌkɪŋ] *n* 1) промока́ние; 2) погруже́ние в во́ду.

duck-legged ['dʌkˌlegd] *a* коротконо́гий; перева́ливающийся на ходу́.

duckling ['dʌklɪŋ] *n* утёнок.

duck's-egg ['dʌkseg] *n* 1) нулево́й счёт (*в кри́кете*); 2) *шк. сленг* нуль, ничего́.

duck-shot ['dʌkʃɔt] *n* ме́лкая дробь.

duckweed ['dʌkwiːd] *n бот.* ря́ска.

ducky [ˈdʌkɪ] *a* ми́лый, тро́гательный (*о ви-де, о́бразе*).

duct [dʌkt] *n* прото́к, кана́л; труба́; lachrymal ~ слёзный прото́к.

ductile [ˈdʌktaɪl] *a* 1) ги́бкий; ко́вкий; тягу́чий; 2) го́дный для ле́пки (*о гли́не и т. п.*); 3) пода́тливый; послу́шный.

ductility [dʌkˈtɪlɪtɪ] *n* 1) ги́бкость; ко́вкость; тягу́честь; 2) пода́тливость; послуша́ние.

dud [dʌd] *n сленг* 1) *pl* оде́жда; лохмо́тья, рвань; 2) неразорва́вшийся снаря́д; 3) неуда́ча; 4) никчёмный челове́к.

dude [djuːd] *n амер. сленг* фат, пижо́н.

dudgeon [ˈdʌdʒən] *n* оби́да; in high ~ с глубо́кой оби́дой, с возмуще́нием.

due I [djuː] *n* 1) до́лжное; то, что принадлежи́т по пра́ву, что сле́дует (*кому́-л.*); to give smb. his ~ отдава́ть до́лжное кому́-л.; 2) долг (*взя́тое взаймы́*); 3) *pl* сбо́ры, нало́ги, по́шлины; 4) *pl* чле́нские взно́сы; Party ~s парти́йные взно́сы.

due II *a* 1) до́лжный; причита́ющийся; to fall (*или* to become) ~ наступа́ть, истека́ть (*о сро́ке*); 2) ожида́емый; назна́ченный; надлежа́щий; in ~ time, in ~ course в своё вре́мя; in ~ form по фо́рме, по всем пра́вилам; 3) *predic* вы́званный, обусло́вленный (*чем-л.— to*).

due III *adv* то́чно, пря́мо.

duel I [ˈdjuːəl] *n* 1) дуэ́ль, поеди́нок; 2) борьба́, состяза́ние.

duel II *v* дра́ться на дуэ́ли.

duet [djuˈet] *n* дуэ́т.

duff [dʌf] *v сленг* 1) фальсифици́ровать; 2) обма́нывать.

duffer [ˈdʌfə] *n* 1) фальсифика́тор; обма́нщик; 2) фальши́вая моне́та; 3) тупи́ца; никчёмный челове́к; 4) бесполе́зная вещь.

dug[1] I [dʌg] *past, p. p. см.* dig II.

dug[2] *n* 1) вы́мя; 2) сосо́к (*живо́тного*).

dug-out [ˈdʌgaut] *n* 1) челно́к, вы́долбленный из бревна́; 2) *воен.* убе́жище, укры́тие, блинда́ж.

duke [djuːk] *n* 1) ге́рцог; 2) *сленг* рука́, кула́к.

dukedom [ˈdjuːkdəm] *n* 1) ге́рцогство; 2) ти́тул ге́рцога.

dulcify [ˈdʌlsɪfaɪ] *v* подсла́щивать.

dulcimer [ˈdʌlsɪmə] *n муз.* цимба́лы.

dull I [dʌl] *a* 1) тупо́й; глу́пый; 2) ту́склый, нея́сный; па́смурный (*о дне*); 3) ску́чный; моното́нный; 4) тупо́й (*нож, край*); 5) приту́пленный; ~ of hearing туго́й на́ ухо; 6) вя́лый (*о торго́вле*); ◇ as ~ as ditch-water невыноси́мо ску́чный.

dull II *v* 1) притупля́ть(ся); 2) де́лать(ся) ту́склым, нея́сным, ску́чным, вя́лым.

dullard [ˈdʌləd] *n* тупи́ца.

dullish [ˈdʌlɪʃ] *a* 1) тупова́тый; 2) скучнова́тый.

duly [ˈdjuːlɪ] *adv* до́лжным о́бразом, пра́вильно; во́время.

dumb I [dʌm] *a* 1) немо́й; 2) безгла́сный; бессло́ве́сный; 3) беззву́чный; 4) молчали́вый; 5) онеме́вший; to strike smb. ~ ошара́шить, огоро́шить кого́-л.; 6) *амер. сленг* глу́пый, бессмы́сленный.

dumb II *n*: the ~ (*употр. как pl*) немы́е.

dumb III *v* заста́вить (за)молча́ть.

dumb-bell I [ˈdʌmbel] *n* 1) *pl* гимнасти́ческие ги́ри, ганте́ли; 2) *амер. сленг* болва́н.

dumb-bell II *v* де́лать упражне́ния с ги́рями.

dumbfound [dʌmˈfaund] *v* порази́ть, ошара́шить, ошеломи́ть.

dumbness [ˈdʌmnɪs] *n* 1) немота́; 2) безмо́лвие.

dumb-waiter [ˈdʌmˈweɪtə] *n* 1) враща́ющийся сто́лик, откры́тая этаже́рка для заку́сок; 2) *амер.* я́щик с по́лками, поднима́емый, как лифт, с этажа́ на эта́ж.

dummy I [ˈdʌmɪ] *n* 1) манеке́н; чу́чело; 2) маке́т; 3) подставно́е лицо́; марионе́тка; игру́шка в чужи́х рука́х; 4) болва́н, тупи́ца; 5) *карт.* «болва́н».

dummy II *a* 1) ло́жный, подде́льный; фикти́вный, подставно́й; 2) уче́бный; 3) *тех.* холосто́й.

dump[1] I [dʌmp] *n* 1) сва́лка; гру́да хла́ма; *амер.* му́сорная ку́ча; 2) *воен.* полево́й склад.

dump[1] II *v* 1) выгружа́ть; сбра́сывать, сва́ливать (*му́сор*); опроки́дывать (*вагоне́тку*); 2) эк. устра́ивать де́мпинг.

dump[2] *n* 1) свинцо́вый кружо́к; фи́шка; 2) *сленг* ме́лкая моне́та; not worth a ~ ничего́ не сто́ит; 3) коро́ты́шка.

dump-car [ˈdʌmpkɑː] *n* опроки́дывающаяся ваго́нетка, ду́мпкар.

dumping [ˈdʌmpɪŋ] *n* 1) вы́грузка; сбра́сывание, сва́ливание; 2) *эк.* де́мпинг, бро́совый э́кспорт.

dumpish [ˈdʌmpɪʃ] *a* уны́лый, печа́льный, гру́стный.

dumpling [ˈdʌmplɪŋ] *n* 1) клёцка; 2) пу́динг; apple ~ я́блоко, запечённое в те́сте; 3) *разг.* коро́тышка (*о челове́ке*).

dumps [dʌmps] *n pl* уны́ние, пода́вленное состоя́ние; in the ~ *разг.* в дурно́м настрое́нии.

dumpy [ˈdʌmpɪ] *a* корена́стый.

dun[1] I [dʌn] *n* серова́то-кори́чневый цвет.

dun[1] II *a* серова́то-кори́чневый.

dun[2] I *n* 1) тре́бование упла́ты до́лга; 2) насто́йчивый креди́тор.

dun[2] II *v* насто́йчиво тре́бовать упла́ты до́лга; надоеда́ть, пристава́ть.

dunce [dʌns] *n* тупи́ца.

dunderhead [ˈdʌndəhed] *n* болва́н.

dune [djuːn] *n* дю́на.

dung[1] I [dʌŋ] *n* помёт, наво́з; удобре́ние.

dung[1] II *v* унаво́живать, удобря́ть.

dung[2] *past, p. p. см.* ding II.

dungaree [ˌdʌŋgəˈriː] *n текст.* хлопчатобума́жная са́ржа.

dung-beetle [ˈdʌŋˌbiːtl] *n* наво́зный жук.

dungeon I [ˈdʌndʒən] *n* подзе́мная темни́ца, тюрьма́.

dungeon II *v* заключа́ть в темни́цу, в тюрьму́.

dunghill [ˈdʌŋhɪl] *n* наво́зная ку́ча.

dungy [ˈdʌŋɪ] *a* наво́зный, гря́зный.

dupable [ˈdjuːpəbl] *a* (легко́) поддаю́щийся обма́ну, сли́шком дове́рчивый.

dupe I [djuːp] *n* 1) обма́нутый челове́к; 2) дове́рчивый челове́к, проста́к.

dupe II *v* обма́нывать, одура́чивать.

dupery [ˈdjuːpərɪ] *n* обма́н, надува́тельство.

duplex [ˈdjuːpleks] *a* двойно́й, двусторо́нний; из двух часте́й.

duplicate[a] I [ˈdjuːplɪkɪt] *n* дублика́т; ко́пия; made in ~ сде́лано в двух экземпля́рах.

duplicate[a] II *a* 1) двойно́й; в двух экземпля́рах; 2) удво́енный; 3) то́чно воспроизводя́щий; 4) запа́сный, запасно́й.

duplicate[b] [ˈdjuːplɪkeɪt] *v* 1) дубли́ровать; 2) удва́ивать; 3) снима́ть ко́пию, де́лать дубле́т.

duplication [ˌdjuːplɪˈkeɪʃən] *n* 1) дубли́рование; 2) удва́ивание; 3) снима́ние ко́пий, размноже́ние; 5) дублика́т, ко́пия.

duplicity [djuːˈplɪsɪtɪ] *n* двули́чность, двуру́шничество.

durability [ˌdjuərəˈbɪlɪtɪ] *n* 1) про́чность; сто́йкость; 2) продолжи́тельность сро́ка слу́жбы; долгове́чность; 3) дли́тельность.

durable [ˈdjuərəbl] *a* 1) про́чный; 2) долговре́менный.

duralumin [djuəˈræljumɪn] *n* дюралюми́ний.

duration [djuəˈreɪʃən] *n* продолжи́тельность; вре́мя; of long ~ долговре́менный; of short ~ кратковре́менный.

duress(e) [djuəˈres] *n* 1) заключе́ние (в тюрьму́), лише́ние свобо́ды; 2) принужде́ние; under ~ по принужде́нию; под давле́нием.

during [ˈdjuərɪŋ] *prep* в тече́ние, в продолже́ние, во вре́мя.

durst [dəːst] *past см.* dare.

dusk I [dʌsk] *n* су́мерки.

dusk II *a поэт.* су́меречный; нея́сный.

dusk III *v поэт.* смерка́ться.

duskiness [ˈdʌskɪnɪs] *n* 1) су́мрак; 2) су́мрачность; 3) сму́глость.

dusky [ˈdʌskɪ] *a* 1) су́меречный; 2) су́мрачный; 3) сму́глый.

dust I [dʌst] *n* 1) пыль; to kick up (*или* to make, to raise) a ~ поднима́ть пыль; *перен. разг.* поднима́ть шум; 2) прах; in the ~ мёртвый (*см. тж.* 3); 3) униже́ние; in the ~ уни́женный (*см. тж.* 2); 4) *бот.* пыльца́; 5) *сленг* де́ньги, презре́нный мета́лл; ◇ to kiss the ~ а) пресмыка́ться; б) потерпе́ть пораже́ние; to bite the ~ упа́сть за́мертво; лежа́ть во пра́хе; to shake the ~ off one's feet отрясти́ прах с ног; to throw ~ into smb.'s eyes вводи́ть в заблужде́ние, втира́ть очки́; пуска́ть пыль в глаза́.

dust II *v* 1) вытира́ть, выбива́ть пыль, чи́стить (*платье*); 2) запыли́ть; покрыва́ть пы́лью; 3) посыпа́ть (*мукой и т. п.*).

dustbin [ˈdʌstbɪn] *n* му́сорный я́щик.

dust-cart [ˈdʌstkɑːt] *n* фурго́н для му́сора.

dust-coat [ˈdʌstkout] *n* пы́льник (*пальто*).

dust-colour [ˈdʌstˌkʌlə] *n* серова́то-кори́чневый цвет.

dust-cover [ˈdʌstˌkʌvə] *n* суперобло́жка.

duster [ˈdʌstə] *n* 1) пы́льная тря́пка; 2) *амер. см.* dust-coat; 3) пылесо́с.

dusting [ˈdʌstɪŋ] *n* 1) стира́ние, смета́ние, выбива́ние пы́ли; 2) *сленг* побо́и; to give a ~ изби́ть, поколоти́ть; 3) *сленг* морска́я ка́чка.

dustman [ˈdʌstmən] *n* му́сорщик.

dustpan [ˈdʌstpæn] *n* сово́к для му́сора.

dust-proof [ˈdʌstpruːf] *a* пыленепроница́емый.

dusty [ˈdʌstɪ] *a* 1) пы́льный; 2) размельчённый, ме́лкий как пыль; 3) сухо́й, неинтере́сный; 4) серова́тый; ◇ not so ~ *разг.* неду́рно, непло́хо.

Dutch I [dʌtʃ] *n* 1): the ~ (*употр. как pl*) нидерла́ндцы; голла́ндцы; 2) нидерла́ндский язы́к;

◇ to beat the ~ превосходи́ть всё; double ~ тараба́рщина.

Dutch II *a* нидерла́ндский; голла́ндский; *амер. тж.* неме́цкий.

Dutchman [ˈdʌtʃmən] *n* 1) нидерла́ндец; голла́ндец; *амер. тж.* немец; 2) голла́ндское су́дно; ◇ I'm a ~ if я не я бу́ду, е́сли не.

Dutchwoman [ˈdʌtʃˌwumən] *n* нидерла́ндка; голла́ндка.

duteous [ˈdjuːtjəs] *a* 1) испо́лненный созна́ния до́лга; послу́шный (*до́лгу*); 2) поко́рный.

dutiable [ˈdjuːtjəbl] *a* подлежа́щий обложе́нию нало́гом *или* по́шлиной.

dutiful [ˈdjuːtɪful] *см.* duteous.

duty [ˈdjuːtɪ] *n* 1) долг, обя́занность; to do (*или* to perform) one's ~ исполня́ть свой долг; honourable ~ почётная обя́занность; as in ~ bound из чу́вства до́лга; 2) слу́жба, служе́бные обя́занности; дежу́рство; field ~ слу́жба в де́йствующей а́рмии; daily ~ су́точное дежу́рство; on ~ при исполне́нии служе́бных обя́занностей; на дежу́рстве; off ~ вне слу́жбы; to do ~ for заменя́ть, замеща́ть; 3) по́шлина; сбор, нало́г; customs duties тамо́женная по́шлина; excess profits ~ нало́г на сверхпри́быль; 4) почте́ние; to present (*или* to send) one's ~ свиде́тельствовать своё почте́ние; 5) *тех.* мо́щность.

duty-free I [ˈdjuːtɪˈfriː] *a* беспо́шлинный.

duty-free II *adv* беспо́шлинно.

duty-paid [ˈdjuːtɪpeɪd] *a* опла́ченный по́шлиной.

dwarf I [dwɔːf] *n* 1) ка́рлик; 2) ка́рликовое живо́тное, расте́ние; 3) *миф.* гном.

dwarf II *a* ка́рликовый.

dwarf III *v* 1) меша́ть ро́сту; 2) подчёркивать незначи́тельность (*чего-л.*) по контра́сту, затмева́ть.

dwarfish [ˈdwɔːfɪʃ] *a* 1) ка́рликовый; 2) недора́звитый.

dwell [dwel] *v* (*past, p. p.* dwelt) 1) жить, обита́ть; находи́ться, пребыва́ть; to ~ in uncertainty быть в нереши́тельности; 2) заде́рживаться, подро́бно остана́вливаться (*на — (up)on*).

dweller [ˈdwelə] *n* жи́тель; жиле́ц, обита́тель.

dwelling [ˈdwelɪŋ] *n* жили́ще, дом.

dwelling-house [ˈdwelɪŋhaus] *n* жило́й дом.

dwelling-place [ˈdwelɪŋpleɪs] *n* местожи́тельство.

dwelt [dwelt] *past, p. p. см.* dwell.

dwindle [ˈdwɪndl] *v* 1) уменьша́ться, сокраща́ться; истоща́ться (*о запа́се и т. п.*); 2) теря́ть значе́ние; снижа́ться (*о ка́честве и т. п.*).

dye I [daɪ] *n* 1) кра́ска; кра́сящее вещество́; краси́тель; 2) окра́ска, цвет; отте́нок; 3) *attr* краси́льный; ◇ of the deepest ~ отъя́вленный, закоренелый.

dye II *v* 1) кра́сить; окра́шивать; 2) окра́шиваться, принима́ть окра́ску.

d'ye [djе] *разг.* = do you.

dye-house [ˈdaɪhaus] *n* краси́льня.

dyeing [ˈdaɪɪŋ] *n* 1) кра́шение, окра́ска; 2) краси́льное де́ло.

dyer [ˈdaɪə] *n* краси́льщик.

dye-stuff [ˈdaɪstʌf] *n* кра́сящее вещество́, краси́тель.

dye-works [ˈdaɪwəːks] *n* краси́льня.

dying I ['daɪɪŋ] n умира́ние, смерть, уга-
са́ние.

dying II a 1) умира́ющий, угаса́ющий; 2) пред-
сме́ртный.

dyke I, II [daɪk] см. dike I, II.

dynamic [daɪ'næmɪk] a 1) динами́ческий;
2) энерги́чный; акти́вный; 3) мед. функциона́ль-
ный.

dynamics [daɪ'næmɪks] n pl 1) дина́мика;
2) дви́жущие си́лы.

dynamite I ['daɪnəmaɪt] n динами́т.

dynamite II v взрыва́ть динами́том.

dynamo ['daɪnəmou] n эл. дина́мо-маши́на.

dynastic [dɪ'næstɪk] a династи́ческий.

dynasty ['dɪnəstɪ] n дина́стия.

dysentery ['dɪsntrɪ] n дизентери́я.

dyspepsia [dɪs'pepsɪə] n диспепси́я.

dyspeptic [dɪs'peptɪk] a 1) страда́ющий пло-
хи́м пищеваре́нием; 2) в пода́вленном состоя́нии.

E

E, e [iː] n 1) 5-я бу́ква англ. алфави́та;
2) муз. но́та ми.

each [iːtʃ] pron ка́ждый; ~ other друг дру́га.

eager ['iːgə] a 1) си́льно, стра́стно жела́ю-
щий (чего-л.); стремя́щийся (к чему-л.— for,
after, about); 2) пы́лкий; 3) энерги́чный.

eagerness ['iːgənɪs] n пыл, рве́ние.

eagle ['iːgl] n 1) орёл; 2) амер. уст.: double ~
моне́та в 20 до́лларов; 3) attr орли́ный.

eagle-owl ['iːgl'aul] n фи́лин.

eaglet ['iːglɪt] n орлёнок.

ear¹ [ɪə] n 1) у́хо; to prick up one's ~s на-
сторожи́ть у́ши, насторожи́ться; to shut one's ~s to
пропуска́ть что-л. ми́мо уше́й; быть глухи́м к чему́-л.;
my ~s are singing у меня́ шуми́т в уша́х; over head
and ~s, head over ~s, up to the ~s по́ у́ши (в рабо́те
и т. п.); to be all ~s внима́тельно слу́шать; he was
all ~s он весь преврати́лся в слух; 2) слух; quick ~
о́стрый слух; to play (to sing) by ~ игра́ть (петь)
по слу́ху; to have a good (bad, poor, no) ~ for
music име́ть хоро́ший (плохо́й) музыка́льный слух;
to give ~ to прислу́шиваться к; to gain (или to
have, to win) the ~ of быть благоскло́нно вы́слу-
шанным; for one's own private ~ по секре́ту; 3)
ушко́; 4) ру́чка (напр. кувши́на); ◊ to give a thick
~ дать здоро́вую оплеу́ху; to set by the ~s пос-
со́рить; to turn a deaf ~ to игнори́ровать, не слу́-
шать, не обраща́ть внима́ния; to have itching ~s
быть па́дким до новосте́й, сенса́ций.

ear² n ко́лос.

ear-drum ['ɪədrʌm] n анат. бараба́нная пере-
по́нка.

ear-flap ['ɪəflæp] n нау́шник (ша́пки).

earful ['ɪəful] n: an ~ of tip-top tunes мно́-
жество са́мых популя́рных мело́дий.

earl [əːl] n граф.

ear-lap ['ɪəlæp] n 1) мо́чка (у́ха); 2) нау́ш-
ник (ша́пки).

earldom ['əːldəm] n 1) ти́тул гра́фа; 2) родо-
во́е, насле́дственное владе́ние гра́фа.

earliness ['əːlɪnɪs] n 1) ра́ннее вре́мя; 2) преж-
девре́менность.

early I ['əːlɪ] a 1) ра́нний; 2) преждевре́менный.

early II adv ра́но; ~ in the day ра́но у́тром;
перен. заблаговре́менно.

earmark I ['ɪəmɑːk] n 1) клеймо́ на у́хе (у жи-
во́тного); 2) отличи́тельный знак; 3) за́гнутый
у́гол страни́цы.

earmark II v 1) клейми́ть (скот); 2) загиба́ть
у́гол страни́цы; 3) ассигнова́ть, выделя́ть; пред-
назнача́ть (для какой-л. це́ли).

earn [əːn] v 1) зараба́тывать; 2) заслу́живать.

earnest¹ I ['əːnɪst] n: in ~ серьёзно, всерьёз;
in real ~, in dead ~ соверше́нно серьёзно.

earnest¹ II a серьёзный.

earnest² n зада́ток; зало́г.

earnings ['əːnɪŋz] n pl за́работок; average ~
сре́дний за́работок.

ear-phone ['ɪəfoun] n нау́шник ра́дио или теле-
фо́на; головно́й телефо́н.

ear-ring ['ɪərɪŋ] n серьга́.

earshot ['ɪəʃɔt] n слы́шимость; within (out
of) ~ в преде́лах (вне преде́лов) слы́шимости.

ear-tab ['ɪətæb] n нау́шник (ша́пки).

earth I [əːθ] n 1) земля́; bitter ~ магне́зия;
2) по́чва; грунт; floating ~ плывуны́; scorched ~
вы́жженная земля́; 3) су́ша; 4) нора́; to take ~,
to go to ~ скры́ться в нору́; перен. пря́таться,
притаи́ться; to run to ~ а) скры́ться в нору́;
б) загна́ть в нору́ (зве́ря); в) обнару́жить; отыс-
ка́ть; добра́ться до су́ти де́ла; to stop an ~ охо́т.
заткну́ть (ли́сью) нору́; 5) эл., ра́дио заземле́-
ние; 6) употребля́ется для усиле́ния вопро́са: how
on ~? каки́м о́бразом?; why on ~? чего ра́ди?,
с какой ста́ти?; 7) attr земно́й; 8) attr земля-
но́й; грунтово́й (о доро́ге); 9) attr эл., ра́дио
заземля́ющий, заземли́тельный; ◊ to burn the ~
нести́сь во весь опо́р.

earth II v 1) зарыва́ть в зе́млю; зака́пывать;
оку́чивать; 2) загоня́ть в нору́; 3) зарыва́ться в
нору́; 4) эл., ра́дио заземля́ть; 5) ав. сажа́ть (самолёт); to be ~ed сде́лать вы́нужденную по-
са́дку.

earth-bound ['əːθbaund] a 1) свя́занный с Землёй, земно́й; 2) напра́вленный к Земле́.

earthen ['əːθən] a 1) земляно́й; 2) гли́няный (об
изде́лиях).

earthenware ['əːθənwɛə] n 1) гли́няная, фая́нсо-
вая посу́да; 2) кера́мика; гонча́рные изде́лия.

earthing ['əːθɪŋ] n эл., ра́дио заземле́ние.

earth-light ['əːθlaɪt] n астр. свече́ние земно́й
атмосфе́ры; пе́пельный свет.

earthly ['əːθlɪ] a 1) земно́й; 2) разг. обыкн. с
отрица́нием: не употр. разг. бесполе́зно; not
an ~ chance ни мале́йшей возмо́жности.

earthquake ['əːθkweɪk] n землетрясе́ние; перен.
(социа́льное) потрясе́ние.

earth-shine ['əːθʃaɪn] см. earth-light.

earthwork ['əːθwəːk] n 1) земляно́е укрепле́ние;
2) pl земляны́е рабо́ты.

earthworm ['əːθwəːm] n земляно́й червь;
перен. низкопокло́нник.

earthy ['əːθɪ] a 1) земляно́й, земли́стый; 2) зем-
но́й, жите́йский; гру́бо материа́льный.

ear-trumpet ['ɪə,trʌmpɪt] n слухова́я тру́бка (для
глухи́х).

ear-wax ['ɪəwæks] *n* ушна́я се́ра.

earwig I ['ɪəwɪg] *n зоол.* уховёртка.

earwig II *v* нашёптывать, наушничать.

ease I [iːz] *n* 1) поко́й; at ~ а) поко́йно, удо́бно, свобо́дно; б) *воен.* во́льно; ill at ~ не по себе́; нело́вко; to set at ~ успоко́ить, ободри́ть; 2) непринуждённость, свобо́да; at heart's ~ по жела́нию; 3) облегче́ние; 4) лёгкость.

ease II *v* 1) облегча́ть (*страдание, тяжесть и т. п.*); успока́ивать (*боль и т. п.*); 2) распуска́ть, ослабля́ть; 3) *шутл.* укра́сть (*что-л.—of*); □ to ~ **down** убавля́ть (*ход*); уменьша́ть (*напряжение, усилие*); to ~ **in** войти́ в строй (*о кораблях*); to ~ **off** а) *см.* to ~ down; б) отстраня́ть; отта́лкивать (*лодку*); в) отходи́ть.

easel ['iːzl] *n* мольбе́рт.

easily ['iːzɪlɪ] *adv* легко́; свобо́дно.

easiness ['iːzɪnɪs] *n* 1) лёгкость; 2) непринуждённость.

east I [iːst] *n* 1) восто́к; *мор.* ост; the East а) Восто́к; б) *амер.* восто́чные шта́ты; Far (Near, Middle) East Да́льний (Бли́жний, Сре́дний) Восто́к; to the ~ (of) к восто́ку (от); 2) восто́чный ве́тер; *мор.* ост.

east II *a* восто́чный.

east III *adv* к восто́ку от, на восто́к от.

East-end ['iːst'end] *n* Йст-Энд, восто́чная (рабо́чая) часть Ло́ндона.

East-ender ['iːst'endə] *n* жи́тель Йст-Энда, пролета́рий.

Easter ['iːstə] *n рел.* 1) па́сха; 2) *attr* пасха́льный.

easterly I ['iːstəlɪ] *a* 1) обращённый, напра́вленный к восто́ку; 2) ду́ющий с восто́ка, восто́чный (*о ветре*).

easterly II *adv* 1) к восто́ку, на восто́к; 2) с восто́ка.

eastern I ['iːstən] *n* (*тж.* Eastern) жи́тель, уроже́нец Восто́ка.

eastern II *a* 1) живу́щий на Восто́ке; 2) восто́чный; 3) обращённый на восто́к.

easterner ['iːstənə] *n* (*тж.* Easterner) 1) жи́тель Восто́ка; 2) жи́тель восто́чной ча́сти США.

easternmost ['iːstənmoust] *a* са́мый восто́чный.

eastward I ['iːstwəd] *n* восто́чное направле́ние.

eastward II *a* напра́вленный на восто́к, к восто́ку.

eastward III *adv* к восто́ку, на восто́к, в восто́чном направле́нии.

eastwards ['iːstwədz] *см.* eastward III.

easy I ['iːzɪ] *a* 1) лёгкий, нетру́дный; ~ of access досту́пный; 2) (с)поко́йный, удо́бный; 3) усту́пчивый, ги́бкий, покла́дистый; ужи́вчивый; to come ~ to не чини́ть препя́тствий, отнести́сь благоскло́нно; 4) свобо́дный (*от страха, страдания и т. п.*); 5) непринуждённый; 6) поло́гий (*о ска́те*); 7) неусто́йчивый (*о рынке*); 8) не име́ющий спро́са (*о товаре*); ◊ ~ on the trigger *амер.* вспы́льчивый, легко́ возбуди́мый.

easy II *adv* 1) легко́, споко́йно; take it ~! а) не торопи́тесь!; б) не волну́йтесь!; не принима́йте бли́зко к се́рдцу!; 2) споко́йно; удо́бно; 3) непринуждённо.

easy III *n разг.* переды́шка, остано́вка; ~ all! переста́ть грести́!

easy-going ['iːzɪˌgouɪŋ] *a* 1) беспе́чный, беззабо́тный; 2) споко́йный (*о лошади*).

eat [iːt] *v* (*past* ate; *p. p.* eaten) есть; to ~ well облада́ть хоро́шим аппети́том; it ~s well э́то вку́сно; to ~ badly есть ма́ло *или* без аппети́та; the biscuit ~s short пече́нье рассыпа́ется во рту; □ to ~ **away** а) съеда́ть; пожира́ть; б) разъеда́ть; разруша́ть; to ~ **in** а) пита́ться у себя́ до́ма; б) въеда́ться; to ~ **into** а) въеда́ться; б) растра́чивать; to ~ **off** отъеда́ть (*о кислоте и т. п.*); to ~ **out** пожира́ть, уничтожа́ть; to ~ **up** съеда́ть, пожира́ть; ◊ to ~ one's heart out мо́лча страда́ть.

eatable ['iːtəbl] *a* съедо́бный.

eatables ['iːtəblz] *n pl разг.* пи́ща, съестны́е припа́сы.

eaten ['iːtn] *p. p. см.* eat.

eater ['iːtə] *n* 1) *разг.* обе́дающий; сидя́щий за столо́м; 2) едо́к; a hearty (a poor) ~ челове́к с хоро́шим (с плохи́м) аппети́том.

eating ['iːtɪŋ] *n* еда́.

eating-house ['iːtɪŋhaus] *n* столо́вая, заку́сочная, рестора́н.

eats [iːts] *n pl амер. сленг* еда́, пи́ща.

eaves [iːvz] *n pl* 1) наве́с кры́ши, стреха́; 2) *поэт.* ве́ки; ресни́цы.

eavesdrop ['iːvzdrɔp] *v* подслу́шивать.

ebb I [eb] *n* 1) отли́в; 2) упа́док.

ebb II *v* 1) отлива́ть, убыва́ть; 2) угаса́ть, ослабева́ть (*часто* to ~ away).

ebb-tide ['eb'taid] *n* отли́в.

ebony I ['ebənɪ] *n* чёрное, эбе́новое де́рево.

ebony II *a* 1) (из) чёрного де́рева, эбе́новый; 2) чёрный.

ebullient [ɪ'bʌljənt] *a* 1) кипя́щий; 2) кипу́чий, по́лный энтузиа́зма; возбуждённый.

eccentric I [ɪk'sentrɪk] *n* 1) стра́нный, эксцентри́чный челове́к; чуда́к; 2) *тех.* эксце́нтрик.

eccentric II *a* 1) стра́нный, эксцентри́чный; 2) *мат., тех.* эксцентри́ческий.

eccentricity [ˌeksen'trɪsɪtɪ] *n* 1) эксцентри́чность; 2) *мат., тех.* эксцентриситет.

ecclesiastic I [ɪˌkliːzɪ'æstɪk] *n* духо́вное лицо́.

ecclesiastic II *a см.* ecclesiastical.

ecclesiastical [ɪˌkliːzɪ'æstɪkəl] *a* духо́вный, церко́вный.

echelon ['eʃəlɔn] *n* 1) *воен.* эшело́н; 2) усту́п; in ~ усту́пами.

echo I ['ekou] *n* 1) э́хо; отголо́сок; 2) подража́ние; 3) подража́тель.

echo II *v* 1) отража́ться (*о звуке*); 2) повторя́ть (*звук — об эхе*); 3) вто́рить; повторя́ть (*чьи-л. слова*); подража́ть.

echo-sounder ['ekouˌsaundə] *n* эхоло́т.

eclectic I [ek'lektɪk] *n* экле́ктик.

eclectic II *a* эклекти́ческий.

eclipse I [ɪ'klɪps] *n* 1) затме́ние; annular (partial, total) ~ кольцеобра́зное (части́чное, по́лное) затме́ние; 2) поте́ря бле́ска, пы́шности; потускне́ние.

eclipse II *v* затмева́ть.

ecliptic [ɪ'klɪptɪk] *n астр.* экли́птика.

ecology [iː'kɔlədʒɪ] *n биол.* эколо́гия.

economic [ˌiːkə'nɔmɪk] *a* 1) хозя́йственный; 2) экономи́ческий; 3) *разг.* эконо́мный, бережли́вый.

economical [,iːkə'nɔmɪkəl] *a* 1) эконо́мный, бережли́вый; 2) экономи́ческий.

economics [,iːkə'nɔmɪks] *n* 1) эконо́мика; наро́дное хозя́йство; 2) полити́ческая эконо́мия.

economist [iˈkɔnəmɪst] *n* 1) экономи́ст; 2) бережли́вый челове́к.

economize [iˈkɔnəmaɪz] *v* эконо́мить; сберега́ть.

economy [iˈkɔnəmɪ] *n* 1) хозя́йство; political ~ полити́ческая эконо́мия; rural ~ се́льское хозя́йство; 2) эконо́мия, бережли́вость; 3) *pl* сбереже́ния.

ecstasy ['ekstəsɪ] *n* экста́з.

ecstatic [eksˈtætɪk] *a* исступлённый; восто́рженный.

eczema ['eksɪmə] *n мед.* экзе́ма.

eddy I ['edɪ] *n* 1) (небольшо́й) водоворо́т; 2) вихрь; вихрево́е движе́ние; клубы́ (*дыма и т. п.*).

eddy II *v* кружи́ться в водоворо́те.

Eden ['iːdn] *n* рай.

edge I [edʒ] *n* 1) край; кро́мка; ~ of a wood опу́шка ле́са; 2) остриё, ле́звие; *перен.* крити́ческое положе́ние, кра́йность; 3) хребе́т, гре́бень, кряж (*горный*); 4) преиму́щество; ◇ on ~ нетерпели́вый; раздражённый; to give the ~ of one's tongue to ре́зко говори́ть с кем-л.; to take the ~ off осла́бить (си́лу, напряже́ние), уме́рить.

edge II *v* 1) точи́ть, отта́чивать; 2) окаймля́ть, обрамля́ть; 3) обреза́ть края́; 4) подстрига́ть (*траву*); □ to ~ **away** отходи́ть осторо́жно, бочко́м; to ~ **into** а) вти́скивать(ся); б) вме́шиваться; to ~ **off** *см.* to ~ away; to ~ **on** подстрека́ть; to ~ **out** а) вытесня́ть; б) выбира́ться.

edge-tool ['edʒˈtuːl] *n* ре́жущий инструме́нт; ◇ to play with ~s ≅ игра́ть с огнём.

edgeways ['edʒweɪz] *adv* 1) остриём, кра́ем (вперёд); 2) край к кра́ю.

edgewise ['edʒwaɪz] *см.* edgeways.

edging ['edʒɪŋ] *n* 1) край; 2) кайма́; окаймле́ние; кант.

edgy ['edʒɪ] *a* 1) о́стрый, заострённый; 2) *жив.* с ре́зкими ко́нтурами; 3) раздражённый.

edible I ['edɪbl] *n обыкн. pl* съедо́бное, съестно́е.

edible II *a* съедо́бный.

edict ['iːdɪkt] *n* эди́кт, ука́з.

edification [,edɪfɪˈkeɪʃən] *n* назида́ние, наставле́ние, поуче́ние.

edifice ['edɪfɪs] *n* зда́ние; сооруже́ние.

edify ['edɪfaɪ] *v* наставля́ть, поуча́ть.

edit ['edɪt] *v* 1) редакти́ровать, подгота́вливать к печа́ти; 2) издава́ть (*книги, газету и т. п.*); 3) монти́ровать (*фильм*).

edition [ɪˈdɪʃən] *n* изда́ние; second (popular) ~ второ́е (общедосту́пное) изда́ние; special ~ экстренный вы́пуск.

editor ['edɪtə] *n* реда́ктор; associate ~ *амер.* помо́щник реда́ктора.

editorial I [,edɪˈtɔːrɪəl] *n* передова́я (статья́).

editorial II *a* редакцио́нный, реда́кторский.

editorialist [,edɪˈtɔːrɪəlɪst] *n амер.* а́втор передови́ц.

editor-in-chief ['edɪtərɪn'tʃiːf] *n* гла́вный реда́ктор.

educate ['edjuːkeɪt] *v* 1) воспи́тывать; дава́ть образова́ние; 2) развива́ть (*способности*); 3) дрессирова́ть (*животных*).

educated ['edjuːkeɪtɪd] *a* 1) образо́ванный; 2) развито́й (*о способности*).

education [,edjuːˈkeɪʃən] *n* 1) воспита́ние; образова́ние; обуче́ние; party ~ партийное просвеще́ние; all-round (trade, primary, higher) ~ разносторо́ннее (профессиона́льное, нача́льное, вы́сшее) образова́ние; compulsory ~ обяза́тельное обуче́ние; nursery ~ дошко́льное воспита́ние; 2) воспита́ние, разви́тие (*способностей, характера*); 3) дрессиро́вка.

educational [,edjuːˈkeɪʃənl] *a* воспита́тельный; образова́тельный; уче́бный, педагоги́ческий.

educative ['edjuːkətɪv] *a* 1) образова́тельный, просвети́тельный; 2) воспи́тывающий, воспита́тельный.

educator ['edjuːkeɪtə] *n* педаго́г; воспита́тель.

educe [iːˈdjuːs] *v* 1) развива́ть, выявля́ть (*способности*); 2) выводи́ть, заключа́ть (*from*); 3) *хим.* выделя́ть.

eduction [iːˈdʌkʃən] *n* 1) выявле́ние; 2) вы́вод; 3) *тех.* вы́пуск; вы́ход.

eel [iːl] *n зоол.* у́горь.

e'en [iːn] *поэт. см.* even[1] III.

e'er [ɛə] *поэт. см.* ever.

eerie ['ɪərɪ] *a* 1) жу́ткий, мра́чный; 2) суеве́рно боязли́вый.

eery ['ɪərɪ] *см.* eerie.

efface [ɪˈfeɪs] *v* стира́ть; *перен. тж.* изгла́живать, вычёркивать (*из памяти и т. п.*); to ~ oneself стушёвываться, отстраня́ться.

effect I [ɪˈfekt] *n* 1) результа́т, сле́дствие; to have ~ поде́йствовать, име́ть жела́тельный результа́т; of no ~ бесполе́зный; безрезульта́тный; to this ~ для э́той це́ли, для э́того; 2) де́йствие, си́ла; действи́тельность; cross ~ обра́тное де́йствие; to give ~ to, to put into ~ вводи́ть, приводи́ть в де́йствие; to take ~, to go into ~ вступа́ть в си́лу (*о законе, правиле и т. п.*); to bring (*или* to carry) into ~ осуществля́ть; in ~ в действи́тельности, в су́щности; 3) эффе́кт, впечатле́ние; calculated for ~ рассчи́танный на эффе́кт; bombshell ~ впечатле́ние разорва́вшейся бо́мбы; 4) содержа́ние, смысл; 5) *pl* иму́щество, пожи́тки.

effect II *v* соверша́ть; производи́ть; выполня́ть; осуществля́ть.

effective I [ɪˈfektɪv] *n воен.* 1) солда́т, го́дный к слу́жбе; 2) *pl* чи́сленный соста́в (*армии*).

effective II *a* 1) де́йствующий, име́ющий си́лу (*о законе, правиле и т. п.*); 2) действи́тельный, эффекти́вный, успе́шный; 3) эффе́ктный, производя́щий впечатле́ние; 4) *тех.* поле́зный (*о пло́щади, действии и т. п.*); 5) го́дный к вое́нной слу́жбе.

effector [ɪˈfektə] *n* исполни́тельный элеме́нт (*в вычисли́тельной те́хнике*).

effectual [ɪˈfektʃuəl] *a* 1) эффекти́вный, достига́ющий це́ли, действи́тельный; 2) *юр.* име́ющий си́лу, действи́тельный.

effectuate [ɪˈfektʃueɪt] *v* соверша́ть, выполня́ть, приводи́ть в исполне́ние.

effeminacy [ɪˈfemɪnəsɪ] *n* же́нственность, изне́женность.

effeminate [ɪˈfemɪnɪt] *a* женственный, женоподобный, изнеженный.

effervescent [ˌefəˈvesnt] *a* шипучий; *перен.* возбуждённый; кипучий.

effete [eˈfiːt] *a* 1) истощённый, слабый; 2) бесплодный; 3) упадочный.

efficacious [ˌefɪˈkeɪʃəs] *a* эффективный; производительный.

efficacy [ˈefɪkəsɪ] *n* эффективность, сила; действенность.

efficiency [ɪˈfɪʃənsɪ] *n* 1) эффективность, действенность; tactical ~ боеспособность; 2) производительность, продуктивность, мощность; 3) умение, (работо)способность; 4) *тех.* коэффициент полезного действия.

efficient [ɪˈfɪʃənt] *a* 1) эффективный, действительный, действенный; 2) квалифицированный; знающий своё дело, умелый.

effigy [ˈefɪdʒɪ] *n* портрет, изображение.

effloresce [ˌefloːˈres] *v* 1) расцветать, зацветать; 2) *геол.* выкристаллизоваться; выветриться; 3) плесневеть.

efflorescence [ˌefloːˈresns] *n* 1) расцвет; 2) *геол.* выветривание кристаллов; 3) плесневение; 4) *мед.* высыпание.

effluence [ˈefluəns] *n* истечение.

effluent I [ˈefluənt] *n* 1) рукав реки; 2) сток.

effluent II *a* вытекающий.

efflux [ˈeflʌks] *n* 1) истечение; утечка; 2) струя выхлопных газов.

effort [ˈefət] *n* 1) усилие, напряжение; 2) попытка; 3) *разг.* достижение.

effortless [ˈefətlɪs] *a* 1) не делающий усилий, пассивный; 2) нетрудный, не требующий усилий.

effrontery [eˈfrʌntərɪ] *n* наглость, бесстыдство.

effulgent [eˈfʌldʒənt] *a* лучезарный.

effuse [eˈfjuːz] *v* изливать, распространять (*свет и т. п.*).

effusion [ɪˈfjuːʒən] *n* 1) пролитие (*крови*); излияние; 2) поток (*слов, стихов и т. п.*).

effusive [ɪˈfjuːsɪv] *a* 1) экспансивный, несдержанный; 2) преувеличенный.

egad [ɪˈɡæd] *int* ей-богу!

egg[1] [eɡ] *n* 1) яйцо; soft(-boiled) ~ яйцо всмятку; hard-boiled ~ крутое яйцо; shady ~ тухлое яйцо; scrambled ~s яичница-болтунья; powdered ~s яичный порошок; ham (bacon) and ~s яичница с ветчиной (с беконом); 2) *сленг:* good ~ а) превосходный человек; б) превосходное дело; в) превосходно!; bad ~ а) непутёвый, никудышный человек; б) гиблое дело; odd ~ чудак; ◇ in the ~ в зачатке, на самой ранней стадии; as sure as ~s is ~s ≅ как дважды два четыре, наверняка; to put all one's ~s in one basket а) рисковать всем, поставить всё на карту; б) поместить все свои деньги в одно предприятие, в один банк.

egg[2] *v*: to ~ on подстрекать, подбивать (*на какой-л. поступок*).

egg-plant [ˈeɡplɑːnt] *n* баклажан.

egg-shaped [ˈeɡʃeɪpt] *a* овальный, яйцевидный.

egg-shell [ˈeɡʃel] *n* 1) яичная скорлупа; 2) *attr* тонкий, прозрачный (*о фарфоре*).

eglantine [ˈeɡləntaɪn] *n* шиповник.

egoism [ˈeɡouɪzəm] *n* эгоизм.

egoist [ˈeɡouɪst] *n* эгоист.

egoistic(al) [ˌeɡouˈɪstɪk(əl)] *a* эгоистичный, эгоистический.

egregious [ɪˈɡriːdʒəs] *a* 1) отъявленный; 2) вопиющий.

egress [ˈiːɡres] *n* 1) выход; 2) право выхода.

egression [iːˈɡreʃən] *n* выход.

egret [ˈiːɡret] *n* 1) белая цапля; 2) эгрет(ка); 3) пушок (*одуванчика*).

Egyptian I [ɪˈdʒɪpʃən] *n* 1) египтянин; египтянка; the ~s египтяне; 2) египетская сигарета; 3) *уст.* цыган; цыганка.

Egyptian II *a* египетский.

eh [eɪ] *int* а?, как?, что (вы сказали)?, не правда ли?; а!, вот как!

eider [ˈaɪdə] *n зоол.* гага.

eider-down [ˈaɪdədaun] *n* 1) гагачий пух; 2) пуховое стёганое одеяло.

eider-duck [ˈaɪdədʌk] *см.* eider.

eight I [eɪt] *num* восемь.

eight II *n* восьмёрка.

eighteen [ˈeɪˈtiːn] *num* восемнадцать.

eighteenth I [ˈeɪˈtiːnθ] *num* восемнадцатый.

eighteenth II *n* восемнадцатая часть.

eighth I [eɪtθ] *num* восьмой.

eighth II *n* восьмая часть.

eighties [ˈeɪtɪz] *n pl* 1) восьмидесятые годы; 2) возраст от 79 до 90 лет.

eightieth I [ˈeɪtɪθ] *num* восьмидесятый.

eightieth II *n* восьмидесятая часть.

eighty [ˈeɪtɪ] *num* восемьдесят.

either I [ˈaɪðə] *pron* 1) каждый (*из двух*); оба, и тот и другой; 2) тот или другой, любой; один из двух, кто-либо (*из двух*).

either II *conj* 1) или; либо; ~ ... or... или...; 2) тоже, также (*при отрицании*); if he does not come I shall not ~ если он не придёт, то и я не приду.

ejaculate [ɪˈdʒækjuleɪt] *v* 1) восклицать; 2) извергать, выделять (*жидкость*).

eject [iːˈdʒekt] *v* 1) выгонять (*с места, должности*), выселять (*from*); 2) извергать, выбрасывать (*дым и т. п.*).

ejection [iːˈdʒekʃən] *n* 1) изгнание; выселение; 2) выбрасывание, извержение; испражнение; 3) извёрженная, выброшенная масса; лава.

eke [iːk] *v*: to ~ out восполнять (*with*); to ~ out one's livelihood ухитряться сводить концы с концами.

el [el] *n амер. разг.* надземная железная дорога (*на эстакадах*).

elaborate[a] [ɪˈlæbərɪt] *a* тщательно разработанный; искусно сделанный; сложный.

elaborate[b] [ɪˈlæbəreɪt] *v* 1) детально разрабатывать, вырабатывать; 2) развивать (*теорию, мысль; on, upon*).

elaboration [ɪˌlæbəˈreɪʃən] *n* разработка; совершенствование.

elapse [ɪˈlæps] *v* проходить, протекать, пролетать (*о времени*).

elastic I [ɪˈlæstɪk] *n* резинка (*шнур или подвязка*).

elastic II *a* эластичный, упругий; *перен.* гибкий; приспосабливающийся.

elasticity [ˌelæsˈtɪsɪtɪ] *n* гибкость, эластичность; *перен. тж.* приспособляемость.

elate I [ɪˈleɪt] *a* в приподнятом настроении.

elate II v 1) поднима́ть настрое́ние; подба́дривать; 2) приводи́ть в восто́рг.

elation [ı'leıʃən] n припо́днятое настрое́ние.

elbow I ['elbou] n 1) ло́коть; at one's ~ под руко́й, ря́дом; out at ~s a) с протёртыми локтя́ми (об одежде); б) бе́дный, пло́хо оде́тый, обо́рванный; 2) тех. коле́но; ◊ to rub ~s with smb. разг. води́ть компа́нию, якша́ться с кем-л.

elbow II v толка́ть локтя́ми; to ~ oneself прота́лкиваться, проти́скиваться (in, into, through).

elbow-room ['elbourum] n просто́р.

elder[1] I ['eldə] n 1) ста́рец; 2) pl ста́рые лю́ди, ста́рши; 3) старе́йшина.

elder[1] II a ста́рший.

elder[2] n бузина́.

elderly ['eldəlı] a пожило́й.

eldest ['eldıst] a (са́мый) ста́рший.

elect I [ı'lekt] n избра́нник; the ~ (употр. как pl) и́збранные.

elect II a 1) и́збранный; 2) наречённая (о невесте).

elect III v 1) выбира́ть; избира́ть; 2) реши́ть, предпоче́сть.

election [ı'lekʃən] n 1) вы́боры; general (periodical) ~ всео́бщие (очередны́е) вы́боры; midterm (амер. special) ~ дополни́тельные вы́боры; the ~ is on иду́т вы́боры; to hold an ~ проводи́ть вы́боры; 2) избра́ние.

electioneer [ı,lekʃə'nıə] v проводи́ть предвы́борную кампа́нию; агити́ровать за кандида́та.

electioneering [ı,lekʃə'nıərıŋ] n предвы́борная кампа́ния.

elective [ı'lektıv] a 1) вы́борный; и́збранный; 2) избира́тельный; 3) име́ющий избира́тельные права́; 4) амер. необяза́тельный.

elector [ı'lektə] n 1) избира́тель; 2) амер. выбо́рщик (избираемый для выборов президента и вице-президента).

electoral [ı'lektərəl] a избира́тельный.

electorate [ı'lektərıt] n избира́тели, континге́нт избира́телей.

electric(al) [ı'lektrık(əl)] a электри́ческий.

electrician [ılek'trıʃən] n 1) электроте́хник; 2) электромонтёр.

electricity [ılek'trısıtı] n электри́чество.

electrification [ı,lektrıfı'keıʃən] n 1) электрифика́ция; 2) электриза́ция.

electrify [ı'lektrıfaı] v 1) электрифици́ровать; 2) электризова́ть; перен. наэлектризова́ть, возбуди́ть.

electrization [ı,lektraı'zeıʃən] n электриза́ция.

electrize [ı'lektraız] см. electrify.

electrocardiogram [ı'lektrou,kɑːdıəgræm] n мед. электрокардиогра́мма.

electrocute [ı'lektrəkjuːt] v 1) казни́ть на электри́ческом сту́ле; 2) уби́ть электри́ческим то́ком.

electrocution [ı,lektrə'kjuːʃən] n казнь на электри́ческом сту́ле.

electrode [ı'lektroud] n электро́д.

electrolysis [ılek'trɔlısıs] n электро́лиз.

electromagnet [ı'lektrou'mægnıt] n электромагни́т.

electromotive [ı'lektroumoutıv] a электродви́жущий.

electron [ı'lektrɔn] n физ. 1) электро́н; 2) attr электро́нный.

electronic [ılek'trɔnık] a электро́нный.

electronics [ılek'trɔnıks] n электро́ника.

electroplate [ı'lektroupleıt] v гальванизи́ровать.

elegance ['elıgəns] n изя́щество, элега́нтность.

elegancy ['elıgənsı] см. elegance.

elegant ['elıgənt] a 1) изя́щный, элега́нтный; 2) разг. превосхо́дный; прекра́сный; лу́чший.

elegiac [,elı'dʒaıək] a элеги́ческий; гру́стный.

elegy ['elıdʒı] n эле́гия.

element ['elımənt] n 1) элеме́нт; 2) pl осно́вы (науки и т. п.); 3) стихи́я; in his ~ в свое́й стихи́и; ≅ как ры́ба в воде́; 4) до́ля, ма́лое коли́чество; 5) воен. подразделе́ние; 6) амер. звено́ (самолётов).

elemental [,elı'mentl] a 1) стихи́йный; 2) нача́льный, основно́й; элемента́рный.

elementary [,elı'mentərı] a 1) нача́льный, первонача́льный; элемента́рный; 2) хим. неразложи́мый.

elephant ['elıfənt] n слон; white ~ бе́лый слон; перен. обремени́тельное иму́щество; ◊ to see the ~ узна́ть жизнь; ви́деть свет.

elephantine [,elı'fæntaın] a слоно́вый; перен. неуклю́жий, громо́здкий.

elevate ['elıveıt] v 1) поднима́ть; 2) возвыша́ть.

elevated I ['elıveıtıd] a 1) по́днятый; 2) возвы́шенный; 3) надзе́мный, на эстака́де (о дороге); 4) разг. подвы́пивший.

elevated II n амер. разг. надзе́мная желе́зная доро́га (на эстакадах).

elevating ['elıveıtıŋ] a подъёмный.

elevation [,elı'veıʃən] n 1) подня́тие; возвыше́ние; 2) возвы́шенность (стиля и т. п.); 3) высота́ (над уровнем моря, над горизонтом); 4) холм, возвы́шенность; 5) тех. про́филь, (вертика́льный) разре́з.

elevator ['elıveıtə] n 1) подъёмник; лифт; 2) элева́тор; 3) ав. руль высоты́.

eleven [ı'levn] num оди́ннадцать.

eleventh I [ı'levnθ] num оди́ннадцатый.

eleventh II n оди́ннадцатая часть.

elf [elf] n (pl elves) 1) миф. эльф; 2) ка́рлик; 3) прока́зник.

elfin I ['elfın] n 1) ка́рлик; малю́тка; 2) прока́зник.

elfin II a волше́бный; относя́щийся к э́льфам.

elfish ['elfıʃ] см. elvish.

elf-lock ['elflɔk] n спу́танные во́лосы.

elicit [ı'lısıt] v 1) выявля́ть, вызыва́ть; извлека́ть; 2) допы́тываться, добива́ться.

elide [ı'laıd] v 1) выпуска́ть, опуска́ть (слог или гласный звук) при произнесе́нии; 2) обходи́ть молча́нием.

eligibility [,elıdʒə'bılıtı] n пра́во быть и́збранным.

eligible ['elıdʒəbl] a 1) име́ющий пра́во быть и́збранным (for); 2) подходя́щий, жела́тельный.

eliminate [ı'lımıneıt] v 1) выбра́сывать, исключа́ть (из — from); 2) уничтожа́ть, упраздня́ть; ликвиди́ровать; 3) мат. приводи́ть уравне́ние к одному́ неизве́стному.

elimination [ı,lımı'neıʃən] n 1) исключе́ние, изгна́ние; 2) уничтоже́ние; упраздне́ние; 3) мат. приведе́ние уравне́ния к одному́ неизве́стному.

elision [ı'lıʒən] n лингв. эли́зия.

élite [eɪ'liːt] *n* отборная часть, цвет (*чего-л. — of*), элита.

elk [elk] *n* лось.

ell¹ [el] *n ист. мера длины* (≅ *113 см*).

ell² *n* крыло дома; *амер.* пристройка.

ellipse [ɪ'lɪps] *n* 1) *мат.* эллипс; 2) *см.* ellipsis.

ellipsis [ɪ'lɪpsɪs] *n* (*pl* ellipses [ɪ'lɪpsiːz]) *лингв.* эллипс.

elliptic(al) [ɪ'lɪptɪk(əl)] *a мат., лингв.* эллиптический.

elm [elm] *n бот.* ильм, вяз.

elocution [ˌeləˈkjuːʃən] *n* ораторское искусство.

elongate ['iːlɔŋgeɪt] *v* 1) удлинять(ся); растягивать(ся); 2) продлить (*срок*).

elope [ɪ'loup] *v* 1) бежать (*с возлюбленным*); 2) скрыться.

eloquence ['eləkwəns] *n* красноречие.

eloquent ['eləkwənt] *a* красноречивый.

else [els] *adv* 1) ещё, кроме; anybody ~ ещё кто-нибудь; who ~? кто ещё?; who ~'s чей; somebody ~'s чей-то, кого-то другого, принадлежащий кому-то другому; what ~ could I say? что ещё (*или* что, кроме этого) я мог сказать?; 2) иначе, или же, в противном случае, а (не) то; run (or) ~ you will be late бегите, а (не) то вы опоздаете.

elsewhere ['els'wɛə] *adv* где-нибудь в другом месте.

elucidate [ɪ'luːsɪdeɪt] *v* проливать свет, разъяснять, объяснять.

elucidation [ɪˌluːsɪ'deɪʃən] *n* разъяснение.

elucidative [ɪ'luːsɪdeɪtɪv] *a* объяснительный, разъяснительный.

elude [ɪ'luːd] *v* избегать, уклоняться, ускользать.

elusion [ɪ'luːʒən] *n* уклонение, увёртка.

elusive [ɪ'luːsɪv] *a* 1) неуловимый, ускользающий; уклончивый; 2) слабый (*о памяти*).

elusory [ɪ'luːsərɪ] *a* ускользающий; неуловимый.

elves [elvz] *pl см.* elf.

elvish ['elvɪʃ] *a* 1) волшебный; 2) крошечный; 3) проказливый.

em- [em-, ɪm-] *pref* фонетический вариант en- *перед* m, b, p.

'em [əm] *разг.* = them.

emaciate [ɪ'meɪʃɪeɪt] *v* изнурять, истощать.

emaciation [ɪˌmeɪsɪ'eɪʃən] *n* изнурение, истощение.

emanate ['eməneɪt] *v* 1) исходить, истекать; 2) происходить (*from*).

emanation [ˌemə'neɪʃən] *n* истечение, испускание, излучение.

emancipate [ɪ'mænsɪpeɪt] *v* освобождать от зависимости и ограничений, эмансипировать.

emancipation [ɪˌmænsɪ'peɪʃən] *n* освобождение, эмансипация.

emasculateᵃ [ɪ'mæskjulɪt] *a* 1) кастрированный; *перен.* выхолощенный; 2) изнеженный.

emasculateᵇ [ɪ'mæskjuleɪt] *v* 1) кастрировать; *перен.* обеднять (*язык*), выхолащивать (*идею и т. п.*); 2) ослаблять, обессиливать; изнеживать.

embalm [ɪm'bɑːm] *v* 1) наполнять благоуханием; 2) бальзамировать (*труп*); *перен.* сохранять от забвения.

embank [ɪm'bæŋk] *v* ограждать дамбами, насыпью.

embankment [ɪm'bæŋkmənt] *n* 1) насыпь; дамба; 2) (каменная) набережная.

embargo I [ɪm'bɑːgou] *n* эмбарго; запрещение; to lay an ~ on налагать запрещение, эмбарго на; to be under an ~ быть под запретом.

embargo II *v* 1) налагать эмбарго (*на суда, торговлю*); 2) задерживать, реквизировать (*суда*).

embark [ɪm'bɑːk] *v* 1) грузить(ся), садиться (на корабль); 2) предпринимать, начинать (*какое-л. дело; in, on, upon*).

embarkation [ˌembɑː'keɪʃən] *n* посадка, погрузка (на корабль).

embarrass [ɪm'bærəs] *v* 1) смущать, приводить в замешательство; 2) затруднять; стеснять; 3) обременять (*долгами*).

embarrassment [ɪm'bærəsmənt] *n* 1) замешательство, смущение; 2) затруднение; 3) запутанность (*в делах, долгах*).

embassy ['embəsɪ] *n* посольство.

embed [ɪm'bed] *v* 1) закапывать, укреплять (*в грунте*); 2) вделывать, заделывать (*во что-л.*); вмазывать; ~ded in concrete забетонированный, заделанный в бетон; 3) врезаться; ~ded in one's recollection (*или* memory) врезавшийся в память; 4) укладывать (*напр., шпалы*).

embellish [ɪm'belɪʃ] *v* украшать; приукрашивать.

ember¹ ['embə] *n обыкн. pl* последние (тлеющие) угольки; горячая зола.

ember² *см.* ember-goose.

ember-goose ['embəguːs] *n зоол.* полярная гагара.

embezzle [ɪm'bezl] *v* присваивать, растрачивать (*чужие деньги, имущество*).

embitter [ɪm'bɪtə] *v* 1) отравлять (*радость и т. п.*); 2) отягчать (*горе и т. п.*); 3) раздражать, озлоблять.

emblazon [ɪm'bleɪzən] *v* расписывать, превозносить.

emblem ['embləm] *n* эмблема, символ.

emblematic(al) [ˌemblɪ'mætɪk(əl)] *a* символический.

emblematize [em'blemətaɪz] *v* служить эмблемой, символизировать.

embodiment [ɪm'bɔdɪmənt] *n* 1) воплощение, олицетворение; 2) объединение; включение; 3) *воен.* формирование.

embody [ɪm'bɔdɪ] *v* 1) воплощать (в себе), олицетворять; 2) воплощать (*в действительность*), облекать в конкретную форму (*мысли и т. п.*); 3) включать; заключать в себе, содержать; 4) *воен.* формировать.

embog [ɪm'bɔg] *v* завязнуть в болоте.

embolden [ɪm'bouldən] *v* придавать храбрости, ободрять.

embosom [ɪm'buzəm] *v* 1) обнимать; 2) окружать.

embosomed [ɪm'buzəmd] *a* окружённый, обрамлённый (*with*); заключённый между (*in*).

emboss [ɪm'bɔs] *v* 1) выбивать, чеканить; 2) украшать рельефом.

embowel [ɪm'bauəl] *v* потрошить.

embrace I [ɪm'breɪs] *n* объятия.

embrace II *v* 1) обнимать(ся); 2) (вос)пользоваться (*случаем, предложением*); 3) охватывать; включать; заключать в себе; 4) принимать (*рели-*

гию, *образ мыслей и т. п.*); 5) избира́ть (*специа́льность*).

embrasure [ɪm'breɪʒə] *n* амбразу́ра.

embrocation [ˌembrou'keɪʃən] *n* растира́ние (*мазь, жидкость*).

embroider [ɪm'brɔɪdə] *v* 1) вышива́ть; 2) приукра́шивать.

embroidery [ɪm'brɔɪdərɪ] *n* 1) вышива́ние; 2) вы́шивка; 3) украше́ние, прикра́сы.

embroil [ɪm'brɔɪl] *v* 1) запу́тывать (*дела, рассказ и т. п.*); 2) впу́тывать (*в неприятности*); 3) ссо́рить (*with*).

embryo I ['embrɪou] *n* заро́дыш, эмбрио́н.

embryo II *a* заро́дышевый, эмбриона́льный.

embryonic [ˌembrɪ'ɔnɪk] *a* эмбриона́льный.

emend [i:'mend] *v* исправля́ть, выправля́ть (*текст*); вноси́ть попра́вки, измене́ния.

emerald I ['emərəld] *n* 1) изумру́д; 2) изумру́дный цвет.

emerald II *a* изумру́дный.

emerge [ɪ'məːdʒ] *v* 1) всплыва́ть; появля́ться; возника́ть; 2) выявля́ться, выясня́ться.

emergence [ɪ'məːdʒəns] *n* 1) появле́ние; выявле́ние.

emergency I [ɪ'məːdʒənsɪ] *n* непредви́денный слу́чай; кра́йняя необходи́мость, кра́йность; on ~, in case of ~ в слу́чае кра́йней необходи́мости.

emergency II *a* 1) запа́сный, запасно́й, вспомога́тельный; 2) авари́йный; 3) неприкоснове́нный (*запас, паёк*); 4) вре́менный (*о постройке и т. п.*); 5) э́кстренный, чрезвыча́йный (*о полномо́чиях, ме́рах*); 6) *ав.* вы́нужденный (*о посадке*).

emeritus [i:'merɪtəs] *a* отставно́й, в отста́вке.

emersion [i:'məːʃən] *n* 1) появле́ние; 2) всплыва́ние, всплы́тие.

emery ['emərɪ] *n* нажда́к.

emetic [ɪ'metɪk] *n* рво́тное (*лека́рство*).

emigrant I ['emɪgrənt] *n* 1) переселе́нец; 2) эмигра́нт.

emigrant II *a* 1) переселе́нческий; 2) эмигри́рующий; эмигра́нтский.

emigrate ['emɪgreɪt] *v* 1) переселя́ть(ся); 2) эмигри́ровать; 3) *разг.* переезжа́ть.

emigration [ˌemɪ'greɪʃən] *n* 1) переселе́ние; 2) эмигра́ция.

eminence ['emɪnəns] *n* 1) высота́; возвыше́ние; возвы́шенность; 2) высо́кое положе́ние; превосхо́дство (*умственное*); of ~ знамени́тый; высо́кого положе́ния; 3) (E.) преосвяще́нство (*титул кардина́ла*).

eminent ['emɪnənt] *a* 1) знамени́тый, выдаю́щийся; 2) возвыша́ющийся; возвы́шенный.

emissary ['emɪsərɪ] *n* эмисса́р.

emission [ɪ'mɪʃən] *n* 1) выделе́ние (*тепла*); излуче́ние (*света*); испуска́ние (*запаха*); 2) *фин.* эми́ссия, вы́пуск (*ценных бумаг, денег и т. п.*); 3) *физ.* эмана́ция электро́нов; 4) *attr* эмиссио́нный.

emissive [ɪ'mɪsɪv] *a* излуча́ющий; выделя́ющий; испуска́ющий.

emit [ɪ'mɪt] *v* 1) издава́ть, испуска́ть (*звук, крик, запах*); 2) выделя́ть (*тепло*); излуча́ть (*свет*); 3) выпуска́ть (*деньги*).

emolument [ɪ'mɔljumənt] *n* дохо́д; за́работок.

emotion [ɪ'mouʃən] *n* си́льное чу́вство, возбужде́ние, душе́вное волне́ние; эмо́ция; with ~ с чу́вством.

emotional [ɪ'mouʃənl] *a* 1) волну́ющий(ся); взволно́ванный; 2) эмоциона́льный.

emotionality [ˌmouʃə'nælɪtɪ] *n* эмоциона́льность.

emperor ['empərə] *n* импера́тор.

emphasis ['emfəsɪs] *n* 1) ударе́ние, акце́нт; 2) подчёркивание; to lay (*или* to put) special ~ уси́ленно подчёркивать, придава́ть осо́бое значе́ние, осо́бую вырази́тельность; 3) ре́зкость ко́нтуров (*в живописи*).

emphasize ['emfəsaɪz] *v* 1) де́лать (осо́бое) ударе́ние (*на слове и т. п.*); 2) подчёркивать, придава́ть осо́бое значе́ние.

emphatic [ɪm'fætɪk] *a* вырази́тельный, подчёркнутый, эмфати́ческий.

emphatically [ɪm'fætɪkəlɪ] *adv* 1) с осо́бенным выраже́нием; 2) подчёркнуто; 3) многозначи́тельно.

Empire [ɑːŋ'pɪə] *n* 1) (стиль) ампи́р; 2) *attr* в сти́ле ампи́р.

empire I ['empaɪə] *n* 1) импе́рия; 2) госпо́дство (*над — over*); ◊ Invisible ~ неви́димая импе́рия, ку-клукс-кла́н.

empire II *a* импе́рский.

empiric I [em'pɪrɪk] *n* 1) эмпи́рик; 2) зна́харь, врач-шарлата́н.

empiric II *a* эмпири́ческий.

empirical [em'pɪrɪkəl] *a* эмпири́ческий.

empiricist [em'pɪrɪsɪst] *n* эмпи́рик.

empirio-criticism [em'pɪrɪou'krɪtɪsɪzəm] *n* эмпириокритици́зм.

emplacement [ɪm'pleɪsmənt] *n* 1) местоположе́ние; ме́сто расположе́ния; 2) *воен.* оруди́йная платфо́рма; огнева́я то́чка.

employ I [ɪm'plɔɪ] *n* слу́жба; to be in the ~ of smb. служи́ть, рабо́тать у кого́-л.

employ II *v* 1) держа́ть на слу́жбе; испо́льзовать, по́льзоваться услу́гами (*кого́-л.*); 2) употребля́ть, испо́льзовать; применя́ть; to ~ oneself (in) занима́ться.

employee [ˌemplɔɪ'iː] *n* слу́жащий.

employer [ɪm'plɔɪə] *n* нанима́тель, работода́тель.

employment [ɪm'plɔɪmənt] *n* 1) слу́жба, рабо́та; заня́тие; 2) примене́ние, испо́льзование; 3) *эк.* за́нятость; full ~ по́лная за́нятость; 4) *attr*: ~ bureau бюро́ по на́йму; ~ agent аге́нт по на́йму.

empoison [ɪm'pɔɪzn] *v* отравля́ть (*тж. перен.*).

emporium [em'pɔːrɪəm] *n* 1) торго́вый центр; 2) *разг.* большо́й магази́н.

empower [ɪm'pauə] *v* 1) уполномо́чивать; 2) дава́ть возмо́жность, пра́во.

empress ['emprɪs] *n* императри́ца.

emptiness ['emptɪnɪs] *n* пустота́.

empty I ['emptɪ] *a* 1) пусто́й; 2) бессодержа́тельный; 3) *разг.* голо́дный.

empty II *v* 1) опорожня́ть, высыпа́ть, вылива́ть; 2) пересыпа́ть, перелива́ть; 3) впада́ть (*о реке; into*); 4) пусте́ть, опорожня́ться.

empty-handed ['emptɪ'hændɪd] *a* с пусты́ми рука́ми.

empty-headed ['emptɪ'hedɪd] *a* пустоголо́вый.

empty-pated ['emptɪ'peɪtɪd] *см.* empty-headed.

empyrean I [ˌempaɪ'riːən] *n* 1) *миф.* эмпире́й; 2) не́бо.

empyrean II *a* небе́сный, заобла́чный.

emu ['iːmjuː] *n* *зоол.* эму́.

emulate ['emjuleɪt] v 1) соревнова́ться; 2) сопе́рничать.

emulation [,emju'leɪʃən] n 1) соревнова́ние; socialist ~ социалисти́ческое соревнова́ние; 2) сопе́рничество.

emulous ['emjuləs] a 1) соревну́ющийся; 2) сопе́рничающий; 3) жа́ждущий чего́-л. (of).

emulsion [ɪ'mʌlʃən] n эму́льсия.

emulsive [ɪ'mʌlsɪv] a эмульсио́нный; масляни́стый.

en- [en-, ɪn-] pref 1) служит для образования переходных гл. от сущ. или прил. и придаёт им значение: а) включения внутрь чего-л.: to encage сажа́ть в кле́тку; б) приведения в какое-л. состояние: to enable дава́ть возмо́жность; to enslave закабаля́ть; 2) служит для образования гл. с соответствующим переходным значением: to enforce принужда́ть, наста́ивать.

enable [ɪ'neɪbl] v дава́ть возмо́жность, пра́во (что-л. сделать).

enact [ɪ'nækt] v 1) предпи́сывать; постановля́ть; 2) представля́ть, игра́ть (роль); 3) обыкн. pass происходи́ть, разы́грываться.

enactment [ɪ'næktmənt] n 1) введе́ние в си́лу (закона); 2) зако́н, указ.

enamel I [ɪ'næməl] n 1) эма́ль; 2) разг. глазу́рь.

enamel II v 1) покрыва́ть эма́лью; 2) покрыва́ть глазу́рью; 3) испещря́ть.

enamo(u)r [ɪ'næmə] v обыкн. pass возбужда́ть любо́вь; to be ~ed of (стра́стно) люби́ть.

encamp [ɪn'kæmp] v располага́ть(ся) ла́герем.

encampment [ɪn'kæmpmənt] n 1) ла́герь, ла́герная стоя́нка; hut ~ бара́чный ла́герь; 2) разби́вка ла́геря.

encase [ɪn'keɪs] v 1) упако́вать, положи́ть в я́щик; 2) облека́ть; ~d in armour зако́ванный в броню́.

encasement [ɪn'keɪsmənt] n упако́вка, футля́р.

enchain [ɪn'tʃeɪn] v 1) зако́вывать; сажа́ть на цепь; 2) прико́вывать (внимание); ско́вывать (чувства); 3) сцепля́ть, соединя́ть.

enchant [ɪn'tʃɑːnt] v очаро́вывать.

enchanter [ɪn'tʃɑːntə] n волше́бник, чароде́й.

enchantment [ɪn'tʃɑːntmənt] n очарова́ние.

enchantress [ɪn'tʃɑːntrɪs] n волше́бница, чароде́йка; перен. тж. обворожи́тельная же́нщина.

encircle [ɪn'sɜːkl] v окружа́ть.

encircling I [ɪn'sɜːklɪŋ] n окруже́ние.

encircling II a охва́тывающий, окружа́ющий.

enclasp [ɪn'klɑːsp] v обхва́тывать, обнима́ть.

enclose [ɪn'klouz] v 1) вкла́дывать (особ. в письмо); 2) прилага́ть; окружа́ть, огора́живать; окаймля́ть; 3) заключа́ть; ограни́чивать.

enclosure [ɪn'klouʒə] n 1) вложе́ние (содержимое пакета); 2) огоро́женное ме́сто; 3) огра́да.

encode [ɪn'koud] v коди́ровать, шифрова́ть.

encoder [ɪn'koudə] n коди́рующее устро́йство.

encompass [ɪn'kʌmpəs] v 1) окружа́ть; 2) содержа́ть, заключа́ть (в себе́).

encore I [ɔŋ'kɔː] int бис!

encore II n вы́зов на «бис»; to give three ~s биси́ровать три ра́за.

encore III v вызыва́ть на «бис», тре́бовать повторе́ния.

encounter I [ɪn'kauntə] n 1) столкнове́ние, схва́тка, сты́чка; 2) неожи́данная встре́ча.

encounter II v 1) ста́лкиваться; име́ть столкнове́ние; 2) (неожи́данно) встре́тить(ся).

encourage [ɪn'kʌrɪdʒ] v 1) ободря́ть; поощря́ть; 2) помога́ть, подде́рживать; спосо́бствовать; 3) подстрека́ть.

encouragement [ɪn'kʌrɪdʒmənt] n 1) ободре́ние; поощре́ние; 2) по́мощь, подде́ржка; 3) подстрека́тельство.

encouraging [ɪn'kʌrɪdʒɪŋ] a ободря́ющий; обнадёживающий.

encroach [ɪn'kroutʃ] v вторга́ться; посяга́ть (на чужую территорию, чужие права; on).

encumber [ɪn'kʌmbə] v 1) затрудня́ть, препя́тствовать; меша́ть; стесня́ть; 2) загроможда́ть; 3) обременя́ть (долгами и т. п.).

encumbrance [ɪn'kʌmbrəns] n 1) препя́тствие, поме́ха; затрудне́ние; 2) бре́мя, обу́за; 3) юр. закладна́я (на имущество).

encyclop(a)edia [en,saɪklou'piːdjə] n энциклопе́дия.

encyclop(a)edic(al) [en,saɪklou'piːdɪk(əl)] a энциклопеди́ческий.

end I [end] n 1) коне́ц; ~ on концо́м к себе́; on ~ стоймя́ (см. тж. ◊); по ~ of без конца́, (бесконе́чно) мно́го, ма́сса (неприятностей, огорчений и т. п.); ~ to ~ непреры́вной це́пью, вплотну́ю; to be at an ~, to come to an ~ приходи́ть к концу́, конча́ться; to the bitter ~ до (са́мого) конца́, до преде́ла; to put an ~ to, to make an ~ of положи́ть коне́ц (чему-л.); 2) оста́ток, обло́мок, обры́вок, обре́зок; 3) результа́т, сле́дствие; in the ~ в коне́чном счёте, в результа́те; 4) смерть; to be near one's ~ умира́ть, быть при́ смерти; 5) цель; to what ~? с како́й це́лью?; to gain one's ~s дости́гнуть це́ли; ◊ ~ on — беспреры́вно, подря́д; the business ~ практи́ческая, наибо́лее ва́жная сторона́ де́ла; at a loose ~ не у дел; at one's wits' ~ в смуще́нии, в замеша́тельстве; озада́ченный; to keep (или to hold) one's ~ up не сдава́ться, стара́ться не па́дать ду́хом; to make both ~s meet своди́ть концы́ с конца́ми; to be at the ~ of one's tether дойти́ до преде́ла; the thin ~ of the wedge скро́мное, но многообеща́ющее нача́ло.

end II v конча́ть(ся) (чем-л. — in); □ to ~ off, to ~ up ока́нчиваться; ◊ to ~ in smoke ко́нчиться ниче́м.

endanger [ɪn'deɪndʒə] v угрожа́ть; подверга́ть опа́сности.

endear [ɪn'dɪə] v внуши́ть любо́вь.

endearment [ɪn'dɪəmənt] n привя́занность; ла́ска, не́жность.

endeavo(u)r I [ɪn'devə] n попы́тка, стара́ние.

endeavo(u)r II v пыта́ться (сделать что-л.); прилага́ть уси́лия, стара́ться.

ending ['endɪŋ] n 1) оконча́ние; 2) attr оконча́тельный, заключи́тельный.

endless ['endlɪs] a бесконе́чный, несконча́емый; бесчи́сленный.

endlong ['endlɔŋ] adv 1) пря́мо, вдоль; 2) стоймя́, вертика́льно.

endmost ['endmoust] a са́мый да́льний.

endorse [ɪn'dɔːs] v 1) де́лать переда́точную на́дпись; индосси́ровать; 2) писа́ть, распи́сываться на оборо́те (документа); 3) подтвержда́ть; одобря́ть.

endorsement [ɪn'dɔːsmənt] n 1) переда́точная

надпись (*на чеке, векселе*); 2) подтверждéние; одобрéние.

endow [ın'dau] *v* 1) обеспéчивать постоя́нным дохóдом; 2) одаря́ть; ~ed with одарённый (*спосóбностями и т. п.*); 3) дава́ть (*привилегии, права; with*).

endowment [ın'daumənt] *n* 1) вклад, пожéртвование; 2) дарова́ние; ◊ ~ with information сообщéние свéдений.

endue [ın'dju:] *v* 1) облача́ть (*with*); 2) одаря́ть, наделя́ть; ~d with одарённый, наделённый.

end-up ['end'ʌp] *a разг.* курнóсый.

endurance [ın'djuərəns] *n* 1) вынóсливость; стóйкость; 2) прóчность.

endure [ın'djuə] *v* 1) выноси́ть; терпéть; 2) продолжа́ться, дли́ться.

endways ['endweız] *adv* концóм вперёд *или* вверх; стóймя.

endwise ['endwaız] *см.* endways.

enema ['enımə] *n мед.* кли́зма.

enemy I ['enımı] *n* 1) враг; bitter ~ злéйший враг; sworn ~ закля́тый враг; the Enemy дья́вол; 2): the ~ (*употр. как pl*) неприя́тель, проти́вник; ◊ to kill the ~ корота́ть врéмя; how goes the ~?, what says the ~? котóрый час?

enemy II *a* врáжеский, неприя́тельский.

energetic [‚enə'dʒetık] *a* энерги́чный.

energetics [‚enə'dʒetıks] *n* энергéтика.

energy ['enədʒı] *n* 1) энéргия, си́ла; atomic ~ áтомная энéргия; 2) *pl* уси́лия.

enervate I ['enə:veıt] *a* слáбый, бесси́льный; рассла́бленный.

enervate II *v* ослабля́ть; расслабля́ть.

enervation [‚enə:'veıʃən] *n* расслаблéние.

enfeeble [ın'fi:bl] *v* ослабля́ть.

enfold [ın'fould] *v* 1) заку́тывать, завёртывать (*in, with*); 2) обнима́ть, обхва́тывать; 3) образóвать скла́дки.

enforce [ın'fɔ:s] *v* 1) принужда́ть, заставля́ть; 2) навя́зывать; 3) проводи́ть в жизнь (*закон*); 4) уси́ливать.

enforcement [ın'fɔ:smənt] *n* принуждéние; давлéние.

enfranchise [ın'fræntʃaız] *v* 1) предоставля́ть избира́тельные права́; 2) предоставля́ть (*гóроду*) прáво представи́тельства в парла́менте; 3) освобожда́ть.

engage [ın'geıdʒ] *v* 1) нанима́ть; зака́зывать зара́нее (*места и т. п.*); 2) занима́ться, быть за́нятым (*тж.* to be ~d in); say I am ~d скажи́те, что я за́нят; to be ~d in medicine занима́ться медици́ной; to ~ in politics пуска́ться в поли́тику; 3) занима́ть, привлека́ть (*внимание и т. п.*); завладева́ть (*вниманием и т. п.*); вовлека́ть (*в разговор*); 4) обя́зываться, свя́зывать себя́ слóвом *или* обяза́тельством (*особ. жениться*); to be ~d быть помóлвленным; 5) *воен.* вступа́ть (*в бой; тж.* to ~ in battle); вводи́ть в дéло, в бой; открыва́ть огóнь (*тж.* to ~ by fire); 6) *тех.* зацепля́ть; включа́ть; □ to ~ for обеща́ть, гаранти́ровать.

engaged [ın'geıdʒd] *a* 1) за́нятый; 2) помóлвленный.

engagement [ın'geıdʒmənt] *n* 1) приглашéние; свида́ние; встрéча; 2) дéло, заня́тие; 3) обяза́тельство; to meet one's ~s выполня́ть обяза́тельства; плати́ть долги́; 4) помóлвка; 5) *воен.* бой, сты́чка.

engaging [ın'geıdʒıŋ] *a* привлека́тельный, очарова́тельный; увлека́тельный.

engender [ın'dʒendə] *v* порожда́ть; вызыва́ть, возбужда́ть.

engine ['endʒın] *n* 1) (парова́я) маши́на; мотóр, дви́гатель; (internal-)combustion ~, explosion ~ дви́гатель внýтреннего сгора́ния; jet ~ реакти́вный дви́гатель; rotary ~ ротацióнная маши́на; 2) парóвоз, локомоти́в; 3) орýдие; срéдство; 4) *attr* паровóзный; 5) *attr* маши́нный; 6) *attr* мотóрный.

engine-crew ['endʒınkru:] *n ж.-д.* паровóзная брига́да.

engine-driver ['endʒın‚draıvə] *n ж.-д.* машини́ст.

engineer I [‚endʒı'nıə] *n* 1) инженéр; civil ~ инженéр-строи́тель; 2) механи́к; 3) машини́ст; 4) *воен.* сапёр; 5) *pl воен.* инженéрно-сапёрные ча́сти; 6) *attr* инженéрный; 7) *attr* сапёрный.

engineer II *v* 1) быть инженéром; 2) проекти́ровать; строи́ть; 3) *разг.* устра́ивать.

engineering [‚endʒı'nıərıŋ] *n* 1) тéхника; agricultural ~ агротéхника; electronic ~ электрóнная тéхника; 2) (инженéрно-)строи́тельное искýсство; 3) машинострóение.

engine-house ['endʒınhaus] *n ж.-д.* паровóзное депó.

engine-plant ['endʒınplɑ:nt] *n* 1) паровозострои́тельный завóд; 2) маши́нная устанóвка.

engine-room ['endʒınrum] *n* маши́нное отделéние.

engird [ın'gə:d] *v* (*past, p. p.* engirded, engirt) опоя́сывать.

engirdle [ın'gə:dl] *см.* engird.

engirt [ın'gə:t] *past, p. p. см.* engird.

English I ['ıŋglıʃ] *n* 1): the ~ (*употр. как pl*) англича́не; 2) англи́йский язы́к; Old ~ древнеанглийский язы́к; Middle ~ среднеанглийский язы́к; in plain ~ пря́мо, откровéнно, без обиняков.

English II *a* англи́йский.

Englishman ['ıŋglıʃmən] *n* англича́нин.

Englishwoman ['ıŋglıʃ‚wumən] *n* англича́нка.

engrain [ın'greın] *v* пропи́тывать (*краской*); *перен.* внедря́ть, укореня́ть.

engrained [ın'greınd] *a* отъя́вленный, закоренéлый.

engrave [ın'greıv] *v* 1) гравирова́ть; рéзать (*по дереву, камню, металлу*); 2) запечатлева́ть (*в па́мяти; оп, upon*).

engraving [ın'greıvıŋ] *n* 1) гравирова́ние; 2) гравю́ра.

engross [ın'grous] *v* завладева́ть (*вниманием, разговором*); поглоща́ть, занима́ть (*чьё-л. внимание, время*); ~ed in smth. погружённый во что-л., поглощённый чем-л.

engrossing [ın'grousıŋ] *a* поглоща́ющий (*время, внимание*); всепоглоща́ющий.

engulf [ın'gʌlf] *v* 1) поглоща́ть; 2) подавля́ть.

enhance [ın'hɑːns] *v* увели́чивать; повыша́ть; уси́ливать.

enigma [ı'nıgmə] *n* зага́дка.

enigmatic(al) [‚enıg'mætık(əl)] *a* зага́дочный.

enjoin [ın'dʒɔın] *v* предпи́сывать; прика́зывать.

enjoy [ın'dʒɔı] *v* 1) получа́ть удовóльствие; весели́ться (*тж.* to ~ oneself); 2) пóльзоваться (*права́ми и т. п.*); обла́дать (*здорóвьем и т. п.*).

enjoyable [ın'dʒɔıəbl] *a* прия́тный.

enjoyment [ɪn'dʒɔɪmənt] *n* 1) наслаждéние, удовóльствие; 2) обладáние.

enkindle [ɪn'kɪndl] *v* зажигáть, воспламенять.

enlace [ɪn'leɪs] *v* обвивáть, опýтывать; окружáть.

enlarge [ɪn'lɑːdʒ] *v* 1) увелúчивать(ся); расширять(ся); 2) распространяться (*о чём-л. — upon*); 3) *фото* увелúчивать.

enlighten [ɪn'laɪtn] *v* 1) осведомлять; 2) просвещáть; 3) *поэт.* проливáть свет.

enlightened [ɪn'laɪtnd] *a* 1) осведомлённый; 2) просвещённый.

enlightenment [ɪn'laɪtnmənt] *n* 1) просвещённость; 2) просвещéние.

enlist [ɪn'lɪst] *v* 1) доброво́льно поступáть на воéнную слýжбу; 2) набирáть, вербовáть (на воéнную слýжбу); 3) заручáться (*содéйствием, поддéржкой*).

enlistee [ˌenlɪs'tiː] *n амер.* поступúвший на воéнную слýжбу.

enliven [ɪn'laɪvn] *v* оживúть, развеселúть.

enmity ['enmɪtɪ] *n* враждéбность, неприязнь; враждá.

ennoble [ɪ'noubl] *v* облагорáживать.

ennui [ɑː'nwiː] *n* скýка.

enormity [ɪ'nɔːmɪtɪ] *n* 1) гнýсность; 2) чудóвищное преступлéние.

enormous [ɪ'nɔːməs] *a* 1) огрóмный, громáдный; 2) ужáсный.

enough I [ɪ'nʌf] *a* достáточный.

enough II *n* достáточное количество; we have ~ of everything у нас всегó довóльно; ~ and to spare бóльше, чем нýжно; I have had ~ of him он мне надоéл, я устáл от негó.

enough III *adv* достáточно, довóльно; sure ~ без сомнéния.

enquire [ɪn'kwaɪə] *см.* inquire.

enquiry [ɪn'kwaɪərɪ] *см.* inquiry.

enrage [ɪn'reɪdʒ] *v* бесúть, приводúть в бéшенство, в ярость.

enrapture [ɪn'ræptʃə] *v* восхищáть.

enrich [ɪn'rɪtʃ] *v* 1) обогащáть; 2) удобрять (*почву*).

enrol(l) [ɪn'roul] *v* 1) вносúть в спúсок (*членов какой-л. организации*); (за)регистрúровать; 2) поступáть на воéнную слýжбу.

enrollee [ɪn'roulɪ] *n амер.* зачúсленный на воéнную слýжбу.

enrolment [ɪn'roulmənt] *n* 1) внесéние в спúсок; регистрáция; 2) приём нóвых члéнов.

enrooted [ɪn'ruːtɪd] *a* вкоренúвшийся.

ensconce [ɪn'skɔns] *v* 1) укрыть(ся); 2) уютно усéсться, устрóиться; 3) *воен.* засéсть.

enshrine [ɪn'ʃraɪn] *v* хранúть, лелéять (*чью-л. память и т. п.*).

enshroud [ɪn'ʃraud] *v* покрывáть, окýтывать.

ensign ['ensaɪn] *n* 1) значóк, эмблéма; 2) знáмя, флаг; 3) знаменóсец; 4) *амер. мор.* (млáдший) лейтенáнт.

ensilage I ['ensɪlɪdʒ] *n с.-х.* 1) сúлос; 2) силосовáние.

ensilage II *v с.-х.* силосовáть.

ensile [en'saɪl] *v с.-х.* силосовáть.

enslave [ɪn'sleɪv] *v* порабощáть; *перен.* дéлать рабóм (*привычки, предрассýдка и т. п.*).

enslavement [ɪn'sleɪvmənt] *n* порабощéние.

ensnare [ɪn'snɛə] *v* поймáть в ловýшку.

ensue [ɪn'sjuː] *v* 1) (по)слéдовать; silence ~d послéдовало молчáние; 2) получáться в результáте, происходúть (*from, on*).

ensuing [ɪn'sjuːɪŋ] *a* 1) (по)слéдующий; 2) вытекáющий.

ensure [ɪn'ʃuə] *v* обеспéчивать, гарантúровать; ручáться.

entail I [ɪn'teɪl] *n* родовóе имéние, майорáт.

entail II *v* 1) влечь за собóй, вызывáть; 2) *юр.* учреждáть заповéдное имýщество, майорáт.

entangle [ɪn'tæŋgl] *v* 1) запýтывать; впýтывать; 2) поймáть в ловýшку.

entanglement [ɪn'tæŋglmənt] *n* 1) затруднéние, затруднúтельное положéние; запýтанность; 2) *воен.* заграждéние, препятствие.

enter ['entə] *v* 1) входúть; вступáть; 2) проникáть; 3) вступáть (*в должность; upon*); поступáть (*в армию, училище и т. п.*); 4) вносúть, запúсывать (*в книги, спúски и т. п.*); регистрúровать; 5) запúсывать(ся) (*для участия в состязáниях и т. п.; for*); □ to ~ into а) вступáть; входúть; б) являться составнóй чáстью; в) разделять, сочýвствовать; to ~ upon а) приступáть, начинáть; б) *юр.* вступáть во владéние.

enteric I [en'terɪk] *n* брюшнóй тиф (*тж.* ~ fever).

enteric II *a* брюшнóй.

enterprise ['entəpraɪz] *n* 1) предприятие; 2) предприúмчивость, смéлость; инициатúва.

enterprising ['entəpraɪzɪŋ] *a* предприúмчивый, инициатúвный.

entertain [ˌentə'teɪn] *v* 1) принимáть, занимáть (*гостéй, посетúтелей*); 2) питáть (*надéжду, сомнéния и т. п.*); 3) принимáть во внимáние, учúтывать.

entertaining [ˌentə'teɪnɪŋ] *a* занимáтельный, интерéсный.

entertainment [ˌentə'teɪnmənt] *n* 1) приём (*гостéй*); звáный вéчер; to give an ~ принимáть гостéй; 2) гостеприúмство; обслýживание (*гостéй, постояльцев*); 3) развлечéние, увеселéние.

enthral(l) [ɪn'θrɔːl] *v* 1) порабощáть; 2) очарóвывать.

enthrone [ɪn'θroun] *v* возводúть на престóл.

enthusiasm [ɪn'θjuːzɪæzəm] *n* энтузиáзм; востóрг; spontaneous ~ úскренний энтузиáзм.

enthusiast [ɪn'θjuːzɪæst] *n* энтузиáст.

enthusiastic [ɪnˌθjuːzɪ'æstɪk] *a* востóрженный.

enthusiastically [ɪnˌθjuːzɪ'æstɪkəlɪ] *adv* 1) востóрженно; с востóргом; 2) с энтузиáзмом.

entice [ɪn'taɪs] *v* соблазнять, увлекáть; перемáнивать; □ to ~ away увлéчь.

enticement [ɪn'taɪsmənt] *n* 1) замáнивание; 2) примáнка, соблáзн; 3) очаровáние.

enticing [ɪn'taɪsɪŋ] *a* соблазнúтельный.

entire I [ɪn'taɪə] *n* 1) (the ~) цéлое; полнотá; 2) некастрúрованное живóтное, *особ.* жеребéц.

entire II *a* 1) пóлный, совершéнный; 2) цéльный, сплошнóй; 3) чúстый, беспрúмесный; 4) некастрúрованный (*о живóтном*).

entirely [ɪn'taɪəlɪ] *adv* 1) всецéло, вполнé, совершéнно; 2) исключúтельно, едúнственно.

entirety [ɪn'taɪətɪ] *n* 1) полнотá, цéльность; in its ~ во всей полнотé, пóлностью; 2) óбщая сýмма; 3) *юр.* совмéстное владéние (*чем-л.*).

entitle [ɪn'taɪtl] *v* 1) давáть прáво; уполномóчивать; to be ~d иметь право (на — to); 2) озаглавливать; давать название, называть.

entity ['entɪtɪ] n 1) сущность, существо; class ~ классовая сущность; 2) что-л. реально существующее, реальность.

entomb [ɪn'tuːm] v 1) погребать; 2) служить гробницей.

entombment [ɪn'tuːmmənt] n погребение.

entomological [ˌentɔmə'lɔdʒɪkəl] a энтомологический.

entomology [ˌentə'mɔlədʒɪ] n энтомология.

entr'acte ['ɔntrækt] n антракт.

entrails ['entreɪlz] n pl внутренности, кишки; перен. недра.

entranceᵃ ['entrəns] n 1) вход; back ~ чёрный ход; по ~ вход воспрещён; to force an ~ врываться (в — into); 2) вступление (в должность, в союз и т. п.; into, upon); 3) выход (актёра на сцену); 4) attr входной; 5) attr вступительный.

entranceᵇ [ɪn'trɑːns] v приводить в состояние восторга, оцепенения, исступления (with).

entrap [ɪn'træp] v поймать в ловушку; обмануть, запутать.

entreat [ɪn'triːt] v умолять, упрашивать.

entreaty [ɪn'triːtɪ] n мольба, просьба.

entrée ['ɔntreɪ] n 1) право входа, доступа; 2) блюдо, подаваемое между рыбой и жарким.

entremets ['ɔntrəmeɪ] n дополнительные овощные и др. блюда (подаваемые после жаркого).

entrench [ɪn'trentʃ] v воен. укреплять траншеями; to ~ oneself окапываться.

entrenchment [ɪn'trentʃmənt] n воен. окоп; полевое укрепление, траншеи.

entrust [ɪn'trʌst] v возлагать; поручать, вверять.

entry ['entrɪ] n 1) вход, вступление; (торжественный) выход; 2) вход (ворота, дверь и т. п.); 3) вестибюль; 4) занесение (в список, в торговые книги); (отдельная) запись; 5) устье (реки); 6) амер. начало (какого-л. периода); 7) юр. вступление во владение.

entwine [ɪn'twaɪn] v 1) вплетать, сплетать; 2) обвивать (with, about, round); 3) обнимать.

entwist [ɪn'twɪst] v обвивать, оплетать.

enumerate [ɪ'njuːməreɪt] v перечислять.

enumeration [ɪˌnjuːmə'reɪʃən] n 1) перечисление; 2) перечень.

enunciate [ɪ'nʌnsɪeɪt] v 1) провозглашать, объявлять; 2) формулировать, излагать (предложение, теорию); 3) произносить (слова).

enure [ɪ'njuə] см. inure.

envelop [ɪn'veləp] v 1) закутывать, завёртывать; 2) окутывать; ~ed in flames охваченный пламенем; ~ed in mystery окутанный тайной; 3) воен. окружать, обходить.

envelope ['envɪloup] 1) обёртка; конверт; 2) оболочка.

envenom [ɪn'venəm] v отравлять.

enviable ['envɪəbl] a завидный; возбуждающий зависть.

envious ['envɪəs] a завистливый.

environ [ɪn'vaɪərən] v окружать.

environment [ɪn'vaɪərənmənt] n окружающая обстановка, окружение, (внешняя) среда.

environs ['envɪrɔnz] n pl 1) окрестности; 2) предместья.

envisage [ɪn'vɪzɪdʒ] v 1) смотреть в лицо (опасности и т. п.); 2) рассматривать (вопрос); 3) предусматривать.

envoy ['envɔɪ] n 1) посланник; special ~ чрезвычайный посланник; 2) агент.

envy I ['envɪ] n 1) зависть; out of ~ из зависти; 2) предмет зависти.

envy II v завидовать.

enwind [ɪn'waɪnd] v обвивать(ся).

enwrap [ɪn'ræp] v завёртывать; окутывать (in, with).

eparchy ['epɑːkɪ] n епархия.

epaulet(te) ['epoulet] n эполет.

ephemera [ɪ'femərə] n 1) зоол. подёнка, однодневка; 2) что-л. мимолётное, скоропреходящее.

ephemeral [ɪ'femərəl] a 1) недолговечный, преходящий, эфемерный; 2) живущий только один или несколько дней (о растениях, насекомых).

epic I ['epɪk] n 1) эпическая поэма; 2) сказание.

epic II a эпический.

epical ['epɪkəl] a эпический.

epicentra [ˌepɪ'sentrə] pl см. epicentrum.

epicentre ['epɪsentə] см. epicentrum.

epicentrum [ˌepɪ'sentrəm] n (pl epicentra) эпицентр (землетрясения).

epicurean I [ˌepɪkjuə'riːən] n эпикуреец.

epicurean II a эпикурейский.

epicycle [ˌepɪ'saɪkl] n мат. эпицикл.

epidemic I [ˌepɪ'demɪk] n эпидемия; to stamp out an ~ ликвидировать эпидемию.

epidemic II a эпидемический.

epidemical [ˌepɪ'demɪkəl] см. epidemic II.

epigram ['epɪgræm] n эпиграмма.

epigraph ['epɪgrɑːf] n эпиграф.

epilogue ['epɪlɔg] n эпилог.

episcopal [ɪ'pɪskəpəl] a епископский; епископальный.

episcopate [ɪ'pɪskəpɪt] n 1) сан епископа; 2) епархия.

episode ['epɪsoud] n эпизод.

episodic(al) [ˌepɪ'sɔdɪk(əl)] a эпизодический; случайный.

epistle [ɪ'pɪsl] n послание.

epistolary [ɪ'pɪstələrɪ] a эпистолярный, в форме письма.

epitaph ['epɪtɑːf] n эпитафия.

epithet ['epɪθet] n эпитет.

epoch ['iːpɔk] n эпоха; glacial ~ ледниковый период.

epoch-making ['iːpɔkˌmeɪkɪŋ] a значительный, эпохальный.

epopee ['epoupiː] n эпопея.

epos ['epɔs] n эпос; эпическая поэма.

equability [ˌekwə'bɪlɪtɪ] n равномерность; уравновешенность.

equable ['ekwəbl] a ровный, равномерный; уравновешенный.

equal I ['iːkwəl] n равный, ровня; he has no ~ ему нет равного.

equal II a 1) равный, одинаковый; равносильный; 2) пригодный, способный; she is not ~ to the task она не справляется с этой работой.

equal III v равняться.

equality [iː'kwɔlɪtɪ] n равенство; равноправие; on an ~ with на равных условиях.

equalization [ˌiːkwəlaɪ'zeɪʃən] *n* ура́внивание, уравне́ние.

equalize ['iːkwəlaɪz] *v* ура́внивать (*with, to*); уравнове́шивать.

equally ['iːkwəlɪ] *adv* равно́, в ра́вной сте́пени.

equanimity [ˌiːkwə'nɪmɪtɪ] *n* хладнокро́вие; невозмути́мость.

equate [ɪ'kweɪt] *v* равня́ть; ура́внивать.

equation [ɪ'kweɪʃən] *n* 1) выра́внивание; 2) *мат.* уравне́ние; simple ~ уравне́ние пе́рвой сте́пени; biquadratic ~ биквадра́тное уравне́ние.

equator [ɪ'kweɪtə] *n* эква́тор.

equatorial [ˌekwə'tɔːrɪəl] *a* экваториа́льный.

equestrian I [ɪ'kwestrɪən] *n* вса́дник.

equestrian II *a* ко́нный.

equi- [iːkwɪ-, ɪkwɪ-] *pref* равно-; equivalent равноце́нный.

equiangular [ˌiːkwɪ'æŋgjulə] *a* *мат.* равноуго́льный.

equilateral ['iːkwɪ'lætərəl] *a* *мат.* равносторо́нний.

equilibrate [ˌiːkwɪ'laɪbreɪt] *v* уравнове́шивать(ся).

equilibration [ˌiːkwɪlaɪ'breɪʃən] *n* 1) уравнове́шивание; 2) равнове́сие.

equilibrist [iː'kwɪlɪbrɪst] *n* канатохо́дец; эквилибри́ст.

equilibrium [ˌiːkwɪ'lɪbrɪəm] *n* равнове́сие.

equinoctial I [ˌɪkwɪ'nɔkʃəl] *n* небе́сный эква́тор; равноде́нственная ли́ния.

equinoctial II *a* равноде́нственный.

equinox ['iːkwɪnɔks] *n* равноде́нствие.

equip [ɪ'kwɪp] *v* снаряжа́ть; оснаща́ть; экипирова́ть; снабжа́ть.

equipage ['ekwɪpɪdʒ] *n* 1) принадле́жности; обору́дование; 2) снаряже́ние, экипиро́вка; 3) экипа́ж, кома́нда.

equipment [ɪ'kwɪpmənt] *n* 1) обору́дование; 2) *воен.* снаряже́ние; 3) *ж.-д.* подвижно́й соста́в.

equitable ['ekwɪtəbl] *a* справедли́вый, беспристра́стный.

equity ['ekwɪtɪ] *n* справедли́вость, беспристра́стность.

equivalence [ɪ'kwɪvələns] *n* равноце́нность, равноси́льность, равнозна́чность, эквивале́нтность.

equivalency [ɪ'kwɪvələnsɪ] *см.* equivalence.

equivalent I [ɪ'kwɪvələnt] *n* эквивале́нт.

equivalent II *a* равноце́нный, равноси́льный, ра́вный по величине́; эквивале́нтный.

equivocal [ɪ'kwɪvəkl] *a* 1) двусмы́сленный; 2) сомни́тельный.

equivoke ['ekwɪvouk] *n* двусмы́сленность, экиво́к; каламбу́р.

equivoque ['ekwɪvouk] *см.* equivoke.

era ['ɪərə] *n* э́ра; эпо́ха.

eradiate [ɪ'reɪdɪeɪt] *v* излуча́ть.

eradiation [ɪˌreɪdɪ'eɪʃən] *n* излуче́ние.

eradicate [ɪ'rædɪkeɪt] *v* вырыва́ть с ко́рнем; *перен.* искореня́ть.

eradication [ɪˌrædɪ'keɪʃən] *n* искорене́ние.

erase [ɪ'reɪz] *v* 1) стира́ть, подчища́ть; 2) изгла́живать (*из памяти*).

eraser [ɪ'reɪzə] *n* ла́стик, рези́нка.

ere I [ɛə] *prep поэт.* до, пе́ред; ~ long вско́ре.

ere II *conj поэт.* пре́жде чем; скоре́е чем.

erect I [ɪ'rekt] *a* 1) прямо́й, вертика́льный; 2) стоя́чий, по́днятый; 3) *уст.* живо́й (*об уме*).

erect II *adv* пря́мо.

erect III *v* 1) стро́ить, осно́вывать; воздвига́ть; 2) создава́ть; 3) выпрямля́ть.

erection [ɪ'rekʃən] *n* 1) выпрямле́ние; 2) сооруже́ние, строе́ние; 3) *тех.* монта́ж, сбо́рка.

eremite ['erɪmaɪt] *n* отше́льник.

Erin ['ɪərɪn] *n поэт.* Ирла́ндия.

ermine ['əːmɪn] *n* горноста́й; .◊ to wear the ~ быть чле́ном верхо́вного суда́.

erode [ɪ'roud] *v* 1) разъеда́ть; разруша́ть (*тка́ни*); 2) *геол.* размыва́ть; выве́тривать.

erosion [ɪ'rouʒən] *n* эро́зия; *перен.* разложе́ние.

erosive [ɪ'rousɪv] *a* 1) разъеда́ющий; 2) вызыва́ющий эро́зию.

erotic [ɪ'rɔtɪk] *a* эроти́ческий.

err [əː] *v* 1) ошиба́ться, заблужда́ться; 2) греши́ть.

errand ['erənd] *n* поруче́ние; to send on an ~ посла́ть с поруче́нием; to run ~s, to go on ~s быть на посы́лках; ◊ a fool's ~ безнадёжное де́ло.

errand-boy ['erəndbɔɪ] *n* ма́льчик-рассы́льный.

errant ['erənt] *a* 1) стра́нствующий; 2) блужда́ющий; 3) заблу́дший.

errata [ɪ'reɪtə] *pl см.* erratum.

erratic [ɪ'rætɪk] *a* 1) неуве́ренный; неусто́йчивый; 2) сумасбро́дный, беспоря́дочный; 3) непра́вильный, оши́бочный.

erratum [ɪ'reɪtəm] *n* (*pl* errata) опеча́тка; опи́ска.

erring ['əːrɪŋ] *a* заблу́дший.

erroneous [ɪ'rounjəs] *a* оши́бочный.

error ['erə] *n* 1) оши́бка; заблужде́ние; to make (*или* to commit) an ~ сде́лать оши́бку; впасть в заблужде́ние; in ~ оши́бочно, по оши́бке; 2) уклоне́ние, отклоне́ние, погре́шность.

erudite ['eruːdaɪt] *a* учёный.

erudition [ˌeruː'dɪʃən] *n* эруди́ция, начи́танность; учёность.

erupt [ɪ'rʌpt] *v* 1) изверга́ться (*о вулка́не*); 2) прорезываться (*о зуба́х*).

eruption [ɪ'rʌpʃən] *n* 1) изверже́ние (*вулка́на*); 2) прорезывание (*зубо́в*); 3) взрыв (*сме́ха, гне́ва и т. п.*); 4) *мед.* сыпь, высыпа́ние.

eruptive [ɪ'rʌptɪv] *a* 1) *геол.* вулкани́ческий, изве́рженный; 2) *мед.* сопровожда́емый сы́пью.

erythrocyte [ɪ'rɪθrəsaɪt] *n* *физиол.* эритроци́т.

escalation [ˌeskə'leɪʃən] *n* эскала́ция, усиле́ние (*войны́, напряжённости*).

escalator ['eskəleɪtə] *n* эскала́тор, дви́жущаяся ле́стница.

escapade [ˌeskə'peɪd] *n* 1) весёлая проде́лка, эскапа́да; 2) побе́г (*из заключе́ния*).

escape I [ɪs'keɪp] *n* 1) бе́гство, побе́г; 2) избавле́ние, спасе́ние; to have a hairbreadth (*или* narrow) ~ едва́ избежа́ть опа́сности, быть на волосо́к от; ejection ~ катапульти́рование; 3) уте́чка (*воды́, га́за, электри́чества*).

escape II *v* 1) бежа́ть (*из заключе́ния*); 2) избежа́ть (*опа́сности*), спасти́сь; отде́латься; 3) ускользну́ть (*о смы́сле и т. п.*); 4) вырыва́ться (*о слова́х, кри́ке, сто́не*); 5) дава́ть уте́чку.

escarp [ɪs'kɑːp] *n* *воен.* эска́рп, круто́й отко́с.

eschew [ɪs'tʃuː] *v* избега́ть, возде́рживаться от.

escort[a] ['eskɔːt] *n* охра́на, конво́й, эско́рт.

escort[b] [ɪs'kɔːt] *v* конвои́ровать, эскорти́ровать, сопровожда́ть.

escutcheon [ɪs'kʌtʃən] *n* щит герба́; a blot on one's ~ *перен.* пятно́ на чьей-л. репута́ции.

Eskimo ['eskɪmou] *n* 1) эскимо́с; эскимо́ска; the ~es эскимо́сы; 2) *attr* эскимо́сский.

especial [ɪs'peʃəl] *a* осо́бенный, специа́льный.

especially [ɪs'peʃəlɪ] *adv* осо́бенно, специа́льно.

espionage [,espɪə'nɑ:ʒ] *n* шпиона́ж.

esplanade [,esplə'neɪd] *n* эсплана́да, площа́дка для прогу́лок.

espouse [ɪs'pauz] *v* 1) жени́ться (*на ком-л.*); 2) выдава́ть за́муж (*io*); 3) признава́ть, подде́рживать.

espy [ɪs'paɪ] *v* 1) уви́деть, зави́деть издалека́; 2) обнару́жить.

Esquimau ['eskɪmou] *см.* Eskimo.

esquire [ɪs'kwaɪə] *n* эсква́йр (*обычно сокращённо ставится после фамилии:* William Jones, Esq.).

essayᵃ ['eseɪ] *n* 1) о́черк; 2) попы́тка; 3) про́ба; о́пыт.

essayᵇ [e'seɪ] *v* 1) испы́тывать, про́бовать; 2) пыта́ться.

essayist ['eseɪɪst] *n* очерки́ст.

essence ['esns] *n* 1) су́щность, существо́; 2) существова́ние; 3) эссе́нция; 4) духи́.

essential I [ɪ'senʃəl] *n* 1) неотъе́млемость, су́щность; 2) *pl* предме́ты пе́рвой необходи́мости (*тж.* ~s of life).

essential II *a* 1) неотъе́млемый, суще́ственный, составля́ющий су́щность (*чего-л.*); 2) эфи́рный, летýчий.

essentiality [ɪ,senʃɪ'ælɪtɪ] *n* су́щность; суще́ственность.

essentially [ɪ'senʃəlɪ] *adv* по существу́.

establish [ɪs'tæblɪʃ] *v* 1) осно́вывать, учрежда́ть; устана́вливать; 2) устра́ивать; to be ~ed a) устра́иваться (*на рабо́те и т. п.*); б) укорени́ться (*об обы́чае и т. п.*); 3) дока́зывать (*факт и т. п.*).

established [ɪs'tæblɪʃt] *a* 1) устано́вленный; 2) упро́чившийся, укорени́вшийся; акклиматизи́ровавшийся; 3) официа́льный, госуда́рственный (*о це́ркви*).

establishment [ɪs'tæblɪʃmənt] *n* 1) установле́ние; основа́ние; введе́ние; 2) учрежде́ние (*госуда́рственное или обще́ственное*); 3) штат (*служащих*); 4) (дома́шнее) хозя́йство.

estate [ɪs'teɪt] *n* 1) име́ние; иму́щество; personal (real) ~ дви́жимое (недви́жимое) иму́щество; 2) сосло́вие; the fourth ~ *шутл.* «четвёртое сосло́вие», пре́сса; 3) *уст.* положе́ние (*в о́бществе*).

esteem I [ɪs'ti:m] *n* уваже́ние.

esteem II *v* 1) уважа́ть, почита́ть; 2) счита́ть, рассма́тривать, оце́нивать.

estimable ['estɪməbl] *a* досто́йный уваже́ния.

estimateᵃ ['estɪmɪt] *n* 1) оце́нка; 2) сме́та; the Estimates прое́кт (госуда́рственного) бюдже́та (*в А́нглии*).

estimateᵇ ['estɪmeɪt] *v* 1) цени́ть, оце́нивать; 2) составля́ть сме́ту; приблизи́тельно подсчи́тывать.

estimation [,estɪ'meɪʃən] *n* 1) оце́нка; мне́ние; in my ~ по моему́ мне́нию; 2) уваже́ние; to hold in ~ уважа́ть; 3) расчёт, подсчёт.

estimator ['estɪmeɪtə] *n* оце́нщик.

Estonian I [es'tounjən] *n* 1) эсто́нец; эсто́нка; the ~s эсто́нцы; 2) эсто́нский язы́к.

Estonian II *a* эсто́нский.

estrange [ɪs'treɪndʒ] *v* отдаля́ть; отстраня́ть, отчужда́ть.

estrangement [ɪs'treɪndʒmənt] *n* отчужде́ние; отчуждённость.

estuary ['estjuərɪ] *n* эстуа́рий; морско́й рука́в.

et cetera, etcetera [ɪt'setrə] *n* 1) и так да́лее, и тому́ подо́бное; 2) *pl* оста́тки; вся́кая вся́чина.

etch [etʃ] *v* гравирова́ть на мета́лле травле́нием.

etcher ['etʃə] *n* гравёр; офорти́ст.

etching ['etʃɪŋ] *n* 1) гравирова́ние на мета́лле травле́нием; 2) гравю́ра на мета́лле, офо́рт.

eternal [i:'tə:nl] *a* ве́чный; *разг. тж.* постоя́нный, неизме́нный.

eternalize [i:'tə:nəlaɪz] *v* увекове́чивать.

eternity [i:'tə:nɪtɪ] *n* ве́чность.

ether ['i:θə] *n* 1) *хим., физ.* эфи́р; 2) *поэт.* не́бо.

ethereal [i:'θɪərɪəl] *a* эфи́рный.

ethereality [i:,θɪərɪ'ælɪtɪ] *n* эфи́рность, лёгкость.

ethic(al) ['eθɪk(əl)] *a* эти́чный; эти́ческий, мора́льный.

ethics ['eθɪks] *n* э́тика, мора́ль.

Ethiopian I [,i:θɪ'oupjən] *n* эфио́п; эфио́пка; the ~s эфио́пы.

Ethiopian II *a* эфио́пский.

ethnic(al) ['eθnɪk(əl)] *a* 1) этни́ческий; 2) язы́ческий.

ethnographic(al) [,eθnə'græfɪk(əl)] *a* этнографи́ческий.

ethnography [eθ'nɔgrəfɪ] *n* этногра́фия.

ethnology [eθ'nɔlədʒɪ] *n* этноло́гия.

etiquette [,etɪ'ket] *n* 1) этике́т; 2) (профессиона́льная) э́тика.

etymologic(al) [,etɪmə'lɔdʒɪk(əl)] *a* этимологи́ческий.

etymology [,etɪ'mɔlədʒɪ] *n* этимоло́гия.

eucalyptus [,ju:kə'lɪptəs] *n* (*pl тж.* eucalypti [,ju:kə'lɪptaɪ]) *бот.* эвкали́пт.

eulogy ['ju:lədʒɪ] *n* хвале́бная речь; панеги́рик.

eunuch ['ju:nək] *n* е́внух.

euphemism ['ju:fɪmɪzəm] *n стил.* эвфеми́зм.

euphonic(al) [ju:'fɔnɪk(əl)] *a* благозву́чный.

euphony ['ju:fənɪ] *n* благозву́чие.

euphuism ['ju:fju:ɪzəm] *n* эвфуи́зм, напы́щенный стиль.

eureka [juə'ri:kə] *int* э́врика!

European I [,juərə'pi:ən] *n* европе́ец; the ~s европе́йцы.

European II *a* европе́йский.

evacuate [ɪ'vækjueɪt] *v* 1) эвакуи́ровать; 2) опоро́жнять; очища́ть (*желу́док*); 3) *тех.* выка́чивать, выса́сывать.

evacuation [ɪ,vækju'eɪʃən] *n* 1) эвакуа́ция; 2) испражне́ние; очище́ние (*желу́дка*).

evacuee [ɪ,vækju'i:] *n* эвакуи́рованный; эвакуи́руемый.

evade [ɪ'veɪd] *v* 1) избега́ть; уклоня́ться (*от отве́та, исполне́ния обя́занностей*); 2) ускольза́ть; 3) не поддава́ться (*уси́лиям, убежде́нию*); 4) обходи́ть (*зако́н, вопро́с*).

evaluate [ɪ'væljueɪt] *v* 1) оце́нивать; выража́ть в ци́фрах.

evaluation [ɪ,vælju'eɪʃən] *n* оце́нка.

evanescent [,i:və'nesnt] *a* 1) мимолётный; 2) *мат.* бесконе́чно ма́лый.

evangelical [,i:væn'dʒelɪkəl] *a* 1) ева́нгельский; 2) евангели́ческий.

evangelist [ɪ'vændʒɪlɪst] *n* евангели́ст.

evaporate [ɪ'væpəreɪt] *v* 1) испаря́ться; *перен. разг.* а) улету́чиваться, исчеза́ть; б) умере́ть; 2) выпа́ривать; обезво́живать.

evaporation [ɪ,væpə'reɪʃən] *n* 1) испаре́ние; 2) парообразова́ние; 3) выпа́ривание; обезво́живание.

evasion [ɪ'veɪʒən] *n* 1) уклоне́ние; 2) уве́ртка.

evasive [ɪ'veɪsɪv] *a* 1) укло́нчивый; 2) неулови́мый.

eve [iːv] *n* 1) кану́н; on the ~ накану́не; Christmas ~ рожде́ственский соче́льник; 2) *поэт.* ве́чер.

even¹ I ['iːvən] *a* 1) ро́вный, гла́дкий; 2) на одно́м у́ровне, вро́вень (*with*); 3) одина́ковый, ра́вный; схо́дный; тако́й же; 4) уравнове́шенный, споко́йный (*о характере*); 5) чётный; ◊ to be (*или* to get) ~ with smb. свести́ счёты с кем-л.

even¹ II *v* 1) равня́ть; ура́внивать (*тж.* to ~ up); 2) выра́внивать, сгла́живать; ◊ to ~ up on *амер.* отплати́ть, отомсти́ть, расквита́ться.

even¹ III *adv* 1) да́же; ~ if, ~ though да́же е́сли, хотя́ бы и; 2) *уст.* как раз, то́чно.

even² *n поэт.* ве́чер.

even-handed ['iːvən'hændɪd] *a* беспристра́стный.

evening ['iːvnɪŋ] *n* 1) ве́чер; *перен.* зака́т жи́зни; 2) ве́чер, вечери́нка; 3) *attr* вече́рний.

even-minded ['iːvən'maɪndɪd] *a* споко́йный, уравнове́шенный.

event [ɪ'vent] *n* 1) слу́чай; собы́тие; in the ~ of в слу́чае, на слу́чай (*чего-л.*); in either ~, at all ~s во вся́ком слу́чае; in that ~ в э́том слу́чае; 2) исхо́д, результа́т; 3) вид спо́рта; но́мер в програ́мме состяза́ний.

eventful [ɪ'ventful] *a* по́лный собы́тий, бога́тый собы́тиями.

eventless [ɪ'ventlɪs] *a* бе́дный собы́тиями.

eventual [ɪ'ventʃuəl] *a* 1) возмо́жный; 2) коне́чный.

eventuality [ɪ,ventʃu'ælɪtɪ] *n* возмо́жность; возмо́жный слу́чай.

eventually [ɪ'ventʃuəlɪ] *adv* в конце́ концо́в, в коне́чном ито́ге.

eventuate [ɪ'ventʃueɪt] *v* 1) разреша́ться, конча́ться (*чем-л.* — *in*); 2) случа́ться, возника́ть.

ever ['evə] *adv* 1) когда́-либо; ~ and anon *уст.* вре́мя от вре́мени; hardly ~ ре́дко; почти́ никогда́; 2) всегда́; for ~ навсегда́; ~ after, ~ since с тех пор (как); Yours ~ пре́данный вам, всегда́ ваш (*в конце письма*); 3) *употребляется для усиле́ния вопроса*: who ~ can it be? да кто же э́то (мо́жет быть)?; why ~ didn't you say so? (да) почему́ же вы так не сказа́ли?; 4) то́лько (*в сравни́тельных предложе́ниях* as... as ~): be as quick as ~ you can поторопи́тесь как то́лько мо́жете; 5): ~ so о́чень, намно́го; it is ~ so much easier э́то гора́здо ле́гче; thank you ~ so much большо́е вам спаси́бо; 6): ~ such *разг.* о́чень; he's ~ such a good fellow он о́чень хоро́ший па́рень.

everglade ['evəgleɪd] *n амер.* боло́тистая ме́стность, места́ми поро́сшая высо́кой траво́й (*особ.* the Everglades в *Ю́жной Флори́де*).

evergreen I ['evəgriːn] *n* вечнозелёное расте́ние.

evergreen II *a* вечнозелёный.

ever-increasing ['evərɪn'kriːsɪŋ] *a* (всё) возраста́ющий.

everlasting I [,evə'lɑːstɪŋ] *n* 1) ве́чность; 2) *бот.*

имморте́ль, бессме́ртник; 3) про́чная шерстяна́я ткань.

everlasting II *a* 1) ве́чный; 2) долгове́чный; 3) постоя́нный, повторя́ющийся.

evermore ['evə'mɔː] *adv* наве́ки, навсегда́.

every ['evrɪ] *a* ка́ждый; ~ now and again, now and then вре́мя от вре́мени; ~ one (of them) ка́ждый (из них); все; ~ so often времена́ми, нерегуля́рно; ~ other a) череду́ющийся; б) все остальны́е; ~ other day че́рез день.

everybody ['evrɪbɒdɪ] *n* все; ка́ждый, вся́кий (челове́к).

everyday ['evrɪdeɪ] *a* ежедне́вный; обы́чный; повседне́вный.

everyone ['evrɪwʌn] *n* все; ка́ждый, вся́кий (челове́к).

everything ['evrɪθɪŋ] *n* всё.

everyway ['evrɪweɪ] *adv* 1) во всех направле́ниях; 2) во всех отноше́ниях.

everywhere ['evrɪwɛə] *adv* (по)всю́ду, везде́.

evict [iː'vɪkt] *v* 1) выселя́ть; 2) оття́гать (по суду́).

eviction [iː'vɪkʃən] *n* 1) выселе́ние; 2) лише́ние иму́щества по суду́.

evidence I ['evɪdəns] *n* 1) очеви́дность; in ~ заме́тный, на виду́; име́ющийся налицо́ (см. *тж.* 3); 2) основа́ние, доказа́тельство, свиде́тельство; direct ~ прямы́е ули́ки; to give (*или* to bear) ~ of smth. свиде́тельствовать, говори́ть о чём-л. (см. *тж.*-3); 3) *юр.* ули́ка; свиде́тельское показа́ние; circumstantial ~ ко́свенные ули́ки; cumulative ~ совоку́пность ули́к; presumptive ~ показа́ния, осно́ванные на дога́дках; to give ~ дава́ть показа́ния (см. *тж.* 2); to call in ~ вызыва́ть в суд (*в ка́честве свиде́теля*); to turn King's (*или* Queen's) ~ вы́дать соуча́стников; in ~ при́нятый в ка́честве доказа́тельства (см. *тж.* 1).

evidence II *v* служи́ть доказа́тельством, дока́зывать; свиде́тельствовать.

evident ['evɪdənt] *a* я́вный, очеви́дный, я́сный.

evidential [,evɪ'denʃəl] *a* осно́ванный на очеви́дности; очеви́дный, я́вный.

evil I ['iːvl] *n* 1) зло; 2) бе́дствие, несча́стье; 3) грех.

evil II *a* 1) злой, зловре́дный; 2) вре́дный; па́губный; 3) дурно́й; недо́брый (*о часе*); злонаме́ренный.

evil-doer ['iːvl'duːə] *n* 1) престу́пник; злоде́й; 2) гре́шник.

evil-minded ['iːvl'maɪndɪd] *a* злой, зло́бный.

evince [ɪ'vɪns] *v* пока́зывать, выка́зывать; проявля́ть.

evoke [ɪ'vouk] *v* 1) вызыва́ть, пробужда́ть (*чу́вства и т. п.*); 2) *юр.* затре́бовать (де́ло) в вы́сшую инста́нцию; 3) вызыва́ть (*духов*).

evolution [,iːvə'luːʃən] *n* 1) разви́тие, эволю́ция; 2) *мат.* извлече́ние ко́рня; 3) *воен., мор.* манёвр, перестрое́ние.

evolutional [,iːvə'luːʃənl] *см.* evolutionary.

evolutionary [,iːvə'luːʃnərɪ] *a* эволюцио́нный.

evolutionism [,iːvə'luːʃənɪzəm] *n* тео́рия эволю́ции.

evolve [ɪ'vɒlv] *v* 1) развёртывать; развива́ть; 2) развива́ться, эволюциони́ровать; 3) выделя́ть (*теплоту́, га́зы*); издава́ть (*за́пах*).

ewe [juː] *n* овца́.

ewer ['juːə] *n* кувши́н.

ex- [eks-, ıks-] *pref со значением*: 1) *удаления из чего-л., нахождения вне чего-л.*: to extract вырывать; exterritorial экстерриториальный; 2) *указания на прежнее звание, положение* экс-, *бывший*; ex-president бывший президент.

exacerbate [eks'æsəːbeıt] *v* 1) обострять (*болезнь и т. п.*); 2) раздражать (*человека*).

exact I [ıg'zækt] *a* точный.

exact II *v* 1) (настоятельно) требовать; вымогать; 2) взыскивать (*from, of*).

exacting [ıg'zæktıŋ] *a* 1) требовательный; 2) чрезмерный, изнуряющий (*о работе и т. п.*).

exaction [ıg'zækʃən] *n* 1) (настоятельное) требование; 2) вымогательство.

exactitude [ıg'zæktıtjuːd] *n* точность.

exactly [ıg'zæktlı] *adv* 1) точно, как раз; 2) именно, совершенно верно (*в ответе*).

exactor [ıg'zæktə] *n* 1) требовательный человек; 2) истец; 3) вымогатель.

exaggerate [ıg'zædʒəreıt] *v* 1) преувеличивать; 2) чрезмерно подчёркивать.

exaggerated [ıg'zædʒəreıtıd] *a* 1) преувеличенный; 2) *мед.* расширенный, увеличенный.

exaggeration [ıg,zædʒə'reıʃən] *n* преувеличение.

exaggerative [ıg'zædʒərətıv] *a* преувеличивающий.

exalt [ıg'zɔːlt] *v* 1) возносить; возвеличивать; 2) превозносить; 3) повышать (*в должности и т. п.*); 4) сгущать, усиливать; 5) возбуждать (*воображение*).

exaltation [,egzɔːl'teıʃən] *n* 1) возвышение, возвеличивание; 2) восторг; экзальтация.

exam [ıg'zæm] *сокр. разг. см.* examination 2).

examinant [ıg'zæmınənt] *n* экзаменатор.

examination [ıg,zæmı'neıʃən] *n* 1) осмотр, освидетельствование; исследование; post-mortem ~ вскрытие (*трупа*); 2) экзамен; competitive ~ конкурсный экзамен; preliminary ~ вступительный экзамен; to take an ~, to go in for an ~ держать экзамен; to pass one's ~ выдержать экзамен; to sit for an ~ сдавать экзамен; to fail in an ~ провалиться на экзамене; 3) допрос.

examinational [ıg,zæmı'neıʃənl] *a* экзаменационный.

examination-paper [ıg,zæmı'neıʃən'peıpə] *n* 1) опросный лист; 2) экзаменационная работа.

examine [ıg'zæmın] *v* 1) рассматривать; 2) осматривать, исследовать; (о)свидетельствовать; 3) экзаменовать; 4) допрашивать, опрашивать.

examinee [ıg,zæmı'niː] *n* экзаменующийся.

examiner [ıg'zæmınə] *n* 1) экзаменующий; экзаменатор; 2) *амер.* ревизор.

example [ıg'zɑːmpl] *n* пример; for ~ например; to give (*или* to set) an ~ показывать, подавать пример; beyond ~, without ~ без прецедента; to make an ~ of наказать в пример другим.

exasperate [ıg'zɑːspəreıt] *v* 1) раздражать, выводить из себя; 2) возбуждать; побуждать (*к чему-л.*); 3) усиливать (*боль и т. п.*).

exasperating [ıg'zɑːspəreıtıŋ] *a* раздражающий, изводящий.

exasperation [ıg,zɑːspə'reıʃən] *n* раздражение.

excavate ['ekskəveıt] *v* 1) выкапывать, вырывать; 2) копать, рыть; 3) *археол.* раскапывать; вести раскопки.

excavation [,ekskə'veıʃən] *n* 1) выкапывание;

2) выдалбливание; 3) выемка грунта, экскавация; 4) вырытая яма, котлован; 5) *археол.* раскопки.

excavator ['ekskəveıtə] *n* 1) экскаватор; walking ~ шагающий экскаватор; 2) землекоп; 3) археолог.

exceed [ık'siːd] *v* 1) превышать; 2) превосходить (*чем-л., в чём-л.— in*); 3) быть невоздержанным.

exceeding [ık'siːdıŋ] *a* огромный, чрезвычайный.

exceedingly [ık'siːdıŋlı] *adv* чрезвычайно, очень.

excel [ık'sel] *v* превосходить (*in, at*); выделяться (*as, at*).

excellence ['eksələns] *n* 1) превосходство; 2) выдающееся качество, мастерство.

excellency ['eksələnsı] *n* превосходительство.

excellent ['eksələnt] *a* превосходный, великолепный, отличный.

except I [ık'sept] *v* 1) исключать; 2) возражать (*against*).

except II *prep* исключая, за исключением, кроме; ~ for если бы не.

excepting [ık'septıŋ] *prep* за исключением, исключая, кроме.

exception [ık'sepʃən] *n* 1) исключение; with the ~ of за исключением; without ~ без исключения; 2) :to take ~ at обижаться на; to take ~ to возражать.

exceptionable [ık'sepʃnəbl] *a* вызывающий возражения; предосудительный.

exceptional [ık'sepʃənl] *a* исключительный, необычный.

exceptive [ık'septıv] *a* 1) исключительный, составляющий исключение; 2) придирчивый.

excerptᵃ ['eksəːpt] *n* выдержка, отрывок.

excerptᵇ [ek'səːpt] *v* делать выдержки, подбирать цитаты.

excerption [ek'səːpʃən] *n* цитата, выдержка.

excess [ık'ses] *n* 1) избыток; излишек; in ~ of больше чем, сверх (*чего-л.*); 2) невоздержанность, излишество; to ~, in ~ до излишества; 3) *pl* эксцесс; выходка; 4) *attr* избыточный, (из)лишний.

excessive [ık'sesıv] *a* чрезмерный; излишний.

exchange I [ıks'tʃeındʒ] *n* 1) обмен; in ~ (for) взамен, в обмен; 2) размен; free ~ свободная валюта; 3) вексельные операции, оплата векселями; 4) биржа; Labour Exchange биржа труда; Stock Exchange фондовая биржа; 5) центральная телефонная станция; 6) *attr* меновой.

exchange II *v* 1) обменивать(ся); 2) разменивать.

exchangeable [ıks'tʃeındʒəbl] *a* годный для обмена.

exchequer [ıks'tʃekə] *n* 1) казначейство, казна; 2) *разг.* средства, финансы.

excise[1] [ek'saız] *v* отрезать; вырезать.

excise[2] I *n* акциз (*тж.* ~ duty).

excise[2] II *v* взимать, налагать акцизный сбор.

excitable [ık'saıtəbl] *a* возбудимый.

excitant I ['eksıtənt] *n* возбуждающее средство.

excitant II *a* возбуждающий.

excitation [,eksı'teıʃən] *n* возбуждение.

excite [ık'saıt] *v* 1) возбуждать; волновать; 2) побуждать; 3) *эл.* возбудить (*ток*).

excitement [ık'saıtmənt] *n* возбуждение, волнение.

exclaim [ıks'kleım] *v* вскрикнуть; воскликнуть;

☐ to ~ **against** ропта́ть, гро́мко обвиня́ть, протестова́ть.

exclamation [ˌekskləˈmeɪʃən] *n* восклица́ние.

exclamatory [eksˈklæmətərɪ] *a* восклица́тельный.

exclude [ɪksˈkluːd] *v* 1) исключа́ть; не допуска́ть (*возможности и т. п.*).

exclusion [ɪksˈkluːʒən] *n* исключе́ние; to the ~ of за исключе́нием.

exclusive [ɪksˈkluːsɪv] *a* 1) исключи́тельный; осо́бый; ~ of исключа́я, не счита́я; 2) разбо́рчивый, предъявля́ющий стро́гие тре́бования; 3) недосту́пный; за́мкнутый; с ограни́ченным до́ступом (*о клу́бе*); 4) *амер.* первокла́ссный.

exclusively [ɪksˈkluːsɪvlɪ] *adv* исключи́тельно, исключа́я.

excrescence [ɪksˈkresns] *n* разраста́ние; наро́ст, ши́шка.

excrete [eksˈkriːt] *v* выделя́ть, изверга́ть.

excretion [eksˈkriːʃən] *n* физиол. выделе́ние.

excretive [eksˈkriːtɪv] *a* спосо́бствующий выделе́нию.

exculpate [ˈekskʌlpeɪt] *v* опра́вдывать, реабили́тировать.

exculpatory [eksˈkʌlpətərɪ] *a* опра́вдывающий; оправда́тельный.

excursion [ɪksˈkəːʃən] *n* 1) экску́рсия; пое́здка; прогу́лка; 2) *attr* экскурсио́нный.

excursionist [ɪksˈkəːʃnɪst] *n* 1) экскурса́нт; 2) тури́ст.

excursive [eksˈkəːsɪv] *a* 1) отклоня́ющийся, блужда́ющий; 2) беспоря́дочный (*о чтении*).

excursus [eksˈkəːsəs] *n* отступле́ние (*от темы, от сути*); э́кскурс.

excusable [ɪksˈkjuːzəbl] *a* извини́тельный, прости́тельный.

excusatory [ɪksˈkjuːzətərɪ] *a* извини́тельный; оправда́тельный.

excuse[a] [ɪksˈkjuːs] *n* 1) извине́ние; оправда́ние; in ~ of в оправда́ние чего́-л.; without ~ без (доста́точных) основа́ний; sorry ~ неуда́чное оправда́ние; 2) отгово́рка; предло́г; lame (*или* poor, thin) ~ сла́бая, неуда́чная отгово́рка; specious ~ благови́дный предло́г.

excuse[b] [ɪksˈkjuːz] *v* 1) извиня́ть, проща́ть; ~ me! извини́те!, прости́те!; 2) опра́вдывать; to ~ oneself извиня́ться, проси́ть проще́ния; 3) освобожда́ть (*от службы, обязанностей, налогов; from*).

exeat [ˈeksɪæt] *n* разреше́ние на кратковре́менный о́тпуск (*в университете, монастыре и т. п.*).

execrable [ˈeksɪkrəbl] *a* отврати́тельный.

execrate [ˈeksɪkreɪt] *v* 1) пита́ть отвраще́ние; 2) призыва́ть прокля́тия, проклина́ть.

executant [ɪgˈzekjutənt] *n* исполни́тель.

execute [ˈeksɪkjuːt] *v* 1) исполня́ть; выполня́ть; 2) приводи́ть в исполне́ние (*приговор и т. п.*); 3) казни́ть; 4) оформля́ть (*документ*).

execution [ˌeksɪˈkjuːʃən] *n* 1) выполне́ние; to carry into ~, to put in ~ осуществля́ть, выполня́ть; 2) исполне́ние; *муз. тж.* мастерство́ исполне́ния; 3) результа́т, де́йствие (*особ. разруши́тельное*); разруше́ние; опустоше́ние; 4) казнь; 5) *юр.* выполне́ние форма́льностей; оформле́ние (*документа*).

executioner [ˌeksɪˈkjuːnə] *n* пала́ч.

executive I [ɪgˈzekjutɪv] *n* 1) исполни́тельная власть; исполни́тельный о́рган; (Chief) Executive

а) президе́нт США; б) губерна́тор шта́та; 2) руководи́тель, администра́тор; 3) *амер.* нача́льник шта́ба; помо́щник команди́ра; ста́рший (*на батаре́е*).

executive II *a* 1) исполни́тельный; 2) администра́торский, организацио́нный.

executor [ɪgˈzekjutə] *n* 1) душеприка́зчик; 2) суде́бный исполни́тель.

exemplar [ɪgˈzemplə] *n* 1) образе́ц; 2) тип, экземпля́р.

exemplary [ɪgˈzemplərɪ] *a* образцо́вый, приме́рный.

exemplify [ɪgˈzemplɪfaɪ] *v* 1) служи́ть приме́ром; 2) приводи́ть приме́р; 3) снима́ть и заверя́ть ко́пию.

exempt I [ɪgˈzempt] *a* свобо́дный, освобождённый (*от налогов и т. п.; from*).

exempt II *v* освобожда́ть.

exemption [ɪgˈzempʃən] *n* освобожде́ние.

exercise I [ˈeksəsaɪz] *n* 1) упражне́ние; заня́тие; 2) трениро́вка; моцио́н; 3) проявле́ние (*терпения и т. п.*); 4) осуществле́ние; 5) *pl* обря́ды, ритуа́л; 6) *pl амер.* пра́зднества, торжества́; 7) *attr* уче́бный, трениро́вочный.

exercise II *v* 1) упражня́ть(ся); 2) трениро́вать(ся); 3) проявля́ть (*терпение, способности*); соблюда́ть (*осторожность*); 4) осуществля́ть; испо́льзовать; 5) *pass* быть обеспоко́енным (*чем-л. — about*).

exert [ɪgˈzəːt] *v* 1) ока́зывать (*действие, влияние и т. п.*); 2) прилага́ть, напряга́ть (*силы*); to ~ oneself стара́ться, прилага́ть уси́лия, напряга́ть си́лы.

exertion [ɪgˈzəːʃən] *n* стара́ние, уси́лие, напряже́ние.

exeunt [ˈeksɪʌnt] *v* «ухо́дят» (*ремарка в пьесе*).

exfoliate [eksˈfoulɪeɪt] *v* шелуши́ться, отсла́иваться.

exhalation [ˌekshəˈleɪʃən] *n* 1) выдыха́ние; вы́дох; 2) испаре́ние; пар, тума́н; 3) взрыв (*гнева и т. п.*).

exhale [eksˈheɪl] *v* 1) выдыха́ть; 2) выделя́ть (*пар*); 3) выделя́ться (*о парах*), испаря́ться; 4) дать вы́ход (*гневу и т. п.*).

exhaust I [ɪgˈzɔːst] *n* тех. 1) вы́пуск; вы́хлоп; 2) *attr* выпускно́й; выхлопно́й.

exhaust II *v* 1) изнуря́ть, истоща́ть; исче́рпывать; выма́тывать (*силы*); 2) опустоша́ть, выче́рпывать; 3) выса́сывать, выка́чивать (*воздух*); выпуска́ть (*пар*).

exhausted [ɪgˈzɔːstɪd] *a* истощённый; изнурённый, изму́ченный.

exhausting [ɪgˈzɔːstɪŋ] *a* утоми́тельный; изнури́тельный.

exhaustion [ɪgˈzɔːstʃən] *n* 1) истоще́ние; изнуре́ние; 2) дистрофи́я; 3) вытя́гивание, выса́сывание; 4) разреже́ние (*воздуха*).

exhaustive [ɪgˈzɔːstɪv] *a* 1) исче́рпывающий; 2) истоща́ющий.

exhibit I [ɪgˈzɪbɪt] *n* 1) экспона́т; 2) вы́ставка; экспози́ция; пока́з; 3) *юр.* веще́ственное доказа́тельство.

exhibit II *v* 1) проявля́ть, пока́зывать; 2) выставля́ть, экспони́ровать.

exhibition [ˌeksɪˈbɪʃən] *n* 1) вы́ставка; 2) проявле́ние; пока́з; to make an ~ of oneself показывать себя с невыгодной стороны; делать из себя посмешище; 3) стипендия.

exhibitioner [,eksɪ'bɪʃnə] *n* стипендиат.

exhibitor [ɪg'zɪbɪtə] *n* экспонент.

exhilarate [ɪg'zɪləreɪt] *v* оживлять; веселить.

exhilarated [ɪg'zɪləreɪtɪd] *a* 1) весёлый; 2) подвыпивший, навеселе.

exhilaration [ɪg,zɪlə'reɪʃən] *n* 1) весёлость; 2) увеселение.

exhort [ɪg'zɔt] *v* увещевать, убеждать; призывать (*к* — *to*).

exhortation [,egzɔ'teɪʃən] *n* 1) увещевание; призыв; 2) проповедь.

exhumation [,ekshju:'meɪʃən] *n* выкапывание трупа, эксгумация.

exigence ['eksɪdʒəns] *n* острая необходимость, крайность.

exigency ['eksɪdʒənsɪ] *см.* exigence.

exigent ['eksɪdʒənt] *a* 1) спешный, срочный; безотлагательный; 2) требовательный.

exigible ['eksɪdʒɪbl] *a* подлежащий взысканию.

exile I ['eksaɪl] *n* 1) изгнание; ссылка; 2) изгнанник; ссыльный.

exile II *v* изгонять; ссылать.

exist [ɪg'zɪst] *v* быть, существовать; жить; находиться.

existence [ɪg'zɪstəns] *n* 1) существование; жизнь; 2) наличие.

existent [ɪg'zɪstənt] *a* 1) существующий; 2) наличный.

existentialism [,ekzɪ'stenʃəlɪzəm] *n* экзистенциализм.

exit I ['eksɪt] *n* 1) выход; 2) уход (*актёра со сцены*); *перен.* смерть; to make one's ~ а) сойти со сцены; б) умереть.

exit II *v* «уходит» (*ремарка в пьесе*).

exodus ['eksədəs] *n* массовый уход, бегство.

exonerate [ɪg'zɔnəreɪt] *v* снять бремя вины, оправдать, реабилитировать.

exoneration [ɪg,zɔnə'reɪʃən] *n* оправдание, реабилитация.

exorbitant [ɪg'zɔbɪtənt] *a* непомерный, чрезмерный.

exosphere ['eksəsfɪə] *n* экзосфера.

exoteric [,eksou'terɪk] *a* (обще)доступный, понятный.

exotic I [eg'zɔtɪk] *n* экзотическое растение (*тж. перен.*).

exotic II *a* экзотический; иноземный.

expand [ɪks'pænd] *v* 1) расширять(ся); увеличивать(ся) (*в объёме*); 2) развивать (*мысль*); 3) *мат.* раскрывать (*формулу*); 4) развивать(ся) (*into*); 5) раскрываться, распускаться (*о почках, бутонах*).

expanse [ɪks'pæns] *n* 1) пространство; протяжение; гладь (*водная*); 2) экспансия; расширение, распространение.

expansibility [ɪks,pænsə'bɪlɪtɪ] *n* растяжимость, расширение.

expansible [ɪks'pænsəbl] *a* растяжимый.

expansion [ɪks'pænʃən] *n* 1) экспансия; 2) расширение, распространение; 3) пространство, протяжение.

expansive [ɪks'pænsɪv] *a* 1) экспансивный, несдержанный; 2) расширяющийся; 3) обширный.

expatriate [eks'pætrɪeɪt] *v* изгонять из отечества; to ~ oneself эмигрировать.

expect [ɪks'pekt] *v* 1) ожидать; 2) рассчитывать, надеяться; 3) *разг.* (пред)полагать.

expectancy [ɪks'pektənsɪ] *n* 1) ожидание; предвкушение; надежда; 2) вероятность (*of*).

expectant [ɪks'pektənt] *a* 1) ожидающий; рассчитывающий (*на что-л.*); 2) выжидательный.

expectation [,ekspek'teɪʃən] *n* 1) ожидание; надежда; beyond ~ сверх ожидания; contrary to ~(s), against ~(s) против ожидания; to answer (*или* to meet, to come up to) one's ~(s) оправдывать надежды, ожидания; 2) *pl* виды на будущее; 3) вероятность.

expectorant I [eks'pektərənt] *n мед.* отхаркивающее средство.

expectorant II *a мед.* отхаркивающий.

expectorate [eks'pektəreɪt] *v* отхаркивать, откашливать.

expedience [ɪks'piːdjəns] *n* целесообразность.

expediency [ɪks'piːdjənsɪ] *см.* expedience.

expedient I [ɪks'piːdjənt] *n* уловка, приём.

expedient II *a* 1) целесообразный; уместный; 2) удобный, выгодный.

expedition [,ekspɪ'dɪʃən] *n* 1) экспедиция; 2) быстрота, поспешность.

expeditionary [,ekspɪ'dɪʃnərɪ] *a* экспедиционный.

expeditious [,ekspɪ'dɪʃəs] *a* быстрый, скорый.

expel [ɪks'pel] *v* 1) выгонять; исключать; 2) выталкивать, выбрасывать.

expend [ɪks'pend] *v* тратить, расходовать.

expenditure [ɪks'pendɪtʃə] *n* 1) расход, трата; 2) расходы.

expense [ɪks'pens] *n* 1) трата; *pl* расходы; heavy ~s большие расходы; at one's ~ за чей-л. счёт; 2) цена, стоимость; at the ~ of his life (health) ценою его жизни (здоровья).

expensive [ɪks'pensɪv] *a* дорогой.

experience I [ɪks'pɪərɪəns] *n* 1) опыт; to know by ~ знать по опыту; to learn by ~ познать на собственном (горьком) опыте; to gather ~ накапливать опыт; to share ~ with smb. делиться опытом с кем-л.; 2) случай; приключение; переживание; a strange (an unpleasant) ~ странный (неприятный) случай.

experience II *v* испытать; узнать по опыту.

experienced [ɪks'pɪərɪənst] *a* опытный.

experiment[a] [ɪks'perɪmənt] *n* опыт, эксперимент.

experiment[b] [ɪks'perɪment] *v* производить опыты, экспериментировать (*on, with*).

experimental [eks,perɪ'mentl] *a* экспериментальный, пробный; подопытный.

experimentalize [eks,perɪ'mentəlaɪz] *v* производить опыты, экспериментировать.

experimentation [eks,perɪmen'teɪʃən] *n* проведение опытов, экспериментирование.

expert I ['ekspət] *n* знаток, специалист, эксперт.

expert II *a* опытный; искусный; квалифицированный.

expiate ['ekspɪeɪt] *v* искупать (*вину*).

expiration [,ekspaɪə'reɪʃən] *n* 1) выдыхание; выдох; 2) окончание; истечение (*срока*).

expiratory [ɪks'paɪərətərɪ] *a* выдыхательный.

expire [ɪks'paɪə] *v* 1) выдыхать; 2) оканчиваться; истекать (*о сроке*); 3) угасать; умирать.

explain [ıks'pleın] *v* объяснять; to ~ oneself объясниться, представить объяснения; □ to ~ away оправдываться.

explanation [ˌekspləˈneıʃən] *n* 1) объяснение; 2) толкование.

explanatory [ıks'plænətərı] *a* объяснительный.

explicable ['eksplıkəbl] *a* объяснимый.

explicate ['eksplıkeıt] *v* развивать (*мысль*); толковать, объяснять.

explicative [eks'plıkətıv] *a* объяснительный.

explicatory [eks'plıkətərı] *см.* explicative.

explicit [ıks'plısıt] *a* 1) ясный, точный; подробный; 2) искренний (*о человеке*).

explode [ıks'ploud] *v* 1) взрывать(ся); *перен.* разражаться (*гневом и т. п.*); 2) подрывать (*устои, веру и т. п.*).

exploit[a] ['eksploıt] *n* подвиг.

exploit[b] [ıks'ploıt] *v* 1) эксплуатировать; использовать (*в своих интересах*); 2) разрабатывать (*копи, месторождения*).

exploitation [ˌeksploıˈteıʃən] *n* 1) эксплуатация; 2) разработка месторождений.

exploiter [ıks'ploıtə] *n* эксплуататор.

exploration [ˌeksplɔːˈreıʃən] *n* исследование; space ~ освоение космоса.

explorative [eks'plɔːrətıv] *a* исследовательский; исследующий.

exploratory [eks'plɔːrətərı] *см.* explorative.

explore [ıks'plɔː] *v* 1) исследовать; 2) *геол., воен.* разведывать.

explorer [ıks'plɔːrə] *n* 1) исследователь; 2) *мед.* зонд.

explosion [ıks'plouʒən] *n* взрыв, вспышка (*тж. перен.*).

explosive I [ıks'plousıv] *n* 1) взрывчатое вещество; 2) *фон.* взрывной согласный.

explosive II *a* 1) взрывчатый; *перен.* вспыльчивый; 2) *фон.* взрывной.

exponent [eks'pounənt] *n* 1) истолкователь; 2) исполнитель (*муз. произведения*); 3) представитель, тип, образец; 4) *мат.* показатель степени.

export[a] ['ekspɔːt] *n* 1) экспорт; 2) *attr* экспортный.

export[b] [eks'pɔːt] *v* экспортировать, вывозить.

exportation [ˌekspɔːˈteıʃən] *n* вывоз, экспортирование.

expose [ıks'pouz] *v* 1) выставлять, подвергать действию (*солнца, света, непогоды и т. п.*); to be ~d to rain находиться под дождём; 2) выставлять (*напоказ, на продажу*); 3) ~d to the East *etc* обращённый на восток *и т. п.*; 4) подвергать (*опасности, случайностям и т. п.*); бросать (*ребёнка*) на произвол судьбы; 5) открывать (*секрет*); 6) разоблачать; 7) *фото* делать выдержку.

exposition [ˌekspəˈzıʃən] *n* 1) описание; объяснение, толкование; 2) выставка; 3) *фото* экспозиция, выдержка.

expositive [eks'pozıtıv] *a* описательный; объяснительный.

expository [eks'pozıtərı] *a* объяснительный.

expostulate [ıks'postʃuleıt] *v* уговаривать, увещевать.

exposure [ıks'pouʒə] *n* 1) незащищённость

(*от опасности, риска, действия света, солнца, непогоды и т. п.*); 2) радиоактивное облучение; 3) оставление (*ребёнка*) на произвол судьбы; 4) выставка (*товаров*); 5) разоблачение; 6) местоположение; вид; the house has a southern ~ дом выходит на юг; 7) *фото* экспозиция.

expound [ıks'paund] *v* 1) излагать; 2) толковать, разъяснять.

express[1] I [ıks'pres] *n* 1) *ж.-д.* экспресс; 2) нарочный, курьер; 3) срочное почтовое отправление; 4) *амер.* срочная пересылка (*товаров, денег*); 5) *амер.* транспортная контора (*тж.* ~ company).

express[1] II *a* 1) специальный; спешный, срочный; 2) *ж.-д.* курьерский; 3) *амер.* транспортный.

express[1] III *v* 1) отправлять срочной почтой; 2) *амер.* пересылать через посредство транспортной конторы; 3) ехать экспрессом.

express[1] IV [ıks'pres] *adv* 1) спешно; 2) с нарочным; 3) экспрессом, курьерским поездом.

express[2] I *a* точный; ясно, определённо выраженный.

express[2] II *v* выражать; to ~ oneself выражать свои мысли, высказываться; to ~ oneself on a subject высказаться по поводу чего-л.

expressible [ıks'presəbl] *a* выражаемый.

expression [ıks'preʃən] *n* 1) выражение; beyond (*или* past) ~ невыразимо; 2) выразительность; 3) вид; выражение лица.

expressive [ıks'presıv] *a* выразительный.

expressly[1] [ıks'preslı] *adv* нарочно; специально.

expressly[2] *adv* точно, ясно, определённо.

expropriate [eks'prouprıeıt] *v* экспроприировать; конфисковать.

expropriation [eksˌprouprıˈeıʃən] *n* экспроприация; конфискация.

expulsion [ıks'pʌlʃən] *n* изгнание; увольнение; исключение (*из школы и т. п.*).

exquisite ['ekskwızıt] *a* 1) превосходный, изысканный; 2) острый (*об ощущении*).

ex-serviceman ['eks'səːvısmən] *n* демобилизованный.

extant [eks'tænt] *a* существующий, сохранившийся до настоящего времени.

extasy ['ekstəsı] *см.* ecstasy.

extemporaneous [eksˌtempəˈreınjəs] *см.* extempore I.

extemporary [ıks'tempərərı] *см.* extempore I.

extempore I [eks'tempərı] *a* импровизированный.

extempore II *adv* экспромтом, без подготовки.

extemporize [ıks'tempəraız] *v* импровизировать.

extend [ıks'tend] *v* 1) протягивать, вытягивать; 2) простираться; тянуться; 3) расширять (-ся); 4) распространять (*влияние*); 5) выказывать (*сочувствие*); оказывать (*покровительство и т. п.*); 6) продлить (*срок*); 7) *воен.* рассыпать (-ся) в цепь; 8) *спорт. разг.* напрягать силы.

extended [ıks'tendıd] *a* 1) протянутый, вытянутый; растянутый; 2) длительный; 3) продолженный; продлённый; 4) протяжённый; 5) *грам.* распространённый.

extensibility [ıksˌtensəˈbılıtı] *n* растяжимость.

extensible [ıks'tensəbl] *a* растяжимый.

extension [ıks'tenʃən] *n* 1) вытягивание; 2) протяжение; протяжённость; 3) расширение; 4) распространение (*сочувствия, влияния и · т. п.*); 5) удлинение; продление; отсрочка.

extensive [ɪks'tensɪv] *a* 1) обширный, пространный; 2) крупный; 3) *с.-х.* экстенсивный.

extent [ɪks'tent] *n* 1) протяжение; пространство; 2) степень; to a great ~ в большой мере, степени; to the full ~ в полной мере; to a certain ~ в известной мере; до некоторой степени; to such an ~ до такой степени, до таких пределов, в такой мере.

extenuate [eks'tenjueɪt] *v* уменьшать (*вину*); стараться найти оправдание.

extenuation [eks,tenju'eɪʃən] *n* извинение; частичное оправдание.

exterior I [eks'tɪərɪə] *n* 1) внешность, наружность; наружная сторона; 2) экстерьер.

exterior II *a* внешний, наружный.

exterminate [eks'tɜːmɪneɪt] *v* искоренять, истреблять.

extermination [eks,tɜːmɪ'neɪʃən] *n* истребление, уничтожение, искоренение; mass ~ массовое уничтожение.

exterminatory [eks'tɜːmɪnətərɪ] *a* истребительный.

external [eks'tɜːnl] *a* внешний; наружный.

externalize [eks'tɜːnəlaɪz] *v* облекать в конкретную форму.

externals [eks'tɜːnlz] *n pl* 1) внешность; 2) внешние обстоятельства; 3) несущественное, внешнее.

exterritorial ['eks,terɪ'tɔːrɪəl] *a* экстерриториальный.

exterritoriality ['eks,terɪ,tɔːrɪ'ælɪtɪ] *n* экстерриториальность.

extinct [ɪks'tɪŋkt] *a* 1) потухший; *перен.* угасший (*о чувстве*); 2) вымерший (*о народе, племени*); пресёкшийся (*о роде*).

extinction [ɪks'tɪŋkʃən] *n* 1) тушение; 2) угасание; потухание; 3) вымирание (*рода*); 4) погашение (*долга*); 5) прекращение (*вражды*).

extinguish [ɪks'tɪŋgwɪʃ] *v* 1) гасить, тушить; 2) затмевать; 3) уничтожать, убивать (*надежду, любовь и т. п.*); подавлять (*способности*); 4) заставить замолчать (*противника*); 5) погашать (*долг*).

extinguisher [ɪks'tɪŋgwɪʃə] *n* (огне)тушитель; гаситель.

extirpate ['ekstɜːpeɪt] *v* 1) вырывать с корнем, искоренять; 2) истреблять; 3) *мед.* удалять.

extirpator ['ekstɜːpeɪtə] *n* 1) искоренитель, истребитель; 2) *с.-х.* экстирпатор, культиватор.

extol [ɪks'tɔl] *v* превозносить, расхваливать.

extort [ɪks'tɔːt] *v* 1) вымогать (*деньги*); 2) выпытывать (*секрет и т. п.*).

extortion [ɪks'tɔːʃən] *n* 1) вымогательство; 2) назначение непомерно высоких цен.

extra I ['ekstrə] *n* 1) что-л. за дополнительную плату; dancing is an ~ за танцы — особая плата; 2) высший сорт; 3) специальный выпуск (*газеты*).

extra II *a* 1) дополнительный, экстренный; 2) высшего качества.

extra III *adv* дополнительно, особо.

extra- ['ekstrə-] *pref* со значением вне-, сверх-, экстра-.

extract[a] ['ekstrækt] *n* 1) экстракт; 2) выдержка (*из книги*).

extract[b] [ɪks'trækt] *v* 1) приготовлять экстракт; выжимать (*сок*); 2) делать выдержки, извлечения (*из книги*); 3) удалять (*зуб*); извлекать (*пулю, пробку и т. п.*); 4) извлекать (*удовольствие, выгоду*); вырывать (*согласие и т. п.*); вытягивать (*информацию*); 5) *мат.* извлекать корень.

extraction [ɪks'trækʃən] *n* 1) извлечение; 2) происхождение; 3) экстракт, эссенция.

extractive I [ɪks'træktɪv] *n* экстракт, извлечение.

extractive II *a* 1) извлекаемый, добываемый; 2) добывающий (*о промышленности*).

extradite ['ekstrədaɪt] *v* выдавать (*преступника*).

extradition [,ekstrə'dɪʃən] *n* выдача (*преступника*).

extraneous [eks'treɪnjəs] *a* чуждый, посторонний.

extraordinary [ɪks'trɔːdnrɪ] *a* 1) необычайный, необыкновенный; удивительный, странный; 2) чрезвычайный, экстраординарный.

extraterrestrial ['ekstrətɪ'restrɪəl] *a* заатмосферный, внеземной; космический.

extravagance [ɪks'trævɪgəns] *n* 1) сумасбродство, нелепость; 2) расточительность; 3) излишество.

extravagancy [ɪks'trævɪgənsɪ] *см.* extravagance.

extravagant [ɪks'trævɪgənt] *a* 1) сумасбродный, нелепый; 2) расточительный; 3) непомерный.

extra-violet ['ekstrə'vaɪəlɪt] *a физ.* ультрафиолетовый.

extreme I [ɪks'triːm] *n* 1) крайность; крайняя степень; to run to an ~, to go to ~s впадать в крайности; in the ~ чрезвычайно, в высшей степени; 2) *обыкн. pl* противоположность; крайность; ~s meet противоположности сходятся; 3) *мат.* крайний член (*пропорции*).

extreme II *a* 1) крайний; дальний; 2) чрезвычайный; 3) экстремистский; 4) последний, предсмертный.

extremely [ɪks'triːmlɪ] *adv* крайне, чрезвычайно; очень.

extremeness [ɪks'triːmnɪs] *n* крайность; крайняя степень.

extremist [ɪks'triːmɪst] *n* сторонник крайних мер, экстремист.

extremity [ɪks'tremɪtɪ] *n* 1) край, конец; оконечность; 2) *pl* конечности; 3) крайность; driven to ~ доведённый до крайности; 4) *обыкн. pl* крайние, чрезвычайные меры.

extricate ['ekstrɪkeɪt] *v* 1) выпутывать; высвобождать; выводить (*из затруднительного положения*); выносить (*раненых*); to ~ oneself а) выпутаться; б) *воен.* оторваться от противника; 2) *хим.* выделять.

extrinsic(al) [eks'trɪnsɪk(əl)] *a* внешний, несвойственный.

extrude [eks'truːd] *v* 1) выталкивать, вытеснять (*from*); 2) выдавливать; штамповать.

extrusion [eks'truːʒən] *n* 1) выталкивание, вытеснение; 2) выдавливание; штамповка.

exuberance [ɪg'zjuːbərəns] *n* изобилие, богатство; избыток.

exuberancy [ɪg'zjuːbərənsɪ] *см.* exuberance.

exuberant [ɪg'zjuːbərənt] *a* 1) обильный, избыточный; 2) пышный, богатый (о *растительности*); 3) бьющий через край (*об энергии и т. п.*); 4) цветущий (*о здоровье*); 5) красочный; 6) многословный.

exudation [ˌeksjuˈdeiʃən] *n* 1) выделение пота; 2) *мед.* экссудат, выпот.

exude [igˈzjuːd] *v* выделять(ся) (*напр., о поте*).

exult [igˈzʌlt] *v* ликовать, торжествовать.

exultant [igˈzʌltənt] *a* ликующий, торжествующий.

exultation [ˌegzʌlˈteiʃən] *n* ликование, торжество.

eye I [ai] *n* 1) глаз; protruding ~s глаза навыкате; saucer ~s круглые глаза, глаза, как плошки; black ~ подбитый глаз; naked ~ невооружённый глаз; shifty ~s бегающие глаза; starry ~s лучистые глаза; swimming ~s глаза, полные слёз; to cast down one's ~s опустить глаза; to screw up one's ~s прищуриться; to shut one's ~s закрывать глаза на что-л.; to be all ~s смотреть во все глаза; up to the ~s in smth. ≅ по уши в чём-л.; to have (*или* to keep) an ~ on следить за; to cock one's ~s подмигивать; to cry one's ~s out выплакать все глаза; to wipe smb.'s ~s a) осушить слёзы кому-л.; б) *сленг* опередить кого-л., «утереть нос» кому-л.; to turn a blind ~ to закрывать глаза на что-л.; 2) зрение; to save one's ~s беречь зрение; 3) взгляд; взор; to clap (*или* to set) one's ~s on увидеть, заметить; to catch one's ~ а) поймать (чей-л.) взгляд; б) привлекать внимание; 4) точка зрения; in the ~ (of) с точки зрения (*кого-л.*); in my ~s по-моему; ушко (*иголки*); петелька; 6) глазок (*для наблюдения*); 7) *бот.* глазок; 8) *горн.* устье шахты; ◊ ~ for ~ око за око; green ~ зависть; mind your ~! глядите в оба!; in my mind's ~ мысленно, в воображении; ~ of the day солнце; in the wind's ~ против ветра; to have an ~ for a) иметь верный глаз; б) иметь способности к чему-л.; to make ~s at smb. делать глазки кому-л.; to cast (*или* to make) sheep's ~s at smb. бросать влюблённые взгляды на кого-л.; to see ~ to ~ with smb. быть полностью согласным с чем-л., разделять взгляды чьи-л. взгляды; to keep one's ~s skinned, to keep an ~ cocked держать ухо востро, смотреть в оба; (oh) my ~(s)! *сленг восклицание удивления*.

eye II *v* (пристально) смотреть, разглядывать; наблюдать.

eyeball [ˈaibɔːl] *n* глазное яблоко.

eyebrow [ˈaibrau] *n* бровь.

eyeful [ˈaiful] *n*: to get an ~ of smth. насмотреться на что-л.

eye-glass [ˈaiglɑːs] *n* 1) *pl* пенсне; очки; лорнет; 2) монокль; 3) линза.

eyehole [ˈaihoul] *n* 1) глазная впадина; 2) глазок, щелка (*для подсматривания*).

eyelash [ˈailæʃ] *n* ресница.

eyelet [ˈailit] *n* 1) ушко, петелька; 2) глазок, щелка; небольшое отверстие.

eyelid [ˈailid] *n* веко; never batted an ~ не заснул ни на минуту; ◊ to hang on by the ~s еле держаться.

eyepiece [ˈaipiːs] *n* окуляр; окулярная трубка.

eyeshot [ˈaiʃɔt] *n* поле зрения.

eyesight [ˈaisait] *n* зрение.

eyesore [ˈaisɔː] *n* что-л. противное, оскорбительное (*для глаза*).

eye-tooth [ˈaituːθ] *n* глазной зуб; ◊ to cut one's eye-teeth сделаться благоразумным.

eyewash [ˈaiwɔʃ] *n* 1) примочка для глаз; 2) *разг.* (грубая) лесть; очковтирательство.

eye-wink [ˈaiwiŋk] *n* 1) взгляд; 2) миг.

eye-witness [ˈaiˌwitnis] *n* очевидец, свидетель.

F

F, f [ef] *n* 1) 6-я буква англ. алфавита; 2) *муз.* нота фа.

fable [ˈfeibl] *n* 1) басня; 2) *собир.* небылицы, ложь; 3) сюжет, фабула.

fabric [ˈfæbrik] *n* 1) ткань, материя; 2) сооружение, здание; 3) остов; структура, устройство; the ~ of society общественный строй; 4) выделка; 5) *attr* тканый.

fabricate [ˈfæbrikeit] *v* 1) фабриковать, выдумывать; 2) подделывать; 3) выделывать, изготовлять; производить; 4) собирать из готовых частей (*напр., дом*).

fabrication [ˌfæbriˈkeiʃən] *n* 1) выдумка; 2) подделка; 3) производство; сооружение.

fabulist [ˈfæbjulist] *n* 1) баснописец; 2) выдумщик.

fabulous [ˈfæbjuləs] *a* 1) легендарный, мифический; баснословный; 2) неправдоподобный, невероятный.

façade [fəˈsɑːd] *n* фасад; *перен.* внешний вид, видимость.

face I [feis] *n* 1) лицо; big ~ лицо с крупными чертами; broad, large ~ круглое, широкое лицо; ~ to ~ лицом к лицу; to one's ~ открыто, в лицо; full ~ анфас; half ~ вполоборота, в профиль; 2) выражение лица, гримаса; а wry ~ гримаса отвращения; искажённое лицо; to pull (*или* to wear) a long ~ иметь печальный *или* мрачный вид; вытянуться (*о лице*); to make (*или* to pull) ~s гримасничать; строить рожи; poker ~ тупое, невыразительное лицо; 3) нахальство, наглость; to have the ~ to say иметь наглость сказать; 4) внешний вид; фасад; лицевая, внешняя сторона, лицо (*ткани*); on the ~ of (it) на первый взгляд; 5) поверхность; 6) циферблат часов; 7): in black (*или* bold) ~ жирным шрифтом; ◊ in the ~ of a) перед лицом чего-л.; б) вопреки; to fly in the ~ of бросать вызов, не считаться, не повиноваться; to save one's ~ сохранить, спасти репутацию; to lose one's ~ потерять репутацию; to set (*или* to put) one's ~ against решительно возражать, противиться; that puts a new ~ on the matter это меняет дело; это другое дело.

face II *v* 1) стоять лицом к, быть обращённым в какую-л. сторону; повернуть(ся) лицом к; стоять перед; 2) встречать смело, не дрогнув; смело смотреть в лицо; 3) отделывать (*платье и т. п.*); облицовывать; полировать; обтачивать; □ to ~ **down** осадить, запугать; to ~ **out** выполнить; б) выдержать.

face-about [ˈfeisəˌbaut] *n* *воен.* поворот кругом.

face-on [ˈfeisˈɔn] *adv* по направлению к, лицом к (*to*).

facer ['feɪsə] *n* 1) удáр в лицó; 2) неожи́данное затруднéние.

facet ['fæsɪt] *n* грань, фацéт.

facetious [fə'siːʃəs] *a* шутли́вый.

facial I ['feɪʃəl] *a* лицевóй.

facial II *n* массáж лицá.

facile ['fæsaɪl] *a* 1) лёгкий; 2) поклáдистый (*о человéке*).

facilitate [fə'sɪlɪteɪt] *v* 1) облегчáть; 2) продвигáть.

facility [fə'sɪlɪtɪ] *n* 1) лёгкость; 2) устýпчивость, поклáдистость; 3) дар, спосóбность; 4) плáвность; бéглость (*речи*); 5) *pl* возмóжности; благоприя́тные услóвия; 6) *pl* удóбства; оборýдование.

facing ['feɪsɪŋ] *n* облицóвка; отдéлка; обтóчка.

facsimile [fæk'sɪmɪlɪ] *n* факси́миле; in ~ а) в ви́де факси́миле; б) в тóчности.

fact [fækt] *n* 1) факт; собы́тие; dry ~s гóлые фáкты; accomplished ~ соверши́вшийся факт; fixed ~ твёрдо устанóвленный факт; to slur a ~ over пройти́ ми́мо фáкта; to accept the ~ примири́ться с фáктом; 2) и́стина, действи́тельность; in ~, in point of ~ действи́тельно, факти́чески.

faction ['fækʃən] *n* 1) фрáкция; 2) кли́ка; 3) разноглáсие, раздóр.

factious ['fækʃəs] *a* фракциóнный.

factitious [fæk'tɪʃəs] *a* искýсственный.

factitive ['fæktɪtɪv] *a грам.* каузáльный.

factor ['fæktə] *n* 1) фáктор; 2) *мат.* мнóжитель; 3) коэффициéнт; 4) агéнт, посрéдник; комиссионéр.

factory ['fæktərɪ] *n* 1) фáбрика; завóд; 2) фактóрия; 3) *attr* фабри́чный.

factotum [fæk'toutəm] *n* 1) фактóтум, довéренное лицó; 2) мáстер на все рýки.

factual ['fæktʃuəl] *a* факти́ческий; реáльный.

faculty ['fækəltɪ] *n* 1) дар, спосóбность; 2) факультéт; 3) преподавáтельский состáв университéта.

fad [fæd] *n* причýда, при́хоть.

fade [feɪd] *v* 1) вя́нуть, увядáть; 2) выцветáть, блёкнуть, теря́ть свéжесть; 3) постепéнно исчезáть; изглáживаться; стирáться, сливáться (*об оттéнках, очертáниях*); ослабевáть, замирáть (*о звýках; тж.* to ~ away); 4) обесцвéчивать; □ to ~ **in** *рáдио, тлв.* а) постепéнно уси́ливаться (*о звýке*); б) становиться отчётливее (*об изображéнии*); to ~ **out** *рáдио, тлв.* а) постепéнно ослабевáть (*о звýке*); б) исчезáть (*об изображéнии*).

fadeaway ['feɪdə,weɪ] *n амер.* исчезновéние.

fag I [fæg] *n* 1) тяжёлая, нýдная рабóта; 2) изнурéние, истощéние; 3) млáдший учени́к, оказывающий услýги стáршим (*в англ. шкóлах*); 4) *сленг* папирóса.

fag II *v* 1) труди́ться, корпéть; 2) утомля́ть(ся) (*тж.* to ~ out); 3) оказывать услýги стáршим товáрищам (*в англ. шкóлах*).

fag-end ['fæg'end] *n* 1) негóдный остáток чегó-л.; 2) окýрок.

fag(g)ot ['fægət] *n* 1) вязáнка хвóроста; 2) *ист.* сожжéние на кострé.

faience [faɪ'ɑːns] *n* фая́нс.

fail I [feɪl] *v* 1) не удавáться; не сбывáться; потерпéть неудáчу; he tried to learn to sing, but he ~ed он прóбовал учи́ться петь, но неудáчно; 2) обманýть ожидáния; 3) провали́ть(ся) на экзáмене; 4) обанкрóтиться; 5) забы́ть, не испóлнить; he ~ed to appear он не появи́лся; don't ~ to let me know не забýдьте

сообщи́ть мне; 6) недоставáть, не хватáть; 7) имéть недостáток в чём-л.; 8) ослабевáть, угасáть, теря́ть си́лы; the sick man's heart was ~ing сéрдце больнóго сдáло.

fail II *n*: without ~ непремéнно, обязáтельно; навернякá.

failing I ['feɪlɪŋ] *n* 1) оши́бка; слáбость, недостáток; 2) слáбость, слáбая стрýнка.

failing II *prep* за неимéнием, за отсýтствием.

failure ['feɪljə] *n* 1) неудáча; провáл; 2) недостáток, отсýтствие чегó-л.; corn ~, crop ~ неурожáй; 3) несостоя́тельность, банкрóтство; 4) неудáчник; неудáвшееся дéло; 5) *тех.* авáрия; 6): heart ~ *мед.* сердéчная недостáточность *или* слáбость.

fain I [feɪn] *a predic* 1) вы́нужденный; she was ~ to keep silence онá былá вы́нуждена молчáть; 2) готóвый сдéлать чтó-л.

fain II *adv* охóтно, с рáдостью; I would ~ go я охóтно пошёл бы, я рад был бы пойти́.

fain III *v*: ~ I, ~s I! чур меня́!

fainéant [,feɪneɪ'ɑːŋ] *n* лентя́й, бездéльник.

faint I [feɪnt] *n* обмóрок; dead ~ глубóкий обмóрок; пóлная потéря сознáния.

faint II *a* 1) слáбый, ослабéвший; to feel ~ чýвствовать дурнотý; to go ~ потеря́ть сознáние; 2) слáбый, нея́сный; смýтный; блéдный; not the ~est hope ни малéйшей надéжды; 3) рóбкий, вя́лый.

faint III *v* 1) пáдать в обмóрок, теря́ть сознáние (*тж.* to ~ away); 2) теря́ть мýжество, ослабевáть.

faint-heart ['feɪnthɑːt] *n* трус, малодýшный человéк.

faint-hearted ['feɪnt'hɑːtɪd] *a* малодýшный, трусли́вый.

fainting-fit ['feɪntɪŋfɪt] *n* обмóрок.

faintly ['feɪntlɪ] *adv* слáбо, едвá.

fair[1] [fɛə] *n* 1) я́рмарка; 2) благотвори́тельный базáр; ◊ vanity fair житéйская суетá.

fair[2] I [fɛə] *a* 1) справедли́вый, чéстный; беспристрáстный; ~ and square откры́тый, чéстный; 2) достáточный, поря́дочный, неплохóй; 3) белокýрый, свéтлый; 4) благоприя́тный, я́сный (*о погóде*); 5) вéжливый; 6) чи́стый, незапя́тнанный; 7) прекрáсный, краси́вый.

fair[2] II *adv* 1) чéстно; пря́мо; я́сно; откры́то; 2) *уст.* вéжливо, любéзно; ◊ ~ and softly! ти́ше!

fair[3] *n*: for ~ действи́тельно.

fair-dealing I ['fɛə,diːlɪŋ] *n* чéстность, прямотá.

fair-dealing II *a* чéстный, прямóй.

fairly ['fɛəlɪ] *adv* 1) справедли́во, беспристрáстно; ~ speaking открóвенно говоря́; 2) совершéнно; 3) снóсно; ~ well неплóхо, довóльно хорошó.

fairy I ['fɛərɪ] *n* фéя; эльф; bad ~ злой гéний.

fairy II *a* волшéбный, скáзочный.

Fairyland ['fɛərɪlænd] *n* скáзочная, волшéбная странá.

fairy-tale ['fɛərɪteɪl] *n* скáзка.

faith [feɪθ] *n* 1) вéра; довéрие; to pin one's ~ to (*или* upon) слéпо вéрить, полагáться; 2) вероисповéдание, рели́гия; 3) вéрность; чéстность; good ~ добросóвестность; bad ~ веролóмство; недобросóвестность; Punic ~ измéна, веролóмство; upon my ~!, in ~! кляну́сь чéстью!; 4) обещáние; обéт; to keep (to break) one's ~ держáть (нарушáть) слóво.

faithful I ['feɪθful] *a* 1) вéрный, прéданный;

2) добросо́вестный; 3) заслу́живающий дове́рия; то́чный, ве́рный.

faithful II *n*: the ~ (*употр. как pl*) ве́рующие; правове́рные.

faithfully ['feɪθfulɪ] *adv* ве́рно; че́стно; yours ~ ≅ с соверше́нным почте́нием (*в письме*).

faithfulness ['feɪθfulnɪs] *n* 1) ве́рность; достове́рность; 2) че́стность.

faithless ['feɪθlɪs] *a* 1) вероло́мный; 2) не заслу́живающий дове́рия; 3) неве́рующий.

fake I [feɪk] *n* 1) подде́лка; фальши́вка; 2) плуто́вство; 3) *attr* подде́льный; фальши́вый.

fake II *v* 1) подде́лывать, фальсифици́ровать, фабрикова́ть (*тж.* to ~ up); 2) дура́чить; 3) прики́дываться (*больны́м и т. п.*), симули́ровать (*боле́знь*).

faker ['feɪkə] *n* 1) моше́нник; обма́нщик; 2) у́личный разно́счик.

fakir ['fɑːkɪə] *n* факи́р.

falcon ['fɔːlkən] *n* со́кол.

falconer ['fɔːlkənə] *n* соко́льничий.

falconry ['fɔːlkənrɪ] *n* соко́линая охо́та.

fall I [fɔːl] *n* 1) паде́ние; *перен. тж.* упа́док; to have a ~ упа́сть; to have a bad ~ нело́вко упа́сть; гро́хнуться; 2) оса́дки; a heavy ~ of rain ли́вень; 3) о́сень (*тж.* ~ of the leaf); 4) *обыкн. pl* водопа́д; 5) укло́н; склон, спуск; 6) *гидр.* высота́ паде́ния (*воды́*).

fall II *v* (*past* fell; *p. p.* fallen) 1) па́дать; пасть (*тж. в бою́*); 2) спада́ть, понижа́ться; стиха́ть; 3) приходи́ться, выпада́ть; to ~ to one's lot выпада́ть на чью-л. до́лю; 4) *как глагол-свя́зка с предикати́вным прил. выража́ет перехо́д из одного́ состоя́ния в друго́е*: to ~ asleep засну́ть; to ~ sick захвора́ть; 5) впада́ть в, доходи́ть до (*какого-л. состоя́ния; in, into*); to ~ into a rage впада́ть в гнев, (раз)гне́ваться; to ~ into error впада́ть в оши́бку, ошиба́ться; to ~ into talk разговори́ться; to ~ in love влюби́ться; 6) вы́тянуться (*о лице́*); 7) руби́ть, вали́ть (*де́рево*); □ to ~ **across** случа́йно встре́тить; to ~ **among** случа́йно попа́сть, очути́ться; to ~ **apart** распада́ться; to ~ **away** а) покида́ть; б) исчеза́ть; в) отпада́ть; г) ча́хнуть; to ~ **back** а) отступа́ть; б) прибега́ть к (по́мощи) (*upon*); to ~ **behind** отстава́ть; остава́ться позади́; to ~ **down** а) упа́сть, пасть ниц; б) *амер.* потерпе́ть неуда́чу; to ~ **for** *разг.* чу́вствовать влече́ние (*к кому́-л.*); поддава́ться (*чему́-л.*); to ~ **in** а) совпада́ть, соотве́тствовать; б) обру́шиваться, прова́ливаться; в) истека́ть (*о сро́ке*); г) случа́йно встре́титься, столкну́ться (*with*); д) согласи́ться, дости́гнуть соглаше́ния (*with*); to ~ **off** а) па́дать, уменьша́ться; б) отпада́ть; в) *мор.* не слу́шаться руля́; to ~ **on** а) напада́ть, вступа́ть в бой; б) набра́сываться (*на еду́*); to ~ **out** а) выпада́ть; б) ссо́риться; в) случа́ться; г) *воен.* выходи́ть из стро́я; ~ out! во́льно!; to ~ **out of** отка́зываться от (*привы́чки и т. п.*); to ~ **over** *амер.* а) споткну́ться; б) увлека́ться; в) to ~ over each other дра́ться, боро́ться, сопе́рничать друг с дру́гом; to ~ **through** потерпе́ть неуда́чу, провали́ться; to ~ **to** а) набра́сываться на что-л.; б) принима́ться за еду́; to ~ **under** подпада́ть; подверга́ться; to ~ **upon** напада́ть, ната́лкиваться на что-л.; ◊ to ~ on one's feet

счастли́во отде́латься; уда́чно вы́йти из тру́дного положе́ния; to ~ to pieces разва́литься; to ~ flat провали́ться, не име́ть успе́ха.

fallacious [fə'leɪʃəs] *a* оши́бочный, ло́жный.

fallacy ['fæləsɪ] *n* 1) оши́бка, заблужде́ние; 2) ло́жный вы́вод.

fall-away ['fɔːlə'weɪ] *n* отделе́ние (*ступе́ни раке́ты*).

fallen ['fɔːlən] *p. p. см.* fall II.

fall-off ['fɔːlɔf] *см.* fall-away.

fall-out ['fɔːlaut] *n* 1) выпаде́ние радиоакти́вных оса́дков; 2) радиоакти́вные оса́дки.

fallow I ['fælou] *n* 1) *с.-х.* пар; 2) необрабо́танная земля́.

fallow II *a* 1) вспа́ханный под пар; 2) необрабо́танный (*о земле́*); 3) неразвито́й (*о челове́ке*).

fallow III *v* поднима́ть целину́.

fallow-deer ['fæloudɪə] *n* лань.

false I [fɔːls] *a* 1) ло́жный; неве́рный, обма́нчивый, оши́бочный; 2) подде́льный; фальши́вый; иску́сственный; 3) нейскренний, вероло́мный.

false II *adv*: to play smb. ~ преда́ть кого-л.; поки́нуть кого-л. в беде́.

falsehood ['fɔːlshud] *n* 1) ложь, непра́вда; 2) лжи́вость.

falseness ['fɔːlsnɪs] *n* 1) оши́бочность; 2) нейскренность, фальши́вость, лжи́вость; 3) вероло́мство.

falsification ['fɔːlsɪfɪ'keɪʃən] *n* фальсифика́ция, подде́лка; искаже́ние (*фа́ктов и т. п.*).

falsify ['fɔːlsɪfaɪ] *v* 1) фальсифици́ровать, подде́лывать; искажа́ть (*фа́кты и т. п.*); 2) обма́нывать (*наде́жды*).

falsity ['fɔːlsɪtɪ] *n* 1) ло́жность; оши́бочность; 2) нейскренность; вероло́мство.

falter ['fɔːltə] *v* 1) спотыка́ться, идти́ неуве́ренно; 2) запина́ться, говори́ть заика́ясь; 3) колеба́ться; дро́гнуть; □ to ~ **out** пробормота́ть.

faltering ['fɔːltərɪŋ] *a* 1) дрожа́щий (*о го́лосе*); 2) запина́ющийся, нереши́тельный; 3) ло́маный (*о языке́*).

fame I [feɪm] *n* изве́стность, сла́ва; репута́ция; ill ~ дурна́я сла́ва, молва́.

fame II *v* прославля́ть.

famed [feɪmd] *a* просла́вленный; изве́стный, знамени́тый.

familiar [fə'mɪljə] *a* 1) бли́зкий; хорошо́ знако́мый, изве́стный; 2) обы́чный; привы́чный; 3) фамилья́рный.

familiarity [fə,mɪlɪ'ærɪtɪ] *n* 1) бли́зость, бли́зкие отноше́ния; 2) хоро́шее знако́мство (*с чем-л.— with*); 3) фамилья́рность.

familiarize [fə'mɪljəraɪz] *v* познако́мить, озна-ко́мить.

family ['fæmɪlɪ] *n* 1) семья́, семе́йство; род; long ~ многоде́тная семья́; 2) *биол.* семе́йство; 3) *лингв.* семья́; 4) *attr* семе́йный, родово́й.

famine ['fæmɪn] *n* го́лод.

famish ['fæmɪʃ] *v* 1) голода́ть (*тж. разг.* to be ~ing); 2) мори́ть го́лодом.

famous ['feɪməs] *a* 1) знамени́тый, изве́стный, сла́вный; 2) *разг.* превосхо́дный.

fan[1] [fæn] *n* 1) ве́ер; 2) вентиля́тор; 3) ло́пасть (*винта́*); крыло́ ветряно́й ме́льницы; 4) *с.-х.* ве́ялка.

fan¹ II *v* 1) обмахивать; 2) *поэт.* обвевать, освежать; 3) *с.-х.* веять.

fan² *n разг.* любитель, энтузиаст; болельщик; поклонник.

fanatic I [fəˈnætɪk] *n* фанатик.

fanatic II *a* фанатический.

fanatical [fəˈnætɪkəl] *см.* fanatic II.

fanaticism [fəˈnætɪsɪzəm] *n* фанатизм.

fancier [ˈfænsɪə] *n* знаток, любитель.

fanciful [ˈfænsɪful] *a* 1) причудливый, прихотливый, капризный; 2) фантастический.

fancy I [ˈfænsɪ] *n* 1) фантазия, воображение; 2) мысленный образ; 3) прихоть, каприз; 4) вкус, пристрастие, склонность; to take a ~ to (*или* for) полюбить; 5) (the ~) энтузиаст; любитель; болельщик.

fancy II *a* 1) фантастический; воображаемый; 2) прихотливый, причудливый; необыкновенный; 3) модный; 4) маскарадный; 5) *амер.* высшего качества; 6) улучшенной породы.

fancy III *v* 1) воображать, представлять себе; ~!, just ~! подумайте (только)!; 2) (пред-)полагать; 3) *refl разг.* быть о себе высокого мнения; 4) любить, нравиться.

fancy-ball [ˈfænsɪˈbɔːl] *n* маскарад, костюмированный бал.

fancy-work [ˈfænsɪwəːk] *n* вышивание; вышивка.

fang [fæŋ] *n* 1) клык; 2) ядовитый зуб (*у змеи*); 3) корень зуба; 4) *тех.* зубец.

fanner [ˈfænə] *n с.-х.* веялка.

fan-tail [ˈfænteɪl] *n* 1) трубастый голубь; 2) зюйдвестка.

fantastic(al) [fænˈtæstɪk(əl)] *a* 1) причудливый, эксцентричный; 2) воображаемый, нереальный.

fantasy [ˈfæntəsɪ] *n* 1) фантазия; 2) каприз.

far I [fɑː] *a* (*compar* farther, further; *superl* farthest, furthest) дальний; отдалённый, далёкий (*тж.* ~ off).

far II *adv* (*compar* farther, further; *superl* farthest, furthest) 1) далеко (*тж.* ~ away, ~ off, ~ out); ~ and near, ~ and wide повсюду; how ~ a) как далеко, куда; б) до какой степени, насколько; ~ in the day к концу дня; 2) гораздо, намного (*тж.* ~ and away); ◇ ~ from it совсем, отнюдь нет; as ~ as a) до; б) насколько; (in) so ~ as до тех пор пока; насколько; so ~ до сих пор; пока; so ~ so good пока всё хорошо; thus ~ до сих пор; ~ gone a) охваченный (*каким-л. чувством*); б) в тяжёлом состоянии (*о больном*); в) очень пьяный.

far III *n* 1) далёкое расстояние; from ~ издали, издалека; 2): by ~ намного, гораздо.

far-away [ˈfɑːrəweɪ] *a* 1) дальний, далёкий; 2) отсутствующий, мечтательный (*о взгляде*).

far-between [ˈfɑːbɪˈtwiːn] *a* редкий.

farce [fɑːs] *n* фарс, шутка.

fare I [fɛə] *n* 1) стоимость проезда, билета; what's the ~ to Leningrad? сколько стоит билет до Ленинграда?; 2) седок, пассажир; 3) пища, питание; bad (*или* poor) ~ плохое питание; homely ~ простая пища.

fare II *v* 1) быть; поживать; how ~s it? как дела?, как поживаете?; 2) питаться, столоваться; 3) *поэт.* путешествовать, ехать (*тж.* to ~ forth);

◇ you may go farther and ~ worse ≅ будьте довольны тем, что имеете.

Far-Eastern [ˈfɑːrˈiːstən] *a* дальневосточный.

farewell I [ˈfɛəˈwel] *n* 1) прощание; to bid ~ прощаться; 2) *attr* прощальный.

farewell II *int* прощайте!, счастливого пути!

far-famed [ˈfɑːˈfeimd] *a* широко известный.

far-fetched [ˈfɑːˈfetʃt] *a* 1) неестественный, натянутый; надуманный; 2) привезённый издалека.

farinaceous [ˌfærɪˈneɪʃəs] *a* мучнистый, мучной.

farl [fɑːl] *n шотл.* тонкая овсяная лепёшка.

farm I [fɑːm] *n* 1) (крестьянское) хозяйство; collective ~ колхоз; state ~ совхоз; individual ~ единоличное (крестьянское) хозяйство; 2) ферма, хутор; milk ~ молочная ферма; poultry ~ птицеферма; 3) питомник, заповедник; silver-fox ~ питомник серебристых лисиц; 4) *см.* farm-house.

farm II *v* 1) обрабатывать землю; 2) сдавать землю в аренду (*тж.* to ~ out).

farmer [ˈfɑːmə] *n* 1) фермер; 2) арендатор; 3) крестьянин; collective ~ колхозник; individual ~ крестьянин-единоличник.

farm-hand [ˈfɑːmhænd] *n* сельскохозяйственный рабочий.

farm-house [ˈfɑːmhaus] *n* жилой дом на ферме, на хуторе.

farming [ˈfɑːmɪŋ] *n* занятие сельским хозяйством; земледелие; high ~ интенсивное земледелие.

farmstead [ˈfɑːmsted] *n* крестьянский двор, ферма со службами.

farmyard [ˈfɑːmjɑːd] *n* двор фермы.

far-reaching [ˈfɑːˈriːtʃɪŋ] *a* далеко идущий, чреватый последствиями.

farrier [ˈfærɪə] *n* 1) ковочный кузнец; 2) *уст.* коновал, ветеринар.

farriery [ˈfærɪərɪ] *n* 1) кузнечное ремесло; 2) кузница; 3) *уст.* ветеринария, ветеринарная хирургия.

farrow¹ I [ˈfærou] *n* опорос.

farrow¹ II *v* пороситься.

farrow² *a* яловая (*о корове*).

far-seeing [ˈfɑːˈsiːɪŋ] *a* дальновидный, предусмотрительный.

far-sighted [ˈfɑːˈsaitɪd] *a* дальнозоркий; *перен.* дальновидный.

far-sightedness [ˈfɑːˈsaitɪdnɪs] *n* дальнозоркость; *перен.* дальновидность.

farther I, II [ˈfɑːðə] *см.* further I, II.

farthermost [ˈfɑːðəmoust] *a* самый дальний.

farthest I [ˈfɑːðɪst] *a* (*superl см.* far I) самый дальний; at (the) ~ самое большее; самое позднее.

farthest II *adv* (*superl см.* far II) дальше всего.

farthing [ˈfɑːðɪŋ] *n* фартинг ($^1/_4$ пенса); ◇ it's not worth a (brass) ~ гроша ломаного не стоит; not to care a (brass) ~ совершенно не интересоваться, наплевать.

fascinate [ˈfæsɪneɪt] *v* очаровывать, пленять; зачаровывать (*взглядом*).

fascination [ˌfæsɪˈneɪʃən] *n* очарование, обаяние.

fascine [fæˈsiːn] *n* фашина.

fascism [ˈfæʃɪzəm] *n* фашизм.

fascist I ['fæʃist] *n* фашист.

fascist II *a* фашистский.

fash I [fæʃ] *n шотл.* беспокойство; мучение; досада.

fash II *v шотл.* беспокоить; мучить; огорчать.

fashion I ['fæʃən] *n* 1) вид, образ; манера; after a ~, in a ~ до некоторой степени, некоторым образом; after the ~ of наподобие; 2) стиль, мода; in ~ в моде; модный; out of ~ старомодный, вышедший из моды; to follow the ~ следовать моде; to be all the ~ быть очень модным, очень распространённым.

fashion II *v* придавать вид, форму; выделывать.

fashionable ['fæʃnəbl] *a* 1) фешенебельный, модный; 2) светский.

fashion-paper ['fæʃən‚peipə] *n* модный журнал.

fast¹ I [fɑːst] *n церк.* пост.

fast¹ II *v* поститься.

fast² I *a* 1) крепкий, прочный, устойчивый; стойкий; to make ~ закреплять; to stand ~ держаться крепко; 2) скорый, быстроходный; 3) показывающий больший вес, неточный (*о весах*); спешащий (*о часах*); 4) беспутный, легкомысленный, фривольный.

fast² II *adv* 1) крепко, сильно, прочно; 2) быстро, скоро, часто; to live ~ прожигать жизнь.

fasten ['fɑːsn] *v* 1) прикреплять, привязывать; связывать, скреплять; 2) укреплять, завинчивать, зажимать; 3) запирать(ся); 4) застёгивать(ся); 5) устремлять, сосредоточивать (*взгляд, мысли; на — on, upon*); 6) приписывать (*кому-л.— on, upon*); 7) ухватиться за, наброситься (*on, upon*): □ to ~ off закреплять (*нитку*); to ~ up закрывать; завязывать, заколачивать.

fastener ['fɑːsnə] *n* 1) запор; задвижка; 2) застёжка; 3) зажим; 4) скрепка (*для бумаг*).

fastidious [fæs'tidiəs] *a* 1) разборчивый, требовательный, привередливый; 2) утончённый.

fat I [fæt] *n* 1) сало, жир; 2) что-л. самое лучшее; 3) *тех.* смазка; 4) *театр.* выигрышное место роли (*тж.* a bit of ~); ◊ to live on the ~ of the land жить в роскоши; the ~ is in the fire *погов.* ≅ быть беде.

fat I *a* 1) жирный, сальный, маслянистый; 2) полный, толстый; 3) откормленный, упитанный; 4) плодородный, тучный (*о земле*); 5) богатый, обильный; 6) выгодный; 7) тупоумный; ◊ to cut it ~ хвастаться, выставлять напоказ.

fat III *v см.* fatten.

fatal ['feitl] *a* 1) фатальный, роковой, неизбежный; 2) смертельный, губительный, пагубный.

fatalism ['feitəlizəm] *n* фатализм.

fatalist ['feitəlist] *n* фаталист.

fatality [fə'tæliti] *n* 1) обречённость; рок; 2) смерть (*на войне, от несчастного случая*); 3) несчастье.

fate I [feit] *n* 1) судьба; рок; to tempt ~ искушать судьбу; to share the same ~ разделить ту же участь; his ~ is sealed его судьба уже решена; 2): the Fates *миф.* парки; 3) гибель, смерть; ◊ as sure as ~ несомненно.

fate II *v* предопределять; he was ~d to do smth. ему было суждено сделать что-л.

fated ['feitid] *a* обречённый.

fateful ['feitful] *a* 1) пророческий; 2) роковой; обречённый; 3) решительный, важный.

fat-guts ['fætgʌts] *n* толстяк.

fat-head ['fæthed] *n* болван.

father I ['fɑːðə] *n* 1) отец; 2) родоначальник; предок; to be gathered to one's ~s отправиться к праотцам, скончаться; 3) автор, творец, основатель; 4) старейший член (*какого-л. общества и т. п.*); 5) священник; ghostly ~ духовник; ◊ Pilgrim Fathers *амер. ист.* первые колонисты в Массачусетсе в 1620 г.

father II *v* 1) производить, порождать; 2) быть *или* считаться отцом, автором, создателем; 3) приписывать отцовство, авторство; возлагать ответственность (*на — on, upon*); 4) усыновлять; отечески заботиться.

fatherhood ['fɑːðəhud] *n* отцовство.

father-in-law ['fɑːðərinlɔː] *n* (*pl* fathers-in-law) свёкор; тесть.

fatherland ['fɑːðəlænd] *n* родина, отечество.

fatherless ['fɑːðəlis] *a* (оставшийся) без отца.

fatherly I ['fɑːðəli] *a* отеческий.

fatherly II *adv* отечески.

fathom I ['fæðəm] *n* морская сажень (= *1,82 м*).

fathom II *v* 1) измерять глубину; 2) вникать, понимать.

fathomless ['fæðəmlis] *a* бездонный; неизмеримый; непроницаемый.

fatigue I [fə'tiːg] *n* 1) утомление; усталость; 2) утомительная работа; 3) *воен.* внестроевой наряд солдата (*тж.* ~ duty).

fatigue II *v* утомлять, изнурять.

fatling ['fætliŋ] *n* откормленное на убой молодое животное.

fatness ['fætnis] *n* 1) полнота, толщина; 2) плодородность, тучность (*земли*).

fatten ['fætn] *v* 1) откармливать (*на убой*); 2) жиреть; 3) удобрять (*землю*).

fatty I ['fæti] *n* толстяк.

fatty II *a* 1) жирный; полный; 2) жировой.

fatuity [fə'tjuːiti] *n* глупость, бессмысленность.

fatuous ['fætjuəs] *a* глупый, бессмысленный; бесполезный.

fat-witted ['fæt‚witid] *a* тупой, глупый.

faucet ['fɔːsit] *n амер.* водопроводный кран; 2) вентиль; втулка.

faugh [fɔː] *int* тьфу!

fault [fɔːlt] *n* 1) недостаток, дефект; to find with ~ жаловаться (*на кого-л.*); придираться (*к кому-л.*); 2) ошибка; промах; вина; in ~ виноват(ый); 3) *спорт.* промах, неправильно поданный мяч; 4) *геол.* разлом, сдвиг, сброс; ◊ to be at ~ а) потерять след; б) быть в затруднении; to a ~ чрезмерно, слишком.

fault-finder ['fɔːlt‚faində] *n* 1) придирчивый человек; 2) *тех.* прибор для определения повреждения, дефектоскоп.

fault-finding I ['fɔːlt‚faindiŋ] *n* 1) придирчивость; 2) *тех.* определение аварии.

fault-finding II *a* придирчивый.

faultless ['fɔːltlis] *a* безупречный.

faulty ['fɔːlti] *a* 1) ошибочный; 2) испорченный, неисправный.

faun [fɔːn] *n миф.* фавн.

fauna [ˈfɔːnə] *n* (*pl тж.* faunae [ˈfɔːniː]) фа́уна.

favor [ˈfeɪvə] *амер. см.* favour.

favour I [ˈfeɪvə] *n* 1) благоскло́нность, располо́жение; ми́лость; to find ~ in the eyes of заслужи́ть' расположе́ние; to curry ~ with заи́скивать, льстить; to look with ~ on относи́ться доброжела́тельно к; by your ~ с ва́шего позволе́ния; 2) покрови́тельство; по́мощь, защи́та; under ~ of the night под покро́вом но́чи; in ~ of а) за, в защи́ту; б) в по́льзу, на счёт (кого́-л.); на и́мя (кого́-л.; *о чеке и т. п.*); 3) одолже́ние; I should esteem it a ~ сочту́ э́то за одолже́ние; 4) *ком.* письмо́; in reply to your ~ of June the 5th в отве́т на ва́ше письмо́ от 5 ию́ня; 5) сувени́р, вещи́ца, да́нная на па́мять; 6) значо́к, розе́тка, бант.

favour II *v* 1) относи́ться благоскло́нно, доброжела́тельно; 2) ока́зывать одолже́ние, любе́зность, внима́ние; ~ me with your attention благоволи́те удели́ть мне внима́ние; 3) покрови́тельствовать; помога́ть, подде́рживать; способствовать; 4) ока́зывать предпочте́ние; быть пристра́стным; 5) *разг.* быть похо́жим (*на кого́-л.*).

favourable [ˈfeɪvərəbl] *a* 1) благоскло́нный, располо́женный; 2) благоприя́тный; подходя́щий, удо́бный.

favoured [ˈfeɪvəd] *a* 1) привилегиро́ванный; most ~ *дип.* наибо́лее благоприя́тствуемый; 2) благода́тный (*о климате и т. п.*); 3) пе́реданный; a letter ~ by Comrade X. письмо́, пе́реданное това́рищем X.

favourite I [ˈfeɪvərɪt] *n* люби́мец; фавори́т.

favourite II *a* люби́мый.

fawn[1] **I** [fɔːn] *n* 1) оленёнок; in ~ сте́льная (*о ланке*); 2) желтова́то-кори́чневый цвет.

fawn[1] **I** *a* желтова́то-кори́чневый.

fawn[2] *v* 1) виля́ть хвосто́м; ласка́ться (*тж.* to ~ on, to ~ upon); 2) подли́зываться, прислу́живаться.

fawn-coloured [ˈfɔːnˌkʌləd] *см.* fawn[1] II.

fawning [ˈfɔːnɪŋ] *a* раболе́пный.

faze [feɪz] *v амер. разг.* досажда́ть, беспоко́ить; расстра́ивать.

fear I [fɪə] *n* 1) страх, боя́знь; in ~ (of) в стра́хе (пе́ред чем-л.); for ~ of из боя́зни, из стра́ха; 2) опасе́ние; по ~ вряд ли; едва́ ли; ◇ without ~ or favour беспристра́стно.

fear II *v* 1) боя́ться; never ~! не бо́йтесь!; 2) опаса́ться (*чего́-л.*); 3) почита́ть.

fearful [ˈfɪəful] *a* 1) ужа́сный, стра́шный; 2) боязли́вый; ро́бкий нереши́тельный.

fearless [ˈfɪəlɪs] *a* бесстра́шный.

fearnought [ˈfɪənɔːt] *n* 1) касто́р (*сукно*); 2) оде́жда из касто́ра; 3) храбре́ц, бесстра́шный челове́к.

fearsome [ˈfɪəsəm] *a* стра́шный, ужа́сный.

feasible [ˈfiːzəbl] *a* 1) возмо́жный, вероя́тный; 2) выполни́мый, осуществи́мый; 3) приго́дный.

feast I [fiːst] *n* 1) пир; банке́т; пра́зднество; 2) пра́здник; 3) наслажде́ние.

feast II *v* 1) пирова́ть; принима́ть, угоща́ть (*гостей*); 2) пра́здновать; 3) наслажда́ться.

feat [fiːt] *n* 1) по́двиг; ~ of arms боево́й по́двиг; 2) иску́сство, ло́вкость, си́ла.

feather I [ˈfeðə] *n* 1) перо́; *pl* опере́ние; to crop smb's ~s *перен.* подре́зать кры́лья кому́-л.; уни́зить кого́-л.; 2) пти́ца, дичь; ◇ a ~ in one's cap предме́т го́рдости; to show the white ~ стру́сить; in high (*или* full) ~ в хоро́шем настрое́нии; в прекра́сном состоя́нии; to singe one's ~s опали́ть себе́ кры́лышки; to cut a ~ а) ре́зать во́ду (*о быстроидущем судне*); б) рисова́ться, выставля́ть что-л. напока́з; пуска́ть пыль в глаза́.

feather II *v* 1) украша́ть пе́рьями; 2) выстила́ть пе́рьями (*гнездо*); 3) оперя́ться.

feather-brained [ˈfeðəbreɪnd] *a* глу́пый, пусто́й, ве́треный.

feathered [ˈfeðəd] *a* 1) укра́шенный, покры́тый пе́рьями; 2) крыла́тый, бы́стрый.

feathering [ˈfeðərɪŋ] *n* 1) опере́ние; 2) *архит.* фесто́н.

feather-weight [ˈfeðəweɪt] *n спорт.* «вес пера́».

feathery [ˈfeðərɪ] *a* 1) покры́тый пе́рьями; 2) име́ющий вид пера́; 3) лёгкий (как пёрышко).

feature I [ˈfiːtʃə] *n* 1) *обыкн. pl* черты́ лица́; 2) осо́бенность, характе́рная черта́; 3) гвоздь (*программы*), боеви́к (*в кино*); 4) статья́ (*в газете или журнале*); 5) полнометра́жный фильм.

feature II *v* 1) быть характе́рной черто́й; 2) рисова́ть, изобража́ть; 3) печа́тать на ви́дном ме́сте (*в газете*); 4) *амер.* пока́зывать (*на экране*), выводи́ть в гла́вной ро́ли.

featureless [ˈfiːtʃəlɪs] *a* невырази́тельный, бесцве́тный.

febrile [ˈfiːbraɪl] *a мед.* лихора́дочный.

February [ˈfebruərɪ] *n* 1) февра́ль; 2) *attr* февра́льский.

feckless [ˈfeklɪs] *a* 1) сла́бый; беспо́мощный; 2) бесполе́зный, тще́тный.

feculent [ˈfekjulənt] *a* му́тный.

fecund [ˈfiːkənd] *a* 1) плодоро́дный; 2) плодови́тый.

fecundity [fiˈkʌndɪtɪ] *n* 1) плодоро́дие; 2) плодови́тость.

fed [fed] *past, p. p. см.* feed[1] II.

federal I [ˈfedərəl] *n* федерали́ст; the Federals «северя́не» (*в гражданской войне 1861—1865 гг. в Америке*).

federal II *a* федера́льный.

federate[a] [ˈfedərɪt] *a* федерати́вный.

federate[b] [ˈfedəreɪt] *v* объединя́ть(ся) на федерати́вных нача́лах.

federation [ˌfedəˈreɪʃən] *n* федера́ция.

federative [ˈfedərətɪv] *a* федерати́вный.

fee I [fiː] *n* 1) вознагражде́ние, гонора́р; (о)пла́та; 2) взнос; admission ~ вступи́тельный взнос; входна́я пла́та; 3) чаевы́е; 4) *ист.* лен, феода́льное поме́стье.

fee II *v* (*past, p. p.* feed) 1) вознагражда́ть, опла́чивать; 2) дава́ть на чай; 3) нанима́ть (*кого́-л.*).

feeble [ˈfiːbl] *a* 1) сла́бый; 2) хи́лый, не́мощный; бле́дный.

feeble-minded [ˈfiːblˈmaɪndɪd] *a* слабоу́мный.

feed[1] **I** [fiːd] *n* 1) пита́ние, пи́ща, корм; фура́ж; off one's ~ без аппети́та; 2) кормле́ние, да́ча (*корма*); 3) *тех.* пита́ние, пода́ча материа́ла; 4) *уст.* вы́гон, па́стбище; out at ~ на подно́жном корму́.

feed[1] **II** *v* (*past, p. p.* fed) 1) корми́ть, дава́ть пи́щу; *тех.* пита́ть; 2) задава́ть корм, ска́рмливать; 3) пасти́ (*скот*); 4) есть; пита́ться, корми́ться (*чем-л. — on, upon*); 5) снабжа́ть (*водой,*

198

топливом, сырьём); □ to ~ **down** стравливать (*пастбище*); to ~ **up** откармливать; усиленно питать; to be fed up *сленг* быть сытым по горло (*with*).

feed[2] *past, p. p. см.* fee II.

feeder ['fiːdə] *n* 1) едок, иждивенец; gross ~, large ~ обжора; 2) детский рожок; 3) детский нагрудник; 4) кормушка; 5) приток (*реки*); канал; 6) *ж.-д.* ветка, вспомогательная линия (*тж.* ~ railway, ~ line); 7) *тех.* подающий механизм.

feel I [fiːl] *n* 1) ощущение, осязание; to have a soapy (greasy) ~ быть мыльным (сальным) на ощупь; cold to the ~ холодный на ощупь; 2) вкус к чему-л.

feel II *v* (*past, p. p.* felt) 1) щупать, ощупывать, нащупывать; осязать; ~ how cold my hands are пощупайте, какие у меня холодные руки; to ~ one's way а) идти ощупью, нащупывать дорогу; б) действовать осторожно, осмотрительно; 2) чувствовать, ощущать; испытывать; to ~ quite oneself быть бодрым; владеть собой; she ~s glad она счастлива, она довольна; to ~ like быть склонным, испытывать желание (*сделать что-л.; часто с последующим pres. p.; см. тж.* 3); I don't ~ like a walk now мне что-то не хочется идти гулять; to ~ like drinking, eating иметь желание попить, поесть; 3) давать ощущение; быть на ощупь; the water ~s so cold вода такая холодная, вода кажется такой холодной; the air ~s cold воздух что-то холодный; to ~ like давать ощущение чего-л. (*см. тж.* 2); it ~s like velvet похоже на бархат; it ~s like rain по-видимому, будет дождь; 4) со)чувствовать, переживать; to ~ a friend's death переживать смерть друга; to ~ the insult deeply остро переживать оскорбление; to ~ deeply for smb. глубоко сочувствовать кому-л.; 5) видеть, сознавать; считать; иметь определённую точку зрения (*на что-л.— about*); I ~ that I ought to say no more я вижу, что больше говорить не должен; □ to ~ **up** быть в состоянии (*сделать что-л.— to*); I don't ~ up to a long hike today я сегодня не способен к длительной прогулке.

feeler ['fiːlə] *n* 1) *зоол.* щупальце, усик; 2) пробный шар, зондирование почвы; 3) *воен. разг.* разведчик.

feeling I ['fiːlɪŋ] *n* 1) ощущение, сознание (*чего-л.— of*); 2) чувство; good ~ дружелюбие; ill ~ враждебность; one's better ~s лучшее, что есть в человеке; 3) волнение, возбуждение; the speech aroused strong ~ on all sides речь вызвала у всех возмущение; I have no ~ about his attack on me я не сержусь на его нападки; 4) настроение; убеждение; мнение; what is your ~ about this idea? как вы находите эту мысль?

feeling II *a* 1) чувствительный; 2) сочувствующий.

feet [fiːt] *pl см.* foot I.

feign [feɪn] *v* 1) выдумывать, придумывать; 2) симулировать; притворяться.

feigningly ['feɪnɪŋlɪ] *adv* притворно.

feint [feɪnt] *n* 1) притворство; to make a ~ of притворяться; 2) *воен.* ложная атака; 3) *attr* притворный, ложный.

feldspar ['feldspɑː] *n мин.* полевой шпат.

felicitate [fɪ'lɪsɪteɪt] *v* поздравлять.

felicitous [fɪ'lɪsɪtəs] *a* подходящий, удачный.

felicity [fɪ'lɪsɪtɪ] *n* 1) счастье; блаженство; 2) удачность, меткость (*выражения*); 3) удачное, подходящее выражение.

feline ['fiːlaɪn] *a* 1) кошачий; 2) хитрый, злобный, коварный.

fell[1] [fel] *n* шкура, мех; ~ of hair нечёсаные волосы, космы.

fell[2] *n* 1) гора (*в названиях*); 2) болотистая местность (*в северной Англии*).

fell[3] *a поэт.* жестокий, ужасный, беспощадный.

fell[4] *v* 1) поражать ударом (*кулака, оружия*); 2) срубать, валить (*дерево*).

fell[5] *past см.* fall II.

fellah ['felə] *n* феллах.

feller ['felə] *сленг см.* fellow 1).

felloe ['felou] *n* обод (*колеса*).

fellow ['felou] *n* 1) человек, парень; poor ~ бедняга; my dear ~, my good ~ дорогой мой; a good ~ славный парень; old ~ старик, старина; 2) товарищ; собрат; 3) (F.) член совета колледжа; 4) (F.) член научного общества; 5) пара, парная вещь; 6) *attr:* ~ soldier соратник, собрат по оружию.

fellow-countryman ['felou'kʌntrɪmən] *n* соотечественник.

fellow-feeling ['felou'fiːlɪŋ] *n* 1) сочувствие, симпатия; 2) общность взглядов *или* интересов.

fellow-passenger ['felou'pæsɪndʒə] *n* спутник.

fellowship ['felouʃɪp] *n* 1) товарищество; 2) братство; сообщничество; 3) чувство товарищества (*тж.* good ~); 4) членство (*в совете колледжа; в научном обществе*).

fellow-traveller ['felou'trævlə] *n* 1) попутчик; 2) *полит.* сочувствующий, попутчик.

felly ['felɪ] *см.* felloe.

felon I ['felən] *n* уголовный преступник.

felon II *a поэт.* жестокий; преступный.

felonious [fɪ'lounjəs] *a* преступный, уголовный.

felony ['felənɪ] *n* уголовное преступление.

felspar ['felspɑː] *см.* feldspar.

felt[1] I [felt] *n* 1) фетр; войлок; 2) *разг.* фетровая шляпа; 3) *attr* фетровый; войлочный.

felt[1] II *v* 1) валять шерсть; 2) покрывать войлоком.

felt[2] *past, p. p. см.* feel II.

felucca [fe'lʌkə] *n* фелюга (*лодка*).

female I ['fiːmeɪl] *n* 1) женщина (*обыкн. пренебр.*); 2) самка; женская особь.

female II *a* 1) женского пола; 2) женский.

femineity [ˌfemɪ'niːɪtɪ] *n* 1) женственность; 2) женоподобность.

feminine ['femɪnɪn] *a* женский; женственный.

fen [fen] *n* болото, топь; the Fens низкая болотистая местность в Кембриджшире и Линкольншире.

fen-berry ['fenˌberɪ] *n* клюква.

fence I [fens] *n* 1) ограда; изгородь, забор; picket ~ частокол; 2) фехтование; 3) *сленг* укрыватель краденого; 4) *сленг* притон для укрывания краденого; ◊ to mend one's ~s *амер.* усиливать свои личные политические позиции; to sit on the ~ выжидать, не становиться ни на чью сто́рону (*в споре и т. п.*); to come down on the right side of the ~ стать на сто́рону победи́теля, сильне́йшей стороны́ (*в споре*).

fence II *v* 1) огора́живать, огражда́ть, окружа́ть (*тж.* to ~ about, in, round, up); 2) защища́ть; 3) фехтова́ть; to ~ with a question пари́ровать вопро́с; уклоня́ться от прямо́го отве́та; 4) брать барье́р (*о лошади*); 5) *сленг* торгова́ть кра́деным.

fence-month ['fensmʌnθ] *см.* fence-season.

fence-season ['fens͵siːzn] *n* вре́мя го́да, когда́ охо́та запрещена́.

fencing ['fensɪŋ] *n* 1) огора́живание; 2) *см.* fence I, 1); 3) фехтова́ние; 4) *сленг* укрыва́тельство кра́деного.

fend [fend] *v* 1) отража́ть, пари́ровать (*тж.* to ~ off, to ~ from); 2) не подпуска́ть, отгоня́ть (*тж.* to ~ away, to ~ from); 3) забо́титься (*for*); he must ~ for himself он до́лжен сам забо́титься о себе́.

fender ['fendə] *n* 1) предохрани́тельная решётка (*на паровозе, трамвае*); огражда́ющий щит; 2) *мор.* кра́нец, прива́льный брус; 3) ками́нная решётка; 4) крыло́ (*автомобиля и т. п.*); 5) *амер.* щито́к от гря́зи (*над колесом автомобиля и т. п.*).

Fenian ['fiːnjən] *n ист.* фе́ний (*член ирландского тайного общества*).

fennel ['fenl] *n* фе́нхель, сла́дкий укро́п.

fenny ['fenɪ] *a* боло́тистый.

feoff [fef] *см.* feud².

feoffee [fe'fiː] *n ист.* владе́лец ле́на, ле́нник.

fermentᵃ ['fəːment] *n* 1) ферме́нт, дро́жжи, заква́ска; 2) возбужде́ние, броже́ние.

fermentᵇ [fəˈment] *v* 1) броди́ть; вызыва́ть броже́ние; 2) волнова́ть(ся); быть в возбужде́нии.

fermentation [͵fəːmen'teɪʃən] *n* 1) броже́ние, фермента́ция; 2) волне́ние, броже́ние.

fern [fəːn] *n бот.* па́поротник.

ferocious [fəˈrouʃəs] *a* ди́кий; свире́пый; жесто́кий.

ferocity [fəˈrɔsɪtɪ] *n* ди́кость; свире́пость; жесто́кость.

ferret¹ I ['ferɪt] *n* 1) хорёк; 2) сы́щик.

ferret¹ II *v* 1) охо́титься с хорько́м; 2) выгоня́ть из норы́ (*from, out of; тж.* to ~ off, away, out); 3) ша́рить, ры́ться (*for; тж.* to ~ about); □ to ~ out разы́скивать; выпы́тывать, разузнава́ть.

ferret² *n* пло́тная тесьма́.

ferriferous [feˈrɪfərəs] *a* содержа́щий желе́зо, желе́зистый.

ferro-concrete ['ferou'kɔŋkriːt] *n* железобето́н.

ferrous ['ferəs] *a хим.* желе́зистый.

ferrule ['feruːl] *n* 1) металли́ческий ободо́к *или* наконе́чник; 2) окружна́я желе́зная доро́га.

ferry I ['ferɪ] *n* перево́з, перепра́ва; паро́м; ◊ to take the ~ умере́ть.

ferry II *v* 1) перевози́ть, переправля́ться (*на лодке, пароме*); 2) *ав.* перегоня́ть (*самолёты*); перебра́сывать, доставля́ть (*по воздуху*).

ferry-boat ['feribout] *n* паро́м.

ferryman ['ferɪmən] *n* перево́зчик, паро́мщик.

fertile ['fəːtaɪl] *a* 1) плодоро́дный, изоби́льный; 2) изобрета́тельный.

fertility [fəˈtɪlɪtɪ] *n* 1) плодоро́дие; 2) бога́тство (*воображения и т. п.*).

fertilization [͵fəːtɪlaɪ'zeɪʃən] *n* 1) удобре́ние (*почвы*); 2) *биол.* оплодотворе́ние; опыле́ние.

fertilize ['fəːtɪlaɪz] *v* 1) удобря́ть (*почву*); 2) *биол.* оплодотворя́ть.

fertilizer ['fəːtɪlaɪzə] *n* удобре́ние.

ferule ['feruːl] *n* лине́йка (*для наказания школьников*); ◊ to be under the ~ of быть в подчине́нии у кого́-л.

fervency ['fəːvənsɪ] *n* пыл, горя́чность; рве́ние.

fervent ['fəːvənt] *a* горя́чий, пы́лкий; ре́вностный.

fervid ['fəːvɪd] *a* горя́чий, пы́лкий.

fervour ['fəːvə] *n* жар, пыл; рве́ние; страсть.

festal ['festl] *a* пра́здничный; ра́достный.

fester I ['festə] *n* нагное́ние.

fester II *v* 1) гнои́ться (*о ране*); вызыва́ть нагное́ние; 2) терза́ть, му́чить.

festival ['festəvəl] *n* 1) пра́зднество; 2) фестива́ль.

festive ['festɪv] *a* пра́здничный; весёлый, ра́достный.

festivity [fes'tɪvɪtɪ] *n* 1) весе́лье; пра́зднование; 2) *обыкн. pl* пра́зднество, торжества́.

festoon I [fes'tuːn] *n* 1) гирля́нда; 2) *архит.* фесто́н.

festoon II *v* украша́ть гирля́ндами, фесто́нами.

fetch¹ I [fetʃ] *n* хи́трость, проде́лка.

fetch¹ II *v* 1) (сходи́ть и) привести́, принести́; to (go and) ~ a doctor сходи́ть за врачо́м; 2) вызыва́ть (*слёзы, вздох и т. п.*); 3) приноси́ть (*доход, деньги*); прода́ть за, вы́ручить; this won't ~ much за э́то мно́го не даду́т; 4) наноси́ть (*удар*); 5) *разг.* очаро́вывать, привлека́ть; □ to ~ away вы́рваться, освободи́ться; to ~ out выявля́ть; to ~ up а) рвать, тошни́ть; б) нагоня́ть, навёрстывать; в) *амер.* заверша́ть, зака́нчивать; ◊ to ~ and carry а) распространя́ть (*новости, слухи*); б) прислу́живать, быть на побегу́шках.

fetch² *n* при́зрак, привиде́ние.

fetching ['fetʃɪŋ] *a разг.* привлека́тельный, очарова́тельный.

fête I [feɪt] *n* 1) пра́здник, пра́зднество; 2) имени́ны.

fête II *v* пра́здновать; че́ствовать.

fetid ['fetɪd] *a* злово́нный.

fetish ['fiːtɪʃ] *n* 1) фети́ш; куми́р; 2) амуле́т.

fetlock ['fetlɔk] *n* щётка (*над копытом лошади*).

fetter I ['fetə] *n обыкн. pl* 1) пу́ты; 2) ножны́е кандалы́; 3) око́вы, у́зы; ра́бство.

fetter II *v* 1) спу́тывать (*лошадь*); 2) ско́вывать; зако́вывать (*в кандалы*); 3) свя́зывать, ско́вывать, стесня́ть.

fettle ['fetl] *n* положе́ние, состоя́ние; in good ~ в хоро́шем состоя́нии.

fetus ['fiːtəs] *см.* foetus.

feud¹ [fjuːd] *n* (насле́дственная) вражда́; blood ~ кро́вная месть, родова́я вражда́; deadly ~ сме́ртельная вражда́.

feud² *n ист.* фео́д, лен.

feudal ['fjuːdl] *a* феода́льный.

feudalism ['fjuːdəlɪzəm] *n* феодали́зм.

feudality [fjuːˈdælɪtɪ] *n* феодали́зм.

feuilleton ['fəːɪtɔːŋ] *n* 1) подвал (*в газете*); 2) фельетон.

fever I ['fiːvə] *n* 1) жар, лихорадочное состояние; лихорадка; brain ~ воспаление мозга; scarlet ~ скарлатина; intermitting ~ перемежающаяся лихорадка; spotted ~ сыпной тиф; typhoid ~ брюшной тиф; yellow ~, jungle ~ жёлтая, тропическая лихорадка; 2) нервное возбуждение.

fever II *v* бросать в жар; лихорадить.

feverish ['fiːvərɪʃ] *a* лихорадочный.

few I [fjuː] *a* немного, немногие; несколько (*тж.* a ~); in ~, in ~ words в немногих словах, вкратце.

few II *n* незначительное число, немногие; the ~ меньшинство, «избранные»; not a ~ много; a good ~ (of) порядочное число; (quite) a ~ *разг.* очень много, значительное количество.

fewness ['fjuːnɪs] *n* немногочисленность.

fez [fez] *n* феска.

fiancé [fɪ'ɑːnseɪ] *n* жених.

fiancée [fɪ'ɑːnseɪ] *n* невеста.

fiasco [fɪ'æskou] *n* неудача, фиаско.

fib¹ I [fɪb] *n разг.* выдумка, враньё.

fib¹ II *v разг.* выдумывать, врать.

fib² I *n спорт.* удар (*в боксе*).

fib² II *v спорт.* наносить удар(ы).

fiber ['faɪbə] *см.* fibre.

fibre ['faɪbə] *n* 1) волокно; жилка; 2) характер, склад характера; of coarse ~ грубый (*о человеке*).

fibred ['faɪbəd] *a* волокнистый.

fibrous ['faɪbrəs] *a* волокнистый; фиброзный.

fibster ['fɪbstə] *n* врунишка.

fickle ['fɪkl] *a* непостоянный, изменчивый.

fiction ['fɪkʃən] *n* 1) беллетристика; 2) вымысел, фикция.

fiction-monger ['fɪkʃən'mʌŋɡə] *n* выдумщик, враль.

fictitious [fɪk'tɪʃəs] *a* фиктивный; вымышленный, воображаемый.

fiddle I ['fɪdl] *n разг.* скрипка; ◊ fit as a ~ в прекрасном настроении; в добром здоровье; as long as a ~ вытянутый, мрачный (*о лице*); to hang up one's ~ оставить работу; выйти на пенсию; to play first ~ играть первую скрипку; занимать первенствующее положение.

fiddle II *v* 1) *разг.* играть на скрипке; 2) бездельничать, заниматься пустяками (*тж.* to ~ about); 3) *сленг* обманывать; he ~d it он скрыл недостачу (*тж.* подделкой счетов).

fiddlededee ['fɪdldɪ'diː] *n* чепуха, вздор.

fiddler ['fɪdlə] *n* 1) скрипач (*особ. уличный*); 2) бездельник; 3) *сленг* монета в 6 пенсов.

fiddlestick ['fɪdlstɪk] *n* смычок.

fiddlesticks ['fɪdlstɪks] *int* вздор, чепуха!

fidelity [fɪ'delɪtɪ] *n* 1) верность, преданность; 2) точность, правильность.

fidget I ['fɪdʒɪt] *n* 1) *обыкн. pl* беспокойное состояние; беспокойные, нервные движения; суетливость; 2) нервный, беспокойный человек.

fidget II *v* 1) беспокойно двигать, вертеться, ёрзать (*часто* to ~ about); 2) волноваться, суетиться; 3) волновать, нервировать.

fidgety ['fɪdʒɪtɪ] *a* суетливый, беспокойный.

fie [faɪ] *int* фу!; ~ upon you! какой стыд!

fief [fiːf] *см.* feud².

field I [fiːld] *n* 1) поле; большое пространство *или* протяжение; ~ of vision, visual ~ поле зрения; 2) месторождение (*см.* coal-field, gold-field, oilfield); 3) спортивная площадка; athletic ~ стадион, спортивная площадка; 4) поле битвы, сражения; сражение; in the ~ в походе, на войне; to keep the ~ вести военные действия; to take the ~ начинать сражение; 5) сфера, область деятельности *или* наблюдения; 6) *спорт.* игроки, участники состязания; участники охоты; 7) *attr* полевой; ◊ fair ~ and no favour равные условия состязания, равные шансы для всех.

field II *v спорт.* отбивать мяч.

field-glass ['fiːldɡlɑːs] *n* полевой бинокль.

Field-Marshal ['fiːld'mɑːʃəl] *n* фельдмаршал.

field-officer ['fiːld,ɔfɪsə] *n* старший офицер.

field-work¹ ['fiːldwəːk] *n воен.* полевое укрепление.

field-work² *n* полевая съёмка, работа в поле (*геолога и т. п.*).

fiend [fiːnd] *n* 1) дьявол; злой дух, демон; 2) *разг.* жертва вредной привычки; drug ~ наркоман; 3) *шутл.* энтузиаст чего-л.; mathematics ~ человек, увлекающийся математикой; fresh-air ~ любитель свежего воздуха.

fiendish ['fiːndɪʃ] *a* дьявольский, жестокий.

fierce [fɪəs] *a* 1) свирепый, лютый, беспощадный; неистовый; 2) сильный; 3) горячий; 4) *амер.* неприятный.

fiery ['faɪərɪ] *a* 1) огненный; пылающий; жгучий; 2) горячий, вспыльчивый; 3) воспламеняющийся.

fifteen ['fɪf'tiːn] *num* пятнадцать.

fifteenth I ['fɪf'tiːnθ] *num* пятнадцатый.

fifteenth II *n* пятнадцатая часть.

fifth I [fɪfθ] *num* пятый.

fifth II *n* пятая часть.

fifties ['fɪftɪz] *n pl* (the ~) 1) пятидесятые годы; 2) возраст от 49 до 60 лет.

fiftieth I ['fɪftɪθ] *num* пятидесятый.

fiftieth II *n* пятидесятая часть.

fifty ['fɪftɪ] *num* пятьдесят.

fifty-fifty I ['fɪftɪ'fɪftɪ] *a* равный; on a ~ basis на равных основаниях.

fifty-fifty II *adv* пополам, поровну; to go ~ делить поровну.

fig¹ [fɪɡ] *n* 1) *см.* fig-tree; 2) фига, винная ягода, инжир; 3) *разг.:* don't care a ~!, a ~ for! наплевать!

fig² I *n* 1) наряд; in full ~ в полном параде; 2) настроение; in good ~ в хорошем настроении.

fig² II *v* наряжать (*обыкн.* to ~ out, to ~ up).

fight I [faɪt] *n* 1) бой, битва, сражение; схватка, драка; *перен.* спор, борьба; ~ for peace борьба за мир; stand-up ~ открытая борьба; sham ~ показной бой (*на манёврах*); военная игра; to spoil for a ~ искать ссоры, лезть в драку; 2) задор; to have ~ in one быть полным задора; to show ~ не поддаваться.

fight II *v* (*past, p. p.* fought) сражаться, биться, вести бой, бороться, драться (*с, против —* with, against; *за —* for); □ to ~ **down** подавить; to ~ **off** побороть (*врага, болезнь*); to ~ **on** продолжать бороться, сражаться; to ~ **out:** to ~ (it) out довести борьбу до конца; ◊ to ~ shy of уклоняться, держаться в стороне.

fighter ['faɪtə] *n* 1) боёц; 2) *ав.* истреби́тель.

fighting I ['faɪtɪŋ] *n* сраже́ние, бой; борьба́; дра́ка; hand-to-hand ~ рукопа́шный бой; house-to-house ~ у́личные бои.

fighting II *a* боево́й.

figment ['fɪgmənt] *n* вы́мысел, плод воображе́ния.

fig-tree ['fɪgtriː] *n* смоко́вница, фи́говое де́рево.

figurative ['fɪgjurətɪv] *a* 1) метафори́ческий, о́бразный; фигура́льный; 2) изобрази́тельный; пласти́ческий.

figure I ['fɪgə] *n* 1) фигу́ра; вне́шний вид, о́блик; 2) фигу́ра, ли́чность; person of ~ выдаю́щаяся, заме́тная ли́чность; 3) ци́фра; double ~s двузна́чные чи́сла; control (*или* key, target) ~s контро́льные ци́фры; he got it at a low (high) ~ он доста́л э́то по дешёвой (дорого́й) цене́; what's the ~? ско́лько сто́ит!; 4) *pl* арифме́тика; 5) *мат.* фигу́ра, те́ло; 6) изображе́ние, портре́т, ста́туя; 7) иллюстра́ция, рису́нок, чертёж (*в книге; сокр.* fig.); 8) риторическая фигу́ра; ~ of speech мета́фора; 9) фигу́ра (*в танцах, на коньках*); ◇ to cut a ~ производи́ть впечатле́ние; игра́ть роль; to cut (*или* to make) a brilliant (poor) ~ представля́ть собо́й великоле́пную (жа́лкую) фигу́ру.

figure II *v* 1) представля́ть себе́ (*часто* to ~ oneself); how do you ~ it out? как вы э́то себе́ представля́ете?; 2) служи́ть си́мволом, прообра́зом; 3) фигури́ровать, игра́ть роль (*as*); 4) изобража́ть (*графически*); 5) обознача́ть ци́фрами; 6) рассчи́тывать, исчисля́ть; □ to ~ **on** рассчи́тывать на; де́лать расчёты; to ~ **out** выража́ться (*в цифрах; at*); to ~ **up** подсчи́тывать.

figured ['fɪgəd] *a* узо́рный, узо́рчатый, фигу́рный.

figure-head ['fɪgəhed] *n* 1) номина́льный нача́льник; подставно́е лицо́; 2) *шутл.* лицо́; 3) изображе́ние фигу́ры на носу́ корабля́.

filament ['fɪləmənt] *n* 1) нить, жи́лка; нитеви́дное волокно́; 2) *эл.* нить, волосо́к нака́ла.

filch [fɪltʃ] *v* укра́сть, стащи́ть.

file¹ I [faɪl] *n* 1) напи́льник; пи́лочка для ногте́й; 2) *сленг* хитре́ц, пройдо́ха, жу́лик (*обыкн.* old ~, deep ~); ◇ to bite (*или* to gnaw) the ~ предприня́ть безнадёжное де́ло.

file¹ II *v* 1) подпи́ливать, шлифова́ть напи́льником; 2) отде́лывать (*стиль и т. п.*); □ to ~ **away** (от)шлифова́ть.

file² I *n* 1) скоросшива́тель; шпи́лька (*для нака́лывания бумаг*); 2) подши́тые бума́ги; де́ло; подши́тый компле́кт газе́т; 3) картоте́ка.

file² II *v* 1) подшива́ть и храни́ть бума́ги; сдава́ть в архи́в; 2) *амер.* подава́ть, представля́ть докуме́нт(ы).

file³ I *n* 1) ряд, шере́нга (*тж. воен.*); in single ~, in Indian ~ гусько́м, зме́йкой; 2) хвост, о́чередь.

file³ II *v* идти́ гусько́м; □ to ~ **away** уходи́ть шере́нгой; to ~ **in** входи́ть шере́нгой; to ~ **off** *см.* to ~ away; to ~ **out** выходи́ть шере́нгой.

filer ['faɪlə] *n* скоросшива́тель, регистра́тор.

filet ['fɪ'leɪ] *n* 1) филе́, филе́йная рабо́та; 2) *кул.* филе́(й).

filial ['fɪljəl] *a* 1) сыно́вний, доче́рний; 2) филиа́льный.

filibuster I ['fɪlɪbʌstə] *n* 1) вое́нный авантюри́ст;

2) *амер. полит.* обструкциони́ст; 3) флибустье́р, пира́т.

filibuster II *v амер. полит.* применя́ть обстру́кцию.

filigree ['fɪlɪgriː] *n* филигра́нь, филигра́нная рабо́та.

filings ['faɪlɪŋz] *n pl* металли́ческие опи́лки.

fill I [fɪl] *n* 1) доста́точное коли́чество (*чтобы наполнить что-л.*); 2) по́лный запа́с; сто́лько, ско́лько хо́чется; to eat (to drink) one's ~ нае́сться досы́та (напи́ться вво́лю); 3) *амер.* на́сыпь.

fill II *v* 1) наполня́ть(ся); заполня́ть(ся); 2) затыка́ть, закла́дывать (*отверстие*); 3) пломби́ровать (*зуб*); 4) име́ться в доста́точном коли́честве; 5) удовлетворя́ть, насыща́ть; 6) занима́ть (*положение*); выполня́ть (*обязанности, поручения*); □ to ~ **in** а) заполня́ть; впи́сывать, вноси́ть; б) залива́ть, засыпа́ть; to ~ **out** расширя́ть(-ся), наполня́ть(ся); to ~ **up** а) наполня́ть(ся); заполня́ть(ся); б) дополня́ть; возмеща́ть (*недоста́ющее*); в) шпаклева́ть.

fillet ['fɪlɪt] *n* 1') у́зкая головна́я повя́зка; 2) *кул.* филе́(й).

filling ['fɪlɪŋ] *n* 1) наполне́ние, насы́пка; 2) запра́вка горю́чим; 3) зубна́я пло́мба; 4) наби́вка; шпаклёвка; 5) начи́нка.

fillip I ['fɪlɪp] *n* 1) щелчо́к; 2) побужде́ние, толчо́к, сти́мул; 3) пустя́к.

fillip II *v* 1) дать щелчо́к, щёлкнуть; 2) подтолкну́ть, напо́мнить.

filly ['fɪlɪ] *n* 1) молода́я кобы́ла; 2) молода́я весёлая де́вушка.

film I [fɪlm] *n* 1) то́нкая оболо́чка; лёгкий слой; перепо́нка; плёнка (*тж. фото*); 2) фильм; adventure ~ приключе́нческий фильм; box-office ~ фильм, де́лающий сбо́ры; crime (*или* whodunit) ~ детекти́вный фильм; nature ~ фильм о приро́де; feature ~ полнометра́жный фильм; 3) *pl* (the ~s) кинокарти́ны, кино́; 4) ды́мка, тума́н; пелена́; 5) то́нкая нить; 6) *attr* кино-.

film II *v* 1) покрыва́ть(ся) плёнкой, оболо́чкой; 2) застила́ться ды́мкой, тума́ном; 3) засня́ть; производи́ть киносъёмку; 4) экранизи́ровать (*лит. произведе́ние*); 5): he ~s (ill) well он (не)фотогени́чен.

filmdom ['fɪlmdəm] *n* кинопромы́шленность.

filmgoer ['fɪlm͵gouə] *n* кинозри́тель; посети́тель кино́.

filter I ['fɪltə] *n* фильтр.

filter II *v* 1) фильтрова́ть, проце́живать; 2) проса́чиваться (*о воде, новостях; тж.* to ~ through, to ~ out).

filth [fɪlθ] *n* 1) грязь; 2) отврати́тельная еда́, отбро́сы; 3) непристо́йность; скверносло́вие.

filthy ['fɪlθɪ] *a* 1) гря́зный, нечи́стый; 2) презре́нный, ни́зкий; 3) развращённый; непристо́йный.

filtrate ['fɪltreɪt] *см.* filter II.

filtration [fɪl'treɪʃən] *n* фильтрова́ние, фильтра́ция.

Fin [fɪn] *см.* Finn.

fin [fɪn] *n* 1) плавни́к; 2) *ав.* киль; 3) *сленг* рука́.

final I ['faɪnl] *n* 1) *спорт.* встре́ча в фина́ле, фина́л; 2) выпускно́й экза́мен.

final II *a* 1) после́дний; коне́чный, заключи́тельный; 2) оконча́тельный, реша́ющий; фина́льный.

finale [fɪˈnɑːlɪ] *n лит., муз.* финáл; grand ～ финáл óперы.

finality [faɪˈnælɪtɪ] *n* 1) закóнченность; окончáтельность; 2) заключéние.

finalize [ˈfaɪnəlaɪz] *v* заверша́ть, доводи́ть до концá.

finally [ˈfaɪnəlɪ] *adv* 1) в концé концóв, в заключéние; 2) окончáтельно.

finance I [faɪˈnæns] *n* 1) финáнсы; 2) *pl* дéньги, дохóды, финáнсы; 3) управлéние финáнсами.

finance II *v* 1) финанси́ровать; 2) занима́ться финáнсовыми операциями.

financial [faɪˈnænʃəl] *a* финáнсовый.

financier [faɪˈnænsɪə] *n* финанси́ст.

finch [fɪntʃ] *n* зя́блик.

find I [faɪnd] *v* (*past, p. p.* found) 1) находи́ть, обнару́живать; to ～ oneself а) очути́ться, оказа́ться; б) найти́ своё призва́ние (*см. тж.* 3); 2) находи́ть, приходи́ть к заключéнию, убежда́ться; 3) снабжа́ть; all found на всём готóвом; to ～ oneself забóтиться о своих ну́ждах, быть на своих харчáх (*см. тж.* 1); 4) *юр.* реша́ть; объявля́ть; □ to ～ **out** (раз)узна́ть, вы́яснить; поня́ть; обнару́жить, откры́ть.

find II *n* нахóдка; откры́тие.

finder [ˈfaɪndə] *n* 1) нашéдший, тот, кто нашёл; 2) *тех.* искáтель; 3) *фото* видоискáтель.

finding [ˈfaɪndɪŋ] *n* 1) нахóдка; откры́тие; 2) определéние (местонахождéния), ориентирóвка; 3) *pl* полу́ченные дáнные; 4) приклáд (*портнóго*); фурниту́ра (*сапóжника*); 5) приговóр (*судá*), верди́кт (*присяжных*).

fine[1] I [faɪn] *n* 1) пéня, штраф; 2) задáток.

fine[1] II *v* налагáть пéню, штраф; штрафовáть.

fine[2] *n*: in ～ в óбщем, слóвом; наконéц.

fine[3] I *a* 1) тóнкий; 2) нéжный, изя́щный, утончённый, краси́вый, делика́тный; 3) чи́стый; очи́щенный; высококáчественный; 4) прекрáсный, превосхóдный; слáвный; 5) я́сный (*о погóде*); 6) мéлкий; 7) блестя́щий, наря́дный; 8) óстрый; 9) тóчный.

fine[3] II *adv* изя́щно, тóнко; прекрáсно; to talk ～ говори́ть остроу́мно.

fine[3] III *n* я́сная погóда.

fine[3] IV *v* дéлать(ся) прозрáчным; очища́ть(ся); □ to ～ **away**, to ～ **down**, to ～ **off** дéлать(ся) тóньше; нежнéе; уменьша́ть(ся), заостря́ть(ся).

fine-drawn [ˈfaɪnˈdrɔːn] *a* тóнкий, иску́сный.

fine-grained [ˈfaɪnˈɡreɪnd] *a* мелкозерни́стый.

finery [ˈfaɪnərɪ] *n* пы́шный наря́д, украшéние; убрáнство.

fine-spun [ˈfaɪnˈspʌn] *a* 1) тóнкий (*о ткáни*); 2) хитросплетённый.

finesse [fɪˈnes] *n* 1) тóнкость; 2) ухищрéние; хи́трость.

finger I [ˈfɪŋɡə] *n* 1) пáлец; little ～ мизи́нец; index (ring) ～ указáтельный (безымя́нный) пáлец; 2) стрéлка, указáтель; ◇ to lay (*или* to put) one's ～ on а) косну́ться больнóго мéста; б) прямо указáть на; to point a ～ of scorn презри́тельно указывать (*на когó-л.— at*); to burn one's ～s обжéчься на чём-л.; to have a ～ in the pie быть замéшанным в дéле; приложи́ть ру́ку к чему́-л.; his ～s are all thumbs он óчень неуклю́ж; to snap one's ～s at смотрéть с презрéнием, плевáть, игнори́ровать; with a wet ～ с лёгкостью;

to twist (*или* to turn) smb. round one's little ～ помыкáть кем-л.; ≅ вить верёвки из когó-л.

finger II *v* 1) трóгать, прикасáться пáльцами; вертéть в пáльцах; 2) брать (взя́тку); воровáть; 3) игрáть (*на муз. инструмéнте*).

finger-alphabet [ˈfɪŋɡərˌælfəbɪt] *n* áзбука глухонемы́х.

finger-ends [ˈfɪŋɡərendz] *pl см.* finger-tips.

finger-language [ˈfɪŋɡəˌlæŋɡwɪdʒ] *см.* finger-alphabet.

finger-mark I [ˈfɪŋɡəmɑːk] *n* 1) след, пятнó от пáльцев; 2) *см.* finger-print.

finger-mark II *v* захватáть пáльцами.

finger-post [ˈfɪŋɡəpoust] *n* указáтельный столб.

finger-print [ˈfɪŋɡəprɪnt] *n* отпечáток пáльца.

finger-tips [ˈfɪŋɡətɪps] *n pl* кóнчики пáльцев; ◇ to have at one's ～ знать как свой пять пáльцев.

finical [ˈfɪnɪkəl] *a* 1) разбóрчивый, приди́рчивый; 2) жемáнный; изы́сканный; 3) причу́дливый.

finicking [ˈfɪnɪkɪŋ] *см.* finical.

finicky [ˈfɪnɪkɪ] *см.* finical.

finis [ˈfaɪnɪs] *n* конéц.

finish I [ˈfɪnɪʃ] *n* 1) конéц, окончáние; фи́ниш; 2) отдéлка; закóнченность.

finish II *v* 1) кончáть(ся), закáнчивать(ся) (*чем-л.— in, by*); 2) заверша́ть, отдéлывать (*тж.* to ～ off, to ～ up); 3) прекращáть(ся); 4) прикóнчить, уби́ть; 5) доконáть (*тж.* to ～ off).

finished [ˈfɪnɪʃt] *a* кóнченый; закóнченный, отдéланный.

finite [ˈfaɪnaɪt] *a* 1) ограни́ченный, имéющий предéл; 2) *грам.* ли́чный (*о глагóле*).

fink [fɪŋk] *n амер. сленг* штрейкбрéхер; шпиóн предпринимáтеля.

Finn [fɪn] *n* финн; the ～s фи́нны.

Finnish I [ˈfɪnɪʃ] *n* фи́нский язы́к.

Finnish II *a* фи́нский.

fiord [fjɔːd] *n* фиóрд.

fir [fəː] *n* 1) пи́хта; 2) ель (*тж.* ～-tree); 3) хвóйный лес.

fir-cone [ˈfəːkoun] *n* елóвая ши́шка.

fire I [ˈfaɪə] *n* 1) огóнь, плáмя; to set ～ разжигáть; поджигáть; to make up the ～ развести́ огóнь, затопи́ть пéчку; to keep up a good ～ поддéрживать си́льный огóнь; to mend the ～ уси́лить огóнь, подбрóсить тóплива; to strike ～ вы́сечь *или* разду́ть огóнь; to poke the ～ мешáть у́гли (кочергóй); on ～ в огнé, в плáмени, горя́щий; *перен.* в возбуждéнии; to set on ～ поджигáть; *перен.* возбуждáть; to catch (*или* to take) ～ загорéться; 2) пожáр; 3) жар, лихорáдка; St. Anthony's ～ рóжистое воспалéние; рóжа; 4) пыл, воодушевлéние; вдохновéние; 5) (оруди́йный) огóнь, стрельбá; concentric ～ сосредотóченный огóнь; running ～ бéглый огóнь; *перен.* град возражéний, крити́ческих замечáний *и т. п.*; under ～ под огнём; 6) *attr* пожáрный; 7) *attr* зажигáтельный; 8) *attr* огнеупóрный; 9) *attr воен.* огневóй; ◇ to shoot ～ сверкáть глазáми; метáть и́скры (*о глазáх*); to hang ～ мéдлить, мéшкать.

fire II *v* 1) поджигáть; зажигáть; 2) воспламеня́ть(ся); взрывáть(ся); 3) воодушевля́ть; разжигáть (*воображéние и т. п.*); 4) стреля́ть, вы́стрелить (*at*); вести́ огóнь; 5) топи́ть (*печь*); 6) прижи-гать; 7) обжига́ть (*кирпичи, посуду*); 8) *разг.* выгоня́ть, увольня́ть; □ to ~ **away** *разг.* начина́ть; ~ **away!** говори́, выкла́дывай!; to ~ **back** *косм.* передава́ть на зе́млю (*фотоснимки*); to ~ **off** вы́палить; to ~ **out** *см.* 8); to ~ **up** вспыли́ть.

fire-alarm ['faɪərəˌlɑːm] *n* 1) пожа́рная трево́га; 2) пожа́рный сигна́л.

fire-arm ['faɪərɑːm] *n обыкн. pl* огнестре́льное ору́жие.

fire-ball ['faɪəbɔːl] *n* 1) метео́р; 2) шарови́дная мо́лния; 3) *воен. ист.* зажига́тельное ядро́.

fire-bomb ['faɪəbɔm] *n* зажига́тельная бо́мба.

fire-brand ['faɪəbrænd] *n* 1) головёшка; 2) зачи́нщик, подстрека́тель.

fire-brick ['faɪəbrɪk] *n* огнеупо́рный кирпи́ч.

fire-brigade ['faɪəbrɪˌɡeɪd] *n* пожа́рная кома́нда.

fire-bug ['faɪəbʌɡ] *n* 1) *зоол.* светля́к; 2) *амер.* поджига́тель.

fire-control ['faɪəkənˌtrəul] *n* 1) борьба́ с лесны́ми пожа́рами; 2) *воен.* управле́ние огнём; 3) *тех.* регулиро́вка горе́ния.

fire-cracker ['faɪəˌkrækə] *n* (ёлочная) хлопу́шка.

fire-damp ['faɪədæmp] *n* рудни́чный газ.

fire-engine ['faɪərˌendʒɪn] *n* пожа́рная маши́на.

fire-escape ['faɪərɪsˌkeɪp] *n* пожа́рная ле́стница.

fire-extinguisher ['faɪərɪksˌtɪŋɡwɪʃə] *n* огнетуши́тель.

fire-fighter ['faɪəˌfaɪtə] *n амер.* (лесной) пожа́рный.

fire-fly ['faɪəflaɪ] *n зоол.* светля́к (*летающий*).

fire-hose ['faɪəhouz] *n* пожа́рный рука́в, шланг.

fire-insurance ['faɪərɪnˌʃuərəns] *n* страхова́ние от огня́.

fireman ['faɪəmən] *n* 1) пожа́рный; 2) кочега́р.

fire-place ['faɪəpleɪs] *n* 1) ками́н, оча́г; 2) *тех.* горн.

fire-plug ['faɪəplʌɡ] *n* пожа́рный кран.

fireproof ['faɪəpruːf] *a* огнеупо́рный.

fire-screen ['faɪəskriːn] *n* огнева́я заве́са.

fireside ['faɪəsaɪd] *n* 1) ме́сто у ками́на; *перен.* дома́шний оча́г; 2) *attr* дома́шний.

fire-warden ['faɪəˌwɔːdn] *n* пожа́рный инспе́ктор *или* объе́здчик (*в лесу*).

firewood ['faɪəwud] *n* дрова́.

firework(s) ['faɪəwɜːk(s)] *n* фейерве́рк.

fire-worshipper ['faɪəˌwɜːʃɪpə] *n* огнепокло́нник.

firing ['faɪərɪŋ] *n* 1) стрельба́; 2) прижига́ние; 3) о́бжиг.

firm¹ [fɜːm] *n* фи́рма.

firm² I *a* 1) твёрдый; про́чный, пло́тный; 2) постоя́нный, неизме́нный; усто́йчивый; непоколеби́мый; 3) насто́йчивый.

firm² II *v* 1) укрепля́ть(ся); уплотня́ть(ся); утрамбо́вывать зе́млю (*после посадки растений*).

firm² III *adv* 1) кре́пко, твёрдо, про́чно; 2) неизме́нно.

firmament ['fɜːməmənt] *n* небе́сный свод.

firmness ['fɜːmnɪs] *n* 1) твёрдость, кре́пость, пло́тность; про́чность; 2) неизме́нность, постоя́нство; непоколеби́мость.

fir-needle ['fɜːˌniːdl] *n* ело́вая *или* сосно́вая игла́, хво́я.

first I [fɜːst] *num* пе́рвый.

first II *a* 1) пе́рвый; ра́нний; 2) пе́рвый, выдаю́щийся; лу́чший.

first III *adv* 1) сперва́, снача́ла; пре́жде всего́ (*тж.* ~ of all, ~ and foremost); ~ and last в о́бщем; ~ or last ра́но и́ли по́здно; 2) скоре́е, предпочти́тельно; 3) впервы́е.

first IV *n* 1) (the ~) пе́рвое число́ (*месяца*); 2) (the ~) пе́рвый (*упомянутый человек или предмет*); 3): at ~ внача́ле, сперва́; from the ~ с (са́мого) нача́ла; from ~ to last с нача́ла до конца́; 4) *pl* первосо́ртные това́ры.

first-born ['fɜːstbɔːn] *n* пе́рвенец.

first-class I ['fɜːst'klɑːs] *a* первокла́ссный, превосхо́дный.

first-class II *adv* 1) превосхо́дно; 2) в пе́рвом кла́ссе (*поезда, парохода*).

first-fruits ['fɜːst'fruːts] *n pl* пе́рвые плоды́.

first-hand I ['fɜːst'hænd] *a* непосре́дственный, из пе́рвых рук.

first-hand II *adv* непосре́дственно, из пе́рвых рук.

firstling ['fɜːstlɪŋ] *n обыкн. pl* пе́рвые плоды́ *или* результа́ты; 2) пе́рвенец (*животного*).

firstly ['fɜːstlɪ] *adv* во-пе́рвых.

first-night ['fɜːst'naɪt] *n театр.* пе́рвое представле́ние, премье́ра.

first-nighter [ˌfɜːst'naɪtə] *n* посети́тель театра́льных премье́р.

first-rate I ['fɜːst'reɪt] *a* первокла́ссный, превосхо́дный.

first-rate II *adv разг.* превосхо́дно.

firth [fɜːθ] *n* 1) морско́й зали́в; морско́й рука́в; 2) у́стье реки́.

fir-tree ['fɜːtriː] *n* ель.

fiscal ['fɪskəl] *a* 1) фиска́льный; 2) фина́нсовый (*о годе*).

fish¹ I [fɪʃ] *n* (*pl тж. без измен.*) 1) ры́ба; to take ~ лови́ть ры́бу; 2) *пренебр.*: poor ~ никчёмный челове́к; cool ~ наха́л; odd ~, queer ~ чуда́к; 3) *attr* ры́бный, ры́бий; 4) *attr* рыболо́вный; ◊ to cry stinking ~ ≅ выноси́ть сор из избы́; to feed the ~es а) утону́ть; б) страда́ть морско́й боле́знью.

fish¹ II *v* 1) лови́ть, уди́ть ры́бу; 2) лови́ть, иска́ть (*в воде; for*); 3) *разг.* стара́ться получи́ть; домога́ться (*чего-л.— for*); □ to ~ **out** а) вы́ловить, перевести́ всю ры́бу (*в пруде, реке и т. п.*); б) выта́скивать; выу́живать, выпы́тывать (*секреты; of*); ◊ to ~ in troubled waters лови́ть ры́бу в му́тной воде́.

fish² *n* фи́шка.

fisher ['fɪʃə] *n* 1) рыба́к, рыболо́в; 2) рыба́чья ло́дка.

fisherman ['fɪʃəmən] *n* рыба́к, рыболо́в.

fishery ['fɪʃərɪ] *n* 1) ры́бная ло́вля, ры́бный про́мысел; 2) то́ня.

fish-hook ['fɪʃhuk] *n* рыболо́вный крючо́к.

fishing ['fɪʃɪŋ] *n* ры́бная ло́вля.

fishing-line ['fɪʃɪŋlaɪn] *n* лёса.

fishing-rod ['fɪʃɪŋrɔd] *n* уди́лище; у́дочка.

fishmonger ['fɪʃˌmʌŋɡə] *n* торго́вец ры́бой.

fish-pond ['fɪʃpɔnd] *n* 1) пруд для разведе́ния ры́бы, садо́к; 2) *шутл.* мо́ре.

fishwife ['fɪʃwaɪf] *n* 1) (у́личная) торго́вка ры́бой; 2) скандали́стка.

fishy ['fɪʃɪ] *a* 1) ры́бий; ры́бный; 2) ры́бный, бога́тый ры́бой; 3) *разг.* сомни́тельный, неправдоподо́бный.

fission ['fıʃən] *n* 1) *биол.* деле́ние кле́тки; 2) расщепле́ние а́тома (*тж.* atom ~); 3) *attr* а́томный (*о бомбе*).

fissure ['fıʃə] *n* 1) тре́щина, расще́лина; изло́м; разры́в; 2) *анат.* изви́лина (*головно́го мо́зга*).

fist I [fıst] *n* 1) кула́к; 2) *разг.* рука́; 3) *шутл.* по́черк; ◊ to grease smb.'s ~ дать взя́тку, «подма́зать» кого́-л.; mailed ~ брониро́ванный кула́к, вое́нная си́ла.

fist II *v* уда́рить кулако́м.

fisticuffs ['fıstıkʌfs] *n pl* кула́чный бой.

fistula ['fıstjulə] *n мед.* фи́стула.

fit¹ [fıt] *n* 1) паракси́зм; припа́док, при́ступ; ~ of epilepsy (hysteria) припа́док эпиле́псии (истери́и); a ~ of nerves a) не́рвный припа́док; б) припа́док я́рости; 2) поры́в; a ~ of energy прили́в эне́ргии; by ~s (and starts) поры́вами; уры́вками; 3) настрое́ние; капри́з; влече́ние; жела́ние; a ~ of indifference состоя́ние безразли́чия, равноду́шия; a scolding (drinking) ~ жела́ние побрани́ться (вы́пить); ◊ to give smb. a ~ (*или* ~s) порази́ть, возмути́ть, оскорби́ть кого́-л.; to beat smb. into ~s легко́ победи́ть, поби́ть кого́-л.; to have a ~ быть о́чень удивлённым, поражённым, возмущённым.

fit² **I** *a* 1) (при)го́дный, подходя́щий; приспосо́бленный; 2) подоба́ющий, досто́йный; it is not ~ не подоба́ет; 3) гото́вый; I am not ~ я не могу́, я не в состоя́нии; 4) здоро́вый, бо́дрый.

fit² **II** *v* 1) соотве́тствовать; годи́ться; подходи́ть (*по хара́ктеру, разме́ру и т. п.*); быть впо́ру; the cap ~s ша́пка впо́ру; *перен.* ≅ не в бровь, а в глаз; 2) приспоса́бливать(ся), прила́живать(ся); 3) устана́вливать, монти́ровать; 4) снабжа́ть (*with*); 5) *амер.* гото́вить (*к поступле́нию в уче́бное заведе́ние*); □ to ~ in a) вставля́ть, приспоса́бливать, пригоня́ть; б) подходи́ть; to ~ on примеря́ть; пригоня́ть друг к дру́гу; to ~ out a) снаряжа́ть, снабжа́ть; экипирова́ть; б) обставля́ть.

fit² **III** *n* 1) приго́нка, приспособле́ние; tight ~ пло́тная приго́нка; 2): to be a bad (an excellent) ~ пло́хо (превосхо́дно) сиде́ть (*о пла́тье*).

fitchew ['fıtʃuː] *n* хорёк.

fitful ['fıtful] *a* су́дорожный; поры́вистый; преры́вистый.

fitness ['fıtnıs] *n* (при)го́дность; уме́стность.

fit-out ['fıtaut] *n разг.* снаряже́ние; обмундирова́ние; экипиро́вка.

fitter ['fıtə] *n* 1) монтёр, устано́вщик; меха́ник; сле́сарь; сбо́рщик; 2) портно́й, производя́щий раскро́й, приме́рку и подго́нку оде́жды.

fitting **I** ['fıtıŋ] *n* 1) прила́живание; приго́нка; приме́рка; 2) устано́вка, сбо́рка, монта́ж; 3) *обыкн. pl тех.* армату́ра, приспособле́ния; принадле́жности, прибо́р(ы).

fitting **II** *a* го́дный, подходя́щий; надлежа́щий.

fitting-shop ['fıtıŋʃɔp] *n* сбо́рочная мастерска́я.

five I [faıv] *num* пять.

five II *n* 1) число́ пять; пятёрка; 2) *pl разг.* пять па́льцев; пятерня́ (*тж.* bunch of ~s); 3) *pl* пятипроце́нтная це́нная бума́га; 4) банкно́т в 5 фу́нтов сте́рлингов *или* 5 до́лларов.

fivefold I ['faıvfould] *a* пятикра́тный.

fivefold II *adv* впя́теро.

fiver ['faıvə] *n разг.* пятёрка (*пять фу́нтов стерлингов или пять до́лларов*).

fix I [fıks] *v* 1) укрепля́ть, закрепля́ть; 2) внедря́ть, вводи́ть; 3) устана́вливать, назнача́ть, фикси́ровать (*срок, це́ну*); 4) отмеча́ть, устана́вливать (*како́е-л. явле́ние*); 5) устремля́ть, сосредото́чивать (*взгляд, мы́сли и т. п.; on, upon*); 6) привлека́ть, остана́вливать (*взгляд, внима́ние и т. п.*); 7) *фото* фикси́ровать, закрепля́ть; 8) де́лать *или* станови́ться жёстким; тверде́ть; 9) сгуща́ть(ся); 10) (*тж.* to ~ up) *амер.* заменя́ет любо́й глаго́л, означа́ющий приготовле́ние, приведе́ние в поря́док и т. п.; вы́бор пра́вильного перевода определя́ется дополне́нием и конте́кстом, *напр.:* to ~ a breakfast пригото́вить за́втрак; to ~ a coat пригото́вить, почи́стить *или* почини́ть пиджа́к; to ~ the fire развести́ ого́нь; to ~ up for the night устро́ить, приюти́ть на́ ночь; □ to ~ on вы́брать, останови́ться на чём-л.; to ~ up *см.* 10); to ~ upon *см.* to ~ on.

fix II *n* 1) диле́мма; затрудни́тельное положе́ние; 2) определе́ние местонахожде́ния (*самолёта, кора́бля*).

fixation [fık'seıʃən] *n* 1) фикса́ция; 2) сгуще́ние; 3) *фото* закрепле́ние.

fixed [fıkst] *a* 1) неподви́жный, постоя́нный, неизме́нный; 2) закреплённый; 3) *хим.* свя́занный; нелету́чий; ◊ well ~ *амер.* обеспе́ченный, состоя́тельный.

fixedly ['fıksıdlı] *adv* 1) при́стально, в упо́р; 2) твёрдо.

fixings ['fıksıŋz] *n pl амер.* 1) снаряже́ние; обору́дование; принадле́жности; 2) отде́лка (*пла́тья*); 3) *кул.* гарни́р.

fixture ['fıkstʃə] *n* 1) что-л. устано́вленное, про́чное; 2) армату́ра; 3) устано́вленная, фикси́рованная величина́; 4) *разг.* лицо́, про́чно обоснова́вшееся в како́м-л. ме́сте; старожи́л; 5) назна́ченный день (*для состяза́ния и т. п.*); 6) *юр.* дви́жимость, продава́емая вме́сте с до́мом, землёй.

fix-up ['fıksʌp] *n амер.* приспособле́ние, устро́йство.

fizgig ['fızgıg] *n* 1) коке́тливая молода́я же́нщина, коке́тка; 2) шути́ха (*фейерве́рк*).

fizz I [fız] *n* 1) шипе́ние; 2) *разг.* шампа́нское.

fizz II *v* шипе́ть, и́скриться (*о вине́*).

fizzle I ['fızl] *n* 1) лёгкое шипе́ние; 2) фиа́ско, неуда́ча.

fizzle II *v* слегка́ шипе́ть; □ to ~ out конча́ться неуда́чей.

fizzy ['fızı] *a* газиро́ванный, шипу́чий.

flabbergast ['flæbəgɑːst] *v* ошеломля́ть, поража́ть.

flabby ['flæbı] *a* 1) отви́слый, вя́лый; 2) сла́бый; слабохара́ктерный.

flaccid ['flæksıd] *см.* flabby.

flag¹ [flæg] *n* 1) зна́мя; 2) флаг, флажо́к; ~ of truce, white ~ бе́лый (парламентёрский) флаг; black ~ a) чёрный (пира́тский) флаг; б) флаг, поднима́емый над тюрьмо́й в знак соверши́вшейся ка́зни; yellow ~ жёлтый (каранти́нный) флаг; to lower one's ~ a) спуска́ть флаг для салю́та; б) сдава́ться; покоря́ться; to hoist (to strike) one's ~ принима́ть (сдава́ть) кома́ндование; 3) *attr* фла́гманский.

flag[1] II *v* 1) поднима́ть флаг; украша́ть фла́гами; 2) сигнализи́ровать фла́гами *или* флажка́ми; □ to ~ **down** останови́ть (*кого-л.*).

flag[2] *n* 1) *бот.* и́рис; шпа́жник; 2) дли́нный и то́нкий лист расте́ния.

flag[3] I *n* 1) ка́менная плита́; 2) *pl см.* flagging[1] 1).

flag[3] II *v* мости́ть, выстила́ть ка́менными плита́ми.

flag[4] *v* 1) пови́снуть, пони́кнуть; 2) ослабева́ть, затиха́ть.

flag-captain ['flæg'kæptɪn] *n* команди́р фла́гманского корабля́.

flagellation [ˌflædʒə'leɪʃən] *n* бичева́ние.

flagging[1] ['flægɪŋ] *n* 1) мостова́я, тротуа́р, пол из ка́менных плит; 2) моще́ние, выстила́ние пли́тами.

flagging[2] *a* слабе́ющий, затиха́ющий.

flagitious [flə'dʒɪʃəs] *a* престу́пный; гну́сный; отврати́тельный, ужа́сный.

flagman ['flægmən] *n* сигна́льщик.

flag-officer ['flæg.ɔfɪsə] *n* адмира́л.

flagon ['flægən] *n* 1) графи́н, кувши́н; 2) больша́я пло́ская буты́ль, фля́га.

flag-pole ['flæg.poul] *n* флагшто́к.

flagrant ['fleɪgrənt] *a* 1) вопию́щий, возмути́тельный; 2) ужа́сный, ужаса́ющий.

flagship ['flægʃɪp] *n* фла́гманский кора́бль.

flagstaff ['flægstɑːf] *n* флагшто́к.

flag-station ['flæg.steɪʃən] *n* остано́вка (по́езда) по тре́бованию.

flagstone ['flægstoun] *n* ка́менная плита́ для моще́ния.

flail I [fleɪl] *n* цеп.

flail II *v* молоти́ть.

flair [fleə] *n* 1) чутьё, нюх; 2) любо́вь, скло́нность.

flak [flæk] *n* 1) зени́тная артилле́рия; 2) ого́нь зени́тной артилле́рии; 3) *attr* противозени́тный, защи́тный.

flake[1] I [fleɪk] *n* 1) лёгкий *или* пуши́стый клочо́к чего́-л.; ~ of snow снежи́нка; ~ of fire и́скра; 2) *pl* хло́пья; 3) чешу́йка; 4) ряд, слой.

flake[1] II *v* 1) па́дать хло́пьями; 2) рассла́иваться (*тж.* to ~ away, to ~ off).

flake[2] *n* суши́лка для ры́бы.

flaky ['fleɪkɪ] *a* 1) хлопьеви́дный; 2) сло́истый; чешу́йчатый.

flam [flæm] *n* вы́думка; ложь.

flamboyant [flæm'bɔɪənt] *a* цвети́стый, я́ркий, вы́чурный.

flame I [fleɪm] *n* 1) пла́мя; the ~s ого́нь; in ~s в огне́; to shoot out ~ изверга́ть пла́мя; 2) фа́кел (*ракетного двигателя*); 3) пыл, страсть; 4) *разг.* предме́т стра́сти; an old ~ of mine моя́ ста́рая любо́вь.

flame II *v* 1) пыла́ть, горе́ть, пламене́ть; 2) воспламеня́ть; 3) вспы́хнуть (*о страсти, лице*); 4) сия́ть, свети́ться; 5) подверга́ться де́йствию огня́ (*напр., для стерилиза́ции*); □ to ~ **out** вспы́хнуть, вспыли́ть; to ~ **up** вспы́хнуть, покрасне́ть.

flameproof ['fleɪmpruːf] *a* невоспламеня́ющийся, огнесто́йкий.

flaming ['fleɪmɪŋ] *a* 1) пыла́ющий; горя́щий; 2) я́ркий, пламене́ющий; 3) жа́ркий; 4) пы́лкий, пла́менный.

flammable ['flæməbl] *a* горю́чий, воспламеня́емый.

flange ['flændʒ] *n* 1) вы́ступ, борт; 2) *тех.* край; закра́ина.

flank I [flæŋk] *n* 1) бок, сторона́; 2) склон (*горы*); 3) боковая́ сторона́ (*здания*); 4) *воен.* фланг; to turn the ~ of обойти́ фланг; *перен.* перехитри́ть (*кого-л.*); разби́ть, опрове́ргнуть (*доводы*); 5) *attr воен.* фланго́вый, фланки́рующий.

flank II *v* 1) располага́ть, находи́ться, быть располо́женным сбо́ку; грани́чить, примыка́ть; 2) *воен.* фланки́ровать.

flannel I ['flænl] *n* 1) флане́ль; 2) *pl* флане́левый (спорти́вный) костю́м; флане́левое бельё; to be awarded one's ~s заслужи́ть пра́во носи́ть цвета́ свое́й кома́нды (*в игре́ в крике́т*).

flannel II *a* флане́левый.

flannel III *v* протира́ть флане́лью.

flannelled ['flænld] *a* во флане́левом костю́ме.

flap I [flæp] *n* 1) что-л., *прикреплённое то́лько с одной стороны, напр.*: две́рца лю́ка, откидна́я доска́ стола́, кла́пан (карма́на), нау́шник, поля́ шля́пы *и т. п.*; 2) лёгкий уда́р, шлепо́к; 3) взмах кры́льев; 4) хлопу́шка (*для мух*); 5) *сленг* страх, смяте́ние; 6) *амер. сленг* возду́шный налёт.

flap II *v* 1) колеба́ть(ся), колыха́ть(ся); развева́ть(ся); 2) свиса́ть; 3) шлёпать, ударя́ть; 4) маха́ть; взма́хивать, хло́пать (*кры́льями*); 5) отгоня́ть (*тж.* to ~ away, to ~ off); □ to ~ **about** *сленг* болта́ть.

flapdoodle ['flæp.duːdl] *n* глу́пости, ерунда́.

flap-eared ['flæpɪəd] *a* вислоу́хий.

flapjack ['flæpdʒæk] *n* блин, ола́дья.

flapper ['flæpə] *n* 1) *см.* flap I, 1) *и* 4); 2) ласт (*моржа, тюленя*); 3) ди́кий утёнок; птене́ц куропа́тки; 4) *разг.* де́вочка-подро́сток; 5) *сленг* рука́; 6) напомина́ние.

flare I [fleə] *n* 1) я́ркий неро́вный свет; сверка́ние; я́ркое пла́мя; 2) вспы́шка (*пламени*); 3) светово́й сигна́л; 4) освети́тельная раке́та; 5) *разг.* хва́стовство; показно́й блеск.

flare II *v* 1) горе́ть, вспы́хивать я́рким пла́менем; сверка́ть; 2) вспы́хнуть, вспыли́ть (*тж.* to ~ up, to ~ out); 3) выступа́ть нару́жу, выдава́ться.

flare-up ['fleər'ʌp] *n* 1) вспы́шка (*пламени, света, гнева и т. п.*); 2) блестя́щий, но непродолжи́тельный успе́х; 3) шу́мная ссо́ра; шу́мное весе́лье.

flaring ['fleərɪŋ] *a* 1) крича́щий, броса́ющийся в глаза́; 2) пыла́ющий; вспы́хивающий.

flash I [flæʃ] *n* 1) вспы́шка, про́блеск; in a ~ в одно́ мгнове́ние; 2) показно́й блеск, хва́стовство; 3) *амер.* кра́ткое телегра́фное сообще́ние (*в газете*); bulletin ~ сво́дка о хо́де вы́боров (*передава́емая по ра́дио*).

flash II *a* 1) показно́й, крича́щий; 2) подде́льный, фальши́вый; 3) воровско́й.

flash III *v* 1) вспы́хивать; пыла́ть; сверка́ть; 2) мелька́ть; промелькну́ть; осени́ть; 3) сообща́ть по телегра́фу; □ to ~ **out**, to ~ **up** вспы́хнуть, вспыли́ть.

flash-light ['flæʃlaɪt] *n* 1) сигна́льный ого́нь; про́блесковый свет мая́ка; 2) карма́нный электри́ческий фона́рь; 3) вспы́шка ма́гния.

flash-point ['flæʃpɔɪnt] *n* температу́ра вспы́шки, то́чка воспламене́ния; ~s of war очаги́ войны́.

flashy ['flæʃɪ] *a* дешёвый, показной; бросающийся в глаза, кричащий.

flask [flɑːsk] *n* 1) фляжка; vacuum ~ термос; 2) оплетённая бутыль; 3) пороховница; 4) *хим.* колба.

flat¹ [flæt] *n* квартира (*расположенная на одном этаже*).

flat² I *n* 1) плоская поверхность; плоскость; 2) равнина, низина; 3) вагон-платформа; 4) плоскодонка; 5) *муз.* бемоль; 6) *театр.* задник; 7) *сленг* простофиля; 8) широкая неглубокая корзина.

flat² II *a* 1) плоский, ровный, гладкий; as ~ as a pancake совершенно плоский; 2) растянувшийся во всю длину, плашмя; to fall ~ не удаться, не иметь успеха, не произвести желаемого действия (*см. тж.* flat² III); 3) мелкий, неглубокий; 4) прямой, ясный, категорический; that's ~ это ясно, окончательно; 5) скучный, вялый, неоживлённый; плоский (*о шутке*); 6) выдохшийся, ослабевший; спустивший воздух (*о шине*); 7) *муз.* бемольный; 8) полосовой (*о железе*).

flat² III *adv* плоско, гладко; to stamp ~ притоптать; 2) плашмя; to fall ~ растянуться (*см. тж.* flat² II); 3) прямо, ясно; как раз; категорически, решительно; ~ and plain напрямик, ясно, точно.

flat-boat ['flætbout] *n* плоскодонная лодка.

flatbottomed ['flæt,bɔtəmd] *a* плоскодонный.

flat-car ['flætkɑː] *n* вагон-платформа.

flat-fish ['flætfɪʃ] *n* плоская рыба (*камбала и т. п.*); ◊ a regular ~ *разг.* настоящий дурак.

flat-foot ['flætfuːt] *n* 1) плоскостопие; 2) *амер. сленг* полисмен, полицейский.

flat-footed I ['flæt,futɪd] *a* 1) страдающий плоскостопием; 2) *амер. сленг* решительный; ◊ to catch ~ a) захватить врасплох; б) застать на месте преступления.

flat-footed II *adv амер. сленг:* to come out ~ твёрдо стоять на своём, решительно поддерживать что-л.

flat-iron ['flæt,aɪən] *n* утюг.

flatly ['flætlɪ] *adv* 1) плоско, ровно, гладко; 2) категорически, решительно; 3) скучно, безжизненно.

flatness ['flætnɪs] *n* 1) плоскость, ровность; 2) безвкусица; 3) скука, уныние; вялость; 4) решительность, прямота; категоричность.

flat-out ['flæt'aut] *n амер. разг.* неудача, провал.

flatten ['flætn] *v* делать(ся) плоским, ровным; выравнивать, разглаживать; □ to ~ out *ав.* выровнять (*самолёт*).

flatter ['flætə] *v* 1) льстить; превозносить; 2): to ~ oneself that льстить себя надеждой, что; сметь думать, что; ласкать (*слух, зрение*).

flatterer ['flætərə] *n* льстец.

flattery ['flætərɪ] *n* лесть.

flattie ['flætɪ] *n сленг* полицейский.

flattop ['flættɔp] *n разг.* авианосец.

flatulent ['flætjulənt] *a* 1) *мед.* вызывающий газы; страдающий газами; 2) напыщенный, надутый, претенциозный.

flatways ['flætweɪz] *adv* плашмя.

flatwise ['flætwaɪz] *см.* flatways.

flaunt [flɔːnt] *v* 1) реять, гордо развеваться (*о*

знамёнах); 2) размахивать (*флагом*); 3) рисоваться, щеголять.

flautist ['flɔːtɪst] *n* флейтист.

flavor I, II ['fleɪvə] *амер. см.* flavour I, II.

flavour I ['fleɪvə] *n* 1) аромат, букет (*вина*); 2) приятный вкус, запах; 3) привкус.

flavour II *v* придавать вкус, приправлять.

flavouring ['fleɪvərɪŋ] *n* (душистая) приправа, специя.

flavourless ['fleɪvəlɪs] *a* 1) безвкусный; 2) без запаха.

flaw¹ I [flɔː] *n* 1) трещина; 2) недостаток, порок, изъян; пятно; брак (*в товаре*); 3) упущение, ошибка, слабое место (*в документе и т. п.*).

flaw¹ II *v* 1) трескаться; вызывать трещины; 2) портить(ся); 3) *юр.* делать недействительным.

flaw² *n* сильный порыв ветра, шквал.

flawless ['flɔːlɪs] *a* безупречный.

flax [flæks] *n* 1) лён; 2) льняное полотно.

flaxen ['flæksən] *a* льняной.

flax-seed ['flæks‚siːd] *n* льняное семя.

flaxy ['flæksɪ] *a* льняной.

flay [fleɪ] *v* 1) сдирать кожу; 2) чистить, снимать кожицу, кору *и т. п.*; 3) резко критиковать, разносить; 4) вымогать; грабить, «драть шкуру».

flea [fliː] *n* блоха; ◊ a ~ in the ear резкий ответ.

flea-bite ['fliːbaɪt] *n* 1) укус блохи; 2) мелкая неприятность.

fleck I [flek] *n* 1) пятнышко, крапинка; веснушка; 2) блик (*солнца, света*); 3) частичка (*чего-л.*).

fleck II *v* покрывать пятнами, испещрять.

flecker ['flekə] *v* испещрять, покрывать пятнами.

fled¹ [fled] *past, p. p. см.* flee.

fled² *past, p. p. см.* fly² 1 6).

fledge [fledʒ] *v* 1) опериться; 2) выращивать птенцов; 3) выстилать пухом и перьями (*гнездо*).

fledg(e)ling ['fledʒlɪŋ] *n* только что оперившийся птенец; *перен.* неопытный юнец.

flee [fliː] *v* (*past, p. p.* fled) 1) убегать, спасаться бегством; 2) избегать, сторониться; 3) *только в past и p. p.* пролететь, промелькнуть, исчезнуть.

fleece I [fliːs] *n* 1) овечья шерсть; руно; 2) облака «барашками»; 3) *текст.* начёс, ворс.

fleece II *v* 1) обирать; вымогать (*деньги*); 2) густо покрывать.

fleecy ['fliːsɪ] *a* 1) шерстистый; покрытый шерстью; 2) курчавый, кудрявый.

fleet¹ [fliːt] *n* 1) флот; флотилия; the ~ военный флот; mercantile (air) ~ торговый (воздушный) флот; 2) парк (*автомобилей, тракторов и т. п.*).

fleet² *n* залив, ручей.

fleet³ I *a* 1) быстрый; 2) *поэт.* быстротечный; 3) мелкий, неглубокий (*о реке и т. п.*).

fleet³ II *v* 1) протекать, миновать, пролетать; 2) скользить мимо.

fleet³ III *adv* неглубоко.

Fleet Street ['fliːt'striːt] *n* Флит-стрит, лондонская пресса (*по названию улицы, где сосредоточены редакции газет*).

Fleming ['flemɪŋ] *n* фламандец.

Flemish I ['flemɪʃ] *n:* the ~ (*употр. как pl*) фламандцы.

Flemish II *a* фламандский.

flesh I [fleʃ] *n* 1) мя́со; те́ло; плоть; proud ~ *мед.* ди́кое мя́со; in ~ в те́ле, по́лный; in the ~ живо́й; во пло́ти; to lose ~ похуде́ть; to put on ~, to pick up ~ (по)толсте́ть, (по)полне́ть; ~ and blood а) плоть и кровь; б) челове́ческая приро́да; живо́й челове́к; в) *attr* живо́й, реа́льный; one's own ~ and blood бли́зкие (ро́дственники), своя́ кровь; 2) род челове́ческий; челове́ческая приро́да; all ~ всё живо́е; сме́ртные; 3) мя́коть (*плода*).

flesh II *v* 1) отка́рмливать; 2) полне́ть; 3) впервы́е обагри́ть кро́вью (*меч*).

fleshings [ˈfleʃɪŋz] *n pl* трико́ теле́сного цве́та.

fleshly [ˈfleʃlɪ] *a* 1) чу́вственный, пло́тский; 2) мирско́й, матери́альный.

flesh-pots [ˈfleʃpɔts] *n pl* жи́зненные бла́га; ро́скошь.

flesh-wound [ˈfleʃwuːnd] *n* пове́рхностная ра́на.

fleshy [ˈfleʃɪ] *a* мяси́стый.

flew [fluː] *past см.* fly² I.

flex I [fleks] *n* эл. ги́бкий шнур.

flex II *v* сгиба́ть, гнуть.

flexibility [ˌfleksɪˈbɪlɪtɪ] *n* ги́бкость; *перен. тж.* пода́тливость, усту́пчивость.

flexible [ˈfleksəbl] *a* ги́бкий; *перен. тж.* пода́тливый, усту́пчивый; легко́ приспособля́ющийся.

flexion [ˈflekʃən] *n* 1) сгиба́ние; 2) изги́б, изо́гнутость; 3) *грам.* фле́ксия.

flexional [ˈflekʃənl] *a* *грам.* флекти́вный.

flexuosity [ˌfleksjuˈɔsɪtɪ] *n* изви́листость; изви́лина.

flexuous [ˈflekʃuəs] *a* 1) изви́листый; 2) коле́блющийся.

flexure [ˈflekʃə] *n* сгиб, изги́б, кривизна́.

flibbertigibbet [ˈflɪbətɪˌdʒɪbɪt] *n* легкомы́сленный, пусто́й болту́н, спле́тник.

flick I [flɪk] *n* 1) щелчо́к; лёгкий уда́р (*хлысто́м и т. п.*); 2) ре́зкое движе́ние, толчо́к; 3) *pl разг.* кинокарти́на; to go to the ~s пойти́ в кино́.

flick II *v* 1) щёлкнуть; стегну́ть; 2) сма́хивать щелчко́м (*пыль, кро́шки и т. п.*); *обыкн.* to ~ away, to ~ off).

flicker I [ˈflɪkə] *n* 1) мерца́ние, коле́блющийся свет; про́блеск; 2) колеба́ние; 3) *pl разг.* кинокарти́на; ◊ without the ~ of an eyebrow ≅ и бро́вью не повёл, и гла́зом не моргну́л.

flicker II *v* 1) мерца́ть, мига́ть; 2) колеба́ться, колыха́ться, дрожа́ть; 3) налета́ть (*о ве́терке*); 4) вспы́хивать и га́снуть (*об огне́, наде́жде*).

flier [ˈflaɪə] *n* 1) лётчик; 2) пти́ца; насеко́мое; 3) быстрохо́дный парохо́д; 4) *амер.* экспре́сс; 5) рыса́к.

flight¹ [flaɪt] *n* 1) полёт; перелёт; non-stop ~ *ав.* беспоса́дочный перелёт; high-speed ~ *ав.* высокоскоростно́й полёт; probing ~ *ав., косм.* про́бный полёт, перелёт; space ~ косми́ческий полёт; free ~ *косм.* свобо́дный полёт; man-in-space ~ полёт челове́ка в ко́смос; 2) бег, тече́ние (*вре́мени*); 3) звено́ (*самолётов*); 4) ста́я (*птиц, насеко́мых*); 5) град (*пуль, стрел*); 6) марш (*ле́стницы; тж.* ~ of stairs); 7) ряд (*барье́ров на скачка́х, шлю́зов*); ◊ in the first (*или* highest) ~ на пе́рвом ме́сте, веду́щий.

flight² *n* бе́гство; побе́г; отступле́ние; to take (to) ~, to betake oneself to ~ обраща́ться в бе́гство, бежа́ть; to put to ~ обраща́ть в бе́гство.

flighty [ˈflaɪtɪ] *a* 1) капри́зный, ве́треный, непо-

сто́янный; 2) поме́шанный, полоу́мный; 3) пугли́вый (*о ло́шади*).

flimsy I [ˈflɪmzɪ] *n* 1) то́нкая бума́га; 2) *сленг* банкно́т, «бума́жка».

flimsy II *a* 1) хру́пкий, непро́чный; 2) неоснова́тельный, пове́рхностный.

flinch [flɪntʃ] *v* 1) отступа́ть; уклоня́ться (*от обя́занностей и т. п.*); 2) вздра́гивать.

fling I [flɪŋ] *n* 1) бросо́к, швыро́к; 2) ре́зкое движе́ние; 3) *разг.* вы́пад, ре́зкое, насме́шливое замеча́ние; to have a ~ at smb. напа́сть на кого́-л.; пройти́сь на чей-л. счёт; 4) поры́в (*весе́лья, гне́ва и т. п.*); to have one's ~ отда́ть дань удово́льствиям, перебеси́ться; ◊ the Highland ~ стреми́тельный шотла́ндский та́нец.

fling II *v* (*past. p. p.* flung) 1) броса́ть(ся), кида́ть(ся); 2) набра́сывать, наки́дывать (*пла́тье и т. п.; on*); 3) заки́дывать (*тж.* to ~ about); 4) испуска́ть, распространя́ть (*за́пах, свет*); □ to ~ about разбра́сывать; to ~ aside отверга́ть, пренебрега́ть; to ~ away а) отбра́сывать; б) бро́ситься вон; to ~ down а) сбра́сывать; б) разруша́ть, губи́ть; to ~ off а) сбра́сывать, стря́хивать; отде́лываться от; б) бро́сить (*замеча́ние*); в) дать выраже́ние (*чему́-л.*); to ~ out а) бро́ситься вон; б) разрази́ться (*бра́нью*); в) брыка́ться; to ~ to захло́пнуть; to ~ up бро́сить, оста́вить; ◊ to ~ up one's heels показа́ть пя́тки, удра́ть; to ~ oneself (up)on smb.'s mercy отда́ться на ми́лость кого́-л.

flint [flɪnt] *n* кре́мень; ◊ to skin a ~ быть скупы́м.

flinty [ˈflɪntɪ] *a* 1) кремни́стый, кремнёвый; 2) жёсткий, суро́вый.

flip I [flɪp] *n* 1) щелчо́к; 2) флип, подслащённый горя́чий напи́ток из сме́си пи́ва со спи́ртом.

flip II *v* щёлкать, слегка́ ударя́ть.

flippancy [ˈflɪpənsɪ] *n* 1) легкомы́слие, ве́треность; 2) непочти́тельность, де́рзость; 3) болтли́вость.

flippant [ˈflɪpənt] *a* 1) легкомы́сленный, ве́треный; 2) непочти́тельный, де́рзкий; 3) болтли́вый.

flipper [ˈflɪpə] *n* плавни́к; пла́вательная перепо́нка.

flirt I [flɜːt] *n* 1) предме́т уха́живания, фли́рта; 2) коке́тка; 3) толчо́к; взмах.

flirt II *v* 1) уха́живать, флиртова́ть (*with*); 2) подта́лкивать.

flirtation [flɜːˈteɪʃən] *n* уха́живание, флирт.

flirtatious [flɜːˈteɪʃəs] *a* коке́тливый, лю́бящий флиртова́ть.

flit [flɪt] *v* 1) порха́ть; 2) пролета́ть, проноси́ться (*ча́сто* to ~ about, by, past, to and fro); 3) переезжа́ть, уезжа́ть.

flitter [ˈflɪtə] *v* порха́ть.

flivver [ˈflɪvə] *n амер. сленг* 1) дешёвый автомоби́ль; 2) неуда́ча.

float I [fləut] *n* 1) поплаво́к; 2) буй; 3) плот, паро́м; 4) плаву́чая ма́сса (*льда и т. п.*); 5) го́нка, сплав (*ле́са*); 6) пузы́рь (*у ры́бы*); 7) пла́вательный пояс; 8): on the ~ на воде́, на плаву́; 9) *обыкн. pl театр.* ра́мпа; 10) поло́к, теле́га; 11) мастеро́к, тёрка (*штукату́ра*).

float II *v* 1) пла́вать, держа́ться на пове́рхности (*воды́ и т. п.*); 2) плыть, нести́сь (*по тече́нию, во́здуху*); *перен.* проноси́ться (*в мы́слях, перед глаза́ми*); 3) затопля́ть, наводня́ть; 4) спуска́ть (на *воду*); 5) снима́ть (*с мели*); 6) сплавля́ть (*лес*); 7) пуска́ть в ход (*предприятие*); 8) выпуска́ть (*заём*); 9) пуска́ть (*слух*).

floatable ['floutəbl] *a* 1) плаву́чий; 2) сплавно́й.

floatage ['floutɪdʒ] *n* 1) плаву́честь; 2) пла́вающие суда́ и ло́дки; 3) пла́вающие обло́мки; 4) надво́дная часть су́дна.

floatation [flou'teɪʃən] *n* 1) пла́вание; 2) *ком.* основа́ние предприя́тия; 3) *горн.* флота́ция.

floating I ['floutɪŋ] *n* пла́вание; free ~ свобо́дное пла́вание (*в состоянии невесомости*).

floating II *a* 1) пла́вающий; 2) плаву́чий; наплавно́й (*о мосте*); 3) перевози́мый мо́рем, морско́й; ~ сargo морско́й груз; 4) изме́нчивый, теку́чий.

floaty ['floutɪ] *a* 1) плаву́чий; 2) лёгкий.

flock[1] [flɔk] *n* 1) пуши́нка, клочо́к (*шерсти и т. п.*); 2) *pl текст.* очёс(ки); 3) *pl хим.* хло́пья.

flock[2] I *n* 1) ста́до (*мелкого рогатого скота или домашней птицы*); 2) ста́я (*птиц*); 3) толпа́ (*людей*); to come in ~s вали́ть толпо́й; 4) де́ти (*в семье*); ученики́ (*учителя*); 5) *церк.* па́ства.

flock[2] II *v* собира́ться, дви́гаться толпо́й; держа́ться вме́сте; стека́ться (*о толпе*).

floe [flou] *n* плаву́чая льди́на (*тж.* ice-floe).

flog [flɔg] *v* 1) поро́ть, сечь; 2) стега́ть, подстёгивать; 3) *сленг* побива́ть, побежда́ть; □ to ~ into вбива́ть, побо́ями внуша́ть (*что-л.*); to ~ out выбива́ть, побо́ями отуча́ть (*от чего-л.*).

flogging ['flɔgɪŋ] *n* по́рка.

flood I [flʌd] *n* 1) наводне́ние; полово́дье; пото́п; пото́к (*тж. перен.*); ~s of rain пото́ки дождя́; a ~ of tears пото́к слёз; the Flood *библ.* всеми́рный пото́п; 2) прили́в; 3) *поэт.* река́, мо́ре, пото́к; ~ and field вода́ и су́ша; ◇ to throw a ~ of light пролива́ть свет.

flood II *v* 1) затопля́ть, наводня́ть; залива́ть; переполня́ть (*водой*); 2) хлы́нуть; 3) ороша́ть.

flood-gate ['flʌdgeɪt] *n* шлюз(ные воро́та).

flood-light I ['flʌdlaɪt] *n* проже́ктор.

flood-light II *v* освеща́ть проже́ктором.

flood-lit ['flʌdlɪt] *a* освещённый проже́ктором.

flood-tide ['flʌdtaɪd] *n* прили́в.

floor I [flɔː] *n* 1) пол; насти́л; corn ~ гумно́, ток; dirt (parqueted) ~ земляно́й (паркéтный) пол; to pace the ~ ходи́ть по ко́мнате взад и вперёд; 2) эта́ж, я́рус; first ~ a) второ́й эта́ж; б) *амер.* пе́рвый эта́ж; 3) места́ чле́нов собра́ния, парла́мента в за́ле заседа́ний; to cross the ~ of the House *парл.* перейти́ из одно́й па́ртии в другу́ю; 4) (the ~) пра́во выступле́ния; to ask (*или* to claim) the ~ проси́ть сло́ва; to have (*или* to take) the ~ выступа́ть, брать сло́во; 5) дно (*моря*).

floor II *v* 1) настила́ть пол; 2) повали́ть, сбить с ног; одоле́ть; 3) смути́ть, поста́вить в тупи́к; 4) посади́ть на ме́сто (*ученика, не знающего урока*).

floor-cloth ['flɔːklɔθ] *n* линоле́ум.

floorer ['flɔːrə] *n* 1) сокруши́тельный уда́р; 2) затрудни́тельное положе́ние; 3) *разг.* тру́дный, озада́чивающий вопро́с.

flooring ['flɔːrɪŋ] *n* 1) насти́л пола; 2) пол.

flop I [flɔp] *n* 1) шлепо́к; 2) *сленг* неуда́ча.

flop II [flɔp] *v* 1) шлёпать(ся); бить(ся); полоскáться (*о парусах*); 2) плюхнуться, шлёпнуться (*тж.* to ~ down); 3) швырну́ть (*тж.* to ~ down); 4) *сленг*

потерпе́ть неуда́чу; 5) переметну́ться (*к другой па́ртии; тж.* to ~ over).

flop III *int* шлёп!

flop-house ['flɔphaus] *n амер.* ночле́жный дом.

floppy ['flɔpɪ] *a* 1) вися́щий, болта́ющийся; 2) лени́вый (*об уме*); 3) небре́жный (*о стиле*).

flora ['flɔːrə] *n* (*pl тж.* florae ['flɔːriː]) фло́ра.

floral ['flɔːrəl] *n* 1) цвето́чный; 2) относя́щийся к фло́ре.

florescence [flɔː'resns] *n* цвете́ние; *перен.* расцве́т.

floriculture ['flɔːrɪkʌltʃə] *n* цветово́дство.

florid ['flɔrɪd] *a* 1) цвети́стый, вы́чурный; 2) крича́щий, показно́й; 3) цвету́щий, румя́ный.

florin ['flɔrɪn] *n* флори́н (*монета*).

florist ['flɔrɪst] *n* 1) торго́вец цвета́ми; 2) цветово́д.

flotilla [flou'tɪlə] *n* флоти́лия.

flotsam ['flɔtsəm] *n* пла́вающие обло́мки; ~ and jetsam a) обло́мки; б) никчёмные лю́ди.

flounce[1] I [flauns] *n* ре́зкое движе́ние.

flounce[1] II *v* броса́ться, мета́ться.

flounce[2] I *n* обо́рка.

flounce[2] II *v* отде́лывать обо́рками.

flounder[1] ['flaundə] *n* пло́ская ры́ба (*мелкая камбала и т. п.*).

flounder[2] *v* 1) бара́хтаться; спотыка́ться; тяжело́, с трудо́м (пере)ступа́ть; 2) де́лать оши́бки, пу́таться (*в делах, словах*).

flour I ['flauə] *n* 1) (пшени́чная) мука́; 2) порошо́к, пу́дра.

flour II *v* 1) посыпа́ть муко́й; 2) *амер.* моло́ть (*зерно*).

flouring-mill ['flauərɪŋˌmɪl] *n амер.* ме́льница.

flourish I ['flʌrɪʃ] *n* 1) завиту́шка; ро́счерк (*пера*); 2) цвети́стое *или* напы́щенное выраже́ние; прикра́сы; 3) разма́хивание (*оружием, руками*); *перен.* хвастовство́, ва́жничанье; 4) *муз.* туш, фанфа́ры; 5): in full ~ в по́лном расцве́те.

flourish II *v* 1) пы́шно расти́; 2) процвета́ть, преуспева́ть; 3) де́лать завиту́шки, ро́счерк (*пером*); 4) выставля́ть напока́з, хва́стать; 5) разма́хивать (*оружием, руками*).

flourishing ['flʌrɪʃɪŋ] *a* 1) здоро́вый, цвету́щий; 2) процвета́ющий.

flourmill ['flauəmɪl] *n* ме́льница.

flout I [flaut] *n* насме́шка, издева́тельство.

flout II *v* насмеха́ться, издева́ться.

flow I [flou] *n* 1) тече́ние; 2) пото́к; струя́; a steady ~ непреры́вный пото́к; 3) прили́в; 4) наплы́в, изоби́лие; ~ of spirits жизнера́достность; ~ of soul серде́чный разгово́р; серде́чные излия́ния; 5) пла́вность ли́ний (*платья, фигуры*).

flow II *v* 1) течь, струи́ться (*тж. перен.*); разлива́ться; 2) прибыва́ть (*о воде*); 3) стека́ться, прибыва́ть; 4) ниспада́ть (*о платье, складках*); 5) *уст.* изоби́ловать (with); □ to ~ down стека́ть; to ~ in впада́ть; стека́ться; to ~ out вытека́ть; происте-ка́ть.

flower I ['flauə] *n* 1) цвето́к; цвету́щее расте́ние; in ~ в цвету́; natural ~s живы́е цветы́; 2) цвет, краса́ (*чего-л. — of*); 3) цвете́ние, расцве́т; 4) *attr* цвето́чный; ◇ to sprinkle the ~s *амер. сленг* дава́ть взя́тки.

flower II *v* 1) цвести́; 2) украша́ть цвета́ми *или* цвето́чным узо́ром.

flowerbed ['flauəbed] *n* клумба.

floweret ['flauərɪt] *n поэт.* цветочек.

flowerpot ['flauəpɔt] *n* цветочный горшок.

flower-show ['flauəʃou] *n* выставка цветов.

flowery ['flauərɪ] *a* 1) покрытый цветами; 2) цветистый.

flowing ['flouɪŋ] *a* 1) текущий; 2) гладкий, плавный.

flown [floun] *p. p. см.* fly² I.

flu [fluː] *сокр. разг. см.* influenza.

fluctuate ['flʌktʃueit] *v* 1) колебаться; быть неустойчивым, нерешительным; 2) колыхать(ся), волновать(ся).

fluctuation [ˌflʌktʃu'eiʃən] *n* 1) колебание; неустойчивость; неуверенность; 2) колыхание.

flue¹ [fluː] *n* пушок; *pl* хлопья.

flue² *n* 1) дымовая труба, дымоход; 2) вытяжная труба, вытяжка.

flue³ *n см.* flu.

flue⁴ *v* расширять (отверстие); расширяться.

fluency ['fluːənsɪ] *n* плавность, беглость (*речи*).

fluent I ['fluːənt] *n мат.* интеграл; переменная величина; функция.

fluent II *a* 1) гладкий, плавный; беглый (*о речи*); 2) свободно, бегло говорящий (*об ораторе и т. п.*).

fluently ['fluːəntlɪ] *adv* плавно, гладко; бегло (*о речи*).

fluff I [flʌf] *n* 1) пух, пушок; ворс; 2) пушистый мех; 3) *театр. сленг* плохо выученная роль.

fluff II *v* 1) ворсить; 2) взбивать, распушать (*тж.* to ~ up, to ~ out); 3) делать или работать кое-как, неумело; (ис)портить (*работу, игру*); 4) *театр. сленг* плохо знать роль.

fluffiness ['flʌfɪnɪs] *n* пушистость, мягкость.

fluffy ['flʌfɪ] *a* пушистый, мягкий.

fluid I ['fluːɪd] *n* жидкая *или* газообразная среда; жидкость; газ.

fluid II *a* жидкий, текучий; газообразный.

fluke I [fluːk] *n* (счастливая) случайность.

fluke II *v* повезти; достигнуть чего-л. благодаря (счастливой) случайности.

flummery ['flʌmərɪ] *n* пустяки, вздор; пустые комплименты.

flung [flʌŋ] *past, p. p. см.* fling II.

flunk I [flʌŋk] *n амер.* провал (*на экзамене*).

flunk II *v амер.* провалиться (*на экзамене*).

flunkey ['flʌŋkɪ] *n презр.* (ливрейный) лакей; *перен.* низкопоклонник, подхалим.

fluorescence [fluə'resns] *n* свечение, флюоресценция.

fluorescent [fluə'resnt] *a* флюоресцирующий; флюоресцентный.

flurry I ['flʌrɪ] *n* 1) сильный порыв ветра; шквал; ливень; снегопад; 2) возбуждение, волнение, оживление.

flurry II *v* волновать, возбуждать; будоражить.

flush¹ I [flʌʃ] *n* 1) внезапный приток воды; 2) внезапная краска, прилив крови (*к лицу*); 3) *поэт.* заря (*тж.* the ~ of dawn); 4) прилив (*радости и т. п.*); 5) наплыв, приток (*товаров и т. п.*); 6) приступ (*лихорадки*); 7) расцвет (*весны, молодости, сил*).

flush¹ II *a* 1) полный (*до берегов*); 2) в уровень, в край, впритык (*with*); 3) *обыкн. predic разг.* изобилующий, богатый (*чем-л. — of*); ~ of money богатый (деньгами); 4) щедрый, расточительный;

flush¹ III *v* 1) броситься в лицо (*о крови, краске*); вспыхнуть, покраснеть; (за)пылать; 2) быстро приливать, хлынуть (*о воде*); затоплять; 3) промывать (*струёй воды*); 4) быть охваченным (*гордостью, радостью; with*); □ to ~ up покраснеть, вспыхнуть.

flush² I *n* стая вспугнутых птиц.

flush² II *v* 1) взлетать, вспархивать; 2) вспугивать, поднимать (*дичь — о собаке*).

flush³ *n* карты одной масти на руках.

fluster I ['flʌstə] *n* волнение, суматоха.

fluster II *v* 1) волновать; 2) волноваться, суетиться; 3) подпоить; 4) подвыпить.

flute [fluːt] *n* флейта.

flutist ['fluːtɪst] *n* флейтист.

flutter I ['flʌtə] *n* 1) порхание; 2) трепетание; 3) трепет, волнение; возбуждение; 4) сенсация; переполох; 5) *разг.* спекуляция, риск (*обыкн. в азартных играх*).

flutter II *v* 1) махать крыльями; порхать, перепархивать; 2) трепетать, дрожать; метаться; 3) развеваться; 4) неровно биться (*о пульсе*); □ to ~ out выпорхнуть.

fluvial ['fluːvjəl] *a* речной.

flux I [flʌks] *n* 1) течение, поток; 2) прилив; 3) движение, смена; in a state of ~ в состоянии изменения.

flux II *v* 1) течь, вытекать, истекать; 2) плавить, растоплять; расплавлять.

fluxible ['flʌksɪbl] *a* плавкий.

fly¹ [flai] *n* муха; ◇ to break (*или* to crush) a ~ (up)on the wheel ≅ стрелять из пушек по воробьям; a ~ in the ointment ≅ ложка дёгтя в бочке мёда; there are no flies on him a) его не проведёшь; он начеку; б) он надёжен, он безупречен.

fly² I *v* (*past* flew; *p. p.* flown) 1) летать; лететь; to ~ high высоко заноситься, быть честолюбивым; 2) мчаться, нестись; 3) заставлять летать; гонять (*голубей*); 4) вести, пилотировать (*самолёт*); 5) развеваться; 6) (*past, p. p.* fled) покидать (*страну и т. п.*); □ to ~ at нападать; to ~ away пролетать; улетать; to ~ into a) впадать (*в гнев, ярость и т. п.*); б) вбежать, влететь (*в комнату*); в): to ~ into pieces разлететься на куски; to ~ off a) убегать; улетать; б) уклоняться; в) слетать, соскакивать (*с чего-л.*); to ~ out разражаться (*бранью, гневом*); to ~ over перепрыгнуть, перемахнуть (*через*); to ~ to бросаться (*к чему-л.*); браться (*за что-л.*); to ~ upon *см.* to ~ at; ◇ ~ in the face of открыто не повиноваться, бросать вызов (*кому-л.*); to let ~ (at) а) стрелять (*в кого-л., что-л.*); б) сильно выругать; to send smb. flying выгнать кого-л.

fly² II *n* 1) полёт, перелёт; 2) одноконный наёмный экипаж; 3) клапан (*кармана*); 4) откидное полотнище (*палатки*); 5) крыло (*ветряка*).

fly³ *a разг.* осмотрительный, хитрый.

fly-away ['flaiəˌwei] *a* 1) развевающийся (*об одежде, волосах*); 2) ветреный, непостоянный; легкомысленный.

fly-bitten ['flaiˌbitn] *a* засиженный мухами.

fly-catcher ['flaiˌkætʃə] *n* 1) мухоловка; 2) мухолов (*птица*); 3) насекомоядное растение.

flyer ['flaiə] *см.* flier.

flying I ['flaiiŋ] *n* 1) полёт(ы); high-altitude ~

высо́тные полёты; blind ~ слепо́й полёт; 2) лётное де́ло.

flying II *a* 1) лета́ющий, лета́тельный; летучий; 2) *ав.* лётный; 3) бы́стрый; мимолётный; 4) развева́ющийся.

fly-leaf ['flaɪliːf] *n полигр.* фо́рзац.

fly-sheet ['flaɪʃiːt] *n* листо́вка.

fly-trap ['flaɪtræp] *n см.* fly-catcher 1) *и* 3).

fly-wheel ['flaɪwiːl] *n тех.* махово́е колесо́.

foal I [foul] *n* жеребёнок; ослёнок; in ~, with ~ жерёбая.

foal II *v* жереби́ться.

foam I [foum] *n* 1) пе́на; 2) мы́ло (*на лошади*); 3) *поэт.* мо́ре; 4) *pl* пенопла́сты.

foam II *v* 1) пе́ниться; 2) быть в мы́ле (*о лошади*); ◇ to ~ at the mouth прийти́ в бе́шенство.

foaming-at-the-mouth ['foumɪŋətðə'mauθ] *a* с пе́ной у рта.

foam-rubber ['foum,rʌbə] *n* пе́нистая *или* гу́бчатая рези́на.

foamy ['foumɪ] *a* 1) пе́нящийся, пе́нистый; 2) взмы́ленный, покры́тый пе́ной.

fob[1] [fɔb] *n* карма́шек для часо́в.

fob[2] *v* обма́нывать, одура́чивать; ☐ to ~ **off** всуча́ть, подсо́вывать.

focal ['foukəl] *a физ.* фо́кусный.

foci ['fousaɪ] *pl см.* focus I.

fo'c's'le ['fouksl] *см.* forecastle.

focus I ['foukəs] *n* (*pl тж.* foci) 1) *физ.* фо́кус; 2) центр, средото́чие.

focus II *v* 1) фокуси́ровать(ся); помеща́ть в фо́кусе; 2) сосредото́чивать(ся) (*на — on*).

fodder I ['fɔdə] *n* фура́ж; корм; ◇ cannon ~ пу́шечное мя́со.

fodder II *v* задава́ть корм.

foe [fou] *n поэт.* враг.

foetus ['fiːtəs] *n* плод, эмбрио́н.

fog[1] I [fɔg] *n* 1) тума́н; мгла; 2) нея́сность, замеша́тельство; 3) *фото* вуа́ль.

fog[1] II *v* 1) оку́тывать(ся) тума́ном; затума́нивать(ся); 2) озада́чивать.

fog[2] I *n* 1) ота́ва; 2) трава́, оста́вшаяся неско́шенной на́ зиму.

fog[2] II *v* 1) оста́вить траву́ неско́шенной на́ зиму; 2) пасти́ скот на ота́ве.

fog-bank ['fɔgbæŋk] *n* густо́й тума́н на мо́ре.

fog-bound ['fɔgbaund] *a* заде́ржанный тума́ном (*о судне*).

fogey ['fougɪ] *n* старомо́дный, отста́лый челове́к (*обыкн.* old ~).

foggy ['fɔgɪ] *a* тума́нный.

fogy ['fougɪ] *см.* fogey.

foible ['fɔɪbl] *n* 1) сла́бость хара́ктера; 2) сла́бая стру́нка, пу́нктик.

foil[1] I [fɔɪl] *n* 1) фо́льга; станио́ль; 2) амальга́ма, зерка́льная наво́дка; 3) контра́ст; 4) *архит.* ли́ственный орна́мент (*в готике*).

foil[1] II *v* подчёркивать, выделя́ть (*что-л.*) контра́стом.

foil[2] I *n* след зве́ря.

foil[2] II *v* 1) сбива́ть со сле́да; 2) одура́чивать, ста́вить в тупи́к; 3) расстра́ивать, срыва́ть пла́ны; 4) отража́ть (*уда́р*); 5) брать верх.

foil[3] *n* рапи́ра.

foist [fɔɪst] *v* 1) всучи́ть; навяза́ть (*on, upon*); 2) всу́нуть, включи́ть (*in, into*).

fold[1] I [fould] *n* 1) заго́н для ове́ц, овча́рня (*обыкн.* sheep-fold); 2) па́ства.

fold[1] II *v* загоня́ть (*ове́ц*).

fold[2] I *n* 1) скла́дка; сгиб; 2) сгиба́ние; 3) *тех.* фальц.

fold[2] II *v* 1) скла́дывать, сгиба́ть, загиба́ть; фальцева́ть; 2) завёртывать; оку́тывать; 3) обхва́тывать; to ~ in arms сжима́ть в объя́тиях; to ~ to one's breast прижа́ть к груди́.

folder ['fouldə] *n* 1) фальцо́вщик; 2) фальцева́льная маши́на; 3) брошю́ра; проспе́кт.

folding ['fouldɪŋ] *a* складно́й; ство́рчатый; откидно́й.

foliage ['foulɪɪdʒ] *n* 1) листва́; 2) ли́ственный орна́мент.

foliate[a] ['foulɪt] *a* 1) листообра́зный; 2) ли́ственный.

foliate[b] ['foulɪeɪt] *v* 1) *архит.* украша́ть ли́ственным орна́ментом; 2) расщепля́ть(ся).

folk [fouk] *n* (*pl тж. без измен.*) 1) лю́ди; родня́; old ~s at home роди́тели; 2) *уст.* наро́д; 3) *attr* наро́дный.

folk-lore ['foukb:] *n* фолькло́р.

follow ['fɔlou] *v* 1) сле́довать, идти́ за; 2) пресле́довать; 3) следи́ть (*глаза́ми*); 4) следи́ть за, сосредото́читься на; 5) понима́ть, ула́вливать смысл; I ~ you я вас понима́ю, я вас слу́шаю; 6) разделя́ть взгля́ды, подде́рживать; 7) занима́ться (*чем-л.*); избира́ть профе́ссию; to ~ the sea стать, быть моряко́м; to ~ the law стать, быть юри́стом; ☐ to ~ **on** продолжа́ть (пре)сле́довать; to ~ **out** а) (пре)сле́довать до конца́; б) осуществля́ть, выполня́ть; to ~ **up** упо́рно (пре)сле́довать, добива́ться; ◇ as ~s как сле́дует ни́же (*при перечислении*); his arguments are as ~s его́ до́воды сле́дующие.

follower ['fɔlouə] *n* 1) сле́дующий (*за кем-л.*); 2) после́дователь, приве́рженец; 3) ухажёр (*служа́нки*).

following I ['fɔlouɪŋ] *n* 1) после́дователи; 2) сви́та; 3) (the ~) сле́дующее; in the ~ ни́же, в дальне́йшем.

following II *a* 1) сле́дующий; после́дующий; 2) попу́тный.

folly ['fɔlɪ] *n* глу́пость; безрассу́дство; дорогосто́ящий капри́з.

foment [fou'ment] *v* 1) класть припа́рку; согрева́ть; 2) подстрека́ть; раздува́ть, разжига́ть (*вражду́ и т. п.*).

fond [fɔnd] *a* 1) не́жный, лю́бящий; to be ~ of люби́ть; 2) чрезме́рно дове́рчивый; 3) безрассу́дный.

fondle ['fɔndl] *v* ласка́ть.

fondly ['fɔndlɪ] *adv* 1) не́жно, с любо́вью; 2) тще́тно; неоснова́тельно.

fondness ['fɔndnɪs] *n* не́жность, любо́вь.

food [fuːd] *n* 1) пи́ща (*тж. перен.*); пита́ние; bad ~ непита́тельная пи́ща; mental ~ пи́ща для ума́; ~ for meditation пи́ща для размышле́ний; ~ for powder пу́шечное мя́со; to punish one's ~ *шутл.* мно́го есть; 2) продово́льствие, проду́кты пита́ния; корм; preserved ~ консе́рвы; processed ~ бакале́я, бакале́йные това́ры; tinned ~ консе́рвы (*в жестя́нках*); infants' ~ де́тская мука́, пита́-

тельная смесь; 3) *attr* продовольственный, пищевой.

food-stuff [ˈfuːdstʌf] *n* пищевой продукт.

fool I [fuːl] *n* 1) дурак, глупец; arrant ~ набитый дурак; solemn ~ дурак с важным видом, напыщенный дурак; a ~ in grain стопроцентный дурак; to be a ~ to быть ничём в сравнении с; to make a ~ of одурачивать (*кого-л.*); 2) шут; to play the ~ валять дурака; ◊ to be a ~ for one's pains напрасно стараться *или* трудиться; остаться в дураках.

fool II *a амер.* глупый, безрассудный; безумный.

fool III *v* 1) одурачивать, обманывать; 2) дурачиться; □ to ~ about a) дурачиться; б) зря болтаться; в) волочиться (*за кем-л.*); to ~ around *амер. см.* to ~ about; to ~ away безрассудно растрачивать (*деньги, время*); упускать (*случай*); to ~ into обманом вовлечь (*во что-л.*); to ~ out of обманом выманить; to ~ with дурачиться, забавляться с кем-л.

foolery [ˈfuːlərɪ] *n* глупость; дурачество.

foolhardiness [ˈfuːlˌhɑːdɪnɪs] *n* безрассудная храбрость.

foolhardy [ˈfuːlˌhɑːdɪ] *a* безрассудно храбрый, отчаянный.

foolish [ˈfuːlɪʃ] *a* глупый, безрассудный.

foolishness [ˈfuːlɪʃnɪs] *n* глупость, безрассудство.

foolproof [ˈfuːlpruːf] *a* 1) несложный, понятный; 2) *тех.* безопасный при неумелом *или* неосторожном обращении.

foot I [fut] *n* (*pl* feet) 1) нога, ступня; on ~ пешком; *перен.* в движении, в ходу; to set ~ ступить, наступить (*на — on*); *перен.* утвердиться; to set on ~ пустить в ход; 2) шаг, походка; light (heavy) feet лёгкие (тяжёлые) шаги; to put one's best ~ forward прибавлять шагу, торопиться; 3) пехота; ~ and horse пехота и кавалерия; 4) фут (*около 30,5 см*); 5) основание; подножие; нижняя часть; at the ~ of the bed в ногах кровати; 6) *лит.* стопа; 7) (*pl* foots) осадок, подонки; 8) *attr* ножной; 9) *attr* пеший; пехотный; 10) *attr* пешеходный; ◊ to have cold feet трусить; не хотеть сражаться; to keep one's feet устоять, удержаться на ногах; to find one's feet стать на́ ноги; утвердиться; to put one's ~ in(to) а) вмешаться; б) влипнуть, сделать оплошность, сесть в лужу; to put one's ~ down занять твёрдую позицию, утвердиться; to be on one's feet а) быть на ногах, оправиться после болезни; б) быть самостоятельным; to set smb. on his feet помочь кому́-л. стать самостоятельным, независимым; to get on one's feet взять слово (*на собрании*).

foot II *v* 1) идти (пешком); to ~ it а) идти пешком; б) танцевать; 2) надвязывать (чулок); 3) подытоживать, подсчитывать; *разг.* заплатить (*по счёту; тж.* to ~ up); □ to ~ up составлять, доходить до (*о сумме, счёте и т. п.*; to).

football [ˈfutbɔːl] *n* 1) футбол (*тж.* association ~); 2) футбольный мяч.

footballer [ˈfutbɔːlə] *n* футболист.

footboard [ˈfutbɔːd] *n* подножка, ступенька.

footboy [ˈfutbɔɪ] *n* мальчик-слуга; посыльный.

footfall [ˈfutfɔːl] *n* звук шагов.

foot-gear [ˈfutgɪə] *n разг.* 1) обувь; 2) чулки, носки.

foot-hill [ˈfuthɪl] *n* предгорье.

foothold [ˈfuthould] *n* 1) точка опоры; to gain a ~ (крепко) обосноваться; 2) *воен.* опорный пункт.

footing [ˈfutɪŋ] *n* 1) точка опоры; опора; основание; to lose one's ~ оступиться; поскользнуться; потерять точку опоры; to regain one's ~ подняться (*после падения*); to gain a ~ а) найти точку опоры; б) приобрести положение в обществе; 2) взаимоотношения; on a friendly ~ в дружеских отношениях (*с кем-л. — with*); on a ~ of equality на равных условиях, на равной ноге (*с кем-л. — with*); 3) итог (*столбца цифр*); ◊ to pay (for) one's ~ сделать вступительный взнос, внести свой пай, свою долю.

footless [ˈfutlɪs] *a* 1) безногий; 2) лишённый основания; поверхностный; 3) *амер.* бесполезный, тщетный.

footlet [ˈfutlɪt] *n* подследник.

footlights [ˈfutlaɪts] *n pl театр.* рампа; to appear before the ~ стать актёром, появиться на сцене.

footman [ˈfutmən] *n* 1) (ливрейный) лакей; 2) *уст.* пехотинец.

foot-mark [ˈfutmɑːk] *n* след (ноги).

foot-note [ˈfutnout] *n* сноска (*внизу страницы*).

foot-passenger [ˈfutˌpæsɪndʒə] *n* пешеход.

foot-path [ˈfutpɑːθ] *n* (пешеходная) дорожка, тропинка.

footprint [ˈfutprɪnt] *n* след (ноги).

foot-race [ˈfutreɪs] *n* состязание в беге *или* ходьбе.

foot-rule [ˈfutruːl] *n* фут (*для измерения*).

foot-soldier [ˈfutˌsouldʒə] *n* пехотинец.

footsore [ˈfutsɔː] *a* со стёртыми ногами.

footstep [ˈfutstep] *n* 1) шаг; 2) звук шагов; поступь; 3) след (ноги); to follow in smb.'s ~s идти по чьим-л. стопам, следовать чьему-л. примеру.

footstool [ˈfutstuːl] *n* 1) скамеечка для ног; 2) *амер.* мир, земля.

foot-wear [ˈfutwɛə] *см.* foot-gear.

fop [fɔp] *n* щёголь, фат, пижон.

foppery [ˈfɔpərɪ] *n* щегольство, фатовство.

foppish [ˈfɔpɪʃ] *a* 1) щегольской; фатоватый; 2) пустой, тщеславный.

for I [fɔː (*сильная форма*), fə (*слабая форма*)] *prep* 1) в пространственном значении указывает на: а) конечную цель движения в, на; I am just starting ~ the South (~ Moscow) я сейчас отбываю на юг (в Москву); this boat is bound ~ Odessa этот корабль держит курс на Одессу; б) *расстояние, на которое данный предмет продвигается; обычно не переводится*: to walk ~ a mile пройти милю; 2) *во временном значении указывает на*: а) *протяжённость, длительность, срок, в течение которого действие происходило или будет происходить в течение*; ~ a week (a year, a month, a fortnight, a few days, some time) в течение недели (года, месяца, двух недель, нескольких дней, некоторого времени); б) *срок, на который рассчитано действие*: на; ~ a week (a year *etc*) на неделю (год *и т. п.*); ~ long надолго; ~ good навсегда; good-bye ~ the present пока до свидания; 3) *указывает на цель, назначение, стремление, склонность* за, ради, для, к; *иногда передаётся дательным падежом*; these apples are ~ sale эти яблоки предназначены для продажи; this book is ~ children эта книга для детéй; I am longing ~ the country я стремлю́сь в дерéвню; this artist has an ear ~ music у э́того музыкáнта хорóший слух; the man ~ the job человéк, как бýдто сóзданный для дáнной рабóты; to go (to send) ~ the doctor сходи́ть (послáть) за врачóм; to go ~ a soldier стать воéнным; ~ my (his, your) sake рáди меня́ (негó, вас); 4) *указывает на причину, повод* от, рáди; to cry (to shout) ~ joy плáкать (кричáть) от рáдости; ~ fun, ~ a joke рáди шýтки, в шýтку; ~ several reasons по мнóгим соображéниям; famous ~ извéстный чем-л.; 5) *указывает на отношение к факту, явлению* к, в отношéнии, по отношéнию к; he has no liking ~ medicine он не лю́бит медици́ну; he does not care ~ doctors он не считáется с врачáми; to give up (a man, a ship, an aeroplane) ~ lost считáть (человéка, парохóд, самолёт) поги́бшим; 6) *указывает на замену, замещение и т. п.* за, вмéсто; how much did you pay ~ this dress? скóлько вы заплати́ли за э́то плáтье?; not ~ the world ни за что на свéте.

for II *conj* так как, потомý что.

forage I [ˈfɔrɪdʒ] *n* 1) фурáж; корм; 2) *воен.* фуражирóвка.

forage II *v* 1) *воен.* фуражи́ровать; 2) разы́скивать (*продовольствие, что-л. необходимое; for, about*); опустошáть.

forasmuch [fərəzˈmʌtʃ] *adv*: ~ as так как, ввидý тогó, что; поскóльку.

foray I [ˈfɔreɪ] *n* набéг, налёт.

foray II *v* дéлать набéг, опустошáть.

forbad, forbade [fɔˈbæd, fəˈbeɪd] *past см.* forbid.

forbear [a] [ˈfɔbɛə] *n обыкн. pl* 1) прéдок; 2) предшéственник.

forbear [b] [fɔˈbɛə] *v* (*past* forbore; *p. p.* forborne) 1) удéрживаться, воздéрживаться (*от — from*); 2) проявля́ть терпéние.

forbearance [fɔˈbɛərəns] *n* терпéние, сдéржанность, вы́держка.

forbid [fəˈbɪd] *v* (*past* forbad, forbade; *p. p.* forbidden) запрещáть; не позволя́ть.

forbidden I [fəˈbɪdn] *p. p. см.* forbid.

forbidden II *a* запрéтный; запрещённый.

forbidding [fəˈbɪdɪŋ] *a* оттáлкивающий; внушáющий отвращéние *или* страх.

forbore [fɔˈbɔ] *past см.* forbear [b].

forborne [fɔˈbɔn] *p. p. см.* forbear [b].

force I [fɔs] *n* 1) си́ла; мощь; driving ~, impelling ~ дви́жущая си́ла; attractive ~ си́ла притяжéния; to come into ~ входи́ть в си́лу; (to remain) in ~ (остáваться) в си́ле, дéйствовать; of no ~ недействи́тельный; 2) наси́лие; by ~ наси́льно, си́лой; 3) *обыкн. pl* (вооружённые) си́лы; air ~ воéнно-воздýшные си́лы; ground ~s, land ~s сухопýтные, назéмные войскá; effective ~s боевóй состáв, кáдровые войскá; missile ~s ракéтно-я́дерные войскá; police ~ the ~ поли́ция; in ~ значи́тельными си́лами; to join ~s соединя́ть си́лы; объединя́ть уси́лия; ◇ by ~ of посрéдством, путём.

force II *v* 1) заставля́ть, принуждáть; вынуждáть; 2) взлáмывать; влáмываться; пробивáться; 3) *воен.* форси́ровать (*реку и т. п.*); 4) наси́ловать, (пере)напрягáть; 5) иску́сственно ускоря́ть (*рост, созревание растений, плодов*); □ to ~ **in** а) продáвить; б) проложи́ть себé путь.

forced [fɔst] *a* 1) принуди́тельный; вы́нужденный; 2) принуждённый, натя́нутый; 3) форси́рованный.

forceful [ˈfɔsful] *a* действи́тельный; убеди́тельный, си́льный.

forceless [ˈfɔslɪs] *a* бесси́льный.

forceps [ˈfɔseps] *n* (*pl без измен. и* forcepses) пинцéт; хирурги́ческие щипцы́.

forcible [ˈfɔsəbl] *a* 1) принуди́тельный, наси́льственный; 2) си́льный, убеди́тельный.

ford I [fɔd] *n* брод.

ford II *v* переходи́ть, переезжáть вброд.

fore I [fɔ] *n мор.* нос, носовáя часть сýдна; ◇ to the ~ тут же, под рукóй; на перéднем плáне, на видý; to come to the ~ вы́двинуться вперёд; *спорт.* вы́йти на пéрвое мéсто.

fore II *a* 1) перéдний; 2) *мор.* носовóй.

fore III *adv* впереди́; ~ and aft *мор.* на носý и на кормé; вдоль всегó сýдна.

fore- [fɔ-] *pref* 1) *с сущ. означает переднюю часть чего-л., что-л. находящееся впереди* перéдний; forepaw перéдняя лáпа; 2) *с гл. означает действие, происходящее ранее обычного срока* пред-; to foretell предскáзывать.

forearm [ˈfɔrɑːm] *n* рукá (*от кисти до локтя*); предплéчье.

forebear [fɔˈbɛə] *см.* forbear [b].

forebode [fɔˈboud] *v* 1) предвещáть; 2) предчýвствовать (*несчастье, беду*).

foreboding [fɔˈboudɪŋ] *n* 1) предзнаменовáние (*обычно плохое*); 2) (дурнóе) предчýвствие.

forecast [a] [ˈfɔkɑːst] *n* предсказáние; прогнóз.

forecast [b] [ˈfɔkɑːst] *v* (*past, p. p.* forecast, forecasted) предскáзывать.

forecasting [ˈfɔkɑːstɪŋ] *n* предсказáние, прогнóз; long-distance ~ долгосрóчный прогнóз (*погоды*).

forecastle [ˈfoukslɪ] *n мор.* полубáк.

foreclose [fɔˈklouz] *v* 1) предрешáть (*вопрос и т. п.*); 2) *юр.* исключáть; лишáть прáва пóльзования, вы́купа.

foredate [fɔˈdeɪt] *v* дати́ровать зáдним числóм.

foredeck [ˈfɔdek] *n мор.* бак.

foredoom [fɔˈduːm] *v* обрекáть.

forefather [ˈfɔˌfɑːðə] *n обыкн. pl* прáотец, прéдок.

forefinger [ˈfɔˌfɪŋgə] *n* указáтельный пáлец.

forefront [ˈfɔfrʌnt] *n* 1) перéд; перéдняя часть; 2) *воен.* передовáя ли́ния (фрóнта); 3) центр дéятельности.

foregather [fɔˈgæðə] *v* 1) собирáться; встречáться; 2) общáться.

forego [fɔˈgou] *v* (*past* forewent; *p. p.* foregone) 1) предшéствовать; 2) откáзываться, воздéрживаться (*от чего-либо*).

foregoing [fɔˈgouɪŋ] *a* предшéствующий; вышеупомя́нутый.

foregone I [fɔˈgɔn] *p. p. см.* forego.

foregone II *a* предрешённый, неизбéжный; предвзя́тый.

foreground [ˈfɔgraund] *n* перéдний план.

forehand [ˈfɔhænd] *a* 1) заблаговрéменный; 2) *спорт.* спрáва (*об ударе в теннисе*).

forehanded [ˈfɔhændɪd] *a* 1) своеврéменный, заблаговрéменный; 2) *амер.* предусмотри́тельный; 3) *амер.* преуспевáющий.

forehead [ˈfɔrɪd] *n* лоб; retreating ~ покáтый лоб.

foreign ['fɔrɪn] *a* 1) иностра́нный; 2) незнако́мый, чужо́й; 3) чу́ждый; 4) посторо́нний.

foreigner ['fɔrɪnə] *n* 1) иностра́нец; 2) посторо́нний (челове́к).

foreknew [fɔː'njuː] *past см.* foreknow.

foreknow [fɔː'nou] *v* (*past* foreknew; *p. p.* foreknown) знать зара́нее; предви́деть.

foreknowledge ['fɔː'nɔlɪdʒ] *n* предви́дение.

foreknown [fɔː'noun] *p. p. см.* foreknow.

foreland ['fɔːlənd] *n* 1) мыс, вы́ступ; 2) прибре́жная полоса́.

forelock ['fɔːlɔk] *n* прядь воло́с на лбу; хохо́л; ◊ to take time (*или* occasion) by the ~ воспо́льзоваться слу́чаем, не упусти́ть моме́нт.

foreman ['fɔːmən] *n* 1) ма́стер; ста́рший рабо́чий; прора́б; деся́тник; 2) *юр.* старшина́ прися́жных.

foremast ['fɔːmɑːst] *n мор.* фок-ма́чта.

foremost I ['fɔːmoust] *a* 1) пере́дний; передово́й, пе́рвый; 2) основно́й, са́мый гла́вный.

foremost II *adv* пре́жде всего́, во-пе́рвых (*тж.* first and ~).

forenoon ['fɔːnuːn] *n* дополу́денное вре́мя, у́тро.

forensic [fə'rensɪk] *a* суде́бный.

foreordain ['fɔːrɔː'deɪn] *v* предопределя́ть.

forepart ['fɔːpɑːt] *n* пере́дняя часть.

forepaw ['fɔːpɔː] *n* пере́дняя ла́па.

fore-ran [fɔː'ræn] *past см.* fore-run.

fore-run [fɔː'rʌn] *v* (*past* fore-ran; *p. p.* fore-run) 1) предше́ствовать; 2) предвеща́ть.

forerunner ['fɔː,rʌnə] *n* 1) предше́ственник; предте́ча; 2) предве́стник.

foresail ['fɔːseɪl] *n мор.* фок.

foresaw [fɔː'sɔː] *past см.* foresee.

foresee [fɔː'siː] *v* (*past* foresaw; *p. p.* foreseen) предви́деть, знать зара́нее.

foreseen [fɔː'siːn] *p. p. см.* foresee.

foreshadow [fɔː'ʃædou] *v* предвеща́ть; служи́ть предостереже́нием, предзнаменова́нием.

foreshortening [fɔː'ʃɔːtnɪŋ] *n* раку́рс.

foresight ['fɔːsaɪt] *n* 1) предви́дение; 2) предусмотри́тельность; 3) му́шка (*ружья́*).

forest I ['fɔrɪst] *n* 1) лес; 2) *attr* лесно́й.

forest II *v* сажа́ть лес; заса́живать ле́сом.

forestall [fɔː'stɔːl] *v* предвосхища́ть; предупрежда́ть.

forester ['fɔrɪstə] *n* 1) лесни́чий; лесни́к; 2) лесно́й жи́тель.

forestry ['fɔrɪstrɪ] *n* 1) лесово́дство; 2) лесни́чество.

foretaste[a] ['fɔːteɪst] *n* предвкуше́ние; to get a ~ of получи́ть представле́ние (*о чём-л.*).

foretaste[b] [fɔː'teɪst] *v* предвкуша́ть.

foretell [fɔː'tel] *v* (*past, p. p.* foretold) предска́зывать.

forethought ['fɔːθɔːt] *n* 1) предусмотри́тельность; 2) попече́ние, забо́та.

foretoken[a] ['fɔːtoukən] *n* предзнаменова́ние.

foretoken[b] [fɔː'toukən] *v* предвеща́ть.

foretold [fɔː'tould] *past, p. p. см.* foretell.

forever [fə'revə] *adv* навсегда́, наве́чно, наве́ки.

forewarn [fɔː'wɔːn] *v* предостерега́ть.

forewent [fɔː'went] *past см.* forego.

foreword ['fɔːwəːd] *n* предисло́вие; введе́ние (*к кни́ге*).

forfeit I ['fɔːfɪt] *n* 1) штраф; 2) распла́та (*за что-л.*); his life was the ~ of his crime он поплати́лся жи́знью за своё преступле́ние; 3) конфиско́ванная вещь; 4) конфиска́ция; наложе́ние штра́фа; 5) фант; *pl* игра́ в фа́нты.

forfeit II *a* конфиско́ванный.

forfeit III *v* 1) потеря́ть (*что-л.*); 2) поплати́ться (*чем-л.*); лиши́ться пра́ва (*на что-л.*).

forfeiture ['fɔːfɪtʃə] *n* 1) поте́ря; конфиска́ция; 2) лише́ние, поте́ря пра́ва (*на что-л.*).

forgather [fɔː'gæðə] *см.* foregather.

forgave [fə'geɪv] *past см.* forgive.

forge[1] I [fɔːdʒ] *n* 1) (кузне́чный) горн; 2) ку́зница.

forge[1] II *v* 1) кова́ть; 2) подде́лывать; 3) фабрикова́ть, выду́мывать.

forge[2] *v* с трудо́м подвига́ться вперёд (*тж.* to ~ ahead).

forger ['fɔːdʒə] *n* 1) кузне́ц; 2) подде́лыватель (*по́дписи, докуме́нта и т. п.*); фальшивомоне́тчик.

forgery ['fɔːdʒərɪ] *n* 1) подде́лка, подло́г; 2) фальши́вый докуме́нт; подло́жная по́дпись.

forget [fə'get] *v* (*past* forgot; *p. p.* forgotten) забыва́ть; to ~ oneself а) забыва́ться, поступа́ть недосто́йно; б) ду́мать о други́х, забыва́я себя́.

forgetful [fə'getful] *a* забы́вчивый.

forgetfulness [fə'getfulnɪs] *n* забы́вчивость.

forget-me-not [fə'getmɪnɔt] *n* незабу́дка.

forgive [fə'gɪv] *v* (*past* forgave; *p. p.* forgiven) проща́ть.

forgiven [fə'gɪvn] *p. p. см.* forgive.

forgiveness [fə'gɪvnɪs] *n* 1) проще́ние; 2) снисходи́тельность; незлопа́мятность.

forgiving [fə'gɪvɪŋ] *a* снисходи́тельный, всепроща́ющий.

forgo [fɔː'gou] (*past* forwent; *p. p.* forgone) *см.* forego 2).

forgone [fɔː'gɔn] *p. p. см.* forgo.

forgot [fə'gɔt] *past см.* forget.

forgotten [fə'gɔtn] *p. p. см.* forget.

fork I [fɔːk] *n* 1) ви́лка; 2) ви́лы; 3) развили́на, разветвле́ние, развило́к (*доро́ги*); 4) рука́в (*реки́*).

fork II *v* 1) поднима́ть ви́лами; 2) разветвля́ться; □ to ~ out, to ~ over *сленг* раскошели́ться.

forked [fɔːkt] *a* 1) раздво́енный; 2) разветвлённый; 3) зигзагообра́зный (*о мо́лнии*).

forlorn [fə'lɔːn] *a* 1) несча́стный; 2) *поэт.* поки́нутый, забро́шенный; 3): ~ hope безнадёжное, ги́блое де́ло.

form I [fɔːm] *n* 1) фо́рма (*тж. грам.*); 2) фигу́ра (*челове́ка*); 3) форма́льность; церемо́ния; поря́док; 4) вид, род; 5) класс (*в шко́ле*); the first ~ мла́дший класс; 6) бланк, образе́ц; 7) оборо́т (*ре́чи*); 8) скаме́йка.

form II *v* 1) формирова́ть; придава́ть, принима́ть фо́рму, вид; 2) образо́вывать, составля́ть; 3) превраща́ться; 4) развива́ть, трениро́вать; 5) *воен.* стро́ить(ся).

formal ['fɔːməl] *a* 1) форма́льный, официа́льный; церемо́нный; 2) вне́шний; 3) пра́вильный, симметри́чный.

formalism ['fɔːməlɪzəm] *n* формали́зм.

formality [fɔː'mælɪtɪ] *n* 1) форма́льность; церемо́ния; 2) соблюде́ние форма́льностей; 3) су́хость; формали́зм.

formation [fɔː'meɪʃən] *n* 1) образова́ние, формирова́ние; 2) поря́док, построе́ние (*войск*); 3) *геол.* форма́ция.

formative ['fɔːmətɪv] *a* 1) образу́ющий; 2) *лингв.* словообразу́ющий.

former ['fɔːmə] *a* 1) пре́жний, бы́вший; проше́дший, да́вний; 2) пе́рвый (*из двух*).

formerly ['fɔːməlɪ] *adv* пре́жде; не́когда.

formication [ˌfɔːmɪ'keɪʃən] *n* мура́шки (*по телу*).

formidable ['fɔːmɪdəbl] *a* 1) значи́тельный, грома́дный; 2) тру́дный; 3) стра́шный, гро́зный.

formless ['fɔːmlɪs] *a* бесфо́рменный.

form-master ['fɔːmˌmɑːstə] *n* кла́ссный наста́вник, руководи́тель.

formula ['fɔːmjulə] *n* (*pl тж.* formulae ['fɔːmjuliː]) 1) фо́рмула; 2) до́гмат (*религии*); 3) пра́вила; 4) предписа́ние, реце́пт.

formulate ['fɔːmjuleɪt] *v* 1) (с)формули́ровать; 2) выража́ть фо́рмулой.

formulation [ˌfɔːmju'leɪʃən] *n* формулиро́вка.

fornication [ˌfɔːnɪ'keɪʃən] *n* незако́нное сожи́тельство; прелюбодея́ние.

forsake [fə'seɪk] *v* (*past* forsook; *p. p.* forsaken) покида́ть, оставля́ть.

forsaken I [fə'seɪkən] *p. p. см.* forsake.

forsaken II *a* бро́шенный, поки́нутый.

forsook [fə'suk] *past см.* forsake.

forsooth [fə'suːθ] *adv ирон.* пра́вда, в са́мом де́ле, пои́стине.

forswear [fɔː'sweə] *v* (*past* forswore; *p. p.* forsworn) 1) наруша́ть кля́тву; отрека́ться; 2): to ~ oneself дава́ть ло́жную кля́тву.

forswore [fɔː'swɔː] *past см.* forswear.

forsworn [fɔː'swɔːn] *p. p. см.* forswear.

fort [fɔːt] *n* форт.

forth [fɔːθ] *adv* 1) вперёд; back and ~ туда́ и сюда́; 2) *выражает выдвижение, вынесение на передний план*: to come ~ вы́ступить (*из шеренги*); вы́йти вперёд; 3) *с некоторыми гл. движения указывает на отъезд, отбытие*: to sail ~ отплы́ть; 4) впредь; from that day ~ впредь, начина́я с того́ дня.

forthcoming I [fɔːθ'kʌmɪŋ] *n* появле́ние; приближе́ние.

forthcoming II *a* предстоя́щий, приближа́ющийся; появля́ющийся.

forthright I ['fɔːθ'raɪt] *a* 1) прямо́й; открове́нный; реши́тельный; 2) ло́вкий.

forthright II *adv* пря́мо, напрями́к.

forthwith ['fɔːθ'wɪθ] *adv* то́тчас, неме́дленно.

forties ['fɔːtɪz] *n pl* (the ~) 1) сороковы́е го́ды; 2) во́зраст от 39 до 50 лет; ◇ the roaring ~ «бу́йные сороковы́е» широ́ты (*область сильных ветров в Атлантическом океане*).

fortieth I ['fɔːtɪɪθ] *num* сороково́й.

fortieth II. *n* сорокова́я часть.

fortification [ˌfɔːtɪfɪ'keɪʃən] *n* 1) фортифика́ция; 2) *pl* укрепле́ния.

fortify ['fɔːtɪfaɪ] *v* укрепля́ть; *перен.* подкрепля́ть.

fortitude ['fɔːtɪtjuːd] *n* си́ла ду́ха, му́жество.

fortnight ['fɔːtnaɪt] *n* две неде́ли; today ~, this day ~ че́рез две неде́ли (*считая с сегодняшнего дня*).

fortnightly I ['fɔːtˌnaɪtlɪ] *a* двухнеде́льный.

fortnightly II *adv* оди́н раз в две неде́ли.

fortress ['fɔːtrɪs] *n* кре́пость; to seize a ~ взять кре́пость.

fortuitous [fɔː'tjuɪtəs] *a* случа́йный.

fortuity [fɔː'tjuːɪtɪ] *n* случа́йность; слу́чай.

fortunate ['fɔːtʃnɪt] *a* счастли́вый; уда́чный; благоприя́тный.

fortunately ['fɔːtʃnɪtlɪ] *adv* 1) к сча́стью; 2) счастли́во.

fortune ['fɔːtʃən] *n* 1) сча́стье; уда́ча, форту́на; good ~ уда́ча, сча́стье; bad ~, ill ~ неуда́ча, несча́стье; to seek one's ~ попыта́ть сча́стья; 2) судьба́; to tell ~s гада́ть, предска́зывать судьбу́; 3) бога́тство; to make a ~ разбогате́ть; a small ~ *разг.* деньжо́нки; to come into a ~ получи́ть насле́дство; to push one's ~ улучша́ть своё благосостоя́ние, де́лать карье́ру (*любыми средствами*).

fortuneless ['fɔːtʃənlɪs] *a* 1) бе́дный, небога́тый; 2) несча́стный, неуда́чливый.

fortune-teller ['fɔːtʃənˌtelə] *n* гада́лка, ворожея́.

forty ['fɔːtɪ] *num* со́рок.

forum ['fɔːrəm] *n* 1) *ист.* фо́рум; 2) суд; the ~ of public opinion суд обще́ственного мне́ния.

forward I ['fɔːwəd] *a* 1) пере́дний; передово́й; 2) преждевре́менно развито́й; 3) ра́нний; скороспе́лый; 4) гото́вый, стремя́щийся (*что-л. сделать*); 5) де́рзкий, развя́зный; 6) *ком.* заблаговре́менный.

forward II *n спорт.* напада́ющий.

forward III *adv* 1) вперёд; 2) впредь.

forward IV *v* 1) препровожда́ть, посыла́ть, отправля́ть; 2) помога́ть, спосо́бствовать; ускоря́ть (*рост и т. п.*).

forwardness ['fɔːwədnɪs] *n* 1) ра́ннее разви́тие, созрева́ние, наступле́ние (*чего-л.*); 2) гото́вность, стремле́ние (*что-л. сделать*); 3) де́рзость, развя́зность.

forwards ['fɔːwədz] *adv* вперёд.

forwent [fɔː'went] *past см.* forgo.

fossick ['fɔsɪk] *v австрал. разг.* ша́рить, иска́ть.

fossil I ['fɔsl] *n* 1) ископа́емое; 2) челове́к с устаре́лыми воззре́ниями.

fossil II *a* 1) ископа́емый; 2) устаре́лый, допото́пный.

foster ['fɔstə] *v* 1) воспи́тывать; выха́живать; 2) благоприя́тствовать; спосо́бствовать; поощря́ть; 3) леле́ять.

foster-brother ['fɔstəˌbrʌðə] *n* сво́дный, моло́чный брат.

foster-child ['fɔstətʃaɪld] *n* приёмыш.

foster-daughter ['fɔstəˌdɔːtə] *n* приёмная дочь.

foster-father ['fɔstəˌfɑːðə] *n* приёмный оте́ц.

foster-mother ['fɔstəˌmʌðə] *n* корми́лица; приёмная мать.

foster-sister ['fɔstəˌsɪstə] *n* сво́дная, моло́чная сестра́.

foster-son ['fɔstəsʌn] *n* приёмный сын.

fought [fɔːt] *past, p. p. см.* fight II.

foul I [faul] *n* 1) наруше́ние пра́вил (*игры, состяза́ний*); 2) столкнове́ние (*лодок, всадников и т. п.*).

foul II *a* 1) гря́зный (*тж. перен.*); загрязнённый, засорённый; 2) *разг.* скве́рный, плохо́й; he is a ~ dancer он плохо́й танцо́р; a ~ journey неуда́чное путеше́ствие; 3) нече́стный; преда́тельский; 4) неприли́чный, непристо́йный; 5) гно́йный, гноя́щийся; зара́зный; обло́женный (*о горле, языке*); 6) сыро́й, гнило́й (*о воздухе и т. п.*); бу́рный; ве́треный (*о погоде*); 7) встре́чный, проти́вный (*о ветре*); 8) обро́сший (*о подводной части судна*).

foul III *v* 1) (за)па́чкать(ся) (*тж. перен.*); засоря́ть(ся); 2) столкну́ться; засто́порить (*дви-*

жение), созда́ть зато́р; 3) *спорт.* нече́стно игра́ть; сде́лать непра́вильный ход.

foul IV *adv* нече́стно, преда́тельски; ◊ to fall (*или* to run) ~ of a) столкну́ться с; б) поссо́риться с.

foulard [fuːˈlɑːd] *n текст.* фуля́р.

foul-mouthed [ˈfaulmauðd] *a* скверносло́вящий.

found[1] [faund] *past, p. p. см.* find I.

found[2] *v* 1) закла́дывать (основа́ние); осно́вывать; 2) учрежда́ть; создава́ть; 3) осно́вываться, быть осно́ванным (*на — on, upon*); well ~ed основа́тельный; ill ~ed неоснова́тельный.

found[3] *v тех.* пла́вить, лить, отлива́ть.

foundation [faunˈdeɪʃən] *n* 1) фунда́мент, основа́ние, осно́ва; to lay ~ закла́дывать фунда́мент; положи́ть нача́ло; 2) основа́ние, учрежде́ние; 3) фонд; 4) учрежде́ние, осно́ванное на чей-л. вклад *или* фонд.

founder[1] [ˈfaundə] *n* основа́тель, учреди́тель.

founder[2] *n* пла́вильщик, лите́йщик.

founder[3] *v* 1) пойти́ *или* пусти́ть ко дну; обва́ливаться; подава́ться, оседа́ть.

foundling [ˈfaundlɪŋ] *n* найдёныш.

foundry [ˈfaundrɪ] *n* 1) лите́йная (мастерска́я); лите́йный заво́д; 2) лите́йное де́ло.

fount [faunt] *n* 1) *поэт.* фонта́н; ключ; исто́чник; 2) *см.* fountain 3).

fountain [ˈfauntɪn] *n* 1) фонта́н; 2) исто́чник (*тж. перен.*); 3) резервуа́р (*лампы, вечного пера*).

fountain-head [ˈfauntɪnˈhed] *n* (перво)исто́чник.

fountain-pen [ˈfauntɪnpen] *n* ве́чное перо́, автомати́ческая ру́чка.

four I [fɔː] *пит* четы́ре.

four II *n* 1) четвёрка; 2) *pl* четырёхпроце́нтная це́нная бума́га; ◊ on all ~s a) на четвере́ньках; б) то́чно совпада́ющий (*с — with*).

fourfold I [ˈfɔːfould] *a* четырёхкра́тный.

fourfold II *adv* вче́тверо.

four-footed [ˈfɔːfutɪd] *a* четвероно́гий.

four-in-hand [ˈfɔːrɪnˈhænd] *n* 1) экипа́ж четвёркой; 2) га́лстук-самовя́з (*с двумя длинными концами*).

four-seater [ˈfɔːsiːtə] *n* четырёхме́стная маши́на.

four-square [ˈfɔːˈskwɛə] *a* 1) квадра́тный; 2) усто́йчивый, основа́тельный.

fourteen [ˈfɔːtiːn] *пит* четы́рнадцать.

fourteenth I [ˈfɔːtiːnθ] *пит* четы́рнадцатый.

fourteenth II *n* четы́рнадцатая часть.

fourth I [fɔːθ] *пит* четвёртый.

fourth II *n* че́тверть, четвёртая часть.

fourthly [ˈfɔːθlɪ] *adv* в-четвёртых.

four-wheeled [ˈfɔːˈwiːld] *a* четырёхколёсный.

fowl I [faul] *n* 1) пти́ца (*тж. собир.*); 2) пету́х, ку́рица; to draw a ~ потроши́ть ку́рицу.

fowl II *v* охо́титься за ди́чью.

fox I [fɔks] *n* 1) лиси́ца, лиса́; arctic ~ песе́ц; silver ~ сере́бристая лиси́ца; a sly ~ хитре́ц; 2) ли́сий мех; 3) *амер. унив. сленг* первоку́рсник; 4) *attr* ли́сий.

fox II *v* 1) хитри́ть, обма́нывать; 2) незаме́тно следи́ть (*за кем-л.*).

fox-earth [ˈfɔksəːθ] *n* ли́сья нора́.

foxed [fɔkst] *a* вы́цветший, покры́тый бу́рыми пя́тнами (*о бумаге*).

foxglove [ˈfɔksglʌv] *n бот.* наперстя́нка.

foxhound [ˈfɔkshaund] *n* англи́йская пора́тая го́нчая.

fox-terrier [ˈfɔksˌterɪə] *n* фокстерье́р.

foxy [ˈfɔksɪ] *a* 1) ли́сий; 2) хи́трый; 3) ры́жий, кра́сно-бу́рый.

foyer [ˈfɔɪeɪ] *n* фойе́.

fracas [ˈfrækɑː] *n* шум, гвалт; шу́мная ссо́ра.

fraction [ˈfrækʃən] *n* 1) дробь; common ~, vulgar ~ проста́я дробь; decimal ~ десяти́чная дробь; proper ~ пра́вильная дробь; 2) часть, части́ца; до́ля.

fractional [ˈfrækʃənl] *a* дро́бный.

fractious [ˈfrækʃəs] *a* капри́зный; раздражи́тельный.

fracture I [ˈfræktʃə] *n* 1) *мед.* перело́м; 2) изло́м; тре́щина.

fracture II *v* 1) лома́ть(ся); 2) раздробля́ть.

fragile [ˈfrædʒaɪl] *a* хру́пкий.

fragility [frəˈdʒɪlɪtɪ] *n* хру́пкость.

fragment [ˈfrægmənt] *n* 1) обло́мок; оско́лок; обры́вок; 2) отры́вок, часть.

fragmentary [ˈfrægməntərɪ] *a* 1) отры́вочный; обры́вочный; 2) *геол.* обло́мочный.

fragrance [ˈfreɪgrəns] *n* арома́т, благоуха́ние.

fragrant [ˈfreɪgrənt] *a* арома́тный, благоуха́ющий; *перен.* прия́тный.

frail[1] [freɪl] *a* 1) хру́пкий; сла́бый, боле́зненный; 2) слабохара́ктерный; мора́льно неусто́йчивый; 3) бре́нный, преходя́щий.

frail[2] *n* корзи́на (*для упаковки фруктов*).

frailty [ˈfreɪltɪ] *n* 1) хру́пкость; сла́бость; 2) бре́нность.

frame I [freɪm] *n* 1) ра́ма; ра́мка; 2) строе́ние; строй; систе́ма; ~ of life о́браз жи́зни; ~ of mind о́браз мы́слей; расположе́ние ду́ха, настрое́ние; to be out of ~ быть не в ду́хе; 3) скеле́т, костя́к; 4) карка́с; сруб; 5) (те́ло)сложе́ние; 6) парнико́вая ра́ма; 7) *кино* кадр; 8) *тех.* фе́рма.

frame II *v* 1) вставля́ть, заключа́ть в ра́му; обрамля́ть, окружа́ть; 2) стро́ить; создава́ть; составля́ть; выраба́тывать; 3) *амер. разг.* ло́жно обвиня́ть; фабрикова́ть, извраща́ть (*тж.* to ~ up); 4) приспособля́ть; предназнача́ть; 5) произноси́ть, стро́ить фра́зу; 6) вообража́ть; 7) развива́ться.

frame-up [ˈfreɪmʌp] *n амер.* подтасо́вка фа́ктов; подстро́енное обвине́ние, провока́ция; (суде́бная) инсцениро́вка.

framework [ˈfreɪmwəːk] *n* 1) ра́ма, обрамле́ние; 2) о́стов, карка́с; сруб; 3) строй; структу́ра; to return into the ~ of воссоедини́ться с.

framing [ˈfreɪmɪŋ] *n* обрамле́ние.

framing-up [ˈfreɪmɪŋˈʌp] *см.* frame-up.

franc [fræŋk] *n* франк (*денежная единица*).

franchise [ˈfræntʃaɪz] *n* 1) привиле́гия; 2) пра́во уча́ствовать в вы́борах.

Franciscan [frænˈsɪskən] *n* франциска́нец (*монах*).

Frank [fræŋk] *n ист.* франк.

frank[1] [fræŋk] *a* открове́нный, и́скренний, откры́тый, прямо́й.

frank[2] *v* отправля́ть франки́рованным письмо́м.

frankfurter [ˈfræŋkfətə] *n* соси́ска.

frankincense [ˈfræŋkɪnˌsens] *n* ла́дан.

frankly [ˈfræŋklɪ] *adv* откры́то, пря́мо; открове́нно (говоря́).

frankness ['fræŋknɪs] *n* откровённость, йскренность.

frantic ['fræntɪk] *a* нейстовый, бёшеный.

fraternal [frə'tə:nl] *a* брáтский.

fraternity [frə'tə:nɪtɪ] *n* брáтство; общйна.

fraternize ['frætənaɪz] *v* братáться.

fratricide ['freɪtrɪsaɪd] *n* 1) братоубийство; 2) братоубийца.

fraud [frɔ:d] *n* 1) обмáн, мошённичество; 2) обмáнщик, мошённик.

fraudulent ['frɔ:djulənt] *a* обмáнный, мошённический.

fraught [frɔ:t] *a predic* пóлный, преисполненный; чревáтый (*with*).

fray[1] [freɪ] *n* шýмная ссóра, дрáка.

fray[2] I *n* обтрёпанные краи чегó-л.; «бахромá» (*на рукавах, брюках*).

fray[2] II *v* обтрёпывать(ся).

frazzle ['fræzl] *n амер.* истрёпанность; worn to a ~ совершённо изнóшенный; to beat to a ~ *сленг* избйть, исколошмáтить.

freak [fri:k] *n* 1) причýда, каприз; выходка, шáлость; 2) урóд (*тж.* ~ of nature); 3) внезáпное прекращéние *или* восстановлéние радиоприёма.

freaked [fri:kt] *a* испещрённый.

freakish ['fri:kɪʃ] *a* капризный; причýдливый.

freckle I ['frekl] *n* веснýшка.

freckle II *v* покрывáть(ся) веснýшками.

free I [fri:] *a* 1) свобóдный; 2) освобождённый; to make (*или* to set) ~ освобождáть; выпускáть на свобóду; ~ of charge бесплáтный; ~ from fear бесстрáшный; 3) добровóльный; 4) вóльный, распýщенный (*о поведении и т. п.*); to make ~ with a) позволáть себé лйшнее; б) вóльно обращáться; свобóдно распоряжáться (*чужими вещами*); 5) бесплáтный; ◊ ~ and easy непринуждённый.

free II *adv* 1) свобóдно; 2) бесплáтно.

free III *v* освобождáть.

freebooter ['fri:,bu:tə] *n* пирáт.

freedman ['fri:dmən] *n* вольноотпýщенник, освобождённый раб.

freedom ['fri:dəm] *n* 1) свобóда; незавйсимость; ~ of speech свобóда слóва; ~ of the press свобóда печáти; 2) свобóдное пóльзование; he has the ~ of the library он имéет свобóдный дóступ в библиотéку; 3) *pl* вóльности.

freedom-loving ['fri:dəm,lʌvɪŋ] *a* свободолюбйвый.

free-hand ['fri:hænd] *a* (сдéланный) от рукй (*о рисунке*); ручнóй (*о работе*).

free-handed ['fri:'hændɪd] *a* щéдрый.

freely ['fri:lɪ] *adv* 1) свобóдно; вóльно; 2) обйльно.

freeman ['fri:mən] *n* 1) свобóдный человéк (*не раб*); 2) свобóдный гражданйн (*города*).

freemason ['fri:,meɪsn] *n* масóн.

free-spoken ['fri:'spoukən] *a* откровéнный, прямóй.

free-thinker ['fri:'θɪŋkə] *n* свободомыслящий, вольнодýмец.

free-will ['fri:'wɪl] *a* добровóльный (*см. тж.* will[1] I).

freeze [fri:z] *v* (*past* froze; *p. p.* frozen) 1) морóзить, заморáживать; *перен.* леденйть; it ~s морóзит; 2) мёрзнуть, замерзáть; коченéть; 3) смерзáться, примерзáть (*to; тж.* to ~ together); □ to

~ **down** замёрзнуть; to ~ **in**: to be frozen in быть затёртым льдáми; to ~ **on** *сленг* крéпко уцепйться, вцепйться (*to*); to ~ **out** *сленг* выжить когó-л., отдéлаться; to ~ **over** замёрзнуть, покрыться льдом; to ~ **up**: to be frozen up застыть, закоченéть.

freezing I ['fri:zɪŋ] *n* 1) замерзáние; застывáние; 2) заморáживание; ~ of wages заморáживание зáработной плáты.

freezing II *a* 1) ледянóй; леденящий; 2) охлаждáющий.

freezing-point ['fri:zɪŋpɔɪnt] *n* тóчка замерзáния.

freight I [freɪt] *n* 1) фрахт; груз; 2) перевóзка грýзов (*по воде, амер. тж. по суше*); 3) стóимость перевóзки; 4) *attr* товáрный.

freight II *v* 1) грузйть (*судно*); 2) фрахтовáть.

freighter ['freɪtə] *n* 1) фрахтóвщик; 2) получáтель *или* отправйтель грýзов; 3) грузовóе сýдно; 4) грузовóй самолёт.

French I [frentʃ] *n* 1): the ~ (*употр. как pl*) францýзы; 2) францýзский язык.

French II *a* францýзский.

Frenchman ['frentʃmən] *n* францýз.

Frenchwoman ['frentʃ,wumən] *n* францýженка.

frenzied ['frenzɪd] *a* 1) бéшеный, взбешённый; 2) ожесточённый, бýрный.

frenzy ['frenzɪ] *n* нейстовство, бéшенство.

frequency ['fri:kwənsɪ] *n* частотá; high ~ высóкая частотá; frame ~ *кино* кáдровая частотá, скóрость киносъёмки.

frequent[a] ['fri:kwənt] *a* 1) чáстый; чáсто повторяющийся *или* встречáющийся; 2) обычный, постоянный.

frequent[b] [fri'kwent] *v* чáсто посещáть.

frequentative [fri'kwentətɪv] *a грам.* многокрáтный.

frequenter [fri'kwentə] *n* завсегдáтай.

frequently ['fri:kwəntlɪ] *adv* 1) чáсто; 2) обычно.

fresco ['freskou] *n* 1) фрéска; 2) фрéсковая живопись.

fresh I [freʃ] *a* 1) свéжий; 2) несолёный, прéсный; 3) нóвый; 4) чйстый, неиспóрченный; неóпытный; 5) крéпкий, сйльный (*о ветре*); 6) *амер.* дéрзкий; 7) *сленг* подвыпивший.

fresh II *adv* тóлько что, недáвно, свеже-.

fresh III *a* свéжесть; прохлáда.

freshen ['freʃn] *v* 1) освежáть (*тж.* to ~ up); 2) свежéть.

freshet ['freʃɪt] *n* 1) струя, потóк прéсной воды, вливáющейся в мóре; 2) пáводок, половóдье.

freshly ['freʃlɪ] *adv* тóлько что, недáвно; свеже- (*обыкн. в сочетании с р. р., напр.:* ~-painted свежевыкрашенный).

freshman ['freʃmən] *n* первокýрсник.

freshwater ['freʃ,wɔ:tə] *a* пресновóдный (*см. тж.* water I).

fret[1] I [fret] *n* орнáмент (*обыкн. прямоугóльный*).

fret[1] II *v* покрывáть резьбóй; украшáть лепным орнáментом.

fret[2] I *n* раздражéние.

fret[2] II *v* 1) подтáчивать, разъедáть; 2) терзáть(ся), мýчить(ся); 3) рябйть (*воду*); покрывáться рябью.

fret[3] *n* лад (*в гитаре и т. п.*).

fretful ['fretful] *a* раздражйтельный.

fret-saw ['fretsɔ:] *n* лобзик.

fretwork ['fretwə:k] *n* резное *или* лепное украшение.

friable ['fraɪəbl] *a* крошащийся; рыхлый.

friar ['fraɪə] *n* 1) монах; 2) *полигр.* белое *или* слабо отпечатавшееся место.

friary ['fraɪərɪ] *n* мужской монастырь.

fricative I ['frɪkətɪv] *n фон.* фрикативный звук.

fricative II *a фон.* фрикативный.

friction ['frɪkʃən] *n* 1) трение; 2) конфликт, трения; 3) *мед.* растирание; вытирание; 4) *тех.* сцепление; 5) *attr* фрикционный.

Friday ['fraɪdɪ] *n* пятница; ◊ Man ~ Пятница (*друг Робинзона Крузо*).

fridge [frɪdʒ] *n разг.* холодильник.

friend [frend] *n* 1) друг; приятель; sworn ~s закадычные друзья; to make ~s with подружиться; 2) знакомый; 3) товарищ, коллега; 4) сторонник, доброжелатель; 5) секундант; 6) (F.) квакер; ◊ a ~ at court влиятельный друг, «рука»; a ~ in need is a ~ indeed *посл.* ≅ друзья познаются в беде.

friendless ['frendlɪs] *a* не имеющий друзей, одинокий.

friendliness ['frendlɪnɪs] *n* дружелюбие.

friendly ['frendlɪ] *a* 1) дружеский, дружественный; 2) дружелюбный; благосклонный; сочувствующий; 3) благотворный, благоприятный.

friendship ['frendʃɪp] *n* 1) дружба; 2) дружелюбие.

frieze [fri:z] *n архит.* фриз.

frigate ['frɪgɪt] *n мор.* фрегат.

frige [frɪdʒ] *см.* fridge.

fright I [fraɪt] *n* 1) испуг; страх; to have a ~ бояться; to give a ~ испугать; to take ~ испугаться; 2) *разг.* страшилище, пугало.

fright II *v поэт.* пугать.

frighten ['fraɪtn] *v* (ис)пугать; to be ~ed испугаться; быть испуганным; to ~ into smth. испугать, страхом довести до чего-л.; to ~ out of smth. запугиванием заставить отказаться от чего-л.; □ to ~ away спугнуть.

frightened ['fraɪtnd] *a* испуганный, напуганный.

frightful ['fraɪtful] *a* 1) страшный, ужасный; 2) безобразный.

frigid ['frɪdʒɪd] *a* 1) холодный; 2) равнодушный, холодный; 3) леденящий.

frigidity [frɪ'dʒɪdɪtɪ] *n* 1) мерзлота; eternal ~ вечная мерзлота; 2) холодность.

frill [frɪl] *n* 1) оборка; 2) *pl* ужимки; важничанье; спесь; to put on ~s важничать; манерничать; 3) *pl* ненужный лоск, украшательство (*лит. стиля и т. п.*).

fringe I [frɪndʒ] *n* 1) бахрома; 2) обрамление; край, кайма; 3) чёлка.

fringe II *v* 1) обшивать, украшать бахромой; 2) обрамлять, окаймлять.

frippery ['frɪpərɪ] *n* 1) дешёвые кричащие украшения; безделушки; 2) легкомысленный поступок.

Frisco ['frɪskou] *n разг. г.* Сан-Франциско.

frisk I [frɪsk] *n* прыжок.

frisk II *v* прыгать, скакать, резвиться.

frisky ['frɪskɪ] *a* весёлый, резвый, игривый.

frith [frɪθ] *см.* firth.

fritter¹ ['frɪtə] *n* оладья (*с яблоками и т. п.*); пончик.

fritter² *v* крошить; □ to ~ away распылять, растрачивать по мелочам.

frivolity [frɪ'vɔlɪtɪ] *n* легкомыслие.

frivolous ['frɪvələs] *a* 1) легкомысленный, пустой, поверхностный; 2) пустяковый.

friz I, II [frɪz] *см.* frizz¹ I, II.

frizz¹ I [frɪz] *n* 1) завиток; 2) вьющиеся волосы.

frizz¹ II *v* 1) завивать мелкими кудряшками; 2) виться.

frizz² *v* шипеть (*на сковороде*).

frizzle¹ I, II ['frɪzl] *см.* frizz¹ I, II.

frizzle² *v* 1) жарить(ся) с шипением; 2) изнемогать от жары.

fro [frou] *adv*: to and ~ туда и обратно, взад и вперёд.

frock [frɔk] *n* 1) платье; 2) *см.* frock-coat; 3) ряса.

frock-coat ['frɔk'kout] *n* сюртук.

frog [frɔg] *n* лягушка.

frog-in-the-throat ['frɔgɪnðə'θrout] *n* хрипота.

frogman ['frɔgmən] *n* 1) аквалангист; 2)· водолаз-разведчик.

frolic I ['frɔlɪk] *n* веселье, проказы.

frolic II *v* веселиться, резвиться, проказничать.

frolicsome ['frɔlɪksəm] *a* резвый, игривый.

from [frɔm (*сильная форма*), frəm (*слабая форма*)] *prep* 1) *в пространственном значении указывает на*: а) *движение, удаление от какого-л. предмета* от, из, с; he is coming ~ Leningrad to-night сегодня вечером он приезжает из Ленинграда; ~ end to end из конца в конец; б) *расстояние от какого-л. предмета* от; we are 50 kilometres ~ Sochi мы находимся в 50-ти километрах от Сочи; 2) *во временном значении указывает на удаление от определённого момента* с, от; ~ the XVI century onwards начиная с XVI века; ~ the very first, ~ the outset с самого начала; ~ the beginning сначала; ~ long ago с давних пор; ~ a child с детства; ~ day to day изо дня в день; ~ of old с далёких времён; издавна; ~ time to time время от времени; 3) *указывает на происхождение, источник* от, из, по; he is ~ Kiev он родом из Киева; I got a letter ~ my friend я получил письмо от своего приятеля; to speak ~ memory говорить по памяти; you cannot always judge ~ appearances нельзя судить только по виду; 4) *указывает на отсчёт от определённой числовой величины* от; we saw ~ 15 to 20 tractors in the field мы увидели в поле от 15 до 20 тракторов; I shall be at the Institute ~ 9 till 3 o'clock я буду в институте от 9 до 3; 5) *указывает на причину, повод для какого-л. действия* из, от, из-за; your friend did it ~ good motives ваш приятель сделал это из хороших побуждений; to suffer ~ cold страдать от холода; 6) *указывает на различие одного предмета или качества от другого* от; not to know black ~ white не отличать белого от чёрного; 7) *указывает на ограничение, отнятие, сокрытие и т. п.* от, у; I prevented him ~ sending this telegram я удержал его от посылки этой телеграммы.

front I [frʌnt] *n* 1) перёд, передняя сторона; in ~ of впереди, перед; to the ~ вперёд (*см.*

тж. 2); to come to the ~ вы́двинуться, обрати́ть на себя́ внима́ние; 2) фронт; to the ~ на фронт (*см. тж.* 1); united ~ еди́ный фронт; popular ~ наро́дный фронт; 3) *архит.* фаса́д; 4) накрахма́ленная мани́шка; 5) *поэт.* чело́, лоб, лицо́; 6) примо́рский бульва́р, на́бережная; 7): to have the ~ to име́ть на́глость (*сделать что-л.*).

front II *a* 1) пере́дний; 2) *фон.* переднеязы́чный; 3) *воен.* фронтово́й.

front III *v* 1) быть обращённым к; выходи́ть на; 2) противостоя́ть; 3) станови́ться, ста́вить во фронт.

frontage ['frʌntɪdʒ] *n* 1) фаса́д; 2) палиса́дник; 3) грани́ца уча́стка (*проходящая по дороге, реке*); 4) *воен.* протяже́ние по фро́нту; ширина́ фро́нта.

frontal ['frʌntl] *a* 1) *анат.* ло́бный; 2) *воен.* лобово́й, фронта́льный.

front-bencher ['frʌnt'bentʃə] *n* член прави́тельства, бы́вший мини́стр *или* ли́дер полити́ческой па́ртии (*занимающий место в первых рядах парламента*).

frontier ['frʌntjə] *n* 1) грани́ца; 2) *attr* пограни́чный.

frontiersman ['frʌntjəzmən] *n* пограни́чный жи́тель.

frontispiece ['frʌntɪspiːs] *n* *архит., полигр.* фронтиспи́с.

frontlet ['frʌntlɪt] *n* 1) повя́зка на лбу; 2) лоб живо́тного; 3) пятно́ на лбу живо́тного.

front-rank ['frʌnt,ræŋk] *a* передово́й.

frost I [frɔst] *n* 1) моро́з; white ~, hoar ~ и́ней, и́зморозь; black ~ си́льный моро́з (*без снега*); sharp ~ си́льный моро́з; ringing ~ треску́чий моро́з; covered with ~ зайндеве́вший, замёрзший (*об окне*); 2) хо́лодность, суро́вость; 3) *разг.* неуда́ча, прова́л.

frost II *v* 1) подмора́живать, покрыва́ть и́неем; 2) расхола́живать; 3) побива́ть моро́зом; 4) покрыва́ть глазу́рью; посыпа́ть са́харной пу́дрой; 5) подко́вывать на зи́мние подко́вы (*с шипами*).

frost-bite ['frɔstbaɪt] *n* отморо́женное ме́сто.

frost-bitten ['frɔst,bɪtn] *a* обморо́женный, отморо́женный.

frosted ['frɔstɪd] *a* 1) покры́тый и́неем; *перен.* тро́нутый седино́й; 2) тро́нутый моро́зом; 3) посы́панный са́харной пу́дрой; покры́тый глазу́рью; 4) ма́товый (*о стекле*).

frost-hardy ['frɔst,hɑːdɪ] *a* морозосто́йкий.

frosting ['frɔstɪŋ] *n* 1) и́ней, лёд на о́кнах; 2) мат на стекле́; 3) глазу́рь.

frost-nailed ['frɔstneɪld] *a* подко́ванный на шипа́х.

frostshoe ['frɔstʃuː] *n* (зи́мняя) подко́ва с шипа́ми.

frosty ['frɔstɪ] *a* 1) моро́зный; *перен.* холо́дный; 2) зайндеве́вший; *перен.* седо́й.

froth I [frɔθ] *n* 1) пе́на; 2) пустяки́; болтовня́.

froth II *v* 1) пе́ниться; покрыва́ться пе́ной; 2) вспе́нивать; 3) взмы́лить(ся) (*о лошади*); 4) пустосло́вить.

frothy ['frɔθɪ] *a* 1) пе́нистый; 2) лёгкий, пусто́й, бессодержа́тельный.

frown I [fraun] *n* 1) сдви́нутые, насу́пленные бро́ви; 2) хму́рый вид, взгляд.

frown II *v* 1) (на)хму́риться, насу́питься;

2) смотре́ть ко́со, неодобри́тельно (*на — at, on, upon*).

frowzy ['frauzɪ] *a* 1) пло́хо па́хнущий; за́тхлый; спёртый; 2) гря́зный, нечистопло́тный; неря́шливый.

froze [frouz] *past см.* freeze.

frozen I ['frouzn] *p. p. см.* freeze.

frozen II *a* 1) заморо́женный, замёрзший; засты́вший; 2) холо́дный, чёрствый.

fructify ['frʌktɪfaɪ] *v* 1) оплодотворя́ть; 2) приноси́ть плоды́.

frugal ['fruːgəl] *a* 1) бережли́вый, эконо́мный; 2) дёшево сто́ящий, скро́мный.

frugality [fruː'gælɪtɪ] *n* 1) бережли́вость, эконо́мность; 2) уме́ренность.

fruit I [fruːt] *n* 1) фрукт; плод; candied ~s цука́ты, заса́харенные фру́кты; 2) *обыкн. pl* плоды́, результа́ты; 3) *attr* фрукто́вый.

fruit II *v* приноси́ть плоды́, плодоноси́ть.

fruitage ['fruːtɪdʒ] *n* 1) фру́кты; плоды́ (*тж. перен.*); 2) (весь) урожа́й (*фруктов, плодов*); 3) плодоноше́ние.

fruitful ['fruːtful] *a* 1) плодоро́дный, плодови́тый; 2) плодотво́рный; 3) вы́годный, поле́зный.

fruitfulness ['fruːtfulnɪs] *n* плодови́тость.

fruition [fruː'ɪʃən] *n* осуществле́ние (*желаний, надежд*).

fruitless ['fruːtlɪs] *a* 1) беспло́дный; 2) бесполе́зный.

fruit-sugar ['fruːt,ʃugə] *n* глюко́за.

fruity ['fruːtɪ] *a* 1) фрукто́вый; 2) сла́дкий, мелоди́чный (*о голосе*).

frustrate [frʌs'treɪt] *v* расстра́ивать, разруша́ть (*планы, замыслы*).

frustration [frʌs'treɪʃən] *n* расстро́йство (*планов*); круше́ние (*надежд*).

fry I [fraɪ] *n* жа́реное; жарко́е.

fry II *v* жа́рить(ся).

fry² *n* ме́лкая рыбёшка; small ~ *пренебр.* ме́лкая со́шка; *шутл.* мелюзга́ (*о детях*).

frying-pan ['fraɪɪŋpæn] *n* сковорода́; ◊ out of the ~ into the fire *посл.* ≅ из огня́ да в полымя́.

fub [fʌb] *см.* fob².

fuddle I ['fʌdl] *n* 1) попо́йка; 2) опьяне́ние.

fuddle II *v* 1) пья́нствовать; напива́ться; 2) напа́ивать; одурма́нивать.

fudge I [fʌdʒ] *n разг.* 1) глу́пости, чушь; вы́думка, «стряпня́»; 2) что-л. сде́ланное кое-ка́к; 3) изве́стия «в после́днюю мину́ту» (*в газетах*); 4) мя́гкая конфе́та.

fudge II *v разг.* 1) сде́лать кое-ка́к; 2) выду́мать, «состря́пать»; 3) помеща́ть «в после́днюю мину́ту» (*в газетах*).

fudge III *int* вздор!, чушь!

fuel I [fjuəl] *n* то́пливо; горю́чее; liquid ~ жи́дкое то́пливо; ◊ to add ~ to the flames (*или* to the fire) подлива́ть ма́сло в ого́нь.

fuel II *v* запаса́ть(ся), снабжа́ть(ся) то́пливом; заправля́ть(ся) горю́чим.

fugacious [fjuː'geɪʃəs] *a* мимолётный.

fugitive I ['fjuːdʒɪtɪv] *n* 1) бегле́ц; 2) бе́женец; 3) дезерти́р.

fugitive II *a* 1) бе́глый, бежа́вший; 2) мимолётный; кра́ткий, быстроте́чный; 3) недолгове́чный, име́ющий вре́менный успе́х.

fugue [fjuːg] *n муз.* фу́га.

fulcrum ['fʌlkrəm] *n* (*pl* fulcra ['fʌlkrə])
1) *физ.* то́чка опо́ры, центр враще́ния; 2) сре́дство для достиже́ния це́ли.

fulfil(l) [ful'fɪl] *v* 1) исполня́ть, выполня́ть, осуществля́ть; 2) заверша́ть.

fulfilment [ful'fɪlmənt] *n* 1) выполне́ние, исполне́ние, осуществле́ние; 2) заверше́ние.

full I [ful] *n* 1) всё; це́лое; I cannot tell you the ~ of it я не могу́ сказа́ть вам всего́ об э́том; in ~ по́лностью; to the ~ вполне́, в по́лной ме́ре; 2) вы́сшая то́чка (*чего-л.*); the moon is past the ~ луна́ на уще́рбе.

full II *a* 1) по́лный; це́лый; напо́лненный; 2) оби́льный; 3) то́лстый, по́лный; 4) широ́кий, свобо́дный (*о платье*); 5) дости́гший вы́сшей то́чки.

full III *adv* 1) по́лностью; вполне́; 2) пря́мо, то́чно; как раз; 3) бо́лее чем доста́точно.

full-back ['fulbæk] *n* защи́тник (*в футбо́ле*).

full-blooded ['ful'blʌdɪd] *a* 1) чистокро́вный; 2) полнокро́вный; 3) си́льный.

full-blown ['ful'bloun] *a* вполне́ распусти́вшийся (*о цветке*).

fuller ['fulə] *n* валя́льщик.

full-face ['ful'feɪs] *adv* повёрнутый анфа́с.

full-fledged ['ful'fledʒd] *a* 1) зако́нченный, сложи́вшийся; вполне́ разви́вшийся; 2) опери́вшийся.

full-length I ['ful'leŋθ] *n* портре́т во весь рост.

full-length II *a* во весь рост (*о портре́те*).

full-length III *adv* во всю длину́.

ful(l)ness ['fulnɪs] *n* 1) полнота́; 2) оби́лие.

full-timer ['ful,taɪmə] *n* 1) рабо́чий, за́нятый по́лный рабо́чий день; 2) учени́к, посеща́ющий все заня́тия.

fully ['fulɪ] *adv* вполне́, соверше́нно, целико́м, по́лностью.

fulminant ['fʌlmɪnənt] *a* молниено́сный.

fulminate ['fʌlmɪneɪt] *v* 1) сверка́ть (*как мо́лния*); 2) мета́ть гро́мы и мо́лнии, громи́ть (*against*).

fulsome ['fulsəm] *a* чрезме́рный (до отвраще́ния) (*о ле́сти и т. п.*).

fumade [fjuː'meɪd] *n* копчу́шка.

fumble ['fʌmbl] *v* 1) ша́рить, нащу́пывать (*for, after*); 2) нело́вко, неуме́ло обраща́ться; 3) мя́млить.

fume I [fjuːm] *n* 1) дым благово́ний; *обыкн. pl* пары́ (*вина и т. п.*); exhaust ~s отрабо́танные, выхлопны́е га́зы; 2) испаре́ние; to send off ~s выделя́ть испаре́ния; 3) возбужде́ние, раздраже́ние; in a ~ в раздраже́нии.

fume II *v* 1) *поэт.* воскуря́ть (*благово́ния*); благоуха́ть; 2) оку́ривать; копти́ть; 3) дыми́ть(ся); испаря́ться, выдыха́ться (*обыкн.* to ~ away); 4) раздража́ться (*at*).

fumigate ['fjuːmɪgeɪt] *v* оку́ривать.

fun [fʌn] *n* 1) весе́лье, заба́ва; what ~! как ве́село!; 2) шу́тка; to make ~ of, to poke ~ at высме́ивать, дразни́ть; подпусти́ть шпи́льку; подшу́чивать (над); for ~, in ~ в шу́тку; he is good (*или* great) ~ он о́чень заба́вен; ◇ like ~ основа́тельно, до конца́, энерги́чно.

function I ['fʌŋkʃən] *n* 1) фу́нкция; 2) *pl* слу-

жебные, профессиона́льные обя́занности; 3) торжество́.

function II *v* функциони́ровать, де́йствовать; 2) выполня́ть фу́нкции, назначе́ние.

functional ['fʌŋkʃənl] *a* функциона́льный.

functionary I ['fʌŋkʃnərɪ] *n* должностно́е лицо́; чино́вник.

functionary II *a* 1) официа́льный; 2) *физиол.* функциона́льный.

fund I [fʌnd] *n* 1) фонд, запа́с; 2) фонд; капита́л; sinking ~ амортизацио́нный капита́л; relief ~ фонд по́мощи; yellow-dog ~, slush ~ су́мма, ассигно́ванная капитали́стами на взя́тки, по́дкупы и т. п.; 3) *pl* де́нежные сре́дства; in ~s бога́тый деньга́ми; при деньга́х; out of ~s без де́нег; 4) *pl* (the ~s) госуда́рственные проце́нтные бума́ги.

fund II *v* 1) вкла́дывать де́ньги в це́нные бума́ги; 2) де́лать запа́с.

fundamental I [,fʌndə'mentl] *n* 1) при́нцип, основно́е пра́вило; 2) *pl* осно́вы.

fundamental II *a* основно́й; суще́ственный.

funeral I ['fjuːnərəl] *n* по́хороны; ◇ that's your ~ *разг.* э́то ва́ше де́ло.

funeral II *a* похоро́нный.

funereal [fjuː'nɪərɪəl] *a* похоро́нный; тра́урный.

fungi ['fʌŋgaɪ] *pl см.* fungus.

fungous ['fʌŋgəs] *a* гу́бчатый, ноздрева́тый.

fungus ['fʌŋgəs] *n* (*pl тж.* fungi) гриб; грибо́к; пле́сень.

funicular I [fjuː'nɪkjulə] *n* фуникулёр (*тж.* ~ railway).

funicular II *a* кана́тный.

funk I [fʌŋk] *n разг.* 1) испу́г; па́ника; blue ~ у́жас; to be in a (blue) ~ тру́сить; 2) трус.

funk II *v разг.* 1) тру́сить; 2) уклоня́ться; 3) внуша́ть страх.

funnel ['fʌnl] *n* 1) воро́нка; 2) дымова́я труба́.

funny¹ ['fʌnɪ] *n* я́лик, душегу́бка.

funny² *a* 1) смешно́й; коми́ческий; 2) стра́нный.

funster ['fʌnstə] *n амер.* шутни́к.

fur I [fəː] *n* 1) мех; шерсть; шку́р(к)а; 2) *обыкн. pl* пушни́на, меха́; 3) *собир.* пушно́й зверь; ~ and feather пушно́й зверь и дичь; hunt ~ за́йцы; 4) налёт (*на языке́ больно́го*); 5) на́кипь (*на сте́нках сосу́да*); оса́док (*в вине́*); ◇ to make the ~ fly подня́ть шум, зате́ять ссо́ру.

fur II *a* пушно́й.

fur III *v* 1) *то́лько р. р.* опуша́ть, подбива́ть ме́хом; 2) покрыва́ть(ся) на́кипью; 3) счища́ть на́кипь; 4) покрыва́ть(ся) налётом (*о языке́ больно́го*).

furbelow ['fəːbɪlou] *n* 1) обо́рка; 2) *pl презр.* тря́пки, наря́ды.

furbish ['fəːbɪʃ] *v* 1) чи́стить, очища́ть; полирова́ть (*тж.* to ~ up); 2) подновля́ть, реставри́ровать (*тж.* to ~ up).

furious ['fjuərɪəs] *a* разъярённый, взбешённый, неи́стовый; fast and ~ бу́йный, шу́мный (*о весе́лье и т. п.*).

furl [fəːl] *v* скла́дывать, свёртывать, ска́тывать, убира́ть (*паруса́*).

furlong ['fəːləŋ] *n* фа́рлонг (= 1/8 ми́ли).

furlough I ['fəːlou] *n* о́тпуск.

furlough II *v* предоставля́ть о́тпуск, увольня́ть в о́тпуск.

furnace ['fə:nɪs] n печь; то́пка; горн; *перен.* горни́ло, испыта́ние.

furnish ['fə:nɪʃ] v 1) снабжа́ть, предоставля́ть; приноси́ть; 2) представля́ть; 3) обставля́ть, меблирова́ть.

furnishings ['fə:nɪʃɪŋz] n pl 1) дома́шние принадле́жности; обстано́вка; 2) обору́дование.

furniture ['fə:nɪtʃə] n 1) ме́бель, обстано́вка; 2) содержи́мое; ~ of one's pockets де́ньги; ~ of one's mind зна́ния.

furred [fə:d] a 1) опушённый, отде́ланный, подби́тый, покры́тый ме́хом; 2) пуши́стый; 3) обло́женный (*о языке*); 4) покры́тый на́кипью.

furrier ['fʌrɪə] n мехови́щк, скорня́к.

furrow I ['fʌrou] n 1) борозда́; 2) глубо́кая морщи́на.

furrow II v 1) паха́ть; де́лать бо́розды; 2) борозди́ть (*море и т. п.*); 3) покрыва́ть морщи́нами.

furrowy ['fʌroui] a морщи́нистый.

furry ['fə:rɪ] a 1) меховой, похо́жий на мех; 2) покры́тый, подби́тый ме́хом.

fur-seal ['fə:si:l] n зоол. ко́тик.

further I ['fə:ðə] adv (compar см. far II) 1) да́льше, да́лее; 2) кро́ме того́; к тому́ же.

further II a (compar см. far I) 1) дальне́йший, поздне́йший; until ~ notice впредь до дальне́йшего уведомле́ния; 2) дополни́тельный, доба́вочный; 3) бо́лее отдалённый.

further III v продвига́ть, спосо́бствовать, соде́йствовать.

furtherance ['fə:ðərəns] n продвиже́ние; соде́йствие.

furthermore ['fə:ðə'mɔ:] adv кро́ме того́, к тому́ же.

furthermost ['fə:ðəmoust] см. farthermost.

furthest I, II ['fə:ðɪst] см. farthest I, II.

furtive ['fə:tɪv] a 1) скры́тый, незаме́тный; та́йный; 2) кра́дущийся; 3) ворова́тый.

furtively ['fə:tɪvlɪ] adv укра́дкой, кра́дучись; скры́тно.

fury ['fjuərɪ] n 1) я́рость, неи́стовство, бе́шенство; in a ~ в бе́шенстве; like ~ неи́стово, си́льно; 2) фу́рия.

furze [fə:z] n бот. дрок.

fuse[1] I [fju:z] n 1) запа́л, бикфо́рдов шнур; фити́ль; 2) воен. заря́дная тру́бка, взрыва́тель.

fuse[1] II v воспламеня́ть.

fuse[2] I n 1) пла́вка; 2) эл. пла́вкий предохрани́тель.

fuse[2] II v пла́вить(ся); расплавля́ть(ся), сплавля́ть(ся); □ to ~ together а) сплавля́ть; б) совмеща́ть.

fuselage ['fju:zɪlɑ:ʒ] n ав. фюзеля́ж.

fusibility [,fju:zə'bɪlɪtɪ] n пла́вкость.

fusible ['fju:zəbl] a пла́вкий.

fusillade I [,fju:zɪ'leɪd] n 1) стрельба́; 2) расстре́л.

fusillade II v 1) обстре́ливать; 2) расстре́ливать.

fusion ['fju:ʒən] n 1) пла́вка; 2) распла́вленная ма́сса; 3) сплав; 4) коали́ция, слия́ние; 5) attr термоя́дерный (*о бомбе*).

fuss I [fʌs] n 1) суматоха, суета́; волне́ние из-за пустяко́в; возбужде́ние; to make a ~ подня́ть шум; шу́мно суети́ться; to kick up a ~ подня́ть сумато́ху.

fuss II v 1) суети́ться, занима́ться пустяка́ми;

волнова́ться из-за пустяко́в; 2) надоеда́ть, беспоко́ить (пустяка́ми); □ to ~ up амер. наряжа́ться.

fussy ['fʌsɪ] a суетли́вый, беспоко́йный.

fussy-pot ['fʌsɪpɔt] n разг. суетли́вый челове́к.

fustian ['fʌstɪən] n 1) бумазе́я; 2) напы́щенный стиль; 3) attr бумазе́йный; 4) attr напы́щенный, претенцио́зный.

fusty ['fʌstɪ] a 1) за́тхлый; спёртый; 2) устаре́вший, старомо́дный.

futile ['fju:taɪl] a 1) бесполе́зный; тще́тный; 2) пусто́й, пове́рхностный.

futility [fju:'tɪlɪtɪ] n 1) тще́тность, бесполе́зность; 2) пусто́та, пове́рхностность.

future I ['fju:tʃə] n 1) бу́дущее, бу́дущность; for the ~, in the ~ впредь, в бу́дущем; 2) *грам.* бу́дущее вре́мя.

future II a бу́дущий.

futurism ['fju:tʃərɪzəm] n футури́зм.

futurity [fju:'tʃuərɪtɪ] n 1) бу́дущее, бу́дущность; 2) рел. загро́бная жизнь.

fuze [fju:z] см. fuse[1] I.

fuzz I [fʌz] n 1) пушо́к, пуши́нка; 2) пуши́стые, пы́шные во́лосы.

fuzz II v 1) разлета́ться (*как пух*); 2) покрыва́ться пуши́нками.

fuzzily ['fʌzɪlɪ] adv нея́сно, сму́тно.

fuzzy ['fʌzɪ] a 1) пуши́стый; 2) запу́шённый; 3) нея́сный, сму́тный; неопределённый; 4) вью́щийся.

fylfot ['fɪlfɔt] n сва́стика.

G

G, g [dʒi:] n 1) 7-я бу́ква англ. алфави́та; 2) муз. но́та соль.

gab[1] I [gæb] n разг. 1) болтовня́; stop your ~! замолчи́те!, переста́ньте болта́ть!; 2) болтли́вость.

gab[1] II v болта́ть.

gab[2] n 1) тех. крюк, ви́лка; 2) зару́бка.

gabardine ['gæbədi:n] см. gaberdine.

gabble I ['gæbl] n 1) болтовня́; 2) бормота́ние, невня́тная речь.

gabble II v 1) болта́ть; 2) бормота́ть, невня́тно говори́ть.

gabbler ['gæblə] n болту́н.

gabby ['gæbɪ] a разг. болтли́вый.

gaberdine ['gæbədi:n] n текст. габарди́н.

gable ['geɪbl] n архит. 1) фронто́н; 2) конёк кры́ши.

gabled ['geɪbld] a остроконе́чный (*о крыше*).

gab-tongue ['gæbtʌŋ] n болту́н.

gaby ['geɪbɪ] n проста́к.

gad[1] [gæd] v 1) шля́ться, шата́ться (*обыкн.* to ~ about, abroad, out); 2) ползти́ (*о растениях*).

gad[2] int выража́ет изумле́ние; by ~! ей-бо́гу!

gadabout ['gædəbaut] n праздношата́ющийся.

gad-fly ['gædflaɪ] n о́вод, слепе́нь; перен. надое́дливый челове́к.

gadget ['gædʒɪt] n разг. 1) приспособле́ние (*в механизме, машине*); 2) спо́соб, приём.

Gael [geɪl] n гэл (*житель горной Шотла́ндии*).

Gaelic I [ˈgeɪlɪk] *n* гэ́льский язы́к.

Gaelic II *a* гэ́льский.

gaff¹ [gæf] *n* острога́.

gaff² *n сленг* дешёвый теа́тр (*тж.* реппу ~); балага́н.

gaffer [ˈgæfə] *n* 1) стари́к; 2) деся́тник.

gag I [gæg] *n* 1) затычка, кляп; 2) *театр.* коми́ческий но́мер; импровиза́ция; отсебя́тина; 3) *парл.* прекраще́ние пре́ний; 4) *сленг* обма́н, хи́трость.

gag II *v* 1) затыка́ть рот (*кому-л.*); 2) заста-́вить замолча́ть; 3) *театр.* вставля́ть отсебя́тину; 4) *сленг* обма́нывать, надува́ть.

gaga [ˈgægɑ] *a сленг* 1) бессмы́сленный; 2) не в своём уме́, рехну́вшийся.

gage¹ I [geɪdʒ] *n* 1) зало́г; 2) вы́зов (*на поеди-нок*); to throw down a ~ бро́сить вы́зов.

gage¹ II *v* 1) руча́ться; 2) *уст.* би́ться об закла́д.

gage² I, II *амер. см.* gauge I, II.

gaggle [ˈgægl] *v* гогота́ть (*о гусях*).

gaiety [ˈgeɪətɪ] *n* 1) весе́лье, весёлость; 2) *pl* развлече́ния; 3) весёлый вид.

gaily [ˈgeɪlɪ] *adv* 1) ве́село; 2) я́рко.

gain I [geɪn] *n* 1) увеличе́ние, прирост; 2) при́-быль; вы́игрыш; 3) за́работок; 4) *pl* дохо́ды; 5) нажи́ва; коры́сть.

gain II *v* 1) зараба́тывать, добыва́ть; 2) получа́ть, приобрета́ть; 3) достига́ть; добива́ться; одержи́вать (*победу*); 4) выи́грывать; 5) извлека́ть по́льзу, вы́году; 6) улучша́ться; 7) идти́ вперёд, спеши́ть (*о часах*); □ to ~ on *см.* to ~ upon; to ~ over убеди́ть, перемани́ть на свою́ сто́рону; to ~ upon a) нагоня́ть, настига́ть; б) сниска́ть расположе́ние; в) захва́тывать постепе́нно часть су́ши (*о море*).

gainful [ˈgeɪnful] *a* сто́ящий, вы́годный; дохо́д-ный, прибыльный.

gainings [ˈgeɪnɪŋz] *n pl* 1) вы́игрыш; 2) за́ра-боток; дохо́д.

gainsaid [geɪnˈsed] *past, p. p. см.* gainsay.

gainsay [geɪnˈseɪ] *v* (*past, p. p.* gainsaid) 1) противоре́чить; 2) отрица́ть.

gainst, 'gainst [geɪnst] *поэт см.* against.

gait [geɪt] *n* 1) похо́дка; 2) аллю́р; 3) *амер.* ско́рость.

gaiters [ˈgeɪtəz] *n pl* гама́ши; ге́тры.

gala [ˈgɑːlə] *n* 1) пра́зднество, торжество́; 2) *attr* пра́здничный, пара́дный.

galantine [ˈgælntiːn] *n* заливно́е (*кушанье*).

galaxy [ˈgæləksɪ] *n* 1) *астр.* Мле́чный Путь; 2) плея́да.

gale [geɪl] *n* 1) си́льный ве́тер; *мор.* бу́ря, шторм; 2) *поэт.* ветеро́к, зефи́р; 3) взрыв сме́ха; 4) *разг.* состоя́ние оживле́ния, весёлость.

gall¹ [gɔːl] *n* 1) желчь; 2) жёлчный пузы́рь; 3) го́речь; зло́ба; раздраже́ние; си́льная оби́да; ~ and wormwood что-л. посты́лое; men who chew their ~ зло́бные, жёлчные лю́ди; 4) *амер.* на́глость.

gall² I *n* натёртое ме́сто, пузы́рь; сса́дина; 2) раздраже́ние (*кожи*).

gall² II *v* 1) натере́ть (*ногу и т. п.*), ссади́ть (*кожу*); 2) раздража́ть, беспоко́ить.

gallant*ᵃ* I [ˈgælənt] *n* све́тский челове́к, кава-ле́р.

gallant*ᵃ* II *a* 1) хра́брый, сме́лый; до́блестный;

2) *поэт.* бо́рзый (*о коне*); 3) *поэт.* велича́вый (*о корабле*); 4) изы́сканно ве́жливый; 5) *уст.* блестя́щий, наря́дный.

gallant*ᵃ* III *v* 1) флиртова́ть (*with*); 2) сопро-вожда́ть (*даму*).

gallant*ᵇ* I [gəˈlænt] *n* покло́нник, любо́вник.

gallant*ᵇ* II *a* 1) гала́нтный, любе́зный (*с жен-щинами*); 2) любо́вный.

gallantry [ˈgæləntrɪ] *n* 1) хра́брость, сме́лость; 2) гала́нтность, учти́вость; 3) любо́вная интри́-га.

gall-bladder [ˈgɔlˌblædə] *n анат.* жёлчный пу-зы́рь.

gallery [ˈgælərɪ] *n* 1) галере́я; 2) прохо́д, коридо́р; 3) *театр.* галёрка; пу́блика на галёрке; to play to the ~ подла́живаться под вкус толпы́; 4) хо́ры, балко́н; the press ~ балко́н для кор-респонде́нтов газе́т (*в англ. пала́те общи́н*); 5) *горн.* штрек.

galley [ˈgælɪ] *n* 1) вельбо́т, ги́чка; 2) *мор.* ка́м-буз; 3) *ист.* гале́ра; *pl* принуди́тельные рабо́ты (*на гале́рах*); 4) *полигр.* набо́рная доска́; вер-ста́тка.

galley-slave [ˈgælɪsleɪv] *n* 1) *ист.* гребе́ц на гале́ре (*раб или ка́торжник*); 2) челове́к, выпол-ня́ющий тяжёлую рабо́ту.

Gallic [ˈgælɪk] *a* га́лльский; францу́зский.

gallicism [ˈgælɪsɪzəm] *n* галлици́зм.

galligaskins [ˌgælɪˈgæskɪnz] *n pl шутл.* широ́-кие брю́ки.

gallipot [ˈgælɪpɔt] *n* небольша́я обли́вна́я ба́нка.

gallivant [ˌgælɪˈvænt] *v* шля́ться, броди́ть.

gallon [ˈgælən] *n* галло́н (*мера жи́дких и сыпу́-чих тел в А́нглии = 4,54 л; в США = 3,78 л*); imperial ~ англи́йский галло́н.

galloon [gəˈluːn] *n* галу́н.

gallop I [ˈgæləp] *n* гало́п; at full ~ во весь опо́р; to go for a ~ пусти́ть ло́шадь в гало́п; скака́ть во весь опо́р.

gallop II *v* 1) скака́ть во весь опо́р; галопи́ро-вать; 2) пуска́ть гало́пом (*ло́шадь*); 3) бы́стро чита́ть, говори́ть (*часто* to ~ over, to ~ through); 4) бы́стро прогресси́ровать (*о боле́зни*).

galloway [ˈgæləweɪ] *n* малоро́слая ло́шадь шотла́ндской поро́ды.

gallows [ˈgæloʊz] *n pl* ви́селица.

gallows-bird [ˈgæloʊzbɜːd] *n* ви́сельник, негодя́й.

gallows-tree [ˈgæloʊztriː] *n* ви́селица.

gall-stone [ˈgɔːlstoun] *n мед.* жёлчный ка́мень.

galoot [gəˈluːt] *n разг.* у́вален.

galop I [ˈgæləp] *n* гало́п (*танец*).

galop II *v* танцева́ть гало́п.

galore [gəˈlɔː] *adv* (*ста́вится по́сле сущ.*) в изоби́лии.

galosh [gəˈlɔʃ] *см.* golosh.

galumph [gəˈlʌmf] *v разг.* пры́гать от ра́дости.

galvanic [gælˈvænɪk] *a* 1) *эл.* гальвани́ческий; 2) принуждённый, неесте́ственный (*о смехе, улы́бке*).

galvanize [ˈgælvənaɪz] *v* 1) *тех., мед.* гальвани-зи́ровать; 2) оцинко́вывать; 3) оживля́ть.

gambade [gæmˈbeɪd] *n* 1) прыжо́к, курбе́т (*ло́шади*); 2) неожи́данная вы́ходка.

gambado [gæmˈbeɪdou] *см.* gambade.

gamble I [ˈgæmbl] *n* 1) аза́ртная игра́; 2) риско́-ванное де́ло; афе́ра.

gamble II *v* 1) игра́ть в аза́ртные и́гры; 2) рискова́ть (*with*); 3) игра́ть, спекули́ровать (*на би́рже*); □ to ~ **away** прои́грывать (*состояние и т. п.*).

gambler ['gæmblə] *n* 1) игро́к, картёжник; 2) моше́нник, афери́ст.

gambol I ['gæmbəl] *n* прыжо́к.

gambol II *v* пры́гать, скака́ть.

game I [geɪm] *n* 1) игра́; ~s of chance аза́ртные и́гры; to play a good (poor) ~ быть хоро́шим (плохи́м) игроко́м; to play the ~ соблюда́ть пра́вила; *перен.* поступа́ть благоро́дно; 2) развлече́ние, заба́ва; 3) шу́тка; to make ~ of высме́ивать; to speak in ~ говори́ть в шу́тку; 4) за́мысел, план; 5) уло́вка, хи́трость; none of your ~s! *разг.* бро́сьте свои́ шту́чки!; you're having a ~ with me вы хоти́те меня́ одура́чить; 6) *спорт.* па́ртия; *pl* состяза́ния, и́гры; the Olympic Games Олимпи́йские и́гры; ◊ the ~ is not worth the candle *погов.* игра́ не сто́ит свеч; the ~ is up ≅ де́ло прои́грано, всё ко́нчено; to have the ~ in one's hands име́ть ко́зыри на рука́х; быть в вы́игрышном положе́нии.

game[1] II *a* 1) задо́рный, бо́йкий; сме́лый; to die ~ умере́ть, но не сда́ться; стоя́ть на́смерть; 2) гото́вый (*на что-л.*); to be ~ for a walk охо́тно пойти́ гуля́ть.

game[1] III *v* игра́ть в аза́ртные и́гры; □ to ~ **away** проигра́ть.

game[2] *n* дичь; fair ~ дичь, на кото́рую разрешено́ охо́титься; *перен.* объе́кт пресле́дования; big ~ кру́пная дичь (*тж. перен.*); ◊ to fly at higher ~ высоко́ ме́тить; заноси́ться; to pull a ~ out of the fire спасти́ положе́ние.

game[3] [geɪm] *a* искале́ченный (*о ноге*).

game-bag ['geɪmbæg] *n* ягдта́ш.

game-cock ['geɪmkɔk] *n* бойцо́вый пету́х.

gamekeeper ['geɪm‚kiːpə] *n* лесни́к, охраня́ющий дичь (*от браконьеров и т. п.*).

game-laws ['geɪmlɔːz] *n pl* пра́вила охо́ты.

gamely ['geɪmlɪ] *adv* сто́йко, бо́дро.

gamesome ['geɪmsəm] *a* игри́вый, шутли́вый; весёлый.

gamester ['geɪmstə] *n* игро́к, картёжник.

gaming-house ['geɪmɪŋhaus] *n* иго́рный дом.

gammer ['gæmə] *n разг.* стару́ха.

gammon[1] I ['gæmən] *n* о́корок.

gammon[1] II *v* копти́ть (*окорок*).

gammon[2] I *n* обма́н, надува́тельство.

gammon[2] II *v* 1) обма́нывать; 2) притворя́ться.

gammon[2] III *int* чушь!, ерунда́!

gamp [gæmp] *n разг.* большо́й зонт.

gamut ['gæmət] *n* 1) *муз.* га́мма; 2) диапазо́н (*голоса*); 3) полнота́, глубина́ (*чего-л.*).

gamy[1] ['geɪmɪ] *a* сме́лый, задо́рный.

gamy[2] *a* 1) име́ющий вкус ди́чи; 2) с душко́м (*о дичи*).

gander ['gændə] *n* 1) гуса́к; 2) дура́к, о́лух.

gang[1] [gæŋ] *n* 1) па́ртия, брига́да, сме́на (*рабочих*); section ~ па́ртия железнодоро́жных рабо́чих (*на путевом участке*); 2) набо́р, компле́кт (*инструментов*).

gang[2] *n* ша́йка, ба́нда.

gang[3] *v шотл.* идти́.

gang-board ['gæŋbɔːd] *n* схо́дни.

ganger[1] ['gæŋə] *n* надсмо́трщик, деся́тник.

ganger[2] *n* пешехо́д.

ganglia ['gæŋglɪə] *pl см.* ganglion.

gangling ['gæŋglɪŋ] *a* неуклю́жий.

ganglion ['gæŋglɪən] *n* (*pl* ganglia) *анат.* 1) не́рвный у́зел; *перен.* центр (*деятельности, интересов*); 2) не́рвная кле́тка.

gang-plank ['gæŋplæŋk] *см.* gang-board.

gangrene ['gæŋgriːn] *n* 1) омертве́ние (*тка́ней организма*), гангре́на; 2) рак (*дерева*).

gangrenous ['gæŋgrɪnəs] *a* омертве́лый, гангрено́зный.

gangster ['gæŋstə] *n* банди́т, га́нгстер.

gangway ['gæŋweɪ] *n* 1) прохо́д (*между рядами кресел*); 2) схо́дни; 3) *стр.* мостки́.

gantry ['gæntrɪ] *n* 1) *тех.* порта́л (*подъёмного крана*); 2) *ж.-д.* сигна́льный мо́стик; 3) подста́вка для бо́чек.

gaol I [dʒeɪl] *n* 1) тюрьма́; 2) тюре́мное заключе́ние.

gaol II *v* сажа́ть в тюрьму́.

gaol-bird ['dʒeɪlbəd] *n* ареста́нт; уголо́вник.

gaoler ['dʒeɪlə] *n* тюре́мный надзира́тель, тюре́мщик.

gap [gæp] *n* 1) брешь, проло́м (*в стене, заборе*); лазе́йка; 2) «окно́» (*в расписании занятий*); 3) пробе́л, про́пуск; to fill up (*или* to stop) the ~ запо́лнить про́пуск, пробе́л; 4) расхожде́ние (*во взглядах и т. п.*); 5) глубо́кое уще́лье; прохо́д (*в горах*); 6) *воен.* разры́в (*линии фронта*); 7) *тех.* зазо́р.

gape I [geɪp] *n* 1) зево́к; the ~s а) зево́та (*болезнь кур*); б) *шутл.* при́ступ зево́ты; 2) изумлённый, недоуме́нный взгляд; 3) отве́рстие; зия́ние.

gape II *v* 1) зева́ть; 2) раскры́ть рот (*от изумле́ния*); смотре́ть рази́нув рот; гла́зеть; 3) зия́ть; □ to ~ **after**, to ~ **for** стра́стно жела́ть чего́-л.; to ~ **(up)on** смотре́ть на что-л., рази́нув рот (*от изумле́ния*).

garage I ['gærɑːʒ] *n* гара́ж.

garage II *v* ста́вить в гара́ж.

garb I [gɑːb] *n* 1) наря́д; 2) национа́льный костю́м; 3) одея́ние (*характерное для определённой профессии*).

garb II *v обыкн. pass* одева́ть, облача́ть.

garbage ['gɑːbɪdʒ] *n* 1) отбро́сы, му́сор; 2) требуха́, вну́тренности; 3) макулату́ра, низкопро́бная литерату́ра.

garble ['gɑːbl] *v* подтасо́вывать, искажа́ть (*факты и т. п.*).

garçon [‚gɑː'sɔŋ] *n* официа́нт.

garden I ['gɑːdn] *n* 1) сад; the ~ of England *перен.* ю́жные райо́ны А́нглии; 2) *pl* парк; 3) огоро́д (*тж.* kitchen-~); 4) *attr* садо́вый, огоро́дный.

garden II *v* разводи́ть сад; занима́ться садово́дством.

gardener ['gɑːdnə] *n* 1) садо́вник; 2) садово́д.

gardening ['gɑːdnɪŋ] *n* садово́дство.

garden-stuff ['gɑːdnstʌf] *n* о́вощи, фру́кты.

gargle I ['gɑːgl] *n* полоска́ние (*для горла*).

gargle II *v* полоска́ть (*горло*).

garish ['gɛərɪʃ] *a* 1) я́ркий, ослепи́тельный; 2) крича́щий (*о платье, красках*); показно́й.

garland I ['gɑːlənd] *n* 1) вено́к; гирля́нда; 2) приз, па́льма пе́рвенства; 3) *уст.* антоло́гия; 4) *уст.* диаде́ма.

garland II *v* украшáть гирляндами, венкóм.

garlic ['gɑːlɪk] *n* чеснóк.

garment ['gɑːmənt] *n* 1) предмéт одéжды; 2) *pl* одéжда; 3) покрóв, одея́ние; ◊ nether ~s *шутл.* брюки.

garner i ['gɑːnə] *n* *поэт.* житница, амбáр; *перен.* хранилище.

garner II *v* склáдывать в амбáр; запасáть; *перен.* хранить (*in*).

garnet ['gɑːnɪt] *n* *мин.* гранáт.

garnish I ['gɑːnɪʃ] *n* 1) украшéния; отдéлка; 2) гарнир.

garnish II *v* 1) украшáть; отдéлывать; 2) гарнировáть (*блюдо*).

garniture ['gɑːnɪtʃə] *n* 1) украшéние; отдéлка; 2) гарнитýра; 3) гарнир.

garret ['gærət] *n* 1) чердáк; мансáрда; from ~ to cellar свéрху дóнизу; по всемý дóму; 2) *сленг* головá, «чердáк».

garrison I ['gærɪsn] *n* гарнизóн.

garrison II *v* 1) стáвить гарнизóн; вводить войскá; 2) назначáть на гарнизóнную слýжбу.

garrulity [gæ'ruːlɪtɪ] *n* говорливость, словоохóтливость; болтливость.

garrulous ['gæruləs] *a* 1) говорливый, словоохóтливый; болтливый; 2) журчáщий (*о ручье*).

garter ['gɑːtə] *n* подвязка; the Garter óрден Подвязки (*высший орден в Англии*).

gas I [gæs] *n* 1) газ; natural (detonating, noble) ~ природный (гремýчий, инéртный) газ; air ~ *тех.* карбюрированный газ; горючая смесь; producer ~ *тех.* генерáторный газ; deceptive ~ *воен.* маскирýющий газ; to turn on the ~ открыть, включить газ; to turn off the ~ закрыть, выключить газ; 2) светильный газ; 3) *воен.* отравляющее веществó; 4) *амер.* бензин; горючее; step on the ~! нажми педáль!, «дай гáзу!»; 5) *разг.* пустóй разговóр, бахвáльство; 6) *горн.* гремýчий *или* рудничный газ; 7) *attr* гáзовый.

gas II *v* 1) заражáть отравляющими веществáми; 2) наполнять гáзом; 3) выделять газ; 4) *амер.* заправляться горючим; 5) *разг.* болтáть пóпусту; бахвáлиться, хвáстаться (*тж.* to ~ away).

gas-alarm ['gæsə'lɑːm] *n* *воен.* химическая тревóга.

gas-bag ['gæsbæg] *n* 1) гáзовый баллóн; 2) *разг.* болтýн; пустозвóн.

gasbracket ['gæs,brækɪt] *n* гáзовый рожóк.

gas-burner ['gæs,bəːnə] *n* гáзовая горéлка.

gas-engine ['gæs,endʒɪn] *n* гáзовый двигатель.

gaseous ['geɪzjəs] *a* газообрáзный; гáзовый.

gas-fitter ['gæs,fɪtə] *n* монтёр по устанóвке гáзовых труб; газопровóдчик.

gash I [gæʃ] *n* глубóкий прорéз; глубóкая рáна.

gash II *v* наносить глубóкую рáну; сильно порéзать.

gas-helmet ['gæs,helmɪt] *n* противогáзовый шлем.

gasification [,gæsɪfɪ'keɪʃən] *n* превращéние в газ; газификáция.

gasify ['gæsɪfaɪ] *v* превращáть в газ; газифицировать.

gas-jet ['gæsdʒet] *n* гáзовый рожóк, горéлка.

gaslight ['gæslaɪt] *n* 1) гáзовое освещéние; 2) гáзовая лáмпа.

gas-mantle ['gæs,mæntl] *n* калильная сéтка.

gas-mask ['gæsmɑːsk] *n* противогáз.

gas-meter ['gæs,miːtə] *n* газомéр; гáзовый счéтчик; ◊ to lie like a ~ ≅ врать как сивый мéрин.

gasolene ['gæsəliːn] *n* 1) газолин; 2) *амер.* бензин.

gasoline ['gæsəliːn] *см.* gasolene.

gasometer [gæ'sɔmɪtə] *n* 1) газомéр; 2) газомéр; гáзовый счéтчик.

gasp I [gɑːsp] *n* затруднённое дыхáние, удýшье; at one's last ~ при послéднем издыхáнии.

gasp II *v* 1) тяжелó дышáть, задыхáться; 2) раскрывáть рот (*от изумления*); □ to ~ **for** стрáстно желáть чегó-л.; to ~ **out** произносить задыхáясь, выпáливать (*слова*).

gasper ['gɑːspə] *n* *сленг* дешёвая папирóса.

gas-plant ['gæs'plɑːnt] *n* 1) гáзовый завóд; 2) газогенерáторная устанóвка.

gas-producer ['gæsprə,djuːsə] *n* газогенерáтор.

gas-proof ['gæspruːf] *a* газонепроницáемый.

gassed [gæst] *a* 1) отрáвленный гáзом; 2) *воен.* поражённый, заражённый отравляющими веществáми.

gas-shell ['gæsʃel] *n* *воен.* химический снаряд.

gas-shelter ['gæs,ʃeltə] *n* газоубéжище.

gas-stove ['gæs'stouv] *n* гáзовая плитá.

gassy ['gæsɪ] *a* 1) похóжий на газ; 2) словоохóтливый; болтливый.

gas-tank ['gæstæŋk] *n* *амер.* 1) бак для горючего, бензобáк; 2) резервуáр для гáза.

gastric ['gæstrɪk] *a* желýдочный.

gas-warfare ['gæs,wɔːfɛə] *n* химическая войнá.

gas-works ['gæswəːks] *n* гáзовый завóд.

gate [geɪt] *n* 1) ворóта, калитка; 2) вход, выход; 3) шлагбáум; 4) шлюз; 5) входнáя плáта; 6) гóрный прохóд; ◊ to get the ~ получить отстáвку; to give the ~ уволить.

gate-crasher ['geɪt,kræʃə] *n* *сленг* 1) «зáяц» (*безбилетный зритель*); 2) незвáный гость.

gatehouse ['geɪthaus] *n* сторóжка у ворóт.

gate-keeper ['geɪt,kiːpə] *n* приврáтник.

gate-post ['geɪtpoust] *n*: between you and me and the ~ мéжду нáми говоря; под стрóгим секрéтом.

gateway ['geɪtweɪ] *n* 1) подворóтня; прохóд; 2) ворóта; a ~ to fame (to knowledge, to success) путь к слáве (к знáниям, к успéху).

gather ['gæðə] *v* 1) собирáть(ся); 2) накоплять, приобретáть; 3) поднимáть (*с земли, пола*); 4) снимáть, собирáть (*урожай*); рвать (*цветы*); собирáть (*ягоды*); 5) мóрщить (*лоб*); 6) собирáть в сбóрку, сбóрить (*платье*); 7) нарывáть; 8) дéлать вывод, заключáть; □ to ~ **up** а) подбирáть; б) суммировать; в) сжимáться; г): to ~ oneself up подтянýться, собрáться с силами.

gathering ['gæðərɪŋ] *n* 1) собрáние, сбóрище; скоплéние; 2) собирáние; комплектовáние; 3) нагноéние, нарыв.

gathers ['gæðəz] *n pl* сбóрки (*на платье*).

gaud [gɔːd] *n* 1) мишурá; безделýшка; 2) *pl* пышные прáзднества.

gaudy I ['gɔːdɪ] *n* 1) пышное прáзднество;

2) юбиле́йный обе́д (*в честь бывших студентов в английских университетах*).

gaudy II *a* 1) я́ркий, крича́щий, безвку́сный (*об одежде*); 2) цвети́стый, витиева́тый (*о стиле*).

gauffer ['gɔːfə] *см.* gof(f)er.

gauge I [geɪdʒ] *n* 1) ме́ра, разме́р; to take the ~ of измеря́ть; 2) кали́бр, шабло́н; 3) *ж.-д.* ширина́ коле́й; broad (narrow) ~ широ́кая (у́зкая) коле́я; 4) измери́тельный прибо́р; 5) крите́рий.

gauge II *v* 1) измеря́ть, вымеря́ть; 2) градуи́ровать, наноси́ть деле́ния; 3) оце́нивать (*характер, поведение человека*).

gauge-glass ['geɪdʒglɑːs] *n* водоме́рное стекло́.

gauging-station ['geɪdʒɪŋ,steɪʃən] *n* гидрометри́ческая ста́нция.

Gaul [gɔːl] *n* 1) *ист.* галл; 2) *шутл.* францу́з.

gaunt [gɔːnt] *a* 1) худо́й, изможде́нный; изнуре́нный; 2) мра́чный (*о местности*).

gauntlet[1] ['gɔːntlɪt] *n* 1) рукави́ца (*шофёра, лётчика и т. п.*); 2) *ист.* перча́тка, ла́тная рукави́ца; to fling (*или* to throw) down the ~ бро́сить вы́зов; to pick (*или* to take) up the ~ приня́ть вы́зов.

gauntlet[2] *n*: to run the ~ проходи́ть сквозь строй; *перен.* подверга́ться ре́зкой кри́тике; быть раскритико́ванным.

gauntry ['gɔːntrɪ] *см.* gantry.

gauze [gɔːz] *n* 1) газ (*ткань*); 2) ма́рля; 3) ды́мка (*в воздухе*); 4) *тех.* металли́ческая се́тка.

gauzy ['gɔːzɪ] *a* то́нкий, просве́чивающий (*о материи*).

gave [geɪv] *past см.* give I.

gavel ['gævl] *n* молото́к (*аукциониста или председателя собрания*).

gawk [gɔːk] *n* остоло́п, простофи́ля.

gawky ['gɔːkɪ] *a* неуклю́жий, засте́нчивый; глупова́тый.

gay [geɪ] *a* 1) весёлый; 2) я́ркий, блестя́щий, пёстрый (*о красках*); 3) беспу́тный.

gaze I [geɪz] *n* при́стальный взгляд.

gaze II *v* при́стально смотре́ть (*на — at, on, upon*), вгля́дываться.

gazebo [gə'ziːbou] *n* 1) да́ча (*с открывающимся вдаль видом*); 2) бельведе́р.

gazelle [gə'zel] *n* газе́ль.

gazette I [gə'zet] *n* 1) прави́тельственный бюллете́нь (*содержащий сообщения о назначениях, награждениях и т. п.*); 2) *уст.* газе́та.

gazette II *v* опублико́вывать в прави́тельственном бюллете́не.

gazetteer [,gæzɪ'tɪə] *n* географи́ческий спра́вочник.

gazogene ['gæzədʒiːn] *n* 1) аппара́т для гази́рования напи́тков; 2) *тех.* газогенера́тор.

gear I [gɪə] *n* 1) механи́зм, аппара́т; прибо́р; landing ~ а) *ав.* поса́дочное устро́йство, шасси́; б) *сленг* но́ги; 2) приспособле́ния; принадле́жности; 3) *тех.* шестерня́, зубча́тая переда́ча; приво́д; in ~ включённый; out of ~ вы́ключенный; *перен.* дезорганизо́ванный; не в поря́дке; 4) *авто* переда́ча; first (second, third) ~ пе́рвая (втора́я, тре́тья) переда́ча; reverse ~ за́дний ход; 5) *мор.* осна́стка; 6) у́пряжь; 7) у́тварь; предме́ты дома́шнего обихо́да.

gear II *v* 1) снабжа́ть приво́дом, переда́чей;

2) приводи́ть в движе́ние (*механизм*); 3) запряга́ть, надева́ть у́пряжь (*часто* to ~ up); □ to ~ down *тех.* замедля́ть движе́ние; to ~ up *тех.* ускоря́ть движе́ние.

gear-box ['gɪəbɔks] *n тех.* коро́бка скоросте́й, коро́бка переда́ч.

gear-case ['gɪəkeɪs] *см.* gear-box.

gearing ['gɪərɪŋ] *n тех.* зубча́тый приво́д, зубча́тая переда́ча.

gear-wheel ['gɪəwiːl] *n* шестерёнка, зубча́тое колесо́.

gee [dʒiː] *int* но! (*понукание лошади*) (*тж.* gee-ho, gee-up, gee-wo).

gee(-gee) ['dʒiː(dʒiː)] *n разг., дет.* лоша́дка.

geese [giːs] *pl см.* goose[1].

geezer ['giːzə] *n сленг* старика́шка; старушо́нка.

gelatin(e) [,dʒelə'tiːn] *n* желати́н; сту́день.

gelatinous [dʒɪ'lætɪnəs] *a* желати́новый; студени́стый.

gelid ['dʒelɪd] *a* ледяно́й, студёный; *перен.* холо́дный, кра́йне сде́ржанный (*о проявлении чувств*).

gem I [dʒem] *n* 1) драгоце́нный ка́мень; самоцве́т; 2) ге́мма; 3) драгоце́нность; *перен. тж.* жемчу́жина.

gem II *v* украша́ть драгоце́нными камня́ми.

geminate I ['dʒemɪneɪt] *a* сдво́енный.

geminate II *v* сдва́ивать, удва́ивать.

gemination [,dʒemɪ'neɪʃən] *n* сдва́ивание, удвое́ние.

gemma ['dʒemə] *n* (*pl* gemmae ['dʒemiː]) *бот.* по́чка.

gemmate ['dʒemeɪt] *v* пуска́ть по́чки.

gemmation [dʒe'meɪʃən] *n* 1) образова́ние по́чек; 2) почкова́ние.

gendarme ['ʒɑːndɑːm] *n* жанда́рм.

gendarmerie [ʒɑːn'dɑːməriː] *n* жандарме́рия.

gender I ['dʒendə] *n* 1) *грам.* род; masculine (feminine, neuter) ~ мужско́й (же́нский, сре́дний) род; 2) *шутл.* пол.

gender II *v поэт.* порожда́ть.

gene [dʒiːn] *n биол.* ген.

genealogical [,dʒiːnjə'lɔdʒɪkəl] *a* генеалоги́ческий.

genealogy [,dʒiːnɪ'ælədʒɪ] *n* родосло́вная, генеало́гия.

genera ['dʒenərə] *pl см.* genus.

general I ['dʒenərəl] *n* генера́л, полково́дец; lieutenant ~ генера́л-лейтена́нт; major ~ генера́л-майо́р; governor ~ губерна́тор коло́нии *или* домини́она.

general II *a* 1) о́бщий, всео́бщий; 2) генера́льный; основно́й; 3) гла́вный, руководя́щий; 4) обы́чный; in ~ вообще́, в о́бщих черта́х.

General-in-Chief ['dʒenərəlɪn'tʃiːf] *n* главнокома́ндующий.

generalissimo [,dʒenərə'lɪsɪmou] *n* генерали́ссимус.

generality [,dʒenə'rælɪtɪ] *n* 1) всео́бщность; 2) неопределённость; 3) *pl* о́бщие места́ (*в речи, суждении и т. п.*); 4) бо́льшая часть; большинство́.

generalization [,dʒenərəlaɪ'zeɪʃən] *n* обобще́ние.

generalize ['dʒenərəlaɪz] *v* 1) обобща́ть; 2) вводи́ть во всео́бщее употребле́ние.

generally ['dʒenərəlı] *adv* 1) обычно; 2) вообще, в общем смысле; в общих чертах; 3) большей частью; 4) широко, в большинстве случаев.

generalship ['dʒenərəlʃıp] *n* 1) звание генерала; 2) военное искусство; 3) (искусное) руководство.

generate ['dʒenəreıt] *v* 1) порождать, вызывать (*чувства*); 2) производить.

generation [ˌdʒenə'reıʃən] *n* 1) зарождение, возникновение; spontaneous ~ самозарождение; 2) поколение; the rising ~ подрастающее поколение, смена; the younger ~ младшее поколение; 3) потомство; род; 4) *тех.* образование (*пара*); генерация.

generative ['dʒenərətıv] *a* производящий, порождающий.

generator ['dʒenəreıtə] *n* 1) производитель; 2) *тех.* источник энергии; генератор.

generic [dʒı'nerık] *a* 1) родовой; характерный для определённого класса, вида (*животных*); 2) общий.

generosity [ˌdʒenə'rɔsıtı] *n* 1) великодушие; благородство (*характера*); 2) щедрость.

generous ['dʒenərəs] *a* 1) великодушный; благородный (*о характере, поступке*); 2) щедрый; 3) обильный; 4) плодородный (*о почве*); 5) густой, насыщенный (*о цвете*); 6) крепкий (*о вине*).

genesis ['dʒenısıs] *n* происхождение, возникновение; генезис.

genet ['dʒenıt] *n* 1) *зоол.* виверра; 2) мех виверры.

genetic(al) [dʒı'netık(əl)] *a* генетический.

genetics [dʒı'netıks] *n* генетика.

geneva [dʒı'niːvə] *n* джин; можжевёловая водка.

genial ['dʒiːnjəl] *a* 1) сердечный, радушный; добрый; доброжелательный; 2) мягкий, тёплый (*о климате*).

geniality [ˌdʒiːnı'ælıtı] *n* 1) сердечность, радушие; доброта; доброжелательность; 2) мягкость (*климата и т. п.*).

genie ['dʒiːnı] *n* (*pl* genii) джин (*дух в арабских сказках*).

genii[1] ['dʒiːnıaı] *pl см.* genie.

genii[2] *pl см.* genius 4).

genista [dʒı'nıstə] *n бот.* дрок.

genital ['dʒenıtl] *a* половой.

genitals ['dʒenıtlz] *n pl* половые органы.

genitive ['dʒenıtıv] *n грам.* родительный падеж.

genius ['dʒiːnjəs] *n* 1) одарённость; гениальность; 2) гений, гениальный человек; 3) дух (*языка, нации и т. п.*); 4) (*pl* genii) дух; evil (good) ~ злой (добрый) дух.

genre [ʒɑːŋr] *n* жанр; манера, стиль.

gent [dʒent] *n разг.* господин, джентльмен.

genteel [dʒen'tiːl] *a ирон.* 1) утончённый (*о манерах*); 2) воспитанный, светский; 3) модный, изящный.

gentility [dʒen'tılıtı] *n ирон.* аристократические замашки; 2) *уст.* родовитость, знатность.

gentle I ['dʒentl] *a* 1) мягкий, добрый, спокойный; кроткий (*о характере*); 2) нежный, ласковый; 3) лёгкий, слабый (*о ветерке*); 4) послушный, смирный (*о животном*); 5) отлогий (*о склоне, спуске*); 6) знатный, родовитый.

gentle II *n* наживка (*для уженья*).

gentlefolk(s) ['dʒentlfouk(s)] *n pl* дворянство, знать.

gentleman ['dʒentlmən] *n* 1) джентльмен, господин (*обращение к мужчине*); 2) благородный, порядочный человек; fine ~ светский человек; 3) *уст.* дворянин; ~ in waiting камергер; ◇ ~ at large человек без определённых занятий; ~ of fortune пират; gentlemen of the long robe судьи; юристы; gentlemen of cloth духовенство; the old ~ *шутл.* дьявол.

gentleman-at-arms ['dʒentlmənət'ɑːmz] *n* лейб-гвардеец.

gentlemanlike ['dʒentlmənlaık] *a* 1) вежливый, благовоспитанный; 2) поступающий по-джентльменски.

gentlemanly ['dʒentlmənlı] *см.* gentlemanlike 2).

gentleness ['dʒentlnıs] *n* 1) мягкость, кротость; 2) отлогость.

gentlewoman ['dʒentlˌwumən] *n* 1) дама, леди; 2) *уст.* дворянка.

gently ['dʒentlı] *adv* 1) мягко, кротко, нежно; 2) спокойно, медленно; ~! тише!, осторожнее!, медленней!; 3) отлого.

gentry ['dʒentrı] *n* мелкопоместное дворянство, джентри.

genuine ['dʒenjuın] *a* 1) подлинный, истинный; 2) искренний.

genus ['dʒiːnəs] *n* (*pl* genera) 1) *биол.* род; 2) сорт.

geodesy [dʒiː'ɔdısı] *n* геодезия.

geographer [dʒı'ɔgrəfə] *n* географ.

geographic(al) [dʒıə'græfık(əl)] *a* географический.

geography [dʒı'ɔgrəfı] *n* 1) география; 2) *attr* географический.

geologic(al) [dʒıə'lɔdʒık(əl)] *a* геологический.

geologist [dʒı'ɔlədʒıst] *n* геолог.

geology [dʒı'ɔlədʒı] *n* 1) геология; 2) *attr* геологический.

geometric(al) [dʒıə'metrık(əl)] *a* геометрический.

geometry [dʒı'ɔmıtrı] *n* геометрия; descriptive ~ начертательная геометрия; plane ~ планиметрия; solid ~ стереометрия.

George [dʒɔːdʒ] *n сленг* автопилот.

Georgian[1] I ['dʒɔːdʒən] *n* 1) грузин; грузинка; the ~s грузины; 2) грузинский язык.

Georgian[1] II *a* грузинский.

Georgian[2] I *n* уроженец штата Джорджия (*в США*).

Georgian[2] II *a* относящийся к штату Джорджия.

Georgian[3] *a* эпохи одного из английских королей Георгов (*XVIII в.*).

geranium [dʒı'reınjəm] *n бот.* герань.

germ I [dʒəːm] *n* 1) зародыш; эмбрион; *бот.* завязь; 2) микроб; 3) зачаток, начало; in ~ в зародыше; в зачаточном состоянии; 4) *attr* бактериологический.

germ II *v* давать ростки, развиваться.

German I ['dʒəːmən] *n* 1) немец; немка; the ~s немцы; 2) немецкий язык.

German II *a* немецкий, германский.

german ['dʒəːmən] *a* родной (*в сочетании с*

brother, sister); двоюродный (*в сочетании с* cousin).

germane [dʒə'meɪn] *a* уместный; имеющий отношение (*к чему-л.— to*).

germinal ['dʒə:mɪnl] *a* зародышевый; зачаточный.

germinate ['dʒə:mɪneɪt] *v* 1) прорастать; давать почки; пускать ростки; 2) вызывать к жизни, порождать; 3) зарождаться.

germination [,dʒə:mɪ'neɪʃən] *n* 1) прорастание; 2) развитие, рост.

gerrymander I ['gerɪmændə] *n* предвыборные махинации (*в буржуазных странах*).

gerrymander II *v* 1) подтасовывать (*результаты выборов*); 2) искажать факты, фальсифицировать.

gerund ['dʒerənd] *n* грам. герундий.

gerund-grinder ['dʒerənd,graɪndə] *n* пренебр. 1) учитель латинского языка; 2) учитель-формалист.

gesso ['dʒesou] *n* гипс (*для скульптурных работ*).

gestation [dʒes'teɪʃən] *n* беременность; период беременности.

gesticulate [dʒes'tɪkjuleɪt] *v* жестикулировать.

gesticulation [dʒes,tɪkju'leɪʃən] *n* жестикуляция.

gesture I ['dʒestʃə] *n* жест; жестикуляция; facial ~ мимика; fine ~ благородный жест, поступок.

gesture II *v* жестикулировать.

get [get] *v* (*past, p. p.* got; *уст. и амер. p. p.* gotten) 1) получать; 2) доставать, добывать; to ~ a living зарабатывать на жизнь; 3) доставлять, приносить; to ~ smb. home отвезти кого-л. домой; 4) добиться; to ~ one's own way добиться своего; поставить на своём; 5) покупать, приобретать; 6) (*с последующим сложным дополнением — сущ. или мест. + Inf*) убедить, заставить (*кого-л. сделать что-л.*); ~ him to go убедите его уйти; 7) схватить (*болезнь*); to ~ the measles заболеть корью; 8) добираться, доезжать; достигать (*места*): to ~ home а) попасть домой; б) попасть в цель; 9) перебираться, переезжать, переходить, переправляться (*через мост, реку; across*); перелезать (*через забор; over*); 10) (*в форме Pres. Perf.*) разг. иметь, обладать (*часто с усечённой формой вспом. гл.* have — 've, has — 's (*в 3-м л. ед. ч.*) является эквивалентом Present гл. to have); I've got a pencil у меня есть карандаш; 11) (*в форме Pres. Perf.+Inf* образует фразовое сказуемое в сочетании с сущ.) быть обязанным; быть должным (*что-л. сделать*); you've got to do it вы должны сделать это; I've got to pass the examination я должен сдать экзамен; 12) (*с Inf смыслового гл. придаёт ему характер однократного действия*): to ~ to know узнать; 13) (*со сложным дополнением — сущ. или мест.+p. р. — обозначает, что действие выполняется кем-л. по желанию действующего лица*) заказать, поручить (*сделать что-л.*); I got a coat made я заказал себе пальто; 14) (*с прил. и p. p.*) становиться, делаться; it is ~ting dark становится темно, темнеет; to ~ done разделаться, покончить (*с чем-л.— with*); 15) улавливать смысл, понимать; 16) ста-

вить в тупик, озадачивать; □ to ~ **about** а) распространяться (*о слухах*); б) переезжать, передвигаться; в) начинать (вы)ходить (*после болезни*); to ~ **abroad** см. to ~ about а); to ~ **across** *разг.* довести (*до сознания кого-л.; to*); to ~ **ahead** обогнать (*в учении, успехах*); to ~ **along** а) жить, поживать; б) делать успехи; в) жить в дружбе, ладить; г): ~ along with you! *разг.* убирайся; to ~ **at** а) добраться; дозвониться (*по телефону*); б) понять, постичь; в) *разг.* подкупить; г) *разг.* высмеять; to ~ **away** а) удирать; отправляться; б) *амер.* авто трогать с места; в) *ав.* взлететь; г): ~ away with you! *шутл.* да ну тебя!; брось болтать чепуху!; д): to ~ away with smth. преуспевать, иметь успех; е): to ~ smth. away убрать, устранить, снять что-л.; to ~ **back** а) вернуться; б) возмещать (*потерю, убыток*); to ~ **by** проходить мимо (*кого-л., чего-л.*); to ~ **down** а) спуститься, сойти; б) снять (*с полки*); в) проглатывать; г) засесть (*за учение и т. п.; to*); to ~ **in** а) влезть, войти; б) пройти на выборах (*о кандидате*); в) вернуть (*долги и т. п.*); г) убирать (*сено, урожай*); д) нанести удар; to ~ **into** надевать, напяливать на себя (*одежду, обувь*); to ~ **off** а) сходить, слезать (*с лошади, трамвая*); б) сбежать; в) спастись, отделаться (*от наказания*); to ~ **on** а) садиться (*на лошадь*); б) надевать; в) приближаться (*о времени*); г) делать успехи; преуспевать; to ~ on well (ill) жить хорошо (плохо); she is ~ting on nicely она поправляется; д) ладить (*with*); е) стареть, стариться; to ~ **out** а) выходить, вылезать (*из — of*); б) доставать, вынимать; в) стать известным (*о секрете*); г) выведывать, разузнавать; д) бросать (*привычку*), избегать (*делать что-л.*); to ~ **over** а) преодолеть (*трудности*); б) оправиться (*от болезни, испуга*); в) разделаться, покончить (*с чем-л.*); to ~ **round** обойти, надуть, провести (*кого-л.*); to ~ **through** а) справиться с чем-л.; сдать экзамен; б) провести *или* пройти (*о законопроекте*); в) разделаться, покончить (*с чем-л.— with*); to ~ **to** приниматься за что-л.; to ~ **together** собирать(ся); to ~ **under** тушить (*пожар*); to ~ **up** а) вставать; подниматься; б) садиться (*в экипаж, на лошадь*); в) организовывать; осуществлять; ставить (*пьесу*); оформлять (*книгу*); г) причёсывать(ся); гримировать(ся); наряжать(ся); д) усиливаться (*о ветре, пожаре*); ◊ to ~ **by** heart выучить наизусть; to ~ **into** one's head а) ударить в голову (*о спиртных напитках*); б) забрать себе в голову; to ~ one's own back on smb. отомстить за обиду; to ~ **off** with a whole skin *погов.* ≅ выйти сухим из воды.

get-at-able [get'ætəbl] *a* доступный.

getaway ['getəweɪ] *n* разг. бегство, побег; to make one's ~ бежать, устроить побег.

getter ['getə] *n* 1) добытчик; приобретатель; 2) *горн.* рудокоп.

get-up ['getʌp] *n* 1) манера одеваться; стиль; 2) оформление (*книги*); 3) постановка (*пьесы*); 4) *амер.* предприимчивость.

gewgaw ['gju:gɔ:] *n* безделушка, мишура.

geyser[a] ['gaɪzə] *n* гейзер.

geyser[b] ['gi:zə] *n* газовая колонка (*в ванне*).

gharry ['gærɪ] *n* наёмный экипаж (*в Индии*).

ghastly I ['gɑːstlɪ] *a* 1) стра́шный, ужа́сный; 2) ме́ртвенно-бле́дный; 3) *разг.* ужаса́ющий, скве́рный; 4) принуждённый (*об улыбке*); криво́й (*об усмешке*).

ghastly II *adv* стра́шно, ужа́сно.

gherkin ['gəːkɪn] *n* корнишо́н.

ghetto ['getou] *n* ге́тто, евре́йский кварта́л.

ghost [goust] *n* 1) привиде́ние, при́зрак; дух; тень (*умершего*); to give up the ~ *уст.* испусти́ть дух, сконча́ться; to raise a (*или* the) ~ вызыва́ть ду́ха; ~s of the past те́ни про́шлого; 2) лёгкий след (*чего-л.*), намёк; the ~ of a smile чуть заме́тная улы́бка; 3) факти́ческий а́втор, та́йно рабо́тающий для друго́го лица́; ◇ the ~ walks *театр. сленг* выпла́чивают зарпла́ту.

ghostly ['goustlɪ] *a* 1) при́зрачный; 2) духо́вный.

ghoul [guːl] *n* вампи́р, вурдала́к.

ghoulish ['guːlɪʃ] *a* отврати́тельный, стра́шный.

GI I ['dʒiːˈaɪ] (*сокр. от* government issue) *n амер.* солда́т.

GI II *a амер.* 1) казённый, вое́нного образца́; 2) арме́йский.

giant I ['dʒaɪənt] *n* велика́н, исполи́н; тита́н.

giant II *a* гига́нтский; исполи́нский; грома́дный.

giantess ['dʒaɪəntɪs] *n* велика́нша.

giantlike ['dʒaɪəntlaɪk] *a* огро́мный, исполи́нский.

giant('s)-stride ['dʒaɪənt(s)'straɪd] *n спорт.* гига́нтские шаги́.

giaour ['dʒauə] *n* гяу́р, неве́рный.

gibber I ['dʒɪbə] *n* невня́тная болтовня́, бормота́ние.

gibber II *v* невня́тно болта́ть, бормота́ть.

gibberish ['dʒɪbərɪʃ] *n* невня́тная речь; тараба́рщина.

gibbet I ['dʒɪbɪt] *n* 1) ви́селица; 2) пове́шение.

gibbet II *v* 1) ве́шать, казни́ть че́рез пове́шение; 2) выставля́ть на позо́р, на посме́шище.

gibbon ['gɪbən] *n зоол.* гиббо́н.

gibbosity [gɪ'bɔsɪtɪ] *n* 1) горба́тость; 2) вы́пуклость..

gibbous ['gɪbəs] *a* 1) горба́тый; 2) вы́пуклый.

gibe I [dʒaɪb] *n* насме́шка.

gibe II *v* насмеха́ться (*над кем-л. — at*).

giblets ['dʒɪblɪts] *n pl* (гуси́ные) потроха́.

giddiness ['gɪdɪnɪs] *n* 1) головокруже́ние; 2) легкомы́слие, ве́треность.

giddy ['gɪdɪ] *a* 1) испы́тывающий головокруже́ние; to feel ~ чу́вствовать головокруже́ние; 2) головокружи́тельный (*об успехе, высоте и т. п.*); 3) легкомы́сленный, ве́треный.

giddy-go-round ['gɪdɪgou,raund] *n* карусе́ль.

gift I [gɪft] *n* 1) пода́рок, дар; I would not have it at a ~ ≅ я э́того и да́ром не возьму́; 2) спосо́бность, дарова́ние; the ~ of the gab дар сло́ва.

gift II *v* одаря́ть, наделя́ть (*чем-л. — with*).

gifted ['gɪftɪd] *a* спосо́бный, одарённый; дарови́тый.

gig¹ [gɪg] *n* 1) кабриоле́т; 2) ги́чка (*узкая, быстроходная лодка*).

gig² *n* острога́.

gigantic [dʒaɪ'gæntɪk] *a* гига́нтский, грома́дный.

giggle I ['gɪgl] *n* хихи́канье.

giggle II *v* хихи́кать.

gig-lamps ['gɪglæmps] *n pl сленг* очки́.

gigolo ['ʒɪgəlou] *n* наёмный партнёр (*в танцах*), жи́голо.

gild¹ [gɪld] *v* 1) золоти́ть, покрыва́ть позоло́той; 2) украша́ть.

gild² *n см.* guild.

gilded ['gɪldɪd] *a* позоло́ченный.

gillᵃ¹ [gɪl] *n обыкн. pl* 1) жа́бры; 2) второ́й подборо́док; ◇ rosy about the ~s здоро́вый, морда́стый.

gillᵃ² *n* 1) леси́стый овра́г; 2) го́рный пото́к.

gillᵇ [dʒɪl] *n* че́тверть пи́нты (*англ.=0,142 л, амер.=0,118 л*).

gillyflower ['dʒɪlɪ,flauə] *n* 1) левко́й; 2) *редко* гвозди́ка.

gilt I [gɪlt] *n* позоло́та; ◇ to take the ~ off the gingerbread ≅ показа́ть что-л. без прикра́с.

gilt II *a* золочёный, позоло́ченный.

gilt-edged ['gɪltedʒd] *a* с золоты́м обре́зом.

gimcrack I ['dʒɪmkræk] *n* безделу́шка, мишура́.

gimcrack II *a* сде́ланный ко́е-ка́к, на ско́рую ру́ку.

gimlet ['gɪmlɪt] *n* бура́вчик.

gimmick ['gɪmɪk] *n амер.* трюк, уло́вка.

gin¹ [dʒɪn] *n* джин, во́дка.

gin² I *n* 1) джин (*хлопкоочистительная машина*); 2) подъёмная лебёдка; во́рот; 3) западня́, сило́к.

gin² II *v* 1) очища́ть хло́пок; 2) лови́ть в западню́.

ginger I ['dʒɪndʒə] *n* 1) имби́рь; to eat the ~ *амер. сленг* ≅ снима́ть пе́нки, брать всё лу́чшее; 2) *разг.* огонёк; воодушевле́ние; «изю́минка»; he wants some ~ ему́ «изю́минки» не хвата́ет; 3) рыжева́тый цвет (*волос*).

ginger II *v* 1) взба́дривать (*лошадь*); 2) *разг.* подстёгивать, подхлёстывать (*тж.* to ~ up).

ginger-beer ['dʒɪndʒə'bɪə] *n* имби́рный лимона́д, имби́рное пи́во.

gingerbread I ['dʒɪndʒəbred] *n* имби́рный пря́ник.

gingerbread II *a* показно́й, пы́шный.

gingerly I ['dʒɪndʒəlɪ] *a* осторо́жный, осмотри́тельный; ро́бкий.

gingerly II *adv* осторо́жно.

gingery ['dʒɪndʒərɪ] *a* 1) имби́рный, пря́ный; 2) раздражи́тельный, вспы́льчивый; 3) рыжева́тый.

gingham ['gɪŋəm] *n* 1) кле́тчатая *или* полоса́тая бума́жная *или* льняна́я мате́рия из кра́шеной пря́жи; 2) *разг.* зо́нтик.

ginny ['dʒɪnɪ] *a* опьянённый, нетре́звый; to get ~ вы́пить, клю́кнуть.

gin-palace ['dʒɪn,pælɪs] *n разг.* тракти́р, таве́рна, пивна́я.

ginseng ['dʒɪnseŋ] *n* женьше́нь.

gin-shop ['dʒɪnʃɔp] *n* ви́нная ла́вка.

gippo ['dʒɪpou] *n воен. разг.* суп, похлёбка; подли́вка.

Gipsy I ['dʒɪpsɪ] *n* 1) цыга́н; цыга́нка; the Gipsies цыга́не; 2) цыга́нский язы́к.

Gipsy II *a* цыга́нский.

giraffe [dʒɪ'rɑːf] *n* жира́ф.

gird¹ [gəːd] *v* (*past, p. p.* girded, girt) 1) прикрепля́ть са́блю, ша́шку к по́ясу; 2) подпоя́сываться; 3) облека́ть вла́стью (*with*); 4) окружа́ть;

5) *поэт.* опоясывать; to ~ oneself up for готовиться к чему-л.

gird² I *n* насмешка.

gird² II *v* насмехаться (*над — at*).

girder ['gə:də] *n* 1) балка; 2) ферма (*моста*); 3) *радио* мачта.

girdle I ['gə:dl] *n* 1) пояс, кушак; under one's ~ на поводу у кого-л.; 2) анат. пояс; 3) кольцо (*на дереве — при кольцевании*).

girdle II *v* 1) подпоясывать; 2) кольцевать (*плодовые деревья*); 3) окружать (*чем-л.— with*).

girl [gə:l] *n* 1) девочка; 2) девушка, молодая женщина; bus ~ кондукторша автобуса; office ~ служащая; shop ~ продавщица; old ~ милая, старушка (*в обращении*); my dear ~ женушка (*в обращении*); the ~s дочери (*в одной семье*); 3) служанка, прислуга; домашняя работница, 4) *разг.* невеста, возлюбленная (*тж.* best ~); ◇ hello ~ *амер. разг.* телефонистка.

girlhood ['gə:lhud] *n* девичество.

girlie ['gə:lɪ] *n* ласк. девочка.

girlish ['gə:lɪʃ] *a* 1) девический; 2) изнеженный, похожий на девочку (*о мальчике*).

girt [gə:t] *past, p. p. см.* gird¹.

girth I [gə:θ] *n* 1) подпруга; 2) обхват; размер (*дерева в обхвате и т. п.*).

girth II *v* 1) подтягивать подпругу; 2) мерить в обхвате; 3) окружать, опоясывать.

gist [dʒɪst] *n* суть, сущность.

give I [gɪv] *v* (*past.* gave; *p. p.* given) 1) давать; даровать, жаловать (*награду, орден, грамоту*); 2) платить; 3) заражать; 4) *в сочетаниях со связанным именным дополнением выражает однократное действие и передаётся русским гл. однократного вида, соответствующим по значению именному дополнению, напр.:* to ~ a look взглянуть; to ~ a sigh вздохнуть; 5) вручать (*послание, записку и т. п.*); 6) передавать (*привет, поклон*); 7) отдавать, посвящать (*жизнь, время, труд*); 8) устраивать, давать (*обед, вечеринку, бал*); 9) высказывать (*свои соображения, своё мнение*); 10) причинять (*беспокойство, неприятности*); 11) выносить (*приговор и т. п.*); 12) подаваться, оседать (*о фундаменте, здании и т. п.*); гнуться (*о дереве, металле*); 13) выходить (*об окне, двери, тж — upon*); вести (*о дороге; к — into*); □ to ~ **away** a) отдавать, дарить; б) раздавать (*призы, деньги*); в) выдавать, предавать (*кого-л.*); разоблачать; г) выдавать (*замуж*); to ~ **back** a) возвращать, отдавать; б) отплатить (*за обиду*); to ~ **forth** a) объявлять; обнародовать; выпускать; б) распускать слух; to ~ **in** a) уступать, сдаваться; б) подавать (*заявление, отчёт и т. п.*); сдавать (*документы*); to ~ **off** испускать; to ~ **out** a) иссякнуть, кончиться (*о запасах, силе*); б) распределять; в) объявлять; г) выпускать, издавать; д) передавать; to ~ **over** a) перестать (*делать что-л.*); бросать (*привычку*); to ~ **up** a) отказаться (*от работы, предложения и т. п.*); б) уступить; to ~ oneself up предаваться (*чему-л.*); в) махнуть рукой (*на что-л.*); to ~ smb. up as dead *или* for dead умереть; б) выдать (*беглеца*); в) признать безнадёжным (*больного*); ◇ to ~ as good as one gets не оставаться в долгу, отвечать тем же; to ~ it smb. hot задавать кому-л. жару, распекать кого-л.

give II *n* эластичность; гибкость; ◇ ~ and take

а) взаимные уступки, компромисс; б) обмен (*мнениями*).

give-away ['gɪvə,weɪ] *n разг.* ненамеренное разоблачение тайны.

given I ['gɪvn] *p. p. см.* give I.

given II *a* 1) данный; 2) приверженный; увлекающийся.

giver ['gɪvə] *n* дающий, раздающий, отдающий (*человек*).

gizzard ['gɪzəd] *n* 1) второй желудок (*у птиц*); 2) *разг.* горло, глотка; to stick in one's ~ стать поперёк горла; ◇ to fret one's ~ волноваться, сходить с ума (*от беспокойства*).

glacé ['glæseɪ] *a* 1) сатинированный (*о ткани*); 2) глазированный, засахаренный.

glacial ['gleɪsjəl] *a* 1) ледниковый; 2) ледяной; холодный, леденящий (*тж. перен.*); 3) *хим.* кристаллизованный.

glacier ['glæsjə] *n* ледник, глетчер.

glad [glæd] *a* 1) *predic* довольный; 2) радостный, утешительный (*об известиях*); 3) яркий.

gladden ['glædn] *v* радовать, веселить.

glade [gleɪd] *n* 1) прогалина, просека, поляна; 2) полоса света, просвет; 3) *амер.* полынья.

gladiator ['glædɪeɪtə] *n* гладиатор.

gladly ['glædlɪ] *adv* с радостью.

gladsome ['glædsəm] *a поэт.* радостный.

Gladstone ['glædstən] *n* 1) кожаный саквояж (*тж.* ~ bag); 2) двухместный экипаж.

glair [glɛə] *n* яичный белок.

glamorous ['glæmərəs] *a* обаятельный, чарующий, пленительный.

glamour I ['glæmə] *n* 1) обаяние, очарование; 2) чары; волшебство; to cast a ~ over очаровать; 3) *attr* обаятельная, очаровательная (*о девушке*).

glamour II *v* зачаровывать, пленять.

glance I [glɑ:ns] *n* 1) быстрый взгляд; at a ~ с одного взгляда; to cast a ~ at бросить быстрый взгляд на; to give a ~ at взглянуть на; to steal a ~ взглянуть украдкой; stealthy ~ взгляд украдкой; 2) вспышка, блеск.

glance II *v* взглянуть (*на — at*) бегло просматривать (*over*); 2) вспыхнуть, блеснуть, сверкнуть (*о свете*); 3) перескакивать (*с одной темы на другую*); 4) скользнуть по поверхности (*о холодном оружии*).

gland¹ [glænd] *n* 1) железа; lachrymal ~ слёзная железа; 2) *pl* шейные железки, гланды.

gland² *n тех.* сальник.

glanders ['glændəz] *n pl вет.* сап.

glandule ['glændjuːl] *n* 1) железка; 2) небольшая опухоль.

glare I [glɛə] *n* 1) яркий свет; ослепительный блеск; 2) блестящая мишура; 3) пристальный *или* свирепый взгляд.

glare II *v* 1) ослепительно сверкать; 2) пристально *или* свирепо смотреть (*на — at*).

glaring ['glɛərɪŋ] *a* 1) яркий, ослепительный (*о свете*); 2) кричащий (*о цвете*); 3) пристальный *или* свирепый (*о взгляде*); 4) грубый (*об ошибке*).

glass I [glɑ:s] *n* 1) стекло; shatter-proof ~ небьющееся стекло; 2) стеклянная посуда; medicine ~ мензурка; 3) стакан, рюмка; *разг.* выпивка; I have had a ~ too much я выпил лишнего; to clink ~es чокаться; to raise one's ~ to smb.'s health поднима́ть бока́л за чье́-л. здоро́вье; 4) парнико́вая ра́ма; 5) ли́нза; телеско́п; бино́кль; микроско́п; баро́метр; 6) зе́ркало; 7) pl очки́; 8) attr стекля́нный.

glass II v 1) отража́ться (как в зеркале); 2) вставля́ть стёкла, остекля́ть; 3) помеща́ть в парни́к.

glass-blower ['glɑːs,blouə] n стеклоду́в.

glass-culture ['glɑːs,kʌltʃə] n парнико́вая культу́ра.

glass-cutter ['glɑːs,kʌtə] n 1) стеко́льщик; 2) алма́з (для резки стекла).

glass-dust ['glɑːsdʌst] n нажда́к.

glassful ['glɑːsful] n стака́н (как мера ёмкости).

glass-house ['glɑːshaus] n 1) тепли́ца; оранжере́я; 2) стеко́льный заво́д.

glass-paper ['glɑːs,peipə] n стекля́нная шку́рка, нажда́чная бума́га.

glass-work ['glɑːswəːk] n 1) стеко́льное произво́дство; 2) pl стеко́льный заво́д.

glassy ['glɑːsi] a 1) зерка́льный (о водной поверхности); 2) стекля́нный, безжи́зненный (о взгляде); 3) облада́ющий сво́йством стекла́.

glaze I [gleiz] n 1) глазу́рь; гля́нец; 2) глази́ро́ванная посу́да.

glaze II v 1) застекля́ть, вставля́ть стёкла; 2) покрыва́ть глазу́рью; 3) тускне́ть, стеклене́ть (о глазах); 4) полирова́ть.

glazier ['gleizjə] n 1) стеко́льщик; 2) гонча́р-глазиро́вщик.

glazy ['gleizi] a 1) глянцеви́тый; 2) ту́склый, остеклене́вший (о глазах).

gleam I [gliːm] n 1) сла́бый свет, о́тблеск, отраже́ние (лучей заходящего солнца); 2) про́блеск, вспы́шка (юмора, надежды).

gleam II v 1) отража́ться от како́го-л. блестя́щего предме́та; 2) свети́ться, мерца́ть.

glean [gliːn] v 1) подбира́ть коло́сья (после жатвы); 2) собира́ть по кро́хам (сведения и т. п.).

gleanings ['gliːniŋz] n pl 1) со́бранные по́сле жа́твы коло́сья; 2) со́бранные фа́кты; обры́вки све́дений, зна́ний.

glee [gliː] n 1) весе́лье, ликова́ние; 2) пе́сня (для нескольких голосов).

gleeful ['gliːful] a весёлый, ра́достный; лику́ющий.

glen [glen] n лощи́на, у́зкая доли́на.

glengarry [glen'gæri] n шотла́ндская ша́пка (с лентами сзади).

glib [glib] a 1) речи́стый, говорли́вый; 2) бо́йкий (о речи).

glide I [glaid] n 1) скольже́ние; пла́вное движе́ние; 2) ав. плани́рование; 3) муз. хромати́ческая га́мма; 4) фон. промежу́точный звук.

glide II v 1) скользи́ть; дви́гаться пла́вно; 2) дви́гаться кра́дучись; 3) проходи́ть незаме́тно, пролета́ть (о времени); 4) ав. плани́ровать.

glider ['glaidə] n ав. планёр.

gliding ['glaidiŋ] n 1) скольже́ние; 2) планери́зм.

glim [glim] n сленг 1) свет; 2) глаз.

glimmer I ['glimə] n 1) мерца́ние, сла́бый свет; 2) сла́бый про́блеск (надежды и т. п.).

glimmer II v мерца́ть, ту́скло свети́ть.

glimpse I [glimps] n 1) мимолётное впечат-

ле́ние; at a ~ с пе́рвого взгля́да; to catch (или to get) a ~ of уви́деть ме́льком; 2) про́блеск.

glimpse II v 1) уви́деть ме́льком; 2) мелька́ть; промелькну́ть.

glint I [glint] n вспы́шка, сверка́ние; я́ркий блеск.

glint II v 1) вспы́хивать, сверка́ть; я́рко блесте́ть; 2) отража́ть (свет).

glissade I [gli'sɑːd] n 1) скольже́ние, соска́льзывание; 2) глиссе́ (в танцах).

glissade II v 1) скользи́ть, соска́льзывать; 2) де́лать глиссе́.

glisten ['glisn] v сверка́ть, блесте́ть; и́скри́ться.

glister ['glistə] v уст. блесте́ть, сверка́ть.

glitter I ['glitə] n 1) блеск, сверка́ние; 2) по́мпа, пы́шность.

glitter II v блесте́ть, сверка́ть; ◊ all is not gold that ~s посл. не всё то зо́лото, что блести́т.

g-load ['dʒiːloud] n косм. перегру́зка.

gloaming ['gloumiŋ] n вече́рние су́мерки.

gloat [glout] v 1) пожира́ть глаза́ми (over, upon); 2) та́йно злора́дствовать; 3) ра́доваться (про себя).

globe [gloub] n 1) шар; the ~ of the eye глазно́е я́блоко; 2) (the ~) земно́й шар; 3) небе́сное те́ло; 4) гло́бус; terrestrial (celestial) ~ географи́ческий (небе́сный) гло́бус; 5) держа́ва (эмблема власти монарха); 6) кру́глый абажу́р; 7) attr шарови́дный, сфери́ческий.

globe-trotter ['gloub,trɔtə] n мно́го путеше́ствовавший челове́к.

globose ['gloubous] a шарови́дный, сфери́ческий.

globular ['glɔbjulə] a шарови́дный, сфери́ческий.

globule ['glɔbjuːl] n 1) ша́рик; шарови́дная части́ца; 2) физиол. кра́сный кровяно́й ша́рик; 3) пилю́ля.

gloom I [gluːm] n 1) мрак; темнота́; 2) уны́ние, мра́чность, пода́вленное настрое́ние.

gloom II v 1) быть в мра́чном настрое́нии, быть в уны́нии; име́ть хму́рый вид; 2) хму́риться, покрыва́ться ту́чами; 3) вызыва́ть уны́ние; омрача́ть.

gloomy ['gluːmi] a 1) мра́чный; 2) угрю́мый; пода́вленный; 3) хму́рый, уны́лый.

glorification [,glɔːrifi'keiʃən] n прославле́ние, восхвале́ние.

glorify ['glɔːrifai] v 1) прославля́ть, восхваля́ть; превозноси́ть; 2) разг. украша́ть.

gloriole ['glɔːrioul] n орео́л, сия́ние.

glorious ['glɔːriəs] a 1) сла́вный, знамени́тый; 2) прекра́сный, чуде́сный, восхити́тельный (тж. ирон.); 3) разг. подвы́пивший.

glory I ['glɔːri] n 1) сла́ва; 2) прославле́ние, триу́мф; 3) великоле́пие, красота́; 4) орео́л, сия́ние; ◊ ~ morning = бот. вьюно́к; Old Glory амер. разг. госуда́рственный флаг США; to go to ~ разг. умере́ть; to send to ~ разг. уби́ть, прико́нчить.

glory II v горди́ться (чем-л. — in).

gloss[1] I [glɔs] n 1) лоск, вне́шний блеск; 2) обма́нчивая нару́жность).

gloss[1] II v 1) наводи́ть лоск, придава́ть блеск; 2) представля́ть в лу́чшем ви́де, све́те (тж. to ~ over).

gloss[2] I n 1) гло́сса, заме́тка на поля́х; толкова́ние; 2) подстро́чник; глосса́рий; 3) истолкова́ние.

gloss[2] II v 1) де́лать заме́тки (на полях); снаб-

жа́ть коммента́рием; 2) неблагоприя́тно истолко́-
вывать.

glossary ['glɔsərı] *n* 1) слова́рь (*приложенный
в конце книги*), глосса́рий; 2) слова́рь специа́льных
те́рминов.

glossology [glɔ'sɔlədʒı] *n* терминоло́гия.

glossy ['glɔsı] *a* блестя́щий, лосня́щийся, гля́нце-
ви́тый.

glottis ['glɔtıs] *n анат.* голосова́я щель.

glove I [glʌv] *n* перча́тка, рукави́ца; to throw
down the ~ бро́сить перча́тку, вы́звать на поеди́-
нок, дуэль; to take up the ~ подня́ть перча́тку,
приня́ть вы́зов (*на дуэль*); ◊ to fit like a ~
быть как раз впо́ру; to take off the ~s пригото́-
виться к бо́ю; to go for the ~s *сленг* лезть на-
проло́м.

glove II *v* надева́ть перча́тки.

glow I [glou] *n* 1) пыл, жар; зной; scorching ~
паля́щий зной; 2) свет, за́рево, о́тблеск (*пожара,
заката*); 3) румя́нец; 4) я́ркость (*красок*);
5) оживлённость; горя́чность; 6) *эл.* свече́ние.

glow II *v* 1) свети́ться; 2) накаля́ться до́красна,
добела́; 3) тлеть; 4) пламене́ть; 5) сгора́ть (*от
страсти, любви*); 6) пыла́ть (*о щеках*); сверка́ть
(*о глазах*); сия́ть (*от радости*).

glower ['glauə] *v* серди́то смотре́ть (*на — at*).

glowing ['glouıŋ] *a* 1) я́рко светя́щийся;
2) раскалённый добела́; 3) горя́чий, пы́лкий;
4) я́ркий (*о красках*); 5) пыла́ющий, горя́щий
(*о щеках*); ~ with health пы́шущий здоро́вьем.

glow-lamp ['gloulæmp] *n* ла́мпа накалива́ния.

glow-worm ['glouwəːm] *n* светля́к.

glucose ['gluːkous] *n* глюко́за.

glue I [gluː] *n* (столя́рный) клей.

glue II *v* 1) кле́ить, приклеи́вать; 2) приклеи́вать-
ся; прилипа́ть, пристава́ть; скле́иваться; в) быть
неотлу́чно (*при ком-л.*).

gluey ['gluːı] *a* кле́йкий, ли́пкий.

glum [glʌm] *a* мра́чный, хму́рый; угрю́мый.

glut I [glʌt] *n* 1) пресыще́ние; 2) избы́ток
(*товаров и т. п.*); 3) изли́шество, неуме́ренность
(*в еде и т. п.*).

glut II *v* 1) насыща́ть; пресыща́ть; удовлет-
воря́ть (*желания и т. п.*); 2) наполня́ть до отка́за;
3) зава́ливать (*товарами*); переполня́ть.

gluten ['gluːtən] *n* клейкови́на.

glutinous ['gluːtınəs] *a* кле́йкий.

glutton ['glʌtn] *n* 1) обжо́ра; 2) жа́дный, не-
насы́тный челове́к; a ~ for work работя́га;
3) *зоол.* росома́ха.

gluttonous ['glʌtnəs] *a* прожо́рливый, ненасы́т-
ный.

gluttony ['glʌtnı] *n* прожо́рливость, ненасы́т-
ность.

glycerin(e) [‚glısə'riːn] *n* глицери́н.

G-man ['dʒiːmæn] *n амер. разг.* аге́нт Феде-
ра́льного бюро́ рассле́дований.

gnarled [nɑːld] *a* 1) узлова́тый; свилева́тый
(*о древесине*); сучкова́тый, криво́й (*о дереве*);
2) углова́тый (*о движениях*); неуклю́жий; 3) уп-
ря́мый, несгово́рчивый.

gnarly ['nɑːlı] *см.* gnarled.

gnash [næʃ] *v* скрежета́ть зуба́ми.

gnat [næt] *n* кома́р; ◊ to strain at a ~ быть
ме́лочным.

gnaw [nɔː] *v* (*p. p.* gnawed, gnawn) 1) грызть,

глода́ть; 2) разъеда́ть (*о кислоте*); 3) подта́чи-
вать (*здоровье*); терза́ть, му́чить.

gnawer ['nɔːə] *n* грызу́н.

gnawn [nɔːn] *p. p. см.* gnaw.

gneiss [naıs] *n геол.* гнейс.

gnome¹ [noum] *n* афори́зм.

gnome² *n* ка́рлик, гном, эльф.

go I [gou] *v* (*past* went; *p. p.* gone) 1) идти́,
ходи́ть; е́хать (*поездом, трамваем и т. п.*); лете́ть
(*самолётом*); who goes there? кто идёт? (*окрик
часового*); 2) уходи́ть, уезжа́ть; отправля́ться
(*тж. о поезде, пароходе*); направля́ться, дви́гаться;
to go for a ride пое́хать, отпра́виться на прогу́лку
(*особ. верхом, на велосипеде или автомобиле*);
to go for a swim пойти́ купа́ться; отпра́виться
на пляж; to go for a walk пойти́ (по)гуля́ть;
let me go! отпусти́те меня́!; 3) (*с последующим
гл. в форме Gerund*) отпра́виться, пое́хать, пойти́;
to go shopping отпра́виться за поку́пками; to go
mushrooming пойти́ за гриба́ми; 4) вести́ (*о дороге, пути*); простира́ться (*в каком-л. направлении*);
пролега́ть, тяну́ться (*о дороге*); 5) быть, находи́ться
в каком-л. состоя́нии; to go hungry быть постоя́нно
голо́дным; she is 7 months gone with child она́ на
седьмо́м ме́сяце бере́менности; 6) быть в ходу́,
в обраще́нии; 7) де́йствовать, рабо́тать (*о машине,
механизме*); ходи́ть (*о часах*); би́ться (*о сердце,
пульсе*); 8) отбива́ть вре́мя, бить (*о часах*); зво-
ни́ть (*о звонке, колоколе*); 9) пройти́, получи́ть
призна́ние (*о плане, проекте*); 10) гласи́ть (*о тексте, статье*); 11) нача́ть издава́ть како́й-л. звук;
зашипе́ть (*о машине*); заскрипе́ть; хло́пнуть
(*о двери*); 12) проходи́ть; рассе́иваться; исче-
за́ть; расходи́ться; 13) умира́ть, ги́бнуть; to go
hence ≅ отпра́виться на тот свет; she is gone
она́ поги́бла; её бо́льше нет (*в живых*); to go
west *сленг* окочу́риться, умере́ть; 14) ло́пнуть, по-
терпе́ть крах (*о банке*); 15) продава́ться (*по
такой-то цене*); 16) теря́ть (*сознание, зрение,
слух*); слабе́ть (*об умственных способностях,
силах*); 17) обру́шиться; оторва́ться, отлома́ться;
откочну́ть; 18) умеща́ть(ся); укла́дываться (*в
чём-л.*); 19) храни́ться (*постоянно*); that book goes
on the second shelf э́та кни́га стои́т на второ́й по́лке;
20) сле́довать определённому о́бразу де́йствий;
21) поступа́ть (*о чём-л. посланном, отправленном*);
22) подходи́ть, быть под стать; 23) *в сочетании с
прил.* означа́ет перехо́д в како́е-л. состоя́ние:
to go sick захвора́ть; 24) передава́ться (*по телеграфу, почте*); 25) спосо́бствовать (*обычно с последующим гл. в Inf*); 26) *употребление оборота*
to be going + Inf *смыслового гл. выражает намерение субъекта совершить действие в ближай-
шем будущем:* I am going to write a book я соби-
ра́юсь, намерева́юсь написа́ть кни́гу; □ to
go **about** а) расха́живать, ходи́ть туда́ и сюда́;
б) принима́ться (*за что-л.*), занима́ться (*чем-л.*);
to go about one's business занима́ться свои́м обы́ч-
ным де́лом; в) циркули́ровать (*о слухах, деньгах*);
to go **ahead** дви́гаться вперёд; идти́ впереди́ (*на
состязании*); go ahead! вперёд!; продолжа́й(те)!; to
go **along** а) продолжа́ть, дви́гаться вперёд; б) со-
провожда́ть (*with*); в): go along with you! *разг.*
что ты!, не расска́зывай ска́зки!; to go **at** а) бро́-
ситься (*на кого-л.*); б) взя́ться, приня́ться (*за
что-л.*); to go **away** уйти́; to go **back** а) возвра-

щаться; б) отказаться (*от чего-л.— on*); в) нарушить (*слово, сделку; on*); to go **behind** пересматривать (*основания, решения*); изучать, рассматривать (*факты и т. п.*); to go **between** посредником; to go **beyond** превышать, превосходить; to go **by** а) проходить (*о времени*); б) руководствоваться (*чем-л.*); to go **down** а) спускаться; б) заходить (*о солнце, луне*); в) (за)тонуть, идти ко дну (*о корабле*); г) быть проглоченным (*о пище*); д) быть принятым, одобренным; е) запоминаться; ж) приходить в упадок; уступать, не выдерживать; з) падать, снижаться (*о ценах*); и) стихать (*о ветре, буре*); к) окончить университет (*в Англии*); to go **for** а) считаться, слыть (*кем-л.*); б) обрушиваться на кого-л.; подвергать критике; в) броситься, напасть (*на кого-л.*); г) иметь цену; to go **for** nothing ничего не стоить; to go **in** а) входить, въезжать; б) спрятаться за тучу (*о солнце, луне*); в) увлекаться (*чем-л.— for*); г) действовать совместно (*с кем-л.— with*); to go **into** а) войти, вступить; заняться какой-л. деятельностью; б) часто посещать, появляться; в) впадать (*в истерику*); приходить (*в ярость*); г) расследовать, рассматривать; to go **off** а) уходить, уезжать, убегать; б) взрываться; выстрелить (*об орудии*); в) раздаться (*о выстреле, гудке и т. п.*); загудеть; г) выпалить (*слова, фразы*); д) вспылить; разозлиться; е) терять сознание; забыться; умереть; ж) успокаиваться (*о боли, волнении*); з) пройти (*о концерте и т. п.*); и) сбыть, продать; to go **on** а) продолжать; б) приближаться (*о времени, возрасте; for*); в) болтать, трещать без умолку; г) проявлять упорство, настойчивость (*в чём-л.— with*); to go **out** а) выходить; б) выйти (*из состава правительства*); в) забастовать; г) выступать в поход; д) погаснуть; е) кончаться (*о месяце, годе*); ж) пойти на заработки; з) *см.* to go down к); to go **over** а) переходить (*на другую сторону*); пересекать; б) перечитывать, пересчитывать, пересматривать; повторять; в) тщательно изучать; г) превосходить; д) перейти из одной партии в другую; переменить веру; е) быть отложенным (*о проекте закона*); ж) *хим.* переходить, превращаться; to go **round** а) обойти кругом; б) заходить в гости запросто; в) хватать на всех; to go **through** а) осматривать (*вещи, багаж*); б) рассматривать (*вопрос, проблему*); в) перенести (*операцию*); г) считывать (*роль*); д) растратить, израсходовать; промотать (*состояние*); е) выдержать определённое число изданий (*о книге*); ж) пройти, быть принятым (*о законопроекте, предложении*); доводить до конца, завершать (*дело, задачу и т. п.; with*); и) упорно работать (*над чем-л.*); to go **to:** go to! ну!; что ж! (*выражает призыв, протест, насмешку*); to go **together** подходить (*один к другому*), сочетаться; to go **under** а) заходить, закатываться (*о солнце*); б) тонуть; в) гибнуть, умирать; г) не выдерживать (*испытаний, страданий*); to go **up** а) подниматься, восходить (*на гору*); б) расти, увеличиваться (*в числе*); повышаться (*о ценах*); в) взорваться; г) *амер.* разориться; д) готовиться к защите диссертации; to go **with** а) соответствовать; согласоваться (*с чем-л.*); б) быть заодно (*с кем-л.*); ◊ it goes without saying само собой разумеется; it goes like this дело обстоит так; to go

right through идти напролом; to go out of one's way стараться изо всех сил; ≅ из кожи (вон) лезть.

go II *n* 1) движение, ход; on the go а) в движении; б) на склоне, на закате (*дней*); в) в пьяном виде; 2) энергия; рвение; воодушевление; 3) *разг.* мода; all the go (очень) в моде; 4) *разг.* обстоятельство, неожиданный поворот дел; a pretty go! хорошенькое дельце!; a near go ≅ на волосок от чего-л.; 5) успех, удача; it's no go! *разг.* полный провал!; ничего не выходит!; 6) соглашение, сделка; is it a go? по рукам?; 7) *разг.* попытка; to have a go at попытаться, рискнуть, попытать счастья; 8) порция вина, кушанья.

goad I [goud] *n* стимул.

goad II *v* подгонять (*стадо*); 2) пробуждать, приводить в бешенство.

go-ahead I ['gouəhed] *n* 1) предприимчивый человек; 2) *разг.* прогресс; движение вперёд.

go-ahead II *a* предприимчивый.

goal [goul] *n* 1) цель; место назначения; 2) *спорт.* ворота; to keep ∼ быть вратарём, стоять в воротах; 3) *спорт.* гол; to make (*или* to score) a ∼ забить гол.

goalkeeper ['goul₁ki:pə] *n спорт.* вратарь.

go-as-you-please ['gouəzju:'pli:z] *a* 1) имеющий произвольную скорость, ритм; лишённый плана; 2) неограниченный (*правилами, законом*), нестеснённый.

goat [gout] *n* 1) козёл; коза; 2) (G.) созвездие Козерога; ◊ to play the giddy ∼ *разг.* валять дурака; to get smb.'s ∼ *сленг* рассердить кого-л.

goatee [gou'ti:] *n* козлиная бородка.

goatish ['goutiʃ] *a* 1) козлиный; 2) похотливый.

goatskin ['goutskɪn] *n* сафьян.

goatsucker ['gout₁sʌkə] *n* козодой (*птица*).

goaty ['gouti] *a* козлиный.

gobble¹ ['gɔbl] *v* есть жадно, быстро; пожирать.

gobble² *v* 1) кулдыкать (*об индюке*); 2) бормотать (*тж.* to ∼ out).

gobelin I ['goubəlɪn] *n* гобелен; ковёр.

gobelin II *a* гобеленовый.

go-between ['goubɪ₁twi:n] *n* посредник.

goblet ['gɔblɪt] *n* кубок, бокал.

goblin¹ ['gɔblɪn] *n* домовой.

goblin² *n разг.* фунт стерлингов.

go-by ['goubaɪ] *n:* to give one the ∼ пройти мимо не поздоровавшись, не обратив внимания.

go-cart ['gouka:t] *n* 1) детская коляска; 2) рамка на колёсах для обучения ходьбе маленьких детей.

god [gɔd] *n* 1) бог, божество; my ∼! боже мой!; ∼ bless me (*или* my life, my soul)! *восклицания, выражающие удивление;* ∼ damn you! *восклицание, выражающее проклятие;* ∼ forbid! боже сохрани!; не дай бог!; избави бог!; household ∼s *миф.* лары и пенаты (*покровители домашнего очага*); 2) *pl театр.* посетители галёрки.

godchild ['gɔdtʃaɪld] *n* крестник, крестница.

goddaughter ['gɔd₁dɔ:tə] *n* крестница.

goddess ['gɔdɪs] *n* богиня.

godfather ['gɔd₁fɑ:ðə] *n* крёстный (отец).

godfearing ['gɔd₁fɪərɪŋ] *a* богобоязненный.

godforsaken ['gɔdfə₁seɪkn] *a разг.* заброшенный, захолустный; забытый.

godless ['gɔdlɪs] *a* безбожный.

godlike ['gɔdlaɪk] *a* божественный; богоподобный.

godliness ['gɔdlɪnɪs] *n* набожность.

godly ['gɔdlɪ] *a* благочестивый.

godmother ['gɔd,mʌðə] *n* крёстная (мать).

godparent ['gɔd,pɛərənt] *n* крёстный (отец), крёстная (мать).

godsend ['gɔdsend] *n* неожиданное счастливое событие; удача, находка.

godson ['gɔdsʌn] *n* крестник.

godspeed ['gɔd'spiːd] *n* пожелание успеха.

goer ['gouə] *n* 1) ходок; a slow ~, a bad ~ плохой ходок; 2) отъезжающий.

gof(f)er ['goufə] *v* гофрировать.

go-getter ['gou'getə] *n амер. разг.* предприимчивый делец.

goggle I ['gɔgl] *a* выпученный (*о глазах*).

goggle II *v* 1) таращить глаза; вращать глазами; 2) смотреть широко раскрытыми глазами.

goggled ['gɔgld] *a* носящий защитные очки, в защитных очках.

goggles ['gɔglz] *n pl* 1) защитные *или* тёмные очки; *сленг* очки; 2) *сленг* глаза навыкате; 3) вертячка (*болезнь овец*).

going ['gouɪŋ] *a* 1) существующий, имеющийся в наличии; 2) действующий, работающий; 3) текущий; 4) *оборот* to be ~ + *Inf* смыслового гл. см. go I, 26).

goings-on ['gouɪŋz'ɔn] *n pl* поведение; повадки; образ жизни.

gold [gould] *n* 1) золото; 2) богатство; сокровища; 3) ценная вещь; 4) золотистый цвет; old ~ цвет червонного золота; 5) центр мишени (*при стрельбе из лука*).

gold II *a* 1) золотой; 2) золотистого цвета.

gold-digger ['gould,dɪgə] *n* 1) золотоискатель; 2) *разг.* авантюристка.

gold-dust ['goulddʌst] *n* золотоносный песок.

golden ['gouldən] *a* 1) золотистый; 2) золотой (*обыкн. перен.*).

gold-fever ['gould,fiːvə] *n* золотая лихорадка; погоня за золотом.

gold-field ['gouldfiːld] *n* 1) золотоносный район; 2) золотой прииск.

goldfinch ['gouldfɪntʃ] *n* 1) *зоол.* щегол; 2) *сленг* золотая монета.

gold-fish ['gouldfɪʃ] *n* золотая рыбка.

goldilocks ['gouldɪlɔks] *n бот.* лютик золотистый.

gold-mine ['gouldmaɪn] *n* золотой прииск; *перен.* «золотое дно».

gold-rush ['gouldrʌʃ] *n* золотая лихорадка.

goldsmith ['gouldsmɪθ] *n* золотых дел мастер.

golf I [gɔlf] *n* гольф.

golf II *v* играть в гольф.

golfer ['gɔlfə] *n* игрок в гольф.

golly ['gɔlɪ] *int амер. разг.*: by ~! ей-богу!, право!

golosh [gə'lɔʃ] *n* галоша.

goluptious [gə'lʌpʃəs] *a шутл.* 1) восхитительный; 2) вкусный.

gondola ['gɔndələ] *n* 1) гондола; 2) корзинка (*воздушного шара*); 3) *амер. ж.-д.* вагон-платформа.

gondolier [,gɔndə'lɪə] *n* гондольер.

gone I [gɔn] *p. p. см.* go I.

gone II *a* 1) утраченный, потерянный; разру-

шенный; 2) ушедший, уехавший; 3) пропащий; 4) прошедший, истёкший; 5) умерший; 6) влюблённый, потерявший голову от любви (*on, upon*).

goner ['gɔnə] *n сленг* конченый, пропащий человек.

gonfalon ['gɔnfələn] *n* знамя; хоругвь.

gong [gɔŋ] *n* гонг.

good I [gud] *a* (*compar* better; *superl* best) 1) хороший; 2) годный; полезный; 3) умелый, способный; ~ at languages способный к языкам; 4) доброкачественный; свежий (*о пище*); 5) добрый, доброжелательный; 6) милый, любезный; be ~ enough будьте так добры; how ~ of you! как мило с вашей стороны!; 7) плодородный (*о почве*); 8) надлежащий, целесообразный; 9) надёжный; подходящий; 10) большой, сильный; *разг.* здоровый, хороший (*о нагоняе*); ◇ to make ~ а) возмещать; б) исполнять (*желание*); to stand ~ оставаться в силе; to be as ~ as one's word держать своё слово.

good II *n* 1) добро; польза; a (fat) lot of ~ масса хорошего; it's no ~ talking бесполезно говорить; what ~ will it do? что пользы в этом?; up to no ~ ни к чему не годный; 2) *pl см.* goods; ◇ for ~ (and all) навсегда, окончательно.

good-bye[a] [gud'baɪ] *n* прощание; to bid (*или* to say) ~ прощаться.

good-bye[b] [gud'baɪ] *int* до свидания!, прощай(те)!

good-fellowship [,gud'felouʃɪp] *n* общительность.

good-for-nothing I ['gudfə,nʌθɪŋ] *n* никчёмный человек; бездельник.

good-for-nothing II *a* никчёмный, ни на что не годный.

good-hearted ['gud'hɑːtɪd] *a* добросердечный.

good-humoured ['gud'hjuːməd] *a* добродушный.

good-looker [,gud'lukə] *n амер. сленг* красавец.

good-looking ['gud'lukɪŋ] *a* красивый, интересный; хорошенький.

goodly ['gudlɪ] *a* 1) красивый, миловидный; 2) внушительный, крупный; значительный.

goodman ['gudmæn] *n уст.* хозяин дома, глава семьи.

good-natured ['gud'neɪtʃəd] *a* добродушный.

goodness ['gudnɪs] *n* 1) доброта, великодушие; любезность; 2) добродетель; 3) ценные свойства; хорошее качество; ◇ ~ gracious! господи! (*восклицание*); for ~'s sake ради бога! ~ knows кто его знает; thank ~! слава богу!

goods [gudz] *n pl* 1) товар(ы); industrial ~ промышленные изделия; consumer ~ предметы широкого потребления; fancy ~ галантерея; б) модный товар; 2) вещи, имущество, пожитки; ~ and chattels *разг.* пожитки, барахло; 3) багаж, груз; 4) *attr* товарный (*о поезде и т. п.*); багажный, грузовой; ◇ a piece of ~ *шутл.* человек, персона.

good-tempered ['gud'tempəd] *a* 1) с хорошим характером; 2) уравновешенный.

goodwife ['gudwaɪf] *n уст.* хозяйка дома.

goodwill ['gud'wɪl] *n* 1) расположение (к —to, towards); доброжелательность; добрая воля; 2) готовность (сделать что-л.); 3) *ком.* престиж фирмы.

goody[1] ['gudɪ] *n обыкн. pl* конфета, сласти.

goody[2] *n уст.* хозяйка, матушка.

goody³ *a* сентимента́льный; ха́нжеский (*тж.* goody-goody).

go-off ['gou'ɔːf] *n* нача́ло, старт; at the first ~ с са́мого нача́ла; с пе́рвой попы́тки.

goofy ['guːfɪ] *a разг.* глу́пый; бестолко́вый; отупе́вший.

goose¹ [guːs] *n* (*pl* geese) 1) гусь; гусы́ня; 2) простофи́ля, проста́к; 3) *attr* гуси́ный; ◊ to give the ~ оши́кать, освиста́ть (*актёра*); the ~ hangs high ≅ всё в поря́дке; де́ло на мази́; all his geese are swans ≅ он (постоя́нно) преувеличи́вает; to cook one's own ~ *посл.* ≅ руби́ть сук, на кото́ром сиди́шь; to kill the ~ that lays the golden eggs *посл.* ≅ уби́ть ку́рицу, несу́щую золоты́е я́йца.

goose² *n* (*pl* gooses) портно́вский утю́г.

gooseberry ['guzbərɪ] *n* крыжо́вник; ◊ old ~ дья́вол, чёрт; to play old ~ производи́ть беспоря́док, сумато́ху; to play ~ ≅ сопровожда́ть влюблённых для прили́чия.

goose-egg ['guːseg] *n* 1) гуси́ное яйцо́; 2) ноль (*в играх*).

goose-flesh ['guːsfleʃ] *n* гуси́ная ко́жа (*от холода, возбуждения*).

goosey ['guːsɪ] *a* глу́пый, тупо́й.

gopher ['goufə] *см.* gof(f)er.

Gordian ['gɔːdjən] *a*: to cut the ~ knot разруби́ть го́рдиев у́зел.

gore¹ [gɔː] *n* запёкшаяся кровь; *поэт.* кровь.

gore² I *n* клин (*в платье и т. п.*).

gore² II *v* вставля́ть клин.

gore³ *v* 1) (за)бода́ть; пронзи́ть; 2) проби́ть (*борт судна*).

gorge I [gɔːdʒ] *n* 1) уще́лье; 2) *уст.* гло́тка, го́рло; my ~ rises at this меня́ от э́того тошни́т; 3) съе́денная пи́ща; 4) зава́л, нагроможде́ние; про́бка; 5) *воен.* го́ржа.

gorge II *v* жа́дно есть; объеда́ться.

gorgeous ['gɔːdʒəs] *a* 1) я́ркий (*об окраске*); 2) пы́шный; великоле́пный; ослепи́тельный; 3) витиева́тый (*о стиле*).

gorget ['gɔːdʒɪt] *n* 1) ожере́лье; 2) цветно́е пятно́ на ше́йке пти́цы; 3) *ист.* ла́тный нагру́дник.

gorgon ['gɔːgən] *n* меге́ра; страши́лище.

gorilla [gə'rɪlə] *n* гори́лла.

gormandize ['gɔːməndaɪz] *v* объеда́ться, обжира́ться.

gorse [gɔːs] *n бот.* дрок.

gory ['gɔːrɪ] *a* 1) окрова́вленный, покры́тый кро́вью; 2) кровопроли́тный; 3) *поэт.* а́лый.

gosh [gɔʃ] *int разг.*: by ~! не мо́жет быть! (*выражение изумления*).

gosling ['gɔzlɪŋ] *n* гусёнок.

gospel ['gɔspəl] *n* 1) ева́нгелие; 2) религио́зные убежде́ния.

gospeller ['gɔspələ] *n* 1) евангели́ст; 2) пропове́дник; hot ~ горя́чий защи́тник.

gossamer ['gɔsəmə] *n* 1) то́нкая мате́рия, газ; 2) паути́нка (*в воздухе*).

gossip I ['gɔsɪp] *n* 1) болтовня́, бесе́да; 2) спле́тня; слу́хи; 3) ку́мушка, спле́тница; спле́тник.

gossip II *v* 1) болта́ть; 2) спле́тничать; передава́ть слу́хи.

gossipy ['gɔsɪpɪ] *a* 1) болтли́вый, лю́бящий посплетничать; 2) пусто́й, пра́здный (*о болтовне*).

got [gɔt] *past, p. p. см.* get.

Goth [gɔθ] *n* 1) *ист.* гот; 2) ва́рвар, ванда́л.

Gothic I ['gɔθɪk] *n* 1) го́тский язы́к; 2) готи́ческий стиль; 3) готи́ческий шрифт.

Gothic II *a* 1) го́тский; 2) готи́ческий; 3) ва́рварский.

go-to-meeting ['goutə'miːtɪŋ] *a шутл.* пра́здничный, лу́чший (*о костюме, шляпе и т. п.*).

gotten ['gɔtn] *уст. и амер. р. р. см.* get.

gourd [guəd] *n* 1) ты́ква; 2) буты́ль из ты́квы.

gourmand I ['guəmənd] *n* 1) гурма́н; ла́комка; 2) обжо́ра.

gourmand II *a* обжо́рливый.

gout [gaut] *n* 1) пода́гра; 2) ка́пля, бры́зги; 3) сгу́сток кро́ви.

gouty ['gautɪ] *a* 1) подагри́ческий; 2) страда́ющий пода́грой.

govern ['gʌvən] *v* 1) управля́ть, пра́вить; 2) регули́ровать; руководи́ть; 3) владе́ть (*собой, своими страстями*); 4) влия́ть на кого́-л.; направля́ть (*течение событий*); определя́ть (*курс, ход дел*); 5) *грам.* управля́ть, тре́бовать согласова́ния.

governable ['gʌvənəbl] *a* послу́шный.

governance ['gʌvənəns] *n* управле́ние, руково́дство.

governess ['gʌvənɪs] *n* гуверна́нтка, воспита́тельница.

governing ['gʌvənɪŋ] *a* пра́вящий.

government ['gʌvnmənt] *n* 1) прави́тельство; the Soviet Government Сове́тское прави́тельство; responsible ~ отве́тственное министе́рство; 2) фо́рма правле́ния; 3) управле́ние; local ~ ме́стное самоуправле́ние; 4) прови́нция (*управляемая губернатором*); 5) *attr* прави́тельственный; госуда́рственный; губерна́торский; ◊ carpet-bag ~ *амер. сленг* прави́тельство полити́ческих авантюри́стов; petticoat ~ же́нское заси́лье.

governmental [,gʌvən'mentl] *a* прави́тельственный, госуда́рственный.

governorᵃ ['gʌvənə] *n* 1) прави́тель; 2) губерна́тор; 3) коменда́нт (*крепости*); 4) *разг.* оте́ц; 5) заве́дующий (*школой, больницей*); 6) *тех.* регуля́тор.

governorᵇ ['gʌvnə] *n разг.* хозя́ин, нанима́тель.

gowk [gauk] *n* 1) *диал.* куку́шка; 2) дура́к, глупе́ц.

gown I [gaun] *n* 1) пла́тье (*женское*); morning ~ хала́т; 2) ма́нтия (*судьи, студента университета и т. п.*); 3) ри́мская то́га.

gown II *v* надева́ть; быть оде́тым; she was perfectly ~ed она́ была́ прекра́сно оде́та.

grab I [græb] *n* 1) бы́строе хвата́тельное движе́ние; 2) захва́т, присвое́ние; 3) хи́щничество; 4) *тех.* ковш; черпа́к; ◊ to get (*или* to have) the ~ on *сленг* име́ть преиму́щество пе́ред кем-л.

grab II *v* 1) внеза́пно схвати́ть; 2) пыта́ться схвати́ть (*at*); 3) присва́ивать, захва́тывать.

grab-all ['græb,ɔːl] *n разг.* су́мка для ме́лких веще́й; 2) *сленг* скря́га.

grabber ['græbə] *n* рвач, хапу́га.

grabble ['græbl] *v* 1) ощу́пывать, нащу́пывать; 2) по́лзать на четвере́ньках (*в поисках чего-л.* for).

grace I [greɪs] *n* 1) привлека́тельность, гра́ция, изя́щество; the Graces *миф.* Гра́ции; 2) такт, прили́чие, любе́зность; with a good ~ любе́зно, охо́тно; with a bad ~, with an ill ~

неохо́тно; беста́ктно; 3) благоскло́нность, благоволе́ние; to be in smb.'s good ~s по́льзоваться чьим-л. расположе́нием; 4) *pl* привлека́тельные сво́йства, ка́чества; 5) ми́лость, милосе́рдие; поми́лование; 6) ми́лость, све́тлость; your ~ ва́ша све́тлость (*обраще́ние к ге́рцогу или архиепи́скопу*); 7) разреше́ние на получе́ние учёной сте́пени (*в англ. университе́тах*); 8) отсро́чка, льго́та; 9) моли́тва (*до и по́сле еды*); 10) *муз.* фиориту́ра; 11) *pl* игра́ в серсо́.

grace II *v* 1) украша́ть (*with*); 2) удоста́ивать, награжда́ть.

grace-cup ['greɪskʌp] *n* заздра́вная ча́ша.

graceful ['greɪsful] *a* 1) грацио́зный, стро́йный; изя́щный; 2) элега́нтный.

graceless ['greɪslɪs] *a* 1) бессты́жий, непристо́йный; испо́рченный, развращённый; 2) *редко* некраси́вый, непривлека́тельный.

gracious I ['greɪʃəs] *a* ми́лостивый, милосе́рдный; 2) прия́тный, до́брый; 3) снисходи́тельный, невзыска́тельный.

gracious II *int:* ~ me! бо́же мой!

gradate [grə'deɪt] *v* 1) располага́ть по степеня́м (*разви́тия и т. п.*); 2) *жив.* переходи́ть от одного́ отте́нка к друго́му.

gradation [grə'deɪʃən] *n* 1) постепе́нность, града́ция; 2) *обыкн. pl* сте́пень, ступе́нь разви́тия; 3) *pl* перехо́дные ступе́ни; 4) *жив.* постепе́нный перехо́д, отте́нок; 5) *лингв.* чередова́ние гла́сных.

grade I ['greɪd] *n* 1) сте́пень, зва́ние; ранг; 2) *амер.* класс (*шко́льный*); 3) *pl* нача́льная шко́ла; 4) *амер.* отме́тка; 5) гра́дус; 6) ка́чество, сорт; 7) *с.-х.* но́вая, улу́чшенная поро́да; 8) *амер. ж.-д.* укло́н; on the down ~ под укло́н; on the up ~ на подъёме; ◇ to make the ~ доби́ться своего́.

grade II *v* 1) располага́ть по степеня́м; 2) сортирова́ть, отбира́ть по сорта́м, катего́риям; 3) распределя́ть по сте́пени интенси́вности (*цве́та, кра́ски*); 4) *амер.* ста́вить отме́тки; 5) *с.-х.* улучша́ть поро́ду скре́щиванием; 6) *ж.-д.* нивели́ровать.

gradient ['greɪdjənt] *n* 1) укло́н, накло́н; 2) *физ.* градие́нт; 3) склоне́ние (*стре́лки баро́метра*).

gradual ['grædjuəl] *a* постепе́нный, после́дова-тельный.

gradually ['grædjuəlɪ] *adv* постепе́нно, ма́ло-пома́лу.

graduateᵃ ['grædjuɪt] *n* 1) име́ющий учёную сте́пень; 2) око́нчивший вы́сшее уче́бное заведе́ние; челове́к с вы́сшим образова́нием; 3) *амер.* око́нчивший любо́е уче́бное заведе́ние; 4) мензу́рка.

graduateᵇ ['grædjueɪt] *v* 1) око́нчить (*уче́бное заведе́ние; from*); 2) градуи́ровать, наноси́ть деле́ния; 3) располага́ть в после́довательном поря́дке; 4) распределя́ть (*нало́ги*); 5) *хим.* сгуща́ть жи́дкость (*выпа́риванием*).

graduation [ˌgrædju'eɪʃən] *n* 1) оконча́ние ку́рса (*в уче́бном заведе́нии; from*); 2) получе́ние учёной сте́пени; 3) града́ция; 4) градуиро́вка (*сосу́да и т. п.*); 5) выпа́ривание (*жи́дкости*).

graft¹ I [grɑːft] *n* 1) черено́к, росто́к; 2) приви́вка (*расте́ния*); 3) *мед.* переса́дка тка́ней.

graft¹ II *v* 1) привива́ть (*расте́ние; in, into, on, upon*); 2) *мед.* переса́живать ткань.

graft² I *n амер. разг.* 1) взя́точничество, систе́ма по́дкупов; 2) взя́тка, по́дкуп.

graft² II *v амер. разг.* дава́ть, брать взя́тки; подкупа́ть.

grafter¹ ['grɑːftə] *n* 1) *с.-х.* приво́й; 2) нож (*садо́вый*).

grafter² *n амер.* взя́точник, моше́нник.

grafting ['grɑːftɪŋ] *n с.-х.* приви́вка; bark ~ приви́вка глазко́м.

grain I [greɪn] *n* 1) зерно́; хле́бные зла́ки; 2) крупи́нка (*са́хара, со́ли и т. п.*), песчи́нка; мельча́йшая части́ца; 3) гран (*едини́ца ве́са =* *0,0648 г*); 4) зерни́стость, грануля́ция; 5) волокно́, жи́лка; фи́бра, ни́тка; dyed in ~ окра́шенный в пря́же; 6) строе́ние, структу́ра (*де́рева, ка́мня*); 7) склад хара́ктера, скло́нность; ◇ against the ~ про́тив ше́рсти; про́тив во́ли, жела́ния; to go against the ~ идти́ вразре́з с чем-л.

grain II *v* 1) дроби́ть; 2) очища́ть ко́жу от ше́рсти; 3) кра́сить под де́рево *или* мра́мор; 4) *уст.* кра́сить.

grainy ['greɪnɪ] *a* зерни́стый, грануля́рован-ный.

gram¹ [græm] *n* ме́лкий горо́шек.

gram² *см.* gramme.

grammar ['græmə] *n* 1) грамма́тика; 2) введе́ние в нау́ку; элеме́нты нау́ки; 3) *attr* граммати́ческий.

grammar-school ['græməskuːl] *n* 1) сре́дняя класси́ческая шко́ла; 2) *амер.* ста́ршие кла́ссы сре́дней шко́лы.

grammatical [grə'mætɪkəl] *a* граммати́ческий; граммати́чески пра́вильный.

gramme [græm] *n* грамм.

gramophone ['græməfoun] *n* граммофо́н, патефо́н.

grampus ['græmpəs] *n* 1) дельфи́н-каса́тка; 2) челове́к с тяжёлым дыха́нием.

granary ['grænərɪ] *n* 1) амба́р; зернохрани́лище; 2) жи́тница, бога́тая хлеборо́дная о́бласть.

grand I [grænd] *a* 1) вели́чественный; грандио́зный; 2) вели́кий (*тж. с ти́тулами*); 3) ва́жный, гла́вный, основно́й; 4) великоле́пный, роско́шный; пы́шный; 5) производя́щий си́льное впечатле́ние, импоза́нтный; 6) возвы́шенный; благоро́дный; 7) зна́тный; 8) ва́жничающий; to do the ~ *разг.* ва́жничать, задава́ться; 9) *разг.* прекра́сный, замеча́тельный; 10) *муз.* большо́й, в.по́лном соста́ве (*об орке́стре*).

grand II *n* 1) роя́ль; 2) *амер. сленг* ты́сяча до́лларов.

grandad ['grændæd] *n разг.* де́душка.

grandchild ['græntʃaɪld] *n* внук, вну́чка.

grand-dad ['grændæd] *см.* grandad.

grand-daughter ['grænˌdɔːtə] *n* вну́чка.

grandee [græn'diː] *n* 1) вельмо́жа, ва́жная персо́на; 2) (*испа́нский*) гранд.

grandeur ['grændʒə] *n* 1) великоле́пие, ро́скошь, пы́шность; 2) благоро́дство; зна́тность; 3) вели́чие.

grandfather ['grændˌfɑːðə] *n* де́душка, дед.

grandiloquence [græn'dɪləkwəns] *n* высокопа́рность, напы́щенность.

grandiloquent [græn'dɪləkwənt] *a* высокопа́рный, напы́щенный.

grandiose ['grændɪous] *a* 1) грандио́зный;

2) производя́щий си́льное впечатле́ние; 3) напы́щенный, претенцио́зный.

grandma ['grænmɑ] см. grandmamma.

grandmamma ['grænmə,mɑ] n разг. ба́бушка.

grandmother ['græn,mʌðə] n ба́бушка; ◊ to teach one's ~ to suck eggs ≅ я́йца ку́рицу не у́чат.

grandpa ['grænpɑ] см. grandpapa.

grandpapa ['grænpə,pɑ] n разг. де́душка.

grandparents ['græn,pɛərənts] n pl де́душка и ба́бушка.

grandsire ['græn,saɪə] n уст. 1) де́душка; стари́к; 2) pl пре́дки.

grandson ['grænsʌn] n внук.

grandstand ['grænd,stænd] a амер. показно́й.

grange [greɪndʒ] n уса́дьба, фе́рма с надво́рными постро́йками.

granite ['grænɪt] n 1) грани́т; 2) attr грани́тный.

granitic [græ'nɪtɪk] a грани́тный.

granny ['grænɪ] n 1) разг. ба́бушка; стару́шка; 2) воен. сленг тяжёлое ору́дие.

grant I [grɑnt] n 1) дар, пода́рок; 2) субси́дия, дота́ция; 3) да́рственная гра́мота; 4) разреше́ние, согла́сие.

grant II v 1) дарова́ть, жа́ловать, дари́ть; 2) дава́ть дота́цию; 3) соглаша́ться, дава́ть согла́сие; 4) разреша́ть, дозволя́ть; 5) допуска́ть; to take for ~ed счита́ть само́ собо́й разуме́ющимся, не тре́бующим доказа́тельств.

grantee [grɑn'tiː] n получа́ющий дар, пожа́лование.

grant-in-aid ['grɑntɪn'eɪd] n субси́дия.

granular ['grænjulə] a зерни́стый; гранули́рованный.

granulate ['grænjuleɪt] v 1) распада́ться на ме́лкие зёрна; 2) дроби́ть, мельчи́ть; 3) гранули́ровать.

granulation [,grænju'leɪʃən] n 1) грануля́ция; гранули́рование; 2) зерне́ние, дробле́ние.

granule ['grænjuːl] n зёрнышко.

grape [greɪp] n 1) виногра́д (о плода́х обыкн. в pl); sour ~s ≅ зе́лен виногра́д; 2) см. grease[a] 4); 3) см. grape-shot.

grape-fruit ['greɪpfruːt] n гре́йпфрут.

grape-shot ['greɪpʃɔt] n воен. ист. карте́чь.

grape-sugar ['greɪpʃugə] n виногра́дный са́хар, глюко́за.

grape-vine ['greɪpvaɪn] n виногра́дная лоза́.

graph [græf] n гра́фик, диагра́мма.

graphic ['græfɪk] a 1) графи́ческий, изобрази́тельный; 2) кра́сочный (в расска́зе); нагля́дный.

graphite ['græfaɪt] n графи́т.

grapnel ['græpnəl] n мор. дрек, ко́шка.

grapple I ['græpl] n 1) ко́шка, крюк; 2) схва́тка, борьба́.

grapple II v сцепи́ться, схвати́ться (в борьбе́); □ to ~ with боро́ться с; пыта́ться преодоле́ть (затрудне́ние) или разреши́ть (зада́чу).

grappling-iron ['græplɪŋ,aɪən] n ко́шка, крюк.

grasp I [grɑsp] n 1) хва́тка; 2) облада́ние, власть; 3) понима́ние, спосо́бность схва́тывания; ◊ within ~ в преде́лах досяга́емости; beyond ~ вне преде́лов досяга́емости.

grasp II v 1) схва́тывать, зажима́ть (в руке́); захва́тывать; 2) ухвати́ться (за — at); 3) кре́пко

держа́ться за что-л.; 4) понима́ть, осознава́ть; усва́ивать.

grasper ['grɑspə] n рвач, хапу́га.

grasping ['grɑspɪŋ] a жа́дный, скупо́й.

grass I [grɑs] n 1) трава́, дёрн; 2) па́стбище; at ~ на подно́жном корму́; перен. без рабо́ты; в о́тпуске, на о́тдыхе; to send to ~ выгоня́ть в по́ле (скот); 3) горн. пове́рхность земли́; ◊ not to let ~ grow under one's feet ≅ не дать мхом порасти́; де́йствовать прово́рно; to go to ~ упа́сть на зе́млю; быть сби́тым с ног.

grass II v 1) порасти́ трава́й; 2) засева́ть траво́й; покрыва́ть дёрном; 3) растяну́ться на траве́; 4) раскла́дывать лён (для отбе́лки); 5) разг. сбива́ть с ног; 6) выгоня́ть в по́ле (скот).

grass-cutter ['grɑs,kʌtə] n газонокоси́лка.

grasshopper ['grɑs,hɔpə] n кузне́чик; амер. тж. саранча́.

grass-snake ['grɑssneɪk] n зоол. уж.

grassy ['grɑsɪ] a 1) покры́тый траво́й; 2) травяно́й; травяни́стый.

grate[1] I [greɪt] n 1) решётка; 2) ками́нная решётка.

grate[1] II v загороди́ть решёткой.

grate[2] v 1) тере́ть (на тёрке); 2) скрести́ с ре́зким зву́ком; 3) скрипе́ть; 4) скрежета́ть (зуба́ми); 5) раздража́юще де́йствовать (на кого́-л.— on, upon).

grateful ['greɪtful] a 1) благода́рный; 2) прия́тный.

gratification [,grætɪfɪ'keɪʃən] n 1) удовлетворе́ние; удово́льствие; 2) вознагражде́ние.

gratify ['grætɪfaɪ] v 1) удовлетворя́ть; ра́довать глаз; доставля́ть удово́льствие; 2) потво́рствовать (капри́зам); 3) уст. вознагражда́ть.

grating ['greɪtɪŋ] n решётка.

gratis ['greɪtɪs] adv беспла́тно, да́ром.

gratitude ['grætɪtjuːd] n благода́рность.

gratuitous [grə'tjuːɪtəs] a 1) беспла́тный; даро́вой; 2) беспричи́нный.

gratuity [grə'tjuːɪtɪ] n 1) де́нежный пода́рок; 2) «чаевы́е»; 3) воен. награ́дные.

gratulatory ['grætjuleɪtərɪ] a поздрави́тельный.

grave[a1] [greɪv] n моги́ла; перен. смерть; to sink into the ~ сойти́ в моги́лу.

grave[a2] a 1) ва́жный, ве́ский; серьёзный; 2) влия́тельный, авторите́тный; 3) степе́нный; вели́чественный; 4) мра́чный, тёмный (о кра́сках); 5) ни́зкий (о то́не).

grave[a3] v (past graved; p. p. graved, graven) 1) высека́ть, выреза́ть; 2) запечатлева́ть (в па́мяти; in, on).

grave[b] [grɑv] a фон. тупо́й (об ударе́нии).

gravel I ['grævəl] n 1) гра́вий; 2) золотоно́сный песо́к; 3) мед. ка́мни (в мочево́м пузыре́).

gravel II v 1) посыпа́ть гра́вием; 2) поража́ть, приводи́ть в замеша́тельство, ста́вить в тупи́к.

graven ['greɪvən] p. p. см. grave[a3].

graver ['greɪvə] n гравёр, ре́зчик.

gravestone ['greɪvstoun] n надгро́бный па́мятник, надгро́бие; моги́льная плита́.

graveyard ['greɪvjɑd] n кла́дбище.

gravid ['grævɪd] a бере́менная.

gravitate ['grævɪteɪt] v 1) физ. притя́гивать(ся); 2) тяготе́ть, стреми́ться (к чему́-л.).

gravitation [͵grævɪ'teɪʃən] *n* *физ.* тяготе́ние, притяже́ние.

gravity ['grævɪtɪ] *n* 1) торже́ственность; 2) ва́жность, серьёзность; 3) сте́пенность, уравнове́шенность; 4) *физ.* си́ла тя́жести; specific ~ уде́льный вес; 5) притяже́ние, тяготе́ние.

gravy ['greɪvɪ] *n* подли́вка; со́ус.

gray I, II, III [greɪ] *см.* grey I, II, III.

graze[1] [greɪz] *v* 1) слегка́ задева́ть, дотра́гиваться (*до чего-л.* — against, along); 2) сдира́ть, натира́ть (*кожу*).

graze[2] *v* 1) пасти́ (*скот*); 2) держа́ть на подно́жном корму́; 3) пасти́сь; щипа́ть траву́.

grazer ['greɪzə] *n* живо́тное на подно́жном корму́.

grazier ['greɪzjə] *n* животново́д; скотово́д.

grease[a] [griːs] *n* 1) жир, са́ло; in ~, in pride of ~, in prime of ~ отко́рмленный на убо́й; 2) топлёное са́ло; 3) сма́зка, сма́зочный материа́л; мазь; 4) *вет.* подсе́д.

grease[b] [griːz] *v* сма́зывать; зама́сливать, заса́ливать.

grease-box ['griːsbɔks] *n* *мех.* маслёнка; бу́кса.

greaser ['griːzə] *n* 1) сма́зчик; 2) кочега́р (*на парохо́де*); 3) *амер. сленг* мексика́нец.

greasy ['griːzɪ] *a* 1) жи́рный, са́льный; 2) ско́льзкий; 3) прито́рный (*в обраще́нии*).

great [greɪt] *a* 1) вели́кий; 2) большо́й, огро́мный (*с оттенком удивле́ния, стра́ха и т. п.*); 3) возвы́шенный (*о це́ли, мы́сли и т. п.*); 4) замеча́тельный, прекра́сный (*о певце́, худо́жнике и т. п.*); 5) си́льный, интенси́вный; 6) дли́тельный, продолжи́тельный, до́лгий; 7) *predic* о́пытный, иску́сный (*в чём-л.* — at); 8) *predic* интересу́ющийся; понима́ющий, разбира́ющийся (*в чём-л.* — on); 9) *разг.* превосхо́дный; that's ~! прекра́сно!, здо́рово!; 10) *в степеня́х родства́* пра-; ~-grandfather пра́дед.

greatcoat ['greɪtkout] *n* 1) пальто́; 2) шине́ль.

great-hearted ['greɪt'hɑːtɪd] *a* великоду́шный.

greatly ['greɪtlɪ] *adv* 1) о́чень; 2) значи́тельно, весьма́; 3) благоро́дно, возвы́шенно.

greatness ['greɪtnɪs] *n* 1) величина́; 2) вели́чие, сла́ва.

greats [greɪts] *n* заключи́тельный экза́мен на сте́пень бакала́вра (*в Оксфо́рдском университе́те*).

greed [griːd] *n* а́лчность, жа́дность.

greediness ['griːdɪnɪs] *n* 1) жа́дность; а́лчность; ску́пость; 2) прожо́рливость.

greedy ['griːdɪ] *a* 1) жа́дный (of, for); 2) скупо́й; 3) прожо́рливый.

Greek I [griːk] *n* 1) грек; греча́нка; the ~s гре́ки; 2) гре́ческий язы́к; ◊ it is ~ to me э́то для меня́ соверше́нно непоня́тно.

Greek II *a* гре́ческий.

green I [griːn] *a* 1) зелёный, ~ with envy позелене́вший от за́висти; 2) покры́тый траво́й, листво́й; зелене́ющий; 3) бле́дный, боле́зненный; 4) расти́тельный (*о пи́ще*); 5) незре́лый, неспе́лый, сыро́й; 6) молодо́й; *перен.* неопы́тный, дове́рчивый; 7) необъе́зженный (*о ло́шади*); 8) све́жий, незажи́вший (*о ра́не*); 9) по́лный сил, цвету́щий.

green II *n* 1) зелёный цвет; 2) зелёная кра́ска; 3) мо́лодость, си́ла; in the ~ в расцве́те сил;

4) расти́тельность; 5) *pl* о́вощи, зе́лень; 6) зелёная лужа́йка; пусты́рь, заро́сший траво́й.

green III *v* 1) зелене́ть; 2) кра́сить в зелёный цвет; 3) *сленг* подшути́ть; □ to ~ out дава́ть ростки́.

greenbacks ['griːnbæks] *n* *pl* *амер.* бума́жные де́ньги, банкно́ты.

greener ['griːnə] *n* *разг.* 1) новичо́к, неопы́тный челове́к; 2) проста́к.

greenery ['griːnərɪ] *n* расти́тельность.

green-eyed ['griːnaɪd] *a* ревни́вый, зави́стливый.

greengage ['griːngeɪdʒ] *n* венге́рка (*сорт слив*).

greengrocer ['griːn͵grousə] *n* продаве́ц овоще́й и фру́ктов; зеленщи́к.

greengrocery ['griːn͵grousərɪ] *n* 1) фрукто́вый, зеленно́й магази́н; 2) фру́кты, зе́лень.

greenhorn ['griːnhɔːn] *n* проста́к, неопы́тный челове́к.

greenhouse ['griːnhaus] *n* оранжере́я, тепли́ца.

greenish ['griːnɪʃ] *a* зеленова́тый.

green-room ['griːnrum] *n* ко́мната о́тдыха (*для актёров*); to talk ~ ≅ спле́тничать о театра́льных дела́х.

greensickness ['griːn͵sɪknɪs] *n* *мед.* бле́дная не́мочь.

greensward ['griːnswɔːd] *n* газо́н, дёрн.

greet [griːt] *v* 1) приве́тствовать, здоро́ваться; 2) встреча́ть (*аплодисме́нтами, возгла́сами и т. п.*); 3) доноси́ться (*о зву́ке*); 4) открыва́ться (*взо́ру*).

greeting ['griːtɪŋ] *n* 1) приве́тствие, покло́н; to extend one's warm ~s передава́ть горя́чие приве́ты; 2) встре́ча (*аплодисме́нтами, возгла́сами*).

gregarious [gre'gɛərɪəs] *a* 1) живу́щий стада́ми, ста́ями; 2) общи́тельный.

gregory-powder ['gregərɪ͵paudə] *n* реве́нный порошо́к (*слаби́тельное*).

grenade [grɪ'neɪd] *n* 1) грана́та; 2) огнетуши́тель.

grenadier [͵grenə'dɪə] *n* гренаде́р.

grew [gruː] *past см.* grow.

grey I [greɪ] *a* 1) се́рый; 2) па́смурный, су́мрачный; 3) мра́чный, уны́лый; 4) седо́й, седе́ющий (*о волоса́х*); to turn ~ седе́ть; 5) пожило́й, о́пытный.

grey II *n* 1) се́рый цвет; 2) се́рый костю́м; 3) су́мрак; 4) ло́шадь се́рой ма́сти.

grey III *v* 1) станови́ться се́рым, седы́м; седе́ть; 2) кра́сить в се́рый цвет.

greybeard ['greɪbɪəd] *n* 1) пожило́й челове́к; стари́к; 2) гли́няный сосу́д (*для спиртны́х напи́тков*).

grey-headed ['greɪ'hedɪd] *a* 1) седоволо́сый; 2) ста́рый, поно́шенный.

grey-hen ['greɪhen] *n* тете́рка.

greyhound ['greɪhaund] *n* 1) борза́я; 2) быстрохо́дный океа́нский парохо́д (*тж.* ocean ~); 3) авто́бус да́льнего сле́дования.

greyish ['greɪɪʃ] *a* 1) серова́тый; 2) седе́ющий; с про́седью.

grid [grɪd] *n* 1) *радио, тлв.* се́тка; 2) *см.* gridiron I).

griddle ['grɪdl] *n* сковоро́дка.

gridiron ['grɪd͵aɪən] *n* 1) решётка; се́тка; ра́шпер; 2) *театр.* колосники; 3) *амер. разг.* футбо́льное по́ле.

grief [griːf] *n* 1) го́ре, огорче́ние; печа́ль; crushing ~ тя́жкое го́ре; 2) беда́, несча́стье; to come to ~ попа́сть в беду́; потерпе́ть неуда́чу; to bring to ~ довести́ до беды́.

grievance ['griːvəns] *n* 1) оби́да, по́вод для недово́льства; 2) жа́лоба.

grieve [griːv] *v* 1) огорча́ть; 2) горева́ть (*at, for, about, over*).

grievous ['griːvəs] *a* 1) го́рестный, печа́льный; приско́рбный; 2) мучи́тельный, гнету́щий; тя́гостный; 3) вопию́щий.

griffin[1] ['grifin] *n* европе́ец, неда́вно прие́хавший в Индию *или* стра́ны Бли́жнего Восто́ка; *перен.* новичо́к.

griffin[2] *n миф.* грифо́н; *перен.* бди́тельный страж, це́рбер.

griffon ['grifən] *см.* griffin[2].

grig [grig] *n* 1) *зоол.* у́горь; 2) сверчо́к; кузне́чик; as lively (*или* merry) as a ~ о́чень весёлый.

grill I [gril] *n* 1) ра́шпер; 2) решётка; 3) жа́реные на ра́шпере ры́ба, мя́со; 4) штёмпель для гаше́ния почто́вых ма́рок.

grill II *v* 1) жа́рить(ся) на ра́шпере; 2) пали́ть, печь (*о солнце*); 3) пе́чься на со́лнце; 4) *амер.* му́чить; допра́шивать; 5) погаша́ть почто́вые ма́рки.

grille [gril] *n* решётка.

grim [grim] *a* 1) жесто́кий, свире́пый; 2) стра́шный, суро́вый; злове́щий; 3) неумоли́мый.

grimace I [gri'meis] *n* грима́са, ужи́мка.

grimace II *v* грима́сничать.

grime I [graim] *n* са́жа, грязь, въе́вшаяся в ко́жу.

grime II *v* па́чкать, грязни́ть.

grimy ['graimi] *a* 1) гря́зный, запа́чканный са́жей, у́глем; 2) сму́глый.

grin I [grin] *n* оска́л зубо́в (*при улыбке*); усме́шка.

grin II *v* 1) ска́лить зу́бы; 2) ухмыля́ться (*чему-л.*— *at*); ◊ to ~ and bear it сто́йко выноси́ть что-л.

grind I [graind] *n* 1) разма́лывание; 2) тяжёлая, однообра́зная рабо́та; what a ~! кака́я ску́ка!, кака́я тоска́!; 3) прогу́лка для моцио́на; 4) ска́чки с препя́тствиями.

grind II *v* (*past, p. p.* ground) 1) моло́ть; разма́лывать (*часто* to ~ down); толо́чь; 2) разжёвывать; 3) угнета́ть, му́чить; 4) точи́ть, отта́чивать; 5) шлифова́ть; 6) ста́чиваться; шлифова́ться; 7) верте́ть ру́чку (*ручно́й ме́льницы, шарма́нки*); игра́ть на шарма́нке (*часто* to ~ out); 8) скрежета́ть зуба́ми; 9) тере́ться обо что-л. со скри́пом; 10) *разг.* зубри́ть; рабо́тать усе́рдно, кропотли́во (*над чем-л.*— *at*); 11) вда́лбливать (*ученику́*).

grinder ['graində] *n* 1) точи́льщик; шлифо́вщик; 2) кофе́йная ме́льница; meat ~ мясору́бка; 3) точи́льный ка́мень; 4) *сленг* зубри́ла; 5) *разг.* репети́тор; 6) коренно́й зуб; *pl разг.* зу́бы.

grindstone ['graindstoun] *n* 1) жёрнов; 2) точи́льный ка́мень.

grip I [grip] *n* 1) схва́тывание, зажа́тие; хва́тка; пожа́тие; close ~ мёртвая хва́тка; a ~

of steel желе́зная хва́тка; to come to ~s схвати́ться (*о борца́х*); 2) спосо́бность поня́ть, охвати́ть; 3) уме́ние завладе́ть внима́нием; 4) ру́чка, рукоя́тка; 5) *см.* gripsack; 6) *тех.* тиски́.

grip II *v* 1) схвати́ть; сжать; 2) кре́пко держа́ть; 3) понима́ть, постига́ть (*умо́м*); 4) овладева́ть внима́нием; 5) затира́ть (*льда́ми*); зажима́ть, захва́тывать.

gripe I [graip] *n* 1) сжа́тие; 2) зажи́м; *перен.* тиски́; 3) рукоя́тка; 4) *pl разг.* ко́лики, спа́змы.

gripe II *v* 1) схва́тывать; сжима́ть; 2) притесня́ть, угнета́ть; 3) вызыва́ть ко́лики.

grippe [grip] *n* грипп.

gripsack ['gripsæk] *n амер.* саквоя́ж.

grisly ['grizli] *a* стра́шный, наводя́щий у́жас.

grist [grist] *n* 1) зерно́ для помо́ла; 2) при́быль, бары́ш; to bring ~ to the mill приноси́ть дохо́д; all is ~ that comes to his mill ≅ он всё испо́льзует, он из всего́ извлека́ет бары́ш; 3) со́лод.

gristle ['grisl] *n анат.* хрящ.

grit[1] [grit] *n* 1) песчи́нки; ме́лкий песо́к; гра́вий; 2) крупнозерни́стый песча́ник; 3) *разг.* твёрдость хара́ктера, вы́держка; ◊ to put ~ in the machine ≅ вставля́ть па́лки в колёса.

grit[2] *v* 1) скрипе́ть; 2) скрежета́ть (*зуба́ми*).

grits [grits] *n pl* овся́ная крупа́.

gritstone ['gritstoun] *см.* grit[1] 2).

gritty ['griti] *a* 1) содержа́щий песо́к; 2) песча́ный; 3) *разг.* реши́тельный, насто́йчивый; сме́лый.

grizzle[1] ['grizl] *n* 1) седо́й челове́к; 2) седо́й пари́к; 3) се́рый цвет; 4) се́рая ло́шадь; 5) необожжённый кирпи́ч.

grizzle[2] *v* 1) рыча́ть, огрыза́ться; 2) капри́зничать (*о де́тях*).

grizzled ['grizld] *a* седе́ющий, с про́седью.

grizzly I ['grizli] *n* североамерика́нский се́рый медве́дь, гри́зли.

grizzly II *a* се́рый, седо́й.

groan I [groun] *n* стон; тяжёлый вздох.

groan II *v* 1) тяжело́ вздыха́ть, стона́ть; о́хать; to ~ inwardly быть расстро́енным; 2) говори́ть со вздо́хами, сто́нами (*ча́сто* to ~ out); □ to ~ down: to ~ down a speaker сто́нами и вздо́хами заста́вить ора́тора замолча́ть; to ~ for жа́ждать чего́-л.; to ~ under страда́ть под тя́жестью чего́-л.

groat [grout] *n* ничто́жная су́мма; ◊ I don't care a ~ мне соверше́нно наплева́ть на э́то.

groats [grouts] *n pl* крупа́ (*обы́кн. овся́ная*).

grocer ['grousə] *n* продаве́ц бакале́йных това́ров, бакале́йщик.

grocery ['grousəri] *n* 1) бакале́йно-гастрономи́ческий магази́н; 2) *pl* бакале́я.

grog [grog] *n* грог, пунш.

groggy ['grogi] *a* 1) пья́ный; 2) нетвёрдый на нога́х; 3) неусто́йчивый.

groin [groin] *n* 1) пах; 2) *архит.* кресто́вый свод.

groom I [grum] *n* 1) ко́нюх; грум; 2) придво́рный; 3) жени́х.

groom II *v* чи́стить ло́шадь, ходи́ть за ло́шадью; well ~ed ухо́женный, вы́холенный.

groomsman ['grumzmən] *n* ша́фер.

groove I [gruːv] *n* 1) вы́емка, жело́бок; паз;

прорез; нарезка; 2) рутина, привычка; заведённый порядок (жизни).

groove II v 1) делать выемку, прорез, нарезку и т. п.; 2) прорывать проход (о реке).

grope [group] v 1) ощупывать; 2) идти ощупью; перен. нащупывать (for).

gropingly ['groupıŋlı] adv на ощупь, ощупью.

gross I [grous] n 1) масса; by the ~ оптом; 2) двенадцать дюжин, гросс (счёт мелких галантерейных и других товаров).

gross II a 1) большой, объёмистый; массивный; 2) тучный, полный; 3) буйный (о растительности); 4) грубый, примитивный, простой (о пище и т. п.); 5) крупный, грубого помола; 6) плотный, тяжёлый (о воздухе); 7) вульгарный, грязный; непристойный, скабрёзный; 8) валовой, оптовый.

grotesque I ['grou'tesk] n 1) гротеск; 2) уродливое, комическое существо, предмет и т. п.

grotesque II a 1) гротескный; 2) абсурдный, нелепый.

grotto ['grɔtou] n грот, пещера.

grouch I [grautʃ] n разг. 1) дурное настроение; 2) брюзга; 3) обида.

grouch II v разг. ворчать.

ground[1] [graund] n 1) земля, почва, грунт; firm ~ суша, твёрдая земля; to break (fresh) ~ а) поднимать целину; перен. прокладывать новые пути; б) расчищать площадку (для строительства); вырыть котлован; to fall to the ~ упасть; перен. рушиться (о надеждах, планах); to till the ~ обрабатывать землю; 2) местность, территория; the ~ dips (или slopes) toward местность имеет наклон к; debatable ~ территория, оспариваемая двумя сторонами; перен. предмет спора; to cover much ~ покрывать расстояние; to gain (или to get) ~ продвигаться вперёд; перен. делать успехи; to give (или to lose) ~ отступать; 3) площадка, участок земли; football ~ футбольное поле; pleasure ~ площадка для игр; 4) плац; аэродром; drill ~ учебный плац; firing ~ артиллерийский полигон; practice ~ а) учебный плац; б) спортплощадка (при школе); to take ~ приземлиться; 5) pl сад, приусадебный участок; 6) партер (в театре); 7) основание, мотив, точка зрения; common (или meeting) ~ общие взгляды, общая платформа; solid ~s (или to hold (или to keep, to stand) one's ~ отстаивать свою позицию; to shift one's ~ изменить свою позицию; 8) дно моря; to take the ~ мор. сесть на мель; to strike ~ налететь на мель; to touch the ~ коснуться дна; перен. дойти до сути дела; 9) pl осадок, гуща; 10) жив. грунт, фон; 11) муз. тема; 12) эл. заземление; 13) attr сухопутный (о птицах); живущий в норах (о зверях); ползучий, карликовый (о растениях); наземный (о войсках); ◊ down to the ~ разг. совершенно, абсолютно, вполне; forbidden ~ запрещённая тема; above ~ живой, в живых; below ~ умерший, усопший; to kiss the ~ простираться ниц; to cut the ~ from under one's feet выбить почву из-под ног у кого-л.; сорвать чьи-л. планы.

ground[1] II v 1) обосновывать (принцип, положение); 2) обучать основам предмета (in); 3) грунтовать; 4) класть, опускать на землю; 5) мор. наскочить на мель; 6) эл. заземлять.

ground[2] past, p. p. см. grind II.

ground-floor ['graund'flɔ:] n нижний, цокольный этаж; ◊ to get in on the ~ оказаться в выигрышном положении.

grounding ['graundıŋ] n 1) обучение основам предмета; 2) заложение основ, базы; 3) грунтовка; 4) эл. заземление.

groundless ['graundlıs] a беспочвенный, лишённый оснований.

groundwork ['graundwə:k] n фундамент, основа.

group I [gru:p] n 1) группа; 2) группировка, фракция; 3) воен. авиагруппа; амер. авиаполк.

group II v 1) группировать(ся) (тж. to ~ together); 2) подбирать цвета, краски; 3) классифицировать.

group-captain ['gru:p,kæptın] n полковник авиации (в Англии).

grouse[1] n (pl без измен.) шотландская куропатка; black ~ тетерев-косач; great ~, wood ~ тетерев-глухарь; white ~ белая куропатка; hazel ~ рябчик.

grouse[2] I n разг. ворчун.

grouse[2] v разг. ворчать.

grove [grouv] n 1) роща, лесок; 2) горн. штольня.

grovel ['grɔvl] v лежать ниц, пресмыкаться, подхалимничать; to lie in the dust and ~ ≅ лизать пятки.

groveller ['grɔvlə] n подхалим, низкопоклонник.

grow [grou] v (past grew; p. p. grown) 1) расти; 2) пускать ростки, давать побеги; 3) усиливаться (о боли и т. п.); увеличивать(ся); to ~ in experience обогащаться опытом; to keep steadily ~ing неуклонно возрастать; 4) как глагол-связка с предикативным прил., наречием и сущ.; часто переводится гл., образованным от прил. становиться, делаться; she grew pale она побледнела; 5) выращивать, культивировать; 6) отращивать (бороду, волосы); □ to ~ down уменьшаться; укорачиваться; to ~ into а) врастать; б) превращаться; to ~ on нравиться всё больше и больше; завладевать (чувствами, привычками кого-л.); to ~ out вырастать из; перерастать (рамки, границы, размеры; of); to ~ out of use выйти из употребления; to ~ over зарастать (травой); to ~ up а) вырастать, становиться взрослым; б) возникать (об обычаях); to ~ upon см. to ~ on.

grower ['grouə] n 1) садовод; плодовод; 2): a free ~ свободно растущее растение; a rank ~ буйно растущее растение.

growing I ['grouıŋ] n рост; выращивание.

growing II a растущий, увеличивающийся; возрастающий (об интересе и т. п.).

growl[1] [graul] n 1) рычание; 2) ворчание; 3) грохот; раскат (грома).

growl II v 1) рычать; 2) ворчать; 3) греметь (о громе).

growler ['graulə] n 1) брюзга, ворчун; 2) небольшой айсберг; 3) амер. сленг кувшин для пива; 4) старомодный четырёхколёсный экипаж.

grown [groun] p. p. см. grow.

grown-up I ['grounʌp] n взрослый (человек).

grown-up II a взрослый.

growth [grouθ] *n* 1) рост, развитие; 2) происхождение; приро́ст; 4) по́росль; second ~ молода́я по́росль ле́са (*после вырубки*); 5) *мед.* новообразова́ние, о́пухоль.

groyne [grɔin] *n* волноре́з.

grub I [grʌb] *n* 1) личи́нка; 2) литерату́рный поде́нщик; 3) *сленг* пи́ща, еда́.

grub II *v* 1) расчища́ть зе́млю; корчева́ть, выко́рчёвывать (*часто* to ~ up, to ~ out); 2) находи́ть, раздобыва́ть (*тж.* to ~ up, to ~ out); *перен.* отка́пывать; 3) ры́ться, копа́ться (*в архивах*); 4) *сленг* корми́ть; есть, пита́ться; □ to ~ away корпе́ть, упо́рно труди́ться.

grubby [ˈgrʌbɪ] *a* 1) гря́зный, чума́зый, неопря́тный; 2) черви́вый.

grudge I [grʌdʒ] *n* недово́льство, недоброжела́тельство; to have a ~ against smb., to bear (*или* to owe) smb. a ~ ≅ име́ть зуб про́тив кого́-л.

grudge II *v* 1) жале́ть (*что-л. для кого́-л.*); do you ~ me it? вам жаль дать мне э́то?; 2) зави́довать; испы́тывать недо́брое чу́вство к кому́-л.

grudgingly [ˈgrʌdʒɪŋlɪ] *adv* неохо́тно, не́хотя.

gruel I [ˈgruəl] *n* жи́дкая (овся́ная) ка́ша, каши́ца; ◊ to get (*или* to have, to take) one's ~ получи́ть взбу́чку, вы́говор; to give smb. his ~ дать взбу́чку.

gruel II *v сленг* 1) отчи́тывать; дава́ть взбу́чку; 2) стро́го нака́зывать.

gruelling [ˈgruəlɪŋ] *амер. см.* gruesome.

gruesome [ˈgruːsəm] *a* стра́шный, ужа́сный, отврати́тельный.

gruff [grʌf] *a* 1) гру́бый; 2) ре́зкий; 3) гру́бый, ни́зкий, си́плый (*о голосе*).

grumble I [ˈgrʌmbl] *n* 1) ворча́ние, воркотня́; 2) ро́пот, недово́льство (*высказываемое вслух*); 3) *pl* дурно́е настрое́ние; 4) гро́хот.

grumble II *v* 1) ворча́ть; жа́ловаться (*на — at, about, over*); 2) грохота́ть.

grumbler [ˈgrʌmblə] *n* ворчу́н, брюзга́.

grumpy [ˈgrʌmpɪ] *a разг.* угрю́мый, серди́тый, сварли́вый, раздражи́тельный.

grunt I [grʌnt] *n* 1) хрю́канье; 2) ворча́ние.

grunt II *v* 1) хрю́кать; 2) ворча́ть.

gryphon [ˈgrɪfən] *см.* griffin[2].

guano [ˈgwɑːnou] *n* гуа́но.

guarantee I [ˌgærənˈtiː] *n* 1) гара́нтия, руча́тельство; 2) зало́г; 3) поручи́тель; 4) тот, кому́ вно́сится зало́г.

guarantee II *v* 1) гаранти́ровать, руча́ться; 2) обеспе́чивать; страхова́ть (*against*); 3) утвержда́ть (*во владении; in*).

guarantor [ˌgærənˈtɔː] *n* поручи́тель.

guaranty [ˈgærəntɪ] *n* 1) гара́нтия, обяза́тельство; 2) зало́г.

guard I [gɑːd] *n* 1) бди́тельность; осторо́жность; to be on ~ быть насторо́же, начеку́; to be off ~ проявля́ть беспе́чность, быть недоста́точно бди́тельным; 2) охра́на, стра́жа, конво́й, карау́л; a ~ of honour почётный карау́л; the advance(d) ~ *воен.* аванга́рд; on ~ *воен.* в карау́ле; на часа́х; to mount (to relieve) ~ вступа́ть в (сменя́ть) карау́л; to station a ~, to set the ~ ста́вить карау́л, часово́го; to stand ~ стоя́ть на часа́х; 3) часово́й, карау́льный, сто́рож; конво́ир; 4) *pl* гва́рдия; Horse Guards ко́нная гва́рдия; 5) предохра-

ни́тельное приспособле́ние; решётка (*каминная*); the ~ of a sword эфе́с (*сабли*); 6) *спорт.* оборони́тельное положе́ние; 7) *ж.-д.* конду́ктор; *амер.* тормозно́й конду́ктор; 8) *attr* сторожево́й, карау́льный.

guard II *v* 1) охраня́ть, защища́ть (*от — from, against*); 2) храни́ть, оберега́ть, предохраня́ть; 3) сторожи́ть, карау́лить; 4) сде́рживать (*мысли, чувства*); 5) принима́ть ме́ры предосторо́жности, остерега́ться, бере́чься (*against*).

guard-boat [ˈgɑːdbout] *n* сторожево́е су́дно.

guard-house [ˈgɑːdhaus] *n* 1) карау́льное помеще́ние; 2) гауптва́хта.

guardian [ˈgɑːdjən] *n* 1) *юр.* опеку́н, попечи́тель; 2) храни́тель.

guardianship [ˈgɑːdjənʃɪp] *n* опе́ка; опеку́нство.

guard-room [ˈgɑːdrum] *см.* guard-house.

guardsman [ˈgɑːdzmən] *n* 1) гварде́ец; 2) *амер.* карау́льный.

gubernatorial [ˌgjuːbənəˈtɔːrɪəl] *a* губерна́торский.

gudgeon [ˈgʌdʒən] *n* 1) пескарь; 2) простофи́ля; «шля́па».

guerdon [ˈgəːdən] *n поэт.* награ́да.

guerilla [gəˈrɪlə] *см.* guerrilla.

guerrilla [gəˈrɪlə] *n* 1) партиза́нская война́ (*тж.* ~ war); 2) партиза́н; 3) партиза́нский отря́д; 4) *attr* партиза́нский.

guess I [ges] *n* предположе́ние, дога́дка; at a ~, by ~ науга́д; предположи́тельно.

guess II *v* 1) предполага́ть; дога́дываться; to keep smb. ~ing *разг.* держа́ть кого́-л. в недоуме́нии; озада́чивать кого́-л.; 2) отга́дывать, уга́дывать; 3) *амер. разг.* полага́ть, счита́ть; I ~ я ду́маю, я полага́ю.

guess-work [ˈgeswəːk] *n* дога́дки, предположе́ния; гада́ние на кофе́йной гу́ще.

guest [gest] *n* 1) гость; 2) постоя́лец (*в гости́нице*); paying ~ пансионе́р; 3) парази́т (*растение, животное*).

guest-room [ˈgestrum] *n* ко́мната для госте́й, прие́зжих.

guffaw I [gʌˈfɔː] *n* хо́хот, го́гот.

guffaw II *v* хохота́ть, гогота́ть.

guidance [ˈgaidəns] *n* руково́дство; води́тельство.

guide I [gaid] *n* 1) проводни́к, гид, экскурсово́д; 2) веду́щий при́нцип; 3) руководи́тель; сове́тчик; 4) руково́дство, посо́бие, уче́бник; путеводи́тель; 5) *воен.* разве́дчик; 6) *тех.* направля́ющая дета́ль.

guide II *v* 1) вести́, быть чьим-л. проводнико́м; 2) руководи́ть, направля́ть; 3) вести́ дела́, быть руководи́телем.

guide-book [ˈgaidbuk] *n* путеводи́тель.

guided [ˈgaidid] *a* управля́емый.

guide-post [ˈgaidpoust] *n* указа́тельный столб (*на перекрёстке*).

guild [gɪld] *n ист.* ги́льдия; цех.

Guildhall [ˈgɪldˈhɔːl] *n* 1) (the ~) ра́туша (*в Ло́ндоне*); 2) *ист.* ме́сто собра́ний ги́льдии, це́ха.

guile [gail] *n* обма́н; веролóмство; кова́рство; full of ~ веролóмный, кова́рный; to get smth. by ~ добы́ть что-л. обма́ном.

guileful [ˈgailful] *a* веролóмный; кова́рный.

guileless [ˈgaillis] *a* простоду́шный.

guillotine I [ˌgɪləˈtiːn] *n* 1) гильоти́на; 2) *тех.* ре́зальная маши́на.

guillotine II *v* гильотини́ровать.

guilt [gɪlt] *n* вина́, вино́вность.

guiltily [ˈgɪltɪlɪ] *adv* винова́то; с винова́тым ви́дом.

guiltless [ˈgɪltlɪs] *a* невино́вный, неви́нный, винова́тый.

guilty [ˈgɪltɪ] *a* 1) вино́вный; (not) ~ (не)вино́вен (*приговор суда*); to plead (not) ~ (не) призна́ть себя́ вино́вным; 2) винова́тый (*о взгляде и т. п.*); 3) престу́пный.

guinea [ˈgɪnɪ] *n* гине́я (*денежная единица= =21 шиллингу*).

guinea-fowl [ˈgɪnɪfaul] *n* цеса́рка.

guinea-pig [ˈgɪnɪpɪg] *n* 1) морска́я сви́нка; 2) *разг.* ми́чман.

guise [gaɪz] *n* 1) нару́жность, о́блик; 2) вид, обма́нчивая вне́шность, ма́ска; предло́г; in (*или* under) the ~ of под ви́дом, под ма́ской; 3) *уст.* привы́чка, мане́ра.

guitar [gɪˈtɑː] *n* гита́ра.

gulch [gʌlʃ] *n амер.* овра́г, уще́лье (*с золотоносной жилой*).

gulf I [gʌlf] *n* 1) морско́й зали́в; 2) про́пасть, бе́здна, пучи́на; 3) водоворо́т; 4) *разг.* дипло́м без отли́чия.

gulf II *v* 1) поглоща́ть; 2) *разг.* присужда́ть дипло́м без отли́чия.

gull¹ [gʌl] *n* ча́йка.

gull² *n* проста́к, простофи́ля.

gullet [ˈgʌlɪt] *n* 1) гло́тка; 2) пищево́д.

gullibility [ˌgʌlɪˈbɪlɪtɪ] *n* дове́рчивость, легкове́рие.

gullible [ˈgʌləbl] *a* дове́рчивый, легкове́рный.

gully [ˈgʌlɪ] *n* 1) лощи́на; размы́тый водо́й овра́г; 2) водосто́чная кана́ва, водосто́к.

gulp [gʌlp] *n* 1) большо́й глото́к; at one ~ одни́м ду́хом, сра́зу; 2) глота́ние.

gulp II *v* 1) прогла́тывать; глота́ть с жа́дностью *или* уси́лием (*тж.* to ~ down); 2) сде́рживать (*волнение, гнев*); глота́ть (*слёзы*); 3) дави́ться, задыха́ться.

gum¹ [gʌm] *n обыкн. pl* десна́.

gum² I *n* 1) каме́дь, гу́мми; 2) *амер. разг.* рези́на; *pl* гало́ши; 3) каме́дное де́рево; 4) смоли́стое выделе́ние; 5) *attr:* ~ arabic гуммиара́бик; ~ elastic рези́на, каучу́к.

gum² II *v* 1) скле́ивать (*тж.* to ~ down, together); 2) выделя́ть каме́дь, смолу́.

gumboil [ˈgʌmbɔɪl] *n мед.* флюс.

gum-boots [ˈgʌmbuːts] *n pl* рези́новые сапоги́.

gummy [ˈgʌmɪ] *a* 1) ли́пкий, кле́йкий; 2) смоли́стый; 3) опу́хший, отёчный.

gumption [ˈgʌmpʃən] *n разг.* нахо́дчивость, сообрази́тельность, практи́ческая смётка, предприи́мчивость.

gumptious [ˈgʌmpʃəs] *a разг.* нахо́дчивый, сообрази́тельный, предприи́мчивый.

gumshoe [ˈgʌmʃuː] *n амер.* 1) *разг.* гало́ша; 2) *сленг* полице́йский, сы́щик; 3) *attr* де́йствующий тайко́м, секре́тно.

gumshoe II *v амер.* кра́сться, идти́ кра́дучись.

gum-tree [ˈgʌmtriː] *n* каме́дное де́рево; эвкали́пт; ◊ up a ~ в тупике́.

gun I [gʌn] *n* 1) ору́дие, пу́шка; 2) пулемёт;

3) ружьё (*охотничье*); карабѝн; *ист.* мушкѐт; double-barrelled ~ двуство́лка; smooth-bore ~ гладкоство́льное ружьё; sporting ~ охо́тничье ружьё; tommy ~ пистоле́т-пулемёт То́мпсона, автома́т; 4) *амер. разг.* револьве́р; 5) оруди́йный вы́стрел; салю́т; 6) стрело́к, охо́тник; 7) *сленг* вор; 8) *attr* оруди́йный, пу́шечный; ◊ to stand (*или* to stick) to one's ~s отста́ивать, сохраня́ть свои́ пози́ции; to blow great ~s реве́ть (*о буре*); big ~, great ~ *разг.* ва́жная персо́на, «ши́шка».

gun II *v* 1) охо́титься; *разг.* стреля́ть; 2) обстре́ливать артиллери́йским огнём.

gunboat [ˈgʌnbout] *n мор.* канонѐрка.

gun-carriage [ˈgʌnˌkærɪdʒ] *n воен.* лафѐт.

gunman [ˈgʌnmən] *n* 1) вооружённый револьве́ром; 2) *амер. разг.* банди́т, уби́йца.

gunner [ˈgʌnə] *n* 1) артиллери́ст; пулемётчик; 2) охо́тник.

gunnery [ˈgʌnərɪ] *n* 1) артиллери́йское де́ло; 2) артиллери́йская стрельба́.

gunny [ˈgʌnɪ] *n* ткань из джу́та, рого́жка.

gunpowder [ˈgʌnˌpaudə] *n* по́рох; white ~ безды́мный по́рох.

gun-room [ˈgʌnrum] *n* 1) каю́т-компа́ния мла́дших офице́ров (*на военных кораблях*); 2) ко́мната для хране́ния охо́тничьих ру́жей.

gun-running [ˈgʌnˌrʌnɪŋ] *n* незако́нный ввоз ору́жия.

gunshot [ˈgʌnʃɒt] *n* 1) да́льность вы́стрела; within ~ на расстоя́нии пу́шечного вы́стрела; out of ~ вне досяга́емости вы́стрела; 2) *ист.* пу́шечное ядро́.

gunsmith [ˈgʌnsmɪθ] *n* оруже́йный ма́стер.

gunstick [ˈgʌnstɪk] *n* шо́мпол.

gurgle [ˈgɜːgl] *n* бу́льканье, журча́ние.

gurgle II *v* бу́лькать, журча́ть.

gush I [gʌʃ] *n* 1) ли́вень; стреми́тельный пото́к (*внезапно образовавшийся*); a ~ of oil нефтяно́й фонта́н; 2) излия́ние (*чувств*); пото́к слов; a ~ of anger вспы́шка гне́ва.

gush II *v* 1) хлы́нуть (*тж.* to ~ out); 2) излива́ть(ся) (*о чувствах*); to ~ into tears зали́ться слеза́ми.

gusher [ˈgʌʃə] *n* 1) словоохо́тливый челове́к, излива́ющийся в свои́х чу́вствах; 2) нефтяно́й фонта́н.

gusset [ˈgʌsɪt] *n* вста́вка, клин.

gust [gʌst] *n* 1) си́льный поры́в (*ветра*); 2) хлы́нувший дождь; 3) вспы́шка (*гнева и т. п.*).

gustation [gʌsˈteɪʃən] *n* про́ба на вкус.

gusto [ˈgʌstou] *n* вкус, смак; интере́с, любо́вь (*к чему-л.*).

gusty [ˈgʌstɪ] *a* поры́вистый; бу́рный, ве́треный.

gut I [gʌt] *n* 1) кишка́; blind ~ слепа́я кишка́; 2) *pl* вну́тренности; 3) *pl разг.* содержа́ние; this has no ~s in it э́то никуда́ не годи́тся; 4) *мед.* кетгу́т; 5) *разг.* си́ла во́ли; бо́дрость ду́ха; he has left half his ~s behind him му́жество почти́ поки́нуло его́; он упа́л ду́хом; 6) струна́ *или* леса́ (*из кишки*); 7) глубо́кий овра́г, у́зкий проли́в.

gut II *v* 1) потроши́ть (*рыбу, дичь и т. п.*); 2) гра́бить, очища́ть; опустоша́ть; выгора́ть (*при пожаре*); 3) усво́ить суть, содержа́ние (*книги*); 4) *разг.* жа́дно есть.

gutta-percha [ˌgʌtəˈpɜːtʃə] *n* гуттапе́рча.

gutter I [ˈgʌtə] *n* 1) водосто́чный жёлоб; 2) сто́чная кана́вка (*вдоль тротуара*); ары́к; 3) подо́нки (*общества*); to rise from the ~ вы́йти из низо́в; 4) *attr* у́личный, бульва́рный.

gutter II *v* 1) де́лать желоба́, кана́вки; 2) стека́ть (*по жёлобу, кана́вке*); 3) оплыва́ть (*о свечке*).

gutter-snipe ['gʌtəsnaɪp] *n* у́личный мальчи́шка, беспризо́рный ребёнок.

guttle ['gʌtl] *v* жа́дно есть, пожира́ть.

guttler ['gʌtlə] *n* обжо́ра.

guttural I ['gʌtərəl] *n фон.* задненёбный звук.

guttural II *a* 1) горта́нный; 2) *фон.* задненёбный.

gutty ['gʌtɪ] *n разг.* гуттапе́рчевый мяч (*для гольфа*).

guy[1] I [gaɪ] *n* 1) *разг.* па́рень, ма́лый; a regular (a wise) ~ сла́вный (у́мный) ма́лый; 2) чу́чело, пу́гало; 3) смешно́ оде́тый челове́к.

guy[1] II *v* 1) выставля́ть на посме́шище; 2) осме́ивать; издева́ться.

guy[2] I *n сленг* побе́г, та́йный ухо́д; to do a ~ исче́знуть, сбежа́ть; to give the ~ to улизну́ть от кого́-л.

guy[2] II *v сленг* удира́ть, убега́ть.

guy[3] I *n мор.* оття́жка, ва́нта, трос.

guy[3] II *v мор.* укрепля́ть оття́жками; расча́ливать.

guzzle ['gʌzl] *v* 1) есть, пить с жа́дностью; 2) пропива́ть, проеда́ть (*деньги и т. п.*).

guzzler ['gʌzlə] *n* пья́ница, обжо́ра.

gym [dʒɪm] *n* 1) *сокр. разг. см.* gymnasium 1); 2) *сокр. разг. см.* gymnastic I.

gymnasium [dʒɪm'neɪzjəm] *n* (*pl тж.* gymnasia [dʒɪm'neɪzɪə]) 1) гимнасти́ческий зал; 2) [*тж.* gɪm'nɑːzɪəm] гимна́зия.

gymnast ['dʒɪmnæst] *n* гимна́ст.

gymnastic [dʒɪm'næstɪk] *n pl* гимна́стика.

gymnastic II *a* гимнасти́ческий.

gynaecological [,gaɪnɪkə'lɔdʒɪkəl] *a* гинекологи́ческий.

gynaecology [,gaɪnɪ'kɔlədʒɪ] *n* гинеколо́гия.

gyp[1] [dʒɪp] *n разг.* слуга́ (*в Ке́мбриджском университете*).

gyp[2] I *n амер. сленг* моше́нник, шу́лер.

gyp[2] II *v амер. сленг* моше́нничать.

H

H, h [eɪtʃ] *n* 8-я бу́ква англ. алфави́та; to drop one's ~'s не произноси́ть h там, где ну́жно.

ha [hɑː] *int* ба! (*выражает удивление, радость*).

haberdasher ['hæbədæʃə] *n* торго́вец галантере́ей *или* мужски́м бельём.

haberdashery ['hæbədæʃərɪ] *n* 1) галантере́я; 2) мужско́е бельё; 3) галантере́йный магази́н.

habiliments [hə'bɪlɪmənts] *n pl* оде́жда.

habit I ['hæbɪt] *n* 1) привы́чка; обы́чай; обыкнове́ние; from ~ по привы́чке; to fall (*или* to get) into the ~ of, to form a ~ усво́ить привы́чку; to break off a ~ бро́сить привы́чку; we are in the ~ of мы привы́кли; ~ is second nature привы́чка — втора́я нату́ра; 2) сложе́ние, телосложе́ние; склад (*ума*); of leap ~ худоща́вый; 3) сво́йство, осо́бенность (*растения, животного*); 4) амазо́нка

(*костюм для верховой езды*); 5) *уст.* оде́жда, пла́тье.

habit II *v обыкн. pass* одева́ть; облача́ть.

habitable ['hæbɪtəbl] *a* го́дный для жилья́; обита́емый.

habitant ['hæbɪtənt] *n* жи́тель.

habitat ['hæbɪtæt] *n* 1) жили́ще; 2) ро́дина (*животного, растения*).

habitation [,hæbɪ'teɪʃən] *n* 1) житьё, прожива́ние; 2) жили́ще; жильё.

habitual [hə'bɪtʃuəl] *a* 1) обы́чный; привы́чный; 2) запра́вский; го́рький (*о пьянице*).

habitually [hə'bɪtʃuəlɪ] *adv* обы́чно; по привы́чке.

habituate [hə'bɪtʃueɪt] *v* 1) приуча́ть; to be ~d привы́кнуть; 2) *амер. разг.* ча́сто посеща́ть.

habitude ['hæbɪtjuːd] *n* 1) привы́чка; скло́нность; 2) сво́йство; конститу́ция (*физическая или психическая*).

habitué [hə'bɪtjueɪ] *n* завсегда́тай, ча́стый посети́тель.

hack[1] I [hæk] *n* 1) ра́на, разре́з; сса́дина от уда́ра; 2) зару́бка, зазу́брина; 3) моты́га, кирка́.

hack[1] II *v* 1) разруба́ть; кромса́ть; 2) зазу́бривать; 3) обтёсывать (*камень*); 4) ударя́ть проти́вника в го́лень (*при игре в футбол*); 5) наноси́ть ре́заную ра́ну; 6) разрыхля́ть (*мотыгой*); разбива́ть (*киркой*); 7) ка́шлять сухи́м ка́шлем.

hack[2] I *n* 1) наёмная ло́шадь; *амер. тж.* наёмный экипа́ж; 2) верхова́я ло́шадь; 3) кля́ча; 4) челове́к, выполня́ющий тяжёлую, ну́дную рабо́ту, поде́нщик.

hack[2] II *v* 1) дава́ть во вре́менное по́льзование (*лошадь*); 2) е́хать верхо́м (*не спеша*); 3) нанима́ть для тяжёлой рабо́ты; 4) опошля́ть.

hackle[1] I ['hækl] *n* 1) гре́бень для льна; 2) пе́рья на ше́е петуха́; ◊ with his ~s up разъярённый.

hackle[1] II *v* чеса́ть лён.

hackle[2] *v* разруба́ть; кромса́ть.

hackly ['hæklɪ] *a* зазу́бренный, шерохова́тый.

hackney I ['hæknɪ] *n* 1) верхова́я ло́шадь; 2) *attr* наёмный.

hackney II *v* де́лать бана́льным, изби́тым.

hackneyed ['hæknɪd] *a* бана́льный, изби́тый.

hack-saw ['hæksɔː] *n тех.* ножо́вка, пила́ (*для металла*).

had [hæd (*сильная форма*), həd, əd (*слабые формы*)] *past, p. p. см.* have I.

haddock ['hædək] *n pl без измен.* пи́кша (*род трески*).

hadn't ['hædnt] *разг.* = had not.

haematic [hɪ'mætɪk] *a мед.* кровяно́й.

haematite ['hemətaɪt] *n мин.* кра́сный железня́к.

haemoglobin [,hiːmou'gloubɪn] *n физиол.* гемоглоби́н.

haemorrhage ['hemərɪdʒ] *n мед.* кровотече́ние; кровоизлия́ние; cerebral ~ кровоизлия́ние в мозг.

haemostatic [,hiːmou'stætɪk] *n* кровооста́навливающее сре́дство.

haft I [hɑːft] *n* рукоя́тка (*кинжала*); эфе́с (*шашки, сабли*); ру́чка (*ножа*).

haft II *v* укрепля́ть на рукоя́тке, наса́живать (*на ручку и т. п.*).

hag [hæg] *n* ве́дьма; карга́.

haggard ['hægəd] *a* измождённый, изму́ченный.

haggle ['hægl] *v* спо́рить (*обыкн. о цене*), торгова́ться (*about, over*).

hagridden ['hæg,rɪdn] *a* мучимый кошмарами.

hail[1] I [heɪl] *n* град.

hail[1] II *v*. 1) сыпаться градом; осыпать градом (*ударов и т. п.*); 2): it is ~ing, it ~s идёт град.

hail[2] I *n* приветствие; оклик; within ~ на расстоянии человеческого голоса.

hail[2] II *v* 1) приветствовать; 2) окликать; 3) провозглашать, объявлять (*кого-л. кем-л.*); ◊ to ~ from приходить, прибывать (*о корабле и т. п.*); б) *разг.* происходить из; where do you ~ from? откуда вы?

hail[2] III *int* привет!

hail-fellow ['heɪl,felou] *n* приятель.

hail-fellow-well-met ['heɪl,felou'wel'met] *a* в приятельских отношениях со всеми.

hailstorm ['heɪlstɔːm] *n* дождь с градом; сильный град.

hair [hɛə] *n* 1) волос; волосы; волосок; iron-grey ~ пепельные волосы; to do one's ~ причёсывать (-ся); his ~ stood on end у него волосы стали дыбом; to lose one's ~ а) полысеть; б) *разг.* рассердиться; 2) щетина, шерсть (*животных*); 3) ворс; 4) *attr* волосяной; ◊ against the ~ против шерсти; to a ~ точь-в-точь; to comb a person's ~ for him давать нагоняй, намылить голову; keep your ~ on! *разг.* спокойно!, не горячитесь!; to split ~s вдаваться в тонкости; спорить о мелочах; to take a ~ of the dog that bit you *разг.* а) опохмеляться; б) клин клином вышибать; not to turn a ~ ≅ и глазом не моргнуть.

hairbreadth ['hɛəbredθ] *n* минимальное расстояние; within a ~ на волосок (*от чего-л.*).

hairbrush ['hɛəbrʌʃ] *n* щётка для волос.

hairclipper ['hɛə,klɪpə] *n* машинка для стрижки волос.

hair-cut ['hɛəkʌt] *n* стрижка.

hair-do ['hɛəduː] *n* разг. причёска.

hairdresser ['hɛə,dresə] *n* парикмахер (*обыкн. дамский*).

hairless ['hɛəlɪs] *a* безволосый, лысый.

hair-line ['hɛəlaɪn] *n* 1) тонкая, волосная линия; 2) бечёвка, леска (*из волоса*); 3) *attr* точный.

hairpin ['hɛəpɪn] *n* 1) шпилька; 2) *attr*: ~ bend крутой поворот дороги (*особ. в горах*).

hair-slide ['hɛəslaɪd] *n* заколка (*для волос*).

hair-splitting ['hɛə,splɪtɪŋ] *n* крохоборство, мелочной педантизм.

hairspring ['hɛəsprɪŋ] *n* волосок, пружинка (*в часах*).

hairy ['hɛərɪ] *a* покрытый волосами, волосатый.

hake [heɪk] *n* (*pl без измен.*) хек (*рыба*).

halberd ['hælbəd] *n ист.* алебарда.

halcyon I ['hælsɪən] *n* зимородок (*птица*).

halcyon II *a*: ~ days тихие, ясные дни.

hale[1] [heɪl] *a* здоровый, сильный; ~ and hearty здоровый и бодрый.

hale[2] *v уст.* тянуть (*силой*).

half I [hɑːf] *n* (*pl* halves) 1) половина; часть; by halves пополам; the larger ~ большая часть; he is older than you by ~ он вдвое старше вас; 2) семестр; ◊ better ~ дражайшая половина; ~ the battle а) полдела; б) залог победы, успеха; to cry halves требовать равной доли; to do a thing by halves делать кое-как; to go halves делить пополам; иметь половину (*в чём-л.*).

half II *a* половинный; частичный.

half III *adv* наполовину, частично; ~ past one половина второго; ◊ not ~ а) совсем не; not ~ bad совсем неплохо; б) *сленг* очень, ужасно.

half-and-half ['hɑːfənd'hɑːf] *a* 1) смешанный в равных количествах; 2) половинчатый.

half-back ['hɑːf'bæk] *n спорт.* полузащитник.

half-baked ['hɑːf'beɪkt] *a* 1) недопечённый; полусырой; 2) недоделанный; непродуманный; 3) незрелый, неопытный.

half-blood ['hɑːfblʌd] *n* 1) брат *или* сестра по одному из родителей; 2) родство по одному из родителей.

half-bred ['hɑːfbred] *a* нечистокровный.

half-breed ['hɑːfbriːd] *n* 1) метис; 2) гибрид.

half-brother ['hɑːf,brʌðə] *n* единокровный *или* единоутробный брат.

half-circle ['hɑːf,sɜːkl] *n* полукруг.

halfcrown ['hɑːf'kraun] *n* полкроны (*до 1970 г. монета в 2½ шиллинга*).

half-done ['hɑːf'dʌn] *a* недоделанный; недоваренный; недожаренный.

half-hearted ['hɑːf'hɑːtɪd] *a* 1) равнодушный; вялый; in a ~ way без всякого воодушевления; 2) малодушный; нерешительный.

half-length ['hɑːf'leŋθ] *n* поясной портрет.

half-mast ['hɑːf'mɑːst] *n*: flags were at ~ флаги были приспущены.

halfpenny ['heɪpnɪ] *n* 1) полпенни (*монета*); 2) *attr* грошовый.

half-price ['hɑːf'praɪs] *adv* за полцены.

half-seas-over ['hɑːfsiːz'ouvə] *a predic разг.* подвыпивший.

half-sister ['hɑːf,sɪstə] *n* единокровная *или* единоутробная сестра.

half-time ['hɑːf'taɪm] *n* 1) сокращённый наполовину рабочий день; 2) *спорт.* половина игры.

half-timer ['hɑːf'taɪmə] *n* 1) работающий неполную рабочую неделю; 2) учащийся, освобождённый от части занятий в школе (*в связи с работой*).

half-tone ['hɑːftoun] *n* 1) *муз., жив.* полутон; 2) *полигр.* автотипия.

half-way I ['hɑːf'weɪ] *a* 1) находящийся на полпути; 2) половинчатый; недостаточный.

half-way II *adv* 1) на полпути; to meet ~ *перен.* идти на компромисс; 2) наполовину.

half-witted ['hɑːf'wɪtɪd] *a* слабоумный; очень глупый.

half-word ['hɑːf'wɜːd] *n* намёк; полуслово, полслова.

half-year ['hɑːf'jɜː] *n* 1) полгода; 2) семестр.

half-yearly I ['hɑːf'jɜːlɪ] *a* полугодовой.

half-yearly II *adv* раз в полгода.

halibut ['hælɪbət] *n* палтус (*рыба*).

hall [hɔːl] *n* 1) зал; 2) общая столовая (*в англ. колледжах*); 3) общественное здание; Town Hall ратуша, муниципалитет; drill ~ манеж; 4) вестибюль, приёмная; холл; *амер. тж.* коридор; 5) помещичий дом (*в Англии*); 6) *амер.* здание школы *или* колледжа.

hallelujah [,hælɪ'luːjə] *int* аллилуйя!

hall-mark I ['hɔːl'mɑːk] *n* 1) пробирное клеймо; проба; 2) отличительный признак, характерное свойство.

hall-mark II *v* 1) ставить пробу; 2) отмечать печатью (*чего-л.*).

hallo(a) I [həˈlou] *int* алло́!, здоро́во!

hallo(a) II *v* оклика́ть.

halloo I [həˈluː] *int* ату́!

halloo II *v* 1) крича́ть ату́, улюлю́кать, натра́вливать соба́к; *перен.* нау́ськивать, подстрека́ть; 2) крича́ть, ау́кать; ◊ don't ~ until you are out of the wood *погов.* ≅ не говори́ гоп, пока́ не переско́чишь.

hallow [ˈhælou] *v* 1) освяща́ть; 2) чтить (как святы́ню).

hallowed [ˈhæloud] *a* свяще́нный.

hallucination [hə,luːsɪˈneɪʃən] *n* галлюцина́ция.

hallway [ˈhɔːl,weɪ] *n амер.* прихо́жая; коридо́р.

halm [hɑːm] *см.* haulm.

halo I [ˈheɪlou] *n* 1) светя́щийся круг, ободо́к (*вокруг солнца, луны*); 2) нимб; ве́нчик; орео́л; сия́ние.

halo II *v* окружа́ть орео́лом.

halt¹ I [hɔːlt] *n* 1) остано́вка; прива́л; at the ~ на ме́сте; to call a ~ назнача́ть прива́л; to bring to a ~ останови́ть, задержа́ть (*движение и т. п.*); to come to a ~ остана́вливаться; 2) трамва́йная остано́вка; *ж.-д.* полуста́нок.

halt¹ II *v* остана́вливать(ся), де́лать прива́л; ~! стой! (*команда*).

halt² *v* 1) колеба́ться, не реша́ться; 2) запина́ться.

halter I [ˈhɔːltə] *n* 1) недоу́здок; 2) верёвка с пе́тлей (*для повешения*); to come to the ~ попа́сть на ви́селицу.

halter II *v* 1) надева́ть недоу́здок, приуча́ть к узде́; 2) ве́шать (*казнить*).

halve [hɑːv] *v* 1) дели́ть попола́м; 2) сокраща́ть наполови́ну.

halves [hɑːvz] *pl см.* half I.

ham [hæm] *n* 1) о́корок, ветчина́; 2) бедро́, ля́жка.

ham-handed [ˈhæmˈhændɪd] *a* неуклю́жий, нескла́дный.

hamlet [ˈhæmlɪt] *n* дереву́шка.

hammer I [ˈhæmə] *n* 1) молото́к, мо́лот; ~ and sickle серп и мо́лот; throwing the ~ *спорт.* мета́ние мо́лота; to bring to the ~ пусти́ть с молотка́, прода́ть на аукцио́не; to come under the ~ пойти́ с молотка́ (*на аукционе*); 2) *воен.* куро́к, уда́рник; ◊ ~ and tongs *разг.* изо всех сил, неща́дно.

hammer II *v* 1) бить (молотко́м), закола́чивать, вбива́ть; 2) стуча́ть, бараба́нить; 3) кова́ть; чека́нить; 4) объявля́ть несостоя́тельным должнико́м; ▢ to ~ at a) упо́рно рабо́тать над чем-л.; б) пристава́ть (назо́йливо); to ~ in, to ~ into вкола́чивать, вбива́ть; вда́лбливать; to ~ out выко́вывать; *перен.* выду́мывать; to ~ together скола́чивать.

hammer-blow [ˈhæməblou] *n* мо́щный, сокруши́тельный уда́р.

hammering [ˈhæmərɪŋ] *n* 1) закола́чивание, вбива́ние; 2) ко́вка, чека́нка; 3) стук, уда́ры; *разг.* побо́и.

hammerman [ˈhæməmən] *n* молотобо́ец.

hammersmith [ˈhæməsmɪθ] *n* кузне́ц.

hammock [ˈhæmək] *n* гама́к; (подвесна́я) ко́йка (*на пароходе*).

hamper¹ [ˈhæmpə] *v* меша́ть, препя́тствовать, затрудня́ть.

hamper² *n* 1) больша́я корзи́на с кры́шкой; 2) паке́т с ла́комствами и съестны́м.

hamstring I [ˈhæmstrɪŋ] *n* подколе́нное сухожи́лие.

hamstring II *v* (*past* hamstringed; *p. p.* hamstrung) 1) подреза́ть сухожи́лия; 2) кале́чить.

hamstrung [ˈhæmstrʌŋ] *p. p. от* hamstring II.

hand I [hænd] *n* 1) рука́ (*кисть руки*); ~ in ~ рука́ об руку; вме́сте; to shake ~s здоро́ваться за́ руку; to clasp smb.'s ~ пожа́ть ру́ку; to offer one's ~ а) протяну́ть ру́ку (*для пожатия*); б) сде́лать предложе́ние (*о браке*); to rub one's ~s потира́ть ру́ки (*от удовольствия*); to join ~s пожима́ть друг дру́гу ру́ки; *перен.* объединя́ться для чего-л.; ~s off! ру́ки прочь!; ~s up! ру́ки вверх!; at ~ под руко́й, тут же; бли́зкий (*тж. о времени*); at first (second) ~ из пе́рвых (вторы́х) рук; by ~ а) от руки́, ручны́м спо́собом; б) с на́рочным; by the ~ за́ руку; from ~ to ~ из рук в ру́ки; on ~ име́ющийся в распоряже́нии, на рука́х; *амер.* под рука́ми; поблизости; on one's ~s а) в чьём-л. распоряже́нии; б) на чьей-л. отве́тственности; в) на чьём-л. попече́нии; to ~ под рука́ми; налицо́; to come to ~ попа́сть в ру́ки; 2) владе́ние, распоряже́ние, власть; to have in ~ а) владе́ть, распоряжа́ться; б) управля́ть; in ~ а) в рука́х, в исполне́нии, в рабо́те; б) рассма́триваемый (*о вопросе, деле и т. п.*); it is no longer in my ~s э́то уже́ не в мое́й вла́сти; to keep in ~ держа́ть в подчине́нии; to get (smth.) off one's ~s изба́виться (от чего-л.), освободи́ться от отве́тственности (за что-л.); to get out of ~ отби́ться от рук; to change ~s переходи́ть из рук в ру́ки; 3) (наёмный) рабо́тник; *pl* рабо́чая си́ла, рабо́чие ру́ки; factory ~ фабри́чный рабо́чий; 4) ло́вкость, уме́ние; 5) исполни́тель, рабо́тник; a good ~ at (*или* in) smth. ло́вкий, иску́сный в чём-л.; an old ~ at smth. о́пытный в чём-л.; 6) по́черк; a legible ~ разбо́рчивый по́черк; 7) по́дпись; to witness the ~ of smb. заве́рить чью-л. по́дпись; 8) пере́дняя ла́па; 9) стре́лка часо́в; 10) сторона́; at the ~s of со стороны́ (*кого-л.*); on the one ~..., on the other ~... с одно́й стороны́..., с друго́й стороны́...; 11) *pl* экипа́ж, кома́нда (*корабля*); 12) *карт.* игро́к; ка́рты в руке́ игрока́; to show one's ~ *перен.* раскры́ть ка́рты; 13) ширина́ ладо́ни (*как мера*); 14) *pl сленг* аплодисме́нты; 15) *attr* ручно́й; ~ and (*или* in) glove with в бли́зких, прия́тельских отноше́ниях; to kiss one's ~ to посыла́ть возду́шные поцелу́и; at any ~ во вся́ком слу́чае; with a high ~ надме́нно, высокоме́рно; to bear (*или* to have) a ~ in уча́ствовать в чём-л.; to turn one's ~ to принима́ться за что-л.; to lay violent ~s on захвати́ть си́лой; to gain the upper ~ одоле́ть, победи́ть; взять верх; to get one's ~ in освои́ться с чем-л., наби́ть ру́ку; to get the better ~ получи́ть преиму́щество, переве́с; to give (to have) a free ~ предоста́вить (име́ть) свобо́ду де́йствий; to live from ~ to mouth а) ко́е-ка́к перебива́ться; жить впро́голодь; б) жить сего́дняшним днём; to have one's ~s full быть о́чень за́нятым, не име́ть свобо́дной мину́ты; to keep ~s in pockets безде́льничать, лоды́рничать; ~s down легко́, с лёгкостью; off ~ а) экспро́мтом, без подгото́вки; б) бесцеремо́нно; небре́жно; ◊ to win ~s down легко́ достига́ть чего́-л.; to feed out of one's ~ быть поко́рным, послу́шным; to grease smb.'s ~ дать взя́тку, «подма́зать».

hand II *v* 1) передавать; вручать; 2) помогать (*войти в вагон*); подсаживать; □ to ~ **down** а) помогать сойти вниз; б) завещать потомству; to ~ **in** вручать, подавать (*заявление*); to ~ **out** а) раздавать; б) высаживать; to ~ **over** передавать другому; to ~ **up** подавать снизу вверх; ◊ to ~ it to smb. воздавать должное кому-л.

handbag ['hændbæg] *n* 1) дамская сумочка; 2) (ручной) чемодан.

hand-barrow ['hænd,bærou] *n* 1) ручная тележка; тачка; 2) носилки.

handbill ['hændbɪl] *n* анонс, афиша.

handbook ['hændbuk] *n* руководство, справочник; указатель.

handcart ['hændkɑːt] *n* ручная тележка, тачка.

handcuff I ['hændkʌf] *n обыкн. pl* наручники.

handcuff II *v* надевать наручники.

handful ['hændful] *n* 1) пригоршня, горсть; 2) небольшое количество, «горсточка» (*людей*); 3) *разг.* «наказание», «беда»; the boy is quite a ~ этот мальчик — чистое наказание.

handglass ['hændglɑːs] *n* 1) ручное зеркало; 2) ручная лупа.

hand-grenade ['hændgrɪˌneɪd] *n* ручная граната.

handgrip ['hændgrɪp] *n* 1) пожатие руки; 2) схватка врукопашную.

handhold ['hændhould] *n* ручка (*за которую можно держать, нести*); то, за что можно ухватиться рукой.

handicap I ['hændɪkæp] *n* 1) *спорт.* гандикап; 2) помеха, затруднение.

handicap II *v* 1) *спорт.* уравнивать силы (*противников*); 2) ставить в невыгодное положение; 3) быть помехой, затруднять.

handicraft ['hændɪkrɑːft] *n* 1) ремесло; ручная работа; 2) ловкость, искусность (*в работе*); 3) *attr* ремесленный; кустарный.

handicraftsman ['hændɪˌkrɑːftsmən] *n* ремесленник.

handily ['hændɪlɪ] *adv* ловко; искусно.

handiness ['hændɪnɪs] *n* 1) ловкость; искусность; 2) лёгкая управляемость; поворотливость.

handiwork ['hændɪwəːk] *n* ручная работа; ручное изделие; рукоделие.

handkerchief ['hæŋkətʃɪf] *n* 1) носовой платок; 2) шейный платок, косынка.

handle I ['hændl] *n* 1) ручка; рукоятка; 2) предлог, повод, удобный случай; to give (*или* to leave) a ~ to доставить случай, дать повод к чему-л.; ◊ a ~ to one's name титул; to go off the ~ выйти из себя.

handle II *v* 1) трогать руками, держать в руках; 2) обращаться, обходиться (*с кем-л., чем-л.*); 3) трактовать; 4) управлять; 5) торговать (*чем-л.*).

handle-bar ['hændlbɑː] *n* руль (*велосипеда, мотоцикла*).

hand-made ['hænd'meɪd] *a* ручной (*работы*).

hand-me-down ['hændmiːˈdaun] *a разг.* 1) готовый (*о платье*); 2) подержанный; поношенный.

hand-on-heart ['hændɔnˈhɑːt] *a* чистосердечный.

hand-organ ['hændˌɔːgən] *n* шарманка.

handout[1] ['hændaut] *n амер.* милостыня, подаяние.

handout[2] *n* текст заявления для печати.

handrail ['hændreɪl] *n* перила; поручень.

handsel ['hænsəl] *n* 1) подарок к Новому году;

2) первый взнос; задаток, залог; 3) предвкушение.

handshake ['hændʃeɪk] *n* рукопожатие.

handsome ['hænsəm] *a* 1) красивый; 2) изрядный, порядочный (*о сумме и т. п.*); 3) щедрый; 4) хороший (*об обращении*); ◊ ~ is that ~ does *погов.* ≅ судят не по словам, а по делам.

handspring ['hændsprɪŋ] *n спорт.* поворот рывком, колесо.

hand-to-hand ['hændtəˈhænd] *a* рукопашный (*о бое*).

handwork ['hændwəːk] *n* ручная работа.

handwriting ['hændˌraɪtɪŋ] *n* почерк.

handy ['hændɪ] *a* 1) ловкий, искусный; 2) имеющийся под рукой; 3) удобный (*для пользования*); to come in ~ пригодиться.

handy-man ['hændɪmən] *n* 1) мастер на все руки; 2) подручный.

hang I [hæŋ] *v* (*past, p. p.* hung) 1) вешать, подвешивать; развешивать; 2) (*past, p. p.* hanged) повесить, казнить; 3) висеть; □ to ~ **about**, *амер.* to ~ **around** а) околачиваться, слоняться; б) надвигаться (*о грозе и т. п.*); to ~ **back** колебаться, не решаться; to ~ **down** свисать, ниспадать; to ~ **on** а) стойко держаться; упорствовать; б) полагаться, рассчитывать на кого-л.; to ~ **out** а) вывешивать (*флаги*); б) высовываться (*из окна*); to ~ **over** нависать; to ~ **together** а) быть заодно, держаться друг друга; б) соответствовать, совпадать; to ~ **up** а) откладывать, приостанавливать; затягивать; б) *разг.* повесить телефонную трубку, прекратить разговор; в) развесить (*картины, бельё*); ◊ to ~ heavy (on one's hands) медленно тянуться (*о времени*); to ~ (up)on smb.'s lips (*или* words) внимать каждому слову; слушать с восторгом; ~ it, ~ you! убирайтесь к чёрту!

hang II *n только sg* 1) вид, манера; mark the ~ of the dress, skirt *etc* обратите внимание на то, как сидит платье, юбка *и т. п.*; 2) *разг.* значение, смысл; to get the ~ of понять, в чём дело; 3) способ действия (*машины и т. п.*); 4) склон, скат; ◊ not a ~ нисколько.

hangar ['hæŋə] *n* ангар; навес.

hangdog I ['hæŋdɔg] *n* мошенник; висельник.

hangdog II *a* 1) низкий, подлый; 2) пристыженный, виноватый (*о виде*).

hanger ['hæŋə] *n* 1) крюк, крючок; 2) вешалка (*у платья*); 3) подвеска.

hanger-on ['hæŋər'ɔn] *n* (*pl* hangers-on) *презр.* 1) прихлебатель; 2) приспешник.

hanging ['hæŋɪŋ] *n* 1) повешение (*казнь*); 2) вешание; подвешивание; 3) *обыкн. pl* занавески, драпировки, портьеры.

hangman ['hæŋmən] *n* палач.

hang-nail ['hæŋneɪl] *n* заусеница.

hang-over ['hæŋˌouvə] *n* 1) пережиток; 2) похмелье.

hank [hæŋk] *n* моток.

hanker ['hæŋkə] *v* жаждать чего-л., стремиться к чему-л., мечтать о чём-л. (*after*).

hanky ['hæŋkɪ] *n разг.* носовой платок.

hanky-panky ['hæŋkɪ'pæŋkɪ] *n разг.* фокусы, плутовство, проделки.

hansel ['hænsəl] *см.* handsel.

hansom ['hænsəm] *n* двухколёсный экипа́ж (*с ме́стом для ку́чера сза́ди*).

hap I [hæp] *n* (счастли́вый) слу́чай.

hap II *v* случа́ться.

haphazard I ['hæp'hæzəd] *n* слу́чай, случа́йность; at ∼, by ∼ случа́йно; наудачу.

haphazard II *a* случа́йный.

haphazard III *adv* случа́йно.

hapless ['hæplıs] *a* несча́стный, злополу́чный.

haply ['hæplı] *adv уст.* 1) случа́йно; 2) мо́жет быть.

happen ['hæpən] *v* 1) случа́ться, происходи́ть; as it ∼s случа́йно; 2) случа́йно оказа́ться; оказа́ваться; 3) име́ть сча́стье, посчастли́виться; □ to ∼ upon натолкну́ться, случа́йно встре́тить.

happening ['hæpnıŋ] *n* слу́чай, собы́тие.

happily ['hæpılı] *adv* 1) сча́стливо; 2) к сча́стью.

happiness ['hæpınıs] *n* сча́стье.

happy ['hæpı] *a* 1) счастли́вый; дово́льный; 2) уда́чный, подходя́щий; 3) *predic* рад, сча́стлив; ◇ as ∼ as the day is long о́чень счастли́вый.

happy-go-lucky I ['hæpıgou,lʌkı] *a* 1) беспе́чный; 2) случа́йный.

happy-go-lucky II *adv* по во́ле слу́чая.

harangue I [hə'ræŋ] *n* (торже́ственная) речь, обраще́ние (*к пу́блике*).

harangue II *v* произноси́ть речь, обраща́ться с ре́чью.

harass ['hærəs] *v* беспоко́ить, не дава́ть поко́я; изма́тывать.

harbinger I ['hɑːbındʒə] *n* предве́стник; ве́стник.

harbinger II *v* возвеща́ть, объявля́ть.

harbor I, II ['hɑːbə] *амер. см.* harbour I, II.

harbour I ['hɑːbə] *n* 1) га́вань; 2) убе́жище, приста́нище.

harbour II *v* 1) станови́ться на я́корь в га́вани; 2) дава́ть убе́жище; укрыва́ть; приюти́ть; 3) тай́ть (*мы́сли*); пита́ть (*чу́вства*).

harbourage ['hɑːbərıdʒ] *n* 1) убе́жище; приста́нище; 2) ме́сто для стоя́нки судо́в.

hard I [hɑːd] *a* 1) твёрдый; жёсткий; ∼ and fast стро́го определённый; твёрдый (*о пра́виле*); 2) тру́дный, тяжёлый (*о рабо́те, времена́х*); 3) си́льный (*о ли́вне, моро́зе*); суро́вый (*о зиме́*); 4) кре́пкий, туго́й; 5) неприя́тный, ре́зкий; 6) чёрствый, безжа́лостный; 7) усе́рдный, рабо́тящий; 8) *амер.* спиртно́й; 9) *фон.* глухо́й (*о зву́ке*); ◇ ∼ of hearing туго́й на́ ухо; to be ∼ on smb. быть несправедли́вым к кому́-л.; to be ∼ up быть в стеснённом, тру́дном положе́нии.

hard II *adv* 1) твёрдо, кре́пко, си́льно; 2) усе́рдно, упо́рно, энерги́чно; 3) с трудо́м; нелегко́; 4) тяжело́, пло́хо; it will go ∼ with him ему́ пло́хо придётся; 5) бли́зко; ∼ by, ∼ at hand совсе́м бли́зко; вслед, по пята́м.

hard III *n* 1) при́стань для ме́лких судо́в; 2) твёрдая площа́дка, доро́жка на боло́те; 3) *сленг* ка́торга.

hard-bitten ['hɑːd'bıtn] *a* 1) огрубе́лый; 2) вынос́ливый, сто́йкий; 3) упо́рный; упря́мый.

hard-boiled ['hɑːd'bɔıld] *a* 1) сва́ренный вкруту́ю; 2) *разг.* круто́й (*о нра́ве*); чёрствый; неподат́ливый (*о челове́ке*); 3) *амер.* практи́чный; иску́шённый, вида́вший ви́ды.

harden ['hɑːdn] *v* 1) де́лать(ся) твёрдым, твер-

дёть; *перен.* закаля́ть(ся); укрепля́ть(ся); 2) ожесточа́ть(ся); станови́ться чёрствым, бесчу́вственным; 3) *тех.* зака́ливать; цементи́ровать.

hard-favoured ['hɑːd'feıvəd] *см.* hard-featured.

hard-featured ['hɑːd'fiːtʃəd] *a* с гру́быми черта́ми лица́.

hard-fisted ['hɑːd'fıstıd] *a* скупо́й.

hard-fought ['hɑːd'fɔːt] *a* ожесточённый, упо́рный (*о бо́е*).

hard-headed ['hɑːd'hedıd] *a* практи́чный, трёзвый; сухо́й.

hard-hearted ['hɑːd'hɑːtıd] *a* безжа́лостный, жесто́кий.

hardihood ['hɑːdıhud] *n* 1) отва́га; сме́лость; 2) де́рзость, на́глость.

hardily ['hɑːdılı] *adv* сме́ло, отва́жно.

hardiness ['hɑːdınıs] *n* 1) кре́пость, выно́сливость; 2) отва́га, де́рзость.

hardly ['hɑːdlı] *adv* 1) едва́, лишь; едва́ ли; не совсе́м; 2) с трудо́м; наси́лу; 3) гру́бо; суро́во, жесто́ко.

hard-mouthed ['hɑːd'mauðd] *a* 1) туго́уздый (*о лоша́ди*); 2) неподат́ливый; 3) ре́зкий, гру́бый.

hardness ['hɑːdnıs] *n* 1) твёрдость; про́чность, кре́пость; 2) тру́дность (*понима́ния, рабо́ты*); суро́вость (*кли́мата*); жёсткость (*воды́*).

hardshell ['hɑːdʃel] *a* непоколеби́мый, непрекло́нный.

hardship ['hɑːdʃıp] *n* лише́ния, нужда́, испыта́ния.

hard-tack ['hɑːdtæk] *n* суха́рь, гале́та.

hard-up ['hɑːd'ʌp] *a* 1) си́льно нужда́ющийся; 2) в затрудни́тельном положе́нии.

hardware ['hɑːdwɛə] *n* скобяны́е изде́лия.

hardwood ['hɑːdwud] *n* твёрдая древеси́на.

hardy[1] ['hɑːdı] *a* 1) выно́сливый, сто́йкий; зимосто́йкий (*о расте́нии*); 2) сме́лый, бесстра́шный.

hardy[2] *n* 1) реза́к, нож, се́чка; 2) долото́, зуби́ло.

hare [hɛə] *n* за́яц; ◇ ∼ and hounds «за́яц и соба́ки» (*назва́ние игры́*); to run with the ∼ and hunt with the hounds ≅ служи́ть и на́шим и ва́шим.

harebell ['hɛəbel] *n бот.* колоко́льчик.

hare-brained ['hɛəbreınd] *a* легкомы́сленный, безрассу́дный.

hare-lip ['hɛə'lıp] *n мед.* за́ячья губа́.

harem ['hɛərem] *n* гаре́м.

haricot ['hærıkou] *n* 1) рагу́; 2) фасо́ль (*тж.* ∼ bean).

hark [hɑːk] *v* слу́шать; ∼! слу́шай!, чу!; *охот.* ищи́!; ◇ to ∼ back to old times возвраща́ться к про́шлому.

harlequin ['hɑːlıkwın] *n* 1) арлеки́н; 2) пая́ц, шут.

harlot ['hɑːlət] *n* проститу́тка.

harlotry ['hɑːlətrı] *n* развра́т.

harm I [hɑːm] *n* вред, уще́рб; зло, оби́да; it will do no ∼ э́то не повреди́т; to do ∼ приноси́ть вред; to get into ∼, to come to ∼ попа́сть в беду́; to keep out of ∼'s way избега́ть (всего́) дурно́го, вре́дного; to think (*или* to mean) no ∼ не име́ть дурны́х наме́рений.

harm II *v* вреди́ть.

harmful ['hɑːmful] *a* вре́дный, опа́сный, па́губный.

harmless ['hɑːmlɪs] *a* безвре́дный, безопа́сный; безоби́дный.

harmonic [hɑː'mɔnɪk] *a* гармони́чный, стро́йный.

harmonica [hɑː'mɔnɪkə] *n* губна́я гармо́ника.

harmonious [hɑː'mounjəs] *a* 1) дру́жный, согла́сный; 2) гармони́чный, гармони́ческий.

harmonium [hɑː'mounjəm] *n* фисгармо́ния.

harmonize ['hɑːmənaɪz] *v* 1) гармони́ровать; 2) приводи́ть в гармо́нию; согласо́вывать; 3) *муз.* аранжи́ровать.

harmony ['hɑːmənɪ] *n* 1) гармо́ния; благозву́чие; 2) гармо́ния, согла́сие; to be in (out of) ~ with smb. быть в согла́сии, ла́дить (не ла́дить) с кем-л.

harness I ['hɑːnɪs] *n* 1) у́пряжь, сбру́я; 2) *ист.* доспе́хи; ◊ in ~ за рабо́той, на рабо́те; to die in ~ умере́ть на своём посту́.

harness II *v* запряга́ть.

harp I [hɑːp] *n* а́рфа.

harp II *v* 1) игра́ть на а́рфе; 2) повторя́ть одно́ и то же, завести́ волы́нку.

harper ['hɑːpə] *n* арфи́ст.

harpist ['hɑːpɪst] *см.* harper.

harpoon I [hɑː'puːn] *n* гарпу́н; острога́.

harpoon II *v* бить гарпуно́м.

harpsichord ['hɑːpsɪkɔːd] *n* клавико́рды; клавеси́н.

harpy ['hɑːpɪ] *n* 1) (H.) *миф.* га́рпия; 2) стяжа́тель, хи́щник.

harridan ['hærɪdən] *n* ста́рая карга́, ве́дьма.

harrier¹ ['hærɪə] *n* го́нчая (*на за́йца*); *pl* сво́ра го́нчих (*с охо́тниками*).

harrier² *n* лунь (*пти́ца*).

harrow I ['hærou] *n* борона́; ◊ under the ~ в беде́.

harrow II *v* 1) борони́ть; 2) причиня́ть боль, ра́нить.

harry ['hærɪ] *v* 1) опустоша́ть, разоря́ть; гра́бить; 2) изводи́ть, му́чить.

harsh [hɑːʃ] *a* 1) ре́зкий, неприя́тный; 2) жёсткий; гру́бый; 3) жесто́кий; бесчу́вственный.

harshness ['hɑːʃnɪs] *n* ре́зкость; гру́бость; жесто́кость.

harslet ['hɑːslɪt] *см.* haslet.

hart [hɑːt] *n* оле́нь (*самец ста́рше пяти́ лет*).

hartal ['hɑːtɑːl] *n* прекраще́ние рабо́ты и торго́вли (*в знак проте́ста или тра́ура в И́ндии*).

hartshorn ['hɑːtshɔːn] *n* 1) оле́ний рог; 2) наша́тырный спирт (*тж.* spirit of ~).

harum-scarum I ['hɛərəm'skɛərəm] *n* безрассу́дный, опроме́тчивый челове́к.

harum-scarum II *a* безрассу́дный, опроме́тчивый.

harvest I ['hɑːvɪst] *n* 1) жа́тва; убо́рка урожа́я; сбор (*плодо́в и т. п.*); 2) результа́ты, плоды́.

harvest II *v* 1) собира́ть урожа́й; жать; 2) пожина́ть (*плоды́*).

harvester ['hɑːvɪstə] *n* 1) жнец; жни́ца; 2) *с.-х.* жа́твенная маши́на, жне́йка-сноповяза́лка.

has [hæz (*си́льная фо́рма*), həz, əz (*сла́бые фо́рмы*)] 3-е л. ед. ч. наст. вр. гл. to have.

has-been ['hæz,biːn] *n разг.* 1) «бы́вший» (челове́к); 2) что-л., вы́шедшее из употребле́ния, устаре́вшее.

hash I [hæʃ] *n* 1) блю́до из ру́бленого мя́са; 2) смесь; 3) меша́нина; пу́таница; to make a ~ of

напу́тать; напо́ртить; ◊ to settle smb.'s ~ разде́латься с кем-л.

hash II *v* 1) руби́ть, кроши́ть (*мя́со*); 2) напу́тать, напо́ртить.

hasher ['hæʃə] *n* мясору́бка.

hashish ['hæʃɪʃ] *n* гаши́ш.

haslet ['heɪzlɪt] *n* жа́реные потроха́.

hasn't ['hæznt] *разг.* = has not.

hasp I [hɑːsp] *n* 1) засо́в, запо́р; 2) застёжка; 3) мото́к.

hasp II *v* запира́ть на засо́в, накла́дывать засо́в.

hassock ['hæsək] *n* 1) поду́шечка (*для коленопреклоне́ния в це́ркви*); 2) пук травы́.

haste I [heɪst] *n* спе́шка, поспе́шность; торопли́вость; in ~ второпя́х, на́скоро, на ско́рую ру́ку; to make ~ спеши́ть, торопи́ться; ◊ more ~, less speed ≅ ти́ше е́дешь, да́льше бу́дешь.

haste II *v см.* hasten.

hasten ['heɪsn] *v* 1) торопи́ть; подгоня́ть; ускоря́ть; 2) спеши́ть, торопи́ться.

hastily ['heɪstɪlɪ] *adv* 1) поспе́шно, торопли́во; на́скоро; 2) необду́манно; 3) запа́льчиво.

hastiness ['heɪstɪnɪs] *n* 1) поспе́шность; 2) необду́манность; 3) вспы́льчивость.

hasty ['heɪstɪ] *a* 1) поспе́шный; бы́стрый, торопли́вый; 2) необду́манный, опроме́тчивый; 3) вспы́льчивый; запа́льчивый.

hat I [hæt] *n* шля́па, ша́пка; tin ~ *воен. сленг* стально́й шлем; cocked ~ треуго́лка; crush ~ складно́й цили́ндр; high (*или* silk, top) ~ цили́ндр; Gipsy ~ широкопо́лая соло́менная шля́па; ~ in hand уни́женно; подобостра́стно; to hang up one's ~ оста́ться, расположи́ться надо́лго; to keep on one's ~ не снима́ть шля́пы; to touch one's ~ to smb. приве́тствовать кого́-л., снима́я шля́пу, здоро́ваться; ◊ a bad ~ *сленг* непутёвый челове́к; to talk through one's ~ *сленг* а) хва́стать; б) нести́ чушь; to pass (*или* to send) round the ~ пусти́ть ша́пку по кру́гу, собира́ть поже́ртвования.

hat II *v* надева́ть шля́пу.

hatch¹ [hætʃ] *n* 1) две́рца; кры́шка лю́ка; люк; under ~es а) под па́лубой; б) в заточе́нии; в) в беде́; г) уме́рший; погребённый; 2) запру́да; шлюзова́я ка́мера.

hatch² I *n* 1) выведе́ние (*цыпля́т*); 2) вы́водок.

hatch² II *v* 1) выси́живать (*цыпля́т*); 2) выводи́ть (*цыпля́т*) в инкуба́торе; 3) вылупля́ться из яйца́; 4) замышля́ть; вына́шивать (*иде́ю и т. п.*); подгота́вливать (*за́говор и т. п.*).

hatch³ I *n* вы́гравированная ли́ния, штрих.

hatch³ II *v* штрихова́ть, гравирова́ть.

hatcher ['hætʃə] *n* 1) насе́дка; 2) инкуба́тор; 3) загово́рщик, интрига́н.

hatchery ['hætʃərɪ] *n* пито́мник (*особ. для разведе́ния рыб*).

hatchet ['hætʃɪt] *n* топо́рик; ◊ to bury the ~ прекрати́ть ра́спри, заключи́ть мир; to dig (*или* to take) up the ~ нача́ть войну́; to throw the ~ преувели́чивать.

hatchet-face ['hætʃɪtfeɪs] *n* дли́нное лицо́ с о́стрыми черта́ми.

hatchetman ['hætʃɪtmən] *n амер.* приспе́шник.

hatchway ['hætʃweɪ] *n* люк.

hate I [heɪt] *n* не́нависть; отвраще́ние.

hate II *v* 1) ненави́деть; 2) *разг.* не терпе́ть, не хоте́ть; I ~ to do it я во́все не хочу́ э́то де́лать.

hateful ['heɪtful] *a* 1) ненави́стный; 2) ненави́дящий.

hater ['heɪtə] *n* ненави́стник.

hatless ['hætlɪs] *a* без шля́пы, с непокры́той голово́й.

hatred ['heɪtrɪd] *n* не́нависть; вражда́.

hat-stand ['hætstænd] *n* ве́шалка для шляп.

hatter ['hætə] *n* 1) шля́пный ма́стер; 2) продаве́ц шляп.

haughtiness ['hɔ:tɪnɪs] *n* высокоме́рие, надме́нность.

haughty ['hɔ:tɪ] *a* высокоме́рный, надме́нный.

haul I [hɔ:l] *n* 1) тя́га, волоче́ние; 2) выта́скивание, вытя́гивание; 3) перево́зка; 4) уло́в; добы́ча; трофе́и; 5) *горн.* отка́тка; 6) *ж.-д.* пробе́г.

haul II *v* 1) тащи́ть, тяну́ть, волочи́ть; 2) перевози́ть; 3) *горн.* отка́тывать; 4) меня́ть направле́ние (*о ветре, судне*).

haulage ['hɔ:lɪdʒ] *n* 1) тя́га; перета́скивание; букси́ровка; 2) перево́зка; 3) сто́имость перево́зки; 4) *горн.* отка́тка.

haulm [hɔ:m] *n* 1) сте́бель; 2) соло́ма (*для крыш*).

haunch [hɔ:ntʃ] *n* 1) бедро́, ля́жка; 2) за́дняя нога́, филе́йная часть (*об оленине и т. п.*).

haunt I [hɔ:nt] *n* 1) ча́сто посеща́емое ме́сто; 2) прито́н.

haunt II *v* 1) ча́сто посеща́ть; 2) пресле́довать (*о мыслях*); упо́рно возвраща́ться (*к чему-л.*); 3) явля́ться (*о привидениях, духах*).

haunted ['hɔ:ntɪd] *a* 1) ча́сто посеща́емый; 2) посеща́емый ду́хами, заколдо́ванный.

haunter ['hɔ:ntə] *n* постоя́нный посети́тель; завсегда́тай.

hautboy ['oubɔɪ] *n* гобо́й.

hauteur [ou'tə:] *n* надме́нность, высокоме́рие.

have I [hæv (*сильная форма*), həv, əv (*слабые формы*)] *v* (*past, p. p.* had) 1) име́ть; 2) *с последующим Inf* быть до́лжным, обя́занным что-л. де́лать; he has to do his work он до́лжен сде́лать свою́ рабо́ту; 3) знать, понима́ть; he has no French он не зна́ет францу́зского языка́; he has your idea он по́нял ва́шу мысль; 4) *с последующим сложным дополнением* отдава́ть, заставля́ть сде́лать что-л.; to ~ a coat altered отда́ть пальто́ в переде́лку; to ~ one's hair cut остри́чь во́лосы; please, ~ the boy bring my books пусть ма́льчик принесёт мои́ кни́ги; 5) пойма́ть; *сленг* обману́ть; the hound has him соба́ка пойма́ла его́; you ~ been had вас обману́ли; 6) говори́ть, выска́зывать; as Shakespeare has it как ска́зано у Шекспи́ра; 7): to ~ dinner обе́дать; to ~ breakfast за́втракать; to ~ tea пить чай; 8): to ~ a walk погуля́ться; to ~ a smoke покури́ть; 9) *употребля́ется как вспомога́тельный гл. для образова́ния сло́жных времён гру́ппы перфе́кта, напр.:* I ~ finished, I had finished я зако́нчил; I shall ~ finished я зако́нчу; □ to ~ **on** носи́ть, быть оде́тым в; to ~ **out:** to ~ out (with) вы́яснить, обсуди́ть что-л. (*в разговоре с кем-л.*); ◊ had rather, had better лу́чше бы, сле́довало бы.

have II [hæv] *n* 1): the ~s and ~-nots иму́щие и неиму́щие; 2) *разг.* обма́н.

haven ['heɪvn] *n* 1) га́вань; 2) убе́жище, приста́нище.

have-on ['hævɔn] *n разг.* обма́н.

haver ['heɪvə] *n обыкн. pl шотл.* болтовня́, бессмы́слица.

haversack ['hævəsæk] *n* (солда́тская) су́мка для прови́зии; вещево́й мешо́к.

havoc ['hævək] *n* разоре́ние, опустоше́ние; разруше́ние; to make ~ of, to play ~ with (*или* among) а) производи́ть беспоря́док, опустоша́ть; б) испо́ртить, подорва́ть (*веру и т. п.*).

haw [hɔ:] *n* 1) я́года боя́рышника; 2) боя́рышник.

hawk[1] I [hɔ:k] *n* со́кол; я́стреб; *перен.* хи́щник.

hawk[1] II *v* 1) охо́титься с со́колом; 2) напада́ть, налета́ть как я́стреб (*at*).

hawk[2] *v* торгова́ть вразно́с; *перен.* распространя́ть (*новости, сплетни*).

hawk[3] *v* отка́шливать(ся), отха́ркивать(ся).

hawker[1] ['hɔ:kə] *n* охо́тник с со́колом.

hawker[2] *n* разно́счик, у́личный торго́вец.

hawk-eyed ['hɔ:kaɪd] *a* име́ющий о́строе зре́ние; *перен.* бди́тельный.

hawser ['hɔ:zə] *n* кана́т, трос.

hawthorn ['hɔ:θɔ:n] *n* боя́рышник.

hay I [heɪ] *n* 1) се́но; to make ~ заготовля́ть, коси́ть и суши́ть се́но; 2) *attr* сенно́й; ◊ to make ~ of напу́тать, напо́ртить; make ~ while the sun shines *посл.* ≈ коси́ коса́, пока́ роса́; to hit the ~ отпра́виться на боку́ю.

hay II *v* коси́ть и суши́ть се́но.

haycock ['heɪkɔk] *n* копна́ се́на.

hay-fork ['heɪfɔ:k] *n* ви́лы.

haying ['heɪɪŋ] *n амер.* сеноко́с.

hayloft ['heɪlɔft] *n* сенова́л.

haymaker ['heɪˌmeɪkə] *n* 1) рабо́чий на сеноко́се; 2) *сленг* си́льный, ошеломля́ющий уда́р.

haymaking ['heɪˌmeɪkɪŋ] *n* сеноко́с.

hayrick ['heɪrɪk] *n* стог се́на.

hayseed ['heɪsi:d] *n амер. разг.* деревéнщина.

haystack ['heɪstæk] *см.* hayrick.

haywire ['heɪwaɪə] *a амер. разг.:* to go ~ помеша́ться, спя́тить.

hazard I ['hæzəd] *n* 1) шанс; 2) риск, опа́сность; at all ~s во что бы то ни ста́ло; to run (*или* to stand) the ~ of рискова́ть (*чем-л.*); 3) аза́ртная игра́; 4) *спорт.* препя́тствие (*в гольфе*).

hazard II *v* 1) рискова́ть, ста́вить на ка́рту; 2) осме́литься.

hazardous ['hæzədəs] *a* риско́ванный, опа́сный.

haze[1] I [heɪz] *n* лёгкий тума́н, ды́мка; *перен.* тума́н в голове́.

haze[1] II *v* затума́нивать.

haze[2] *v* 1) *мор.* изнуря́ть рабо́той; 2) *амер.* дразни́ть, пристава́ть.

hazel I ['heɪzl] *n* оре́шник.

hazel II *a* све́тло-кори́чневый; ка́рий.

hazel-hen ['heɪzlhen] *n* ря́бчик.

hazel-nut ['heɪzlnʌt] *n* оре́х.

haziness ['heɪzɪnɪs] *n* тума́нность.

hazy ['heɪzɪ] *a* тума́нный; подёрнутый ды́мкой; сму́тный.

H-bomb ['eɪtʃ'bɔm] *n* водоро́дная бо́мба.

he [hi:] *pron pers* он.

he- [hɪ-] *pref.* прибавля́емый к существи́тель-

ным для обозначения самца животного: he-goat козёл.

head I [hed] *n* 1) голова; to shake one's ~ качать головой; to hang down one's ~ вешать голову, унывать; to raise one's ~ появляться; to hide one's ~ скрываться, прятаться (*от стыда*); 2) (*pl без измен.*) голова скота; twenty ~ of cattle двадцать голов скота; 3) глава, руководитель; 4) ум, способности; he has a good ~ on his shoulders у него хорошая голова; 5) головка (*винта*), шляпка (*гвоздя*); 6) верхушка, верхняя часть; крышка; 7) головка нарыва; to gather ~ созревать (*о нарыве*); 8) высшая точка, кризис; to bring to a ~ обострять; to come (*или* to draw) to a ~ назреть; подойти к развязке; достигнуть критической точки; 9) передняя, головная часть (*процессии и т. п.*); at the ~ of во главе; 10) кочан; 11) пена; 12) изголовье; 13) исток реки, ручья; 14) мыс; 15) нос (*судна*); 16) лицевая сторона монеты; 17) рубрика; раздел; подзаголовок; 18) ударная *или* режущая часть инструмента; 19) *тех.* давление; напор; ◇ ~ first, ~ foremost a) головой вперёд; б) очертя голову; to make ~ продвигаться; to make ~ against сопротивляться; ~ of hair шапка волос; ~ over ears по уши; ~ over heels вверх тормашками, кувырком; кубарем; ~s or tails ≅ орёл или решка; cannot make ~ or tail of it не могу ничего понять; to eat one's ~ off не оправдывать своей работой стоимости содержания; by the ~ and ears насильно, «за волосы» (*притянуть*); to keep one's ~ сохранять спокойствие; to keep one's ~ above water быть вне опасности, избежать финансовой катастрофы; to turn smb.'s ~ кружить голову кому-л.; to lay ~s together совещаться; off one's ~ вне себя; to go off one's ~ потерять голову; to go to the ~ ударить в голову (*опьянить*); out of one's ~ потерявший голову; обезумевший; to put out of one's ~ выбросить из головы, забыть; over one's ~ а) выше чьего-л. понимания; б) через голову кого-л.; two ~s are better than one ≅ ум хорошо, а два лучше.

head II *a* 1) главный; ведущий; 2) передовой; 3) головной, передний.

head III *v* 1) возглавлять; руководить; 2) направлять(ся); держать курс (*на — for*); 3) озаглавливать; 4) брать начало; вытекать; 5) формировать (*крону, колос*); 6) достигать высшей *или* критической точки; 7) *спорт.* играть головой; □ to ~ back, to ~ off преграждать .(*путь*), препятствовать.

headache ['hedeɪk] *n* головная боль; bad (*или* splitting, violent) ~ сильная головная боль.

headband ['hedbænd] *n* головная повязка, лента.

head-dress ['heddres] *n* 1) головной убор; 2) причёска.

header ['hedə] *n* 1) *спорт.* прыжок в воду вниз головой; 2) *с.-х.* хедер (*комбайна*).

headgear ['hedgɪə] *n* головной убор.

heading ['hedɪŋ] *n* 1) заголовок; надпись; cross ~ подзаголовок (*в газетной статье*); to come (*или* to fall) under two ~s делиться на две группы, категории; 2) курс (*корабля, самолёта*); 3) *горн.* штольня, забой.

head-in-the-sand ['hedɪnðə,sænd] *a:* ~ policy страусовая политика.

headland ['hedlənd] *n* 1) мыс; 2) незапаханный край поля.

headless ['hedlɪs] *a* 1) не имеющий головы, верхушки; 2) безголовый, безмозглый; 3) без руководителя, без главы.

headlight ['hedlaɪt] *n* фара (*автомобиля*); фонарь (*паровоза*).

head-line I ['hedlaɪn] *n* заголовок.

head-line II *v* озаглавить, дать заголовок.

head-liner ['hed,laɪnə] *n* *разг.* ведущий актёр, исполнитель, лектор (*имя которого на афише пишется крупными буквами*).

headlong I ['hedlɔŋ] *a* 1) стремительный; 2) опрометчивый; 3) *поэт.* крутой, отвесный.

headlong II *adv* 1) головой вперёд; 2) стремглав, очертя голову.

headman ['hed'mæn] *n* 1) вождь (*племени и т. п.*); 2) десятник.

head-master ['hed'mɑːstə] *n* директор школы.

head-mistress ['hed'mɪstrɪs] *n* директор школы (*женщина*).

headmost ['hedmoust] *a* передовой, передний.

head-nurse ['hednəːs] *n* старшая сестра (*в больнице и т. п.*).

head-on ['hed'ɔn] *adv* головой, передней частью.

headphones ['hedfounz] *n pl* головной телефон, (радио)наушники.

head-piece ['hedpiːs] *n* 1) шлем; 2) ум, смекалка; 3) умница; 4) заставка (*в книге*).

headquarters ['hed'kwɔːtəz] *n* штаб, штаб-квартира; главное управление, центр; General Headquarters ставка, главное командование.

headsman ['hedzmən] *n* палач.

headstall ['hedstɔːl] *n* недоуздок.

headstone ['hedstoun] *n* могильный камень, надгробие.

headstrong ['hedstrɔŋ] *a* упрямый, своевольный.

head-voice ['hedvɔɪs] *n* высокий голос.

headwater ['hed,wɔːtə] *n* 1) *pl* воды с верховья; исток (*реки*); 2) *гидр.* верхний горизонт воды.

headway ['hedweɪ] *n* (про)движение вперёд; *перен.* прогресс, успех.

head-work ['hedwəːk] *n* умственная работа.

heady ['hedɪ] *a* 1) стремительный; опрометчивый; 2) опьяняющий, крепкий.

heal [hiːl] *v* 1) лечить, излечивать (*of*); 2) заживать (*о ране*); оправляться, вылечиваться.

heal-all ['hiːlˌɔːl] *n* универсальное средство, панацея.

healer ['hiːlə] *n* исцелитель.

healing I ['hiːlɪŋ] *n* 1) лечение; 2) заживление (*раны*).

healing II *a* лечебный, целебный.

health [helθ] *n* 1) здоровье; to drink smb.'s ~, to drink a ~ to smb. пить за чьё-л. здоровье; to propose the ~ of провозглашать тост за; 2) *attr* гигиенический; санитарный.

healthful ['helθful] *a* здоровый, полезный для здоровья, целебный.

healthy ['helθɪ] *a* 1) здоровый; 2) полезный для здоровья.

heap I [hiːp] *n* 1) груда, куча; 2) *разг.* масса; множество; a ~ of people масса народа; ~s of times мно́го раз, о́чень ча́сто; ◊ struck (*или* knocked) all of a ~ *разг.* поражённый, ошеломлённый.

heap II *v* 1) нагроможда́ть; собира́ть в ку́чу, нака́пливать (*часто* to ~ up, to ~ together); 2) нагружа́ть (*with*); 3) осыпа́ть (*наградами, оскорблениями; кого-л. — upon*).

heaps [hiːps] *adv*: he is ~ better *разг.* ему́ мно́го лу́чше.

hear [hɪə] *v* (*past, p. p.* heard) 1) слы́шать; 2) слу́шать, внима́ть; выслу́шивать (*тж.* to ~ out); 3) услы́шать, узна́ть (*o — of, about; тж.* to get to ~); 4) получа́ть изве́стие (*from*); 5) *юр.* слу́шать де́ло.

heard [həːd] *past, p. p. см.* hear.

hearer ['hɪərə] *n* слу́шатель.

hearing ['hɪərɪŋ] *n* 1) слух; in smb.'s ~ в чьём-л. прису́тствии; out of ~ так далеко́, что нельзя́ расслы́шать; 2) слу́шание, выслу́шивание; to give both sides a ~ выслу́шивать о́бе сто́роны; 3) *юр.* слу́шание *или* разбо́р де́ла.

hearken ['hɑːkən] *v* слу́шать, выслу́шивать.

hearsay ['hɪəseɪ] *n* 1) слух, молва́; 2) *attr* осно́ванный на слу́хах.

hearse [həːs] *n* катафа́лк.

heart [hɑːt] *n* 1) се́рдце; *перен. тж.* душа́; single ~ простоду́шие, прямоду́шие; after one's (own) ~ по со́бственному жела́нию, по́ се́рдцу; at ~, in one's ~ of ~s в глубине́ души́; в душе́; from one's ~ и́скренне, от души́; to cry one's ~ out вы́плакаться; to have no ~ быть бессерде́чным; to have at ~ быть заинтересо́ванным; it breaks my ~ у меня́ се́рдце разрыва́ется; to set one's ~ on стреми́ться к чему́-л., жела́ть чего́-л. всем се́рдцем; to take to ~ принима́ть бли́зко к се́рдцу; with a heavy (*или* leaden) ~ с тяжёлым се́рдцем; with all one's ~, with one's whole ~ от всего́ се́рдца, от всей души́; with half a ~ неохо́тно; her ~ went out to the child она́ была́ полна́ сочу́вствия и жа́лости к ребёнку; 2) суть, су́щность; to get to the ~ of a subject добра́ться до са́мой су́ти де́ла; 3) сердцеви́на; ядро́; in the ~ of the forest в глубине́ ле́са; 4) хра́брость, му́жество; to pluck up (*или* to take) ~ подбодри́ться, собра́ться с ду́хом; to lose ~ потеря́ть му́жество, бо́дрость ду́ха; приуны́ть; out of ~ в уны́нии; в плохо́м настрое́нии; his ~ failed him у него́ упа́ло се́рдце; 5) *ласк.*: dear ~, sweet ~ дорого́й, -а́я, ми́лый, -ая; 6) *pl карт.* че́рви ◊ ~ and soul со всей эне́ргией; to have one's ~ in one's boots стру́сить; to have one's ~ in one's mouth си́льно испуга́ться, растеря́ться; to have one's ~ (*или* one's ~ is) in the right place име́ть до́брые (*или* хоро́шие) наме́рения; to wear one's ~ on one's sleeve не отлича́ться сде́ржанностью, не уме́ть скрыва́ть свои́ чу́вства; by ~ наизу́сть.

heart-ache ['hɑːteɪk] *n* душе́вная боль, скорбь.

heart-beat ['hɑːtbiːt] *n* 1) пульса́ция, бие́ние се́рдца; 2) волне́ние.

heart-breaking ['hɑːtˌbreɪkɪŋ] *a* 1) душераздира́ющий; 2) *разг.* ску́чный, ну́дный.

heart-broken ['hɑːtˌbroukən] *a* уби́тый го́рем; с разби́тым се́рдцем.

heartburn ['hɑːtbəːn] *n* изжо́га.

heart-burning ['hɑːtˌbəːnɪŋ] *n* ре́вность; за́висть; доса́да.

heart-disease ['hɑːtdɪˌziːz] *n* боле́знь се́рдца; поро́к се́рдца.

-hearted [-'hɑːtɪd] *в сложных словах переводится в зависимости от первой части слова, напр.*: good-hearted добросерде́чный; light-hearted беспе́чный, весёлый.

hearten ['hɑːtn] *v* (*тж.* to ~ up) 1) ободря́ть; подбодря́ть; 2) приободри́ться, воспря́нуть ду́хом.

heart-felt ['hɑːtfelt] *a* и́скренний.

hearth [hɑːθ] *n* 1) оча́г; печь, ками́н; 2) дома́шний оча́г; 3) под пе́чи.

hearth-rug ['hɑːθrʌg] *n* ко́врик пе́ред ками́ном.

hearthside ['hɑːθsaɪd] *n*: at the ~ у ками́на; у дома́шнего очага́.

heartily ['hɑːtɪlɪ] *adv* 1) и́скренне, серде́чно, тепло́; 2) охо́тно; усе́рдно; to set to work ~ усе́рдно взя́ться за рабо́ту; to eat ~ есть с аппети́том; 3) о́чень; соверше́нно; he is ~ tired он о́чень уста́л.

heartiness ['hɑːtɪnɪs] *n* 1) и́скренность, серде́чность; 2) кре́пость, си́ла.

heartless ['hɑːtlɪs] *a* бессерде́чный, безжа́лостный.

heart-rending ['hɑːtˌrendɪŋ] *a* душераздира́ющий.

heartsease ['hɑːtsiːz] *n* аню́тины гла́зки.

heartsick ['hɑːtsɪk] *a* удручённый, пода́вленный.

heart-strings ['hɑːtstrɪŋz] *n pl* глубоча́йшие чу́вства, стру́ны се́рдца.

heart-to-heart ['hɑːttəˌhɑːt] *a*: ~ talk разгово́р по душа́м.

hearty ['hɑːtɪ] *a* 1) и́скренний, серде́чный; тёплый, дру́жеский; 2) кре́пкий, бо́дрый; 3) оби́льный (*o еде*).

heat I [hiːt] *n* 1) теплота́, жара́, жар; *тех.* нагре́в, нака́л; latent ~ скры́тая теплота́; red (white) ~ кра́сное (бе́лое) кале́ние; blazing ~, parching ~ паля́щий зной; 2) пыл, жар, горя́чность; fever ~ жар, лихора́дочное состоя́ние; in the ~ of the fight в пылу́, в разга́ре бо́я; at white ~ в разга́ре; 3): in a dead ~ ра́зом; at a ~ за оди́н раз; в оди́н приём; 4) *амер.* допро́с с пристра́стием; to turn (*или* to put) on the ~ *разг.* допра́шивать с пристра́стием; 5) пери́од те́чки (*у животных*).

heat II *v* 1) нагрева́ть (ся), накаля́ть (ся) (*тж.* to ~ up); 2) разогрева́ть (*пищу; тж.* to ~ up); 3) топи́ть; 4) воспламени́ть; разгорячи́ть (ся).

heated ['hiːtɪd] *a* разгорячённый, возбуждённый.

heat-engine ['hiːtˌendʒɪn] *n* теплово́й дви́гатель.

heater ['hiːtə] *n* 1) гре́лка; 2) печь, радиа́тор; 3) кипяти́льник.

heath [hiːθ] *n* 1) степь, равни́на, поро́сшая ве́реском; 2) ве́реск.

heath-bell ['hiːθbel] *n* цвето́к ве́реска.

heath-berry ['hiːθˌberɪ] *n* черни́ка и други́е я́годы, расту́щие среди́ ве́реска.

heath-cock ['hiːθkɔk] *n* те́терев.

heathen I ['hiːðən] *n* язы́чник.

heathen II *a* язы́ческий.

heathenish ['hiːðənɪʃ] *a* 1) язы́ческий; 2) ва́рварский.

heathenism ['hiːðənɪzəm] *n* 1) язы́чество; 2) ва́рварство.

heather ['heðə] *n* вереск.

heath-hen ['hiːθhen] *n* тетёрка.

heating I ['hiːtɪŋ] *n* 1) нагревание; нагрев; накал; 2) отопление; central ~ центральное отопление.

heating II *a* 1) согревающий; 2) отопительный.

heat-lightning ['hiːtˌlaɪtnɪŋ] *n* зарница.

heat-spot ['hiːtspɔt] *n* веснушка.

heave I [hiːv] *n* 1) подъём, вздымание; ~ of the sea волнение на море; 2) рвота; 3) *pl* вет. запал.

heave II *v* (*past, p. p.* heaved, hove) 1) поднимать; тянуть (*якорь, канат*); перемещать (*тяжести*); 2) поворачиваться, идти (*о судне*); 3) вздыматься; подниматься и опускаться (*о волнах*); 4) испускать, издавать (*звук*); 5) тужиться (*при рвоте*); 6) *разг.* бросать; □ to ~ to *мор.* ложиться в дрейф, лежать в дрейфе; останавливаться; ◊ ~ ho! дружно!, взяли! (*восклицание при подъёме якоря и т. п.*); to ~ in sight показаться на горизонте.

heaven ['hevn] *n* небо, небеса; ◊ by ~s! ей-богу!; thank ~! слава богу!; good ~s! боже мой!; to move ~ and earth ≅ пустить всё в ход, поднять всех на ноги.

heavenly ['hevnlɪ] *a* 1) небесный; *перен. тж.* божественный; 2) *разг.* восхитительный.

heavily ['hevɪlɪ] *adv* 1) тяжело; 2) тягостно; 3) сильно.

heaviness ['hevɪnɪs] *n* 1) тяжесть; большой вес; 2) удручённое состояние, уныние.

heavy I ['hevɪ] *a* 1) тяжёлый; 2) сильный (*о дожде и т. п.*); бурный (*о море*); 3) нагруженный; отяжелевший; 4) обильный, богатый (*об урожае и т. п.*); 5) труднопереносимый; 6) труднопроходимый (*о дороге*); 7) мрачный; печальный; 8) скучный, тупой.

heavy II *adv* тяжело; сильно; to hang ~ медленно тянуться (*о времени*); to sit ~ оп тяготить.

heavy-duty ['hevɪ'djuːtɪ] *a* *тех.* тяжёлого типа; высокомощный.

heavy-handed ['hevɪ'hændɪd] *a* 1) нескладный, неуклюжий; 2) жестокий, деспотический.

heavy-hearted ['hevɪ'hɑːtɪd] *a* с тяжёлым сердцем, печальный.

heavy-laden ['hevɪ'leɪdn] *a* 1) тяжело нагруженный; 2) с тяжёлым сердцем, подавленный.

heavy-weight ['hevɪweɪt] *n* *спорт.* тяжеловес.

Hebrew I ['hiːbruː] *n* 1) еврей; 2) древнееврейский язык, иврит.

Hebrew II *a* (древне)еврейский.

heckle ['hekl] *v* забрасывать вопросами.

hectare ['hektɑː] *n* гектар.

hectic I ['hektɪk] *n* 1) чахоточный больной; 2) чахоточный румянец, жар.

hectic II *a* 1) чахоточный; 2) лихорадочный; 3) *разг.* беспорядочный, сумбурный.

hector I ['hektə] *n* хвастун; забияка.

hector II *v* задирать (*кого-л.*); грозиться.

hectowatt ['hektəˌwɔt] *n* эл. гектоватт.

he'd [hiːd] *разг.* = he had, he would.

hedge I [hedʒ] *n* 1) (живая) изгородь; ограда; 2) преграда; препятствие.

hedge II *v* 1) огораживать(ся) изгородью; 2) ограждать себя от возможных потерь; 3) уклоняться от прямого ответа; □ to ~ in сжиматься со всех сторон, окружать; to ~ off отгораживать.

hedgehog ['hedʒhɔg] *n* 1) ёж; *амер. тж.* дикобраз; 2) неуживчивый человек.

hedgerow ['hedʒrou] *n* ряд кустов, деревьев; живая изгородь.

heed I [hiːd] *n* внимание; внимательное отношение; to give (*или* to pay, to take) ~ to обращать внимание на, уделять внимание; to take no ~ of не обращать внимания.

heed II *v* обращать внимание; слушать внимательно.

heedful ['hiːdful] *a* внимательный; заботливый.

heedless ['hiːdlɪs] *a* 1) невнимательный; 2) небрежный; необдуманный, неосторожный.

hee-haw I ['hiː'hɔː] *n* 1) крик осла; 2) громкий глупый смех.

hee-haw II *v* 1) кричать (*об осле*); 2) громко хохотать.

heel[1] I [hiːl] *n* 1) пятка; at ~, at (*или* on, upon) one's ~s по пятам, следом; under the ~ of под пятой кого-л.; 2) каблук; to click one's ~s щёлкать, приступать каблуками; down at ~ а) стоптанный (*об обуви*); б) неряшливо *или* очень бедно одетый; 3) остаток чего-л. (*корка сыра, хлеба*); 4) *амер. сленг* подлец, мерзавец; 5) *тех.* пята, грань, ребро; ◊ ~ of Achilles ахиллесова пята, уязвимое место; to cool (*или* to kick) one's ~s дожидаться; to lay (*или* to clap) by the ~s поймать, задержать, арестовать; to show a clean pair of ~s, to take to one's ~s удирать, улепётывать.

heel[1] II *v* 1) приступать каблуками (*в танце*); 2) прибивать каблуки; 3) следовать по пятам.

heel[2] I *n* *мор.* крен.

heel[2] II *v* *мор.* кренить(ся); накреняться.

heeler ['hiːlə] *n* *амер.* 1) приспешник политического деятеля; 2) *сленг* доносчик, предатель.

heeltap ['hiːltæp] *n* 1) набойка на каблуке; 2) недопитый стакан; no ~s! пить до дна!

heft I [heft] *n* *амер.* вес; тяжесть.

heft II *v* *амер.* определять вес чего-л. (*приподнимая на руке*).

hefty ['heftɪ] *a* *разг.* большой, здоровенный.

hegemonic [ˌhiːgɪ'mɔnɪk] *a* руководящий, ведущий.

hegemony [hiː'geməni] *n* гегемония.

heifer ['hefə] *n* тёлка.

heigh [heɪ] *int* эй!

heigh-ho ['heɪ'hou] *int восклицание, выражающее удивление, радость, досаду.*

height [haɪt] *n* 1) высота, вышина; рост; average ~ средний рост; to be... in ~ иметь... в вышину; at a ~ of на высоте; giddy ~ головокружительная высота; 2) возвышенность, холм; 3) вершина, высшая точка, высшая степень; in the ~ of в разгаре.

heighten ['haɪtn] *v* повышать(ся); увеличивать(ся); усиливать(ся).

heinous ['heɪnəs] *a* отвратительный; ужасный.

heir [εə] *n* наследник.

heirdom ['εədəm] *n* наследование.

heiress ['εərɪs] *n* наследница.

heirloom ['εəluːm] *n* 1) фамильная вещь; 2) наследственная черта; 3) наследие.

held [held] *past, p. p. см.* hold[1] II.

helicab ['helɪkæb] *n* пассажирский вертолёт.

helical ['helɪkl] *a* спира́льный; винтово́й.

helices ['helɪsiːz] *pl см.* helix.

helicopter ['helɪkɔptə] *n* вертолёт, гелико́птер.

heliograph ['hiːliougrɑːf] *n* гелио́граф.

heliotrope ['heljətroup] *n бот.* гелиотро́п.

heliport ['helɪpɔːt] *n* вертолётная ста́нция.

helium ['hiːljəm] *n хим.* ге́лий.

helix ['hiːlɪks] *n* (*pl* helices) 1) спира́ль(ная ли́ния); 2) ули́тка; 3) *архит.* завито́к.

hell [hel] *n* 1) ад; 2) (иго́рный) прито́н; ◇ a ~ of a noise а́дский шум; to raise ~ шуме́ть, буя́нить; to move ~ пусти́ть всё в ход; ~! чёрт возьми́!; like ~ отча́янно; go to ~! иди́(те) к чёрту!; what the ~ do you want? како́го чёрта вам ну́жно?

he'll [hiːl] *разг.* = he will.

Hellas ['helæs] *n* Элла́да.

hell-cat ['helkæt] *n* мега́ра.

Hellene ['heliːn] *n* э́ллин; грек.

Hellenic I [he'liːnɪk] *n* гре́ческий язы́к.

Hellenic II *a* э́ллинский; гре́ческий.

hellish ['helɪʃ] *a* а́дский; проти́вный.

hello ['he'lou] *int* приве́т!

helm[1] [helm] *n* руль; штурва́л; *перен.* власть, управле́ние; the ~ of state а) бразды́ правле́ния; б) прави́тельство страны́; the man at the ~ рулево́й; ко́рмчий; to answer the ~ слу́шаться руля́.

helm[2] *n уст., поэт.* шлем.

helmet ['helmɪt] *n* 1) шлем, ка́ска; 2) *тех.* колпа́к.

helmsman ['helmzmən] *n* рулево́й, ко́рмчий.

helot ['helət] *n* раб, ило́т.

help I [help] *n* 1) по́мощь; can I be of any ~ to you? не могу́ ли я быть вам чем-нибудь поле́зен (*или* помо́чь вам)?; 2) сре́дство; спасе́ние; there's no ~ for it э́тому нельзя́ помо́чь; 3) помо́щник; 4) *амер.* прислу́га, дома́шняя рабо́тница; mother's ~ бо́нна.

help II *v* 1) помога́ть; 2) передава́ть, раздава́ть (*кушанье за столом; to*); please ~ yourself to what you like best бери́те, пожа́луйста, что вам бо́льше нра́вится; 3) удержа́ться, воздержа́ться; he could not ~ believing her он не мог не пове́рить ей; she could not ~ crying она́ не могла́ удержа́ться от слёз; 4): don't do more than you can ~ не де́лайте ничего́ сверх необходи́мого, сде́лайте то́лько са́мое необходи́мое; don't be longer than you can ~ не остава́йтесь до́льше, чем необходи́мо; □ to ~ **down** помо́чь сойти́; to ~ **forward** а) вести́ вперёд; б) продвига́ть (*дело*); to ~ **in** помо́чь войти́, ввести́; to ~ **into** а) помо́чь войти́; б) помо́чь наде́ть, пода́ть (*пальто и т. п.*); to ~ **off** а) помо́чь вы́путаться, вы́свободить; б) помо́чь снять что-л.; to ~ **on** пода́ть пальто́, помо́чь оде́ться; to ~ **out** а) вы́ручить; б) помо́чь вы́йти; to ~ **through** соде́йствовать выполне́нию чего́-л.; to ~ **up** помо́чь встать, подня́ться.

helper ['helpə] *n* помо́щник.

helpful ['helpful] *a* поле́зный.

helpfully ['helpfulɪ] *adv* 1) с большо́й по́льзой; 2) услу́жливо; любе́зно; с гото́вностью.

helping ['helpɪŋ] *n* 1) по́мощь; 2) по́рция (*кушанья*).

helpless ['helplɪs] *a* беспо́мощный.

helpmate ['helpmeɪt] *n* помо́щник, това́рищ; подру́га.

helpmeet ['helpmiːt] *см.* helpmate.

helter-skelter I ['heltə'skeltə] *n* беспоря́док, суматоха.

helter-skelter II *adv* в беспоря́дке, как попа́ло.

helve [helv] *n* рукоя́тка; топори́ще.

hem[a] **I** [hem] *n* рубе́ц, край, кро́мка, кайма́.

hem[a] **II** *v* подруба́ть; □ to ~ **about**, to ~ **in**, to ~ **round** заключа́ть, окружа́ть, окаймля́ть.

hem[b] **I** [mm] *int* гм!

hem[b] **II** *v* произноси́ть «гм», пока́шливать, прочища́ть го́рло; to ~ and haw запина́ться, мя́млить; не реша́ться, колеба́ться.

he-man ['hiːmæn] *n разг.* настоя́щий мужчи́на.

hemisphere ['hemɪsfɪə] *n* полуша́рие; cerebral ~s полуша́рия головно́го мо́зга.

hemistich ['hemɪstɪk] *n* полусти́шие.

hemlock ['hemlɔk] *n* 1) *бот.* болиголо́в; 2) тсу́га (*хвойное дерево в Америке и Азии*).

hemoglobin [ˌhiːmou'gloubɪn] *см.* haemoglobin.

hemorrhage ['hemərɪdʒ] *см.* haemorrhage.

hemp [hemp] *n* 1) конопля́; пенька́; Indian ~ инди́йская конопля́, гаши́ш; 2) *шутл.* верёвка, пе́тля.

hempen ['hempən] *a* пенько́вый; конопля́ный.

hem-stitch I ['hemstɪtʃ] *n* мере́жка; ажу́рная стро́чка.

hem-stitch II *v* де́лать мере́жку, ажу́рную стро́чку.

hen [hen] *n* 1) ку́рица; clucking ~ клу́ш(к)а; 2) са́мка (*некоторых птиц*); ◇ like a ~ with one chicken хлопотли́во.

henbane ['henbeɪn] *n бот.* белена́.

hence I [hens] *adv* 1) отсю́да; 2) с э́тих пор; с э́того вре́мени; many years ~ че́рез мно́го лет; 3) сле́довательно, потому́.

hence II *int* прочь!, убира́йся!

henceforth ['hens'fɔːθ] *adv* с э́того вре́мени; впредь.

henceforward ['hens'fɔːwəd] *см.* henceforth.

henchman ['hentʃmən] *n* 1) сторо́нник, приве́рженец; 2) приспе́шник, прихвостень; 3) *ист.* оружено́сец, паж.

hen-coop ['henkuːp] *n* кле́тка для кур.

hen-harrier ['hen'hærɪə] *n* лунь (*птица*).

hen-hearted ['hen'hɑːtɪd] *a* малоду́шный.

henna I ['henə] *n* хна.

henna II *a* краснова́то-кори́чневый.

henna III *v* окра́шивать хной.

hen-pecked ['henpekt] *a* находя́щийся под башмако́м у жены́.

hepatic [hɪ'pætɪk] *a* 1) печёночный; 2) поле́зный для пе́чени; 3) кори́чневый.

heptagon ['heptəgən] *n мат.* семиуго́льник.

her I [həː] *pron pers* 1) (*косв. п. от* she) её, ей, е́ю; о ней; have you seen ~? ви́дели ли вы её?; give ~ да́йте ей; 2) *разг.* она́; it's ~ э́то она́.

her II *pron poss* её; it is ~ book э́то её кни́га.

herald I ['herəld] *n* ве́стник; *ист.* геро́льд.

herald II *v* 1) сообща́ть, возвеща́ть; 2) вводи́ть (*кого-л.* в ко́мнату).

heraldic [he'rældɪk] *a* геральди́ческий.

heraldry ['herəldrɪ] *n* гера́льдика.

herb [həːb] *n* трава́; расте́ние (*особ. лекарственное*).

herbaceous [həː'beɪʃəs] *a* травяно́й; травяни́стый.

herbage ['hə:bɪdʒ] *n собир.* тра́вы; травяно́й покро́в.

herbarium [hə:'bɛərɪəm] *n* герба́рий.

herbivorous [hə:'bɪvərəs] *a* травоя́дный.

Herculean [,hə:kju'li:ən] *a* 1) геркуле́совский; о́чень си́льный; 2) о́чень тру́дный.

herd I [hə:d] *n* 1) ста́до; *перен.* толпа́; 2) пасту́х; 3) *attr* ста́дный (*об инстинкте*).

herd II *v* 1) ходи́ть ста́дом (*with*); *перен.* толпи́ться; 2) пасти́; □ to ~ **together** сбива́ться в ку́чу.

herdsman ['hə:dzmən] *n* пасту́х.

here [hɪə] *adv* 1) здесь, тут; ~ and there там и сям; ~ and there and everywhere повсю́ду; neither ~ nor there некста́ти, ни к селу́ ни к го́роду; 2) сюда́; 3) вот; ~ they are вот и они́; ◊ ~ below на э́том све́те, в э́той жи́зни; ~ goes! нача́ли!, начнём!, пошли́!; ~'s to you! за ва́ше здоро́вье!

hereabout(s) ['hɪərə,baut(s)] *adv* где́-то здесь, поблизости.

hereafter I [hɪər'a:ftə] *n* бу́дущее.

hereafter II *adv* в бу́дущем.

hereat [hɪər'æt] *adv уст.* при сём; при э́том.

hereby ['hɪə'baɪ] *adv* 1) настоя́щим; э́тим, сим; 2) таки́м о́бразом.

hereditary [hɪ'redɪtərɪ] *a* 1) насле́дственный; 2) традицио́нный (*в данной семье, в роду*).

heredity [hɪ'redɪtɪ] *n* насле́дственность.

herein ['hɪər'ɪn] *adv* при сём; в э́том.

hereinafter ['hɪərɪn'a:ftə] *adv* ни́же, в дальне́йшем (*в документах*).

hereof [hɪər'ɔv] *adv* 1) об э́том; 2) отсю́да, из э́того.

hereon [hɪər'ɔn] *adv* 1) на э́том; 2) вслед за э́тим; по́сле э́того.

here's [hɪəz] *разг.* = here is.

heresy ['herəsɪ] *n* е́ресь.

heretic ['herətɪk] *n* ерети́к.

heretical [hɪ'retɪkəl] *a* ерети́ческий.

hereto ['hɪə'tu:] *adv уст.* к э́тому, к тому́ (же).

heretofore ['hɪətu'fɔ:] *adv* пре́жде, до сих по́р.

hereupon ['hɪərə'pɔn] *adv* 1) по́сле э́того; 2) всле́дствие э́того.

herewith ['hɪə'wɪð] *adv* 1) при сём (*прилагается*); 2) настоя́щим (*сообщается и т. п.*).

heritable ['herɪtəbl] *a* 1) насле́дственный; насле́дуемый; 2) могу́щий насле́довать.

heritage ['herɪtɪdʒ] *n* насле́дство; насле́дие.

hermetic [hə:'metɪk] *a* пло́тно закры́тый, гермети́ческий.

hermit ['hə:mɪt] *n* отше́льник.

hermitage ['hə:mɪtɪdʒ] *n* жили́ще отше́льника; уединённое жили́ще.

hero ['hɪərou] *n* геро́й; Hero of the Soviet Union Геро́й Сове́тского Сою́за; Hero of Socialist Labour Геро́й Социалисти́ческого Труда́.

heroic I [hɪ'rouɪk] *a* 1) герои́ческий, геро́йский; 2) высокопа́рный, напы́щенный (*о языке*).

heroic II *n* 1) пятисто́пный ямб; 2) *pl* высокопа́рный стиль, язы́к.

heroin ['herouɪn] *n* герои́н.

heroine ['herouɪn] *n* герои́ня.

heroism ['herouɪzəm] *n* герои́зм, геро́йство.

heron ['herən] *n* ца́пля.

herpes ['hə:pi:z] *n мед.* лиша́й.

herring ['herɪŋ] *n* сельдь; red ~ копчёная сельдь.

herring-bone ['herɪŋboun] *n* 1) «ёлочка», вы́шивка *или* шов «ёлочкой»; 2) подъём «ёлочкой» (*на лыжах*); 3) кла́дка кирпиче́й в «ёлочку».

hers [hə:z] *pron poss* её; this book is ~ э́та кни́га её.

herself [hə:'self] *pron* 1) *refl* себя́, самоё себя́, -сь; she asks ~ a question она́ задаёт себе́ вопро́с, она́ спра́шивает самоё себя́; she works for ~ она́ рабо́тает на себя́; she has hurt ~ она́ уши́блась; she is talking to ~ она́ разгова́ривает сама́ с собо́й; 2) *употребляется для усиления* сама́; she told me so ~ она́ сама́ мне так сказа́ла; 3): she did it all by ~ она́ де́лала э́то сама́ (одна́); by ~ отде́льно; одино́ко, самостоя́тельно; she lives by ~ она́ живёт одино́ко; ◊ she is not ~ она́ сама́ не своя́; she came to ~ она́ пришла́ в себя́.

Hertz [hə:ts] *n* герц (*единица частоты*).

he's [hi:z] *разг.* = he is, he has.

hesitant ['hezɪtənt] *a* нереши́тельный, колеблю́щийся.

hesitate ['hezɪteɪt] *v* 1) колеба́ться, не реша́ться; 2) запина́ться, заика́ться.

hesitatingly ['hezɪteɪtɪŋlɪ] *adv* нереши́тельно.

hesitation [,hezɪ'teɪʃən] *n* 1) колеба́ние, нереши́тельность; сомне́ние; неохо́та; 2) заика́ние.

heterodox ['hetərədɔks] *a* неортодокса́льный, ерети́ческий.

heterogeneous ['hetərou'dʒi:njəs] *a* разноро́дный.

hew [hju:] *v* (*past* hewed; *p. p.* hewed, hewn) 1) руби́ть, разруба́ть; 2) обтёсывать; □ to ~ **down** сруба́ть; to ~ **off** отруба́ть; *горн.* отбива́ть; to ~ **out** высека́ть, выруба́ть.

hewer ['hju:ə] *n* 1) дровосе́к; 2) каменотёс; 3) *горн.* забо́йщик.

hewn [hju:n] *p. p. см.* hew.

hexagon ['heksəgən] *n мат.* шестиуго́льник.

hexameter [hek'sæmɪtə] *n* гекза́метр.

hey [heɪ] *int* 1) эй! (*оклик*); 2) а? (*выражает вопрос и т. п.*).

hey-day ['heɪdeɪ] *int восклицание, выражающее радость, удивление.*

heyday ['heɪdeɪ] *n* расцве́т, зени́т, апоге́й.

hiatus [haɪ'eɪtəs] *n* 1) пробе́л, про́пуск; 2) *лингв.* зия́ние.

hibernate ['haɪbə:neɪt] *v* 1) зимова́ть; 2) проводи́ть зи́му в спя́чке (*о животных*); 3) пребыва́ть в безде́йствии.

hibernation [,haɪbə:'neɪʃən] *n* 1) зимо́вка; 2) зи́мняя спя́чка.

Hibernian I [haɪ'bə:njən] *n поэт.* ирла́ндец.

Hibernian II *a поэт.* ирла́ндский.

hiccup I ['hɪkʌp] *n* ико́та.

hiccup II *v* ика́ть.

hick [hɪk] *n амер. разг.* се́льский жи́тель; «деревёнщина».

hid [hɪd] *past, p. p. см.* hide[2].

hidden I ['hɪdn] *a* скры́тый; та́йный.

hidden II *p. p. см.* hide[2].

hide[1] I [haɪd] *n* шку́ра, ко́жа; raw ~ сыромя́тная, недублёная ко́жа; ◊ ~ and hair цели́ком, по́лностью, без оста́тка; to tan smb.'s ~ отколоти́ть кого́-л.

hide[1] II *v разг.* вы́пороть, отколоти́ть.

hide[2] *v* (*past* hid; *p. p.* hid, hidden) пря́тать(ся); скрыва́ть(ся).

hide-and-seek [ˈhaɪdəndˈsiːk] *n* (игра́ в) пря́тки.

hidebound [ˈhaɪdbaund] *a* 1) о́чень худо́й (*о скоте́*); 2) ограни́ченный, с у́зким кругозо́ром; педанти́чный.

hideous [ˈhɪdɪəs] *a* 1) проти́вный, отврати́тельный; 2) стра́шный, ужа́сный.

hiding[1] [ˈhaɪdɪŋ] *n* побо́и; to give a good ~ хороше́нько отколоти́ть.

hiding[2] *n* 1) скрыва́ние; сокры́тие; in ~ скрыва́ясь, в бега́х; 2) та́йное убе́жище.

hiding-place [ˈhaɪdɪŋpleɪs] *n* потаённое ме́сто; тайни́к.

hie [haɪ] *v поэт.* бы́стро идти́, спеши́ть.

hierarchy [ˈhaɪərɑːkɪ] *n* иера́рхия.

hieroglyph [ˈhaɪərəglɪf] *n* иеро́глиф.

hieroglyphic [ˌhaɪərəˈglɪfɪk] *a* иероглифи́ческий.

hieroglyphics [ˌhaɪərəˈglɪfɪks] *n pl* иеро́глифика.

higgle [ˈhɪgl] *v* 1) торгова́ться; 2) торгова́ть вразно́с.

higgledy-piggledy I [ˈhɪgldɪˈpɪgldɪ] *n* полне́йший беспоря́док.

higgledy-piggledy II *a* беспоря́дочный, спу́танный.

higgledy-piggledy III *adv* в беспоря́дке, как попа́ло.

higgler [ˈhɪglə] *n* разно́счик.

high I [haɪ] *a* 1) высо́кий; возвы́шенный; 2) вы́сший, гла́вный, верхо́вный; 3) си́льный; 4) дорого́й (*о цена́х и т. п.*); 5) роско́шный; 6) высо́кий, ре́зкий (*о зву́ке*); 7) *фон.* ве́рхний; 8) слегка́ испо́рченный (*о мя́се, дичи*); 9) наивы́сший, кра́йний; it is ~ time to go давно́ пора́ идти́; ◊ ~ and dry а) вы́брошенный на бе́рег (*о су́дне*); б) поки́нутый в беде́; в) отстаю́щий от собы́тий, жи́зни; ~ and low (лю́ди) вся́кого зва́ния (*см. тж.* high II ◊); ~ and mighty высокоме́рный.

high II *adv* 1) высоко́; 2) си́льно; в высо́кой сте́пени; кра́йне; 3) до́рого; 4) ре́зко (*о зву́ке*); ◊ to stand ~ быть в почёте; ~ and low везде́, повсю́ду (*см. тж.* high I ◊); to run ~ а) подыма́ться, вздыма́ться (*о мо́ре*); б) возбужда́ться.

highball [ˈhaɪbɔːl] *n амер. разг.* «ха́йбол» (*виски с содо́вой*).

high-blown [ˈhaɪˌbloun] *a* 1) си́льно разду́тый; 2) напы́щенный.

high-born [ˈhaɪbɔːn] *a* зна́тного происхожде́ния.

high-bred [ˈhaɪbred] *a* 1) поро́дистый, хоро́шей поро́ды; 2) хорошо́ воспи́танный.

highbrow [ˈhaɪbrau] *n* челове́к, кича́щийся (мни́мой) учёностью, высо́кой интеллектуа́льностью.

high-coloured [ˈhaɪˈkʌləd] *a* 1) румя́ный; 2) я́ркий, живо́й (*об описа́нии*); 3) преувели́ченный.

higher-up [ˈhaɪərˈʌp] *n амер. разг.* ва́жная персо́на, «ши́шка».

high-falutin [ˈhaɪfəˈluːtɪn] *a* напы́щенный.

high-flier [ˈhaɪˈflaɪə] *см.* high-flyer.

high-flown [ˈhaɪfloun] *a* напы́щенный.

high-flyer [ˈhaɪˈflaɪə] *n* честолю́бец.

high-frequency [ˈhaɪˈfriːkwənsɪ] *a* высо́кой частоты́, коротково́лновый.

high-grade [ˈhaɪgreɪd] *a* высокосо́ртный, высокока́чественный.

high-handed [ˈhaɪˈhændɪd] *a* вла́стный; своево́льный.

high-hat [ˈhaɪˈhæt] *n амер.* 1) ва́жная персо́на; 2) зано́счивый челове́к.

highland [ˈhaɪlənd] *n обыкн. pl* го́рная страна́; the Highlands се́верная, гори́стая часть Шотла́ндии.

Highlander [ˈhaɪləndə] *n* 1) го́рец; 2) шотла́ндский го́рец.

highlight I [ˈhaɪlaɪt] *n обыкн. pl* 1) световой эффе́кт (*в жи́вописи, фотогра́фии*); 2) основно́й *или* са́мый интере́сный моме́нт; ◊ to be in the ~ быть в це́нтре внима́ния.

highlight II *v* выдвига́ть на пе́рвый план; придава́ть большо́е значе́ние.

highly [ˈhaɪlɪ] *adv* 1) о́чень, весьма́; си́льно; 2) благоприя́тно, благоскло́нно; положи́тельно.

high-minded [ˈhaɪˈmaɪndɪd] *a* благоро́дный, высоконра́вственный.

highness [ˈhaɪnɪs] *n* 1) высота́; возвы́шенность; 2) высо́кая сте́пень чего́-л.; 3) (H.) высо́чество (*ти́тул*).

high-pitched [ˈhaɪˈpɪtʃt] *a* 1) высо́кий, ре́зкий (*о зву́ке, го́лосе*); 2) высо́кий и круто́й (*о кры́ше*); 3) возвы́шенный.

high-pressure [ˈhaɪˈpreʃə] *a* 1) рабо́тающий под высо́ким давле́нием (*о маши́не и т. п.*); 2) насто́йчивый, агресси́вный; 3) интенси́вный, напряжённый.

high-road [ˈhaɪˈroud] *см.* highway.

high-rolling [ˈhaɪˈroulɪŋ] *n амер.* мотовство́, расточи́тельность.

high-scaler [ˈhaɪˌskeɪlə] *n* верхола́з.

high-sounding [ˈhaɪˌsaundɪŋ] *a* гро́мкий, пы́шный.

high-speed [ˈhaɪˈspiːd] *a* быстрохо́дный; скоростно́й.

high-spirited [ˈhaɪˈspɪrɪtɪd] *a* 1) сме́лый; горя́чий, пы́лкий; 2) в хоро́шем настрое́нии.

high-stepper [ˈhaɪˈstepə] *n разг.* карьери́ст.

high-strung [ˈhaɪstrʌŋ] *a* чувстви́тельный; не́рвный.

high-up [ˈhaɪˈʌp] *a* 1) высоко́ располо́женный; 2) высокопоста́вленный.

highway [ˈhaɪweɪ] *n* 1) больша́я доро́га, шоссе́; 2) гла́вный путь; *перен.* прямо́й путь (*к чему́-л.*).

highwayman [ˈhaɪweɪmən] *n* разбо́йник с большо́й доро́ги.

hijack [ˈhaɪdʒæk] *v* 1) огра́бить автомоби́ль, торго́вый фурго́н *и т. п.* на доро́ге; 2) захвати́ть, угна́ть самолёт.

hike I [haɪk] *n* 1) *разг.* прогу́лка, путеше́ствие пешко́м; похо́д; 2) *воен.* марш в пе́шем строю́.

hike II *v* 1) *разг.* ходи́ть пешко́м, гуля́ть; 2) бродя́жничать; 3) *воен.* идти́ в пе́шем строю́.

hilarious [hɪˈlɛərɪəs] *a* весёлый, шу́мный.

hilarity [hɪˈlærɪtɪ] *n* шу́мное весе́лье, весёлость.

hill I [hɪl] *n* 1) холм, возвы́шенность, го́рка; 2) ку́ча.

hill II *v* 1) насыпа́ть ку́чу; 2) оку́чивать (*расте́ния*).

hillock [ˈhɪlək] *n* хо́лмик; буго́р.

hillside [ˈhɪlˈsaɪd] *n* склон холма́; косого́р.

hilly [ˈhɪlɪ] *a* холми́стый.

hilt [hɪlt] *n* рукоятка; эфес; (up) to the ~ a) по рукоятку; б) вполне, целиком и полностью.

him [hɪm] *pron pers* (*косв. п. от* he) 1) его, ему, им, о нём; 2) *разг.* он; that's ~ это он.

himself [hɪm'self] *pron* 1) *refl* себя, самого себя, -ся; he persuaded ~ он убеждал самого себя; he works for ~ он работает на себя; he hurt ~ он ушибся; he is talking to ~ он разговаривает сам с собой; 2) *употребляется для усиления* сам; he told so ~ он сам так сказал; 3): he did it all by ~ он делал это сам (один); by ~ отдельно; одиноко; самостоятельно; he lives by ~ он живёт одиноко; ◊ he is not ~ он сам не свой; he came to ~ он пришёл в себя.

hind¹ [haɪnd] *n* 1) батрак, работник на ферме; 2) *презр.* деревенщина.

hind² *n* самка оленя.

hind³ *a* задний.

hinderᵃ ['haɪndə] *a* задний.

hinderᵇ ['hɪndə] *v* мешать, препятствовать; служить помехой.

Hindi ['hɪn'diː] *n* язык хинди.

hindmost ['haɪndmoust] *a* 1) самый задний; 2) самый отдалённый.

Hindoo I, II ['hɪn'duː] *см.* Hindu I, II.

hindrance ['hɪndrəns] *n* препятствие, помеха.

hindsight ['haɪndsaɪt] *n* 1) непредусмотрительность; 2) *воен.* прицел.

Hindu I ['hɪn'duː] *n* индус.

Hindu II *a* индусский.

Hindustani I [ˌhɪndu'staːnɪ] *n* (язык) хиндустани.

Hindustani II *a* индийский.

hinge I [hɪndʒ] *n* 1) шарнир, петля; 2) суть; стержень, ось; ◊ off the ~s в беспорядке, в расстройстве.

hinge II *v* 1) привешивать, прикреплять на шарнирах *или* петлях; 2) висеть, вращаться на шарнирах *или* петлях; 3) зависеть (*от чего-л.* — on).

hint I [hɪnt] *n* намёк; a broad ~ ясный намёк; to drop (*или* to give) a delicate (*или* gentle) ~ тонко намекнуть; to take a ~ понять намёк.

hint II *v* намекать (*на что-л.* — that, at).

hinterland ['hɪntəlænd] *n* 1) район(ы) вглубь от прибрежной полосы *или* границы; *воен.* глубокий тыл; 2) район, тяготеющий к какому-л. центру.

hintingly ['hɪntɪŋlɪ] *adv* в виде намёка.

hip¹ [hɪp] *n* бедро; ◊ to have smb. on the ~ держать кого-л. в руках; полностью подчинить кого-л.; to smite ~ and thigh разбить наголову.

hip² *n* ягода шиповника.

hip³ I *n разг.* уныние, меланхолия.

hip³ II *v разг.* повергать в уныние.

hip⁴ *int*: ~, ~, hurrah! гип, гип, ура!

hip-bath ['hɪpbɑːθ] *n* поясная ванна.

hippo ['hɪpou] *сокр. разг. см.* hippopotamus.

hippodrome ['hɪpədroum] *n* 1) ипподром; 2) цирк.

hippopotamus [ˌhɪpə'pɒtəməs] *n* (*pl тж.* hippopotami [ˌhɪpə'pɒtəmaɪ]) гиппопотам, бегемот.

hire I ['haɪə] *n* 1) наём, прокат; to let out on ~ сдавать внаём; давать напрокат; 2) плата за наём.

hire II *v* нанимать; □ to ~ out сдавать внаём, давать напрокат.

hireling ['haɪəlɪŋ] *n* наёмник, наймит.

hire-purchase ['haɪə'pəːtʃəs] *n* продажа, покупка, приобретение в рассрочку.

hire-system ['haɪə'sɪstɪm] *см.* hire-purchase.

hirsute ['həːsjuːt] *a* волосатый; косматый.

his [hɪz] *pron poss* его; принадлежащий ему; ~ book его книга; it is ~ это его.

hiss I [hɪs] *n* свист, шипение.

hiss II *v* 1) свистеть, шипеть; 2) освистывать; □ to ~ away, to ~ down, to ~ off освистать, прогнать (*со сцены и т. п.*).

hist [sːt, hɪst] *int* тише!; тс!

historian [hɪs'tɔːrɪən] *n* историк.

historic [hɪs'tɔrɪk] *a* исторический, имеющий историческое значение.

historical [hɪs'tɔrɪkəl] *a* исторический, исторически установленный (*о факте и т. п.*).

historiography [hɪstɔːrɪ'ɔgrəfɪ] *n* историография.

history ['hɪstərɪ] *n* история.

histrionic [ˌhɪstrɪ'ɔnɪk] *a* 1) актёрский; сценический; 2) театральный, неестественный; 3) лицемерный.

histrionics [ˌhɪstrɪ'ɔnɪks] *n pl* 1) театральное представление; 2) театральное искусство; 3) театральность; искусственность.

hit I [hɪt] *n* 1) удар, толчок; 2) попадание; full ~ прямое попадание; 3) успех, удача; a lucky ~ неожиданный успех; the new play was the ~ of the season новая пьеса была гвоздём сезона; 4) спектакль, фильм *и т. п.*, пользующийся успехом; smash(ing) ~ нашумевший фильм; 5) сатирический выпад; нападки (at).

hit II *v* (*past, p. p.* hit) 1) ударять, поражать; to ~ a man when he's down бить лежачего (*тж. перен.*); 2) ударяться; сталкиваться; 3) попадать в цель; *перен.* задевать (за живое); to ~ it попасть в точку; 4) (случайно) найти, напасть (*на мысль*; *upon*); встретить; 5) уловить (*сходство*); □ to ~ off подражать; копировать; to ~ out наносить удары, бросаться на кого-л.; ◊ to ~ it off ладить (*с кем-л.* — with).

hit-and-miss ['hɪtən'mɪs] *a* неточный.

hitch I [hɪtʃ] *n* 1) толчок; 2) *мор.* узел, петля; 3) зацепка; 4) задержка, помеха; without a ~ совершенно гладко, без помех.

hitch II *v* 1) подталкивать, подтягивать, тащить; 2) зацеплять(ся), закреплять(ся); 3) сцеплять, скреплять; привязывать (*лошадь*); 4) *амер. сленг* жениться; 5) *сленг см.* hitch-hike.

hitch-hike ['hɪtʃhaɪk] *v амер.* путешествовать на попутных машинах.

hither ['hɪðə] *adv* сюда; ~ and thither (и) туда и сюда.

hitherto ['hɪðə'tuː] *adv* до настоящего времени, до сих пор.

hive I [haɪv] *n* 1) улей; пчелиный рой; 2) людской муравейник.

hive II *v* 1) сажать в улей; *перен.* поселить, приютить; 2) роиться; 3) жить вместе, обществом.

hives [haɪvz] *n pl* сыпь, крапивница.

ho [hou] *int* эй!

hoar I [hɔː] *n* 1) иней; 2) густой туман; 3) старость.

hoar II *a* 1) покрытый инеем, побелевший; 2) седой.

hoard I [hɔːd] *n* 1) запас(ы), что-л. накопленное, припрятанное; 2) подбор фактов.

hoard II *v* запасать; копить, припрятывать.

hoarder ['hɔːdə] *n* скопидом; запасливый человек.

hoarding ['hɔːdɪŋ] *n* 1) временный забор вокруг стройки; 2) щит для афиш.

hoar-frost ['hɔːfrɔst] *n* иней, изморозь.

hoarse [hɔːs] *a* хриплый, охрипший; to cry (to talk) oneself ~ докричаться (договориться) до хрипоты.

hoary ['hɔːrɪ] *a* 1) седой; 2) древний, старый.

hoax I [houks] *n* обман, хитрость, трюк.

hoax II *v* обмануть, провести, подшутить.

hob [hɔb] *n* 1) полка в камине для подогревания пищи; 2) гвоздь, колышек для обозначения мишени (*в игре*); 3) ступица колеса; 4) *тех.* бесконечный винт.

hobble I ['hɔbl] *n* 1) хромота, прихрамывание; 2) неловкое, затруднительное положение; 3) путы.

hobble II *v* 1) прихрамывать, хромать; ковылять; 2) запинаться; 3) стреножить лошадь.

hobbledehoy ['hɔbldɪ'hɔɪ] *n* неуклюжий подросток.

hobby ['hɔbɪ] *n* 1) конёк, хобби; to ride (*или* to mount) a ~ сесть на своего (любимого) конька; 2) *см.* hobby-horse.

hobby-horse ['hɔbɪhɔːs] *n* лошадка (*игрушка*), палочка с лошадиной головой; конь-качалка.

hobgoblin ['hɔb,gɔblɪn] *n* 1) бесёнок, чертёнок; домовой; 2) пугало, призрак.

hobnail ['hɔbneɪl] *n* сапожный гвоздь с большой шляпкой.

hob-nob ['hɔbnɔb] *v* 1) выпивать вместе; 2) *разг.* водиться, дружить.

hobo ['houbou] *n* амер. бродяга; странствующий рабочий.

hock¹ I, II [hɔk] *см.* hough I, II.

hock² *n* рейнвейн (*вино*).

hock³ I *n* сленг залог, заклад; in ~ а) в закладе; б) в тюрьме.

hock³ II *v* сленг закладывать (*вещь*).

hockey ['hɔkɪ] *n* хоккей.

hock-shop ['hɔkʃɔp] *n* сленг ломбард.

hocus ['houkəs] *v* 1) обманывать, одурачивать; 2) одурманивать наркотиками.

hocus-pocus I ['houkəs'poukəs] *n* фокус; проделка.

hocus-pocus II *v* проделать фокус, одурачить.

hod [hɔd] *n* стр. лоток (*для кирпичей, извести*); творило.

hodge-podge ['hɔdʒpɔdʒ] *см.* hotchpotch.

hodman ['hɔdmən] *n* 1) подручный каменщика; 2) подсобный рабочий; 3) литературный подёнщик.

hoe I [hou] *n* мотыга.

hoe II *v* мотыжить, разрыхлять землю.

hoe-cake ['houkeɪk] *n* амер. кукурузная лепёшка.

hog I [hɔg] *n* 1) свинья; боров; 2) амер. свинина; 3) годовалая овца; 4) грубый, грязный человек; 5) тех. прогиб; искривление; 6) щётка, скребок; ◇ to bring ~s to a bad market обмануться в расчёте, просчитаться; to go the whole ~

а) делать что-л. основательно; доводить что-л. до конца; б) идти на всё, ни перед чем не останавливаться.

hog II *v* 1) выгибать(ся); искривляться; 2) чистить (*щёткой, скребком*).

hogback ['hɔgbæk] *n* гряда гор с острым гребнем.

hoggish ['hɔgɪʃ] *a* 1) свинский, грязный; 2) жадный.

hogshead ['hɔgzhed] *n* 1) большая бочка; 2) мера жидкости (*около 238 л*).

hog-wash ['hɔgwɔʃ] *n* помои.

hoist I [hɔɪst] *n* 1) подъём, поднятие; 2) подъёмник, лифт; 3) лебёдка.

hoist II *v* поднимать (*флаг, паруса, груз*).

hoist-bridge ['hɔɪstbrɪdʒ] *n* подъёмный мост.

hoity-toity I ['hɔɪtɪ'tɔɪtɪ] *a* 1) обидчивый; 2) надменный; важничающий; 3) редк. резвый, игривый.

hoity-toity II *int* ирон. скажите пожалуйста!

hold¹ I [hould] *n* 1) захват, взятие; держание; владение; to catch (*или* to take) ~ of smth. ухватиться за что-л.; овладевать чем-л.; to leave ~ of, to relinquish one's ~ выпускать из рук; 2) власть; влияние; to get a firm ~ of прочно завладеть; 3) ушко, захват; 4) понимание, улавливание.

hold¹ II *v* (*past, p. p.* held) 1) держать(ся), удерживать(ся); 2) выдерживать; 3) вмещать; содержать, заключать в себе; 4) иметь; владеть; 5) иметь силу (*о законе и т. п.*); this rule will ~ in all cases это правило относится ко всем случаям; 6) сдерживать, останавливать; 7) считать, полагать; □ to ~ back а) удерживать(ся) (*от чего-л.— from*); б) воздерживаться (*from*); в) скрывать, утаивать; to ~ by придерживаться (*решения и т. п.*); слушаться (*совета*); to ~ down подавлять, подчинять; to ~ forth а) предлагать; б) разглагольствовать; to ~ in сдерживать(ся); to ~ off а) не подпускать (*близко*); б) задерживать, откладывать; to ~ on а) держаться (*крепко*) за что-л.; б) продолжать делать что-л., упорствовать; to ~ out а) протягивать (*руку*); б) подавать (*надежду*); в) выдержать, выстоять; to ~ over а) откладывать; б) оставлять в должности; to ~ up а) держаться за что-л.; б) придерживаться чего-л.; to ~ together объединяться; to ~ up а) выставлять (напоказ); б) поддерживать, подпирать; в) задерживать, останавливать; амер. разг. остановить силой и ограбить; to ~ with соглашаться; одобрять; ◇ hard! стой!

hold² *n* трюм.

holdall ['houldɔːl] *n* 1) вещевой мешок; сумка; 2) ящик для инструментов.

holdback ['houldbæk] *n* помеха, препятствие.

holder ['houldə] *n* 1) держатель, владелец; арендатор; 2) оправа; 3) ручка, рукоятка.

holdfast ['houldfɑːst] *n* 1) захват; in one's ~ в руках; to lose one's ~ выпустить из рук; 2) тех. скоба, крюк; анкерная плита; 3) столярные тиски.

holding ['houldɪŋ] *n* 1) участок земли (*особ. арендованный*); 2) владение (*ценными бумагами, акциями*); арендное владение; 3) удерживание, задерживание, закрепление.

hold-up ['houldʌp] *n* разг. 1) налёт, ограбление; 2) остановка, задержка (*в движении транспорта*).

hole I [houl] *n* 1) дыра, отверстие; 2) углубление, яма; скважина; 3) ямка, лунка для мяча; 4) пещера;. нора; 5) захолустье; «дыра»; 6) *разг.* затруднительное положение; in a ~ в затруднительном положении; ◊ to pick ~s in придираться; to make a ~ in опустошить (*запасы, сбережения и т. п.*).

hole II *v* 1) прорезать, пробивать отверстия; продырявить; 2) загонять шар в лунку; 3) зарываться, уходить в нору; 4) загнать (*зверя*) в нору.

hole-and-corner ['houlənd'kɔːnə] *a разг.* тайный, скрытый.

holer ['houlə] *n горн.* забойщик; бурильщик.

holey ['houlı] *a* дырявый.

holiday ['hɔlədı] *n* 1) праздник; день отдыха; нерабочий день; to make a ~ прекращать работу; 2) *pl* каникулы; 3) отпуск (*служащего*); on (a) ~ в отпуске; walking ~ отпуск, проведённый в турпоходе; 4) *attr* праздничный; каникулярный; ◊ blind man's ~ *шутл.* сумерки.

holidayer ['hɔlədeıə] *n* 1) отдыхающий, гуляющий; 2) отпускник.

holiday-maker ['hɔlədı,meıkə] *n* отдыхающий, гуляющий.

holiness ['houlınıs] *n* святость; His Holiness его святейшество (*титул папы*).

holland ['hɔlənd] *n* 1) холст, полотно; brown ~ небелёное суровое полотно; 2) *pl* голландская водка, джин.

Hollander ['hɔləndə] *n* голландец.

holler ['hɔlə] *v сленг* кричать.

hollo(a) I ['hɔlou] *n* крик, окрик.

hollo(a) II *v* 1) кричать; 2) звать собак.

hollo(a) III *int* эй!

hollow I ['hɔlou] *n* 1) впадина, углубление, выемка; 2) полость; пустота; 3) лощина; 4) дупло.

hollow II *a* 1) полый; пустой; пустотелый; 2) имеющий форму чаши, миски; глубокий (*о посуде*); 3) ввалившийся, впалый; 4) глухой (*о звуке, тоне*); 5) пустой, несерьёзный; неискренний; 6) голодный.

hollow III *v* 1) выдалбливать (*тж.* to ~ out); 2) подмывать (*берег*).

hollow IV *adv разг.* совершенно; здорово.

hollow-eyed ['hɔlouaıd] *a* с ввалившимися *или* глубоко сидящими глазами.

hollow-hearted ['hɔlou'hɑːtıd] *a* неискренний.

holly ['hɔlı] *n бот.* остролист.

hollyhock ['hɔlıhɔk] *n бот.* мальва.

holm[1] [houm] *n* 1) островок на реке, озере; 2) пойма.

holm[2] *n* каменный дуб.

holm-oak ['houm'ouk] *см.* holm[2].

holocaust ['hɔləkɔːst] *n* 1) (само)сожжение; 2) гибель, уничтожение; world ~ мировая бойня (*о первой мировой войне*).

holster ['houlstə] *n* кобура.

holt [hoult] *n поэт.* 1) роща; 2) лесистый холм.

holy ['houlı] *a* святой, священный.

holystone I ['houlıstoun] *n* песчаник (*для чистки палубы*); пемза.

holystone II *v* чистить, драить (*палубу*).

homage ['hɔmıdʒ] *n* 1) уважение, почтение; to do ~, to pay ~ оказывать внимание; свидетельствовать почтение; 2) *ист.* принесение феодальной присяги.

home I [houm] *n* 1) дом; at ~ дома; to feel at ~ быть как дома; make yourself at ~ будьте как дома; he is from ~ его нет дома; 2) родина; to fight for one's ~ сражаться за родину; 3) метрополия; 4) домашний очаг; семья, родные; have you news from ~? имеете ли вы вести от своих (*или* из дому)?; 5) приют; a ~ for the blind приют для слепых; ◊ to be at ~ (at, in, on, with) хорошо знать (*что-л.*); harvest ~ праздник урожая.

home II *a* 1) домашний; семейный; родной; 2) внутренний (*о торговле и т. п.*); отечественный (*о товарах и т. п.*); 3) обратный (*о поездке и т. п.*).

home III *v* 1) возвращаться домой (*особ. о почтовом голубе*); 2) предоставлять дом (*кому-л.*).

home IV *adv* 1) дома; домой; на родину; 2) в цель, в точку; to strike ~ попасть в точку, задеть за живое; 3) до отказа, до упора; до конца; до места, на место; to drive ~ а) забить до конца (*гвоздь*); б) доводить до успешного конца; в) убедить, втолковать; ◊ to bring ~ убедить, втолковать; to come ~ to доходить (*до кого-л.*), быть понятным; nothing to write ~ about *разг.* ничего особенного, ничего интересного.

homebody ['houm,bɔdı] *n* домосед, -ка; a regular ~ заядлый домосед.

home-bred ['houm'bred] *a* доморощенный; простой.

home-coming ['houm,kʌmıŋ] *n* возвращение домой.

home-felt ['houmfelt] *a* (глубоко) прочувствованный.

home-keeping ['houm,kiːpıŋ] *a* домоседливый.

homeless ['houmlıs] *a* бездомный, бесприютный.

homelike ['houmlaık] *a* домашний, привычный, уютный.

homeliness ['houmlınıs] *n* 1) домашний уют; привычная обстановка; 2) простота; примитивность; 3) невзрачность.

homely ['houmlı] *a* 1) домашний, уютный; 2) простой, повседневный; скромный; 3) некрасивый, невзрачный.

home-made ['houm'meıd] *a* домашнего производства; сделанный кустарным способом.

Home Rule ['houmruːl] *n ист.* гомруль (*буржуазно-националистическое движение в Ирландии*).

home-sick ['houmsık] *a* тоскующий по родине, по дому.

home-sickness ['houm,sıknıs] *n* тоска по родине, ностальгия.

homespun I ['houmspʌn] *n* домотканая материя.

homespun II *a* 1) домотканый; 2) доморощенный, простой.

homestead ['houmsted] *n* 1) дом с участком и службами; усадьба; ферма; 2) *амер.* участок поселенца.

home-thrust ['houm'θrʌst] *n* удáчный удáр, удáр, достигший цéли.

homeward I ['houmwəd] *a* ведущий, идущий к дóму, домóй.

homeward II *adv* к дóму, домóй.

homeward-bound ['houmwəd'baund] *a* возвращáющийся домóй, на рóдину (*о корáбле*).

homewards ['houmwədz] *см.* homeward II.

home-work ['houmwə:k] *n* 1) домáшняя рабóта (*особ. шкóльника*); 2) надóмная рабóта.

homicidal [,hɔmɪ'saɪdl] *a* убийственный; смертонóсный.

homicide ['hɔmɪsaɪd] *n* 1) убийца; 2) убийство.

homily ['hɔmɪlɪ] *n* прóповедь; поучéние.

homing I ['houmɪŋ] *n ав., косм.* (само-)наведéние.

homing II *a* возвращáющийся домóй; почтóвый (*о гóлубе*).

hominy ['hɔmɪnɪ] *n* мамалыга.

homoeopathy [,houmɪ'ɔpəθɪ] *n* гомеопáтия.

homogeneous [,hɔmə'dʒi:njəs] *a* однорóдный.

homograph ['hɔmougrɑːf] *n лингв.* омóграф.

homologous [hɔ'mɔləgəs] *a* соотвéтственный.

homonym ['hɔmənɪm] *n* 1) *лингв.* омóним; 2) тёзка.

homophone ['hɔməfoun] *n лингв.* омофóн.

homy ['houmɪ] *a* домáшний; напоминáющий роднóй дом.

hone I [houn] *n* точильный кáмень; оселóк.

hone II *v* точить.

honest ['ɔnɪst] *a* 1) чéстный; 2) правдивый; искренний; I shall be ~ with you я бýду с вáми откровéнен, я скажý вам прямо; 3) настоящий, нефальсифицированный.

honesty ['ɔnɪstɪ] *n* 1) чéстность; 2) правдивость, прямотá.

honey ['hʌnɪ] *n* 1) мёд; 2) слáдость; 3) *разг.* голýбчик, дýшенька.

honey-bee ['hʌnɪbiː] *n* (рабóчая) пчелá.

honeycomb I ['hʌnɪkoum] *n* 1) (медóвые) сóты; 2) *тех.* рáковина (*на отливке*).

honeycomb II *a* сóтовый; ячéистый, ноздревáтый.

honeycomb III *v* продырявить, изрешетить.

honey-dew ['hʌnɪdjuː] *n* 1) медвяная росá; 2) *поэт.* нектáр; 3) табáк, пропитанный патóкой.

honeyed ['hʌnɪd] *a* медóвый, слáдкий (*как мёд*); *перен.* льстивый.

honeymoon I ['hʌnɪmuːn] *n* медóвый мéсяц.

honeymoon II *v* проводить медóвый мéсяц (*in, at*).

honey-mouthed ['hʌnɪ,mauðd] *a* медоточивый, сладкоречивый.

honeysuckle ['hʌnɪ,sʌkl] *n бот.* жимолость.

honied ['hʌnɪd] *см.* honeyed.

honk I [hɔŋk] *n* 1) крик диких гусéй; 2) автомобильный гудóк.

honk II *v* 1) кричáть (*о диких гусях*); 2) сигнáлить, гудéть (*об автомобиле*).

honor I, II ['ɔnə] *амер. см.* honour I, II.

honorable ['ɔnərəbl] *амер. см.* honourable.

honorarium [,ɔnə'rɛərɪəm] *n* (*pl тж.* honoraria [,ɔnə'rɛərɪə]) гонорáр.

honorary ['ɔnərərɪ] *a* 1) почётный; 2) являющийся дéлом чéсти; 3) исполняющий обязанности без вознаграждéния.

honorific [,ɔnə'rɪfɪk] *a* выражáющий почтéние, почтительный.

honour I ['ɔnə] *n* 1) честь; слáва; in ~ в честь; (up)on my (word of) ~ чéстное слóво; 2) почёт, уважéние; to give (*или* to pay, to do) ~ окáзывать уважéние, свидéтельствовать почтéние; 3) хорóшая репутáция; дóброе имя; 4) благорóдство; 5) *pl* пóчести; нагрáды; military ~s вóинские пóчести; 6) *pl унив.* отличие; 7) (H.): Your Honour! вáша честь!, вáша милость!; ◊ ~s of war почётные услóвия сдáчи; to be an ~ to one's school (family) дéлать честь своéй шкóле (семьé); to do the ~s of the house принимáть, занимáть гостéй.

honour II *v* 1) уважáть, почитáть, чтить; 2) удостáивать (*чего-л.— with*); 3) платить в срок (*по вéкселю*).

honourable ['ɔnərəbl] *a* 1) благорóдный; 2) чéстный; 3) уважáемый, почтéнный; 4) почётный.

hood I [hud] *n* 1) капюшóн; кáпор; 2) колпáк; крышка, чехóл; 3) верх экипáжа; верх кýзова (*автомобиля*); 4) *тех.* капóт (*двигателя*).

hood II *v* 1) покрывáть капюшóном, колпакóм и т. п.; 2) закрывáть, прятать.

hoodie ['hudɪ] *n* сéрая ворóна.

hoodlum ['huːdləm] *n амер. разг.* хулигáн.

hoodoo I ['huːduː] *n амер.* 1) кто-л., что-л., приносящие несчáстье; 2) несчáстье, бедá.

hoodoo II *v амер.* приносить несчáстье; сглáзить.

hoodwink ['hudwɪŋk] *v* 1) завязывать глазá; 2) обмáнывать.

hoof I [huːf] *n* (*pl тж.* hooves) 1) копыто; on the ~ живóй, живьём (*о скоте*); cloven ~ раздвóенное копыто; 2) *шутл.* ногá (*человéка*); ◊ to show the cloven ~ проявлять дурнóй харáктер.

hoof II *v* 1) бить копытом; 2) *разг.* выгнать, уволить (*тж.* to ~ out); 3) идти пешкóм.

hoofed [huːft] *a* копытный (*о живóтном*).

hook I [huk] *n* 1) крюк; крючóк; ~ and eye крючóк (*застёжка*); 2) багóр; 3) серп; pruning ~ садóвый нож; 4) крутóй изгиб; излучина; 5) ловýшка, западня; примáнка; 6) *сленг* жýлик, вор; ◊ by ~ or by crook так или инáче, во что бы то ни стáло; ~ не мáльчик, так кáтаньем; to drop (*или* to pop) off the ~s *сленг* сыгрáть в ящик, отпрáвиться на тот свет; to go off the ~s *разг.* а) рехнýться, свихнýться; б) умерéть; off the ~s а) расстрóенный; б) сбившийся с пути; on one's own ~ по сóбственному почину; на свою отвéтственность; with a ~ at the end с (мысленной) оговóркой.

hook II *v* 1) зацеплять (*крюкóм*); надевáть, навéшивать (*на крюк*); 2) застёгивать(ся) (*о крючкáх*); 3) ловить (*рыбу*); *перен.* поймáть на ýдочку, подцепить; 4) *сленг* красть; 5): to ~ it *сленг* удрáть, смыться; □ to ~ in заполучить; to ~ out выведать.

hookah ['hukə] *n* кальян.

hooked [hukt] *a* 1) крючковáтый; кривóй; 2) имéющий крючóк *или* крючки; 3) *амер.* (с)вязанный крючкóм.

hooker ['hukə] *n* рыболóвное сýдно.

hook-nosed ['huk'nouzd] *a* с крючковáтым *или* орлиным нóсом.

hook-up ['hukʌp] *n* 1) сцепле́ние, соедине́ние; 2) *радио разг.* одновре́менная переда́ча одно́й програ́ммы по не́скольким ста́нциям.

hook-worm ['hukwə:m] *n* глист.

hooky ['hukı] *n*: to play ~ *амер. сленг* безде́льничать, прогу́ливать (*занятия в школе*).

hooligan ['hu:lıgən] *n* хулига́н.

hoop¹ I [hu:p] *n* 1) о́бруч; о́бод; to trundle a ~ ката́ть о́бруч (*детский*); 2) воро́та (*в крокете*).

hoop¹ II *v* набива́ть о́бручи; скрепля́ть обруча́ми.

hoop² I *n* 1) крик, ги́канье; 2) ка́шель (*как при коклюше*).

hoop² II *v* ги́кать.

hooper ['hu:pə] *n* бо́ндарь, боча́р.

hooping-cough ['hu:pıŋkɔf] *n* коклю́ш.

hoopoe ['hu:pu:] *n* удо́д (*птица*).

hoop-skirt ['hu:pskə:t] *n* кринoли́н, фи́жмы.

hoot I [hu:t] *n* 1) крик совы́; 2) кри́ки, улюлю́канье; 3) звук гудка́, рожка́ *и т. п.*; ◊ I don't care (*или* give) a ~ *разг.* мне на э́то наплева́ть.

hoot II *v* 1) крича́ть (*о сове*); 2) гуде́ть, свисте́ть (*о гудке, сирене*); 3) крича́ть (*на кого-л.— at*); улюлю́кать; to ~ with laughter хохота́ть во всё го́рло; □ to ~ **after** гна́ться за кем-л. с кри́ками, пресле́довать кого́-л.; to ~ **away**, to ~ **off**, to ~ **out** вы́гнать кри́ками.

hooter ['hu:tə] *n* гудо́к, сире́на.

hooves [hu:vz] *pl см.* hoof I.

hop¹ I [hɔp] *n* хмель (*растение*).

hop¹ II *v* собира́ть хмель.

hop² I *n* 1) прыжо́к, скачо́к; пры́ганье; 2) *разг.* та́нец, та́нцы; 3) *ав. разг.* полёт на коро́ткое расстоя́ние.

hop² II *v* 1) пры́гать, скака́ть на одно́й ноге́, подпры́гивать; 2) перепры́гивать (*over*); 3) *разг.* танцева́ть, пляса́ть; □ to ~ **off** *ав.* взлета́ть, отрыва́ться от земли́; ◊ ~ it! *разг.* убира́йся!

hope I [houp] *n* наде́жда; forlorn ~ безнадёжное де́ло; to be past (*или* beyond) ~ быть в безнадёжном положе́нии; in vain ~ тще́тно; to resign all ~ оста́вить вся́кую наде́жду; to elevate ~s возбужда́ть наде́жды; to pin one's ~s on возлага́ть наде́жды на кого́-л.

hope II *v* 1) наде́яться; I ~ so наде́юсь, что э́то так; I ~ not наде́юсь, что э́того не бу́дет; to ~ against hope наде́яться, не име́я для э́того основа́ний; 2) ожида́ть, предвкуша́ть (*обыкн.* to ~ for).

hoped-for ['houptfɔ:] *a* стра́стно ожида́емый; жела́нный; long ~ долгожда́нный.

hopeful I ['houpful] *n* челове́к, подаю́щий наде́жды.

hopeful II *a* 1) по́лный наде́жд, надеющийся; 2) подаю́щий больши́е наде́жды, многообеща́ющий.

hopefulness ['houpfulnıs] *n* оптими́зм.

hopeless ['houplıs] *a* 1) потеря́вший наде́жду, отча́явшийся; 2) безнадёжный, безвы́ходный.

hopelessness ['houplısnıs] *n* безнадёжность.

hop-o'-my-thumb ['hɔpəmı'θʌm] *n* ка́рлик; ма́льчик с па́льчик.

hopper¹ ['hɔpə] *n* собира́тель хме́ля.

hopper² *n* 1) прыгу́н; 2) пры́гающее насеко́мое;

3) *тех.* засыпна́я воро́нка; 4) ваго́н с опроки́дывающимся ку́зовом.

hopscotch ['hɔpskɔtʃ] *n* «кла́ссы» (*детская игра*).

hoptoad ['hɔptoud] *n амер.* жа́ба.

horde I [hɔ:d] *n* 1) орда́; 2) ша́йка, вата́га; 3) *обыкн. pl амер.* мно́жество; толпа́ (*народа*); 4) ста́я; рой.

horde II *v* собира́ться то́лпами.

horizon [hə'raızn] *n* 1) горизо́нт; 2) (у́мственный) кругозо́р.

horizontal I [,hɔrı'zɔntl] *n* горизонта́ль.

horizontal II *a* горизонта́льный.

hormone ['hɔ:moun] *n физиол.* гормо́н.

horn I [hɔ:n] *n* 1) рог; 2) *pl* ро́жки (*улитки*); у́сики (*насекомого*); 3) рожо́к (*муз. инструмент*); гудо́к; охо́тничий рог; to wind a ~ игра́ть на рожке́; 4) ру́пор; 5) *тех.* вы́ступ, шип; рыча́г; 6) *attr* рогово́й; ◊ ~ of plenty рог изоби́лия; on the ~s of a dilemma в затрудни́тельном положе́нии; to draw (*или* to pull) in one's ~s съёжиться, присми́реть; to show (*или* to put out, to thrust forth) the ~s приня́ть оборони́тельное положе́ние; to raise the ~s горди́ться.

horn II *v* забода́ть; ◊ to ~ in *разг.* вме́шиваться.

hornbeam ['hɔ:nbi:m] *n* граб (*дерево*).

horned [hɔ:nd] *a* рога́тый.

hornet ['hɔ:nıt] *n зоол.* ше́ршень.

hornpipe ['hɔ:npaıp] *n* 1) волы́нка (*муз. инструмент*); 2) матро́сский та́нец.

horn-rimmed ['hɔ:n,rımd] *a* в рогово́й опра́ве.

horny ['hɔ:nı] *a* 1) рогово́й; 2) име́ющий рог(а́); 3) мозо́листый.

horny-handed ['hɔ:nı'hændıd] *a* с мозо́листыми рука́ми.

horrible ['hɔrəbl] *a* 1) стра́шный, ужа́сный; 2) проти́вный, отврати́тельный.

horrid ['hɔrıd] *a* 1) ужа́сный; стра́шный; 2) *разг.* о́чень неприя́тный, проти́вный.

horrific [hɔ'rıfık] *a* ужаса́ющий.

horrify ['hɔrıfaı] *v* 1) ужаса́ть; пуга́ть, страши́ть; 2) шоки́ровать.

horror ['hɔrə] *n* 1) у́жас; си́льный страх; 2) отвраще́ние (*к чему-л.— of*); ◊ the ~s припа́док бе́лой горя́чки.

horror-stricken ['hɔrə,strıkən] *a* поражённый у́жасом, в у́жасе.

horror-struck ['hɔrə,strʌk] *см.* horror-stricken.

hors-d'oeuvre [ɔ:'də:vr] *n* заку́ска.

horse I [hɔ:s] *n* 1) ло́шадь, конь; a half-bred ~ ло́шадь-полукро́вка; riding (draught) ~ верхова́я (ломова́я) ло́шадь; to take ~ сесть на ло́шадь; е́хать на ло́шади; to ride a ~ to death загна́ть ло́шадь; to ~! по ко́ням!, сади́сь!; iron ~ парово́з; танк; 2) *собир.* ко́нница, кавале́рия; ~ and foot ко́нница и пехо́та; light ~ лёгкая кавале́рия; 3) конь (*гимнастический*); 4) ра́ма, стано́к, подста́вка; 5) *attr* ко́нный; ко́нский; *перен.* гру́бый, живо́тный; ◊ to be on (*или* to mount, to ride) the high ~ ва́жничать; to flog a dead ~ занима́ться бесполе́зным де́лом; white ~s бара́шки (*на море*); dark ~ «тёмная лоша́дка»; a ~ of another colour совсе́м друго́е де́ло; don't look a gift ~ in the mouth дарёному коню́ в зу́бы не смо́трят.

horse II *v* 1) сесть, вскочи́ть на ло́шадь; е́хать верхо́м; 2) взвали́ть *или* посади́ть на ло́шадь; 3) поставля́ть лошаде́й.

horseback I ['hɔːsbæk] *n*: on ~ верхо́м.

horseback II *adv* амер. верхо́м (*на лошади*).

horseborne ['hɔːsbɔːn] *a* вью́чный.

horse-box ['hɔːsbɔks] *n* ваго́н для лошаде́й.

horse-breeding ['hɔːs'briːdɪŋ] *n* 1) конево́дство; 2) *attr* конево́дческий.

horse-chestnut ['hɔːs'tʃesnʌt] *n* ко́нский кашта́н.

horse-cloth ['hɔːsklɔθ] *n* попо́на.

horse-collar ['hɔːs'kɔlə] *n* хому́т.

horse-comb ['hɔːskoum] *n* скребни́ца.

horse-coper ['hɔːs,koupə] *см.* horse-dealer.

horse-cover ['hɔːs,kʌvə] *см.* horse-cloth.

horse-dealer ['hɔːs,diːlə] *n* бары́шник.

horse-drawn ['hɔːsdrɔːn] *a* на ко́нной тя́ге.

horseflesh ['hɔːsfleʃ] *n* 1) кони́на; 2) *собир.* ко́нский соста́в.

horse-fly ['hɔːsflaɪ] *n* слепе́нь.

horse-hair ['hɔːshɛə] *n* 1) ко́нский во́лос; 2) *attr* из ко́нского во́лоса.

horse-laugh ['hɔːslɑːf] *n* гру́бый, гро́мкий смех.

horseless ['hɔːslɪs] *a* безлоша́дный.

horseman ['hɔːsmən] *n* вса́дник; нае́здник; кавалери́ст.

horsemanship ['hɔːsmənʃɪp] *n* иску́сство верхово́й езды́.

horse-marines ['hɔːsmə,riːnz] *n pl*: tell that to the ~! *разг.* вздор!; расска́зывай(те) э́то кому́-нибудь друго́му!; ври бо́льше!

horseplay ['hɔːspleɪ] *n* шу́мная игра́, гру́бое развлече́ние.

horsepower ['hɔːs,pauə] *n тех.* 1) лошади́ная си́ла; мо́щность; indicated ~ индика́торная (номина́льная) мо́щность; 2) ко́нный приво́д.

horse-race ['hɔːsreɪs] *n* ска́чки.

horse-radish ['hɔːs,rædɪʃ] *n* хрен.

horse-sense ['hɔːssens] *n разг.* грубова́тый здра́вый смысл.

horseshoe ['hɔːʃuː] *n* подко́ва.

horseshoer ['hɔːʃuə] *n* ко́вочный кузне́ц.

horsewhip I ['hɔːswɪp] *n* хлыст.

horsewhip II *v* хлеста́ть.

horsewoman ['hɔːs,wumən] *n* вса́дница; нае́здница.

horsy ['hɔːsɪ] *a* 1) ко́нский, лошади́ный; 2) увлека́ющийся лошадьми́, ко́нным спо́ртом.

horticulture ['hɔːtɪkʌltʃə] *n* садово́дство.

hose I [houz] *n* 1) шланг, рука́в, кишка́ (*для поливки*); 2) *собир.* чулки́.

hose II *v* полива́ть из шла́нга, из кишки́.

hosier ['houʒə] *n* торго́вец трикота́жем.

hosiery ['houʒərɪ] *n собир.* чуло́чные изде́лия, трикота́ж.

hospice ['hɔspɪs] *n* 1) гости́ница (*особ. монастырская*); 2) бога́дельня, прию́т.

hospitable ['hɔspɪtəbl] *a* гостеприи́мный.

hospital ['hɔspɪtl] *n* 1) го́спиталь, больни́ца; field ~ полево́й го́спиталь; to walk the ~s проходи́ть пра́ктику в больни́це (*о студенте*); lying-in ~ роди́льный дом; 2) *attr* госпита́льный; санита́рный.

hospitality [,hɔspɪ'tælɪtɪ] *n* гостеприи́мство, раду́шие.

hospitalize ['hɔspɪtəlaɪz] *v* госпитализи́ровать, помеща́ть в больни́цу.

host[1] [houst] *n* 1) мно́жество; толпа́; 2) *уст.* по́лчище, во́йско; ◇ the ~s of heaven, the heavenly ~s а) небе́сные свети́ла; б) а́нгелы, си́лы небе́сные; а ~ in himself оди́н сто́ит мно́гих.

host[2] *n* 1) хозя́ин; 2) хозя́ин гости́ницы; ◇ to reckon without one's ~ просчита́ться.

hostage ['hɔstɪdʒ] *n* 1) зало́жник; 2) зало́г.

hostel ['hɔstəl] *n* общежи́тие.

hostess ['houstɪs] *n* хозя́йка.

hostile I ['hɔstaɪl] *n* враг.

hostile II *a* 1) вра́жеский, неприя́тельский; 2) вражде́бный.

hostility [hɔs'tɪlɪtɪ] *n* 1) вражде́бность; 2) состоя́ние войны́; 3) *pl* вое́нные де́йствия; to open hostilities нача́ть вое́нные де́йствия.

hostler ['ɔslə] *n* ко́нюх (*на постоялом дворе*).

hot I [hɔt] *a* 1) горя́чий; жа́ркий; I am ~ мне жа́рко; he goes ~ and cold его́ броса́ет то в жар, то в хо́лод; 2) разгорячённый; раздражённый, возбуждённый; to get ~ разгорячи́ться, разволнова́ться; 3) пы́лкий, увлека́ющийся (*чем-л. — on*); 4) о́стрый, пря́ный; 5) све́жий (*о новостях и т. п.*).

hot II *adv* 1) горячо́, жа́рко; 2) возбуждённо, раздражённо; 3) пы́лко; ◇ to give it smb. ~ *разг.* зада́ть пе́рцу; to get it ~ получи́ть хоро́ший нагоня́й.

hotbed ['hɔtbed] *n* 1) парни́к; 2) расса́дник, оча́г (*болезни и т. п.; of*).

hot-blooded ['hɔt'blʌdɪd] *a* пы́лкий, стра́стный.

hot-brained ['hɔt,breɪnd] *см.* hot-headed.

hotchpot ['hɔtʃpɔt] *см.* hotchpotch.

hotchpotch ['hɔtʃpɔtʃ] *n* 1) рагу́ из овоще́й с мя́сом; 2) вся́кая вся́чина, винегре́т.

hotel [hou'tel] *n* оте́ль, гости́ница, to put up at a ~ останови́ться в гости́нице.

hotfoot I ['hɔtfut] *v разг.* нести́сь, мча́ться.

hotfoot II *adv разг.* бы́стро; поспе́шно; to chase ~ пресле́довать по пята́м; to come down ~ примча́ться.

hothead ['hɔthed] *n* горя́чая голова́ (*о человеке*).

hot-headed ['hɔt'hedɪd] *a* горя́чий, вспы́льчивый; опроме́тчивый.

hothouse ['hɔthaus] *n* тепли́ца, оранжере́я.

hot-pot ['hɔtpɔt] *n* тушёное мя́со с карто́фелем.

hotspur ['hɔtspə] *n* горя́чий, вспы́льчивый челове́к.

Hottentot ['hɔtntɔt] *n* готтенто́т.

hough I [hɔk] *n* поджи́лки, коле́нное сухожи́лие (*животного*).

hough II *v* подреза́ть поджи́лки.

hound I [haund] *n* 1) охо́тничья соба́ка; the ~s сво́ра го́нчих; to follow the ~s, to ride to ~s охо́титься с го́нчими; 2) негодя́й, соба́ка.

hound II *v* охо́титься с го́нчими, трави́ть соба́ками; *перен.* натра́вливать, нау́ськивать; выжива́ть кого́-л.; to ~ to death сжить со све́та; □ to ~ on подстрека́ть.

hour ['auə] *n* 1) час; вре́мя; business ~s, office ~s часы́ рабо́ты (*учреждений, магазинов и т. п.*); labour ~s рабо́чее вре́мя; breakfast ~ вре́мя за́втрака; dinner ~ обе́денное вре́мя;

consulting ~s приёмные часы́ (у врача́); the off ~s свобо́дные часы́; ~s of market часы́ торго́вли; at a good ~ во́время, кста́ти; by the ~ по часа́м (рабо́тать и т. п.); in a good (evil) ~ в до́брый (недо́брый) час; 2): to keep early (или good) ~s встава́ть или ложи́ться ра́но; to keep late (или bad) ~s встава́ть или ложи́ться по́здно; the small ~s вре́мя по́сле полу́ночи; dead ~s глухи́е ночны́е часы́; rush ~s часы́-пик; ◊ at the eleventh ~ в после́дний моме́нт.

hour-circle ['auə'sə:kl] *n* меридиа́н.

hour-glass ['auəglɑːs] *n* песо́чные часы́.

hour-hand ['auəhænd] *n* часова́я стре́лка.

houri ['huərɪ] *n* гу́рия; краса́вица.

hourly I ['auəlɪ] *a* 1) (по)часово́й; ежеча́сный; 2) (о́чень) ча́стый; непреста́нный.

hourly II *adv* ежеча́сно; ча́сто; непреста́нно.

house I [haus] *n* 1) дом; зда́ние; жили́ще; a detached ~ особня́к; apartment ~ многокварти́рный дом; poultry ~ пти́чник; 2) дом, семья́, хозя́йство; ~ and home дом, дома́шний ую́т; to keep ~ вести́ хозя́йство; to keep the ~ (постоя́нно) сиде́ть до́ма, не выходи́ть; to keep open ~ жить откры́тым до́мом, принима́ть большо́е о́бщество; 3) дом, дина́стия, род; 4) (*тж.* the H.) пала́та (парла́мента); the Upper House ве́рхняя пала́та; of two ~s двухпала́тный; the House of Commons пала́та о́бщин (в А́нглии); the House of Lords пала́та ло́рдов (в А́нглии); the House of Representatives пала́та представи́телей (в США); to be in the ~ заседа́ть в парла́менте; to make a House обеспе́чить кво́рум (в пала́те о́бщин); 5) торго́вая фи́рма; publishing ~ изда́тельство; 6) теа́тр; аудито́рия; пу́блика; settlement ~ *амер.* конце́ртный зал, ме́стный теа́тр (в поселе́нии); a full ~ по́лный сбор; to bring down the ~ вы́звать гром аплодисме́нтов; 7) представле́ние; сеа́нс в кино́; 8) оте́ль, гости́ница (*тж.* ~ of entertainment); a half-way ~ а) придоро́жная гости́ница; б) компроми́сс; 9) бар; a public ~ тракти́р; barrel ~ *амер.* пивна́я; ви́нный погребо́к; 10) (the H.) *разг.* (ло́ндонская) би́ржа; 11) (the H.) *разг.* рабо́тный дом; 12) *attr* дома́шний; ◊ the narrow ~ моги́ла; like a ~ on fire легко́ и бы́стро; a ~ of ill fame публи́чный дом.

house II *v* 1) предоставля́ть жили́ще, поселя́ть; помеща́ть, размеща́ть; 2) поселя́ться, жить в до́ме; помеща́ться, размеща́ться.

houseboat ['hausbout] *n* ло́дка, приспосо́бленная для жилья́.

housebreaker ['haus,breɪkə] *n* 1) взло́мщик, граби́тель; 2) рабо́чий по сно́су домо́в.

houseful ['hausful] *n* по́лный дом.

household I ['haushould] *n* 1) семья́, домоча́дцы, дома́шние; 2) дома́шнее хозя́йство.

household II *a* дома́шний, семе́йный.

householder ['haushouldə] *n* 1) съёмщик кварти́ры; 2) глава́ семьи́.

housekeeper ['haus,kiːpə] *n* эконо́мка, домоправи́тельница.

housekeeping ['haus,kiːpɪŋ] *n* дома́шнее хозя́йство; домово́дство.

houseless ['hauslɪs] *a* бездо́мный.

housemaid ['hausmeɪd] *n* го́рничная.

housemaster ['haus,mɑːstə] *n* заве́дующий пансио́ном при шко́ле.

housemates ['hausmeɪts] *n pl* жильцы́.

house-physician ['hausfɪ,zɪʃən] *n* врач, живу́щий при больни́це.

house-top ['haustɔp] *n* кры́ша; to cry (или to proclaim) from the ~s провозглаша́ть во всеуслы́шание.

house-warming ['haus,wɔːmɪŋ] *n* пра́зднование новосе́лья.

housewife[a] ['hauswaif] *n* хозя́йка до́ма, дома́шняя хозя́йка.

housewife[b] ['hʌzɪf] *n* рабо́чая шкату́лка (с принадле́жностями для шитья́).

housewifely ['hauswaiflɪ] *a* дома́шний; хозя́йственный; домови́тый.

housework ['hauswəːk] *n* дома́шняя рабо́та.

housing[1] ['hauzɪŋ] *n* 1) снабже́ние, обеспе́чение жили́щем; 2) убе́жище, прию́т; 3) *собир.* дома́, жили́щный фонд; жили́щное строи́тельство; 4) *тех.* кожу́х, футля́р, коро́бка; 5) ни́ша, вы́емка.

housing[2] *n* попо́на.

hove [houv] *past, p. p. см.* heave II.

hovel ['hɔvəl] *n* 1) лачу́га, хиба́рка; 2) наве́с.

hover ['hɔvə] *v* 1) пари́ть (о пти́це; *тж.* to ~ over); порха́ть (о ба́бочке); верт́еться, суети́ться (вокру́г, о́коло — about, around); 3) быть в нереши́тельности, колеба́ться.

how [hau] *adv* 1) как?, каки́м о́бразом?; ~ can it be done? как э́то мо́жно сде́лать?; ~ did it happen? как э́то случи́лось?; ~ so? как так?; 2) (на)ско́лько; ~ far is it? далеко́ ли э́то?; 3) как, что; tell him ~ to do it скажи́те ему́, как э́то сде́лать; 4) как (при восклица́нии); ~ far it is! как э́то далеко́!; ~ absurd! кака́я чепуха́!; ~ kind of you! как э́то ми́ло с ва́шей стороны́!; 5) почему́?; ~ is it you don't want to go? почему́ вы не хоти́те идти́?; ◊ ~ are you? как пожива́ете?; ~ do you do? здра́вствуйте!; ~ now? что э́то зна́чит?; and ~! *амер. разг.* ещё как!, ещё бы!, о́чень да́же!

how-d'ye-do ['haudɪ'duː] *n разг.* затрудни́тельное или щекотли́вое положе́ние; here's a nice ~! хоро́шенькая исто́рия!, вот тебе́ и на!

however I [hau'evə] *adv* как бы ни; ско́лько бы ни.

however II *conj* тем не ме́нее, несмотря́ на.

howitzer ['hauɪtsə] *n* га́убица.

howl I [haul] *n* 1) вой, завыва́ние; 2) стон, крик; 3) *радио* свист.

howl II *v* 1) выть, завыва́ть; 2) гро́мко стона́ть, крича́ть (от бо́ли); □ to ~ **down** заглуша́ть (во́ем, кри́ком).

howler ['haulə] *n* 1) пла́кальщик; 2) *разг.* грубе́йшая оши́бка; 3) реву́н (обезья́на); 4) *тех.* реву́н; ◊ to come a ~ попа́сть в беду́.

howling ['haulɪŋ] *a* 1) во́ющий; 2) мра́чный, уны́лый; 3) *сленг* ужа́сный; вопию́щий.

howsoever ['hausou'evə] *adv* как бы ни.

hoy[1] [hɔɪ] *n* небольшо́е берегово́е су́дно.

hoy[2] *int* эй!

hoyden ['hɔɪdn] *n* сорване́ц (о де́вочке).

hub[1] [hʌb] *n* 1) сту́пица колеса́; вту́лка; 2) центр (внима́ния, интере́сов и т. п.); ~ of the universe центр мирозда́ния, пуп земли́.

hub[2] *n см.* hubby.

hubbub ['hʌbʌb] *n* шум, гам, гул голосо́в.

hubby ['hʌbɪ] *n разг.* муженёк.

huckleberry [ˈhʌklbèrɪ] *n* черни́ка; red ~ брус-ни́ка.

huckster I [ˈhʌkstə] *n* 1) у́личный *или* мелочно́й торго́вец; 2) бары́шник; торга́ш.

huckster II *v* 1) занима́ться мелочно́й торго́влей; 2) торгова́ться.

huddle I [ˈhʌdl] *n* 1) гру́да, ку́ча; 2) толпа́; 3) беспоря́док, сумато́ха; 4) *амер. разг.* та́йное совеща́ние.

huddle II *v* 1) толпи́ться, тесни́ться (*тж.* to ~ together); вали́ть толпо́й; 2) сва́ливать в беспоря́дке, укла́дывать ко́е-ка́к; 3) де́лать что-л. на ско́рую ру́ку, ко́е-ка́к; 4) сверну́ться «кала́чиком», съёжиться (*тж.* to ~ up); to ~ oneself up in a corner заби́ться в у́гол; 5) набра́сывать, наки́дывать на себя́ (*оде́жду; on*).

hue¹ [hjuː] *n* цвет, оттéнок.

hue² *n*: ~ and cry кри́ки «карау́л!», «держи́!»; пого́ня (*за кем-л.*); to raise a ~ and cry подня́ть трево́гу.

huff I [hʌf] *n* вспы́шка гне́ва, раздраже́ния; to get into a ~ раздража́ться.

huff II *v* 1) задира́ть; серди́ть, раздража́ть; 2) подстрека́ть, принужда́ть (*угро́зами*); 3) обижа́ть(ся); оскорбля́ть(ся).

huffy [ˈhʌfɪ] *a* 1) оби́женный; 2) оби́дчивый; раздражи́тельный.

hug I [hʌg] *n* 1) кре́пкое объя́тие; to give a ~ обня́ть; 2) сжа́тие, хва́тка.

hug II *v* 1) кре́пко обнима́ть, сжима́ть в объя́тиях; 2) держа́ться (*бе́рега и т. п.*); 3) ав.: to ~ the ground лете́ть бре́ющим полётом; ◊ to ~ oneself on (*или* for) smth. быть дово́льным, поздравля́ть себя́ с чем-л.

huge [hjuːdʒ] *a* огро́мный, грома́дный, гига́нтский.

hugely [ˈhjuːdʒlɪ] *adv* о́чень; чрезвыча́йно.

hugger-mugger I [ˈhʌgəˌmʌgə] *n* 1) та́йна, секре́т; in ~ тайко́м, укра́дкой; 2) беспоря́док.

hugger-mugger II *a* 1) та́йный; 2) беспоря́дочный.

hugger-mugger III *v* 1) де́лать тайко́м, скрыва́ть; 2) зама́лчивать, замя́ть (*де́ло*); 3) де́лать беспоря́дочно, ко́е-ка́к.

hugger-mugger IV *adv* 1) та́йно, укра́дкой; 2) беспоря́дочно; ко́е-ка́к.

huguenot [ˈhjuːgənɔt] *n ист.* гугено́т.

hulk [hʌlk] *n* 1) неповоро́тливое су́дно; 2) ко́рпус ста́рого *или* него́дного корабля́; 3) неуклю́жий челове́к; 4) что-л. громо́здкое, нескла́дное.

hulking [ˈhʌlkɪŋ] *a* громо́здкий, неуклю́жий.

hull¹ I [hʌl] *n* шелуха́, скорлупа́, ко́жа.

hull¹ II *v* очища́ть от шелухи́, лущи́ть.

hull² I *n* 1) ко́рпус (*корабля́, та́нка*); 2) ав. фюзеля́ж.

hull² II *v* проби́ть снаря́дом ко́рпус корабля́.

hullabaloo [ˌhʌləbəˈluː] *n* шум, гам, кри́ки.

hulled [hʌld] *a* лущёный, очи́щенный.

hullo [ˈhʌˈlou] *int* алло́!

hum¹ I [hʌm] *n* жужжа́ние, гуде́ние; глухо́й шум, гул.

hum¹ II *v* 1) жужжа́ть, гуде́ть; 2) напева́ть; мурлы́кать; 3) говори́ть запина́ясь; to ~ and haw мя́млить, тяну́ть; 4) *разг.* проявля́ть акти́вность, оживле́ние.

hum² *int* гм!

hum³ *n см.* humbug I.

human I [ˈhjuːmən] *a* челове́ческий; людско́й; сво́йственный челове́ку.

human II *n* челове́к, сме́ртный.

humane [hjuːˈmeɪn] *a* 1) гума́нный, челове́чный; 2) гуманита́рный (*о нау́ке*); изя́щный (*о слове́сности*).

humanism [ˈhjuːmənɪzəm] *n* 1) гумани́зм; 2) гума́нность.

humanitarian I [hjuːˌmænɪˈtɛrɪən] *n* 1) гумани́ст; 2) филантро́п.

humanitarian II *a* гума́нный, человеколюби́вый.

humanity [hjuːˈmænɪtɪ] *n* 1) челове́чество, челове́ческий род; 2) челове́ческая приро́да; 3) гума́нность, человеколю́бие; доброта́; 4) *pl* (the humanities) гуманита́рные нау́ки.

humanize [ˈhjuːmənaɪz] *v* 1) де́лать (бо́лее) челове́чным; очелове́чивать; 2) станови́ться гума́нным; 3) смягча́ть, де́лать нежне́е (*о то́не*).

humankind [ˈhjuːmənˈkaɪnd] *n* челове́чество, челове́ческий род.

humanly [ˈhjuːmənlɪ] *adv* по-челове́чески; человеколюби́во.

humble I [ˈhʌmbl] *a* 1) скро́мный; 2) просто́й; бе́дный; 3) поко́рный, смире́нный.

humble II *v* 1) унижа́ть; 2) смиря́ть.

humble-bee [ˈhʌmblbiː] *n* шмель.

humbug I [ˈhʌmbʌg] *n* 1) обма́н; притво́рство; 2) обма́нщик; лицеме́р; 3) вздор, бессмы́слица.

humbug II *v* обма́нывать; обма́ном вовлека́ть (*into*); выма́нивать (*out of*).

humbug III *int* чепуха́!, ерунда́!

humdrum I [ˈhʌmdrʌm] *n* 1) однообра́зие, ску́ка; 2) бана́льность, о́бщее ме́сто; 3) ску́чный челове́к.

humdrum II *a* 1) ску́чный, однообра́зный; 2) заура́дный; 3) бана́льный.

humdrum III *v* говори́ть ску́чно, бана́льно.

humid [ˈhjuːmɪd] *a* сыро́й; вла́жный.

humidify [hjuːˈmɪdɪfaɪ] *v* увлажня́ть.

humidity [hjuːˈmɪdɪtɪ] *n* сы́рость; вла́жность.

humiliate [hjuːˈmɪlieɪt] *v* унижа́ть; оскорбля́ть.

humiliation [hjuːˌmɪlɪˈeɪʃən] *v* униже́ние; оскорбле́ние.

humility [hjuːˈmɪlɪtɪ] *n* 1) скро́мность; 2) смире́ние, поко́рность; кро́тость.

humming-bird [ˈhʌmɪŋbəːd] *n* коли́бри.

humming-top [ˈhʌmɪŋtɔp] *n* волчо́к, юла́.

hummock [ˈhʌmək] *n* 1) хо́лмик; буго́р; 2) (ледяно́й) то́рос.

humor I, II [ˈhjuːmə] *амер. см.* humour I, II.

humorist [ˈhjuːmərɪst] *n* юмори́ст.

humorous [ˈhjuːmərəs] *a* 1) юмористи́ческий; 2) смешно́й, заба́вный.

humour I [ˈhjuːmə] *n* 1) ю́мор; шутли́вость; чу́вство ю́мора; dry ~ мане́ра говори́ть смешны́е ве́щи невозмути́мо споко́йным то́ном; 2) настрое́ние; нрав, хара́ктер; скло́нность, расположе́ние (*к чему́-л. — for*); in good (bad, ill) ~ в хоро́шем (дурно́м) настрое́нии; out of ~ не в ду́хе, недово́льный; серди́тый.

humour II *v* 1) потака́ть кому́-л.; балова́ть; 2) приноравли́ваться, быть усту́пчивым.

humoursome [ˈhjuːməsəm] *a* 1) капри́зный;

своенра́вный; 2) раздражи́тельный, брюзгли́вый.

hump I [hʌmp] *n* 1) горб; 2) буго́р(о́к); 3) *разг.* дурно́е, мра́чное настрое́ние; хандра́; to give smb. the ~ нагоня́ть тоску́ на кого́-л.

hump II *v* 1) го́рбиться; 2) приводи́ть *или* приходи́ть в дурно́е настрое́ние.

humpback ['hʌmpbæk] *n* 1) горб; 2) горбу́н, горбу́нья.

hump-backed ['hʌmpbækt] *a* горба́тый.

humph [mm, hʌmf] *int* гм!

humpty-dumpty ['hʌmptɪ'dʌmptɪ] *n* коротышка.

Hun [hʌn] *n ист.* гунн; *перен.* дика́рь, ва́рвар.

hunch I [hʌntʃ] *n* 1) горб; 2) то́лстый кусо́к, ломо́ть; 3) *амер. разг.* подозре́ние; предчу́вствие; to have a ~ that подозрева́ть, что; оn a ~ по подозре́нию, на основа́нии подозре́ния.

hunch II *v* го́рбиться; изгиба́ться.

hunch-back ['hʌntʃbæk] *n* горбу́н.

hundred I ['hʌndrəd] *num* сто.

hundred II *n* со́тня; число́ сто; by the ~ со́тнями; in ~s по со́тням (*счита́ть и т. п.*); ◇ one ~ per cent на сто проце́нтов, вполне́.

hundredfold I ['hʌndrədfould] *a* стокра́тный.

hundredfold II *adv* во́ сто крат.

hundred-percent ['hʌndrədpə'sent] *a разг.* стопроце́нтный, соверше́нный, зако́нченный.

hundred-percenter ['hʌndrədpə'sentə] *n амер.* ура́-патрио́т.

hundredth I ['hʌndrədθ] *num* со́тый.

hundredth II *n* со́тая часть.

hundredweight ['hʌndrədweit] *n* це́нтнер (*в Англии*=50,8 *кг, в США*=45,3 *кг*).

hung [hʌŋ] *past, p. p. см.* hang I.

Hungarian I [hʌŋ'gεərɪən] *n* 1) венгр, венге́рец; венге́рка; the ~s ве́нгры; 2) венге́рский язы́к.

Hungarian II *a* венге́рский.

hunger I ['hʌŋgə] *n* 1) го́лод; keen ~ си́льный го́лод; to stay ~ *разг.* замори́ть червячка́; утоли́ть го́лод; 2) си́льное жела́ние, жа́жда чего́-л. (*after, for*); ◇ ~ is the best relish го́лод — лу́чший по́вар.

hunger II *v* 1) быть голо́дным, чу́вствовать го́лод; 2) си́льно жела́ть, жа́ждать чего́-л. (*after, for*); 3) принужда́ть го́лодом (*into, out of*).

hunger-strike I ['hʌŋgəstraik] *n* голодо́вка (*заключённых*).

hunger-strike II *v* объявля́ть голодо́вку.

hungrily ['hʌŋgrɪlɪ] *adv* жа́дно, с жа́дностью.

hungry ['hʌŋgrɪ] *a* 1) голо́дный; голода́ющий; to go ~ быть постоя́нно голо́дным; 2) си́льно жела́ющий, жа́ждущий чего́-л. (*for*); 3) ску́дный, то́щий (*о по́чве*); ◇ ~ as a hunter ≅ голо́дный как волк.

hunk [hʌŋk] *n разг.* большо́й кусо́к, ломо́ть.

hunks [hʌŋks] *n* скря́га.

hunky-dory [,hʌŋkɪ'dourɪ] *a амер. разг.* первокла́ссный, отли́чный.

hunt I [hʌnt] *n* 1) охо́та; 2) по́иски (*for*).

hunt II *v* 1) охо́титься; иска́ть, стара́ться доста́ть (*for*); 3) трави́ть, пресле́довать, гнать; □ to ~ after гоня́ться; иска́ть; to ~ away прогоня́ть; to ~ down вы́следить; пойма́ть; загна́ть; to ~ out вы́искать, откопа́ть; to ~ up иска́ть.

hunter ['hʌntə] *n* 1) охо́тник; 2) гу́нтер (*охот-*

ничья ло́шадь); 3) охо́тничья соба́ка; 4) карма́нные часы́ с кры́шкой.

hunting ['hʌntɪŋ] *n* 1) охо́та; 2) *attr* охо́тничий.

hunting-box ['hʌntɪŋbɔks] *n* охо́тничий до́мик.

huntsman ['hʌntsmən] *n* охо́тник.

hurdle I ['hə:dl] *n* 1) перено́сная загоро́дка, плете́нь; 2) препя́тствие, барье́р (*тж. перен.*).

hurdle II *v* 1) огора́живать плетнём; 2) переска́кивать (*через барьер, препятствие*); *перен.* преодолева́ть.

hurdle-race ['hə:dlreis] *n* 1) ска́чки с препя́тствиями; 2) барье́рный бег.

hurdy-gurdy ['hə:di,gə:dɪ] *n* шарма́нка.

hurl I [hə:l] *n* си́льный бросо́к.

hurl II *v* броса́ть (с си́лой); швыря́ть; мета́ть (*копьё*); to ~ oneself бро́ситься (*на — at, upon*).

hurly-burly ['hə:lɪ,bə:lɪ] *n* 1) перепо́лох, сумато́ха; шум; смяте́ние; 2) *attr* шу́мный, по́лный суеты́ (*о городе и т. п.*).

hurrah I [hu'rɑ:] *n* ура́.

hurrah II *v* крича́ть ура́.

hurrah III *int* ура́!

hurray I, II, III [hu'rei] *см.* hurrah I, II, III.

hurricane ['hʌrɪkən] *n* урага́н, бу́ря.

hurried ['hʌrɪd] *a* торопли́вый, бы́стрый, поспе́шный.

hurriedly ['hʌrɪdlɪ] *adv* поспе́шно, торопли́во.

hurry I ['hʌrɪ] *n* 1) спе́шка; торопли́вость, поспе́шность; in a ~ a) второпя́х; на́скоро; б) *разг.* охо́тно; легко́; to be in a ~ торопи́ться, спеши́ть; по ~ не к спе́ху; 2) нетерпе́ние, нетерпели́вое жела́ние (*сделать, получить что-либо*).

hurry II *v* 1) торопи́ть(ся); спеши́ть; подгоня́ть; ~ up! поторопи́сь!; 2) де́лать что-л. поспе́шно *или* о́чень бы́стро; поспе́шно вта́скивать (*в — into*); to ~ into action *воен.* поспе́шно броса́ть в бой; to ~ out of sight поспе́шно спря́тать; □ to ~ away, to ~ off поспе́шно уйти́, уе́хать, увезти́, унести́; to ~ over, to ~ through сде́лать ко́е-ка́к, второпя́х.

hurry-scurry I ['hʌrɪ'skʌrɪ] *n* беспоря́дочная спе́шка, суета́.

hurry-scurry II *a* суетли́вый.

hurry-scurry III *v* де́лать на́спех, суети́ться.

hurry-scurry IV *adv* ко́е-ка́к, как попа́ло.

hurst [hə:st] *n* 1) хо́лмик; 2) леси́стый холм; ро́ща; 3) о́тмель.

hurt I [hə:t] *n* 1) уши́б, ра́на, поврежде́ние; 2) уще́рб, вред, зло; 3) оби́да.

hurt II *v* (*past, p. p.* hurt) 1) причиня́ть боль; ушиби́ть, повреди́ть; to get ~ ушиби́ться, пора́ниться; 2) причиня́ть вред, уще́рб; 3) обижа́ть; де́лать бо́льно, задева́ть; 4) *разг.* боле́ть.

hurtful ['hə:tful] *a* вре́дный.

hurtle ['hə:tl] *v* 1) *уст.* ударя́ться (*обо что-л.*), ната́лкиваться (*на — against*); ста́лкиваться (*с — together*); 2) лете́ть, нести́сь с шу́мом, сви́стом; 3) стреми́тельно направля́ться, броса́ться.

husband I ['hʌzbənd] *n* 1) муж; 2) *уст.* хозя́ин.

husband II *v* 1) относи́ться по-хозя́йски, эконо́мить, бере́чь; 2) *уст.* обраба́тывать зе́млю, паха́ть.

husbandry ['hʌzbəndrɪ] *n* 1) эконо́мия, береж-

ли́вость; 2) заня́тие се́льским хозя́йством; земле-
де́лие; animal ~ животново́дство.

hush I [hʌʃ] *n* тишина́, молча́ние.

hush II *v* 1) заста́вить замолча́ть; успока́ивать;
водворя́ть тишину́; 2) замолча́ть, ути́хнуть; □
to ~ **up** зама́лчивать, скрыва́ть; замя́ть; *разг.*
засекре́тить.

hush III *int* ти́ше!, тс!

hushaby [ˈhʌʃəbaɪ] *int* баю-ба́й.

hush-hush I [ˈhʌʃˈhʌʃ] *a разг.* не подлежа́щий
разглаше́нию, засекре́ченный.

hush-hush II *v разг.* засекре́чивать.

hush-money [ˈhʌʃˌmʌnɪ] *n* взя́тка за молча́ние.

husk I [hʌsk] *n* шелуха́, скорлупа́; нару́жная
оболо́чка.

husk II *v* очища́ть от шелухи́, лущи́ть.

huskily [ˈhʌskɪlɪ] *adv* хри́пло, хри́плым го́ло-
сом.

husky[1] I [ˈhʌskɪ] *a* 1) покры́тый шелухо́й;
2) сухо́й (*как шелуха́*); 3) охри́пший, си́плый;
4) *разг.* ро́слый и си́льный.

husky[1] II *n разг.* ро́слый и си́льный челове́к.

husky[2] *n* ла́йка (*соба́ка*).

hussar [huˈzɑː] *n* гуса́р.

hussy [ˈhʌsɪ] *n* 1) де́рзкая девчо́нка; 2) по-
таску́шка.

hustings [ˈhʌstɪŋz] *n* 1) избира́тельная, пред-
вы́борная кампа́ния; 2) *амер.* трибу́на на пред-
вы́борном ми́тинге.

hustle I [ˈhʌsl] *n* 1) толкотня́; у́личное движе́-
ние, оживле́ние; 2) *разг.* энерги́чная де́ятель-
ность.

hustle II *v* 1) толка́ть(ся); тесни́ть(ся); 2) то-
ропи́ть, подгоня́ть; 3) заставля́ть, принужда́ть
(*into*); вта́лкивать; 4) торопи́ться, суети́ться;
5) *разг.* де́йствовать бы́стро, энерги́чно; □ to ~
away оттесни́ть, отбро́сить; to ~ **through** прота́л-
киваться, пробива́ться.

hustler [ˈhʌslə] *n* энерги́чный, напо́ристый
челове́к.

hut I [hʌt] *n* 1) хи́жина; хиба́рка; 2) *воен.*
бара́к.

hut II *v* 1) помеща́ть в бара́ки; 2) жить в бара́-
ках.

hutch [hʌtʃ] *n* 1) кле́тка для кро́ликов; 2) я́щик,
ларь; 3) *разг.* лачу́га, хиба́рка.

huzza [huˈzɑː] *n, v* I, II, III [huˈzɑː] *см.* hurrah I, II, III.

huzzy [ˈhʌzɪ] *см.* hussy.

hyacinth [ˈhaɪəsɪnθ] *n* гиаци́нт.

hyaena [haɪˈiːnə] *см.* hyena.

hybrid I [ˈhaɪbrɪd] *n* гибри́д; по́месь.

hybrid II *a* гибри́дный, сме́шанный.

hybridization [ˌhaɪbrɪdaɪˈzeɪʃən] *n* скре́щивание,
гибридиза́ция.

hydra [ˈhaɪdrə] *n* ги́дра.

hydrangea [haɪˈdreɪndʒə] *n* горте́нзия.

hydrant [ˈhaɪdrənt] *n* водоразбо́рный кран,
-ная коло́нка.

hydrate [ˈhaɪdreɪt] *n хим.* гидра́т; ~ of lime
гашёная и́звесть.

hydraulic [haɪˈdrɔːlɪk] *a* гидравли́ческий.

hydraulics [haɪˈdrɔːlɪks] *n* гидра́влика.

hydro [ˈhaɪdrou] *сокр. см.* hydropathic I.

hydrocarbon [ˌhaɪdrouˈkɑːbən] *n* углеводоро́д.

hydroelectric [ˈhaɪdrouɪˈlektrɪk] *a* гидро-
электри́ческий.

hydrogen [ˈhaɪdrɪdʒən] *n* 1) водоро́д; heavy ~
тяжёлый водоро́д, дейте́рий; 2) *attr* водоро́дный.

hydropathic I [ˌhaɪdrəˈpæθɪk] *n* водолече́бница.

hydropathic II *a* водолече́бный.

hydropathy [haɪˈdrɔpəθɪ] *n* водолече́ние.

hydrophobia [ˌhaɪdrəˈfoubjə] *n* водобоя́знь,
бе́шенство.

hydroplane [ˈhaɪdrꞓupleɪn] *n* 1) гли́ссер;
2) гидропла́н.

hydropsy [ˈhaɪdrɔpsɪ] *n мед.* водя́нка.

hydrostatics [ˌhaɪdrouˈstætɪks] *n* гидроста́тика.

hydroxide [haɪˈdrɔksaɪd] *n хим.* во́дная о́кись,
гидроо́кись.

hyena [haɪˈiːnə] *n* гие́на.

hygiene [ˈhaɪdʒiːn] *n* гигие́на.

hygienic(al) [haɪˈdʒiːnɪk(əl)] *a* гигиени́ческий;
здоро́вый.

hymen [ˈhaɪmen] *n анат.* де́вственная плева́.

hymeneal [ˌhaɪmeˈniːəl] *a* бра́чный.

hymn I [hɪm] *n* церко́вный гимн.

hymn II *v* петь ги́мны; славосло́вить.

hyper- [ˈhaɪpə-] *pref со значением увеличенного,
повышенного количества, силы и т. п.* сверх-, повы́-
шенный, увели́ченный; hypersensitive сверхчув-
стви́тельный.

hyperbole [haɪˈpəːbəlɪ] *n* преувеличе́ние, гипе́р-
бола.

hyperborean I [ˌhaɪpəbɔːˈriːən] *n поэт.* гипербо-
ре́ец, жи́тель кра́йнего се́вера.

hyperborean II *a поэт.* се́верный, гиперборе́й-
ский.

hypercritical [ˈhaɪpəˈkrɪtɪkəl] *a* сли́шком стро́-
гий, приди́рчивый.

hypersonic [ˈhaɪpəˈsounɪk] *a* сверхзвуково́й;
ультразвуково́й.

hypertension [ˈhaɪpəˈtenʃən] *n* повы́шенное кро-
вяно́е давле́ние.

hypertrophy [haɪˈpəːtrəfɪ] *n* гипертрофи́я.

hyphen I [ˈhaɪfən] *n* дефи́с, соедини́тельная чёрточка (-).

hyphen II *v* писа́ть че́рез дефи́с.

hyphenate [ˈhaɪfəneɪt] *см.* hyphen II.

hypnosis [hɪpˈnousɪs] *n* гипно́з.

hypnotic I [hɪpˈnɔtɪk] *n* 1) загипнотизи́рованный
челове́к; 2) снотво́рное сре́дство.

hypnotic II *a* 1) гипноти́ческий; 2) снотво́рный.

hypnotist [ˈhɪpnətɪst] *n* гипнотизёр.

hypnotize [ˈhɪpnətaɪz] *v* гипнотизи́ровать.

hypo- [ˈhaɪpou-] *pref со значением уменьшён-
ного количества, ослабленной силы и т. п.* под-,
гипо-, ипо-; hypodermic подко́жный; hypophysis ги-
пофи́з.

hypochondria [ˌhaɪpouˈkɔndrɪə] *n* мра́чное, по-
да́вленное состоя́ние, ипохо́ндрия.

hypocrisy [hɪˈpɔkrəsɪ] *n* лицеме́рие, притво́рство;
ха́нжество.

hypocrite [ˈhɪpəkrɪt] *n* лицеме́р; ханжа́.

hypocritical [ˌhɪpəˈkrɪtɪkəl] *a* лицеме́рный, при-
тво́рный; ха́нжеский.

hypodermatic I, II [ˌhaɪpoudəˈmætɪk] *амер. см.*
hypodermic I, II.

hypodermic I [ˌhaɪpəˈdəːmɪk] *n* подко́жное впры́-
скивание.

hypodermic II *a* подко́жный.

hypotenuse [haɪˈpɔtɪnjuːz] *n мат.* гипотену́за.

hypothec [hɪˈpɔθek] *n* ипоте́ка; закладна́я.

hypothecate [haɪ'pɔθɪkeɪt] *v* закла́дывать (*недви́жимость*).

hypothesis [haɪ'pɔθɪsɪs] *n* (*pl* hypotheses [haɪ'pɔθɪsiːz]) гипо́теза, предположе́ние.

hypothetic(al) [,haɪpou'θetɪk(əl)] *a* предположи́тельный, гипотети́ческий.

hy-spy ['haɪ'spaɪ] *n* игра́ в пря́тки, «па́лочка-выруча́лочка».

hysteria [hɪs'tɪərɪə] *n* истери́я.

hysterical [hɪs'terɪkəl] *a* истери́ческий, истери́чный.

hysterics [hɪs'terɪks] *n* исте́рика.

I

I¹, i [aɪ] *n* 9-я бу́ква англ. алфави́та; ◊ to dot one's i's ста́вить то́чки над i.

I² *pron pers* я.

iambi [aɪ'æmbaɪ] *pl см.* iambus.

iambic I [aɪ'æmbɪk] *n* ямби́ческий стих.

iambic II *a* ямби́ческий.

iambus [aɪ'æmbəs] *n* (*pl тж.* iambi) ямб.

ibidem [ɪ'baɪdem] *adv* там же.

ice I [aɪs] *n* 1) лёд; drifting ~ плаву́чий, дрейфу́ющий лёд; to break the ~ разби́ть лёд; *перен.* сде́лать пе́рвый шаг, положи́ть нача́ло; on thin ~ *перен.* в затрудни́тельном, щекотли́вом положе́нии; 2) моро́женое; 3) (са́харная) глазу́рь; 4) *attr* ледяно́й; ледо́вый; ◊ to cut no ~ а) не име́ть значе́ния; б) де́йствовать впусту́ю.

ice II *v* 1) замора́живать; ~d up затёртый льда́ми; 2) покрыва́ть(ся) льдом; 3) покрыва́ть са́харной глазу́рью.

ice-age ['aɪseɪdʒ] *n* леднико́вый пери́од.

ice-axe ['aɪsæks] *n* ледору́б.

iceberg ['aɪsbəːg] *n* а́йсберг.

iceblink ['aɪsblɪŋk] *n* о́тблеск льда.

ice-boat ['aɪsbout] *n* 1) бу́ер (*сани с парусом*); 2) ледоко́л.

ice-bound ['aɪsbaund] *a* затёртый льда́ми.

ice-box ['aɪsbɔks] *n амер. разг.* холоди́льник.

ice-breaker ['aɪs,breɪkə] *n* ледоко́л.

ice-cake ['aɪskeɪk] *n* плаву́чая льди́на.

ice-cream ['aɪs'kriːm] *n* моро́женое.

ice-drift ['aɪsdrɪft] *n* 1) дрейф льда; 2) торо́сы.

ice-field ['aɪsfiːld] *n* ледяно́е по́ле.

ice-floe ['aɪsflou] *n* 1) плаву́чая льди́на; 2) *attr:* the ~ drifting expedition экспеди́ция на дрейфу́ющей льди́не.

ice-house ['aɪshaus] *n* 1) льдохрани́лище; 2) ледяно́й дом.

Icelander ['aɪsləndə] *n* исла́ндец; исла́ндка; the ~s исла́ндцы.

Icelandic I [aɪs'lændɪk] *n* исла́ндский язы́к.

Icelandic II *a* исла́ндский.

iceman ['aɪsmæn] *n* 1) поля́рный путеше́ственник, поля́рник; 2) альпини́ст; 3) моро́женщик; *амер.* продаве́ц льда.

ice-pack ['aɪspæk] *n* торо́систый *или* па́ковый лёд.

ice-yacht ['aɪsjɔt] *см.* ice-boat 1).

icicle ['aɪsɪkl] *n* сосу́лька.

icily ['aɪsɪlɪ] *adv* хо́лодно.

icon ['aɪkɔn] *n* 1) ико́на; 2) изображе́ние, портре́т; ста́туя.

icy ['aɪsɪ] *a* 1) ледяно́й, холо́дный; 2) покры́тый льдом.

I'd [aɪd] *разг.* = I would, I should, I had.

idea [aɪ'dɪə] *n* 1) поня́тие, представле́ние; to have an ~ of име́ть поня́тие, представле́ние о; not the remotest (*или* the faintest) ~ ни мале́йшего представле́ния; to give a slight ~ дать о́бщее представле́ние; I had no ~ you were there я и не подозрева́л, что вы бы́ли там; 2) мысль, иде́я; fixed ~ навя́зчивая иде́я; 3) воображе́ние, фанта́зия; what an ~! что за мысль!, что за фанта́зия!; what's the big ~? каку́ю ещё глу́пость вы заду́мали?

ideal I [aɪ'dɪəl] *n* идеа́л, соверше́нство; beau ~ образе́ц соверше́нства.

ideal II *a* 1) идеа́льный, соверше́нный; 2) вообража́емый, нереа́льный.

idealism [aɪ'dɪəlɪzəm] *n* идеали́зм.

idealist [aɪ'dɪəlɪst] *n* идеали́ст.

idealistic [aɪ,dɪə'lɪstɪk] *a* идеалисти́ческий.

idealization [aɪ,dɪəlaɪ'zeɪʃən] *n* идеализа́ция.

idealize [aɪ'dɪəlaɪz] *v* идеализи́ровать.

idem ['aɪdem] *n* то же (са́мое); тот же (*автор кни́ги*).

identic(al) [aɪ'dentɪk(əl)] *a* 1) тот же (са́мый) (*об одно́м предме́те*); 2) одина́ковый, тожде́ственный, иденти́чный (*with*).

identification [aɪ,dentɪfɪ'keɪʃən] *n* 1) отождествле́ние; 2) опозна́ние; установле́ние ли́чности, по́длинности; 3) *attr* опознава́тельный, для опознава́ния.

identify [aɪ'dentɪfaɪ] *v* 1) устана́вливать тожде́ство (*with*); 2) опознава́ть, устана́вливать ли́чность; распознава́ть; to ~ oneself назва́ть себя́, предъяви́ть удостовере́ние ли́чности; 3) отождествля́ться; солидаризи́роваться; to ~ oneself with примкну́ть (*к па́ртии*), присоедини́ться (*к поли́тике и т. п.*).

identity [aɪ'dentɪtɪ] *n* 1) тожде́ственность, иденти́чность; 2) ли́чность, индивидуа́льность; 3) по́длинность; 4) *мат.* тожде́ство.

ideological [,aɪdɪə'lɔdʒɪkəl] *a* идеологи́ческий.

ideologist [,aɪdɪ'ɔlədʒɪst] *n* идео́лог.

ideology [,aɪdɪ'ɔlədʒɪ] *n* идеоло́гия; Marxist ~ маркси́стская идеоло́гия.

idiom ['ɪdɪəm] *n лингв.* 1) идио́ма, идиомати́ческое выраже́ние; 2) диале́кт, го́вор, наре́чие; local ~ ме́стный диале́кт.

idiomatic [,ɪdɪə'mætɪk] *a лингв.* 1) идиомати́ческий; 2) ме́стный, диалекта́льный; 3) разгово́рный.

idiosyncrasy [,ɪdɪə'sɪŋkrəsɪ] *n мед.* идиосинкрази́я.

idiot ['ɪdɪət] *n* идио́т, дура́к.

idiotic [,ɪdɪ'ɔtɪk] *a* идио́тский.

idle I ['aɪdl] *a* 1) незаня́тый, нерабо́тающий, безде́йствующий; to lie ~ лежа́ть без употребле́ния; to stand ~ не рабо́тать (*о фа́брике и т. п.*); 2) лени́вый, пра́здный; 3) бесполе́зный, тще́тный; 4) пусто́й, неоснова́тельный; 5) холосто́й (*о хо́де маши́ны*).

idle II *v* 1) лени́ться, безде́льничать; to ~ away the time проводи́ть (*вре́мя, жизнь*) в безде́йствии, в безде́лье; 2) *тех.* рабо́тать на холосто́м ходу́; враща́ться вхолосту́ю; □ to ~ over рабо́тать заме́дленным те́мпом; рабо́тать вхолосту́ю.

idleness ['aɪdlɪnɪs] n 1) лень, пра́здность, безде́лье; 2) отсу́тствие рабо́ты, безрабо́тица; 3) безде́йствие.

idler ['aɪdlə] n 1) лентя́й, безде́льник; 2) *тех.* направля́ющее колесо́ (*гусеницы*); направля́ющий шкив.

idly ['aɪdlɪ] *adv* лени́во; пра́здно.

idol ['aɪdl] n и́дол, куми́р.

idolater [aɪ'dɔlətə] n 1) идолопокло́нник; 2) покло́нник, обожа́тель.

idolatry [aɪ'dɔlətrɪ] n 1) идолопокло́нство; 2) обожа́ние, поклоне́ние.

idyll ['ɪdɪl] n иди́ллия.

idyllic [aɪ'dɪlɪk] a идилли́ческий.

if I [ɪf] *conj* слу́жит *для выраже́ния*: 1) *усло́вия, предположе́ния* е́сли; I should do it if I were you я бы сде́лал так, е́сли бы был на ва́шем ме́сте; 2) *стремле́ния, жела́ния* е́сли бы; if I only knew! е́сли бы я то́лько знал!; 3) *повто́рности де́йствия* вся́кий раз как; if I do not understand I ask questions вся́кий раз, как я не понима́ю, я спра́шиваю; 4) *лёгкого сомне́ния — с предше́ствующим* as как бу́дто; as if he did not hear about it! как бу́дто он не слы́шал об э́том!; 5) *явля́ется вво́дным сло́вом в ко́св. вопро́се* ли; I do not know if he understands the text я не зна́ю, понима́ет ли он текст.

if II n: if ifs and ans were pots and pans *погов.* ≅ е́сли бы да кабы́.

iffy ['ɪfɪ] a *амер.* неопределённый.

igneous ['ɪgnɪəs] a 1) о́гненный, огнево́й; 2) *геол.* изве́рженный; вулкани́ческого происхожде́ния.

ignis fatuus ['ɪgnɪs'fætjuəs] n блужда́ющий огонёк; *перен.* обма́нчивая наде́жда.

ignite [ɪg'naɪt] v 1) зажига́ть(ся), воспламеня́ть(ся); загора́ться; 2) раскаля́ть.

igniter [ɪg'naɪtə] n воспламени́тель, зажига́тель.

ignition [ɪg'nɪʃən] n 1) воспламене́ние; зажига́ние; вспы́шка; 2) прока́ливание.

ignoble [ɪg'noubl] a ни́зкий, по́длый; неблагоро́дный.

ignominious [,ɪgnə'mɪnɪəs] a позо́рный, бесче́стный.

ignominy ['ɪgnəmɪnɪ] n 1) бесче́стье, позо́р; 2) бесче́стное, посты́дное поведе́ние.

ignoramus [,ɪgnə'reɪməs] n неве́жда.

ignorance ['ɪgnərəns] n 1) незна́ние, неве́дение (*of*); 2) неве́жество.

ignorant ['ɪgnərənt] a 1) не зна́ющий; не осведомлённый (*of, in*); 2) неве́жественный.

ignore [ɪg'nɔ:] v 1) не принима́ть в расчёт; игнори́ровать; юр. отклоня́ть.

il- [ɪl-] *pref со значе́нием отрица́ния того́, что вы́ражено ко́рнем сло́ва; встреча́ется то́лько в слова́х, ко́рни кото́рых начина́ются с* l не-; illogical нелоги́чный.

ill I [ɪl] n 1) зло; вред; 2) *pl* несча́стья, невзго́ды, бе́ды.

ill II a 1) *predic* больно́й; to be ~ быть больны́м; to fall (*или* to be taken) ~ заболе́ть; 2) плохо́й; несоверше́нный; 3) дурно́й; вре́дный; 4) злой; вражде́бный.

ill *adv* 1) пло́хо; неблагоприя́тно; to speak ~ of пло́хо говори́ть, отзыва́ться о ком-л.; to take a thing ~ пло́хо приня́ть что-л.; оби́деться на что-л.; 2) едва́ (ли), с трудо́м; ~ provided пло́хо снабжённый, необеспе́ченный.

ill-advised ['ɪləd'vaɪzd] a неблагоразу́мный.

ill-affected ['ɪlə'fektɪd] a неблагожела́тельный, нерасполо́женный (*к кому́-л.*).

ill-bred ['ɪl'bred] a пло́хо воспи́танный, невоспи́танный, гру́бый.

ill-breeding ['ɪl'bri:dɪŋ] n невоспи́танность; плохи́е мане́ры; гру́бость.

ill-conditioned ['ɪlkən'dɪʃənd] a 1) злой, сварли́вый; 2) в плохо́м состоя́нии; неиспра́вный.

ill-disposed ['ɪldɪs'pouzd] a 1) злой; 2) недоброжела́тельный (*к — towards*).

illegal [ɪ'li:gəl] a 1) нелега́льный; 2) противозако́нный.

illegibility [ɪ,ledʒɪ'bɪlɪtɪ] n неразбо́рчивость, неудобочита́емость.

illegible [ɪ'ledʒəbl] a неразбо́рчивый, неудобочита́емый.

illegitimacy [,ɪlɪ'dʒɪtɪməsɪ] n незако́нность.

illegitimate I [,ɪlɪ'dʒɪtɪmɪt] a 1) незако́нный; 2) незаконнорождённый; 3) непра́вильный (*о вы́воде*).

illegitimate II v объявля́ть незако́нным.

ill-fated ['ɪl'feɪtɪd] a злополу́чный; несчастли́вый; принося́щий несча́стье.

ill-favoured ['ɪl'feɪvəd] a 1) некраси́вый; 2) неприя́тный, отта́лкивающий.

ill-founded ['ɪl'faundɪd] a необосно́ванный.

ill-gotten ['ɪl'gɔtn] a доста́вшийся нече́стным путём.

ill-humoured ['ɪl'hju:məd] a в плохо́м настрое́нии.

illiberal [ɪ'lɪbərəl] a 1) отста́лый; ограни́ченный; 2) нетерпи́мый; 3) гру́бый, ни́зкий; 4) скупо́й.

illicit [ɪ'lɪsɪt] a 1) незако́нный; запрещённый.

illiteracy [ɪ'lɪtərəsɪ] n негра́мотность.

illiterate I [ɪ'lɪtərɪt] n 1) негра́мотный (челове́к); 2) неу́ч.

illiterate II a 1) негра́мотный; 2) необразо́ванный.

ill-judged ['ɪl'dʒʌdʒd] a 1) неблагоразу́мный; 2) несвоевре́менный.

ill-mannered ['ɪl'mænəd] a невоспи́танный, гру́бый.

ill-natured ['ɪl'neɪtʃəd] a гру́бый; зло́бный.

illness ['ɪlnɪs] n боле́знь.

illogical [ɪ'lɔdʒɪkəl] a нелоги́чный.

ill-omened ['ɪl'oumend] a злове́щий, предвеща́ющий несча́стье.

ill-spoken ['ɪl'spoukən] a по́льзующийся дурно́й репута́цией.

ill-starred ['ɪl'stɑ:d] a злополу́чный; неуда́чливый; роди́вшийся под несчастли́вой звездо́й.

ill-tempered ['ɪl'tempəd] a раздражи́тельный.

ill-timed ['ɪl'taɪmd] a несвоевре́менный.

ill-treat ['ɪl'tri:t] v пло́хо, жесто́ко обраща́ться.

illuminant I [ɪ'lju:mɪnənt] n 1) освети́тельный прибо́р, материа́л; 2) исто́чник све́та.

illuminant II a освети́тельный; освеща́ющий.

illuminate [ɪ'lju:mɪneɪt] v 1) освеща́ть; озаря́ть; 2) просвеща́ть; 3) пролива́ть свет на, разъясня́ть; 4) устра́ивать иллюмина́цию; 5) украша́ть (*ру́копись*) цветны́ми рису́нками.

illumination [ɪ,lju:mɪ'neɪʃən] n 1) освеще́ние; 2) освещённость, я́ркость; 3) *обыкн. pl* иллюмина́ция; 4) цветны́е рису́нки (*в ру́кописи*).

illuminator [ɪ,lju:mɪ'neɪtə] n 1) иллюмина́тор;

2) освети́тель, рефле́ктор; 3) худо́жник-иллюстра́тор.

illumine [ɪˈljuːmɪn] v 1) освеща́ть; озаря́ть, броса́ть свет; 2) просвеща́ть.

ill-use [ˈɪlˈjuːz] *см.* ill-treat.

illusion [ɪˈluːʒən] n 1) иллю́зия; обма́н чувств; мира́ж; 2) прозра́чный тюль.

illusionist [ɪˈluːʒənɪst] n 1) мечта́тель; 2) иллюзиони́ст, фо́кусник.

illusive [ɪˈluːsɪv] a обма́нчивый, иллюзо́рный.

illusory [ɪˈluːsərɪ] *см.* illusive.

illustrate [ˈɪləstreɪt] v иллюстри́ровать; поясня́ть.

illustration [ˌɪləsˈtreɪʃən] n 1) иллюстра́ция, рису́нок; 2) приме́р.

illustrative [ˈɪləstreɪtɪv] a иллюстрати́вный, поясни́тельный.

illustrator [ˈɪləstreɪtə] n иллюстра́тор.

illustrious [ɪˈlʌstrɪəs] a знамени́тый; просла́вленный.

ill-will [ˈɪlˈwɪl] n недоброжела́тельство; зла́я во́ля.

I'm [aɪm] *разг.* = I am.

im-¹ [ɪm-] *pref со значением включения внутрь, нахождения внутри чего-л.; используется для образования переходных глаголов, корни которых начинаются с m, b, p:* to imbed вставля́ть, вреза́ть, вде́лывать.

im-² *pref со значением отрицания того, что выражено корнем слова; встречается только в словах, корни которых начинаются с m, b, p:* immoral амора́льный; imperishable неруши́мый; ве́чный; непо́ртящийся.

image I [ˈɪmɪdʒ] n 1) о́браз, изображе́ние; 2) отраже́ние (*в зеркале*); 3) подо́бие; he is the very ~ of his father он вы́литый оте́ц; 4) мета́фора; to speak in ~s говори́ть о́бразно; 5) ико́на.

image II v 1) изобража́ть; создава́ть о́браз; отобража́ть; 2) представля́ть себе́, вызыва́ть в воображе́нии; 3) отража́ть (*как в зеркале*).

imaginable [ɪˈmædʒɪnəbl] a вообрази́мый.

imaginary [ɪˈmædʒɪnərɪ] a вообража́емый; мни́мый.

imagination [ɪˌmædʒɪˈneɪʃən] n воображе́ние; фанта́зия.

imaginative [ɪˈmædʒɪnətɪv] a 1) облада́ющий бога́тым воображе́нием; 2) бога́тый поэти́ческими о́бразами, о́бразный.

imagine [ɪˈmædʒɪn] v 1) представля́ть себе́, вообража́ть; 2) предполага́ть, ду́мать.

imbecile I [ˈɪmbɪsiːl] n 1) слабоу́мный; идио́т; 2) глупе́ц.

imbecile II a 1) слабоу́мный; 2) глу́пый, неразу́мный.

imbecility [ˌɪmbɪˈsɪlɪtɪ] n 1) слабоу́мие; 2) глу́пость; неразу́мный посту́пок.

imbibe [ɪmˈbaɪb] v 1) впи́тывать, вса́сывать; 2) поглоща́ть; вдыха́ть; 3) усва́ивать, ассимили́ровать.

imbroglio [ɪmˈbrouljou] n сло́жная ситуа́ция; пу́таница.

imbrue [ɪmˈbruː] v обагри́ть, запятна́ть (*кро́вью*).

imbue [ɪmˈbjuː] v 1) пропи́тывать, насыща́ть; 2) окра́шивать; 3) наполня́ть (*чу́вством*).

imitate [ˈɪmɪteɪt] v 1) подража́ть, копи́ровать;

2) передра́знивать; 3) имити́ровать, подде́лывать.

imitation [ˌɪmɪˈteɪʃən] n 1) подража́ние; 2) подде́лка, имита́ция; 3) *attr* иску́сственный, подде́льный.

imitative [ˈɪmɪtətɪv] a 1) подража́тельный; 2) изобрази́тельный; 3) иску́сственный, подде́льный.

imitator [ˈɪmɪteɪtə] n подража́тель.

immaculate [ɪˈmækjulɪt] a 1) чи́стый; незапя́тнанный; 2) безупре́чный (*часто ирон.*); 3) непоро́чный.

immaterial [ˌɪməˈtɪərɪəl] a 1) несуще́ственный; 2) бестеле́сный, невеще́ственный.

immature [ˌɪməˈtjuə] a незре́лый; не(до)разви́вшийся; ра́нний.

immaturity [ˌɪməˈtjuərɪtɪ] n незре́лость.

immeasurable [ɪˈmeʒərəbl] a неизмери́мый, грома́дный.

immediate [ɪˈmiːdjət] a 1) непосре́дственный, прямо́й (*о взаимоотношениях, действиях*); 2) ближа́йший; 3) неме́дленный, безотлага́тельный; сро́чный.

immediately [ɪˈmiːdjətlɪ] adv 1) неме́дленно; 2) непосре́дственно.

immemorial [ˌɪmɪˈmɔːrɪəl] a незапа́мятный.

immense [ɪˈmens] a 1) огро́мный, грома́дный, необъя́тный; 2) *разг.* замеча́тельный, великоле́пный.

immensely [ɪˈmenslɪ] adv чрезвыча́йно, о́чень.

immensity [ɪˈmensɪtɪ] n грома́дность, необъя́тность.

immerse [ɪˈməːs] v 1) погружа́ть; 2) вовлека́ть; запу́тывать.

immersion [ɪˈməːʃən] n погруже́ние.

immigrant I [ˈɪmɪgrənt] n иммигра́нт; переселе́нец.

immigrant II a иммигри́рующий; переселя́ющийся.

immigrate [ˈɪmɪgreɪt] v иммигри́ровать; переселя́ть(ся).

immigration [ˌɪmɪˈgreɪʃən] n иммигра́ция; переселе́ние.

imminence [ˈɪmɪnəns] n угро́за, бли́зость (*чего-л.*).

imminent [ˈɪmɪnənt] a бли́зкий, угрожа́ющий; надвига́ющийся.

immobile [ɪˈmoubaɪl] a неподви́жный; недви́жимый.

immobility [ˌɪmouˈbɪlɪtɪ] n неподви́жность.

immobilize [ɪˈmoubɪlaɪz] v 1) де́лать неподви́жным; ско́вывать; остана́вливать; 2) изыма́ть из обраще́ния (*монету*).

immoderate [ɪˈmɔdərɪt] a неуме́ренный, чрезме́рный.

immodest [ɪˈmɔdɪst] a 1) нескро́мный, неприли́чный; 2) на́глый, бессты́дный.

immodesty [ɪˈmɔdɪstɪ] n 1) нескро́мность, неприли́чие; 2) на́глость, бессты́дство.

immolate [ˈɪmouleɪt] v приноси́ть в же́ртву.

immolation [ˌɪmouˈleɪʃən] n же́ртва; жертвоприноше́ние.

immoral [ɪˈmɔrəl] a безнра́вственный.

immorality [ˌɪməˈrælɪtɪ] n безнра́вственность.

immortal [ɪˈmɔːtl] a бессме́ртный; неувяда́емый.

immortality [ˌɪmɔːˈtælɪtɪ] n бессме́ртие.

immortalize [ɪˈmɔːtəlaɪz] *v* обессме́ртить.

immovability [ɪˌmuːvəˈbɪlɪtɪ] *n* неподви́жность; недви́жимость; 2) споко́йствие, бесстра́стие; 3) непоколеби́мость.

immovable [ɪˈmuːvəbl] *a* 1) неподви́жный; недви́жимый; 2) споко́йный, бесстра́стный; 3) непоколеби́мый; 4) недви́жимый (*об имуществе*).

immovables [ɪˈmuːvəblz] *n pl* недви́жимое иму́щество, недви́жимость.

immune [ɪˈmjuːn] *a* невоспри́имчивый, облада́ющий иммуните́том (*к — from, against, to*).

immunity [ɪˈmjuːnɪtɪ] *n* 1) иммуните́т, невоспри́имчивость (*к — from*); 2) освобожде́ние (*от платежа, налога*).

immure [ɪˈmjuə] *v* 1) заключа́ть в тюрьму́; to ~ oneself запере́ться в четырёх стена́х; 2) замуро́вывать.

immutable [ɪˈmjuːtəbl] *a* неизме́нный; непрело́жный.

imp [ɪmp] *n* чертёнок, бесёнок.

impact[a] [ˈɪmpækt] *n* 1) уда́р, толчо́к (*on, against*); столкнове́ние; 2) возде́йствие, влия́ние.

impact[b] [ɪmˈpækt] *v* пло́тно сжима́ть, про́чно укрепля́ть (*into, in*).

impair [ɪmˈpɛə] *v* ослабля́ть; вреди́ть; по́ртить.

impale [ɪmˈpeɪl] *v* 1) пронза́ть; to ~ oneself upon наскочи́ть, напоро́ться; 2) сажа́ть на́ кол.

impalpable [ɪmˈpælpəbl] *a* 1) неосяза́емый; 2) непостижи́мый.

impart [ɪmˈpɑːt] *v* 1) наделя́ть; 2) сообща́ть (*новости и т. п.*).

impartial [ɪmˈpɑːʃəl] *a* беспристра́стный, справедли́вый.

impartiality [ɪmˌpɑːʃɪˈælɪtɪ] *n* беспристра́стие, справедли́вость.

impassable [ɪmˈpɑːsəbl] *a* непроходи́мый; непрое́зжий.

impasse [æmˈpɑːs] *n* тупи́к; *перен. тж.* безвы́ходное положе́ние.

impassible [ɪmˈpæsɪbl] *a* 1) нечувстви́тельный; бесчу́вственный; 2) бесстра́стный.

impassioned [ɪmˈpæʃənd] *a* охва́ченный стра́стью; стра́стный.

impassive [ɪmˈpæsɪv] *a* 1) безмяте́жный, споко́йный; 2) бесстра́стный; 3) нечувстви́тельный; бесчу́вственный.

impatience [ɪmˈpeɪʃəns] *n* нетерпе́ние.

impatient [ɪmˈpeɪʃənt] *a* 1) нетерпели́вый; 2) нетерпи́мый, раздражи́тельный; 3) горя́щий жела́нием (*сделать что-л.*).

impeach [ɪmˈpiːtʃ] *v* 1) подверга́ть сомне́нию; 2) порица́ть, обвиня́ть (*of, with*); 3) *юр.* предъявля́ть обвине́ние в госуда́рственном преступле́нии.

impeachment [ɪmˈpiːtʃmənt] *n* 1) порица́ние; обвине́ние; 2) *юр.* привлече́ние к суду́ за госуда́рственное преступле́ние.

impeccable [ɪmˈpekəbl] *n* непогреши́мый; безупре́чный.

impecunious [ˌɪmpɪˈkjuːnjəs] *a* нужда́ющийся, не име́ющий де́нег.

impede [ɪmˈpiːd] *v* меша́ть, препя́тствовать.

impediment [ɪmˈpedɪmənt] *n* поме́ха, препя́тствие; an ~ in one's speech заика́ние.

impel [ɪmˈpel] *v* 1) побужда́ть; 2) продвига́ть, толка́ть; приводи́ть в движе́ние.

impellent I [ɪmˈpelənt] *n* дви́жущая си́ла.

impellent II *a* побужда́ющий, дви́гающий.

impend [ɪmˈpend] *v* надвига́ться; угрожа́ть, нависа́ть (*over*).

impendence [ɪmˈpendəns] *n* бли́зость, угро́за (*чего-л.*).

impending [ɪmˈpendɪŋ] *a* надвига́ющийся, угрожа́ющий, неминуемый.

impenetrable [ɪmˈpenɪtrəbl] *a* 1) непроница́емый; 2) непроходи́мый; 3) непостижи́мый; 4) *воен.* непробива́емый.

impenitent [ɪmˈpenɪtənt] *a* нераска́янный, нераска́явшийся.

imperative I [ɪmˈperətɪv] *n грам.* повели́тельное наклоне́ние.

imperative II *a* 1) вла́стный, повели́тельный; 2) настоя́тельный, неотло́жный; 3) *грам.* повели́тельный.

imperceptible [ˌɪmpəˈseptəbl] *a* незаме́тный; незначи́тельный.

imperfect I [ɪmˈpɜːfɪkt] *n грам.* проше́дшее несоверше́нное вре́мя.

imperfect II *a* 1) непо́лный, недоста́точный; 2) несоверше́нный, дефе́ктный; 3) *грам.* обознача́ющий незако́нченное де́йствие.

imperfection [ˌɪmpəˈfekʃən] *n* 1) неполнота́; несоверше́нство; 2) недоста́ток.

imperial I [ɪmˈpɪərɪəl] *n* 1) эспаньо́лка (*бородка*); 2) империа́л, верх (*дилижанса, омнибуса и т. п.*).

imperial II *a* 1) импе́рский; 2) импера́торский; 3) вы́сший, верхо́вный; 4) вели́чественный; великоле́пный; 5) устано́вленный, станда́ртный (*об англ. мерах*).

imperialism [ɪmˈpɪərɪəlɪzəm] *n* империали́зм.

imperialist [ɪmˈpɪərɪəlɪst] *n* 1) империали́ст; 2) *attr* империалисти́ческий.

imperialistic [ɪmˌpɪərɪəˈlɪstɪk] *a* империалисти́ческий.

imperil [ɪmˈperɪl] *v* подверга́ть опа́сности.

imperious [ɪmˈpɪərɪəs] *a* 1) вла́стный, повели́тельный; 2) настоя́тельный.

imperishable [ɪmˈperɪʃəbl] *a* 1) ве́чный, неруши́мый; 2) непо́ртящийся.

impermeable [ɪmˈpɜːmjəbl] *a* непроница́емый.

impermissible [ˌɪmpəˈmɪsəbl] *a* непозволи́тельный.

impersonal [ɪmˈpɜːsnl] *a* 1) безли́чный (*тж. грам.*); 2) объекти́вный, беспристра́стный.

impersonate [ɪmˈpɜːsəneɪt] *v* 1) олицетворя́ть, воплоща́ть; 2) исполня́ть, игра́ть роль (*кого-л.*); 3) выдава́ть себя́ (*за кого-л.*).

impersonation [ɪmˌpɜːsəˈneɪʃən] *n* 1) олицетворе́ние, воплоще́ние; 2) исполне́ние ро́ли (*кого-л.*); 3) стремле́ние вы́дать себя́ (*за кого-л.*).

impertinence [ɪmˈpɜːtɪnəns] *n* 1) де́рзость; наха́льство; 2) неуме́стность.

impertinent [ɪmˈpɜːtɪnənt] *a* 1) де́рзкий; наха́льный; 2) неуме́стный; не относя́щийся к де́лу; 3) неле́пый.

imperturbability [ˈɪmpɜːˌtɜːbəˈbɪlɪtɪ] *n* невозмути́мость, споко́йствие.

imperturbable [ˌɪmpɜːˈtɜːbəbl] *a* невозмути́мый, споко́йный.

impervious [ɪmˈpɜːvjəs] *a* 1) непроница́емый, непроходи́мый (*to*); 2) невоспри́имчивый; ~ to argument глухо́й .к угово́рам, не поддаю́щийся убежде́ниям.

impetuosity [ɪmˌpetjuˈɔsɪtɪ] *n* стреми́тельность.

impetuous [ɪmˈpetjuəs] *a* 1) стреми́тельный, поры́вистый; 2) запа́льчивый, необду́манный.

impetus [ˈɪmpɪtəs] *n* дви́жущая си́ла; побужде́ние, толчо́к, и́мпульс, сти́мул; to put fresh ~ вдохну́ть но́вые си́лы.

impiety [ɪmˈpaɪətɪ] *n* 1) неве́рие; 2) непочти́тельность, неуваже́ние.

impinge [ɪmˈpɪndʒ] *v* 1) ударя́ться (*o — on, upon*); 2) покуша́ться (*на — on, upon*).

impious [ˈɪmpɪəs] *a* не(благо)чести́вый.

impish [ˈɪmpɪʃ] *a* прока́зливый.

implacability [ɪmˌplækəˈbɪlɪtɪ] *n* неумоли́мость; непримири́мость.

implacable [ɪmˈplækəbl] *a* неумоли́мый; непримири́мый.

implant [ɪmˈplɑːnt] *v* насажда́ть; *перен. тж.* внедря́ть.

implement[a] [ˈɪmplɪmənt] *n* ору́дие, инструме́нт; принадле́жность.

implement[b] [ˈɪmplɪment] *v* 1) приводи́ть в исполне́ние, выполня́ть; 2) снабжа́ть, обеспе́чивать инструме́нтами.

implicate [ˈɪmplɪkeɪt] *v* 1) спу́тывать; 2) вовлека́ть, впу́тывать; to be ~d in быть заме́шанным в; 3) подразумева́ть, заключа́ть в себе́.

implication [ˌɪmplɪˈkeɪʃən] *n* 1) (со)уча́стие, заме́шанность; прича́стность; 2) подразумева́емое; 3) смысл, значе́ние; by ~ по смы́слу; 4) вы́вод, заключе́ние.

implicit [ɪmˈplɪsɪt] *a* 1) подразумева́емый; нея́сно вы́раженный; 2) безотчётный, слепо́й (*о ве́ре, повинове́нии и т. п.*).

implore [ɪmˈplɔː] *v* умоля́ть, упра́шивать.

imply [ɪmˈplaɪ] *v* 1) зна́чить, заключа́ть в себе́; 2) подразумева́ть; намека́ть.

impolite [ˌɪmpəˈlaɪt] *a* неве́жливый, неучти́вый.

impolitic [ɪmˈpɔlɪtɪk] *a* 1) неполити́чный; 2) беста́ктный.

imponderability [ɪmˌpɔndərəˈbɪlɪtɪ] *n* невесо́мость.

imponderable [ɪmˈpɔndərəbl] *a* 1) невесо́мый; лёгкий; 2) не поддаю́щийся учёту.

import[a1] [ˈɪmpɔːt] *n* 1) ввоз, и́мпорт; 2) *обыкн. pl* ввози́мые, и́мпортные това́ры; 3) *attr* и́мпортный, ввозно́й.

import[a2] *n* 1) смысл, значе́ние; 2) ва́жность.

import[b1] [ɪmˈpɔːt] *v* 1) ввози́ть, импорти́ровать; 2) привноси́ть, вкла́дывать (*чу́вства, мы́сли и т. п.*).

import[b2] *v* 1) означа́ть, подразумева́ть; выража́ть; 2) име́ть значе́ние, ва́жность.

importance [ɪmˈpɔːtəns] *n* ва́жность, большо́е значе́ние, значи́тельность; to be of ~ име́ть значе́ние; to be of no ~ не име́ть значе́ния; to attach ~ придава́ть (большо́е) значе́ние, счита́ть ва́жным.

important [ɪmˈpɔːtənt] *a* ва́жный, значи́тельный.

importation [ˌɪmpɔːˈteɪʃən] *n* ввоз, и́мпорт.

importunate [ɪmˈpɔːtjunɪt] *a* 1) насто́йчивый; 2) назо́йливый; 3) настоя́тельный, безотлага́тельный.

importune [ɪmˈpɔːtjuːn] *v* домога́ться, надоеда́ть про́сьбами.

importunity [ˌɪmpɔːˈtjuːnɪtɪ] *n* назо́йливость, надое́дливость; *pl* насто́йчивые про́сьбы.

impose [ɪmˈpouz] *v* 1) налага́ть (*обяза́тельство*); облага́ть (*нало́гом, по́шлиной; on*); 2) вынужда́ть (*к чему́-л.*); 3) обма́ном всучи́ть (*on, upon*); 4) импони́ровать, производи́ть впечатле́ние.

imposing [ɪmˈpouzɪŋ] *a* производя́щий си́льное впечатле́ние, внуши́тельный.

imposition [ˌɪmpəˈzɪʃən] *n* 1) нало́г; обложе́ние (*нало́гом*); 2) доба́вочный уро́к, штрафна́я рабо́та (*наказа́ние в англ. шко́лах*); 3) обма́н, моше́нничество.

impossibility [ɪmˌpɔsəˈbɪlɪtɪ] *n* 1) невозмо́жность; 2) невозмо́жное.

impossible [ɪmˈpɔsəbl] *a* невозмо́жный.

impostor [ɪmˈpɔstə] *n* 1) самозва́нец; 2) обма́нщик, моше́нник, плут.

imposture [ɪmˈpɔstʃə] *n* обма́н, плутовство́, моше́нничество.

impotent [ˈɪmpətənt] *a* бесси́льный, сла́бый; беспо́мощный.

impound [ɪmˈpaund] *v* 1) конфискова́ть; 2) загоня́ть (*скот*); 3) запира́ть, заключа́ть.

impoverish [ɪmˈpɔvərɪʃ] *v* 1) доводи́ть до нищеты́, разоря́ть; 2) истоща́ть (*по́чву, си́лы*); 3) обедня́ть, де́лать ску́чным, бесцве́тным.

impracticable [ɪmˈpræktɪkəbl] *a* 1) неосуществи́мый; 2) неподатливый; 3) непроходи́мый, непрое́зжий.

impractical [ɪmˈpræktɪkəl] *a амер.* 1) непракти́чный; него́дный; 2) *см.* impracticable 1).

imprecate [ˈɪmprɪkeɪt] *v* призыва́ть несча́стья, прокля́тия (*на кого́-л. — upon*).

imprecation [ˌɪmprɪˈkeɪʃən] *n* прокля́тие.

impregnability [ɪmˌpregnəˈbɪlɪtɪ] *n* непристу́пность; неуязви́мость.

impregnable [ɪmˈpregnəbl] *a* непристу́пный; непоколеби́мый; неуязви́мый.

impregnate[a] [ɪmˈpregnɪt] *a* 1) бере́менная; 2) оплодотворённый; 3) пропи́танный (*with*).

impregnate[b] [ˈɪmpregneɪt] *v* 1) оплодотворя́ть; 2) наполня́ть, пропи́тывать (*with*).

impregnation [ˌɪmpregˈneɪʃən] *n* 1) зача́тие; оплодотворе́ние; 2) пропи́тывание.

impresario [ˌɪmpreˈsɑːrɪou] *n* (*pl тж.* impresari [ˌɪmpreˈsɑːriː]) импреса́рио, антрепренёр.

impress[a] [ˈɪmpres] *n* печа́ть, отпеча́ток (*тж. перен.*).

impress[b1] [ɪmˈpres] *v* 1) отпеча́тывать, печа́тать; ста́вить печа́ть (*on*); 2) клейми́ть, штемпелева́ть (*чем-л. — with*); 3) внуша́ть, влия́ть (*on*); 4) поража́ть, производи́ть глубо́кое впечатле́ние.

impress[b2] *v* реквизи́ровать (*для обще́ственных нужд*).

impressible [ɪmˈpresəbl] *a* впечатли́тельный; восприи́мчивый.

impression [ɪmˈpreʃən] *n* 1) впечатле́ние; sharp ~ си́льное впечатле́ние; auditive (visual) ~ слухово́е (зри́тельное) впечатле́ние, восприя́тие; under the ~ (of) под впечатле́нием; to convey the ~ создава́ть впечатле́ние; 2) отпеча́ток; 3) о́ттиск; 4) печа́ть, печа́тание; тисне́ние; 5) изда́ние.

impressionable [ɪmˈpreʃnəbl] *a* впечатли́тельный, восприи́мчивый.

impressionism [ɪmˈpreʃnɪzəm] *n иск.* импрессиони́зм.

impressionist [ɪm'preʃnɪst] *n иск.* импрессиони́ст.

impressive [ɪm'presɪv] *a* вырази́тельный; производя́щий глубо́кое впечатле́ние, тро́гательный.

imprest ['ɪmprest] *n* подотчётная су́мма.

imprimatur [ˌɪmprɪ'meɪtə] *n* 1) са́нкция; одобре́ние; 2) официа́льное разреше́ние (*печа́тать кни́гу и т. п.*).

imprintᵃ ['ɪmprɪnt] *n* 1) отпеча́ток; штамп; 2) *полигр.* выходны́е да́нные (*тж.* publisher's ~, printer's ~).

imprintᵇ [ɪm'prɪnt] *v* 1) отпеча́тывать (*on, with*); 2) оставля́ть след; запечатлева́ть.

imprison [ɪm'prɪzn] *v* заключа́ть в тюрьму́.

imprisonment [ɪm'prɪznmənt] *n* (тюре́мное) заключе́ние.

improbability [ɪmˌprɔbə'bɪlɪtɪ] *n* неправдоподо́бие.

improbable [ɪm'prɔbəbl] *a* неправдоподо́бный.

improbity [ɪm'proubɪtɪ] *n* нече́стность.

impromptu I [ɪm'prɔmptjuː] *n* экспро́мт; импровиза́ция.

impromptu II *a* импровизи́рованный.

impromptu III *adv* экспро́мтом, без подгото́вки.

improper [ɪm'prɔpə] *a* 1) непра́вильный; 2) неуме́стный; 3) непристо́йный, неприли́чный.

impropriety [ˌɪmprə'praɪətɪ] *n* 1) непра́вильность; 2) неуме́стность; 3) наруше́ние обы́чаев, прили́чий.

improvable [ɪm'pruːvəbl] *a* 1) могу́щий быть улу́чшенным, усоверше́нствованным; 2) удо́бный, приго́дный для обрабо́тки (*о земле́*).

improve [ɪm'pruːv] *v* 1) улучша́ть(ся), (у)соверше́нствовать(ся); to ~ in health поправля́ться; 2) (вос)по́льзоваться (*слу́чаем*); 3) повыша́ться в цене́; □ to ~ **away** пыта́ясь улу́чшить, испо́ртить де́ло; to ~ **upon** улучша́ть.

improvement [ɪm'pruːvmənt] *n* улучше́ние; усоверше́нствование.

improvident [ɪm'prɔvɪdənt] *a* 1) непредусмотри́тельный; 2) расточи́тельный.

improvisation [ˌɪmprəvaɪ'zeɪʃən] *n* импровиза́ция.

improvisator [ɪm'prɔvɪzeɪtə] *n* импровиза́тор.

improvise ['ɪmprəvaɪz] *v* импровизи́ровать.

imprudence [ɪm'pruːdəns] *n* неблагоразу́мие, опроме́тчивость; неосторо́жность.

imprudent [ɪm'pruːdənt] *a* неблагоразу́мный, опроме́тчивый; неосторо́жный.

impudence ['ɪmpjudəns] *n* де́рзость; бессты́дство.

impudent ['ɪmpjudənt] *a* де́рзкий; бессты́дный.

impugn [ɪm'pjuːn] *v* оспа́ривать, опроверга́ть.

impulse ['ɪmpʌls] *n* толчо́к; побужде́ние; поры́в, и́мпульс.

impulsion [ɪm'pʌlʃən] *n* и́мпульс, побужде́ние.

impulsive [ɪm'pʌlsɪv] *a* 1) импульси́вный, поры́вистый; 2) побужда́ющий; *тех.* де́йствующий под влия́нием толчка́.

impulsively [ɪm'pʌlsɪvlɪ] *adv* 1) под влия́нием мину́ты; 2) под впечатле́нием; поры́висто.

impunity [ɪm'pjuːnɪtɪ] *n* безнака́занность; with ~ безнака́занно.

impure [ɪm'pjuə] *a* 1) нечи́стый; гря́зный; 2) сме́шанный, с при́месью.

impurity [ɪm'pjuərɪtɪ] *n* 1) нечистота́; 2) при́месь.

imputation [ˌɪmpjuː'teɪʃən] *n* 1) обвине́ние; вмене́ние в вину́; 2) пятно́, тень (*на репута́ции*).

impute [ɪm'pjuːt] *v* 1) припи́сывать (*кому́-л.*); 2) вменя́ть в вину́.

in I [ɪn] *prep* 1) *в простра́нственном значе́нии указывает на нахожде́ние в преде́лах или внутри чего́-л.* (*в том числе́ в преде́лах большо́го го́рода*; *см.* at 1, в) *в*(о), *на*; in the USSR (Moscow, the capital, the country, the house, the street, the garden, the yard) в СССР (Москве́, столи́це, дере́вне, до́ме, на у́лице, в саду́, во дворе́); in the cosmos в ко́смосе; 2) *во временно́м значе́нии указывает на: а) пери́од бо́льше часа в; перево́дится тж. наре́чиями:* in the morning (afternoon, evening) у́тром (по́сле полу́дня, ве́чером); in summer (autumn, winter, spring) ле́том (о́сенью, зимо́й, весно́й); in January (March *etc*) в январе́ (ма́рте *и т. д.*); in 1961 в 1961 г.; in the XX century в XX ве́ке; *б) пери́од вре́мени, по проше́ствии или в тече́ние кото́рого бу́дет происходи́ть де́йствие в* тече́ние, за, че́рез; I will come to see you in a week я навещу́ вас че́рез неде́лю; the boy did the task in an hour ма́льчик вы́полнил зада́ние за час; 3) *выража́ет: а) состоя́ние, в кото́ром нахо́дится предме́т или сопу́тствующие де́йствию обстоя́тельства в, на, у; перево́дится тж. наре́чиями:* in difficulties (danger, distress, sorrow, mourning, need, earnest, fact, fun) в затрудни́тельном положе́нии (опа́сности, беде́, го́ре, тра́уре, нужде́, серьёзно, факти́чески, в шу́тку); in office (power, practice, use, fashion) на слу́жбе (у вла́сти, на пра́ктике, в употребле́нии, в ходу́, в мо́де); *б) вне́шнее оформле́ние предме́та в; перево́дится тж. наре́чиями:* in black (white, silk) в чёрном (бе́лом, шелку́); in pen (pencil, ink, black and white) перо́м (карандашо́м, в карандаше́, черни́лами, чёрным по бе́лому); *в) разделе́ние, расчлене́ние на ча́сти на;* to cut in pieces ре́зать на куски́; *г) отноше́ние одного́ числа́ к друго́му на, к;* one in every ten оди́н из десяти́, оди́н на де́сять; one in a hundred оди́н на со́тню.

in II *adv* внутри́; внутрь; in and out туда́ и сюда́; ◊ in at one ear and out at the other *посл.* ≅ в одно́ у́хо вошло́, в друго́е вы́шло.

in III *n*: the ~s полити́ческая па́ртия у вла́сти; ~s and outs а) все вхо́ды и вы́ходы; б) дета́ли; подного́тная; в) прави́тельство и оппозицио́нные па́ртии.

in-¹ [ɪn-] *pref со значе́нием включе́ния внутрь, нахожде́ния внутри́ чего́-л.:* inland вну́тренняя часть страны́; *испо́льзуется та́кже для образова́ния перехо́дных глаго́лов:* to trust ве́рить, to intrust вверя́ть.

in-² *pref со значе́нием отрица́ния того́, что вы́ражено ко́рнем сло́ва; встреча́ется в слова́х, ко́рни кото́рых начина́ются с любо́го зву́ка, кро́ме* l, m, b, p *и* r (*см.* il-, im-², ir-) не-, без-; бес-; inorganic неоргани́ческий.

inability [ˌɪnə'bɪlɪtɪ] *n* неспосо́бность; невозмо́жность.

inaccessibility ['ɪnækˌsesə'bɪlɪtɪ] *n* недосту́пность, непристу́пность.

inaccessible [ˌɪnæk'sesəbl] *a* недосту́пный, недосяга́емый, непристу́пный.

inaccuracy [ɪn'ækjurəsɪ] *n* 1) нето́чность; 2) оши́бка.

inaccurate [ın'ækjurıt] *a* 1) неточный; 2) ошибочный.

inaction [ın'ækʃən] *n* бездействие; инертность.

inactive [ın'æktıv] *a* бездеятельный; инертный.

inactivity [ˌınæk'tıvıtı] *n* бездеятельность; инертность.

inadequacy [ın'ædıkwəsı] *n* 1) несоответствие (*чему-л.*); 2) недостаточность.

inadequate [ın'ædıkwıt] *a* 1) не отвечающий требованиям, назначению; 2) недостаточный; 3) непропорциональный; неадекватный.

inadmissible [ˌınəd'mısəbl] *a* недопустимый, неприемлемый.

inadvertence [ˌınəd'vəːtəns] *n* 1) невнимательность; небрежность; 2) оплошность; 3) неумышленность.

inadvertency [ˌınəd'vəːtənsı] *см.* inadvertence.

inadvertent [ˌınəd'vəːtənt] *a* 1) невнимательный; небрежный; 2) неумышленный, нечаянный.

inalienable [ın'eıljənəbl] *a* неотъемлемый.

inalterable [ın'ɔːltərəbl] *a* неизменный, неизменяемый.

inane I [ı'neın] *n* (the ~) пустота, бесконечное пространство.

inane II *a* 1) пустой, бессодержательный; 2) бессмысленный.

inanimate [ın'ænımıt] *a* 1) неодушевлённый; неживой; безжизненный; 2) скучный.

inanimation [ınˌænı'meıʃən] *n* 1) неодушевлённость; 2) безжизненность.

inanity [ı'nænıtı] *n* 1) пустота, бессодержательность; 2) бессмысленность.

inapplicable [ın'æplıkəbl] *a* неприменимый, несоответствующий, неподходящий.

inappreciable [ˌınə'priːʃəbl] *a* 1) незаметный; не принимаемый в расчёт, незначительный; 2) неоценимый, бесценный.

inappreciation [ˌınəˌpriːʃı'eıʃən] *n* недооценка.

inapprehensible [ınˌæprı'hensəbl] *a* непостижимый.

inapproachable [ˌınə'proutʃəbl] *a* недоступный; недостижимый.

inappropriate [ˌınə'prouprııt] *a* неподходящий; несоответствующий; неуместный.

inapt [ın'æpt] *a* 1) неискусный; неспособный; 2) неподходящий.

inaptitude [ın'æptıtjuːd] *n* 1) неспособность; неумение; 2) несоответствие.

inarticulate [ˌınɑː'tıkjulıt] *a* 1) нечленораздельный; невнятный; бессвязный; 2) косноязычный; немой.

inasmuch [ınəz'mʌtʃ] *adv*: ~ as ввиду того, что; так как.

inattention [ˌınə'tenʃən] *n* невнимание; невнимательность.

inattentive [ˌınə'tentıv] *a* невнимательный.

inaudible [ın'ɔːdəbl] *a* неслышный; невнятный.

inaugurate [ı'nɔːgjureıt] *v* 1) торжественно открывать (*памятник, выставку и т. п.*); 2) торжественно вводить в должность *и т. п.*); 3) начинать.

inauguration [ıˌnɔːgju'reıʃən] *n* 1) торжественное открытие; 2) торжественное вступление в должность.

inauspicious [ˌınɔːs'pıʃəs] *a* неблагоприятный, не предвещающий хорошего.

inborn [ın'bɔːn] *a* врождённый.

inbound ['ınbaund] *a* прибывающий, прилетающий из-за границы (*о корабле, самолёте*).

inbreathe ['ın'briːð] *v* вдыхать; *перен.* вдохнуть в кого-л. (*силы, надежду*).

inbred ['ın'bred] *a* 1) врождённый; 2) рождённый от родителей, состоящих в родстве.

incalculable [ın'kælkjuləbl] *a* 1) неисчислимый, несметный; 2) не поддающийся предварительному учёту; 3) ненадёжный (*о человеке*).

incandescence [ˌınkæn'desns] *n* накал, накаливание; белое каление; *перен.* жар, пыл.

incandescent [ˌınkæn'desnt] *a* 1) пылающий, раскалённый, накалённый; 2) ослепительный, сверкающий.

incapability [ınˌkeıpə'bılıtı] *n* неспособность.

incapable [ın'keıpəbl] *a* неспособный (*к, на* — *of*).

incapacitate [ˌınkə'pæsıteıt] *v* 1) сделать неспособным; вывести из строя; 2) *юр.* лишать права; to be ~d from voting лишаться права голоса.

incapacity [ˌınkə'pæsıtı] *n* 1) неспособность (*к* — *for*); 2) *юр.* неправоспособность.

incarnate[a] [ın'kɑːnıt] *a* воплощённый.

incarnate[b] ['ınkɑːneıt] *v* воплощать.

incarnation [ˌınkɑː'neıʃən] *n* воплощение.

incendiarism [ın'sendjərızəm] *n* 1) поджог; 2) подстрекательство.

incendiary I [ın'sendjərı] *n* 1) поджигатель; 2) подстрекатель.

incendiary II *a* 1) поджигающий; 2) подстрекающий; 3) *воен.* зажигательный.

incense[a] I ['ınsens] *n* ладан, фимиам.

incense[a] II *v* кадить; курить фимиам.

incense[b] [ın'sens] *v* сердить, раздражать, приводить в негодование.

incentive I [ın'sentıv] *n* побудительная причина, побуждение.

incentive II *a* побудительный.

inception [ın'sepʃən] *n* 1) начало; 2) получение учёной степени.

inceptive [ın'septıv] *a* 1) начинающий(ся), начальный; 2) *грам.* начинательный.

incertitude [ın'səːtıtjuːd] *n* неуверенность, неопределённость.

incessant [ın'sesnt] *a* непрекращающийся, непрерывный; беспрестанный.

incest ['ınsest] *n* кровосмешение.

inch[1] I [ıntʃ] *n* 1) дюйм (= *2,5 см*); every ~ целиком, с ног до головы; 2) малое количество, малость; безделица; ~ by ~es постепенно, понемножку; мало-помалу; within an ~ of близко, на волосок от; 3) *pl* рост; a man of your ~es человек вашего роста.

inch[1] II *v* медленно двигаться (*тж.* to ~ one's way forward); □ to ~ along *амер. сленг* делать медленные, но верные успехи.

inch[2] *n диал.* (маленький) островок.

inchoate I ['ınkoueıt] *a* 1) зачаточный, рудиментарный; 2) только что начатый.

inchoate II *v* 1) начинать; 2) давать начало, порождать.

incidence ['ınsıdəns] *n* 1) охват; сфера действия; 2) падение, наклон, скос.

incident I ['ınsıdənt] *n* 1) случай, происшествие; инцидент; 2) эпизод (*в поэме, пьесе*).

incident II *a* 1) присущий (*to*); 2) падающий (*о луче, свете и т. п.; upon*).

271

incidental [ˌɪnsɪ'dentl] *a* 1) случа́йный, побо́чный; 2) прису́щий, сопу́тствующий.

incidentally [ˌɪnsɪ'dentlɪ] *adv* случа́йно.

incinerate [ɪn'sɪnəreɪt] *v* сжига́ть; испепеля́ть.

incinerator [ɪn'sɪnəreɪtə] *n* 1) мусоросжига́тельная печь; 2) кремато́рий.

incipient [ɪn'sɪpɪənt] *a* начина́ющийся; нача́льный.

incise [ɪn'saɪz] *v* 1) надреза́ть; вреза́ть; насека́ть; 2) выреза́ть, гравирова́ть.

incision [ɪn'sɪʒən] *n* 1) разре́з, надре́з; насе́чка; 2) *хим.* растворе́ние.

incisive [ɪn'saɪsɪv] *a* 1) ре́жущий; о́стрый; 2) проница́тельный; 3) ко́лкий; ре́зкий; 4) *хим.* растворя́ющий.

incisor [ɪn'saɪzə] *n* резе́ц, пере́дний зуб.

incite [ɪn'saɪt] *v* 1) возбужда́ть; 2) побужда́ть; понужда́ть, подстрека́ть.

incitement [ɪn'saɪtmənt] *n* 1) возбужде́ние; 2) побужде́ние, подстрека́тельство; 3) побуди́тельная причи́на; сти́мул.

incivility [ˌɪnsɪ'vɪlɪtɪ] *n* неве́жливость.

inclement [ɪn'klemənt] *a* суро́вый, холо́дный (*о кли́мате, пого́де*).

inclinable [ɪn'klaɪnəbl] *a* скло́нный, располо́женный (*к чему́-л.— to*).

inclination [ˌɪnklɪ'neɪʃən] *n* 1) накло́н, наклоне́ние; скат; 2) скло́нность, наклонность (*to, for*); 3) отклоне́ние, склоне́ние (*магни́тной стре́лки*).

incline I [ɪn'klaɪn] *n* накло́н; накло́нная пло́скость.

incline I *v* 1) наклоня́ть(ся), склоня́ть(ся); 2) быть скло́нным, располо́женным (*к чему́-л.*).

inclose [ɪn'klouz] *см.* enclose.

inclosure [ɪn'klouʒə] *см.* enclosure.

include [ɪn'kluːd] *v* заключа́ть, содержа́ть (в себе́); включа́ть.

including [ɪn'kluːdɪŋ] *prep* включа́я, в том числе́.

inclusion [ɪn'kluːʒən] *n* включе́ние.

inclusive [ɪn'kluːsɪv] *a* включа́ющий в себя́, содержа́щий; pages 5 to 25 ~ страни́цы от 5 до 25 включи́тельно.

incognito I [ɪn'kɔgnɪtou] *n* инко́гнито.

incognito II *adv* инко́гнито, под чужи́м и́менем.

incognizable [ɪn'kɔgnɪzəbl] *a* непознава́емый.

incoherence [ˌɪnkou'hɪərəns] *n* несвя́зность; бессвя́зность; непосле́довательность.

incoherent [ˌɪnkou'hɪərənt] *a* несвя́зный; бессвя́зный; непосле́довательный.

incombustible [ˌɪnkəm'bʌstəbl] *a* негорю́чий, несгора́емый, огнесто́йкий.

income ['ɪnkəm] *n* дохо́д, прихо́д; за́работок.

incomer ['ɪnˌkʌmə] *n* 1) входя́щий; воше́дший; 2) пришёлец; иммигра́нт; 3) прее́мник.

income-tax ['ɪnkəmtæks] *n* подохо́дный нало́г.

incoming I ['ɪnˌkʌmɪŋ] *n* 1) прибы́тие; *обыкн. pl* дохо́ды.

incoming II *a* 1) прибыва́ющий; 2) сменя́ющий, сле́дующий (*оди́н за други́м*); 3) поступа́ющий (*о платеже́, дохо́де*).

incommensurable [ˌɪnkə'menʃərəbl] *a* 1) несоизмери́мый; несоразме́рный (*с — with*); 2) *мат.* иррациона́льный.

incommensurate [ˌɪnkə'menʃərɪt] *a* несоразме́рный; несоизмери́мый (*с — with, to*).

incommode [ˌɪnkə'moud] *v* беспоко́ить, меша́ть.

incommodious [ˌɪnkə'moudjəs] *a* неудо́бный.

incommunicable [ˌɪnkə'mjuːnɪkəbl] *a* непередава́емый.

incommunicative [ˌɪnkə'mjuːnɪˌkeɪtɪv] *a* необщи́тельный.

incomparable [ɪn'kɔmpərəbl] *a* 1) беспод́обный, несравне́нный; 2) несравни́мый (*с — with, to*).

incompatible [ˌɪnkəm'pætəbl] *a* несовмести́мый.

incompetence [ɪn'kɔmpɪtəns] *n* 1) некомпете́нтность; 2) *юр.* неправоспосо́бность.

incompetent [ɪn'kɔmpɪtənt] *a* 1) некомпете́нтный, несве́дущий; 2) *юр.* неправоспосо́бный.

incomplete [ˌɪnkəm'pliːt] *a* 1) непо́лный; 2) незако́нченный, незавершённый; 3) несоверше́нный.

incomprehensible [ɪnˌkɔmprɪ'hensəbl] *a* непоня́тный, непостижи́мый.

incomprehension [ɪnˌkɔmprɪ'henʃən] *n* непонима́ние.

incompressible [ˌɪnkəm'presəbl] *a* несжима́емый, несжима́ющийся.

incomputable [ˌɪnkəm'pjuːtəbl] *a* бесчи́сленный, неисчисли́мый.

inconceivable [ˌɪnkən'siːvəbl] *a* 1) непостижи́мый, невообрази́мый; 2) *разг.* невероя́тный.

inconclusive [ˌɪnkən'kluːsɪv] *a* неубеди́тельный; нереша́ющий.

incondite [ɪn'kɔndɪt] *a* неотде́ланный (*о лит. произведе́нии и т. п.*).

incongruity [ˌɪnkɔŋ'gruːɪtɪ] *n* 1) несоотве́тствие; несовмести́мость; 2) неле́пость, неуме́стность.

incongruous [ɪn'kɔŋgruəs] *a* 1) несоотве́тственный; несовмести́мый (*with*); 2) неуме́стный, неле́пый.

inconsecutive [ˌɪnkən'sekjutɪv] *a* непосле́довательный.

inconsequence [ɪn'kɔnsɪkwəns] *n* непосле́довательность.

inconsequent [ɪn'kɔnsɪkwənt] *a* непосле́довательный; нелоги́чный.

inconsequential [ɪnˌkɔnsɪ'kwenʃəl] *см.* inconsequent.

inconsiderable [ˌɪnkən'sɪdərəbl] *a* незначи́тельный, нева́жный.

inconsiderate [ˌɪnkən'sɪdərɪt] *a* 1) невнима́тельный, нечу́ткий; 2) необду́манный, неосмотри́тельный, опроме́тчивый.

inconsistent [ˌɪnkən'sɪstənt] *a* 1) несовмести́мый; несообра́зный; 2) противоречи́вый; 3) непостоя́нный, неусто́йчивый.

inconsolable [ˌɪnkən'souləbl] *a* безуте́шный.

inconspicuous [ˌɪnkən'spɪkjuəs] *a* незаме́тный, не броса́ющийся в глаза́, не привлека́ющий внима́ния.

inconstant [ɪn'kɔnstənt] *a* 1) непостоя́нный; изме́нчивый, неусто́йчивый; 2) нерегуля́рный.

incontestable [ˌɪnkən'testəbl] *a* неоспори́мый, неопровержи́мый, бесспо́рный.

incontinence [ɪn'kɔntɪnəns] *n* 1) невоздержа́нность; 2) несде́ржанность.

incontinent [ɪn'kɔntɪnənt] *a* 1) невоздержа́нный; 2) несде́ржанный.

incontinently [ɪn'kɔntɪnəntlɪ] *adv* то́тчас, неме́дленно.

incontrovertible [ˌɪnkɔntrə'vəːtəbl] *a* неоспори́мый, неопровержи́мый, бесспо́рный.

inconvenience [ˌɪnkən'viːnjəns] *n* неудо́бство; to put to ~ затрудня́ть, причиня́ть неудо́бство.

inconvenient [ˌɪnkən'viːnjənt] *a* 1) неудобный; неловкий; беспокойный; 2) неподходящий, неприличный.

inconvertible [ˌɪnkən'vɜːtəbl] *a* 1) не подлежащий обмену (*на золото*); неразменный; 2) необратимый.

inconvincible [ˌɪnkən'vɪnsəbl] *a* не поддающийся убеждению.

incoordination [ˌɪnkouˌɔːdɪ'neɪʃən] *n* несогласованность.

incorporate[a] [ɪn'kɔːpərɪt] *a* соединённый, объединённый.

incorporate[b] [ɪn'kɔːpəreɪt] *v* 1) соединять(ся), объединять(ся); 2) смешивать(ся) (*c — with*); 3) включать в число членов; вводить в состав.

incorporation [ɪnˌkɔːpə'reɪʃən] *n* 1) объединение; 2) корпорация; 3) включение в число членов; введение в состав.

incorporeal [ˌɪnkɔː'pɔːrɪəl] *a* невещественный; бесплотный.

incorrect [ˌɪnkə'rekt] *a* 1) неверный, неправильный; ошибочный; 2) неисправный; 3) некорректный.

incorrigible [ɪn'kɔrɪdʒəbl] *a* неисправимый.

incorruptible [ˌɪnkə'rʌptəbl] *a* 1) неподкупный; 2) непортящийся; 3) нетленный.

increase[a] ['ɪnkriːs] *n* 1) рост, увеличение, возрастание; wage ~ повышение заработной платы; to be on the ~ расти; 2) прирост, прибавление.

increase[b] [ɪn'kriːs] *v* расти, возрастать; увеличивать(ся); повышать(ся).

increasing [ɪn'kriːsɪŋ] *a* возрастающий, увеличивающийся.

increasingly [ɪn'kriːsɪŋlɪ] *adv* всё более и более; во всё возрастающем размере.

incredibility [ɪnˌkredɪ'bɪlɪtɪ] *n* невероятность, неправдоподобие.

incredible [ɪn'kredəbl] *a* невероятный, неправдоподобный.

incredulity [ˌɪnkrɪ'djuːlɪtɪ] *n* недоверчивость.

incredulous [ɪn'kredjuləs] *a* недоверчивый.

increment ['ɪnkrɪmənt] *n* 1) возрастание, увеличение; 2) прирост; прибыль.

incriminate [ɪn'krɪmɪneɪt] *v* обвинять (*в преступлении*), инкриминировать; вменять в вину.

incriminatory [ɪn'krɪmɪnətərɪ] *a* обвинительный.

incrustation [ˌɪnkrʌs'teɪʃən] *n* 1) инкрустация; 2) кора; корка; 3) *тех.* накипь.

incubate ['ɪnkjubeɪt] *v* 1) высиживать, выводить цыплят; сидеть на яйцах; 2) вынашивать (*идею и т. п.*).

incubation [ˌɪnkju'beɪʃən] *n* 1) высиживание, выведение цыплят; 2) *мед.* инкубационный период.

incubator ['ɪnkjubeɪtə] *n* инкубатор.

inculcate ['ɪnkʌlkeɪt] *v* внедрять, внушать (*in, upon*).

inculcation [ˌɪnkʌl'keɪʃən] *n* внедрение, внушение.

inculpate ['ɪnkʌlpeɪt] *v* 1) обвинять; 2) изобличать.

incumbent [ɪn'kʌmbənt] *a* 1) лежащий, давящий (*на — on*); 2) возложенный (*на кого-л.— upon*); обязательный; it is ~ on you to warn them вам надлежит предостеречь их.

incunabula [ˌɪnkjuː'næbjulə] *n pl* инкунабулы, первопечатные книги.

incur [ɪn'kɜː] *v* 1) подвергаться чему-л.; навле-

кать; 2) влезать (*в долги*); 3) нести (*убытки, потери*).

incurability [ɪnˌkjuərə'bɪlɪtɪ] *n* 1) неизлечимость; 2) неискоренимость.

incurable I [ɪn'kjuərəbl] *n* неизлечимый больной.

incurable II *a* 1) неизлечимый; 2) неискоренимый.

incuriosity [ɪnˌkjuərɪ'ɔsɪtɪ] *n* отсутствие любопытства, любознательности.

incurious [ɪn'kjuərɪəs] *a* 1) нелюбопытный, нелюбознательный; 2) невнимательный; 3) неинтересный; not ~ небезынтересный.

incursion [ɪn'kɜːʃən] *n* 1) набег, нападение; 2) вторжение; нашествие.

incurved ['ɪnkɜːvd] *a* вогнутый.

indebted [ɪn'detɪd] *a* 1) должный (*кому-л.*), в долгу (*у кого-л.— to*); 2) обязанный (*кому-л., чему-л.— to; чем-л.— for*).

indebtedness [ɪn'detɪdnɪs] *n* задолженность; долг (*тж. перен.*).

indecency [ɪn'diːsnsɪ] *n* неприличие, непристойность.

indecent [ɪn'diːsnt] *a* неприличный, непристойный; неподобающий.

indecision [ˌɪndɪ'sɪʒən] *n* нерешительность.

indecisive [ˌɪndɪ'saɪsɪv] *a* 1) нерешительный; 2) нерешающий; 3) неопределённый, нерешённый, неясный.

indeclinable [ˌɪndɪ'klaɪnəbl] *a грам.* несклоняемый.

indecorous [ɪn'dekərəs] *a* неприличный, неблагопристойный; дурного вкуса.

indecorum [ˌɪndɪ'kɔːrəm] *n* нарушение приличий.

indeed [ɪn'diːd] *adv* 1) действительно, в самом деле; he was ~ a remarkable man он был действительно замечательным человеком; who is this comrade X? — Who is he, ~? кто этот товарищ X? — Кто он, в самом деле?; 2) в самом деле?, неужели?; 3) *служит для усиления*: this is quick work, ~! вот это быстро сделано!; yes, ~! ну да!, да, конечно!; по, ~! конечно, нет!

indefatigable [ˌɪndɪ'fætɪgəbl] *a* неутомимый, неослабный.

indefeasible [ˌɪndɪ'fiːzəbl] *a* неотъемлемый; непреложный, нерушимый.

indefinable [ˌɪndɪ'faɪnəbl] *a* неопределённый.

indefinite [ɪn'defɪnɪt] *a* 1) неопределённый; 2) неограниченный.

indelible [ɪn'delɪbl] *a* несмываемый, нестираемый; неизгладимый.

indelicacy [ɪn'delɪkəsɪ] *n* неделикатность, нескромность, бестактность.

indelicate [ɪn'delɪkɪt] *a* неделикатный, нескромный, бестактный.

indemnify [ɪn'demnɪfaɪ] *v* 1) обезопасить, застраховать (*от — from, against*); 2) возмещать, компенсировать (*за — for*); 3) освободить от наказания (*за — for*).

indemnity [ɪn'demnɪtɪ] *n* 1) гарантия от ущерба, потерь; 2) возмещение, компенсация; 3) контрибуция.

indent I [ɪn'dent] *n* 1) зубец, вырез; выемка; 2) *полигр.* абзац, отступ; 3) клеймо; отпечаток; 4) письменное требование, заявка; заказ.

indent II *v* 1) зазубривать, выдалбливать, вырезать, насекать (*зубцами*); 2) *полигр.* делать абзац, о́тступ; 3) реквизи́ровать; 4) предъявля́ть о́рдер, тре́бование (кому́-л.— иро́п; на что-л.— for).

indentation [ˌindenˈteiʃən] n 1) зубе́ц, вы́рез; 2) полигр. абза́ц, о́тступ; 3) изви́лина, углубле́ние (берега).

indented [inˈdentid] a зубча́тый; зазу́бренный.

indention [inˈdenʃən] см. indentation.

indenture [inˈdentʃə] n пи́сьменный догово́р, контра́кт.

independence [ˌindiˈpendəns] n незави́симость, самостоя́тельность.

independent [ˌindiˈpendənt] a незави́симый, самостоя́тельный.

indescribable [ˌindisˈkraibəbl] a неопису́емый.

indestructible [ˌindisˈtrʌktəbl] a неразруши́мый, неруши́мый.

indeterminable [ˌindiˈtəːminəbl] a неопредели́мый.

indeterminate [ˌindiˈtəːminit] a 1) неопределённый, нея́сный; 2) нерешённый.

indetermination [ˈindiˌtəːmiˈneiʃən] n 1) неопределённость; 2) нереши́тельность.

index I [ˈindeks] n (pl тж. indices) 1) и́ндекс; 2) (алфави́тный) указа́тель; 3) стре́лка; 4) указа́тельный па́лец (тж. ~ finger); 5) мат. показа́тель сте́пени.

index II v 1) снабжа́ть указа́телем; 2) заноси́ть в указа́тель.

Indiaman [ˈindjəmæn] n торго́вое су́дно Ост-и́ндской компа́нии.

Indian I [ˈindjən] n 1) инди́ец; индиа́нка; the ~s инди́йцы; 2) индее́ц; the ~s инде́йцы; Red ~ красноко́жий индее́ц; 3) европе́ец, до́лго жи́вший в Инди́и.

Indian II a 1) инди́йский; 2) инде́йский.

india-rubber [ˈindjəˈrʌbə] n 1) каучу́к, рези́на; 2) рези́нка для стира́ния, ла́стик; 3) attr рези́новый.

indicate [ˈindikeit] v 1) ука́зывать, пока́зывать; означа́ть; 2) обознача́ть; 3) мед. тре́бовать (лече́ния и т. п.); предпи́сывать; 4) тех. измеря́ть мо́щность (маши́ны) индика́тором.

indicated [ˈindikeitid] a тех. индика́торный.

indication [ˌindiˈkeiʃən] n 1) указа́ние, показа́ние (прибора); 2) приме́та, симпто́м, знак.

indicative I [inˈdikətiv] n грам. изъяви́тельное наклоне́ние.

indicative II a 1) ука́зывающий, пока́зывающий (на — of); 2) грам. изъяви́тельный.

indicator [ˈindikeitə] n 1) индика́тор; указа́тель; 2) счётчик; 3) стре́лка цифербла́та.

indicatory [inˈdikətəri] a указа́тельный, ука́зывающий.

indices [ˈindisiːz] pl см. index I.

indict [inˈdait] v предъявля́ть обвине́ние.

indictable [inˈdaitəbl] a подлежа́щий суде́бному пресле́дованию.

indictment [inˈdaitmənt] n обвини́тельный акт; to bring in an ~ обвини́ть в чём-л.

indifference [inˈdifrəns] n 1) равноду́шие; безразли́чие; 2) незначи́тельность, малова́жность.

indifferent [inˈdifrənt] a 1) равноду́шный; безразли́чный; 2) беспристра́стный; 3) посре́дственный; нева́жный, незначи́тельный; 4) хим., эл. нейтра́льный.

indigence [ˈindidʒəns] n нужда́, бе́дность.

indigene [ˈindidʒiːn] n тузе́мец; ме́стный жи́тель.

indigenous [inˈdidʒinəs] a тузе́мный; ме́стный; приро́дный.

indigent [ˈindidʒənt] a нужда́ющийся, бе́дный.

indigested [ˌindiˈdʒestid] a 1) непереваренный (желудком); 2) непроду́манный, нея́сный.

indigestible [ˌindiˈdʒestibl] a неудобовари́мый.

indigestion [ˌindiˈdʒestʃən] n расстро́йство, несваре́ние желу́дка.

indignant [inˈdignənt] a негоду́ющий, возмущённый.

indignation [ˌindigˈneiʃən] n негодова́ние, возмуще́ние.

indignity [inˈdigniti] n пренебреже́ние, неуваже́ние.

indirect [ˌindiˈrekt] a 1) непрямо́й; око́льный (о пути); укло́нчивый (об ответе); 2) ко́свенный (тж. грам.); 3) побо́чный.

indiscernible [ˌindiˈsəːnəbl] a незаме́тный, неразличи́мый.

indiscreet [ˌindisˈkriːt] a 1) неблагоразу́мный; 2) необду́манный, неосторо́жный; 3) нескро́мный.

indiscrete [inˈdiskriːt] a неразделённый, нерасчленённый.

indiscretion [ˌindisˈkreʃən] n 1) неосторо́жность, опроме́тчивость; 2) нескро́мность; 3) невежливость.

indiscriminate [ˌindisˈkriminit] a 1) неразбо́рчивый; 2) сме́шанный, беспоря́дочный.

indiscrimination [ˈindisˌkriмиˈneiʃən] n неразбо́рчивость.

indispensable [ˌindisˈpensəbl] a 1) необходи́мый; 2) обяза́тельный (о правиле и т. п.).

indispose [ˌindisˈpouz] v 1) вызыва́ть недомога́ние; to be ~d быть нездоро́вым; 2) де́лать неприго́дным, неспосо́бным (к чему-л.— for); 3) отвраща́ть (от), восстана́вливать (против — towards, from).

indisposition [ˌindispəˈziʃən] n 1) недомога́ние, нездоро́вье; 2) нерасположе́ние, нежела́ние; 3) отвраще́ние (to, towards).

indisputable [ˌindisˈpjuːtəbl] a неоспори́мый, бесспо́рный.

indissoluble [ˌindiˈsɔljubl] a 1) неразры́вный, нерасторжи́мый; 2) хим. нераствори́мый, неразложи́мый.

indistinct [ˌindisˈtiŋkt] a 1) нея́сный, сму́тный; неотчётливый; 2) невня́тный.

indistinctive [ˌindisˈtiŋktiv] a нехаракте́рный, нетипи́чный.

indistinguishable [ˌindisˈtiŋgwiʃəbl] a неразличи́мый.

indivertible [ˌindiˈvəːtibl] a неотврати́мый.

individual I [ˌindiˈvidjual] n 1) отде́льное лицо́, индиви́дуум; ли́чность; 2) о́собь.

individual II a 1) индивидуа́льный, ли́чный; 2) характерный, осо́бенный; 3) отде́льный, ча́стный; едини́чный; одино́чный.

individualism [ˌindiˈvidjuəlizəm] n индивидуали́зм.

individualist [ˌindiˈvidjuəlist] n индивидуали́ст.

individuality [ˌindiˌvidjuˈæliti] n индивидуа́льность.

individualization [ˌindiˌvidjuəlaiˈzeiʃən] n обособле́ние, индивидуализа́ция.

individualize [ˌindiˈvidjuəlaiz] v 1) придава́ть

индивидуа́льный хара́ктер; 2) то́чно, дета́льно определя́ть, устана́вливать.

individually [ˌɪndɪˈvɪdjuəlɪ] *adv* обосо́бленно; в отде́льности.

indivisibility [ˈɪndɪˌvɪzɪˈbɪlɪtɪ] *n* недели́мость.

indivisible I [ˌɪndɪˈvɪzəbl] *n* бесконе́чно ма́лая, недели́мая часть, величина́.

indivisible II *a* недели́мый, бесконе́чно ма́лый.

Indo-Chinese [ˈɪndoutʃaɪˈniːz] *a* индокита́йский.

indocile [ɪnˈdousaɪl] *a* непоко́рный, непослу́шный.

indoctrinate [ɪnˈdɔktrɪneɪt] *v* 1) обуча́ть, инструкти́ровать; 2) внедря́ть, внуша́ть (*идеи; with*).

Indo-European [ˈɪndouˌjuərəˈpiːən] *a* индоевропе́йский.

indolence [ˈɪndələns] *n* ле́ность, пра́здность.

indolent [ˈɪndələnt] *a* 1) лени́вый, пра́здный; 2) *мед.* безболе́зненный.

indomitable [ɪnˈdɔmɪtəbl] *a* неукроти́мый; упо́рный, упря́мый.

Indonesian I [ˌɪndouˈniːʒən] *n* индонези́ец; индонези́йка; the ~s индонези́йцы.

Indonesian II *a* индонези́йский.

indoor [ˈɪndɔː] *a* ко́мнатный, в закры́том помеще́нии; кла́ссный (*о занятиях, обучении*).

indoors [ˈɪnˈdɔːz] *adv* (внутри́) до́ма, в помеще́нии; to stay ~ не выходи́ть, остава́ться до́ма.

indorsation [ˌɪndɔːˈseɪʃən] *см.* endorsement.

indorse [ɪnˈdɔːs] *см.* endorse.

indorsee [ˌɪndɔːˈsiː] *n* ком. индосса́т.

indorsement [ɪnˈdɔːsmənt] *см.* endorsement.

indraft [ˈɪndrɑːft] *см.* indraught.

indraught [ˈɪndrɑːft] *n* прито́к (*воздуха, воды и т. п.*).

indubitable [ɪnˈdjuːbɪtəbl] *a* несомне́нный.

induce [ɪnˈdjuːs] *v* 1) побужда́ть, заставля́ть; 2) вызыва́ть; стимули́ровать; 3) *эл.* индукти́ровать.

inducement [ɪnˈdjuːsmənt] *n* побужде́ние; побуди́тельная причи́на, сти́мул.

induct [ɪnˈdʌkt] *v* 1) устра́ивать, водворя́ть (*into*); 2) зачисля́ть, официа́льно вводи́ть в до́лжность; *амер. воен.* зачисля́ть на слу́жбу; 3) вводи́ть, посвяща́ть; 4) *эл.* индукти́ровать.

inductee [ˌɪndʌkˈtiː] *n* амер. новобра́нец.

induction [ɪnˈdʌkʃən] *n* 1) вступле́ние, введе́ние; 2) официа́льное введе́ние в до́лжность; *амер. воен.* зачисле́ние на слу́жбу; 3) *лог.* инду́кция; 4) *attr* индукцио́нный; 5) *attr амер.* призывно́й.

inductive [ɪnˈdʌktɪv] *a* 1) *лог.* индукти́вный; 2) *эл.* индукцио́нный; 3) вса́сывающий.

inductor [ɪnˈdʌktə] *n* инду́ктор.

indue [ɪnˈdjuː] *см.* endue.

indulge [ɪnˈdʌldʒ] *v* 1) предава́ться (*чему-л.— in*); позволя́ть себе́ (удово́льствие); to ~ in rowing увлека́ться гре́блей; 2) потво́рствовать, балова́ть; 3) доставля́ть удово́льствие.

indulgence [ɪnˈdʌldʒəns] *n* 1) снисхожде́ние, снисходи́тельность; терпи́мость; 2) потво́рство, потака́ние (*свои́м сла́бостям*); 3) льго́та; привиле́гия; ми́лость; 4) отсро́чка (*платежа*); 5) *церк.* индульге́нция.

indulgent [ɪnˈdʌldʒənt] *a* 1) снисходи́тельный; терпи́мый; 2) потво́рствующий.

indurate [ˈɪndjuəreɪt] *v* 1) де́лать(ся) твёрдым; затвердева́ть; 2) де́латься бесчу́вственным; черстве́ть.

induration [ˌɪndjuəˈreɪʃən] *n* 1) затвердо́ние; 2) огрубе́ние, чёрствость.

industrial I [ɪnˈdʌstrɪəl] *n* 1) промы́шленник; 2) *pl* а́кции промы́шленных предприя́тий.

industrial II *a* 1) индустриа́льный, промы́шленный; 2) произво́дственный.

industrialist [ɪnˈdʌstrɪəlɪst] *n* промы́шленник.

industrialization [ɪnˌdʌstrɪəlaɪˈzeɪʃən] *n* индустриализа́ция.

industrious [ɪnˈdʌstrɪəs] *a* трудолюби́вый, усе́рдный, приле́жный.

industry [ˈɪndəstrɪ] *n* 1) промы́шленность, индустри́я; home (large-scale, light, foodstuff) ~ оте́чественная (кру́пная, лёгкая, пищева́я) промы́шленность; basic ~, heavy ~ тяжёлая промы́шленность; domestic ~, handicraft ~ куста́рная промы́шленность; 2) прилежа́ние.

indwell [ˈɪnˈdwel] *v* (*past, p. p.* indwelt) жить, постоя́нно пребыва́ть.

indweller [ˈɪnˈdwelə] *n* жи́тель, обита́тель.

indwelt [ˈɪnˈdwelt] *past, p. p. см.* indwell.

inebriate[a] I [ɪˈniːbrɪɪt] *n* пья́ница.

inebriate[a] II *a* пья́ный, опьяне́вший.

inebriate[b] [ɪˈniːbrɪeɪt] *v* опьяня́ть, пьяни́ть.

inedibility [ɪnˌedɪˈbɪlɪtɪ] *n* несъедо́бность.

inedible [ɪnˈedɪbl] *a* несъедо́бный.

inedited [ɪnˈedɪtɪd] *a* неи́зданный.

ineffable [ɪnˈefəbl] *a* несказа́нный.

ineffaceable [ˌɪnɪˈfeɪsəbl] *a* неизглади́мый.

ineffective [ˌɪnɪˈfektɪv] *a* 1) недействи́тельный, безрезульта́тный; не даю́щий эффе́кта; не достига́ющий це́ли; 2) неспосо́бный, неуме́лый.

ineffectual [ˌɪnɪˈfektʃuəl] *a* беспло́дный, безрезульта́тный.

inefficacious [ˌɪnefɪˈkeɪʃəs] *a* недействи́тельный, неэффекти́вный.

inefficiency [ˌɪnɪˈfɪʃənsɪ] *n* 1) неспосо́бность; неуме́лость; 2) безрезульта́тность, неэффекти́вность.

inefficient [ˌɪnɪˈfɪʃənt] *a* 1) неспосо́бный; неуме́лый; 2) неквалифици́рованный; 3) безрезульта́тный; неэффекти́вный; непроизводи́тельный.

inelegant [ɪnˈelɪgənt] *a* неизя́щный, безвку́сный.

ineligible [ɪnˈelɪdʒəbl] *a* 1) неподходя́щий, него́дный; 2) не могу́щий быть и́збранным.

inept [ɪˈnept] *a* 1) неподходя́щий, неуме́стный; 2) глу́пый.

ineptitude [ɪˈneptɪtjuːd] *n* 1) неуме́стность; 2) неспосо́бность, неуме́лость; глу́пость.

inequality [ˌɪniːˈkwɔlɪtɪ] *n* 1) нера́венство; 2) ра́зница, разли́чие; 3) неро́вность (*пове́рхности*).

inequilateral [ˌɪnɪkwɪˈlætərəl] *a* неравносторо́нний.

inequitable [ɪnˈekwɪtəbl] *a* несправедли́вый.

inequity [ɪnˈekwɪtɪ] *n* несправедли́вость.

ineradicable [ˌɪnɪˈrædɪkəbl] *a* неискорени́мый.

inerrable [ɪnˈerəbl] *a* непогреши́мый.

inerrancy [ɪnˈerənsɪ] *n* непогреши́мость.

inert [ɪˈnəːt] *a* 1) ине́ртный; 2) вя́лый, бездея́тельный.

inertia [ɪˈnəːʃjə] *n* 1) *физ.* ине́рция, си́ла ине́рции; 2) вя́лость; ине́ртность.

inessential [ˈɪnɪˈsenʃəl] *a* несуще́ственный.

inestimable [ɪnˈestɪməbl] *a* неоцени́мый.

inevitability [ɪnˌevɪtəˈbɪlɪtɪ] *n* неизбе́жность.

inevitable [ɪnˈevɪtəbl] *a* 1) неизбе́жный, неминуе́мый; 2) *разг.* неизме́нный.

inexact [ˌɪnɪgˈzækt] *a* неточный.

inexactitude [ˌɪnɪgˈzæktɪtjuːd] *n* неточность.

inexcusable [ˌɪnɪksˈkjuːzəbl] *a* непростительный.

inexhaustible [ˌɪnɪgˈzɔːstəbl] *a* 1) неисчерпаемый, неистощимый; 2) неутомимый.

inexorable [ɪnˈeksərəbl] *a* безжалостный, неумолимый; непреклонный.

inexpedient [ˌɪnɪksˈpiːdjənt] *a* нецелесообразный, невыгодный; несоответствующий (*обстоятельствам*).

inexpensive [ˌɪnɪksˈpensɪv] *a* недорогой, дешёвый.

inexperience [ˌɪnɪksˈpɪərɪəns] *n* неопытность.

inexperienced [ˌɪnɪksˈpɪərɪənst] *a* неопытный.

inexpert [ˌɪneksˈpəːt] *a* 1) неумелый, неискусный; 2) несведущий, неопытный.

inexpiable [ɪnˈekspɪəbl] *a* 1) неискупимый (*о вине*); 2) неумолимый.

inexplicable [ɪnˈeksplɪkəbl] *a* необъяснимый.

inexplicit [ˌɪnɪksˈplɪsɪt] *a* неясный, неопределённый.

inexpressible [ˌɪnɪksˈpresəbl] *a* невыразимый.

inexpressibles [ˌɪnɪksˈpresəblz] *n pl* *шутл.* штаны, «невыразимые».

inexpressive [ˌɪnɪksˈpresɪv] *a* невыразительный.

inextinguishable [ˌɪnɪksˈtɪŋgwɪʃəbl] *a* неугасимый.

inextricable [ɪnˈekstrɪkəbl] *a* сложный, запутанный, неразрешимый, безвыходный.

infallibility [ɪnˌfælɪˈbɪlɪtɪ] *n* непогрешимость.

infallible [ɪnˈfæləbl] *a* 1) непогрешимый; 2) верный, безошибочный.

infamous [ˈɪnfəməs] *a* 1) позорный, постыдный; 2) бесчестный, низкий.

infamy [ˈɪnfəmɪ] *n* 1) позор, бесчестие; 2) позорное, бесчестное поведение; 3) низость.

infancy [ˈɪnfənsɪ] *n* 1) младенчество; 2) *юр.* несовершеннолетие.

infant I [ˈɪnfənt] *n* 1) младенец, ребёнок; 2) *юр.* несовершеннолетний.

infant II *a* детский, младенческий.

infanticide [ɪnˈfæntɪsaɪd] *n* 1) детоубийство; 2) детоубийца.

infantile [ˈɪnfəntaɪl] *a* 1) младенческий, детский; 2) начальный, в начальной стадии.

infantine [ˈɪnfəntaɪn] *см.* infantile.

infantry [ˈɪnfəntrɪ] *n* 1) пехота; 2) *attr* пехотный.

infantryman [ˈɪnfəntrɪmən] *n* пехотинец.

infatuate [ɪnˈfætjueɪt] *v* увлекать, кружить голову.

infatuation [ɪnˌfætjuˈeɪʃən] *n* 1) слепое увлечение; ослепление; 2) влюблённость.

infect [ɪnˈfekt] *v* заражать.

infectible [ɪnˈfektəbl] *a* подверженный заразе, восприимчивый к заразе.

infection [ɪnˈfekʃən] *n* 1) заражение; 2) инфекция, зараза; 3) заразительность.

infectious [ɪnˈfekʃəs] *a* 1) инфекционный, заразный; 2) заразительный.

infective [ɪnˈfektɪv] *см.* infectious.

infer [ɪnˈfəː] *v* 1) заключать, выводить; 2) значить; подразумевать.

inference [ˈɪnfərəns] *n* вывод, заключение.

inferior I [ɪnˈfɪərɪə] *n* подчинённое лицо, подчинённый.

inferior II *a* 1) низший (*по положению, чину*); 2) плохой, низкого качества; 3) нижний.

inferiority [ɪnˌfɪərɪˈɔrɪtɪ] *n* более низкое положение, качество.

infernal [ɪnˈfəːnl] *a* 1) адский; 2) дьявольский.

inferno [ɪnˈfəːnou] *n* ад, преисподняя.

infertile [ɪnˈfəːtaɪl] *a* бесплодный; неплодородный.

infertility [ˌɪnfəˈtɪlɪtɪ] *n* бесплодие; неплодородие.

infest [ɪnˈfest] *v* нападать; заполнять; кишеть.

infidelity [ˌɪnfɪˈdelɪtɪ] *n* 1) неверность, измена; conjugal ~ супружеская измена; 2) неверие.

infiltrate [ˈɪnfɪltreɪt] *v* 1) просачиваться, проникать; 2) фильтровать.

infiltration [ˌɪnfɪlˈtreɪʃən] *n* 1) просачивание, проникновение (*жидкости и т. п.*); 2) *мед.* инфильтрация; инфильтрат.

infinite I [ˈɪnfɪnɪt] *n*: the ~ бесконечное пространство; the Infinite бог.

infinite II *a* 1) бесконечный; безграничный; 2) несметный; 3) *грам.* неопределённый (*о глаголе*).

infinitesimal I [ˌɪnfɪnɪˈtesɪməl] *n* бесконечно малая величина.

infinitesimal II *a* бесконечно малый.

infinitive I [ɪnˈfɪnɪtɪv] *n* *грам.* неопределённая форма глагола, инфинитив; split ~ неопределённая форма глагола с отделённой от него частицей to (*напр.*: no one claims to completely understand it никто не утверждает, что вполне понимает это).

infinitive II *a* *грам.* неопределённый.

infinity [ɪnˈfɪnɪtɪ] *n* бесконечность; безграничность.

infirm [ɪnˈfəːm] *a* 1) немощный, дряхлый; 2) слабый, нерешительный.

infirmary [ɪnˈfəːmərɪ] *n* госпиталь, лазарет.

infirmity [ɪnˈfəːmɪtɪ] *n* 1) немощность, дряхлость; 2) физический *или* моральный недостаток; 3) слабохарактерность; ~ of purpose слабость воли.

inflame [ɪnˈfleɪm] *v* 1) зажигать(ся), воспламенять(ся), вспыхивать; 2) *мед.* воспаляться.

inflammable I [ɪnˈflæməbl] *n* легковоспламеняющееся вещество.

inflammable II *a* 1) воспламеняющийся, воспламеняемый; 2) легко возбуждающийся, возбудимый.

inflammation [ˌɪnfləˈmeɪʃən] *n* 1) воспламенение; 2) *мед.* воспаление.

inflammatory [ɪnˈflæmətərɪ] *a* 1) возбуждающий; 2) *мед.* воспалительный.

inflate [ɪnˈfleɪt] *v* 1) надувать; наполнять газом, воздухом; 2) наполнять (*важностью, гордостью*; *with*); 3) вздувать цены; 4) *эк.* производить инфляцию.

inflated [ɪnˈfleɪtɪd] *a* надутый, напыщенный.

inflation [ɪnˈfleɪʃən] *n* 1) надувание; наполнение газом; 2) вздутие; 3) *эк.* инфляция.

inflect [ɪnˈflekt] *v* 1) сгибать; 2) *грам.* изменять окончание слова; склонять; спрягать; 3) *муз.* модулировать.

inflection [ɪnˈflekʃən] *см.* inflexion.

inflective [ɪnˈflektɪv] *a* *грам.* изменяемый; склоняемый; спрягаемый.

inflexible [ɪnˈfleksəbl] *a* негнущийся, несгибаемый, негибкий; *перен.* непреклонный; суровый.

inflexion [ɪnˈflekʃən] *n* 1) сгибание; 2) *грам.* флексия; 3) *муз.* модуляция.

inflexional [ɪnˈflekʃənl] *a лингв.* изменяющий окончание; флективный.

inflict [ɪnˈflɪkt] *v* 1) наносить (*удар, ущерб и т. п.*); 2) причинять (*боль, горе и т. п.*); 3) налагать (*взыскание*).

inflow [ˈɪnflou] *n* 1) впадение; 2) приток, наплыв.

inflowing I [ˈɪnflouɪŋ] *n* впадение.

inflowing II *a* впадающий, втекающий.

influence I [ˈɪnfluəns] *n* влияние, (воз)действие (*на — upon, over, with*).

influence II *v* (по)влиять, воздействовать.

influent I [ˈɪnfluənt] *n* приток (*реки*).

influent II *a* втекающий, впадающий.

influential [ˌɪnfluˈenʃəl] *a* влиятельный.

influenza [ˌɪnfluˈenzə] *n мед.* инфлюэнца, грипп.

influx [ˈɪnflʌks] *n* 1) впадение (*в реку*); 2) приток, наплыв.

inform [ɪnˈfɔːm] *v* 1) сообщать, информировать, уведомлять; 2) осведомлять; 2) наполнять (*воодушевлением и т. п.*); 3) обвинять; подавать в суд (*на кого-л.— against*).

informal [ɪnˈfɔːml] *a* 1) неофициальный, неформальный; 2) разговорный (*о стиле*).

informality [ˌɪnfɔːˈmælɪtɪ] *n* отступление от формы; несоблюдение формальностей, церемоний.

informant [ɪnˈfɔːmənt] *n* осведомитель; доносчик.

information [ˌɪnfəˈmeɪʃən] *n* 1) сообщение, информация; 2) известия, новости; 3) знание, осведомлённость; 4) *юр.* обвинение, жалоба; 5) *attr* информационный.

informative [ɪnˈfɔːmətɪv] *a* 1) информационный; 2) поучительный.

informed [ɪnˈfɔːmd] *a* 1) знающий; образованный; 2) осведомлённый.

informer [ɪnˈfɔːmə] *n* 1) сообщающий, осведомляющий; 2) осведомитель; доносчик.

infraction [ɪnˈfrækʃən] *n* нарушение.

infra-red [ˈɪnfrəˈred] *a физ.* инфракрасный.

infrasonic [ˈɪnfrəˈsɔnɪk] *a физ.* ультразвуковой.

infrequent [ɪnˈfriːkwənt] *a* редкий, нечастый.

infringe [ɪnˈfrɪndʒ] *v* нарушать (*закон, обещание и т. п.*).

infuriate [ɪnˈfjuərɪeɪt] *v* приводить в ярость, в бешенство.

infuse [ɪnˈfjuːz] *v* 1) вливать (*into*); *перен.* возбуждать, вселять (*надежду и т. п.; into*); 2) настаивать (*чай, травы*).

infusion [ɪnˈfjuːʒən] *n* 1) вливание; *перен.* внушение, вселение (*надежды и т. п.*); 2) настой; 3) примесь.

infusoria [ˌɪnfjuːˈzɔːrɪə] *n pl зоол.* инфузории.

ingathering [ˈɪnˌgæðərɪŋ] *n* сбор урожая.

ingenious [ɪnˈdʒiːnjəs] *a* изобретательный; остроумный.

ingenuity [ˌɪndʒɪˈnjuːɪtɪ] *n* изобретательность; остроумие.

ingenuous [ɪnˈdʒenjuəs] *a* 1) открытый, чистосердечный; 2) бесхитростный, простой.

ingest [ɪnˈdʒest] *v* проглатывать.

inglorious [ɪnˈglɔːrɪəs] *a* бесславный, позорный.

ingoing I [ˈɪnˌgouɪŋ] *n редк.* 1) вхождение, вступление; 2) плата за оборудование и ремонт арендуемого помещения, взимаемая вперёд.

ingoing II *a* входящий, вступающий.

ingot [ˈɪŋgət] *n* слиток, брусок.

ingraft [ɪnˈgrɑːft] *v бот.* прививать (*тж. перен.*).

ingrained [ɪnˈgreɪnd] *a* 1) укоренившийся; застарелый; 2) проникший, впитавшийся; 3) *геол.* вкрапленный.

ingrate [ɪnˈgreɪt] *a* неблагодарный.

ingratiate [ɪnˈgreɪʃɪeɪt] *v* стараться понравиться; to ~ oneself with smb. снискать чьё-л. расположение.

ingratitude [ɪnˈgrætɪtjuːd] *n* неблагодарность.

ingredient [ɪnˈgriːdjənt] *n* составная часть, ингредиент.

ingress [ˈɪngres] *n* 1) вход, доступ; 2) право входа, доступа.

ingulf [ɪnˈgʌlf] *см.* engulf.

inhabit [ɪnˈhæbɪt] *v* населять; жить, проживать (*где-л.*).

inhabitant [ɪnˈhæbɪtənt] *n* житель; обитатель; жилец (*дома*).

inhalation [ˌɪnhəˈleɪʃən] *n* 1) вдыхание; 2) *мед.* ингаляция.

inhale [ɪnˈheɪl] *v* 1) вдыхать; 2) затягиваться (*при курении*).

inhaler [ɪnˈheɪlə] *n* 1) *мед.* ингалятор; 2) респиратор.

inhere [ɪnˈhɪə] *v* 1) быть присущим (*кому-л., чему-л.— in*); 2) принадлежать (*о правах*).

inherent [ɪnˈhɪərənt] *a* присущий; неотъемлемый.

inherit [ɪnˈherɪt] *v* (у)наследовать.

inheritable [ɪnˈherɪtəbl] *a* 1) наследственный; 2) имеющий права на наследство.

inheritance [ɪnˈherɪtəns] *n* 1) (у)наследование; 2) наследство; 3) наследственность.

inheritor [ɪnˈherɪtə] *n* наследник.

inhibit [ɪnˈhɪbɪt] *v* 1) сдерживать; *физиол.* задерживать, тормозить.

inhibited [ɪnˈhɪbɪtɪd] *a* сдержанный; замкнутый.

inhibition [ˌɪnhɪˈbɪʃən] *n* 1) сдерживание, подавление; 2) *физиол.* задерживание, торможение.

inhospitable [ɪnˈhɔspɪtəbl] *a* негостеприимный.

inhospitality [ˈɪnˌhɔspɪˈtælɪtɪ] *n* негостеприимство.

inhuman [ɪnˈhjuːmən] *a* 1) бесчеловечный; 2) не свойственный человеку; нечеловеческий.

inhumanity [ˌɪnhjuːˈmænɪtɪ] *n* бесчеловечность, жестокость.

inimical [ɪˈnɪmɪkəl] *a* 1) враждебный, неприязненный (*to*); 2) вредный (*to*).

inimitable [ɪˈnɪmɪtəbl] *a* неподражаемый.

iniquitous [ɪˈnɪkwɪtəs] *a* 1) несправедливый; 2) беззаконный.

iniquity [ɪˈnɪkwɪtɪ] *n* 1) большая несправедливость; 2) беззаконие; зло.

initial I [ɪˈnɪʃəl] *a* (перво)начальный.

initial II *v* ставить инициалы.

initials [ɪˈnɪʃəlz] *n pl* инициалы.

initiate^a [ɪ'nɪʃɪɪt] *a* 1) посвящённый (*в тайну*); 2) принятый (*в общество*).

initiate^b [ɪ'nɪʃɪeɪt] *v* 1) начинать, приступать (*к чему-л.*); быть инициатором (*чего-л.*); 2) посвящать (*в тайну; in*); 3) принимать, вводить (*в общество; into*).

initiation [ɪ,nɪʃɪ'eɪʃən] *n* 1) посвящение (*в тайну*); 2) принятие, введение (*в общество*); 3) *attr* вступительный (*о членском взносе*).

initiative I [ɪ'nɪʃɪətɪv] *n* инициатива; to take the ~ взять инициативу.

initiative II *a* начальный.

inject [ɪn'dʒekt] *v* 1) впрыскивать, вводить (*в — into*); 2) *амер.* вставлять (*замечание и т. п.*).

injection [ɪn'dʒekʃən] *n* 1) инъекция, впрыскивание; 2) лекарство для впрыскивания.

injudicious [,ɪndʒuː'dɪʃəs] *a* необдуманный, неблагоразумный.

injunction [ɪn'dʒʌŋkʃən] *n* 1) приказание; 2) (судебное) предписание *или* запрещение (*чего-л.*).

injure ['ɪndʒə] *v* 1) портить, вредить; повреждать; 2) обижать; 3) ушибать, ранить.

injurious [ɪn'dʒuərɪəs] *a* 1) несправедливый; 2) оскорбительный; 3) вредный.

injury ['ɪndʒərɪ] *n* 1) вред; повреждение; 2) ранение; ушиб; 3) несправедливость; оскорбление; обида.

injustice [ɪn'dʒʌstɪs] *n* несправедливость; you do him an ~ вы несправедливы к нему.

ink I [ɪŋk] *n* 1) чернила; India (n) ~ китайская тушь; 2) типографская краска (*тж.* printer's ~).

ink II *v* пачкать, мазать чернилами, краской.

ink-jerker ['ɪŋk,dʒəːkə] *амер. см.* ink-slinger.

inkling ['ɪŋklɪŋ] *n* намёк; лёгкое подозрение (*of*).

ink-slinger ['ɪŋk,slɪŋə] *n презр.* писака.

inkstand ['ɪŋkstænd] *n* чернильница; письменный прибор.

ink-well ['ɪŋkwel] *n* чернильница (*вделанная в стол или парту*).

inky ['ɪŋkɪ] *a* 1) испачканный чернилами, в чернилах; 2) чернильный; 3) чёрный.

inlaid I ['ɪn'leɪd] *past, p. p. см.* inlay^b.

inlaid II *a* мозаичный, инкрустированный.

inland^a ['ɪnlənd] *n* внутренняя территория страны (*удалённая от моря или границ*).

inland II *a* 1) расположенный внутри страны; 2) внутренний.

inland^b [ɪn'lænd] *adv* внутрь, внутри страны.

in-law ['ɪnlɔː] *n обыкн. pl* родственник со стороны мужа *или* жены.

inlay^a ['ɪnleɪ] *n* инкрустация, мозаика.

inlay^b ['ɪn'leɪ] *v* (*past, p. p.* inlaid) 1) покрывать инкрустацией, мозаикой; 2) вставлять; выкладывать, выстилать.

inlet ['ɪnlet] *n* 1) небольшой залив, бухта; 2) *тех.* впуск, впускное отверстие; 3) *эл.* ввод; 4) *attr* впускной.

inly ['ɪnlɪ] *adv поэт.* внутренне, глубоко; искренне.

inlying ['ɪn,laɪɪŋ] *a* лежащий внутри, внутренний.

inmate ['ɪnmeɪt] *n* 1) жилец; житель; обитатель; 2) находящийся в тюрьме, больнице *и тому подобное*.

inmost ['ɪnmoust] *a* глубочайший; сокровенный.

inn [ɪn] *n* 1) гостиница, постоялый двор; 2): the Inns of Court четыре юридические корпорации, готовящие адвокатов.

innate ['ɪ'neɪt] *a* врождённый.

inner ['ɪnə] *a* внутренний.

innermost ['ɪnəmoust] *см.* inmost.

innings ['ɪnɪŋz] *n* (*pl без измен.*) 1) *спорт* (очередная) подача мяча; 2) период нахождения у власти (*политической партии, деятеля*); ◊ a good long ~ полоса удач; you had your ~ ваше время прошло.

innkeeper ['ɪn,kiːpə] *n* хозяин гостиницы, постоялого двора.

innocence ['ɪnəsns] *n* 1) невинность; простота, наивность; 2) невиновность.

innocent I ['ɪnəsnt] *n* 1) невинный младенец (*тж. шутл. о взрослом*); 2) простофиля.

innocent II *a* 1) невиновный (*of*); 2) невинный; наивный; простодушный; 3) *разг.* лишённый (*чего-л. — of*).

innocuous [ɪ'nɔkjuəs] *a* безвредный.

innovate ['ɪnouveɪt] *v* вводить новшества, изменения.

innovation [,ɪnou'veɪʃən] *n* нововведение, новшество; новаторство.

innovator ['ɪnouveɪtə] *n* новатор; рационализатор.

innoxious [ɪ'nɔkʃəs] *a* безвредный.

innuendo [,ɪnju:'endou] *n* косвенный намёк.

innumerable [ɪ'nju:mərəbl] *a* неисчислимый, бесчисленный, несметный.

inobservance [,ɪnəb'zəːvəns] *n* 1) невнимание; невнимательность; 2) пренебрежение (*к законам, обычаям и т. п.*).

inoccupation ['ɪn,ɔkju'peɪʃən] *n* незанятость, праздность.

inoculate [ɪ'nɔkjuleɪt] *v* 1) прививать, делать (предохранительную) прививку; 2) внушать, прививать.

inoculation [ɪ,nɔkju'leɪʃən] *n* 1) прививка; 2) привитие (*навыков и т. п.*).

inoffensive [,ɪnə'fensɪv] *a* 1) безобидный; безвредный; 2) неоскорбительный.

inofficial [,ɪnə'fɪʃəl] *a* неофициальный.

inoperable [ɪn'ɔpərəbl] *a мед.* неоперабельный.

inoperative [ɪn'ɔpərətɪv] *a* 1) недействующий; бездеятельный; 2) не имеющий силы (*о законе*).

inopportune [ɪn'ɔpətju:n] *a* несвоевременный.

inordinate [ɪ'nɔːdɪnɪt] *a* 1) чрезмерный; 2) беспорядочный.

inorganic [,ɪnɔː'gænɪk] *a* 1) неорганический; 2) чуждый.

in-patient ['ɪn,peɪʃənt] *n* стационарный больной.

inquest ['ɪnkwest] *n юр.* следствие, дознание.

inquietude [ɪn'kwaɪɪtjuːd] *n* беспокойство.

inquire [ɪn'kwaɪə] *v* 1) узнавать, спрашивать; 2) наводить справки, осведомляться (*у — of; о — after, for*); 3) исследовать, расследовать (*что-л. — into*).

inquiry [ɪn'kwaɪərɪ] *n* 1) вопрос, расспросы, наведение справок; to make inquiries наводить справки; 2) допрос; расследование, следствие;

to prosecute an ~ вести расследование; 3) исследование.

inquisition [ˌɪnkwɪˈzɪʃən] *n* 1) следствие, расследование; 2) (the I.) инквизиция.

inquisitive [ɪnˈkwɪzɪtɪv] *a* 1) любознательный, пытливый; 2) любопытный.

inquisitor [ɪnˈkwɪzɪtə] *n* 1) судебный следователь; 2) инквизитор.

inroad [ˈɪnroud] *n* 1) вторжение; нашествие; 2) посягательство.

inrush [ˈɪnrʌʃ] *n* 1) напор, натиск; 2) обвал; 3) прорыв.

insalubrious [ˌɪnsəˈluːbrɪəs] *a* вредный для здоровья, нездоровый.

insane [ɪnˈseɪn] *a* душевнобольной; *перен.* сумасшедший, безрассудный.

insanitary [ɪnˈsænɪtərɪ] *a* антисанитарный.

insanity [ɪnˈsænɪtɪ] *n* умопомешательство.

insatiable [ɪnˈseɪʃjəbl] *a* ненасытный, жадный (*of*).

insatiate [ɪnˈseɪʃɪɪt] *см.* insatiable.

inscribe [ɪnˈskraɪb] *v* 1) вписывать, писать, надписывать; 2) начертать на камне, металле (*имя, надпись*); 3) врезаться (*в память*), запечатлеть(ся) (*в памяти*).

inscription [ɪnˈskrɪpʃən] *n* надпись.

inscrutable [ɪnˈskruːtəbl] *a* 1) непостижимый, таинственный; 2) непроницаемый (*о выражении лица*).

insect[1] [ˈɪnsekt] *n* 1) насекомое; 2) ничтожество.

insect[2] *n амер. разг.* межведомственный национальный центр контроля и наблюдения за космическим пространством.

insecticide [ɪnˈsektɪsaɪd] *n* средство от насекомых, инсектицид.

insectivorous [ˌɪnsekˈtɪvərəs] *a зоол.* насекомоядный.

insecure [ˌɪnsɪˈkjuə] *a* 1) ненадёжный; 2) небезопасный.

insecurity [ˌɪnsɪˈkjuərɪtɪ] *n* 1) ненадёжность; 2) опасное положение.

inseminate [ɪnˈsemɪneɪt] *v* сеять, насаждать (*in*).

insensate [ɪnˈsenseɪt] *a* 1) бесчувственный; 2) неодушевлённый; 3) бессмысленный, неразумный.

insensibility [ɪnˌsensəˈbɪlɪtɪ] *n* 1) бессознательное состояние, обморок; 2) бесчувственность; 3) равнодушие (*to*).

insensible [ɪnˈsensəbl] *a* 1) без сознания, в обмороке; 2) безразличный, бесчувственный; 3) незаметный, неощутимый; нечувствительный.

insensitive [ɪnˈsensɪtɪv] *a* нечувствительный.

inseparable [ɪnˈsepərəbl] *a* 1) неразлучный; 2) неотделимый.

insert I [ˈɪnsəːt] *n* вставка, вклейка.

insert II *v* 1) вставлять; 2) помещать (*статью, объявление*); 3) вносить (*исправления и т. п.*); наносить (*на карту*).

insertion [ɪnˈsəːʃən] *n* 1) вставление, помещение; 2) добавление, вставка (*в рукопись, корректуру*); 3) прошивка.

inset[a] [ˈɪnset] *n* 1) *полигр.* вклейка, вкладка; вкладные листы; 2) вставка (*в платье*).

inset[b] [ˈɪnset] *v* 1) вставлять; 2) *полигр.* делать вкладки, вклейки.

inshore I [ˈɪnˈʃɔː] *a* прибрежный.

inshore II *adv* близко к берегу.

inside I [ˈɪnˈsaɪd] *n* 1) внутренняя сторона, часть; внутренность; the ~ of a week середина недели; the ~ of a book содержание книги; 2) изнанка; ~ out наизнанку; 3) *разг.* внутренности, желудок.

inside II *a* 1) внутренний; 2) скрытый; секретный.

inside III *adv* внутрь, внутри; ~ of a week в пределах недели; please step ~ входите, пожалуйста.

inside IV *prep* внутрь, внутри, с внутренней стороны, на внутренней стороне.

insider [ˈɪnˈsaɪdə] *n* 1) свой человек; член (*общества или организации*); 2) посвящённый в тайну.

insidious [ɪnˈsɪdɪəs] *a* 1) коварный, предательский; 2) скрытый; незаметно подкрадывающийся (*напр., о болезни*).

insight [ˈɪnsaɪt] *n* проницательность, проникновение (*into*); понимание, интуиция.

insignia [ɪnˈsɪgnɪə] *n pl* 1) знаки отличия; 2) значки; 3) *воен.* знаки различия.

insignificance [ˌɪnsɪgˈnɪfɪkəns] *n* 1) незначительность; маловажность; 2) бессодержательность.

insignificant [ˌɪnsɪgˈnɪfɪkənt] *a* 1) незначительный, неважный; ничтожный; 2) бессодержательный.

insincere [ˌɪnsɪnˈsɪə] *a* неискренний.

insincerity [ˌɪnsɪnˈserɪtɪ] *n* неискренность.

insinuate [ɪnˈsɪnjueɪt] *v* 1) сеять, вселять (*сомнение, недоверие и т. п.*); 2) *refl* вкрадываться, втираться (*into*); to ~ oneself into smb.'s favour втереться кому-л. в доверие; 3) инсинуировать, намекать.

insinuation [ɪnˌsɪnjuˈeɪʃən] *n* 1) инсинуация; 2) вкрадчивость.

insipid [ɪnˈsɪpɪd] *a* 1) безвкусный, пресный; *перен.* скучный, неинтересный; 2) безжизненный, вялый.

insist [ɪnˈsɪst] *v* настаивать (*на — on, upon*).

insistence [ɪnˈsɪstəns] *n* 1) настойчивость; 2) настояние, требование.

insistency [ɪnˈsɪstənsɪ] *см.* insistence.

insistent [ɪnˈsɪstənt] *a* настойчивый.

insolation [ˌɪnsouˈleɪʃən] *n* инсоляция; воздействие солнечных лучей.

insolence [ˈɪnsələns] *n* высокомерие; дерзость, наглость.

insolent [ˈɪnsələnt] *a* 1) высокомерный; дерзкий, наглый; 2) оскорбительный, обидный.

insoluble [ɪnˈsɔljubl] *a* 1) нерастворимый; 2) неразрешимый.

insolvent I [ɪnˈsɔlvənt] *n* несостоятельный должник; банкрот.

insolvent II *a* несостоятельный.

insomnia [ɪnˈsɔmnɪə] *n* бессонница.

insomuch [ˌɪnsouˈmʌtʃ] *adv*: ~ that настолько, что.

inspect [ɪnˈspekt] *v* 1) осматривать; рассматривать; 2) инспектировать; 3) наблюдать, надзирать.

inspection [ɪnˈspekʃən] *n* 1) осмотр, освидетельствование; 2) инспектирование; 3) наблюдение, надзор.

inspector [ın'spektə] *n* 1) инспе́ктор; 2) контролёр, ревизо́р; 3) наблюда́тель, надзира́тель.

inspiration [ˌınspə'reıʃən] *n* 1) вдохнове́ние; to draw ~ че́рпать вдохнове́ние; 2) вдохнови́тель; вдохновля́ющая иде́я; 3) вдыха́ние.

inspire [ın'spaıə] *v* 1) вдохновля́ть, вооодушевля́ть; 2) внуша́ть (*чувство и т. п.*); 3) та́йно внуша́ть; инспири́ровать; 4) вдыха́ть.

inspirit [ın'spırıt] *v* вдохну́ть (*жизнь, мужество и т. п.*); ободри́ть.

instability [ˌınstə'bılıtı] *n* 1) неусто́йчивость; 2) непостоя́нство.

install [ın'stɔːl] *v* 1) водворя́ть, помеща́ть, устра́ивать; 2) устана́вливать; монти́ровать; проводи́ть (*электричество и т. п.*).

installation [ˌınstə'leıʃən] *n* 1) водворе́ние, устро́йство; 2) устано́вка; прово́дка; монта́ж, сбо́рка.

instalment [ın'stɔːlmənt] *n* отде́льный вы́пуск *или* часть (*книги*); (очередно́й) взнос (*в части́чное погаше́ние*); by ~s a) в рассро́чку; б) частя́ми, отде́льными вы́пусками (*о книге*).

instance I ['ınstəns] *n* 1) приме́р; for ~ наприме́р; 2) отде́льный слу́чай; in this ~ в э́том слу́чае; in the first ~ снача́ла, сперва́, в пе́рвую о́чередь; 3) настоя́ние, тре́бование; at the ~ of по настоя́нию, по тре́бованию.

instance II *v* 1) приводи́ть в ка́честве приме́ра; 2) служи́ть приме́ром.

instant I ['ınstənt] *n* мгнове́ние, моме́нт; this ~ сейча́с; on the ~ неме́дленно, то́тчас; the ~ (that)... как то́лько...

instant II *a* 1) спе́шный, неотло́жный; 2) неме́дленный; 3) теку́щий, теку́щего ме́сяца; the 1st inst.(ant) 1-го сего́ ме́сяца.

instantaneous [ˌınstən'teınjəs] *a* 1) мгнове́нный, момента́льный; 2) одновреме́нный.

instantly ['ınstəntlı] *adv* то́тчас, неме́дленно.

instead [ın'sted] *adv* вме́сто, взаме́н; ~ of going (reading *etc*) вме́сто того́, что́бы пойти́ (чита́ть *и т. п.*); ~ of me (him *etc*) вме́сто меня́ (него́ *и т. п.*).

instep ['ınstəp] *n* подъём (*ноги́, обу́ви*).

instigate ['ınstıgeıt] *v* 1) побужда́ть; 2) подстрека́ть, провоци́ровать.

instigation [ˌınstı'geıʃən] *n* подстрека́тельство.

instil(l) [ın'stıl] *v* 1) внуша́ть, привива́ть (*привы́чки, взгля́ды и т. п.*); 2) нака́пать (*лекарство*).

instinct[a] ['ınstıŋkt] *n* 1) инсти́нкт; herd ~ ста́дное чу́вство; 2) врождённое чутьё; интуи́ция.

instinct[b] [ın'stıŋkt] *a predic* по́лный, (пре)испо́лненный (*чего-л.* — *with*).

instinctive [ın'stıŋktıv] *a* инстинкти́вный, бессозна́тельный.

institute I ['ınstıtjuːt] *n* институ́т.

institute II *v* 1) учрежда́ть, осно́вывать; вводи́ть; 2) возбужда́ть (*де́ло*); начина́ть, назнача́ть (*рассле́дование и т. п.*).

institution [ˌınstı'tjuːʃən] *n* 1) установле́ние, учрежде́ние (*чего-л.* — *of*); 2) институ́т (*общественный*); 3) учрежде́ние; о́бщество; scholastic ~ уче́бное заведе́ние.

instruct [ın'strʌkt] *v* 1) обуча́ть, инструкти́ровать (*in*); 2) дава́ть инстру́кции, указа́ния, распоряже́ния; 3) сообща́ть, информи́ровать.

instruction [ın'strʌkʃən] *n* 1) обуче́ние, инструкти́рование; 2) *pl* инстру́кции, директи́вы; 3) *attr* уче́бный.

instructional [ın'strʌkʃənl] *a* уче́бный.

instructive [ın'strʌktıv] *a* 1) инструкти́вный; 2) поучи́тельный.

instructor [ın'strʌktə] *n* 1) инстру́ктор, руководи́тель; 2) *амер.* преподава́тель вы́сшего уче́бного заведе́ния.

instrument I ['ınstrumənt] *n* 1) инструме́нт; *перен.* ору́дие (*чего-л.*); stringed ~s стру́нные инструме́нты; 2) *тех.* прибо́р; 3) *юр.* докуме́нт.

instrument II *v муз.* инструментова́ть.

instrumental [ˌınstru'mentl] *a* 1) инструмента́льный; 2) (дости́гнутый, соверше́нный) при по́мощи прибо́ров, по прибо́рам; 3) спосо́бствующий (*чему-л.*); to be ~ in smth. спосо́бствовать, соде́йствовать чему́-л.; 4) *грам.* инструмента́льный, твори́тельный (*о падеже*).

instrumentality [ˌınstrumen'tælıtı] *n* сре́дство, спо́соб; посре́дство; by the ~ of че́рез посре́дство, посре́дством.

instrumentation [ˌınstrumen'teıʃən] *n* 1) *муз.* инструменто́вка; 2) *тех.* аппарату́ра; 3) *тех.* оснаще́ние аппарату́рой, инструме́нтами.

insubordinate [ˌınsə'bɔːdnıt] *a* непоко́рный; недисциплини́рованный.

insubordination ['ınsəˌbɔːdı'neıʃən] *n* неподчине́ние, неповинове́ние, ослуша́ние.

insubstantial [ˌınsəb'stænʃəl] *a* неоснова́тельный; *поэт.* нереа́льный, иллюзо́рный.

insufferable [ın'sʌfərəbl] *a* 1) нестерпи́мый; 2) нетерпи́мый, недопусти́мый.

insufficiency [ˌınsə'fıʃənsı] *n* недоста́точность.

insufficient [ˌınsə'fıʃənt] *a* недоста́точный; неудовлетвори́тельный, непо́лный.

insufflate ['ınsʌfleıt] *v* вдува́ть.

insular I ['ınsjulə] *n* островитя́нин.

insular II *a* 1) островно́й; 2) сво́йственный островитя́нам; *перен.* ограни́ченный, у́зких взгля́дов.

insulate ['ınsjuleıt] *v* 1) изоли́ровать; 2) образова́ть о́стров.

insulating ['ınsjuleıtıŋ] *a тех.* изоляцио́нный, изоли́рующий.

insulation [ˌınsju'leıʃən] *n* 1) изоля́ция, обособле́ние; 2) *тех.* изоляцио́нный материа́л.

insulator ['ınsjuleıtə] *n* изоля́тор.

insulin ['ınsjulın] *n фарм.* инсули́н.

insult[a] ['ınsʌlt] *n* оскорбле́ние; to swallow an ~ проглоти́ть оби́ду.

insult[b] [ın'sʌlt] *v* оскорбля́ть, наноси́ть оскорбле́ние.

insuperable [ın'sjuːpərəbl] *a* непреодоли́мый.

insupportable [ˌınsə'pɔːtəbl] *a* невыноси́мый, нестерпи́мый.

insurance [ın'ʃuərəns] *n* 1) страхова́ние; 2) страхова́я пре́мия, су́мма; 3) *attr* страхово́й.

insure [ın'ʃuə] *v* 1) (за)страхова́ть(ся); 2) обеспе́чивать.

insurgent I [ın'sɜːdʒənt] *n* повста́нец.

insurgent II *a* повста́нческий; восста́вший.

insurmountable [ˌınsɜː'mauntəbl] *a* непреодоли́мый.

insurrection [ˌınsə'rekʃən] *n* 1) восста́ние; 2) мяте́ж, бунт.

insurrectional [ˌɪnsəˈrekʃənl] *a* 1) повста́нческий; 2) мяте́жный.

insurrectionist [ˌɪnsəˈrekʃnɪst] *n* повста́нец.

insusceptible [ˌɪnsəˈseptəbl] *a* нечувстви́тельный, невоспри́имчивый.

intact [ɪnˈtækt] *a* нетро́нутый, неповреждённый, це́лый.

intake [ˈɪnteɪk] *n* 1) впуск; 2) впускно́е, входно́е отве́рстие; 3) поглоще́ние, потребле́ние; 4) *attr* впускно́й; приёмный.

intangible [ɪnˈtændʒəbl] *a* 1) неосяза́емый; 2) неулови́мый; 3) непостижи́мый.

integer [ˈɪntɪdʒə] *n* це́лое число́.

integral I [ˈɪntɪɡrəl] *n* мат. интегра́л.

integral II *a* 1) неотъе́млемый; 2) по́лный, це́лый; 3) *мат.* интегра́льный.

integrate [ˈɪntɪɡreɪt] *v* 1) составля́ть це́лое; соединя́ть; 2) *мат.* интегри́ровать.

integrity [ɪnˈteɡrɪtɪ] *n* 1) полнота́, це́лостность; 2) че́стность; прямота́; 3) чистота́.

integument [ɪnˈteɡjumənt] *n* нару́жный покро́в, оболо́чка.

intellect [ˈɪntɪlekt] *n* ум, интелле́кт; the great ~s of the age вели́кие умы́ совреме́нности.

intellection [ˌɪntɪˈlekʃən] *n* у́мственная де́ятельность, интелле́кт.

intellective [ˌɪntɪˈlektɪv] *a* у́мственный, мысли́тельный.

intellectual I [ˌɪntɪˈlektʃuəl] *n* 1) мы́слящий челове́к; интеллиге́нт; 2) *pl* (the ~s) интеллиге́нция.

intellectual II *a* 1) у́мственный; интеллектуа́льный; 2) мысли́тельный; мы́слящий; у́мный (*о лице и т. п.*).

intelligence[1] [ɪnˈtelɪdʒəns] *n* 1) ум; у́мственные спосо́бности; superior (average) ~ хоро́шие (сре́дние) у́мственные спосо́бности; 2) смышлё́ность; поня́тливость.

intelligence[2] *n* 1) све́дения, изве́стия, информа́ция; 2) агенту́рная разве́дка; 3) *attr* разве́дывательный.

intelligencer [ɪnˈtelɪdʒənsə] *n* та́йный аге́нт, осведоми́тель; шпио́н.

intelligent [ɪnˈtelɪdʒənt] *a* 1) у́мный; 2) смышлё́ный.

intelligentsia [ɪnˌtelɪˈdʒentsɪə] *n* интеллиге́нция.

intelligible [ɪnˈtelɪdʒəbl] *a* поня́тный, вразуми́тельный.

intemperance [ɪnˈtempərəns] *n* 1) неуме́ренность, невоздё́ржанность; 2) пья́нство.

intemperate [ɪnˈtempərɪt] *a* 1) невоздё́ржанный; несде́ржанный; 2) си́льно пью́щий.

intend [ɪnˈtend] *v* 1) намерева́ться, предполага́ть (*сделать что-л.*); 2) предназнача́ть; 3) подразумева́ть.

intense [ɪnˈtens] *a* 1) си́льный, интенси́вный; 2) напряжённый; 3) ре́вностный; 4) впечатли́тельный.

intensification [ɪnˌtensɪfɪˈkeɪʃən] *n* усиле́ние, интенсифика́ция.

intensify [ɪnˈtensɪfaɪ] *v* уси́ливать(ся).

intension [ɪnˈtenʃən] *n* 1) напряже́ние, уси́лие; 2) напряжённость.

intensity [ɪnˈtensɪtɪ] *n* си́ла, интенси́вность; напряже́ние.

intensive [ɪnˈtensɪv] *a* 1) интенси́вный, напряжённый, глубо́кий; 2) *грам.* усили́тельный.

intent I [ɪnˈtent] *n* наме́рение; ◊ to all ~s and purposes а) в су́щности; б) во всех отноше́ниях.

intent II *a* 1) внима́тельный, при́стальный; насто́йчивый; 2) наме́ренный (*что-л. сделать*); скло́нный (*к чему-л.— on*).

intention [ɪnˈtenʃən] *n* наме́рение, у́мысел; за́мысел; our ~ is мы намерева́емся, предполага́ем; without ~ неумы́шленно.

intentional [ɪnˈtenʃənl] *a* умы́шленный, преднаме́ренный.

inter [ɪnˈtə:] *v* хорони́ть.

inter- [ˈɪntə-, ˈɪntə:-] *pref* 1) меж-, между-; interdental межзу́бный (*о звуке*); 2) взаимо-; interplay взаимоде́йствие, взаимосвя́зь; 3) пере-; to intermingle переме́шивать.

interact[a] [ˈɪntərækt] *n* 1) антра́кт; 2) интерлю́дия, интерме́дия.

interact[b] [ˌɪntərˈækt] *v* взаимоде́йствовать, де́йствовать друг на дру́га.

interaction [ˌɪntərˈækʃən] *n* взаимоде́йствие.

interblend [ˌɪntə:ˈblend] *v* сме́шивать(ся).

interbreed [ˌɪntə:ˈbri:d] *v* скре́щивать(ся) (*о живо́тных*).

intercede [ˌɪntə:ˈsi:d] *v* хода́тайствовать, заступа́ться (*за кого-л.— for, перед кем-л.— with*).

intercept [ˌɪntə:ˈsept] *v* 1) перехва́тывать (*письмо́, самолё́ты и т. д.*); 2) остана́вливать, заде́рживать; прегражда́ть, отреза́ть путь; 3) прерыва́ть, выключа́ть (*ток, свет, во́ду и т. п.*); 4) *мат.* отложи́ть отре́зок на ли́нии двумя́ то́чками.

interception [ˌɪntə:ˈsepʃən] *n* 1) перехва́т(ыва-ние); 2) прегражде́ние.

interchange[a] [ˈɪntə:ˈtʃeɪndʒ] *n* 1) обме́н; 2) переста́новка, перемеще́ние; 3) сме́на, чередова́ние.

interchange[b] [ˌɪntə:ˈtʃeɪndʒ] *v* 1) обме́ниваться; 2) переставля́ть, перемеща́ть; 3) чередова́ть(ся).

interchangeable [ˌɪntə:ˈtʃeɪndʒəbl] *a* замени́мый; взаимозаменя́емый.

intercollegiate [ˈɪntə:kəˈli:dʒɪɪt] *a* (между)шко́льный (*о спорти́вном состяза́нии*).

intercommunicate [ˌɪntə:kəˈmju:nɪkeɪt] *v* сообща́ться друг с дру́гом, ме́жду собо́й.

intercommunication [ˈɪntə:kəˌmju:nɪˈkeɪʃən] *n* связь, сноше́ние, обще́ние, сообще́ние.

intercommunion [ˌɪntə:kəˈmju:njən] *n* взаимосвя́зь.

interconnect [ˈɪntə:kəˈnekt] *v* свя́зывать(ся), соединя́ть(ся).

intercourse [ˈɪntə:kɔ:s] *n* обще́ние; связь, сноше́ния.

interdependence [ˌɪntə:dɪˈpendəns] *n* взаимозави́симость, взаимосвя́зь.

interdependent [ˌɪntə:dɪˈpendənt] *a* взаимозави́симый; зави́сящий оди́н от друго́го.

interdict[a] [ˈɪntə:dɪkt] запреще́ние, запре́т.

interdict[b] [ˌɪntə:ˈdɪkt] *v* 1) запреща́ть, воспреща́ть; 2) уде́рживать (*from*); 3) отлуча́ть (от це́ркви).

interdictory [ˌɪntə:ˈdɪktərɪ] *a* запрети́тельный.

interest I [ˈɪntrɪst] *n* 1) интере́с; to take ~ интересова́ться (*чем-л.— in*); 2) заинтересо́ванность, дóля (*в чём-л.*); 3) вáжность, значéние; of no little ~ немаловáжный; 4) процéнт(ы); simple (compound) ~ просты́е (слóжные) процéнты; rate of ~ процéнтная стáвка; with ~ с процéнтами; *перен.* с лихвóй; 5) влия́ние (*на когó-л.* — with); 6) лúца, объединённые óбщностью интерéсов; the business ~s все крýпные фúрмы вмéсте взя́тые; the landed ~ землевладéльцы.

interest II *v* интересовáть; заинтересóвывать.

interested ['ıntrıstıd] *a* заинтересóванный (*в чём-л.* — in).

interesting ['ıntrıstıŋ] *a* интерéсный.

interfere [,ıntə'fıə] *v* 1) мешáть; служúть помéхой, препя́тствовать; 2) вмéшиваться (in); 3) стáлкиваться (with).

interference [,ıntə'fıərəns] *n* 1) вмешáтельство; 2) помéха, препя́тствие; 3) *радио* помéхи.

interflow[a] ['ıntəflou] *n* слия́ние.

interflow[b] [,ıntə'flou] *v* сливáться.

interfuse [,ıntə'fjuːz] *v* смéшивать(ся), перемéшивать(ся).

intergrowth ['ıntə,grouθ] *n* прорастáние.

interim ['ıntərım] *n* 1) промежýток врéмени, врéмя мéжду...; in the ~ тем врéменем; at ~ врéменно исполня́ющий обя́занности; *attr* врéменный, промежýточный; предварúтельный.

interior I [ın'tıərıə] *n* 1) внýтренняя часть, сторонá; 2) внýтренняя óбласть страны́; 3) внýтренние делá (страны́); 4) *разг.* внýтренности, желýдок; 5) *иск.* интерьéр.

interior II *a* внýтренний.

interjacent [,ıntə'dʒeısnt] *a* промежýточный.

interject [,ıntə'dʒekt] *v* прерывáть замечáнием, вставля́ть замечáние.

interjection [,ıntə'dʒekʃən] *n* 1) восклицáние; 2) *грам.* междомéтие.

interlace [,ıntə'leıs] *v* переплетáть(ся), сплетáть(-ся).

interlard [,ıntə'lɑːd] *v* пересыпáть, уснащáть (*речь, письмó инострáнными словáми и т. п.*).

interline[1] [,ıntə'laın] *v* подбивáть (*одéжду*) вáтой, стáвить дополнúтельную подклáдку.

interline[2] *v* впúсывать мéжду строк.

interlinear [,ıntə'lınıə] *a* междустрóчный; подстрóчный.

interlock [,ıntə'lɔk] *v* сцепля́ть(ся), соединя́ть(-ся).

interlocution [,ıntəlou'kjuːʃən] *n* бесéда, собесéдование.

interlocutor [,ıntə'lɔkjutə] *n* собесéдник.

interlope [,ıntə'loup] *v* 1) вмéшиваться в чужúе делá; 2) занимáться контрабáндой.

interloper [,ıntə'loupə] *n* человéк, вмéшивающийся в чужúе делá (*обыкн. рáди вы́годы*).

interlude ['ıntəluːd] *n* 1) антрáкт; промежýток; 2) *театр.* интермéдия; 3) *муз.* интерлю́дия; 4) фарс, комéдия.

intermarriage [,ıntə'mærıdʒ] *n* 1) брак мéжду лúцами рáзных национáльностей; 2) *разг.* брак мéжду рóдственниками.

intermarry ['ıntə'mærı] *v* 1) породнúться; смешáться (*о рáсах, племенáх*); 2) вступáть в брак (*о рóдственниках*).

intermeddle [,ıntə'medl] *v* вмéшиваться (*во что-л.* — with, in).

intermedia [,ıntə'miːdıə] *pl см.* intermedium.

intermediary I [,ıntə'miːdjərı] *n* посрéдник.

intermediary II *a* 1) посрéднический; 2) промежýточный.

intermediate[a] [,ıntə'miːdjət] *a* промежýточный.

intermediate[b] [,ıntə'miːdıeıt] *v* быть посрéдником (*мéжду* — between).

intermediation ['ıntə,miːdı'eıʃən] *n* посрéдничество.

intermediator [,ıntə'miːdıeıtə] *n* посрéдник.

intermedium [,ıtə'miːdıəm] *n* (*pl тж.* intermedia) посрéдство.

interment [ın'təːmənt] *n* погребéние.

interminable [ın'təːmınəbl] *a* бесконéчный.

intermingle [,ıntə'mıŋgl] *v* 1) смéшивать(ся), перемéшивать(ся); 2) общáться.

intermission [,ıntə'mıʃən] *n* 1) переры́в; останóвка; пáуза; without ~ беспреры́вно; 2) *амер.* антрáкт; 3) *шк.* перемéна; 4) *мед.* перебóй (*пýльса*).

intermit [,ıntə'mıt] *v* прервáть(ся), останóвить (-ся).

intermittent ['ıntə'mıtənt] *a* перемежáющийся; преры́вистый; с перебóями.

intermix [,ıntə'mıks] *v* смéшивать(ся).

intermixture [,ıntə'mıkstʃə] *n* смéшение; смесь.

intern[1] [ın'təːn] *v* интернúровать.

intern[2] *n* *амер.* интéрн (*студéнт или молодóй врач, рабóтающий в больнúце*).

internal [ın'təːnl] *a* 1) внýтренний; 2) душéвный, сокровéнный.

International [,ıntə'næʃənl] *n* Интернационáл (*организáция*).

international [,ıntə'næʃənl] *a* междунарóдный, интернационáльный.

Internationale [,ıntənæʃə'nɑːl] *n* Интернационáл (*гимн*).

internationalism [,ıntə'næʃnəlızəm] *n* интернационалúзм.

internationalize [,ıntə'næʃnəlaız] *v* 1) дéлать (-ся) интернационáльным; 2) стáвить (*территóрию, странý*) под контрóль рáзных госудáрств.

internationally [,ıntə'næʃnəlı] *adv* всемúрно; во всём мúре.

interne [ın'təːn] *см.* intern[2].

internecine [,ıntə'niːsaın] *a* 1) междоусóбный; 2) смертонóсный, истребúтельный.

internee [,ıntəː'niː] *n* интернúрованный.

internment [ın'təːnmənt] *n* интернúрование.

interpellate [ın'təːpeleıt] *v* дéлать запрóс (*в парлáменте*).

interpellation [ın,təːpe'leıʃən] *n* запрóс (*в парлáменте*).

interplanetary [,ıntə'plænıtərı] *a* межпланéтный.

interplay ['ıntə'pleı] *n* взаимодéйствие.

interpolate [ın'təːpouleıt] *v* интерполúровать; дéлать встáвки в текст чужóй рýкописи.

interpose [,ıntə'pouz] *v* 1) вставля́ть; вводúть; 2) становúться мéжду; вклúниваться; 3) смéшиваться; 4) прерывáть (*замечáниями и т. п.*).

interpret [ın'təːprıt] *v* 1) толковáть, истолкóвывать; 2) переводúть (*ýстно*); быть перевóдчиком (*ýстным*).

interpretation [ın,təːprı'teıʃən] *n* толковáние, объяснéние, истолковáние.

interpretative [ın'təːprıtətıv] *a* объяснúтельный.

interpreter [ɪn'tɜːprɪtə] *n* 1) истолкова́тель; 2) (у́стный) перево́дчик.

interregnum [ˌɪntə'regnəm] *n* (*pl тж.* interregna [ˌɪntə'regnə]) междуца́рствие.

interrelated ['ɪntəːrɪ'leɪtɪd] *a* взаимосвя́занный.

interrelation ['ɪntəːrɪ'leɪʃən] *n* взаимоотноше́ние, взаимосвя́зь.

interrogate [ɪn'terəgeɪt] *v* 1) спра́шивать; опра́шивать; 2) допра́шивать.

interrogation [ɪnˌterə'geɪʃən] *n* 1) вопро́с; 2) допро́с.

interrogative [ˌɪntə'rɔgətɪv] *a* вопроси́тельный (*тж. грам.*).

interrogatory I [ˌɪntə'rɔgetərɪ] *n* 1) вопро́с; 2) допро́с; 2) опро́сный лист.

interrogatory II *a* вопроси́тельный.

interrupt [ˌɪntə'rʌpt] *v* 1) прерыва́ть; 2) препя́тствовать, меша́ть.

interruption [ˌɪntə'rʌpʃən] *n* 1) переры́в; преры-ва́ние; 2) остано́вка; 3) *тех.* разры́в, разъедине́ние; наруше́ние.

intersect [ˌɪntəː'sekt] *v* пересека́ть(ся); перекре́-щивать(ся); скре́щивать(ся).

intersection [ˌɪntəː'sekʃən] *n* 1) пересече́ние; 2) то́чка пересече́ния.

intersperse [ˌɪntəː'spəːs] *v* 1) рассе́ивать, разбра́-сывать, рассыпа́ть (*среди, между — among, be-tween*); 2) разнообра́зить, пересыпа́ть (*чем-л.— with*).

interstellar ['ɪntəː'stelə] *a* межзвёздный.

interstice [ɪn'təːstɪs] *n* 1) промежу́ток; 2) щель, расще́лина.

intertwine [ˌɪntəː'twaɪn] *v* переплета́ть(ся).

intertwist [ˌɪntəː'twɪst] *v* скру́чивать(ся); пере-кру́чивать(ся).

interurban [ˌɪntər'əːbən] *a* междугоро́дный.

interval ['ɪntəvəl] *n* 1) промежу́ток, интерва́л; at ~s a) с промежу́тками; б) тут и там; в) вре́мя от вре́мени; 2) переры́в, па́уза; 3) *муз.* интер-ва́л.

intervene [ˌɪntəː'viːn] *v* 1) вме́шиваться; всту-па́ться (*in*); 2) лежа́ть, быть располо́женным (*между — between*); 3) происходи́ть (*в определён-ный промежу́ток времени*).

intervention [ˌɪntəː'venʃən] *n* 1) вмеша́тельство; 2) интерве́нция.

interventionist [ˌɪntəː'venʃənɪst] *n* интерве́нт.

interview I ['ɪntəvjuː] *n* 1) встре́ча; бесе́да, раз-гово́р (*с глазу на глаз*); 2) интервью́.

interview II *v* бесе́довать; интервью́и́ровать.

interweave [ˌɪntəː'wiːv] *v* (*past* interwove; *p. p.* interwoven) 1) вотка́ть, затка́ть; 2) переплета́ть; вплета́ть.

interwove [ˌɪntə'wouv] *past см.* interweave.

interwoven [ˌɪntə'wouvn] *p. p. см.* interweave.

intestate [ɪn'testɪt] *n* уме́рший без завеща́ния.

intestinal [ɪn'testɪnl] *a* кише́чный.

intestine I [ɪn'testɪn] *n обыкн. pl* кишки́, кише́ч-ник; small (large) ~ то́нкая (то́лстая) кишка́.

intestine II *a* вну́тренний, междоусо́бный.

intimacy ['ɪntɪməsɪ] *n* бли́зость, инти́мность.

intimateᵃ I ['ɪntɪmɪt] *n* бли́зкий друг.

intimateᵃ II *a* 1) сокрове́нный; 2) инти́мный, ли́ч-ный; 3) бли́зкий; хорошо́ знако́мый.

intimateᵇ ['ɪntɪmeɪt] *v* 1) ста́вить в изве́стность; сообща́ть; 2) намека́ть, подразумева́ть.

intimation [ˌɪntɪ'meɪʃən] *n* 1) сообще́ние, извеще́-ние; указа́ние; 2) намёк.

intimidate [ɪn'tɪmɪdeɪt] *v* пуга́ть; запу́гивать.

intimidation [ɪnˌtɪmɪ'deɪʃən] *n* 1) запу́гивание; 2) запу́ганность.

intimity [ɪn'tɪmɪtɪ] *n* 1) инти́мность; 2) уединён-ность.

into ['ɪntu (*сильная форма*), 'ɪntə (*слабая фор-ма*)] *prep* 1) *в пространственном значении указы-вает на движение внутрь ограниченного простран-ства* в, на; ~ the house (the garden, the under-ground) в дом (в сад, в метро́); 2) *указывает на включение в пределы чего-л.* в; a few students more were included ~ the list ещё не́сколько студе́нтов бы́ли включены́ в спи́сок; 3) *указывает на переход в новое состояние, качество, форму* в; this house has been converted ~ a hospital э́тот дом был пре-вращён в больни́цу; 4) *указывает на деление на части* на; he divided his plot ~ two equal parts он раз-дели́л свой уча́сток на две ра́вные ча́сти.

intolerable [ɪn'tɔlərəbl] *a* невыноси́мый, нестер-пи́мый.

intolerance [ɪn'tɔlərəns] *n* нетерпи́мость.

intolerant [ɪn'tɔlərənt] *a* нетерпи́мый.

intonation [ˌɪntou'neɪʃən] *n* 1) интона́ция; моду-ля́ция (*голоса*); 2) пе́ние речитати́вом; произнесе́-ние нараспе́в.

intone [ɪn'toun] *v* 1) интони́ровать; модули́ро-вать (*голос*); 2) петь речитати́вом; произноси́ть нараспе́в.

intoxicant I [ɪn'tɔksɪkənt] *n* опьяня́ющий напи́-ток.

intoxicant II *a* опьяня́ющий.

intoxicate [ɪn'tɔksɪkeɪt] *v* опьяня́ть; возбужда́ть.

intoxicated [ɪn'tɔksɪkeɪtɪd] *a* 1) пья́ный; 2) опья-нённый, возбуждённый.

intoxication [ɪnˌtɔksɪ'keɪʃən] *n* 1) опьяне́ние; возбужде́ние; 2) *мед.* интоксика́ция, отравле́ние.

intra- ['ɪntrə-] *pref* внутри-; intracellular вну-трикле́точный.

intractable [ɪn'træktəbl] *a* 1) непоко́рный, труд-новоспиту́емый; неподатливый; 2) труднообраба́-тываемый; 3) не поддаю́щийся лече́нию.

intramural ['ɪntrə'mjuərəl] *a* (происходя́щий) в стена́х (*дома, школы и т. п.*).

intransigent I [ɪn'trænsɪdʒənt] *n* 1) полити́ческий де́ятель, не изменя́ющий свои́м при́нципам; 2) не-примири́мый республика́нец.

intransigent II *a* непримири́мый, непрекло́нный.

intransitive [ɪn'trɑːnsɪtɪv] *a* непереходный (*о гла-голе*).

intrench [ɪn'trentʃ] *см.* entrench.

intrepid [ɪn'trepɪd] *a* бесстра́шный, неустраши́-мый.

intrepidity [ˌɪntrɪ'pɪdɪtɪ] *n* бесстра́шие, неустра-ши́мость.

intricacy ['ɪntrɪkəsɪ] *n* запу́танность, сло́жность; пу́таница.

intricate ['ɪntrɪkɪt] *a* запу́танный, сло́жный.

intrigue I [ɪn'triːg] *n* интри́га.

intrigue II *v* 1) интригова́ть (*против — against*); 2) име́ть любо́вную интри́гу (*with*); 3) вызыва́ть интере́с, любопы́тство.

intrinsic [ɪn'trɪnsɪk] *a* вну́тренний; прису́щий, сво́йственный (*чему-л.*).

intro- ['ɪntrə-] *pref со значением движения, вне-*

сения, введения внутрь: to introspect заниматься самоанализом.

introduce [ˌɪntrə'djuːs] *v* 1) вводить; 2) представлять (*кому-л. — to*); знакомить (*с кем-л. — to*); 3) вносить на рассмотрение, обсуждение (*вопрос, законопроект и т. п.*).

introduction [ˌɪntrə'dʌkʃən] *n* 1) введение; внесение; 2) (официальное) представление, знакомство; рекомендация; 3) нововведение; 4) предисловие, введение.

introductory [ˌɪntrə'dʌktərɪ] *a* вводный, вступительный; предварительный.

introspect [ˌɪntrou'spekt] *v* заниматься самоанализом.

introspection [ˌɪntrou'spekʃən] *n* самоанализ, самонаблюдение.

introspective [ˌɪntrou'spektɪv] *a* занимающийся самоанализом, самонаблюдением.

introvert[a] ['ɪntrouvəːt] *n* человек, сосредоточенный на своём внутреннем мире.

introvert[b] [ˌɪntrou'vəːt] *v* сосредоточиваться на самом себе.

intrude [ɪn'truːd] *v* 1) вторгаться (*into*); 2) навязывать(ся) (*upon*).

intruder [ɪn'truːdə] *n* 1) захватчик; 2) человек, присваивающий чужие права; 3) навязчивый человек.

intrusion [ɪn'truːʒən] *n* 1) вторжение (*into*); 2) присвоение чужих прав; 3) навязывание (*своего мнения и т. п.; upon*).

intrusive [ɪn'truːsɪv] *a* навязчивый.

intrust [ɪn'trʌst] *амер. см.* entrust.

intuition [ˌɪntjuː'ɪʃən] *n* интуиция, чутьё.

intuitive [ɪn'tjuːɪtɪv] *a* интуитивный.

inundate ['ɪnʌndeɪt] *v* наводнять, затоплять.

inundation [ˌɪnʌn'deɪʃən] *n* наводнение, затопление.

inure [ɪ'njuə] *v* 1) закалять, приучать (*к чему-л. — to*); 2) служить на пользу; 3) *юр.* вступать в силу, быть действительным.

invade [ɪn'veɪd] *v* 1) вторгаться; захватывать; 2) овладевать, заполнять, нахлынуть (*о чувстве и т. п.*); 3) посягать (*на чьи-л. права*).

invader [ɪn'veɪdə] *n* интервент, захватчик; оккупант.

invalid[a] I ['ɪnvəliːd] *n* больной.

invalid[a] II ['ɪnvəliːd] *a* 1) больной, нетрудоспособный; 2) (предназначенный) для больных.

invalid[b] [ˌɪnvə'liːd] *v* 1) делать(ся) больным, нетрудоспособным; 2) признавать негодным к службе (*по состоянию здоровья*).

invalid[c] [ɪn'vælɪd] *a* недействительный, не имеющий законной силы.

invalidate [ɪn'vælɪdeɪt] *v* делать недействительным, лишать законной силы.

invalidation [ɪn,vælɪ'deɪʃən] *n* лишение законной силы.

invaluable [ɪn'væljuəbl] *a* неоценимый.

invariability [ɪn,vɛərɪə'bɪlɪtɪ] *n* неизменяемость, неизменность.

invariable [ɪn'vɛərɪəbl] *a* 1) неизменяемый, неизменный; 2) *мат.* постоянный.

invasion [ɪn'veɪʒən] *n* 1) вторжение, нашествие; 2) посягательство (*на чьи-л. права*).

invasive [ɪn'veɪsɪv] *a* 1) вторгающийся; захватнический; 2) посягающий (*на чьи-л. права*).

invective [ɪn'vektɪv] *n обыкн. pl* брань; ругательства.

inveigh [ɪn'veɪ] *v* нападать, ругать, поносить.

inveigle [ɪn'viːgl] *v* заманивать, соблазнять, совращать.

invent [ɪn'vent] *v* 1) изобретать; 2) придумывать; выдумывать.

invention [ɪn'venʃən] *n* 1) изобретение; 2) выдумка; 3) изобретательность.

inventive [ɪn'ventɪv] *a* изобретательный.

inventor [ɪn'ventə] *n* 1) изобретатель; 2) выдумщик.

inventory I ['ɪnvəntrɪ] *n* 1) инвентарь; 2) предметы, внесённые в инвентарь; 3) инвентаризация.

inventory II *v* вносить в инвентарь; инвентаризировать.

inveracity [ˌɪnvə'ræsɪtɪ] *n* лживость.

inverse I ['ɪnvəːs] *n* противоположность; обратный порядок.

inverse II *a* обратный; противоположный.

inversion [ɪn'vəːʃən] *n* 1) перевёртывание; перевёрнутость; 2) *грам.* инверсия.

invert [ɪn'vəːt] *v* 1) переворачивать, перевёртывать, опрокидывать; 2) переставлять, менять местами.

invertebrate I [ɪn'vəːtɪbrɪt] *n* беспозвоночное (животное).

invertebrate II *a* беспозвоночный; *перен.* бесхребетный, бесхарактерный.

invest [ɪn'vest] *v* 1) помещать, вкладывать (*деньги*); 2) одевать, окутывать (*with, in*); 3) облекать (*полномочиями и т. п.; in, with*); 4) *воен.* окружить, обложить (*крепость и т. п.*).

investigate [ɪn'vestɪgeɪt] *v* 1) расследовать; 2) исследовать.

investigation [ɪn,vestɪ'geɪʃən] *n* 1) расследование; следствие; 2) исследование.

investigator [ɪn'vestɪgeɪtə] *n* 1) исследователь, испытатель; 2) следователь.

investigatory [ɪn'vestɪgeɪtərɪ] *a* исследовательский.

investiture [ɪn'vestɪtʃə] *n* 1) облечение (*властью*); введение в должность, во владение; 2) награждение.

investment [ɪn'vestmənt] *n* 1) (капитало)вложение, помещение денег; 2) вклад; 3) предприятие *или* бумаги, в которые вложены деньги; 4) облечение (*полномочиями и т. п.*); 5) *воен.* осада, блокада.

investor [ɪn'vestə] *n* вкладчик.

inveterate [ɪn'vetərɪt] *a* закоренелый; заядлый.

invidious [ɪn'vɪdɪəs] *a* 1) оскорбительный, возмутительный (*о поведении, обращении и т. п.*); 2) ненавистный.

invigorate [ɪn'vɪgəreɪt] *v* 1) придавать силы, укреплять; 2) воодушевлять.

invigorative [ɪn'vɪgərətɪv] *a* бодрящий, укрепляющий.

invincibility [ɪn,vɪnsɪ'bɪlɪtɪ] *n* непобедимость.

invincible [ɪn'vɪnsəbl] *a* непобедимый.

inviolable [ɪn'vaɪələbl] *a* нерушимый.

invisibility [ɪn,vɪzə'bɪlɪtɪ] *n* невидимость.

invisible [ɪn'vɪzəbl] *a* невидимый.

invitation [ˌɪnvɪ'teɪʃən] *n* приглашение.

invite [ɪn'vaɪt] *v* 1) приглашать; просить; 2) возбуждать, привлекать, побуждать.

inviting [ɪn'vaɪtɪŋ] *a* соблазнительный, привлекательный.

invocation [ˌɪnvou'keɪʃən] *n* 1) *поэт.* призыв, обращение к музе; 2) заклинание.

invoice ['ɪnvɔɪs] *n* накладная, фактура.

invoke [ɪn'vouk] *v* 1) призывать; 2) взывать (*о помощи, защите*); 3) вызывать заклинанием.

involuntary [ɪn'vɔləntərɪ] *a* невольный; непроизвольный.

involve [ɪn'vɔlv] *v* 1) окутывать; 2) вовлекать, впутывать; запутывать; 3) включать в себя; 4) влечь за собой; 5) закручивать спиралью.

invulnerable [ɪn'vʌlnərəbl] *a* неуязвимый.

inward I ['ɪnwəd] *a* 1) внутренний; направленный, обращённый внутрь; 2) умственный, духовный.

inward II *adv* 1) внутрь; 2) внутренно.

inwardly ['ɪnwədlɪ] *adv* 1) внутри; внутрь; 2) внутренне; про себя.

inwards I ['ɪnwədz] *n pl* внутренности.

inwards II *adv* 1) внутрь; 2) внутренне.

iodine ['aɪədiːn] *n* йод.

ion ['aɪən] *n физ.* ион.

Ionic [aɪ'ɔnɪk] *a* ионический.

ionic [aɪ'ɔnɪk] *a физ.* ионный.

ionosphere [aɪ'ɔnəsfɪə] *n* ионосфера.

iota [aɪ'outə] *n* йота, малая величина.

ir- [ɪr-] *pref* со значением отрицания того, что выражено корнем слова; встречается только в словах, корни которых начинаются с r: irreconcilable непримиримый.

Iraki I, II [ɪ'rɑːkɪ] *см.* Iraqi I, II.

Iranian I [aɪ'reɪnjən] *n* 1) житель Ирана, иранец; иранка; the ~s иранцы; 2) персидский язык.

Iranian II *a* иранский, персидский.

Iraqi I [ɪ'rɑːkɪ] *n* житель Ирака.

Iraqi II *a* иракский.

irascible [ɪ'ræsɪbl] *a* раздражительный, вспыльчивый.

irate [aɪ'reɪt] *a* гневный; разгневанный, сердитый.

ire ['aɪə] *n поэт.* гнев.

ireful ['aɪəful] *a* гневный.

iridescence [ˌɪrɪ'desns] *n* радужность; переливчатость.

iridescent [ˌɪrɪ'desnt] *a* радужный; переливчатый.

iris¹ ['aɪərɪs] *n* радужная оболочка (*глаза*).

iris² *n бот.* ирис.

Irish I ['aɪərɪʃ] *n* 1): the ~ (*употр. как pl*) ирландцы; 2) ирландский язык.

Irish II *a* ирландский.

Irishman ['aɪərɪʃmən] *n* ирландец.

Irishwoman ['aɪərɪʃˌwumən] *n* ирландка.

irk [əːk] *v уст.* надоедать, раздражать.

irksome ['əːksəm] *a* утомительный, скучный, докучливый.

iron I ['aɪən] *n* 1) *хим.* железо; 2) чёрный металл, *напр.* железо, чугун, сталь; cast ~ чугун; as hard as ~ твёрдый как сталь; *перен. тж.* жестокий, суровый; 3) железное изделие; 4) утюг; 5) *pl* цепи, оковы; in ~s в кандалах; 6) *pl* стремена; ◊ strike while the ~ is hot *посл.* куй железо, пока горячо; (too) many ~s in the fire (слишком) много дел одновременно.

iron II *a* железный.

iron III *v* 1) гладить, утюжить; 2) крыть железом; 3) заковывать; □ to ~ out сглаживать, улаживать.

iron-clad I ['aɪənklæd] *n* броненосец.

iron-clad II *a* бронированный.

ironic(al) [aɪ'rɔnɪk(əl)] *a* иронический.

ironing ['aɪənɪŋ] *n* глажение, утюжка.

ironmonger ['aɪənˌmʌŋgə] *n* торговец скобяными изделиями.

ironside ['aɪənsaɪd] *n* 1) отважный, бесстрашный человек; 2) (I.) *pl ист.* «Железнобокие» (*о войсках Кромвеля*).

ironworks ['aɪənwəːks] *n* железоделательный *или* чугуноплавильный завод.

ironyᵃ ['aɪənɪ] *a* железный; железистый.

ironyᵇ ['aɪərənɪ] *n* ирония.

irradiance [ɪ'reɪdjəns] *n* излучение; сияние.

irradiant [ɪ'reɪdjənt] *a* излучающий; сияющий, светящийся.

irradiate [ɪ'reɪdɪeɪt] *v* 1) освещать, озарять; 2) излучать; 3) проливать свет (*на что-л.*).

irradiation [ɪˌreɪdɪ'eɪʃən] *n* 1) блеск, сияние, свечение; 2) освещение, озарение; 3) *физ.* иррадиация; излучение.

irrational I [ɪ'ræʃənl] *n мат.* иррациональное число.

irrational II *a* 1) неразумный; нерациональный; 2) *мат.* иррациональный.

irrationality [ɪˌræʃə'nælɪtɪ] *n* 1) неразумность, нелогичность; нерациональность; 2) *мат.* иррациональность.

irreclaimable [ˌɪrɪ'kleɪməbl] *a* 1) неисправимый; негодный; 2) безвозвратный.

irrecognizable [ɪ'rekəgnaɪzəbl] *a* неузнаваемый.

irreconcilable [ɪ'rekənsaɪləbl] *a* 1) непримиримый; 2) несовместимый, противоречивый (*о мыслях и т. п.*).

irrecoverable [ˌɪrɪ'kʌvərəbl] *a* непоправимый; безвозвратный.

irredeemable [ˌɪrɪ'diːməbl] *a* 1) безнадёжный; непоправимый; 2) не подлежащий обмену на звонкую монету (*о бумажных деньгах*).

irreducible [ˌɪrɪ'djuːsəbl] *a* 1) неуменьшаемый; 2) непревратимый (*в иное состояние и т. п.*); 3) *мат.* несократимый; 4) *мед.* невправимый.

irrefutable [ɪ'refjutəbl] *a* неопровержимый.

irregular [ɪ'regjulə] *a* 1) неправильный (*тж. грам.*); нерегулярный; 2) незаконный; нарушающий правила, форму; 3) неровный (*о поверхности*); 4) несимметричный; 5) неравномерный; 6) *воен.* нерегулярный.

irregularity [ɪˌregju'lærɪtɪ] *n* 1) неправильность; нарушение правил; 2) неровность (*поверхности*); 3) несимметричность; 4) неравномерность, нерегулярность.

irregulars [ɪ'regjuləz] *n pl* нерегулярные войска.

irrelevance [ɪ'relɪvəns] *n* 1) неуместность; 2) не относящийся к делу вопрос *и т. п.*

irrelevant [ɪ'relɪvənt] *a* неуместный, не относящийся к делу.

irremediable [ˌɪrɪ'miːdjəbl] *a* 1) непоправимый; 2) неизлечимый, неисцелимый.

irremissible [ˌɪrɪ'mɪsɪbl] *a* 1) непростительный; 2) обязательный.

irremovable [ˌɪrɪ'muːvəbl] *a* 1) неустранимый; 2) несменяемый (*по должности*).

irreparable [ɪˈrepǝrǝbl] *a* непоправимый, невозвратимый.

irreplaceable [ˌɪrɪˈpleɪsǝbl] *a* незаменимый.

irrepressible [ˌɪrɪˈpresǝbl] *a* неугомонный, неукротимый; неудержимый.

irreproachable [ˌɪrɪˈprǝutʃǝbl] *a* безупречный, безукоризненный.

irresistible [ˌɪrɪˈzɪstǝbl] *a* непреодолимый.

irresolute [ɪˈrezǝluːt] *a* нерешительный.

irresolution [ˌɪˌrezǝˈluːʃǝn] *n* нерешительность.

irrespective [ˌɪrɪsˈpektɪv] *a* безотносительный; независимый (*от чего-л.*).

irresponsibility [ˈɪrɪsˌpɔnsǝˈbɪlɪtɪ] *n* безответственность.

irresponsible [ˌɪrɪsˈpɔnsǝbl] *a* 1) неответственный; 2) безответственный.

irresponsive [ˌɪrɪsˈpɔnsɪv] *a* не отвечающий, не реагирующий (*на — to*).

irretrievable [ˌɪrɪˈtriːvǝbl] *a* непоправимый; невознаградимый.

irreverent [ɪˈrevǝrǝnt] *a* непочтительный.

irreversible [ˌɪrɪˈvǝːsǝbl] *a* 1) неопрокидывающийся; 2) необратимый; 3) непреложный, нерушимый.

irrevocable [ɪˈrevǝkǝbl] *a* 1) бесповоротный, окончательный; 2) *см.* irreversible 3).

irrigate [ˈɪrɪgeɪt] *v* 1) орошать; 2) *мед.* промывать.

irrigation [ˌɪrɪˈgeɪʃǝn] *n* 1) орошение, ирригация; 2) *мед.* промывание.

irrigative [ˈɪrɪgǝtɪv] *a* оросительный, ирригационный.

irritable [ˈɪrɪtǝbl] *a* 1) раздражительный; 2) воспалённый, раздражённый.

irritant I [ˈɪrɪtǝnt] *n* раздражающее средство.

irritant II *a* раздражающий.

irritate [ˈɪrɪteɪt] *v* раздражать.

irritation [ˌɪrɪˈteɪʃǝn] *n* раздражение.

irritative [ˈɪrɪteɪtɪv] *a* раздражающий.

is [ɪz] *3-е л. ед. ч. наст. вр. изъяв. накл. гл.* to be.

isinglass [ˈaɪzɪŋglɑːs] *n* 1) рыбий клей; 2) *разг.* слюда.

Islam [ˈɪzlɑːm] *n* ислам.

Islamite I [ˈɪzlǝmaɪt] *n* мусульманин.

Islamite II *a* мусульманский.

island [ˈaɪlǝnd] *n* 1) остров; coastal (*или* offshore) ~s прибрежные острова; 2) *attr* островной.

islander [ˈaɪlǝndǝ] *n* островитянин.

isle [aɪl] *n поэт.* остров (*тж. в геогр. названиях*); ◇ the Emerald Isle Ирландия.

islet [ˈaɪlɪt] *n* островок.

isn't [ˈɪznt] *разг.* = is not.

isolate [ˈaɪsǝleɪt] *v* 1) изолировать, обособлять; 2) *хим.* выделять (*из смеси*).

isolation [ˌaɪsǝˈleɪʃǝn] *n* 1) изоляция, изолирование; 2) уединение.

isolationism [ˌaɪsǝˈleɪʃnɪzǝm] *n полит.* изоляционизм.

isolator [ˈaɪsǝleɪtǝ] *n* изолятор.

isotherm [ˈaɪsǝuθǝːm] *n* изотерма.

isotope [ˈaɪsǝutǝup] *n физ.* изотоп.

Israelite I [ˈɪzrɪǝlaɪt] *n* израильтянин, еврей.

Israelite II *a* израильский, еврейский.

issue I [ˈɪsjuː] *n* 1) вытекание, истечение; выделение; 2) выход(ное отверстие); 3) выпуск (*газет,*

денег, займа и т. п.*); издание; government ~ казённого образца; 4) устье реки; 5) исход, результат; in the ~ в конечном счёте, в итоге; 6) потомство, дети; without ~ бездетный; 7) спорный вопрос; разногласие; at ~ а) в разногласии, в ссоре (*о людях*); б) нерешённый, спорный (*о вопросе, деле и т. п.*); to take ~ расходиться, быть в противоречии; to join ~ а) приступить к прениям; б) заспорить.

issue II *v* 1) выходить, исходить, вытекать; 2) происходить, получаться в результате чего-л. (*from*); кончаться, иметь результатом (*in*); 3) выпускать; издавать; 4) снабжать, выдавать.

isthmus [ˈɪsmǝs] *n* перешеек.

it I [ɪt] *pron pers* 1) он, она, оно (*о предметах и животных*); 2) это; 3) *при безл. гл. и оборотах не переводится*: it is never late to mend исправить никогда не поздно; it is easy (difficult, early, late, time, cold, warm, chilly, hot) легко (трудно, рано, поздно, пора, холодно, тепло, прохладно, жарко); it drizzles моросит; 4) *в качестве дополнения вместе с глаголами образует разговорные идиомы*: to come it strong зайти слишком далеко; хватить через край; быть очень напористым.

it II *n* 1) *разг.* верх совершенства, идеал; she has it она очень привлекательна, в ней есть «изюминка»; to be it быть выдающимся (*в чём-л.*); to think one is it *амер.* много о себе воображать; 2) *амер. сленг* простофиля, дурак; ◇ in for it в затруднительном положении; на волосок от.

Italian I [ɪˈtæljǝn] *n* 1) итальянец; итальянка; the ~s итальянцы; 2) итальянский язык.

Italian II *a* итальянский.

italics [ɪˈtælɪks] *n pl* курсив(ный шрифт).

itch I [ɪtʃ] *n* 1) зуд; 2) чесотка; 3) страстное стремление (*к — for*).

itch II *v* 1) чесаться, вызывать зуд; 2) нетерпеливо желать; my fingers ~ to be at him у меня руки чешутся задать ему трёпку.

itchy [ˈɪtʃɪ] *a* вызывающий зуд; зудящий.

item I [ˈaɪtem] *n* 1) пункт, параграф, статья; 2) вопрос (*на повестке дня*); номер (*программы*); 3) новость, сообщение (*в газете*).

item II *adv* тоже.

iterate [ˈɪtǝreɪt] *v* повторять.

iteration [ˌɪtǝˈreɪʃǝn] *n* повторение.

itinerant [ɪˈtɪnǝrǝnt] *a* 1) странствующий; 2) объезжающий свой округ.

itinerary I [aɪˈtɪnǝrǝrɪ] *n* 1) маршрут; 2) путеводитель; 3) путевые заметки.

itinerary II *a* путевой, дорожный.

itinerate [ɪˈtɪnǝreɪt] *v* 1) странствовать; 2) объезжать свой округ (*о проповеднике и т. д.*).

it's [ɪts] *разг.* = it is.

its [ɪts] *pron poss* принадлежащий ему, ей; его, её; свой, своя, своё, свои.

itself [ɪtˈself] *pron refl* 1) сам, само, сама; by ~ само собой; 2) себя; -ся, -сь.

I've [aɪv] *разг.* = I have.

ivory [ˈaɪvǝrɪ] *n* 1) слоновая кость; 2) *pl разг.* предметы из слоновой кости: игральные кости, бильярдные шары, клавиши и т. п.; 3) *сленг* зубы; to show one's ivories *разг.* смеяться, скалить зубы; 4) цвет слоновой кости; 5) *attr* (из) слоновой кости; 6) *attr* цвета слоновой кости.

ivy [ˈaɪvɪ] *n бот.* плющ.

J

J, j [dʒeɪ] *n* 10-я буква *англ. алфавита.*

jab I [dʒæb] *n* 1) удáр; пинóк; толчóк; 2) *воен.* удáр штыкóм; кóлющий удáр.

jab II *v* 1) толкáть; пихáть; 2) вонзáть, втыкáть (*into*); 3) колóть (*штыкóм*).

jabber I ['dʒæbə] *n* 1) болтовня, трескотня; 2) бормотáние.

jabber II *v* 1) болтáть, таратóрить, трещáть; 2) бормотáть, бубни́ть.

Jack [dʒæk] *n разг.*: ~ and Gill (*или* Jill) пáрень и дéвушка; ~ of all trades на все рýки мáстер; ~ Frost ≅ Морóз Крáсный Нос; ~ in office высокомéрный чинóвник; бюрокрáт; ~ Ketch палáч; before you could say ~ Robinson ≅ в два счёта; и áхнуть не успéл.

jack[1] I [dʒæk] *n* 1) человéк, пáрень; every man ~ всякий и кáждый; yellow ~ жёлтая лихорáдка; 2) матрóс (*тж.* ~ tar); 3) *карт.* валéт; 4) *тех.* домкрáт, рычáг; 5) *сленг* воéнный полицéйский.

jack[1] II *v* поднимáть домкрáтом (*тж.* to ~ up).

jack[2] *n мор.* гюйс, флаг; Union Jack британский национáльный флаг; to have a ~ up с пóднятым флáгом.

Jack-a-dandy [,dʒækə'dændɪ] *n* франт, дéнди.

jackal I ['dʒækɔːl] *n* 1) шакáл; 2) человéк, выполняющий для другóго черновýю рабóту.

jackal II *v* исполнять черновýю рабóту.

jackanapes ['dʒækəneɪps] *n* 1) дéрзкий ребёнок; 2) нахáл; 3) щёголь, фат.

jackass ['dʒækæs] *n* 1) осёл; 2) дурáк, болвáн.

jackboot ['dʒækbuːt] *n* сапóг выше колéн; *ист.* ботфóрт.

jackdaw ['dʒækdɔː] *n* гáлка.

jacket ['dʒækɪt] *n* 1) жакéт; кýртка; френч; cork ~ прóбковый спасáтельный жилéт; Eton ~ корóткая кýртка; Norfolk ~ тужýрка (*с поясом*); френч; round ~ полуфрáк; strait ~ а) смири́тельная рубáшка; б) *амер. воен. сленг* ки́тель; to dust smb.'s ~ поколоти́ть когó-л.; 2) шкýра (*животного*); 3) кожурá (*картофеля*); 4) пáпка, облóжка (*книги*); 5) *тех.* кожýх (*машины*).

jacketed ['dʒækɪtɪd] *a* 1) одéтый в кýртку; одéтая в жакéт; 2) *тех.* обши́тый; облóженный.

jack-in-the-box ['dʒækɪnðəbɔks] *n* 1) ящик с выскáкивающей фигýркой (*игрушка*); 2) вид фейервéрка.

jack-knife ['dʒæknaɪf] *n* складнóй нож.

jack-o'-lantern ['dʒækə,læntən] *n* блуждáющий огонёк.

Jack-pudding ['dʒæk'pudɪŋ] *n* шут, фигляр.

jack-towel ['dʒæk,tauəl] *n* полотéнце (*для общего пользования на ролике*).

jade[1] I [dʒeɪd] *n* 1) кляча; 2) *шутл.* озорни́ца; saucy ~ нахáлка.

jade[1] II *v* 1) заéздить (*лошадь*); 2) измýчить (*человека*).

jade[2] *n мин.* нефри́т.

jaded ['dʒeɪdɪd] *a* заéзженный, измýченный.

jag I [dʒæg] *n* 1) óстрый выступ, зубéц; óстрая вершина (*скалы, утёса*); 2) зазýбрина.

jag II *v* дéлать зазýбрины, вырезáть зубцáми *или* фестóнами; □ to ~ up *сленг* наложи́ть взыскáние.

jagged ['dʒægɪd] *a* зубчáтый, зазýбренный.

jaggy ['dʒægɪ] *см.* jagged.

jaguar ['dʒægjuə] *n* ягуáр.

jail I [dʒeɪl] *n* 1) тюрьмá; 2) (*без артикля*) тюрéмное заключéние.

jail II *v* заключáть в тюрьмý.

jailbird ['dʒeɪlbəd] *n* арестáнт; уголóвник, престýпник-рецидиви́ст.

jailer ['dʒeɪlə] *n* тюрéмщик.

jalousie ['ʒæluːziː] *n* стáвни, жалюзи́.

jam[1] [dʒæm] *n* варéнье; джем; real ~ *сленг* настоящее удовóльствие, и́стинное наслаждéние.

jam[2] I *n* 1) сжáтие, зажимáние; 2) защемлéние; 3) толпá, дáвка; загромождéние, затóр; traffic ~ «прóбка» (*в уличном движении*); 4) *амер. разг.* затрудни́тельное положéние; 5) заедáние, перебóи в рабóте (*машины и т. п.*); 6) *радио* помéхи при приёме.

jam[2] II *v* 1) зажимáть, сжимáть, сти́скивать; 2) защемлять; 3) вти́скивать (*into*); 4) набивáть (-ся) биткóм; 5) загромождáть, запрýживать (*проход, улицу и т. п.*); 6) *тех.* закли́нивать; 7) *радио* мешáть рабóте другóй радиостáнции; заглушáть или искажáть радиопередáчу.

jamb [dʒæm] *n* 1) косяк (*окна, двери*); 2) *pl* боковые стéнки камина.

jamboree [,dʒæmbə'riː] *n разг.* 1) вечери́нка, пирýшка; 2) слёт бойскáутов.

jangle I ['dʒæŋgl] *n* 1) рéзкий звук, шум, гам; 2) звон (*колоколов*).

jangle II *v* 1) издавáть рéзкие звýки; 2) говори́ть грóмко, рéзко.

janitor ['dʒænɪtə] *n* 1) швейцáр; приврáтник; 2) *амер.* двóрник; стóрож.

January ['dʒænjuərɪ] *n* 1) январь; 2) *attr* янвáрский.

Jap [dʒæp] *n разг.* япóнец.

japan I [dʒə'pæn] *n* 1) чёрный лак; 2) лакирóванная япóнская вéщица.

japan II *v* покрывáть чёрным лáком.

Japanese I [,dʒæpə'niːz] *n* 1) япóнец; япóнка; the ~ (*употр. как pl*) япóнцы; 2) япóнский язык.

Japanese II *a* япóнский.

jape I [dʒeɪp] *n* шýтка.

jape II *v* шути́ть.

jar[1] [dʒɑː] *n* 1) кувши́н, бáнка; 2) *эл.* лéйденская бáнка.

jar[2] I *n* 1) дрожáние; дребезжáние; рéзкий дребезжáщий звук; 2) нéрвное потрясéние, шок; 3) несоглáсие, дисгармóния; 4) ссóра.

jar[2] II *v* 1) дребезжáть; 2) дéйствовать на нéрвы, корóбить (*on*); 3) не согласовáться, дисгармони́ровать; 4) спóрить, ссóриться.

jar[3] *n*: on the ~ *разг.* приоткрытый.

jargon ['dʒɑːgən] *n* 1) жаргóн; 2) тарабáрщина.

jargonize ['dʒɑːgənaɪz] *v* 1) говори́ть на жаргóне; 2) пересыпáть речь профессионáльными тéрминами.

jasmin(e) ['dʒæsmɪn] *n* жасми́н.

jasper ['dʒæspə] *n мин.* яшма.

jaundice I ['dʒɔːndɪs] *n* 1) *мед.* желтýха, разли́тие жёлчи; yellow ~ тропи́ческая (жёлтая) лихорáдка; 2) жёлчность; злóбность; 3) зáвисть; рéвность.

jaundice II *v* 1) вызывáть желтýху; 2) *обыкн. р. р.* возбуди́ть зáвисть, рéвность.

jaundiced [ʹdʒɔ:ndɪst] *a* зави́стливый, ревни́вый; пристра́стный.

jaunt I *n* увесели́тельная пое́здка.

jaunt II *v* отправля́ться в увесели́тельную пое́здку.

jauntiness [ʹdʒɔ:ntɪnɪs] *n* 1) беспе́чность; оживлённость; весёлость; 2) самодово́льство.

jaunting-car [ʹdʒɔ:ntɪŋkɑ:] *n* двухколёсный экипа́ж (*распространённый в Ирландии*).

jaunty [ʹdʒɔ:ntɪ] *a* 1) беспе́чный; оживлённый; весёлый, бо́йкий; 2) самодово́льный.

Javanese I [͵dʒɑ:vəʹni:z] *n* 1) ява́нец; ява́нка; the ~ (*употр. как pl*) ява́нцы; 2) ява́нский язы́к.

Javanese II *a* ява́нский.

javelin [ʹdʒævlɪn] *n* мета́тельное копьё, дро́тик.

jaw I [dʒɔ:] *n* 1) че́люсть; lantern ~ впа́лые щёки, у́зкое худо́е лицо́; 2) *pl* рот, пасть; in the ~s of death в когтя́х сме́рти; 3) *pl* тесни́на; у́зкий вы́ход (*из долины, залива и т. п.*); 4) *pl* тиски́, клёщи; 5) *разг.* болтли́вость; hold your ~! придержи́ свой язы́к!; не болта́й ли́шнего!; 6) ску́чное нравоуче́ние.

jaw II *v разг.* вести́ ску́чный, ну́дный разгово́р; 2) отчи́тывать, де́лать вы́говор.

jaw-bone [ʹdʒɔ:boun] *n* челюстна́я кость.

jaw-breaker [ʹdʒɔ:͵breɪkə] *n разг.* труднопроизноси́мое сло́во.

jay [dʒeɪ] *n* 1) со́йка (*птица*); 2) глу́пый болту́н; пустосло́в.

jay-walker [ʹdʒeɪ͵wɔ:kə] *n разг.* неосторо́жный пешехо́д.

jazz I [dʒæz] *n* 1) джаз; 2) джа́зовая му́зыка; 3) шу́мное поведе́ние; 4) *амер.* эне́ргия.

jazz II *a* нестро́йный (*о звуках*); я́ркий, крича́щий (*о красках и т. п.*); вульга́рный.

jazz III *v* 1) исполня́ть джа́зовую му́зыку; 2) танцева́ть под джаз.

jealous [ʹdʒeləs] *a* 1) зави́стливый; подозри́тельный; недоброжела́тельный; to be ~ of smb. а) зави́довать кому́-л.; б) относи́ться с подозре́нием к кому́-л.; в) ревнова́ть к кому́-л.; 2) ревни́вый; to be ~ ревнова́ть; 3) ре́вностный; забо́тливый.

jealousy [ʹdʒeləsɪ] *n* 1) ре́вность, ревни́вость; 2) за́висть; подозри́тельность.

jean [dʒeɪn] *n* пло́тная хлопчатобума́жная ткань.

jeans [dʒi:nz] *n pl* джи́нсы (*брюки*).

jeep [dʒi:p] *n амер.* а́вто джип.

jeer I [dʒɪə] *n* насме́шка, глумле́ние.

jeer II *v* высме́ивать, насмеха́ться, глуми́ться (*над — at*); to ~ at smb. зло подшу́чивать над кем-л.

Jehu [ʹdʒi:hju:] *n шутл.* возни́ца, извозчик.

jejune [dʒɪʹdʒu:n] *a* 1) худо́й, то́щий; ску́дный; 2) беспло́дный (*о почве*); 3) ску́чный; сухо́й, неинтере́сный.

jelly I [ʹdʒelɪ] *n* 1) желе́; 2) сту́день, заливно́е.

jelly II *v* застыва́ть (*о желе и т. п.*).

jelly-fish [ʹdʒelɪfɪʃ] *n* 1) меду́за; 2) *амер.* бесхара́ктерный, мягкоте́лый челове́к.

jemmy [ʹdʒemɪ] *n* 1) воровско́й лом, «фо́мка»; отмы́чка; 2) бара́нья голова́ (*кушанье*).

jenny [ʹdʒenɪ] *n тех.* 1) подъёмный кран, лебёдка; 2) пряди́льная маши́на (*тж.* spinning-jenny).

jenny-ass [ʹdʒenɪæs] *n* осли́ца.

jeopardize [ʹdʒepədaɪz] *v* подверга́ть опа́сности, рискова́ть (*чем-л.*).

jeopardy [ʹdʒepədɪ] *n* опа́сность, риск.

jeremiad [͵dʒerɪʹmaɪəd] *n* го́рькая жа́лоба.

jerk¹ I [dʒə:k] *n* 1) толчо́к, рыво́к; дёрганье; 2) су́дорожное подёргивание; the ~s конву́льсии.

jerk¹ II *v* 1) ре́зко толка́ть; 2) дви́гаться ре́зкими толчка́ми; дёргать (*о поезде и т. п.*); 3) говори́ть отры́висто.

jerk² *v* вя́лить мя́со дли́нными то́нкими куска́ми.

jerky [ʹdʒə:kɪ] *a* 1) отры́вистый; 2) тря́ский; даю́щий ре́зкие толчки́.

Jerry [ʹdʒerɪ] *n воен. сленг* не́мец, фриц.

jerry-building [ʹdʒerɪ͵bɪldɪŋ] *n* непро́чная постро́йка.

jerry-built [ʹdʒerɪbɪlt] *a* постро́енный на ско́рую ру́ку, кое-ка́к.

jersey [ʹdʒə:zɪ] *n* 1) нате́льная фуфа́йка; вя́заный жаке́т; 2) джерси́ (*вязаная ткань*); 3) пла́тье, ко́фточка *и т. д.* из джерси́.

jessamine [ʹdʒesəmɪn] *см.* jasmin(e).

jest I [dʒest] *n* 1) шу́тка; лёгкая насме́шка; подшу́чивание; in ~ в шу́тку; 2) посме́шище; a standing ~ предме́т постоя́нных насме́шек.

jest II *v* 1) шути́ть, подшу́чивать; 2) насмеха́ться.

jest-book [ʹdʒestbuk] *n* собра́ние шу́ток, анекдо́тов.

jester [ʹdʒestə] *n* 1) шутни́к; 2) шут, кло́ун.

Jesuit [ʹdʒezjuɪt] *n* 1) иезуи́т; 2) лицеме́р.

jet¹ I [dʒet] *n* 1) *мин.* гага́т, чёрный янта́рь; 2) блестя́щий чёрный цвет.

jet² I *n* 1) струя́ (*воды, пара, газа*); 2) *тех.* форсу́нка; сопло́; 3) *тех.* ли́тник; 4) *разг.* реакти́вный самолёт; straight ~ реакти́вный самолёт (без пропе́ллера); 5) *attr* реакти́вный.

jet² II *v* бить струёй.

jet-black [ʹdʒetʹblæk] *a* чёрный как смоль.

jet-fighter [ʹdʒet͵faɪtə] *n* реакти́вный истреби́тель.

jet-propelled [ʹdʒetprəʹpeld] *a* с реакти́вным дви́гателем (*о самолёте и т. п.*).

jetsam [ʹdʒetsəm] *n* груз, сбро́шенный с корабля́ во вре́мя бу́ри и приби́тый к бе́регу.

jettison I [ʹdʒetɪsn] *n* выбра́сывание гру́за за борт.

jettison II *v* 1) выбра́сывать груз за борт; 2) отде́латься (*от чего-л.*).

jetty¹ [ʹdʒetɪ] *n* 1) мол, при́стань; 2) плоти́на, да́мба.

jetty² *a* чёрный как смоль.

Jew [dʒu:] *n* евре́й; the ~ (*употр. как pl*) евре́и.

jewel I [ʹdʒu:əl] *n* 1) драгоце́нный ка́мень; to set a ~ вставля́ть драгоце́нный ка́мень в опра́ву; 2) драгоце́нность; це́нная вещь; 3) сокро́вище.

jewel II *v* 1) украша́ть драгоце́нными камня́ми; 2) вставля́ть ка́мни (*в часовой механизм*).

jeweller [ʹdʒu:ələ] *n* ювели́р.

jewel(le)ry [ʹdʒu:əlrɪ] *n* 1) драгоце́нности; ювели́рные изде́лия; 2) ювели́рное де́ло.

Jewess [ʹdʒu:ɪs] *n* евре́йка.

Jewish [ʹdʒu:ɪʃ] *a* евре́йский.

jib¹ I [dʒɪb] *n* 1) *мор.* кли́вер; 2) *тех.* попере́чина, уко́сина; стрела́ кра́на; ◊ the cut of his ~ его́ вне́шний вид.

jib¹ II *v мор.* перебрасывать (*парус*).

jib² *v* упираться (*о лошади*); артачиться; □ to ~ at сомневаться, колебаться.

jibber ['dʒɪbə] *n* норовистая лошадь.

jibe¹ I, II [dʒaɪb] *см.* gibe I, II.

jibe² *v амер.* соответствовать, совпадать.

jiff(y) ['dʒɪf(ɪ)] *n разг.* мгновение, миг; in a ~ в один миг; wait half a ~ подождите минутку.

jig¹ I [dʒɪg] *n* 1) матрица; шаблон; 2) мелкий инструмент.

jig¹ II *v* 1) промывать руду; 2) сортировать.

jig² I *n* джига (*танец*).

jig² II *v* 1) танцевать джигу; 2) быстро двигаться взад и вперёд; to ~ up and down in excitement метаться из угла в угол от волнения.

jiggery-pokery ['dʒɪgərɪ'poukərɪ] *n разг.* ерунда, чепуха.

jiggle ['dʒɪgl] *v* покачивать.

jig-saw ['dʒɪgsɔ:] *n* машинная пила-ножовка.

Jill [dʒɪl] *n* девушка.

jilt I [dʒɪlt] *n* кокетка, обманщица.

jilt II *v* обманывать; обольщать.

Jim Crow ['dʒɪm'krou] *n амер. презр.* Джим Кроу (*кличка, даваемая неграм американскими расистами*).

jimmy ['dʒɪmɪ] *амер. см.* jemmy.

jingle I ['dʒɪŋgl] *n* 1) звяканье, побрякивание; 2) созвучие, аллитерация.

jingle II *v* 1) позвякивать, побрякивать; 2) изобиловать аллитерациями.

jingo I ['dʒɪŋgou] *n* ура-патриот; шовинист.

jingo II *a* шовинистический.

jingoism ['dʒɪŋgouɪzəm] *n* ура-патриотизм, шовинизм.

jinks [dʒɪŋks] *n:* high ~ шумное веселье.

jitney ['dʒɪtnɪ] *n амер. разг.* 1) пять центов; 2) дешёвое маршрутное такси; 3) *attr* третьесортный, дешёвый.

jitters ['dʒɪtəz] *n pl разг.* нервное возбуждение; to have the ~ нервничать.

jittery ['dʒɪtərɪ] *a разг.* нервный, нервничающий.

jiu-jitsu [dʒu:'dʒɪtsu:] *n* джиу-джитсу (*японская борьба*).

job¹ I [dʒɔb] *n* 1) работа, труд; занятие; bonus (fat) ~ сдельная (доходная) работа; odd ~s случайная работа; by the ~ сдельно, аккордно; 2) дело; bad ~ гиблое дело; неудача; good ~ хорошее состояние дел; 3) *разг.* место, служба, должность; out of ~ без работы; 4) урок, задание; 5) недобросовестная сделка, махинация; 6) использование своего положения в личных интересах; ◊ to do a person's ~ разорить человека.

job¹ II *v* 1) работать нерегулярно, случайно; 2) работать сдельно; 3) брать *или* давать напрокат (*лошадь, экипаж и т. п.*); 4) спекулировать, быть маклером; 5) заключать недобросовестные сделки, устраивать аферы; 6) злоупотреблять своим положением.

job² I *n* тычок, рывок, толчок.

job² II *v* 1) колоть; пырнуть, ткнуть; 2) рвануть лошадь за удила.

jobation [dʒou'beɪʃən] *n* выговор, длинное нравоучение.

jobber ['dʒɔbə] *n* 1) маклер, комиссионер; спекулянт; 2) человек, имеющий случайную работу;

3) недобросовестный делец.

jobbery ['dʒɔbərɪ] *n* 1) использование служебного положения в корыстных целях; 2) сомнительные операции; спекуляция.

jobless ['dʒɔblɪs] *a* безработный.

jobmaster ['dʒɔb,ma:stə] *n* человек, дающий напрокат экипажи и лошадей.

jockey I ['dʒɔkɪ] *n* 1) жокей; 2) *attr* жокейский.

jockey II *v* перехитрить, обмануть; □ to ~ into обманом, хитростью склонить к чему-л.; to ~ out хитростью, обманом получить что-л.

jocko ['dʒɔkou] *n* шимпанзе; *разг.* обезьяна.

jocose [dʒə'kous] *a* шутливый; игривый; обладающий юмором.

jocosity [dʒou'kɔsɪtɪ] *n* шутливость; игривость, юмор.

jocular ['dʒɔkjulə] *a* весёлый; шутливый, юмористический.

jocund ['dʒɔkənd] *a* 1) весёлый; радостный, оживлённый; 2) приятный.

jocundity [dʒou'kʌndɪtɪ] *n* весёлость, оживлённость.

Joe [dʒou] *n:* not for ~! ни за что!; ~ Miller избитая шутка, избитый анекдот.

jog I [dʒɔg] *n* 1) толчок, подталкивание; 2) медленная ходьба; медленная, тряская езда; 3) лёгкая рысь; 4) *амер.* неровность.

jog II *v* 1) толкать, подталкивать; 2) помогать кому-л. припомнить; 3) ехать не спеша, трястись; тащиться (*часто* to ~ on, to ~ along); 4) медленно развиваться; matters ~ along somehow дела кое-как идут.

joggle I ['dʒɔgl] *n* лёгкий толчок; встряхивание.

joggle II *v* 1) толкать, подталкивать; трясти; 2) двигаться толчками.

jogtrot ['dʒɔg'trɔt] *n* 1) рысца; 2) однообразие, рутина.

John [dʒɔn] *n употр. для образования прозвищ, напр.:* ~ Bull английский народ; типичный англичанин.

johnny ['dʒɔnɪ] *n* 1) *разг.* парень, малый; 2) щёголь.

johnny-cake ['dʒɔnɪ,keɪk] *n* маисовая лепёшка (*в США*); пшеничная лепёшка (*в Австралии*).

join I [dʒɔɪn] *n* соединение; точка, линия, плоскость соединения.

join II *v* 1) соединять(ся); присоединять(ся); 2) связывать (*дружбой, работой*); 3) объединять (-ся); 4) вступать в члены (*партии, союза и т. п.*); 5) поступить (*на военную службу*); прибыть в часть; 6) записываться (*в библиотеку*); 7) впадать (*о ручье, речке*); 8) быть смежным; граничить; 9) встретить; нагнать; □ to ~ up *разг.* поступить на военную службу.

joiner ['dʒɔɪnə] *n* 1) столяр; 2) строгальный станок; 3) *амер.* общительный человек.

joinery ['dʒɔɪnərɪ] *n* 1) столярное ремесло; 2) столярные изделия; 3) столярная мастерская.

joint I [dʒɔɪnt] *n* 1) место соединения, стык; 2) *анат.* сустав; сочленение; out of ~ вывихнутый; *перен.* не в порядке; 3) часть разрубленной туши (*нога, лопатка и т. п.*); 4) *амер. разг.* тайный притон; 5) *бот.* узел; 6) *тех.* шарнир, паз, шов.

joint II *a* 1) общий, совместный; соединённый; 2) акционерный (*о капитале*); 3) комбинированный.

joint III *v* 1) сочленя́ть; пригоня́ть (*две части*); 2) расчленя́ть, разнима́ть.

jointly [ʹdʒɔıntlı] *adv* совме́стно, сообща́.

joint-stock [ʹdʒɔıntstɔk] *a* акционе́рный.

jointure I [ʹdʒɔıntʃə] *n* иму́щество, име́ние, запи́санное на и́мя жены́; вдо́вья часть насле́дства.

jointure II *v* вы́делить часть иму́щества, насле́дства жене́.

joist [dʒɔıst] *n* ба́лка, перекла́дина, стропи́ло.

joke I [dʒouk] *n* 1) шу́тка; the best of the ~ са́мая заба́вная часть, са́мая соль; the ~ of the town посме́шище го́рода; to crack (*или* to cut, to spring) ~s отпуска́ть шу́тки; to see a ~ понима́ть шу́тку; practical ~ зла́я шу́тка, сы́гранная с кем-л.; in ~ в шу́тку; it is no (*или* beyond a) ~ э́то не шу́тка, де́ло серьёзное; 2) остро́та; 3) курьёзный, смешно́й слу́чай.

joke II *v* шути́ть, подшу́чивать; дразни́ть; joking apart шу́тки в сто́рону.

joker [ʹdʒoukə] *n* 1) шутни́к, насме́шник; 2) *сленг* челове́к, па́рень; 3) джо́кер (*в поке́ре*).

joky [ʹdʒoukı] *a* шутли́вый; шу́точный.

jollify [ʹdʒɔlıfaı] *v* 1) весели́ться; 2) кути́ть, бра́жничать.

jollity [ʹdʒɔlıtı] *n* 1) весе́лье, ра́дость; 2) пра́зднество.

jolly I [ʹdʒɔlı] *a* 1) весёлый, оживлённый; ра́достный; 2) *разг.* сла́вный, прия́тный; преле́стный; 3) пра́здничный, торже́ственно-ра́достный; 4) слегка́ навеселе́, подвы́пивший.

jolly II *adv разг.* о́чень; ~ fine о́чень хорошо́.

jolly-boat [ʹdʒɔlıbout] *n* четвёрка (*шлю́пка*).

jolt I [dʒoult] *n* толчо́к, тря́ска.

jolt II *v* 1) трясти́, потря́хивать; подбра́сывать; 2) е́хать по тря́ской доро́ге, трясти́сь (*тж.* to ~ along).

jolterhead [ʹdʒoultəhed] *n* о́лух, болва́н.

jolty [ʹdʒoultı] *a* тря́ский.

jonquil [ʹdʒɔŋkwıl] *n* 1) *бот.* нарци́сс; 2) све́тло-жёлтый, па́левый цвет.

jorum [ʹdʒɔːrəm] *n* больша́я ча́ша, *особ.* ча́ша с пу́ншем.

josh [dʒɔʃ] *n амер. сленг* доброду́шная шу́тка.

joss [dʒɔs] *n* кита́йский и́дол.

joss-house [ʹdʒɔshaus] *n* кита́йский храм, куми́рня.

jostle I [ʹdʒɔsl] *n* толчо́к; столкнове́ние; толкотня́.

jostle II *v* толка́ть(ся), пиха́ть(ся); □ to ~ against натолкну́ться на кого́-л.; to ~ away вы́толкнуть; to ~ through проти́скиваться.

jot I [dʒɔt] *n*: not a ~ ни на йо́ту, ни ка́пли.

jot II *v* кра́тко записа́ть, наброса́ть (*тж.* to ~ down).

jotting [ʹdʒɔtıŋ] *n* кра́ткая, бе́глая за́пись.

joule [dʒuːl] *n эл.* джо́уль.

journal [ʹdʒəːnl] *n* 1) журна́л (*преиму́щественно науч́ный*); 2) дневни́к; the Journals *парл.* протоко́лы заседа́ний; 3) *мор.* судово́й журна́л; 4) *тех.* ше́йка (*ва́ла и оси́*); ца́пфа.

journalese [ˏdʒəːnəʹliːz] *n* газе́тный стиль.

journalism [ʹdʒəːnəlızəm] *n* профе́ссия журнали́ста.

journalist [ʹdʒəːnəlıst] *n* 1) журнали́ст; 2) реда́ктор журна́ла.

journalistic [ˏdʒəːnəʹlıstık] *a* журна́льный, относя́щийся к журнали́стике.

journey I [ʹdʒəːnı] *n* 1) пое́здка, прогу́лка; путеше́ствие (*сухопу́тное*); interplanetary ~ межпланѐтное путеше́ствие; pleasure ~ увесели́тельная пое́здка; to (under)take a ~ предприня́ть пое́здку, путеше́ствие; I wish you a good, pleasant ~! счастли́вого пути́!; to be on a ~ путеше́ствовать; to go on (*или* to make) a ~ отправля́ться в путеше́ствие; 2) рейс.

journey II *v* путеше́ствовать; соверша́ть пое́здку.

journeyman [ʹdʒəːnımən] *n* 1) квалифици́рованный рабо́чий; 2) *уст.* подёнщик, подмасте́рье; 3) наёмник.

joust [dʒaust] *n ист.* турни́р, ры́царский поеди́нок.

Jove [dʒouv] *n* 1) *миф.* Юпи́тер; by ~! ей-бо́гу!, кляну́сь!; 2) *поэт.* плане́та Юпи́тер.

jovial [ʹdʒouvjəl] *a* весёлый, игри́вый; общи́тельный.

joviality [ˏdʒouvıʹælıtı] *n* весёлость, игри́вость; общи́тельность.

jowl [dʒaul] *n* 1) че́люсть; челюстна́я кость; 2) щека́.

joy I [dʒɔı] *n* ра́дость, удово́льствие; весе́лье; for ~, with ~ от ра́дости; to the ~ of к ра́дости (*кого́-л.*); I wish you ~ поздравля́ю вас.

joy II *v поэт.* ра́довать(ся), весели́ть(ся).

joy-bells [ʹdʒɔıbelz] *p pl* колоко́льный звон по слу́чаю ра́достного собы́тия (*побе́ды и т. п.*).

joyful [ʹdʒɔıful] *a* по́лный ра́дости, весе́лья; дово́льный, счастли́вый.

joyless [ʹdʒɔılıs] *a* безра́достный.

joyous [ʹdʒɔıəs] *a* весёлый, ра́достный.

joy-ride [ʹdʒɔıraıd] *n разг.* увесели́тельная пое́здка на чужо́й маши́не (*соверша́емая тайко́м*).

J-pen [ʹdʒeıʹpen] *n* перо́ «ро́ндо».

jubilance [ʹdʒuːbıləns] *n* ликова́ние.

jubilant [ʹdʒuːbılənt] *a* лику́ющий.

jubilate [ʹdʒuːbıleıt] *v* ликова́ть, торжествова́ть.

jubilation [ˏdʒuːbıʹleıʃən] *n* ликова́ние.

jubilee [ʹdʒuːbıliː] *n* юбиле́й; пра́зднество.

Judaic [dʒuːʹdeıık] *a* иуде́йский, евре́йский.

judas [ʹdʒuːdəs] *n* 1) (J.) преда́тель; 2) глазо́к (*в две́ри*).

judge I [dʒʌdʒ] *n* 1) судья́; ~ advocate вое́нный прокуро́р; Judge Advocate General нача́льник вое́нно-юриди́ческой слу́жбы, генера́льный прокуро́р; 2) арби́тр, экспе́рт; 3) знато́к, цени́тель.

judge II *v* 1) суди́ть, выноси́ть пригово́р; 2) вести́ сле́дствие; 3) реша́ть вопро́с; 4) счита́ть, полага́ть; to ~ by appearances суди́ть по вне́шнему ви́ду; 5) осужда́ть, порица́ть.

judgematic(al) [dʒʌdʒʹmætık(əl)] *a разг.* рассуди́тельный, здравомы́слящий.

judgement [ʹdʒʌdʒmənt] *n* 1) пригово́р, реше́ние суда́; to pass ~ выноси́ть реше́ние, пригово́р; ~ by default реше́ние в по́льзу истца́ (*за нея́вкой отве́тчика*); 2) наказа́ние, ка́ра; 3) сужде́ние, мне́ние; in my ~ по-мо́ему; 4) здра́вый смысл, проница́тельность.

judgement-day [ʹdʒʌdʒməntdeı] *n рел.* день стра́шного суда́.

judgment [ʹdʒʌdʒmənt] *см.* judgement.

judicature [ʹdʒuːdıkətʃə] *n* 1) трибуна́л;

2) су́дьи (*как корпора́ция*); 3) правосу́дие, суд; 4) отправле́ние правосу́дия.

judicial [dʒuːˈdɪʃəl] *a* 1) суде́бный; суде́йский; 2) крити́ческий; беспристра́стный.

judiciary [dʒuːˈdɪʃɪərɪ] *n собир.* су́дьи; суде́йская корпора́ция.

judicious [dʒuːˈdɪʃəs] *a* разу́мный, здравомы́слящий, рассуди́тельный.

jug¹ I [dʒʌg] *n* 1) кувши́н; 2) *разг.* тюрьма́, «куту́зка» (*тж.* stone-jug).

jug¹ II *v* 1) сажа́ть в тюрьму́; 2) туши́ть (*заячье, кроличье мясо*).

jug² I *n* щёлканье соловья́.

jug² II *v* щёлкать (*о соловье*).

jugful [ˈdʒʌgful] *n* по́лный кувши́н (*чего-л.*).

jugged [dʒʌgd] *a* зубча́тый.

juggins [ˈdʒʌgɪnz] *n сленг* дура́к.

juggle I [ˈdʒʌgl] *n* 1) фо́кус; трюк; 2) обма́н, плутовство́.

juggle II *v* 1) пока́зывать фо́кусы; 2) извраща́ть (*факты, слова; with*); 3) надува́ть, обма́нывать; to ~ a person out of a thing обма́ном вы́манить у кого́-л. каку́ю-л. вещь; to ~ a thing away обма́ном завладе́ть ве́щью.

juggler [ˈdʒʌglə] *n* 1) фо́кусник; 2) шарлата́н, моше́нник.

jugglery [ˈdʒʌglərɪ] *n* 1) пока́зывание фо́кусов; 2) шарлата́нство, моше́нничество.

Jugoslav I [ˈjuːgouˈslɑːv] *n* югосла́в, жи́тель Югосла́вии.

Jugoslav II *a* югосла́вский.

juice [dʒuːs] *n* 1) сок; digestive ~ пищеваρи́тельный сок; gastric ~ желу́дочный сок; 2) су́щность (*чего-л.*); 3) *разг.* электроэне́ргия; 4) *разг.* бензи́н.

juicy [ˈdʒuːsɪ] *a* 1) со́чный; 2) сыро́й (*о пого́де*); 3) *разг.* интеллектуа́льно ра́звитый; интере́сный; 4) *разг.* колори́тный; я́ркий.

julep [ˈdʒuːlep] *n* 1) лека́рственное питьё; 2) *амер.* охлаждённая во́дка с пря́ностями.

July [dʒuːˈlaɪ] *n* 1) ию́ль; 2) *attr* ию́льский.

jumble I [ˈdʒʌmbl] *n* 1) беспоря́дочная смесь, ку́ча; 2) беспоря́док; толчея́.

jumble II *v* 1) дви́гаться в беспоря́дке; 2) толка́ться; □ to ~ **up** сме́шивать(ся), перепу́тывать(ся).

jumble-sale [ˈdʒʌmblseɪl] *n* прода́жа по дешёвке на благотвори́тельном база́ре.

jumble-shop [ˈdʒʌmblʃɔp] *n* ла́вка, где прода́ются разнообра́зные това́ры.

jumbo [ˈdʒʌmbou] *n* большо́й неуклю́жий челове́к *или* живо́тное; гига́нт; коло́сс.

jump I [dʒʌmp] *n* 1) прыжо́к, скачо́к; high (long, standing, running) ~ прыжо́к в высоту́ (в длину́, с ме́ста, с разбе́га); 2) вздра́гивание (*от неожи́данности*); the ~s *разг.* бе́лая горя́чка; 3) внеза́пное повыше́ние (*цен, температу́ры и т. п.*); a ~ in prices ре́зкий подъём цен; 4) бы́стрый перехо́д (*разгово́ра, мы́сли и т. п.*).

jump II *v* 1) пры́гать, скака́ть; to ~ for joy пры́гать от ра́дости; 2) вска́кивать; подска́кивать, подпры́гивать; вздра́гивать; to ~ to one's feet бы́стро встать, вскочи́ть на́ ноги; 3) переска́кивать; перепры́гивать (*тж.* to ~ over); 4) повыша́ться (*о цена́х и т. п.*); 5) приня́ть с ра́достью, ухвати́ться за (*предложе́ние и т. п.*);

at); 6) набро́ситься (*на кого-л.— on*); 7) совпада́ть, согласо́вываться, сходи́ться (*together, with*); 8) сходи́ть (*с рельсов*); 9) бы́стро пробежа́ть (*место в книге*); 10) подбра́сывать, кача́ть; 11) заста́вить пры́гать; □ to ~ **down** а) соскочи́ть, спры́гнуть; б) помо́чь спры́гнуть; to ~ **in**, to ~ **into** вскочи́ть (*куда-л.*); to ~ **out** вы́скочить, вы́прыгнуть; to ~ **over** перепры́гивать; to ~ **up** вска́кивать; ◊ to ~ out of one's skin a) быть вне себя́ от ра́дости; б) подскочи́ть от испу́га; to be ~ed into заста́вить сде́лать что-л. обма́нным путём; to ~ **down** one's throat *разг.* энерги́чно возража́ть кому́-л.; to ~ to conclusions де́лать поспе́шные вы́воды.

jumper¹ [ˈdʒʌmpə] *n* 1) прыгу́н, скаку́н; 2) парашюти́ст; 3) пры́гающее насеко́мое (*блоха́, кузне́чик и т. п.*); 4) *амер.* сала́зки.

jumper² *n* 1) дже́мпер; 2) паруси́новая блу́за (*матро́сская*).

jumpy [ˈdʒʌmpɪ] *a* 1) раздражи́тельный, нерво́зный; 2) де́йствующий на не́рвы.

junction [ˈdʒʌŋkʃən] *n* 1) соедине́ние, стык; то́чка соедине́ния; 2) *ж.-д.* у́зел; узлова́я ста́нция; 3) ме́сто слия́ния (*рек*); скре́щивание (*доро́г*); распу́тье, перекрёсток.

juncture [ˈdʒʌŋktʃə] *n* 1) соедине́ние, сочлене́ние; ме́сто соедине́ния; 2) стече́ние обстоя́тельств; положе́ние дел; at this ~ в э́тот моме́нт; при э́том положе́нии дел; at a critical ~ в крити́ческом положе́нии, в крити́ческий моме́нт.

June [dʒuːn] *n* 1) ию́нь; 2) *attr* ию́ньский.

jungle [ˈdʒʌŋgl] *n* 1) джу́нгли; the law of the ~ зако́н джу́нглей; 2) за́росли, де́бри; 3) *attr* живу́щий в джу́нглях; ◊ hobo ~ ночле́жка (*для безрабо́тных и бродя́г в США*).

jungly [ˈdʒʌŋglɪ] *a* покры́тый густы́ми за́рослями, джу́нглями.

junior I [ˈdʒuːnjə] *n* 1) мла́дший (*по во́зрасту, по служе́бному положе́нию*); 2) студе́нт мла́дшего ку́рса; *амер.* студе́нт предпосле́днего ку́рса.

junior II *a* мла́дший (*по во́зрасту, положе́нию*).

juniority [ˌdʒuːnɪˈɔrɪtɪ] *n* мла́дший во́зраст.

juniper [ˈdʒuːnɪpə] *n* можжеве́льник.

junk¹ [dʒʌŋk] *n* 1) утильсырьё, старьё; отбро́сы; 2) ломо́ть (*хлеба*); кусо́к (*чего-л.*); 3) чурба́н, коло́да; 4) *мор. разг.* солони́на.

junk² *n* джо́нка, сампа́н (*кита́йское плоскодо́нное су́дно*).

junket I [ˈdʒʌŋkɪt] *n* 1) сла́дкий творо́г с муска́тным оре́хом и сли́вками; 2) пир, пи́ршество; пикни́к.

junket II *v* пирова́ть; устра́ивать пикни́к.

junk-shop [ˈdʒʌŋkʃɔp] *n* ла́вка ста́рых веще́й, материа́лов.

junta [ˈdʒʌntə] *n полит.* ху́нта.

Jupiter [ˈdʒuːpɪtə] *n* 1) *миф.* Юпи́тер; by ~! ей-бо́гу!; 2) плане́та Юпи́тер.

jurat [ˈdʒuəræt] *n* ста́рший член муниципалите́та (*в А́нглии*).

juridical [dʒuəˈrɪdɪkəl] *a* юриди́ческий, суде́йский; суде́бный; зако́нный.

jurisdiction [ˌdʒuərɪsˈdɪkʃən] *n* 1) отправле́ние правосу́дия; 2) юрисди́кция; 3) о́бласть, террито́рия, на кото́рую распространя́ется юрисди́кция.

jurisprudence ['dʒuərɪs,pruːdəns] *n* законоведение, юриспруденция; medical ~ судебная медицина.

jurisprudent I ['dʒuərɪs,pruːdənt] *n* юрист, правовед.

jurisprudent II *a* сведущий в законах.

jurist ['dʒuərɪst] *n* юрист.

juror ['dʒuərə] *n* 1) член жюри; 2) присяжный (заседатель).

jury ['dʒuərɪ] *n* 1) присяжные, суд присяжных; common ~ суд присяжных по гражданским и уголовным делам; grand ~ большое жюри (*решающее вопрос о предании кого-л. суду*); coroner's ~ понятые при расследовании случаев скоропостижной смерти; 2) жюри (*по присуждению премий, выигрышей и т. п.*).

jury-box ['dʒuərɪbɔks] *n* место присяжных в суде.

juryman ['dʒuərɪmən] *n* 1) присяжный; 2) член жюри.

just[1] I [dʒʌst] *a* 1) справедливый, правильный; 2) заслуженный, должный; 3) верный, точный.

just[1] II *adv* 1) как раз; именно; ~ as you say как раз так, как вы говорите; ~ about here где-то здесь; 2) только что; ~ now только сейчас, только что; ~ then в тот самый момент; 3) *разг.* вполне, совсем, совершенно; решительно; определённо; 4) едва, еле-еле; 5): ~ shut the door! пожалуйста, закройте дверь!; ~ listen to her! вы только послушайте её!; ~ a moment, please! минуточку!

just[2] *см.* joust.

justice ['dʒʌstɪs] *n* 1) справедливость; to do ~ а) воздавать должное (*человеку*); б) отдать честь (*кушанью*), отведать; 2) правосудие; to administer ~ отправлять правосудие; 3) судья (*особ. в верховном суде Англии*); Justice of the Peace мировой судья; 4) член городского магистра (*в Англии*).

justifiability [,dʒʌstɪfaɪə'bɪlɪtɪ] *n* законность; позволительность.

justifiable ['dʒʌstɪfaɪəbl] *a* могущий быть оправданным.

justification [,dʒʌstɪfɪ'keɪʃən] *n* 1) оправдание, реабилитация; извинение; 2) подтверждение, подкрепление (*фактами*).

justificatory ['dʒʌstɪfɪkeɪtərɪ] *a* оправдательный.

justify ['dʒʌstɪfaɪ] *v* 1) оправдывать (*человека, поступок*); извинять; 2) подтверждать, подкреплять (*фактами*).

jut I [dʒʌt] *n* выступ.

jut II *v* выступать, выдаваться (*тж.* to ~ out).

Jute [dʒuːt] *n ист.* ют; племя ютов (*одно из древненегерманских племён*).

jute [dʒuːt] *n* 1) джут; 2) *attr* джутовый.

juvenescence [,dʒuːvɪ'nesns] *n* юность, молодость.

juvenile I ['dʒuːvɪnaɪl] *n* юноша, подросток.

juvenile II *a* 1) юношеский, молодой, юный; 2) предназначенный для юношества.

juxtapose ['dʒʌkstəpouz] *v* помещать рядом; сопоставлять.

juxtaposition [,dʒʌkstəpə'zɪʃən] *n* сопоставление.

K

K, k [keɪ] *n* 11-я буква англ. алфавита.

kail [keɪl] *см.* kale.

kale [keɪl] *n* 1) кудрявая капуста; 2) суп с кудрявой капустой.

kali ['kælɪ] *n хим.* поташ, щёлок.

kalium ['keɪlɪəm] *n хим.* калий.

Kanaka ['kænəkə, kə'nækə] *n* 1) канак (*житель тихоокеанских островов*); 2) рабочий сахарных плантаций (*в Австралии*).

kangaroo [,kæŋgə'ruː] *n* 1) кенгуру; 2) *pl сленг* акции западноавстралийских рудников; 3) биржевики, спекулирующие на этих акциях.

kaolin ['keɪəlɪn] *n* каолин.

Kazakh I [kɑː'zɑːk] *n* 1) казах; казашка; the ~ (*употр. как pl*) казахи; 2) казахский язык.

Kazakh II *a* казахский.

keel I [kiːl] *n* киль (*корабля*); *поэт.* корабль; false ~ фальшкиль; on an even ~ не качаясь из стороны в сторону; to lay down a ~ заложить судно.

keel II *v* килевать корабль; переворачивать килем вверх; □ to ~ **over** опрокидывать(ся).

keen [kiːn] *a* 1) острый; 2) сильный, резкий; 3) живой (*об интересе и т..п.*); проницательный (*об уме, взгляде*); 4) тонкий (*о слухе*); 5) строгий (*о критике*); 6) пронизывающий (*о ветре*); 7) энергичный; 8) страстно желающий, стремящийся к; увлекающийся; to be ~ on страстно желать чего-л.; увлекаться чем-л.; ◊ ~ as mustard охваченный энтузиазмом.

keen-set ['kiːn'set] *a* 1) голодный; 2) сильно желающий (*чего-л.— for*).

keep I [kiːp] *n* 1) содержание, прокорм; to earn one's ~ зарабатывать себе на пропитание; in good (low) ~ в хорошем (плохом) состоянии; 2) главная башня (*в замке*); цитадель; ◊ for ~s *разг.* навсегда.

keep II *v* (*past, p. p.* kept) 1) держать, иметь (*птицу, скот и т. п.*); you may ~ this это вам (*о подарке*); 2) держать (*слово*), исполнять (*обещание*); 3) хранить, сохранять; to ~ in mind помнить; he ~s nothing from me он ничего не скрывает от меня; 4) соблюдать (*обычаи, законы*); 5) справлять (*праздники*); 6) содержать (*семью*); 7) иметь (*лавочку, магазин*); we don't ~ it (them) мы этого товара не держим; 8) вести (*дневник, счета и т. п.*); 9) управлять, вести; 10) охранять, защищать; 11) задерживать; I won't ~ you long я вас долго не задержу; 12) находиться, держаться; to ~ indoors сидеть, находиться дома; to ~ well up держаться впереди; 13) держать(ся), сохранять(ся) (*в определённом положении, состоянии*); the meat will not ~ long мясо долго не пролежит; 14) *с формами причастия настоящего времени глаголов указывает на продолжающийся характер действия, напр.:* he ~s talking он продолжает говорить; он всё время говорит; □ to ~ **away** а) остерегаться (*собаки, огня и т. п.*); б) держаться в отдалении; в) убирать, прятать (*от кого-л.— from*); to ~ **back** а) удерживать; задерживать; ~ back! не подходите!; б) скрывать (*факты и т. п.*); to ~ **down** а) держать в подчинении, угнетать;

б) подавля́ть (*восста́ние, чу́вство*); в) не дава́ть развива́ться; to ~ **from** возде́рживаться от чего́-л.; to ~ smb. from (+ *Gerund смыслового гл.*) не дава́ть возмо́жности кому́-л. (*сде́лать что-л.*); to ~ **in** а) сде́рживать (*чу́вства*); б) оставля́ть по́сле уро́ков (*шко́льника*); в) подде́рживать (*ого́нь*); г): ~ **in**! не выходи́те!; д): to ~ **in** with smb. остава́ться в хоро́ших отноше́ниях с кем-л.; to ~ **off** а) держа́ть(ся) в отдале́нии; не подпуска́ть; ~ **off**! наза́д!; б) возде́рживаться; to ~ **on** (+ *Gerund смыслового гл.*) продолжа́ть (*де́лать что-л.*); всё вре́мя занима́ться чем-л.; to ~ **on** reading продолжа́ть чита́ть; to ~ **out** а) не допуска́ть, не впуска́ть; не позволя́ть; б) не вме́шиваться, оставля́ть в стороне́; to ~ **to** а) приде́рживаться чего́-л.; не отклоня́ться (*от те́мы и т. п.*); б) ограни́чиваться чем-л.; to ~ **together** остава́ться, держа́ться вме́сте; to ~ **under** держа́ть в подчине́нии; to ~ **up** а) подде́рживать; не дава́ть снижа́ться (*це́нам*); б) не дава́ть тону́ть; в) держа́ться бо́дро; г): to ~ **up** to date пополня́ть после́дними да́нными; д) приде́рживаться (*обы́чаев*); е) не отстава́ть, поспева́ть (*with*); ◊ to ~ **on** at a person *разг.* постоя́нно отчи́тывать, брани́ть кого́-л.

keeper [ˈkiːpə] *n* 1) храни́тель, сто́рож; *мор.* днева́льный; zoo ~ рабо́тник зоопа́рка; 2) *в сло́жных слова́х име́ет значе́ние* хозя́ин, владе́лец, *напр.*: innkeeper хозя́ин гости́ницы; shopkeeper владе́лец магази́на; 3) санита́р (*в сумасше́дшем до́ме*).

keeping [ˈkiːpɪŋ] *n* 1) владе́ние, содержа́ние; 2) хране́ние; охра́на, попече́ние; in safe ~ в безопа́сности; в сохра́нности; 3) согла́сие, согласова́ние; гармо́ния; in ~ with в согла́сии с; out of ~ with при отсу́тствии согла́сия с; несогласо́ванно.

keeping-room [ˈkiːpɪŋrum] *n амер.* гости́ная, о́бщая ко́мната.

keepsake [ˈkiːpseɪk] *n* 1) пода́рок на па́мять; 2) *уст.* альбо́м с иллюстра́циями; 3) *attr* сентимента́льный.

keg [keg] *n* бочо́нок (*ёмкостью до 10 галло́нов*).

Kelt [kelt] *см.* Celt.

ken I [ken] *n* зна́ние, у́мственный кругозо́р; beyond my ~ вы́ше моего́ понима́ния.

ken II *v шотл.* (*past, p. p.* kent) узнава́ть; знать.

kennel[1] I [ˈkenl] *n* 1) соба́чья конура́; 2) лачу́га, хиба́рка.

kennel[1] II *v* 1) помеща́ть в хиба́рку, в лачу́гу; загоня́ть в конуру́; 2) жить в конуре́.

kennel[2] *n* сток, водосто́чная кана́ва.

kent [kent] *past, p. p. см.* ken II.

Kentish [ˈkentɪʃ] *a* ке́нтский.

kept [kept] *past, p. p. см.* keep II.

kerb [kəːb] *n* 1) край тротуа́ра; 2) *attr* у́личный.

kerb-stone [ˈkəːbstoun] *n* бордю́рный ка́мень.

kerchief [ˈkəːtʃɪf] *n* головно́й плато́к, косы́нка.

kerchiefed [ˈkəːtʃɪft] *a* покры́тый платко́м, косы́нкой.

kernel [ˈkəːnl] *n* 1) зерно́, ядро́ (*оре́ха и т. п.*); зёрнышко; *перен.* суть де́ла; 2) *филос.* рациона́льное зерно́.

kerosene [ˈkerəsiːn] *n* кероси́н.

kersey [ˈkəːzɪ] *n* гру́бая шерстяна́я ткань в ру́бчик.

ketch [ketʃ] *n* двухма́чтовое па́русное су́дно.

ketchup [ˈketʃəp] *n* ке́тчуп (*о́стрый тома́тный со́ус*).

kettle [ˈketl] *n* металли́ческий ча́йник; the ~ began to sing ча́йник зашуме́л; ◊ a pretty (*или* a nice) ~ of fish неразбери́ха; ≅ «весёленькая исто́рия».

kettle-drum [ˈketldrʌm] *n* лита́вра.

key[1] I [kiː] *n* 1) ключ; to get (*или* to have) the ~ of the street ≅ оказа́ться без кро́ва, оста́ться на у́лице; golden (*или* silver) ~ взя́тка, по́дкуп; 2) разга́дка (*к реше́нию чего́-л.*); 3) подстро́чный перево́д; собра́ние отве́тов к зада́чам и т. п.; 4) *муз.* ключ, тона́льность; реги́стр, высота́ то́на; all in the same ~ *перен.* всё в том же то́не (ду́хе, сти́ле); in minor ~ *перен.* в мино́рном то́не; to speak in a high (low) ~ говори́ть высо́ким (ни́зким) го́лосом; 5) кла́виша; 6) *эл.* ключ, кно́пка; telegraph ~ ключ Мо́рзе; 7) *тех.* клин; шпо́нка; закре́п; 8) *attr* гла́вный, веду́щий, кома́ндный.

key[1] II *v* 1) запира́ть на ключ; 2) настра́ивать (*муз. инструме́нт*); 3) закли́нивать, закрепля́ть кли́ном, шпо́нкой (*тж.* to ~ in, to ~ on); □ to ~ **up** подба́дривать кого́-л.

key[2] *n* риф; о́тмель.

keyboard [ˈkiːbɔːd] *n* 1) клавиату́ра; 2) *эл.* коммута́тор; распредели́тельная доска́.

keyhole [ˈkiːhoul] *n* замо́чная сква́жина.

key-note [ˈkiːnout] *n* 1) *муз.* основно́й тон, тона́льность; 2) лейтмоти́в; основна́я мысль.

key-ring [ˈkiːrɪŋ] *n* кольцо́ для ключе́й.

keystone [ˈkiːstoun] *n* 1) *архит.* замко́вый *или* ключево́й ка́мень (*сво́да или а́рки*); 2) краеуго́льный ка́мень; основно́й при́нцип.

khaki I [ˈkɑːkɪ] *n* 1) ха́ки (*мате́рия защи́тного цве́та*); 2) фо́рменная оде́жда из ха́ки.

khaki II *a* защи́тного цве́та, цве́та ха́ки, коричнева́то-зелёный.

khan [kɑːn] *n* хан.

kibe [kaɪb] *n* отморо́женное ме́сто, преврати́вшееся в я́зву; ◊ to tread on one's ~s наступи́ть на люби́мую мозо́ль; заде́ть кого́-л. за живо́е.

kick I [kɪk] *n* 1) уда́р ного́й, брыка́нье; пино́к; more ~s than halfpence бо́льше кри́тики, чем похвалы́; to get the ~ а) получи́ть пино́к; б) быть уво́ленным; 2) *разг.* си́ла сопротивле́ния; *амер.* проте́ст; he has no ~ left он весь вы́дохся, обесси́лел; 3) *разг.* ра́достное волне́ние, возбужде́ние; 4) отда́ча (*ружья́*); 5) *спорт.* уда́р; penalty ~ одиннадцатиметро́вый (штрафно́й) уда́р; 6) футболи́ст (*обыкн. с* good *или* bad).

kick II *v* 1) брыка́ть(ся), ляга́ть(ся); бить ного́й; to ~ **downstairs** спусти́ть с ле́стницы; 2) отдава́ть (*о ружье́*); 3) *разг.* сканда́лить, бузи́ть; выража́ть недово́льство, возража́ть (*тж.* to ~ against, to ~ at); 4) подпры́гивать (*о мяче́*); 5) *спорт.* забива́ть гол; □ to ~ **back** а) отплати́ть; б) отдава́ть (*о ружье́*); to ~ **off** а) сбро́сить (*ту́фли*); б) нача́ть игру́ в футбо́л; уда́рить мяч; to ~ **out** вы́гнать, вы́ставить (*кого́-л.*); to ~ **up** поднима́ть (*пыль, шум, сканда́л*); ◊ to ~ **upstairs** дать почётную отста́вку.

kicker ['kɪkə] *n* 1) скандалист, бузотёр; 2) брыкливая лошадь; 3) футболист, подающий мяч.

kickshaw ['kɪkʃɔ:] *n* 1) *пренебр.* лакомство; 2) пустяк, безделушка.

kid[1] I [kɪd] *n* 1) козлёнок; 2) лайка (*кожа*); 3) *разг.* ребёнок; детка (*в обращении*); 4) *attr* лайковый.

kid[1] II *v* ягниться.

kid[2] I *n сленг* обман, надувательство.

kid[2] II *v сленг* обманывать, надувать.

kiddy ['kɪdɪ] *n разг.* ребёнок, малыш.

kid-glove ['kɪdglʌv] *n* 1) лайковая перчатка; 2) *презр.* белоручка; 3) *attr* мягкий, осторожный.

kidnap ['kɪdnæp] *v* 1) похищать (*детей*); насильно увозить; умыкать (*невесту*).

kidnapper ['kɪdnæpə] *n* похититель (*особ. детей*).

kidney ['kɪdnɪ] *n анат.* почка; floating ~ блуждающая почка; 2) характер, тип, род; 3) *attr* почечный; похожий на почку.

kill I [kɪl] *v* 1) убивать; 2) губить, уничтожать, проваливать (*законопроект*); 3) бить, резать (*скот*); 4) заглушать (*о звуках*); глушить; 5) сильно поразить; восхитить; □ to ~ **off** отделаться от кого-л., уничтожить, убить.

kill II *n* убийство; to turn in for the ~ принять участие в убийстве, быть соучастником убийства; to move in for the ~ *перен.* приготовиться к последнему удару.

killer ['kɪlə] *n* убийца.

killing ['kɪlɪŋ] *a* 1) убийственный, смертоносный; 2) уморительный; восхитительный.

killjoy ['kɪldʒɔɪ] *n* нудный, скучный человек, брюзга.

kiln [kɪln] *n* печь для обжига и сушки (*извести, кирпича*).

kilo ['ki:lou] *n амер.* 1) килограмм, кило; 2) километр.

kilogram(me) ['kɪləgræm] *n* килограмм.

kilometer ['kɪlə,mi:tə] *амер. см.* kilometre.

kilometre ['kɪlə,mi:tə] *n* километр.

kilt I [kɪlt] *n* юбка (*шотландского горца или стрелка*).

kilt II *v* 1) подтыкать подол; 2) закладывать в складки.

kiltie ['kɪltɪ] *n* шотландский солдат в национальном костюме.

kin I [kɪn] *n* 1) род, семья; 2) родня, родственники; родство; of ~ сродни; next of ~ близкий родственник.

kin II *a predic* родственный; ~ to родственный; подобный, похожий.

kinchin ['kɪntʃɪn] *n сленг* ребёнок.

kind[1] [kaɪnd] *n* 1) род, семейство; human ~ человеческий род; 2) порода (*животных*); 3) разряд, класс; разновидность; 4) сорт, тип, сорт; of a better ~ лучшего сорта; усовершенствованного типа; smth. of the ~ что-л. в этом роде; coffee of a ~ плохой сорт кофе; what ~ of? что за...?; nothing of the ~ ничего подобного: these ~ of men *разг.* такого типа люди; he is a ~ of он что-то вроде; all ~s of всякого рода; 5) природа, натура, сущность; to act after one's ~ быть верным себе (*в поступках*); 6) качество, характер; to differ in ~, not merely in degree различаться по качеству, а не только по степени; ◊ in

~ натурой; to repay one's insolence in ~ отплатить тем же; a ~ of *разг.* несколько, отчасти, как будто.

kind[2] *a* 1) милый, славный; добрый, сердечный; it is ~ of you это очень мило с вашей стороны; 2) внимательный (*к кому-л.*); любезный; be so ~ as to будьте так любезны; 3) податливый, послушный.

kindergarten ['kɪndə,gɑ:tn] *n* детский сад.

kind-hearted ['kaɪnd'hɑ:tɪd] *a* добрый, мягкосердечный.

kindle ['kɪndl] *v* 1) зажигать, поджигать; 2) разжигать (*страсть*); возбуждать; 3) загораться, вспыхивать.

kindliness ['kaɪndlɪnɪs] *n* 1) доброта; 2) добрый поступок.

kindling ['kɪndlɪŋ] *n* 1) растопка; 2) разжигание.

kindly I ['kaɪndlɪ] *a* 1) добрый, благожелательный; 2) мягкий, приятный (*о климате*).

kindly II *adv* доброжелательно, любезно; ~ show me the way будьте любезны, скажите, как пройти; would you ~ tell me the time? скажите, пожалуйста, который час?

kindness ['kaɪndnɪs] *n* 1) доброта; 2) одолжение; любезность; внимание (*к кому-л.*); have the ~ ... будьте любезны...; 3) доброе дело.

kindred I ['kɪndrɪd] *n* 1) кровное родство; 2) родня; 3) род; клан; 4) сходство характеров.

kindred II *a* 1) родственный; 2) сходный, похожий.

kine [kaɪn] *уст. поэт. pl см.* cow[1].

kinema ['kɪnɪmə] *см.* cinema.

kinetics [kaɪ'netɪks] *n* динамика.

king [kɪŋ] *n* 1) король, царь; the ~ of beasts царь зверей, лев; the ~ of birds орёл; ~ of terrors смерть; ◊ oil ~ нефтяной король.

kingdom ['kɪŋdəm] *n* королевство, царство; the United Kingdom Соединённое королевство; ◊ gone to ~ come *разг.* ушедший на тот свет, умерший.

kingfisher ['kɪŋ,fɪʃə] *n* зимородок.

kinglet ['kɪŋlɪt] *n презр.* царёк.

kingly ['kɪŋlɪ] *a* 1) величественный; 2) королевский; царственный.

kink I [kɪŋk] *n* 1) перекручивание, петля; узел; 2) завиток (*волос*); 3) судорога, спазм(а).

kink II *v* свёртывать(ся) в петлю, перекрутить(ся).

kinky ['kɪŋkɪ] *a* вьющийся, курчавый.

kinsfolk ['kɪnzfouk] *n pl* родственники, родня.

kinship ['kɪnʃɪp] *n* 1) родство; 2) сходство.

kinsman ['kɪnzmən] *n* родственник, родич.

kinswoman ['kɪnz,wumən] *n* родственница.

kiosk [kɪ'ɔsk] *n* киоск.

kip [kɪp] *n сленг* ночлежка.

kipper I ['kɪpə] *n* копчёная рыба.

kipper II *v* коптить, солить рыбу.

Kirghiz I ['kə:gɪz] *n* 1) киргиз; киргизка; the ~ (*употр. как pl*) киргизы; 2) киргизский язык.

Kirghiz II *a* киргизский.

kiss I [kɪs] *n* поцелуй; to give a ~ поцеловать; to steal (*или* to snatch) a ~ сорвать поцелуй; to wave (*или* to throw, to blow) a ~ послать воздушный поцелуй.

kiss II *v* 1) целовать; 2) слегка касаться.

kit[1] [kɪt] *n* 1) ранец, вещевой мешок; 2) багаж; 3) снаряжение; 4) кадка; 5) набор инструментов (*рабочего*); 6) ящик для инструментов (*рабочего*).

kit[2] *n сокр. разг. см.* kitten I.

kit-bag ['kɪtbæg] *n* вещевой мешок.

kitchen ['kɪtʃɪn] *n* кухня; public ~ общественная столовая (*для безработных*).

kitchener ['kɪtʃɪnə] *n* кухонная плита.

kitchen-garden ['kɪtʃɪn'gɑːdn] *n* огород.

kitchen-maid ['kɪtʃɪnmeɪd] *n* судомойка.

kitchen-stuff ['kɪtʃɪnstʌf] *n* продукты, *особ.* овощи, необходимые для готовки.

kite [kaɪt] *n* 1) бумажный змей; to fly a ~ пускать змея; *перен.* пускать пробный шар; 2) коршун; 3) хищный человек, рвач; 4) жулик, шулер; 5) *карт.* подложный вексель.

kith [kɪθ] *n*: ~ and kin знакомые и родственники.

kithless ['kɪθlɪs] *a* безродный.

kitten I ['kɪtn] *n* котёнок.

kitten II *v* котиться.

kittle ['kɪtl] *a* щепетильный, обидчивый; «трудный» (*в обращении*).

kitty ['kɪtɪ] *n* 1) киса (*в обращении к кошке*); 2) *карт.* банк.

kloof [kluːf] *n* ущелье.

knack [næk] *n* 1) умение, сноровка; 2) приём; 3) привычка.

knacker ['nækə] *n* 1) скупщик (*старых домов, пароходов на слом, старых лошадей на мясо*); 2) живодёр.

knacky ['nækɪ] *a* ловкий, умелый; находчивый.

knag [næg] *n* сук.

knaggy ['nægɪ] *a* сучковатый.

knap [næp] *v* разбивать щебень; дробить камень.

knapsack ['næpsæk] *n* рюкзак; ранец.

knar [nɑː] *n* нарост, узел (*на стволе дерева*).

knave [neɪv] *n* 1) негодяй; жулик, плут; 2) *карт.* валет.

knavery ['neɪvərɪ] *n* жульничество, мошенничество.

knavish ['neɪvɪʃ] *a* жульнический, плутовской.

knead [niːd] *v* 1) месить (*тесто, глину*); смешивать; 2) массировать, разминать; 3) формировать (*характер*).

kneading-trough ['niːdɪŋtrɔf] *n* квашня.

knee [niː] *n* 1) колено; to bring smb. to his ~s *перен.* поставить кого-л. на колени; to go on one's ~s становиться на колени; he felt his ~s give у него подкосились ноги; up to one's ~s по колено; 2) наколенник; 3) *тех.* соединительное колено; 4) *attr* коленный; ◊ to give a ~ to поддерживать, оказывать поддержку.

knee-breeches ['niːˌbrɪtʃɪz] *n pl* бриджи.

knee-cap ['niːkæp] *n* 1) *анат.* коленная чашка; 2) наколенник.

knee-deep ['niːˈdiːp] *a* по колено.

knee-joint ['niːdʒɔɪnt] *n* коленный сустав.

kneel [niːl] *v* (*past, p. p.* knelt) 1) становиться на колени; 2) стоять на коленях (*перед кем-л.— to*).

knee-pan ['niːpæn] *см.* knee-cap 1).

knell I [nel] *n* 1) погребальный звон; 2) предвестие смерти, гибели.

knell II *v* 1) звонить при похоронах; 2) звучать зловеще; предвещать (*смерть*).

knelt [nelt] *past, p. p. см.* kneel.

knew [njuː] *past см.* know I.

Knickerbocker ['nɪkəbɔkə] *n* уроженец *или* житель Нью-Йорка (*особ. голландского происхождения*).

knickerbockers ['nɪkəbɔkəz] *n pl.* бриджи.

knickers ['nɪkəz] *разг. см.* knickerbockers.

knick-knack ['nɪknæk] *n* 1) безделушка, украшение; 2) лакомство.

knick-knackery ['nɪknækərɪ] *n* всякие безделушки, мишура.

knife I [naɪf] *n* (*pl* knives) 1) нож, ножик; to play a good ~ and fork есть с аппетитом; to put a ~ into smb. зарезать, заколоть кого-л.; 2) хирургический нож, скальпель; the ~ *разг.* хирургическая операция; 3) сечка; 4) *тех.* струг, резец; 5) *attr* ножевой; ◊ to get a ~ into smb. иметь зуб против кого-л.; резко выказывать свою неприязнь к кому-л.; before you can say ~ немедленно, моментально; ≅ и ахнуть не успел.

knife II *v* резать, колоть ножом; наносить удар ножом.

knife-edge ['naɪfedʒ] *n* 1) остриё ножа; 2) опорная призма (*весов и т. п.*).

knife-grinder ['naɪfˌgraɪndə] *n* 1) точильщик; 2) точильный камень.

knife-switch ['naɪfswɪtʃ] *n эл.* рубильник.

knight I [naɪt] *n* 1) рыцарь; 2) человек, имеющий звание "knight" (*титул, даваемый за личные заслуги перед англ. короной*); 3) кавалер одного из высших английских орденов; Knight of the Bath кавалер ордена Бани; 4) *шахм.* конь.

knight II *v* возводить в рыцарское достоинство.

knight-errant [naɪt'erənt] *n* странствующий рыцарь.

knightly I ['naɪtlɪ] *a* рыцарский.

knightly II *adv* по-рыцарски.

knit [nɪt] *v* (*past, p. p.* knitted, knit) 1) вязать (*чулки и т. п.*); 2) срастаться; 3) сращивать(ся), скреплять(ся); 4) соединять(ся) спаивать(ся) (*тж.* to ~ together); 5) хмурить брови; □ to ~ up а) поднимать спущенные петли; штопать; б) заканчивать (*спор и т. п.*).

knitted ['nɪtɪd] *a* вязаный, трикотажный.

knitter ['nɪtə] *n* 1) трикотажная машина; 2) вязальщик, -ица.

knitting ['nɪtɪŋ] *n* вязание, вязка.

knitting-needle ['nɪtɪŋˌniːdl] *n* вязальная спица, игла.

knit-wear ['nɪtweə] *n собир.* трикотаж.

knit-work ['nɪtwəːk] *n* 1) трикотажные изделия; 2) вязание.

knives [naɪvz] *pl см.* knife I.

knob [nɔb] *n* 1) шишка, выпуклость; 2) ручка (*двери и т. п.*); 3) набалдашник; 4) кусок (*сахара, угля и т. п.*); 5) *тех.* ручка, головка, кнопка; thumb ~ кнопка (*шариковой ручки*); 6) *сленг* голова, башка.

knobble ['nɔbl] *n* маленькая шишка, выпуклость.

knobby ['nɔbɪ] *a* шишкова́тый, покры́тый ши́шками.

knobstick ['nɔbstɪk] *n* 1) па́лка с набалда́шником, дуби́нка; 2) *разг.* штрейкбре́хер.

knock I [nɔk] *n* 1) уда́р; 2) стук (*в дверь*); 3) перебо́и (*в машине*); ◇ to get the ~ *разг.* а) лиши́ться ме́ста, рабо́ты; б) *театр.* быть пло́хо при́нятым пу́бликой.

knock II *v* 1) ударя́ть(ся); би́ть(ся), разбива́ть(ся); to ~ to pieces разбива́ть вдре́безги; to ~ home про́чно забива́ть; 2) стуча́ть(ся) (*в дверь*; *тж.* to ~ at the door); колоти́ть; 3) *разг.* ошеломля́ть, поража́ть, изумля́ть; 4) *амер. разг.* критикова́ть; придира́ться; □ to ~ about а) вести́ разгу́льный о́браз жи́зни; б) болта́ться (*по свету*); стра́нствовать; в) бить, колоти́ть; to ~ against а) налете́ть, наскочи́ть, наткну́ться (*на кого-л.*); б) уда́риться, сту́кнуться; to ~ down а) сбить с ног (*ударом, выстрелом*); б) слома́ть, снести́ (*дом*); в) уда́ром молотка́ объявля́ть вещь про́данной; г) разбира́ть на ча́сти (*машину для перевозки*); д) *разг.* сбива́ть це́ны; е) *амер. сленг* прикарма́нить (*деньги*); to ~ in, to ~ into а) взлома́ть (*дверь, ящик и т. п.*); б) вбива́ть; to ~ off а) стряхну́ть; б) сба́вить (*цену*); в) прекрати́ть рабо́ту; г) поспе́шно зако́нчить, бы́стро отде́латься; д) создава́ть стихи́ экспро́мтом; to ~ out а) выбива́ть, выкола́чивать (*тж. курительную трубку*); б) одолева́ть, побежда́ть; в) нокаути́ровать (*в боксе*); г) потрясти́, порази́ть; to ~ together а) сту́кать(ся), ста́лкивать(ся); б) скола́чивать на ско́рую ру́ку; to ~ under покоря́ться, подчиня́ться; to ~ up а) уда́ром подбро́сить вверх; б) на́скоро устра́ивать, скола́чивать; в) подня́ть, разбуди́ть (*стуком в дверь*); г) изму́чить, утоми́ть; to be ~ed up быть утомлённым, изму́ченным; быть соверше́нно без сил; ◇ to ~ into a cocked hat исколошма́тить; to ~ into the middle of next week ≅ «всы́пать по пе́рвое число́».

knockabout I ['nɔkəbaut] *n* гру́бый фарс.

knockabout II *a* 1) шу́мный, бу́рный (*о представлении*); 2) веду́щий стра́нствующий о́браз жи́зни; 3) рабо́чий, доро́жный (*о костюме*).

knock-down I ['nɔk'daun] *n* 1) *спорт.* нокда́ун; 2) кре́пкое пи́во.

knock-down II *a* 1) сокруши́тельный (*об ударе*); 2) са́мый ни́зкий, минима́льный (*о цене на аукцио́не*); 3) разбо́рный (*о машине и т. п.*).

knocker ['nɔkə] *n* молото́чек на две́ри (*вместо звонка*); ◇ up to the ~ *сленг* а) «с иголо́чки»; б) в соверше́нстве.

knock-out ['nɔkaut] *n* 1) *спорт.* нока́ут; 2) соглаше́ние ме́жду уча́стниками аукцио́на о поку́пке веще́й по ни́зким це́нам; 3) *амер. сленг* сног-сшиба́тельный успе́х.

knoll [noul] *n* холмик, бугоро́к.

knot I [nɔt] *n* 1) у́зел; 2) бант; 3) у́зы; 4) затрудне́ние; загво́здка; Gordian ~ го́рдиев у́зел; to cut the ~ разруба́ть у́зел; 5) *бот.* у́зел, наро́ст; сучо́к; 6) гру́ппа, ку́чка (*людей*); 7) *мор.* у́зел (*мера длины = 1,853 м*).

knot II *v* завя́зывать узло́м.

knotty ['nɔtɪ] *a* 1) узлова́тый; сучкова́тый; 2) запу́танный, тру́дный.

knout I [naut] *n* кнут.

knout II *v* бить кнуто́м.

know I [nou] *v* (*past* knew, *p. p.* known) 1) знать; быть знако́мым; to ~ by sight (by name) знать в лицо́ (по и́мени); to ~ what's what *разг.* быть себе́ на уме́; знать что к чему́; to get to ~ узна́ть, услы́шать; to ~ smb. in the flesh знать кого́-л. при жи́зни; 2) уме́ть (де́лать что-л.); 3) узнава́ть; отлича́ть, различа́ть (*from*).

know II *n*: to be in the ~ быть в ку́рсе де́ла.

know-all ['nou'ɔːl] *n* всезна́йка.

know-how ['nouhau] *n* о́пыт, сноро́вка, уме́ние.

knowing ['nouɪŋ] *a* 1) зна́ющий, уме́лый; 2) ло́вкий; хи́трый; 3) *разг.* мо́дный.

knowingly ['nouɪŋlɪ] *adv* 1) созна́тельно; 2) уме́ло, ло́вко.

knowledge ['nɔlɪdʒ] *n* 1) позна́ния, зна́ния; his ~ of literature его́ позна́ния в литерату́ре; patchy ~ случа́йные, обры́вочные зна́ния; 2) осведомлённость; to come to one's ~ сде́латься изве́стным кому́-л.; to my ~ наско́лько я зна́ю; without my ~ без моего́ ве́дома; 3) знако́мство; 4) нау́ка; branches of ~ о́трасли нау́ки.

known I [noun] *p. p. см.* know I.

known II *a* изве́стный; internationally ~ име́ющий мирово́е и́мя, всеми́рно изве́стный (*об учёном, арти́сте и т. п.*).

know-nothing ['nou,nʌθɪŋ] *n* 1) неве́жда, несве́дущий челове́к; 2) *филос.* агно́стик.

knuckle I ['nʌkl] *n* 1) суста́в па́льца, костя́шка; 2) но́жка (*телячья, свиная*); 3) *тех.* шарни́р.

knuckle II *v* ударя́ть костя́шками па́льцев; □ to ~ down: to ~ down to work энерги́чно взя́ться за рабо́ту; to ~ under уступа́ть, подчиня́ться.

knucklebone ['nʌklboun] *n* 1) ба́бка; 2) *pl* игра́ в ба́бки.

knuckle-duster ['nʌkl,dʌstə] *n* касте́т.

knur(r) [nəː] *n* у́зел; наро́ст (*на дереве*).

kodak I ['koudæk] *n* фотоаппара́т (*системы Кодак*).

kodak II *v* де́лать момента́льные фотосни́мки; *перен. разг.* бы́стро схва́тывать, я́рко обрисо́вывать.

kolkhoz [kɔl'kɔːz] *n* 1) колхо́з; 2) *attr* колхо́зный.

Komsomol ['kɔmsɔmɔl] *n* 1) комсомо́л; 2) комсомо́лец; 3) *attr* комсомо́льский.

kopeck ['koupek] *см.* copeck.

Korean I [kə'rɪən] *n* 1) коре́ец; корея́нка; the ~s коре́йцы; 2) коре́йский язы́к.

Korean II *a* коре́йский.

kotow I, II ['kou'tau] *см.* kowtow I, II.

kowtow I ['kau'tau] *n* ни́зкий покло́н; *перен.* раболе́пие.

kowtow II *v* ни́зко кла́няться (*касаясь голово́й земли́*); *перен.* раболе́пствовать.

kraal [krɑːl] *n* огоро́женный тузе́мный посёлок, краа́ль (*в Южной Африке*).

Kremlin ['kremlɪn] *n* 1) Кремль; 2) *attr* кремлёвский.

kudos ['kjuːdɔs] *n разг.* сла́ва.

Ku-Klux-Klan ['kjuːklʌks'klæn] *n* ку-клукс-кла́н (*реакцио́нная фаши́стская организа́ция в США*).

L

L, l [el] *n* 12-я буква англ. алфавита.

la [lɑː] *n муз.* ля.

lab [læb] *сокр. разг. см.* laboratory.

label I ['leɪbl] *n* ярлы́к; этике́тка; field ~ поме́та (*в словаре*).

label II *v* 1) прикрепля́ть ярлы́к, этике́тку; *перен.* прикле́ить ярлы́к; 2) относи́ть к какой-л. катего́рии.

labial I ['leɪbjəl] *n фон.* губно́й звук.

labial II *a* губно́й.

labialization [ˌleɪbɪəlaɪˈzeɪʃən] *n фон.* лабиализа́ция.

labiodental I ['leɪbɪouˈdentl] *n фон.* гу́бно-зубно́й звук.

labiodental II *a фон.* гу́бно-зубно́й.

labor I, II ['leɪbə] *амер. см.* labour I, II.

laboratory [ləˈbɔrətərɪ] *n* лаборато́рия.

laborious [ləˈbɔːrɪəs] *a* 1) тру́дный; трудоёмкий; 2) трудолюби́вый; 3) вы́мученный (*о стиле*).

labour I ['leɪbə] *n* 1) труд; surplus ~ *полит. эк.* приба́вочный труд; lost ~ напра́сный труд; тще́тные уси́лия; hard ~ ка́торжные рабо́ты; juvenile ~ труд подро́стков; forced ~ принуди́тельный труд; 2) рабо́чий класс; рабо́чая си́ла; труд; Labour and Capital труд и капита́л; 3) ро́ды; родовы́е му́ки; to be in ~ роди́ть, му́читься ро́дами; 4) *attr* трудово́й; рабо́чий; 5) *attr* лейбори́стский; ◇ ~ of love бескоры́стный труд.

labour II *v* 1) труди́ться; 2) прилага́ть уси́лия; добива́ться (*for или* to + *Inf*); to ~ for peace добива́ться ми́ра; 3) продвига́ться с трудо́м; 4) быть в затрудне́нии, в трево́ге; 5) тща́тельно, кропотли́во разраба́тывать.

Labour Day ['leɪbəˈdeɪ] *n* День труда́ (*в США — первый понедельник сентября*).

laboured ['leɪbəd] *a* 1) тру́дный; доста́вшийся с трудо́м; 2) затруднённый (*о дыхании*); 3) вы́мученный (*о стиле*).

labourer ['leɪbərə] *n* неквалифици́рованный рабо́чий, чернорабо́чий.

Labourist ['leɪbərɪst] *см.* Labourite.

Labourite ['leɪbəraɪt] *n полит.* лейбори́ст.

labour-market ['leɪbəˌmɑːkɪt] *n* ры́нок труда́.

Labour-Party ['leɪbəˈpɑːtɪ] *n* лейбори́стская па́ртия.

labour-saving ['leɪbəˌseɪvɪŋ] *a* эконо́мящий труд (*о приспособлении и т. п.*); рационализа́торский.

labyrinth ['læbərɪnθ] *n* лабири́нт.

lace I [leɪs] *n* 1) кру́жево; 2) шнуро́к, тесьма́; 3) галу́н (*обыкн.* gold ~).

lace II *v* 1) шнурова́ть; 2) затя́гиваться в корсе́т; 3) отде́лывать (*кружевом, тесьмой и т. п.*); обшива́ть (*галуном*); 4) подбавля́ть спиртны́е напи́тки в чай, ко́фе; 5) бить, хлеста́ть.

lacerate ['læsəreɪt] *v* 1) раздира́ть, разрыва́ть; 2) терза́ть (*сердце, чувства*); 3) кале́чить.

lachrymal ['lækrɪməl] *a* слёзный (*о железе, протоке и т. п.*).

lachrymatory ['lækrɪmətərɪ] *a* слезоточи́вый (*о газе*).

lachrymose ['lækrɪmous] *a* слезли́вый, плакси́вый.

lacing ['leɪsɪŋ] *n* 1) шнур; шнуро́вка; 2) шнурова́ние.

lack I [læk] *n* недоста́ток, отсу́тствие (*чего-л.* — of); for ~ of за недоста́тком, за отсу́тствием; по ~ оби́лие.

lack II *v* 1) испы́тывать недоста́ток, нужда́ться; не име́ть; 2) не хвата́ть, недостава́ть; he is ~ing ему́ недостаёт, ему́ не хвата́ет.

lackadaisical [ˌlækəˈdeɪzɪkəl] *a* то́мный, жема́нный; сентимента́льный.

lacker I, II ['lækə] *см.* lacquer I, II.

lackey I ['lækɪ] *n* лаке́й.

lackey II *v* лаке́йствовать, уго́дничать.

lackland ['lækˌlænd] *a* безземе́льный.

lacklustre ['lækˌlʌstə] *a* ту́склый (*о глазах, взгляде*).

laconic [ləˈkɔnɪk] *a* лакони́чный, кра́ткий.

laconism ['lækənɪzəm] *n* лакони́зм.

lacquer I ['lækə] *n* 1) лак; политу́ра; 2) *собир.* лак, лакиро́ванные изде́лия.

lacquer II *v* покрыва́ть ла́ком, лакирова́ть.

lacquey I, II ['lækɪ] *см.* lackey I, II.

lactation [lækˈteɪʃən] *n* 1) кормле́ние гру́дью; 2) выделе́ние молока́.

lactic ['læktɪk] *a хим.* моло́чный.

lactiferous [lækˈtɪfərəs] *a* выделя́ющий молоко́, мле́чный сок.

lactose ['læktouz] *n* моло́чный са́хар, лакто́за.

lacuna [ləˈkjuːnə] *n* (*pl тж.* lacunae [ləˈkjuːniː]) 1) пробе́л, про́пуск; 2) углубле́ние, впа́дина (*в кости, ткани*).

lacy ['leɪsɪ] *a* кружевно́й.

lad [læd] *n* ма́льчик, ю́ноша; па́рень.

ladder ['lædə] *n* 1) ле́стница (*приставная, верёвочная*); *мор.* трап; 2) сре́дство для достиже́ния успе́ха; 3) спусти́вшаяся петля́ (*на чулке*).

laddie ['lædɪ] *n* мальчуга́н, парни́шка.

lade [leɪd] *v* (*past* laded; *p. p.* laded, laden) грузи́ть, нагружа́ть.

laden I ['leɪdn] *p. p. см.* lade.

laden II *a* гружёный, нагру́женный (*with*); заста́вленный (*посудой, кушаньями*); гну́щийся под тя́жестью (*плодов*); *перен.* обременённый; пода́вленный.

lading ['leɪdɪŋ] *n* 1) погру́зка; 2) груз; 3) фрахт.

ladle I ['leɪdl] *n* больша́я ло́жка; ковш, черпа́к; soup ~ разлива́тельная ло́жка, полови́ник.

ladle II *v* че́рпать, перелива́ть; □ to ~ **out** а) разлива́ть; б) раздава́ть.

lady ['leɪdɪ] *n* 1) да́ма; госпожа́; my ~ суда́рыня (*обращение*); 2) (L.) ле́ди (*титул знатной дамы*); 3) да́ма се́рдца, возлю́бленная; 4) *разг.* жена́; 5) *в некоторых сочетаниях обозначает существо женского пола, напр.:* ~-doctor же́нщина-врач; ~-cat ко́шка.

lady-bird ['leɪdɪbəːd] *n* бо́жья коро́вка.

lady-bug ['leɪdɪbʌg] *амер. см.* lady-bird.

lady-help ['leɪdɪˈhelp] *n* эконо́мка.

lady-in-waiting ['leɪdɪɪnˈweɪtɪŋ] *n* (*pl* ladies-in-waiting) фре́йлина.

lady-killer ['leɪdɪˌkɪlə] *n* сердцее́д.

ladylike ['leɪdɪlaɪk] *a* 1) с хоро́шими мане́рами, воспи́танная; 2) же́нственный, изне́женный (*о мужчине*).

lady-love ['leɪdɪlʌv] *n* возлю́бленная.

ladyship ['leɪdɪʃɪp] *n* 1) положе́ние, зва́ние ле́ди; 2): your (her) ~ ва́ша (её) ми́лость (*в обраще́нии, упомина́нии*).

lady's-maid ['leɪdɪzmeɪd] *n* го́рничная, камери́стка.

lag[1] I [læg] *n* отстава́ние, запа́здывание.

lag[1] II *v* отстава́ть, запа́здывать, тащи́ться (*тж.* to ~ behind).

lag[2] I *n сленг* ка́торжник.

lag[2] II *v сленг* 1) ссыла́ть на ка́торгу; 2) аресто́вывать, заде́рживать.

lag[3] I *n* 1) боча́рная клёпка; 2) деревя́нная пла́нка.

lag[3] II *v* 1) обшива́ть пла́нками; 2) покрыва́ть терми́ческой изоля́цией.

laggard I ['lægəd] *n* 1) у́валень; 2) безде́льник.

laggard II *a* медли́тельный, вя́лый.

lagoon [lə'guːn] *n* лагу́на.

lagune [lə'guːn] *см.* lagoon.

laic I ['leɪɪk] *n* миря́нин.

laic II *a* све́тский; мирско́й.

laicize ['leɪɪsaɪz] *v* секуляризи́ровать (*изыма́ть из ве́дения духове́нства*).

laid [leɪd] *past, p. p. см.* lay[1] I.

lain [leɪn] *p. p. см.* lie[2] I.

lair [lɛə] *n* 1) берло́га, ло́говище, нора́; 2) заго́н для скота́.

laird [lɛəd] *n шотл.* поме́щик.

laity ['leɪɪtɪ] *n собир.* 1) миря́не; 2) непрофессиона́лы; профа́ны.

lake [leɪk] *n* о́зеро; The Great Lakes Вели́кие озёра (*Ве́рхнее, Гуро́н, Мичига́н, Эри, Онта́рио*); The Lakes *см.* lake-country.

lake-country [ˌleɪk'kʌntrɪ] *n* страна́ озёр.

lake-land ['leɪklænd] *см.* lake-country.

lakelet ['leɪklɪt] *n* озерцо́.

laky ['leɪkɪ] *a* озёрный, со мно́жеством озёр.

lam [læm] *v сленг* бить, колоти́ть.

lama[1] ['lɑːmə] *n* ла́ма (*будди́йский мона́х*).

lama[2] *n см.* llama.

lamb I [læm] *n* 1) ягнёнок; *перен.* а́гнец, ове́чка; like a ~ поко́рно, безро́потно; 2) мя́со молодо́го бара́шка; ◊ one's ewe ~ еди́нственное дитя́, еди́нственное сокро́вище.

lamb II *v* ягни́ться.

lambency ['læmbənsɪ] *n* сверка́ние, блеск.

lambent ['læmbənt] *a* 1) мерца́ющий; светя́щийся (*о не́бе*); 2) лучи́стый, сверка́ющий (*о глаза́х*); 3) блестя́щий (*об остроу́мии и т. п.*).

lambkin ['læmkɪn] *n* ягнёночек.

lamblike ['læmlaɪk] *a* кро́ткий; неви́нный.

lambrequin [ˌlæmbəkɪn] *n* ламбреке́н.

lambskin ['læmskɪn] *n* мерлу́шка.

lame I [leɪm] *a* 1) хромо́й; уве́чный; ~ of (*или* in) a leg хрома́ющий на одну́ но́гу; 2) неуда́чный, неудовлетвори́тельный, неубеди́тельный (*о до́воде, объясне́нии*); 3) непра́вильный, непо́лный (*о разме́ре стиха́*).

lame II *n*: the ~ (*употр. как pl*) хромы́е.

lame III *v* уве́чить, кале́чить.

lamely ['leɪmlɪ] *adv* 1) прихра́мывая; 2) запина́ясь, смуща́ясь.

lameness ['leɪmnɪs] *n* хромота́.

lament I [lə'ment] *n* 1) стена́ние; сето́вание, жа́лоба; 2) эле́гия; погреба́льная песнь.

lament II *v* 1) го́рько жа́ловаться, сето́вать; 2) опла́кивать; горева́ть.

lamentable ['læməntəbl] *a* 1) прискорбный; плаче́вный; 2) *презр.* жа́лкий.

lamentation [ˌlæmən'teɪʃən] *n* жа́лобы, сето́вания, плач.

laminate ['læmɪneɪt] *v* 1) расщепля́ть(ся) на то́нкие слои́, пласти́нки; 2) прока́тывать в листы́ (*о мета́лле*); 3) покрыва́ть листовы́м мета́ллом.

laminated ['læmɪneɪtɪd] *a* листово́й; пласти́нчатый; сло́истый.

lamination [ˌlæmɪ'neɪʃən] *n* рассло́ение; распа́щивание, раска́тывание.

lamp I [læmp] *n* 1) ла́мпа; фона́рь; *перен.* све́точ; red ~ а) кра́сный фона́рь на желе́зной доро́ге как сигна́л опа́сности; б) кра́сный свет у кварти́ры врача́ *или* у две́ри апте́ки; standard ~ торше́р; 2) *поэт.* свети́ло; ◊ to smell of the ~ быть вы́мученным (*о сти́ле, слоге*).

lamp I *v* 1) освеща́ть; 2) свети́ть.

lampblack ['læmpblæk] *n* (ла́мповая) ко́поть, са́жа.

lamp-burner ['læmpˌbəːnə] *n* ла́мповая горе́лка.

lamp-chimney ['læmpˌtʃɪmnɪ] *n* ла́мповое стекло́.

lamp-holder ['læmpˌhouldə] *n* патро́н (*ла́мпочки*).

lamplighter ['læmpˌlaɪtə] *n* фона́рщик; ◊ like a ~ о́чень бы́стро.

lampoon I [læm'puːn] *n* зла́я сати́ра; памфле́т; па́сквиль.

lampoon II *v* писа́ть памфле́т(ы), па́сквили.

lampooner [læm'puːnə] *n* памфлети́ст; пасквиля́нт.

lampoonist [læm'puːnɪst] *см.* lampooner.

lamppost ['læmppoust] *n* фона́рный столб; ◊ between you and me and the ~ ≅ ме́жду на́ми (говоря́).

lamprey ['læmprɪ] *n* мино́га.

lamp-shade ['læmpʃeɪd] *n* абажу́р.

lamp-socket ['læmpˌsɔkɪt] *см.* lamp-holder.

Lancaster ['læŋkəstə] *n*: House of ~ *ист.* дина́стия Ланка́стеров, А́лая ро́за.

lance I [lɑːns] *n* 1) пи́ка, копьё; to break a ~ (with) лома́ть ко́пья, спо́рить (*с кем-л.*); 2) острога́; 3) ланце́т.

lance II *v* 1) пронза́ть пи́кой; 2) вскрыва́ть ланце́том.

lance-corporal ['lɑːnsˌkɔːpərəl] *n воен.* мла́дший капра́л.

lancer ['lɑːnsə] *n* 1) *воен.* ула́н; 2) *pl* лансье́ (*стари́нный та́нец*); 3) *сленг* про́мах.

lance-sergeant ['lɑːnsˌsɑːdʒənt] *n* мла́дший сержа́нт.

lancet ['lɑːnsɪt] *n* ланце́т.

lancinating ['lɑːnsɪneɪtɪŋ] *a* о́стрый, дёргающий (*о бо́ли*).

land I [lænd] *n* 1) земля́, су́ша (*тж.* dry ~); on ~ на су́ше; to go (*или* to travel) by ~ е́хать по су́ше; to reach ~ дости́гнуть бе́рега, приста́ть к бе́регу; to come to ~ войти́ в га́вань; 2) страна́; госуда́рство; native ~ ро́дина, отчи́зна; 3) по́чва; droughty ~ засу́шливые зе́мли; fat (poor) ~ плодоро́дная (ску́дная) по́чва; 4) земе́льная со́бственность; *pl* поме́стья; 5) *attr* сухопу́тный; 6) *attr* земе́льный; ◊ ~ of cakes Шотла́ндия; ~ of promise *библ.* земля́ обетова́нная; the Holy

Land Палести́на; the ~ of Nod ца́рство сна; how the ~ lies как обстоя́т дела́.

land II *v* 1) выса́живать(ся) на бе́рег; прича́ливать; 2) прибыва́ть; достига́ть (*какого-л. места*); 3) *ав.* приземля́ться, сади́ться; 4) приводи́ть к чему́-л.; to ~ in difficulties ста́вить в затрудни́тельное положе́ние; 5) наноси́ть уда́р; попада́ть; 6) выта́скивать на бе́рег (*рыбу*); *перен.* пойма́ть, заполучи́ть.

land-agent [ˈlænd͵eidʒənt] *n* 1) комиссионе́р по прода́же земе́льной со́бственности; 2) управля́ющий име́нием.

land-bank [ˈlændbæŋk] *n* земе́льный банк.

land-breeze [ˈlændbriːz] *n* берегово́й ве́тер, бриз.

landed [ˈlændid] *a* 1) земе́льный; 2) владе́ющий земе́льной со́бственностью.

landfall [ˈlændfɔːl] *n* 1) о́ползень; 2) *мор.* подхо́д к бе́регу.

land-grabbing [ˈlænd͵græbiŋ] *a* захва́тнический.

landholder [ˈlænd͵houldə] *n* аренда́тор *или* владе́лец земе́льного уча́стка.

landing [ˈlændiŋ] *n* 1) вы́садка на бе́рег; ме́сто вы́садки; 2) *воен.* деса́нт; 3) *ав.* приземле́ние, поса́дка; emergency (soft) ~ вы́нужденная (мя́гкая) поса́дка; 4) *ав.* поса́дочная площа́дка; 5) ле́стничная площа́дка; 6) *attr воен.* деса́нтный; 7) *attr. ав.* поса́дочный.

landing-net [ˈlændiŋ͵net] *n* рыболо́вный сачо́к.

landing-party [ˈlændiŋ͵pɑːti] *n* деса́нт, деса́нтный отря́д.

landing-place [ˈlændiŋ͵pleis] *n* 1) ме́сто вы́садки; при́стань; 2) *ав.* поса́дочная площа́дка.

landing-stage [ˈlændiŋ͵steidʒ] *n* при́стань.

land-jobber [ˈlænd͵dʒɔbə] *n* спекуля́нт земе́льными уча́стками.

landlady [ˈlæn͵leidi] *n* 1) владе́лица до́ма (*сдаю́щая кварти́ры*); 2) хозя́йка гости́ницы, пансио́на *и т. п.*; 3) поме́щица.

land-law [ˈlændlɔː] *n обыкн. pl* зако́н(ы) о земе́льной со́бственности.

landless [ˈlændlis] *a* безземе́льный.

land-locked [ˈlændlɔkt] *a* окружённый су́шей; закры́тый (*о гава́ни*).

landloper [ˈlænd͵loupə] *см.* landlouper.

landlord [ˈlænlɔːd] *n* 1) (кру́пный) землевладе́лец, поме́щик; 2) владе́лец до́ма (*сдаю́щий кварти́ры*); 3) хозя́ин гости́ницы, пансио́на.

landlordism [ˈlænlɔːdizəm] *n* 1) систе́ма кру́пного ча́стного землевладе́ния; 2) идеоло́гия кру́пных землевладе́льцев.

landlouper [ˈlænd͵loupə] *n* бродя́га.

landlubber [ˈlænd͵lʌbə] *n мор. разг.* новичо́к в морско́м де́ле.

landmark [ˈlændmɑːk] *n* 1) ориенти́р; 2) поворо́тный пункт, ве́ха (*в исто́рии, жи́зни*); 3) межево́й знак; ве́ха.

landmine [ˈlændmain] *n воен.* фуга́с.

landocracy [lænˈdɔkrəsi] *n* земе́льная аристокра́тия, землевладе́льцы.

land-on [ˈlændˈɔn] *v ав.* приземля́ться, де́лать поса́дку.

landowner [ˈlænd͵ounə] *n* землевладе́лец.

landowning I [ˈlænd͵ouniŋ] *n* землевладе́ние.

landowning II *a* землевладе́льческий.

landrail [ˈlændreil] *n* коросте́ль.

landscape [ˈlænskeip] *n* ландша́фт, пейза́ж.

landscape-gardening [ˈlænskeip͵gɑːdniŋ] *n* плани́ровка садо́в, па́рков *и т. п.*

landscape-painter [ˈlænskeip͵peintə] *n* пейзажи́ст.

land-slide [ˈlændslaid] *n* 1) о́ползень; обва́л; 2) ре́зкое измене́ние в обще́ственном мне́нии, в распределе́нии голосо́в ме́жду па́ртиями.

landslip [ˈlændslip] *n* о́ползень.

landsman [ˈlændzmən] *n* не моря́к, сухопу́тный жи́тель.

land-surveyor [ˈlændsəːˈveiə] *n* землеме́р.

land-tax [ˈlændtæks] *n* поземе́льный нало́г.

landward(s) [ˈlændwəd(z)] *adv* к бе́регу.

lane [lein] *n* 1) доро́жка, тропи́нка (*обыкн. между изгоро́дями*); 2) переу́лок; у́зкая у́лица; ~s and alleys закоу́лки; 3) прохо́д (*между ряда́ми*); 4) морска́я тра́сса; ◊ hunger ~ «доро́га го́лода», безрабо́тица; red ~ *сленг* го́рло.

language [ˈlæŋgwidʒ] *n* язы́к; речь; native (living, dead) ~ родно́й (живо́й, мёртвый) язы́к; finger ~ *см.* finger-language; sign ~ язы́к же́стов; abusive (*или* bad, warm) ~ брань; foul ~ скверносло́вие, strong ~ си́льные выраже́ния.

languid [ˈlæŋgwid] *a* вя́лый, сла́бый; безжи́зненный; ску́чный.

languish [ˈlæŋgwiʃ] *v* 1) вя́нуть, слабе́ть, ча́хнуть; 2) томи́ться, тоскова́ть (*for*); изнемога́ть; 3) принима́ть то́мный вид.

languor [ˈlæŋgə] *n* 1) вя́лость, апати́чность; уста́лость; 2) то́мность; 3) безде́йствие, засто́й.

lank [læŋk] *a* 1) худоща́вый, высо́кий и то́нкий; 2) дли́нный и мя́гкий (*о траве́ и т. п.*); 3) гла́дкий, прямо́й (*о волоса́х*).

lanky [ˈlæŋki] *a* долговя́зый.

lantern [ˈlæntən] *n* 1) фона́рь; *перен.* свето́ч; blind ~, dark ~ потайно́й фона́рь; magic ~ волше́бный фона́рь; parish ~ *шутл.* луна́; 2) светова́я ка́мера маяка́; 3) *архит.* фона́рь.

lanyard [ˈlænjəd] *n* 1) реме́нь, шнур (*для свистка́, бино́кля*); 2) *мор.* тро́совый та́лреп.

lap[1] I [læp] *n* 1) пола́, фа́лда; скла́дка (*оде́жды*); подо́л; кла́пан (*карма́на*); 2) коле́ни; 3) лощи́на, уще́лье; 4) круг, ра́унд (*в состяза́нии*); 5) *тех.* перекры́тие, накла́дка; откидно́й кла́пан; ◊ in Fortune's ~ в полосе́ сча́стья, уда́чи.

lap[1] II *v* 1) загиба́ть, скла́дывать; завёртывать; оку́тывать; охва́тывать; 2) перекрыва́ть; 3) выдава́ться, свиса́ть.

lap[2] I [læp] *n* 1) лака́ние; 2) жи́дкая пи́ща (*для соба́к*); *сленг* «помо́и», сла́бый напи́ток; 4) плеск (*волн*).

lap[2] II *v* 1) лака́ть; 2) жа́дно пить (*тж.* to ~ up, to ~ down); *перен.* упива́ться чем-л.; 3) плеска́ться о́ бе́рег (*о волна́х*).

lap-dog [ˈlæpdɔg] *n* ко́мнатная соба́чка.

lapel [ləˈpel] *n* отворо́т, ла́цкан.

lapidary I [ˈlæpidəri] *n* грани́льщик; гравёр по ка́мню.

lapidary II *a* 1) вы́гравированный на ка́мне; 2) сжа́тый, лапида́рный (*о сти́ле*).

lapidate [ˈlæpideit] *v* побива́ть камня́ми.

lapis lazuli [͵læpisˈlæzjulai] *n* ля́пис-лазу́рь.

Laplander [ˈlæplændə] *n* саа́ми, лопа́рь; лопа́рка; the ~s саа́ми, лопари́.

Lapp [læp] *см.* Laplander.

Lappish I ['læpıʃ] *n* язы́к саа́ми.

Lappish II *a* саа́мский, лопа́рский.

lapse I [læps] *n* 1) оши́бка; опи́ска; упуще́-ние; погре́шность; 2) прегреше́ние; отклоне́ние (от пра́вильного пути́); 3) тече́ние (*времени, воды́*); 4) истече́ние сро́ка; поте́ря пра́ва (*на владе́-ние и т. п.*).

lapse II *v* 1) отклоня́ться от пра́вильного пу-ти́; 2) пасть (*нра́вственно*); 3) впада́ть (*в како́е-л. состоя́ние*); 4) истека́ть (*о сро́ке*); теря́ть си́лу; переходи́ть к друго́му владе́льцу; 5) проходи́ть, исчеза́ть (*постепе́нно*).

lapwing ['læpwıŋ] *n* чи́бис.

larcenous ['lɑːsınəs] *a* воровско́й.

larceny ['lɑːsnı] *n* воровство́; petty ~ ме́лкое воровство́.

larch [lɑːtʃ] *n* ли́ственница.

lard I [lɑːd] *n* свино́е са́ло; лярд.

lard II *v* 1) шпигова́ть; 2) уснаща́ть (*мета-фо́рами и т. п.*).

larder ['lɑːdə] *n* кладова́я.

lardy ['lɑːdı] *a* жи́рный, са́льный.

Lares ['lɛəriːz] *n pl миф., поэт.* ла́ры; ~ and Penates ла́ры и пена́ты, дома́шний оча́г.

large I [lɑːdʒ] *a* 1) большо́й; кру́пный; зна-чи́тельный; многочи́сленный (*о населе́нии и т. п.*); 2) широ́кий (*о взгля́дах, толкова́нии*); 3) *уст.* ще́дрый, великоду́шный.

large II *n*: at ~ а) в це́лом; во всём объёме; б) на свобо́де; to set at ~ освободи́ть, вы́пус-тить на свобо́ду; в) подро́бно, простра́нно (*рас-сказа́ть, описа́ть*); г) вообще́ говоря́; без опре-делённой це́ли; promises made at ~ неопределён-ные обеща́ния; in ~ в большо́м масшта́бе.

large III *adv* 1) широко́; простра́нно; 2) хваст-ли́во.

large-handed ['lɑːdʒ'hændıd] *a* ще́дрый.

large-hearted ['lɑːdʒ'hɑːtıd] *a* великоду́шный.

large-leaved ['lɑːdʒ'liːvd] *a* с больши́ми ли́стьями (*о де́реве*).

largely ['lɑːdʒlı] *adv* 1) широко́; в большо́м, широ́ком масшта́бе; 2) в значи́тельной сте́пени, в большо́й ме́ре; 3) оби́льно; ще́дро.

large-minded ['lɑːdʒ'maındıd] *a* с широ́кими взгля́дами; терпи́мый.

largeness ['lɑːdʒnıs] *n* 1) большо́й, кру́пный разме́р; (больша́я) величина́; 2) широта́ взгля́-дов; 3) ще́дрость; великоду́шие.

large-scale ['lɑːdʒskeıl] *a* кру́пный (*о промы́ш-ленности и т. п.*).

largess(e) ['lɑːdʒes] *n уст.* 1) ще́дрость; 2) ще́д-рый дар.

lariat I ['lærıət] *n* арка́н; лассо́.

lariat II *v* лови́ть арка́ном.

lark[1] [lɑːk] *n* жа́воронок.

lark[2] I *n* весёлая шу́тка; ша́лость, прока́за; for a ~ шу́тки ра́ди.

lark[2] II *v* шути́ть; весели́ться, резви́ться.

larky ['lɑːkı] *a* весёлый, лю́бящий шу́тки, прока́зы.

larrikin ['lærıkın] *n* хулига́н.

larrup ['lærəp] *v разг.* бить, колоти́ть.

larva ['lɑːvə] *n* (*pl* larvae ['lɑːviː]) 1) ли-чи́нка; 2) голова́стик.

larval ['lɑːvəl] *a* личи́ночный, в ста́дии личи́нки.

laryngitis [ˌlærın'dʒaıtıs] *n мед.* ларинги́т.

larynx ['lærıŋks] *n* горта́нь.

lascivious [lə'sıvıəs] *a* сладостра́стный, по-хотли́вый.

laser ['leızə] *n физ.* ла́зер.

lash I [læʃ] *n* 1) плеть, хлыст; реме́нь (*кнута́*); 2) уда́р хлысто́м, плётью; the ~ по́рка; 3) рес-ни́ца; 4) *мор.* найто́в.

lash II *v* 1) хлеста́ть, стега́ть; *перен.* бичева́ть; высме́ивать; 2) понужда́ть, подгоня́ть; 3) доводи́ть (*до бе́шенства и т. п.; to, into*); 4) брани́ться; 5) привя́зывать (*to, on*); связы-вать (*тж.* to ~ together); □ to ~ **out** а) внеза́пно лягну́ть; ки́нуться; б) разрази́ться (*бра́нью и т. п.*).

lasher ['læʃə] *n* запру́да.

lashing ['læʃıŋ] *n* 1) по́рка; наказа́ние, нагоня́й; 2) верёвка, реме́нь (*для привя́зывания*); 3) привя́зывание, вя́зка; 4) *pl разг.* мно́жество, ма́сса (*чего́-л. — of*).

lass [læs] *n* 1) де́вушка; 2) возлю́бленная.

lassie ['læsı] *n ласк.* 1) де́вушка, де́вочка; 2) ми́лочка, ду́шечка.

lassitude ['læsıtjuːd] *n* уста́лость; вя́лость.

lasso I ['læsou] *n* арка́н, лассо́.

lasso II *v* лови́ть арка́ном.

last[1] I [lɑːst] *n* 1) что-л. после́днее по вре́-мени; in my ~ в моём после́днем письме́; my ~ мой мла́дший сын; to breathe one's ~ испусти́ть после́дний вздох, умере́ть; the ~, this ~ после́д-ний из упомя́нутых; 2) коне́ц; at ~ наконе́ц; to the ~, till the ~ а) до конца́; б) до сме́рти; his ~ его́ смерть, его́ после́дние часы́, мину́ты; the ~ of *амер.* коне́ц (*го́да, ме́сяца, пери́ода и т. п.*).

last[1] II *a* 1) после́дний; оконча́тельный; ~ but one предпосле́дний, ~ but two тре́тий с конца́; ~ but not least после́днее, но не ме́нее ва́ж-ное; 2) про́шлый; ~ year про́шлый год; ~ week про́шлая неде́ля; ~ Monday про́шлый понеде́ль-ник; 3) кра́йний, чрезвыча́йный; 4) нежела́тель-ный; he's the ~ man I wanted to see его́ я ме́ньше всего́ хоте́л бы ви́деть; 5) *superl см.* late I.

last[1] III *adv* 1) в после́дний раз; на после́д-нем ме́сте, в конце́ (*при перечисле́нии и т. п.*); 2) *superl см.* late II.

last[2] I *v* 1) продолжа́ться, дли́ться; 2) быть доста́точным, хвата́ть; it will ~ me a month мне хва́тит э́того на ме́сяц; 3) сохраня́ться; держа́ться; носи́ться (*о тка́ни*).

last[2] II *n* выно́сливость, вы́держка.

last[3] *n* коло́дка (*сапо́жная*); ◊ to stick to one's ~ занима́ться свои́м де́лом, не вме́шивать-ся в чужи́е дела́.

last[4] *n* ласт (*ме́ра*).

lasting ['lɑːstıŋ] *a* 1) продолжи́тельный, дли́-тельный; 2) про́чный, постоя́нный; неизме́нный.

lastly ['lɑːstlı] *adv* на после́днем ме́сте, в конце́, наконе́ц, под коне́ц (*при перечисле́нии*).

latch I [lætʃ] *n* 1) щеко́лда, затво́р; за-дви́жка; 2) америка́нский замо́к.

latch II *v* запира́ть(ся).

latch-key ['lætʃkiː] *n* 1) ключ от америка́н-ского замка́; 2) отмы́чка.

late I [leıt] *a* (*compar* later, latter; *superl* latest, last) 1) по́здний (*о вре́мени, пери́оде; тж. о цвета́х, фру́ктах*); 2) запозда́вший, запозда́-

лый; to be ~ опозда́ть; it is too ~ to go тепе́рь уже́ по́здно идти́; 3) неда́вний, после́дний; of ~ years за (*или* в) после́дние го́ды; 4) поко́йный, уме́рший; бы́вший.

late II *adv* (*compar* later; *superl* latest, last) 1) по́здно; early or ~ ра́но йли по́здно; better ~ than never лу́чше по́здно, чем никогда́; 2) неда́вно, за после́днее вре́мя (*тж.* of ~).

lateen [lə'tiːn] *a* треуго́льный (*о парусе*).

lately ['leɪtlɪ] *adv* неда́вно; за после́днее вре́мя.

lateness ['leɪtnɪs] *n* запозда́лость; опозда́ние.

latent ['leɪtənt] *a* скры́тый; в скры́том состоя́нии.

later I ['leɪtə] *a* (*compar см.* late I) бо́лее по́здний.

later II *adv* (*compar см.* late II) по́зже; ~ on поздне́е, пото́м; no ~ than yesterday не да́лее, как вчера́.

lateral ['lætərəl] *a* 1) боково́й; попере́чный; горизонта́льный; 2) побо́чный; второстепе́нный.

latest I ['leɪtɪst] *a* (*superl см.* late I) са́мый по́здний; са́мый све́жий (*об известиях и т. п.*).

latest II *adv superl см.* late II.

latex ['leɪteks] *n* ла́текс, мле́чный сок (*каучуконосов*).

lath I [lɑːθ] *n* пла́нка; дра́нка; ре́йка.

lath II *v* прибива́ть пла́нки.

lathe [leɪð] *n* тока́рный стано́к.

lather I ['lɑːðə] *n* 1) мы́льная пе́на; 2) пе́на, мы́ло (*на лошади*).

lather II *v* 1) намы́ливать(ся); 2) взмы́ливаться (*о лошади*); 3) *разг.* бить, колоти́ть.

lathery ['lɑːðərɪ] *a* 1) намы́ленный, в мы́льной пе́не; 2) взмы́ленный, в мы́ле (*о лошади*); 3) *разг.* ду́тый, нереа́льный.

lathi ['lɑːtiː] *n* око́ванная желе́зом дуби́нка (*оружие в Индии*).

lathy ['lɑːθɪ] *a* долговя́зый; худо́й.

Latin I ['lætɪn] *n* лати́нский язы́к, латы́нь; ◊ thieves' ~ воровско́й жарго́н.

Latin II *a* 1) лати́нский; 2) рома́нский (*о народе, языке*).

latitude ['lætɪtjuːd] *n* 1) *геогр.* широта́; low ~s тропи́ческие широ́ты; 2) широта́ взгля́дов; терпи́мость; 3) *шутл.* (больша́я) ширина́; обши́рность.

latrine [lə'triːn] *n* отхо́жее ме́сто, убо́рная (*в ла́гере, бараке*).

latter ['lætə] *a* 1) *compar см.* late I; 2) .неда́вний, после́дний; 3) после́дний, второ́й (*из упомяну́тых*).

latter-day ['lætə'deɪ] *a* совреме́нный, нове́йший.

latterly ['lætəlɪ] *adv* 1) неда́вно; 2) к концу́, под коне́ц (*жизни и т. п.*).

lattice ['lætɪs] *n* 1) решётка; 2) *attr* решётчатый.

latticed ['lætɪst] *a* решётчатый.

Latvian I ['lætvɪən] *n* 1) латы́ш; латы́шка; the ~s латыши́; 2) латы́шский язы́к.

Latvian II *a* латви́йский.

laud I [lɔːd] *n* хвала́; хвале́бный гимн.

laud II *v* хвали́ть, восхваля́ть.

laudable ['lɔːdəbl] *a* 1) похва́льный; 2) *мед.* доброка́чественный.

laudanum ['lɔdnəm] *n* насто́йка о́пия.

laudation [lɔ'deɪʃən] *n* восхвале́ние.

laudatory ['lɔːdətərɪ] *a* хвале́бный.

laugh I [lɑːf] *n* смех; to give a ~, to break into a ~ рассмея́ться; to raise a ~ вы́звать смех; to

have (*или* to get) the ~ of smb. восторжествова́ть над кем-л.

laugh II *v* смея́ться; to ~ to scorn высме́ивать; □ to ~ at a) смея́ться, насмеха́ться; б) улыба́ться кому́-л.; to ~ away рассе́ять, прогна́ть сме́хом (*скуку, уны́ние*); to ~ down заглуши́ть сме́хом, заста́вить замолча́ть (*оратора и т. п.*); to ~ off отшути́ться; to ~ out (of) а) насме́шками отучи́ть (*от привы́чки и т. п.*); б) насме́шками вы́гнать; to ~ over обсужда́ть в шутли́вом то́не; ◊ to ~ in one's sleeve ≅ смея́ться в кула́к, исподтишка́; he ~s best who ~s last *посл.* хорошо́ смеётся тот, кто смеётся после́дним.

laughable ['lɑːfəbl] *a* смешно́й, заба́вный; коми́чный.

laughing ['lɑːfɪŋ] *a* 1) смею́щийся, улыба́ющийся, весёлый; 2) смешно́й.

laughing-gas ['lɑːfɪŋ'gæs] *n* веселя́щий газ.

laughing-stock ['lɑːfɪŋstɔk] *n* посме́шище.

laughter ['lɑːftə] *n* смех; хо́хот; shrill ~ зво́нкий смех.

launch[1] I [lɔːntʃ] *n* спуск су́дна на́ воду.

launch[1] II *v* 1) спуска́ть су́дно на́ воду; 2) запуска́ть (*ракету*); выпуска́ть (*стрелу́, торпе́ду*); 3) пуска́ть в ход, начина́ть; 4) броса́ть(ся) (*в ата́ку*); наноси́ть (*уда́р*); 5) разрази́ться (*бра́нью; тж.* to ~ out); 6) пусти́ться (*в разгово́р, спор; into; тж.* to ~ out); □ to ~ out отпра́виться, пусти́ться в путь.

launch[2] *n* 1) барка́с; 2) мото́рная ло́дка.

launching ['lɔːntʃɪŋ] *n* 1) спуск су́дна на́ воду; 2) броса́ние, мета́ние; 3) за́пуск (*ракеты и т. п.*); test ~ про́бный за́пуск.

launder ['lɔːndə] *v* 1) стира́ть (*бельё*); 2) стира́ться (*хорошо, плохо* — *о ткани*).

laundress ['lɔːndrɪs] *n* пра́чка.

laundry ['lɔːndrɪ] *n* 1) пра́чечная; 2) бельё (*для стирки или из стирки*).

laureate ['lɔːrɪɪt] *n* лауреа́т; Lenin Prize Laureate лауреа́т Ле́нинской пре́мии.

laurel I ['lɔrəl] *n* 1) лавр; 2) *обыкн. pl* ла́вры; лавро́вый вено́к; to reap (*или* to win) ~s пожина́ть ла́вры; to rest on one's ~s почи́ть на ла́врах.

laurel II *v* венча́ть лавро́вым венко́м.

lava ['lɑːvə] *n* ла́ва.

lavatory ['lævətərɪ] *n* убо́рная, туале́тная ко́мната.

lave [leɪv] *v поэт.* 1) мыть; 2) смыва́ть (*о ручье и т. п.*).

lavender ['lævɪndə] *n* лава́нда; to lay up in ~ а) перекла́дывать лава́ндой (*бельё и т. п.*); б) приберега́ть на бу́дущее.

laverock ['lævərək] *поэт. см.* lark[1].

lavish I ['lævɪʃ] *a* 1) ще́дрый; расточи́тельный; 2) оби́льный.

lavish II *v* 1) быть ще́дрым, расточи́тельным; 2) расточа́ть.

lavishness ['lævɪʃnɪs] *n* 1) ще́дрость; расточи́тельность; 2) оби́лие.

law [lɔː] *n* 1) зако́н; пра́вило; electoral ~ избира́тельный зако́н; martial ~ вое́нное положе́ние; 2) пра́во; юриспруде́нция; ~ and order правопоря́док; common ~ а) непи́санный зако́н; б) обы́чное пра́во; civil (international) ~ гражда́нское (междунаро́дное) пра́во; to read ~ изуча́ть пра́во; 3) профе́ссия юри́ста; to practise ~ быть юри́-

стом; 4) суд, судéбный процéсс; to go to ~ подáть в суд; to have (*или* to take) the ~ of smb. привлекáть когó-л. к судý; to take the ~ into one's own hands распрáвиться без судá; Lynch ~ линчевáние, суд Лйнча, самосýд; 5) *спорт.* преимýщество (*предоставляемое в состязании и т. п.*); *перен.* отсрóчка; поблáжка; ◊ periodic ~ периодйческая система элемéнтов Менделéева); to lay down the ~ говорйть безапелляциóнно, не допускáть возражéний; necessity knows no ~ *посл.* для нуждьí нет закóна.

law-abiding ['lɔːəˌbaɪdɪŋ] *a* подчиняющийся закóнам, законопослýшный.

law-breaker ['lɔːˌbreɪkə] *n* правонарушйтель.

law-court ['lɔːˌkɔːt] *n* суд.

lawful ['lɔːful] *a* закóнный.

lawgiver ['lɔːˌgɪvə] *n* законодáтель.

lawless ['lɔːlɪs] *a* 1) беззакóнный; 2) необýзданный.

lawlessness ['lɔːlɪsnɪs] *n* произвóл, беззакóние.

law-maker ['lɔːˌmeɪkə] *n* законодáтель.

lawn[1] [lɔːn] *n* батйст.

lawn[2] *n* лужáйка, газóн.

lawn-mower ['lɔːnˌmouə] *n* газонокосйлка.

lawny[1] ['lɔːnɪ] *a* батйстовый.

lawny[2] *a* со мнóжеством лужáек, газóнов.

lawsuit ['lɔːsjuːt] *n* судéбный процéсс.

law-term ['lɔːtəːm] *n* 1) юридйческий тéрмин; 2) перйод судéбных сéссий.

lawyer ['lɔːjə] *n* 1) адвокáт; юрйст; 2) законовéд.

lax [læks] *a* 1) вялый, слáбый; 2) небрéжный; неряшливый; 3) расхлябанный; 4) неплóтный.

laxative I ['læksətɪv] *n* слабйтельное (*срéдство*).

laxative II *a* слабйтельный.

laxity ['læksɪtɪ] *n* 1) вялость, слáбость; 2) расхлябанность, распýщенность; 3) неточность, неопределённость.

lay[1] I [leɪ] *v* (*past, p. p.* laid) 1) класть; положйть; 2) возлагáть (*надежды*); 3) повалйть; примять (*траву и т. п.*); прибйть (*пыль*); to ~ low а) повалйть, опрокйнуть; б) унйзить; 4) накрывáть (*стол*); 5) приводйть в какóе-л. состояние; положéние; to ~ bare обнажáть, открывáть, покáзывать; to ~ open открывáть, оставлять незащищённым; to ~ smb. under obligation обязывать когó-л.; to ~ under necessity вынуждáть; 6) нестйсь (*о курице; тж.* to ~ eggs); 7) припйсывать (*что-л. кому-л.*); предъявлять (*обвинéние*); налагáть (*взыскание и т. п.*); 8) успокáивать, утешáть; 9) *разг.* держáть пари, бйться об заклáд; □ to ~ about: to ~ about one наносйть удáры напрáво и налéво; ~ aside а) откладывать в стóрону, отбрáсывать; б) откладывать приберегáть; to ~ by см. to ~ aside б); to ~ down а) укладывать; б) сложйть (*оружие, полномóчия*); отказываться (*от дóлжности и т. п.*); в) оставлять (*надéжду и т. п.*); в) составлять, набрáсывать (*план*); г) излагáть; to ~ in а) запасáть; б) *разг.* «всыпать»; to ~ into см. to ~ in б); to ~ off а) снимáть (*одéжду*); б) откладывать (*в стóрону*); в) *амер.* увольнять; г) прекращáть рабóту; □ to ~ on а) облагáть (*налóгом и т. п.*); б) накладывать (*крáску и т. п.*); в) *разг.* наносйть (*удáры*); to ~ out а) выкладывать, выставлять (*напокáз*); б) планйровать (*расположéние чего-л.*); в) *разг.* сбить с ног; вывести

из стрóя (*в футбóле и т. п.*); г) трáтить, расхóдовать дéньги; д) положйть на стол (*покóйника*); е): to ~ oneself out старáться, из кóжи лезть; to ~ up копйть, откладывать про запáс; ◊ to ~ to heart принимáть блйзко к сéрдцу; to ~ it on thick грýбо льстить, захвáливать; «пересáливать».

lay[1] II *n* 1) (рас)положéние чегó-л.; 2) *сленг* род занятий, пóприще.

lay[2] *past см.* lie[2] I.

lay[3] *n* 1) (кóроткая) пéсенка; 2) пéние птиц.

lay[4] *a* 1) свéтский, мирскóй; 2) непрофессионáльный.

lay-by ['leɪbaɪ] *n* площáдка при магистрáли для стоянки автомашйн.

layer[a1] ['leɪə] *n* 1) слой, пласт; 2) *бот.* отвóдок.

layer[a2] *n*: this hen is a good (bad) ~ эта кýрица хорошó (плóхо) несётся.

layer[b] ['leə] *v* разводйть отвóдками (*растéния*).

layer-cake ['leɪəkeɪk] *n* слоёный торт; слоёный пирóг.

layette [leɪ'et] *n* придáное новорождённого.

lay-figure ['leɪˌfɪgə] *n* 1) манекéн (*худóжника*); 2) ничтóжество (*о человéке*); 3) неправдоподóбный персонáж; нереáльный óбраз.

layman ['leɪmən] *n* 1) мирянин; 2) неспециалйст.

lay-off ['leɪɔːf] *n* 1) приостанóвка произвóдства; 2) вынужденная безрабóтица; 3) увольнéние.

lay-out ['leɪaut] *n* 1) план, разбйвка (*сáда и т. д.*); 2) положéние дел; 3) *амер.* оборýдование; 4) набóр инструмéнтов; 5) макéт (*кнйги, газéты и т. п.*).

laze [leɪz] *v разг.* ленйться, бездéльничать, лóдырничать (*тж.* to ~ away).

laziness ['leɪzɪnɪs] *n* лéность; лень.

lazy ['leɪzɪ] *a* ленйвый.

lazy-bones ['leɪzɪbounz] *n разг.* лентяй.

lea [liː] *n* 1) *поэт.* луг, пóле; 2) *с.-х.* пар, пóле под пáром.

leach I [liːtʃ] *n* 1) рапá, рассóл; 2) щёлок.

leach II *v* выщелáчивать.

lead[a] [led] *n* 1) свинéц; white ~ свинцóвые белйла; red ~ сýрик; 2) *мор.* лот; to cast (*или* to heave) the ~ промéрить глубинý; 3) *pl полигр.* шпóны; 4) *pl* свинцóвые пóлосы для покрытия крыши; 5) *attr* свинцóвый; ◊ to swing the ~ *сленг* уклоняться от рабóты, симулйруя болéзнь.

lead[b] I [liːd] *n* 1) руковóдство, инициатйва; to take the ~ брать на себя руковóдство, инициатйву; 2) примéр; to follow the ~ of слéдовать чьемý-л. примéру; to give smb. a ~ показáть комý-л. примéр; 3) указáние, дирéктива; 4) пéрвенство, пéрвое мéсто; in the ~ во главé (*процéссии, колóнны*); 5) *театр.* глáвная роль; исполнйтель (-ница) глáвной рóли; 6) *карт.* пéрвый ход; it is your ~ ваш ход, вам начинáть; 7) дорóжка; 8) поводóк (*для собáк*); 9) *тех.* шаг *или* ход винтá; 10) *эл.* прóвод; 11) *геол.* жйла.

lead[b] II *v* (*past, p. p.* led) 1) вестй; to ~ the way идтй во главé, вестй за собóй; to ~ nowhere ни к чемý не приводйть; to ~ astray сбить с путй йстинного; 2) руководйть, возглавлять; 3) приводйть; 4) идтй пéрвым (*в состязáнии*); 5) *карт.* ходйть; □ to ~ away уводйть; увлекáть; to ~ back отводйть назáд; to ~ off а) начинáть; открывáть (*прéния, бал и т. п.*); б) отводйть, отклонять;

отвраща́ть; to ~ **out** выводи́ть; to ~ **out of** выходи́ть (*о комнатах*); to ~ **up** (*to*) а) приводи́ть к чему́-л.; б) подготовля́ть к чему́-л.; наводи́ть разгово́р на что-л.

leaden ['ledn] *a* 1) свинцо́вый; 2) се́рый (*о небе*); 3) тяжёлый.

leader ['liːdə] *n* 1) руководи́тель, вождь; ли́дер; pioneer ~ пионервожа́тый; 2) вожа́к; 3) дирижёр; ре́гент (*хора*); 4) передова́я статья́; 5) пере́дняя ло́шадь (*в упряжке*); 6) *эл.* про́вод, проводни́к; 7) водосто́чный кана́л, жёлоб; 8) гла́вный побе́г (*растения*).

leaderette [ˌliːdəˈret] *n* коро́ткая редакцио́нная заме́тка (*в газете*).

leadership ['liːdəʃɪp] *n* руково́дство.

leading ['liːdɪŋ] *a* 1) веду́щий; руководя́щий; передово́й; головно́й (*о корабле, отряде*); ~ man (lady) исполни́тель(ница) гла́вной ро́ли; 2) *тех.* веду́щий, направля́ющий; ходово́й.

leading-strings ['liːdɪŋstrɪŋz] *n pl* помо́чи; in ~ *перен.* на поводу́.

lead-off ['liːdɔːf] *n* нача́ло.

leaf I [liːf] *n* (*pl* **leaves**) 1) лист; 2) листва́; to come into ~, to put forth leaves покрыва́ться листво́й, распуска́ться (*о деревьях*); in ~ распусти́вшийся (*о деревьях и т. п.*); 3) лист (*книги*); страни́ца; loose ~ вкладно́й лист; 4) ство́рка (*двери*); откидна́я доска́; 5) *attr* листово́й; ◇ to turn over a new ~ нача́ть но́вую жизнь; to take a ~ out of smb.'s book сле́довать чьему́-л. приме́ру, подража́ть кому́-л.

leaf II *v* 1) покрыва́ться листво́й; 2) перели́стывать.

leafage ['liːfɪdʒ] *n* листва́.

leaf-bud ['liːfbʌd] *n* листова́я по́чка.

leafless ['liːflɪs] *a* безли́стный.

leaflet ['liːflɪt] *n* 1) листо́вка; 2) ли́стик, листо́чек, листо́к.

leafstalk ['liːfstɔːk] *n* черешо́к.

leafy ['liːfɪ] *a* покры́тый ли́стьями.

league¹ ['liːg] *n* лье (*мера длины*).

league² I *n* сою́з, ли́га; in ~ with в сою́зе с.

league² II *v* объединя́ть(ся); образова́ть сою́з.

leaguer ['liːgə] *n* член ли́ги *или* сою́за.

leak I [liːk] *n* течь, уте́чка; to spring a ~, to start a ~ дать течь.

leak II *v* 1) дава́ть течь, пропуска́ть во́ду; 2) проса́чиваться; □ to ~ **out** проса́чиваться, вытека́ть; *перен.* обнару́живаться, станови́ться изве́стным (*о секрете и т. п.*).

leakage ['liːkɪdʒ] *n* 1) уте́чка, проса́чивание; 2) обнаруже́ние (*секрета и т. п.*).

leaky ['liːkɪ] *a* 1) име́ющий течь; неплотный; 2) не уме́ющий храни́ть секре́ты.

lean¹ I [liːn] *n* по́стное мя́со.

lean¹ II *a* 1) худо́й, то́щий; as ~ as a rake худ как ще́пка; 2) нежи́рный; по́стный; 3) ску́дный.

lean² I *v* (*past, p. p.* **leaned, leant**) 1) наклоня́ться; сгиба́ться; 2) опира́ться; прислоня́ть(ся) (*on, against*); 3) полага́ться (*на — on, upon*); 4) склоня́ться, име́ть скло́нность, тенде́нцию (*к чему́-л.— to, towards*); ◇ ~ over backward ударя́ться в другу́ю кра́йность.

lean² II *n* накло́н.

leaning ['liːnɪŋ] *n* скло́нность.

leant [lent] *past, p. p. см.* lean² I.

lean-to ['liːnˈtuː] *n* пристро́йка (*к зданию*); наве́с.

leap I [liːp] *n* прыжо́к, скачо́к; a ~ into the cosmos прыжо́к в ко́смос; a ~ in the dark прыжо́к в неизве́стность, риско́ванный шаг; by ~s and bounds с большо́й быстрото́й.

leap II *v* (*past, p. p.* **leapt, leaped**) пры́гать, скака́ть; перепры́гивать (*тж.* to ~ over).

leap-day ['liːpdeɪ] *n* 29 февраля́ (*см. тж.* leap--year).

leap-frog ['liːpfrɔg] *n* чехарда́.

leapt [lept] *past, p. p. см.* leap II.

leap-year ['liːpjɑː] *n* високо́сный год.

learn [ləːn] *v* (*past, p. p.* **learnt, learned**) 1) учи́ться; учи́ть что-л.; научи́ться чему́-л.; to ~ by heart, to ~ by rote учи́ть наизу́сть; 2) узнава́ть; 3) *уст., шутл.* учи́ть кого́-л.

learnedᵃ ['ləːnɪd] *a* учёный.

learnedᵇ [ləːnt] *past, p. p. см.* learn.

learner ['ləːnə] *n* уча́щийся, учени́к.

learning ['ləːnɪŋ] *n* 1) уче́ние; 2) учёность; образова́ние.

learnt [ləːnt] *past, p. p. см.* learn.

lease I [liːs] *n* 1) аре́нда; сда́ча внаём; by ~, on ~ в аре́нду, на усло́виях аре́нды; 2) аре́ндный до́говор; ◇ a fresh ~ of power продле́ние президе́нтских полномо́чий; to take a new ~ of life воспря́нуть ду́хом, верну́ться к жи́зни.

lease II *v* сдава́ть *или* брать в аре́нду.

leasehold I ['liːshould] *n* арендо́ванное иму́щество.

leasehold II *a* арендо́ванный.

leaseholder ['liːshouldə] *n* аренда́тор; съёмщик.

leash I [liːʃ] *n* 1) сво́ра, реме́нь; to hold in ~ *перен.* держа́ть на при́вязи, сде́рживать; 2) *охот.* сво́ра из трёх соба́к.

leash II *v* держа́ть на при́вязи.

least I [liːst] *n* ма́лое коли́чество; са́мое ме́ньшее; the ~ you must do са́мое ме́ньшее, что вы должны́ сде́лать; at (the) ~ по кра́йней ме́ре; in the ~ по ме́ньшей ме́ре; not in the ~ ничу́ть, ниско́лько; to say the ~ of it мя́гко выража́ясь.

least II *a* (*superl см.* little II) наиме́ньший, мале́йший.

least III *adv* (*superl см.* little III) в наиме́ньшей сте́пени.

leather I ['leðə] *n* 1) ко́жа; patent ~ лакиро́ванная ко́жа; 2) ко́жаные изде́лия; 3) реме́нь; 4) *pl* ко́жаные штаны́; 5) *pl* кра́ги; 6) *сленг* футбо́льный мяч; 7) *attr* ко́жаный.

leather II *v* 1) покрыва́ть, обшива́ть ко́жей; 2) поро́ть ремнём.

leatherette [ˌleðəˈret] *n* иску́сственная ко́жа.

leather-head ['leðəhed] *n* болва́н.

leathering ['leðərɪŋ] *n* 1) *тех.* ко́жаная наби́вка; 2) по́рка (*ремнём*); to give smb. a ~ вы́пороть кого́-л.

leathern ['leðəːn] *a* ко́жаный.

leathery ['leðərɪ] *a* 1) похо́жий на ко́жу; 2) жёсткий (*о мясе*).

leave¹ I [liːv] *n* 1) разреше́ние, позволе́ние; by (*или* with) your ~ с ва́шего разреше́ния; 2) о́тпуск (*тж.* ~ of absence); on ~ в о́тпуске; on sick ~ в о́тпуске по боле́зни; 3) отъе́зд, ухо́д; проща́ние; to take one's ~ уезжа́ть; проща́ться (*с кем-л. — of*); ◇ to take French ~ уйти́ не про-

щаясь; to take ~ of one's senses потерять рассу́-
док.

leave¹ II *v* (*past, p. p.* left) 1) уезжа́ть; уходи́ть;
отходи́ть (*о по́езде*); 2) оставля́ть; покида́ть;
3) предоставля́ть; ~ it to me предоста́вьте э́то
мне; I ~ it to you предоставля́ю вам (*реша́ть, де́-
лать и т. п.*); it ~s much to be desired оставля́ет же-
ла́ть мно́гого; 4) оставля́ть в том же состоя́нии;
the story left him cool расска́з его́ не тро́нул; to ~
undone (unsaid) так и не сде́лать (не сказа́ть); ~
it at that! *разг.* оста́вьте!, дово́льно!; 5) оставля́ть
в насле́дство; □ to ~ **behind** а) оставля́ть, забы-
ва́ть (*где-л.*); б) опережа́ть; превосходи́ть; to ~
off перестава́ть, броса́ть привы́чку; **to** ~ **off** smoking бро́сить кури́ть; to ~ **out** пропуска́ть; упу-
ска́ть; to ~ **over** откла́дывать; ◇ to ~ smb. to
himself (*или* to his own devices) предоста́вить
кого́-л. самому́ себе́.

leave² *v* покрыва́ться листво́й.

leaven I ['levn] *n* дро́жжи, заква́ска; *перен.* воз-
де́йствие, влия́ние.

leaven II *v* ста́вить на дрожжа́х; *перен.* возде́й-
ствовать.

leaves [liːvz] *pl см.* leaf I.

leavings ['liːvɪŋz] *n pl* оста́тки, отбро́сы.

lecherous ['letʃərəs] *a* распу́тный.

lechery ['letʃərɪ] *n* распу́тство.

lection ['lekʃən] *n* 1) чте́ние; 2) разночте́ние,
вариа́нт.

lecture I ['lektʃə] *n* 1) ле́кция; to give (*или* to
deliver) a ~ чита́ть ле́кцию; 2) вы́говор; нота́ция;
to give (*или* to read) smb. a ~ де́лать вы́говор
кому́-л., отчи́тывать кого́-л.

lecture II *v* чита́ть ле́кцию, ле́кции; 2) де́лать вы́-
говор, отчи́тывать.

lecturer ['lektʃərə] *n* 1) ле́ктор; 2) преподава́тель
(*университе́та*); 3) чита́ющий нота́ции.

lecturing ['lektʃərɪŋ] *n*: to do ~ чита́ть ле́кции.

led [led] *past, p. p. см.* lead⁶ II.

ledge [ledʒ] *n* 1) вы́ступ, край, борт; карни́з;
2) риф; *горн.* ру́дная жи́ла.

ledger ['ledʒə] *n* 1) *бухг.* гла́вная кни́га, гросс-
бу́х; 2) *амер.* кни́га за́писи а́ктов гражда́нского со-
стоя́ния; 3) *стр.* попере́чная ба́лка; лёжень; плита́;
4) моги́льная плита́.

ledger-bait ['ledʒəbeɪt] *n* нажи́вка.

lee [liː] *n* 1) подве́тренная сторона́; 2) защи́та;
under the ~ of под защи́той (*чего́-л.*); 3) *attr*
подве́тренный.

leech [liːtʃ] *n* 1) пия́вка; to stick like a ~ при-
ста́ть как пия́вка; 2) кровопи́йца, вымога́тель.

leek [liːk] *n* лук-поре́й (*тж. как национа́льная
эмбле́ма Уэ́льса*); ◇ to eat the (*или* one's) ~
проглоти́ть оби́ду.

leer I [lɪə] *n* хи́трый, зло́бный взгляд и́скоса.

leer II *v* хи́тро, зло́бно смотре́ть.

leery [']ɪərɪ] *a сленг* хи́трый.

lees [liːz] *n pl* 1) оста́тки; оса́док на дне; to drink
(*или* to drain) to the ~ вы́пить всё; *перен.* испи́ть
ча́шу до дна; 2) подо́нки.

leeward I ['liːwəd] *n* подве́тренная сторона́.

leeward II *a* подве́тренный.

leeward III *adv* под ве́тер, под ве́тром.

leeway ['liːweɪ] *n* 1) *ав.* снос (самолёта) ве́тром;
2) *мор.* дрейф (су́дна) под ве́тер; 3): to make up ~
вы́йти из затрудни́тельного положе́ния.

left¹ I [left] *n* 1) ле́вая сторона́; ле́вая рука́;
воен. ле́вый фланг; to keep to the ~ держа́ться ле́вой
стороны́; over the ~! *разг.* как раз наоборо́т!;
2): the Left (*употр. как pl*) *полит.* ле́вые.

left¹ II *a* ле́вый.

left¹ III *adv* нале́во, сле́ва; ~ about face! *воен.*
(нале́во) круго́м!

left² *past, p. p. см.* leave¹ II.

left-hand ['lefthænd] *a* 1) ле́вый; 2) сде́ланный
ле́вой руко́й; 3) *тех.* с ле́вым хо́дом (о винте́).

left-handed ['left'hændɪd] *a* 1) де́лающий всё ле́-
вой руко́й; 2) сде́ланный ле́вой руко́й; 3) неуклю́-
жий, нескла́дный; 4) двусмы́сленный, сомни́тель-
ный (о комплиме́нте и т. п.).

left-hander ['left'hændə] *n* 1) левша́; 2) уда́р ле́-
вой руко́й.

leftist ['leftɪst] *n полит.* член ле́вой па́ртии, ле́-
вый.

leftmost ['left‚məust] *a* са́мый ле́вый.

left-over ['left‚əuvə] *n амер.* 1) оста́ток; 2) пере-
жи́ток.

leftward I ['leftwəd] *a* 1) ле́вый (о настрое́ниях);
2) лева́цкий.

leftward II *adv см.* leftwards.

leftwards ['leftwədz] *adv* сле́ва, вле́во.

left-wing ['left‚wɪŋ] *a* ле́вый, прогресси́вный.

leg I [leg] *n* 1) нога́; to stretch one's ~s размя́ть
но́ги, пройти́сь; to give smb. a ~ up помо́чь кому́-л.
взобра́ться *или* преодоле́ть препя́тствие; to keep
one's ~s (у)держа́ться на нога́х; to run off one's
~s сби́ться с ног; to take to one's ~s удра́ть, уле-
петну́ть; to stand on one's own ~s стоя́ть на свои́х
нога́х, быть незави́симым; to set smb. on his ~s по-
мо́чь кому́-л. стать на́ ноги, стать самостоя́тель-
ным; 2) но́жка; сто́йка, подста́вка; *перен.* опо́ра;
3) штани́на; 4) *тех.* коле́но; 5) сторона́ треуго́ль-
ника (*кро́ме основа́ния*); 6) *сленг* жу́лик, моше́н-
ник; 7) эта́п путеше́ствия, полёта; ◇ to pull smb.'s
~ *разг.* одура́чить кого́-л., подшути́ть над кем-л.;
to shake a ~ *разг.* танцева́ть.

leg II *v*: to ~ it ходи́ть, шага́ть; «отмаха́ть».

legacy ['legəsɪ] *n* насле́дство; насле́дие.

legal ['liːgəl] *a* 1) юриди́ческий; 2) зако́нный;
узако́ненный; 3) лега́льный.

legality [liː'gælɪtɪ] *n* зако́нность.

legalize ['liːgəlaɪz] *v* узако́нивать, легализова́ть.

legateᵃ ['legɪt] *n* 1) лега́т, па́пский посо́л; 2) *уст.*
представи́тель.

legateᵇ [lɪ'geɪt] *v* завеща́ть.

legatee [‚legə'tiː] *n* насле́дник.

legation [lɪ'geɪʃən] *n* (дипломати́ческая) ми́ссия.

leg-bail ['leg'beɪl] *n*: to give ~ удра́ть,
скры́ться.

legend ['ledʒənd] *n* 1) леге́нда; 2) на́дпись (на
моне́те, меда́ли и т. п.).

legendary ['ledʒəndərɪ] *a* легенда́рный.

legerdemain ['ledʒədə'meɪn] *n* 1) ло́вкость рук,
фо́кусы; 2) ло́вкий обма́н.

leggings ['legɪŋz] *n pl* гама́ши; кра́ги.

leggy ['legɪ] *a* длинноно́гий.

legibility [‚ledʒɪ'bɪlɪtɪ] *n* чёткость (по́черка,
шри́фта).

legible ['ledʒəbl] *a* чёткий, разбо́рчивый.

legion ['liːdʒən] *n* легио́н; *перен.* мно́жество; ◇
Legion of Honour о́рден Почётного легио́на (во
Фра́нции).

legionary I [ˈliːdʒənərɪ] *n* легионе́р.

legionary II *a* легионе́рский.

legislate [ˈledʒɪsleɪt] *v* издава́ть зако́ны.

legislation [ˌledʒɪsˈleɪʃən] *n* законода́тельство; labour ~ трудово́е законода́тельство.

legislative [ˈledʒɪslətɪv] *a* законода́тельный.

legislator [ˈledʒɪsleɪtə] *n* законода́тель.

legislature [ˈledʒɪsleɪtʃə] *n* законода́тельная власть.

legist [ˈliːdʒɪst] *n* законове́д, правове́д.

legitimacy [lɪˈdʒɪtɪməsɪ] *n* зако́нность; узако́ненность.

legitimateᵃ [lɪˈdʒɪtɪmɪt] *a* 1) зако́нный; узако́ненный; пра́вильный; 2) законнорождённый.

legitimateᵇ [lɪˈdʒɪtɪmeɪt] *v* 1) узако́нивать; 2) усыновля́ть.

legitimation [lɪˌdʒɪtɪˈmeɪʃən] *n* 1) узаконе́ние; 2) усыновле́ние.

legman [ˈlegmən] *n* амер. сленг репортёр.

leg-pull [ˈlegpul] *n* попы́тка одура́чить, обману́ть кого́-л.

leguminous [leˈɡjuːmɪnəs] *a* бот. стручко́вый, бобо́вый.

leisure [ˈleʒə] *n* 1) досу́г; at ~ на досу́ге; 2) *attr* свобо́дный, неза́нятый (о времени и т. п.).

leisured [ˈleʒəd] *a* досу́жий, пра́здный.

leisurely I [ˈleʒəlɪ] *a* неторопли́вый, споко́йный.

leisurely II *adv* не спеша́, споко́йно; обду́манно.

lemon [ˈlemən] *n* 1) лимо́н; 2) лимо́нный цвет; 3) сленг некраси́вая де́вушка; 4) *attr* лимо́нный; лимо́нного цве́та; ◇ to hand smb. a ~ разг. обману́ть, наду́ть кого́-л.

lemonade [ˌleməˈneɪd] *n* лимона́д.

lemon-drop [ˈlemədrɔp] *n* лимо́нный ледене́ц.

lemony [ˈlemənɪ] *a* лимо́нный.

lemur [ˈliːmə] *n* зоол. лему́р.

lend [lend] *v* (*past, p. p.* lent) 1) дава́ть взаймы́, ода́лживать; дава́ть на вре́мя; ссужа́ть де́ньги под проце́нты; 2) придава́ть (достоинство, очарова́ние); 3) дава́ть, предоставля́ть (помощь и т. п.); 4): to ~ itself быть приго́дным; to ~ oneself приспоса́бливаться к чему́-л.

lender [ˈlendə] *n* заимода́вец.

length [leŋθ] *n* 1) длина́; at full ~ а) во всю длину́, растяну́вшись; б) со все́ми подро́бностями; to measure one's ~ растяну́ться во весь рост; 2) расстоя́ние; 3) продолжи́тельность, дли́тельность; of some ~ дово́льно дли́тельный; in ~ of time с тече́нием вре́мени, со вре́менем; 4) фон. долгота́ гла́сного; 5) отре́зок, кусо́к; ◇ at ~ а) наконе́ц; б) подро́бно, со все́ми дета́лями; to go all ~s (или to great ~s, to any ~) идти́ на всё, ни пе́ред чем не остана́вливаться; to keep smb. at arm's ~ держа́ть кого́-л. на почти́тельном расстоя́нии.

lengthen [ˈleŋθən] *v* удлиня́ть(ся); □ to ~ out чрезме́рно затя́гивать, растя́гивать.

lengthways [ˈleŋθweɪz] *adv* в длину́; вдоль.

lengthwise I [ˈleŋθwaɪz] *a* продо́льный.

lengthwise II *adv* в длину́, вдоль.

lengthy [ˈleŋθɪ] *a* сли́шком дли́нный, растя́нутый (о речи и т. п.).

lenience [ˈliːnjəns] *n* мя́гкость, снисходи́тельность.

leniency [ˈliːnjənsɪ] *см.* lenience.

lenient [ˈliːnjənt] *a* мя́гкий, снисходи́тельный.

Leninism [ˈlenɪnɪzəm] *n* ленини́зм.

Leninist I [ˈlenɪnɪst] *n* ле́нинец.

Leninist II *a* ле́нинский.

Leninite [ˈlenɪnaɪt] *см.* Leninist I.

lenitive I [ˈlenɪtɪv] *n* успока́ивающее сре́дство.

lenitive II *a* успокои́тельный; мягчи́тельный.

lenity [ˈlenɪtɪ] *n* 1) снисходи́тельность; 2) кро́тость.

lens [lenz] *n* 1) ли́нза; опти́ческое стекло́; 2) анат. хруста́лик гла́за (тж. crystalline ~).

lent¹ [lent] *n* церк. вели́кий пост.

lent² *past, p. p. см.* lend.

lenten [ˈlentən] *a* 1) великопо́стный; 2) по́стный (тж. перен.).

lentil [ˈlentɪl] *n* чечеви́ца.

leonine [ˈliːənaɪn] *a* льви́ный.

leopard [ˈlepəd] *n* леопа́рд; ◇ can the ~ change his spots? посл. ≅ горба́того моги́ла испра́вит.

leopardess [ˈlepədɪs] *n* са́мка леопа́рда.

leper [ˈlepə] *n* прокажённый.

leprosy [ˈleprəsɪ] *n* мед. прока́за.

leprous [ˈleprəs] *a* прокажённый.

lesion [ˈliːʒən] *n* 1) поврежде́ние, пораже́ние (органа, ткани); 2) юр. убы́ток, вред.

less I [les] *n* ме́ньшее коли́чество, ме́ньшая су́мма; in ~ than no time в мгнове́ние о́ка.

less II *a* (*compar см.* little II) ме́ньший.

less III *adv* (*compar см.* little III) ме́ньше, ме́нее; none the ~ тем не ме́нее.

less IV *prep* без; a month ~ three days ме́сяц без трёх дней.

lessee [leˈsiː] *n* съёмщик, аренда́тор.

lessen [ˈlesn] *v* 1) уменьша́ть(ся); 2) преуменьша́ть (заслуги, достоинства).

lesser [ˈlesə] *a* (*compar см.* little II) ме́ньший.

lesson [ˈlesn] *n* 1) уро́к; to do (или to make) ~s гото́вить уро́ки; to say one's ~ отвеча́ть уро́к; to give (to take) ~s дава́ть (брать) уро́ки; 2) *pl* заня́тия; 3) нота́ция; to give smb. a ~ прочесть кому́-л. нота́цию; 4) уро́к, предостереже́ние; 5) церк. отры́вок из би́блии, чита́емый во вре́мя слу́жбы.

lesson II *v* отчи́тывать, чита́ть нота́цию.

lessor [leˈsɔː] *n* сдаю́щий в аре́нду.

lest [lest] *conj* 1) что́бы не; be careful ~ you fall from the tree будь осторо́жен, что́бы не упа́сть с де́рева; 2) как бы не; I was afraid ~ he should be late я боя́лся, как бы он не опозда́л.

let I [let] *v* (*past, p. p.* let) 1) позволя́ть; пуска́ть; дава́ть; to ~ be не вме́шиваться, не обраща́ть внима́ния; to ~ drop (или fall) роня́ть; to ~ go а) освобожда́ть; отпуска́ть; б) выпуска́ть из рук; в) выбра́сывать из головы́; to ~ it go at that придётся останови́ться на э́том; to ~ oneself go дать себе́ во́лю, увле́чься; to ~ hear (или know) дать знать; to ~ slip неча́янно проговори́ться; оговори́ться; to ~ see показа́ть; 2) сдава́ть внаём; the house is to (be) ~ дом сдаётся; to ~ сдаётся (надпись); 3) в повел. накл. употребля́ется как вспом. гл., выража́ющий пожела́ние, приказа́ние и т. п.: ~ us go пойдём(те); ~ every man do his duty пусть ка́ждый выполня́ет свой долг; ~ you and me try дава́йте попро́буем; ~ AB be equal to CD пусть AB равно́ CD; □ to ~ **down** а) опуска́ть; спуска́ть вниз; б) обижа́ть; унижа́ть; to ~ smb. down easily (или gently) стара́ться не сли́шком оби́деть кого́-л.; быть снисходи́тельным к кому́-л.; в) разочаро́вывать, обескура́живать; г) покида́ть в беде́; to ~ in впуска́ть; to ~ into знако́мить с чем-л., посвяща́ть (*в секрет и т. п.*); to ~ off а) отпуска́ть, проща́ть; б) разряди́ть (ружьё); вы́стрелить; to ~ on а) притворя́ться, де́лать вид; б) *разг.* открыва́ть, выдава́ть (секре́т); to ~ out б) выпуска́ть; б) выдава́ть (*секрет и т. п.*); в) де́лать ши́ре, выпуска́ть (*платье*); г) сдава́ть внаём; to ~ up *амер. разг.* прекраща́ть (-ся).

let II *n* сда́ча внаём.

lethal ['li:θəl] *a* смерте́льный; смертоно́сный (*об оружии*).

lethargic [le'θɑːdʒɪk] *a* 1) летарги́ческий; 2) со́нный, вя́лый.

lethargy ['leθədʒɪ] *n* 1) летарги́я; 2) вя́лость, инéртность, апа́тия.

Lethe ['li:θɪ] *n миф., поэт.* Ле́та.

let-off ['let‚ɔːf] *n* проще́ние.

Lett [let] *n* 1) латы́ш; латы́шка; the ~s латыши́; 2) латы́шский язы́к.

letter I ['letə] *n* 1) бу́ква; capital (small, initial) ~ прописна́я (строчна́я, нача́льная) бу́ква; the ~ of the law бу́ква зако́на; ~ for ~ досло́вно, то́чно; to the ~ соверше́нно то́чно; in ~ and in spirit по фо́рме и по существу́; 2) *полигр.* ли́тера; 3) письмо́; посла́ние; registered (dead) ~ заказно́е (не доста́вленное адреса́ту) письмо́; ~ of credit аккредити́в; ~ of attorney дове́ренность; ~s of credence *дип.* вери́тельные гра́моты; ~s patent жа́лованная гра́мота; пате́нт; 4) *pl* литерату́ра; литерату́рное образова́ние.

letter II *v* 1) помеча́ть бу́квами; 2) вытисня́ть бу́квы, загла́вие на переплёте.

letter-box ['letəbɔks] *n* почто́вый я́щик.

letter-card ['letəkɑːd] *n* откры́тка, письмо́-секре́тка.

letter-case ['letəkeɪs] *n* бума́жник.

lettered ['letəd] *a* 1) (литерату́рно) образо́ванный; начи́танный; 2) с тиснёным загла́вием на переплёте; 3) ли́терный, обозна́ченный бу́квой.

letter-friend ['letəfrend] *n* друг по перепи́ске.

letterhead ['letəhed] *n* печа́тный заголо́вок на почто́вой бума́ге.

lettering ['letərɪŋ] *n* (печа́тная) на́дпись; тисне́ние.

letter-paper ['letə‚peɪpə] *n* почто́вая бума́га.

letter-perfect ['letə'pəːfɪkt] *a театр.* твёрдо зна́ющий свою́ роль.

letterpress ['letəpres] *n* печа́тный текст (*в книге с иллюстрациями*); in ~ в тéксте.

Lettish I ['letɪʃ] *n* латы́шский язы́к.

Lettish II *a* латы́шский.

lettuce ['letɪs] *n* сала́т, латýк.

let-up ['let‚ʌp] *n* приостано́вка, прекраще́ние.

leucocyte ['ljuːkəsaɪt] *n физиол.* лейкоци́т.

lev [lev] *n* (*pl* leva ['levə]) лев (*денежная едини́ца Болгарии*).

levant [lɪ'vænt] *v* скры́ться, сбежа́ть, не уплати́в долго́в.

levee[1] ['levɪ] *n* 1) приём во дворце́; вы́ход (*короля*); 2) приём госте́й.

levee[2] I *n амер.* 1) да́мба (*для защиты от наводне́ния*); 2) при́стань.

levee[2] II *v амер.* стро́ить да́мбы.

level I ['levl] *n* 1) у́ровень; on a ~ with на одно́м у́ровне с; sea ~ у́ровень мо́ря; to find one's own ~ а) знать своё ме́сто; б) найти́ себе́ ра́вных; to bring smb. to his ~ поста́вить кого́-л. на ме́сто; 2) равни́на; пло́ская горизонта́льная пове́рхность; dead ~ а) равни́на; б) посре́дственность; 3) ватерпа́с; нивели́р; у́ровень (*инструмент*); ◊ on the ~ че́стно.

level II *a* 1) пло́ский, ро́вный; горизонта́льный; на одно́м у́ровне (*c — with*); 2) равноме́рный; ра́вный; одина́ковый; 3) уравнове́шенный, споко́йный; ◊ to do one's ~ best сде́лать всё возмо́жное.

level III *v* 1) выра́внивать; сгла́живать; to ~ to (*или* with) the ground сровня́ть с землёй; to ~ up (down) повыша́ть (понижа́ть) (при выра́внивании); 2) наводи́ть (*оружие; at*); наце́ливать, направля́ть (*удар, сатиру; at, against*); 3) нивели́ровать, ура́внивать.

level-headed ['levl'hedɪd] *a* уравнове́шенный, здравомы́слящий.

lever I ['liːvə] *n* рыча́г.

lever II *v* поднима́ть рычаго́м.

leverage ['liːvərɪdʒ] *n* 1) систе́ма рычаго́в; 2) подъёмная си́ла (*рычага*); 3) сре́дство для достиже́ния це́ли.

leveret ['levərɪt] *n* зайчо́нок.

leviathan [lɪ'vaɪəθən] *n* 1) *библ.* левиафа́н; 2) грома́дина (*особ. о корабле*).

levin ['levɪn] *n поэт.* мо́лния.

levitation [‚levɪ'teɪʃən] *n* взлёт, подъём.

levity ['levɪtɪ] *n* легкомы́слие.

levy I ['levɪ] *n* 1) сбор, взима́ние (*податей, нало́гов*); су́мма сбо́ра; 2) набо́р рекру́тов; новобра́нцы; ополче́ние; ~ in mass поголо́вный набо́р (всех мужчи́н, го́дных к вое́нной слу́жбе); national ~ наро́дное ополче́ние.

levy II *v* 1) собира́ть, взима́ть (*налоги, контрибу́цию*); 2) облага́ть (*налогом и т. п.*); 3) набира́ть (*рекрутов*); 4) вести́ (*войну*).

lewd [luːd] *a* 1) непристо́йный, неприли́чный; 2) похотли́вый.

lewisite ['luːɪsaɪt] *n хим.* люизи́т.

lexical ['leksɪkəl] *a* 1) лекси́ческий; 2) слова́рный.

lexicographer [‚leksɪ'kɔgrəfə] *n* лексико́граф, состави́тель словаре́й.

lexicography [‚leksɪ'kɔgrəfɪ] *n* лексикогра́фия, составле́ние словаре́й.

lexicology [‚leksɪ'kɔlədʒɪ] *n* лексиколо́гия.

lexicon ['leksɪkən] *n* слова́рь.

liability [‚laɪə'bɪlɪtɪ] *n* 1) отве́тственность; 2) *pl* обяза́тельства; задо́лженность; долги́; to meet one's liabilities покры́ть задо́лженность; 3) подве́рженность, скло́нность; 4) *амер.* поме́ха.

liable ['laɪəbl] *a* 1) обя́занный (*to+Inf*); свя́занный обяза́тельством; отве́тственный (*за — for*); 2) подве́рженный (*болезни и т. п.*); подлежа́щий; ~ for service in the armed forces военнообя́занный; 3) вероя́тный, возмо́жный; difficulties are ~ to occur тру́дности, вероя́тно, встре́тятся; glass is ~ to break стекло́ легко́ лома́ется.

liaise [lɪ'eɪz] *v* устана́вливать *или* подде́рживать связь.

liaison [liː'eɪzɔ̃] *n* 1) (любо́вная) связь; 2) *воен.* связь взаимоде́йствия; 3) *attr* относя́щийся к (во́йскам) свя́зи (*об офицере, авиации*).

liana [lɪ'ɑːnə] *n* лиа́на.

liar ['laɪə] *n* лгун; ◊ ~s have need of good memories *посл.* лжецам надо иметь хорошую память.

libation [laɪ'beɪʃən] *n* возлияние; *шутл.* выпивка.

libel I ['laɪbəl] *n* клевета.

libel II *v* клеветать.

libeller ['laɪblə] *n* клеветник.

libellous ['laɪbləs] *a* клеветнический.

liberal I ['lɪbərəl] *n* 1) либерал; 2) (L.) *полит.* либерал, член партии либералов.

liberal II *a* 1) либеральный; 2) щедрый; великодушный; 3) обильный; 4) свободомыслящий; 5) гуманитарный.

liberalism ['lɪbərəlɪzəm] *n* либерализм.

liberality [,lɪbə'rælɪtɪ] *n* 1) щедрость; 2) широта взглядов; терпимость.

liberate ['lɪbəreɪt] *v* 1) освобождать; 2) *хим.* выделять.

liberation [,lɪbə'reɪʃən] *n* 1) освобождение; 2) *хим.* выделение.

liberator ['lɪbəreɪtə] *n* освободитель.

libertine I ['lɪbə:taɪn] *n* 1) распутник; 2) вольнодумец; 3) *ист.* вольноотпущенник.

libertine II *a* 1) распущенный, безнравственный; 2) свободомыслящий; 3) *ист.* вольноотпущенный.

liberty ['lɪbətɪ] *n* 1) свобода; civil liberties гражданские свободы; ~ of the press (of speech, of conscience) свобода печати (слова, совести); at ~ свободный, на свободе; to set at ~ выпускать на свободу; 2) вольность; to take the ~ to do (*или* of doing) smth. позволить себе сделать что-л.; to take liberties with smb. позволять себе вольности с кем-л.; 3) *pl* привилегии.

liberty-man ['lɪbətɪmæn] *n* моряк, уволенный на берег.

librarian [laɪ'brɛərɪən] *n* библиотекарь.

library ['laɪbrərɪ] *n* 1) библиотека; free ~ бесплатная библиотека; lending ~, circulating ~ библиотека с выдачей книг на дом; reference ~ справочная библиотека; walking ~ *шутл.* «ходячая энциклопедия»; *attr* библиотечный.

libretto [lɪ'bretou] *n* либретто.

lice [laɪs] *pl см.* louse.

licence ['laɪsəns] *n* 1) разрешение, лицензия; удостоверение, патент; driving ~ водительские права; 2) вольность; своеволие.

license I ['laɪsəns] *см.* licence.

license II *v* разрешать; давать право, патент, лицензию.

licensed ['laɪsənst] *a* 1) имеющий разрешение, право, лицензию на что-л.; 2) признанный (*о писателе и т. п.*); 3) привилегированный.

licensee [,laɪsən'si:] *n* лицо, имеющее разрешение, патент, лицензию.

licentious [laɪ'senʃəs] *a* распущенный, безнравственный.

lichen ['laɪkən] *n* 1) лишай; 2) *бот.* лишайник.

lick I [lɪk] *n* 1) облизывание; 2) незначительное количество, капелька, кусочек чего-л.; 3) *сленг* короткий сильный удар; 4) *сленг* шаг; at a great ~, at full ~ быстрым шагом; ◊ a ~ and a promise *разг.* a) быстрое, небрежное умывание; б) кое-как сделанная работа.

lick II *v* 1) лизать, облизывать; to ~ one's chops (*или* lips) облизывать(ся), предвкушать что-л.; 2) *разг.* бить; 3) *разг.* побивать, превосходить;

4) *разг.* спешить; ◊ to ~ into shape придать надлежащий вид, привести в порядок.

lickerish ['lɪkərɪʃ] *a* 1) любящий полакомиться; жадный, падкий (*до чего-л., на что-л.*); 2) распутный.

licking ['lɪkɪŋ] *n разг.* 1) побои; нагоняй; 2) поражение (*в игре, состязании*).

lickspittle ['lɪkspɪtl] *n* подхалим.

lid [lɪd] *n* 1) крышка; колпак; 2) веко (*тж.* eyelid); to narrow one's ~s прищуриться.

Lido ['li:dou] *n* (плавательный) бассейн на открытом воздухе.

lie[1] I [laɪ] *n* ложь, обман; to tell a ~ солгать; it is a simple ~ это просто ложь; to give smb. the ~ обвинять, уличать кого-л. во лжи; to give the ~ to smth. показывать ложность чего-л., опровергать; ◊ white ~ невинная, извинительная ложь.

lie[1] II *v* (*pres. p.* lying) 1) лгать; 2) быть обманчивым (*о наружности, виде*).

lie[2] I *v* (*past* lay; *p. p.* lain; *pres. p.* lying) 1) лежать; 2) покоиться (*в могиле*); 3) быть расположенным (*о городе, озере и т. п.*); 4) находиться, быть (*в каком-л. состоянии, положении*); to ~ low а) лежать распростёртым; б) *разг.* скрываться, таиться; 5) заключаться (*в чём-л. — in*); as far as in me ~s... насколько я могу...; всё, что в моих силах; it ~s with you (to do, to decide) ваше дело (делать, решать); 6) *юр.* быть законным, допустимым; □ to ~ **back** откинуться (*на спинку и т. п.*); to ~ **by** оставаться без употребления; б) отдыхать; to ~ **down** ложиться; прилечь; to take it lying down принимать покорно; to ~ **in** а) лежать в родах; б) *воен.* лежать в засаде; to ~ **over** откладывать(ся); отсрочивать(ся); to ~ **up** а) лежать в кровати, не выходить из комнаты (*из-за болезни*); б) стоять в стороне, отстраняться; в) стоять в доке (*о корабле*); ◊ to ~ on the bed one has made *посл.* ≅ что посеешь, то и пожнёшь; to ~ to one's work налегать на работу, усердствовать.

lie[2] II *n* (рас)положение; направление; the ~ of the land характер местности; *перен.* положение вещей.

lief [li:f] *adv* охотно.

liege I [li:dʒ] *n ист.* 1) сеньор; 2) вассал.

liege II *a ист.* 1) сеньориальный; 2) вассальный.

liegeman ['li:dʒmæn] *n* 1) *ист.* вассал; 2) послушный исполнитель, последователь.

lien [lɪən] *n* право наложения ареста на имущество должника.

lieu [lju:] *n*: in ~ of вместо.

lieutenant [lef'tenənt, *амер.* lju:'tenənt] *n* 1) лейтенант; 2) заместитель, помощник; агент.

lieutenant-colonel [lef'tenənt'kə:nl] *n* подполковник.

lieutenant-governor[a] [lef'tenənt'gʌvənə] *n* губернатор провинции (*в англ. колониях*).

lieutenant-governor[b] [lju:'tenənt'gʌvənə] *n амер.* вице-губернатор (*штата*).

life [laɪf] *n* (*pl* lives) 1) жизнь; for ~ (на) всю жизнь; to see ~ повидать свет, узнать жизнь; to bring (to come) to ~ привести (прийти) в себя (*после обморока*); to lay down one's ~ отдать свою жизнь; to lose one's ~ погибнуть; to take smb.'s ~ убить кого-л.; to take one's own ~ покончить (жизнь) самоубийством; upon (*или* 'pon) my ~!

клянусь жизнью!; to pawn one's ~ ручаться жизнью; 2) образ жизни; regular ~ регулярный образ жизни; stirring ~ деятельная жизнь, занятость; 3) жизнеописание, биография; 4) живость, воодушевление; full of ~ полный жизни; to be the ~ (или ~ and soul) of the party быть душой общества; to put ~ into one's work работать с душой; 5) натура; натуральная величина; to the ~ точно; as large as ~ в натуральную величину; 6) долговечность, срок службы машины и т. п.; ◊ still ~ натюрморт; I cannot for the ~ of me хоть убей, не могу; to lead a cat and a dog ~ погов. жить как кошка с собакой; while there is ~ there is hope посл. пока человек жив, он надеется.

lifebelt ['laɪfbelt] n спасательный пояс.

life-blood ['laɪfblʌd] n 1) поэт. кровь; 2) источник силы, жизни.

life-boat ['laɪfbout] n спасательная лодка.

lifebuoy ['laɪfbɔɪ] см. lifebelt.

life-giving ['laɪf,gɪvɪŋ] a живительный, животворный.

life-guard ['laɪfgɑːd] n 1) личная охрана; 2) спасатель.

life-jacket ['laɪf,dʒækɪt] n спасательный жилет или пояс.

lifeless ['laɪflɪs] a 1) неживой; безжизненный; 2) бездыханный, мёртвый; 3) скучный.

life-like ['laɪflaɪk] a словно живой.

life-line ['laɪflaɪn] n спасательная верёвка.

lifelong ['laɪflɔŋ] a пожизненный; на всю жизнь (о друге); в течение всей жизни.

life-office ['laɪf,ɔfɪs] n контора по страхованию жизни.

life-preserver ['laɪfprɪ,zəːvə] n 1) спасательный пояс; 2) дубинка.

lifer ['laɪfə] n сленг приговорённый к пожизненному заключению.

life-size(d) ['laɪf'saɪz(d)] a в натуральную величину.

lifetime ['laɪftaɪm] n продолжительность жизни; the chance of one's ~ возможность, которая бывает раз в жизни.

life-work ['laɪfwəːk] n труд или дело всей жизни.

lift I [lɪft] n 1) поднятие, подъём; to give smb. a ~ a) подсадить, подвезти кого-л.; б) помочь кому-л.; 2) подъёмник, лифт; 3) подъёмная сила; 4) возвышенность; ◊ dead ~ непосильная задача.

lift II v 1) поднимать (тж. to ~ off, to ~ up); 2) подниматься; возвышаться; 3) рассеиваться (о тумане, мраке); 4) копать (картофель и т. п.); 5) разг. красть (особ. скот); совершать плагиат.

ligament ['lɪgəmənt] n анат. связка.

ligature I ['lɪgətʃuə] n 1) связь; 2) мед. лигатура, нитка для перевязки (кровеносного сосуда); 3) полигр. лигатура; 4) муз. легато.

ligature II v перевязывать (кровеносный сосуд).

light I [laɪt] n 1) свет; освещение; дневной свет; in a good ~ при хорошем освещении, хорошо видный; to bring to ~ выявлять; выводить на чистую воду; to come to ~ обнаруживаться; родиться, появиться на свет; to stand in smb.'s ~ заслонять кому-л. свет; перен. стоять на дороге, мешать кому-л.; to throw (или to shed) ~ пролить свет (на что-л. — ирон.); 2) огонь; свеча, лампа, маяк и т. п.; to strike a ~ зажечь спичку; to give the green ~ амер. открыть путь; floating ~ пла-

вучий маяк; before the ~s разг. на сцене, перед рампой; 3) просвет, окно; 4) светило; перен. знаменитость; 5) pl (умственные) способности; 6) сведения, информация; 7) точка зрения, аспект; 8) pl сленг глаза; ◊ northern ~s, polar ~s северное сияние; to see the red ~ чувствовать приближение опасности.

light¹ II a светлый.

light¹ III v (past, p. p. lit, lighted) 1) освещать(-ся); осветить(ся); 2) зажигать(ся); □ to ~ up a) закуривать; б) зажигать свет; в) загораться (о глазах, лице).

light² a 1) лёгкий; легковесный; 2) незначительный; to make ~ of не придавать значения, относиться несерьёзно; 3) нетрудный, лёгкий; 4) легкомысленный; беспечный, весёлый; 5) рыхлый (о почве).

light³ v (past, p. p. lit, lighted) 1) сходить, спускаться (тж. to ~ down, to ~ off); опускаться, садиться на что-л. (о птице, бабочке; on, upon); 2) неожиданно натолкнуться на что-л. (on, upon).

lighten¹ ['laɪtn] v 1) освещать; 2) светлеть, светиться; 3) сверкать; it ~ed сверкнула молния.

lighten² v 1) облегчать; делать(ся) более лёгким; 2) смягчать (наказание); 3) поднимать настроение.

lighter¹ ['laɪtə] n 1) зажигалка (тж. cigar ~, cigarette ~); 2) тех. запал.

lighter² n мор. лихтер.

light-fingered ['laɪt,fɪŋgəd] a 1) ловкий; 2) вороватый.

light-footed ['laɪt,futɪd] a быстроногий; проворный.

light-headed ['laɪt'hedɪd] a 1) пустой, легкомысленный; 2) чувствующий головокружение; в бреду.

light-hearted ['laɪt'hɑːtɪd] a беспечный, весёлый.

lighthouse ['laɪthaus] n маяк.

lightly ['laɪtlɪ] adv 1) слегка, едва; 2) легко, без усилий; 3) беспечно, весело; 4) несерьёзно, необдуманно.

light-minded ['laɪt'maɪndɪd] a легкомысленный.

lightness ['laɪtnɪs] n 1) лёгкость; 2) беспечное, весёлое настроение; 3) легкомыслие.

lightning ['laɪtnɪŋ] n молния; heat (или sheet, summer) ~ зарница; like ~ с быстротой молнии, молниеносно.

lightning-bug ['laɪtnɪŋbʌg] n светляк.

lightning-conductor ['laɪtnɪŋkən,dʌktə] n молниеотвод.

lightning-rod ['laɪtnɪŋrɔd] см. lightning-conductor.

lightship ['laɪtʃɪp] n плавучий маяк.

lightsome¹ ['laɪtsəm] a 1) лёгкий, грациозный; 2) весёлый, радостный, быстрый.

lightsome² a светлый, яркий.

light-weight I ['laɪtweɪt] n 1) человек ниже среднего веса; спорт. легковес; 2) несерьёзный, поверхностный человек.

light-weight II a 1) ниже среднего веса; 2) легковесный.

lignite ['lɪgnaɪt] n бурый уголь, лигнит.

likable ['laɪkəbl] см. likeable.

like¹ I [laɪk] n нечто подобное, похожее, равное, одинаковое; and the ~ и тому подобное; or the ~ или что-либо подобное; did you ever see the ~ of it? видели ли вы что-либо подобное?; will never do the ~ again никогда не бу́ду де́лать подо́бных веще́й; ◊ cures ~ ≅ клин кли́ном вышиба́ют; to requite (*или* to return) ~ for ~ ≅ отплати́ть той же моне́той.

like[1] **II** *a* 1) похо́жий, подо́бный; something ~ 100 roubles о́коло 100 рубле́й; what is he (it) ~? что он (э́то) собо́й представля́ет?; 2) одина́ковый, ра́вный; 3) вероя́тный, возмо́жный.

like[1] **III** *adv* 1) так, подо́бно э́тому; 2): very ~, ~ enough весьма́ вероя́тно, возмо́жно; 3) *сленг* так сказа́ть.

like[2] **I** *n* обыкн. *pl* симпа́тии; скло́нности, влече́ния; ~s and dislikes симпа́тии и антипа́тии.

like[2] **II** *v* люби́ть, нра́виться; I ~ him он мне нра́вится; I should ~ я бы хоте́л; as you ~ как вам уго́дно.

likeable ['laɪkəbl] *a* прия́тный, привлека́тельный.

likelihood ['laɪklɪhud] *n* вероя́тность; in all ~ по всей вероя́тности.

likely **I** ['laɪklɪ] *a* 1) вероя́тный; 2) подходя́щий; спосо́бный (*о челове́ке*).

likely **II** *adv* вероя́тно (обыкн. most ~, very ~); as ~ as not вполне́ вероя́тно.

liken ['laɪkən] *v* сра́внивать; находи́ть схо́дство, уподобля́ть (*to*).

likeness ['laɪknɪs] *n* 1) схо́дство (*ме́жду* — *between*; с — *to*); 2) подо́бие; портре́т; speaking ~ вы́литый портре́т; то́чная ко́пия; 3) о́браз; личи́на; in the ~ of a friend под личи́ной дру́га; in the ~ of a bird в о́бразе пти́цы (*в ска́зках*).

likewise ['laɪkwaɪz] *adv* подо́бно; та́кже, то́же.

liking ['laɪkɪŋ] *n* 1) расположе́ние, любо́вь; a ~ for children любо́вь к де́тям; 2) скло́нность, вкус (*к чему́-л.* — *for*); to one's ~ по вку́су (*кому́-л.*).

lilac **I** ['laɪlək] *n* сире́нь.

lilac **II** *a* сире́невый.

Lilliputian **I** [ˌlɪlɪ'pjuːʃjən] *n* лилипу́т.

Lilliputian **II** *a* кро́шечный.

lilt **I** [lɪlt] *n* жива́я, весёлая пе́сенка.

lilt **II** *v* петь жи́во, ве́село.

lily ['lɪlɪ] *n* 1) ли́лия; tiger (Easter) ~ кра́сная (бе́лая) ли́лия; water ~ водяна́я ли́лия, кувши́нка; lent ~ жёлтый нарци́сс; 2) *attr* бе́лый, лиле́йный.

lily-livered ['lɪlɪˌlɪvəd] *a* трусли́вый.

lily-of-the-valley ['lɪlɪəvðə'vælɪ] *n* ла́ндыш.

lily-white ['lɪlɪ'waɪt] *a* лиле́йно-бе́лый.

limb[1] [lɪm] *n* 1) коне́чность, член (*те́ла*); 2) сук, ве́тка; 3) *разг.* непослу́шный ребёнок, не́слух; ◊ a ~ of the law *шутл.* блюсти́тель поря́дка, страж зако́на (*об адвока́те, полице́йском*).

limb[2] *n* 1) край, диск (*со́лнца, луны́*); 2) лимб (*круг с деле́ниями*); 3) часть, дета́ль.

limber[1] ['lɪmbə] *n воен.* передо́к (*ору́дия*).

limber[1] **II** *a* 1) ги́бкий; 2) прово́рный.

limber[2] **II** *v* де́лать(ся) ги́бким.

limbo ['lɪmbou] *n* 1) тюрьма́, заточе́ние; 2) забве́ние, забро́шенность; 3) *рел.* преддве́рие а́да.

lime[1] **I** [laɪm] *n* и́звесть; burnt ~ негашёная и́звесть; slack(ed) ~ гашёная и́звесть.

lime[1] **II** *v* 1) бели́ть и́звестью; 2) удобря́ть и́звестью.

lime[2] *n* разнови́дность лимо́на.

lime[3] *n* ли́па.

lime-juice ['laɪmdʒuːs] *n* лимо́нный сок.

limekiln ['laɪmkɪln] *n* печь для о́бжига и́звести.

limelight ['laɪmlaɪt] *n*: in the ~ на виду́, в це́нтре внима́ния.

Limerick ['lɪmərɪk] *n* шу́точное стихотворе́ние.

limestone ['laɪmstoun] *n* известня́к.

lime-tree ['laɪmtriː] *n* ли́па.

limey ['laɪmɪ] *n амер. сленг* англича́нин.

limit **I** ['lɪmɪt] *n* преде́л, грани́ца; to set a ~ установи́ть преде́л; положи́ть коне́ц; within ~s в преде́лах, уме́ренно; without ~ безграни́чно.

limit **II** *v* ограни́чивать.

limitary ['lɪmɪtərɪ] *a* 1) ограни́ченный; 2) ограни́чительный; 3) пограни́чный.

limitation [ˌlɪmɪ'teɪʃən] *n* 1) ограниче́ние; 2) ограни́ченность; 3) преде́л; преде́льный срок; 4) *pl* недоста́тки.

limited ['lɪmɪtɪd] *a* ограни́ченный.

limitless ['lɪmɪtlɪs] *a* безграни́чный; беспреде́льный.

limousine ['lɪmuːziːn] *n* закры́тый автомоби́ль, лимузи́н.

limp[1] **I** [lɪmp] *n* хромота́, прихра́мывание; to have a bad ~ си́льно хрома́ть; to walk with a ~ прихра́мывать.

limp[1] **II** *v* хрома́ть, прихра́мывать; идти́ с трудо́м.

limp[2] *a* мя́гкий, нежёсткий (*о воротничке, переплёте книги*); *перен.* сла́бый, вя́лый.

limpid ['lɪmpɪd] *a* прозра́чный.

limy ['laɪmɪ] *a* 1) известко́вый; 2) кле́йкий.

linage ['laɪnɪdʒ] *n* 1) число́ строк в печа́тной страни́це; 2) постро́чная опла́та.

linchpin ['lɪntʃpɪn] *n* чека́ (*колеса́*).

linden ['lɪndən] *n* ли́па.

line[1] **I** [laɪn] *n* 1) ли́ния, черта́; 2) *pl* очерта́ния, ко́нтур; 3) верёвка, шнур; про́вод; 4) борозда́; морщи́на; 5) грани́ца, преде́л; border ~, ~ of demarcation демаркацио́нная ли́ния; to draw the ~ at провести́ грани́цу; *перен.* положи́ть преде́л чему́-л.; 6) ряд, верени́ца; *амер. тж.* о́чередь, хвост; assembly ~ сбо́рочный конве́йер; 7) строка́; to drop a few ~s черкну́ть не́сколько строк; 8) стро́чка стихо́в, стих; *pl* стихи́; 9) *pl театр.* ре́плика; слова́ ро́ли; 10) леса́ (*удочки*); 11) эква́тор; 12) железнодоро́жная *или* парохо́дная ли́ния; branch ~ ж.-д. ве́тка; 13) ли́ния (*телефо́нная, телегра́фная и т. п.*); ~ engaged!, ~ busy! за́нято! (*отве́т телефони́стки*); the ~ is bad пло́хо слы́шно; hold the ~! не ве́шайте тру́бки!; 14) *воен.* ли́ния фро́нта; развёрнутый строй; шере́нга; 15) род заня́тий, специа́льность; that is not in (*или* out of) my ~ э́то не по мое́й специа́льности; 16) о́браз де́йствий, ли́ния поведе́ния; направле́ние, устано́вка; to take a strong ~ де́йствовать энерги́чно; in ~ with в согла́сии с; в соотве́тствии с; to come into ~ with smb. согласи́ться с кем-л., присоедини́ться к кому́-л.; 17) происхожде́ние, родосло́вная; male (female) ~ мужска́я (же́нская) ли́ния; 18) *pl* судьба́, рок; hard ~s несча́стная судьба́; 19) ли́ния (*ме́ра длины́* =¹/₁₂ *дю́йма*); 20) *pl разг.* свиде́тельство о бра́ке (*тж.* marriage ~s); ◊ all along the ~ во всём, по всех отноше́ниях; to get a ~ (*o* — *on*); to toe the ~ а) встать на ста́ртовую черту́; б) подчиня́ться дисципли́не, стро́го приде́рживаться пра́вил.

line[1] **II** *v* 1) проводи́ть ли́нии; линова́ть; отмеча́ть черто́й; 2) выстра́ивать(ся) в ряд; 3) стоя́ть, тяну́ться вдоль чего́-л. (*тж.* to ~ up); □ to ~

through вычёркивать; to ~ up а) строиться, выстраиваться; б) стоять в очереди; в) размежёвываться.

line[2] *v* 1) класть на подкладку; подбивать; 2) обивать, обшивать изнутри; 3) *разг.* наполнять, набивать; 4) служить подкладкой; 5) облицовывать.

lineage ['lɪnɪɪdʒ] *n* 1) происхождение, родословная; 2) род.

lineal ['lɪnɪəl] *a* 1) линейный; 2) происходящий по прямой линии от кого-л. (*о потомке*).

lineament ['lɪnɪəmənt] *n обыкн. pl* 1) черты (лица); 2) отличительная черта.

linear ['lɪnɪə] *a* 1) линейный; 2) узкий и длинный.

lined [laɪnd] *a* изборождённый морщинами, морщинистый.

lineman ['laɪnmən] *n* 1) *амер.* линейный монтёр; 2) *см.* linesman 1.

linen I ['lɪnɪn] *n* 1) холст, полотно; 2) бельё; ◊ to wash one's dirty ~ in public ≅ выносить сор из избы.

linen II *a* льняной.

liner[1] ['laɪnə] *n* рейсовый самолёт *или* пароход, лайнер.

liner[2] *n тех.* прокладка; вкладыш; втулка.

linesman ['laɪnzmən] *n* 1) *ж.-д.* путевой обходчик; 2) *спорт.* судья на линии.

line-up ['laɪnʌp] *n разг.* 1) соотношение, размежевание (*сил*); 2) *спорт.* расположение игроков перед началом игры.

ling [lɪŋ] *n* вереск.

linger ['lɪŋgə] *v* 1) задерживаться, оставаться; 2) мешкать, медлить; 3) (медленно) тянуться (*о времени*); 4) терять время зря; возиться (*с — over, upon*); 5) затягиваться (*о болезни*); 6) влачить жалкое существование (*тж.* to ~ out one's life).

lingerie ['lænʒəriː] *n* 1) женское бельё; 2) полотняные изделия.

lingering ['lɪŋgərɪŋ] *a* 1) медлительный; 2) томительный; 3) затяжной (*о болезни*).

lingo ['lɪŋgou] *n* 1) *презр.* иностранный язык; 2) профессиональный жаргон.

lingual ['lɪŋgwəl] *n* 1) *анат.* язычный; 2) *лингв.* языковой.

linguist ['lɪŋgwɪst] *n* языковед, лингвист.

linguistic [lɪŋ'gwɪstɪk] *a* языковедческий, лингвистический.

linguistics [lɪŋ'gwɪstɪks] *n* языкознание, языковедение, лингвистика.

liniment ['lɪnɪmənt] *n* жидкая мазь (*для растирания*).

lining ['laɪnɪŋ] *n* 1) подкладка; 2) *тех.* обкладка, обивка, облицовка.

link[1] I [lɪŋk] *n* 1) (связующее) звено; связь; missing ~ недостающее звено; to establish close ~s установить тесную связь; 2) *pl* узы; 3) *обыкн. pl* запонка (*тж.* cuff-links); 4) петля (*в вязанье*).

link[1] II *v* 1) соединять, связывать (*to; тж.* to ~ together); 2) включать(ся); 3) примыкать (*к — on, in*); 4) брать под руку.

link[2] *n* факел.

links [lɪŋks] *n pl* 1) дюны; 2) поле для игры в гольф.

link-up ['lɪŋkʌp] *n косм.* стыковка.

linnet ['lɪnɪt] *n* коноплянка (*птица*).

linoleum [lɪ'nouljəm] *n* линолеум.

linotype ['laɪnoutaɪp] *n полигр.* линотип.

linseed ['lɪnsiːd] *n* 1) льняное семя; 2) *attr* льняной.

linsey-woolsey ['lɪnzɪ'wulzɪ] *n* грубая полушерстяная ткань.

lint [lɪnt] *n* корпия.

lintel ['lɪntl] *n* перемычка окна *или* двери.

liny ['laɪnɪ] *a* морщинистый.

lion ['laɪən] *n* 1) лев; 2) знаменитость; 3) *pl* достопримечательности.

lioness ['laɪənɪs] *n* львица.

lion-hearted ['laɪən,hɑːtɪd] *a* храбрый, смелый.

lion-hunter ['laɪən,hʌntə] *n* 1) охотник на львов; 2) человек, гоняющийся за знаменитостями.

lionize ['laɪənaɪz] *v* 1) носиться с кем-л. как со знаменитостью; 2) показывать достопримечательности.

lip I [lɪp] *n* 1) губа; cleft ~ *мед.* заячья губа; to curl one's ~ презрительно кривить рот; 2) край (*сосуда, раны*); 3) *сленг* дерзость, нахальство; none of your ~! без дерзостей!; ◊ stiff upper ~ упорство; выносливость; to keep (*или* to carry) a stiff upper ~ а) сохранять мужество; б) упорствовать, упрямиться.

lip II *a* 1) губной; 2) неискренний; только на словах.

lip III *v* касаться губами.

lip-deep ['lɪpdiːp] *a* неискренний.

lip-language ['lɪp,læŋgwɪdʒ] *n* умение (*глухонемого*) понимать речь по движению губ.

lipsalve ['lɪpsɑːv] *n* гигиеническая губная помада, мазь; *перен.* лесть.

lip-service ['lɪp,sɜːvɪs] *n* неискренние излияния.

lipstick ['lɪpstɪk] *n* губная помада.

liqueur [lɪ'kjuə] *n* ликёр.

liquid I ['lɪkwɪd] *n* 1) жидкость; 2) *фон.* плавный звук.

liquid II *a* 1) жидкий; текучий; водянистый (*о глазах*); 2) неустойчивый, непостоянный; 3) прозрачный, светлый; 4) *фон.* плавный; 5) *фин.* легко реализуемый, ликвидный.

liquidate ['lɪkwɪdeɪt] *v* 1) ликвидировать; 2) выплатить, погасить (*долг*); 3) *разг.* прикончить; положить конец; избавиться от; 4) обанкротиться (*о фирме и т. п.*).

liquidation [,lɪkwɪ'deɪʃən] *n* 1) ликвидация; уничтожение; избавление от чего-л.; 2) выплата, погашение (*долга*); 3) банкротство; to go into ~ обанкротиться.

liquor[a] I ['lɪkə] *n* 1) (спиртной) напиток; hard ~ крепкий спиртной напиток; in ~, the worse for ~ подвыпивший; 2) отвар.

liquor[a] II *v* 1) *разг.* выпивать (*тж.* to ~ up); 2) смазывать (*кожу*) салом.

liquor[b] ['lɪkwɔː] *n фарм.* раствор.

lira ['lɪərə] *n* (*pl тж.* lire ['lɪərɪ]) лира (*денежная единица Италии*).

lisp I [lɪsp] *n* 1) шепелявость; 2) лепет; 3) шорох, шелест.

lisp II *v* 1) шепелявить; 2) лепетать (*о детях*).

lissom(e) ['lɪsəm] *a* 1) гибкий; 2) проворный.

list[1] I [lɪst] *n* 1) список; перечень; the active ~ *воен.* кадровый состав; the retired ~ список отставных офицеров; duty ~ расписание (дежурств); subscription ~ подписной лист; black ~

чёрный спи́сок; 2) край, кро́мка, кайма́; 3) *pl* аре́на борьбы́; *ист.* аре́на турни́ра.

list[1] II *v* вноси́ть в спи́сок, запи́сывать; перечисля́ть.

list[2] I *n* крен, накло́н; to have (*или* to take) a ~ накрени́ться.

list[2] II *v* накрени́ться, наклони́ться.

listen ['lɪsn] *v* 1) слу́шать; прислу́шиваться (к чему́-л. — *to, for*); 2) внима́тельно выслу́шивать; 3) слу́шаться; уступа́ть (*про́сьбе и т. п.*); □ to ~ in а) слу́шать ра́дио; б) подслу́шивать.

listener ['lɪsnə] *n* 1) слу́шатель; to be a good ~ уме́ть слу́шать; 2) *воен.* слуха́ч.

listless ['lɪstlɪs] *a* равноду́шный, безразли́чный, апати́чный.

lit[1] [lɪt] *past, p. p. см.* light[1] III.

lit[2] *past, p. p. см.* light[3].

liter ['liːtə] *амер. см.* litre.

literacy ['lɪtərəsɪ] *n* гра́мотность.

literal ['lɪtərəl] *a* 1) буква́льный; досло́вный, то́чный; 2) бу́квенный; 3) сухо́й; педанти́чный.

literally ['lɪtərəlɪ] *adv* 1) досло́вно, сло́во в сло́во; то́чно, буква́льно; 2) без преувеличе́ния.

literary ['lɪtərərɪ] *a* литерату́рный; а́вторский (*о пра́ве*).

literate I ['lɪtərɪt] *n* гра́мотный *или* образо́ванный челове́к.

literate II *a* гра́мотный; образо́ванный.

literature ['lɪtərɪtʃə] *n* литерату́ра.

lithe [laɪð] *a* ги́бкий.

lithograph I ['lɪθəɡrɑːf] *n* литогра́фия, литогра́фский о́ттиск.

lithograph II *v* литографи́ровать.

lithography [lɪˈθɔɡrəfɪ] *n* литогра́фия (*спо́соб печа́ти*).

Lithuanian I [ˌlɪθjuːˈeɪnjən] *n* 1) лито́вец; лито́вка; the ~s лито́вцы; 2) лито́вский язы́к.

Lithuanian II *a* лито́вский.

litigant ['lɪtɪɡənt] *n* сторона́ (*в суде́бном проце́ссе*).

litigate ['lɪtɪɡeɪt] *v* 1) суди́ться с кем-л.; 2) оспа́ривать (*на суде́*).

litigation [ˌlɪtɪˈɡeɪʃən] *n* тя́жба; спор.

litigious [lɪˈtɪdʒəs] *a* сутя́жнический.

litmus ['lɪtməs] *n хим.* 1) ла́кмус; 2) *attr* ла́кмусовый (*о бума́ге*).

litre ['liːtə] *n* литр.

litter[1] ['lɪtə] *n* 1) паланки́н; 2) носи́лки.

litter[2] I *n* 1) сор, му́сор; 2) беспоря́док; 3) подсти́лка (*для скота́*); 4) помёт (*припло́д свине́й, соба́к и др. живо́тных*).

litter[2] II *v* 1) сори́ть, разбра́сывать; 2) подстила́ть (*соло́му и т. п.; тж.* to ~ down); 3) пороси́ться, щени́ться *и т. п.*

litter-box ['lɪtəbɔks] *n* у́рна (*для му́сора*).

littery ['lɪtərɪ] *a* замусо́ренный.

little I ['lɪtl] *n* 1) немно́гое; ко́е-что; небольшо́е коли́чество; a ~ немно́го; not a ~ совсе́м нема́ло; ~ or nothing почти́ ничего́; he did what ~ he could он сде́лал то немно́гое, что мог; after a ~ немно́го спустя́; for a ~ ненадо́лго; by ~ and ~, by ~ and ~ постепе́нно, ма́ло-пома́лу; in ~ в небольшо́м масшта́бе; в миниатю́ре; to make ~ of быть невысо́кого мне́ния о, не придава́ть большо́го значе́ния (*чему́-л.*); 2) (the ~) «ма́ленькие лю́ди»; ◊ from ~ up *амер.* с де́тства.

little II *a* (*compar* less, lesser; *superl* least) 1) ма́ленький, ма́лый, небольшо́й; 2) незначи́тельный; несуще́ственный; 3) ме́лкий, ни́зкий, ме́лочный.

little III *adv* 1) (*compar* less; *superl* least) немно́го, ма́ло; 2) совсе́м не; he ~ knows он не зна́ет во́все.

littleness ['lɪtlnɪs] *n* 1) незначи́тельность; небольшо́й разме́р; небольша́я сте́пень; 2) ме́лочность; ограни́ченность.

littoral I ['lɪtərəl] *n* побере́жье; примо́рский райо́н.

littoral II *a* прибре́жный.

liturgy ['lɪtədʒɪ] *n* ме́сса; литурги́я.

livable ['lɪvəbl] *a* 1) го́дный для житья́, жилья́; 2) сно́сный; 3) ужи́вчивый, общи́тельный.

live[a] [lɪv] *v* жить; существова́ть; to ~ to be old дожи́ть до ста́рости; to ~ high жить широко́; to ~ by one's labour жить свои́м трудо́м; to ~ on vegetables пита́ться овоща́ми; □ to ~ in име́ть жильё по ме́сту рабо́ты; to ~ on (продолжа́ть) жить; to ~ out вы́жить, пережи́ть; to ~ through пережи́ть; to ~ up (*to*) жить согла́сно чему́-л. (*при́нципам, убежде́ниям и т. п.*); ◊ ~ and learn! век живи́ — век учи́сь!

live[b] [laɪv] *a* 1) живо́й; 2) настоя́щий, реа́льный; актуа́льный (*о вопро́се, про́сьбе*); 3) энерги́чный, живо́й, горя́чий; 4) непога́сший, горя́щий; де́йствующий; 5) заря́женный; 6) *радио, тлв.* передаю́щийся без за́писи на плёнку.

liveable ['lɪvəbl] *см.* livable.

livelihood ['laɪvlɪhud] *n* сре́дства к существова́нию; to pick up a ~ зараба́тывать на пропита́ние.

liveliness ['laɪvlɪnɪs] *n* жи́вость; оживле́ние.

livelong ['lɪvlɔŋ] *a поэт.* весь, це́лый (*о дне, но́чи*).

lively ['laɪvlɪ] *a* 1) живо́й, по́лный жи́зни; оживлённый, весёлый; 2) си́льный, я́ркий (*об описа́нии, впечатле́нии и т. п.*); ◊ to make things ~ for smb. зада́ть жа́ру кому́-л.

liven ['laɪvn] *v* оживля́ть(ся) (*тж.* to ~ up).

liver[1] ['lɪvə] *n* 1) *анат.* пе́чень; 2) печёнка (*пи́ща*).

liver[2] *n:* good ~ а) доброде́тельный челове́к; б) гурма́н; жуи́р; a free ~ живу́щий в своё удово́льствие; a close ~ скупе́ц.

liver-coloured ['lɪvəˌkʌləd] *a* краснова́то-кори́чневого цве́та.

liveried ['lɪvərɪd] *a* в ливре́е.

liverish ['lɪvərɪʃ] *a разг.* 1) страда́ющий боле́знью пе́чени; 2) жёлчный, раздражи́тельный.

livery ['lɪvərɪ] *n* 1) ливре́я; 2) *ист.* костю́м чле́на ги́льдии; 3) *поэт.* наря́д; покро́в; winter ~ of birds зи́мнее опере́ние птиц; 4) пла́тная коню́шня.

lives [laɪvz] *pl см.* life.

live-stock ['laɪvstɔk] *n* дома́шний скот; живо́й инвента́рь.

livid ['lɪvɪd] *a* 1) мёртвенно-бле́дный (*о лице́*); 2) *разг.* о́чень зло́й.

living I ['lɪvɪŋ] *n* 1) жизнь, о́браз жи́зни; житьё; high ~ жизнь на широ́кую но́гу; plain ~ проста́я, скро́мная жизнь; 2) сре́дства к существова́нию; to make (*или* to earn) one's ~ зараба́тывать на жизнь.

living II *a* 1) живо́й, живу́щий; совреме́нный; 2) о́чень похо́жий, живо́й, вы́литый.

living-room ['lıvıŋrum] *n* общая комната, столовая, гостиная.

lizard ['lızəd] *n* ящерица.

'll [l] *разг. сокр. от* shall *или* will *после* I, you, he *и т. д.*

llama ['lɑːmə] *n зоол.* лама.

load I [loud] *n* 1) груз; нагрузка; тяжесть; *перен.* бремя; dead ~ а) мёртвый груз; тара; б) *ав.* собственный вес; 2) *pl разг.* множество, избыток (*of*); 3) *воен.* заряд.

load II *v* 1) грузить; нагружать; *перен.* обременять; 2) осыпать (*подарками, похвалами и т. п.*); 3) заряжать (*оружие*).

loader ['loudə] *n* 1) грузчик; 2) погрузочное приспособление; 3) *воен.* заряжающий (*номер*).

loading ['loudıŋ] *n* 1) погрузка; 2) груз, нагрузка; 3) *воен.* заряжание.

load-pack ['loudpæk] *n* вьюк.

loadstar ['loudstɑː] *см.* lodestar.

loaf[1] [louf] *n* (*pl* loaves) 1) каравай, буханка хлеба; булка; the ~ хлеб; 2) голова сахару (*тж.* sugar-loaf); 3) кочан (*капусты*); 4) *сленг* голова.

loaf[2] I *n* бездельничанье.

loaf[2] II *v* 1) бездельничать; 2) слоняться.

loafer ['loufə] *n* бездельник.

loam [loum] *n* 1) жирная глина; clay ~ жирный суглинок; sandy ~ супесь; 2) формовочная глина.

loamy ['loumı] *a* глинистый.

loan I [loun] *n* 1) заём; state (domestic) ~ государственный (внутренний) заём; on ~ взаймы; 2) заимствование (*о слове, обычае*).

loan II *v* 1) предоставлять заём, давать взаймы; 2) заимствовать (*слово*).

loan-word ['lounwəːd] *n* заимствованное слово.

loath [louθ] *a predic* несклонный, нежелающий; to be ~ не хотеть; nothing ~ охотно, без всяких возражений.

loathe [louð] *v* 1) чувствовать отвращение; 2) *разг.* не любить.

loathsome ['louðsəm] *a* отвратительный, противный.

loaves [louvz] *pl см.* loaf[1].

lob [lɔb] *v* 1) тяжело, неуклюже ходить *или* бегать; 2) высоко подбрасывать мяч (*в теннисе и т. п.*).

lobby I ['lɔbı] *n* 1) вестибюль; коридор; фойе; 2) кулуары (*парламента*); 3) лобби, группа лиц, «обрабатывающая» членов парламента в пользу какого-л. законопроекта.

lobby II *v* воздействовать на членов парламента, «обрабатывать».

lobe [loub] *n* 1) мочка уха (*тж.* ~ of the ear); 2) доля; ~ of the lung лёгочная доля.

lobster ['lɔbstə] *n* омар, рак; ◊ red as a ~ красный как рак.

lobster-eyed ['lɔbstəraıd] *a* пучеглазый.

local[1] I ['loukəl] *n* 1) пригородный поезд; 2) местный житель; 3) местная партийная *или* профсоюзная организация; 4) местные новости (*в газете*); 5) *разг.* местный трактир.

local[1] II *a* 1) местный; 2) распространённый *или* встречающийся только местами (*обыкн.* quite ~, very ~).

local[2] *см.* locale.

locale [lou'kɑːl] *n* место (*действия*).

localism ['loukəlızəm] *n* 1) местный патрио-

тизм; местные интересы; 2) *лингв.* местное выражение, провинциализм.

locality [lou'kælıtı] *n* 1) место, местность; местоположение; 2) населённый пункт; 3) *обыкн. pl* окрестности; 4) способность ориентироваться на местности.

localize ['loukəlaız] *v* 1) ограничивать распространение, локализовать; 2) определять местонахождение; относить к определённому месту.

locate [lou'keıt] *v* 1) располагать; поселять; to be ~d (in) а) жить (в); б) быть расположенным (в); 2) обнаруживать, определять место, местонахождение.

location [lou'keıʃən] *n* 1) местоположение; 2) размещение, поселение; 3) местожительство; 4) обнаружение, определение места (*чего-л.*); 5) *кино* натура.

locative ['lɔkətıv] *n грам.* местный падеж.

loch [lɔk] *n шотл.* 1) озеро; 2) узкий морской залив.

lock[1] [lɔk] *n* 1) локон; *pl тж.* волосы; 2) пучок, клок (*шерсти, волос и т. д.*).

lock[2] I *n* 1) замок; запор; Yale ~ американский замок; under ~ and key под замком; 2) замок (*ружья*); 3) шлюз; плотина; 4) затор (*в уличном движении*); 5) чека (*колеса*); ◊ ~, stock and barrel целиком, полностью.

lock[2] II *v* 1) запирать(ся) на замок; 2) соединять(ся), сцеплять(ся); 3) шлюзовать; □ to ~ away спрятать под замок, запереть; to ~ in, to ~ into а) запирать, замыкать; б) зажимать; to ~ out а) запирать, не впускать; б) объявлять локаут; to ~ up а) запирать; б) заключать (*в тюрьму и т. п.*); в) утаивать (*факты и т. п.*).

locker ['lɔkə] *n* запирающийся шкафчик, ящик; ◊ Davy Jones's ~ *мор. сленг* могила в море; to go to Davy Jones's ~ утонуть.

locket ['lɔkıt] *n* медальон.

lock-gate ['lɔk'geıt] *n* шлюзные ворота.

lock-keeper ['lɔk¸kiːpə] *n* сторож шлюза.

lock-out ['lɔkaut] *n* локаут.

locksmith ['lɔksmıθ] *n* слесарь.

lock-stitch ['lɔkstıtʃ] *n* машинный шов.

lock-up ['lɔkʌp] *n* 1) арестантская камера; тюрьма; 2) время окончания работы, занятий (*в учреждениях и в школах*); время закрытия магазинов; 3) мёртвый капитал; 4) *attr* запирающийся.

locomotion [¸loukə'mouʃən] *n* передвижение.

locomotive I ['loukə¸moutıv] *n* паровоз, тепловоз, локомотив.

locomotive II *a* движущий(ся).

locum ['loukəm] *n*: to do ~s временно замещать, исполнять обязанности (*врача, священника*); ~ tenens временный заместитель.

locust[1] ['loukəst] *n* саранча.

locust[2] *n* белая акация.

locution [lou'kjuːʃən] *n* оборот речи; идиома.

lode [loud] *n* (рудная) жила; залежь.

lodestar ['loudstɑː] *n* Полярная звезда; *перен.* путеводная звезда.

lodge I [lɔdʒ] *n* 1) сторожка; помещение привратника, швейцара; 2) (охотничий) домик; 3) *амер.* палатка индейцев, вигвам; 4) масонская ложа; 5) нора (*выдры*); хатка (*бобра*); берлога.

lodge II *v* 1) размести́ть(ся); посели́ть(ся); приюти́ть; 2) помеща́ть, класть; 3) всади́ть (*пу́лю*); 4): to ~ in the memory запечатле́ть в па́мяти; 5) застря́ть (*о пуле*); 6) подава́ть (*жалобу, заявление*); 7): to ~ power with (*или* in the hands of) smb. облека́ть кого́-л. вла́стью; 8) приби́ть (*ветром*); поле́чь от ве́тра (*о посевах и т. п.*).

lodgement ['lɔdʒmənt] *см.* lodgment.

lodger ['lɔdʒə] *n* жиле́ц.

lodging ['lɔdʒɪŋ] *n* 1) жили́ще; 2) *обыкн. pl* (снима́емая) ко́мната, ко́мнаты, кварти́ра; dry ~ ко́мната без пита́ния.

lodging-house ['lɔdʒɪŋhaus] *n* меблиро́ванные ко́мнаты; common ~ ночле́жный дом.

lodgment ['lɔdʒmənt] *n* 1) жили́ще, помеще́ние; прию́т; 2) про́чное положе́ние; опо́ра; 3) скопле́ние чего́-л.; зато́р; 4) пода́ча (*заявления, жалобы*); 5) *воен.* захва́т и заня́тие пози́ции; to find a ~ обоснова́ться, закрепи́ться.

loess [lɜːs] *n геол.* лёсс.

loft I [lɔft] *n* 1) черда́к; 2) сенова́л; 3) хо́ры (*в церкви*); *амер.* галере́я (*в торговом помещении*); 4) голубя́тня; 5) уда́р вверх (*в гольфе*).

loft II *v* 1) держа́ть голубе́й; 2) посыла́ть мяч вверх (*в гольфе*).

loftiness ['lɔftɪnɪs] *n* 1) больша́я высота́; 2) возвы́шенность (*идеалов и т. п.*); 3) высокоме́рие, надме́нность; 4) вели́чественность; ста́тность.

lofty ['lɔftɪ] *a* 1) о́чень высо́кий; 2) возвы́шенный; 3) высокоме́рный; надме́нный; 4) вели́чественный; ста́тный.

log I [lɔg] *n* 1) бревно́; коло́да; чурба́н; 2) *мор. лаг;* 3) *см.* log-book 1).

log II *v* 1) руби́ть лес; рабо́тать на лесозагото́вках; 2) вноси́ть в ва́хтенный журна́л; □ to ~ off выкорчёвывать.

logarithm ['lɔɡərɪθəm] *n мат.* логари́фм.

log-book ['lɔgbuk] *n* 1) ва́хтенный *или* бортово́й журна́л; 2) формуля́р (*самолёта, автомашины*).

logged [lɔgd] *a* 1) насы́щенный, пропи́танный водо́й; 2) расчи́щенный от ле́са.

logger ['lɔgə] *n амер.* лесору́б.

loggerhead ['lɔgəhed] *n* 1) непропорциона́льно больша́я голова́; пти́ца с непоме́рно большо́й голово́й; 2) *уст.* о́лух, болва́н; ◊ to be at ~s ссо́риться; to fall to ~s дра́ться.

logging ['lɔgɪŋ] *n* 1) лесозагото́вка; 2) *см.* log-rolling.

logic ['lɔdʒɪk] *n* ло́гика.

logical ['lɔdʒɪkəl] *a* 1) логи́ческий; 2) логи́чный, после́довательный.

log-rolling ['lɔgroulɪŋ] *n амер.* 1) перека́тка брёвен; 2) взаи́мные услу́ги (*обыкн. в политике*); взаи́мное восхвале́ние.

loin [lɔɪn] *n* 1) *pl* поясни́ца; 2) филе́йная часть (*туши*); ◊ to gird up one's ~s собра́ться с си́лами, подгото́виться (*к чему-л.*).

loin-cloth ['lɔɪnklɔθ] *n* набе́дренная повя́зка.

loiter ['lɔɪtə] *v* 1) слоня́ться без де́ла; 2) ме́шкать; замина́ться.

loll [lɔl] *v* 1) сиде́ть разваля́сь, стоя́ть в лени́вой по́зе; 2) высо́вывать язы́к (*обыкн.* to ~ out); 3) высо́вываться (*о языке*).

lollipop ['lɔlɪpɔp] *n обыкн. pl* леденец, конфе́та.

Londoner ['lʌndənə] *n* ло́ндонец.

lone [loun] *a* 1) одино́кий; *шутл.* незаму́жняя; 2) уединённый.

loneliness ['lounlɪnɪs] *n* одино́чество.

lonely ['lounlɪ] *a* 1) одино́кий; 2) уединённый; пусты́нный.

lonesome ['lounsəm] *a* 1) одино́кий, тоску́ющий; 2) тоскли́вый, уны́лый.

long[1] I [lɔŋ] *a* 1) дли́нный; 2) до́лгий (*тж. фон.*); продолжи́тельный; 3) име́ющий (таку́ю-то) длину́ *или* продолжи́тельность; a mile ~ длино́й в одну́ ми́лю; an hour ~ продолжа́ющийся час; 4) ме́дленный, медли́тельный; how ~ you are! как вы копа́етесь!; he is very ~ in coming он о́чень до́лго не идёт; he will not be ~ in coming он не заме́длит прийти́.

long[1] II *adv* 1) до́лго; as ~ as, so ~ as пока́; ~ live..! да здра́вствует..!; 2) давно́; ~ after спустя́ мно́го вре́мени; ~ before задо́лго до; ~ ago, ~ since давны́м-давно́; уже́; ◊ so ~ *разг.* до свида́ния.

long[1] III *n* 1) до́лгий срок, до́лгий промежу́ток вре́мени; before ~ ско́ро; for ~ надо́лго; will not take ~ не займёт мно́го вре́мени; 2) *фон.* до́лгий гла́сный; 3) до́лгий слог; ◊ the ~ and the short of it коро́че говоря́.

long[2] *v* 1) стра́стно жела́ть, жа́ждать (*чего-л.— for, to*); 2) тоскова́ть.

long-ago I ['lɔŋə'gou] *n* далёкое про́шлое; да́вние времена́.

long-ago II *a* давнопроше́дший, далёкий.

long-bow ['lɔŋbou] *n* большо́й лук (*оружие*); ◊ to draw (*или* to pull) the ~ расска́зывать небыли́цы.

long-distance ['lɔŋ'distəns] *a* 1) да́льний; отдалённый; 2) междугоро́дный (*о телефонном разговоре*); 3) долгосро́чный (*о прогнозе погоды*).

long-drawn(-out) ['lɔŋ'drɔːn(aut)] *a* (сли́шком) затяну́вшийся.

longevity [lɔn'dʒevɪtɪ] *n* долгове́чность.

longevous [lɔn'dʒiːvəs] *a* долгове́чный.

long-headed ['lɔŋ'hedɪd] *a* проница́тельный; хи́трый.

longing I ['lɔŋɪŋ] *n* си́льное жела́ние, стремле́ние (*к чему-л.— for*).

longing II *a* си́льно жела́ющий, жа́ждущий.

longitude ['lɔndʒɪtjuːd] *n геогр.* долгота́.

longitudinal [,lɔndʒɪ'tjuːdɪnl] *a* 1) продо́льный; 2) *геогр.* относя́щийся к долготе́.

long-lived ['lɔŋ'lɪvd] *a* долгове́чный.

long-nosed ['lɔŋnouzd] *a* длинноно́сый; *перен.* любопы́тный, проны́рливый.

long-playing ['lɔŋpleɪŋ] *a* долгоигра́ющий (*о пластинке*).

long-range ['lɔŋ'reɪndʒ] *a* да́льнего де́йствия; да́льний; дальнобо́йный (*об орудии*).

longshoreman ['lɔŋ,ʃɔːmən] *n* 1) порто́вый гру́зчик; 2) прибре́жный рыба́к.

long-sighted ['lɔŋ'saɪtɪd] *a* 1) дальнозо́ркий; 2) дальнови́дный.

longspun ['lɔŋspʌn] *a* растя́нутый, несконча́емый.

long-standing ['lɔŋ'stændɪŋ] *a* давни́шний.

long-suffering I ['lɔŋ'sʌfərɪŋ] *n* долготерпе́ние.

long-suffering II *a* многострада́льный.

long-term [ˈlɔŋˈtəːm] *a* долгосро́чный; дли́тельный.

long-tongued [ˈlɔŋˈtʌŋd] *a* болтли́вый.

longueurs [ˌlɔŋˈgəːz] *n pl* длинно́ты (*в рома́не, пье́се и т. п.*).

longways [ˈlɔŋweɪz] *adv* в длину́.

long-winded [ˈlɔŋˈwɪndɪd] *a* 1) спосо́бный до́лго бежа́ть, не задыха́ясь; 2) многоречи́вый, ску́чный.

longwise [ˈlɔŋwaɪz] *см.* longways.

looby [ˈluːbɪ] *n* ду́рень.

loofah [ˈluːfɑː] *n бот.* люфа́.

look I [luk] *n* 1) взгляд; a blank (longing) ~ бессмы́сленный (тоску́ющий) взгляд; to give a ~ посмотре́ть, взгляну́ть; to give a ~ in загляну́ть, зайти́ мимохо́дом; to give smb. a searching ~ посмотре́ть испыту́юще на кого́-л.; to have a ~ а) ознако́миться; б) посмотре́ть (*на — at*); 2) *обыкн. pl* выраже́ние (*лица́, глаз*); нару́жность, вид; good ~s красота́, милови́дность.

look II *v* 1) смотре́ть, гляде́ть; *перен.* быть внима́тельным, следи́ть; to ~ ahead a) смотре́ть вперёд; б) ду́мать о бу́дущем; ~ ahead! береги́сь!; 2) вы́глядеть, име́ть вид; to ~ like быть похо́жим; to ~ oneself again прийти́ в себя́, опра́виться; that ~s heavy по ви́ду *или* на вид э́то тяжело́; it would ~ as if... похо́же на то, что...; 3) выходи́ть на (*о ко́мнате, о́кнах; into, onto*); □ to ~ **about** a) огля́дываться; б) осма́триваться, ориенти́роваться; в) иска́ть; to ~ **after** a) присма́тривать за кем-л., чем-л.; забо́титься; б) провожа́ть глаза́ми; to ~ **at** смотре́ть; обраща́ть внима́ние; it is fair (*или* good) to ~ at прия́тно смотре́ть; to ~ **down** смотре́ть свысока́ (*on, upon*); презира́ть; to ~ **for** a) иска́ть; б) ожида́ть, наде́яться; to ~ **forward** ожида́ть, предвкуша́ть (*to*); to ~ in загля́нуть, зайти́; to ~ **into** a) загля́дывать внутрь чего́-л.; б) рассма́тривать, иссле́довать (*вопро́с и т. п.*); to ~ **on** наблюда́ть; быть (то́лько) зри́телем; to ~ **out** a) быть насторо́же; б) выходи́ть на (*об о́кнах и т. п.; on, over*); в) подыска́ть, высма́тривать (*for*); to ~ **over** a) просма́тривать; б) пропусти́ть, не заме́тить; в) проща́ть, смотре́ть сквозь па́льцы; to ~ **round** a) огля́дываться круго́м; б) обду́мать всё предвари́тельно; to ~ **through** просма́тривать; *перен.* ви́деть кого́-л. наскво́зь; to ~ **to** a) забо́титься; следи́ть за чем-л.; б) рассчи́тывать, наде́яться на; to ~ **up** a) иска́ть (*в справо́чнике*); б) смотре́ть вверх; to ~ smb. up and down сме́рить кого́-л. взгля́дом; to ~ up to smb. уважа́ть кого́-л., относи́ться с почте́нием; ◇ ~ alive! живе́й!; ~ before you leap бу́дьте осмотри́тельны, осторо́жны; ~ here! послу́шай (-те)!; ~ sharp! смотри́(те) в о́ба!; don't ~ a gift horse in the mouth даре́ному коню́ в зу́бы не смо́трят; to ~ at him судя́ по его́ ви́ду.

looker-on [ˈlukərˈɔn] *n* (*pl* lookers-on) зри́тель, наблюда́тель; ◇ lookers-on see most of the game ≅ со стороны́ видне́е.

look-in [ˈlukˈɪn] *n* 1) бы́стрый взгляд; 2) коро́ткое посеще́ние; 3): to have a ~ *спорт.* име́ть ша́нсы на успе́х.

looking-glass [ˈlukɪŋglɑːs] *n* зе́ркало.

look-out [ˈlukˈaut] *n* 1) бди́тельность; on the ~ for насторо́же; *воен.* на стра́же; to keep a ~ стоя́ть на карау́ле, на стра́же; 2) наблюда́тель-

ный пост; 3) наблюда́тель; 4) вид (*на мо́ре, го́род и т. п.*); 5) ви́ды, перспекти́вы.

look-see [ˌlukˈsiː] *n сленг* бе́глый взгляд.

loom¹ [luːm] *n* 1) тка́цкий стано́к; 2) валёк весла́.

loom² *v* 1) нея́сно вырисо́вываться, ма́ячить; 2) нависа́ть, угрожа́ть (*over*).

loon [luːn] *n* гага́ра.

loop I [luːp] *n* пе́тля; *ав.* мёртвая пе́тля; пе́тля Не́стерова; to ~ the ~ *ав.* де́лать мёртвую пе́тлю.

loop II *v* де́лать пе́тлю; закрепля́ть пе́тлей.

loop-aerial [ˈluːpˈɛərɪəl] *n ра́дио* ра́мочная анте́нна.

loop-hole [ˈluːphoul] *n* 1) бойни́ца, амбразу́ра; 2) лазе́йка.

loose I [luːs] *a* 1) свобо́дный; to let ~ выпуска́ть, освобожда́ть; 2) незакреплённый, ненатя́нутый; осла́бленный, развя́занный; болта́ющийся; 3) широ́кий, просто́рный (*об оде́жде*); 4) нето́чный, неопределённый; расплы́вчатый; 5) ры́хлый (*о по́чве*); неплотный (*о тка́ни и т. п.*); 6) небре́жный, неря́шливый; 7) распу́щенный (*о челове́ке*); 8) *тех.* холосто́й.

loose II *adv* 1) свобо́дно; 2) широ́ко; 3) нето́чно.

loose III *n*: to give (a) ~ to one's feelings дать вы́ход, во́лю чу́вствам.

loose IV *v* 1) освобожда́ть, дава́ть во́лю; 2) развя́зывать, распуска́ть, ослабля́ть; отпуска́ть; 3) вы́стрелить.

loosen [ˈluːsn] *v* 1) ослабля́ть(ся); 2) развя́зывать, распуска́ть; 3) разжима́ть; расша́тывать; 4) ослабля́ть (*дисципли́ну и т. п.*); 5) разрыхля́ть; 6) вызыва́ть де́йствие (*кише́чника*).

loot I [luːt] *n* 1) добы́ча; награ́бленное добро́; 2) незако́нные дохо́ды чино́вников.

loot II гра́бить.

lop¹ I [lɔp] *n* ве́тки, су́чья.

lop¹ II *v* 1) отреза́ть, обруба́ть ве́тки, су́чья; 2) очища́ть де́рево от су́чьев (*обыкн.* to ~ off, to ~ away); 3) обкорна́ть; 4) отруба́ть (*го́лову, ру́ку*); 5) сокраща́ть, уре́зывать.

lop² *v* 1) свива́ть; 2) опуска́ть (*у́ши*); 3) дви́гаться неуклю́же; □ to ~ **about** слоня́ться (*без де́ла*).

lope I [loup] *n* прыжки́, скачки́ (*особ. живо́тных*).

lope II *v* бежа́ть вприпры́жку.

lop-eared [ˈlɔpɪəd] *a* вислоу́хий.

loppings [ˈlɔpɪŋz] *n pl* обру́бленные ве́тки, су́чья.

lop-sided [ˈlɔpˈsaɪdɪd] *a* 1) кривобо́кий; 2) однобо́кий; неравноме́рный; несимметри́чный.

loquacious [louˈkweɪʃəs] *a* болтли́вый; говорли́вый.

loquacity [louˈkwæsɪtɪ] *n* болтли́вость.

lord I [lɔːd] *n* 1) лорд; пэр; член пала́ты ло́рдов; First Lord of the Admiralty морско́й мини́стр (*в А́нглии до 1964 г.*); Lords *разг.* пала́та ло́рдов; my Lord [mɪˈlɔːd] мило́рд (*как обраще́ние*); 2) господи́н, хозя́ин; повели́тель; коро́ль, магна́т (*промы́шленности*); ~ of the manor владе́лец поме́стья; 3) бог; ◇ to live like a ~ жить в ро́скоши; to act the ~ кома́ндовать, распоряжа́ться.

lord II *v*: to ~ it (over) разы́грывать ло́рда, ва́жничать; вести́ себя́ самовла́стно.

lordliness ['lɔːdlɪnɪs] *n* 1) высокоме́рие; 2) великоле́пие, пы́шность.

lordly I ['lɔːdlɪ] *a* 1) высокоме́рный; вла́стный (*о тоне и т. п.*); 2) ба́рственный, ва́жный.

lordly II *adv* 1) го́рдо, надме́нно; 2) по-ба́рски.

lordship ['lɔːdʃɪp] *n* 1) власть, госпо́дство; 2): your (his) ~ ва́ша (его́) све́тлость (*в обраще́нии, при упомина́нии*).

lore [lɔː] *n* (по)зна́ния (*в како́й-л. о́бласти*).

lorgnette [lɔːˈnjet] *n* 1) лорне́т; 2) театра́льный бино́кль.

lorry I ['lɔrɪ] *n* 1) грузови́к; 2) *ж.-д.* платфо́рма (*ваго́н*); 3) поло́к; подво́да.

lorry II *v* путеше́ствовать *или* перевози́ть на грузовика́х.

lorry-hop ['lɔrɪhɔp] *v* путеше́ствовать, по́льзуясь попу́тными грузовика́ми.

lose [luːz] *v* (*past, p. p.* lost) 1) теря́ть; лиша́ться; утра́чивать; 2) упуска́ть (*возмо́жность, слу́чай*); 3) прои́грывать; 4) терпе́ть поте́ри, убы́ток, уще́рб (*от — by*); 5) *pass* погиба́ть; пропада́ть; 6) вызыва́ть поте́рю, причиня́ть уще́рб; 7): to ~ oneself заблуди́ться; to ~ oneself in погрузи́ться во что-л.; 8) отстава́ть (*о часа́х*).

loser ['luːzə] *n* теря́ющий, прои́грывающий; проигра́вший; a good ~ переноси́щий про́игрыш ве́село, бо́дро; the ~ must pay проигра́вший пла́тит; to come off a ~ проигра́ть, оста́ться в про́игрыше.

losings ['luːzɪŋz] *n pl* поте́ри.

loss [lɔs] *n* 1) поте́ря, утра́та; уро́н; to have a ~, to meet with a ~ понести́ поте́рю; 2) убы́ток; про́игрыш; dead ~ чи́стый убы́ток; to sell at a ~ продава́ть в убы́ток; ◊ to be at a ~ быть в затрудне́нии, в замеша́тельстве.

lost [lɔst] *past, p. p. см.* lose.

lot I [lɔt] *n* 1) жре́бий; *перен.* судьба́, у́часть; to cast (to draw) ~s броса́ть (тяну́ть) жре́бий; the ~ fell upon me жре́бий пал на меня́; to cast (*или* to throw) in one's ~ with smb. раздели́ть судьбу́ с кем-л.; 2) уча́сток (земли́); parking ~ *амер.* стоя́нка автомоби́лей; 3) гру́ппа люде́й, компа́ния; 4) па́ртия (*това́ров, предме́тов*); 5) *разг.* ма́сса, большо́е коли́чество; a ~ of мно́го; ~s and ~s of огро́мное коли́чество чего́-л; a fat ~ *сленг* о́чень мно́го; *ирон.* о́чень ма́ло; ◊ a bad ~ плохо́й челове́к.

lot II *v* 1) дели́ть на ча́сти, разбива́ть на уча́стки (*тж.* to ~ out); 2) рассчи́тывать (*на что-л.— ирон*).

lotion ['loʊʃən] *n* 1) примо́чка; лосьо́н; 2) *сленг* спиртно́й напи́ток.

lottery ['lɔtərɪ] *n* лотере́я.

lotto ['lɔtoʊ] *n* лото́.

lotus ['loʊtəs] *n* ло́тос.

lotus-eater ['loʊtəsˌiːtə] *n* пра́здный мечта́тель.

loud I [laud] *a* 1) гро́мкий; зву́чный; 2) шу́мный; шумли́вый; 3) крича́щий (*о цве́те, наря́де*).

loud II *adv* гро́мко.

loud-coloured ['laudˈkʌləd] *a* крича́щий (*о цве́те тка́ни, оде́жды*).

loudly ['laudlɪ] *adv* 1) гро́мко; шу́мно; 2) крича́ще (*оде́тый и т. п.*).

loud-mouth ['laudmauθ] *n* крику́н.

loud speaker ['laudˈspiːkə] *n* громкоговори́тель; репроду́ктор.

lough [lɔk] *n ирл.* о́зеро; зали́в.

lounge I [laundʒ] *n* 1) пра́здное времяпрепровожде́ние; 2) ко́мната о́тдыха; 3) кре́сло, шезло́нг.

lounge II *v* 1) сиде́ть разваля́сь, отдыха́ть; 2) слоня́ться, безде́льничать.

lounge-chair ['laundʒˌtʃeə] *n* (удо́бное) кре́сло.

lounger ['laundʒə] *n* празднoшата́ющийся; безде́льник.

lounge-suit ['laundʒˌsjuːt] *n* пиджа́чная па́ра.

lour ['lauə] *см.* lower[b].

louse [laus] *p* (*pl* lice) вошь.

lousy ['lauzɪ] *a* 1) вши́вый; 2) *разг.* ни́зкий, гну́сный; 3): ~ with по́лный, перепо́лненный; ~ with money о́чень бога́тый.

lout [laut] *n* грубы́й, неотёсанный челове́к.

loutish ['lautɪʃ] *a* грубы́й, неотёсанный.

lovable ['lʌvəbl] *a* ми́лый, привлека́тельный.

love I [lʌv] *n* 1) любо́вь; cupboard ~ любо́вь по расчёту; 2) влюблённость; to be in ~ with быть влюблённым в кого́-л.; to fall in ~ with влюби́ться в кого́-л.; to declare one's ~ объясни́ться в любви́; to make ~ to уха́живать за кем-л.; in ~ with влюблённый; 3) предме́т любви́; возлю́бленный, -ная; 4) *разг.* что-л. о́чень привлека́тельное; 5) *спорт.* нуль; ◊ for the ~ of ра́ди, во и́мя; for ~ or money любо́й цено́й; not for ~ or money ни за что, ни за каки́е де́ньги; to give (to send) one's ~ to smb. передава́ть (посыла́ть) приве́т кому́-л.; to play for ~ игра́ть не на де́ньги; there's no ~ lost between them они́ недолю́бливают друг дру́га.

love II *v* 1) люби́ть; 2) .хоте́ть, жела́ть; I would so ~ to see you again я рад был бы уви́деть вас сно́ва; ◊ ~ me, ~ my dog лю́бишь меня́, люби́ и мою́ соба́ку.

love-affair ['lʌvəˌfeə] *n* любо́вная интри́га, рома́н.

love-bird ['lʌvbəːd] *n* ма́ленький попуга́й я́ркой окра́ски.

love-child ['lʌvtʃaild] *n* дитя́ любви́ (*о внебра́чном ребёнке*).

loveless ['lʌvlɪs] *a* 1) без любви́ (*о бра́ке*); 2) нелюбя́щий; 3) нелюби́мый.

loveliness ['lʌvlɪnɪs] *n* очарова́ние, привлека́тельность; красота́.

lovelock ['lʌvlɔk] *n* ма́ленький ло́кон, спуска́ющийся на лоб.

love-lorn ['lʌvlɔːn] *a* 1) страда́ющий от безнадёжной любви́; 2) поки́нутый (*люби́мым челове́ком*).

lovely ['lʌvlɪ] *a* 1) преле́стный, очарова́тельный; 2) ми́лый, любе́зный, прия́тный; 3) *разг.* восхити́тельный.

love-making ['lʌvˌmeikɪŋ] *n* уха́живание.

love-match ['lʌvmætʃ] *n* брак по любви́.

lover ['lʌvə] *n* 1) любо́вник; возлю́бленный; *pl* влюблённые; plighted ~s помо́лвленные; 2) люби́тель (*чего́-л.— of*); 3) приве́рженец; ~s of peace сторо́нники ми́ра.

lovesick ['lʌvsɪk] *a* снеда́емый любо́вью, томя́щийся от любви́.

loving ['lʌvɪŋ] *a* лю́бящий, не́жный; пре́данный.

loving-cup ['lʌvɪŋ'kʌp] *n* круговая чаша.

low[1] I [lou] *a* 1) низкий; низменный; 2) слабый; подавленный, пониженный; to bring ~ подавлять, унижать; to feel ~ чувствовать себя подавленным; 3) скудный, недостаточный (*о запасах и т. п.*); ограниченный; 4) тихий (*о голосе*); низкий (*о ноте*); 5) вульгарный, низменный; низкий, подлый; ◊ in ~ water в бедственном *или* тяжёлом положении.

low[1] II *adv* 1) низко; низменно; 2) скудно; в бедности; 3) тихо; слабо.

low[2] I *n* мычание.

low[2] II *v* мычать.

low-born ['lou'bɔːn] *n* низкого происхождения.

low-bred ['lou'bred] *a* невоспитанный, неотёсанный.

lowbrow ['loubrau] *n разг.* человек, не претендующий на высокий интеллектуальный уровень.

low-browed ['loubraud] *a* 1) низколобый, узколобый; 2) нависший (*о скалах*); 3) с низким входом, мрачный (*о здании*).

low-down ['loudaun] *a разг.* 1) низкий, подлый; 2) грубый, вульгарный.

lower[a] I ['louə] *a* (*compar см.* low[1] I) низший; нижний.

lower[a] II *v* 1) снижать(ся), понижать(ся); опускать(ся); 2) спускать (*шлюпку, парус, флаг*); 3) уменьшать(ся); 4) подавлять, унижать.

lower[b] ['lauə] *v* 1) хмуриться (*at, on, upon*); 2) темнеть, покрываться тучами (*о небе*).

lowermost ['louəmoust] *a* самый нижний.

low-grade[1] ['lou'greid] *n* пологий подъём.

low-grade[2] *a* низкосортный, низкопробный.

lowland ['loulənd] *n обыкн. pl* низменность, низина; the Lowlands южная, равнинная часть Шотландии.

lowlander ['louləndə] *n* 1) житель низин; 2) (L.) житель юга Шотландии.

lowly I ['louli] *a* скромный; смиренный.

lowly II *adv* скромно.

low-paid ['lou'peid] *a* низкооплачиваемый.

low-powered ['lou'pauəd] *a тех.* маломощный; малолитражный (*об автомобиле*).

low-spirited ['lou'spiritid] *a* подавленный, удручённый.

loyal ['lɔiəl] *a* верный, лояльный; преданный.

loyalty ['lɔiəlti] *n* верность, лояльность; преданность.

lozenge ['lɔzindʒ] *n* 1) ромб; 2) таблетка.

L. s. d., £.s.d. ['eles'diː] *n* фунты стерлингов, шиллинги и пенсы; *разг.* деньги.

lubber ['lʌbə] *n* увалень.

lubberly I ['lʌbəli] *a* неуклюжий, нескладный.

lubberly II *adv* неуклюже; неумело.

lubricant I ['luːbrikənt] *n* смазочный материал, смазка.

lubricant II *a* смазочный; для смазки.

lubricate ['luːbrikeit] *v* 1) смазывать (*машину и т. п.*); 2) *разг.* «подмазать».

lubrication [‚luːbri'keiʃən] *n* смазка, смазывание (*машины*).

lubricator ['luːbrikeitə] *n* 1) маслёнка; 2) смазчик; 3) смазочное вещество.

lubricous ['luːbrikəs] *a* 1) гладкий, скользкий; *перен.* увёртливый; 2) похотливый.

luce [luːs] *n* щука.

lucent ['luːsnt] *a* 1) светящийся; яркий; 2) прозрачный, просвечивающий.

lucerne [luː'səːn] *n бот.* люцерна.

lucid ['luːsid] *a* 1) ясный, прозрачный; *поэт.* светлый, яркий; 2) понятный, ясный (*о рассуждении и т. п.*).

lucidity [luː'siditi] *n* 1) ясность, прозрачность; 2) понятность.

luck [lʌk] *n* счастье; удача; судьба; bad ~, ill ~ несчастье, неудача; a real piece of bad ~ полная неудача; страшное невезение; rough ~ горькая доля; good ~ удача, счастливый случай; good ~! счастливо!, желаю успеха!; by (good) ~ по счастью; for ~! на счастье!; his ~ held счастье ему улыбалось; to try one's ~ попытать счастья; ◊ worse ~ *разг.* к несчастью; as ~ would have it а) как нарочно; б) к счастью; devil's own ~ необыкновенная удача; ≅ чертовски везёт; down on one's ~ *сленг* а) в беде, в несчастье; б) на мели, без денег.

luckily ['lʌkili] *adv* к счастью; по счастью.

luckless ['lʌklis] *a* несчастливый, незадачливый; злополучный.

lucky ['lʌki] *a* 1) счастливый, удачный; удачливый; 2) приносящий счастье; 3) случайный.

lucrative ['luːkrətiv] *a* прибыльный, доходный, выгодный.

lucre ['luːkə] *n* прибыль, барыш; выгода; ◊ filthy ~ презренный металл.

ludicrous ['luːdikrəs] *a* нелепый, смешной.

lug[1] I [lʌg] *n* 1) волочение; 2) дёрганье; 3) *pl амер. разг.* важничанье; to put on ~s важничать, напускать на себя важность.

lug[1] II *v* 1) тащить(ся); волочить(ся); 2) дёргать (*at*); □ to ~ away утаскивать; увлекать за собой; to ~ in, to ~ into *разг.* приплести ни к селу ни к городу; to ~ off *см.* to ~ away; to ~ out вытаскивать; вынимать (*из ножен*).

lug[2] *n тех.* ушко, проушина; зажим; ручка.

luggage ['lʌgidʒ] *n* багаж; чемоданы, саквояжи *и т. п.*; to register ~ сдавать багаж; 2) *attr* багажный.

lugubrious [luː'gjuːbriəs] *a* печальный, траурный.

lukewarm ['luːkwɔːm] *a* 1) тепловатый; 2) равнодушный.

lull I [lʌl] *n* (временное) затишье, успокоение.

lull II *v* 1) убаюкивать; 2) успокаивать (*боль*); 3) усыплять (*подозрения*); 4) успокаиваться, затихать (*о буре и т. п.*).

lullaby ['lʌləbai] *n* колыбельная песня.

lumber[1] I ['lʌmbə] *n* 1) лесоматериалы; 2) громоздкие ненужные вещи, хлам.

lumber[1] II *v* 1) заготавливать лес; 2) загромождать; сваливать в беспорядке.

lumber[2] *v* громыхать, проезжать с грохотом (*тж.* to ~ along, by, past).

lumbering ['lʌmbəriŋ] *n* лесоразработки.

lumberman ['lʌmbəmən] *n* 1) лесоруб; 2) лесопромышленник.

lumber-mill ['lʌmbəmil] *n* лесопильный завод.

lumber-room ['lʌmbərum] *n* чулан.

lumberyard ['lʌmbər‚jɑːd] *n амер.* лесной склад.

luminary ['luːminəri] *n* светило.

luminescence [,luːmɪ'nesns] *n* свече́ние.

luminous ['luːmɪnəs] *a* 1) светя́щийся, све́тлый; 2) я́сный, поня́тный.

lump I [lʌmp] *n* 1) ком; глы́ба; a ~ in the throat комо́к в го́рле; 2) гру́да; ку́ча; in the ~ о́птом, гурто́м, огу́лом; *перен.* в це́лом; 3) буго́р, вы́ступ; о́пухоль, ши́шка; 4) чурба́н, дуби́на, тупи́ца.

lump II *v* 1) сме́шивать, сва́ливать в (одну́) ку́чу (*with*; *тж.* to ~ together); брать огу́лом, без разбо́ра; 2): to ~ it *разг.* мири́ться с чем-л.; «проглоти́ть»; □ to ~ **along** тяжело́ ступа́ть; to ~ **down** гру́зно сади́ться, опуска́ться.

lumper ['lʌmpə] *n* гру́зчик.

lumping ['lʌmpɪŋ] *a* 1) *разг.* огро́мный; 2) по́лный, хоро́ший (*о весе*); 3) тяжёлый (*о по́ступи*).

lumpish ['lʌmpɪʃ] *a* 1) тяжёлый; неуклю́жий; 2) тупо́й, глупы́й.

lumpy ['lʌmpɪ] *a* комкова́тый; буго́рчатый.

lunacy ['luːnəsɪ] *n* 1) сумасше́ствие, безу́мие; 2) *юр.* невменя́емость; 3) *разг.* безу́мие, больша́я глу́пость.

lunar ['luːnə] *a* лу́нный.

lunatic I ['luːnətɪk] *n* сумасше́дший, поме́шанный.

lunatic II *a* 1) сумасше́дший, безу́мный; 2) глу́пый.

lunation [luː'neɪʃən] *n* лу́нный ме́сяц.

lunch I [lʌntʃ] *n* ленч, второ́й за́втрак; *амер.* лёгкая заку́ска; to have (*или* to take) ~ за́втракать; заку́сывать; basket ~ пикни́к.

lunch II *v* 1) за́втракать; заку́сывать; 2) угоща́ть за́втраком.

luncheon ['lʌntʃən] *n* за́втрак.

lung [lʌŋ] *n* 1) лёгкое; the ~s лёгкие; good ~s *перен.* си́льный го́лос; 2) *pl*: the ~s of London зелёный масси́в Ло́ндона.

lunge I [lʌndʒ] *n* 1) ко́рда; 2) мане́ж.

lunge II *v* гоня́ть на ко́рде (*ло́шадь*).

lunge 2 I *n* 1) уда́р (*рапи́рой и т. п.*); вы́пад (*при уда́ре*); 2) толчо́к, стреми́тельное движе́ние.

lunge 2 II *v* 1) наноси́ть уда́р; де́лать вы́пад; 2) устреми́ться, ри́нуться.

lungful ['lʌŋful] *n*: to get a ~ of fresh air вдохну́ть по́лной гру́дью; надыша́ться све́жим во́здухом.

lupus ['luːpəs] *n* *мед.* волча́нка.

lurch 1 I [ləːtʃ] *n* 1) крен (*су́дна*); 2) ша́ткая похо́дка.

lurch 1 II *v* 1) крени́ться; 2) идти́ шата́ясь.

lurch 2 *n*: to leave smb. in the ~ поки́нуть кого́-л. в беде́.

lurcher ['ləːtʃə] *n* 1) вори́шка, жу́лик; 2) шпио́н.

lure I [ljuə] *n* 1) собла́зн; 2) *охот.* ва́бик; прима́нка.

lure II *v* 1) завлека́ть; соблазня́ть; 2) *охот.* прима́нивать.

lurid ['ljuərɪd] *a* 1) мёртвенно-бле́дный, посине́вший; 2) стра́шный, злове́щий, мра́чный.

lurk I [ləːk] *n* 1): on the ~ та́йно высма́тривая, подстерега́я; 2) *разг.* обма́н, подло́г.

lurk II *v* 1) скрыва́ться (в заса́де); 2) таи́ться; остава́ться незаме́ченным.

lurking-place ['ləːkɪŋpleɪs] *n* потаённое ме́сто; убе́жище.

luscious ['lʌʃəs] *a* 1) со́чный, арома́тный; 2) прито́рный; 3) перегру́женный (*метафо́рами, эпи́тетами*).

lush 1 [lʌʃ] *a* со́чный; бу́йный (*о расти́тельности*).

lush 2 I *n* сленг спиртны́е напи́тки.

lush 2 II *v* сленг 1) выпива́ть; 2) подпа́ивать.

lust I [lʌst] *n* 1) вожделе́ние; 2) страсть (*к чему́-л.— of, for*).

lust II *v* 1) испы́тывать вожделе́ние; 2) стра́стно жела́ть (*чего́-л.— after, for*).

lustful ['lʌstful] *a* похотли́вый, сладостра́стный.

lustiness ['lʌstɪnɪs] *n* си́ла, бо́дрость, кре́пость.

lustre ['lʌstə] *n* 1) блеск; лоск, гля́нец; 2) сла́ва, вели́чие; to add (*или* to give) ~ to, to shed (*или* to throw) ~ on придава́ть блеск чему́-л.; прославля́ть; 3) лю́стра.

lustreless ['lʌstəlɪs] *a* ту́склый; ма́товый (*о кра́ске*).

lustrous ['lʌstrəs] *a* блестя́щий; глянцеви́тый.

lusty ['lʌstɪ] *a* си́льный, кре́пкий, здоро́вый.

lute [luːt] *n* лю́тня.

Lutheran I ['luːθərən] *n* лютера́нин.

Lutheran II *a* лютера́нский.

luxuriance [lʌg'zjuərɪəns] *n* 1) изоби́лие; пы́шность; 2) бога́тство (*воображе́ния и т. п.*).

luxuriant [lʌg'zjuərɪənt] *a* 1) бога́тый, оби́льный; плодоро́дный; 2) бу́йный, пы́шный (*о расти́тельности*); 3) цвети́стый (*о сло́ге*).

luxuriate [lʌg'zjuərɪeɪt] *v* 1) бу́йно, пы́шно расти́; 2) наслажда́ться (*чем-л.— in, on*); роско́шествовать.

luxurious [lʌg'zjuərɪəs] *a* 1) роско́шный; пы́шный; 2) лю́бящий ро́скошь, расточи́тельный.

luxury ['lʌkʃərɪ] *n* 1) ро́скошь; 2) предме́т ро́скоши; 3) большо́е удово́льствие, наслажде́ние.

lycée ['liːseɪ] *n* лице́й (*сре́дняя шко́ла во Фра́нции*).

Lyceum [laɪ'sɪəm] *n* лекто́рий; чита́льня.

lye [laɪ] *n* щёлок.

lying 1 I ['laɪɪŋ] *n* ложь, лжи́вость.

lying 1 II *a* ло́жный, обма́нчивый.

lying 1 III *pres. p.* см. lie 1 II.

lying 2 I *n* 1) лежа́ние; 2) ме́сто для лежа́ния, «ло́же».

lying 2 II *a* лежа́щий, лежа́чий.

lying 2 III *pres. p.* см. lie 2 I.

lying-in ['laɪɪŋ'ɪn] *n* ро́ды.

lymph [lɪmf] *n* *физиол.* ли́мфа.

lymphatic [lɪm'fætɪk] *a* 1) *физиол.* лимфати́ческий; 2) флегмати́чный.

lynch [lɪntʃ] *v* линчева́ть.

lynx [lɪŋks] *n* *зоол.* рысь.

lynx-eyed ['lɪŋksaɪd] *a* с о́стрым зре́нием.

lyre ['laɪə] *n* ли́ра.

lyre-bird ['laɪəbəːd] *n* пти́ца-ли́ра.

lyric I ['lɪrɪk] *n* 1) лири́ческое стихотворе́ние; 2) *pl* ли́рика.

lyric II *a* лири́ческий.

lyrical ['lɪrɪkəl] *a* 1) лири́ческий; 2) восто́рженный; эмоциона́льный.

lyricism ['lɪrɪsɪzəm] *n* лири́зм.

lyrist *a* ['lɪrɪst] *n* ли́рик.

lyrist *b* ['laɪərɪst] *n* игра́ющий на ли́ре.

M

M, m [em] *n* 13-я буква англ. алфавита.

ma [mɑː] *n разг.* ма́ма.

ma'am [mæm] *сокр. см.* madam.

macabre [mə'kɑːbr] *a* мра́чный, ужа́сный.

macaco [mə'keɪkou] *n* мака́ка.

macadam I [mə'kædəm] *n* щебень (*для моще́ния*).

macadam II *a* шоссе́йный; шосси́рованный (щебнем).

macadamize [mə'kædəmaɪz] *v* мости́ть щебнем.

macaroni [ˌmækə'rounɪ] *n* 1) макаро́ны; 2) франт, хлыщ (*в Англии в XVIII в.*).

macaroon [ˌmækə'ruːn] *n* минда́льное пече́нье.

mace[1] [meɪs] *n* 1) *ист.* булава́; 2) жезл.

mace[2] *n* муска́тный оре́х.

macerate ['mæsəreɪt] *v* 1) разма́чивать, размягча́ть; растворя́ть; 2) изнуря́ть, истоща́ть.

maceration [ˌmæsə'reɪʃən] *n* 1) размягче́ние, разма́чивание; 2) изнуре́ние, истоще́ние.

machination [ˌmækɪ'neɪʃən] *n* махина́ция.

machine [mə'ʃiːn] *n* 1) маши́на, инструме́нт; механи́зм; centrifugal ~ центрифу́га; calculating ~ счётная маши́на; kneading ~ тестомеша́лка; mincing ~ мясору́бка; talking ~ фоно́граф; 2) автомаши́на; велосипе́д; самолёт; 3) челове́к, де́йствующий маши́нально *или* рабо́тающий как маши́на; 4) аппара́т (*организацио́нный, госуда́рственный*); state ~ госуда́рственный аппара́т; 5) *амер.* организа́ция *или* па́ртия, контроли́рующая полити́ческую жизнь страны́; 6) *attr* маши́нный.

machine-gun I [mə'ʃiːngʌn] *n* 1) пулемёт; 2) *attr* пулемётный.

machine-gun II *v* обстре́ливать из пулемёта.

machine-gunner [mə'ʃiːnˌgʌnə] *n* пулемётчик.

machinery [mə'ʃiːnərɪ] *n* 1) маши́ны; маши́нное обору́дование; 2) дета́ли маши́н; механи́змы; 3) аппара́т (*госуда́рственный и т. п.*).

machinist [mə'ʃiːnɪst] *n* 1) машини́ст; меха́ник; 2) сле́сарь; 3) машинострои́тель.

mackerel ['mækrəl] *n* макре́ль, ску́мбрия (*рыба*).

mackintosh ['mækɪntɔʃ] *n* 1) макинто́ш, непромока́емое пальто́; 2) прорези́ненная ткань.

mad I [mæd] *a* 1) сумасше́дший, безу́мный; to go ~ сойти́ с ума́; to drive (*или* to send) smb. ~ своди́ть с ума́; to like ~ *разг.* как сумасше́дший (*бежа́ть, крича́ть и т. п.*); 2) бе́шеный; 3) поме́шанный на чём-л., увлечённый чем-л. (*after, about, for, on*); 4) сумасбро́дный, безрассу́дный; 5) *разг.* о́чень серди́тый; to get ~ рассерди́ться; don't be ~ at me не серди́тесь на меня́; 6) бу́йно весёлый; ◊ ~ as a hatter, ~ as a March hare спя́тивший.

mad II *v* 1) своди́ть, сходи́ть с ума́; 2) *разг.* выводи́ть из себя́.

madam ['mædəm] *n* суда́рыня, мада́м.

madcap ['mædkæp] *n* 1) сумасбро́д; сорвиголова́; 2) *attr* сумасбро́дный.

madden ['mædn] *v* 1) своди́ть, сходи́ть с ума́; 2) раздража́ть.

made I [meɪd] *past, p. p. см.* make I.

made II *a* 1) сде́ланный, пригото́вленный; де-

жу́рный (*о блю́де*); 2) сло́женный (*обыкн. в сочета́ниях*): well-made хорошо́ сло́женный; stoutly-made то́лстый *и т. п.*).

made-up ['meɪd'ʌp] *a* 1) иску́сственный; 2) составно́й; со́бранный.

madhouse ['mædhaus] *n* сумасше́дший дом.

madman ['mædmən] *n* сумасше́дший, безу́мец.

madness ['mædnɪs] *n* 1) сумасше́ствие, безу́мие; 2) бе́шенство.

madwoman ['mædˌwumən] *n* сумасше́дшая, безу́мная.

maelstrom ['meɪlstroum] *n* водоворо́т, вихрь (*тж. перен.*).

mag[1] [mæg] *n сленг* полпе́нни.

mag[2] *n разг.* 1) болту́н(ья); 2) болтовня́.

magazine [ˌmægə'ziːn] *n* 1) (периоди́ческий) журна́л; 2) артиллери́йский склад; 3) *тех.* магази́н; 4) *attr* магази́нный.

maggot ['mægət] *n* 1) личи́нка; 2) блажь, причу́да (*тж. a* ~ in one's brain).

maggoty ['mægətɪ] *a* 1) черви́вый; 2) с причу́дами, блажно́й.

Magi ['meɪdʒaɪ] *n pl библ.* волхвы́, ма́ги.

magic I ['mædʒɪk] *n* 1) ма́гия, колдовство́, волшебство́; 2) ча́ры, очарова́ние.

magic II *a* волше́бный, маги́ческий.

magical ['mædʒɪkəl] *см.* magic II.

magician [mə'dʒɪʃən] *n* волше́бник, маг.

magisterial [ˌmædʒɪs'tɪərɪəl] *a* 1) суде́йский; 2) повели́тельный, вла́стный; 3) авторите́тный.

magistracy ['mædʒɪstrəsɪ] *n* 1) магистрату́ра; 2) до́лжность судьи́.

magistral I [mə'dʒɪstrəl] *n* магистра́ль, магистра́льная ли́ния.

magistral II *a* 1) повели́тельный; авторите́тный; 2) гла́вный; магистра́льный.

magistrate ['mædʒɪstrɪt] *n* 1) (мирово́й) судья́; police ~ представи́тель суда́ при поли́ции; 2) член магистра́та (*в Англии*).

Magna C(h)arta ['mægnə'kɑːtə] *n ист.* Вели́кая ха́ртия во́льностей (*1215 г.*).

magnanimity [ˌmægnə'nɪmɪtɪ] *n* великоду́шие.

magnanimous [mæg'nænɪməs] *a* великоду́шный.

magnate ['mægneɪt] *n* магна́т; oil ~ нефтяно́й коро́ль.

magnesia [mæg'niːʃə] *n хим.* о́кись ма́гния, жжёная магне́зия.

magnesium [mæg'niːzjəm] *n хим.* ма́гний.

magnet ['mægnɪt] *n* магни́т.

magnetic [mæg'netɪk] *a* 1) магни́тный; 2) привлека́тельный; притяга́тельный.

magnetics [mæg'netɪks] *n физ.* магнети́зм.

magnetism ['mægnɪtɪzəm] *n* 1) магнети́зм; притяже́ние; terrestrial ~, earth ~ земно́й магнети́зм; permanent ~ оста́точный магнети́зм; 2) ли́чное обая́ние; привлека́тельность.

magnetize ['mægnɪtaɪz] *v* 1) намагни́чивать(ся); 2) гипнотизи́ровать; 3) притя́гивать, привлека́ть.

magnification [ˌmægnɪfɪ'keɪʃən] *n* увеличе́ние; усиле́ние.

magnificence [mæg'nɪfɪsns] *n* великоле́пие.

magnificent [mæg'nɪfɪsnt] *a* 1) великоле́пный, вели́чественный; 2) *разг.* прекра́сный, изуми́тельный.

magnifier ['mægnɪfaɪə] *n* 1) лу́па; 2) *радио* усили́тель.

magnify ['mægnɪfaɪ] *v* 1) увели́чивать; 2) преувели́чивать.

magnifying ['mægnɪfaɪɪŋ] *a* увеличи́тельный.

magnitude ['mægnɪtjuːd] *n* 1) величина́; 2) ва́жность.

magnolia [mæg'nouljə] *n* магно́лия.

magpie ['mægpaɪ] *n* 1) соро́ка; 2) болту́н(ья).

Magyar I ['mægjɑː] *n* 1) венгр, венге́рец; мадья́р; венге́рка; мадья́рка; the '~s ве́нгры, венге́рцы; мадья́ры; 2) венге́рский язы́к.

Magyar II *a* венге́рский.

Maharaja(h) [,mɑːhə'rɑːdʒə] *n* магара́джа.

mahogany [mə'hɔgənɪ] *n* кра́сное де́рево.

Mahometan I, II [mə'hɔmɪtən] *см.* Mohammedan I, II.

maid [meɪd] *n* 1) де́вушка; old ~ ста́рая де́ва; ~ of honour а) фре́йлина; б) подру́жка неве́сты; 2) служа́нка; го́рничная.

maiden I ['meɪdn] *n* 1) де́вушка; 2) ста́рая де́ва.

maiden II *a* 1) де́вичий; 2) чи́стый, де́вственный; 3) пе́рвый; неиспро́бованный; ~ flight пе́рвый полёт (*самолёта*); ~ speech пе́рвая речь (*нового члена парламента*).

maidenhood ['meɪdnhud] *n* деви́чество.

maidenly ['meɪdnlɪ] *a* де́вичий, деви́ческий.

maid-of-all-work ['meɪdəvɔːl'wəːk] *n* одна́ прислу́га.

maidservant ['meɪd,səːvənt] *n* служа́нка.

mail¹ I [meɪl] *n* 1) по́чта; *fap* ~ пи́сьма от покло́нников, боле́льщиков; 2) су́мка с по́чтой; 3) почто́вый по́езд (*тж.* ~ train); 4) *attr* почто́вый.

mail¹ II *v* посыла́ть по по́чте, по́чтой.

mail² I *n* броня́, до́спех; кольчу́га (*тж.* chain-mail, ring-mail).

mail² II *v* покрыва́ть, одева́ть бронёй.

mail-boat ['meɪlbout] *n* почто́вый парохо́д.

mail-cart ['meɪlkɑːt] *n* 1) почто́вая каре́та; 2) де́тская коля́ска.

mail-coach ['meɪl'koutʃ] *см.* mail-cart 1).

maillot [maɪ'jou] *n* 1) трико́ (*акробатов, танцоров и т. п.*); 2) же́нский купа́льный костю́м (*без бретелек*).

maim [meɪm] *v* кале́чить, уве́чить.

main I [meɪn] *n* 1) гла́вное; in the ~ в основно́м; 2) магистра́ль; 3) *поэт.* откры́тое мо́ре.

main II *a* 1) гла́вный, основно́й; важне́йший; 2) бо́льший, сильне́йший.

mainland ['meɪnlənd] *n* матери́к; контине́нт.

mainly ['meɪnlɪ] *adv* 1) бо́льшей ча́стью; 2) гла́вным о́бразом.

mainmast ['meɪnmɑːst] *n* мор. грот-ма́чта.

mainsail ['meɪnseɪl] *n* мор. грот.

mainspring ['meɪnsprɪŋ] *n* ходова́я пружи́на (*часового механизма*); *перен.* дви́жущая си́ла.

mainstay ['meɪnsteɪ] *n* мор. гро́та-шта́г; *перен.* гла́вная подде́ржка, опло́т.

maintain [men'teɪn] *v* 1) подде́рживать; 2) содержа́ть; 3) сохраня́ть; 4) ока́зывать (*сопротивление, поддержку*); отста́ивать; 5) утвержда́ть (*that*); 6) продолжа́ть; вести́.

maintenance ['meɪntɪnəns] *n* 1) подде́ржка, подержа́ние; 2) содержа́ние; сре́дства к существо-

ва́нию; 3) утвержде́ние; 4) *тех.* обслу́живание; 5) *attr* обслу́живающий; ремо́нтный.

maize [meɪz] *n* 1) кукуру́за, ма́ис; 2) жёлтый цвет.

majestic [mə'dʒestɪk] *a* вели́чественный.

majesty ['mædʒɪstɪ] *n* 1) вели́чественность, вели́чие; 2) вели́чество (*титул*).

majolica [mə'jɔlɪkə] *n* майо́лика.

major¹ I ['meɪdʒə] *n* совершенноле́тний (*в Англии — 21 г.*).

major¹ II *a* 1) гла́вный, основно́й; 2) бо́льший; 3) ста́рший; 4) *муз.* мажо́рный.

major² *n* майо́р; drum ~ ста́рший бараба́нщик, тамбурмажо́р.

major-domo ['meɪdʒə'doumou] *n* дворе́цкий, мажордо́м.

majority [mə'dʒɔrɪtɪ] *n* 1) большинство́; ~ of votes большинство́ голосо́в; absolute ~ абсолю́тное большинство́; marginal ~, overwhelming ~ подавля́ющее большинство́; bare ~, narrow ~ незначи́тельное большинство́; to gain (*или* to carry) the ~ получи́ть большинство́ голосо́в; the ~ has it при́нято большинство́м голосо́в; 2) совершенноле́тие; 3) чин, зва́ние майо́ра; ◊ to join the ~ умере́ть.

make I [meɪk] *v* (*past, p. p.* made) 1) сде́лать; соверша́ть; производи́ть; 2) гото́вить, приготовля́ть; убира́ть, приводи́ть в поря́док; 3) составля́ть, равня́ться; образо́вывать; 2 and 3 = 5 два плюс три равня́ется пяти́; 5) станови́ться, стать; сде́латься; 6) *с Inf без* to заставля́ть, побужда́ть; ~ him repeat it заста́вьте его́ повтори́ть э́то; 7) зараба́тывать; 8) предполага́ть; what bird do you ~ that to be? как вы ду́маете, кака́я э́то пти́ца?; 9) успе́ть, поспе́ть; дости́гнуть (*тж.* to ~ it); 10) дви́гаться, отправля́ться; he made towards the town он напра́вился к го́роду; 11) получа́ть; 12) *с прямым дополнением, выраженным сущ., образует устойчивые словосочетания, которые приводятся в словаре при соответствующих сущ., напр.:* to ~ way *см.* way *и т. д.*; □ to ~ **against** быть неблагоприя́тным, говори́ть не в по́льзу (*кого-л.*); to ~ **away** а) убежа́ть, поспеш
́ть прочь; б) изба́виться, отде́латься, уби́ть (*with*); to ~ away with himself поко́нчить жизнь самоуби́йством; в) испо́льзовать, исче́рпать (*with*); to ~ **for** а) соде́йствовать; б) направля́ться в; в) напада́ть; to ~ **off** удра́ть, скры́ться; to ~ **out** а) составля́ть (*документ*); выпи́сывать (*чек*); б) дока́зывать; в) понима́ть; уясня́ть себе́; г) разбира́ть, различа́ть; to ~ **over** а) передава́ть; б) переде́лывать; to ~ **up** а) пополня́ть, возмеща́ть, компенси́ровать; навёрстывать; б) составля́ть, собира́ть; в) гримирова́ть(ся); г) выду́мывать; д) устра́ивать, ула́живать; е) мири́ться; let us ~ it up дава́йте забу́дем э́то, дава́йте поми́римся; ж) реша́ть; з) шить, кройть; и) *полигр.* верста́ть; к) заи́скивать, лебези́ть (*перед кем-л. — to*); ◊ to ~ believe де́лать вид, притворя́ться; вообража́ть себя́ (*кем-л.*); to ~ do дово́льствоваться (*чем-л.*).

make II *n* 1) вид, сорт, ма́рка; 2) стиль, фасо́н; do you like the ~ of that coat? нра́вится ли вам фасо́н э́того пальто́?; 3) склад хара́ктера; 4) произво́дство, рабо́та; is this your own ~? э́то ва́ша рабо́та?; 5) разви́тие, проце́сс; ◊ on the ~

сленг а) корьíстный; стремя́щийся к наживе; б) делающий карье́ру.

make-believe I ['meɪkbɪ,liːv] *n* 1) воображе́ние; фанта́зия; 2) притво́рство; предло́г.

make-believe II *a* 1) воображаемый; 2) притво́рный.

makepeace ['meɪkpiːs] *n* примири́тель, миротво́рец.

maker ['meɪkə] *n* созда́тель, творе́ц.

makeshift ['meɪkʃɪft] *n* 1) заме́на, временное сре́дство; 2) *attr* импровизи́рованный, временный, заменяющий что-л.

make-up ['meɪkʌp] *n* 1) грим, косме́тика; to wear ~ употребля́ть косме́тику; 2) грим и костю́м (*актёра*); 3) соста́в; 4) нату́ра, склад (*характера*); people of a nervous ~ не́рвные лю́ди; 5) вы́думка; 6) *полигр.* вёрстка.

makeweight ['meɪkweɪt] *n* дове́сок, доба́вка.

making ['meɪkɪŋ] *n* 1) изготовле́ние, произво́дство; in the ~ в проце́ссе рабо́ты, созда́ния; that was the ~ of him э́то созда́ло ему́ успе́х; благодаря́ э́тому он вы́двинулся; 2) изде́лие; 3) *pl* зада́тки; 4) *pl* зарабо́ток; 5) *pl амер. разг.* таба́к и бума́га для самокру́ток.

mal- [mæl-] *pref со значением* плохо́й, несправедли́вый, непра́вильный; maladjusted пло́хо приспосо́бленный, при́гнанный; maladminister пло́хо управля́ть.

malady ['mælədɪ] *n* боле́знь.

malaria [mə'lɛərɪə] *n* маляри́я.

malarial [mə'lɛərɪəl] *a* маляри́йный.

Malay I [mə'leɪ] *n* 1) мала́ец; the ~s мала́йцы; 2) мала́йский язы́к.

Malay II *a* мала́йский.

Malayan I, II [mə'leɪən] *см.* Malay I, II.

malcontent ['mælkən,tent] *a* недово́льный.

male I [meɪl] *n* 1) мужчи́на; 2) саме́ц.

male II *a* мужско́й.

male- ['mælɪ-, mə'le-] *pref со значением* зло-; malefaction злодея́ние.

malediction [,mælɪ'dɪkʃən] *n* прокля́тие.

malefactor ['mælɪfæktə] *n* злоумы́шленник, престу́пник.

maleficent [mə'lefɪsnt] *a* па́губный, вре́дный; вредоно́сный.

malevolence [mə'levələns] *n* недоброжела́тельство; злора́дство.

malevolent [mə'levələnt] *a* недоброжела́тельный; злора́дный.

malfeasance [mæl'fiːzəns] *n юр.* 1) должностно́е преступле́ние; наруше́ние обще́ственного дове́рия; 2) злодея́ние.

malformation ['mælfɔː'meɪʃən] *n* уро́дство.

malformed [mæl'fɔːmd] *a* уро́дливый, бесфо́рменный.

malice ['mælɪs] *n* 1) зло́ба; зло́бность; to bear ~ (to) име́ть злы́е, престу́пные наме́рения; 2) *юр.* престу́пное наме́рение.

malicious [mə'lɪʃəs] *a* 1) злой; 2) преднаме́ренный.

malign I [mə'laɪn] *a* 1) вре́дный; злока́чественный; 2) зло́бный; зло́стный.

malign II *v* злосло́вить; клевета́ть.

malignant [mə'lɪgnənt] *a* 1) зло́бный, зло́стный; 2) зловре́дный; 3) *мед.* злока́чественный.

malignity [mə'lɪgnɪtɪ] *n* 1) зло́бность; 2) зловре́дность; 3) *мед.* злока́чественность.

malinger [mə'lɪŋgə] *v* симули́ровать.

malingerer [mə'lɪŋgərə] *n* симуля́нт.

mallard ['mæləd] *n* ди́кая у́тка.

malleability [,mælɪə'bɪlɪtɪ] *n* 1) ко́вкость; 2) пода́тливость; усту́пчивость.

malleable ['mælɪəbl] *a* 1) ко́вкий (*о металле*); 2) пода́тливый; усту́пчивый.

mallet ['mælɪt] *n* деревя́нный молото́к.

mallow ['mælou] *n бот.* ма́льва.

malnutrition ['mælnjuː'trɪʃən] *n* плохо́е пита́ние, недоеда́ние.

malpractice ['mæl'præktɪs] *n* 1) незако́нные де́йствия; 2) небре́жность, невнима́ние (*врача к пациенту*).

malt I [mɔːlt] *n* 1) со́лод; 2) *attr* солодо́вый.

malt II *v* 1) солоди́ть; 2) солоде́ть.

Maltese I ['mɔːl'tiːz] *n* мальти́ец; the ~ (*употр. как pl*) мальти́йцы.

Maltese II *a* мальти́йский.

Malthusian I [mæl'θjuːzjən] *n* мальтузиа́нец.

Malthusian II *a* мальтузиа́нский.

maltreat [mæl'triːt] *v* пло́хо, жесто́ко обраща́ться.

maltreatment [mæl'triːtmənt] *n* плохо́е обраще́ние.

mam(m)a [mə'mɑː] *n дет.* ма́ма.

mammal ['mæməl] *n* (*pl* mammalia [mæ'meɪljə]) млекопита́ющее.

mammon ['mæmən] *n* мамо́н(а), де́ньги.

mammoth I ['mæməθ] *n* ма́монт.

mammoth II *a* грома́дный, гига́нтский.

mammy ['mæmɪ] *n* 1) *дет.* ма́ма, ма́мочка; 2) *амер.* ня́ня-негритя́нка; 3) *амер.* ста́рая негритя́нка.

man I [mæn] *n* (*pl* men) 1) челове́к; any ~ любо́й челове́к; по ~ никто́; (all) to a ~ все до одного́, все без исключе́ния; old ~ стари́к; оте́ц; дружи́ще; men of the other days лю́ди друго́й эпо́хи; the right ~ in the right place челове́к на своём ме́сте, подходя́щий челове́к; 2) *во фразеологических сочетаниях* челове́к: а) *как общественный деятель или представитель профессии*: Party ~ член па́ртии; public ~ обще́ственный де́ятель; ~ of letters писа́тель; учёный; men of the pen литерату́рные рабо́тники; ~ of science учёный; ~ of business, business ~ деле́ц, коммерса́нт; ~ of property состоя́тельный челове́к, со́бственник; City ~ фина́нсист, коммерса́нт; medical ~ врач; leading ~ актёр, игра́ющий гла́вную роль; one-dollar-a-year ~ *амер.* кру́пный деле́ц, рабо́тающий в прави́тельственных о́рганах и официа́льно получа́ющий оди́н до́ллар в год; plain-clothes ~ сы́щик; переоде́тый полице́йский; old-clothes ~ старьёвщик; б) *как обладатель качеств*: ~ of genius гениа́льный челове́к; ~ of distinction (*или* of mark, of note) выдаю́щийся, знамени́тый челове́к; ~ of vision проница́тельный челове́к; ~ of principle принципиа́льный челове́к; ~ of no principles беспринци́пный челове́к; ~ of tact такти́чный челове́к; ~ of ideas изобрета́тельный, нахо́дчивый челове́к; a ~ with plenty of guts челове́к с си́льной во́лей; men of the day изве́стные лю́ди; ~ of sense разу́мный челове́к; ~ of no scruples недобросо́вестный, бессо́вестный челове́к; deep ~ хи́трый челове́к;

self-made ~ человек, выбившийся самостоятельно в люди; the wild men a) дикари; б) люди крайних убеждений; wise ~ мудрец; маг, волшебник; ~ of iron железный человек, человек с железной волей; bad ~ *амер.* головорез, отчаянный человек; ~ of pleasure сластолюбец; ~ in the street обыкновенный человек, обыватель; ~ of the world a) светский человек; б) человек, умудрённый опытом; ~ about town светский человек; прожигатель жизни; family ~ семейный человек; семьянин; домосед; ~ of feeling сентиментальный человек; ~ of blood неистовый человек; ~ of impulse импульсивный человек; ~ of family знатный человек; *амер.* семейный человек; right-hand ~ правая рука (*о человеке*); to be one's own ~ быть независимым, самостоятельным; 3) мужчина; муж; ~ and wife муж и жена; be a ~!, play the ~! будь смел!, будь мужчиной!; lady's ~ дамский угодник; fancy ~ жених, возлюбленный; *сленг* сутенёр; best ~ шафер; 4) рабочий; service ~ монтёр; 5) слуга; I'm your ~! я к вашим услугам!; я согласен!; 6) *pl* солдаты; матросы; 7) пешка (*в шахматах*); шашка; ◊ iron ~ *амер. шутл.* доллар; the outer ~ наружность, костюм; the inner ~ душа; *шутл.* желудок; to refresh one's inner ~ заморить червячка, поесть; the nether ~ *шутл.* ноги; good ~! здорово!; здравствуй!; snow ~ снежная баба, снежный болван; ~ of straw a) соломенное чучело; б) фиктивный противник; в) ненадёжный человек.

man II *v* 1) укомплектовывать людьми, персоналом; 2) подбодрять; to ~ oneself взять себя в руки.

manacle I ['mænəkl] *n обыкн. pl* наручники; ручные кандалы; *перен.* путы; препятствие.

manacle II *v* надевать наручники; *перен.* связывать; препятствовать.

manage ['mænɪdʒ] *v* 1) управлять; заведовать, руководить; 2) уметь обращаться с, владеть (*оружием, инструментом и т. п.*); 3) устраивать(ся); 4) ухитряться; 5) справляться.

manageable ['mænɪdʒəbl] *a* 1) поддающийся управлению; 2) выполнимый; 3) смирный, послушный; 4) сговорчивый, податливый.

management ['mænɪdʒmənt] *n* 1) управление; руководство; 2) (the ~) дирекция, правление; 3) умение владеть (*инструментом*); умение справляться (*с работой*).

manager ['mænɪdʒə] *n* 1) управляющий, заведующий; директор; 2) хозяин; хозяйка.

managing ['mænɪdʒɪŋ] *a* 1) руководящий, заведующий; 2) деловой, энергичный; 3) экономный; скупой.

mandarin¹ ['mændərɪn] *n* 1) *ист.* мандарин (*китайский чиновник*); 2) косный, отсталый руководитель.

mandarin² *n* 1) мандарин (*плод*); 2) оранжевый цвет.

mandarine ['mændərɪːn] *см.* mandarin².

mandatary ['mændətərɪ] *n полит.* мандатарий.

mandate I ['mændeɪt] *n* 1) мандат; 2) наказ (*избирателей*).

mandate II *v* передавать (*страну*) под мандат другого государства.

mandated ['mændeɪtɪd] *a* подмандатный.

mandatory I ['mændətərɪ] *n см.* mandatary.

mandatory II *a* 1) мандатный; 2) повелительный; принудительный, обязательный.

mandolin ['mændəlɪn] *n* мандолина.

mandoline [,mændə'liːn] *см.* mandolin.

mandrill ['mændrɪl] *n зоол.* мандрил.

mane [meɪn] *n* грива.

man-eater ['mæn,iːtə] *n* людоед.

manège [mæ'neɪʒ] *n* 1) манеж; 2) верховая езда.

maneuver I, II [mə'nuːvə] *см.* manoeuvre I, II.

manful ['mænful] *a* мужественный; решительный.

manganese [,mæŋgə'niːz] *n хим.* марганец.

manganic [mæŋ'gænɪk] *a хим.* марганцевый, марганцовый.

mange [meɪndʒ] *n* чесотка; парша.

mangel(-wurzel) ['mæŋgl('wəːzl)] *n* кормовая свёкла.

manger ['meɪndʒə] *n* ясли, кормушка.

mangle¹ ['mæŋgl] *v* 1) рубить, кромсать; 2) калечить; 3) искажать (*слова, текст и т. п.*).

mangle² I *n* каток (*для белья*).

mangle² II *v* катать бельё.

mango ['mæŋgou] *n бот.* манго.

mangrove ['mæŋgrouv] *n* 1) мангровое дерево; 2) *pl* мангровые леса.

mangy ['meɪndʒɪ] *a* 1) чесоточный; паршивый; 2) грязный; потрёпанный.

manhandle ['mæn,hændl] *v* 1) передвигать, переносить, грузить (*вручную*); 2) *разг.* грубо обращаться, третировать.

manhole ['mænhoul] *n* 1) люк; 2) смотровое отверстие.

manhood ['mænhud] *n* 1) возмужалость; зрелость; 2) мужество; 3) мужское население (*страны*).

mania ['meɪnjə] *n* мания.

maniac I ['meɪnɪæk] *n* маньяк.

maniac II *a* помешанный.

maniacal [mə'naɪəkəl] *a* маниакальный.

manicure I ['mænɪkjuə] *n* 1) маникюр; 2) *см.* manicurist.

manicure II *v* делать маникюр.

manicurist ['mænɪkjuərɪst] *n* маникюрша.

manifest I ['mænɪfest] *n* декларация судового груза.

manifest II *a* ясный, очевидный.

manifest III *v* 1) ясно показывать; делать очевидным; проявлять; 2) доказывать; 3) обнародовать; издать манифест; 4) заносить в декларацию судового груза; 5) появляться (*о привидении*).

manifestation [,mænɪfes'teɪʃən] *n* 1) проявление; доказательство; 2) манифестация; 3) обнародование.

manifesto [,mænɪ'festou] *n* манифест; the Communist Manifesto Манифест Коммунистической партии.

manifold I ['mænɪfould] *n* 1) копия (*документа и т. п.*); 2) *тех.* трубопровод.

manifold II *a* 1) многообразный, разнородный; 2) многочисленный.

manifold III *v* размножать (*документ*).

manikin ['mænɪkɪn] *n* 1) манекен; 2) человечек, карлик.

manipulate [mə'nɪpjuleɪt] *v* 1) умело обращать-

ся; уме́ло управля́ть; манипули́ровать; 2) подта-
со́вывать, подде́лывать.

manipulation [mə,nɪpjuˈleɪʃən] *n* 1) манипуля́-
ция; обраще́ние; 2) подтасо́вка.

manipulator [məˈnɪpjuleɪtə] *n* манипуля́тор; пе-
реда́ющий ключ (*телегра́фа, ра́дио*).

mankind[a] [mænˈkaɪnd] *n* челове́чество; чело-
ве́ческий род.

mankind[b] [ˈmænkaɪnd] *n* мужчи́ны.

manlike [ˈmænlaɪk] *a* 1) мужско́й, подоба́ющий
мужчи́не; 2) мужеподо́бный.

manliness [ˈmænlɪnɪs] *n* му́жественность.

manly [ˈmænlɪ] *a* 1) му́жественный; 2) муже-
подо́бный.

man-made [ˈmænˈmeɪd] *a* иску́сственный, со́з-
данный рука́ми челове́ка.

manna [ˈmænə] *n* ма́нна небе́сная.

manna-croup [ˈmænəˈkruːp] *n* ма́нная крупа́.

manned [mænd] *a* 1) укомплекто́ванный (*пер-
со́налом*); 2) пилоти́руемый (*о лета́тельном ап-
пара́те*).

mannequin [ˈmænɪkɪn] *n* 1) манеке́н; 2) мане-
ке́нщица.

manner [ˈmænə] *n* 1) спо́соб, о́браз де́йствий;
~ of life о́браз жи́зни; 2) мане́ра; 3) *pl* обы́чаи,
нра́вы; 4) *pl* мане́ры; уме́ние держа́ть себя́; he has
по ~s он пло́хо воспи́тан; 5) иск. стиль, мане́-
ра (*худо́жника*); ~ of execution мане́ра исполне́-
ния; 6) род, сорт; all ~ of всевозмо́жные; по ~
of никако́й; ◊ in a ~ в не́котором смы́сле; до из-
ве́стной сте́пени; in a ~ of speaking так сказа́ть;
in a promiscuous ~ науда́чу; by no ~ (of means)
ни в ко́ем слу́чае.

mannerism [ˈmænərɪzəm] *n* 1) мане́рность;
2) иск. маньери́зм.

mannerliness [ˈmænəlɪnɪs] *n* ве́жливость, воспи́-
танность.

mannerly [ˈmænəlɪ] *a* ве́жливый, воспи́танный.

mannish [ˈmænɪʃ] *a* 1) мужеподо́бный; 2) муж-
ско́й.

manoeuvre I [məˈnuːvə] *n* 1) манёвр; 2) *pl воен.,
мор.* манёвры; 3) интри́га.

manoeuvre II *v* 1) *воен., мор.* проводи́ть манёвры; 2) маневри́ровать.

man-of-war [ˈmænəvˈwɔː] *n* (*pl* men-of-war) вое́-
нный кора́бль.

manor [ˈmænə] *n* поме́стье.

manor-house [ˈmænəhaus] *n* поме́щичий дом.

manorial [məˈnɔːrɪəl] *a* манориа́льный.

man-o'-war [ˈmænəˈwɔː] *см.* man-of-war.

manpower [ˈmæn,pauə] *n* 1) рабо́чая си́ла; ра-
бо́чие; 2) ли́чный соста́в.

manse [mæns] *n* дом свяще́нника.

mansion [ˈmænʃən] *n* большо́й дом; особня́к.

Mansion-house [ˈmænʃənhaus] *n*: the ~ офи-
циа́льная резиде́нция лорд-мэ́ра в Ло́ндоне.

manslaughter [ˈmæn,slɔːtə] *n* 1) человекоуби́й-
ство; 2) *юр.* непредумы́шленное уби́йство.

mantelpiece [ˈmæntlpiːs] *n* 1) облицо́вка ками́на;
по́лка над ками́ном.

mantis [ˈmæntɪs] *n зоол.* богомо́л.

mantle I [ˈmæntl] *n* 1) наки́дка; *перен.* покро́в;
2) *тех.* кали́льная се́тка.

mantle II *v* 1) покрыва́ть, оку́тывать; 2) крас-
не́ть (*о лице́*); прилива́ть к лицу́ (*о кро́ви*);
3) покрыва́ться на́кипью.

man-trap [ˈmæntræp] *n* лову́шка, западня́.

manual I [ˈmænjuəl] *n* 1) руково́дство; наставле́-
ние; уче́бник; 2) клавиату́ра (*орга́на*).

manual II *a* 1) ручно́й; 2) физи́ческий (*о рабо́-
те*); физи́ческого труда́ (*о лю́дях*).

manufactory [,mænjuˈfæktərɪ] *n* фа́брика.

manufacture I [,mænjuˈfæktʃə] *n* 1) произво́д-
ство; фабрика́ция; 2) *pl* изде́лия, фабрика́ты.

manufacture II *v* производи́ть, выде́лывать; фаб-
рикова́ть.

manufacturer [,mænjuˈfæktʃərə] *n* 1) фабрика́нт,
предпринима́тель; 2) изготови́тель, производи́-
тель.

manufacturing [,mænjuˈfæktʃərɪŋ] *n* 1) обраба́-
тывающая промы́шленность; 2) произво́дство; вы́-
делка; обрабо́тка.

manumission [,mænjuˈmɪʃən] *n ист.* 1) освобож-
де́ние от ра́бства; 2) во́льная, отпускна́я.

manure I [məˈnjuə] *n* наво́з, удобре́ние.

manure II *v* удобря́ть, унаво́живать (*зе́млю*).

manuscript I [ˈmænjuskrɪpt] *n* ру́копись.

manuscript II *a* рукопи́сный.

Manx I [mæŋks] *n*: the ~ (*употр. как pl*)
жи́тели о-ва Мэн.

Manx II *a* с о-ва Мэн.

Manxman [ˈmæŋksmən] *n* жи́тель о-ва Мэн.

many I [ˈmenɪ] *n* мно́жество; мно́гие; the ~
большинство́; a good ~ поря́дочное коли́чество,
поря́дочно; a great ~ грома́дное коли́чество; мно́-
жество.

many II *a* (*compar* more; *superl* most) мно́-
гие, мно́го; as ~ сто́лько же; as ~ again вдво́е;
ещё сто́лько же; not so ~ as ме́ньше, чем; how ~?
ско́лько?; one too ~ ли́шний, нежела́тельный; to
be one too ~ for превосходи́ть, быть сильне́е,
иску́снее, умне́е (*кого́-л.*).

Maori [ˈmaurɪ] *n* 1) мао́ри; 2) язы́к мао́ри.

map I [mæp] *n* 1) ка́рта (*географи́ческая и т. п.*);
celestial ~ ка́рта звёздного не́ба; contour (ed) ~
ко́нтурная ка́рта; circulation ~ доро́жная ка́рта (с
указа́нием маршру́тов); 2) план; ◊ off the ~
разг. устаре́вший, не име́ющий значе́ния; on the ~
ва́жный, значи́тельный.

map II *v* наноси́ть на ка́рту; ▢ to ~ out пла-
ни́ровать, распределя́ть.

maple [ˈmeɪpl] *n* клён.

maple-leaf [ˈmeɪplliːf] *n* клено́вый лист (*тж. как
эмбле́ма Кана́ды*).

mar [mɑː] *v* по́ртить; ◊ to make or ~ *погов.*
≅ ли́бо пан, ли́бо пропа́л.

Marathon [ˈmærəθən] *n спорт.* марафо́нский
бег (*тж.* ~ race).

maraud [məˈrɔːd] *v* мародёрствовать.

marauder [məˈrɔːdə] *n* мародёр.

marauding I [məˈrɔːdɪŋ] *n* мародёрство.

marauding II *a* мародёрский, хи́щнический.

marble I [ˈmɑːbl] *n* 1) мра́мор; 2) *pl* скульпту́-
ра из мра́мора; 3) *pl* (мра́морные) ша́рики (*де́т-
ская игра́*); 4) *attr* мра́морный.

March [mɑːtʃ] *n* 1) март; 2) *attr* ма́ртов-
ский.

march[1] I [mɑːtʃ] *n* 1) *воен.* марш, перехо́д;
forced ~ форси́рованный марш; 2) похо́д; hunger
~ голо́дный похо́д (*безрабо́тных*); 3) ход, разви́-
тие (*собы́тий, нау́ки и т. п.*); 4) *муз.* марш; dead ~
похоро́нный марш; ◊ to steal a ~ on smb. a)

(незаметно) опередить кого́-л.; б) обману́ть чью-л. бди́тельность.

march¹ II *v* 1) марширова́ть; 2) дви́гать(ся); to ~ ahead идти́ вперёд; □ to ~ off а) выступа́ть; уходи́ть; б) уводи́ть; отводи́ть; to ~ on продвига́ться вперёд; to ~ out выходи́ть, выступа́ть; выводи́ть (*войска*).

march² I *n обыкн. pl* грани́ца; пограни́чная полоса́.

march² II *v* грани́чить.

marchioness [ˈmɑːʃənɪs] *n* марки́за (*в Англии*).

mare [mɛə] *n* кобы́ла; ◇ on Shanks's ≅ на свои́х на двои́х, пешко́м; the grey ~ is the better horse ≅ (она́) де́ржит му́жа под башмако́м; the two-legged ~ ви́селица.

mare's-nest [ˈmɛəznest] *n* иллю́зия, заблужде́ние; to find a ~ ≅ попа́сть па́льцем в не́бо.

margarine [ˌmɑːdʒəˈriːn] *n* маргари́н.

marge¹ [mɑːdʒ] *n поэт.* край, грань.

marge² *n разг.* маргари́н.

margin [ˈmɑːdʒɪn] *n* 1) по́ле (*страни́цы*); 2) край, грань; 3) бе́рег; 4) опу́шка (*ле́са*); 5) запа́с (*вре́мени, де́нег*); wide ~ of бо́льше, чем ну́жно (*вре́мени и т. п.*); ~ of safety *тех.* надёжность; запа́с про́чности; 6) ра́зница ме́жду себесто́имостью и прода́жной цено́й; ◇ by a narrow ~ е́ле-е́ле, с трудо́м.

marginal [ˈmɑːdʒɪnəl] *a* 1) кра́йний; 2) напи́санный, сде́ланный на поля́х (*кни́ги*).

marguerite [ˌmɑːɡəˈriːt] *n* маргари́тка.

marigold [ˈmærɪɡould] *n бот.* ноготки́.

marihuana [ˌmærɪˈ(h)wɑːnə] *n* марихуа́на.

marijuana [ˌmærɪˈ(h)wɑːnə] *см.* marihuana.

marine I [məˈriːn] *n* 1) флот; merchant ~, mercantile ~ торго́вый флот; 2) моря́к; the ~s морска́я пехо́та; ◇ tell that to the ~s ври бо́льше!, расска́зывай ска́зки!

marine II *a* 1) морско́й; 2) фло́тский.

mariner [ˈmærɪnə] *n* моря́к; матро́с.

marital [ˈmærɪtl] *a* 1) супру́жеский, му́жнин; 2) бра́чный.

maritime [ˈmærɪtaɪm] *a* 1) морско́й; 2) примо́рский; берегово́й.

marjoram [ˈmɑːdʒərəm] *n бот.* майора́н.

mark¹ I [mɑːk] *n* 1) знак; ~ of interrogation вопроси́тельный знак; 2) ме́тка; отпеча́ток; след; пятно́; mother's ~ ро́динка; high-water ~ у́ровень прили́ва; *перен.* наивы́сший преде́л, наибо́льшая высота́; 3) при́знак, показа́тель; 4) знак, клеймо́; 5) отме́тка, балл; bad (good) ~ плоха́я (хоро́шая) отме́тка; his ~ in arithmetic was 5 у него́ пятёрка по арифме́тике; 6) цель, мише́нь; to hit (to miss) the ~ попа́сть в цель (промахну́ться); beside (*или* wide of) the ~ ми́мо це́ли; *перен.* не по существу́; некста́ти; 7) изве́стность; to make one's ~ доби́ться изве́стности; of ~ изве́стный (*о челове́ке*); 8) но́рма, у́ровень; below the ~ пло́хо, ни́же сре́днего (*о ка́честве*); не на высоте́ (*положе́ния*); up to the ~ хоро́ший, удовлетвори́тельный; не на высоте́; 9) крест (*вме́сто по́дписи*); ◇ bless (*или* save) the ~ а) с позволе́ния сказа́ть; б) бо́же сохрани́; easy ~ *амер. сленг* проста́к; to toe the ~ а) встать на ста́ртовую черту́; стать в шере́нгу; б) стро́го выполня́ть свои́ обя́занности, подчиня́ться приказа́ниям; to overstep the ~ перейти́ грани́цы дозво́ленного.

mark¹ II *v* 1) ста́вить знак; штемпелева́ть; марки́ровать; ме́тить (*бельё*); 2) ста́вить балл, отме́тку (*уча́щемуся*); 3) оставля́ть след, пятно́; 4) отмеча́ть; характеризова́ть; замеча́ть; 5) выставля́ть це́ну (*на това́ре*); □ to ~ **down** указа́ть (на това́ре) сни́женную це́ну; to ~ **off** разделя́ть; разграни́чивать; to ~ **out** размеча́ть; отделя́ть; предназнача́ть; to ~ **up** указа́ть (на това́ре) повы́шенную це́ну.

mark² *n* ма́рка (*де́нежная едини́ца ГДР, ФРГ*).

marked [mɑːkt] *a* 1) заме́ченный, отме́ченный; 2) заме́тный; 3) ви́дный, изве́стный; 4) клеймёный, заклеймённый.

marker [ˈmɑːkə] *n* 1) маркёр; 2) клеймо́вщик; 3) закла́дка (*в кни́ге*).

market I [ˈmɑːkɪt] *n* 1) ры́нок; stiff (sensitive) ~ *эк.* усто́йчивый (неусто́йчивый) ры́нок; (European) Common Market *эк.* (Европе́йский) «О́бщий ры́нок»; to glut the ~ зава́ливать ры́нок това́рами; 2) торго́вля; сбыт; to come into the ~ поступа́ть в прода́жу; to put on the ~ пуска́ть в прода́жу; 3) спрос; to find a ~ по́льзоваться спро́сом; 4) цена́; курс; to play the ~ игра́ть на би́рже; 5) *амер.* продово́льственный магази́н; 6) *attr* ры́ночный, база́рный; ◇ to make a ~ of променя́ть (*что-л.*) на ху́дшее.

market II *v* 1) торгова́ть *или* покупа́ть на ры́нке; 2) продава́ть.

marketable [ˈmɑːkɪtəbl] *a* 1) хо́дкий; 2) прода́жный, иду́щий в прода́жу.

market-day [ˈmɑːkɪtdeɪ] *n* база́рный день.

marketing [ˈmɑːkɪtɪŋ] *n* 1) торго́вля; 2) предме́т торго́вли.

market-place [ˈmɑːkɪtpleɪs] *n* база́рная пло́щадь.

markka [ˈmɑːkə] *n* ма́рка (*де́нежная едини́ца Финля́ндии*).

marksman [ˈmɑːksmən] *n* ме́ткий стрело́к, сна́йпер.

marl I [mɑːl] *n* ме́ргель; известко́вая гли́на.

marl II *v* удобря́ть ме́ргелем.

marmalade [ˈmɑːməleɪd] *n* мармела́д, пови́дло.

marmoset [ˈmɑːməzet] *n* марты́шка.

marmot [ˈmɑːmət] *n* суро́к.

maroon¹ I [məˈruːn] *n* кашта́новый цвет.

maroon¹ *n* кашта́новый, кашта́нового цве́та.

maroon² *v* 1) выса́живать и поселя́ть на необита́емом о́строве *или* в безлю́дной ме́стности (*в наказа́ние*); 2) безде́льничать.

marquee [mɑːˈkiː] *n* больша́я пала́тка, тент.

marquis [ˈmɑːkwɪs] *n* марки́з.

marquise [mɑːˈkiːz] *n* марки́за.

marriage [ˈmærɪdʒ] *n* 1) заму́жество; жени́тьба; брак; ~ of convenience брак по расчёту; companionable ~ брак по договорённости (*зара́нее огова́риваются коли́чество дете́й и усло́вия разво́да*); to contract a ~ заключа́ть брак; 2) сва́дьба; 3) те́сный сою́з; соедине́ние, сочета́ние; 4) стыко́вка (*ступе́ней раке́ты*).

married [ˈmærɪd] *a* жена́тый; заму́жняя; to get ~ жени́ться; вы́йти за́муж.

marrow [ˈmærou] *n* 1) ко́стный мозг; to the ~ (of one's bones) до мо́зга косте́й; spinal ~ спинно́й мозг; 2) су́щность; гла́вное; 3) кабачо́к (*о́вощ; тж.* vegetable ~).

marrowbone [ˈmærouboun] *n* 1) мозгова́я кость; 2) *pl шутл.* коле́ни; down on your ~s! на коле́ни!, проси́ проще́ния!; ◊ to ride in the ~ coach идти́ пешко́м, е́хать «на свои́х на двои́х».

marry ['mærɪ] v 1) жени́ть(ся); выходи́ть, выдава́ть за́муж; to ~ smb. off вы́дать за́муж кого́-л.; жени́ть кого́-л.; to be married to smb. быть жена́тым на ком-л.; быть за́мужем за кем-л.; to get married to smb. жени́ться на ком-л., вы́йти за́муж за кого́-л.; 2) соединя́ть, сочета́ть.

Mars [mɑːs] n астр., миф. Марс.

Marseillaise [ˌmɑːsə'leɪz] n марселье́за.

marsh [mɑːʃ] n 1) боло́то; 2) боло́тистая ме́стность; 3) attr боло́тный; боло́тистый.

marshal I ['mɑːʃəl] n 1) ма́ршал; 2) церемонийме́йстер; 3) амер. нача́льник поли́ции; суде́бный исполни́тель; provost ~ нача́льник вое́нной поли́ции.

marshal II v 1) приводи́ть в поря́док; 2) располага́ть в определённом поря́дке; выстра́ивать (войска́, проце́ссию); 3) торже́ственно вводи́ть.

marshy ['mɑːʃɪ] a боло́тистый.

marsupial I [mɑː'sjuːpjəl] n су́мчатое живо́тное.

marsupial II a зоол. су́мчатый.

mart [mɑːt] n 1) торго́вый центр; 2) аукцио́нный зал; 3) поэт. я́рмарка, ры́нок.

marten ['mɑːtɪn] n куни́ца.

martial ['mɑːʃəl] a 1) вое́нный; 2) вои́нственный.

Martian I ['mɑːʃjən] n марсиа́нин, жи́тель Ма́рса.

Martian II a марсиа́нский.

martin ['mɑːtɪn] n городска́я ла́сточка.

martyr I ['mɑːtə] n му́ченик.

martyr II v преда́ть му́ченической сме́рти; му́чить.

martyrdom ['mɑːtədəm] n 1) му́ченичество; 2) муче́ние, му́ка.

marvel I ['mɑːvəl] n чу́до, изуми́тельная вещь.

marvel II v удивля́ться, поража́ться.

marvellous ['mɑːvɪləs] a чуде́сный, необыкнове́нный, изуми́тельный.

Marxian I ['mɑːksjən] n маркси́ст.

Marxian II a маркси́стский.

Marxism ['mɑːksɪzəm] n маркси́зм.

Marxism-Leninism ['mɑːksɪzəm'lenɪnɪzəm] n маркси́зм-ленини́зм.

Marxist I ['mɑːksɪst] n маркси́ст.

Marxist II a маркси́стский.

marzipan [ˌmɑːzɪ'pæn] n марципа́н.

mascot ['mæskət] n талисма́н; челове́к или вещь, принося́щие сча́стье.

masculine I ['mɑːskjulɪn] n 1) грам. мужско́й род; 2) сло́во мужско́го ро́да.

masculine II a 1) мужско́й; 2) му́жественный, си́льный; 3) мужеподо́бный.

maser ['meizə] n физ. ма́зер.

mash¹ I [mæʃ] n 1) су́сло; 2) тёплое по́йло из отрубе́й, зерна́ и т. п.; 3) карто́фельное пюре́; 4) меша́нина.

mash¹ II v 1) зава́ривать со́лод; 2) разда́вливать, размина́ть.

mash² I n разг. предме́т любви́, обожа́ния; возлю́бленный, возлю́бленная.

mash² II v разг. прельща́ть; to be ~ed on быть влюблённым в

mask I [mɑːsk] n 1) ма́ска; перен. тж. личи́на; 2) противога́з (тж. gas-mask).

mask II v 1) маскирова́ть(ся); 2) скрыва́ть (чу́вства), притворя́ться.

masked [mɑːskt] a 1) переоде́тый, маскиро́ванный; 2) воен. замаскиро́ванный.

mason ['meɪsn] n 1) ка́менщик; 2) масо́н.

masonic [mə'sɔnɪk] a масо́нский.

masonry ['meɪsnrɪ] n ка́менная или кирпи́чная кла́дка.

masquerade I [ˌmæskə'reɪd] n маскара́д.

masquerade II v 1) (за)маскирова́ться; 2) притворя́ться.

mass¹ I [mæs] n 1) ма́сса; confused ~ беспоря́дочная ма́сса; in the ~ в це́лом; 2) большо́е коли́чество чего́-л.; the (great) ~ of бо́льшая часть; he is a ~ of bruises он весь в синяка́х; 3) pl (наро́дные) ма́ссы, наро́д; 4) attr ма́ссовый.

mass¹ II v 1) собира́ть(ся) в ку́чу; 2) сосредото́чить, стяну́ть (войска́).

mass² n ме́сса (церк. слу́жба).

massacre I ['mæsəkə] n резня́, избие́ние.

massacre II v устра́ивать резню́; убива́ть.

massage I ['mæsɑːʒ] n масса́ж.

massage II v масси́ровать.

masseur [mæ'səː] n массажи́ст.

masseuse [mæ'səːz] n массажи́стка.

massif ['mæsiːf] n го́рный масси́в.

massive ['mæsɪv] a 1) масси́вный; 2) си́льный; масси́рованный.

massy ['mæsɪ] a масси́вный; тяжёлый.

mast [mɑːst] n ма́чта; Venetian ~ разноцве́тная ма́чта (для украше́ния у́лиц); ◊ to serve (или to sail) before the ~ быть просты́м матро́сом.

master I ['mɑːstə] n 1) хозя́ин; господи́н; to be ~ of владе́ть, облада́ть; to be one's own ~ быть самостоя́тельным; 2) учи́тель; дире́ктор (шко́лы, колле́джа); head ~ дире́ктор, нача́льник (уче́бного заведе́ния); 3) вели́кий худо́жник, ма́стер; old ~s а) ста́рые мастера́; б) карти́ны ста́рых мастеро́в; 4) ма́стер; квалифици́рованный рабо́чий; past ~ знато́к своего́ де́ла, специали́ст; ~ of fence иску́сный фехтова́льщик; перен. спо́рщик; to make oneself ~ of доби́ться соверше́нства в чём-л., овладе́ть чем-л.; 5) капита́н торго́вого су́дна (тж. ~ mariner); 6) маги́стр (учёное зва́ние); 7) при обраще́нии к ю́ношам см. mister; 8) attr гла́венствующий, превосходя́щий; гла́вный; ◊ Master of Ceremonies а) церемонийме́йстер; б) амер. конфера́нсье.

master II v 1) подчини́ть себе́; 2) владе́ть, овладе́ть (чу́вствами, языко́м и т. п.); 3) преодолева́ть (тру́дности); 4) руководи́ть, управля́ть.

masterful ['mɑːstəful] a 1) вла́стный; 2) мастерско́й.

master-key ['mɑːstəkiː] n отмы́чка.

masterly I ['mɑːstəlɪ] a мастерско́й.

masterly II adv мастерски́.

masterpiece ['mɑːstəpiːs] n замеча́тельное произведе́ние иску́сства, шеде́вр.

mastership ['mɑːstəʃɪp] n 1) мастерство́; 2) главе́нство; 3) до́лжность, обя́занности учи́теля, дире́ктора.

master-stroke ['mɑːstəstrouk] n мастерско́й, ло́вкий ход.

mastery ['mɑːstərɪ] n 1) госпо́дство, власть; 2) мастерство́; соверше́нное владе́ние (чем-л.).

mastic ['mæstɪk] n 1) смола́ масти́кового де́рева; 2) масти́ковое де́рево; 3) бле́дно-жёлтый цвет.

masticate ['mæstɪkeɪt] v жева́ть.

masticatory ['mæstɪkətərɪ] *a* жева́тельный.

mastiff ['mæstɪf] *n* масти́ф (*порода собак*).

mastodon ['mæstədɔn] *n* мастодо́нт.

mat¹ I [mæt] *n* 1) цино́вка; полови́к, мат; on the ~ *сленг* в беде́; to leave on the ~ *сленг* отказа́ть в приёме, в разгово́ре; 2) подста́вка (*под лампу, блюдо и т. п.*); 3) ком, спу́танный клок (*волос, травы*).

mat¹ II *v* 1) устила́ть, покрыва́ть ма́тами; 2) спу́таться, сваля́ться (*о волосах и т. п.; тж.* to ~ together).

mat² I *n* 1) паспарту́; 2) ма́товая отде́лка *или* кра́ска.

mat² II *a* ма́товый; ту́склый.

match¹ [mætʃ] *n* спи́чка (*тж.* safety ~); to strike a ~ чи́ркать спи́чкой; заже́чь спи́чку.

match² I *n* 1) па́ра; ро́вня; па́рная *или* подходя́щая (*по качеству*) вещь; he is no ~ for her он ей не па́ра; 2) брак, па́ртия; to make a ~ вступи́ть в брак; 3) состяза́ние, матч; return ~ рева́нш.

match² II *v* 1) подбира́ть (под па́ру); 2) жени́ть; выдава́ть за́муж; 3) равня́ться; подходи́ть (*по характеру, качеству, цвету и т. п.*); 4) противопоставля́ть, сра́внивать (*with*); 5) состяза́ться.

match-box ['mætʃbɔks] *n* спи́чечная коро́бка.

matchless ['mætʃlɪs] *a* несравнённый, несравни́мый, бесподо́бный.

matchwood ['mætʃwud] *n* спи́чечная соло́мка; ◊ to make ~ of разби́ть, расколоти́ть вдре́безги.

mate¹ I [meɪt] *n* 1) (со)това́рищ; room ~ това́рищ по ко́мнате; 2) супру́г(а); 3) саме́ц; са́мка; 4) помо́щник, подру́чный; 5) *мор.* помо́щник капита́на.

mate¹ II *v* 1) сочета́ть(ся) бра́ком; 2) спа́ривать(ся) (*о птицах*); 3) обраща́ться (*with*).

mate² I *n* шахм. мат.

mate² II *v* шахм. сде́лать мат.

mater ['meɪtə] *n* шк. сленг мать.

material I [mə'tɪərɪəl] *n* 1) материа́л; raw ~s сырьё; 2) *текст.* мате́рия; 3) *pl* принадле́жности; writing ~s пи́сьменные принадле́жности.

material II *a* 1) материа́льный; 2) суще́ственный.

materialism [mə'tɪərɪəlɪzəm] *n* материали́зм; dialectical ~ диалекти́ческий материали́зм; historical ~ истори́ческий материали́зм.

materialist I [mə'tɪərɪəlɪst] *n* материали́ст.

materialist II *a* материалисти́ческий; ~ conception of history материалисти́ческое понима́ние исто́рии.

materialistic [mə,tɪərɪə'lɪstɪk] *a* материалисти́ческий.

materialize [mə'tɪərɪəlaɪz] *v* 1) осуществля́ть (-ся); претворя́ть(ся) в жизнь; 2) материализова́ть(ся).

maternal [mə'tə:nl] *a* 1) матери́нский; 2) с матери́нской стороны́ (*о родне*).

maternity [mə'tə:nɪtɪ] *n* матери́нство.

mathematical [,mæθɪ'mætɪkəl] *a* 1) математи́ческий; 2) то́чный.

mathematician [,mæθɪmə'tɪʃən] *n* матема́тик.

mathematics [,mæθɪ'mætɪks] *n* матема́тика (*тж.* pure ~); applied ~, mixed ~ прикладна́я матема́тика.

matinée ['mætɪneɪ] *n* дневно́й спекта́кль; дневно́й конце́рт.

matins ['mætɪnz] *n pl* 1) церк. (за)у́треня;

2) *поэт.* у́треннее щебета́ние птиц; to be at ~ петь у́треннюю пе́сню (*о птицах*).

matrass ['mætrəs] *n* ко́лба.

matriarchy ['meɪtrɪɑːkɪ] *n* матриарха́т.

matrices ['meɪtrɪsiːz] *pl см.* matrix.

matricide ['meɪtrɪsaɪd] *n* 1) матереуби́йство; 2) матереуби́йца.

matriculate [mə'trɪkjuleɪt] *v* принима́ть *или* быть при́нятым в вы́сшее уче́бное заведе́ние.

matriculation [mə,trɪkju'leɪʃən] *n* приня́тие, зачисле́ние в вы́сшее уче́бное заведе́ние.

matrimonial [,mætrɪ'mounjəl] *a* супру́жеский.

matrimony ['mætrɪmənɪ] *n* брак, супру́жество.

matrix ['meɪtrɪks] *n* (*pl тж.* matrices) *тех.* ма́трица; фо́рма.

matron ['meɪtrən] *n* 1) заму́жняя же́нщина; матро́на; 2) заве́дующая хозя́йством (*школы и т. п.*); эконо́мка.

matted ['mætɪd] *a* 1) спу́танный (*о волосах*); 2) покры́тый цино́вками, полови́ками.

matter I ['mætə] *n* 1) де́ло, вопро́с; су́щность, содержа́ние; a ~ of fact действи́тельность; as a ~ of fact на са́мом де́ле, факти́чески; ~ of course де́ло есте́ственное, само́ собо́ю разуме́ющееся; as a ~ of course как не́что само́ собо́ю разуме́ющееся; ~ of life and death вопро́с жи́зни и сме́рти; a ~ of argument спо́рный вопро́с; ~ of habit де́ло привы́чки; ~ of opinion спо́рный вопро́с; it is no laughing ~ э́то не шу́тка, здесь смея́ться не́чему; a ~ of two days вопро́с, де́ло двух дней; to push the ~ through доводи́ть де́ло до конца́; 2) основа́ние, по́вод; 3) вещество́; grey ~ се́рое вещество́ мо́зга; *разг.* ум; dead ~ неоргани́ческое вещество́; 4) материа́л; printed ~ печа́тный материа́л; postal ~ почто́вое отправле́ние; 5) *филос.* мате́рия; 6) *мед.* гной; ◊ what is the ~? в чём де́ло?, что случи́лось?; what is the ~ with you? что с ва́ми?; no ~ ничего́, нева́жно, всё равно́; it is (*или* makes) no ~ нева́жно, не име́ет значе́ния; for that ~, for the ~ of that что каса́ется э́того, в э́том отноше́нии; in the ~ of что каса́ется, в вопро́се о; to take ~s easy не волнова́ться, не обраща́ть внима́ния; not to mince the ~ говори́ть пря́мо, без обиняко́в.

matter II *v* 1) име́ть значе́ние; it doesn't ~ э́то нева́жно, не име́ет значе́ния; 2) выделя́ть гной, гно́иться.

matter-of-course ['mætərəv'kɔːs] *a* само́ собо́ю разуме́ющийся; есте́ственный.

matter-of-fact ['mætərəv'fækt] *a* сухо́й, лишённый воображе́ния, прозаи́ческий.

matting ['mætɪŋ] *n* цино́вка; рого́жа.

mattock ['mætək] *n* моты́га; кирка́.

mattress ['mætrɪs] *n* матра́ц, тюфя́к; (inner-) spring ~ пружи́нный матра́ц.

mature I [mə'tjuə] *a* 1) зре́лый; созре́вший; 2) хорошо́ проду́манный; 3) подлежа́щий опла́те (*ввиду наступившего срока платежа — о векселе*).

mature II *v* 1) созрева́ть; 2) доводи́ть до соверше́нства; разраба́тывать; 3) наступа́ть (*о сроке платежа*).

maturity [mə'tjuərɪtɪ] *n* 1) зре́лость; 2) заверше́нность; 3) срок платежа́ по ве́кселю.

maudlin ['mɔːdlɪn] *a* слезли́вый, расчу́вствовавшийся; сентимента́льный.

maul I [mɔːl] *n* деревя́нный молото́к; колоту́шка.

maul II *v* 1) кале́чить; терза́ть; 2) жесто́ко критиковать; 3) грубо, небрежно, неумело обращаться.

maunder ['mɔːndə] v 1) бессвязно говорить, бормотать; 2) действовать, двигаться неуверенно, бесцельно.

mausoleum [ˌmɔːsəˈlɪəm] n мавзолей.

mauve [mouv] a розовато-лиловый.

mavis ['meɪvɪs] n поэт. певчий дрозд.

mawkish ['mɔːkɪʃ] a 1) неприятный на вкус; 2) сентиментальный.

maxim ['mæksɪm] n принцип; правило поведения; copy-book ~s прописные истины.

maximum I ['mæksɪməm] n максимум.

maximum II a максимальный.

May [meɪ] n 1) май; the First of ~ Первое мая; 2) (m.) расцвет жизни; 3) attr майский; 4) attr первомайский.

may [meɪ] v (past might) модальный гл., входящий в состав сложного модального сказуемого мочь, иметь разрешение (последующий смысловой гл. употребляется без частицы to: you ~ take this book вы можете взять эту книгу; отриц. и вопр. формы употребляются без гл. to do: ~ I come in? разрешите войти?; ~ I ask? можно спросить?) 1) указывает на возможность: it ~ be возможно (что), может быть (что); it ~ rain tomorrow возможно, завтра будет дождь, завтра может пойти дождь; the train ~ be late поезд, возможно, опоздает, поезд может опоздать; 2) выражает просьбу или позволение: ~ I go now? могу я теперь уйти?; you ~ go вы можете уйти; в повел. накл. выражает пожелание: ~ you be very happy желаю вам много счастья; 4) в вопр. предложениях указывает на неуверенность: who ~ that be? кто бы это мог быть?

maybe ['meɪbiː] adv может быть.

May Day ['meɪdeɪ] n Первое мая, первомайский праздник.

mayor [mɛə] n мэр (города); Lord ~ лорд-мэр, мэр г. Лондона.

maypole ['meɪpoul] n 1) майское дерево (украшенный цветами столб, вокруг которого пляшут 1-го Мая в Англии); 2) разг. верзила.

maze I [meɪz] n 1) лабиринт; 2) путаница; to be in a ~ быть в затруднении.

maze II v поставить в затруднительное положение.

mazy ['meɪzɪ] a запутанный.

me [miː] pron pers (косв. п. от I) 1) мне, меня; 2) разг. я; it's me это я.

mead[1] [miːd] n поэт. луг.

mead[2] n мёд (напиток).

meadow ['medou] n луг.

meager ['miːgə] амер. см. meagre.

meagre ['miːgə] a 1) худой; тощий; 2) скудный, ограниченный; 3) бедный, бессодержательный.

meal[1] I [miːl] n 1) еда; 2) завтрак, обед, ужин; evening ~ ужин; square ~ сытный обед; to have a stand-up ~ закусить на ходу, перекусить.

meal[1] II v есть, принимать пищу.

meal[2] n мука; whole ~ непросеянная мука.

mealtime ['miːltaɪm] n обеденное время, время принятия пищи.

mealy ['miːlɪ] a 1) мучной; 2) мучнистый; 3) (запачканный) в муке; 4) бледный; 5) рыхлый; 6) см. mealy-mouthed.

mealy-mouthed ['miːlɪmauðd] a льстивый, сладкоречивый.

mean[1] I [miːn] n 1) середина; the happy ~, the golden ~ золотая середина; 2) мат. среднее число; arithmetical ~ среднее арифметическое; 3) обыкн. pl способ, средство; ~s of communication средства сообщения; by ~s of посредством, при помощи; by all ~s во что бы то ни стало; конечно; by any ~s каким бы то ни было образом; by fair ~s or foul всеми средствами; правдами и неправдами; by some ~s (or other) так или иначе; by no ~s отнюдь не; никоим образом; 4) pl (денежные) средства; private ~s личные средства, личное состояние.

mean[1] II a средний.

mean[2] a 1) посредственный, плохой, слабый; 2) незначительный; захудалый; 3) скромный; смущающийся; to feel ~ чувствовать себя неловко; 4) нечестный, подлый, низкий, гадкий; 5) скупой.

mean[3] v (past, p. p. meant) 1) значить, означать, иметь значение; what does it ~? что это значит?; 2) предназначать(ся); 3) думать, подразумевать; what do you ~? что вы имеете в виду?; что вы хотите сказать?; 4) иметь в виду, намереваться; to ~ well (ill) иметь хорошие (плохие) намерения.

meander I [mɪˈændə] n 1) pl извилины (дороги, реки); 2) архит. меандр.

meander II v 1) извиваться (о реке, дороге); 2) бродить без цели (тж. to ~ along); 3) вести пустую болтовню.

meaning I ['miːnɪŋ] n значение; смысл.

meaning II a значащий; (много)значительный, выразительный.

meaningless ['miːnɪŋlɪs] a бессмысленный.

meanly ['miːnlɪ] adv 1) подло, низко; гадко; 2) слабо, посредственно.

meanness ['miːnnɪs] n 1) низость, подлость; 2) посредственность.

meant [ment] past, p. p. см. mean[3].

meantime I ['miːntaɪm] n: in the ~ тем временем, между тем.

meantime II adv тем временем, между тем.

meanwhile I, II ['miːnˈwaɪl] см. meantime I, II.

measles ['miːzlz] n 1) корь; German ~ краснуха; 2) вет. финноз.

measly ['miːzlɪ] a 1) заражённый трихинами или финнами (о мясе); 2) разг. жалкий, ничтожный.

measurable ['meʒərəbl] a измеримый.

measurably ['meʒərəblɪ] adv значительно.

measure I ['meʒə] n 1) мера; dry ~s меры сыпучих тел; linear ~s, long ~s меры длины; liquid ~s меры жидкостей; square ~s меры поверхности; short ~ недомер; full ~ полная мера; beyond ~, out of ~ чрезмерно; in a ~, in some ~ отчасти; до некоторой степени; in a great (или large) ~ в большой степени; to set ~s to поставить предел, ограничить; 2) мерка; to take smb.'s ~ а) снять мерку с кого-л.; б) раскусить кого-л., оценить чьи-л. способности, возможности; to make to ~ сделать по мерке; 3) мерило; 4) мера, мероприятие; precautionary ~s меры предосторожности; to take ~s принимать меры; 5) мат. делитель; greatest common ~ общий наибольший делитель; 6) поэт. метр, размер; 7) муз. такт.

measure II v 1) мерить, измерять; отмерять (тж. to ~ off); 2) снимать мерку (для платья); 3) оценивать (*положение, характер и т. п.*); to ~ with one's eye смёрить взгля́дом; 4) поме́ряться си́лами (*with*); 5) име́ть разме́ры; □ to ~ out отмеря́ть, выдава́ть по ме́рке; to ~ up (*to, with*) а) достига́ть; б) соотве́тствовать; в) опра́вдывать (*наде́жды*).

measured ['meʒəd] *a* 1) изме́ренный; 2) разме́ренный, ме́рный, ритми́чный; 3) взве́шенный, обду́манный.

measureless ['meʒəlɪs] *a* неизмери́мый.

measurement ['meʒəmənt] *n* 1) измере́ние; 2) разме́ры; *pl* систе́ма мер.

meat [mi:t] *n* 1) мя́со (*тж.* butcher's ~); chilled ~ моро́женое мя́со; 2) *уст.* пи́ща; еда́; green ~ зе́лень, о́вощи; 3) содержа́ние; full of ~ содержа́тельный (*о книге и т. п.*); ◊ to be ~ and drink to smb. доставля́ть огро́мное удово́льствие; ≅ хле́бом не корми́.

meat-chopper ['mi:t,tʃɔpə] *n* мясору́бка.

meaty ['mi:tɪ] *a* мяси́стый; *перен.* содержа́тельный.

meccano [mə'kɑːnou] *n* констру́ктор (*детская игру́шка*).

mechanic [mɪ'kænɪk] *n* меха́ник; ремёсленник, мастерово́й.

mechanical [mɪ'kænɪkəl] *a* 1) маши́нный; 2) механи́ческий; 3) машина́льный; 4) *филос.* механисти́ческий.

mechanician [,mekə'nɪʃən] *n* 1) машинострои́тель; 2) констру́ктор.

mechanics [mɪ'kænɪks] *n* меха́ника; fine ~ то́чная меха́ника.

mechanism ['mekənɪzəm] *n* 1) механи́зм; устро́йство; структу́ра; 2) те́хника (*напр., музыка́нта*); 3) *филос.* механици́зм.

mechanize ['mekənaɪz] *v* механизи́ровать.

medal ['medl] *n* меда́ль; о́рден.

medalled ['medld] *a* 1) награждённый меда́лью, о́рденом; 2) укра́шенный, уве́шанный меда́лями, ордена́ми.

medallion [mɪ'dæljən] *n* медальо́н.

meddle ['medl] *v* вме́шиваться (*не в своё дело; in, with*).

meddler ['medlə] *n* надое́дливый, вме́шивающийся во всё челове́к.

meddlesome ['medlsəm] *a* надое́дливый, вме́шивающийся не в свои́ дела́.

media ['mi:djə] *pl см.* medium I.

mediaeval [,medɪ'i:vəl] *см.* medieval.

medial ['mi:djəl] *a* сре́дний, среди́нный.

median I ['mi:djən] *n мат.* медиа́на.

median II *a* сре́дний, среди́нный.

mediateᵃ ['mi:dɪɪt] *a* промежу́точный.

mediateᵇ ['mi:dɪeɪt] *v* 1) служи́ть свя́зью, посре́дником (*между*); 2) занима́ть промежу́точное положе́ние.

mediation [,mi:dɪ'eɪʃən] *n* посре́дничество.

medical I ['medɪkəl] *n разг.* студе́нт-ме́дик.

medical II *a* 1) медици́нский, враче́бный; 2) терапевти́ческий.

medicament [me'dɪkəmənt] *n* лека́рство.

medicate ['medɪkeɪt] *v* 1) лечи́ть, пи́чкать (лека́рствами); 2) пропи́тывать (лека́рством).

medicinal [me'dɪsɪnl] *a* целе́бный; лече́бный; лека́рственный.

medicine ['medsɪn] *n* 1) медици́на; aerospace ~

авиацио́нно-косми́ческая медици́на; 2) лека́рство; patent ~, proprietory ~ патенто́ванное сре́дство; a ~ of great virtue хорошо́ де́йствующее лека́рство; 3) колдовство́; заклина́ние; 4) амуле́т.

medicine-man ['medsɪnmæn] *n* зна́харь, колду́н, шама́н.

medieval [,medɪ'i:vəl] *a* средневеко́вый.

mediocre ['mi:dɪoukə] *a* посре́дственный.

mediocrity [,mi:dɪ'ɔkrɪtɪ] *n* посре́дственность.

meditate ['medɪteɪt] *v* 1) размышля́ть (*о чём-л.— on, upon*); 2) замышля́ть.

meditation [,medɪ'teɪʃən] *n* 1) размышле́ние; разду́мье; 2) созерца́ние.

meditative ['medɪtətɪv] *a* 1) заду́мчивый; 2) созерца́тельный.

mediterranean [,medɪtə'reɪnjən] *a* 1) средиземно-мо́рский; 2) вну́тренний (*о мо́ре*).

medium I ['mi:djəm] *n* (*pl тж.* media) 1) сре́дство; through (*или* by) the ~ of посре́дством, че́рез посре́дство; mass media сре́дства ма́ссовой информа́ции; 2) *физ.* среда́; 3) обстано́вка; усло́вия (*жи́зни*); 4) середи́на, промежу́точная ступе́нь; 5) раствори́тель (*кра́сок*); 6) ме́диум.

medium II *a* сре́дний, уме́ренный.

medley I ['medlɪ] *n* 1) смесь; 2) сме́шанное о́бщество; 3) *муз.* попурри́.

medley II *a* сме́шанный.

medley III *v* сме́шивать, переме́шивать.

meed [mi:d] *n поэт.* награ́да.

meek [mi:k] *a* мя́гкий, кро́ткий; скро́мный.

meerschaum ['mɪəʃəm] *n* пе́нковая тру́бка.

meet I [mi:t] *v* (*past, p. p.* met) 1) встреча́ть(ся); собира́ться (*тж.* to ~ together); well met! добро́ пожа́ловать!, рад на́шей встре́че!; 2) знако́мить (-ся); ~ comrade S позво́льте познако́мить вас с това́рищем С.; 3) идти́ навстре́чу; удовлетворя́ть (*жела́ния и т. п.*); 4) сходи́ться; 5) опла́чивать (*обяза́тельства, счета́ и т. п.*); □ to ~ with а) встре́титься с; натолкну́ться на; б) испыта́ть, подве́ргнуться.

meet II *n* ме́сто сбо́ра.

meeting ['mi:tɪŋ] *n* 1) ми́тинг; собра́ние, заседа́ние; general ~ о́бщее собра́ние; mass ~ ма́ссовый ми́тинг; plenary ~ плена́рное заседа́ние; Summit ~ совеща́ние на вы́сшем у́ровне; to hold (to proclaim) a ~ проводи́ть (запреща́ть) собра́ние; 2) встре́ча; 3) дуэ́ль; 4) *ж.-д.* разъе́зд.

megaphone ['megəfoun] *n* мегафо́н, ру́пор.

megrim ['mi:grɪm] *n* 1) мигре́нь; 2) при́хоть, причу́да; 3) *pl* уны́ние, плохо́е настрое́ние.

melancholic [,melən'kɔlɪk] *a* уны́лый, гру́стный; меланхоли́ческий.

melancholy I ['melənkəlɪ] *n* уны́ние, грусть; меланхо́лия.

melancholy II *a* гру́стный, уны́лый; меланхоли́ческий.

mêlée ['meleɪ] *n* 1) схва́тка, сва́лка; 2) жа́ркий спор.

meliorate ['mi:lɪəreɪt] *v* 1) улучша́ть(ся); 2) *с.-х.* мелиори́ровать.

meliorative ['mi:lɪəreɪtɪv] *a* 1) улучша́ющий; 2) *с.-х.* мелиорати́вный.

mellifluous [me'lɪfluəs] *a* медото́чивый, сладкоре́чивый.

mellow I ['melou] *a* 1) сла́дкий и со́чный, зре́лый (*о плода́х*); 2) вы́держанный (*о вине*); 3) плодоро́дный, жи́рный (*о почве*); 4) мя́гкий, со́чный (*о голосе, цвете и т. п.*); 5) добродушный; умудрённый (*годами, опытом*); 6) *разг.* подвыпивший.

mellow II *v* 1) созрева́ть; де́лать(ся) спе́лым, со́чным; 2) смягча́ть(ся).

melodious [mɪˈloudjəs] *a* 1) мелоди́чный; 2) музыка́льный.

melodrama [ˈmeləˌdrɑːmə] *n* 1) мелодра́ма; 2) театра́льность (*жестов, слов и т. п.*).

melody [ˈmelədɪ] *n* 1) мело́дия; 2) мелоди́чность.

melon [ˈmelən] *n* ды́ня; water ~ арбу́з.

melt I [melt] *n* 1) распла́вленный мета́лл; 2) пла́вка (*количество металла*).

melt II *v* 1) та́ять; to ~ into rain разрази́ться дождём (*о туче*); to ~ into tears распла́каться; 2) пла́вить(ся), растопля́ть(ся); 3) растворя́ться; 4) слива́ться (*об очертаниях*); 5) смягча́ть(ся), слабе́ть; □ to ~ **away** (рас)та́ять; исчеза́ть вдали́; to ~ **down** расплавля́ть; растворя́ть; to ~ **out** выплавля́ть.

melting I [ˈmeltɪŋ] *n* 1) пла́вка; 2) та́яние.

melting II *a* 1) пла́вящийся; 2) не́жный, мя́гкий; чувстви́тельный; 3) тро́гательный.

melting-point [ˈmeltɪŋpɔint] *n* то́чка плавле́ния.

member [ˈmembə] *n* 1) член; Member of Parliament член парла́мента; private ~ of Parliament рядово́й член парла́мента, т. е. не член прави́тельства; corresponding ~ член-корреспонде́нт; unruly ~ *шутл.* язы́к; 2) *тех.* элеме́нт, дета́ль.

membership [ˈmembəʃɪp] *n* 1) чле́нство; 2) коли́чество чле́нов; 3) *attr* чле́нский.

membrane [ˈmembrein] *n* 1) *анат.* плёнка, оболо́чка, плева́, перепо́нка; 2) *тех.* мембра́на.

membran(e)ous [memˈbrein(j)əs] *a* перепо́нчатый; плёночный.

memento [mɪˈmentou] *n* напомина́ние.

memoir [ˈmemwɑː] *n* 1) мемуа́ры, запи́ски, воспомина́ния; 2) *pl* (авто)биогра́фия; 3) *pl* учёные запи́ски (*общества*).

memorable [ˈmemərəbl] *a* па́мятный, незабве́нный.

memorandum [ˌmeməˈrændəm] *n* (*pl тж.* memoranda [ˌmeməˈrændə]) 1) заме́тка, па́мятка; 2) меморандум.

memorial I [mɪˈmɔːriəl] *n* 1) па́мятник (*в честь события, деятеля*); 2) *pl* воспомина́ния; хро́ника; 3) пети́ция.

memorial II *a* па́мятный, мемориа́льный, в па́мять (*чего-л.*).

memorize [ˈmeməraiz] *v* 1) увекове́чивать; 2) запомина́ть; зау́чивать.

memory [ˈmemərɪ] *n* 1) па́мять; запомина́ние; great ~ блестя́щая па́мять; elusive ~, short ~ сла́бая, коро́ткая па́мять; retentive ~ хоро́шая па́мять; in ~ of в па́мять (*кого-л., чего-л.*); to commit to ~ запомина́ть, зау́чивать наизу́сть; to escape one's ~ улету́читься из па́мяти; to jog one's ~ помога́ть кому́-л. припо́мнить; within the ~ of men, within living ~ на па́мяти живу́щих; 2) воспомина́ние; 3) *тех.* запомина́ющее устро́йство.

men [men] *pl см.* man I.

menace I [ˈmenəs] *n* угро́за; standing ~ ве́чная угро́за.

menace II *v* угрожа́ть.

menacingly [ˈmenəsɪŋlɪ] *adv* угрожа́юще.

menagerie [mɪˈnædʒərɪ] *n* звери́нец.

mend I [mend] *n* запла́та, зашто́панная дыра́; ◇ on the ~ на попра́вку, на улучше́ние (*о здоровье, делах и т. п.*).

mend II *v* 1) што́пать; поправля́ть, чини́ть; ремонти́ровать; 2) улучша́ть(ся), поправля́ться (*о здоровье*); 3) ускоря́ть (*шаг*); 4): to ~ the fire усилить ого́нь, подбро́сить то́плива.

mendacious [menˈdeiʃəs] *a* лжи́вый.

mender [ˈmendə] *n* 1) тот, кто чи́нит, што́пает, исправля́ет; 2) ремо́нтный ма́стер.

mendicant I [ˈmendikənt] *n* ни́щий; ни́щенствующий мона́х.

mendicant II *a* ни́щенствующий (*обыкн. о мона́хах*).

menfolk [ˈmenfouk] *n pl разг.* мужско́е населе́ние; мужско́й соста́в (*семьи, компании и т. п.*).

menial I [ˈmiːnjəl] *n презр.* слуга́; лаке́й.

menial II *a* 1) гру́бый (*о работе*); 2) лаке́йский, рабо́ле́пный.

meningitis [ˌmenɪnˈdʒaitis] *n мед.* менинги́т.

mensuration [ˌmensjuəˈreiʃən] *n* измере́ние.

mental [ˈmentl] *a* 1) у́мственный; 2) мы́сленный, производи́мый в уме́; 3) психи́ческий.

mentality [menˈtælɪtɪ] *n* 1) склад ума́; 2) спосо́бность мышле́ния; 3) умонастрое́ние.

mentally [ˈmentəlɪ] *adv* мы́сленно.

menthol [ˈmenθɔl] *n хим.* менто́л.

mention I [ˈmenʃən] *n* упомина́ние; намёк.

mention II *v* упомина́ть; don't ~ it не ·сто́ит (благода́рности, извине́ния); not to ~ не говоря́ уже́ о.

mentor [ˈmentɔː] *n* наста́вник, ме́нтор.

menu [ˈmenjuː] *n* меню́.

mercantile [ˈməːkəntail] *a* 1) торго́вый, комме́рческий; 2) торга́шеский, ме́лочный.

mercenary I [ˈməːsɪnərɪ] *n* наёмник.

mercenary II *a* 1) наёмный; 2) коры́стный; торга́шеский.

mercer [ˈməːsə] *n* торго́вец шёлком.

mercery [ˈməːsərɪ] *n* торго́вля шёлком.

merchandise [ˈməːtʃəndaiz] *n* това́ры.

merchant I [ˈməːtʃənt] *n* 1) опто́вый торго́вец, коммерса́нт, купе́ц; 2) *амер.* ла́вочник.

merchant II *a* торго́вый, комме́рческий.

merchantman [ˈməːtʃəntmən] *n* торго́вый кора́бль.

merciful [ˈməːsiful] *a* милосе́рдный; жа́лостливый; сострада́тельный.

merciless [ˈməːsilis] *a* безжа́лостный.

mercurial I [məːˈkjuəriəl] *n* рту́тный препара́т.

mercurial II *a* 1) рту́тный; 2) живо́й, подви́жный.

Mercury [ˈməːkjurɪ] *n астр., миф.* Мерку́рий.

mercury [ˈməːkjurɪ] *n* 1) ртуть; 2) рту́тный препара́т; 3) *attr* рту́тный.

mercy [ˈməːsɪ] *n* 1) ми́лость; милосе́рдие; сострада́ние; проще́ние; to cry (*или* to beg) for ~ проси́ть проще́ния, снисхожде́ния, поща́ды; at the ~ of во вла́сти (*кого-л., чего-л.*); to show ~ проявля́ть ми́лость, снисхожде́ние (*к кому-л.*); to have ~ (up)on щади́ть; 2) уда́ча.

mere[1] [mɪə] *n* о́зеро, пруд.

mere[2] *a* су́щий; я́вный, просто́й.

merely [ˈmɪəlɪ] *adv* про́сто, то́лько.

meretricious [ˌmerɪˈtrɪʃəs] *a* 1) показно́й, крича́щий; мишу́рный; 2) распу́тный.

merge [məːdʒ] *v* 1) поглоща́ть; 2) слива́ть(ся), соединя́ть(ся).

meridian I [mə'rɪdɪən] *n* 1) меридиа́н; 2) зени́т; 3) расцве́т (*жизни*).

meridian II *a* 1) полу́денный; (находя́щийся) в зени́те; 2) вы́сший, кульминацио́нный.

meridional [mə'rɪdɪənl] *a* меридиона́льный.

merino [mə'riːnou] *n* 1) мерино́с (*порода овец*); 2) мерино́совая шерсть; 3) *attr* мерино́совый.

merit I ['merɪt] *n* 1) заслу́га; to make a ~ of ста́вить себе́ в заслу́гу; 2) досто́инство; ка́чество.

merit II *v* заслу́живать.

meritorious [,merɪ'tɔːrɪəs] *a* заслу́живающий похвалы́, награ́ды; похва́льный.

mermaid ['məːmeɪd] *n* руса́лка.

merman ['məːmæn] *n* водяно́й.

merrily ['merɪlɪ] *adv* ве́село, оживлённо.

merriment ['merɪmənt] *n* весе́лье.

merry ['merɪ] *a* 1) весёлый; to make ~ весели́ться; to make ~ over потеша́ться, смея́ться (*над кем-л., чем-л.*); 2) *уст.* прия́тный; 3) *разг.* навеселе́; подвы́пивший.

merry-go-round ['merɪgou,raund] *n* 1) карусе́ль; 2) *разг.* кольцева́я тра́нспортная развя́зка; 3) вихрь (*удовольствий и т. п.*).

merry-maker ['merɪ,meɪkə] *n* весельча́к; заба́вник.

merry-making ['merɪ,meɪkɪŋ] *n* весе́лье; заба́ва, поте́ха.

mésalliance [me'zælɪəns] *n* нера́вный брак, меза́льянс.

mesh I [meʃ] *n* 1) пе́тля, яче́йка, отве́рстие (*сети, решета и т. п.*); 2) *pl* се́ти; *перен. тж.* западня́; 3): in ~ *тех.* в сцепле́нии.

mesh II *v* 1) пойма́ть в се́ти; 2) *тех.* зацепля́ть(ся).

meshy ['meʃɪ] *a* се́тчатый; яче́истый.

mesmerism ['mezmərɪzəm] *n* 1) гипноти́зм; 2) гипно́з.

mesmerize ['mezməraɪz] *v* гипнотизи́ровать.

meson ['miːzɔn] *n физ.* мезо́н.

mesosphere [,mesou'sfɪə] *n* мезосфе́ра.

mess¹ I [mes] *n* 1) о́бщий стол, о́бщее пита́ние; it's time to go to ~ пора́ идти́ к столу́; 2) каю́т-компа́ния; 3) *attr* столо́вый.

mess¹ II *v* обе́дать совме́стно, за о́бщим столо́м.

mess² I *n* 1) беспоря́док; пу́таница, кутерьма́; неприя́тность; to make a ~ произвести́ беспоря́док, пу́таницу; in a ~ а) в беспоря́дке; б) в неприя́тном положе́нии; to get into a ~ попа́сть в беду́; a jolly ~ I am in! ну и попа́л же я в переде́лку!; 2) похлёбка; болту́шка (*для собак*).

mess² II *v* 1) производи́ть беспоря́док, пу́таницу; 2) па́чкать; 3) по́ртить де́ло; 4) лоды́рничать, рабо́тать с ленцо́й (*часто* to ~ about).

message I ['mesɪdʒ] *n* 1) сообще́ние, донесе́ние; письмо́, запи́ска; to go on a ~ отпра́виться с донесе́нием, с поруче́нием; to deliver (to leave) a ~ принести́ (оста́вить) письмо́, запи́ску; there is a ~ for you а) для вас есть письмо́, запи́ска; б) вам проси́ли переда́ть; 2) ми́ссия; 3) *амер.* посла́ние президе́нта конгре́ссу.

message II *v* 1) посыла́ть сообще́ние, донесе́ние; 2) передава́ть сигна́лами, сигнализи́ровать.

messenger ['mesɪndʒə] *n* 1) по́сланный, посы́льный; ве́стник; 2) предве́стник.

messmate ['mesmeɪt] *n* однока́шник; сотрапе́зник.

Messrs ['mesəz] *n pl* господа́ (*ставится перед фами́лиями владе́льцев фи́рмы*).

messy ['mesɪ] *a* 1) гря́зный; 2) беспоря́дочный.

met [met] *past, p. p. см.* meet I.

metabolism [me'tæbəlɪzəm] *n* обме́н веще́ств.

metal I ['metl] *n* 1) мета́лл; ferrous ~s чёрные мета́ллы; Britannia ~, white ~ бе́лый мета́лл, имита́ция серебра́; yellow ~ лату́нь; 2) щебень; *ж.-д.* балла́ст (*тж.* road-metal); 3) *pl* ре́льсы; 4) *attr* металли́ческий; ◇ heavy ~ тяжёлая арти́ллерия.

metal II *v* 1) покрыва́ть, обшива́ть мета́ллом; 2) мости́ть щебнем.

metalled ['metld] *a* шосси́рованный, шоссе́йный.

metallic [mɪ'tælɪk] *a* металли́ческий.

metallurgical [,metə'lɑːdʒɪkəl] *a* металлурги́ческий.

metallurgist [me'tælədʒɪst] *n* металлу́рг.

metallurgy [me'tælədʒɪ] *n* металлу́ргия.

metamorphose [,metə'mɔːfouz] *v* превраща́ть, обраща́ть (*в* — into); изменя́ть.

metamorphosis [,metə'mɔːfəsɪs] *n* (*pl* metamorphoses [,metə'mɔːfəsiːz]) метаморфо́за; превраще́ние.

metaphor ['metəfə] *n* мета́фора.

metaphorical [,metə'fɔrɪkəl] *a* метафори́ческий.

metaphysical [,metə'fɪzɪkəl] *a* метафизи́ческий.

metaphysics [,metə'fɪzɪks] *n* метафи́зика.

mete¹ [miːt] *n* 1) грани́ца; 2) пограни́чный столб или знак.

mete² *v поэт.* 1) измеря́ть; 2) отмеря́ть, распределя́ть (*тж.* to ~ out); 3) назнача́ть (*награду, наказание*).

meteor ['miːtjə] *n* 1) метео́р; 2) *attr* метео́рный.

meteoric [,miːtɪ'ɔrɪk] *a* 1) метеори́ческий; метео́рный; 2) атмосфе́рный, атмосфери́ческий; 3) бы́стрый, блиста́тельный (*об успехе, карьере*).

meteorite ['miːtjəraɪt] *n* 1) метеори́т; 2) *attr* метеори́тный.

meteorological [,miːtjərə'lɔdʒɪkəl] *a* метеорологи́ческий; атмосфери́ческий.

meteorology [,miːtjə'rɔlədʒɪ] *n* 1) метеороло́гия; 2) метеорологи́ческие усло́вия.

meter¹ ['miːtə] *n* счётчик; измери́тель.

meter² *n амер. см.* metre¹.

methane ['meθeɪn] *n хим.* мета́н.

method ['meθəd] *n* 1) ме́тод, спо́соб; dialectical ~ диалекти́ческий ме́тод; 2) систе́ма; поря́док.

methodical [mɪ'θɔdɪkəl] *a* 1) методи́чный, методи́ческий; 2) системати́ческий.

methyl ['meθɪl] *n хим.* 1) мети́л; 2) *attr* мети́ловый.

meticulous [mɪ'tɪkjuləs] *a* ме́лочный; дото́шный.

metre¹ ['miːtə] *n* метр.

metre² *n* метр, разме́р, ритм (*в стихосложе́нии*).

metric ['metrɪk] *a* метри́ческий.

metrical ['metrɪkəl] *a* 1) метро́вый; 2) измери́тельный; 3) метри́ческий.

metropolis [mɪ'trɔpəlɪs] *n* 1) столи́ца; the ~ Ло́ндон; 2) метропо́лия; 3) центр де́ятельности.

metropolitan I [,metrə'pɔlɪtən] *n* 1) жи́тель столи́цы; 2) архиепи́скоп; митрополи́т.

metropolitan II *a* 1) столи́чный; 2) епархиа́льный.

mettle ['metl] *n* 1) хара́ктер, темпера́мент; 2) пыл, рве́ние; to be on one's ~ проявля́ть пыл;

делать всё возможное; 3) храбрость, мужество; ◇ to put smb. on his ~ a) испытывать чьё-л. мужество, выносливость; б) воодушевить кого-л., пробудить рвение в ком-л.

mettlesome ['metlsəm] *a* смелый, рьяный.

mew[1] I, II [mju:] *см.* miaow I, II.

mew[2] *n* чайка (*тж.* sea-mew).

mew[3] I *n* клетка (*для сокола*).

mew[3] II *v* 1) сажать в клетку; 2) запирать, заключать в тюрьму (*тж.* to ~ up).

mewl [mju:l] *v* 1) мяукать; 2) хныкать.

mews [mju:z] *n* стойла; конюшни.

Mexican I ['meksɪkən] *n* мексиканец; the ~s мексиканцы.

Mexican II *a* мексиканский.

mezzanine ['mezəni:n] *n* 1) антресоли; 2) *театр.* помещение под сценой.

mi [mi:] *n муз.* ми.

miaow I [mi:'au] *n* мяуканье.

miaow II *v* мяукать.

mica ['maɪkə] *n* слюда.

mice [maɪs] *pl см.* mouse[a].

microbe ['maɪkroub] *n* микроб.

microbiology ['maɪkroubaɪ'ɔlədʒɪ] *n* микробиология.

microclimate ['maɪkrou'klaɪmɪt] *n* микроклимат.

microcosm ['maɪkroukɔzəm] *n* 1) микрокосм; 2) миниатюрное изображение.

microfilm I ['maɪkroufɪlm] *n* микроплёнка.

microfilm II *v* снимать на микроплёнку.

micro-organism ['maɪkrou'ɔ:gənɪzəm] *n* микроорганизм.

microphone ['maɪkrəfoun] *n* микрофон.

microscope ['maɪkrəskoup] *n* микроскоп; electron(ic) ~ электронный микроскоп.

microscopic(al) [,maɪkrəs'kɔpɪk(əl)] *a* микроскопический.

mid I [mɪd] *a* средний, срединный.

mid II *prep см.* amid.

midday ['mɪdeɪ] *n* 1) полдень; 2) *attr* полуденный.

middle I ['mɪdl] *n* середина.

middle II *a* средний.

middle-aged ['mɪdl'eɪdʒd] *a* пожилой, средних лет.

middleman ['mɪdlmæn] *n* посредник; комиссионер.

middling I ['mɪdlɪŋ] *a* 1) средний; 2) второстепенный, посредственный.

middling II *adv* так себе, средне.

middlings ['mɪdlɪŋz] *n pl* второсортный товар.

middy ['mɪdɪ] *разг. см.* midshipman.

midge [mɪdʒ] *n* мошка.

midget ['mɪdʒɪt] *n* 1) крошка, карлик; 2) миниатюрная фотокарточка; 3) *амер.* мошкара.

midland I ['mɪdlənd] *n* 1) внутренняя, центральная часть страны; 2) *pl* (the Midlands) центральные графства Англии.

midland II *a* 1) средний, центральный; 2) удалённый от моря.

midmost ['mɪdmoust] *a* центральный.

midnight ['mɪdnaɪt] *n* 1) полночь; 2) непроглядная тьма; 3) *attr* полуночный; тёмный.

midriff ['mɪdrɪf] *n анат.* диафрагма.

midship ['mɪdʃɪp] *n* средняя часть корабля.

midshipman ['mɪdʃɪpmən] *n* корабельный гардемарин.

midst I [mɪdst] *n* середина; in the ~ of среди, между; in our (your) ~ среди нас (вас), в нашей (вашей) среде.

midst II *prep см.* amidst.

midsummer ['mɪd,sʌmə] *n* середина лета; летнее солнцестояние (*21 июня*); Midsummer day Иванов день (*24 июня*).

midway ['mɪd'weɪ] *adv* на полпути.

midwife ['mɪdwaɪf] *n* акушерка, повивальная бабка.

midwinter ['mɪd'wɪntə] *n* середина зимы; зимнее солнцестояние (*21 декабря*).

mien [mi:n] *n* 1) манера; вид, наружность; 2) мина, выражение лица.

might[1] [maɪt] *past см.* may.

might[2] *n* сила; могущество; with ~ and main изо всех сил.

might-have-been ['maɪthəv,bi:n] *n* 1) упущенная возможность; 2) неудачник.

mightily ['maɪtɪlɪ] *adv* 1) сильно; 2) *разг.* очень, чрезвычайно.

mightiness ['maɪtɪnɪs] *n* 1) мощность; 2) величие.

mighty I ['maɪtɪ] *a* 1) сильный; мощный; могущественный; 2) массивный; 3) *разг.* громадный.

mighty II *adv разг.* очень; that is ~ easy это очень легко.

mignonette [,mɪnjə'net] *n* резеда.

migraine ['mi:greɪn] *n* мигрень.

migrant I ['maɪgrənt] *n* 1) переселенец; 2) перелётная птица.

migrant II *a* 1) кочующий; 2) перелётный.

migrate [maɪ'greɪt] *v* 1) переселяться; мигрировать; 2) совершать перелёт (*о птицах*).

migration [maɪ'greɪʃən] *n* 1) переселение; миграция; 2) перелёт (*птиц*).

migratory ['maɪgrətərɪ] *a* 1) кочующий; 2) перелётный; 3) *мед.* блуждающий.

mike[1] I [maɪk] *n* безделье; to do a ~ бездельничать.

mike[1] II *v* бездельничать, отлынивать от работы.

mike[2] *n разг.* микрофон.

milage ['maɪlɪdʒ] *см.* mileage.

milch [mɪltʃ] *a* молочный (*о скоте*); дойная (*о корове*).

mild [maɪld] *a* 1) мягкий; 2) слабый (*о пиве, лекарстве и т. п.*); неострый (*о пище*); 3) тихий, кроткий (*о человеке*).

mildew ['mɪldju:] *n* 1) мильдью (*болезнь растений*); 2) плесень.

mildly ['maɪldlɪ] *adv* мягко; кротко; to put it ~ мягко выражаясь.

mildness ['maɪldnɪs] *n* 1) мягкость; 2) слабость; 3) вялость.

mile [maɪl] *n* миля; a long ~ добрая миля; ◇ ~s better (easier) много лучше (легче).

mileage ['maɪlɪdʒ] *n* 1) расстояние в милях; 2) число пройденных миль; 3) проездные деньги.

milepost ['maɪlpoust] *n* мильный столб.

milestone ['maɪlstoun] *n* мильный камень; *перен.* веха (*в жизни, истории*).

militant ['mɪlɪtənt] *a* 1) воинствующий; 2) воинственный.

militarism ['mɪlɪtərɪzəm] *n* милитаризм.

militarist ['mılıtərıst] *n* милитари́ст.

militarization [,mılıtəraı'zeıʃən] *n* милитариза́ция.

militarize ['mılıtəraız] *v* 1) милитаризи́ровать; 2) военизи́ровать.

military I ['mılıtərı] *n* (the ~) *собир.* вое́нные.

military II *a* вое́нный, во́инский.

militate ['mılıteıt] *v* 1) воева́ть; 2) говори́ть, свиде́тельствовать про́тив (*об уликах, доказательствах и т. п.*; against).

milk I [mılk] *n* 1) молоко́; new ~ парно́е молоко́; desiccated ~ сухо́е молоко́; pigeon's ~ ≅ «пти́чье молоко́»; 2) мле́чный сок (*растений*); 3) *attr* моло́чный.

milk II *v* 1) дои́ть; 2) дава́ть молоко́ (*о скоте*); 3) извлека́ть вы́году, эксплуати́ровать; 4) *сленг* перехва́тывать (*телеграфные, телефонные сообщения*).

milk-and-water ['mılkən'wɔtə] *a* 1) сла́бый; 2) безли́чный; безво́льный.

milker ['mılkə] *n* 1) доя́р; доя́рка; 2) дои́льная маши́на; 3) до́йная коро́ва.

milkmaid ['mılkmeıd] *n* 1) доя́рка; 2) моло́чница.

milkman ['mılkmən] *n* 1) продаве́ц молока́; 2) доя́р.

milksop ['mılksɔp] *n* не́женка, «сосуно́к»; бесхара́ктерный челове́к, «ба́ба».

milk-white ['mılkwaıt] *a* моло́чно-бе́лый.

milky ['mılkı] *a* 1) моло́чный; 2) облачный, тума́нный.

mill I [mıl] *n* 1) ме́льница; 2) заво́д, фа́брика; 3) *спорт.* кула́чный бой; 4) *сленг* тюрьма́; 5) *attr* ме́льничный; 6) *attr* фабри́чный, заводски́й; ◇ to go through the ~ пройти́ суро́вую шко́лу, мно́го испыта́ть (*в жизни*).

mill II *v* 1) моло́ть; ру́шить (*зерно*); дроби́ть (*руду*); 2) сбива́ть (*в пену*); 3) бить, тузи́ть; 4) беспоря́дочно кружи́ть (*о стаде, толпе; тж.* to ~ about).

millboard ['mılbɔd] *n* то́лстый карто́н.

millennium [mı'lenıəm] *n* тысячеле́тие.

miller ['mılə] *n* ме́льник; ◇ to drown the ~ си́льно разба́вить водо́й (*спиртное, чай*).

millet ['mılıt] *n* про́со.

mill-hand ['mılhænd] *n* фабри́чный рабо́чий.

milliard ['mıljɑd] *n* миллиа́рд.

milligramme ['mılıgræm] *n* миллигра́мм.

millimetre ['mılı,miːtə] *n* миллиме́тр.

milliner ['mılınə] *n* моди́стка.

millinery ['mılınərı] *n* 1) да́мские шля́пы (*как товар*); 2) магази́н, мастерска́я да́мских шляп.

million ['mıljən] *n* 1) миллио́н; 2) (the ~) мно́жество, ма́сса.

millionaire [,mıljə'neə] *n* миллионе́р.

mill-pond ['mılpɔnd] *n* ме́льничный пруд.

millstone ['mılstoun] *n* жёрнов; ◇ to see far into a ~ быть о́чень проница́тельным.

mime [maım] *v* изобража́ть мими́чески.

mimeograph I ['mımıəgræf] *n* мимео́граф.

mimeograph II *v* размножа́ть (*документы*).

mimic I ['mımık] *n* подража́тель, имита́тор.

mimic II *a* 1) подража́тельный; 2) подде́льный.

mimic III *v* 1) передра́знивать; подража́ть; 2) походи́ть на.

mimicry ['mımıkrı] *n* 1) имити́рование; 2) *биол.* мимикри́я.

mince I [mıns] *n* фарш.

mince II *v* 1) руби́ть, кроши́ть (*мясо*); 2) смягча́ть (*слова*); 3) говори́ть, дви́гаться жема́нно.

mincemeat ['mınsmiːt] *n* 1) мясно́й фарш; 2) начи́нка из изю́ма, минда́ля и са́хара; ◇ to make ~ of преврати́ть в котле́ту, уничто́жить, разгроми́ть (*противника*).

mincing ['mınsıŋ] *a* жема́нный.

mind I [maınd] *n* 1) па́мять; воспомина́ние; to bear (*или* to keep) in ~ по́мнить, име́ть в виду́; to go (*или* to pass) out of ~ быть забы́тым; ускользну́ть из па́мяти; to call to ~ припомина́ть; to bring to ~ вспомина́ть; 2) мне́ние; мысль; взгляд, о́браз мы́слей; to be of one ~ (with) быть того́ же мне́ния (как и); разделя́ть мне́ние (кого́-л.); to my ~ по моему́ мне́нию; to alter (*или* to change) one's ~ переду́мать, измени́ть своё мне́ние; to speak one's ~ вы́сказаться открове́нно; on one's ~ на уме́, в мы́слях; to cross one's ~ прийти́ в го́лову, на ум; to disburden one's ~ вы́сказаться, отвести́ ду́шу; to make up one's ~ (to) а) реши́ть (*что-л.*); б) примири́ться (*с чем-л.*); 3) ум, ра́зум; *перен.* мысли́тель; daring ~ де́рзкий ум; сме́лое воображе́ние; spacious ~ широ́кий кругозо́р; to be in one's right ~ быть в здра́вом уме́; the great ~s of the world вели́кие умы́ челове́чества; 4) наме́рение, жела́ние; to have a (good) ~ (to + Inf) име́ть (большо́е) жела́ние (*что-л. сделать*); to have half a ~ (to + Inf) быть не прочь (*что-л. сделать*); to be in a good ~ твёрдо реши́ть, намерева́ться; to be in two ~s не реша́ться, колеба́ться; to set one's ~ on о́чень жела́ть; to know one's own ~ знать чего́ хо́чешь, не колеба́ться; 5) дух, душа́.

mind II *v* 1) по́мнить; 2) забо́титься, занима́ться чем-л.; 3) обраща́ть внима́ние, придава́ть значе́ние; never ~! ничего́!, не беда́!, всё равно́!; 4) остерега́ться, бере́чься; 5) возража́ть; if you don't ~ е́сли вы не возража́ете; would you ~ ringing пожа́луйста, позвони́те; I don't ~ it нет, ниско́лько.

minded ['maındıd] *a* располо́женный (*что-л. сделать*).

-minded [-maındıd] *в сложных словах:* high-minded великоду́шный; small-minded ме́лочный.

mindful ['maındful] *a* внима́тельный, забо́тливый (of).

mindless ['maındlıs] *a* 1) бессмы́сленный; 2) не ду́мающий (*о чём-л. — of*), не счита́ющийся (*с чем-л. — of*).

mine[1] [maın] *pron poss* мой, моя́, моё; мои́.

mine[2] I *n* 1) рудни́к, копь; при́иск; исто́чник; 3) *воен.* ми́на; 4) *ист.* подко́п.

mine[2] II *v* 1) разраба́тывать рудни́к, добыва́ть руду́ (*и т. п.*); 2) подка́пываться; подрыва́ть (*репутацию и т. п.*); 3) мини́ровать.

minefield ['maınfiːld] *n* ми́нное по́ле; ми́нное загражде́ние.

minelayer ['maın,leıə] *n* *мор.* ми́нный загради́тель.

miner ['maınə] *n* 1) горня́к, горнорабо́чий; шахтёр; 2) *воен.* минёр.

mineral I ['mınərəl] *n* 1) минера́л; 2) *pl* поле́зные ископа́емые; 3) *pl разг.* минера́льная вода́.

mineral II *a* 1) минера́льный; 2) неоргани́ческий.

mineralogy [,mɪnə'rælədʒɪ] *n* минерало́гия.

minesweeper ['maɪn,swiːpə] *n мор.* ми́нный тра́льщик.

minethrower ['maɪn,θrouə] *n* миномёт.

minever ['mɪnɪvə] *n* горноста́й (*мех*).

mineworker ['maɪn,wɜːkə] *см.* miner 1).

mingle ['mɪŋgl] *v* 1) сме́шивать(ся); to ~ in (*или* with) the crowd сме́шаться с толпо́й; 2) враща́ться (*в обществе и т. п.*), обща́ться (*с кем-л.— in, with*).

miniature I ['mɪnjətʃə] *n* миниатю́ра.

miniature II *a* миниатю́рный.

miniature III *v* изобража́ть в миниатю́ре.

mini-car ['mɪnɪkɑː] *n* малолитра́жный автомоби́ль, малолитра́жка.

minikin I ['mɪnɪkɪn] *n* кро́шечное существо́.

minikin II *a* 1) кро́шечный; 2) жема́нный, мане́рный.

minima ['mɪnɪmə] *pl см.* minimum.

minimize ['mɪnɪmaɪz] *v* преуменьша́ть.

minimum ['mɪnɪməm] *n* (*pl* minima) 1) ми́нимум; 2) *attr* минима́льный.

mining ['maɪnɪŋ] *n* 1) го́рное де́ло; го́рная промы́шленность; 2) *воен.* ми́нное де́ло; 3) *attr* го́рный; ру́дный; бурово́й.

minion ['mɪnjən] *n* 1) люби́мец, фавори́т; ~ of fortune ба́ловень судьбы́; 2) креату́ра, послу́шное ору́дие (*кого-л.*).

mini-skirt ['mɪnɪskɜːt] *n* ми́ни-ю́бка.

minister I ['mɪnɪstə] *n* 1) мини́стр; cabinet ~ член кабине́та мини́стров; prime ~ премье́р-мини́стр; 2) *дип.* посла́нник; ~ plenipotentiary полномо́чный представи́тель; resident ~ дипломати́ческий представи́тель; 3) свяще́нник.

minister II *v* прислу́живать, помога́ть (*to*).

ministerial [,mɪnɪs'tɪərɪəl] *a* 1) министе́рский; 2) подде́рживающий прави́тельство; 3) служе́бный, подчинённый; 4) свяще́ннический; па́стырский.

ministry ['mɪnɪstrɪ] *n* 1) министе́рство; 2) кабине́т мини́стров; 3) духове́нство; 4) служе́ние.

miniver ['mɪnɪvə] *см.* minever.

mink [mɪŋk] *n зоол.* но́рка.

minnow ['mɪnou] *n* 1) песка́рь, голья́н; ме́лкая пресново́дная ры́ба; 2) мелюзга́.

minor I ['maɪnə] *n* 1) *муз.* мино́рный ключ, мино́р; 2) подро́сток, несовершенноле́тний; 3) *ист.* франциска́нский мона́х, минори́т.

minor II *a* 1) ме́ньший; незначи́тельный, второстепе́нный; ма́лый (*о планетах*); 2) *муз.* мино́рный (*тж. перен.*); 3) мла́дший (*из двух братьев в школе*).

minority [maɪ'nɔrɪtɪ] *n* 1) ме́ньшее число́; меньшинство́; national ~ национа́льное меньшинство́; 2) несовершенноле́тие.

minster ['mɪnstə] *n* 1) (кафедра́льный) собо́р; 2) монасты́рская це́рковь.

minstrel ['mɪnstrəl] *n* 1) менестре́ль; поэ́т, певе́ц; 2) *pl* исполни́тели негритя́нских пе́сен (*загримиро́ванные не́грами*).

mint¹ [mɪnt] *n* 1) *бот.* мя́та; 2) *attr* мя́тный.

mint² I *n* 1) моне́тный двор; 2) больша́я су́мма де́нег (*тж.* a ~ of money); 3) происхожде́ние, исто́чник.

mint² II *v* 1) чека́нить; 2) выду́мывать, изобрета́ть.

minuend ['mɪnjuend] *n мат.* уменьша́емое.

minuet [,mɪnju'et] *n* менуэ́т.

minus I ['maɪnəs] *n* ми́нус, знак ми́нуса.

minus II *a* 1) лишённый (*чего-л.*); 2) отрица́тельный (*о величине, заря́де и т. п.*).

minus III *prep* ми́нус, без.

minuscule [mɪ'nʌskjuːl] *n* строчна́я бу́ква.

minuteᵃ I ['mɪnɪt] *n* 1) мину́та; the ~ (that) как то́лько; on (*или* to) the ~ мину́та в мину́ту; 2) запи́ска, заме́тка, набро́сок; 3) *pl* протоко́л (*заседа́ния, собра́ния*); to keep the ~ вести́ протоко́л.

minuteᵃ II *v* 1) рассчи́тывать вре́мя; 2) набра́сывать на́черно; 3) протоколи́ровать, вести́ протоко́л; □ to ~ down записа́ть, заме́тить себе́.

minuteᵇ [maɪ'njuːt] *a* 1) ме́лкий, мельча́йший; 2) незначи́тельный; 3) то́чный, тща́тельный, подро́бный.

minute-hand ['mɪnɪthænd] *n* мину́тная стре́лка.

minutelyᵃ I ['mɪnɪtlɪ] *a* ежемину́тный.

minutelyᵃ II *adv* ежемину́тно.

minutelyᵇ I [maɪ'njuːtlɪ] *a* то́чный; дета́льный.

minutelyᵇ II *adv* то́чно; дета́льно.

minuteness [maɪ'njuːtnɪs] *n* 1) то́чность, тща́тельность; подро́бность; 2) ма́лость.

minutiae [maɪ'njuːʃiː] *n pl* ме́лочи, дета́ли.

minx [mɪŋks] *n* 1) де́рзкая девчо́нка; 2) коке́тка; шалу́нья; 3) распу́тница.

miracle ['mɪrəkl] *n* 1) чу́до; to a ~ удиви́тельно хорошо́; 2) средневеко́вая мисте́рия (*тж.* ~ play).

miraculous [mɪ'rækjuləs] *a* сверхъесте́ственный; чуде́сный; удиви́тельный.

mirage ['mɪrɑːʒ] *n* мира́ж.

mire I ['maɪə] *n* 1) боло́то, тряси́на; to find oneself (*или* to stick) in the ~ оказа́ться в затрудни́тельном положе́нии; 2) грязь; to drag through the ~ облива́ть гря́зью, поро́чить.

mire II *v* 1) завя́знуть в боло́те, тряси́не; *перен.* оказа́ться в затрудни́тельном положе́нии; 2) забры́згивать гря́зью; *перен.* черни́ть.

mirror I ['mɪrə] *n* 1) зе́ркало (*тж. перен.*); false ~ криво́е зе́ркало; 2) зерка́льная пове́рхность; 3) отображе́ние.

mirror II *v* отража́ть, отобража́ть.

mirth [mɜːθ] *n* весе́лье, ра́дость.

mirthful ['mɜːθful] *a* весёлый, ра́достный.

miry ['maɪərɪ] *a* 1) то́пкий; 2) гря́зный.

mis- [mɪs-] *pref со знач.:* а) *неправильности:* misprint опеча́тка; misdeed злодея́ние; опло́шность; б) *отрица́ния:* mistrust недове́рие.

misadventure ['mɪsəd'ventʃə] *n* несча́стье, несча́стный слу́чай.

misanthrope ['mɪzənθroup] *n* человеконенави́стник; мизантро́п.

misapply ['mɪsə'plaɪ] *v* 1) непра́вильно употребля́ть; 2) злоупотребля́ть.

misapprehend ['mɪs,æprɪ'hend] *v* превра́тно поня́ть.

misapprehension ['mɪs,æprɪ'henʃən] *n* заблужде́ние; недоразуме́ние.

misappropriation ['mɪsə,prouprɪ'eɪʃən] *n* незако́нное присвое́ние.

misbehave ['mɪsbɪ'heɪv] *v* пло́хо себя́ вести́.

misbehaviour ['mɪsbɪ'heɪvjə] *n* плохо́е поведе́ние.

misbelief ['mɪsbɪ'liːf] *n* заблужде́ние.

misbeliever [ˈmɪsbɪˈliːvə] n еретик.

miscalculate [ˈmɪsˈkælkjuleɪt] v просчитаться; ошибиться в расчёте.

miscalculation [ˈmɪsˌkælkjuˈleɪʃən] n просчёт, ошибка в расчёте.

miscall [ˈmɪsˈkɔːl] v 1) называть не тем именем; 2) *диал.* бранить, ругать.

miscarriage [mɪsˈkærɪdʒ] n 1) неудача, ошибка; 2) недоставка по адресу; 3) выкидыш, аборт.

miscarry [mɪsˈkærɪ] v 1) потерпеть неудачу; 2) затеряться, не дойти до адресата; 3) выкинуть; сделать выкидыш.

miscellanea [ˌmɪsɪˈleɪnɪə] n pl 1) (литературная) смесь; 2) сборник.

miscellaneous [ˌmɪsɪˈleɪnjəs] a 1) разнообразный, разный; 2) разносторонний (*о человеке*).

miscellany [mɪˈselənɪ] n 1) смесь; 2) сборник.

mischance [mɪsˈtʃɑːns] n неудача; by ~ к несчастью, по несчастной случайности.

mischief [ˈmɪstʃɪf] n 1) вред, повреждение; to make ~ вредить; ссорить; to do smb. a ~ *разг.* ранить, обидеть кого-л.; the ~ of it is that... беда в том, что...; to play the ~ with a) повредить; б) спутать, привести в беспорядок; 2) шалости, проказы; озорство; full of ~ озорной, бедовый; 3) озорник, шалун; 4): where the ~ have you been? *разг.* ≅ где, чёрт возьми, ты был?

mischief-maker [ˈmɪstʃɪfˌmeɪkə] n интриган.

mischievous [ˈmɪstʃɪvəs] a 1) вредный; 2) непослушный, озорной (*о ребёнке*).

misconceive [ˌmɪskənˈsiːv] v 1) иметь неправильное представление; 2) превратно, неправильно понимать, истолковывать.

misconception [ˈmɪskənˈsepʃən] n 1) неправильное представление, понимание; 2) недоразумение.

misconduct[a] [ˈmɪsˈkɔndəkt] n 1) дурное поведение; 2) супружеская неверность; 3) плохое обращение (*с чем-л.*).

misconduct[b] [ˈmɪskənˈdʌkt] v 1) плохо вести себя; 2) нарушать супружескую верность; 3) плохо обращаться (*с чем-л.*).

misconstruction [ˈmɪskənsˈtrʌkʃən] n 1) неверное истолкование; 2) неправильное построение.

misconstrue [ˈmɪskənˈstruː] v неправильно истолковывать.

miscount I [ˈmɪsˈkaunt] n неправильный подсчёт, просчёт.

miscount II v неправильно подсчитывать, просчитаться.

miscreant I [ˈmɪskrɪənt] n 1) негодяй; 2) *уст.* еретик.

miscreant II a 1) испорченный; 2) *уст.* еретический.

misdeal [ˈmɪsˈdiːl] v (*past, p. p.* misdealt) 1) неправильно поступать; 2) неправильно сдавать (*карты*), подтасовывать.

misdealing [ˈmɪsˈdiːlɪŋ] n нечестный поступок; беспринципное поведение.

misdealt [ˈmɪsˈdelt] *past, p. p. см.* misdeal.

misdeed [ˈmɪsˈdiːd] n 1) злодеяние; преступление; 2) оплошность.

misdemeanour [ˌmɪsdɪˈmiːnə] n (судебно наказуемый) поступок.

misdirect [ˈmɪsdɪˈrekt] v 1) неверно направить; давать неправильные указания; 2) отправить не по адресу.

misdirection [ˈmɪsdɪˈrekʃən] n неправильное указание; неверное направление.

misdoing [ˈmɪsˈduːɪŋ] *см.* misdeed.

miser [ˈmaɪzə] n скряга, скупец.

miserable [ˈmɪzərəbl] a 1) жалкий, несчастный; 2) плохой, ненастный (*о погоде*); 3) бедный, убогий, скудный.

miserably [ˈmɪzərəblɪ] *adv* 1) убого, бедно; 2) ужасающе, очень.

miserliness [ˈmaɪzəlɪnɪs] n скупость.

miserly [ˈmaɪzəlɪ] a скупой.

misery [ˈmɪzərɪ] n 1) несчастье, страдание; to be in (*или* to suffer) ~ from toothache мучиться зубной болью; 2) нищета, бедность, убогость.

misfeasance [ˈmɪsˈfiːzəns] n *юр.* злоупотребление властью.

misfire I [ˈmɪsˈfaɪə] n 1) осечка; 2) незапуск (*двигателя*).

misfire II v дать осечку.

misfit I [ˈmɪsfɪt] n плохо сидящее платье; *перен.* человек не на своём месте, неподходящий человек.

misfit II v плохо сидеть (*о платье*).

misfortune [mɪsˈfɔːtʃən] n несчастье, неудача.

misgave [mɪsˈgeɪv] *past см.* misgive.

misgive [mɪsˈgɪv] v (*past* misgave; *p. p.* misgiven) вызывать дурные предчувствия, внушать опасения.

misgiven [mɪsˈgɪvn] *p. p. см.* misgive.

misgiving [mɪsˈgɪvɪŋ] n опасение, предчувствие.

misgovern [ˈmɪsˈgʌvən] v плохо управлять.

misguide [mɪsˈgaɪd] v вводить в заблуждение.

mishandle [ˈmɪsˈhændl] v плохо обращаться.

mishap [ˈmɪshæp] n неудача.

mishear [mɪsˈhɪə] v (*past, p. p.* misheard) ослышаться.

misheard [mɪsˈhəːd] *past, p. p. см.* mishear.

misinform [ˈmɪsɪnˈfɔːm] v дезинформировать.

misinformation [ˌmɪsɪnfəˈmeɪʃən] n дезинформация.

misinterpret [ˈmɪsɪnˈtəːprɪt] v неправильно, неверно истолковывать.

misjudge [ˈmɪsˈdʒʌdʒ] v недооценивать; неверно судить (*о ком-л., о чём-л.*).

mislaid [mɪsˈleɪd] *past, p. p. см.* mislay.

mislay [mɪsˈleɪ] v (*past, p. p.* mislaid) затерять; положить не на место.

mislead [mɪsˈliːd] v (*past, p. p.* misled) вводить в заблуждение.

misled [mɪsˈled] *past, p. p. см.* mislead.

mismanage [ˈmɪsˈmænɪdʒ] v плохо управлять (*чем-л.*).

misnomer [ˈmɪsˈnoumə] n неправильное употребление имени *или* термина.

misplace [ˈmɪsˈpleɪs] v 1) положить, поставить не на место; 2) доверить(ся) кому-л., не заслуживающему доверия.

misprint I [ˈmɪsˈprint] n опечатка.

misprint II v 1) неправильно напечатать; 2) сделать опечатку.

mispronunciation [ˈmɪsprəˌnʌnsɪˈeɪʃən] n неправильное произношение.

misquote [ˈmɪsˈkwout] v неправильно цитировать.

misread [ˈmɪsˈriːd] v (*past, p. p.* misread [ˈmɪsˈred]) неправильно читать, неправильно толковать.

misrepresent [ˈmɪsˌreprɪˈzent] *v* искажа́ть, представля́ть в ло́жном све́те.

misrepresentation [ˈmɪsˌreprɪzenˈteɪʃən] *n* искаже́ние, представле́ние в ло́жном све́те.

misrule [ˈmɪsˈruːl] *n* 1) плохо́е (у)правле́ние; 2) беспоря́док.

miss[1] [mɪs] *n* мисс, ба́рышня.

miss[2] I *n* 1) про́мах; 2) отсу́тствие; ◊ to give smth. a ~ избега́ть чего́-л.; a lucky ~ счастли́вое избавле́ние.

miss[2] II *v* 1) промахну́ться, не дости́чь це́ли (*тж. перен.*); 2) упусти́ть (*возмо́жность*); 3) пропусти́ть; прогляде́ть; не услы́шать; не заста́ть; опозда́ть (*на поезд и т. п.*); 4) скуча́ть, чу́вствовать отсу́тствие (*кого́-л., чего́-л.*); 5) избежа́ть; ☐ to ~ out вы́пустить, опусти́ть (*слово, стро́чку и т. п.*).

mis-shapen [ˈmɪsˈʃeɪpən] *a* уро́дливый.

missile I [ˈmɪsaɪl] *n* (мета́тельный) снаря́д; раке́та; реакти́вный снаря́д; guided ~ управля́емый снаря́д; bumper ~ двухступе́нчатая раке́та.

missile II *a* 1) мета́тельный; 2) раке́тный, реакти́вный.

missing [ˈmɪsɪŋ] *a* недостаю́щий; отсу́тствующий; пропа́вший.

mission [ˈmɪʃən] *n* 1) ми́ссия; trade ~ торго́вое представи́тельство; 2) призва́ние; 3) зада́ча, зада́ние, поруче́ние.

missionary I [ˈmɪʃnərɪ] *n* миссионе́р.

missionary II *a* миссионе́рский.

missive [ˈmɪsɪv] *n* официа́льное письмо́; посла́ние.

mis-spell [ˈmɪsˈspel] *v* (*past, p. p.* mis-spelt) писа́ть с оши́бками.

mis-spelt [ˈmɪsˈspelt] *past, p. p. см.* mis-spell.

mis-spend [ˈmɪsˈspend] *v* (*past, p. p.* mis-spent) зря тра́тить.

mis-spent [ˈmɪsˈspent] *past, p. p. см.* mis-spend.

mis-state [ˈmɪsˈsteɪt] *v* (с)де́лать ло́жное заявле́ние, ло́жно свиде́тельствовать.

mis-statement [ˈmɪsˈsteɪtmənt] *n* ло́жное заявле́ние.

mis-step [ˈmɪsˈstep] *v* оступи́ться.

mist I [mɪst] *n* тума́н; ды́мка; и́зморось; Scotch ~ густо́й тума́н с и́зморосью.

mist II *v* 1) застила́ть, оку́тывать тума́ном; 2) застила́ть слеза́ми; 3): it is ~ing мороси́т.

mistake I [mɪsˈteɪk] *n* оши́бка, заблужде́ние; by ~ по оши́бке; to make a ~ ошиби́ться; to make a big ~ сде́лать, допусти́ть кру́пную оши́бку; and no ~, to make no ~ несомне́нно; непреме́нно, обяза́тельно.

mistake II *v* (*past* mistook; *p. p.* mistaken) 1) ошиба́ться, заблужда́ться; you are ~n вы ошиба́етесь; 2) обману́ться; перепу́тать; (оши́бочно) приня́ть за.

mistaken I [mɪsˈteɪkən] *p. p. см.* mistake II.

mistaken II *a* 1) оши́бочный; 2) неуме́стный.

mister [ˈmɪstə] *n* (*сокр.* Mr) ми́стер, господи́н (*ста́вится перед фами́лией*).

mistimed [ˈmɪsˈtaɪmd] *a* сде́ланный, ска́занный не во́время *или* некста́ти.

mistiness [ˈmɪstɪnɪs] *n* тума́нность.

mistletoe [ˈmɪsltou] *n бот.* оме́ла.

mistook [mɪsˈtuk] *past см.* mistake II.

mistreat [mɪsˈtriːt] *амер. см.* maltreat.

mistreatment [mɪsˈtriːtmənt] *амер. см.* maltreatment.

mistress [ˈmɪstrɪs] *n* 1) хозя́йка; 2) мастери́ца (*в како́м-л. де́ле*), специали́стка; 3) учи́тельница; head ~ нача́льница, заве́дующая (*уче́бным заведе́нием*); 4) влады́чица; 5) возлю́бленная, любо́вница; 6) (*сокр.* Mrs [ˈmɪsɪz]) ми́ссис, госпожа́ (*ста́вится перед фами́лией заму́жней же́нщины*).

mistrust I [ˈmɪsˈtrʌst] *n* недове́рие, подозре́ние.

mistrust II *v* не доверя́ть, подозрева́ть.

mistrustful [mɪsˈtrʌstful] *a* недове́рчивый, подозри́тельный.

misty [ˈmɪstɪ] *a* 1) тума́нный; 2) затума́ненный; 3) сму́тный, нея́сный.

misunderstand [ˈmɪsʌndəˈstænd] *v* (*past, p. p.* misunderstood) непра́вильно поня́ть, истолкова́ть.

misunderstanding [ˈmɪsʌndəˈstændɪŋ] *n* 1) непра́вильное понима́ние; 2) недоразуме́ние; 3) размо́лвка.

misunderstood [ˈmɪsʌndəˈstud] *past, p. p. см.* misunderstand.

misuse[a] [ˈmɪsˈjuːs] *n* 1) непра́вильное употребле́ние; 2) плохо́е обраще́ние; 3) злоупотребле́ние.

misuse[b] [ˈmɪsˈjuːz] *v* 1) непра́вильно употребля́ть; 2) пло́хо обраща́ться; 3) злоупотребля́ть.

mite [maɪt] *n* 1) полу́шка; not a ~ *разг.* во́все нет, совсе́м нет; 2) ле́пта; 3) кро́шка, ребёнок.

mitigate [ˈmɪtɪgeɪt] *v* 1) смягча́ть; 2) ослабля́ть; уменьша́ть.

mitigation [ˌmɪtɪˈgeɪʃən] *n* 1) смягче́ние; 2) облегче́ние; ослабле́ние; уменьше́ние.

mitt [mɪt] *n* 1) *см.* mitten 1), 2); 2) *pl разг.* боксёрские перча́тки; 3) *сленг* рука́, кула́к; ◊ to tip one's ~ a) здоро́ваться; б) угада́ть чьи-л. наме́рения.

mitten [ˈmɪtn] *n* 1) ва́режка; рукави́ца; 2) мите́нка (*же́нская перча́тка без па́льцев*); ◊ to give the ~ a) отказа́ть (*жениху́*); б) уво́лить с рабо́ты.

mix [mɪks] *v* 1) меша́ть; сме́шивать(ся); 2) сходи́ться; обща́ться; they do not ~ well они́ не подхо́дят друг дру́гу; они́ не ла́дят друг с дру́гом; ☐ to ~ up a) хорошо́ переме́шивать; б) спу́тать, перепу́тать; в) впу́тывать; to be ~ed up быть заме́шанным (*во что-л.*).

mixed [mɪkst] *a* 1) сме́шанный; 2) *разг.* одуре́вший, опьяне́вший.

mixer [ˈmɪksə] *n* 1) *тех.* меша́лка, смеси́тель, ми́ксер; 2) *разг.*: good (bad) ~ общи́тельный (необщи́тельный) челове́к.

mix-in [ˈmɪksˈɪn] *n разг.* дра́ка, потасо́вка.

mixture [ˈmɪkstʃə] *n* 1) сме́шивание; 2) смесь; 3) миксту́ра.

mix-up [ˈmɪksˈʌp] *n разг.* 1) потасо́вка, дра́ка; 2) неразбери́ха.

miz(z)en [ˈmɪzn] *n мор.* биза́нь.

mizzle I [ˈmɪzl] *n* и́зморось, ме́лкий дождь.

mizzle II *v*: it ~s мороси́т.

moan I [moun] *n* стон.

moan II *v* 1) стона́ть; 2) опла́кивать; жа́ловаться.

moat I [mout] *n* ров, напо́лненный водо́й.

moat II *v* окружа́ть рвом.

mob I [mɔb] *n* 1) толпа́; 2) сбо́рище; 3) *сленг* ша́йка воро́в; swell ~ шика́рно оде́тые карма́нные во́ры.

mob II *v* 1) окружа́ть толпо́й; 2) толпи́ться.

mobile ['moubaɪl] *a* 1) подвижнóй; 2) измéнчивый; гúбкий (*об уме*); 3) *воен.* мобúльный; лёгкий (*об артиллерии*); 4) манёвренный (*о войне*).

mobility [mou'bɪlɪtɪ] *n* 1) подвúжность; мобúльность; 2) измéнчивость, непостоянство.

mobilization [,moubɪlaɪ'zeɪʃən] *n* мобилизáция.

mobilize ['moubɪlaɪz] *v* мобилизовáть.

moccasin ['mɔkəsɪn] *n* мокасúн.

mocha ['moukə] *n* мóкко (*тж.* Mocha coffee).

mock I [mɔk] *a* 1) лóжный; мнúмый; притвóрный; 2) фальшúвый, поддéльный; имитúрующий; 3) инсценúрованный.

mock II *v* 1) насмехáть(ся) (*at*); высмéивать; 2) дразнúть; передрáзнивать; 3) обмáнывать (*надежды и т. п.*).

mocker ['mɔkə] *n* 1) насмéшник; 2) пересмéшник (*птица*).

mockery ['mɔkərɪ] *n* 1) осмеяние; насмéшка; издевáтельство; 2) посмéшище.

mocking-bird ['mɔkɪŋbəːd] *n* пересмéшник (*птица*).

mock-up ['mɔkʌp] *n* макéт, модéль.

modal ['moudl] *a* *грам.* модáльный.

mode [moud] *n* 1) вид, спóсоб, мéтод; 2) обычай; óбраз (дéйствий); ~ of life óбраз жúзни; 3) обычай, мóда; 4) *грам.* наклонéние; 5) *муз.* тонáльность.

model I ['mɔdl] *n* 1) модéль; 2) *разг.* тóчная кóпия; 3) образéц; 4) натýрщик, -ица; 5) манекéн; живáя модéль; 6) *attr* образцóвый, примéрный.

model II *v* 1) модéлировать; 2) создавáть по образцý (*after, on, upon*); 3) оформлять.

moderateᵃ I ['mɔdərɪt] *n* *полит.* оппортунúст; «умéренный».

moderateᵃ II *a* 1) умéренный; 2) воздéржанный; выдержанный (*о характере*); 3) срéдний, посрéдственный (*о качестве*); 4) *полит.* оппортунистúческий; «умéренный».

moderateᵇ ['mɔdəreɪt] *v* 1) умерять; смягчáть; сдéрживать; 2) становúться мягче, ровнéе; смягчáться; 3) затихáть, стихáть.

moderation [,mɔdə'reɪʃən] *n* 1) умéренность; in ~ умéренно; 2) воздержáние; 3) сдéрживание; 4) выдержка (*характера*); 5) *pl* пéрвый публúчный экзáмен на стéпень бакалáвра (*в Оксфорде*).

moderator ['mɔdəreɪtə] *n* 1) регулятор; 2) арбúтр; посрéдник; 3) экзаменáтор.

modern I ['mɔdən] *n* совремéнный человéк.

modern II *a* 1) совремéнный; 2) нóвый (*о языках, учении и т. п.*).

modernism ['mɔdənɪzəm] *n* модернúзм.

modernize ['mɔdənaɪz] *v* модернизúровать.

modest ['mɔdɪst] *a* 1) скрóмный; 2) умéренный.

modesty ['mɔdɪstɪ] *n* 1) скрóмность; 2) умéренность.

modification [,mɔdɪfɪ'keɪʃən] *n* 1) (видо)изменéние; 2) *лингв.* перегласóвка, умляут.

modify ['mɔdɪfaɪ] *v* 1) (видо)изменять; 2) смягчáть; 3) *грам.* определять; 4) *лингв.* смягчáть умляутом.

modish ['moudɪʃ] *a* мóдный.

modulate ['mɔdjuleɪt] *v* модулúровать.

modulation [,mɔdju'leɪʃən] *n* модуляция.

Mogul I [mou'gʌl] *n* монгóл; the Great (*или* Grand) ~ *ист.* Велúкий Могóл.

Mogul II *a* монгóльский.

mohair ['mouhɛə] *n* 1) ангóрская шерсть; 2) *текст.* мóгер, мохéр.

Mohammedan I [mou'hæmɪdən] *n* магометáнин; магометáнка.

Mohammedan II *a* магометáнский.

Mohican ['mouɪkən] *n* могикáнин.

moiety ['mɔɪətɪ] *n* *юр.* половúна.

moil I [mɔɪl] *n* тяжёлая, изнурúтельная рабóта; *перен.* мучéние, мýка.

moil II *v* выполнять тяжёлую рабóту (*тж.* to toil and ~).

moire [mwɑ:] *n* муáр (*ткань*).

moiré ['mwɑːreɪ] *a* муáровый.

moist [mɔɪst] *a* 1) сырóй, влáжный; мокровáтый; 2) дождлúвый.

moisten ['mɔɪsn] *v* смáчивать; увлажнять(ся).

moisture ['mɔɪstʃə] *n* влáга, сырость; влáжность.

molar I ['moulə] *n* кореннóй зуб.

molar II *a* коренной (*о зубе*).

molasses [mə'læsɪz] *n* пáтока, мелáсса.

mold [mould] *см.* mould.

Moldavian I [mɔl'deɪvjən] *n* 1) молдавáнин; молдавáнка; the ~s молдавáне; 2) молдáвский язык.

Moldavian II *a* молдáвский.

molder ['mouldə] *см.* moulder.

molding ['mouldɪŋ] *см.* moulding.

moldy ['mouldɪ] *см.* mouldy.

mole¹ [moul] *n* рóдинка.

mole² *n* 1) крот; 2) *attr* кротóвый.

mole³ *n* 1) мол; 2) дáмба.

molecular [mou'lekjulə] *a* молекулярный.

molecule ['mɔlɪkjuːl] *n* молéкула.

molehill ['moulhɪl] *n* кротóвина.

moleskin ['moulskɪn] *n* 1) кротóвый мех; 2) *текст.* молескúн.

molest [mou'lest] *v* приставáть, досаждáть.

molestation [,moules'teɪʃən] *n* приставáние.

mollification [,mɔlɪfɪ'keɪʃən] *n* успокоéние, смягчéние.

mollify ['mɔlɪfaɪ] *v* успокáивать, смягчáть.

mollusc ['mɔləsk] *n* моллюск.

mollusk ['mɔləsk] *см.* mollusc.

molly-coddle I ['mɔlɪkɔdl] *n* нéженка.

molly-coddle II *v* нéжить, баловáть.

molten ['moultən] *a* 1) литóй; 2) расплáвленный.

moment ['moumənt] *n* 1) момéнт; миг, мгновéние; at any ~ в любóе врéмя, всегдá; at the ~ в настоящее врéмя, сейчáс; at that ~ в то врéмя, тогдá; at odd ~s в свобóдное врéмя, мéжду дéлом; in a ~ в одúн миг, óчень скóро; one ~, half a ~ сейчáс, сию минýту; the ~ (that) как тóлько; this ~ а) немéдленно, тóтчас; б) тóлько что; to the ~ тóчно; 2) вáжность; of great ~ вáжный; of no ~ невáжный.

momenta [mou'mentə] *pl см.* momentum.

momentary ['mouməntərɪ] *a* 1) момéнтáльный, мгновéнный; 2) преходящий; кратковрéменный.

momently ['moumantlɪ] *adv* 1) с минýты на минýту; 2) ежеминýтно; 3) на мгновéние.

momentous [mou'mentəs] *a* вáжный; имéющий большóе значéние (*в настоящий момент*).

momentum [mou'mentəm] *n* (*pl* momenta) 1) движущая сила; импульс, толчок; 2) *физ., мех.* количество движения; инерция; скорость движения.

monarch ['mɔnək] *n* монарх; *перен.* царь.

monarchic(al) [mɔ'nɑːkɪk(əl)] *a* монархический.

monarchist ['mɔnəkɪst] *n* монархист.

monarchy ['mɔnəkɪ] *n* монархия; constitutional ~, limited ~ конституционная, ограниченная монархия.

monastery ['mɔnəstərɪ] *n* монастырь (*мужской*).

monastic I [mə'næstɪk] *n* монах.

monastic II *a* 1) монашеский; 2) монастырский.

Monday ['mʌndɪ] *n* понедельник; Black ~ *шк.* первый день после каникул.

monetary ['mʌnɪtərɪ] *a* 1) денежный; 2) монетный.

money ['mʌnɪ] *n* 1) деньги; ~ of account расчётная денежная единица; good ~ высокая ставка, высокая заработная плата; even ~ круглая сумма; ready ~ наличные деньги; odd ~ сдача; остаток; hot ~ а) деньги, добытые нечестным путём; б) «горячие» деньги (*капитал, вывозимый за границу из опасения его обесценения, налогового обложения и т. п.*); to make ~ заработать деньги; разбогатеть; to coin ~ быстро разбогатеть; to put ~ into вкладывать деньги в; to put ~ aside, to save ~ откладывать, копить деньги; to put ~ on делать ставку, ставить на (*лошадь*); to raise ~ добывать деньги; 2) *attr* денежный; финансовый; ◇ for my ~ ... на мой взгляд..., насколько я понимаю...

money-bag ['mʌnɪbæg] *n* 1) мешок для денег; 2) денежный мешок, богач; 3) *pl* богатство.

money-box ['mʌnɪbɔks] *n* копилка.

money-grubber ['mʌnɪˌgrʌbə] *n* стяжатель; скряга.

money-lender ['mʌnɪˌlendə] *n* ростовщик.

monger ['mʌŋgə] *n* торговец (*обыкн. в сложных словах*); ironmonger торговец железом; fishmonger торговец рыбой.

Mongol I ['mɔŋgɔl] *n* монгол; монголка; the ~s монголы.

Mongol II *a* монгольский.

Mongolian [mɔŋ'gouljən] *n* 1) *см.* Mongol I; 2) монгольский язык.

mongoose ['mɔŋguːs] *n* *зоол.* мангуста.

mongrel I ['mʌŋgrəl] *n* дворняжка; 2) помесь.

mongrel II *a* нечистокровный.

monitor ['mɔnɪtə] *n* 1) старший ученик, наблюдающий за порядком в младшем классе; староста в классе; 2) наставник; советчик; 3) *тех.* монитор; корректирующее *или* управляющее устройство.

monk [mʌŋk] *n* монах.

monkey I ['mʌŋkɪ] *n* 1) обезьяна; 2) *шутл.* шалун, баловник; 3) *сленг* 500 фунтов стерлингов; *амер.* 500 долларов; ◇ to put his ~ up разозлить кого-л.; to get one's ~ up разозлиться; to play ~ валять дурака.

monkey II *v* 1) передразнивать; подшучивать; 2) дурачиться.

monkey-business ['mʌŋkɪˌbɪznɪs] *n* *разг.* бессмысленная, бесполезная работа.

monkeyish ['mʌŋkɪʃ] *a* 1) обезьяний; 2) шаловливый.

monkey-wrench ['mʌŋkɪrentʃ] *n* раздвижной гаечный ключ.

monkish ['mʌŋkɪʃ] *a* монашеский.

mono- ['mɔnə-] *pref* со значением одно-, моно-; monobasic *хим.* одноосновный; monoplane моноплан.

monocle ['mɔnɔkl] *n* монокль.

monogamy [mə'nɔgəmɪ] *n* единобрачие.

monogram ['mɔnəgræm] *n* монограмма.

monograph ['mɔnəgrɑːf] *n* монография.

monolithic [ˌmɔnou'lɪθɪk] *a* монолитный.

monologue ['mɔnələg] *n* монолог.

monoplane ['mɔnəpleɪn] *n* моноплан.

monopolist [mə'nɔpəlɪst] *n* 1) монополист; 2) сторонник системы монополий; 3) *attr* монополистический.

monopolization [məˌnɔpəlaɪ'zeɪʃən] *n* монополизация.

monopolize [mə'nɔpəlaɪz] *v* монополизировать.

monopoly [mə'nɔpəlɪ] *n* 1) монополия; 2) *attr* монопольный.

monosyllabic ['mɔnəsɪ'læbɪk] *a* односложный.

monosyllable ['mɔnəˌsɪləbl] *n* односложное слово.

monotone I ['mɔnətoun] *n* монотонность.

monotone II *v* монотонно читать, говорить, петь.

monotonous [mə'nɔtnəs] *a* монотонный; однообразный, скучный.

monotony [mə'nɔtnɪ] *n* монотонность; однообразие, скука.

monsoon [mɔn'suːn] *n* 1) муссон (*ветер*); 2) дождливый сезон.

monster I ['mɔnstə] *n* 1) чудовище; 2) урод.

monster II *a* исполинский, громадный.

monstrosity [mɔns'trɔsɪtɪ] *n* 1) чудовищность; 2) чудовище.

monstrous ['mɔnstrəs] *a* 1) чудовищный; 2) уродливый; 3) исполинский, громадный; 4) *разг.* нелепый, абсурдный.

montage [mɔn'tɑːʒ] *n* *кино* монтаж, монтирование.

month [mʌnθ] *n* месяц; this day ~ через месяц; ◇ a ~ of Sundays бесконечно долгий срок, никогда.

monthly I ['mʌnθlɪ] *n* ежемесячный журнал.

monthly II *a* (еже)месячный.

monthly III *adv* ежемесячно.

monument ['mɔnjumənt] *n* памятник, монумент.

monumental [ˌmɔnju'mentl] *a* 1) монументальный; 2) изумительный; 3) увековечивающий.

moo I [muː] *n* мычание.

moo II *v* мычать.

mood[1] [muːd] *n* настроение; расположение; in the ~ в настроении; расположенный (*что-л. делать*); in no ~ не в настроении; нерасположенный.

mood[2] *n* 1) *грам.* наклонение; 2) *муз.* тональность.

moody ['muːdɪ] *a* 1) неровный, непостоянный (*о характере*); 2) угрюмый, невесёлый; в плохом настроении.

moon I [muːn] *n* 1) луна, месяц; full ~ полнолуние; полная луна; half ~ полумесяц; new ~ новолуние; молодой месяц; mock ~ ложная луна; 2) *астр.* спутник; 3) лунный месяц; 4) *поэт.* *см.* month; ◇ to cry for the ~ желать невозмо́жного; once in a blue ~ о́чень ре́дко; в ко́и-то ве́ки; to cover with the ~ *сленг* спать под откры́тым не́бом в па́рке (*о безрабо́тных*); to shoot the ~ *сленг* но́чью съе́хать с кварти́ры, чтобы уклони́ться от упла́ты долго́в.

moon II *v* 1) дви́гаться, де́йствовать, как во сне (*тж.* to ~ about); 2) бесце́льно, бесполе́зно прово́дить вре́мя (*тж* to ~ away).

moonbeam ['mu:nbi:m] *n* луч луны́; полоса́ лу́нного све́та.

moon-blindness ['mu:n,blaɪndnɪs] *n мед.* кури́ная слепота́.

mooncalf ['mu:nkɑ:f] *n* дурачо́к.

moonlight ['mu:nlaɪt] *n* 1) лу́нный свет; 2) *attr* лу́нный, освещённый луно́й.

moonlit ['mu:nlɪt] *a* освещённый луно́й.

moonshine ['mu:nʃaɪn] *n* 1) лу́нный свет; 2) вздор; 3) *амер. разг.* самого́н.

moonshiner ['mun,ʃaɪnə] *n амер. разг.* 1) самого́нщик; 2) контрабанди́ст, ввозя́щий спирт.

moonship ['mu:nʃɪp] *n* косми́ческий кора́бль для полётов на Луну́.

moonstruck ['mu:nstrʌk] *a* поме́шанный, ненорма́льный.

Moor [muə] *n* 1) марокка́нец; 2) *ист.* мавр.

moor[1] [muə] *n* (боло́тистая) ме́стность, поро́сшая ве́реском.

moor[2] *v* прича́лить; пришвартова́ться.

moorings ['muərɪŋz] *n pl мор.* 1) мёртвые якоря́; 2) ме́сто стоя́нки.

Moorish ['muərɪʃ] *a* маврита́нский.

moorland ['muələnd] *n* ме́стность, поро́сшая ве́реском.

moot I [mu:t] *a* спо́рный.

moot II *v* ста́вить вопро́с на обсужде́ние, обсужда́ть.

mop[1] I [mɔp] *n* 1) шва́бра; 2) ко́смы (*воло́с*).

mop[1] II *v* 1) мыть пол шва́брой; подтира́ть; 2) вытира́ть (*слёзы, пот*); □ ~ up а) *разг.* пожира́ть, поглоща́ть; б) вытира́ть; осуша́ть; в) *разг.* уничтожа́ть, прика́нчивать; г) *воен.* очи́стить от неприя́теля.

mop[2] I *n*: ~s and mows грима́сы.

mop[2] II *v*: to ~ and mow грима́сничать.

mope I [moup] *n* 1) хандря́щий челове́к; 2) *pl* (the ~s) хандра́.

mope II *v* хандри́ть.

moped ['mouped] *n* велосипе́д с мото́ром.

mopish ['moupɪʃ] *a* уны́лый, хандря́щий.

moraine [mə'reɪn] *n геол.* море́на, леднико́вое отложе́ние.

moral I ['mɔrəl] *n* 1) мора́ль; 2) *pl* нра́вственность; нра́вы; ◊ the very ~ of *разг.* то́чная ко́пия, вы́литый портре́т.

moral II *a* 1) мора́льный; нра́вственный; 2) доброде́тельный; 3) нравоучи́тельный.

morale [mɔ'rɑ:l] *n* мора́льное состоя́ние.

moralist ['mɔrəlɪst] *n* 1) морали́ст; 2) доброде́тельный челове́к.

morality [mə'rælɪtɪ] *n* 1) мора́ль, э́тика; 2) нравоуче́ние; copy-book ~ прописна́я мора́ль; 3) *pl* нра́вственное поведе́ние.

moralize ['mɔrəlaɪz] *v* 1) морализи́ровать; 2) извлека́ть мора́ль, уро́к; 3) исправля́ть нра́вы.

morally ['mɔrəlɪ] *adv* 1) мора́льно; нра́вствен-

но; 2) в нра́вственном отноше́нии; 3) факти́чески, в су́щности.

morass [mə'ræs] *n* боло́то; тряси́на.

moratorium [,mɔrə'tɔ:rɪəm] *n* морато́рий.

morbid ['mɔːbɪd] *a* 1) боле́зненный; 2) патологи́ческий.

morbidity [mɔː'bɪdɪtɪ] *n* 1) боле́зненность; 2) заболева́емость.

mordant I ['mɔːdənt] *n* протра́ва.

mordant II *a* 1) е́дкий; разъеда́ющий; 2) ко́лкий, язви́тельный, саркасти́ческий.

more I [mɔː] *a* 1) (*compar см.* much II, many II) бо́льший; 2) ещё; two ~ ещё два; bring some ~ water принеси́те ещё воды́.

more II *adv* 1) (*compar см.* much III) бо́льше, бо́лее; the ~ the better чем бо́льше, тем лу́чше; the ~... the ~... чем бо́льше..., тем бо́льше...; the ~ he gets, the ~ he wants чем бо́льше он име́ет, тем бо́льше ему́ ну́жно; ~ or less а) бо́лее и́ли ме́нее; б) приблизи́тельно; he is no ~ его́ нет бо́льше, он у́мер; 2) *слу́жит для образова́ния сравн. ст. прил. и наре́чий:* ~ easily ле́гче; ~ truly верне́е, точне́е *и т. д.*; 3) опя́ть, сно́ва; ещё; once ~ ещё раз; never ~ никогда́; ◊ what is ~ что ещё важне́е; и вдоба́вок.

moreover [mɔː'rouvə] *adv* кро́ме того́, бо́лее того́.

morganatic [,mɔːgə'nætɪk] *a* морганати́ческий.

morgue [mɔːg] *n* морг.

moribund ['mɔrɪbʌnd] *a* умира́ющий; угаса́ющий.

morion ['mɔrɪən] *n ист.* шиша́к.

Mormon ['mɔːmən] *n* мормо́н; *перен.* многожёнец.

morn [mɔːn] *n поэт.* у́тро.

morning ['mɔːnɪŋ] *n* 1) у́тро; good ~ здра́вствуйте, с до́брым у́тром; 2) *поэт.* у́тренняя заря́; 3) *attr* у́тренний.

Morning Star ['mɔːnɪŋ'stɑː] *n* «Мо́рнинг стар» (*прогресси́вная англи́йская газе́та*).

morocco [mə'rɔkou] *n* 1) сафья́н; 2) *attr* сафья́новый.

moron ['mɔrən] *n* слабоу́мный.

morose [mə'rous] *a* мра́чный, угрю́мый.

morphia ['mɔːfjə] *см.* morphine.

morphine ['mɔːfiːn] *n* мо́рфий.

morphological [,mɔːfə'lɔdʒɪkəl] *a* морфологи́ческий.

morphology [mɔː'fɔlədʒɪ] *n* морфоло́гия.

morrow ['mɔrou] *n* 1) *уст.* у́тро; good ~ здра́вствуйте, с до́брым у́тром; 2) (the ~) сле́дующий день; on the ~ of... вслед за..., по́сле..., по оконча́нии...

morse [mɔːs] *n* морж.

morsel ['mɔːsəl] *n* кусо́чек.

mortal I ['mɔːtl] *n* сме́ртный, челове́к.

mortal II *a* 1) сме́ртный; 2) смерте́льный; 3) ужа́сный (*о бо́ли*); 4) *разг.* си́льный; ужа́сный; 5) *разг.* смерте́льно ску́чный.

mortality [mɔː'tælɪtɪ] *n* 1) сме́ртность; 2) смерте́льность; 3) *собир.* лю́ди, сме́ртные.

mortally ['mɔːtəlɪ] *adv* смерте́льно.

mortar I ['mɔːtə] *n* 1) известко́вый раство́р; 2) сту́пка; 3) *воен.* морти́ра; миномёт.

mortar II *v* скрепля́ть известко́вым раство́ром.

mortar-board ['mɔːtəbɔːd] *n* головно́й убо́р англи́йских профессоро́в и студе́нтов.

mortgage I ['mɔːgɪdʒ] *n* 1) заклад; 2) закладная.

mortgage II *v* 1) закладывать; 2) ручаться.

mortician [mɔ'tɪʃən] *n амер.* владелец похоронного бюро.

mortification [‚mɔːtɪfɪ'keɪʃən] *n* 1) унижение; обида; 2) подавление (*чувства*); умерщвление (*плоти*); 3) *мед.* омертвение.

mortify ['mɔːtɪfaɪ] *v* 1) унижать; обижать; 2) подавлять (*чувства, страсти и т. п.*); умерщвлять (*плоть*); 3) *мед.* омертветь.

mortuary I ['mɔːtjuərɪ] *n* морг, покойницкая.

mortuary II *a* похоронный.

mosaic I [mə'zeɪɪk] *n* мозаика.

mosaic II *a* мозаичный.

Moslem I ['mɔzlem] *n* мусульманин.

Moslem II *a* мусульманский.

mosque [mɔsk] *n* мечеть.

mosquito [məs'kiːtou] *n* 1) комар; москит; 2) *attr* противомоскитный.

mosquito-craft [məs'kiːtoukrɑːft] *n* торпедный катер; торпедные катера.

mosquito-fleet [məs'kiːtoufliːt] *n* «москитный» флот, торпедные катера.

moss I [mɔs] *n* 1) мох; 2) торфяник, торфяное болото.

moss II *v* зарастать мхом, быть покрытым мхом.

mossy ['mɔsɪ] *a* мшистый.

most I [moust] *a* (*superl см.* much II, many II) наибольший.

most II *adv* (*superl см.* much III) 1) больше всего; 2) *служит для образования превосх. ст. прил. и наречий:* ~ certain(ly) вне всякого сомнения; 3) очень, весьма; 4): ten at ~ не больше десяти; самое большее десять; this is at ~ a folly это не более чем глупость.

most III *n* большая часть; наибольшее количество; at the ~ самое большее; ~ of them большинство, большая часть из них; to make the ~ of использовать наилучшим образом.

mostly ['moustlɪ] *adv* большею частью, обычно, главным образом.

mote [mout] *n* пылинка.

motel [mou'tel] *n* мотель, гостиница для автомобилистов.

motet [mou'tet] *n* песнопение.

moth [mɔθ] *n* 1) моль; 2) мотылёк.

moth-eaten ['mɔθ‚iːtn] *a* изъеденный молью; *перен.* допотопный, устаревший.

mother[1] I ['mʌðə] *n* 1) мать; expectant ~ будущая мать, беременная женщина; new ~ *разг.* роженица, молодая мать; 2) инкубатор (*тж.* artificial ~); 3) *attr* родной (*о языке, стране*); 4) *attr* врождённый, природный.

mother[1] II *v* 1) усыновлять; заботиться как мать; 2) приписывать (авторство) кому-л.

mother[2] I *n* маточный раствор.

motherhood ['mʌðəhud] *n* материнство.

mother-in-law ['mʌðərɪnlɔː] *n* (*pl* mothers-in-law) тёща; свекровь.

motherland ['mʌðəlænd] *n* отечество, родина.

motherless ['mʌðəlɪs] *a* лишённый матери, без матери.

motherly ['mʌðəlɪ] *a* материнский.

mother-of-pearl I ['mʌðərəv'pəːl] *n* перламутр.

mother-of-pearl II *a* перламутровый.

motif [mou'tiːf] *n* основная идея, лейтмотив.

motion I ['mouʃən] *n* 1) движение; ход; seesaw ~ колебательное движение; to set (*или* to put) in ~ приводить в движение; 2) телодвижение, жест; 3) побуждение; of one's own ~ по собственному побуждению, добровольно; 4) предложение (*на собрании*); to bring forward a ~ вносить предложение; to carry (to reject) the ~ принять (отклонить) предложение; 5) *юр.* запрос в суд.

motion II *v* показывать жестом.

motional ['mouʃənl] *a* двигательный; движущий.

motionless ['mouʃənlɪs] *a* неподвижный; без движения.

motion-picture ['mouʃən'pɪktʃə] *n* кинокартина; фильм; кино.

motivate ['moutɪveɪt] *v* 1) побуждать; 2) служить поводом; 3) мотивировать.

motive I ['moutɪv] *n* 1) мотив, побуждение, повод; 2) *см.* motif.

motive II *a* 1) движущий; 2) двигательный.

motive III *v см.* motivate.

motiveless ['moutɪvlɪs] *a* не имеющий основания, беспочвенный.

motley I ['mɔtlɪ] *n* 1) невозможная смесь; 2) *ист.* шутовской костюм; to wear the ~ быть шутом.

motley II *a* разноцветный; пёстрый.

motor I ['moutə] *n* 1) мотор; to cut the ~ *разг.* заглушить мотор; выключить мотор (*автомашины*); 2) двигатель (*внутреннего сгорания*); 3) автомобиль; 4) *анат.* двигательный мускул; двигательный нерв.

motor II *a* 1) двигательный; 2) моторный.

motor III *v* ехать, везти на автомобиле.

motorcade ['moutəkeɪd] *n разг.* вереница, кортеж автомобилей.

motor-car ['moutəkɑː] *n* 1) легковой автомобиль; 2) *амер.* моторный вагон.

motor-cycle ['moutə‚saɪkl] *n* мотоцикл.

motoring ['moutərɪŋ] *n* 1) автомобильное дело; 2) автомобильный спорт.

motorist ['moutərɪst] *n* автомобилист.

motorize ['moutəraɪz] *v* моторизировать.

motorman ['moutəmən] *n* 1) (вагоно)вожатый; 2) машинист.

mottle I ['mɔtl] *n* крапинка.

mottle II *v* испещрять.

mottled ['mɔtld] *a* 1) крапчатый; 2) покрытый пятнами; испещрённый.

motto ['mɔtou] *n* 1) девиз; 2) эпиграф.

mould[1] I [mould] *n* 1) почва; 2) взрыхлённая земля; 3) *поэт.* прах; man of ~ простой смертный.

mould[1] II *v* рыхлить, насыпать землю; ▫ to ~ up окучивать.

mould[2] I *n* 1) (литейная) форма; шаблон; 2) формочка (*для пудинга и т. п.*); 3) отливка; 4) склад характера; ◊ cast in the same ~ одинаковый, похожий, такой же; cast in a different ~ непохожий, совсем другой.

mould[2] II *v* 1) формовать; отливать в форму; 2) делать по шаблону; создавать по образцу (*on, upon*); 3) формировать характер; 4) превращать в (*into*).

mould[3] I *n* плесень.

mould[3] II *v* плесневеть.

moulder[1] ['mouldə] *v* рассыпаться, разрушаться, разлагаться (*тж. перен.; часто* to ~ away).

moulder² *n* литейщик; формовщик; *перен.* создатель, творец.

moulding ['mouldɪŋ] *n* 1) отливка; 2) обыкн. *pl* архит. лепное украшение; 3) багет, лепная рама.

mouldy ['mouldɪ] *a* 1) заплесневелый; *перен.* устарелый; to go ~ заплесневеть; 2) *разг.* скучный, утомительный.

moult I [moult] *n* линька.

moult II *v* линять (*о птицах*).

mound¹ [maund] *n* насыпь; холм; курган; могильный холм.

mound² *n* держава (*эмблема*).

mount¹ I [maunt] *n* гора, холм.

mount¹ II *v* 1) подниматься; повышаться; 2) всходить, влезать; 3) приливать к лицу (*о крови*).

mount² I *n* верховая лошадь.

mount² II *v* 1) садиться, сажать верхом; садиться (*в машину*); 2) снабжать верховыми лошадьми.

mount³ I *n.* 1) установка, монтирование; 2) оправа (*камня и т. п.*).

mount³ II *v* 1) устанавливать, монтировать; 2) оправлять, вставлять в оправу, в раму; 3) оформлять (*спектакль*); 4) набивать (*чучело*).

mountain ['mauntɪn] *n* 1) гора; 2) масса, множество; 3) *attr* (на)горный; ◊ to remove ~s сдвинуть гору, сделать чудо; to make ~s out of mole-hills *посл.* ≅ делать из мухи слона.

mountaineer [,mauntɪ'nɪə] *n* 1) горец; 2) альпинист.

mountaineering [,mauntɪ'nɪərɪŋ] *n* альпинизм.

mountainous ['mauntɪnəs] *a* 1) гористый; 2) громадный.

mountain-range ['mauntɪnreɪndʒ] *n* горная цепь.

mountebank ['mauntɪbæŋk] *n* шарлатан.

mounted ['mauntɪd] *a* верховой, конный.

mounting¹ ['mauntɪŋ] *n* 1) установка, монтаж; 2) оправа; 3) набивка (*чучела*).

mounting² *n* посадка на лошадь, в машину.

mourn [mɔːn] *v* оплакивать; грустить.

mourner ['mɔːnə] *n* 1) присутствующий на похоронах; 2) плакальщик.

mournful ['mɔːnful] *a* печальный; мрачный; траурный.

mourning ['mɔːnɪŋ] *n* 1) траур; to go into ~ надеть траур; in ~ а) в трауре; б) подбитый (*о глазе*); в) грязный (*о ногтях*); 2) *attr* траурный.

mouseᵃ [maus] *n* (*pl* mice) мышь; harvest ~ полевая мышь.

mouseᵇ [mauz] *v* 1) ловить мышей; 2) выслеживать.

mousetrap ['maustræp] *n* мышеловка.

moustache [məs'tɑːʃ] *n* усы.

mouthᵃ [mauθ] *n* 1) рот; уста; by ~ устно; from ~ to ~ из уст в уста; hold your ~! *груб.* замолчи!, заткнись!; 2) едок (*входное, выходное*) отверстие; 4) устье (*реки*); 5) гримаса; 6) *сленг* нахальство; ◊ hard ~ тугоуздая лошадь; to flap one's ~ болтать; down in the ~ в унынии, в плохом настроении; to give ~ давать голос (*о собаке*); to open one's ~ wide заломить цену.

mouthᵇ [mauð] *v* 1) изрекать, торжественно говорить; 2) брать в рот; 3) впадать (*о реке*); 4) гримасничать; 5) приучать лошадь к узде.

mouthful ['mauθful] *n* кусок (*который можно взять в рот за один раз*); глоток; ◊ to say a ~ сказать что-л. важное.

mouth-organ ['mauθ,ɔːgən] *n* губная гармоника.

mouthpiece ['mauθpiːs] *n* 1) мундштук; 2) глашатай; выразитель (*мнения, интересов партии, класса и т. п.*).

movable ['muːvəbl] *a* 1) подвижной; передвижной; 2) движимый (*об имуществе*).

movables ['muːvəblz] *n pl* движимость, движимое имущество.

move I [muːv] *n* 1) ход (*в игре*); 2) движение, действие; *перен.* поступок; шаг; on the ~ а) на ходу; б) в движении, в развитии; to make a ~ а) отправляться; б) предпринимать что-л.; в) вставать из-за стола; to get a ~ on *разг.* торопиться, спешить; 3) переезд (*на другую квартиру*).

move II *v* 1) двигать(ся), передвигать(ся); 2) перевозить, переезжать; 3) вращаться (*в обществе*); 4) (рас)трогать; вызывать (*смех, гнев и т. п.*); 5) побуждать; 6) вносить (*предложение*); 7) расти; развиваться; 8) действовать, предпринимать (*что-л.*); nobody seems willing to in the matter никто не хочет вмешиваться в дело; □ to ~ **about,** to ~ **away** переходить, переезжать с места на место; to ~ **back** пятиться; идти задним ходом; to ~ **down** опускать, спускать; to ~ **in** а) въезжать (*куда-л.*); б) вдвигать; to ~ **off** отодвигать; to ~ **on** а) предложить уйти, пройти; б) переменить положение (*тела*); to ~ **out** а) выводить; выдвигать; б) выезжать (*из дома, квартиры*); to ~ **up** а) пододвигать; б) подтягивать(ся).

moveless ['muːvlɪs] *a* неподвижный.

movement ['muːvmənt] *n* 1) движение; in and out ~ возвратно-поступательное движение; spontaneous ~ порыв; 2) передвижение; 3) *ком.* оживление; 4) переезд; 5) ход (*машины, механизма*); 6) *муз.* темп, ритм.

mover ['muːvə] *n* 1) двигатель; движущая сила; 2) инициатор; автор.

movies ['muːvɪz] *n pl разг.* кино.

moving ['muːvɪŋ] *a* 1) движущий(ся); 2) трогательный, волнующий.

mowᵃ I [mou] *n* 1) стог, скирда; 2) сеновал.

mowᵃ II *v* (*past* mowed; *p. p.* mowed, mown) косить; □ to ~ **down,** to ~ **off** скашивать, выкашивать.

mowᵇ I [mau] *n* гримаса.

mowᵇ II *v* гримасничать.

mower ['mouə] *n* 1) косец, косарь; 2) (сено)косилка, жнейка.

mown [moun] *p. p. см.* mow ᵃ II.

Mr ['mɪstə] *сокр. см.* mister.

Mrs ['mɪsɪz] *сокр. см.* mistress.

much I [mʌtʃ] *n* многое; to make ~ of быть высокого мнения о, ценить; носиться с кем-л., чем-л.; not ~ of a... плохой, неважный; not ~ of a painter плохой художник; not ~ of a hat неважная шляпа; с позволения сказать, шляпа.

much II *a* (*compar* more; *superl* most) 1) много; how ~? а) сколько?; б) какая цена?; сколько стоит?; 2) большой; to be too ~ for быть не по силам; half as ~ в полтора раза больше.

much III *adv* (*compar* more; *superl* most) 1) очень; 2) почти; ~ of a size (height *etc*) почти того же разме́ра (той же высоты́ *и т. п.*); I thought as ~ я так и ду́мал, я э́того и ожида́л; 3) мно́го, гора́здо, бо́льше (*служит для усиления сравн. ст.*); ~ better гора́здо, мно́го лу́чше; ◊ as ~ as to say как бы жела́я сказа́ть.

mucilage ['mjuːsɪlɪdʒ] *n* 1) слизь; 2) кле́йкое вещество́ (*растений*); расти́тельный клей.

muck I [mʌk] *n* 1) наво́з; 2) грязь; 3) *разг.* ме́рзость.

muck II *v* 1) унаво́живать; 2) па́чкать, грязни́ть; □ to ~ **about** *сленг* слоня́ться; to ~ **up** *разг.* испо́ртить.

mucker ['mʌkə] *n сленг* 1) тяжёлое паде́ние; *перен.* больша́я неуда́ча; to come a ~ попа́сть в беду́; to go a ~ сли́шком мно́го истра́тить; 2) непоря́дочный, нече́стный челове́к.

muck-rake ['mʌkreɪk] *n* 1) гра́бли для наво́за; 2) люби́тель гря́зных спле́тен.

muckworm ['mʌkwəːm] *n* 1) наво́зный червь; 2) стяжа́тель.

mucous ['mjuːkəs] *a* сли́зистый.

mucus ['mjuːkəs] *n* слизь.

mud [mʌd] *n* грязь, сля́коть; to stick in the ~ завя́знуть; *перен.* отста́ть от жи́зни.

muddle I ['mʌdl] *n* беспоря́док; пу́таница; to make a ~ of спу́тать, перепу́тать (*что-л.*).

muddle II *v* 1) пу́тать, вноси́ть беспоря́док (*тж.* to ~ up, to ~ together); 2) неуме́ло рабо́тать, де́лать кое-ка́к; 3) опьяня́ть, одурма́нивать; □ to ~ **away** зря тра́тить; to ~ **on** де́йствовать наобу́м, без пла́на; to ~ **through** кое-ка́к довести́ де́ло до конца́.

muddle-headed ['mʌdl,hedɪd] *a* глу́пый, тупо́й, бестолко́вый.

muddy I ['mʌdɪ] *a* 1) гря́зный, в грязи́, запа́чканный; 2) му́тный; ту́склый; 3) помути́вшийся (*о рассудке*); 4) хри́плый (*о голосе*).

muddy II *v* 1) па́чкать в грязи́, забры́згивать гря́зью; 2) (за)мути́ть.

mudguard ['mʌdgɑːd] *n* крыло́, щито́к от гря́зи (*у автомобиля*).

muff[1] [mʌf] *n* му́фта.

muff[2] I *n* 1) нело́вкий, неуклю́жий челове́к; «шля́па»; 2) про́мах.

muff[2] II *v* промахну́ться, прома́зать.

muffin ['mʌfɪn] *n* кру́глая бу́лочка.

muffle ['mʌfl] *v* 1) заку́тывать, уку́тывать (*часто* to ~ up); 2) заглуша́ть, подавля́ть (*крик и т. п.*).

muffler ['mʌflə] *n* 1) шарф, кашне́; 2) *тех.* глуши́тель; 3) *муз.* сурди́нка; 4) боксёрская перча́тка.

mufti ['mʌftɪ] *n* шта́тское пла́тье; in ~ не в фо́рме, в шта́тском.

mug[1] [mʌg] *n* 1) кру́жка; 2) *сленг* мо́рда; рот.

mug[2] *n разг.* проста́к, новичо́к.

mug[3] I *n сленг* зубри́ла.

mug[3] II *v сленг* зубри́ть.

mug[4] *v сленг* грима́сничать.

muggy ['mʌgɪ] *a* тёплый, вла́жный (*о погоде*); удушли́вый, спёртый (*о воздухе*).

mulatto I [mjuːˈlætou] *n* мула́т(ка).

mulatto II *a* оли́вковый, сму́глый.

mulberry ['mʌlbərɪ] *n* 1) *бот.* шелкови́ца; 2) *attr* тёмно-кра́сный.

mulch I [mʌlʃ] *n с.-х.* му́льча.

mulch II *v с.-х.* мульчи́ровать.

mulct I [mʌlkt] *n* штраф.

mulct II *v* 1) штрафова́ть; 2) отнима́ть; лиша́ть (*чего-л.* — of).

mule[1] [mjuːl] *n* 1) мул; 2) тупи́ца, осёл; упря́мец; 3) гибри́д, по́месь.

mule[2] *n* дома́шняя ту́фля без за́дника.

muleteer [,mjuːlɪˈtɪə] *n* пого́нщик му́лов.

mulish ['mjuːlɪʃ] *a* упря́мый (как осёл).

mull[1] I [mʌl] *n* пу́таница.

mull[1] II *v* пу́тать, спу́тать.

mull[2] *v амер. разг.* обду́мывать, размышля́ть; «мере́кать».

mull[3] *n текст.* мусли́н.

mull[4] *v* подогрева́ть вино́ с пря́ностями.

mullet ['mʌlɪt] *n*: red ~ барабу́лька (*рыба*); grey ~ кефа́ль (*рыба*).

multi- ['mʌltɪ-] *pref со значением* много-; multicellular *биол.* многокле́точный.

multiengined ['mʌltɪ'endʒɪnd] *a* многомото́рный.

multifarious [,mʌltɪˈfɛərɪəs] *a* разнообра́зный.

multiform ['mʌltɪfɔːm] *a* многообра́зный.

multiman ['mʌltɪmən] *a* многоме́стный.

multimillionaire ['mʌltɪmɪljəˈnɛə] *n* мультимиллионе́р.

multinomial [,mʌltɪˈnoumɪəl] *n мат.* многочле́н.

multiple I ['mʌltɪpl] *n мат.* кра́тное число́; least common ~ о́бщее наиме́ньшее кра́тное.

multiple II *a* 1) многочи́сленный; многокра́тный; 2) составно́й; соединённый; 3) *мат.* кра́тный.

multiplex ['mʌltɪpleks] *a* 1) сло́жный; 2) многокра́тный.

multiplicand [,mʌltɪplɪˈkænd] *n мат.* мно́жимое.

multiplication [,mʌltɪplɪˈkeɪʃən] *n* 1) *мат.* умноже́ние; 2) увеличе́ние.

multiplicity [,mʌltɪˈplɪsɪtɪ] *n* разнообра́зие; сло́жность; the ~ of многочи́сленность.

multiplier ['mʌltɪplaɪə] *n* мно́житель, коэффицие́нт.

multiply ['mʌltɪplaɪ] *v* 1) увели́чивать(ся); 2) размножа́ть(ся); 3) *мат.* умножа́ть, мно́жить.

multitude ['mʌltɪtjuːd] *n* 1) мно́жество; большо́е число́; 2) толпа́; the ~ ма́ссы.

multitudinous [,mʌltɪˈtjuːdɪnəs] *a* многочи́сленный.

mum[1] I [mʌm] *a predic* молчали́вый; to keep ~ молча́ть, пома́лкивать; to sit ~ сиде́ть мо́лча.

mum[1] II *int* тс!, ти́ше!; ~'s the word! пома́лкивай!

mum[1] III *v* игра́ть в пантоми́ме.

mum[2] *n разг.* ма́ма.

mumble I ['mʌmbl] *n* ша́мканье, бормота́ние.

mumble II *v* 1) бормота́ть, ша́мкать; 2) с трудо́м жева́ть.

mummery ['mʌmərɪ] *n* 1) пантоми́ма; 2) *презр.* «представле́ние», «спекта́кль».

mummify ['mʌmɪfaɪ] *v* 1) превраща́ть в му́мию; 2) высу́шивать; смо́рщивать(ся).

mummy[1] ['mʌmɪ] *n* 1) му́мия; 2) му́мия (*кори́чневая краска*).

mummy[2] *n* ма́ма.

mumps [mʌmps] *n* 1) сви́нка (*болезнь*); 2) хандра́; плохо́е настрое́ние.

munch [mʌntʃ] *v* ча́вкать.

mundane ['mʌndeɪn] *a* све́тский, мирско́й; земно́й.

municipal [mjuːˈnɪsɪpəl] *a* 1) муниципа́льный, городско́й, коммуна́льный; 2) самоуправля́ющийся.

municipality [mjuːˌnɪsɪˈpælɪtɪ] *n* 1) го́род, месте́чко с самоуправле́нием; 2) муниципалите́т.

munificence [mjuːˈnɪfɪsns] *n* ще́дрость.

munificent [mjuːˈnɪfɪsnt] *a* ще́дрый.

munition I [mjuːˈnɪʃən] *n обыкн. pl* вое́нные запа́сы; снаряже́ние.

munition II *v* снабжа́ть а́рмию.

mural I [ˈmjuərəl] *n* стенна́я жи́вопись, фре́ска.

mural II *a* стенно́й.

murder I [ˈmɜːdə] *n* (преднаме́ренное) уби́йство; judicial ~ юриди́ческое уби́йство; суде́бная оши́бка; ◇ to cry (blue) ~ подня́ть трево́гу; завопи́ть; ~ will out *посл.* ≅ ши́ла в мешке́ не утаи́шь.

murder II *v* 1) убива́ть, соверша́ть уби́йство; 2) губи́ть, кове́ркать.

murderer [ˈmɜːdərə] *n* уби́йца.

murderous [ˈmɜːdərəs] *a* 1) уби́йственный; смертоно́сный; 2) крова́вый, кровожа́дный.

murk I [mɜːk] *n поэт.* темнота́, мрак.

murk II *a поэт.* тёмный, мра́чный.

murky [ˈmɜːkɪ] *a* тёмный, су́мрачный; па́смурный.

murmur I [ˈmɜːmə] *n* 1) журча́ние; шо́рох; жужжа́ние; 2) приглушённые голоса́; шёпот; 3) ворча́ние.

murmur II *v* 1) журча́ть; шелесте́ть; жужжа́ть; 2) шепта́ть; 3) ворча́ть, ропта́ть (*на — at, against*).

murrain [ˈmʌrɪn] *n* чума́ (рога́того скота́).

muscle [ˈmʌsl] *n* 1) му́скул; мы́шца; facial ~ лицево́й му́скул; 2) (физи́ческая) си́ла.

Muscovite I [ˈmʌskəvaɪt] *n* 1) москви́ч(ка); 2) *уст.* ру́сский.

Muscovite II *a уст.* ру́сский.

muscular [ˈmʌskjulə] *a* 1) му́скульный; 2) му́скулистый.

muse¹ [mjuːz] *n* (the ~) му́за.

muse² I *n уст.* заду́мчивость.

muse² II *v* 1) мечта́ть; заду́мываться, размышля́ть (*над — on, upon, over*); 2) мечта́тельно смотре́ть (*на — on*).

museum [mjuːˈzɪəm] *n* музе́й.

mush [mʌʃ] *n* 1) мя́коть; ка́шица; 2) *амер.* ка́ша.

mushroom I [ˈmʌʃrum] *n* 1) гриб; 2) бы́стрый рост, разви́тие; 3) *attr* грибно́й; 4) *attr* быстрорасту́щий.

mushroom II *v* 1) собира́ть грибы́; 2) *амер.* бы́стро расти́; 3) *амер.* распространя́ться (*об огне́*).

music [ˈmjuːzɪk] *n* 1) му́зыка; to set to ~ положи́ть на му́зыку; 2) но́ты; 3) *уст.* орке́стр; ◇ to face the ~ безбоя́зненно встре́тить кри́тику, тру́дности, не дро́гнуть.

musical [ˈmjuːzɪkəl] *a* 1) музыка́льный; 2) мелоди́чный.

musician [mjuːˈzɪʃən] *n* 1) музыка́нт; 2) компози́тор.

musing [ˈmjuːzɪŋ] *n* заду́мчивость, мечта́тельность; глубо́кое разду́мье.

musk [mʌsk] *n* 1) му́скус; 2) за́пах му́скуса; 3) *attr* му́скусный.

muskeg [ˈmʌskeg] *n* торфяно́е боло́то; топь.

musket [ˈmʌskɪt] *n ист.* мушке́т.

musketeer [ˌmʌskɪˈtɪə] *n ист.* мушкетёр.

musketry [ˈmʌskɪtrɪ] *n* 1) руже́йный ого́нь; 2) стрелко́вое де́ло.

musk-rat [ˈmʌskræt] *n зоол.* онда́тра.

Muslim I, II [ˈmʌslɪm] *см.* Moslem I, II.

muslin [ˈmʌzlɪn] *n* 1) кисея́; a bit of ~ *разг.* же́нщина, де́вушка; 2) *амер.* миткаль.

musquash [ˈmʌskwɔʃ] *см.* musk-rat.

muss I [mʌs] *n амер. разг.* пу́таница, беспоря́док.

muss II *v амер. разг.* приводи́ть в беспоря́док, пу́тать (*обыкн.* to ~ up).

mussel [ˈmʌsl] *n* двуство́рчатая ра́ковина.

Mussulman I [ˈmʌslmən] *n* (*pl* Mussulmans) мусульма́нин.

Mussulman II *a* мусульма́нский.

must¹ [mʌst] *v* (*past* must) *модальный гл.*, входя́щий в соста́в сло́жного мода́льного сказу́емого 1) до́лжен, обя́зан (*после́дующий смыслово́й гл. употр. без части́цы* to: you ~ study well вы должны́ хорошо́ учи́ться; *отриц. и вопр. фо́рмы употр. без гл.* to do: ~ you go to the library? No, I ~ not вы должны́ идти́ в библиоте́ку? — Нет, не до́лжен); 1) *выража́ет обяза́нность*: I ~ keep my promise я до́лжен вы́полнить своё обеща́ние; you ~ have known quite well what I meant вы прекра́сно зна́ли, что я хоте́л сказа́ть; 2) *ука́зывает на неизбе́жность*: all men ~ die все лю́ди сме́ртны; 3) *выража́ет необходи́мость*: one ~ eat to live чтобы жить, ну́жно есть; I ~ away я до́лжен е́хать, отправля́ться; we ~ see what can be done посмо́трим, что мо́жно сде́лать; you ~ know до́лжен вам сказа́ть; I ~ ask you for your name позво́льте узна́ть ва́шу фами́лию; 4) *выража́ет уве́ренность, ука́зывает на очеви́дность*: one ~ be crazy to talk so на́до быть сумасше́дшим, чтобы так говори́ть; you ~ have heard about it вы, вероя́тно, об э́том слы́шали; you ~ have caught the train if you had run вы бы успе́ли на по́езд, е́сли бы побежа́ли; 5) *ука́зывает на доса́дную случа́йность*: just as I was busiest, he ~ come worrying me! и на́до же бы́ло ему́ помеша́ть мне в то вре́мя, когда́ я был так за́нят!

must² *n* пле́сень.

mustache [məsˈtɑːʃ] *см.* moustache.

mustachioed [məsˈtɑːʃɪəd] *a* уса́тый.

mustang [ˈmʌstæŋ] *n* муста́нг.

mustard [ˈmʌstəd] *n* 1) горчи́ца; 2) *attr* горчи́чный.

muster I [ˈmʌstə] *n* смотр, осмо́тр, перекли́чка; to pass ~ оказа́ться го́дным, вы́держать испыта́ние.

muster II *v* собира́ть(ся).

muster-roll [ˈmʌstəˈroul] *n воен.* спи́сок ли́чного соста́ва.

mustn't [ˈmʌsnt] *разг.* = must not.

musty [ˈmʌstɪ] *a* 1) заплёсневелый; за́тхлый; 2) устаре́лый, ко́сный.

mutable [ˈmjuːtəbl] *a* изме́нчивый, переме́нчивый.

mutation [mjuːˈteɪʃən] *n* 1) измене́ние; 2) превра́тность; 3) *биол.* мута́ция; 4) *фон.* перегласо́вка; умля́ут.

mute I [mjuːt] *n* 1) немо́й (челове́к); 2) *фон.* взрывно́й согла́сный; 3) *театр.* стати́ст; 4) фа́кельщик (*похоро́нной проце́ссии*); 5) *муз.* сурди́нка.

mute II *a* 1) немо́й; 2) безмо́лвный, молчали́вый;

3) *фон.* взрывной (*о согласном*); непроизносимый (*о букве*).

mute III *v муз.* надевать сурдинку; with ~d strings под сурдинку.

mutilate ['mjuːtɪleɪt] *v* 1) калечить, увечить; 2) портить; искажать (*смысл*).

mutilation [ˌmjuːtɪ'leɪʃən] *n* 1) увечье; 2) искажение.

mutineer [ˌmjuːtɪ'nɪə] *n* мятежник.

mutinous ['mjuːtɪnəs] *a* мятежный.

mutiny I ['mjuːtɪnɪ] *n* мятеж; восстание.

mutiny II *v* поднять мятеж; восстать, взбунтоваться.

mutter I ['mʌtə] *n* 1) бормотание; 2) ворчание.

mutter II *v* 1) бормотать; 2) ворчать (*на — against, at*); 3) говорить тихо, невнятно; *перен.* говорить по секрету.

mutton ['mʌtn] *n* 1) баранина; 2) *attr* бараний.

mutton-chop ['mʌtn'tʃɔp] *n* 1) баранья котлета; 2) *pl* бачки.

mutual ['mjuːtʃuəl] *a* 1) взаимный; обоюдный; 2) общий.

mutuality ['mjuːtʃu'ælɪtɪ] *n* взаимность; обоюдность; взаимная зависимость.

muzzle I ['mʌzl] *n* 1) морда (*животного*); 2) жерло, дуло; 3) намордник.

muzzle II *v* 1) надевать намордник; 2) заставить (за)молчать.

my [maɪ] *pron poss* мой, моя, моё; мой.

myope ['maɪoup] *n* близорукий человек.

myopia [maɪ'oupjə] *n* близорукость.

myriad I ['mɪrɪəd] *n* мириады, громадное число.

myriad II *a* бесчисленный, несметный.

myrrh [məː] *n* мирра (*благовоние*).

myrtle ['məːtl] *n бот.* мирт.

myself [maɪ'self] *pron* 1) *refl* себя, меня, -ся; 2) *употр. для усиления* сам; I did it ~ я это сам сделал.

mysterious [mɪs'tɪərɪəs] *a* таинственный.

mystery ['mɪstərɪ] *n* 1) тайна; to make a ~ of сделать секрет из; 2) *церк.* таинство; 3) *ист.* мистерия.

mystic I ['mɪstɪk] *n* мистик.

mystic II *a* мистический, таинственный.

mystical ['mɪstɪkəl] *см.* mystic II.

mysticism ['mɪstɪsɪzəm] *n* мистицизм.

mystification [ˌmɪstɪfɪ'keɪʃən] *n* мистификация.

mystify ['mɪstɪfaɪ] *v* 1) мистифицировать; обманывать; 2) окружать таинственностью.

mystique [mɪs'tiːk] *n* мистика.

myth [mɪθ] *n* 1) миф(ы); 2) мифическое лицо, событие *и т. п.*

mythical ['mɪθɪkəl] *a* мифический, легендарный.

mythological [ˌmɪθə'lɔdʒɪkəl] *a* мифологический.

mythology [mɪ'θɔlədʒɪ] *n* мифология.

N

N, n [en] *n* 1) *14-я буква англ. алфавита*; 2) *мат.* неопределённая величина.

nab¹ [næb] *n* курок.

nab² *v разг.* поймать, схватить на месте преступления; арестовать.

nabob ['neɪbɔb] *n* набоб.

nacelle [nɑ'sel] *n* открытая кабина (*самолёта*); корзина (*аэростата*); гондола (*дирижабля*).

nadir ['neɪdɪə] *n* 1) *астр.* надир; 2) период крайнего упадка.

nag¹ [næg] *n разг.* 1) небольшая верховая лошадь, пони; 2) кляча.

nag² *v* придираться (*к кому-л. — at*); донимать придирками.

nagger ['nægə] *n* придира, ворчун; сварливая женщина.

naïf [nɑ'iːf] *см.* naïve.

nail¹ [neɪl] *n* ноготь; коготь.

nail² I *n* гвоздь; ◊ on the ~ тотчас же; right as ~s совершенно правильно; to hit the (right) ~ on the head попасть в точку, угадать; hard as ~s закалённый; to fight tooth and ~ сражаться с ожесточением.

nail² II *v* 1) забивать гвозди; прибивать гвоздями; 2) приковывать (*внимание*); 3) *разг.* схватить, поймать, арестовать, задержать; 4) *разг.* обнаружить, «накрыть»; to be ~ed попасться (*в чём-л.*); □ to ~ at пригвоздить; to ~ down прибивать (*гвоздями*); *перен.* прижать к стене (*кого-л.*); to ~ together (*наскоро*) сколачивать; to ~ up заколачивать.

nail-brush ['neɪlbrʌʃ] *n* щётка для ногтей.

nailing I ['neɪlɪŋ] *a разг.* первоклассный; превосходный.

nailing II *adv сленг* превосходно.

naïve, naive [nɑ'iːv, neɪv] *a* 1) наивный, простоватый; 2) безыскусственный.

naïveté [nɑ'iːvteɪ] *см.* naïvety.

naïvety, naivety [nɑ'iːvtɪ, 'neɪvtɪ] *n* 1) наивность, простоватость; 2) безыскусственность.

naked ['neɪkɪd] *a* 1) голый; обнажённый, нагой; 2) лишённый листвы, растительности *и т. п.*; 3) явный, открытый; неприкрашенный; 4) невооружённый (*о глазе*); 5) неизолированный (*о проводе*).

namby-pamby I ['næmbɪ'pæmbɪ] *n* сентиментальность; жеманство.

namby-pamby II *a* сентиментальный; жеманный.

name I [neɪm] *n* 1) имя; first ~, Christian ~, *амер.* given ~ имя (*в отличие от фамилии*); pet ~ ласкательное имя; in the ~ of от имени, именем; во имя; to go by (*или* under) the ~ of слыть, быть известным как...; to use smb.'s ~ сослаться на кого-л.; 2) фамилия; maiden ~ девичья фамилия; what is your ~? как ваша фамилия?; assumed ~ псевдоним; please put my ~ down for a ticket пожалуйста, запишите меня на билет; to put one's ~ to the message подписываться под воззванием; to send in one's ~ записываться (*на конкурс и т. п.*); 3) название, наименование; in ~ по названию (*а не по существу*); 4) репутация; bad ~, ill ~ плохая репутация; 5) великий человек; the great ~s of history исторические личности; 6) *грам.* имя существительное; common ~ имя нарицательное; proper ~ имя собственное; ◊ to call ~s ругать кого-л., обзывать.

name II *v* 1) называть, давать имя; to ~ after smb. называть в честь кого-л.; 2) указывать, назначать (*день, цену*).

name-day ['neɪmdeɪ] *n* именины.

nameless ['neɪmlɪs] *a* 1) безымянный; аноним-

ный; 2) неизве́стный; 3) не поддаю́щийся описа́-
нию, отврати́тельный; 4) невырази́мый; несказа́н-
ный.

namely ['neɪmlɪ] *adv* а и́менно, то́ есть.

namesake ['neɪmseɪk] *n* тёзка.

nankeen [næŋ'kiːn] *n* 1) на́нка (*грубая хлопчато-
бумажная ткань*); 2) *pl* на́нковые брю́ки.

nanny ['nænɪ] *n дет.* ня́ня.

nanny(-goat) ['nænɪ(gout)] *n* коза́.

nap¹ I [næp] *n* дремо́та, коро́ткий сон; to have
(*или* to snatch, to take) a ~ вздремну́ть, соснуть;
to steal a ~ вздремну́ть укра́дкой.

nap¹ II *v* дрема́ть, вздремну́ть; to be caught
~ping быть засти́гнутым враспло́х.

nap² *n* ворс (*на сукне*).

nap³ *n*: to go ~ оп поста́вить всё на ка́рту.

napalm ['neɪpɑːm] *n* 1) напа́лм; 2) *attr* напа́лмо-
вый.

nape [neɪp] *n* заты́лок; за́дняя часть ше́и (*обыкн.*
~ of the neck).

napery ['neɪpərɪ] *n* столо́вое бельё.

naphtha ['næfθə] *n* 1) нефть; 2) кероси́н.

napkin ['næpkɪn] *n* 1) салфе́тка; to lay up in a ~
≅ положи́ть под спуд; не употребля́ть; 2) пелёнка;
подгу́зник.

napoo [næ'puː] *int воен. сленг* нет!, пропа́л!,
исче́з!, ко́нчено!

narcissus [nɑː'sɪsəs] *n* (*pl тж.* narcissi [nɑː'sɪsaɪ])
нарци́сс.

narcosis [nɑː'kousɪs] *n* нарко́з.

narcotic I [nɑː'kɔtɪk] *n* наркоти́ческое сре́дство;
нарко́тик.

narcotic II *a* наркоти́ческий; усыпля́ющий.

nark [nɑːk] *n сленг* сы́щик, шпик.

narrate [næ'reɪt] *v* повествова́ть, расска́зывать.

narration [næ'reɪʃən] *n* повествова́ние, рас-
ска́з.

narrative I ['nærətɪv] *n* по́весть, расска́з; повe-
ствова́ние.

narrative II *a* повествова́тельный.

narrator [næ'reɪtə] *n* расска́зчик.

narrow I ['nærou] *a* 1) у́зкий (*тж. перен.*);
2) те́сный; 3) ограни́ченный; тру́дный; 4) немно́го
превыша́ющий (*в численном отношении*); 5) тща́-
тельный, подро́бный; стро́гий (*об осмотре и т. п.*);
6) скупо́й; расчётливый.

narrow II *v* 1) су́живать(ся); 2) ограни́чивать.

narrow III *n обыкн. pl* у́зкая часть (*пролива,
реки*); тесни́на.

narrow-gauge ['nærougeɪdʒ] *a* узкоколе́йный.

narrowly ['næroulɪ] *adv* 1) тща́тельно, подро́бно;
при́стально; 2) чуть-чу́ть, едва́; 3) у́зко, те́сно.

narrow-minded ['nærou'maɪndɪd] *a* ограни́чен-
ный, недалёкий, с предрассу́дками.

narrowness ['nærounɪs] *n* у́зость.

nasal I ['neɪzəl] *n фон.* носово́й звук.

nasal II *a* 1) носово́й; 2) гнуса́вый.

nasalize ['neɪzəlaɪz] *v фон.* произноси́ть в нос.

nascent ['næsnt] *a* рожда́ющийся, появля́ю-
щийся, образу́ющийся.

nasturtium [nəs'təːʃəm] *n* настурция.

nasty ['nɑːstɪ] *a* 1) отврати́тельный; проти́вный;
ужа́сный, ме́рзкий (*о зрелище, виде*); 2) неприли́ч-
ный, гря́зный; 3) га́дкий, своенра́вный, злой; don't
be ~! не капри́зничай!, не злись!; to turn ~ разо-
зли́ться; 4) сыро́й (*о почве*); скве́рный, нена́стный

(*о погоде*); 5) бу́рный (*о море*); 6) угрожа́ющий,
опа́сный, тяжёлый (*о болезни и т. п.*).

natal ['neɪtl] *a* относя́щийся к рожде́нию.

natality [neɪ'tælɪtɪ] *n* рожда́емость, есте́ствен-
ный приро́ст населе́ния.

natation [neɪ'teɪʃən] *n* пла́вание.

nation ['neɪʃən] *n* 1) на́ция, наро́д; freedom-
-loving ~s свободолюби́вые наро́ды; United Nations Объединённые На́ции; 2) наро́дность; нацио-
на́льность; 3) госуда́рство, страна́; peace-loving
~s миролюби́вые стра́ны.

national I ['næʃənl] *n обыкн. pl* соотече́ственник,
согражда́нин.

national II *a* 1) национа́льный; наро́дный; 2) го-
суда́рственный.

nationalism ['næʃnəlɪzəm] *n* национали́зм.

nationalist I ['næʃnəlɪst] *n* национали́ст.

nationalist II *a* националисти́ческий.

nationality [,næʃə'nælɪtɪ] *n* 1) национа́льность;
национа́льная принадле́жность; what is his ~? кто
он по национа́льности?; 2) наро́дность; 3) нацио-
на́льные черты́.

nationalization [,næʃnəlaɪ'zeɪʃən] *n* национали-
за́ция.

nationalize ['næʃnəlaɪz] *v* 1) де́лать наро́дным
достоя́нием; национализи́ровать; 2) принима́ть
в по́дданство.

nation-wide ['neɪʃənwaɪd] *a* общенаро́дный, все-
наро́дный.

native I ['neɪtɪv] *n* 1) уроже́нец (*of*); 2) тузе́мец;
3) ме́стное расте́ние *или* живо́тное.

native II *a* 1) родно́й, роди́мый; 2) приро́дный,
прирождённый; врождённый; 3) ме́стный; тузе́м-
ный; to go ~ переня́ть ме́стные обы́чаи; 4) иско́н-
ный, урождённый; 5) есте́ственный, чи́стый; само-
ро́дный.

native-born ['neɪtɪv'bɔːn] *a* тузе́мный.

natrium ['neɪtrɪəm] *n хим.* на́трий.

natron ['neɪtrən] *n хим.* натр; со́да; углеки́слый
на́трий.

natty ['nætɪ] *a* 1) аккура́тно сши́тый, изя́щный;
2) ло́вкий, иску́сный.

natural I ['nætʃrəl] *n* 1) одарённый челове́к,
саморо́док; 2) *муз.* бека́р; знак бека́ра; 3) идио́т
от рожде́ния; дурачо́к.

natural II *a* 1) есте́ственный; приро́дный; 2) ре-
а́льный; настоя́щий; 3) непринуждённый; 4) обы́ч-
ный; норма́льный, натура́льный; 5) прису́щий
(*кому-л.*), врождённый; it comes ~ to him a) э́то
получа́ется у него́ есте́ственно; б) э́то ему́ легко́
даётся; 6) побо́чный, внебра́чный (*о ребёнке*).

naturalism ['nætʃrəlɪzəm] *n* натурали́зм.

naturalist ['nætʃrəlɪst] *n* 1) естествоиспыта́тель;
био́лог; 2) натурали́ст (*в искусстве*).

naturalistic [,nætʃrə'lɪstɪk] *a* натуралисти́че-
ский.

naturalization [,nætʃrəlaɪ'zeɪʃən] *n* 1) натурали-
за́ция; 2) акклиматиза́ция (*растений, животных*);
3) введе́ние но́вых слов (*в язык*).

naturalize ['nætʃrəlaɪz] *v* 1) натурализова́ть(ся)
(*об иностранце*); 2) акклиматизи́ровать (*растения,
животных*); 3) вводи́ть но́вые слова́ (*в язык*).

naturally ['nætʃrəlɪ] *adv* 1) есте́ственно; 2) ко-
не́чно; 3) по приро́де.

nature ['neɪtʃə] *n* 1) приро́да; 2) су́щность,
основно́е сво́йство; in the ~ of things в приро́де ве-

щей; неизбе́жно; in the course of ∼ при есте́ственном хо́де веще́й; 3) хара́ктер, прирождённые ка́чества; by ∼ по приро́де; against ∼ противоесте́ственный; 4) нрав, нату́ра; good ∼ доброду́шие; ill ∼ злой хара́ктер; 5) *иск.* нату́ра; to draw from ∼ рисова́ть с нату́ры; 6) род, сорт, тип.

naught [nɔːt] *n* 1) нуль; 2) *уст.* ничто́; to set at ∼ ≅ ни в грош не ста́вить; to bring to ∼ свести́ на нет; to come to ∼ свести́сь к нулю́.

naughty [ˈnɔːtɪ] *a* 1) непослу́шный, шаловли́вый; 2) неприли́чный, непристо́йный.

nausea [ˈnɔːsjə] *n* 1) тошнота́; морска́я боле́знь; 2) отвраще́ние.

nauseate [ˈnɔːsɪeɪt] *v* 1) вызыва́ть отвраще́ние; 2) чу́вствовать тошноту́, отвраще́ние.

nauseous [ˈnɔːsjəs] *a* отврати́тельный; тошнотво́рный.

nautical [ˈnɔːtɪkəl] *a* морско́й, морехо́дный.

naval [ˈneɪvəl] *a* (вое́нно-)морско́й; фло́тский.

nave[1] [neɪv] *n* архит. неф.

nave[2] *n* 1) ступи́ца (*колеса́*); 2) *тех.* втулка (*колеса*).

navel [ˈneɪvəl] *n* пупо́к, пуп; *перен.* центр (*чего́-л.*).

navigable [ˈnævɪɡəbl] *a* 1) судохо́дный; 2) го́дный для морско́го пла́вания; 3) управля́емый (*об аэроста́те*).

navigate [ˈnævɪɡeɪt] *v* 1) пла́вать (*на корабле́*); лета́ть (*на самолёте*); 2) управля́ть (*кораблём, самолётом*); *перен.* проводи́ть (*законопроект в парла́менте*).

navigation [ˌnævɪˈɡeɪʃən] *n* 1) навига́ция; судохо́дство; inland ∼ речно́е судохо́дство; aerial ∼ воздухопла́вание; 2) кораблевожде́ние (*наука*).

navigator [ˈnævɪɡeɪtə] *n* 1) *мор., ав.* штурман; 2) морепла́ватель.

navvy [ˈnævɪ] *n* 1) землеко́п; 2) землечерпа́лка.

navy [ˈneɪvɪ] *n* 1) вое́нно-морско́й флот; the Royal Navy брита́нский флот; 2) *поэт.* эска́дра, флоти́лия; 3) адмиралте́йство; 4) *attr* вое́нно-морско́й.

navy-blue [ˈneɪvɪˈbluː] *a* тёмно-си́ний.

naw [nɔː] *adv разг.* нет.

nawab [nəˈwɔːb] *см.* nabob.

nay I [neɪ] *n* отрица́тельный отве́т, «нет»; отка́з; he will not take ∼ он не при́мет отка́за; yea and ∼ и да и нет; to say smb. ∼ отказа́ть кому́-л.

nay II *adv* 1) бо́лее того́; да́же; 2) *уст.* нет; ну что ж.

Nazi [ˈnɑːtsɪ] *n* 1) наци́ст, фаши́ст; 2) *attr* наци́стский, фаши́стский.

Nazism [ˈnɑːtsɪzəm] *n* наци́зм, фаши́зм.

neap I [niːp] *n* квадрату́рный, наиме́ньший прили́в.

neap II *v* 1) убыва́ть (*о прили́ве*); 2): to be ∼ed оказа́ться на мели́.

near I [nɪə] *a* 1) бли́зкий; ∼ and dear бли́зкий и дорого́й; 2) ближа́йший (*о вре́мени*); 3) близлежа́щий; кратча́йший, прямо́й (*о пути́*); 4) кропотли́вый (*о хара́ктере рабо́ты*); 5) ле́вый (*о ноге́ ло́шади, колесе́ экипа́жа*); 6) скупо́й, прижи́мистый.

near I *v* приближа́ться, подходи́ть.

near III *adv* 1) бли́зко, поблизости; по́дле; far and ∼ везде́, повсю́ду; to come ∼, to draw ∼ приближа́ться; ∼ by побли́зости; ∼ at hand a) под руко́й; бли́зко; б) ско́ро; 2) почти́, чуть не.

near IV *prep* 1) о́коло, во́зле (*кого́-л. или како́го-л. предме́та, ме́ста и т. п.*); 2) к, о́коло (*о вре́мени*).

near-by [ˈnɪəbaɪ] *a* близлежа́щий, сосе́дний.

nearly [ˈnɪəlɪ] *adv* 1) почти́; 2) о́коло, приблизи́тельно; 3) бли́зко.

nearness [ˈnɪənɪs] *n* бли́зость.

near-sighted [ˈnɪəˈsaɪtɪd] *a* близору́кий (*см. тж.* sight I).

near-sightedness [ˈnɪəˈsaɪtɪdnɪs] *n* близору́кость.

near-silk [ˈnɪəsɪlk] *n* 1) иску́сственный шёлк; 2) *attr* сде́ланный из иску́сственного шёлка.

neat[1] [niːt] *a* 1) аккура́тный, опря́тный; 2) изя́щный; скро́мный; 3) чёткий, я́сный (*о пла́не, схе́ме*); 4) отто́ченный, лакони́ческий (*о сти́ле*); 5) ло́вкий, иску́сный.

neat[2] *n* 1) бык, коро́ва; 2) *собир.* кру́пный рога́тый скот.

neath I, II [niːθ] *уст. см.* beneath I, II.

neat-handed [ˈniːtˈhændɪd] *a* ло́вкий, иску́сный.

nebulous [ˈnebjuləs] *a* 1) сму́тный, нея́сный; тума́нный; 2) о́блачный.

necessarily [ˈnesɪsərɪlɪ] *adv* обяза́тельно, непреме́нно.

necessary I [ˈnesɪsərɪ] *n* 1) необходи́мое; 2) *pl* предме́ты пе́рвой необходи́мости (*тж.* the necessaries of life); 3) *амер.* убо́рная.

necessary II *a* 1) необходи́мый, ну́жный; 2) неизбе́жный.

necessitate [nɪˈsesɪteɪt] *v* 1) вызыва́ть необходи́мость, де́лать необходи́мым; 2) вынужда́ть.

necessitous [nɪˈsesɪtəs] *a* бе́дный, нужда́ющийся.

necessity [nɪˈsesɪtɪ] *n* 1) необходи́мость, нужда́; logical ∼ логи́ческая необходи́мость; to urge the ∼ of наста́ивать на необходи́мости чего́-л., ссыла́ться на необходи́мость; to be under the ∼ of doing smth. быть вы́нужденным сде́лать что-л.; 2) *pl* предме́ты пе́рвой необходи́мости (*тж.* prime necessities); 3) неизбе́жность; of ∼ неизбе́жно; 4) *обыкн. pl* нужда́, бе́дность, стеснённые обстоя́тельства; to be in ∼ быть в нужде́; ◇ ∼ is the mother of invention *посл.* необходи́мость — мать изобрета́тельности.

neck [nek] *n* 1) ше́я; to break one's ∼ сверну́ть себе́ ше́ю (*при паде́нии*); to get it in the ∼ *разг.* а) получи́ть по ше́е; б) получи́ть вы́говор; to put one's ∼ into the noose ≅ самому́ лезть в пе́тлю; ∼ and ∼ *спорт.* голова́ в го́лову; to risk one's ∼ рискова́ть свое́й голово́й; to save one's ∼ уйти́ це́лым и невреди́мым; 2) во́рот, горлови́на; 3) го́рлышко (*буты́лки*); 4) гриф (*скри́пки, виолонче́ли и т. п.*); 5) у́зкая часть (*чего́-л.*); прохо́д, проли́в; 6) переше́ек, коса́; мыс; a narrow ∼ of land переше́ек; 7) *анат.* ше́йка; 8) *attr* ше́йный; ◇ a stiff ∼ упо́рство, упря́мство; to break the ∼ of вы́полнить бо́льшую часть де́ла; ∼ or nothing ≅ ли́бо пан, ли́бо пропа́л; to turn (*или* to throw) out smb. ∼ and crop реши́тельно вы́ставить, вы́гнать кого́-л. вон.

neckband [ˈnekbænd] *n* во́рот (*руба́шки*).

neckcloth [ˈnekklɔθ] *n уст.* га́лстук; ше́йный плато́к.

neckerchief [ˈnekətʃɪf] *n* ше́йный плато́к, косы́нка.

necklace [ˈneklɪs] *n* ожере́лье.

necklet [ˈneklɪt] *n* 1) ожере́лье; 2) горже́тка.

neck-piece ['nek͵piːs] *n* горжётка.

necktie ['nektaɪ] *n* гáлстук.

neckwear ['nekwɛə] *n собир.* воротнички, гáлстуки, шáрфы.

necrology [ne'krɔlədʒɪ] *n* 1) некролóг; 2) спúсок умéрших.

nectar ['nektə] *n* 1) нектáр; цветóчный сок; 2) чудéсный напúток; 3) газирóванная водá.

Neddy ['nedɪ] *n разг.* óслик.

née [neɪ] *a* урождённая (*ставится после фамилии замужней женщины*: Mrs Thomson, née Sedley).

need I [niːd] *n* 1) нáдобность, нуждá, потрéбность; if ~ be (*или* were) éсли нýжно, éсли потрéбуется; there is no ~ to do it нет нáдобности, не нýжно дéлать э́то; he had ~ ему́ слéдовало бы; to meet the ~s удовлетворя́ть потрéбности; to be in ~ of, to have ~ of нуждáться в чём-л.; to stand in ~ нуждáться (*в чём-л. — of*); 2) бéдность, нищетá, нуждá.

need II *v* 1) нуждáться в чём-л.; имéть нáдобность, потрéбность; 2) трéбоваться; 3) слéдовать, быть дóлжным (*в 3-ем л. ед. ч.* need; *в отриц. и вопр. предложениях последующий Inf употр. без* to); you ~ not go there вам не слéдует éздить тудá; he ~ not have done it ему́ не слéдовало дéлать э́того.

needful I ['niːdful] *a* необходúмый, потрéбный.

needful II *n* (the ~) *сленг* дéньги.

needle I ['niːdl] *n* 1) иглá, игóлка; to ply one's ~ занимáться шитьём, шить; to look for a ~ in a haystack (*или* in a bundle of hay) искáть игóлку в стóге сéна; занимáться безнадёжным дéлом; as sharp as a ~ ≅ а) óстрый как брúтва; б) проницáтельный; 2) спúца *или* крючóк (*для вязания*); 3) стрéлка (*компаса или телеграфного аппарата*); 4) иглá (*хвойного дерева*); 5) обелúск; 6) островокóнечная вершúна (*горы*); 7) шпиль (*башни, колокóльни*); 8) *мин.* игóльчатый кристáлл; 9) (the ~) *сленг* нéрвный припáдок, раздражéние; to get (*или* to have) the ~ — быть в нéрвном состоя́нии; 10) *attr* игóльный; игóльчатый; 11) *attr* швéйный.

needle II *v* 1) шить, зашивáть иглóй; 2) протúскиваться, проникáть сквозь; 3) *мин.* кристаллизовáться úглами.

needle-case ['niːdlkeɪs] *n* игóльник.

needle-lace ['niːdlleɪs] *n* крýжево, вя́заное крючкóм.

needless ['niːdlɪs] *a* ненýжный; бесполéзный; ~ to say... не говоря́ ужé о...

needlewoman ['niːdl͵wumən] *n* портнúха, швея́.

needlework ['niːdlwəːk] *n* шитьё; вышивáние.

needments ['niːdmənts] *n pl* всё необходúмое (*в дорогу*).

needs [niːdz] *adv* по необходúмости; непремéнно, обязáтельно.

needy ['niːdɪ] *a* нуждáющийся, бéдствующий.

ne'er [nɛə] *поэт. см.* never 1).

ne'er-do-weel I, II ['nɛəduː͵wiːl] *см.* ne'er-do-well I, II.

ne'er-do-well I ['nɛəduː͵wel] *n* бездéльник.

ne'er-do-well II *a* никудá не гóдный.

nefarious [nɪ'fɛərɪəs] *a* гнýсный, нúзкий, сквéрный.

negate [nɪ'geɪt] *v* 1) отрицáть; 2) отвергáть.

negation [nɪ'geɪʃən] *n* 1) отрицáние; 2) отрицáтельная величинá.

negative I ['negətɪv] *n* 1) отрицáние; отрицáтельный отвéт, факт, харáктер, персонáж *и т. п.*; to return a ~ сказáть «нет»; in the ~ отрицáтельно; 2) откáз, несоглáсие; 3) запрéт, вéто; 4) *грам.* отрицáтельная частúца; 5) *мат.* отрицáтельная величинá; 6) *фото* негатúв; 7) *эл.* отрицáтельный пóлюс, катóд.

negative II *a* 1) отрицáтельный; 2) *фото* негатúвный; обрáтный (*об изображении*).

negative III *v* 1) откáзывать, наклáдывать запрéт, вéто; 2) опровергáть; 3) нейтрализовáть (*действие чего-л.*).

negatory ['negətərɪ] *a* отрицáтельный.

neglect I [nɪ'glekt] *n* 1) пренебрежéние; небрéжность; 2) запýщенность, забрóшенность.

neglect II *v* 1) не обращáть внимáния на; проявля́ть мáло забóты; 2) запускáть (*дела, занятия и т. п.*); пренебрегáть.

neglectful [nɪ'glektful] *a* 1) небрéжный; невнимáтельный, пренебрежúтельный; 2) нерадúвый; беззабóтный.

négligé ['neglɪʒeɪ] *n* дáмский халáт; домáшнее плáтье.

negligence ['neglɪdʒəns] *n* 1) небрéжность, нерадúвость; 2) халáтность; 3) неря́шливость.

negligent ['neglɪdʒənt] *a* 1) небрéжный, нерадúвый; 2) халáтный, беспéчный.

negligible ['neglɪdʒəbl] *a* незначúтельный; не принимáемый во внимáние.

negotiable [nɪ'gouʃjəbl] *a* 1) могýщий стать предмéтом сдéлки; 2) проходúмый (*о дорогах*); достýпный (*о вершинах*).

negotiant [nɪ'gouʃɪənt] *n* негоциáнт; оптóвый торгóвец, совершáющий крýпные сдéлки.

negotiate [nɪ'gouʃɪeɪt] *v* 1) вестú переговóры; обсуждáть услóвия; догорáриваться (*с кем-л. о чём-л. — with*); 2) договорúться, совершúть (*сделку и т. п.*); 3) пускáть в обращéние (*вексель и т. п.*); 4) преодолевáть (*трудности и т. п.*).

negotiation [nɪ͵gouʃɪ'eɪʃən] *n* 1) переговóры; обсуждéние услóвий; ~s are under way ведýтся переговóры; protracted ~s затянýвшиеся переговóры; 2) преодолéние (*затруднений*).

negotiator [nɪ'gouʃɪeɪtə] *n* лицó, ведýщее переговóры; посрéдник.

Negress ['niːgrɪs] *n* негритя́нка.

Negrillo [ne'grɪlou] *n* негр кáрликового плéмени (*в Африке*).

Negrito [ne'griːtou] *n* негритóс (*Малайского архипелага*).

Negro I ['niːgrou] *n* негр; the ~es нéгры.

Negro II *a* негритя́нский.

neigh I [neɪ] *n* ржáние.

neigh II *v* ржать.

neighbour I ['neɪbə] *n* 1) сосéд, сосéдка; 2) сосéдний, находя́щийся ря́дом предмéт; 3) *attr* сосéдский; сосéдний.

neighbour II *v* гранúчить с; находúться у сáмого крáя (*upon*).

neighbourhood ['neɪbəhud] *n* 1) сосéдство; 2) окрéстности, окрýга; 3) сосéди; 4) *уст.* добрососéдские отношéния (*тж.* good ~); 5) блúзость; in the ~ of а) поблúзости, по сосéдству с; б) приблизúтельно, óколо.

neighbouring [ˈneɪbərɪŋ] *a* сосе́дний, сме́жный.

neighbourly [ˈneɪbəlɪ] *a* доброcосе́дский, дру́жественный.

neither I [ˈnaɪðə, *амер.* ˈniːðə] *a* никако́й, ни оди́н (из).

neither II *adv* 1) ни...; ~ ... nor ни... ни; it is ~ hot nor cold ни жа́рко ни хо́лодно; 2) та́кже не (*в отриц. предложениях*); he cannot swim ~ can his brother он не уме́ет пла́вать, и его́ брат та́кже; ~ do I и я та́кже (*после гл. в отриц. форме*).

neither III *pron* ни тот ни друго́й.

neither IV *conj уст.* ни.

nenuphar [ˈnenjufɑː] *n* водяна́я ли́лия.

neologism [niːˈɔlədʒɪzəm] *n* неологи́зм.

neon [ˈniːən] *n хим.* 1) нео́н; 2) *attr* нео́новый.

nephew [ˈnevjuː, *амер.* ˈnefjuː] *n* племя́нник.

nepotism [ˈnepətɪzəm] *n* кумовство́, семе́йственность.

Neptune [ˈneptjuːn] *n астр., миф.* Непту́н.

nereid [ˈnɪərɪɪd] *n миф.* нереи́да.

nerve I [nəːv] *n* 1) нерв; *pl* не́рвность, не́рвное состоя́ние; afferent ~s центростреми́тельные (*или* чувстви́тельные) не́рвы; efferent ~s дви́гательные не́рвы; visual (sympathetic) ~ зри́тельный (симпати́ческий) нерв; to get on one's ~s де́йствовать на не́рвы; to set one's ~s on edge раздража́ть кого́-л.; iron ~s, ~s of steel желе́зные не́рвы; to suffer from ~s страда́ть расстро́йством не́рвной систе́мы; 2) прису́тствие ду́ха, му́жество, самооблада́ние; to have the ~ to do smth. име́ть му́жество сде́лать что-л. (*см. тж.* 4); to lose one's ~ потеря́ть му́жество; 3) си́ла, эне́ргия; to strain every ~ напря́чь все си́лы; приложи́ть все уси́лия; 4) *разг.* на́глость, наха́льство; to have the ~ to do smth. име́ть наха́льство сде́лать что-л. (*см. тж.* 2); 5) *бот., зоол.* жи́лка; 6) *attr* не́рвный.

nerve II *v* придава́ть си́лу, хра́брость; to ~ oneself собра́ться с си́лами.

nerveless [ˈnəːvlɪs] *a* 1) лишённый не́рвов; 2) сла́бый, вя́лый, лишённый бо́дрости.

nervous [ˈnəːvəs] *a* 1) не́рвный; 2) нерви́рующий, де́йствующий на не́рвы; 3) возбуди́мый; взволно́ванный; 4) вырази́тельный (*о стиле*).

nervy [ˈnəːvɪ] *a* 1) *разг.* не́рвный, возбуждённый; 2) *сленг* хра́брый, сме́лый; 3) *сленг* самоуве́ренный; самонадея́нный; 4) *поэт.* му́скулистый, си́льный.

ness [nes] *n* мыс.

nest I [nest] *n* 1) гнездо́; hornet's ~ оси́ное гнездо́; to bring a hornet's ~ about one's ears, to stir up a hornet's ~ потрево́жить оси́ное гнездо́ (*тж. перен.*); 2) вы́водок (*птиц, живо́тных*); 3) ую́тный уголо́к, гнёздышко; 4) прито́н; 5) лабири́нт (*переу́лков*); ◊ to foul one's own ~ ≅ выноси́ть сор из избы́; to feather one's ~ ≅ набива́ть себе́ карма́н; богате́ть.

nest II *v* 1) вить гнездо́; гнезди́ться; 2) охо́титься за гнёздами (*тж.* to go ~ ing); 3) вставля́ть оди́н предме́т в друго́й.

nestle [ˈnesl] *v* 1) удо́бно, ую́тно уса́живаться (*in, into, among; тж.* to ~ down); 2) прильну́ть, прижа́ться (*к — to*); 3) юти́ться, укрыва́ться.

nestling [ˈneslɪŋ] *n* пте́нчик; малы́ш.

net I [net] *n* 1) сеть; се́ти, тенёта; to cast a ~ закидывать сеть; 2) се́тка; 3) паути́на; 4) западня́.

net II *v* 1) лови́ть сетя́ми; расставля́ть се́ти

(*тж. перен.*); 2) покрыва́ть се́тью; 3) попа́сть в се́тку (*о мяче*); 4) плести́ се́ти.

net² I *n* чи́стый дохо́д.

net² II *a* чи́стый, не́тто (*о ве́се, дохо́де*).

net² III *v* получа́ть *или* приноси́ть чи́стый дохо́д.

nether [ˈneðə] *a уст., шутл.* 1) ни́жний; 2) а́дский, подзе́мный.

Netherlander [ˈneðələndə] *n* нидерла́ндец.

Netherlandish [ˈneðələndɪʃ] *a* нидерла́ндский.

nethermost [ˈneðəmoust] *a* са́мый ни́жний.

nettle I [ˈnetl] *n* 1) крапи́ва; small ~ жгу́чая крапи́ва; to grasp the ~ *перен.* сме́ло преодолева́ть тру́дности; 2) *attr* крапи́вный.

nettle II *v* 1) обжига́ть крапи́вой; 2) раздража́ть, злить.

nettle-rash [ˈnetlræʃ] *n мед.* крапи́вная лихора́дка.

network [ˈnetwəːk] *n* 1) сеть, се́тка; 2) сеть (*желе́зных доро́г, кана́лов и т. п.*).

neuralgia [njuəˈrældʒə] *n* невралги́я.

neurasthenia [ˌnjuərəsˈθiːnjə] *n* неврастени́я.

neuritis [njuəˈraɪtɪs] *n мед.* неври́т.

neurosis [njuəˈrousɪs] *n* невро́з.

neurotic [njuəˈrɔtɪk] *a* не́рвный, невроти́ческий.

neuter I [ˈnjuːtə] *n* 1) *грам.* сре́дний род; существи́тельное, прилага́тельное, местоиме́ние сре́днего ро́да; 2) *грам.* непереходный глаго́л; 3) кастри́рованное живо́тное.

neuter II *a* 1) сре́днего ро́да; 2) непереходный (*о глаго́ле*); 3) кастри́рованный, беспло́дный; 4) *ре́дко* нейтра́льный; to stand ~ остава́ться нейтра́льным.

neutral I [ˈnjuːtrəl] *n* 1) нейтра́льное госуда́рство; 2) граждани́н нейтра́льного госуда́рства.

neutral II *a* 1) нейтра́льный; 2) сре́дний; промежу́точный, неопределённый (*о цве́те*); 3) беспо́лый.

neutrality [njuːˈtrælɪtɪ] *n* нейтралите́т; armed ~ вооружённый нейтралите́т.

neutralize [ˈnjuːtrəlaɪz] *v* 1) объявля́ть нейтра́льным; 2) нейтрализова́ть; обезвре́живать; 3) *воен.* подавля́ть огнём.

neutron [ˈnjuːtrɔn] *n физ.* нейтро́н.

never [ˈnevə] *adv* 1) никогда́; well, I ~!, I ~ did! никогда́ ничего́ подо́бного не (ви́дел, говори́л и т. п.); will he ~ come! да когда́ же он придёт наконе́ц!; 2) *разг. употр. для усиле́ния отрица́ния*: ~ a one ни оди́н; ~ fear не беспоко́йтесь, бу́дьте уве́рены; 3) *разг.* коне́чно нет; не мо́жет быть; 4) ни ра́зу; ◊ ~ mind! ничего́!, пустяки́!; не беспоко́йтесь!; ~ so как бы ни.

nevermore [ˈnevəˈmɔː] *adv* никогда́ (бо́льше).

nevertheless [ˌnevəðəˈles] *adv* тем не ме́нее; несмотря́ на; одна́ко.

new I [njuː] *a* 1) но́вый; 2) ино́й, друго́й; 3) неда́вний, неда́внего происхожде́ния; 4) све́жий; парно́й (*о молоке́*); молодо́й (*о вине́, карто́феле, месяце*); 5) совреме́нный; нове́йший; после́дний (*о мо́де*); 6) передово́й; 7) незнако́мый; 8) вновь и́збранный (*парла́мент и т. п.*).

new II *adv* ново-, свеже-, вновь, неда́вно (*обычно в сло́жных слова́х, напр.*: ~-born новорождённый; ~-mown свежеско́шенный; ~-built вновь вы́строенный и т. п.).

new-blown [ˈnjuːbloun] *a* то́лько что расцве́тший.

new-born ['njuːbɔːn] *a* 1) новорождённый; 2) возрождённый.

new-built ['njuːbɪlt] *a* 1) вновь выстроенный; 2) перестроенный.

new-comer ['njuːˌkʌmə] *n* 1) вновь прибывший; 2) незнакомец.

new-fallen ['njuːˌfɔːlən] *a* только что выпавший (*о снеге*).

new-fangled ['njuːˌfæŋgld] *a пренебр.* новомодный.

new-fashioned ['njuːˈfæʃənd] *a* модный, новомодный.

new-found ['njuːfaund] *a* вновь обретённый.

Newfoundland [njuːˈfaundlənd] *n* ньюфаундлёнд, водолаз (*порода собак*).

Newgate ['njuːgɪt] *n* 1) ньюгейтская долговая тюрьма (*разрушена в 1902 г.*); 2) *attr* ньюгейтский.

newish ['njuːɪʃ] *a* довольно новый.

new-laid ['njuːleɪd] *a* свежеснесённый (*о яйце*).

newly ['njuːlɪ] *adv* 1) недавно, только что; 2) вновь, заново.

newness ['njuːnɪs] *n* новизна.

news [njuːz] *n* известия, новости (*обыкн. с гл. в ед. ч.*); what's the ~ ?, is there any ~? что нового?; frontpage ~ газетная сенсация; distressing ~ печальные новости; hot (stale) ~ свежие (устаревшие) новости; that is no ~ это не ново; to break the ~ смягчать дурные вести, осторожно сообщать; that ~ will keep эту новость можно сообщить потом; ◇ no ~ is good ~ *посл.* отсутствие вестей — само по себе хорошая весть; bad ~ travels quickly, ill ~ flies fast *посл.* ≅ худые вести не лежат на месте.

news-agent ['njuːzˌeɪdʒənt] *n* газетчик (*имеющий киоск*).

news-boy ['njuːzbɔɪ] *n* газетчик, разносчик газет.

newscast ['njuːzkɑːst] *n* передача последних известий по радио.

newscaster ['njuːzˌkɑːstə] *n* радиокомментатор; диктор последних известий.

news-dealer ['njuːzˌdiːlə] *амер. см.* news-agent.

news-man ['njuːzmən] *n* 1) *см.* news-boy; 2) *разг.* корреспондент газеты.

newsmonger ['njuːzˌmʌŋgə] *n* сплетник, -ица.

newspaper ['njuːsˌpeɪpə] *n* 1) газета; 2) *attr* газетный.

newsprint ['njuːzprɪnt] *n* газетная бумага.

news-reel I ['njuːzriːl] *n* кинохроника, киножурнал.

news-reel II *v* сниматься в кинохронике.

news-room ['njuːzrum] *n* 1) читальня, читальный зал; 2) *амер.* отдел новостей (*в газете, на радио и т. п.*).

news-sheet ['njuːzʃiːt] *n* 1) газета; 2) листовка.

news-stand ['njuːzstænd] *n* 1) газетный киоск; 2) *амер.* книжный киоск.

newsy I ['njuːzɪ] *n амер. разг. см.* news-boy.

newsy II *a разг.* богатый новостями или сплетнями.

newt [njuːt] *n* тритон.

new-year's ['njuːˈjəːz] *a* новогодний (*см. тж.* year).

New Yorker ['njuːˈjɔːkə] *n* житель Нью-Йорка.

next I [nekst] *a* 1) следующий; 2) ближайший,

соседний; ~ of kin ближайший родственник; ~ to nothing почти ничего; 3) будущий.

next II *adv* затем, потом; what ~? что же дальше?

next III *prep* рядом, около; he placed his chair ~ hers он поставил свой стул рядом с её (*стулом*).

next IV *n* следующий, ближайший человек *или* предмет; ~ please! следующий, пожалуйста!; I will tell you in my ~ я расскажу вам в следующем письме.

next-door ['nekst'dɔː] *a* ближайший, соседний.

nexus ['neksəs] *n* 1) связь, узы; 2) *грам.* нексус.

Niagara [naɪˈægərə] *n*: to shoot ~ решиться на отчаянный шаг.

nib [nɪb] *n* 1) перо; остриё пера; 2) остриё, острый конец (*предмета*).

nibble ['nɪbl] *v* 1) есть маленькими кусочками; 2) откусывать; щипать (*at*); 3) не решаться, колебаться.

niblick ['nɪblɪk] *n* клюшка (*для игры в гольф*).

nibs [nɪbz] *n сленг*: his ~ их милость.

nice [naɪs] *a* 1) приятный, милый, славный, хороший; 2) любезный, внимательный (*в обращении*); тактичный; 3) хорошенький, изящный; сделанный со вкусом; 4) точный, тонкий, чувствительный (*о механизме*); 5) острый, тонкий (*о слухе, зрении и т. п.*); 6) изысканный (*о стиле, манерах*); 7) щепетильный; скрупулёзный; 8) привередливый, придирчивый; 9) тщательный, аккуратный; 10) вкусный, сладкий (*о пище*); 11) щекотливый (*о вопросе и т. п.*); 12) *уст.* своенравный, глупый.

nice-looking ['naɪsˌlukɪŋ] *a* миловидный; привлекательный.

nicely ['naɪslɪ] *adv* 1) хорошо, мило, любезно; 2) тонко, деликатно; 3) *разг.* как раз; it will suit me ~ это мне как раз подойдёт.

nicety ['naɪsɪtɪ] *n* 1) точность; to a ~ точно, впору, как раз; 2) *pl* тонкости, мелкие детали; 3) утончённость; изящество; 4) разборчивость, щепетильность; 5) *уст.* лакомство.

niche [nɪtʃ] *n* 1) ниша; 2) убежище.

Nick [nɪk] *n*: Old ~ дьявол.

nick I [nɪk] *n* 1) заметка, метка; зарубка; 2) щербина (*в посуде*); 3) точный момент времени; in the very ~ of time как раз вовремя.

nick II *v* 1) делать метки, зарубки; 2) попасть в точку, угадать; 3) поспеть вовремя (*на поезд и т. п.*); 4) арестовать, задержать (*преступника*); 5) *разг.* обмануть, надуть; 6) *разг.* украсть, стащить.

nickel I ['nɪkl] *n* 1) *хим.* никель; 2) *амер.* монета в 5 центов; 3) *attr* никелевый.

nickel II *v* никелировать.

nicker ['nɪkə] *v* 1) ржать; 2) хохотать, гоготать.

nick-nack ['nɪknæk] *n* безделушка, украшение.

nickname I ['nɪkneɪm] *n* 1) прозвище; 2) уменьшительное имя.

nickname II *v* давать прозвище.

niddle-noddle ['nɪdlˌnɔdl] *см.* nid-nod.

nid-nod ['nɪdˌnɔd] *v* кивать.

niece [niːs] *n* племянница.

nifty I ['nɪftɪ] *n амер. разг.* остроумное замечание; острое словцо.

nifty II *a амер. разг.* изящный; стильный.

niggard I ['nɪgəd] *n* скряга.

niggard II *a* скупой, скаредный.

niggardly I [ˈnɪgədlɪ] *a* 1) скупой; 2) скудный.

niggardly II *adv* 1) скупо; 2) скудно.

nigger [ˈnɪgə] *n* (*слово, используемое американскими расистами*) негр; темнокожий.

nigh I [naɪ] *a уст., поэт.* близкий, ближний.

nigh II *adv уст., поэт.* поблизости, рядом.

night [naɪt] *n* 1) ночь; in the ~, at ~ ночью; by ~ в течение ночи; all ~ long всю ночь напролёт; starlight ~ звёздная ночь; good ~! спокойной ночи!; to bid good ~ пожелать спокойной ночи; to have (*или* to pass) a good (bad) ~ хорошо (плохо) спать ночь; to make a ~ of it прокутить всю ночь; to stay over ~ переночевать; ~ and day и днём и ночью; Arabian ~s сказки «Тысяча и одной ночи»; 2) вечер; last ~ вчера вечером; the ~ before last позавчера вечером; first ~ первое представление, премьера; a ~ out a) вечеринка; б) выходной вечер (*у прислуги*); 3) сумерки, темнота, мрак; to go forth into the ~ исчезнуть во мраке; 4) *attr* ночной, вечерний.

night-bird [ˈnaɪtbəːd] *n* 1) ночная птица; 2) ночной гуляка; полуночник.

night-blindness [ˈnaɪtˌblaɪndnɪs] *n* куриная слепота.

night-cap [ˈnaɪtkæp] *n* 1) ночной колпак; 2) стаканчик спиртного на ночь.

night-club [ˈnaɪtklʌb] *n* ночной клуб.

night-dress [ˈnaɪtdres] *n* ночная сорочка (*женская, детская*).

nightfall [ˈnaɪtfɔːl] *n* сумерки.

night-gown [ˈnaɪtgaun] *см.* night-dress.

night-hag [ˈnaɪthæg] *n* кошмар.

nightingale [ˈnaɪtɪŋgeɪl] *n* 1) соловей; 2) *attr* соловьиный.

nightjar [ˈnaɪtdʒɑː] *n* козодой (*птица*).

night-light [ˈnaɪtlaɪt] *n* ночник.

night-long I [ˈnaɪtlɔŋ] *a* длящийся всю ночь.

night-long II *adv* в течение всей ночи, всю ночь.

nightly I [ˈnaɪtlɪ] *a* 1) ночной; 2) еженощный.

nightly II *adv* ночью, по ночам, еженощно.

nightmare [ˈnaɪtmeə] *n* кошмар.

night-rider [ˈnaɪtˌraɪdə] *n амер.* конный налётчик.

night-school [ˈnaɪtskuːl] *n* вечерняя школа, вечерние курсы.

night-shirt [ˈnaɪtʃəːt] *n* ночная рубашка (*мужская*).

night-soil [ˈnaɪtsɔɪl] *n* нечистоты.

night-stool [ˈnaɪtstuːl] *n* ночной горшок, судно.

night-suit [ˈnaɪtsjuːt] *n* пижама.

night-time [ˈnaɪttaɪm] *n* ночное время, ночь; in the ~ ночью.

night-walker [ˈnaɪtˌwɔːkə] *n* 1) ночной бродяга; 2) проститутка; 3) лунатик.

night-watch [ˈnaɪtˈwɔtʃ] *n* 1) ночной дозор; 2) ночной дозорный; 3) ночная вахта.

night-wear [ˈnaɪtweə] *n* ночное бельё.

nigrescent [naɪˈgresənt] *a* черноватый, чернеющий.

nil [nɪl] *n* нуль (*особ. при счёте в играх*).

nimbi [ˈnɪmbaɪ] *pl см.* nimbus.

nimble [ˈnɪmbl] *a* 1) быстрый, прыткий; лёгкий

(*в движениях*); шустрый; 2) живой, сообразительный.

nimbus [ˈnɪmbəs] *n* (*pl тж.* nimbi) 1) нимб, сияние, ореол; 2) *метеор.* дождевые облака.

niminy-piminy [ˈnɪmɪnɪˈpɪmɪnɪ] *a* жеманный, чопорный, натянутый.

nincompoop [ˈnɪnkəmpuːp] *n* дурачок, простак, «шляпа».

nine I [naɪn] *num* девять.

nine II *n* девятка; ◊ the Nine *миф.* девять муз; up to the ~s совершенно; чрезвычайно; dressed up to the ~s расфранчённый.

ninefold I [ˈnaɪnfould] *a* девятикратный.

ninefold II *adv* в девять раз.

ninepins [ˈnaɪnpɪnz] *n* кегли.

nineteen [ˈnaɪnˈtiːn] *num* девятнадцать; ◊ to go (*или* to talk) ~ to the dozen трещать, болтать без устали.

nineteenth I [ˈnaɪnˈtiːnθ] *num* девятнадцатый.

nineteenth II *n* девятнадцатая часть.

nineties [ˈnaɪntɪz] *n pl* (the ~) 1) девяностые годы; 2) возраст между 89 и 100 годами.

ninetieth I [ˈnaɪntɪθ] *num* девяностый.

ninetieth II *n* девяностая часть.

ninety [ˈnaɪntɪ] *num* девяносто.

ninny [ˈnɪnɪ] *n* дурак, простофиля.

ninth I [naɪnθ] *num* девятый.

ninth II *n* девятая часть.

nip[1] I [nɪp] *n* 1) щипок; укус; 2) едкое замечание; колкость; 3) резкое воздействие (*мороза, ветра*).

nip[1] II *v* 1) щипать; кусать; укусить, тяпнуть (*о собаке*); 2) прищемить, зажать; 3) побить (*морозом*); 4) пресечь, прекратить развитие; 5) *разг.* стащить, стянуть; □ to ~ along *разг.* спешить, торопиться; to ~ away *разг.* ускользнуть, смыться; to ~ in вмешаться в разговор; to ~ off а) отщипнуть, откусить; б) удрать.

nip[2] *n* небольшой кусок (*пищи*); глоток (*спиртного*); to freshen the ~ *разг.* опохмеляться.

nipper [ˈnɪpə] *n* 1) «кусака»; 2) клешня (*краба, рака*); 3) *pl* пенсне; 4) *pl* острогубцы, кусачки, клещи; 5) *разг.* мальчик, парень, подручный; 6) *сленг* беспризорный; 7) *pl сленг* ручные кандалы.

nipping [ˈnɪpɪŋ] *a* 1) морозный; резкий (*о ветре*); 2) едкий, колкий.

nipple [ˈnɪpl] *n* 1) сосок (*груди*); 2) соска; 3) бугор, сопка; 4) пузырь (*в стекле, металле*).

nippy [ˈnɪpɪ] *a* 1) *см.* nipping 1); 2) *разг.* проворный, прыткий.

nisei [ˈniːˈseɪ] *n амер.* американец японского происхождения.

niter [ˈnaɪtə] *амер. см.* nitre.

nitrate I [ˈnaɪtreɪt] *n хим.* соль азотной кислоты, нитрат.

nitrate II *v хим.* нитрировать.

nitre [ˈnaɪtə] *n хим.* селитра.

nitric [ˈnaɪtrɪk] *a хим.* азотный.

nitrite [ˈnaɪtraɪt] *n хим.* соль азотистой кислоты.

nitrogen [ˈnaɪtrɪdʒən] *n хим.* 1) азот; 2) *attr* азотный.

nitrogenous [naɪˈtrɔdʒɪnəs] *a хим.* азотный.

nitrous [ˈnaɪtrəs] *a хим.* азотистый.

nitwit [ˈnɪtwɪt] *n амер. сленг* дурак; простофиля.

nix[1] I [nɪks] *n сленг* нуль, ничего.

nix[1] II *adv сленг* нет.

nix² *int* ти́хо!, осторо́жно! (*знак предупреждения об опасности*).

nix³ *n фольк.* водяно́й.

nixie ['nɪksɪ] *n фольк.* руса́лка.

no I [nou] *n* 1) отрица́ние; отка́з; two noes make a yes два отрица́ния равны́ утвержде́нию; 2) *pl* голосу́ющие про́тив; the noes have it большинство́ про́тив.

no II *a* 1) никако́й; it is no joke э́то совсе́м не шу́тка; in no time бы́стро, в оди́н моме́нт; 2) не (*придаётся противоположное значение последующему сущ.*); he is no genius он далеко́ не ге́ний; 3) *выражает запрещение*: no talking! не разгова́ривать!; no larks! шу́тки в сто́рону!; 4) *в сочетании с отглагольным сущ. выражает невозможность*: there is no knowing... нельзя́ знать..., никто́ не смо́жет сказа́ть...

no III *part* нет.

no IV *adv* не (*при степенях сравнения*); the weather is no better today than it was yesterday сего́дня пого́да не лу́чше, чем вчера́; he is no more его́ нет в живы́х.

nob [nɔb] *n сленг* 1) голова́; башка́; 2) «ши́шка», ва́жная осо́ба; высокопоста́вленное лицо́; 3) *карт.* козырно́й вале́т.

nobble ['nɔbl] *v сленг* 1) испо́ртить ло́шадь (*перед скачками*); 2) подкупи́ть; 3) обма́нывать, жу́льничать; 4) укра́сть; 5) пойма́ть (*преступника*).

nobby ['nɔbɪ] *a сленг* мо́дный, шика́рный, элега́нтный.

nobility¹ [nou'bɪlɪtɪ] *n* благоро́дство; великоду́шие.

nobility² *n* дворя́не, дворя́нство; the ~ титуло́ванная аристокра́тия (*в Англии*).

noble I ['noubl] *a* 1) благоро́дный; великоду́шный; 2) вели́чественный, ста́тный, велича́вый; 3) прекра́сный, превосхо́дный; 4) зна́тный, титуло́ванный; 5) *хим.* ине́ртный (*о газе*); 6) благоро́дный (*о металле*).

noble II *n см.* nobleman.

nobleman ['noublmən] *n* дворяни́н; пэр (*в Англии*).

noble-minded ['noubl'maɪndɪd] *a* великоду́шный, благоро́дный.

noblewoman ['noubl,wumən] *n* дворя́нка.

nobly ['noublɪ] *adv* 1) благоро́дно; 2) прекра́сно, превосхо́дно.

nobody ['noubədɪ] *n* 1) никто́; 2) челове́к, не име́ющий ве́са в о́бществе; ничто́жество.

nocturnal [nɔk'tə:nl] *a* ночно́й.

nocturne ['nɔktə:n] *n* 1) *муз.* ноктю́рн; 2) *жив.* ночно́й пейза́ж.

nod I [nɔd] *n* 1) киво́к; 2) клева́ние но́сом; дремо́та.

nod II *v* 1) кива́ть голово́й (*тж. в знак согласия*); 2) клева́ть но́сом, дрема́ть; 3) прозева́ть что-л.; 4) наклоня́ться, кача́ться (*о деревьях*); 5) грози́ть обва́лом; покоси́ться (*о зданиях*).

nodal ['noudl] *a* центра́льный, узлово́й.

noddle ['nɔdl] *n разг.* башка́.

noddy ['nɔdɪ] *n* 1) проста́к, дура́к; 2) *зоол.* глу́пая кра́чка.

node [noud] *n* 1) у́зел, узлова́я то́чка (*тж. физ., мат.*); 2) *мед.* наро́ст, утолще́ние; 3) *астр.* то́чка пересече́ния орби́т.

nodus ['noudəs] *n* (*pl* nodi ['noudaɪ]) 1) у́зел; 2) сло́жное сплете́ние обстоя́тельств; 3) завя́зка (*интриги*).

nog¹ [nɔg] *n* 1) го́голь-мо́голь; 2) кре́пкое пи́во.

nog² *n* клин, деревя́нный гвоздь.

noggin ['nɔgɪn] *n* 1) небольша́я кру́жка; 2) че́тверть пи́нты (*мера жидкости*).

no-go ['nou'gou] *n* затрудни́тельное положе́ние, тупи́к.

nohow ['nouhau] *adv* ника́к, нико́им о́бразом.

noise I [nɔɪz] *n* 1) шум, гро́хот, крик, гвалт; to make a ~ шуме́ть, крича́ть; to make a ~ in the world заста́вить говори́ть о себе́, нашуме́ть; 2) звук; 3) *уст.* слух, молва́; ◊ a big ~ *амер. разг.* «ши́шка», хозя́ин.

noise II *v* 1) обнаро́довать; разгласи́ть (*тж. to ~ abroad*); 2) *редк.* шуме́ть, крича́ть.

noiseless ['nɔɪzlɪs] *a* 1) бесшу́мный; 2) беззву́чный, безмо́лвный.

noisome ['nɔɪsəm] *a* 1) неприя́тный, скве́рный (*о запахе*); 2) вре́дный, нездоро́вый.

noisy ['nɔɪzɪ] *a* 1) шу́мный; галдя́щий; 2) шумли́вый; 3) крича́щий, я́ркий (*о цвете, костюме и т. п.*).

nomad I ['nɔməd] *n* 1) коче́вник; 2) бродя́га, стра́нник.

nomad II *a* 1) кочево́й; 2) бродя́чий.

nomadic [nou'mædɪk] *a* 1) кочево́й; 2) бродя́чий.

nomenclature [nou'menklətʃə] *n* номенклату́ра.

nominal ['nɔmɪnl] *a* 1) номина́льный; 2) именно́й (*тж. грам.*); 3) усло́вный (*о судебном приговоре*).

nominally ['nɔmɪnəlɪ] *adv* номина́льно.

nominate ['nɔmɪneɪt] *v* 1) выдвига́ть, выставля́ть кандида́та; 2) назнача́ть (*на должность*).

nomination [,nɔmɪ'neɪʃən] *n* 1) выставле́ние кандида́та (*на выборах*); 2) назначе́ние (*на должность*); 3) пра́во назначе́ния *или* выставле́ния кандида́та.

nominative I ['nɔmɪnətɪv] *n грам.* имени́тельный паде́ж.

nominative II *a* 1) *грам.* имени́тельный; 2) назна́ченный (*на должность*).

nominee [,nɔmɪ'ni:] *n* кандида́т (*на должность или на избрание*).

non- [nɔn-] *pref придаёт сущ. и прил. отриц. смысл*: edible съедо́бный; non-edible несъедо́бный.

nonage ['nounɪdʒ] *n* несовершенноле́тие; незре́лость.

non-aggression ['nɔnəg'reʃən] *n* ненападе́ние (*см. тж.* pact).

non-aggressive ['nɔnəg'resɪv] *a* неагресси́вный.

non-attendance ['nɔnə'tendəns] *n* непосеще́ние заня́тий.

non-belligerent ['nɔnbɪ'lɪdʒərənt] *a* невою́ющий, не находя́щийся в состоя́нии войны́.

nonchalance ['nɔnʃələns] *n* 1) беззабо́тность, беспе́чность; небре́жность; 2) безразли́чие; бесстра́стность.

nonchalant ['nɔnʃələnt] *a* 1) беззабо́тный, беспе́чный; небре́жный; 2) безразли́чный; бесстра́стный.

non-com [,nɔn'kɔm] *n воен. разг.* сержа́нт.

non-combatant ['nɔn'kɔmbətənt] *a* нестроево́й (*о солдате*).

non-committal I ['nɔnkə'mɪtl] *n* укло́нчивость.

non-committal II *a* уклончивый.

non-conductor ['nɔnkən,dʌktə] *n физ.* непроводник; диэлектрик; изолятор.

nonconformist ['nɔnkən'fɔːmist] *n* сектант, диссидент.

non-co-operation ['nɔnkou,ɔpə'reiʃən] *n* политика бойкота.

nondescript I ['nɔndiskript] *n* нечто неопределённое, ни то ни сё.

nondescript II *a* неописуемый, трудно определимый.

none I [nʌn] *pron* никто, ничто; ◇ ~ of that! чтоб этого больше не было!; прекратите это!; ~ but только.

none II *adv* нисколько, совсем не, вовсе не; ~ the less тем не менее; нисколько не меньше; I am ~ the better for it мне от этого нисколько не легче.

non-effective I [,nɔni'fektiv] *n* человек, не годный к военной службе.

non-effective II *a* непригодный.

nonentity [nɔ'nentiti] *n* 1) несуществующая вещь; 2) небытие; 3) ничтожный человек, ничтожество.

non-essential ['nɔni'senʃəl] *a* несущественный, неважный.

non-ferrous [nɔn'ferəs] *a* цветной (*о металле*).

nonfulfilment ['nɔnful'filmənt] *n* невыполнение.

non-interference ['nɔn,intə'fiərəns] *n* невмешательство.

non-intervention ['nɔn,intə:'venʃən] *n* невмешательство.

non-lending ['nɔn'lendiŋ] *a* без выдачи (книг) на дом.

non-metal ['nɔn,metl] *n* металлоид.

non-party ['nɔn'pɑːti] *a* беспартийный.

non-persistent ['nɔnpə'sistənt] *a* нестойкий (*о газе*).

nonplus I ['nɔn'plʌs] *n* замешательство; затруднительное положение; at a ~ в тупике.

nonplus II *v* приводить в замешательство, ставить в тупик.

non-productive [,nɔnprə'dʌktiv] *a* 1) непроизводящий; 2) непроизводительный.

nonproliferation ['nɔnprə,lifə'reiʃən] *n* нераспространение; nuclear ~ нераспространение ядерного оружия.

non-resistant I [,nɔnri'zistənt] *n* непротивленец.

non-resistant II *a* не оказывающий сопротивления, несопротивляющийся.

nonsense I ['nɔnsəns] *n* 1) вздор, ерунда, чепуха; arrant ~ сущий вздор; clotted ~, flat ~ совершенная чепуха *или* ерунда; stark ~ чистейший вздор; to talk ~ говорить глупости; 2) бессмысленные поступки; 3) абсурд, абсурдность; 4) пустяки.

nonsense II *int* глупости!; чушь!, ерунда!

nonsensical [nɔn'sensikəl] *a* нелепый, бессмысленный.

non-stop ['nɔn'stɔp] *a* 1) беспосадочный (*о перелёте*); 2) безостановочный; прямого сообщения (*о поезде*).

nonsuch ['nʌnsʌtʃ] *n* образец (*совершенства*).

non-suit I ['nɔn'sjuːt] *n юр.* прекращение иска.

non-suit II *v юр.* прекращать дело.

non-union [nɔn'juːnjən] *a* не состоящий членом профсоюза, не связанный с профсоюзом.

non-unionist ['nɔn'juːnjənist] *n* не член профсоюза.

noodle[1] ['nuːdl] *n* лапша.

noodle[2] *n сленг* 1) голова, башка; 2) простак, «шляпа».

nook [nuk] *n* 1) укромный уголок; 2) глухое, удалённое место; 3) закоулок; 4) бухточка.

noon [nuːn] *n* 1) полдень; at ~ в полдень; high ~ самый полдень; *перен.* лучшая часть чего-л., расцвет; 2) *поэт.* полночь.

noonday ['nuːndei] *n* 1) полдень, время около полудня; 2) *attr* полуденный.

nooning ['nuːniŋ] *n* 1) полдень; 2) полуденный перерыв (*для еды или отдыха*); 3) отдых, еда (*в полдень*).

noontide ['nuːntaid] *n* 1) полдень; *перен.* расцвет, зенит (*жизни, деятельности и т. п.*); 2) *поэт.* полночь; 3) полуденный прилив.

noontime ['nuːntaim] *n* полдень.

noose I [nuːs] *n* 1) петля, лассо, аркан; 2) ловушка, силок.

noose II *v* 1) поймать арканом, силком; заманить в ловушку; 2) повесить (*преступника*).

nor [nɔː] *conj* 1) ни (*как коррелят к предшествующему* neither); he could neither read ~ write он не мог ни читать ни писать; 2) *поэт.* ни (*как коррелят при опущенном предшествующем* neither); he ~ I was there ни его, ни меня не было там; 3) ни (*как коррелят к следующему* nor, *вместо* neither); ~ he ~ I was there ни его, ни меня там не было; 4) и... не, также... не (*как продолжение выражения отрицания после отриц. предложений, содержащих* not, no, never *и т. п.*); he left and I never saw him again — did I regret it он уехал, я больше его не видел и не жалел об этом; 5) также, тоже... не (*после утвердительных предложений употр. для подтверждения мысли, выраженной отрицательно*); they are happy, ~ shall we mourn они счастливы, и мы также не будем горевать.

Nordic ['nɔːdik] *a* северный, скандинавский.

nor'-easter ['nɔː'riːstə] *см.* north-easter.

norland ['nɔːlənd] *n* северный район (*какой-л. страны*).

norm [nɔːm] *n* норма, образец.

normal I ['nɔːməl] *n* 1) нормальное состояние; нормальный тип, размер, образец; 2) *мат.* перпендикуляр; 3) *мед.* нормальная температура; 4) *хим.* нормальный раствор.

normal II *a* 1) нормальный; обыкновенный, обычный; 2) средний, среднеарифметический; 3) *мат.* перпендикулярный.

normalcy ['nɔːməlsi] *см.* normality.

normality [nɔː'mæliti] *n* нормальность; нормальное, обычное состояние.

normalize ['nɔːməlaiz] *v* 1) нормировать; 2) нормализовать.

normally ['nɔːməli] *adv* нормально; обыкновенно, обычно, как правило.

Norman I ['nɔːmən] *n* 1) норманец; 2) *ист.* норманн; 3) нормандский диалект (*тж.* ~ French официальный язык Англии XII—XIV вв.).

Norman II *a* 1) нормандский; 2) *ист.* норманнский.

Norse I [nɔːs] *n* 1) норвежцы; 2) древние норвежцы *или* древние скандинавы; 3) древненорвежский язык.

Norse II *a* 1) норве́жский; 2) древненорве́жский; 3) древнескандина́вский.

Norseman ['nɔːsmən] *n* 1) норве́жец; 2) дре́вний скандина́в.

north I [nɔːθ] *n* 1) се́вер; *мор.* норд; magnetic ~ се́верный магни́тный по́люс; и́стинный се́вер; 2) се́верный ве́тер.

north II *a* 1) се́верный; 2) обращённый на се́вер.

north III *adv* к се́веру, на се́вер, в се́верном направле́нии; ~ of се́вернее (*чего-л.*).

north-east I ['nɔːθ'iːst] *n* се́веро-восто́к; *мор.* норд-о́ст.

north-east II *a* се́веро-восто́чный.

north-east III *adv* к се́веро-восто́ку.

north-easter [nɔːθ'iːstə] *n* си́льный се́веро-восто́чный ве́тер, норд-о́ст.

north-easterly I [nɔːθ'iːstəlı] *a* се́веро-восто́чный, ду́ющий с се́веро-восто́ка (*о ветре*).

north-easterly II *adv* с се́веро-восто́ка; к се́веро-восто́ку.

north-eastward I ['nɔːθ'iːstwəd] *n* се́веро-восто́к.

north-eastward II *a* располо́женный в се́веро-восто́чном направле́нии; се́веро-восто́чный.

north-eastward III *adv* к се́веро-восто́ку, на се́веро-восто́к.

north-eastwards [nɔːθ'iːstwədz] *см.* north-eastward III.

norther ['nɔːðə] *n* си́льный се́верный ве́тер.

northerly I ['nɔːðəlı] *a* 1) обращённый, напра́вленный к се́веру; 2) ду́ющий с се́вера, се́верный (*о ветре*).

northerly II *adv* 1) к се́веру, на се́вер; 2) с се́вера.

northern I ['nɔːðən] *n* жи́тель се́вера (*какой-л. страны*).

northern II *a* се́верный, обращённый на се́вер.

northerner ['nɔːðənə] *n* жи́тель се́вера, северя́нин.

northernmost ['nɔːðənmoust] *a* са́мый се́верный.

northing ['nɔːθıŋ] *n* отклоне́ние к се́веру.

Northland ['nɔːθlənd] *n* 1) се́верные райо́ны (*страны*); 2) скандина́вский полуо́стров.

Northman ['nɔːθmən] *n* 1) норве́жец; 2) жи́тель Скандина́вии; 3) дре́вний скандина́в.

north-polar ['nɔːθ'poulə] *a* се́верный, поля́рный, аркти́ческий.

Northumbria [nɔː'θʌmbrıə] *n* 1) Норту́мберленд; 2) *ист.* Норту́мбрия.

Northumbrian I [nɔː'θʌmbrıən] *n* 1) нортумбри́ец; 2) *ист.* норту́мбрский диале́кт; 3) се́верный диале́кт (*современного англ. языка*).

Northumbrian II *a* норту́мбрский.

northward I ['nɔːθwəd] *n* се́верное направле́ние.

northward II *a* напра́вленный на се́вер, к се́веру.

northward III *adv* к се́веру, на се́вер.

northwardly I ['nɔːθwədlı] *a* се́верный (*о ветре*).

northwardly II *adv* к се́веру, на се́вер.

northwards ['nɔːθwədz] *см.* northward III.

north-west I ['nɔːθ'west] *n* се́веро-за́пад; *мор.* норд-ве́ст.

north-west II *a* се́веро-за́падный.

north-west III *adv* к се́веро-за́паду.

north-wester ['nɔːθ'westə] *n* си́льный се́веро-за́падный ве́тер, норд-ве́ст.

north-westerly I ['nɔːθ'westəlı] *a* се́веро-за́падный, ду́ющий с се́веро-за́пада (*о ветре*).

north-westerly II *adv* с се́веро-за́пада; к се́веро-за́паду.

north-westward I ['nɔːθ'westwəd] *n* се́веро-за́пад.

north-westward II *a* располо́женный в се́веро-за́падном направле́нии; се́веро-за́падный.

north-westward III *adv* к се́веро-за́паду, на се́веро-за́пад.

north-westwards ['nɔːθ'westwədz] *см.* north-westward III.

Norwegian I [nɔː'wiːdʒən] *n* 1) норве́жец; норве́жка; the ~s норве́жцы; 2) норве́жский язы́к.

Norwegian II *a* норве́жский.

nor'-wester [nɔː'westə] *n* 1) *см.* north-wester; 2) стака́н спиртно́го; 3) клеёнчатая ша́пка, зюйд-ве́стка.

nose I [nouz] *n* 1) нос; to pull a long ~ *разг.* показа́ть «нос»; to blow one's ~ сморка́ться; to cock one's ~ задира́ть нос, задава́ться; to count (*или* to tell) ~s *разг.* подсчи́тывать голоса́; производи́ть подсчёт прису́тствующих; to poke (*или* to thrust) one's ~ into сова́ть свой нос, вме́шиваться; to speak through the ~ говори́ть в нос; 2) обоня́ние; чутьё, нюх; to have a good ~ име́ть хоро́шее чутьё (*тж. перен.*); to follow one's ~ а) руково́дствоваться ню́хом, чутьём; б) идти́ пря́мо вперёд; 3) но́сик (*чайника*); го́рлышко, ры́льце; 4) нос, передняя часть (*корабля, самолёта*); 5) *сленг* осведоми́тель; 6) *геогр.* мыс, нос; ◊ big ~s запра́вилы; to bite (*или* to snap) one's ~ off гру́бо отве́тить, огрызну́ться; to lead by the ~ вести́ кого́-л. на поводу́; to pay through the ~ плати́ть бе́шеные де́ньги; to put one's ~ out of joint ≅ а) вы́жить кого́-л.; б) расстро́ить чьи-л. пла́ны; to hold (*или* to keep, to put) a person's ~ to the grindstone заставля́ть кого́-л. рабо́тать без о́тдыха; to turn up one's ~ at относи́ться с презре́нием к, вороти́ть нос от; to wipe another's ~ надува́ть, обма́нывать кого́-л.; under one's ~ у себя́ под но́сом, пря́мо перед собо́й; to cut off one's ~ to spite one's face ≅ повреди́ть, напа́костить себе́.

nose II *v* 1) ню́хать, чу́ять, чу́вствовать за́пах; 2) тяну́ть но́сом, вдыха́ть но́сом; 3) проню́хать, разню́хать (*тж.* ~ out); 4) вы́следить (*after, for*); 5) сова́ть нос в чужи́е дела́ (*about, into*); 6) осторо́жно продвига́ться вперёд (*о лодке, корабле́*).

nosebag ['nouzbæg] *n* 1) то́рба; 2) *сленг* противога́з.

nosedive I ['nouzdaıv] *n* 1) *ав.* пики́рование; to fall into a ~ пики́ровать; 2) неожи́данное нападе́ние.

nosedive II *v ав.* пики́ровать.

nosegay ['nouzgeı] *n* буке́т цвето́в.

nose-piece ['nouzpiːs] *n* 1) нахра́пник (*уздечки*); 2) *тех.* наконе́чник, сопло́; брандспо́йт.

noserag ['nouzræg] *n разг.* носово́й плато́к.

nosey ['nouzı] *см.* nosy.

nostalgia [nɔs'tældʒıə] *n* тоска́ по ро́дине, ностальги́я.

nostril ['nɔstrıl] *n* ноздря́.

nostrum ['nɔstrəm] *n* 1) патенто́ванное лека́рство; панаце́я от всех боле́зней; сна́добье; 2) излю́бленный приём (*полит. партии*).

nosy ['nouzı] *a* 1) носа́тый; 2) *разг.* любопы́тный, сую́щий всю́ду свой нос; 3) ду́рно па́хнущий.

not [nɔt] *adv* не, нет; ни; ◇ ~ at all совсе́м не, отню́дь не; во́все нет; ~ in the least ничу́ть, ниско́лько; ~ a bit of it ниско́лько; ~ but, ~ but that, ~ but what хотя́; не то что́бы; ~ half a) совсе́м не; б) *сленг* о́чень, ужа́сно; ~ once nor twice ча́сто; ~ a few мно́го; мно́гие; ~ for the world ни за что на све́те; ~ worth a button ≅ ло́маного гроша́ не сто́ит.

notability [ˌnoutə'bılıtı] *n* 1) изве́стность; знамени́тость; 2) изве́стный, знамени́тый челове́к.

notable I ['noutəbl] *n* 1) знамени́тый, выдаю́щийся челове́к; 2) *ист.* нота́бль.

notable II *a* 1) выдаю́щийся; 2) значи́тельный, заме́тный; 3) практи́чный, хозя́йственный (*о же́нщине*).

notarial [nou'tɛərıəl] *a* нотариа́льный.

notarize ['noutəraız] *v* нотариа́льно заверя́ть (*догово́р и т. п.*).

notary ['noutərı] *n* нота́риус (*тж.* ~ public).

notation [nou'teıʃən] *n* 1) систе́ма обозначе́ния, за́писи; musical ~ но́тная за́пись; 2) за́пись, запи́сывание.

notch I [nɔtʃ] *n* 1) зару́бка, зазу́брина, наре́зка; 2) *тех.* вы́емка; про́резь; 3) *амер.* сте́пень, у́ровень.

notch II *v* де́лать зару́бки; наноси́ть ме́тки, ме́тить.

note I [nout] *n* 1) *обыкн. pl* заме́тка, за́пись; to make (*или* to take) a ~ of smth. приня́ть что-л. к све́дению; to take ~s of a lecture записа́ть ле́кцию; to compare ~s обме́ниваться взгля́дами, мне́ниями; 2) (дипломати́ческая) но́та; 3) запи́ска, распи́ска; ~ of hand, promissory ~ долгово́е обяза́тельство; circular ~ аккредити́в; treasury ~ казначе́йский биле́т; 4) примеча́ние, сно́ска; 5) значи́тельность, изве́стность; репута́ция; 6) но́тка, тон; to change one's ~ измени́ть тон; заговори́ть по-друго́му; 7) *муз.* но́та; 8) пе́ние, крик, ка́рканье (*птиц*); 9) сигна́л; a ~ of warning предупрежде́ние; 10) знак; ~ of exclamation восклица́тельный знак; ~ of interrogation вопроси́тельный знак.

note II *v* 1) запи́сывать, заноси́ть в тетра́дку, записну́ю кни́жку *и т. п.*; 2) упомина́ть; отмеча́ть; 3) замеча́ть, примеча́ть; 4) ука́зывать, обознача́ть; 5) анноти́ровать.

note-book ['noutbuk] *n* записна́я кни́жка.

noted ['noutıd] *a* знамени́тый, изве́стный (*for*).

note-paper ['nout͵peıpə] *n* почто́вая бума́га.

note-shaver ['nout͵ʃeıvə] *n* *амер. сленг* ростовщи́к.

noteworthy ['nout͵wə:ðı] *a* достопримеча́тельный; досто́йный внима́ния.

nothing I ['nʌθıŋ] *n* 1) ноль; 2) ничто́; пустя́к; ~ of the kind, ~ of the sort ничего́ подо́бного; ~ doing *разг.* ничего́ не вы́йдет; «но́мер не пройдёт»; ничего́ не поде́лаешь; all to ~ всё ни к чему́; to come to ~ ко́нчиться ниче́м; 3) *pl* пустяки́, ме́лочи; the little ~s of life ме́лочи жи́зни; 4) небытие́, нере́альность; ◇ ~ venture ~ have *посл.* ≅ волко́в боя́ться — в лес не ходи́ть.

nothing II *adv* ниско́лько, совсе́м нет.

nothingness ['nʌθıŋnıs] *n* 1) ничто́жество; 2) пустяки́; 3) небытие́, нере́альность.

notice I ['noutıs] *n* 1) извеще́ние, уведомле́ние, сообще́ние; calling-up ~ пове́стка о призы́ве в а́рмию; to come to smb.'s ~ стать изве́стным кому́-л.; to give ~ сообща́ть, уведомля́ть; to have ~ знать, име́ть све́дения; to send a ~ посла́ть извеще́ние, уведомле́ние; at (*или* on) short ~ то́тчас же; at a moment's ~ неме́дленно; 2) предупрежде́ние; to give smb. a week's ~ предупреди́ть кого́-л. за неде́лю; 3) объявле́ние; obituary ~ объявле́ние о сме́рти; некроло́г; to post (to paste up) a ~ пове́сить (раскле́ить) объявле́ние; till further ~ до осо́бого распоряже́ния; 4) наблюде́ние; внима́ние; to come into ~ привле́чь внима́ние; to bring smth. to smb.'s ~ предлага́ть что-л. чьему́-л. внима́нию; обрати́ть чьё-л. внима́ние на что-л.; to take no ~ of не обраща́ть внима́ния на; beneath one's ~ не заслу́живающий чьего́-л. внима́ния; 5) обозре́ние, реце́нзия.

notice II *v* 1) замеча́ть, обраща́ть внима́ние; 2) отмеча́ть, упомина́ть; 3) предупрежда́ть; 4) дава́ть обзо́р, рецензи́ровать.

noticeable ['noutısəbl] *a* заме́тный, приме́тный.

notice-board ['noutısbɔ:d] *n* доска́ объявле́ний.

notifiable ['noutıfaıəbl] *a* подлежа́щий регистра́ции (*об инфекцио́нном заболева́нии*).

notification [ˌnoutıfı'keıʃən] *n* 1) уведомле́ние, извеще́ние; 2) объявле́ние.

notify ['noutıfaı] *v* 1) извеща́ть, уведомля́ть; 2) доводи́ть до всео́бщего све́дения, объявля́ть.

notion ['nouʃən] *n* 1) поня́тие, представле́ние; I have not the haziest (*или* slightest) ~ of what he means я не име́ю ни мале́йшего представле́ния о том, что́ он име́ет в виду́; 2) взгляд, то́чка зре́ния, мне́ние; 3) иде́я, мысль; 4) наме́рение; 5) остроу́мное приспособле́ние, прибо́р *и т. п.*; 6) *pl амер.* галантере́я.

notional ['nouʃənl] *a* 1) познава́емый; содержа́щий мысль; 2) умозри́тельный, отвлечённый; 3) вообража́емый; 4) *грам.* зна́чимый, смыслово́й.

notoriety [ˌnoutə'raıətı] *n* 1) изве́стность; 2) дурна́я сла́ва; 3) челове́к, по́льзующийся дурно́й сла́вой.

notorious [nou'tɔːrıəs] *a* 1) изве́стный; 2) отъя́вленный; заве́домый; неисправи́мый.

notwithstanding I [ˌnɔtwıθ'stændıŋ] *prep* несмотря́ на, вопреки́.

notwithstanding II *adv* тем не ме́нее, одна́ко.

nought [nɔ:t] *n* 1) ничто́; to bring to ~ своди́ть на нет; to come to ~ сойти́ на нет; to set at ~ ни во что́ не ста́вить; 2) ничто́жество (*о челове́ке*); 3) *мат.* ноль; ~s and crosses кре́стики и но́лики (*игра́*).

noun [naun] *n грам.* и́мя существи́тельное; collective ~ и́мя существи́тельное собира́тельное; common ~ и́мя существи́тельное нарица́тельное; verbal ~ отглаго́льное существи́тельное.

nourish ['nʌrıʃ] *v* 1) пита́ть, корми́ть; 2) леле́ять (*наде́жду*).

nourishing ['nʌrıʃıŋ] *a* пита́тельный.

nourishment ['nʌrıʃmənt] *n* 1) пита́ние; 2) пи́ща.

novel[1] ['nɔvəl] *n* 1) рома́н; dime ~ дешёвый приключе́нческий рома́н; problem ~ тенденцио́зный рома́н; 2) по́весть, нове́лла.

novel[2] *a* но́вый, неизве́данный.

novelese [ˌnɔvə'liːz] *n* язы́к и стиль рома́на.

novelette [ˌnɔvə'let] *n* небольша́я нове́лла; расска́з, по́весть.

novelist ['nɔvəlıst] *n* писа́тель-романи́ст.

novelty ['nɔvəltɪ] n 1) новизна; 2) новинка, новшество; 3) новость.

November [nou'vembə] n 1) ноябрь; 2) attr ноябрьский.

novice ['nɔvɪs] n 1) новичок; 2) послушник, -ица; 3) новообращённый.

now I [nau] adv 1) теперь, сейчас; 2) тотчас же, сию же минуту; 3) тогда, в то время (в рассказе); 4): ~ then! ну!; послушайте!; ◊ every ~ and then то и дело; ~ and again иногда; ~ and then время от времени; just ~ только что; ~... ~ то... то; he says ~ one thing ~ another он говорит то одно, то другое.

now II conj когда, раз; ~ you are here, why not stay? раз вы уже здесь, почему бы не остаться?

now III n данный момент; настоящее время; before ~ раньше; by ~ к настоящему моменту; till ~ до настоящего момента.

nowaday ['nauədeɪ] a теперешний.

nowadays I ['nauədeɪz] n настоящее время.

nowadays II adv теперь, в настоящее время; в наши дни.

noway ['nouweɪ] adv ни в коем случае.

nowhere ['nouwɛə] adv нигде, никуда.

nowise ['nouwaɪs] adv никоим образом; отнюдь не.

noxious ['nɔkʃəs] a вредный; пагубный, нездоровый.

nozzle ['nɔzl] n 1) носик (чайника); 2) розетка (подсвечника); 3) тех. выпускное отверстие; брандспойт; 4) сленг нос.

n't [nt] разг. = not.

nth [enθ] a энный; to the nth (degree) до любых пределов.

nuance [njuː'ɑːns] n оттенок, нюанс.

nub [nʌb] n 1) шишка, утолщение; 2) кусок, комок (угля); 3) амер. разг. суть, соль (рассказа).

nubbin ['nʌbɪn] n амер. 1) кусочек, комочек; 2) небольшой незрелый початок кукурузы.

nubble ['nʌbl] см. nub 1), 2).

nubia ['njuːbjə] n женский шерстяной шарф.

nuclear ['njuːklɪə] a 1) ядерный, содержащий ядро; 2) атомный.

nucleate ['njuːklɪeɪt] v образовывать ядро.

nucleus ['njuːklɪəs] n (pl тж. nuclei ['njuːklɪaɪ]) 1) ядро, ячейка; 2) серое вещество (головного мозга); 3) центр, зародыш.

nude I [njuːd] n 1) обнажённая фигура (в скульптуре, живописи); 2) pl тонкие чулки, «паутинка».

nude II a 1) голый; обнажённый, нагой; 2) телесного цвета (о чулках); 3) юр. недействительный.

nudge I [nʌdʒ] n лёгкий толчок.

nudge II v слегка подталкивать (локтем).

nudity ['njuːdɪtɪ] n нагота.

nugatory ['njuːgətərɪ] a 1) пустячный; не имеющий никакой цены; 2) тщетный, напрасный.

nugget ['nʌgɪt] n самородок (золота).

nuisance ['njuːsns] n 1) неприятность, досада; what a ~! какая досада!; 2) неприятный, надоедливый человек; to make a ~ of oneself надоедать; he is a perfect ~ он страшно надоедлив; 3): public ~ нарушение или нарушитель общественного порядка.

null [nʌl] a predic 1) недействительный; ~ and void недействительный; юр. не имеющий силы; 2) невыразительный (о лице).

nullah ['nʌlə] n инд. 1) русло реки (обыкн. высохшее); 2) овраг; 3) поток, ручей.

nullification [ˌnʌlɪfɪ'keɪʃən] n аннулирование.

nullify ['nʌlɪfaɪ] v аннулировать; делать недействительным.

nullity ['nʌlɪtɪ] n 1) ничтожество; 2) ничтожность; 3) юр. недействительность; ~ of marriage недействительность брака.

numb I [nʌm] a 1) онемелый, оцепенелый; 2) окоченелый.

numb II v вызывать онемение или окоченение; перен. поражать.

number I ['nʌmbə] n 1) число, количество; broken ~ дробь; even ~ чётное число; odd ~ нечётное число; prime ~ простое число; whole ~s целые числа; a ~ of целый ряд, много; quite a ~ целый ряд; without ~ бесчисленный; 2) сумма, итог; цифра; 3) номер; serial ~ порядковый номер; to take the ~ of the car записать номер машины; 4) выпуск, номер (газеты, журнала); back ~ старый номер (газеты, журнала); перен. отсталый человек; 5) pl большое количество; in ~s в большом количестве; 6) грам. числительное; cardinal ~s количественные числительные; ordinal ~s порядковые числительные; 7) грам. число; 8) pl поэт. размер, ритм; стихи; ◊ his ~ goes up сленг он кончается, умирает; to lose the ~ of one's mess воен. умереть.

number II v 1) иметь номер; 2) нумеровать; 3) воен. рассчитываться; 4) числиться, быть в числе (among); 5) насчитывать; 6) считать; □ to ~ off делать перекличку по номерам.

numberless ['nʌmbəlɪs] a 1) бесчисленный, неисчислимый; 2) не имеющий номера.

numbness ['nʌmnɪs] n онемение, оцепенение; окоченение.

numerable ['njuːmərəbl] a исчислимый, поддающийся счёту.

numeral I ['njuːmərəl] n 1) грам. имя числительное; cardinal ~ количественное числительное; ordinal ~ порядковое числительное; 2) цифра.

numeral II a числовой; цифровой.

numerary ['njuːmərərɪ] a числовой.

numeration [ˌnjuːmə'reɪʃən] n 1) исчисление, счёт; decimal ~ десятичная система счисления; 2) нумерация.

numerator ['njuːməreɪtə] n 1) мат. числитель; 2) вычислитель; нумератор.

numerical [njuː'merɪkəl] a числовой; цифровой.

numerous ['njuːmərəs] a многочисленный.

numismatics [ˌnjuːmɪz'mætɪks] n нумизматика.

numskull ['nʌmskʌl] n болван, тупица; дурацкая башка.

nun [nʌn] n монахиня.

nunnery ['nʌnərɪ] n женский монастырь.

nuptial ['nʌpʃəl] a брачный, свадебный.

nuptials ['nʌpʃəlz] n pl свадьба.

nurse I [nəːs] n 1) кормилица; няня; 2) медицинская сестра (тж. trained ~); 3): the ~ of liberty колыбель свободы.

nurse II v 1) кормить, выкармливать (ребёнка); 2) нянчить; 3) ухаживать (за больным); 4) выращивать (растение); 5) лелеять (надежду); 6) питать, таить (злобу и т. п.).

nurse-child ['nəːstʃaɪld] n питомец; приёмыш.

nurseling ['nəːslɪŋ] см. nursling.

nurse-maid ['nə:smeid] *n* няня.

nursery ['nə:srı] *n* 1) детская (*комната*); 2) (детские) ясли (*тж.* public ~); 3) питомник; 4) инкубатор; 5) садок (*для рыб*).

nursling ['nə:slıŋ] *n* 1) грудной ребёнок; 2) питомец; 3) молодое растение.

nurture I ['nə:tʃə] *n* 1) воспитание, обучение; 2) выращивание; 3) питание; пища.

nurture II *v* 1) обучать, воспитывать; 2) выращивать; вынашивать (*план и т. п.*); 3) питать.

nut [nʌt] *n* 1) орех; 2) *сленг* голова, «котелок»; off one's ~ а) сумасшедший; б) *сленг* человек; «тип»; 4) *сленг* фат, щёголь; 5) гайка; ◊ a hard ~ to crack а) трудная задача, трудное дело; б) «трудный человек»; to be ~s on а) очень любить что-л.; б) знать что-л. как свои пять пальцев.

nutcrackers ['nʌt,krækəz] *n pl* щипцы для орехов.

nutmeg ['nʌtmeg] *n* мускатный орех.

nutria ['njuːtrıə] *n* 1) *зоол.* нутрия; 2) мех-нутрии.

nutrient ['njuːtrıənt] *a* питательный.

nutriment ['njuːtrımənt] *n* питательное вещество; пища; корм.

nutrition [njuˈtrıʃən] *n* 1) питание; 2) пища; корм.

nutritious [njuˈtrıʃəs] *a* питательный.

nutritive I ['njuːtrıtıv] *n* питательное вещество.

nutritive II *a* 1) питательный; 2) пищевой.

nuts [nʌts] *int* глупости!, ерунда!, вздор!

nutshell ['nʌtʃel] *n* ореховая скорлупа; ◊ in a ~ кратко, в двух словах.

nutting ['nʌtıŋ] *n* собирание орехов.

nut-tree ['nʌttriː] *n* орешник.

nutty ['nʌtı] *a* 1) имеющий вкус ореха; вкусный; 2) интересный, пикантный; 3) *разг.* нарядный, щегольской; 4) *разг.* увлекающийся (*чем-л. — upon*); 5) *сленг* ненормальный, не в своём уме.

nuzzle ['nʌzl] *v* 1) водить носом, нюхать (*о собаках*); 2) рыть землю (*носом, рылом*); 3) совать нос, морду (*at, against, into*); 4) тереться носом, мордой обо что-л.; 5) свернуться в клубок; прикорнуть; уютно улечься.

nylon ['naılən] *n* 1) нейлон; 2) *pl* нейлоновые чулки.

nymph [nımf] *n* 1) *миф.* нимфа; 2) *поэт.* красивая, изящная девушка; 3) личинка (*насекомого*).

O

O, o[1] [ou] *n* 15-я буква англ. алфавита; an o, a round o круг.

o[2] *int:* O dear me! о боже!

oafish ['oufıʃ] *a* глупый, нескладный.

oak [ouk] *n* 1) дуб; dwarf ~ карликовый дуб; 2) древесина дуба; изделие из дуба; дубовая мебель; bog ~ морёный дуб; 3) *attr* дубовый.

oak-apple ['ouk,æpl] *см.* oak-gall.

oaken ['oukən] *a* дубовый.

oak-gall ['oukgɔːl] *n* чернильный орешек.

oakum ['oukəm] *n* пакля.

oar I [ɔː] *n* 1) весло; to pull an ~ грести; to rest

on one's ~s сушить вёсла; отдыхать; *перен.* почивать на лаврах; 2) гребец; a good (practised) ~ хороший (опытный) гребец; ◊ to have an ~ in every man's boat вмешиваться в чужие дела; to put one's ~ in *разг.* вмешаться (*в разговор и т. п.*).

oar II *v* грести.

oared [ɔːd] *a* имеющий вёсла; гребной.

oarlock ['ɔːlɔk] *n* уключина.

oarsman ['ɔːzmən] *n* гребец.

oasis [ouˈeısıs] *n* (*pl* oases [ouˈeısiːz]) оазис.

oat [out] *n обыкн. pl* овёс; ◊ to feel one's ~s *амер. разг.* а) быть весёлым, оживлённым; б) чувствовать свою силу; to sow one's wild ~s отдать дань юношеским увлечениям; перебеситься; to smell one's ~s напрячь последние силы (*когда близка цель*).

oatcake ['outkeık] *n* овсяная лепёшка.

oaten ['outn] *a* 1) овсяный; 2) соломенный.

oath [ouθ] *n* 1) клятва; присяга; ~ of allegiance клятва в верности; to administer an ~ приводить к присяге; on ~ под присягой; to make (*или* to swear, to take) an ~ дать клятву; 2) проклятия, ругательства.

oath-breaking ['ouθ,breıkıŋ] *n* нарушение клятвы *или* присяги.

oatmeal ['outmiːl] *n* 1) толокно; 2) овсянка, овсяная каша.

obduracy ['ɔbdjurəsı] *n* 1) чёрствость; ожесточение; 2) упрямство.

obdurate ['ɔbdjurıt] *a* 1) чёрствый; ожесточённый; 2) упрямый.

obedience [əˈbiːdjəns] *n* послушание, повиновение; in ~ to согласно.

obedient [əˈbiːdjənt] *a* послушный; покорный.

obeisance [ouˈbeısəns] *n* 1) почтение, уважение; to do (*или* to make, to pay) ~ to выражать почтение; 2) почтительный поклон.

obelisk ['ɔbılısk] *n* 1) обелиск; 2) *полигр.* знак ссылки.

obese [ouˈbiːs] *a* жирный, полный, тучный.

obesity [ouˈbiːsıtı] *n* полнота, тучность.

obey [əˈbeı] *v* слушаться, повиноваться; подчиняться, выполнять (*приказание и т. п.*).

obituary I [əˈbıtjuərı] *n* некролог.

obituary II *a* некрологический.

object[a] ['ɔbdʒıkt] *n* 1) предмет; объект; 2) цель, намерение; my ~ in coming here цель моего приезда сюда; 3) *грам.* дополнение; direct (indirect) ~ прямое (косвенное) дополнение; prepositional ~ предложное дополнение; 4) *разг.* человек *или* вещь смешного, жалкого вида; what on ~ you are! какой (ужасный) вид у тебя!

object[b] [əbˈdʒekt] *v* 1) возражать (*против чего-л.*), протестовать (*against, to*); 2) не любить (*чего-л.*), не переносить.

object-finder ['ɔbdʒıkt,faındə] *n фото* видоискатель.

object-glass ['ɔbdʒıktglɑːs] *n* объектив.

objection [əbˈdʒekʃən] *n* 1) возражение; протест; to take ~ возражать; 2) нелюбовь, неодобрение.

objectionable [əbˈdʒekʃnəbl] *a* 1) нежелательный, вызывающий возражения; 2) неприятный; неудобный.

objective I [əbˈdʒektıv] *n* 1) цель, стремление; 2) *грам.* объектный падеж; 3) объектив; 4): military ~ военный объект.

objective II *a* 1) объекти́вный; 2) действи́тельный, реа́льный; 3) *грам.* относя́щийся к дополне́нию.

objectivity [,ɔbdʒek'tɪvɪtɪ] *n* объекти́вность; Olympian ~ по́лная беспристра́стность, объекти́вность.

objectless ['ɔbdʒɪktlɪs] *a* беспредме́тный, бесце́льный.

object-lesson ['ɔbdʒɪkt,lesn] *n* нагля́дный уро́к (*тж. перен.*).

objector [əb'dʒektə] *n* возража́ющий; conscientious ~ челове́к, отка́зывающийся от вое́нной слу́жбы по полити́ческим *или* религио́зным моти́вам.

objurgate ['ɔbdʒəgeɪt] *v* попрека́ть; жури́ть.

objurgation [,ɔbdʒə'geɪʃən] *n* попрёк, уко́р.

objurgatory [əb'dʒəgətərɪ] *a* укори́зненный.

oblation [ou'bleɪʃən] *n* 1) жертвоприноше́ние, же́ртва; 2) поже́ртвование.

obligate ['ɔblɪgeɪt] *v* обя́зывать.

obligation [,ɔblɪ'geɪʃən] *n* 1) обяза́тельство; to undertake ~s брать на себя́ обяза́тельства; 2) обя́занность; to be under (an) ~ to smb. быть обя́занным кому́-л., быть в долгу́ перед кем-л.; 3) принуди́тельная си́ла, обяза́тельность (*закона, догово́ра и т. п.*); of ~ обяза́тельный.

obligatory [ɔ'blɪgətərɪ] *a* 1) обяза́тельный; 2) обя́зывающий, принужда́ющий.

oblige [ə'blaɪdʒ] *v* 1) обя́зывать; заставля́ть; 2) де́лать одолже́ние.

obliging [ə'blaɪdʒɪŋ] *a* обяза́тельный, любе́зный.

oblique I [ə'bli:k] *a* 1) накло́нный; косо́й; 2) око́льный, непрямо́й; 3) *грам.* ко́свенный (*о падеже́, ре́чи*).

oblique II *v* отклоня́ться.

obliquity [ə'blɪkwɪtɪ] *n* 1) косо́е направле́ние; 2) отклоне́ние от прямо́го пути́.

obliterate [ə'blɪtəreɪt] *v* 1) вычёркивать, стира́ть; 2) уничтожа́ть; изгла́живать.

obliteration [ə,blɪtə'reɪʃən] *n* 1) уничтоже́ние; вычёркивание; 2) забве́ние.

oblivion [ə'blɪvɪən] *n* забве́ние; to fall (*или* to pass, to sink) into ~ быть пре́данным забве́нию.

oblivious [ə'blɪvɪəs] *a* 1) забы́вчивый, непо́мнящий; забыва́ющий (of); 2) даю́щий забве́ние.

oblong ['ɔblɔŋ] *a* продолгова́тый; удлинённый.

obloquy ['ɔbləkwɪ] *n* 1) оскорбле́ние; злосло́вие; 2) позо́р.

obnoxious [əb'nɔkʃəs] *a* проти́вный, несно́сный.

oboe ['oubou] *n* гобо́й.

obscene [ɔb'si:n] *a* непристо́йный, неприли́чный.

obscenity [ɔb'si:nɪtɪ] *n* непристо́йность.

obscure I [əb'skjuə] *a* 1) тёмный, мра́чный; 2) нея́сный; непоня́тный; сму́тный (*об о́бразе, представле́нии*); 3) скры́тый, глубо́кий (*о значе́нии*); 4) неизве́стный, незаме́тный; безве́стный.

obscure II *v* 1) затемня́ть; 2) затмева́ть; помрача́ть; 3) де́лать нея́сным; затрудня́ть понима́ние.

obscurity [əb'skjuərɪtɪ] *n* 1) тьма, темнота́, мрак; 2) нея́сность, непоня́тность; 3) неизве́стность, безве́стность.

obsequies ['ɔbsɪkwɪz] *n pl* обря́д погребе́ния, по́хороны.

obsequious [əb'si:kwɪəs] *a* раболе́пный, зайски́вающий.

observable [əb'zə:vəbl] *a* 1) (легко́) заме́тный, приме́тный; 2) (досто)примеча́тельный.

observance [əb'zə:vəns] *n* 1) соблюде́ние (*зако́на, обы́чая и т. п.*); 2) обря́д, ритуа́л.

observant [əb'zə:vənt] *a* 1) наблюда́тельный; внима́тельный; 2) соблюда́ющий (*зако́ны, пра́вила*).

observation [,ɔbzə'veɪʃən] *n* 1) наблюде́ние; to keep under ~ следи́ть, держа́ть под наблюде́нием; 2) наблюда́тельность; 3) замеча́ние, выска́зывание; 4) *attr* для наблюде́ний; наблюда́тельный (*о пу́нкте и т. п.*).

observatory [əb'zə:vətrɪ] *n* 1) обсервато́рия; mountain top ~ го́рная обсервато́рия; 2) наблюда́тельный пункт.

observe [əb'zə:v] *v* 1) наблюда́ть, замеча́ть; следи́ть за чем-л.; изуча́ть; 2) соблюда́ть (*зако́ны, обы́чаи и т. п.*); 3) де́лать замеча́ние, выска́зывать; it will be ~d сле́дует заме́тить.

observer [əb'zə:və] *n* 1) наблюда́тель; 2) тот, кто соблюда́ет (*зако́ны, пра́вила и т. п.*), выполня́ет (*обеща́ния*); 3) обозрева́тель (*в газе́те*).

observing [əb'zə:vɪŋ] *a* наблюда́тельный.

obsess [əb'ses] *v* овладе́ть, обуя́ть (*о стра́хе*); пресле́довать (*о мы́сли*).

obsession [əb'seʃən] *n* 1) одержи́мость; наважде́ние; 2) навя́зчивая иде́я.

obsolescent [,ɔbsə'lesnt] *a* выходя́щий из употребле́ния; отжива́ющий.

obsolete ['ɔbsəli:t] *a* 1) устаре́лый; вы́шедший из употребле́ния; 2) *биол.* рудимента́рный.

obstacle ['ɔbstəkl] *n* препя́тствие, поме́ха; to overcome (*или* to surmount) ~s преодолева́ть препя́тствия; to throw ~s in smb.'s way чини́ть препя́тствия кому́-л.

obstinacy ['ɔbstɪnəsɪ] *n* упря́мство; упо́рство.

obstinate ['ɔbstɪnɪt] *a* упря́мый; упо́рный; ~ as a mule упря́мый как осёл.

obstreperous [əb'strepərəs] *a* шумли́вый; беспоко́йный.

obstruct [əb'strʌkt] *v* 1) загражда́ть путь, препя́тствовать движе́нию; меша́ть; 2) устра́ивать обстру́кцию.

obstruction [əb'strʌkʃən] *n* 1) загражде́ние, заку́порка; препя́тствие, поме́ха; 2) обстру́кция.

obstructive [əb'strʌktɪv] *a* 1) препя́тствующий, меша́ющий; 2) обструкцио́нный.

obtain [əb'teɪn] *v* 1) получа́ть, достава́ть; приобрета́ть; 2) доби́ться, дости́гнуть; 3) быть при́знанным; применя́ться.

obtainable [əb'teɪnəbl] *a* достижи́мый, досту́пный.

obtrude [əb'tru:d] *v* навя́зывать(ся).

obtruncate [əb'trʌŋkeɪt] *v* обреза́ть, среза́ть верху́шку.

obtrusive [əb'tru:sɪv] *a* навя́зчивый.

obturate ['ɔbtjuəreɪt] *v* затыка́ть, заку́поривать.

obturator ['ɔbtjureɪtə] *n* 1) зaты́чка; 2) *фото* затво́р.

obtuse [əb'tju:s] *a* 1) тупо́й; 2) бестолко́вый, глу́пый.

obverse I ['ɔbvə:s] *n* лицева́я сторона́ (*моне́ты, меда́ли и т. п.*).

obverse II *a* лицево́й, пере́дний.

obviate ['ɔbvɪeɪt] *v* избега́ть, уклоня́ться (*от чего́-л.*); устраня́ть.

obvious ['ɔbvɪəs] *a* очеви́дный, я́сный, я́вный.

occasion I [ə'keɪʒən] *n* 1) слу́чай, возмо́жность;

on ~ при слу́чае; on the ~ of по слу́чаю; to improve (*или* to seize) the ~, to take ~ (вос)-по́льзоваться слу́чаем; (up)on all ~s во вся́ком слу́чае; 2) обстоя́тельство; 3) по́вод, причи́на; to give ~ to дава́ть по́вод для, вызыва́ть (*что-л.*); there is no ~ for... нет основа́ния для...; 4) собы́тие; to celebrate the ~ отме́тить, отпра́здновать э́то собы́тие; this is a great ~ э́то большо́е собы́тие; 5) *pl уст.* дела́; ◊ to rise to the ~ оказа́ться на высоте́ положе́ния.

occasion II *v* дава́ть по́вод, вызыва́ть; служи́ть причи́ной; that is what ~ed me to be late вот почему́ я опозда́л.

occasional [ə'keɪʒənl] *a* 1) случа́йный; случа́ющийся иногда́; ре́дкий; 2) приуро́ченный к определённому моме́нту *или* собы́тию.

occasionally [ə'keɪʒnəlɪ] *adv* случа́йно; и́зредка; вре́мя от вре́мени.

Occident ['ɔksɪdənt] *n* (the~) За́пад, стра́ны За́пада.

Occidental [ˌɔksɪ'dentl] *n* жи́тель За́пада.

occidental [ˌɔksɪ'dentl] *a* за́падный.

occlude [ɔ'kluːd] *v* 1) заку́поривать, закрыва́ть (*отве́рстие, поры*); 2) *хим.* поглоща́ть (*газы*).

occult [ɔ'kʌlt] *a* 1) та́йный, сокрове́нный; 2) таи́нственный, оккульти́ный.

occupancy ['ɔkjupənsɪ] *n* 1) заня́тие, завладе́ние; 2) вре́менное владе́ние, аре́нда.

occupant ['ɔkjupənt] *n* 1) жиле́ц, обита́тель; 2) вре́менный владе́лец; 3) оккупа́нт.

occupation [ˌɔkju'peɪʃən] *n* 1) заня́тие; профе́ссия; 2) вре́менное по́льзование; 3) оккупа́ция, заня́тие.

occupational [ˌɔkjuː'peɪʃənl] *a* профессиона́льный.

occupier ['ɔkjupaɪə] *n* 1) жиле́ц; 2) аренда́тор, вре́менный владе́лец.

occupy ['ɔkjupaɪ] *v* 1) завладе́ть, заня́ть; оккупи́ровать; 2) занима́ть (*дом, помеще́ние*); арендова́ть; 3) занима́ть (*до́лжность*); 4) занима́ть (*вре́мя, внима́ние*); to ~ oneself with smth. занима́ться чем-л.

occur [ə'kəː] *v* 1) име́ть ме́сто, случа́ться; 2) приходи́ть на ум *или* в го́лову; it ~red to me мне пришло́ в го́лову, мне предста́вилось; 3) встреча́ться, име́ться; 4) *геол.* залега́ть.

occurrence [ə'kʌrəns] *n* 1) слу́чай, происше́ствие; an everyday ~ обы́чное явле́ние; to be of common (*или* of frequent) ~ быть ча́стым, обы́чным явле́нием; 2) местонахожде́ние; 3) *геол.* месторожде́ние.

ocean ['ouʃən] *n* 1) океа́н; 2) мно́жество, ма́сса; 3) *attr* океа́нский.

ocean-going ['ouʃən͵gouɪŋ] *a* океа́нский (*о парохо́де*).

oceanic [ˌouʃɪ'ænɪk] *a* океа́нский, океани́ческий.

ochre ['oukə] *n* 1) о́хра; 2) жёлтый цвет; 3) *сленг* де́ньги, зо́лото.

o'clock [ə'klɔk]: what ~ is it? кото́рый час?; it is two ~ два часа́.

octagon ['ɔktəgən] *n* восьмиуго́льник.

octave ['ɔktɪv] *n* 1) *муз.* окта́ва; 2) восьмисти́шие; 3) ви́нная бо́чка (*ёмкостью о́коло 61 л*).

octavo [ɔk'teɪvou] *n* форма́т (*кни́ги*) в ⅛ листа́.

October [ɔk'toubə] *n* 1) октя́брь; 2) *attr* октя́брь-

ский; the Great ~ Socialist Revolution Вели́кая Октя́брьская социалисти́ческая револю́ция.

octogenarian I [ˌɔktoudʒɪ'nɛərɪən] *n* восьмидеся-тиле́тний челове́к.

octogenarian II *a* восьмидесятиле́тний.

octopus ['ɔktəpəs] *n* осьмино́г, спрут.

ocular I ['ɔkjulə] *n* окуля́р.

ocular II *a* 1) глазно́й; 2) нагля́дный (*о доказа́тельстве и т. п.*).

oculist ['ɔkjulɪst] *n* окули́ст.

odd [ɔd] *a* 1) нечётный; ~ and even чёт и не́чет; 2) ли́шний; twenty ~ два́дцать с ли́шним; 3) стра́нный, необы́чный, чудно́й; 4) непа́рный (*о перча́тке, чулке́ и т. п.*); разро́зненный (*о тома́х изда́ния*); 5) случа́йный (*о рабо́те, за́работке*); 6) свобо́дный, неза́нятый (*о вре́мени и т. п.*).

odd-come-short ['ɔdkʌm'ʃɔːt] *n* оста́ток.

odd-come-shortly ['ɔdkʌm'ʃɔːtlɪ] *n* (в) ближа́й-ший день; one of these odd-come-shortlies вско́ре.

oddity ['ɔdɪtɪ] *n* 1) стра́нность, чудакова́тость; 2) чуда́к, стра́нный челове́к; 3) стра́нный слу́чай, удиви́тельная вещь.

oddly ['ɔdlɪ] *adv* стра́нно; чудно́; ~ enough как э́то ни стра́нно.

oddments ['ɔdmənts] *n pl* оста́тки; разро́зненные предме́ты.

odds [ɔdz] *n pl* (*употр. тж как sg*) 1) ра́зница; нера́венство; to make ~ even уничто́жить ра́зницу; 2) преиму́щество; 3) ша́нсы; long (short) ~ нера́вные (почти́ ра́вные) ша́нсы; the ~ are that it will rain вероя́тно, пойдёт дождь; 4) разногла́сие; to be at ~ не ла́дить; ссо́риться (*из-за чего-л.—about*); ◊ ~ and ends оста́тки; ра́зные ме́лочи.

ode [oud] *n* о́да.

odious ['oudjəs] *a* 1) ненави́стный; отврати́тель-ный; 2) одио́зный.

odium ['oudjəm] *n* 1) не́нависть; 2) уко́р, упрёк; позо́р; 3) одио́зность.

odor ['oudə] *амер. см.* odour.

odoriferous [ˌoudə'rɪfərəs] *a* благоуха́ющий; души́стый.

odorous ['oudərəs] *a* паху́чий; благоуха́ющий.

odour ['oudə] *n* 1) за́пах; арома́т; *перен.* душо́к; 2) сла́ва, репута́ция; to be in good (bad) ~ with smb. быть в (не)ми́лости у кого́-л.

of [ɔv (*си́льная фо́рма*), əv (*сла́бая фо́рма*)] *prep* ука́зывает на: 1) *принадле́жность лицу́ или предме́ту:* the towns of our country города́ на́шей страны́; 2) *а́вторство:* the works of Dickens произведе́ния Ди́ккенса; 3) *часть от це́лого:* a pound of sugar фунт са́хару; many of us мно́гие из нас; member of congress член конгре́сса; 4) *материа́л, из кото́рого что-л. сде́лано* из; a house of bricks ка́мен-ный дом; 5) *причи́ну* от; he died of hunger (of chole-ra, of his wounds) он у́мер от го́лода (от холе́ры, от ран); 6) *происхожде́ние, исто́чник* из, у; he comes of a worker's family он происхо́дит из рабо́чей семьи́; he asked a question of me он спроси́л у меня́; 7) *ка́чество или свойство:* man of tact такти́чный челове́к; man of genius гениа́льный челове́к; man of distinction выдаю́щийся, знамени́тый челове́к; 8) *вре́мя:* of an evening ка́к-нибудь ве́чером; of late неда́вно; of old давно́; all of a sudden вдруг; за́пно; 9) *содержи́мое како́го-л. вмести́лища:* a glass of milk стака́н молока́; a pail of water ведро́ воды́.

off [ɔːf] *adv* ука́зывает на: 1) *удале́ние:* a long

way ~ далеко; ~ with you! прочь!; 2) *снятие предмета одежды*: hats ~! шапки долой!; ~ with your hat! снимите шляпу!; 3) *прекращение или законченный характер действия*: to break ~ negotiations прервать переговоры; the contest came ~ on the day fixed состязание произошло в назначенный день; 4) *выключение какого-л. аппарата, механизма из действия*: turn ~ the gas! выключи(те) газ!; switch ~ the light! выключи(те) свет!; 5) *состояние человека*: this man is well ~ это обеспеченный человек; your friend is badly ~ ваш приятель беден; ◊ ~ and on время от времени.

off II *prep указывает на*: 1) *удаление с поверхности предмета* с; the plate fell ~ the table тарелка упала со стола; 2) *отклонение от нормы*: ~ one's balance потерявший равновесие; ~ colour имеющий нездоровый вид; 3) *неучастие в чём-л.*: he is ~ gambling он не принимает участия в игре; 4) *расстояние* от; a village some kilometres ~ the main road посёлок в нескольких километрах от большой дороги; ~ the coast неподалёку от берега.

off III *a* 1) свободный (*о времени, часах*); 2) дальний; 3) неурожайный (*о годе*); 4) мёртвый (*о сезоне*); 5) боковой (*об улице*); 6) правый (*о стороне*); 7) обращённый в сторону моря (*о борте корабля*); 8) несвежий (*о пище*); 9) маловероятный (*о случае*); 10) плохо себя чувствующий.

off IV *v разг.* прекращать (*переговоры*).

offal [ˈɔfəl] *n* 1) потроха; требуха; 2) отбросы; 3) падаль.

offcast [ˈɔːfkɑːst] *a* отвергнутый.

offence [əˈfens] *n* 1) обида, оскорбление; no ~ (was) meant (я) не хотел вас обидеть; ничего обидного здесь нет; to give ~ обижать; to take ~ обижаться (*на — at*); 2) нападение; *воен.* наступление; 3) преступление, правонарушение; нарушение (*правил и т. n.*); to commit an ~ against совершить преступление против чего-л.

offenceless [əˈfenslɪs] *a* безобидный.

offend [əˈfend] *v* 1) обижать, оскорблять; причинить неприятность; to be ~ed быть обиженным; 2) погрешить (*против закона, совести и т. n.; against*).

offender [əˈfendə] *n* 1) обидчик; оскорбитель; 2) правонарушитель, преступник; juvenile ~ малолетний преступник.

offensive I [əˈfensɪv] *n воен.* наступление; to take the ~ перейти в наступление; *перен.* занять агрессивную позицию.

offensive II *a* 1) оскорбительный, обидный; 2) неприятный, противный (*о запахе*); 3) наступательный; агрессивный.

offer I [ˈɔfə] *n* предложение; ◊ on ~ (имеется) в продаже.

offer II [ˈɔfə] *v* 1) предлагать; 2) пытаться, пробовать; 3) оказывать (*сопротивление*); 4) представляться (*о случае, возможности*); 5) приносить (*жертвы*).

offering [ˈɔfərɪŋ] *n* 1) предложение; 2) подношение; 3) жертвоприношение.

offertory [ˈɔfətərɪ] *n* пожертвования, собранные в церкви.

offhand I [ˈɔːfhænd] *a* 1) сделанный без подготовки, экспромтом; 2) бесцеремонный.

offhand II *adv* 1) экспромтом; тотчас; 2) бесцеремонно.

offhandedly [ˈɔːfˈhændɪdlɪ] *adv* бесцеремонно; небрежно.

office [ˈɔfɪs] *n* 1) должность; an honorary ~ почётная должность; to hold ~ занимать пост; to take ~ вступить в должность; to get (*или* to come) into ~ принять дела; приступать к исполнению обязанностей; to be in ~ быть у власти; 2) обязанность; функция; 3) контора, канцелярия; editorial ~ редакция; publishing ~ издательство; private ~ личный кабинет; inquiry ~ справочное бюро; 4) управление, ведомство; министерство; Foreign and Commonwealth Office Министерство иностранных дел и по делам Содружества (*в Англии*); Home Office Министерство внутренних дел (*в Англии*); Record Office государственный архив; Holy Office *ист.* инквизиция; 5) услуга; an ill ~ плохая услуга; 6) *pl* службы, подсобные помещения; 7) церковная служба; обряд; the last ~s похоронный обряд; 8) *сленг.* намёк.

office-boy [ˈɔfɪsbɔɪ] *n* посыльный, рассыльный.

officer I [ˈɔfɪsə] *n* 1) чиновник; должностное лицо; государственный служащий; returning ~ *парл.* чиновник, проводящий выборы; police ~ полицейский; custom-house ~ таможенный чиновник; 2) офицер; liaison ~ офицер связи; ~ of the day, orderly ~ дежурный офицер; non-commissioned ~ военнослужащий сержантского состава; 3) капитан торгового судна.

officer II *v обыкн. pass* 1) укомплектовать офицерским составом; 2) командовать.

official I [əˈfɪʃəl] *n* чиновник, должностное лицо; служащий (*государственный, банковский*).

official II *a* 1) официальный; 2) служебный; 3) формальный.

officialdom [əˈfɪʃəldəm] *n* 1) бюрократизм; 2) *собир.* чиновничество; официальные лица.

officially [əˈfɪʃəlɪ] *adv* официально.

officiate [əˈfɪʃɪeɪt] *v* 1) исполнять обязанности (*кого-л. — as*); to ~ as host быть за хозяина; 2) совершать богослужение.

officious [əˈfɪʃəs] *a* 1) назойливый; навязчивый; угодливый; 2) официозный.

offing [ˈɔfɪŋ] *n* взморье; морская даль; in the ~ а) недалеко, неподалёку; б) в недалёком будущем.

offish [ˈɔfɪʃ] *a разг.* 1) нелюдимый; замкнутый; 2) чопорный.

off-print [ˈɔːfprɪnt] *n* (отдельный) оттиск (*статьи и т. n.*).

offscourings [ˈɔːfˌskauərɪŋz] *n pl* отбросы.

offset I [ˈɔfset] *n* 1) *см.* offshoot; 2) возмещение, компенсация; 3) уступ.

offset II *v* 1) возмещать, компенсировать; 2) сводить баланс.

offshoot [ˈɔːfʃuːt] *n* 1) побег; ответвление; отпрыск; отрог.

off-shore [ˈɔfʃɔː] *a* 1) направляющийся от берега, с берега; 2) находящийся далеко от берега.

off-side [ˈɔːfsaɪd] *n спорт.* (положение) вне игры.

offspring [ˈɔːfsprɪŋ] *n* 1) отпрыск, потомок; 2) плод, результат (*чего-л.*).

offspur [ˈɔːfspə] *n* отрог.

oft [ɔft] *adv поэт.* часто.

often [ˈɔfn] *adv* часто; ~ and ~ весьма часто.

oftentimes [ˈɔfntaɪmz] *adv* часто, много раз.

oft-recurring [ˈɔftrɪˈkəːrɪŋ] *a* часто повторяющийся.

ogle I ['ougl] *n* влюблённый взгляд.

ogle II *v* бросáть влюблённые взгля́ды; стрóить глáзки.

ogre ['ougə] *n* великáн-людоéд.

ogress ['ougrıs] *n* великáнша-людоéдка.

oh [ou] *int* о!

ohm [oum] *n эл.* ом.

oil I [ɔıl] *n* 1) мáсло (*растительное или мине-
ральное*); essential ~s, volatile ~s эфи́рные, ле-
тýчие маслá; cod-liver ~ ры́бий жир; blasting ~
нитроглицери́н; 2) нефть; to strike ~ найти́ нефтянóй истóчник; *перен.* сдéлать вы́годное дéло;
3) *жив.* мáсло; to paint in ~s писáть мáслом;
4) смáзочный материáл; ◊ ~ of birch ≅ берёзо-
вая кáша, пóрка; to pour ~ on the flame подливáть
мáсла в огóнь; to pour ~ on troubled waters
умиротворя́ть, успокáивать; to burn the midnight
~ рабóтать по ночáм.

oil II *v* смáзывать; *перен.* «подмáзать», дать
взя́тку.

oil-bearing ['ɔıl‚bɛərıŋ] *a* нефтенóсный.

oilcake ['ɔılkeık] *n* жмых.

oilcan ['ɔılkæn] *n тех.* маслёнка.

oilcloth ['ɔılklɔθ] *n* клеёнка.

oil-colour ['ɔıl‚kʌlə] *n обыкн. pl* мáсляная крáска.

oil-derrick ['ɔıl‚derık] *n* нефтянáя вы́шка.

oiler ['ɔılə] *n* 1) нефтеналивнóе сýдно; 2) смáзчик; 3) *тех.* маслёнка.

oilfield ['ɔılfiːld] *n* 1) месторождéние нéфти;
2) нефтянóй прóмысел.

oil-fuel ['ɔılfjuəl] *n* жи́дкое тóпливо.

oilman ['ɔılmən] *n* 1) продавéц мáсляных крáсок, москатéльщик; 2) смáзчик.

oil-paint ['ɔıl'peınt] *см.* oil-colour.

oil-painting ['ɔıl'peıntıŋ] *n* 1) жи́вопись мáслом;
2) карти́на, напи́санная мáслом.

oil-paper ['ɔıl‚peıpə] *n* промáсленная бумáга,
вощáнка.

oil-silk ['ɔılsılk] *n* водооттáлкивающая шёлковая ткань.

oilskin ['ɔılskın] *n* 1) клеёнка; 2) *pl* клеёнчатый
костю́м.

oilstone ['ɔılstoun] *n* оселóк, точи́льный кáмень.

oil-well ['ɔılwel] *n* нефтянáя сквáжина.

oily ['ɔılı] *a* 1) мáсляный; маслянистый, жи́р-
ный; 2) елéйный.

ointment ['ɔıntmənt] *n* мазь; помáда.

O. K. I ['ou'keı] *n разг.* одобрéние.

O. K. II *a predic разг.* всё в поря́дке; хорошó.

O. K. III *v* (*past, p. p.* O. K.'d; *pres. p.* O. K.'ing)
разг. одобря́ть.

old I [ould] *a* 1) стáрый; to get (*или* to grow) ~
стáриться; 2) стáрческий; старообрáзный; 3): how
~ is he? скóлько емý лет?; he is ten years ~ емý
дéсять лет; 4) стари́нный; дáвний; 5) прéжний; бы́в-
ший; прóшлый; 6) закоренéлый (*in, at*); 7) *разг.*
придаёт сущ. ласкáтельное значéние: ~ boy дру-
жи́ще; ~ man старинá; 8) *сленг придаёт сущ.
усилительное значéние:* to have a good ~ time
хорошó повесели́ться; ◊ as ~ as the hills старó
как мир.

old II *n* 1): the ~ (*употр. как pl*) старики́;
2) дáвнее прóшлое; дрéвность; of ~ в прéжнее
врéмя; в старинý; from ~ of йстари.

olden I ['ouldən] *a* дáвний; былóй.

---

olden II *v* старéть; стáриться.

old-fashioned ['ould'fæʃənd] *a* 1) устарéлый;
стари́нный; 2) старомóдный.

oldish ['ouldıʃ] *a* старовáтый.

oldster ['ouldstə] *n разг.* пожилóй человéк.

old-time ['ouldtaım] *a* стари́нный, прéжних времён.

old-timer ['ould'taımə] *n* старожи́л.

old-world ['ouldwəːld] *a амер.* относя́щийся
к Стáрому Свéту.

olfactory I [ɔl'fæktərı] *n обыкн. pl* óрган обоня́-
ния.

olfactory II *a* обоня́тельный.

oligarchy ['ɔlıɡɑːkı] *n* олигáрхия.

olio ['ouliou] *n* 1) смесь; вся́кая вся́чина; меша-
ни́на; 2) *муз.* попурри́; 3) кýшанье из мя́са с ово-
щáми.

olive I ['ɔlıv] *n* 1) оли́ва, масли́на; 2) *см.* olive-
-branch; 3) оли́вковый цвет.

olive II *a* оли́вковый, оли́вкового цвéта.

olive-branch ['ɔlıvbrɑːntʃ] *n* оли́вковая ветвь
(*как символ мира*); to hold out the ~ дéлать ми́р-
ные предложéния.

olive-oil ['ɔlıv'ɔıl] *n* провáнское мáсло.

olive-wood ['ɔlıvwud] *n* оли́вковая рóща.

olympiad [ou'lımpıæd] *n* олимпиáда.

Olympic [ou'lımpık] *a* олимпи́йский.

omega ['oumıɡə] *n* омéга (*см. тж.* alpha).

omelet(te) ['ɔmlıt] *n* омлéт, яи́чница.

omen I ['oumen] *n* предзнаменовáние, знак; to
be of good (bad) ~ служи́ть хорóшей (дурнóй) при-
мéтой.

omen II *v* служи́ть предзнаменовáнием; предвещáть.

ominous ['ɔmınəs] *a* зловéщий; угрожáющий.

omission [ou'mıʃən] *n* прóпуск; упущéние,
оплóшность.

omit [ou'mıt] *v* 1) пропускáть; не включáть;
2) упускáть; пренебрегáть; to ~ to do (*или* doing)
smth. не сдéлать чегó-л.

omnibus I ['ɔmnıbəs] *n* 1) óмнибус; 2) автóбус.

omnibus II *a* 1) охвáтывающий нéсколько раздé-
лов *или* пýнктов (*о резолюции и т. п.*); 2) общe-
достýпный.

omnipotent [ɔm'nıpətənt] *a* всемогýщий.

omnipresent ['ɔmnı'prezənt] *a* вездесýщий.

omniscient [ɔm'nısıənt] *a* всевéдущий.

omnivorous [ɔm'nıvərəs] *a* 1) всея́дный (*тж.
перен.*); 2) всепожирáющий.

on I [ɔn] *prep* 1) *в пространственном значении
указывает: а) на нахождéние на повéрхности, другого предмета на*; the table-cloth and dishes are on
the table скáтерть и посýда на столé; is on board
ship он на бортý корабля́; б) *на нахождéние около
какого-л. водного пространства* на, у; the town lies
on the Volga (on the coast of the Black Sea, on lake
Michigan) гóрод располóжен на Вóлге (на берегý
Чёрного мóря, на берегý óзера Мичигáн); в) *на
направление, цель движения* на; the boy threw the
ball on the ground мáльчик брóсил мяч нá пол;
2) *во временном значении указывает: а) на опредe-
лённый день недели* в; we hope to see you on Sunday
мы надéемся ви́деть вас в воскресéнье; on
another day в другóй день; on any day в любóй день;
б) *на определённую дату месяца, года*: on the 7th of
November 7 ноября́; в) *на часть дня, при котором*

имеется дата: on the morning of the 7th of November утром 7 ноября; г) *на последовательность, очерёдность наступления действий* по, после; on arrival we went to see the sights of the town по прибытии мы отправились осматривать достопримечательности города; 3) *указывает на состояние, характер действия* в, на; on leave в отпуске; on trial на испытании; on the trial под следствием; to be on strike бастовать; on the move а) на ходу; б) в движении, в развитии; to be on the spree кутить; to be on the committee быть членом комиссии; on trust на веру; on speaking terms знакомый с кем-л.; on a friendly footing на короткой (дружеской) ноге; 4) *указывает цель или назначение действия*; on purpose нарочно, намеренно; on business по делу; 5) *указывает исходные основания, причину, источник:* on a new principle на новых основах, принципах; on that ground на этом основании; on the faith полагаясь (*на что-л. — of*); on my account или за мой счёт; on an annuity на ежегодную ренту; on his income на свой доход; on a pension на пенсию.

on II *adv указывает:* 1) на продолжение действия, выраженного глаголом: to read (to write, to walk) on продолжать читать (писать, шагать); go on! продолжайте! 2) на включение какого-л. аппарата, механизма в действие: turn on the gas! включи(те) газ!; switch on the current! включи(те) ток!; 3) на наличие какой-л. одежды на ком-л.: what had he on? во что он был одет?, что было на нём?; he had a new blue coat (gloves, his brown hat) on он был в новом синем пальто (в перчатках, в коричневой шляпе), на нём было новое синее пальто (перчатки, коричневая шляпа).

once I [wʌns] *n* один раз; for this (*или* that) ~ на этот раз; ~ is enough достаточно одного раза.

once II *adv* 1) (один) раз; ~ again, ~ more ещё раз; ~ or twice раз; несколько раз; б) иногда; ~ in a while, ~ and again иногда; время от времени; ~ every day раз в день; ~ for all раз навсегда; more than ~ не раз, неоднократно; not ~ ни разу, никогда; 2) некогда, когда-то; однажды; ~ upon a time there was (*или* there lived) ≅ жил-был когда-то; 3) если только; стоит только; ~ he understands... если только он поймёт..., стоит только ему понять...; ◊ at ~ тотчас, сразу, немедленно; all at ~ а) внезапно, неожиданно; б) все вместе, все сразу.

once-over [wʌns,ouvə] *n амер. разг.* беглый просмотр.

oncoming I ['ɔn,kʌmɪŋ] *n* приближение.

oncoming II *a* надвигающийся, приближающийся.

one I [wʌn] *пит* один; ◊ ~ or two немного, несколько; ~ too many слишком много; number ~ сам, собственная персона.

one II *n* 1) единица, (число) один; write down three ~s напишите три единицы; ~ by ~ один за другим, друг за другом; поодиночке; ~ and all все вместе и каждый в отдельности; at ~ в согласии, единодушно; 2) *слово-заместитель определяемого; ставится во избежание повторения упомянутого сущ.:* have you a knife? I have ~ есть у вас нож? У меня есть; a new law and an old ~ новый закон и старый; 3) :the little ~s дети; the great ~s and the little ~s большие и малые; my little ~ дитя моё.

one III *a* 1) один; первый; chapter ~ глава пер-

вая; 2) единственный; the ~ way to do it единственный способ сделать это; ~ in a thousand очень редкий, один на тысячу; 3) единый; with ~ voice единодушно; 4) одинаковый, такой же; it is all ~ безразлично; одинаково; 5) неопределённый, какой-то; ~ fine morning в одно прекрасное утро; I met him ~ night я встретил его как-то вечером.

one IV *pron* 1) некто, кто-то; is he ~ that can be trusted? он такой человек, на которого можно положиться?; 2) *безл.:* ~ never knows what may happen никогда не знаешь, что может случиться; how can ~ do it? как это можно сделать?

one-aloner [ˈwʌnəˈlounə] *n* совершенно одинокий человек; одиночка.

one-eyed [ˈwʌnˈaɪd] *a* одноглазый.

onefold [ˈwʌn,fould] *a* простой, несложный.

one-horse(d) [ˈwʌnˈhɔːs(t)] *a* 1) одноконный; 2) *разг.* маломощный; 3) мелкий, незначительный.

one-idea'd [ˈwʌnaɪˈdɪəd] *a* узкий, ограниченный (*о человеке*).

one-legged [ˈwʌnˈlegd] *a* 1) одноногий; 2) однобокий, односторонний.

oneness [ˈwʌnnɪs] *n* 1) единство; 2) тождество; 3) исключительность.

oner [ˈwʌnə] *n разг.* 1) замечательный чем-л. человек или предмет; a ~ at «специалист», знаток, дока; 2) сильный удар; 3) явная ложь.

onerous [ˈɔnərəs] *a* обременительный; тягостный.

oneself [wʌnˈself] *pron refl* (самого) себя; -ся; to do for ~ делать для себя; to keep ~ to ~ быть замкнутым, необщительным; to hurt ~ ушибиться.

one-sided [ˈwʌnˈsaɪdɪd] *a* 1) однобокий; кривобокий; 2) односторонний; ограниченный; 3) пристрастный, предубеждённый.

one-time [ˈwʌnˈtaɪm] *a* былой; прошлый.

one-track [ˈwʌnˈtræk] *a* 1) одноколейный; 2) ограниченный, узкий.

one-way [ˈwʌnˈweɪ] *a* односторонний (*о движении и т. п.*).

onfall [ˈɔn,fɔːl] *n* нападение.

onion [ˈʌnjən] *n* лук; луковица.

on-looker [ˈɔn,lukə] *n* зритель; (случайный) свидетель; наблюдатель.

only I [ˈounlɪ] *a* единственный; one and ~ один единственный.

only II *adv* только; исключительно, единственно; лишь; not ~ не только; if ~ если бы только; ~ just только что; ~ not чуть не, едва не; ~ too glad очень рад; ~ think! подумать только!

only III *conj* но, только; ~ that если бы не то, что.

onrush [ˈɔnrʌʃ] *n* натиск; атака.

onset [ˈɔnset] *n* 1) атака, нападение; натиск; 2) начало; at the first ~ сразу же; to give a fresh ~ сделать новую попытку.

onslaught [ˈɔnslɔːt] *n* атака; нападение.

onto [ˈɔntu] *prep* на; to throw a ball ~ the roof бросить мяч на крышу; to get ~ a horse сесть на лошадь.

onus [ˈounəs] *n* бремя; ответственность.

onward I [ˈɔnwəd] *a* продвигающийся, идущий вперёд; прогрессивный; the ~ movement движение вперёд.

onward II *adv* вперёд; дальше; you are so far ~ of your way вы зашли так далеко.

onwards ['ɔnwədz] *adv* вперёд; дальше.

oof [uːf] *n сленг* деньги, богатство.

ooze I [uːz] *n* 1) жидкая грязь; ил; 2) медленное выделение влаги.

ooze II *v* медленно течь *или* вытекать; сочиться (*о крови, гное*); *перен.* исчезать, покидать; his courage ~d away вся его храбрость пропала; the secret ~d out тайна раскрылась.

oozy ['uːzɪ] *a* илистый, тинистый; вязкий.

opacity [ou'pæsɪtɪ] *n* 1) непрозрачность; acoustic ~ звуконепроницаемость; 2) затенённость, темнота; 3) неясность, смутность (*образа*).

opal ['oupəl] *n мин.* опал.

opaque [ou'peɪk] *a* 1) непрозрачный; свето-непроницаемый; 2) неясный, смутный; 3) тупой, глупый.

ope [oup] *поэт. см.* open III.

open I ['oupən] *a* 1) открытый; раскрывшийся (*о цветке*); to do ~ открывать, раскрывать; to break (*или* to throw, to burst, to fling, to fly) ~ распахивать (*дверь и т. п.*); to cut ~, to tear ~ распечатывать (*письмо, пакет и т. п.*); 2) доступный, открытый (*о собрании и т. п.*); 3) откровенный, искренний; открытый (*о лице*); to be ~ with smb. быть откровенным с кем-л.; 4) открытый, явный; 5) свободный (*о пути*); очистившийся ото льда (*о реке и т. п.*); 6) мягкий (*о погоде, зиме*).

open II *n* (the ~) открытый воздух, открытое пространство; to come into the ~ *перен.* высказаться, быть откровенным.

open III *v* 1) открывать(ся), раскрывать(ся); вскрывать(ся) (*о нарыве*); 2) начинать(ся); открывать(ся) (*о собрании, прениях*); □ to ~ into сообщаться (*о комнатах*); вести в (*о двери*); to ~ on (*to*) выходить на (*об окнах, комнатах и т. п.*); to ~ out a) раскрывать, развёртывать; б) расправлять (*крылья — о птице*); to ~ up a) открывать доступ чему-л.; б) раскрывать, обнаруживать.

open-air ['oupn'ɛə] *a* (находящийся) на открытом воздухе.

open-armed ['oupən'ɑːmd] *a* с распростёртыми объятиями.

opencast ['oupənkɑːst] *n горн.* 1) открытая выработка, карьер; 2) *attr* (добытый) открытым способом.

open-eared ['oupən'ɪəd] *a* внимательно слушающий.

open-eyed ['oupn'aɪd] *a* 1) с широко раскрытыми глазами; удивлённый; 2) бдительный.

open-handed ['oupn'hændɪd] *a* щедрый; великодушный.

open-hearted ['oupən,hɑːtɪd] *a* чистосердечный.

opening I ['oupnɪŋ] *n* 1) отверстие; щель; расщелина; 2) начало, вступление, вступительная часть; 3) открытие (*съезда, выставки и т. п.*); 4) вакансия; 5) удачное стечение обстоятельств, возможность; 6) *шахм.* дебют.

opening II *a* 1) первый, начальный; 2) вступительный; открывающий; 3) исходный.

openly ['oupnlɪ] *adv* 1) открыто; публично; 2) откровенно.

open-minded ['oupn'maɪndɪd] *a* 1) с широким кругозором; 2) непредубеждённый, справедливый.

openness ['oupnnɪs] *n* 1) откровенность, прямота; 2) явность.

open-work ['oupnwəːk] *n* ажурная строчка.

opera ['ɔpərə] *n* опера.

opera-glass(es) ['ɔpərəglɑːs(ɪz)] *n* (театральный) бинокль.

opera-hat ['ɔpərəhæt] *n* складной цилиндр.

opera-house ['ɔpərəhaus] *n* оперный театр.

operate ['ɔpəreɪt] *v* 1) действовать; работать; 2) управлять машиной, приводить в действие; 3) оказывать действие, действовать (*о лекарстве и т. п.*); 4) оперировать; to be ~d on for appendicitis прооперироваться по поводу аппендицита; 5) эксплуатировать, разрабатывать.

operatic ['ɔpə'rætɪk] *a* оперный.

operating ['ɔpəreɪtɪŋ] *a амер.:* ~ costs текущие расходы.

operating-table ['ɔpəreɪtɪŋ,teɪbl] *n* операционный стол.

operating-theatre ['ɔpəreɪtɪŋ,θɪətə] *n* операционная (*для показательных операций*).

operation [,ɔpə'reɪʃən] *n* 1) действие; работа; операция; in ~ в действии; 2) процесс; 3) операция (*хирургическая*); 4) *мат.* действие; 5) эксплуатация, разработка; 6) управление (*предприятием и т. п.*).

operational [,ɔpə'reɪʃənl] *a эк.* эксплуатационный (*о расходах, стоимости*).

operative I ['ɔpərətɪv] *n* (фабричный) рабочий.

operative II *a* 1) действующий (*о законе и т. п.*); действительный; 2) оперативный; 3) операционный.

operator ['ɔpəreɪtə] *n* 1) хирург; 2) рабочий, обслуживающий машину *или* станок; 3) оператор; телеграфист; радист; ◊ big ~s *амер.* крупные чиновники; высокие должностные лица.

operetta [,ɔpə'retə] *n* оперетта.

opine [ou'paɪn] *v* полагать, высказывать мнение.

opinion [ə'pɪnjən] *n* мнение; public ~ общественное мнение; in my ~ по моему мнению; to be of (the) ~ that... полагать, что...; to have no ~ of быть невысокого мнения о; to act up to one's ~s поступать согласно своим убеждениям; ◊ ~s differ *погов.* ≅ о вкусах не спорят.

opinionated [ə'pɪnjəneɪtɪd] *a* самоуверенный; упрямый.

opium ['oupjəm] *n* опиум.

opium-eater ['oupjəm,iːtə] *n* курильщик опиума.

opponent I [ə'pounənt] *n* противник; оппонент.

opponent II *a* враждебный; несогласный.

opportune ['ɔpətjuːn] *a* 1) благоприятный, подходящий (*о моменте и т. п.*); 2) уместный, своевременный.

opportunism ['ɔpətjuːnɪzəm] *n* оппортунизм.

opportunist ['ɔpətjuːnɪst] *n* оппортунист.

opportunity [,ɔpə'tjuːnɪtɪ] *n* удобный случай; (благоприятная) возможность; to improve (*или* to take, to seize) the ~ воспользоваться случаем; to lose an ~, to let an ~ slip упустить возможность, случай.

oppose [ə'pouz] *v* 1) сопротивляться, противиться; возражать, отклонять (*резолюцию*); 2) противопоставлять; 3) мешать, препятствовать.

opposite I ['ɔpəzɪt] *n* противоположность; direct ~ полная противоположность.

opposite II *a* 1) противополо́жный; 2) располо́женный напро́тив.

opposite III *adv* напро́тив; про́тив.

opposite IV *prep* напро́тив; про́тив.

opposition [‚ɔpə'zıʃən] *n* 1) сопротивле́ние, противоде́йствие; 2) оппози́ция; 3) противополо́жность, контра́ст; 4) *астр.* противостоя́ние.

oppress [ə'pres] *v* 1) угнета́ть, притесня́ть; 2) удруча́ть, угнета́ть; to feel ~ed быть пода́вленным.

oppression [ə'preʃən] *n* 1) угнете́ние, притесне́ние; 2) пода́вленность, угнетённое состоя́ние.

oppressive [ə'presıv] *a* 1) гнету́щий; тя́гостный; 2) суро́вый, деспоти́ческий.

oppressor [ə'presə] *n* угнета́тель, притесни́тель.

opprobrious [ə'proubrıəs] *a* оскорби́тельный; позо́рный.

opprobrium [ə'proubrıəm] *n* позо́р.

optic ['ɔptık] *a* глазно́й, зри́тельный.

optical ['ɔptıkəl] *a* зри́тельный; опти́ческий.

optics ['ɔptıks] *n* о́птика.

optimism ['ɔptımızəm] *n* оптими́зм.

optimist ['ɔptımıst] *n* оптими́ст.

optimistic [‚ɔptı'mıstık] *a* оптимисти́ческий.

optimum ['ɔptıməm] *n* 1) совоку́пность наибо́лее благоприя́тных усло́вий, о́птимум; 2) *attr* оптима́льный.

option ['ɔpʃən] *n* 1) вы́бор; 2) пра́во, свобо́да вы́бора.

optional ['ɔpʃənl] *a* необяза́тельный, факульта́тивный.

opulence ['ɔpjuləns] *n* состоя́тельность, бога́тство.

opulent ['ɔpjulənt] *a* 1) состоя́тельный, бога́тый; 2) пы́шный.

or [ɔ:] *conj* и́ли; or else ина́че; either... or и́ли... и́ли.

oracle ['ɔrəkl] *n* 1) ора́кул; 2) предсказа́ние, прорица́ние.

oracular [ɔ'rækjulə] *a* 1) проро́ческий; му́дрый; 2) зага́дочный, нея́сный.

oral I ['ɔ:rəl] *n разг.* у́стный экза́мен.

oral II *a* 1) у́стный; слове́сный; 2) *мед.* ора́льный, ротово́й.

orally ['ɔ:rəlı] *adv* у́стно.

orange I ['ɔrındʒ] *n* 1) апельси́н; blood ~ королёк; 2) апельси́нное де́рево; 3) ора́нжевый цвет.

orange II *a* ора́нжевый.

orange-blossom ['ɔrındʒ‚blɔsəm] *n* 1) помера́нцевые цветы́; 2) флёрдора́нж (*украшение невесты*).

orange-peel ['ɔrındʒpiːl] *n* 1) апельси́нная ко́рка; 2) апельси́нный цука́т.

orangery ['ɔrındʒərı] *n* оранжере́я.

orang-outang, orang-utan ['ɔ:rəŋ'uːtæŋ, 'ɔ:rəŋ'uːtæn] *n* орангута́нг.

orate [ɔ:'reıt] *v шутл.* ора́торствовать, разглаго́льствовать.

oration [ɔ:'reıʃən] *n* 1) речь (*публичная*); 2) *грам.:* direct ~ пряма́я речь; indirect ~ ко́свенная речь.

orator ['ɔrətə] *n* ора́тор.

oratorical [‚ɔrə'tɔrıkəl] *a* 1) ора́торский; 2) рито́рический.

oratorio [‚ɔrə'tɔ:rıou] *n муз.* орато́рия.

oratory[1] ['ɔrətərı] *n* 1) красноре́чие; ора́торское иску́сство; 2) рито́рика.

oratory[2] *n* часо́вня; моле́льня.

orb [ɔːb] *n* 1) шар; сфери́ческое те́ло; 2) небе́сное свети́ло; 3) орби́та; 4) глазно́е я́блоко; *поэт.* глаз.

orbit I ['ɔːbıt] *n* 1) орби́та; circular (planned, predicted) ~ кругова́я (за́данная, расчётная) орби́та; to put in ~ вы́вести на орби́ту; 2) оборо́т (*вокруг Земли*); 3) глазна́я впа́дина.

orbit II *v* 1) выводи́ть на орби́ту; 2) выходи́ть на орби́ту; 3) дви́гаться по орби́те.

orbital ['ɔːbıtəl] *a* орбита́льный, соверша́емый по орби́те.

orchard ['ɔːtʃəd] *n* фрукто́вый сад.

orchestra ['ɔːkıstrə] *n* 1) орке́стр; 2) ме́сто для орке́стра в теа́тре; 3) *амер.* парте́р (*тж.* ~ stalls).

orchestral [ɔ:'kestrəl] *a* оркестро́вый.

orchestrate ['ɔːkıstreıt] *v* оркестрова́ть, инструментова́ть.

orchestration [‚ɔːkes'treıʃən] *n* оркестро́вка, инструменто́вка.

orchid ['ɔːkıd] *n* орхиде́я.

ordain [ɔ:'deın] *v* 1) посвяща́ть в духо́вный сан; 2) предпи́сывать; распоряжа́ться.

ordeal [ɔ:'diːl] *n* 1) тяжёлое испыта́ние; 2) *ист.* «суд бо́жий».

order I ['ɔːdə] *n* 1) поря́док; после́довательность; 2) чистота́, поря́док; испра́вность; out of ~ не в поря́дке; to put in ~ приводи́ть в поря́док; to get out of ~ испо́ртиться; in bad ~ неиспра́вный; 3) поря́док, споко́йствие; to keep ~ соблюда́ть поря́док; to come to ~ успоко́иться, угомони́ться (*об учащихся*); perfect ~ по́лный поря́док; 4) поря́док (*собрания и т. п.*); уста́в, регла́мент; standing ~s уста́в; регла́мент; ~ of the day пове́стка дня (*собрания*); 5) класс о́бщества, социа́льная гру́ппа; 6) о́рден; 7) духо́вный сан; to take holy ~s стать духо́вным лицо́м; 8) сте́пень, ранг; 9) *мат.* сте́пень; 10) *биол.* отря́д; поря́док; 11) прика́з; распоряже́ние; by ~ по прика́зу; under the ~s of под кома́ндой (*кого-л.*); 12) зака́з; to ~ на зака́з; on ~ зака́зано (*но ещё не доста́влено*); 13) о́рдер; postal ~, money ~ почто́вый де́нежный перево́д; 14) *воен.* строй; open ~ разо́мкнутый строй; ◊ apple-pie ~ образцо́вый поря́док; in ~ that с тем, что́бы; in ~ to для того́, что́бы.

order II *v* 1) прика́зывать; предпи́сывать; распоряжа́ться; 2) зака́зывать; 3) приводи́ть в поря́док; 4) назнача́ть, пропи́сывать (*лекарство*); 5) предопределя́ть; □ to ~ about кома́ндовать, помыка́ть.

orderliness ['ɔːdəlınıs] *n* аккура́тность, поря́док.

orderly I ['ɔːdəlı] *n* 1) *воен.* ордина́рец, связно́й; санита́р (*в госпитале*); 2) убо́рщик у́лиц.

orderly II *a* 1) аккура́тный, опря́тный; в по́лном поря́дке; 2) хоро́шего поведе́ния; дисциплини́рованный; 3) пра́вильный, регуля́рный; 4) *воен.* дежу́рный.

ordinal I ['ɔːdınl] *n* поря́дковое числи́тельное.

ordinal II *a* поря́дковый.

ordinance ['ɔːdınəns] *n* 1) ука́з, декре́т; постановле́ние; 2) обря́д.

ordinary ['ɔːdnrı] *a* 1) обы́чный, обыкнове́нный, норма́льный; out of the ~ необы́чный; исключи́тельный; 2) зауря́дный, посре́дственный.

ordination [ˌɔːdɪ'neɪʃən] *n* посвящение в духовный сан.

ordnance ['ɔːdnəns] *n* артиллерийские орудия; артиллерия.

ordure ['ɔːdjuə] *n* 1) навоз; грязь; 2) непристойность.

ore [ɔː] *n* руда; mineral ~ руда, содержащая минерал(ы).

ore-dressing ['ɔːˌdresɪŋ] *n* обработка *или* обогащение руд.

organ ['ɔːgən] *n* 1) орган; sense ~s органы чувств; ~s of speech органы речи; ~s of digestion органы пищеварения; reproductional ~s органы размножения; 2) орган, учреждение; ~s of government органы государственного управления; 3) *муз.* орган; reed ~, American ~ фисгармония; mouth ~ губная гармоника; 4) газета, журнал.

organ-blower ['ɔːgənˌblouə] *n* раздувальщик мехов (*органа*).

organic [ɔː'gænɪk] *a* органический.

organism ['ɔːgənɪzəm] *n* организм.

organist ['ɔːgənɪst] *n* органист.

organization [ˌɔːgənaɪ'zeɪʃən] *n* 1) организация; 2) устройство, структура.

organize ['ɔːgənaɪz] *v* организовать.

organized ['ɔːgənaɪzd] *a* 1) организованный; ~ labour члены профсоюза; 2): ~ matter живая материя.

organizer ['ɔːgənaɪzə] *n* организатор.

organ-loft ['ɔːgənlɔft] *n* галерея в церкви для органа.

orgy ['ɔːdʒɪ] *n* оргия.

oriel ['ɔːrɪəl] *n* закрытый балкон; *архит.* эркер, фонарь.

Orient ['ɔːrɪənt] *n* (the ~) Восток, страны Востока.

orient I ['ɔːrɪənt] *a* 1) восточный; 2) блестящий, яркий; 3) восходящий (*о солнце*).

orient II *v* 1) определять местонахождение, ориентировать; to ~ oneself ориентироваться; 2) располагать фасадом на восток.

Oriental [ˌɔːrɪ'entl] *n* житель Востока.

oriental [ˌɔːrɪ'entl] *a* восточный.

orientalist [ˌɔːrɪ'entəlɪst] *n* востоковед.

orientate ['ɔːrɪenteɪt] *v* ориентировать(ся).

orientation [ˌɔːrɪen'teɪʃən] *n* ориентация; ориентирование.

orifice ['ɔrɪfɪs] *n* 1) отверстие; 2) устье, выход; проход.

origin ['ɔrɪdʒɪn] *n* 1) начало, источник; the ~ of a disease происхождение болезни; 2) происхождение; of humble ~ незнатного происхождения.

original I [ə'rɪdʒənl] *n* 1) оригинал, подлинник; 2) чудак, оригинал.

original II *a* 1) первоначальный; 2) подлинный; 3) оригинальный, новый, свежий.

originality [əˌrɪdʒɪ'nælɪtɪ] *n* 1) подлинность; 2) оригинальность, новизна, свежесть.

originally [ə'rɪdʒnəlɪ] *adv* 1) первоначально; 2) оригинально; 3) по происхождению.

originate [ə'rɪdʒɪneɪt] *v* 1) происходить, брать начало, возникать (*from, in*); 2) порождать, создавать, давать начало.

origination [əˌrɪdʒɪ'neɪʃən] *n* 1) начало, происхождение; 2) порождение.

originator [ə'rɪdʒɪneɪtə] *n* 1) автор, создатель; изобретатель; 2) инициатор.

oriole ['ɔːrɪoul] *n* иволга.

orlop ['ɔːlɔp] *n мор.* кубрик, нижняя палуба.

ornament[a] ['ɔːnəmənt] *n* украшение, орнамент.

ornament[b] ['ɔːnəmənt] *v* украшать.

ornamental [ˌɔːnə'mentl] *a* служащий украшением, декоративный.

ornamentation [ˌɔːnəmen'teɪʃən] *n* 1) украшение (*действие*); 2) украшения.

ornate [ɔː'neɪt] *a* 1) с украшениями; 2) витиеватый (*о стиле*).

orphan I ['ɔːfən] *n* сирота.

orphan II *a* сиротский.

orphan III *v* лишать родителей, делать сиротой.

orphanage ['ɔːfənɪdʒ] *n* 1) сиротство; 2) приют для сирот.

orphaned ['ɔːfənd] *a* осиротевший; осиротелый.

orphanhood ['ɔːfənhud] *n* сиротство.

orrery ['ɔrərɪ] *n* планетарий.

orthodox ['ɔːθədɔks] *a* ортодоксальный.

orthodoxy ['ɔːθədɔksɪ] *n* ортодоксальность.

orthoepy ['ɔːθouepɪ] *n лингв.* орфоэпия.

orthographic [ˌɔːθə'græfɪk] *a* орфографический.

orthography [ɔː'θɔgrəfɪ] *n* орфография, правописание.

oscillate ['ɔsɪleɪt] *v* качать(ся); колебаться (*тж. перен.*).

oscillation [ˌɔsɪ'leɪʃən] *n* качание, колебание.

osier ['ouʒə] *n* 1) ива; ивовая лоза; 2) *attr* ивовый.

osseous ['ɔsɪəs] *a* 1) костистый; 2) костный.

ossification [ˌɔsɪfɪ'keɪʃən] *n* окостенение.

ossify ['ɔsɪfaɪ] *v* костенеть.

ossuary ['ɔsjuərɪ] *n* 1) склеп; 2) кремационная урна.

ostensible [ɔs'tensəbl] *a* мнимый; показной.

ostentation [ˌɔsten'teɪʃən] *n* выставление напоказ, хвастовство.

ostentatious [ˌɔsten'teɪʃəs] *a* показной; нарочитый.

ostler ['ɔslə] *n* конюх.

ostracism ['ɔstrəsɪzəm] *n* остракизм.

ostracize ['ɔstrəsaɪz] *v* подвергать остракизму.

ostrich ['ɔstrɪtʃ] *n* страус.

other I ['ʌðə] *a* 1) другой, иной; none ~ than никто иной; 2) с *сущ. во мн. ч.* остальные; ~ pupils остальные ученики.

other II *pron* другой; one or ~ тот или другой.

other III *adv* иначе; he could not do ~ than he did он не мог поступить иначе.

otherwise ['ʌðəwaɪz] *adv* 1) иначе, иным способом *или* образом; по-другому; 2) в других отношениях; 3) или же, иначе, в противном случае.

otherwise-minded ['ʌðəwaɪzˌmaɪndɪd] *a* инакомыслящий.

other-worldly ['ʌðəˌwəːldlɪ] *a* «не от мира сего»; 2) потусторонний.

otter ['ɔtə] *n* выдра.

Ottoman I ['ɔtəmən] *n* турок.

Ottoman II *a* турецкий.

ottoman ['ɔtəmən] *n* диван, оттоманка.

ought [ɔːt] *v* *употр. перед др. гл. для выражения долженствования или большей вероятности:* you ~ to go there вы должны были пойти туда;

it ~ not to be allowed этого не следует разрешать; it ~ to be a fine day tomorrow завтра, должно быть, будет хороший день.

ounce¹ [auns] n 1) (сокр. oz) унция (= 28,3 г); 2) капля, чуточка.

ounce² n барс.

our [′auə] pron poss наш, наша, наше, наши; ~ book наша книга.

ours [′auəz] pron poss 1) наш; this book is ~ эта книга наша; 2) замещает сущ.: ~ is a large room наша комната большая; ~ will come later наши придут позже.

ourself, ourselves [‚auə′self, ‚auə′selvz] pron 1) refl себя; самих себя, -сь; we cannot see ourselves as others see us мы не видим себя, как другие нас видят; 2) употребляется для усиления (мы) сами; we ourselves will do the work мы сами сделаем эту работу.

oust [aust] v выгонять, вытеснять, занимать чьё-л. место.

out I [aut] prep 1) в пространственном значении указывает на: а) положение вне чего-л. из; he took a pencil ~ of his pocket он вынул карандаш из кармана; б) движение за пределы чего-л. из; they went ~ of the room они вышли из комнаты; 2) указывает на материал, из которого сделан предмет: this house is made ~ of brick этот дом сделан из кирпича; 3) указывает на целое или группу, из которой выделяется часть: two students ~ of fifteen were absent двое студентов из пятнадцати отсутствовали.

out II adv указывает на: 1) действие, направленное наружу; обыкн. переводится глаголом с приставкой вы-; to go ~ выходить; to take ~ вынимать; to fly ~ вылетать; he is ~ его нет дома; the girl is ~ девушка выезжает в свет; his arm is ~ у него вывихнута рука; the secret is ~ секрет раскрыт; the book is ~ книга вышла из печати; the flowers (leaves) are ~ цветы (листья) распустились; 2) совершенный характер действия: to fill ~ заполнять; расширять(ся); 3) причину, основание, цель действия: he acted ~ of pity (~ of curiosity, ~ of jealousy, ~ of gratitude, ~ of spite, ~ of good nature, ~ of kindness) он действовал из жалости (из любопытства, из ревности, из благодарности, из желания сделать наперекор, назло, из добрых чувств, по доброте душевной); 4) отсутствие признака, выраженного сущ.: ~ of date устаревший; ~ of colour выцветший, выгоревший; ~ of shape бесформенный; ~ of wear вышедший из моды; ~ of coal (wood) без угля (дров); ~ of health больной; ~ of heart а) в унынии; б) обескураженный; ~ of patience потерявший всякое терпение; ~ of mind а) из памяти вон; б) забытый; to be ~ of one's mind быть не в своём уме; ~ of place а) неуместный, неподходящий; б) безработный; ~ of work безработный; ~ of time не в такт.

out III n 1) разг.: at ~s with everybody со всеми в ссоре, на ножах; 2) лазейка, путь к отступлению.

out IV a 1) наружный, внешний; 2) находящийся вне игры.

out V int вон!, прочь!; ~ upon you! уст. стыд и срам!

out- [aut-] pref 1) глаголам придаёт значение превосходства пере-; outshout перекричать; outrun перегнать, обогнать; 2) глаголам придаёт значение завершённости вы-; outflow вытекать; outspeak высказывать(ся); 3) сущ. и прил. придаёт значение: а) выхода, проявления: outburst взрыв чувств; б) отдалённости: outlying отдалённый.

outage [′autɪdʒ] n 1) простой, остановка работы; 2) утечка; 3) выпускное отверстие.

out-and-away [′autəndə′weɪ] adv намного.

out-and-out [′autənd′aut] a полный, совершённый; категорический (об отказе и т. п.).

outbade [aut′beɪd] past см. outbid.

outbalance [aut′bæləns] n перевешивать; превосходить.

outbid [aut′bɪd] v (past outbid, outbade; p. р. outbid, outbidden) предлагать более высокую цену (чем другие).

outbidden [aut′bɪdn] p. р. см. outbid.

outboard [′aut‚bɔːd] adv за бортом.

outbound [′autbaund] a 1) отбывающий; идущий в море (о корабле); улетающий за границу (о самолёте); 2) отправляемый, подлежащий отправке (о грузе).

outbrave [aut′breɪv] v 1) превосходить мужеством; 2) не побояться; выдержать (что-л.).

outbreak [′autbreɪk] n 1) взрыв, вспышка (гнева и т. п.); начало (революции, забастовки, войны); 2) восстание, возмущение.

outbuilding [′aut‚bɪldɪŋ] n 1) пристройка; 2) pl службы.

outburst [′autbəːst] n 1) взрыв, вспышка; 2) поток (слёз).

outcast I [′autkɑːst] n изгнанник.

outcast II a 1) изгнанный, отверженный; 2) бездомный, бесприютный.

outclass [aut′klɑːs] v превосходить.

outcome [′autkʌm] n 1) результат; последствие; исход; 2) выход, выпускное отверстие.

outcry I [′autkraɪ] n 1) крик; выкрик; 2) протест.

outcry II v 1) кричать, выкрикивать; 2) протестовать.

outdated [aut′deɪtɪd] a устарелый.

outdid [aut′dɪd] past см. outdo.

outdistance [aut′dɪstəns] v обогнать, перегнать.

outdo [aut′duː] v (past outdid; p. р. outdone) превзойти.

outdone [aut′dʌn] p. р. см. outdo.

outdoor [′autdɔː] a (находящийся или происходящий) вне дома, на открытом воздухе.

outdoors [′aut′dɔːz] adv на открытом воздухе, вне дома.

outdrive [aut′draɪv] v (past outdrove; p. р. outdriven) обогнать.

outdriven [aut′drɪvn] p. р. см. outdrive.

outdrove [aut′drouv] past см. outdrive.

outer [′autə] a 1) наружный, внешний; 2) космический (о пространстве); 3) филос. объективный.

outermost [′autəmoust] a самый дальний, самый отдалённый (от центра).

outface [aut′feɪs] v 1) смутить дерзким взглядом; 2) держаться вызывающе.

outfall [′autfɔːl] n исток (реки).

outfield [′autfiːld] n 1) отдалённое поле; 2) часть поля, отдалённая от воротцев (в крикете).

out-fight [aut'faıt] *v* 1) *воен.* побеждать в бою; 2) иметь перевес над противником.

out-fighting [aut'faıtıŋ] *n воен.* бой на дальних подступах.

outfit I ['autfıt] *n* 1) снаряжение; обмундирование; 2) оборудование; 3): mental and moral ~ умственные и нравственные качества.

outfit II *v* снаряжать; снабжать оборудованием.

outflank [aut'flæŋk] *v* выйти во фланг (*противнику*); *перен.* обойти, перехитрить (*кого-л.*).

outflew [aut'fluː] *past см.* outfly.

outflow[a] ['autflou] *n* 1) истечение, выход; 2) исток (*реки*).

outflow[b] [aut'flou] *v* вытекать.

outflown [aut'floun] *p. p. см.* outfly.

outfly [aut'flaı] *v* (*past* outflew; *p. p.* outflown) обогнать (*в полёте*).

outgeneral [aut'dʒenərəl] *v* победить превосходством тактики.

outgiving ['aut,gıvıŋ] *n* высказывание, заявление.

outgo[a] ['autgou] *n* 1) выход, уход, отправление; 2) расход, издержки.

outgo[b] [aut'gou] *v* (*past* outwent; *p. p.* outgone) превзойти; опередить.

outgoing ['aut,gouıŋ] *a* уходящий, отбывающий, отъезжающий.

outgoings ['aut,gouıŋz] *n pl* издержки.

outgone [aut'gɔn] *p. p. см.* outgo[b].

outgrew [aut'gruː] *past см.* outgrow.

outgrow [aut'grou] *v* (*past* outgrew; *p. p.* outgrown) 1) перерасти (*кого-л., что-л.*); вырасти (*из платья*); 2) отделаться с возрастом от привычки, увлечения *и т. п.*

outgrown [aut'groun] *p. p. см.* outgrow.

outgrowth ['autgrouθ] *n* 1) отросток; отпрыск; 2) нарост; 3) продукт, результат.

outhouse ['authaus] *n* 1) надворное строение; 2) флигель.

outing ['autıŋ] *n* (загородная) прогулка.

out-jockey [aut'dʒɔkı] *v разг.* перехитрить.

outlaid [aut'leıd] *past, p. p. см.* outlay[b].

outlandish [aut'lændıʃ] *a* 1) заморский, чужеземный; 2) диковинный, странный.

outlast [aut'lɑːst] *v* 1) продолжаться дольше чем...; 2) прожить дольше чем..., пережить что-л.

outlaw I ['autlɔː] *n* 1) человек вне закона, отверженный; изгнанник; 2) бандит, разбойник.

outlaw II *v* 1) объявлять кого-л. вне закона; изгонять; 2) *амер.* лишать законной силы.

outlawry ['autlɔːrı] *n* объявление вне закона, изгнание.

outlay[a] ['autleı] *n* 1) издержки, расходы, затраты; 2) смета.

outlay[b] [aut'leı] *v* (*past, p. p.* outlaid) расходовать, тратить.

outlet ['autlet] *n* 1) выходное *или* выпускное отверстие; 2) выход (*тж. перен.*); выпуск; сток; to find an ~ for one's energies найти выход своей энергии.

outline I ['autlaın] *n* 1) очертание, контур; 2) набросок, эскиз; очерк; in ~ в общих чертах; 3) *pl* основы.

outline II *v* 1) нарисовать контур; 2) обрисовать, наметить в общих чертах; сделать набросок.

outlive [aut'lıv] *v* пережить (*кого-л., что-л.*).

outlook ['autluk] *n* 1) вид; 2) перспектива; виды на будущее; 3) наблюдательный пункт; 4) точка зрения; world ~ мировоззрение.

outlying ['aut,laııŋ] *a* 1) отдалённый, далёкий; 2) наружный.

outmarch ['aut'mɑːtʃ] *v* опередить.

outmatch [aut'mætʃ] *v* превосходить.

outnumber [aut'nʌmbə] *v* превосходить численно.

out-of-date ['autəv'deıt] *a* устарелый; старомодный.

out-of-door(s) I ['autəv'dɔːz] *a см.* outdoor.

out-of-door(s) II *adv см.* outdoors.

out-of-the-way ['autəvðə'weı] *a* 1) отдалённый, труднодоступный (*о селении и т. п.*); 2) необычный, странный.

out-of-work ['autəv'wəːk] *a* безработный.

outpace [aut'peıs] *v* обгонять, опережать.

out-patient ['aut,peıʃənt] *n* амбулаторный больной.

outplay [aut'pleı] *v* обыграть.

outpost ['autpoust] *n* 1) аванпост; 2) сторожевая застава; 3) отдалённое поселение.

outpour[a] ['autpɔː] *n* излияние.

outpour[b] [aut'pɔː] *v* 1) выливать; 2) изливать.

outpouring [aut'pɔːrıŋ] *n обыкн. pl* излияние (*чувств*).

output ['autput] *n* 1) продукция; выпуск; 2) *тех.* производительность.

outrage I ['autreıdʒ] *n* 1) нарушение закона *или* чьих-л. прав; 2) насилие; 3) оскорбление; надругательство.

outrage II *v* 1) нарушать закон, права; 2) производить насилие; 3) оскорбить; надругаться.

outrageous [aut'reıdʒəs] *a* 1) неистовый; 2) оскорбительный; возмутительный.

outran [aut'ræn] *past см.* outrun.

outrank [aut'ræŋk] *v* превосходить.

out-relief ['autrı,liːf] *n* пособие неимущим (*не живущим в домах призрения*).

outridden [aut'rıdn] *p. p. см.* outride.

outride [aut'raıd] *v* (*past* outrode; *p. p.* outridden) 1) перегнать; 2) выдержать (*шторм, несчастье*).

outright[a] ['autraıt] *a* совершенный, полный, отъявленный.

outright[b] [aut'raıt] *adv* 1) вполне, совершенно; 2) раз навсегда; 3) прямо, открыто.

outrival [aut'raıvəl] *v* превзойти.

outrode [aut'roud] *past см.* outride.

outrun [aut'rʌn] *v* (*past* outran; *p. p.* outrun) 1) обогнать, опередить; 2) убежать от кого-л.; 3) переходить все границы.

outrunner ['aut,rʌnə] *n* 1) скороход; 2) пристяжная лошадь; 3) собака-вожак (*в упряжке*).

outsat [aut'sæt] *past, p. p. см.* outsit.

outset ['autset] *n* отправление; начало; at the ~ вначале; from the ~ с самого начала.

outshine [aut'ʃaın] *v* затмить.

outside I ['aut'saıd] *n* 1) наружная сторона; 2) наружность, внешность; 3) внешний мир; from the ~ извне, из внешнего мира; 4) крайняя степень; at the ~ самое большее, в лучшем случае.

outside II *a* 1) наружный, внешний; 2) посторонний; 3) крайний, предельный, наибольший; 4) крайний (*о месте*).

outside III *adv* 1) снаружи, извне; наружу; ~ and in снаружи и внутри; 2) на (открытом) воздухе, на дворе.

outside IV *prep* вне, за пределами, за пределы; ~ the door за дверью; ~ the house вне дома; у дома, перед домом; that is ~ my plans это не входит в мои планы; ~ the range за пределами досягаемости.

outsider [ˈautˈsaɪdə] *n* 1) посторонний человек; не член (*организации и т. п.*); 2) *спорт.* аутсайдер; 3) *разг.* невоспитанный человек.

outsit [autˈsɪt] *v* (*past, p. p.* outsat) пересидеть (*кого-л.*); засидеться.

outsized [ˈautsaɪzd] *a* больше обычного размера.

outskirts [ˈautskəːts] *n pl* 1) окраина; предместье; окрестности; 2) опушка леса.

outsmart [autˈsmɑːt] *v амер. разг.* перехитрить.

outspoken [autˈspoukən] *a* 1) откровенный, прямой; 2) высказанный, выраженный.

outspread I [ˈautˈspred] *n* распространение.

outspread II *a* распростёртый; расстилающийся.

outspread III *v* (*past, p. p.* outspread) 1) распространять(ся); 2) простираться, расстилаться.

outstanding [autˈstændɪŋ] *a* 1) выдающийся; (хорошо) известный; 2) неуплаченный (*о долге и т. п.*); 3) невыполненный; неразрешённый (*о вопросе, споре*).

outstay [autˈsteɪ] *v* 1) засиживаться, оставаться слишком долго; 2) выдержать, выстоять.

outstep [autˈstep] *v* переступать границы; выходить за пределы.

outstretched [autˈstretʃt] *a* 1) протянутый (*о руке и т. п.*); 2) растянутый, растянувшийся.

outstrip [autˈstrɪp] *v* 1) обгонять, опережать; 2) превосходить в чём-л.

out-talk [autˈtɔːk] *v* заговорить (*кого-л.*); не дать сказать слова (*другому*).

out-top [autˈtɔp] *v* быть выше; *перен.* превосходить.

outvoice [autˈvɔɪs] *v* 1) перекричать; 2) переубедить.

outvote [autˈvout] *v* получить большее количество голосов.

outwalk [autˈwɔːk] *v* идти быстрее *или* дальше кого-л.

outward I [ˈautwəd] *a* 1) внешний, наружный; 2) направленный наружу; 3) видимый.

outward II *adv* наружу, вне, за пределы.

outward-bound [ˈautwədˈbaund] *a* отплывающий за границу (*о корабле*).

outwardly [ˈautwədlɪ] *adv* внешне, по виду.

outwards [ˈautwədz] *adv* наружу, вне, за пределы.

outwash [autˈwɔʃ] *v* отмывать.

outwear [autˈwɛə] *v* (*past* outwore; *p. p.* outworn); 1) изнашивать; 2) истощать (*терпение и т. п.*); 3) сохраняться, носиться дольше (*об одежде*).

outweigh [autˈweɪ] *v* быть тяжелее, превосходить по весу; *перен.* перевешивать.

outwent [autˈwent] *past см.* outgo[b].

outwit [autˈwɪt] *v* перехитрить, провести кого-л.

outwore [autˈwɔː] *past см.* outwear.

outwork[a] [ˈautwəːk] *n* 1) *воен.* внешнее, передовое укрепление; 2) работа вне мастерской.

outwork[b] [autˈwəːk] *v* работать лучше *или* быстрее кого-л.

outworn I [autˈwɔːn] *p. p. см.* outwear.

outworn II *a* 1) изношенный; негодный к употреблению; 2) устарелый (*о взглядах, обычаях*); 3) избитый (*о цитате и т. п.*); 4) изнурённый.

ouzel [ˈuːzl] *n* дрозд.

oval I [ˈouvəl] *n* овал.

oval II *a* овальный.

ovation [ouˈveɪʃən] *n* овация.

oven [ˈʌvn] *n* печь.

over I [ˈouvə] *prep* 1) *в пространственном значении указывает на:* а) *положение над другим предметом* над; a red flag flies ~ the building of the Supreme Soviet красный флаг развевается над зданием Верховного Совета; б) *движение поверх чего-л.* через; the boy got ~ the fence and jumped ~ the brooklet мальчик перелез через изгородь и перепрыгнул через ручеёк; в) *положение поперёк чего-л., протяжение от одного конца, края до другого* через; there are many bridges ~ the Thames через Темзу много мостов; г) *местоположение по ту сторону реки, улицы, залива, моря и т. п.* по ту сторону, за; the school ~ the street школа на той стороне улицы; ~ the sea по ту сторону океана, за океаном, за морем; he lives ~ the way он живёт через дорогу; д) *движение в разных направлениях* по; he has travelled ~ the whole country он путешествовал по всей стране; е) *распространение по территории* по; wheat is grown all ~ Australia пшеницу сеют по всей Австралии; 2) *указывает на количественное превышение* свыше, больше; ~ 562 million свыше 562 миллионов; 3) *указывает на промежуток времени, в течение которого происходило действие* за; he should pack up ~ night if he had to start early in the morning ему следовало собраться за ночь, если он должен был выехать рано утром; 4) *указывает на связь между действием и предметом, сопутствующим действию* за; у; на; ~ a bottle за бутылкой (вина); they were sitting ~ a fire они сидели у огня, у камина; 5) *служит для связи между гл. и соответствующими дополнениями:* the meeting was presided ~ by a representative of the Soviet Peace Committee на собрании председательствовал представитель Советского комитета защиты мира.

over II *adv* 1) *указывает на движение через что-л.; часто переводится гл. с приставкой пере-;* to jump ~ перепрыгивать; to sail ~ переплыть (*на судне*); when are you coming ~ to see us? когда вы приедете к нам в гости?; 2) *указывает на доведение действия до конца:* to read a book ~ прочесть книгу до конца; 3) *указывает на повторение с изменением:* the translation is badly done, it must be done ~ перевод сделан плохо, его нужно переделать; 4) *указывает на прекращение действия:* the lesson (the meeting) is ~ занятие (собрание) окончено; it is all ~ with him с ним всё кончено; его пришёл конец; 5) *указывает на передачу чего-л. одним лицом другому:* we have handed ~ the package to his son мы передали посылку его сыну; 6) *в сочетаниях:* ~ again опять, повторно; ~ and above в добавление, к тому же.

over III *n* 1) излишек; приплата; 2) *воен.* перелёт.

over IV *a* 1) верхний; 2) вышестоящий; 3) излишний, избыточный; 4) чрезмерный.

over- ['ouvə-] *pref со значением* сверх-, над-, пере-, чрезмерно.

overact [,ouvər'ækt] *v* переигрывать (роль).

overall I ['ouvərɔːl] *n* (рабочий) халат, спецодежда; *pl* широкие рабочие брюки; комбинезон.

overall II *a* общий, предельный (*о размерах и т. п.*).

overarch [,ouvər'ɑːtʃ] *v* 1) покрывать сводом; 2) образовывать свод, арку.

overate [,ouvər'eɪt] *past см.* overeat.

overawe [,ouvər'ɔː] *v* внушать благоговейный страх.

overbalance I [,ouvə'bæləns] *n* перевес.

overbalance II *v* 1) перевешивать; превосходить (*по весу, значению и т. п.*); 2) вывести из равновесия.

overbear [,ouvə'bɛə] *v* (*past* overbore; *p. p.* overborne) 1) осилить; превозмочь, подавить; 2) превосходить.

overbearing [,ouvə'bɛərɪŋ] *a* властный; повелительный (*о тоне*).

overblown ['ouvə'bloun] *a* 1) отцветающий; 2) пронёсшийся (*о буре и т. п.*).

overboard ['ouvəbɔːd] *adv* за борт; man ~! человек за бортом!; to throw ~ выбросить за борт (*тж. перен.*).

overbold ['ouvə'bould] *a* слишком смелый, дерзкий.

overbore [,ouvə'bɔː] *past см.* overbear.

overborne [,ouvə'bɔːn] *p. p. см.* overbear.

overbrim [,ouvə'brɪm] *v* переливать(ся) через край; переполнять(ся).

overburden [,ouvə'bəːdn] *v* перегружать.

overcame [,ouvə'keɪm] *past см.* overcome.

overcast I ['ouvə'kɑːst] *a* покрытый облаками; пасмурный (*о погоде*).

overcast II *v* (*past, p. p.* overcast) 1) покрывать (-ся); затемнять, затенять; 2) зашивать через край.

overcharge I ['ouvə'tʃɑːdʒ] *n* 1) слишком высокая цена; 2) *эл.* перезаряд(ка); 3) *воен.* усиленный заряд.

overcharge II *v* 1) запрашивать чрезмерную цену; 2) *эл.* перезаряжать; 3) *воен.* заряжать усиленным зарядом; 4) перегружать (*чрезмерно*).

overcloud [,ouvə'klaud] *v* застилать(ся) облаками; *перен.* омрачать(ся).

overcoat ['ouvəkout] *n* пальто.

overcome [,ouvə'kʌm] *v* (*past* overcame; *p. p.* overcome) 1) побороть, победить, преодолеть; 2) охватить, обуять (*о чувстве*); ~ by а) охваченный; б) измученный (*голодом и т. п.*).

overcrop [,ouvə'krɔp] *v* истощать землю.

overcrowd [,ouvə'kraud] *v* 1) переполнять (*помещение и т. п.*); 2) толпиться.

overcrowded [,ouvə'kraudɪd] *a* переполненный (*о театре, вагоне*).

overdid [,ouvə'dɪd] *past см.* overdo.

overdo [,ouvə'duː] *v* (*past* overdid; *p. p.* overdone) 1) переборщить; переусердствовать; 2) преувеличивать, утрировать; 3) пережарить.

overdone[a] [,ouvə'dʌn] *p. p. см.* overdo.

overdone[b] ['ouvə'dʌn] *a* 1) преувеличенный, утрированный; 2) пережаренный.

overdose[a] ['ouvədous] *n* слишком большая доза.

overdose[b] ['ouvə'dous] *v* давать слишком большую дозу.

overdraft ['ouvədrɑːft] *n* превышение своего кредита в банке.

overdraw ['ouvə'drɔː] *v* (*past* overdrew; *p. p.* overdrawn) 1) превысить кредит в банке; 2) преувеличивать; утрировать.

overdrawn ['ouvə'drɔːn] *p. p. см.* overdraw.

overdress ['ouvə'dres] *v* одеваться слишком нарядно *или* кричаще.

overdrew ['ouvə'druː] *past см.* overdraw.

overdrive ['ouvə'draɪv] *v* (*past* overdrove; *p. p.* overdriven) 1) переутомить, изнурить; 2) загнать (*лошадь*).

overdriven ['ouvə'drɪvn] *p. p. см.* overdrive.

overdrove ['ouvə'drouv] *past см.* overdrive.

overdue ['ouvə'djuː] *a* 1) запоздалый, запоздавший; the train is ~ поезд запаздывает; 2) просроченный.

overeat ['ouvər'iːt] *v* (*past* overate; *p. p.* overeaten) объедаться.

overeaten ['ouvər'iːtn] *p. p. см.* overeat.

overestimate[a] ['ouvər'estɪmɪt] *n* 1) слишком высокая оценка; 2) раздутая смета.

overestimate[b] ['ouvər'estɪmeɪt] *v* 1) переоценивать; 2) составлять раздутую смету.

overfed ['ouvə'fed] *past, p. p. см.* overfeed.

overfeed ['ouvə'fiːd] *v* (*past, p. p.* overfed) 1) перекармливать; 2) объедаться.

overflight ['ouvəflaɪt] *n* полёт над чужой территорией; перелёт границы.

overflow[a] ['ouvəflou] *n* 1) переливание через край; 2) разлив, наводнение; 3) избыток.

overflow[b] [,ouvə'flou] *v* 1) переливаться через край, вытекать; 2) разливаться (*о реке*); 3) затоплять; 4) переполнять; 5): to ~ with smth. быть переполненным чем-л.

overflyer ['ouvə,flaɪə] *n* нарушитель границы (*о самолёте, лётчике*).

overfulfilment ['ouvəful'fɪlmənt] *n* перевыполнение.

overgrew ['ouvə'gruː] *past см.* overgrow.

overgrow ['ouvə'grou] *v* (*past* overgrew; *p. p.* overgrown) 1) расти слишком быстро; заглушать (*о растениях*); 2): to ~ one's clothes вырасти из платья.

overgrown I ['ouvə'groun] *p. p. см.* overgrow.

overgrown II *a* 1) заросший; 2) переросший.

overgrowth ['ouvəgrouθ] *n* 1) чрезмерный, беспорядочный рост; 2) нарост.

overhang[a] ['ouvəhæŋ] *n* выступ, навес.

overhang[b] ['ouvə'hæŋ] *v* (*past, p. p.* overhung) 1) свешиваться, нависать; угрожать.

overhaul[a] ['ouvəhɔːl] *n* тщательный осмотр.

overhaul[b] [,ouvə'hɔːl] *v* 1) тщательно осматривать; нагонять.

overhead I ['ouvə'hed] *a* 1) верхний, надземный; 2) накладной (*о расходах*).

overhead II *adv* наверху, на верхнем этаже.

overhear [,ouvə'hɪə] *v* (*past, p. p.* overheard) 1) подслушивать; 2) нечаянно услышать.

overheard [,ouvə'həːd] *past, p. p. см.* overhear.

overheat I ['ouvə'hiːt] *n* перегрев.

overheat II *v* перегревáть(ся).

overhung ['ouvə'hʌŋ] *past, p. p. см.* overhang[b].

over-indulge [,ouvərın'dʌldʒ] *v* позволя́ть сли́шком мнóго, злоупотребля́ть (*обыкн. удовóльствиями*).

overjoy [,ouvə'dʒɔı] *v* осчастли́вить, безмéрно обрáдовать.

overjoyed [,ouvə'dʒɔıd] *a* óчень довóльный; рáдостный, счастли́вый.

overlabour ['ouvə'leıbə] *v* 1) переутомля́ть рабóтой; 2) сли́шком тщáтельно отдéлывать.

overladen ['ouvə'leıdn] *a* перегрýженный.

overlaid [,ouvə'leıd] *past, p. p. см.* overlay[b].

overlain ['ouvə'leın] *p. p. см.* overlie.

overland[a] ['ouvəlænd] *a* сухопýтный.

overland[b] [,ouvə'lænd] *adv* по сýше, на сýше.

overlap [,ouvə'læp] *v* 1) части́чно покрывáть, перекрывáть; 2) части́чно совпадáть.

overlay[a] ['ouvəleı] *n* покры́шка.

overlay[b] [,ouvə'leı] *v* (*past, p. p.* overlaid) покрывáть (*крáской и т. п.*).

overlay[c] ['ouvə'leı] *past см.* overlie.

overleaf ['ouvə'li:f] *adv* на оборóте (*страни́цы*).

overleap [,ouvə'li:p] *v* 1) перепры́гивать, перескáкивать; 2) пропускáть.

overlie ['ouvə'laı] *v* (*past* overlay; *p. p.* overlain) лежáть на чём-л., над чем-л.

overlive ['ouvə'lıv] *v* 1) пережи́ть когó-л.; 2) прожигáть жизнь.

overload[a] ['ouvəloud] *n* перегрýзка.

overload[b] ['ouvə'loud] *v* перегружáть.

overlook [,ouvə'luk] *v* 1) возвышáться (*над гóродом и т. п.*); 2) смотрéть на что-л. свéрху; 3) выходи́ть на...; the window ~s the sea из окнá открывáется вид нá море; 4) пропусти́ть, прогляди́ть; 5) прощáть, смотрéть сквозь пáльцы; 6) следи́ть, внимáтельно наблюдáть; 7) сглáзить.

overly ['ouvəlı] *adv разг.* чрезмéрно, сли́шком.

overman ['ouvəmæn] *n* 1) «сверхчеловéк»; 2) *горн.* деся́тник; штéйгер.

overmaster [,ouvə'mɑːstə] *v* 1) покоря́ть, побеждáть; 2) овладéть всецéло (*о чýвстве*).

overmatch [,ouvə'mætʃ] *v* превосходи́ть (*когó-л. чем-л.*).

overmature ['ouvəmə'tjuə] *a* перезрéлый.

overmuch ['ouvə'mʌtʃ] *adv* чрезмéрно, сли́шком мнóго.

over-nice ['ouvə'naıs] *a* 1) сли́шком разбóрчивый; 2) изощрённый.

overnight I ['ouvə'naıt] *a* происходи́вший наканýне вéчером.

overnight II *adv* наканýне вéчером; с вéчера (и всю ночь); to stay ~ провести́ ночь; переночевáть.

overpaid ['ouvə'peıd] *past, p. p. см.* overpay.

overpass [,ouvə'pɑːs] *v* 1) переходи́ть, пересекáть (*грани́цу и т. п.*); 2) превосходи́ть, превышáть; 3) оставля́ть без внимáния, проходи́ть ми́мо.

overpast ['ouvə'pɑːst] *a* прóшлый, давнó прошéдший.

overpay ['ouvə'peı] *v* (*past, p. p.* overpaid) переплáчивать.

overpeopled ['ouvə'pi:pld] *a* перенаселённый.

over-persuade ['ouvəpə'sweıd] *v* переубеди́ть, склони́ть к чемý-л.

overplus ['ouvəplʌs] *n* избы́ток, изоби́лие.

overpoise I ['ouvə'pɔız] *n* перевéс.

overpoise II *v* перевéшивать.

overpopulation ['ouvə,pɔpju'leıʃən] *n* перенаселённость.

overpower [,ouvə'pauə] *v* подавля́ть, побеждáть.

overpowering [,ouvə'pauərıŋ] *a* 1) непреодоли́мый; 2) подавля́ющий.

over-production ['ouvəprə'dʌkʃən] *n* перепроизвóдство.

overran [,ouvə'ræn] *past см.* overrun.

overrate ['ouvə'reıt] *v* переоцéнивать.

overreach [,ouvə'ri:tʃ] *v* 1) растяну́ть(ся); 2) превы́сить (*полномóчия и т. п.*); 3) перехитри́ть, обману́ть; to ~ oneself просчитáться, обману́ться; 4) *refl* засекáться (*о лóшади*).

overridden [,ouvə'rıdn] *p. p. см.* override.

override [,ouvə'raıd] *v* (*past* overrode; *p. p.* overridden) 1) переéхать, задави́ть лóшадью; 2) попирáть (ногáми); 3) отвергáть, не принимáть во внимáние; 4) загнáть (*лóшадь*).

overrode [,ouvə'roud] *past см.* override.

overrule [,ouvə'ru:l] *v* 1) госпóдствовать; *перен.* брать верх над кем-л.; 2) быть сильнéе, перевéшивать; 3) отвергáть, отклоня́ть (*предложéние, дóвод и т. п.*); 4) считáть недействи́тельным.

overrun [,ouvə'rʌn] *v* (*past* overran; *p. p.* overrun) 1) переливáться чéрез край; *перен.* распространя́ться (*за предéлы*); наводня́ть; 2) переходи́ть грани́цы; 3) *обыкн. pass* зарастáть (*сорнякáми; with*); 4) опустошáть (*странý — о неприя́теле*).

oversaw ['ouvə'sɔː] *past см.* oversee.

oversea(s) I ['ouvə'siː(z)] *a* замóрский, заграни́чный; внéшний (*о торгóвле*).

oversea(s) II *adv* зá морем, чéрез мóре; to go ~ éхать зá море.

oversee ['ouvə'siː] *v* (*past* oversaw; *p. p.* overseen) надзирáть, наблюдáть за кем-л., чем-л.

overseen ['ouvə'siːn] *p. p. см.* oversee.

overseer ['ouvəsıə] *n* надзирáтель, надсмóтрщик.

overset ['ouvə'set] *v* (*past, p. p.* overset) 1) нарушáть, расстрáивать; 2) опроки́дывать.

overshadow [,ouvə'ʃædou] *v* 1) затемня́ть, затеня́ть; 2) затмевáть.

overshoe ['ouvə'ʃuː] *n* галóша, бóтик.

overshoot ['ouvə'ʃuːt] *v* (*past, p. p.* overshot) промахну́ться (*при стрельбé*); *перен.* зайти́ сли́шком далекó; преувели́чить.

overshot ['ouvə'ʃɔt] *past, p. p. см.* overshoot.

oversight ['ouvəsaıt] *n* 1) недосмóтр; оплóшность; 2) надзóр; to be under the ~ of smb. быть под надзóром когó-л.

over-simplify [,ouvə'sımplıfaı] *v* упрощáть; понимáть упрощённо.

oversleep [,ouvə'sliːp] *v* (*past, p. p.* overslept) проспáть, заспáться.

oversleeve ['ouvə'sliːv] *n* нарукáвник.

overslept ['ouvə'slept] *past, p. p. см.* oversleep.

overspend ['ouvə'spend] *v* (*past, p. p.* overspent) трáтить, расхóдовать сли́шком мнóго.

overspent ['ouvə'spent] *past, p. p. см.* overspend.

overspread [ˌouvə'spred] *v* (*past; p. p.* overspread) 1) разбрасывать; 2) покрывать; 3) простирать(ся); 4) распространять(ся).

overstate ['ouvə'steɪt] *v* преувеличивать.

overstatement ['ouvə'steɪtmənt] *n* преувеличение.

overstay ['ouvə'steɪ] *v* задержаться, засидеться.

overstep ['ouvə'step] *v* переступить, перешагнуть; *перен.* переходить границы.

overstock I ['ouvə'stɔk] *n* излишний запас, избыток.

overstock II *v* делать излишний запас; забивать (*напр., товаром*).

overstrainᵃ ['ouvəstreɪn] *n* чрезмерное напряжение.

overstrainᵇ ['ouvə'streɪn] *v* перенапрягать; переутомлять.

overstrung ['ouvə'strʌŋ] *a* слишком напряжённый.

overt ['ouvəːt] *a* открытый, явный, нескрываемый.

overtake [ˌouvə'teɪk] *v* (*past* overtook; *p. p.* overtaken) 1) догнать, наверстать; 2) застигнуть (*врасплох*); 3) овладевать; ~n by (*или* with) fear охваченный страхом.

overtaken [ˌouvə'teɪkən] *p. p. см.* overtake.

overtax ['ouvə'tæks] *v* 1) облагать чрезмерным налогом; 2) обременять чрезмерно.

overthrew ['ouvə'θruː] *past см.* overthrowᵇ.

overthrowᵃ ['ouvəθrou] *n* 1) ниспровержение, свержение; 2) расстройство (*планов и т. п.*).

overthrowᵇ [ˌouvə'θrou] *v* (*past* overthrew; *p. p.* overthrown) 1) низвергать, свергать; опрокидывать; 2) побеждать; уничтожать.

overthrown [ˌouvə'θroun] *p. p. см.* overthrowᵇ.

overtime I ['ouvətaɪm] *n* сверхурочное время.

overtime II *adv* сверхурочно.

overtone ['ouvətoun] *n муз.* обертон.

overtook [ˌouvə'tuk] *past см.* overtake.

overtop ['ouvə'tɔp] *v* 1) превышать, быть выше; 2) превосходить; затмевать.

overture ['ouvətʃuə] *n* 1) *обыкн. pl* начало переговоров; (официальное) предложение; 2) *муз.* увертюра.

overturnᵃ ['ouvətəːn] *n* 1) ниспровержение, свержение; поражение; 2) *амер.* переворот.

overturnᵇ [ˌouvə'təːn] *v* 1) опрокидывать(ся); 2) падать; 3) ниспровергать, свергать; наносить поражение.

overvalue I ['ouvə'væljuː] *n* переоценка, (слишком) высокая оценка.

overvalue II *v* переоценивать, высоко оценивать; придавать слишком большое значение.

overwatched [ˌouvə'wɔtʃt] *a* изнурённый чрезмерным бодрствованием *или* бессонницей.

overweening [ˌouvə'wiːnɪŋ] *a* высокомерный; самонадеянный; самоуверенный.

overweigh ['ouvə'weɪ] *v* быть тяжелее, чем...; перевешивать.

overweightᵃ ['ouvəweɪt] *n* 1) излишек веса; 2) перевес, преобладание.

overweightᵇ [ˌouvə'weɪt] *a predic* выше положенного веса.

overweightᶜ [ˌouvə'weɪt] *v обыкн. p. p.* слишком обременять, перегружать (*чем-либо — with*).

overwhelm [ˌouvə'welm] *v* 1) заливать, затоплять; *перен.* забрасывать (*вопросами и т. п.*); 2) овладевать, переполнять (*о чувстве*); 3) сокрушать, подавлять; 4) ошеломлять, поражать.

overwhelming [ˌouvə'welmɪŋ] *a* 1) несметный; 2) непреодолимый; 3) подавляющий (*о большинстве и т. п.*); решительный (*о победе*).

overworkᵃ ['ouvəwəːk] *n* 1) сверхурочная работа; 2) перегрузка, перенапряжение.

overworkᵇ ['ouvə'wəːk] *v* 1) слишком долго *или* тяжело работать; переутомляться (*тж.* to ~ oneself); 2) переутомлять.

overwrought ['ouvə'rɔːt] *a* 1) переутомлённый (работой); 2) возбуждённый, взвинченный; 3) тщательно отделанный.

owe [ou] *v* 1) быть должным кому-л.; 2) быть в долгу перед кем-л.; быть обязанным кому-либо.

owing ['ouɪŋ] *a* 1) должный; причитающийся; 2) обязанный кому-л.; 3) происходящий от; 4): ~ to благодаря, вследствие.

owl [aul] *n* сова; ◊ to send ~s to Athens возить сов в Афины; ≅ ездить в Тулу со своим самоваром.

owlet ['aulɪt] *n* молодая сова, совёнок.

owl-light ['aullaɪt] *n* сумерки.

own I [oun] *a* 1) свой собственный; with one's ~ eyes собственными глазами; 2) родной (*об отце, брате и т. п.*).

own II *n*: to hold one's ~ стоять на своём; отстаивать свою точку зрения; on one's ~ *разг.* самостоятельно.

own III *v* 1) иметь, владеть; 2) признавать(ся); he ~s himself indebted он признаёт себя обязанным; he ~s you are right он признаёт, что вы правы; to ~ to smth. признаваться в чём-л.; □ to ~ up *разг.* а) откровенно признаваться; б) покорно соглашаться.

owner ['ounə] *n* владелец, собственник; хозяин; factory ~ фабрикант; joint ~ совладелец; the ~ *сленг.* капитан.

ownerless ['ounəlɪs] *a* беспризорный, не имеющий хозяина; бесхозный.

ownership ['ounəʃɪp] *n* 1) собственность; владение; 2) право собственности.

ox [ɔks] *n* (*pl.* oxen) бык; вол; ◊ the black ox а) старость; б) несчастье.

oxalic [ɔk'sælɪk] *a хим.* щавелевый.

oxbow ['ɔksbou] *n* ярмо.

oxen ['ɔksən] *n* 1) *pl см.* ox; 2) рогатый скот.

ox-eyed ['ɔksaɪd] *a* большеглазый, волоокий.

oxford ['ɔksfəd] *n* 1) полуботинок; 2) стальной цвет.

oxherd ['ɔkshəːd] *n* пастух.

oxhide ['ɔkshaɪd] *n* воловья шкура.

oxidation [ˌɔksɪ'deɪʃən] *n* окисление.

oxide ['ɔksaɪd] *n* окись; carbonic ~ окись углерода.

oxidize ['ɔksɪdaɪz] *v* окислять(ся).

oxygen ['ɔksɪdʒən] *n* 1) кислород; 2) *attr* кислородный.

oxygenous [ɔk'sɪdʒɪnəs] *a* кислородный.

oyster ['ɔɪstə] *n* устрица; ◊ close (*или* dumb) as an ~ ≅ нем как рыба.

ozone ['ouzoun] *n хим.* озон.

ozonize ['ouzənaɪz] *v* озонировать.

P

P, p [pːː] *n* 16-я буква англ. алфавита; ◇ to mind one's P's and Q's соблюдать осторожность *или* приличия.

pa [pɑ] *n разг.* папа.

pace^a I [peɪs] *n* 1) шаг; длина шага; to mend one's ~ ускорять шаг; 2) скорость; темп; to go the ~ а) идти, ехать с большой скоростью; б) тратить много денег, транжирить; to keep ~ with идти в ногу с кем-л.; поспевать за кем-л.; to hit the ~ мчаться; *перен.* прожигать жизнь; at a quick (*или* great) ~ очень быстро; at a slow ~ очень медленно; at a snail's ~ черепашьим шагом; to put on ~ прибавить шагу; 3) походка, поступь; 4) аллюр, иноходь; 5) ступенька; ◇ to put smb. through his ~s подвергнуть кого-л. испытанию.

pace^a II *v* 1) шагать; расхаживать; 2) мерить шагами (*тж.* to ~ out, to ~ off); 3) идти шагом (*о лошади*); идти иноходью; 4) задавать темп (*в состязании*).

pace^b ['peɪsɪ] *prep* с позволения кого-л.

pacer ['peɪsə] *n* иноходец.

pacha ['pɑʃə] *см.* pasha.

pacific [pə'sɪfɪk] *a* 1) мирный; 2) мирно настроенный, спокойный; 3) (P.) тихоокеанский.

pacification [ˌpæsɪfɪ'keɪʃən] *n* 1) умиротворение, успокоение; 2) восстановление мира, спокойствия (*в стране*).

pacificism [pə'sɪfɪsɪzəm] *см.* pacifism.

pacifico [pə'sɪfɪkou] *n разг.* мирный, мирно настроенный человек.

pacifier ['pæsɪfaɪə] *n* 1) успокоитель; 2) успокаивающее средство; 3) пустышка, кольцо (*для грудных детей*).

pacifism ['pæsɪfɪzəm] *n* пацифизм.

pacifist ['pæsɪfɪst] *n* пацифист.

pacify ['pæsɪfaɪ] *v* 1) успокаивать, умиротворять; укрощать (*гнев*); восстанавливать мир, спокойствие (*в стране*).

pack I [pæk] *n* 1) тюк, кипа, связка; пакет; пачка (*папирос*); 2) *воен.* сумка, ранец; 3) шайка, банда (*воров и т. п.*); 4) свора (*собак*); стая (*волков*); 5) множество, масса; a ~ of lies сплошная ложь; a ~ of nonsense сплошная чушь; 6) колода (*карт*); 7) масса плавучего льда; 8) *attr* вьючный; 9) *attr* упаковочный.

pack II *v* 1) упаковывать, запаковывать; 2) укладывать (*в дорогу; тж.* to ~ up); 3) заполнять, забивать (*пространство; with*); 4) набивать (*чемодан и т. п.*); 5) консервировать (*продукты*); 6) навьючивать (*животное*); 7) собираться в стаи (*о волках*); 8) быстро собраться и уехать; 9) заполнять своими сторонниками (*собрание, суд и т. п.; with*); □ to ~ off выпроваживать, прогонять; to ~ up *разг.* прекратить работу.

package I ['pækɪdʒ] *n* 1) посылка; сверток; тюк; 2) упаковка; 3) место (*багажа*).

package II *v амер.* упаковывать.

pack-animal ['pæk,ænɪməl] *n* вьючное животное.

packer ['pækə] *n* 1) упаковщик; 2) упаковочная машина.

packet ['pækɪt] *n* 1) пакет, связка; пачка (*конвертов, папирос*); 2) *см.* packet-boat.

packet-boat ['pækɪtbout] *n* почтовый пароход, пакетбот.

pack-horse ['pækhɔːs] *n* вьючная лошадь.

packing ['pækɪŋ] *n* 1) упаковка, укупорка; 2) упаковочный материал; ~ not included цена без упаковки; 3) *тех.* набивка, прокладка.

packman ['pækmən] *n* разносчик, коробейник.

packsack ['pæksæk] *n* рюкзак.

pack-saddle ['pæk,sædl] *n* вьючное седло.

packthread ['pækθred] *n* бечёвка, шпагат.

pact [pækt] *n* договор, пакт; Pact of Peace Пакт Мира; non-aggression ~ договор о ненападении; to enter into ~ заключить договор.

pad I [pæd] *n* 1) мягкая прокладка; 2) мягкое седло; седёлка; 3) подушка (*для печати*); 4) бювар; 5) подушечка (*на подошве некоторых животных*); 6) лапа (*зайца, лисицы и т. п.*); 7) *косм.* стартовый стол (*тж.* launching ~, firing ~).

pad II *v* 1) заполнять мягкой прокладкой; 2) подбивать ватой; обивать чем-л. мягким; 3) растягивать (*рассказ и т. п.; тж.* to ~ out).

padding ['pædɪŋ] *n* 1) набивочный материал; 2) многословие.

paddle¹ I ['pædl] *n* 1) весло (*с широкой лопастью*); 2) лопасть (*гребного колеса*); 3) гребля; 4) валёк (*для стирки белья*); 5) *зоол.* плавник; ласт; плавательная перепонка; 6) *pl* ласты (*аквалангиста*).

paddle¹ II *v* грести одним веслом; плыть на байдарке.

paddle² *v* 1) шлёпать по воде (*босыми ногами*), бултыхаться в воде; плескаться; 2) играть пальцами (*in, on, about*); 3) ковылять (*о ребёнке*).

paddle-wheel ['pædlwiːl] *n* гребное колесо (*парохода*).

paddock ['pædək] *n* 1) выгон, загон; лужайка (*при ипподроме*); 2) *австрал.* поле, участок земли.

paddy¹ ['pædɪ] *n* 1) рис (*на корню или в шелухе*); 2) *attr* рисовый (*о поле*).

paddy² *n см.* paddywhack 1).

paddywhack ['pædɪwæk] *n* 1) *разг.* гнев, ярость; 2) *амер.* шлепок.

Padishah ['pɑːdɪʃɑ] *n* падишах.

padlock I ['pædlɔk] *n* висячий замок.

padlock II *v* запирать на висячий замок.

pagan I ['peɪgən] *n* язычник.

pagan II *a* языческий.

page¹ I [peɪdʒ] *n* 1) страница; specimen ~ пробная страница; front ~ первая страница (*газеты*); title ~ титульный лист.

page¹ II *v* нумеровать страницы.

page² I *n* 1) мальчик-слуга; 2) паж.

page² II *v* 1) сопровождать в качестве пажа; 2) *амер.* вызывать кого-л., выкликая фамилию.

pageant ['pædʒənt] *n* 1) инсценировка; живая картина; 2) маскарад; 3) красивое зрелище; пышная процессия; карнавальное шествие; 4) *ист.* подвижная сцена (*на колёсиках*).

pageantry ['pædʒəntrɪ] *n* 1) блеск, шик, помпа; 2) видимость, блеф.

pah [pɑ] *int* фу!

paid [peɪd] *past, p. p. см.* pay¹ II.

paid-up ['peɪd'ʌp] *a* уплаченный, внесённый (*о деньгах*).

pail [peɪl] *n* 1) ведро́, бадья́; ка́дка; 2) *мор.* бак.

pailful ['peɪlful] *n* по́лное ведро́ (*чего-л.*).

paillasse [pæl'jæs] *n* соло́менный тюфя́к.

pain I [peɪn] *n* 1) боль, страда́ние; severe ~ о́страя боль; to stand the ~ выноси́ть боль; I have a ~ in my ear у меня́ боли́т у́хо; 2) огорче́ние, го́ре; he is in great ~ у него́ большо́е го́ре; 3) *pl* уси́лия, стара́ния; for my ~s за труды́, в награ́ду; to save one's ~s эконо́мить свой труд, свои́ си́лы; to spare no ~s не жале́ть свои́х сил, трудо́в; to take great ~s прилага́ть все уси́лия; to be at the ~s doing smth. стара́ться де́лать что-л.; 4) наказа́ние; on (*или* under) ~ of death под стра́хом сме́ртной ка́зни; ~s and penalties взыска́ния и наказа́ния; ◊ по ~s no gains *посл.* ≅ под лежа́чий ка́мень вода́ не течёт.

pain II *v* 1) причиня́ть боль, страда́ния; 2) боле́ть.

painful ['peɪnful] *a* 1) боле́зненный; мучи́тельный; 2) тя́гостный, тяжёлый; 3) тру́дный.

pain-killer ['peɪn,kɪlə] *n* болеутоля́ющее сре́дство.

painless ['peɪnlɪs] *a* безболе́зненный.

painstaking ['peɪnz,teɪkɪŋ] *a* стара́тельный, кропотли́вый.

paint I [peɪnt] *n* 1) кра́ска; окра́ска; dazzle ~ *мор.* маскиро́вочная окра́ска; камуфля́ж; 2) *pl* кра́ски; 3) румя́на.

paint II *v* 1) кра́сить, окра́шивать; 2) писа́ть кра́сками, рисова́ть; 3) опи́сывать в я́рких кра́сках; to ~ in bright colours приукра́шивать; представля́ть в ро́зовом све́те; not so black as he is ~ed ≅ не так плох, как его́ изобража́ют; 4) кра́сить(ся), румя́нить(ся); □ to ~ out закра́шивать (*надпись и т. п.*).

paintbrush ['peɪntbrʌʃ] *n* кисть.

painted ['peɪntɪd] *a* окра́шенный, цветно́й.

painter[1] ['peɪntə] *n* 1) худо́жник, живопи́сец; animal ~ анимали́ст; landscape ~ пейзажи́ст; portrait ~ портрети́ст; 2) маля́р.

painter[2] *n мор.* (носово́й) фа́линь; to cut the ~ *перен.* порва́ть связь, отдели́ться.

painting ['peɪntɪŋ] *n* 1) жи́вопись, ро́спись; genre (landscape, easel, mural) ~ жа́нровая (пейзажная, станко́вая, фре́сковая) жи́вопись; 2) карти́на; 3) окра́ска, покра́ска; 4) маля́рное де́ло.

pair I [pɛə] *n* 1) па́ра; in ~s па́рами; a ~ of compasses ци́ркуль; 2) супру́жеская чета́; the happy ~ молодожёны; 3) *pl* партнёры (*в картах*); 4) *парл.* два чле́на оппозицио́нных па́ртий, не уча́ствующие в голосова́нии по соглаше́нию; 5) сме́на, брига́да (*рабочих*); 6) *attr* па́рный.

pair II *v* 1) соединя́ть(ся) по́ двое; 2) спа́ривать(ся); 3) сочета́ться бра́ком; □ to ~ off дели́ться попа́рно; *разг.* жени́ться, вы́йти за́муж (*with*).

pajamas [pə'dʒɑːməz] *см.* pyjamas.

Pakistani I [,pækɪs'tɑːnɪ] *n* пакиста́нец.

Pakistani II *a* пакиста́нский.

pal I [pæl] *n разг.* 1) това́рищ, прия́тель; 2) соуча́стник.

pal II *v разг.* подружи́ться (*тж.* to ~ up).

palace ['pælɪs] *n* 1) дворе́ц; 2) роско́шный дом, особня́к; 3) *attr* дворцо́вый.

palankeen [,pælən'kiːn] *n* паланки́н, носи́лки.

palatability [,pælətə'bɪlɪtɪ] *n* прия́тный вкус; *перен.* прия́тность.

palatable ['pælətəbl] *a* вку́сный, пика́нтный; *перен.* прия́тный.

palatal I ['pælətl] *n фон.* палата́льный звук.

palatal II *a* 1) нёбный; 2) *фон.* палата́льный.

palatalization ['pælətəlaɪ'zeɪʃən] *n фон.* смягче́ние (*согласных*), палатализа́ция.

palatalize ['pælətəlaɪz] *v фон.* смягча́ть, палатализова́ть.

palate ['pælɪt] *n* 1) нёбо; hard (soft) ~ твёрдое (мя́гкое) нёбо; cleft ~ *мед.* во́лчья пасть; 2) вкус, аппети́т; 3) скло́нность, интере́с.

palatial [pə'leɪʃəl] *a* 1) дворцо́вый; 2) роско́шный, велича́ственный.

palaver I [pə'lɑːvə] *n* 1) перегово́ры (*между путешественниками и туземцами*); 2) пуста́я болтовня́; 3) лесть.

palaver II *v* 1) болта́ть; 2) льстить, говори́ть льсти́во.

pale[1] I [peɪl] *a* 1) бле́дный; 2) ту́склый, нея́ркий (*о свете, цвете и т. п.*).

pale[1] II *v* 1) бледне́ть; 2) тускне́ть.

pale[2] I [peɪl] *n* 1) кол; 2) *редко* огра́да, частоко́л; 3) грани́ца, преде́лы.

pale[2] II *v* обноси́ть огра́дой, частоко́лом.

paled [peɪld] *a* огоро́женный (*частоколом*).

pale-face ['peɪlfeɪs] *n* бледноли́цый, бе́лый челове́к.

palette ['pælɪt] *n* пали́тра.

palfrey ['pɔːlfrɪ] *n уст., поэт.* верхова́я ло́шадь.

paling ['peɪlɪŋ] *n* 1) забо́р, частоко́л, тын; 2) *собир.* ко́лья.

palisade I [,pælɪ'seɪd] *n* 1) палиса́д, частоко́л; 2) *pl амер.* гряда́ скал.

palisade II *v* обноси́ть забо́ром, частоко́лом, ты́ном.

palish ['peɪlɪʃ] *a* бледнова́тый.

pall[1] I [pɔːl] *n* 1) покро́в (*на гробе*); 2) пелена́, заве́са; покро́в; 3) ма́нтия.

pall[1] II *v* покрыва́ть; оку́тывать.

pall[2] *v* 1) надоеда́ть, станови́ться утоми́тельным; 2) насыща́ть, пресыща́ть (*тж.* to ~ on).

pallet ['pælɪt] *n* 1) соло́менный тюфя́к; 2) ко́йка.

palliasse [pæl'jæs] *см.* paillasse.

palliate ['pælɪeɪt] *v* 1) облегча́ть (*боль*); 2) извиня́ть, смягча́ть (*обиду, вину*); опра́вдывать (*преступление*).

palliation [,pælɪ'eɪʃən] *n* 1) вре́менное облегче́ние (*боли*); 2) смягче́ние, извине́ние (*обиды, вины*); опра́вдание (*преступления*).

palliative I ['pælɪətɪv] *n* паллиати́в, полуме́ра.

palliative II *a* 1) паллиати́вный; 2) смягча́ющий.

pallid ['pælɪd] *a* мёртвенно-бле́дный.

pallidness ['pælɪdnɪs] *n* мёртвенная бле́дность.

pall-mall ['pel'mel] *n* стари́нная игра́ в шары́.

pallor ['pælə] *n* бле́дность.

palm[1] I [pɑːm] *n* 1) ладо́нь; to grease (*или* to oil) smb.'s ~ «подма́зать», дать взя́тку; to have an itching ~ охо́тно брать взя́тки; 2) ло́пасть (*весла*); ла́па (*якоря*).

palm[1] II *v* 1) пря́тать в руке́; 2) тро́гать, гла́дить ладо́нью; 3) подкупа́ть, дава́ть взя́тку; □ ~ off всуча́ть, подсо́вывать (*кому-л. — on, upon*).

palm[2] *n* 1) па́льма, па́льмовое де́рево; 2) пальмовая ветвь; *перен.* побе́да, триу́мф; to bear (*или* to carry off) the ~ получи́ть па́льму пе́рвенства; одержа́ть побе́ду; to yield the ~ уступи́ть па́льму пе́рвенства (*кому-л.— to*); призна́ть себя́ побеж-дённым; 3) *attr* па́льмовый.

palmetto [pæl'metou] *n* пальме́тто; ка́рликовая па́льма.

palmful ['pɑːmful] *n* горсть (*чего-л.*).

palmy ['pɑːmɪ] *a* 1) цвету́щий, процвета́ющий; 2) бога́тый па́льмами.

palpable ['pælpəbl] *a* 1) ощути́мый, осяза́емый; 2) очеви́дный, я́вный.

palpate ['pælpeɪt] *v* ощу́пывать.

palpitant ['pælpɪtənt] *a* трепе́щущий.

palpitate ['pælpɪteɪt] *v* 1) пульси́ровать, би́ться (*о сердце*); 2) дрожа́ть, трепета́ть.

palpitation [,pælpɪ'teɪʃən] *n* 1) пульса́ция, сердцебие́ние; 2) трепета́ние.

palsy I ['pɔːlzɪ] *n* парали́ч.

palsy II *v* парализова́ть.

palter ['pɔːltə] *v* 1) криви́ть душо́й; уви́ливать, хитри́ть; 2) торгова́ться; 3) занима́ться пустяка́ми.

paltry ['pɔːltrɪ] *a* 1) ме́лкий, незначи́тельный, ничто́жный; 2) жа́лкий; 3) презре́нный.

pampas ['pæmpəs] *n pl* пампа́сы.

pamper ['pæmpə] *v* 1) балова́ть, изне́живать.

pamphlet ['pæmflɪt] *n* 1) брошю́ра; 2) памфле́т.

pamphleteer I [,pæmflɪ'tɪə] *n* памфлети́ст.

pamphleteer II *v* писа́ть памфле́ты.

pan I [pæn] *n* 1) сковорода́; 2) кастрю́ля; 3) ча́шка (*весов*); 4) металли́ческий сосу́д, таз *и т. п.*; 5) *тех.* поддо́н; коры́то; лото́к.

pan II *v* 1) промыва́ть (*золотоно́сный песо́к*); 2) *разг.* зада́ть жа́ру; ре́зко критикова́ть; □ to ~ out a) намыва́ть зо́лото; б) преуспева́ть; в) уда-ва́ться, устра́иваться.

panacea [,pænə'sɪə] *n* универса́льное сре́дство, панаце́я.

panache [pə'næʃ] *n* 1) султа́н (*украшение на шлеме*); 2) рисо́вка, щегольство́.

panama [,pænə'mɑː] *n* пана́ма (*тж.* ~ hat); 2) *разг.* кру́пное моше́нничество.

pancake ['pænkeɪk] *n* блин, ола́дья.

pancreas ['pæŋkrɪəs] *n* поджелу́дочная железа́.

pandemonium [,pændɪ'mounjəm] *n* ад кроме́ш-ный; «вавило́нское столпотворе́ние».

pander I ['pændə] *n* 1) посо́бник; 2) сво́дник.

pander II *v* 1) сво́дничать; 2) потво́рствовать.

pandowdy [pæn'daudɪ] *n амер.* я́блочный пу́-динг.

pane [peɪn] *n* 1) око́нное стекло́; 2) пане́ль; 3) грань (*бриллианта, гайки*).

paned [peɪnd] *a* со стёклами, остеклённый.

panegyric I [,pænɪ'dʒɪrɪk] *n* (по)хвала́, панеги́-рик.

panegyric II *a* хвале́бный.

panel I ['pænl] *n* 1) пане́ль; филёнка; 2) то́нкая доска́ для жи́вописи; 3) вста́вка друго́го материа́ла *или* цве́та в пла́тье; 4) фотосни́мок большо́го форма́та; 5) спи́сок прися́жных; прися́жные; 6) *тех.* прибо́рная *или* распредели́тельная доска́.

panel II *v* 1) обшива́ть пане́лями; 2) отде́лывать пла́тье вста́вкой друго́го цве́та; 3) включа́ть в спи́сок прися́жных.

panelling ['pænlɪŋ] *n* пане́льная обши́вка.

panful ['pænful] *n* по́лная кастрю́ля, сковорода́ (*чего-л.*).

pang [pæŋ] *n* 1) о́страя боль; 2) *pl* угрызе́ния (*совести*).

panhandle ['pæn,hændl] *n* 1) ру́чка сковороды́, кастрю́ли; 2) *амер.* у́зкий вы́ступ террито́рии ме́жду двумя́ други́ми террито́риями.

panic I ['pænɪk] *n* па́ника; seized by ~ охва́чен-ный па́никой.

panic II *a* пани́ческий.

panic III *v* 1) впада́ть в па́нику; 2) *амер. сленг* держа́ть зри́телей в напряже́нии.

panicky ['pænɪkɪ] *a разг.* пани́ческий.

panic-monger ['pænɪk,mʌŋgə] *n* паникёр.

panic-stricken ['pænɪk,strɪkən] *a* охва́ченный па́никой; в па́нике.

panne [pæn] *n* панба́рхат.

pannier ['pænɪə] *n* корзи́на (*особ. вьючная*).

pannikin ['pænɪkɪn] *n* ми́сочка; кру́жка.

panoplied ['pænəplɪd] *a* во всеору́жии.

panoply ['pænəplɪ] *n* доспе́хи.

panorama [,pænə'rɑːmə] *n* панора́ма.

pan-pipe [,pænpaɪp] *n* свире́ль.

pansy ['pænzɪ] *n бот.* аню́тины гла́зки.

pant I [pænt] *n* 1) тяжёлое дыха́ние; 2) пыхте́-ние; 3) бие́ние (*сердца*).

pant II *v* 1) тяжело́ дыша́ть; 2) пыхте́ть; 3) стра́-стно жела́ть чего́-л.; 4) си́льно би́ться, трепета́ть (*о сердце*); 5) говори́ть задыха́ясь; выпа́ливать (*обыкн.* to ~ out).

pantalet(te)s [,pæntə'lets] *n pl* де́тские *или* да́м-ские панталоны.

pantaloon [,pæntə'luːn] *n* 1) *ист.* рейту́зы; 2) *амер.* брю́ки.

panther ['pænθə] *n зоол.* 1) панте́ра; 2) *амер.* пу́ма, кугуа́р; 3) леопа́рд.

pantile ['pæntaɪl] *n* голла́ндская, желобча́тая черепи́ца.

pantomime ['pæntəmaɪm] *n* пантоми́ма.

pantry ['pæntrɪ] *n* 1) кладова́я, чула́н; 2) бу-фе́тная.

pants [pænts] *n pl* 1) кальсо́ны; 2) *амер. разг.* брю́ки.

pants suit ['pæntssjuːt] *n амер.* брю́чный костю́м (*женский*).

panzer ['pæntsə] *a* бронета́нковый.

pap [pæp] *n* ка́шка, каши́ца.

papa [pə'pɑː] *n дет.* па́па.

papacy ['peɪpəsɪ] *n* па́пство.

papal ['peɪpəl] *a* па́пский.

paper ['peɪpə] *n* 1) бума́га; carbon ~ копиро-ва́льная бума́га, *разг.* копи́рка; gelatine ~ фото-бума́га; India ~ то́нкая про́чная тря́пичная бу-ма́га; plotting (brown, litmus) ~ миллиметро́вая (обёрточная, ла́кмусовая) бума́га; to commit to ~ запи́сать, зафикси́ровать; to put on ~ запи́сывать; 2) газе́та; 3) докуме́нт; *pl* ли́чные докуме́нты; bal-lot (*или* voting) ~ избира́тельный бюллете́нь; walk-ing ~s рабо́чие бума́ги (*выдаваемые подростку, достигшему 14 лет*); to send in one's ~s посла́ть свои́ докуме́нты (*напр., в учебное заведение*); б) пода́ть в отста́вку; 4) нау́чный докла́д, статья́; 5) *собир.* векселя́, банкно́ты, бума́жные де́ньги; 6) обо́и; 7) *сленг* контрама́рка; 8) *attr* бума́жный; 9) *attr* существу́ющий то́лько на бума́ге; 10) *attr* газе́тный.

paper II *v* 1) завёртывать в бума́гу; 2) окле́ивать (*обо́ями*); 3) *ре́дко* писа́ть на бума́ге.

paper-back [ˈpeɪpəbæk] *n* дешёвая кни́га, журна́л в мя́гкой обло́жке.

paper-hanger [ˈpeɪpəˌhæŋə] *n* обо́йщик.

paper-hangings [ˈpeɪpəˌhæŋɪŋz] *n pl* обо́и.

paper-knife [ˈpeɪpənaɪf] *n* разрезно́й нож.

paper-mill [ˈpeɪpəmɪl] *n* бума́жная фа́брика.

paper-weight [ˈpeɪpəweɪt] *n* пресс-папье́.

papery [ˈpeɪpərɪ] *a* похо́жий на бума́гу, то́нкий.

papier-mâché [ˈpæpjeɪˈmɑːʃeɪ] *n* папье́-маше́.

papoose [pəˈpuːs] *n* инде́йский ребёнок.

paprika [ˈpæprɪkə] *n* кра́сный пе́рец.

Papuan I [ˈpæpjuən] *n* папуа́с; папуа́ска; the ~s папуа́сы.

Papuan II *a* папуа́сский.

papyrus [pəˈpaɪərəs] *n* (*pl* papyri [pəˈpaɪəraɪ]) 1) папи́рус; 2) *attr* папи́русный.

par[1] [pɑː] *n* 1) ра́венство; on a ~ (with) наравне́, на ра́вных нача́лах (с); 2) номина́льная сто́имость; above (below) ~ вы́ше (ни́же) номина́льной сто́имости (*см. тж.* 3); at ~ по номина́льной сто́имости; 3) норма́льное коли́чество, ка́чество, состоя́ние; on a ~ в сре́днем; above (below) ~ вы́ше (ни́же) норма́льного (*см. тж.* 2); I feel below ~ мне не по себе́; 4) *attr* норма́льный, сре́дний.

par[2] *n сокр. разг. см.* paragraph I, 3).

parable [ˈpærəbl] *n* при́тча, иносказа́ние; to take up one's ~ заговори́ть нравоучи́тельным то́ном.

parabola [pəˈræbələ] *n мат.* пара́бола.

parabolic [ˌpærəˈbɔlɪk] *a* 1) иносказа́тельный; 2) *мат.* параболи́ческий.

parachute I [ˈpærəʃuːt] *n* 1) парашю́т; 2) *attr* парашю́тный.

parachute II *v* спуска́ть(ся) с парашю́том.

parachute-jumper [ˈpærəʃuːtˌdʒʌmpə] *n* парашюти́ст.

parade I [pəˈreɪd] *n* 1) пара́д войск; 2) пока́з, вы́ставка; to make a ~ of щеголя́ть чем-л., выставля́ть напока́з; beauty ~ ко́нкурс красоты́; ~ of words краси́вые слова́; 3) плац; 4) ме́сто для гуля́нья; 5) гуля́ющая пу́блика; 6) *амер.* проце́ссия, ше́ствие.

parade II *v* 1) *воен.* стро́иться; идти́ стро́ем; 2) выставля́ть напока́з; 3) разгу́ливать, ше́ствовать.

parade-ground [pəˈreɪdgraund] *n* уче́бный плац.

paradigm [ˈpærədaɪm] *n* 1) *грам.* паради́гма; 2) образе́ц, приме́р.

paradise [ˈpærədaɪs] *n* 1) рай; a fool's ~ нереа́льный мир, призра́чное сча́стье; 2) *театр.* галёрка.

paradox [ˈpærədɔks] *n* парадо́кс.

paradoxical [ˌpærəˈdɔksɪkəl] *a* парадокса́льный.

paraffin I [ˈpærəfɪn] *n* 1) парафи́н; 2) парафи́новое ма́сло; 3) *attr* парафи́новый.

paraffin II *v* покрыва́ть парафи́ном.

paragon [ˈpærəgən] *n* образе́ц (соверше́нства).

paragraph I [ˈpærəgrɑːf] *n* 1) абза́ц; 2) пара́граф; 3) газе́тная заме́тка.

paragraph II *v* 1) дели́ть на абза́цы; 2) писа́ть *или* публикова́ть заме́тку.

parallel I [ˈpærəlel] *n* 1) паралле́ль; соотве́тствие, анало́гия; to draw a ~ between проводи́ть паралле́ль ме́жду чем-л. *или* кем-л., сра́внивать; 2) паралле́льная ли́ния; 3) *эл.* паралле́льное соедине́ние; 4) *полигр.* знак ‖.

parallel II *a* 1) паралле́льный; 2) подо́бный, схо́дный.

parallel III *v* 1) проводи́ть паралле́ль, сра́внивать; 2) соотве́тствовать; 3) *эл.* соединя́ть паралле́льно.

paralyse [ˈpærəlaɪz] *v* парализова́ть.

paralysis [pəˈrælɪsɪs] *n* (*pl* paralyses [pəˈrælɪsiːz]) парали́ч.

paralytic I [ˌpærəˈlɪtɪk] *n* парали́тик.

paralytic II *a* парали́чный.

paramount [ˈpærəmaunt] *a* верхо́вный; вы́сший; важне́йший, первостепе́нный.

paramour [ˈpærəmuə] *n* любо́вник; любо́вница.

parapet [ˈpærəpɪt] *n* 1) парапе́т, пери́ла; 2) *воен.* бру́ствер.

paraph I [ˈpærəf] *n* ро́счерк.

paraph II *v* парафи́ровать (*догово́р*).

paraphrase I [ˈpærəfreɪz] *n* переска́з, парафра́з(а).

paraphrase II *v* переска́зывать, парафрази́ровать.

parasite [ˈpærəsaɪt] *n* парази́т, туне́ядец.

parasitic [ˌpærəˈsɪtɪk] *a* паразити́ческий.

parasitism [ˈpærəsaɪtɪzəm] *n* паразити́зм.

parasol [ˌpærəˈsɔl] *n* зо́нтик (*от со́лнца*).

parataxis [ˌpærəˈtæksɪs] *n грам.* бессою́зное подчине́ние *или* сочине́ние.

paratrooper [ˈpærətruːpə] *n* парашюти́ст-деса́нтник.

paratroops [ˈpærətruːps] *n pl* парашю́тно-деса́нтные войска́.

paratyphoid [ˈpærəˈtaɪfɔɪd] *n мед.* парати́ф.

parboil [ˈpɑːbɔɪl] *v* 1) обва́ривать кипятко́м; 2) перегрева́ть.

parcel I [ˈpɑːsl] *n* 1) паке́т; свёрток; у́зел; 2) посы́лка; 3) па́ртия (*това́ра*); 4) уча́сток (*земли́*); 5) гру́ппа люде́й; ку́ча веще́й.

parcel II *v* 1) дели́ть на ча́сти, дроби́ть (*обыкн.* to ~ out); 2) завёртывать в паке́т, свёрток; свя́зывать в у́зел.

parch [pɑːtʃ] *v* 1) слегка́ поджа́ривать; 2) суши́ть, высу́шивать; 3) запека́ться (*о губа́х*); пересыха́ть (*о го́рле, языке́*); □ to ~ up высыха́ть, со́хнуть.

parched [pɑːtʃt] *a* запёкшийся (*о губа́х*).

parching [ˈpɑːtʃɪŋ] *a* паля́щий.

parchment [ˈpɑːtʃmənt] *n* 1) пергаме́нт; 2) ру́копись на пергаме́нте; 3) пергаме́нтная бума́га.

pard [pɑːd] *n амер. сленг* партнёр.

pardon I [ˈpɑːdn] *n* 1) проще́ние, извине́ние; I beg your ~ прости́те!, извини́те!; 2) *юр.* поми́лование; general ~ амни́стия; free ~ по́лное проще́ние, поми́лование; 3) *ист.* па́пская индульге́нция.

pardon II *v* 1) проща́ть, извиня́ть; ~ me! прошу́ проще́ния!, извини́те меня́!; 2) (по)ми́ловать.

pardonable [ˈpɑːdnəbl] *a* извини́тельный, прости́тельный.

pardoner [ˈpɑːdnə] *n ист.* продаве́ц индульге́нций.

pare [pɛə] *v* 1) чи́стить (*карто́фель*); среза́ть кожуру́; 2) подреза́ть но́гти; □ to ~ away *см.* to ~ off; to ~ down сокраща́ть, уре́зывать (*расхо́ды*); to ~ off среза́ть.

parent [ˈpɛərənt] *n* 1) оте́ц, мать; *pl* роди́тели; 2) пре́док; 3) производи́тель; 4) исто́чник; 5) *attr* ро́дственный (*о языке́*); 6) *attr* исхо́дный.

parentage ['pɛərəntɪdʒ] *n* происхождéние, лúния родствá.

parental [pə'rentl] *a* родúтельский; отцóвский; матерúнский (*о чувстве*); рóдственный.

parenthesis [pə'renθɪsɪs] *n* (*pl* parentheses [pə'renθɪsiːz]) 1) грам. ввóдное слóво *или* предложéние; 2) *pl* крýглые скóбки; 3) интермéдия.

parenthetic(al) [,pærən'θetɪk(əl)] *a* 1) ввóдный, заключённый в скóбки; 2) встáвленный мимохóдом.

parenthood ['pɛərənthud] *n* отцóвство, матерúнство.

par excellence [pɑːr'eksəlɑːns] *adv* по преимýществу; глáвным óбразом.

pariah ['pærɪə] *n* пáрия.

paring ['pɛərɪŋ] *n* 1) срéзывание; 2) *pl* обрéзки, очúстки.

parish ['pærɪʃ] *n* 1) церкóвный прихóд; 2) óкруг (*тж.* civil ~); 3) прихожáне; 4) *attr* прихóдский; ◊ to go on the ~ получáть пособие по бéдности.

parishioner [pə'rɪʃənə] *n* прихожáнин, -нка.

Parisian I [pə'rɪzjən] *n* парижáнин, -нка.

Parisian II *a* парúжский.

parity ['pærɪtɪ] *n* 1) рáвенство; 2) соотвéтствие, аналóгия; 3) эк. паритéт, равноцéнность.

park I [pɑːk] *n* 1) парк (*тж. автомобильный, артиллерийский и т. п.*); national ~ заповéдник; the Park Гáйд-парк (*в Лондоне*); 2) *амер.* высокогóрная долúна.

park II *v* 1) разбивáть парк, огорáживать под парк; 2) стáвить в парк (*автомашины*); no ~ing (allowed) стоянка автомашúн воспрещáется; 3) *разг.* оставлять; 4) *воен.* стáвить на стоянку.

parkland ['pɑːklænd] *n* лесúстый учáсток, используемый как парк.

parkway ['pɑːkweɪ] *n* *амер.* обсáженная дерéвьями дорóга.

parky ['pɑːkɪ] *a* *разг.* прохлáдный (*о воздухе*).

parlance ['pɑːləns] *n* манéра говорúть, выражáться; in common ~ в просторéчии; in legal ~ на юридúческом языкé.

parlay I ['pɑːleɪ] *n* *амер.* парú.

parlay II *v* *амер.* держáть парú, стáвить на (*во время состязания*).

parley I ['pɑːlɪ] *n* встрéча, конферéнция (*воюющих сторон*); переговóры; to beat (*или* to sound) a ~ *воен.* давáть сигнáл о желáнии вестú переговоры.

parley II *v* 1) вестú переговóры, договáриваться; 2) говорúть, изъясняться (*на чужом языке*).

parliament ['pɑːləmənt] *n* 1) парлáмент; to go into ~, to come to ~ стать членом парлáмента; to sit in ~ быть членом парлáмента; 2) *attr* парлáментский.

parliamentarian I [,pɑːləmən'tɛərɪən] *n* 1) член парлáмента; парламентáрий; 2) *ист.* сторóнник парлáмента (*в эпоху гражданской войны в Англии в XVII веке*).

parliamentarian II *a* парлáментский.

parliamentary [,pɑːlə'mentərɪ] *a* 1) парлáментский; парламентáрный; 2) *разг.* вéжливый.

parlo(u)r ['pɑːlə] *n* 1) гостúная, óбщая кóмната; 2) кóмната óтдыха; 3) приёмная (*в гостинице*); 4) *амер.* зал, ателье, кабинéт.

parlo(u)rmaid ['pɑːləmeɪd] *n* гóрничная.

parly ['pɑːlɪ] *n* слéнг (*сокр. от* parliamentary train) дешёвый пóезд 3-го клáсса.

parochial [pə'roukjəl] *a* 1) прихóдский; 2) мéстный, ýзкий, огранúченный.

parodist ['pærədɪst] *n* пародúст.

parody I ['pærədɪ] *n* парóдия.

parody II *v* пародúровать.

parole I [pə'roul] *n* 1) чéстное слóво, обещáние; on ~ (взятый) на порýки, (освобождённый) услóвно; 2) *воен.* парóль.

parole II *v* освобождáть под чéстное слóво.

parolee [pə,rou'liː] *n* освобождённый под чéстное слóво.

paroxysm ['pærəksɪzəm] *n* пароксúзм, припáдок, прúступ.

parquet I ['pɑːkeɪ] *n* 1) паркéт; 2) *амер.* перéдние ряды́ партéра; 3) *attr* паркéтный.

parquet II *v* настилáть паркéт.

parquetry ['pɑːkɪtrɪ] *n* паркéт.

parricide ['pærɪsaɪd] *n* 1) отцеубúйца; 2) измéнник рóдины; 3) отцеубúйство; 4) измéна рóдине.

parrot I ['pærət] *n* попугáй.

parrot II *v* повторять как попугáй.

parrotry ['pærətrɪ] *n* бессмы́сленное повторéние чужúх слов.

parry I ['pærɪ] *n* парúрование, отражéние удáра.

parry II *v* отражáть, парúровать (*удар*).

parse [pɑːz] *v* дéлать граммати́ческий разбóр.

parsimonious [,pɑːsɪ'mounjəs] *a* 1) бережлúвый, экономный; 2) скупóй.

parsimony ['pɑːsɪmənɪ] *n* 1) бережлúвость, эконóмия; 2) скýпость.

parsing ['pɑːzɪŋ] *n* граммати́ческий разбóр.

parsley ['pɑːslɪ] *n* бот. петрýшка.

parsnip ['pɑːsnɪp] *n* бот. пастернáк.

parson ['pɑːsn] *n* свящéнник, пáстор.

part I [pɑːt] *n* 1) часть; a great ~ бóльшая часть; the better ~ дóбрая половúна, большинствó; in ~ чáстью; for the most ~ бóльшей чáстью; глáвным óбразом; обы́чно; ~ and parcel неотъéмлемая часть; ~ of speech грам. часть рéчи; 2) часть тéла; óрган; the ~s половы́е óрганы; 3) часть (*в книге*); вы́пуск; 4) учáстие, дóля; to bear (*или* to take) ~ in принимáть учáстие в чём-л.; 5) сторонá (*в споре и т. п.*); for my ~ что касáется меня, с моéй стороны́; on the ~ of от úмени; to take the ~ of стать на стóрону когó-л.; to take ~ with поддéрживать когó-л.; 6) обя́занность, дéло; I have done my ~ я сдéлал своё дéло; 7) роль; to act (*или* to play) a ~ а) игрáть роль; б) притворяться; pale ~ незначúтельный, не производящий никакóго впечатлéния; 8) запаснáя часть; 9) муз. пáртия, гóлос; 10) *pl* мéстность, край; in these ~s в этих краях; 11) *pl* уст. спосóбности; a man of ~s спосóбный человéк; ◊ to take in bad ~ обúдеться; to have neither ~ nor lot in не имéть ничегó óбщего с.

part II *v* 1) делúть(ся); разделять(ся); расступáться (*о толпе*); 2) расставáться, расходúться; 3) дéлать пробóр (*в волосах*); 4) уезжáть; 5) умирáть; □ to ~ from уйтú; расстáться с кем-л.; to ~ with a) расстáться; б) отпускáть (*прислугу*).

partake [pɑː'teɪk] *v* (*past* partook; *p. p.* partaken) 1) принимáть учáстие (*в чём-л.* — in, of); разделять (*с кем-л.* — with); 2) *разг.* отвéдать, вы́пить, съесть (*что-л.* — of); 3) воспóльзоваться (*гостеприимством; of*); 4) имéть харáктер (*чего-л.* — of); отзывáть (*чем-л.* — of).

partaken [pɑː'teɪkən] *p. p. см.* partake.

partaker [pɑː'teɪkə] *n* участник.

parted ['pɑːtɪd] *a* разделённый, разлучённый.

parterre [pɑː'tɛə] *n* 1) партéр; 2) *амер.* задние ряды партéра, амфитеáтр; 3) цветнúк.

partial ['pɑːʃəl] *a* 1) частúчный, непóлный; чáстный; 2) неравнодýшный (*к — to*); 3) пристрáстный.

partiality [ˌpɑːʃɪ'ælɪtɪ] *n* 1) пристрáстие; 2) склóнность.

participant [pɑː'tɪsɪpənt] *n* участник.

participate [pɑː'tɪsɪpeɪt] *v* 1) принимáть учáстие, учáствовать (*in*); 2) разделять (*рáдость, труд*; *in*).

participation [pɑːˌtɪsɪ'peɪʃən] *n* учáстие; соучáстие.

participator [pɑː'tɪsɪpeɪtə] *n* участник.

participial [ˌpɑːtɪ'sɪpɪəl] *a грам.* причáстный.

participle ['pɑːtsɪpl] *n грам.* причáстие; past ~ причáстие прошéдшего врéмени; present ~ причáстие настоящего врéмени.

particle ['pɑːtɪkl] *n* 1) частúца; ~ of dust пылúнка; 2) *грам.* неизменяемая частúца; прéфикс, сýффикс.

particoloured ['pɑːtɪˌkʌləd] *a* пёстрый, разноцвéтный.

particular I [pə'tɪkjulə] *n* 1) детáль, подрóбность; in ~ в чáстности; в осóбенности, осóбенно; to go into ~s вдавáться в подрóбности; 2) *pl* подрóбный отчёт; to give all the ~s давáть подрóбный отчёт; 3) *pl* обстоятельства.

particular II *a* 1) осóбый, осóбенный; 2) отдéльный, определённый; специфúческий, достопримечáтельный; 3) исключúтельный; блúзкий (*о друге*); 4) подрóбный, детáльный, обстоятельный; 5) требовательный, разбóрчивый (*в едé и т. п.*); привередливый; 6) тщáтельный; to be ~ in one's speech óчень следúть за своéй рéчью.

particularism [pə'tɪkjulərɪzəm] *n* 1) исключúтельная привéрженность (*к комý-л., чемý-л.*); 2) *полит.* сепаратúзм.

particularity [pəˌtɪkju'lærɪtɪ] *n* 1) осóбенность, подрóбность; спецúфика; 2) обстоятельность; тщáтельность.

particularize [pə'tɪkjuləraɪz] *v* вдавáться в подрóбности.

particularly [pə'tɪkjulərlɪ] *adv* 1) óчень; 2) осóбенно, в осóбенности; 3) подрóбно, в подрóбностях; 4) в чáстности.

parting I ['pɑːtɪŋ] *n* 1) расставáние, разлýка; отъéзд; *перен. уст.* смерть; 2) прощáние; at ~ на прощáние; 3) разделéние; разветвлéние (*дорóги*); 4) пробóр.

parting II *a* 1) прощáльный; 2) уходящий, умирáющий; 3) угасáющий, склоняющийся к вéчеру (*о дне*); 4) разделяющий; разветвляющийся, расходящийся (*о дорóге*).

partisan [ˌpɑːtɪ'zæn] *n* 1) сторóнник, привéрженец; 2) партизáн; 3) *attr* партизáнский.

partisanship [ˌpɑːtɪ'zænʃɪp] *n* привéрженность.

partition I [pɑː'tɪʃən] *n* 1) расчленéние; разделéние; 2) отделéние (*в ящике столá, в шкафý*); ячéйка; 3) перегорóдка, перебóрка; внýтренняя стенá (*в дóме*).

partition II *v* расчленять, разделять; □ to ~ off отгораживать перегорóдкой.

partitive I ['pɑːtɪtɪv] *n грам.* разделúтельное слóво.

partitive II *a грам.* разделúтельный, партитúвный.

partly ['pɑːtlɪ] *adv* 1) частúчно; 2) отчáсти.

partner I ['pɑːtnə] *n* 1) участник, -ица (*чего-л. — in, of*); товáрищ (*по дéлу, рабóте; with*); 2) пáйщик, компаньóн; senior ~ главá фúрмы; 3) муж, женá; 4) партнёр.

partner II *v* 1) быть партнёром; 2) дéлать (*чьим-л.*) партнёром.

partnership ['pɑːtnəʃɪp] *n* 1) учáстие; 2) товáрищество, компáния.

partook [pɑː'tuk] *past см.* partake.

part-owner ['pɑːtˌoʊnə] *n* совладéлец.

partridge ['pɑːtrɪdʒ] *n* куропáтка.

part-time ['pɑːt'taɪm] *adv*: to be employed ~ быть на почасовóй оплáте, не имéть пóлной рабóчей нагрýзки.

party¹ ['pɑːtɪ] *n* 1) пáртия; the Communist Party of the Soviet Union Коммунистúческая пáртия Совéтского Союза; 2) *attr* партúйный.

party² *n* 1) компáния; 2) приём гостéй, вéчер; вечерúнка; to have a ~ принимáть гостéй; dinner ~ гóсти, собрáвшиеся к обéду; dancing ~ вечерúнка с танцами; stag ~ холостяцкая вечерúнка; to give a ~ устрáивать вéчер, вечерúнку; 3) отряд, комáнда; 4) *юр.* сторонá; 5) (со)учáстник.

pasha ['pɑːʃə] *n* пашá.

pass I [pɑːs] *n* 1) прохóд; 2) ущéлье; 3) перевáл; 4) сдáча экзáмена на «удовлетворúтельно»; to get (*или* to take) a ~ получúть «удовлетворúтельно» (*на экзáмене*); 5) критúческое положéние; a pretty ~ сквéрный оборóт (*дел*); 6) прóпуск; *воен.* увольнúтельная (*запúска*); 7) (бесплáтный) билéт; контрамáрка; boarding ~ посáдочный талóн (*на самолёт*); 8) фарвáтер; 9) *карт.* пас; 10) выпад (*в фехтовáнии*); ◊ to bring to ~ совершáть, осуществлять; to come to ~ случáться, происходúть.

pass II *v* 1) проходúть, проезжáть, двúгаться, пролетáть (*мúмо чего-л. — by*; *чéрез что-л. — across, over*); 2) переходúть, пересекáть, переезжáть; переправлять(ся); перевáливать (*чéрез гóры*); 3) сдавáть (*экзáмен*); 4) стáвить отмéтку; пропускáть (*экзаменýющегося*); that won't ~! это не пройдёт!; 6) проводúть (*врéмя, лéто и т. п.*); 7) проходúть (*о врéмени*); 8) передавáть; 9) превращáться, переходúть (*из однóго состояния в другóе*); 10) происходúть, случáться; 11) превышáть, выходúть за предéлы; 12) принимáть (*закóн, резолюцию*); получáть одобрéние (*законодáтельного óргана*); 13) выносúть (*решéние, пригово́р; оп, *ирон*); 14) пускáть в обращéние; 15) быть в обращéнии; 16) уходúть, исчезáть, приходúть к концý; кончáться; умирáть; 17) пропускáть, не замечáть; 18) проводúть (*рукóй*); 19) *карт., спорт.* пасовáть; □ to ~ away а) скончáться, умерéть; б) исчéзнуть; to ~ by а) проходúть мúмо; б) оставлять без внимáния; to ~ for считáться, слыть кем-л.; to ~ into превращáться, переходúть; дéлаться; to ~ off а) постепéнно проходúть (*об ощущéниях*); б) хорошó пройтú (*о мероприятиях, событиях*); в) пронестúсь, пройтú (*о дождé, бýре*); г) сбывáть, подсóвывать (*ирон*); д) выдавáть (*себя, когó-л. за — for, as*); to ~ on проходúть *или* передавáть дáльше; переходúть (*к другóму* *вопросу*); ~ on please! проходи́те!, не остана́вливайтесь!; to ~ **out** a) успе́шно пройти́ (*курс обучения*); б) сбыть, прода́ть (*товар*); в) *амер. сленг* потеря́ть созна́ние; «окочу́риться», умере́ть; to ~ **over** a) не замеча́ть, не обраща́ть внима́ния; б) умере́ть, сконча́ться; в) *хим.* дистилли́роваться; to ~ **round** a) передава́ть друг дру́гу; б) обма́тывать; обводи́ть; to ~ **through** a) пережива́ть (*время, период*); б) просе́ивать, процежи́вать; в) продева́ть; ◊ to ~ **by the name of** быть изве́стным под и́менем; to ~ **in one's checks** *сленг* умере́ть.

passable ['pɑːsəbl] *a* 1) проходи́мый; прое́зжий; 2) сно́сный, удовлетвори́тельный.

passably ['pɑːsəblɪ] *adv* доста́точно, поря́дочно.

passage I ['pæsɪdʒ] *n* 1) прохо́д, прое́зд; 2) перее́зд, рейс, пое́здка (*по мо́рю*); 3) пла́та за прое́зд; to take one's ~ купи́ть биле́т на парохо́д; 4) перелёт (*птиц*); 5) коридо́р, пасса́ж; доро́га, путь; кана́л; 6) перева́л; перепра́ва; 7) до́ступ, вход, вы́ход; пра́во прохо́да; 8) ход, тече́ние (*событий, времени*); 9) происше́ствие; 10) перехо́д, превраще́ние; 11) утвержде́ние (*зако́на*); 12) *pl* столкнове́ние; сты́чка; to have stormy ~s with име́ть с кем-л. кру́пный разгово́р; 13) отры́вок (*из книги и т. п.*).

passage II *v* соверша́ть перее́зд; пересека́ть (*море, канал и т. п.*).

passage-way ['pæsɪdʒweɪ] *n* прохо́д; коридо́р; пасса́ж.

passbook ['pɑːsbuk] *n* 1) ба́нковская кни́жка; 2) *амер.* забо́рная кни́жка.

passenger ['pæsɪndʒə] *n* 1) пассажи́р; 2) пу́тник; 3) *attr* пассажи́рский.

passer-by ['pɑːsə'baɪ] *n* (*pl* passers-by ['pɑːsəz'baɪ]) прохо́жий.

passing I ['pɑːsɪŋ] *n*: in ~ мимохо́дом.

passing II *a* 1) (ско́ро)преходя́щий; мимолётный; 2) бе́глый, случа́йный.

passing III *adv уст.* чрезвыча́йно.

passingly ['pɑːsɪŋlɪ] *adv* мимохо́дом, кста́ти.

passion ['pæʃən] *n* 1) си́льное чу́вство (*радости, горя и т. п.*); 2) страсть, пыл; 3) увлече́ние, любо́вь (*for*); 4) вспы́шка гне́ва, при́ступ; to fly into a ~ разозли́ться, прийти́ в я́рость; to be in a ~ быть в гне́ве; серди́ться.

passionate ['pæʃənɪt] *a* 1) горя́чий, пы́лкий; 2) стра́стный, влюблённый; 3) вспы́льчивый, невы́держанный.

passion-flower ['pæʃən,flauə] *n бот.* страстоцве́т.

passionless ['pæʃənlɪs] *a* бесстра́стный; невозмути́мый, холо́дный.

passive I ['pæsɪv] *n грам.* страда́тельный зало́г.

passive II *a* 1) пасси́вный, ине́ртный; безде́ятельный; 2) поко́рный; 3) *грам.* страда́тельный.

passkey ['pɑːskiː] *n* отмы́чка.

passport ['pɑːspɔːt] *n* 1) па́спорт; 2) ли́чные ка́чества.

password ['pɑːswɜːd] *n* паро́ль.

past I [pɑːst] *n* 1) про́шлое; the shadowy ~, the dim and distant ~ далёкое про́шлое; 2) *грам.* фо́рма проше́дшего вре́мени.

past II *a* 1) про́шлый, мину́вший; исте́кший; бы́вший; 2) *грам.* проше́дший.

past III *adv* ми́мо.

past IV *prep* 1) за, по́сле; he is ~ sixty ему́ за шестьдеся́т; ~ noon по́сле полу́дня; 2) за, ми́мо;

---

the house is ~ the library дом нахо́дится за библиоте́кой; 3) сверх, свы́ше.

paste I [peɪst] *n* 1) те́сто (*сдо́бное*); 2) пастила́, халва́; 3) па́ста, масти́ка; 4) клей, кле́йстер; 5) стекло́видная ма́сса.

paste II *v* скле́ивать; накле́ивать; обкле́ивать (*with*); □ to ~ **up** раскле́ивать.

pasteboard ['peɪstbɔːd] *n* 1) карто́н; 2) *сленг* визи́тная ка́рточка; 3) *сленг* железнодоро́жный биле́т; 4) *attr* карто́нный; 5) *attr* непро́чный.

pastel [pæs'tel] *n* 1) пасте́ль; 2) си́няя кра́ска (*из вайды*).

pastime ['pɑːstaɪm] *n* прия́тное времяпрепровожде́ние, развлече́ние; игра́.

pastiness ['peɪstɪnɪs] *n* кле́йкость, ли́пкость.

pastor ['pɑːstə] *n* па́стор.

pastoral I ['pɑːstərəl] *n* пастора́ль.

pastoral II *a* 1) пасту́шеский; 2) пастора́льный.

pastorate ['pɑːstərɪt] *n* 1) па́сторство; 2) *собир.* па́сторы.

pastry ['peɪstrɪ] *n* конди́терские изде́лия (*пирог, пиро́жное, торт*).

pasturage ['pɑːstjurɪdʒ] *n* 1) па́стбище; 2) подно́жный корм; 3) пастьба́.

pasture I ['pɑːstʃə] *n* 1) подно́жный корм; 2) па́стбище, вы́гон.

pasture II *v* пасти́(сь).

pasty[a] ['peɪstɪ] *a* 1) тестообра́зный; 2) одутлова́тый, бле́дный (*тж.* ~-faced).

pasty[b] ['pæstɪ] *n* 1) паште́т; 2) пиро́г.

pat[1] I [pæt] *n* 1) похло́пывание; 2) хло́панье, шлёпанье; 3) кусо́к (*сбитого масла*).

pat[1] II *v* 1) слегка́ похло́пывать; погла́живать; 2) пригла́живать; *амер.* слегка́ прито́пывать.

pat[2] *adv* 1) как раз; то́чка в то́чку; to come ~ подоспе́ть во́время; 2): to stand ~ держа́ться своего́ реше́ния; вести́ свою́ ли́нию.

patch I [pætʃ] *n* 1) запла́та; 2) пла́стырь; 3) повя́зка (*на глазу*); 4) му́шка (*на лице*); 5) лоску́т; обры́вок; 6) кусо́к, небольшо́й уча́сток (*земли*); 7) пятно́; ◊ not a ~ on ничто́ в сравне́нии.

patch II *v* лата́ть; ста́вить запла́ты; □ to ~ **up** a) чини́ть на ско́рую ру́ку; заде́лывать; б) ула́живать (*ссору*).

patchwork ['pætʃwɜːk] *n* 1) одея́ло, покры́шка и т. п. из разноцве́тных лоскуто́в; 2) мешани́на; 3) *attr* лоску́тный; пёстрый.

patchy ['pætʃɪ] *a* 1) пятни́стый; 2) разношёрстный; неодноро́дный; 3) случа́йный, обры́вочный (*о знаниях*).

pate [peɪt] *n разг.* 1) голова́, башка́; 2) маку́шка, те́мя; 3) *шутл.* ум.

patency ['peɪtənsɪ] *n* я́вность, очеви́дность.

patent I ['peɪtənt] *n* 1) пате́нт; дипло́м; 2) знак, печа́ть (*ума, гениальности*).

patent II *a* 1) откры́тый; очеви́дный, я́вный; 2) име́ющий пате́нт, дипло́м; 3) патенто́ванный; 4) лакиро́ванный (*об обуви, коже*); 5) *разг.* оригина́льный, остроу́мный.

patent III *v* получа́ть, выдава́ть пате́нт.

patentee [,peɪtən'tiː] *n* владе́лец пате́нта.

patent-leather ['peɪtənt'leðə] *a* лакиро́ванный.

paternal [pə'tɜːnl] *a* 1) отцо́вский; 2) оте́ческий; 3) ро́дственный по отцу́.

paternity [pə'tɜːnɪtɪ] *n* 1) отцо́вство; 2) происхожде́ние по отцу́; 3) а́вторство.

path [pɑːθ] *n* 1) тропа́, тропи́нка, доро́жка; 2) бегова́я доро́жка; трек; 3) путь; to cross smb.'s ~ стать кому́-л. поперёк доро́ги; 4) ли́ния де́йствия *или* поведе́ния.

pathetic [pəˈθetik] *a* патети́ческий, тро́гательный.

pathetics [pəˈθetiks] *n* патэ́тика.

pathfinder [ˈpɑːθˌfaində] *n* следопы́т.

pathless [ˈpɑːθlis] *a* 1) бездоро́жный; 2) непрото́рённый; неиссле́дованный.

pathos [ˈpeiθɔs] *n* па́фос.

pathway [ˈpɑːθwei] *n* 1) тропа́, тропи́нка; доро́жка; путь; 2) мостки́.

patience [ˈpeiʃəns] *n* 1) терпе́ние; I am out of (*или* I have no) ~ with him я потеря́л вся́кое терпе́ние с ним; 2) насто́йчивость; 3) пасья́нс; to play ~ раскла́дывать пасья́нс.

patient I [ˈpeiʃənt] *n* пацие́нт, больно́й.

patient II *a* 1) терпели́вый; 2) упо́рный; насто́йчивый; 3) допуска́ющий (*of*).

patio [ˈpætiou] *n* вну́тренний дво́рик.

patriarch [ˈpeitriɑːk] *n* 1) глава́ ро́да, общи́ны, семьи́; 2) патриа́рх; 3) родонача́льник; основа́тель.

patriarchal [ˌpeitriˈɑːkəl] *a* 1) патриарха́льный; 2) патриа́рший.

patriarchy [ˈpeitriɑːki] *n* 1) патриарха́т; 2) патриа́рхия.

patrician I [pəˈtriʃən] *n* 1) *ист.* патри́ций; 2) аристокра́т.

patrician II *a* 1) патрициа́нский; 2) аристократи́ческий.

patricide [ˈpætrisaid] *n* 1) отцеуби́йство; 2) отцеуби́йца.

patrimony [ˈpætriməni] *n* 1) родово́е поме́стье; 2) насле́дство.

patriot [ˈpeitriət] *n* патрио́т.

patriotic [ˌpætriˈɔtik] *a* патриоти́ческий.

patriotism [ˈpætriətizəm] *n* патриоти́зм; Soviet ~ сове́тский патриоти́зм.

patrol I [pəˈtroul] *n* 1) патрули́рование; 2) патру́ль; карау́л; дозо́р, разъе́зд; on ~ в дозо́ре; 3) *attr* патру́льный, дозо́рный.

patrol II *u* патрули́ровать; обходи́ть дозо́ром.

patrolman [pəˈtroulmæn] *n амер.* 1) полице́йский; 2) патру́льный, дозо́рный.

patron [ˈpeitrən] *n* 1) покрови́тель, патро́н; шеф; 2) постоя́нный покупа́тель, клие́нт; 3) засту́пник.

patronage [ˈpætrənidʒ] *n* 1) покрови́тельство, засту́пничество; 2) ше́фство; 3) пра́во назначе́ния на до́лжность; 4) постоя́нные покупа́тели, клиенту́ра; 5) фина́нсовая подде́ржка (*частных учрежде́ний, предприя́тий*); 6) покрови́тельственный вид; снисходи́тельное отноше́ние.

patronize [ˈpætrənaiz] *v* 1) покрови́тельствовать, опека́ть; 2) быть постоя́нным покупа́телем, клие́нтом; 3) ока́зывать фина́нсовую подде́ржку (*ча́стным учрежде́ниям, предприя́тиям*); 4) относи́ться покрови́тельственно, снисходи́тельно.

patronymic [ˌpætrəˈnimik] *n* 1) о́тчество; 2) родово́е и́мя; 3) фами́лия.

patten [ˈpætn] *n* деревя́нный башма́к.

patter[1] I [ˈpætə] *n* 1) стук (*дождя́, ка́пель*); 2) топота́нье.

patter[1] II *v* 1) бараба́нить, стуча́ть (*о дожде́, ка́плях*); 2) топота́ть (*о ребёнке*).

patter[2] I *n* 1) жарго́н, арго́; 2) бы́страя речь, скорогово́рка.

patter[2] II *v* говори́ть скорогово́ркой; тарато́рить.

pattern I [ˈpætən] *n* 1) образе́ц, обра́зчик; 2) моде́ль; 3) вы́кройка; to take a ~ of снять вы́кройку (*с чего́-л.*); 4) рису́нок, узо́р (*на мате́рии и т. п.*); 5) *амер.* отре́з (*на пла́тье*); 6) *тех.* фо́рма; шабло́н; 7) *attr* приме́рный, образцо́вый.

pattern II *v* 1) украша́ть узо́ром; 2) де́лать по образцу́, копи́ровать (*after, on, upon*).

patty [ˈpæti] *n* пирожо́к; лепёшечка.

paucity [ˈpɔːsiti] *n* малочи́сленность, ма́лое коли́чество.

paunch I [pɔːntʃ] *n* 1) живо́т, брю́хо; 2) пе́рвый желу́док (*у жва́чных*).

paunch II *v* потроши́ть.

paunchy [ˈpɔːntʃi] *a* то́лстый, с брюшко́м.

pauper [ˈpɔːpə] *n* бедня́к.

pauperism [ˈpɔːpərizəm] *n* кра́йняя бе́дность, нищета́; паупери́зм.

pauperize [ˈpɔːpəraiz] *v* доводи́ть до нищеты́.

pause I [pɔːz] *n* 1) остано́вка, па́уза; переды́шка; переры́в; 2) замеша́тельство; to give ~ to приводи́ть в замеша́тельство; at ~ в нереши́тельности; 3) *лит.* цезу́ра; 4) *муз.* ферма́та.

pause II *v* 1) остана́вливаться, де́лать па́узу, переды́шку; to ~ upon smth. задержа́ться на чём-л.; 2) находи́ться в нереши́тельности, ме́длить.

pave [peiv] *v* 1) мости́ть; настила́ть (*пол*); 2) устила́ть (*цвета́ми и т. п.*).

pavement [ˈpeivmənt] *n* 1) тротуа́р; crazy ~ садо́вая доро́жка (*вы́ложенная пли́тками непра́вильной фо́рмы*); 2) моза́ичный пол; 3) *амер.* мостова́я; 4) материа́л для моще́ния.

pavilion I [pəˈviljən] *n* 1) павильо́н; 2) пала́тка, шатёр; 3) госпита́льный бара́к.

pavilion II *v* 1) укрыва́ть(ся) (*в павильо́не, пала́тке и т. п.*); 2) стро́ить павильо́ны; разбива́ть пала́тки.

paving [ˈpeiviŋ] *n* 1) мостова́я; 2) материа́л для моще́ния.

paw I [pɔː] *n* 1) ла́па; 2) *разг.* рука́.

paw II *v* 1) тро́гать, скрести́ ла́пой; 2) бить копы́том; 3) *разг.* хвата́ть; обла́пить (*тж.* to ~ over).

pawn[1] [pɔːn] *n шахм.* пе́шка (*тж. перен. о челове́ке*).

pawn[2] I *n* зало́г, закла́д; at ~, in ~ в закла́де.

pawn[2] II *v* 1) закла́дывать, отдава́ть в зало́г; 2) руча́ться (*че́стью и т. п.*).

pawnbroker [ˈpɔːnˌbroukə] *n* хозя́ин ломба́рда; ростовщи́к.

pawnee [pɔːˈniː] *n* закла́дчик.

pawnshop [ˈpɔːnʃɔp] *n* ломба́рд.

pax [pæks] *int шк.* чур-чура́!

pay[1] I [pei] *n* 1) зарпла́та, жа́лованье; окла́д; full ~ по́лная ста́вка; half ~ полста́вки; take-home ~ *амер.* зарпла́та за вы́четом нало́гов и т. п.; in the ~ of на жа́лованье у кого́-л.; на́нятый кем-л.; 2) посо́бие; dismissal ~, severancy ~ выходно́е посо́бие; strike ~ посо́бие, выдава́емое профсою́зом бастую́щим; 3) пла́та, вы́плата, упла́та; back ~ *амер.* заде́ржка в вы́плате зарпла́ты; 4) отпла́та, возме́здие; 5) *attr* пла́тный; платёжный.

pay[1] II *v* (*past, p. p.* paid) 1) плати́ть; 2) вознагражда́ть, опла́чивать; 3) выпла́чивать (*долг, су́мму, вы́куп*); 4) окупа́ться, быть вы́годным; приноси́ть дохо́д (*о це́нных бума́гах*); 5) возмеща́ть;

who breaks ~s виновный расплачивается; 6) обращать (внимание; на — to); оказывать (почтение); говорить (комплименты); 7) наносить (визит), посещать; □ to ~ **back** а) выплачивать, возвращать (деньги); б) отплачивать; to ~ smb. back in his own coin отплатить той же монетой; не остаться в долгу; to ~ **down** платить наличными; to ~ **for** а) оплачивать; б) поплатиться; to ~ **in** вносить деньги на свой текущий счёт; to ~ **off** а) расплачиваться сполна; б) увольнять (рабочих, матросов); в) отплатить; to ~ **out** а) выплачивать; б) smb. out отплатить кому-л.; в) мор. травить (канат); to ~ **up** выплачивать сполна; ◊ to ~ for a dead horse платить впустую; to ~ for one's whistle расплачиваться за свою прихоть.

pay² v мор. смолить.

payable ['peɪəbl] a 1) подлежащий уплате; 2) выгодный; доходный.

paybox ['peɪbɔks] n амер. (театральная) касса.

pay-day ['peɪdeɪ] n день выдачи жалованья; платёжный день.

payee [peɪ'iː] n получатель (денег); предъявитель чека, векселя.

payer ['peɪə] n плательщик.

paying ['peɪɪŋ] a выгодный, доходный.

payload ['peɪloud] n полезный груз.

paymaster ['peɪˌmɑːstə] n кассир, казначей; ~ general главный казначей.

payment ['peɪmənt] n 1) платёж, уплата; cash ~ наличный расчёт; ~ in kind платёж натурой; 2) вознаграждение; возмездие.

pay-off ['peɪˌɔːf] n амер. 1) выплата жалованья; 2) время выплаты жалованья; 3) разг. развязка (событий); финал.

pay-office ['peɪˌɔfɪs] n касса.

pay-out ['peɪˌaut] n выплата.

pay-roll ['peɪroul] амер. 1) см. pay-sheet; 2): inflated ~ раздутые штаты.

pay-sheet ['peɪʃiːt] n платёжная ведомость.

pea [piː] n 1) горох; split ~s лущёный горох; sweet ~ душистый горошек; 2) горошина; as like as two ~s ≅ похожи как две капли воды; 3) attr гороховый.

peace [piːs] n 1) мир; at ~ в мире (с кем-л. — with); universal ~ всеобщий мир, мир во всём мире; dependable (или lasting, durable) ~ прочный мир; to ensure ~ обеспечивать мир; to preserve ~ отстаивать мир, сохранять мир; to struggle for ~ бороться за мир; to make ~ а) заключать мир; б) помириться; to make one's ~ with помириться с; ~ with honour почётный мир; 2) спокойствие, порядок; ~! тише!, замолчите!; to break the ~ поднимать скандал, ссору; нарушать порядок; to keep the ~ сохранять спокойствие, не нарушать порядка; не поднимать скандала; leave me in ~! оставь(те) меня в покое!; ~ of mind спокойствие духа; 3) тишина; покой; to hold one's ~ (про)молчать; 4) attr мирный.

peaceable ['piːsəbl] a мирный, миролюбивый.

peaceful ['piːsful] a мирный, спокойный.

peace-lover ['piːsˌlʌvə] n сторонник мира.

peace-loving ['piːsˌlʌvɪŋ] a миролюбивый.

peacemaker ['piːsˌmeɪkə] n миротворец.

peace-pipe ['piːspaɪp] n трубка мира.

peace-time ['piːstaɪm] n 1) мирное время; 2) attr

относящийся к мирному времени; мирного времени.

peach¹ [piːtʃ] n 1) персик; 2) персиковое дерево; 3) сленг «первый сорт»; красавица.

peach² v сленг доносить (на сообщника; against, on, upon).

peach-coloured ['piːtʃˌkʌləd] a персикового цвета.

peach-tree ['piːtʃtriː] n персиковое дерево.

peachy ['piːtʃɪ] a 1) похожий на персик; 2) разг. прелестный, замечательный.

peacock I ['piːkɔk] n 1) павлин; 2) attr павлиний.

peacock II v важничать, чваниться; задаваться.

peacockery ['piːkɔkərɪ] n чванство; позёрство.

peafowl ['piːfaul] n павлин, пава.

peahen ['piː'hen] n пава.

pea-jacket ['piːˌdʒækɪt] n 1) мор. бушлат; 2) тужурка.

peak¹ [piːk] n 1) пик, остроконечная вершина; 2) высшая точка; максимум (кривой); 3) козырёк (фуражки, кепки); 4) клинышек (бороды).

peak² v слабеть, чахнуть; ~ and pine чахнуть и томиться.

peaked¹ [piːkt] a остроконечный.

peaked² a осунувшийся; заострившийся (о чертах лица).

peal I [piːl] n 1) звон колоколов, трезвон; 2) подбор колоколов; 3) удар, раскат (грома); взрыв (смеха); грохот (орудий).

peal II v 1) раздаваться; греметь; трезвонить; 2) возвещать трезвоном (тж. to ~ out).

peanut ['piːnʌt] n земляной орех, арахис.

pear [peə] n 1) груша; 2) грушевое дерево; 3) attr грушевый.

pearl I [pəːl] n 1) жемчуг; жемчужина, перл; Venetian ~ искусственный жемчуг; 2) перламутр; 3) капля росы; слеза; 4) крупинка, зёрнышко; 5) attr жемчужный; перламутровый; 6) attr перловый (о крупе); ◊ to cast (или to throw) ~s before swine посл. метать бисер перед свиньями.

pearl II v 1) украшать жемчугом; 2) добывать жемчуг; 3) выступать каплями; ~ed with dew покрытый каплями росы.

pearl-barley ['pəːl'bɑːlɪ] n перловая крупа.

pearl-diver ['pəːlˌdaɪvə] n искатель, ловец жемчуга.

pearly ['pəːlɪ] a 1) жемчужный; 2) усыпанный жемчугом.

peart [pɪət] a диал. 1) оживлённый, весёлый; 2) ловкий.

pear-tree ['peətriː] n грушевое дерево.

peasant ['pezənt] n 1) крестьянин; medium ~ крестьянин-середняк; poor ~ крестьянин-бедняк; 2) attr крестьянский; сельский.

peasantry ['pezəntrɪ] n крестьянство.

pease [piːz] n 1) собир. горох; 2) attr гороховый.

pease-pudding ['piːzˌpudɪŋ] n гороховое пюре.

peat [piːt] n 1) торф; 2) attr торфяной.

peatbog ['piːtbɔg] n торфяник, торфяное болото.

peatery ['piːtərɪ] n торфяные разработки.

peatmoss ['piːt'mɔs] n торфяной мох.

peaty ['piːtɪ] a торфяной.

pebble I ['pebl] n 1) голыш, галька; 2) горный хрусталь; 3) линза (из горного хрусталя).

pebble II v посыпать галькой.

pebbly ['peblɪ] a покрытый галькой.

peccable ['pekəbl] a грешный, греховный.

peccant ['pekənt] *a* 1) грехо́вный; 2) боле́зненный; 3) детони́рующий (*о струнах*).

peck[1] [pek] *n* 1) че́тверть бу́шеля (*мера сыпучих тел*); 2) мно́жество, ма́сса; a ~ of troubles ма́сса неприя́тностей.

peck[2] I *n* 1) клево́к; 2) *шутл.* лёгкий поцелу́й; 3) *сленг* пи́ща.

peck[2] II *v* 1) клева́ть; 2) долби́ть, прода́лбливать; 3) *разг.* есть понемно́гу, отщи́пывать (*at*).

pecker ['pekə] *n* 1) *сленг* нос; клюв; keep your ~ up! крепи́сь!, не унывай!; 2) кирка́.

peckish ['pekıʃ] *a разг.* голо́дный; to feel ~ проголода́ться.

pectoral ['pektərəl] *a* 1) грудно́й (*тж. о голосе*); 2) нагру́дный.

peculiar I [pɪ'kjuːljə] *n* 1) индивидуа́льное сво́йство, осо́бенность; 2) ли́чная со́бственность.

peculiar II *a* 1) характе́рный, осо́бенный; 2) ли́чный, со́бственный; индивидуа́льный; 3) необы́чный, стра́нный, своеобра́зный.

peculiarity [pɪ,kjuːlɪ'ærɪtɪ] *n* 1) осо́бенность; 2) ли́чное ка́чество, сво́йство; 3) характе́рная черта́; 4) стра́нность; своеобра́зие.

pecuniary [pɪ'kjuːnjərɪ] *a* де́нежный.

pedagogic(al) [,pedə'gɔdʒɪk(əl)] *a* педагоги́ческий.

pedagogics [,pedə'gɔdʒɪks] *n* педаго́гика.

pedagogue ['pedəgɔg] *n* 1) учи́тель; педаго́г; 2) педа́нт.

pedagogy ['pedəgɔgɪ] *n* педаго́гика.

pedal I ['pedl] *n* педа́ль; ножно́й рыча́г.

pedal II *a* 1) педа́льный; 2) *анат., зоол.* ножно́й.

pedal III *v* 1) нажима́ть педа́ль; рабо́тать педа́лями; 2) *разг.* е́хать на велосипе́де.

pedant ['pedənt] *n* 1) педа́нт; 2) доктринёр.

pedantic [pɪ'dæntɪk] *a* педанти́чный.

pedantry ['pedəntrɪ] *n* педанти́зм.

peddle ['pedl] *v* 1) торгова́ть ме́лким това́ром, торгова́ть вразно́с; 2) разме́ниваться на ме́лочи; занима́ться мелоча́ми.

peddler ['pedlə] *см.* pedlar.

peddlery ['pedlərɪ] *см.* pedlary.

peddling ['pedlɪŋ] *a* ме́лкий, ме́лочный, пустяко́вый.

pedestal ['pedɪstl] *n* 1) пьедеста́л; подста́вка; 2) ба́за, основа́ние.

pedestrian I [pɪ'destrɪən] *n* пешехо́д.

pedestrian II *a* 1) пе́ший, пешехо́дный; 2) ску́чный.

pedigree ['pedɪgriː] *n* 1) родосло́вная; 2) происхожде́ние; 3) этимоло́гия (*слова*); 4) *attr* племенно́й.

pedigreed ['pedɪgriːd] *a* поро́дистый.

pediment ['pedɪmənt] *n архит.* фронто́н.

pedlar ['pedlə] *n* разно́счик, коробе́йник.

pedlary ['pedlərɪ] *n* 1) торго́вля вразно́с; 2) ме́лкий това́р.

peek I [piːk] *n* взгляд укра́дкой; бы́стрый взгляд.

peek II *v* 1) загля́дывать (*тж.* to ~ in); 2) выгля́дывать (*тж.* to ~ out).

peel[1] I [piːl] *n* кожура́, шелуха́; ко́жица, ко́рка; candied ~ цука́т.

peel[1] II *v* 1) снима́ть кожуру́, ко́жицу; чи́стить (*фрукты, овощи*); 2) лупи́ться, сходи́ть, шелуши́ться (*о коже; тж.* to ~ off).

peel[2] *n* пе́карская лопа́та.

peeler[1] ['piːlə] *n:* potato ~ картофелечи́стка.

peeler[2] *n сленг* полице́йский.

peeling ['piːlɪŋ] *n* кожура́, очи́стки.

peep[1] I [piːp] *n* 1) взгляд укра́дкой; to get a ~ of уви́деть; to have (*или* to take) a ~ at взгляну́ть на; 2) про́блеск; the ~ of day, the ~ of dawn рассве́т; 3) щель, просве́т.

peep[1] II *v* 1) смотре́ть сквозь ма́ленькое отве́рстие (*through*); подгля́дывать; 2) бро́сить бе́глый взгляд (*на что-л. —* at); 3) выгля́дывать, прогля́дывать (*о солнце*); 4) проявля́ться (*о качестве; часто* to ~ out); □ to ~ **into** загля́дывать, заходи́ть (*куда-л.*); to ~ **out** выгля́дывать.

peep[2] I *n* писк; чири́канье.

peep[2] II *v* 1) пища́ть; чири́кать; 2) говори́ть то́неньким голоско́м.

peeper[1] ['piːpə] *n* 1) согляда́тай, шпик; 2) *сленг* глаз.

peeper[2] *n* пискý́н.

peep-hole ['piːphoul] *n* смотрово́е отве́рстие; глазо́к.

peer[1] [pɪə] *v* 1) всма́триваться, вгля́дываться (*at, into, through*); 2) пока́зываться, выгля́дывать (*о солнце*).

peer[2] I *n* ро́вня; without ~ несравне́нный.

peer[2] II *v* равня́ться (*с кем-л.*), быть ра́вным (*кому-л.*).

peer[3] I *n* пэр, лорд; член пала́ты ло́рдов.

peer[3] II *v* де́лать пэ́ром.

peerage ['pɪərɪdʒ] *n* 1) сосло́вие пэ́ров, знать; 2) зва́ние пэ́ра; 3) родосло́вная кни́га пэ́ров.

peeve I [piːv] *n* раздража́ющее обстоя́тельство; my pet ~ «люби́мая мозо́ль», больно́е ме́сто.

peeve II *v* раздража́ть.

peeved [piːvd] *a разг.* раздражённый.

peevish ['piːvɪʃ] *a* 1) ворчли́вый, сварли́вый; раздражи́тельный; 2) капри́зный, неужи́вчивый.

peg I [peg] *n* 1) ко́лышек; деревя́нный гвоздь; 2) ве́шалка; крючо́к (*вешалки*); off the ~ гото́вый (*о платье*); 3) коло́к (*муз. инструме́нта*); 4) ви́ски или конья́к с со́довой; 5) *разг.* деревя́нная нога́; 6) *тех.* вту́лка, заты́чка; ◊ a round ~ in a square hole челове́к, находя́щийся не на своём ме́сте; не подходя́щий к да́нной рабо́те челове́к; a ~ to hang a thing on a) причи́на; по́вод (*для оправда́ния и т. п.*); б) те́ма (*для разгово́ра*); to come down a ~ сба́вить тон; to take smb. down a ~ or two осади́ть, сбить спесь с кого́-л.

peg II *v* 1) забива́ть ко́лышек, деревя́нный гвоздь (*обыкн.* to ~ down, in, out); 2) держа́ть це́ну на одно́м у́ровне; 3) *разг.* це́литься; швыря́ть, броса́ть (*тж.* to ~ at); to ~ **away** упо́рно рабо́тать, корпе́ть (*над чем-л. —* at); добива́ться; to ~ **down** a) закрепля́ть ко́лышками; б) свя́зывать; to ~ **out** a) размеча́ть ко́лышками (*участок земли*); б) *разг.* умере́ть.

pegging ['pegɪŋ] *n* 1) закрепле́ние ко́лышками; 2) стабилиза́ция (*цен*).

peg-top ['pegtɔp] *n* юла́, волчо́к.

pejorative ['piːdʒərətɪv] *a* уничижи́тельный.

pelargonium [,pelə'gounjəm] *n* гера́нь; пеларго́ния.

pelerine ['peləriːn] *n* пелери́на.

pelf [pelf] *n презр.* де́ньги, «презре́нный мета́лл»; бога́тство.

pelican ['pelɪkən] *n* пелика́н.

pelisse [pe'liːs] *n* 1) длинная дамская накидка на меху; 2) детское пальто.

pellet ['pelɪt] *n* 1) шарик, катышек (*из бумаги, хлеба*); 2) пуля; дробинка; 3) пилюля.

pell-mell I ['pel'mel] *n* беспорядок; неразбериха; мешанина.

pell-mell II *a* беспорядочный.

pell-mell III *adv* в беспорядке, кое-как; вперемешку.

pellucid [pe'ljuːsɪd] *a* 1) прозрачный; 2) ясный.

pelt[1] I [pelt] *n* 1) сильный удар; попадание; 2): at full ~ полным ходом.

pelt[1] II *v* 1) забрасывать (*камнями и т. п.*); *перен.* обрушиваться на кого-л.; 2) лить (*о дожде; тж.* to ~ down); 3) *амер.* спешить.

pelt[2] *n* шкура; кожа.

pelting ['peltɪŋ] *a* проливной.

peltry ['peltrɪ] *n* пушной товар, пушнина.

pelvis ['pelvɪs] *n* (*pl* pelves ['pelviːz]) *анат.* таз.

pen[1] I [pen] *n* 1) перо (*писчее*); ручка с пером; рейсфедер (*чертёжный*); ~ and ink письменные принадлежности; to put ~ to paper взяться за перо; начать писать; 2) литературный труд; стиль; to live by one's ~ жить литературным трудом; fluent ~ лёгкий, бойкий стиль; to wield a (skilful) ~ владеть пером, обладать литературным талантом; 3) писатель; the best ~s of the day лучшие писатели современности.

pen[1] II *v* 1) писать (*пером*); 2) сочинять, составлять.

pen[2] I *n* 1) загон (*для скота, птицы*); 2) помещение для арестованных (*при полицейском участке*).

pen[2] II *v* 1) загонять (*скот*); 2) держать в закрытом месте (*часто* to ~ up, to ~ in).

penal ['piːnl] *a* 1) уголовный; 2) каторжный (*о работах*); 3) подлежащий наказанию, наказуемый (*о преступлении*).

penalize ['piːnəlaɪz] *v* 1) наказывать; штрафовать (*тж. спорт.*); 2) ставить в невыгодное положение.

penalty ['penltɪ] *n* 1) наказание; взыскание; on ~, under ~ под страхом наказания; to pay the ~ отбывать наказание; 2) *спорт.* штраф.

pen-and-ink ['penənd'ɪŋk] *a* сделанный пером (*о рисунке*); написанный пером.

pence [pens] *n pl см.* penny 1); school ~ еженедельный взнос за обучение в начальной школе; ◊ take care of the ~ and the pounds will take care of themselves *посл.* береги пенсы, а фунты сами себя сберегут; ≅ копейка рубль бережёт.

penchant ['рaːŋʃaŋ] *n* склонность (к кому-л., к чему-л. — for); a slight ~ небольшое увлечение.

pencil I ['pensl] *n* 1) карандаш; lead (indelible) ~ простой (химический) карандаш; in ~ написанный карандашом, в карандаше; 2) кисть (*художника*); *перен.* манера писать; 3) *физ.* узкий параллельный пучок лучей.

pencil II *v* 1) писать карандашом; рисовать; 2) раскрашивать карандашами; тушевать.

pencil-case ['penslkeɪs] *n* пенал.

pencraft ['penkrɑːft] *n* 1) искусство письма; 2) литературный стиль.

pendant I ['pendənt] *n* 1) брелок, подвеска, кулон; 2) пара (*к какому-л. предмету*); 3) *мор.* вымпел.

pendant II *a см.* pendent II.

pendent I ['pendənt] *n см.* pendant 1.

pendent II *a* 1) висящий, висячий; свисающий; 2) ожидающий решения, нерешённый; 3) *грам.* незаконченный (*о предложении*).

pending I ['pendɪŋ] *a* 1) нерешённый, ожидаемый; 2) висящий; 3) неминуемый.

pending II *prep* 1) в продолжение, в течение; 2) до, вплоть до; в ожидании.

pendulous ['pendjuləs] *a* 1) висящий; подвешенный; 2) качающийся.

pendulum ['pendjuləm] *n* 1) маятник; 2) неустойчивый человек.

penetrable ['penɪtrəbl] *a* проницаемый.

penetrate ['penɪtreɪt] *v* 1) проникать; 2) проходить, входить (*into, through, to*); 3) пронизывать, пропитывать (*чем-л.* — with); 4) глубоко трогать; 5) постигать, понимать; вникать.

penetrating ['penɪtreɪtɪŋ] *a* 1) проницательный; 2) пронзительный.

penetration [,penɪ'treɪʃən] *n* 1) проникновение; 2) проницаемость; 3) проницательность; 4) *воен.* наступление с целью прорыва.

penetrative ['penɪtrətɪv] *a* 1) проникающий; 2) пронзительный, резкий (*о звуке*); 3) проницательный.

pen-friend ['penfrend] *n* друг по переписке.

penguin ['peŋgwɪn] *n* 1) пингвин; 2) *ав.* учебный макет самолёта.

penholder ['pen,houldə] *n* ручка (*для пера*).

peninsula [pɪ'nɪnsjulə] *n* полуостров.

peninsular [pɪ'nɪnsjulə] *a* полуостровной.

penitence ['penɪtəns] *n* раскаяние; покаяние.

penitent I ['penɪtənt] *n* кающийся грешник.

penitent II *a* кающийся.

penitential [,penɪ'tenʃəl] *a* покаянный.

penitentiary I [,penɪ'tenʃərɪ] *n* 1) исправительный дом; 2) *амер.* каторжная тюрьма.

penitentiary II *a* исправительный.

penknife ['pennaɪf] *n* перочинный нож.

penman ['penmən] *n* 1) каллиграф, писец; 2) писатель.

penmanship ['penmənʃɪp] *n* 1) каллиграфия, чистописание; 2) почерк; 3) стиль *или* манера писателя.

pen-name ['penneɪm] *n* псевдоним.

pennant ['penənt] *n* 1) *мор.* вымпел; 2) *амер.* знамя (*приз в состязании*).

pennies ['penɪz] *pl см.* penny.

penniless ['penɪlɪs] *a* безденежный; нуждающийся, бедный.

penn'orth ['penəθ] *см.* penny-worth.

penny ['penɪ] *n* 1) (*pl* pence — *о денежной сумме*; pennies — *об отдельных монетах*) пенни, пенс (= $1/100$ ф. ст., до 1971 г.= $1/12$ шиллинга); 2) (*pl* pennies) *амер.* монета в 1 цент; ◊ a pretty ~ кругленькая сумма; изрядная сумма; in for a ~, in for a pound *посл.* ≅ назвался груздём, полезай в кузов; not a ~ to bless oneself with ни гроша за душой; to turn an honest ~ подрабатывать; a ~ for your thoughts! о чём призадумались?

penny-a-liner ['penɪə'laɪnə] *n* наёмный писака.

penny-wise ['penɪ'waɪz] *a* мелочный; ~ and pound-foolish скупой в мелочах и расточительный в крупных делах.

penny-worth ['penəθ] *n* 1) небольшое количество товара; not a ~ ни чуточки, ни капельки; 2):

a good (bad) ~ хоро́шая (плоха́я) сде́лка; 3) *attr* грошо́вый.

pension I [ˈpenʃən] *n* 1) пе́нсия, посо́бие; old--age ~ пе́нсия по ста́рости; 2) пансио́н.

pension II *v* назнача́ть пе́нсию; □ to ~ off увольня́ть на пе́нсию.

pensionary I [ˈpenʃənərɪ] *n* пенсионе́р.

pensionary II *a* пенсио́нный.

pensioner [ˈpenʃənə] *n* 1) пенсионе́р; 2) студе́нт, опла́чивающий обуче́ние и содержа́ние.

pensive [ˈpensɪv] *a* 1) заду́мчивый, мечта́тельный; 2) печа́льный.

pent [pent] *a* за́пертый, заключённый.

penta- [ˈpentə-] *pref* пяти-; pentagon пятиуго́льник.

Pentagon [ˈpentəgən] *n* Пентаго́н, вое́нное мини́стерство США; *перен.* америка́нский милитари́зм.

pentathlon [penˈtæθlən] *n спорт.* пятибо́рье.

penthouse [ˈpenthaus] *n* наве́с.

pent-up [ˈpentʌp] *a* скры́тый; сде́рживаемый (*о чувстве*).

penult(imate) I [pɪˈnʌlt(ɪmɪt)] *n* предпосле́дний слог.

penult(imate) II *a* предпосле́дний.

penurious [pɪˈnjuərɪəs] *a* 1) бе́дный, ску́дный; 2) ска́редный, скупо́й.

penury [ˈpenjurɪ] *n* 1) кра́йняя бе́дность; безде́нежье; 2) недоста́ток (*of*).

peon [ˈpiːən] *n* батра́к, подёнщик (*в Латинской Аме́рике*).

peonage [ˈpiːənɪdʒ] *n* батра́чество; кабала́.

peony [ˈpɪənɪ] *n бот.* пио́н.

people I [ˈpiːpl] *n* 1) наро́д, на́ция; 2) (*употр. как pl*) лю́ди; населе́ние; жи́тели; working ~ трудя́щиеся; big ~ изве́стные лю́ди; ~ of good will лю́ди до́брой во́ли; young ~ молодёжь; country ~ дереве́нские жи́тели; little ~ детвора́; professional ~ лю́ди определённой профе́ссии; the little ~, the good ~ фе́и, э́льфы; ~ say... говоря́т...; to poll ~ проводи́ть рефере́ндум; most ~ большинство́; 3) (*употр. как pl*) родны́е, ро́дственники; my ~ мои́ ро́дственники, родны́е.

people II *v* заселя́ть; населя́ть.

pep I [pep] *n разг.* бо́дрость ду́ха, эне́ргия, си́ла.

pep II *v*: to ~ up вселя́ть бо́дрость ду́ха.

pepper I [ˈpepə] *n* 1) пе́рец; *перен.* острота́; 2) вспы́льчивость.

pepper II *v* 1) пе́рчить; 2) осыпа́ть.

pepper-and-salt I [ˈpepərəndˈsɔːlt] *n* шерстяна́я мате́рия с и́скрой.

pepper-and-salt II *a* 1) кра́пчатый; 2) с про́седью (*о волоса́х*).

pepperbox [ˈpepəbɔks] *n* 1) пе́речница; 2) *шутл.* ба́шенка.

pepper-castor [ˈpepəˌkɑːstə] *n* пе́речница.

peppercorn [ˈpepəkɔːn] *n* перчи́нка, зёрнышко пе́рца.

peppermint [ˈpepəmɪnt] *n* 1) *бот.* пе́речная мя́та; 2) мя́тная лепёшка.

peppery [ˈpepərɪ] *a* 1) напе́рченный, о́стрый, е́дкий; 2) вспы́льчивый, раздражи́тельный.

peppy [ˈpepɪ] *a сленг* энерги́чный.

peptic [ˈpeptɪk] *a* пищевари́тельный.

per [pɜː] *prep* 1) по, че́рез, посре́дством; ~ post по по́чте; ~ steamer парохо́дом; 2) в, на ,(*ука́зывает на определённый срок*); ~ annum в год;

3) на; ~ capita на челове́ка, на ду́шу; 4) за; ~ yard за ярд.

peradventure I [pərədˈventʃə] *n уст.* неизве́стность; сомни́тельный факт; beyond ~, without ~ вне вся́кого сомне́ния.

peradventure II *adv уст.* возмо́жно, мо́жет быть; if ~ е́сли бы; lest ~ что́ бы ни случи́лось.

perambulate [pəˈræmbjuleɪt] *v* 1) ходи́ть взад и вперёд, расха́живать; 2) объезжа́ть (*террито́рию*); обходи́ть грани́цы (*владе́ний*).

perambulator [ˈpræmbjuleɪtə] *n* де́тская коля́ска.

perceivable [pəˈsiːvəbl] *a* заме́тный, ощути́мый.

perceive [pəˈsiːv] *v* 1) осознава́ть, понима́ть; постига́ть, воспринима́ть; 2) ощуща́ть, чу́вствовать.

per cent [pəˈsent] *n* проце́нт; three ~ три проце́нта.

percentage [pəˈsentɪdʒ] *n* проце́нт; проце́нтное отноше́ние.

percept [ˈpɜːsept] *n филос.* объе́кт *или* результа́т восприя́тия.

perceptible [pəˈseptəbl] *a* 1) заме́тный; ощути́мый; 2) познава́емый.

perception [pəˈsepʃən] *n* 1) восприя́тие; позна́ние; 2) понима́ние.

perceptive [pəˈseptɪv] *a* воспринима́ющий, познаю́щий.

perceptivity [ˌpɜːsepˈtɪvɪtɪ] *n* восприи́мчивость.

perch[1] I [pɜːtʃ] *n* 1) насе́ст, жёрдочка; 2) *разг.* высо́кое *или* про́чное положе́ние; come off your ~! не задава́йтесь!, не ва́жничайте!; 3) ме́ра длины́ (= 5,03 м).

perch[1] II *v* 1) сади́ться на насе́ст; сиде́ть на ве́тке, жёрдочке (*о пти́цах*); 2) взобра́ться, вскара́бкаться; 3) помеща́ть высоко́; 4) *обыкн. p. p.* находи́ться, располага́ться на возвы́шенности.

perch[2] *n* о́кунь.

perchance [pəˈtʃɑːns] *adv уст.* возмо́жно, мо́жет быть; случа́йно.

percolate [ˈpɜːkəleɪt] *v* 1) проце́живать, фильтрова́ть; 2) проса́чиваться.

percolator [ˈpɜːkəleɪtə] *n* 1) фильтр; цеди́лка; си́течко; 2) кофе́йник с си́течком.

percuss [pəˈkʌs] *v мед.* выстуки́вать.

percussion [pəˈkʌʃən] *n* 1) уда́р (*одного́ тела о друго́е*); столкнове́ние, сотрясе́ние; 2) *мед.* выстуки́вание; 3) *attr* уда́рный, взрывно́й; разрывно́й (*о пу́ле*).

percussive [pəˈkʌsɪv] *a* уда́рный.

perdition [pəˈdɪʃən] *n* прокля́тие, поги́бель.

perdu(e) [pəˈdjuː] *a* скры́тый, укры́тый; притаи́вшийся; to lie ~ лежа́ть в заса́де; притаи́ться.

perdurable [pəˈdjuərəbl] *a* ве́чный, постоя́нный.

peregrinate [ˈperɪɡrɪneɪt] *v шутл.* стра́нствовать, путеше́ствовать.

peremptory [pəˈremptərɪ] *a* 1) не допуска́ющий возраже́ний; безапелляцио́нный; 2) повели́тельный, вла́стный.

perennial I [pəˈrenjəl] *n бот.* многоле́тнее расте́ние.

perennial II *a* 1) круглогоди́чный; 2) непересыха́ющий (*о реке́ и т. п.*); 3) неувяда́емый, ве́чный; 4) многоле́тний (*о расте́нии*).

perfect[a] I [ˈpɜːfɪkt] *n грам.* перфе́кт, соверше́нная фо́рма (*глаго́ла*).

perfect[a] II *a* 1) соверше́нный, безупре́чный; 2) зако́нченный; це́льный; 3) то́чный; абсолю́тный; 4) хорошо подготовленный; 5) настоящий, истинный; 6) прекрасный (*о погоде*); 7) *грам.* перфектный.

perfect[b] [pə'fekt] *v* 1) совершенствовать; улучшать; 2) завершать, заканчивать.

perfection [pə'fekʃən] *n* 1) совершенствование; 2) законченность; совершенство; to ~ в совершенстве; 3) *pl* достоинства, совершенства; 4) завершение.

perfectly ['pəːfɪktlɪ] *adv* совершенно; вполне; отлично.

perfidious [pəː'fɪdɪəs] *a* предательский, вероломный.

perfidy ['pəːfɪdɪ] *n* предательство, вероломство.

perforate ['pəːfəreɪt] *v* 1) просверливать, пробуравливать, пробивать (*отверстия*); 2) проникать (*into, through*).

perforation [,pəːfə'reɪʃən] *n* 1) просверливание, пробуравливание, пробивание (*отверстий*); 2) отверстие.

perforce [pə'fɔːs] *adv* по необходимости; волей-неволей.

perform [pə'fɔːm] *v* 1) выполнять (*обещание, приказание и т. п.*); совершать; 2) представлять, играть, исполнять (*роль, муз. произведение*).

performance [pə'fɔːməns] *n* 1) исполнение, выполнение; 2) подвиг; 3) *театр.* представление, спектакль.

performer [pə'fɔːmə] *n* исполнитель.

perfume[a] ['pəːfjuːm] *n* 1) аромат, запах; 2) духи.

perfume[b] [pə'fjuːm] *v* надушить.

perfumer [pə'fjuːmə] *n* парфюмер.

perfumery [pə'fjuːmərɪ] *n* парфюмерия.

perfunctory [pə'fʌŋktərɪ] *a* небрежный, поверхностный.

perfuse [pə'fjuːz] *v* 1) обрызгивать, опрыскивать; 2) заливать (*о свете*).

pergola ['pəːgələ] *n* беседка *или* крытая аллея из вьющихся растений.

perhaps [pə'hæps, præps] *adv* может быть, возможно.

peri ['pɪərɪ] *n* 1) *миф.* пери; 2) красавица.

peril I ['perɪl] *n* опасность; риск; at your ~ на ваш страх и риск; in ~ of с риском; at the ~ of с опасностью.

peril II *v* подвергать опасности.

perilous ['perɪləs] *a* опасный, рискованный.

period ['pɪərɪəd] *n* 1) период; 2) время, эпоха; 3) цикл, круг; 4) *грам.* период, законченное предложение; 5) точка; to put a ~ to поставить точку; положить конец (*чему-л.*); 6) *pl* менструации.

periodic [,pɪərɪ'ɔdɪk] *a* 1) периодический; 2) циклический.

periodical I [,pɪərɪ'ɔdɪkəl] *n* журнал, периодическое издание.

periodical II *a* периодический.

periphery [pə'rɪfərɪ] *n* периферия, окружность.

periphrastic [,perɪ'fræstɪk] *a* иносказательный.

periscope ['perɪskoup] *n* перископ.

perish ['perɪʃ] *v* 1) погибать, умирать; 2) *обыкн.* *pass* страдать (*от холода и т. п.*).

perishable ['perɪʃəbl] *a* 1) бренный, непрочный; 2) скоропортящийся.

perishables ['perɪʃəblz] *n pl* скоропортящийся товар, груз.

periwig ['perɪwɪg] *n* парик.

periwigged ['perɪwɪgd] *a* в парике.

perjure ['pəːdʒə] *v*: to ~ oneself лжесвидетельствовать; нарушать клятву.

perjured ['pəːdʒəd] *a* виновный в клятвопреступлении.

perjurer ['pəːdʒərə] *n* клятвопреступник; -ица.

perjury ['pəːdʒərɪ] *n* 1) клятвопреступление, лжесвидетельство; 2) вероломство.

perk [pəːk] *v* 1) задирать нос, поднимать голову (*тж.* to ~ up); 2): to ~ oneself up прихорашиваться; оживляться.

perky ['pəːkɪ] *a* 1) весёлый, бойкий; 2) дерзкий; наглый, самоуверенный.

permanence ['pəːmənəns] *n* постоянство; неизменность.

permanency ['pəːmənənsɪ] *n* 1) постоянство; 2) постоянная работа, должность.

permanent ['pəːmənənt] *a* 1) постоянный, неизменный; перманентный; 2) остаточный.

permanently ['pəːmənəntlɪ] *adv* постоянно, неизменно.

permeable ['pəːmjəbl] *a* проницаемый.

permeant ['pəːmɪənt] *a* проницаемый, пропускающий.

permeate ['pəːmɪeɪt] *v* 1) проходить (*сквозь какую-л. массу*), проникать; 2) распространяться (*among, through*).

permissible [pə'mɪsəbl] *a* позволительный, допустимый.

permission [pə'mɪʃən] *n* разрешение, позволение.

permissive [pə'mɪsɪv] *a* допускающий, дозволяющий, разрешающий.

permit[a] ['pəːmɪt] *n* 1) пропуск; 2) разрешение.

permit[b] [pə'mɪt] *v* 1) разрешать, позволять; 2) давать возможность; weather ~ting если погода будет благоприятствовать; to ~ of (*of*).

permittance [pə'mɪtəns] *n* 1) *уст.* разрешение, позволение; 2) *эл.* проводимость; 3) *эл.* ёмкость.

permutation [,pəːmjuː'teɪʃən] *n* 1) перемена, изменение; 2) *мат.* перестановка.

pernicious [pəː'nɪʃəs] *a* вредный, вредоносный; гибельный, пагубный.

pernickety [pə'nɪkɪtɪ] *a разг.* 1) привередливый; 2) суетливый; 3) щекотливый.

perorate ['perəreɪt] *v* 1) ораторствовать, разглагольствовать; 2) резюмировать, делать заключение.

peroration [,perə'reɪʃən] *n* 1) разглагольствование; 2) заключение, конец речи.

peroxide [pə'rɔksaɪd] *n хим.* перекись.

perpendicular I [,pəːpən'dɪkjulə] *n* 1) перпендикуляр; отвес; out of ~ невертикальный, не под прямым углом; 2) *сленг* еда стоя.

perpendicular II *a* перпендикулярный, отвесный, вертикальный.

perpetrate ['pəːpɪtreɪt] *v* совершать (*преступление*).

perpetrator ['pəːpɪtreɪtə] *n* нарушитель, преступник.

perpetual [pə'petʃuəl] *a* 1) вечный, постоянный; 2) пожизненный; 3) *разг.* постоянный, нескончаемый (*о потоке и т. п.*).

perpetuate [pə'petjueɪt] *v* увековечивать.

perpetuity [,pəːpɪ'tjuːɪtɪ] *n* 1) вечность; in ~ навсегда, навеки; 2) пожизненная рента.

perplex [pə'pleks] *v* 1) ошеломлять, сбивать с толку; 2) вносить путаницу, запутывать.

perplexed [pə'plekst] *a* 1) ошеломлённый, сбитый с толку, растерянный; 2) запутанный, сложный.

perplexity [pə'pleksɪtɪ] *n* 1) растерянность; сильное смущение; 2) затруднение, дилемма.

perquisite ['pɜːkwɪzɪt] *n* приработок.

perquisition [ˌpɜːkwɪ'zɪʃən] *n* 1) тщательный обыск; 2) опрос; расследование.

perry ['perɪ] *n* грушевый сидр.

persecute ['pɜːsɪkjuːt] *v* 1) преследовать, подвергать гонениям (*за убеждения и т. п.*); 2) надоедать, приставать (*с вопросами и т. п.*).

persecution [ˌpɜːsɪ'kjuːʃən] *n* преследование, гонение.

persecutor ['pɜːsɪkjuːtə] *n* преследователь, гонитель.

perseverance [ˌpɜːsɪ'vɪərəns] *n* упорство, настойчивость.

persevere [ˌpɜːsɪ'vɪə] *v* 1) добиваться своего, настаивать (*на — in*); 2) проявлять упорство, настойчивость.

persevering [ˌpɜːsɪ'vɪərɪŋ] *a* настойчивый, упорный.

Persian I ['pɜːʃən] *n* 1) перс; персиянка; the ~s персы; 2) персидский язык.

Persian II *a* персидский.

persiflage [ˌpeəsɪ'flɑːʒ] *n* лёгкая шутка, подшучивание.

persist [pə'sɪst] *v* 1) упорствовать (*in*); 2) оставаться, сохраняться.

persistence [pə'sɪstəns] *n* 1) упорство, настойчивость; 2) выносливость; 3) постоянство.

persistency [pə'sɪstənsɪ] *см.* persistence.

persistent [pə'sɪstənt] *a* 1) упорный, настойчивый; 2) стойкий, живучий; 3) постоянный.

person ['pɜːsn] *n* 1) человек, особа, лицо; личность; in (one's own) ~ лично, сам; not a single ~ ни одной души, никого; to accept the ~ of, to accept ~s относиться лицеприятно; проявлять пристрастное отношение; squeezable ~s податливый человек; displaced ~s перемещённые лица; 2) внешность; he has a fine ~ он красив; 3) персонаж, действующее лицо; 4) *грам.* лицо; 5) *зоол.* особь; ◊ to have a ~ in one's pocket иметь кого-л. в своей власти.

personable ['pɜːsnəbl] *a* красивый, представительный.

personage ['pɜːsnɪdʒ] *n* 1) выдающаяся фигура, личность; 2) человек, особа; 3) действующее лицо, персонаж.

personal I ['pɜːsnl] *a* 1) личный (*тж. грам.*); to become ~ переходить на личности; 2) *юр.* движимый (*об имуществе*).

personal II *n* *амер.* заметка в газете (*о каком-л. человеке*).

personality [ˌpɜːsə'nælɪtɪ] *n* 1) личность, индивидуальность; 2) личные свойства; особенности характера; 3) *обыкн. pl* выпад (*против кого-л.*).

personalize ['pɜːsənəlaɪz] *v* олицетворять.

personally ['pɜːsnəlɪ] *adv* лично, сам; что касается меня; ~ I differ from you что касается меня, то я расхожусь с вами во мнении.

personalty ['pɜːsnltɪ] *n* *юр.* движимое имущество.

personification [pɜːˌsɔnɪfɪ'keɪʃən] *n* олицетворение; воплощение.

personify [pɜː'sɔnɪfaɪ] *v* олицетворять; воплощать.

personnel [ˌpɜːsə'nel] *n* личный состав, персонал.

perspective I [pə'spektɪv] *n* 1) перспектива; 2) вид, горизонт.

perspective II *a* перспективный.

perspicacious [ˌpɜːspɪ'keɪʃəs] *a* проницательный.

perspicacity [ˌpɜːspɪ'kæsɪtɪ] *n* проницательность.

perspicuity [ˌpɜːspɪ'kjuːɪtɪ] *n* 1) ясность, понятность; 2) прозрачность; 3) проницательность.

perspicuous [pə'spɪkjuəs] *a* 1) ясный, понятный; 2) ясно выражающий свои мысли; 3) прозрачный.

perspiration [ˌpɜːspə'reɪʃən] *n* 1) потение; 2) пот, испарина.

perspire [pəs'paɪə] *v* потеть; покрываться испариной.

persuade [pə'sweɪd] *v* 1) убедить (*of, that*); 2) уговорить (*to + Inf, into*); отговорить (*from, out of*).

persuader [pə'sweɪdə] *n* убеждающий, уговаривающий.

persuasion [pə'sweɪʒən] *n* 1) убеждение; 2) убедительность; 3) вероисповедание; 4) *шутл.* сорт, класс.

persuasive I [pə'sweɪsɪv] *n* побуждение.

persuasive II *a* убедительный.

pert [pɜːt] *a* 1) дерзкий, нахальный; 2) бойкий, развязный.

pertain [pɜː'teɪn] *v* 1) относиться, иметь отношение (*к — to*); 2) принадлежать (*to*).

pertinacious [ˌpɜːtɪ'neɪʃəs] *a* 1) упрямый; 2) упорный.

pertinacity [ˌpɜːtɪ'næsɪtɪ] *n* упрямство, неуступчивость.

pertinent ['pɜːtɪnənt] *a* подходящий; уместный; относящийся к делу; по существу.

perturb [pə'tɜːb] *v* 1) беспокоить, волновать; смущать; 2) приводить в смятение.

perturbation [ˌpɜːtə'beɪʃən] *n* 1) беспокойство, волнение; 2) пертурбация.

peruke [pə'ruːk] *n* парик.

perusal [pə'ruːzəl] *n* внимательное чтение; прочтение.

peruse [pə'ruːz] *v* внимательно читать; *перен.* рассматривать.

Peruvian I [pə'ruːvjən] *n* перуанец; перуанка; the ~s перуанцы.

Peruvian II *a* перуанский.

pervade [pə'veɪd] *v* наполнять, пропитывать (*ароматом и т. п.*); распространяться.

perverse [pə'vɜːs] *a* 1) своенравный, капризный; несговорчивый; 2) извращённый, порочный.

perversion [pə'vɜːʃən] *n* извращение.

perversity [pə'vɜːsɪtɪ] *n* 1) своенравие; несговорчивость; 2) извращённость, порочность.

pervertᵃ ['pɜːvɜːt] *n* 1) извращённый человек; 2) отступник, ренегат.

pervertᵇ [pə'vɜːt] *v* 1) совращать; 2) вводить в заблуждение; 3) извращать.

pervious ['pɜːvjəs] *a* 1) проницаемый, пропускающий (*влагу*); 2) поддающийся (*влиянию и т. п.*).

peseta [pə'setə] *n* песета (*испанская монета*).

pesky ['peskɪ] *a* *амер. сленг* беспокойный, надоедливый.

pest [pest] *n* 1) бич, язва; 2) надоедливый

человек; 3) паразит, вредитель; 4) *уст.* чума, мор.

pester ['pestə] *v* докучать, надоедать.

pest-house ['pesthaus] *n* чумной барак.

pestiferous [pes'tifərəs] *a* 1) вредный, вредоносный; 2) заразный; 3) *разг.* надоедливый, докучливый.

pestilence ['pestiləns] *n* 1) бубонная чума; мор; 2) поветрие, эпидемия.

pestilent ['pestilənt] *a* 1) вредоносный; пагубный; 2) смертельный, ядовитый; 3) *разг.* надоедливый.

pestle I ['pesl] *n* пестик (*ступки*).

pestle II *v* толочь.

pet[^1] I [pet] *n* 1) любимец, баловень; 2) любимое животное; любимая вещь; 3) *attr* любимый.

pet[^1] II *v* баловать, ласкать.

pet[^2] *n* скверное настроение; to be in a ~ быть в дурном настроении.

petal ['petl] *n* *бот.* лепесток.

Peter ['pi:tə]: to rob ~ to pay Paul облагодетельствовать одного за счёт другого.

peter ['pi:tə] *v* *сленг*: to ~ out истощаться, иссякать.

petersham ['pi:təʃəm] *n* 1) толстое сукно; 2) пальто (*из толстого сукна*).

petition I [pi'tiʃən] *n* 1) прошение, просьба, петиция; to present a ~ подавать просьбу, петицию; 2) молитва.

petition II *v* просить, ходатайствовать; подавать прошение.

petitioner [pi'tiʃnə] *n* проситель; *юр.* истец.

petrel ['petrəl] *n* *зоол.* буревестник.

petrifaction [,petri'fækʃən] *n* 1) окаменение; 2) окаменелость.

petrify ['petrifai] *v* 1) окаменевать; 2) остолбенеть; 3) поражать, ошеломлять.

petrol ['petrəl] *n* 1) бензин, газолин; 2) *attr* бензиновый.

petroleum [pi'trouljəm] *n* нефть.

petticoat ['petikout] *n* 1) нижняя юбка; детская юбочка; 2) *шутл.* женщина, девушка; *pl* женский пол; 3) *attr* женский.

pettifog ['petifɔg] *v* 1) заниматься крючкотворством; 2) вздорить по пустякам.

pettifogger ['petifɔgə] *n* крючкотвор, интриган.

pettifogging ['petifɔgiŋ] *a* низкий, мелочный, ничтожный.

pettish ['petiʃ] *a* раздражительный, обидчивый.

petty ['peti] *a* мелкий; мелочный; пустяковый; ничтожный.

petulance ['petjuləns] *n* раздражительность; обидчивость.

petulant ['petjulənt] *a* раздражительный; обидчивый.

petunia [pi'tju:njə] *n* *бот.* петуния.

pew [pju:] *n* 1) скамья в церкви; 2) *разг.* сиденье; take a ~ садитесь.

pewter ['pju:tə] *n* 1) олово; сплав олова со свинцом; 2) оловянная посуда; 3) *attr* оловянный.

phantasy ['fæntəsi] *см.* fantasy.

phantom ['fæntəm] *n* 1) призрак, привидение; 2) иллюзия; 3) *attr* призрачный, иллюзорный.

Pharaoh ['fɛərou] *n* *ист.* фараон.

Pharisee ['færisi:] *n* фарисей, ханжа.

pharmacist ['fɑːməsist] *n* *амер.* фармацевт.

pharmacy ['fɑːməsi] *n* 1) фармацевтика; 2) аптека.

pharos ['fɛərɔs] *n* *поэт.* маяк, светоч.

pharynx ['færiŋks] *n* *анат.* глотка.

phase [feiz] *n* фаза.

pheasant ['feznt] *n* *зоол.* фазан.

phenomena [fi'nɔminə] *pl см.* phenomenon.

phenomenal [fi'nɔminl] *a* необычайный, феноменальный.

phenomenon [fi'nɔminən] *n* (*pl* phenomena) 1) явление; 2) необыкновенное явление; феномен.

phew [fju:] *int* фу!, тьфу!; ну и ну!

phial ['faiəl] *n* склянка, пузырёк.

philander [fi'lændə] *v* флиртовать, ухаживать.

philanderer [fi'lændərə] *n* ухажёр, волокита.

philanthropy [fi'lænθrəpi] *n* филантропия.

philharmonic [,filɑː'mɔnik] *a* филармонический; музыкальный (*об обществе*).

Philistine I ['filistain] *n* филистер; обыватель, мещанин.

Philistine II *a* филистерский; обывательский, мещанский.

philological [,filə'lɔdʒikəl] *a* языковедческий, филологический.

philologist [fi'lɔlədʒist] *n* языковед, филолог.

philology [fi'lɔlədʒi] *n* языкознание, филология.

philosopher [fi'lɔsəfə] *n* философ.

philosophic(al) [,filə'sɔfik(əl)] *a* философский.

philosophize [fi'lɔsəfaiz] *v* философствовать.

philosophy [fi'lɔsəfi] *n* философия; Marxist-Leninist ~ марксистско-ленинская философия; moral ~ этика; natural ~ физика.

phiz [fiz] *n* *разг.* физиономия.

phlegm [flem] *n* 1) мокрота, слизь; 2) флегматичность, вялость.

phlegmatic [fleg'mætik] *a* флегматичный, вялый.

phlox [flɔks] *n* *бот.* флокс.

phoenix ['fi:niks] *n* 1) *миф.* феникс; 2) образец совершенства.

phone[^1] I [foun] *n* *разг.* телефон, телефонная трубка; by (*или* over) the ~ по телефону; on the ~ у телефона; to answer the ~ ответить по телефону; to get smb. on the ~ дозвониться кому-л.; to hang up the ~ повесить трубку.

phone[^1] II *v* *разг.* телефонировать.

phone[^2] *n* *фон.* фона, звук речи.

phoneme ['founi:m] *n* *лингв.* фонема.

phonemic [fou'ni:mik] *a* фонематический.

phonetic [fou'netik] *a* фонетический.

phonetician [,founi'tiʃən] *n* фонетист.

phonetics [fou'netiks] *n* 1) фонетика; фонетическая система (*данного языка*); 2) *pl* произношение; his ~ are good у него хорошее произношение.

phoney I, II ['founi] *см.* phony I, II.

phonic ['founik] *a* звуковой, речевой.

phonograph ['founəgrɑːf] *n* фонограф.

phonology [fou'nɔlədʒi] *n* фонология.

phony I ['founi] *n* *разг.* 1) подделка; 2) жулик, обманщик; he wasn't a ~ он ведь не врал.

phony II *a* *разг.* поддельный; мошеннический; дутый (*об акциях*).

phosphate ['fɔsfeit] *n* *хим.* фосфат.

phosphoric [fɔsˈfɔrɪk] *a* 1) *хим.* фо́сфорный; 2) фосфори́ческий (*о свете*).

phosphorous [ˈfɔsfərəs] *a хим.* фо́сфористый.

phosphorus [ˈfɔsfərəs] *n* фо́сфор.

photo [ˈfoutou] *разг. см.* photograph I.

photocell [ˈfoutəsel] *n* фотоэлеме́нт.

photograph I [ˈfoutəgrɑːf] *n* фотока́рточка, фотогра́фия.

photograph II *v* фотографи́ровать, снима́ть.

photographer [fəˈtɔgrəfə] *n* фото́граф.

photographic [ˌfoutəˈgræfɪk] *a* фотографи́ческий.

photography [fəˈtɔgrəfɪ] *n* фотогра́фия.

photosensitive [ˌfoutəˈsensɪtɪv] *a* светочувстви́тельный.

phrase I [freɪz] *n* 1) выраже́ние, оборо́т (*часто фразеологический*), словосочета́ние; stock ~, set ~ усто́йчивое словосочета́ние; 2) фразиро́вка, стиль (*речи*); in simple ~ просты́м языко́м; 3) *муз.* фра́за; 4) *pl* пусты́е слова́.

phrase II *v* 1) выража́ть слова́ми; 2) *муз.* фрази́ровать.

phrase-book [ˈfreɪzbuk] *n* слова́рь идио́м.

phrase-monger [ˈfreɪzˌmʌŋgə] *n* фразёр.

phraseological [ˌfreɪzɪəˈlɔdʒɪkəl] *a* фразеологи́ческий.

phraseology [ˌfreɪzɪˈɔlədʒɪ] *n* фразеоло́гия.

phut [fʌt] *adv*: to go ~ ло́пнуть, потерпе́ть крах, ко́нчиться ниче́м.

physic I [ˈfɪzɪk] *n* 1) медици́на; 2) *разг.* лека́рство; 3) *сленг* взбу́чка.

physic II *v* 1) лечи́ть; 2) *сленг* всы́пать, зада́ть жа́ру.

physical [ˈfɪzɪkəl] *a* физи́ческий; материа́льный, теле́сный.

physician [fɪˈzɪʃən] *n* врач, до́ктор; consulting ~ врач-консульта́нт.

physicist [ˈfɪzɪsɪst] *n* фи́зик.

physics [ˈfɪzɪks] *n* фи́зика.

physiological [ˌfɪzɪəˈlɔdʒɪkəl] *a* физиологи́ческий.

physiologist [ˌfɪzɪˈɔlədʒɪst] *n* физио́лог.

physiology [ˌfɪzɪˈɔlədʒɪ] *n* физиоло́гия.

physique [fɪˈziːk] *n* телосложе́ние; вне́шность.

pianist [ˈpjænɪst] *n* пиани́ст(ка).

piano [ˈpjænou] *n* фортепья́но; рояль; grand ~ роя́ль; cottage ~, upright ~ пиани́но; to play the ~ игра́ть на роя́ле.

piano-organ [ˈpjænouˌɔːgən] *n* шарма́нка.

piano-player [ˈpjænouˌpleɪə] *n* 1) пиани́ст; 2) пиано́ла.

piazza [pɪˈætsə] *n* 1) пло́щадь (*часто базарная*); 2) *амер.* вера́нда.

pibroch [ˈpiːbrɔk] *n муз.* 1) шотла́ндская воды́нка; 2) вариа́ция для воды́нки.

picaresque [ˌpɪkəˈresk] *a* авантю́рный, плутовско́й (*о романе*).

picaroon I [ˌpɪkəˈruːn] *n* 1) плут; 2) банди́т; пира́т; 3) пира́тское су́дно.

picaroon II *v* соверша́ть пира́тские набе́ги.

piccaninny I [ˈpɪkənɪnɪ] *n* негритёнок.

piccaninny II *a* ма́ленький.

piccolo [ˈpɪkəlou] *n муз.* ма́лая фле́йта.

pick¹ [pɪk] *v* 1) выбира́ть, отбира́ть; подбира́ть; to ~ and choose быть разбо́рчивым; 2) собира́ть, рвать (*цветы, фрукты и т. п.*); 3) бура́вить, сверли́ть; 4) ковыря́ть, выко́выривать; 5) чи́стить (*ягоды*); обдира́ть, очища́ть; ощи́пывать (*птицу*);

6) обгла́дывать (*кость*); 7) клева́ть (*зёрна*); есть (*маленькими кусочками*); 8) обворо́вывать, очища́ть (*карманы*); 9) взла́мывать (*замок*); открыва́ть отмы́чкой; 10) *амер.* перебира́ть (*струны*); □ to ~ at придира́ться, ворча́ть, пили́ть; to ~ off а) перестре́ливать (*одного за другим*); б) отрыва́ть; to ~ on *разг.* а) докуча́ть; б) дразни́ть; критикова́ть; to ~ out а) выбира́ть; б) вырыва́ть; в) различа́ть; г) понима́ть, схва́тывать (*смысл, значение*); д) подбира́ть (*по слуху*); е) оттеня́ть; to ~ up а) разрыхля́ть (*землю*); б) поднима́ть (*с пола, с земли*); подбира́ть; в) подхвати́ть (*слова, выражения*); г) приня́ть пасса́жиров (*о поезде*); д) собра́ть (*сведения*); е) зараба́тывать (*на пропитание*); ж) «пойма́ть» (*по радио, прожектором*); приня́ть (*изображение, снимок из космоса*); з) попра́виться, вы́здороветь; и) ускоря́ть (*движение*); к) заезжа́ть (*за кем-л.*); л) познако́миться; *разг.* подружи́ться (*с кем-л.— with*).

pick² *n* 1) вы́бор; take your ~! выбира́йте!; 2): the ~ of the basket что-л. са́мое отбо́рное, са́мое лу́чшее; 3) удар.

pick³ *n* 1) кирка́, кайла́; 2) зубочи́стка.

pick-a-back [ˈpɪkəbæk] *adv* на спине́, за плеча́ми.

pickaninny I, II [ˈpɪkənɪnɪ] *см.* piccaninny I, II.

pickax(e) I [ˈpɪkæks] *n* кирка́, кайла́.

pickax(e) II *v* рабо́тать кирко́й.

picked [pɪkt] *a* отбо́рный, ото́бранный.

picket I [ˈpɪkɪt] *n* 1) кол; 2) пике́т; 3) пике́тчик; 4) *воен.* (сторожева́я) заста́ва.

picket II *v* 1) огора́живать; 2) привя́зывать к колу́; 3) выставля́ть пике́ты; 4) *воен.* охраня́ть, пикети́ровать.

picking [ˈpɪkɪŋ] *n* 1) собира́ние, отбо́р; 2) *pl* оста́тки, объе́дки; 3) *pl* ме́лкая пожи́ва; ~ and stealing ме́лкая кра́жа.

pickle I [ˈpɪkl] *n* 1) рассо́л; у́ксус для марина́да; 2) *обыкн. pl* соле́нья, марина́д; марино́ванные огурцы́; пи́кули; 3) неприя́тное положе́ние; to be in a sad ~ попа́сть в беду́; 4) *разг.* озорно́й ребёнок.

pickle II *v* марино́вать.

picklock [ˈpɪklɔk] *n* 1) взло́мщик; 2) отмы́чка.

pick-me-up [ˈpɪkmiːʌp] *n* возбужда́ющее сре́дство.

pickpocket [ˈpɪkˌpɔkɪt] *n* вор-карма́нник; beware of ~s! остерега́йтесь воро́в!

pick-up [ˈpɪkʌp] *n* 1) *авто* пика́п; 2) *разг.* случа́йное знако́мство; 3) ада́птер, звукоснима́тель.

picnic I [ˈpɪknɪk] *n* 1) пикни́к (*амер. тж.* basket ~); 2) прия́тное времяпрепровожде́ние; по ~ не шу́тка, нелёгкое де́ло.

picnic II *v* принима́ть уча́стие в пикнике́.

picric [ˈpɪkrɪk] *a хим.* пикри́новый.

pictorial I [pɪkˈtɔːrɪəl] *n* иллюстри́рованный журна́л.

pictorial II *a* 1) иллюстри́рованный; 2) живопи́сный; изобрази́тельный; 3) графи́ческий.

picture I [ˈpɪktʃə] *n* 1) карти́на, карти́нка, изображе́ние; to fire back ~s посыла́ть фотосни́мки на зе́млю; to frame a ~ вставля́ть карти́ну в ра́мку; 2) портре́т; 3) о́браз; *перен.* живо́е описа́ние; 4) воплоще́ние (*здоровья и т. п.*); 5) *pl* кинокарти́на (*тж.* moving ~s); 6) то́чная ко́пия (*кого-л.*).

picture II v 1) писа́ть (кра́сками); рисова́ть; 2) опи́сывать; 3) вообража́ть, представля́ть себе́ (тж. to ~ to oneself).

picture-book ['pɪktʃəbuk] n де́тская кни́жка с карти́нками.

picture-card ['pɪktʃəkɑːd] n фигу́рная ка́рта (коро́ль, да́ма, вале́т).

picture-gallery ['pɪktʃə,gælərɪ] n карти́нная галере́я.

picturesque [,pɪktʃə'resk] a 1) живопи́сный; 2) о́бразный; я́ркий, цвети́стый; 3) колори́тный.

picture-writing ['pɪktʃə,raɪtɪŋ] n иероглифи́ческое письмо́.

piddling ['pɪdlɪŋ] a пустяко́вый, ме́лкий, ничто́жный.

pie[1] [paɪ] n 1) пиро́г; shepherd's ~ картофе́льная запека́нка с мя́сом; 2) амер. торт, сла́дкий пиро́г; Eskimo ~ эскимо́ (моро́женое); ◊ ~ in the sky амер. что-л. несбы́точное; to eat humble ~ смиря́ться, покоря́ться; унижа́ться.

pie[2] n соро́ка.

piebald I ['paɪbɔːld] n пе́гая ло́шадь.

piebald II a пе́гий; перен. пёстрый; разношёрстный.

piece I [piːs] n 1) кусо́к, часть, уча́сток; a ~ of ground уча́сток земли́; a ~ of water пруд, озерко́; a bad ~ of road плохо́й, разби́тый уча́сток доро́ги; ~ by ~ по куска́м, постепе́нно; частя́ми; by the ~ за шту́ку; поштучно; сде́льно, за вы́полненную рабо́ту; to take to ~s разобра́ть на ча́сти; to pick to ~s разбира́ть на ча́сти; распа́рывать; перен. подверга́ть кри́тике; 2) обло́мок, обры́вок; a ~ of paper клочо́к бума́ги; to break to ~s разби́ть вдре́безги; to come (или to go) to ~s треща́ть по всем швам, разлете́ться на куски́; разби́ться вдре́безги; to tear to ~s разорва́ть на клочки́; 3) произведе́ние, пье́са, карти́на; a ~ of art худо́жественное произведе́ние; a ~ of music музыка́льное произведе́ние; a ~ of poetry стихотворе́ние; a ~ of painting карти́на; museum ~ музе́йная вещь или ре́дкость (тж. перен.); conversation ~ жа́нровая карти́на; dramatical ~ дра́ма, драмати́ческое произведе́ние; costume ~ театр. истори́ческая пье́са; 4) отде́льный предме́т, шту́ка; a ~ of furniture часть обстано́вки (отде́льная вещь: стул, стол и т. п.); a ~ of plate посу́дина; a ~ of wall-paper руло́н обо́ев; 5) образе́ц; факт; посту́пок; a ~ of folly сумасше́дший посту́пок; a ~ of impertinence наха́льный, де́рзкий посту́пок; 6) ша́хматная фигу́ра; 7) моне́та (тж. a ~ of money); 8) воен. огнево́е сре́дство (пулемёт, винто́вка и т. п.; тж. a ~ of ordnance); field ~ полево́е ору́дие; 9) амер. музыка́льный инструме́нт; 10) вста́вка, запла́та; ◊ a ~ of advice сове́т; a ~ of news но́вость; a ~ of luck уда́ча; a ~ of work (отде́льно вы́полненная) рабо́та; all of a ~ схо́дный, одного́ ка́чества; to cut to ~s a) жесто́ко раскритикова́ть; б) воен. разгроми́ть войска́; to pull to ~s раскритикова́ть; «разде́лать под оре́х»; to give a ~ of one's mind вы́сказаться напрями́к; отчита́ть (кого́-л.).

piece II v 1) чини́ть, лата́ть (пла́тье); 2) соединя́ть, собира́ть по кусо́чкам; комбини́ровать; ▢ to ~ down надставля́ть (оде́жду); to ~ on прила́живать (к чему́-л.—to); to ~ out составля́ть це́лое (из часте́й); комбини́ровать; to ~ together соединя́ть; to ~ up лата́ть.

piecemeal I ['piːsmiːl] a части́чный, постепе́нный.

piecemeal II adv 1) части́чно, постепе́нно; 2) поштучно; 3) сде́льно.

piece-work ['piːswəːk] n сде́льная рабо́та.

pied [paɪd] a пёстрый, пятни́стый.

pier [pɪə] n 1) мол, волноре́з; 2) мор. пирс; 3) при́стань; 4) сва́я, бык (моста́); 5) просте́нок.

pierce [pɪəs] v 1) пронза́ть, протыка́ть, прока́лывать; 2) пробура́вливать; сверли́ть; 3) проводи́ть (тунне́ль); 4) проника́ть; 5) выгля́дывать из-за туч (о со́лнце); 6) наруша́ть (тишину́), проре́зать (во́здух); 7) прони́зывать (о хо́лоде); 8) воен. прорыва́ть (ли́нию фро́нта).

piercing ['pɪəsɪŋ] a 1) пронзи́тельный (о кри́ке); 2) о́стрый (о бо́ли, чу́встве); 3) прони́зывающий (о взгля́де, хо́лоде); 4) воен. бронебо́йный.

pier-glass ['pɪəglɑːs] n трюмо́.

piety ['paɪətɪ] n благоче́стие, на́божность.

piffle I ['pɪfl] n разг. болтовня́, глу́пость, ерунда́.

piffle II v разг. говори́ть глу́пости, болта́ть.

pig I [pɪg] n 1) свинья́ (тж. перен. о челове́ке); sucking ~ поросёнок; 2) свини́на; порося́тина; roast ~ жа́реный поросёнок; 3) до́лька (апельси́на); 4) тех. чу́шка, болва́нка; 5) ж.-д. толка́ч; 6) воен. сленг аэроста́т загражде́ния; ◊ cold ~ облива́ние холо́дной водо́й (что́бы разбуди́ть); ~s might fly посл. ≅ быва́ет, что и коро́вы лета́ют; to buy a ~ in a poke посл. ≅ покупа́ть кота́ в мешке́; to make a ~ of oneself обжира́ться.

pig II v 1) пороси́ться; 2) жить в грязи́.

pigeon ['pɪdʒɪn] n 1) го́лубь; голу́бка; homing ~ почто́вый го́лубь; 2) проста́к, «шля́па»; to pluck a ~ обобра́ть простака́.

pigeon-breasted ['pɪdʒɪn,brestɪd] a с кури́ной гру́дью (о челове́ке).

pigeon-hearted ['pɪdʒɪn'hɑːtɪd] a трусли́вый; ро́бкий.

pigeon-hole I ['pɪdʒɪnhoul] n 1) голуби́ное гнездо́; 2) отделе́ние пи́сьменного стола́ (для бума́г).

pigeon-hole II v раскла́дывать, классифици́ровать по докуме́нты; перен. «класть под сукно́».

pigeonry ['pɪdʒɪnrɪ] n голубя́тня.

piggery ['pɪgərɪ] n свина́рник, хлев.

piggish ['pɪgɪʃ] a 1) сви́нский; 2) гря́зный; 3) жа́дный; 4) упря́мый.

piggy ['pɪgɪ] n сви́нка, поросёнок.

piggy-wiggy ['pɪgɪ,wɪgɪ] n 1) сви́нка, поросёнок; 2) грязну́ля (о ребёнке); 3) игра́ в чижи́.

pigheaded ['pɪg'hedɪd] a упря́мый, тупо́й.

pig-iron ['pɪg,aɪən] n чугу́н в чу́шках.

pigmy ['pɪgmɪ] см. pygmy.

pignut ['pɪgnʌt] n земляно́й оре́х.

pigskin ['pɪgskɪn] n 1) свина́я ко́жа; 2) разг. седло́; 3) амер. разг. футбо́льный мяч.

pigsty ['pɪgstaɪ] n свина́рник.

pigtail ['pɪgteɪl] n коси́чка, коса́.

pike[1] [paɪk] n щу́ка.

pike[2] I n 1) пи́ка; копьё; 2) остриё, шип.

pike[2] II v зака́лывать (пи́кой, копьём).

pike[3] n см. turnpike.

piker ['paɪkə] n амер. разг. осторо́жный или ро́бкий деле́ц, игро́к.

pikestaff ['paɪkstɑːf] n дре́вко пи́ки.

pilaster [pɪ'læstə] n архит. пиля́стра.

pilchard ['pɪltʃəd] *n* сарди́н(к)а.

pile¹ I [paɪl] *n* 1) ку́ча, гру́да; шта́бель; 2) ки́па, па́чка; 3) *разг.* мно́жество, ма́сса; 4) грома́дное зда́ние; грома́да; 5) *разг.* состоя́ние; to make one's ~ сколоти́ть состоя́ние; 6) я́дерный реа́ктор (*тж.* atomic ~); 7) *эл.* батаре́я.

pile¹ II *v* скла́дывать в ку́чу, гру́ду; нагроможда́ть; *перен.* собира́ть, нака́пливать (*тж.* to ~ up); ◇ to ~ it on *разг.* преувели́чивать.

pile² I *n* сва́я.

pile² II *v* вбива́ть сва́и.

pile³ *n* 1) ворс; 2) шерсть; во́лос, пух.

pile⁴ *n мед.* 1) геморроида́льная ши́шка; 2) *pl* геморро́й.

piled [paɪld] *a* ворси́стый.

pilfer ['pɪlfə] *v* ворова́ть, таска́ть; стяну́ть.

pilferage ['pɪlfərɪdʒ] *n* ме́лкая кра́жа.

pilferer ['pɪlfərə] *n* ме́лкий жу́лик.

pilgrim ['pɪlgrɪm] *n* 1) пало́мник, пилигри́м; 2) стра́нник.

pilgrimage ['pɪlgrɪmɪdʒ] *n* 1) пало́мничество; 2) дли́тельное путеше́ствие.

pill I [pɪl] *n* 1) пилю́ля, табле́тка; 2) *разг.* неприя́тный челове́к; 3) *разг.* мяч, шар; 4) *pl* билья́рд; ◇ to gild the ~ позолоти́ть пилю́лю; a bitter (*или* hard) ~ to swallow тя́гостная необходи́мость; a ~ to cure an earthquake ≅ «ка́пля в мо́ре».

pill II *v* 1) дава́ть пилю́ли; 2) *сленг* забаллоти́ровать.

pillage I ['pɪlɪdʒ] *n* 1) грабёж, мародёрство; 2) добы́ча, награ́бленные ве́щи.

pillage II *v* гра́бить, мародёрствовать.

pillar ['pɪlə] *n* 1) столб, коло́нна; 2) опо́ра, столп; ◇ from ~ to post взад и вперёд, туда́ и сюда́; из одного́ положе́ния в друго́е.

pillar-box ['pɪləbɔks] *n* почто́вый я́щик.

pillbox ['pɪlbɔks] *n* 1) коро́бочка для пилю́ль, табле́ток; 2) *шутл.* кро́шечный до́мик; ма́ленький экипа́ж; 3) *воен.* дот.

pillion ['pɪljən] *n* 1) седе́льная поду́шка; 2) за́днее сиде́нье (*мотоцикла*).

pillory I ['pɪlərɪ] *n* позо́рный столб; to put in the ~ выставля́ть на посме́шище; to be put (*или* set) in the ~ быть вы́ставленным к позо́рному столбу́.

pillory II *v* 1) ста́вить к позо́рному столбу́; 2) выставля́ть на посме́шище.

pillow ['pɪlou] *n* 1) поду́шка; 2) *тех.* подкла́дка, вкла́дыш.

pillow-case ['pɪloukeɪs] *n* на́волочка.

pillow-slip ['pɪlouslɪp] *см.* pillow-case.

pillowy ['pɪlouɪ] *a* мя́гкий; усту́пчивый.

pilot I ['paɪlət] *n* 1) ло́цман, рулево́й; 2) пило́т, лётчик; 3) (о́пытный) проводни́к; 4) *тех.* вспомога́тельный механи́зм; 5) *attr* рулево́й, штурма́нский; ◇ to drop the ~ отве́ргнуть ве́рного сове́тчика.

pilot II *v* 1) вести́, управля́ть; пилоти́ровать; 2) быть проводнико́м, направля́ть.

pilotage ['paɪlətɪdʒ] *n* 1) веде́ние корабля́; ло́цманское де́ло; 2) *ав.* пилоти́рование; пилота́ж; 3) ло́цманский сбор.

pilot-cloth ['paɪlətklɔθ] *n* то́лстое си́нее сукно́.

pilot-engine ['paɪlət,endʒɪn] *n* 1) маневро́вый локомоти́в; 2) *ж.-д.* снегоочисти́тель.

pilot-house ['paɪləthaus] *n мор.* рулева́я ру́бка.

pimp I [pɪmp] *n* сво́дник.

pimp II *v* сво́дничать.

pimping ['pɪmpɪŋ] *a* 1) ме́лкий; 2) сла́бый, боле́зненный.

pimple ['pɪmpl] *n* пры́щик; goose ~s гуси́ная ко́жа.

pimpled ['pɪmpld] *a* прыща́вый.

pin I [pɪn] *n* 1) була́вка, шпи́лька; 2) *pl сленг* но́ги; he is quick on his ~s он бы́стро хо́дит (*или* бе́гает); 3) ке́гля; 4) *муз.* коло́к; 5) бочо́нок (= 4¹⁄₂ *галло́на*); 6) *тех.* ца́пфа; шкво́рень; ше́йка; ◇ in a merry ~ в весёлом настрое́нии; I don't care a ~ мне наплева́ть; you might have heard a ~ fall ≅ слы́шно бы́ло, как му́ха пролети́т; to be on ~s and needles ≅ сиде́ть как на иго́лках; not a ~ to choose between them ≅ их друг от дру́га не отличи́шь.

pin II *v* 1) прика́лывать, пришпи́ливать (*к чему́-л.— to*); ска́лывать (*обыкн.* to ~ together); to ~ smb. to the wall пригвозди́ть к стене́ (*шашкой*); *перен.* припере́ть к стене́; 2) прока́лывать; 3) свя́зывать (*обеща́нием и т. п.*; *часто* to ~ down).

pinafore ['pɪnəfɔ:] *n* пере́дник (*де́тский*); фа́ртук.

pince-nez ['pɛːnsneɪ] *n* пенсне́.

pincers ['pɪnsəz] *n pl* 1) щипцы́, кле́щи; пинце́т; 2) *зоол.* клешни́.

pinch I [pɪntʃ] *n* 1) щипо́к; 2) щепо́тка (*соли и т. п.*); 3) кра́йняя нужда́; at a ~ в кра́йнем слу́чае; 4) *сленг* кра́жа; 5) *сленг* аре́ст, налёт.

pinch II *v* 1) ущипну́ть, прищеми́ть; 2) щипа́ть (*о моро́зе*); 3) му́читься (*го́лодом*); 4) сжима́ть, жать (*об о́буви*); 5) искривля́ться, искажа́ться (*о ли е*); 6) скупи́ться; 7) уреза́ть, ограни́чивать; 8) *сленг* стащи́ть, укра́сть; 9) *сленг* арестова́ть.

pinchbeck ['pɪntʃbek] *n* 1) томпа́к; 2) фальши́вые драгоце́нности, подде́льная вещь; 3) *attr* подде́льный.

pinchers ['pɪntʃəz] *n pl* кле́щи, щипцы́.

pine¹ [paɪn] *n* 1) сосна́; 2) *разг.* анана́с; 3) *attr* сосно́вый.

pine² *v* 1) ча́хнуть (*тж.* to ~ away); томи́ться (*for*); 2) жа́ждать, изныва́ть, тоскова́ть (*по чему́-л.—after*).

pineapple ['paɪn,æpl] *n* 1) анана́с; 2) *воен. сленг* ручна́я грана́та, «лимо́нка»; 3) *attr* анана́сный.

pine-cone ['paɪnkoun] *n* сосно́вая ши́шка.

pinery ['paɪnərɪ] *n* 1) сосно́вое насажде́ние; 2) анана́сная тепли́ца.

pinfold ['pɪnfould] *n* заго́н для скота́.

ping I [pɪŋ] *n* свист (*пу́ли*).

ping II *v* свисте́ть.

ping-pong ['pɪŋpɔŋ] *n* пинг-по́нг (*насто́льный те́ннис*).

pin-head ['pɪnhed] *n* 1) була́вочная голо́вка; 2) *сленг* тупи́ца, дура́к.

pinion¹ ['pɪnjən] *n* 1) оконе́чность пти́чьего крыла́; 2) перо́; 3) *поэт.* крыло́.

pinion² *n* 1) *тех.* шестерня́; зубча́тое колесо́; 2) *ист.* зубе́ц стены́.

pink¹ I [pɪŋk] *n* 1) ро́зовый цвет; 2) *бот.* гвозди́ка; 3) (the ~) образе́ц, соверше́нство; the ~ of health воплоще́ние здоро́вья; the ~ of perfection верх соверше́нства; in the ~ *разг.* в расцве́те сил, здоро́вья.

pink[1] II *a* ро́зовый.

pink[2] *v* 1) протыка́ть, прока́лывать; 2) украша́ть ды́рочками, зубца́ми (to ~ out).

pinkish ['pɪŋkɪʃ] *a* розова́тый.

pinnace ['pɪnɪs] *n ист.* команди́рский ка́тер.

pinnacle ['pɪnəkl] *n* 1) бельведе́р, шпиц; 2) высокого́рная верши́на; 3) кульминацио́нный пункт.

pinny ['pɪnɪ] *n дет.* переде́дничек.

pint [paɪnt] *n* пи́нта (*мера ёмкости = 0,57 л*).

pinto ['pɪntou] *a амер.* пе́гий, пятни́стый.

pin-up ['pɪnʌp] *n* фотогра́фия хоро́шенькой де́вушки, кинозвезды́ *и т. п.*, прикреплённая на стене́ (*тж.* ~ girl).

piny ['paɪnɪ] *a* 1) изоби́лующий со́снами; 2) сосно́вый.

pioneer I [,paɪə'nɪə] *n* 1) пионе́р (*член пионерской организации*); 2) пионе́р, пе́рвый поселе́нец; 3) *воен.* сапёр; 4) инициа́тор; 5) *attr* пионе́рский; 6) *attr воен.* сапёрный.

pioneer II *v* 1) прокла́дывать путь; 2) быть пионе́ром.

pious ['paɪəs] *a* набо́жный, благочести́вый.

pip[1] ['pɪp] *n* 1) очко́ (*в домино, картах*); 2) звёздочка (*на погонах*).

pip[2] *n*: to have the ~ *сленг* быть не в ду́хе, быть в плохо́м настрое́нии.

pip[3] *n* ко́сточка, зёрнышко (*плода*).

pip[4] *v* пища́ть, чири́кать.

pip[5] *v разг.* 1) подстрели́ть; 2) положи́ть коне́ц; 3) расстро́ить (*планы*); 4) забаллоти́ровать.

pipage ['paɪpɪdʒ] *n* перека́чка по трубопрово́ду (*нефти и т. п.*).

pipe[1] I [paɪp] *n* 1) труба́, трубопрово́д; the ~s радиа́тор; 2) тру́бка (*курительная*); clay ~ гли́няная тру́бка; to smoke the ~ of peace вы́курить тру́бку ми́ра, прийти́ к соглаше́нию; 3) свире́ль, ду́дка, фле́йта; *pl* духовы́е инструме́нты; 4) пе́ние, свист (*птиц*); 5) *pl* дыха́тельные пути́; ◊ put that in your ~ and smoke it *разг.* ≅ над э́тим сто́ит поду́мать.

pipe[1] II *v* 1) игра́ть (*на свирели, дудке и т. п.*); 2) издава́ть ре́зкий звук, свисте́ть; 3) прокла́дывать тру́бы; 4) пуска́ть по труба́м; 5) украша́ть ка́нтом; 6) *мор.* вызыва́ть ду́дкой, свиста́ть; □ to ~ **away** *мор.* дава́ть сигна́л к отплы́тию; to ~ **down** сни́зить тон, стать ме́нее самоуве́ренным; to ~ **up** заигра́ть; запе́ть; заговори́ть.

pipe[2] *n* ви́нная бо́чка (= 105 галло́нов).

pipeclay ['paɪpkleɪ] *n* 1) мя́гкая бе́лая гли́на; 2) *attr* сде́ланный из бе́лой гли́ны.

pipeful ['paɪpful] *n* по́лная тру́бка (*табаку*).

pipeline ['paɪplaɪn] *n* трубопрово́д; нефтепрово́д.

piper ['paɪpə] *n* ду́дочник, флейти́ст; ◊ to pay the ~ брать на себя́ расхо́ды.

piping I ['paɪpɪŋ] *n* 1) игра́ (*на дудке и т. п.*); 2) насви́стывание; писк; 3) пе́ние птиц; 4) тру́бы; трубопрово́д; 5) са́харный узо́р (*на торте*); 6) кант (*на одежде*).

piping II *a* пискли́вый; ◊ ~ hot *разг.* о́чень горя́чий; све́женький; ≅ с пы́лу, с жа́ру.

pipkin ['pɪpkɪn] *n* гли́няный горшо́чек, ми́ска.

pipy ['paɪpɪ] *a* 1) тру́бчатый; 2) ре́зкий, зы́чный.

piquancy ['pi:kənsɪ] *n* пика́нтность, острота́.

piquant ['pi:kənt] *a* пика́нтный, о́стрый.

pique I [pi:k] *n* размо́лвка, оби́да, раздраже́ние;

in a fit of ~ в поры́ве раздраже́ния; out of ~ с доса́ды, со зло́сти.

pique II *v* 1) уколо́ть, заде́ть (*самолюбие*), уязви́ть; 2) возбужда́ть (*интерес, любопытство*); 3): to ~ oneself on чва́ниться, «задава́ться»; 4) *ав.* пики́ровать.

piquet [pɪ'ket] *n карт.* пике́т.

piracy ['paɪərəsɪ] *n* 1) пира́тство; 2) наруше́ние а́вторского пра́ва.

pirate I ['paɪərɪt] *n* 1) пира́т; пира́тский кора́бль; 2) наруши́тель а́вторского пра́ва.

pirate II *v* 1) занима́ться пира́тством; 2) самово́льно переиздава́ть.

piratic(al) [paɪ'rætɪk(əl)] *a* пира́тский.

pirogue [pɪ'roug] *n* пиро́га (*лодка*).

pish [pɪʃ] *int* фи!

pistachio [pɪs'tɑ:ʃɪou] *n* 1) фиста́шка; 2) фиста́шковое де́рево; 3) фиста́шковый цвет; 4) *attr* фиста́шковый (*о цвете*).

pistil ['pɪstɪl] *n бот.* пе́стик.

pistol ['pɪstl] *n* пистоле́т, револьве́р; silenced ~ бесшу́мный пистоле́т.

piston ['pɪstən] *n* 1) по́ршень; 2) писто́н, кла́пан (*духового инструмента*); 3) *attr* поршнево́й.

piston-rod ['pɪstənrɔd] *n тех.* шату́н.

pit[1] I [pɪt] *n* 1) я́ма; углубле́ние; впа́дина; air ~ возду́шная я́ма; the ~ of the stomach подло́жечная я́мка; to dig a ~ for smb. *перен.* рыть кому́-л. я́му; 2) ша́хта, копь; карье́р; шурф; 3) западня́; 4) (the ~) ад, преиспо́дняя; 5) парте́р (*обычно ряды за креслами*); 6) пу́блика парте́ра; 7) ряби́на, о́спина (*на коже*); 8) *амер.* отде́л това́рной би́ржи; 9) аре́на (*для петушиного боя*); 10) *уст.* тюрьма́, острог.

pit[1] II *v* 1) рыть я́мы; 2) закла́дывать в я́мы для хране́ния (*овощи*); 3) покрыва́ться о́спинами; 4) выступа́ть оди́н про́тив друго́го.

pit[2] I *n амер.* ко́сточка (*фруктовая*).

pit[2] II *v амер.* вынима́ть ко́сточку.

pit-a-pat ['pɪtə'pæt] *adv*: his heart went ~ се́рдце затрепета́ло; his feet went ~ у него́ но́ги подкоси́лись.

pitch[1] I [pɪtʃ] *n* 1) высота́ (*тона, звука и т. п.*); у́ровень, сте́пень, си́ла; absolute ~ абсолю́тный слух; to rise to a deafening ~ сде́латься оглуши́тельным (*о шуме и т. п.*); 2) килева́я ка́чка; to give a ~ зары́ться но́сом (*о корабле*); 3) бросо́к; 4) накло́н, скат; пока́тость; 5) па́ртия това́ра; 6) постоя́нное ме́сто (*уличного торговца*); 7) *спорт.* центра́льная часть кри́кетного по́ля.

pitch[1] II *v* 1) разбива́ть (*палатку, лагерь*); 2) броса́ть, мета́ть; подава́ть (*мяч*); 3) *муз.* придава́ть определённую высоту́; 4) испы́тывать килеву́ю ка́чку (*о корабле*); □ to ~ **in** *разг.* энерги́чно бра́ться за что-л.; to ~ **into** *разг.* а) набра́сываться, напада́ть; б) жа́дно есть; to ~ **upon** случа́йно выбира́ть.

pitch[2] I *n* смола́, дёготь, вар.

pitch[2] II *v* смоли́ть.

pitch-black ['pɪtʃ'blæk] *a* чёрный как смоль.

pitch-dark ['pɪtʃ'dɑ:k] *a* тёмный, «хоть глаз вы́коли».

pitched [pɪtʃt] *a*: ~ battle реши́тельное сраже́ние.

pitcher[1] ['pɪtʃə] *n* кувши́н; ◊ the ~ goes often to the well *погов.* повади́лся кувши́н по во́ду ходи́ть;

little ~s have long ears *погов.* маленькие дети слышат много лишнего.

pitcher[2] *n спорт.* подающий мяч.

pitchfork ['pɪtʃfɔːk] *n* вилы; ◊ it rains ~s льёт как из ведра.

pitchy ['pɪtʃɪ] *a* 1) смолистый; 2) смоляной; 3) чёрный.

piteous ['pɪtɪəs] *a* жалкий, достойный сожаления.

pitfall ['pɪtfɔːl] *n* ловушка, западня.

pith [pɪθ] *n* 1) сердцевина, мякоть (*растения*); 2) спинной мозг; 3) суть, существо (*дела*); the ~ and marrow of смая суть чего-л.; 4) сила, энергия.

pithless ['pɪθlɪs] *a* 1) без сердцевины; *перен.* слабый, мягкий; бесхарактерный; 2) бессодержательный.

pithy ['pɪθɪ] *a* 1) с сердцевиной; *перен.* сильный, энергичный; 2) выразительный (*о стиле*).

pitiable ['pɪtɪəbl] *a* жалкий, несчастный; ничтожный.

pitiful ['pɪtɪful] *a* 1) жалкий, вызывающий жалость; 2) сострадательный; 3) ничтожный, презренный.

pitiless ['pɪtɪlɪs] *a* безжалостный.

pitman ['pɪtmən] *n* 1) (*pl* pitmen) шахтёр; 2) (*pl* pitmans) *тех.* шатун.

pit-pat ['pɪt'pæt] *см.* pit-a-pat.

pittance ['pɪtəns] *n* 1) небольшое жалованье, гроши; 2) скудный доход; a mere ~ жалкая подачка.

pitter-patter I ['pɪtə,pætə] *n* мелькание (*света*); частое постукивание (*дождя*).

pitter-patter II *adv* быстро, непрерывно.

pity I ['pɪtɪ] *n* жалость, сожаление; to have (*или* to take) ~ on smb. сжалиться над кем-л.; it is a (great) ~ (очень) жаль; what a ~! как жаль!; for ~'s sake! умоляю вас!; the ~ of it! очень жаль!

pity II *v* жалеть, соболезновать.

pityingly ['pɪtɪɪŋlɪ] *adv* с сожалением, с жалостью.

pivot I ['pɪvət] *n* 1) точка опоры (*или* вращения); 2) стержень, шкворень; 3) основа, центр.

pivot II *v* 1) вращаться вокруг оси; вертеться; 2) снабжать стержнем.

pivotal ['pɪvətl] *a* 1) осевой, стержневой; 2) основной, центральный.

pixy ['pɪksɪ] *n* фея.

placable ['plækəbl] *a* кроткий, незлопамятный; благодушный.

placard I ['plækɑːd] *n* плакат, афиша.

placard II *v* 1) развешивать, расклеивать (*плакаты*); 2) рекламировать (*плакатами*).

placate [plə'keɪt] *v* 1) успокаивать; умиротворять; 2) *амер.* заручиться поддержкой.

place I [pleɪs] *n* 1) место; attendant's ~ рабочее место; natal ~ место рождения; to give ~ to уступать место, давать место; to take ~ иметь место, случаться, происходить; to take the ~ of заменить (*кого-л., что-л.*); in ~ of вместо; in the first ~ первым делом; in ~ уместный, подходящий; out of ~ а) неуместный, неподходящий; б) безработный; 2) сиденье, место (*в экипаже, за столом и т. п.*); to engage (*или* to secure) ~s заказать билеты; 3) дом, жилище; загородный дом; 4) населённый пункт, местечко, посёлок, город; 5) долж-

ность; положение; 6) площадь (*в названиях*); ◊ to keep smb. in his ~ держать кого-л. в узде; не давать зазнаваться; there is no ~ like home *посл.* ≅ в гостях хорошо, а дома лучше.

place II *v* 1) помещать, размещать, ставить, класть; 2) устраивать на место, должность; 3) определять место, положение; 4) *спорт.* присудить призовое место.

place-hunter ['pleɪs,hʌntə] *n* карьерист.

placeman ['pleɪsmən] *n* чиновник, «чинуша».

placid ['plæsɪd] *a* спокойный, мирный, безмятежный.

placidity [plæ'sɪdɪtɪ] *n* спокойствие, безмятежность.

placket ['plækɪt] *n* 1) разрез (*в юбке, рубашке*); 2) карман (*в юбке*).

plafond [plɑ'fɔŋ] *n архит.* плафон.

plage [plɑːʒ] *n* 1) взморье, песчаный пляж; 2) морской курорт.

plagiarism ['pleɪdʒjərɪzəm] *n* плагиат.

plagiarist ['pleɪdʒərɪst] *n* плагиатор.

plagiarize ['pleɪdʒəraɪz] *v* заниматься плагиатом.

plague I [pleɪg] *n* 1) бедствие, бич, наказание; a ~ of rats нашествие крыс; 2) *разг.* неприятность, беспокойство; 3) чума, мор; bubonic ~ бубонная чума; pneumonic ~ лёгочная чума; ◊ ~ on him! чтоб ему пусто было!

plague II *v* 1) *разг.* беспокоить, мучить, надоедать, докучать; 2) зачумлять; 3) насылать бедствие.

plaguesome ['pleɪgsəm] *a разг.* досадный, надоедливый.

plaguy I ['pleɪgɪ] *a* надоедливый, докучливый; неприятный.

plaguy II *adv* очень, чрезвычайно.

plaice [pleɪs] *n* камбала.

plaid [plæd] *n* 1) плед; shepherd's ~ клетчатый плед; 2) шотландка (*ткань*).

plain[1] I [pleɪn] *a* 1) ясный, очевидный, понятный; as ~ as a pikestaff ясный как день, очевидный; 2) простой, без претензий; обыкновенный; 3) гладкий, без рисунка (*о ткани*); 4) ровный (*о местности*); 5) откровенный, прямой; to be ~ with говорить откровенно с кем-л.; 6) некрасивый (*о лице*).

plain[1] II *adv* 1) чётко, разборчиво; 2) откровенно.

plain[2] *n* 1) равнина; 2) *pl* степи; *амер.* прерии.

plainly ['pleɪnlɪ] *adv* откровенно; прямо, без обиняков.

plainsman ['pleɪnzmən] *n* житель равнины.

plain-song ['pleɪnsɔŋ] *n* простое хоровое пение.

plain-spoken ['pleɪn'spoukən] *a* прямой, откровенный.

plaint [pleɪnt] *n* 1) *поэт.* жалоба, стенание; плач; 2) *юр.* иск.

plaintiff ['pleɪntɪf] *n юр.* истец; истица.

plaintive ['pleɪntɪv] *a* жалобный, заунывный; траурный.

plait I [plæt, *амер.* pleɪt] *n* 1) коса (*волос*); 2) складка (*на платье*).

plait II *v* заплетать.

plan I [plæn] *n* 1) план; to hit upon a ~ придумать план; 2) проект, замысел; 3) чертёж, схема.

plan II *v* 1) плани́ровать; составля́ть план; проекти́ровать; 2) стро́ить пла́ны; намерева́ться; затева́ть; 3) *амер.* наде́яться, ожида́ть.

plane¹ I [pleɪn] *n* 1) самолёт; hospital ~ санита́рный самолёт; pursuit ~ самолёт-истреби́тель; 2) пло́скость; 3) у́ровень; 4) крыло́ самолёта.

plane¹ II *a* пло́ский, ро́вный.

plane¹ III *v* скользи́ть; *ав.* плани́ровать.

plane² I *n* руба́нок, фуга́нок.

plane² II *v* 1) строга́ть; выра́внивать; 2) скобли́ть; □ to ~ **away**, to ~ **down** состру́гивать.

plane³ *n* плата́н, чина́ра.

planeload ['pleɪnloud] *n* компле́кт пассажи́ров в самолёте.

planet ['plænɪt] *n* плане́та.

planetarium [,plænɪ'tɛərɪəm] *n* планета́рий.

planetary ['plænɪtərɪ] *a* 1) плане́тный; 2) блужда́ющий.

planet-struck ['plænɪt,strʌk] *a* пани́ческий; в па́нике.

plangent ['plændʒənt] *a* 1) с шу́мом разбива́ющийся о бе́рег (*о волнах*); 2) гу́лкий.

plank I [plæŋk] *n* 1) (обшивна́я) доска́, пла́нка; 2) пункт парти́йной програ́ммы.

plank II *v* 1) обшива́ть (*доска́ми*); 2) *сленг* выкла́дывать, плати́ть (*тж.* to ~ **down**); 3) *амер.* жа́рить (*на па́лочках*).

planking ['plæŋkɪŋ] *n* доща́тая обши́вка.

planner ['plænə] *n* планиро́вщик; ◊ war ~s поджига́тели войны́.

plant¹ I [plɑːnt] *n* расте́ние; са́женец, расса́да; garden ~ садо́вое расте́ние; in ~ расту́щий, в соку́; to lose ~ засыха́ть.

plant¹ II *v* 1) сажа́ть (*расте́ния*); заса́живать (*with*); 2) внедря́ть (*иде́и, взгля́ды*); насажда́ть (*при́нципы и т. п.*); 3) выпуска́ть малько́в (*для разведе́ния*); 4) устана́вливать; водружа́ть (*зна́мя*); 5) осно́вывать (*коло́нию*); заселя́ть; □ to ~ **out** выса́живать в грунт.

plant² *n* 1) устано́вка, обору́дование; 2) заво́д, фа́брика.

plant³ I *n сленг* 1) надува́тельство, моше́нничество; 2) сы́щик.

plant³ II *v сленг* 1) пря́тать (*добы́чу*); 2) устра́ивать (*махина́ции*).

plantain ['plæntɪn] *n бот.* подоро́жник.

plantation [plæn'teɪʃən] *n* 1) планта́ция; 2) насажде́ние; 3) *ист.* коло́ния.

planter ['plɑːntə] *n* 1) планта́тор; 2) *с.-х.* сажа́лка.

plant-louse ['plɑːnt'laus] *n* тля.

plaque [plɑːk] *n* таре́лка (*как украше́ние*).

plash¹ I [plæʃ] *n* 1) всплеск; 2) лу́жа.

plash¹ II *v* плеска́ть(ся).

plash² *v* плести́ (*плете́нь*); переплета́ть (*ве́тви*).

plashy ['plæʃɪ] *a* 1) боло́тистый, сыро́й; 2) плеска́ющийся.

plasma ['plæzmə] *n* 1) *физиол.* пла́зма; 2) *биол.* протопла́зма; 3) *мин.* зелёный халцедо́н.

plaster I ['plɑːstə] *n* 1) штукату́рка; the ~ of Paris алеба́стр; гипс; 2) пла́стырь; mustard ~ горчи́чник.

plaster II *v* 1) штукату́рить; 2) покрыва́ть, зама́зывать (*алеба́стром*); 3) гру́бо льстить; to ~ with praise осыпа́ть похвала́ми; 4) накла́дывать пла́стырь.

plasterer ['plɑːstərə] *n* штукату́р.

plastic I ['plæstɪk] *n* 1) пластма́сса; 2) пла́стика; пласти́чность.

plastic II *a* 1) пласти́ческий; 2) лепно́й, скульпту́рный; 3) пласти́чный, ги́бкий.

plasticine ['plæstɪsiːn] *n* пластили́н.

plasticity [plæs'tɪsɪtɪ] *n* пласти́чность, ги́бкость.

plastron ['plæstrən] *n* 1) *ист.* ла́тный нагру́дник; 2) мани́шка.

plat I [plæt] *n* 1) (небольшо́й) уча́сток земли́; 2) *амер.* план, ка́рта.

plat II *v амер.* снима́ть план.

platan ['plætən] *см.* plane³.

plate I [pleɪt] *n* 1) таре́лка; 2) посу́да, серви́ровка; 3) пласти́нка; доще́чка (*тж. на двери́ с фами́лией*); 4) эста́мп; гравю́ра; 5) иллюстра́ция (*на отде́льном листе́*); 6) фотопласти́нка; 7) *полигр.* стереоти́п, печа́тная фо́рма; 8) *эл.* ано́д; 9) приз, ку́бок; 10) вставна́я че́люсть.

plate II *v* 1) брони́ровать, покрыва́ть бронёй; 2) золоти́ть, серебри́ть, никелирова́ть; 3) *полигр.* стереотипи́ровать.

plateau ['plætou] *n* (*pl тж.* plateaux) плато́, плоскогорье.

plateful ['pleɪtful] *n* по́лная таре́лка (*чего́-л.*).

platform ['plætfɔːm] *n* 1) платфо́рма; перро́н; 2) трибу́на; сце́на; 3) площа́дка (*ле́стницы, ваго́на и т. п.*); space ~ косми́ческая ста́нция (*или* платфо́рма); 4) полити́ческая платфо́рма, пози́ция; 5) оруди́йная площа́дка; 6) пло́ская возвы́шенность.

plating ['pleɪtɪŋ] *n* никелиро́вка, золоче́ние, серебре́ние.

platinum ['plætɪnəm] *n хим.* 1) пла́тина; 2) *attr* пла́тиновый.

platitude ['plætɪtjuːd] *n* бана́льность, по́шлость.

platitudinous [,plætɪ'tjuːdɪnəs] *a* по́шлый, пло́ский.

platoon [plə'tuːn] *n* 1) *воен.* взвод; 2) (полице́йский) отря́д.

plaudits ['plɔːdɪts] *n pl* рукоплеска́ния, аплодисме́нты; ова́ции.

plausibility [,plɔːzə'bɪlɪtɪ] *n* вероя́тность, правдоподо́бие.

plausible ['plɔːzəbl] *a* 1) вероя́тный, правдоподо́бный; 2) уме́ющий внуша́ть дове́рие.

play I [pleɪ] *n* 1) игра́; to be at ~ игра́ть; out of ~ вне игры́; fair ~ че́стный посту́пок; the ~ of fancy игра́ воображе́ния; ~ of words пустосло́вие, игра́ слова́ми; ~ on words игра́ слов, каламбу́р; a child's ~ пустяко́вое де́ло; «де́тская игра́»; 2) пье́са, спекта́кль; to go to the ~ идти́ в теа́тр; to produce a ~ (по)ста́вить пье́су; how long will this ~ run? как до́лго бу́дет идти́ э́та пье́са?; miracle ~ средневеко́вая мисте́рия; 3) шу́тка, каламбу́р; in ~ в шу́тку; 4) де́йствие, движе́ние; to bring (*или* to call) into ~ приводи́ть в де́йствие, пуска́ть в ход; to come into ~ вступа́ть в де́йствие, начина́ть де́йствовать; to make ~ де́йствовать реши́тельно; 5) перели́вы (*кра́сок*); плеск (*воды́*); 6) просто́р, свобо́да де́йствий.

play II *v* 1) игра́ть; to ~ **high** *см.* high II ◊; to ~ **fair** поступа́ть че́стно; to ~ **foul** поступа́ть нече́стно, жу́льничать; to ~ **into** smb.'s hands игра́ть на́ руку кому́-л.; to ~ **(up)on** smb.'s feelings игра́ть на чьих-л. чу́вствах; to ~ smb. false преда́ть кого́-л.; поки́нуть кого́-л. в беде́; to ~ fast and loose вести́ себя́ безотве́тственно; не выполня́ть обяза́тельств; вести́ двойну́ю игру́; 2) исполня́ть (*роль, муз. произведение*); 3) выезжа́ть на гастро́ли; 4) забавля́ться, резви́ться; 5) ходи́ть (*шашкой, картой*); 6) свобо́дно дви́гаться (*о механизме*); 7) приводи́ть в де́йствие; 8) бить (*о фонтане*); 9) перелива́ться (*о свете, красках*); □ to ~ off a) разы́грывать, дура́чить (*кого́-л.*); б) натра́вливать; to ~ off one person against another стра́вливать кого́-л.; to ~ **out**: to be ~ed out вы́дохнуться (*о человеке*); to ~ up a) де́ятельно уча́ствовать (*в разговоре, действиях*); б): to ~ smb. up a) дразни́ть, издева́ться над кем-л.; б) *амер.* испо́льзовать (*кого́-л.*); в): to ~ up to поды́грывать; *перен.* подли́зываться к кому́-л.

playable ['pleɪəbl] *a* го́дный, подходя́щий для игры́.

play-actor ['pleɪˌæktə] n 1) *пренебр.* актёр; 2) неи́скренний челове́к.

play-bill ['pleɪbɪl] *n* афи́ша; програ́мма (*театра́льная*).

play-book ['pleɪbuk] *n* сбо́рник пьес.

play-boy ['pleɪbɔɪ] *n* пове́са.

play-day ['pleɪdeɪ] *n* 1) пра́здник (*для шко́льников*); 2) нерабо́чий день (*из-за отсутствия работы*).

played-out ['pleɪd'aut] *a разг.* измо́танный, вы́дохшийся.

player ['pleɪə] *n* 1) игра́ющий; игро́к; 2) актёр; музыка́нт; 3) пиано́ла.

playfellow ['pleɪˌfelou] *n* друг де́тства; (со)това́рищ.

play-field ['pleɪfiːld] *n* спорти́вная площа́дка.

playful ['pleɪful] *a* 1) игри́вый; шаловли́вый; 2) шутли́вый; ирони́ческий.

playfulness ['pleɪfulnɪs] *n* игри́вость.

playgame ['pleɪgeɪm] *n*: it is a ~! э́то ерунда́!, пусто́е де́ло!

playgoer ['pleɪˌgouə] *n* театра́л; зри́тель.

playground ['pleɪgraund] *n* площа́дка (*для игр*), спорти́вная площа́дка.

playhouse ['pleɪhaus] *n* 1) драмати́ческий теа́тр; 2) *амер.* игру́шечный до́мик; 3) *амер.* до́мик для игр (*на детской площадке*).

playing-card ['pleɪɪŋ'kɑːd] *n* игра́льная ка́рта.

playing-field ['pleɪɪŋfiːld] *n* спорти́вная площа́дка, стадио́н.

playlet ['pleɪlɪt] *n* небольша́я пье́са.

playmate ['pleɪmeɪt] *n* 1) друг де́тства; 2) партнёр (*в спортивных играх*).

plaything ['pleɪθɪŋ] *n* игру́шка.

playtime ['pleɪtaɪm] *n* вре́мя о́тдыха, развлече́ния.

playwright ['pleɪraɪt] *n* драмату́рг.

plea [pliː] *n* 1) оправда́ние; 2) до́вод; 3) заявле́ние (*защитника или подсудимого*); to hold ~s подава́ть в суд; 4) про́сьба; мольба́; a ~ for mercy про́сьба о поми́ловании.

plead [pliːd] *v* 1) обраща́ться с про́сьбой; 2) ходáтайствовать (*за кого́-л.— for*); 3) отста́ивать (*что-л.— for*); выступа́ть про́тив (*чего́-л.— against*); 4) де́лать заявле́ние (*на суде*); to ~ (not) guilty (не) призна́ть себя́ вино́вным; 5) выступа́ть в ка́честве адвока́та; защища́ть; 6) ссыла́ться на.

pleader ['pliːdə] *n* защи́тник, адвока́т.

pleading ['pliːdɪŋ] *n* 1) засту́пничество, хода́тайство; 2) *pl юр.* состяза́тельные бума́ги; 3) *юр.* заявле́ние истца́ и отве́тчика; 4) *юр.* судогово́ре́ние.

pleasant ['pleznt] *a* 1) прия́тный; 2) сла́вный, ми́лый; 3) хоро́ший (*о погоде*); 4) весёлый, оживлённый; 5) *уст.* шутли́вый.

pleasantly ['plezntlɪ] *adv* 1) любе́зно; 2) ве́село.

pleasantness ['plezntnɪs] *n* 1) прия́тность; 2) прия́тные ка́чества.

pleasantry ['plezntrɪ] *n* 1) доброду́шная шу́тка; ю́мор; 2) шутли́вое замеча́ние;·коми́ческая вы́ходка.

please [pliːz] *v* 1) нра́виться; 2) *pass:* to be ~d with быть дово́льным чем-л.; as ~d as Punch чрезвыча́йно дово́лен; 3) угожда́ть; ра́довать; 4) соблаговоли́ть; изво́лить; 5): (if you) ~ пожа́луйста; in his pocket, if you ~, was a letter!·в его́ карма́не, изво́лите ли ви́деть, бы́ло письмо́!

pleasing ['pliːzɪŋ] *a* 1) прия́тный, доставля́ющий удово́льствие; 2) привлека́тельный, нра́вящийся.

pleasurable ['pleʒərəbl] *a* доставля́ющий удово́льствие, наслажде́ние; прия́тный.

pleasure I ['pleʒə] *n* 1) удово́льствие, наслажде́ние; развлече́ние; it gives me much ~ э́то доставля́ет мне большо́е удово́льствие; to take ~ in наслажда́ться, испы́тывать удово́льствие; may we have the ~ of your company? a) разреши́те соста́вить вам компа́нию!; б) позво́льте вас пригласи́ть!; it's a ~ не сто́ит благода́рности, пожа́луйста (*в ответ на благодарность*); 2) во́ля, соизволе́ние; at ~ по жела́нию; 3) *attr* увесели́тельный.

pleasure II *v* 1) наслажда́ться, испы́тывать удово́льствие; 2) *разг.* иска́ть развлече́ний.

pleasure-boat ['pleʒəbout] *n* прогу́лочная шлю́пка, прогу́лочный ка́тер.

pleasure-ground ['pleʒəgraund] *n* 1) площа́дка для игр; спортплоща́дка; 2) парк.

pleat I [pliːt] *n* скла́дка.

pleat II *v* де́лать скла́дки.

pleb [pleb] *разг. см.* plebeian I.

plebeian I [plɪ'biːən] *n* плебе́й.

plebeian II *a* плебе́йский.

plebiscite ['plebɪsɪt] *n* плебисци́т.

pledge I [pledʒ] *n* 1) зало́г, закла́д; to put in ~ заложи́ть; to take out of ~ вы́купить из закла́да; the ~ of love, the ~ of union плод любви́, ребёнок; 2) поручи́тельство; 3) тост; 4) (торже́ственное) обеща́ние; заро́к; under ~ of secrecy заро́к сохрани́ть та́йну; election ~s предвы́борные обеща́ния; to take the ~ дать заро́к воздержа́ния.

pledge II *v* 1) закла́дывать; 2) руча́ться; обеща́ть; 3) обя́зываться; 4) пить за здоро́вье (*кого́-л.*).

plenary ['pliːnərɪ] *a* 1) по́лный, абсолю́тный, неограни́ченный; 2) плена́рный (*о заседании*).

plenipotent [plə'nɪpətənt] *см.* plenipotentiary II.

plenipotentiary I [ˌplenɪpə'tenʃərɪ] *n* полномо́чный представи́тель.

plenipotentiary II *a* полномо́чный.

plenitude ['plenɪtjuːd] *n* 1) полнота́; изоби́лие; 2) расцве́т (*сил*).

plenteous ['plentjəs] *a* оби́льный; урожа́йный.

plentiful ['plentiful] *a* 1) оби́льный, изоби́льный; 2) бога́тый (*чем-л.*); 3) плодоро́дный.

plenty I ['plentı] *n* 1) обилие, изобилие; ~ of много; ~ more ещё очень много; 2) избыток; in ~ в избытке.

plenty II *adv* вполне, довольно.

plenum ['pli:nəm] *n* пленум.

pleura ['pluərə] *n* плевра.

pleurisy ['pluərısı] *n мед.* плеврит.

pliability [,plaıə'bılıtı] *n* 1) гибкость; 2) уступчивость, податливость.

pliable ['plaıəbl] *a* 1) гибкий; 2) податливый, уступчивый.

pliant ['plaıənt] *a* 1) гибкий; 2) мягкий, уступчивый.

pliers ['plaıəz] *n pl* плоскогубцы.

plight[1] [plaıt] *n* бедственное, тяжёлое положение; in a sad (*или* sorry) ~ в тяжёлом состоянии; in an evil ~ в скверном положении; in a wretched ~ в бедственном положении.

plight[2] I *n* 1) обещание; 2) помолвка.

plight[2] II *v* 1) давать обещание; 2) помолвить.

plinth [plınθ] *n* плинтус; цоколь.

plod I [plɔd] *n* 1) тяжёлый труд; 2) тяжёлая походка.

plod II *v* 1) брести, тащиться (*часто* to ~ along); 2) корпеть (*над чем-л.* — at).

plodder ['plɔdə] *n разг.* усидчивый человек.

plodding ['plɔdıŋ] *a* усидчивый, трудолюбивый, работающий много.

plop I [plɔp] *n* всплеск; шлёпанье (*по воде*).

plop II *v* бултыхнуться, шлёпнуться (*в воду*).

plop III *int* бултых!, шлёп!

plosion ['plouʒən] *n фон.* взрыв.

plosive I ['plousıv] *n фон.* взрывной согласный.

plosive II *a фон.* взрывной (*о согласном звуке*).

plot[1] I [plɔt] *n* фабула, сюжет.

plot[1] II *v* набрасывать сюжет.

plot[2] I *n* заговор; to discover a ~ раскрыть заговор; to nip a ~ пресечь заговор.

plot[2] II *v* 1) замышлять, интриговать, строить козни; 2) устраивать заговор.

plot[3] I *n* 1) участок (*земли*); a potato ~ картофельное поле; 2) *амер.* план, чертёж.

plot[3] II *v* 1) составлять план, чертёж; 2) наносить на карту, чертёж; 3) делить землю на участки (*тж.* to ~ out).

plotter ['plɔtə] *n* заговорщик; интриган.

plough I [plau] *n* 1) плуг; 2) снегоочиститель; 3) пашня; 4) *сленг* провал (*на экзамене*); 5) (the P.) Большая Медведица (*созвездие*).

plough II *v* 1) пахать; 2) проводить борозду; 3) бороздить (*море и т. п.*); рассекать (*волны*); 4) *разг.* провалиться (*на экзамене*), «засыпаться»; □ to ~ **through** a) продвигаться с трудом; б) одолеть (*книгу*); to ~ **up** взрыхлять (*землю*); вспахивать.

ploughman ['plaumən] *n* пахарь.

ploughshare ['plauʃɛə] *n с.-х.* лемех.

plow I, II [plau] *амер. см.* plough I, II.

pluck I [plʌk] *n* 1) дерганье; 2) потроха, ливер; 3) мужество, отвага; full of ~ отважный.

pluck II *v* 1) собирать, рвать (*цветы*); 2) ощипывать (*птицу*); 3) выдёргивать (*волосы*); 4) *разг.* обобрать, ограбить; 5) *разг.* провалить (*на экзамене*), «засыпать»; 6) перебирать (*струны*); 7) хвататься за (*at*); □ to ~ **away** выдирать, выдёргивать; to ~ **out**, to ~ **up** *уст.* вырывать; искоренять.

plucky ['plʌkı] *a* отважный, смелый.

plug I [plʌg] *n* 1) затычка; пробка; 2) *эл.* штепсель; 3) запальная свеча; 4) прессованный табак (*для жевания*); 5) *амер. разг.* кляча.

plug II *v* 1) затыкать; закупоривать; 2) *разг.* усидчиво работать; корпеть (*тж.* to ~ away); 3) *разг.* ударять, стрелять; □ to ~ **in** вставлять штепсель; to ~ **up** закупоривать.

plug-switch ['plʌgswıtʃ] *n* штепсельный выключатель.

plug-ugly ['plʌg,ʌglı] *n амер. разг.* хулиган.

plum [plʌm] *n* 1) слива; French ~ чернослив; 2) сливовое дерево; 3) изюм; 4) тёмно-фиолетовый цвет; 5) *разг.* лакомый кусочек; 6) *attr* сливовый.

plumage ['plu:mıdʒ] *n* оперение.

plumb I [plʌm] *n* 1) грузило; 2) отвес, ватерпас; out of ~ неперпендикулярно; невертикально.

plumb II *a* 1) вертикальный; отвесный; 2) истинный.

plumb III *v* 1) ставить по отвесу; 2) паять; 3) измерять глубину.

plumb IV *adv* 1) вертикально; 2) точно, правильно; 3) *амер. сленг* совершенно, абсолютно.

plumbago [plʌm'beıgou] *n* 1) графит; 2) рисунок в карандаше.

plumbeous ['plʌmbıəs] *a* свинцовый, свинцового цвета.

plumber ['plʌmə] *n* 1) водопроводчик; 2) паяльщик.

plumbery ['plʌmərı] *n* 1) водопроводное дело; 2) паяльная мастерская.

plumbic ['plʌmbık] *a хим.* свинцовый.

plumbing ['plʌmıŋ] *n* 1) водопроводное дело; 2) водопровод, водопроводная система; 3) измерение глубины; забрасывание лота.

plumbum ['plʌmbəm] *n* свинец.

plum-duff ['plʌmdʌf] *n* пудинг с коринкой.

plume I [plu:m] *n* 1) перо; in borrowed ~s ≅ «в павлиньих перьях»; 2) султан, плюмаж.

plume II *v* 1) оправлять перья (*о птице*); 2) украшать перьями, плюмажем; 3): to ~ oneself on кичиться, задирать нос.

plummet ['plʌmıt] *n* 1) свинцовый отвес; 2) грузило (*удочки*).

plummy ['plʌmı] *a разг.* завидный; хороший, выгодный.

plump[1] I [plʌmp] *a* полный, толстый, пухлый.

plump[1] II *v* полнеть, толстеть (*тж.* to ~ up, to ~ out); □ to ~ **up** взбивать (*подушки*).

plump[2] I *n* неожиданное падение.

plump[2] II *a* прямой, категорический.

plump[2] III *v* 1) грохнуться, шлёпнуться; 2) голосовать только за одного кандидата (*на выборах*); 3) вваливаться (*часто* upon, into); нагрянуть.

plump[2] IV *adv* 1) внезапно; 2) прямо, напрямик.

plum-pudding ['plʌm'pudıŋ] *n* (рождественский) пудинг.

plumy ['plu:mı] *a* 1) покрытый перьями; 2) украшенный султаном, плюмажем.

plunder I ['plʌndə] *n* 1) грабёж, разграбление; 2) добыча; награбленное имущество.

plunder II *v* грабить; расхищать.

plunderer ['plʌndərə] *n* грабитель.

plunge I [plʌndʒ] *n* 1) погружение, окунание;

2) ныря́ние; ◇ to take the ~ сде́лать реши́тельный шаг.

plunge II *v* 1) погружа́ть(ся), окуна́ть(ся); 2) вонза́ть (*кинжал, шпагу*); 3) вверга́ть (*в войну, нищету*); доводи́ть (*до нищеты*); 4) ныря́ть; 5) броса́ться вперёд; 6) *разг.* аза́ртно игра́ть; рискова́ть; 7) залеза́ть в долги́; 8) обрыва́ться (*о скале, дороге*).

plunger ['plʌndʒə] *n* 1) *разг.* аза́ртный игро́к; 2) водола́з; 3) *тех.* плу́нжер, ска́льчатый по́ршень.

plunging ['plʌndʒɪŋ] *a* 1) ныря́ющий, погружа́ющийся; 2) *воен.* навесно́й (*об огне*).

plunk I [plʌŋk] *n* звон (*струн*).

plunk II *v* 1) перебира́ть (*струны*); 2) звене́ть (*о струне*); 3) шлёпаться; 4) *разг.* провали́ться, «засы́паться» (*на экзамене*).

pluperfect I ['pluː'pəːfɪkt] *n грам.* предпрошéдшая фо́рма проше́дшего вре́мени.

pluperfect II *a грам.* предпрошéдший.

plural I ['pluərəl] *n грам.* мно́жественное число́.

plural II *a* мно́жественный; многочи́сленный.

plurality [pluə'rælɪtɪ] *n* 1) мно́жественность; 2) большинство́ голосо́в; 3) совмести́тельство.

plus I [plʌs] *n* 1) знак плюс; 2) положи́тельная величина́.

plus II *a* 1) доба́вочный; 2) положи́тельный (*о величине, электри́ческом заря́де*).

plus III *prep* плюс.

plus-fours ['plʌs'fɔːz] *n pl* брю́ки гольф.

plush [plʌʃ] *n* 1) плюш, плис; 2) *attr* плю́шевый, пли́совый.

plushy ['plʌʃɪ] *a* барха́тистый.

plutocracy [pluː'tɔkrəsɪ] *n* плутокра́тия.

plutocrat ['pluːtəkræt] *n* плутокра́т.

pluviometer [ˌpluːvɪ'ɔmɪtə] *n* дождеме́р.

pluvious ['pluːvjəs] *a* дождли́вый.

ply[1] [plaɪ] *v* 1) усе́рдно рабо́тать; занима́ться (*рабо́той, ремесло́м*); 2) по́тчевать, угоща́ть; 3) засыпа́ть (*вопро́сами*); 4) подбра́сывать (*дрова́*); 5) подхлёстывать (*лошаде́й*); 6) курси́ровать (*о парохо́де, автомоби́ле*); 7) *мор.* лави́ровать.

ply[2] *n* 1) скла́дка; слой; 2) вито́к (*верёвки*); 3) скло́нность, жи́лка, спосо́бность.

ply-wood ['plaɪwud] *n* фане́ра.

pneumatic I [njuː'mætɪk] *n* пневмати́ческая ши́на.

pneumatic II *a* пневмати́ческий, возду́шный.

pneumatics [njuː'mætɪks] *n* пневма́тика.

pneumonia [njuː'mounjə] *n* воспале́ние лёгких, пневмони́я.

poach[1] [poutʃ] *v* вари́ть я́йца без скорлупы́.

poach[2] *v* 1) занима́ться браконье́рством, незако́нно охо́титься; 2) вме́шиваться; to ~ on smb.'s preserves вме́шиваться в чьи-л. дела́; 3) выта́птывать (*траву́*) на чужо́й земле́; 4) мять (*гли́ну*).

pock [pɔk] *n* о́спина.

pocket I ['pɔkɪt] *n* 1) карма́н; карма́шек; to have smb. in one's ~ держа́ть кого́-л. под свои́м влия́нием; to pick a ~ вы́тащить, укра́сть из карма́на; 2) де́ньги; empty ~(s) безде́нежье; deep ~(s) состоя́тельность; to be in ~ нажи́ть де́ньги; to be out of ~ потеря́ть де́ньги (*в сде́лке*); терпе́ть убы́тки; 3) мешо́к; 4) лу́за (*билья́рда*); 5) ларь, бу́нкер; 6) *ав.* возду́шная я́ма; 7) *горн.* карма́н, гнездо́; 8) *attr* карма́нный.

pocket II *v* 1) класть в карма́н; 2) присва́ивать;

прикарма́нивать; 3) загоня́ть шар (*в лу́зу*); 4) *амер.* положи́ть под сукно́.

pocket-book ['pɔkɪtbuk] *n* 1) карма́нная записна́я кни́жка; 2) бума́жник.

pocketful ['pɔkɪtful] *a* по́лный карма́н (*чего́-л.*).

pocket-knife ['pɔkɪtnaɪf] *n* карма́нный нож.

pocket-money ['pɔkɪtˌmʌnɪ] *n* карма́нные де́ньги.

pock-mark ['pɔkmɑːk] *n* ряби́на (*на лице́*).

pock-marked ['pɔkmɑːkt] *a* рябо́й.

pod[1] I [pɔd] *n* 1) стручо́к; 2) ко́кон.

pod[1] II *v* 1) лущи́ть, шелуши́ть; 2) покрыва́ться стручка́ми.

pod[2] *n* 1) небольшо́е ста́до (*кито́в, морже́й*); 2) ста́йка (*птиц*).

podded ['pɔdɪd] *a* 1) стручко́вый; 2) состоя́тельный, зажи́точный.

podgy ['pɔdʒɪ] *a разг.* ни́зенький и то́лстый.

poem ['pouɪm] *n* 1) стихотворе́ние; 2) поэ́ма.

poesy ['pouɪzɪ] *n* поэ́зия.

poet ['pouɪt] *n* поэ́т; ~ laureate поэ́т-лауреа́т; придво́рный поэ́т; lake ~s поэ́ты «озёрной шко́лы» (*Во́рдсворт, Ко́льридж, Са́ути*).

poetaster [ˌpouɪ'tæstə] *n* рифмоплёт.

poetess ['pouɪtɪs] *n* поэте́сса.

poetic(al) [pou'etɪk(əl)] *a* поэти́ческий; стихотво́рный.

poetics [pou'etɪks] *n* поэ́тика.

poetry ['pouɪtrɪ] *n* поэ́зия, стихи́.

poignancy ['pɔɪnənsɪ] *n* 1) острота́; 2) ко́лкость; пика́нтность; 3) ре́зкость (*бо́ли*); 4) прони ца́тельность; острота́ (*пережива́ний, воспомина́ний*).

poignant ['pɔɪnənt] *a* 1) о́стрый; 2) ко́лкий; е́дкий; 3) ре́зкий (*о бо́ли*); 4) го́рький (*о слеза́х*); мучи́тельный (*о воспомина́ниях*); 5) проница́тельный; 6) живо́й (*об интере́се*).

poignantly ['pɔɪnəntlɪ] *adv* 1) о́стро, ко́лко, е́дко; 2) мучи́тельно.

point I [pɔɪnt] *n* 1) то́чка; five ~ seven (5.7) пять це́лых семь деся́тых; ~ of interrogation вопроси́тельный знак; ~ of view то́чка зре́ния; 2) ме́сто, пункт; a ~ of departure отправно́й пункт; cardinal ~s стра́ны све́та; 3) остриё; ко́нчик (*иглы́*); *перен.* грань; at the ~ of the sword вооружённой си́лой, огнём и мечо́м; at the ~ of накану́не, на гра́ни; at the ~ of death при́ смерти; to be on the ~ of + *Gerund* смыслово́го *гл.* собира́ться сде́лать что-л. в ближа́йшем бу́дущем; we are on the ~ of leaving for the Soviet Union мы вско́ре уезжа́ем в Сове́тский Сою́з; 4) выдаю́щаяся часть; мыс; верши́на (*горы́*); 5) суть де́ла; «соль» расска́за; the ~ in question те́ма разгово́ра, обсужде́ния; to come to the ~ дойти́ до су́ти де́ла; to speak to the ~ говори́ть на те́му, по существу́ де́ла; away from (*или* off, beside) the ~ не на те́му, не по существу́; at all ~s во всех отноше́ниях; a ~ of honour де́ло че́сти; I see your ~ я понима́ю, что вы хоти́те сказа́ть (*или* что вы име́ете в виду́); in ~ of fact действи́тельно, факти́чески; in ~ of в отноше́нии, что каса́ется; 6) моме́нт; отде́льная сторона́ како́го-л. явле́ния; to touch upon some ~s in the report затро́нуть в докла́де не́которые моме́нты; 7) черта́; ка́чество; what is his strong ~? в чём он силён?; to make a ~ of + *Gerund* смыслово́го *гл.* положи́ть себе́ за пра́вило; I make a ~ of getting up early я, как пра́вило, встаю ра́но; 8) деле́ние (*термо́метра, ко́мпаса и т. п.*); ~s of the compass ру́мбы (*ка́ждое из 32 деле́ний на кру́ге ко́мпаса*); 9) очко́; to give ~s to smb. дава́ть не́сколько очко́в вперёд (*тж. перен.*); to gain one's ~ доби́ться своего́; дости́гнуть це́ли; 10) *ж.-д.* стре́лочный перево́д; 11) *воен.* головно́й дозо́р; 12) *охот.* сто́йка; to come to a ~ де́лать сто́йку.

point II *v* 1) ука́зывать, пока́зывать (*на — at, to*); 2) наводи́ть (*ору́жие, телеско́п; на — at*); 3) ука́зывать направле́ние (*to*); 4) говори́ть, свиде́тельствовать (*o — to*); 5) точи́ть (*каранда́ш*); 6) расставля́ть зна́ки препина́ния; 7) *охот.* де́лать сто́йку (*о соба́ке*); □ to ~ out ука́зывать; пока́зывать; обраща́ть внима́ние.

point-blank I ['pɔɪnt'blæŋk] *a* 1) произведённый прямо́й наво́дкой (*о вы́стреле*); 2) реши́тельный, категори́ческий.

point-blank II *adv* 1) в упо́р; прямо́й наво́дкой; to fire ~ вы́стрелить в упо́р; 2) реши́тельно, категори́чески, наотре́з.

point-duty ['pɔɪnt,djuːtɪ] *n* регули́рование движе́ния (*на перекрёстках у́лиц*).

pointed ['pɔɪntɪd] *a* 1) остроконе́чный; 2) *архит.* стре́льчатый (*об а́рках, сво́дах*); 3) о́стрый, крити́ческий (*о замеча́нии*); 4) наведённый (*об ору́жии*); 5) подчёркнутый.

pointedly ['pɔɪntɪdlɪ] *adv* 1) о́стро; 2) стара́ясь подчеркну́ть; с осо́бенным выраже́нием; многозначи́тельно.

pointer ['pɔɪntə] *n* 1) стре́лка (*весо́в, часо́в*), указа́тель; ука́зка; 2) по́йнтер (*поро́да соба́к*); 3) намёк; 4) *воен.* наво́дчик.

pointless ['pɔɪntlɪs] *a* 1) неостроу́мный, пло́ский (*об анекдо́те, расска́зе*); 2) бессмы́сленный, бесце́льный; сде́ланный невпопа́д; 3) *спорт.* не вы́игравший ни одного́ очка́, име́ющий ноль на своём счету́; 4) тупо́й.

pointsman ['pɔɪntsmən] *n* 1) стре́лочник; 2) регулиро́вщик.

poise I [pɔɪz] *n* 1) равнове́сие; 2) уравнове́шенность; стаби́льность; 3) поса́дка головы́; оса́нка; 4) нереши́тельность.

poise II *v* 1) баланси́ровать, держа́ть равнове́сие; 2) находи́ться в равнове́сии; 3) уравнове́шивать (*в во́здухе*).

poison I ['pɔɪzn] *n* 1) яд; отра́ва; to hate like ~ бе́шено ненави́деть; 2) *attr* ядови́тый; 3) *attr* отравля́ющий (*о вещество́*).

poison II *v* 1) отравля́ть, трави́ть; 2) *воен.* заража́ть (*ме́стность*); 3) по́ртить, развраща́ть.

poisoner ['pɔɪznə] *n* отрави́тель.

poisoning ['pɔɪznɪŋ] *n* 1) отравле́ние; 2) *воен.* заражé́ние (*ме́стности*); 3) по́рча, развраще́ние.

poisonous ['pɔɪznəs] *a* 1) ядови́тый; 2) *разг.* отврати́тельный.

poke I [pouk] *n* 1) толчо́к, тычо́к; 2) *разг.* ло́дырь, копу́ша.

poke II *v* 1) ты́кать (*па́льцем, па́лкой*), сова́ть (*тж.* to ~ in, up, down); to ~ and pry сова́ть нос не в своё де́ло; to ~ smb. in the ribs слегка́ подта́лкивать; 2) меша́ть (*кочерго́й*); □ to ~ about проявля́ть любопы́тство; to ~ into иссле́довать, разузнава́ть; to ~ through проткну́ть.

poker[1] ['poukə] *n* кочерга́; by the holy ~ шуто́чная кля́тва.

pocker[2] *n карт.* по́кер.

poker-work ['poukəwɜːk] *n* выжига́ние по де́реву.

pok(e)y ['poukɪ] *a* 1) убо́гий, те́сный; 2) неопределённый, случа́йный (*о заня́тии*); 3) безвку́сный, неря́шливый (*об оде́жде*); 4) *амер. разг.* медли́тельный, лени́вый.

polar ['poulə] *a* 1) поля́рный; 2) по́люсный; 3) диаметра́льно противополо́жный.

polarity [pou'lærɪtɪ] *n* 1) *физ.* поля́рность; 2) соверше́нная противополо́жность.

Pole [poul] *n* поля́к; по́лька; the ~s поля́ки.

pole[1] [poul] *n* 1) шест, жердь; 2) столб; under bare ~s a) *мор.* со спу́щенными паруса́ми; б) доведённый до кра́йности (*о челове́ке*); 3) баго́р; 4) ды́шло.

pole[2] *n* по́люс; Arctic (*или* North) ~ Се́верный по́люс; Antarctic (*или* South) ~ Ю́жный по́люс; celestial ~ *астр.* по́люс ми́ра; magnetic ~ магни́тный по́люс; ◊ as far apart as the ~s диаметра́льно противополо́жные.

pole-ax(e) I ['poulæks] *n* 1) *ист.* берды́ш, секи́ра; 2) реза́к (*мясника́*).

pole-ax(e) II *v* наноси́ть уда́р, убива́ть берды́шом, секи́рой.

polecat ['poulkæt] *n* хорёк.

polemic(al) [pə'lemɪk(əl)] *a* полеми́ческий.

polemics [pə'lemɪks] *n* поле́мика.

pole-star ['poulstɑː] *n* Поля́рная звезда́; *перен.* путево́дная звезда́.

police I [pə'liːs] *n* 1) поли́ция; the ~ (*употр. как pl*) полице́йские; mounted ~ ко́нная поли́ция; military ~ вое́нная поли́ция; 2) *attr* полице́йский.

police II *v* подде́рживать поря́док (*в стране́, го́роде*); *перен.* управля́ть.

police-court [pə'liːskɔːt] *n* полице́йский суд (*в Англии*).

policeman [pə'liːsmən] *n* полице́йский, полисме́н.

police-station [pə'liːs'steɪʃən] *n* полице́йский уча́сток.

policy[1] ['pɔlɪsɪ] *n* 1) поли́тика; peace ~ ми́рная поли́тика, поли́тика ми́ра; tough ~ твёрдая поли́тика; a ~ of grab поли́тика захва́тов; a give-and-take ~ поли́тика взаи́мных усту́пок; for reasons of ~ по полити́ческим соображе́ниям; 2) ли́ния поведе́ния, курс; 3) *pl* полити́ческий курс; 4) целесообра́зность, благоразу́мие, дальнови́дность; 5) хи́трость, ло́вкость.

policy[2] *n* 1) по́лис (*страхово́й*); 2) *амер.* аза́ртная игра́.

policy-holder ['pɔlɪsɪ,houldə] *n* владе́лец *или* держа́тель страхово́го по́лиса.

Polish I ['poulɪʃ] *n* по́льский язы́к.

Polish II *a* по́льский.

polish I ['pɔlɪʃ] *n* 1) полиро́вка; 2) лак, политу́ра; мазь для чи́стки; shoe ~ крем для о́буви; 3) лоск; изы́сканность (*мане́р*).

polish II *v* 1) полирова́ть; шлифова́ть; чи́стить о́бувь; 2) отде́лывать (*тж.* to ~ away, off, out); 3) станови́ться гла́дким, шлифо́ванным; 4) улучша́ться (*тж.* to ~ up); □ to ~ off *разг.* разде́латься; бы́стро спра́виться, поко́нчить.

polished ['pɔlɪʃt] *a* 1) полиро́ванный; 2) изы́сканный, элега́нтный; 3) глянцеви́тый.

polite [pə'laɪt] *a* 1) ве́жливый, воспи́танный; 2) изя́щный (*о литерату́ре*); класси́ческий (*об образова́нии*); 3) изы́сканный (*об о́бществе*).

politeness [pə'laɪtnɪs] *n* вежливость, воспитанность.

politic ['pɔlɪtɪk] *a* 1) разумный; обдуманный; 2) ловкий, хитрый; политичный.

political [pə'lɪtɪkəl] *a* политический; государственный.

politician [,pɔlɪ'tɪʃən] *n* 1) политик; государственный деятель; 2) *амер. презр.* политикан.

politico [pə'lɪtɪkou] *n презр.* политикан.

politics ['pɔlɪtɪks] *n* 1) политика; to talk ~ обсуждать вопросы политики; to go into ~ посвятить себя политической деятельности; 2) политические убеждения; what are your ~? каких политических убеждений вы придерживаетесь?

polity ['pɔlɪtɪ] *n* 1) государственное устройство; 2) государство.

Poll [pɔl] *n* попугай, «попка».

pollᵃ I [poul] *n* 1) список избирателей; 2) регистрация избирателей; 3) голосование; баллотировка; 4) число поданных голосов; a heavy (light) ~ высокий (низкий) процент участия в выборах; public opinion ~ опрос общественного мнения; 5) *pl амер.* избирательный пункт; 6) *шутл.* голова, затылок.

pollᵃ II *v* 1) регистрировать избирателей; 2) голосовать; 3) подсчитывать голоса; 4) подстригать.

pollᵇ [pɔl] *n*: the ~ *унив. сленг* студенты, окончившие Кембриджский университет без отличия; to go out in the ~ получить степень без отличия.

pollard ['pɔləd] *n* подстриженное дерево.

pollen ['pɔlɪn] *n бот.* пыльца.

polling ['poulɪŋ] *n* голосование; gallop ~ *амер.* опрос населения с целью выявления общественного мнения.

polling-booth ['poulɪŋbuːð] *n* кабина для голосования.

polling-centre ['poulɪŋ,sentə] *n* избирательный пункт, участок.

pollster ['poulstə] *n* человек, проводящий опрос общественного мнения.

poll-tax ['poultæks] *n* подушный налог.

pollute [pə'luːt] *v* 1) осквернять; 2) загрязнять; 3) развращать.

pollution [pə'luːʃən] *n* 1) осквернение; 2) загрязнение; 3) *физиол.* поллюция.

polo ['poulou] *n спорт.* поло; water ~ водное поло.

polonium [pə'lounɪəm] *n хим.* полоний.

poltroon [pɔl'truːn] *n* трус.

poly- ['pɔlɪ-] *pref со значением* много-; polychrome полихромный, многоцветный.

polychromatic [,pɔlɪkrə'mætɪk] *a* многоцветный, многокрасочный.

polygamy [pɔ'lɪgəmɪ] *n* многобрачие, полигамия.

polyphony [pə'lɪfənɪ] *n муз., фон.* полифония.

polysemantic ['pɔlɪsɪ'mæntɪk] *a* многозначный.

polysemy ['pɔlɪsɪmɪ] *n* многозначность.

polysyllabic ['pɔlɪsɪ'læbɪk] *a* многосложный.

polysyllable ['pɔlɪ,sɪləbl] *n* многосложное слово.

polytechnic I [,pɔlɪ'teknɪk] *n* политехникум.

polytechnic II *a* политехнический.

polyvalent [pɔ'lɪvələnt] *a хим.* многовалентный.

pomade [pə'mɑːd] *n* помада.

pomegranate ['pɔm,grænɪt] *n бот.* гранат.

Pomeranian [,pɔmə'reɪnjən] *n* шпиц (*порода собак*).

pomp [pɔmp] *n* пышность, помпа.

pomposity [pɔm'pɔsɪtɪ] *n* напыщенность, помпезность.

pompous ['pɔmpəs] *a* 1) напыщенный; 2) пышный, помпезный.

poncho ['pɔntʃou] *n* пончо (*южноамериканский плащ*).

pond I [pɔnd] *n* 1) пруд; водоём, бассейн; the ~ catches пруд замёрз; 2) садок (*для разведения рыбы*).

pond II *v* запруживать.

ponder ['pɔndə] *v* размышлять; тщательно обдумывать; взвешивать (*тж.* to ~ on, to ~ over).

ponderable ['pɔndərəbl] *a* весомый, материальный.

ponderous ['pɔndərəs] *a* 1) увесистый; 2) тяжеловесный; 3) тяжёлый (*о стиле*); нудный.

ponderously ['pɔndərəslɪ] *adv* тяжело, тяжеловесно.

pongee [pɔn'dʒiː] *n* чесуча (*ткань*).

pontiff ['pɔntɪf] *n* 1) папа (римский); 2) архиерей; 3) первосвященник.

pontoon¹ [pɔn'tuːn] *n* 1) понтон; понтонный мост; 2) плавучий док; 3) кессон; 4) поплавок (*гидросамолёта*).

pontoon² *n карт.* двадцать одно, «очко».

pony I ['pounɪ] *n* 1) пони; 2) *сленг* 25 фунтов стерлингов; 3) *амер.* шпаргалка; 4) *разг.* стопка вина.

pony II *v амер.* готовить уроки по шпаргалке.

poodle ['puːdl] *n* пудель.

pooh [pu] *int* фу!, вздор!, чепуха!

pooh-pooh [puː'puː] *v* высмеивать; отзываться с презрением.

pool¹ [puːl] *n* 1) лужа; 2) небольшой пруд; 3) омут; 4) бассейн; swimming ~ плавательный бассейн; the Pool название Темзы на протяжении нескольких миль ниже Лондонского моста.

pool² I *n* 1) соглашение между предпринимателями для устранения конкуренции; 2) объединение капиталов (*в интересах финансовых кругов*); 3) бюро; translator's ~ бюро переводчиков; typist ~ машинное бюро; motor ~ *амер.* автопарк; 4) *карт.* пулька; 5) пул (*американский вид бильярда*).

pool² II *v* 1) обмениваться (*опытом, информацией и т. п.*); 2) объединять капиталы; 3) организовывать дело на паях.

poolroom ['puːlrum] *n амер.* помещение для игры в пул.

poop¹ I [puːp] *n* корма, ют.

poop¹ II *v* 1) захлёстывать корму (*о волне*); 2) зачерпнуть кормой.

poop² *n сленг* дурень, балда.

poor I [puə] *a* 1) бедный, неимущий; 2) несчастный, бедный, вызывающий сожаление; 3) плохой (*о знаниях, специалисте и т. п.*); 4) дешёвый, незатейливый, простой; 5) жалкий, невзрачный; 6) неплодородный, тощий (*о почве*); 7) низкий, плохой (*об урожае, качестве*); 8) скудный, ничтожный (*о заработке и т. п.*); недостаточный (*о пище*); 9) бледный, слабый (*о речи, выступ-*

лении); малоинтере́сный; ◇ as ~ as a church mouse *погов.* ≅ бе́ден как церко́вная кры́са.

poor II *n*: the ~ (*употр. как pl*) беднота́, бе́дные, неиму́щие.

poor-house ['puəhaus] *n* богаде́льня; рабо́тный дом.

poor-law ['puəlɔ:] *n* зако́н об оказа́нии по́мощи бе́дным.

poorly I ['puəlɪ] *a*: she is very ~ today ей сего́дня о́чень нездоро́вится, ей не по себе́.

poorly II *adv* пло́хо, недоста́точно; нева́жно; he is very ~ off его́ де́нежные дела́ пло́хи.

poorness ['puənɪs] *n* ску́дость (*тж. почвы*); недоста́точность.

poor-spirited ['puə'spɪrɪtɪd] *a* трусли́вый, малоду́шный.

pop[1] I [pɔp] *n* 1) отры́вистый звук (*как от выскочившей пробки*); 2) вы́стрел; 3) *разг.* шипу́чий напи́ток; 4) *сленг*: in ~ в закла́де.

pop[1] II *v* 1) хло́пнуть, вы́стрелить (*тж. о бутылке с шипучим напитком*); 2) тре́скаться (*о каштанах и т. п.*); 3) неожи́данно появи́ться, прийти́; to ~ in and out бе́гать взад и вперёд; 4) су́нуть (*into*); 5) *сленг* заложи́ть, отда́ть в закла́д; □ to ~ in загляну́ть.

pop[1] III *adv* неожи́данно, внеза́пно; to go ~ взорва́ться.

pop[1] IV *int* хлоп!

pop[2] I *n разг.* популя́рный конце́рт.

pop[2] II *a разг.* популя́рный.

pop-corn ['pɔpkɔn] *n* возду́шная кукуру́за.

pope [poup] *n* 1) па́па (*ри́мский*); 2) свяще́нник.

pop-gun ['pɔpgʌn] *n* 1) хлопу́шка (*игрушка*); 2) духово́е ружьё.

popinjay ['pɔpɪndʒeɪ] *n* фат, щёголь.

poplar ['pɔplə] *n* то́поль; trembling ~ оси́на.

poplin ['pɔplɪn] *n* попли́н (*ткань*).

popover ['pɔp,ouvə] *n* по́нчик.

popple I ['pɔpl] *n* плеска́ние, плеск.

popple II *v* 1) плеска́ться; 2) бурли́ть, вскипа́ть (*о воде*).

poppy ['pɔpɪ] *n* 1) мак; 2) *attr* ма́ковый.

poppy-cock ['pɔpɪkɔk] *n амер. разг.* ерунда́, чушь.

populace ['pɔpjuləs] *n* просто́й наро́д.

popular ['pɔpjulə] *a* 1) наро́дный; 2) популя́рный; he is ~ with the students он по́льзуется популя́рностью среди́ студе́нтов; 3) общедосту́пный.

popularity [,pɔpju'lærɪtɪ] *n* популя́рность.

popularize ['pɔpjuləraɪz] *v* популяризи́ровать.

popularly ['pɔpjuləlɪ] *adv* всем наро́дом; всенаро́дно.

populate ['pɔpjuleɪt] *v* населя́ть; заселя́ть; densely (scarcely) ~d гу́сто- (ре́дко-, ма́ло-) населённый.

population [,pɔpju'leɪʃən] *n* 1) населе́ние, жи́тели; resident (floating, surplus) ~ постоя́нное (теку́щее, избы́точное) населе́ние; 2) заселе́ние.

populous ['pɔpjuləs] *a* густонаселённый, лю́дный.

porcelain ['pɔ:slɪn] *n* 1) фарфо́р; 2) фарфо́ровая вещь; 3) *attr* фарфо́ровый.

porch [pɔ:tʃ] *n* 1) по́ртик, кры́тая галере́я; 2) подъе́зд, крыльцо́; 3) *амер.* вера́нда, терра́са.

porcine ['pɔ:saɪn] *a* свино́й.

porcupine ['pɔ:kjupaɪn] *n* дикобра́з.

pore[1] [pɔ:] *v* 1) размышля́ть (*над чем-л. — over, on, upon*); 2) сосредото́ченно гляде́ть (*на что-л. — at*); 3) вчи́тываться.

pore[2] *n* по́ра; отве́рстие.

pork [pɔ:k] *n* 1) свини́на; 2) *attr* сде́ланный из свини́ны, свино́й.

porky ['pɔ:kɪ] *a* 1) свино́й; 2) *разг.* жи́рный, мяси́стый.

porosity [pɔ:'rɔsɪtɪ] *n* по́ристость.

porous ['pɔ:rəs] *a* по́ристый.

porpoise ['pɔ:pəs] *n* дельфи́н.

porridge ['pɔrɪdʒ] *n* (овся́ная) ка́ша; ◇ to keep one's breath to cool one's ~ пома́лкивать, держа́ть своё мне́ние при себе́.

porringer ['pɔrɪndʒə] *n* ми́сочка.

port[1] [pɔ:t] *n* 1) порт, га́вань; free ~ откры́тый порт; close ~ порт на реке́; ~ of destination (*или* of entry, of call) порт назначе́ния; treaty ~ порт, откры́тый для торго́вли в си́лу междунаро́дных соглаше́ний; 2) прию́т, убе́жище; any ~ in a storm ≅ в беде́ любо́й вы́ход хоро́ш; 3) *attr* портово́й.

port[2] I *n* 1) *мор.* порт, по́ртик (*отверстие в борту*); viewing ~ *косм.* иллюмина́тор; 2) ле́вый борт; 3) *attr* ле́вый.

port[2] II *v мор.* класть (*руля́*) нале́во.

port[3] *n* оса́нка, мане́ра держа́ться.

port[4] *n* портве́йн.

portability [,pɔ:tə'bɪlɪtɪ] *n* портати́вность.

portable ['pɔ:təbl] *a* 1) портати́вный, перено́сный; разбо́рный; 2) дви́жимый (*об имуществе*).

portage I ['pɔ:tɪdʒ] *n* 1) перево́зка, транспорти́ровка; прово́з; 2) во́лок; 3) сто́имость перево́зки.

portage II *v* переправля́ть во́локом.

portal ['pɔ:tl] *n* 1) порта́л, гла́вный вход; 2) та́мбур (*дверей*); 3) воро́та; 4) *attr* порта́льный.

portative ['pɔ:tətɪv] *a* портати́вный, передвижно́й.

portend [pɔ:'tend] *v* предвеща́ть.

portent ['pɔ:tent] *n* 1) предзнаменова́ние; 2) чу́до.

portentous [pɔ:'tentəs] *a* 1) предска́зывающий дурно́е, злове́щий; 2) порази́тельный; необыкнове́нный; 3) ва́жный, напы́щенный (*о человеке*).

porter[1] ['pɔ:tə] *n* 1) носи́льщик; гру́зчик; 2) *амер.* проводни́к (*спального вагона*).

porter[2] *n* швейца́р; привра́тник.

porter[3] *n* по́ртер, чёрное пи́во.

porter-house ['pɔ:təhaus] *n* пивна́я, таве́рна.

portfolio [pɔ:t'fouljou] *n* 1) портфе́ль; 2) па́пка, «де́ло»; 3) *разг.* до́лжность мини́стра; 4) *амер.* портфе́ль це́нных бума́г (*банка*).

porthole ['pɔ:thoul] *n* (бортово́й) иллюмина́тор.

portico ['pɔ:tɪkou] *n* по́ртик, кры́тая галере́я.

portière [pou'tjɛə] *n* портье́ра.

portion I ['pɔ:ʃən] *n* 1) часть, до́ля; 2) по́рция; 3) прида́ное; 4) уде́л, у́часть.

portion II *v* 1) дели́ть на ча́сти; 2) выделя́ть часть, до́лю; 3) наделя́ть прида́ным; обеспе́чивать; □ to ~ out производи́ть разде́л (*имущества*).

portionless ['pɔ:ʃənlɪs] *a* не име́ющий насле́дства, прида́ного.

portliness ['pɔːtlɪnɪs] *n* 1) солидность; представительность; 2) тучность, полнота.

portly ['pɔːtlɪ] *a* 1) солидный, крупный (*о человеке*); 2) представительный, осанистый.

portmanteau [pɔːt'mæntou] *n* (*pl тж.* portmanteaux) чемодан.

portrait ['pɔːtrɪt] *n* 1) портрет; full-length ~ портрет во весь рост; half-length ~ поясной портрет; kit-cat ~ портрет, немного меньше поясного; he has got his ~ taken он снялся; 2) изображение, описание.

portraitist ['pɔːtrɪtɪst] *n* портретист.

portraiture ['pɔːtrɪtʃə] *n* 1) портретная живопись; 2) портрет(ы); 3) изображение.

portray [pɔː'treɪ] *v* 1) рисовать портрет; 2) изображать, описывать.

portrayal [pɔː'treɪəl] *n* 1) рисование (*портрета*); 2) изображение, описание.

portreeve ['pɔːtriːv] *n* 1) *ист.* мэр города; 2) помощник мэра.

Portuguese I [,pɔːtjuˈgiːz] *n* 1) португалец; португалка; the ~ (*употр. как pl*) португальцы; 2) португальский язык.

Portuguese II *a* португальский.

pose[1] I [pouz] *n* 1) поза; 2) позирование.

pose[1] II *v* 1) ставить (*вопрос, задачу*); 2) установить (*предмет*), поставить в определённую позу (*натурщика*); 3) принять позу, вид (*кого-л.* — as).

pose[2] *v* поставить в тупик, озадачить.

poser ['pouzə] *n* трудный вопрос.

poseur [pou'zəː] *n* позёр.

position I [pə'zɪʃən] *n* 1) (место)положение; in (out of) ~ на (не на) месте; 2) позиция; 3) состояние; in a ~ to do в состоянии сделать (*что-л.*); 4) должность; место; 5) отношение (*к чему-л.* — on); 6) *attr* позиционный (*о войне*).

position II *v* 1) ставить, помещать; 2) определять местоположение.

positive I ['pɔzɪtɪv] *n* 1) *грам.* положительная степень; 2) *мат.* положительное количество; 3) *фото* позитив.

positive II *a* 1) положительный; позитивный; 2) уверенный; самоуверенный; 3) *разг.* явный, абсолютный; 4) *грам.* положительный (*о степени*).

positively ['pɔzətɪvlɪ] *adv* безусловно; категорически, решительно.

possess [pə'zes] *v* 1) владеть, обладать; to ~ oneself of завладеть, овладеть чем-л.; to be ~ed of иметь, обладать; 2) овладевать, захватывать (*о чувстве и т. п.*); what ~es you? что на тебя нашло?

possessed [pə'zest] *a* одержимый; ненормальный, рехнувшийся.

possession [pə'zeʃən] *n* 1) владение, обладание; in ~ of владеющий чем-л.; in the ~ of находящийся в чьём-л. владении; to come into (*или* to take) ~ of вступить во владение, стать владельцем; 2) *pl* владения, собственность; имущество; 3) зависимая территория.

possessive I [pə'zesɪv] *n* *грам.* притяжательный падеж.

possessive II *a* 1) собственнический; 2) *грам.* притяжательный.

possessor [pə'zesə] *n* владелец, обладатель.

possibility [,pɔsə'bɪlɪtɪ] *n* возможность, вероятность.

possible ['pɔsəbl] *a* 1) возможный, вероятный; is it ~? не может быть! (*выражение удивления*); if (it is) ~ если возможно; 2) *разг.* сносный, терпимый.

possibly ['pɔsəblɪ] *adv* возможно, по возможности.

possum ['pɔsəm] *n разг.* опоссум; ◊ to play ~ а) прикидываться больным *или* мёртвым; б) обманывать кого-л.

post[1] I [poust] *n* 1) столб, кол; starting ~ столб у старта; winning ~ столб у финиша; the frontier ~ пограничный столб; 2) свая, подпорка.

post[1] II *v* расклеивать объявления *или* афиши (*обыкн.* to ~ up); объявлять.

post[2] I *n* 1) почта; by ~ почтой, по почте; by return ~ с обратной почтой; military ~ полевая почта; 2) почтовое отделение; 3) доставка почты; general ~ первая почта; 4) *уст.* почтовая станция; 5) *attr* почтовый.

post[2] II *v* 1) отправить по почте; опустить в почтовый ящик; 2) *уст.* ехать на почтовых; 3) спешить, торопиться; 4) *бухг.* переносить запись в гроссбух (*тж.* to ~ up); 5) доставлять самые последние известия *или* новости, информировать (*тж.* to ~ up).

post[2] III *adv* 1) почтой; 2) *уст.* на почтовых; 3) спешно.

post[3] I *n* 1) пост, должность; 2) *воен.* пост; 3) *воен.* форт, укрепление; 4) *амер. воен.* гарнизон; постоянная стоянка.

post[3] II *v* располагать, расставлять (*солдат и т. п.*).

post[4] *prep* после.

post- [poust-] *pref* со значением после.

postage ['poustɪdʒ] *n* стоимость почтового отправления; inland ~ внутренний почтовый тариф.

postal I ['poustəl] *n амер.* открытка.

postal II *a* почтовый.

post-bag ['poustbæg] *n* сумка почтальона.

post-boy ['poustbɔɪ] *n* 1) почтальон; 2) форейтор.

postcard ['poustkɑːd] *n* почтовая открытка.

post-chaise ['poustʃeɪz] *n* почтовая карета.

poster[1] ['poustə] *n* плакат, афиша; to post up a ~ вывесить плакат.

poster[2] *n* почтовая лошадь.

posterior I [pɔs'tɪərɪə] *n обыкн. pl* зад.

posterior II *a* 1) последующий, позднейший (*to*); 2) задний.

posterity [pɔs'terɪtɪ] *n* потомство; потомки.

post-free ['poust'friː] *adv* пересылка бесплатно.

postgraduate ['poust'grædjuɪt] *n* 1) аспирант; 2) *attr* аспирантский.

post-haste ['poust'heɪst] *adv* весьма спешно.

posthumous ['pɔstjuməs] *a* 1) посмертный; 2) рождённый после смерти отца.

postil(l)ion [pəs'tɪljən] *n* форейтор.

postman ['poustmən] *n* почтальон.

postmark I ['poustmɑːk] *n* почтовый штемпель.

postmark II *v* штемпелевать (*письмо*).

postmaster ['poust,mɑːstə] *n* почтмейстер; Postmaster General министр почт.

postmeridian ['poustmə'rɪdɪən] *a* послеполуденный.

post meridiem ['poustmə'rɪdɪəm] *adv* после полудня (*сокр.* p. m.).

post-mortem I ['poust'mɔːtem] *n* вскрытие (*трупа*).

post-mortem II *a* посмертный.

post-obit [,poust'ɔbɪt] *n* обязательство уплатить кредитору по получении наследства.

post-office ['poust,ɔfɪs] *n* 1) почта, почтовое отделение; 2) *attr* почтовый.

post-paid ['poust'peɪd] *a* с оплаченными почтовыми расходами.

postpone [poust'poun] *v* откладывать, отсрочивать.

postponement [poust'pounmənt] *n* отсрочка.

postposition ['poustpə'zɪʃən] *n* 1) помещение позади; 2) *грам.* постпозиция.

postprandial [poust'prændɪəl] *a* *шутл.* послеобеденный.

post-rider ['poust,raɪdə] *n* почтальон (*развозящий почту верхом или на велосипеде*).

postscript ['pousskrɪpt] *n* постскриптум.

postulate ['pɔstjuleɪt] *v* требовать, обусловливать.

posture I ['pɔstʃə] *n* 1) поза, положение; 2) состояние.

posture II *v* 1) ставить в позу; 2) принять позу, положение; позировать.

post-war ['poust'wɔː] *a* послевоенный.

posy ['pouzɪ] *n* 1) букет цветов; 2) *уст.* девиз (*на кольце*).

pot I [pɔt] *n* 1) горшок, котелок; кружка; 2) *спорт. разг.* кубок; 3) напиток; 4) колпак дымовой трубы; ◇ big ~ важная персона; the ~ calls the kettle black *погов.* ≅ не смейся горох, не лучше бобов; to keep the ~ boiling a) зарабатывать на пропитание; б) продолжать заниматься своим делом; to make the ~ boil ≅ зарабатывать себе на кусок хлеба; to go to ~ *разг.* a) разориться, «вылететь в трубу»; б) пойти насмарку; in one's ~s пьян как стелька; a ~ of money большая сумма денег.

pot II *v* 1) класть в горшок *или* в котелок; 2) варить, тушить; консервировать; 3) сажать в горшок (*цветы*); 4) загонять в лузу (*шар*); 5) застрелить в упор.

potash ['pɔtæʃ] *n хим.* поташ.

potassic [pə'tæsɪk] *a хим.* калийный.

potassium [pə'tæsjəm] *n хим.* калий.

potation [pou'teɪʃən] *n* 1) питьё, выпивка; 2) спиртной напиток.

potato [pə'teɪtou] *n* 1) картофель, new ~es молодой картофель; sweet ~ .батат, сладкий картофель; ~es boiled in their jackets картофель «в мундире»; 2) *attr* картофельный; ◇ small ~es пустяки.

pot-boiler ['pɔt,bɔɪlə] *n* *разг.* 1) халтура; 2) халтурщик.

potency ['poutənsɪ] *n* сила, могущество.

potent ['poutənt] *a* 1) могущественный; 2) сильнодействующий; 3) убедительный.

potentate ['poutənteɪt] *n* властелин, монарх.

potential I [pə'tenʃəl] *n* потенциал.

potential II *a* возможный, потенциальный.

potentiality [pə,tenʃɪ'ælɪtɪ] *n* возможность, потенциальность.

potentially [pə'tenʃəlɪ] *adv* возможно.

pot-herb ['pɔthəːb] *n разг.* овощ, зелень.

pot-hole ['pɔthoul] *n* рытвина.

pot-house ['pɔthaus] *n* пивная.

potion ['pouʃən] *n* 1) питьё; 2) зелье.

potsherd ['pɔtʃəːd] *n* черепок.

potter[1] ['pɔtə] *n* гончар, горшечник.

potter[2] *v* 1) лодырничать, работать, спустя рукава; 2) убивать время.

pottery ['pɔtərɪ] *n* 1) глиняная посуда; 2) гончарное дело; 3) гончарная мастерская.

potty ['pɔtɪ] *a разг.* 1) мелкий, незначительный; 2) лёгкий, пустячный; 3) чудаковатый.

pot-valiant ['pɔt,væljənt] *a* храбрый во хмелю.

pouch I [pautʃ] *n* 1) мешочек, сумка; *воен.* подсумок; 2) кисет; 3) *уст.* кошелёк.

pouch II *v* 1) класть в карман *или* в мешок; 2) прикарманить; 3) плохо сидеть, висеть мешком.

pouf [puːf] *n* пуф, пуфик.

poult [poult] *n* цыплёнок; индюшонок.

poulterer ['poultərə] *n* торговец домашней птицей.

poultice I ['poultɪs] *n* припарка.

poultice II *v* класть припарку.

poultry ['poultrɪ] *n* домашняя птица.

pounce I [pauns] *n* 1) внезапный налёт, прыжок; 2) коготь (*ястреба и т. п.*).

pounce II *v* 1) налетать, накидываться; ринуться; 2) схватить когтями.

pound[1] [paund] *n* 1) фунт (*англ.* = 453,6 *г*); 2) фунт стерлингов (*тж.* ~ sterling).

pound[2] *v* 1) колотить; дубасить; to ~ out (a tune) on the piano колотить по роялю; 2) колотиться (*о сердце*); 3) обстреливать, бомбардировать (*at, on*); 4) толочь; 5) продвигаться с трудом (*along*).

pound[3] I *n* загон (*для скота*).

pound[3] II *v* 1) загонять (*в загон*); 2) заключать в тюрьму.

pounder[1] ['paundə] *n* пестик (*ступки*).

pounder[2] *n* предмет весом в один фунт.

pour [pɔː] *v* 1) лить(ся); it is ~ing wet льёт как из ведра; 2) наливать (*into*); 3) одаривать, осыпать (*подарками и т. п.*; *тж.* to ~ down, out, forth); □ to ~ forth извергать (*слова*); to ~ in a) сыпаться (*о новостях и т. п.*); б) валить (*о дыме, о толпе*); to ~ out a) разливать (*чай, вино*); б) *см.* to ~ in б); to ~ through литься сквозь (*о свете*).

pourparler [puə'pɑːleɪ] *n обыкн. pl* (предварительные) переговоры.

pout I [paut] *n:* to be in the ~s дуться.

pout II *v* надувать губы; дуться.

pouter ['pautə] *n* надутый, вечно недовольный человек.

poverty ['pɔvətɪ] *n* 1) бедность; to sink into ~ впадать в нищету; 2) скудость; оскудение.

poverty-stricken ['pɔvetɪ,strɪkn] *a* 1) бедный; впавший в нищету; 2) выхолощенный (*о языке*).

powder I ['paudə] *n* 1) порошок, пыль; 2) пудра; 3) порох; brown ~ бурый дымный порох; blasting ~ минный порох; smokeless ~ бездымный порох; ◇ not worth ~ and shot ≅ ломаного гроша не стоит.

powder II *v* 1) толочь, превращать в порошок; 2) пудрить(ся); 3) посыпать порошком.

powder-flask ['paudəflɑːsk] *n* пороховница.

powder-magazine ['paudəmægə,ziːn] *n* пороховой погреб; *мор.* крюйт-камера.

powder-mill ['paudəmɪl] *n* пороховой завод.

powder-puff ['paudərʌf] *n* пуховка.

powdery ['paudərɪ] *a* 1) рассыпчатый, порошкообразный; 2) покрытый пудрой, порошком.

power ['pauə] *n* 1) сила, энергия; electric ~ электроэнергия; holding ~ способность удерживать (*атомы, молекулы*); locomotive ~ движущая сила; 2) мощность, производительность; the mechanical ~s простые машины; 3) питание (*аппаратуры, агрегата*); 4) держава; the Great Powers *или* the first-rate Powers великие державы; a naval ~ морская держава; signatory Powers страны, подписавшие договор, соглашение; 5) (государственная) власть; Soviet Power Советская власть; sovereign (*или* supreme) ~ верховная власть; in ~ у власти; 6) полномочия; ~ of attorney полномочие; доверенность; emergency ~s чрезвычайные полномочия; 7) могущество, власть; 8) *часто pl* способности, возможности; purchasing ~ покупательная способность; it is out of my ~ это не в моих возможностей; I'll do all in my ~ я сделаю всё, что в моих силах, всё, что возможно; 9) *разг.* масса, множество; a ~ of money уйма денег; 10) *мат.* степень; 64 is the 6th ~ of two 64 представляет собой два в шестой степени; 11) *attr* силовой, энергетический; моторный.

power-boat ['pauəbout] *n* моторный катер.

powerful ['pauəful] *a* 1) сильный, могучий, мощный; 2) могущественный; 3) сильнодействующий; 4) яркий (*о речи, описании*).

power-house ['pauəhaus] *n* электростанция.

powerless ['pauəlɪs] *a* бессильный.

power-plant ['pauəplɑːnt] *n* силовая установка.

power-shovel ['pauə,ʃʌvl] *n* экскаватор.

power-station ['pauə,steɪʃən] *n* электростанция.

powwow I ['pauwau] *n* 1) церемония заклинания (*у индейцев*); 2) собрание (*индейцев*); 3) *амер. шутл.* собрание, совещание.

powwow II *v* устраивать совещание; вести переговоры.

practicable ['præktɪkəbl] *a* 1) осуществимый, реальный; 2) проходимый, проезжий.

practical ['præktɪkəl] *a* 1) практический; 2) практичный; полезный; 3) фактический, настоящий.

practically[a] ['præktɪkəlɪ] *adv* практически.

practically[b] ['præktɪklɪ] *adv* 1) фактически, на деле; 2) почти.

practice I ['præktɪs] *n* 1) практика; to put into ~ осуществить, ввести в обиход, в обращение; 2) обычай, привычка; 3) практика; навык, тренировка; to be out of ~ не иметь опыта, практики (*в чём-л.*); 4) практика, работа по специальности; 5) *обыкн. pl* делишки, махинации; sharp ~ мошенничество; corrupt ~s взяточничество; discreditable ~s тёмные дела; 6) *воен.* учебная стрельба; musketry ~ обучение стрельбе из винтовки; ◊ ~ makes perfect *посл.* ≅ навык мастера ставит.

practice II *v амер. см.* practise.

practician [præk'tɪʃən] *n* практик.

practise ['præktɪs] *v* 1) упражнять(ся), тренировать(ся), практиковать(ся); 2) применять; □ to ~ **upon** злоупотреблять; надувать (*кого-л.*).

practitioner [præk'tɪʃnə] *n* практикующий врач *или* юрист; general ~ врач общей практики (*терапевт и хирург*).

pragmatic [præg'mætɪk] *a филос.* прагматический.

pragmatical [præg'mætɪkəl] *a* 1) догматичный; 2) назойливый.

pragmatism ['prægmətɪzəm] *n* 1) *филос.* прагматизм; 2) догматизм; 3) назойливость.

prairie ['prɛərɪ] *n* 1) прерия, степь; 2) *attr* степной, живущий в прерии.

prairie-schooner ['prɛərɪ'skuːnə] *n амер.* фургон переселенцев.

praise I [preɪz] *n* 1) похвала; beyond ~ выше всякой похвалы; 2) восхваление; to sing the ~s of неустанно хвалить, восхвалять.

praise II *v* 1) хвалить; to ~ to the skies восхвалять, превозносить до небес; 2) возносить хвалу, восхвалять.

praiseworthy ['preɪz,wəːðɪ] *a* достойный похвалы, похвальный.

pram[a] [præm] *n разг.* детская коляска.

pram[b] [prɑːm] *n* плоскодонное судно.

prance I [prɑːns] *n* скачок, курбет.

prance II *v* 1) гарцевать, становиться на дыбы; 2) ходить гоголем, задаваться.

prandial ['prændɪəl] *a шутл.* обеденный.

prank[1] [præŋk] *n* проделка, трюк, шалость; to play ~s откалывать штуки, резвиться.

prank[2] *v* 1) крикливо одеваться, разряжаться (*тж.* to ~ out, to ~ up); 2) пускать пыль в глаза.

prankish ['præŋkɪʃ] *a* шаловливый; озорной.

prate I [preɪt] *n* пустословие.

prate II *v* нести чепуху, пустословить.

prattle I ['prætl] *n* 1) лепет; 2) болтовня.

prattle II *v* 1) лепетать; 2) болтать.

prattler ['prætlə] *n* 1) ребёнок (*младшего возраста*); 2) болтун, говорун.

pray [preɪ] *v* 1) молиться (*за кого-л.* — for); past ~ing for а) безнадёжно болен; б) на грани катастрофы; 2) умолять; просить; ~! пожалуйста!, прошу вас!

prayer[a] [prɛə] *n* 1) молитва; to say one's ~s молиться; 2) просьба.

prayer[b] ['preɪə] *n* 1) молящийся; 2) проситель.

prayer-book ['prɛəbuk] *n* молитвенник.

pre- [priː-] *pref со значением* до-, пред-; заранее; pre-war довоенный; pre-establish устанавливать заранее.

preach [priːtʃ] *v* проповедовать.

preacher ['priːtʃə] *n* проповедник.

preachment ['priːtʃmənt] *n разг.* проповедь (*особ. скучная*), нравоучение.

preamble [priː'æmbl] *n* 1) преамбула; 2) вступление, предисловие.

pre-arranged ['priːə'reɪndʒd] *a* заранее подготовленный, запланированный; плановый.

precarious [prɪ'kɛərɪəs] *a* 1) случайный; неопределённый; 2) ненадёжный; рискованный; 3) необоснованный.

precaution [prɪ'kɔːʃən] *n* 1) предосторожность; мера предосторожности; to take ~s принять меры предосторожности (*против чего-л.* — against); Air-Raid ~s гражданская ПВО; 2) предостережение.

precautionary [prɪ'kɔːʃnərɪ] *a* предупредительный.

precautious [prɪˈkɔːʃəs] *a* осторо́жный, бди́-
тельный.

precede [priːˈsiːd] *v* 1) предше́ствовать, стоя́ть
пе́ред чем-л., впереди́ кого́-л.; ~d by во главе́
(*чего-л.*); 2) занима́ть бо́лее высо́кое положе́-
ние (*по должности, званию*).

precedence [priːˈsiːdəns] *n* 1) предше́ствование;
2) бо́лее высо́кое положе́ние (*по должности, званию и т. п.*); старшинство́; to take (*или* to
have) ~ of превосходи́ть по до́лжности, зва́нию.

precedent[a] [ˈpresidənt] *n* прецеде́нт.

precedent[b] [priːˈsiːdənt] *a* предше́ствующий.

preceding [priːˈsiːdɪŋ] *a* предше́ствующий.

precept [ˈpriːsept] *n* 1) пра́вило, указа́ние;
2) *юр.* предписа́ние; 3) за́поведь.

preceptor [priːˈseptə] *n* наста́вник.

precinct [ˈpriːsɪŋkt] *n* 1) террито́рия, прилега́ю-
щая к зда́нию; 2) *pl* окре́стности; 3) *амер.* из-
бира́тельный уча́сток; 4) *амер.* полице́йский уча́с-
ток.

precious I [ˈpreʃəs] *a* 1) драгоце́нный; 2) до-
рого́й; люби́мый; my ~ мой ми́лый; 3) отбо́рный,
краси́вый; 4) *разг. для усиления:* he has got into
a ~ mess он попа́л в весьма́ тру́дное положе́ние.

precious II *adv разг.* о́чень; здо́рово.

precipice [ˈpresipis] *n* про́пасть; обры́в.

precipitance [priːˈsipitəns] *см.* precipitancy.

precipitancy [priːˈsipitənsi] *n* 1) стреми́тель-
ность; 2) опроме́тчивость.

precipitant [priːˈsipitənt] *a* 1) стреми́тельный;
2) опроме́тчивый.

precipitate[a] I [priːˈsipitit] *n хим.* оса́док.

precipitate[a] II *a* 1) стреми́тельный; 2) опро-
ме́тчивый, неосмотри́тельный.

precipitate[b] [priːˈsipiteit] *v* 1) низверга́ть; 2) уско-
ря́ть; 3) *хим.* осажда́ть(ся); 4) выпада́ть (*об
осадках*); 5) бро́ситься.

precipitation [priˌsipiˈteiʃən] *n* 1) стреми́тель-
ность; 2) паде́ние; 3) *хим.* осажде́ние; 4) выпа-
де́ние оса́дков.

precipitous [priˈsipitəs] *a* обры́вистый; круто́й;
отве́сный.

précis [ˈpreisiː] *n* конспе́кт.

precise [priˈsais] *a* 1) то́чный, определённый;
2) аккура́тный, пунктуа́льный; 3) тща́тельный;
4) щепети́льный; педанти́чный.

precisely [priˈsaisli] *adv* 1) то́чно, как раз;
определённо; 2) педанти́чно.

precision [priˈsiʒən] *n* 1) то́чность, аккура́т-
ность; чёткость; 2) ме́ткость.

preclude [priˈkluːd] *v* 1) устраня́ть, предотвра-
ща́ть; 2) меша́ть (*from*).

precocious [priˈkouʃəs] *a* скороспе́лый; преж-
девре́менный; 2) развито́й не по года́м (*о ребёнке*).

precocity [priˈkɔsiti] *n* ра́ннее разви́тие.

preconceived [ˈpriːkənˈsiːvd] *a* предвзя́тый.

preconception [ˈpriːkənˈsepʃən] *n* 1) предвзя́тое
мне́ние; 2) предви́дение.

precursor [priːˈkəːsə] *n* 1) предте́ча, предше́ст-
венник; 2) предве́стник.

precursory [priːˈkəːsəri] *a* предвеща́ющий (*of*).

predacious [priˈdeiʃəs] *a* хи́щный.

predator [ˈpredətə] *n* хи́щник.

predatory [ˈpredətəri] *a* 1) хи́щный; 2) гра-
би́тельский, хи́щнический.

predecessor [ˈpriːdisesə] *n* 1) предше́ственник;
2) пре́док.

predestination ˈ[priːˌdestiˈneiʃən] *n* предопреде-
ле́ние.

predestine [priːˈdestin] *v* предопределя́ть.

predicament [priˈdikəmənt] *n* 1) неприя́тное по-
ложе́ние; затрудне́ние; what a ~! кака́я доса́да!;
2) *лог.* катего́рия.

predicant [ˈpredikənt] *n* пропове́дник.

predicate[a] [ˈpredikit] *n грам.* сказу́емое, пре-
дика́т.

predicate[b] [ˈpredikeit] *v* 1) утвержда́ть, объяв-
ля́ть; 2) *грам.* предици́ровать.

predication [ˌprediˈkeiʃən] *n* 1) утвержде́ние;
2) *грам.* предика́ция.

predicative I [priˈdikətiv] *n грам.* именна́я
часть составно́го сказу́емого.

predicative II *a грам.* предикати́вный.

predict [priˈdikt] *v* предска́зывать.

prediction [priˈdikʃən] *n* предсказа́ние.

predilection [ˌpriːdiˈlekʃən] *n* пристра́стие, скло́н-
ность (*к чему-л.— for*).

predispose [ˈpriːdisˈpouz] *v* 1) предрасполага́ть;
2) склоня́ть (*к чему-л.— to*).

predisposition [ˈpriːˌdispəˈziʃən] *n* 1) предрас-
положе́ние; 2) скло́нность.

predominance [priˈdɔminəns] *n* преоблада́ние,
госпо́дство.

predominant [priˈdɔminənt] *a* преоблада́ющий,
госпо́дствующий, домини́рующий.

predominate [priˈdɔmineit] *v* преоблада́ть; гос-
по́дствовать (*над — over*).

pre-eminent [priːˈeminənt] *a* выдаю́щийся.

pre-empt [priːˈempt] *v* приобрета́ть ра́ньше дру-
ги́х.

preen [priːn] *v* чи́стить (*перья*) клю́вом; to ~
oneself прихора́шиваться.

pre-establish [ˌpriːisˈtæbliʃ] *v* устана́вливать за-
ра́нее.

prefab [ˈpriːfæb] *n разг.* разбо́рный дом.

prefabricate [ˈpriːˈfæbrikeit] *v* 1) изготовля́ть за-
ра́нее; 2) изготовля́ть заводски́м спо́собом.

preface I [ˈprefis] *n* 1) предисло́вие; проло́г;
вво́дная часть; 2) введе́ние.

preface II *v* писа́ть предисло́вие; дать преди-
сло́вие.

prefatory [ˈprefətəri] *a* вво́дный, вступи́тель-
ный.

prefect [ˈpriːfekt] *n* 1) префе́кт; 2) *шк.* ста́р-
ший учени́к (*следящий за дисципли́ной*).

prefecture [ˈpriːfektʃuə] *n* префекту́ра.

prefer [priˈfəː] *v* 1) предпочита́ть; отда́ть пред-
почте́ние (*чему-л.*); 2) повыша́ть (*по слу́жбе*).

preferable [ˈprefərəbl] *a* предпочти́тельный.

preferably [ˈprefərəbli] *adv* предпочти́тельно,
лу́чше.

preference [ˈprefərəns] *n* 1) предпочте́ние; 2)
преиму́щественное пра́во; 3) льго́тная тамо́женная
по́шлина.

preferential [ˌprefəˈrenʃəl] *a* 1) по́льзующийся
предпочте́нием; 2) льго́тный (*о пошлинах*).

preferment [priˈfəːmənt] *n* 1) предпочте́ние;
2) продвиже́ние по слу́жбе, повыше́ние.

prefix[a] [ˈpriːfiks] *n грам.* пре́фикс, приста́вка.

prefix[b] [priːˈfiks] *v* 1) предпосла́ть; 2) присоеди-
ни́ть в ви́де пре́фикса.

pregnable ['pregnəbl] *a* ненадёжно укреплённый; уязви́мый.

pregnancy ['pregnənsɪ] *n* 1) бере́менность; 2) чрева́тость; 3) бога́тство (*воображения*).

pregnant ['pregnənt] *a* 1) бере́менная; 2) чрева́тый (*последствиями*); 3) бога́тый (*мыслями, идея-ми*); творческий (*об уме*).

prehistoric ['pri:hɪs'tɔrɪk] *a* доистори́ческий.

prejudge ['pri:'dʒʌdʒ] *v* 1) выноси́ть реше́ние до суда́; 2) предреша́ть.

prejudice I ['predʒudɪs] *n* 1) предубежде́ние; 2) предрассу́док; 3) вред, ущерб; in ~ of, to the ~ of в ущерб; without ~ to без ущерба для кого́-л.

prejudice II *v* 1) предубежда́ть; 2) наноси́ть ущерб, причиня́ть вред.

prejudicial ['predʒu'dɪʃəl] *a* вредный, па́губный.

prelate ['prelɪt] *n* прела́т; *амер.* свяще́нник.

preliminary I [prɪ'lɪmɪnərɪ] *n* 1) подготови́тельное мероприя́тие; 2) *pl* предвари́тельные переговоры.

preliminary II *a* предвари́тельный, прелимина́рный.

prelude I ['prelju:d] *n* 1) вступле́ние (*к чему-л. — to, of*); 2) *муз.* прелю́дия.

prelude II *v* служи́ть вступле́нием.

premature [,premə'tjuə] *a* преждевре́менный; поспе́шный, скороспе́лый.

premeditated [pri:'medɪteɪtɪd] *a* преднаме́ренный; обду́манный зара́нее.

premeditation [pri:,medɪ'teɪʃən] *n* преднаме́ренность.

premier I ['premjə] *n* премье́р-мини́стр.

premier II *a* пе́рвый.

première ['premjɛə] *n* премье́ра.

premise[a] ['premɪs] *n* 1) предпосы́лка; 2) *pl юр.* преа́мбула; 3) *pl* помеще́ние, дом (*с прилегающими пристройками и участком земли*); ◇ to be drunk on the ~s распи́вочно; to be drunk to the ~s ≅ допи́ться до чёртиков.

premise[b] [prɪ'maɪz] *v* предпосыла́ть.

premium ['pri:mjəm] *n* 1) награ́да, пре́мия; to put a ~ on поощря́ть; 2) пла́та (*за обучение и т. п.*); 3) страхова́я пре́мия; *фин.* лаж; at a ~ вы́ше номина́ла; *перен.* в ходу́, в мо́де.

premonition [,pri:mə'nɪʃən] *n* 1) предупрежде́ние; 2) предчу́вствие.

premonitory [prɪ'mɔnɪtərɪ] *a* предваря́ющий, предостерега́ющий.

prentice ['prentɪs] *n разг.* подмасте́рье.

preoccupation [pri:,ɔkju'peɪʃən] *n* 1) заня́тие ме́ста и т. п. ра́ньше друго́го; 2) озабо́ченность; поглощённость (*чем-л.*).

preoccupied [pri:'ɔkjupaɪd] *a* поглощённый мы́слями; озабо́ченный.

preoccupy [pri:'ɔkjupaɪ] *v* 1) заня́ть, захвати́ть ра́нее други́х; 2) занима́ть, поглоща́ть внима́ние.

pre-ordain ['pri:ɔ:'deɪn] *v* предопределя́ть.

prep[1] I [prep] *n шк. разг.* приготовле́ние уро́ков; 2) приготови́тельная шко́ла.

prep[1] II *a разг.* приготови́тельный.

prep[2] *n сокр. см.* preposition.

preparation [,prepə'reɪʃən] *n* 1) приготовле́ние; to make ~s гото́виться; проводи́ть подгото́вку (*к чему-л. — for*); in ~ for имея в виду́; 2) под-

готовка; выполне́ние дома́шних зада́ний; 3) препара́т.

preparative I [prɪ'pærətɪv] *n* подготови́тельный эта́п; подготови́тельный проце́сс.

preparative II *a* подготови́тельный, подгота́вливающий.

preparatory I [prɪ'pærətərɪ] *n* приготови́тельная шко́ла.

preparatory II *a* 1) вступи́тельный; 2) подготови́тельный; приготови́тельный.

preparatory III *adv* пре́жде чем, до того́ как (*to*).

prepare [prɪ'pɛə] *v* гото́вить(ся), приготавливать(ся), подготавливать(ся).

preparedness [prɪ'pɛədnɪs] *n* гото́вность.

prepay ['pri:'peɪ] *v* плати́ть вперёд.

preponderance [prɪ'pɔndərəns] *n* 1) переве́с; 2) превосхо́дство.

preponderant [prɪ'pɔndərənt] *a* переве́шивающий, преоблада́ющий.

preponderate [prɪ'pɔndəreɪt] *v* 1) переве́шивать, име́ть переве́с (*over*); 2) превосходи́ть, превыша́ть (*over*); преоблада́ть.

preposition [,prepə'zɪʃən] *n грам.* предло́г.

prepositional [,prepə'zɪʃənl] *a* предло́жный.

prepossess [,pri:pə'zes] *v* 1) внуша́ть (*чувство*); 2) овладева́ть (*о чувстве, мысли*); 3) предрасполага́ть.

prepossessing [,pri:pə'zesɪŋ] *a* располага́ющий.

prepossession [,pri:pə'zeʃən] *n* 1) предубежде́ние; 2) предрасположе́ние.

preposterous [prɪ'pɔstərəs] *a* 1) неле́пый, абсу́рдный; 2) превра́тный; 3) нерациона́льный.

prerogative [prɪ'rɔgətɪv] *n* 1) прерогати́ва; исключи́тельное пра́во.

presage I ['presɪdʒ] *n* 1) предчу́вствие; 2) предзнаменова́ние, предсказа́ние.

presage II *v* 1) предчу́вствовать; име́ть предчу́вствие; 2) предвеща́ть; знаменова́ть; 3) предска́зывать.

presbyter ['prezbɪtə] *n* свяще́нник.

Presbyterian I [,prezbɪ'tɪərɪən] *n* пресвитериа́нин.

Presbyterian II *a* пресвитериа́нский.

presbytery ['prezbɪtərɪ] *n* дом католи́ческого свяще́нника.

preschool ['pri:'sku:l] *a* дошко́льный.

prescind [prɪ'sɪnd] *v* 1) отделя́ть; 2) отвлека́ть (*от чего-л. — from*); 3) абстраги́ровать.

prescribe [prɪs'kraɪb] *v* 1) предпи́сывать; 2) пропи́сывать (*лекарство; кому-л. — to, for; против чего-л. — for*).

prescript ['pri:skrɪpt] *n* предписа́ние.

prescription [prɪs'krɪpʃən] *n* 1) реце́пт; to write (*или* to make out) a ~ вы́писать реце́пт; 2) предпи́сывание; предписа́ние.

prescriptive [prɪs'krɪptɪv] *a* даю́щий директи́вы, предписа́ния, инстру́кции.

presence ['prezns] *n* 1) прису́тствие, нали́чие; the ~ of mind прису́тствие ду́ха; 2) оса́нка, вне́шний вид.

presence-chamber ['prezns'tʃeɪmbə] *n* приёмная.

present[a1] I ['preznt] *n* 1) настоя́щее вре́мя; at ~ тепе́рь, в да́нное вре́мя; for the ~ на э́тот раз, пока́; these ~s *шут.* настоя́щий, да́нный докуме́нт; 2) *грам.* фо́рма настоя́щего вре́мени; Present Continuous конкре́тная фо́рма настоя́щего вре́мени: I am reading я чита́ю (*в момент выска-*

зывания); Present Indefinite общая форма настоящего времени: I read я читаю (*это моё обыкновение*); Present Perfect совершённая форма настоящего времени: I have read я прочёл (*и поэтому знаю содержание*); Historic Present историческое настоящее.

present^{a1} II *a* 1) *predic* присутствующий; to be ~ присутствовать; to be ~ to the imagination жить в воображении; to be ~ to the mind быть незабываемым; 2) нынешний, настоящий; современный; 3) данный, этот самый.

present^{a2} *n* подарок; to make a ~ of подарить что-л.

present^b [prɪˈzent] *v* 1) дарить (*что-л.— with*); 2) подавать; передавать на рассмотрение (*заявление, послание и т. п.*); 3) представлять (*кого-л. кому-л.— to*); to ~ oneself явиться, прийти; 4) ставить (*пьесу*); 5) являться, представлять (*собой*); 6) слать, посылать (*благодарность, привет*).

presentable [prɪˈzentəbl] *a* приличный; презентабельный.

presentation [ˌprezenˈteɪʃən] *n* 1) представление (*кого-л. кому-л.— to*); 2) *театр.* представление; 3) преподнесение (*подарка*); 4) подарок, подношение.

present-day [ˈprezntˈdeɪ] *a* современный.

presentee [ˌpreznˈtiː] *n* 1) получатель подарка; 2) лицо, представляемое ко двору короля.

presentiment [prɪˈzentɪmənt] *n* предчувствие.

presentive [prɪˈzentɪv] *a* знаменательный, предметный (*о словах*).

presently [ˈprezntlɪ] *adv* 1) вскоре, немного времени спустя; 2) сейчас.

presentment [prɪˈzentmənt] *n* 1) представление, спектакль; 2) изображение, описание; 3) *юр.* заявление присяжных.

preservation [ˌprezəˈveɪʃən] *n* 1) сохранение, предохранение; 2) сохранность; 3) консервирование.

preservative I [prɪˈzəːvətɪv] *n* предохранительное средство.

preservative II *a* предохранительный.

preserve I [prɪˈzəːv] *n* 1) *pl* консервы; варенье; 2) заповедник.

preserve II *v* 1) хранить (*овощи, продукты*); 2) консервировать; варить варенье; 3) сохранять, оберегать; 4) охранять от браконьеров.

preserved [prɪˈzəːvd] *a* консервированный.

preside [prɪˈzaɪd] *v* председательствовать (*на — at, over*).

presidency [ˈprezɪdənsɪ] *n* 1) президентство; 2) председательство; 3) *ист.* округ (*в Индии*).

president [ˈprezɪdənt] *n* 1) президент; (vice-) ~ elect (вице-)президент, избранный, но ещё не вступивший в должность; 2) председатель; 3) *ист.* губернатор (*колонии*).

presidential [ˌprezɪˈdenʃəl] *a* президентский.

presidio [prɪˈsɪdɪou] *n* форт.

presidium [prɪˈsɪdɪəm] *n* президиум; The Presidium of the Supreme Soviet of the USSR Президиум Верховного Совета СССР.

press^1 I [pres] *n* 1) печать, пресса; yellow (gutter) ~ жёлтая (бульварная) пресса; 2) печатный станок; to be in the ~ быть в печати; 3) типография; 4) работник печати; 5) пресс,

тиски; 6) давка, свалка; 7) толпа; 8) спешка; большое количество срочной работы; 9) шкаф.

press^1 II *v* 1) жать, сжимать, прижимать; 2) сплющить, прессовать; 3) выжимать; 4) настаивать; to ~ hard настоятельно требовать; 5) торопить (*с — for*); to be ~ed for time располагать незначительным временем, очень торопиться; 6) навязывать (*кому-л.— upon*); 7) гладить (*утюгом*); □ to ~ **down** толкать; to ~ **forward** устремляться вперёд; to ~ **out** выжимать; to ~ **to** вынуждать, заставлять.

press^2 *v* 1) вербовать насильно; 2) реквизировать.

press-agency [ˈpresˌeɪdʒənsɪ] *n* газетное агентство.

press-agent [ˈpresˌeɪdʒənt] *n* агент по рекламе (*спектаклей, концертов и т. п.*).

press-conference [ˈpresˈkɔnfərəns] *n* пресс-конференция.

press-corrector [ˈpreskəˈrektə] *n* корректор.

press-gallery [ˈpresˈɡælərɪ] *n* места для репортёров (*в парламенте*).

pressing [ˈpresɪŋ] *a* 1) срочный, неотложный; 2) настоятельный; 3) настойчивый.

pressman [ˈpresmən] *n* 1) печатник; 2) журналист, газетчик.

pressure [ˈpreʃə] *n* 1) давление; high (low) ~ высокое (низкое) давление; 2) гнёт, давление; financial ~ денежные затруднения; under ~ под давлением, не по собственному желанию; to bring ~ to bear upon, to put ~ upon оказывать давление на кого-л.; 3) сжатие, прессование; 4) *эл.* напряжение.

pressurized [ˈpreʃəraɪzd] *a* герметический, герметизированный.

prestige [presˈtiːʒ] *n* престиж.

presumable [prɪˈzjuːməbl] *a* возможный, вероятный.

presumably [prɪˈzjuːməblɪ] *adv* вероятно; предположительно.

presume [prɪˈzjuːm] *v* 1) (пред)полагать; 2) осмелиться, позволить себе; □ to ~ **(up)on** полагаться (*на что-л.*).

presumedly [prɪˈzjuːmɪdlɪ] *adv* вероятно; предположительно.

presumption [prɪˈzʌmpʃən] *n* 1) предположение; 2) *юр.* презумпция; 3) самонадеянность.

presumptive [prɪˈzʌmptɪv] *a* предполагаемый, предположительный.

presumptuous [prɪˈzʌmptʃuəs] *a* самонадеянный, наглый.

presuppose [ˌpriːsəˈpouz] *v* 1) предполагать; 2) требовать в качестве условия.

pretence [prɪˈtens] *n* 1) притворство; false ~s обман, притворство; 2) отговорка, предлог; under the ~ of под предлогом; 3) претензия, требование; 4) претенциозность.

pretend [prɪˈtend] *v* 1) притворяться, делать вид; 2) претендовать, иметь виды (*на — to*).

pretended [prɪˈtendɪd] *a* притворный, лицемерный.

pretender [prɪˈtendə] *n* 1) притворщик, лицемер; 2) претендент.

pretense [prɪˈtens] *см.* pretence.

pretension [prɪˈtenʃən] *n* 1) претензия; притязание; 2) претенциозность.

pretentious [prɪ'tenʃəs] *a* претенциозный.

preterit(e) ['pretərɪt] *n грам.* форма прошедшего времени.

pretext ['priːtekst] *n* предлог, отговорка.

prettiness ['prɪtɪnɪs] *n* прелесть, миловидность.

pretty I ['prɪtɪ] *a* 1) привлекательный, прелестный; 2) хорошенький (*о женщинах, детях*); as ~ as paint хороша как картинка; 3) мелодичный, красивый (*о песне*); 4) приятный; 5) *разг.* значительный, изрядный; кругленький (*о сумме денег*).

pretty II *n* 1): my ~ душка (*в обращении*); 2) *pl* красивые вещи, платья.

pretty III *adv разг.* вполне, довольно, достаточно; ~ much почти.

prevail [prɪ'veɪl] *v* 1) преобладать; господствовать; 2) быть распространённым; 3) одолевать; превозмогать; □ to ~ (up)on убедить, уговорить.

prevailing [prɪ'veɪlɪŋ] *a* 1) преобладающий, господствующий; 2) распространённый.

prevalence ['prevələns] *n* 1) распространение; 2) преобладание, господство.

prevalent ['prevələnt] *a* 1) преобладающий; 2) широко распространённый.

prevaricate [prɪ'værɪkeɪt] *v* говорить уклончиво, кривить душой.

prevent [prɪ'vent] *v* 1) предотвращать, предупреждать; 2) мешать, препятствовать (*чему-л. from*).

prevention [prɪ'venʃən] *n* предотвращение, предупреждение; ~ of accidents техника безопасности; ◊ ~ is better than cure *посл.* предупреждение лучше лечения.

preventive I [prɪ'ventɪv] *n* предохранительная мера; профилактическое средство.

preventive II *a* 1) предохранительный, профилактический; 2) превентивный.

preview ['priːvjuː] *n* 1) (предварительный) просмотр (*фильма*); public ~ общественный просмотр; 2) показ кадров будущего фильма.

previous I ['priːvjəs] *a* 1) предыдущий, предшествующий (*to*); 2) предварительный; преждевременный; 3) *разг.* поспешный, скорый.

previous II *adv*: ~ to до, прежде, ранее.

previously ['priːvjəslɪ] *adv* предварительно, заранее.

prevision [priː'vɪʒən] *n* предвидение.

pre-war ['priː'wɔː] *a* довоенный.

prey I [preɪ] *n* 1) добыча; 2) жертва; to fall a ~ to пасть жертвой (*чего-л.*).

prey II *v* 1) охотиться, ловить (*свою жертву*); 2) грабить; 3) обманывать, вымогать; 4) подтачивать (*здоровье*).

price I [praɪs] *n* 1) цена; cash ~ продажная цена (*наличными деньгами*); ceiling (exorbitant, fixed) ~s вздутые (непомерные, твёрдые) цены; cost ~ себестоимость; to pay a heavy ~ дорого заплатить (*за — for*); spot ~ цена за наличный расчёт; trade ~ фабричная цена; to cut ~s снижать цены; at any ~ любой ценой, во что бы то ни стало; 2) ценность; above (*или* beyond, without) ~ бесценный.

price II *v* оценивать; назначать цену.

price-cutting ['praɪs‚kʌtɪŋ] *n* снижение цен.

priceless ['praɪslɪs] *a* 1) бесценный; неоценимый; 2) *сленг* бесподобный.

price-list ['praɪslɪst] *n* прейскурант.

prick I [prɪk] *n* 1) остриё; 2) шип (*розы*); 3) укол, прокол; the ~s of conscience угрызения совести; ◊ to kick against the ~s ≅ лезть на рожон.

prick II *v* 1) колоть(ся); 2) прокалывать, накалывать; 3) мучить, терзать (*об угрызениях совести*); 4) накалывать (*узор*); делать разметки (*на полотне*); 5) *уст.* пришпоривать (*коня*); □ to ~ off, to ~ out пикировать рассаду; to ~ up а) поднимать уши (*о собаке и т. п.*); б) настораживаться.

prick-eared ['prɪk'ɪəd] *a* со стоячими ушами (*о собаке*).

prick-ears ['prɪk'ɪəz] *n pl* стоячие уши (*у собаки*); *перен.* «ушки на макушке».

prickle I ['prɪkl] *n* 1) шип, колючка; 2) «иголки» по телу.

prickle II *v* 1) колоть; 2) вызывать колющую боль; 3) подстрекать.

prickly ['prɪklɪ] *a* колючий.

pride I [praɪd] *n* 1) гордость; to take a ~ in smth. а) гордиться чем-л.; б) находить удовольствие в чём-л.; 2) чувство собственного достоинства; false ~ чванство; 3) расцвет (*сил и т. п.*); the ~ of the morning утренний туман; ◊ to put one's ~ in one's pocket проглотить обиду.

pride II *v*: to ~ oneself (up)on гордиться (*кем-л., чем-л.*).

priest [priːst] *n* 1) священник; 2) жрец.

prig I [prɪg] *n* 1) педант, формалист; 2) *сленг* вор.

prig II *v сленг* воровать.

priggish ['prɪgɪʃ] *a* 1) педантичный; 2) самодовольный.

prim I [prɪm] *a* чопорный; натянутый; ~ and proper жеманный.

prim II *v* принимать чопорный, официальный вид.

primacy ['praɪməsɪ] *n* 1) первенство; 2) сан архиепископа.

primal ['praɪməl] *a* 1) примитивный, первобытный; 2) главный, основной.

primary I ['praɪmərɪ] *n* 1) основной цвет; 2) *амер.* предвыборное собрание избирателей одной партии; 3) *эл.* первичная обмотка; 4) *астр.* планета.

primary II *a* 1) первичный, начальный; 2) основной, главный; 3) первостепенный.

primate ['praɪmɪt] *n* архиепископ.

prime[1] I [praɪm] *n* 1) расцвет; in the ~ of life в расцвете сил; 2) начало, весна; раннее утро; the ~ of the year весна.

prime[1] II *a* 1) важнейший; 2) главный; 3) превосходный; лучший, высшего качества; 4) основной, первичный.

prime[2] *v* 1) вставлять (*запал, взрыватель*); 2) *тех.* заливать (*мотор перед пуском*); 3) *разг.* накормить, напоить досыта; ~d with hearty meal плотно поевши; 4) инструктировать, подготавливать кого-л. заранее; 5) грунтовать.

primer[1] ['praɪmə] *n* 1) букварь; учебник для начинающих; 2) молитвенник.

primer[2] *n* капсюль; запал.

primeval [praɪ'miːvəl] *a* первобытный.

priming ['praɪmɪŋ] *n жив.* грунтовка; грунт.

primitive I ['prɪmɪtɪv] *n* 1) примитив; 2) примитивист.

primitive II *a* 1) примитивный; 2) первобытный; 3) простой, обычный; 4) основной.

primordial [praɪ'mɔːdjəl] *a* изначальный, исконный.

primp [prɪmp] *v амер.* наряжать(ся).

primrose ['prɪmrouz] *n* 1) *бот.* первоцвет, примула; 2) *attr* бледно-жёлтый.

prince [prɪns] *n* принц; *ист.* государь; князь; the Prince of Wales принц Уэльский (*наследный принц в Англии*).

princeling ['prɪnslɪŋ] *n презр.* князёк.

princely ['prɪnslɪ] *a* 1) великолепный, роскошный; 2) царственный.

princess [prɪn'ses] *n* принцесса; княгиня; княжна; ~ royal старшая дочь короля.

principal I ['prɪnsəpəl] *n* 1) глава, начальник; 2) директор (*школы*); 3) главное действующее лицо; 4) *юр.* главный виновник; 5) *эк.* основной капитал.

principal II *a* 1) главный; основной; важнейший; 2) ведущий.

principality [ˌprɪnsɪ'pælɪtɪ] *n* княжество; the Principality Уэльс.

principally ['prɪnsəplɪ] *adv* главным образом, большей частью.

principle ['prɪnsəpl] *n* 1) принцип; закон; unanimity ~ принцип единогласия; the ~ of relativity теория относительности; on ~ из принципа; in ~ в принципе; of ~ принципиальный; of no ~s беспринципный; 2) (перво)причина; основа; 3) *хим.* составная часть, элемент.

prink [prɪŋk] *v* наряжаться, прихорашиваться.

print¹ I [prɪnt] *n* 1) отпечаток, след; 2) печатание; to be in ~ выйти из печати; to be out of ~ быть распроданной (*о книге*); 3) *амер.* печатное издание; газета; 4) шрифт; печать; blue ~ синька, светокопия; 5) гравюра, эстамп; 6) *фото* отпечаток (*с негатива*).

print¹ II *v* 1) печатать (*книгу, газету*); издавать; 2) запечатлевать(ся); 3) *фото* отпечатывать(ся).

print² I *n* ситец.

print² II *v* набивать (*ситец*).

printer¹ ['prɪntə] *n* печатник, типограф.

printer² *n текст.* набойщик.

printing ['prɪntɪŋ] *n* 1) печатание; 2) печатное издание.

printing-house ['prɪntɪŋhaus] *n* типография.

printing-press ['prɪntɪŋˌpres] *n* печатный станок.

print-shop ['prɪntʃɔp] *n* магазин гравюр.

print-works ['prɪntwəːks] *n* ситценабивная фабрика.

prior¹ ['praɪə] *a* предшествующий; ~ to раньше, прежде, до.

prior² *n* настоятель, аббат.

priority [praɪ'ɔrɪtɪ] *n* 1) старшинство, приоритет; 2) порядок срочности; очередность; to take ~ of предшествовать.

priory ['praɪərɪ] *n* монастырь.

prism ['prɪzəm] *n* призма.

prison ['prɪzn] *n* тюрьма; to break ~ бежать из тюрьмы; to put to ~ посадить в тюрьму; to cast into ~ бросить в тюрьму.

prison-breaker ['prɪznˌbreɪkə] *n* бежавший из тюрьмы.

prisoner ['prɪznə] *n* 1) заключённый, арестованный; ~ of State, State ~ политический заключённый; to be a ~ to one's chair быть прикованным к креслу; to be kept a close ~ находиться в строгой изоляции; 2) (военно)пленный (*тж.* ~ of war); to take (*или* to make) smb. ~ взять кого-л. в плен.

privacy ['praɪvəsɪ] *n* 1) уединение, одиночество; уединённость; to keep ~ не вмешиваться в чужие дела, стоять в стороне; 2) тайна, секретность.

private I ['praɪvɪt] *n* рядовой, солдат.

private II *a* 1) частный, личный; 2) уединённый; 3) тайный, конфиденциальный; секретный; in ~ а) частным образом; б) по секрету; в) наедине; to keep smth. ~ держать что-л. в тайне.

privateer [ˌpraɪvə'tɪə] *n мор.* капер.

privation [praɪ'veɪʃən] *n* лишения, нужда.

privilege I ['prɪvɪlɪdʒ] *n* привилегия, преимущество; to be a ~ доставлять исключительное наслаждение, удовольствие.

privilege II *v* давать привилегию; освобождать от чего-л.

privileged ['prɪvɪlɪdʒd] *a* привилегированный.

privy ['prɪvɪ] *a* 1) тайный, секретный; 2) частный; 3) уединённый, скрытый; ◊ to be ~ to быть причастным к.

prize¹ I [praɪz] *n* 1) приз, премия; the Lenin Prize Ленинская премия; the International Lenin Peace Prize Международная Ленинская премия за укрепление мира между народами; 2) награда; 3) выигрыш; the ~ of life жизненные блага; 4) *attr* премированный, удостоенный премии.

prize¹ II *v* 1) высоко ценить; оценивать.

prize² *n* 1) *мор.* трофей; захваченное судно; to become a ~ of быть захваченным; to make (a) ~ of захватить; 2) *attr* призовой.

prize-fighter ['praɪzˌfaɪtə] *n* боксёр-профессионал.

prizewinner ['praɪzˌwɪnə] *n* 1) лауреат; Lenin ~ лауреат Ленинской премии; 2) премированный.

pro [prou] *n разг.* специалист.

pro- [prou-] *pref* 1) *со значением* сторонник; 2) *со значением* заместитель; pro-rector проректор.

probability [ˌprɔbə'bɪlɪtɪ] *n* вероятность; возможность; in all ~ по всей вероятности; there is no ~ (*или* that) совершенно невероятно, что...; the ~ is that по-видимому.

probable ['prɔbəbl] *a* 1) вероятный, возможный; 2) предполагаемый; 3) правдоподобный.

probably ['prɔbəblɪ] *adv* вероятно.

probate I ['proubɪt] *n* 1) *юр.* официальное утверждение завещания; 2) заверенная копия завещания.

probate II *v* утверждать завещание.

probation [prə'beɪʃən] 1) испытание, стажировка; 2) испытательный срок; *юр.* условное освобождение.

probationary [prə'beɪʃnərɪ] *a* испытательный.

probationer [prə'beɪʃnə] *n* 1) испытуемый; стажёр; 2) *юр.* условно осуждённый.

probe I [proub] *n* 1) зонд; space ~ космический зонд; 2) *амер.* расследование; 3) *косм.* автоматическая научно-исследовательская станция; Venusian ~ косми́ческая раке́та для изуче́ния Вене́ры.

probe II *v* 1) зонди́ровать; 2) рассле́довать.

probity ['proubiti] *n* че́стность, неподку́пность.

problem ['prɔbləm] *n* пробле́ма; зада́ча (*тж. мат.*); to solve a ~ реша́ть зада́чу.

problematic(al) [,prɔblɪ'mætɪk(əl)] *a* проблемати́чный; спо́рный; сомни́тельный.

procedure [prə'siːdʒə] *n* 1) процеду́ра; 2) о́браз де́йствий; поведе́ние.

proceed [prə'siːd] *v* 1) продолжа́ть; let us now ~! бу́дем продолжа́ть!; 2) возобновля́ть (*дело, игру*); приня́ться за; how shall we ~? как мы начнём?; 3) отправля́ться в путь; 4) переходи́ть (*к чему-л.*); 5) поступа́ть, вести́ себя́; 6) раздава́ться, исходи́ть (*откуда-л.— from*); возника́ть (*о болезнях*); происходи́ть; 7) *юр.* возбужда́ть де́ло (*против — against*); 8) получа́ть учёную сте́пень.

proceeding [prə'siːdɪŋ] *n* 1) посту́пок; 2) *pl* судопроизво́дство, веде́ние де́ла; to take legal ~s возбуди́ть де́ло; 3) *pl* труды́. (*учёного общества*); дела́; протоко́лы.

proceeds ['prousiːdz] *n pl* вы́ручка, дохо́д.

processᵃ ['prouses] *n* 1) проце́сс; to be in ~ происходи́ть, име́ть ме́сто; to be in ~ of *показыва́ет продолжающееся действие:* the house is in ~ of construction дом сейча́с стро́ится; 2) ме́тод, техноло́гический проце́сс, спо́соб; 3) *юр.* вы́зов в суд, судебное предписа́ние.

processᵇ [prə'ses] *v* 1) подверга́ть технологи́ческому проце́ссу; обраба́тывать; 2) *юр.* возбужда́ть де́ло, проце́сс.

processing [prə'sesɪŋ] *n* перерабо́тка (пищевы́х) проду́ктов.

procession I [prə'seʃən] *n* проце́ссия.

procession II *v* уча́ствовать в проце́ссии.

proclaim [prə'kleɪm] *v* 1) объявля́ть; 2) провозглаша́ть; 3) объявля́ть на чрезвыча́йном положе́нии (*город, район*); 4) запреща́ть (*собра́ние*).

proclamation [,prɔklə'meɪʃən] *n* 1) объявле́ние; 2) провозглаше́ние.

proclivity [prə'klɪvɪtɪ] *n* скло́нность.

procrastinate [prou'kræstɪneɪt] *v* откла́дывать, ме́длить.

procrastination [prou,kræstɪ'neɪʃən] *n* промедле́ние.

procreate ['proukrɪeɪt] *v* порожда́ть.

procreation [,proukrɪ'eɪʃən] *n* порожде́ние.

procure [prə'kjuə] *v* 1) обеспе́чивать, достава́ть; заготовля́ть; 2) *уст.* причиня́ть; вызыва́ть (*смерть*); 3) сво́дничать.

prod I [prɔd] *n* 1) тычо́к, пино́к; a ~ with a bayonet уда́р штыко́м; 2) пробо́йник, ши́ло.

prod II *v* 1) ты́кать; коло́ть; 2) подгоня́ть; подстрека́ть.

prodigal I ['prɔdɪgəl] *n* мот, расточи́тель.

prodigal II *a* 1) расточи́тельный; 2) ще́дрый (*на что-л. — of*); 3) изоби́льный.

prodigality [,prɔdɪ'gælɪtɪ] *n* 1) расточи́тельность; 2) изоби́лие.

prodigious [prə'dɪdʒəs] *a* 1) огро́мный, невероя́тный; 2) удиви́тельный, изуми́тельный.

prodigy ['prɔdɪdʒɪ] *n* 1) одарённый челове́к; 2) чу́до.

produceᵃ ['prɔdjuːs] *n* 1) проду́кция, проду́кт; 2) результа́т.

produceᵇ [prə'djuːs] *v* 1) производи́ть, выраба́тывать; 2) написа́ть, изда́ть (*книгу*); 3) (по)ста́вить (*пьесу, кинокартину*); 4) предъявля́ть (*билеты, доказа́тельства и т. п.*); 5) вынима́ть, достава́ть; 6) *мат.* проводи́ть, продолжа́ть (*линию*).

producer [prə'djuːsə] *n* 1) производи́тель; 2) режиссёр; постано́вщик; 3) *тех.* генера́тор; 4) *attr.* генера́торный.

producible [prə'djuːsəbl] *a* производи́мый.

product ['prɔdəkt] *n* 1) проду́кт, изде́лие; фабрика́т; 2) результа́т; 3) *хим.* проду́кт реа́кции; 4) *мат.* произведе́ние.

production [prə'dʌkʃən] *n* 1) произво́дство; изготовле́ние; вы́работка; commodity ~ това́рное произво́дство; 2) проду́кция, това́ры; пода́ча (*нефтяной скважины*); 3) произведе́ние (*литературы, искусства*); 4) постано́вка (*пьесы, кинокарти́ны*).

productive [prə'dʌktɪv] *a* 1) производи́тельный; продукти́вный; 2) плодоро́дный; 3) плодови́тый; 4) плодотво́рный (*о влиянии*).

productivity [,prɔdʌk'tɪvɪtɪ] *n* продукти́вность, производи́тельность; ~ of labour производи́тельность труда́.

profanation [,prɔfə'neɪʃən] *n* опошле́ние, профана́ция.

profane I [prə'feɪn] *a* 1) све́тский, мирско́й; 2) непосвящённый; 3) язы́ческий; 4) нечести́вый, непристо́йный.

profane II *v* оскверня́ть.

profess [prə'fes] *v* 1) выража́ть (*мнение, удовлетворе́ние*); 2) откры́то признава́ть, заявля́ть; 3) испове́довать (*веру*); 4) де́лать вид, прики́дываться; 5) занима́ться како́й-л. де́ятельностью; 6) преподава́ть.

professedly [prə'fesɪdlɪ] *adv* я́вно, откры́то.

profession [prə'feʃən] *n* 1) профе́ссия; legal ~ профе́ссия юри́ста; liberal ~s свобо́дные профе́ссии; 2) лю́ди одно́й профе́ссии; the ~ *сленг* актёры; 3) призна́ние (*в своих чувствах*); the ~s of friendship увере́ния в дру́жбе; the ~s of love излия́ния в любви́; 4) вероиспове́дание.

professional I [prə'feʃənl] *n* 1) специали́ст; 2) профессиона́л.

professional II *a* 1) профессиона́льный; 2) обу́ченный, име́ющий профе́ссию *или* специа́льность.

professor [prə'fesə] *n* 1) профе́ссор; 2) *разг.* инстру́ктор, тре́нер.

professorial [,prɔfe'sɔːrɪəl] *a* профе́ссорский.

professorship [prə'fesəʃɪp] *n* профессу́ра.

proffer I ['prɔfə] *n* предложе́ние.

proffer II *v* предлага́ть.

proficiency [prə'fɪʃənsɪ] *n* о́пытность, сноро́вка, уме́ние.

proficient I [prə'fɪʃənt] *n* специали́ст; знато́к.

proficient II *a* о́пытный, уме́лый, иску́сный (*в чем-л. — in, at*).

profile I ['proufiːl, *амер. тж.* 'proufaɪl] *n* 1) про́филь, очерта́ние; 2) габари́т, ко́нтур.

profile II *v* изобража́ть в про́филе *или* в разре́зе.

profit I ['prɔfɪt] *n* 1) вы́года, по́льза; to make a ~ on извлека́ть вы́году; 2) *обыкн. pl* дохо́д(ы), при́быль, бары́ш; gross ~s валово́й дохо́д; net ~

чи́стый дохо́д; to split the ~s подели́ть дохо́ды; 3) проце́нты, начисле́ния.

profit II *v* 1) получа́ть по́льзу; 2) приноси́ть вы́году; 3) воспо́льзоваться (*чем-л.*— *by*).

profitable ['prɒfɪtəbl] *a* 1) вы́годный, дохо́дный, при́быльный; 2) поле́зный.

profiteer I [ˌprɒfɪ'tɪə] *n* спекуля́нт; war ~s спекули́рующие на войне́, поджига́тели войны́.

profiteer II *v* спекули́ровать.

profligacy ['prɒflɪgəsɪ] *n* распу́тство.

profligate I ['prɒflɪgɪt] *n* распу́тник.

profligate II *a* 1) распу́тный; 2) расточи́тельный.

profound [prə'faund] *a* 1) глубо́кий; 2) по́лный, абсолю́тный; 3) му́дрый, дальнови́дный; 4) ни́зкий (*о поклоне*); 5) проникнове́нный.

profoundness [prə'faundnɪs] *см.* profundity.

profundity [prə'fʌndɪtɪ] *n* 1) глубина́; 2) про́пасть.

profuse [prə'fjuːs] *a* 1) оби́льный; изоби́льный; бога́тый (*чем-л.*); чрезме́рный; 2) ще́дрый (*на что-л.*— *in*, *of*).

profusely [prə'fjuːslɪ] *adv* оби́льно, чрезме́рно.

profusion [prə'fjuːʒən] *n* 1) оби́лие, бога́тство, избы́ток; 2) чрезме́рная ро́скошь; 3) ще́дрость; расточи́тельность.

progeny ['prɒdʒɪnɪ] *n* 1) пото́мок, пото́мство; 2) после́дователи, ученики́.

prognosis [prɒg'nousɪs] *n* (*pl* prognoses [prɒg'nousiːz]) прогно́з.

prognostic I [prəg'nɒstɪk] *n* предве́стие, предсказа́ние.

prognostic II *a* предвеща́ющий.

program(me) ['prougræm] *n* 1) програ́мма, план; what is the ~? чем мы займёмся?; 2) *attr* програ́ммный.

progress[a] ['prougres] *n* 1) прогре́сс; движе́ние вперёд; рост, разви́тие; to be in ~ a) развива́ться; б) вести́сь (*о следствии и т. п.*); 2) продвиже́ние; *перен. тж.* успе́хи; to make ~ де́лать успе́хи; 3) тече́ние вре́мени, собы́тий.

progress[b] [prə'gres] *v* 1) прогресси́ровать; развива́ться; 2) продвига́ться вперёд; 3) де́лать успе́хи.

progression [prə'greʃən] *n* 1) продвиже́ние; движе́ние вперёд; 2) *мат.* прогре́ссия; arithmetical ~ арифмети́ческая прогре́ссия; geometric(al) ~ геометри́ческая прогре́ссия.

progressionist [prə'greʃnɪst] *n* сторо́нник прогре́сса.

progressist [prə'gresɪst] *n* прогресси́ст.

progressive I [prə'gresɪv] *n* прогресси́вный де́ятель.

progressive II *a* 1) прогресси́вный; 2) поступа́тельный; 3) прогресси́рующий, возраста́ющий.

prohibit [prə'hɪbɪt] *v* 1) запреща́ть; 2) не дава́ть (*делать что-л.; from*).

prohibition [ˌprouɪ'bɪʃən] *n* запре́т, запреще́ние (*особ. продажи спиртных напитков*).

prohibitive [prə'hɪbɪtɪv] *a* 1) запрети́тельный (*о пошлине и т. п.*); 2) запреща́ющий, препя́тствующий.

project[a] ['prɒdʒekt] *n* прое́кт; план; предложе́ние; to start a ~ вы́двинуть прое́кт *или* предложе́ние; 2) стро́йка, строи́тельство.

project[b] [prə'dʒekt] *v* 1) проекти́ровать; 2) со-

ставля́ть, обду́мывать (*план*); 3) отбра́сывать, отража́ть (*тень, луч света*); 4) выбра́сывать, выпуска́ть (*снаряд*); 5) выдава́ться, выступа́ть.

projectile[a] ['prɒdʒɪktaɪl] *n* снаря́д (*бомба, грана́та, пуля*).

projectile[b] [prə'dʒektaɪl] *a* мета́тельный.

projection [prə'dʒekʃən] *n* 1) проекти́рование; прое́кт; 2) прое́кция; 3) вы́ступ; выдаю́щаяся часть.

projector [prə'dʒektə] *n* 1) проекти́ровщик; 2) прожёктер; 3) проекцио́нный, «волше́бный» фона́рь.

proletarian I [ˌproule'tɛərɪən] *n* пролета́рий.

proletarian II *a* пролета́рский.

proletariat(e) [ˌproule'tɛərɪət] *n* пролетариа́т.

prolific [prə'lɪfɪk] *a* 1) плодоро́дный; 2) плодови́тый; 3) изоби́лующий (*чем-л.— in*, *of*).

prolix ['proulɪks] *a* ну́дный, тягу́чий; многосло́вный.

prologue ['proulɒg] *n* проло́г.

prolong [prə'lɒŋ] *v* 1) продлева́ть; 2) продо́лжить (*линию*).

prolongation [ˌproulɒŋ'geɪʃən] *n* 1) продле́ние; отсро́чка; пролонга́ция; 2) продолже́ние (*линии*).

prolonged [prə'lɒŋd] *a* 1) дли́тельный; 2) затяну́вшийся (*о посещении и т. п.*).

promenade I [ˌprɒmɪ'nɑːd, *амер. тж.* prɒmɪ'neɪd] *n* 1) прогу́лка; гуля́нье; 2) ме́сто для гуля́нья; 3) *разг.* бал, та́нцы; 4) *attr* прогу́лочный (*о палубе*).

promenade II *v* 1) прогу́ливаться; разгу́ливать; 2) выводи́ть на прогу́лку.

prominence ['prɒmɪnəns] *n* 1) выдаю́щееся положе́ние; to give ~ to продвига́ть; 2) вы́ступ; 3) вы́пуклость, неро́вность.

prominency ['prɒmɪnənsɪ] *n* заме́тное, ви́дное положе́ние.

prominent ['prɒmɪnənt] *a* 1) выдаю́щийся; 2) выступа́ющий, торча́щий; 3) ви́дный, изве́стный.

promiscuity [ˌprɒmɪs'kjuːɪtɪ] *n* 1) разноро́дность; разношёрстность; 2) сме́шанный хара́ктер (*чего-л.*); 3) беспоря́дочность.

promiscuous [prə'mɪskjuəs] *a* 1) разноро́дный; разношёрстный; 3) совме́стный (*о купании*); 4) беспоря́дочный; 5) *разг.* случа́йный.

promise I ['prɒmɪs] *n* 1) обеща́ние; to break one's ~ не сдержа́ть обеща́ния; to keep one's ~ сдержа́ть обеща́ние; испо́лнить обе́щанное; to give (*или* to make) a ~ дать обеща́ние; to go back on one's ~ нару́шать обеща́ние; 2) перспекти́ва; of great ~ подаю́щий наде́жды, многообеща́ющий.

promise II *v* 1) обеща́ть; 2) *только в 1 л.* уверя́ю вас; it was not so easy, I ~ you э́то бы́ло не так легко́, уверя́ю вас; 3) подава́ть наде́жды.

promising ['prɒmɪsɪŋ] *a* подаю́щий наде́жды; the weather looks ~ пого́да обеща́ет быть хоро́шей.

promissory ['prɒmɪsərɪ] *a* 1) содержа́щий обеща́ние; 2) долгово́й (*об обязательстве*).

promontory ['prɒməntrɪ] *n* мыс.

promote [prə'mout] *v* 1) повыша́ть, продвига́ть (*по службе*); 2) производи́ть в чин; 3) помога́ть, соде́йствовать, спосо́бствовать; 4) *шк.* переводи́ть в сле́дующий класс; 5) *шахм.* продвига́ть (*пешку*); 6) *хим.* ускоря́ть (*реакцию*).

promoter [prə'moutə] *n* 1) лицо, способствующее развитию науки, искусства *и т. п.*; покровитель; патрон; 2) *хим.* активатор.

promotion [prə'mouʃən] *n* 1) производство в чин; 2) содействие; 3) продвижение (*по службе и т. п.*); 4) *шк.* перевод в следующий класс.

prompt I [prɔmpt] *a* 1) быстрый; незамедлительный; 2) проворный; 3) подлежащий немедленной оплате *или* доставке (*о товаре*).

prompt II *v* 1) толкать, побуждать; 2) подсказывать; 3) *театр.* суфлировать.

prompt-box ['prɔmptbɔks] *n* суфлёрская будка.

prompter ['prɔmptə] *n* 1) суфлёр; 2) побудитель к действию, «толкач».

prompting ['prɔmptiŋ] *n* побуждение.

promptitude ['prɔmptitjuːd] *n* 1) быстрота; проворство; 2) аккуратность (*в платежах*).

promulgate ['prɔməlgeit] *v* 1) объявлять, обнародовать, опубликовывать (*закон, указ*); 2) распространять (*учение, веру*).

promulgation [‚prɔməl'geiʃən] *n* обнародование, опубликование (*закона, указа*).

prone [proun] *a* 1) распростёртый, лежащий ничком; 2) *predic* склонный.

prong I [prɔŋ] *n* 1) зуб(ец); 2) вилы.

prong II *v* 1) проткнуть; 2) поворачивать вилами.

pronominal [prə'nɔminl] *a грам.* местоименный.

pronoun ['prounaun] *n* местоимение; demonstrative (indefinite, interrogative, personal, possessive, relative) ~ указательное (неопределённое, вопросительное, личное, притяжательное, относительное) местоимение.

pronounce [prə'nauns] *v* 1) произносить, выговаривать; 2) заявлять, объявлять; 3) высказываться (*о — on, за — for; против — against; в пользу — in favour of*).

pronounceable [prə'naunsəbl] *a* произносимый.

pronounced [prə'naunst] *a* 1) резко выраженный; 2) определённый, явный.

pronouncement [prə'naunsmənt] *n* 1) объявление решения *или* приговора; 2) официальное заявление.

pronunciation [prə‚nʌnsi'eiʃən] *n* произношение, выговор.

proof I [pruːf] *n* 1) доказательство; 2) испытание, проба; 3) *мат.* проверка; 4) крепость (*спирта*); 5) *полигр.* корректура; гранка; galley ~s гранки; press ~ сводка; ◊ the ~ of the pudding is in the eating *посл.* ≅ всё проверяется практикой.

proof II *a* 1) непроницаемый; непробиваемый; 2) не поддающийся (*лести, подкупу и т. п.*); неподкупный; 3) установленной крепости (*о спирте*).

proof-read ['pruːf‚riːd] *v* читать гранки; держать корректуру.

proof-reader ['pruːf‚riːdə] *n* корректор.

proof-sheet ['pruːfʃiːt] *n* корректурный оттиск, лист.

prop I [prɔp] *n* 1) подпорка, подставка; 2) опора (*тж. перен.*).

prop II *v* подпирать, поддерживать (*тж.* to ~ up).

propaganda [‚prɔpə'gændə] *n* пропаганда; smear ~ клеветническая пропаганда.

propagandist [‚prɔpə'gændist] *n* пропагандист.

propagate ['prɔpəgeit] *v* 1) размножать(ся); разводить; 2) распространять(ся); 3) *физ.* передавать (*звук, свет, тепло*) на расстояние.

propagation [‚prɔpə'geiʃən] *n* 1) размножение; разведение; 2) распространение.

propel [prə'pel] *v* 1) двигать вперёд; приводить в движение; 2) стимулировать.

propeller [prə'pelə] *n* 1) *ав.* воздушный винт; 2) *мор.* гребной винт.

propensity [prə'pensiti] *n* склонность, предрасположение (*к чему-л.— to*).

proper ['prɔpə] *a* 1) присущий, свойственный; 2) подходящий, надлежащий; правильный; 3) пристойный, приличный; 4) точный, истинный; 5) *разг.* основательный, настоящий; 6) собственный; 7) *уст.* красивый.

properly ['prɔpəli] *adv* 1) как следует; должным образом, правильно; 2) прилично; 3) *разг.* здорово, хорошенько; 4) собственно, строго говоря; ~ speaking собственно говоря.

propertied ['prɔpətid] *a* имущий.

property ['prɔpəti] *n* 1) собственность, имущество; immovable ~ недвижимое имущество; personal ~, portable ~ движимое имущество; landed ~ земельная собственность, private ~ частная собственность; a ~ земельная собственность, имение; literary ~ авторское право; 2) свойство, качество; 3) *pl театр.* бутафория.

prophecy ['prɔfisi] *n* пророчество.

prophesy ['prɔfisai] *v* пророчить, предсказывать.

prophet ['prɔfit] *n* 1) пророк; 2) предсказатель.

prophetic(al) [prə'fetik(əl)] *a* пророческий.

propinquity [prə'piŋkwiti] *n* близость, (с)родство.

propitiate [prə'piʃieit] *v* 1) умиротворять; 2) умилостивлять.

propitious [prə'piʃəs] *a* 1) благоприятный; 2) благосклонный.

proportion I [prə'pɔːʃən] *n* пропорция, (со)отношение; in ~ to соразмерно; out of ~ несоизмеримо; несоразмерно.

proportion II *v* соразмерять (*с чем-л.— to*).

proportional I [prə'pɔːʃənl] *n мат.* член пропорции.

proportional II *a* пропорциональный.

proportionate[a] [prə'pɔːʃnit] *a* пропорциональный, соразмерный.

proportionate[b] [prə'pɔːʃneit] *v* соразмерять, делать пропорциональным.

proposal [prə'pouzəl] *n* предложение; to make a ~ внести предложение.

propose [prə'pouz] *v* 1) предложить, предлагать; вносить предложение; 2) представлять (*кандидата на должность*); 3) предполагать, намереваться; строить планы; 4) делать предложение (*о браке; to*); 5) загадывать (*загадку*); 6) провозглашать тост.

proposition [‚prɔpə'ziʃən] *n* 1) предложение; 2) утверждение; 3) *разг.* предприятие, дело; 4) *мат.* теорема; доказательство теоремы; ◊ he is a tough ~ с ним трудно иметь дело.

propound [prə'paund] *v* 1) выдвигать (*теорию, проблему*); 2) ставить на обсуждение (*план, вопрос*); 3) загадывать (*загадку*).

proprietary I [prə'praiətəri] *n* право собственности.

proprietary II *a* 1) собственнический; составляющий собственность; 2) патенто́ванный (*о лека́рствах*).

proprietor [prə'praıətə] *n* владе́лец, со́бственник; хозя́ин; landed ~ землевладе́лец.

proprietress [prə'praıətrıs] *n* со́бственница, владе́лица; хозя́йка.

propriety [prə'praıətı] *n* 1) присто́йность, прили́чие; the proprieties a) прили́чия; б) *сленг* бутафо́рия; 2) уме́стность.

propulsion [prə'pʌlʃən] *n* 1) толчо́к; движе́ние вперёд; 2) дви́жущая си́ла; jet ~ реакти́вный дви́гатель.

propulsive [prə'pʌlsıv] *a* 1) приводя́щий в движе́ние; 2) побужда́ющий.

prorogation [,prourə'geıʃən] *n* переры́в в рабо́те парла́мента.

prorogue [prə'roug] *v* 1) откла́дывать (*се́ссию парла́мента*); 2) отсро́чить.

pros [prouz] *n*: the ~ and cons до́воды за и про́тив.

prosaic [prou'zeıık] *a* 1) прозаи́ческий; 2) повседне́вный, ску́чный.

proscenium [prou'si:njəm] *n* (*pl* proscenia [prou'si:njə]) авансце́на.

proscribe [prous'kraıb] *v* 1) объявля́ть вне зако́на; изгоня́ть, высыла́ть; 2) запреща́ть; 3) *уст.* оглаша́ть (*фами́лии престу́пников*).

proscription [prous'krıpʃən] *n* 1) объявле́ние вне зако́на, проскри́пция; изгна́ние; 2) запреще́ние; 3) *уст.* оглаше́ние (*фами́лий престу́пников*).

prose I [prouz] *n* 1) про́за; 2) повседне́вность; про́за жи́зни; 3) *attr* прозаи́ческий.

prose II *v* 1) писа́ть про́зой; 2) говори́ть ну́дно, ску́чно.

prosecute ['prɔsıkju:t] *v* 1) вести́ (*заня́тия, рассле́дование, торго́влю*); проводи́ть; 2) пресле́довать суде́бным поря́дком.

prosecution [,prɔsı'kju:ʃən] *n* 1) веде́ние (*заня́тий, рассле́дования, торго́вли*); 2) *юр.* суде́бное пресле́дование; 3) (the ~) *юр.* обвине́ние (*сторона́ в суде́бном проце́ссе*).

prosecutor ['prɔsıkju:tə] *n* 1) обвини́тель; public ~ прокуро́р; 2) исте́ц.

proselyte ['prɔsılaıt] *n* новообращённый.

proselytize ['prɔsılıtaız] *v* обраща́ть в свою́ ве́ру.

prosit ['prousıt] *int* за ва́ше здоро́вье!

prosody ['prɔsədı] *n* *лит.* просо́дия.

prospect[a] ['prɔspekt] *n* 1) вид, карти́на приро́ды, панора́ма; 2) перспекти́ва; 3) *обыкн.* *pl* пла́ны, ви́ды на бу́дущее; cheerful (gloomy) ~s блестя́щие (мра́чные) перспекти́вы; what are your ~s for today? что вы собира́етесь де́лать сего́дня? 4) *амер.* предполага́емый клие́нт; 5) *геол., горн.* разве́дка, изыска́ние.

prospect[b] [prəs'pekt] *v* иссле́довать; де́лать изыска́ния.

prospective [prəs'pektıv] *a* бу́дущий, ожида́емый.

prospector [prəs'pektə] *n* *геол., горн.* разве́дчик, изыска́тель; золотоиска́тель.

prospectus [prəs'pektəs] *n* проспе́кт (*кни́ги, изда́ния*).

prosper ['prɔspə] *v* преуспева́ть, процвета́ть; де́лать успе́хи.

prosperity [prɔs'perıtı] *n* 1) процвета́ние, благо-

де́нствие; благосостоя́ние; 2) *pl* благоприя́тные обстоя́тельства.

prosperous ['prɔspərəs] *a* 1) цвету́щий, процвета́ющий; 2) име́ющий уда́чу, успе́шный; 3) зажи́точный, состоя́тельный; 4) благоприя́тный; попу́тный (*о ве́тре*).

prosthesis ['prɔsθısıs] *n* 1) проте́з; 2) *лингв.* проте́за.

prostitute I ['prɔstıtju:t] *n* 1) проститу́тка; 2) найми́т; прода́жный челове́к.

prostitute II *v* 1) занима́ться проститу́цией; 2) проститу́ировать, изменя́ть свои́м убежде́ниям.

prostitution [,prɔstı'tju:ʃən] *n* 1) проститу́ция; 2) проститу́ирование.

prostrate[a] ['prɔstreıt] *a* 1) распростёртый, пове́рженный; 2) изможде́нный, обесси́левший; в простра́ции.

prostrate[b] [prɔs'treıt] *v* 1) поверга́ть (*на зе́млю*); to ~ oneself па́дать ниц (*before, at*); *перен.* унижа́ться; 2) истоща́ть, изнуря́ть; 3) доводи́ть до отча́яния.

prostration [prɔs'treıʃən] *n* 1) пове́рженное состоя́ние; 2) изнеможе́ние, истоще́ние; упа́док сил; простра́ция.

prosy ['prouzı] *a* 1) прозаи́ческий; 2) прозаи́чный, бана́льный; утоми́тельный.

protagonist [prou'tægənıst] *n* 1) гла́вный геро́й (*лит. произведе́ния*); 2) актёр, игра́ющий гла́вную роль; 3) побо́рник.

protasis ['prɔtəsıs] *n* (*pl* protases ['prɔtəsi:z]) *грам.* часть усло́вного предложе́ния, содержа́щая усло́вие.

protect [prə'tekt] *v* 1) защища́ть (*от — from; про́тив — against*); оборонять; 2) предохраня́ть; 3) покрови́тельствовать.

protection [prə'tekʃən] *n* 1) защи́та, оборо́на; 2) предохране́ние; 3) охра́на; labour ~ охра́на труда́; 4) охра́нная гра́мота; 5) покрови́тельство; 6) *см.* protectionism.

protectionism [prə'tekʃənızəm] *n* *эк.* протекциони́зм.

protective [prə'tektıv] *a* 1) защи́тный, охра́нный; 2) предохрани́тельный; 3) покрови́тельственный; защити́тельный.

protector [prə'tektə] *n* 1) защи́тник; 2) покрови́тель, храни́тель; 3) *ист.* ре́гент; Lord Protector лорд-проте́ктор (*ти́тул Кро́мвеля*); 4) *тех.* предохрани́тель.

protectorate [prə'tektərıt] *n* протектора́т.

protectorship [prə'tektəʃıp] *n* 1) протектора́т; 2) покрови́тельство.

protein ['prouti:n] *n* 1) протеи́н, бело́к.

protest[a] ['proutest] *n* проте́ст; under ~ про́тив во́ли; наси́льно; to enter (*или* to make, to lodge) a ~ заявля́ть, подава́ть проте́ст; 2) опротесто́вание (*ве́кселя*).

protest[b] [prə'test] *v* 1) протестова́ть, возража́ть; 2) опротесто́вывать (*ве́ксель*); 3) торже́ственно заявля́ть; I ~ я заверя́ю вас.

protestant ['prɔtıstənt] *n* *рел.* 1) протеста́нт; 2) *attr* протеста́нтский.

protestation [,proutes'teıʃən] *n* 1) торже́ственное завере́ние, заявле́ние; 2) *ре́дко* проте́ст; возраже́ние.

protocol I ['proutəkɔl] *n* 1) протоко́л; 2) дополни́тельное междунаро́дное соглаше́ние;

3) *дип.* прелиминарный договор, соглашение; 4) правила этикета.

protocol II *v* протоколировать, вести протокол.

proton ['proutən] *n физ.* протон.

protract [prə'trækt] *v* 1) растягивать; 2) медлить; тянуть (*время*); 3) чертить (*план*).

protracted [prə'træktɪd] *a* 1) затянувшийся; 2) длительный; затяжной.

protraction [prə'trækʃən] *n* 1) проволочка, промедление; 2) нанесение на план; вычерчивание.

protractor [prə'træktə] *n* 1) *тех.* транспортир, угломер; 2) *анат.* разгибательная мышца.

protrude [prə'truːd] *v* 1) выдаваться, торчать; 2) высовывать (*язык*).

protruding [prə'truːdɪŋ] *a* 1) торчащий, выдающийся, выступающий вперёд; 2) высунутый наружу.

protrusion [prə'truːʒən] *n* 1) выступ; 2) высовывание.

protrusive [prə'truːsiv] *a* 1) выступающий, торчащий; 2) выдающийся вперёд.

protuberance [prə'tjuːbərəns] *n* 1) выпуклость; 2) опухоль; 3) *астр.* протуберанец.

protuberant [prə'tjuːbərənt] *a* выпуклый, выдающийся вперёд.

proud [praud] *a* 1) гордый; to be ~ of гордиться (*чем-л., кем-л.*); 2) надменный, высокомерный; 3) самодовольный; ~ as Punch преисполненный самодовольства; as ~ as a peacock важный, гордый, как павлин; 4) довольный; you do me ~ *сленг* вы мне оказываете много чести; 5) горделивый, величавый; великолепный (*о вещах*); 6) горячий, ретивый (*о коне*).

proud-spirited ['praud'spiritid] *a* гордый, заносчивый.

prove [pruːv] *v* 1) доказывать; 2) испытывать; пробовать; 3) *с последующим Inf смыслового гл.* оказаться, оказываться; the report ~d to be very interesting доклад оказался очень интересным; 4) удостоверять; 5) *юр.* утверждать (*завещание*); 6) *мат.* проверять.

provenance ['provinəns] *n* происхождение, источник; its ~ is doubtful сомнительного происхождения; to settle the ~ of установить происхождение, источник.

provender ['provində] *n* корм.

provenience [prou'viːniəns] *см.* provenance.

proverb ['provəb] *n* пословица; поговорка.

proverbial [prə'vəːbjəl] *a* вошедший в пословицу; широко известный; легендарный.

provide [prə'vaid] *v* 1) обеспечивать, снабжать; 2) доставлять, давать; 3) заготавливать; 4) предусматривать; 5) принимать меры (for).

provided [prə'vaidid] *conj* при условии; лишь бы; если только; в том случае если.

providence ['providəns] *n* 1) предусмотрительность; 2) бережливость; 3) (P.) провидение.

provident ['providənt] *a* 1) предусмотрительный; 2) осторожный; бережливый, расчётливый.

providential [.provi'denʃəl] *a* 1) счастливый; 2) предопределённый.

provider [prə'vaidə] *n* поставщик.

providing [prə'vaidiŋ] *conj* при условии, учитывая.

province ['provins] *n* 1) область, провинция; 2) *pl* периферия, удалённая от центра местность; 3) сфера деятельности, компетенция; 4) область знаний; 5) епархия.

provincial I [prə'vinʃəl] *n* провинциал.

provincial II *a* провинциальный.

provincialism [prə'vinʃəlizəm] *n* провинциализм.

provinciality [prə,vinʃi'æliti] *n* провинциальность.

provision I [prə'viʒən] *n* 1) заготовление, заготовка; 2) снабжение, обеспечение; to make ~ обеспечивать; 3) *pl* съестные припасы, провиант; 4) постановление; мера предосторожности (*против чего-л.* — against); 5) *юр.* положение (*договора и т. п.*).

provision II *v* снабжать продовольствием.

provisional [prə'viʒənl] *a* 1) временный; 2) предварительный.

proviso [prə'vaizou] *n* оговорка, условие.

provisory [prə'vaizəri] *a* 1) временный; 2) условный.

provocation [.provə'keiʃən] *n* 1) вызов; побуждение; подстрекательство; 2) провокация; 3) раздражение.

provocative I [prə'vɔkətiv] *n* 1) возбуждающее средство; 2) возбудитель; раздражитель.

provocative II *a* 1) раздражающий; 2) вызывающий (*о поведении и т. п.*); 3) возбуждающий, стимулирующий (*интерес, любопытство*).

provoke [prə'vouk] *v* 1) вызывать, возбуждать; 2) провоцировать; 3) раздражать, сердить, злить; 4) побуждать.

provoking [prə'voukiŋ] *a* досадный, неприятный.

provost[a] ['provəst] *n* 1) ректор (*колледжа*); 2) *шотл.* мэр города.

provost[b] [prə'vou] *n* офицер военной полиции.

prow [prau] *n* 1) нос (*корабля, самолёта*); 2) *поэт.* судно, корабль.

prowess ['prauis] *n* доблесть, удаль.

prowl I [praul] *v* красться, пробираться (*к добыче*); *перен.* пролезть, втереться.

prowl II *n*: on the ~ крадучись.

proximate ['prɔksimit] *a* ближайший, непосредственный.

proximity [prɔk'simiti] *n* близость; ~ of blood кровное родство.

proximo ['prɔksimou] *adv* следующего месяца; on the 1st ~ первого числа следующего месяца.

proxy ['prɔksi] *n* 1) передача голоса, полномочий; доверенность (*на право голосования и т. п.*); by ~ по доверенности; 2) заместитель; 3) уполномоченный; to be (*или* to stand) ~ for быть чьим-л. уполномоченным.

prude [pruːd] *n* 1) жеманница; 2) не в меру щепетильная женщина.

prudence ['pruːdəns] *n* 1) осторожность, осмотрительность; 2) благоразумие, рассудительность; 3) расчётливость, бережливость.

prudent ['pruːdənt] *a* 1) осторожный, осмотрительный; 2) благоразумный, рассудительный; 3) расчётливый, бережливый.

prudery ['pruːdəri] *n* притворная стыдливость; излишняя щепетильность.

prudish ['pruːdiʃ] *a* 1) щепетильный, стыдливый; 2) жеманный.

prune I [pruːn] *n* 1) чернослив; 2) красновато-

-лило́вый цвет; ◇ ~s and prism жема́нство, ма-
не́рность в ре́чи.

prune II *v* 1) обреза́ть, подстрига́ть (*деревья
и т. п.*); 2) сокраща́ть (*расходы*); 3) упроща́ть
(*стиль; обыкн.* to ~ away, to ~ down).

Prussian I ['prʌʃən] *n* пруссáк.

Prussian II *a* прýсский.

prussic ['prʌsɪk] *см.* acid I.

pry¹ I [praɪ] *n* любопы́тный челове́к (*тж.*
Paul Pry).

pry¹ II *v* 1) смотре́ть внима́тельно, с любопы́т-
ством; 2) подгля́дывать, подсма́тривать (*тж.* to ~
about); 3) сова́ть нос (*в чужие дела; into*);
допы́тываться.

pry² *v* поднима́ть *или* вскрыва́ть при по́мощи
рычага́.

prying ['praɪɪŋ] *a* 1) пытли́вый; 2) назо́йливо
любопы́тный.

psalm [sɑːm] *n* псало́м.

pseudo ['psjuːdou] *a* фальши́вый, подде́льный,
притво́рный.

pseudo- ['psjuːdou-] *pref* ложно-, псевдо-.

pseudonym ['psjuːdənɪm] *n* псевдони́м.

pshaw I [pʃɔː] *int* фи!

pshaw II *v* выража́ть пренебреже́ние; фы́ркать.

psychiatrist [saɪˈkaɪətrɪst] *n* психиа́тр.

psychic ['saɪkɪk] *a* психи́ческий.

psychological [ˌsaɪkəˈlɔdʒɪkəl] *a* психологи́чес-
кий.

psychologist [saɪˈkɔlədʒɪst] *n* психо́лог.

psychology [saɪˈkɔlədʒɪ] *n* психоло́гия.

ptarmigan ['tɑːmɪgən] *n* куропа́тка; rock ~ го́р-
ная куропа́тка.

pub [pʌb] *n разг.* пивна́я, кабачо́к.

puberty ['pjuːbətɪ] *n* полова́я зре́лость.

public I ['pʌblɪk] *n* 1) пýблика, наро́д; general ~
широ́кая пýблика; in ~ откры́то, публи́чно; 2)
обще́ственность; 3) *разг.* пивна́я, таве́рна.

public II *a* 1) обще́ственный; 2) (обще)наро́д-
ный; 3) коммуна́льный; 4) публи́чный, общедостýп-
ный; 5) откры́тый, гла́сный.

publican ['pʌblɪkən] *n* 1) тракти́рщик; 2) от-
кýпщик (*в древнем Риме*).

publication [ˌpʌblɪˈkeɪʃən] *n* 1) опубликова́ние;
оглаше́ние; 2) изда́ние (*книги, журнала, газеты*);
публика́ция.

publicist ['pʌblɪsɪst] *n* 1) публици́ст; корреспон-
де́нт газе́ты; 2) *юр.* специали́ст по междунаро́д-
ному пра́ву.

publicity [pʌbˈlɪsɪtɪ] *n* 1) гла́сность; to give ~
to предава́ть гла́сности; 2) рекла́ма.

publicize ['pʌblɪsaɪz] *v* 1) реклами́ровать;
2) разглаша́ть; 3) оповеща́ть; извеща́ть.

publicly ['pʌblɪklɪ] *adv* публи́чно; откры́то.

publish ['pʌblɪʃ] *v* 1) обнаро́довать; оглаша́ть;
2) издава́ть, опублико́вывать.

publisher ['pʌblɪʃə] *n* изда́тель.

publishing ['pʌblɪʃɪŋ] *a:* ~ house, ~ office
изда́тельство.

publishment ['pʌblɪʃmənt] *n* 1) изда́ние, вы́ход
в свет; 2) опубликова́ние.

pucker I ['pʌkə] *n* 1) морщи́на, скла́дка;
2) *разг.* раздражённое состоя́ние.

pucker II *v* 1) мо́рщить(ся); 2) де́лать скла́дки.

puckery ['pʌkərɪ] *a* 1) смо́рщенный; 2) раздра-
жа́ющий.

puckish ['pʌkɪʃ] *a* прока́зливый; шаловли́вый;
озорно́й.

pud [pʌd] *n дет.* рýчка, ла́пка.

pudding ['pudɪŋ] *n* пýдинг; hasty ~ заварно́й
пýдинг; black ~ кровяна́я колбаса́; Yorkshire ~
пиро́г из взби́того те́ста (*с куском жареного
мяса*).

puddle I ['pʌdl] *n* 1) лýжица; 2) гли́няная
обма́зка.

puddle II *v* 1): to be ~d покрыва́ться лýжами;
2) мути́ть во́ду; бара́хтаться в воде́; 3) смуща́ть,
сбива́ть с то́лку; 4) меси́ть грязь; 5) меси́ть (*глину*); 6) обкла́дывать (*глиной*); 7) пудлингова́ть
(*железо*); 8) трамбова́ть.

puddly ['pʌdlɪ] *a* покры́тый лýжами.

pudgy ['pʌdʒɪ] *a* то́лстый, пýхлый.

pueblo [puˈeblou] *n* 1) посёлок инде́йцев;
2) жи́тель инде́йской дере́вни.

puerile ['pjuəraɪl] *a* ребя́ческий.

puff I [pʌf] *n* 1) дунове́ние (*ветра*); 2) поры́в,
струя́ во́здуха; 3) дымо́к; клуб (*дыма, пара*);
4) пухо́вка; 5) сло́йка, слоёный пирожо́к; 6) буф
(*отделка у платья*); 7) пухо́вое стёганое одея́ло;
8) крикли́вая рекла́ма.

puff II *v* 1) дуть коро́ткими поры́вами; 2) пых-
те́ть; to ~ and blow (*или* pant) тяжело́ дыша́ть,
пыхте́ть; to be ~ed запыха́ться; 3) пуска́ть клýбы
(*дыма*); 4) кури́ть (*сигару*); попы́хивать (*сигарой*); to ~ at a pipe попы́хивать трýбкой; 5) ки-
чи́ться, ва́жничать; 6) чрезме́рно расхва́ливать;
реклами́ровать; □ to ~ **away** сдува́ть; to ~ **out**
а) задува́ть, гаси́ть (*свечу*); б) выбива́ться поры́-
вами, клуба́ми; to ~ **up** поднима́ться клуба́ми
(*о дыме и т. п.*).

puff-ball ['pʌfbɔːl] *n* дождеви́к (*гриб*).

puff-box ['pʌfbɔks] *n* пýдреница.

puffed-up ['pʌftʌp] *a* надме́нный, кичли́вый.

puffy ['pʌfɪ] *a* 1) одутлова́тый; 2) поры́вистый
(*о ветре*); 3) запыха́вшийся; 4) *редко* кичли́-
вый; 5) напы́щенный; высокопа́рный.

pug [pʌg] *n* 1) мопс, мо́ська; 2) курно́сый нос.

pugilism ['pjuːdʒɪlɪzəm] *n* бокс; кула́чный бой.

pugilist ['pjuːdʒɪlɪst] *n* боксёр.

pugnacious [pʌgˈneɪʃəs] *a* драчли́вый.

pukka ['pʌkə] *a инд.* полнове́сный, полноце́нный.

pule [pjuːl] *v* хны́кать; пища́ть.

pull I [pul] *n* 1) тя́га; си́ла тя́ги; a dead ~ нап-
ра́сное уси́лие; to give a ~ at дёрнуть; 2) глото́к;
to take a ~ at (за)глотнýть; 3) шнуро́к, рýчка
(*звонка*); 4) гребля́; to go for a short ~ поката́-
ться (немно́го) на ло́дке; 5) *разг.* проте́кция;
6) преимýщество; to have the ~ of име́ть преимýщество пе́ред кем-л.

pull II *v* 1) тянýть, тащи́ть; 2) дёргать; to ~
smb. by the ear отодра́ть кого́-л. за́ уши; 3) притя́-
гивать; 4) надвига́ть, натя́гивать; 5) звони́ть (*в
звонок*); 6) грести́, идти́ на вёслах; 7) грима́с-
ничать, стро́ить ро́жи; 8) останови́ть ло́шадь
(*натянув вожжи*); 9) затя́гиваться (*папиросой*);
10) *спорт.* отбива́ть, посыла́ть мяч (*влево —
в крикете, гольфе*); □ to ~ **about** грýбо обра-
ща́ться; to ~ **at** а) дёргать; стара́ться сдви́нуть
(*дёргая к себе*); б) затя́гиваться (*папиросой,
сигарой*); в) тянýть (*из бутылки*); to ~ **down**
а) сноси́ть (*дом*); б) обескура́живать; в) изнуря́ть,
ослабля́ть; to ~ **in** а) оса́живать (*лошадь*);

б) сокраща́ть (*расходы*); to ~ off а) выи́грывать (*приз, состяза́ние*); б) стащи́ть, ски́нуть (*одежду, обувь*); в) удаля́ться; to ~ off the road съезжа́ть с доро́ги; to ~ out а) выта́скивать; вырыва́ть (*растение*); выщи́пывать (*перья, пух*); удаля́ть (*зуб*); б) отходи́ть (*от ста́нции — о по́езде*); в) вы́йти на вёслах; to ~ over а) надева́ть (*че́рез го́лову*); б) перета́скивать; to ~ through спра́виться (*с боле́знью, тру́дностями*); преодоле́ть; to ~ together а) рабо́тать дру́жно; б); to ~ oneself together собра́ться с си́лами; взять себя́ в ру́ки; to ~ up а) останови́ть (*ло́шадь, экипа́ж*); б) продвига́ться вперёд (*в состяза́нии*); в) выдёргивать.

pullet ['pulıt] *n* моло́дка (*ку́рица*).

pulley ['pulı] *n* шкив; блок, во́рот; driving ~ приводно́й шкив.

Pullman ['pulmən] *n* спа́льный ваго́н.

pull-over ['pul,ouvə] *n* пуло́вер, сви́тер.

pulmonary ['pʌlmənərı] *a* лёгочный.

pulp I [pʌlp] *n* 1) мя́коть (*плода́*); 2) бума́жная, древе́сная ма́сса; 3) пу́льпа (*зу́ба*).

pulp II *v* превраща́ть(ся) в мя́гкую ма́ссу.

pulpit ['pulpıt] *n* 1) ка́федра (*проповедника*); 2) *pl собир.* пропове́дники.

pulpy ['pʌlpı] *a* мя́гкий, мяси́стый.

pulsate [pʌl'seıt] *v* пульси́ровать, би́ться.

pulse I [pʌls] *n* 1) пульс; to feel the ~ щу́пать пульс; *перен.* разузнава́ть наме́рения; 2) бие́ние (*се́рдца, жи́зни*); 3) вибра́ция; 4) ритм уда́ров (*вёсел и т. п.*); 5) чу́вство, настрое́ние; to stir one's ~s поднима́ть настрое́ние.

pulse II *v* пульси́ровать; би́ться (*о се́рдце и т. п.*).

pulverize ['pʌlvəraız] *v* 1) растира́ть, размельча́ть, превраща́ть(ся) в порошо́к; 2) распыля́ть (-ся); 3) разбива́ть (*до́воды проти́вника*).

pulverizer ['pʌlvəraızə] *n* 1) распыли́тель; пульвериза́тор; 2) форсу́нка.

puma ['pjuːmə] *n зоол.* пу́ма.

pumice(-stone) I ['pʌmıs(stoun)] *n* пе́мза.

pumice(-stone) II *v* тере́ть, чи́стить пе́мзой.

pummel ['pʌml] *v* бить кулака́ми, тузи́ть.

pump I [pʌmp] *n* 1) насо́с; air ~ возду́шный насо́с; 2) водока́чка.

pump I II *v* 1) кача́ть (*насо́сом*); to ~ hard накача́ть ши́ну до отка́за; to ~ dry вы́качать до́суха; 2) наполня́ть во́здухом (*лёгкие и т. п.*); нагнета́ть во́здух; 3) всади́ть (*пу́лю в кого́-л. — into*); 4) выу́живать све́дения; выве́дывать (*у кого́-л. — out of*); □ to ~ out выка́чивать; to ~ up нака́чивать (*во́ду*).

pump² *n* (лакиро́ванная) ба́льная ту́фля.

pumpkin ['pʌmpkın] *n* ты́ква.

pump-room ['pʌmprum] *n* 1) кио́ск с минера́льной водо́й; 2) насо́сное отделе́ние.

pun [pʌn] *n* игра́ слов; каламбу́р; to perpetrate a ~ сочини́ть каламбу́р.

Punch [pʌntʃ] *n* 1) Петру́шка; ~ and Judy *де́йствующие ли́ца ку́кольной коме́дии*); 2) «Панч» (*назва́ние англ. юмористи́ческого журна́ла*).

punch¹ I [pʌntʃ] *n* 1) уда́р кулако́м; 2) *разг.* си́ла, эффе́кт.

punch¹ II *v* ударя́ть кулако́м.

punch² *n* 1) пунш; 2) *attr* пу́ншевый.

punch³ I *n* компо́стер.

punch³ II *v* компости́ровать, пробива́ть отве́рстия.

punctilious [pʌŋk'tılıəs] *a* педанти́чный, щепети́льный.

punctual ['pʌŋktʃuəl] *a* то́чный, пунктуа́льный.

punctuality [,pʌŋktʃu'ælıtı] *n* то́чность, пунктуа́льность.

punctuate ['pʌŋktʃueıt] *v* 1) расставля́ть зна́ки препина́ния; 2) прерыва́ть, перемежа́ть.

punctuation [,pʌŋktʃu'eıʃən] *n* расстано́вка зна́ков препина́ния, пунктуа́ция.

puncture I ['pʌŋktʃə] *n* 1) проко́л (*ши́ны и т. п.*); 2) пробо́й (*изоля́ции*).

puncture II *v* 1) прока́лывать (*ши́ну и т. п.*); пробива́ть (*отве́рстие*); 2) ло́пнуть (*о ши́не*).

pundit ['pʌndıt] *n* 1) учёный инду́с, па́ндит; 2) *шутл.* учёный муж.

pungency ['pʌndʒənsı] *n* е́дкость, острота́.

pungent ['pʌndʒənt] *a* е́дкий, о́стрый.

punish ['pʌnıʃ] *v* 1) нака́зывать; налага́ть взыска́ние; 2) *разг.* суро́во обраща́ться с кем-л.; зада́ть пе́рцу; 3) *разг.* изнуря́ть.

punishable ['pʌnıʃəbl] *a* заслу́живающий наказа́ния.

punishment ['pʌnıʃmənt] *n* наказа́ние; corporal ~ теле́сное наказа́ние; to commute the ~ смягча́ть наказа́ние; to set a ~ налага́ть взыска́ние.

punitive ['pjuːnıtıv] *a* кара́тельный.

punster ['pʌnstə] *n* остря́к.

punt¹ I [pʌnt] *n* плоскодо́нная ло́дка.

punt¹ II *v* плыть на плоскодо́нке (*отта́лкиваясь шесто́м*).

punt² I *n спорт.* выбива́ние мяча́ из рук (*вратарём*).

punt² II *v спорт.* вы́бить мяч из рук.

puny ['pjuːnı] *a* ма́ленький, хи́лый, тщеду́шный.

pup¹ I [pʌp] *n* 1) щено́к; to sell smb. a ~ *разг.* наду́ть, одура́чивать (*кого́-л.*); 2) детёныш (*волчо́нок, лисёнок, тюленёнок*); 3) самонаде́янный молодо́й челове́к.

pup II *v* щени́ться.

pupil¹ ['pjuːpl] *n* 1) учени́к, уча́щийся; 2) воспи́танник; 3) практика́нт.

pupil² *n* зрачо́к.

pupil(l)age ['pjuːpılıdʒ] *n* 1) малоле́тство; 2) учени́чество.

pupil(l)ary¹ ['pjuːpıları] *a* 1) учени́ческий; 2) находя́щийся под опе́кой.

pupil(l)ary² *a* зрачко́вый.

puppet ['pʌpıt] *n* 1) ку́кла, марионе́тка; 2) *attr* ку́кольный (*о теа́тре*); марионе́точный (*о прави́тельстве*).

puppet-play ['pʌpıtpleı] *n* ку́кольный спекта́кль.

puppetry ['pʌpıtrı] *n* 1) ку́кольная коме́дия; 2) лицеме́рие, ха́нжество.

puppet-show ['pʌpıtʃou] *n* ку́кольный теа́тр.

puppy ['pʌpı] *n* 1) щено́к; 2) детёныш; 3) фат, ветрого́н; 4) самонаде́янный юне́ц, молокосо́с.

purblind ['pəːblaınd] *a* 1) подслепова́тый; 2) недальнови́дный, тупо́й.

purchasable ['pəːtʃəsəbl] *a* прода́жный.

purchase I ['pəːtʃəs] *n* 1) поку́пка; 2) ку́пленная вещь; 3) годово́й дохо́д (*с земли́*); 4) вы́игрыш в си́ле; преиму́щество.

purchase II *v* 1) покупа́ть, закупа́ть; 2) приобрета́ть; 3) *тех.* поднима́ть (*рычаго́м, лебёдкой*).

pure [pjuə] *a* 1) чи́стый; беспри́месный; 2) чисто-кро́вный; 3) настоя́щий, чисте́йший; 4) просто́й (*о стиле*); 5) отчётливый, я́сный (*о звуке, ноте*); 6) целому́дренный, непоро́чный; безупре́чный; 7) свобо́дный (*от — from*).

purely ['pjuəlɪ] *adv* 1) исключи́тельно, по́лностью, целико́м; 2) соверше́нно, вполне́.

purgative I ['pə:gətɪv] *n* слаби́тельное (*лекарство*).

purgative II *a* 1) *мед.* слаби́тельный; очисти́тельный; 2) очища́ющий.

purgatorial [,pə:gə'tɔ:rɪəl] *a* очисти́тельный, искупи́тельный.

purgatory I ['pə:gətərɪ] *n* чисти́лище.

purgatory II *a* очисти́тельный.

purge I [pə:dʒ] *n* 1) очище́ние; чи́стка (*тж. политическая*); 2) *мед.* слаби́тельное.

purge II *v* 1) очища́ть (*от чего-л.— from*); освобожда́ть, избавля́ть (*от кого-л.— of*); 2) проводи́ть чи́стку (*партии и т. п.*); 3) дава́ть слаби́тельное; 4) сла́бить; □ to ~ **away** счища́ть; вычища́ть; to ~ **out** прочища́ть.

purification [,pjuərɪfɪ'keɪʃən] *n* очи́стка; очище́ние.

purifier ['pjuərɪfaɪə] *n тех.* очисти́тель.

purify ['pjuərɪfaɪ] *v* очища́ть(ся) (*от чего-л.— of, from*).

purist ['pjuərɪst] *n* пури́ст.

Puritan ['pjuərɪtən] *n* 1) пурита́нин; 2) (p.) свято́ша; 3) *attr* пурита́нский.

Puritanism ['pjuərɪtənɪzəm] *n* 1) пурита́нство; 2) (p.) стро́гие нра́вы.

purity ['pjuərɪtɪ] *n* 1) чистота́; 2) неви́нность, непоро́чность; 3) про́ба (*драгоценных металлов*).

purl[1] I [pə:l] *n* журча́ние.

purl[1] II *v* журча́ть.

purl[2] I *n* 1) галу́н; 2) оборо́тное двухлицево́е вяза́ние.

purl[2] II *v* 1) украша́ть галуно́м; 2) вяза́ть оборо́тной двухлицево́й вя́зкой.

purlieu ['pə:lju:] *n* 1) *pl* предме́стье, при́город; 2) *pl* трущо́бы; 3) окра́ина, опу́шка (*леса*); *ист.* земля́, прилега́ющая к короле́вскому ле́су.

purple I ['pə:pl] *n* 1) багря́ный, пурпу́рный цвет; 2) фиоле́товый цвет; 3) порфи́ра; 4) сан кардина́ла.

purple II *a* 1) багря́ный, пурпу́рный; тёмно-кра́сный; 2) фиоле́товый; 3) *поэт.* ца́рский; 4) пы́шный.

purple III *v* багрове́ть; де́лать(ся) тёмно-кра́сным.

purport I ['pə:pət] *n* 1) о́бщее содержа́ние, смысл; 2) *юр.* текст докуме́нта.

purport II *v* 1) говори́ть, свиде́тельствовать (*о чём-л.*); 2) означа́ть, подразумева́ть.

purpose I ['pə:pəs] *n* 1) цель, назначе́ние; nefarious ~s гну́сные це́ли; to the ~ кста́ти, к де́лу; beside the ~ нецелесообра́зно; of set ~ с умы́слом; on ~ наро́чно; наме́ренно; to answer (*или* to serve) the ~ отвеча́ть це́ли, своему́ назначе́нию; годи́ться; for that ~ с э́той це́лью; 2) успе́х, результа́т; to good ~ с больши́м успе́хом; to little ~ с ма́лым успе́хом, с ма́лым результа́том; to no ~ безрезульта́тно; напра́сно; to some ~ с не́которым успе́хом.

purpose II *v* намерева́ться; to be ~d *уст.* име́ть наме́рение.

purposeful ['pə:pəsful] *a* 1) име́ющий наме́рение; целеустремлённый; 2) умы́шленный, преднаме́ренный.

purposeless ['pə:pəslɪs] *a* 1) бесце́льный; 2) без вся́кого наме́рения; 3) бесполе́зный.

purposely ['pə:pəslɪ] *adv* преднаме́ренно; наро́чно.

purr I [pə:] *n* мурлы́канье.

purr II *v* мурлы́кать.

purse I [pə:s] *n* 1) кошелёк; мошна́; 2) де́ньги; fat (*или* long, heavy) ~ доста́ток; обеспе́ченность; light ~ бе́дность; the public ~ казна́; to button up one's ~ скупи́ться, ска́редничать; to have a common ~ име́ть о́бщие сре́дства; to line one's ~ ≅ набива́ть свой кошелёк; to open one's ~ раскоше́ливаться; 3) де́нежные фо́нды; to make up a ~ собра́ть де́ньги (*по подписке*); 4) де́нежный приз, пре́мия; to give (*или* to put up) a ~ присужда́ть пре́мию, дава́ть приз.

purse II *v* мо́рщить(ся).

purse-proud ['pə:spraud] *a* зазна́вшийся (*от своего богатства*).

pursuance [pə'sju:əns] *n* выполне́ние, исполне́ние; in ~ of во исполне́ние (*чего-л.*), согла́сно (*чему-л.*).

pursuant [pə'sju:ənt] *adv*: ~ to согла́сно чему́-л.

pursue [pə'sju:] *v* 1) пресле́довать; бежа́ть за кем-л.; гна́ться; 2) пресле́довать цель; 3) сле́довать; 4) де́йствовать (*по плану*); 5) занима́ться (*чем-л.*); име́ть профе́ссию; 6) вести́ (*следствие*); 7) продолжа́ть (*обсуждение, поездку, путешествие*).

pursuer [pə'sju:ə] *n* 1) пресле́дующий; 2) гони́тель; 3) *юр.* исте́ц.

pursuit [pə'sju:t] *n* 1) пресле́дование; пого́ня; in ~ of в по́исках; в пого́не за, пресле́дуя; 2) заня́тие; daily ~s повседне́вные заня́тия, дела́.

pursy[1] ['pə:sɪ] *a* 1) страда́ющий оды́шкой; 2) ту́чный.

pursy[2] *a* зазна́вшийся.

purulent ['pjuərulənt] *a* гно́йный, гноя́щийся.

purvey [pə'veɪ] *v* 1) обеспе́чивать (*провиантом*); снабжа́ть (*продуктами*); 2) заготовля́ть.

purveyance [pə'veɪəns] *n* 1) запа́сы; 2) загото́вка.

purveyor [pə'veɪə] *n* поставщи́к, загото́витель (*продуктов*).

purview ['pə:vju:] *n* 1) круг (*деятельности, забот*); сфе́ра, компете́нция; 2) обзо́р; 3) кругозо́р; 4) статья́ зако́на.

pus [pʌs] *n* гной.

push I [puʃ] *n* 1) толчо́к; уда́р; to give the ~ толкну́ть, пихну́ть; to get the ~ получи́ть отста́вку; 2) кно́пка; 3) уси́лие; энерги́чная попы́тка; to make a ~ из ко́жи лезть; 4) напо́р; на́тиск; 5) реши́тельный моме́нт; 6) эне́ргия, предприи́мчивость; 7) *воен.* наступле́ние, продвиже́ние вперёд.

push II *v* 1) толка́ть; прота́лкивать; 2) проби-ва́ться, проти́скиваться; 3) осуществля́ть нажи́м (*на кого-л.*); понужда́ть (*кого-л. к чему-л.— to*); 4) ускоря́ть (*ход событий*); 5) реклами́ровать (*товары*); 6): to be ~ed for располага́ть ма́лым коли́чеством (*времени, денег*); 7) притесня́ть, торопи́ть (*должника*); □ to ~ **along** а) торопи́ться; б) спеши́ть зако́нчить (*работу*); to ~ **aside** устраня́ть (*препя́тствия*); to ~ **away** отта́лкивать; to ~ **forward** торопи́ться; стреми́ться вперёд; to ~ **in** приближа́ться к бе́регу (*о ло́дке*); to ~ **off** а) отта́лкиваться от бе́рега, отча́ливать; б) *разг.* смота́ться, исче́знуть; to ~ **on** устремля́ться вперёд; to ~ **out** а) дава́ть ростки́ (*о расте́нии*); б) выступа́ть, выдава́ться (*о мы́се и т. п.*); to ~ **through** прота́лкивать(ся).

push-button [ˈpuʃˌbʌtn] *n* 1) кно́пка (*выключа́теля*); 2) *attr* кно́почный (*об управле́нии*); 3) *attr* «кно́почный» (*о войне́*).

push-cart [ˈpuʃkɑ:t] *n* ручна́я теле́жка.

pusher [ˈpuʃə] *n* 1) толка́ч; 2) самоуве́ренный, напо́ристый челове́к.

pushing [ˈpuʃiŋ] *a* энерги́чный, предприи́мчивый.

push-over [ˈpuʃˌouvə] *n* *амер. разг.* 1) пустяко́вое де́ло; 2) сла́бый игро́к.

puss [pus] *n* 1) ко́шечка; a ~ in the corner «ко́шка в углу́» (*де́тская игра́*); 2) за́яц; 3) *разг.* коке́тливая де́вушка, же́нщина; sly ~ коке́тка.

pussy [ˈpusi] *n* 1) ки́ска; 2) мя́гкий, пуши́стый предме́т.

pussy-cat [ˈpusikæt] *n* ки́ска, ко́шечка.

pussyfoot I [ˈpusifut] *n* *амер. разг.* осторо́жный челове́к.

pussyfoot II *v* 1) идти́ кра́дущейся, коша́чьей похо́дкой; 2) *амер. разг.* де́йствовать осторо́жно, с огля́дкой.

pustular [ˈpʌstjulə] *a* прыщева́тый.

put [put] *v* (*past, p. p.* put); 1) класть, положи́ть, (по)ста́вить; to ~ to bed укла́дывать спать; to ~ smb. in charge of ста́вить во главе́; to ~ into one's head внуши́ть кому́-л.; to ~ into shape придава́ть фо́рму; 2) приводи́ть (*в како́е-л. состоя́ние*); to ~ in order приводи́ть в поря́док; to ~ smb. at his ease дать кому́-л. почу́вствовать себя́ непринуждённо; 3) помеща́ть; сажа́ть (*в тюрьму́, сумасше́дший дом и т. п.*); 4) выража́ть; to ~ it in black and white запи́сывать чёрным по бе́лому; излага́ть (*пи́сьменно*); to ~ into words выража́ть слова́ми; to ~ (words) to music переложи́ть (слова́) на му́зыку; 5) переводи́ть (*с одного́ языка́ на друго́й; from... into*); 6) счита́ть; исчисля́ть, определя́ть (*величину́ и т. п. во сто́лько-то едини́ц; at*); 7) применя́ть, прилага́ть; 8) ста́вить (*на рассмотре́ние; for*); задава́ть (*вопро́с*); 9) облага́ть (*нало́гом; on*); 10) *мор.* заходи́ть в порт (*о корабле́*); □ to ~ **about** а) *разг.* (о)беспоко́ить; встрево́жить, испуга́ть; б) распространя́ть (*слух и т. п.*); в) *мор.* сде́лать поворо́т; лечь на друго́й галс; to ~ **across** перевози́ть, переправля́ть (*на паро́ме, ло́дке*); to ~ **aside** а) откла́дывать; б) копи́ть (*де́ньги*); в) отводи́ть (*до́вод*); to ~ **away** а) убира́ть (*что-л.*); пря́тать; б) *разг.* съеда́ть, пожира́ть (*пи́щу*); в) *разг.* сажа́ть (*в тюрьму́, сумасше́дший дом*); г) откла́дывать (*сбереже́ния*); д) *мор.* отча́ливать; to ~ **back** а) положи́ть, поста́вить обра́тно (*на пре́жнее ме́сто*); б) верну́ться в га́вань (*о корабле́*); в) передвига́ть наза́д (*стре́лки часо́в*); to ~ **by** а) откла́дывать (*де́ньги*); б) избега́ть (*разгово́ра*); to ~ **down** а) запи́сывать; б) подавля́ть (*восста́ние*); в) заста́вить замолча́ть; г) относи́ть, припи́сывать (*чему́-л.— to*);

д) запи́сывать, относи́ть на чей-л. счёт; to ~ **forth** а) напряга́ть (*си́лы*); б) пуска́ть (*побе́ги*); to ~ **forward** выдвига́ть (*тео́рию*); to ~ **in** а) вставля́ть (*стёкла, слова́ в разгово́р*); б) *разг.* выполня́ть (*рабо́ту*); в) проводи́ть вре́мя (*за каки́м-л. де́лом*); г) подава́ть (*жа́лобу*); предъявля́ть (*прете́нзию*); д) запряга́ть (*лошаде́й*); е) *разг.* выступа́ть кандида́том (*far*); to ~ **in for** а post иска́ть ме́ста, рабо́ты; ж) *мор.* входи́ть в га́вань; to ~ **off** а) откла́дывать (*де́ло, заня́тие*); б) передвига́ть (*шля́пу, пальто́*); в) отгова́ривать (*от чего́-л.— from*); г) отде́лываться (*от кого́-л.*); to ~ off with a jest отде́латься шу́ткой; д) *мор.* отча́ливать; to ~ **on** а) надева́ть; б) передвига́ть вперёд (*стре́лки часо́в*); в) принима́ть вид; напуска́ть на себя́ (*ва́жность и т. п.*); to ~ **out** а) выгоня́ть, выставля́ть; б) выкла́дывать (*ве́щи*); в) вы́вихнуть (*ру́ку, но́гу*); г) туши́ть, гаси́ть, выключа́ть (*газ, свет и т. п.*); д) раздража́ть; меша́ть; е) выходи́ть в мо́ре; to ~ **through** а) *разг.* вы́полнить (*рабо́ту, поста́вленную зада́чу*); б) соедини́ть (*по телефо́ну*); to ~ **together** а) сопоставля́ть; б) компили́ровать; в) собира́ть (*меха́низм*); to ~ **up** а) раскрыва́ть (*зо́нтик*); б) приюти́ть; в) стро́ить; воздвига́ть (*зда́ние*); г) устана́вливать (*до́ску, решётку и т. п.*); д) выве́шивать (*фла́ги, объявле́ния*); е) дать, сде́лать объявле́ние (*о прода́же*); ж) подыма́ть це́ну; з) уложи́ть, запакова́ть; и) вложи́ть в но́жны (*меч, са́блю*); к) останови́ться (*где-л. вре́менно; at*); л) терпе́ть, мири́ться (*с чем-л.— with*); to ~ **upon** а) обременя́ть; б) обма́нывать; ◇ to ~ smb. off his guard усыпи́ть чью-л. бди́тельность; to ~ smb. on his guard предостерега́ть кого́-л.; never ~ off till tomorrow what you can do today *посл.* не откла́дывай на за́втра то́, что мо́жно сде́лать сего́дня.

putrefaction [ˌpjuːtriˈfækʃən] *n* гние́ние.

putrefy [ˈpjuːtrifai] *v* гнить.

putrescent [pjuːˈtresnt] *a* гнию́щий.

putrid [ˈpjuːtrid] *a* 1) гнило́й; разлага́ющийся; 2) воню́чий; 3) испо́рченный.

putridity [pjuːˈtriditi] *n* гниль, гни́лость.

puttee [ˈpʌti] *n* 1) обмо́тка (*для ног*); 2) кра́га.

putter [ˈpʌtə] *v* труди́ться впусту́ю (*над чем-л.— over*); □ to ~ **about** броди́ть без це́ли.

putty I [ˈpʌti] *n* зама́зка; шпаклёвка; строи́тельный раство́р.

putty II *v* шпаклева́ть; зама́зывать о́кна (*тж.* to ~ up).

put-up [ˈputˌʌp] *a* *разг.* заду́манный; сплани́рованный зара́нее.

puzzle I [ˈpʌzl] *n* 1) недоуме́ние; 2) замеша́тельство; 3) неразреши́мый вопро́с; 4) зага́дка; головоло́мка; cross-word ~ кроссво́рд.

puzzle II *v* 1) поста́вить в тупи́к; приводи́ть в недоуме́ние; 2) запу́тывать; 3) лома́ть го́лову (*над чем-л.— over*); □ to ~ **out** разобра́ться в чём-л.; распу́тать.

puzzlement [ˈpʌzlmənt] *n* замеша́тельство; смуще́ние.

puzzling [ˈpʌzliŋ] *a* приводя́щий в замеша́тельство; сбива́ющий с то́лку.

pygmy [ˈpigmi] *n* пигме́й.

pyjamas [pəˈdʒɑːməz] *n pl* пижа́ма.

pyramid [ˈpirəmid] *n* пирами́да.

pyramidal [pɪ'ræmɪdl] a пирамида́льный.
pyre ['paɪə] n погреба́льный костёр.

Q

Q, q [kjuː] n 17-я бу́ква англ. алфави́та.
quack[1] I [kwæk] n кря́канье (уток).
quack[1] II v 1) кря́кать; 2) треща́ть, болта́ть.
quack[2] n 1) зна́харь; шарлата́н; 2) attr шарлата́нский.
quackery ['kwækərɪ] n шарлата́нство.
quadrangle ['kwɔ,dræŋgl] n 1) четырёхуго́льник; 2) четырёхуго́льный двор.
quadrant ['kwɔdrənt] n квадра́нт, че́тверть кру́га, се́ктор в 90°.
quadrate I ['kwɔdrɪt] n квадра́т.
quadrate II a квадра́тный; прямоуго́льный.
quadrature ['kwɔdrətʃə] n квадрату́ра.
quadrilateral I [,kwɔdrɪ'lætərəl] n четырёхуго́льник.
quadrilateral II a четырёхсторо́нний.
quadrille [kwə'drɪl] n кадри́ль.
quadruped ['kwɔdruped] n четвероно́гое (живо́тное).
quadruple I ['kwɔdrupl] n учетверённое коли́чество.
quadruple II a 1) учетверённый; 2) состоя́щий из четырёх часте́й; 3) четырёхсторо́нний (о соглаше́нии).
quadruple III v учетверя́ть.
quadruplets ['kwɔdruplɪts] n pl четверня́.
quaff [kwɑːf] v пить больши́ми глотка́ми, за́лпом.
quag [kwæg] см. quagmire.
quaggy ['kwægɪ] a 1) то́пкий; болоти́стый; 2) дря́блый.
quagmire ['kwægmaɪə] n боло́то, тряси́на (тж. перен.).
quail[1] [kweɪl] n пе́репел.
quail[2] v испуга́ться, стру́сить; дро́гнуть.
quaint [kweɪnt] a 1) привлека́тельный, заба́вный; 2) необы́чный, стра́нный.
quake I [kweɪk] n 1) дрожа́ние, дрожь; 2) землетрясе́ние.
quake II v дрожа́ть, трясти́сь; to ~ with fear дрожа́ть от стра́ха.
Quaker ['kweɪkə] n ква́кер.
quaky ['kweɪkɪ] a дрожа́щий.
qualification [,kwɔlɪfɪ'keɪʃən] n 1) квалифика́ция; 2) ограниче́ние; огово́рка; 3) (избира́тельный) ценз; age (educational, electoral, property) ~ возрастно́й (образова́тельный, избира́тельный, иму́щественный) ценз; residential ~ ценз осе́длости.
qualified ['kwɔlɪfaɪd] a 1) подходя́щий; приго́дный; 2) ограни́ченный; 3) сде́ржанный.
qualifier ['kwɔlɪfaɪə] n грам. определи́тель.
qualify ['kwɔlɪfaɪ] v 1) гото́вить(ся) (к чему́-л. — for); 2) ограни́чивать; 3) квалифици́ровать, определя́ть (как — as); 4) видоизменя́ть, смягча́ть; 5) разбавля́ть (спирт и т. п.).
qualitative ['kwɔlɪtətɪv] a ка́чественный.
quality ['kwɔlɪtɪ] n 1) ка́чество; сорт; high (poor) ~ вы́сшее (плохо́е) ка́чество; of good ~

высо́кого ка́чества; 2) сво́йство; 3) хоро́шее ка́чество, высокосо́ртность.
qualm [kwɔːm] n 1) при́ступ тошноты́; 2) при́ступ малоду́шия или растёрянности; 3) сомне́ния, колеба́ния; ~s of conscience угрызе́ния со́вести.
quandary ['kwɔndərɪ] n затрудни́тельное положе́ние.
quanta ['kwɔntə] pl см. quantum.
quantitative ['kwɔntɪtətɪv] a коли́чественный.
quantity ['kwɔntɪtɪ] n 1) коли́чество; negligible ~ а) незначи́тельное коли́чество; б) челове́к, с кото́рым не счита́ются; 2) большо́е коли́чество; in quantities в большо́м коли́честве, ма́ссами; 3) мат. величина́; unknown ~ неизве́стная величина́, неизве́стное; 4) фон. долгота́ зву́ка.
quantum ['kwɔntəm] n (pl quanta) 1) коли́чество, су́мма; 2) до́ля, части́ца; 3) физ. квант; 4) attr: ~ theory ква́нтовая тео́рия.
quarantine I ['kwɔrəntiːn] n каранти́н.
quarantine II v подверга́ть каранти́ну.
quarrel I ['kwɔrəl] n ссо́ра; раздо́ры; спор; to pick (или to seek) а ~ иска́ть по́вод для ссо́ры, придира́ться; ◊ to take up another's ~ приня́ть чью-л. сто́рону в спо́ре.
quarrel II v 1) ссо́риться; спо́рить; 2) придира́ться, брани́ться; ◊ to ~ with one's bread and butter идти́ про́тив со́бственных интере́сов.
quarrelsome ['kwɔrəlsəm] a вздо́рный; драчли́вый; задири́стый.
quarry[1] I ['kwɔrɪ] n 1) каменоло́мня, карье́р; 2) исто́чник све́дений.
quarry[1] II v 1) разраба́тывать карье́р, добыва́ть ка́мень; 2) ры́ться (в кни́гах и т. п.).
quarry[2] n добы́ча (на охо́те); перен. наме́ченная же́ртва.
quart [kwɔːt] n 1) ква́рта (= ¹/₄ галло́на = = 1,14 л); 2) сосу́д ёмкостью в 1 ква́рту; ◊ to try to put a ~ into a pint pot ≅ пыта́ться сде́лать невозмо́жное.
quarter I ['kwɔːtə] n 1) че́тверть (чего-л. — of); 2) че́тверть ча́са; а ~ to one без че́тверти час; 3) кварта́л (года); 4) страна́ све́та; 5) ме́сто, сторона́; from every ~, from all ~s со всех сторо́н; from no ~ ниотку́да, ни с чьей стороны́; 6) кварта́л (города); 7) pl кварти́ра, помеще́ние; to take up one's ~s поселя́ться; at close ~s в те́сном сосе́дстве; 8) pl воен. кварти́ры, каза́рмы; 9) поща́да; to give no ~ не дава́ть поща́ды; 10) че́тверть ту́ши; hind ~s за́дняя часть; ◊ not a ~ so good as далеко́ не так хоро́ш как; to come to close ~s а) сцепи́ться в спо́ре; б) схвати́ться врукопа́шную.
quarter II v 1) дели́ть на четы́ре ча́сти; 2) четвертова́ть; 3) расквартиро́вывать; 4) квартирова́ть (at).
quarter-day ['kwɔːtədeɪ] n пе́рвый день кварта́ла (срок платеже́й).
quarter-deck ['kwɔːtədek] n мор. 1) ют; 2) шка́нцы.
quarterly I ['kwɔːtəlɪ] n журна́л, выходя́щий раз в три ме́сяца.
quarterly II a кварта́льный, трёхме́сячный.
quarterly III adv раз в три ме́сяца, покварта́льно.
quartermaster ['kwɔːtə,mɑːstə] n 1) воен. квартирме́йстер; 2) мор. старшина́-рулево́й.

quartern ['kwɔːtən] *n* 1) че́тверть пи́нты; 2) станда́ртная буха́нка хле́ба (*4 фунта*).

quarter-sessions ['kwɔːtəˈseʃənz] *n pl* се́ссия мировы́х суде́й (*раз в три месяца*).

quartet(te) [kwɔːˈtet] *n муз.* кварте́т.

quarto ['kwɔːtou] *n* 1) че́тверть листа́; 2) кни́га форма́том в ¹/₄ листа́.

quartz [kwɔːts] *n мин.* кварц.

quash [kwɔʃ] *v* 1) аннули́ровать, отменя́ть (*приговор и т. п.*); 2) подавля́ть (*восстание и т. п.*).

quasi ['kwɑːzɪ] *adv* как бу́дто; как бы; я́кобы; почти́.

quaver I ['kweɪvə] *n* 1) дрожа́ние го́лоса; 2) трель.

quaver II *v* 1) дрожа́ть (*о голосе*); 2) говори́ть дрожа́щим го́лосом; 3) выводи́ть тре́ли.

quavery ['kweɪvərɪ] *a* дрожа́щий.

quay [kiː] *n* мол, прича́л; на́бережная.

queasy ['kwiːzɪ] *a* 1) вызыва́ющий тошноту́; 2) испы́тывающий тошноту́ *или* недомога́ние; 3) сла́бый (*о желудке*); 4) привере́дливый, разбо́рчивый.

queek [kwiːk] *v* крича́ть (*о сове*).

queen I [kwiːn] *n* 1) короле́ва; 2) *карт.* да́ма; 3) *шахм.* ферзь; 4) ма́тка (*у пчёл*).

queen II *v* 1): to ~ it a) держа́ться короле́вой; б) возглавля́ть, заправля́ть (*о женщине*); 2) *шахм.* проводи́ть *или* проходи́ть в ферзи́.

queenly ['kwiːnlɪ] *a* короле́вский, ца́рственный.

queer I [kwɪə] *a* 1) стра́нный; чудакова́тый; 2) сомни́тельный, подозри́тельный; there is something ~ about it что́-то здесь нела́дно, подозри́тельно; 3) чу́вствующий дурноту́ *или* недомога́ние; ◊ in Queer street *разг.* а) в долга́х; б) в беде́.

queer II *v разг.* по́ртить.

quell [kwel] *v* подавля́ть (*страх, сопротивление*).

quench [kwentʃ] *v* 1) гаси́ть, туши́ть; 2) утоля́ть (*жажду*); 3) подавля́ть (*чувство*); 4) охлажда́ть (*пыл*); 5) зака́ливать (*сталь*).

quenchless ['kwentʃlɪs] *a* неугаси́мый; неутоли́мый.

querulous ['kwerʊləs] *a* брюзгли́вый, недово́льный; раздражи́тельный.

query I ['kwɪərɪ] *n* 1) вопро́с; 2) вопроси́тельный знак.

query II *v* 1) спра́шивать, осведомля́ться; 2) выража́ть сомне́ние, подверга́ть сомне́нию; 3) ста́вить вопроси́тельный знак.

quest I [kwest] *n* по́иски; in ~ of в по́исках чего́-л., кого́-л.

quest II *v* производи́ть по́иски, разы́скивать.

question I ['kwestʃən] *n* 1) вопро́с; leading (nice, poignant, needling) ~ наводя́щий (щекотли́вый, о́стрый, язви́тельный) вопро́с; indirect (*или* oblique) ~ ко́свенный вопро́с; dumb ~ *разг.* глу́пый вопро́с; to put a ~ задава́ть вопро́с; to parry a ~ уклоня́ться от отве́та (*на вопрос*); ask no ~s не задава́йте вопро́сов; 2) обсужда́емый вопро́с, де́ло, пробле́ма; vexed ~ спо́рный вопро́с; it is not the ~ де́ло не в э́том; beside the ~ не по существу́ (вопро́са); the ~ of the hour актуа́льный, злободне́вный вопро́с; to initiate (to settle) a ~ подня́ть, возбуди́ть (реши́ть) вопро́с; to beg the ~ уклони́ться от реше́ния вопро́са; a matter

in ~ обсужда́емый вопро́с; a person in ~ тот, о ком идёт речь; 3) сомне́ние; beyond (*или* out of, without) ~ вне сомне́ния; to call in ~ подверга́ть сомне́нию; оспа́ривать; ◊ out of the ~ не мо́жет быть и ре́чи; to pop the ~ сде́лать предложе́ние о бра́ке.

question II *v* 1) спра́шивать, ста́вить вопро́сы; 2) допра́шивать; 3) сомнева́ться, подверга́ть сомне́нию; 4) иссле́довать, стара́ться распозна́ть.

questionable ['kwestʃənəbl] *a* сомни́тельный, подозри́тельный.

questioner ['kwestʃənə] *n* интервьюе́р, корреспонде́нт.

questionless I ['kwestʃənlɪs] *a* несомне́нный, бесспо́рный.

questionless II *adv* несомне́нно.

question-mark ['kwestʃənmɑːk] *n* вопроси́тельный знак, знак вопро́са.

questionnaire [ˌkwestʃəˈneə] *n* анке́та, вопро́сник.

queue I [kjuː] *n* 1) коса́ (*волос*); 2) о́чередь, хвост; to stand in ~ стоя́ть в о́череди.

queue II *v* 1) заплета́ть ко́су; 2) стоя́ть в о́череди; станови́ться в о́чередь.

quibble I ['kwɪbl] *n* 1) игра́ слов, каламбу́р; 2) уве́ртка, уклоне́ние (*от вопроса*); софи́зм.

quibble II *v* уклоня́ться от су́ти вопро́са.

quick I [kwɪk] *a* 1) бы́стрый; ско́рый; to be ~ спеши́ть; be ~! живо!, поторопи́тесь!; 2) живо́й, прово́рный; ~ to understand поня́тливый, сообрази́тельный; ~ to sympathize отзы́вчивый; ~ to take offence оби́дчивый; ~ of apprehension бы́стро, живо схва́тывающий.

quick II *n* 1) чувстви́тельное ме́сто; to cut to the ~ заде́ть за живо́е; to the ~ до мо́зга косте́й, до глубины́ души́; 2) *уст.* живо́й; the ~ and the dead живы́е и мёртвые.

quick III *adv* бы́стро; живо.

quicken ['kwɪkən] *v* 1) ускоря́ть(ся); 2) оживля́ть(ся); 3) разжига́ть.

quickie ['kwɪkɪ] *n разг.* халту́ра, на́спех вы́пущенная проду́кция (*о фильме, книге и т. п.*).

quicklime ['kwɪklaɪm] *n* негашёная и́звесть.

quickly ['kwɪklɪ] *adv* бы́стро; ско́ро.

quickness ['kwɪknɪs] *n* 1) быстрота́; 2) сообрази́тельность, нахо́дчивость.

quicksand ['kwɪksænd] *n* зыбу́чий песо́к.

quickset ['kwɪkset] *n* жива́я и́згородь.

quicksilver ['kwɪkˌsɪlvə] *n* ртуть.

quickwitted ['kwɪkˈwɪtɪd] *a* смышлёный, сообрази́тельный, нахо́дчивый.

quid¹ [kwɪd] *n* кусо́к прессо́ванного табака́ для жева́ния.

quid² *n* (*pl без измен.*) *сленг* совере́н *или* фунт сте́рлингов.

quiddity ['kwɪdɪtɪ] *n* 1) су́щность, суть; 2) софи́зм.

quidnunc ['kwɪdnʌŋk] *n* спле́тник, болту́н.

quiescence [kwaɪˈesns] *n* поко́й; неподви́жность; пасси́вность.

quiescent [kwaɪˈesnt] *a* неподви́жный; безде́йствующий; пасси́вный.

quiet I ['kwaɪət] *n* поко́й, тишина́, споко́йствие; безмо́лвие; on the ~ а) в тиши́; б) в та́йне; тайко́м.

quiet II *a* 1) ти́хий, споко́йный; неслы́шный,

бесшу́мный; keep ~! не шуми́те!; замолчи́те!; 2) споко́йный, ми́рный; 3) скро́мный (*об образе жизни*); 4) нея́ркий (*о красках*); 5) скры́тый; укро́мный; to keep smth. ~ ума́лчивать о чём-л.; скрыва́ть что-л.

quiet III *v* успока́ивать(ся); □ to ~ **down** утиха́ть.

quieten [ˈkwaɪətn] *v* успока́ивать(ся); утиха́ть.

quietly [ˈkwaɪətlɪ] *adv* ти́хо, споко́йно.

quietness [ˈkwaɪətnɪs] *n* споко́йствие, тишина́, поко́й.

quietude [ˈkwaɪɪtjuːd] *n* поко́й, тишина́, мир.

quietus [kwaɪˈiːtəs] *n* ухо́д из жи́зни, коне́ц, смерть.

quill I [kwɪl] *n* 1) пти́чье перо́; 2) (гуси́ное) перо́ для письма́; to drive a ~ быть писа́телем; 3) игла́ дикобра́за; 4) *тех.* шпу́ля.

quill II *v* 1) гофрирова́ть; 2) нама́тывать на кату́шку.

quill-driver [ˈkwɪlˌdraɪvə] *n шутл.* писа́ка; журнали́ст.

quilt I [kwɪlt] *n* стёганое одея́ло.

quilt II *v* 1) стега́ть (*одея́ло*); 2) *разг.* компили́ровать.

quince [kwɪns] *n* айва́.

quincentenary [ˌkwɪnsenˈtiːnərɪ] *n* пятисотле́тие.

quinine [kwɪˈniːn] *n* хини́н.

quinquagenarian I [ˌkwɪŋkwədʒɪˈnɛərɪən] *n* пятидесятиле́тний челове́к.

quinquagenarian II *a* пятидесятиле́тний.

quinsy [ˈkwɪnzɪ] *n* ангина.

quint [kwɪnt] *n муз.* кви́нта.

quintal [ˈkwɪntl] *n* це́нтнер.

quintessence [kwɪnˈtesns] *n* квинтэссе́нция.

quintet(te) [kwɪnˈtet] *n муз.* квинте́т.

quintuple I [ˈkwɪntjupl] *a* 1) пятикра́тный; 2) состоя́щий из пяти́ часте́й.

quintuple II *v* увели́чивать(ся) в пять раз.

quintuplets [ˈkwɪntjuplɪts] *n pl* пять близнецо́в.

quip [kwɪp] *n* 1) остро́та; эпигра́мма; 2) уве́ртка; софи́зм.

quire[1] [ˈkwaɪə] *n* 1) десть (*бума́ги*); 2) сфальцо́ванный печа́тный лист; in ~s несброшюро́ванный, в листа́х.

quire[2] I, II *см.* choir I, II.

quirk [kwɜːk] *n* 1) вы́верт, выкрута́сы; 2) завито́к, ро́счерк пера́; 3) остроу́мное замеча́ние; каламбу́р; 4) уве́ртка.

quirt I [kwɜːt] *n амер.* ара́пник.

quirt II *v амер.* хлеста́ть ара́пником.

quit I [kwɪt] *n* ухо́д с рабо́ты, со слу́жбы.

quit II *a predic* свобо́дный, отде́лавшийся (*от чего-л., кого-л.*); to be (*или* to get) ~ of освободи́ться, отде́латься.

quit III *v* 1) покида́ть, оставля́ть; 2) *амер.* броса́ть, прекраща́ть (*работу и т. п.*); 3) *поэт.* плати́ть; отпла́чивать, воздава́ть.

quitclaim I [ˈkwɪtkleɪm] *n* отка́з от пра́ва.

quitclaim II *v* отка́зываться от пра́ва.

quite [kwaɪt] *adv* 1) вполне́, соверше́нно, совсе́м, всеце́ло; oh, ~! о да!, вполне́!; 2) о́чень; ~ a long time ago о́чень давно́; 3) в не́которой сте́пени, дово́льно; it is ~ hot дово́льно жа́рко.

quits [kwɪts] *a predic:* to be ~ расквита́ться;

быть в расчёте; to cry ~ а) расквита́ться; б) пойти́ на мирову́ю, согласи́ться.

quittance [ˈkwɪtəns] *n* 1) квита́нция; 2) опла́та, возмеще́ние.

quitter [ˈkwɪtə] *n сленг* челове́к, легко́ броса́ющий на́чатое, не выполня́ющий своего́ до́лга.

quiver[1] I [ˈkwɪvə] *n* дрожь, тре́пет.

quiver[1] II *v* дрожа́ть, трепета́ть, трясти́сь; to ~ with excitement дрожа́ть от возбужде́ния.

quiver[2] *n* колча́н; ◊ an arrow left in one's ~ сре́дство, оста́вшееся про запа́с.

quiverful [ˈkwɪvəful] *n* 1) по́лный колча́н стрел; 2) *шутл.* больша́я семья́.

qui vive [kiːˈviːv] *n:* on the ~ насторо́же, начеку́.

quixotism, quixotry [ˈkwɪksətɪzəm, ˈkwɪksətrɪ] *n* донкихо́тство.

quiz[1] I [kwɪz] *n* 1) насме́шка; шу́тка, мистифика́ция; 2) насме́шник.

quiz[1] II *v* 1) шути́ть; насмеха́ться, подшу́чивать; 2) смотре́ть с любопы́тством на кого́-л.

quiz[2] I *n амер.* прове́рка зна́ний, опро́с; прове́рочные вопро́сы.

quiz[2] II *v амер.* проверя́ть зна́ния, проводи́ть испыта́ние.

quizzical [ˈkwɪzɪkəl] *a* 1) насме́шливый; шутли́вый; 2) чудакова́тый.

quod I [kwɔd] *n сленг* тюрьма́.

quod II *v сленг* сажа́ть в тюрьму́.

quoin [kɔɪn] *n* 1) вне́шний у́гол зда́ния; 2) углово́й ка́мень кла́дки; 3) клин.

quondam [ˈkwɔndæm] *a* бы́вший.

quorum [ˈkwɔːrəm] *n* кво́рум.

quota [ˈkwoutə] *n* до́ля, часть, кво́та.

quotation [kwouˈteɪʃən] *n* 1) цита́та; outworn ~s зата́сканные цита́ты; 2) цити́рование; 3) котиро́вка, курс.

quote I [kwout] *n* 1) *разг.* цита́та; 2) *pl* кавы́чки.

quote II *v* 1) цити́ровать; ссыла́ться на кого́-л.; 2) назнача́ть це́ну, коти́ровать.

quoth [kwouθ] *v уст.* сказа́л, сказа́ла.

quotidian [kwɔˈtɪdɪən] *a* 1) ежедне́вный; 2) бана́льный.

quotient [ˈkwouʃənt] *n мат.* ча́стное.

R

R, r [ɑː] *n* 18-я бу́ква англ. алфави́та; ◊ the three R's *разг.* чте́ние, письмо́, арифме́тика (reading, (w)riting, (a)rithmetic).

rabbet [ˈræbɪt] *n* желобо́к, вы́емка.

rabbit I [ˈræbɪt] *n* 1) кро́лик; *перен. разг.* трус; 2) *разг.* плохо́й игро́к.

rabbit II *v* охо́титься на кро́ликов.

rabbit-hole [ˈræbɪthoul] *n* кро́личья но́рка.

rabbit-hutch [ˈræbɪthʌtʃ] *n* кле́тка для дома́шних кро́ликов.

rabbit-warren [ˈræbɪtˌwɔrɪn] *n* кро́личий садо́к.

rabble [ˈræbl] *n* 1) толпа́; 2) (the ~) сброд.

rabid [ˈræbɪd] *a* 1) я́ростный, неи́стовый; 2) бе́шеный (*о собаке и т. п.*).

rabidity [ræˈbɪdɪtɪ] *n* я́рость, неи́стовство.

rabies [ˈreɪbiːz] *n* бе́шенство, водобоя́знь.

raccoon [rəˈkuːn] *см.* racoon.

race[1] I [reɪs] *n* 1) состязáние в бéге; гóнки; the ~s скáчки; obstacle ~s скáчки с препятствиями; 2) бы́стрый ход, бы́строе движéние; 3) бы́строе *или* си́льное течéние; поток; 4) жи́зненный путь; ◊ armaments ~, arms ~ гóнка вооружéний.

race[1] II *v* 1) бы́стро дви́гаться, бежáть; 2) состязáться в скóрости; 3) гнать (*лóшадь, маши́ну*).

race[2] *n* 1) рáса; the human ~ человéчество; 2) потóмство, род; 3) порóда; сорт; род; 4) осóбый аромáт (*вина*).

race[3] *n* кóрень.

race-card ['reɪskɑːd] *n* прогрáмма скáчек.

racecourse ['reɪskɔːs] *n* беговáя дорóжка; скаковóй круг, ипподрóм.

race-hatred ['reɪs,heɪtrɪd] *n* национáльная враждá.

racehorse ['reɪshɔːs] *n* скаковáя лóшадь.

race-meeting ['reɪs,miːtɪŋ] *n* день скáчек.

racer ['reɪsə] *n* 1) учáстник гóнок *или* скáчек; 2) беговáя лóшадь; 3) гóночная маши́на, яхта *и т. п.*

rachitis [ræ'kaɪtɪs] *n* рахи́т.

racial ['reɪʃəl] *a* рáсовый.

racialism ['reɪʃəlɪzəm] *n* раси́зм.

racism ['reɪsɪzəm] *см.* racialism.

rack[1] I [ræk] *n* 1) кормýшка; 2) вéшалка; 3) пóлка *или* сéтка для вещéй (*в вагóне*); 4) решётка; 5) *тех.* зубчáтая рéйка; 6) рáма; стóйка; штати́в; 7) *ист.* ды́ба; *перен.* пы́тка, мучéние; to be on the ~ мýчиться.

rack[1] II *v* 1) класть на пóлку *или* в сéтку; 2) мýчить, пытáть; 3) напрягáть; изнурять.

rack[2] *n*: to go to ~ and ruin поги́бнуть.

racket[1] ['rækɪt] *n* ракéтка (*для тéнниса*).

racket[2] I *n* 1) шум, гам; 2) развлечéния; рассéянный óбраз жи́зни; to go on the ~ усилéнно развлекáться; 3) улóвка, комбинáция; 4) *амер.* шантáж, вымогáтельство; ◊ to stand the ~ (of) а) оплáчивать расхóды; расплáчиваться за что-л.; б) брать на себя отвéтственность *или* вину́; в) мири́ться с послéдствиями.

racket[2] II *v* 1) производи́ть шум, беспорядок; 2) вести́ рассéянный óбраз жи́зни.

racketeer [,rækɪ'tɪə] *n амер.* вымогáтель; банди́т, гáнгстер.

racketeering [,rækɪ'tɪərɪŋ] *n амер.* бандити́зм; вымогáтельство.

rackety ['rækɪtɪ] *a* шýмный, беспорядочный.

rack-rent I ['rækrent] *n* непомéрная арéндная плáта.

rack-rent II *v* взимáть óчень высóкую арéндную плáту.

rack-wheel ['rækwiːl] *n* зубчáтое колесó.

racoon [rə'kuːn] *n* енóт.

racquet ['rækɪt] *см.* racket[1].

racy ['reɪsɪ] *a* 1) характéрный; с óсобым вкýсом *или* зáпахом (*о фрýктах и т. п.*); 2) си́льный, живóй, энерги́чный; ◊ ~ of the soil а) нарóдный, простóй; б) колори́тный (*о рéчи и т. п.*).

radar ['reɪdə] *n* 1) радáр; 2) радиолокáция.

radial ['reɪdjəl] *a* 1) радиáльный; лучи́стый; 2) *анат.* лучевóй.

radiance ['reɪdjəns] *n* 1) сияние; 2) великолéпие, блеск.

radiancy ['reɪdjənsɪ] *см.* radiance.

radiant ['reɪdjənt] *a* 1) лучи́стый, излучáющий; 2) сияющий, лучезáрный.

radiate[a] ['reɪdɪɪt] *a* лучи́стый; лучевóй.

radiate[b] ['reɪdɪeɪt] *v* 1) излучáть (*свет, теплó*); сиять; 2) излучáться, исходи́ть; 3) расходи́ться рáдиусами (из цéнтра).

radiation [,reɪdɪ'eɪʃən] *n* 1) излучéние (*тж. перен.*); лучеиспускáние; радиáция; 2) *attr* свя́занный с радиáцией; лучевóй (*о болéзни*).

radiator ['reɪdɪeɪtə] *n* радиáтор.

radical I ['rædɪkəl] *n* 1) *хим.* радикáл; 2) *мат.* знак кóрня; кóрень; 3) *полит.* радикáл.

radical II *a* 1) кореннóй, основнóй; радикáльный, пóлный; 2) *мат.* относя́щийся к кóрню; 3) *полит.* радикáльный.

radicalism ['rædɪkəlɪzəm] *n полит.* радикали́зм.

radii ['reɪdɪaɪ] *pl см.* radius.

radio I ['reɪdɪou] *n* 1) рáдио; 2) радиоприёмник; 3) радиогрáмма.

radio II *v* передавáть по рáдио.

radio- ['reɪdɪou-] *в слóжных словáх* радио-.

radio-active ['reɪdɪou'æktɪv] *a* радиоакти́вный.

radio-activity ['reɪdɪouæk'tɪvɪtɪ] *n* радиоакти́вность.

radiogram ['reɪdɪougræm] *n* 1) радиогрáмма; 2) рентгéновский сни́мок.

radio-location ['reɪdɪoulou'keɪʃən] *n* радиолокáция.

radioman ['reɪdɪoumən] *n разг.* ради́ст.

radio-telegram ['reɪdɪou'telɪgræm] *n* радиотелегрáмма.

radish ['rædɪʃ] *n* реди́ска.

radium ['reɪdjəm] *n хим.* рáдий.

radius ['reɪdjəs] *n* (*pl тж.* radii) 1) рáдиус; 2) спи́ца (*колесá*); 3) *анат.* лучевáя кость.

raffish ['ræfɪʃ] *a* беспýтный.

raffle I ['ræfl] *n* лотерéя.

raffle II *v* 1) разы́грывать в лотерéе; 2) учáствовать в лотерéе.

raft[1] I [rɑːft] *n* 1) плот; 2) парóм.

raft[1] II *v* 1) гнать плоты́; сплавля́ть лес; 2) переправля́ть(ся) на парóме.

raft[2] *n амер. разг.* мнóжество; мáсса.

rafter[1] ['rɑːftə] *n см.* raftsman.

rafter[2] *n стр.* стропи́ло.

raftsman ['rɑːftsmən] *n* 1) плотовщи́к; 2) парóмщик.

rag[1] [ræg] *n* 1) тря́пка; лоскýт; обры́вок; клочóк; 2) *pl* тряпьё; лохмóтья; in ~s в лохмóтьях, обóрванный; 3) незначи́тельное коли́чество; not a ~ of ни кáпли, ничегó; 4) *пренебр.* тря́пка, лоскýт (*о флáге, пáрусе*); листóк (*о газéте*); 5) *attr* тряпи́чный; ◊ to chew the ~ *разг.* завести́ волы́нку; ворчáть, пили́ть когó-л.

rag[2] I *n* шýмное весéлье; шýтки.

rag[2] II *v* 1) дразни́ть; подшýчивать; 2) шумéть, бушевáть.

ragamufin ['rægəmʌfɪn] *n* оборвáнец.

rag-and-bone-man [,rægən'bounmæn] *n* старьёвщик.

rag-bolt ['rægboult] *n* 1) *тех.* áнкерный болт; 2) уклю́чина.

rage I [reɪdʒ] *n* 1) я́рость, неи́стовство; to fly into a ~ прийти́ в я́рость; 2) *разг.* óбщее увлечéние, мóда; to be all the ~ быть óчень мóдным.

rage II *v* 1) беси́ться; 2) бушевáть, неи́стовствовать; свире́пствовать (*об эпидемии и т. п.*); to ~ itself out зати́хнуть, прекрати́ться (*о буре и тому подобное*).

ragged ['rægɪd] *a* 1) рва́ный; изо́рванный (*об одежде*); 2) обо́рванный, оде́тый в лохмо́тья; 3) неаккура́тный; запу́щенный (*о саде*); 4) шерохова́тый, неро́вный; 5) рва́ный (*о ране*).

raggery ['rægərɪ] *n разг.* «тря́пки», пла́тья.

raging ['reɪdʒɪŋ] *a* 1) я́ростный; 2) си́льный (*о боли и т. п.*).

ragman ['rægmən] *n* старьёвщик.

ragout ['ræguː] *n* рагу́.

ragtag ['rægtæg] *n разг.* сброд.

ragtime ['rægtaɪm] *n* 1) синкопи́рованный плясово́й ритм; 2) *attr* смехотво́рный.

raid I [reɪd] *n* налёт, набе́г; рейд.

raid II *v* соверша́ть налёт *или* набе́г; производи́ть обла́ву; вторга́ться.

raider ['reɪdə] *n* 1) уча́стник налёта *или* набе́га; 2) *воен.* рейдер; 3) *ав.* самолёт, соверша́ющий налёт.

rail¹ I [reɪl] *n* 1) пери́ла; огра́да; 2) рельс; to get (*или* to run) off the ~s сойти́ с ре́льсов; off the ~s а) соше́дший с ре́льсов; б) вы́битый из колеи́; 3) железнодоро́жный путь; by ~ по желе́зной доро́ге; 4) перекла́дина, попере́чина, брус; 5) ве́шалка; ◇ to sit on the ~ *амер.* выжида́ть, колеба́ться.

rail¹ II *v* 1) огора́живать; 2) прокла́дывать ре́льсы; 3) путеше́ствовать по желе́зной доро́ге; □ to ~ in огороди́ть; to ~ off отгороди́ть.

rail² *v* руга́ть, брани́ть; упрека́ть; придира́ться.

rail³ *n* коросте́ль, дерга́ч.

railing ['reɪlɪŋ] *n* огра́да; пери́ла.

raillery ['reɪlərɪ] *n* доброду́шное подшу́чивание.

railroad I ['reɪlroud] *n амер.* 1) желе́зная доро́га; 2) *attr* железнодоро́жный.

railroad II *v амер.* 1) путеше́ствовать *или* перевози́ть по желе́зной доро́ге; 2) стро́ить желе́зную доро́гу; 3) *разг.* прота́лкивать, проводи́ть в спе́шном поря́дке (*дело, закон; through*); 4) *разг.* водворя́ть (*кого-л. куда-л.; to, into*); 5) *сленг* сажа́ть в тюрьму́ (*по ложному обвинению*).

railway I ['reɪlweɪ] *n* 1) желе́зная доро́га; aerial ~ подвесна́я доро́га; elevated (circular) ~ надзе́мная (окружна́я) желе́зная доро́га; 2) *attr* железнодоро́жный.

railway II *v* 1) путеше́ствовать по желе́зной доро́ге; 2) стро́ить желе́зную доро́гу.

railwayman ['reɪlweɪmən] *n* железнодоро́жный слу́жащий.

railway-yard ['reɪlweɪˌjɑːd] *n* сортиро́вочная ста́нция, железнодоро́жный парк.

raiment ['reɪmənt] *n поэт.* оде́жда, одея́ние.

rain I [reɪn] *n* 1) дождь; pouring ~, pelting ~ проливно́й дождь; the ~s пери́од тропи́ческих дожде́й, дождли́вый сезо́н; ~ or shine в любу́ю пого́ду; to be caught in the ~ попа́сть под дождь, быть засти́гнутым дождём; to keep the ~ out укры́ться от дождя́; 2) пото́к, руче́й (*слёз*); град (*ударов, пуль*).

rain II *v* 1): it ~s, it is ~ing идёт дождь; 2) ли́ть(ся); сы́пать(ся) (*в большом количестве*); ◇ it never ~s but it pours *посл.* ≅ пришла́ беда́, отворя́й воро́та; беда́ (никогда́) не прихо́дит одна́.

rainbow ['reɪnbou] *n* 1) ра́дуга; 2) *attr* ра́дужный, краси́вый.

raincoat ['reɪnkout] *n* непромока́емый плащ.

raindrop ['reɪndrɔp] *n* дождева́я ка́пля.

rainfall ['reɪnfɔːl] *n* 1) ли́вень; 2) коли́чество оса́дков.

rain-gauge ['reɪngeɪdʒ] *n метео.* дождеме́р.

rainless ['reɪnlɪs] *a* засу́шливый; без дождя́.

rainproof ['reɪnpruːf] *a* непромока́емый.

rain-storm ['reɪnstɔːm] *n* ли́вень с урага́ном.

raintight ['reɪntaɪt] *см.* rainproof.

rain-water ['reɪnˌwɔːtə] *n* дождева́я вода́.

rain-worm ['reɪnwɔːm] *n* дождево́й червь.

rainy ['reɪnɪ] *a* 1) дождли́вый; 2) дождево́й (*о тучах и т. п.*); ◇ for a ~ day на чёрный день.

raise I [reɪz] *n* 1) подъём; 2) повыше́ние; увеличе́ние.

raise II *v* 1) поднима́ть; 2) воздвига́ть; 3) буди́ть; 4) повыша́ть (*по должности*); выдвига́ть; 5) повыша́ть (*заработную плату и т. п.*); 6) повыша́ть (*голос*); 7) расти́ть; выра́щивать; 8) вызыва́ть, возбужда́ть; порожда́ть; 9) собира́ть (*войско, налоги*); 10) издава́ть (*возглас, крик*); 11) добыва́ть, извлека́ть (*из земли*); 12) снима́ть (*осаду, блокаду*); ◇ to ~ from the dead верну́ть к жи́зни.

raisin ['reɪzn] *n* изю́м.

rajah ['rɑːdʒə] *n* ра́джа.

rake¹ I [reɪk] *n* гра́бли.

rake¹ II *v* 1) сгреба́ть; зара́внивать гра́блями; 2) собира́ть (*обыкн.* to ~ up, to ~ together); 3) тща́тельно иска́ть, ры́ться (*among, in*); □ to ~ in загреба́ть де́ньги; to ~ out выгреба́ть; *перен.* добыва́ть с трудо́м; to ~ up сгреба́ть; вороши́ть (*тж. перен.*).

rake² I *n* пове́са; распу́тник.

rake² II *v* повесничать.

rake-off ['reɪkˌɔf] *n амер. разг.* 1) незако́нная при́быль (*участника в деле*); взя́тка; 2) до́ля посре́дника.

raker ['reɪkə] *n* 1) гра́бли; 2) рабо́тающий гра́блями.

rakish¹ ['reɪkɪʃ] *a* распу́тный; распу́щенный.

rakish² *a* 1) быстрохо́дный (*о корабле*); 2) щегольско́й.

rally¹ I ['rælɪ] *n* 1) объедине́ние; 2) собра́ние; слёт; *амер.* ма́ссовый ми́тинг; 3) восстановле́ние (*сил*).

rally¹ II *v* 1) собира́ть(ся) вновь; воссоедини́ть (-ся); сплоти́ть(ся); 2) оправля́ться (*от болезни и т. п.*); 3) приходи́ть на по́мощь.

rally¹ *v* шути́ть, подшу́чивать над кем-л.

ram I [ræm] *n* 1) бара́н; 2) тара́н; 3) (R.) Ове́н (*созвездие*).

ram II *v* 1) уда́рить(ся); вреза́ться; 2) тара́нить; 3) забива́ть, вкола́чивать; to ~ into smb., to ~ it home вбива́ть в го́лову.

ramble I ['ræmbl] *n* прогу́лка, пое́здка.

ramble II *v* 1) броди́ть; 2) переска́кивать с предме́та на предме́т (*в разговоре*).

rambler ['ræmblə] *n* 1) праздношата́ющийся; 2) ползу́чее расте́ние.

rambling ['ræmblɪŋ] *a* 1) слоня́ющийся; бродя́чий; 2) разбро́санный, постро́енный без пла́на;

3) бессвя́зный (*о разговоре, рассказе*); 4) ползу́чий (*о растении*).

ramification [ˌræmɪfɪˈkeɪʃən] *n* 1) разветвле́ние; ответвле́ние; 2) *собир.* ве́тви де́рева.

ramify [ˈræmɪfaɪ] *v* разветвля́ться.

rammer [ˈræmə] *n* 1) *тех.* трамбо́вка; ба́ба; 2) *воен.* шо́мпол; 3) *сленг.* рука́.

rammish [ˈræmɪʃ] *a* ду́рно па́хнущий.

ramp¹ I [ræmp] *n* 1) накло́нная пло́скость; скат; 2) *разг.* вспы́шка гне́ва.

ramp¹ II *v* 1) стоя́ть на за́дних ла́пах (*о геральдическом льве и т. п.*); 2) принима́ть угрожа́ющую по́зу; 3) *обыкн. шутл.* пры́гать, броса́ться в я́рости; бушева́ть; 4) бу́йно расти́ (*о растениях*).

ramp² I *n сленг* 1) вымога́тельство; 2) грабёж.

ramp² II *v сленг* 1) вымога́ть; 2) гра́бить.

rampage I [ræmˈpeɪdʒ] *n* неи́стовство, я́рость, бу́йство; on the ~ в я́рости.

rampage II *v* неи́стовствовать, бу́йствовать.

rampageous [ræmˈpeɪdʒəs] *a* неи́стовый, бу́йный.

rampancy [ˈræmpənsɪ] *n* неи́стовство.

rampant [ˈræmpənt] *a* 1) стоя́щий на за́дних ла́пах (*о геральдическом льве и т. п.*); 2) неи́стовый; разъярённый; 3) бу́йно разро́сшийся (*о растениях*); 4) весьма́ распространённый, процвета́ющий (*о пороках и т. п.*).

rampart I [ˈræmpɑːt] *n* 1) (крепостно́й) вал; 2) опло́т, защи́та.

rampart II *v* защища́ть, укрепля́ть ва́лом.

ramrod [ˈræmrɔd] *n* шо́мпол..

ramshackle [ˈræmˌʃækl] *a* ве́тхий.

ran [ræn] *past см.* run II.

ranch I [rɑːntʃ] *n* ра́нчо, (скотово́дческая) фе́рма.

ranch II *v* жить на фе́рме; занима́ться ското-во́дством.

rancher [ˈrɑːntʃə] *n* 1) хозя́ин ра́нчо; 2) рабо́тник на ра́нчо.

ranchman [ˈrɑːntʃmən] *см.* rancher.

rancid [ˈrænsɪd] *a* прого́рклый; проту́хший.

rancidity [rænˈsɪdɪtɪ] *n* прого́рклость.

rancidness [ˈrænsɪdnɪs] *см.* rancidity.

rancorous [ˈræŋkərəs] *a* зло́бный; вражде́б-ный.

rancour [ˈræŋkə] *n* зло́ба; вражда́.

random I [ˈrændəm] *n*: at ~ случа́йно, науга́д, наобу́м.

random II *a* случа́йный; беспоря́дочный; шально́й (*о пуле*).

ranee [rɑːˈniː] *n* супру́га ра́джи.

rang [ræŋ] *past см.* ring² II.

range I [reɪndʒ] *n* 1) ряд, ли́ния; 2) па́стбище; 3) о́бласть распростране́ния (*растения, живот-ного*); зо́на, сфе́ра; 4) амплиту́да; диапазо́н, преде́лы; 5) протяже́ние, простра́нство; ~ of vision кругозо́р, по́ле зре́ния; 6) ра́диус де́йствия; да́льность, диста́нция (*стрельбы*); out of ~ вне дося-га́емости; 7) плита́ (*кухонная*); 8) стре́льбище, полиго́н.

range II *v* 1) выстра́ивать(ся) в ряд; ста́вить в поря́дке; 2) классифици́ровать; 3): to ~ oneself присоединя́ться, примыка́ть; 4) броди́ть, стран-ствовать, скита́ться (*по — over, through*); 5) пере-ходи́ть с одного́ на друго́е (*о разговоре*); 6) про-стира́ться (*от... до*); 7) колеба́ться (*в известных преде́лах*); 8) встреча́ться (*в определённых гра-*

ницах — *о растении, животном*); 9) *воен.* при-стре́ливаться; бить (*на определённое расстояние — об орудии*).

range-finder [ˈreɪndʒˌfaɪndə] *n воен.* дально-ме́р.

ranger [ˈreɪndʒə] *n* 1) бродя́га; стра́нник; 2) лес-ни́чий; 3) ко́нный полице́йский; 4) *pl амер.* деса́нтно-диверсио́нные ча́сти.

rangy [ˈreɪndʒɪ] *a* 1) бродя́чий; блужда́ющий; 2) стро́йный, му́скулистый; 3) обши́рный, про-стра́нный.

rank¹ I [ræŋk] *n* 1) ряд; шере́нга; 2) зва́ние, чин; honorary ~ почётное зва́ние; 3) ранг, катего́рия, разря́д; 4): the ~s, the ~ and file рядово́й со-ста́в, рядовы́е; to rise from the ~s a) *воен.* выд-винуться из рядовы́х в офице́ры; б) *разг.* вы́йти в лю́ди; to reduce to the ~s разжа́ловать в рядо-вы́е; 5) высо́кое положе́ние; (the) ~ and fashion вы́сшее о́бщество.

rank¹ II *v* 1) стро́ить(ся) в шере́нгу; выстра́и-вать(ся) в ряд; 2) распределя́ть, классифици́ро-вать; 3) счита́ться; he ~s among the best writers его́ счита́ют одни́м из лу́чших писа́телей; 4) за-нима́ть (*определённое*) положе́ние; to ~ high (low) занима́ть высо́кое (ни́зкое) положе́ние; 5) быть вы́ше (*по чину, званию*).

rank² *a* 1) роско́шный, бу́йный (*о раститель-ности*); 2) заро́сший; 3) плодоро́дный, ту́чный (*о почве*); 4) прого́рклый, проту́хший; 5) отъ-я́вленный; су́щий, соверше́нный; 6) гру́бый, про-ти́вный.

ranker [ˈræŋkə] *n* офице́р, вы́служившийся из рядовы́х.

rankle [ˈræŋkl] *v* причиня́ть боль; му́чить, терза́ть (*о воспоминании и т. п.*).

ransack [ˈrænsæk] *v* 1) иска́ть, обы́скивать; ры́ться (*в поисках чего-л*); 2) гра́бить.

ransom I [ˈrænsəm] *n* вы́куп.

ransom II *v* 1) выкупа́ть; освобожда́ть за вы́куп; 2) тре́бовать вы́купа (*за кого-л*); 3) искупа́ть.

rant I [rænt] *n* напы́щенная речь; гро́мкие слова́.

rant II *v* 1) говори́ть напы́щенно; 2) бахва́литься.

ranunculus [rəˈnʌŋkjuləs] *n* (*pl тж.* ranunculi [rəˈnʌŋkjulaɪ]) *бот.* лю́тик

rap¹ I [ræp] *n* 1) (лёгкий) уда́р; 2) лёгкий стук; a ~ on the door стук в дверь.

rap¹ II *v* 1) слегка́ ударя́ть; 2) стуча́ть, простуки-вать; 3) ре́зко отве́тить; □ to ~ out гру́бо кри́кнуть, га́ркнуть (*на кого-л*.).

rap² *n*: not a ~ ни гроша́; not worth a ~ ничего́ не сто́ящий, никчёмный; I don't care a ~ мне наплева́ть.

rapacious [rəˈpeɪʃəs] *a* 1) хи́щный; 2) жа́дный.

rapacity [rəˈpæsɪtɪ] *n* жа́дность.

rape I [reɪp] *n* 1) похище́ние; 2) изнаси́лование.

rape II *v* 1) похища́ть; 2) наси́ловать.

rapid I [ˈræpɪd] *a* 1) бы́стрый, ско́рый; 2) круто́й (*о склоне*).

rapid II *n обыкн. pl* стремни́на; поро́ги реки́.

rapidity [rəˈpɪdɪtɪ] *n* быстрота́, ско́рость.

rapier [ˈreɪpɪə] *n* рапи́ра.

rapine [ˈræpaɪn] *n* грабёж.

rapprochement [ræˈprɔʃmɑːŋ] *n* сближе́ние, возобновле́ние дру́жеских отноше́ний.

rapt [ræpt] *a* 1) восхищённый, в восто́рге; 2) пог-лощённый, увлечённый; 3) похи́щенный.

rapture [ˈræptʃə] *n* 1) восто́рг; восхище́ние;

to be in ~s быть в восторге; to go into ~s прийти в восторг; 2) похищение.

rapturous ['ræptʃərəs] *a* восторженный.

rara avis ['rɛərə'eivis] *n* редкость, диковинка.

rare[1] I [rɛə] *a* 1) редкий, редкостный; необычный; особенный; 2) замечательный, исключительный (*о памяти, способностях*); 3) разрежённый, негустой; 4) инертный (*о газе*).

rare[1] II *adv разг.* исключительно.

rare[2] *a амер.* недожаренный, недоваренный.

rarefaction [,rɛəri'fækʃən] *n* разрежение; разжижение.

rarefy ['rɛərifai] *v* 1) разрежать(ся); разжижать(ся); 2) очищать.

rarely ['rɛəli] *adv* 1) редко, нечасто; 2) необычайно, исключительно.

rarity ['rɛəriti] *n* 1) редкость; 2) редкое явление; 3) разрежённость (*воздуха и т. п.*).

rascal ['rɑːskəl] *n* мошенник.

rascality [rɑs'kæliti] *n* мошенничество.

rash[1] [ræʃ] *a* стремительный; поспешный; опрометчивый.

rash[2] *n* сыпь.

rasher ['ræʃə] *n* тонкий ломтик ветчины (*для жаренья*).

rashness ['ræʃnis] *n* стремительность; опрометчивость.

rasp I [rɑːsp] *n* 1) рашпиль; 2) дребезжание; резкий, скребущий звук.

rasp II *v* 1) скрести, тереть; подпиливать; 2) дребезжать; 3) раздражать, резать ухо; 4) пиликать.

raspberry ['rɑːzbəri] *n* 1) малина; 2) *сленг* звук или жест, выражающий презрение; to give (*или* to hand) smb. a ~ обидеть, оскорбить кого-либо.

raspberry-cane ['rɑːzbərikein] *n обыкн. pl* малинник.

rasping ['rɑːspiŋ] *n обыкн. pl тех.* стружка.

rat I [ræt] *n* 1) крыса; 2) дезертир; перебежчик; 3) *сленг*: ~s! вздор!, ерунда!; ◇ as wet as a ~, like a drowned ~ а) насквозь промокший; б) в жалком виде; to have ~s in the attic *сленг* чердак не в порядке; винтиков не хватает; to smell a ~ чуять недоброе; подозревать.

rat II *v* 1) истреблять крыс; 2) дезертировать; изменить (*партии, делу*).

ratable ['reitəbl] *a* подлежащий обложению (налогами).

rat-catcher ['ræt,kætʃə] *n* крысолов.

ratchet ['rætʃit] *n тех.* храповик.

rate[1] I [reit] *n* 1) ставка; тариф; норма; the ~s of wages ставки заработной платы; flat ~ *эк.* единообразная ставка (*налогов и т. п.*); ~ of exchange валютный курс; ~ of surplus value *полит. эк.* норма прибавочной стоимости; average ~ of profit *полит. эк.* средняя норма прибыли; 2) коэффициент; процент; доля; at the ~ in количестве...; 3) темп, скорость; at the ~ of... an hour со скоростью... в час; 4) цена; the regular ~ обычная, нормальная цена; at the ~ of... по (*такой-то*) цене; 5) разряд, класс; сорт; ◇ at any ~ во всяком случае; по меньшей мере; at that ~ в таком случае; at this ~ таким образом; если так.

rate[1] II *v* 1) оценивать, определять, устанавливать; 2) считать; he was ~d one of the bravest men

он считался одним из самых храбрых; 3) облагать налогом.

rate[2] *v* бранить(ся).

rateable ['reitəbl] *см.* ratable.

ratepayer ['reit,peiə] *n* налогоплательщик.

rather ['rɑːðə] *adv* 1) охотнее, лучше, предпочтительнее; I would ~ go today than tomorrow я бы лучше (*или* охотнее) пошёл сегодня, чем завтра; 2) вернее, скорее, правильнее; 3) до некоторой степени, немного, пожалуй; he was ~ tired он порядком устал; 4): ~! *разг.* о да!, да, конечно! (*в ответ*); ◇ the ~ that... тем более, что...

ratification [,rætifi'keiʃən] *n* ратификация, подписание (*договора и т. п.*).

ratify ['rætifai] *v* утверждать; ратифицировать, подписывать (*договор и т. п.*).

rating[1] ['reitiŋ] *n* 1) оценка; определение класса *или* разряда; 2) класс, разряд; ранг; положение; 3) обложение налогом; 4) *тех., эк.* мощность; производительность.

rating[2] *n* выговор, нагоняй.

ratio ['reiʃiou] *n* отношение, пропорция, соотношение.

ration I ['ræʃən] *n* 1) паёк; порция; *воен.* рацион; emergency ~, the iron ~ неприкосновенный запас; 2) *pl* провизия; 3) *attr* пайковый.

ration II *v* 1) выдавать пайки, снабжать продовольствием; 2) нормировать выдачу какого-л. продукта.

rational ['ræʃənl] *a* разумный; рациональный, целесообразный.

rationalism ['ræʃnəlizəm] *n* рационализм.

rationalist I ['ræʃnəlist] *n* рационалист.

rationalist II *a* рационалистический.

rationalistic [,ræʃnə'listik] *a* рационалистический.

rationality [,ræʃə'næliti] *n* разумность, рациональность.

rationalization [,ræʃnəlai'zeiʃən] *n* 1) рационализация; 2) *мат.* освобождение от иррациональности.

rationalize ['ræʃnəlaiz] *v* 1) рационализировать; 2) объяснять рационалистически; 3) *мат.* освобождать от иррациональности.

ration-book ['ræʃənbuk] *n* продовольственная книжка.

ration-card ['ræʃənkɑːd] *n* продовольственная карточка.

rationing ['ræʃniŋ] *n* нормирование продуктов.

ratsbane ['rætsbein] *n* 1) отрава для крыс; 2) ядовитое растение.

rat-tat [,ræt'tæt] *n* (громкий) стук в дверь.

rattle I ['rætl] *n* 1) треск, грохот; дребезжание; 2) шум, суматоха; 3) погремушка; 4) трещотка (*ночного сторожа*); 5) *разг.* болтун, пустомеля.

rattle II *v* 1) трещать; грохотать, громко стучать; дребезжать; 2) двигаться, падать с грохотом; 3) громко и быстро говорить, трещать; «отбарабанить» (*урок, стихи и т. п.*); 4) *разг.* смущать; раздражать; to get ~d нервничать, терять спокойствие.

rattle-box ['rætlbɔks] *n* 1) детская погремушка; 2) *разг.* болтун, трещотка.

rattlebrained ['rætlbreind] *a* пустоголовый.

rattleheaded ['rætl,hedid] *см.* rattle-brained.

rattler ['rætlə] *n* 1) болтун, пустомеля; 2) что-л.

грохочущее; старый экипаж, поезд, пулемёт *и т. п.*; 3) *амер. разг.* гремучая змея; 4) необыкновенное происшествие, сенсация; 5) *разг.* яркий образец (*чего-л.*).

rattlesnake ['rætlsneɪk] *n* гремучая змея.

rattling I ['rætlɪŋ] *a* 1) грохочущий, шумный; 2) сильный (*о ветре, дожде*); быстрый (*о походке*); 3) *разг.* великолепный.

rattling II *adv* очень, чрезвычайно.

rat-trap ['rættræp] *n* крысоловка.

raucous ['rɔːkəs] *a* хриплый.

ravage I ['rævɪdʒ] *n* 1) опустошение, разорение; 2) *pl* разрушительное действие.

ravage II *v* опустошать, разорять.

rave [reɪv] *v* 1) бредить, говорить бессвязно; 2) говорить восторженно (*about, of*); 3) неистовствовать; реветь, бушевать (*о ветре и т. п.*).

ravel I ['rævəl] *n* 1) путаница; узел; 2) обрывок (*нитки и т. п.*).

ravel II *v* 1) распутывать; разрывать; (*часто* to ~ out*); 2) протираться (*о ткани*); 3) запутывать(ся), усложнять(ся).

ravelin ['rævlɪn] *n* равелин.

raven^a I ['reɪvn] *n* ворон.

raven^a II *a* вороной, чёрный.

raven^b ['rævn] *v* 1) грабить; 2) искать добычу; 3) (жадно) пожирать; иметь волчий аппетит.

ravenous ['rævɪnəs] *a* 1) хищный; 2) жадный; прожорливый; 3) грабительский.

ravin ['rævɪn] *n поэт.* грабёж.

ravine [rə'viːn] *n* глубокое ущелье; лощина; овраг.

raving I ['reɪvɪŋ] *n часто pl* бред.

raving II *a* бредовой.

ravish ['rævɪʃ] *v* 1) восхищать; приводить в восторг; 2) *уст., поэт.* похищать; 3) насиловать.

ravishing ['rævɪʃɪŋ] *a* восхитительный.

ravishment ['rævɪʃmənt] *n* 1) восхищение, восторг; 2) *уст., поэт.* похищение; 3) изнасилование.

raw I [rɔː] *a* 1) сырой; 2) недоваренный; непропечённый; недожаренный; 3) необработанный; 4) неопытный; необученный; 5) сырой, промозглый (*о погоде*); холодный (*о ветре*); 6) с ободранной кожей, *перен.* чувствительный, 7) кровоточащий (*о ране*); 8) *амер. сленг* нечестный.

raw II *n* 1) сырьё; 2) ссадина; больное место; to touch smb. on the ~ задеть кого-л. за живое.

raw III *v* сдирать кожу.

raw-boned ['rɔːbound] *a* очень худой, костлявый.

rawhide ['rɔːhaɪd] *a* (сделанный) из сыромятной кожи.

rawness ['rɔːnɪs] *n* 1) необработанность; 2) неопытность; 3) больное место; 4) сырость (*на улице*).

ray¹ I [reɪ] *n* 1) луч; gamma ~s гамма-лучи, гамма-излучение; cosmic ~s космические лучи, космическое излучение; 2) проблеск; a ~ of hope проблеск надежды.

ray¹ II *v* 1) излучать(ся); 2) расходиться лучами; 3) облучать.

ray² *n* скат (*рыба*).

rayon ['reɪɒn] *n* искусственный шёлк, вискоза.

raze [reɪz] *v* 1) разрушать до основания, сносить; to ~ to the ground стереть с лица земли; сровнять с землёй; 2) вычёркивать, стирать (*обыкн. перен.*).

razor ['reɪzə] *n* бритва; safety ~ безопасная бритва.

razor-back ['reɪzəbæk] *n* полосатик (*кит*).

razor-edge ['reɪzər'edʒ] *n* 1) остриё бритвы; острый край; 2) резкая грань; 3) опасное положение.

re [riː] *n муз.* ре.

re- [riː-] *pref указывает:* а) *на повторение действия, выраженного основным гл.*: to reprint перепечатать; to re-read перечитать, вновь прочесть; б) *на возобновление действия, выраженного основным словом:* to renew возобновлять; в) *на возвращение в прежнее состояние:* to recall отзывать; to reimport ввозить обратно.

reach I [riːtʃ] *n* 1) протягивание (*руки и т. п.*); 2) досягаемость; within (out of) ~ в пределах (вне пределов) досягаемости; within easy ~ поблизости, недалеко (от); 3) круг (понимания); охват, кругозор; it is beyond my ~ мне это недоступно, непонятно; 4) протяжение, пространство; a ~ of woodland широкая полоса лесов.

reach II *v* 1) протягивать; вытягивать (*часто* to ~ out); to ~ for smth. протягивать руку за чем-л.; 2) передавать, подавать; 3) доставать, брать (*с полки и т. п.*); 4) доезжать; достигать, доходить; 5) составлять (*сумму*); 6) простираться; 7) застать; настигнуть; 8) трогать; оказывать влияние; □ to ~ after тянуться за чем-л.; *перен.* стремиться к чему-л.

reach-me-down I ['riːtʃmɪ'daun] *n* готовое платье.

reach-me-down II *a* готовый (*о платье*).

react [riː'ækt] *v* 1) реагировать; 2) (воз)действовать (*на — on, upon*); 3) *хим.* вызывать реакцию; 4) противодействовать (*against*); оказывать сопротивление.

re-act ['riː'ækt] *v* повторить, сделать ещё раз.

reactance [riː'æktəns] *n эл.* реактивное сопротивление.

reaction¹ [riː'ækʃən] *n* 1) реакция; chain ~ цепная реакция; 2) взаимодействие; 3) воздействие, влияние; 4) противодействие; 5) слабость, реакция (*после напряжения и т. п.*); 6) *attr* реактивный.

reaction² *n полит.* реакция.

reactionary¹ [riː'ækʃnərɪ] *a* обратный, дающий обратную реакцию.

reactionary² I *n полит.* реакционер.

reactionary² II *a полит.* реакционный.

reactionist [riː'ækʃənɪst] *см.* reactionary² I.

reactive [riː'æktɪv] *a* 1) реагирующий; 2) противодействующий; 3) реактивный.

reactor [riː'æktə] *n физ.* реактор, атомный котёл.

read^a I [riːd] *v* (*past, p. p.* read [red]) 1) читать; to ~ aloud, to ~ out читать вслух; to ~ to oneself читать про себя; to ~ oneself hoarse дочитаться до хрипоты; 2) понимать; 3) изучать; to ~ up for examinations готовиться к экзаменам; to ~ for a doctorate готовить докторскую диссертацию (*in*); 4) объяснять, истолковывать; разгадывать (*сон, загадку*); 5) гласить (*о цитате, документе*); показывать (*о приборе*); to ~ untrue показывать неверно; □ to ~ on продолжать читать; читать дальше; to ~ over прочесть вновь, перечитать; to ~ through прочесть; ◊ to ~ between lines читать между строк.

read^a II *n* чтение; to have a good (a short) ~ почитать как следует (немного, недолго).

read^b I [red] *past, p. p.* см. read^a I.

read^b II *a* начитанный, знающий, образованный.

readable ['riːdəbl] *a* 1) легко читающийся, интересный; 2) чёткий; удобочитаемый.

readdress ['riːə'dres] *v* переадресовать.

reader ['riːdə] *n* 1) читатель; любитель чтения; gentle ~ благосклонный читатель (*в обращении автора*); 2) читающий; 3) чтец; лектор; 4) корректор; 5) рецензент (*издательства*); 6) хрестоматия.

readily ['redɪlɪ] *adv* 1) охотно, быстро, с готовностью; 2) легко; без труда.

readiness ['redɪnɪs] *n* 1) готовность, охота; 2) подготовленность, состояние готовности; 3) находчивость, быстрота; 4) согласие.

reading ['riːdɪŋ] *n* 1) чтение; close ~ внимательное чтение; 2) публичное чтение; лекция; 3) начитанность, знания; of vast ~ начитанный; 4) вариант текста, разночтение; 5) толкование, понимание; 6) показание (*прибора*); 7) чтение законопроекта в парламенте; the first (second, third) ~ первое, (второе, третье) чтение.

reading-desk ['riːdɪŋdesk] *n* пюпитр.

reading-glass ['riːdɪŋglɑːs] *n* увеличительное стекло.

reading-lamp ['riːdɪŋlæmp] *n* настольная лампа.

reading-room ['riːdɪŋrum] *n* читальный зал, читальня.

readjust ['riːə'dʒʌst] *v* переделывать, приспособлять; исправлять.

readjustment ['riːə'dʒʌstmənt] *n* переделка, приспособление; исправление.

ready I ['redɪ] *a* 1) готовый; 2) *predic* согласный, готовый (*на что-л. или сделать что-л.*); 3) быстрый; проворный; 4) легкодоступный, находящийся под рукой; наличный (*о деньгах*); ~ at hand тут же, под рукой.

ready II *v* готовить, подготавливать.

ready-made ['redɪ'meɪd] *a* 1) готовый (*о платье*); 2) шаблонный, стандартный (*о мнении, мысли*).

reaffirm ['riːə'fəːm] *v* подтверждать (снова).

reagent [riː'eɪdʒənt] *n хим.* реактив, реагент.

real^a I ['rɪəl] *a* 1) действительный, реальный; настоящий, подлинный; истинный; 2) недвижимый (*об имуществе*).

real^a II *adv разг.* очень.

real^b [reɪ'ɑːl] *n ист.* реал (*испанская монета*).

realism ['rɪəlɪzəm] *n* реализм; socialist ~ социалистический реализм.

realist ['rɪəlɪst] *n* реалист.

realistic [rɪə'lɪstɪk] *a* реалистичный; реалистический.

reality [riː'ælɪtɪ] *n* реальность; действительность; истинность; подлинность; in ~ на самом деле, в действительности.

realizable ['rɪəlaɪzəbl] *a* 1) осуществимый; 2) поддающийся пониманию.

realization [ˌrɪəlaɪ'zeɪʃən] *n* 1) осуществление; реализация; 2) понимание, осознание; to have a true (*или* a full) ~ of smth. ясно сознавать что-л.; вполне отдавать себе отчёт в чём-л.; 3) реализация, продажа.

realize ['rɪəlaɪz] *v* 1) понимать, осознавать; ясно

представлять себе; 2) осуществлять, выполнять; 3) реализовать; продавать; 4) получать прибыль; 5) приносить доход.

really ['rɪəlɪ] *adv* действительно, на самом деле; право.

realm [relm] *n* 1) королевство; *перен.* царство; 2) область, сфера.

realty ['rɪəltɪ] *n* недвижимое имущество.

ream¹ [riːm] *n* стопа (*бумаги*).

ream² *v тех.* рассверливать, развёртывать.

reamer ['riːmə] *n тех.* развёртка.

reanimate ['riː'ænɪmeɪt] *v* 1) оживлять, возвращать к жизни; 2) воодушевлять.

reap [riːp] *v* жать, снимать урожай; *перен.* пожинать плоды; ◊ to ~ as one has sown что посеешь, то и пожнёшь; to ~ where one has not sown пожинать плоды чужого труда.

reaper ['riːpə] *n* 1) жнец; жница; 2) жатвенная машина, жатка.

reaping-hook ['riːpɪŋ'huk] *n* серп.

reaping-machine ['riːpɪŋmə,ʃiːn] *см.* reaper 2).

reappear ['riːə'pɪə] *v* снова показываться, вновь появляться.

rear¹ [rɪə] *v* 1) поднимать; возносить; 2) воздвигать (*памятник и т. п.*); 3) воспитывать; выращивать; 4) становиться на дыбы (*тж.* to ~ up).

rear² *n* 1) тыл; to bring up the ~ замыкать шествие; in (the) ~ в тылу; 2) задняя сторона; задний конец; а (*или* in) the ~ of the house а) позади дома; б) в задней части дома; 3) спина; 4) *attr* задний; тыловой.

rear-admiral ['rɪə'ædmərəl] *n* контр-адмирал.

rear-guard ['rɪəgɑːd] *n* арьергард.

rearm ['riː'ɑːm] *v* перевооружать(ся).

rearmament ['riː'ɑːməmənt] *n* перевооружение.

rearmost ['rɪəmoust] *a* самый задний, последний.

rearrange ['riːə'reɪndʒ] *v* 1) снова устроить, наладить; 2) устроить, расположить по-новому.

rearward I ['rɪəwəd] *n* замыкающая часть; арьергард; тыл.

rearward II *a* задний; тыльный.

rearward III *adv* назад; в тыл.

rearwards ['rɪəwədz] *adv* назад; в тыл; в сторону тыла.

reason I ['riːzn] *n* 1) причина, основание; соображение; довод; объяснение, оправдание; to give (*или* to tell) one's ~s сообщить свои соображения; to discover good ~s найти хорошее объяснение; by ~ of по причине; with ~ не без основания; 2) разум, рассудок; здравый смысл; in ~ (благо-)разумный, рассудительный; beyond ~ неблагоразумный; to bring to ~ образумить; to come to ~ образумиться; to lose one's ~ потерять рассудок; to listen to ~, to hear ~ прислушаться к голосу рассудка; it stands to ~ это разумно, это совершенно ясно.

reason II *v* 1) рассуждать (*about, of, upon*); 2) *обыкн. p. p.* обдумывать; 3) убеждать, уговаривать (*тж.* to ~ into); разубеждать (*в чём-л.— out of*); □ to ~ out продумать до конца.

reasonable ['riːznəbl] *a* 1) (благо)разумный; 2) умеренный; приемлемый; сносный.

reasonably ['riːznəblɪ] *adv* разумно; обоснованно.

reasoning I ['riːznɪŋ] *n* 1) размышление; рассуждение; 2) объяснение; аргументация.

reasoning II *a* спосо́бный рассужда́ть, мы́слящий.

reassert [ˌriːəˈsəːt] *v* заверя́ть, подтвержда́ть.

reassurance [ˌriːəˈʃuərəns] *n* увере́ние, заверённие, увещева́ние.

reassure [ˌriːəˈʃuə] *v* увещева́ть, убежда́ть, заверя́ть.

reave [riːv] *v* (*past, p. p.* reft) 1) похища́ть, отнима́ть; 2) гра́бить.

reaver [ˈriːvə] *n* граби́тель.

rebate[a] [ˈriːbeɪt] *n* ски́дка, усту́пка.

rebate[b] [rɪˈbeɪt] *v* де́лать ски́дку *или* усту́пку.

rebel[a] [ˈrebl] *n* 1) повста́нец; бунтовщи́к; 2) *attr* повста́нческий (*об отря́де, а́рмии*); мяте́жный.

rebel[b] [rɪˈbel] *v* 1) восстава́ть (*против — against*); 2) ока́зывать сопротивле́ние; протестова́ть; 3) *разг.* возмуща́ться.

rebellion [rɪˈbeljən] *n* 1) восста́ние; 2) сопротивле́ние; возмуще́ние.

rebellious [rɪˈbeljəs] *a* 1) мяте́жный; бунта́рский; 2) недисциплини́рованный; непослу́шный (*о ребёнке*).

rebind [ˈriːˈbaɪnd] *v* (*past, p. p.* rebound) переплета́ть (*кни́гу*).

rebirth [ˈriːˈbəːθ] *n* возрожде́ние; *перен. тж.* второ́е рожде́ние.

reborn [ˈriːˈbɔːn] *a* возрождённый.

rebound[a] [ˈriːˈbaund] *past, p. p.* см. rebind.

rebound[b] I [rɪˈbaund] *n* отско́к, отда́ча, рикоше́т; to hit on the ~ бить *или* ударя́ть рикоше́том.

rebound[b] II *v* 1) отска́кивать; рикоше́тировать; отпря́нуть; 2) име́ть обра́тное де́йствие.

rebuff I [rɪˈbʌf] *n* 1) ре́зкий отка́з *или* отве́т; отпо́р; 2) неуда́ча (*неожи́данная*).

rebuff II *v* 1) дава́ть отпо́р; ре́зко отка́зывать; 2) *воен.* отража́ть ата́ку.

rebuilt [ˈriːˈbɪlt] *a* за́ново отстро́енный, восстано́вленный.

rebuke I [rɪˈbjuːk] *n* 1) упрёк; without ~ безупре́чный; 2) замеча́ние, вы́говор.

rebuke II *v* упрека́ть; де́лать вы́говор.

rebus [ˈriːbəs] *n* ре́бус.

rebut [rɪˈbʌt] *v* 1) дава́ть отпо́р, отража́ть; отверга́ть; 2) опроверга́ть.

rebuttal [rɪˈbʌtəl] *n* опроверже́ние.

recalcitrant [rɪˈkælsɪtrənt] *a* непоко́рный; непослу́шный.

recall I [rɪˈkɔːl] *n* 1) отозва́ние (*депута́та, посла́*); 2) *воен.* сигна́л к возвраще́нию; 3) *амер.* отбо́й; 4): beyond ~, past ~ а) невосстанови́мое, непоправи́мое; б) забы́тое.

recall II *v* 1) отзыва́ть; вызыва́ть обра́тно; 2) вспомина́ть; напомина́ть, воскреша́ть в па́мяти; 3) брать обра́тно; 4) отменя́ть (*прика́з, зака́з*); 5) *воен.* призыва́ть (*запасны́х*).

recant [rɪˈkænt] *v* отка́зываться (*от мне́ния, убежде́ния*), отрека́ться.

recantation [ˌriːkænˈteɪʃən] *n* отрече́ние.

recapitulate [ˌriːkəˈpɪtjuleɪt] *v* резюми́ровать, сумми́ровать.

recapitulation [ˈriːkəˌpɪtjuˈleɪʃən] *n* вы́вод, резюме́.

recapitulative [ˌriːkəˈpɪtjulətɪv] *a* конспекти́вный (*об обзо́ре и т. п.*).

recapture [ˈriːˈkæptʃə] *v* отби́ть, захвати́ть обра́тно.

recast I [ˈriːˈkɑːst] *n* прида́ние но́вой фо́рмы; переде́лка.

recast II *v* (*past, p. p.* recast) 1) *тех.* перелива́ть, отлива́ть за́ново; 2) придава́ть но́вую фо́рму; переде́лывать; to ~ a play за́ново поста́вить пье́су, перераспредели́ть ро́ли (*ме́жду актёрами*).

recede [riːˈsiːd] *v* 1) удаля́ться, отходи́ть; ретирова́ться; to ~ into the background отступа́ть на за́дний план; 2) отка́зываться (*от догово́ра и т. п.*); 3) убыва́ть, идти́ на у́быль (*о воде́*); 4) па́дать (*в цене́ и т. п.*).

receipt I [rɪˈsiːt] *n* 1) получе́ние; on ~ по получе́нии; 2) распи́ска (в получе́нии); квита́нция; 3) *обы́кн. pl* прихо́д; ~s and expenses прихо́д и расхо́д; 4) реце́пт (*кулина́рный*).

receipt II *v* дава́ть распи́ску в получе́нии.

receipt-book [rɪˈsiːtbuk] *n* квитанцио́нная кни́жка.

receive [rɪˈsiːv] *v* 1) получа́ть; принима́ть; 2) воспринима́ть (*но́вые иде́и, сообще́ние*); 3) принима́ть (*госте́й*).

received [rɪˈsiːvd] *a* общепри́нятый; общепри́знанный.

receiver [rɪˈsiːvə] *n* 1) получа́тель; 2) *тех.* приёмник; 3) радиоприёмник; 4) телефо́нная тру́бка; 5) суде́бный исполни́тель.

receiving-order [rɪˈsiːvɪŋˌɔːdə] *n* исполни́тельный лист.

receiving-set [rɪˈsiːvɪŋset] *n* радиоприёмник.

recency [ˈriːsnsɪ] *n* новизна́, све́жесть.

recension [rɪˈsenʃən] *n* 1) просмо́тр те́кста; 2) просмо́тренный текст.

recent [ˈriːsnt] *a* неда́вний; но́вый, све́жий, совреме́нный.

recently [ˈriːsntlɪ] *adv* неда́вно.

receptacle [rɪˈseptəkl] *n* 1) коро́бка, я́щик; мешо́к; 2) вмести́лище, храни́лище.

reception [rɪˈsepʃən] *n* 1) приём; приня́тие; получе́ние; warm ~ горя́чий приём; 2) приём (*госте́й*), встре́ча, вечери́нка; 3) восприя́тие.

receptive [rɪˈseptɪv] *a* 1) воспри́мчивый; 2) рецепти́вный.

receptivity [ˌriːsepˈtɪvɪtɪ] *n* 1) воспри́мчивость; 2) ёмкость.

recess I [rɪˈses] *n* 1) углубле́ние, ни́ша; in the ~ of a cave в глубине́ пеще́ры; 2) укро́мное ме́сто; тайни́к; 3) переры́в в заня́тиях; кани́кулы; 4) *амер.* (больша́я) переме́на (*в шко́ле*).

recess II *v* 1) де́лать углубле́ние, выреза́ть; 2) помеща́ть в укро́мном ме́сте; 3) отодвига́ть наза́д; 4) де́лать переры́в в заня́тиях.

recession [rɪˈseʃən] *n* 1) удале́ние; ухо́д; 2) углубле́ние.

recessive [rɪˈsesɪv] *a* удаля́ющийся, отступа́ющий (наза́д).

recipe [ˈresɪpɪ] *n* 1) реце́пт; 2) предписа́ние; 3) сре́дство; спо́соб де́йствий.

recipient I [rɪˈsɪpɪənt] *n* 1) получа́тель; 2) *мед.* реципие́нт.

recipient II *a* 1) принима́ющий; 2) воспри́мчивый.

reciprocal I [rɪˈsɪprəkəl] *a* 1) взаи́мный, обою́дный; отве́тный; 2) соотве́тственный, эквивале́нтный; 3) *грам.* взаи́мный (*о местоиме́ниях*).

reciprocal II *n* *мат.* обра́тная величина́, обра́тная дробь.

reciprocate [rɪ'sɪprəkeɪt] v 1) отпла́чивать; отвеча́ть взаи́мностью; 2) обме́ниваться (любе́зностями, услу́гами); 3) дви́гать(ся) попереме́нно взад и вперёд (напр., о по́ршне).

reciprocation [rɪ,sɪprə'keɪʃən] n 1) отве́тное де́йствие; 2) взаи́мный обме́н; 3) возвра́тно-поступа́тельное движе́ние.

reciprocity [,resɪ'prɔsɪtɪ] n 1) взаи́мность; 2) взаимоде́йствие; 3) взаи́мный обме́н (услу́гами, привиле́гиями).

recital [rɪ'saɪtl] n 1) подро́бный расска́з, описа́ние, изложе́ние; 2) конце́рт (одного́ исполни́теля или одного́ компози́тора).

recitation [,resɪ'teɪʃən] n 1) амер. у́стный отве́т; у́стный опро́с (ученико́в, студе́нтов); 2) деклама́ция; публи́чное чте́ние.

recitative [,resɪtə'ti:v] n речитати́в.

recite [rɪ'saɪt] v 1) расска́зывать; отвеча́ть уро́к; 2) декламирова́ть, чита́ть наизу́сть; 3) перечисля́ть.

reciter [rɪ'saɪtə] n 1) деклама́тор, чтец; 2) хрестома́тия для деклама́ции.

reck [rek] v 1) обыкн. в отриц. предложе́ниях принима́ть во внима́ние, обраща́ть внима́ние; he ~ed not of the danger он пренебрега́л опа́сностью; 2) обыкн. в вопр. предложе́ниях име́ть значе́ние, зна́чить; what ~s it? како́е э́то име́ет значе́ние?; what ~s him that..? како́е ему́ де́ло, что..?

reckless ['reklɪs] a безрассу́дный; опроме́тчивый; не ду́мающий (о чём-л. — of).

reckon ['rekən] v 1) счита́ть, рассчи́тывать, подсчи́тывать (тж. to ~ up); 2) счита́ть (кем-л., чем-л.); рассма́тривать; to be ~ed счита́ться, рассчи́тывать (на кого́-л. что-л. — on, upon); 4) ду́мать, полага́ть; □ to ~ among, to ~ in причисля́ть к; включа́ть; to ~ with а) счита́ться с кем-л., с чем-л.; б) рассчи́тываться, распла́чиваться (по счета́м).

reckoning ['rekənɪŋ] n 1) счёт, расчёт; вычисле́ние; by my ~ по моему́ расчёту; to be out in one's ~s оши́биться в расчётах; to make no ~ of не принима́ть в расчёт, не придава́ть значе́ния; 2) распла́та; 3) счёт (осо́б. в гости́нице); 4) определе́ние местонахожде́ния корабля́.

reclaim I [rɪ'kleɪm] v 1) исправля́ть; восстана́вливать; 2) поднима́ть (новь); 3) тре́бовать обра́тно.

reclaim II n: beyond ~, past ~ неисправи́мый.

reclamation [,reklə'meɪʃən] n 1) исправле́ние; 2) мелиора́ция; 3) подъём (нови); 4) реклама́ция, заявле́ние прете́нзий.

réclame [reɪ'klɑːm] n рекла́ма.

recline [rɪ'klaɪn] v 1) отки́дываться наза́д; прислоня́ться; приле́чь; опира́ться; 2) полага́ться (на — on, upon); 3) отки́дывать (го́лову).

recluse I [rɪ'klu:s] n отше́льник, затво́рник.

recluse II a 1) уединённый; 2) живу́щий в уедине́нии.

recognition [,rekəg'nɪʃən] n 1) узнава́ние; опозна́ние; 2) призна́ние; to win ~ from заслужи́ть призна́ние (об актёре и т. п.).

recognizance [rɪ'kɔgnɪzəns] n 1) обяза́тельство (да́нное суду́); 2) зало́г.

recognize ['rekəgnaɪz] v 1) узнава́ть; 2) признава́ть; 3) выража́ть призна́ние, одобре́ние.

recoil I [rɪ'kɔɪl] n 1) отда́ча (ружья́); отка́т (ору́дия); 2) отвраще́ние; у́жас (перед чем-л.).

recoil II v 1) отскочи́ть, отпря́нуть; отшатну́ться; 2) отдава́ть (о ружье́); отка́тываться (об ору́дии); 3) чу́вствовать отвраще́ние; испы́тывать у́жас (перед чем-л.).

recollect [,rekə'lekt] v вспомина́ть.

re-collect ['ri:kə'lekt] v 1) собира́ть вновь; 2): to ~ oneself прийти́ в себя́, опо́мниться, опра́виться.

recollection [,rekə'lekʃən] n воспомина́ние; па́мять; a dim ~, hazy ~ сму́тное воспомина́ние; within one's ~ на чьей-л. па́мяти; to the best of my ~ наско́лько я по́мню.

recommend [,rekə'mend] v 1) рекомендова́ть; сове́товать; представля́ть (к награ́де и т. п.; for); 2) поруча́ть кому́-л., отдава́ть на попече́ние; 3) говори́ть в по́льзу (кого́-л., чего́-л.).

recommendation [,rekəmen'deɪʃən] n 1) рекоменда́ция; сове́т; представле́ние (к награ́де и т. п.; for); 2) ка́чества, говоря́щие в по́льзу (кого́-л., чего́-л.).

recommendatory [,rekə'mendətərɪ] a рекоменда́тельный.

recompense I ['rekəmpens] n вознагражде́ние; компенса́ция.

recompense II v вознагражда́ть; компенси́ровать.

reconcilable ['rekənsaɪləbl] a примири́мый; совмести́мый.

reconcile ['rekənsaɪl] v 1) примиря́ть; to ~ oneself, to be ~d (при)мири́ться с чем-л.; 2) ула́живать (спо́ры и т. п.); 3) согласова́ть (мне́ния и т. п.).

reconcilement ['rekənsaɪlmənt] n 1) примире́ние; 2) ула́живание; 3) согласова́ние (мне́ний и т. п.).

reconciliation [,rekənsɪlɪ'eɪʃən] n примире́ние.

recondite [rɪ'kɔndaɪt] a 1) глубо́кий, глубокомы́сленный; 2) нея́сный, тёмный.

recondition [,ri:kən'dɪʃən] v 1) переде́лывать, перестра́ивать; 2) восстана́вливать си́лы.

reconnaissance [rɪ'kɔnɪsəns] n 1) разве́дка; рекогносциро́вка; 2) разве́дывательный отря́д; 3) attr разве́дывательный.

reconnoitre [,rekə'nɔɪtə] v разве́дывать; производи́ть разве́дку или рекогносциро́вку.

reconsider ['ri:kən'sɪdə] v пересма́тривать (за́ново).

reconstruct ['ri:kəns'trʌkt] v 1) перестра́ивать; реконструи́ровать; 2) восстана́вливать, воссозда́вать.

reconstruction ['ri:kəns'trʌkʃən] n 1) перестро́йка; реконстру́кция; реорганиза́ция; 2) восстановле́ние.

record[a] ['rekɔ:d] n 1) за́пись; протоко́л; отчёт; on ~ запи́санный, зарегистри́рованный; занесённый в протоко́л; off the ~ а) неофициа́льно; б) неофициа́льный; не подлежа́щий оглаше́нию в печа́ти; personnel ~ спи́сок ли́чного соста́ва; 2) мемуа́ры, за́писки; ле́топись собы́тий; 3) да́нные или све́дения о ком-л., о чём-л.; voting ~s результа́ты голосова́ния; a good (bad) ~ хоро́шая (плоха́я) репута́ция; ~ of service, service ~ послужно́й спи́сок; 4) реко́рд; to beat (или to break, to cut) the ~ поби́ть реко́рд; 5) па́мятник

про́шлого, свиде́тельство (чего-л.); 6) граммо-
фо́нная пласти́нка; за́пись на пласти́нке; long-
-playing ~ долгоигра́ющая пласти́нка; 7) attr
реко́рдный.

record[b] [rɪ'kɔːd] v 1) запи́сывать, регистри́ро-
вать; заноси́ть (в спи́сок, протоко́л); протоколи́-
ровать; 2) увекове́чивать; 3) запи́сывать на
пласти́нку, на плёнку.

recorder [rɪ'kɔːdə] n 1) регистра́тор; протоко-
ли́ст; учётчик; 2) самопи́шущий, регистри́рующий
прибо́р; 3) кино звукозапи́сывающий аппара́т;
4) рико́рдер (ти́тул судьи́ в не́которых города́х).

recordist [rɪ'kɔːdɪst] n звукоопера́тор.

recount [rɪ'kaunt] v расска́зывать, излага́ть
собы́тия.

re-count ['riː'kaunt] v пересчи́тывать.

recoup [rɪ'kuːp] v 1) компенси́ровать, возме-
ща́ть; 2) юр. уде́рживать (из су́ммы).

recourse [rɪ'kɔːs] n 1) обраще́ние за по́мощью;
to have ~ to обраща́ться за по́мощью, прибе-
га́ть к по́мощи; 2) прибе́жище.

recover [rɪ'kʌvə] v 1) получа́ть обра́тно, обре-
та́ть сно́ва; наверста́ть (поте́рянное вре́мя);
to ~ oneself, to ~ consciousness прийти́ в созна́-
ние; опо́мниться; to ~ one's legs встать на́ ноги
(по́сле паде́ния); 2) выздора́вливать, оправля́ть-
ся (от боле́зни; from); 3) юр. выи́грывать про-
це́сс; 4) воен. отби́ть, вновь овладе́ть; 5) тех.
восстана́вливать.

recovered [rɪ'kʌvəd] a вы́здорове́вший, опра́-
ви́вшийся.

recovery [rɪ'kʌvərɪ] n 1) выздоровле́ние;
2) восстановле́ние; возвраще́ние (утра́ченного,
поте́рянного); возмеще́ние; 3) тех. регенера́ция.

recreancy ['rekrɪənsɪ] n поэт. 1) тру́сость,
малоду́шие; 2) отсту́пничество, изме́на.

recreant I ['rekrɪənt] n поэт. 1) трус; 2) отсту́п-
ник, изме́нник.

recreant II a поэт. 1) трусли́вый, малоду́шный;
2) преда́тельский, изме́ннический.

recreate ['rekrɪeɪt] v 1) отдыха́ть, освежа́ться,
восстана́вливать си́лы; 2) развлека́ть(ся).

recreation [,rekrɪ'eɪʃən] n 1) о́тдых, восста-
новле́ние сил; 2) развлече́ние, и́гры.

recreative [,riːkrɪ'eɪtɪv] a 1) освежа́ющий,
восстана́вливающий; 2) занима́тельный.

recrudescence [,riːkruː'desns] n но́вая вспы́шка
(боле́зни и т. п.), рециди́в.

recruit I [rɪ'kruːt] n 1) новобра́нец, рекру́т;
2) но́вый член (о́бщества, клу́ба).

recruit II v 1) вербова́ть, набира́ть (в а́рмию,
флот); 2) привлека́ть к уча́стию; пополня́ть
(свои́ ряды́); 3) укрепля́ть (здоро́вье, си́лы).

recruital [rɪ'kruːtəl] n набо́р; вербо́вка; рекру-
ти́рование.

recruitment [rɪ'kruːtmənt] n 1) набо́р новобра́н-
цев; 2) пополне́ние (рядо́в); 3) укрепле́ние
(здоро́вья).

rectangle ['rek,tæŋgl] n прямоуго́льник.

rectangular [rek'tæŋgjulə] a прямоуго́льный.

rectification [,rektɪfɪ'keɪʃən] n 1) исправле́ние;
2) хим. очи́стка, ректифика́ция; 3) эл. выпрямле́-
ние (то́ка); 4) ра́дио детекти́рование.

rectifier ['rektɪfaɪə] n 1) хим. очисти́тель,
ректифика́тор; 2) эл. выпрями́тель (то́ка);
3) ра́дио детектор.

rectify ['rektɪfaɪ] v 1) исправля́ть, выправля́ть;
2) хим. очища́ть, ректифици́ровать; 3) эл. выпрям-
ля́ть (ток); 4) ра́дио детекти́ровать.

rectilineal [,rektɪ'lɪnɪəl] a прямолине́йный.

rectilinear [,rektɪ'lɪnɪə] см. rectilineal.

rectitude ['rektɪtjuːd] n 1) прямота́, че́стность;
высо́кая нра́вственность; 2) справедли́вость.

rector ['rektə] n 1) ре́ктор; 2) прихо́дский
свяще́нник.

rectorship ['rektəʃɪp] n до́лжность ре́ктора.

rectory ['rektərɪ] n дом прихо́дского свяще́н-
ника.

recumbent [rɪ'kʌmbənt] a лежа́щий, откину́в-
шийся.

recuperate [rɪ'kjuːpəreɪt] v 1) выздора́вливать;
восстана́вливать си́лы; 2) тех. восстана́вливать,
регенери́ровать.

recuperation [rɪ,kjuːpə'reɪʃən] n 1) выздоровле́-
ние; восстановле́ние сил; 2) тех. восстановле́ние,
регенера́ция.

recur [rɪ'kəː] v 1) возвраща́ться (мы́сленно
и́ли в разгово́ре; к — to); 2) (сно́ва) приходи́ть
в го́лову; 3) повторя́ться, происходи́ть вновь.

recurrence [rɪ'kʌrəns] n возвраще́ние; повторе́-
ние.

recurrent [rɪ'kʌrənt] a 1) повторя́ющийся,
периоди́ческий; 2) мед. рецидив́ный, возвра́тный.

recurve [riː'kəːv] v загиба́ться наза́д.

red[1] I [red] a 1) кра́сный; 2) румя́ный (о ще-
ка́х, лице́); 3) ры́жий (о волоса́х); 4) покрасне́в-
ший; ~ with anger покрасне́вший от гне́ва;
◇ to see ~ рассвире́петь, обезу́меть от я́рости;
not a ~ cent амер. нет ни гроша́.

red[1] II n 1) кра́сный цвет; 2) су́рик; 3): the
Reds pl амер. красноко́жие, инде́йцы.

red[2] I n: the Reds pl поли́т. революционе́ры,
кра́сные.

red[2] II a поли́т. революцио́нный, кра́сный.

redbait ['red,beɪt] v амер. пресле́довать про-
гресси́вные элеме́нты.

redbaiting ['red,beɪtɪŋ] n амер. пресле́дование,
тра́вля прогресси́вных элеме́нтов.

redbreast ['redbrest] n мали́новка (пти́ца).

redcoat ['redkout] n брита́нский солда́т.

redden ['redn] v 1) окра́шивать(ся) в кра́сный
цвет; 2) красне́ть.

reddish ['redɪʃ] a краснова́тый.

redeem [rɪ'diːm] v 1) выкупа́ть (зало́женное
иму́щество); выпла́чивать (долг по закладно́й);
2) возмеща́ть; 3) искупа́ть (вину́, грехи́); исправ-
ля́ть (оши́бку); 4) выполня́ть (обеща́ние и т. п.);
5) спаса́ть, выкупа́ть.

redeemer [rɪ'diːmə] n 1) спаси́тель, избави́тель;
2) искупи́тель.

redemption [rɪ'dempʃən] n 1) вы́куп; вы́плата;
2) искупле́ние; 3) освобожде́ние; спасе́ние.

red-handed ['red'hændɪd] a 1) с окрова́влен-
ными рука́ми; 2): to catch (и́ли to take) ~ пой-
ма́ть на ме́сте преступле́ния.

red-hot ['red'hɒt] a 1) накалённый докрасна́;
2) горя́чий, пла́менный; возбуждённый.

re-did ['riː'dɪd] past см. re-do.

redintegrate [re'dɪntɪgreɪt] v восстана́вливать
(це́лостность, еди́нство); воссоединя́ть.

redistribute ['riːdɪs'trɪbjuːt] v перераспреде-
ля́ть.

redistribution ['riː͵dıstrı'bjuːʃən] *n* перераспределе́ние, переде́л.

red-letter ['red'letə] *a* пра́здничный (*о дне*); *перен.* па́мятный, счастли́вый.

redness ['rednıs] *n* краснота́.

re-do ['riː'duː] *v* (*past* re-did; *p. p.* re-done) де́лать за́ново, переде́лывать.

redolence ['redouləns] *n* благоуха́ние, арома́т.

redolent ['redoulənt] *a* 1) паху́чий; арома́тный, благоуха́ющий; си́льно па́хнущий (*чем-л.— of*); 2) вызыва́ющий воспомина́ние (*о чём-л.—of*).

re-done ['riː'dʌn] *p. p. см.* re-do.

redouble ['rı'dʌbl] *v* 1) удва́ивать(ся), си́льно увели́чивать(ся); 2) усугубля́ть(ся); 3) скла́дывать вдво́е.

redoubt [rı'daut] *n воен.* реду́т.

redoubtable [rı'dautəbl] *a* гро́зный, опа́сный (*о враге и т. п.*).

redound [rı'daund] *v* спосо́бствовать, соде́йствовать; that ~s to his honour э́то де́лает ему́ честь.

redress I [rı'dres] *n* 1) исправле́ние, восстановле́ние; 2) возмеще́ние, удовлетворе́ние.

redress II *v* 1) исправля́ть, восстана́вливать; 2) загла́живать (*вину*); удовлетворя́ть.

redskin ['redskın] *n* североамерика́нский инде́ец, красноко́жий.

reduce [rı'djuːs] *v* 1) уменьша́ть, понижа́ть, ослабля́ть; сокраща́ть (*расходы и т. п.*); 2) *разг.* худе́ть; 3) снижа́ть (*в зва́нии, чине и т. п.*); 4) доводи́ть (*до слёз, кра́йности, нищеты́; to*); 5) приводи́ть в определённое состоя́ние; to ~ to silence заста́вить замолча́ть; to ~ to order привести́ в поря́док; 6) обраща́ть; превраща́ть; to ~ to writing изложи́ть в пи́сьменной фо́рме; 7) покоря́ть, побежда́ть; 8) вправля́ть (*вы́вих*).

reduction [rı'dʌkʃən] *n* 1) уменьше́ние, сокраще́ние; сниже́ние (*цен и т. п.*); ~ of arms, ~ of armaments сокраще́ние вооруже́ний; 2) доведе́ние (*до чего-л.— to*); 3) сниже́ние (*в зва́нии, чине и т. п.*); 4) превраще́ние; измене́ние фо́рмы или состоя́ния; 5) приведе́ние дробе́й к одному́ знамена́телю; 6) покоре́ние, подавле́ние; 7) вправле́ние (*вы́виха*); 8) уме́ньшенная ко́пия (*карти́ны, ка́рты*).

redundance [rı'dʌndəns] *n* 1) избы́ток, чрезме́рность; 2) многосло́вие.

redundancy [rı'dʌndənsı] *см.* redundance.

redundant [rı'dʌndənt] *a* 1) изли́шний; чрезме́р-, ный; 2) многосло́вный.

reduplicate [rı'djuːplıkeıt] *v* удва́ивать; повторя́ть.

reduplication [rı͵djuːplı'keıʃən] *n* удвое́ние; повторе́ние.

red-wing ['redwıŋ] *n* дрозд.

reed [riːd] *n* 1) тростни́к, камы́ш; 2) тростни́к или соло́ма для крыш; 3) свире́ль; 4) язычо́к (*в муз. инструме́нте*); the ~s язычко́вые музыка́льные инструме́нты; ◊ a broken (*или* bruised) ~ а) ненадёжный челове́к; б) непро́чная вещь.

reeded ['riːdıd] *a* 1) заро́сший камышо́м *или* тростнико́м; 2) кры́тый тростнико́м; 3) *муз.* язычко́вый.

reed-pipe ['riːdpaıp] *n* 1) свире́ль; 2) язычко́вая тру́бка орга́на.

reedy ['riːdı] *a* 1) заро́сший тростнико́м; 2) тростнико́вый; 3) стро́йный (как тростни́к); 4) пронзи́тельный.

reef[1] [riːf] *n* 1) риф, подво́дная скала́; 2) золотоно́сная жи́ла.

reef[2] I *n мор.* риф (*на па́русе*); to take in a ~ а) брать ри́фы; б) де́йствовать осторо́жно, осмотри́тельно.

reef[2] II *v мор.* брать ри́фы.

reek I [riːk] *n* 1) пар, дым, чад; 2) дурно́й за́пах; вонь.

reek II *v* 1) дыми́ться, чади́ть; 2) пло́хо па́хнуть, воня́ть (*чем-л.— of*); he ~s of tobacco от него́ рази́т табако́м; 3): to ~ with sweat облива́ться по́том; ~ing with blood окрова́вленный.

reeky ['riːkı] *a* 1) дымя́щийся; 2) ды́мный, закопчённый.

reel[1] I [riːl] *n* 1) кату́шка, шпу́лька; 2) руле́тка; 3) *кино* кату́шка для фи́льма; часть кинофи́льма; a picture in six ~s карти́на в шести́ частя́х; ◊ (right) off the ~ без переры́ва, безостано́вочно, подря́д.

reel[1] II *v* нама́тывать; □ to ~ off говори́ть *или* писа́ть бы́стро, не остана́вливаясь.

reel[2] I *n* 1) колеба́ние, шата́ние; without a ~ or a stagger без вся́ких колеба́ний; 2) бы́стрый та́нец.

reel[2] II *v* 1) кружи́ться, верте́ться; to ~ before one's eyes заверте́ться, поплы́ть пе́ред глаза́ми; 2) чу́вствовать головокруже́ние; 3) кача́ться; покачну́ться (*от уда́ра*); 4) шата́ться, идти́ шата́ясь; 5) танцева́ть бы́стрый та́нец.

re-elect ['riːı'lekt] *v* переизбира́ть, избира́ть сно́ва.

re-election ['riːı'lekʃən] *n* переизбра́ние, втори́чное избра́ние.

re-establish ['riːıs'tæblıʃ] *v* восстана́вливать.

refection [rı'fekʃən] *n* заку́ска.

refectory [rı'fektərı] *n* столо́вая (*в шко́ле, университе́те*); тра́пезная (*в монастыре́*).

refer [rı'fəː] *v* 1) отсыла́ть (*к — to*), направля́ть (*за информа́цией, по́мощью и ' т. п.*); 2) передава́ть на рассмотре́ние; I ~ it to you предоставля́ю э́то вам (реша́ть); 3) наводи́ть спра́вку, справля́ться (*чему-л.*); 4) припи́сывать (*чему-л.*); объясня́ть (*чем-л.*); 5) ссыла́ться (*на кого-л., что-л.*); упомина́ть; 6) относи́ться, име́ть отноше́ние (*к кому-л., чему-л.*).

referee I [͵refə'riː] *n* 1) трете́йский судья́; 2) *спорт.* судья́.

referee II *v спорт.* быть судьёй.

reference I ['refrəns] *n* 1) ссы́лка; сно́ска; cross ~ перекрёстная ссы́лка; paginal ~ ссы́лка на страни́цу; to make ~ to ссыла́ться на; with ~ to ссыла́ясь на; 2) спра́вка; for ready ~ для удо́бства наведе́ния спра́вок; 3) упомина́ние; намёк; to make no ~ to не упомина́ть о чём-л.; 4) рекоменда́ция; to give good ~s предста́вить хоро́шие рекоменда́ции; 5) лицо́, даю́щее рекоменда́цию; 6) отноше́ние; in ~ to, with ~ to относи́тельно, что каса́ется; without ~ to безотноси́тельно к, незави́симо от; 7) переда́ча на рассмотре́ние; отсы́лка к друго́му лицу́ *или* в другу́ю инста́нцию.

reference II *v* снабжа́ть (текст) ссы́лками.

referendum [ˌrefəˈrendəm] *n полит.* референдум.

refillᵃ [ˈriːfɪl] *n* дополнение, пополнение; ~ of fuel заправка горючим.

refillᵇ [ˈriːfɪl] *v* наполнять вновь; пополнять(ся) (*горючим*).

refine [rɪˈfaɪn] *v* 1) очищать(ся); рафинировать; 2) делать(ся) более изящным, утончённым; 3) совершенствовать(ся); 4) вдаваться в тонкости.

refined [rɪˈfaɪnd] *a* 1) очищенный, рафинированный; 2) изысканный, изящный (*о манерах*); утончённый.

refinement [rɪˈfaɪnmənt] *n* 1) очищение, рафинирование; отделка, обработка; 2) изящество (*манер*); утончённость, изысканность; 3) усовершенствование.

refinery [rɪˈfaɪnərɪ] *n* очистительный завод.

refit I [ˈriːfɪt] *n* 1) ремонт, починка; 2) снаряжение (*корабля и т. п.*).

refit II *v* 1) ремонтировать; 2) снаряжать заново (*корабль и т. п.*).

reflect [rɪˈflekt] *v* 1) отражать (*свет, звук*); 2) отражаться; давать отражение, образ (*о зеркале*); 3) отражать, изображать (*в литературе и т. п.*); 4) бросать тень (*на — on, upon*); отражаться (*на — on, upon*); 5) размышлять, раздумывать.

reflection [rɪˈflekʃən] *n* 1) отражение; отсвет; отблеск; 2) отражение, образ (*в литературе и т. п.*); 3) размышление; раздумье; соображение, мысль; on ~ подумав; по зрелом размышлении; 4) пятно, тень; to cast ~s бросать тень на; 5) порицание, осуждение; 6) *физиол.* способность образования рефлексов.

reflective [rɪˈflektɪv] *a* 1) отражающий; 2) мыслящий, склонный к размышлениям; 3) задумчивый (*о взгляде, виде*).

reflector [rɪˈflektə] *n* рефлектор.

reflex I [ˈriːfleks] *n* 1) отражение, образ; отблеск, отсвет; 2) *физиол.* рефлекс; conditioned (unconditioned) ~ условный (безусловный) рефлекс.

reflex II *a* 1) отражённый; представляющий собой реакцию; 2) рефлекторный; непроизвольный.

reflexion [rɪˈflekʃən] *см.* reflection.

reflexive I [rɪˈfleksɪv] *n грам.* 1) возвратный глагол; 2) возвратное местоимение.

reflexive II *a грам.* возвратный.

reflux [ˈriːflʌks] *n* отлив.

reforest [riːˈfɔrɪst] *v* насаждать леса, восстанавливать лесные массивы.

reformᵃ I [rɪˈfɔːm] *n* реформа, преобразование; улучшение; currency ~ денежная реформа.

reformᵃ II *v* 1) преобразовывать, реформировать; улучшать; 2) улучшаться, исправляться.

reformᵇ [ˈriːˈfɔːm] *v* 1) переделывать; формировать заново; 2) *воен.* перестраивать(ся).

reformation [ˌrefəˈmeɪʃən] *n* 1) преобразование; 2) улучшение, исправление; 3) (the R.) *ист.* Реформация.

reformative· [rɪˈfɔːmətɪv] *a* 1) преобразующий, реформирующий; 2) исправительный.

reformatory I [rɪˈfɔːmətərɪ] *n* исправительное заведение для малолетних преступников.

reformatory II *a* исправительный.

reformed [rɪˈfɔːmd] *a* 1) исправленный, преобразованный; 2) исправившийся.

reformer [rɪˈfɔːmə] *n* 1) преобразователь, реформатор; 2) сторонник реформ.

reformist [rɪˈfɔːmɪst] *n полит.* реформист.

refract [rɪˈfrækt] *v физ.* преломлять (*лучи*).

refraction [rɪˈfrækʃən] *n физ.* преломление.

refractive [rɪˈfræktɪv] *a* преломляющий.

refractory I [rɪˈfræktərɪ] *n* огнеупорный строительный материал.

refractory II *a* 1) упрямый, упорный; 2) огнеупорный, огнестойкий; тугоплавкий; 3) упорный, трудно поддающийся лечению.

refrain¹ [rɪˈfreɪn] *v* 1) удерживать (*от чего-л. — from*); сдерживать; 2) удержаться (*от чего-л. — from*); воздержаться; he could not ~ from saying он не мог не сказать.

refrain² *n* припев, рефрен.

refresh [rɪˈfreʃ] *v* 1) освежать; оживлять, подкреплять; to ~ oneself освежиться, подкрепиться (*едой, питьём*); 2) возобновлять запасы, припасы; 3) подновлять, подправлять.

refresher [rɪˈfreʃə] *n* 1) освежающий напиток; что-л. освежающее; 2) напоминание; 3) *разг.* выпивка.

refreshment [rɪˈfreʃmənt] *n* 1) подкрепление; восстановление сил, отдых; 2) *обыкн. pl* освежающие напитки, закуска.

refrigerant I [rɪˈfrɪdʒərənt] *n* 1) охлаждающее средство, охладитель; 2) жаропонижающее средство.

refrigerant II *a* охлаждающий.

refrigerate [rɪˈfrɪdʒəreɪt] *v* охлаждать; замораживать.

refrigeration [rɪˌfrɪdʒəˈreɪʃən] *n* охлаждение; замораживание.

refrigerator [rɪˈfrɪdʒəreɪtə] *n* холодильник.

reft [reft] *past, p. p. см.* reave.

refuel [ˈriːˈfjuəl] *v* пополнять(ся) горючим, топливом.

refuge [ˈrefjuːdʒ] *n* 1) убежище; *перен.* прибежище; пристанище; to take ~ in lying прибегнуть ко лжи; to take ~ in silence отмалчиваться; 2) «островок безопасности» (*на улице с большим движением*).

refugee [ˌrefjuˈdʒiː] *n* 1) беженец; 2) эмигрант.

refulgent [rɪˈfʌldʒənt] *a* сияющий; лучезарный.

refundᵃ [ˈriːfʌnd] *n* возвращение (*денег*); возмещение (*расходов*).

refundᵇ [ˈriːˈfʌnd] *v* возвращать (*деньги*); возмещать (*расходы*).

refusal [rɪˈfjuːzəl] *n* 1) отказ; flat (*или* plump, square) ~ категорический отказ; weak ~ нерешительный отказ; to take no ~ не принимать отказа, быть очень настойчивым; 2) право первого выбора; to have (to give) the ~ иметь (предоставлять) право выбирать первым.

refuseᵃ [ˈrefjuːs] *n* отбросы; остатки; мусор; отходы.

refuseᵇ [rɪˈfjuːz] *v* 1) отказывать; отвергать; 2) отказываться; отрицать.

refutation [ˌrefjuˈteɪʃən] *n* опровержение.

refute [rɪˈfjuːt] *v* опровергать.

regain [rɪˈgeɪn] *v* 1) вернуть себе, вновь приобрести; восстановить (*здоровье*); 2) достигать (*берега и т. п.*); 3) *воен.* снова завладеть.

regal ['riːgəl] *a* 1) королевский; 2) царственный; царский.

regale I [rɪ'geɪl] *n* угощение; пир.

regale II *v* 1) угощать, потчевать; пировать; 2) услаждать, ласкать (*слух и т. п.*); to ~ oneself наслаждаться.

regalia [rɪ'geɪljə] *n pl* регалии.

regard I [rɪ'gɑːd] *n* 1) взгляд, взор; 2) внимание, уважение; забота; to pay ~ to оказывать почтение кому-л.; out of ~ for you из уважения к вам; to pay no ~ to не считаться с, не обращать внимания на; without ~ to не обращая внимания на; не соблюдая (*чего-л.*); to have ~ for считаться (*с желаниями, чувствами*); 3) *pl* привет, поклон; to send one's ~s передавать привет; best ~s, kind ~s сердечный привет; 4) отношение; in this ~ в этом отношении; in ~ to, with ~ to по отношению к, относительно, что касается, по поводу; 5) оценка, хорошее мнение; to have high ~ for считать хорошим; высокого ставить.

regard II *v* 1) смотреть на, наблюдать; 2) считать, рассматривать; she ~s him as among her friends она считает его своим другом; to ~ in the light (*или* under the aspect) of рассматривать в свете чего-л., с точки зрения чего-л.; 3) *обыкн. с отрицанием* принимать во внимание; обращать внимание; уважать (*мнение, совет*); he is much ~ed он пользуется большим уважением; 4) относиться, касаться; as ~s что касается; that ~s you это касается вас, это относится к вам.

regardful [rɪ'gɑːdful] *a* внимательный, заботливый.

regarding [rɪ'gɑːdɪŋ] *prep* относительно; о, об.

regardless I [rɪ'gɑːdlɪs] *a* не обращающий внимания, не считающийся (*с чем-л.* — of); ~ of danger равнодушный к опасности.

regardless II *adv* не обращая внимания, не думая; ~ of невзирая на, не считаясь с.

regatta [rɪ'gætə] *n* парусные *или* гребные гонки.

regency ['riːdʒənsɪ] *n* регентство.

regenerate[a] [rɪ'dʒenərɪt] *a* 1) возрождённый; 2) преобразованный; улучшенный.

regenerate[b] [rɪ'dʒenəreɪt] *v* 1) перерождать(ся); возрождать(ся); 2) порождать снова; 3) *тех.* восстанавливать, регенерировать.

regeneration [rɪˌdʒenə'reɪʃən] *n* 1) возрождение; 2) *тех.* восстановление, регенерация.

regenerative [rɪ'dʒenərətɪv] *a* 1) возрождающий(ся), восстанавливающий(ся); 2) *тех.* регенеративный.

regenerator [rɪ'dʒenəreɪtə] *n тех.* преобразователь; регенератор.

regent ['riːdʒənt] *n* 1) регент; 2) *амер.* член правления (университета).

regicide ['redʒɪsaɪd] *n* 1) цареубийца; 2) цареубийство.

régime, regime [reɪ'ʒiːm] *n* режим, строй.

regimen ['redʒɪmən] *n* 1) *уст.* правление; система правления; 2) *мед.* режим; диета; 3) *грам.* управление.

regiment I ['redʒɪmənt] *n* 1) полк; 2) *обыкн. pl* множество.

regiment II *v* 1) формировать полк; 2) организовать, распределять по группам.

regimental [ˌredʒɪ'mentl] *a* полковой.

regimentals [ˌredʒɪ'mentlz] *n pl* полковая форма.

region ['riːdʒən] *n* 1) область; район; край; страна; *перен.* область, сфера; the lower ~s, the nether ~s а) преисподняя, ад; б) *уст.* подвальный этаж; the upper ~s небеса; in the ~ of поблизости; 2): the ~ of the heart область сердца; the abdominal ~ брюшная полость.

regional ['riːdʒənl] *a* областной; районный; местный; региональный.

register I ['redʒɪstə] *n* 1) журнал (*записей*); список, опись, реестр; ~ of births, marriages and burials книга записи актов гражданского состояния; 2) заслонка; 3) *муз.* регистр; 4) *тех.* счётчик, счётный механизм; cash ~ кассовый аппарат; 5) *attr* регистрационный; регистрирующий.

register II *v* 1) заносить в список, записывать; регистрировать(ся); to ~ oneself вносить своё имя в список; 2) показывать, отмечать (*о приборе*); 3) отправлять заказным (*письмо и т. п.*); 4) *разг.* выражать, показывать, проявлять; 5) запечатлевать(ся).

registration [ˌredʒɪs'treɪʃən] *n* регистрация; запись.

registry ['redʒɪstrɪ] *n* 1) регистратура; 2) регистрация; запись; 3) журнал записей; реестр.

regnant ['regnənt] *a* 1) царствующий; 2) преобладающий; широко распространённый.

regress[a] ['riːgres] *n* 1) возвращение, возврат; обратное движение; 2) регресс, упадок.

regress[b] [rɪ'gres] *v* 1) двигаться назад; 2) регрессировать.

regression [rɪ'greʃən] *n* 1) возвращение к прежнему состоянию; 2) регресс.

regressive [rɪ'gresɪv] *a* обратный, регрессивный.

regret I [rɪ'gret] *n* 1) сожаление; раскаяние; печаль; with much ~, with many ~s с большим сожалением; 2) *обыкн. pl* извинения; to express ~ (for) извиняться, просить прощения (за).

regret II *v* 1) сожалеть; 2) горевать; 3) раскаиваться.

regretful [rɪ'gretful] *a* 1) полный сожаления; опечаленный; 2) раскаивающийся; полный раскаяния.

regrettable [rɪ'gretəbl] *a* прискорбный.

regrouping ['riːˈgruːpɪŋ] *n* перегруппировка.

regular I ['regjulə] *a* 1) регулярный, систематический; правильный; нормальный; 2) *грам., мат.* правильный; 3) обычный; очередной; 4) квалифицированный; профессиональный; 5) *разг.* настоящий, сущий; 6) официальный; формальный; 7) *воен.* кадровый.

regular II *n* 1) солдат регулярной армии; кадровый военный; 2) монах.

regularity [ˌregju'lærɪtɪ] *n* правильность, регулярность; порядок, система.

regulate ['regjuleɪt] *v* регулировать; упорядочивать; 2) приспосабливать (*к требованиям, условиям*); соразмерять; 3) выверять, регулировать (*механизм и т. п.*).

regulation [ˌregju'leɪʃən] *n* 1) регулирование;

приведе́ние в поря́док; урегули́рование; 2) пра́вило, предписа́ние; 3) *pl* уста́в, наставле́ние; инстру́кция; 4) *attr* пра́вильный; устано́вленного образца́; фо́рменный.

regulative [ˈregjulətɪv] *a* регули́рующий.

regulator [ˈregjuleɪtə] *n* 1) регулиро́вщик; 2) регуля́тор.

rehabilitate [ˌriːəˈbɪlɪteɪt] *v* 1) реабилити́ровать; восстана́вливать (*в права́х, до́лжности, чи́не и т. п.*); 2) восстана́вливать; реконструи́ровать; реставри́ровать.

rehabilitation [ˈriːəˌbɪlɪˈteɪʃən] *n* 1) реабилита́ция; восстановле́ние (*в права́х, до́лжности, чи́не и т. п.*); 2) восстановле́ние; реконстру́кция; реставра́ция.

rehearsal [rɪˈhəːsəl] *n* 1) репети́ция; dress ~ генера́льная репети́ция; 2) повторе́ние, переска́з.

rehearse [rɪˈhəːs] *v* 1) репети́ровать; 2) повторя́ть; переска́зывать.

rehouse [ˈriːˈhauz] *v* переселя́ть в но́вые дома́.

reign I [reɪn] *n* 1) ца́рствование; 2) ца́рская *или* короле́вская власть; 3) власть, ца́рство (*напр., зако́на*).

reign II *v* 1) ца́рствовать; 2) цари́ть, госпо́дствовать.

reimburse [ˌriːɪmˈbəːs] *v* возмеща́ть.

rein I [reɪn] *n* по́вод, поводья́; во́жжи; *перен.* узда́; to draw ~ (*или* the ~s) а) останови́ть ло́шадь; б) сде́рживать; to give the horse ~ (*или* the ~s) отпусти́ть поводья́; to give ~ (*или* the ~s) to one's imagination дать во́лю воображе́нию; with a loose ~ отпусти́в поводья́; *перен.* без стро́гостей, мя́гко; the ~s of government бразды́ правле́ния; to keep a tight ~ (on) держа́ть в узде́; to take the ~s взять на себя́ руково́дство.

rein II *v* пра́вить (*ло́шадью*); *перен.* управля́ть; □ to ~ back а) остана́вливать (*ло́шадь*); б) сде́рживать; to ~ in остана́вливать; уде́рживать; to ~ up *см.* to ~ back.

reincarnation [ˈriːɪnkɑːˈneɪʃən] *n* перевоплоще́ние.

reindeer [ˈreɪndɪə] *n* се́верный оле́нь.

reinforce [ˌriːɪnˈfɔːs] *v* подкрепля́ть, укрепля́ть; уси́ливать.

reinforcement [ˌriːɪnˈfɔːsmənt] *n* 1) усиле́ние; укрепле́ние; 2) *обыкн. pl* подкрепле́ние, пополне́ние; 3) *тех.* армату́ра.

reinless [ˈreɪnlɪs] *a* без поводье́в; *перен.* без узды́, без контро́ля.

reinstate [ˌriːɪnˈsteɪt] *v* 1) восстана́вливать в пре́жнем положе́нии, в права́х *и т. п.*; 2) восстана́вливать (*поря́док*); 3) поправля́ть (*здоро́вье*).

reinsurance [ˈriːɪnˈʃuərəns] *n* перестрахо́вка.

reissue [ˈriːˈɪsjuː] *v* выпуска́ть сно́ва; переиздава́ть (*кни́гу*).

reiterate [riːˈɪtəreɪt] *v* повторя́ть (*многокра́тно*).

reiteration [riːˌɪtəˈreɪʃən] *n* повторе́ние (*многокра́тное*); переле́в.

reject I [rɪˈdʒekt] *v* 1) отбра́сывать, забрако́вывать; 2) отка́зывать(ся); отверга́ть; отклоня́ть (*предложе́ние, по́мощь*); 3) изверга́ть; изрыга́ть.

reject II *n* 1) него́дный к вое́нной слу́жбе; 2) уценённый това́р.

rejectee [ˌriːdʒekˈtiː] *n амер.* него́дный к вое́нной слу́жбе.

rejection [rɪˈdʒekʃən] *n* 1) отка́з; отклоне́ние, неприня́тие; 2) брако́вка; призна́ние него́дным (*к вое́нной слу́жбе*); 3) изверже́ние.

rejector [rɪˈdʒektə] *n тех.* отража́тель.

rejects [rɪˈdʒekts] *n pl* брак; отбро́сы.

rejoice [rɪˈdʒɔɪs] *v* ра́довать(ся); весели́ть(ся); to ~ at (*или* in) smth. наслажда́ться чем-л., ра́доваться чему́-л.

rejoicing [rɪˈdʒɔɪsɪŋ] *n* 1) сча́стье, ра́дость; 2) *обыкн. pl* пра́зднование, весе́лье.

re-join [ˈriːˈdʒɔɪn] *v* присоединя́ться к кому́-л., чему́-л.; возвраща́ться (*в свою́ часть и т. п.*).

rejoin [rɪˈdʒɔɪn] *v* отвеча́ть, возража́ть.

rejoinder [rɪˈdʒɔɪndə] *n* отве́т, возраже́ние.

rejunction [ˈriːˈdʒʌŋkʃən] *n* присоедине́ние, возвраще́ние (*к кому́-л., чему́-л.*).

rejuvenate [rɪˈdʒuːvɪneɪt] *v* омола́живать(ся).

rejuvenation [rɪˌdʒuːvɪˈneɪʃən] *n* 1) омоложе́ние; 2) восстановле́ние сил, здоро́вья.

rejuvenescent [ˌriːdʒuːvɪˈnesnt] *a* 1) молоде́ющий; 2) придаю́щий си́лы, жи́вость.

rekindle [ˈriːˈkɪndl] *v* разжига́ть сно́ва; *перен.* возбужда́ть (*наде́жды и т. п.*).

re-laid [ˈriːˈleɪd] *past, p. p. см.* re-lay.

relapse I [rɪˈlæps] *n* повторе́ние, рециди́в.

relapse II *v* впада́ть сно́ва (*в како́е-л. состоя́ние*); заболева́ть; возвраща́ться (*к ду́рной привы́чке и т. п.*); to ~ into silence замо́лкнуть.

relate [rɪˈleɪt] *v* 1) расска́зывать; 2) свя́зывать, устана́вливать связь *или* отноше́ние ме́жду чем-л.; 3): to be ~d быть свя́занным; состоя́ть в родстве́; distantly ~d да́льние ро́дственники; pretty nearly ~d бли́зкая родня́; 4) относи́ться, име́ть отноше́ние, каса́ться (*to*).

relation [rɪˈleɪʃən] *n* 1) *обыкн. pl* отноше́ние, соотноше́ние, связь; business ~s деловы́е отноше́ния, делова́я связь; strained ~s натя́нутые отноше́ния; ~s of production произво́дственные отноше́ния; ~s of production произво́дственные отноше́ния; with ~ to принима́я во внима́ние; to have no ~ to the question не относи́ться к (да́нному) вопро́су; to be out of all ~s (*to*) не име́ть никако́го отноше́ния (*к чему́-л.*) *или* значе́ния (*для чего́-л.*); 2) расска́з, повествова́ние, изложе́ние; 3) ро́дственник; ро́дственница; 4) родство́.

relationship [rɪˈleɪʃənʃɪp] *n* 1) родство́; 2) *собир.* родня́, ро́дственники; 3) связь, отноше́ние.

relative I [ˈrelətɪv] *n* 1) ро́дственник; ро́дственница; a remote ~ да́льний ро́дственник; 2) *грам.* относи́тельное местоиме́ние.

relative II *a* 1) относи́тельный, сравни́тельный; 2) свя́занный (*друг с дру́гом*), взаи́мный; соотве́тственный; 3) *грам.* относи́тельный.

relatively [ˈrelətɪvlɪ] *adv* 1) относи́тельно, по по́воду; 2) относи́тельно, сравни́тельно; 3) соотве́тственно.

relativity [ˌreləˈtɪvɪtɪ] *n* 1) относи́тельность; 2) тео́рия относи́тельности.

relax [rɪˈlæks] *v* 1) ослабля́ть, уменьша́ть напряже́ние, расслабля́ть; 2) отдыха́ть; 3) смягча́ть(ся); де́латься ме́нее стро́гим (*о дисципли́не и т. п.*); 4) слабе́ть.

relaxation [ˌriːlækˈseɪʃən] *n* 1) ослабле́ние, уменьше́ние напряже́ния; 2) смягче́ние (*наказа-*

ния и т. п.); ослабле́ние (*дисципли́ны*); 3) переды́шка; 4) развлече́ние.

relay^a I [ˈriˈleɪ] *n* 1) сме́на (*солда́т, рабо́чих*); 2) подста́ва, сме́на (*лошаде́й*).

relay^a II *v* сменя́ть; обеспе́чивать сме́ной.

relay^b I [ˈriˈleɪ] *n* 1) *эл.* реле́; 2) *ра́дио* трансля́ция.

relay^b II *v* 1) передава́ть (*да́льше*); 2) *ра́дио* трансли́ровать.

re-lay [ˈriˈleɪ] *v* (*past, p. p.* re-laid) перекла́дывать, класть сно́ва.

relay-race [ˈriˈleɪreɪs] *n* эстафе́тный бег.

relay-station [ˈriˈleɪˌsteɪʃən] *n* *ра́дио* ретрансляцио́нная ста́нция.

release I [rɪˈliːs] *n* 1) освобожде́ние; 2) облегче́ние (*бо́ли и т. п.*); 3) *тех.* разъедине́ние; расцепле́ние; выключа́ющий механи́зм; 4) отбо́й; 5) сбра́сывание (*авиабо́мб*).

release II *v* 1) освобожда́ть (*from*); выпуска́ть на во́лю; 2) вы́пустить в свет (*кни́гу*); опубликова́ть (*заявле́ние и т. п.*); вы́пустить на экра́н (*фильм*); 3) отпуска́ть, (вы)пуска́ть; сбра́сывать (*авиабо́мбы*); to ~ oneself высвобожда́ться; 4) отка́зываться (*от прав и т. п.*); освобожда́ть (*от обеща́ния, обяза́тельства и т. п.*); проща́ть (*долг*); 5) *тех.* разобща́ть, расцепля́ть; 6) *ав.* раскрыва́ть (*пара-шю́т*).

relegate [ˈrelɪgeɪt] *v* 1) высыла́ть, изгоня́ть; 2) разжа́ловать; «сдава́ть в архи́в»; 3) передава́ть (*де́ло, вопро́с для исполне́ния, реше́ния*).

relegation [ˌrelɪˈgeɪʃən] *n* 1) вы́сылка, изгна́ние; 2) разжа́лование; 3) переда́ча (*де́ла и т. п.*).

relent [rɪˈlent] *v* смягча́ться.

relentless [rɪˈlentlɪs] *a* 1) неумоли́мый, безжа́лостный; 2) неуста́нный; неотсту́пный.

relevance [ˈrelɪvəns] *n* уме́стность.

relevancy [ˈrelɪvənsɪ] *см.* relevance.

relevant [ˈrelɪvənt] *a* уме́стный; относя́щийся к де́лу.

reliability [rɪˌlaɪəˈbɪlɪtɪ] *n* 1) надёжность; достове́рность (*све́дений и т. п.*); 2) про́чность.

reliable [rɪˈlaɪəbl] *a* 1) надёжный; заслу́живающий дове́рия; достове́рный; 2) про́чный.

reliance [rɪˈlaɪəns] *n* 1) дове́рие, уве́ренность (*on, upon, in*); to have (*или* to feel) ~ upon пита́ть дове́рие к кому́-л.; 2) наде́жда, опо́ра; расчёт (*на что-л.*); to place ~ in (*или* on) наде́яться, полага́ться на; 3) испо́льзование; extensive ~ широ́кое примене́ние.

reliant [rɪˈlaɪənt] *a* 1) уве́ренный; 2) самоуве́ренный, самонаде́янный.

relic [ˈrelɪk] *n обыкн. pl* 1) след, оста́ток; пережи́ток; 2) *рел.* мо́щи; 3) рели́квия; 4) *pl геол.* рели́кт.

relief^1 [rɪˈliːf] *n* 1) облегче́ние (*бо́ли, страда́ния и т. п.*); утеше́ние; to bring (*или* to give) ~ приноси́ть облегче́ние; 2) по́мощь; посо́бие; 3) освобожде́ние (*от рабо́ты, от упла́ты штра́фа*); 4) сме́на (*дежу́рных, карау́льных*); in the ~ при сме́не, во вре́мя сме́ны; 5) переме́на, разнообра́зие.

relief^2 *n* 1) релье́ф (*изображе́ние*); low ~ барелье́ф; in ~ вы́пуклый, релье́фный; 2) релье́ф ме́стности; 3) релье́фность, я́ркость; 4) *attr* релье́фный.

relieve^1 [rɪˈliːv] *v* 1) облегча́ть; уменьша́ть, ослабля́ть (*напряже́ние*); успока́ивать (*трево́гу*);

2) освобожда́ть (*от чего́-л.*); увольня́ть; 3) сменя́ть (*дежу́рного и т. п.*); 4) приходи́ть на по́мощь, выруча́ть; 5) вноси́ть разнообра́зие, оживля́ть.

relieve^2 *v* де́лать релье́фным.

religion [rɪˈlɪdʒən] *n* рели́гия.

religious [rɪˈlɪdʒəs] *a* религио́зный.

relinquish [rɪˈlɪŋkwɪʃ] *v* 1) оставля́ть (*наде́жду*); броса́ть (*привы́чку*); отка́зываться (*от чего́-л.*); 2) уступа́ть, передава́ть (*кому́-л.*).

relish I [ˈrelɪʃ] *n* 1) (прия́тный) вкус; при́вкус; 2) припра́ва; 3) пристра́стие, вкус (*к чему́-л.*); скло́нность; with a great ~ с удово́льствием, с наслажде́нием; 4) привлека́тельность; to lose its ~ теря́ть свою́ пре́лесть.

relish II *v* 1) придава́ть вкус; приправля́ть; 2) находи́ть вку́сным, смакова́ть; получа́ть удово́льствие (*от чего́-л.*); he did not ~ the prospect of... ему́ не улыба́лась перспекти́ва...; 3) име́ть при́вкус, отзыва́ться (*чем-л. — of*).

reload [ˈriˈloud] *v* 1) перегружа́ть; нагружа́ть сно́ва; 2) перезаряжа́ть.

reluctance [rɪˈlʌktəns] *n* неохо́та; отвраще́ние; with ~ неохо́тно, не́хотя.

reluctant [rɪˈlʌktənt] *a* 1) де́лающий с неохо́той; 2) неохо́тный; вы́нужденный (*о согла́сии и т. п.*); 3) сопротивля́ющийся; не поддаю́щийся (*лече́нию*).

reluctantly [rɪˈlʌktəntlɪ] *adv* неохо́тно, с неохо́той; не жела́я того́.

rely [rɪˈlaɪ] *v* полага́ться (*на — on, upon*); доверя́ть; you may ~ upon it вы мо́жете быть уве́рены в э́том; I ~ upon your word я вам доверя́ю.

remade [ˈriˈmeɪd] *past p. p. см.* remake.

remain I [rɪˈmeɪn] *n обыкн. pl* 1) оста́ток; оста́тки; 2) рели́квии; следы́ про́шлого; 3) пережи́тки; 4) посме́ртные произведе́ния; литерату́рное насле́дство; 5) оста́нки.

remain II *v* оста́ваться.

remainder I [rɪˈmeɪndə] *n* 1) оста́ток, оста́тки; остально́е, остальны́е; 2) *attr* оста́вшийся; остально́й.

remainder II *v* распродава́ть оста́тки тиража́ кни́ги (*по дешёвой цене́*).

remake [ˈriˈmeɪk] *v* (*past, p. p.* remade) переде́лывать, де́лать за́ново.

reman [ˈriˈmæn] *v* 1) *воен.* укомплекто́вывать, подкрепля́ть людьми́; 2) подбодря́ть, вселя́ть му́жество.

remand I [rɪˈmɑːnd] *n* 1) возвраще́ние (*заключённого*) под стра́жу; 2) *воен.* отчисле́ние; исключе́ние из спи́сков; 3) *attr:* ~ home дом предвари́тельного заключе́ния.

remand II *v* 1) возвраща́ть (*заключённого*) под стра́жу; to ~ for court martial преда́ть вое́нному суду́; 2) *воен.* отчисля́ть.

remark I [rɪˈmɑːk] *n* 1) замеча́ние; opening ~s предвари́тельные замеча́ния; to make no ~ ничего́ не сказа́ть; 2) заме́тка; 3) примеча́ние.

remark II *v* 1) замеча́ть, отмеча́ть; наблюда́ть; 2) сде́лать замеча́ние, вы́сказаться (*о чём-л., по по́воду чего́-л. — on, upon*).

remarkable [rɪˈmɑːkəbl] *a* замеча́тельный, выдаю́щийся (*чем-л. — for*).

remarkably [rɪˈmɑːkəblɪ] *adv* замеча́тельно; необыкнове́нно.

remediable [rɪ'miːdjəbl] *a* поправимый; излечимый.

remedial [rɪ'miːdjəl] *a* 1) лечебный, излечивающий; облегчающий; 2) ремонтный.

remedy I ['remɪdɪ] *n* 1) лекарство; средство (*тж. перен.*); 2) возмещение.

remedy II *v* 1) вылечивать; 2) исправлять; 3) возмещать.

remember [rɪ'membə] *v* 1) помнить; вспоминать; to ~ oneself опомниться; 2) передавать привет; ~ me kindly to them пожалуйста, передайте им привет от меня; 3) упоминать в завещании, завещать; 4) дарить; давать на чай.

remembrance [rɪ'membrəns] *n* 1) воспоминание; память; in ~ of в память; 2) *pl* привет; give my ~s to your parents передайте от меня привет вашим родителям; 3) подарок на память, сувенир.

remind [rɪ'maɪnd] *v* напоминать.

reminder [rɪ'maɪndə] *n* напоминание; gentle ~ намёк.

remindful [rɪ'maɪndful] *a* напоминающий; вызывающий воспоминания.

reminiscence [ˌremɪ'nɪsns] *n* 1) воспоминание; память о (*of*); 2) *pl* воспоминания, мемуары.

reminiscent [ˌremɪ'nɪsnt] *a* 1) напоминающий (*о прошлом; of*); вызывающий воспоминания; 2) (*часто*) вспоминающий (*прошлое*); склонный к воспоминаниям.

remiss [rɪ'mɪs] *a* 1) невнимательный, небрежный; 2) слабый; вялый.

remissible [rɪ'mɪsɪbl] *a* простительный, позволительный.

remission [rɪ'mɪʃən] *n* 1 прощение; 2) освобождение от наказания, от уплаты долгов; отмена *или* смягчение (*приговора*); 3) уменьшение, ослабление (*боли, напряжения*).

remissive [rɪ'mɪsɪv] *a* 1) прощающий; освобождающий; 2) ослабляющий, уменьшающий.

remit [rɪ'mɪt] *v* 1) прощать; 2) отменять *или* смягчать (*приговор, наказание*); 3) уменьшать (-ся), ослаблять(ся) (*об усилиях, напряжении и т. п.*); 4) пересылать; переводить по почте (*деньги*); 5) *юр.* передавать в другую инстанцию; откладывать на более поздний срок.

remittance [rɪ'mɪtəns] *n* 1) перевод, пересылка (*денег*); *воен.* перевод (денег) по аттестату; 2) переводимые деньги.

remittee [ˌrɪmɪ'tiː] *n* получатель денег по переводу *или* по аттестату.

remittent [rɪ'mɪtənt] *a* перемежающийся (*о лихорадке*).

remnant ['remnənt] *n* 1) остаток; 2) пережиток.

remodel ['riː'mɔdl] *v* реконструировать; переделывать.

remonstrance [rɪ'mɔnstrəns] *n* протест, возражение.

remonstrate [rɪ'mɔnstreɪt] *v* 1) протестовать, возражать (*against*); 2) убеждать, увещевать (*with*).

remorse [rɪ'mɔːs] *n* 1) угрызение совести; раскаяние; 2) сожаление; жалость; without ~ безжалостно, беспощадно.

remorseful [rɪ'mɔːsful] *a* 1) полный раскаяния; 2) сострадательный; полный сожаления.

remorseless [rɪ'mɔːslɪs] *a* безжалостный, беспощадный.

remote [rɪ'mout] *a* 1) дальний, отдалённый; далёкий (*по времени*); дальний (*о родстве*); 2) незначительный, малый; 3) *тех.* действующий на расстоянии (*о приборе*); дистанционный (*об управлении и т. п.*).

remount[a] ['riː'maunt] *n* 1) запасная лошадь; 2) *воен.* ремонтная лошадь; конский ремонт.

remount[b] [riː'maunt] *v* *воен.* ремонтировать (*кавалерию*).

removable [rɪ'muːvəbl] *a* 1) подвижной, съёмный; 2) сменяемый; устранимый.

removal [rɪ'muːvəl] *n* 1) удаление; уборка (*со стола и т. п.*); 2) перемещение; переезд (*в другое помещение и т. п.*); 3) смещение (*с должности*); 4) устранение.

remove I [rɪ'muːv] *v* 1) уносить; убирать (*со стола и т. п.*); снимать (*шляпу, пальто*); to ~ oneself удаляться, уходить; 2) перемещать; 3) переезжать; 4) смещать (*с должности*), увольнять; 5) удалять, устранять; избавляться (*от кого-л., чего-л.*); 6) выводить (*пятна*).

remove II *n* 1) удаление, отдаление; степень отдаления; at every ~ с каждым шагом; 2) степень родства; 3) перевод ученика в следующий класс; to get one's ~ быть переведённым в следующий класс; 4) класс (*в некоторых англ. школах*); 5) смена блюд (*за столом*).

removed [rɪ'muːvd] *a* удалённый; отдалённый; уединённый; ◊ once ~ двоюродный; twice ~ троюродный.

remover [rɪ'muːvə] *n* 1) перевозчик мебели (*тж.* furniture ~); 2) пятновыводитель; ink ~ средство для удаления чернильных пятен.

remunerate [rɪ'mjuːnəreɪt] *v* вознаграждать; оплачивать, компенсировать.

remuneration [rɪˌmjuːnə'reɪʃən] *n* вознаграждение; воздаяние; оплата, компенсация.

remunerative [rɪ'mjuːnərətɪv] *a* 1) (щедро) вознаграждающий; 2) выгодный, хорошо оплачиваемый.

renaissance [rə'neɪsəns] *n* 1) (R.) эпоха Возрождения, Ренессанс; 2) возрождение, оживление; 3) (R.) *attr* относящийся к эпохе Возрождения.

renal ['riːnəl] *a* почечный.

rename ['riː'neɪm] *v* переименовать.

renascence [rɪ'næsns] *n* 1) возрождение, возобновление; 2) (R.) *см.* renaissance 1).

renascent [rɪ'næsnt] *a* возрождающийся.

rencounter I [ren'kauntə] *n* 1) столкновение, стычка; дуэль; 2) (случайная) встреча.

rencounter II *v* столкнуться, встретиться.

rend [rend] *v* (*past, p. p.* rent) 1) разрывать, раздирать, рвать; отрывать (*насильно*); 2) расщеплять, раскалывать.

render ['rendə] *v* 1) отдавать; воздавать; 2) оказывать (*услугу, помощь*); 3) представлять (*объяснение, отчёт, основания*); 4) превращать, делать; to ~ active активизировать; to ~ helpless делать беспомощным; to ~ liable подвергать (*опасности, риску и т. п.*); 5) изображать, воспроизводить; исполнять (*роль*); 6) переводить (*на другой язык*); 7) платить (*дань и т. п.*); 8) штукатурить; 9) топить (*жир*).

rendering ['rendərɪŋ] *n* 1) перевод; 2) толкование (*образа, произведения*); исполнение (*роли*); 3) оказание услуги, помощи *и т. п.*

rendezvous I ['rɔndɪvuː] *n* 1) свида́ние; 2) ме́сто свида́ния; ме́сто встреч; 3) *воен.* ме́сто сбо́ра.

rendezvous II *v* встреча́ться в назна́ченном ме́сте.

rendition [ren'dɪʃən] *n* 1) перево́д; толкова́ние (*образа, роли, муз. произведения*); 2) *редко* переда́ча, вы́дача (*преступника другому государству*).

renegade I ['renɪgeɪd] *n* ренега́т, изме́нник; отсту́пник.

renegade II *a* преда́тельский, изме́ннический.

renew [rɪ'njuː] *v* 1) обновля́ть; восстана́вливать, реставри́ровать; to ~ oneself возрожда́ться; 2) возобновля́ть (*аренду, подписку, знакомство*).

renewal [rɪ'njuːəl] *n* 1) возрожде́ние, восстановле́ние; 2) возобновле́ние; повторе́ние; the ~ of hostilities возобновле́ние вое́нных де́йствий.

renounce [rɪ'nauns] *v* отка́зываться (*от прав, требований и т. п.*); отрека́ться; отверга́ть, отклоня́ть; не признава́ть.

renouncement [rɪ'naunsmənt] *n* отка́з; отрече́ние.

renovate ['renouveɪt] *v* поправля́ть, подновля́ть, освежа́ть.

renovation [,renou'veɪʃən] *n* восстановле́ние; реконстру́кция.

renown [rɪ'naun] *n* сла́ва, изве́стность.

renowned [rɪ'naund] *a* знамени́тый, просла́вленный, изве́стный.

rent[1] I [rent] *n* 1) разре́з; дыра́, проре́ха; разры́в (*тж. перен.*); 2) рассе́лина, щель, тре́щина.

rent[1] II *past, p. p. см.* rend.

rent[2] I *n* 1) аре́ндная пла́та; кварти́рная пла́та; 2) ре́нта; land ~ земе́льная ре́нта; life ~ пожи́зненная ре́нта; 3) наём; for ~ внаём; напрока́т.

rent[2] II *v* 1) нанима́ть; 2) сдава́ть в аре́нду; дава́ть напрока́т; 3) сдава́ться (в аре́нду); the house ~s for... a year дом сдаётся за... в год.

rental ['rentl] *n* аре́ндная пла́та.

renter ['rentə] *n* 1) съёмщик; аренда́тор; 2) сдаю́щий в аре́нду.

rent-free I ['rent'friː] *a* освобождённый от аре́ндной *или* кварти́рной пла́ты.

rent-free II *adv* без аре́ндной *или* кварти́рной пла́ты.

rentier ['rɔntɪeɪ] *n* рантье́.

renunciation [rɪ,nʌnsɪ'eɪʃən] *n* отка́з (*от прав, имущества и т. п.*); отрече́ние.

reopen ['riː'oupən] *v* открыва́ть(ся) вновь.

reorganization ['riː,ɔːgənaɪ'zeɪʃən] *n* реорганиза́ция, преобразова́ние.

reorganize ['riː'ɔːgənaɪz] *v* реорганизова́ть, преобразова́ть.

rep[1] [rep] *n* репс (*материя*).

rep[2] *n сленг* репети́ция.

repaid ['riː'peɪd] *past, p. p. см.* repay.

repair[1] I [rɪ'peə] *n* 1) *часто pl* ремо́нт; почи́нка; under ~ в ремо́нте; permanent ~ теку́щий ремо́нт; 2) го́дность; испра́вность; in good ~ в по́лной испра́вности; in bad ~ в неиспра́вном состоя́нии; to keep in ~ содержа́ть в испра́вности; beyond ~ соверше́нно него́дный; out of ~ неиспра́вный, нужда́ющийся в ремо́нте; 3) *attr* ремо́нтный.

repair[1] II *v* 1) ремонти́ровать, исправля́ть, починя́ть; 2) возмеща́ть; 3) исправля́ть (*ошибку, несправедливость*).

repair[2] *v* 1) отправля́ться, направля́ться (*куда-л., к кому-л.*); 2) прибега́ть (*к — to*).

repairable [rɪ'peərəbl] *a* поддаю́щийся ремо́нту.

repairman [rɪ'peəmæn] *n* сле́сарь-ремо́нтник.

reparable ['repərəbl] *a* поправи́мый.

reparation [,repə'reɪʃən] *n* 1) исправле́ние, приведе́ние в испра́вное состоя́ние; 2) *pl* возмеще́ние; репара́ции.

repartee [,repɑː'tiː] *n* 1) остроу́мный отве́т; 2) остроу́мие, нахо́дчивость.

repast [rɪ'pɑːst] *n* 1) еда́ (*обед, ужин и т. п.*); 2) пи́ршество.

repatriate [riː'pætrɪeɪt] *v* возвраща́ть на ро́дину, репатрии́ровать.

repatriation ['riː,pætrɪ'eɪʃən] *n* возвраще́ние на ро́дину, репатриа́ция.

repay ['riː'peɪ] *v* (*past, p. p.* repaid) 1) отдава́ть долг; 2) отпла́чивать; 3) возмеща́ть, вознагражда́ть.

repayable [riː'peɪəbl] *a* подлежа́щий упла́те *или* возмеще́нию.

repayment [riː'peɪmənt] *n* 1) отпла́та; 2) возмеще́ние, вознагражде́ние.

repeal I [rɪ'piːl] *n* отме́на, аннули́рование.

repeal II *v* отменя́ть, аннули́ровать.

repeat I [rɪ'piːt] *v* 1) повторя́ть; тверди́ть; to ~ oneself повторя́ться; 2) говори́ть наизу́сть; репети́ровать; 3) повторя́ться, (вновь) случа́ться; on ~ed occasions неоднокра́тно.

repeat II *n* 1) повторе́ние; 2) исполне́ние на бис.

repeatedly [rɪ'piːtɪdlɪ] *adv* повто́рно; неоднокра́тно, не́сколько раз.

repeater [rɪ'piːtə] *n* 1) тот, кто повторя́ет, де́лает что-л. повто́рно; 2) *амер. разг.* студе́нт-второго́дник; 3) рецидиви́ст; 4) магази́нная винто́вка; 5) *мат.* непреры́вная дробь; 6) часы́ с репети́цией.

repel [rɪ'pel] *v* 1) отража́ть (*атаку неприятеля*); отгоня́ть, отта́лкивать; отверга́ть (*предложение, просьбу*); 2) внуша́ть отвраще́ние; вызыва́ть неприя́знь; 3) *физ.* отта́лкивать.

repellent [rɪ'pelənt] *a* отта́лкивающий, отврати́тельный; неприя́тный (*о манере*).

repent [rɪ'pent] *v* сожале́ть, сокруша́ться (*о чём-л.*); ка́яться.

repentance [rɪ'pentəns] *n* раска́яние; сожале́ние.

repentant [rɪ'pentənt] *a* раска́ивающийся; сожале́ющий.

repercussion [,riːpə'kʌʃən] *n* 1) отда́ча (*в орудии*); 2) о́тзвук, э́хо (*тж. перен.*).

repertoire ['repətwɑː] *n* репертуа́р.

repertory ['repətɪ] *n* 1) репертуа́р; 2) склад; запа́с; 3) спра́вочник, сбо́рник.

repetition [,repɪ'tɪʃən] *n* 1) повторе́ние; 2) повторе́ние наизу́сть; 3) репети́ция; 4) ко́пия; подража́ние.

repetitious [,repɪ'tɪʃəs] *a* повторя́ющийся, надое́дливый.

repine [rɪ'paɪn] *v* ропта́ть, се́товать (*at, against*).

replace [rɪ'pleɪs] *v* 1) ста́вить, класть обра́тно *или* на ме́сто; 2) заменя́ть, замеща́ть; impossible to ~ незамени́мый; 3) возмеща́ть, восстана́вливать (*что-л. утраченное*).

replaceable [rɪ'pleɪsəbl] *a* замени́мый.

replacement [rɪ'pleɪsmənt] *n* 1) заме́на, замеще́ние; 2) *воен.* пополне́ние.

replenish [rɪ'plenɪʃ] v снóва наполня́ть; пополня́ть; подбра́сывать (*дрова в печь*).

replenishment [rɪ'plenɪʃmənt] n наполне́ние; пополне́ние.

replete [rɪ'pliːt] a 1) напо́лненный, перепо́лненный; по́лный (*чего-л.*); 2) хорошо́ снабжённый, обеспе́ченный.

repletion [rɪ'pliːʃən] n переполне́ние.

replica ['replɪkə] n ко́пия, репроду́кция (*карти́ны*).

reply I [rɪ'plaɪ] n отве́т; in ~ в отве́т; ~ paid с опла́ченным отве́том.

reply II v отвеча́ть (*на — to; вместо, за кого-л. — for*).

report I [rɪ'pɔːt] n 1) отчёт, отчётный докла́д; 2) *воен.* донесе́ние; ра́порт; 3) слух, молва́; the ~ has it that... говоря́т, что...; mere ~ то́лько слух; 4) репута́ция; 5) та́бель успева́емости (*в школе*); 6) звук вы́стрела, вы́стрел.

report II v 1) расска́зывать, сообща́ть; опи́сывать; it is ~ed сообща́ется; 2) докла́дывать; представля́ть отчёт; 3) *воен.* доноси́ть; рапортова́ть; to ~ oneself ill пода́ть ра́порт о боле́зни; 4) явля́ться; to ~ for work явля́ться на рабо́ту; 5) составля́ть отчёт (*для газеты*); дава́ть о́тзыв; 6) выдвига́ть обвине́ние (*против кого-л.*).

reporter [rɪ'pɔːtə] n 1) репортёр; 2) докла́дчик.

repose[1] [rɪ'pouz] v: to ~ confidence in, to ~ trust in *или* on доверя́ть(ся) (*кому-л.*), полага́ться (*на кого-л., что-л.*).

repose[2] I n 1) поко́й, о́тдых, сон; 2) споко́йствие; 3) непринуждённость; to have ~ of manner держа́ться непринуждённо, свобо́дно.

repose[2] II v 1) отдыха́ть, спать (*тж.* to ~ oneself); 2) поко́иться, лежа́ть; класть (*голову*); 3) осно́вываться, держа́ться (*на чём-л. — on*).

repository [rɪ'pɔzɪtərɪ] n 1) склад; храни́лище; вмести́лище; 2) носи́тель (*чего-л.*).

reprehend [,reprɪ'hend] v де́лать вы́говор, жури́ть, отчи́тывать.

reprehensible [,reprɪ'hensəbl] a досто́йный порица́ния; предосуди́тельный.

reprehension [,reprɪ'henʃən] n порица́ние, осужде́ние.

represent [,reprɪ'zent] v 1) представля́ть, изобража́ть; 2) представля́ть себе́, вообража́ть; 3) исполня́ть (роль), изобража́ть; 4) быть представи́телем, представля́ть.

representation [,reprɪzen'teɪʃən] n 1) изображе́ние; представле́ние; 2) представи́тельство; permanent ~ *дип.* постоя́нное представи́тельство; adequate ~ соотве́тственное представи́тельство.

representative I [,reprɪ'zentətɪv] n 1) представи́тель; делега́т; уполномо́ченный; 2) образе́ц; типи́чный представи́тель (*вида животных и т. п.*); 3) член пала́ты представи́телей (*в США*).

representative II a 1) представля́ющий, изобража́ющий; 2) характе́рный, типи́чный; показа́тельный; 3) *полит.* представи́тельный.

repress [rɪ'pres] v 1) подавля́ть (*восстание и т. п.*); 2) сде́рживать (*слёзы и т. п.*).

repression [rɪ'preʃən] n 1) подавле́ние; репре́ссия; 2) сде́рживание (*чувств и т. п.*).

repressive [rɪ'presɪv] a репресси́вный.

reprieve I [rɪ'priːv] n 1) отсро́чка в исполне́нии пригово́ра; 2) вре́менное облегче́ние, переды́шка.

reprieve II v 1) отсро́чивать исполне́ние пригово́ра; 2) дава́ть переды́шку, вре́менное облегче́ние.

reprimand I ['reprɪmɑːnd] n вы́говор.

reprimand II v де́лать *или* объявля́ть вы́говор.

reprint I ['riːprɪnt] n 1) но́вое изда́ние, переизда́ние; перепеча́тка; 2) отде́льный о́ттиск (*статьи и т. п.*).

reprint II v выпуска́ть но́вое изда́ние, переиздава́ть; перепеча́тывать.

reprisal [rɪ'praɪzəl] n репресса́лия.

reproach I [rɪ'proutʃ] n 1) упрёк, уко́р; to heap ~es on, to hurl ~es at осыпа́ть упрёками кого́-л.; 2) позо́р; without ~ безупре́чный; to bring ~ on позо́рить (*кого-л.*).

reproach II v упрека́ть, укоря́ть.

reproachful [rɪ'proutʃful] a 1) укори́зненный; 2) недосто́йный, посты́дный.

reproachfully [rɪ'proutʃfulɪ] adv укори́зненно; с уко́ром.

reprobate I ['reproubeɪt] n негодя́й, подле́ц.

reprobate II a по́длый, ни́зкий, безнра́вственный.

reprobate III v осужда́ть, порица́ть.

reprobation [,reprou'beɪʃən] n осужде́ние, порица́ние.

reproduce [,riːprə'djuːs] v 1) размножа́ться; 2) воспроизводи́ть; 3) де́лать ко́пию.

reproducer [,riːprə'djuːsə] n 1) репроду́ктор, громкоговори́тель; 2) воспроизводи́тель.

reproduction [,riːprə'dʌkʃən] n 1) размноже́ние; 2) воспроизведе́ние; 3) ко́пия, репроду́кция; 4) *эк.* воспроизво́дство; ~ on a large scale расши́ренное воспроизво́дство.

reproductive [,riːprə'dʌktɪv] a воспроизводи́тельный.

reproof [rɪ'pruːf] n упрёк; вы́говор; with ~ с укори́зной.

reprove [rɪ'pruːv] v упрека́ть; брани́ть; де́лать вы́говор.

reptile I ['reptaɪl] n пресмыка́ющееся; *перен.* подхали́м; ни́зкий, по́длый челове́к.

reptile II a 1) пресмыка́ющийся (*тж. перен.*); 2) по́длый; прода́жный (*о прессе*).

republic [rɪ'pʌblɪk] n респу́блика; People's ~ наро́дная респу́блика.

republican I [rɪ'pʌblɪkən] n 1) республика́нец; 2) (R.) *амер.* член республика́нской па́ртии.

republican II a республика́нский.

repudiate [rɪ'pjuːdɪeɪt] v 1) отрека́ться (*от чего-л., кого-л.*); 2) отверга́ть, не признава́ть (*теорию, доктрину*); 3) отка́зываться (*от уплаты долга, от выполнения обязательства*); 4) разводи́ться.

repudiation [rɪ,pjuːdɪ'eɪʃən] n 1) отрече́ние; отка́з; отрица́ние; 2) отка́з (*от уплаты долга, выполнения обязательства*); 3) разво́д.

repugnance [rɪ'pʌgnəns] n 1) отвраще́ние; антипа́тия; 2) противоре́чие; несовмести́мость.

repugnancy [rɪ'pʌgnənsɪ] *см.* repugnance.

repugnant [rɪ'pʌgnənt] a 1) отврати́тельный, невыноси́мый (*to*); 2) испы́тывающий отвраще́ние, антипа́тию (*to*); 3) несовмести́мый, противоре́чащий (*with, to*).

repulse I [rɪ'pʌls] n 1) отраже́ние (*атаки и т. п.*); отпо́р; 2) отка́з.

repulse II v 1) отража́ть, отбива́ть (*атаку*);

2) опроверга́ть (*обвинение*); 3) отверга́ть; отта́лкивать.

repulsion [rɪ'pʌlʃən] *n* 1) отвраще́ние; антипа́тия; 2) *физ.* отта́лкивание.

repulsive [rɪ'pʌlsɪv] *a* 1) отврати́тельный, отта́лкивающий; 2) отража́ющий; 3) отверга́ющий.

reputable ['repjutəbl] *a* почте́нный, уважа́емый.

reputation [ˌrepjuː'teɪʃən] *n* репута́ция; до́брое и́мя; to stab one's ~ повреди́ть свое́й репута́ции; to have a ~ for wit сла́виться остроу́мием; to live up to one's ~ не роня́ть своего́ до́брого и́мени; оправда́ть ожида́ния.

repute I [rɪ'pjuːt] *n* репута́ция; о́бщее мне́ние; according to ~ по о́бщему мне́нию; по слу́хам; to be in ~ сла́виться, быть изве́стным; of ~ изве́стный, знамени́тый; bad ~ дурна́я сла́ва.

repute II *v обыкн. pass* счита́ть, полага́ть.

reputed [rɪ'pjuːtɪd] *a* 1) по́льзующийся хоро́шей репута́цией; изве́стный; 2) счита́ющийся (*кем-л.*), предполага́емый.

request I [rɪ'kwest] *n* 1) про́сьба; тре́бование, зая́вка; запро́с; at ~ по про́сьбе; по тре́бованию; to make a ~ обрати́ться с про́сьбой, сде́лать запро́с; to comply with one's ~ удовлетвори́ть чью-л. про́сьбу; 2) спрос; in great ~ в большо́м ходу́, популя́рный.

request II *v* 1) проси́ть; запра́шивать; 2) предлага́ть (*исполнить что-л.*).

requiem ['rekwɪem] *n* ре́квием.

require [rɪ'kwaɪə] *v* 1) тре́бовать, прика́зывать; 2) нужда́ться, име́ть на́добность; it ~d all his courage пона́добилось всё его́ му́жество.

requirement [rɪ'kwaɪəmənt] *n* 1) тре́бование; необходи́мое усло́вие; 2) потре́бность, нужда́.

requisite I ['rekwɪzɪt] *n* то, что необходи́мо.

requisite II *a* необходи́мый, потре́бный, тре́буемый.

requisition I [ˌrekwɪ'zɪʃən] *n* 1) тре́бование, зая́вка; 2) реквизи́ция.

requisition II *v* реквизи́ровать.

requital [rɪ'kwaɪtl] *n* 1) вознагражде́ние, воздая́ние; 2) возме́здие.

requite [rɪ'kwaɪt] *v* 1) отпла́чивать, воздава́ть; 2) отомсти́ть.

rescind [rɪ'sɪnd] *v* отменя́ть, аннули́ровать.

rescript ['riːskrɪpt] *n* 1) ука́з, рескри́пт; 2) что-л. перепи́санное.

rescue I ['reskjuː] *n* 1) спасе́ние, избавле́ние; to the ~ на по́мощь, на вы́ручку; 2) *attr* спаса́тельный.

rescue II *v* спаса́ть, избавля́ть; выруча́ть.

rescuer ['reskjuə] *n* спаси́тель, избави́тель.

research I [rɪ'səːtʃ] *n* 1) иссле́дование; изыска́ние, изуче́ние; 2) тща́тельные по́иски; 3) иссле́довательская рабо́та; 4) *attr* иссле́довательский.

research II *v* иссле́довать; занима́ться иссле́дованиями (*into*).

researcher [rɪ'səːtʃə] *n* иссле́дователь.

reseda ['resɪdə] *n* резеда́.

resemblance [rɪ'zembləns] *n* схо́дство; to bear (*или* to show) ~ име́ть схо́дство, быть похо́жим.

resemble [rɪ'zembl] *v* быть похо́жим, походи́ть на что-л.

resent [rɪ'zent] *v* негодова́ть, возмуща́ться; обижа́ться.

resentful [rɪ'zentful] *a* 1) возмущённый; оби́женный; 2) злопа́мятный, оби́дчивый.

resentment [rɪ'zentmənt] *n* негодова́ние; чу́вство оби́ды.

reservation [ˌrezə'veɪʃən] *n* 1) огово́рка; without ~ безогово́рочно; with ~ of за исключе́нием (*чего-л.*); огово́рив (*что-л.*); with the mental ~ поду́мав про себя́; 2) ума́лчивание; сокры́тие; 3) сде́ржанность; 4) *амер.* предвари́тельный зака́з (*мест на парохо́де, в теа́тре, гости́нице и т. п.*); резерви́рование; 5) *амер.* зара́нее зака́занное ме́сто (*на парохо́де, в гости́нице и т. п.*); 6) сохране́ние в запа́се, про запа́с; 7) *амер.* резерви́рованный для како́й-л. це́ли земе́льный уча́сток; Indian ~s террито́рии, отведённые для инде́йцев в США; резерва́ции.

reserve I [rɪ'zəːv] *n* 1) запа́с; резе́рв (*тж. воен.*); in ~ в запа́се; 2) запове́дник; a forest ~ лесно́й запове́дник; 3) огово́рка, усло́вие; исключе́ние, изъя́тие; without ~ без исключе́ний, безусло́вно; 4) сде́ржанность; осторо́жность; 5) скры́тность, за́мкнутость; 6) сокры́тие; умолча́ние; to speak without ~ говори́ть откры́то, ничего́ не скрыва́я; 7) *attr* запа́сный, запасно́й, резе́рвный.

reserve II *v* 1) запаса́ть, откла́дывать; сберега́ть, сохраня́ть (*про запа́с*); 2) откла́дывать на бу́дущее; переноси́ть; 3) резерви́ровать, оставля́ть в резе́рве; огова́ривать (*пра́во и т. п.*); 4) зака́зывать зара́нее.

reserved [rɪ'zəːvd] *a* 1) резе́рвный, запа́сный; 2) зака́занный зара́нее; 3) сде́ржанный; осторо́жный; 4) за́мкнутый, необщи́тельный.

reservedly [rɪ'zəːvɪdlɪ] *adv* сде́ржанно, осторо́жно.

reservist [rɪ'zəːvɪst] *n* резерви́ст.

reservoir ['rezəvwɑː] *n* 1) резервуа́р; храни́лище (*воды́, не́фти*); 2) запа́с; склад, сокро́вищница.

reset ['riː'set] *v* (*past, p. p.* reset) 1) вновь устана́вливать; 2) (вновь) вставля́ть в опра́ву; 3) вправля́ть (*сло́манную ру́ку и т. п.*).

reside [rɪ'zaɪd] *v* 1) жить, прожива́ть (*где-л. — in, at*); 2) находи́ться, быть (*в чём-л. — in*); быть прису́щим, сво́йственным (*кому-л., чему-л. — in*).

residence ['rezɪdəns] *n* 1) местожи́тельство; жили́ще; резиде́нция; 2) прожива́ние, пребыва́ние; to take up one's ~ посели́ться.

resident I ['rezɪdənt] *n* 1) (постоя́нный) жи́тель; 2) резиде́нт.

resident II *a* живу́щий (*где-л., при ком-л., чём-л.*); постоя́нный (*о населе́нии и т. п.*).

residential [ˌrezɪ'denʃəl] *a* состоя́щий из жилы́х домо́в (*о райо́не го́рода*).

residua [rɪ'zɪdjuə] *pl см.* residuum.

residual I [rɪ'zɪdjuəl] *n* оста́ток, ра́зность.

residual II *a* 1) остаю́щийся, оста́вшийся; 2) оста́точный.

residue ['rezɪdjuː] *n* 1) оста́ток; 2) оса́док.

residuum [rɪ'zɪdjuəm] *n* (*pl* residua) 1) оста́ток; 2) *хим.* оса́док.

resign [rɪ'zaɪn] *v* 1) отка́зываться (*от до́лжности*); уходи́ть *или* подава́ть в отста́вку; слага́ть с себя́ (*обя́занности и т. п.*); 2): to ~ oneself подчини́ться, покоря́ться (*кому-л., чему-л. — to*); примиря́ться (*с чем-л. — to*).

resignation [ˌrezɪg'neɪʃən] *n* 1) отка́з от до́лжности, ухо́д в отста́вку; отста́вка; 2) заявле́ние об отста́вке; to send in (*или* to tender) one's ~ пода́ть заявле́ние об отста́вке; 3) поко́рность, смире́ние.

resigned [rɪˈzaɪnd] *a* поко́рный, смире́нный, безро́потный.

resilience [rɪˈzɪlɪəns] *n* упру́гость, эласти́чность.

resiliency [rɪˈzɪlɪənsɪ] *см.* resilience.

resilient [rɪˈzɪlɪənt] *a* 1) упру́гий, эласти́чный; 2) жизнера́достный, неунываю́щий.

resin I [ˈrezɪn] *n* смола́.

resin II *v* смоли́ть.

resinous [ˈrezɪnəs] *a* смоли́стый.

resist [rɪˈzɪst] *v* 1) сопротивля́ться, проти́виться; 2) противостоя́ть; вы́держать, устоя́ть про́тив чего́-л., кого́-л.; 3) *обыкн. с отрица́нием* удержа́ться, воздержа́ться; he could not ~ laughing он не мог удержа́ться от сме́ха.

resistance [rɪˈzɪstəns] *n* 1) сопротивле́ние; противоде́йствие; to offer ~ ока́зывать сопротивле́ние; 2) сопротивля́емость; the ~ to wear сопротивле́ние изно́су; 3) эл. сопротивле́ние.

resistant [rɪˈzɪstənt] *a* сопротивля́ющийся; сто́йкий, про́чный.

resistless [rɪˈzɪstlɪs] *a* 1) непреодоли́мый; 2) неспосо́бный сопротивля́ться.

resoluble [rɪˈzɔljubl] *a* раствори́мый; разложи́мый.

resolute [ˈrezəluːt] *a* реши́тельный; твёрдый, непоколеби́мый.

resolution [ˌrezəˈluːʃən] *n* 1) реше́ние; резолю́ция; to make a ~ реши́ть, приня́ть реше́ние; to pass (*или* to take, to adopt) a ~ приня́ть реше́ние, резолю́цию; 2) реши́тельность, реши́мость, твёрдость; 3) разложе́ние (на составны́е ча́сти); 4) раство́р; 5) разбо́рка, демонта́ж.

resolve I [rɪˈzɔlv] *n* 1) реше́ние; 2) *поэт.* реши́тельность, твёрдость хара́ктера; сме́лость; of great ~ сме́лый и реши́тельный.

resolve II *v* 1) реша́ть(ся), принима́ть реше́ние; to be ~d твёрдо реши́ть; 2) реша́ть голосова́нием; 3) разреша́ть (*сомне́ния и т. п.*); 4) распада́ться; разлага́ть(ся); растворя́ть(ся).

resolved [rɪˈzɔlvd] *a* реши́тельный, твёрдый.

resonance [ˈrezənəns] *n* резона́нс.

resonant [ˈrezənənt] *a* 1) звуча́щий, раздаю́щийся; 2) с хоро́шим резона́нсом.

resort I [rɪˈzɔːt] *n* 1) обраще́ние (*за по́мощью*); примене́ние (*како́го-л. сре́дства*); the ~ to force примене́ние си́лы, наси́лия; without ~ to force не прибега́я к наси́лию; 2) прибе́жище; утеше́ние, наде́жда; in the last ~, as a last ~ в кра́йнем слу́чае, как после́днее сре́дство; 3) посеща́емое ме́сто; health ~ куро́рт; summer ~ да́чное ме́сто.

resort II *v* 1) прибега́ть к чему́-л., обраща́ться к кому́-л. (*за по́мощью и т. п.; to*); 2) (*ча́сто*) посеща́ть.

resound [rɪˈzaund] *v* 1) звуча́ть (*гро́мко*), раздава́ться (*о зву́ках*); оглаша́ться (*зву́ками чего́-л.*); 2) отража́ть, повторя́ть звук; 3) греме́ть (*о сла́ве, и́мени*); 4) прославля́ть.

resource [rɪˈzɔːs] *n* 1) *обыкн. pl* сре́дства, ресу́рсы; natural ~s есте́ственные бога́тства; 2) спо́соб, сре́дство; 3) времяпрепровожде́ние, развлече́ние; 4) нахо́дчивость; изобрета́тельность; of ~ изобрета́тельный; нахо́дчивый.

resourceful [rɪˈzɔːsful] *a* нахо́дчивый, сообрази́тельный; ло́вкий.

respect I [rɪsˈpekt] *n* 1) уваже́ние; почте́ние (*к кому́-л. — for*); to pay one's ~s ока́зывать почте́ние; give my ~s to переда́йте мой приве́т; out of ~ to из уваже́ния к кому́-л.; 2) отноше́ние; in this ~ в э́том отноше́нии; in other ~s в други́х отноше́ниях, в остально́м; in all ~s во всех отноше́ниях; in no ~ ни в како́м отноше́нии; in ~ of что каса́ется; with ~ to a) принима́я во внима́ние *или* учи́тывая; б) что каса́ется; without ~ to не принима́я во внима́ние.

respect II *v* уважа́ть, почита́ть; щади́ть (*чу́вства*).

respectability [rɪsˌpektəˈbɪlɪtɪ] *n* 1) почте́нность; 2) поря́дочность, че́стность.

respectable [rɪsˈpektəbl] *a* 1) почте́нный; поря́дочный; 2) дово́льно хоро́ший, прили́чный, прие́млемый; 3) поря́дочный (*по величине́, коли́честву*).

respectful [rɪsˈpektful] *a* почти́тельный; ве́жливый.

respectfully [rɪsˈpektfulɪ] *adv* почти́тельно; yours ~ с почте́нием (*в письме́*).

respecting [rɪsˈpektɪŋ] *prep* относи́тельно.

respective [rɪsˈpektɪv] *a* соотве́тственный; the men retired to their ~ homes лю́ди разошли́сь по свои́м дома́м.

respectively [rɪsˈpektɪvlɪ] *adv* 1) что каса́ется ка́ждого в отде́льности; 2) в ука́занном поря́дке, соотве́тственно.

respiration [ˌrespəˈreɪʃən] *n* дыха́ние.

respirator [ˈrespəreɪtə] *n* 1) респира́тор; 2) противога́з.

respiratory [rɪsˈpaɪərətərɪ] *a* дыха́тельный.

respire [rɪsˈpaɪə] *v* 1) дыша́ть; 2) переводи́ть дыха́ние.

respite I [ˈrespaɪt] *n* 1) переды́шка; 2) отсро́чка (*наказа́ния*).

respite II *v* 1) дава́ть переды́шку; 2) предоставля́ть отсро́чку; приостана́вливать.

resplendence [rɪsˈplendəns] *n* великоле́пие, блеск.

resplendent [rɪsˈplendənt] *a* блиста́тельный, сверка́ющий, великоле́пный; to be ~ with блиста́ть, сверка́ть чем-л.

respond [rɪsˈpɔnd] *v* 1) отвеча́ть; 2) удовлетворя́ть (*тре́бованиям и т. п.; to*); 3) отплати́ть (*чем-л. — with*); 4) реаги́ровать; to ~ to treatment (to the medicine) поддава́ться лече́нию (де́йствию лека́рства).

respondent I [rɪsˈpɔndənt] *n* отве́тчик.

respondent II *a* 1) реаги́рующий; 2) отзы́вчивый; 3) выступа́ющий отве́тчиком.

response [rɪsˈpɔns] *n* 1) отве́т; in ~ to в отве́т на; in ~ to a signal по сигна́лу; 2) о́тклик; реа́кция; popular ~ о́тклики обще́ственности.

responsibility [rɪsˌpɔnsəˈbɪlɪtɪ] *n* 1) отве́тственность; on one's own ~ на свою́ отве́тственность, на свой страх и риск; 2) обя́занности, обяза́тельства.

responsible [rɪsˈpɔnsəbl] *a* 1) отве́тственный (*пе́ред — to; за — for*); обя́занный; to be ~ нести́ отве́тственность (*за что-л. — for*); 2) созна́тельный, разу́мный; досто́йный дове́рия.

responsive [rɪsˈpɔnsɪv] *a* 1) отве́тный (*о взгля́де и т. п.*); 2) отзы́вчивый, чувстви́тельный.

rest[1] I [rest] *n* 1) о́тдых, поко́й; сон; at ~ а) в поко́е; б) неподви́жный; мёртвый; to have (*или* to take) ~ отдохну́ть; to set at ~ a) успока́ивать; б) ула́живать (*вопрос и т. п.*); 2) неподви́жность; to bring to ~ остана́вливать (*экипаж и т. п.*); 3) переры́в; па́уза (*тж. муз.*); 4) подста́вка, опо́ра; упо́р; сто́йка; 5) ме́сто для о́тдыха; 6) моги́ла; смерть; to go to one's long ~ умере́ть, засну́ть наве́ки.

rest[1] **II** *v* 1) отдыха́ть; лежа́ть (споко́йно); поко́иться; дава́ть о́тдых; not let smb. ~ не дава́ть кому́-л. поко́я; 2) прислоня́ться, опира́ться (*on, against*); 3) полага́ться; возлага́ть (*наде́жды; in*); 4) остана́вливаться, быть прико́ванным (*о взгля́де, мы́слях и т. п.; on*); 5) пребыва́ть, находи́ться; принадлежа́ть; in people's democracies government ~s with the people в стра́нах наро́дной демокра́тии власть принадлежи́т наро́ду.

rest[2] **I** *n* (the ~) оста́ток; остально́е, остальны́е; all the ~, the ~ of it всё остально́е, всё про́чее.

rest[2] **II** *v* остава́ться; ◊ it ~s with you to decide реше́ние за ва́ми.

restate ['riː'steɪt] *v* вновь заявля́ть.

restaurant ['restərɔːŋ] *n* рестора́н.

rest-cure ['restkjuə] *n* лече́ние поко́ем, по́лный поко́й.

rest-day ['restdeɪ] *n* день о́тдыха.

restful ['restful] *a* 1) успокои́тельный, успока́ивающий; 2) споко́йный, ти́хий.

rest-home ['resthoum] *n* дом о́тдыха.

rest-house ['resthaus] *n* гости́ница для путеше́ственников.

resting-place ['restɪŋpleɪs] *n* 1) ме́сто о́тдыха; 2) площа́дка на ле́стнице; ◊ last ~ моги́ла.

restitution [ˌrestɪ'tjuːʃən] *n* 1) возвраще́ние (*утра́ченного, о́тнятого*); 2) возмеще́ние; удовлетворе́ние; to make ~ возмеща́ть убы́тки; 3) восстановле́ние.

restive ['restɪv] *a* 1) своенра́вный, упря́мый; беспоко́йный; 2) норови́стый (*о ло́шади*).

restless ['restlɪs] *a* 1) беспоко́йный; 2) неспоко́йный, неугомо́нный, нетерпели́вый.

restock ['riː'stɔk] *v* пополня́ть запа́с.

restoration [ˌrestə'reɪʃən] *n* 1) восстановле́ние; реставра́ция; 2) реконстру́кция; 3) возобновле́ние.

restorative **I** [rɪs'tɔrətɪv] *n* *мед.* тонизи́рующее, укрепля́ющее лека́рство.

restorative **II** *a* укрепля́ющий (*здоро́вье*).

restore [rɪs'tɔː] *v* 1) восстана́вливать; реставри́ровать, реконструи́ровать; to be ~d to health вы́здороветь; 2) возвраща́ть, возмеща́ть (*кому́-л.—to*).

restorer [rɪs'tɔrə] *n* 1) реставра́тор; 2) восстанови́тель (*тж.* hair ~).

restrain [rɪs'treɪn] *v* 1) сде́рживать, обу́здывать; 2) уде́рживать, подавля́ть; ограни́чивать; 3) подверга́ть заключе́нию, заде́рживать.

restrained [rɪs'treɪnd] *a* 1) сде́ржанный; 2) ограни́ченный.

restraint [rɪs'treɪnt] *n* 1) сде́ржанность, за́мкнутость; стро́гость; 2) стесне́ние, ограниче́ние; 3) задержа́ние, заключе́ние (*в тюрьму́ и т. п.*); to be under ~ находи́ться в сумасше́дшем до́ме; to put under ~ брать под стра́жу; 4) сде́рживающее нача́ло; without ~ свобо́дно, безуде́ржно.

restrict [rɪs'trɪkt] *v* ограни́чивать.

restriction [rɪs'trɪkʃən] *n* ограниче́ние.

restrictive [rɪs'trɪktɪv] *a* 1) ограничи́тельный; 2) сде́рживающий.

result **I** [rɪ'zʌlt] *n* 1) результа́т, сле́дствие; исхо́д; without ~ безрезульта́тно; as a ~ of в результа́те; 2) ито́г (*вычисле́ний*).

result **II** *v* 1) проистека́ть, происходи́ть в результа́те; 2) конча́ться чем-л., приводи́ть к чему́-л., име́ть результа́том (*in*); to ~ in complete failure око́нчиться по́лной неуда́чей.

resultant **I** [rɪ'zʌltənt] *n* *физ.* равноде́йствующая.

resultant **II** *a* 1) проистека́ющий (*из чего́-л.*); получа́ющийся в результа́те; 2) *физ.* равноде́йствующий.

resume [rɪ'zjuːm] *v* 1) возобновля́ть; продолжа́ть (*по́сле переры́ва*); 2) принима́ть обра́тно; сно́ва занима́ть (*места́ и т. п.*); 3) верну́ться (*к пре́жнему состоя́нию, настрое́нию*); 4) подводи́ть ито́г, сумми́ровать, резюми́ровать.

résumé ['rezjuːmeɪ] *n* ито́г; сво́дка; резюме́.

resumption [rɪ'zʌmpʃən] *n* 1) возобновле́ние; продолже́ние (*по́сле переры́ва*); the ~ of hostilities возобновле́ние вое́нных де́йствий; 2) возвраще́ние (*к чему́-л.*); the ~ of duties возвраще́ние к исполне́нию обя́занностей; 3) получе́ние обра́тно.

resumptive [rɪ'zʌmptɪv] *a* сумми́рующий, обобща́ющий.

resurgent [rɪ'səːdʒənt] *a* 1) возрожда́ющийся (*о наде́жде, чу́встве*); 2) оправля́ющийся, ожива́ющий.

resurrect [ˌrezə'rekt] *v* *разг.* 1) воскреса́ть; 2) воскреша́ть (*обы́чай и т. п.*); 3) выка́пывать (*из моги́лы, из-под земли́*).

resurrection [ˌrezə'rekʃən] *n* 1) воскресе́ние (*из мёртвых*); 2) воскреше́ние, восстановле́ние (*обы́чая и т. п.*); 3) выка́пывание (*тру́пов*).

resuscitate [rɪ'sʌsɪteɪt] *v* 1) воскреша́ть, оживля́ть; приводи́ть в чу́вство; 2) воскреса́ть.

retail[a] **I** ['riːteɪl] *n* 1) ро́зничная прода́жа; by ~ в ро́зницу; 2) *attr* ро́зничный.

retail[a] **II** *adv* в ро́зницу.

retail[b] **II** [riː'teɪl] *v* 1) продава́ть(ся) в ро́зницу; 2) переска́зывать, повторя́ть (*слу́хи, но́вости*).

retailer [riː'teɪlə] *n* 1) ро́зничный торго́вец, ла́вочник; 2) болту́н, спле́тник.

retain [rɪ'teɪn] *v* 1) уде́рживать, подпира́ть; 2) сохраня́ть; 3) по́мнить; 4) нанима́ть за определённую пла́ту (*обы́кн. адвока́та*).

retainer [rɪ'teɪnə] *n* 1) *ист.* слуга́; васса́л; *перен.* приве́рженец; 2) предвари́тельный гонора́р адвока́ту.

retaliate [rɪ'tælɪeɪt] *v* 1) отпла́чивать, отвеча́ть тем же; 2) предъявля́ть встре́чное обвине́ние; 3) *эк.* применя́ть репресса́лии.

retaliation [rɪˌtælɪ'eɪʃən] *n* отпла́та, воздая́ние, возме́здие.

retaliatory [rɪ'tælɪətərɪ] *a* отве́тный.

retard [rɪ'tɑːd] *v* 1) замедля́ть, заде́рживать; тормози́ть (*разви́тие и т. п.*); 2) запа́здывать, отстава́ть.

retardation [ˌriːtɑː'deɪʃən] *n* 1) замедле́ние, заде́ржка; поме́ха, препя́тствие; 2) запа́здывание, отстава́ние.

retch [riːtʃ] *v* рыга́ть; ту́житься (*при рво́те*).

retention [rɪ'tenʃən] *n* 1) уде́рживание; сохране́ние; 2) заде́ржка (*мочи́*).

retentive [rɪ'tentɪv] *a* 1) (хорошо́) уде́рживающий, сохраня́ющий; 2) хоро́ший (*о памяти*).

reticence ['retɪsəns] *n* 1) сде́ржанность, скры́тность; молчали́вость; 2) ума́лчивание.

reticent ['retɪsənt] *a* сде́ржанный, скры́тный; молчали́вый.

reticulate [rɪ'tɪkjulɪt] *a* се́тчатый.

reticule ['retɪkjuːl] *n* да́мская су́мочка.

retina ['retɪnə] *n* сетча́тка (*глаза*).

retinue ['retɪnjuː] *n* сви́та.

retire [rɪ'taɪə] *v* 1) уходи́ть, удаля́ться; 2) уходи́ть в отста́вку; 3) уединя́ться; to ~ into oneself уйти́ в себя́; 4) ложи́ться спать (*тж.* to ~ to rest, to bed, for the night); 5) *воен.* отходи́ть, отступа́ть; отводи́ть наза́д; 6) увольня́ть(ся); 7) *эк.* изыма́ть из обраще́ния.

retired [rɪ'taɪəd] *a* 1) отставно́й, в отста́вке; 2) уединённый; скры́тый; 3) за́мкнутый, скры́тный.

retirement [rɪ'taɪəmənt] *n* 1) отста́вка; ухо́д с рабо́ты; 2) уедине́ние; уединённая жизнь; 3) *воен.* отхо́д, отступле́ние.

retiring [rɪ'taɪərɪŋ] *a* 1) сде́ржанный; скро́мный, засте́нчивый; 2) скло́нный к уедине́нию.

retiring-room [rɪ'taɪərɪŋrum] *n* убо́рная.

retort[1] I [rɪ'tɔːt] *n* возраже́ние; остроу́мная ре́плика.

retort[1] II *v* 1) (ре́зко) возража́ть; пари́ровать; 2) отвеча́ть тем же; бить проти́вника его́ же ору́жием.

retort[2] I *n хим.* рето́рта.

retort[2] II *v хим.* перегоня́ть.

retouch I ['riːtʌtʃ] *n* ре́тушь, ретуши́рование.

retouch I *v* ретуши́ровать; подправля́ть (*карти́ну и т. п.*).

retrace [rɪ'treɪs] *v* 1) проследи́ть (*тече́ние, ход чего́-л. до нача́ла, исто́чника*); восстанови́ть в па́мяти; 2) возвраща́ться (по про́йденному пути́).

retract [rɪ'trækt] *v* 1) втя́гивать (*ко́гти и т. п.*); оття́гивать, отводи́ть наза́д; 2) брать обра́тно (*слова́ и т. п.*); отменя́ть; отрека́ться, отпира́ться.

retraction [rɪ'trækʃən] *n* 1) втя́гивание (*ко́гтей и т. п.*); отведе́ние наза́д; сокраще́ние, сжа́тие; 2) отрече́ние, отка́з (*от свои́х слов и т. п.*).

retreat I [rɪ'triːt] *n* 1) отступле́ние; отхо́д; 2) сигна́л к отступле́нию; отбо́й; to sound a ~ бить отбо́й; to beat a ~ *перен.* бить отбо́й, отступа́ть; 3) уединённое ме́сто; убе́жище, приста́нище; 4) уедине́ние.

retreat II *v* 1) отступа́ть, отходи́ть; 2) удаля́ться; 3) уступа́ть.

retrench [rɪ'trentʃ] *v* сокраща́ть, уре́зывать.

retrenchment [rɪ'trentʃmənt] *n* сокраще́ние расхо́дов.

retrial ['riːtraɪəl] *n* пересмо́тр суде́бного де́ла.

retribution [ˌretrɪ'bjuːʃən] *n* заслу́женное наказа́ние, возме́здие.

retributive [rɪ'trɪbjutɪv] *a* кара́ющий, кара́тельный.

retrievable [rɪ'triːvəbl] *a* восстанови́мый; поправи́мый.

retrieval [rɪ'triːvəl] *n* 1) возвраще́ние; 2) восстановле́ние; выздоровле́ние.

retrieve I [rɪ'triːv] *v* 1) находи́ть (*поте́рянное*); возвраща́ть (*себе́*); обрета́ть (*вновь*); 2) восстана́вливать, поправля́ть (*дела́ и т. п.*); 3) исправ-

ля́ть (*оши́бку*); спаса́ть (*положе́ние*); 4) находи́ть и приноси́ть (*дичь — о соба́ке*).

retrieve II *n*: beyond ~, past ~ безвозвра́тно; непоправи́мо.

retriever [rɪ'triːvə] *n* охо́тничья соба́ка.

retroaction [ˌretrou'ækʃən] *n* обра́тное де́йствие.

retroactive [ˌretrou'æktɪv] *см.* retrospective.

retrograde I ['retrougreɪd] *a* 1) напра́вленный наза́д; *воен.* отступа́тельный; 2) реакцио́нный.

retrograde II *v* 1) отступа́ть, отходи́ть; 2) регресси́ровать.

retrogression [ˌretrou'greʃən] *n* 1) обра́тное движе́ние; 2) регре́сс; упа́док.

retrogressive [ˌretrou'gresɪv] *a* 1) возвраща́ющийся обра́тно; 2) регресси́рующий.

retro-rocket ['retrou'rɔkɪt] *n* тормозна́я раке́та.

retrospect ['retrouspekt] *n* взгляд наза́д, в про́шлое; in ~ ретроспекти́вно.

retrospective [ˌretrou'spektɪv] *a* 1) ретроспекти́вный; 2) относя́щийся к про́шлому; 3) *юр.* име́ющий обра́тную си́лу.

return I [rɪ'tən] *n* 1) возвраще́ние; обра́тный путь; by ~ (of post) обра́тной по́чтой; 2) возвра́т, отда́ча; *перен.* отпла́та, воздая́ние; in ~ в обме́н, в опла́ту; 3) дохо́д, при́быль (*от чего́-л.*); оборо́т (*капита́ла*); 4) отчёт; (отчётные) све́дения; popular vote ~ результа́ты о́бщего голосова́ния (*избира́телей*); 5) возвраще́ние, отве́т; 6) *attr* обра́тный; 7) *attr* отве́тный; в отве́т; many happy ~s (of the day)! ≅ поздравля́ю с днём рожде́ния!

return II *v* 1) возвраща́ться, идти́ обра́тно; 2) повторя́ться (*о при́ступе боле́зни*); возвраща́ться (*к те́ме и т. п.*); 3) отвеча́ть, возража́ть; 4) возвраща́ть, отдава́ть, отпла́чивать; отвеча́ть (*чем-л. на что-л.*); 5) дава́ть отчёт, докла́дывать; 6) избира́ть (*в парла́мент*); 7) приноси́ть (*дохо́д, при́быль*).

returnee [ˌrɪtəː'niː] *n* возвраща́ющийся в часть (*по́сле госпита́ля*); (вновь) при́званный на действи́тельную слу́жбу.

reunion ['riː'juːnjən] *n* 1) воссоедине́ние; 2) о́бщая встре́ча; a family ~ сбор всей семьи́.

reunite ['riːjuː'naɪt] *v* 1) воссоединя́ть(ся); 2) собира́ться вме́сте, встреча́ться.

rev I [rev] *n разг.* оборо́т.

rev II *v разг.* враща́ть(ся); верте́ть(ся); □ to ~ **up** увели́чивать ско́рость, число́ оборо́тов.

revamp [rɪ'væmp] *v амер.* починя́ть, поправля́ть, ремонти́ровать.

reveal [rɪ'viːl] *v* 1) пока́зывать, обнару́живать; 2) открыва́ть, разоблача́ть; выдава́ть (*секре́т*).

reveille [rɪ'vælɪ] *n воен.* побу́дка; у́тренняя заря́.

revel I ['revl] *n* 1) (бу́йное) весе́лье; 2) *pl* пиру́шка.

revel II *v* 1) пирова́ть, кути́ть; 2) весели́ться; 3) наслажда́ться (*чем-л.— in*).

revelation [ˌrevɪ'leɪʃən] *n* 1) откры́тие, обнаруже́ние; 2) открове́ние.

revelry ['revlrɪ] *n* бу́йное весе́лье; разгу́л.

revenge I [rɪ'vendʒ] *n* 1) месть, мще́ние; to take (one's) ~ on smb. отомсти́ть кому́-л.; in ~ в отме́стку; 2) рева́нш; to give smb. his ~ дать возмо́жность отыгра́ться.

revenge II *v* мстить; to ~ oneself on smb. отомстить кому-л.

revengeful [rɪ'vendʒful] *a* мстительный.

revenger [rɪ'vendʒə] *n* мститель.

revenge-seeker [rɪ'vendʒ'si:kə] *n* реваншист.

revenue ['revɪnju:] *n* 1) (годовой) доход; государственный доход; 2) *pl* доходные статьи; 3) департамент налогов и сборов.

reverberate [rɪ'və:bəreɪt] *v* 1) отражать(ся); отдаваться (*о звуке*); 2) *тех.* плавить (*в отражательной печи*).

reverberation [rɪ,və:bə'reɪʃən] *n* 1) отражение; 2) эхо, отзвук.

revere [rɪ'vɪə] *v* чтить, уважать; благоговеть.

reverence I ['revərəns] *n* 1) почтение, уважение; благоговение; 2) низкий поклон; 3) *уст., шутл.*: your ~ ваше преподобие (*обращение к священнику*).

reverence II *v* почитать, чтить.

reverend ['revərənd] *a* 1) почтенный, уважаемый; 2) (R.) преподобный (*как обращение к священнику*).

reverent ['revərənt] *a* почтительный; благоговейный.

reverential [,revə'renʃəl] *см.* reverent.

reverie ['revərɪ] *n* 1) мечты; to be lost in ~ мечтать; 2) мечтание; 3) *муз.* фантазия.

reversal [rɪ'və:səl] *n* 1) изменение; перемена (*места, направления*); перестановка (*в обратном порядке*); 2) отмена, уничтожение.

reverse I [rɪ'və:s] *n* 1) противоположное, обратное; quite the ~ полная противоположность; 2) обратная сторона; the ~ of the medal оборотная сторона медали (*тж. перен.*); 3) перемена к худшему; превратности (*судьбы*); неудача; *воен.* поражение; to have (*или* to sustain) a ~ потерпеть поражение; 4) задний *или* обратный ход; in ~, on the ~ задним ходом.

reverse II *a* обратный; противоположный; on the ~ side на обороте.

reverse III *v* 1) поворачивать (*в обратную сторону*); выворачивать (*наизнанку*); переворачивать; 2) менять направление (*движения, вращения*); давать обратный *или* задний ход; 3) опрокидывать; 4) отменять, аннулировать.

reversible [rɪ'və:səbl] *a* 1) обратимый; 2) двусторонний (*о ткани*).

reversion [rɪ'və:ʃən] *n* 1) возвращение (*к прежнему состоянию*); 2) *юр.* обратный переход имущественных прав к первоначальному собственнику; 3) *биол.* атавизм.

revert [rɪ'və:t] *v* 1) возвращаться (*к прежнему состоянию и т. п.*); to ~ to the ranks быть разжалованным в рядовые; 2) возвращаться к прежнему владельцу.

revery ['revərɪ] *см.* reverie.

revet [rɪ'vet] *v тех.* облицовывать.

revetment [rɪ'vetmənt] *n* облицовка.

review I [rɪ'vju:] *n* 1) рассмотрение; обзор; обозрение; to come under ~ подвергаться рассмотрению, изучению; 2) просмотр; проверка; 3) рецензия; критическая статья; 4) периодический журнал; 5) *воен.* смотр, парад; 6) пересмотр (*судебного дела, своих позиций*).

review II *v* 1) обозревать; 2) (снова) просматривать; проверять; 3) делать обзор; рецензиро-

вать; 4) *воен.* делать смотр, принимать парад; 5) пересматривать (*судебное дело, свои позиции*).

reviewer [rɪ'vju:ə] *n* обозреватель; рецензент.

revile [rɪ'vaɪl] *v* ругать(ся).

revise I [rɪ'vaɪz] *n* вторая корректура; сверка.

revise II *v* 1) проверять и исправлять; 2) менять, пересматривать (*убеждения и т. п.*); перерабатывать.

reviser [rɪ'vaɪzə] *n* ревизионный корректор.

revision [rɪ'vɪʒən] *n* 1) пересмотр; осмотр; ревизия; 2) просмотренное и исправленное издание.

revisionism [rɪ'vɪʒənɪzəm] *n полит.* ревизионизм.

revisory [rɪ'vaɪzərɪ] *a* ревизионный.

revival [rɪ'vaɪvəl] *n* 1) возрождение; оживление; 2) возобновление (*постановки и т. п.*); восстановление.

revive [rɪ'vaɪv] *v* 1) приходить *или* приводить в чувство; 2) оживать, воскресать (*о надеждах и т. п.*); 3) оживлять, возрождать; восстанавливать (*обычай, моду*); возобновлять (*постановку и т. п.*).

revivify [ri:'vɪvɪfaɪ] *v* оживлять.

revocable ['revəkəbl] *a* подлежащий отмене.

revocation [,revə'keɪʃən] *n* отмена, аннулирование.

revoke [rɪ'vouk] *v* 1) отменять (*закон*); 2) брать назад (*обещание*).

revolt I [rɪ'voult] *n* 1) восстание; мятеж; in ~ охваченный восстанием; 2) *уст.* отвращение.

revolt II *v* 1) восставать, поднимать восстание; 2) отворачиваться с возмущением *или* отвращением; 3) возмущать, отталкивать.

revolting [rɪ'voultɪŋ] *a* отвратительный, отталкивающий.

revoluble [rɪ'vɔljubl] *a* вращающийся.

revolution[1] [,revə'lu:ʃən] *n* 1) революция; the Great October Socialist Revolution Великая Октябрьская социалистическая революция; 2) переворот; industrial ~ промышленный переворот.

revolution[2] *n* 1) вращение; 2) оборот; ~s per minute число оборотов в минуту; 3): the ~ of the seasons смена времён года.

revolutionary I [,revə'lu:ʃnərɪ] *n* революционер.

revolutionary II *a* революционный.

revolutionism [,revə'lu:ʃnɪzəm] *n* революционность.

revolutionist [,revə'lu:ʃnɪst] *n* революционер.

revolutionize [,revə'lu:ʃnaɪz] *v* 1) революционизировать; 2) производить коренную ломку.

revolve [rɪ'vɔlv] *v* 1) вращать(ся); вертеться (*о колёсах и т. п.*); 2) периодически сменяться (*о временах года*); 3) обдумывать, обмозговывать.

revolver [rɪ'vɔlvə] *n* 1) револьвер; 2) *тех.* барабан.

revolving [rɪ'vɔlvɪŋ] *a* 1) вращающийся; поворотный; 2) обращающийся (*о суммах*).

revue [rɪ'vju:] *n театр.* эстрадное обозрение, ревю.

revulsion [rɪ'vʌlʃən] *n* 1) внезапное резкое изменение (*чувств и т. п.*); to undergo a ~ резко измениться; 2) отвращение; 3) *мед.* отвлечение боли.

reward I [rɪ'wɔ:d] *n* 1) награда; награждение; as a ~ for в награду за; 2) вознаграждение; воздаяние.

reward II *v* 1) награждáть; 2) воздавáть; вознаграждáть.

rewarding [rɪˈwɔːdɪŋ] *a* стóящий; is it so ~ (to be, to do etc)? так ли хорошó, стóит ли (это дéлать и т. п.)?

reword [riːˈwəːd] *v* 1) вýразить другúми словáми или в другóй фóрме; 2) повторúть.

rewrite [riːˈraɪt] *v* (past rewrote; p. p. rewritten) переписáть.

rewritten [ˈriːˈrɪtn] *p. p. см.* rewrite.

rewrote [ˈriːˈrout] *past. см.* rewrite.

Reynard [ˈrenəd, ˈreɪnɑːd] *n* Лисá (в фольклóре).

rhapsody [ˈræpsədɪ] *n* 1) рапсóдия; 2) востóрженное выскáзывание, напыщенная речь; to go into rhapsodies over smth. восхищáться чем-л.

rheostat [ˈriːoustæt] *n эл.* реостáт.

rhetoric [ˈretərɪk] *n* ритóрика.

rhetorical [rɪˈtɔrɪkəl] *a* риторúческий.

rheumatic I [ruːˈmætɪk] *n* 1) ревмáтик; 2) *pl разг.* ревматúзм.

rheumatic II *a* ревматúческий.

rheumatism [ˈruːmətɪzəm] *n* ревматúзм.

rhino [ˈraɪnou] *n разг.* 1) носорóг; 2) автомобúль-амфúбия.

rhinoceros [raɪˈnɔsərəs] *n* носорóг.

rhomb [rɔm] *n* ромб.

rhombic [ˈrɔmbɪk] *a* ромбúческий.

rhombus [ˈrɔmbəs] *n* ромб.

rhubarb [ˈruːbɑːb] *n* ревéнь.

rhumb [rʌm] *n мор.* румб.

rhyme I [raɪm] *n* 1) рúфма; double (*или* female, feminine) ~ жéнская рúфма; single (*или* male, masculine) ~ мужскáя рúфма; 2) рифмóванные стихú; ◊ neither ~ nor reason ни склáду ни лáду; without ~ or reason без всякого смысла.

rhyme II *v* 1) рифмовáть(ся); 2) писáть рифмóванные стихú.

rhymed [raɪmd] *a* рифмóванный.

rhymer [ˈraɪmə] *n* рифмоплёт.

rhymester [ˈraɪmstə] *см.* rhymer.

rhythm [ˈrɪðəm] *n* 1) ритм; 2) размéр (стихá).

rhythmic(al) [ˈrɪðmɪk(əl)] *a* ритмúческий; ритмúчный, мéрный.

rib [rɪb] *n* 1) ребрó; short (*или* false, floating) ~ лóжное ребрó; 2) *шутл.* женá; 3) (óстрый) край, ребрó (чего-л.); 4) рýбчик (на ткáни); 5) *тех.* флáнец, бýртик; 6) жúлка (листá); 7) *ав.* нервюра; 8) *мор.* шпангóут.

ribald I [ˈrɪbəld] *n* грубиян; сквернослóв.

ribald II *a* грýбый, неприлúчный, непристóйный.

ribaldry [ˈrɪbəldrɪ] *n* сквернослóвие; непристóйное поведéние.

riband I, II [ˈrɪbənd] *см.* ribbon I, II.

ribbed [rɪbd] *a* ребрúстый; рифлёный, с насéчкой.

ribbon I [ˈrɪbən] *n* 1) лéнта; ýзкая полосá; typewriter ~ лéнта для пúшущей машúнки; 2) *pl* клóчья; ~s of mist клóчья тумáна; torn to ~s разóрванный в клóчья; 3) *pl* вóжжи; to handle (*или* to take) the ~s прáвить; 4) *attr* лéнточный; из лéнт(ы).

ribbon II *v* украшáть лéнтами.

rice [raɪs] *n* 1) рис; 2) *attr* рúсовый.

rice-paper [ˈraɪsˌpeɪpə] *n* рúсовая бумáга.

rice-water [ˈraɪsˌwɔːtə] *n* рúсовый отвáр.

rich I [rɪtʃ] *a* 1) богáтый (чем-л. — in); 2) обúльный, изобúлующий; 3) плодорóдный (о пóчве); 4) жúрный; сдóбный; густóй (о молокé); 5) цéнный (о мысли, предложéнии); 6) густóй, сóчный, яркий (о крáсках); густóй, глубóкий (о гóлосе, тóне).

rich II *n*: the ~ (*употр. как pl*) богачú, богáтые.

riches [ˈrɪtʃɪz] *n pl* 1) богáтство; 2) обúлие.

richly [ˈrɪtʃlɪ] *adv* 1) богáто, роскóшно; 2) вполнé, основáтельно; пóлностью (заслужúть, отплатúть и т. п.).

richness [ˈrɪtʃnɪs] *n* 1) богáтство (чего-л.); 2) плодорóдие (пóчвы); 3) яркость (крáсок, впечатлéний); 4) жúрность, сóчность (пúщи).

rick I [rɪk] *n* стог.

rick II *v* склáдывать в стог.

rickets [ˈrɪkɪts] *n мед.* рахúт.

rickety [ˈrɪkɪtɪ] *a* 1) рахитúчный; слáбый (о здорóвье); 2) шáткий, неустóйчивый (о мéбели); непрóчный.

rickshaw [ˈrɪkʃɔː] *n* рúкша.

ricochet I [ˈrɪkəʃet] *n* рикошéт.

ricochet II бить рикошéтом.

rid [rɪd] *v* (past, p. p. rid, ridded) освобождáть, избавлять (от чего-л. — of); to get ~ of избавляться, отдéлываться от чего-л., когó-л.

riddance [ˈrɪdəns] *n* избавлéние (от чего-л., когó-л.); устранéние; to make a good ~ счáстливо избáвиться, отдéлаться.

ridden [ˈrɪdn] *p. p. см.* ride II.

-ridden [-rɪdn] *в сложных словáх означáет* под влáстью чего-л.; одержúмый чем-л.; fear-ridden охвáченный стрáхом.

riddle[1] I [ˈrɪdl] *n* загáдка; to read (*или* to solve) a ~ разгадáть загáдку.

riddle[1] II *v* 1) говорúть загáдками; 2) отгáдывать (загáдки); разгáдывать.

riddle[2] I *n* 1) решетó, сúто, грóхот; 2) экрáн, щит.

riddle[2] II *v* 1) просéивать; *перен.* проверять прáвильность (доказáтельств и т. п.); 2) изрешетúть (пýлями); 3) забрáсывать вопрóсами, возражéниями.

ride I [raɪd] *n* 1) прогýлка (верхóм, на велосипéде); to give smb. a ~ прокатúть когó-л.; to have a ~, to go for a ~ прокатúться; 2) ездá, поéздка; to steal a ~ проéхать зáйцем; 3) дорóга (для катáния, езды).

ride II *v* (past rode; p. p. ridden) 1) éхать верхóм; 2) сидéть верхóм (на чём-л.); 3) éхать (в поéзде, автомобúле и т. п.); 4) плыть; скользúть (по волнáм); нестúсь; to ~ at anchor стоять на якоре; 5) управлять (особ. жестóко); 6) угнетáть; обуревáть, овладевáть; □ to ~ at направлять на; to ~ down a) нагнáть, догнáть когó-л. верхóм; б) сшибúть с ног, задавúть; to ~ out благополýчно перенестú (шторм — о корáбле); ◊ to ~ for a fall a) нестúсь во весь опóр; б) дéйствовать безрассýдно, опромéтчиво.

rider [ˈraɪdə] *n* 1) всáдник; наéздник; 2) дополнéние, попрáвка (к докумéнту и т. п.).

riderless [ˈraɪdəlɪs] *a* без всáдника.

ridge I [rɪdʒ] *n* 1) грéбень горы; гóрный хребéт; 2) конёк (крыши); 3) бороздá, грéбень борозды; грядка; 4) рýбчик (на матéрии); тóлстая крóмка; край, ребрó.

ridge II v образо́вывать бо́розды *или* скла́дки; морщи́ть; топо́рщить(ся).

ridged [rɪdʒd] a остроконе́чный.

ridicule I [ˈrɪdɪkjuːl] n насме́шка, осмея́ние; to hold up to ~ де́лать посме́шищем, высме́ивать.

ridicule II v высме́ивать, поднима́ть на́ смех.

ridiculous [rɪˈdɪkjuləs] a смешно́й, смехотво́рный, неле́пый.

riding [ˈraɪdɪŋ] n верхова́я езда́.

riding-breeches [ˈraɪdɪŋˌbrɪtʃɪz] n pl бри́джи для верхово́й езды́.

riding-habit [ˈraɪdɪŋˌhæbɪt] n амазо́нка (*же́нский костюм для верховой езды*).

riding-hag [ˈraɪdɪŋhæg] n разг. кошма́р.

rife [raɪf] a predic 1) ча́стый, обы́чный; распространённый; to be (*или* to grow, to wax) ~ станови́ться обы́чным; 2) по́лный (*чего-л.*), изоби́лующий; ~ with rumours по́лный слу́хов.

riffle [ˈrɪfl] n 1) тех. желобо́к, кана́вка; 2) амер. стремни́на.

riff-raff I [ˈrɪfræf] n отбро́сы, подо́нки.

riff-raff II a разг. никчёмный, никуда́ не го́дный.

rifle[1] I [ˈraɪfl] n 1) винто́вка; 2) pl воен. стрелки́, стрелко́вая часть; 3) attr руже́йный, винто́вочный; стрелко́вый.

rifle[1] II v 1) нареза́ть кана́л ствола́ (*винтовки и т. п.*); 2) стреля́ть из винто́вки.

rifle[2] v 1) гра́бить, красть; 2) обдира́ть (*кору и т. п.*).

rifleman [ˈraɪflmən] n стрело́к.

rifle-range [ˈraɪflreɪndʒ] n 1) тир, стре́льбище; 2) см. rifle-shot 3).

rifle-shot [ˈraɪflʃɔt] n 1) вы́стрел из винто́вки; 2) (хоро́ший) стрело́к из винто́вки; 3) да́льность (руже́йного) вы́стрела.

rifling [ˈraɪflɪŋ] n наре́зка (*в стволе оружия*).

rift I [rɪft] n 1) тре́щина; щель; рассе́лина; разры́в; a ~ in the clouds просве́т ме́жду ту́чами; 2) уще́лье; ◊ a ~ in the lute нача́ло разла́да, «тре́щинка».

rift II v раска́лывать(ся), расщепля́ть(ся).

rig[1] I [rɪg] n 1) снаряже́ние; осна́стка; сна́сти; 2) разг. оде́жда; наря́д; вне́шний вид; 3) экипа́ж, вы́езд; 4) с.-х. борозда́.

rig[1] II v снаряжа́ть; оснаща́ть; □ to ~ **out** а) снаряжа́ть; б) наряжа́ть; ~ged out разоде́тый; to ~ **up** а) см. to ~ out; б) снаряжа́ть *или* стро́ить на́спех.

rig[2] I n проде́лка; прока́за; to run the ~ прока́зничать; to run the ~ upon smb. сыгра́ть с кем-л. шу́тку.

rig[2] II v прока́зничать; выки́дывать шту́ки; 2): to ~ the market иску́сственно повыша́ть *или* понижа́ть це́ны.

rigger [ˈrɪgə] n авиамеха́ник.

rigging [ˈrɪgɪŋ] n 1) мор. снаряже́ние, сна́сти; 2) разг. пла́тья, «тря́пки».

right[1] I [raɪt] n 1) пра́во; справедли́вое тре́бование (to); to demand (*или* to maintain) one's ~, to stand upon one's ~ отста́ивать свои́ права́; to reserve the ~ сохраня́ть за собо́й пра́во; ~s and duties права́ и обя́занности; by ~ of по пра́ву (*чего-л.*); to be in the ~ быть пра́вым; 2) справедли́вость; пра́вильность; to do smb. ~ отдава́ть

кому́-л. до́лжное, справедли́вость; 3) pl и́стинное положе́ние, действи́тельные фа́кты; ◊ to set (*или* to put) smth. to ~s навести́ поря́док, привести́ в поря́док.

right[1] II a 1) пра́вый; пра́вильный; ве́рный; справедли́вый; to do what is ~ поступа́ть справедли́во; to be ~ быть пра́вым; to put ~ исправля́ть; to put one ~ with smb. оправда́ть кого́-л. в чьих-л. глаза́х; 2) подходя́щий; надлежа́щий; the ~ book та кни́га, кото́рая нужна́; the ~ man (for) подходя́щий челове́к; как раз тот челове́к, кото́рый ну́жен; not the ~ man не тот (челове́к) (*который нужен, который подразумевается*); 3) лицево́й (*о стороне ткани*); 4) уме́стный; 5) здоро́вый; испра́вный; в хоро́шем состоя́нии, в поря́дке; to feel all ~ чу́вствовать себя́ хорошо́; to look all ~ вы́глядеть хорошо́, быть здоро́вым; 6) прямо́й (*о линии, угле*).

right[1] III v 1) выпрямля́ть(ся); выправля́ть; 2) исправля́ть(ся); to ~ oneself реабилити́ровать себя́.

right[1] IV adv 1) пра́вильно; справедли́во; надлежа́щим *или* до́лжным о́бразом; 2) пря́мо; ~ along не остана́вливаясь, неукло́нно; ~ on пря́мо вперёд; 3) то́чно, как раз; ~ in the middle то́чно на середи́не; ~ opposite как раз *или* пря́мо напро́тив; ~ now сейча́с же, то́тчас же, в э́тот моме́нт; ~ in the eye, ~ in the face пря́мо в глаза́, в лицо́; 4) о́чень.

right[2] I n 1) пра́вая сторона́; пра́вая рука́; to keep to the ~ держа́ться пра́вой стороны́; to the ~ напра́во (*куда*); on the ~ напра́во (*где*); (the Rights) pl полит. пра́вые.

right[2] II a 1) пра́вый (*о руке, стороне*); 2) полит. пра́вый, консервати́вный.

right[2] III adv напра́во; ~ and left во все сто́роны.

right-about [ˈraɪtəbaut] n: to send (to the) ~ (*или* ~s) прогна́ть, вы́проводить.

right-angled [ˈraɪtˌæŋgld] a прямоуго́льный.

right-down [ˈraɪtdaun] a разг. соверше́нный; отъя́вленный.

righteous [ˈraɪtʃəs] a 1) справедли́вый; 2) пра́ведный.

rightful [ˈraɪtful] a 1) зако́нный; 2) справедли́вый; 3) принадлежа́щий по пра́ву.

right-hand [ˈraɪthænd] a пра́вый, находя́щийся спра́ва.

right-hander [ˈraɪtˈhændə] n разг. уда́р пра́вой руко́й.

rightly [ˈraɪtlɪ] adv 1) пра́вильно; 2) справедли́во; 3) ве́рно; до́лжным о́бразом.

rigid [ˈrɪdʒɪd] a 1) жёсткий; негну́щийся; твёрдый; 2) стро́гий (*о правиле, режиме и т. п.*); 3) непрекло́нный; сто́йкий.

rigidity [rɪˈdʒɪdɪtɪ] n 1) жёсткость; твёрдость; 2) стро́гость; 3) сто́йкость, непрекло́нность.

rigmarole [ˈrɪgməroul] n 1) болтовня́, вздор; 2) attr вздо́рный, бессвя́зный.

rigor[a] [ˈraɪgɔː] n 1) озно́б.

rigor[b] амер. см. rigour.

rigorism [ˈrɪgərɪzəm] n стро́гость, ригори́зм.

rigorous [ˈrɪgərəs] a 1) стро́гий; 2) то́чный; 3) суро́вый (*о климате, погоде и т. п.*).

rigour [ˈrɪgə] n 1) стро́гость; 2) суро́вость (*зимы, климата и т. п.*).

rile [raɪl] *v разг.* 1) мутить (*воду и т. п.*); 2) сердить, раздражать.

rill [rɪl] *n* ручеёк.

rim I [rɪm] *n* ободок, край; кайма; обод (*колеса*); кольцо, круг.

rim II *v* 1) окаймлять, окружать; 2) снабжать ободом.

rime¹ I, II [raɪm] *см.* rhyme I, II.

rime² I *n обыкн. поэт.* иней; изморозь.

rime² II *обыкн. поэт.* покрывать инеем.

rimer [ˈraɪmə] *см.* reamer.

rimless [ˈrɪmlɪs] *a* без обода, без оправы.

-rimmed [-rɪmd] *в сложных словах* в оправе; gold-rimmed в золотой оправе.

rimy [ˈraɪmɪ] *a* покрытый инеем, заиндевевший.

rind [raɪnd] *n* 1) кожура; кора; 2) корка.

ring¹ [rɪŋ] *n* 1) кольцо; ободок; обруч; круг; wedding ~ обручальное кольцо; ~s of tree годичные кольца (*дерева*); livid ~s синие круги (*под глазами*); ~s of smoke клубы дыма; split ~ разрезное кольцо (для ключей); 2) арена (*тж.* circus ~); площадка (*для борьбы*), ринг; 3) объединение торговцев для контроля над рынком; 4) клика; 5) шайка, банда; ◊ to make ~s round smb. превзойти, опередить, обогнать кого-л.

ring² I *n* 1) звон; 2) звонок; to give a ~ позвонить; loud ~ громкий звонок; 3) звук; the ~ of one's voice звук голоса; to have the ~ of truth звучать правдиво; ◊ to have the true ~ быть настоящим, подлинным.

ring² II *v* (*past* rang, rung; *p. p.* rung) 1) звенеть; звучать; оглашаться (*звуками*); раздаваться (*о звуке*); to ~ true (false) звучать искренне (фальшиво); 2) звонить; □ to ~ for вызывать звонком; to ~ in вводить, представлять (*кого-л.*); to ~ off давать отбой (*по телефону*); to ~ up звонить, вызывать по телефону.

ring-dove [ˈrɪŋdʌv] *n* вяхирь (*голубь*).

ringer [ˈrɪŋə] *n* 1) звонок; 2) тот, кто звонит; 3) звонарь; 4) *разг.* первоклассная вещь.

ring-fence [ˈrɪŋfens] *n* ограда.

ringing I [ˈrɪŋɪŋ] *n* 1) звон; трезвон; 2) вызов.

ringing II *a* 1) звонкий, звучный, громкий; 2) трескучий (*о морозе*).

ringleader [ˈrɪŋˌliːdə] *n* главарь, зачинщик, вожак.

ringlet [ˈrɪŋlɪt] *n* 1) колечко; 2) локон.

ring-mail [ˈrɪŋmeɪl] *n* кольчуга.

ringworm [ˈrɪŋwəːm] *n мед.* стригущий лишай.

rink I [rɪŋk] *n* каток.

rink II *v* кататься на роликах.

rinse I [rɪns] *n* полоскание; to give a ~ прополоскать.

rinse II *v* 1) полоскать; промывать; 2) *разг.* запивать. (*еду*).

riot I [ˈraɪət] *n* 1) бунт; 2) нар шение общественного порядка, тишины; 3) раз. л; необузданность; to run ~ а) вести себя буйно; б) свирепствовать (*о болезни*); в) буйно разрастись.

riot II *v* 1) принимать участие в бунте; 2) буйствовать; шуметь; предаваться (*разгулу и т. п.*).

rioter [ˈraɪətə] *n* бунтовщик.

riotous [ˈraɪətəs] *a* буйный; шумный, шумливый.

rip¹ I [rɪp] *n* разрыв, разрез; распоротый шов.

rip¹ II *v* 1) рвать, разрывать, распарывать; 2) рваться, пороться; лопаться; раскалываться; 3) распиливать (*вдоль*); □ to ~ off сдирать, отдирать; to ~ out а) выдирать, вырывать; б) испускать (*крик*); в) отпускать (*ругательство*); to ~ up а) распарывать; вскрывать; б) бередить (*старые раны*); ◊ to let things ~ не вмешиваться (*в ход событий*).

rip² *n* 1) кляча; 2) распутник.

ripe [raɪp] *a* спелый, зрелый; готовый; to be ~ наступить (*о времени*).

ripen [ˈraɪpən] *v* зреть, созревать.

ripeness [ˈraɪpnɪs] *n* 1) зрелость; 2) законченность.

riposte I [rɪˈpoust] *n* ответный выпад (*в фехтовании*); *перен.* ответный удар; находчивый ответ.

riposte II *v* парировать удар.

ripping I [ˈrɪpɪŋ] *a разг.* великолепный, превосходный.

ripping II *adv разг.*: ~ good очень хороший, великолепный.

ripple I [ˈrɪpl] *n* 1) рябь (*на воде*); 2) волнистость (*волос*); 3) журчание.

ripple II *v* 1) покрывать(ся) рябью; рябить; 2) журчать.

ripply [ˈrɪplɪ] *a* 1) покрытый рябью; 2) волнистый.

riprap [ˈrɪpræp] *n* мелкий щебень.

rip-saw [ˈrɪpsɔː] *n* продольная пила.

rise I [raɪz] *n* 1) подъём; повышение; увеличение; the ~ to power приход к власти; to be on the ~ повышаться (*о ценах и т. п.*); *перен.* идти в гору; 2) восход (*солнца*); 3) происхождение, начало; to have (*или* to take) ~ in (*или* from) начинаться с чего-л., иметь началом что-л.; происходить из чего-л.; to give ~ to а) вызывать что-л., давать повод к чему-л.; б) давать начало (*реке*); в) порождать; 4) возвышенность, холм; подъём горы; sharp ~ крутой подъём; a ~ in the road подъём дороги; 5) выход на поверхность; обнаружение; ◊ to get (*или* to take) a ~ out of smb. раздразнить кого-л., вывести кого-л. из себя.

rise II *v* (*past* rose; *p. p.* risen) 1) подниматься, вставать; 2) в(о)сходить (*о солнце*); 3) увеличиваться, возрастать; повышаться (*о ценах и т. п.*); 4) подниматься, подходить (*о тесте*); 5) возвышаться, быть выше (*тж.* to ~ above); 6) приобретать вес (*в обществе*); to ~ in the world преуспевать; 7) восставать; противиться; to ~ in rebellion восстать; to ~ in arms восстать с оружием в руках; 8) брать начало, возникать; 9) выходить на поверхность; □ to ~ to а) достигать, быть равным; б) удовлетворять, отвечать (*требованиям и т. п.*).

risen [ˈrɪzn] *p. p. см.* rise II.

risibility [ˌrɪzɪˈbɪlɪtɪ] *n* смешливость.

risible [ˈrɪzɪbl] *a* 1) смешливый; 2) смешной; смехотворный.

rising I [ˈraɪzɪŋ] *n* 1) вставание; 2) восход (*солнца*); 3) поднятие; повышение; возвышение; 4) восстание.

rising II *a* 1) поднимающийся; возрастающий; подрастающий; 2) преуспевающий; 3) приближающийся (*к определённому возрасту*).

risk I [rɪsk] *n* риск; at the ~ of one's own life с риском для жизни, рискуя жизнью; to run the ~, to run ~s подвергаться риску; рисковать; to take the ~ of рискнуть; there is the ~ of his catching cold он рискует простудиться.

risk II *v* 1) рисковать; to ~ one's health рисковать здоровьем; 2) идти на риск; отваживаться; to ~ failure быть готовым к неудаче.

riskiness ['rɪskɪnɪs] *n* рискованность, опасность.

risky ['rɪskɪ] *a* рискованный, опасный.

rissole ['rɪsoul] *n* пирожок с мясной *или* рыбной начинкой, обжаренный в масле.

rite [raɪt] *n* обряд; ритуал; burial ~s, funeral ~s похоронные обряды; the ~s of hospitality обычаи гостеприимства.

ritual I ['rɪtjuəl] *n* 1) ритуал; 2) *церк.* требник.

ritual II *a* обрядовый; ритуальный.

rival I ['raɪvəl] *n* 1) соперник; конкурент; 2) *воен.* противник.

rival II *a* соперничающий; конкурирующий.

rival III *v* соперничать; конкурировать.

rivalry ['raɪvəlrɪ] *n* соперничество; конкуренция.

rive I [raɪv] *n* трещина; щель.

rive II *v* (*past* rived; *p. p.* rived, riven) раскалывать(ся); расщеплять(ся); разрывать(ся).

riven ['rɪvən] *p. p. см.* rive II.

river ['rɪvə] *n* 1) река; поток; to cross the ~ переправиться через реку; *перен.* преодолеть препятствие; 2) *attr* речной.

river-basin ['rɪvə,beɪsn] *n* бассейн реки.

river-bed ['rɪvə'bed] *n* русло реки.

river-horse ['rɪvəhɔːs] *n* гиппопотам.

riverside ['rɪvəsaɪd] *n* 1) берег (реки); прибрежная полоса; 2) *attr* (находящийся) на берегу, прибрежный.

rivet I [rɪvɪt] *n* заклёпка.

rivet II *v* 1) клепать, заклёпывать; 2) приковывать (*взор, внимание*).

rivulet ['rɪvjulɪt] *n* ручеёк, речушка.

roach¹ [routʃ] *n* плотва.

roach² *n* *амер.* таракан.

road [roud] *n* 1) дорога; путь; on the ~ в дороге, в пути; на пути (*к чему-л.*); to be in the ~, to get in one's ~ стать (кому-л.) поперёк дороги; to take the ~ отправиться в путь; arterial ~ магистраль; dirt ~ грунтовая дорога; country ~ просёлочная дорога; royal ~ to лёгкий путь к чему-л.; 2) улица; to cross the ~ перейти улицу; 3) *pl* *мор.* рейд; 4) *attr* дорожный.

road-bed ['roudbed] *n* полотно дороги.

road-book ['roudbuk] *n* путеводитель.

road-hog ['roudhɔg] *n* «лихач» (*о шофёре*).

road-house ['roudhaus] *n* гостиница, закусочная, буфет (*при дороге*).

road-metal ['roud,metl] *n* щебень.

road-side I ['roudsaɪd] *n* край, обочина дороги.

road-side II *a* придорожный.

roadstead ['roudsted] *n* *мор.* рейд.

roadster ['roudstə] *n* 1) *авто* родстер (*тип кузова*); 2) экипаж для дальних поездок; 3) опытный путешественник.

roadway ['roudweɪ] *n* шоссе; мостовая; проезжая часть дороги.

roam I [roum] *n* странствование; скитание.

roam II *v* бродить; странствовать; скитаться.

roan I [roun] *n* чалая лошадь.

roan II *a* чалый.

roar I [rɔː] *n* 1) рёв, рычание; шум (*ветра*); a ~ (*или* ~s) of laughter взрыв(ы) смеха; 2) грохот.

roar II *v* 1) реветь, орать, рычать; to ~ with laughter хохотать во всё горло; 2) грохотать; 3) бушевать (*о буре*).

roaring I ['rɔːrɪŋ] *n* рёв, шум.

roaring II *a* 1) шумный; буйный; 2) живой; кипучий.

roast I [roust] *n* жареное, жаркое; ◊ to rule the ~ задавать тон; верховодить.

roast II *a* жареный.

roast III *v* 1) жарить(ся); печь(ся); греть(ся); to ~ oneself at the fire греться у огня; 2) *разг.* высмеивать, издеваться; 3) *амер. разг.* бранить; критиковать; 4) *тех.* обжигать; выжигать.

roaster ['roustə] *n* 1) жаровня; *тех.* обжигательная печь; 3) что-л., подходящее для жаренья (*цыплёнок и т. п.*).

roasting-jack ['roustɪŋdʒæk] *n* вертел.

rob [rɔb] *v* 1) обкрадывать, грабить; 2) отнимать; лишать чего-л.

robber ['rɔbə] *n* грабитель, разбойник.

robbery ['rɔbərɪ] *n* грабёж, кража.

robe I [roub] *n* 1) мантия; широкая одежда; the long ~ мантия судьи, адвоката; 2) халат; 3) *амер.* (меховая) полость.

robe II *v* надевать; облачать(ся).

robin ['rɔbɪn] *n* малиновка.

robot ['roubɔt] *n* 1) робот, автомат со сложными функциями; 2) автоматический сигнал уличного движения; 3) *attr* автоматический.

robust [rə'bʌst] *a* 1) здоровый, сильный, крепкий; 2) здравый, ясный (*об уме*).

roc [rɔk] *n* рух (*сказочная птица*).

rock¹ [rɔk] *n* 1) утёс, скала; the Rock Гибралтар; 2) горная порода; 3) *амер.* камень; ◊ (up-) on the ~s ≅ «на мели».

rock² *v* 1) качать(ся); трясти(сь); 2) укачивать, убаюкивать.

rock³ *n* *уст.* прялка.

rock-bottom ['rɔk'bɔtəm] *n* 1) самая низкая точка; основание; 2) *attr разг.* самый низкий (*о цене*).

rocker ['rɔkə] *n* 1) кресло-качалка; 2) качалка (*колыбели*).

rocket I ['rɔkɪt] *n* 1) ракета; braking (crewless, cosmic, high altitude, multistage, sounding) ~ тормозная (непилотируемая, космическая, высотная, многоступенчатая, зондирующая) ракета; carrier ~ ракетоноситель; 2) *сленг* нагоняй; to give smb. a ~ отчитать кого-л. как следует; 3) *attr* ракетный; реактивный.

rocket II *v* 1) взлетать (*как ракета*); 2) пускать ракеты.

rocketry ['rɔkɪtrɪ] *n* ракетная техника.

rock-hewn ['rɔkhjuːn] *a* высеченный из камня.

rocking-chair ['rɔkɪŋtʃeə] *n* кресло-качалка.

rocking-horse ['rɔkɪŋhɔːs] *n* (игрушечная) лошадь-качалка.

rock-oil ['rɔkɔɪl] *n* нефть.

rock-salt ['rɔk'sɔːlt] *n* каменная соль.

rock-tar ['rɔktɑ] *см.* rock-oil.

rocky[1] [ˈrɔkɪ] a 1) скалистый; каменистый; 2) твёрдый; непоколебимый.

rocky[2] a 1) неустойчивый, качающийся (о столе и т. п.); to be ~ качаться; 2) пошатнувшийся (о здоровье, положении).

rod [rɔd] n 1) прут; жезл; стержень; брус; 2) розга; перен. наказание; the ~ порка; to kiss the ~ покорно переносить наказание; to make smb. kiss the ~ заставить просить прощения; принудить к покорности; 3) удочка; 4) мера длины (≅ 5 м); 5) тех. рейка; штанга; 6) амер. сленг револьвер; ◊ to spare the ~ and spoil the child ≅ баловством портить ребёнка.

rode [roud] past см. ride II.

rodent [ˈroudənt] n грызун.

rodeo [rouˈdeiou] n амер. 1) загон для клеймения скота; 2) состязание ковбоев в верховой езде, родео.

roe[1] [rou] n косуля.

roe[2] n икра (рыбья).

roentgen [ˈrɔntjən] n физ. 1) рентген; 2) attr рентгеновский.

rogue [roug] n 1) жулик, мошенник; негодяй; 2) шутл. плутишка, проказник; to play the ~ проказничать.

roguery [ˈrougərɪ] n 1) мошенничество; жульничество; 2) проказы.

roguish [ˈrougɪʃ] a 1) жуликоватый; 2) шаловливый, проказливый.

roil [rɔɪl] v 1) мутить (воду и т. п.); взбалтывать; 2) раздражать; досаждать.

roily [ˈrɔɪlɪ] a мутный.

roister [ˈrɔɪstə] v бесчинствовать.

roistering I [ˈrɔɪstərɪŋ] n бесчинство.

roistering II a шумный; буйный.

role [roul] n 1) роль; 2) функция.

roll I [roul] n 1) свиток; свёрток; рулон; катышек; воен. скатка; 2) список; реестр; ведомость; to call the ~ делать перекличку, вызывать по списку; to be on the ~s быть внесённым в список; состоять в списке; ~ of honour список убитых на войне; 3) булочка; 4) катание; вращение; качка; 5) раскат (грома и т. п.); 6) ролик; цилиндр; 7) походка вразвалку.

roll II [roul] v 1) катить(ся); вертеть(ся); вращать (-ся); 2) катать(ся); 3) свёртывать, скатывать; 4) качаться; волноваться (о море); 5) укатывать (дорогу); 6) прокатывать (металл); 7) раскатывать (тесто); 8) греметь, грохотать (о громе и т. п.); 9) проходить, уходить (о годах и т. п.); □ to ~ **away** а) откатывать(ся); б) рассеиваться (о тумане); to ~ **back** откатывать(ся) назад; to ~ **in** а) сходиться в большом количестве; б) прийти, появиться неожиданно; to ~ **on** лететь (о времени); to ~ **out** раскатывать; to ~ **over** а) перекатывать(ся); б) опрокинуть; to ~ **up** а) свёртывать(ся); завёртывать(ся); to ~ oneself up закутаться, завернуться (во что-л. — in); б) разг. появиться (на сцене); в) разг. появиться внезапно.

roll-call [ˈroulkɔːl] n перекличка.

roll-collar [ˈroul‚kɔlə] n отложной воротничок.

roller [ˈroulə] n 1) ролик; вал; цилиндр; 2) каток (дорожный); 3) волна, бурун; 4) attr тех. роликовый; вальцовый.

roller-skate I [ˈroulə‚skeɪt] n ролики.

roller-skate II v кататься на роликах.

roller-towel [ˈroulə‚tauəl] n полотенце на ролике.

rollick [ˈrɔlik] v веселиться; резвиться.

rolling I [ˈroulɪŋ] n бортовая качка.

rolling II a холмистый.

rolling-mill [ˈroulɪŋmɪl] n тех. прокатный стан.

rolling-pin [ˈroulɪŋpɪn] n скалка.

rolling-stock [ˈroulɪŋstɔk] n ж.-д. подвижной состав.

roly-poly I [ˈroulɪˈpoulɪ] n 1) пудинг с вареньем; 2) «пышка» (о ребёнке).

roly-poly II a пухлый, толстый (о ребёнке).

Romaic I [rouˈmeiɪk] n новогреческий язык.

Romaic II a новогреческий.

Roman I [ˈroumən] n 1) римлянин; 2) католик; 3) прямой светлый шрифт.

Roman II a 1) римский; 2) латинский (об алфавите); 3) католический; 4) прямой светлый (о шрифте).

Romance I [rəˈmæns] n романские языки.

Romance II a романский.

romance I [rəˈmæns] n 1) поэма или роман о рыцарях; рыцарский роман; 2) романтическая история; 3) романтика; 4) выдумка, небылица.

romance II v преувеличивать, сочинять; фантазировать.

romantic I [rəˈmæntɪk] n романтик.

romantic II a романтический; романтичный.

romanticism [rəˈmæntɪsɪzəm] n романтизм.

romanticist [rəˈmæntɪsɪst] n романтик.

Romany I [ˈrɔmənɪ] n 1) цыган; цыганка; the ~ собир. цыгане; 2) цыганский язык.

Romany II a цыганский.

romp I [rɔmp] n 1) шалун, сорванец; 2) шумная игра, возня.

romp II v поднимать возню, возиться.

rompers [ˈrɔmpəz] n pl детский комбинезон.

rood [ruːd] n 1) четверть акра; not a ~ ни клочка земли; 2) уст. распятие, крест.

roof I [ruːf] n 1) крыша, кровля; перен. кров; curb ~, gable ~ двускатная крыша; terraced ~ плоская крыша; the ~ of the world «крыша мира» (о горной цепи); the ~ of the mouth нёбо; under one's ~ в своём доме; 2) ав. абсолютный потолок; 3) горн. кровля, потолок (выработки); 4) империал (дилижанса).

roof II v покрывать (крышей); настилать крышу.

roofer [ˈruːfə] n кровельщик.

roofing [ˈruːfɪŋ] n 1) кровельный материал; кровля; 2) кровельные работы.

roofless [ˈruːflɪs] a 1) не имеющий крыши (о доме); 2) бездомный, не имеющий крова.

rook[1] [ruk] n шахм. ладья.

rook[2] I [ruk] n 1) грач; 2) мошенник, шулер.

rook[2] II v обманывать, мошенничать; нечестно играть (в карты, кости).

rookery [ˈrukərɪ] n 1) грачевник; 2) птичий базар; 3) группа ветхих домишек; трущобы; 4) густонаселённый дом; 5) притон (воровской, игорный).

rookie [ˈrukɪ] n сленг рекрут, новобранец.

rooky [ˈrukɪ] амер. см. rookie.

room I [rum] n 1) комната; refreshment ~ буфет; consulting ~ кабинет врача; operating ~

операцио́нная; reception ~ гости́ная, приёмная; single ~ ко́мната на одного́ челове́ка; local ~ отде́л ме́стных новосте́й (*в реда́кции газеты*); to share a ~ with жить в одно́й ко́мнате с кем-л.; to do one's ~ убира́ть ко́мнату; to keep one's ~ не выходи́ть из ко́мнаты; 2) *pl* помеще́ние, кварти́ра; 3) простра́нство, ме́сто; there is ~ for one more in the car в маши́не есть ме́сто ещё для одного́ челове́ка; to make ~ for посторони́ться, дать ме́сто; no ~ to move не́где поверну́ться; there is plenty of ~ here здесь мно́го ме́ста; 4) возмо́жность; there is. no ~ for doubt нет основа́ний сомнева́ться; there is ~ for improvement есть возмо́жность улучше́ния, усоверше́нствования; ◊ in the ~ of вме́сто; your ~ is better than your company лу́чше бы вы ушли́.

room II *v* занима́ть ко́мнату, жить в ко́мнате; to ~ with жить с кем-л. (*в одно́й ко́мнате*).

roomer ['rumə] *n* амер. жиле́ц.

roomful ['rumful] *n* по́лная ко́мната.

roominess ['rumınıs] *n* вмести́тельность.

rooming-house ['rumıŋhaus] *n* амер. меблиро́ванные ко́мнаты.

room-mate ['rummeıt] *n* това́рищ по ко́мнате.

roomy ['rumı] *a* вмести́тельный, просто́рный.

roost I [ru:st] *n* насе́ст; at ~ на насе́сте; *перен.* в посте́ли; to go to ~ удаля́ться на поко́й; ◊ to rule the ~ верхово́дить.

roost II *v* уса́живаться на насе́ст; *перен.* устра́иваться на́ ночь.

rooster ['ru:stə] *n* пету́х.

root I [ru:t] *n* 1) ко́рень; to strike (*или* to take) ~ пуска́ть ко́рни, укореня́ться (*тж. перен.*); a ~ of mountain подно́жие горы́; 2) *обыкн. pl* корнепло́ды; 3) причи́на, исто́чник; the ~ of the matter существо́ де́ла; 4) *мат.* ко́рень; square (cube) ~ квадра́тный (куби́ческий) ко́рень; ◊ ~ and branch а) по́лностью, всё целико́м; б) тща́тельно, основа́тельно.

root II *v* 1) пуска́ть ко́рни; *перен.* укореня́ться; 2) прико́вывать (*к ме́сту*); 3) рыть зе́млю, подрыва́ть ко́рни (*о свиньях*); 4) иска́ть, ры́ться; 5) *амер. разг.* приве́тствовать, шу́мно одобря́ть; □ to ~ **out**, to ~ **up** вырыва́ть с ко́рнем; выкорчёвывать, искореня́ть.

rooted ['ru:tıd] *a* 1) укорени́вшийся; про́чный; 2) глубо́кий (*о чу́встве*).

rootlet ['ru:tlıt] *n* корешо́к.

rooty ['ru:tı] *a* со мно́жеством корне́й.

rope I [roup] *n* 1) верёвка, кана́т; on the ~ свя́занные верёвкой (*об альпини́стах*); 2) ни́тка; вя́занка; a ~ of pearls ни́тка же́мчуга; a ~ of onions свя́зка лу́ка; 3) тягу́чая кле́йкая жи́дкость; 4) *attr* кана́тный, верёвочный; ◊ the ~ пове́шение; a ~ of sand ненадёжная связь (*или* опо́ра); to show smb. the ~s ввести́ кого́-л. в курс де́ла; to know the ~s хорошо́ ориенти́роваться в чём-л.; to be at the end of one's ~ исто́щить все си́лы, исчерпа́ть все возмо́жности; to give smb. ~ дава́ть свобо́ду де́йствий; on the high ~ в припо́днятом настрое́нии.

rope II *v* 1) свя́зывать верёвкой; привя́зывать, закрепля́ть кана́том; 2) тяну́ть на верёвке, кана́те; 3) лови́ть арка́ном; 4) густе́ть, станови́ться кле́йким; □ to ~ **in** втя́гивать, вовлека́ть; to ~ **off** оцепля́ть кана́том.

rope-dancer ['roup,da:nsə] *n* кана́тный плясу́н.

rope-ladder ['roup,lædə] *n* верёвочная ле́стница.

rope-walker ['roup,wɔːkə] *n* канатохо́дец.

rope-way ['roupweı] *n* кана́тная доро́га.

ropy ['roupı] *a* тягу́чий, кле́йкий, ли́пкий.

rosary ['rouzərı] *n* 1) чётки; 2) роза́рий.

rose¹ I [rouz] *n* 1) ро́за; ро́зовый куст; 2) ро́зовый цвет; 3) розе́тка; ◊ a ~ without a thorn ро́за без шипо́в, необыкнове́нная уда́ча; not all ~s не всё хорошо́, не всё гла́дко; under the ~ по секре́ту, тайко́м; to gather (life's) ~s срыва́ть цветы́ удово́льствий.

rose¹ II *a* ро́зовый.

rose² *past. см.* rise II.

roseate ['rouzııt] *a* ро́зовый; *перен.* ра́достный, све́тлый.

rose-bud ['rouzbʌd] *n* буто́н ро́зы.

rose-coloured ['rouz,kʌləd] *a* 1) ро́зовый; 2) ра́дужный; 3) привлека́тельный.

rose-leaf ['rouzli:f] *n* лепесто́к ро́зы.

rosemary ['rouzmərı] *n* розмари́н.

roseola [rou'zi:ələ] *n* красну́ха (*боле́знь*).

rose-tree ['rouztri:] *n* ро́зовый куст.

rosette [rou'zet] *n* розе́тка.

rose-water ['rouz,wɔːtə] *n* 1) ро́зовая вода́; 2) прито́рная любе́зность; 3) *attr* сентимента́льный.

rosewood ['rouzwud] *n* палиса́ндровое де́рево.

rosin I ['rɔzın] *n* смола́, канифо́ль.

rosin II *v* натира́ть канифо́лью.

roster ['roustə] *n* 1) спи́сок; 2) *воен.* расписа́ние дежу́рств, спи́сок наря́дов.

rostrum ['rɔstrəm] *n* (*pl тж.* rostra ['rɔstrə]) 1) трибу́на; ка́федра; 2) клюв; 3) нос корабля́.

rosy ['rouzı] *a* 1) ро́зовый; румя́ный; цвету́щий; 2) я́ркий, све́тлый; *перен.* ра́дужный.

rot I [rɔt] *n* 1) гние́ние, гниль; 2) *разг.* вздор, ерунда́; perfect ~, tommy ~ су́щий вздор; don't talk ~ не болта́йте вздо́ра; 3) неуда́ча.

rot II *v* 1) гнить, по́ртиться; *перен.* разлага́ться; 2) гнои́ть; по́ртить; 3) *сленг* подшу́чивать, дразни́ть; □ to ~ **away** погиба́ть.

rotary ['routərı] *a* враща́тельный; ротацио́нный.

rotate [rou'teıt] *v* 1) враща́ть(ся); 2) сменя́ть(ся) по о́череди; чередова́ть(ся).

rotation [rou'teıʃən] *n* 1) враще́ние; 2) чередова́ние; периоди́ческое повторе́ние; ~ of crops, crop ~ севооборо́т; by ~, in ~ по о́череди; попереме́нно.

rotational [rou'teıʃənl] *a* 1) враща́ющийся; 2) переме́нный, череду́ющийся.

rotative ['routətıv] *см.* rotational.

rotatory ['routətərı] *a* враща́тельный; враща́ющийся.

rote [rout] *n*: by ~ наизу́сть, на па́мять.

rotor ['routə] *n тех.* ро́тор; колесо́ турби́ны.

rotten ['rɔtn] *a* 1) гнило́й; испо́рченный; ту́хлый (*о яйце́*); 2) него́дный; сла́бый; 3) безнра́вственный, по́длый, ни́зкий.

rottenness ['rɔtnnıs] *n* 1) гни́лость; испо́рченность; 2) ни́зость (*поведе́ния и т. п.*); нече́стность.

rotter ['rɔtə] *n сленг* дрянь (*о челове́ке*).

rotund [rou'tʌnd] *a* 1) округлённый; кру́глый; по́лный, пу́хлый; 2) зву́чный; полнозву́чный; 3) витиева́тый (*о сти́ле*).

rouble ['ru:bl] *n* рубль.

rouge I [ru:ʒ] *n* 1) румя́на; 2) губна́я пома́да.

rouge II *v* 1) румя́ниться; 2) кра́сить гу́бы.

rough I [rʌf] *a* 1) гру́бый; 2) неро́вный, шерохова́тый; пересечённый (*о местности*); 3) бу́рный (*о море*); ре́зкий (*о ветре*); 4) просто́й; неотде́ланный, необрабо́танный; черново́й; приблизи́тельный; ~ and ready сде́ланный ко́е-ка́к; 5) неве́жливый, неделика́тный; 6) тяжёлый, опа́сный (*о путешествии и т. п.*); 7) косма́тый; 8) те́рпкий; 9) ре́жущий у́хо (*о звуке*).

rough II *n* 1) неро́вность (*местности*); 2) гру́бость; неотде́ланность; in the ~ в незако́нченном *или* сыро́м ви́де; 3) грубия́н, хулига́н.

rough III *v* 1) де́лать вчерне́; 2): to ~ it обходи́ться без удо́бств; □ to ~ in, to ~ out набра́сывать (*вчерне*); to ~ up a) взъеро́шивать; б) раздража́ть (*кого-л.*).

rough IV *adv* гру́бо; ре́зко.

roughage ['rʌfɪdʒ] *n амер.* гру́бые корма́.

roughcast I ['rʌfkɑːst] *n* гру́бая штукату́рка.

roughcast II *a* 1) гру́бо оштукату́ренный; 2) сде́ланный на́черно.

roughcast III *v* 1) штукату́рить; 2) де́лать вчерне́; набра́сывать (*план и т. п.*).

roughen ['rʌfn] *v* де́лать(ся) гру́бым; грубе́ть.

rough-hew ['rʌf'hjuː] *v* обтёсывать гру́бо.

rough-house ['rʌfhaus] *v сленг* сканда́лить, буя́нить.

roughly ['rʌflɪ] *adv* гру́бо; ~ speaking гру́бо говоря́.

rough-neck ['rʌfnek] *n амер. сленг* 1) буя́н, хулига́н; 2) *attr* хулига́нский.

rough-rider ['rʌf,raɪdə] *n* бере́йтор.

roughshod ['rʌfʃɔd] *a* подко́ванный на шипа́х; ◊ to ride ~ over тира́нить.

roulette [ru:'let] *n* руле́тка (*игра*).

Roumanian I [ru:'meɪnjən] *n* 1) румы́н; румы́нка; the ~s румы́ны; 2) румы́нский язы́к.

Roumanian II *a* румы́нский.

round I [raund] *n* 1) круг; 2) обхо́д (*патруля, сто́рожа*); объе́зд (*врача́*); прогу́лка; to go (*или* to make) the ~ обходи́ть; to go for a ~ идти́ на прогу́лку; 3) кругово́е движе́ние; цикл; 4) тур; ра́унд; 5) залп; вы́стрел; 6) патро́н; 7) ступе́нька (*ле́стницы*); 8) хорово́д; 9) сфе́ра; круг (*интере́сов, обя́занностей*); daily ~ ежедне́вные дела́, заня́тия, обя́занности; ◊ a ~ of cheers (*или* of applause) взрыв аплодисме́нтов.

round II *a* 1) кру́глый; кругово́й; шарообра́зный; 2) по́лный; кру́гленький (*о су́мме*); 3) открове́нный, прямо́й (*о выска́зывании*); 4) че́стный (*о сде́лке и т. п.*); 5) мя́гкий, прия́тный (*о го́лосе*); 6) округлённый, закруглённый.

round III *v* 1) закругля́ть; округля́ть(ся); 2) огиба́ть; обходи́ть круго́м; облета́ть; 3) зака́нчивать (*тж.* to ~ out); □ to ~ off a) округля́ть, закругля́ть; б) зака́нчивать; to ~ on *разг.* доноси́ть; to ~ up a) сгоня́ть (*скот*); б) окружа́ть, производи́ть обла́ву.

round IV *adv* 1) со всех сторо́н, вокру́г; ~ about вокру́г да о́коло; 2) круго́м; око́льным путём; 3) обра́тно; 4) в окру́жности, в обхва́те; ◊ taking it all ~ рассма́тривая со всех сторо́н.

round V *prep* 1) вокру́г; ~ the world вокру́г све́та; ~ the corner за́ угол; за угло́м; 2) по; ~ the garden по са́ду.

roundabout I ['raundəbaut] *n* 1) око́льный путь; 2) карусе́ль; 3) *амер.* ку́ртка.

roundabout II *a* 1) око́льный, кру́жный, обхо́дный; 2) по́лный, то́лстый.

roundelay ['raundɪleɪ] *n* 1) коро́ткая пе́сенка с припе́вом; 2) пе́ние пти́цы; 3) хорово́дный та́нец.

roundhead ['roundhed] *n ист.* круглоголо́вый.

round-house ['raundhaus] *n* 1) кормова́я ру́бка; 2) *амер.* парово́зное депо́.

roundish ['raundɪʃ] *a* окру́глый, кругова́тый.

roundly ['raundlɪ] *adv* 1) кру́гло; 2) по́лностью; основа́тельно; оконча́тельно; 3) пря́мо; ре́зко, открове́нно.

roundsman ['raundzmən] *n амер.* полице́йский инспе́ктор.

round-trip ['raundtrɪp] *n амер.* экскурсио́нная пое́здка (*обыкн. по кольцево́му маршру́ту*).

round-up ['raundʌp] *n* 1) округле́ние, закругле́ние; 2) заго́н скота́ (*для осмо́тра*); 3) обла́ва; 4) обзо́р новосте́й (*по ра́дио, в газе́те*); press ~ обзо́р печа́ти.

rouse [rauz] *v* 1) буди́ть; 2) пробужда́ться (*тж.* to ~ up); 3) побужда́ть; возбужда́ть; to ~ oneself встряхну́ться; 4) вспугну́ть (*дичь и т. п.*).

roustabout ['roustə,baut] *n амер.* рабо́чий (*на при́стани, на парохо́де*).

rout[1] I [raut] *n* разгро́м, пораже́ние; беспоря́дочное бе́гство; to put to ~ разгроми́ть, обрати́ть в бе́гство.

rout[1] II *v* разбива́ть на́голову, обраща́ть в бе́гство.

rout[2] *n* 1) пиру́шка; шу́мное сбо́рище; 2) *уст.* ра́ут, зва́ный ве́чер.

rout[3] *v* 1) подрыва́ть ко́рни (*о свинье́*); выка́пывать; 2) выта́скивать (*тж.* to ~ out).

route I [ru:t] *n* маршру́т, путь, направле́ние, курс; en ~ по пути́.

route II *v* направля́ть (*по определённому маршру́ту*).

routine [ru:'ti:n] *n* 1) устано́вленный поря́док; установи́вшаяся пра́ктика; определённый режи́м; 2) шабло́н, рути́на; 3) *attr* определённый, устано́вленный.

rove [rouv] *v* 1) броди́ть; скита́ться; стра́нствовать; 2) блужда́ть (*о взгля́де*).

rover ['rouvə] *n* 1) скита́лец; стра́нник; 2) морско́й разбо́йник, пира́т; 3) ста́рший бойска́ут; 4) «разбо́йник» (*в кроке́те*).

row[a1] I [rou] *n* ряд; in a ~ в ряд; in ~s ряда́ми; ◊ a hard ~ to hoe *амер.* тру́дная зада́ча, «кре́пкий оре́шек».

row[a2] I *n* 1) гребля́; прогу́лка в ло́дке; to go for a ~ пое́хать ката́ться на ло́дке.

row[a2] II *v* 1) грести́; 2) перевози́ть в ло́дке; □ to ~ **down** перегна́ть на ло́дке.

row[b] I [rau] *n разг.* 1) шум; ссо́ра; сканда́л; дра́ка; what's all this ~ about? в чём де́ло?, что там за шум?; to have a ~ шуме́ть, спо́рить; ссо́риться; to kick up a ~ подня́ть шум; затея́ть дра́ку *или* ссо́ру; 2) нагоня́й; to get into a ~ получи́ть нагоня́й.

row[b] II *v разг.* 1) де́лать вы́говор; руга́ть; 2) сканда́лить.

rowan ['rauən] n рябина.

row-boat ['roubout] n гребная лодка.

rowdy I ['raudɪ] n хулиган, буян; грубиян.

rowdy II a буйный; грубый.

rower ['rouə] n гребец.

rowing[a] ['rouɪŋ] n гребля.

rowing[b] ['rauɪŋ] n выговор, нагоняй.

rowlock ['rɔlək] n уключина.

royal ['rɔɪəl] a 1) королевский; 2) британский (о флоте, войсках и т. п.); 3) великолепный; царственный.

royalist I ['rɔɪəlɪst] n 1) роялист; 2) амер. твердолобый.

royalist II a роялистский; монархический.

royalty ['rɔɪəltɪ] n 1) королевская власть; 2) величие, царственность; 3) член(ы) королевской семьи; 4) обыкн. pl королевские привилегии; 5) плата землевладельцу за разработку недр; 6) авторский гонорар.

rub I [rʌb] n 1) трение; 2) натирание; стирание; the ~ of a brush чистка щёткой; to give a ~ потереть; 3) затруднение, помеха; there is the ~ вот в чём затруднение, загвоздка; 4) язвительное замечание, насмешка.

rub II v 1) тереть(ся); 2) натирать; 3) стирать (что-л.; тж. to ~ out); 4) соприкасаться; задевать; 5) раздражать; □ to ~ along a) ладить, уживаться; б) продвигаться с трудом, продираться; to ~ away стирать(ся); to ~ down а) вытирать досуха; б) сглаживать; to ~ in а) втирать; б) вдалбливать; повторять, подчёркивать; to ~ off стирать, вытирать; to ~ through протирать (сквозь сито и т. п.); to ~ up а) полировать; б) освежать в памяти.

rub-a-dub ['rʌbə'dʌb] n барабанный бой.

rubber[1] I ['rʌbə] n 1) резина, каучук; 2) резинка; 3) pl резиновые изделия; 4) pl галоши; 5) массажист; 6) приспособление для натирания, вытирания.

rubber[1] II a резиновый; прорезиненный.

rubber[1] III v покрывать резиной, прорезинивать.

rubber[2] n карт. роббер.

rubberized ['rʌbəraɪzd] a прорезиненный.

rubberneck I ['rʌbənek] n разг. любопытный человек.

rubberneck II v разг. любопытствовать, вытягивать шею (стараясь увидеть).

rubber-tree ['rʌbətri:] n каучуконос.

rubber-vine ['rʌbəvaɪn] см. rubber-tree.

rubbish ['rʌbɪʃ] n 1) мусор, хлам; 2) вздор, ерунда; 3) сленг деньги.

rubbishy ['rʌbɪʃɪ] a никуда не годный, дряннóй.

rubble ['rʌbl] n 1) бут, булыжник; 2) галька, валун.

rube [ru:b] n амер. разг. деревенщина.

rubicund ['ru:bɪkənd] a румяный.

ruble ['ru:bl] см. rouble.

rubric ['ru:brɪk] n рубрика, заголовок.

ruby I ['ru:bɪ] n 1) рубин; 2) красный цвет; ◊ above rubies неоценимый, бесценный.

ruby II a рубиновый; красный.

ruche [ru:ʃ] n рюш.

ruck[1] I [rʌk] n складка, морщина.

ruck[1] II v морщить(ся).

ruck[2] I n 1) толпа; давка; 2) вздор, чепуха.

ruck[2] II v толпиться.

rucksack ['ruksæk] n походный мешок, рюкзак.

ruction ['rʌkʃən] n обыкн. pl разг. 1) беспокойство, волнение; 2) беспорядки, волнения.

rudder ['rʌdə] n 1) руль; elevating ~ ав. руль высоты; 2) руководящий принцип.

rudderless ['rʌdəlɪs] a без руля; перен. без руководства.

ruddy ['rʌdɪ] a 1) румяный, красный; 2) цветущий (о здоровье).

rude [ru:d] a 1) грубый, неотёсанный; невоспитанный; 2) сильный; резкий; 3) неотделанный; 4) примитивный; 5) внезапный.

rudeness ['ru:dnɪs] n грубость.

rudiment ['ru:dɪmənt] n 1) pl начатки; элементарные принципы; 2) рудиментарный, зачаточный или недоразвитый орган.

rudimentary [,ru:dɪ'mentərɪ] a 1) элементарный; 2) зачаточный, недоразвитый, рудиментарный.

rue[1] [ru:] v (со)жалеть; раскаиваться; печалиться, горевать.

rue[2] n бот. рута.

rueful ['ru:ful] a 1) печальный; унылый; 2) жалкий, жалобный.

ruefully ['ru:fulɪ] adv 1) печально; уныло; 2) с сожалением; с сочувствием.

ruff[1] [rʌf] n брыжи.

ruff[2] n ёрш (рыба).

ruffian I ['rʌfjən] n хулиган; негодяй, головорез.

ruffian II a хулиганский; грубый.

ruffle I ['rʌfl] n 1) гофрированная манжетка, оборка; 2) рябь; 3) суматоха, волнение; ссора.

ruffle II v 1) морщить; ерошить (волосы); топорщить(ся); 2) рябить (воду); 3) гофрировать, собирать в сборки; 4) нарушать спокойствие, раздражать; 5) трепыхаться; 6) хорохориться.

ruffler ['rʌflə] n разг. 1) хвастун; 2) задира; хулиган.

rug [rʌg] n 1) ковёр; 2) плед.

Rugby ['rʌgbɪ] n спорт. регби (тж. ~ football).

rugged ['rʌgɪd] a 1) неровный, шероховатый, шершавый; пересечённый (о местности); 2) грубый, морщинистый (о лице); 3) неотделанный; 4) суровый; резкий; 5) яростный; 6) тяжёлый, трудный (о жизни); 7) амер. сильный, крепкий.

rugose ['ru:gous] a морщинистый.

ruin I [ruɪn] n 1) гибель; разорение; крушение; крах; to bring to ~ погубить; разорить; 2) обыкн. pl развалина, руина; in ~s в развалинах.

ruin II v 1) разорять; разрушать; to ~ oneself а) разоряться; б) губить себя; 2) губить; портить.

ruination [ruɪ'neɪʃən] n гибель; крушение; полное разорение.

ruinous ['ruɪnəs] a 1) гибельный, губительный, разрушительный; разорительный; 2) разрушенный; развалившийся.

rule I [ru:l] n 1) правило; принцип; норма; as a ~ как правило, обычно; by ~ по правилам; general ~ общее правило; ~ of three мат. тройное правило; ~s of the game правила игры; ~ of the road правила движения по дорогам; ~ of thumb приближённый подсчёт; ≅ на глазóк; to make it a ~ взять за прáвило; 2) правлéние, власть; влады́чество; the ~ of the people народовлáстие; 3) постановлéние судá *или* судьи́; 4) устáв (*общества, ордена*); 5) линéйка; 6) *полигр.* линéйка, шпон.

rule II *v* 1) прáвить, управля́ть; влáствовать; 2) постановля́ть, устанáвливать прáвило; решáть (*that*); 3) линовáть, графи́ть; 4) стоя́ть на определённом у́ровне (*о ценах*); □ to ~ **out** исключáть.

ruler[1] ['ru:lə] *n* линéйка.

ruler[2] *n* прави́тель.

ruling I ['ru:lɪŋ] *n* 1) управлéние; 2) постановлéние; судéбное решéние.

ruling II *a* прáвящий; госпóдствующий.

rum[1] [rʌm] *n* 1) ром; 2) *амер.* спиртнóе.

rum[2] *a разг.* стрáнный; to feel ~ чýвствовать себя́ не в своéй тарéлке.

rumble[1] I ['rʌmbl] *n* 1) громыхáние, грóхот; 2) дополни́тельное сидéнье *или* мéсто для багажá в зáдней чáсти экипáжа; 3) *амер. авто* откиднóе сидéнье.

rumble[1] II *v* громыхáть, грохотáть.

rumble[2] *v сленг* проникáть в сáмую суть; ви́деть насквóзь.

rumble-tumble ['rʌmbl,tʌmbl] *n* 1) тря́ска; 2) громóздкий тря́ский экипáж.

ruminant I ['ru:mɪnənt] *n* жвáчное живóтное.

ruminant II *a* 1) жвáчный; 2) задýмчивый; вдýмчивый.

ruminate ['ru:mɪneɪt] *v* 1) жевáть жвáчку; 2) раздýмывать, размышля́ть (*о чём-л.— on, about, over, of*).

rumination [,ru:mɪ'neɪʃən] *n* 1) жевáние жвáчки; 2) размышлéние.

rummage I ['rʌmɪdʒ] *n* 1) тщáтельные пóиски; óбыск, обшáривание; 2) хлам.

rummage II *v* 1) ры́ться, перерывáть, шáрить (*in*); 2) обнарýживать, вытáскивать, вынимáть (*тж.* to ~ out, to ~ up).

rummage-sale ['rʌmɪdʒ'seɪl] *n* распродáжа случáйных вещéй (*с благотворительной целью*).

rummer ['rʌmə] *n* кýбок.

rummy ['rʌmɪ] *см.* rum[2].

rumor I, II ['ru:mə] *амер. см.* rumour I, II.

rumour I ['ru:mə] *n* слух, молвá, тóлки; discrepant ~s противорéчивые слýхи; ~s are about (*или* afloat) хóдят слýхи; there is a ~... говоря́т...

rumour II *v* распространя́ть слýхи, расскáзывать нóвости; it is ~ed that... хóдят слýхи, что...

rump [rʌmp] *n* 1) огýзок; 2) (the R.) *ист.* остáтки Дóлгого парлáмента, «охвóстье».

rumple ['rʌmpl] *v* мять, приводи́ть в беспоря́док.

rumpus ['rʌmpəs] *n разг.* шум, гам, ссóра.

run I [rʌn] *n* 1) бег; пробéг; (крáткая) поéздка; at a ~ бегóм; on the ~ в движéнии; на ходý; б) поспéшно отступáя; в) в бегáх; to come on the ~ прийти́ в движéние; to go for a ~ пробежáться; to take a ~ разбежáться; 2) течéние; направлéние, тендéнция; the ~ of events ход *или* течéние собы́тий; at a ~ подря́д; at (*или* in) the long ~ в концé концóв, впослéдствии; to keep on the ~ не давáть останови́ться; 3) пробéг; прогóн; 4) пери́од врéмени; a ~ of (good) luck

счастли́вая полосá, полосá удáч; a ~ of wet weather пери́од дождéй; to have a long ~ быть дóлго в ходý; 5) разрешéние пóльзоваться чем-л.; the ~ of a library разрешéние пóльзоваться библиотéкой; 6) спрос; 7) ряд, сéрия; the play had a ~ of 50 nights пьéса шла 50 раз подря́д; 8) срéдний ýровень; the common ~, the ~ of mankind обыкновéнные лю́ди; out of the ~ необы́чный, из ря́да вон выходя́щий; 9) стáя (*рыб*); 10) загóн (*для скота, домашней птицы*); 11) *амер.* (небольшóй) потóк, ручéй; 12) рулáда; 13) *амер.* спусти́вшаяся пéтля на чулкé; ◇ to go with a ~ ≅ идти́ глáдко, как по мáслу.

run II *v* (*past* ran; *p. p.* run) 1) бéгать, бежáть; 2) дви́гаться, ходи́ть; плыть, курси́ровать; кати́ться; 3) бы́стро распространя́ться; 4) течь, ли́ться; расплывáться (*о чернилах*); приливáть (*о крови*); to ~ with быть зáлитым чем-л.; 5) расти́, ви́ться (*о ползучих растениях*); 6) тянýться, простирáться, проходи́ть (*о линиях и т. п.*); 7) гласи́ть (*о документе, тексте*); the letter ~s thus в письмé скáзано слéдующее; 8) вращáться, рабóтать (*о машине, моторе*); дéйствовать; 9) подвергáться; 10) *как глагол-связка в составном сказуемом:* to ~ cold похолодéть; to ~ dry высыхáть; иссякáть; to ~ mad сходи́ть с умá; to ~ high a) вздымáться (*о волнах*); волновáться (*о море*); б) разгорáться (*о страстях*); to ~ low a) понижáться, опускáться; б) истощáться, иссякáть; 11) выставля́ть свою́ кандидатýру; 12) проби́ть(ся); to ~ a blockade прорвáть блокáду; 13) гнать, подгоня́ть; 14) втыкáть, вонзáть (*в — into*); вдевáть (*нитку*); удáрять (*обо что-л.— against*); 15) плáвить, лить (*металл*); 16) вести́ (*дело*), управля́ть (*предприятием и т. п.*); 17) преслéдовать, трави́ть (*зверя*); □ to ~ **about** a) суети́ться; бéгать тудá и сюдá; б) рези́ться (*о детях*); to ~ **across** натолкнýться, случáйно встрéтиться; to ~ **after** a) *разг.* бéгать, ухáживать за кем-л.; б) преслéдовать; to ~ **against** столкнýться с чем-л., кем-л., натолкнýться на; to ~ **at** набрóситься, наки́нуться на когó-л.; to ~ **away with** убегáть, уноси́ что-л. *или* похи́тив когó-л.; to ~ **down** a) останáвливаться (*о механизме, часах*); б) догнáть, насти́гнуть; в) *разг.* изничтóжить; г) истощáть(ся), изнуря́ть(ся); д) опроки́дывать; е) задави́ть, переéхать; to ~ **for** догоня́ть, бежáть за чем-л.; to ~ for it *разг.* удирáть, спасáться; to ~ **in** a) навести́ть, загляну́ть; б) *разг.* задержáть, арестовáть; в) соглашáться; сходи́ться, совпадáть (*with*); to ~ **into** a) наéхать, наскочи́ть; натолкнýться; столкнýться; б) достигáть, доходи́ть до; the book has ~ into six editions кни́га вы́держала шесть издáний; в) впадáть, попадáть (*в какое-л. положение*); to ~ into debt влезáть в долги́; to ~ into mischief попадáть в бедý; to ~ **off** убежáть, удрáть; to ~ off the rails сходи́ть с рéльсов; to ~ **on** a) продолжáть; б) *полигр.* набирáть в подбóр; to ~ **out** a) кончáться, истекáть; б) выступáть (*о строении и т. п.*); to ~ **over** a) переéхать, задави́ть; б) переливáться чéрез край; в) просмáтривать, перели́стывать; to ~ **through** a) бéгло, бы́стро просмотрéть; б) проколóть; в) промотáть (*состояние*); г) зачеркнýть; to ~ **to** достигáть (*суммы, степени*); to ~ to extremes впада́ть в кра́йности; to ~ **up** а) доходи́ть, достига́ть (до — to); б) (бы́стро) съе́здить (в го́род и т. п.); в) поднима́ть(ся); расти́.

runabout I ['rʌnəbaut] n 1) бродя́га, праздношата́ющийся; 2) небольшо́й автомоби́ль; 3) мото́рная ло́дка.

runabout II а бродя́чий.

runaway I ['rʌnəweɪ] n бегле́ц, дезерти́р.

runaway II v сбежа́вший; бе́глый.

run-down I ['rʌndaun] n 1) уменьше́ние чи́сленности (особ. войск); 2) кра́ткое изложе́ние.

run-down II а 1) изнурённый, истощённый; 2) захуда́лый, жа́лкий.

runes [ruːnz] n pl ру́ны.

rung[1] [rʌŋ] past, p. p. см. ring[2] II.

rung[2] n 1) ступе́нька (стремя́нки); 2) перекла́дина; 3) спи́ца колеса́.

runic ['ruːnɪk] а руни́ческий.

runlet ['rʌnlɪt] n ручеёк.

runnel ['rʌnl] n 1) небольшо́й ручей; 2) кана́ва.

runner ['rʌnə] n 1) бегу́н; relay ~ уча́стник эстафе́ты; 2) посы́льный, гоне́ц; 3) контрабанди́ст; 4) доро́жка (из полотна́, кру́жев); 5) по́лоз (сане́й); 6) сте́лющийся побе́г (с корня́ми); 7) тех. бегуно́к, ро́лик, като́к.

runner-up ['rʌnər'ʌp] n уча́стник состяза́ния, заня́вший второ́е ме́сто.

running I ['rʌnɪŋ] n 1) бег, бе́ганье; беготня́; 2) течь, выделе́ние; 3) рабо́та, ход (маши́ны, мото́ра); движе́ние, де́йствие; ◊ to be in the ~ име́ть ша́нсы на вы́игрыш; to be out of the ~ не име́ть ша́нсов на вы́игрыш; to make good one's ~ не отстава́ть (от други́х); to take up the ~ брать инициати́ву.

running II а 1) бегу́щий, теку́щий; пла́вный; 2) теку́чий; гноя́щийся (о ра́не и т. п.); слезя́щийся (о глаза́х); 3) бегово́й; 4) после́довательный, продолжа́ющийся непреры́вно; for three days ~ три дня подря́д.

running-board ['rʌnɪŋbɔːd] n подно́жка (автомоби́ля и т. п.).

running-title ['rʌnɪŋ'taɪtl] n полигр. колонти́тул.

run-out ['rʌn,aut] n 1) вы́ход; вы́пуск; 2) ав. разбе́г.

runt [rʌnt] n 1) малоро́слое живо́тное; 2) челове́к небольшо́го ро́ста, коротышка.

run-up ['rʌn,ʌp] n разбе́г.

runway ['rʌnweɪ] n 1) доро́жка, прохо́д; тропи́нка к водопо́ю (для живо́тных); 2) ав. взлётно-поса́дочная доро́жка; 3) ж.-д. подъездно́й путь.

rupee [ruː'piː] n ру́пия (денежная единица Индии, Пакистана и т. п.).

rupture I ['rʌptʃə] n 1) перело́м; 2) разры́в (тж. перен.); 3) мед. гры́жа; прободе́ние.

rupture II v прорыва́ть (оболо́чку); разрыва́ть (тж. перен.— отноше́ния и т. п.).

rural ['ruərəl] а се́льский, дереве́нский.

ruse [ruːz] n уло́вка, хи́трость; ~ of war вое́нная хи́трость.

rush[1] [rʌʃ] n 1) тростни́к, камы́ш; 2) соверше́нный пустя́к, ме́лочь; is not worth a ~ ни гроша́ не сто́ит; not to care a ~ не придава́ть никако́го значе́ния, не обраща́ть внима́ния; 3) attr тростнико́вый, камышо́вый.

rush[2] I n 1) напо́р, на́тиск, наплы́в; а ~ of wind поры́в ве́тра; а ~ of blood прили́в кро́ви; 2) стреми́тельная ата́ка, бросо́к; 3) спе́шка; стреми́тельный темп; 4): it is a regular ~ э́то фо́рменная обира́ловка; 5) attr спе́шный, сро́чный; ◊ ~ of armaments го́нка вооруже́ний.

rush[2] II v 1) броса́ться, нести́сь, мча́ться, устремля́ться; хлы́нуть; 2) де́йствовать о́чень или сли́шком поспе́шно; to ~ to a conclusion де́лать поспе́шный вы́вод; 3) воен. стреми́тельно продвига́ться; 4) торопи́ть, тащи́ть; 5) дуть поры́вами (о ве́тре); 6) разг. обдира́ть (покупа́теля).

rush-hours ['rʌʃ,auəz] n pl часы́ пик.

rushy ['rʌʃɪ] а 1) заро́сший тростнико́м, камышо́м; 2) тростнико́вый.

rusk [rʌsk] n суха́рь.

russet I ['rʌsɪt] n 1) краснова́то-кори́чневый цвет; 2) гру́бая краснова́то-кори́чневая ткань; 3) кори́чные я́блоки (сорт).

russet II а краснова́то-кори́чневый.

Russian I ['rʌʃən] n 1) ру́сский; ру́сская; the ~s ру́сские; 2) ру́сский язы́к.

Russian II а ру́сский.

rust I [rʌst] n 1) ржа́вчина; 2) бот. ржа, головня́.

rust II v 1) ржа́веть; де́латься ржа́вым; 2) по́ртиться, притупля́ться (от безде́йствия).

rust-free ['rʌstfriː] а нержаве́ющий.

rustic I ['rʌstɪk] n се́льский жи́тель, крестья́нин.

rustic II а 1) се́льский, дереве́нский; 2) просто́й; простова́тый; 3) гру́бый, нескла́дный, неотёсанный.

rusticate ['rʌstɪkeɪt] v 1) отправля́ть в дере́вню; 2) жить в дере́вне; 3) исключа́ть вре́менно из университе́та, колле́джа.

rusticity [rʌs'tɪsɪtɪ] n 1) простота́, безыску́сственность; 2) дереве́нские нра́вы.

rustiness ['rʌstɪnɪs] n ржа́вость; ржа́вчина.

rustle I ['rʌsl] n ше́лест, шо́рох; шурша́ние.

rustle II v 1) шелесте́ть; шурша́ть; 2) амер. разг. де́йствовать бы́стро, энерги́чно; 3) амер. красть (скот и т. п.).

rustler ['rʌslə] n амер. 1) энерги́чный, живо́й челове́к; 2) конокра́д.

rustless ['rʌstlɪs] а нержаве́ющий.

rustproof ['rʌstpruːf] см. rust-free.

rusty[1] ['rʌstɪ] а 1) ржа́вый, заржа́вленный; 2) цве́та ржа́вчины; порыже́вший; 3) запу́щенный; ◊ to turn ~ наду́ться, разозли́ться, вспыли́ть.

rusty[2] а прого́рклый.

rut I [rʌt] n 1) коле́я, борозда́; 2) привы́чка; 3) тех. вы́емка, паз, фальц.

rut II v оставля́ть коле́й.

rutabaga [,ruːtə'beɪgə] n амер. брю́ква.

ruthless ['ruːθlɪs] а безжа́лостный; жесто́кий.

rye [raɪ] n 1) рожь; 2) амер. хле́бная во́дка; 3) attr ржано́й.

rye-bread ['raɪbred] n ржано́й хлеб.

ryot ['raɪət] n инди́йский крестья́нин, земледе́лец.

S

S, s [es] n 19-я бу́ква англ. алфави́та.

's [z, s] разг. сокращённая фо́рма: 1) has в фо́рме Present Perfect: he's done it=he has done it он сделал э́то; 2) is *в фо́рме Continuous или глаго́ла-свя́зки в сло́жном сказу́емом*: he's going to Leningrad tonight=he is going to Leningrad tonight он е́дет в Ленингра́д сего́дня ве́чером; it's time to go to school = it is time to go to school пора́ идти́ в шко́лу; 3) us *фо́рма ко́св. п. ли́чного мест.* we мы: let's speak English = let us speak English дава́йте говори́ть по-англи́йски.

saber I, II ['seibə] *амер. см.* sabre I, II.

sable¹ ['seibl] *n* 1) со́боль; 2) собо́лий мех.

sable² *a поэт.* тёмный, чёрный, мра́чный, тра́урный.

sabotage I ['sæbətɑːʒ] *n* 1) сабота́ж; 2) диве́рсия.

sabotage II *v* саботи́ровать.

saboteur [,sæbə'təː] *n* 1) сабота́жник; 2) диверса́нт, вреди́тель.

sabre I ['seibə] *n* са́бля; ша́шка; the ~ вое́нная си́ла, вое́нная власть; to rattle the ~ бряца́ть ору́жием.

sabre II *v* руби́ть са́блей, ша́шкой.

saccharin ['sækərin] *n* сахари́н.

saccharineᵃ ['sækərin] *n см.* saccharin.

saccharineᵇ ['sækərain] *a* са́харный.

sachem ['seitʃəm] *n* 1) вождь (*у не́которых инде́йских племён*); 2) ва́жная персо́на.

sack¹ I [sæk] *n* 1) мешо́к, куль; 2) сак (*пальто́*); ◇ to get the ~ быть уво́ленным; to give the ~ уво́лить; a sad ~ *амер.* челове́к, постоя́нно всё пу́тающий; «вели́кий пу́таник».

sack¹ II *v* 1) класть в мешо́к, куль; 2) *разг.* увольня́ть.

sack² I *n* разграбле́ние, грабёж; to put to ~ подверга́ть разграбле́нию (*побеждённый го́род*).

sack² II *v* гра́бить, подверга́ть разграбле́нию.

sackcloth ['sækklɔθ] *n* мешкови́на; дерю́га; гру́бый холст; ◇ in ~ and ashes ≅ посы́пав главу́ пе́плом; по́лный ско́рби.

sackful ['sækful] *n* по́лный мешо́к (*чего́-л.*).

sacking ['sækiŋ] *n* 1) мешкови́на; 2) увольне́ние; bombshell ~s внеза́пные увольне́ния.

sacral ['seikrəl] *a* обря́довый.

sacrament ['sækrəmənt] *n* 1) *церк.* та́инство, прича́стие; 2) знак, си́мвол; 3) обе́т, кля́тва.

sacramental [,sækrə'mentl] *a* 1) свяще́нный; заве́тный; 2) торже́ственный.

sacred ['seikrid] *a* 1) свяще́нный, свято́й; 2) духо́вный (*о му́зыке*); 3) неприкоснове́нный; 4) посвящённый (*кому́-л.— to*).

sacrifice I ['sækrifais] *n* 1) же́ртва; the great ~, last ~ смерть в бою́ за ро́дину; at a ~ в убы́ток; 2) жертвоприноше́ние.

sacrifice II *v* 1) приноси́ть же́ртву; 2) же́ртвовать; to ~ oneself же́ртвовать собо́й.

sacrificial [,sækri'fiʃəl] *a* же́ртвенный.

sacrilege ['sækrilidʒ] *n* святота́тство, кощу́нство.

sad [sæd] *a* 1) печа́льный, уны́лый; опеча́ленный; 2) доса́дный (*об оши́бке и т. п.*); 3) ту́склый, тёмный, мра́чный (*о цве́те*); 4) отъя́вленный, неисправи́мый (*о челове́ке*).

sadden ['sædn] *v* опеча́лить(ся).

saddle I ['sædl] *n* 1) седло́; to be in the ~ е́хать верхо́м; *перен.* а) руководи́ть, верши́ть дела́ми; б) быть в по́лной гото́вности; 2) чересседе́льник; 3) седлови́на (*горы́*); ◇ to put the ~ on the right

(wrong) horse ≅ обвиня́ть кого́ (не) сле́дует, обвиня́ть (не) справедли́во.

saddle II *v* 1) седла́ть (*ло́шадь*); оседла́ть; 2) обременя́ть (*кого́-л. чем-л. — with*); 3) взва́ливать (*вину́ на кого́-л.— upon*).

saddle-bag ['sædlbæg] *n* седе́льный вьюк, перемётная сума́.

saddle-bow ['sædlbou] *n* седе́льная лука́.

saddle-cloth ['sædlklɔθ] *n* чепра́к, потни́к.

saddle-horse ['sædlhɔːs] *n* верхова́я ло́шадь.

saddler ['sædlə] *n* шо́рник.

sadness ['sædnis] *n* печа́ль, уны́ние; огорче́ние.

safe¹ [seif] *a* 1) невреди́мый, це́лый; ~ and sound жив-здоро́в; цел и невреди́м; 2) безопа́сный, не внуша́ющий опасе́ний; благополу́чный; 3) надёжный, внуша́ющий дове́рие, ве́рный; it is ~ to say мо́жно с уве́ренностью сказа́ть; 4) осторо́жный, осмотри́тельный.

safe² *n* 1) сейф; несгора́емый шкаф; 2) чула́н, я́щик; холоди́льный шкаф (*для хране́ния проду́ктов*).

safeblower ['seif,blouə] *n амер.* взло́мщик сейфов.

safebreaker ['seif,breikə] *n амер.* взло́мщик сейфов.

safe-conduct ['seif'kɔndəkt] *n* охра́нное свиде́тельство; про́пуск.

safeguard I ['seifgɑːd] *n* 1) охра́на; ме́ра предосторо́жности; гара́нтия; 2) про́пуск; 3) предохрани́тельное приспособле́ние.

safeguard II *v* 1) охраня́ть; предохраня́ть; 2) обеспе́чивать, гаранти́ровать.

safely ['seifli] *adv* 1) в сохра́нности; в безопа́сности; 2) благополу́чно.

safety ['seifti] *n* 1) безопа́сность; сохра́нность; невреди́мость; ~ first! «соблюда́йте осторо́жность!» (*при перехо́де у́лицы*); in ~ в безопа́сности; в надёжном ме́сте; at ~ на предохрани́теле (*об ору́жии*); with ~ без ри́ска; to play for ~ избега́ть ри́ска; не хоте́ть рискова́ть; 2) предохрани́тельные приспособле́ния; 3) *attr* безопа́сный; предохрани́тельный.

safety-belt ['seiftibelt] *n* 1) спаса́тельный по́яс (*на воде́*); 2) *ав.* привязно́й реме́нь.

safety-catch ['seiftikætʃ] *см.* safety-lock.

safety-lamp ['seiftilæmp] *n* безопа́сная ла́мпа.

safety-lock ['seiftilɔk] *n* предохрани́тельный болт, предохрани́тель.

safety-match ['seiftimætʃ] *n* (безопа́сная) спи́чка.

safety-pin ['seiftipin] *n* англи́йская була́вка.

safety-valve ['seiftivælv] *n* предохрани́тельный кла́пан.

sag [sæg] *v* 1) обвиса́ть; провиса́ть; оседа́ть; прогиба́ться; 2) *амер.* спада́ть, ослабева́ть; 3) па́дать (*о цене́*); 4) *мор.* отклоня́ться от ку́рса.

saga ['sɑːgə] *n* са́га, сказа́ние.

sagacious [sə'geiʃəs] *a* 1) проница́тельный; прозорли́вый; 2) сообрази́тельный, смышлёный; 3) у́мный (*о живо́тном*).

sagacity [sə'gæsiti] *n* 1) проница́тельность, острота́ ума́; 2) сообрази́тельность, смышлёность, смека́лка; 3) *pl* о́стрые, ме́ткие замеча́ния.

sage I [seidʒ] *n* мудре́ц.

sage II *a* му́дрый; рассуди́тельный; здра́вый.

Sahib ['sɑːhib] *n* са(г)и́б.

said [sed] *past, p. p. см.* say I.

saiga ['saɪgə] *n зоол.* сайга́(к).

sail I [seɪl] *n* 1) па́рус, паруса́; lateen ~ треуго́льный па́рус; (in) full ~ на всех паруса́х; to set ~ подня́ть паруса́; отпра́виться в пла́вание (*куда-л.* — *for*); under ~ с по́днятыми паруса́ми; to take in ~ а) убра́ть паруса́; б) уме́рить свой пыл; to trim the ~s to the wind *перен.* держа́ть нос по ве́тру; 2) морско́е путеше́ствие, пое́здка; to go for a ~ прое́хаться по́ морю; соверши́ть пое́здку по́ морю; 3) па́русные суда́, па́русное су́дно; 4) крыло́ (*ветряно́й ме́льницы*).

sail II *v* 1) идти́ (*о корабле́*); 2) плыть, идти́ под паруса́ми; to ~ under false colours *перен.* действовать под чужи́м и́менем; 3) пари́ть в во́здухе (*о птицах*); плыть (*об облака́х*); 4) вести́; управля́ть (*кораблём, самолётом*); 5) входи́ть пла́вно с ва́жным ви́дом (*куда-л. — into*); □ to ~ **in** а) входи́ть в порт, га́вань; б) реши́тельно взя́ться (*за что-л.*); вмеша́ться; to ~ **into** *разг.* набро́ситься (*на кого-л.*).

sailboat ['seɪlbout] *n амер.* па́русное су́дно; па́русная ло́дка.

sail-cloth ['seɪlklɔθ] *n* паруси́на.

sailer ['seɪlə] *n* па́русное су́дно; па́русник.

sailing ['seɪlɪŋ] *n* 1) пла́вание под паруса́ми; 2) отплы́тие; 3) *pl* расписа́ние движе́ния парохо́дов; 4) па́русный спорт; 5) кораблевожде́ние; 6) *attr* па́русный; 7) *attr* относя́щийся к расписа́нию; ◊ it will be all plain ~ ≅ всё пойдёт как по ма́слу.

sailing-ship ['seɪlɪŋʃɪp] *см.* sailing-vessel.

sailing-vessel ['seɪlɪŋˌvesl] *n* па́русное су́дно.

sailor ['seɪlə] *n* 1) моря́к; матро́с; a ~ before the mast (рядово́й) матро́с; I am a good (bad) ~ я хорошо́ (пло́хо) переношу́ пое́здки по́ морю; 2) *attr* морско́й, матро́сский.

saint [seɪnt, *перед именем со́бственным* snt, sɪnt] *n* свято́й (*сокр.* St., S.).

sake [seɪk] *n* 1): for the ~ of ра́ди; для; for my ~ ра́ди меня́; for mercy's ~, for goodness' ~, for heaven's ~ ра́ди бо́га; for conscience' ~ для успокое́ния со́вести; for pity's ~! умоля́ю вас!; 2): for the ~ of glory из-за сла́вы; for the ~ of making money из-за де́нег.

saké ['sɑːkɪ] *n* саке́ (*япо́нская во́дка*).

salable ['seɪləbl] *a* 1) хо́дкий (*о това́ре*); 2) схо́дный (*о цене́*).

salad ['sæləd] *n* 1) лату́к, сала́т; 2) сала́т; винегре́т; to dress the ~ запра́вить сала́т, винегре́т; 3) *attr* сала́тного цве́та, светло-зелёный.

salad-oil ['sæləd‚ɔɪl] *n* расти́тельное ма́сло, прова́нское ма́сло.

salamander ['sælə‚mændə] *n* 1) *зоол.* салама́ндра; 2) жаро́вня.

salaried ['sælərɪd] *a* получа́ющий жа́лованье, окла́д; находя́щийся на жа́лованье, окла́де.

salary ['sælərɪ] *n* жа́лованье, окла́д; to draw one's ~ получи́ть жа́лованье.

sale [seɪl] *n* 1) прода́жа; white ~ прода́жа белья́; remnant ~ распрода́жа оста́тков; to be for (*или* on) ~ продава́ться, поступи́ть в прода́жу; to have a good ~ име́ть хоро́ший сбыт, бы́стро продава́ться; there is no ~ for these goods э́тот това́р не идёт; 2) аукцио́н; to put up for ~ продава́ть с молотка́; 3) распрода́жа по дешёвым це́нам

(*в конце́ сезо́на*); spring (summer, winter) ~s весе́нняя (ле́тняя, зи́мняя) распрода́жа това́ров.

saleable ['seɪləbl] *см.* salable.

salesclerk ['seɪlzklɑːk] *n амер.* продаве́ц (*в универма́ге*).

salesgirl ['seɪlzgəːl] *n* продавщи́ца.

saleslady ['seɪlzˌleɪdɪ] *n амер. разг.* продавщи́ца.

salesman ['seɪlzmən] *n* 1) продаве́ц; 2) *амер.* коммивояжёр.

salesmanship ['seɪlzmənʃɪp] *n* уме́ние торгова́ть.

salespeople ['seɪlzˌpiːpl] *n pl собир.* продавцы́.

saleswoman ['seɪlzˌwumən] *n* продавщи́ца.

salience ['seɪljəns] *n* вы́ступ; вы́пуклость, релье́ф.

saliency ['seɪljənsɪ] *см.* salience.

salient I ['seɪljənt] *n* вы́ступ, выдаю́щаяся вперёд часть (*до́ма, бе́рега и т. п.*).

salient II *a* 1) выдаю́щийся (*о черта́х хара́ктера и т. п.*); 2) выступа́ющий, торча́щий; 3) вы́пуклый.

salineᵃ [sə'laɪn] *n* 1) солонча́к, солёное о́зеро; 2) *хим.* соль.

salineᵇ ['seɪlaɪn] *a* 1) солёный; 2) соляно́й, солево́й.

saliva [sə'laɪvə] *n* слюна́.

sallow¹ ['sælou] *n* и́ва, лоза́.

sallow² *a* боле́зненный, желтова́тый (*о цве́те лица́*).

sally I ['sælɪ] *n* 1) *воен.* вы́лазка; 2) пое́здка, прогу́лка (*за́ город*); 3) вспы́шка (*гне́ва*); 4) остроу́мная ре́плика.

sally II *v* 1) де́лать вы́лазку (*ча́сто to ~ out*); 2) *разг.* отпра́виться на экску́рсию, на прогу́лку (*ча́сто to ~ forth, to ~ out*).

salmon I ['sæmən] *n* 1) ло́сось, ры́ба семе́йства лососёвых (*сёмга, горбу́ша и др.*); 2) лососи́на.

salmon II *a* ора́нжево-ро́зовый.

salon ['sælɔːŋ] *n* 1) сало́н; 2) худо́жественный сало́н.

saloon [sə'luːn] *n* 1) зал, приёмная; shaving (hair-dresser's) ~ мужско́й (да́мский) зал (*в парикма́херской*); 2) рестора́н; 3) каю́т-компа́ния (*на корабле́*); 4) *ж.-д.* сало́н-ваго́н; 5) *амер.* бар; 6) закры́тый автомоби́ль.

salt I [sɔːlt] *n* 1) соль; I am not made of ~ ≅ я не са́харный, не раста́ю; in ~ просо́ленный; засо́ленный; to earn one's ~ зараба́тывать себе́ на пропита́ние; to eat smb.'s ~ а) быть в гостя́х у кого́-л.; б) быть нахле́бником у кого́-л.; he is not worth his ~ он ни на что не го́ден; above (below) the ~ на пере́днем (да́льнем) конце́ стола́; 2) *разг.* быва́лый моря́к; old ~ морско́й волк; 3) остроу́мие, изю́минка; Attic ~ то́нкое остроу́мие; ◊ to cast (*или* to lay, to put) ~ on the tail of пойма́ть, излови́ть.

salt II *a* 1) солёный; 2) засо́ленный; 3) е́дкий, о́стрый (*о ре́чи, замеча́нии*).

salt III *v* 1) соли́ть; 2) заса́ливать, консерви́ровать; □ to ~ **away** копи́ть (*де́ньги*).

salt-cellar ['sɔːlt‚selə] *n* соло́нка.

salted ['sɔːltɪd] *a* 1) посо́ленный, засо́ленный; 2) *разг.* о́пытный; прожжённый.

salt-marsh ['sɔːltmɑːʃ] *n* солонча́к.

saltpeter ['sɔːlt‚piːtə] *n амер. см.* saltpetre.

saltpetre ['sɔːlt‚piːtə] *n* сели́тра.

salt-water ['sɔːlt‚wɔːtə] *a* солёный, морско́й (*о воде́*).

saltworks ['sɔːltwəːks] *n* соляно́й заво́д.

salty ['sɔːltɪ] *a* 1) солёный; 2) е́дкий, о́стрый (*о замечании, слове*).

salubrious [sə'luːbrɪəs] *a* здоро́вый, поле́зный для здоро́вья.

salutary ['sæljutərɪ] *a* благотво́рный, целе́бный.

salutation [ˌsæljuː'teɪʃən] *n* приве́тствие.

salute I [sə'luːt] *n* 1) приве́тствие; to imprint a chaste ~ запечатле́ть поцелу́й; 2) салю́т; 3) *воен.* отда́ние че́сти.

salute II *v* 1) здоро́ваться, приве́тствовать; 2) *воен.* отдава́ть честь, приве́тствовать; салютова́ть; 3) *уст.* целова́ть.

salvage I ['sælvɪdʒ] *n* 1) спасе́ние иму́щества (*на море или во время пожара*); to make ~ of спаса́ть (*имущество*); 2) спасённое иму́щество; 3) вознагражде́ние (*за спасённое имущество*); 4) *воен.* сбор трофе́ев; трофе́и.

salvage II *v* 1) спаса́ть иму́щество (*на море, от пожара*); 2) *воен.* собира́ть трофе́и.

salvation [sæl'veɪʃən] *n* спасе́ние.

salveᵃ I [sɑːv] *n* 1) *поэт.* целе́бная мазь; 2) успока́ивающее сре́дство; *перен.* цели́тельный бальза́м.

salveᵃ II *v* 1) *уст.* сма́зывать (*мазью*); 2) сгла́живать (*трудности*); 3) сгла́живаться (*о недостатках*); 4) загла́живать (*вину*); 5) успока́ивать (*совесть*).

salveᵇ [sælv] *v* спаса́ть иму́щество (*на море, от огня*).

salveᶜ ['sælvɪ] *int* здоро́во! (*приветствие при встрече*).

salver ['sælvə] *n* подно́с.

salvo ['sælvou] *n* 1) залп (*орудий*); 2) взрыв, гром (*аплодисментов*).

same I [seɪm] *a* 1) тот же са́мый, та же са́мая, то же са́мое; all the ~ а) тем не ме́нее, всё же; б) безразли́чно; it is all the ~ to me мне всё равно́; much the ~ почти́ одно́ и то же; just the ~ одно́ и то же; one and the ~ тот же са́мый; 2) одина́ковый, схо́дный; тожде́ственный, подо́бный.

same II *pron:* and never found (met) the ~ again так и не нашёл (не встре́тил) его́.

sameness ['seɪmnɪs] *n* 1) схо́дство; единообра́зие; тожде́ственность, подо́бие; 2) однообра́зие, моното́нность.

sample I ['sɑːmpl] *n* 1) образе́ц; обра́зчик; моде́ль; про́ба; 2) *attr* служа́щий образцо́м.

sample II *v* собира́ть образцы́, брать обра́зчик, про́бу.

sampler ['sɑːmplə] *n* 1) обра́зчик; 2) *тех.* моде́ль.

sanative ['sænətɪv] *a* целе́бный, лече́бный, оздоровля́ющий.

sanatorium [ˌsænə'tɔːrɪəm] *n* (*pl тж.* sanatoria [ˌsænə'tɔːrɪə]) санато́рий.

sanatory ['sænətərɪ] *см.* sanative.

sanctified ['sæŋktɪfaɪd] *a* 1) освящённый; 2) ха́нжеский.

sanctify ['sæŋktɪfaɪ] *v* 1) освяща́ть; 2) посвяща́ть; 3) очища́ть (*от порока*); 4) благословля́ть; санкциони́ровать.

sanctimonious [ˌsæŋktɪ'mounjəs] *a* ха́нжеский.

sanctimony ['sæŋktɪmənɪ] *n* ха́нжество.

sanction I ['sæŋkʃən] *n* 1) са́нкция, утвержде́ние; 2) одобре́ние (*чего-л.*); 3) *часто pl* са́нкция; кара́тельная ме́ра.

sanction II *v* 1) утверди́ть, санкциони́ровать; 2) одо́брить.

sanctuary ['sæŋktʃuərɪ] *n* 1) святи́лище; свята́я святы́х; 2) убе́жище; to break ~ наруша́ть пра́во неприкосновённости убе́жища; to take ~ иска́ть убе́жища; 3) запове́дник.

sanctum ['sæŋktəm] *n* 1) *см.* sanctuary 1); 2) кабине́т.

sand I [sænd] *n* 1) песо́к; fine ~ ме́лкий песо́к; built on ~ постро́енный на песке́, непро́чный; 2) *pl* пески́, песча́ная пусты́ня; 3) *pl* песча́ный пляж; о́тмель; 4) *pl* вре́мя жи́зни; the ~s are running out вре́мя подхо́дит к концу́; после́дние мину́ты истека́ют; 5) *амер. разг.* сме́лость, отва́га; твёрдость хара́ктера; 6) песо́чный цвет; ◊ to plough the ~(s) *погов.* ≅ решето́м во́ду носи́ть.

sand II *v* 1) посыпа́ть песко́м; 2) полирова́ть, шлифова́ть песко́м.

sandal¹ ['sændl] *n* санда́лия.

sandal² *n* *см.* sandalwood.

sandalwood ['sændlwud] *n* санда́ловое де́рево.

sandbag ['sændbæg] *n* мешо́к с песко́м (*для балласта*).

sand-bank ['sændbæŋk] *n* песча́ная о́тмель, коса́.

sand-blast ['sændblɑːst] *v* шлифова́ть, очища́ть песко́м.

sandboy ['sændbɔɪ] *n:* as jolly as a ~ ≅ ве́сел как молодо́й ме́сяц.

sand-glass ['sændglɑːs] *n* песо́чные часы́.

sandpaper ['sændˌpeɪpə] *n* нажда́чная бума́га.

sandstone ['sændstoun] *n* песча́ник.

sand-storm ['sændstɔːm] *n* саму́м, песча́ная бу́ря.

sandwich I ['sænwɪdʒ] *n* са́ндвич, бутербро́д.

sandwich II *v* помеща́ть ме́жду двумя́ предме́тами.

sandwich-man ['sænwɪdʒmæn] *n* челове́к-рекла́ма.

sandy ['sændɪ] *a* 1) песча́ный; песо́чный; 2) рыжева́тый; 3) непро́чный, неусто́йчивый.

sane [seɪn] *a* 1) здра́вый (*о суждении*); 2) здоро́вый (*о психике*); норма́льный; 3) здравомы́слящий.

sang [sæŋ] *past см.* sing II.

sang-froid ['sɑːŋ'frwɑː] *n* хладнокро́вие; вы́держка.

sanguinary ['sæŋgwɪnərɪ] *a* 1) кровопроли́тный; 2) кровожа́дный; 3) крова́вый (*о законе*).

sanguine ['sæŋgwɪn] *a* 1) сангвини́ческий, живо́й, жизнера́достный; 2) оптимисти́ческий; 3) румя́ный; цвету́щий.

sanguineous [sæŋ'gwɪnɪəs] *a* 1) кровяно́й; 2) крова́во-кра́сный; 3) полнокро́вный.

sanitaria [ˌsænɪ'teərɪə] *pl см.* sanitarium.

sanitarian I [ˌsænɪ'teərɪən] *n* санита́рный инспе́ктор.

sanitarian II *a* санита́рный.

sanitarium [ˌsænɪ'teərɪəm] *n* (*pl тж.* sanitaria) *амер. см.* sanatorium.

sanitary ['sænɪtərɪ] *a* санита́рный, гигиени́ческий.

sanitation [ˌsænɪ'teɪʃən] *n* 1) оздоровле́ние, улучше́ние санита́рных усло́вий; 2) санита́рия.

sanity ['sænɪtɪ] *n* 1) норма́льное психи́ческое состоя́ние; 2) здравомы́слие; здра́вый ум.

sank [sæŋk] *past см.* sink¹.

Sanskrit ['sænskrɪt] *n* санскри́т.

Santa Claus [ˌsæntəˈklɔːz] *n* Са́нта Кла́ус, дед-моро́з.

sap¹ I [sæp] *n* 1) сок расте́ний; 2) живу́честь, жизнеспосо́бность; 3) *поэт.* кровь; 4) *разг.* дура́к.

sap¹ *v* истоща́ть си́лы.

sap² I *n воен.* са́па, транше́я.

sap² II *v* 1) подводи́ть са́пу; де́лать подко́п; 2) подка́пываться (*под кого-л.*); 3) мини́ровать (*стену, скалу*); 4) подта́чивать (*здоровье*); 5) подмыва́ть (*о воде, прибое, приливе*); 6) *сленг* корпе́ть над кни́гами.

saphead [ˈsæphed] *n разг.* «глу́пая башка́», балда́.

sapheaded [ˈsæpˌhedɪd] *a* глу́пый, придуркова́тый.

sapid [ˈsæpɪd] *a* 1) вку́сный, аппети́тный; 2) живо́й, интере́сный, содержа́тельный (*о разговоре*).

sapient [ˈseɪpjənt] *a ирон.* му́дрый, му́дрствующий.

sapless [ˈsæplɪs] *a* 1) истощённый, худосо́чный; 2) вя́лый, бесцве́тный.

sapling [ˈsæplɪŋ] *n* 1) молодо́е де́ревце; 2) молодо́е существо́.

sapphire I [ˈsæfaɪə] *n* сапфи́р.

sapphire II *a* сапфи́ровый.

sappy [ˈsæpɪ] *a* 1) со́чный (*о растении*); 2) по́лный сил, эне́ргии; 3) *разг.* глу́пый.

sarcasm [ˈsɑːkæzəm] *n* сарка́зм.

sarcastic [sɑːˈkæstɪk] *a* саркасти́ческий.

sarcophagus [sɑːˈkɔfəgəs] *n* (*pl* sarcophagi [sɑːˈkɔfəgaɪ]) саркофа́г.

sardine [sɑːˈdiːn] *a* сарди́нка; packed like ~s ≅ как сельди́ в бо́чке.

sardonic [sɑːˈdɔnɪk] *a* сардони́ческий.

sash [sæʃ] *n* око́нный переплёт.

sash-window [ˈsæʃˌwɪndou] *n* подъёмное окно́.

sat [sæt] *past, p. p. см.* sit.

Satan [ˈseɪtən] *n* сатана́.

satanic [səˈtænɪk] *a* сатани́нский, дья́вольский.

satchel [ˈsætʃəl] *n* су́мка, ра́нец.

sate¹ [seɪt] *v* насыща́ть; пресыща́ть.

sate² *уст. past, p. p. см.* sit.

sateen [sæˈtiːn] *n* сати́н.

satellite [ˈsætəlaɪt] *n* 1) сателли́т; *перен. тж.* после́дователь; 2) *астр.* спу́тник; Venusian ~ спу́тник Вене́ры.

satiate I [ˈseɪʃɪeɪt] *a поэт.* пресы́щенный.

satiate II *v* насыща́ть.

satiety [səˈtaɪətɪ] *n* пресы́щенность, пресыще́ние; насыще́ние.

satin [ˈsætɪn] *n* 1) атла́с; 2) *attr* атла́сный.

satire [ˈsætaɪə] *n* сати́ра.

satiric(al) [səˈtɪrɪk(əl)] *a* сатири́ческий.

satirist [ˈsætərɪst] *n* сати́рик.

satirize [ˈsætəraɪz] *v* высме́ивать.

satisfaction [ˌsætɪsˈfækʃən] *n* 1) удовлетворе́ние; to demand ~ тре́бовать дуэ́ли *или* извине́ния; to give ~ дать удовлетворе́ние, удовлетвори́ть; it would be a ~ to me мне бу́дет прия́тно; 2) упла́та, погаше́ние до́лга; in ~ of в упла́ту обяза́тельств; 4) искупле́ние.

satisfactory [ˌsætɪsˈfæktərɪ] *a* удовлетвори́тельный, доста́точный; отвеча́ющий, соотве́тствующий тре́бованиям.

satisfy [ˈsætɪsfaɪ] *v* 1) удовлетворя́ть; to be satisfied быть дово́льным, удовлетвори́ться (*чем-л.—*

with); 2) соотве́тствовать, отвеча́ть (*требова-ниям*); 3) выпла́чивать (*долг*); 4) утоля́ть (*голод, любопытство и т. п.*); 5) убежда́ть (*в чём-л.— of*); to ~ oneself убеди́ться.

saturate [ˈsætʃəreɪt] *v* 1) насыща́ть; 2) пропи́тывать.

saturated [ˈsætʃəreɪtɪd] *a* 1) насы́щенный; 2) пропи́танный; 3) я́ркий (*о цвете*).

saturation [ˌsætʃəˈreɪʃən] *n* насыще́ние, насы́щенность.

Saturday [ˈsætədɪ] *n* 1) суббо́та; 2) *attr* суббо́тний.

Saturn [ˈsætən] *n астр., миф.* Сату́рн.

saturnine [ˈsætəːnaɪn] *a* мра́чный.

satyr [ˈsætə] *n* сати́р.

sauce I [sɔːs] *n* 1) со́ус; припра́ва; poignant ~ о́стрый со́ус; 2) пика́нтность; 3) *разг.* на́глость, де́рзость; none of your ~! не наха́льничай!; 4) *амер.* фрукто́вое пюре́, пови́дло; ◇ what's ~ for the goose is ~ for the gander *посл.* ≅ что хорошо́ для одного́, то годи́тся и для друго́го.

sauce II *v* 1) полива́ть со́усом; 2) придава́ть пика́нтность; приправля́ть остроу́мием; 3) *разг.* говори́ть де́рзко, дерзи́ть.

sauce-boat [ˈsɔːsbout] *n* со́усник.

saucebox [ˈsɔːsbɔks] *n разг.* нагле́ц, наха́л(ка).

saucepan [ˈsɔːspən] *n* кастрю́ля.

saucer [ˈsɔːsə] *n* блю́дце; поддо́нник.

saucy [ˈsɔːsɪ] *a* 1) на́глый, наха́льный; 2) живо́й, бо́йкий; 3) *разг.* щегольско́й, мо́дный.

saunter I [ˈsɔːntə] *n* прогу́лка.

saunter II *v* прогу́ливаться, проха́живаться.

sausage [ˈsɔsɪdʒ] *n* 1) колбаса́; соси́ска; 2) «колбаса́», аэроста́т наблюде́ния.

savage I [ˈsævɪdʒ] *n* 1) дика́рь, тузе́мец; 2) гру́бый, жесто́кий челове́к.

savage II *a* 1) ди́кий, ва́рварский; 2) жесто́кий; 3) *разг.* взбешённый.

savagery [ˈsævɪdʒərɪ] *n* 1) ди́кость; 2) жесто́кость.

savannah [səˈvænə] *n* сава́нна.

save I [seɪv] *v* 1) спаса́ть; 2) храни́ть, сохраня́ть, бере́чь; to ~ oneself бере́чь свои́ си́лы; ~ me from ..! нет уж, увольте меня́ от ..!; 3) откла́дывать, сберега́ть (*деньги*); 4) эконо́мить; откла́дывать, копи́ть; 5) избавля́ть (*от чего-л.— from*); 6) отбива́ть нападе́ние (*в футболе*); □ to ~ up копи́ть (*деньги*).

save II *prep* кро́ме, исключа́я; ~ and except за исключе́нием, не счита́я.

save-all [ˈseɪvɔːl] *n* спецоде́жда, комбинезо́н, хала́т.

saver [ˈseɪvə] *n* 1) спаси́тель (*душ*); 2) эконо́мный челове́к; 3) вещь, механи́зм, сберега́ющие вре́мя.

saving I [ˈseɪvɪŋ] *n* 1) эконо́мия; 2) *pl* сбереже́ния.

saving II *a* 1) эконо́мный; бережли́вый; 2) спаси́тельный; 3) *юр.* содержа́щий огово́рку.

saving III *prep* исключа́я; ~ your presence (*или* reverence) извини́те за выраже́ние.

savings-bank [ˈseɪvɪŋzbæŋk] *n* сберега́тельная ка́сса.

savio(u)r [ˈseɪvjə] *n* спаси́тель.

savo(u)r I [ˈseɪvə] *n* 1) вкус, при́вкус; 2) *уст.* арома́т, за́пах; 3) отличи́тельное ка́чество, свойство; 4) интере́с, острота́, смак; 5) репута́ция.

savo(u)r II *v* 1) дава́ть вкус, при́вкус; име́ть вкус, при́вкус; 2) отдава́ть (*чем-л.* — of); 3) смакова́ть; отве́дывать.

savoury I ['seɪvərɪ] *n* о́страя заку́ска.

savoury II *a* 1) вку́сный; 2) пика́нтный; о́стрый (*на вкус*); прия́тный.

savoy [sə'vɔɪ] *n* саво́йская капу́ста.

savvy I ['sævɪ] *n сленг* понима́ние, сообрази́тельность, ра́зум.

savvy II *v сленг*: ~? поня́тно?; по ~ не понима́ю; не понима́ешь *и т. п.*

saw[1] I [sɔː] *n* пила́; circular ~ кру́глая пила́; to set a ~ направля́ть пилу́.

saw[1] II *v* (*past* sawed; *p. p.* sawed, sawn) пили́ть, распи́ливать.

saw[2] *past см.* see[1].

saw[3] *n* погово́рка, выраже́ние.

sawdust ['sɔːdʌst] *n* опи́лки.

saw-horse ['sɔːhɔːs] *n* ко́злы (*для пилки*).

sawmill ['sɔːmɪl] *n* лесопи́льный заво́д, лесопи́лка.

sawn [sɔːn] *p. p. см.* saw[1] II.

sawyer ['sɔːjə] *n* 1) пи́льщик; 2) *амер.* коря́га (*в реке*).

Saxon I ['sæksn] *n* 1) *ист.* сакс, англоса́кс; 2) саксо́нец; 3) (англо)саксо́нский язы́к.

Saxon II *a* (англо)саксо́нский.

Saxony ['sæksnɪ] *n* то́нкая шерсть *или* шерстяна́я мате́рия.

saxophone ['sæksəfoun] *n муз.* саксофо́н.

say I [seɪ] *v* (*past, p. p.* said) 1) сказа́ть, говори́ть; I ~! послу́шайте!; you don't ~ so! не мо́жет быть!; ~ no more! хва́тит!, доста́точно!; easier said than done ле́гче сказа́ть, чем сде́лать; least said soonest mended разгово́ры то́лько вредя́т де́лу; no sooner said than done ≅ ска́зано — сде́лано; I should ~ я ду́маю, я полага́ю; that is to ~ то есть; they ~ говоря́т (*тж. как вводное слово*); not to ~ чтобы не сказа́ть (бо́льше); 2) выража́ть, сообща́ть, заявля́ть; 3) чита́ть (*стихотворе́ние*); отвеча́ть (*урок*); 4): ~ five roubles о́коло пяти́ рубле́й; ◊ that goes without ~ing само́ собо́й разуме́ется.

say II *n* 1) мне́ние; to have one's ~ вы́сказаться; 2): it is now my ~ тепе́рь моя́ о́чередь говори́ть.

saying ['seɪɪŋ] *n* погово́рка; as the ~ is (*или* goes) как говори́тся; there is no ~ тру́дно сказа́ть.

say-so ['seɪˌsou] *n разг.* 1) утвержде́ние, сообще́ние (*отдельного лица*); 2) оконча́тельное мне́ние; 3) приказа́ние.

scab I [skæb] *n* 1) штрейкбре́хер; преда́тель; 2) *уст.* негодя́й, мерза́вец; 3) струп (*на ране*); 4) парша́, чесо́тка; 5) *attr* штрейкбре́херский, прода́жный.

scab II *v* 1) быть штрейкбре́хером; 2) покрыва́ться паршо́й.

scabbard I ['skæbəd] *n* но́жны.

scabbard II *v* вкла́дывать в но́жны.

scabby ['skæbɪ] *a* 1) покры́тый паршо́й, чесо́ткой; 2) шелуди́вый; 3) *разг.* парши́вый.

scabrous ['skeɪbrəs] *a* 1) шерохова́тый; 2) затрудни́тельный; 3) скабрёзный.

scaffold I ['skæfəld] *n* 1) леса́ (*строительные*); 2) эшафо́т, пла́ха; to go to the ~ сложи́ть го́лову

на пла́хе; to send to the ~ приговори́ть к сме́ртной ка́зни; 3) помо́ст, трибу́на.

scaffold II *v* ста́вить леса́, эшафо́т, помо́ст.

scaffolding ['skæfəldɪŋ] *n* леса́ (*строительные*).

scalawag ['skæləwæg] *n* 1) *разг.* негодя́й, прохво́ст; 2) *амер. ист.* урожёнец ю́жных шта́тов, подде́рживавший северя́н.

scald[1] I [skɔːld] *n* ожо́г.

scald[1] II *v* 1) обва́ривать, ошпа́ривать (*тж.* to ~ out); 2) обвари́ться, ошпа́риться; 3) пастеризова́ть (*молоко*).

scald[2] *n* скальд, поэ́т.

scale[1] I [skeɪl] *n* 1) разме́р; масшта́б; large ~ кру́пный масшта́б; on a large (*или* vast) ~ в больши́х масшта́бах; on a small ~ в небольши́х масшта́бах; on the widest ~ в широ́ких масшта́бах; to no ~ не по масшта́бу; 2) шкала́; sliding ~ скользя́щая шкала́; high (low) in the ~ высо́кое (ни́зкое) положе́ние на шкале́; 3) *муз.* га́мма; 4) лине́йка (*с делениями*); 5) *мат.* систе́ма счисле́ния; decimal ~ десяти́чная систе́ма счисле́ния; 6) *уст.* ле́стница, ступе́нь.

scale[1] II *v* 1) взбира́ться (*по ступеням, лестнице*); 2) де́лать по масшта́бу; измеря́ть по масшта́бу; □ to ~ **down** уменьша́ть, снижа́ть (*о зарплате*); to ~ **up** повыша́ть (*о ценах*).

scale[2] I *n* 1) ча́ш(к)а весо́в; to hold the ~s even быть справедли́вым, беспристра́стным; to turn the ~ at ве́сить (*столько-то*); to turn (*или* to tip) the ~ склони́ть ча́шу весо́в; реши́ть исхо́д де́ла; 2) *pl* весы́ (*тж.* a pair of ~s).

scale[2] II *v* 1) ве́шать, взве́шивать; 2) ве́сить.

scale[3] I *n* 1) чешуя́; чешу́йка; 2) *часто pl* пелена́; ~s fell from his eyes пелена́ спа́ла с его́ глаз; 3) на́кипь; окали́на.

scale[3] II *v* 1) снима́ть, соска́бливать чешую́; 2) шелуши́ть(ся); 3) покрыва́ть(ся) на́кипью.

scaled [skeɪld] *a* 1) чешу́йчатый; 2) покры́тый на́кипью.

scallawag ['skæləwæg] *см.* scalawag.

scallop ['skɔləp] *n* 1) ра́ковина; 2) *pl* фесто́ны, зубцы́.

scalp I [skælp] *n* 1) скальп; to take one's ~ *перен.* победи́ть кого́-л.; 2) *амер.* лёгкая нажи́ва.

scalp II *v* 1) скальпи́ровать; 2) *амер.* спекули́ровать; нажива́ться.

scaly ['skeɪlɪ] *a* 1) чешу́йчатый; 2) покры́тый на́кипью; 3) *сленг* ме́рзкий, презре́нный.

scamp[1] *n* [skæmp] *n* негодя́й; a thorough ~ никчёмный челове́к.

scamp[2] *v* рабо́тать небре́жно.

scamper I ['skæmpə] *n* 1) бы́стрый бег; 2) бе́глое, невнима́тельное чте́ние.

scamper II *v* бежа́ть стремгла́в; улепётывать.

scan [skæn] *v* 1) внима́тельно рассма́тривать; разгля́дывать; 2) бе́гло просма́тривать; 3) сканди́ровать.

scandal ['skændl] *n* 1) позо́р, позо́рный посту́пок; what a ~! како́й позо́р!; 2) спле́тни; to talk ~ спле́тничать; 3) недосто́йный челове́к; 4) сканда́л.

scandalize ['skændəlaɪz] *v* возмуща́ть, шоки́ровать.

scandalmonger ['skændlˌmʌŋgə] *n* спле́тник.

scandalous ['skændələs] *a* 1) позо́рный, позо́рящий; 2) оскорби́тельный, сканда́льный; 3) клеветни́ческий; 4) лю́бящий поспле́тничать.

Scandinavian I [ˌskændɪ'neɪvjən] *n* скандинáв; уроженец *или* житель Скандинáвии.

Scandinavian II *a* скандинáвский.

scant [skænt] *a* скýдный, недостáточный; to be ~ of не хватáть, недоставáть; ~ of breath задыхáющийся.

scanty ['skæntɪ] *a* 1) скýдный; ограниченный; 2) убóгий.

scape [skeɪp] *см.* escape II.

scapegoat ['skeɪpgout] *n* козёл отпущéния.

scapegrace ['skeɪpgreɪs] *n* шалопáй, повéса.

scar[1] I [skɑː] *n* 1) шрам, рубéц; 2) пятнó (*позóра*).

scar[1] II *v* 1) покрывáться рубцáми; 2) зарубцевáться.

scar[2] *n* 1) утёс, скалá; 2) подвóдная скалá, риф.

scaramouch ['skærəmautʃ] *n уст.* 1) шут, пая́ц; 2) хвастливый трус; бездéльник.

scarce I [skɛəs] *a* 1) скýдный, имéющийся в небольшóм колѝчестве; 2) рéдкий; to make oneself ~ а) рéдко покáзываться; б) держáться в отдалéнии; в) удрáть, испарѝться.

scarce II *adv* едвá.

scarcely ['skɛəslɪ] *adv* 1) едвá; 2) вряд ли; ~ enough вряд ли хвáтит; ~ ever не всегдá; 3) не совсéм.

scarcity ['skɛəsɪtɪ] *n* 1) скýдость; недостáточность; дефицит; 2) рéдкость.

scare I [skɛə] *n* внезáпный испýг; ýжас; пáника.

scare II *v* 1) пугáть, приводѝть в ýжас; he was ~d out of his seven senses ≅ он был напýган дó смерти; 2) отпýгивать (*птиц*); ⬜ to ~ away спугнýть, отпугнýть.

scarecrow ['skɛəkrou] *n* пýгало.

scaremonger ['skɛəˌmʌŋgə] *n* паникёр.

scarf [skɑːf] *n* (*pl тж.* scarves) 1) шарф, кашнé; 2) гáлстук.

scarify ['skɛərɪfaɪ] *v* 1) *мед.* дéлать насéчки, надрéзы; 2) сурóво критиковáть; 3) оскорблять чьи-л. чýвства; 4) *с.-х.* разрыхлять, рыхлить (*пóчву*).

scarlet I ['skɑːlɪt] *n* áлый цвет.

scarlet II *a* áлый.

scarp [skɑːp] *n* 1) крутóй склон; откóс; 2) *воен.* эскáрп.

scarves [skɑːvz] *pl см.* scarf.

scary ['skɛərɪ] *a разг.* 1) жýткий, вызывáющий испýг; 2) пуглѝвый.

scathe I [skeɪð] *n* ущéрб, вред; without ~ невредѝмый.

scathe II *v* причинять ущéрб, вредить.

scatheless ['skeɪðlɪs] *a обыкн. predic* невредѝмый.

scatter ['skætə] *v* 1) рассыпáть; разбрáсывать; расшвѝривать; 2) посыпáть (*чем-л. — with*); 3) брызгать; разбрызгивать; 4) развéивать; 5) раздавáть (*богáтства*); 6) бросáться, сорить (*деньгáми*); 7) разгонять (*облакá и т. п.*); 8) рассéиваться (*о толпé, облакáх*); 9): to be ~ed рассéиваться (*о надéждах, плáнах и т. п.*).

scatter-brain ['skætəbreɪn] *n* вертопрáх.

scatter-brained ['skætəbreɪnd] *a* легкомѝсленный, вéтреный.

scattered ['skætəd] *a* 1) разбрóсанный (*о домáх, предмéтах*); 2) отдéльный, разрóзненный; 3) рассéянный (*об облакáх*).

scaur [skɔː] *см.* scar[2].

scavenge ['skævɪndʒ] *v* убирáть мýсор (*с улиц*).

scavenger ['skævɪndʒə] *n* мýсорщик.

scavenging ['skævɪndʒɪŋ] *n* убóрка мýсора.

scenario [sɪ'nɑːrɪou] *n* сценáрий.

scene [siːn] *n* 1) мéсто дéйствия, арéна; the ~ is laid in дéйствие происхóдит в; 2) событие, происшéствие; 3) скандáл; сцéна; to make a ~ устрáивать сцéну; 4) явлéние, сцéна (*часть пьéсы*); crowd ~ мáссовая сцéна; 5) декорáция; side ~ кулѝса; behind the ~s за кулѝсами; 6) зрéлище, вид; a striking ~ потрясáющее зрéлище; a ~ of destruction картѝна разрушéния; 7) *уст.* сцéна, эстрáда; to quit the ~ *перен.* умерéть.

scene-painter ['siːnˌpeɪntə] *n* худóжник-декорáтор.

scenery ['siːnərɪ] *n* 1) декорáции; 2) óбщий вид; картѝна; пейзáж.

scene-shifter ['siːnˌʃɪftə] *n* рабóчий сцéны.

scenic ['siːnɪk] *a* 1) живопѝсный; 2) театрáльный, сценѝческий.

scent I [sent] *n* 1) зáпах; 2) духѝ; to put some ~ (по)душить (*духáми*); to wear ~ употреблять духѝ, душѝться; 3) след; off the ~ не по слéду; по непрáвильному слéду; blazing ~, hot ~ горячий след; false ~ лóжный след; to be on the right ~ быть на прáвильном путѝ; напáсть на прáвильный след; to put (*или* to throw) one off the ~ напрáвить по лóжному слéду; 4) нюх, чутьё.

scent II *v* 1) обонять; 2) чýять; 3) душѝть (*духáми*); 4) пáхнуть (*чем-л. — of*); ⬜ ~ out разузнáть, разнюхать.

sceptic ['skeptɪk] *n* скéптик.

sceptical ['skeptɪkəl] *a* скептѝческий.

scepticism ['skeptɪsɪzəm] *n* скептицѝзм.

sceptre ['septə] *n* скѝпетр.

schedule I ['ʃedjuːl, *амер.* 'skedjuːl] *n* 1) катáлог, пéречень; 2) óпись, инвентáрь; 3) расписáние, таблѝца, грáфик.

schedule II *v* 1) вносѝть в катáлог, óпись *и т. п.*; 2) планѝровать; 3) составлять расписáние, грáфик.

scheme I [skiːm] *n* 1) план, проéкт; прогрáмма дéйствий; 2) схéма; 3) построéния (*наýчные*); систéма (*воззрéний и т. п.*); 4) диагрáмма, кáрта; 5) *pl* интрѝги, прóиски.

scheme II *v* 1) строить плáны; составлять проéкты; 2) интриговáть, замышлять.

schemer ['skiːmə] *n* 1) интригáн; 2) прожектёр.

schism ['sɪzəm] *n церк.* раскóл.

schismatic I [sɪz'mætɪk] *n* раскóльник.

schismatic II *a* раскóльнический.

scholar ['skɔlə] *n* 1) *уст.* учáщийся; 2) учёный; 3) стипендиáт; 4) *разг.* грамотéй.

scholarly ['skɔləlɪ] *a* эрудѝрованный, учёный.

scholarship ['skɔləʃɪp] *n* 1) учёность, эрудѝция; 2) стипéндия.

scholastic I [skə'læstɪk] *n* 1) схолáст; 2) педáнт.

scholastic II *a* 1) учéбный; шкóльный; 2) схоластѝческий; 3) педантѝчный.

school I [skuːl] *n* 1) шкóла; continuation ~ дополнѝтельная шкóла (*для пополнéния образовá-*

ния по выходе из начальной школы); elementary (*или* primary) ~, *амер.* grade ~ нача́льная шко́ла; grammar ~ сре́дняя шко́ла (*типа гимназии в Англии*); higher grade ~ по́лная сре́дняя шко́ла; secondary ~, *амер.* high ~ сре́дняя шко́ла; industrial ~, *амер.* trade ~ (профессиона́льно-) техни́ческое учи́лище, ремесленное училище; infant ~ приготови́тельная шко́ла (*для детей 5—7 лет в Англии*); modern secondary ~ непо́лная сре́дняя шко́ла (*1—5 классы в Англии*); modern technical ~ сре́дняя шко́ла (*с техническим уклоном в Англии*); normal ~ педагоги́ческое учи́лище *или* техникум; public ~ а) класси́ческая гимна́зия; б) закры́тая сре́дняя шко́ла (*в Англии*); в) государственная беспла́тная шко́ла (*в США*); vocational ~ профессиона́льная шко́ла; nursery ~s де́тские сады́; approved ~ госуда́рственная шко́ла для малоле́тних правонаруши́телей; to attend ~ посеща́ть школу; to be at ~ учи́ться в шко́ле; to leave ~ око́нчить шко́лу; to put (*или* to send) to ~ отда́ть в шко́лу; there will be no ~ today сего́дня не бу́дет заня́тий; 2) шко́ла (*в науке, литературе, искусстве*); of the old ~ старомо́дный; 3) уча́щиеся (*одной школы*); 4) класс (*помещение*); 5) *attr* уче́бный, шко́льный.

school II *v* 1) обуча́ть, тренирова́ть; 2) де́лать вы́говор, отчи́тывать.

school-book ['skuːlbuk] *n* шко́льный уче́бник.

schoolboy ['skuːlbɔi] *n* шко́льник, учени́к.

schoolfellow ['skuːl,felou] *n* шко́льный това́рищ.

schoolgirl ['skuːlgəːl] *n* шко́льница, учени́ца.

schoolhouse ['skuːlhaus] *n* зда́ние школы.

schooling ['skuːliŋ] *n* 1) обуче́ние; 2) образова́ние; 3) преподава́ние; 4) вы́говор, нравоуче́ние.

school-ma'am ['skuːlmæm] *n разг.* шко́льная учи́тельница.

schoolman ['skuːlmən] *n* 1) шко́льный учи́тель; 2) схола́ст.

schoolmaster ['skuːl,mɑːstə] *n* шко́льный учи́тель, педаго́г.

school-mate ['skuːlmeit] *n* соучени́к, однока́шник.

schoolmistress ['skuːl,mistris] *n* шко́льная учи́тельница.

schoolroom ['skuːlrum] *n* класс, кла́ссная ко́мната.

school-teacher ['skuːl,tiːtʃə] *n* шко́льный учи́тель, шко́льная учи́тельница.

school-time ['skuːltaim] *n* 1) часы́ заня́тий (*в школе*); 2) го́ды уче́ния, шко́льные го́ды.

school-yard ['skuːljɑːd] *n* спортплоща́дка (*при школе*), шко́льный двор.

schooner[1] ['skuːnə] *n* 1) шху́на; 2) *амер.* фурго́н переселе́нцев.

schooner[2] *n амер. разг.* большо́й стака́н (*для пива*).

schwa [ʃwɑː] *n фон.* шва, нейтра́льный гла́сный [ə].

science ['saiəns] *n* 1) нау́ка; о́трасль нау́ки; exact ~ то́чная нау́ка; applied ~ прикладна́я нау́ка; pure ~ «чи́стая» нау́ка; natural ~ есте́ственные нау́ки; social ~ обще́ственные нау́ки; space ~s косми́ческие нау́ки; 2) ло́вкость, уме́ние.

scientific [,saiən'tifik] *a* 1) нау́чный; учёный; 2) иску́сный, уме́лый.

scientifically [,saiən'tifikəli] *adv* с нау́чной то́чки зре́ния, нау́чно, с нау́чных пози́ций.

scientist ['saiəntist] *n* учёный; Honoured Scientist заслу́женный де́ятель нау́ки; top ~s веду́щие учёные страны́.

scimitar ['simitə] *n* крива́я са́бля, ятага́н.

scintilla [sin'tilə] *n* и́скра; крупи́нка; not a ~ of ни ка́пли.

scintillate ['sintileit] *v* и́скриться; мерца́ть.

scintillation [,sinti'leiʃən] *n* 1) сверка́ние, мерца́ние; 2) вспы́шка.

scion ['saiən] *n* 1) побе́г, черено́к (*растения*); 2) пото́мок, о́трыск (*кого-л.— of*).

scissor ['sizə] *v* ре́зать но́жницами; □ to ~ out вы́резать (*ножницами*).

scissors ['sizəz] *n pl* но́жницы (*тж.* a pair of ~).

scobs [skɔbz] *n pl* опи́лки.

scoff I [skɔf] *n* насме́шка; the ~ of посме́шище.

scoff II *v* 1) говори́ть, выска́зываться ирони́чески; 2) насмеха́ться (*над — at*); осме́ивать.

scoffer ['skɔfə] *n* насме́шник.

scold I [skould] *n* сварли́вая же́нщина.

scold II *v* брани́ть, руга́ть, отчи́тывать.

scolding ['skouldiŋ] *n* 1) пробо́рка, нагоня́й; 2) брань.

sconce[1] [skɔns] *n шутл.* «башка́», «черепо́к».

sconce[2] *n* подсве́чник, канделя́бр.

scon(e) [skɔn] *n* пшени́чная *или* ячме́нная лепёшка; dropped ~ *амер.* кру́глый хлебе́ц.

scoop I [skuːp] *n* 1) сово́к; 2) ковш (*экскаватора*); 3) ло́жечка (*хирургический инструмент*); 4) котлова́н, я́ма; 5) черпа́ние; 6) *разг.* большо́й куш (*денег*); 7) сенсацио́нная но́вость (*в газете*).

scoop II *v* брать (*совком*); забира́ть (*ковшом*); че́рпать; □ to ~ in собира́ть; to ~ out вычёрпывать; to ~ up поднима́ть.

scoot [skuːt] *v разг.* сорва́ться с ме́ста; бежа́ть стремгла́в.

scooter ['skuːtə] *n* 1) де́тский самока́т; 2) мотороллер (*тж.* motor ~); 3) ску́тер.

scope [skoup] *n* 1) кругозо́р, разма́х; 2) сфе́ра де́йствий; 3) компете́нция; beyond my ~ вне мое́й компете́нции.

scorbutic I [skɔː'bjuːtik] *n* цинго́тный больно́й.

scorbutic II *a* цинго́тный.

scorch I [skɔːtʃ] *n* 1) ожо́г; 2) *разг.* бе́шеная езда́.

scorch II *v* 1) опаля́ть; пали́ть (*о солнце*); 2) подгора́ть; 3) коро́биться (*от жары*); 4) *разг.* мча́ться, нести́сь с бе́шеной ско́ростью (*об автомобиле и т. п.*).

scorcher ['skɔːtʃə] *n* 1) жа́ркий, зно́йный день; 2) *разг.* лиха́ч (*о водителе и т. п.*).

scorching ['skɔːtʃiŋ] *a* 1) паля́щий, зно́йный; 2) жесто́кий, уничтожа́ющий (*о критике, ответе и т. п.*).

score I [skɔː] *n* 1) счёт очко́в (*в спортивных играх*); 2) табли́ца вы́игранных очко́в; to keep the ~ вести́ счёт; 3) причи́на, основа́ние; on the ~ of всле́дствие, по причи́не; 4) отме́тка, зару́бка, ме́тка; 5) острота́ на чужо́й счёт; to be fond of making ~s остри́ть на чей-л. счёт; 6) уда́ча; what a ~! как повезло́!; 7) *pl* мно́жество, ма́сса; ~s of people мно́го наро́ду; 8) два деся́тка, два́дцать; 9) *муз.* партиту́ра; ◊ to pay off (*или* to settle) old ~s сводить старые счёты; to quit ~s with расквитаться с кем-л.; rejected on the ~ of absurdity отклонено по причине явного абсурда; to go off at ~s (*или* at full ~) приняться с жаром за что-л.

score II *v* 1) делать отметки, зарубки; 2) вести счёт выигрышей; 3) записывать на чей-л. счёт; 4) выигрывать; иметь успех, удачу; you have ~d вам повезло; 5) *амер.* резко критиковать; 6) *муз.* оркестровать; □ to ~ **off** *разг.* одержать верх, переспорить; to ~ **out** зачеркнуть, вымарать; to ~ **under** подчёркивать; to ~ **up** подсчитывать (*очки в игре и т. п.*).

scorer ['skɔːrə] *n* маркёр, счётчик (*в спортивных играх*).

scorn I [skɔːn] *n* 1) презрение, пренебрежение; to think ~ of презирать; 2) насмешка, издёвка; 3) объект презрения; he is a ~ to, he is the ~ of его презирают, над ним насмехаются.

scorn II *v* 1) презирать; пренебрегать; to ~ to do smth. не унижаться до чего-л., не позволять себе сделать что-л.; 2) насмехаться, глумиться (*над — at*).

scornful ['skɔːnful] *a* презрительный; насмешливый.

scorpion ['skɔːpjən] *n* 1) скорпион; 2) (S.) Скорпион (*созвездие*).

Scot [skɔt] *n* 1) шотландец; 2) *ист.* скотт (*кельт*).

scot [skɔt] *n ист.* налог, подать; to pay ~ and lot платить все налоги; *перен.* нести бремя.

Scotch I [skɔtʃ] *n* 1): the ~ (*употр. как pl*) шотландцы; 2) шотландский диалект; 3) *разг.* шотландское виски.

Scotch II *a* шотландский.

scotch I [skɔtʃ] *n* 1) надрез, заметка, метка; 2) клин.

scotch II *v* 1) ранить, калечить; 2) делать заметку, надрез; надрезать; 3) уничтожать, ликвидировать.

Scotchman ['skɔtʃmən] *n* шотландец.

Scotchwoman ['skɔtʃˌwumən] *n* шотландка, уроженка Шотландии.

scot-free ['skɔt'friː] *a* 1) невредимый, безнаказанный; to get off ~, to go ~ остаться безнаказанным; 2) *редко* освобождённый от налога.

Scotia ['skouʃə] *n поэт.* Шотландия.

Scotland Yard ['skɔtlənd'jɑːd] *n* 1) Скотленд-ярд (*центральное управление полиции и сыскного отделения в Лондоне*); 2) полиция.

Scots I [skɔts] *n* шотландский язык.

Scots II *a* шотландский.

Scotsman ['skɔtsmən] *см.* Scotchman.

Scotswoman ['skɔts,wumən] *см.* Scotchwoman.

Scottish I, II ['skɔtiʃ] *см.* Scotch I 1), II.

scoundrel ['skaundrəl] *n* подлец, мерзавец.

scour¹ I ['skauə] *n* чистка; to give it a ~ основательно чистить; отчистить.

scour¹ II *v* чистить; □ to ~ **away**, to ~ **off**, to ~ **out** отчистить, оттереть.

scour² *v* 1) рыскать (*по — about*); 2) прочёсывать (*лес, местность*).

scourge I [skəːdʒ] *n* 1) *уст.* плеть; 2) бич; бедствие, кара; ◇ the white ~ туберкулёз.

scourge II *v* 1) бичевать; 2) карать, подвергать наказанию.

scout¹ I [skaut] *n* 1) разведчик (*тж. о самолёте и корабле*); boy ~ бойскаут; 2) *амер. разг.* малый, парень; 3) служитель (*в Оксфордском университете*).

scout¹ II *v* 1) разведывать; 2) наблюдать, осматривать.

scout² *v* отвергать с негодованием, презрением.

scouting ['skautiŋ] *n* разведка, разведывание.

scow [skau] *n* шаланда.

scowl I [skaul] *n* мрачный вид; нахмуренный взгляд.

scowl II *v* 1) хмуриться (*at, on*); 2) иметь угрожающий вид.

scrabble I [skræbl] *n* каракули.

scrabble II *v* 1) царапать, скрести; 2) писать каракулями.

scrag I [skræg] *n* 1) шея бараньей *или* телячьей туши; 2) *сленг* шея; 3) кощей; «кожа да кости».

scrag II *v разг.* 1) вешать (*казнить*); 2) свернуть шею (*кому-л.*).

scraggy ['skrægi] *a* тощий, сухопарый.

scram [skræm] *v амер. разг.* удрать, выбраться.

scramble I ['skræmbl] *n* 1) карабканье; 2) свалка, схватка.

scramble II *v* 1) карабкаться; 2) драться за захват (*чего-л.— for*); 3) беспорядочно собирать (*часто* to ~ up); 4) делать яичницу-болтунью.

scrannel ['skrænl] *a уст.* 1) скрипучий; 2) тощий, худощавый.

scrap¹ I [skræp] *n* 1) кусок; 2) клочок, обрывок (*бумаги*); лоскуток (*материи*); 3) *pl* объёдки; отбросы; 4) вырезка (*из газеты, журнала*); 5) *pl* металлический лом, скрап.

scrap¹ II *v* 1) ломать на мелкие куски; разламывать; превращать в утиль; 2) выбрасывать как утиль; отдавать на слом.

scrap² I *n разг.* скандал, потасовка.

scrap² II *v разг.* устраивать скандал, потасовку.

scrap-book ['skræpbuk] *n* альбом (*с вырезками из газет и т. п.*).

scrape I [skreip] *n* 1) царапина; 2) скрип пера; 3) шарканье (*ногой*); 4) затруднение, неприятное положение; to be in a ~ быть в затруднительном положении; to get into a ~ попасть в неприятное положение; 5) очистка, соскабливание, отскабливание.

scrape II *v* 1) скоблить; скрести; 2) тереть(ся) (*обо что-л.—against*); 3) пилякать (*на скрипке*); 4) скаредничать, экономить; □ to ~ **away**, to ~ **down**, to ~ **off** отскабливать, отскребать, отчищать; to ~ **out** выскабливать, выскребать; to ~ **through** а) с трудом пробраться; б) еле-еле сдать (*экзамен*); to ~ **together**, to ~ **up** наскребать, накапливать (*с большим трудом*).

scrape-penny ['skreip,peni] *n* скряга.

scraper ['skreipə] *n* 1) скребок; 2) железка (*для очистки обуви*); 3) *тех.* скрепер.

scrap-heap ['skræphiːp] *n* куча (*лома и т. п.*); свалка (*отбросов*).

scrappy¹ ['skræpi] *a* 1) обрывочный, отрывочный; бессвязный; 2) лоскутный.

scrappy² *a сленг* скандальный, склочный.

scratch I [skrætʃ] *n* 1) царапина; 2) росчерк (*пера*); 3) почёсывание; зуд; 4) царапанье; 5) *спорт.* черта, отмечающая старт; from ~ с самого начала.

scratch II *a разг.* 1) случа́йный; 2) разношёрстный, сбо́рный.

scratch III *v* 1) цара́пать, оцара́пать; расцара́пать; 2) чеса́ть(ся), скрести́(сь); 3) чи́ркать; 4) вычёркивать; 5) скрипе́ть (*о перьях*); □ to ~ along *сленг* перебива́ться; to ~ off, to ~ out вычёркивать; to ~ together, to ~ up наскрести́.

scratchy ['skrætʃɪ] *a* 1) небре́жный, гру́бый (*о рисунке*); 2) цара́пающий (*о пере*); 3) случа́йный, пло́хо подо́бранный, сбо́рный.

scrawl I [skrɔːl] *n* кара́кули.

scrawl II *v* писа́ть кара́кулями.

scrawny ['skrɔːnɪ] *a амер. разг.* худо́й, то́щий, худоща́вый.

screak I [skriːk] *n* 1) визг; 2) скрип.

screak II [*v*] 1) визжа́ть; 2) скрипе́ть.

scream I [skriːm] *n* 1) пронзи́тельный крик (*от боли, испуга*); вопль; визг; взви́згивание; 2) ре́зкий звук, лязг; 3) *сленг* умо́ра, поте́ха; 4) взрыв хо́хота; ~s of laughter неудержи́мый хо́хот.

scream II *v* 1) вскри́кнуть, взви́згнуть (*от боли, испуга*); 2) зареве́ть (*о свистке, сире́не*); 3) говори́ть, петь (*с напряже́нием в го́лосе; тж.* to ~ out); 4): to ~ with laughter хохота́ть, гогота́ть.

screamer ['skriːmə] *n сленг* 1) *амер.* сенсацио́нный заголо́вок; 2) потряса́ющий, удиви́тельный факт; умори́тельное происше́ствие; 3) *амер.* восклица́тельный знак.

screaming ['skriːmɪŋ] *a* 1) крича́щий (*тж. о кра́сках*); 2) умори́тельный, коми́ческий.

screamy ['skriːmɪ] *a* экспанси́вный, истери́чный.

screech I [skriːtʃ] *n* 1) крик (*ужаса, я́рости*); 2) злове́щий крик, звук.

screech II *v* 1) закрича́ть (*от ужаса, я́рости*); 2) злове́ще крича́ть.

screech-owl ['skriːtʃaul] *n* 1) уша́стая сова́; 2) предве́стник дурно́го.

screed [skriːd] *n* 1) ну́дная речь, ну́дное повествова́ние; 2) утоми́тельная цита́та.

screen I [skriːn] *n* 1) ши́рма; 2) экра́н; 3) щит, доска́ (*для объявле́ний*); 4) перегоро́дка; window ~ око́нная решётка; 5) заве́са; 6) покро́в, прикры́тие; under the ~ of night под покро́вом но́чи; 7) решето́, си́то (*для угля́, песка́*); 8) *воен.* охране́ние, прикры́тие; заве́са.

screen II *v* 1) прикрыва́ть, укрыва́ть; защища́ть (*от уда́ра, хо́лода*); 2) демонстри́ровать (*на экра́не*); 3) производи́ть киносъёмку; экранизи́ровать; 4) составля́ть сцена́рий (*кинофи́льма*); 5) просе́ивать (*через решето́*).

screw I [skruː] *n* 1) винт; male ~, external ~ болт, шуру́п; female ~, internal ~ га́йка; endless ~, perpetual ~ *тех.* червя́к; there is a ~ loose somewhere а) что́-то не в поря́дке, что́-то нела́дно; б) «ви́нтика не хвата́ет» (*о челове́ке*); to put the ~ on *перен.* «нажа́ть» на кого́-л.; 2) *ав.* (возду́шный) винт; *мор.* (гребно́й) винт; 3) поворо́т винта́; 4) фу́нтик табака́, со́ли; 5) *разг.* скря́га; an old ~, a regular ~ скупердя́й; 6) кля́ча; an old ~ ста́рая кля́ча, одёр; 7) *разг.* жа́лованье.

screw II *v* 1) приви́нчивать, зави́нчивать; 2) враща́ться винтообра́зно; 3) заставля́ть, принужда́ть; 4) прибедня́ться; □ to ~ down ока́зывать нажи́м, заставля́ть; to ~ out вымога́ть (*согла́сие, де́ньги и т. п.; of*); to ~ up а) завин-

ти́ть; подтя́гивать (*струну́; дисципли́ну*); б) скла́дывать (*гу́бы ба́нтиком*); в) щу́рить (*глаза́*).

screw-ball I ['skruːbɔːl] *n* сумасбро́д.

screw-ball II *a* сумасбро́дный; эксцентри́чный.

screwdriver ['skruːˌdraɪvə] *n* отвёртка.

screwed [skruːd] *a* 1) приви́нченный, зави́нченный; 2) име́ющий винтову́ю наре́зку; 3) *сленг* навеселе́; подвы́пивший.

screw-nut ['skruːnʌt] *n* га́йка.

scribble I ['skrɪbl] *n* 1) кара́кули; 2) небре́жно напи́санная заме́тка и т. п.

scribble II *v* писа́ть кара́кулями, неразбо́рчиво, небре́жно.

scribbler ['skrɪblə] *n* писа́ка, бумагомара́тель.

scribe [skraib] *n* 1) пи́сарь, перепи́счик; 2) грамоте́й; I am no great ~ я не ма́стер писа́ть; 3) *разг.* писа́тель.

scrimmage ['skrɪmɪdʒ] *n* сва́лка, потасо́вка.

scrimpy ['skrɪmpɪ] *a* ску́дный, ограни́ченный.

scrimshank ['skrɪmʃæŋk] *v разг.* уклоня́ться от обя́занностей.

scrip [skrɪp] *n* 1) распи́ска, квита́нция; 2) клочо́к бума́ги.

script [skrɪpt] *n* 1) по́черк; 2) ру́копись; 3) ско́ропись; 4) *театр.* текст пье́сы; 5) киносцена́рий.

scriptural ['skrɪptʃərəl] *a* библе́йский.

scripture ['skrɪptʃə] *n* свяще́нное писа́ние, би́блия.

script-writer ['skrɪptˌraɪtə] *n* сценари́ст.

scrivener ['skrɪvnə] *n уст.* нота́риус; пи́сарь.

scroll [skroul] *n* 1) сви́ток (*пергаме́нта, папи́руса*); 2) *поэт.* спи́сок; 3) *архит.* завито́к.

scroop I ['skruːp] *n* скрип.

scroop II *v* скрипе́ть.

scrouge [skraudʒ, skruːdʒ] *v разг.* толпи́ться, дави́ться.

scrounge [skraundʒ] *v разг.* 1) вы́просить, вы́клянчить; 2) стащи́ть.

scrub¹ I [skrʌb] *n* чи́стка щёткой.

scrub¹ II *v* 1) тере́ть, чи́стить щёткой; 2) *тех.* промыва́ть (*газ*).

scrub² *n* 1) куста́рник; за́росли куста́рника; 2) поро́сшая куста́рником ме́стность; 3) малоро́слое живо́тное; 4) ничто́жный челове́к; 5) *спорт.* второ́й соста́в бейсбо́льной *или* футбо́льной кома́нд.

scrubber ['skrʌbə] *n* скребо́к.

scrubby ['skrʌbɪ] *a* 1) низкоро́слый; 2) поро́сший куста́рником; 3) недора́звитый; захуда́лый, жа́лкий.

scrubwoman ['skrʌbˌwumən] *n амер.* убо́рщица, подёнщица.

scruff [skrʌf] *n*: to take (*или* to seize) by the ~ of the neck схвати́ть за ши́ворот.

scrummage ['skrʌmɪdʒ] *см.* scrimmage.

scrumptious ['skrʌmpʃəs] *a* чуде́сный, превосхо́дный, отме́нный.

scrunch I [skrʌntʃ] *n* хруст; потре́скивание.

scrunch II *v* хрусте́ть, потре́скивать.

scruple I ['skruːpl] *n* 1) сомне́ния, колеба́ния; to have little ~ испы́тывать сла́бые угрызе́ния со́вести; не постесня́ться (*сде́лать что-л.*); to have ~s стесня́ться (*сде́лать что-л.*); to make no ~s to do smth. не постесня́ться сде́лать что-л.; he did it without ~ он сде́лал э́то не моргну́в гла́зом; of no ~s недобросо́вестный, бессо́вестный; 2) скру́пул (= *20 гра́нам*).

scruple II *v* колебáться, стесняться; не решáться; he does not ~ to say он не постесняется сказáть; he would ~ to lie он не позвóлит себé солгáть.

scrupulous [ˈskruːpjuləs] *a* 1) щепетúльный; 2) сóвестливый, добросóвестный; 3) скрупулёзный, тщáтельный.

scrutineer [ˌskruːtɪˈnɪə] *n* контролёр (*на выборах*).

scrutinize [ˈskruːtɪnaɪz] *v* критúчески рассмáтривать, изучáть, тщáтельно исслéдовать.

scrutiny [ˈskruːtɪnɪ] *n* 1) критúческое рассмотрéние; внимáтельное изучéние, разбóр; 2) испытýющий взгляд; 3) провéрка на выборах.

scud I [skʌd] *n* 1) стремúтельный бег; 2) несýщиеся облакá.

scud II *v* 1) скользúть, мчáться; 2) нестúсь (*об облаках*).

scuff I [skʌf] *n* домáшняя тýфля (*без задника*).

scuff II *v* 1) волочúть нóгу, шáркать ногáми; 2) протерéться, износúться.

scuffle I [ˈskʌfl] *n* дрáка, потасóвка.

scuffle II *v* дрáться.

scull I [skʌl] *n* 1) кормовóе веслó; 2) ялик, тýзик.

scull II *v* грестú пáрными вёслами.

scullery [ˈskʌlərɪ] *n* помещéние для мытья посýды.

sculp [skʌlp] *v разг.* ваять, лепúть, высекáть.

sculptor [ˈskʌlptə] *n* скýльптор.

sculpture I [ˈskʌlptʃə] *n* скульптýра; извая́ние.

sculpture II *v* ваять, высекáть, лепúть.

scum I [skʌm] *n* 1) пéна, нáкипь; 2) подóнки (*общества*).

scum II *v* 1) снимáть пéну; 2) пéниться, покрывáться пéной.

scummy [ˈskʌmɪ] *a* пéнистый.

scurf [skəːf] *n* 1) пéрхоть; 2) налёт, отложéния; 3) инкрустáция (*на металле*).

scurrile [ˈskʌrɪl] *см.* scurrilous.

scurrility [skʌˈrɪlɪtɪ] *n* 1) грýбое, непристóйное шутовствó; 2) непристóйное, оскорбúтельное замечáние.

scurrilous [ˈskʌrɪləs] *a* 1) грýбый, оскорбúтельный; 2) шутовскóй; насмéшливый.

scurry I [ˈskʌrɪ] *n* 1) беготня́, суетá; 2) внезáпный лúвень, снегопáд.

scurry II *v* бéгать, суетúться; сновáть взад и вперёд.

scurvied [ˈskəːvɪd] *a* цингóтный.

scurvy[1] [ˈskəːvɪ] *n* цингá.

scurvy[2] *a* 1) нúзкий, пóдлый; 2) презрéнный, омерзúтельный.

scutage [ˈskjuːtɪdʒ] *n ист.* щитовóй сбор.

scutcheon [ˈskʌtʃən] *n* щит гербá.

scutter [ˈskʌtə] *v* удирáть, улепётывать.

scuttle[1] I [ˈskʌtl] *n* 1) ведрó для ýгля; 2) колúчество ýгля (*равное ведру*).

scuttle[2] I *n* 1) тороплúвая похóдка; 2) стремúтельное бéгство.

scuttle[2] II *v* стремúтельно бежáть, удирáть.

scuttle[3] I *n* 1) *мор.* люк; 2) отвéрстие (*в крыше, в борту корабля*).

scuttle[3] II *v* пробивáть борт *или* днúще.

scuttle-butt [ˈskʌtlbʌt] *n* 1) *мор.* бóчка для прéсной воды́; 2) *амер. сленг* слух, сплéтня.

scythe I [saɪð] *n с.-х.* косá.

scythe II *v с.-х.* косúть.

sea [siː] *n* 1) мóре, океáн; at ~ в открытом мóре; to be at ~ *перен.* быть в тупикé, не знать, что дéлать; by ~ мóрем; by the ~ у мóря; on the ~ а) в мóре; б) на морскóм берегý; on the open ~ в открытом мóре; across (*или* beyond, over) the ~(s) зá морем, за океáном; choppy ~ неспокóйное мóре; closed ~ внýтреннее, закрытое мóре; heavy ~ бýрное мóре; the high ~ открытое мóре; the narrow ~s Ла-Мáнш и Ирлáндское мóре; rolling ~ волнýющееся мóре; ~s mountains high разбушевáвшееся мóре; proud ~ вздымáющееся мóре; serene ~ безмятéжное мóре; the ~s went high мóре разбушевáлось; the four ~s моря, омывáющие Великобритáнию (*Атлантический океан, Ирландское море, Северное море, пролив Ла-Манш*); to follow the ~ стать морякóм; to go to ~ а) отпрáвиться в плáвание; б) стать морякóм; to put (out) to ~ выходúть в мóре; пускáться в плáвание; to take the ~ держáть курс в открытое мóре; 2) морскáя волнá, вал; beam ~ боковáя волнá; a ~ struck us волнá захлестнýла нас; to ship a ~ черпнýть воды́ (*о лодке*); 3) мнóжество, мáсса; a ~ of fire мóре огня́; a ~ of faces мóре голóв; a ~ of troubles бéздна несчáстий; 4) *attr* морскóй; примóрский; океáнский; ◇ half ~s over ≅ подвыпивший, под мýхой.

seaboard [ˈsiːbɔːd] *n* 1) морскóе побережье; бéрег мóря; примóрье; 2) *attr* примóрский; прибрéжный.

sea-born [ˈsiːbɔːn] *a поэт.* 1) рождённый у мóря; 2) порождённый мóрем.

sea-borne [ˈsiːbɔːn] *a* доставляемый мóрем, морскúм путём.

sea-calf [ˈsiːkɑːf] *n* тюлéнь.

sea-dog [ˈsiːdɔg] *n* 1) стáрый моряк; «морскóй волк»; 2) тюлéнь.

seafarer [ˈsiːˌfɛərə] *n поэт.* моряк, мореплáватель.

seafaring I [ˈsiːˌfɛərɪŋ] *n* 1) профéссия морякá; 2) морскóе плáвание, путешéствие.

seafaring II *a* морехóдный.

sea-girt [ˈsiːgəːt] *a* окружённый, опоясанный мóрем.

seagoing [ˈsiːˌgouɪŋ] *a* 1) океáнский, дáльнего плáвания (*о судне*); 2) морехóдный.

sea-gull [ˈsiːgʌl] *n* чáйка.

sea-horse [ˈsiːhɔːs] *n* 1) морж; 2) морскóй конёк.

sea-king [ˈsiːkɪŋ] *n* кóнунг, вúкинг.

seal[1] I [siːl] *n* 1) печáть; Great Seal большáя госудáрственная печáть (*в Англии*); Privy Seal а) мáлая госудáрственная печáть; б) лорд хранúтель печáти (*в Англии*); to receive (to return) the ~s занять (остáвить) пост лóрда-кáнцлера *или* минúстра; to set one's ~ приложúть печáть (*к чему-л.* — to); удостовéрить; under the ~ of secrecy с услóвием сохранúть тáйну; 2) плóмба, клеймó; 3) *тех.* изоляция.

seal[1] II *v* 1) приложúть печáть; скрепúть печáтью; 2) запечáтать (*тж.* to up); 3) решúть бесповорóтно (*чью-л. судьбу*); 4) запечатлевáть; 5) налагáть отпечáток; 6) закрывáть; изолúровать; замáзывать (*окно*); затыкáть (*трубу*).

seal² *n* 1) тюле́нь; морско́й ко́тик; 2) ко́тиковый мех; 3) *attr* ко́тиковый.

sealery ['siːlərɪ] *n* ле́жбище тюле́ней, морски́х ко́тиков.

sealing-wax ['siːlɪŋwæks] *n* сургу́ч.

seal-ring ['siːlrɪŋ] *n* пе́рстень с печа́ткой.

sealskin ['siːlskɪn] *n* 1) ко́тиковый мех; 2) тюле́нья ко́жа.

seam I [siːm] *n* 1) шов; 2) шрам, рубе́ц.

seam II *v* 1) сшива́ть; 2) покрыва́ть(ся) морщи́нами.

seamaid ['siːmeɪd] *n поэт.* руса́лка; морска́я де́ва.

seaman ['siːmən] *n* матро́с; моря́к.

seamanship ['siːmənʃɪp] *n* мореxо́дное иску́сство; иску́сство кораблевожде́ния.

sea-mark ['siːmɑːk] *n* береговой знак; мая́к.

sea-mew ['siːmjuː] *n* ча́йка.

seamstress ['semstrɪs] *n* портни́ха, швея́.

seamy ['siːmɪ] *a* 1) со шва́ми (нару́жу); 2) неприя́тный, непригля́дный.

Seanad Eireann ['sænəd'eərɪn] *n* Ве́рхняя пала́та (*Ирла́ндской Респу́блики*).

séance ['seɪɑːns] *n* 1) сеа́нс; 2) заседа́ние.

seaplane ['siːpleɪn] *n* гидросамолёт.

seaport ['siːpɔːt] *n* 1) морско́й порт; 2) примо́рский го́род.

sear I [sɪə] *n* ожо́г.

sear II *a поэт.* сухо́й, увя́дший.

sear III *v* 1) опаля́ть; 2) прижига́ть; 3) притупля́ть (*боль*); 4) высу́шивать, иссуша́ть; 5) со́хнуть, увяда́ть.

search I [səːtʃ] *n* 1) по́иски; to be in ~ of разы́скивать; иска́ть что-л.; to make a ~ производи́ть ро́зыски (*чего-л. — for*); 2) о́быск.

search II *v* 1) иска́ть, производи́ть ро́зыски (*чего-л. — for*); 2) обы́скивать, производи́ть о́быск; 3) иссле́довать, зонди́ровать (*рану*); 4) осма́тривать (*вещи в тамо́жне*); 5) прохва́тывать (*о хо́лоде, ве́тре*); □ to ~ out выи́скивать; обнару́живать.

searching ['səːtʃɪŋ] *a* 1) тща́тельный, доскона́льный (*об осмотре, исследовании*); 2) проница́тельный, испыту́ющий (*о взгляде*); 3) прони́зывающий, ре́зкий (*о ветре*).

searchlight ['səːtʃlaɪt] *n* 1) проже́ктор; 2) луч проже́ктора; 3) *attr* прожёкторный.

search-warrant ['səːtʃˌwɔrənt] *n* о́рдер на о́быск.

sea-scape ['siːskeɪp] *n* морско́й пейза́ж.

seashore ['siːʃɔː] *n* морско́й бе́рег, побере́жье.

seasick ['siːsɪk] *a* страда́ющий морско́й боле́зню; to be ~ страда́ть морско́й боле́знью.

seasickness ['siːˌsɪknɪs] *n* морска́я боле́знь.

seaside ['siːsaɪd] *n* 1) бе́рег мо́ря, примо́рье, примо́рский край; 2) *attr* примо́рский.

season¹ I ['siːzn] *n* 1) вре́мя го́да; сезо́н; пора́; in ~ са́мое вре́мя (*фру́ктам, ры́бе и т. п.*); out of ~ не вре́мя (*фру́ктам и т. п.*); the holiday ~ вре́мя, перио́д кани́кул; theatrical ~ театра́льный сезо́н; the off (*или* dead, dull) ~ мёртвый сезо́н; silly ~ зати́шье в пре́ссе; close ~ вре́мя, когда́ охо́та запрещена́; shooting ~ вре́мя, когда́ охо́та разрешена́; for a ~ в тече́ние не́которого вре́мени; 3) *attr* сезо́нный.

season¹ II *v* 1) созрева́ть, поспева́ть; 2) выдер-

живать (*вино и т. п.*); 3) закаля́ть (*войска́, люде́й*).

season² *v* 1) приправля́ть, придава́ть вкус, остроту́; 2) подправля́ть, украша́ть (*речь*).

seasonable ['siːznəbl] *a* 1) по сезо́ну; 2) подходя́щий, своевре́менный.

seasonal ['siːzənl] *a* сезо́нный.

seasoned ['siːznd] *a* 1) вы́держанный (*о вине и т. п.*); 2) закалённый, быва́лый.

seasoning ['siːznɪŋ] *n* припра́ва.

seat¹ I [siːt] *n* 1) сиде́нье; стул, кре́сло; garden ~ а) садо́вая скаме́йка; б) сиде́нье наверху́ авто́буса, тролле́йбуса; jump ~ откидно́е сиде́нье; take a ~! сади́тесь!; to keep one's ~ оста́ться сиде́ть; не встать; please keep your ~ сиди́те, пожа́луйста!; 2) ме́сто (*в театре, поезде, парла́менте*); take your ~s! займи́те ва́ши места́! (*предупрежде́ние пе́ред отхо́дом поезда*); please keep this ~ for me пожа́луйста, скажи́те, что э́то ме́сто за́нято; to book (*или* to secure) ~s купи́ть, заказа́ть биле́ты (*в театр, на конце́рт; for*); to take a ~ купи́ть биле́т в теа́тр (*на что-л. — for*); to contest a ~ вести́ борьбу́ за ме́сто в парла́менте; to win a ~ доби́ться ме́ста в парла́менте; to lose one's ~ не быть переи́збранным в парла́мент; to take a back ~ *амер. перен.* стушева́ться.

seat¹ II *v* 1) сажа́ть, предлага́ть сесть; pray be ~ed! прошу́ сади́ться!; to be ~ed сиде́ть; 2) устро́иться, обоснова́ться; 3) вмеща́ть; име́ть сто́лько-то мест; 4) проводи́ть (*кандида́та в парла́мент*).

seat² I *n* 1) местонахожде́ние; местопребыва́ние; местожи́тельство; 2) центр; county ~ *амер.* окружно́й центр; a ~ of learning центр нау́ки; 3) расса́дник (*боле́зни и т. п.*); 4) уса́дьба.

seat² II *v* быть располо́женным; размеща́ться.

seat-belt ['siːtbelt] *n ав.* привязно́й ремёнь.

sea-wall ['siːwɔːl] *n* да́мба.

seaward I ['siːwəd] *a* напра́вленный к мо́рю, в сто́рону мо́ря.

seaward II *adv* в направле́нии мо́ря, к мо́рю, в сто́рону мо́ря.

seawards ['siːwədz] *см.* seaward II.

seaweed ['siːwiːd] *n* морска́я во́доросль.

seaworthy ['siːwəːðɪ] *a* го́дный для пла́вания; хорошо́ оснащённый.

secant I ['siːkənt] *n мат.* 1) секу́щая; 2) се́канс.

secant II *a* пересека́ющий.

secede [sɪ'siːd] *v* вы́йти из соста́ва (*союза, общества*); вы́делиться.

secession [sɪ'seʃən] *n* 1) вы́ход из соста́ва (*союза, общества и т. п.*); отделе́ние, отпаде́ние; 2) *ист.* попы́тка вы́хода 11 ю́жных шта́тов из соста́ва США в 1860—1861 гг.

seclude [sɪ'kluːd] *v* 1) уединя́ться; 2) изоли́ровать; отделя́ть (*от чего-л. — from*).

secluded [sɪ'kluːdɪd] *a* уединённый, изоли́рованный.

seclusion [sɪ'kluːʒən] *n* 1) уедине́ние, одино́чество; изоля́ция; 2) уединённое ме́сто.

seclusive [sɪ'kluːsɪv] *a* 1) стремя́щийся к уедине́нию; 2) изоли́рующий.

second¹ ['sekənd] *n* секу́нда, моме́нт, мгнове́ние.

second² I *n* 1) помо́щник; сле́дующий по ра́нгу; 2) получи́вший второ́й приз; 3) секунда́нт; 4) *pl* товары второго сорта; 5) *муз.* второй голос; альт.

second² II *v* 1) поддерживать, оказывать содействие; I ~ your motion я голосую за ваше предложение; 2) помогать.

second² III *num* второй; in the ~ place во-вторых.

second² IV *a* 1) второстепенный; 2) худший (*по качеству*); меньший (*по значению*); ~ to none непревзойдённый.

second² V *adv* вторым номером (*в состязании*); во второй группе.

secondary ['sekəndərı] *a* 1) вторичный; 2) второстепенный; 3) средний (*об образовании, школе*).

second-class ['sekənd'klɑ:s] *a* второразрядный; второстепенный; второго класса.

seconder ['sekəndə] *n* лицо, поддерживающее предложение (*на собрании, заседании*).

second-hand ['sekənd'hænd] *a* поддержанный (*о вещах*); 2) полученный из вторых рук (*о сведениях, новостях*); 3) букинистический.

secondly ['sekəndlı] *adv* во-вторых.

second-rate ['sekənd'reit] *a* 1) второразрядный; второсортный; 2) посредственный (*о человеке*).

secrecy ['si:krısı] *n* 1) секретность, конспирация; in strict ~ в строгом секрете, под строжайшим секретом; 2) умение сохранять тайну; 3) скрытность; 4) уединение, изоляция.

secret I ['si:krıt] *n* секрет, тайна; in ~ по секрету; в секретном порядке; an open ~ секрет полишинеля; to be in the ~ быть посвящённым в тайну; to let smb. into the ~ посвятить кого-л. в тайну; to keep a ~ сохранять секрет, не разглашать тайны.

secret II *a* 1) секретный; top ~ совершенно секретно (*надпись на документах*); 2) тайный; скрытый; 3) потайной (*о двери, шкафе и т. п.*); 4) уединённый (*о месте*), укромный; 5) скрытный.

secretaire [,sekrı'tɛə] *n* секретер, бюро, письменный стол.

secretariat [,sekrə'tɛərıət] *n* секретариат.

secretary¹ ['sekrətrı] *n* 1) секретарь; ~ general генеральный секретарь; permanent ~ непременный секретарь; private ~ личный секретарь; 2) министр; Secretary of State министр (*в Англии*); государственный секретарь, министр иностранных дел (*в США*); Secretary of State for Foreign Affairs министр иностранных дел (*в Англии*); the Secretary of War *уст.* военный министр (*в США*); the Home Secretary министр внутренних дел.

secretary² *n амер. см.* secretaire.

secrete [sı'kri:t] *v* 1) прятать; 2) *физиол.* выделять (*о железах*).

secretion [sı'kri:ʃən] *n* 1) сокрытие; 2) *физиол.* секреция, выделение; internal ~ внутренняя секреция.

sect [sekt] *n* секта.

sectarian I [sek'tɛərıən] *n* сектант.

sectarian II *a* сектантский.

sectarianism [sek'tɛərıənızəm] *n* сектантство.

section I ['sekʃən] *n* 1) отрезок, сегмент; отдельная деталь (*машины*); 2) раздел (*книги*); параграф; 3) *амер.* район, участок (*площадью в 1 кв. милю*); квартал (*города*); 4) сечение, разрез; cross ~ поперечное сечение; 5) срез; 6) секция; отсек; landing ~ спускаемый аппарат

(*кабина космонавта*); the orbital ~ орбитальный отсек; 7) *воен.* отделение (*в пехоте*); взвод (*в кавалерии*); 8) *амер.* спальное купе.

section II *v* делить на части; подразделять.

sectional ['sekʃnl] *a* 1) секционный; 2) местный, групповой; 3) разборный.

sector ['sektə] *n* сектор, участок.

secular ['sekjulə] *a* 1) светский, мирской; 2) вековой, происходящий раз в сто лет.

secularize ['sekjuləraız] *v* секуляризировать.

secure I [sı'kjuə] *a* 1) безопасный; 2) надёжный; верный; 3) уверенный; to be ~ быть уверенным (*в чём-л. — of*); 4) незыблемый, прочный; 5) обеспеченный (*о победе, результате*); 6) хорошо охраняемый (*о пленных, арестованных*).

secure II *v* 1) обеспечить (*победу, успех*); 2) обезопасить; 3) гарантировать; страховать; 4) достать, раздобыть; 5) запереть на замок (*дверь, ворота*); 6) схватить, посадить под стражу.

security [sı'kjuərıtı] *n* 1) безопасность; 2) порука, поручительство; 3) уверенность; 4) гарантия; залог; to give ~ давать залог (*подо что-л. — for*); 5) *pl* ценные бумаги.

sedan [sı'dæn] 1) *авто* седан; 2) *уст.* портшёз.

sedate [sı'deıt] *a* спокойный, уравновешенный; степенный.

sedative I ['sedətıv] *n мед.* успокаивающее средство.

sedative II *a* успокаивающий; болеутоляющий.

sedentary ['sedntərı] *a* сидячий (*об образе жизни*).

sedge [sedʒ] *n бот.* осока.

sediment ['sedımənt] *n* осадок; гуща.

sedition [sı'dıʃən] *n* призыв к мятежу, бунту.

seditious [sı'dıʃəs] *a* мятежный, бунтарский.

seduce [sı'dju:s] *v* обольщать, соблазнять.

seduction [sı'dʌkʃən] *n* соблазн, обольщение.

seductive [sı'dʌktıv] *a* соблазнительный, обольстительный.

sedulity [sı'dju:lıtı] *n* прилежание, усердие.

sedulous ['sedjuləs] *a* прилежный, усидчивый; усердный.

see¹ [si:] *v* (*past* saw; *p. p.* seen) 1) (у)видеть, (по)глядеть; (по)смотреть; let me ~ (your book, your picture *etc*) покажите мне (вашу книгу, ваш портрет *и т. п.*); he ~s double у него в глазах двоится; 2) видеться, увидеться, встретиться; to come to ~ прийти в гости; to go to ~ пойти в гости; 3) понимать, разуметь! I ~! да, понимаю!; don't you ~? разве не ясно?, разве не понятно?; let me ~ дайте мне подумать; as I ~ it как я это понимаю; as far as I can ~ насколько я понимаю; насколько я могу судить; 4) испытать, пережить; he (she) will never ~ 40, 50... again ≅ ему (ей) уже за 40, 50... лет; 5) (по-) советоваться, (про)консультироваться (*с врачом и т. д.*); 6) провожать; I will ~ you home я провожу вас до дому; to ~ smb. (to the theatre, to the train *etc*) проводить кого-л. (в театр, на поезд *и т. п.*); to ~ **about** проследить (*за каким-л. делом*), распорядиться (*относительно чего-л.*); позаботиться (*о чём-л.*); 6) рассмотреть, продумать; to ~ **after** смотреть (*за кем-л.*), ухаживать; присматривать (*за чем-л.*); to ~ **in** встречать (*Новый год*); to ~ **into** вникать (*во* *что-л.*), рассма́тривать (*вопрос*); to ~ **off** провожа́ть (*уезжающего*); to ~ **out** а) проводи́ть до двере́й; б) пережи́ть; в) досиде́ть до конца́; to ~ **over** осма́тривать (*помещение*); to ~ **through** а) ви́деть наскво́зь; б) доводи́ть до конца́; в): to ~ smb. through помога́ть кому́-л. в чём-л.; to ~ **to** присма́тривать (*за кем-л., чем-л.*); позабо́титься (*о чём-л.*); постере́чь.

see² *n* епа́рхия.

seed I [siːd] *n* 1) се́мя; *собир.* семена́; to sow the ~s of discord (*или* dissension) *перен.* се́ять семена́ раздо́ра; to go (*или* to run) to ~ пойти́ в семена́; *перен.* опусти́ться; to set ~s се́ять семена́; 2) зерно́; 3) пото́мство; to raise up ~ име́ть пото́мство.

seed II *v* 1) пойти́ в се́мя; 2) роня́ть (*семена*); 3) се́ять; засе́ять (*поле*); 4) очища́ть от зёрнышек (*фрукты, изюм*).

seed-bed ['siːd‚bed] *n* парни́к; гря́дка с расса́дой.

seeder ['siːdə] *n* 1) се́ятель; 2) се́ялка (разбросна́я); 3) маши́на для удале́ния семя́н.

seeding-machine ['siːdɪŋmə'ʃiːn] *n* се́ялка.

seedling ['siːdlɪŋ] *n* се́янец, расса́да.

seedsman ['siːdzmən] *n* торго́вец семена́ми.

seed-time ['siːdtaɪm] *n* вре́мя се́ва.

seedy ['siːdɪ] *a* 1) напо́лненный семена́ми; 2) *разг.* поно́шенный; потрёпанный; 3) *разг.* нездоро́вый; to feel ~ пло́хо себя́ чу́вствовать; to look ~ пло́хо вы́глядеть.

seeing ['siːɪŋ] *conj* принима́я во внима́ние, учи́тывая; поско́льку.

seek [siːk] *v* (*past, p. p.* sought) 1) иска́ть, разы́скивать; 2) пыта́ться, стара́ться (*с последую́щим Inf*); □ to ~ **after**, to ~ **for** добива́ться (*чего-л.*); to be much sought after по́льзоваться успе́хом; быть в большо́м ходу́; to ~ **through** обы́скивать (*место и т. п.*).

seem [siːm] *v* 1) каза́ться; it ~s to me мне ка́жется; 2) *личная форма гл.* to seem + *Inf другого гл. переводится по-русски сложноподчинённым предложением с формой кажется в главном предложении и личной формой другого гл. в придаточном предложении*: he ~s to live in here ка́жется, он живёт здесь.

seeming ['siːmɪŋ] *a* ка́жущийся, мни́мый, притво́рный.

seemingly ['siːmɪŋlɪ] *adv* по-ви́димому, су́дя по ви́ду.

seemly ['siːmlɪ] *a* прили́чный; благопристо́йный; подоба́ющий.

seen [siːn] *p. p. см.* see¹.

seep [siːp] *v* проса́чиваться, течь.

seer-off ['sɪər‚ɔf] *n* провожа́ющий.

seesaw I ['siː‚sɔː] *n* 1) кача́ние на доске́; to play (at) ~ кача́ться на доске́ (*о детях*); 2) де́тские каче́ли; 3) колеба́ния; 4) *attr* неусто́йчивый, коле́блющийся.

seesaw II *v* 1) кача́ться на доске́; 2) кача́ться из стороны́ в сто́рону; 3) колеба́ться.

seesaw III *adv* вверх и вниз, взад и вперёд; to go ~ колеба́ться.

seethe [siːð] *v* (*past, p. p.* seethed; *уст. past* sod; *p. p.* sodden) 1) кипе́ть; бурли́ть; 2) вздыма́ться, пе́ниться.

segment ['segmənt] *n* 1) отре́зок; 2) до́ля (*апельси́на*); 3) *мат.* сегме́нт.

segregateᵃ ['segrɪgɪt] *a* отде́льный, одино́чный.

segregateᵇ ['segrɪgeɪt] *v* отделя́ть(ся), выделя́ть(ся).

segregation [‚segrɪ'geɪʃən] *n* 1) отделе́ние; выделе́ние; 2) изоля́ция; сегрега́ция.

seigneur [seɪn'jəː] *см.* seignior.

seignior ['seɪnjə] *n ист.* синьо́р, феода́л.

seigniorage ['seɪnjərɪdʒ] *n ист.* 1) пра́во феода́ла; 2) по́шлина на пра́во чека́нки моне́ты.

seigniory ['seɪnjərɪ] *n ист.* феода́льное владе́ние.

seine [seɪn] *n* кошелько́вый не́вод.

seismic ['saɪzmɪk] *a* сейсми́ческий.

seize [siːz] *v* 1) схвати́ть; схва́тывать; 2) захвати́ть, завладе́ть (*городом, кораблём и т. п.*); конфискова́ть; 3) поня́ть, ухвати́ть (*смысл, мысль*); 4) *обыкн. pass* охвати́ть, обуя́ть (*о па́нике, стра́хе*); 5) воспо́льзоваться (*случаем*); 6) *мор.* найто́вить.

seizure ['siːʒə] *n* 1) конфиска́ция, наложе́ние аре́ста; 2) захва́т; овладе́ние; 3) припа́док; апоплекси́ческий уда́р.

seldom ['seldəm] *adv* ре́дко.

select I [sɪ'lekt] *v* отбира́ть, подбира́ть, сортирова́ть.

select II *a* отбо́рный, и́збранный; исключи́тельный.

selection [sɪ'lekʃən] *n* 1) отбо́р, подбо́р; 2) набо́р (*веще́й, предме́тов*); 3) и́збранные произведе́ния; 4) *биол.* отбо́р, селе́кция.

selective [sɪ'lektɪv] *a* 1) отбо́рочный; 2) селекцио́нный; 3) избира́тельный, селекти́вный.

self I [self] *n* (*pl* selves) со́бственное «я»; я сам; my own ~ моё «я»; second ~ второ́е «я»; пра́вая рука́; one's better ~ лу́чшее, что есть в челове́ке; ◇ ~ comes first ≅ своя́ руба́шка бли́же к те́лу.

self II *a* 1) сплошно́й, одноро́дный (*о цвете*); 2) *прибавляется к притяжательным мест.* my, your *или к личным мест. в объектном падеже* him, her, *образуя соответствующие возвратные мест. ед. ч.*: myself я сам, меня́ (себя́); yourself вы са́ми, вас сами́х (*об одном лице*) *и т. п.*

self- [self-] *pref* само-.

self-acting ['self'æktɪŋ] *a* автомати́ческий.

self-assertion ['selfə'səːʃən] *n* защи́та свои́х прав, тре́бований.

self-centered ['self'sentəd] *a* эгоисти́чный.

self-collected ['selfkə'lektɪd] *a* 1) споко́йный, невозмути́мый; 2) со́бранный.

self-conceit ['selfkən'siːt] *n* самомне́ние, зано́счивость.

self-conceited ['selfkən'siːtɪd] *a* зано́счивый, с самомне́нием; самоуве́ренный.

self-conscious ['self'kɔnʃəs] *a* 1) засте́нчивый; смущённый; 2) отдаю́щий себе́ отчёт (*в свои́х мы́слях, де́йствиях*).

self-consistent ['selfkən'sɪstənt] *a* логи́ческий; це́льный, логи́чески вы́держанный.

self-contained ['selfkən'teɪnd] *a* 1) за́мкнутый, необщи́тельный; 2) самостоя́тельный, не зави́сящий (*от различных фа́ктов*); 3) обеспе́чивающий себя́ всем необходи́мым.

self-criticism ['self'krɪtɪsɪzəm] *n* самокри́тика.

self-denial ['selfdɪ'naɪəl] *n* самоотрече́ние.

self-determination ['selfdɪ‚təːmɪ'neɪʃən] *n* 1) самоопределе́ние; 2) реши́тельность.

self-determined ['selfdɪ'təːmɪnd] *a* независимый, самостоятельный.

self-educated ['self'edjukeɪtɪd] *a* выучившийся самостоятельно.

self-governed ['self'gʌvənd] *a* имеющий самоуправление; свободный.

self-governing ['self'gʌvənɪŋ] *a* самоуправляющийся.

self-government ['self'gʌvnmənt] *n* самоуправление; автономия, самостоятельность.

self-importance ['selfɪm'pɔːtəns] *n* самомнение, важничанье.

self-interest ['self'ɪntrɪst] *n* 1) эгоизм; 2) личный интерес.

selfish ['selfɪʃ] *a* эгоистичный.

selfishness ['selfɪʃnɪs] *n* эгоизм.

self-loading ['self'loudɪŋ] *a* самозарядный, .автоматический (*о винтовке, орудии*).

self-made ['self'meɪd] *a* обязанный всем самому себе.

self-opinion ['selfə'pɪnjən] *n* самомнение; самоувереность.

self-opinionated ['selfə'pɪnjəneɪtɪd] *a* самоуверенный, упрямый.

self-possessed ['selfpə'zest] *a* владеющий собой, хладнокровный, спокойный.

self-possession ['selfpə'zeʃən] *n* самообладание, хладнокровие.

self-propelled ['selfprə'peld] *a* самоходный; самодвижущийся.

self-recording ['selfrɪ'kɔːdɪŋ] *a* самозаписывающий, самопишущий.

self-regard ['selfrɪ'gɑːd] *n* 1) эгоизм; 2) самоуважение.

self-reliant ['selfrɪ'laɪənt] *a* уверенный в себе.

self-sacrifice ['self'sækrɪfaɪs] *n* самопожертвование.

selfsame ['selfseɪm] *a* тот же самый.

self-seeker ['self'siːkə] *n* своекорыстный человек.

self-seeking I ['self'siːkɪŋ] *n* своекорыстие.

self-seeking II *a* своекорыстный.

self-service ['self'səːvɪs] *n* самообслуживание.

self-starter ['self'stɑːtə] *n тех.* автоматический стартер; самопуск.

self-study ['self'stʌdɪ] *n* самостоятельное изучение.

self-styled ['self'staɪld] *a* самозванный.

self-taught ['self'tɔːt] *a* обучившийся самостоятельно.

self-teaching ['self'tiːtʃɪŋ] *см.* textbook.

self-will ['self'wɪl] *n* своеволие.

self-willed ['self'wɪld] *a* своевольный, упрямый.

self-winding ['self'waɪndɪŋ] *a* с автоматическим заводом.

sell [sel] *v* (*past, p. p.* sold) 1) продать, продавать; 2) торговать; 3) предавать (*дело, интересы и т. п.*); 4) ходко идти (*о товаре*); продаваться; 5) *сленг* надувать, обжуливать; □ to ~ **off** распродать (*остатки*); ¹to ~ **out** а) распродавать; б) продаваться; to ~ **up** продавать с торгов.

seller ['selə] *n* 1) продавец; продавщица; 2) продаваемый товар; best ~ а) ходкий товар; б) пользующаяся успехом (*книга*).

sell-out ['sel,aut] *n* 1) *амер. разг.* распродажа;

2) *разг.* пьеса, выставка, пользующаяся большим успехом; 3) измена, предательство.

selves [selvz] *pl* 1) *см.* self I; 2) прибавляется с *мест.* our, your, them, *образуя соответствующие возвратные мест. мн. ч.*: ourselves мы сами, нас самих; yourselves вы сами, вас самих; themselves они сами, их самих.

semantic [sɪ'mæntɪk] *a лингв.* семантический.

semantics [sɪ'mæntɪks] *n лингв.* семантика, семасиология.

semaphore I ['seməfɔː] *n* семафор.

semaphore II *v* сигнализировать; сигналить.

semasiology [sɪ,meɪsɪ'ɔlədʒɪ] *n лингв.* семасиология.

semblance ['sembləns] *n* 1) видимость; under the ~ of под видом; to put on a ~ of надеть личину, сделать вид; 2) сходство, подобие; a feeble ~ of слабое подобие; 3) внешний вид.

semester [sɪ'mestə] *n* 1) семестр; 2) *attr* семестровый.

semi- ['semɪ] *pref* полу-.

semicircle ['semɪ,səːkl] *n* полукруг.

semicolon ['semɪ'koulən] *n* точка с запятой.

semi-colonial ['semɪkə'lounjəl] *a* полуколониальный.

semifinal ['semɪ'faɪnl] *n спорт.* полуфинал.

seminar ['seminɑː] *n* семинар.

seminary ['seminərɪ] *n* 1) семинария (*духовная*); 2) питомник; *перен.* рассадник.

semi-official ['semɪə'fɪʃəl] *a* полуофициальный.

Semite ['siːmaɪt] *n* семит.

Semitic I [sɪ'mɪtɪk] *n* семитские языки.

Semitic II *a* семитский.

semivowel ['semɪ'vauəl] *n фон.* полугласный (звук).

semolina [,semə'liːnə] *n* манная крупа.

sempstress ['sempstrɪs] *см.* seamstress.

senate ['senɪt] *n* 1) сенат; 2) совет (*в университетах*).

senator ·['senətə] *n* сенатор.

senatorial [,senə'tɔːrɪəl] *a* 1) сенаторский; 2) *амер.* имеющий право избирать сенаторов.

send [send] *v* (*past, p. p.* sent) 1) посылать, послать, отправлять (*за кем-л., чем-л.— for*); to ~ flying обратить в бегство; отбросить; to ~ to the chair *амер.* приговорить к казни на электрическом стуле; 2) бросать, пускать (*мяч и т. п.*); 3) испускать (*свет, запах*); издавать (*звук*)); 4) *радио* передавать; □ to ~ **away** а) посылать; б) прогонять; увольнять; to ~ **down** а) отчислять (*из университета*); б) снижать (*цены, температуру*); to ~ **forth** а) испускать; издавать; б) *in* присылать (*счёт, экспонат*); подавать (*заявление*); to ~ **off** а) отсылать (*письмо, посылку и т. п.*); б) выделять (*испарения*); в) провожать; г) прогонять; to ~ **on** отправлять, отсылать заранее; to ~ **out** а) отправлять; б) посылать (*приглашения*); в) испускать, излучать; издавать (*звук*); г) распускаться (*о деревьях*); to ~ **up** а) повышать (*цены, температуру*); б) подавать (*еду*); в) отправлять (*в высшую инстанцию*).

sender ['sendə] *n* 1) отправитель; 2) телеграфный аппарат, передатчик.

send-off ['send'ɔf] *n разг.* 1) проводы; 2) почин; to give a ~ сделать почин; 3) хвалебная рецензия.

senescent [se'nesənt] *a* стареющий.

seneschal ['senıʃəl] *n* *ист.* сенешáль.

senile ['si:naıl] *a* стáрческий; дря́хлый.

senility [sı'nılıtı] *n* стáрость; дря́хлость, одряхлéние.

senior I ['si:njə] *n* 1) стáрший (*по возрасту, положению*); 2) *амер.* ученúк выпускнóго клáсса; студéнт послéднего кýрса.

senior II *a* стáрший.

seniority ['si:nı'ɔrıtı] *n* старшинствó.

sensation [sen'seıʃən] *n* 1) ощущéние; чýвство; 2) сенсáция; to make a great ~ произвестú сенсáцию; the latest ~ «гвоздь сезóна».

sensational [sen'seıʃənl] *a* сенсациóнный.

sensation-monger [sen'seıʃən'mʌŋgə] *n* распространúтель сенсациóнных слýхов.

sense I [sens] *n* 1) чýвство, ощущéние; the five ~s óрганы чувств; to have keen (*или* quick) ~s обладáть óстрым восприя́тием; a ~ of duty чýвство дóлга; a ~ of humour чýвство ю́мора; a ~ of pain ощущéние бóли; ~ of proportion чýвство мéры; 2) *pl* рáзум, рассýдок; сознáние; to be out of one's ~s рехнýться, свихнýться; to lose one's ~s быть не в своём умé; to come to one's ~s прийтú в себя́; *перен.* образýмиться; 3) здрáвый смысл; common (*или* sound, good) ~ здрáвый смысл, практúческая смётка; to talk ~ говорúть разýмно, дéльно; to have the ~ (*of или* to + *Inf*) быть достáточно разýмным, чтóбы...; 4) смысл, значéние; strict ~ тóчный смысл; literal ~ буквáльный смысл; in a good (bad) ~ в хорóшем (плохóм) смы́сле слóва; to make no ~ не имéть никакóго смы́сла; to make ~ of поня́ть смысл, значéние; in a ~ в извéстном смы́сле; in no ~ ни в какóм отношéнии; 5) мнéние, суждéние (*коллектива*); to take the ~ of the meeting определúть мнéние собрáния голосовáнием.

sense II *v* 1) чýвствовать, ощущáть; 2) понимáть.

senseless ['senslıs] *a* 1) без сознáния, бесчýвственный, бездыхáнный; to knock ~ оглушúть (*удáром*); 2) бессмы́сленный, глýпый.

sensibility ['sensı'bılıtı] *n* 1) чувствúтельность, восприúмчивость; 2) *pl* эмоционáльность; 3) *pl* обúдчивость; 4) тóчность, чувствúтельность (*прибóра*).

sensible ['sensəbl] *a* 1) разýмный, рассудúтельный; 2) осознаю́щий; to be ~ of чýвствовать, осознавáть; 3) ощутúмый, замéтный.

sensitive ['sensıtıv] *a* 1) чувствúтельный; восприúмчивый; 2) обúдчивый, легкó реагúрующий; 3) чувствúтельный (*о прибóрах*); 4) светочувствúтельный (*о бумáге*).

sensitivity ['sensı'tıvıtı] *n* чувствúтельность.

sensory ['sensərı] *a* чувствúтельный.

sensual ['senʃuəl] *a* чýвственный; похотлúвый; сладострáстный.

sensuality ['senʃu'ælıtı] *n* чýвственность.

sensuous ['senʃuəs] *a* 1) чýвственный (*о восприятии*); 2) эстетúческий.

sent [sent] *past, p. p. см.* send.

sentence I ['sentəns] *n* 1) предложéние (*граммáтическое*); complex ~ сложноподчинённое предложéние; compound ~ сложносочинённое предложéние; 2) приговóр; nominal ~, probationary ~ услóвный приговóр; severe ~ сурóвый приговóр; to pass ~ выносúть приговóр (*кому-л.*

— *upon*); to serve a ~ отбывáть наказáние; 3) *уст.* изречéние.

sentence II *v* приговáривать, осуждáть.

sententious [sen'tenʃəs] *a* изобúлующий афорúзмами, нравоучúтельный, поучúтельный.

sentient ['senʃənt] *a* чýвствующий, ощущáющий.

sentiment ['sentımənt] *n* 1) чýвство; 2) мнéние, отношéние; 3) проявлéние чувств; 4) сентиментáльность.

sentimental ['sentı'mentl] *a* чувствúтельный; сентиментáльный.

sentimentality ['sentımen'tælıtı] *n* сентиментáльность.

sentinel ['sentınl] *n* 1) часовóй; to stand ~ over стоя́ть на часáх; охраня́ть; 2) *поэт.* страж.

sentry ['sentrı] *n* часовóй; дежýрный; караýльный; to keep ~ охраня́ть, стоя́ть на часáх; дежýрить; to carry off a ~ «снять», захватúть часовóго; to relieve ~ сменя́ть караýл.

sentry-box ['sentrıbɔks] *n* бýдка часовóго.

separable ['sepərəbl] *a* отделúмый.

separate[a] ['seprıt] *a* 1) отдéльный; раздéльный; 2) изолúрованный; 3) разлúчный; 4) сепарáтный.

separate[b] ['sepəreıt] *v* 1) отделя́ть(ся); 2) разъединя́ть(ся); 3) разлучáться, расставáться; расходúться (*о супрýгах*); 4) разнимáть; 5) разлагáть(ся) (*на части*); 6) сортировáть, отсéивать.

separation ['sepə'reıʃən] *n* 1) отделéние, разделéние; разъединéние; 2) разлýка; 3) *юр.* развóд.

separatist ['sepərətıst] *n* сторóнник отделéния, сепаратúст.

separative ['sepərətıv] *a* стремя́щийся к отделéнию.

sepoy ['si:pɔı] *n* *ист.* сипáй.

September [səp'tembə] *n* 1) сентя́брь; 2) *attr* сентя́брьский.

septennial [sep'tenjəl] *a* 1) происходя́щий одúн раз в семь лет; 2) семилéтний.

septic I ['septık] *n* септúческое срéдство.

septic II *a* септúческий.

sepulcher ['sepəlkə] *см.* sepulchre.

sepulchral [sı'pʌlkrəl] *a* 1) могúльный; погребáльный; 2) замогúльный; глухóй (*о гóлосе*).

sepulchre ['sepəlkə] *n* гробнúца; могúла.

sepulture ['sepəltʃə] *n* 1) погребéние; 2) *уст.* гробнúца.

sequel ['si:kwəl] *n* 1) продолжéние; in the ~ затéм, впослéдствии; 2) послéдующие собы́тия; 3) результáт, слéдствие.

sequence ['si:kwəns] *n* 1) послéдовательность; the ~ of events ход собы́тий; ~ of tenses *грам.* согласовáние времён; in ~ подря́д, одúн за другúм; 2) поря́док слéдования, ряд; 3) (по)слéдствие, результáт.

sequent ['si:kwənt] *a* 1) послéдующий, слéдующий; 2) послéдовательный.

sequential [sı'kwenʃəl] *a* 1) послéдовательный; 2) слéдующий (*из чего-л.*); вытекáющий.

sequester [sı'kwestə] *v* *юр.* налагáть секвéстр; конфисковáть.

sequoia [sı'kwɔıə] *n* *бот.* секвóйя, мáмонтово дéрево.

sera ['sıərə] *pl см.* serum.

serape [se'rɑpı] *n* шаль я́ркого цвéта.

Serb [sɔːb] *см.* Serbian I.

Serbian I ['sɔːbjən] *n* 1) серб; сербка; the ~s сербы; 2) сербский язык.

Serbian II *a* сербский.

sere [sɪə] *a* сухой, увядший.

serenade I [ˌserɪ'neɪd] *n* серенада.

serenade II *v* исполнять серенаду.

serene [sɪ'riːn] *a* 1) спокойный, безмятежный; all ~ *сленг* всё в порядке; 2) чистый; безоблачный, ясный; прозрачный (*о воздухе*).

sereneness [sɪ'riːnnɪs] *n* 1) спокойствие; 2) чистота, прозрачность (*неба, воздуха*).

serenity [sɪ'renɪtɪ] *n* 1) спокойствие, безмятежность; 2) безоблачность; чистота (*неба, воздуха*); 3) светлость (*титул*).

serf [sɜːf] *n* 1) крепостной (*крестьянин*); 2) раб.

serfdom ['sɜːfdəm] *n* 1) крепостное право; 2) рабство.

serge [sɜːdʒ] *n* саржа (*ткань*).

sergeant ['sɑːdʒənt] *n* 1) сержант; ~ major старшина; 2) *см.* serjeant.

serial I ['sɪərɪəl] *n* 1) продолжающееся издание; 2) роман в нескольких выпусках; многосерийный фильм, сериал.

serial II *a* 1) выходящий выпусками; 2) серийный; 3) порядковый (*о числе, номере*).

series ['sɪəriːz] *n* 1) ряд, серия; infinite ~ бесконечный ряд; in ~ а) последовательно, по порядку; б) *эл.* соединённый последовательно; 2) комплект (*газеты, журнала и т. п.*).

serious ['sɪərɪəs] *a* 1) серьёзный, глубокомысленный; 2) важный; 3) вызывающий опасение (*о болезни*).

seriously ['sɪərɪəslɪ] *adv* серьёзно.

seriousness ['sɪərɪəsnɪs] *n* серьёзность; важность (*положения*).

serjeant ['sɑːdʒənt] *n* судебный пристав; Common Serjeant судейский чиновник.

Serjeant-at-arms ['sɑːdʒəntət'ɑːmz] *n* парламентский пристав.

sermon ['sɜːmən] *n* проповедь.

serous ['sɪərəs] *a* сывороточный.

serpent ['sɜːpənt] *n* 1) змея; 2) предатель.

serpentine ['sɜːpəntaɪn] *a* 1) змейный; 2) змеевидный; 3) предательский.

serried ['serɪd] *a* сомкнутый, плечом к плечу.

serum ['sɪərəm] *n* (*pl тж.* sera) *физиол.* сыворотка.

servant ['sɜːvənt] *n* 1) слуга, служанка; general ~ домашняя работница; 2) служащий; civil ~ государственный служащий; public ~ должностное лицо; your obedient ~ ваш покорный слуга (*в конце письма*).

servant-girl ['sɜːvəntgɜːl] *n* служанка.

servant-maid ['sɜːvəntmeɪd] *n* служанка.

serve [sɜːv] *v* 1) служить; работать (*на кого-л.*); to ~ as служить в качестве 2) проходить службу (*в армии, флоте и т. п.*); 3) оказать услугу; 4) подходить, годиться; it will ~ а) подойдёт; б) этого достаточно, хватит; 5) подавать (*кушанье к столу*); 6) обслуживать; 7) обходиться (*с кем-л.*); 8) благоприятствовать (*о погоде*); 9) отбывать (*наказание, срок службы и т. п.*); 10) подавать (*мяч в теннисе*); □ to ~ **for** годиться (*для чего-л.*); to ~ **out** а) раздавать, выдавать (*паёк и т. п.*); б) отплатить, наказать;

to ~ **round** обносить, угощать (*гостей*); to ~ **up** подавать на стол; to ~ **with:** to ~ smb. with обслуживать кого-л., подавать кому-л. (*пищу*); ◇ it ~s him right! так ему и надо!

service I ['sɜːvɪs] *n* 1) служба; off ~ *воен.* вне службы, не при исполнении служебных обязанностей; on ~ *воен.* на службе, при исполнении служебных обязанностей; civil ~ государственная, гражданская служба; colour ~ действительная военная служба (*в Англии*); compulsory ~ воинская повинность; diplomatic ~ дипломатическая деятельность; national ~ воинская повинность; secret ~ разведывательная служба; selective ~ *амер.* воинская повинность для отдельных граждан (*по отбору*); to see ~ а) быть опытным служакой; б) изнашиваться; 2) обслуживание, сервис; maid ~ обслуживание стиркой; public ~ коммунальные услуги; medical ~ медицинская служба; photocopy ~ микрофильмирование; in my ~ у меня в услужении; 3) движение; regular ~ регулярное движение; railway ~ железнодорожное движение; shuttle ~ двусторонее движение транспорта; steamboat ~ пароходное движение; 4) услуга, одолжение; I am at your ~ к вашим услугам; to do a ~ оказать услугу; to do ~ сослужить службу; to be of ~ быть полезным; can I be of ~ to you? чем могу быть полезен?; yeoman's ~ помощь в нужде; 5) сервиз; dinner (tea) ~ обеденный (чайный) сервиз; 6) *рел.* служба; 7) *воен.* род войск; the senior ~ английский военно-морской флот (*в отличие от армии*); 8) подача мяча (*в теннисе*); 9) *attr* служебный.

service II *v* 1) обслуживать; 2) заправлять (*горючим*).

serviceable ['sɜːvɪsəbl] *a* 1) полезный; пригодный; 2) прочный; ноский (*о материи*); 3) *уст.* внимательный, обходительный.

serviceman ['sɜːvɪsmən] *n* военнослужащий.

service-pipe ['sɜːvɪspaɪp] *n* водопроводная *или* газопроводная труба.

serviette [ˌsɜːvɪ'et] *n* салфетка.

servile ['sɜːvaɪl] *a* 1) раболепный, льстивый; 2) рабский, подобострастный.

servility [sə'vɪlɪtɪ] *n* раболепство; подобострастие.

servitor ['sɜːvɪtə] *n* *уст.* слуга; приближённый.

servitude ['sɜːvɪtjuːd] *n* 1) рабство; порабощение; *перен.* зависимость; 2) отбытие наказания; penal ~ каторжные работы.

sesame ['sesəmɪ] *n* *бот.* кунжут.

session ['seʃən] *n* 1) заседание; to be in ~ заседать; general ~s заседания коллегии мировых судей (*в Англии, в графствах 4 раза в год*); petty ~s заседания коллегии мировых судей (*для разбора мелких дел*); executive ~ *амер.* а) закрытое заседание; б) конфиденциальная встреча; 2) сессия; 3) *амер.* учебный год; summer ~ летние курсы (*при учебном заведении*).

sessional ['seʃənl] *a* сессионный.

set[1] I [set] *v* (*past, p. p.* set) 1) класть, ставить, помещать; 2) приводить в какое-л. состояние; to ~ in order (in motion) приводить в порядок (в движение); to ~ on foot пустить в ход; to ~ at liberty, to ~ free освобождать, выпускáть на свобóду; to ~ fair устанáвливаться (*о погóде*); 3) принимáться (*за дело, рабóту и т. п.; to*); 4) сажáть (*растéние*); 5) прилагáть (*знáния, умéние к чему́-л.— to*); 6) прикла́дывать (*печать*); 7) стáвить (*пóдпись, фами́лию*); 7) захо-ди́ть, сади́ться (*о сóлнце, лунé*); 8) стáвить (*задáчу*), выдвигáть (*проблéму*); 9) подавáть (*примéр*); 10) подымáть (*парусá*); 11) возлагáть (*надéжды; на — on, упон*); 12) вправля́ть (*кость, сустáв*); 13) вставля́ть (*в рáму, в опрáву*); 14) направля́ть (*пилу́*), прáвить (*бри́тву*); 15) *полигр.* набирáть; 16) выставля́ть (*в кáчестве модéли*); 17) налагáть (*взыскáние*); 18) назна-чáть (*цéну на что-л.— on*); 19) расставля́ть (*караýл, часовы́х*); 20) переклáдывать (*на мýзыку; to*); 21) сти́скивать (*зýбы*); 22) сажáть (*кýрицу на яйца*); 23) затвердевáть; густéть, застывáть (*о сли́вках, желе́ и т. п.*); 24) дéлать стóйку (*о собáке*); 25) сидéть (*о плáтье*); 26) усыпáть (*чем-л.— with*); 27) *с гл. в фóрме Gerund обозначáет начáло дéйствия, внезáпность наступи́в-шего дéйствия:* to ~ smb. laughing рассмеши́ть когó-л.; to ~ going пусти́ть, привести́ в движéние; □ to ~ **about** а) приступáть (*к чему́-л.*); предпринимáть шаги́ (*в отношéнии чегó-л.*); б) распространя́ть; to ~ **against** настрóить прó-тив, восстанови́ть; to ~ **apart** а) приберегáть; б) отделя́ть; to ~ **aside** а) отклáдывать в стóрону, приберегáть; б) отвергáть, не принимáть в расчёт; в) отмени́ть, аннули́ровать (*постановлéние*); to ~ at бро́ситься (*на когó-л.*); to ~ **back** а) останови́ть (*движéние*); воспрепя́тствовать; б) отводи́ть (*стрéлку часóв*); to ~ **before** изло-жи́ть, предстáвить (*фáкты*); to ~ **by** отклáдывать; приберегáть; to ~ **down** а) выса́живать (*на останóвке*); б) запи́сывать; в) рассмáтривать, считáть (*кем-л., чем-л.— as*); г) припи́сывать; д) излагáть в пи́сьменной фóрме; to ~ **forth** а) излагáть; б) отправля́ться (*в путешéствие*); в) издáть, опубликовáть; to ~ **forward** а) про-двигáть, поддéрживать; б) выдвигáть; в) отправ-ля́ться в путь; to ~ **in** наступáть (*о сезóне, погóде*); устанáвливаться (*о мóдах, погóде*); to ~ **off** а) украшáть; б) оттеня́ть; в) *см.* to ~ forth б); г) взрывáть; запускáть (*ракéту и т. п.*); д): to ~ one off побуждáть (*к чему́-л.*); е) отделя́ть (*запятóй и т. п.*); ж) оттеня́ть, подчёркивать; to ~ **on** а) натрáвливать; б) брóситься (*на когó-л.*); to ~ **out** а) выставля́ть на продáжу; б) расставля́ть; развéшивать; в) вы́ехать; вы́ле-теть (*на самолёте*); to ~ **over** постáвить во главé; to ~ начинáть, принимáться (*за рабóту, еду́ и т. п.*); to ~ **up** а) воздвигáть, устанáвливать (*столб, колóнну, стáтую*); б) учреждáть, осно-вывать; в) начинáть (*дéло*); г) стать, сдéлаться (*торгóвцем, бýлочником и т. п.; as*); д) выдвигáть, развивáть (*теóрию*); е) попрáвиться (*пóсле болéзни*); ж) предъявля́ть претéнзии (*на что-л.— for*); з): to be ~ up задирáть нос, заноси́ться; to ~ **upon** брóситься, атаковáть.

set¹ II *n* 1) направлéние (*течéния, вéтра*); 2) напрáвленность (*мнéния, суждéния*); 3) посáд-ка (*головы́*); 4) декорáции (*to*); 5) стóйка (*собáки*); 6) росто́к, побéг (*растéния*); 7) *поэт.* захóд (*сóлн-ца*); ◊ to make a dead ~ at а) рéзко напада́ть (*на когó-л.*); б) старáться (*завоевáть довéрие*).

set¹ III *a* 1) зарáнее назнáченный; предписан-ный, устанóвленный; 2) засты́вший (*об улы́бке, взгля́де*); 3) реши́тельный (*о харáктере*); 4) твёр-дый (*о мнéнии, взгля́дах, ценáх*); 5) установи́в-шийся (*о погóде*); 6) свернýвшийся (*о молокé*); 7) затвердéвший (*о цемéнте*).

set² *n* 1) набóр (*предмéтов*); комплéкт (*инстру-мéнтов, книг*); a ~ of drawing instruments готовáльня; dinner ~ обéденный серви́з; toilet ~ туалéтный прибóр; 2) грýппа, круг лиц; literary ~ литератýрные круги́; the smart ~ мóдная пýбли-ка; 3) аппарáт; receiving ~ радиоприёмник.

set-back [ˈsetbæk] *n* 1) задéржка; препя́тствие; 2) поражéние, фиáско; to suffer a ~ потерпéть поражéние.

set-down [ˈsetˈdaun] *n* отпóр, рéзкий откáз.

set-off [ˈsetˈɔːf] *n* 1) противовéс; контрáст; 2) *стр.* вы́ступ.

set-out [setˈaut] *n* 1) начáло; 2) вы́ставка, витри́на.

settee [seˈtiː] *n* дивáн.

setter [ˈsetə] *n* сéттер (*порóда собáк*).

setting [ˈsetiŋ] *n* 1) окружéние, обрамлéние; окружáющая прирóда; 2) опрáва; 3) *театр.* постанóвка; декорáции и костю́мы; 4) *муз.* мýзыка на словá; 5) захóд (*сóлнца*).

settle [ˈsetl] *v* 1) устрáивать (*делá*); 2) решáть (*вопрóс*); it's ~d! решенó и подпи́сано!; 3) догo-вáриваться (*тж.* to ~ on); назначáть (*врéмя, цéну*); 4) опла́чивать, закрывáть (*счёт*); 5) посe-ля́ться, обосновáться; 6) заселя́ть, колонизи́-ровать; 7) усáживаться, устрáиваться (*в крéсле, на дивáне и т. п.; тж.* to ~ oneself down); 8) успокóиться; угомони́ться; he can't ~ to anything он не мóжет ничéм заня́ться; 9) разре-шáть (*сомнéния*); 10) улéчься, осéсть (*о пы́ли*); 11) осéсть (*о дóме*); 12) мéдленно погружáться (*о корáбле*); 13) завещáть (*комý-л.— on*); □ to ~ **down** принимáться, брáться (*за какóе-л. дéло; to*); to ~ down to married life обзавести́сь семьёй; to ~ **out** осаждáться, выпадáть в осáдок; to ~ **up** закóнчить дéнежные расчёты.

settlement [ˈsetlmənt] *n* 1) урегули́рование, разрешéние (*вопрóса*); 2) устрóйство; postwar ~ послевоéнное устрóйство; 3) заселéние, колониза́-ция; 4) колóния, поселéние; 5) посёлок, дерéвня; 6) *ист.* сéттльмент (*европéйский квартáл в нéкото-рых городáх стран Востóка*); ◊ marriage ~ акт распоряжéния имýществом по слýчаю заклю-чéния брáка.

settler [ˈsetlə] *n* 1) поселéнец; 2) *разг.* решáю-щий удáр; 3) *разг.* решáющий дóвод.

settling [ˈsetliŋ] *n* 1) осáдка; 2) *pl* осáдок.

set-to [ˈsetˈtuː] *n разг.* 1) дрáка, схвáтка; 2) спор.

set-up [ˈsetʌp] *n* 1) организáция, устрóйство; структýра; 2) осáнка; 3) *амер.* состязáние, матч (*организóванные в расчёте на лёгкую побéду*).

seven I [ˈsevn] *num* семь.

seven II *n* семёрка.

sevenfold I [ˈsevnfould] *a* семикрáтный.

sevenfold II *adv* в семикрáтном размéре; в семь раз.

seventeen [ˈsevnˈtiːn] *num* семнáдцать; sweet ~ расцвéт мóлодости.

seventeenth I [ˈsevnˈtiːnθ] *num* семнáдцатый.

seventeenth II *n* семнáдцатая часть.

seventh I ['sevnθ] *num* седьмóй.

seventh II *n* седьмáя часть.

seventies ['sevntız] *n pl* (the ~) 1) семидесятые гóды; 2) вóзраст мéжду 69 и 80 годáми.

seventieth I ['sevntııθ] *num* семидесятый.

seventieth II *n* однá семидесятая часть.

seventy ['sevntı] *num* сéмьдесят.

sever ['sevə] *v* 1) рассекáть, разрезáть; 2) разрывáть (*связи, отношéния*); 3) разделять (-ся); разъединять(ся); to ~ oneself отделиться, отколóться (*от* — *from*).

severable ['sevərəbl] *a* отделимый.

several I ['sevrəl] *pron* 1) нéсколько; 2) нéкоторые.

several II *a* 1) осóбый; 2) отдéльный; 3) различный.

severally ['sevrəlı] *adv* 1) отдéльно, пóрознь; 2) соотвéтственно.

severance ['sevərəns] *n* 1) отделéние, разъединéние; 2) разрыв (*отношéний, связей*).

severe [sı'vıə] *a* 1) стрóгий (*о взгляде, дисциплине, критике и т. п.*); to be ~ upon рéзко критиковáть; 2) сурóвый (*о пригóворе, лицé, погóде и т. п.*); 3) серьёзный (*о болéзни*); сильный, óстрый (*о бóли*); 4) тяжёлый (*о потéрях, испытáнии*); жестóкий (*о конкурéнции и т. п.*); высóкий (*о трéбованиях*); 5) стрóгий (*о стиле, красотé, простотé*); 6) éдкий, саркастический (*о замечáнии*).

severely [sı'vıəlı] *adv* 1) стрóго; сурóво; серьёзно; 2) тяжелó.

severity [sı'verıtı] *n* 1) стрóгость (*взгляда, стиля и т. п.*); 2) *pl* стрóгости (*о мероприятиях, дисциплине*); 3) сурóвость (*пригóвора, погóды и т. п.*); 4) остротá (*бóли*); 5) тóчность.

sew [sou] *v* (*p. p.* sewn, sewed) шить; зашивáть, пришивáть; □ to ~ **down** пришивáть; to ~ **in** вшивáть; to ~ **on** *см.* to ~ down; to ~ **together** сшивáть; to ~ **up** зашивáть.

sewage ['sjuːıdʒ] *n* стóчные вóды.

sewer I ['sjuə] *n* канализациóнная трубá; стóчная трубá.

sewer II *v* канализировать.

sewerage ['sjuərıdʒ] *n* канализáция.

sewing ['souıŋ] *n* шитьё.

sewing-machine ['souıŋmə,ʃiːn] *n* швéйная машина.

sewn [soun] *p. p. см.* sew.

sex [seks] *n* 1) биол. пол; the ~ *шутл.* жéнщины; the fair (*или* gentle) ~ прекрáсный пол, жéнщины; the softer (*или* weaker) ~ слáбый пол, жéнщины; the stronger (*или* sterner) ~ мужчины; 2) *разг.* половáя жизнь, половые отношéния.

sextant ['sekstənt] *n* секстáнт.

sexton ['sekstən] *n* церкóвный стóрож, пономáрь.

sexual ['seksuəl] *a* половóй, сексуáльный.

shabbiness ['ʃæbınıs] *n* убóгость; невзрáчность.

shabby ['ʃæbı] *a* 1) поношенный, потёртый, затáсканный (*об одéжде*); убóгий, запущенный (*о жилище*); 2) бéдно одéтый, обносившийся; 3) низкий, некрасивый (*о постýпках*).

shack [ʃæk] *n* лачýга, хибáрка.

shackle I ['ʃækl] *n pl* кандалы; ýзы; óковы (*тж. перен.*); the ~s of convention услóвности; ограничéния.

shackle II *v* закóвывать (*в кандалы*); *перен.* скóвывать; обуздывать; сдéрживать.

shade I [ʃeıd] *n* 1) тень; to cast (*или* to put, to throw) into the ~ затмевáть; 2) затенённое мéсто; 3) *pl* сýмрак; 4) оттéнок, нюáнс (*цвéта, значéния*); различие (*во мнéниях*); 5) привидéние, призрак; the ~s of night ночные призраки; the ~s of death тéни усóпших; 6) абажýр; 7) *амер.* штóра (*тж.* window ~); 8) защитное стеклó (*на оптическом инструмéнте*).

shade II *v* 1) затенять; 2) защищáть (*от свéта, сóлнца*); заслонять; 3) омрачáть; 4) затушёвывать; 5) незамéтно переходить (*в другóй цвет; into*); исчезáть (*тж.* to ~ off, to ~ away); 6) смягчáть окрáску, цвет (*тж.* to ~ down); 7) *амер.* слегкá уступáть (*в цené*).

shading ['ʃeıdıŋ] *n* 1) слáбый оттéнок, нюáнс; 2) затенéние.

shadow I ['ʃædou] *n* 1) тень (*от предмéтов*); deep ~s тёмные, густые тéни; to cast (*или* to throw) ~s отбрáсывать тень; 2) *pl* сýмрак, полумрáк; 3) сень, покрóв; 4) призрак; he is a mere ~ of his former self от негó остáлась лишь однá тень; 5) лёгкий намёк, тень (*сомнéния и т. п.*); 6) постоянный спýтник, «тень»; 7) соглядáтай.

shadow II *v* 1) затенять, отбрáсывать тень; 2) омрачáть; 3) защищáть, заслонять (*от сóлнца, свéта*); 4) слéдовать по пятáм (*о сыщиках, шпиóнах*); выслéживать; 5) предскáзывать, предрекáть (*тж.* to ~ forth).

shadowland ['ʃædoulənd] *n* цáрство тéней.

shadowy ['ʃædouı] *a* 1) тенистый, затенённый; 2) тумáнный, неясный; смýтный; 3) призрачный.

shady ['ʃeıdı] *a* 1) тенистый; 2) призрачный, неясный; 3) *разг.* тёмный (*о делáх, личностях*); ◊ to keep ~ держáться в тени, в сторонé.

shaft [ʃɑːft] *n* 1) дрéвко (*копья, пики*); 2) *поэт.* копьё, стрелá; 3) рýчка, рукоятка; 4) злóбный выпад, насмéшка; a random ~ а) бесцéльный выстрел; б) необдýманное замечáние; 5) луч (*свéта*); 6) вспышка (*мóлнии*); 7) оглóбля; 8) колóнна; обелиск; 9) *горн.* шáхта; 10) *тех.* вал, ось.

shag [ʃæg] *n* 1) густáя шевелюра; 2) махóрка.

shaggy ['ʃægı] *a* 1) космáтый, лохмáтый; 2) волосáтый; 3) с начёсом (*о ткáни*).

shagreen [ʃæ'griːn] *n* шагрéнь (*сорт кóжи*).

shake I [ʃeık] *n* 1) встряска, сотрясéние; 2) дрожáние; вибрáция; all of a ~ дрожá; 3) рукопожáтие; 4) кивóк (*головы*); a ~ of the head покáчивание головóй (*в знак отрицáния*); 5) толчóк, удáр; 6) *разг.* землетрясéние; 7) трéщина (*в землé, дéреве*); 8) *муз.* трель; 9) *разг.* мгновéние; in half a ~ моментáльно.

shake II *v* (*past* shook; *p. p.* shaken) 1) трясти; 2) дрожáть (*от волнéния, хóлода*); 3) качáться, покáчиваться (*грозя падéнием*); 4) раскáчиваться; 5) размáхивать; 6) потрясáть; 7) качáть (*головóй*); 8) поколебáть, ослáбить; 9) *муз.* выводить трéли; □ to ~ **down** а) трясти (*плоды с дéрева*); б) сносить (*дом*); в) утрясáть(ся); г) освóиться, сжиться; д) *сленг* вымогáть (*дéньги*); to ~ **off** а) стряхивать (*пыль*); б) отдéлываться (*от болéзни, от назóйливого человéка*); to ~ **out** а) вытряхивать; б) развёртывать (*пáрус, флаг*); to ~ **up** а) встряхивать, взбáлтывать; б) расшевелить.

shakedown ['ʃeɪk'daun] *n* 1) постéль на полу́ (*из соломы и т. п.*); to give a ~ *разг.* приюти́ть, устро́ить на ночлéг; 2) *амер.* вымога́тельство (*денег*).

shaken ['ʃeɪkən] *p. p. см.* shake II.

shake-up ['ʃeɪk'ʌp] *n* по́лная смéна персона́ла; чи́стка (*государственного аппарата в США*).

shaking ['ʃeɪkɪŋ] *n* 1) сотрясéние; 2) кача́ние; пока́чивание; 3) при́ступ маляри́и; лихора́дка.

shako ['ʃækou] *n воен.* ки́вер.

shaky ['ʃeɪkɪ] *a* 1) ша́ткий; неусто́йчивый; непро́чный; 2) дрожа́щий; трясу́щийся; to feel ~ чу́вствовать себя́ пло́хо; 3) ненадёжный, колéблющийся.

shale [ʃeɪl] *n* гли́нистый сла́нец.

shall [ʃæl (*сильная форма*), ʃəl, ʃl (*слабые формы*)] *v* (*past* should) 1) *как вспом. гл. используется для образования форм будущего времени 1-го л. ед. и мн. ч.*: in summer I ~ go to the seaside лéтом я поéду на мо́ре; 2) *как модальный гл. используется со смысловым гл. для образования модального сказуемого 2-го и 3-го л. и выражает намерение, уверенность, приказание, долженствование*: he ~ come tomorrow он до́лжен приéхать за́втра.

shallop ['ʃæləp] *n поэт.* чёлн, ладья́.

shallow I ['ʃælou] *n* мелково́дье; о́тмель.

shallow II *a* 1) мéлкий (*о реке, тарелке*); 2) неглубо́кий, повéрхностный (*об уме, человеке*).

shallow III *v* мелéть.

shalt [ʃælt] *поэт.* 2-е л. ед. ч. от shall.

sham I [ʃæm] *n* 1) поддéлка; 2) симуля́нт; притво́рщик; 3) мошéнник; 4) притво́рство, обма́н, фи́кция.

sham II *a* поддéльный; притво́рный; фикти́вный.

sham III *v* дéлать вид; притворя́ться, прики́дываться.

shamble¹ ['ʃæmbl] *n pl* 1) бо́йня (*тж. перен.*); 2) мясно́й ларёк.

shamble² I *n* ша́ркающая похо́дка.

shamble² II *v* ша́ркать (*ногами*).

shame I [ʃeɪm] *n* 1) стыд; it's a ~! сты́дно!; what a ~! како́й стыд!, како́й позо́р!; for ~! сты́дно!; howling ~ стыд и срам; ~ on you! как вам не сты́дно!; past ~ бессты́дный; to cry ~ upon изоблича́ть; стыди́ть; 2) позо́р; срам; to put to ~ посрами́ть, опозо́рить; to think ~ презира́ть.

shame II *v* 1) стыди́ть; 2) (о)позо́рить, (по)срами́ть; 3) *уст.* стыди́ться.

shamefaced ['ʃeɪmfeɪst] *a* застéнчивый, ро́бкий; стыдли́вый.

shameful ['ʃeɪmful] *a* посты́дный, позо́рный.

shameless ['ʃeɪmlɪs] *a* бессты́дный; цини́чный.

shammer ['ʃæmə] *n* симуля́нт, притво́рщик.

shammy ['ʃæmɪ] *n* за́мша.

shampoo I [ʃæm'puː] *n* 1) мытьё головы́; 2) шампу́нь.

shampoo II *v* мыть го́лову.

shamrock ['ʃæmrɔk] *n бот.* кисли́ца; трили́стник (*тж. как национальная эмблема Ирландии*).

shandrydan ['ʃændrɪdæn] *n* рыдва́н; *шутл.* колыма́га.

shanghai [ʃæŋ'haɪ] *v сленг* завербова́ть матро́са на кора́бль в пья́ном ви́де.

shank [ʃæŋk] *n* 1) го́лень (*ноги*); 2) стéржень; стéбель; ◇ to go on Shanks's pony (*или* mare) ≅ идти́ пешко́м, на свои́х двои́х.

shan't [ʃɑːnt] *разг.* = shall not.

shanty¹ ['ʃæntɪ] *n* лачу́га, хиба́рка.

shanty² *n* хорова́я пéсня матро́сов (*во время работы*).

shape I [ʃeɪp] *n* 1) фо́рма; to take ~ приня́ть фо́рму; 2) очерта́ние; вид; 3) фигу́ра; о́браз; обли́чие, подо́бие; 4) образéц, модéль, шабло́н; 5) при́зрак; 6) *разг.* состоя́ние, положéние; in bad ~ в плохо́м состоя́нии; in any ~ во вся́ком слу́чае.

shape II *v* 1) придава́ть *или* принима́ть фо́рму; to ~ into smth. придава́ть фо́рму чего́-л.; 2) создава́ть; 3) выража́ть слова́ми; 4) приспоса́бливать; □ to ~ **up** *разг.* принима́ть определённую фо́рму.

shapeless ['ʃeɪplɪs] *a* бесфо́рменный.

shapely ['ʃeɪplɪ] *a* 1) стро́йный, хорошо́ сложённый; 2) пра́вильной фо́рмы.

shard [ʃɑːd] *n* 1) надкры́лье (*жука*); 2) черепо́к, оско́лок.

share¹ I [ʃeə] *n* 1) часть, до́ля; lion's ~ льви́ная до́ля; to fall to one's ~ приходи́ться на чью-л. до́лю; 2) уча́стие; 3) пай; on ~s на пая́х; to go ~s дели́ть (*с кем-л.; что-л.— in*); 4) а́кция.

share¹ II *v* 1) дели́ть, распределя́ть; 2) владéть совмéстно; дели́ть (*что-л. с кем-л.— with*); 3) принима́ть уча́стие, имéть до́лю (*в чём-л.— in*).

share² *n* лéмех.

sharecropper ['ʃeə,krɔpə] *n амер.* аренда́тор-испо́льщик.

shareholder ['ʃeə,houldə] *n* акционéр, па́йщик.

shark I [ʃɑːk] *n* 1) аку́ла; 2) хи́щник (*о человеке*); вымога́тель; мошéнник.

shark II *v* 1) пожира́ть; 2) мошéнничать; занима́ться вымога́тельством.

sharp¹ I [ʃɑːp] *a* 1) о́стрый; 2) круто́й (*о повороте, склоне*); 3) рéзко очéрченный, отчётливый (*о контурах, линиях*); 4) си́льный (*о впечатлении*); 5) пронзи́тельный (*о крике, голосе*); 6) прони́зывающий (*о ветре*); си́льный (*о моро́зе*); 7) рéзкий (*о боли*); 8) грубый (*о словах*); 9) стро́гий (*о выговоре*); 10) жесто́кий (*о борьбе*); упо́рный (*о состязании*); 11) чу́ткий, то́нкий (*о слухе, восприятии*); хоро́ший (*о зрении*); 12) язви́тельный; злой (*о языке*); 13) остроу́мный (*о замечании*); as ~ as a needle ≅ а) о́стрый как бри́тва; б) проница́тельный; 14) шу́стрый (*о ребёнке*); сообрази́тельный; 15) хи́трый, ло́вкий, проны́рливый.

sharp¹ II *adv* 1) ро́вно, то́чно; at five o'clock ~ ро́вно в 5 часо́в; 2) осторо́жно; look ~! осторо́жно!, береги́сь!; 3) кру́то, рéзко.

sharp² I *n* 1) *муз.* диéз; 2) *разг.* жу́лик, плут; 3) *амер. шутл.* знато́к.

sharp² II *a* сли́шком высо́кий (*о тоне*).

sharp³ II *v* плутова́ть.

sharpen ['ʃɑːpən] *v* 1) точи́ть; заостря́ть; 2) чини́ть (*карандаш*); 3) улучша́ть (*аппетит*).

sharper ['ʃɑːpə] *n* жу́лик, плут; шу́лер.

sharp-set ['ʃɑːp'set] *a* о́чень голо́дный, проголода́вшийся.

sharpshooter ['ʃɑːp,ʃuːtə] *n* мéткий стрело́к, сна́йпер.

sharp-sighted ['ʃɑːp'saɪtɪd] *a* 1) имéющий о́строе зрéние; 2) проница́тельный, сообрази́тельный.

sharp-witted [ˈʃɑːpˈwitid] *a* 1) ýмный, проница́тельный; 2) остроýмный.

shatter [ˈʃætə] *v* 1) разбива́ть; 2) расша́тывать (*здоровье, нервы*); 3) расстра́ивать (*планы*); разруша́ть наде́жды; 4) разбива́ться, разлета́ться вдре́безги.

shave I [ʃeɪv] *n* 1) бритьё; to have a ~ побри́ться; 2): close (*или* narrow, near) ~ почти́ немину́емая ги́бель; it was a close ~ он был на волосо́к от сме́рти; he missed it by a close (*или* narrow) ~ он чуть бы́ло не поги́б.

shave II *v* (*past* shaved; *p. p.* shaved, shaven) 1) брить(ся); to get ~d побри́ться (*у парикма́хера*); 2) строга́ть; 3) подстрига́ть; 4) пройти́ ми́мо, едва́ не заде́в.

shaven [ˈʃeɪvn] *p. p.* см. shave II.

shaver [ˈʃeɪvə] *n* 1) плут; 2) *разг.* юне́ц, парнёк (*обыкн.* young ~).

shaving [ˈʃeɪvɪŋ] *n* 1) бритьё; 2) *pl* стру́жки.

shaving-brush [ˈʃeɪvɪŋbrʌʃ] *n* ки́сточка для бритья́.

shawl [ʃɔːl] *n* шаль.

she [ʃiː] *pron pers* она́.

she- [ʃɪ-] *pref,* прибавля́емый к сущ. для обозначе́ния са́мки живо́тного: she-ass осли́ца, she-wolf волчи́ца.

sheaf I [ʃiːf] *n* (*pl* sheaves) 1) сноп; 2) вяза́нка.

sheaf II *v* вяза́ть (*снопы*).

shear I [ʃɪə] *n* 1) стри́жка; 2) *pl* но́жницы; 3) *pl* ре́жущая маши́на.

shear II *v* (*past* sheared, *уст.* shore; *p. p.* shorn, *редко* sheared) 1) стричь (*овец*); 2) ре́зать; 3) обдира́ть как ли́пку; 4) *поэт.* руби́ть (*о мече́*).

sheath [ʃiːθ] *n* (*pl* sheaths [ʃiːðz]) 1) но́жны; 2) футля́р; 3) *анат.* оболо́чка; 4) *тех.* обши́вка; кожу́х.

sheathe [ʃiːð] *v* 1) вкла́дывать в но́жны; 2) класть в футля́р; 3) *тех.* обшива́ть.

sheathing [ˈʃiːðɪŋ] *n* обши́вка.

sheave[1] [ʃiːv] *v* вяза́ть (*снопы*).

sheave[2] *n* 1) шпу́лька, кату́шка; 2) *тех.* шкив, блок.

sheaves [ʃiːvz] *pl* см. sheaf I.

shed[1] [ʃed] *n* 1) наве́с; 2) сара́й; сенова́л; 3) анга́р, гара́ж.

shed[2] *v* (*past, p. p.* shed) 1) лить, пролива́ть (*слёзы, кровь, свет*); 2) роня́ть (*ли́стья*); теря́ть (*во́лосы, шерсть, перья, зу́бы*); 3) сбра́сывать (*оде́жду, ко́жу*); 4) издава́ть (*звук*); испуска́ть (*благоуха́ние*); излуча́ть (*свет, тепло́*); 5) распространя́ть (*влия́ние*); расточа́ть (*ми́лости*); 6) бить (*о фонта́не*).

sheen I [ʃiːn] *n* 1) блеск; гля́нец; сия́ние; 2) роско́шный наря́д.

sheen II *a уст.* блестя́щий, прекра́сный.

sheen III *v* блесте́ть, сия́ть.

sheep [ʃiːp] *n* (*pl без измен.*) 1) овца́, бара́н; 2) шевро́ (*сорт ко́жи*); 3) засте́нчивый челове́к, тихо́ня; ◊ black ~ негодя́й; Neptune's ~ бара́шки (*на мо́ре*).

sheep-dog [ˈʃiːpdɔg] *n* овча́рка.

sheep-fold [ˈʃiːpfould] *n* заго́н (*для ове́ц*); овча́рня.

sheepish [ˈʃiːpɪʃ] *a* 1) засте́нчивый; ро́бкий; мя́гкий (*по хара́ктеру*); 2) глупова́тый.

sheep's-head [ˈʃiːpshed] *n* «бара́нья голова́», дура́к.

sheepskin [ˈʃiːpskɪn] *n* 1) овчи́на; 2) мерлу́шка; 3) перга́мент; бара́нья ко́жа; 4) *амер. разг.* дипло́м.

sheep-walk [ˈʃiːpwɔːk] *n* ове́чье па́стбище.

sheer[1] I [ʃɪə] *a* 1) я́вный, абсолю́тный; полне́йший (*о неве́жестве и т. п.*); 2) прозра́чный, просве́чивающий (*о мате́рии*); 3) чи́стый, без при́меси; 4) круто́й, отве́сный.

sheer[1] II *adv* 1) соверше́нно, абсолю́тно; 2) отве́сно.

sheer[2] *v* свора́чивать (*с пути́, ку́рса*); отклоня́ться (*тж.* to ~ away); □ to ~ off расста́ться; удали́ться.

sheet[1] I [ʃiːt] *n* 1) простыня́; between the ~s в посте́ли; 2) лист (*желе́за, стекла́, бума́ги*); 3) *pl* страни́цы кни́ги; 4) газе́та; 5) язы́к (*пла́мени*); 6) во́дное простра́нство; снежная равни́на; 7) *геол.* пласт; ◊ a clean ~ безупре́чное про́шлое; to come down in ~s лить как из ведра́ (*о дожде́*); to stand in a white ~ откры́то ка́яться.

sheet[1] II *v* 1) покрыва́ть (*простынёй, сне́гом и т. п.*); 2) *тех.* покрыва́ть листа́ми.

sheet[2] I *n мор.* шкот; ◊ three ~s in the wind (*или* in the wind's eye) *разг.* вдрызг пья́ный.

sheet[2] II *v мор.* выбира́ть шко́ты.

sheet-anchor [ˈʃiːtˌæŋkə] *n* 1) *мор.* запа́сный я́корь; 2) после́днее прибе́жище; после́дняя наде́жда.

sheeted [ˈʃiːtɪd] *a* покры́тый.

sheeting [ˈʃiːtɪŋ] *n* 1) покры́тие; 2) широ́кая мате́рия (*для простынь*).

sheik(h) [ʃeɪk, *амер.* ʃiːk] *n* шейх.

shelf [ʃelf] *n* (*pl* shelves) 1) по́лка; to be laid (*или* put) on the ~ *перен.* получи́ть отста́вку; быть сда́нным в архи́в; 2) усту́п; 3) риф, (от)ме́ль.

shell I [ʃel] *n* 1) ра́ковина, раку́шка; to go into one's ~ замкну́ться в себе́; to come out of one's ~ *перен.* разговори́ться, разболта́ться; 2) скорлупа́ (*яйца́, оре́ха*); шелуха́; оболо́чка; 3) снаря́д, грана́та; blind ~ неразорва́вшийся снаря́д; star ~ освети́тельный снаря́д; 4) ги́льза (*патро́на*); 5) па́нцирь, щит (*черепа́хи*).

shell II *v* 1) снима́ть скорлупу́; лущи́ть; вынима́ть из ра́ковины; 2) обстре́ливать (*снаря́дами*); бомбарди́ровать; □ to ~ off шелуши́ться; to ~ out а) *разг.* раскоше́ливаться; б) *воен.* вы́бить артиллери́йским огнём.

shellfire [ˈʃelˌfaɪə] *n* артиллери́йский ого́нь, обстре́л.

shell-fish [ˈʃelfɪʃ] *n* во́дное живо́тное, име́ющее па́нцирь (*черепа́ха, краб и т. д.*).

shelling [ˈʃelɪŋ] *n* артиллери́йский обстре́л.

shell-proof [ˈʃelpruːf] *a* брониро́ванный; не пробива́емый снаря́дами и т. п.

shell-shock [ˈʃelʃɔk] *n* конту́зия, шок.

shell-shocked [ˈʃelʃɔkt] *a* конту́женный.

shelter I [ˈʃeltə] *n* 1) убе́жище, прию́т; 2) укры́тие; прикры́тие; bomb-proof ~ бомбоубе́жище; under the ~ of под прикры́тием; под защи́той; to find ~ найти́ убе́жище, укры́ться; to take ~ укры́ться; *перен.* прибега́ть (*к чему́-л.* — in).

shelter II *v* 1) прикрыва́ть, защища́ть; служи́ть прикры́тием; 2) укрыва́ть, дава́ть прию́т; 3) укрыться; to ~ oneself under (*или* behind) а) укрыться; б) прикрываться, прятаться зá спину (*кого-л.*).

shelve¹ [ʃelv] *v* 1) расставлять (*книги на полках*); 2) делать полки (*в шкафу, буфете*); 3) откладывать, «класть под сукнó»; 4) увольнять.

shelve² *v* иметь отлóгий спуск; спускáться отлóго.

shelves [ʃelvz] *pl см.* shelf.

shenanigan [ʃɪ'nænɪgən] *n часто pl разг.* 1) ерундá, чепухá; 2) обмáн.

shepherd I ['ʃepəd] *n* 1) пастýх; 2) пáстырь.

shepherd II *v* 1) пасти овéц; 2) присмáтривать, забóтиться (*о ком-л.*).

shepherd-dog ['ʃepəd͵dɔg] *n* овчáрка.

shepherdess ['ʃepədɪs] *n* пастýшка.

sherd [ʃəːd] *см.* shard.

sheriff ['ʃerɪf] *n* шерúф.

sherry ['ʃerɪ] *n* хéрес (*винó*).

shew [ʃou] *v* (*past* shewed; *p. p.* shewn) *уст. см.* show II.

shewn [ʃoun] *p. p. см.* shew.

shibboleth ['ʃɪbəleθ] *n* 1) примéта для опознáния; 2) парóль.

shield I [ʃiːld] *n* 1) щит; 2) защúта, защúтник.

shield II *v* защищáть; прикрывáть (*щитóм и т. п.*).

shift I [ʃɪft] *n* 1) перестанóвка, передвижéние; 2) (*рабóчая*) смéна; day ~ дневнáя (нóчнáя) смéна; 3) смéна, перемéна; a ~ of clothes смéна бельá; a ~ of crops севооборóт; 4) рабóчий день; 5) сдвиг; the Great Vowel Shift *лингв.* велúкий сдвиг глáсных; 6) улóвка; увéртка; a mere ~ пустóй предлóг; to make ~ обойтúсь (*при помощи чего-л.— with; без чего-л.— without*); 7) *уст.* сорóчка.

shift II *v* 1) перемещáть(ся); 2) (пере)менять; заменять (*одно другим; for*); 3) переклáдывать (*с одного лица на другое — обвинéние и т. п.*); 4) изворáчиваться; to~ for oneself обходúться свóими сúлами; 5) *тех.* менять, переключáть скóрости (*в автомобúле*); 6) *лингв.* переходúть (*в другой звук*).

shiftless ['ʃɪftlɪs] *a* 1) беспомóщный; 2) неумéлый.

shift-over ['ʃɪftouvə] *n* перехóд; ~ to a shorter workday перехóд на сокращённый рабóчий день.

shifty ['ʃɪftɪ] *a* 1) нахóдчивый; изобретáтельный; 2) изворóтливый, продувнóй; 3) перемéнчивый; ненадёжный; 4) бегáющий (*о глазáх*).

shilling ['ʃɪlɪŋ] *n* шúллинг (*англ. монета =* ¹/₂₀ *фунта стéрлингов; чеканилась до 1971 г.*); ◊ long ~s хорóший зáработок; to cut off with a ~ лишúть наслéдства.

shilly-shally I ['ʃɪlɪ͵ʃælɪ] *n* нерешúтельность; колебáние.

shilly-shally II *a* нерешúтельный.

shilly-shally III *v* проявлять нерешúтельность, колебáться.

shimmer I ['ʃɪmə] *n* слáбый óтблеск; мерцáние.

shimmer II *v* давáть óтблеск; мерцáть.

shimmery ['ʃɪmərɪ] *a* мерцáющий; дающий óтблеск.

shimmy ['ʃɪmɪ] *n разг.* рубáшка.

shin I [ʃɪn] *n* гóлень.

shin II *v* карáбкаться (*тж.* to ~ up).

shin-bone ['ʃɪnboun] *n* большеберцóвая кость.

shindy ['ʃɪndɪ] *n разг.* 1) потасóвка, возня; скандáл; 2) *амер.* вечерúнка с тáнцами.

shine I [ʃaɪn] *n* 1) сияние, свет; 2) сóлнечное сияние; 3) блеск; to put a good ~ on навестú блеск, глянец; to take the ~ out of затмúть когó-л.; to give a ~ начúстить (*обувь*); 4) *разг.* шум, гам, скандáл.

shine II *v* (*past, p. p.* shone) 1) светúть, сиять; 2) блестéть, сверкáть; светúться; to ~ with health дышáть здорóвьем; 3) блистáть (*в обществе, раз-говоре*); 4) *амер. разг.* чúстить, начищáть (*обувь*).

shiner ['ʃaɪnə] *n* 1) *разг.* чúстильщик (*обуви*); 2) *pl разг.* лакирóванные тýфли; 3) *разг.* монéта; 4) *pl разг.* дéньги; 5) *сленг* подбúтый глаз.

shingle¹ I ['ʃɪŋgl] *n* 1) *pl* дрáнка; 2) корóткая стрúжка; 3) *амер. разг.* дощéчка (*с фамúлией*).

shingle¹ II *v* 1) крыть дрáнкой (*крышу*); 2) корóтко стричь (*вóлосы*).

shingle² *n* гáлька.

shining ['ʃaɪnɪŋ] *a* 1) сияющий, яркий; 2) блестящий.

shinny ['ʃɪnɪ] *n* хоккéй (*с упрощёнными прáвилами*).

shiny ['ʃaɪnɪ] *a* 1) сóлнечный; 2) яркий, блестящий, глянцевúтый; 3) лоснящийся.

ship I [ʃɪp] *n* 1) корáбль, сýдно, парохóд; on board (the) ~ на бортý корабля; to take (the) ~ сесть на корáбль, отпрáвиться в плáвание; the ~ of the line линéйный корáбль; the ~ of the desert верблюд; 2) *сленг* гóночная лóдка; 3) *амер.* самолёт; 4) *attr* корабéльный; судовóй, парохóдный.

ship II *v* 1) грузúть (*товáры*); производúть посáдку (*пассажúров*); 2) перевозúть, отправлять; 3) нанимáть(ся) (*на судно*).

shipboard ['ʃɪpbɔːd] *n* борт корабля; on ~ на бортý корабля, на корабле́.

shipbuilder [͵ʃɪp'bɪldə] *n* кораблестроúтель; судострóитель.

shipman ['ʃɪpmən] *n уст.* моряк.

shipmaster ['ʃɪp͵mɑːstə] *n* 1) капитáн корабля; 2) шкúпер.

shipmate ['ʃɪpmeɪt] *n* товáрищ по слýжбе (*на корабле*); товáрищ по плáванию.

shipment ['ʃɪpmənt] *n* 1) грýзы, товáры; 2) отпрáвка, погрýзка (*товáров*); 3) перевóзка, достáвка (*грýзов*).

shipowner ['ʃɪp͵ounə] *n* судовладéлец.

shipper ['ʃɪpə] *n* отправúтель (*грýзов*); поставщúк.

shipping ['ʃɪpɪŋ] *n* 1) торгóвые судá; торгóвый флот; 2) погрýзка (*грýзов*); 3) перевóзка (*грýзов*) мóрем, по воде́.

shipshape ['ʃɪpʃeɪp] *a predic* в пóлном порядке.

shipwreck I ['ʃɪprek] *n* 1) кораблекрушéние; 2) облóмки корабля; 3) крушéние (*надéжд и т. п.*).

shipwreck II *v* 1) вызвать кораблекрушéние; to be ~ed потерпéть кораблекрушéние; 2) разрушáть (*надéжды и т. п.*).

shipwright ['ʃɪpraɪt] *n* корабéльный плóтник.

ship-yard ['ʃɪpjɑːd] *n* верфь.

shirk [ʃəːk] *v* саботúровать; увúливать, уклоняться (*от работы, обязанностей*).

shirker ['ʃəːkə] *n* саботáжник.

shirt [ʃəːt] *n* 1) мужская рубашка, сорочка; boiled ~ крахмальная рубашка; *перен.* элегантный, вылощенный человек; 2) блузка; ◇ to have one's ~ out выйти из себя; to keep one's ~ on сохранять спокойствие; he has not a ~ on his back ≅ у него нет (ни) гроша за душой.

shirting ['ʃəːtɪŋ] *n* материал на мужские рубашки.

shiver[1] I ['ʃɪvə]. *n* дрожь, трепет; to get (*или* to have) the ~s чувствовать дрожь; this gives me the ~s *шутл.* от этого у меня мурашки забегали; от этого меня в дрожь бросает.

shiver[1] II *v* 1) дрожать (*от холода, страха; with*); 2) трепетать.

shiver[2] I *n обыкн. pl* обломок, осколок; to break to ~s разлететься вдребезги.

shiver[2] II *v* разбиваться, разлетаться на куски.

shivery[1] ['ʃɪvərɪ] *a* 1) дрожащий, трепещущий; 2) пугливый.

shivery[2] *a* хрупкий, ломкий.

shoal[1] I [ʃoul] *n* 1) мелкое место, мелководье; 2) песчаная отмель; 3) *обыкн. pl* скрытая опасность.

shoal[1] II *a* мелкий, мелководный.

shoal[1] III *v* мелеть.

shoal[2] I *n* 1) косяк, стая (*рыб*); 2) масса (*людей*).

shoal[2] II *v* 1) собираться стаями, косяками (*о рыбе*); 2) толпиться (*о людях*).

shock[1] I· [ʃɔk] *n* 1) удар; толчок; electric ~ удар электрического разряда; 2) потрясение, шок; 3) *attr* ударный.

shock[1] II *v* 1) поражать; потрясать; 2) возмущать, шокировать.

shock[2] I *n* копна.

shock[2] II *v* ставить в копны, скирдовать.

shock[3] I *n* 1) копна волос; 2) мохнатая собака.

shock[3] II *a* мохнатый.

shock-absorber ['ʃɔkəb,sɔːbə] *n тех.* амортизатор.

shocker ['ʃɔkə] *n* бульварный роман.

shocking I ['ʃɔkɪŋ] *a* возмутительный, ужасный, потрясающий.

shocking II *adv* ужасно, очень.

shod [ʃɔd] *past, p. p. см.* shoe II.

shoddy I ['ʃɔdɪ] *n* 1) искусственная шерсть; 2) хлам.

shoddy II *a* 1) поддельный, искусственный; 2) дрянной.

shoe I [ʃuː] *n* 1) ботинок, полуботинок, туфля; Oxford ~ полуботинок; to be in another's ~s оказаться в чьём-л. положении; to shake in one's ~s трястись от страха; to know where the ~ pinches знать по опыту, в чём трудность; that's where the ~ pinches ≅ вот в чём дело, трудность; вот где собака зарыта; 2) подкова; 3) наконечник; 4) *тех.* колодка, башмак; 5) железный полоз; ◇ to wait for dead men's ~s ждать наследства; to lick smb.'s ~s ≅ лизать кому-л. пятки.

shoe II *v* (*past, p. p.* shod) 1) обувать; 2) подковывать.

shoeblack ['ʃuːblæk] *n* чистильщик сапог.

shoe-lace ['ʃuːleɪs] *n* шнурок для ботинок.

shoemaker ['ʃuː,meɪkə] *n* сапожник.

shoe-string ['ʃuːstrɪŋ] *n* шнурок для ботинок.

shoe-tree ['ʃuːtriː] *n* колодка.

shone [ʃɔn, *амер.* ʃoun] *past, p. p. см.* shine II.

shoo [ʃuː] *v* вспугивать, прогонять.

shook [ʃuk] *past см.* shake II.

shoot I [ʃuːt] *n* 1) побег, росток; 2) состязание в стрельбе; 3) наклонный сток; жёлоб, лоток; 4) выезд на охоту.

shoot II *v* (*past, p. p.* shot) 1) стрелять (*из ружья, винтовки и т. п.; во что-л.— at*); 2) застрелить (*тж.* to ~ dead); to ~ oneself застрелиться; 3) засыпать (*вопросами*); 4) охотиться; to go ~ing ходить на охоту; 5) пронестись, промчаться (*мимо — past; через — through, over*); 6) испускать (*свет*); 7) давать, пускать (*ростки, побеги*); 8) *кино, фото* заснять; 9) бросать (*игральные кости*); 10) отодвигать, задвигать (*засов*); 11) определять высоту (*солнца*); 12) *спорт.* посылать мяч; □ to ~ **ahead** вырваться вперёд, опередить своих противников (*в состязании*); to ~ **away** расстрелять (*все патроны*); to ~ **down** застрелить; сбить (*снарядом*); to ~ **forth** а) пронестись, промелькнуть; б) прорастать; распускаться (*о почках*); давать (*побеги*); to ~ **in** пристреливаться; to ~ **out** а) выдаваться (*о мысе, косе*); б) извергать, выбрасывать; в) вылетать; г) пускать (*ростки, побеги*); to ~ **up** а) быстро расти; расти как на дрожжах; б) возвышаться (*о вершине*); в) вздыматься (*о пламени*); г) *амер.* терроризировать стрельбой.

shooter ['ʃuːtə] *n* 1) стрелок; 2) огнестрельное оружие; ◇ square ~ *разг.* честный человек.

shooting ['ʃuːtɪŋ] *n* 1) стрельба; 2) охота; 3) право охоты; 4) *кино* съёмка; 5) острая, внезапная боль.

shop I [ʃɔp] *n* 1) магазин, лавка; chemist's ~ аптека; barrel ~ пивная; curiosity ~ антикварный магазин; to come to the wrong ~ обратиться не по адресу; to shut up ~ свернуть дело, закончить что-л.; to talk ~ затрагивать узкопрофессиональные темы во время общего разговора; 2) мастерская; цех; assembly ~, adjusting ~ сборочный цех; valet ~ мастерская (*или* комбинат) бытового обслуживания; 3) *амер.* небольшое кафе, ресторанчик.

shop II *v* делать покупки.

shop-assistant ['ʃɔpə,sɪstənt] *n* продавец.

shop-girl ['ʃɔpɡəːl] *n* продавщица.

shopkeeper ['ʃɔp,kiːpə] *n* владелец магазина; лавочник.

shopman ['ʃɔpmən] *n* 1) продавец; 2) хозяин магазина.

shopper ['ʃɔpə] *n* покупатель.

shopping ['ʃɔpɪŋ] *n:* to do ~ делать покупки; to go (out) ~ отправиться за покупками.

shoppy ['ʃɔpɪ] *a разг.* профессиональный (*о разговоре*).

shop-steward ['ʃɔpstjuəd] *n* делегат от рабочих (*для переговоров с предпринимателем*); фабрично-заводской староста.

shopwalker ['ʃɔp,wɔːkə] *n* дежурный администратор (*в большом магазине*).

shore[1] [ʃɔː] *n* 1) берег моря; to go on ~ сойти на берег; 2) край; my native ~ мой край родной; 3) прибрежные воды; in ~ в прибрежных водах.

shore[2] I *n* подпорка.

shore² II *v* ста́вить подпо́рки, подпира́ть (*тж.* to ~ up).

shore³ *уст. past см.* shear II.

shoreline ['ʃɔːlaɪn] *n* берегова́я ли́ния.

shoreward ['ʃɔːwəd] *adv* по направле́нию к бе́регу.

shorn I [ʃɔːn] *p. p. см.* shear II.

shorn II *a* остри́женный, сре́занный, подре́занный.

short I [ʃɔːt] *a* 1) коро́ткий, кра́ткий; 2) ни́зкий (*о росте*); 3) сла́бый (*о памяти, зрении*); 4) вспы́льчивый (*о характере*); 5) недоста́точный, ску́дный; име́ющийся в ма́лом коли́честве; to be ~ of ощуща́ть, име́ть недоста́ток в чём-л.; I am ~ of money у меня́ не хвата́ет де́нег; to come ~ (of) а) не хвата́ть; б) получи́ть ма́лую вы́году; to fall ~, to drop ~ а) не хвата́ть; б) не долета́ть до це́ли, дава́ть недолёт; в) не достига́ть це́ли; обману́ть чьи-л. ожида́ния; to feel ~ чу́вствовать себя́ пода́вленным; to run ~ of не хвати́ть, истощи́ться; to be ~ of breath задыха́ться; 6) ре́зкий, отры́вистый, сухо́й (*об ответе, приёме, обраще́нии*); 7) хру́пкий, ло́мкий (*о металле*); 8) рассы́пчатый, песо́чный (*о печенье*); 9) *сленг* кре́пкий (*о напитке*).

short II *adv* 1) внеза́пно, сра́зу; to cut smb. ~ ре́зко прерва́ть кого́-л.; 2) не доезжа́я; ~ of the town недалеко́ от го́рода; 3) кра́тко.

short III *n* 1) *фон.* кра́ткий гла́сный звук; 2) *pl* тру́сики; 3) *воен.* недолёт (*о снаряде*); 4) *эл. разг.* коро́ткое замыка́ние; 5) короткометра́жный фильм; 6): for ~ для кра́ткости; in ~ вкра́тце, одни́м сло́вом.

shortage ['ʃɔːtɪdʒ] *n* недоста́ток, нехва́тка.

shortbread ['ʃɔːtbred] *n* песо́чное пече́нье.

shortcake ['ʃɔːtkeɪk] *см.* shortbread.

short-circuit ['ʃɔːt'sɜːkɪt] *v* эл. сде́лать коро́ткое замыка́ние, замкну́ть накоро́тко.

shortcoming [ʃɔːt'kʌmɪŋ] *n* недоста́ток, дефе́кт.

shorten ['ʃɔːtn] *v* 1) сокраща́ть(ся), укора́чивать(ся); 2) свёртывать (*паруса*).

shorthand I ['ʃɔːthænd] *n* стеногра́фия.

shorthand II *a* стенографи́ческий.

short-handed ['ʃɔːt'hændɪd] *a* испы́тывающий *или* име́ющий недоста́ток в рабо́чей си́ле.

shortish ['ʃɔːtɪʃ] *a* короткова́тый.

short-lived ['ʃɔːt'lɪvd] *a* кратковре́менный, мимолётный.

shortly ['ʃɔːtlɪ] *adv* 1) вско́ре; 2) ко́ротко, вкра́тце; 3) ре́зко, су́хо.

short-sighted ['ʃɔːt'saɪtɪd] *a* 1) близору́кий; 2) недальнови́дный.

short-spoken ['ʃɔːt'spoukən] *a* лакони́чный; кра́ткий.

short-tempered ['ʃɔːt'tempəd] *a* вспы́льчивый.

short-term ['ʃɔːtɜːm] *a* краткосро́чный.

short-wave ['ʃɔːt'weɪv] *a* радио коротково́лновый.

short-winded ['ʃɔːt'wɪndɪd] *a* страда́ющий оды́шкой.

shot¹ [ʃɔt] *n* 1) вы́стрел; звук вы́стрела; point-blank ~ вы́стрел в упо́р; without firing a ~ не сде́лав ни одного́ вы́стрела; 2) пу́шечное ядро́; пу́ля; 3) стрело́к; a crack ~, a sure ~ ме́ткий стрело́к; 4) (*pl без измен.*) дроби́нка, дробь (*для стрельбы*); small ~ дробь; 5) попы́тка; to have (*или* to take, to try) a ~ попыта́ться (сде-

лать что-л.; *at*); 6) дога́дка; to make a good (bad) ~ (не) угада́ть, (не) разгада́ть; 7) *кино* кадр; 8) фотосни́мок; ◇ by a long ~ намно́го, в значи́тельной сте́пени; like a ~ в два счёта; not a ~ in the locker ни копе́йки де́нег.

shot² *n* счёт (*в гости́нице*); to pay one's ~ рассчита́ться, расплати́ться (*по счёту*).

shot³ *past, p. p. см.* shoot II; ◇ I'll be ~! не мо́жет быть!, неуже́то!

shot-gun ['ʃɔtgʌn] *n* охо́тничье ружьё.

should [ʃud (*си́льная фо́рма*), ʃəd (*сла́бая фо́рма*)] 1) *past см.* shall; 2) *как вспомога́тельный гл. употр.*: а) *в фо́рме Conditional 1-го л. обо́их чисе́л для выраже́ния усло́вности*: I ~ be very glad if you could tell me his address я был бы о́чень рад, е́сли бы вы сообщи́ли мне его́ а́дрес; б) *в фо́рме Future in the Past 1-го л. обо́их чисе́л для выраже́ния бу́дущего де́йствия, о кото́ром говори́лось в про́шлом*: I said we ~ visit the place next week я сказа́л, что мы посети́м э́то ме́сто на сле́дующей неде́ле; 3) *как мода́льный гл. выража́ет рекоменда́цию, сове́т, увещева́ние*: you ~ not do that вам не сле́довало бы де́лать э́того; she ~ be more attentive at her lessons ей сле́довало бы быть бо́лее внима́тельной на уро́ках; 4) *с эмоциона́льной окра́ской выража́ет удивле́ние, возмуще́ние, ра́дость, огорче́ние*: why ~ I do it? а заче́м мне э́то де́лать?; 5) *с после́дующей фо́рмой Perfect Infinitive выража́ет*: а) *в утверди́тельном предложе́нии, что де́йствие не́ было вы́полнено*: you ~ have come yesterday вам ну́жно было бы прийти́ вчера́; б) *в отрица́тельном предложе́нии, что де́йствие бы́ло вы́полнено, одна́ко оно́ рассма́тривается как нежела́тельное*: you shouldn't have told him that вам не сле́довало бы говори́ть ему́ об э́том.

shoulder I ['ʃouldə] *n* 1) плечо́; лопа́тка; door-wide ~s ≅ коса́я са́жень в плеча́х; round ~s суту́лые пле́чи; суту́лость; to put out (*или* to disloeate) one's ~ вы́вихнуть плечо́; to shrug one's ~s пожима́ть плеча́ми; ~ to ~ а) плечо́м к плечу́; б) соедини́нными уси́лиями; 2) усту́п; 3) обо́чина (*доро́ги*); ◇ to give smb. the cold ~ оказа́ть холо́дный приём; хо́лодно встре́тить, приня́ть; to put (*или* to set) one's ~ to the wheel принале́чь, сде́лать уси́лие; straight from the ~ сплеча́, без увёрток; to rub ~s with якша́ться с кем-л.; to go over the left ~ пойти́ пра́хом; пойти́ вкривь и вкось.

shoulder II *v* 1) взва́ливать на пле́чи; 2) брать на себя́ (*отве́тственность, рабо́ту и т. п.*); 3) толка́ть(ся); прота́лкивать(ся).

shoulder-belt ['ʃouldəbelt] *n* 1) пе́ревязь (*че́рез плечо́*); 2) *воен.* (плечева́я) портупе́я.

shoulder-blade ['ʃouldəbleɪd] *n* анат. лопа́тка.

shoulder-strap ['ʃouldəstræp] *n* воен. пого́н.

shouldn't ['ʃudnt] *разг. =* should not.

shout I [ʃaut] *n* гро́мкий крик; во́зглас; вы́крик.

shout II *v* 1) гро́мко крича́ть; крича́ть (*на кого́-л.— at, кому́-л.— to*); 2) звать (*кого́-л.— at*); подзыва́ть (*кого́-л.— for*); 3): to ~ with laughter гро́мко смея́ться; □ to ~ **down** кри́ками заста́вить (*ора́тора*) замолча́ть.

shouting ['ʃautɪŋ] *n* 1) кри́ки; 2) во́згласы (*одобре́ния и т. п.*).

shove [ʃʌv] *v* 1) су́нуть, ткнуть, пихну́ть (*куда́-л.*); 2) толка́ть, пиха́ть (*кого́-л.*); □ to ~

off a) отта́лкивать(ся) (*от берега*), отшварто́вываться; б) *разг.* смыва́ться, удира́ть.

shovel I [ˈʃʌvl] *n* 1) лопа́та; сово́к; 2) ковш (*экскаватора*); scoop ~ землечерпа́лка, экскава́тор.

shovel II *v* 1) сгреба́ть; 2) копа́ть, рыть.

show I [ʃou] *n* 1) пока́з, пока́зывание; the ~ of hands подня́тие рук (*при голосовании*); in dumb ~ зна́ками, с по́мощью зна́ков; 2) вы́ставка; 3) вид, зре́лище; 4) ви́димость, обма́нчивый вид; to make a ~ of де́лать вид; to do smth. for ~ сде́лать что-л. для ви́димости; 5) *разг.* организа́ция, предприя́тие; to run the ~ быть во главе́ (*чего-л.*); 6) *разг.* удо́бный слу́чай; to get a fair ~ име́ть удо́бный слу́чай; 7) *разг.* спекта́кль; ◇ to give the ~ away выдава́ть секре́т.

show II *v* (*past* showed; *p. p.* shown; *иногда пишется* shew, shewed, shewn) 1) пока́зывать; демонстри́ровать; 2) предъявля́ть, представля́ть (*документ*); 3) проявля́ть (*чувства*); 4) провожа́ть, проводи́ть (*куда-л.*); 5) быть ви́димым, заме́тным; 6) *разг.* устра́ивать (*выставку, спекта́кль*); □ to ~ **in** ввести́, провести́ в помеще́ние; to ~ **off** a) пуска́ть пыль в глаза́; задава́ться; рисова́ться; б) представля́ть в вы́годном све́те; to ~ **out** выводи́ть, провожа́ть из помеще́ния; to ~ **over**, to ~ **round** пока́зывать (*город, музей и т. п.*); to ~ **up** a) разоблача́ть; изоблича́ть; б) выдава́ться; в) выявля́ться; г) объяви́ться, появи́ться.

show-boat [ˈʃoubout] *n амер.* плаву́чий теа́тр.

show-case [ˈʃoukeɪs] *n* витри́на.

show-down [ˈʃoudaun] *n* 1) раскры́тие карт; 2) раскры́тие свои́х возмо́жностей, ресу́рсов *и т. п.*; 3) *амер. разг.* открове́нный обме́н мне́ниями.

shower I [ˈʃauə] *n* 1) ли́вень (*тж.* a ~ of rain); 2) си́льный снегопа́д; 3) пото́к (*слёз*); 4) град (*пуль, вопросов*); 5) душ; ◇ a ~ of gifts мно́жество пода́рков; in ~s во мно́жестве.

shower II *v* 1) ли́ть(ся) ли́внем; 2) засыпа́ть (*вопросами, подарками*).

shower-bath [ˈʃauəbɑːθ] *n* душ.

showman [ˈʃoumən] *n* 1) устро́итель вы́ставки; 2) хозя́ин ци́рка, балага́на *и т. п.*

showmanship [ˈʃoumənʃɪp] *n* уме́ние привле́чь внима́ние, показа́ть това́р лицо́м.

shown [ʃoun] *p. p. см.* show II.

show-off [ˈʃouˌɔf] *n* 1) рисо́вка, жема́нство; 2) *разг.* позёр.

show-room [ˈʃourum] *n* вы́ставочный зал; демонстрацио́нный зал (*образцов товаров и т. п.*).

show-window [ˈʃouˈwɪndou] *n* витри́на.

showy [ˈʃoui] *a* 1) пы́шный (*о цветах*); 2) я́ркий, крича́щий (*о платье*).

shrank [ʃræŋk] *past см.* shrink.

shrapnel [ˈʃræpnl] *n* шрапне́ль.

shred I [ʃred] *n* лоску́т, тря́пка, обры́вок; to cut to ~s ре́зать на куски́; to tear to ~s рвать на куски́, рвать в кло́чья.

shred II *v* (*past. p. p.* shredded, *уст.* shred) 1) кромса́ть, рвать, драть (*на куски*); 2) се́чься, располза́ться (*о материи*); □ to ~ **away** рассе́иваться (*о дыме*).

shrew [ʃruː] *n* стропти́вая, сварли́вая же́нщина.

shrewd [ʃruːd] *a* 1) проница́тельный; то́нкий

(*об уме*); 2) *уст.* хи́трый, зло́бный; 3) ре́зкий, прони́зывающий (*о ветре, холоде*).

shrewish [ˈʃruːɪʃ] *a* сварли́вый.

shriek I [ʃriːk] *n* пронзи́тельный крик; визг.

shriek II *v* пронзи́тельно крича́ть, вопи́ть, ора́ть.

shrill I [ʃrɪl] *a* 1) пронзи́тельный, ре́зкий; 2) душераздира́ющий.

shrill II *v* пронзи́тельно крича́ть, визжа́ть.

shrimp [ʃrɪmp] *n* 1) креве́тка; 2) малю́тка, ка́рлик; 3) ничто́жество (*о человеке*).

shrine [ʃraɪn] *n* 1) гробни́ца; 2) храм, алта́рь; 3) ме́сто поклоне́ния, святы́ня.

shrinedom [ˈʃraɪndəm] *n* люби́тели па́мятников старины́.

shrink [ʃrɪŋk] *v* (*past* shrank; *p. p.* shrunk) 1) сади́ться (*о материи*); сжима́ться (*от холода*); to ~ at a touch сжима́ться, мо́рщиться от прикоснове́ния; 2) отпря́нуть, отскочи́ть наза́д; 3) избега́ть, уклоня́ться (*от чего-л. — from*); to ~ from society избега́ть о́бщества; I ~ from telling her у меня́ не хвата́ет ду́ху сказа́ть ей; ◇ to ~ into oneself уйти́ в себя́.

srinkage [ˈʃrɪŋkɪdʒ] *n* 1) сокраще́ние, сжа́тие; 2) усу́шка, утру́ска, уса́дка.

shrive [ʃraɪv] *v* (*past* shrived, shrove; *p. p.* shrived, shriven) испове́доваться, ка́яться.

shrivel [ˈʃrɪvl] *v* (*тж.* to ~ up) 1) сжима́ться, ссыха́ться, свёртываться (*от жары, засухи, мороза*); 2) скрю́чиваться.

shriven [ˈʃrɪvn] *p. p. см.* shrive.

shroud I [ʃraud] *n* 1) са́ван; 2) пелена́, покро́в, заве́са; under a ~ of mystery под покро́вом та́йны; 3) *pl мор.* ва́нты.

shroud II *v* 1) завёртывать в са́ван; 2) скрыва́ть; 3) оку́тывать, заку́тывать.

shrove [ʃrouv] *past см.* shrive.

Shrovetide [ˈʃrouvtaɪd] *n* ма́сленица.

shrub [ʃrʌb] *n* куст.

shrubbery [ˈʃrʌbərɪ] *n* куста́рник.

shrubby [ˈʃrʌbɪ] *a* 1) поро́сший куста́рником; 2) куста́рниковый.

shrug I [ʃrʌg] *n* пожима́ние (*плечами*).

shrug II *v* пожима́ть (*плечами*).

shrunk [ʃrʌŋk] *p. p. см.* shrink.

shrunken [ˈʃrʌŋkən] *a* дря́блый, смо́рщенный (*от старости*).

shuck I [ʃʌk] *n амер.* 1) шелуха́; 2) ра́ковина (*устрицы*); ◇ not worth ~s! ло́маного гроша́ не сто́ит!, чепуха́!

shuck II *v амер.* очища́ть от шелухи́.

shudder I [ˈʃʌdə] *n* содрога́ние.

shudder II *v* содрога́ться; I ~ to think я содрога́юсь при мы́сли.

shuffle I [ˈʃʌfl] *n* 1) ша́ркающая, нетвёрдая похо́дка; 2) тасова́ние (*карт*); 3) уве́ртка, уло́вка; 4) переме́на мест.

shuffle II *v* 1) ша́ркать (*ногами*); 2) уви́ливать, уве́ртываться (*от чего-л. — out of*); 3) виля́ть, хитри́ть; 4) тасова́ть (*карты*); 5) меня́ться места́ми; 6) ёрзать (*на стуле*); 7) сме́шивать в ку́чу; □ to ~ **off** a) швырну́ть в сто́рону; б) изба́виться, отде́латься.

shuffler [ˈʃʌflə] *n* 1) тасу́ющий ка́рты; 2) пройдо́ха.

shun [ʃʌn] *v* избега́ть, остерега́ться.

'shun [ʃʌn] *int воен.* сми́рно!

shunt I [ʃʌnt] *n* 1) перевод, переключение; 2) ж.-д. перевод на запасный путь; 3) ж.-д. стрелка.

shunt II *v* 1) сворачивать; отклоняться (*от пути*); 2) разг. откладывать (*обсуждение, проект*); 3) ж.-д. переводить на запасный путь.

shut I [ʃʌt] *v* (*past. p. p.* shut) 1) закрывать(ся); 2) затворять (*дверь, окно и т. п.*); 3) заключать, сажать (*во что-л. — into*); 4) не впускать (*в помещение; out of*); □ to ~ **down** а) останавливать(ся) (*о заводе, предприятии*); б) прекратить работу; to ~ **in** а) запереть (*где-л.*); б): to be ~ in быть окружённым (*горами, домами*); в) заслонять, загораживать; to ~ **into** прищемить, защемить; to ~ **off** а) выключать (*пар, воду, ток*); б) изолировать (*от кого-л. — from*); в) вешать (*телефонную трубку*); to ~ **out** не впускать, не допускать; to ~ **up** а) запирать (*двери и т. п.*); б) закрыть (*магазин и т. п.*); в) заключать (*в тюрьму; in*); г) разг. (заставить) замолчать; ~ up! замолчи!

shut II *a* закрытый; запертый.

shut-down [ˈʃʌt,daun] *n* 1) закрытие, остановка (*завода, предприятия*); 2) выключение.

shut-in I [ˈʃʌt,ɪn] *n* амер. постельный больной.

shut-in II *a* находящийся в больнице.

shut-off [ˈʃʌt,ɔːf] *n* выключатель.

shutter I [ˈʃʌtə] *n* 1) ставень; to put up the ~s перен. закончить работу; закрыть предприятие; 2) заслонка, задвижка; 3) затвор (*фотоаппарата*).

shutter II *v* закрывать ставнями.

shuttle I [ˈʃʌtl] *n* 1) челнок (*ткацкого станка, швейной машины*); 2) амер. пригородный поезд.

shuttle II *v* двигаться взад и вперёд.

shuttle-train [ˈʃʌtltreɪn] *n* пригородный поезд.

shy[1] I [ʃaɪ] *a* 1) застенчивый; робкий, нерешительный; to be ~ of не решаться (*сделать что-л.*); 2) пугливый (*о животном*); 3) недоверчивый; 4) амер. сленг недостаточный.

shy[1] II *v* 1) отпрянуть, отскочить; 2) броситься в сторону (*о лошади и т. п.*); □ to ~ **away** избегать, уклоняться; to ~ away from contact не вступать в общение, в контакт с незнакомыми людьми (*на улице, в поезде, троллейбусе*).

shy[2] I *n* разг. 1) бросок; 2) попытка; to have a ~ at попытаться.

shy[2] II *v* разг. швырять; бросать.

Siamese I [,saɪəˈmiːz] *n см.* Thai.

Siamese II *a* сиамский.

sibilant I [ˈsɪbɪlənt] *n* фон. свистящий *или* шипящий звук.

sibilant II *a* фон. свистящий *или* шипящий (*о звуке*).

sick [sɪk] *a* 1) больной; to fall (*или* to go, to turn) ~ захворать; 2) чувствующий тошноту; to be ~, to feel ~ а) чувствовать тошноту; б) амер. быть больным; 3) разг. уставший, измученный; to be ~ ɔi smth. пресытиться чем-л.; I am ~ of... мне надоело...; I am ~ and tired of it мне это осточертело; to be ~ at heart тосковать, кручиниться; to be ~ for a sight of home тосковать по дому.

sick-bed [ˈsɪkbed] *n* постель больного.

sicken [ˈsɪkn] *v* 1) болеть, заболевать; 2) чувствовать отвращение, тошноту (*к чему-л. — at*);

3) вызывать тошноту, отвращение; 4) утомляться (*от чего-л. — of*); 5) чахнуть (*о растении*).

sickening [ˈsɪknɪŋ] *a* 1) отвратительный; 2) чахлый.

sickle [ˈsɪkl] *n* серп.

sick-leave [ˈsɪkliːv] *n* 1) отпуск по болезни; 2) бюллетень, больничный лист.

sick-list [ˈsɪkˈlɪst] *n* 1) список больных; 2) больничный лист; on ~ на бюллетене.

sickly [ˈsɪklɪ] *a* 1) болезненный; больной (*о виде и т. п.*); 2) нездоровый (*о местности и т. п.*); 3) тошнотворный; 4) теплящийся (*об огне, свете*); 5) блёклый (*о цвете*).

sickness [ˈsɪknɪs] *n* 1) болезнь, заболевание; radiation ~ лучевая болезнь; falling ~ падучая (болезнь), эпилепсия; 2) тошнота.

side I [saɪd] *n* 1) сторона; blank ~ слабая сторона; blind ~ слабое место (*у человека*); the right ~ of cloth лицевая сторона материи; the seamy (*или* the wrong) ~ of cloth изнанка; on all ~s со всех сторон; on both ~s с каждой стороны; с обеих сторон; on the right (*или* on the sunny) ~ of forty моложе сорока лет; под сорок лет; on the shady ~ of forty старше сорока лет; за сорок лет; to get on the right ~ of smb. заслужить чью-л. благосклонность; to look on the sunny ~ of things смотреть бодро на жизнь; to take ~s примкнуть (*к кому-л. — with*); стать на чью-л. сторону; 2) стена (*комнаты*); стенка (*ящика и т. п.*); 3) склон (*горы, холма*); 4) поле (*страницы*); 5) бок; to shake (to split) one's ~s трястись (надрываться) от смеха; by the ~ of рядом, поблизости; ~ by ~ рядом, бок о бок; 6) линия (*родства*); distaff ~, spindle ~ женская линия (*рода*); spear ~ мужская линия (*рода*); 7) разг. чванство, зазнайство; to put on ~ задаваться; 8) *attr* боковой; 9) *attr* побочный.

side II *v* стать на чью-л. сторону (*with*).

sideboard [ˈsaɪdbɔːd] *n* 1) буфет, сервант; 2) подсобный столик (*в столовой*).

side-car [ˈsaɪdkɑː] *n* коляска (*мотоцикла*).

sidehill [ˈsaɪdhɪl] *n* амер. склон, скат (*горы*).

sidelight [ˈsaɪdlaɪt] *n* 1) свет, идущий сбоку; 2) случайная информация; сведения, проливающие свет на что-л.; 3) иллюминатор; 4) боковое окно; 5) мор. отличительный огонь.

side-line [ˈsaɪdlaɪn] *n* 1) боковая линия; 2) побочная работа, занятие.

sidelong I [ˈsaɪdlɔŋ] *a* косой, направленный в сторону.

sidelong II *adv* вкось.

sidereal [saɪˈdɪərɪəl] *a* звёздный (*о годе, часе и т. п.*).

side-saddle [ˈsaɪd,sædl] *n* дамское седло.

side-slip I [ˈsaɪdslɪp] *n* скольжение.

side-slip II *v* 1) скользить вбок; 2) ав. скользить на крыло.

side-splitting [ˈsaɪd,splɪtɪŋ] *a* уморительный.

side-step [ˈsaɪdstep] *v* 1) отступить в сторону; 2) увиливать, уклоняться.

side-track I [ˈsaɪdtræk] *n* ж.-д. запасный путь.

side-track II *v* 1) ж.-д. переводить на запасный путь; 2) откладывать (*рассмотрение чего-л.*); 3) уводить в сторону, отвлекать (*от — from*).

side-view [ˈsaɪdvjuː] *n* профиль, вид сбоку.

sidewalk [ˈsaɪdwɔːk] *n* амер. тротуар.

sideward I ['saɪdwəd] *a* напра́вленный в сто́рону.

sideward II *adv* в сто́рону, вбок, вкось.

side-way I ['saɪdweɪ] *n* 1) боковая тропи́нка; 2) око́льный путь.

side-way II *adv* в сто́рону.

sideways I ['saɪdweɪz] *a* напра́вленный в сто́рону.

sideways II *adv* 1) в сто́рону; 2) бо́ком.

side-wind ['saɪdwɪnd] *n* посторо́ннее влия́ние.

side-winder ['saɪd,wɪndə] *n разг.* ошеломля́ющий уда́р (*нанесённый сбоку*).

siding ['saɪdɪŋ] *n* 1) *ж.-д.* запа́сный путь, ве́тка; 2) *амер.* обши́вка (*здания*).

sidle ['saɪdl] *v* (под)ходи́ть бочко́м (*to; тж.* to ~ up).

sidy ['saɪdɪ] *a разг.* претенцио́зный, с претéнзией на (*что-л.*).

siege I [siːdʒ] *n* 1) оса́да; to lay ~ а) нача́ть оса́ду (*чего-л.— to*); б) *разг.* приуда́рить, нача́ть уха́живать (*за кем-л.— to*); to raise the ~ снять оса́ду; to stand a ~ выде́рживать оса́ду; 2) *уст.* сиде́нье; трон; 3) *attr* оса́дный.

siege II *v уст.* осади́ть.

siege-gun ['siːdʒɡʌn] *n ист.* оса́дное ору́дие.

sienna [sɪ'enə] *n* сие́на (*краска*).

sierra [sɪ'ərə] *n* го́рная цепь.

siesta [sɪ'estə] *n* послеобе́денный о́тдых, сие́ста.

sieve I [sɪv] *n* 1) решето́; си́то; like a ~ *перен.* дыря́вая как решето́ (*о голове*); 2) болту́н.

sieve II *v* просе́ивать (*сквозь сито, решето*).

sift [sɪft] *v* 1) просе́ивать (*сквозь сито, решето*); 2) посыпа́ть (*сахаром и т. п.*); 3) внима́тельно иссле́довать, изуча́ть (*факты, данные и т. п.*); 4) се́яться, па́дать (*о дожде и т. п.*).

sigh I [saɪ] *n* вздох; a ~ of relief вздох облегче́ния; to fetch a ~ вздохну́ть; to heave a ~ тяжело́ вздохну́ть.

sigh II *v* 1) вздыха́ть, вздохну́ть; 2) тоскова́ть (*о ком-л., о чём-л.— for*); сокруша́ться; 3) гуде́ть, шуме́ть (*о ветре*).

sight I [saɪt] *n* 1) зре́ние; keen ~ о́строе зре́ние; long ~ дальнозо́ркость; near ~, short ~ близору́кость; second ~ яснови́дение; 2) по́ле зре́ния; to catch (*или* to get) ~ of уви́деть, заме́тить; to come into ~ показа́ться, появи́ться; to lose ~ of потеря́ть из ви́ду; at ~, on ~ при ви́де; at first ~ с пе́рвого взгля́да; to know by ~ знать в лицо́; in one's ~ а) в чьих-л. глаза́х; б) на чьих-л. глаза́х; in ~ а) в виду́ (*берега, города и т. п.*); б) в перспекти́ве; out of ~ вне по́ля зре́ния; out of my ~! прочь с глаз мои́х!; within ~ в преде́лах ви́димости; 3) вид, зре́лище; a grand (memorable) ~ вели́чественное (па́мятное) зре́лище; nasty ~ ужа́сное, мёрзкое зре́лище; a sorry ~ печа́льное зре́лище; to make a ~ of oneself де́лать из себя́ посме́шище; 4) *pl* достопримеча́тельности; to see the ~s осма́тривать достопримеча́тельности; 5) прице́л; to take a careful ~ тща́тельно прице́ливаться; 6) *разг.* мно́жество; ма́сса; ◇ to play at ~ игра́ть с листа́; out of ~ out of mind *посл.* ≅ с глаз доло́й — из се́рдца вон.

sight II *v* 1) заме́тить, разгляде́ть, вы́смотреть; 2) производи́ть наблюде́ния (*с помощью*

инструме́нтов*); 3) наводи́ть (*оружие, орудие*); брать прице́л.

sightless ['saɪtlɪs] *a* 1) слепо́й, лишённый зре́ния; 2) неви́димый, незри́мый.

sightly ['saɪtlɪ] *a* ви́дный; краси́вый.

sightseeing I ['saɪt,siːɪŋ] *n* осмо́тр достопримеча́тельностей; to go ~ осма́тривать достопримеча́тельности.

sightseeing II *a* экскурсио́нный (*об автомоби́ле*).

sightseer ['saɪt,siːə] *n* тури́ст (*осма́тривающий достопримеча́тельности*).

sign I [saɪn] *n* 1) знак; manual ~ собственноручная по́дпись; the negative ~ знак «ми́нус»; *разг. шутл.* ничто́, ничего́; the positive ~ знак «плюс»; unlike ~s *мат.* зна́ки «плюс» и «ми́нус»; to give a ~ пода́ть знак; 2) при́знак; to show ~s подава́ть при́знаки (*жизни, роста и т. п.*); 3) си́мвол, усло́вный знак; ~s of the times знаме́ние вре́мени; 4) вы́веска; 5) *мед.* симпто́м; 6) *след.*

sign II *v* 1) подпи́сывать(ся); 2) де́лать знак; подава́ть сигна́л руко́й (*кому-л.— for*); □ to ~ away отка́зываться (*в чью-л. по́льзу*); to ~ off *амер. радио* объявля́ть о конце́ переда́чи, о прекраще́нии рабо́ты радиоста́нции; to ~ on а) наня́ть (*на работу*); б) дать подписку о согла́сии рабо́тать; to ~ up подписа́ть контра́кт (*о поступле́нии на работу*).

signal I ['sɪɡnl] *n* 1) сигна́л; visual ~ светово́й, опти́ческий сигна́л; ~ of distress сигна́л бе́дствия; 2) знак; to make a ~ пода́ть знак, сигна́л; 3) *ж.-д.* семафо́р.

signal II *a* 1) сигна́льный; 2) блестя́щий, выдаю́щийся (*о побе́де, успе́хе*).

signal III *v* дава́ть сигна́л, сигнализи́ровать.

signal-book ['sɪɡnlbuk] *n* код, сигна́льная кни́га.

signal-box ['sɪɡnlbɔks] *n ж.-д.* сигна́льная бу́дка; блокпо́ст.

signally ['sɪɡnəlɪ] *adv* блестя́щим о́бразом, на ре́дкость.

signal-man ['sɪɡnlmən] *n* сигна́льщик.

signatory I ['sɪɡnətərɪ] *n* сторона́, подписа́вшая до́говор, соглаше́ние.

signatory II *a* подписа́вший (*договор, соглаше́ние*).

signature ['sɪɡnɪtʃə] *n* 1) по́дпись; to bear the ~ име́ть по́дпись; 2) *полигр.* сигнату́ра; 3) *муз.* ключ.

signboard ['saɪnbɔːd] *n* вы́веска.

signer ['saɪnə] *n* лицо́, сторона́, страна́ (*подписа́вшая договор, соглаше́ние*).

signet I ['sɪɡnɪt] *n* 1) печа́тка; 2) печа́ть.

signet II *v* прикла́дывать (*печать*).

significance [sɪɡ'nɪfɪkəns] *n* 1) значе́ние (*фа́кта, собы́тия*); of no ~ не име́ющий значе́ния; 2) ва́жность, значи́тельность; 3) вырази́тельность.

significant [sɪɡ'nɪfɪkənt] *a* 1) ва́жный, суще́ственный; знамена́тельный; 2) многозначи́тельный; вырази́тельный.

signification [,sɪɡnɪfɪ'keɪʃən] *n* 1) значе́ние, смысл; 2) значи́мость.

significative [sɪɡ'nɪfɪkətɪv] *a* ука́зывающий (*на что-л.— of*); свиде́тельствующий (*о чём-л.— of*); означа́ющий.

signify ['sɪgnɪfaɪ] *v* 1) выража́ть, выка́зывать; 2) означа́ть, зна́чить; 3) име́ть значе́ние, игра́ть роль; what does it ~? а) како́е э́то име́ет значе́ние?; б) что э́то зна́чит?; 4) ука́зывать, предвеща́ть.

signpost ['saɪnpoust] *n* указа́тельный столб.

silage ['saɪlɪdʒ] *n* си́лос.

silence I ['saɪləns] *n* 1) тишина́, безмо́лвие; dead ~, haunted ~ мёртвая тишина́; in ~ в тишине́; бесшу́мно; 2) молча́ние; to break (to keep) ~ нару́шить (храни́ть) молча́ние; to put to ~ заста́вить замолча́ть; 3) забве́ние; to pass into ~ быть пре́данным забве́нию; ◊ ~ gives consent *погов.* ≅ молча́ние — знак согла́сия.

silence II *v* 1) заста́вить замолча́ть; заглуши́ть; 2) успоко́ить; убаю́кать.

silence III *int* молча́ть!, ти́ше!

silencer ['saɪlənsə] *n* 1) глуши́тель; 2) *муз.* модера́тор.

silent ['saɪlənt] *a* 1) ти́хий, безмо́лвный; бесшу́мный; 2) молчали́вый; 3) немо́й; 4) ума́лчивающий; 5) поту́хший, неде́йствующий (*о вулка́не*); 6) непроизноси́мый (*о бу́квах*).

silhouette I [ˌsɪluːˈet] *n* силуэ́т.

silhouette II *v* вырисо́вываться на фо́не (*чего́-л.*).

silica ['sɪlɪkə] *n мин.* кремнезём, кварц.

silicon ['sɪlɪkən] *n хим.* кре́мний.

silk [sɪlk] *n* 1) шёлк; 2) шёлковое пла́тье; 3) *pl* шелка́; 4) *attr* шёлковый.

silken ['sɪlkən] *a* 1) шелкови́стый; 2) *уст.* шёлковый; 3) наря́дный, шика́рный; 4) мя́гкий, вкра́дчивый.

silk-mill ['sɪlkmɪl] *n* шелкопряди́льная фа́брика.

silk-stocking ['sɪlk'stɔkɪŋ] *n* 1) аристокра́т; 2) *attr* привилегиро́ванный, аристократи́ческий.

silkworm ['sɪlkwəːm] *n* шелкови́чный червь.

silky ['sɪlkɪ] *a* 1) шелкови́стый, мя́гкий; 2) вкра́дчивый.

sill [sɪl] *n* 1) поро́г (*две́ри, шлю́за*); 2) подоко́нник (*см. тж.* window-sill).

silly I ['sɪlɪ] *n разг.* дура́к.

silly II *a* 1) глу́пый; неразу́мный; 2) слабоу́мный.

silo I ['saɪlou] *n* 1) си́лос; 2) си́лосная я́ма; 3) *attr* си́лосный.

silo II *v* силосова́ть.

silt [sɪlt] *n* ил.

silvan ['sɪlvən] *a* 1) лесно́й; 2) леси́стый.

silver I ['sɪlvə] *n* 1) серебро́; German ~ мельхио́р; 2) сере́бряные де́ньги; 3) сере́бряная посу́да; 4) *attr* сере́бряный; серебри́стый; седо́й (*о волоса́х*).

silver II *v* 1) серебри́ть(ся); 2) покрыва́ть (зе́ркало) амальга́мой.

silver-fir ['sɪlvəfəː] *n* пи́хта.

silver-tongued ['sɪlvə'tʌŋd] *a* сладкозву́чный; красноречи́вый.

silverware ['sɪlvəˌwεə] *n* сере́бряные изде́лия.

silvery ['sɪlvərɪ] *a* 1) серебри́стый; 2) чи́стый (*о зву́ке, го́лосе*).

similar ['sɪmɪlə] *a* 1) схо́жий, похо́жий; 2) подо́бный (*тж. мат.*); схо́дный; одина́ковый.

similarity [ˌsɪmɪˈlærɪtɪ] *n* 1) схо́дство; 2) подо́бие (*тж. мат.*).

similarly ['sɪmɪləlɪ] *adv* так же, подо́бным о́бразом.

simile ['sɪmɪlɪ] *n* сравне́ние (*речева́я фигу́ра*).

similitude [sɪˈmɪlɪtjuːd] *n* 1) схо́дство; о́браз, подо́бие; to assume the ~ приня́ть о́браз, вид (*кого́-л.— of*); 2) сравне́ние (*речева́я фигу́ра*).

simitar ['sɪmɪtə] *см.* scimitar.

simmer I ['sɪmə] *n* закипа́ние.

simmer II *v* 1) закипа́ть; бу́лькать; 2) с трудо́м сде́рживать (*гнев, смех*); □ to ~ **down** а) перестава́ть кипе́ть; б) остыва́ть (*о гне́ве*).

simon-pure ['saɪmən'pjuə] *a* настоя́щий, по́длинный.

simoom [sɪˈmuːm] *n* саму́м.

simp [sɪmp] *n амер. разг.* проста́к, «шля́па».

simper I ['sɪmpə] *n* глу́пая, самодово́льная улы́бка.

simper II *v* глу́по улыба́ться.

simple ['sɪmpl] *a* 1) просто́й, несло́жный; 2) пра́вильный (*о дро́би*); однозна́чный (*о числе́*); 3) прямо́й, че́стный; 4) простоду́шный, наи́вный; 5) незамыслова́тый, незате́йливый; 6) незна́тный; 7) я́вный, и́стинный.

simple-hearted ['sɪmpl'hɑːtɪd] *a* простоду́шный.

simple-minded ['sɪmpl'maɪndɪd] *a* 1) бесхи́тростный; 2) тупова́тый; глупова́тый.

simpleton ['sɪmpltən] *n* проста́к, недалёкий челове́к.

simplicity [sɪmˈplɪsɪtɪ] *n* 1) простота́; 2) незате́йливость; 3) бесхи́тростность, простоду́шие; 4) тупова́тость.

simplification [ˌsɪmplɪfɪˈkeɪʃən] *n* упроще́ние.

simplify ['sɪmplɪfaɪ] *v* упроща́ть.

simply ['sɪmplɪ] *adv* 1) про́сто, про́сто-на́просто; то́лько; 2) простоду́шно, бесхи́тростно; 3) незате́йливо; 4) абсолю́тно.

simulate ['sɪmjuleɪt] *v* 1) симули́ровать, притворя́ться; 2) походи́ть (*на что-л.*).

simulation [ˌsɪmjuˈleɪʃən] *n* симуля́ция, притво́рство.

simultaneous [ˌsɪməlˈteɪnjəs] *a* одновреме́нный.

simultaneousness [ˌsɪməlˈteɪnjəsnɪs] *n* одновреме́нность.

sin I [sɪn] *n* 1) грех; deadly ~, mortal ~ сме́ртный грех; 2) просту́пок, наруше́ние (*зако́на, при́нципов*); besetting ~ основно́й недоста́ток, поро́к; ◊ in ~ в незако́нном бра́ке.

sin II *v* (со)греши́ть.

since I [sɪns] *adv* 1) с тех пор; с того́ вре́мени; ever ~ с того́ вре́мени, с тех пор; I have not seen her ~ я её не ви́дел с тех пор; 2) зате́м; 3) тому́ наза́д; it is a yeag ~ э́то бы́ло год тому́ наза́д.

since II *prep* 1) с (*тако́го-то вре́мени*): ~ yesterday со вчера́шнего дня; ~ last year с про́шлого го́да; 2) со вре́мени; по́сле.

since III *conj* 1) с тех пор как; 2) так как, поско́льку.

sincere [sɪnˈsɪə] *a* 1) чистосерде́чный, и́скренний; 2) неподде́льный.

sincerely [sɪnˈsɪəlɪ] *adv* чистосерде́чно, и́скренне; Yours ~ и́скренне Ваш (*фо́рмула ве́жливости в конце́ письма́*).

sincerity [sɪnˈserɪtɪ] *n* чистосерде́чность, и́скренность.

sine [saɪn] *n мат.* си́нус.

sinecure ['saɪnɪkjuə] *n* синеку́ра.

sinew ['sɪnjuː] *n* 1) сухожи́лие; 2) *pl* мускулату́ра; 3) *pl* (дви́жущие) си́лы.

sinewy ['sɪnjuːɪ] *a* 1) жи́листый, му́скулистый; 2) вырази́тельный, я́ркий (*о стиле, языке*).

sinful ['sɪnful] *a* гре́шный.

sing I [sɪŋ] *n* 1) пе́ние; 2) *разг.* спе́вка; 3) звон (*в ушах*); шум (*ветра*); свист (*пули*).

sing II *v* (*past* sang; *p. p.* sung) 1) петь, распева́ть; to ~ flat (sharp) петь ни́же (вы́ше), чем ну́жно, фальши́вить; to ~ small *перен.* сба́вить тон; to ~ smb. to sleep убаю́кать кого́-л.; 2) воспева́ть (*of*); 3) шуме́ть, гуде́ть (*о ветре, лесе и т. п.*); жужжа́ть (*о пчеле*); свисте́ть (*о пуле и т. п.*); 4) звене́ть (*в ушах*); □ to ~ out вскри́кивать, выкри́кивать; to ~ up (за)пе́ть гро́мче.

singe I [sɪndʒ] *n* пове́рхностный ожо́г.

singe II *v* 1) опаля́ть, обжига́ть; 2) спали́ть, подпали́ть; 3) запятна́ть (*репутацию*).

singer ['sɪŋə] *n* 1) певе́ц, певи́ца; 2) поэ́т; 3) пе́вчая пти́ца.

Singhalese I [ˌsɪŋhə'liːz] *n* 1) синга́лец; синга́лка; the ~ (*употр. как pl*) синга́льцы; 2) синга́льский язы́к.

Singhalese II *a* синга́льский.

single I ['sɪŋgl] *a* 1) оди́н, еди́нственный; not a ~ ни оди́н; 2) рассчи́танный на одного́; отде́льный (*о комнате, кровати и т. п.*); 3) одино́кий; 4) холосто́й, незаму́жняя; 5) и́скренний, прямо́й; 6) *уст.* сре́дней кре́пости (*о пиве и т. п.*).

single II *v* выбира́ть; отбира́ть (*тж.* to ~ out).

single- ['sɪŋgl-] *pref* одно-.

single-breasted ['sɪŋgl'brestɪd] *a* однобо́ртный (*о пальто и т. п.*).

single-handed ['sɪŋgl'hændɪd] *a* 1) рабо́тающий без посторо́нней по́мощи; 2) однору́кий.

single-hearted ['sɪŋgl'hɑːtɪd] *a* прямоду́шный, чистосерде́чный.

single-minded ['sɪŋgl'maɪndɪd] *a* 1) целеустремлённый; 2) и́скренний.

singleness ['sɪŋglnɪs] *n* одино́чество; ~ of purpose целеустремлённость.

single-phase ['sɪŋgl'feɪz] *a* *эл.* однофа́зный.

singlet ['sɪŋglɪt] *n* фуфа́йка.

singly ['sɪŋglɪ] *adv* 1) поодино́чке, отде́льно; 2) в одино́чку, без чужо́й по́мощи.

Sing Sing ['sɪŋ,sɪŋ] *n* Синг-Си́нг (*тюрьма в Нью-Йорке*).

singsong I ['sɪŋsɒŋ] *n* 1) импровизи́рованный конце́рт; 2) моното́нное чте́ние, деклама́ция.

singsong II *a* моното́нный, однообра́зный.

singular I ['sɪŋgjulə] *n* *грам.* еди́нственное число́.

singular II *a* 1) необыкнове́нный, чрезвыча́йный; 2) стра́нный, чудно́й; 3) *грам.* еди́нственный; 4) отде́льный.

singularity [ˌsɪŋgju'lærɪtɪ] *n* 1) осо́бенность, своеобра́зие; 2) специфи́чность.

Sinhalese I, II [ˌsɪŋhə'liːz] *см.* Singhalese I, II.

sinister ['sɪnɪstə] *a* 1) злове́щий; 2) дурно́й; 3) бе́дственный, ги́бельный, па́губный (*to*).

sinistrous ['sɪnɪstrəs] *a* 1) злове́щий; 2) злополу́чный.

sink¹ [sɪŋk] *v* (*past* sank; *p. p.* sunk) 1) (по)топи́ть; (по)тону́ть; to ~ or to swim ≅ и́ли пан и́ли пропа́л; была́ не была́; to ~ at sight *мор.* топи́ть без предупрежде́ния; 2) погружа́ть(ся) (*в воду, сон, забвение; into*); опусти́ться (*в крес-*

ло, на дива́н; *into*); 3) клони́ться, опуска́ться (*к горизонту*); 4) спада́ть (*о приливе, уровне воды и т. п.*); понижа́ться (*о местности*); 5) затопи́ть (*местность*); 6) оседа́ть (*о здании*); 7) ослабева́ть, теря́ть (*силы*); ги́бнуть; he is ~ing fast он бы́стро опуска́ется, ги́бнет; 8) падать (*о цене, стоимости, барометре*); 9) затиха́ть (*о ветре, звуке*); понижа́ть (*голос*); опуска́ть (*голову, глаза*); 10) теря́ть (*капитал*); 11) рыть (*колодец, шахту*); прокла́дывать (*трубу*); 12) впада́ть (*в нищету*); 13) вва́ливаться (*о глазах, щеках*); 14) погря́знуть (*в грехах*); 15) скрыва́ть (*имя и т. п.*); 16) игнори́ровать.

sink² *n* 1) ра́ковина (*водопроводная*); 2) ни́зкое ме́сто, низи́на; 3) сто́чная труба́; 4) прито́н, верте́п.

sinking ['sɪŋkɪŋ] *n* 1) потопле́ние; 2) погруже́ние; 3) оседа́ние (*местности, здания*).

sinking-fund ['sɪŋkɪŋfʌnd] *n* амортизацио́нный фонд.

sinless ['sɪnlɪs] *a* безгре́шный.

sinner ['sɪnə] *n* гре́шник, гре́шница.

Sinn Fein ['ʃɪn'feɪn] *n* Шинфе́йн (*националисти́ческая организа́ция Ирла́ндии*).

sinologist [sɪ'nɒlədʒɪst] *n* китаи́ст, сино́лог.

sinology [sɪ'nɒlədʒɪ] *n* китаеве́дение, синоло́гия.

sinuous ['sɪnjuəs] *a* 1) изви́листый; с изги́бами; 2) волокни́стый.

Sioux [suː] *n* сиу (*индеец одного из северо-американских племён*); the ~ (*употр. как pl*) сиу.

sip I [sɪp] *n* ма́ленький глото́к.

sip II *v* потя́гивать, пить ма́ленькими глотка́ми.

siphon ['saɪfən] *n* сифо́н.

sipid ['sɪpɪd] *a* прия́тный (*на вкус*); вку́сный.

sipper ['sɪpə] *n* соло́минка (*через которую пьют напитки*).

sir [sə] *n* господи́н, сэр (*как обращение*); Dear Sir Ми́лостивый госуда́рь (*формальное обращение в письме*).

sire ['saɪə] *n* 1) *поэт.* оте́ц, пре́док; 2) ва́ше вели́чество; 3) саме́ц.

siren ['saɪərɪn] *n* сире́на.

sirloin ['səːlɔɪn] *n* филе́й.

siskin ['sɪskɪn] *n* чиж.

sissy ['sɪsɪ] *n* *амер. разг.* 1) не́женка; «ба́ба»; 2) де́вочка; «сестрёнка».

sister ['sɪstə] *n* 1) сестра́ (*тж. медицинская*); full ~, ~ german родна́я сестра́; 2) *attr* сестри́нский; 3) *attr* ро́дственный (*о народах*); одноти́пный (*о судах, учебных заведениях*).

sister-in-law ['sɪstərɪnlɔː] *n* (*pl* sisters-in-law) неве́стка, золо́вка.

sisterly ['sɪstəlɪ] *a* сестри́нский.

sit [sɪt] *v* (*past, p. p.* sat, *уст.* sate) 1) сиде́ть; you'll get ~! *разг.* я тебе́ покажу́!, вот подожди́!; 2) заседа́ть (*о парламенте, суде и т. п.*); 3) сиде́ть (*на яйцах*); 4) пози́ровать (*for*); 5) годи́ться, быть впо́ру (*о платье*); 6) занима́ть до́лжность (*в суде и т. п.*); □ to ~ down а) сади́ться; б) сади́ться обе́дать, есть; в): to ~ down before обложи́ть (*город, крепость*); to ~ down under стерпе́ть (*обиду, оскорбление*); to ~ for а) быть депута́том в парла́менте (*от какого-л. округа, партии*); б): to ~ for an examination сдава́ть экза́мен; to ~ **in** смотре́ть за ребёнком в отсу́тствие роди́телей; to ~ **on** а) быть чле́ном (*комиссии*); б) вести́ рассле́дование; в) *разг.* сбить спесь; to ~ **out** а) не уча́ствовать (*в танцах*); б) досиде́ть (*до конца спектакля*); в) пересиде́ть (*посетите́лей*); to ~ **through** вы́сидеть (*до конца*); to ~ **up** а) заси́живаться; не ложи́ться спать; ждать до по́здней но́чи (*кого-л.— for*); б) приподня́ться (*в постели*); в) *разг.* дать встря́ску; ~ up straight! сиди́те пря́мо!; to ~ **upon** см. to ~ on.

sit-down ['sɪt,daun] *n* италья́нская забасто́вка.

sit-downer ['sɪt,daunə] *n* уча́стник италья́нской забасто́вки.

site [saɪt] *n* 1) местоположе́ние; 2) ме́сто, уча́сток; construction ~ строи́тельная площа́дка; landing ~ поса́дочная площа́дка; район поса́дки; launching ~ космодро́м.

sitter ['sɪtə] *n* 1) лицо́, остаю́щееся до́ма с детьми́; 2) нату́рщик; 3) насе́дка; 4) *разг.* лёгкая рабо́та.

sitting ['sɪtɪŋ] *n* 1) заседа́ние; 2) сеа́нс; 3) сиде́ние; at a ~ в оди́н присе́ст.

sitting-room ['sɪtɪŋrum] *n* гости́ная.

situate ['sɪtjueɪt] *v* располага́ть, размеща́ть; to be ~d находи́ться, быть располо́женным.

situated ['sɪtjueɪtɪd] *a* располо́женный, размещённый; находя́щийся; ~ as I am в моём положе́нии.

situation [,sɪtju'eɪʃən] *n* 1) местоположе́ние, расположе́ние; 2) ме́стность; 3) состоя́ние; положе́ние (*дел и т. п.*); strong ~ о́страя ситуа́ция (*в лит. произведе́нии*); a tense ~ напряжённое положе́ние; to feel out the ~ зонди́ровать по́чву; to save the ~ спаса́ть положе́ние; to wake up to the ~ осозна́ть всю серьёзность обстано́вки; 4) ме́сто, до́лжность; to find a ~ устро́иться на ме́сто.

six I [sɪks] *num* шесть.

six II *n* шестёрка; ◊ at ~es and sevens а) вверх дном, в беспоря́дке; б) в по́лном разногла́сии.

sixpence ['sɪkspəns] *n* моне́та в шесть пе́нсов; полуши́ллинга (*чека́нилась до 1971 г.*); ◊ it doesn't matter a ~ ≅ ло́маного гроша́ не сто́ит; not a ~ to scratch with ≅ ни гроша́ в карма́не.

sixteen ['sɪks'tiːn] *num* шестна́дцать.

sixteenth I ['sɪks'tiːnθ] *num* шестна́дцатый.

sixteenth II *n* одна́ шестна́дцатая часть.

sixth I [sɪksθ] *num* шесто́й.

sixth II *n* одна́ шеста́я часть.

sixties ['sɪkstɪz] *n pl* (the ~) 1) шестидеся́тые го́ды; 2) во́зраст ме́жду 59 и 70 года́ми.

sixtieth I ['sɪkstɪθ] *num* шестидеся́тый.

sixtieth II *n* одна́ шестидеся́тая часть.

sixty ['sɪkstɪ] *num* шестьдеся́т; ◊ like ~ *амер. сленг* ужа́сно, о́чень си́льно.

sizable ['saɪzəbl] *a* значи́тельный; большо́го разме́ра, объёмистый.

size I [saɪz] *n* 1) разме́р, величина́; of vast ~ больши́х разме́ров; 2) форма́т; cabinet ~ каби́нетный форма́т; 3) объём, вмести́мость; 4) ме́рка; to take the ~ of сме́рить; обме́рить; 5) но́мер (*обуви, перчаток и т. п.*); 6) *полигр.* кегль; ◊ that's about the ~ of it *разг.* вот таковы́ дела́.

size II *v* 1) сортирова́ть по разме́ру; 2) изго-

товля́ть по определённому разме́ру; □ to ~ **up** а) определя́ть разме́р; б) подходи́ть по разме́ру; в) *разг.* составля́ть сужде́ние (*о человеке и т. п.*).

sizzle I ['sɪzl] *n* шипе́ние.

sizzle II *v* 1) шипе́ть; 2) *разг.*: it ~s па́рит, печёт.

skald [skɔːld] см. scald[2].

skate[1] I [skeɪt] *n спорт.* конёк.

skate[1] II *v* ката́ться на конька́х; to go ~ing ката́ться на конька́х.

skate[2] *n*: cheap ~ *амер.* ме́лкая душо́нка, ничто́жество.

skater ['skeɪtə] *n* 1) конькобе́жец; 2) ката́ющийся на конька́х; are you the ~? вы ката́етесь на конька́х?

skating ['skeɪtɪŋ] *n* ката́ние на конька́х.

skating-rink ['skeɪtɪŋrɪŋk] *n* като́к.

skedaddle [skɪ'dædl] *v разг.* удира́ть, улепётывать.

skeleton ['skelɪtn] *n* 1) скеле́т; 2) карка́с, осно́ва; 3) набро́сок; ◊ family ~, ~ in the cupboard семе́йная та́йна; a ~ at the feast ≅ челове́к, по́ртящий всем настрое́ние; ~ of one and half a dozen of the other ≅ хрен ре́дьки не сла́ще.

skeptic ['skeptɪk] см. sceptic.

sketch I [sketʃ] *n* 1) набро́сок, эски́з; to take a ~ зарисова́ть, сде́лать зарисо́вку; 2) бе́глый о́черк, кра́ткая заме́тка (*о событиях*); 3) *театр.* скетч; 4) *разг.* чу́чело горо́ховое.

sketch II *v* 1) де́лать набро́сок, эски́з; 2) писа́ть заме́тку.

sketch-book ['sketʃbuk] *n* альбо́м.

sketchy ['sketʃɪ] *a* 1) отры́вочный; 2) пове́рхностный; 3) лёгкий (*о еде*).

skew I [skjuː] *a* косо́й; раско́сый.

skew II *v* 1) отклоня́ться, свора́чивать в сто́рону; 2) смотре́ть и́скоса; 3) искажа́ть, извраща́ть.

skewbald ['skjuːbɔːld] *a* пе́гий.

skewer I ['skjuə] *n* ве́ртел.

skewer II *v* наса́живать на ве́ртел.

skew-eyed ['skjuːaɪd] *a* косогла́зый.

ski I [skiː] *n* лы́жа.

ski II *v* (*past, p. p.* ski'd) ходи́ть на лы́жах.

ski'd [skiːd] *past. p. p. см.* ski II.

skid I [skɪd] *n* 1) скольже́ние в сто́рону, буксова́ние; to go into a ~ нача́ть скользи́ть; забуксова́ть; 2) тормозно́й башма́к; 3) *ав.* хвостово́й косты́ль.

skid II *v* 1) скользи́ть в сто́рону, буксова́ть; 2) тормози́ть.

skier ['skiːə] *n* лы́жник.

skiff [skɪf] *n* ло́дка, я́лик.

skiing ['skiːɪŋ] *n* ката́ние, ходьба́ на лы́жах; to go ~ ката́ться на лы́жах.

skilful ['skɪlful] *a* ло́вкий, иску́сный, уме́лый.

skilfulness ['skɪlfulnɪs] *n* ло́вкость, уме́ние.

skill [skɪl] *n* 1) мастерство́, иску́сство, уме́ние; 2) квалифика́ция (*рабочих*).

skilled [skɪld] *a* 1) уме́лый, ло́вкий; 2) квалифици́рованный.

skillet ['skɪlɪt] *n* 1) сковорода́; 2) кастрю́ля с дли́нной ру́чкой.

skillful ['skɪlful] *амер. см.* skilful.

skim [skɪm] *v* 1) снима́ть (*пену, сливки и т. п.*); 2) просма́тривать, бе́гло прочи́тывать (*through*); 3) скользи́ть, едва́ каса́ться (*поверхности; along*, over); 4) броса́ть (*камешки по пове́рхности воды*).

skimmer ['skɪmə] *n* шумо́вка.

skimming ['skɪmɪŋ] *n* 1) скольже́ние; 2) пове́рхностное чте́ние; 3) *pl* отбро́сы; ока́лина, шлак.

skimp [skɪmp] *v* 1) ску́дно снабжа́ть; 2) эконо́мить; урéзывать; скáредничать.

skimpy ['skɪmpɪ] *a* 1) ску́дный; 2) бережли́вый; скáредный.

skin I [skɪn] *n* 1) кóжа, шкýра; ~ and bone ≅ кóжа да кóсти, исхудáвший; stripped to the ~ а) раздéтый донагá; б) обóбранный до ни́тки; wet to the ~ промóкший до костéй; to be in smb.'s ~ быть в чьей-л. шкýре; to change one's ~ *перен.* перекрáситься; to have a thick ~ быть толстокóжим; to have a thin ~ быть оби́дчивым, чувстви́тельным (*к критике и т. п.*); to jump out of one's ~ быть вне себя́ (*от радости, изумления*); to keep a whole ~ уйти́ цéлым и невреди́мым; to save one's ~ спасáть свою́ шкýру; 2) кожурá (*плодов*); плёнка (*на жидкости*); оболóчка; 3) мех (*для вина*); бурдю́к; 4) *сленг* скря́га; ◇ by (*или* with) the ~ of one's teeth едвá-едвá, éле-éле.

skin II *v* 1) сдирáть (*кóжу, шелухý, шкýру*); 2) стáскивать (*фуфáйку и т. п.*); 3) *разг.* обдирáть как ли́пку; обобрáть дóчиста; 4) (*обыкн.* to ~ over) покрывáться (*кóжицей*); зарубцóвываться (*о ране*).

skin-deep I ['skɪn'diːp] *a* пове́рхностный.

skin-deep II *adv* пове́рхностно.

skinflint ['skɪnflɪnt] *n* скря́га.

skin-game ['skɪngeɪm] *n разг.* 1) жу́льничество, обмáн; 2) нечéстная игрá.

skin-grafting ['skɪn,grɑːftɪŋ] *n мед.* пересáдка, трансплантáция кóжи.

skinner ['skɪnə] *n* скорня́к.

skinny I ['skɪnɪ] *a* худóй, исхудáлый.

skinny II *n разг.* худы́шка.

skip¹ I [skɪp] *n* 1) скачóк, прыжóк; подпры́гивание; 2) пры́гающая похóдка; 3) перепры́гивание с мéста на мéсто; 4) прóпуск (*при чтении*).

skip¹ II *v* 1) подпры́гивать, подскáкивать; to ~ out of the way отскочи́ть в стóрону; 2) перескáкивать (*с одной темы на другую*); 3) опускáть (*часть текста при чтении*); 4) *амер. разг.* удрáть (*тж.* to ~ off); 5) *шк.* перескочи́ть (*через класс*); 6) отскáкивать рикошéтом; □ to ~ across, to ~ over *разг.* съéздить, проéхаться (*куда-л.— to*).

skip² *см.* skipper 2).

skipper ['skɪpə] *n* 1) капитáн (*торгового корабля*); 2) *спорт. разг.* капитáн комáнды.

skirmish I ['skəːmɪʃ] *n* сты́чка, столкновéние.

skirmish II *v* сражáться мéлкими отря́дами.

skirr I [skəː] *n* шум (*машин*).

skirr II *v* бы́стро бéгать, сновáть, носи́ться.

skirt I [skəːt] *n* 1) ю́бка; hobble ~ у́зкая ю́бка; divided ~ широ́кие брю́ки; 2) полá, подóл; 3) *pl* край, окрáина; on the ~s of на окрáине; на опу́шке (*леса*); 4) *сленг* жéнщина, дéвушка; ◇ to clear the ~s of smb. смыть позóрное пятнó.

skirt II *v* 1) быть располóженным на окрáине, лежáть на опу́шке, грани́чить; 2) опоя́сывать; 3) проходи́ть вдоль кра́я, грани́цы.

skirting-board ['skəːtɪŋbɔːd] *n* пли́нтус.

skit [skɪt] *n* 1) шу́тка, парóдия; 2) скетч.

skittish ['skɪtɪʃ] *a* 1) игри́вый, весёлый; 2) пугли́вый (*о лошади*).

skittle I ['skɪtl] *n pl* кéгли; ◇ ~s! ерундá!, чушь!

skittle II *v:* ~ away *разг.* растрáтить, растранжи́рить.

skittle-alley ['skɪtl,ælɪ] *n* кегельбáн.

skulk I [skʌlk] *n* симуля́нт.

skulk II *v* 1) притаи́ться; 2) симули́ровать; 3) крáсться.

skull [skʌl] *n* 1) чéреп; 2) *разг.* бáшка; to have a thick ~ *перен.* имéть «мéдный» лоб, быть тупоголóвым.

skull-cap ['skʌlkæp] *n* ермóлка, тюбетéйка.

skunk I [skʌŋk] *n* 1) *зоол.* воню́чка, скунс; 2) ску́нсовый мех; 3) *разг.* подлéц, дрянь (*о человеке*).

skunk II *v амер. сленг* обыгрáть в пух и (в) прах.

sky [skaɪ] *n* 1) нéбо, небесá; leaden ~ свинцóвое нéбо; mackerel ~ нéбо в барáшках; out of a clear ~ ≅ как снег нá голову, совершéнно неожи́данно; the ~ grew deeper нéбо потемнéло; to praise (*или* to laud) to the skies восхваля́ть, превозноси́ть до небéс; 2) *часто pl* погóда, кли́мат.

sky-blue ['skaɪ'bluː] *a* лазу́рный.

sky-high ['skaɪ'haɪ] *adv* óчень высокó.

skylark I ['skaɪlɑːk] *n* жáворонок.

skylark II *v* резви́ться, проказничать.

skylight ['skaɪlaɪt] *n* 1) стекля́нная кры́ша; вéрхний свет; 2) световóй люк.

sky-line ['skaɪlaɪn] *n* 1) горизóнт, ли́ния горизóнта; 2) очертáния (*на фоне неба*).

skyman ['skaɪmən] *n разг.* лётчик.

skyrocket I ['skaɪ,rɔkɪt] *n* сигнáльная ракéта.

skyrocket II *v* 1) устремля́ться ввысь; 2) *амер.* бы́стро расти́ (*о ценах и т. п.*).

sky-scraper ['skaɪ,skreɪpə] *n* 1) небоскрёб; 2) высóтный дом.

sky-writing ['skaɪ,raɪtɪŋ] *n* 1) дымовáя нáдпись (*вычéрчиваемая самолётом*); 2) возду́шная реклáма.

slab [slæb] *n* 1) плитá (*каменная*); 2) ломóть (*хлеба и т. п.*); 3) *стр.* горбы́ль.

slack¹ I [slæk] *n* 1) зати́шье в торгóвле; 2) бездéйствие; 3) *pl* широ́кие брю́ки.

slack¹ II *a* 1) мéдлительный; 2) лени́вый; разбóлтанный; 3) свобóдный; ненатя́нутый; 4) расхля́банный (*о дисциплине*); 5) вя́лый (*о торговле*); 6) расслабля́ющий (*о погоде*).

slack¹ III *v* 1) *разг.* распускáться, лóдырничать; 2) утоля́ть (*жажду*); 3) гаси́ть (*известь*); 4) утихáть, стихáть (*о ветре*); 5) идти́ вя́ло (*о торговле*); □ to ~ off ослабля́ть (*напряжение*); остывáть (*о рвении*); to ~ up сбавля́ть, замедля́ть ход (*о поезде*).

slack² *n* у́гольная пыль.

slacken ['slækən] *v* 1) замедля́ть; 2) ослабля́ть; 3) слабéть; 4) станови́ться вя́лым (*о торговле*); 5) разбáлтываться.

slacker ['slækə] *n разг.* 1) лóдырь, прогу́льщик; 2) дезерти́р.

slag [slæg] *n* шлак.

slain [sleɪn] *p. p. см.* slay.

slake [sleɪk] *v* 1) утоля́ть (*жажду*); удовлетворя́ть (*желание*); 2) гаси́ть (*известь*).

slam¹ I [slæm] *n* 1) захлóпывание (*двери*); хлóпанье (*дверьми*); 2) *амер. сленг* стрóгая кри́тика.

slam[1] II v 1) хло́пать (дверьми и т. п.); 2) амер. сленг раскритикова́ть; □ to ~ **down** а) захло́пнуть (дверь, окно); б) швырну́ть с шу́мом.

slam[2] n карт. шлем.

slander I ['slɑːndə] n клевета́; спле́тня.

slander II v клевета́ть; спле́тничать; злосло́вить.

slanderer ['slɑːndərə] n клеветни́к.

slanderous ['slɑːndərəs] a клеветни́ческий.

slang [slæŋ] n 1) сленг, жарго́н; 2) attr относя́щийся к сле́нгу.

slank [slæŋk] уст. past см. slink.

slant I [slɑːnt] n 1) укло́н; накло́н; склон; on the ~ в накло́нном положе́нии; 2) амер. то́чка зре́ния; 3) амер. разг. взгляд.

slant II a накло́нный.

slant III v име́ть укло́н, накло́н.

slanting ['slɑːntɪŋ] a накло́нный, косо́й.

slantwise I ['slɑːntwaɪz] a накло́нный.

slantwise II adv под укло́н, накло́нно; ко́со.

slap I [slæp] n шлепо́к; a ~ in the eye (или face) пощёчина; перен. ре́зкий отпо́р.

slap II v шлёпать; хло́пать; □ to ~ **down** положи́ть с шу́мом (книгу, журнал), хло́пнуть (чем-л.).

slap III adv разг. пря́мо; to run ~ into smb. налете́ть с разма́ху на кого́-л.

slap-bang ['slæp'bæŋ] adv со всего́ разма́ху; с шу́мом.

slapdash I ['slæpdæʃ] a поспе́шный, необду́манный.

slapdash II adv поспе́шно, необду́манно.

slapjack ['slæpdʒæk] n амер. блин, ола́дья.

slapstick ['slæpstɪk] n 1) хлопу́шка; 2) фарс (тж. ~ comedy).

slash I [slæʃ] n 1) уда́р сплеча́, ре́зкий уда́р; 2) разре́з, ра́на; 3) про́резь; 4) вы́рубка; 5) обыкн. pl амер. боло́тистое ме́сто, топь.

slash II v 1) руби́ть (шашкой); 2) хлеста́ть; 3) среза́ть (косой), коси́ть; 4) де́лать про́рези, разре́зы; 5) ре́зко критикова́ть, бичева́ть.

slashing I ['slæʃɪŋ] n ру́бка (шашкой); се́ча.

slashing II a 1) стреми́тельный; сокруши́тельный; 2) ре́зкий, уничтожа́ющий (о критике).

slat I [slæt] n перекла́дина; пла́нка.

slat II v класть перекла́дины.

slate I [sleɪt] n 1) сла́нец, ши́фер; 2) гри́фельная доска́; to clean the ~ расквита́ться; ликвиди́ровать пре́жние обяза́тельства; 3) амер. предвари́тельный спи́сок кандида́тов (на выборах); ◊ to have a ~ loose быть у́мственно неполноце́нным.

slate II v 1) крыть ши́фером (крышу); 2) вноси́ть в спи́сок кандида́тов; 3) амер. разг. выдвига́ть (на должность и т. п.); 4) разноси́ть, де́лать вы́говор; ре́зко критикова́ть.

slate-pencil ['sleɪt'pensl] n гри́фель.

slattern ['slætən] n неря́ха.

slatternly I ['slætənlɪ] a неря́шливый.

slatternly II adv неря́шливо.

slaughter I ['slɔːtə] n 1) кровопроли́тие, резня́; wholesale ~ ма́ссовая резня́; 2) убо́й (скота).

slaughter II v устра́ивать резню́; реза́ть; убива́ть.

slaughter-house ['slɔːtəhaus] n бо́йня.

Slav I [slɑːv] n славяни́н; славя́нка; the ~s славя́не.

Slav II a славя́нский.

slave I [sleɪv] n раб, нево́льник.

slave II v рабо́тать как раб.

slave-driver ['sleɪv‚draɪvə] n 1) надсмо́трщик над нево́льниками; 2) эксплуата́тор.

slave-holder ['sleɪv‚houldə] n рабовладе́лец.

slaver[a] ['sleɪvə] n 1) работорго́вец; 2) нево́льничье су́дно.

slaver[b] I ['slævə] n 1) слюна́; 2) глу́пая болтовня́; 3) неприкры́тая лесть.

slaver[b] II v 1) пуска́ть слюну́; 2) льстить.

slavery ['sleɪvərɪ] n 1) ра́бство; wage ~ наёмное ра́бство; chattel ~ систе́ма ра́бского труда́; 2) тяжёлый труд.

slavey ['slævɪ] n сленг служа́нка (в Англии).

Slavic I ['slævɪk] n гру́ппа славя́нских языко́в.

Slavic II a славя́нский.

Slavonian I [slə'vounɪən] n 1) слове́нец; 2) славяни́н.

Slavonian II a 1) слове́нский; 2) славя́нский.

Slavonic I, II [slə'vɔnɪk] см. Slavic I, II.

slay [sleɪ] v (past slew; p. p. slain) избива́ть, убива́ть.

sleazy ['sliːzɪ] a непро́чный, то́нкий.

sled I, II [sled] см. sledge[1] I, II.

sledge[1] I [sledʒ] n са́ни; саля́зки.

sledge[1] II v 1) е́хать в саня́х; 2) перевози́ть на саня́х.

sledge[2] n кузне́чный мо́лот, кува́лда.

sledge-hammer I ['sledʒ‚hæmə] n см. sledge[2].

sledge-hammer II a мо́щный.

sledge-hammer III v бить мо́лотом.

sleek I [sliːk] a 1) гла́дкий; лосня́щийся; 2) ухо́женный, хо́леный; 3) вкра́дчивый (о манерах), еле́йный (о словах, речи).

sleek II v пригла́живать, прили́зывать.

sleeky ['sliːkɪ] a 1) гла́дкий, прили́занный; 2) хи́трый.

sleep I [sliːp] n 1) сон; beauty ~ ра́нний сон (до полуночи); dead (или deep, profound) ~ глубо́кий сон; sound ~ кре́пкий сон; light ~ лёгкий сон; broken ~ чу́ткий сон; soft ~ прия́тный, споко́йный сон; to drop off to ~ а) пойти́ спать; б) задрема́ть; to go to ~ засну́ть; in one's ~ во сне; to get a ~ сосну́ть, вздремну́ть; to put to ~ укла́дывать спать; to send smb. to ~ усыпи́ть; to sink into a deep ~ кре́пко засну́ть; to sleep the ~ of the just ≅ спать сном пра́ведника; 2) спя́чка, сонли́воеть; winter ~ зи́мняя спя́чка; to fall on ~ засну́ть ве́чным сном; ◊ to have a ~ on it ≅ у́тро вечера мудрене́е.

sleep II v (past, p. p. slept) 1) спать; to ~ like a log (или top) спать как уби́тый; to ~ with one eye open чу́тко спать; 2) (пере)ночева́ть; 3) разг. помеща́ть (на ночь); предоста́вить ночле́г; □ to ~ **away** проспа́ть; to ~ a) заспа́ться; б) только pass быть за́нятым (о постели и т. п.); his bed was not slept in last night вчера́ он не ночева́л до́ма; to ~ **off** а) отоспа́ться; б) проспа́ться; to ~ **on**, to ~ **over**, to ~ **upon** отложи́ть до за́втра (рассмотрение дела и т. п.).

sleeper ['sliːpə] n 1) спя́щий (челове́к); light (heavy) ~ чу́тко (кре́пко) спя́щий челове́к; poor ~ челове́к, страда́ющий бессо́нницей; 2) со́ня; 3) ж.-д. шпа́ла; 4) спа́льный ваго́н; palace ~ сленг това́рный ваго́н.

sleepiness ['sliːpɪnɪs] n сонли́вость.

sleeping-bag ['sli:pɪŋbæg] *n* (меховой) спа́льный мешо́к.

sleeping-car ['sli:pɪŋkɑ:] *n* спа́льный ваго́н.

sleepless ['sli:plɪs] *a* 1) бессо́нный; 2) бди́тельный, бо́дрствующий; 3) неугомо́нный, мяте́жный (*об океане, море*).

sleep-walker ['sli:pwɔ:kə] *n* луна́тик.

sleepy ['sli:pɪ] *a* 1) со́нный, сонли́вый; спя́щий; to be ~ хоте́ть спать; 2) лени́вый; 3) безжи́зненный, ти́хий (*о городе, улице*); 4) нагоня́ющий сон; 5) снотво́рный (*о лекарстве*).

sleepyhead ['sli:pɪhed] *n* со́ня.

sleet I [sli:t] *n* дождь со сне́гом, крупа́; 2) ледяна́я ко́рка (*на деревьях, проволоке и т. п.*).

sleet II *v*: it ~s идёт дождь со сне́гом.

sleeve I [sli:v] *n* 1) рука́в; up one's ~ под рука́ми, гото́вый; to turn up one's ~ а) засучи́ть рукава́; б) пригото́виться (*к действию, работе и т. п.*); 2) *тех.* му́фта; втулка; ◇ to have smth. up one's ~ а) быть себе́ на уме́; б) име́ть, держа́ть что-л. про запа́с.

sleeve II *v* 1) приде́лывать рукава́; 2) *тех.* скрепля́ть му́фтой.

sleigh I [sleɪ] *n* са́ни, са́нки.

sleigh II *v* е́хать в саня́х.

sleight-of-hand ['slaɪtəv'hænd] *n* ло́вкость рук, жонглёрство.

slender ['slendə] *a* 1) то́нкий, стро́йный, грацио́зный; 2) сла́бый (*о надежде, звуке*); скудный (*о заработке, пище*).

slept [slept] *past, p. p. см.* sleep II.

sleuth I [slu:θ] *n* 1) *разг.* сы́щик; 2) соба́ка-ище́йка.

sleuth II *v* высле́живать.

sleuth-hound ['slu:θ'haund] *см.* sleuth I.

slew¹ [slu:] *past см.* slay.

slew² I *n* поворо́т; враще́ние.

slew² II *v* враща́ть(ся), повора́чивать(ся).

slew³ *n амер.* за́водь.

slew⁴ *n амер. разг.* мно́жество, ма́сса.

slice I [slaɪs] *n* 1) ло́мтик (*хлеба, ветчины и т. п.*); 2) часть; 3) широ́кий нож.

slice II *v* 1) ре́зать ло́мтиками; 2) разреза́ть (*волны*); 3) *спорт.* «прома́зать».

slick I [slɪk] *a разг.* 1) гла́дкий; 2) ло́вкий, бы́стрый; 3) хи́трый; 4) ско́льзкий.

slick II *adv разг.* гла́дко; без перебо́ев; пря́мо.

slicker ['slɪkə] *n амер.* 1) плащ; 2) *разг.* жу́лик.

slid [slɪd] *past, p. p. см.* slide II.

slidden ['slɪdn] *p. p. см.* slide II.

slide I [slaɪd] *n* 1) скольже́ние; 2) като́к; го́рка для ката́ния; 3) диапозити́в; 4) предме́тное стекло́ (*микроскопа*); 5) *тех.* скользя́щая часть механи́зма; 6) о́ползень.

slide II *v* (*past slid; p. p.* slid, slidden); 1) скользи́ть; кати́ться (*по льду, снегу*); *перен.* ускольза́ть; 2) проскользну́ть (*в комнату и т. п.; in*); 3) поскользну́ться; буксова́ть (*об автомобиле*); □ to ~ away ускользну́ть; to ~ over слегка́ затро́нуть.

sliding-rule ['slaɪdɪŋ'ru:l] *n* логарифми́ческая, счётная лине́йка.

slight I [slaɪt] *n* 1) оскорби́тельное равноду́шие; невнима́ние; 2) игнори́рование.

slight II *a* 1) сла́бый (*о запахе, привкусе и т. п.*); 2) незначи́тельный, нева́жный, пустяко́вый; 3) лёг-

кий (*об испуге, ранении, оби́де и т. д.*); 4) гру́бый (*о наброске, очерке*); 5) то́нкий, хру́пкий.

slight III *v* относи́ться с невнима́нием; трети́ровать.

slim [slɪm] *a* 1) то́нкий, изя́щный, стро́йный; 2) хру́пкий (*о телосложении*); 3) сла́бый (*об извинении*); 4) незначи́тельный, ску́дный; 5) хи́трый, продувно́й.

slime I [slaɪm] *n* 1) ли́пкая грязь, ил; 2) слизь.

slime II *v* покрыва́ть ли́пкой гря́зью.

slimsy ['slɪmzɪ] *a амер.* непро́чный, хру́пкий.

slimy ['slaɪmɪ] *a* 1) и́листый, гря́зный; 2) сли́зистый, ско́льзкий; 3) рабо́лепный, еле́йный.

sling I [slɪŋ] *n* 1) реме́нь; кана́т; ля́мки; 2) пере́вязь; 3) рога́тка; праща́; 4) бросо́к, уда́р.

sling II *v* (*past, p. p.* slung) 1) мета́ть, броса́ть; 2) класть на пе́ревязь (*руку*); 3) ве́шать че́рез плечо́ (*винтовку*); 4) тащи́ть с по́мощью ля́мок.

slingshot ['slɪŋʃɔt] *n* рога́тка (*для стрельбы́*).

slink [slɪŋk] *v* (*past slunk, уст.* slank; *p. p.* slunk) идти́ кра́дучись, кра́сться (*обыкн.* to ~ away, off, by).

slip¹ I [slɪp] *n* 1) скольже́ние; 2) оши́бка, про́мах; a ~ of the pen опи́ска; a ~ of the tongue обмо́лвка, огово́рка; 3) побе́г; to give smb. the ~ сбежа́ть, удра́ть от кого́-л.; 4) ли́фчик; 5) да́мская комбина́ция; 6) на́волочка; 7) сво́ра соба́к; 8) *мор.* э́ллинг, ста́пель; 9) смеще́ние (*почвы*).

slip¹ II *v* 1) скользи́ть; 2) поскользну́ться, оступи́ться; 3) ускольза́ть; let ~ упуска́ть (*случай и т. п.*); 4) исчеза́ть; улету́читься (*из памяти; from*); проноси́ться (*о времени*); 5) сде́лать оши́бку; 6) су́нуть (*руку куда́-л.; что-л. в руку*); 7) спуска́ть (*собак*); □ to ~ away а) удали́ться, уйти́ (*не попрощавшись*); б) проноси́ться, лете́ть (*о времени*); to ~ in а) вкра́сться (*об ошибке*); б) незаме́тно войти́; to ~ off а) скинуть, сбро́сить (*одежду*); б) соскользну́ть; to ~ on наки́нуть, натяну́ть (*одежду*); to ~ out вы́скользнуть; to ~ up *разг.* ошиби́ться, сде́лать оши́бку.

slip² I *n* 1) побе́г (*растения*); черено́к; bastard ~ отро́сток от ко́рня; *перен.* внебра́чный ребёнок; 2) *поэт.* о́тпрыск; 3) у́зкая поло́ска (*леса, земли, бумаги*); 4) *полигр.* гра́нка; 5) *амер.* дли́нная скамья́; 6) ка́рточка (*регистрационная и т. п.*); rejection ~ пи́сьменный отка́з (*автору от редакции*); to get the pink ~ *перен.* получи́ть увольне́ние.

slip² II *v* черенкова́ть.

slip-on I ['slɪp,ɔn] *n* свобо́дное пла́тье.

slip-on II *a* свобо́дный, широ́кий (*о платье*).

slip-over ['slɪp,ouvə] *a* надева́ющийся че́рез го́лову.

slipper ['slɪpə] *n* 1) дома́шняя ту́фля; 2) *тех.* тормозно́й башма́к.

slippery ['slɪpərɪ] *a* 1) ско́льзкий; ~ as an eel увёртливый, изворо́тливый; 2) ненадёжный; неусто́йчивый; 3) нечёткий, нея́сный.

slippy ['slɪpɪ] *a разг.* 1) ско́льзкий; увёртливый; 2) ги́бкий (*об уме*).

slipshod ['slɪpʃɔd] *a* 1) неря́шливо, пло́хо обу́тый; 2) небре́жный, неря́шливый.

slipslop ['slɪpslɔp] *n разг.* 1) бурда́, по́йло; 2) пуста́я болтовня́; перелива́ние из пусто́го в поро́жнее.

slip-up ['slɪp,ʌp] *n разг.* оши́бка.

slit I [slɪt] *n* прорезь; щель.

slit II *v* 1) делать разрез; 2) резать в длину.

slither ['slɪðə] *v разг.* скользить, скатываться.

sliver I ['slɪvə] *n* щепка, лучина.

sliver II *v* откалывать(ся), расщеплять(ся).

slobber I ['slɔbə] *n* 1) слюни; 2) сентиментальная болтовня.

slobber II *v* 1) пустить слюни; слюнявить; 2) ныть; 3) делать кое-как.

slobbery ['slɔbərɪ] *a* слюнявый.

slog [slɔg] *v* 1) сильно ударить; 2) упорно трудиться (*тж.* to ~ away, to ~ on).

slogan ['slougən] *n* лозунг.

sloop [slu:p] *n* шлюп; ~ of war малый корвет.

slop[1] [slɔp] *v* разливать, расплёскивать (*тж.* to ~ about, to ~ out); □ to ~ **over** сентиментальничать; ныть.

slop[2] *n сленг.* полицейский.

slope I [sloup] *n* 1) склон; скат; наклон, откос; a slight (steep) ~ пологий (крутой) склон; 2) гора для катания.

slope II *v* 1) опускаться; подниматься (*о местности*); 2) *сленг* удрать.

sloppy ['slɔpɪ] *a* 1) мокрый, слякотный; 2) грязный, забрызганный грязью; 3) водянистый; 4) *разг.* небрежный, неряшливый; 5) *разг.* сентиментальный.

slops[1] [slɔps] *n pl* помои.

slops[2] *n pl* 1) готовое платье (*дешёвое*); 2) *уст.* широкие штаны.

slop-shop ['slɔpʃɔp] *n* магазин готового платья.

slot [slɔt] *n* прорез, щель; отверстие (*для опускания монеты*).

sloth [slouθ] *n* 1) лень, нерадение; 2) ленивец (*животное*).

slothful ['slouθful] *a* ленивый, нерадивый.

slot-machine ['slɔtmə‚ʃi:n] *n* автомат (*торговый, игорный*).

slouch I [slautʃ] *n* 1) сутулость; to have a ~ сутулиться; 2) неуклюжий человек; 3) опущенные поля (*шляпы*).

slouch II *v* 1) сутулиться; 2) свисать; опускаться (*о полях шляпы*).

slough[a] [slau] *n* 1) трясина; топь; 2) депрессия.

slough[b] [slu:] *n амер.* болотистый пруд.

slough[c] I [slʌf] *n* 1) сброшенная кожа (*змеи*); 2) забытая привычка.

slough[c] II *v* 1) линять, шелушиться, сбрасывать (*кожу; тж.* to ~ off); 2) избавляться (*от привычки; тж.* to ~ off).

Slovak I ['slouvæk] *n* 1) словак; словачка; the ~s словаки; 2) словацкий язык.

Slovak II *a* словацкий.

Slovene I ['slouvi:n] *n* 1) словенец; словенка; the ~ словенцы; 2) словенский язык.

Slovene II *a* словенский.

slovenly I ['slʌvnlɪ] *a* неряшливый, нечистоплотный.

slovenly II *adv* неряшливо.

slow I [slou] *a* 1) медленный; 2) медлительный, неторопливый; ~ of speech говорящий медленно; (as) ~ as a snail ≅ очень медленный, идущий черепашьим шагом; to be ~ отставать (*о часах*); to go ~ быть, стать осмотрительным, осторожным; 3) тупой, бестолковый; 4) идущий с малой скоростью (*о поезде, пароходе*); 5) вялый

(*о торговле*); 6) неинтересный (*об игре*); скучный.

slow II *adv* медленно.

slow III замедлять(ся) (*тж.* to ~ down, to ~ up).

slowcoach ['sloukoutʃ] *n* 1) тупой *или* медлительный человек, тугодум; 2) отсталый человек.

slow-poke ['sloupouk] *n амер. разг.* копуша.

slow-witted ['slou‚wɪtɪd] *a* тупой, бестолковый.

sludge [slʌdʒ] *n* 1) грязь, топь; 2) плавающий лёд; «сало»; 3) отстой.

sludgy ['slʌdʒɪ] *a* грязный, топкий; илистый.

slue I, II [slu:] *см.* slew[2] I, II.

slug[1] [slʌg] *n* 1) слизняк; 2) пуля; 3) *амер.* жетон в 5 центов (*для телефона-автомата*).

slug[2] *амер. см.* slog.

sluggard ['slʌgəd] *n* лентяй, лежебока.

sluggish ['slʌgɪʃ] *a* медлительный.

sluice I [slu:s] *n* 1) шлюз; 2) отводной канал; 3) промывка.

sluice II *v* 1) спускать воду; 2) отводить воду шлюзами; 3) мыть, промывать (*потоком воды*).

sluice-gate ['slu:s‚geɪt] *n* щитовой затвор (*шлюза*).

slum [slʌm] *n обыкн. pl* трущоба.

slumber I ['slʌmbə] *n часто pl* сон; дремота (*тж. поэт.*); leaden ~ тяжёлый сон.

slumber II *v* 1) спать, дремать; □ to ~ **away** проспать, даром потерять время.

slumberous ['slʌmbərəs] *a* 1) сонный; 2) навевающий сон, дремоту; 3) тихий, сонный (*о городке и т. п.*).

slump I [slʌmp] *n* резкое падение (*цен, спроса, интереса*); кризис.

slump II *v* 1) резко падать (*о ценах, спросе, интересе*); 2) тяжело падать; 3) провалиться (*в снег, болото и т. п.*).

slung [slʌŋ] *past, p. p. см.* sling II.

slunk [slʌŋk] *past, p. p. см.* slink.

slur I [slə:] *n* 1) проглатывание звуков; слияние; 2) пятно на репутации; to bring (*или* to cast, to put, to throw) a ~ порочить (*кого-л.— upon*); 3) *муз.* легато.

slur II *v* 1) проглатывать (*слова, звуки*); произносить невнятно; 2) *уст.* относиться с пренебрежением; порочить; □ to ~ **over** не обратить внимания; пропустить мимо ушей.

slush I [slʌʃ] *n* 1) талый снег; жидкая грязь; слякоть; 2) *разг.* сентиментальная болтовня.

slush II *v* 1) обрызгать (*грязью, талым снегом*); 2) смазывать; цементировать.

slushy ['slʌʃɪ] *a* 1) грязный; 2) слякотный; мокрый (*о снеге*).

slut [slʌt] *n* 1) неряха, грязнуля; 2) *шутл.* девчонка.

sluttish ['slʌtɪʃ] *a* неряшливый, нечистоплотный, неопрятный.

sly [slaɪ] *a* 1) хитрый; лукавый; 2) тайный; скрытый; on the ~ тайком.

slyboots ['slaɪbu:ts] *n разг.* хитрец, плут.

smack[1] I [smæk] *n* 1) вкус, привкус; 2) небольшое количество (*еды*); кусочек, капля (*чего-л.*).

smack¹ II *v* 1) иметь вкус, привкус; отдавать чем-л.; 2) смахивать (*на кого-л., что-л. — of*).

smack² I *n* 1) чмоканье; 2) звонкий поцелуй; 3) шлепок; ◇ a ~ in the eye a) неожиданная задержка; б) неожиданное разочарование.

smack² II *v* 1) чмокать; 2) шлёпать (*ладонью*); щёлкать (*хлыстом*).

smack² III *adv разг.* 1) прямо; в самую точку; 2) с треском.

smack³ *n* рыболовное судно.

small I [smɔːl] *a* 1) маленький; 2) тонкий, узкий; 3) короткий (*о времени и т. п.*); 4) небольшой (*о количестве*); 5) мелкий (*о фермерах, торговцах*); 6) неважный, незначительный; 7) скромный; 8) низкий (*о душевных качествах*); 9) пристыженный, униженный; to feel ~ чувствовать себя неловко, быть подавленным, униженным; to look ~ иметь глупый вид; 10) тихий; небольшой (*о голосе*); 11) слабый (*о пиве*); 12) пустой, бессодержательный (*о разговоре*).

small II *n*: the ~ of the back поясница.

small III *adv*: to beat ~ толочь.

small-arms [ˈsmɔːlˈɑːmz] *n* стрелковое оружие.

smallholder [ˈsmɔːlˈhouldə] *n* мелкий собственник.

smallish [ˈsmɔːlɪʃ] *a* малюсенький.

small-minded [ˈsmɔːlˈmaɪndɪd] *a* эгоистичный; мелочный.

smallpox [ˈsmɔːlpɔks] *n* оспа.

smart¹ I [smɑːt] *n* 1) жгучая боль; 2) жгучее чувство (*обиды, огорчения, горя*).

smart¹ II *a* 1) жгучий, острый (*о боли, чувстве*); 2) сильный (*об ударе, стычке*); 3) энергичный, быстрый (*о людях*); 4) умный, сообразительный; (as) ~ as paint очень сообразительный, ловкий; 5) проницательный; 6) остроумный; 7) изящный, элегантный; 8) модный, щеголеватый; 9) *разг.* значительный, порядочный (*о размерах и т. п.*).

smart¹ III *v* 1) болеть; жечь (*о боли*); причинять боль; 2) оскорблять (*чувства*); мучить (*об обиде, оскорблении*); □ to ~ for поплатиться за что-л.

smart² *adv* нарядно, изящно; щеголевато.

smarten [ˈsmɑːtn] *v* прихорашиваться, принаряжаться (*тж.* to ~ up).

smartness [ˈsmɑːtnɪs] *n* нарядность; изящество.

smash I [smæʃ] *n* 1) битьё (*посуды и т. п.*); 2) столкновение, катастрофа; 3) банкротство; to go to ~ a) разориться, обанкротиться; б) разлететься вдребезги; 4) разгром (*противника*).

smash II *v* 1) бить(ся), разбивать(ся) вдребезги (*тж.* to ~ down, in, up); 2) *разг.* сильно ударить; 3) разгромить (*противника*); 4) врезаться (*куда-л.; into*); 5) пробивать путь (*тж.* to ~ through, to ~ along); 6) обанкротиться, разориться.

smasher [ˈsmæʃə] *n разг.* 1) тяжёлый, сокрушительный удар; 2) убедительный довод.

smash-up [ˈsmæʃˌʌp] *n* полный разгром.

smatter [ˈsmætə] *v* знать что-л. поверхностно.

smatterer [ˈsmætərə] *n* дилетант.

smattering [ˈsmætərɪŋ] *n* поверхностные знания; дилетантство.

smear I [smɪə] *n* пятно.

smear II *v* 1) пачкать, мазать; 2) смазывать (*что-л. — on; чем-л. — with*); 3) растекаться (*о чернилах, жире*).

smeary [ˈsmɪərɪ] *a* 1) грязный; 2) замазанный, запачканный.

smell I [smel] *n* 1) запах; cold ~ слабый запах; fragrant ~ благоухание, аромат; disgusting ~, nasty ~ противный запах, вонь; a ~ of powder *перен.* боевой опыт; 2) обоняние; чутьё; 3): to take a ~ at it понюхать.

smell II *v* (*past, p. p.* smelled, smelt) 1) нюхать, ощущать запах; 2) пахнуть (*чем-л. — of*); to ~ sweet приятно пахнуть; to ~ of the candle (*или* of the lamp, *о* слоге и т. п.); □ to ~ **about** разнюхивать; to ~ **at** водить носом, нюхать, чуять; to ~ **out** разнюхать, обнаружить по запаху; учуять (*что-л*); to ~ **round** разузнавать, разнюхивать.

smelling-salts [ˈsmelɪŋsɔːlts] *n* нюхательная соль.

smelly [ˈsmelɪ] *a разг.* зловонный, вонючий.

smelt¹ [smelt] *past, p. p. см.* smell II.

smelt² *v* расплавлять, плавить; выплавлять (*металл*).

smelt³ *n* корюшка (*рыба*).

smelter [ˈsmeltə] *n* 1) плавильщик; 2) плавильня.

smeltery [ˈsmeltərɪ] *n* плавильня.

smile I [smaɪl] *n* улыбка; to give a ~ улыбнуться; forced ~ вынужденная, натянутая улыбка; timid (sarcastic) ~ робкая (саркастическая) улыбка; to be all ~s иметь сияющий вид, сиять.

smile II *v* 1) улыбаться (*чему-л., кому-л. — at*); 2) благоприятствовать (*кому-л., чему-л. — upon*); 3) выражать улыбкой (*одобрение, сочувствие*); □ to ~ **away** улыбкой развеять грусть и т. п.

smiling [ˈsmaɪlɪŋ] *a* 1) улыбающийся, приветливый; 2) ласковый.

smirch I [smɜːtʃ] *n* пятно (*обыкн. перен.*).

smirch II *v* пятнать, пачкать.

smirk I [smɜːk] *n* самодовольная *или* глупая улыбка.

smirk II *v* самодовольно *или* глупо улыбаться.

smit [smɪt] *p. p. см.* smite.

smite [smaɪt] *v* (*past* smote; *p. p.* smitten, *редко* smit) *поэт.* 1) поражать, ударять, наносить удар; 2) сразить (*любовью, страстью и т. п.*); 3) убивать; □ to ~ **off** отсекать (*саблей, шашкой*).

smith [smɪθ] *n* кузнец.

smithereens [ˌsmɪðəˈriːnz] *n pl* осколки, черепки; to break (*или* to smash) into ~ разбивать(ся) вдребезги.

smithery [ˈsmɪðərɪ] *n* 1) кузнечное дело; 2) кузнечные изделия.

smithy [ˈsmɪðɪ] *n* 1) кузница; 2) кузнечный горн.

smitten I [ˈsmɪtn] *p. p. см.* smite.

smitten II *a* 1) поражённый (*болезнью, ужа-*

com; with); 2) разби́тый (параличом); 3) охва́ченный (страхом и т. п.); 4) сражённый (любовью, красотой и т. п.).

smock I [smɔk] n 1) рабо́чий хала́т, спецо́вка; 2) уст. же́нская соро́чка.

smock II v 1) надева́ть хала́т; 2) украша́ть сбо́рками.

smock-frock ['smɔk'frɔk] n рабо́чий хала́т, спецо́вка.

smoke I [smouk] n 1) дым; 2) ко́поть; 3) куре́ние; to have a ~ покури́ть; 4) разг. сигаре́та, папиро́са; 5) attr дымово́й; ◊ ~ without fire погов. нет ды́ма без огня́; from ~ into smother погов. ≅ из огня́ да в по́лымя; to end (или to go up) in ~ ко́нчиться ниче́м; to raise a big ~ амер. подня́ть шум, нача́ть буя́нить; like ~ сленг без сучка́, без задо́ринки; как по ма́слу.

smoke II v 1) дыми́ть(ся); 2) кури́ть; to ~ like a chimney мно́го кури́ть, непреста́нно дыми́ть; 3) кури́ться (о вулкане); 4) копти́ть (что-л.); оку́ривать; 5) дава́ть ко́поть; □ to ~ out выку́ривать.

smoke-ball ['smoukbɔ:l] n дымово́й снаря́д, дымова́я бо́мба.

smoke-dried ['smouk'draid] a копчёный.

smokeless ['smouklis] a безды́мный.

smoker ['smouka] n 1) куря́щий; кури́льщик; I'm not much of a ~ я ма́ло курю́; heavy (или big, great, good) ~ зая́длый кури́льщик; 2) ваго́н для куря́щих; 3) конце́рт, на кото́ром разреша́ется кури́ть.

smoke-screen ['smoukskri:n] n дымова́я заве́са.

smoking-carriage ['smoukiŋ,kæridʒ] n ваго́н для куря́щих.

smoking-compartment ['smoukiŋkəm,pɑ:tmənt] n купе́ для куря́щих.

smoking-room ['smoukiŋ,rum] n кури́тельная (ко́мната).

smoky ['smouki] a 1) ды́мный; 2) ды́мчатый (о цвете); 3) копти́щий; 4) закопчённый.

smolder ['smoulda] см. smoulder.

smooth I [smu:ð] a 1) ро́вный, гла́дкий; 2) споко́йный (о море); 3) благополу́чный (о перее́зде, путеше́ствии); 4) бесперебо́йный; 5) уравнове́шенный, споко́йный (о характере); 6) пла́вный (о речи); мя́гкий (о звуке и т. п.); 7) вкра́дчивый (о манерах); 8) хорошо́ вы́мешанный (о тесте); 9) фон. непридыха́тельный.

smooth II v 1) сде́лать ро́вным, гла́дким; обстрога́ть; 2) прила́живать; 3) успока́ивать; 4) ула́живать; □ to ~ away сгла́живать; to ~ down успока́ивать(ся); to ~ over устраня́ть разногла́сия.

smooth III adv 1) ро́вно, гла́дко; 2) споко́йно; 3) бесперебо́йно.

smooth IV n: to give one's hair a ~ пригла́дить во́лосы.

smoothen ['smu:ðn] v сгла́живать; смягча́ть.

smoothfaced ['smu:ðfeist] a 1) гла́дко вы́бритый; 2) гла́дкий (о материи); 3) лицеме́рный.

smoothly ['smu:ðli] adv 1) гла́дко, ро́вно; 2) безотка́зно; разг. хорошо́, благополу́чно.

smooth-tongued ['smu:ðtʌŋd] a сладкоречи́вый, льсти́вый.

smote [smout] past см. smite.

smother ['smʌðə] v 1) (за)души́ть; 2) задохну́ться; 3) туши́ть (огонь); 4) замя́ть (дело,

сканда́л); замолча́ть (факт); 5) подавля́ть (чу́вство, зевок); 6) осыпа́ть (подарками, поцелуями).

smoulder ['smoulda] v 1) тлеть; 2) таи́ться (о ненависти, недовольстве); 3) горе́ть (скрытой ненавистью, злобой).

smudge I [smʌdʒ] n 1) пятно́ (грязи, жира); 2) е́дкий дым; 3) костёр (от москитов, комаров).

smudge II v 1) сажа́ть пятна; ма́зать, па́чкать; 2) оку́ривать.

smudgy ['smʌdʒi] a 1) гря́зный, вы́мазанный; 2) е́дкий, ды́мный.

smug [smʌg] a 1) самодово́льный; 2) элега́нтный.

smuggle ['smʌgl] v 1) занима́ться контраба́ндой; 2) принести́, унести́, положи́ть тайко́м; □ to ~ in ввози́ть контраба́ндой; to ~ out вывози́ть контраба́ндой.

smuggler ['smʌglə] n контрабанди́ст.

smut I [smʌt] n 1) са́жа; грязь; 2) непристо́йности.

smut II v па́чкать, грязни́ть.

smutch I [smʌtʃ] n 1) грязь; 2) пятно́.

smutch II v па́чкать, ма́зать.

smutty ['smʌti] a 1) чума́зый, гря́зный; 2) непристо́йный.

snack [snæk] n 1) лёгкая заку́ска; to have a ~ перекуси́ть; 2) часть, до́ля; to go ~s дели́ться, брать свою́ до́лю; ~s! чур, по́ровну!

snaffle I ['snæfl] n тре́нзель; to ride smb. on the ~ ≅ держа́ть кого́-л. в узде́.

snaffle II v 1) пра́вить (лошадью); 2) сленг стяну́ть, укра́сть.

snag [snæg] n 1) коря́га; сучо́к; 2) вы́ступ; 3) разг. препя́тствие.

snaggy ['snægi] a 1) сучкова́тый; 2) зава́ленный, усе́янный коря́гами; 3) торча́щий.

snail [sneil] n 1) ули́тка; 2) у́валень, лежебо́ка; 3) тех. спира́ль.

snail-paced ['sneilpeist] a медли́тельный, нетороплы́вый (в ходьбе, движе́ниях).

snake I [sneik] n змея; a ~ in the grass ≅ змея подколо́дная; неви́димый враг; скры́тая опа́сность; a ~ in one's bosom ≅ «змея на груди́», неблагода́рный челове́к; ◊ to have (или to see) ~s in one's boots ≅ допи́ться до бе́лой горя́чки; to raise (или to wake) ~s устро́ить сканда́л.

snake II v 1) извива́ться (как змея); 2) амер. разг. тащи́ть, волочи́ть (груз); □ to ~ out дви́гаться ре́зкими толчка́ми.

snaky ['sneiki] a 1) змеи́ный; 2) киша́щий зме́ями; 3) змееви́дный; 4) ядови́тый, вре́дный (о челове́ке); кова́рный.

snap I [snæp] n 1) щёлканье (пальцами, кнуто́м); 2) сухо́й треск; 3) защёлка, щеко́лда; 4) жи́вость, я́ркость (стиля); 5) разг. эне́ргия, предприи́мчивость; 6) ре́зкие слова́; ре́зкий отве́т; 7) кратковре́менное похолода́ние (тж. cold ~); 8) момента́льный сни́мок; 9) сухо́е пече́нье; 10) сленг лёгкая нажи́ва; лёгкий за́работок.

snap II a поспе́шный; скоропали́тельный; внеза́пный, неожи́данный.

snap III v 1) щёлкать (пальцами, кнуто́м); 2) затреща́ть, тре́снуть; звя́кнуть; 3) защёлкнуть; 4) сверкну́ть (о глазах); 5) де́лать момента́льные сни́мки; 6) ца́пнуть, укуси́ть (кого-л. — at); 7) набро́ситься (с вы́говором, возраже́нием; на ко-

го-л.— at); 8) приня́ть поспе́шное реше́ние; □ to ~ **out** вы́палить (*фразу и т. п.*); to ~ **up** а) схвати́ть, пойма́ть; б) расхвата́ть (*билеты и т. п.*); в) перебива́ть (*говорящего*).

snap IV *adv* неожи́данно, вдруг, внеза́пно.

snappish ['snæpɪʃ] *a* 1) злой, куса́ющийся (*о собаке*); 2) приди́рчивый (*о человеке*); брюзгли́вый.

snappy ['snæpɪ] *a* 1) име́ющий хва́тку; энерги́чный; 2) *разг.* живо́й, оживлённый; 3) потре́скивающий (*об огне*).

snapshot I ['snæpʃɔt] *n* 1) момента́льный сни́мок; 2) вы́стрел (*не це́лясь*).

snapshot II *v* де́лать момента́льный сни́мок.

snare I [snɛə] *n* западня́, лову́шка; to lay а ~ расставля́ть лову́шку (*для кого-л.— for*).

snare II *v* пойма́ть в лову́шку.

snarl¹ I [snɑːl] *n* 1) рыча́ние; 2) ворча́ние; серди́тое замеча́ние.

snarl¹ II *v* рыча́ть, огрыза́ться; □ to ~ **out** прорыча́ть.

snarl² I *n* 1) спу́танные во́лосы; 2) запу́танное положе́ние.

snarl² II *v* спу́тать; запу́тать.

snatch I [snætʃ] *n* 1) рыво́к (*чтобы схвати́ть*); to make а ~ стара́ться схвати́ть (*что-л.— at*); to work by ~es рабо́тать уры́вками; 2) обры́вок (*разговора, песни и т. п.*); 3) моме́нт, мину́тка; to get а ~ of sleep урва́ть мину́тку для сна.

snatch II *v* схвати́ть (*что-л.— at*); хвата́ть; □ to ~ **away** уноси́ть (*кого-л.; о сме́рти*); to ~ **off** сорва́ть (*шля́пу с головы́*); to ~ **out** вы́хватить (*из рук и т. п.; of*).

snatchy ['snætʃɪ] *a* 1) отры́вистый; отры́вочный; 2) судоро́жный.

sneak I [sniːk] *n* доно́счик; сплётник; *шк. сленг* я́бедник.

sneak II *v* 1) кра́сться, подкра́дываться; 2) доноси́ть; *шк. сленг* я́бедничать; 3) *разг.* (у)тащи́ть, (у)красть; □ to ~ **away** ускользну́ть, вы́скользнуть; to ~ **in** бесшу́мно войти́.

sneaker ['sniːkə] *n* 1) *pl амер.* та́почки (*спорти́вные*); 2) доно́счик; сплётник.

sneaky ['sniːkɪ] *a* 1) трусли́вый; 2) по́дленький.

sneer I [snɪə] *n* 1) усме́шка; 2) насме́шливое замеча́ние; насме́шка.

sneer II *v* 1) насмеха́ться (*над — at*); высме́ивать; to ~ smb. down засмея́ть кого́-л.; 2) усмеха́ться.

sneeze I [sniːz] *n* чиха́нье.

sneeze II *v* чиха́ть; not to be ~d at *разг.* то, чего нельзя́ не учи́тывать.

snick I [snɪk] *n* надре́з.

snick II *v* надре́зать.

snicker I ['snɪkə] *n* ти́хое ржа́ние.

snicker II *v* ти́хо ржать.

sniff I [snɪf] *n* 1) сопе́ние; фы́рканье; 2) вдох (*че́рез нос*).

sniff II *v* 1) сопе́ть; фы́ркать; 2) чу́ять, ню́хать; 3) втя́гивать но́сом (*воздух*), вдыха́ть (*тж.* to ~ up); 4) фы́ркать (*в знак презре́ния*); выража́ть презре́ние (*кому-л.— at*).

sniffle ['snɪfl] *v* шмы́гать но́сом.

sniffy ['snɪfɪ] *a разг.* 1) презри́тельный; 2) ду́рно па́хнущий.

snigger I ['snɪgə] *n* хихи́канье.

snigger II *v* хихи́кать.

snip I [snɪp] *n* 1) надре́з; 2) обре́зок; 3) *pl* но́жницы (*для ре́зки мета́лла*); 4) *разг.* портно́й; 5) незначи́тельный челове́к, «пусто́е ме́сто».

snip II *v* разреза́ть но́жницами (*at; тж.* to ~ off).

snipe I [snaɪp] *n* бека́с; ◇ what а ~ you were in that matter! ≅ како́го дурака́ ты сваля́л!

snipe II *v* 1) охо́титься на бека́сов; 2) стреля́ть из укры́тия (*at*).

sniper ['snaɪpə] *n* ме́ткий стрело́к, сна́йпер.

snippet ['snɪpɪt] *n* 1) обре́зок, кусо́к; 2) *pl* обры́вки (*све́дений и т. п.*).

snippy ['snɪpɪ] *a* 1) ре́зкий, гру́бый; 2) отры́вочный.

snivel I ['snɪvl] *n* хны́канье, нытьё.

snivel II *v* хны́кать, ныть.

snob [snɔb] *n* сноб.

snobbery ['snɔbərɪ] *n* сноби́зм.

snood [snuːd] *n* 1) се́тка для воло́с; 2) ле́нта (*на голове́*).

snook [snuːk] *n*: to cock (*или* to cut, to make) а ~ показа́ть дли́нный нос.

snoop [snuːp] *v* 1) *сленг* стащи́ть, стяну́ть; 2) *амер. разг.* сова́ть нос в чужи́е дела́, выню́хивать (*часто* to ~ around).

snoot [snuːt] *n разг.* 1) нос; 2) ро́жа.

snooze I [snuːz] *n разг.* коро́ткий сон.

snooze II *v разг.* вздремну́ть.

snore I [snɔː] *n* храп.

snore II *v* храпе́ть (*о челове́ке*).

snort I [snɔːt] *n* фы́рканье; пыхте́ние.

snort II *v* 1) фы́ркать; храпе́ть (*о маши́не*); 2) пыхте́ть (*о маши́не*); 3) *разг.* смея́ться, фы́ркать (*в лицо́; тж.* to ~ out).

snorter ['snɔːtə] *n разг.* 1) что-л. выдаю́щееся, сногсшиба́тельное; 2) жесто́кий уко́р.

snotty ['snɔtɪ] *a груб.* сопли́вый.

snout [snaut] *n* 1) мо́рда, ры́ло; 2) *тех.* сопло́.

snow I [snou] *n* 1) снег; powder ~ ме́лкий снег; heavy ~ си́льный снег; we shall have ~ пойдёт снег; to be caught in the ~ попа́сть в сне́жный зано́с, в мете́ль; 2) седина́; белизна́; 3) *сленг* кока́ин; 4) *attr* сне́жный.

snow II *v* 1): it ~s, it is ~ing снег идёт; 2) сы́паться (*обыкн.* to ~ in); 3): to be ~ed in (*или* up, under) а) быть занесённым сне́гом; б) быть ошело́млённым.

snowball ['snoubɔːl] *n* сне́жный ком; снежо́к; to play ~s игра́ть в снежки́.

snow-bound ['snoubaund] *a* 1) занесённый сне́гом; заснеженный; 2) заде́ржанный сне́жными зано́сами.

snow-capped ['snoukæpt] *a* покры́тый сне́гом (*о верши́не горы́*).

snow-clad ['snouklæd] *a* покры́тый сне́гом.

snow-drift ['snoudrɪft] *n* сне́жный сугро́б.

snowdrop ['snoudrɔp] *n* подсне́жник.

snowfall ['snoufɔːl] *n* 1) снегопа́д; 2) коли́чество сне́га (*вы́павшее в определённом райо́не*).

snow-flake ['snoufleɪk] *n* снежи́нка; *pl* хло́пья сне́га.

snowman ['snoumən] *n*: Abominable Snowman «сне́жный челове́к».

snowplough ['snou'plau] *n* снегоочисти́тель.

snow-shoes ['snouʃuːz] *n pl* снегосту́пы (*род лыж*).

snow-slide ['snouslaid] *n* снежный обва́л.

snow-slip ['snouslip] *см.* snow-slide.

snow-storm ['snoustɔːm] *n* мете́ль, бура́н.

snow-white ['snou'wait] *a* белосне́жный.

snowy ['snoui] *a* 1) сне́жный; 2) белосне́жный; чи́стый; 3) покры́тый, занесённый сне́гом.

snub[1] I [snʌb] *n* вы́говор, пробо́рка.

snub[1] II *v* пробира́ть, отчи́тывать.

snub[2] *a* курно́сый, вздёрнутый (*о носе*).

snub-nosed ['snʌbnouzd] *a* курно́сый.

snuff[1] I [snʌf] *n* 1) нюхательный таба́к; 2) понюшка табаку́; to take ~ нюхать таба́к; ◊ to give one ~ дать нагоня́й; up to ~ «тёртый кала́ч».

snuff[1] II *v* 1) вдыха́ть; 2) нюхать, обню́хивать; 3) нюхать таба́к; 4) выража́ть презре́ние (*к кому-л., чему-л.— at*).

snuff[2] I *n* нага́р (*на свече*).

snuff[2] II *v* снима́ть нага́р; □ to ~ out a) заду́ть свечу́; б) *разг.* умере́ть.

snuff-box ['snʌfbɔks] *n* табаке́рка.

snuffle I ['snʌfl] *n* 1) сопе́ние; 2) гнуса́вость; 3) *pl* на́сморк.

snuffle II *v* 1) сопе́ть; 2) говори́ть в нос, гнуса́вить.

snuffy ['snʌfi] *a* 1) пожелте́вший; 2) нюхающий таба́к; 3) раздражи́тельный, серди́тый.

snug I [snʌg] *a* 1) ую́тный; as ~ as a bug in a rug о́чень ую́тно; 2) удо́бный (*о помеще́нии*); 3) прилега́ющий (*о пла́тье*); 4) прили́чный (*о сре́дствах, капита́ле*); 5) скры́тый; to lie ~ спря́таться, укры́ться.

snug II *v* ую́тно устро́иться, усе́сться, улё́чься.

snug III *adv* ую́тно, удо́бно.

snuggery ['snʌgəri] *n* 1) ую́тная ко́мната; 2) удо́бное ме́сто.

snuggle ['snʌgl] *v* 1) прильну́ть; прижа́ть(ся); 2) ую́тно усе́сться, сверну́ться (*тж.* to ~ down).

so I [sou] *adv указывает на:* а) *подтверждение предшествующего высказывания* так; I think so, I believe so да!; хорошо́!; and so on, and so forth и так да́лее, и тому́ подо́бное; if so! раз так!; б) *сомнение или отрицание предшествующего высказывания:* I don't think so нет; вряд ли; is that so? ра́зве?; в) *степень или насыщенность данным качеством* так, столь; you are so kind! вы так любе́зны!; so so та́к себе, ничего́ себе́; so far до сих пор; пока́; г) *сравнение, выступая первым элементом корреляции* насколько; so far as... насколько...; so far as I know насколько я знаю; so long as поско́льку, если то́лько; д) *усиление предшеству́ющего высказывания* та́кже; you are a student and so am I вы студе́нт, и я та́кже; you will learn English and so shall I вы бу́дете учи́ться англи́йскому языку́, и я та́кже; е) *вывод или заключение из предше́ствующего высказывания* так, так что; it was raining, and so I could not go out шёл дождь, так что я не мог вы́йти; ж) *подытоживание сказанного ранее* ита́к; so you are going to the South ита́к, вы е́дете на юг; з) *усиление предшествующего слова* же; how so? как же э́то?, как же так?; why so? почему́ же?; и) *приблизительное количество* приблизи́тельно; a week or so ago приблизи́тельно неде́лю тому́ наза́д; к) *цель действия, выраженного в предше́ствующем предложении* с тем чтобы; I tell you that so as to avoid further explanation я говорю́ вам

э́то с тем, чтобы избежа́ть дальне́йших объясне́ний.

so II *conj разг.* сле́довательно; поэ́тому (*тж.* so that); my train was late so I could not come sooner по́езд опозда́л, поэ́тому я не мог прие́хать ра́ньше.

so III *pron обычно в качестве дополнения* к to say, to think э́то; I told you so я вам сказа́л об э́том; you don't say so! не мо́жет быть!; что вы говори́те!

so IV *int* так!, ла́дно!, хва́тит!

soak I [souk] *n* 1) впи́тывание, вса́сывание; 2) *австрал.* ни́зкое *или* заболо́ченное ме́сто.

soak II *v* 1) пропи́тывать; прома́чивать; to be ~ed in пропи́тываться; to be ~ed to the skin ≅ промо́кнуть до косте́й; 2) впи́тывать(ся), вса́сывать(ся); 3) отмока́ть; 4) проса́чиваться (*куда́-л.— into; сквозь что-л.— through*); 5) *разг.* отколоти́ть, вздуть; 6) *разг.* пить го́рькую, пья́нствовать; 7) *сленг* выжима́ть (*де́ньги*); □ to ~ up вбира́ть в себя́, впи́тывать.

soaker ['soukə] *n* 1) проливно́й дождь, ли́вень; 2) *разг.* го́рький пья́ница.

so-and-so ['souənsou] *n* тако́й-то (*вместо имени или фамилии*).

soap I [soup] *n* 1) мы́ло; soft ~ а) жи́дкое мы́ло; б) льсти́вые ре́чи; 2) *амер.* де́ньги (*использованные для полити́ческих махина́ций*); 3) *разг.* лесть.

soap II *v* 1) мы́лить, намы́ливать; 2) *разг.* льстить.

soap-box I ['soupbɔks] *n* 1) мы́льница; 2) *амер.* импровизи́рованная трибу́на.

soap-box II *v амер.* митингова́ть; ора́торствовать.

soap-bubble ['soup,bʌbl] *n* мы́льный пузы́рь.

soap-stone ['soupstoun] *n* тальк.

soap-suds ['soupsʌdz] *n pl* мы́льная пе́на; обмы́лки.

soapy ['soupi] *a* 1) мы́льный; 2) покры́тый мы́лом, пе́ной; 3) *разг.* вкра́дчивый, льсти́вый.

soar [sɔː] *v* 1) вспа́рхивать; 2) пари́ть (*в во́здухе; перен. в облака́х*); 3) *ав.* плани́ровать; 4) вздыма́ться, поднима́ться ввысь; 5) повыша́ться, взлета́ть (*о це́нах*).

sob I [sɔb] *n* рыда́ние; всхли́пывание; to give a ~ всхли́пнуть.

sob II *v* рыда́ть, всхли́пывать; □ to ~ out говори́ть с рыда́ниями.

sober I ['soubə] *a* 1) тре́звый; 2) здра́вый, рассуди́тельный; 3) уме́ренный; 4) споко́йный (*тж. о цве́те, кра́сках*).

sober II *v* вытрезвля́ть(ся) (*тж.* to ~ down).

sober-minded ['soubə,maindid] *a* тре́звый (*о сужде́ниях, де́йствиях*); уравнове́шенный.

sobriety [sou'braiəti] *n* 1) тре́звость; 2) уравнове́шенность; рассуди́тельность.

sobriquet ['soubrikei] *n* про́звище, кли́чка.

sob-stuff ['sɔbstʌf] *n амер.* сентимента́льный расска́з.

so-called ['sou'kɔːld] *a* так называ́емый.

soccer ['sɔkə] *n разг.* футбо́л.

sociability [,souʃə'biliti] *n* обща́тельность.

sociable ['souʃəbl] *a* 1) обща́тельный; 2) дру́жеский.

social I ['souʃəl] *a* 1) обще́ственный, социа́льный; 2) социалисти́ческий; 3) обща́тельный; 4) све́тский (*об этике́те*).

social II *n разг.* вечери́нка; сбо́рище.

social-democracy [ˈsouʃəldɪˌmɔkrəsɪ] *n* социал-демократия.

social-democrat [ˈsouʃəlˌdeməkræt] *n* социал-демократ.

social-democratic [ˈsouʃəlˌdemə'krætɪk] *a* социал-демократический.

socialism [ˈsouʃəlɪzəm] *n* социализм; ~ means peace социализм — это мир.

socialist I [ˈsouʃəlɪst] *n* социалист.

socialist II *a* социалистический.

socialistic [ˌsouʃə'lɪstɪk] *a* социалистический.

socialite [ˈsouʃəlaɪt] *n амер. разг.* лицо, занимающее видное место в обществе.

sociality [ˌsouʃɪ'ælɪtɪ] *n* общественный инстинкт.

socialize [ˈsouʃəlaɪz] *v* обобществлять.

society [sə'saɪətɪ] *n* 1) общество (*тж. научное*); socialist (communist) ~ социалистическое (коммунистическое) общество; 2) общественность; 3) «свет», светское общество; to get into ~ быть принятым в обществе; to go into ~ появляться в обществе.

sociologist [ˌsousɪ'ɔlədʒɪst] *n* социолог.

sociology [ˌsousɪ'ɔlədʒɪ] *n* социология.

sock¹ [sɔk] *n* 1) носок; 2) стелька.

sock² *I n сленг:* to give smb. ~(s) отдуть кого-л.; to pull up one's ~s напрячь все силы.

sock² II *v разг.* сильно ударить, хватить.

sock² III *adv разг.* прямо; hit me ~ in the eye ударил меня прямо в глаз.

sock³ *n с.-х.* лемех, сошник.

socket [ˈsɔkɪt] *n* 1) углубление, гнездо; 2) патрон (*электрической лампы*); 3) глазная впадина.

socle [ˈsɔkl] *n* цоколь; основание (*колонны*); пьедестал (*памятника*).

sod¹ I [sɔd] *n* 1) дёрн; 2) *поэт.* земля; the old ~ родимая сторонка; under the ~ в могиле.

sod¹ II *v* обкладывать дёрном.

sod² *ист. past см.* seethe.

soda [ˈsoudə] *n* 1) сода; 2) каустическая сода; едкий натр; 3) натрий (*в хим. формулах*); 4) содовая вода.

soda-pop [ˈsoudəpɔp] *n разг.* содовая вода.

soda-water [ˈsoudəˌwɔːtə] *см.* soda. 4).

sodden¹ I [ˈsɔdn] *a* 1) пропитанный; 2) промокший; 3) сырой (*о хлебе*); 4) отупевший (*от пьянства*).

sodden¹ II *v* подмачивать(ся); мокнуть.

sodden² *уст. p. p. см.* seethe.

sodium [ˈsoudjəm] *n хим.* 1) натрий; 2) натр; ~ chlorate хлористый натр; поваренная соль.

sofa [ˈsoufə] *n* диван.

soft I [sɔft] *a* 1) мягкий; (as) ~ as butter (*или* down, silk, velvet) ≅ мягкий как воск (*или* пух); to boil ~ варить всмятку; 2) приятный, спокойный (*о сне, дремоте*); 3) нежный, мелодичный (*о звуке, голосе*); 4) неяркий (*о свете, красках*); рассеянный (*о свете*); неясный (*об очертаниях, линиях*); 5) слабый (*о ветре*); небольшой (*о дожде*); тёплый (*о климате*); влажный, сырой (*о воздухе*); 6) утешительный, сочувственный (*о словах, речах*); влюблённый (*о взгляде*); 7) чувствительный, впечатлительный (*о людях*); 8) слабый, слабого здоровья (*о человеке*); 9) лёгкий (*о работе, наживе*); 10) неустойчивый, бесхарактерный, поддающийся влиянию; 11) неконтрастный (*о фотоснимке*); 12) *фон.* палатализованный, смягчённый

(*о согласных*); 13) ковкий, гибкий (*о металле*); 14) безалкогольный (*о напитках*).

soft II *adv* мягко.

soft III *int* тише!

soften [ˈsɔfn] *v* размягчать(ся), смягчать(ся).

soft-headed [ˈsɔftˌhedɪd] *a* глупый, придурковатый.

softhearted [ˈsɔftˈhɑːtɪd] *a* отзывчивый, мягкосердечный.

softly [ˈsɔftlɪ] *adv* 1) мягко, нежно; 2) тихо, тихим голосом.

soft-spoken [ˈsɔftˌspoukən] *a* 1) нежный, тихий (*о голосе*); 2) сладкоречивый.

softy [ˈsɔftɪ] *n разг.* 1) слабохарактерный человек; 2) дурак.

soggy [ˈsɔgɪ] *a* 1) мокрый, промокший насквозь; 2) сырой, непропечённый (*о хлебе*).

soil¹ [sɔɪl] *n* почва; земля; one's native ~ родина; alkali ~s солончаки; poor ~ тощая, плохая почва; productive ~ плодородная почва; rich ~ жирная почва; unbroken ~, virgin ~ целина; новь; permanently frozen ~ вечная мерзлота; to scarify the ~ разрыхлять, рыхлить почву.

soil² I *n* 1) пятно; 2) грязь (*тж. перен.*); 3) удобрение, компост.

soil² II *v* пачкать(ся), грязнить(ся); марать(ся).

soil-pipe [ˈsɔɪlpaɪp] *n* сточная, канализационная труба.

soirée [ˈswɑːreɪ] *n* вечеринка.

sojourn I [ˈsɔdʒəːn, *амер.* ˈsoudʒən] *n* временное пребывание; посещение.

sojourn II *v* гостить, временно жить (*где-л.— at, in; среди кого-л.— among; с кем-л.— with*).

sol [sɔl] *n* нота соль.

solace I [ˈsɔləs] *n* утешение.

solace II *v* утешать.

solar [ˈsoulə] *a астр.* солнечный.

solarium [sou'lɛərɪəm] *n* (*pl* solaria [sou'lɛərɪə]) солярий.

sold [sould] *past, p. p. см.* sell.

solder I [ˈsɔldə] *n* припой, спайка; *перен.* объединение, слияние.

solder II *v* паять, спаивать.

soldier I [ˈsouldʒə] *n* 1) солдат; военный, военнослужащий; disabled ~ инвалид войны; old ~ старый солдат; бывалый человек; tin ~ а) оловянный солдатик; б) солдат бездействующей армии; to play at ~s играть в солдатики; to go for a ~ вступить в армию; 2) полководец; great ~ великий полководец; 3) *сленг* копчёная селёдка.

soldier II *v* служить в армии.

soldierly [ˈsouldʒəlɪ] *a* мужественный, храбрый.

soldiery [ˈsouldʒərɪ] *n* 1) военные; 2) военщина.

sole¹ [soul] *a* 1) единственный; 2) исключительный.

sole² I *n* 1) подошва (*ноги*); 2) подмётка; 3) нижняя часть чего-л.

sole² II *v* ставить подмётки.

solecism [ˈsɔlɪsɪzəm] *n* 1) грамматическая ошибка; 2) нарушение правил (*поведения*).

solely [ˈsoullɪ] *adv* единственно; только, исключительно.

solemn [ˈsɔləm] *a* 1) торжественный; пышный; 2) формальный (*о процедуре, актах*); важный.

solemnity [sə'lemnɪtɪ] *n* 1) торжественность; 2) *обыкн. pl* торжества; торжественная церемония (*по случаю какого-л. события*); 3) *юр.* форма́льность.

solicit [sə'lısıt] *v* 1) хода́тайствовать, испра́шивать; 2) тре́бовать (*что-л.— for; от кого-л.— of*); 3) пристава́ть (*на у́лице*).

solicitation [sə‚lısı'teıʃən] *n* 1) хода́тайство, испра́шивание; 2) тре́бование; 3) пристава́ние (*на у́лице*).

solicitor [sə'lısıtə] *n* 1) хода́тай; 2) стря́пчий, пове́ренный.

Solicitor-General [sə'lısıtə'dʒenərəl] *n* 1) замести́тель мини́стра юсти́ции, защища́ющий интере́сы госуда́рства в суде́бных проце́ссах; 2) *амер.* гла́вный прокуро́р (*некоторых штатов*).

solicitous [sə'lısıtəs] *a* 1) беспоко́ящийся, забо́тящийся (*о — about*); 2) стремя́щийся (*к чему-л.— of*); 3) жела́ющий (*что-л. сделать*); 4) внима́тельный (*к чему-л.*).

solicitude [sə'lısıtjuːd] *n* 1) озабо́ченность, обеспоко́енность; 2) *pl* забо́ты, хло́поты.

solid I ['sɔlıd] *n* 1) *физ.* твёрдое те́ло; 2) *мат.* геометри́ческое те́ло.

solid II *a* 1) твёрдый; to become ~ затвердева́ть, тверде́ть; 2) кре́пкий, про́чный; 3) соли́дный; 4) сплошно́й; це́лый; 5) чи́стый (*о металле*); 6) основа́тельный, убеди́тельный (*об аргументе, доводе и т. п.*); 7) единоду́шный; сплочённый; 8) *мат.* простра́нственный, куби́ческий.

solidarity [‚sɔlı'dærıtı] *n* солида́рность.

solidity [sə'lıdıtı] *n* 1) твёрдость; 2) про́чность; солида́рность.

soliloquize [sə'lıləkwaız] *v* 1) говори́ть с сами́м собо́й; 2) произноси́ть моноло́г.

soliloquy [sə'lıləkwı] *n* 1) разгово́р с сами́м собо́й; 2) моноло́г.

solitary I ['sɔlıtərı] *n* отше́льник, -ица.

solitary II *a* 1) одино́кий; живу́щий одино́ко; 2) уединённый; забро́шенный; забы́тый; 3) едини́чный.

solitude ['sɔlıtjuːd] *n* 1) одино́чество; уедине́ние; забро́шенность; 2) забы́тое, забро́шенное ме́сто.

solo I ['soulou] *n муз.* со́ло; со́льный но́мер.

solo II *a муз.* со́льный.

soloist ['soulouıst] *n* соли́ст.

solstice ['sɔlstıs] *n астр.* солнцестоя́ние; the summer (winter) ~ ле́тнее (зи́мнее) солнцестоя́ние.

solubility [‚sɔlju'bılıtı] *n* раствори́мость.

soluble ['sɔljubl] *a* 1) раствори́мый; 2) разреши́мый.

solution [sə'luːʃən] *n* 1) разреше́ние (*проблемы, вопроса*); 2) реше́ние (*задачи, уравнения, примера*); 3) *хим.* раство́р; 4) оконча́ние боле́зни, разреше́ние.

solvable ['sɔlvəbl] *a* 1) разреши́мый; име́ющий реше́ние; 2) *хим.* раствори́мый.

solve [sɔlv] *v* 1) реша́ть (*задачу, уравнение*); 2) разреша́ть (*проблему, вопрос*).

solvency ['sɔlvənsı] *n* платёжеспосо́бность.

solvent I ['sɔlvənt] *n* раствори́тель.

solvent II *a* 1) платёжеспосо́бный; 2) растворя́ющий.

sombre ['sɔmbə] *a* 1) мра́чный; тёмный; 2) уны́лый, угрю́мый.

sombrero [sɔm'brɛərou] *n* сомбре́ро (*широкополая шляпа*).

some I [sʌm (*сильная форма*), səm (*слабая форма*)] *a* 1) не́который, не́кий; 2) не́сколько; 3) *с числительными* приблизи́тельно, о́коло; 4) *амер. разг.* значи́тельный, си́льный.

some II *pron* 1) *обычно указывает на часть от целого* ско́лько-нибудь, не́которое коли́чество; give me ~ bread да́йте мне хле́ба; 2) ко́е-кто́, не́которые.

some III *adv* до не́которой сте́пени.

somebody I ['sʌmbədı] *pron* кто́-то, кто́-нибудь; не́кто; ~ else кто́-либо друго́й.

somebody II *n* ва́жная персо́на.

someday ['sʌm‚deı] *adv* когда́-нибудь; в оди́н прекра́сный день.

somehow ['sʌmhau] *adv* ка́к-нибудь; каки́м-либо о́бразом, путём; ~ or other так и́ли ина́че.

someone ['sʌmwʌn] *pron* кто́-то, кто́-нибудь; не́кто.

somersault I ['sʌməsɔːlt] *n* 1) кувырка́нье; акроба́тический трюк; 2) по́лный переворо́т (*во мнениях и т. п.*).

somersault II *v* кувырка́ться.

something ['sʌmθıŋ] *pron* что́-либо; что́-нибудь; ~ else что́-нибудь ещё; ~ like не́что вро́де, не́что напомина́ющее; here is ~ for yourself спаси́бо за услу́гу; to be up to ~ затева́ть, замышля́ть что́-то недо́брое; there is ~ in it в э́том есть до́ля и́стины.

sometime I ['sʌmtaım] *a* пре́жний, бы́вший.

sometime II *adv* когда́-нибудь, когда́-либо.

sometimes ['sʌmtaımz] *adv* иногда́, времена́ми.

someway ['sʌmweı] *adv* каки́м-либо о́бразом, ка́к-нибудь.

somewhat I ['sʌmwɔt] *n* не́которая часть, ко́е-что́.

somewhat II *adv* до не́которой сте́пени; отча́сти.

somewhere ['sʌmwɛə] *adv* 1) где́-нибудь; где́-то; ~ else где́-нибудь в друго́м ме́сте; 2) куда́-нибудь, куда́-то; ~ else куда́-нибудь в друго́е ме́сто.

somnambulist [sɔm'næmbjulıst] *n* луна́тик.

somniferous [sɔm'nıfərəs] *a* снотво́рный, усыпля́ющий.

somnolent ['sɔmnələnt] *a* 1) сонли́вый, дрёмлющий; 2) снотво́рный.

son [sʌn] *n* 1) сын; ~ and heir ста́рший сын; the prodigal ~ *библ.* блу́дный сын; ~ of a bitch *груб.* су́кин сын; мерза́вец; ~ of a gun презре́нный челове́к; ~ of shame внебра́чный сын; ~ of the soil ме́стный урожене́ц; ~ of toil тру́женик; 2) зять.

sonant ['sounənt] *n фон.* зво́нкий согла́сный.

song [sɔŋ] *n* 1) пе́сня; ~ and dance шуми́ха, свистопля́ска; swan ~ лебеди́ная пе́сня (*тж. перен.*); to burst (forth) (*или* to break) into ~ запе́ть; to give a ~ спеть; to buy (to sell) for a ~ купи́ть (прода́ть) за бесце́нок; to go for a ~ идти́ за бесце́нок; to sing another ~ *перен.* запе́ть по-ино́му; to render a ~ испо́лнить пе́сню; to set a ~ to music положи́ть пе́сню на му́зыку; 2) пе́ние.

song-bird ['sɔŋbəːd] *n* пе́вчая пти́ца; певу́нья.

songster ['sɔŋstə] *n* 1) певе́ц; 2) пе́вчая пти́ца.

songstress ['sɔŋstrıs] *n* певи́ца.

son-in-law ['sʌnınlɔː] *n* (*pl* sons-in-law) зять.

sonnet ['sɔnıt] *n* соне́т.

sonny ['sʌnı] *n разг.* сыно́к, сыни́шка.

sonority [sə'nɔrıtı] *n* зво́нкость.

sonorous [sə'nɔːrəs] *a* 1) зво́нкий, зву́чный; 2) *фон.* соно́рный; 3) высокопа́рный, напы́щенный.

soon [suːn] *adv* 1) скоро, в ско́ром вре́мени; вско́ре; as ~ as как то́лько; as ~ as possible при пе́рвой возмо́жности; at the ~est са́мое ра́ннее; (just) as ~, as ~ as not так же, столь же охо́тно; 2) ра́но; the ~er the better чем ра́ньше (скоре́й), тем лу́чше; no ~er said than done ≅ ска́зано — сде́лано; ~er or later ра́но и́ли по́здно.

soot I [sut] *n* са́жа.

soot II *v* покрыва́ть са́жей.

sooth [suːθ] *n уст.* и́стина; ~ to say по пра́вде сказа́ть; in (good) ~ пои́стине.

soothe [suːð] *v* 1) успока́ивать, утеша́ть; 2) облегча́ть (*боль, горе*).

soother ['suːðə] *n* пусты́шка (*для грудны́х дете́й*).

soothsay ['suːθ,seɪ] *v* предска́зывать.

soothsayer ['suːθ,seɪə] *n* предсказа́тель.

sooty ['sutɪ] *a* 1) запа́чканный са́жей; в са́же; 2) чёрный как са́жа.

sop I [sɔp] *n* 1) кусо́к хле́ба (*намо́ченный в подли́ве и т. п.*); a ~ in the pan поджа́ренный хлеб; 2) взя́тка; пода́чка.

sop II *v* 1) пропи́тывать (*хлеб подли́вкой и т. п.*); 2) промо́кнуть; промочи́ть; □ to ~ up впи́тывать (*во́ду*).

sophisticate [sə'fɪstɪkeɪt] *v* 1) извраща́ть, подде́лывать; 2) фальсифици́ровать.

sophisticated [sə'fɪstɪkeɪtɪd] *a* искушённый в жите́йских дела́х, о́пытный.

sophistication [sə,fɪstɪ'keɪʃən] *n* 1) софи́стика; 2) фальсифика́ция.

sophomore ['sɔfəmɔː] *n амер.* 1) студе́нт-второку́рсник; 2) *пренебр.* самоуве́ренный неве́жда.

soporific I [,soupə'rɪfɪk] *n* нарко́тик.

soporific II *a* снотво́рный.

sopping ['sɔpɪŋ] *a* промо́кший наскво́зь.

soppy ['sɔpɪ] *a* 1) мо́крый; 2) сыро́й, дождли́вый; 3) сентимента́льный, слезли́вый.

soprano [sə'prɑːnou] *n* сопра́но.

sorcerer ['sɔːsərə] *n* колду́н; чароде́й.

sorcery ['sɔːsərɪ] *n* колдовство́; волшебство́.

sordid ['sɔːdɪd] *a* 1) гря́зный; 2) нече́стный, по́длый; 3) коры́стный.

sore I [sɔː] *n* больно́е ме́сто, боля́чка; нагное́ние; я́зва; ра́на; an open ~ *перен.* обще́ственное зло; to re-open old ~s береди́ть ста́рые ра́ны.

sore II *a* 1) больно́й; to feel ~ боле́ть; 2) воспалённый (*о го́рле, глаза́х*); 3) раздража́ющий, тя́гостный (*об ощуще́ниях, пережива́ниях*); to be ~ ре́зко реаги́ровать (*на что-л.— about*); 4) тяжёлый (*об уча́сти, нужде́*).

sore III *adv* весьма́, чрезвыча́йно.

sorrel[1] ['sɔrəl] *n* щаве́ль.

sorrel[2] I *n* гнеда́я ло́шадь.

sorrel[2] II *a* гнедо́й.

sorrow I ['sɔrou] *n* 1) го́ре, скорбь, печа́ль; keen ~ глубо́кая скорбь; 2) сожале́ние; 3) *ча́сто pl* огорче́ния.

sorrow II *v* горева́ть, скорбе́ть (*о чём-л.— at, for, over*).

sorrowful ['sɔrəful] *a* 1) ско́рбный; уби́тый го́рем; 2) огорчи́тельный, печа́льный; 3) тра́урный, зауны́вный.

sorry ['sɔrɪ] *a* 1) *predic* сожале́ющий; to be (*или* to feel) ~ жале́ть (*кого-л., что-л.— for*); I am ~! винова́т!, прости́те!; I am so ~! мне так жаль!;

2) несча́стный, жа́лкий; 3) гру́стный, печа́льный; уны́лый.

sort I [sɔːt] *n* 1) вид, род, класс; сорт; what ~ of что за; како́й, кака́я, како́е; nothing of the ~! ничего́ подо́бного!; some ~ of како́й-либо; of all ~s вся́кого ро́да; of ~s в не́котором ро́де; a good ~ *разг.* до́брый ма́лый; the better ~ *разг.* выдаю́щиеся лю́ди; 2) ка́чество, хара́ктер; 3) мане́ра, спо́соб; in some ~ до не́которой сте́пени; ◊ after a ~ а) по о́бразу и подо́бию; б) до не́которой сте́пени; to be out of ~s а) быть не в ду́хе; б) нева́жно себя́ чу́вствовать.

sort II *v* сортирова́ть; □ to ~ out а) рассортиро́вывать; б) отбира́ть; в) относи́ть (*к определённому кла́ссу, гру́ппе; with*).

sortie ['sɔːtiː] *n* 1) *воен.* вы́лазка; 2) *ав.* вы́лет.

sot [sɔt] *n* го́рький пья́ница.

sottish ['sɔtɪʃ] *a* спи́вшийся.

soubriquet ['suːbrɪˌkeɪ] *см.* sobriquet.

sough I [sau] *n* ше́лест; вой (*ве́тра*).

sough II *v* шелесте́ть; завыва́ть (*о ве́тре*).

sought [sɔːt] *past, p. p. см.* seek.

soul [soul] *n* 1) душа́, дух; twin ~ ро́дственная душа́; upon my ~! че́стное сло́во!; кляну́сь!; bless my ~ го́споди! (*восклица́ние, выража́ющее удивле́ние*); to be the ~ of быть душо́й (*чего-л.*); to have no ~ быть безду́шным, бесстра́стным; to possess one's ~ владе́ть собо́й; to unbosom (*или* to unbutton) one's ~ откры́ть свою́ ду́шу; he cannot call his ~ his own он себе́ не хозя́ин; 2) челове́к, существо́; good ~ хоро́ший челове́к; be a good ~ and help me *разг.* будь дру́гом, помоги́ мне; dear ~ дружи́ще, старина́; decent ~ прили́чный челове́к; honest ~ че́стный челове́к; kind ~ до́брая душа́; poor ~ бедня́к; simple ~ наи́вный челове́к; worthy ~ досто́йный челове́к; I did not see a ~ я не ви́дел ни души́; 3) воплоще́ние; су́щность, осно́ва.

soulful ['soulful] *a* эмоциона́льный, сентимента́льный.

soulless ['soullɪs] *a* безду́шный.

sound[1] I [saund] *n* звук; шум; within ~ of на расстоя́нии зву́ка, в преде́лах слы́шимости; speech ~ звук ре́чи; sweet ~ прия́тный, не́жный звук.

sound[1] II *v* 1) звуча́ть, раздава́ться; to be ~ed произноси́ться (*о зву́ке*); 2) игра́ть (*на духово́м инструме́нте*); звони́ть (*в ко́локол*); 3) дава́ть сигна́л; труби́ть; 4) выслу́шивать (*больно́го*); 5) разноси́ть (*но́вости и т. п.*).

sound[2] I *a* 1) здоро́вый; as ~ as a roach, as ~ as a bell соверше́нно здоро́вый; ~ in life and limb цел и невреди́м; 2) надёжный; 3) здра́вый (*о сужде́нии, до́воде*); 4) кре́пкий (*о сне*); 5) испра́вный (*о механи́зме*); 6) серьёзный (*об учёном*); 7) суро́вый, жесто́кий (*о наказа́нии*).

sound[2] II *adv* кре́пко; здра́во.

sound[3] *v* 1) изме́рять глубину́ (*ло́том*); 2) иссле́довать зо́ндом (*ра́ну*); 3) зонди́ровать, стара́ться вы́яснить (*мне́ние и т. п.; тж.* to ~ out); 4) ныря́ть (*осо́б. о ки́те*).

sound[4] *n* у́зкий проли́в.

sound-film ['saundfɪlm] *n* звуково́й фильм.

sounding-balloon ['saundɪŋbə'luːn] *n ме́тео* шар-зо́нд.

soundless ['saundlɪs] *a* беззву́чный.

soundproof ['saundpruːf] *a* звуконепроница́емый.

soup [suːp] *n* суп; a thick (clear) ~ крéпкий, навáристый (жúдкий) суп.

soup-plate [ˈsuːppleɪt] *n* глубóкая тарéлка.

sour I [ˈsauə] *a* 1) кúслый; (as) ~ as vinegar óчень кúслый; 2) прокúсший; 3) раздражúтельный; сердúтый.

sour II *v* 1) прокисáть; кúснуть (*тж. перен.*); 2) заквáшивать.

source [sɔːs] *n* 1) истóчник; ~ of information истóчник свéдений; 2) истóк, верхóвье; 3) ключ, роднúк; 4) начáло; истóчник, (перво)причúна.

souse I [saus] *n* 1) прыжóк в вóду; 2) солéнье, маринáд, рассóл; 3) *разг.* пьянúца.

souse II *v* 1) окунáть(ся); 2) окáчивать; 3) мариновáть, солúть; 4) *разг.* напúться пья́ным.

.south I [sauθ] *n* 1) юг; *мор.* зюйд; 2) ю́жный вéтер; 3) (the ~) ю́жные края́, стрáны, райóны.

south II *a* 1) ю́жный; 2) обращённый на юг.

south III *adv* к ю́гу, на юг, в ю́жном направлéнии; to go ~ éхать, летéть на юг.

south-east I [ˈsauθˈiːst] *n* ю́го-востóк; *мор.* зюйд--óст.

south-east II *a* ю́го-востóчный.

south-east III *adv* к ю́го-востóку, в ю́го-востóчном направлéнии; с ю́го-востóка.

south-easter [sauθˈiːstə] *n* ю́го-востóчный вéтер, зюйд-óст.

south-easterly I [sauθˈiːstəlɪ] *a* ю́го-востóчный, ду́ющий с ю́го-востóка (*о ветре*).

south-easterly II *adv* с ю́го-востóка; к ю́го-востóку.

souther [ˈsauðə] *n* ю́жный вéтер.

southerly I [ˈsʌðəlɪ] *a* 1) обращённый, напрáвленный к ю́гу; 2) ду́ющий с ю́га, ю́жный (*о ветре*).

southerly II *adv* 1) к ю́гу, на юг; 2) с ю́га.

southern [ˈsʌðən] *a* ю́жный.

southerner [ˈsʌðənə] *n* южáнин.

southernly [ˈsʌðənlɪ] *a* ю́жный.

southernmost [ˈsʌðənmoust] *a* сáмый ю́жный.

southing [ˈsauðɪŋ] *n* отклонéние к ю́гу.

southmost [ˈsauθmoust] *a* сáмый ю́жный.

southward I [ˈsauθwəd] *n* ю́жное направлéние.

southward II *a* 1) иду́щий на юг; 2) обращённый на юг, к ю́гу.

southward III *adv* в ю́жном направлéнии; к ю́гу, на юг.

southwardly I [ˈsauðwədlɪ] *a* ю́жный (*о ветре*).

southwardly II *adv* к ю́гу, на юг.

southwards [ˈsauθwədz] *см.* southward III.

south-west I [ˈsauθˈwest] *n* ю́го-зáпад; *мор.* зюйд-вéст.

south-west II *a* ю́го-зáпадный.

south-west III *adv* к ю́го-зáпаду, в ю́го-зáпадном направлéнии; с ю́го-зáпада.

south-wester [sauθˈwestə] *n* 1) сúльный ю́го--зáпадный вéтер, зюйд-вéст; 2) зюйдвéстка (*матрóсская шáпка*).

south-westerly I [sauθˈwestəlɪ] *a* ю́го-зáпадный, ду́ющий с ю́го-зáпада (*о ветре*).

south-westerly II *adv* с ю́го-зáпада; к ю́го-зáпаду.

souvenir [ˈsuːvənɪə] *n* сувенúр.

sovereign I [ˈsɔvrɪn] *n* 1) монáрх; 2) суверéнное госудáрство; 3) соверéн (*золотáя англ. монéта в 1 фунт стéрлингов; чекáнилась до 1971 г.*).

sovereign II *a* 1) верхóвный, суверéнный; 2) вы́с-

ший (*об авторитéте, влáсти*); 3) наивы́сший, наибóльший; 4) дéйственный (*о лекáрстве*); 5) беспредéльный (*о презрéнии*).

sovereignty [ˈsɔvrəntɪ] *n* 1) верхóвная власть; 2) суверенитéт; 3) суверéнное госудáрство.

Soviet I [ˈsouvɪet] *n*: the Supreme ~ of the USSR Верхóвный Совéт СССР; the ~ *разг.* Совéтский Сою́з; town ~ городскóй совéт; village ~ сельсовéт.

Soviet II *a* совéтский.

sow[a] [sou] *v* (*past.* sowed; *p. p.* sowed, sown) 1) сéять; засевáть; 2) распространя́ть, сéять (*слухи и т. п.*).

sow[b] [sau] *n* свинья́; ◇ to have (*или* to get, to take) the wrong ~ by the ear попáсть пáльцем в нéбо, ошибúться.

sower [ˈsouə] *n* 1) сéятель; 2) сéялка.

sowing-machine [ˈsouɪŋməˌʃiːn] *n* сéялка.

sown [soun] *p. p. см.* sow[a].

soy [sɔɪ] *n* 1) сóя; 2) сóевый боб; 3) *attr* сóевый.

spa [spɑː] *n* 1) минерáльный истóчник; 2) курóрт с минерáльным истóчником.

space I [speɪs] *n* 1) прострáнство; протяжéние; infinite ~ бесконéчное прострáнство; evacuated ~ разрежённый вóздух; empty ~ безвоздýшное прострáнство; open ~s откры́тые прострáнства; пустыри́; 2) космúческое прострáнство; кóсмос; to walk in ~ выходúть в откры́тый кóсмос; 3) объём; 4) мéсто, сидéнье (*в поéзде, самолёте*); 5) расстоя́ние; 6) промежýток (*врéмени*); 7) момéнт; мгновéние; after a short ~ вскóре; 8) *муз.* интервáл; 9) *attr* космúческий.

space II *v* 1) оставля́ть промежýтки; 2) расставля́ть с промежýтками.

spaceborne [ˈspeɪsbɔːn] *p. p.*: he was ~ он находúлся в кóсмосе.

spacecraft [ˈspeɪskrɑːft] *n* космúческий корáбль.

spaced-out [ˈspeɪstaut] *a* дáнный вразря́дку (*о тéксте*).

space-flight [ˈspeɪsˈflaɪt] *n* космúческий полёт; полёт в кóсмос; manned ~ полёт человéка в кóсмос.

space-laboratory [ˈspeɪsləˈbɔrɪtrɪ] *n* космúческая лаборатóрия.

spaceless [ˈspeɪslɪs] *a* лишённый простóра; бесконéчный (*о горизóнте*).

spaceman [ˈspeɪsmən] *n* космонáвт; dummy ~ груз, имитúрующий вес человéка.

spaceship [ˈspeɪsʃɪp] *n* космúческий корáбль; multi-seat ~ многомéстный космúческий корáбль.

spacious [ˈspeɪʃəs] *a* 1) простóрный; вместúтельный; обшúрный; 2) широкий (*о кругозóре, размáхе и т. п.*).

spade[1] I [speɪd] *n* 1) лопáта; зáступ; 2) *воен.* сóшник орудúя; ◇ to call a ~ a ~ называ́ть вéщи своúми именáми.

spade[1] II *v.* копáть лопáтой, зáступом.

spade[2] *n обыкн. pl карт.* пúки.

spadeful [ˈspeɪdful] *n* пóлная лопáта.

spadger [ˈspædʒə] *n сленг* воробéй.

spake [speɪk] *уст. past см.* speak.

spall I [spɔːl] *n* оскóлок (*кáмня*).

spall II *v* 1) дробúть на мéлкие куски́; 2) разлетáться на мéлкие куски́.

span[1] I [spæn] *n* 1) миг, мгновéние; 2) корóткое расстоя́ние; пядь (= *9 дюймам*); 3) пролёт (*моста*); 4) ширина́ (*реки, канала*); протяжённость (*моста*); 5) ж.-д. перего́н; 6) *ав.* разма́х кры́льев; 7) *мат.* хо́рда дуги́.

span[1] II *v* 1) измеря́ть (*расстояние*); 2) измеря́ть пя́дями; 3) обня́ть за та́лию; 4) протяну́ться (*через реку — о мосте*); 5) соединя́ть (*берега реки*); 6) охва́тывать (*о времени*); 7) *муз.* взять (*окта́ву*).

span[2] *n* упря́жка па́рой.

span[3] *уст. past см.* spin I.

spangle I ['spæŋgl] *n* 1) блёстка; 2) блестя́щая ка́пля.

spangle II *v* 1) украша́ть блёстками; 2) усе́ивать (*звёздами и т. п.*); 3) поблёскивать, сверка́ть.

Spaniard ['spænjəd] *n* испа́нец; испа́нка.

spaniel ['spænjəl] *n* 1) спание́ль (*порода собак*); 2) подли́за, подхали́м; a tame ~ низкопокло́нник, льстец.

Spanish I ['spænɪʃ] *n* 1): the ~ (*употр. как pl*) испа́нцы; 2) испа́нский язы́к.

Spanish II *a* испа́нский.

spank I [spæŋk] *n* шлепо́к.

spank II *v* шлёпать; □ to ~ **along** нести́сь (*о лошади, судне*).

spanking ['spæŋkɪŋ] *a* 1) бы́стрый, быстрохо́дный; 2) све́жий, си́льный (*о ветре*); 3) *разг.* превосхо́дный, замеча́тельный.

spanner ['spænə] *n тех.* га́ечный ключ.

span-new ['spæn'njuː] *a* но́венький, с иго́лочки.

spar[1] [spɑː] *n* 1) брус, перекла́дина; 2) *ав.* лонжеро́н; 3) *мор.* рангоу́т.

spar[2] I *n* 1) бокс; состяза́ние по бо́ксу; 2) спор, препира́тельство.

spar[2] II *v* 1) дра́ться на кула́чках (*с кем-л.— at*); бокси́ровать; 2) дра́ться шпо́рами (*о петухах*); 3) препира́ться, спо́рить.

spar[3] *n мин.* полево́й шпат; flour ~ плавико́вый шпат.

spare I [spɛə] *a* 1) запа́сный; запасно́й; 2) свобо́дный (*о времени*); 3) худо́й, худоща́вый; 4) ску́дный (*о пище*); 5) расчётливый, эконо́мный.

spare II *v* 1) (по)щади́ть; if I am ~d е́сли мне суждено́ ещё прожи́ть; 2) избавля́ть (*от волнения, беспокойства; from*); 3) уделя́ть (*время, внимание, беречь*; 5) эконо́мить, бере́чь; 5) уд́ожи́ть; 6) выделя́ть (*для чего-л.— for*); 7) обходи́ться без чего-л.; возде́рживаться от чего-л.

sparing ['spɛərɪŋ] *a* 1) эконо́мный (*в чём-л.— in*); 2) бережли́вый; 2) скупо́й (*на слова; of*); 3) снисходи́тельный; 4) ску́дный.

spark[1] I [spɑːk] *n* 1) и́скра; 2) вспы́шка, про́блеск; the ~ of life при́знаки жи́зни, жизнеспосо́бность; not a ~ of interest ни мале́йшего интере́са; 3) *pl сленг* ради́ст; ◊ to strike ~s out of извлека́ть поле́зные да́нные из.

spark[1] II *v* 1) дава́ть и́скры; 2) и́скриться; 3) вспы́хивать.

spark[2] I *n* 1) франт, щёголь; 2) ухажёр.

spark[2] II *v* 1) щеголя́ть; 2) уха́живать.

sparkle I ['spɑːkl] *n* 1) и́скорка; 2) блеск, сверка́ние; 3) жи́вость, оживлённость.

sparkle II *v* 1) и́скри́ться; 2) сверка́ть; 3) игра́ть, и́скриться (*о вине*); 4) быть оживлённым.

sparkling ['spɑːklɪŋ] *a* 1) сверка́ющий; и́скрящийся; 2) шипу́чий, искри́стый (*о вине*).

sparrow ['spærou] *n* воробе́й.

sparrow-grass ['spærougrɑːs] *n разг.* спа́ржа.

sparse [spɑːs] *a* 1) ре́дкий (*о населении и т. п.*); жи́дкий (*о волосах*); 2) разбро́санный; 3) ску́дный.

Spartan I ['spɑːtən] *n* спарта́нец.

Spartan II *a* спарта́нский.

spasm ['spæzəm] *n* 1) спа́зма, су́дорога; 2) взрыв гне́ва.

spasmodic [spæz'mɔdɪk] *a* су́дорожный.

spat[1] I [spæt] *n амер.* 1) размо́лвка; 2) шлепо́к, зво́нкий уда́р.

spat[1] II *v амер.* 1) ссо́риться, перебра́ниваться; 2) поколоти́ть.

spat[2] *past, p. p. см.* spit[1] II.

spat[3] *n pl* ге́тры.

spate [speɪt] *n* 1) внеза́пное наводне́ние; 2) внеза́пный ли́вень; *перен.* пото́к.

spatial ['speɪʃəl] *a* простра́нственный.

spatter I ['spætə] *n* 1) бры́зги; 2) бры́зганье; забры́згивание.

spatter II *v* 1) бры́згать; забры́згивать; 2) разбры́згивать; 3) очерни́ть, оклевета́ть.

spatterdashes ['spætə,dæʃɪz] *n pl* ге́тры.

spawn I [spɔːn] *n* 1) икра́; 2) *бот.* мице́лий; 3) *презр.* отро́дье; исча́дие.

spawn II *v* 1) мета́ть икру́; 2) порожда́ть; 3) (рас)плоди́ться.

speak [spiːk] *v* (*past* spoke, *уст.* spake; *p. p.* spoken) 1) говори́ть; разгова́ривать (*с кем-л.— with; по делу — to; о чём-л.— about, of*); to ~ **by the book** говори́ть как по-пи́саному; to ~ (smb.) **fair** говори́ть любе́зно (*с кем-л.*); to ~ **well** отзыва́ться хорошо́ (*о ком-л.— of*); 2) уме́ть говори́ть (*на каком-л. языке*); 3) выступа́ть с ре́чью; 4) выступа́ть (*в защиту кого-л.— for*); 5) име́ть значе́ние, означа́ть; 6): **broadly** ~ing вообще́ говоря́; **frankly** ~ing открове́нно говоря́; **properly** ~ing называ́я ве́щи свои́ми имена́ми, со́бственно говоря́; **roughly** ~ing гру́бо говоря́, приблизи́тельно; **strictly** ~ing стро́го говоря́; 7) заговори́ть (*об орудиях*); 8) *мор.* оклика́ть (*другое судно*); □ to ~ **for** говори́ть от и́мени; to ~ **out** а) выска́зываться открове́нно; б) говори́ть гро́мко; **please** ~ **out!** говори́те громче́! to ~ **to** а) обраща́ться (*к кому-л.*); б) предостерега́ть, убежда́ть; в) подтвержда́ть; to ~ **up** а) заговори́ть гро́мко; б) не удержа́ться и вы́сказаться.

speak-easy ['spiːk,iːzɪ] *n амер. сленг* бар (*незако́нно торгу́ющий спиртны́ми напи́тками*).

speaker ['spiːkə] *n* 1) ора́тор; glib (prosaic) ~ речи́стый (ску́чный) ора́тор; 2): the Speaker спи́кер (*председа́тель пала́ты общи́н в А́нглии, председа́тель пала́ты представи́телей в США*); 3) *радио* ди́ктор; 4) громкоговори́тель.

speaking I ['spiːkɪŋ] *n* речь; выска́зывание.

speaking II *a* 1) говоря́щий; 2) кра́йне вырази́тельный; 3) деклама́торский.

speaking-tube ['spiːkɪŋtjuːb] *n* мегафо́н, перегово́рная тру́бка.

spear[1] I [spɪə] *n* 1) копьё, дро́тик; 2) *поэт.* копьено́сец; 3) острога́.

spear[1] II *v* 1) пронза́ть (*копьём*); 2) бить острого́й; 3) вонза́ться.

spear[2] I *n* 1) росто́к; побе́г; 2) о́стрый лист (*травы*).

spear[2] II *v* 1) дава́ть ростки́; 2) выходи́ть в тру́бку (*о злаках*).

spearhead ['spɪəhed] *n* остриё (*копья*).

spearman ['spɪəmən] *n* копьено́сец.

special I ['speʃəl] *n* 1) э́кстренный вы́пуск (*газеты*); 2) по́езд специа́льного назначе́ния.

special II *a* 1) осо́бый, осо́бенный; 2) специа́льный; 3) э́кстренный; 4) чрезвыча́йный (*о после, уполномоченном*); 5) определённый.

specialist ['speʃəlɪst] *n* специали́ст.

speciality [,speʃɪ'ælɪtɪ] *n* 1) специа́льность; to make a ~ специализи́роваться (*в чём-л.— of*); 2) осо́бая черта́ (*характера и т. п.*); осо́бенность; 3) осо́бое замеча́ние, подро́бность (*в документе*).

specialize ['speʃəlaɪz] *v* 1) специализи́роваться; 2) ограни́чивать; 3) приспоса́бливать(ся) к осо́бым усло́виям.

specialty ['speʃəltɪ] *n* 1) специа́льность; 2) предме́т *или* вещь вы́сшего ка́чества.

specie ['spiːʃiː] *n* зво́нкая моне́та; in ~ а) нату́рой; б) нали́чными деньга́ми.

species ['spiːʃiːz] *n* (*pl без измен.*) 1) класс, род, тип; 2) биол. вид; 3) разнови́дность.

specific I [spɪ'sɪfɪk] *n* 1) специа́льное сообще́ние; 2) *мед.* специа́льное сре́дство, лека́рство.

specific II *a* 1) осо́бый, специфи́ческий; 2) характе́рный; 3) *биол.* видово́й; 4) определённый; 5) *физ.* уде́льный (*о весе*).

specification [,spesɪfɪ'keɪʃən] *n* 1) специфика́ция; 2) дета́ли (*договора, соглашения*).

specify ['spesɪfaɪ] *v* 1) специа́льно упомина́ть, называ́ть; 2) отмеча́ть, ука́зывать; 3) придава́ть осо́бый хара́ктер, осо́бые черты́; 4) дава́ть специфика́цию.

specimen ['spesɪmɪn] *n* 1) образчик, экземпля́р; образе́ц; 2) *разг.* субъе́кт; a queer ~ чуда́к, «тип».

specious ['spiːʃəs] *a* 1) благови́дный; 2) обма́нчивый, показно́й; 3) правдоподо́бный.

speck I [spek] *n* 1) пя́тнышко; 2) части́ца.

speck II *v* пятна́ть.

speckle I ['spekl] *n* пя́тнышко, ме́тка (*на коже*).

speckle II *v* пятна́ть.

speckled ['spekld] *a* 1) кра́пчатый; в кра́пинку; 2) пёстрый, рябо́й (*о курах*).

specs [speks] *n pl разг.* очки́, пенсне́.

spectacle ['spektəkl] *n* зре́лище, сце́на; a lamentable (moving, sad) ~ плаче́вное (тро́гательное, жа́лкое) зре́лище; to make a ~ of oneself обраща́ть на себя́ внима́ние.

spectacled ['spektəkld] *a* 1) в очка́х; 2) очко́вый (*о змее*).

spectacles ['spektəklz] *n pl* 1) очки́; 2) цветны́е стёкла (*семафора*); ◊ to look through rose-coloured ~ смотре́ть сквозь ро́зовые очки́; to see everything through rose-coloured ~ ви́деть всё в ро́зовом све́те.

spectacular [spek'tækjulə] *a* 1) эффе́ктный; 2) захва́тывающий.

spectator [spek'teɪtə] *n* зри́тель, наблюда́тель, очеви́дец.

specter ['spektə] *амер. см.* spectre.

spectra ['spektrə] *pl см.* spectrum.

spectral ['spektrəl] *a* 1) при́зрачный; 2) *физ.* спектра́льный.

spectre ['spektə] *n* 1) при́зрак, привиде́ние; 2) предчу́вствие (*беды*).

spectrum ['spektrəm] *n* (*pl* spectra) *физ.* спектр.

specular ['spekjulə] *a* 1) зерка́льный; 2) отража́ющий (*о поверхности*).

speculate ['spekjuleɪt] *v* 1) размышля́ть, разду́мывать; 2) спекули́ровать.

speculation [,spekju'leɪʃən] *n* 1) размышле́ние; обду́мывание; 2) рассмотре́ние; 3) спекуля́ция, спекули́рование.

speculative ['spekjulətɪv] *a* 1) умозри́тельный, мысли́тельный; 2) спекуляти́вный.

speculator ['spekjuleɪtə] *n* 1) мысли́тель; 2) спекуля́нт.

sped [sped] *past, p. p. см.* speed II.

speech [spiːtʃ] *n* 1) речь, речева́я де́ятельность; reported ~ несо́бственная пряма́я речь; 2) выступле́ние, речь, докла́д; maiden ~ пе́рвое выступле́ние (*в парламенте и т. п.*); policy ~ програ́ммная речь; a ponderous ~ ну́дный докла́д; to deliver (*или* to make) a ~ произноси́ть речь; 3) *театр.* ре́плика; 4) го́вор, диале́кт; 5) мане́ра говори́ть; 6) *attr* речево́й; ◊ ~ is silver but silence is gold ≅ сло́во — серебро́, молча́ние — зо́лото.

speech-day ['spiːtʃdeɪ] *n* акт, а́ктовый день (*в учебном заведении*).

speechless ['spiːtʃlɪs] *a* 1) лиши́вшийся ре́чи; онеме́вший; 2) безмо́лвный, молчали́вый; 3) онеме́вший (*от ужаса и т. п.*).

speed I [spiːd] *n* ско́рость, быстрота́; high ~ максима́льная ско́рость, бы́стрый ход; at full ~ на по́лной ско́рости; по́лным хо́дом; full ~ ahead! по́лный (ход) вперёд! (*команда*); to put in the first (second) ~ включи́ть пе́рвую (втору́ю) ско́рость; with ~ бы́стро; at (*или* with) lightning ~ с быстрото́й мо́лнии; to gather ~ уско́рить ход; набира́ть ско́рость.

speed II *v* (*past, p. p.* sped) 1) продвига́ть, соде́йствовать; 2) спеши́ть; 3) ускоря́ть (*часто* to ~ up); 4) увели́чивать (*выпуск продукции*); ◊ to ~ well преуспева́ть.

speedboat ['spiːdbout] *n* быстрохо́дная мото́рная ло́дка.

speedily ['spiːdɪlɪ] *adv* бы́стро, ско́ро, поспе́шно.

speediness ['spiːdɪnɪs] *n* поспе́шность.

speedometer [spɪ'dɔmɪtə] *n* спидо́метр.

speed-up ['spiːdʌp] *n* 1) ускоре́ние; 2) потого́нная систе́ма повыше́ния производи́тельности труда́ (*в капиталистических странах*).

speedway ['spiːdweɪ] *n* го́ночный трек.

speedy ['spiːdɪ] *a* 1) бы́стрый, ско́рый; 2) прово́рный; 3) поспе́шный.

spell[1] [spel] *v* (*past, p. p.* spelt, spelled) 1) называ́ть по бу́квам; 2) образо́вывать слова́ (*по буквам*); 3) чита́ть по склада́м (*тж.* to ~ out); 4) означа́ть; 5) намека́ть.

spell[2] *n* 1) вре́мя, пери́од; a hot ~ пери́од жары́; a cold ~ похолода́ние; a ~ of fine weather пери́од хоро́шей пого́ды; 2) коро́ткий промежу́ток вре́мени; for a ~ на вре́мя; to give smb. a ~ дать кому́-л. переды́шку; 3) припа́док, при́ступ (*кашля, болезни, смеха и т. п.*).

spell[3] *n* 1) ча́ры; заклина́ние; 2) очарова́ние, обая́ние; under a ~ зачаро́ванный; to cast a ~ очарова́ть (*кого-л.— on*).

spellbind ['spelbaɪnd] *v* (*past, p. p.* spellbound) очаро́вывать.

spellbinder ['spel,baɪndə] *n разг.* ора́тор, владе́ющий свое́й аудито́рией.

spellbound I ['spelbaund] *past, p. p. см.* spellbind.

spellbound II *a* очаро́ванный, засты́вший, ошело́млённый.

speller[1] ['spelə] *n амер.* нача́льный уче́бник орфогра́фии.

speller[2] *n* рабо́тающий сде́льно.

spelling ['spelɪŋ] *n* 1) правописа́ние, орфогра́фия; 2) написа́ние по бу́квам.

spelling-book ['spelɪŋbuk] *n амер.* сбо́рник упражне́ний по правописа́нию.

spelt [spelt] *past, p. p. см.* spell[1].

spencer ['spensə] *n* коро́ткий жаке́т.

spend [spend] *v* (*past, p. p.* spent) 1) тра́тить, растра́чивать; 2) расхо́довать; 3) проводи́ть (*вре́мя*); 4) истощи́ться, исся́кнуть; 5) успоко́иться (*о бу́ре и т. п.*).

spender ['spendə] *n* растра́тчик, мот, транжи́ра.

spendthrift ['spendθrɪft] *n* мот.

spent I [spent] *past, p. p. см.* spend.

spent II *a* 1) истощённый; 2) исся́кший; 3) вы́дохшийся (*о челове́ке*).

sperm [spəːm] *n биол.* спе́рма.

sphere [sfɪə] *n* 1) шар; 2) земно́й шар, гло́бус; 3) сфе́ра; по́ле де́ятельности; 4) компете́нция; out of my ~ вне мое́й компете́нции; 5) (социа́льная) среда́.

spherical ['sferɪkəl] *a* 1) шарообра́зный; шарово́й; 2) сфери́ческий.

sphinx [sfɪŋks] *n* (*pl тж.* sphinges ['sfɪndʒɪz]) сфинкс.

spice I [spaɪs] *n* 1) спе́ция, пря́ность; 2) *собир.* спе́ции; 3) *поэт.* пря́ный за́пах; 4) пика́нтность, изю́минка; 5) при́вкус, отте́нок.

spice II *v* 1) приправля́ть; 2) придава́ть пика́нтность.

spicery ['spaɪsərɪ] *n* 1) спе́ции, пря́ности; 2) пря́ный арома́т.

spick [spɪk] *a:* ~ and span щегольско́й, с иго́лочки.

spicy ['spaɪsɪ] *a* 1) пря́ный; 2) аромати́чный; 3) о́стрый, пика́нтный; 4) неприли́чный, непристо́йный; 5) *сленг* вспы́льчивый.

spider ['spaɪdə] *n* 1) пау́к; *перен. тж.* интрига́н; 2) тага́н; 3) опры́скиватель.

spidery ['spaɪdərɪ] *a* паукообра́зный.

spiffy ['spɪfɪ] *a сленг* элега́нтный; изя́щный.

spigot ['spɪgət] *n* 1) втУлка; 2) *амер.* кран.

spike I [spaɪk] *n* 1) остриё; 2) гвоздь, косты́ль; 3) шип (*на подо́шве*); 4) ко́лос; 5) рог (*молодо́го оле́ня*).

spike II *v* забива́ть гвоздь, косты́ль.

spiky ['spaɪkɪ] *a* остроконе́чный, заострённый.

spile I [spaɪl] *n* 1) заты́чка; 2) сва́я.

spile II *v* 1) затыка́ть; 2) забива́ть сва́и.

spiling ['spaɪlɪŋ] *n* сва́и.

spill[1] I [spɪl] *n* 1) разбры́згивание, бры́зги; 2) разли́тая жи́дкость; 3) *разг.* паде́ние (*седока́ из седла́ и т. п.*).

spill[1] II *v* (*past, p. p.* spilled, spilt) 1) пролива́ть(ся); разлива́ть(ся); 2) рассыпа́ть; 3) *разг.* сбро́сить, вы́бросить (*седока́ из седла́*).

spill[2] *n* 1) лучи́на; 2) скру́ченный кусо́к бума́ги; 3) заты́чка.

spilt [spɪlt] *past, p. p. см.* spill[1] II.

spin I [spɪn] *v* (*past* spun, *уст.* span; *p. p.* spun) 1) прясть, сучи́ть; 2) плести́ (*паути́ну и т. п.*); заплета́ть; 3) крути́ть, пуска́ть волчко́м; to send smb. ~ning отшвырну́ть кого́-л.; 4) расска́зывать (*занима́тельную исто́рию, по́весть*); 5) бы́стро е́хать, бежа́ть; 6) кружи́ться (*о голове́*); 7): to be spun *разг.* «засы́паться» (*на экза́мене*).

spin II *n* 1) верче́ние, круже́ние; 2) *ав.* што́пор; ◇ to go for a ~, to take a ~ прокати́ться.

spinach ['spɪnɪdʒ] *n* шпина́т.

spinage ['spɪnɪdʒ] *см.* spinach.

spinal ['spaɪnl] *a анат.* спинно́й.

spindle I ['spɪndl] *n* 1) веретено́; 2) ме́ра пря́жи (≅ 14 000 *м*); 3) *тех.* ось, вал махови́ка.

spindle II *a* 1) веретенообра́зный; 2) относя́щийся к же́нской ли́нии (*ро́да*).

spindle III *v* вытя́гиваться (*о расте́нии, подро́стке*).

spindlelegs ['spɪndllegz] *разг. см.* spindle-shanks.

spindle-shanks ['spɪndlʃæŋks] *n разг.* долговя́зый челове́к.

spindling ['spɪndlɪŋ] *a* дли́нный и то́нкий.

spindrift ['spɪndrɪft] *n* бры́зги морско́й воды́.

spine [spaɪn] *n* 1) позвоно́чник; 2) конёк (*кры́ши*); 3) шип, игла́, колю́чка; 4) корешо́к (*кни́ги*).

spineless ['spaɪnlɪs] *a* беспозвоно́чный; *перен.* бесхребе́тный, бесхара́ктерный; мягкоте́лый.

spinner ['spɪnə] *n* 1) пряди́льщик, -ица; 2) пряди́льная маши́на.

spinney ['spɪnɪ] *n* за́росли; подле́сок.

spinning ['spɪnɪŋ] *n* пряде́ние.

spinning-jenny ['spɪnɪŋ,dʒenɪ] *n* пряди́льная маши́на.

spinning-wheel ['spɪnɪŋwiːl] *n* пря́лка.

spinster ['spɪnstə] *n* 1) *разг.* ста́рая де́ва; *юр.* незаму́жняя же́нщина; 2) пря́ха.

spiny ['spaɪnɪ] *a* колю́чий, в колю́чках, в шипа́х.

spiracle ['spaɪərəkl] *n* отду́шина.

spiral I ['spaɪərəl] *n* спира́ль; heating ~ змееви́к.

spiral II *a* винтово́й, спира́льный; винтообра́зный.

spiral III *v* стреми́тельно расти́ (*о це́нах*).

spirant I ['spaɪərənt] *n фон.* фрикати́вный согла́сный, спира́нт.

spirant II *a фон.* фрикати́вный.

spire[1] ['spaɪə] *n* 1) шпиль; остриё; 2) пик; остроконе́чная верши́на; 3) росто́к, побе́г.

spire[2] ['spaɪə] *n* 1) спира́ль; 2) вито́к (*спира́ли*).

spirit I ['spɪrɪt] *n* 1) дух; unbending (unbroken) ~ непрекло́нный (несло́мленный) дух; public (team) ~ дух патриоти́зма (коллективи́зма); to summon (*или* to pluck) up ~ собра́ться с ду́хом; 2) привиде́ние; 3) фе́я, эльф; 4) воодушевле́ние, жар; to put ~ into smth. вноси́ть жи́вость, оживле́ние во что-л.; вдохну́ть жизнь во что-л.; to speak with ~ говори́ть с жа́ром; 5) *обыкн. pl* настрое́ние; animal ~ жизнера́достность; good, high ~s хоро́шее, бо́дрое настрое́ние; bad (low) ~ плохо́е (пода́вленное) настрое́ние; my ~ sank я упа́л ду́хом; out of ~ не в настрое́нии; to keep up one's ~ а) бодри́ться; б) ободря́ть; 6) хра́брость, задо́р; 7) хара́ктер; 8) челове́к (*с точки зрения характера, поведения и т. п.*); 9) *хим.* эссе́нция; 10) *pl* спирт; to drink ~s пить спиртны́е напи́тки.

spirit II *v* 1) воодушевля́ть; 2) толка́ть (*на что-л.— on*); побужда́ть (*к чему-л.— at*); □ to ~ **away**, to ~ **off** таи́нственно похи́тить.

spirited ['spɪrɪtɪd] *a* 1) живо́й, оживлённый; 2) сме́лый (*об атаке*); бо́йкий (*об ответе*); 3) энерги́чный; 4) горя́чий (*о лошади*).

spiritual ['spɪrɪtʃuəl] *a* 1) духо́вный; 2) воодушевлённый, одухотворённый; 3) свяще́нный, церко́вный.

spirituous ['spɪrɪtʃuəs] *a* спиртно́й; алкого́льный.

spiry¹ ['spaɪərɪ] *a* шпилеви́дный, остроконе́чный.

spiry² *a* 1) спира́льный, вито́й; 2) вью́щийся.

spit¹ I [spɪt] *n* 1) плево́к; слюна́ (*выплюнутая*); 2) *разг.* вы́литый портре́т; 3) небольшо́й дождь *или* снег.

spit¹ II *v* (*past, p. p.* spat) 1) плева́ть (*на — at, on; перен. тж. ирон.*); 2) бры́згать слюно́й, плева́ться; 3) мороси́ть; 4) шипе́ть (*о кошке*); □ to ~ **at** проявля́ть вражде́бность (*к кому-л.*); to ~ **out** а) изрыга́ть прокля́тия; б) выплёвывать; ~ **it out!** *сленг* говори́те гро́мче!

spit² I *n* 1) ве́ртел; 2) коса́ (*на море*); стре́лка, дли́нная о́тмель.

spit² II *v* 1) наса́живать на ве́ртел; 2) проколо́ть, пронзи́ть.

spite I [spaɪt] *n* злоба, зло́бное чу́вство; from pure ~, out of ~ со зло́сти; из жела́ния сде́лать напереко́р; he has a ~ against me у него́ зуб про́тив меня́; ◇ in ~ of несмотря́ на, вопреки́.

spite II *v* досажда́ть, де́лать на́зло.

spiteful ['spaɪtful] *a* 1) зло́бный; 2) злора́дный, недоброжела́тельный; 3) язви́тельный.

spitfire ['spɪtfaɪə] *n* вспы́льчивый челове́к.

spittle ['spɪtl] *n* слюна́; плево́к.

spittoon [spɪ'tuːn] *n* плева́тельница.

spiv [spɪv] *n разг.* пройдо́ха.

splash I [splæʃ] *n* 1) разбры́згивание; 2) всплеск; 3) бры́зги; 4) пятно́ (*от грязи*); 5) сноп (*света*); ◇ to make a ~ наде́лать шу́му, произвести́ сенса́цию.

splash II *v* 1) бры́згать(ся); плеска́ть(ся); 2) разлета́ться бры́згами; 3) распле́скивать; 4) шлёпать (*по грязи, воде*).

splash-board ['splæʃbɔːd] *n* крыло́ (*автомобиля, экипажа и т. п.*).

splashy ['splæʃɪ] *a* 1) забры́зганный; 2) пятни́стый; 3) *разг.* показно́й.

splay I [spleɪ] *n* амбразу́ра.

splay II *a* 1) вы́тянутый; 2) косо́й; раско́сый.

splay-foot ['spleɪfut] *n* косола́пость.

spleen [spliːn] *n* 1) *анат.* селезёнка; 2) мра́чное настрое́ние, хандра́; 3): to vent one's ~ upon smb. изли́ть на кого́-л. всю зло́бу, жёлчь; to act out of ~ де́лать что-л. со зло́сти.

spleenful ['spliːnful] *a* мра́чный, жёлчный, раздражи́тельный.

splendent ['splendənt] *a* блестя́щий, я́ркий; сверка́ющий.

splendid ['splendɪd] *a* 1) роско́шный, великоле́п-

ный; 2) замеча́тельный, прекра́сный; 3) лучеза́рный; 4) *разг.* первокла́ссный, первосо́ртный; 5) выдаю́щийся (*о способностях*).

splendiferous [splen'dɪfərəs] *a разг.* великоле́пный, превосхо́дный.

splendour ['splendə] *n* 1) великоле́пие, ро́скошь; 2) пы́шность; 3) я́ркость; колори́тность; 4) блеск.

splenic ['splenɪk] *a* селезёночный.

splice I [splaɪs] *n* 1) сплета́ние (*концов каната*); 2) сра́щивание (*концов досок*).

splice II *v* 1) сплета́ть (*концы каната*); 2) сра́щивать (*концы досок*); 3) *разг.* вступа́ть в брак; to get ~d жени́ться, вы́йти за́муж.

splint I [splɪnt] *n* 1) *мед.* лубо́к, ши́на; 2) лубо́к (*для плетения корзин, стульев и т. п.*).

splint II *v мед.* накла́дывать лубо́к, ши́ну.

splinter I ['splɪntə] *n* 1) оско́лок, обло́мок; 2) ще́пка, лучи́на; 3) зано́за; to run a ~ занози́ть.

splinter II *v* раска́лывать(ся), расщепля́ть(ся).

split I [splɪt] *n* 1) расщепле́ние, раска́лывание; 2) раско́л, разры́в (*в отношениях между людьми*); 3) тре́щина, рассе́лина, щель; 4) слоёное изде́лие из фру́ктов, моро́женого, оре́хов *и т. п.*

split II *a* расщеплённый, раско́лотый; раздро́бленный.

split III *v* 1) расщепля́ть; 2) рассла́ивать; 3) отка́лывать; открыва́ть; 4) дроби́ть (*силы*); 5) раска́лываться, рассла́иваться; 6) тре́скаться, растре́скиваться; 7) разбива́ться, разла́мываться; 8) раска́лываться, распада́ться (*на группы, фракции; on*); 9) распи́ть (*бутылку вина*); 10): to ~ with smb. поссо́риться с кем-л.; to~ with laughter расхохота́ться; □ to ~ **off** отка́лываться, отла́мываться; to ~ **up** раска́лываться, разла́мываться.

splitting I ['splɪtɪŋ] *n* расщепле́ние; atom ~ расщепле́ние а́тома.

splitting II *a* 1) оглуши́тельный; 2) си́льный (*о головной боли*); 3) головокружи́тельный (*о скорости*); 4) раско́льнический (*о деятельности, тактике*).

splodge I, II [splɔdʒ] *см.* splotch I, II.

splotch I [splɔtʃ] *n* гря́зное пятно́.

splotch II *v* па́чкать.

splurge I [spləːdʒ] *n разг.* бахва́льство, хвастовство́.

splurge II *v разг.* форси́ть, хва́статься, бахва́литься.

splutter I ['splʌtə] *n* 1) бы́страя, невня́тная речь; 2) спор; препира́ния; 3) сумато́ха; 4) разбры́згивание; бры́зги.

splutter II *v* 1) говори́ть запина́ясь (*от волнения*); 2) бры́згать (*слюной*); 3) обры́згивать, забры́згивать; 4) шипе́ть (*о жидкости*).

spoil I [spɔɪl] *n* 1) добы́ча, награ́бленное; 2) *pl воен.* трофе́и; the ~s of war вое́нная добы́ча; 3) нако́пленное добро́; це́нности; 4) *pl амер.* до́лжности (*получаемые представителями победившей партии*).

spoil II *v* (*past, p. p.* spoiled, *уст.* spoilt) 1) по́ртить(ся), испо́ртить(ся); 2) балова́ть (*ребёнка*); 3) огра́бить, обобра́ть (*противника*); расхища́ть, раста́скивать; ◇ to ~ for a fight лезть в дра́ку.

spoilage ['spɔɪlɪdʒ] *n* 1) по́рча; 2) испо́рченный това́р.

spoilsman ['spɔɪlzmən] *n амер.* человек, получающий должность за политические услуги.

spoilt [spɔɪlt] *уст. past, p. p. см.* spoil II.

spoke[1] [spouk] *n* 1) спица (*колеса*); 2) перекладина (*приставной лестницы*); ◊ a ~ in one's wheel помеха; to put a ~ in smb.'s wheel ≅ ставить палки в колёса, мешать.

spoke[2] *past см.* speak.

spoken I ['spoukən] *p. p. см.* speak.

spoken II *a* разговорный (*о стиле*).

spokesman ['spouksmən] *n* 1) делегат, представитель; 2) оратор; 3) диктор.

spoliation [ˌspouli'eɪʃən] *n* 1) ограбление; 2) захват, конфискация (*судов нейтральных государств*); 3) *юр.* уничтожение, порча документа.

sponge I [spʌndʒ] *n* 1) губка; 2) губчатое вещество; 3) обмывание, обтирание; 4) *разг.* паразит (*о человеке*); ◊ to chuck (*или* to throw) up the ~ признать себя побеждённым; to pass the ~ over предать забвению.

sponge II *v* 1) стирать губкой; 2) жить на чужой счёт; поживиться (*на чужой счёт*); 3) собирать губки; □ to ~ away *см.* to ~ off; to ~ **down**: to ~ oneself down мыться губкой; to ~ **off** вытирать губкой; to ~ **on** жить паразитом, паразитировать; to ~ **out** стирать губкой; to ~ **up** впитывать; вбирать.

sponge-cake ['spʌndʒ'keɪk] *n* бисквит.

sponge-down ['spʌndʒ'daun] *n* обтирание (*губкой*).

sponger ['spʌndʒə] *n* паразит (*о человеке*).

spongy ['spʌndʒɪ] *n* 1) губчатый; 2) пористый.

sponsor I ['spɔnsə] *n* 1) поручитель; 2) фирма, субсидирующая в своих целях радио, концертные выступления; 3) устроитель, организатор; 4) крёстный отец; крёстная мать.

sponsor II *v* 1) ручаться (*за кого-л.*— for); быть ответственным (*за что-л.*— for); 2) поддерживать (*резолюцию и т. п.*); 3) устраивать, организовывать (*митинг и т. п.*); 4) субсидировать.

sponsorship ['spɔnsəʃɪp] *n* поручительство.

spontaneity [ˌspɔntə'niːɪtɪ] *n* самопроизвольность, спонтанность.

spontaneous [spɔn'teɪnjəs] *a* 1) самопроизвольный, спонтанный; стихийный; 2) добровольный; 3) непосредственный, непроизвольный.

spoof I [spuːf] *n сленг* обман, надувательство.

spoof II *v сленг* обманывать, надувать.

spook [spuːk] *n шутл.* привидение.

spool I [spuːl] *n* катушка; шпулька.

spool II *v* наматывать на катушку, шпульку.

spoon[1] I [spuːn] *n* 1) ложка; tea ~ чайная ложка; 2) лопасть весла (*широкая и изогнутая*); ◊ wooden ~ a) последнее место (*в соревнованиях*); б) человек, занявший последнее место (*в соревнованиях*); to be born with a silver ~ in one's mouth *погов.* ≅ родиться в сорочке.

spoon[1] II *v* черпать ложкой (*обыкн.* to ~ up, to ~ out).

spoon[2] *n сленг* 1) простак; 2) влюблённый; to be ~s влюбиться (*в кого-л.*— on); to be on the ~ ухаживать за.

spooney I, II ['spuːnɪ] *см.* spoony I, II.

spoon-fed ['spuːnfed] *a* 1) питающийся с ложки (*о больном*); 2) тщательно опекаемый, охраняемый; 3) *сленг* избалованный.

spoonful ['spuːnful] *n* полная ложка (*чего-л.*).

spoony I ['spuːnɪ] *n* сентиментальный влюблённый, вздыхатель; 2) простак; простофиля.

spoony II *a* 1) влюблённый; 2) глупый, одуревший.

spoor I [spuə] *n* след (*зверя*).

spoor II *v* идти по следу.

sporadic [spə'rædɪk] *a* нерегулярный, спорадический.

spore [spɔː] *n бот.* спора.

sport I [spɔːt] *n* 1) спорт; вид спорта; athletic ~s атлетика; to go in for ~s заниматься спортом; to have good ~ хорошо поохотиться; 2) *pl* спортивные состязания; 3) развлечение; what ~! как интересно!; they thought it a great ~ (это) им казалось очень забавным; 4) шутка, насмешка; in ~, for ~ шутки ради; to make ~ (of) высмеивать; 5) посмешище; 6) игрушка (*судьбы и т. п.*); 7) *разг.* спортсмен; 8) *разг.* славный малый; 9) *спорт.* болельщик; 10) фат, щёголь.

sport II *a* 1) спортивный; 2) верхний (*об одежде*).

sport III *v* 1) заниматься спортом; 2) развлекаться; проводить время; 3) играть, резвиться; 4) высмеивать; 5) *разг.* щеголять (*чем-л. или в чём-л.*); □ to ~ **away** растрачивать, проматывать.

sportdom ['spɔːtdəm] *n* мир спорта.

sporting ['spɔːtɪŋ] *a* 1) занимающийся *или* интересующийся спортом; 2) спортивный; 3) рискованный.

sportive ['spɔːtɪv] *a* 1) резвый, игривый; 2) сделанный в шутку; 3) спортивный.

sports [spɔːts] *см.* sport II.

sportsman ['spɔːtsmən] *n* 1) спортсмен; keen ~ страстный спортсмен; 2) добряк; шутник; 3) *attr* спортсменский.

sportsmanlike ['spɔːtsmənlaɪk] *a* спортсменский.

sportsmanship ['spɔːtsmənʃɪp] *n* спортивная ловкость.

sportswoman ['spɔːts,wumən] *n* спортсменка.

sporty ['spɔːtɪ] *a разг.* 1) показной; щегольской; 2) лихой, удалой.

spot I [spɔt] *n* 1) пятно (*тж. перен.*); пятнышко, крапинка; without a ~ in one's reputation с незапятнанной репутацией; 2) место; on the ~ немедленно, тут же; на месте; to be present on the ~ присутствовать, быть очевидцем; быть тут как тут; blind ~ a) мёртвая точка; б) *радио* зона молчания; solitary ~ уединённое место; raw ~ больное место; tender ~ чувствительное место; weak ~ слабое место; to touch the ~ попасть в цель, в точку; 3) *разг.* чуточка, капелька; ◊ to put on the ~ *разг.* поставить в неловкое, затруднительное положение.

spot II *a* наличный, имеющийся на складе.

spot III *v* 1) пятнать (*тж. перен.*); пачкать; покрывать(ся) пятнами; this silk ~s with water на этом шёлке остаются пятна от воды; 2) *разг.* узнать; заметить; опознать; 3) *воен.* корректировать стрельбу.

spotless ['spɔtlɪs] *a* безупречный; незапятнанный.

spotlight I ['spɔtlaɪt] *n* 1) *театр.* прожектор (*для подсветки*); 2) центр внимания; to be in the ~ быть в центре внимания.

spotlight II *v* осветить прожёктором, ярким светом; оттенить.

spotted ['spɔtɪd] *a* 1) пятнистый, пёстрый; 2) запятнанный.

spotter ['spɔtə] *n* 1) контролёр; 2) *воен.* корректировщик.

spotty ['spɔtɪ] *a* 1) крапчатый, пятнистый; 2) неровный (*о характере*); 3) неодинаковый (*о качестве*).

spousal ['spauzəl] *a* свадебный, брачный.

spouse [spauz] *n* супруг; супруга.

spout I [spaut] *n* 1) носик (*чайника и т. п.*); горлышко; 2) водосточная труба; 3) струя воды; 4) жёлоб; выпускное отверстие; 5) *разг.*: up the ~ в закладе, в залоге; to put up the ~ закладывать (*вещи*).

spout II *v* 1) выпускать струю; бить струёй; 2) *разг.* ораторствовать; разглагольствовать; 3) извергать (*лаву*).

sprain I [spreɪn] *n* растяжение (*сухожилия*).

sprain II *v* растянуть (*сухожилие*).

sprang [spræŋ] *past см.* spring² III.

sprat [spræt] *n* 1) шпрота; 2) малыш; ◊ to risk (*или* to throw) a ~ to catch a whale (*или* a herring) *погов.* рисковать малым, чтобы получить многое.

sprawl [sprɔːl] *v* 1) растянуться (*на земле*), упасть; to send smb. ~ing сбить кого-л. с ног; 2) развалиться, сидеть развалясь; 3) расползаться во все стороны.

sprawly ['sprɔːlɪ] *a* 1) ползучий; 2) раскинувшийся.

spray¹ I [spreɪ] *n* 1) струя воды; 2) брызги; водяная пыль; 3) пульверизатор; 4) град (*пуль*).

spray¹ II *v* 1) разбрызгивать, распылять (*жидкость*); 2) обрызгивать (*растение*).

spray² *n* побег; вéточка.

sprayer ['spreɪə] *n* опрыскиватель.

spread I [spred] *n* 1) распространение; 2) протяжение, протяжённость; the wide ~ of the country широкие просторы; 3) размах; 4) покрывало; 5) *разг.* угощение; a great ~ пирушка; 6) *амер.* масло, джем и т. п. (*то, что мажется на хлеб*); 7) объявление (*длиной в несколько газетных столбцов*).

spread II *v* (*past, p. p.* spread) 1) расстилать (*скатерть и т. п.*); раскладывать (*карту*); 2) расправлять (*крылья*); 3) распространять(ся); 4) разбрасывать (*сено, навоз и т. п.*); 5) намазывать, покрывать слоем (*масла, варенья*); 6) расстилаться (*о виде, панораме*); 7) разводить руками; □ to ~ out a) расстилать; б) разбрасывать.

spread III *a* усеянный (*чем-л. — with*).

spread-eagle ['spred,iːgl] *a амер. разг.* высокопарный; ура-патриотический, хвастливый.

spree [spriː] *n* 1) веселье, резвость; шалость; what a ~! как весело!; 2) кутёж, попойка; to go on the ~ кутить.

sprig [sprɪg] *n* 1) вéточка, росток; 2) узор из цветущих вéточек; 3) *обыкн. презр.* отпрыск, отродье; 4) штифт.

sprightly I ['spraɪtlɪ] *a* 1) оживлённый, весёлый; 2) живой.

sprightly II *adv* 1) вéсело; 2) живо.

spring¹ [sprɪŋ] *n* 1) весна; *перен. тж.* начало, расцвет; 2) *attr* весенний.

spring² I *n* 1) прыжок, скачок; 2) эластичность, упругость; 3) пружина; 4) рессора.

spring² II *a* 1) упругий; 2) пружинный.

spring² III *v* (*past* sprang, sprung; *p. p.* sprung) 1) прыгать, подпрыгивать; подскакивать; to ~ to one's feet вскочить на ноги; to ~ up into the air подскочить в воздух; 2) прорастать, давать ростки; 3) возникать, появляться; 4) подниматься, возвышаться; 5) бросаться, приливать (*о крови*); 6) пружинить; захлопываться (*благодаря пружине*); 7) происходить (*из семьи, рода; from*); 8) вспугивать (*дичь*); 9) коробиться (*о досках*); 10) взрывать (*мину*); 11) отпускать (*шутку*); 12) давать (*трещину, течь*); □ to ~ at наброситься на кого-л.; to ~ up а) возникать (*об обычае*); б) расти, появляться (*о цветах, почках и т. п.*); to ~ upon *см.* to ~ at.

spring³ I *n* 1) источник, ключ, родник; 2) *attr* родниковый.

spring³ II *v* бить (*об источнике, роднике*).

spring-board ['sprɪŋbɔːd] *n* трамплин.

springhead ['sprɪŋhed] *n* источник.

springtide ['sprɪŋtaɪd] *n поэт.* весна.

springtime ['sprɪŋtaɪm] *n* 1) весна, весенний сезон; 2) ранний период.

springy ['sprɪŋɪ] *a* 1) эластичный, упругий; 2) пружинящий.

sprinkle I ['sprɪŋkl] *n* мелкий дождь; a ~ of snow лёгкий снежок, пороша.

sprinkle II *v* 1) брызгать, обрызгивать; 2) посыпать (*порошком*); 3) накрапывать.

sprinkler ['sprɪŋklə] *n* опрыскиватель; street ~ поливочная машина.

sprint I [sprɪnt] *n* спринт, бег на короткую дистанцию.

sprint II *v* бежать на короткую дистанцию.

sprinter ['sprɪntə] *n* спринтер, бегун на короткие дистанции.

sprite [spraɪt] *n* эльф, фея.

sprout I [spraut] *n* 1) росток; побег; 2) *pl* брюссельская капуста (*тж.* Brussels ~s).

sprout II *v* 1) давать ростки, побеги; прорастать (*тж.* to ~ up); 2) быстро развиваться.

spruce¹ I [spruːs] *a* щеголеватый, нарядный.

spruce¹ II *v* наряжаться, рядиться (*тж.* to ~ up).

spruce² *n* ель, хвойное (дéрево).

sprung [sprʌŋ] *past, p. p. см.* spring² III.

spry [spraɪ] *a* 1) живой; сообразительный; 2) проворный, шустрый.

spume I [spjuːm] *n* пена.

spume II *v* пениться.

spun [spʌn] *past, p. p. см.* spin I.

spunk [spʌŋk] *n* 1) мужество; 2) энергия, пыл; 3) трут.

spunky ['spʌŋkɪ] *a* энергичный; горячий, пылкий.

spur I [spəː] *n* 1) шпора (*тж.* у петуха); he needs the ~ *перен.* он нуждается в палке; to put (*или* to set) ~s to пришпоривать; to win one's ~s а) *ист.* получить звание рыцаря; б) отличиться; 2) стимул, побуждение; 3) отрог, уступ; ◊ on the ~ of the moment под влиянием минуты.

spur II *v* 1) пришпоривать; 2): to be ~red on быть побуждаемым, подстрекаемым.

spurious ['spjuərɪəs] *a* 1) подложный, поддельный; 2) *биол.* ложный.

spurn I [spəːn] *n* презрительное отношение.

spurn II *v* оттолкнуть, отпихнуть с презрением (*ногой*).

spurt I [spəːt] *n* 1) сильная струя; 2) взрыв (*чувства и т. п.*); 3) внезапное усилие, рывок.

spurt II *v* 1) бить струёй; 2) делать внезапное усилие, рывок; □ to ~ **out** а) бить струёй; б) выбрасывать (*пламя*); to ~ **up** бить, выбрасывать струю.

sputnik ['sputnɪk] *n* астр. спутник; a round-about ~ маневрирующий спутник.

sputter I ['sрʌtə] *n* 1) шипенье (*свечи, дров*); 2) бессвязная речь; 3) брызги.

sputter II *v* 1) шипеть (*о свече, дровах*); 2) говорить бессвязно; 3) плеваться, брызгать слюной.

spy I [spaɪ] *n* 1) шпион; 2) тайный агент; 3) наблюдение (*за кем-л.*).

spy II *v* 1) шпионить; 2) выслеживать, выведывать; □ to ~ **into** тайно расследовать; to ~ **on** тайно наблюдать, следить (*за кем-л.*); to ~ **out** а) разведывать (*местность*); разузнавать; б) разглядеть, обнаружить, увидеть; to ~ **upon** см. to ~ on.

spyglass ['spaɪɡlɑːs] *n* подзорная труба.

squab I [skwɔb] *n* 1) неоперившийся птенец; 2) приземистый, коренастый человек; 3) туго набитая подушка.

squab II *a* 1) приземистый; коренастый; толстый; 2) неоперившийся.

squabble I ['skwɔbl] *n* перебранка, мелкая ссора.

squabble II *v* вздорить, пререкаться, ссориться из-за пустяков.

squabby ['skwɔd] *a* приземистый; коренастый.

squad [skwɔd] *n* 1) отряд; police ~ отряд полиции; flying ~ летучий отряд; 2) бригада (*рабочих*); 3) воен. отделение; awkward ~ разг. новобранцы, «команда неуклюжих».

squadron ['skwɔdrən] *n* 1) воен. эскадрон; дивизион; 2) мор. эскадра; 3) ав. авиаотряд; эскадрилья.

squadron-leader ['skwɔdrən‚liːdə] *n* майор авиации.

squalid ['skwɔlɪd] *a* 1) грязный, запущенный; 2) убогий, нищенский, жалкий; 3) опустившийся.

squall[1] I [skwɔːl] *n* 1) шквал, вихрь; white ~ внезапный шквал (*в тропических районах*); look out for ~s перен. берегись опасности; 2) разг. шум, сумятица.

squall[1] II *v* дуть порывами.

squall[2] I *n* писк, визг.

squall[2] II *v* пищать, визжать.

squally ['skwɔːlɪ] *a* 1) бурный, порывистый (*о ветре*); 2) разг. угрожающий, опасный.

squalor ['skwɔlə] *n* 1) грязь, запустение; 2) убогость, нищета.

squander I ['skwɔndə] *n* растрата; растрачивание.

squander II *v* растрачивать, расточать; □ to ~ **away** проматывать.

square I [skwɛə] *n* 1) квадрат; 2) прямоугольник; 3) площадь; 4) сквер; 5) квадратный кусок (*чего-л.*); 6) мат. квадрат числа; 7) квартал (*города*); 8) воен. каре; ◇ on the ~ прямо, открыто, без обмана.

square II *a* 1) квадратный; 2) прямоугольный; 3) перпендикулярный (*к чему-л. — with, to*);

4) правильный, точный, ровный; сбалансированный; 5) разг. честный, прямой; 6) категорический (*об отказе*); 7) разг. плотный, сытный (*о еде, обеде и т. п.*): ◇ to get ~ with свести счёты; everything is now ~ всё в порядке.

square III *v* 1) мат. возводить в квадрат; 2) придавать форму квадрата; 3) сбалансировать; сводить (*счёты*); 4) согласовывать, увязывать, сообразовывать (*to, with*); 5) сходиться, совпадать; 6) удовлетворять (*кредиторов*); 7) сленг подкупать.

square IV *adv* 1) в квадрате; 2) перпендикулярно; 3) честно, прямо.

square-built ['skwɛəbɪlt] *a* коренастый, широкоплечий.

square-toes ['skwɛə'touz] *n* 1) старомодный человек; 2) педант.

squash I [skwɔʃ] *n* 1) сутолока, толчея; толпа; 2) пюре (*фруктовое*); lemon ~ содовая вода с лимонным соком.

squash II *v* 1) давить, мять; 2) толпиться; 3) заставить замолчать; оборезать (*кого-л.*).

squashy ['skwɔʃɪ] *a* мягкий, мясистый.

squat I [skwɔt] *n* сидение на корточках.

squat II *a* коренастый, приземистый.

squat III *v* 1) сидеть на корточках (*тж.* to ~ **down**); 2) свернуться в клубок (*о животных*); сжаться, съёжиться; 3) селиться на чужой земле; 4) селиться на государственной земле (*в Австралии*).

squatter ['skwɔtə] *n* 1) сидящий на корточках; 2) поселенец; 3) овцевод (*в Австралии*).

squatty ['skwɔtɪ] *a* приземистый, коренастый.

squaw [skwɔː] *n* индианка.

squawk I [skwɔːk] *n* 1) резкий крик (*птицы*); 2) сленг стенание, жалоба.

squawk II *v* 1) пронзительно кричать; 2) сленг стенать, жаловаться.

squeak I [skwiːk] *n* 1) писк (*мыши*); 2) скрип (*двери*); 3) случай, удача; to have a close (*или* narrow, tight) ~ of it быть на волосок (*от гибели*).

squeak II *v* 1) пищать (*о мыши*); скрипеть (*о двери*); 2) сленг ябедничать, доносить.

squeaker ['skwiːkə] *n* 1) птенец; 2) сленг доносчик.

squeaky ['skwiːkɪ] *a* 1) писклявый; 2) скрипучий.

squeal I [skwiːl] *n* 1) визг; 2) сленг доносчик.

squeal II *v* 1) визжать; 2) сленг доносить; 3) сленг разоблачать, раскрывать (*секрет*).

squeamish ['skwiːmɪʃ] *a* 1) щепетильный, педантичный; 2) разборчивый, привередливый (*особ. в еде*); 3) болезненный, слабый (*о желудке*); to feel ~ чувствовать тошноту.

squeezable ['skwiːzəbl] *a* податливый, уступчивый.

squeeze I [skwiːz] *n* 1) сжатие; пожатие; to give a light ~ слегка сжать, пожать; 2) давка; to have a tight ~ сидеть в тесноте; 3) разг. затруднительное положение; in a tight ~ в тяжёлом положении; money ~ денежные, финансовые затруднения; 4) выжимки; 5) факсимиле; 6) разг. вымогательство; шантаж.

squeeze II *v* 1) сжимать, сдавливать; стискивать; 2) выжимать (*тж.* to ~ **out**); 3) втискивать, впи-хивать; 4) вымога́ть; шантажи́ровать; 5) получа́ть факси́миле, о́ттиск; 6) проти́скиваться (*through*).

squelch I [skweltʃ] *n* 1) хлю́панье; 2) грязь; 3) *разг.* уничтожа́ющий отве́т.

squelch II *v* 1) хлю́пать по гря́зи; 2) *разг.* «обре́зать», заста́вить замолча́ть.

squib I [skwɪb] *n* 1) эпигра́мма; е́дкое замеча́ние; 2) петара́да.

squib II *v* писа́ть эпигра́ммы.

squiffy ['skwɪfɪ] *a сленг* подвы́пивший.

squint I [skwɪnt] *n* 1) косогла́зие; раско́сость; 2) взгляд укра́дкой; to have (*или* to take) a ~ взгляну́ть, погляде́ть.

squint II *a* косогла́зый; раско́сый.

squint III *v* 1) коси́ть (*глаза́ми*); 2) смотре́ть и́скоса (*на кого́-л.— at*); 3) смотре́ть укра́дкой (*на кого́-л.— at*); подсма́тривать (*через что́-л.— through*).

squint-eyed ['skwɪntaɪd] *a* 1) косо́й; 2) подозри́тельный; злове́щий, злоде́йский.

squire ['skwaɪə] *n* 1) сквайр (*поме́щик в Англии*); 2) *амер.* мирово́й судья́ (*тж. как обраще́ние*); 3) молодо́й дворяни́н.

squireling ['skwaɪəlɪŋ] *n* ме́лкий поме́щик.

squirm [skwəːm] *v* извива́ться как червя́к; ко́рчиться.

squirrel ['skwɪrəl, *амер.* 'skəːrəl] *n* 1) бе́лка; 2) *attr* бе́личий; ◊ like a ~ in a cage ≅ как бе́лка в колесе́.

squirt I [skwəːt] *n* 1) шприц; 2) струя́ (*воды*); 3) *разг.* незначи́тельный челове́к.

squirt II *v* 1) пуска́ть струю́; бить струёй; 2) забры́згивать.

St [sənt, sɪnt, snt] *см.* saint.

stab I [stæb] *n* 1) уда́р (*кинжа́лом, штыко́м и т. п.*); a ~ in the back уда́р в спи́ну; преда́тельское нападе́ние; 2) ко́лотая ра́на; 3) внеза́пная о́страя боль.

stab II *v* 1) наноси́ть уда́р, ра́нить (*кинжа́лом, штыко́м; at*); 2) зака́лывать; 3) вонза́ть (*во что́-л.— into*); to ~ in the back всади́ть нож в спи́ну; нанести́ преда́тельский уда́р.

stability [stə'bɪlɪtɪ] *n* 1) про́чность; 2) усто́йчивость, стаби́льность.

stabilization [ˌsteɪbɪlaɪ'zeɪʃən] *n* стабилиза́ция.

stabilize ['steɪbɪlaɪz] *v* стабилизи́ровать(ся).

stabilizer ['steɪbɪlaɪzə] *n ав.* стабилиза́тор.

stable[1] ['steɪbl] *a* 1) про́чный, сто́йкий; 2) усто́йчивый, стаби́льный; 3) постоя́нный.

stable[2] I *n* коню́шня.

stable[2] II *v* помеща́ть, ста́вить в коню́шню.

stable-man ['steɪblmən] *n* ко́нюх.

stack I [stæk] *n* 1) стог (*се́на*); скирда́; 2) ки́па (*бума́г*); 3) *pl* книгохрани́лище; 4) ку́ча, гру́да; a ~ of wood поле́нница (*дров*); 5) дымова́я труба́; ряд труб; 6) *разг.* мно́жество, ма́сса; a whole ~ of work ма́сса рабо́ты; 7) *воен.* винто́вки, соста́вленные в ко́злы; 8) ме́ра дров *или* у́гля (*около 3 м³*).

stack II *v* 1) навива́ть стог; ста́вить в скирды́; копни́ть; 2) громозди́ть, нагроможда́ть.

stackyard ['stækjɑːd] *n* гумно́.

stadium ['steɪdjəm] *n* (*pl тж.* stadia ['steɪdɪə]) стадио́н.

staff[1] I [stɑːf] *n* 1) штат, персона́л; on the ~ в шта́те; editorial ~ редакцио́нная колле́гия;

the ~ of a newspaper сотру́дники газе́ты; 2) *воен.* штаб; General Staff генера́льный штаб; 3) *attr* шта́тный; *воен.* штабно́й.

staff[1] II *v* обеспе́чивать персона́лом.

staff[2] *n* (*pl* staves) 1) па́лка, по́сох; 2) жезл (*си́мвол вла́сти, почётного положе́ния*); 3) дре́вко; ensign ~ кормово́й флагшто́к; 4) опо́ра, осно́ва; 5) *муз.* но́тные лине́йки; ◊ the ~ of life хлеб.

stag I [stæg] *n* 1) оле́нь-саме́ц; 2) *амер. разг.* холостя́к; 3) биржево́й спекуля́нт.

stag II *a* холостя́цкий.

stag III *v* спекули́ровать (*на би́рже*).

stage[1] [steɪdʒ] *n* 1) ста́дия; initial (final) ~ нача́льная (коне́чная) ста́дия; 2) пери́од; 3) фа́за; эта́п; ~ of development эта́п разви́тия; 4) ступе́нь раке́ты.

stage[2] I *n* 1) сце́на, эстра́да, подмо́стки; to be on the ~ быть актёром, актри́сой; to go on the ~ стать актёром, актри́сой, пойти́ на сце́ну; to leave (*или* to quit) the ~ уйти́ со сце́ны; *перен.* умере́ть; to take the ~ уйти́ под аплодисме́нты; 2) теа́тр, драмати́ческое иску́сство; сцени́ческое иску́сство; 3) каре́та, дилижа́нс; 4) платфо́рма; landing ~ при́стань; 5) остано́вка; 6) перего́н, перее́зд; by easy ~s не торопя́сь.

stage[2] II *v* ста́вить (*пье́су*); инсцени́ровать.

stage-coach ['steɪdʒkoutʃ] *n* дилижа́нс, почто́вая каре́та.

stagecraft ['steɪdʒkrɑːft] *n* сцени́ческое иску́сство.

stage-door ['steɪdʒdɔː] *n* служе́бный, актёрский вход в теа́тр.

stagehand ['steɪdʒhænd] *n* рабо́чий сце́ны.

stage-manager ['steɪdʒˌmænɪdʒə] *n* режиссёр.

stage-name ['steɪdʒneɪm] *n* театра́льный псевдони́м.

stagger I ['stægə] *n* 1) пошату́вание; 2) *pl* головокруже́ние.

stagger II ['stægə] *v* 1) идти́ пошату́ваясь, пока́чиваться; 2) дро́гнуть (*о войска́х*); 3) колеба́ться, испы́тывать колеба́ния; 4) расшата́ть; 5) порази́ть, ошеломи́ть; 6) располага́ть зигза́гами; 7) вызыва́ть колеба́ния, сомне́ния.

staging ['steɪdʒɪŋ] *n* 1) постано́вка (*пье́сы*); 2) *стр.* леса́; 3) курси́рование (*дилижа́нсов*).

stagnant ['stægnənt] *a* 1) стоя́чий, засто́йный (*о воде́*); 2) ине́ртный; ко́сный, тупо́й.

stagnate ['stægneɪt] *v* 1) заста́иваться (*о воде́, во́здухе*); 2) (за)косне́ть.

stagy ['steɪdʒɪ] *a* театра́льный, сцени́ческий.

staid [steɪd] *a* степе́нный, благоразу́мный; уравнове́шенный; положи́тельный.

stain I [steɪn] *n* 1) пятно́ (*тж. перен.*); 2) (о)кра́ска; 3) кра́сящее вещество́.

stain II *v* 1) покрыва́ть пя́тнами; па́чкать; 2) кра́сить, окра́шивать; 3) броса́ть тень, позо́рить; пятна́ть.

stainless ['steɪnlɪs] *a* 1) незапя́тнанный, чи́стый; 2) безупре́чный; 3) нержаве́ющий (*о ста́ли*).

stair [steə] *n* 1) ступе́нька (*ле́стницы*); 2) марш (*ле́стницы*); below ~s в полуподва́льном помеще́нии; the top ~ but one предпосле́дний эта́ж; 3) *обыкн. pl* ле́стница; winding ~ винтова́я ле́стница.

staircase ['steəkeɪs] *n* 1) ле́стница; corkscrew ~, spiral ~ винтова́я ле́стница; moving ~ экскала-

тор; principal ~ пара́дная ле́сница; 2) ле́стнич-
ная кле́тка.

stairway ['stɛəweɪ] *n* ле́стница; ле́стничная кле́т-
ка.

stake[1] I [steɪk] *n* 1) столб, кол; at the ~ у по-
зо́рного столба́; 2) сожже́ние на костре́.

stake[1] II *v* 1) отмеча́ть ко́льями; 2) подде́ржи-
вать сто́йками; □ to ~ **down** укрепля́ть сто́й-
ками, ко́льями; to ~ **in** окружа́ть ко́льями; to ~
off, to ~ **out** отмеча́ть грани́цу чего́-л. ве́хами;
to ~ **up** загора́живать ко́льями.

stake[2] I *n* 1) ста́вка (*в игре, на бегах и т. п.*);
for high ~s по большо́й (ста́вке); for low ~s
по ма́ленькой (ста́вке); to be at ~ быть поста́в-
ленным на ка́рту; to put at ~, to set on ~ ста́вить
на ка́рту; 2) пре́мия, приз (*на скачках и т. п.*);
3) до́ля капита́ла в предприя́тии.

stake[2] II *v* ста́вить на ка́рту; рискова́ть чем-л.

stalactite ['stæləktaɪt] *n геол.* сталакти́т.

stalagmite ['stæləgmaɪt] *n геол.* сталагми́т.

stale I [steɪl] *a* 1) чёрствый, засо́хший (*о хлебе*);
2) вы́дохшийся, безвку́сный (*о пиве*); 3) устаре́в-
ший, изби́тый, бана́льный (*о шутке*); 4) потеря́в-
ший све́жесть, си́лу и т. п.; 5) спёртый, тяжёлый
(*о воздухе*).

stale II *v* 1) утра́чивать све́жесть, новизну́;
2) вы́сыхать.

stalemate ['steɪlmeɪt] *n* 1) *шахм.* пат; 2) тупи́к,
безвы́ходное положе́ние.

stalk[1] [stɔːk] *n* 1) сте́бель; 2) фабри́чная труба́.

stalk[2] *v* 1) ше́ствовать; 2) подкра́дываться.

stalking-horse ['stɔːkɪŋhɔːs] *n* пуста́я отгово́рка,
предло́г.

stall[1] I [stɔːl] *n* 1) сто́йло; 2) коню́шня, хлев;
3) кио́ск, ларёк, пала́тка; 4) *pl* места́ в парте́ре
(*первые ряды*).

stall[1] II *v* 1) ста́вить в сто́йло; 2) остана́вливать,
заде́рживать; 3) застрева́ть (*в грязи*).

stall[2] I *n разг.* уве́ртка.

stall[2] II *v разг.* 1) вводи́ть в заблужде́ние;
2) уклоня́ться, обма́нывать.

stallion ['stæljən] *n* жеребе́ц.

stalwart I ['stɔːlwət] *n* 1) челове́к кре́пкого
здоро́вья; 2) сто́йкий член па́ртии.

stalwart II *a* 1) ро́слый, дю́жий, здоро́вый;
2) си́льный, му́жественный; 3) сто́йкий, непоколе-
би́мый.

stamen ['steɪmən] *n* (*pl тж.* stamina) *бот.* ты-
чи́нка.

stamina[1] ['stæmɪnə] *n pl* запа́с жи́зненных сил;
жи́зненная эне́ргия; выно́сливость.

stamina[2] *n pl см.* stamen.

stammer I ['stæmə] *n* заика́ние.

stammer II *v* 1) заика́ться; 2) запина́ться (*от
волнения*); □ to ~ **out** произноси́ть запина́ясь.

stammerer ['stæmərə] *n* заи́ка.

stamp[1] I [stæmp] *n* то́панье (*ногами*).

stamp[1] II *v* 1) топта́ть, выта́птывать; 2) то́пать,
топота́ть (*ногами*); to ~ **out** of a room вы́бежать
с то́потом из ко́мнаты; 3) толо́чь; □ to ~ **down**
притопта́ть; to ~ **out** а) подавля́ть (*восстание*);
б) ликвиди́ровать (*эпидемию*).

stamp[2] I *n* 1) штемпель; печа́ть; postage ~ поч-
то́вая ма́рка; trading ~ торго́вая ма́рка; 2) отпе-
ча́ток; 3) клеймо́, пло́мба.

stamp[2] II *v* 1) ста́вить штемпель, печа́ть; 2) при-

кле́ивать ма́рку; 3) характеризова́ть (*человека*).

stamp-collector ['stæmpkə,lektə] *n* филатели́ст.

stamp-duty ['stæmp,djuːtɪ] *n* ге́рбовый сбор.

stampede I [stæm'piːd] *n* пани́ческое бе́гство.

stampede II *v* 1) броса́ться врассыпну́ю; бежа́ть
в па́нике; 2) обраща́ть в пани́ческое бе́гство.

stanch [stɑːntʃ] *см.* staunch.

stand I [stænd] *n* 1) остано́вка; to be at a ~
быть в тупике́; to put smb. at a ~ поста́вить
кого́-л. в тупи́к; to come to a ~ останови́ться;
to bring to a ~ останови́ть; 2) ме́сто, пози́ция; to
take one's ~ a) заня́ть ме́сто, расположи́ться;
б) осно́вываться (*на чём-л. — on*); опира́ться;
3) стоя́нка (*такси и т. п.*); 4) подста́вка, сто́йка,
этаже́рка; 5) кио́ск, пала́тка; 6) сопротивле́ние;
to make a ~ а) сопротивля́ться (*кому-л. —
against*); б) вы́ступить, стать на защи́ту (*кого-л.—
for*); 7) трибу́на, места́ для зри́телей (*тж.*
grand ~); 8) хлеб на корню́.

stand II *v* (*past, p. p.* stood) 1) стоя́ть; 2) остана́-
вливаться; ~ and deliver! ру́ки вверх!; 3) быть
располо́женным, помеща́ться; 4) держа́ться; 5) по-
ста́вить, помести́ть; 6) прислоня́ть (*к чему-л. —
against*); 7) выноси́ть, выде́рживать (*холод, испытание*); 8) переноси́ть (*человека, манеры, шутки*);
9) быть действи́тельным (*о договоре*); 10) обстоя́ть
(*о делах*); how matters ~ ? как обстоя́т дела́?;
11) не выгора́ть (*об окраске, цвете*); 12) быть
кандида́том (*на должность; for*); 13) угоща́ть,
нести́ расхо́ды (*по угощению*); 14) *в сочетании
с прил. и прич. прош. вр. означает какое-л.
состояние:* to ~ idle не рабо́тать (*о фабрике, заводе*); to ~ convicted (condemned) быть осуждён-
ным (приговорённым); □ to ~ **against** сопро-
тивля́ться; to ~ **aloof** держа́ться пода́ль, в сто-
роне́; не вме́шиваться во что-л.; to ~ **apart** стоя́ть
в стороне́, находи́ться пода́ль; to ~ **aside** отойти́
в сто́рону; to ~ **back** а) держа́ться позади́;
б) отступи́ть; to ~ **behind** отстава́ть; to ~ **between** быть посре́дником; to ~ **by** а) подде́ржи-
вать, стоя́ть за что-л.; б) остава́ться ве́рным (*до-
говору, обещанию*); в) быть зри́телем, свиде́телем;
to ~ **for** а) стоя́ть за что-л., подде́рживать;
б) означа́ть, символизи́ровать; to ~ **in** стои́ть;
б) принима́ть уча́стие; в) *мор.* заходи́ть в порт;
to ~ **off** а) держа́ться на расстоя́нии; б) выходи́ть
в мо́ре; to ~ **on** а) зави́сеть от чего́-л.; б) соб-
люда́ть до мелоче́й; в) тре́бовать уваже́ния (*к пра-
вам, достоинству*); г) *мор.* держа́ться пре́жнего
ку́рса; to ~ **out** а) выдава́ться; б) выделя́ться, вы-
рисо́вываться (*на фоне чего-л.; against*); в) упо́р-
ствовать, наста́ивать; г) выходи́ть в мо́ре; to ~
over откла́дывать (*заседание, рассмотрение*);
to ~ **up** а) встава́ть; б) стоя́ть, боро́ться (*за
что-л. — for*); to ~ **upon** наста́ивать; ◊ it ~s to
reason э́то соверше́нно я́сно, бесспо́рно, очеви́дно;
to ~ to lose идти́ на ве́рное пораже́ние; to ~ to
win име́ть все ша́нсы на вы́игрыш.

standard I ['stændəd] *n* 1) станда́рт, типово́й
образе́ц; мери́ло; но́рма; the ~ of living жи́знен-
ный у́ровень; the ~ of culture культу́рный у́ро-
вень; the ~ of education образова́тельный у́ро-
вень; 2) курс (*валютной системы*); gold ~ по зо-
лото́му ку́рсу; 3) зна́мя, флаг; 4) сто́йка.

standard II *a* 1) станда́ртный, типово́й; образцо́вый; 2) стаби́льный (*об учебнике*); 3) стоя́чий; 4) шта́мбовый (*о растениях*).

standard-bearer [ˈstændəd͵bɛərə] *n* знамено́сец.

standardize [ˈstændədaɪz] *v* стандартизи́ровать.

stand-by [ˈstændbaɪ] *n* 1) горя́чий сторо́нник; 2) опо́ра.

standee [stænˈdiː] *n амер. разг.* стоя́щий пассажи́р *и т. п.*

stand-in [ˈstændɪn] *n* подме́на, заме́на (*актёра*).

standing I [ˈstændɪŋ] *n* 1) положе́ние; social ~ социа́льное положе́ние; of good ~ занима́ющий хоро́шую до́лжность; of high ~ высокопоста́вленный; 2) дли́тельность; продолжи́тельность; of long ~ а) дли́тельный, давни́шний; б) застаре́лый (*о болезни*).

standing II *a* 1) стоя́щий; 2) постоя́нный, устано́вленный; 3) *воен.* регуля́рный; 4) неизме́нный (*о пище*); 5) неистощи́мый.

stand-offish [ˈstændˈɔfɪʃ] *a* холо́дный, сде́ржанный.

standpoint [ˈstændpɔɪnt] *n* то́чка зре́ния.

standstill [ˈstændstɪl] *n* 1) зати́шье; 2) остано́вка; безде́йствие; засто́й; to be at a ~ быть в безде́йствии, засто́е; to come to a ~ останови́ться, засто́порить; зайти́ в тупи́к; to bring to a ~ останови́ть, засто́порить.

stand-up [ˈstændʌp] *a* 1) стоя́чий (*о воротнике*); 2) откры́тый (*о борьбе*); 3) стоя, на ходу́ (*о еде*).

stank [stæŋk] *past см.* stink II.

stannic [ˈstænɪk] *a* оловя́нный.

stanza [ˈstænzə] *n* строфа́, станс.

staple[1] I [ˈsteɪpl] *n* 1) скре́пка (*для сшивания бумаг*); 2) скоба́, крюк.

staple[1] II *v* скрепля́ть.

staple[2] I *n* 1) основно́й проду́кт (*производимый в данной местности*); 2) гла́вный предме́т торго́вли; това́ры (*имеющие постоянный спрос*); 3) гла́вная, основна́я черта́; the ~ of conversation основна́я те́ма разгово́ра; 4) *текст.* ка́чество волокна́.

staple[2] II *a* гла́вный, основно́й.

staple[2] III *v* сортирова́ть, отбира́ть.

star I [stɑː] *n* 1) звезда́, звёздочка; свети́ло; fixed ~ неподви́жная звезда́; shooting ~, falling ~ па́дающая звезда́; метео́р; guiding ~ *перен.* путево́дная звезда́; the Red Star о́рден Кра́сной Звезды́; ~s and stripes национа́льный флаг США; I saw ~s у меня́ и́скры из глаз посы́пались; 2) судьба́, рок; his ~ has (*или* is) set его́ звезда́ закати́лась; his ~ is in the ascendant его́ звезда́ восхо́дит; to thank (*или* to bless) one's ~s благословля́ть судьбу́; to trust one's ~s ве́рить в свою́ звезду́; 3) знамени́тость, знамени́тый актёр *или* актри́са; кинозвезда́; 4) *attr* звёздный.

star II *v* 1) украша́ть звёздами; 2) *театр.* быть веду́щим актёром; то ~ игра́ть гла́вную роль.

starboard I [ˈstɑːbəd] *n мор.* 1) пра́вый борт су́дна; 2) *attr* правобортово́й.

starboard II *v мор.* класть руль напра́во.

starch I [stɑːtʃ] *n* 1) крахма́л; 2) церемо́нность, чо́порность; 3) *амер. разг.* жи́зненная эне́ргия; живу́честь.

starch II *v* крахма́лить (*тж.* to ~ up).

starchy [ˈstɑːtʃɪ] *a* 1) содержа́щий крахма́л; 2) накрахма́ленный; 3) чо́порный; мане́рный.

stare I [stɛə] *n* 1) изумлённый взгляд; взгляд широко́ раскры́тых глаз; cold ~ холо́дный взгляд;

glassy ~ безжи́зненный, стекля́нный взгляд; stony ~ ка́менный, тяжёлый взгляд; vacant ~ отсу́тствующий взгляд; 2) при́стальный взгляд; де́рзкий взгляд.

stare II *v* 1) смотре́ть изумлённо *или* при́стально; тара́щить глаза́ (*на что-л.*— at; от изумления, испуга; with); to ~ down (*или* out) of countenance смути́ть кого́-л. при́стальным взгля́дом; to ~ smb. in the face a) уста́виться на кого́-л.; б) быть очеви́дным, я́вным (*о факте*); в) быть немину́емым, неотврати́мым (*о волосах, перьях*); 2) топо́рщиться (*о волосах, перьях*).

starfish [ˈstɑːfɪʃ] *n зоол.* морска́я звезда́.

star-gazer [ˈstɑː͵ɡeɪzə] *n шутл.* 1) звездочёт; 2) мечта́тель.

staring [ˈstɛərɪŋ] *a* крича́щий, я́ркий, броса́ющийся в глаза́.

stark I [stɑːk] *a* 1) абсолю́тный, по́лный; 2) окоченѐвший.

stark II *adv* соверше́нно.

starlet [ˈstɑːlɪt] *n* звёздочка.

starlight [ˈstɑːlaɪt] *n* 1) свет звёзд; by ~ при звёздах; 2) *attr* звёздный.

starling [ˈstɑːlɪŋ] *n* скворе́ц.

starlit [ˈstɑːlɪt] *a* звёздный, освещённый звёздами.

starred [stɑːd] *a* 1) усе́янный, усы́панный звёздами; 2) укра́шенный звездо́й; 3) с отме́тиной на лбу (*о животном*).

starry [ˈstɑːrɪ] *a* 1) усе́янный звёздами; 2) звёздный; 3) лучи́стый.

star-spangled [ˈstɑː͵spæŋɡld] *a* сия́ющий, усе́янный звёздами.

star-studded [ˈstɑː͵stʌdɪd] *a* усы́панный звёздами.

start I [stɑːt] *n* 1) отправле́ние, нача́ло движе́ния; *спорт.* старт; 2) нача́ло; to make a ~ нача́ть, приступи́ть; to make a good ~ положи́ть хоро́шее нача́ло; to give a ~ in life *перен.* помо́чь встать на́ ноги; 3) вздра́гивание (*от испуга*); to awake with a ~ внеза́пно просну́ться; to give smb. a ~ заста́вить кого́-л. вздро́гнуть; напуга́ть кого́-л.; 4) рыво́к; 5) преиму́щество (*перед кем-л.*— of); you have got the ~ of me у вас есть преиму́щество пе́редо мной.

start II *v* 1) отправля́ться, уезжа́ть (*куда-л.*— for); 2) начина́ть жизнь, карье́ру (*тж.* to ~ out); 3) начина́ть (*дело, разговор и т. п.*); приступа́ть к чему́-л.; to ~ with... нача́ть с того́...; 4) начина́ться (*о процессе, спектакле и т. п.*); 5) пуска́ть (*машину*); тро́гать(ся) с ме́ста (*о поезде, трамвае и т. п.*); 6) вздро́гнуть; 7) бро́ситься; вы́скочить; 8) вскочи́ть; to ~ in one's seat привскочи́ть на сту́ле; 9) учрежда́ть (*газету, журнал*); 10) открыва́ть (*магазин*); 11) покоро́биться (*о дереве*); 12) спугну́ть (*дичь*); подня́ть (*зверя*); 13) *ав.* взлета́ть; □ to ~ **aside** отскочи́ть в сто́рону; to ~ **back** отпря́нуть, отскочи́ть наза́д; to ~ **in** начина́ть, принима́ться за что-л.; to ~ **out** собира́ться сде́лать что-л.; to ~ **up** a) вскочи́ть; б) возни́кнуть, появля́ться (*об идее*).

starter [ˈstɑːtə] *n* ста́ртер.

starting [ˈstɑːtɪŋ] *a* 1) отправно́й (*о пункте*); 2) пусково́й (*о механизме*).

startle I [ˈstɑːtl] *n*: with a ~ в испу́ге, вздро́гнув.

startle II *v* 1) поража́ть, ужаса́ть; 2) напуга́ть; 3) вздра́гивать (*от ужаса*).

startler ['stɑːtlə] *n* 1) сенсацио́нное сообще́ние, сенса́ция.

startling ['stɑːtlɪŋ] *a* ужаса́ющий, потряса́ющий; порази́тельный.

starvation [stɑːˈveɪʃən] *n* 1) голода́ние; го́лод; 2) голодо́вка; 3) голо́дная смерть.

starve [stɑːv] *v* 1) голода́ть, жить впро́голодь; умира́ть от го́лода; I am simply starving я ужа́сно го́лоден; 2) мори́ть го́лодом; *перен.* истоща́ть; to ~ to death замори́ть до́ смерти; to ~ into surrender взять измо́ром; 3) жа́ждать (*чего-л.— for*).

starveling ['stɑːvlɪŋ] *n* замо́рыш.

state[1] I [steɪt] *n* 1) состоя́ние, положе́ние; weightless ~ состоя́ние невесо́мости; the ~ of emergency чрезвыча́йное положе́ние; the ~ of mind душе́вное состоя́ние; the ~ of life о́браз жи́зни, укла́д жи́зни; what a ~ you are in! в како́м вы ви́де!; 2) фо́рма, структу́ра, фа́за; in liquid ~ в жи́дком состоя́нии; in nascent ~ *хим.* в моме́нт образова́ния; 3) великоле́пие, пы́шность; in great ~ о́чень торже́ственно, с большо́й по́мпой; to lie in ~ быть вы́ставленным для проща́ния (*о покойнике*); to receive in ~ устра́ивать торже́ственный приём.

state[1] II *a* 1) торже́ственный; пара́дный; 2) церемониа́льный.

state[2] *v* 1) сообщи́ть, заяви́ть; 2) формули́ровать, констати́ровать; 3) излага́ть.

state[3] I *n* 1) госуда́рство; socialist ~ социалисти́ческое госуда́рство; buffer ~ бу́ферное госуда́рство; 2) штат; States General *ист.* Генера́льные шта́ты; the States Соединённые Шта́ты (*Америки*); Federal States Федера́льные шта́ты (*в гражданской войне 1861—1865 гг. в Аме́рике*); ◊ the Empire State штат Нью-Йо́рк.

state[3] II *a* 1) госуда́рственный; 2) относя́щийся к шта́ту (*в отличие от* federal).

statecraft ['steɪtkrɑːft] *n* уме́ние управля́ть госуда́рством.

stated ['steɪtɪd] *a* 1) устано́вленный; 2) определённый.

stately ['steɪtlɪ] *a* вели́чественный; велича́вый.

statement ['steɪtmənt] *n* 1) сообще́ние; заявле́ние; утвержде́ние; to make a ~ сде́лать сообще́ние, сообщи́ть; (официа́льно) заяви́ть; specific ~ определённо сформули́рованное утвержде́ние; a sweeping ~ огу́льное утвержде́ние; 2) официа́льный отчёт; бюллете́нь.

stateroom ['steɪtrum] *n* 1) пара́дный зал (*для торжественных приёмов*); 2) отде́льная каю́та; 3) *амер.* отде́льное купе́.

statesman ['steɪtsmən] *n* 1) госуда́рственный де́ятель; 2) *амер.* полити́ческий де́ятель.

station I ['steɪʃən] *n* 1) ме́сто, местоположе́ние, пункт; polling ~ избира́тельный уча́сток; clearing ~ эвакуацио́нный пункт; dressing ~ перевя́зочный пункт; lifeboat ~ спаса́тельная ста́нция; postal ~ *амер.* почто́вое отделе́ние; service ~ а) бензоколо́нка; б) электроремо́нтная мастерска́я; в) радиомастерска́я; 2) железнодоро́жная ста́нция; junction ~ узлова́я ста́нция; railway ~ вокза́л; *радио* ста́нция; radar ~ радиолокацио́нная ста́нция; wireless ~ радиоста́н-

ция; 4) остано́вка (трамва́я), стоя́нка автомоби́лей; 5) полице́йский уча́сток (*тж.* police-station); 6) *воен.* форт, пост; *мор.* вое́нно-морска́я ба́за (*тж.* naval ~); 7) ста́нция; astronomical ~ астрономи́ческая обсервато́рия; launch ~, take-off ~ пускова́я ста́нция; observing ~ ста́нция для наблюде́ния; refuelling ~ запра́вочная ста́нция; 8) овцево́дческая фе́рма (*в Австралии*); 9) обще́ственное положе́ние; in a humble ~ скро́много доста́тка (*о человеке*); 10) *attr* станцио́нный.

station II *v* 1) ста́вить, помеща́ть (*куда-л.*); 2) *воен.* размеща́ть, располага́ть.

stationary ['steɪʃnərɪ] *a* 1) неподви́жный; непередвижно́й, непереносный; 2) постоя́нный; усто́йчивый; 3) стациона́рный; 4) позицио́нный (*о войне*); 5) ме́стный (*о войсках*).

stationer ['steɪʃnə] *n* 1) торго́вец канцеля́рскими принадле́жностями; 2) *уст.* книгоизда́тель.

stationery ['steɪʃnərɪ] *n* 1) канцеля́рские принадле́жности; 2) почто́вая бума́га; 3) писчебума́жный магази́н.

station-house ['steɪʃənhaus] *n* зда́ние поли́ции.

station-master ['steɪʃənˌmɑːstə] *n* нача́льник ста́нции.

statistical [stəˈtɪstɪkəl] *a* статисти́ческий.

statistician [ˌstætɪsˈtɪʃən] *n* стати́стик.

statistics [stəˈtɪstɪks] *n* стати́стика.

statuary I ['stætjuərɪ] *n* 1) скульпту́ра; 2) ску́льптор.

statuary II *a* скульпту́рный.

statue ['stætjuː] *n* ста́туя, извая́ние.

statuette [ˌstætjuˈet] *n* статуэ́тка.

stature ['stætʃə] *n* 1) рост; of high (mean) ~ высо́кого (сре́днего) ро́ста; to grow in ~ расти́; 2) высота́ (*предмета*); 3) ва́жность; це́нность.

status ['steɪtəs] *n* 1) положе́ние, состоя́ние дел; 2) обще́ственное положе́ние; 3) юриди́ческое положе́ние, ста́тус.

statute ['stætjuːt] *n* 1) законода́тельный акт, стату́т, узаконе́ние; 2) уста́в (*учреждения, учебного заведения*).

statute-book ['stætjuːtbuk] *n* свод зако́нов.

statutory ['stætjutərɪ] *a* устано́вленный зако́ном, узако́ненный.

staunch[1] [stɔːntʃ] *a* 1) ве́рный, пре́данный, лоя́льный; 2) твёрдый, сто́йкий, непоколеби́мый; 3) непроница́емый (*для жидкости*); 4) упо́рный (*о сопротивлении*).

staunch[2] *v* остана́вливать (*кровь*).

stave I [steɪv] *n* 1) боча́рная доска́, клёпка; 2) перекла́дина (*приставной лестницы*); 3) строфа́ (*стихотворения*); 4) *муз.* но́тные лине́йки.

stave II *v* (*past, p. p.* stove) 1) to ~ in проломи́ть (*бочку, лодку и т. п.*); to ~ off а) отвести́ (*опасность*); предотврати́ть (*болезнь*); б) оття́гивать (*платежи, выполнение работы*).

staves [steɪvz] *pl см.* staff[2].

stay[1] I [steɪ] *n* 1) пребыва́ние; срок пребыва́ния; to make a ~ пробы́ть, погости́ть; to make a short ~ пробы́ть недо́лго; 2) остано́вка, стоя́нка; 3) *юр.* приостано́вка судопроизво́дства.

stay[1] II *v* 1) остава́ться, пребыва́ть; ~ a moment побу́дьте ещё немно́го; 2) останови́ться, жить, гости́ть (*где-л.— at; у кого-л.— with*); 3) *разг.* вы́держать, вы́носить; 4) *юр.* приостана́вливать судопроизво́дство; 5) утоля́ть (*голод*); 6) оста-

ваться (*на обед, спектакль; for*); □ to ~ **away**
не приходи́ть, не явля́ться (*куда-л.— from*);
to ~ **in** сиде́ть до́ма, не выходи́ть; to ~ **on** задержа́ться, пробы́ть до́льше, чем предполага́лось;
to ~ **out** a) отсу́тствовать (*не быть до́ма*); быть
в гостя́х; б) пересиде́ть (*других госте́й*); to ~ **up**
дожида́ться прихо́да (*не ложа́сь спать*).

stay² **I** *n* 1) подпо́рка; 2) *pl* корсе́т
(*тж.* a pair of ~s); 3) опо́ра, подде́ржка; 4) *мор.*
штаг; ле́ер (*для па́руса*); in ~s в бейдеви́нд.

stay² **II** *v* 1) подпира́ть (*тж.* to ~ **up**); 2) поддержи́вать, подкрепля́ть тро́сами (*часто* to ~ **up**); 4) *мор.* де́лать поворо́т овершта́г.

stay-at-home **I** [ˈsteɪəthoum] *n* домосе́д.

stay-at-home **II** *a* домосе́длlivый.

stayer [ˈsteɪə] *n* выно́сливый челове́к *или* живо́тное.

stead [sted] *n:* in my (his, your *etc*) ~ вме́сто
меня́ (него́, вас *и т. п.*); to stand smb. in good ~
сослужи́ть слу́жбу, оказа́ться поле́зным кому́-л.

steadfast [ˈstedfəst] *a* 1) усто́йчивый; про́чный;
2) сто́йкий, непоколеби́мый, твёрдый; 3) неподви́жный, при́стальный (*о взгля́де*).

steady **I** [ˈstedɪ] *a* 1) усто́йчивый, надёжный;
2) постоя́нный; упо́рный; 3) равноме́рный, непреры́вный; 4) установи́вшийся, сложи́вшийся (*об
убежде́ниях*); 5) уравнове́шенный; ро́вный (*в обраще́нии*); 6) че́стный, тре́звый; 7) при́стальный
(*о взгля́де*); 8) неукло́нный; твёрдый (*о руке́, руково́дстве*); 9): keep her ~! та́к держа́ть! (*кома́нда*); ~! осторо́жнее!

steady **II** *v* стабилизи́ровать(ся), де́лать(ся)
усто́йчивым.

steak [steɪk] *n* то́нкий кусо́к (*мя́са, ры́бы, тж.
жа́реный*).

steal **I** [stiːl] *n* 1) кра́жа, покра́жа; 2) *разг.*
кра́деная вещь; 3) *разг.* вещь, доста́вшаяся с
больши́м трудо́м.

steal **II** *v* (*past* stole; *p. p.* stolen) 1) красть,
укра́сть, утащи́ть (*у кого́-л. — from*); ворова́ть;
2) доби́ться чего́-л. тайко́м; 3) похища́ть;
4) кра́дучись войти́ (*куда́-л.— into*); □ to ~
away незаме́тно ускользну́ть, исче́знуть; to ~
by проскользну́ть; пролете́ть (*о года́х*); to ~ **in**
a) незаме́тно войти́; б) вкра́сться (*в дове́рие*);
to ~ **out** улизну́ть; to ~ **past** проскользну́ть;
to ~ **up** подкра́сться.

stealing [ˈstiːlɪŋ] *n* 1) воровство́; 2) *pl* кра́деные
ве́щи.

stealth [stelθ] *n:* by ~ укра́дкой, втихомо́лку,
тайко́м.

stealthily [ˈstelθɪlɪ] *adv* укра́дкой, та́йно, втихомо́лку.

stealthy [ˈstelθɪ] *a* 1) та́йный, скры́тый;
2) бесшу́мный (*о шага́х*).

steam **I** [stiːm] *n* 1) пар; with full ~ on a) на
всех пара́х; б) со всех ног; to blow off ~ выпуска́ть
пар; to get up ~ разводи́ть пары́; *перен.* развива́ть эне́ргию; to let off ~ спуска́ть пар; *перен.*
дать вы́ход свои́м чу́вствам; to put on ~ подба́вить па́ру; to turn on ~ впусти́ть пар; to shut
off ~ закры́ть пар; dead ~ отрабо́танный пар;
dry ~ сухо́й пар; live ~ све́жий пар; saturated
~, wet ~ насы́щенный пар; 2) испаре́ние;
3) *разг.* си́ла, эне́ргия; 4) *attr* парово́й; приводи́мый в движе́ние па́ром.

steam **II** *v* 1) дава́ть пар; 2) превраща́ться в пар;
3) поднима́ться (*о па́ре, испаре́ниях*); 4) запотева́ть, отпотева́ть; 5) дви́гаться (*под де́йствием
па́ра*); 6) вари́ть на пару́, туши́ть; □ to ~
ahead, to ~ **along** продвига́ться вперёд (*энерги́чно*); to ~ **away** a) идти́ хоро́шим хо́дом; б) выкипа́ть; to ~ **into**: to ~ into the harbour входи́ть
в порт, га́вань; to ~ **out**: to ~ out of the harbour
выходи́ть из по́рта, га́вани.

steamboat [ˈstiːmbout] *n* парохо́д.

steam-boiler [ˈstiːmˌbɔɪlə] *n* парово́й котёл.

steam-engine [ˈstiːmˌendʒɪn] *n* парова́я маши́на;
парово́й дви́гатель.

steamer [ˈstiːmə] *n* 1) парохо́д; 2) котёл для
ва́рки на пару́.

steam-gauge [ˈstiːmgeɪdʒ] *n* мано́метр.

steam-navvy [ˈstiːmˌnævɪ] *n* землечерпа́лка.

steam-roller [ˈstiːmˌroulə] *n* парово́й като́к.

steamship [ˈstiːmʃɪp] *n* парохо́д.

steamy [ˈstiːmɪ] *a* 1) парообра́зный; 2) отпотéвший, запоте́вший.

steed [stiːd] *n поэт.* конь; gallant ~ бо́рзый
конь.

steel **I** [stiːl] *n* 1) сталь; stainless ~ нержаве́ющая сталь; 2) *поэт.* меч, шпа́га; cold ~ холо́дное
ору́жие; 3) планше́тка (*в корсе́те*).

steel **II** *a* стально́й; *перен.* жесто́кий, неумоли́мый.

steel **III** *v* 1) покрыва́ть ста́лью; 2) закаля́ть;
ожесточа́ть; to ~ oneself a) ожесточа́ться, закаля́ться (*против чего́-л.— against*); б) приуча́ть
себя́ (*к чему́-л.— to*).

steel-clad [ˈstiːlklæd] *a* зако́ванный в броню́,
покры́тый бронёй.

steelworks [ˈstiːlwəːks] *n* сталелите́йный заво́д.

steely [ˈstiːlɪ] *a* 1) стально́й; сде́ланный из
ста́ли; 2) твёрдый как сталь; непрекло́нный.

steep **I** [stiːp] *a* 1) круто́й, отве́сный; 2) *разг.*
невероя́тный, чрезме́рный; непоме́рный.

steep **II** *n* крутизна́; круча́.

steep **III** *v* 1) выма́чивать, пропи́тывать жи́дкостью;
2) наста́ивать (*чай и т. п.*); 3) погружа́ть; *перен.*
уходи́ть с голово́й (*в нау́ку и т. п.*); 4) погря́знуть
(*в предрассу́дках и т. п.*).

steepen [ˈstiːpən] *n* станови́ться кру́че.

steeple [ˈstiːpl] *n* 1) колоко́льня, ба́шня со
шпи́лем; 2) шпиль.

steeplechase [ˈstiːpltʃeɪs] *n* ска́чки с препя́тствиями; бег по пересечённой ме́стности.

steeple-jack [ˈstiːpldʒæk] *n* верхола́з.

steer¹ [stɪə] *v* 1) управля́ть (*автомоби́лем*);
вести́ (*кора́бль*); 2) держа́ть курс; направля́ть;
to ~ clear of избега́ть; 3) слу́шаться управле́ния;
4) *разг.* заправля́ть, руководи́ть.

steer² *n* бычо́к, молодо́й вол.

steerage [ˈstɪərɪdʒ] *n* 1) рулево́е устро́йство;
2) управле́ние (*корабля́*); 3) помеще́ние для
па́лубных пассажи́ров; четвёртый класс.

steering-wheel [ˈstɪərɪŋwiːl] *n ав., мор.* штурва́л.

steersman [ˈstɪəzmən] *n* 1) рулево́й; шту́рман;
2) води́тель.

steeve **I** [stiːv] *n* подъёмный кран.

steeve **II** *v* пло́тно загружа́ть.

stellar [ˈstelə] *a* звёздный.

stem¹ **I** [stem] *n* 1) сте́бель; ствол; 2) черено́к;
3) но́жка (*рю́мки*); 4) голо́вка (*карма́нных часо́в*); 5) род, пле́мя; 6) *грам.* осно́ва (*сло́ва*);

7) нос (*корабля*); from ~ to stern от но́са до кормы́; *перен.* от нача́ла до конца́; наскво́зь.

stem¹ II *v* происходи́ть, брать нача́ло (*от — from*).

stem² *v* 1) остана́вливать; 2) запру́живать; 3) затыка́ть, заде́лывать (*дыру, отверстие*); 4) идти́, дви́гаться про́тив тече́ния, ве́тра *и т. п.*; *перен. тж.* сопротивля́ться.

stench [stentʃ] *n* вонь, злово́ние.

stencil I ['stensl] *n* трафаре́т, шабло́н.

stencil II *v* раскра́шивать (*по шабло́ну*).

stenographer [ste'nɔgrəfə] *n* стенографи́ст(ка).

stenography [ste'nɔgrəfi] *n* стеногра́фия.

stentorian [sten'tɔːriən] *a* громово́й, зы́чный (*о го́лосе*).

step I [step] *n* 1) шаг; *перен. тж.* посту́пок; ме́ра; in ~ в но́гу; out of ~ не в но́гу; ~ by ~ шаг за ша́гом; in his ~s *перен.* по его́ стопа́м; to keep ~ (with) идти́ в но́гу; поспева́ть за кем-л.; to break ~ сби́ться с ноги́, идти́ не в но́гу; to take ~s принима́ть ме́ры, предпринима́ть шаги́; false ~ оши́бка, ло́жный шаг; 2) *pl* шаги́, звук шаго́в; 3) след ноги́; 4) па (*в та́нцах*); 5) ступе́нька; подно́жка; 6) ранг, чин; 7) ступе́нь (*многоступе́нчатой раке́ты*).

step II *v* 1) шага́ть, ступа́ть; де́лать шаги́; to ~ it а) идти́, ходи́ть; б) танцева́ть; to ~ after smb. сле́довать за кем-л., идти́ по стопа́м кого́-л.; to ~ back а) сде́лать шаг наза́д, отступи́ть; б) верну́ться; 2) измеря́ть шага́ми; 3) де́лать па (*в та́нцах*); ☐ to ~ aside отойти́ в сто́рону, посторони́ться; *перен.* уступи́ть кому́-л. доро́гу; to ~ down спусти́ться, сойти́ (*вниз*); to ~ forth а) сде́лать шаг вперёд; подви́нуться, вы́ступить вперёд; б) вы́йти (*из — from*); to ~ forward *см.* to ~ forth а); to ~ in, to ~ into а) входи́ть, вступа́ть; б) вступа́ться, вме́шиваться (*во что-л.*); to ~ off а) сходи́ть (*с парохо́да, самолёта*); б) *амер. сленг* сде́лать оши́бку; в) умере́ть; to ~ out а) выходи́ть; б) шага́ть, спеши́ть; to ~ over перешагну́ть, переступи́ть; пройти́ че́рез; to ~ short не рассчита́ть ша́га; to ~ up а) поднима́ться; б) подходи́ть; в) продвига́ть; г) увели́чивать; ◊ to ~ on it *сленг* спеши́ть; поддáть хóду; поднажа́ть.

stepbrother ['step,brʌðə] *n* сво́дный брат.

stepchild ['steptʃaild] *n* па́сынок, па́дчерица.

stepdaughter ['step,dɔːtə] *n* па́дчерица.

stepfather ['step,fɑːðə] *n* о́тчим.

step-ladder ['step,lædə] *n* ле́стница-стремя́нка.

stepmother ['step,mʌðə] *n* ма́чеха.

steppe [step] *n* степь.

stepsister ['step,sistə] *n* сво́дная сестра́.

stepson ['stepsʌn] *n* па́сынок.

stereometry [,stiəri'ɔmitri] *n* стереоме́трия.

stereoscope ['stiəriəskoup] *n* стереоско́п.

stereoscopic [,stiəriəs'kɔpik] *a* стереоскопи́ческий.

stereotype I ['stiəriətaip] *n* стереоти́п.

stereotype II *a* стереоти́пный.

stereotype III *v* 1) стереотипи́ровать; 2) печа́тать со стереоти́па.

sterile ['sterail] *a* 1) беспло́дный; 2) стери́льный.

sterility [ste'riliti] *n* 1) беспло́дие; 2) стери́льность.

sterilization [,sterilai'zeiʃən] *n* стерилиза́ция.

sterilize ['sterilaiz] *v* стерилизова́ть.

sterling ['stəːliŋ] *a* 1) полнове́сный, полноце́нный; £5 ~ пять фу́нтов сте́рлингов; 2) первокла́ссный; надёжный; 3) *эк.* сте́рлинговый; в фу́нтах сте́рлингов.

stern¹ [stəːn] *a* 1) стро́гий, суро́вый; 2) непрекло́нный, неумоли́мый.

stern² *n* 1) *мор.* корма́; 2) хвост (*живо́тного, осо́б. го́нчей*); 3) *attr мор.* кормово́й, за́дний.

stevedore ['stiːvidɔː] *n* портóвый гру́зчик.

stew I [stjuː] *n* 1) тушёное мя́со *или* ры́ба; 2) волне́ние; to be in a ~ быть в волне́нии, в раздраже́нии; быть, сиде́ть как на иго́лках; to get into a ~ разволнова́ться.

stew II *v* 1) туши́ть(ся); вари́ть(ся) на сла́бом огне́; 2) изнемога́ть от жары́; ◊ to ~ in one's own juice а) вари́ться в со́бственном соку́; б) пожина́ть плоды́ соде́янного.

steward ['stjuəd] *n* 1) стю́ард, официа́нт (*на парохо́де, самолёте*); 2) заве́дующий хозя́йством, эконо́м; 3) управля́ющий (*до́мом, име́нием*); 4) распоряди́тель (*ба́ла, ска́чек, вы́ставки и т. п.*).

stewardess ['stjuədis] *n* го́рничная, официа́нтка (*на парохо́де*); стюарде́сса, бортпроводни́ца (*на самолёте*).

stew-pan ['stjuːpæn] *n* кастрю́ля для туше́ния (*мя́са, овоще́й и т. п.*).

stick I [stik] *n* 1) па́лка, па́лочка; walking ~ трость, тро́сточка; he wants a ~ *перен.* он заслу́живает па́лки; ~ of chocolate пли́тка шокола́да; 2) ру́чка, рукоя́тка; 3) жезл, по́сох; 4) дирижёрская па́лочка; 5) *разг.* дура́к, тупи́ца, дуби́на; ◊ to hop the ~ внеза́пно умере́ть; to cut one's ~ уйти́, удра́ть; in a cleft ~ в безвы́ходном положе́нии, в тупике́.

stick II *v* (*past, p. p.* stuck) 1) втыка́ть, вонза́ть; утыка́ть; наса́живать; 2) коло́ть, зака́лывать; 3) сова́ть, помеща́ть, ста́вить; 4) кле́ить, прикле́ивать; закле́ивать(ся); 5) пристава́ть, прилипа́ть; 6) держа́ться (*чего-л.*), упо́рствовать (*в чём-л*); быть ве́рным (*дру́гу, до́лгу, сло́ву и т. п.*; *to*); 7) завя́знуть; застрева́ть (*тж.* to ~ fast); to ~ in, to ~ indoors all day торча́ть до́ма це́лый день; to ~ upon one's memory оста́ться, запечатле́ться в па́мяти; 8) *сленг* терпе́ть, сноси́ть; to ~ it (out) терпели́во вы́держать, снести́; 9) упо́рно, насто́йчиво продолжа́ть (*что-л. — at*); to ~ at a piece of work упо́рно продолжа́ть рабо́тать; 10) колеба́ться (*перед — at*); to ~ at trifles остана́вливаться на мелоча́х; to ~ at nothing ни пе́ред чем не остана́вливаться; ☐ to ~ on: to ~ it on *сленг* а) назнача́ть сли́шком высо́кую це́ну; б) преувели́чивать; to ~ out а) выcóвывать(ся); выпя́чивать(ся); торча́ть; б) наста́ивать (*на чём-л. — for*); to ~ up а) торча́ть, выдава́ться; б) ста́вить торчко́м; в) *сленг* ста́вить в тупи́к; stuck up в замеша́тельстве; г) (о)гра́бить; д) защища́ть (*for*); е) ока́зывать сопротивле́ние (*to*).

sticker ['stikə] *n* *разг.* 1) колю́чка, шип; 2) клей, кле́йкое вещество́; 3) афи́ша; 4) приве́рженец; 5) засиде́вшийся гость; 6) залежа́вшийся това́р; 7) бастý́ющий рабо́чий.

stickiness ['stikinis] *n* ли́пкость.

sticking-plaster ['stikiŋ,plɑːstə] *n* ли́пкий пла́стырь.

stickler [ˈstɪklə] *n* 1) упря́мый спо́рщик; 2) я́рый сторо́нник; защи́тник.

sticky [ˈstɪkɪ] *a* 1) ли́пкий, кле́йкий; 2) ду́шный; 3) непреклóнный; 4) *сленг* неприя́тный; he'll come to a ~ end он пло́хо кóнчит.

stiff I [stɪf] *a* 1) жёсткий, тугóй; твёрдый; неги́бкий, негну́щийся; 2) окостенéвший, окоченéвший, одеревенéлый; I feel ~ у меня́ нóет всё тéло; 3) свя́занный (*о движениях*); принуждённый, натя́нутый; официáльный; 4) реши́тельный, непреклóнный; упóрный; 5) трýдный, нелёгкий; 6) си́льный (*о ветре*); 7) крутóй (*о подъёме*); 8) крéпкий (*о напитке*); 9) высóкий, чрезмéрный (*о цене*); 10) густóй, нежи́дкий; ◊ ~ as a ramrod чóпорный, надмéнный.

stiff II *n сленг* 1) *pl* цéнные бумáги; 2) фальши́вая банкнóта; 3) труп; 4) *амер.* неисправи́мый человéк.

stiffen [ˈstɪfn] *v* 1) дéлать(ся) туги́м; придавáть *или* приобретáть жёсткость; 2) (о)коченéть; (о)костенéть; (о)деревенéть; 3) подкрепля́ть; уси́ливать(ся); 4) густéть, сгущáть.

stiff-necked [ˈstɪfˈnekt] *a* упря́мый.

stifle [ˈstaɪfl] *v* 1) души́ть; 2) подавля́ть; 3) гаси́ть; *перен.* замя́ть (*дело*); 4) задыхáться.

stifling [ˈstaɪflɪŋ] *a* ду́шный.

stigma [ˈstɪgmə] *n* пятнó, позóр.

stigmata [ˈstɪgmətə] *n pl мед., рел.* сти́гмы, стигмáты.

stigmatize [ˈstɪgmətaɪz] *v* (за)клейми́ть, (о)позóрить.

stile [staɪl] *n* приступóк, ступéньки у стены́ *или* забóра.

stiletto [stɪˈletou] *n* стилéт.

still I [stɪl] *a* 1) ти́хий, бесшýмный; to keep ~ не шумéть; 2) спокóйный; неподви́жный; to stand ~ останови́ться.

still II *n* 1) тишинá; in the ~ of the night в ночнóй тиши́; 2) фотографи́ческий сни́мок; кадр.

still III *v* успокáивать, унимáть.

still IV *adv* 1) до сих пóр; всё ещё; 2) всё же, тем не мéнее, однáко; 3) *при сравн. ст.* ещё; ~ more ещё бóльше.

still² I *n* 1) перегóнный куб; дистилля́тор; 2) винокýренный завóд.

still² II *v* 1) перегоня́ть; дистилли́ровать; 2) опресня́ть.

still-born [ˈstɪlbɔːn] *a* мертворождённый.

stillness [ˈstɪlnɪs] *n* тишинá; спокóйствие.

still-room [ˈstɪlrum] *n* 1) кладовáя; 2) помещéние для перегóнки.

stilted [ˈstɪltɪd] *a* ходýльный, напы́щенный.

stilts [stɪlts] *n pl* 1) ходýли; 2) *амер. сленг* нóги.

stimulant I [ˈstɪmjulənt] *n* 1) возбуждáющее срéдство; 2) спиртнóй напи́ток; 3) сти́мул.

stimulant II *a* возбуждáющий; стимули́рующий.

stimulate [ˈstɪmjuleɪt] *v* 1) побуждáть, возбуждáть, стимули́ровать; 2) поощря́ть.

stimulation [ˌstɪmjuˈleɪʃən] *n* 1) побуждéние, возбуждéние; 2) поощрéние.

stimulus [ˈstɪmjuləs] *n* (*pl* stimuli [ˈstɪmjulaɪ]) 1) побуди́тельная причи́на, сти́мул; under the ~ of hunger побуждáемый гóлодом, под влия́нием гóлода; 2) возбуди́тель.

sting I [stɪŋ] *n* 1) жáло; 2) *бот.* жгýчий волосóк; 3) укýс (*змеи, насекóмого*); 4) ожóг (*крапи́вой*);

5) жгýчая боль; ~s of hunger мýки гóлода; ~s of remorse угрызéния сóвести; 6) остротá, си́ла; 7) кóлкость.

sting II *v* (*past, p. p.* stung) 1) жáлить; 2) жечь, обжигáть (*о крапи́ве, пéрце и т. п.*); 3) причиня́ть *или* испы́тывать óструю боль; to be stung by remorses мýчиться угрызéниями сóвести; 4) *сленг* (обмáном) вовлéчь в расхóд, «нагрéть»; he was stung for a fiver егó нагрéли на пятёрку.

stinginess [ˈstɪndʒɪnɪs] *n* скáредность, скýпость.

stinging [ˈstɪŋɪŋ] *a* жáлящий; жгýчий; язви́тельный.

stingy [ˈstɪndʒɪ] *a* скупóй, скáредный.

stink I [stɪŋk] *n* вонь, зловóние.

stink II *v* (*past* stank, stunk; *p. p.* stunk) 1) воня́ть; издавáть зловóние; 2) *сленг* учýять; □ to ~ out выгоня́ть, выкýривать.

stint I [stɪnt] *n* 1) ограничéние, предéл; without ~ свобóдно, без ограничéний; 2) (урóчная) рабóта; to do one's daily ~ сдéлать дневнýю рабóту.

stint II *v* ограни́чивать, урéзывать (*в чём-л. — in*).

stipend [ˈstaɪpend] *n* 1) жáлованье; 2) стипéндия.

stipulate [ˈstɪpjuleɪt] *v* 1) обуслóвливать, стáвить услóвием; 2) выговáривать (*что-л. — for*).

stipulation [ˌstɪpjuˈleɪʃən] *n* услóвие, соглашéние.

stir I [stəː] *n* 1) движéние; no ~ in the air вóздух неподви́жен; 2) суетá, суматóха; to make a ~, to create a ~ надéлать шýму, произвести́ сенсáцию; 3) размéшивание, помéшивание; to give the fire a ~ помéшивать огóнь (*в печке*).

stir II *v* 1) дви́гать(ся); шевели́ть(ся); 2) мешáть, размéшивать, помéшивать; 3) возбуждáть, волновáть; □ to ~ up а) размéшивать хорошéнько; взбáлтывать; he wants ~ring up егó нýжно расшевели́ть, раскачáть; б) возбуждáть (*любопы́тство*); в) раздувáть (*ссору*).

stir-about I [ˈstəːrəˌbaut] *n* овся́ная кáша.

stir-about II *a* шýмный, суетли́вый.

stirrer-up [ˈstəːrərˈʌp] *n* 1) винóвник; 2) возбуди́тель.

stirring [ˈstəːrɪŋ] *a* 1) подвижнóй, дéятельный; 2) волнýющий, возбуждáющий.

stirrup [ˈstɪrəp] *n* стрéмя.

stitch I [stɪtʃ] *n* 1) стежóк; шов; пéтля (*в вязáнии*); buttonhole ~ пéтельный шов; herring-bone ~ стежóк ёлочкой; chain ~ тáмбурная стрóчка; to take up (to drop) a ~ подня́ть (спусти́ть) пéтлю; to put ~es in наложи́ть швы; to take out the ~es снять швы; he has not a dry ~ on him на нём нет сухóй ни́тки, он промóк насквóзь; to have not a ~ on быть совершéнно гóлым; 2) óстрая боль, колотьé.

stitch II *v* 1) шить; 2) вышивáть; □ to ~ up зашивáть.

stiverᵃ [ˈstaɪvə] *n*: not (worth) a ~ ни грошá (не стóит); not to care a ~ совершéнно не беспокóиться, не интересовáться, «наплевáть».

stiverᵇ [ˈstɪvə] *v* ерóшить (*волосы*).

stoat¹ [stout] *n* горностáй.

stoat² *v* штуковáть.

stock¹ [stɔk] *n* 1) глáвный ствол (*дéрева*); 2) *с.-х.* подвóй; 3) род, семья́, происхождéние;

of a good ~ из хорошей семьи; 4) порода; 5) основная часть; опора, подпора; ~ of rifle ложе винтовки; 6) ручка, рукоятка, черенок; 7) основной материал, сырьё; 8) крепкий бульон (*из костей*); 9) *pl мор.* стапель; to have on the ~s работать над чем-л.; 10) *pl ист.* колодки; ◇ gazing ~ посмешище; lock, ~ and barrel все поголовно, полностью; ~s and stones а) неодушевлённые предметы; б) скучные люди, «истуканы».

stock² **I** *n* 1) запас; фонд; to have (*или* to keep) in ~ иметь в запасе, в продаже; out of ~ распродано; to lay in a ~ делать запасы; 2) государственные бумаги, фонды; акции; the ~s государственный долг; inscribed ~ именные акции; to sell out ~ продавать ценные бумаги; to sell out ~ продавать ценные бумаги; акционерный капитал (*тж.* joint ~); 4) инвентарь; live ~ *см.* live-stock; dead ~ мёртвый инвентарь; to take ~ производить переучёт, инвентаризировать; to take ~ of приглядываться (*к кому-л.*); знакомиться (*с чем-л.*); to put (*или* to take) ~ in доверять кому-л.; 5) *амер.* скот; ◇ ~ and block а) всё имущество; б) целиком.

stock² **II** *a* 1) готовый, имеющийся наготове; 2) избитый, банальный.

stock² **III** *a* 1) снабжать (*товаром, инвентарём и т. п.*); 2) иметь на складе, в продаже.

stockade I [stɔˈkeid] *n* частокол.

stockade II *v* окружать, обносить частоколом.

stock-breeder [ˈstɔkˌbriːdə] *n* животновод, скотовод.

stockbroker [ˈstɔkˌbroukə] *n* биржевой маклер.

stock-farm [ˈstɔkfɑːm] *n* скотоводческая ферма; животноводческое хозяйство.

stockholder [ˈstɔkˌhouldə] *n* 1) акционер; 2) *австрал.* скотовод.

stock-house [ˈstɔkhaus] *n австрал.* скотный двор.

stockiness [ˈstɔkinis] *n* приземистость, коренастость.

stockinet [ˌstɔkiˈnet] *n* трикотажная ткань.

stocking [ˈstɔkiŋ] *n* чулок.

stockinged [ˈstɔkiŋd] *a* в чулках.

stock-in-trade [ˈstɔkinˈtreid] *n* 1) оборудование; торговый инвентарь; 2) основной капитал; 3) запас товаров; 4) обычный, шаблонный запас фраз, аргументов.

stockjobber [ˈstɔkˌdʒɔbə] *n* 1) биржевой спекулянт; 2) *амер.* биржевой маклер.

stocklist [ˈstɔklist] *n* биржевой бюллетень.

stockman [ˈstɔkmən] *n* скотовод.

stockpile [ˈstɔkpail] *v* накоплять.

stockpiling [ˈstɔkˌpailiŋ] *n* накопление.

stockrider [ˈstɔkˌraidə] *n австрал.* верховой погонщик скота.

stock-still [ˈstɔkˈstil] *a* неподвижный, как вкопанный.

stocky [ˈstɔki] *a* приземистый, коренастый.

stockyard [ˈstɔkjɑːd] *n* 1) скотный двор; 2) скотопригонный двор.

stodge I [stɔdʒ] *n сленг* тяжёлая *или* сытная пища.

stodge II *v сленг* жадно есть.

stodgy [ˈstɔdʒi] *a* 1) тяжёлый (*о пище*); 2) тяжёлый, тяжеловесный (*о стиле*); скучный (*о книге*).

stoic I [ˈstouik] *n* стоик.

stoic II *a* стоический.

stoical [ˈstouikəl] *a* стоический.

stoicism [ˈstouisizəm] *n* стоицизм.

stoke [stouk] *v* 1) подбрасывать топливо; поддерживать огонь (*в топке*); 2) *шутл.* набивать (*рот*).

stokehold [ˈstoukhould] *n* топка; котельное отделение (*парохода*).

stokehole [ˈstoukhoul] *n* 1) *см.* stokehold; 2) место кочегара перед топкой.

stoker [ˈstoukə] *n* 1) кочегар; истопник; 2) механическая топка.

stole¹ [stoul] *n* меховая горжетка, боа.

stole² *past см.* steal II.

stolen [ˈstoulən] *p. p. см.* steal II.

stolid [ˈstɔlid] *a* вялый, флегматичный; тупой.

stomach I [ˈstʌmək] *n* 1) желудок; to turn one's ~ вызывать тошноту; 2) живот; 3) аппетит; to stay one's ~ утолить голод; заморить червячка; 4) *разг.* вкус, расположение (*к чему-л.* — for); to have no ~ for не иметь желания (*сделать что-л.*); 5) proud ~ high ~ высокомерие.

stomach II *v* есть с аппетитом; *перен. разг.* терпеть, выносить; I cannot ~ it я и это не перевариваю, не выношу этого.

stone I [stoun] *n* 1) камень; meteoric ~ метеорит; precious ~ драгоценный камень; head ~ краеугольный камень; not a ~ was left standing камня на камне не осталось; to leave no ~ unturned сделать всё возможное, испробовать все средства; to break ~s зарабатывать на жизнь тяжёлым трудом; to harden into ~ окаменеть; 2) градина; 3) косточка (*плода*); 4) (*pl без измен.*) стоун (*мера веса* ≅ *6,35 кг*); 5) литографский камень; ◇ rolling ~ беспокойный, непостоянный человек, «перекати-поле»; a rolling ~ gathers no moss *посл.* катящийся камень не обрастает мхом; to mark with a white ~ отметить, ознаменовать радостный день.

stone II *a* каменный.

stone III *v* 1) мостить, облицовывать камнем; 2) вынимать косточку (*из плода*); 3) побивать камнями.

stone-blind [ˈstounˈblaind] *a* совершенно слепой.

stone-broke [ˈstounˈbrouk] *a* совершенно разорённый.

stone-cold [ˈstounˈkould] *a* холодный (как камень).

stone-dead [ˈstounˈded] *a* мёртвый.

stone-deaf [ˈstounˈdef] *a* совершенно глухой.

stone-jug [ˈstoundʒʌg] *n сленг* тюрьма.

stone-mason [ˈstounˌmeisn] *n* каменщик.

stone-pit [ˈstounpit] *n* каменоломня.

stoneware [ˈstounwɛə] *n* глиняная посуда, гончарные изделия.

stonework [ˈstounwəːk] *n* каменная кладка.

stony [ˈstouni] *a* 1) каменистый; 2) каменный, твёрдый.

stony-broke [ˈstounibrouk] *см.* stone-broke.

stood [stud] *past, p. p. см.* stand II.

stooge I [stuːdʒ] *n сленг* 1) посмешище; 2) подпевала, подголосок, приспешник; 3) подставное лицо; 4) неопытный лётчик.

stooge II *v сленг:* to ~ about, to ~ around слоняться, шататься; to ~ into неожиданно попасть; to ~ off еле унести ноги.

stool I [stuːl] *n* 1) табурет; piano ~ (вертя-щийся) стул для роя́ля; 2) скаме́ечка для ног; 3) отво́док, ко́рень, пень; 4) *мед.* стул.

stool II *v* 1) пуска́ть побе́ги; 2) испражня́ться.

stool-pigeon ['stuːl‚pɪdʒɪn] *n* 1) го́лубь-мано́к; 2) провока́тор, осведоми́тель.

stoop¹ I [stuːp] *n* 1) суту́лость; 2) *уст.* паде́ние.

stoop¹ II *v* 1) наклоня́ть(ся), нагиба́ть(ся); *перен.* а) снисходи́ть; удоста́ивать; б) унижа́ться; 2) суту́лить(ся); 3) *уст.* устремля́ться вниз.

stoop² *n амер.* крыльцо́ со ступе́ньками, откры́тая вера́нда.

stop I [stɔp] *n* 1) остано́вка; заде́ржка, па́уза; to bring to a ~ останови́ть; to be at a ~ останови́ться; не быть в состоя́нии продолжа́ть; to come to a ~, to make a ~ останови́ться; 2) прекраще́ние, коне́ц; to put a ~ to положи́ть коне́ц чему́-л.; зако́нчить; 3) *грам.* знак препина́ния; full ~ то́чка; to come to a full ~ *перен.* останови́ться; переста́ть; зайти́ в тупи́к; 4) *муз.* кла́пан; кла́виша; педа́ль; лад; 5) *фон.* взрывно́й согла́сный.

stop II *v* 1) остана́вливать(ся); to ~ dead, to ~ short а) внеза́пно, кру́то останови́ться; б) стать в тупи́к; 2) прекраща́ть(ся), конча́ть(ся); do not ~! продолжа́йте!; 3) *разг.* остава́ться; пробы́ть; жить, гости́ть; to ~ at home оста́ться до́ма; 4) заде́рживать; прегражда́ть; 5) уде́рживать (*от чего-л.* — from); 6) уре́зывать; to ~ out of one's salary удержа́ть из зарпла́ты; 7) отража́ть, отбива́ть (*удар, атаку*); 8) затыка́ть, заку́поривать, заде́лывать; пломбирова́ть (*зуб*); 9) *муз.* зажима́ть струну́, кла́пан *или* ве́нтиль инструме́нта; ◻ to ~ by зайти́, зае́хать (*за — for*); to ~ in *амер.* зайти́; to ~ off, to ~ over *амер.* останови́ться, сде́лать остано́вку; to ~ up а) затыка́ть; б) не ложи́ться спать.

stopgap ['stɔpgæp] *n* 1) заты́чка; 2) вре́менный замести́тель.

stop-off ['stɔpɔːf] *n амер.* остано́вка (*в пути*).

stop-over ['stɔpouvə] *см.* stop-off.

stoppage ['stɔpɪdʒ] *n* 1) остано́вка, заде́ржка; 2) забасто́вка, прекраще́ние рабо́ты.

stopper ['stɔpə] *n* заты́чка, про́бка.

stopping ['stɔpɪŋ] *n* зубна́я пло́мба.

stopple I ['stɔpl] *n* про́бка; заты́чка.

stopple II *v* затыка́ть про́бкой, заку́поривать.

stop-press ['stɔppres] *n* э́кстренное сообще́ние (*помещаемое в газете во время печатания*).

stop-watch ['stɔpwɔtʃ] *n* секундоме́р.

storage ['stɔːrɪdʒ] *n* 1) склад(ы́), храни́лище; 2) хране́ние; cold ~ хране́ние в холоди́льниках; 3) цена́, опла́та за хране́ние; 4) накопле́ние; аккумули́рование; 5) запомина́ющее устро́йство (*тж.* magnetic ~).

store I [stɔː] *n* 1) запа́с; изоби́лие; emergency ~ неприкоснове́нный запа́с; to have in ~ име́ть в запа́се, нагото́ве, про запа́с; tomorrow has a surprise in ~ for you за́втра вас ожида́ет сюрпри́з; 2) *pl* иму́щество; запа́сы; припа́сы; 3) магази́н; *амер.* ла́вка; *pl* большо́й универса́льный магази́н; 4) склад; 5) значе́ние, ва́жность; to set ~ by придава́ть большо́е значе́ние; 6) *attr* запа́сный; оставля́емое про запа́с; 7) *attr* гото́вый (*о платье*).

store II *v* 1) запаса́ть, нака́пливать; отка́дывать (*тж.* to ~ up); 2) снабжа́ть; наполня́ть; 3) сда-

ва́ть на хране́ние *или* на склад; 4) содержа́ть, вмеща́ть.

storehouse ['stɔːhaus] *n* склад; *перен.* сокро́вищница.

storekeeper ['stɔː‚kiːpə] *n* 1) кладовщи́к; 2) *амер.* ла́вочник.

storeman ['stɔːmən] *n* кладовщи́к; заве́дующий скла́дом.

store-room ['stɔːrum] *n* кладова́я, цейхга́уз.

storey ['stɔːrɪ] *n* эта́ж; upper ~ ве́рхний эта́ж; *шутл.* голова́, башка́; he is a little wrong in the upper ~ он немно́го не в своём уме́.

storeyed ['stɔːrɪd] *a* 1) име́ющий этажи́; 2) *в сочетании с числительным* -эта́жный; three-storeyed трёхэта́жный.

storied¹ ['stɔːrɪd] *a см.* storeyed.

storied² *a* легенда́рный.

stork [stɔːk] *n* а́ист.

storm I [stɔːm] *n* 1) бу́ря; *перен.* волне́ние, смяте́ние; to ride out the ~ благополу́чно перенести́ шторм (*о корабле*); *перен.* отде́латься благополу́чно; 2): а ~ of ма́сса, мно́жество; 3) пото́к (*слёз*); взрыв (*аплодисментов, негодования и т. п.*); град (*пуль, оскорблений и т. п.*); урага́н (*снарядов*); 4) *воен.* штурм, при́ступ; to take by ~ взять при́ступом; 5) *attr воен.* штурмово́й; уда́рный (*о части*).

storm II *v* 1) бушева́ть (*перен. тж.* to ~ at); 2) *воен.* брать при́ступом.

storm-beaten ['stɔːm‚biːtn] *a* 1) потрёпанный бу́рями (*о корабле*); *перен.* мно́го переживший, изве́давший жите́йские бу́ри; 2) обве́тренный.

storm-bird ['stɔːmbəːd] *n* буреве́стник.

stormbound ['stɔːmbaund] *a* заде́ржанный што́рмом, бу́рей.

storm-cloud ['stɔːmklaud] *n* грозова́я ту́ча.

storm-finch ['stɔːmfɪntʃ] *см.* storm-bird.

stormovik ['stɔːməvɪk] *n ав.* штурмови́к.

storm-petrel ['stɔːm‚petrəl] *см.* storm-bird.

stormy ['stɔːmɪ] *a* 1) бу́рный; 2) предвеща́ющий бу́рю.

story¹ ['stɔːrɪ] *n* 1) расска́з; повествова́ние, исто́рия (*жизни, событий*); to make a long ~ short коро́че говоря́; it is quite another ~ now тепе́рь совсе́м друго́е де́ло, тепе́рь друго́й разгово́р; as the ~ goes как говоря́т; according to his ~ по его́ слова́м; 2) расска́з, по́весть, ска́зка, леге́нда; short ~ коро́ткий расска́з, новелла; cock-and-bull ~ небыли́цы; a gross ~ a naughty ~ неприли́чный анекдо́т; 3) газе́тный материа́л; 4) сюже́т, те́ма, фа́була; 5) *дет.* ложь, вы́думка; oh, you ~! ах ты лгуни́шка!

story² *n см.* storey.

story-book ['stɔːrɪbuk] *n* сбо́рник расска́зов, ска́зок; ска́зки.

story-teller ['stɔːrɪ‚telə] *n* 1) ска́зочник; 2) лгуни́шка.

stout I [staut] *a* 1) то́лстый, по́лный; 2) кре́пкий, про́чный; пло́тный; 3) отва́жный, сме́лый; сто́йкий.

stout II *n* кре́пкий по́ртер.

stoutness ['stautnɪs] *n* 1) полнота́, ту́чность; 2) кре́пость, про́чность; 3) отва́га; хра́брость.

stove¹ [stouv] *n* печь, пе́чка; плита́ (*кухонная*).

stove² *past, p. p. см.* stave II.

stow [stou] *v* 1) укла́дывать, скла́дывать; 2) наполня́ть, набива́ть; 3) *сленг* прекраща́ть;

☐ to ~ **away** a) убира́ть, пря́тать; б) плыть на парохо́де «за́йцем».

stowaway ['stouəweı] *n* безбиле́тный пассажи́р, «за́яц» (*на парохо́де*).

straddle ['strædl] *v* 1) расставля́ть но́ги; ходи́ть, расставля́я но́ги; стоя́ть, сиде́ть, расста́вив но́ги; 2) сиде́ть верхо́м; 3) не примыка́ть ни к одно́й стороне́ (*в споре и т. п.*); вести́ двойну́ю игру́.

straddle-back ['strædlbæk] *adv* расста́вив но́ги; to carry ~ переноси́ть на зако́рках.

strafe I [strɑːf] *n разг.* 1) урага́нный ого́нь; 2) наказа́ние.

strafe II *v разг.* 1) бомбардирова́ть, обстре́ливать; наноси́ть пораже́ние; 2) разноси́ть, руга́ть.

straggle ['strægl] *v* 1) идти́, брести́ в беспоря́дке; отстава́ть; 2) быть разбро́санным (*в беспорядке*).

straggler ['stræglə] *n* 1) отста́вший, отби́вшийся (*солдат и т. д.*); 2) *сленг* бродя́га.

straight I [streıt] *a* 1) прямо́й; 2) че́стный, и́скренний; 3) достове́рный, надёжный; 4) *амер.* ве́рный, пре́данный (*своей партии*); 5) *амер.* неразба́вленный; 6) умы́шленно невырази́тельный (*о лице*).

straight II *n* прямота́; прямизна́; the ~ *амер.* пра́вда; on the ~ про́мо; out of ~ ко́со, кри́во.

straight III *adv* 1) про́мо; ~ from the horse's mouth про́мо со станка́; све́женький, то́лько что изгото́вленный; 2) ме́тко; ~ off, ~ away сра́зу; ~ out напрями́к.

straighten ['streıtn] *v* 1) выпрямля́ть(ся), распрямля́ть(ся); 2) приводи́ть в поря́док; 3) *амер. сленг* исправля́ться.

straightforward I [streıt'fɔːwəd] *a* 1) че́стный, открове́нный; 2) прямо́й.

straightforward II *adv* про́мо.

straightway ['streıtweı] *adv* то́тчас.

strain I [streın] *n* 1) напряже́ние; to bear the ~ выде́рживать напряже́ние; 2) натяже́ние; растяже́ние; 3) *тех.* деформа́ция; 4) *обыкн. pl* напе́в, мело́дия; зву́ки (*музыки*); 5) тон, стиль (*речи*); 6) скло́нность, накло́нность; 7) происхожде́ние; поро́да, кровь; 8) насле́дственность.

strain II *v* 1) напряга́ть(ся); натя́гивать(ся); растя́гивать(ся); to ~ at the oars налега́ть на вёсла; to ~ after smth. добива́ться чего́-л., стреми́ться к чему́-л.; 2) злоупотребля́ть; превыша́ть (*власть, права и т. п.*); 3) искажа́ть; подтасо́вывать, допуска́ть натя́жку (*в толковании и т. п.*); 4) прижима́ть; сжима́ть (*в объятиях*); 5) проце́живать; фильтрова́ть; 6) *тех.* деформи́ровать; ☐ to ~ **off** проце́живать, отце́живать.

strained [streınd] *a* 1) напряжённый; 2) натя́нутый, неесте́ственный; 3) проце́женный, профильтро́ванный.

strainer ['streınə] *n* фильтр, си́то.

strait I [streıt] *n* 1) у́зкий проли́в; 2) *обыкн. pl* стеснённое (*материа́льное*) положе́ние.

strait II *a* 1) у́зкий; 2) стро́гий.

straiten ['streıtn] *v* стесня́ть; ограни́чивать.

strait-laced ['streıtleıst] *a* стро́гий; стро́гих пра́вил; нетерпи́мый.

strand[1] I [strænd] *n* бе́рег.

strand[1] II *v* 1) сесть, посади́ть на мель; 2) вы́бросить(ся) на бе́рег.

strand[2] *n* 1) прядь (*волос, каната и т. п.*); 2) ни́тка бус; 3) черта́ хара́ктера.

stranded ['strændıd] *a* в стеснённых обстоя́тельствах, «на мели́».

strange [streındʒ] *a* 1) стра́нный, необы́чный; I feel ~ мне не по себе́; 2) незнако́мый, неизве́стный; 3) чужо́й; чу́ждый; 4) иностра́нный.

stranger ['streındʒə] *n* 1) посторо́нний челове́к; to make a ~ of хо́лодно обойти́сь с кем-л.; to make no ~ of серде́чно обойти́сь с кем-л.; 2) незнако́мец; he is a ~ to me я его́ не зна́ю; он мне незнако́м; the little ~ новорождённый; 3) иностра́нец; 4) челове́к, чу́ждый чему́-л.; a ~ to fear (челове́к) чу́ждый стра́ху.

strangle ['stræŋgl] *v* 1) души́ть; *перен. тж.* подавля́ть; 2) жать, дави́ть (*о воротнике*).

stranglehold ['stræŋglhould] *n* 1) удуше́ние; подавле́ние; 2) мёртвая хва́тка; 3) безвы́ходное положе́ние.

strangulation [ˌstræŋgjuˈleıʃən] *n* 1) удуше́ние; 2) *мед.* ущемле́ние (*грыжи*).

strap I [stræp] *n* 1) реме́нь, ремешо́к; 2) поло́ска (*материи, металла*); скре́па; 3) *воен.* пого́н (*тж.* shoulder-strap); 4) (the ~) по́рка ремнём.

strap II *v* 1) стя́гивать, скрепля́ть ремня́ми; 2) бить ремнём; 3) пра́вить (*бритву*).

straphanger ['stræpˌhæŋə] *n* пассажи́р, стоя́щий и держа́щийся за реме́нь.

strapping ['stræpıŋ] *a* ро́слый.

strata ['strɑːtə] *pl см.* stratum.

stratagem ['strætıdʒəm] *n* хи́трость; уло́вка.

strategic(al) [strəˈtiːdʒık(əl)] *a* 1) стратеги́ческий; стратеги́чески ва́жный; 2) операти́вный.

strategist ['strætıdʒıst] *n* страте́г.

strategy ['strætıdʒı] *n* 1) *воен.* страте́гия; операти́вное иску́сство; 2) веде́ние опера́ций.

stratification [ˌstrætıfıˈkeıʃən] *n геол.* напласто-ва́ние, залега́ние.

stratify ['strætıfaı] *v* насла́иваться, напласто́-вываться.

stratochamber ['strætouˌtʃæmbə] *n* барока́мера.

stratosphere ['strætousfıə] *n* стратосфе́ра.

stratum ['strɑːtəm] *n* (*pl* strata) 1) *геол.* пласт, напластова́ние; 2) слой (*общества*).

straw I [strɔː] *n* 1) соло́ма; соло́мка; соло́минка; 2) пустя́к, ме́лочь; not to care a ~ относи́ться безразли́чно; not worth a ~ ничего́ не стоя́щий; ◇ the last ~ ≅ после́дняя ка́пля (перепо́лнившая ча́шу).

straw II *a* соло́менный.

strawberry ['strɔːbərı] *n* 1) клубни́ка; земляни́ка; wild ~ лесна́я земляни́ка; 2) *attr* клубни́чный; земляни́чный.

straw-coloured ['strɔːˌkʌləd] *a* соло́менного цве́-та.

stray I [streı] *n* 1) беспризо́рный ребёнок; 2) отби́вшееся от ста́да живо́тное; 3) *юр.* вы́морочное иму́щество; 4) *pl радио* поме́хи.

stray II *a* 1) заблуди́вшийся; 2) бездо́мный, бродя́чий; 3) бессвя́зный (*о мыслях и т. п.*); 4) случа́йный; шально́й (*о пуле*).

stray III *v* 1) блужда́ть; 2) заблуди́ться; отклони́ться, сби́ться (*с прямого пути; тж. перен.*); 3) отби́ться (*от стада*).

streak I [striːk] *n* 1) полоса́, просло́йка, прожи́лка; the silver ~ *разг.* Ла-Ма́нш; ~ of lightning мо́лния; вспы́шка мо́лнии; 2) черта́, черто́чка (*характера*); he has a ~ of humour in him в нём есть юмористическая жилка.

streak II *v* 1) проводить полосы; прочертить (*о молнии*); ~ed with dirt испачканный грязью; 2) промчаться, промелькнуть.

streaky ['striːkɪ] *a* полосатый; слоистый, с прослойками.

stream I [striːm] *n* 1) река; ручей; up (down) ~ вверх (вниз) по реке, по течению; to whip the ~ забрасывать удочку; 2) течение; to go with (against) the ~ плыть по течению (против течения); the ~ of thought ход мысли; 3) поток; a ~ (*или* ~s) of tears потоки слёз; ~s of people толпы людей.

stream II *v* 1) течь, литься, струиться; выливаться; 2) развеваться; 3) лить, струить, источать; □ to ~ **back** отхлынуть; откатиться.

streamer ['striːmə] *n* 1) узкая, длинная лента; 2) вымпел; 3) столб северного сияния; 4) *амер.* газетный заголовок во всю ширину полосы.

streamlet ['striːmlɪt] *n* ручеёк.

streamline I ['striːmlaɪn] *a* обтекаемый.

streamline II *v* 1) придавать обтекаемую форму; 2) рационализировать.

streamlined ['striːmlaɪnd] *a* обтекаемый (*тж. перен.*).

streamliner ['striːm,laɪnə] *n* машина (*автомобиль, локомотив и т. п.*) обтекаемой формы.

street [striːt] *n* 1) улица; main ~ главная улица; side ~ переулок; off ~ боковая улица; back ~ глухая, отдалённая улица; to live in the ~ редко бывать дома; to take to the ~s выходить на улицы (*в знак протеста*); 2) *attr* уличный; ◊ not in the same ~ with *разг.* несравненно ниже, хуже; easy ~ богатство.

street-car ['striːtkɑː] *n* трамвай.

strength [streŋθ] *n* 1) сила; to gather ~ накапливать силы; on the ~ of в силу, на основании (*чего-л.*); the ~ of the working class lies in unity сила рабочего класса в единстве; 2) прочность, крепость; 3) сопротивление; ~ of materials *тех.* сопротивление материалов; 4) *воен.* сила; численность; in full ~ в полном составе; on the ~ в составе, в штате; 5) крепость (*чая, вина и т. п.*).

strengthen ['streŋθən] *v* усиливать(ся); укреплять(ся).

strenuous ['strenjuəs] *a* 1) сильный; энергичный; 2) напряжённый; трудный.

stress I [stres] *n* 1) давление, нажим; напряжение; under the ~ of fear (of weather) под влиянием страха (непогоды); under the ~ of poverty под гнётом нищеты; 2) ударение; to lay ~ on подчёркивать, придавать особое значение.

stress II *v* 1) подчёркивать; ставить ударение; 2) *тех.* подвергать давлению, напряжению.

stretch I [stretʃ] *n* 1) растягивание, вытягивание; натяжение; напряжение, усилие; to give a ~ a) вытянуться; б) потянуться; on the ~ в напряжении; with every faculty on the ~ напрягая все способности; a ~ of authority превышение власти; 2) протяжение, протяжённость; пространство; 3) отрезок (*времени*); at a ~ без перерыва, подряд; 4) *сленг* срок (тюремного заключения).

stretch II *v* 1) растягивать(ся); вытягивать(ся); натягивать(ся); to ~ oneself потягиваться; 2) напрягать(ся); превышать; 3) преувеличивать, лгать (*тж.* to ~ the truth); 4) простираться(ся), тянуть(ся); □ to ~ **out** а) протянуть (*руки, ногу*); б) вытягивать, удлинять.

stretched [stretʃt] *a* распростёртый.

stretcher ['stretʃə] *n* 1) носилки; 2) *сленг* преувеличение, натяжка, ложь.

strew [struː] *v* (*past* strewed; *p. p.* strewed, strewn) 1) посыпать, усыпать; 2) рассыпать; разбрасывать; 3) разбрызгивать.

strewn [struːn] *p. p. см.* strew.

stricken I ['strɪkən] *уст. p. p. см.* strike² I.

stricken II *a* 1) поражённый, охваченный (*тж. в сложных словах, напр.:* terror-stricken охваченный ужасом; poverty-stricken бедствующий); ~ with fever в лихорадке; ~ with paralysis разбитый параличом; ~ in years обременённый годами; 2) разбитый (*о сердце*).

strict [strɪkt] *a* 1) строгий; 2) точный, определённый.

stricture ['strɪktʃə] *n* 1) *обыкн. pl* строгая критика; критическое замечание; 2) *мед.* сужение (*сосудов и т. п.*).

stridden ['strɪdn] *p. p. см.* stride II.

stride I [straɪd] *n* 1) шаг; to take in ~ а) преодолеть без усилия; б) *воен.* захватить одним броском; 2) *pl* успехи.

stride II *v* (*past* strode; *p. p.* stridden) 1) шагать; 2) перешагнуть; 3) сидеть верхом.

strident ['straɪdnt] *a* резкий, скрипучий.

strife [straɪf] *n* борьба, спор.

strike¹ I [straɪk] *a* забастовка, стачка; general ~ всеобщая забастовка, стачка; ballot ~ бойкот выборов; sit-down ~ сидячая забастовка; sit-in (*или* stay-in, stay-down) ~ забастовка, когда бастующие отказываются покинуть помещение; slow-down ~ итальянская забастовка; to go on ~, to come out on ~ объявлять забастовку, забастовать; to be out on ~ бастовать; to stage a ~ проводить забастовку; token ~, sympathetic ~ стачка солидарности.

strike¹ II *v* (*past, p. p.* struck) бастовать, проводить забастовку, стачку.

strike² I *v* (*past, p. p.* struck; *уст. p. p.* stricken) 1) ударять, наносить удар(ы); 2) поражать; 3) прийти на ум, осенить; 4) производить впечатление; how does it ~ you? что вы об этом думаете?; 5) бить, звонить (*о часах*); ударять (*по струнам*); 6) зажигать (*спичку или спичкой*); высекать (*огонь*); 7) удариться обо что-л.; наскочить на что-л.; 8) наткнуться, натолкнуться на, найти (*воду, нефть и т. п.*); 9) направляться (*тж.* to ~ out); пускаться, углубляться (*куда-л.; into*); to ~ to the left (right) повернуть налево (направо); to ~ across переправляться (*через*); 10) пронзать, вонзать; 11) пронизывать, проникать; пускать корни; 12) выбивать, чеканить; 13) спускать (*флаг*); сдаваться; 14) свёртывать (*палатку*); □ to ~ **aside** отбивать; парировать (*удар*); to ~ **back** наносить ответный удар; to ~ **down** а) отбивать, парировать удар; б) свалить с ног; сразить; to ~ **in** вмешаться (*в разговор*) to ~ **off** а) отрубать; б) *полигр.* отпечатывать; в) вычёркивать; г) свора́чивать (*в сто́рону*); д) откомандиро́вывать; освобожда́ть (*от рабо́ты*); to ~ **out** вычёркивать; б) направля́ться; отправля́ться; в) уда́рить спле́ча́; г) приду́мать (*план*); to ~ out a line for oneself быть оригина́льным; оригина́льничать; to ~ **through** зачёркивать, перечёркивать; to ~ **up** а) отбива́ть, пари́ровать (*уда́р*); б) бы́стро *или* случа́йно завяза́ть знако́мство; в) заигра́ть (*об орке́стре*); to ~ **upon** а) па́дать (*о све́те*); б) доноси́ться (*о зву́ке*).

strike² II *n амер.* 1) нахо́дка, откры́тие (*не́фти, зо́лота и т. п.*); 2) фина́нсовая уда́ча.

strike-breaker ['straɪkˌbreɪkə] *n* штрейкбре́хер.

striker¹ ['straɪkə] *n* забасто́вщик.

striker² *n* 1) молотобо́ец; 2) *воен.* уда́рник.

striking ['straɪkɪŋ] *a* 1) порази́тельный; рази́тельный (*о схо́дстве*); 2) *воен.* уда́рный.

string I [strɪŋ] *n* 1) струна́; the ~s стру́нные инструме́нты (*в орке́стре*); to touch the ~s игра́ть (*на а́рфе, гита́ре и т. п.*); to touch a ~ *перен.* затро́нуть стру́нку; to harp on one (*или* on the same) ~ тверди́ть одно́ и то́ же; 2) верёвка, бечёвка; тесёмка, завя́зка; to pull the ~s *перен.* быть скры́тым вдохнови́телем (*чего́-л.*); нажима́ть та́йные пружи́ны; to have smb. on a ~ влия́ть на кого́-л., име́ть кого́-л. в своём подчине́нии; 3) тетива́ (*лу́ка*); to have two ~s to one's bow *перен.* име́ть вы́бор; име́ть дополни́тельный ресу́рс; first ~ гла́вный ресу́рс; second ~ а) допо́лни́тельный ресу́рс; б) *теа́тр.* дублёр; 4) ряд, верени́ца; ~ of people верени́ца люде́й; ~ of burst пулемётная о́чередь; 5) ни́тка (*бус и т. п.*); ~ of pearls ни́тка же́мчуга; 6) волокно́, жи́лка.

string II *v* (*past, p. p.* strung) 1) завя́зывать, свя́зывать; 2) напряга́ть, натя́гивать; *перен.* взви́нчивать; 3) наниза́ть (*бу́сы*); 4) *амер. разг.* обману́ть; □ to ~ **out** растя́гивать(ся); to ~ **up** а) взви́нчивать, напряга́ть (*не́рвы и т. п.*); б) *сленг* вздёрнуть (*на ви́селице*).

stringed [strɪŋd] *a* стру́нный.

stringency ['strɪndʒənsɪ] *n* 1) стро́гость; 2) стеснённые де́нежные обстоя́тельства.

stringent ['strɪndʒənt] *a* 1) стро́гий, строжа́йший; 2) стеснённый (*в деньга́х*); 3) напряжённый (*о де́нежном ры́нке*).

stringy ['strɪŋɪ] *a* 1) волокни́стый, жи́листый; 2) тягу́чий, густо́й.

strip¹ [strɪp] *n* 1) у́зкая поло́ска (*бума́ги, мате́рии и т. п.*); 2) у́зкая полоса́, небольшо́й уча́сток (*земли́, са́да и т. п.*); landing ~ взлёт-но-поса́дочная доро́жка; 3) страни́чка ю́мора (*в газе́те, журна́ле; тж.* comic ~); ◊ to .tear a ~ off smb. разнести́ кого́-л., дать хоро́ший нагоня́й кому́-л.

strip² *v* 1) сдира́ть, обдира́ть; обнажа́ть; 2) отнима́ть, гра́бить, обдира́ть; 3) раздева́ть(ся), обнажа́ть(ся); to be ~ped of leaves стоя́ть го́лыми (*о дере́вьях*); 4) *воен., мор.* разоружа́ть; □ to ~ **off** сдира́ть, соска́бливать, счища́ть.

stripe [straɪp] *n* 1) полоса́; 2) *воен.* наши́вка; лампа́с; to get (*to lose*) one's ~s быть произве́дённым (разжа́лованным); 3) *pl* по́рка; 4) *pl разг.* тигр; ◊ of every ~ всех масте́й.

striped [straɪpt] *a* полоса́тый.

stripling ['strɪplɪŋ] *n* ю́ноша, подро́сток.

strip-tease ['strɪptiːz] *n театр.* стрипти́з.

strive [straɪv] *v* (*past* strove; *p. p.* striven) 1) стара́ться, прилага́ть уси́лия; to ~ for peace боро́ться за мир; стреми́ться к ми́ру; 2) боро́ться (*про́тив чего́-л.— with, against*).

striven ['strɪvn] *p. p. см.* strive.

strivings ['straɪvɪŋz] *n pl* уси́лия.

strode [stroud] *past см.* stride II.

stroke¹ [strouk] *n* 1) уда́р; finishing ~ а) реша́ющий, роково́й уда́р; б) реша́ющий до́вод; 2) уда́р; при́ступ (*боле́зни*); he had a ~ (of paralysis) его́ разби́л парали́ч; heat ~ теплово́й уда́р; 3) взмах (*весла́, кры́льев и т. п.*); piston ~ *тех.* ход по́ршня; with a ~ of the pen одни́м ро́счерком пера́; 4) штрих, черта́; 5) ход, приём; a ~ of luck уда́ча; a ~ of diplomacy дипломати́ческий ход; 6) бой (*часо́в*); on the ~ of time как раз во́время; he was there on the ~ он яви́лся во́время; 7) *спорт.* загребно́й.

stroke² I *n* погла́живание.

stroke² II *v* гла́дить; проводи́ть руко́й (*по чему́-л.*); to ~ smb. the wrong way *перен.* раздража́ть кого́-л., гла́дить про́тив ше́рсти; □ to ~ **down** успоко́ить.

stroll I [stroul] *n* прогу́лка; to take a ~, to go for a ~ прогу́ливаться.

stroll II *v* 1) гуля́ть, прогу́ливаться; 2) стра́нствовать, дава́я представле́ния.

stroller ['stroulə] *n* гуля́ющий.

strong I [strɔŋ] *a* 1) си́льный; 2) кре́пкий; 3) про́чный; усто́йчивый; твёрдый (*об убежде́ниях*); 4) здоро́вый; энерги́чный; 5) гро́мкий (*о го́лосе*); 6) кре́пкий, спиртно́й (*о напи́тках*); о́стрый (*о сы́ре и т. п.*); 7) стро́гий, круто́й; реши́тельный; 8) *грам.* си́льный, с чередова́нием гла́сного (*о глаго́ле*).

strong II *n*: the ~ (*употр. как pl*) 1) си́льные, власть иму́щие; 2) здоро́вые.

strong III *adv разг.* си́льно, реши́тельно; to come it ~ зайти́ сли́шком далеко́; to be going ~ чу́вствовать себя́ си́льным, бо́дрым.

strong-box ['strɔŋbɔks] *n* несгора́емый шкаф *или* я́щик.

stronghold ['strɔŋhould] *n* опло́т, тверды́ня.

strong-room ['strɔŋrum] *n* стальна́я ка́мера (*ба́нка*).

strontium ['strɔnʃɪəm] *n хим.* стро́нций.

strop I [strɔp] *n* 1) реме́нь (*для пра́вки бритв*); 2) *мор.* строп.

strop II *v* пра́вить бри́тву.

strophe ['stroufɪ] *n* строфа́.

strove [strouv] *past см.* strive.

struck¹ [strʌk] *past, p. p. см.* strike² I.

struck² I *past, p. p. см.* strike¹ II.

struck² II *a* охва́ченный забасто́вкой; закры́тый по слу́чаю забасто́вки (*о предприя́тии*).

structural ['strʌktʃərəl] *a* 1) структу́рный; конструкти́вный; 2) строи́тельный.

structure ['strʌktʃə] *n* 1) структу́ра; устро́йство; ~ of society строй о́бщества; social ~ социа́льный строй; the ~ of a language строй языка́; 2) зда́ние, сооруже́ние.

struggle I ['strʌgl] *n* 1) борьба́; class ~ кла́ссовая борьба́; ~ for peace борьба́ за мир; life and death ~ борьба́ не на жизнь, а на сме́рть; 2) напряже́ние, уси́лие.

struggle II *v* 1) боро́ться; 2) би́ться, отбива́ться; сража́ться; 3) стара́ться, де́лать уси́лия; 4) пробива́ться (*through*).

strum I [strʌm] *n* бренча́ние.

strum II *v* бренча́ть.

strung [strʌŋ] *past, p. p. см.* string II.

strut¹ I [strʌt] *n* ва́жная, го́рдая по́ступь.

strut¹ II *v* го́рдо выступа́ть, ходи́ть с ва́жным ви́дом.

strut² I *n* сто́йка, подпо́ра.

strut² II *v* подпира́ть.

strychnin [ˈstrɪknɪn] *n* стрихни́н.

strychnine [ˈstrɪkniːn] *см.* strychnin.

stub I [stʌb] *n* 1) пень; 2) обло́мок (*зуба*); огры́зок (*карандаша*); 3) оку́рок.

stub II *v* 1) выкорчёвывать, вырыва́ть с ко́рнем; 2) загаси́ть (*папиро́су, сига́ру*), придави́в коне́ц (*тж.* to ~ out).

stubble [ˈstʌbl] *n* 1) жнивьё, стерня́; 2) ко́ротко остри́женные во́лосы; 3) небри́тая борода́, «щети́на».

stubborn [ˈstʌbən] *a* упря́мый; упо́рный.

stubbornly [ˈstʌbənlɪ] *adv* упо́рно; упря́мо; с (тем же) упря́мством.

stubbornness [ˈstʌbənnɪs] *n* упря́мство; упо́рство.

stubby [ˈstʌbɪ] *a* коро́ткий и то́лстый; корена́стый.

stucco I [ˈstʌkou] *n* штукату́рка.

stucco II *v* штукату́рить.

stuck [stʌk] *past, p. p. см.* stick II.

stuck-up [ˈstʌkˈʌp] *a* высокоме́рный; зано́счивый.

stud¹ I [stud] *n* 1) пу́говица, за́понка; 2) гвоздь (*с большо́й шля́пкой*).

stud¹ II *v* 1) обива́ть гвоздя́ми (*для украше́ния*); 2) усе́ивать, уса́живать.

stud² *n* 1) коню́шни (*скаковы́х лошаде́й*); 2) ко́нный заво́д.

student [ˈstjuːdənt] *n* 1) студе́нт; 2) изуча́ющий что-л.

stud-farm [ˈstʌdfɑːm] *n* ко́нный заво́д.

stud-horse [ˈstʌdhɔːs] *n* племенно́й жеребе́ц.

studied [ˈstʌdɪd] *a* 1) обду́манный; умы́шленный; де́ланный; 2) начи́танный.

studio [ˈstjuːdɪou] *n* 1) сту́дия, ателье́; 2) радиосту́дия; киносту́дия; телесту́дия.

studious [ˈstjuːdjəs] *a* 1) приле́жный; усе́рдный; 2) забо́тливый.

study I [ˈstʌdɪ] *n* 1) изуче́ние, иссле́дование; заня́тие (нау́кой); to make a ~ of тща́тельно изуча́ть; иссле́довать; the ~ of mathematics заня́тия матема́тикой; 2) предме́т изуче́ния; 3) предме́т, досто́йный внима́ния *или* наблюде́ния; предме́т, вызыва́ющий интере́с; it was a perfect ~ на э́то сто́ило посмотре́ть; 4) предме́т забо́т, стара́ния; 5) о́черк; 6) *иск.* этю́д, набро́сок; эски́з; 7) *муз.* этю́д; 8) рабо́чий кабине́т; ◇ in a brown ~ в глубо́кой заду́мчивости, в разду́мье.

study II *v* 1) изуча́ть, иссле́довать; рассма́тривать; 2) занима́ться, учи́ться; 3) забо́титься, стреми́ться, стара́ться; □ to ~ out выясня́ть; to ~ up гото́виться к экза́мену.

stuff I [stʌf] *n* 1) вещество́, материа́л; raw ~ сырьё; green (*или* garden) ~ о́вощи, зе́лень; doctors' ~ *разг.* лека́рство; he has good ~ in

him, в нём мно́го хоро́шего; 2) шерстяна́я мате́рия; 3) дрянь, хлам (*тж.* poor ~, sorry ~); ~ and nonsense! чепуха́!; small ~ пустяки́, ме́лочи жи́зни; to write sad ~ скве́рно писа́ть, писа́ть дрянны́е кни́ги.

stuff II *v* 1) затыка́ть; набива́ть; 2) начиня́ть, фарширова́ть; 3) засо́вывать, впи́хивать, вти́скивать; 4) объеда́ться, жа́дно есть; 5) *разг.* обма́нывать.

stuffing [ˈstʌfɪŋ] *n* 1) наби́вка (*матра́ца, поду́шки и т. п.*); 2) начи́нка.

stuffy [ˈstʌfɪ] *a* 1) ду́шный; спёртый; 2) стро́гий, щепети́льный.

stultify [ˈstʌltɪfaɪ] *v* 1) выставля́ть в смешно́м *или* глу́пом ви́де; 2) своди́ть на нет (*уси́лия, достиже́ния*).

stumble I [ˈstʌmbl] *n* запи́нка, заде́ржка; оши́бка.

stumble II *v* 1) спотыка́ться; 2) запина́ться; 3) ошиба́ться; заблужда́ться в чём-л. (*at*); □ to ~ **across** наткну́ться на что-л., случа́йно найти́ что-л.; to ~ **along** ковыля́ть, идти́ спотыка́ясь; to ~ **upon** наткну́ться на что-л.

stumbling-block [ˈstʌmblɪŋblɔk] *n* ка́мень преткнове́ния.

stump I [stʌmp] *n* 1) пень; 2) обру́бок; обло́мок; огры́зок; 3) оку́рок; 4) *pl шутл.* но́ги; to stir one's ~s дви́гаться, пошеве́ливаться; 5) импровизи́рованная трибу́на (*на ми́тинге*); to be on the ~ вести́ полити́ческую агита́цию.

stump II *v* 1) *разг.* ста́вить в тупи́к; I'm ~ed я теря́юсь, не зна́ю, что отве́тить, де́лать *и т. п.*; 2) объезжа́ть (*страну́, о́круг и т. п.*) с це́лью агита́ции; □ to ~ **about**, to ~ **along** тяжело́ ступа́ть; to ~ **up** a) переплати́ть; б) вы́ложить де́ньги.

stumpy [ˈstʌmpɪ] *a* коро́ткий и то́лстый; корена́стый, призе́мистый.

stun [stʌn] *v* оглуша́ть, ошеломля́ть.

stung [stʌŋ] *past, p. p. см.* sting II.

stunk [stʌŋk] *past, p. p. см.* stink II.

stunning [ˈstʌnɪŋ] *a* 1) ошеломля́ющий; 2) *разг.* очарова́тельный; 3) *разг.* сногсшиба́тельный, порази́тельный.

stunt¹ I [stʌnt] *n* остано́вка, заде́ржка в ро́сте.

stunt¹ II *v* остана́вливать, заде́рживать рост.

stunt² I *n разг.* трюк.

stunt² II *v* де́лать трю́ки (*осо́б. о фигу́рах вы́сшего пилота́жа*).

stupe¹ [stjuːp] *n* припа́рка.

stupe² *n сленг* дура́к, болва́н, идио́т.

stupefaction [ˌstjuːpɪˈfækʃən] *n* оцепене́ние, остолбене́ние.

stupefy [ˈstjuːpɪfaɪ] *v* 1) изумля́ть, ошеломля́ть; 2) притупля́ть ум.

stupendous [stjuːˈpendəs] *a* изуми́тельный, выдаю́щийся.

stupid [ˈstjuːpɪd] *a* 1) тупо́й; глу́пый; 2) оцепене́лый; отупе́лый.

stupidity [stjuːˈpɪdɪtɪ] *n* ту́пость, глу́пость.

stupor [ˈstjuːpə] *n* оцепене́ние; бесчу́вственное состоя́ние.

sturdy [ˈstəːdɪ] *a* 1) си́льный; 2) кре́пкий; 3) сто́йкий, упо́рный.

sturgeon [ˈstəːdʒən] *n* осётр.

stutter I [ˈstʌtə] *n* заика́ние.

stutter II *v* заикаться; запинаться; □ to ~ **out** произнести запинаясь.

stutterer ['stʌtərə] *n* заика.

sty[1] [staɪ] *n* ячмень (*на глазу*).

sty[2] *n* свиной хлев.

style [staɪl] *n* 1) стиль; the pointed(-arch) ~ готический стиль; Gregorian ~, new ~ новый стиль (*календаря*); 2) направление, школа (*в искусстве*); 3) манера, стиль (*исполнения*); 4) изящество, элегантность, шик; блеск; to live in grand ~ жить на широкую ногу; 5) род, сорт; 6) гравировальная игла; 7) *уст.* стиль (*палочка для писания*).

stylish ['staɪlɪʃ] *a* шикарный; элегантный.

suasion ['sweɪʒən] *n* уговоры, увещевание (*тж.* moral ~).

suave [swɑːv] *a* мягкий; учтивый; вкрадчивый.

suavity ['swævɪtɪ] *n* мягкость; учтивость; вкрадчивость.

sub- [sʌb-] *pref* указывает на: а) *положение ниже чего-л., под чем-л.*: subway подземная железная дорога, подземный ход; б) *более мелкое подразделение, низший чин, калибр и т. п.*: sublieutenant младший лейтенант; subcommittee подкомиссия; в) *недостаточное количество вещества в данном соединении*: subchloride закись хлора; suboxide закись.

subaltern ['sʌbltən] *n* младший офицер.

subclass ['sʌbklɑːs] *n биол.* подкласс.

subcommittee ['sʌbkə,mɪtɪ] *n* подкомиссия.

subconscious ['sʌb'kɒnʃəs] *a* подсознательный.

subdivide ['sʌbdɪ'vaɪd] *v* подразделять(ся).

subdivision ['sʌbdɪ,vɪʒən] *n* подразделение.

subdue [səb'djuː] *v* 1) подавлять; подчинять, покорять; 2) смягчать, ослаблять, приглушать (*звук и т. п.*); понижать (*настроение и т. п.*).

subject[a] I ['sʌbdʒɪkt] *n* 1) тема, сюжет, содержание; предмет (*разговора, исследования и т. п.*); te(t)chy ~ щекотливая тема; to keep to the ~ держаться темы; to traverse a ~ обсудить вопрос со всех сторон; to dismiss the ~ прекратить обсуждение вопроса; to wander from the ~ отклоняться от темы; to change the ~ переменить разговор, тему разговора; on the ~ of на тему, по поводу; 2) причина, повод к чему-л. (*for*); 3) *грам.* подлежащее; 4) подданный; 5) субъект (*тж. филос.*).

subject[a] II *a* 1) подверженный (*to*); ~ to damage подверженный порче; 2) подлежащий (*to*); the arrangement is ~ to your approval дело подлежит вашему утверждению; 3) подвластный, подчинённый; 4) подопытный.

subject[b] [səb'dʒekt] *v* 1) подчинять, покорять; 2) подвергать (*воздействию, влиянию и т. п.; to*).

subjection [səb'dʒekʃən] *n* 1) покорение; 2) подчинение; зависимость.

subjective I [sʌb'dʒektɪv] *n грам.* именительный падеж.

subjective II *a* 1) субъективный; 2) *грам.* свойственный подлежащему; 3) *грам.* именительный (*о падеже*).

subjectivity [,sʌbdʒek'tɪvɪtɪ] *n* субъективность.

subject-matter [,sʌbdʒɪkt,mætə] *n* содержание; сюжет.

subjugate ['sʌbdʒugeɪt] *v* покорять, подчинять, порабощать.

subjugation [,sʌbdʒuˈgeɪʃən] *n* покорение, подчинение.

subjunctive I [səb'dʒʌŋktɪv] *n грам.* сослагательное наклонение.

subjunctive II *a* сослагательный.

sublimate[a] ['sʌblɪmɪt] *n* сулема (*тж.* corrosive ~).

sublimate[b] ['sʌblɪmeɪt] *v хим.* сублимировать, возгонять; *перен.* возвышать, идеализировать.

sublime[1] I [sə'blaɪm] *n*: the ~ возвышенное, великое; from the ~ to the ridiculous от великого до смешного.

sublime[1] II *a* 1) высокий, возвышенный; 2) грандиозный, величественный.

sublime[2] *v см.* sublimate[b].

subliminal [sʌb'lɪmɪnl] *a* подсознательный.

submachine-gun ['sʌbmə'ʃiːngʌn] *n воен.* пистолет-пулемёт; автомат.

submarine I ['sʌbməriːn] *n* подводная лодка (*тж.* ~ boat).

submarine II *a* подводный.

submarine III *v* потопить подводной лодкой.

submerge [səb'mɜːdʒ] *v* 1) затоплять; 2) погружать(ся).

submerged I [səb'mɜːdʒd] *a* 1) затопленный; 2) погружённый.

submerged II *n*: the ~ наибеднейшая и обездоленная часть населения (*тж.* the ~ tenth).

submergence [səb'mɜːdʒəns] *n* 1) затопление; 2) погружение в воду.

submersion [səb'mɜːʃən] *см.* submergence.

submission [səb'mɪʃən] *n* 1) покорность; подчинение; with all due ~ с должным уважением; 2) передача, представление (*на рассмотрение, экспертизу*).

submissive [səb'mɪsɪv] *a* покорный, кроткий, смиренный.

submit [səb'mɪt] *v* 1) покоряться, подчиняться; 2) передавать, представлять (*на рассмотрение, экспертизу*); 3) (почтительно) указывать, утверждать; that, I ~, is a false inference смею утверждать, что это неправильный вывод.

subordinate[a] I [sə'bɔːdnɪt] *n* подчинённое лицо, подчинённый.

subordinate[a] II *a* 1) подчинённый; 2) второстепенный; 3) *грам.* придаточный (*о предложении*).

subordinate[b] [sə'bɔːdɪneɪt] *v* подчинять.

subordination [sə,bɔːdɪ'neɪʃən] *n* подчинение; повиновение; субординация.

suborn [sʌ'bɔːn] *v* подкупать; склонять (*к преступлению*).

subpoena I [səb'piːnə] *n* повестка, вызов в суд.

subpoena II *v* вызывать в суд.

subscribe [səb'skraɪb] *v* 1) подписать своё имя; подписываться (*тж. на газету, журнал; to*); 2) подписать(ся), пожертвовать (*деньги на что-л.*); 3) присоединяться (*к — to*).

subscriber [səb'skraɪbə] *n* подписчик.

subscription [səb'skrɪpʃən] *n* 1) подписка; 2) подпись (*на документе*); 3) подписание; 4) *attr* подписной, осуществлённый по подписке.

subsequent ['sʌbsɪkwənt] *a* последующий; ~ ирон являющийся результатом.

subsequently [ˈsʌbsɪkwəntlɪ] *adv* впоследствии, потом.

subserve [səbˈsəːv] *v* содействовать.

subservience [səbˈsəːvjəns] *n* 1) полезность; 2) раболепие, подхалимство.

subservient [səbˈsəːvjənt] *a* 1) содействующий; служащий средством; 2) раболепный.

subside [səbˈsaɪd] *v* 1) спадать, понижаться (*о воде, температуре*); 2) оседать (*о почве, постройке и т. п.*); опускаться; he ~d into an armchair он опустился в кресло; 3) утихать, успокаиваться (*о буре, возбуждении*).

subsidence [səbˈsaɪdəns] *n* 1) понижение, падение (*уровня воды, температуры*); 2) оседание (*грунта*).

subsidiary I [səbˈsɪdjərɪ] *n* филиал.

subsidiary II *a* 1) вспомогательный, дополнительный; второстепенный; 2) субсидируемый.

subsidize [ˈsʌbsɪdaɪz] *v* субсидировать.

subsidy [ˈsʌbsɪdɪ] *n* денежное ассигнование; дотация; субсидия.

subsist [səbˈsɪst] *v* 1) жить, существовать; 2) содержать.

subsistence [səbˈsɪstəns] *n* 1) существование; 2) средства к существованию (*тж.* means of ~).

subsoil [ˈsʌbsɔɪl] *n* 1) подпочва; 2) *attr* подпочвенный.

substance [ˈsʌbstəns] *n* 1) вещество, материя, субстанция; 2) сущность, суть, существо, основание; in ~ в главном, по существу (*вопроса и т. п.*); 3) содержание; 4) реальная ценность; 5) состояние, богатство.

substantial [səbˈstænʃəl] *a* 1) существенный; заметный; 2) реальный; фактический; вещественный; 3) прочный, крепкий; 4) состоятельный.

substantiate [səbˈstænʃɪeɪt] *v* приводить достаточные основания, доказательства.

substantive I [ˈsʌbstəntɪv] *n грам.* имя существительное.

substantive II *a* 1) самостоятельный, независимый; 2) *грам.:* ~ verb глагол to be.

substation [sʌbˈsteɪʃən] *n* подстанция.

substitute I [ˈsʌbstɪtjuːt] *n* 1) замена; заменитель; суррогат; 2) заместитель.

substitute II *v* 1) заменять; замещать; 2) подменять.

substitution [ˌsʌbstɪˈtjuːʃən] *n* замена, замещение.

substratum [ˈsʌbˈstrɑːtəm] *n* (*pl* substrata [ˈsʌbˈstrɑːtə]) нижний слой; основание.

substruction [sʌbˈstrʌkʃən] *n* фундамент, основание.

substructure [ˈsʌbˌstrʌktʃə] *см.* substruction.

subtend [sʌbˈtend] *v геом.* стягивать; противолежать.

subterfuge [ˈsʌbtəfjuːdʒ] *n* увёртка, уловка.

subterranean [ˌsʌbtəˈreɪnjən] *a* 1) подземный; 2) скрытый, тайный.

subtle [ˈsʌtl] *a* 1) нежный; тонкий, неуловимый; 2) острый; тонкий (*об уме, чувствах и т. п.*); 3) утончённый; 4) искусный; 5) хитрый, коварный; вкрадчивый.

subtlety [ˈsʌtltɪ] *n* 1) нежность; тонкость; неуловимость; 2) утончённость; 3) тонкое различие; 4) искусность; 5) хитрость, коварство.

subtract [səbˈtrækt] *v мат.* вычитать.

subtraction [səbˈtrækʃən] *n мат.* вычитание.

subtrahend [ˈsʌbtrəhend] *n мат.* вычитаемое.

subtropical [ˈsʌbˈtrɔpɪkəl] *a* субтропический.

suburb [ˈsʌbəːb] *n* 1) пригород; *pl* предместья; окрестности; 2) *attr* пригородный.

suburban [səˈbəːbən] *a* пригородный.

subversion [sʌbˈvəːʃən] *n* ниспровержение, свержение; разрушение.

subversive [sʌbˈvəːsɪv] *a* разрушительный; гибельный; *перен.* подрывной.

subvert [sʌbˈvəːt] *v* свергать, ниспровергать; разрушать; *перен.* подрывать.

subway [ˈsʌbweɪ] *n* 1) тоннель; подземный переход; 2) *амер.* метрополитен.

succeed [səkˈsiːd] *v* 1) следовать за, сменять; наследовать; 2) иметь успех; удаваться; преуспевать (*в чём-л.*— in + Gerund); I ~ed мне удалось.

success [səkˈses] *n* 1) успех, удача; big (giddy) ~ крупный (головокружительный) успех; ill ~ неуспех; неудача; to score a great ~ иметь большой успех; 2): this book is a ~ эта книга — удача автора; эта книга имеет успех; he was a great ~ as an actor он был замечательным актёром.

successful [səkˈsesful] *a* 1) удачный; 2) счастливый, удачливый.

succession [səkˈseʃən] *n* 1) последовательность; непрерывный ряд; in ~ подряд; 2) преемственность; 3) право наследования; порядок престолонаследия.

successive [səkˈsesɪv] *a* последующий; последовательный; следующий один за другим.

successor [səkˈsesə] *n* преемник, наследник.

succinct [səkˈsɪŋkt] *a* сжатый, краткий.

succor [ˈsʌkə] I, II *амер. см.* succour I, II.

succotash [ˈsʌkətæʃ] *n амер.* блюдо из зелёной кукурузы и фасоли.

succour I [ˈsʌkə] *n* помощь.

succour II *v* помогать, приходить на помощь.

succulence [ˈsʌkjuləns] *n* сочность.

succulent [ˈsʌkjulənt] *a* сочный.

succumb [səˈkʌm] *v* 1) уступить, прекратить сопротивление; не выдержать; 2) умереть.

such I [sʌtʃ] *a* такой; ~ as такой как; как например (*см. тж.* II).

such II *pron* таковой; ~ as *поэт.* те кто (*см. тж.* I); as ~ как таковой; all ~ такие люди; and ~ и тому подобные.

such-and-such [ˈsʌtʃənsʌtʃ] *a* такой-то.

suck I [sʌk] *n* 1) сосание; to give a ~ кормить грудью; 2) глоток; 3) засасывание, всасывание; 4) *шк. сленг* неудача, разочарование; 5) *pl шк. сленг* сласти.

suck II *v* сосать; высасывать; посасывать (*трубку; at*); □ to ~ in а) всасывать, впитывать; б) засасывать; to ~ out а) высасывать; б) извлекать (*пользу*); to ~ up а) всасывать; поглощать; б) *сленг* подлизываться (*к — at*).

sucker [ˈsʌkə] *n* 1) сосунок; 2) *разг.* паразит; 3) *амер. разг.* молокосос, простак; 4) *амер. разг.* леденец на палочке; 5) присоска, присосок; 6) *тех.* поршень насоса.

sucking [ˈsʌkɪŋ] *a* 1) грудной (*о ребёнке*); 2) начинающий, неопытный; 3) всасывающий.

suckle [ˈsʌkl] *v* кормить (*грудью*); вскармливать.

suckling ['sʌklɪŋ] *n* сосунок; грудной ребёнок; *перен.* молокосос.

suction ['sʌkʃən] *n* 1) сосание; всасывание; поглощение; присасывание; 2) *attr* всасывающий; *тех.* впускной.

sudden I ['sʌdn] *a* внезапный; неожиданный; he is ~ in his movements он очень резок, стремителен в своих движениях.

sudden II *n*: (all) of a ~, on a ~ вдруг, внезапно.

suddenly ['sʌdnlɪ] *adv* вдруг, внезапно.

suds [sʌdz] *n pl* мыльная вода.

sue [sjuː] *v* 1) преследовать судом, возбуждать судебное дело; 2) просить; □ to ~ out выхлопотать (*в суде*).

suède [sweɪd] *n* 1) замша; 2) *attr* замшевый.

suet [sjuɪt] *n* почечное *или* нутряное сало.

suffer ['sʌfə] *v* 1) страдать; испытывать (*боль, горе и т. п.*); претерпевать; 2) допускать, терпеть, сносить, переносить; 3) *уст.* быть казнённым.

sufferance ['sʌfərəns] *n* 1) *уст.* попустительство; 2) терпимость; on ~ из милости; he is here on ~ его здесь только терпят.

suffering ['sʌfərɪŋ] *n* страдание; protracted ~s долгие страдания.

suffice [sə'faɪs] *v* хватать, быть достаточным; удовлетворять; ~ it to say that... достаточно сказать, что...

sufficiency [sə'fɪʃənsɪ] *n* достаточность.

sufficient I [sə'fɪʃənt] *n разг.* достаточное количество.

sufficient II *a* достаточный.

suffix ['sʌfɪks] *n грам.* суффикс, окончание.

suffocate ['sʌfəkeɪt] *v* 1) задыхаться; 2) душить, удушать.

suffocation [,sʌfə'keɪʃən] *n* 1) удушье; 2) удушение.

suffrage ['sʌfrɪdʒ] *n* 1) избирательное право; право голоса; adult ~ право голоса для лиц, достигших совершеннолетия; universal ~ всеобщее избирательное право; household ~ право голоса для съёмщиков квартир; 2) одобрение, согласие.

suffragette [,sʌfrə'dʒet] *n* суфражистка.

suffuse [sə'fjuːz] *v* заливать (*слезами*); покрывать (*румянцем и т. п.*).

sugar I ['ʃugə] *n* 1) сахар; cane (beet) ~ тростниковый (свекловичный) сахар; powdered ~, castor ~ сахарная пудра; granulated ~ сахарный песок; loaf ~ рафинад; lump ~ колотый *или* пилёный сахар; 2) лесть; 3) *хим.* сахароза.

sugar II *v* 1) подслащивать; обсахаривать; 2) льстить.

sugar-basin ['ʃugə,beɪsn] *n* сахарница.

sugar-beet ['ʃugəbiːt] *n* сахарная свёкла.

sugar-bowl ['ʃugəboul] *n* сахарница.

sugar-cane ['ʃugəkeɪn] *n* сахарный тростник.

sugar-loaf ['ʃugəlouf] *n* голова сахару.

sugarplum ['ʃugəplʌm] *n* круглый леденец.

sugar-tongs ['ʃugətɔŋz] *n pl* щипчики для сахара.

sugary ['ʃugərɪ] *a* 1) сахарный; 2) сахаристый; 3) льстивый, приторный, сладкий.

suggest [sə'dʒest] *v* 1) предлагать, советовать; 2) предполагать, допускать; it will not be ~ed трудно допустить; 3) внушать, наводить на мысль;

намекать, подсказывать; does it ~ nothing to you? разве это вам ничего не говорит?

suggestion [sə'dʒestʃən] *n* 1) совет, предложение; намёк; to make a ~ подать мысль; сделать предложение; 2) внушение; full of ~ многозначительный, наводящий на размышления.

suggestive [sə'dʒestɪv] *a* 1) вызывающий мысли, заставляющий думать; 2) соблазнительный, вызывающий неподобающие мысли.

suicidal [sjuɪ'saɪdl] *a* убийственный; губительный, гибельный.

suicide ['sjuɪsaɪd] *n* 1) самоубийство; to commit ~ покончить жизнь самоубийством; 2) самоубийца.

suit[1] [sjuːt] *n* 1) костюм, тройка (*тж.* ~ of clothes); sack ~ (пиджачный) костюм; dress ~ фрак; two-piece (three-piece) ~ женский костюм из двух (трёх) предметов; space ~ космический костюм; a ~ of dittos полный костюм (*из одного материала*); 2) комплект, набор; out of ~s разрозненный; 3) *карт.* масть; long (short) ~ сильная (слабая) масть; to follow ~ ходить в масть; *перен.* следовать примеру, подражать.

suit[2] *n* 1) прошение, просьба, ходатайство; 2) *юр.* тяжба, судебное дело; to bring a ~ against предъявить иск; 3) сватовство, ухаживание.

suit[3] *v* 1) годиться, соответствовать; удовлетворять (требованиям); ~ yourself поступайте как вам угодно; to ~ oneself выбирать по вкусу; that will ~ это подходит, это (меня) устраивает; it does not ~ me это меня не устраивает; 2) быть к лицу; 3) приспосабливать.

suitable ['sjuːtəbl] *a* подходящий, годный.

suitcase ['sjuːtkeɪs] *n* чемодан.

suite [swiːt] *n* 1) набор, комплект; гарнитур; ~ of rooms а) ряд комнат, анфилада комнат; б) комнаты (*в гостинице и т. п.*), занимаемые одним лицом; 2) *муз.* сюита; 3) свита.

suited ['sjuːtɪd] *a* подходящий, годный; соответствующий (*to, for*).

suitor ['sjuːtə] *n* 1) проситель; 2) кавалер, поклонник; 3) *юр.* истец.

sulfur I, II, III ['sʌlfə] *см.* sulphur I, II, III.

sulk I [sʌlk] *n обыкн. pl* плохое настроение (*тж.* a fit of ~s); he is in the ~s он сердит, он в плохом настроении.

sulk II *v* 1) сердиться, дуться; 2) говорить сердито.

sulky I ['sʌlkɪ] *n* одноколка.

sulky II *a* мрачный, хмурый, угрюмый; сердитый.

sullen ['sʌlən] *a* угрюмый, мрачный; замкнутый.

sullens ['sʌlənz] *n pl*: the ~ плохое настроение.

sully ['sʌlɪ] *v* умалять, принижать; пачкать, пятнать.

sulphate ['sʌlfeɪt] *n* соль серной кислоты; сульфат.

sulphur I ['sʌlfə] *n* 1) сера; 2) зеленовато-жёлтый цвет.

sulphur II *a* зеленовато-жёлтый.

sulphur III *v* окуривать серой.

sulphuric [sʌl'fjuərɪk] *a* серный.

sulphurous ['sʌlfərəs] *a* 1) сернистый; 2) зеленовато-жёлтый.

sultan ['sʌltən] *n* султа́н.

sultana [səl'taːnə] *n* 1) султа́нша; 2) ме́лкий изю́м без ко́сточек.

sultriness ['sʌltrɪnɪs] *n* духота́.

sultry ['sʌltrɪ] *a* ду́шный (*о погоде, атмосфере*), зно́йный.

sum I [sʌm] *n* 1) су́мма, о́бщий ито́г, о́бщее коли́чество; ~ total о́бщая су́мма; in a lump ~ единовре́менно (*об уплате*); 2) су́щность, суть; in ~ в о́бщем, в ито́ге, ко́ротко говоря́; 3) арифмети́ческая зада́ча; to do a ~, to do ~s реша́ть зада́чу, зада́чи; he did a rapid ~ in his head он бы́стро реши́л зада́чу в уме́; he is good at ~s он силён в арифме́тике.

sum II *v* подводи́ть ито́г (*часто* to ~ up); □ to ~ up сумми́ровать; резюми́ровать.

summarily ['sʌmərɪlɪ] *adv* кра́тко, вкра́тце.

summarize ['sʌməraɪz] *v* сумми́ровать; резюми́ровать, подводи́ть ито́г.

summary I ['sʌmərɪ] *n* кра́ткое изложе́ние, сво́дка, конспе́кт.

summary II *a* 1) кра́ткий, сжа́тый; 2) ско́рый, уско́ренный.

summer ['sʌmə] *n* 1) ле́то; high ~ (в) разга́р ле́та; Indian ~, St. Martin's ~, St. Luke's ~ тёплые сухи́е дни по́здней о́сени; ≅ «ба́бье ле́то»; 2) год (жи́зни); a child of ten ~s ребёнок десяти́ лет; 3) *attr* ле́тний.

summer-house ['sʌməhaus] *n* бесе́дка.

summer-time ['sʌmətaɪm] *n* ле́тнее вре́мя, ле́тний пери́од.

summit ['sʌmɪt] *n* 1) верши́на; *перен. тж.* верх, преде́л; 2) совеща́ние, конфере́нция на вы́сшем у́ровне; to break up (*или* to disrupt, to torpedo, to wreck) the ~ сорва́ть (торпеди́ровать, провали́ть) совеща́ние, конфере́нцию в верха́х.

summitology [ˌsʌmɪ'tɔlədʒɪ] *n* исто́рия конфере́нций на вы́сшем у́ровне.

summon ['sʌmən] *v* 1) вызыва́ть (*особ. в суд*); призыва́ть; 2) созыва́ть (*собрание*); 3) предлага́ть сда́ться, тре́бовать сда́ться; □ to ~ up собра́ться (*с духом, с силами*).

summons I ['sʌmənz] *n* 1) вы́зов, приглаше́ние яви́ться (*особ. в суд*); суде́бная пове́стка; 2) предложе́ние сда́ться.

summons II *v* вызыва́ть пове́сткой.

sumptuary ['sʌmptʃuərɪ] *a* регули́рующий расхо́ды.

sumptuous ['sʌmptʃuəs] *a* роско́шный, великоле́пный.

sun I [sʌn] *n* 1) со́лнце; the midnight ~ полуно́чное со́лнце; mock ~ *астр.* ло́жное со́лнце; to shoot the ~ определя́ть высоту́ со́лнца; under the ~ под со́лнцем, на земле́; against the ~ про́тив часово́й стре́лки; with the ~ по часово́й стре́лке; his ~ is set вре́мя его́ ко́нчилось, его́ звезда́ закати́лась; to take the ~ а) загора́ть; б) определя́ть высоту́ со́лнца; 2) *поэт.* день, год; 3) *attr* со́лнечный; ◊ to have been out in the ~, to have the ~ in one's eyes быть подвы́пившим.

sun II *v* 1) выставля́ть на со́лнце; подверга́ть де́йствию со́лнца; 2) загора́ть (*тж.* to ~ oneself).

sunbeam ['sʌnbiːm] *n* со́лнечный луч.

sun-blind ['sʌnblaɪnd] *n* тент.

sunburn ['sʌnbəːn] *n* зага́р.

sunburnt ['sʌnbəːnt] *a* загоре́лый.

sundae ['sʌndeɪ] *n амер.* моро́женое с фру́ктами и оре́хами.

Sunday ['sʌndɪ] *n* 1) воскресе́нье; Show ~ после́днее воскресе́нье пе́ред а́ктом (*в Оксфордском университете*); 2) *attr* воскре́сный; ◊ when three ~s come together никогда́.

Sunday-school ['sʌndɪˌskuːl] *n* воскре́сная шко́ла.

sunder ['sʌndə] *v* разделя́ть, разъединя́ть, разлуча́ть.

sundew ['sʌndjuː] *n бот.* рося́нка, мухоло́вка.

sun-dial ['sʌndaɪəl] *n* со́лнечные часы́.

sundown ['sʌndaun] *n* зака́т, захо́д со́лнца.

sundries ['sʌndrɪz] *n pl* вся́кая вся́чина, ра́зное.

sundry ['sʌndrɪ] *a* разли́чный, ра́зный; all and ~ все вме́сте и ка́ждый в отде́льности.

sun-fish ['sʌnfɪʃ] *n* луна́-ры́ба.

sunflower ['sʌnˌflauə] *n* подсо́лнух, подсо́лнечник.

sung [sʌŋ] *p. p. см.* sing II.

sun-glasses ['sʌnˌɡlɑːsɪz] *n pl* защи́тные очки́ (*от солнца*).

sun-hunter ['sʌnˌhʌntə] *n* люби́тель загора́ть.

sunk I [sʌŋk] *p. p. см.* sink[1].

sunk II *a* погружённый, пото́пленный.

sunken ['sʌŋkən] *a* 1) погружённый, зато́пленный; затону́вший; 2) осе́вший; 3) впа́лый (*о щека́х*); запа́вший (*о глазах*).

sunless ['sʌnlɪs] *a* лишённый со́лнца.

sunlight ['sʌnlaɪt] *n* со́лнечный свет.

sunlit ['sʌnlɪt] *a* освещённый со́лнцем.

sunny ['sʌnɪ] *a* со́лнечный; *перен.* ра́достный, весёлый.

sun-rays ['sʌnreɪz] *n pl мед.* ква́рцевая ла́мпа, ква́рцевые лучи́.

sunrise ['sʌnraɪz] *n* восхо́д со́лнца.

sun-seeker ['sʌnˌsiːkə] *см.* sun-hunter.

sunset ['sʌnset] *n* 1) захо́д со́лнца; зака́т; 2) *attr* зака́тный; *перен.* прекло́нный (*о возрасте*).

sunshade ['sʌnʃeɪd] *n* зо́нтик (*от солнца*).

sunshine ['sʌnʃaɪn] *n* 1) со́лнечный свет; 2) я́сная пого́да; *перен.* ра́дость, весе́лье.

sun-spot ['sʌnspɔt] *n* 1) пятно́ (*на солнце*); 2) весну́шка.

sunstroke ['sʌnstrouk] *n* со́лнечный уда́р.

sunsuit ['sʌnsjuːt] *n* лёгкое ле́тнее пла́тье.

sun-tan ['sʌntæn] *n* зага́р; to get a ~ загоре́ть.

sun-up ['sʌnˌʌp] *n* восхо́д со́лнца.

sup I [sʌp] *n* глото́к.

sup II *v* 1) хлеба́ть; отхлёбывать; 2) у́жинать; 3) корми́ть у́жином; 4) съесть за у́жином (*тж.* to ~ off, to ~ on).

super I ['sjuːprə] *n разг.* 1) *театр.* стати́ст; 2) *театр.* актёр на выходны́е ро́ли; 3) незначи́тельный, ли́шний челове́к; 4) первокла́ссный това́р; 5) *кино см.* superfilm.

super II *a* великоле́пный, первокла́ссный.

super- ['sjuːprə-] *pref указывает на:* а) *превосходство или преобладание в качестве, размере, степени и т. п.* сверх-; superfine сверхтонкий, превосхо́дный; б) *положение над чем-л.* над-; superstructure надстро́йка; в) *наличие данного вещества в избытке в каком-л. соединении:* superphosphate суперфосфа́т.

superannuate [ˌsjuːprə'rænjueɪt] *v* 1) увольня́ть по ста́рости; переводи́ть на пе́нсию; 2) исключа́ть из шко́лы неуспева́ющих переро́стков.

superannuated [ˌsjuːpə'rænjueɪtɪd] *a* 1) престаре́лый; 2) устаре́лый, вы́шедший из употребле́ния.

superannuation [ˌsjuːpəˌrænju'eɪʃən] *n* 1) преде́льный во́зраст; 2) увольне́ние по ста́рости *или* за вы́слугой лет; 3) назначе́ние пе́нсии (по ста́рости).

superb [sjuː'pəːb] *a* великоле́пный; прекра́сный; превосхо́дный; роско́шный.

supercargo ['sjuːpəˌkɑːgou] *n мор.* ве́дающий гру́зом на су́дне.

supercilious [ˌsjuːpə'sɪlɪəs] *a* высокоме́рный, надме́нный.

superficial [ˌsjuːpə'fɪʃəl] *a* пове́рхностный; неглубо́кий, вне́шний.

superfilm ['sjuːpəˌfɪlm] *n кино* боеви́к.

superfine ['sjuːpə'faɪn] *a* 1) вы́сшего со́рта, лу́чшего ка́чества; 2) утончённейший.

superfluity [ˌsjuːpə'fluːɪtɪ] *n* 1) оби́лие; 2) избы́ток, изли́шек; 3) изли́шество.

superfluous [sjuː'pəːfluəs] *a* изли́шний, нену́жный, чрезме́рный.

superhuman [ˌsjuːpə'hjuːmən] *a* сверхчелове́ческий.

superimpose ['sjuːpərɪm'pouz] *v* накла́дывать.

superintend [ˌsjuːpərɪn'tend] *v* 1) управля́ть, заве́довать; 2) наблюда́ть, контроли́ровать.

superintendence [ˌsjuːpərɪn'tendəns] *n* 1) заве́дование, управле́ние; 2) контро́ль, надзо́р.

superintendent [ˌsjuːpərɪn'tendənt] *n* 1) нача́льник, заве́дующий; 2) полице́йский инспе́ктор.

superior I [sjuː'pɪərɪə] *n* 1) нача́льник, вышестоя́щий; нача́льство; 2) превосходя́щий кого́-л. в чём-л.; he has no ~ in courage никто́ не превосхо́дит его́ в хра́брости; 3) (S.) настоя́тель (-ница) (*монастыря́*).

superior II *a* 1) вы́сший, ста́рший, вышестоя́щий; 2) превосхо́дный; лу́чший; превосходя́щий; вы́сшего ка́чества; 3) недосту́пный (*чему-л.*), стоя́щий вы́ше (*предрассу́дков и т. п.*).

superiority [sjuːˌpɪərɪ'ɔrɪtɪ] *n* 1) старшинство́; 2) превосхо́дство; переве́с.

superlative I [sjuː'pəːlətɪv] *n грам.* превосхо́дная сте́пень.

superlative II *a* 1) высоча́йший; велича́йший; 2) *грам.* превосхо́дный (*о степени*).

superman ['sjuːpəmæn] *n* сверхчелове́к.

supernatural [ˌsjuːpə'nætʃrəl] *a* сверхъесте́ственный.

supernumerary I [ˌsjuːpə'njuːmərərɪ] *n* 1) сверхшта́тный рабо́тник; 2) *театр.* стати́ст.

supernumerary II *a* сверхшта́тный; дополни́тельный.

superprofit ['sjuːpə'prɔfɪt] *n* сверхприбыль.

superscribe ['sjuːpə'skraɪb] *v* надпи́сывать; адресова́ть.

superscription [ˌsjuːpə'skrɪpʃən] *n* на́дпись; а́дрес.

supersede [ˌsjuːpə'siːd] *v* 1) заменя́ть, смеща́ть (*рабо́тника*); 2) обходи́ть (*при повыше́нии по слу́жбе или награжде́нии*); 3) занима́ть чьё-л. ме́сто; вытесня́ть.

supersonic ['sjuːpə'sɔnɪk] *a* сверхзвуково́й.

supersound [ˌsjuːpə'saund] *n физ.* ультразву́к.

superstition [ˌsjuːpə'stɪʃən] *n* суеве́рие.

superstitious [ˌsjuːpə'stɪʃəs] *a* суеве́рный.

superstructure ['sjuːpəˌstrʌktʃə] *n* надстро́йка;

a ~ on the basis *филос.* надстро́йка над ба́зисом.

supertax ['sjuːpətæks] *n* нало́г на сверхприбыль.

supervene [ˌsjuːpə'viːn] *v* сле́довать за; вытека́ть из.

supervention [ˌsjuːpə'venʃən] *n* (по)сле́дствие, результа́т.

supervise ['sjuːpəvaɪz] *v* 1) надзира́ть, наблюда́ть (*за чем-л.*); 2) просма́тривать; 3) заве́довать.

supervision [ˌsjuːpə'vɪʒən] *n* 1) наблюде́ние, надзо́р; 2) просмо́тр; 3) заве́дование; under the ~ of в ве́дении, под руково́дством кого́-л.

supervisor ['sjuːpəvaɪzə] *n* 1) надсмо́трщик, наблюда́тель; 2) контролёр; 3) *амер.* инспе́ктор (*шко́лы*).

supine[a] ['sjuːpaɪn] *n грам.* супи́н.

supine[b] [sjuː'paɪn] *a* 1) лежа́щий на́взничь; 2) лени́вый; ко́сный.

supper ['sʌpə] *n* у́жин; ◇ the Last Supper та́йная ве́черя.

supplant [sə'plɑːnt] *v* выжива́ть, вытесня́ть.

supple I ['sʌpl] *a* 1) ги́бкий; 2) усту́пчивый, пода́тливый; 3) уго́дливый, льсти́вый.

supple II *v* де́лать(ся) ги́бким, пода́тливым.

supplement[a] ['sʌplɪmənt] *n* дополне́ние, добавле́ние; приложе́ние.

supplement[b] ['sʌplɪment] *v* дополня́ть, пополня́ть.

supplemental [ˌsʌplɪ'mentl] *a* дополни́тельный.

supplementary [ˌsʌplɪ'mentərɪ] *a* дополни́тельный.

suppliant I ['sʌplɪənt] *n* проси́тель.

suppliant II *a* проси́тельный, умоля́ющий.

supplicate ['sʌplɪkeɪt] *v* 1) проси́ть, умоля́ть (*о чём-л. — for; кого-л. — to*).

supplication ['sʌplɪ'keɪʃən] *n* мольба́, про́сьба.

supply[a] I [sə'plaɪ] *n* 1) снабже́ние, поста́вка; подво́з; 2) запа́с; an inexhaustible ~ неисчерпа́емый запа́с; 3) *эк.* предложе́ние; ~ and demand спрос и предложе́ние; 4) *pl* припа́сы, продово́льствие; 5) *pl* де́нежная по́мощь, содержа́ние; 6) *pl* ассигнова́ния, утверждённые парла́ментом; 7) (вре́менный) замести́тель.

supply[a] II *v* 1) снабжа́ть; поставля́ть, доставля́ть; подава́ть; 2) обеспе́чивать, удовлетворя́ть (*потре́бность и т. п.*); восполня́ть (*недоста́ток и т. п.*); 3) замеща́ть.

supply[b] ['sʌplɪ] *adv* 1) ги́бко; 2) льсти́во.

support I [sə'pɔːt] *n* 1) подде́ржка; to give ~ to поддержа́ть; to gain (*или* to get, to obtain) ~ получи́ть подде́ржку; 2) опо́ра; опло́т; 3) подпо́рка, подста́вка.

support II *v* 1) подде́рживать; 2) выде́рживать, выноси́ть; 3) содержа́ть (*семью́*); 4) подде́рживать, подкрепля́ть (*до́воды и т. п.*).

supporter [sə'pɔːtə] *n* 1) сторо́нник, приве́рженец; peace ~ сторо́нник ми́ра; 2) опо́ра, корми́лец (*семьи́*); 3) же́ртвователь.

suppose [sə'pouz] *v* 1) предполага́ть; 2) полага́ть, допуска́ть, ду́мать; what do you ~ he meant? как вы ду́маете, что он име́л в виду́?; I ~ полага́ю, что так, вероя́тно; ◇ в *Imp выража́ет предложе́ние:* ~ we went for a walk? а не пойти́ ли нам прогуля́ться?

supposed [sə'pouzd] *a* мни́мый, предполага́емый.

supposedly [sə'pouzıdlı] *adv* возможно, предположительно.

supposition [,sʌpə'zıʃən] *n* предположение.

supposititious [sə,pozı'tıʃəs] *a* подложный.

suppress [sə'pres] *v* 1) подавлять; 2) запрещать (*газету, книгу и т. п.*); 3) замалчивать, скрывать (*факты, правду и т. п.*).

suppression [sə'preʃən] *n* 1) подавление; 2) запрещение (*газеты, книги*); 3) замалчивание.

suppurate ['sʌpjuəreıt] *v* гноиться.

suppuration [,sʌpjuə'reıʃən] *n* нагноение.

supremacy [sju'preməsı] *n* верховенство; верховная власть.

supreme [sju'priːm] *a* 1) верховный, высший; 2) величайший; 3) крайний.

surcease [sə'siːs] *n* передышка; перерыв, прекращение.

surcharge[a] ['səːtʃɑːdʒ] *n* 1) перегрузка; добавочная нагрузка; 2) перерасход; 3) дополнительная плата; 4) штраф, пеня.

surcharge[b] [sə'tʃɑːdʒ] *v* 1) перегружать; 2) взыскивать (*пеню и т. п.*).

surcingle ['səːsıŋgl] *n* подпруга.

sure I [ʃuə] *a* 1) уверенный; to stand ~ твёрдо стоять (*на ногах*); ~ of убеждённый в чём-л.; ~ of oneself самоуверенный; are you ~? вы уверены?; he feels (*или* is) ~ of success он уверен в успехе; 2) верный, надёжный; несомненный; he is ~ to come он обязательно придёт; be ~ to tell me all the news непременно расскажите мне все новости; to be ~ несомненно, конечно; to be ~ she is not a beauty! конечно, она не красавица!; well I'm ~!, well to be ~! вот те раз!; однако!; to make ~ а) убедиться, удостовериться; б) обеспечить; slow and ~ медленно, но верно.

sure II *adv* конечно, несомненно; as ~ as верно как; ~ enough в действительности, на самом деле; конечно.

sure III *int* безусловно, несомненно.

surely ['ʃuəlı] *adv* 1) несомненно; наверно; конечно; 2) уверенно.

surety ['ʃuətı] *n* 1) поручитель; to stand ~ for брать на поруки, ручаться за кого-л.; 2) уверенность; of a ~ наверно, несомненно; 3) залог.

surf [səːf] *n* бурун.

surface I ['səːfıs] *n* 1) поверхность; specular ~ отражающая поверхность; 2) внешняя сторона, внешность; on the ~ внешне, на первый взгляд; 3) *attr* поверхностный; внешний.

surface II *v* 1) отделывать поверхность; обтёсывать; 2) всплывать на поверхность (*о подводной лодке*).

surface-man ['səːfısmən] *n* ж.-д. путевой сторож, обходчик.

surfboard ['səːfbɔːd] *n* спорт. доска для катания на волнах.

surfeit I ['səːfıt] *n* 1) неумеренность (*особ. в питье и пище*); 2) пресыщение, пресыщенность.

surfeit II *v* 1) перекармливать; 2) объедаться; 3) пресыщаться.

surfing ['səːfıŋ] *n* спорт. катание на волнах.

surge I [səːdʒ] *n* 1) большая волна, волнение; волны; 2) поэт. море; 3) астр. резкое увеличение (*солнечной активности*).

surge II *v* 1) вздыматься (*о волнах*); волноваться (*о ниве*); 2) приливать и отливать (*о тол-*

пе); 3) подниматься, нахлынуть (*о чувствах*); □ to ~ forward устремиться, ринуться вперёд.

surgeon ['səːdʒən] *n* 1) хирург; veterinary ~ ветеринар; 2) военный врач.

surgery ['səːdʒərı] *n* 1) хирургия; 2) хирургический кабинет; приёмная хирурга.

surgical ['səːdʒıkəl] *a* хирургический.

surly ['səːlı] *a* угрюмый, неприветливый.

surmise[a] ['səːmaız] *n* предположение, догадка.

surmise[b] [sə'maız] *v* предполагать, высказывать догадку; подозревать.

surmount [sə'maunt] *v* 1) преодолевать; 2) увенчивать, покрывать.

surname I ['səːneım] *n* 1) фамилия; 2) прозвище.

surname II *v* давать прозвище.

surpass [sə'pɑːs] *v* 1) превосходить, превышать; 2) перегонять.

surplus ['səːpləs] *n* 1) излишек, избыток, остаток; 2) *attr* излишний, избыточный; добавочный, прибавочный.

surprise I [sə'praız] *n* 1) удивление; 2) неожиданность; внезапность; by ~ неожиданно, врасплох; to take by ~ захватить врасплох; 3) сюрприз; to spring ~s делать сюрпризы; 4) *attr* внезапный, неожиданный.

surprise II *v* 1) удивлять; поражать, ошеломлять; I'm ~d at you! вы меня удивляете!; 2) захватить врасплох; to ~ in the act захватить, накрыть на месте преступления; 3): to ~ into (doing) smth. вынудить, принудить к чему-л. (*застав врасплох*).

surprising [sə'praızıŋ] *a* неожиданный; удивительный.

surrealism [sə'rıəlızəm] *n* сюрреализм.

surrender I [sə'rendə] *n* 1) сдача, капитуляция; ~ at discretion сдача на милость победителя; unconditional ~ безоговорочная капитуляция; 2) отказ (*от чего-л.*).

surrender II *v* 1) сдавать(ся), капитулировать; 2) отказываться от чего-л.; 3) уступать, поддаваться.

surreptitious [,sʌrəp'tıʃəs] *a* тайный; сделанный тайком, исподтишка.

surrey ['sʌrı] *n* лёгкий двухместный экипаж.

surrogate ['sʌrəgıt] *n* 1) заменитель; 2) заместитель.

surround [sə'raund] *v* окружать, обступать; *воен.* осаждать.

surroundings [sə'raundıŋz] *n pl* 1) окрестности, окружающая местность; 2) окружение, среда.

surtax I ['səːtæks] *n* добавочный налог.

surtax II *v* облагать добавочным налогом.

surveillance [sə'veıləns] *n* надзор, наблюдение.

survey[a] ['səːveı] *n* 1) обзор; осмотр; 2) обследование; 3) отчёт об обследовании; 4) (топографическая) съёмка; 5) план, карта; 6) топографическое управление.

survey[b] [sə'veı] *v* 1) обозревать; осматривать; 2) обследовать; 3) производить (топографическую) съёмку, изыскания, исследования.

surveyor [sə'veıə] *n* 1) инспектор, контролёр; 2) землемер; топограф.

survival [sə'vaıvəl] *n* 1) выживание; the ~ of the fittest *биол.* естественный отбор; 2) пережиток.

survive [sə'vaıv] *v* 1) выжить; уцелеть; 2) пережить (*современников, события и т. п.*).

survivor [sə'vaɪvə] *n* оставшийся в живых, уцелевший.

susceptibility [sə,septə'bɪlɪtɪ] *n* 1) впечатлительность; восприимчивость; чувствительность; 2) *pl* больное место, чувствительная струнка.

susceptible [sə'septəbl] *a* 1) впечатлительный; восприимчивый; 2) влюбчивый; 3) *predic* чувствительный, подверженный (*чему-л.* — to); 4) допускающий (*что-л.* — of).

suspect[a] [səs'pekt] *v* 1) подозревать; 2) сомневаться (*в чём-л.*).

suspect[b] I ['sʌspekt] *a predic* подозрительный, подозреваемый.

suspect[b] II *n* подозреваемый; подозрительный человек.

suspend [səs'pend] *v* 1) вешать, подвешивать; 2) откладывать; приостанавливать, (временно) прекращать; 3) (временно) отрешать, отстранять (*от должности и т. п.*); 4) (временно) лишать ученика права посещать школу (*в наказание за проступок*).

suspended [səs'pendɪd] *a* 1) подвешенный, висящий; 2) подвесной, висячий; 3) *хим.* взвешенный; 4) приостановленный, отложенный; 5) отстранённый (*от должности*); 6) лишённый права посещать школу.

suspender [səs'pendə] *n* 1) подвязка (*тж.* sock ~); 2) *pl* подтяжки, помочи; лямки.

suspense [səs'pens] *n* неизвестность, ожидание.

suspension [səs'penʃən] *n* 1) подвешивание, подвеска; 2) (временное) прекращение, приостановка; 3) отстранение, отрешение (*от должности*); 4) *attr* подвесной, висячий.

suspension-bridge [səs'penʃənbrɪdʒ] *n* висячий мост.

suspicion [səs'pɪʃən] *n* 1) подозрение; on ~ по подозрению; above ~ выше подозрения; under ~ под подозрением; 2) чуточка, оттенок, намёк.

suspicious [səs'pɪʃəs] *a* подозрительный.

suspiciousness [səs'pɪʃəsnɪs] *n* подозрительность.

sustain [səs'teɪn] *v* 1) поддерживать; 2) выдерживать; 3) понести (*потерю*); потерпеть (*поражение и т. п.*); подвергнуться.

sustained [səs'teɪnd] *a* непрерывный, длительный, долгий; устойчивый.

sustenance ['sʌstɪnəns] *n* 1) питательность; 2) пища; средства к существованию.

suture ['sjuːtʃə] *n* 1) шов; 2) *мед.* наложение шва; 3) *мед.* нить для сшивания раны.

suzerain ['suːzəreɪn] *n* 1) сюзерен; 2) сюзеренное государство.

suzerainty ['suːzəreɪntɪ] *n* 1) протекторат; 2) власть сюзерена.

swab I [swɔb] *n* швабра.

swab II *v*: to ~ down мыть шваброй; to ~ up подтирать шваброй.

swaddle ['swɔdl] *v* пеленать.

swag [swæg] *n* 1) *австрал.* котомка, узелок с вещами; 2) *сленг* добыча грабителя; *перен.* доходы от взяток *или* политических махинаций.

swagger I ['swægə] *n* 1) важный вид; чванство; 2) развязность, нахальство.

swagger II *a* (подчёркнуто) щегольской, шикарный.

swagger III *v* 1) ходить с важным видом; важничать; 2) хвастаться (about).

swagman ['swægmən] *n австрал.* свэгмен (*сезонный рабочий, кочующий безработный и т. д.*).

swain [sweɪn] *n* 1) деревенский парень; 2) *шутл.* обожатель, поклонник; 3) пастушок (*в пасторали*).

swallow[1] I ['swɔlou] *n* 1) глоток; 2) глотка.

swallow[1] II *v* 1) глотать, проглатывать; 2) поглощать (*тж.* to ~ up); 3) принимать на веру; he will ~ anything you tell him он поверит всему, что вы ему скажете.

swallow[2] *n* ласточка.

swallow-tailed ['swɔlouteɪld] *a* с раздвоенным хвостом.

swam [swæm] *past. см.* swim II.

swamp I [swɔmp] *n* 1) болото, топь; 2) *attr* болотный.

swamp II *v* 1) заливать, затоплять; заболачивать; 2) засыпать, заваливать (*письмами, работой и т. п.*).

swampy ['swɔmpɪ] *a* болотистый.

swan [swɔn] *n* лебедь; black ~ чёрный лебедь; *перен.* странное явление; ◊ the Swan of Avon Шекспир.

swank I [swæŋk] *n разг.* хвастовство, бахвальство.

swank II *a разг.* хвастать, бахвалиться.

swanky ['swæŋkɪ] *a разг.* 1) шикарный; 2) кичливый.

swan's-down ['swɔnzdaun] *n* 1) лебяжий пух; 2) вигоневая ткань.

swap I, II [swɔp] *см.* swop I, II.

sward [swɔːd] *n* газон; дёрн.

swarm[1] I [swɔːm] *n* 1) стая; рой; толпа; *pl тж.* масса, множество; 2) пчелиный рой.

swarm[1] II *v* 1) толпиться, двигаться толпами; 2) кишеть, изобиловать (*чем-либо* — with); 3) роиться.

swarm[2] *v* лезть, взбираться, карабкаться на (*тж.* to ~ up).

swart [swɔːt] *уст. см.* swarthy.

swarthy ['swɔːðɪ] *a* смуглый, темнолицый.

swash I [swɔʃ] *n* 1) плеск; 2) сильное течение.

swash II *v* 1) плескать(ся); 2) *уст.* сильно ударить.

swashbuckler ['swɔʃ,bʌklə] *n* 1) головорез, хулиган; 2) хвастун, пустозвон.

swat [swɔt] *v* шлёпнуть, хлопнуть.

swath [swɔːθ] *n* полоса скошенной травы, овса *и т. п.*; прокос; in ~s последовательными рядами.

swathe I [sweɪð] *n* бинт, повязка.

swathe II *v* 1) бинтовать; обматывать; 2) закутывать.

sway I [sweɪ] *n* 1) качание, колебание; взмах; 2) правление; власть, влияние; господство; to hold ~ over господствовать, управлять; 3) тенденция.

sway II *v* 1) качать(ся), колебать(ся); 2) иметь влияние на; 3) управлять, править; властвовать.

swear [sweə] *v* (*past* swore; *p. p.* sworn) 1) клясться; божиться; ручаться; 2) принимать присягу, присягать; 3) приводить к присяге; заставлять поклясться (*в чём-л.* — to); 4) (об)ругать; ругаться; □ to ~ by слепо верить, иметь веру (*во что-л.*); enough to ~ by незначительное количество; to ~ in приводить к присяге; to ~ off зарека́ться, дава́ть заро́к (*не де́лать чего́-л.*); to ~ to утвержда́ть под прися́гой.

sweat I [swet] *n* 1) пот, испа́рина; in a ~, all of a ~ а) весь в поту́; б) в трево́ге, в беспоко́йстве; в нетерпе́нии; running (*или* dripping, wet) with ~ облива́ясь по́том; by (*или* in) the ~ of one's brow в по́те лица́ своего́; 2) *разг.* тяжёлый труд; 3) запотева́ние, выделе́ние и осажде́ние вла́ги на пове́рхности чего́-л.

sweat II *v* 1) поте́ть; to ~ with fear облива́ться холо́дным по́том (*от страха*); 2) запотева́ть, сыре́ть; выделя́ть вла́гу; 3) *разг.* труди́ться; поте́ть (*над чем-л.*); 4) эксплуати́ровать; 5) заста́вить поте́ть; 6) загна́ть (*ло́шадь*); 7) *тех.* припа́ивать (in, on).

sweater ['swetə] *n* 1) сви́тер; 2) эксплуата́тор.

sweat-shop ['swetʃɔp] *n разг.* предприя́тие, применя́ющее потого́нную систе́му труда́.

sweaty ['swetɪ] *a* 1) по́тный; запоте́вший; 2) вызыва́ющий пот, тру́дный (*о рабо́те*).

Swede [swiːd] *n* швед; шве́дка; the ~s шве́ды.

Swedish I ['swiːdɪʃ] *n* шве́дский язы́к.

Swedish II *a* шве́дский.

sweep I [swiːp] *n* 1) вымета́ние, подмета́ние; чи́стка; to give a ~ мести́, смета́ть; to make a clean ~ of по́лностью отде́латься от кого́-л., чего́-л.; 2) трубочи́ст (*тж.* chimney-sweep); 3) разма́х; *перен. тж.* распростране́ние, разви́тие (*боле́зни и т. п.*); with one ~ одни́м взма́хом, одни́м движе́нием; the great ~ of modern research большо́й разма́х нау́чных иссле́дований; 4) охва́т, преде́лы; within the ~ of the eye наско́лько мо́жно охвати́ть гла́зом; в преде́лах ви́димости; 5) движе́ние, тече́ние; 6) поворо́т; изги́б; 7) протяже́ние, пролёт.

sweep II *v* (*past, p. p.* swept) 1) мести́, подмета́ть; чи́стить; очища́ть; 2) смета́ть; сноси́ть, уноси́ть; увлека́ть; 3) проноси́ться; нести́сь; мча́ться; to ~ past проходи́ть, проноси́ться ми́мо; 4) обру́шиваться на что-л.; проноси́ться над чем-л. (*о бу́ре*); 5) проводи́ть (*по чему́-л.*), каса́ться (*чего́-л.*); 6) ва́жно, велича́во выступа́ть; she swept out of the room она́ вели́чественно вы́плыла из ко́мнаты; 7) тяну́ться, простира́ться; 8) охва́тывать; быть охва́ченным; 9) оки́дывать взгля́дом, озира́ть; □ to ~ **away** а) смета́ть; б) уноси́ть (*об эпиде́мии, пото́ке и т. п.*).

sweeper ['swiːpə] *n* 1) мете́льщик, подмета́льщик; 2) *мор.* тра́льщик.

sweeping I ['swiːpɪŋ] *n* 1) подмета́ние, смета́ние; 2) *pl* сор, му́сор.

sweeping II *a* 1) широ́кий, радика́льный, реши́тельный; 2) огу́льный; 3) стреми́тельный; бы́стрый.

sweep-net ['swiːpnet] *n* нево́д.

sweepstake(s) ['swiːpsteɪk(s)] *n* игра́ на ска́чках.

sweet I [swiːt] *n* 1) *обыкн. pl* конфе́та; 2) сла́дкое (блю́до); 3) *обыкн. pl* арома́т; 4) сла́дость, прия́тность; 5) *pl* ра́дости, наслажде́ния; 6) возлю́бленный, -ная.

sweet II *a* 1) сла́дкий; 2) арома́тный, души́стый; 3) све́жий, неиспо́рченный; to keep the room ~ хорошо́ прове́тривать ко́мнату; 4) пре́сный, несолёный; 5) не́жный, мелоди́чный; прия́тный; 6) ми́лый, ла́сковый; привлека́тельный; а ~ one а) пре́лесть, ми́лочка; б) *сленг* си́льный уда́р кулако́м; ◇ to be ~ (up)on быть влюблённым.

sweetbrier ['swiːtˌbraɪə] *n* шипо́вник.

sweeten ['swiːtn] *v* подсла́щивать.

sweetheart ['swiːthɑːt] *n* возлю́бленный, -ная.

sweetish ['swiːtɪʃ] *a* сладкова́тый.

sweetmeat ['swiːtmiːt] *n* конфе́та.

sweetness ['swiːtnɪs] *n* 1) сла́дость; 2) прия́тность.

sweet-shop ['swiːtʃɔp] *n* конди́терская.

sweet-william ['swiːtˌwɪljəm] *n* туре́цкая гвозди́ка.

swell I [swel] *n* 1) вы́пуклость; возвыше́ние; 2) о́пухоль; утолще́ние; 3) зыбь, волне́ние; ground ~ мёртвая зыбь; 4) *муз.* нараста́ние и ослабле́ние зву́ка; 5) *разг.* франт, щёголь; све́тский челове́к; 6) *разг.* выдаю́щийся челове́к (*в како́й-л. о́бласти*); ши́шка.

swell II *a разг.* 1) шика́рный; 2) великоле́пный, отли́чный, замеча́тельный.

swell III *v* (*past* swelled; *p. p.* swelled, swollen) 1) пу́хнуть, распуха́ть; 2) раздува́ть(ся), вздува́ть(ся), надува́ть(ся); 3) поднима́ться; 4) уси́ливаться, увели́чиваться; нараста́ть (*о зву́ке*).

swelling I ['swelɪŋ] *n* 1) о́пухоль; 2) вы́пуклость.

swelling II *a* 1) вздыма́ющийся; 2) нараста́ющий; 3) напы́щенный, высокопа́рный.

swelter I ['sweltə] *n* зной, духота́.

swelter II *v* изнемога́ть от духоты́ и зно́я.

swept [swept] *past, p. p. см.* sweep II.

swerve I ['swəːv] *n* поворо́т, отклоне́ние (в сто́рону).

swerve II *v* отклоня́ть(ся), свора́чивать в сто́рону.

swift I [swɪft] *a* ско́рый, бы́стрый; ~ to anger вспы́льчивый.

swift II *adv* бы́стро, ско́ро.

swift-handed ['swɪft'hændɪd] *a* ло́вкий, бы́стрый.

swiftness ['swɪftnɪs] *n* быстрота́.

swig I [swɪg] *n* глото́к (*спиртно́го*).

swig II *v* потя́гивать вино́.

swill I [swɪl] *n* 1) ополаскивание, облива́ние (*водо́й*); 2) свино́е пи́то, помо́и.

swill II *v* 1) ополаскивать; обмыва́ть, облива́ть (*водо́й; ча́сто* to ~ out); 2) пить с жа́дностью.

swim I [swɪm] *n* 1) пла́вание; let's have a ~ пойдёмте купа́ться; an early ~ ра́ннее купа́ние; to take a ~ вы́купаться; 2) *спорт.* запла́в; 3) за́водь, изоби́лующая ры́бой; ◇ to be in (out of) the ~ быть (не) в ку́рсе де́ла.

swim II *v* (*past* swam; *p. p.* swum) 1) пла́вать, плыть; переплыва́ть; to sink or ~! ≅ была́ не была́!; будь что бу́дет!; 2) заставля́ть плыть; переправля́ть вплавь; 3) залива́ться, наполня́ться; ~ming eyes глаза́, по́лные слёз; 4) кружи́ться (*о голове́*); плыть пе́ред глаза́ми.

swimmer ['swɪmə] *n* 1) плове́ц; 2) поплаво́к.

swimmingly ['swɪmɪŋlɪ] *adv* гла́дко, без поме́х.

swindle I ['swɪndl] *n* обма́н, надува́тельство.

swindle II *v* 1) обма́нывать, надува́ть; 2) обма́ном выма́нивать.

swindler ['swɪndlə] *n* моше́нник, обма́нщик.

swine [swaɪn] *n* (*pl без изме́н.*) свинья́.

swineherd ['swaɪnhəːd] *n* свинопа́с.

swing I [swɪŋ] *n* 1) кача́ние, колеба́ние; разма́х; взмах; in full ~ по́лным хо́дом; в по́лном поря́дке; успе́шно; 2) каче́ли; 3) ритм; 4) сдвиг, измене́ние (*вле́во, впра́во*).

swing II *v* (*past, p. p.* swung) 1) кача́ть(ся);

колеба́ть(ся); колыха́ть(ся); развева́ться; 2) маха́ть, разма́хивать; 3) подве́шивать, ве́шать; висе́ть; 4) идти́ ме́рным ша́гом (*тж.* to ~ along, by, past); 5) повора́чивать(ся), поверну́ть(ся) (*тж.* to ~ round); □ to ~ to захло́пывать(ся).

swinish [ˈswaɪnɪʃ] *a* сви́нский, гря́зный.

swinishness [ˈswaɪnɪʃnɪs] *n* сви́нство.

swipe I [swaɪp] *n* си́льный уда́р.

swipe II *v разг.* 1) си́льно уда́рить; 2) (у)кра́сть.

swipes [swaɪps] *n pl* плохо́е пи́во.

swirl I [swəːl] *n* 1) водоворо́т; 2) круже́ние, завихре́ние; вихрь; 3) воро́нки (*на воде*); 4) след на воде́ (*от лодки и т. п.*).

swirl II *v* 1) образо́вывать водоворо́т; 2) кружи́ться в водоворо́те; 3) оставля́ть след на воде́.

swish I [swɪʃ] *n* взмах (*трости, косы*) со свистом.

swish II *v* 1) рассека́ть во́здух со сви́стом; 2) сечь ро́згой; □ to ~ off сбива́ть (*тростью и т. п., напр., цветы*).

Swiss I [swɪs] *n* швейца́рец; the ~ (*употр. как pl*) швейца́рцы.

Swiss II *a* швейца́рский.

switch I [swɪtʃ] *n* 1) прут; хлыст; 2) *эл.* выключа́тель; переключа́тель; коммута́тор; 3) *ж.-д.* стре́лка; 4) фальши́вая коса́.

switch II *v* 1) стега́ть пруто́м, хлысто́м; 2) разма́хивать; 3) бы́стро поверну́ть; 4) *эл.* переключа́ть, выключа́ть; 5) *ж.-д.* переводи́ть по́езд на другой путь; *перен.* направля́ть (*разговор и т. п.*) в другу́ю сто́рону; to ~ to a new line of talk переключи́ться на другу́ю те́му; □ to ~ off вы́ключить ток, свет, ра́дио; разъедини́ть, дать отбо́й (*по телефо́ну*); to ~ on а) включи́ть ток, свет, ра́дио; б) соедини́ть телефо́нного абоне́нта.

switch-board [ˈswɪtʃbɔːd] *n эл.* распредели́тельный щит.

switch-man [ˈswɪtʃmən] *n* стре́лочник.

switch-plug [ˈswɪtʃplʌg] *n* штепсель выключа́теля.

swob I, II [swɔb] *см.* swab I, II.

swollen [ˈswoulən] *p. p. см.* swell III.

swoon I [swuːn] *n* о́бморок.

swoon II *v* 1) теря́ть созна́ние; па́дать в о́бморок; 2) замира́ть (*о звуке*).

swoop I [swuːp] *n* внеза́пное нападе́ние.

swoop II *v* 1) налета́ть; броса́ться, устремля́ться (*на добычу и т. п.*); 2) *разг.* захвати́ть с налёта (*обыкн.* to ~ up); □ to ~ down а) устремля́ться (*на добычу*); б) *ав.* пики́ровать.

swop I [swɔp] *n разг.* 1) (товаро)обме́н; 2): heart ~ переса́дка се́рдца.

swop II *v разг.* 1) обме́нивать(ся), меня́ть(ся); 2) производи́ть переса́дку (*сердца и т. п.*).

sword [sɔːd] *n* 1) меч; ша́шка, са́бля, шпа́га; cavalry ~ кавалери́йская са́бля, ша́шка; duelling ~ рапи́ра; to draw (*или* to unsheathe) the ~ обнажи́ть меч; *перен.* нача́ть войну́; to sheathe the ~ вложи́ть меч в но́жны; *перен.* ко́нчить войну́; to measure (*или* to cross) ~s with скрести́ть мечи́, поме́ряться си́лами; to put to the ~ уби́ть на войне́; преда́ть мечу́, истреби́ть; казни́ть; 2) (the ~) война́; 3) (the ~) вое́нная мощь.

sword-belt [ˈsɔːdbelt] *n* портупе́я.

sword-fish [ˈsɔːdfɪʃ] *n* меч-ры́ба.

sword-hilt [ˈsɔːdhɪlt] *n* эфе́с.

sword-rattling [ˈsɔːdˈrætlɪŋ] *n* бряца́ние ору́жием.

swore [swɔː] *past см.* swear.

sworn [swɔːn] *p. p. см.* swear.

swum [swʌm] *p. p. см.* swim II.

swung [swʌŋ] *past, p. p. см.* swing II.

sycamore [ˈsɪkəmɔː] *n* 1) я́вор (*тж.* ~ maple); *амер.* плата́н, чина́ра; 2) ту́товая смоко́вница (*тж.* ~ fig).

sycophant [ˈsɪkəfənt] *n* льстец, низкопокло́нник.

syllabic [sɪˈlæbɪk] *a* слогово́й.

syllable [ˈsɪləbl] *n* слог; open (closed) ~ откры́тый (закры́тый) слог; not a ~! ни зву́ка!, ти́ше!

syllabus [ˈsɪləbəs] *n* (*pl тж.* syllabi [ˈsɪləbaɪ]) 1) програ́мма (*обучения*); расписа́ние; 2) конспе́кт, план.

syllogism [ˈsɪlədʒɪzəm] *n* силлоги́зм.

sylvan [ˈsɪlvən] *a* лесно́й, леси́стый.

symbol [ˈsɪmbəl] *n* 1) си́мвол, эмбле́ма; 2) обозначе́ние; знак.

symbolic(al) [sɪmˈbɔlɪk(əl)] *a* символи́ческий.

symbolism [ˈsɪmbəlɪzəm] *n* символи́зм.

symbolize [ˈsɪmbəlaɪz] *v* 1) символизи́ровать; 2) символи́чески изобража́ть.

symmetrical [sɪˈmetrɪkəl] *a* симметри́чный.

symmetry [ˈsɪmɪtrɪ] *n* 1) симметри́я; 2) соразме́рность.

sympathetic [ˌsɪmpəˈθetɪk] *a* 1) сочу́вственный, сочу́вствующий; 2) симпати́чный; 3) симпати́ческий.

sympathize [ˈsɪmpəθaɪz] *v* 1) симпатизи́ровать, сочу́вствовать (*кому-л.— with*); 2) выража́ть симпа́тию, сочу́вствие (*кому-л.— with*).

sympathizer [ˈsɪmpəθaɪzə] *n* сторо́нник; сочу́вствующий.

sympathy [ˈsɪmpəθɪ] *n* 1) взаимопонима́ние; симпа́тия; 2) сочу́вствие (*with*); сострада́ние (*for*).

symphony [ˈsɪmfənɪ] *n* симфо́ния.

symposium [sɪmˈpouzjəm] *n* (*pl* symposia [sɪmˈpouzɪə]) 1) обсужде́ние, собесе́дование; симпо́зиум; 2) сбо́рник стате́й на одну́ те́му.

symptom [ˈsɪmptəm] *n* при́знак, симпто́м.

symptomatic [ˌsɪmptəˈmætɪk] *a* симптомати́ческий.

synchronize [ˈsɪŋkrənaɪz] *v* 1) происходи́ть одновре́менно; совпада́ть по вре́мени; 2) устана́вливать одновре́менность (*событий*); 3) сверя́ть (*часы*); 4) пока́зывать одно́ вре́мя (*о часах*).

synchronous [ˈsɪŋkrənəs] *a* одновре́менный, синхро́нный.

syndicalism [ˈsɪndɪkəlɪzəm] *n* синдикали́зм.

syndicate [ˈsɪndɪkɪt] *n* синдика́т.

synonym [ˈsɪnənɪm] *n* сино́ним.

synonymous [sɪˈnɔnɪməs] *a* синоними́ческий.

synopsis [sɪˈnɔpsɪs] *n* (*pl* synopses [sɪˈnɔpsiːz]) обзо́р; конспе́кт.

syntax [ˈsɪntæks] *n* синтаксис.

synthesis [ˈsɪnθɪsɪs] *n* (*pl* syntheses [ˈsɪnθɪsiːz]) си́нтез.

synthetic [sɪnˈθetɪk] *a* синтети́ческий.

syphon [ˈsaɪfən] *см.* siphon.

Syrian I [ˈsɪrɪən] *n* сири́ец; сири́йка; the ~s сири́йцы.

Syrian II *a* сири́йский.

syringe I [ˈsɪrɪndʒ] *n* 1) шприц; hypodermic ~

шприц для подкожных впрыскиваний; 2) спринцовка; 3) пожарный насос.

syringe II *v* 1) впрыскивать; 2) спринцевать; промывать.

syrup ['sɪrəp] *n* 1) сироп; 2) патока; golden ~ светлая патока.

system ['sɪstɪm] *n* 1) система; ~ of government государственный строй, система правления; grammatical ~ of a language грамматический строй языка; speed-up ~, sweating ~ потогонная система; truck ~ оплата труда (рабочих) товарами; spoils ~ *амер.* система использования служебного положения для предоставления государственных должностей сторонникам победившей партии; 2): railway ~ сеть железных дорог; железнодорожная сеть; automatic orientation ~ автоматическая система ориентации; emergency escape ~ аварийная система спасения; docking ~ система стыковки (*космических кораблей*); river ~ система рек; mountain ~ горный хребет; solar ~ солнечная система; nervous ~ нервная система; 3) организм.

systematic [ˌsɪstɪ'mætɪk] *a* систематический.

systematize ['sɪstɪmətaɪz] *v* систематизировать.

T

T, t [tiː] *n* 20-я буква англ. алфавита; ◊ (right) to a T точь-в-точь; совершенно; в совершенстве; как раз; в точности; to cross the t's ≅ ставить точки над i.

tab [tæb] *n* 1) петелька, ушко; 2) наушник (*на шапке; тж.* ear-tab); 3) *разг.* счёт; учёт; чек; to keep ~ (s) on вести счёт, учёт; *перен.* следить (*за — on*).

tabard ['tæbəd] *n ист.* короткий плащ.

tabby ['tæbɪ] *n* 1) полосатая кошка; 2) сплетница; 3) муар.

tabernacle ['tæbə‚nækl] *n* 1) палатка, шатёр; 2) молельня.

table I ['teɪbl] *n* 1) стол; dining ~, dining-room ~ обеденный стол; 2) еда, трапеза; to be at ~ сидеть за обедом, ужином *и т. п.*; to lay (*или* to spread) the ~ накрывать на стол; to clear the ~ убрать со стола; 3) общество за столом; 4) таблица; табель; расписание; ~ of contents оглавление; multiplication ~ таблица умножения; mortality ~s статистика смертности (*по возрастам*); 5) плоская поверхность; горное плато; 6) дощечка; скрижаль; 7) *attr* столовый; ◊ to turn the ~s а) поменяться ролями; б) отплатить той же монетой.

table II *v* класть на стол; to ~ a motion поставить на обсуждение предложение; 2) составлять таблицу, расписание; 3) откладывать в долгий ящик.

tableau ['tæblou] *n* (*pl* tableaux) 1) картина; яркое изображение; 2) живая картина.

table-cloth ['teɪblklɔθ] *n* скатерть.

table-flap ['teɪblflæp] *n см.* table-leaf 2).

table-knife ['teɪblnaɪf] *n* столовый нож.

tableland ['teɪbllænd] *n* плоскогорье, плато.

table-leaf ['teɪbliːf] *n* 1) вкладная доска раздвижного стола; 2) откидная доска стола.

table-linen ['teɪbl‚lɪnɪn] *n* столовое бельё.

table-napkin ['teɪbl‚næpkɪn] *n* (столовая) салфетка.

table-spoon ['teɪblspuːn] *n* столовая ложка.

tablet ['tæblɪt] *n* 1) дощечка (*с надписью*); 2) блокнот; 3) таблетка (*лекарства*); 4) кусок (*мыла и т. п.*).

table-talk ['teɪbltɔːk] *n* застольная беседа.

table-ware ['teɪblwɛə] *n* столовый прибор (*вилки, ложки и т. п.*).

tabling ['teɪblɪŋ] *n* 1) составление таблицы, расписания; 2) откладывание, затягивание.

tabloid ['tæblɔɪd] *n* 1) табличка; 2) таблетка; 3) *амер.* бульварная газета.

taboo I [tə'buː] *n* запрещение, табу; запрет.

taboo II *a predic* запрещённый; священный.

taboo III *v* запрещать; налагать табу.

tabor ['teɪbə] *n* маленький барабан.

tabouret ['tæbərɪt] *n* 1) скамеечка; табурет; 2) пяльцы.

tabu I, II, III [tə'buː] *см.* taboo I, II, III.

tabular ['tæbjulə] *a* 1) табличный, в виде таблиц; 2) плоский; 3) слоистый, пластинчатый.

tabulate ['tæbjuleɪt] *v* располагать в виде таблиц; сводить в таблицу.

tabulation [ˌtæbju'leɪʃən] *n* составление таблиц.

tabulator ['tæbjuleɪtə] *n* табулятор, приспособление для печатания таблиц.

tacit ['tæsɪt] *a* 1) молчаливый (*о согласии, одобрении*); безмолвный; 2) не выраженный словами, подразумеваемый.

taciturn ['tæsɪtəːn] *a* молчаливый.

tack[1] I [tæk] *n* 1) гвоздь с широкой шляпкой; кнопка; 2) смётывание; стежки; 3) политическая линия, курс; 4) *мор.* галс (*направление*); 5) срок аренды; 6) липкость, клейкость.

tack[1] II *v* 1) прикреплять (*гвоздиками, кнопками; тж.* to ~ down); прибивать; 2) смётывать на живую нитку; 3) добавлять, присоединять (*to, on*); 4) *мор.* поворачивать на другой галс; 5) менять курс, линию поведения.

tack[2] *n* пища, еда; hard ~ сухарь; soft ~ мягкий хлеб.

tackle I ['tækl] *n* 1) принадлежности; оборудование; 2) *мор.* снасти; такелаж; 3) *тех.* полиспаст, система блоков.

tackle II *v* 1) закреплять; привязывать; 2) схватывать, захватывать; 3) браться за что-л. энергично (*to*); 4) биться над чем-л.

tacky ['tækɪ] *a* клейкий; тягучий.

tact [tækt] *n* 1) такт; тактичность; 2) *муз.* такт.

tactful ['tæktful] *a* тактичный.

tactical ['tæktɪkəl] *a* 1) *воен.* тактический; боевой; 2) ловкий.

tactics ['tæktɪks] *n* 1) тактика; "scorched earth" ~ тактика «выжженной земли»; 2) ловкость.

tactile ['tæktaɪl] *a* осязательный; осязаемый.

tactless ['tæktlɪs] *a* бестактный.

Tadjik I [tɑː'dʒɪk] *n* 1) таджик; таджичка; the ~ (*употр. как pl*) *собир.* таджики; 2) таджикский язык.

Tadjik II *a* таджикский.

tadpole ['tædpoul] *n* головастик.

taffeta ['tæfɪtə] *n* тафта.

taffy ['tæfɪ] *см.* toffee.

tag I [tæg] *n* 1) металлический наконечник (*на

шнурке и т. п.); петля, ушко́; 2) ярлы́к, этике́тка; би́рка; 3) изби́тая фра́за; цита́та; 4) сброд; 5) игра́ в са́лки, пятна́шки.

tag II *v* 1) прикрепля́ть ярлы́к, этике́тку, ушко́; 2) сле́довать по пята́м; 3) пойма́ть игра́ющего (*в салки*).

tail I [teɪl] *n* 1) хвост; 2) ни́жняя за́дняя часть чего́-л.; ~ of a cart задо́к теле́ги; 3) коса́, коси́чка; 4) сви́та; 5) о́чередь, «хвост»; 6) *pl разг.* фрак; 7) *ав.* хвостово́е опере́ние; 8) *attr* за́дний; хвостово́й; ◊ ~s up *разг.* в припо́днятом настрое́нии; to turn ~ обрати́ться в бе́гство; with the ~ between the legs поджа́в хвост, стру́сив.

tail II *v* 1) сле́довать по пята́м; 2) отруба́ть хвост; обрыва́ть хвости́ки (*ягод*); □ to ~ after неотсту́пно сле́довать (*за кем-л.*); to ~ away отстава́ть; to ~ on присоединя́ть(ся); to ~ out улизну́ть.

tail-board [ˈteɪlbɔːd] *n* откидно́й борт (*грузови́ка*), откидно́й задо́к (*теле́ги*).

tail-coat [ˈteɪlˈkout] *n разг.* фрак.

tail-end [ˈteɪlˈend] *n* коне́ц; хвост (*проце́ссии*).

tailings [ˈteɪlɪŋz] *n pl* оста́тки; отбро́сы.

tailless [ˈteɪllɪs] *a* бесхво́стый.

tail-light [ˈteɪllaɪt] *n* 1) *авто, ж.-д.* за́дний фона́рь; 2) *ав.* хвостово́й ого́нь.

tailor I [ˈteɪlə] *n* портно́й.

tailor II *v* рабо́тать портны́м, портня́жничать; шить (*костю́мы, пальто́*); well ~ed a) хорошо́ сши́тый (*о костю́ме и т. п.*); б) хорошо́ оде́тый (*о челове́ке*).

tailor-made [ˈteɪləmeɪd] *a* мужско́го покро́я.

tailpiece [ˈteɪlpiːs] *n* 1) заключи́тельная часть чего́-л.; 2) *полигр.* концо́вка.

tail-plane [ˈteɪlpleɪn] *n ав.* стабилиза́тор.

tail-skid [ˈteɪlskɪd] *n ав.* скольже́ние на хвост.

tail-slide [ˈteɪlslaɪd] *см.* tail-skid.

tail-spin [ˈteɪlspɪn] *n ав.* што́пор; to fall into a ~ войти́ в што́пор.

tail-wind [ˈteɪlwɪnd] *n* попу́тный ве́тер.

taint I [teɪnt] *n* 1) пятно́ (позо́ра); следы́ гние́ния, разруше́ния; without any ~ of без те́ни чего́-л.; 2) испо́рченность; заражённость.

taint II *v* по́ртить(ся); заража́ть(ся).

taintless [ˈteɪntlɪs] *a* безупре́чный.

take I [teɪk] *v* (*past* took; *p. p.* taken) 1) брать, взять; 2) отвози́ть, отводи́ть (*куда́-л.*); 3) захва́тывать си́лой, брать в плен; лови́ть; 4) получа́ть; принима́ть; 5) есть, пить; 6) тре́бовать (*вре́мени, терпе́ния и т. п.*); 7) пленя́ть, увлека́ть, нра́виться; име́ть успе́х; 8) выбира́ть (*путь, спо́соб*); 9) нанима́ть, снима́ть (*кварти́ру и т. п.*); 10) понима́ть, полага́ть; предполага́ть; do you ~ me? вы меня́ по́няли?; to ~ smb. to be a clever man счита́ть кого́-л. у́мным челове́ком; to ~ for принима́ть за, ошиба́ться (*приня́в за друго́е*); 11) восприни-ма́ть; подверга́ться; поддава́ться полиро́вке; отде́лке; 12) де́йствовать, ока́зывать де́йствие; 13) *тех.* тверде́ть, схва́тываться (*о цеме́нте и т. п.*); 14) с прямы́м дополне́нием, вы́раженным сущ., образу́ет усто́йчивые словосочета́ния, кото́рые даю́тся при соотве́тствующих сущ., напр.: to ~ measures *см.* measure; to ~ fire *см.* fire и т. д.; □ to ~ aback ошеломи́ть; захвати́ть враспло́х; to ~ across переправля́ть; to ~ after походи́ть на кого́-л.; быть похо́жим; to ~ apart разби-

ра́ть (*механи́зм и т. п.*); to ~ away убира́ть, удаля́ть; уноси́ть; to ~ back брать наза́д; to ~ down a) снима́ть (*с по́лки, с ве́шалки и т. п.*); б) запи́сывать (*под дикто́вку*); в) сноси́ть, разруша́ть; г) прогла́тывать (*с трудо́м*); д) сбива́ть спесь; е) понижа́ть, уменьша́ть, ослабля́ть; ж) разбира́ть (*маши́ну и т. п.*); to ~ from a) отнима́ть; б) умаля́ть; в) *мат.* вычита́ть; to ~ in a) принима́ть (*го́стя*); брать (*жильца́*); б) включа́ть, содержа́ть; охва́тывать; в) понима́ть, постига́ть; признава́ть (*ве́рным, пра́вильным*); г) су́живать, ушива́ть; свёртывать; убира́ть (*паруса́*); д) to be ~ in *разг.* быть обма́нутым, попа́сться; to ~ into: to ~ into one's head забра́ть себе́ в го́лову; наду́мать; to ~ off a) снима́ть; to ~ oneself off снима́ться с ме́ста, уходи́ть; б) уменьша́ть, сбавля́ть; вычита́ть; в) *разг.* подража́ть; передра́знивать; г) *ав.* взлета́ть, отрыва́ться (*от земли́, воды́*); *спорт. тж.* отта́лкиваться; д) вскочи́ть, подпры́гнуть; to ~ on a) принима́ть *или* брать на себя́; б) начина́ть; *воен.* открыва́ть ого́нь по; в) станови́ться популя́рным; име́ть успе́х; г) *разг.* расстра́иваться, огорча́ться бо́льше, чем сле́дует, принима́ть бли́зко к се́рдцу; to ~ out a) вынима́ть; б) выводи́ть на прогу́лку; пригласи́ть, повести́ (*в теа́тр и т. п.*); в) выпи́сывать (*цита́ты и т. п.*); to ~ over a) принима́ть от друго́го (*до́лжность и т. п.*); сменя́ть, идти́ на сме́ну; б) переправля́ть, перевози́ть; to ~ to a) пристрасти́ться (*к чему́-л.*); б) прибега́ть к чему́-л.; обраща́ться к чему́-л.; to ~ to one's bed заболе́ть, слечь в посте́ль; to ~ to one's heels удира́ть, улепётывать; to ~ to the road сде́латься бродя́гой, бродя́чим музыка́нтом и т. п.; to ~ up a) поднима́ть (*тж.* наве́рх); б) поглоща́ть, впи́тывать; в) занима́ть, заполня́ть (*ме́сто, вре́мя*); г) начина́ть; предпринима́ть; д) плати́ть, распла́чиваться; е) испра́вить (*оши́бку*); ула́дить (*ссо́ру*); ж) сближа́ться с кем-л., влюбля́ться (*with*); з) быть дово́льным, удовлетворя́ться (*with*); ◊ to ~ for granted допуска́ть; счита́ть дока́занным *или* дозво́ленным; to ~ smth. in hand принима́ться за что́-л.; предпринима́ть; to ~ it переноси́ть наказа́ние, несча́стье и т. п., не сдава́ясь, не па́дая ду́хом.

take II *n* 1) уло́в (*ры́бы и т. п.*); 2) сбор (*театра́льный*); *pl* бары́ш; 3) *кино* часть сце́ны, засня́тая за оди́н приём.

take-in [ˈteɪkˈɪn] *n разг.* обма́н.

taken [ˈteɪkən] *p. p. см.* take I.

take-off [ˈteɪkɔːf] *n* 1) *разг.* подража́ние; карикату́ра; 2) *ав.* взлёт, отры́в от земли́, подъём; *спорт. тж.* толчо́к, прыжо́к.

taking I [ˈteɪkɪŋ] *n* 1) захва́т, овладе́ние; 2) *pl* бары́ш; 3) *разг.* волне́ние, возбужде́ние.

taking II *a* 1) привлека́тельный; 2) зара́зный.

talc [tælk] *n* тальк.

tale [teɪl] *n* 1) по́весть, расска́з; a tall ~ — невероя́тная исто́рия; it tells its own ~ э́то говори́т само́ за себя́; 2) вы́думка, ба́сня; old wives' ~s ба́бьи ска́зки; 3) спле́тня; to tell ~s a) спле́тничать; б) доноси́ть; 4) число́, коли́чество; the ~ is complete все в сбо́ре, все налицо́; ◊ to tell ~s out of school не доноси́ть сор из избы́.

talebearer [ˈteɪlˌbɛərə] *n* 1) спле́тник; 2) доно́счик, я́бедник.

talent [ˈtælənt] *n* тала́нт.

talented ['tæləntɪd] *a* тала́нтливый, одарённый.

talentless ['tæləntlɪs] *a* безда́рный, лишённый тала́нта.

taleteller ['teɪl,telə] *n* 1) расска́зчик; 2) вы́думщик; 3) спле́тник.

talisman ['tælɪzmən] *n* талисма́н.

talk I [tɔːk] *n* 1) разгово́р; бесе́да (*тж. передава́емая по ра́дио*); small ~ пуста́я болтовня́, пусто́й разгово́р; town ~ городски́е пересу́ды, спле́тни; 2) *pl* перегово́ры; 3) слу́х(и); there is a ~ of... говоря́т, что..., хо́дят слу́хи, что...; 4) предме́т разгово́ра, обсужде́ния; ◊ all ~ and no cider *погов.* ≅ шу́му мно́го, а то́лку ма́ло.

talk II *v* 1) говори́ть; разгова́ривать (*о ком-л., чём-л.— about, of*; *с кем-л.— with*); обрати́ться (*к кому-л.— to*); to ~ Russian разгова́ривать, говори́ть по-ру́сски; it is much ~ed of об э́том мно́го говоря́т; ~ing of а) кста́ти; б) по по́воду, относи́тельно; to ~ from the point отвле́чься в сто́рону (*от вопро́са и т. п.*); to ~ against time говори́ть, чтобы заня́ть вре́мя (*об ора́торе*); 2) погова́ривать; распространя́ть слу́хи; 3) выгова́ривать (*кому-л.— to*); 4) обсужда́ть; совеща́ться; □ to ~ away продолжа́ть говори́ть, заговори́ться; to ~ back возража́ть, не соглаша́ться, не повинова́ться; to ~ down перекрича́ть кого́-л.; to ~ into уговори́ть, убеди́ть; вовле́чь во что-л.; to ~ off: to ~ one's head off заговори́ть кого́-л.; to ~ out отговори́ть, разубеди́ть (*в чём-л.— of*); to ~ over а) обсужда́ть; б) уговори́ть, переубеди́ть; to ~ round а) исче́рпать те́му; б) переубеди́ть; to ~ up а) говори́ть сме́ло и пря́мо; б) хвали́ть, похва́ливать; ◊ to ~ to smb. like a Dutch uncle учи́ть уму́-ра́зуму, оте́чески наставля́ть кого́-л.

talkative ['tɔːkətɪv] *a* разгово́рчивый; болтли́вый.

talkee-talkee ['tɔːkɪ'tɔːkɪ] *n* 1) бесконе́чная болтовня́; 2) ло́маный язы́к.

talker ['tɔːkə] *n* 1) говоря́щий; бесе́дующий; 2) говору́н; болту́н; great ~ люби́тель поболта́ть.

talkies ['tɔːkɪz] *n pl сленг* звуково́е кино́.

talking ['tɔːkɪŋ] *a* 1) говоря́щий; 2) болтли́вый; 3) вырази́тельный.

talking-to ['tɔːkɪŋtuː] *n* вы́говор.

tall [tɔːl] *a* 1) высо́кий; 2) возвы́шенный; 3) *разг.* чрезме́рный; невероя́тный; 4) *predic* высото́й, ро́стом; he is six feet ~ он шести́ фу́тов ро́стом.

tallboy ['tɔːlbɔɪ] *n* 1) высо́кий комо́д; 2) бока́л на высо́кой но́жке.

tallow I ['tælou] *n* 1) са́ло, жир; rendered ~ топлёное са́ло; 2) *attr* са́льный.

tallow II *v* сма́зывать (са́лом); пропи́тывать жи́ром.

tallowy ['tælouɪ] *a* са́льный, жи́рный.

tally I ['tælɪ] *n* 1) би́рка; ярлы́к; 2) едини́ца счёта; 3) дублика́т, ко́пия.

tally II *v* 1) подсчи́тывать; 2) соотве́тствовать, совпада́ть; согласо́вываться (*с чем-л.— with*); 3) прикрепля́ть ярлы́к.

tally-ho I ['tælɪ'hou] *v* нау́ськивать.

tally-ho II *int охот.* ату́!

tallyman ['tælɪmən] *n* торго́вец, продаю́щий по образца́м с рассро́чкой платежа́.

talon ['tælən] *n* 1) ко́готь; 2) дли́нный но́готь.

tamable ['teɪməbl] *a* укроти́мый; поддаю́щийся дрессиро́вке.

tambour I ['tæmbuə] *n* 1) небольшо́й бараба́н; 2) пя́льцы для вышива́ния; 3) та́мбур.

tambour II *v* вышива́ть на пя́льцах.

tambourine [,tæmbə'riːn] *n* бу́бен.

tame I [teɪm] *a* 1) ручно́й, приручённый; 2) поко́рный, пасси́вный; мя́гкий; 3) ску́чный, неинтере́сный; привы́чный, бана́льный.

tame II *v* 1) укроща́ть; прируча́ть; дрессирова́ть; 2) смиря́ть(ся), смягча́ть(ся); 3) подавля́ть, угнета́ть (*чу́вство и т. п.*).

tameless ['teɪmlɪs] *a* неукроти́мый; ди́кий.

tamer ['teɪmə] *n* 1) укроти́тель; дрессиро́вщик; 2) усмири́тель.

Tammany ['tæmənɪ] *n* (*тж.* ~ Hall) организа́ция демократи́ческой па́ртии в Нью-Йо́рке (*изве́стная систе́мой по́дкупов, шанта́жа*).

tam-o'-shanter [,tæmə'ʃæntə] *n* бере́т (*шотла́ндский*).

tamp [tæmp] *v* трамбова́ть.

tamper ['tæmpə] *v* 1) вме́шиваться, сова́ться (*with*); тро́гать (*то, что не сле́дует*); 2) подкупа́ть; подгова́ривать; 3) подде́лывать.

tampon I ['tæmpən] *n мед.* тампо́н.

tampon II *v мед.* вставля́ть тампо́н; тампони́ровать.

tamtam ['tæmtæm] *см.* tomtom.

tan I [tæn] *n* 1) толчёная дубо́вая кора́; 2) рыжева́то-кори́чневый цвет; 3) зага́р.

tan II *a* рыжева́то-кори́чневый.

tan III *v* 1) дуби́ть (*ко́жу*); 2) загора́ть; 3) *разг.* дуба́сить.

tandem I ['tændəm] *n* 1) упря́жка цу́гом; экипа́ж, запряжённый па́рой лошаде́й цу́гом; 2) велосипе́д-та́ндем.

tandem II *adv* цу́гом, гусько́м.

tang¹ [tæŋ] *n* ре́зкий привку́с; осо́бый вкус; *перен.* осо́бая пре́лесть, арома́т.

tang² I *n* звон; ре́зкий звук.

tang² II *v* звене́ть.

tang³ *n* вы́ступ; сте́ржень клинка́ *или* инструме́нта.

tangent I ['tændʒənt] *n мат.* 1) каса́тельная; 2) та́нгенс; ◊ to fly (*или* to go) off at a ~ внеза́пно отклоня́ться (*от те́мы и т. п.*).

tangent II *a мат.* каса́тельный.

tangerine ['tændʒə'riːn] *n* мандари́н.

tangibility [,tændʒɪ'bɪlɪtɪ] *n* 1) осяза́емость; 2) реа́льность.

tangible ['tændʒəbl] *a* 1) осяза́емый; 2) реа́льный; 3) ощути́тельный, заме́тный.

tangle I ['tæŋgl] *n* 1) спу́танный клубо́к; 2) пу́таница; 3) род кру́пных морски́х во́дорослей.

tangle II *v* запу́тывать(ся).

tangly ['tæŋglɪ] *a* 1) запу́танный; 2) покры́тый во́дорослями.

tank¹ I [tæŋk] *n* 1) резервуа́р; цисте́рна, бак; 2) бассе́йн, водоём, пруд.

tank¹ II *v* помеща́ть в резервуа́р; храни́ть в резервуа́ре.

tank² *n воен.* 1) танк; amphibian ~ та́нк-амфи́бия; 2) *attr* та́нковый.

tankage ['tæŋkɪdʒ] *n* 1) ёмкость резервуа́ра, цисте́рны *и т. п.*; 2) хране́ние в цисте́рнах (*не́фти и т. п.*); 3) пла́та за хране́ние.

tankard ['tæŋkəd] *n* больша́я кру́жка (*с кры́шкой*).

tank-car ['tæŋkkæ] n амер. вагон-цистерна.

tanker ['tæŋkə] n 1) танкер, (нефте)наливное судно; 2) самолёт-заправщик.

tankette [tæŋ'ket] n танкетка.

tankman ['tæŋkmæn] n танкист.

tanner[1] ['tænə] n дубильщик.

tanner[2] n сленг монета в 6 пенсов.

tannery ['tænərı] n кожевенный завод.

tannin ['tænın] n таннин, дубильная кислота.

tantalize ['tæntəlaız] v мучить.

tantamount ['tæntəmaunt] a predic равноценный; равносильный.

tantrum ['tæntrəm] n разг. вспышка гнева; приступ дурного настроения.

tap[1] I [tæp] n 1) лёгкий стук или удар; to give a ~ похлопать, пошлёпать; 2) pl сигнал тушить огни (в казармах и т. п.).

tap[1] II v стучать; постучать (в дверь); слегка ударять, постукивать; to ~ on the shoulder похлопать по плечу; □ to ~ in простукивать, прощупывать.

tap[2] I n 1) кран; затычка (в бочке с вином); on ~ распивочно, из бочки; to leave a ~ running оставить кран открытым; 2) сорт, марка (вина, пива); 3) эл. отвод, ответвление.

tap[2] II v 1) починать бочонок; 2) делать прокол (для выпускания жидкости); делать надрез на дереве; 3) выпрашивать, вымогать (деньги и т. п.; for); 4) выявлять, находить (ресурсы и т. п.); 5) перехватывать телеграфные или телефонные сообщения; 6) тех. нарезать внутреннюю резьбу.

tape I [teıp] n 1) тесьма; лента; 2) телеграфная лента; 3) спорт. финишная ленточка; at the ~ на финише; 4) см. tape-line; 5) ферромагнитная лента (магнитофона); to play back the ~ перематывать обратно ферромагнитную ленту; 6) сленг спиртной напиток; ◊ red ~ волокита; бюрократизм; формализм.

tape II v 1) связывать тесьмой; 2) обматывать лентой; 3) записывать на магнитную плёнку; 4) сленг раскусить кого-л., узнать цену кому-л.

tape-line ['teıplaın] n рулетка; мерная лента.

tape-measure ['teıp‚meʒə] см. tape-line.

taper I ['teıpə] n 1) тонкая свеча; 2) слабый свет; 3) конус.

taper II a 1) суживающийся к концу; конусообразный; конический; 2) тонкий и длинный (о пальцах руки).

taper III v 1) суживать(ся); 2) придавать коническую форму.

tapestry I ['tæpıstrı] n 1) гобелен; 2) обивка, обои.

tapestry II v 1) украшать гобеленами; 2) обивать (комнату и т. п.).

tapeworm ['teıpwɜːm] n мед. ленточный червь, солитёр.

tapioca [‚tæpı'oukə] n тапиока (крупа).

tapir ['teıpə] n зоол. тапир.

tapist ['teıpıst] n бюрократ, формалист.

taproom ['tæprum] n бар (в гостинице и т. п.).

tap-root ['tæpruːt] n бот. главный корень.

tapster ['tæpstə] n буфетчик.

tar[1] I [tɑː] n дёготь; жидкая смола; гудрон.

tar[1] II v обмазывать дёгтем; покрывать гудроном; смолить; ◊ ~red with the same brush (или stick) ≅ одним миром мазаны; одного поля ягода.

tar[2] n разг. моряк, матрос.

tarantula [tə'ræntjulə] n тарантул (паук).

tarboosh [tɑː'buːʃ] n феска.

tar-brush ['tɑːbrʌʃ] n кисть для смазки дёгтем; ◊ to have a touch of the ~ презр. иметь примесь негритянской крови.

tardiness ['tɑːdınıs] n 1) медлительность; 2) опоздание.

tardy ['tɑːdı] a 1) запоздалый; поздний; 2) медлительный; медленный; 3) отстающий, отсталый.

tare[1] [teə] n бот. вика.

tare[2] I n 1) тара; вес тары; 2) скидка на тару.

tare[2] II v 1) определять вес тары; 2) делать скидку на тару.

target ['tɑːgıt] n 1) цель, мишень (тж. перен.); off the ~ мимо цели; 2) план, задание; 3) уст. небольшой круглый щит.

tariff I ['tærıf] n 1) тариф; пошлина; railway ~ железнодорожный тариф; retaliatory ~ репрессивные пошлины; 2) расценка.

tariff II v производить оценку; устанавливать расценку.

tarn [tɑːn] n небольшое горное озеро.

tarnish I ['tɑːnıʃ] n 1) тусклость; 2) пятно.

tarnish II v 1) лишать(ся) блеска; тускнеть; 2) запятнать, опорочить.

tarpaulin [tɑː'pɔːlın] n 1) непромокаемый брезент; 2) матросская непромокаемая шапка или куртка; 3) редко матрос, моряк.

tarradiddle ['tærədıdl] n разг. ложь, выдумка.

tarry[a] ['tærı] v 1) медлить, мешкать; 2) задерживаться, временно жить, оставаться (at, in); 3) ждать, дожидаться (for).

tarry[b] ['tɑːrı] a покрытый или вымазанный дёгтем.

tart[1] [tɑːt] a 1) кислый; терпкий; 2) резкий; едкий.

tart[2] n пирог с фруктами или вареньем; торт.

tart[3] n разг. 1) разбитная женщина; 2) проститутка.

tartan ['tɑːtən] n клетчатая шерстяная материя, шотландка.

Tartar I ['tɑːtə] n 1) татарин; татарка; the ~s татары; 2) татарский язык.

Tartar II a татарский.

tartar ['tɑːtə] n винный камень.

task I [tɑːsk] n задание, задача; урок, работа; to set a ~ поставить задачу (перед кем-л.— before); ~ in hand a) начатая работа; б) непосредственная задача; ◊ to take to ~ бранить, делать выговор.

task II v давать задание; задавать работу, урок; 2) обременять, перегружать.

task-force ['tɑːskfɔːs] n воен. (временная) оперативная группа.

taskmaster ['tɑːsk‚mɑːstə] n бригадир, десятник.

taskwork ['tɑːskwɜːk] n урочная работа.

tassel ['tæsəl] n 1) кисточка (украшение); 2) закладка (в книге).

taste I [teıst] n 1) вкус; привкус (чего-л.); to the ~ на вкус; 2) вкус, склонность (к чему-л.— for); discriminating ~ тонкий вкус; to one's ~ по вкусу; 3) маленький кусочек; проба; перен. первое знакомство с чем-л.; a ~ чуточку; to give one a ~ of давать некоторое представление о чём-л.; ◊ ~s differ погов. ≅ о вкусах не спорят.

taste II *v* 1) пробовать; отведывать; *перен.* вкусить, испытать; 2) чувствовать вкус; 3) иметь вкус, привкус; to ~ sweet (bitter, sour) иметь сладкий (горький, кислый) вкус.

tasteful ['teɪstful] *a* 1) сделанный со вкусом; 2) обладающий вкусом.

tasteless ['teɪstlɪs] *a* 1) безвкусный; 2) лишённый вкуса; 3) дурного тона.

taster ['teɪstə] *n* дегустатор.

tastily ['teɪstɪlɪ] *adv разг.* со вкусом, изящно.

tasty ['teɪstɪ] *a* 1) вкусный; 2) *разг.* со вкусом (*сделанный*).

tat [tæt] *см.* tit².

Tatar I, II ['tɑːtə] *см.* Tartar I, II.

tatter I ['tætə] *n* 1) лоскут, тряпка, *pl* лохмотья, рвань; 2) старьёвщик.

tatter II *v* износить, превратить в лохмотья.

tatterdemalion [,tætədə'meɪljən] *n* оборванец.

tattered ['tætəd] *a* оборванный, в лохмотьях.

tatting ['tætɪŋ] *n* плетёное кружево.

tattle I ['tætl] *n* болтовня; сплетни.

tattle II *v* болтать; судачить; сплетничать.

tattler ['tætlə] *n* болтун; сплетник.

tattoo¹ I [tə'tuː] *n воен.* сигнал вечерней зари; to beat (*или* to sound) the ~ бить, играть зорю; ◊ to beat the devil's ~ барабанить пальцами по столу.

tattoo¹ II *v*) *воен.* играть зорю; 2) барабанить пальцами по столу.

tattoo² I *n* татуировка.

tattoo² II *v* татуировать.

taught [tɔːt] *past, p. p. см.* teach.

taunt I [tɔːnt] *n* 1) язвительное замечание; насмешка; 2) предмет насмешек.

taunt II *v* насмехаться; язвить.

tauntingly ['tɔːntɪŋlɪ] *adv* 1) язвительно; насмешливо; 2) с упрёком.

taut [tɔːt] *a* 1) туго натянутый; упругий; 2) напряжённый, взволнованный; 3) подтянутый, аккуратный; 4) строгий.

tauten ['tɔːtn] *v* натягивать(ся) туго.

tautology [tɔː'tɔlədʒɪ] *n* тавтология.

tavern ['tævən] *n* 1) трактир, кабачок; таверна; 2) небольшая гостиница.

tawdry ['tɔːdrɪ] *a* яркий, кричащий, безвкусный.

tawny ['tɔːnɪ] *a* рыжевато-коричневый; золотистый.

tax I [tæks] *n* 1) налог; direct (indirect) ~ прямой (косвенный) налог; to levy ~es взимать налоги; income ~ подоходный налог; 2) бремя; напряжение, нагрузка; испытание; тяжёлая обязанность.

tax II *v* 1) облагать налогом; 2) обременять; испытывать (*терпение и т. п.*); 3) чрезмерно напрягать; утомлять; 4) обвинять; упрекать; 5) *разг.* спрашивать цену; what will you ~ me? сколько это мне будет стоить?

taxable ['tæksəbl] *a* подлежащий обложению налогом.

taxation [tæk'seɪʃən] *n* 1) обложение налогом; взимание налога; 2) размер, сумма налога.

tax-collector ['tækskə,lektə] *n* сборщик налогов.

tax-dodger ['tæks,dɔdʒə] *n разг.* уклоняющийся от уплаты налогов.

tax-free ['tæks'friː] *a* освобождённый от налогов.

taxi I ['tæksɪ] *n* такси.

taxi II *v* 1) ехать *или* везти на такси; 2) *ав.* рулить.

taxi-cab ['tæksɪkæb] *см.* taxi I.

taxi-dancer ['tæksɪ,dɑːnsə] *n* профессиональный партнёр *или* партнёрша (*в дансинге и т. п.*).

taxidermist ['tæksɪdə:mɪst] *n* набивальщик чучел.

taximeter ['tæksɪ,miːtə] *n* таксометр, счётчик (*такси*).

taxing ['tæksɪŋ] *n* обложение налогом.

taxpayer ['tæks,peɪə] *n* налогоплательщик.

tea [tiː] *n* 1) чай; five-o'clock ~ дневной чай (*обыкн. в 5 часов*); high ~ вечерний чай с закуской; to draw ~ дать чаю настояться; 2) крепкий отвар; beef ~ крепкий мясной бульон.

tea-caddy ['tiː,kædɪ] *n* чайница.

tea-cake ['tiːkeɪk] *n* пирожное к чаю.

teach [tiːtʃ] *v* (*past, p. p.* taught) 1) учить; обучать; преподавать; давать уроки; 2) приучать; 3) проучить.

teacher ['tiːtʃə] *n* учитель(ница), преподаватель(ница); certificated ~ дипломированный учитель.

teaching ['tiːtʃɪŋ] *n* 1) обучение; преподавание; 2) *часто pl* учение, доктрина.

tea-cloth ['tiːklɔθ] *n* 1) чайная скатерть; 2) чайное полотенце.

teacup ['tiːkʌp] *n* чайная чашка.

tea-garden ['tiː,gɑːdn] *n* ресторанчик с садом.

teak [tiːk] *n бот.* тик.

tea-kettle ['tiː,ketl] *n* небольшой чайник (*для кипячения воды*).

tea-leaf ['tiːliːf] *n* 1) чайный лист; 2) *pl* спитой чай.

team I [tiːm] *n* 1) упряжка (*лошадей, волов*); 2) спортивная команда; home ~ команда хозяев поля; 3) бригада (*рабочих*); экипаж (*судна и т. п.*); 4) *воен.* расчёт; команда, экипаж.

team II *v* 1) запрягать (*лошадей и т. п.*); 2) объединяться в бригаду, команду и т. п.

teamster ['tiːmstə] *n* возница; погонщик.

teamwise ['tiːmwaɪz] *adv* бригадами, бригадным методом.

team-work ['tiːmwə:k] *n* совместная бригадная работа.

tea-party ['tiː,pɑːtɪ] *n* 1) званый чай; 2) общество, приглашённое на чай.

tea-pot ['tiːpɔt] *n* чайник (*для заварки*).

tearᵃ I [teə] *n* 1) разрыв, разрез; дыра; ~ and wear износ, изнашивание; 2) *амер. сленг* кутёж.

tearᵃ II *v* (*past* tore; *p. p.* torn) 1) рвать; разрывать, раздирать (*тж. перен.*); to ~ (in) to pieces изорвать в клочья; to ~ it *разг.* расстроить все планы; 2) сильно оцарапать, поранить; 3) рваться, изнашиваться; 4) мчаться; □ to ~ **about** носиться; to ~ **along** броситься, устремиться; to ~ **at** тянуть с силой, дёргать; to ~ **away** отрывать; to ~ oneself away (с трудом) оторваться; to ~ **down** срывать; сносить (*постройку*); to ~ **from** отнимать (*силой*), вырывать (*у кого-л.*); to ~ **up** изорвать, изодрать.

tearᵇ [tɪə] *n* слеза; *перен.* капля (*росы*); scalding (poignant, crocodile) ~s жгучие (горькие, крокодиловы) слёзы; to shed ~s проливать слёзы; in (a flood of) ~s в слезах, плача.

tear-drop ['tɪədrɔp] *n* слеза; ~s капли слёз.

tearful ['tɪəful] a 1) плачущий, проливающий слёзы; 2) печальный (о событии, новости).

tearfully ['tɪəfulɪ] adv со слезами, печально.

tear-gas ['tɪə'gæs] n слезоточивый газ.

tearing ['tɛərɪŋ] a разг. стремительный; неистовый, бурный.

tearless ['tɪəlɪs] a 1) без слёз; 2) бесчувственный.

tea-room ['tiːrum] n кафе.

tear-stained ['tɪəsteɪnd] a заплаканный (о лице).

tease I [tiːz] n разг. любитель подразнить; задира, приставала.

tease II v 1) дразнить; 2) приставать, надоедать; 3) просить, выпрашивать; 4) чесать (шерсть, лён); 5) ворсить (сукно).

teaser ['tiːzə] n 1) задира, приставала; 2) попрошайка; 3) разг. головоломка, трудная задача.

tea-service ['tiːˌsɜːvɪs] см. tea-set.

tea-set ['tiːset] n чайный сервиз.

tea-spoon ['tiːspuːn] n чайная ложка.

tea-spoonful ['tiːspuːnˌful] n полная чайная ложка (чего-л.).

teat [tiːt] n сосок.

tea-things ['tiːθɪŋz] n pl чайный сервиз.

tea-tray ['tiːtreɪ] n чайный поднос.

tea-urn ['tiːəːn] n 1) бак для кипячения воды; 2) самовар.

technic(al) ['teknɪk(əl)] a технический.

technicality [ˌteknɪ'kælɪtɪ] n техническая сторона (дела и т. п.); техническое свойство.

technician [tek'nɪʃən] n специалист (в технике, своего дела).

technics ['tekniks] n техника; технические науки.

technique [tek'niːk] n техника (исполнения); технические приёмы.

technocracy [tek'nɔkrəsɪ] n технократия.

technology [tek'nɔlədʒɪ] n 1) технические науки; 2) технология; 3) техника; rocket ~ ракетная техника.

techy ['tetʃɪ] a 1) обидчивый; раздражительный; 2) норовистый (о лошади).

tectonic [tek'tɔnɪk] a 1) геол. структурный; тектонический; 2) архитектурный.

tectonics [tek'tɔniks] n строительное искусство.

ted [ted] v ворошить (сено).

tedder ['tedə] n с.-х. сеноворошилка.

Teddy bear ['tedɪ'bɛə] n мишка, плюшевый медведь (игрушка).

tedious ['tiːdjəs] a скучный; утомительный.

tedium ['tiːdjəm] n скука.

tee I [tiː] n мишень (в играх), метка для мяча в гольфе.

tee II v класть мяч для первого удара; □ to ~ off, to ~ up делать первый удар (в гольфе).

teem [tiːm] v 1) изобиловать (чем-л. — with); кишеть; 2) быть плодородным, плодовитым.

teen-ager ['tiːnˌeɪdʒə] n подросток (от 13 до 19 лет).

teens [tiːnz] n pl возраст от 13 до 19 лет; she is in her ~ ей нет ещё 20.

teeny ['tiːnɪ] a крошечный.

teeter I ['tiːtə] n детские качели.

teeter II v качаться (на качелях).

teeth [tiːθ] pl см. tooth I.

teethe [tiːð] v прорезываться (о зубах).

teetotaller [tiː'toutlə] n трезвенник.

teetotum ['tiːtou'tʌm] n волчок.

tegument ['tegjumənt] n покров, оболочка.

tehee I [tiː'hiː] n хихиканье.

tehee II v хихикать.

telecast I ['telɪkɑːst] n телевизионная передача.

telecast II v передавать по телевидению; вести телевизионную передачу.

telecommunication ['telɪkəˌmjuːnɪ'keɪʃən] n дальняя связь.

telecontrol ['telɪkən'troul] n телеуправление.

telegram ['telɪgræm] n телеграмма.

telegraph I ['telɪgrɑːf] n 1) телеграф; 2) attr телеграфный; ◊ bush ~ сленг неофициальный или тайный источник информации.

telegraph II v телеграфировать.

telegrapher [tɪ'legrəfə] см. telegraphist.

telegraphic [ˌtelɪ'græfɪk] a телеграфный.

telegraphist [tɪ'legrəfɪst] n телеграфист.

telegraph-pole ['telɪgrɑːfpoul] n телеграфный столб.

telegraph-wire ['telɪgrɑːfˌwaɪə] n телеграфный провод.

telephone I ['telɪfoun] n 1) телефон; 2) attr телефонный.

telephone II v телефонировать, звонить по телефону.

telephonist [tɪ'lefənɪst] n телефонист(ка).

telephony [tɪ'lefənɪ] n телефония; wireless ~ радиотелефония, беспроволочная телефония.

telescope I ['telɪskoup] n телескоп.

telescope II v врезаться, сталкиваться (о вагонах при крушении).

telescopic [ˌtelɪs'kɔpɪk] a 1) телескопический; 2) видимый через телескоп; 3) выдвижной.

teleview ['telɪvjuː] v смотреть телевизионную передачу.

televiewer ['telɪvjuːə] n телевизионный зритель, телезритель.

televise ['telɪvaɪz] v передавать по телевидению.

television ['telɪˌvɪʒən] n телевидение.

televisor ['telɪvaɪzə] n телевизор.

tell [tel] v (past, p. p. told) 1) говорить, сказать; высказывать; I told him я сказал ему; I was told мне сказали, я слышал; 2) рассказывать; don't ~ me, never ~ me вы мне не говорите, не рассказывайте сказок; 3) приказывать; do as you are told делайте, как вам приказано; 4) отличать; различать (тж. to ~ apart, to ~ from); to ~ one from the other отличать одного от другого; and how do you ~ them? как вы их различаете?; 5) считать, пересчитывать; all told включая (или считая) всех, всё; 6) объяснять, указывать (дорогу, способ и т. п.); 7) производить действие; сказываться (на — on, upon); the long strain was ~ing on his health длительное напряжение сказалось на его здоровье; 8) сообщать; выдавать секрет; □ to ~ off а) отбирать, выделять; б) воен. производить строевой расчёт; наряжать; назначать; в) разг. выругать, отделать; to ~ on разг. ябедничать; to ~ over считать.

tellable ['teləbl] a такой, который можно или стоит рассказать.

teller ['telə] n 1) рассказчик; 2) счётчик голосов; 3) кассир (в банке); 4) воен. диктор ПВО.

telling ['telɪŋ] *a* 1) значи́тельный; многозначи́тельный; *разг.* основа́тельный; 2) вырази́тельный.

telling-off ['telɪŋ'ɔf] *n разг.* вы́говор, нагоня́й.

telltale I ['telteɪl] *n* 1) спле́тник; болту́н; 2) доно́счик; 3) *тех.* сигна́льное устро́йство.

telltale II *a* 1) преда́тельский; 2) выба́лтывающий (*секреты и т. п.*); 3) *тех.* контро́льный, сигна́льный.

telly ['telɪ] *n разг.* 1) телеви́дение; 2) телеви́зор.

temerity [tɪ'merɪtɪ] *n* 1) опроме́тчивость; безрассу́дство; 2) отва́га.

temper I ['tempə] *n* 1) нрав, хара́ктер; темпера́мент; 2) настрое́ние; in a good ~ в хоро́шем, споко́йном настрое́нии; in a bad ~ в плохо́м настрое́нии, расстро́енный; to keep (*или* to control) one's ~ владе́ть собо́й; to lose one's ~ вы́йти из себя́; out of ~ раздражённый, серди́тый; quick ~, short ~ вспы́льчивость; горя́чность; 3) раздраже́ние, гнев; to show ~ проявля́ть раздраже́ние; to get (*или* to fly) into a ~ (about) рассерди́ться (на); 4) смесь, соста́в сме́си; 5) *тех.* о́тпуск (*металла*).

temper II *v* 1) смягча́ть; умеря́ть, регули́ровать; 2) де́лать смесь; 3) *тех.* отпуска́ть (*металл*); закаля́ть (*тж. перен.*).

tempera ['tempərə] *n жив.* те́мпера.

temperament ['tempərəmənt] *n* темпера́мент.

temperamental [ˌtempərə'mentl] *a* 1) темпера́ментный; 2) сво́йственный определённому темпера́менту.

temperance ['tempərəns] *n* 1) уме́ренность; сде́ржанность; 2) воздержа́ние от спиртны́х напи́тков.

temperate ['tempərɪt] *a* 1) уме́ренный (*о кли́мате*); 2) сде́ржанный.

temperature ['temprɪtʃə] *n* температу́ра; to take one's ~ изме́рить температу́ру; he has a ~ *разг.* у него́ повы́шенная температу́ра.

tempest I ['tempɪst] *n* бу́ря; a ~ of anger бу́рный гнев, вспы́шка гне́ва; ◇ ~ in a tea-pot бу́ря в стака́не воды́.

tempest II *v* бушева́ть.

tempestuous [tem'pestjuəs] *a* бу́рный; бу́йный.

Templar ['templə] *n ист.* тамплие́р, хра́мовник.

temple[1] [templ] *n* храм.

temple[2] *n* висо́к.

templet ['templɪt] *n* шабло́н, кали́бр.

tempo ['tempou] *n* темп.

temporal[1] ['tempərəl] *a* 1) вре́менный, преходя́щий; 2) све́тский, мирско́й.

temporal[2] *a анат.* висо́чный.

temporary I ['tempərərɪ] *n* вре́менный рабо́чий *или* служа́щий.

temporary II *a* вре́менный.

temporize ['tempəraɪz] *v* 1) выжида́ть, стара́ться вы́играть вре́мя; ме́длить; 2) приспоса́бливаться к обстоя́тельствам, ко вре́мени.

tempt [tempt] *v* 1) искуша́ть, соблазня́ть чем-л.; 2) привлека́ть, прельща́ть; 3) *уст.* испы́тывать, проверя́ть.

temptation [temp'teɪʃən] *n* искуше́ние; собла́зн.

tempter ['temptə] *n* искуси́тель; the Tempter сатана́.

tempting ['temptɪŋ] *a* соблазни́тельный, зама́нчивый.

temptress ['temptrɪs] *n* искуси́тельница.

ten I [ten] *num* де́сять; ~ to one де́сять ша́нсов про́тив одного́; почти́ наверняка́.

ten II *n* 1) деся́ток; in ~s деся́тками; 2) *карт.* деся́тка.

tenable ['tenəbl] *a* 1) про́чный, усто́йчивый; 2) *воен.* обороноспосо́бный; 3) логи́чный, после́довательный.

tenacious [tɪ'neɪʃəs] *a* 1) це́пкий, кре́пкий; 2) упо́рный, сто́йкий; ~ of life живу́чий; 3) вя́зкий, ли́пкий.

tenacity [tɪ'næsɪtɪ] *n* 1) це́пкость; 2) упо́рство, сто́йкость; 3) вя́зкость, ли́пкость.

tenancy ['tenənsɪ] *n* 1) аре́нда; 2) арендо́ванное помеще́ние, арендо́ванная земля́; 3) срок аре́нды.

tenant I ['tenənt] *n* 1) нанима́тель, аренда́тор, съёмщик (*помещения*); 2) жиле́ц, обита́тель.

tenant II *v* арендова́ть, нанима́ть.

tenantless ['tenəntlɪs] *a* не сда́нный (*внаём*), свобо́дный, неза́нятый.

tenantry ['tenəntrɪ] *n собир.* аренда́торы.

tench [tenʃ] *n* линь (*рыба*).

.tend[1] [tend] *v* 1) направля́ться; вести́ к чему́-л.; клони́ться к чему́-л.; 2) име́ть *или* проявля́ть тенде́нцию (*к чему́-л.— to*); 3) склоня́ться; име́ть скло́нность.

tend[2] *v* 1) забо́титься (*о ком-л., о чём-л.*); смотре́ть за кем-л.; уха́живать (*за больны́м, за ребёнком, за растениями*); 2) обслу́живать (*маши́ну, стано́к*).

tendance ['tendəns] *n* забо́та о чём-л.; присмо́тр; ухо́д за кем-л., уход-л.

tendency ['tendənsɪ] *n* 1) тенде́нция; скло́нность; 2) накло́нность.

tendentious [ten'denʃəs] *a* тенденцио́зный.

tender[1] ['tendə] *a* 1) не́жный; 2) сла́бый (*о здоро́вье*); 3) мя́гкий; 4) чувстви́тельный; 5) щекотли́вый (*о вопро́се, теме и т. п.*); 6) не́жный; ла́сковый, лю́бящий.

tender[2] *n* лицо́, выполня́ющее определённую фу́нкцию (*обыкн. с предшествующим сущ., напр.:* baby ~ ня́ня; invalid ~ сиде́лка *и т. п.*).

tender[3] *n* 1) *ж.-д.* те́ндер; 2) *мор.* посы́льное су́дно.

tender[4] I *n* 1) предложе́ние (*услуг и т. п.*); 2) заявле́ние о чём-л., зая́вка; 3) представле́ние де́нег (*в уплату долга и т. п.*).

tender[4] II *v* 1) предлага́ть, представля́ть (*заявле́ние, смету и т. п.*); 2) де́лать зая́вку.

tenderfoot ['tendəfut] *n разг.* новичо́к; новоприбы́вший (*в колонию и т. п.*); не привы́кший к тру́дностям, не́женка.

tender-hearted ['tendə'hɑːtɪd] *a* мягкосерде́чный, не́жный, чувстви́тельный.

tenderling ['tendəlɪŋ] *n* не́женка.

tenderloin ['tendələin] *n* вы́резка, филе́йная часть.

tenderness ['tendənɪs] *n* не́жность; мя́гкость.

tendon ['tendən] *n анат.* сухожи́лие.

tendril ['tendrɪl] *n бот.* у́сик.

tenebrous ['tenɪbrəs] *a* тёмный, мра́чный.

tenement ['tenɪmənt] *n* 1) кварти́ра, дом (*снима́емый у хозя́ина*); 2) помеще́ние *или* земля́, сдава́емые в аре́нду; 3) многокварти́рный дом (*с дешёвыми квартирами*).

tenet ['ti:net] *n* принцип, догма.

tenfold I ['tenfould] *a* десятикратный.

tenfold II *adv* вдесятеро.

tenner ['tenə] *n разг.* десятка; банкнот в 10 фунтов, *амер.* в 10 долларов.

tennis ['tenıs] *n спорт.* теннис; lawn ~ лаун-теннис; table ~ настольный теннис; пинг-понг.

tenon I ['tenəp] *n тех.* шип.

tenon II *v тех.* нарезать шипы; соединять на шипах.

tenor[1] ['tenə] *n* 1) течение, направление; the ~ of one's life уклад жизни; 2) общий смысл, значение; содержание.

tenor[2] *n* 1) *муз.* тенор; 2) *attr муз.* теноровый.

tense[1] [tens] *n грам.* время; Present Indefinite ~ общая форма настоящего времени; Present Continuous ~ конкретная форма настоящего времени; Present Perfect ~ совершённая форма настоящего времени; Past Indefinite ~ общая форма прошедшего времени; Past Continuous ~ конкретная форма прошедшего времени; Past Perfect ~ совершённая форма прошедшего времени; пред-прошедшее время; Future Indefinite ~ общая форма будущего времени; Future Continuous ~ конкретная форма будущего времени; Future Perfect ~ совершённая форма будущего времени.

tense[2] I *a* 1) натянутый; 2) напряжённый.

tense[2] II *v* 1) натягивать(ся); 2) напрягать(ся).

tensile ['tensail] *a* растяжимый.

tension ['tenʃən] *n* 1) натяжение, натягивание; 2) напряжение; напряжённое состояние; to ease (*или* to lessen, to decrease, to reduce, to relax) ~ ослабить напряжение; 3) натянутость, неловкость.

tent[1] I [tent] *n* палатка, шатёр; to pitch a ~ ставить палатку; to pitch one's ~ *перен.* поселяться.

tent[1] II *v* разбить палатки, расположиться в палатках.

tent[2] I *n* тампон.

tent[2] II *v* вставлять тампон.

tentacle ['tentəkl] *n* 1) *зоол.* щупальце; 2) *бот.* чувствительный волосок.

tentative I ['tentətıv] *n* попытка, проба; опыт.

tentative II *a* пробный; опытный, экспериментальный.

tent-cloth ['tentkləθ] *n* парусина, брезент, палаточная ткань.

tenterhooks ['tentəhuks] *n pl.:* to be on ~ мучиться, сидеть как на иголках.

tenth I [tenθ] *num* десятый.

tenth II *n* десятая часть; ◊ the submerged ~ наибеднейшая и обездоленная часть населения.

tenuity [te'nju:ıtı] *n* 1) незначительность; тонкость; 2) разрежённость (*воздуха*); 3) бедность; скудость; 4) простота (*стиля и т. п.*).

tenuous ['tenjuəs] *a* 1) незначительный, очень тонкий (*тж. о различии и т. п.*); 2) разрежённый (*о воздухе*).

tenure ['tenjuə] *n* 1) владение, право владения; 2) пребывание (*в должности и т. п.*); 3) срок владения; срок пребывания (*в должности*).

tepee ['ti:pi:] *n* вигвам североамериканских индейцев.

tepid ['tepıd] *a* тепловатый; *перен.* прохладный, холодный.

tercet ['tə:sıt] *n* 1) *лит.* трёхстишие; терцина; 2) *муз.* терцет.

term I [tə:m] *n* 1) срок; определённый период; 2) семестр; lent ~ весенний семестр; 3) термин; *pl* выражения; legal ~s юридические термины; in round ~s в сильных выражениях; in set ~s определённо; in flattering ~s в лестных выражениях; in ~s of на языке (*чего-л., кого-л.*), с точки зрения; 4) статья, пункт; *pl* условия (*договора, соглашения, мира*); to come to ~s with прийти к соглашению с кем-л.; to bring to ~s заставить принять условия; to make ~s договориться с кем-л.; inclusive ~s цена, включающая все услуги (*в гостинице и т. п.*); 5) (личные) отношения; on good (bad) ~s в хороших (плохих) отношениях; on friendly ~s в приятельских отношениях; not to be on speaking ~s with быть в ссоре, не разговаривать друг с другом; 6) предел, граница; 7) *мат.* член; 8) сессия (*суда*).

term II *v* называть; выражать; определять.

termagant I ['tə:məgənt] *n* сварливая, грубая женщина.

termagant II *a* сварливый, крикливый.

terminable ['tə:mınəbl] *a* ограниченный сроком.

terminal I ['tə:mınl] *n* 1) конечный пункт; конечная станция; 2) конечный слог; конечное слово; 3) экзамен в конце семестра; 4) *эл.* клемма; ввод; вывод.

terminal II *a* 1) конечный, концевой; заключительный; 2) предельный; пограничный; 3) семестровый.

terminate ['tə:mıneıt] *v* 1) положить конец, предел; 2) кончать(ся), заканчивать(ся), завершать(ся) (*чем-л.— in*); 3) ограничивать; быть ограниченным.

termination [,tə:mı'neıʃən] *n* 1) окончание, конец; завершение; 2) истечение срока; предел; 3) *тех.* конечное устройство.

termini ['tə:mınaı] *pl см.* terminus.

terminology [,tə:mı'nɔlədʒı] *n* терминология.

terminus ['tə:mınəs] *n* (*pl тж.* termini) 1) конечная станция; 2) предел, граница; 3) конец, цель.

termite ['tə:maıt] *n зоол.* термит.

termless ['tə:mlıs] *a* неограниченный; бессрочный.

ternary I ['tə:nərı] *n* число три, тройка.

ternary II *a* тройной.

terrace I ['terəs] *n* 1) терраса; 2) уступ; 3) плоская крыша; 4) ряд домов; улица (*расположенная по склону*).

terrace II *v* располагать уступами, террасами.

terracotta ['terə'kɔtə] *n* 1) терракота; 2) *attr* терракотовый.

terrain ['tereın] *n* местность.

terrapin ['terəpın] *n* 1) североамериканская водяная черепаха; 2) «черепаха» (*машина-амфибия*).

terrestrial [tı'restrıəl] *a* 1) земной; 2) наземный; сухопутный.

terrible ['terəbl] *a* 1) страшный, ужасный; 2) *разг.* сильный, страшный (*о морозе, ветре и т. п.*).

terrier ['terıə] *n* 1) терьер (*собака*); 2) *разг.* солдат территориальной армии.

terrific [tə'rıfık] *a* 1) ужасающий; 2) *разг.* страшный, ужасный.

terrify ['terɪfaɪ] v сильно пугать, устрашать, ужасать.

territorial I [ˌterɪ'tɔːrɪəl] a 1) (обыкн. Т.) территориальный; 2) земельный.

territorial II n солдат территориальной армии.

territory ['terɪtərɪ] n 1) территория; земля; перен. область, сфера (науки и т. п.); 2) амер. территория, не имеющая прав штата.

terror ['terə] n 1) страх, ужас; 2) террор; 3) лицо или вещь, внушающие страх; ◇ holy ~, perfect ~ шутл. зануда.

terror-haunted ['terəˌhɔːntɪd] a преследуемый страхом.

terrorist ['terərɪst] n террорист.

terrorize ['terəraɪz] v терроризировать.

terror-stricken, terror-struck ['terəˌstrɪkən, 'terəstrʌk] a поражённый ужасом.

terse [tɜːs] a сжатый и выразительный (о стиле и т. п.).

tertiary ['tɜːʃərɪ] a геол. третичный.

tesselated ['tesɪleɪtɪd] a мозаичный.

test I [test] n 1) испытание; проба; проверка; atomic ~ испытание атомного оружия; to put to the (или a) ~ подвергнуть испытанию; to stand the ~ выдержать испытание; 2) мерило, критерий; means ~ проверка нуждаемости (человека, обращающегося за пособием); 3) мед. исследование, анализ; 4) хим. реакция; 5) attr испытательный, пробный; контрольный, проверочный.

test II v 1) подвергать испытанию, проверке; испытывать, проверять; 2) производить опыты.

Testament ['testəmənt] n: the Old ~ Ветхий завет; the New ~ Новый завет.

testament ['testəmənt] n завещание.

testamentary [ˌtestə'mentərɪ] a 1) завещательный; 2) переданный по завещанию.

testate ['testɪt] a оставивший завещание; to die ~ умереть, оставив завещание.

testator [tes'teɪtə] n завещатель.

testatrix [tes'teɪtrɪks] n завещательница.

tester ['testə] n испытатель.

testify ['testɪfaɪ] v 1) свидетельствовать; давать показания (в пользу — to; против кого-л., чего-л. — against); утверждать; 2) (торжественно) заявлять; 3) служить доказательством, свидетельствовать; 4) проявлять (желание, намерение).

testily ['testɪlɪ] adv раздражительно, вспыльчиво.

testimonial [ˌtestɪ'mounjəl] n 1) свидетельство, аттестат; рекомендация; 2) приветственный адрес, подношение.

testimony ['testɪmənɪ] n 1) утверждение; юр. показание; to bear ~ свидетельствовать; 2) доказательство, свидетельство; in ~ of в качестве доказательства; to produce ~ представлять доказательства; 3): the Testimonies pl библ. скрижали.

test-paper ['testˌpeɪpə] n лакмусовая бумага.

test-pilot ['testˌpaɪlət] n лётчик-испытатель.

test-tube ['testtjuːb] n пробирка.

testy ['testɪ] a раздражительный, вспыльчивый.

tetchy ['tetʃɪ] см. techy.

tether I ['teðə] n привязь, путы; перен. предел; ограничение; to come to the end of one's ~ дойти до точки, исчерпать все средства, все возможности.

tether II v привязывать (пасущееся животное); перен. ограничивать, держать в известных пределах.

tetragon ['tetrəgən] n мат. четырёхугольник; regular ~ квадрат.

tetter ['tetə] n лишай, экзема.

Teuton ['tjuːtən] n тевтон, германец.

Teutonic I [tjuː'tɔnɪk] n ист. германский язык.

Teutonic II a ист. германский; тевтонский.

text [tekst] n 1) текст; advanced ~s более трудные тексты; 2) тема, предмет; to stick to one's ~ придерживаться темы; 3) крупный почерк или шрифт; German ~ готический шрифт; 4) учебник.

textbook ['tekstbuk] n учебник; self-teaching ~ самоучитель.

texter ['tekstə] n составитель рекламы.

text-hand ['teksthænd] n крупный почерк или шрифт.

textile I ['tekstaɪl] n обыкн. pl текстильные изделия, ткани.

textile II a 1) текстильный; 2) ткацкий.

textual ['tekstjuəl] a 1) текстовой, относящийся к тексту; 2) текстуальный, буквальный.

texture ['tekstʃə] n 1) ткань; coarse ~ грубая ткань; fine ~ тонкая ткань; 2) качество, плотность ткани; 3) расположение частей; строение, структура.

Thai [taɪ] n 1) таец; тайка; the ~(s) тайцы; 2) тайский язык.

Thames [temz] n Темза; ◇ he will never set the ~ on fire ≅ он пороху не выдумает.

than [ðæn (сильная форма), ðən (слабая форма)] conj выражает сравнение чем; he is taller ~ his sister он выше своей сестры (чем сестра); you know better ~ I do вы знаете лучше, чем я; how else can we come ~ by train? как ещё мы можем приехать, если не поездом?

thane [θeɪn] n ист. тан (титул).

thank [θæŋk] v благодарить (за — for); ~ you благодарю; to have oneself to ~ быть самому виноватым.

thankful ['θæŋkful] a благодарный.

thankless ['θæŋklɪs] a 1) неблагодарный; 2) безвозмездный.

thanks [θæŋks] n pl благодарность; спасибо; to return ~ а) (от)благодарить; б) отвечать на тост; ~ to благодаря; ~ to you благодаря вам; ~ to your efforts благодаря вашим стараниям.

thanksgiving ['θæŋksˌgɪvɪŋ] n благодарственный молебен.

thankworthy ['θæŋkˌwəːðɪ] a заслуживающий благодарности.

thatᵃ I pron 1) [ðæt] demonstr (pl those) служит: а) для указания на отдалённый по месту предмет тот, та, то; you see ~ house over the river вы видите тот дом за рекой; б) для указания на отдалённое во времени явление, событие, действие тот, та, то; этот, эта, это; ~ night we could not sleep в ту (эту) ночь мы не могли спать; в) для противоположения this; this book is interesting, ~ book is thrilling эта книга интересная, та книга захватывающая; 2) [ðət] rel служит: а) для выражения подлежащего или дополнения в относительном придаточном предложении тот, который;

та, которая; то, которое; the man ~ is standing there... человек, который стоит там...; the book ~ I am reading... книга, которую я читаю...; б) *для выражения предложного дополнения с предлогом, отнесённым на конец предложения:* the man ~ I spoke of... человек, о котором я говорил...; 3) *слово-заместитель сущ.; по-русски сущ. обычно повторяется:* the climate here is like ~ of France здешний климат похож на климат Франции.

thatᵃ **II** *adv* столь, так; ~ much так много; ~ far настолько далеко.

thatᵇ [ðæt] *conj* служит для введения различных придаточных предложений то, что; что; для того, чтобы; so ~ так, что; in order ~ для того, чтобы.

thatch I [θætʃ] *n* 1) соломенная *или* тростниковая крыша; 2) *разг.* волосы (*особ. густые*).

thatch II *v* крыть соломой *или* тростником.

thaw I [θɔ:] *n* таяние, оттепель; *перен.* теплота, сердечность.

thaw II *v* 1) таять; 2) оттаивать; *перен.* становиться теплее, сердечнее.

theᵃ [*под ударением* ði:; *в неударном положении перед согласной* ðə, *перед гласной* ðɪ] *определённый член, артикль* — *служебное слово, с помощью которого говорящий выделяет в своей речи возникшие в его сознании единичные понятия, составляющие часть ранее выделенного общего понятия:* the book книга (*т. е. один конкретный представитель ранее выделенной общей категории книг*); *помимо этого определённый член показывает:* a) *что данное единичное понятие употреблено в речи вместо соответствующего общего понятия:* the dog is a domestic animal собака (*всякая собака, в том числе и данная*) — домашнее животное; б) *что прил. употреблено в значении сущ. собирательного:* the poor бедные; the blind слепые; в) *что данное сущ., выражающее более частное конкретное понятие, употреблено для выражения явления в целом:* the saddle верховая езда (*при более частом значении — седло*).

theᵇ [ðə] *adv* употр. *в качестве коррелята при степенях сравнения* чем... тем...; the sooner, the better чем скорей, тем лучше.

theater ['θɪətə] *амер. см.* theatre.

theatre ['θɪətə] *n* 1) театр; the ~ of war театр военных действий; 2) аудитория в виде амфитеатра; 3) драматическая литература, пьесы; good ~ сценичный; 4) *attr* театральный.

theatre-goer ['θɪətə,gouə] *n* театрал.

theatrical [θɪ'ætrɪkəl] *a* 1) театральный; драматический (*о труппе*); сценический; 2) театральный, напыщенный, искусственный; показной.

theatricals [θɪ'ætrɪkəlz] *n pl* 1) спектакли (*особ. любительские*); 2) театральное дело.

thee [ði:] *pron pers* (*косв. падеж от* thou) тебя.

theft [θeft] *n* 1) воровство; 2) кража.

their [ðeə] *pron poss* их; свой; ~ books are on the table их книги на столе; they do ~ lessons они делают свои уроки.

theirs [ðeəz] *pron poss* 1) *predic* их; this book is ~, not ours это их книга, не наша; 2) *замещает сущ.:* our room is small, ~ is large наша комната маленькая, их (комната) большая.

them [ðem] *pron pers* (*косв. падеж от* they) их; им; by ~ ими; to ~ им; with ~ с ними; of ~ их; о них; из них.

thematic [θɪ'mætɪk] *a* тематический; предметный (*о каталоге*).

theme [θi:m] *n* 1) тема, предмет (*разговора, сочинения*); 2) *обыкн. амер.* школьное сочинение или его тема; 3) *грам.* основа; 4) *муз.* тема.

themselves [ðəm'selvz] *pron* 1) *refl* себя, -ся, -сь; себе; they hurt ~ они ушиблись; they have built ~ a house они выстроили себе дом; 2) *употр. для усиления* сами; the teachers ~ say учителя сами говорят; they wanted it ~ они сами этого хотели; ◊ by ~ a) самостоятельно, без чьей-л. помощи; б) одни (*без кого-л.*).

then I [ðen] *adv* 1) тогда, в то время; 2) потом; 2) кроме того; к тому же.

then II *conj* 1) в таком случае; 2) кроме того.

then III *a* тогдашний.

then IV *n:* by ~ к тому времени; since ~ с того времени; every now and ~ время от времени; то и дело.

thence [ðens] *adv* 1) отсюда, из этого (следует); поэтому; 2) оттуда; we went to Moscow, ~ we went to Leningrad мы поехали в Москву, оттуда в Ленинград; 3) с того времени.

thenceforth ['ðens'fɔ:θ] *adv* с того, с этого времени; впредь.

thenceforward ['ðens'fɔ:wəd] *adv* с этого времени; впредь.

theocracy [θɪ'ɔkrəsɪ] *n* теократия.

theologian [θɪə'loudʒjən] *n* богослов.

theology [θɪ'ɔlədʒɪ] *n* богословие.

theorem ['θɪərem] *n* теорема.

theoretic(al) [θɪə'retɪk(əl)] *a* теоретический.

theorist ['θɪərɪst] *n* теоретик.

theorize ['θɪəraɪz] *v* теоретизировать.

theory ['θɪərɪ] *n* теория; Marxist-Leninist ~ марксистско-ленинская теория.

therapeutics [,θerə'pju:tɪks] *n* терапия.

therapy ['θerəpɪ] *см.* therapeutics.

there I [ðeə] *adv* 1) там; are you ~? вы слушаете? (*по телефону*); 2) туда; ~ and back туда и обратно; 3) здесь, тут; 4) *с гл.* to be: ~ is, ~ are есть, имеется, имеются; ◊ ~ and then тотчас же, на месте.

there II *n* (*после предлога*): from ~ оттуда; up to ~ до того места; near ~ поблизости, в тех местах.

there III *int* вот; ну; ~ is a good boy (*или* fellow *etc*)! вот молодец!, вот хорошо!; ~ it is! вот так так!; ~ you are! вот вы где!; вот и вы!; ~!, ~ ! ну, ну, полно!

thereabout(s) ['ðeərəbaut(s)] *adv* 1) поблизости; 2) около этого, приблизительно.

thereafter [ðeər'ɑ:ftə] *adv* 1) с тех пор; с того, с этого времени; 2) согласно этому.

thereat [ðeər'æt] *adv* 1) там; 2) в то время; при этом; 3) поэтому.

thereby ['ðeə'baɪ] *adv* 1) посредством этого; таким образом; 2) в связи с этим; вследствие этого.

therefor [ðeə'fɔ:] *adv уст.* для этого.

therefore ['ðeəfɔ:] *adv* поэтому; потому; следовательно; вследствие.

therefrom [ðeə'frɔm] *adv* оттуда.

therein [ðeər'ɪn] *adv* 1) здесь, там, в нём, в этом; 2) в этом отношении.

thereof [ðɛərʹɔv] *adv* 1) этого; того; 2) из этого; из того.

thereon [ðɛərʹɔn] *adv* 1) на нём, на ней *и т. п.*; 2) после того, вслед за тем.

there's [ðɛəz] *разг.* = there is.

thereto [ðɛəʹtuː] *adv* 1) к нему, к ней *и т. п.*; 2) к тому же, кроме того, вдобавок.

thereupon [ʹðɛərəʹrɔn] *adv* 1) на нём, на ней *и т. п.*; 2) вслед за тем; после того; 3) вследствие этого; поэтому.

therewith [ðɛəʹwɪð] *adv уст.* 1) с этим; при этом; к тому же; 2) тотчас, немедленно.

therewithal [ˌðɛəwɪʹðɔːl] *adv* при этом, к тому же, вдобавок.

therm [θəːm] *n* единица теплоты, калория.

thermal [ʹθəːməl] *a* 1) термический, тепловой; 2) горячий (*об источнике и т. п.*).

thermic [ʹθəːmɪk] *a* термический, тепловой.

thermodynamics [ʹθəːmoudaɪʹnæmɪks] *n* термодинамика.

thermometer [θəʹmɔmɪtə] *n* термометр, градусник.

thermo-nuclear [ʹθəːmouʹnjuːklɪə] *a* термоядерный.

thermos [ʹθəːmɔs] *n* термос.

thermostat [ʹθəːmoustæt] *n* термостат.

thermotechnics [ʹθəːmouˌteknɪks] *n* теплотехника.

thesaurus [θiːʹsɔːrəs] *n* 1) сокровищница (*знаний и т. п.*); 2) толковый словарь; энциклопедия.

these [ðiːz] *pl см.* this.

thesis [ʹθiːsɪs] *n* (*pl* theses [ʹθiːsiːz]) 1) тезис; 2) диссертация; to maintain a ~ for a degree защищать диссертацию; 3) школьное сочинение.

thews [θjuːz] *n pl* 1) мускулы; 2) (мускульная) сила.

they [ðeɪ] *pron pers* они; ~ say говорят; ~ who те, кто.

thick I [θɪk] *a* 1) толстый; a foot ~ толщиной в один фут; 2) плотный; густой (*о волосах, лесе и т. д.*); частый; ~ with полный чего-л.; 3) густой, тягучий (*о жидкости*); 4) мутный, туманный; тусклый; 5) хриплый; 6) тупой, глупый; 7) *разг.* близкий, интимный; 8) жирный (*о почерке, шрифте*); ◊ that is a bit ~ *разг.* это уж чересчур; это невыносимо; ~ as thieves ≅ водой не разольёшь.

thick II *n* 1) чаща; *перен.* гуща; in the ~ of it а) в самой гуще; б) в разгаре; 2) *разг.* тупица; ◊ through ~ and thin несмотря на все препятствия; не колеблясь, стойко.

thick III *adv* 1) плотно; густо, часто; 2) обильно; 3) неясно, хрипло; ◊ ~ and fast быстро, стремительно, одно за другим.

thick-and-thin [ʹθɪkənʹθɪn] *a* стойкий, непоколебимый; преданный (до конца).

thicken [ʹθɪkən] *v* 1) делать(ся) более густым; густеть; 2) становиться неясным, мутным; 3) расти (*о толпе*); 4) *шутл.* усложняться.

thicket [ʹθɪkɪt] *n* чаща, заросли.

thickhead [ʹθɪkhed] *n* тупица.

thick-headed [ʹθɪkʹhedɪd] *a* тупоголовый; глупый.

thickness [ʹθɪknɪs] *n* 1) толщина; 2) густота, плотность; 3) слой.

thickset [ʹθɪkʹset] *a* 1) коренастый; 2) густо посаженный.

thick-skinned [ʹθɪkʹskɪnd] *a* толстокожий; нечувствительный.

thick-skulled [ʹθɪkʹskʌld] *a* тупой, глупый.

thick-witted [ʹθɪkʹwɪtɪd] *a* тупоголовый; глупый.

thief [θiːf] *n* (*pl* thieves) вор.

thieve [θiːv] *v* красть, воровать.

thievery [ʹθiːvərɪ] *n* воровство; a ~ кража.

thieves [θiːvz] *pl см.* thief.

thievish [ʹθiːvɪʃ] *a* 1) вороватый; 2) воровской.

thigh [θaɪ] *n* бедро.

thigh-bone [ʹθaɪboun] *n* берцовая кость.

thill [θɪl] *n* оглобля.

thimble [ʹθɪmbl] *n* 1) напёрсток; 2) наконечник.

thimbleful [ʹθɪmblful] *n разг.* капелька, глоточек.

thin I [θɪn] *a* 1) тонкий; 2) худой, худощавый; ~ as a lath худой, как щепка; 3) редкий (*о волосах*); 4) немногочисленный (*о публике, населении*); редкий (*о населении*); 5) жидкий, водянистый, слабый; 6) слабый, недостаточный; неосновательный; скудный; 7) разрежённый (*о воздухе, газах*); 8) *разг.* неприятный; ◊ that is too ~ ≅ белыми нитками шито.

thin II *v* 1) делать(ся) тонким; худеть; 2) редеть; □ to **down** худеть; to ~ **out** прореживать (*растения*).

thine [ðaɪn] *pron уст.* твой.

thin-faced [ʹθɪnfeɪst] *a* с тонкими чертами лица.

thing [θɪŋ] *n* 1) вещь, предмет; the outward ~s окружающий мир; good ~s лакомства; the ~, the right ~, the very ~, quite the ~ как раз то, что надо; not quite the ~ to do а) не совсем то, что надо; б) не совсем прилично; to be (*или* to feel) not quite the ~ не по себе, чувствовать себя неважно; the last ~ а) последнее слово (*в науке и т. п.*; *in*); б) в последнюю очередь, напоследок; в) совершенно неожиданно; to know a ~ or two а) знать кое-что, догадываться кой о чём; б) быть проницательным; to make a good ~ of it извлекать пользу из чего-л.; 2) *ласково или презр. о живом существе*: little ~ малютка; old ~ голубчик, голубушка; poor ~ бедняжка; dumb ~ бессловесное животное, существо; a mean ~ подлая тварь; 3) дело, факт; событие; обстоятельство; above all ~s прежде всего, самое важное; first ~ первым делом, первым долгом; other ~s being equal при прочих равных условиях; a strange ~ странное дело, что-то странное; ~s look promising положение обнадёживающее; 4) *pl* вещи, багаж; (личные) принадлежности; 5) одежда; to take off one's ~s снять пальто, раздеться; 6) литературное *или* музыкальное произведение; ◊ to see ~s бредить, галлюцинировать; no such ~ ничего подобного; and ~s и так далее; of all ~s вот тебе и на! для one ~ во-первых.

think [θɪŋk] *v* (*past. p. p.* thought) 1) думать; мыслить; обдумывать; to ~ twice хорошенько подумать (*прежде чем сделать*); to ~ aloud думать вслух; 2) считать, полагать; to ~ little of а) быть невысокого мнения о; б) не придавать большого значения; to ~ much (*или* well) of быть высокого мнения о, высоко ценить; to ~ better of а) передумать; переменить мнение о чём-л.;

б) быть лу́чшего мне́ния о ком-л.; 3) понима́ть, представля́ть (себе́); I cannot ~ what you mean не могу́ поня́ть, что вы хоти́те сказа́ть; 4) намерева́ться; име́ть в виду́; □ to ~ **back** стара́ться вспо́мнить, восстанови́ть в па́мяти; to ~ **of** приду́мать; to ~ **out** продума́ть; найти́ реше́ние; to ~ **over** обду́мать, обсуди́ть; to ~ **up** изобрести́, приду́мать (об отгово́рке, предло́ге и т. п.); to ~ **with** быть одного́ мне́ния с кем-л.; ◊ to ~ no end of о́чень высоко́ цени́ть кого́-л.

thinkable ['θɪŋkəbl] a мы́слимый.

thinker ['θɪŋkə] n мысли́тель.

thinking I ['θɪŋkɪŋ] n 1) размышле́ние; обду́мывание; 2) мне́ние; представле́ние; to my ~ по моему́ мне́нию.

thinking II a мы́слящий, разу́мный.

thin-skinned ['θɪn'skɪnd] a 1) с то́нкой ко́жей; 2) чувстви́тельный; оби́дчивый.

third I [θəːd] пит тре́тий.

third II n 1) треть; тре́тья часть; 2) муз. те́рция.

third-rate ['θəːd'reɪt] a третьесо́ртный, нева́жный.

third-rater ['θəːd'reɪtə] n разг. ничто́жество.

thirst I [θəːst] n жа́жда.

thirst II v хоте́ть пить; испы́тывать жа́жду; перен. жа́ждать чего́-л.

thirsty ['θəːstɪ] a 1) томи́мый жа́ждой; испы́тывающий жа́жду; перен. жа́ждущий чего́-л.; he is ~ он хо́чет пить; 2) вызыва́ющий жа́жду; 3) пересо́хший; иссо́хший.

thirteen ['θəː'tiːn] пит трина́дцать.

thirteenth I ['θəː'tiːnθ] пит трина́дцатый.

thirteenth II n трина́дцатая часть.

thirties ['θəːtɪz] n pl (the ~) 1) тридца́тые го́ды; 2) во́зраст от 29 до 40 лет.

thirtieth I ['θəːtɪɪθ] пит тридца́тый.

thirtieth II n тридца́тая часть.

thirty ['θəːtɪ] пит три́дцать.

this [ðɪs] pron demonstr (pl these) э́тот, э́та, э́то; ◊ ~ much сто́лько, так мно́го.

thistle ['θɪsl] n бот. тата́рник; чертополо́х (тж. как национа́льная эмбле́ма Шотла́ндии).

thistly ['θɪslɪ] a 1) заро́сший чертополо́хом; 2) колю́чий.

thither ['ðɪðə] adv уст. туда́.

tho, tho' I, II [ðou] см. though I, II.

thole [θoul] n уклю́чина.

thong [θɔŋ] n реме́нь; плеть.

thorax ['θɔːræks] n грудна́я кле́тка.

thorn [θɔːn] n 1) шип; колю́чка; to be (или to sit) on ~s сиде́ть как на иго́лках; 2) боя́рышник, колю́чий куста́рник; 3) назва́ние руни́ческой бу́квы, соотве́тствующей th; ◊ a ~ in-one's side (или in the flesh) исто́чник раздраже́ния, неприя́тности; ≅ бельмо́ на глазу́.

thorny ['θɔːnɪ] a 1) колю́чий; с шипа́ми; 2) тру́дный; терни́стый; 3) щекотли́вый (о те́ме и т. п.).

thorough ['θʌrə] a по́лный, соверше́нный; основа́тельный, доскона́льный.

thoroughbred I ['θʌrəbred] n 1) чистокро́вное, поро́дистое живо́тное (особ. о ло́шади); 2) разг. хорошо́ воспи́танный челове́к.

thoroughbred II a 1) чистокро́вный, поро́дистый; 2) разг. хорошо́ воспи́танный.

thoroughfare ['θʌrəfɛə] n 1) прохо́д, прое́зд;

"No Thoroughfare" «Прое́зд закры́т», «Прохо́д воспрещён» (на́дпись); 2) широ́кая у́лица, доро́га.

thoroughgoing ['θʌrə͵gouɪŋ] a 1) иду́щий напроло́м, до конца́; прямолине́йный; 2) радика́льный.

thoroughly ['θʌrəlɪ] adv вполне́, до конца́; основа́тельно, доскона́льно.

thoroughness ['θʌrənɪs] n основа́тельность, доскона́льность.

thoroughpaced ['θʌrəpeɪst] a соверше́нный; отъя́вленный.

those [ðouz] pl см. that[a] I.

thou [ðau] pron pers уст., поэт. ты.

though I [ðou] conj 1) хотя́ бы; as ~ как бу́дто, сло́вно.

though II adv одна́ко; всё-таки.

thought[1] [θɔːt] n 1) мысль; мышле́ние; at the ~ of (или that) при мы́сли о; to collect (или to compose) one's ~s собра́ться с мы́слями; (lost) in ~ погружённый в размышле́ния; (up)on second ~s по зре́лом размышле́нии; 2) забо́та; внима́тельность; to show some ~ for smb. прояви́ть внима́ние к кому́-л.; to take ~ поду́мать, позабо́титься (о ком-л.); 3) наме́рение; зате́я; no ~ of и в мы́слях не́ было; 4): a ~ чу́точку; a ~ more немно́жко бо́льше; a ~ better чуть-чу́ть полу́чше, полегче.

thought[2] past, p. p. см. think.

thoughtful ['θɔːtful] a 1) ду́мающий, мы́слящий; заду́мавшийся; he was ~ for a while and then replied он поду́мал немно́го и зате́м отве́тил; 2) глубокомы́сленный; глубо́кий, содержа́тельный (о кни́ге и т. п.); 3) забо́тливый, внима́тельный (к кому́-л. — of).

thoughtfully ['θɔːtfulɪ] adv 1) заду́мчиво; 2) глубокомы́сленно; с глубокомы́сленным ви́дом.

thoughtless ['θɔːtlɪs] a 1) безду́мный, беспе́чный; 2) необду́манный (об отве́те, посту́пке); 3) невнима́тельный (к други́м).

thought-reading ['θɔːt͵riːdɪŋ] n чте́ние чужи́х мы́слей.

thousand I ['θauzənd] пит ты́сяча.

thousand II n ты́сяча; перен. мно́жество; a ~ and one разг. мно́го, ма́сса.

thousandfold I ['θauzəndfould] a в ты́сячу раз бо́льший; тысячекра́тный.

thousandfold II adv в ты́сячу раз бо́льше.

thousandth I ['θauzəntθ] пит ты́сячный.

thousandth II n ты́сячная часть.

thraldom ['θrɔːldəm] n ра́бство; порабоще́ние.

thrall I [θrɔːl] n 1) раб; 2) ра́бство.

thrall II v порабоща́ть.

thrash [θræʃ] v 1) молоти́ть; 2) разг. бить, колоти́ть; 3) разг. победи́ть (в состяза́нии), поби́ть; □ to ~ **out** тща́тельно обсужда́ть; выясня́ть (вопро́с и т. п.); ◊ to ~ over old straw ≅ толо́чь во́ду в сту́пе.

thrasher ['θræʃə] n 1) молоти́льщик; 2) молоти́лка; цеп.

thrashing ['θræʃɪŋ] n 1) молотьба́; 2) разг. побо́и, взбу́чка.

thread I [θred] n 1) ни́тка; перен. нить; to hang by a ~ держа́ться на ни́точке, висе́ть на волоске́; to lose the ~ потеря́ть нить (разгово́ра, расска́за и т. п.); to resume (или to pick up) the ~s of возобнови́ть знако́мство (с кем-л.); the fatal ~, the ~ of life нить жи́зни; 2) резьба́, винтова́я наре́зка; ◊ ~ and thrum всё вме́сте, и хоро́шее и дурно́е.

thread II v 1) продева́ть ни́тку (в иголку); 2) нани́зывать (бусы и т. п.); 3) пробира́ться; проти́скиваться; 4) нареза́ть (резьбу́), снабжа́ть резьбо́й.

threadbare ['θredbɛə] a 1) потёртый, изно́шенный; 2) о́чень бе́дно оде́тый; обноси́вшийся; 3) изби́тый (о шутке и т. п.).

threaded ['θredɪd] a с наре́зкой, с резьбо́й, нарезно́й.

threader ['θredə] n винторе́зный стано́к.

threadlike ['θredlaɪk] a 1) нитеви́дный; 2) волокни́стый.

thread-needle ['θred,niːdl] n «ручеёк» (название детской игры).

thready ['θredɪ] a 1) нитеви́дный, то́нкий; 2) волокни́стый.

threat [θret] n угро́за.

threaten ['θretn] v 1) грози́ть, угрожа́ть; 2) предвеща́ть.

threatening ['θretnɪŋ] a угрожа́ющий, грозя́щий; нави́сший.

threatful ['θretful] a гро́зный.

three I [θriː] num три.

three II n тро́йка; in ~s по три.

three-cornered ['θriː'kɔːnəd] a 1) треуго́льный; 2) нескла́дный, углова́тый.

three-decker ['θriː'dekə] n 1) трёхпа́лубное су́дно; 2) трило́гия, трёхто́мный рома́н.

threefold I ['θriːfould] a утро́енный, тройно́й.

threefold II adv втро́йне.

three-handed ['θriː'hændɪd] a с уча́стием трёх игроко́в.

three-lane ['θriːleɪn] n у́лица с движе́нием тра́нспорта в три ря́да.

three-legged ['θriː'legd] a трёхно́гий.

three-master ['θriː'mɑːstə] n трёхма́чтовый кора́бль.

threepence ['θrepəns] n три пе́нса; моне́та в три пе́нса.

threepenny ['θrepənɪ] a сто́имостью в три пе́нса, грошо́вый.

three-per-cents [,θriːpə'sents] n pl трёхпроце́нтные облига́ции.

three-ply I ['θriːplaɪ] n трёхсло́йная фане́ра.

three-ply II a трёхсло́йный.

three-quarter ['θriː'kwɔːtə] a 1) трёхчетвертно́й; 2) с поворо́том лица́ в три че́тверти (о портрете).

threescore ['θriː'skɔː] n шестьдеся́т.

threnode, threnody ['θriːnəd, 'θriːnədɪ] n похоро́нная песнь, надгро́бный плач.

thresh [θreʃ] см. thrash I.

thresher ['θreʃə] см. thrasher 2).

threshing-floor ['θreʃɪŋflɔː] n ток, гумно́.

threshing-machine ['θreʃɪŋmə,ʃiːn] n молоти́лка.

threshold ['θreʃhould] n поро́г; перен. тж. преддве́рие; on the ~ of revolution на поро́ге револю́ции, накану́не револю́ции.

threw [θruː] past см. throw I.

thrice [θraɪs] adv уст. 1) три́жды; 2) в вы́сшей сте́пени.

thrift [θrɪft] n 1) эконо́мность, бережли́вость; 2) процвета́ние; зажи́точность.

thriftless ['θrɪftlɪs] a неэконо́мный, расточи́тельный.

thrifty ['θrɪftɪ] a 1) эконо́мный, бережли́вый; 2) процвета́ющий; зажи́точный.

thrill I [θrɪl] n 1) дрожь, тре́пет; (ра́достное) волне́ние, возбужде́ние; 2) сленг сенса́ция.

thrill II v 1) вызыва́ть или испы́тывать тре́пет, волне́ние; to ~ with joy (за)трепета́ть от ра́дости; 2) дрожа́ть (от страха, радости и т. п.).

thriller ['θrɪlə] n разг. сенсацио́нный (особ. детекти́вный) рома́н или фильм; «боеви́к».

thrilling ['θrɪlɪŋ] a волну́ющий, захва́тывающий.

thrill-thirsty ['θrɪl'θɜːstɪ] a лю́бящий сенса́ции или детекти́вы.

thrive [θraɪv] (past throve; p. p. thriven) 1) процвета́ть, преуспева́ть; 2) богате́ть, нажива́ться; 3) (бу́йно) расти́, расцвета́ть, хорошо́ развива́ться.

thriven ['θrɪvn] p. p. см. thrive.

thro, thro' I, II, III [θruː] = through I, II, III.

throat [θrout] n 1) го́рло, гло́тка, горта́нь; a ~ of brass гро́мкий, гру́бый го́лос; to clear one's ~ отка́шляться; he has a sore ~ у него́ боли́т го́рло; 2) у́зкий прохо́д, у́зкое отве́рстие; ◊ to cut one's own ~ губи́ть, разоря́ть себя́; to cut another's ~ губи́ть, разоря́ть кого́-л.

throaty ['θroutɪ] a горта́нный; горлово́й; хри́плый.

throb I [θrɔb] n 1) бие́ние, пульса́ция; 2) тре́пет, волне́ние.

throb II v 1) си́льно би́ться, пульси́ровать; 2) трепета́ть, волнова́ться.

throe I [θrou] n обыкн. pl 1) си́льная боль, му́ка; in the ~s of в му́ках; 2) аго́ния; 3) родовы́е му́ки.

throe II v страда́ть, му́читься.

throne I [θroun] n 1) трон, престо́л; to ascend the ~ вступи́ть на престо́л; 2) короле́вская власть.

throne II v 1) возводи́ть на престо́л; 2) восседа́ть.

throng I [θrɔŋ] n толпа́, толчея́; скопле́ние (наро́да).

throng II v толпи́ться; вали́ть толпо́й; переполня́ть (театр, улицу).

throstle ['θrɔsl] n пе́вчий дрозд.

throttle I ['θrɔtl] n 1) разг. гло́тка, го́рло; 2) тех. дро́ссель, регуля́тор.

throttle II v 1) души́ть; 2) задыха́ться; 3) тех. дроссели́ровать; мять (пар); □ to ~ down уме́ньшить газ.

through I [θruː] prep 1) че́рез, сквозь; по; в; 2) че́рез посре́дство; из (какого-л. источника); от (кого-л.); 3) из-за; благодаря́; всле́дствие; 4) в продолже́ние, в тече́ние; ~ the night всю ночь напролёт; 5) включи́тельно; May 15 ~ June 15 с 15-го ма́я по 15-е ию́ня (включи́тельно).

through II a 1) прямо́й, беспереса́дочный; сквозно́й, прямо́го сообще́ния (о вагоне, поезде); 2) свобо́дный (о проходе и т. п.).

through III adv 1) наскво́зь; to be wet ~ промо́кнуть наскво́зь; 2) от нача́ла до конца́; to read a book ~ проче́сть всю кни́гу; to be ~ with smth. поко́нчить с чем-л.

through-and-through ['θruːən'θruː] adv соверше́нно, до конца́, вполне́.

throughout I [θru:'aut] *adv* 1) во всех отношениях; 2) на всём протяжении; 3) повсюду, везде.

throughout II *prep* через; по всему; в продолжение (*всего времени и т. п.*).

through-put ['θru:put] *n* пропускная способность.

throve [θrouv] *past см.* thrive.

throw I [θrou] *v* (*past* threw; *p. p.* thrown) 1) бросать (*тж. перен. — свет, тень, взгляд*); кидать, швырять; метать; to ~ oneself бросаться, кидаться; 2) сбрасывать (*всадника*); класть на обе лопатки (*в борьбе; тж. перен.*); 3) менять (*кожу — о змее*); 4) (внезапно или быстро) приводить (*в какое-л. состояние*); to ~ into disorder (into confusion) приводить в беспорядок (в смятение); 5) *разг.* потрясать; 6) крутить (*пряжу*), сучить; 7) метать (детёнышей) (*о кроликах и т. п.*); □ to ~ **about** разбрасывать; to ~ **aside** отбрасывать, отстранять; to ~ **away** выбрасывать; тратить зря; to ~ **back** а) отбрасывать назад; б) отвергать (резко); to ~ **down** а) сбрасывать; опрокидывать; б) ниспровергать; в) сносить (*здание*); to ~ **in** а) добавлять; б) вставлять (*замечание*); в) *тех.* включать; to ~ **off** а) отбрасывать; отвергать; б) смещать, свергать; в) отвлекать; г) *разг.* сказать вскользь, между прочим; бросить (*замечание и т. п.*); д) сбросить (*пальто и т. п.*); е) избавиться (*от болезни, неприятности*); to ~ **on** набросить, накинуть (*пальто и т. п.*); to ~ **out** а) выбрасывать; б) выставлять, выгонять; в) испускать; г) *тех.* выключать, разъединять; to ~ **over** а) бросать (*за ненадобностью, негодностью*); б) покидать (*друзей*); в) *тех.* переключать; переводить; to ~ **up** а) поднимать (*руки*); вскидывать (*глаза, голову*); б) спешно возводить (*здание, укрепления*); в) отказаться от, бросить (*дело, занятие*); г) извергать; *разг.* рвать.

throw II *n* 1) бросание, бросок; дальность броска, размах; discus ~ метание диска; at a stone's ~ на расстоянии брошенного камня; недалеко; 2) *спорт.* падение (*при борьбе*); 3) *тех.* ход; the ~ of the piston ход поршня; the ~ of the pointer отклонение стрелки.

throw-back ['θroubæk] *n* 1) регресс; возврат к прошлому; 2) атавизм.

throw-down ['θroudaun] *n* 1) поражение; 2) ниспровержение; 3) отказ; отклонение (*предложения*).

thrower ['θrouə] *n* гранатомётчик.

thrown I [θroun] *p. p. см.* throw I.

thrown II *a* кручёный (*о шёлке и т. п.*).

thru I, II, III [θru:] *амер. см.* through I, II, III.

thrum[1] [θrʌm] *n* бахрома; незатканный конец основы.

thrum[2] I *n* бренчание.

thrum[2] II *v* 1) бренчать, тренькать; 2) барабанить пальцами.

thrush[1] [θrʌʃ] *n* дрозд.

thrush[2] *n* молочница, стоматит.

thrust I [θrʌst] *n* 1) толчок; 2) удар; выпад (*против кого-л.*); a home ~ меткий удар; 3) опора; упор; 4) *тех.* нагрузка, давление; напор.

thrust II *v* (*past, p. p.* thrust) 1) толкать; бросать (*с силой*); to ~ oneself бросаться, ус-

тремляться; проталкиваться; to ~ oneself forward «вылезать», стараться обратить на себя внимание; 2) колоть, пронзать; 3) вколачивать; 4) протискиваться; врываться; □ to ~ **aside** отталкивать; отбрасывать, отвергать; to ~ **from** сбрасывать; to ~ **in(to)** а) вталкивать, всовывать; совать; б) вонзать; to ~ oneself into втираться; навязываться; to ~ **on** понуждать; побуждать; to ~ **out** выгонять, выселять; to ~ **through** а) пронзать; прокалывать; б) пробивать(ся); to ~ **together** сжимать; to ~ **upon** навязывать (*силой*).

thud I [θʌd] *n* глухой звук (*при падении*).

thud II *v* свалиться, упасть с глухим шумом.

thug [θʌg] *n* головорез, разбойник.

thumb [θʌm] *n* большой палец (*руки*); ◊ under smb.'s ~ под влиянием кого-л., во власти кого-л.; to twiddle one's ~s бездельничать.

thumb II *v* 1) неуклюже, неловко делать что-л.; 2) загрязнить, захватать; 3) *разг.:* to ~ a ride остановить проезжающий автомобиль, подняв большой палец.

thumb-mark ['θʌmmɑːk] *n* следы пальцев (*на страницах книги*).

thumb-screw ['θʌmskru:] *n* 1) *тех.* винт с накатанной головкой; винт-барашек; 2) *ист.* орудие пытки (*сжимавшее большой палец*).

thumb-tack ['θʌmtæk] *n амер.* чертёжная кнопка.

thump I [θʌmp] *n* тяжёлый удар (*особ. кулаком*); глухой звук (*удара*).

thump II *v* 1) наносить тяжёлый удар; колотить; 2) стучать (*кулаком*); 3) производить глухой звук; падать тяжело (*с глухим шумом*); 4) тяжело, глухо биться (*о сердце*).

thumping I [θʌmpiŋ] *a разг.* громадный.

thumping II *adv разг.* очень, чертовски.

thunder I [θʌndə] *n* 1) гром; 2) грохот; шум; 3) *pl* угрозы.

thunder II *v* 1) греметь; it ~s гром гремит; 2) грохотать, производить шум; 3) метать громы и молнии, грозить.

thunderbolt ['θʌndəboult] *n* вспышка молнии и удар грома; *перен.* гром среди ясного неба.

thunderclap ['θʌndəklæp] *n* удар грома.

thundercloud ['θʌndəklaud] *n* грозовая туча.

thunderer ['θʌndərə] *n* громовержец.

thundering ['θʌndəriŋ] *a* 1) громоподобный, оглушительный; 2) *разг.* громадный; ужасный.

thunderous ['θʌndərəs] *a* 1) грозовой; 2) громовой, громоподобный.

thunder-peal ['θʌndəpi:l] *n* удар *или* раскат грома.

thunderstorm ['θʌndəstɔːm] *n* гроза.

thunderstruck ['θʌndəstrʌk] *a* ошеломлённый; как громом поражённый.

thundery ['θʌndəri] *a* грозовой.

Thursday ['θəːzdi] *n* четверг.

thus [ðʌs] *adv* так, таким образом; так что; ~ and ~ так-то и так-то; ~ far до сих пор; до этого места; ~ much столько.

thwack I [θwæk] *n* удар (*палкой*).

thwack II *v* ударять, бить.

thwart I [θwɔːt] *n* 1) банка, сиденье гребца; 2) распор.

'thwart II *a* 1) попере́чный; 2) несгово́рчивый.

thwart III *v* 1) перечить; 2) препя́тствовать; меша́ть; расстра́ивать *(пла́ны и т. п.)*.

thy [ðaɪ] *pron poss уст.* твой.

thyme [taɪm] *n бот.* тимья́н.

thyroid ['θaɪrɔɪd] *n* щитови́дная железа́.

thyself [ðaɪ'self] *pron refl уст.* ты сам; себя́.

tibia ['tɪbɪə] *n (pl* tibiae ['tɪbiː]) *анат.* большеберцо́вая кость.

tic [tɪk] *n мед.* тик.

tick¹ I [tɪk] *n* 1) ти́канье; to *(или* on) the ~ то́чно, пунктуа́льно; 2) отме́тка, значо́к V, «пти́чка»; 3) *разг.* мгнове́ние, моме́нт.

tick¹ II *v* 1) ти́кать; 2) ста́вить значо́к V, отмеча́ть «пти́чкой»; □ to ~ off *разг.* разруга́ть, «отде́лать»; to ~ out выстуки́вать *(об аппара́те)*; to ~ over а) поверну́ть *(рыча́г, ру́чку)*; б) рабо́тать на холосто́м ходу́.

tick² *n* 1) чехо́л *(матра́ца, поду́шки)*; 2) тик *(мате́рия)*.

tick³ I *n разг.* креди́т; to buy on ~ покупа́ть в креди́т; to run ~ име́ть креди́т.

tick³ II *v разг.* брать, отпуска́ть в креди́т.

tick⁴ *n* клещ.

ticker ['tɪkə] *n* 1) *разг.* часы́; 2) *разг.* телегра́фный аппара́т; 3) *эл.* прерыва́тель; 4) *ра́дио* ти́ккер.

ticket I ['tɪkɪt] *n* 1) биле́т; commutator ~ *амер.* сезо́нный биле́т; return ~ обра́тный биле́т; through ~ биле́т прямо́го сообще́ния; produce your ~s! предъяви́те ва́ши биле́ты!; 2) ярлы́к; price ~ этике́тка с цено́й; 3) *амер.* спи́сок кандида́тов како́й-л. па́ртии на вы́борах; mixed ~ спи́сок кандида́тов ра́зных па́ртий; to be ahead (behind) of one's ~ получи́ть наибо́льшее (наиме́ньшее) коли́чество голосо́в по спи́ску свое́й па́ртии; to vote the straight ~ голосова́ть за кандида́тов одно́й па́ртии; 4) ка́рточка, удостовере́ние; квита́нция; ~ of discharge увольни́тельное свиде́тельство; pawn ~ зало́говая квита́нция; 5) объявле́ние *(о сда́че внаём)*; ◊ that's the ~ *разг.* как раз то, что на́до; not quite the ~ *разг.* не совсе́м то.

ticket II *v* прикрепля́ть ярлы́к, этике́тку.

ticket-of-leave ['tɪkɪtəv'liːv] *a:* ~ man досро́чно освобождённый.

ticking ['tɪkɪŋ] *n* тик *(мате́рия)*.

tickle I ['tɪkl] *n* щеко́тка.

tickle II *v* 1) щекота́ть; чу́вствовать щекота́ние; my nose ~s у меня́ щеко́чет в носу́; 2) забавля́ть, весели́ть, доставля́ть удово́льствие; to ~ to death а) умори́ть со́ смеху; б) си́льно обра́довать; she was ~d pink она́ была́ стра́шно дово́льна.

tickler ['tɪklə] *n* тру́дная зада́ча; головоло́мка.

ticklish ['tɪklɪʃ] *a* 1) щекотли́вый, смешли́вый; 2) оби́дчивый; чувстви́тельный; 3) щекотли́вый, делика́тный *(о вопро́се и т. п.)*.

tick-tack ['tɪk'tæk] *n разг.* 1) ти́канье; тик-та́к; 2) часы́.

tidal ['taɪdl] *a* 1) свя́занный с прили́вом и отли́вом; 2) приходя́щий во вре́мя прили́ва *(о парохо́де)*.

tidbit ['tɪdbɪt] *см.* titbit.

tiddly-winks ['tɪdlɪwɪŋks] *n pl* игра́ в бло́шки.

tide I [taɪd] *n* 1) прили́в и отли́в; the high

(low) ~ вы́сшая (ни́зшая) то́чка прили́ва *или* отли́ва; ~ is falling (rising) вода́ убыва́ет (прибыва́ет); 2) пото́к, тече́ние; направле́ние; to go with the ~ плыть по тече́нию; the ~ has turned сча́стье измени́ло; 3) *уст.* вре́мя го́да, пери́од, сезо́н; ◊ war ~s ве́сти, сообще́ния с фро́нта.

tide II *v* плыть по тече́нию; □ to ~ over а) помога́ть *(перенести́ что-л.)*; б): to ~ over a difficulty преодоле́ть затрудне́ние.

tidewater ['taɪd͵wɔːtə] *n* 1) во́ды прили́ва; 2) морско́й бе́рег; 3) *attr* прибре́жный, примо́рский.

tidiness ['taɪdɪnɪs] *n* опря́тность.

tidings ['taɪdɪŋz] *n pl* но́вости, изве́стия, ве́сти.

tidy I ['taɪdɪ] *a* 1) опря́тный, аккура́тный; в поря́дке, чи́стый *(о ко́мнате и т. п.)*; 2) *разг.* поря́дочный, изря́дный.

tidy II *n* 1) салфе́точка *(на спи́нке мя́гкой ме́бели и т. п.)*; 2) де́тский пере́дник; 3) корзи́нка и т. п. *(для мелоче́й)*.

tidy III *v* убира́ть, приводи́ть в поря́док *(тж.* ~ up).

tie I [taɪ] *n* 1) верёвка, шнуро́к, тесьма́; 2) связь, скре́па; у́зел, соедине́ние; *перен.* у́зы; the ~s of friendship у́зы дру́жбы; 3) га́лстук; 4) горже́тка; 5) попере́чина, соедини́тельная сто́йка; *амер.* шпа́ла; 6) ра́вный счёт *(голосо́в; очко́в в игре́)*; ничья́; 7) *муз.* ли́га.

tie II *v* 1) свя́зывать; завя́зывать; шнурова́ть *(боти́нки)*; 2) скрепля́ть, стя́гивать; 3) стесня́ть, свя́зывать, обя́зывать; ~d to time ограни́ченный вре́менем, сро́ком; 4) сравня́ть счёт; сыгра́ть вничью́; □ to ~ in свя́зываться *(с — with)*; to ~ up а) поста́вить в затрудни́тельное положе́ние; б) объединя́ться, соединя́ть уси́лия *(with)*.

tier*ᵃ* ['taɪə] *n* де́тский фа́ртук.

tier*ᵇ* I [tɪə] *n* 1) я́рус, ряд; 2) бу́хта *(кана́та)*.

tier*ᵇ* II *v* располага́ть я́русами.

tierce [tɪəs] *n* 1) бо́чка *(о́коло 200 л)*; 2) *муз.* те́рция; 3) *карт.* три ка́рты одно́й ма́сти.

tie-up ['taɪʌp] *n* 1) связь; 2) вре́менная приостано́вка рабо́ты; *амер.* забасто́вка.

tie-wig ['taɪwɪg] *n* пари́к с коси́чкой.

tiff¹ I [tɪf] *n* размо́лвка; сты́чка, ссо́ра.

tiff¹ II *v* слегка́ повздо́рить; ду́ться, серди́ться.

tiff² I *n* глото́к спиртно́го.

tiff² II *v* пить небольши́ми глотка́ми, потя́гивать.

tiffin ['tɪfɪn] *n* за́втрак, заку́ска *(на Восто́ке)*.

tig I [tɪg] *n* 1) прикоснове́ние; 2) игра́ в «са́лки».

tig II *v* 1) прикаса́ться, тро́гать; 2) «са́лить».

tiger ['taɪgə] *n* 1) тигр; American ~ ягуа́р; 2) задира, хулига́н; 3) *амер. сленг* во́згласы одобре́ния.

tiger-moth ['taɪgəmɔθ] *n* ночна́я ба́бочка.

tight I [taɪt] *a* 1) пло́тный, компа́ктный; сжа́тый; 2) туго́й; ту́го завя́занный *(об узле́)*; ту́го натя́нутый; 3) непроница́емый *(для воды́, во́здуха и т. п.)*; 4) пло́тно прилега́ющий; те́сный *(об оде́жде, о́буви)*; 5) ску́дный, недоста́точный *(о сре́дствах)*; 6) *разг.* скупо́й; 7) тру́дный, затрудни́тельный; 8) сде́ржанный *(в обраще́нии)*; 9) *разг.* аккура́тный, опря́тный; 10) *разг.* пья́ный.

tight II *adv* 1) пло́тно; 2) ту́го; 3) кре́пко *(держа́ться и т. п.)*; 4) те́сно.

tighten ['taɪtn] *v* 1) сжимáть; натя́гивать; подтя́гивать (*туже*); 2) натя́гиваться; сжимáться.

tight-fisted ['taɪt‚fɪstɪd] *a* скупóй.

tightrope ['taɪtroup] *n* тýго натя́нутые канáт *или* прóволока.

tights [taɪts] *n pl* трикó.

tight-wad ['taɪtwɔd] *n амер.* скря́га, скупéц.

tigress ['taɪgrɪs] *n* тигрúца.

tike [taɪk] *см.* tyke.

tilbury ['tɪlbərɪ] *n уст.* тильбю́ри, лёгкий двухколёсный экипáж.

tilde [tɪld] *n* знак тúльды (~).

tile I [taɪl] *n* 1) черепúца; 2) кáфель, изразéц (*тж.* Dutch ~); 3) гончáрная трубá (*дренáжная*); 4) *разг.* цилúндр (*шля́па*).

tile II *v* крыть черепúцей.

tiling ['taɪlɪŋ] *n* черепúчная крóвля.

till¹ I [tɪl] *prep* 1) *указывает на временнóй предéл какóго-л. дéйствия* до; ~ now до сих пóр; ~ then до тех пóр; 2) *в отриц. предложéнии указывает предéл врéмени, до котóрого дéйствие не совершáлось* не рáньше; he didn't come ~ today до сегóдняшнего дня егó ещё нет.

till¹ II *conj* покá, до тех пор покá; we laughed ~ the tears ran down мы смея́лись до слёз.

till² *n* дéнежный я́щик, кáсса.

till³ *v* воздéлывать (зéмлю), пахáть.

tillable ['tɪləbl] *a* пáхотный.

tillage ['tɪlɪdʒ] *n* 1) обрабóтка земли́; 2) воздéланная земля́, пáшня.

tiller¹ ['tɪlə] *n* 1) земледéлец; 2) *с.-х.* культивáтор.

tiller² I *n* побéг, отрóсток.

tiller² II *v* пускáть побéги.

tilt¹ I [tɪlt] *n* 1) наклóн(ное положéние); крен; склон; откóс; 2) нападéние с копьём, пúкой наперевéс; ◊ at full ~ изо всех сил.

tilt¹ II *v* 1) наклоня́ть(ся); крени́ть(ся); 2) нападáть с копьём, пúкой наперевéс; 3) опрокúдывать(ся); □ to ~ **against**, to ~ **at** борóться с кем-л., чем-л.; *перен.* ломáть кóпья.

tilt² *n* брезéнтовый навéс (*над лóдкой, телéгой*).

tilth [tɪlθ] *n* 1) обрабóтка земли́; 2) воздéланная земля́, пáшня.

tilt-yard ['tɪltjɑːd] *n ист.* арéна для турни́ров.

timber I ['tɪmbə] *n* 1) лесоматериáл; строевóй лес; 2) бревнó, бáлка; 3) *разг.* спúчка.

timber II *v* 1) стрóить из дéрева; 2) плóтничать; столя́рничать.

timbered ['tɪmbəd] *a* 1) деревя́нный, из дéрева; 2) леси́стый, покры́тый лéсом.

timber-toes ['tɪmbətouz] *n pl шутл.* 1) человéк с деревя́нной ногóй; 2) человéк с тяжёлой пóступью.

timbre ['tæmbə] *n* тембр.

timbrel ['tɪmbrəl] *n* бýбен, тамбури́н.

time I [taɪm] *n* 1) врéмя; what ~ is it? котóрый час?; the ~ of (the) day врéмя дня, час; to know the ~ of the day *перен.* быть себé на умé; dinner ~ врéмя обéда; in ~ порá; high ~ сáмое врéмя, как раз, давнó порá; at ~s временáм; времен ами; from ~ to ~ иногдá; врéмя от врéмени; in (good) ~ своеврéменно, вóвремя; all in good ~ всё в своё врéмя; in bad ~ пóздно; in a short ~ в скóром врéмени; for a short ~ на корóткое врéмя; the ~ is ripe for it настáло

врéмя; пришлó врéмя; in ~ по ~ необыкновéнно бы́стро, мгновéнно; at ~ по ~ никогдá; some ~ or other когдá-нибудь; at the same ~ в тó же врéмя, вмéсте с тем; on full ~ с пóлным рабóчим врéменем; получáющий зарплáту за пóлный рабóчий день; on short ~ с непóлным рабóчим врéменем; рабóтающий непóлную рабóчую недéлю; to have a good ~ прия́тно провести́ врéмя; to have a high ~ хорошó провести́ врéмя, повесели́ться; to have a rough ~ терпéть лишéния; to idle (*или* to loiter away, to squander) ~ дáром трáтить врéмя, бездéльничать; to while away the ~ коротáть врéмя; to potter away one's ~ убивáть врéмя; idle ~ *тех.* простóй в рабóте; to gain ~ сэконóмить, вы́играть врéмя; to observe ~ быть óчень тóчным, пунктуáльным; to make ~ наверстáть потéрянное врéмя; ~ presses врéмя не ждёт; at the ~ being в настоя́щий момéнт; take your ~! не спеши́те!, не торопи́тесь!; at odd ~s мéжду дéлом; 2) перúод, порá; in winter ~ зимóй, в зúмнее врéмя; 3) срок; ~ is up срок истёк; to see one's ~ out отслужи́ть весь срок; to do ~ *разг.* отбывáть срок (*заключéния*); 4) *обыкн. pl* эпóха, временá; Shakespeare's ~s эпóха Шекспи́ра; ~ of peace ми́рное врéмя; stirring ~s богáтое собы́тиями врéмя; to go with the ~ идти́ в нóгу со врéменем, с эпóхой; before the (*или* one's) ~ передовóй; behind the (*или* one's) ~ отстáлый; hard ~s тяжёлые временá; ~ out of mind (в) незапáмятные временá; ~ to come бýдущее; бýдущие временá; 5) век, жизнь; it will last my ~ на мой век хвáтит; 6) вóзраст; at his ~ of life в егó гóды, в егó вóзрасте; 7) раз; every ~ кáждый раз, всегдá; at one ~ рáзом; five ~s six is thirty $5 \times 6 = 30$; ten ~s bigger (better *etc*) в дéсять раз бóльше (лýчше *и т. п.*); ~ after ~ раз за рáзом; повтóрно; ~ and again неоднокрáтно; чáсто; ~s out of number бесчи́сленное колúчество раз; 8) темп; такт; ритм; to beat ~ отбивáть такт; to keep ~ а) идти́ вéрно (*о часáх*); б) соблюдáть, выдéрживать темп, ритм; in (out of) ~ (не) в такт.

time II *v* 1) (удáчно) выбирáть врéмя; 2) назначáть врéмя; 3) рассчи́тывать по врéмени, согласóвывать, соразмеря́ть; well ~d хорошó рассчи́танный, своеврéменный; 4) засекáть врéмя; хрономети́ровать; 5) отбивáть такт.

time-bill ['taɪmbɪl] *см.* time-table.

time-bomb ['taɪmbɔm] *n* бóмба замéдленного дéйствия.

time-expired ['taɪmɪks‚paɪəd] *a воен.* отслужи́вший свой срок.

time-fuse ['taɪmfjuːz] *n воен.* дистанциóнная трýбка; запáл.

time-honoured ['taɪm‚ɔnəd] *a* освящённый векáми.

timekeeper ['taɪm‚kiːpə] *n* 1) тáбельщик; 2) *спорт.* хронометри́ст; 3) часы́; хронóметр.

timekeeping ['taɪm‚kiːpɪŋ] *n* хронометрáж.

time-lag ['taɪmlæg] *n* промежýток врéмени мéжду причи́ной и результáтом *или* слéдствием.

timeless ['taɪmlɪs] *a* 1) несвоеврéменный; 2) *поэт.* вéчный; вневрéменный.

timely I ['taɪmlɪ] *a* своеврéменный.

timely II *adv* 1) вóвремя; своеврéменно; 2) рáно; заблаговрéменно.

timepiece ['taɪmpiːs] *n* часы́.

time-server ['taɪmˌsəːvə] *n* приспособле́нец; оппортуни́ст.

time-serving I ['taɪmˌsəːvɪŋ] *n* приспособле́нчество; оппортуни́зм.

time-serving II *a* приспособля́ющийся; оппортунисти́ческий.

time-study ['taɪmˌstʌdɪ] *n* хронометра́ж.

time-table ['taɪmˌteɪbl] *n* 1) расписа́ние; 2) гра́фик.

time-work ['taɪmwəːk] *n* подённая *или* почасова́я рабо́та.

time-worn ['taɪmwɔːn] *a* изно́шенный; обветша́лый.

timid ['tɪmɪd] *a* ро́бкий; несме́лый.

timidity [tɪ'mɪdɪtɪ] *n* ро́бость.

timing I ['taɪmɪŋ] *n* 1) вы́бор вре́мени; расчёт вре́мени; регули́рование; 2) синхро́нность.

timing II *a* регули́рующий; распредели́тельный.

timorous ['tɪmərəs] *a* ро́бкий, боязли́вый.

timothy(-grass) ['tɪməθɪ(grɑːs)] *n бот.* тимофе́евка лугова́я.

tin I [tɪn] *n* 1) о́лово; 2) жесть; 3) жестя́нка, консе́рвная ба́нка; 4) *сленг* де́ньги; 5) *воен. сленг* танк.

tin II *a* 1) оловя́нный; 2) *разг.* нева́жный, не особе́нно хоро́ший.

tin III *v* 1) луди́ть, покрыва́ть о́ловом; 2) консерви́ровать.

tincture I ['tɪŋktʃə] *n* 1) *фарм.* насто́йка, тинкту́ра; 2) отте́нок (*цвета*); 3) при́вкус.

tincture II *v* 1) окра́шивать; придава́ть отте́нок (*чего-л.*); придава́ть при́вкус; 2) пропи́тывать.

tinder ['tɪndə] *n* 1) трут; фити́ль; 2) сухо́е гнило́е де́рево.

tindery ['tɪndərɪ] *a* 1) легковоспламеня́ющийся; 2) вспы́льчивый.

tine [taɪn] *n* зубе́ц (*вил, бороны*); остриё.

ting I [tɪŋ] *n* ре́зкий звук, звон.

ting II *v* звене́ть.

tinge I [tɪndʒ] *n* 1) лёгкая окра́ска; отте́нок; 2) при́месь; при́вкус.

tinge II *v* 1) слегка́ окра́шивать; 2) придава́ть отте́нок, при́вкус; 3) чуть-чу́ть изменя́ть.

tingle I ['tɪŋgl] *n* ощуще́ние зво́на в уша́х, пока́лывания (*в онеме́вших чле́нах*), пощи́пывания (*на моро́зе*).

tingle II *v* 1) испы́тывать звон в уша́х, пока́лывание (*в онеме́вших чле́нах*), пощи́пывание (*на моро́зе*); 2) звене́ть; 3) дрожа́ть, трепета́ть (*от чего-л.— with*).

tinker I ['tɪŋkə] *n* 1) ме́дник, луди́льщик; 2) плохо́й рабо́тник, «сапо́жник»; 3) плоха́я рабо́та.

tinker II *v* 1) пая́ть, луди́ть; починя́ть; 2) пло́хо рабо́тать, по́ртить; чини́ть ко́е-как; to ~ away with (*или* at) smth. вози́ться с чем-л.

tinkle I ['tɪŋkl] *n* звон (*колоко́льчика и т. п.*); звя́канье.

tinkle II *v* звене́ть; звони́ть; звя́кать.

tinkler ['tɪŋklə] *n разг.* колоко́льчик.

tinman ['tɪnmən] *n* жестя́н(щ)ик.

tinned [tɪnd] *a* 1) консерви́рованный (*о проду́ктах*); 2) покры́тый сло́ем о́лова.

tin-opener ['tɪnˌoupnə] *n* консе́рвный нож.

tin-plate ['tɪnpleɪt] *n* жесть.

tinsel I ['tɪnsəl] *n* 1) фо́льга; 2) блёстки, мишура́; 3) показно́й блеск; 4) *attr* мишу́рный; показно́й.

tinsel II *v* украша́ть блёстками, мишуро́й.

tin-smith ['tɪnsmɪθ] *n* жестя́н(щ)ик.

tint I [tɪnt] *n* отте́нок, тон; the autumn ~s осе́нние кра́ски.

tint II *v* слегка́ окра́шивать; придава́ть отте́нок.

tinware ['tɪnwɛə] *n* жестяны́е изде́лия; оловя́нная посу́да.

tiny ['taɪnɪ] *a* о́чень ма́ленький, кро́шечный.

tip[1] I [tɪp] *n* 1) ко́нчик; коне́ц; верши́на (*горы*); on the ~ of the (*или* one's) tongue на языке́, на ко́нчике языка́; on the ~s of one's toes на цы́почках; 2) наконе́чник.

tip[1] II *v* 1) снабжа́ть наконе́чником; надева́ть наконе́чник; 2) среза́ть верху́шки (*дере́вьев, кусто́в*); 3) стричь (*во́лосы*).

tip[2] I *n* 1) лёгкое прикоснове́ние; толчо́к (*небольшо́й*); 2) накло́н; 3) ме́сто сва́лки.

tip[2] II *v* 1) слегка́ ударя́ть, прикаса́ться; 2) наклоня́ть(ся); 3) опроки́дывать; сва́ливать; сбра́сывать; опорожня́ть; □ to ~ out выва́ливать(ся); to ~ over опроки́дывать(ся); to ~ up а) опроки́дывать; б) отки́дывать (*сиде́нье и т. п.*).

tip[3] I *n* 1) чаевы́е; 2) намёк; сове́т, предупрежде́ние; take my ~ послу́шайтесь меня́; the straight ~ надёжный сове́т; 3) ча́стная информа́ция, све́дения (*о беговы́х лошадя́х, биржевы́х сде́лках*).

tip[3] II *v* 1) дава́ть «на чай»; угоща́ть; 2) сообща́ть, передава́ть ча́стную информа́цию; □ to ~ off намека́ть, предупрежда́ть.

tip-cart ['tɪpkɑːt] *n* опроки́дывающаяся теле́жка.

tipcat ['tɪpkæt] *n* игра́ в чижи́.

tip-off ['tɪp'ɔf] *n* намёк; предупрежде́ние; to give the ~ вы́дать.

tip-over ['tɪp'ouvə] *a* опроки́дывающийся.

tippet ['tɪpɪt] *n* 1) капюшо́н; 2) паланти́н.

tipple I ['tɪpl] *n* спиртно́й напи́ток.

tipple II *v* пить, выпива́ть, пья́нствовать.

tippler ['tɪplə] *n* пья́ница.

tipster ['tɪpstə] *n* «жучо́к» (*на ска́чках*).

tipsy ['tɪpsɪ] *a* подвы́пивший.

tiptoe I ['tɪptou] *n* ко́нчики па́льцев, цы́почки; on ~ на цы́почках; *перен.* укра́дкой; to be on ~ with curiosity сгора́ть от любопы́тства.

tiptoe II *v* 1) ходи́ть на цы́почках; 2) кра́сться.

tiptop I ['tɪp'tɔp] *n* вы́сшая то́чка, верши́на, преде́л.

tiptop II *a разг.* превосхо́дный, первокла́ссный.

tiptop III *adv* превосхо́дно, великоле́пно.

tirade [taɪ'reɪd] *n* тира́да.

tire[1] I ['taɪə] *n* 1) ши́на; flat ~ спу́щенная ши́на; 2) о́бод колеса́.

tire[1] II *v* надева́ть ши́ну (*на колесо́*).

tire[2] *v* 1) утомля́ть (*тж.* to ~ out); 2) утомля́ться, устава́ть; 3) надое́сть, прискучи́ть; I am ~d of мне надое́ло, наску́чило.

tired ['taɪəd] *a* уста́лый, утомлённый; пресы́щенный; ~ out изнурённый, изму́ченный.

tireless ['taɪəlɪs] *a* неутоми́мый; неуста́нный.

tiresome ['taɪəsəm] *a* 1) утоми́тельный; 2) надое́дливый; ну́дный, ску́чный.

tiring-house ['taɪərɪŋhaus] *см.* tiring-room.

tiring-room ['taɪərɪŋrum] *n уст.* артисти́ческая убо́рная.

tiro ['taɪərou] *n* новичо́к.

'tis [tɪz] *разг.* = it is.

tissue ['tɪsjuː] *n* 1) ткань; conjunctive ~, connective ~ соедини́тельная ткань; 2) сплете́ние (*выдумок, лжи*); 3) *см.* tissue-paper.

tissue-paper ['tɪsjuːˌpeɪpə] *n* мя́гкая папиро́сная бума́га.

tit[1] [tɪt] *n* сини́ца.

tit[2] *n*: ~ for tat о́ко за о́ко, зуб за́ зуб.

tit[3] *n* сосо́к.

Titan ['taɪtən] *n* тита́н, коло́сс; исполи́н.

titanic [taɪ'tænɪk] *a* титани́ческий, колосса́льный.

titanium [taɪ'teɪnjəm] *n хим.* тита́н.

titbit ['tɪtbɪt] *n* 1) ла́комый кусо́чек; 2) интере́сная но́вость.

tithe I [taɪð] *n* 1) деся́тая часть; 2) незначи́тельная до́ля; not a ~ of то́лько ничто́жная до́ля (*чего-л.*); 3) церко́вная десяти́на.

tithe II *v* 1) упла́чивать церко́вную десяти́ну; 2) облага́ть церко́вной десяти́ной.

titillate ['tɪtɪleɪt] *v* щекота́ть, прия́тно возбужда́ть.

titivate ['tɪtɪveɪt] *v разг.* оправля́ть (*волосы, платье*), приводи́ть себя́ в поря́док, прихора́шиваться.

titlark ['tɪtlɑːk] *n* лугово́й жа́воронок.

title ['taɪtl] *n* 1) загла́вие, назва́ние; заголо́вок; 2) на́дпись, титр (*в кино*); 3) ти́тул; зва́ние; 4) пра́во на что-л.; докуме́нт, удостоверя́ющий тако́е пра́во.

titled ['taɪtld] *a* титуло́ванный.

title-page ['taɪtlpeɪdʒ] *n полигр.* ти́тульный лист.

title-role ['taɪtlroul] *n* загла́вная роль.

titmouse ['tɪtmaus] *n* (*pl* titmice ['tɪtmaɪs]) сини́ца.

titter I ['tɪtə] *n* хихи́канье.

titter II *v* хихи́кать.

tittle ['tɪtl] *n* 1) мале́йшая части́ца, чу́точка; not a ~ of ни ка́пли, ни на́ волос; to a ~ то́чь-в-то́чь; 2) то́чка, чёрточка (*над буквой*).

tittle-tattle I ['tɪtlˌtætl] *n* болтовня́, пустосло́вие; спле́тни.

tittle-tattle II *v* болта́ть, пустосло́вить; спле́тничать.

tittup I ['tɪtəp] *n* 1) шу́мное весе́лье; пля́ски; подпры́гивание; 2) семеня́щая похо́дка; 3) лёгкий гало́п.

tittup II *v* 1) подпры́гивать; весели́ться; 2) семени́ть нога́ми; 3) идти́ гало́пом (*о лошади*).

titubate ['tɪtjubeɪt] *v* запина́ться, заика́ться.

titular I ['tɪtjulə] *n* лицо́, нося́щее номина́льный ти́тул.

titular II *a* 1) нося́щий ти́тул; 2) номина́льный.

titulary ['tɪtjuləri] *см.* titular II.

tizzy ['tɪzɪ] *n разг.* шестипе́нсовик (*монета*).

to[a] I [tu (*сильная форма*), tu (*слабая форма перед гласным*), tə (*слабая форма перед согласным*)] *prep* 1) *в пространственном значении указывает на:* а) *направление движения к определённому предмету* в, на, к; I am going to school (to the university, to the post-office, to the factory *etc*) я иду́ в шко́лу (в университе́т, на по́чту, на фа́брику *и т. п.*); he is going to the concert (to the theatre, to the ball, to the country, to my friend's place *etc*) он е́дет на конце́рт (в теа́тр, на бал, в дере́вню, к моему́ прия́телю *и т. п.*); б) *цель, назначение движения* на; we are going to the rescue мы отправля́емся спаса́ть; в) *предел движения* на, до; we climbed to the very top of the hill мы взобрали́сь на са́мую верши́ну горы́; г) *прикрепление к какому-л. предмету* к; to a post к столбу́; to a gate к воро́там; to the mast к ма́чте; 2) *указывает на лицо, по отношению к которому что-л. совершается; по-русски передаётся дательным падежом:* I sent a letter to your neighbour я посла́л письмо́ ва́шему сосе́ду; 3) *указывает на предел, границу во времени, количестве, числе:* to this day до настоя́щего вре́мени; it's ten to twelve now сейча́с без десяти́ двена́дцать; 4) *указывает на состояние или результат, к которому приводит данное действие:* to fall to decay (*или* to ruin, to pieces) разва́ливаться, распада́ться на куски́; to crumble to dust рассыпа́ться в прах; to run to seed идти́ в се́мя *и т. п.*; 5) *указывает на числовое отношение или пропорцию:* the score was 1 to 3 *спорт.* со счётом 1:3.

to[a] II *part* 1) *частица, служащая показателем инфинитива, напр.:* to take брать; to go идти́; 2) *перед инфинитивом выражает цель, назначение, следствие и т. п. для того, чтобы; с тем, чтобы;* to know English well one must read much чтобы хорошо́ знать англи́йский язы́к, ну́жно мно́го чита́ть; 3) *употр. как заместитель предикативного инфинитива; по-русски не переводится:* "Will you join us?" she asked. I said I'd be delighted to «Вы присоедини́тесь к нам?» — спроси́ла она́. Я сказа́л, что бу́ду о́чень рад.

to[b] [tuː] *adv* 1) *выражает:* а) *приведение в закрытое состояние:* pull the shutters to закро́йте ста́вни; б) *приведение в сознание:* after he came to по́сле того́, как он пришёл в себя́; 2): to and fro туда́ и сюда́; взад и вперёд.

toad [toud] *n* жа́ба; *перен.* га́дина.

toad-eater ['toudˌiːtə] *n* льстец, низкопокло́нник.

toad-eating I ['toudˌiːtɪŋ] *n* низкопокло́нство.

toad-eating II *a* уго́дливый, льсти́вый.

toadstool ['toudstuːl] *n* пога́нка.

toady I ['toudɪ] *n* льстец, низкопокло́нник.

toady II *v* льстить, низкопокло́нничать.

toast[1] I [toust] *n* ло́мтики хле́ба, подрумя́ненные на огне́, то́сты.

toast[1] II *v* 1) подрумя́нивать хлеб; 2) суши́ться, гре́ться (*у огня*).

toast[2] I *n* 1) тост, предложе́ние то́ста; to give (*или* to propose) a ~ предлага́ть тост; 2) лицо́, собы́тие, в честь кото́рого предлага́ется тост.

toast[2] II *v* предлага́ть тост за чьё-л. здоро́вье, пить за чьё-л. здоро́вье.

toaster ['toustə] *n* то́стер.

toast-master ['toustˌmɑːstə] *n* лицо́, провозглаша́ющее то́сты (*на официальном приёме*); тамада́.

tobacco [tə'bækou] *n* таба́к.

tobacco-box [tə'bækouˌbɔks] *n* табаке́рка.

tobacco-pipe [təˈbækoupaıp] *n* трубка.

tobacco-pouch [təˈbækoupautʃ] *n* кисёт.

to-be [təˈbiː] *a* будущий.

toboggan I [təˈbɔgən] *n* тобогган, сани.

toboggan II *v* кататься на санях (*с горы*).

toby[1] [ˈtoubı] *n* пивная кружка (*изображающая толстяка в треуголке*).

toby[2] I *n сленг* грабёж на большой дороге.

toby[2] II *v сленг* грабить на большой дороге.

toco [ˈtoukou] *n сленг* наказание, порка.

tocsin [ˈtɔksın] *n* 1) набат; 2) набатный колокол.

tod [tɔd] *n диал.* лисица.

today, to-day I [təˈdeı] *n* сегодняшний день; сегодня; of ~ современный.

today, to-day II *adv* 1) сегодня; 2) в наше время, теперь.

toddle I [ˈtɔdl] *n* 1) ковыляние; 2) *разг.* прогулка.

toddle II *v* 1) ковылять; 2) *разг.* прогуливаться, бродить.

toddler [ˈtɔdlə] *n* ребёнок, начинающий ходить.

toddy [ˈtɔdı] *n* 1) пунш; 2) пальмовый сок.

to-do [təˈduː] *n* суета, суматоха; to make a ~ суетиться.

toe I [tou] *n* 1) палец на ноге; great ~ большой палец; little ~ мизинец; to toast one's ~s греть ноги; носок обуви, чулка; to turn one's ~s out (in) выворачивать ноги носками наружу (внутрь); 3) передняя часть копыта; загиб подковы; 4) *тех.* пята; ◊ to tread on smb.'s ~s наступить на любимую мозоль, больно задеть; to step on smb.'s ~ наступать на ноги кому-л.; обижать кого-л.; to turn up one's ~s (to the daisies) *сленг* протянуть ноги, умереть.

toe II *v* 1) дотронуться носком; 2) надвязывать носок (*чулка*); □ to ~ out ставить носки врозь.

toe-cap [ˈtoukæp] *n* носок башмака, сапога.

toff [tɔf] *n разг.* фат, франт.

toffee, toffy [ˈtɔfı] *n* конфета (*из сахара и масла*).

tog I [tɔg] *n обыкн. pl разг.* одежда.

tog II *v разг.* одевать; to ~ oneself up (*или* out) наряжаться.

toga [ˈtougə] *n* 1) тога; 2) официальная одежда.

together [təˈgeðə] *adv* 1) вместе; сообща; 2) друг с другом; 3) одновременно; 4) непрерывно; подряд; for hours ~ часами, несколько часов подряд; for weeks ~ несколько недель подряд, неделями; ◊ ~ with вместе с (тем), наряду с.

toil I [tɔıl] *n* тяжёлый труд.

toil II *v* 1) трудиться; делать тяжёлую, утомительную работу; 2) с трудом идти, тащиться.

toiler [ˈtɔılə] *n* труженик; рабочий.

toilet [ˈtɔılıt] *n* 1) туалёт, одевание; 2) костюм; принадлежности туалета; 3) туалетный столик (*с зеркалом*); 4) *амер.* уборная, ванная.

toilful [ˈtɔılful] *см.* toilsome.

toilless [ˈtɔıllıs] *a* нетрудный, неутомительный.

toils [tɔılz] *n pl* сети; западня, ловушка; in the ~ беспомощный (*в трудном положении, в беде*).

toilsome [ˈtɔılsəm] *a* трудный, утомительный.

token [ˈtoukən] *n* 1) знак; символ; in ~ of в знак (*чего-л.*); as a ~ of в знак; на память; 2) признак, примета; 3) подарок на память; 4) жетон, талон.

told [tould] *past, p. p. см.* tell.

tolerable [ˈtɔlərəbl] *a* 1) терпимый; сносный; допустимый; 2) вполне удовлетворительный, довольно хороший.

tolerance [ˈtɔlərəns] *n* 1) терпимость; 2) *тех.* допуск.

tolerant [ˈtɔlərənt] *a* 1) терпимый (*о человеке*); 2) хорошо переносящий какое-л. лекарство *или* яд.

tolerate [ˈtɔləreıt] *v* 1) терпеть, выносить; 2) позволять, допускать.

toleration [ˌtɔləˈreıʃən] *n* терпимость.

toll[1] I [toul] *n* 1) колокольный звон, благовест; 2) похоронный звон.

toll[1] II *v* 1) мерно ударять в колокол, благовестить; 2) звонить (по покойнику).

toll[2] I *n* 1) пошлина, сбор; *перен.* дань; 2) удержание части зерна за помол; to take ~ of удерживать часть чего-л.

toll[2] II *v* взимать сбор, пошлину.

tollable [ˈtouləbl] *a* облагаемый пошлиной, сбором; подлежащий пошлине, сбору.

tollage [ˈtoulıdʒ] *n* взимание *или* уплата пошлины, сбора.

toll-bar [ˈtoulbɑː] *n* застава, шлагбаум (*где взимается сбор*).

toll-gate [ˈtoulgeıt] *см.* toll-bar.

tollhouse [ˈtoulhaus] *n* контора у заставы, где взимается дорожный сбор.

tol-lol [ˌtɔlˈlɔl] *a разг.* сносный, приличный.

toluene [ˈtɔljuiːn] *n хим.* толуол.

Tom [tɔm] *n* 1): ~ Thumb мальчик с пальчик; Blind ~ игра в жмурки; ~, Dick and Harry всякий, каждый; 2) кот; 3) название большого колокола *или* орудия.

tomahawk I [ˈtɔməhɔːk] *n* томагавк; ◊ to bury the ~ заключить мир.

tomahawk II *v* 1) ударять, убивать томагавком; 2) сильно критиковать.

tomato [təˈmɑːtou] *n* помидор, томат.

tomb [tuːm] *n* 1) могила; 2) надгробный памятник, надгробие.

tomboy [ˈtɔmbɔı] *n* девочка с мальчишескими ухватками, сорванец.

tombstone [ˈtuːmstoun] *n* надгробный камень, надгробие.

tom-cat [ˈtɔmkæt] *n* кот.

tome [toum] *n* том, книга (*большая*).

tomfool I [ˈtɔmˈfuːl] *n* 1) дурак, дурень; 2) шут, фигляр; 3) *attr* дурацкий, бессмысленный.

tomfool II *v* дурачиться, валять дурака.

tomfoolery [tɔmˈfuːlərı] *n* шутовство, фиглярство.

Tommy [ˈtɔmı] *n* Томми (*прозвище английского солдата*).

tommy [ˈtɔmı] *n* 1) булочка, хлеб; soft ~ мягкий хлеб (*в противоположность сухарям, галетам и т. п.*); 2) пища; 3) частичная оплата товарами вместо денег.

tommy-gun [ˈtɔmıgʌn] *n* пистолёт-пулемёт.

tommy-shop [ˈtɔmıʃɔp] *n* лавка, где рабочим выдаются товары вместо зарплаты.

tomnoddy ['tɔm,nɔdɪ] *n* ду́рень, простофи́ля.

tomorrow, to-morrow I [tə'mɔrou] *n* за́втрашний день.

tomorrow, to-morrow II *adv* за́втра; наза́втра.

tomtit ['tɔm'tɪt] *n* сини́ца.

tomtom ['tɔmtɔm] *n* тамта́м (*барабан*).

ton [tʌn] *n* 1) то́нна; metric ~ метри́ческая то́нна (*1000 кг*); displacement ~ то́нна водоизмеще́ния; 2) *разг.* тя́жесть; ма́сса; ~s of people ма́сса наро́ду.

tonality [tou'nælɪtɪ] *n* тона́льность.

tone I [toun] *n* 1) тон; deep ~, low ~ ни́зкий тон; high ~, thin ~ высо́кий тон; angry ~ серди́тый тон; heart ~s *мед.* то́ны се́рдца; 2) тон, стиль, хара́ктер; 3) *мед.* то́нус; 4) *жив.* града́ция тоно́в; преоблада́ющий тон; 5) интона́ция, модуля́ция (*голоса*).

tone II *v* 1) гармони́ровать; 2) придава́ть (определённый) тон (*звуку или краске*); (ви́до)изменя́ть тон (*окраски*); 3) настра́ивать; □ to ~ **down** а) смягча́ть (*тон, краски*); б) смягча́ться, ослабева́ть; to ~ **up** уси́ливать(ся); повыша́ть тон чего-л.

toneless ['tounlɪs] *a* невырази́тельный; равноду́шный.

tonga ['tɔŋɡə] *n* лёгкая двуко́лка (*в Индии*).

tongs [tɔŋz] *n pl* щипцы́; кле́щи.

tongue [tʌŋ] *n* 1) язы́к; dirty (*или* foul, furred) ~ обло́женный язы́к; to put out one's ~ пока́зывать язы́к; his ~ failed him у него́ отня́лся язы́к; ~ is too long for his teeth у него́ сли́шком дли́нный язы́к; to wag one's ~ болта́ть (языко́м); to have a loose ~ быть болтли́вым; 2) речь, язы́к; the mother ~ родно́й язы́к; glib ~ бо́йкая речь; 3) язы́к (*как блюдо*); smoked ~ копчёный язы́к; 4) что-л., име́ющее фо́рму языка́, напомина́ющее язы́к; язычо́к (*духового инструмента, обуви*); ~s of flame языки́ пла́мени; the ~ of land *геогр.* коса́; 5) ды́шло; 6) стре́лка (*весов*); 7) *эл.* я́корь; ◇ he has a ready ~ ≅ он за сло́вом в карма́н не поле́зет; to hold one's ~ молча́ть, пома́лкивать; держа́ть язы́к за зуба́ми; to have too much ~ ≅ что на уме́, то и на языке́.

tongueless ['tʌŋlɪs] *a* не име́ющий языка́, без языка́; неспосо́бный говори́ть.

tongue-tied ['tʌŋtaɪd] *a* косноязы́чный.

tongue-twister [,tʌŋ'twɪstə] *n* скороговорка.

tonic I ['tɔnɪk] *n* 1) *мед.* укрепля́ющее сре́дство; 2) *муз.* основно́й тон, тона́льность.

tonic II *a* 1) *мед.* тонизи́рующий, укрепля́ющий; 2) *муз.* тони́ческий.

tonight, to-night I [tə'naɪt] *n* сего́дняшний ве́чер; наступа́ющая ночь.

tonight, to-night II *adv* сего́дня ве́чером; сего́дня но́чью.

tonjon ['tɔndʒɔn] *n* паланки́н (*в Индии*).

tonnage ['tʌnɪdʒ] *n* 1) тонна́ж; водоизмеще́ние; 2) грузова́я по́шлина.

tonometer [tou'nɔmɪtə] *n* 1) *муз.* камерто́н; 2) *мед.* прибо́р для измере́ния кровяно́го давле́ния, тоно́метр.

tonsil ['tɔnsl] *n* миндалеви́дная железа́.

tonsillitis [,tɔnsɪ'laɪtɪs] *n* *мед.* воспале́ние минда́лин, тонзилли́т.

tonsure I ['tɔnʃə] *n* тонзу́ра.

tonsure II *v* выбрива́ть тонзу́ру.

tony ['tounɪ] *a* *амер.* изы́сканный; аристократи́ческий.

too [tuː] *adv* 1) сли́шком; ~ good to be true *разг.* сли́шком хорошо́, что́бы пове́рить; it is ~ much of a good thing ≅ хороше́нького понемно́жку; none ~ pleasant не сли́шком прия́тный; 2) *разг.* о́чень; I am only ~ glad я о́чень рад; 3) та́кже, то́же, ра́вным о́бразом; к тому́ же; take the others ~ возьми́те и остальны́е.

took [tuk] *past* см. take I.

tool I [tuːl] *n* 1) (рабо́чий) инструме́нт; *перен.* ору́дие, сре́дство; edged ~ см. edge-tool; 2) *тех.* резе́ц; 3) стано́к; ◇ to play with edged ~s ≅ игра́ть с огнём.

tool II *v* 1) обраба́тывать мета́лл резцо́м; обтёсывать, отде́лывать; 2) вытисня́ть узо́р (*на переплёте*); 3) *разг.* е́хать *или* везти́ в экипа́же.

tooling ['tuːlɪŋ] *n* (золото́е) тисне́ние (*на переплёте*).

toot I [tuːt] *n* 1) звук рожка́, гудо́к; 2) *амер.* кутёж, весе́лье.

toot II *v* труби́ть в рог, рожо́к; дава́ть гудо́к.

tooth I [tuːθ] *n* (*pl* teeth) 1) зуб; calf's (second) teeth моло́чные (постоя́нные) зу́бы; false (natural) teeth вставны́е («сво́и») зу́бы; a loose ~ шата́ющийся зуб; to fill (*или* to stop) a ~ пломби́ровать зуб; to have a ~ out, to pull a ~ вы́дернуть, удали́ть зуб; to crown a ~ поста́вить коро́нку на зуб; to grit the teeth скрежета́ть зуба́ми; to cut a ~ проре́зываться (*о зубе*); 2) зуб, зубе́ц; ◇ to cast (*или* to throw) smth. in smb.'s teeth броса́ть упрёк в лицо́; ~ and nail изо всех сил; реши́тельно, упо́рно (*сопротивля́ться и т. п.*); to show one's teeth огрызну́ться; to set (*или* to clench) one's teeth сти́снуть зу́бы; to set one's (*или* the) teeth on edge де́йствовать на не́рвы, раздража́ть; in the teeth of напереко́р; sweet ~ сласте́на; to have a sweet ~ люби́ть сла́дкое.

tooth II *v* 1) снабжа́ть зубца́ми; нареза́ть зубцы́; 2) сцепля́ться (*зубца́ми*).

toothache ['tuːθeɪk] *n* зубна́я боль.

tooth-brush ['tuːθbrʌʃ] *n* зубна́я щётка.

tooth-comb ['tuːθkoum] *n* ча́стый гре́бень.

toothed [tuːθt] *a* зубча́тый.

toothful ['tuːθful] *n* глото́к (*обыкн. спиртного*).

toothless ['tuːθlɪs] *a* беззу́бый.

tooth-paste ['tuːθpeɪst] *n* зубна́я па́ста.

toothpick ['tuːθpɪk] *n* 1) зубочи́стка; 2) *сленг* дуби́нка.

tooth-powder ['tuːθ,paudə] *n* зубно́й порошо́к.

toothsome ['tuːθsəm] *a* прия́тный на вкус.

tootle I ['tuːtl] *n* звук трубы́, фле́йты.

tootle II *v* труби́ть; игра́ть на фле́йте.

top I [tɔp] *n* 1) верху́шка, верши́на; маку́шка; the ~ of the head те́мя; from ~ to toe с головы́ до ног; 2) ве́рхняя часть, верх (*экипа́жа, страни́цы*); кры́шка (*кастрю́ли*); to go up ~ подня́ться на второ́й эта́ж авто́буса; to go over the ~ *воен.* идти́ в ата́ку (*из транше́й*); 4) вы́сшая сте́пень; at the ~ of one's voice во весь го́лос; 5) шпиц, шпиль; 6) *горн.* кро́вля (*пласта*); верх, у́стье (*ша́хты*); 7) вы́сшее, пе́рвое ме́сто; the ~ of the class пе́рвый учени́к в кла́ссе; to take the ~ of the table сиде́ть во главе́ стола́; 8) *обыкн. pl* ботва́ (*корнепло́дов*); 9) *pl* отворо-ты (*сапог*); высо́кие сапоги́; 10) *мор.* марс, топ.

top[1] II *a* 1) ве́рхний, вы́сший; 2) максима́льный (*о скорости и т. п.*).

top[1] III *v* 1) покрыва́ть (*сверху*); ~ped with snow покры́тый сне́гом; со сне́жной верши́ной (*о горе*); 2) среза́ть верху́шку (*дерева и т. п.*); *перен. разг.* обезгла́вить; пове́сить; 3) достига́ть верши́ны; подня́ться на верши́ну; 4) поднима́ться, возвыша́ться; 5) превосходи́ть; перекрыва́ть; 6) превыша́ть; достига́ть како́й-л. величины́, ро́ста, ве́са; □ to ~ off отде́лывать; to ~ up а) наполня́ть (*доверху*); долива́ть; б) заверша́ть, уве́нчивать.

top[2] *n* волчо́к (*игрушка*); ◊ old ~ *сленг* старина́ (*обращение*); to sleep like a ~ спать как уби́тый.

topaz ['toupæz] *n* топа́з.

top-boots ['top'buːts] *n pl* высо́кие сапоги́ с отворо́тами.

topcoat ['top'kout] *n* пальто́.

top-dress ['top'dres] *v с.-х.* обкла́дывать, покрыва́ть наво́зом.

tope [toup] *v* пья́нствовать.

topee ['toupiː] *см.* topi.

toper ['toupə] *n* пья́ница.

topfull ['topful] *a* по́лный до краёв, до́верху.

top-heavy ['top'hevɪ] *a* 1) переве́шивающий в ве́рхней ча́сти; неусто́йчивый; 2) подвы́пивший.

top-hole ['top'houl] *a разг.* первокла́ссный, превосхо́дный.

topi ['toupɪ] *n* тропи́ческий шлем (*от солнца*).

topic ['topɪk] *n* те́ма, предме́т (*обсуждения и т. п.*).

topical ['topɪkəl] *a* 1) злободне́вный, актуа́льный; 2) ме́стный, ме́стного значе́ния.

topknot ['topnot] *n* 1) чуб, хохоло́к (*на голове*); 2) пучо́к пе́рьев, лент (*на макушке*); 3) *разг.* голова́.

topless ['toplɪs] *a* о́чень высо́кий.

top-liner ['top'laɪnə] *n амер.* популя́рный актёр, «звезда́».

toplofty ['top'loftɪ] *a разг.* напы́щенный.

topmast ['topmɑːst] *n мор.* сте́ньга.

topmost ['topmoust] *a* 1) са́мый ве́рхний; 2) са́мый ва́жный.

topography [tə'pogrəfɪ] *n* топогра́фия.

topper ['topə] *n разг.* 1) превосхо́дный челове́к; 2) превосхо́дная вещь; 3) цили́ндр (*шляпа*).

topping I ['topɪŋ] *n* 1) ве́рхняя часть, верху́шка; 2) удале́ние верху́шки (*дерева и т. п.*); 3) *pl* сре́занные ча́сти (*дерева и т. п.*).

topping II *a* 1) превосходя́щий (*других*), выдаю́щийся; возвыша́ющийся; 2) *амер.* высокоме́рный; 3) *разг.* отли́чный.

topple ['topl] *v* 1) вали́ть(ся), опроки́дывать(ся); 2) грози́ть паде́нием.

topsail ['topsl] *n мор.* ма́рсель.

topsyturvy I ['topsɪ'təːvɪ] *n* беспоря́док, неразбери́ха, кутерьма́.

topsyturvy II *a* 1) переве́рнутый вверх дном; 2) беспоря́дочный, хаоти́чный.

topsyturvy III *v* переве́ртывать всё вверх дном.

topsyturvy IV *adv* вверх дном, ши́ворот-навы́ворот.

tor [toː] *n* скали́стая верши́на.

torch [toːtʃ] *n* 1) фа́кел; *перен.* све́точ; electric ~ карма́нный электри́ческий фона́рь; 2) пая́льная ла́мпа; ◊ to hand on the ~ передава́ть (*молоды́м*) тради́ции и т. п.

torchlight ['toːtʃlaɪt] *n* свет фа́кела; свет электри́ческого фонаря́.

tore [toː] *past см.* tear[a] II.

toreador ['toːrɪədɔː] *n* тореадо́р.

torment[a] ['toːmənt] *n* 1) муче́ние, му́ка; 2) исто́чник, причи́на му́ки.

torment[b] [toː'ment] *v* 1) му́чить, причиня́ть страда́ния; 2) досажда́ть, раздража́ть.

tormentor [toː'mentə] *n* 1) мучи́тель; 2) колёсная борона́.

tormentress [toː'mentrɪs] *n* мучи́тельница.

torn [toːn] *p. p. см.* tear[a] II.

tornado [toː'neɪdou] *n* си́льный урага́н, смерч; *перен.* взрыв, бу́ря (*аплодисментов и т. п.*).

torpedo I [toː'piːdou] *n* 1) торпе́да; 2) *ж.-д.* сигна́льная петарда́; 3) электри́ческий скат (*рыба*); 4) *attr* торпе́дный.

torpedo II *v* подорва́ть торпе́дой; *перен.* уничто́жить, взорва́ть.

torpedo-boat [toː'piːdoubout] *n* миноно́сец; motor ~ торпе́дный ка́тер.

torpedo-net [toː'piːdounet] *n* противоми́нная сеть.

torpedo-plane [toː'piːdouplein] *n* самолёт-торпедоно́сец.

torpid ['toːpɪd] *a* 1) онеме́лый, оцепене́лый; 2) находя́щийся в спя́чке (*о животном*); 3) вя́лый, апати́чный.

torpor ['toːpə] *n* 1) оцепене́ние, онеме́лость; 2) вя́лость, апа́тия.

torque [toːk] *n* 1) *археол.* кручёное ожере́лье; 2) *тех.* скру́чивающее уси́лие.

torrefy ['torɪfaɪ] *v* 1) обжига́ть; 2) суши́ть.

torrent ['torənt] *n* пото́к (*тж. перен.*).

torrid ['torɪd] *a* жа́ркий, зно́йный; вы́жженный со́лнцем.

torsion ['toːʃən] *n* круче́ние; скру́чивание.

torso ['toːsou] *n* ту́ловище; торс (*статуи*).

tortoise ['toːtəs] *n* черепа́ха.

tortoise-shell ['toːtəʃel] *n* 1) щит черепа́хи (*тж. как материал*); 2) *attr* черепа́ховый.

tortuous ['toːtjuəs] *a* 1) изви́листый; 2) укло́нчивый; нея́сный (*об ответе, доводе*); 3) кова́рный.

torture I ['toːtʃə] *n* пы́тка; to put to the ~ подверга́ть пы́тке.

torture II *v* 1) пыта́ть, подверга́ть пы́тке; 2) му́чить; раздража́ть; 3) искажа́ть.

torturer ['toːtʃərə] *n* мучи́тель; пала́ч.

Tory ['toːrɪ] *n* то́ри, консерва́тор; high ~ кра́йний консерва́тор.

tosh [toʃ] *n разг.* вздор, ерунда́, чепуха́.

toss I [tos] *n* 1) броса́ние, мета́ние, подбра́сывание; the ~ of the coin жеребьёвка; to win (to lose) the ~ (не) угада́ть, како́й стороно́й упа́ла моне́та; 2) вски́дывание (*головы*); 3) толчо́к, сотрясе́ние; 4) волне́ние, смяте́ние; 5) to take a ~ упа́сть (*особ. с лошади*).

toss II *v* 1) кида́ть, броса́ть, мета́ть; 2) подбра́сывать, швыря́ть (*судно*); носи́ться (*по волнам*); 3) поднима́ться и опуска́ться, вздыма́ться; 4) (беспоко́йно) мета́ться (*о больном*); 5) вски́дывать *(голову)*; 6) сбрасывать *(седока)*; □ to ~ **off** выпивать залпом; to ~ **up** a) подбрасывать; б) вскидывать *(голову)*; в) бросать монету.

toss-up ['tɔsʌp] *n* бросание монеты, жеребьёвка; it is a ~ это ещё вопрос.

tossy ['tɔsɪ] *a* дерзкий, бойкий.

tot¹ [tɔt] *n* 1) маленький ребёнок, крошка; 2) *разг.* маленькая рюмка *(вина и т. п.)*.

tot² I *n разг.* сумма *или* сложение нескольких чисел.

tot² II *v разг.* складывать, суммировать *(обыкн.* to ~ up).

total I ['toutl] *n* целое, сумма; итог; the grand ~ общий итог.

total II *a* 1) весь, целый, общий; полный; 2) суммарный; совокупный; 3) всеобщий; тотальный *(о войне)*.

total III *v* 1) подводить итог, суммировать, подсчитывать; 2) насчитывать(ся), составлять *(число)*; 3) доходить до, равняться *(о сумме)*.

totalitarian [,toutælɪ'tɛərɪən] *a* тоталитарный; тотальный *(о войне)*.

totality [tou'tælɪtɪ] *n* вся сумма, всё количество целиком.

totalizator ['toutəlaɪzeɪtə] *n* тотализатор.

totalizer ['toutəlaɪzə] *см.* totalizator.

tote¹ [tout] *сокр. разг. см.* totalizator.

tote² *v амер.* 1) везти, нести, тащить; 2) подвозить; 3) тянуть.

totem ['toutəm] *n* тотем.

totter ['tɔtə] *v* 1) шататься, пошатываться; идти неверной походкой, ковылять; 2) быть неустойчивым, угрожать падением.

tottery ['tɔtərɪ] *a* шаткий, неустойчивый, грозящий падением.

touch I [tʌtʃ] *n* 1) прикосновение; 2) соприкосновение; общение; in ~ with в контакте с; to keep in ~ держать, поддерживать связь; to gain ~ прийти в соприкосновение; 3) осязание; to the ~ на ощупь; 4) штрих; to put the finishing ~ отделывать, заканчивать; personal ~ индивидуальные особенности, характерные черты *(человека)*; 5) оттенок, налёт *(грусти и т. п.)*; 6) манера, приёмы *(художника и т. п.)*; 7) *муз.* туше; 8) испытание; пробный камень; to put *(или* to bring) to the ~ подвергнуть испытанию; 9) лёгкий приступ *(болезни)*; 10) «салки» *(детская игра)*; 11) пространство за боковыми линиями *(футбольного поля)*.

touch II *v* 1) (при)касаться, притрагиваться; трогать; осязать; 2) соприкасаться; 3) касаться *(темы, вопроса)*, затрагивать *(тему и т. п.)*; 4) касаться, иметь отношение к кому-л., чему-л.; 5) трогать, волновать; задевать за живое *(тж.* to ~ to the quick); 6) доставать (до); 7) сравниться; 8) *pass* начать портиться; ~ed with frost тронутый морозом *(о растении)*; 9) поражать; □ *сленг* занимать, получать обманным путём; □ to ~ **at** заходить *(в порт)*; to ~ **down** приземлиться, коснуться земли; to ~ **off** a) сделать набросок; уловить сходство; б) выпалить *(из орудия)*; в) вызвать *(скандал и т. п.)*; г) дать отбой; to ~ **on** затрагивать, касаться вкратце; to ~ **up** поправить *(рисунок и т. п. несколькими штрихами)*; отделать.

touchable ['tʌtʃəbl] *a* осязаемый.

touch-and-go I ['tʌtʃən'gou] *n* ненадёжное, рискованное дело, положение.

touch-and-go II *a* ненадёжный; рискованный, опасный.

touch-down ['tʌtʃdaun] *n ав.* посадка; soft ~ мягкая посадка; to make a ~ совершать посадку.

touched [tʌtʃt] *a predic* 1) взволнованный, тронутый; 2) помешанный, «тронутый»; ◊ ~ in the wind страдающий одышкой.

touching I ['tʌtʃɪŋ] *a* трогательный.

touching II *prep* относительно, касательно *(тж.* as ~).

touch-me-not ['tʌtʃmɪ,nɔt] *n* недотрога.

touchstone ['tʌtʃstoun] *n* 1) пробирный камень; оселок; 2) критерий, стандарт.

touchwood ['tʌtʃwud] *n* трут.

touchy ['tʌtʃɪ] *a* обидчивый; слишком чувствительный.

tough I [tʌf] *a* 1) плотный; упругий; тугой; жёсткий *(о мясе и т. п.)*; 2) вязкий; 3) прочный, крепкий; 4) трудный *(для выполнения)*; 5) упрямый, несговорчивый; 6) упорный, стойкий, выносливый; 7) *амер.* хулиганский.

tough II *n амер.* хулиган; бандит.

toughen ['tʌfn] *v* делать(ся) плотным, тугим, жёстким, трудным.

toupee ['tuːpeɪ] *n* 1) хохолок; тупей; 2) небольшой парик.

tour I [tuə] *n* 1) путешествие, турне; экскурсия, поездка; 2) тур, объезд; обход *(караула и т. п.)*; 3) круг *(обязанностей и т. п.)*; цикл.

tour II [tuə] *v* 1) совершать путешествие, турне; 2) производить объезд, обход.

tourer ['tuərə] *n* туристский автомобиль; открытый легковой автомобиль.

touring I ['tuərɪŋ] *n* туризм.

touring II *a* туристский.

tourist ['tuərɪst] *n* турист, путешественник.

tournament ['tuənəmənt] *n* турнир.

tourney I ['tuənɪ] *n* (средневековый) турнир.

tourney II *v* сражаться на турнире.

tourniquet ['tuənɪkeɪ] *n мед.* турникет, жгут.

tousle ['tauzl] *v* ерошить; растрепать.

tousy ['tauzɪ] *a* взъерошенный, растрёпанный.

tout I [taut] *n* 1) человек, навязывающий свой товар *или* услуги; 2) человек, сообщающий сведения о скаковых лошадях.

tout II *v* 1) навязывать товар; 2) назойливо предлагать что-л.; 3): to ~ (round) for smth. настойчиво добиваться чего-л. *(особ. сведений о скаковых лошадях)*.

tow¹ I [tou] *n* 1) буксировка; 2) буксир; буксирный канат; in ~ на буксире; to have *(или* to take) in ~ брать на буксир; to have smb. in ~ а) иметь кого-л. на своём попечении; б) иметь кого-л. в числе сопровождающих *или* поклонников; 3) *attr* буксирный.

tow¹ II *v* буксировать; тянуть, тащить.

tow² *n* 1) очёски льна, кудель; 2) пакля.

towage ['touɪdʒ] *n* 1) буксировка; 2) оплата буксировки.

toward [tə'wɔːd] *см.* towards.

towards [tə'wɔːdz] *prep указывает на:* 1) *направление к предмету* в, к, в направлении; we travelled ~ the north мы двигались в северном направлении, к северу; your house looks ~ the lake ваш дом выходит фасадом на озеро; 2) *отношение к чему-л. или кому-л.* к, по отношению к; what is your attitude

~ my proposal? каково́ ва́ше отноше́ние к моему́ предложе́нию?; you should be respectful ~ your parents, polite ~ everybody вы должны́ быть почти́тельны к свои́м роди́телям, ве́жливы по отноше́нию ко всем; 3) *приближе́ние к определённой то́чке во вре́мени* к, о́коло; ~ morning (noon, evening) к утру́ (полу́дню, ве́черу); 4) *цель соверше́ния де́йствия* с це́лью, для; to give money ~ smb.'s expenses дать де́ньги на чьи-л. расхо́ды.

tow-boat ['toubout] *n* букси́рный парохо́д.

towel I ['tauəl] *n* полоте́нце; roller ~ полоте́нце на ро́лике; ◊ to throw in the ~ признава́ть себя́ побеждённым; an oaken ~ дуби́нка.

towel II *v* 1) вытира́ть полоте́нцем; 2) *сленг* бить, колоти́ть.

towel-horse ['tauəlhɔːs] *n* ве́шалка для полоте́нца.

tower I ['tauə] *n* ба́шня; вы́шка; ◊ a ~ of strength надёжный защи́тник.

tower II *v* высится, возвыша́ться (*над чем-л.* — over); □ to ~ **above** превосходи́ть (*ростом, умо́м*).

towering ['tauərɪŋ] *a* 1) высо́кий, вы́сящийся; возвыша́ющийся над (*чем-л.*); вздыма́ющийся; 2) неи́стовый, ужа́сный.

towing-line ['touɪŋlaɪn] *n* бечева́, букси́рный кана́т.

towing-rope ['touɪŋroup] *см.* towing-line.

town [taun] *n* 1) го́род; home ~ родно́й го́род; county ~ гла́вный го́род гра́фства (*в А́нглии*); corporate ~ го́род, име́ющий самоуправле́ние; out of ~ а) в дере́вне; б) в отъе́зде; 2) *attr* городско́й; ◊ ~ and gown студе́нты и профессора́ Оксфо́рдского *или* Ке́мбриджского университе́тов и жи́тели О́ксфорда *или* Ке́мбриджа; to paint the ~ red *сленг* дебоши́рить.

town-planning ['taun,plænɪŋ] *n* планиро́вка городо́в.

townsfolk ['taunzfouk] *n pl* горожа́не, городски́е жи́тели.

township ['taunʃɪp] *n* 1) райо́н го́рода; при́город; 2) городско́е управле́ние; 3) *ист.* церко́вный прихо́д; 4) *амер.* месте́чко.

townsman ['taunzmən] *n* 1) горожа́нин; 2) жи́тель того́ же го́рода.

townspeople ['taunz,piːpl] *см.* townsfolk.

tow-path ['toupɑːθ] *n* бечевни́к (*доро́га*).

tow-plane ['toupleɪn] *n* самолёт-буксиро́вщик.

tow-rope ['touroup] *n* 1) букси́рный кана́т; 2) *ав.* гайдро́п.

tow-row ['tourou] *n* шум, гам.

toxaemia [tɔk'siːmɪə] *n* зараже́ние кро́ви.

toxic I ['tɔksɪk] *n* яд.

toxic II *a* ядови́тый.

toxicology [,tɔksɪ'kɔlədʒɪ] *n* уче́ние о я́дах и отравле́ниях, токсиколо́гия.

toxin ['tɔksɪn] *n* токси́н, ядови́тое вещество́.

toy I [tɔɪ] *n* 1) игру́шка; заба́ва; to make a ~ of забавля́ться чем-л.; 2) безделу́шка; 3) что-л. ма́ленькое, незначи́тельное; a ~ of a dog соба́чо́нка; 4) *attr* игру́шечный; ненастоя́щий.

toy II *v* игра́ть, забавля́ться.

toyshop ['tɔɪʃɔp] *n* магази́н игру́шек.

trace¹ I [treɪs] *n* 1) след; 2) черта́; 3) *амер.* тропи́нка; 4) незначи́тельное коли́чество, следы́; 5) чертёж на ка́льке.

trace¹ II *v* 1) наме́тить, наброса́ть, начерти́ть (*план и т. п.*); 2) де́лать ко́пию, кальки́ровать; 3) следи́ть; вы́следить; проследи́ть; 4) усмотре́ть; различи́ть.

trace² *n* постро́мка; ◊ to kick over the ~s взбунтова́ться.

tracer¹ ['treɪsə] *n* 1) трасси́рующий снаря́д (*тж.* ~ shell); 2) ме́ченый а́том (*тж.* ~ element); 3) чертёжник-копиро́вщик; 4) иссле́дователь.

tracer² *n* пристяжна́я ло́шадь.

tracer-bullet ['treɪsə,bulɪt] *n* трасси́рующая пу́ля.

tracery ['treɪsərɪ] *n* узо́р, рису́нок; орна́мент.

trachea [trə'kiːə] *n анат.* трахе́я.

tracing ['treɪsɪŋ] *n* 1) чертёж на ка́льке; 2) копи́рование; 3) трассиро́вка; 4) за́пись самопи́шущего прибо́ра; 5) просле́живание; выслеживание.

tracing-paper ['treɪsɪŋ,peɪpə] *n* воско́вка, ка́лька.

track I [træk] *n* 1) след; to be in the ~ идти́ по стопа́м, сле́довать приме́ру; to be on the ~ а) пресле́довать; б) напа́сть на след; to keep ~ of сле́дить за разви́тием чего́-л.; to lose ~ of потеря́ть след; потеря́ть нить; to cover up one's ~s замета́ть следы́; 2) тропа́, просёлочная доро́га; путь; the beaten ~ прото́ренный, изби́тый путь; рути́на; 3) *ж.-д.* ре́льсовый путь, коле́я; single (double) ~ одноколе́йный (двухколе́йный) путь; off the ~ а) соше́дший с ре́льсов (*о по́езде*); б) уклони́вшийся от те́мы; в) сби́вшийся с пути́; to leave the ~ сойти́ с ре́льсов (*о по́езде*); 4) *спорт.* лыжня́; running ~ бегова́я доро́жка; 5) гу́сеничная ле́нта (*тра́ктора, та́нка*).

track II *v* 1) следи́ть; высле́живать; 2) прокла́дывать путь; намеча́ть курс; 3) оставля́ть следы́; насле́дить; 4) тяну́ть бечево́й; 5) кати́ться по коле́е (*о колёсах*).

trackage ['trækɪdʒ] *n* 1) ре́льсовые пути́; сеть желе́зных доро́г; 2) о́бщая протяжённость желе́зных доро́г.

tracker ['trækə] *n* 1) охо́тник-следопы́т; 2) бурла́к; 3) букси́р; 4) филёр, сы́щик.

trackless ['træklɪs] *a* 1) бездоро́жный; 2) непрото́ренный; 3) безре́льсовый.

trackwalker ['træk,wɔːkə] *n амер. ж.-д.* путево́й обхо́дчик.

trackway ['trækweɪ] *n* 1) тропи́нка; 2) коле́йная доро́га.

tract¹ [trækt] *n* тракта́т; брошю́ра.

tract² *n* 1) полоса́ (*земли́, воды́, ле́са*); простра́нство; 2) путь, тракт; the digestive ~ пищевари́тельный тракт; 3) *уст.* (непреры́вный) пери́од вре́мени.

tractable ['træktəbl] *a* 1) легко́ поддаю́щийся обрабо́тке; 2) послу́шный, сгово́рчивый, мя́гкий.

tractate ['trækteɪt] *n* тракта́т.

traction ['trækʃən] *n* тя́га.

tractor ['træktə] *n* 1) тра́ктор; caterpillar ~ гу́сеничный тра́ктор; 2) *ав.* самолёт с тя́нущим винто́м.

trade I [treɪd] *n* 1) заня́тие; ремесло́; by ~ по профе́ссии; what ~ are you?, what is your ~? чем вы занима́етесь?; 2) *разг.* (the ~) сосло́вие торго́вцев; купцы́, торго́вцы (*в како́й-л. о́трасли*); ли́ца одно́й профе́ссии; to be in the ~ быть торго́вцем, име́ть магази́н; 3) торго́вля; home (*или* domestic, inland) ~ вну́тренняя торго́вля; foreign (*или* oversea) ~ внешняя торговля; free ~ свободная торговля; a roaring ~ оживлённая, бойкая торговля; 4) розничная торговля; 5) *attr* торговый.

trade II *v* 1) торговать (*чем-л.— in*; *с кем-л.— with*); 2) использовать в своих интересах (*on, upon*); 3) обменивать(ся).

Trade Board ['treɪd͵bɔːd] *n* объединённый совет представителей предпринимателей и рабочих.

trade-mark ['treɪd'mɑːk] *n* фабричная марка.

trader ['treɪdə] *n* 1) торговец (*особ. оптовый*); 2) торговое судно.

tradesfolk ['treɪdzfouk] *см.* tradespeople.

tradesman ['treɪdzmən] *n* 1) торговец, лавочник; 2) ремесленник.

tradespeople ['treɪdz͵piːpl] *n pl* купцы, торговцы, лавочники; торговое сословие.

tradeswoman ['treɪdz͵wumən] *n* торговка, лавочница.

trade union ['treɪd͵juːnjən] *n* профсоюз; тред-юнион.

trade-unionism [͵treɪd'juːnjənɪzəm] *n* тред-юнионизм.

trade-unionist [͵treɪd'juːnjənɪst] *n* член тред-юниона, профсоюза.

trade-wind ['treɪdwɪnd] *n* пассатный ветер.

tradition [trə'dɪʃən] *n* 1) традиция; 2) предание.

traditional [trə'dɪʃənl] *a* традиционный; основанный на обычае.

traditionally [trə'dɪʃənlɪ] *adv* по традиции.

traditionary [trə'dɪʃnərɪ] *см.* traditional.

traduce [trə'djuːs] *v* клеветать; злословить.

traffic I ['træfɪk] *n* 1) движение (*уличное, железнодорожное и т. п.*); транспорт, перевозки; 2) торговля.

traffic II ['træfɪk] *v* торговать (*чем-л.— in*).

traffic-light ['træfɪklaɪt] *n* светофор.

tragedian [trə'dʒiːdjən] *n* 1) актёр-трагик, трагический актёр; 2) автор трагедии.

tragedienne [trə͵dʒiːdɪ'en] *n* трагическая актриса.

tragedy ['trædʒɪdɪ] *n* трагедия.

tragic(al) ['trædʒɪk(əl)] *a* 1) трагический; трагедийный; 2) ужасный; катастрофический.

tragicomedy ['trædʒɪ'kɔmɪdɪ] *n* трагикомедия.

tragicomic(al) ['trædʒɪ'kɔmɪk(əl)] *a* трагикомический.

trail I [treɪl] *n* 1) след (*человека, животного*; *тж. перен.*); to be on the ~, to follow the ~ выслеживать, идти по следу; 2) тропинка; тропа; to blaze the ~ намечать, прокладывать путь; 3) хобот лафета; 4) *бот.* стелющийся побег.

trail II *v* 1) выслеживать, идти по следу; 2) тащить(ся), тянуть(ся), волочить(ся); 3) буксировать; 4) свисать (*сзади*); 5) потоптать (*траву*).

trailer ['treɪlə] *n* 1) тот, кто тащит, тянет, идёт по следу; 2) прицеп; 3) стелющееся растение; 4) *кино* анонс, киноафиша.

train[1] I [treɪn] *n* 1) поезд; by ~ поездом, по железной дороге; fast (slow) ~ скорый (пассажирский) поезд; through ~ поезд прямого сообщения; boat ~ поезд, согласованный с расписанием пароходов; local ~ пригородный поезд; baggage (*или* goods, freight) ~ товарный поезд; mixed ~ товаро-пассажирский поезд; owl ~ *амер.* ночной поезд; armoured ~ бронепоезд; hospital ~ санитарный поезд; down ~ поезд, идущий из Лондона (*или из центра*); up ~ поезд,

идущий в Лондон (*или в центр*); parliamentary ~ дешёвый поезд 3-го класса; to take the ~ сесть в поезд; поехать на поезде; to lose one's ~ опоздать на поезд; to catch (*или* to nick) the ~ поспеть на поезд; 2) процессия; свадебный поезд; 3) караван; *воен.* обоз; 4) свита; 5) цепь, ряд, вереница; 6) шлейф (*платья*); хвост (*павлина, кометы*); хобот (*лафета*); 7) *тех.* зубчатая передача; система шестерён; ◇ in ~ в (полной) готовности.

train[1] II *v* 1) ехать поездом; 2) *разг.* водиться (*с кем-л.— with*).

train[2] *v* 1) учить, воспитывать; приучать к дисциплине; 2) тренировать(ся); подготавливать(ся); 3) дрессировать (*животных*); 4) направлять; *воен.* наводить.

train-bearer ['treɪn͵bɛərə] *n* паж.

trained [treɪnd] *a* 1) обученный, подготовленный; 2) тренированный; 3) дрессированный (*о животных*); выезженный (*о лошади*).

trainee [treɪ'niː] *n* проходящий подготовку, обучение, тренировку.

trainer ['treɪnə] *n* 1) тренер; инструктор; 2) дрессировщик.

train-ferry ['treɪn͵ferɪ] *n* железнодорожный паром (*для перевозки поезда*).

training ['treɪnɪŋ] *n* 1) подготовка, (практическое) обучение; тренировка; under ~ проходящий подготовку; 2) дрессировка; 3) *attr* учебный; тренировочный.

training-college ['treɪnɪŋ͵kɔlɪdʒ] *n* педагогический институт, учительский институт.

training-school ['treɪnɪŋskuːl] *см.* training-college.

training-ship ['treɪnɪŋʃɪp] *n* учебное судно.

trainman ['treɪnmən] *n амер.* кондуктор.

trainmaster ['treɪn͵mɑːstə] *n амер.* начальник поезда.

train-oil ['treɪnɔɪl] *n* ворвань.

train-service ['treɪn͵səːvɪs] *n ж.-д.* служба движения.

trait [treɪ, *амер.* treɪt] *n* 1) штрих, чёрточка; 2) черта (*лица, характера*).

traitor ['treɪtə] *n* предатель, изменник.

traitorous ['treɪtərəs] *a* предательский, вероломный.

traitress ['treɪtrɪs] *n* предательница.

trajectory ['trædʒɪktərɪ] *n* траектория.

tram I [træm] *n* 1) трамвай; to take a ~ сесть в трамвай; ехать на трамвае; to get off the ~ сойти с трамвая; 2) *горн.* вагонетка.

tram II *v* 1) ехать в трамвае; 2) *горн.* откатывать на вагонетках.

tram-car ['træmkɑː] *n* трамвай.

tram-line ['træmlaɪn] *n* трамвайная линия.

trammel I ['træməl] *n* 1) невод; трал; 2) сетка для ловли птиц; 3) *pl* путы; препятствие.

trammel II *v* 1) ловить неводом, сетью; 2) сдерживать, стеснять, мешать; служить препятствием.

tramp I [træmp] *n* 1) бродяга; странник; 2) путешествие пешком; 3) (the ~) звук тяжёлых шагов; 4) *мор.* грузовое судно, не совершающее регулярных рейсов.

tramp II *v* 1) бродяжничать; странствовать; 2) идти пешком; бродить; 3) тяжело ступать, топать.

trample I ['træmpl] *n* 1) топта́ние; 2) то́панье; 3) попира́ние.

trample II *v* 1) топта́ть (*траву*); раста́птывать; дави́ть (*виноград*); 2) тяжело́ ступа́ть; то́пать; 3) подавля́ть, попира́ть (*on*).

tramway ['træmwei] *см.* tram-line.

trance [trɑːns] *n* 1) транс; 2) экста́з.

tranquil ['træŋkwil] *a* споко́йный.

tranquillity [træŋ'kwiliti] *n* споко́йствие.

trans- [trænz-] *pref* за-, через-, транс-; по ту сто́рону.

transact [træn'zækt] *v* (про)вести́ (де́ло); выполня́ть, соверша́ть.

transaction [træn'zækʃən] *n* 1) (про)веде́ние (де́ла); выполне́ние; 2) де́ло; сде́лка; 3) *pl* труды́, протоко́лы (*научного общества*).

transatlantic ['trænzət'læntik] *a* трансатланти́ческий.

transceiver [træn'siːvə] *n радио* приёмопередатчик.

transcend [træn'send] *v* 1) переступа́ть преде́лы, грани́цы; 2) превосходи́ть, превыша́ть.

transcendental [ˌtrænsen'dentl] *a* 1) *филос.* трансцендента́льный; 2) нея́сный.

transcontinental ['trænzˌkɔnti'nentl] *a* трансконтинента́льный.

transcribe [træns'kraib] *v* 1) перепи́сывать; 2) транскриби́ровать; 3) *муз.* перелага́ть (*для другого голоса, инструмента*), транспони́ровать; 4) *радио* запи́сывать на плёнку (*для передачи*); передава́ть по ра́дио грамза́пись.

transcript ['trænskript] *n* ко́пия.

transcription [træns'kripʃən] *n* 1) перепи́сывание; 2) транскри́пция; транскриби́рование; 3) ко́пия; 4) *радио* грамза́пись.

transfer[a] ['trænsfəː] *n* 1) перено́с; 2) переда́ча; ~ of authority переда́ча прав *или* полномо́чий; 3) перево́д; to carry out a ~ офо́рмить перево́д; ~ to the reserve *воен.* перево́д в запа́с; 4) переводна́я карти́нка; 5) перево́д рису́нка *и т. п.* на другу́ю пове́рхность; 6) *ж.-д.* переса́дка.

transfer[b] [træns'fəː] *v* 1) переноси́ть, переме́щать; 2) передава́ть; 3) переводи́ть; 4) переса́живаться (*на другой трамвай и т. п.*); де́лать переса́дку (*на железной дороге*); 5) переводи́ть рису́нок *и т. п.* на другу́ю пове́рхность.

transferable [træns'fəːrəbl] *a* допуска́ющий переда́чу.

transferee [ˌtrænsfəˈriː] *n* лицо́, кото́рому передаётся что-л. *или* пра́во на что-л.

transference ['trænsfərəns] *n* 1) перено́с, перенесе́ние; 2) переда́ча; 3) перево́д.

transfiguration [ˌtrænsfigjuə'reiʃən] *n* видоизмене́ние; преобразова́ние; преображе́ние.

transfigure [træns'figə] *v* видоизменя́ть; преобразо́вывать, преобража́ть.

transfix [træns'fiks] *v* пронза́ть; прока́лывать; *перен.* прикова́ть к ме́сту; парализова́ть.

transform [træns'fɔːm] *v* 1) преобразо́вывать; трансформи́ровать; to ~ beyond recognition сде́лать неузнава́емым; 2) превраща́ть.

transformation [ˌtrænsfə'meiʃən] *n* 1) преобразова́ние; трансформа́ция; превраще́ние; 3) пари́к (*женский*).

transformer [træns'fɔːmə] *n* 1) преобразова́тель; 2) *эл.* трансформа́тор.

transfuge [træns'fjuːdʒ] *n* перебе́жчик.

transfuse [træns'fjuːz] *v* 1) перелива́ть; *перен.* передава́ть (*свой энтузиазм и т. п.*); 2) *мед.* де́лать перелива́ние (*крови*); 3) пропи́тывать; прони́зывать.

transfusion [træns'fjuːʒən] *n* перелива́ние; ~ of blood перелива́ние кро́ви.

transgress [træns'gres] *v* 1) переступа́ть (*границы и т. п.*); наруша́ть (*закон и т. п.*); 2) греши́ть.

transgression [træns'greʃən] *n* 1) наруше́ние (*закона и т. п.*); просту́пок; оши́бка; 2) грех; вина́; 3) *геол.* трансгре́ссия.

transgressor [træns'gresə] *n* 1) правонаруши́тель; 2) гре́шник.

tranship [træn'ʃip] *см.* trans-ship.

transience ['trænziəns] *n* скоротечность; мимолётность.

transient ['trænziənt] *a* 1) преходя́щий; мимолётный; скоротечный; кратковре́менный; 2) *амер.* проезжа́ющий, прое́зжий; 3) случа́йный, вре́менный (*о рабочем*); 4) *хим.* нестойкий (*об отравляющем веществе и т. п.*).

transit ['trænsit] *n* 1) прохожде́ние; прое́зд; in ~ в пути́; 2) транзи́т; перево́зка; 3) *астр.* прохожде́ние (*через меридиан*); 4) теодоли́т; 5) *attr* транзи́тный.

transit-duty ['trænsitˌdjuːti] *n* транзи́тная по́шлина.

transition [træn'siʒən] *n* 1) перехо́д; перемеще́ние; ~ from quantity to quality *филос.* перехо́д коли́чества в ка́чество; 2) переме́на; измене́ние; 3) *attr* перехо́дный.

transitional [træn'siʒənl] *a* перехо́дный; промежу́точный.

transitive ['trænsitiv] *a грам.* перехо́дный.

transitory ['trænsitəri] *a* преходя́щий; мимолётный.

translatable [træns'leitəbl] *a* (легко) переводи́мый.

translate [træns'leit] *v* 1) переводи́ть (*на другой язык*; *from — into*); 2) объясня́ть, толкова́ть; 3) *радио* трансли́ровать; передава́ть; 4) *сленг* переде́лывать, переши́вать из ста́рого.

translation [træns'leiʃən] *n* 1) перево́д; close ~, near ~ то́чный перево́д; loose ~ во́льный перево́д; authorized ~ авторизо́ванный перево́д; 2) объясне́ние, толкова́ние; 3) *радио* трансля́ция; 4) перемеще́ние, перенесе́ние; 5) *сленг* переде́лка из ста́рого.

translator [træns'leitə] *n* перево́дчик.

transliteration [ˌtrænzlitə'reiʃən] *n* транслитера́ция.

translucent [trænz'luːsnt] *a* просве́чивающий; полупрозра́чный.

transmigrate ['trænzmaigreit] *v* переселя́ть(ся).

transmigration [ˌtrænzmai'greiʃən] *n* переселе́ние.

transmission [trænz'miʃən] *n* 1) переда́ча; трансми́ссия; radio ~ радиопереда́ча; 2) пересы́лка; 3) *attr* переда́точный; трансмиссио́нный.

transmit [trænz'mit] *v* передава́ть; пересыла́ть.

transmittal [trænz'mitl] *n* переда́ча, пересы́лка.

transmitter [trænz'mitə] *n* 1) переда́точный механи́зм; (радио)переда́тчик; 2) микрофо́н; 3) отправи́тель.

transmogrify [trænz'mɔgrɪfaɪ] v шутл. превращать (таинственным образом).

transmutation [ˌtrænzmjuː'teɪʃən] n превращение; the ~s of fortune превратности судьбы.

transmute [trænz'mjuːt] v превращать.

transoceanic ['trænzˌouʃɪ'ænɪk] a 1) заокеанский; 2) пересекающий океан, трансокеанский.

transom ['trænsəm] n поперечина, перекладина; переплёт окна.

transparency [træns'pɛərənsɪ] n прозрачность.

transparent [træns'pɛərənt] a 1) прозрачный; 2) ясный (о стиле и т. п.); 3) разг. откровенный, прямой.

transpiration [ˌtrænspɪ'reɪʃən] n испарина.

transpire [træns'paɪə] v 1) испаряться; проступать в виде капель пота; 2) просачиваться (о газе и т. п.); 3) обнаруживаться; становиться известным; оказываться; 4) разг. случаться.

transplant [træns'plɑːnt] v 1) пересаживать (растения); 2) переселять; 3) мед. делать пересадку кожи, ткани.

transportᵃ ['trænspɔːt] n 1) транспорт; перевозка; 2) транспортные средства; 3) часто pl увлечение, восторг, восхищение; 4) attr транспортный.

transportᵇ [træns'pɔːt] v 1) перевозить; транспортировать; 2) ссылать (на каторгу); высылать; 3) pass приводить в состояние восторга, восхищения; увлекать; ~ed with joy не помня себя от радости; ~ed with anger вне себя от гнева.

transportable [træns'pɔːtəbl] a транспортабельный.

transportation [ˌtrænspɔː'teɪʃən] n 1) перевозка, транспортировка; 2) перевозочные средства; automobile ~ автотранспорт; 3) высылка; 4) attr перевозочный, транспортный.

transpose [træns'pouz] v 1) перемещать; переставлять; менять порядок; 2) муз. транспонировать.

transposition [ˌtrænspə'zɪʃən] n 1) перемещение; перестановка; изменение порядка (слов и т. п.); 2) муз. транспонировка.

trans-ship [træns'ʃɪp] v перегружать (на другое судно и т. п.).

trans-shipment [træns'ʃɪpmənt] n перегрузка (на другое судно и т. п.).

transuranic [ˌtrænsjuə'reɪnɪk] a хим. трансурановый.

transversal I [trænz'vəːsəl] n пересекающая линия.

transversal II a поперечный.

transverse I ['trænzvəːs] a поперечный.

transverse II adv поперёк.

trap¹ I [træp] n 1) ловушка, западня; капкан; силок; мышеловка; to set (или to lay) a ~ ставить ловушку, капкан; to fall into a ~ попасть в ловушку; перен. тж. попасться на удочку; 2) откидная дверца; опускная дверца люка; 3) лестница-стремянка; 4) дренажная труба; 5) коляска; повозка; 6) сленг полицейский.

trap¹ II v 1) поймать в ловушку; ловить, задерживать; 2) ставить капканы; 3) заманивать.

trap² I n 1) pl личные вещи, пожитки; 2) попона.

trap² II v наряжать; украшать.

trapdoor ['træp'dɔː] n люк.

trapeze [trə'piːz] n спорт. трапеция.

trapezium [trə'piːzjəm] n мат. трапеция.

traphole ['træphoul] n волчья яма.

trapper ['træpə] n охотник, ставящий капканы (на пушного зверя).

trappings ['træpɪŋz] n pl 1) конское снаряжение; 2) амуниция; 3) парадный мундир; 4) украшения.

trappy ['træpɪ] a разг. предательский; опасный.

trapse [treɪps] v шататься без дела, шляться.

trash [træʃ] n 1) отбросы; мусор; хлам; макулатура; 2) дрянь; ◊ white ~ амер. презр. бедняки из белого населения Южных штатов.

trashy ['træʃɪ] a дрянной.

trauma ['trɔːmə] n мед. травма; рана.

traumatic [trɔː'mætɪk] a мед. травматический.

travail I ['træveɪl] n 1) родовые муки; 2) тяжёлый труд.

travail II v 1) мучиться в родах; 2) (тяжело) трудиться.

travel I ['trævl] n 1) путешествие; 2) pl описание путешествия; 3) движение, передвижение, ход.

travel II v 1) путешествовать; ехать; 2) передвигаться; двигаться; 3) переходить от предмета к предмету (о взгляде); перебирать (в уме, в памяти); 4) перемещаться; распространяться (о свете, звуке).

travelled ['trævld] a 1) много путешествовавший; опытный, бывалый; 2) часто посещаемый (путешественниками); 3) проезжий (о дороге).

traveller ['trævlə] n 1) путешественник; путник; commercial ~ коммивояжёр; 2) тех. бегунок; ходовой ролик.

travelling I ['trævlɪŋ] n путешествие.

travelling II a 1) путешествующий; странствующий; 2) подвижной; передвижной (о библиотеке, выставке); походный (о кухне и т. п.).

travelling-bag ['trævlɪŋbæg] n (дорожный) несессер.

travelling-dress ['trævlɪŋdres] n дорожный костюм.

travelogue ['trævəloug] n 1) лекция о путешествиях с показом диапозитивов или фильма; 2) фильм о путешествиях.

traverse I ['trævəːs] n 1) поперечина, перекладина; поперечная линия; 2) препятствие; 3) воен. траверс; 4) воен. горизонтальная наводка; 5) юр. отрицание (утверждения противной стороны).

traverse II a поперечный.

traverse III v 1) пересекать; переходить, переправляться (через); 2) обсуждать; 3) возражать, противоречить; юр. отрицать (см. I, 5).

travesty I ['trævɪstɪ] n пародия.

travesty II v представлять пародию; пародировать.

travois [trə'vwɑː] n повозка (индейцев).

trawl I [trɔːl] n 1) грунтовой невод; 2) трал.

trawl II v 1) тащить (сети) по дну; 2) тралить.

trawler ['trɔːlə] n тральщик.

tray [treɪ] n 1) поднос, лоток; 2) мелкое корыто.

treacherous ['tretʃərəs] a предательский, вероломный; коварный.

treachery ['tretʃərɪ] n предательство, вероломство.

treacle I ['triːkl] n патока.

treacle II v намазывать патокой.

treacly ['triːklɪ] a 1) паточный; 2) приторный.

tread I [tred] n 1) поступь, походка; шаги;

2) ступе́нька; 3) о́бод колеса́; 4) ширина́ хо́да, ширина́ колеи́.

tread II *v* (*past* trod; *p. p.* trodden) 1) ступа́ть; шага́ть, идти́; to ~ in smb.'s (foot)steps идти́ по чьим-л. стопа́м, сле́довать чьему́-л. приме́ру; 2) топта́ть, наступа́ть ного́й; дави́ть; *перен.* попира́ть; to ~ under foot попира́ть нога́ми, топта́ть; 3) протопта́ть (*тропинку и т. п.*); □ to ~ **down** растопта́ть, затопта́ть; to ~ **in** вта́птывать; to ~ **on** сле́довать непосре́дственно за; to ~ on (*или* upon) the heels of smb. сле́довать по пята́м за кем-л.; to ~ **out** а) дави́ть, выжима́ть (*сок — нога́ми*); б) туши́ть (*огонь*); в) *воен.* подавля́ть; to ~ **upon** *см.* to ~ on; ◇ to ~ lightly де́йствовать осторо́жно; to ~ on air ≅ ног под собо́й не чу́ять (*от ра́дости*).

treadle I ['tredl] *n* педа́ль.

treadle II *v* рабо́тать педа́лью.

treason ['tri:zn] *n* изме́на; high ~ госуда́рственная изме́на.

treasonable ['tri:znəbl] *a* изме́ннический, преда́тельский.

treasure I ['treʒə] *n* сокро́вище; buried ~ клад.

treasure II *v* 1) храни́ть как сокро́вище; 2) высоко́ цени́ть; дорожи́ть.

treasure-house ['treʒəhaus] *n* сокро́вищница; храни́лище.

treasurer ['treʒərə] *n* казначе́й.

treasury ['treʒəri] *n* 1) (Т.) казначе́йство; 2) сокро́вищница.

Treasury bench ['treʒəri'bentʃ] *n* скамья́ мини́стров (*в английском парламенте*).

treat I [tri:t] *n* 1) удово́льствие, наслажде́ние; развлече́ние; 2) угоще́ние; a Dutch ~ *разг.* угоще́ние, при кото́ром ка́ждый пла́тит за себя́; to stand ~ *разг.* угоща́ть, плати́ть за други́х.

treat II *v* 1) обраща́ться, обходи́ться; to ~ kindly хорошо́ обраща́ться; to ~ as a child обраща́ться как с ребёнком; 2) рассма́тривать, тракто́вать; рассужда́ть; 3) обраба́тывать (*чем-л.— with*); подверга́ть де́йствию (*чего-л.— with*); 4) лечи́ть (*от чего-л.— for*; *чем-л.— with*); 5) угоща́ть (*чем-л.— to*); 6) пригласи́ть (*в театр и т. п.*); 7) вести́ перегово́ры, догова́риваться.

treatise ['tri:tiz] *n* тракта́т.

treatment ['tri:tmənt] *n* 1) обраще́ние (*с кем-л.*), обхожде́ние; 2) обрабо́тка (*чем-л.*); 3) лече́ние.

treaty ['tri:ti] *n* (междунаро́дный) догово́р; nuclear non-proliferation ~ догово́р о нераспростране́нии я́дерного ору́жия; the test-ban ~ догово́р о запреще́нии испыта́ний (*ядерного оружия*); to be in ~ with находи́ться в догово́рных отноше́ниях с кем-л.

treble I ['trebl] *n* 1) тройно́е коли́чество; 2) *муз.* ди́скант.

treble II *a* 1) тройно́й, троекра́тный, утро́енный; 2) дисканто́вый.

treble III *v* утра́ивать(ся).

tree I [tri:] *n* 1) де́рево; hollow ~ дупли́стое де́рево; 2) коло́дка (*сапожная*); 3) *сленг* ви́селица; ◇ family ~ родосло́вное де́рево; up a ~ в безвы́ходном положе́нии; at the top of the ~ на верши́не мастерства́, карье́ры.

tree II *v* 1) загна́ть на де́рево; *перен.* загна́ть в тупи́к; 2) натя́гивать на коло́дку.

tree-frog ['tri:frog] *n* древе́сная лягу́шка.

treeless ['tri:lis] *a* безле́сный, без дере́вьев, лишённый расти́тельности, го́лый (*о земельном участке*).

tree-toad ['tri:toud] *см.* tree-frog.

trefoil ['trefoil] *n* 1) трили́стник; кле́вер; 2) *архит.* орна́мент в ви́де трили́стника.

trek I [trek] *n* 1) похо́д, перехо́д; марш; to go on the ~ выступа́ть в похо́д; 2) переселе́ние (*особ. в фургонах*).

trek II *v* 1) де́лать перехо́д, соверша́ть марш; 2) переселя́ться.

trellis ['trelis] *n* решётка; шпале́ра.

tremble I ['trembl] *n* дрожь; дрожа́ние.

tremble II *v* дрожа́ть; трепета́ть; to ~ all over дрожа́ть всем те́лом; содрога́ться; to ~ with fear дрожа́ть от стра́ха; to ~ for smb. беспоко́иться о ком-л., дрожа́ть за кого́-л.; to ~ to think трепета́ть при одно́й мы́сли.

tremendous [tri'mendəs] *a* 1) ужа́сный; стра́шный; 2) потряса́ющий; огро́мный.

tremor ['tremə] *n* дрожь.

tremulous ['tremjuləs] *a* 1) дрожа́щий; 2) тре́петный; ро́бкий.

trench I [trentʃ] *n* 1) кана́ва, ров; 2) транше́я; око́п; 3) *attr* транше́йный, око́пный.

trench II *v* 1) рыть кана́вы, транше́и, око́пы; 2) вска́пывать; 3) посяга́ть (*на — upon*); □ to ~ **about**, to ~ **around** ока́пываться.

trenchant ['trentʃənt] *a* 1) ре́жущий, о́стрый; 2) ко́лкий, язви́тельный; рази́щий (*о слове и т. п.*).

trench-bomb ['trentʃbɔm] *n* ручна́я грана́та.

trencher ['trentʃə] *n* доска́ для хле́ба.

trend I [trend] *n* о́бщее направле́ние, тенде́нция.

trend II *v* 1) име́ть тенде́нцию, быть напра́вленным (*в определённую сторону*); 2) отклоня́ться, склоня́ться; клони́ться.

trepan [tri'ræn] *v мед.* трепани́ровать.

trepidation [,trepi'deiʃən] *n* тре́пет; дрожь.

trespass I ['trespəs] *n* 1) наруше́ние грани́ц; 2) просту́пок; прегреше́ние; 3) злоупотребле́ние.

trespass II *v* 1) наруша́ть грани́цы (*on, upon*); 2) соверша́ть просту́пок, прегреше́ние (*against*); 3) злоупотребля́ть (*терпением, гостеприимством; on, upon*).

trespasser ['trespəsə] *n* 1) наруши́тель грани́ц; 2) правонаруши́тель.

tress [tres] *n* 1) ло́кон; коса́; 2) *pl* распу́щенные во́лосы.

tressed [trest] *a* 1) с ко́сами; 2) заплетённый (*в косу*); завито́й (*локонами*).

trestle [tresl] *n* ко́злы, подста́вка; эстака́да.

trews [tru:z] *n pl* кле́тчатые штаны́ (*шотл. горцев*).

trey [trei] *n* тро́йка (*в картах*); три очка́ (*на игральных костях*).

triad ['traiəd] *n* триа́да.

trial ['traiəl] *n* 1) испыта́ние, о́пыт, про́ба; on ~ на испыта́нии; 2) пережива́ние, испыта́ние; злоключе́ние; 3) суде́бное разбира́тельство; суде́бный проце́сс, суд; state ~ суд над госуда́рственным престу́пником; to bring to ~, to put on ~ привлека́ть к суду́; to hold a ~ вести́ суде́бный проце́сс; to stand one's ~ быть под судо́м; 4) попы́тка; покуше́ние; 5) искуше́ние; 6) *attr* про́бный; испыта́тельный.

triangle ['traiæŋgl] *n* треуго́льник.

triangular [traɪˈæŋɡjulə] *a* треуго́льный.

tribal [ˈtraɪbəl] *a* племенно́й; родово́й.

tribe [traɪb] *n* 1) пле́мя; клан; род; nomad ~s кочевы́е племена́, коче́вники; 2) *разг.* компа́ния, гру́ппа; 3) *биол.* три́ба.

tribesman [ˈtraɪbzmən] *n* член ро́да (*того же*); соро́дич, соплеме́нник.

tribrach [ˈtrɪbræk] *n лит.* трибра́хий.

tribulation [ˌtrɪbjuˈleɪʃən] *n* го́ре, напа́сть.

tribunal [traɪˈbjuːnl] *n* 1) суд; трибуна́л; 2) ме́сто судьи́.

tribune[1] [ˈtrɪbjuːn] *n* трибу́н.

tribune[2] *n* трибу́на.

tributary I [ˈtrɪbjutərɪ] *n* 1) да́нник; 2) прито́к (*реки*).

tributary II *a* 1) платя́щий дань; подчинённый; 2) вспомога́тельный; второстепе́нный; 3) явля́ющийся прито́ком.

tribute [ˈtrɪbjuːt] *n* дань; to lay under ~ наложи́ть дань; to pay a ~ плати́ть дань; *перен.* отдава́ть дань (*уважения, восхищения*); floral ~s цвето́чные подноше́ния.

trice[1] [traɪs] *n* мгнове́ние; at a ~, in a ~ в оди́н миг, мгнове́нно.

trice[2] *v* подтя́гивать и привя́зывать (*парус; обыкн.* to ~ up).

tricentenary [ˈtraɪsenˈtiːnərɪ] *n* трёхсотле́тие.

trick I [trɪk] *n* 1) хи́трость, обма́н; to play smb. a ~ обману́ть, наду́ть кого́-л.; to play a nasty ~ сде́лать га́дость кому́-л.; 2) шу́тка, ша́лость; to serve smb. a ~ сыгра́ть шу́тку с кем-л.; dirty ~s, shabby ~s га́дкие шу́тки; по́длая вы́ходка; ~ of the senses обма́н чувств; ~s of fortune превра́тности судьбы́; 3) фо́кус, трюк, «шту́ка»; 4) уло́вка; ло́вкий приём; I know a ~ worth two of that я зна́ю сре́дство получше; 5) характе́рная осо́бенность; мане́ра; чёрточка; 6) *карт.* взя́тка; 7) безделу́шка; игру́шка.

trick II *v* 1) обма́нывать, надува́ть; выма́нивать (out of); 2) наряжа́ть, украша́ть.

trickery [ˈtrɪkərɪ] *n* надува́тельство, обма́н; 2) хи́трость; ло́вкая проде́лка.

trickle I [ˈtrɪkl] *n* стру́йка.

trickle II *v* течь то́нкой стру́йкой, (про)сочи́ться (*тж.* to ~ out); ка́пать.

trickster [ˈtrɪkstə] *n* обма́нщик.

tricksy [ˈtrɪksɪ] *a* шаловли́вый, игри́вый.

tricky [ˈtrɪkɪ] *a* 1) хи́трый; ло́вкий; ненадёжный; 2) сло́жный, тру́дный, мудрёный.

tricot [ˈtrɪkou] *n* 1) трико́ (*материя*); 2) трикота́жное бельё.

tricycle [ˈtraɪsɪkl] *n* трёхколёсный велосипе́д.

trident [ˈtraɪdənt] *n* трезу́бец.

tried I [traɪd] *p. p. см.* try I.

tried II *a* испы́танный, ве́рный, прове́ренный.

triennial I [traɪˈenjəl] *n* 1) трёхле́тие; 2) трёхле́тняя годовщи́на.

triennial II *a* 1) продолжа́ющийся три го́да, трёхле́тний; 2) повторя́ющийся че́рез три го́да.

trier [ˈtraɪə] *n* стара́тельный, добросо́вестный рабо́тник.

trifle I [ˈtraɪfl] *n* 1) пустя́к; ме́лочь; 2) незначи́тельное коли́чество; a ~ немно́жко, слегка́; бискви́т с кре́мом.

trifle II *v* 1) занима́ться пустяка́ми; вести́ себя́ легкомы́сленно; 2) тра́тить понапра́сну (*время,*

си́лы; *тж.* to ~ away); 3) шути́ть; he is not a man to ~ with с ним шу́тки пло́хи; 4) верте́ть в рука́х; тереби́ть.

trifling [ˈtraɪflɪŋ] *a* 1) пустя́чный, пустяко́вый; 2) неинтере́сный, несто́ящий.

trig[1] I [trɪɡ] *n* щёголь, фат.

trig[1] II *a* 1) наря́дный; 2) подтя́нутый; опря́тный; 3) кре́пкий; здоро́вый.

trig[2] I *n* то́рмоз, подкла́дка под колёса.

trig[2] II *v* тормози́ть, остана́вливать.

trig[3] *n шк.* тригономе́трия.

trigger [ˈtrɪɡə] *n* 1) защёлка; 2) *воен.* спусково́й крючо́к.

trigonometry [ˌtrɪɡəˈnɔmɪtrɪ] *n* тригономе́трия.

trihedral [traɪˈhiːdrəl] *a мат.* трёхгра́нный, трёхсторо́нний.

trilateral [traɪˈlætərəl] *a* трёхсторо́нний.

trilby [ˈtrɪlbɪ] *n* мя́гкая фе́тровая шля́па (*мужская*).

trilingual [traɪˈlɪŋɡwəl] *a* трёхъязы́чный; говоря́щий на трёх языка́х.

trill I [trɪl] *n* 1) трель; 2) вибри́рующее г.

trill II *v* 1) выводи́ть тре́ли; 2) произноси́ть г с вибра́цией.

trillion [ˈtrɪljən] *n* триллио́н; *амер.* биллио́н.

trilogy [ˈtrɪlədʒɪ] *n* трило́гия.

trim I [trɪm] *n* 1) поря́док; состоя́ние гото́вности; in good ~ в хоро́шем состоя́нии; in fighting ~ в боево́й гото́вности; in flying ~ гото́вый к полёту; 2) наря́д; украше́ние; отде́лка; 3) *мор.* размеще́ние гру́за и т. п. на су́дне.

trim II *a* 1) приведённый в поря́док; 2) аккура́тный, подтя́нутый; наря́дный; 3) в состоя́нии гото́вности.

trim III *v* 1) приводи́ть в поря́док; 2) отде́лывать; украша́ть; 3) подреза́ть (*фитиль лампы*); подстрига́ть; подра́внивать; 4) *разг.* отчи́тывать, де́лать вы́говор; 5) приспоса́бливаться; колеба́ться ме́жду противополо́жными па́ртиями; 6) *сленг* вымога́ть де́ньги; 7) *мор., ав.* уравнове́шивать.

trimester [traɪˈmestə] *n* триме́стр; трёхме́сячный срок.

trimmer [ˈtrɪmə] *n* приспособле́нец.

trimming [ˈtrɪmɪŋ] *n* 1) отде́лка (*платья*); украше́ние; 2) *pl* припра́ва, гарни́р; 3) *pl* армату́ра; 4) *pl* дополни́тельная опла́та, дополни́тельный за́работок; 5) *тех.* зачи́стка, выра́внивание.

trinket [ˈtrɪŋkɪt] *n* безделу́шка; брело́к.

trinomial I [traɪˈnoumjəl] *n мат.* трёхчле́н.

trinomial II *a мат.* трёхчле́нный.

trio [ˈtriːou] *n* 1) *муз.* три́о; 2) *шутл.* тро́е, тро́йка (*людей*); 3) *ав.* «тро́йка», звено́ из трёх самолётов.

trip I [trɪp] *n* 1) пое́здка, путеше́ствие, экску́рсия; рейс; полёт; pleasure ~ увесели́тельная прогу́лка; a round ~ пое́здка, рейс, полёт туда́ и обра́тно; to make ~s курси́ровать; to take a ~ съе́здить, прое́хаться; 2) лёгкая бы́страя похо́дка; 3) ло́жный шаг, оши́бка; ля́псус; 4) «подно́жка»; 5) *тех.* защёлка, соба́чка.

trip II *v* 1) идти́ легко́ и бы́стро; 2) споткну́ться (*тж. перен.*); сде́лать опло́шность; 3) подста́вить но́жку (*тж. перен.*); 4) опроки́дывать; 5) пойма́ть на оши́бке; 6) сцепля́ть; расцепля́ть, выключа́ть.

tripartite [traɪˈpɑːtaɪt] *a* состоя́щий из трёх часте́й.

tripe [traɪp] *n* 1) рубец (*кушанье*); 2) *разг.* ерунда́, чепуха́.

triple I [ˈtrɪpl] *a* тройно́й; утро́енный.

triple II *v* утра́ивать(ся).

triplet [ˈtrɪplɪt] *n* 1) тро́йка (*три предмета, лица*); 2) тро́йня.

triplicate[a] [ˈtrɪplɪkɪt] *a* тройно́й.

triplicate[b] [ˈtrɪplɪkeɪt] *v* утра́ивать; составля́ть в трёх экземпля́рах *или* ко́пиях.

tripod [ˈtraɪpɔd] *n* 1) трено́га; трено́жник; стол на трёх но́жках; 2) *attr* трёхно́гий.

tripper [ˈtrɪpə] *n разг.* экскурса́нт, тури́ст.

tripping [ˈtrɪpɪŋ] *a* быстроно́гий; с лёгкой похо́дкой.

trippingly [ˈtrɪpɪŋlɪ] *adv* 1) бы́стро и легко́ (*ходить, двигаться*); 2) бо́йко, свобо́дно (*говорить*).

triptych [ˈtrɪptɪk] *n жив.* три́птих.

trishaw [ˈtraɪʃɔː] *n* велори́кша.

trisyllabic [ˌtraɪsɪˈlæbɪk] *a* трёхсло́жный.

trite [traɪt] *a* бана́льный, изби́тый.

tritium [ˈtrɪtɪəm] *n хим.* три́тий.

triumph I [ˈtraɪəmf] *n* триу́мф; побе́да; торже́ство; easy ~ лёгкая побе́да; in ~ а) лику́я; б) торже́ственно.

triumph II *v* 1) торжествова́ть побе́ду; побе́дить; восторжествова́ть (*об идеях*).

triumphal [traɪˈʌmfəl] *a* триумфа́льный.

triumphant [traɪˈʌmfənt] *a* 1) торжеству́ющий; 2) победоно́сный.

trivet [ˈtrɪvɪt] *n* тага́н; ◇ as right as a ~ в по́лном поря́дке.

trivia [ˈtrɪvɪə] *n pl* пустяки́, ме́лочи.

trivial [ˈtrɪvɪəl] *a* 1) обы́денный; тривиа́льный; бана́льный; 2) ме́лкий, незначи́тельный.

triviality [ˌtrɪvɪˈælɪtɪ] *n* 1) тривиа́льность; 2) незначи́тельность; ме́лочи.

trochaic I [trouˈkeɪɪk] *n лит.* хоре́й.

trochaic II *a лит.* хореи́ческий.

troche [trouʃ] *n* табле́тка.

trochee [ˈtroukiː] *n лит.* хоре́й.

trod [trɔd] *past см.* tread II.

trodden [ˈtrɔdn] *p. p. см.* tread II.

troglodyte [ˈtrɔglədaɪt] *n* 1) пеще́рный жи́тель, троглоди́т; *перен.* отше́льник; 2) человекообра́зная обезья́на.

Trojan I [ˈtroudʒən] *n ист.* троя́нец; *перен.* сме́лый челове́к.

Trojan II *a ист.* троя́нский; *перен.* сме́лый.

troll[1] [troul] *v* 1) распева́ть, петь; 2) лови́ть ры́бу на блесну́.

troll[2] *n миф.* тролль.

trolley [ˈtrɔlɪ] *n* 1) теле́жка (разно́счика); 2) ваго́нетка; 3) *эл.* конта́ктный ро́лик; 4) трамва́й.

trolley-car [ˈtrɔlɪkɑː] *n амер.* трамва́й.

trollop [ˈtrɔləp] *n* 1) неря́ха; 2) проститу́тка.

trombone [trɔmˈboun] *n муз.* тромбо́н.

troop I [truːp] *n* 1) *pl* войска́; armoured ~s бронета́нковые войска́; household ~s гва́рдия, гварде́йские ча́сти; to pass ~s in review производи́ть смотр войска́м; with ~s строево́й (*об офице́ре*); 2) толпа́; ма́сса; 3) ста́я; ста́до; 4) взвод; батаре́я; эскадро́н.

troop II *v* 1) собира́ться (*толпо́й*); 2) дви́гаться (*стро́ем*); 3) *воен.* разделя́ть на взво́ды.

troop-carrier [ˈtruːpˌkærɪə] *n* тра́нспортно-деса́нтный самолёт.

trooper [ˈtruːpə] *n* 1) кавалери́ст; танки́ст; 2) ко́нный полице́йский; 3) кавалери́йская ло́шадь; 4) войсково́й тра́нспорт.

troop-horse [ˈtruːphɔːs] *n* строева́я кавалери́йская ло́шадь.

troop-ship [ˈtruːpʃɪp] *n* тра́нспорт для перево́зки войск.

trope [troup] *n лит.* троп.

trophy [ˈtroufɪ] *n* трофе́й.

tropic [ˈtrɔpɪk] *n* 1) тро́пик; the ~s тро́пики (*зона*); ~ of Cancer тро́пик Ра́ка; ~ of Capricorn тро́пик Козеро́га; 2) *attr* тропи́ческий.

tropical[1] [ˈtrɔpɪkəl] *a* тропи́ческий.

tropical[2] *a лит.* фигура́льный; о́бразный.

troposphere [ˈtrɔpousfɪə] *n* тропосфе́ра.

trot I [trɔt] *n* 1) рысь; бы́стрый шаг (*челове́ка*); торопли́вая похо́дка; a round ~ кру́пная рысь; at the ~ ры́сью, на рыся́х; 2) ребёнок, кото́рый у́чится ходи́ть; 3) стару́ха, ста́рая карга́; 4) *амер. сленг.* подстро́чник, шпарга́лка; ◇ to keep smb. on the ~ не дава́ть поко́я.

trot II *v* 1) идти́ ры́сью; пуска́ть ры́сью; 2) бежа́ть, спеши́ть; □ to ~ about бе́гать, суети́ться; to ~ out а) пока́зывать (*ло́шадь*) на рыси́; б) пока́зывать (*това́ры и т. п.*); ◇ to ~ smb. round *разг.* води́ть кого́-л.; пока́зывать кому́-л. (*го́род и т. п.*).

trotter [ˈtrɔtə] *n* 1) рыса́к; 2) *pl* но́жки (*бара́ньи и пр. как блю́до*); 3) *pl сленг* но́ги (*челове́ка*).

trouble I [ˈtrʌbl] *n* 1) беспоко́йство; волне́ние, трево́га; to give ~ причиня́ть беспоко́йство, затрудне́ния; 2) неприя́тность, беда́; in ~ в беде́; to get into ~ попа́сть в беду́; to ask (*или* to look) for ~ *разг.* лезть на рожо́н; 3) забо́ты, хло́поты; уси́лия; to take the ~ труди́ться, взять на себя́ труд; to take much ~ стара́ться, хлопота́ть; 4) волне́ния, беспоря́дки; 5) боле́знь; heart ~ боле́знь се́рдца; 6) *тех.* неиспра́вность; поме́ха, заде́ржка.

trouble II *v* 1) беспоко́ить(ся); волнова́ть(ся); трево́жить(ся); 2) пристава́ть, надоеда́ть; 3) му́чить, не дава́ть поко́я (*о бо́ли и т. п.*); 4) затрудня́ть; утомля́ть (*рабо́той и т. п.*); 5) *тех.* наруша́ть; поврежда́ть.

troublesome [ˈtrʌblsəm] *a* 1) причиня́ющий беспоко́йство; 2) тру́дный, хло́потный; 3) беспоко́йный (*о ребёнке, больно́м*); 4) мучи́тельный (*о ка́шле и т. п.*); 5) назо́йливый.

trough [trɔf] *n* 1) коры́то; кормушка; 2) квашня́; 3) жёлоб, лото́к; 4) впа́дина, котлови́на.

trounce [trauns] *v* 1) бить, поро́ть; 2) наноси́ть тяжёлое пораже́ние; 3) де́лать вы́говор, нака́зывать.

troupe [truːp] *n* тру́ппа.

trouper [ˈtruːpə] *n* актёр, член тру́ппы; ◇ a good ~ работя́га.

trousers [ˈtrauzəz] *n pl* брю́ки.

trousseau [ˈtruːsou] *n* (*pl тж.* trousseaux) прида́ное.

trout [traut] *n* (*pl без измен.*) форе́ль; rainbow ~ ра́дужная форе́ль.

trowel I [ˈtrauəl] *n* 1) лопа́тка (*штукату́ра*); to lay on with a ~ гу́сто нама́зывать; *перен.* гру́бо льстить; 2) садо́вый сово́к.

trowel II *v* накла́дывать *или* разгла́живать лопа́ткой (*штукату́рку*).

troy [trɔɪ] *n* система́ мер ве́са для зо́лота и серебра́.

truant I ['truːənt] *n* лентя́й, безде́льник; прогу́льщик; to play ~ прогуля́ть, пропусти́ть заня́тия в шко́ле.

truant II *a* лени́вый; пра́здный.

truce [truːs] *n* 1) переми́рие; 2) коне́ц, прекраще́ние; 3) переды́шка; зати́шье.

truck¹ I [trʌk] *n* 1) ме́на, обме́н; сде́лка; 2) мелочно́й това́р; 3) систе́ма опла́ты нату́рой; 4) *амер.* о́вощи; 5) *разг.* хлам, нену́жные ве́щи; ◊ to have no ~ with smb. не име́ть де́ла с кем-л., не име́ть ничего́ о́бщего с кем-л.

truck¹ II *v* 1) обме́нивать; вести́ мену́ю торго́влю; 2) плати́ть нату́рой, това́рами.

truck² I *n* 1) грузово́й автомоби́ль, грузови́к; 2) ваго́н-платфо́рма; 3) теле́жка; вагоне́тка; 4) ро́лик.

truck² II *v* перевози́ть на платфо́рмах, на грузовика́х.

truck-farmer ['trʌkˌfɑːmə] *n* *амер.* огоро́дник.

truckle ['trʌkl] *v* раболе́пствовать.

truckle-bed ['trʌklbed] *n* крова́ть-раскладу́шка.

truckler ['trʌklə] *n* подхали́м.

truck-trailer ['trʌkˌtreɪlə] *n* грузови́к с прице́пом.

truculent ['trʌkjulənt] *a* свире́пый, жесто́кий; ва́рварский.

trudge I [trʌdʒ] *n* утоми́тельная прогу́лка; тру́дный путь.

trudge I *v* идти́ с трудо́м; тащи́ться (*через си́лу*).

trudgen ['trʌdʒən] *n* пла́вание во́льным сти́лем.

true I [truː] *a* 1) ве́рный, пра́вильный; и́стинный; it is not ~ э́то непра́вда; is it ~? пра́вда?; to come ~ сбыва́ться; 2) ве́рный, пре́данный; 3) настоя́щий, по́длинный; 4) пра́вильный, то́чный (*о ко́пии и т. п.*); 5) зако́нный, действи́тельный; соотве́тствующий но́рме, пра́вилу и т. п.; 6) правди́вый; непритво́рный.

true II *v* (по)ста́вить пра́вильно, в пра́вильное положе́ние; □ to ~ up выверя́ть; выра́внивать.

true III *adv* 1) ве́рно; 2) то́чно; 3) правди́во.

true-blue I ['truːbluː] *n* ре́вностный сторо́нник, приве́рженец.

true-blue II *a* ве́рный, ре́вностный.

true-born ['truːbɔːn] *a* чистокро́вный.

true-bred ['truːbred] *a* 1) хорошо́ воспи́танный; 2) *см.* true-born.

true-love ['truːlʌv] *n* возлю́бленный, -ая; люби́мый, -ая.

truffle ['trʌfl] *n* трю́фель.

truism ['truːɪzəm] *n* трюи́зм.

truly ['truːlɪ] *adv* 1) правди́во; и́скренне; 2) то́чно; 3) пра́вильно; и́стинно; 4) ве́рно, лоя́льно; пре́данно; 5) действи́тельно, пои́стине; ◊ yours ~ пре́данный вам (*в конце́ письма́*).

trump¹ I [trʌmp] *n* ко́зырь (*тж. перен.*); to play a ~ козырну́ть; to turn up ~s око́нчиться благополу́чно, оберну́ться лу́чше, чем ожида́ли; to play one's last ~ прибе́гнуть к после́днему сре́дству; 2) *разг.* сла́вный па́рень.

trump¹ II *v* козыря́ть; бить ко́зырем; □ to ~ up выду́мывать, фабрикова́ть.

trump² *n* *уст., поэт.* 1) труба́; 2) тру́бный звук; ◊ the last ~, the ~ of doom *библ.* коне́ц све́та.

trumpery I ['trʌmpərɪ] *n* мишура́; хлам.

trumpery II *a* мишу́рный, показно́й; него́дный.

trumpet I ['trʌmpɪt] *n* 1) труба́; 2) слухова́я тру́бка; 3) тру́бный звук; 4) растру́б; 5) ру́пор; ◊ to blow one's own ~ хва́статься, похваля́ться.

trumpet II *v* 1) труби́ть; *перен.* возвеща́ть; разглаша́ть повсю́ду, расска́зывать; 2) реве́ть (*о слоне́*).

trumpet-call ['trʌmpɪtkɔːl] *n* зву́ки трубы́; сигна́л на трубе́; *перен.* призы́в к де́йствию.

trumpeter ['trʌmpɪtə] *n* труба́ч; ◊ to be one's own ~ хва́статься, похваля́ться.

truncated ['trʌŋkeɪtɪd] *a* *мат.* усечённый (*о ко́нусе, пирами́де*).

truncheon I ['trʌntʃən] *n* 1) па́лочка полице́йского; дуби́нка; 2) (ма́ршальский) жезл.

truncheon II *v* бить (*па́лкой, дуби́нкой*).

trundle I ['trʌndl] *n* колёсико, ро́лик.

trundle II *v* кати́ть(ся).

trunk [trʌŋk] *n* 1) ствол; 2) ту́ловище; 3) *архит.* гла́вный ко́рпус; сте́ржень коло́нны; 4) доро́жный сунду́к, чемода́н; 5) хо́бот слона́; 6) *pl* спорти́вные трусы́; 7) магистра́ль (*железнодоро́жная, телефо́нная, телегра́фная*); 8) *сленг* пень, болва́н; 9) *attr* гла́вный; магистра́льный.

trunk-call ['trʌŋkkɔːl] *n* вы́зов по междугоро́дному телефо́ну.

trunnion ['trʌnjən] *n* *тех.* ца́пфа.

truss I [trʌs] *n* 1) свя́зка (*се́на, соло́мы*); 2) *стр.* фе́рма; стропи́ло; 3) *мед.* банда́ж.

truss II *v* 1) свя́зывать, скрепля́ть; 2) *стр.* подде́рживать стропи́лами, фе́рмами.

trust¹ I [trʌst] *n* 1) ве́ра; дове́рие; to have (*или* to put, to repose) ~ in доверя́ть; to take on ~ принима́ть на ве́ру; 2) наде́жда, упова́ние; 3) креди́т; on ~ в долг, в креди́т; 4) опе́ка, опеку́нство; 5) дове́ренное иму́щество; что-л., вве́ренное попече́нию; 6) взя́тое на себя́ обяза́тельство, отве́тственность; 7) управле́ние по дове́ренности.

trust¹ II *a* дове́ренный.

trust¹ III *v* 1) доверя́ть, ве́рить (*в — in*); 2) полага́ться; доверя́ться; 3) вверя́ть, поруча́ть попече́нию; 4) наде́яться, полага́ть; 5) дава́ть в креди́т.

trust² *n* трест.

trust-deed ['trʌstdiːd] *n* *юр.* дове́ренность.

trustee [trʌs'tiː] *n* 1) попечи́тель; опеку́н; 2) дове́ренное лицо́.

trusteeship [trʌs'tiːʃɪp] *n* опе́ка, опеку́нство; попечи́тельство.

trustful ['trʌstful] *a* дове́рчивый.

trustiness ['trʌstɪnɪs] *n* ве́рность, лоя́льность; надёжность.

trustless ['trʌstlɪs] *a* ненадёжный; неве́рный (*о челове́ке*); вероло́мный.

trustworthy ['trʌstˌwəːðɪ] *a* заслу́живающий дове́рия.

trusty I ['trʌstɪ] *n* заключённый, по́льзующийся привиле́гиями за образцо́вое поведе́ние.

trusty II *a* *шутл.* ве́рный, надёжный; че́стный.

truth [truːθ] *n* 1) пра́вда; и́стина; home ~ го́рькая и́стина; naked ~, simple ~ чи́стая пра́вда; unvarnished ~ неприкра́шенная и́стина; in ~ пои́стине, действи́тельно; to tell the ~ а) говори́ть пра́вду; б) по пра́вде говоря́, призна́ться; to stretch the ~ преувели́чивать; to question the ~ of сомнева́ться в и́стинности чего́-л.; 2) правди́вость, и́скренность; 3) то́чность, соотве́тствие.

truthful [ˈtruːθful] *a* 1) правди́вый (*о человеке*); 2) ве́рный, пра́вильный.

truthless [ˈtruːθlɪs] *a* 1) неве́рный, ло́жный; 2) ненадёжный.

try I [traɪ] *v* 1) про́бовать; 2) испы́тывать, подверга́ть испыта́нию; де́лать о́пыты; проверя́ть; 3) пыта́ться, стара́ться; 4) утомля́ть (*зре́ние и т. п.*); 5) испы́тывать (*чьё-л. терпе́ние*); 6) суди́ть; подверга́ть суду́; рассле́довать; 7) очища́ть (*мета́ллы; тж.* to ~ out); □ to ~ for добива́ться, иска́ть (*рабо́ту, ме́сто*); to ~ on а) примеря́ть; б) *разг.* испы́тывать чью-л. вы́держку; to ~ out тща́тельно иссле́довать, прове́рить.

try II *n* 1) попы́тка; to have a ~ at попыта́ться; 2) испыта́ние; to give (it) a ~ испы́тывать; испро́бовать (*что-л.*); to give smb. a ~ дать кому́-л. возмо́жность испыта́ть, испро́бовать что-л.; дать возмо́жность прове́рить себя́.

trying [ˈtraɪɪŋ] *a* 1) тру́дный, утоми́тельный (*о пое́здке и т. п.*); тяжёлый (*о положе́нии и т. п.*); ~ to the health вре́дный для здоро́вья; 2) ску́чный; раздража́ющий; невыноси́мый.

try-on [ˈtraɪˈɒn] *n* 1) приме́рка; 2) *разг.* попы́тка обману́ть.

tryst [traɪst] *n* 1) свида́ние, усло́вленная встре́ча; to keep (to break) ~ прийти́ (не прийти́) на свида́ние; 2) ме́сто встре́чи.

tsar [zɑː] *см.* czar.

tsetse [ˈtsetsɪ] *n* му́ха цеце́.

tub I [tʌb] *n* 1) уша́т, бадья́, лоха́нь; 2) ка́дка; 3) *разг.* ва́нна, купа́ние в ва́нне; 4) *разг.* ло́дка (*особ. ста́рая*).

tub II *v* 1) мы́ть(ся) в ва́нне; 2) сажа́ть расте́ния в ка́дку.

tubby [ˈtʌbɪ] *a* бочкообра́зный; то́лстый, кру́глый (*о человеке*).

tube I [tjuːb] *n* 1) труба́, тру́бка; 2) тю́бик (*па́сты, кре́ма и т. п.*); 3) *радио* электро́нная ла́мпа; 4) метрополите́н (*в Ло́ндоне*).

tube II *v* 1) заключа́ть в трубу́; 2) снабжа́ть труб(к)ами.

tuber [ˈtjuːbə] *n* клу́бень.

tubercle [ˈtjuːbəːkl] *n* 1) *бот.* бугоро́к; клубенёк, 2) *мед.* туберкулёзный бугоро́к.

tubercular [tjuːˈbəːkjulə] *a* туберкулёзный.

tuberculosis [tjuːˌbəːkjuˈlousɪs] *n* туберкулёз.

tuberose [ˈtjuːbərouz] *n* *бот.* тубероза.

tuberous [ˈtjuːbərəs] *a* 1) *бот.* клу́бневый; 2) буго́рчатый; шишкова́тый.

tubing [ˈtjuːbɪŋ] *n* 1) *собир.* тру́бы; трубопрово́д; 2) *тех.* тю́бинг.

tub-thumper [ˈtʌbˌθʌmpə] *n* шумли́вый, напы́щенный ора́тор.

tubular [ˈtjuːbjulə] *a* тру́бчатый; цилиндри́ческий.

tuck I [tʌk] *n* 1) (попере́чная) скла́дка (*на пла́тье*); 2) *сленг* еда́; сла́сти.

tuck II *v* 1) де́лать скла́дки; стя́гивать, собира́ть; 2) подбира́ть под себя́; подтыка́ть; подсо́вывать; □ to ~ away запря́тать; to ~ in *сленг* есть; to ~ into засо́вывать; to ~ up засу́чивать (*рукава́*); подвёртывать, подбира́ть (*подо́л*).

tucker¹ [ˈtʌkə] *n* 1) (кружевно́й) воротни́к, косы́нка; 2) *сленг* еда́.

tucker² *v* *амер. сленг* утомля́ть, изма́тывать.

tuck-in [ˈtʌkˈɪn] *n* *сленг* вку́сная сы́тная еда́.

tuck-shop [ˈtʌkʃəp] *n* *сленг* конди́терская.

Tuesday [ˈtjuːzdɪ] *n* вто́рник.

tuft [tʌft] *n* 1) пучо́к (*пе́рьев, воло́с, тра́вы*); 2) боро́дка кли́нышком; 3) гру́ппа кусто́в.

tug I [tʌg] *n* 1) тя́нущее *или* дёргающее уси́лие; рыво́к; to give a ~ потяну́ть, дёрнуть; 2) букси́р(ное су́дно); 3) постро́мка.

tug II *v* 1) тащи́ть, тяну́ть; дёргать (*изо всех сил*; *at*); 2) букси́ровать.

tugboat [ˈtʌgbout] *n* букси́рное су́дно.

tuition [tjuːˈɪʃən] *n* 1) обуче́ние; 2) пла́та за обуче́ние.

tulip [ˈtjuːlɪp] *n* тюльпа́н.

tulle [tjuːl] *n* тюль (*мате́рия*).

tumble I [ˈtʌmbl] *n* 1) паде́ние; 2) кувырка́нье; 3) беспоря́док.

tumble II *v* 1) па́дать (*споткну́вшись*); 2) опроки́дывать(ся); 3) кувырка́ться; 4) верте́ться, мета́ться (*в крова́ти*); 5) броса́ться; 6) кати́ться; 7) приводи́ть в беспоря́док; мять; еро́шить (*во́лосы*); □ to ~ in a) вва́ливаться; б) *разг.* ложи́ться спа́ть; to ~ out выска́кивать (*из посте́ли и т. п.*); to ~ to *разг.* поня́ть.

tumbledown [ˈtʌmbldaun] *a* ве́тхий, полуразру́шенный.

tumbler [ˈtʌmblə] *n* 1) бока́л; 2) акроба́т; 3) го́лубь-верту́н; 4) *тех.* опроки́дыватель.

tumble-weed [ˈtʌmblwiːd] *n* *бот.* перекати́-по́ле.

tumescent [tjuːˈmesənt] *a* припу́хший.

tumid [ˈtjuːmɪd] *a* 1) опу́хший, распу́хший; 2) напы́щенный.

tummy [ˈtʌmɪ] *n* *разг.* живо́тик.

tumor [ˈtjuːmə] *амер. см.* tumour.

tumour [ˈtjuːmə] *n* о́пухоль; malignant ~ злока́чественная о́пухоль.

tumuli [ˈtjuːmjulaɪ] *pl см.* tumulus.

tumult [ˈtjuːmʌlt] *n* 1) шум, сумато́ха; 2) смяте́ние, волне́ние.

tumultuary [tjuːˈmʌltjuərɪ] *a* шу́мный, бу́йный; беспоря́дочный.

tumultuous [tjuːˈmʌltjuəs] *a* 1) *см.* tumultuary; 2) возбуждённый, взволно́ванный.

tumulus [ˈtjuːmjuləs] *n* (*pl* tumuli) моги́льный холм, курга́н.

tun I [tʌn] *n* больша́я бо́чка.

tun II *v* храни́ть, держа́ть в бо́чке.

tuna [ˈtjuːnə] *n* туне́ц (*ры́ба*).

tune I [tjuːn] *n* 1) мело́дия, моти́в; to change one's ~ to sing another ~ *перен.* запе́ть друго́е, измени́ть тон, заговори́ть по-друго́му; 2) тон, звук; 3) строй, настро́енность; *перен.* согла́сие, гармо́ния; in ~ a) настро́енный (*о роя́ле*); б) в тон (*о пе́нии*); out of ~ a) расстро́енный (*о роя́ле*); б) не в тон (*о пе́нии*); out of ~ with a) не в ла́ду с.

tune II *v* 1) настра́ивать; 2) звуча́ть; □ to ~ in *радио* настра́ивать(ся) на длину́ волны́; to ~ up a) настра́ивать (*инструме́нты*); б) нача́ть игра́ть, петь; в) *шутл.* нача́ть пла́кать (*о ребёнке*); г) нала́живать (*рабо́ту и т. п.*).

tuneful [ˈtjuːnful] *a* мелоди́чный; гармони́чный.

tuneless [ˈtjuːnlɪs] *a* 1) немелоди́чный; нестро́йный; 2) беззву́чный; 3) глухо́й (*о го́лосе*); 4) молчали́вый.

tuner [ˈtjuːnə] *n* настро́йщик.

tungsten [ˈtʌŋstən] *n* *хим.* вольфра́м.

tunic [ˈtjuːnɪk] *n* 1) мунди́р; ки́тель (*солда́та,*

офицера); 2) туни́ка; 3) *биол.* оболо́чка; 4) *бот.* туни́ка, нару́жная оболо́чка.

tuning ['tjuːnɪŋ] *n* настро́йка; регулиро́вка.

tuning-fork ['tjuːnɪŋfɔːk] *n* камерто́н.

tunnel I ['tʌnl] *n* 1) тунне́ль; 2) *горн.* што́льня; прохо́д; 3) *воен.* ми́нная галере́я; 4) дымохо́д, труба́, воро́нка.

tunnel II *v* проводи́ть тунне́ль.

tunny ['tʌnɪ] *n* туне́ц (*рыба*).

turban ['təːbən] *n* тюрба́н, чалма́.

turbid ['təːbɪd] *a* 1) му́тный (*о жидкости*); 2) тума́нный, нея́сный.

turbine ['təːbɪn] *n* турби́на; steam ~ парова́я турби́на.

turbogenerator ['təːbouˈdʒenəreɪtə] *n тех.* турбогенера́тор.

turbo-jet ['təːbouˈdʒet] *a* турбореакти́вный.

turbo-prop ['təːbouˈprɔp] *см.* turbo-jet.

turbot ['təːbət] *n* па́лтус (*рыба*).

turbulence ['təːbjuləns] *n* 1) беспоря́док; 2) волне́ние; бу́рность.

turbulent ['təːbjulənt] *a* 1) беспоко́йный, бу́рный; бу́йный; 2) *физ.* вихрево́й, турбуле́нтный.

tureen [təˈriːn] *n* супова́я ми́ска.

turf I [təːf] *n* 1) дёрн; 2) торф; 3) (the ~) ска́чки; 4) (the ~) бегова́я доро́жка (*на ипподроме*).

turf II *v* покрыва́ть, обкла́дывать дёрном; □ to ~ out *сленг* выбра́сывать.

turgid ['təːdʒɪd] *a* 1) опу́хший; взду́вшийся; 2) напы́щенный, высокопа́рный (*о языке, стиле*).

Turk [təːk] *n* 1) ту́рок; турча́нка; the ~s ту́рки; Young ~ *ист.* младоту́рок; 2) магомета́нин.

turkey ['təːkɪ] *n* 1) индю́к, индю́шка; 2) инде́йка (*как блюдо*); ◊ to talk ~ *амер.* говори́ть серьёзно.

turkey-cock ['təːkɪkɔk] *n* индю́к; *перен.* наду́тый, ва́жничающий челове́к.

Turkish I ['təːkɪʃ] *n* туре́цкий язы́к.

Turkish II *a* туре́цкий.

Turkman ['təːkmən] *n* 1) туркме́н; the Turkmen туркме́ны; 2) туркме́нский язы́к.

Turkmen ['təːkmən] *a* туркме́нский.

Turkoman ['təːkəmən] *см.* Turkman.

turmoil ['təːmɔɪl] *n* смяте́ние, сумато́ха; беспоря́док.

turn I [təːn] *n* 1) оборо́т; a ~ of the wheel оборо́т колеса́; to take a bad ~ принима́ть дурно́й оборо́т (*о делах и т. п.*); 2) поворо́т; a ~ to the left поворо́т нале́во; at every ~ на ка́ждом шагу́, повсю́ду; 3) переме́на, измене́ние; to take a ~ for the better измени́ться к лу́чшему; попра́виться; 4) о́чередь; by ~s, in ~, ~ and ~ about по о́череди; out of ~ не в о́чередь, не по поря́дку; to take ~s череду́ваться, сменя́ться; 5) услу́га; посту́пок; to do smb. a good ~ оказа́ть кому́-л. хоро́шую услу́гу; to do smb. an ill ~ повреди́ть кому́-л.; оказа́ть медве́жью услу́гу; 6) прогу́лка, пое́здка; to go for a ~, to take a ~ прогуля́ться; 7) стиль; мане́ра; хара́ктер; склад (*ума*); 8) *разг.* не́рвное потрясе́ние; to give a ~ си́льно взволнова́ть; перепуга́ть; 9) оборо́т (*речи*); 10) возмо́жность; удо́бный слу́чай; to serve a ~ годи́ться, подходи́ть; ◊ to a ~ то́чно; как раз как ну́жно; one good ~ deserves another *посл.* услу́га за услу́гу.

turn II *v* 1) враща́ть(ся); верте́ть(ся); 2) повора́чивать(ся); повёртывать(ся); 3) направля́ть, об-

раща́ть (*внимание и т. п.*); 4) *как глагол-связка с предикативным прил. и наречием; часто переводится гл., образованным от прил.* станови́ться, де́латься; to ~ pale бледне́ть; 5) изменя́ться; 6) переводи́ть (*на другой язык*); 7) переде́лывать; 8) по́ртиться; скиса́ть; 9) превраща́ть(ся); 10) вывора́чивать наизна́нку; перелицо́вывать; 11) перевёртывать(ся); 12) вызыва́ть отвраще́ние; 13) обта́чивать на тока́рном станке́; □ to ~ **about** обёртываться; поверну́ть(ся) круго́м; to ~ **adrift** покида́ть; оставля́ть на произво́л судьбы́; to ~ **again** возвраща́ться; to ~ **against** а) восста́ть, воспроти́виться; б) восстанови́ть про́тив; испо́льзовать про́тив кого́-л.; to ~ **aside** отводи́ть; отвраща́ть; отклоня́ть(ся); to ~ **away** а) отвора́чиваться; б) прогоня́ть; увольня́ть; to ~ **back** а) прогоня́ть; б) возвраща́ться; поверну́ть обра́тно; to ~ **down** а) загиба́ть, подвёртывать; б) убавля́ть (*свет*); в) подавля́ть; г) отверга́ть; to ~ **in** а) зайти́ мимохо́дом, заверну́ть; б) *разг.* ложи́ться спать; to ~ **into** превраща́ть(ся) во что-л.; to ~ **off** а) закрыва́ть (*кран*); выключа́ть (*свет, газ*); б) увольня́ть; в) сде́лать, доде́лать; г) *сленг* пове́сить; to ~ **on** а) открыва́ть (*кран*); включа́ть (*свет, газ*); б) зави́сеть; в) относи́ться враждебно, напада́ть; to ~ **out** а) вывора́чивать; б) выключа́ть, туши́ть (*свет*); в) выгоня́ть; г) вы́пускать, производи́ть (*изделия*); д) име́ть результа́том, конча́ться; ока́зываться; е) выводи́ть; выходи́ть; ж) *разг.* встава́ть (*с посте́ли*); to ~ **over** а) передава́ть; б) перевёртывать(ся); в) обду́мывать, взве́шивать; г) переверну́ться; to ~ **round** а) оберну́ться; б) измени́ть взгля́ды, убежде́ния; to ~ **to** а) приня́ться за что-л.; б) обрати́ться к кому́-л.; в) приводи́ть к чему́-л., име́ть результа́том; to ~ **up** а) поднима́ть вверх; б) появля́ться внеза́пно.

turnabout ['təːnəˌbaut] *n* карусе́ль.

turncoat ['təːnkout] *n* ренега́т; перебе́жчик.

turn-down ['təːnˌdaun] *a* отложно́й (*о воротнике*).

turner ['təːnə] *n* то́карь.

turnery ['təːnərɪ] *n* 1) тока́рное де́ло, ремесло́; 2) тока́рная мастерска́я; 3) тока́рные изде́лия.

turning I ['təːnɪŋ] *n* 1) поворо́т; перекрёсток; излу́чина (*реки*); 2) обто́чка; тока́рная рабо́та; 3) *воен.* обхо́д фла́нга.

turning II *a* 1) поворо́тный; 2) враща́ющий(ся).

turning-point ['təːnɪŋpɔɪnt] *n* поворо́тный пункт; реша́ющий моме́нт; перело́м, кри́зис.

turnip ['təːnɪp] *n* ре́па; French ~ брю́ква; Swedish ~ турне́пс.

turnkey ['təːnkiː] *n* тюре́мщик, надзира́тель.

turn-out ['təːnˈaut] *n* 1) сбор (*войск' и т. п.*); собра́ние; 2) вы́пуск проду́кции; 3) вы́езд (*экипаж и т. п.*); 4) забасто́вка.

turnover I ['təːnˌouvə] *n* 1) оборо́т (*товаров, средств*); labour ~ теку́честь рабо́чей си́лы; 2) опроки́дывание; 3) пиро́г *или* торт с на́чинкой.

turnover II *a* отложно́й (*о воротнике*).

turnpike ['təːnpaɪk] *n* 1) заста́ва (*где взимается сбор*); 2) *амер.* больша́я доро́га, больша́к.

turn-round ['təːnraund] *n* оборо́т су́дна (*время разгрузки и новой погрузки в порту*).

turn-screw ['təːnskruː] *n* отвёртка.

turnstile ['təːnstaɪl] *n* турнике́т.

turn-table ['tə:n,teɪbl] *n* 1) ж.-д. поворо́тный круг; 2) диск (*патефо́на*).

turn-up ['tə:n'ʌp] *n* 1) шум, суматóха; 2) неожи́данное появле́ние; 3) отворóт (*брюк*).

turpentine ['tə:pəntaɪn] *n* скипида́р.

turpitude ['tə:pɪtjuːd] *n* ни́зость; позóрное поведе́ние.

turps [tə:ps] *n разг.* скипида́р.

turquoise ['tə:kwɑːz] *n* 1) бирюза́; 2) *attr* бирюзóвый.

turret ['tʌrɪt] *n* 1) ба́шенка; 2) *воен.* ба́шня (*орудийная или пулемётная*); *ав.* туре́ль; 3) *attr* ба́шенный.

turtle[1] ['tə:tl] *n см.* turtle-dove.

turtle[2] *n* черепа́ха; ◊ to turn ~ опроки́нуть(-ся); пойти́ ко дну.

turtle-dove ['tə:tldʌv] *n* гóрлица.

tusk I [tʌsk] *n* клык, би́вень.

tusk II *v* ра́нить клыкóм.

tussle I ['tʌsl] *n* борьба́; дра́ка.

tussle II *v* боро́ться; дра́ться.

tussock ['tʌsək] *n* 1) трава́, расту́щая пучкóм; кóчка; 2) хохолóк.

tussore ['tʌsɔ:] *n* 1) туссóр (*шёлк*); 2) шелкови́чный червь.

tut I [tʌt] *v* выража́ть нетерпе́ние, досáду *или* неодобре́ние (*восклица́нием*).

tut II *int* восклица́ние, выражающее нетерпе́ние, досаду или неодобре́ние.

tutelage ['tjuːtɪlɪdʒ] *n* 1) опеку́нство; опéка; 2) нахожде́ние под опéкой; 3) обуче́ние.

tutelar ['tjuːtɪlə] *см.* tutelary.

tutelary ['tjuːtɪlərɪ] *a* 1) опеку́нский; 2) охраня́ющий; опека́ющий.

tutor I ['tjuːtə] *n* 1) дома́шний учи́тель; репети́тор; self-help ~ самоучи́тель; 2) руководи́тель гру́ппы студе́нтов (*в университе́те, колле́дже*); 3) *юр.* опеку́н.

tutor II *v* 1) обуча́ть, дава́ть урóки; 2) наставля́ть; to ~ oneself сде́рживать себя́.

tutoress ['tjuːtərɪs] *n* 1) наста́вница, воспита́тельница; учи́тельница; 2) *юр.* опеку́нша.

tutorial [tjuː'tɔːrɪəl] *a* 1) наста́внический; 2) опеку́нский.

tutorship ['tjuːtəʃɪp] *n* дóлжность, обя́занности учи́теля, наста́вника, опекуна́.

tuxedo [tʌk'siːdou] *n амер.* смóкинг.

twaddle I ['twɔdl] *n* болтовня́, пустослóвие.

twaddle II *v* болта́ть, пустослóвить.

twain [tweɪn] *n уст.* два, двóе; па́ра; in ~ на́двое, попола́м; на ча́сти, на куски́.

twang I [twæŋ] *n* 1) ре́зкий звеня́щий звук (*натянутой струны и т. п.*); 2) гнуса́вый гóлос, гóвор.

twang II *v* 1) звене́ть (*как натянутая струна*); 2) гнуса́вить.

'twas [twɔz] *разг.* = it was.

tweak I [twiːk] *n* щипóк.

tweak II *v* ущипну́ть.

tweed [twiːd] *n* 1) твид (*материя*); 2) костю́м из тви́да.

tweedledum ['twiːdl'dʌm] *n:* ~ and tweedledee двойники́.

'tween [twiːn] *разг.* = between.

tweeny ['twiːnɪ] *n разг.* служа́нка, помога́ющая други́м слу́гам.

tweet I [twiːt] *n* щéбет, чири́канье (*птиц*).

tweet II *v* щебета́ть, чири́кать.

tweezers ['twiːzəz] *n pl* пинцéт.

twelfth I [twelfθ] *num* двена́дцатый.

twelfth II *n* двена́дцатая часть.

twelve [twelv] *num* двена́дцать.

twelvemonth ['twelvmʌnθ] *n* год, 12 мéсяцев.

twelver ['twelvə] *n сленг* ши́ллинг.

twenties ['twentɪz] *n pl* (the ~) 1) двадца́тые гóды; от 19 до 30 лет.

twentieth I ['twentɪɪθ] *num* двадца́тый.

twentieth II *n* двадца́тая часть.

twenty ['twentɪ] *num* два́дцать.

'twere [twə:] *разг.* = it were.

twerp [twə:p] *n сленг* грубия́н.

twice [twaɪs] *adv* два́жды; вдвóе; ~ two is four два́жды два — четы́ре; ~ as good вдвóе лу́чше.

twiddle ['twɪdl] *v* 1) верте́ть (*в рука́х*); 2) безде́льничать.

twig[1] [twɪg] *n* вéточка, пру́тик; ◊ to hop the ~ внеза́пно умере́ть.

twig[2] *v разг.* 1) понима́ть; 2) внима́тельно наблюда́ть, замеча́ть, ула́вливать.

twilight I ['twaɪlaɪt] *n* су́мерки; су́мрак.

twilight II *a* су́меречный, нея́сный.

twill I [twɪl] *n* са́ржа, твил.

twill II *v* ткать са́ржу, твил.

'twill [twɪl] *разг.* = it will.

twin I [twɪn] *n* 1) *обыкн. pl* близнецы́; двóйня; 2) двойни́к; 3) па́рная вещь.

twin II *a* двойнóй; состоя́щий из двух часте́й; па́рный; сдвóенный, спа́ренный.

twine I [twaɪn] *n* 1) бечёвка, шпага́т; 2) круче́ние, скру́чивание.

twine II *v* 1) вить; сплета́ть, свива́ть; плести́; 2) ви́ться, обвива́ться.

twin-engined ['twɪn'endʒɪnd] *a* двухмотóрный (*о самолёте*).

twiner ['twaɪnə] *n* вьюнóк, вью́щееся расте́ние.

twinge I [twɪndʒ] *n* при́ступ бóли; ~s of conscience угрызéния сóвести.

twinge II *v* чу́вствовать *или* вызыва́ть óструю боль.

twinkle I ['twɪŋkl] *n* 1) сверка́ние, мерца́ние; мига́ние; 2) мелька́ние; 3) блеск в глаза́х; a mischievous ~ in the eyes озорны́е и́скорки в глаза́х.

twinkle II *v* 1) мерца́ть, сверка́ть; мига́ть; 2) мелька́ть.

twinkling ['twɪŋklɪŋ] *n* 1) мгновéние; in a ~ в однó мгновéние; in the ~ of an eye в мгновéние óка; 2) мерца́ние.

twirl I [twə:l] *n* 1) враще́ние; круче́ние; 2) вихрь, вихревóе движе́ние.

twirl II *v* 1) верте́ть; кружи́ть (*в танце*); 2) крути́ть.

twist I [twɪst] *n* 1) изги́б, поворóт; кривизна́; 2) кручёная нить; шнур; верёвка; 3) круче́ние, скру́чивание; суче́ние; 4) твист (*танец*); 5) витóй хлеб; 6) искривле́ние; искаже́ние; ~ of the tongue косноязы́чие; 7) вы́вих; 8) (*стра́нная*) осóбенность; 9) *разг.* хорóший аппети́т; 10) *тех.* шаг винтовóй наре́зки, ход (*винта*); ◊ ~ of the wrist лóвкость рук, провóрство, сноро́вка.

twist II *v* 1) вить, свива́ть; сплета́ть; 2) ви́ться, извива́ться; 3) крути́ть, скру́чивать; сучи́ть; 4) вертёть, повора́чивать; 5) искажа́ть; искривля́ть; вывора́чивать; 6) изгиба́ть(ся); 7) *разг.* выду́мывать, «накру́чивать»; 8) обма́нывать.

twister ['twɪstə] *n* 1) сучи́льщик; 2) сучи́льная маши́на; 3) шёнкель; 4) *разг.* вы́думка, ложь, преувеличе́ние; 5) *разг.* обма́нщик, лгун; 6) тру́дная зада́ча.

twit I [twɪt] *n* 1) упрёк; 2) насме́шка; ко́лкость; «шпи́лька».

twit II *v* 1) упрека́ть, попрека́ть; 2) насмеха́ться, говори́ть ко́лкости; поддра́знивать.

twitch I [twɪtʃ] *n* 1) подёргивание, су́дорога; 2) дёрганье.

twitch II *v* 1) дёргать(ся); подёргиваться; 2) выдёргивать (*from*); тащи́ть (*за что-л.*— *at*).

twitter I ['twɪtə] *n* 1) щебет, чири́канье; 2) возбужде́ние, волне́ние; in a ~ трепеща́, в возбужде́нии.

twitter II *v* 1) щебета́ть, чири́кать; 2) дрожа́ть, трепета́ть от волне́ния.

two I [tuː] *num* два; ~ and ~, ~ by ~ по́ двое, попа́рно; in ~ a) на́двое, попола́м; б) врозь, отде́льно; ◊ to be ~ a) расходи́ться во мне́ниях; б) быть в ссо́ре; в) находи́ться в противоре́чии; to put ~ and ~ together сде́лать вы́вод, сообрази́ть что к чему́.

two II *n* два; дво́йка, па́ра; дво́е; in ~ twos *разг.* неме́дленно, в два счёта.

two-decker ['tuːˈdekə] *n* двухпа́лубное су́дно.

two-edged ['tuːˈedʒd] *a* обоюдоо́стрый.

two-engined ['tuːˈendʒɪnd] *a* двухмото́рный.

two-faced ['tuːfeɪst] *a* двули́чный.

twofold I ['tuːfould] *a* двойно́й, удво́енный, двукра́тный.

twofold II *adv* вдво́е; вдвойне́.

two-handed ['tuːˈhændɪd] *a* 1) двуру́чный (*о мече*); 2) для двои́х (*об игре*).

two-leaved ['tuːˈliːvd] *a* двуство́рчатый (*о двери и т. п.*).

two-man ['tuːmən] *a* двухме́стный.

two-master ['tuːˌmɑːstə] *n* двухма́чтовое су́дно.

twopence ['tʌpəns] *n* (моне́та в) два пе́нса.

twopenny ['tʌpnɪ] *a* двухпе́нсовый; *перен.* дешёвый, дрянно́й, него́дный.

twopenny II *n* дешёвое пи́во.

two-ply ['tuːplaɪ] *a* двойно́й; двусло́йный.

two-seater ['tuːˈsiːtə] *n* двухме́стный автомоби́ль, самолёт.

two-sided ['tuːˈsaɪdɪd] *a* двусторо́нний.

'twould [twud] *разг.* = it would.

tycoon [taɪˈkuːn] *n* *амер. разг.* промы́шленный магна́т.

tyke [taɪk] *n* 1) дворня́жка; 2) *разг.* гру́бый, неотёсанный челове́к.

tympanum ['tɪmpənəm] *n* (*pl* тж. tympana ['tɪmpənə]) *анат.* 1) бараба́нная перепо́нка; 2) сре́днее у́хо.

type I [taɪp] *n* 1) тип; типи́чный образе́ц *или* представи́тель; 2) си́мвол; прообраз; 3) *полигр.* ли́тера; шрифт; in black (*или* bold, fat) ~ жи́рным шрифтом.

type II *v* писа́ть на маши́нке.

typescript I ['taɪpskrɪpt] *n* ру́копись на маши́нке.

typescript II *a* машинопи́сный.

type-setter ['taɪpˌsetə] *n* 1) набо́рщик; 2) лино́тип.

type-setting ['taɪpˈsetɪŋ] *n полигр.* 1) набо́р (*процесс*); 2) *attr* набо́рный.

typewrite ['taɪpraɪt] *v* писа́ть на маши́нке.

typewriter ['taɪpˌraɪtə] *n* 1) пи́шущая маши́нка; 2) *редко см.* typist.

typewriting ['taɪpˌraɪtɪŋ] *n* 1) перепи́ска на маши́нке; 2) машинопись.

typewritten ['taɪpˌrɪtn] *a* машинопи́сный, напеча́танный на маши́нке.

typhoid I ['taɪfɔɪd] *n* брюшно́й тиф.

typhoid II *a* тифо́зный.

typhoon [taɪˈfuːn] *n* тайфу́н.

typhous ['taɪfəs] *a* тифо́зный.

typhus ['taɪfəs] *n* сыпно́й тиф.

typical ['tɪpɪkəl] *a* типи́чный, типи́ческий.

typify ['tɪpɪfaɪ] *v* служи́ть типи́чным приме́ром, образцо́м.

typing ['taɪpɪŋ] *n* перепи́ска на маши́нке.

typist ['taɪpɪst] *n* машини́стка.

typographer [taɪˈpɔgrəfə] *n* печа́тник.

typographic(al) [ˌtaɪpəˈgræfɪk(əl)] *a* типогра́фский; книгопеча́тный.

typography [taɪˈpɔgrəfɪ] *n* книгопеча́тание, полиграфи́я.

tyrannical [tɪˈrænɪkəl] *a* тирани́ческий.

tyrannize ['tɪrənaɪz] *v* тира́нить; тира́нствовать.

tyranny ['tɪrənɪ] *n* 1) тирани́я; деспоти́зм; 2) тира́нство; жесто́кость.

tyrant ['taɪərənt] *n* тира́н; де́спот.

tyre I, II ['taɪə] *см.* tire[1] I, II.

tyro ['taɪərou] *см.* tiro.

tzar [zɑː] *см.* czar.

Tzigane I [tsɪˈgɑːn] *n* цыга́н; цыга́нка.

Tzigane II *a* цыга́нский.

U

U, u [juː] *n* 21-я бу́ква англ. алфави́та.

ubiquitous [juːˈbɪkwɪtəs] *a* вездесу́щий.

U-boat ['juːbout] *n* герма́нская подво́дная ло́дка.

udder ['ʌdə] *n* вы́мя.

uglify ['ʌglɪfaɪ] *v* уро́довать, обезобра́живать.

ugly ['ʌglɪ] *a* 1) безобра́зный; 2) га́дкий, проти́вный; 3) угрожа́ющий, опа́сный; 4) зло́бный, серди́тый (*о выражении лица, взгляде*).

uhlan ['uːlɑːn] *n* ула́н.

Ukrainian I [juːˈkreɪnjən] *n* 1) украи́нец; украи́нка; the ~s украи́нцы; 2) украи́нский язы́к.

Ukrainian II *a* украи́нский.

ukulele [ˌjuːkəˈleɪlɪ] *n* гава́йская гита́ра.

ulcer ['ʌlsə] *n* я́зва.

ulcerate ['ʌlsəreɪt] *v* 1) изъязвля́ть; 2) покрыва́ться я́звами; 3) губи́ть, по́ртить.

ulcered ['ʌlsəd] *a* изъязвлённый; я́звенный.

ullage ['ʌlɪdʒ] *n* уте́чка.

ulna ['ʌlnə] *n* (*pl* ulnae ['ʌlniː]) локтева́я кость.

ulster ['ʌlstə] *n* дли́нное свобо́дное пальто́.

ulterior [ʌlˈtɪərɪə] *a* 1) отдалённый, лежа́щий по ту сто́рону; 2) скры́тый, нея́сный, неви́дный.

ultimate ['ʌltɪmɪt] *a* 1) после́дний; коне́чный; оконча́тельный; 2) преде́льный; максима́льный, кра́йний; 3) основно́й.

ultimately [ˈʌltɪmɪtlɪ] *adv* 1) в коне́чном счёте, в конце́ концо́в; 2) оконча́тельно.

ultimatum [ˌʌltɪˈmeɪtəm] *n* ультима́тум.

ultimo [ˈʌltɪmou] *adv* истёкшего ме́сяца.

ultra I [ˈʌltrə] *n* челове́к кра́йних взгля́дов, у́льтра, фана́тик.

ultra II *a* кра́йний.

ultra- [ˈʌltrə-] *pref* ультра-; сверх-; кра́йне.

ultrasonic [ˈʌltrəˈsɔnɪk] *a* сверхзвуково́й.

ultrasound [ˈʌltrəˈsaund] *n* ультразву́к.

ultra-violet [ˈʌltrəˈvaɪəlɪt] *a* ультрафиоле́товый.

umber I [ˈʌmbə] *n* у́мбра (*краска*).

umber II *a* кори́чневый.

umbrage [ˈʌmbrɪdʒ] *n* 1) оби́да; чу́вство оби́ды; to give ~ оби́деть; to take ~ оби́деться (*на — at*); 2) *поэт.* тень; сень.

umbrageous [ʌmˈbreɪdʒəs] *a* 1) оби́дчивый; 2) тени́стый.

umbrella [ʌmˈbrelə] *n* 1) зо́нт(ик); 2) *разг.* параш́ют.

umbrella-stand [ʌmˈbreləstænd] *n* подста́вка для зо́нтиков.

umbrella-tree [ʌmˈbrelətriː] *n* североамерика́нская магно́лия.

umiak [ˈuːmɪæk] *n* эскимо́сская ло́дка из шкур.

umlaut [ˈumlaut] *n лингв.* умля́ут.

umpire I [ˈʌmpaɪə] *n* 1) посре́дник, трете́йский судья́; 2) *спорт.* судья́.

umpire II *v* быть посре́дником, судьёй.

umpteen [ˈʌmptiːn] *a разг.* мно́го.

un- [ʌn-] *pref* 1) с гл. *обозначает действие, обратное тому, которое выражено простым гл.*: to unbutton расстёгивать; to undress раздева́ться; to undo распоро́ть; 2) *с гл., образованными от сущ., выражает устранение того, что выражено в сущ.*: to unbonnet обнажа́ть го́лову (*в знак приветствия*); to unleash спусти́ть с це́пи (*собаку*); 3) *прил. и образованным от них сущ. и наречиям придаёт значение, обратное значению простого прил.; по-русски чаще всего передаётся приставками не- и без-;* unarmed невооружённый; uncultivated невозде́ланный; unmerciful безжа́лостный; 4) *сущ. придаёт отриц. значение:* unemployment безрабо́тица; unsuccess неуда́ча.

unabashed [ˈʌnəˈbæʃt] *a* 1) (ничу́ть) не смути́вшийся, не растеря́вшийся; 2) ни ка́пли не испуга́вшийся.

unable [ʌnˈeɪbl] *a* не могу́щий, не уме́ющий, неспосо́бный; to be ~ не быть в состоя́нии.

unabridged [ˈʌnəˈbrɪdʒd] *a* по́лный, без сокраще́ний.

unacceptable [ˈʌnəkˈseptəbl] *a* неприе́млемый; нежела́тельный.

unaccomplished [ˈʌnəˈkɒmplɪʃt] *a* 1) незако́нченный, незавершённый; 2) неотёсанный.

unaccountable [ˈʌnəˈkauntəbl] *a* 1) необъясни́мый, безотчётный; 2) безотве́тственный.

unaccustomed [ˈʌnəˈkʌstəmd] *a* 1) не привы́кший (*к чему-л. — to*); 2) необы́чный; непривы́чный.

unachievable [ˈʌnəˈtʃiːvəbl] *a* недостижи́мый.

unacknowledged [ˈʌnəkˈnɔlɪdʒd] *a* 1) непри́знанный; незаме́ченный; 2) оста́вшийся без отве́та (*о письме и т. п.*).

unadvised [ˈʌnədˈvaɪzd] *a* поспе́шный, неблагоразу́мный, неосмотри́тельный.

unadvisedly [ˈʌnədˈvaɪzɪdlɪ] *adv* неблагоразу́мно, необду́манно, неосмотри́тельно.

unaffected[a] [ˈʌnəˈfektɪd] *a* незатро́нутый, непострада́вший.

unaffected[b] [ˈʌnəˈfektɪd] *a* и́скренний, непосре́дственный, просто́й.

unaided [ʌnˈeɪdɪd] *a* 1) без по́мощи, без подде́ржки; самостоя́тельный; 2) невооружённый (*о глазе*).

unalloyed [ˈʌnəˈlɔɪd] *a* 1) беспри́месный, чи́стый; 2) неомрачённый.

unalterable [ʌnˈɔːltərəbl] *a* неизме́нный.

unamendable [ˈʌnəˈmendəbl] *a* неисправи́мый; непоправи́мый.

un-American [ˈʌnəˈmerɪkən] *a* антиамерика́нский.

unanimity [ˌjuːnəˈnɪmɪtɪ] *n* единоду́шие.

unanimous [juːˈnænɪməs] *a* единоду́шный, единогла́сный.

unannounced [ˈʌnəˈnaunst] *a* без объявле́ния; без доклада.

unanticipated [ˈʌnænˈtɪsɪpeɪtɪd] *a* непредусмо́тренный, непредви́денный.

unappeasable [ˈʌnəˈpiːzəbl] *a* неутоли́мый; *перен. тж.* непримири́мый (*о вражде и т. п.*).

unapproachable [ˌʌnəˈproutʃəbl] *a* 1) непристу́пный, недосту́пный; 2) недостижи́мый; 3) несравни́мый, бесподо́бный.

unapt [ʌnˈæpt] *a* 1) неуме́лый, неспосо́бный; 2) несклонный; 3) неподходя́щий.

unarm [ʌnˈɑːm] *v* 1) разоружа́ть(ся); 2) обезору́живать.

unarmed [ʌnˈɑːmd] *a* невооружённый; безору́жный.

unartful [ʌnˈɑːtful] *a* безыску́сственный.

unasked [ʌnˈɑːskt] *a* непро́шенный.

unassuming [ˈʌnəˈsjuːmɪŋ] *a* скро́мный; непритяза́тельный.

unauthorized [ʌnˈɔːθəraɪzd] *a* 1) неразрешённый; 2) неправомо́чный.

unavailing [ˈʌnəˈveɪlɪŋ] *a* бесполе́зный; безуспе́шный, тще́тный.

unavoidable [ˌʌnəˈvɔɪdəbl] *a* неизбе́жный, немину́емый.

unaware I [ˈʌnəˈwɛə] *a predic* не зна́ющий, не подозрева́ющий чего-л.; to be ~ of ничего́ не знать о чём-л.

unaware II *adv см.* unawares.

unawares [ˈʌnəˈweəz] *adv* 1) неожи́данно, без предупрежде́ния; to take (*или* to catch) ~ засти́гнуть враспло́х; 2) неча́янно, неумы́шленно; не сознава́я, не отдава́я себе́ отчёта.

unbaked [ˈʌnˈbeɪkt] *a* 1) невы́печенный; *перен. разг.* незре́лый, неопери́вшийся; 2) без чьей-л. подде́ржки.

unbalanced [ʌnˈbælənst] *a* неуравнове́шенный (*о человеке, характере*).

unbar [ʌnˈbɑː] *v* отпира́ть; открыва́ть (*тж. перен.*).

unbearable [ʌnˈbɛərəbl] *a* невыноси́мый.

unbecoming [ˈʌnbɪˈkʌmɪŋ] *a* 1) неподходя́щий; не к лицу́; 2) неприли́чный; неуме́стный.

unbelief [ˈʌnbɪˈliːf] *n* неве́рие.

unbelievable [ˌʌnbɪˈliːvəbl] *a* невероя́тный.

unbend [ʌnˈbend] *v* (*past, p. p.* unbent) 1) выпрямля́ть(ся); 2) дава́ть о́тдых; ослабля́ть напряжéние; 3) вести себя непринуждённо, приветливо.

unbending [ʌnˈbendɪŋ] *a* 1) негнущийся; 2) несгибаемый, непреклонный; 3) простой, непринуждённый.

unbent [ʌnˈbent] *past, p. p. см.* unbend.

unbeseeming [ˌʌnbɪˈsiːmɪŋ] *a* неприличный, неуместный.

unbias(s)ed [ʌnˈbaɪəst] *a* беспристрастный.

unbidden [ʌnˈbɪdn] *a* 1) непрошенный, незваный; 2) добровольный.

unbind [ʌnˈbaɪnd] *v* (*past, p. p.* unbound) 1) развязывать; 2) распускать (*волосы и т. п.*); 3) освобождать (*от обязательств и т. п.*).

unbleached [ʌnˈbliːtʃt] *a* небелёный, суровый (*о холсте*).

unblemished [ʌnˈblemɪʃt] *a* безупречный; незапятнанный.

unblessed [ʌnˈblest] *a* злополучный, несчастный.

unblushing [ʌnˈblʌʃɪŋ] *a* бесстыдный, беззастенчивый, наглый.

unborn [ʌnˈbɔːn] *a* ещё не родившийся; ещё не существующий; будущий.

unbosom [ʌnˈbuzəm] *v* открывать (*тайну*); изливать (*чувства*); to ~ oneself to smb. открывать свою душу кому-л.

unbound [ʌnˈbaund] *past, p. p. см.* unbind.

unbounded [ʌnˈbaundɪd] *a* безграничный, беспредельный; безмерный.

unbridled [ʌnˈbraɪdld] *a* необузданный; разнузданный; распущенный.

unbroken [ʌnˈbroukən] *a* 1) целый, неразбитый; 2) непрерывный; ненарушенный; 3) необъезженный (*о лошади*).

unbuckle [ʌnˈbʌkl] *v* расстёгивать (*пряжку, застёжку*).

unburden [ʌnˈbɜːdn] *v* снимать бремя, тяжесть; облегчать (*душу*); to ~ oneself отвести душу.

unbutton [ʌnˈbʌtn] *v* расстёгивать (*пуговицы*).

uncalled-for [ʌnˈkɔːldfɔː] *a* 1) непрошенный, незваный; нежеланный; 2) неуместный; ничем не вызванный.

uncanny [ʌnˈkænɪ] *a* жуткий; таинственный; страшный.

uncap [ʌnˈkæp] *v* 1) снимать крышку, открывать; 2) снимать шляпу; 3) *воен.* вынимать капсюль.

uncared-for [ʌnˈkɛədfɔː] *a* заброшенный.

uncase [ʌnˈkeɪs] *v* вынимать из ящика, футляра, чехла; снимать чехол (*с чего-л.*); распаковывать.

unceasing [ʌnˈsiːsɪŋ] *a* непрекращающийся, непрерывный; непрестанный.

uncertain [ʌnˈsɜːtn] *a* 1) точно не известный, неопределённый; 2) ненадёжный, изменчивый; 3) неуверенный, сомневающийся.

uncertainty [ʌnˈsɜːtntɪ] *n* 1) неуверенность; сомнения; 2) ненадёжность; неустойчивость; 3) неизвестность, неопределённость.

unchain [ʌnˈtʃeɪn] *v* 1) спускать с цепи; 2) освобождать (*от цепей, оков, рабства*).

uncivil [ʌnˈsɪvl] *a* невоспитанный; грубый, невежливый.

unclasp [ʌnˈklɑːsp] *v* 1) отстёгивать (*пряжку и т. п.*); 2) разжимать (*объятия*); выпускать (*из рук*).

uncle [ʌŋkl] *n* 1) дядя; 2) *шутл.* ростовщик; ◊ Uncle Sam *разг.* дядя Сэм, Соединённые Штаты.

unclean [ʌnˈkliːn] *a* грязный; нечистый, дурной.

unclose [ʌnˈklouz] *v* открывать(ся).

uncoil [ʌnˈkɔɪl] *v* разматывать(ся); раскручивать(ся).

uncoined [ʌnˈkɔɪnd] *a* 1) нечеканный; 2) непритворный, подлинный.

uncomfortable [ʌnˈkʌmfətəbl] *a* 1) неудобный, неприятный; 2) испытывающий неудобство; стеснённый.

uncomfortably [ʌnˈkʌmfətəblɪ] *adv* 1) неудобно, неловко; 2) с неудовольствием, недовольно.

uncommon I [ʌnˈkɔmən] *a* необыкновенный, редкий, замечательный.

uncommon II *adv разг.* очень, чрезвычайно.

uncompromising [ʌnˈkɔmprəmaɪzɪŋ] *a* не идущий на компромиссы; непреклонный, стойкий.

unconcern [ˌʌnkənˈsɜːn] *n* 1) беззаботность; 2) равнодушие, безразличие.

unconcerned [ˌʌnkənˈsɜːnd] *a* 1) беззаботный; ~ about smth. не думающий о чём-л.; 2) равнодушный, невозмутимый; ~ with smth. не интересующийся чем-л.; 3) непринуждённый (*о манере и т. п.*).

unconditional [ˌʌnkənˈdɪʃənl] *a* безусловный; безоговорочный.

unconditioned [ˌʌnkənˈdɪʃənd] *a* 1) неограниченный; необусловленный; неоговорённый; 2) неоспоримый; абсолютный.

unconnected [ˌʌnkəˈnektɪd] *a* 1) не связанный, отдельный; 2) не имеющий (родственных) связей; 3) бессвязный.

unconquerable [ʌnˈkɔŋkərəbl] *a* непобедимый.

unconscionable [ʌnˈkɔnʃnəbl] *a* 1) бессмысленный; чрезмерный; 2) бессовестный.

unconscious I [ʌnˈkɔnʃəs] *a* 1) бессознательный; потерявший сознание; 2) не сознающий чего-л.; 3) невольный; нечаянный.

unconscious II *n* (the ~) подсознательное.

unconstitutional [ˌʌnˌkɔnstɪˈtjuːʃənl] *a* 1) неконституционный; 2) противоречащий конституции.

unconstrained [ˌʌnkənˈstreɪnd] *a* 1) добровольный; без принуждения; 2) нерастерявшийся, спокойный.

uncontrollable [ˌʌnkənˈtrouləbl] *a* 1) не поддающийся контролю; 2) неудержимый.

uncork [ʌnˈkɔːk] *v* 1) откупоривать; 2) *разг.* давать выход, волю (*чувствам*).

uncountable [ʌnˈkauntəbl] *a* неисчислимый, бесчисленный.

uncouple [ʌnˈkʌpl] *v* разъединять; отцеплять; выключать.

uncouth [ʌnˈkuːθ] *a* 1) неуклюжий, несклáдный; грубый (*о манерах и т. п.*); 2) *редко* странный.

uncover [ʌnˈkʌvə] *v* 1) снимать крышку, покров; 2) открывать; обнажать (*голову; тж.* to ~ oneself); 3) обнаруживать, раскрывать.

unction [ʌŋkʃən] *n* 1) втирание мази; 2) мазь; 3) набожность, елейность; 4) пыл, рвение.

unctuous [ʌŋktjuəs] *a* 1) маслянистый; жирный; 2) елейный.

uncurl [ʌnˈkɜːl] *v* развиваться (*о локонах*).

undamped ['ʌn'dæmpt] *a радио* недемпфированный.

undated ['ʌn'deɪtɪd] *a* недатированный.

undaunted [ʌn'dɔːntɪd] *a* неустрашимый; бесстрашный.

undeceive ['ʌndɪ'siːv] *v* выводить из заблуждения.

undecided ['ʌndɪ'saɪdɪd] *a* 1) нерешённый, неустановленный; 2) нерешительный; 3) неясно выраженный.

undecipherable ['ʌndɪ'saɪfərəbl] *a* 1) не поддающийся расшифровке; 2) неразборчивый.

undeniable [ˌʌndɪ'naɪəbl] *a* 1) неоспоримый, несомненный; 2) великолепный, превосходный.

under I ['ʌndə] *prep* 1) *в пространственном значении указывает на:* а) *положение под данным предметом* под (*с тв. п.*); ~ a table (a tree) под столом (деревом); б) *направленность действия куда-л. вниз, ниже кого-л., чего-л.* под (*с вин. п.*); put the basket ~ the table поставь(те) корзину под стол; в) *положение одного предмета относительно другого предмета* ниже (*с род. п.*); to hit a man ~ the belt ударить человека ниже пояса; 2) *указывает на отнесение к определённой графе, рубрике и т. п.* под, к; the use of this verb goes ~ point five употребление этого глагола относится к пункту пятому; 3) *указывает на условия, при которых совершается действие* при, под, на; ~ fire под обстрелом; ~ cover под прикрытием; ~ sail под парусами; ~ heavy penalty под страхом наказания; ~ the circumstances при этих условиях; ~ consideration на рассмотрении; ~ the breath шёпотом; 4) *указывает на более низкую величину, цену, низкое качество* ниже; the child is ~ five ребёнку нет ещё пяти лет; you cannot buy this coat (hat, umbrella) ~ so many roubles (pounds) вы не можете (нельзя) купить это пальто (шляпу, зонтик) меньше, чем за столько-то рублей (фунтов стерлингов); 5) *указывает на строй, правителя, при котором происходит действие* при; ~ capitalism при капитализме; ~ Peter I при Петре I.

under II *a* 1) нижний; 2) нижестоящий; низший.

under III *adv указывает на:* 1) *более низкое положение по сравнению с другим предметом* внизу, ниже; 2) *движение вниз* вниз; 3) *с гл.* to bring, to keep, to knock, to get *и т. п. выражает ослабление действия, сведение действия к нулю:* the fire has been got ~ пожар был потушен.

under- ['ʌndə-] *pref присоединяется:* 1) *к сущ., образуя имена сущ., наречия и прил. со значением:* а) *находящийся ниже,* под; underclothes нижнее бельё; underground подземный; underwater подводный; б) *находящийся ниже по своему положению;* undersecretary заместитель министра; undergraduate студент последнего курса; 2) *к прил., гл. и производным от них со значением недостаточной степени качества или выполнения действия по сравнению с простым словом:* underripe не совсем спелый; to underestimate недооценивать; to underpay оплачивать по пониженной ставке, низко оплачивать.

underact ['ʌndər'ækt] *v* исполнять *или* играть роль слабо, блёдно.

underbade ['ʌndə'beɪd] *past см.* underbid.

underbid ['ʌndə'bɪd] *v (past* underbade, under-

bid; *p. p.* underbidden, underbid) сбивать цену, предлагать меньше (*на аукционе*).

underbidden ['ʌndə'bɪdn] *p. p. см.* underbid.

underbred ['ʌndə'bred] *a* невоспитанный, грубый.

underbrush ['ʌndəbrʌʃ] *n* подлесок; мелкий лес; кустарник.

undercarriage ['ʌndə,kærɪdʒ] *n ав.* шасси.

underclothes ['ʌndəklouðz] *n pl* нижнее бельё.

undercurrent ['ʌndə,kʌrənt] *n* низовое *или* подводное течение; *перен.* скрытая тенденция.

undercut[a] ['ʌndəkʌt] *n* 1) вырезка (*часть туши*); 2) удар снизу вверх; 3) *спорт.* подсечка.

undercut[b] ['ʌndə'kʌt] *v* 1) подрезать; 2) сбивать цену, продавать по более низкой цене (*чем конкурент*).

underdeveloped ['ʌndədɪ'veləpt] *a* недоразвитый; ~ countries слаборазвитые страны.

underdid ['ʌndə'dɪd] *past см.* underdo.

underdo ['ʌndə'duː] *v (past* underdid; *p. p.* underdone) недожаривать.

underdog ['ʌndədɔg] *n* 1) побеждённая сторона; 2) очень бедный, несчастный человек.

underdone ['ʌndə'dʌn] *p. p. см.* underdo.

underestimate[a] ['ʌndər'estɪmɪt] *n* недооценка.

underestimate[b] ['ʌndər'estɪmeɪt] *v* недооценивать.

under-expose ['ʌndərɪks'pouz] *v фото* недодержать.

underfoot [ˌʌndə'fut] *adv* под ногами, на земле.

undergo [ˌʌndə'gou] *v (past* underwent; *p. p.* undergone) подвергаться, испытывать, переносить.

undergone [ˌʌndə'gɔn] *p. p. см.* undergo.

undergraduate [ˌʌndə'grædjuɪt] *n* студент последнего курса.

underground[a] I ['ʌndəgraund] *n* (the ~) метрополитен.

underground[a] II *a* подземный; *перен.* подпольный; тайный.

underground[b] [ˌʌndə'graund] *adv* под землёй; *перен.* подпольно; тайно; нелегально.

undergrowth ['ʌndəgrouθ] *n* подлесок; подрост.

underhand I ['ʌndəhænd] *a* тайный, закулисный.

underhand II *adv* тайно, за спиной.

underlaid [ˌʌndə'leɪd] *past, p. p. см.* underlay[2].

underlain [ˌʌndə'leɪn] *p. p. см.* underlie.

underlay[1] [ˌʌndə'leɪ] *past см.* underlie.

underlay[2] *v (past, p. p.* underlaid) подкладывать; подпирать.

underlie [ˌʌndə'laɪ] *v (past* underlay; *p. p.* underlain) 1) лежать под чем-л.; находиться внизу; 2) лежать в основе (*чего-л.*); крыться (*под чем-л.*).

underline[a] ['ʌndəlaɪn] *n* 1) подпись под рисунком, чертежом (*в книге*); 2) *театр.* анонс о готовящейся постановке (*внизу афиши*); 3) *полигр.* линия, подчёркивающая слово.

underline[b] [ˌʌndə'laɪn] *v* подчёркивать.

underling ['ʌndəlɪŋ] *n обыкн. презр.* мелкая сошка, мелкий чиновник.

underlying [ˌʌndə'laɪɪŋ] *a* 1) основной; 2) расположенный внизу.

undermentioned [ˌʌndə'menʃənd] *a* нижеупомянутый.

undermine [ˌʌndə'maɪn] *v* 1) подкапывать; делать подкоп; 2) минировать; 3) подмывать (*берег*); 4) разрушать, подрывать.

undermost [ˈʌndəmoust] *a* ˋ1) самый нижний; 2) низший.

underneath I [ˌʌndəˈniːθ] *adv* 1) внизу, вниз; 2) в основе.

underneath II *prep* под.

underpaid [ˈʌndəˈpeɪd] *past, p. p. см.* underpay.

underpass [ˈʌndəpɑːs] *n амер.* подземный переход, тоннель.

underpay [ˈʌndəˈpeɪ] *v* (*past, p. p.* underpaid) низко оплачивать, оплачивать по пониженной ставке.

underpopulated [ˈʌndəˈpɔpjuleɪtɪd] *a* малонаселённый.

underrate [ˌʌndəˈreɪt] *v* недооценивать; преуменьшать.

under-secretary [ˈʌndəˈsekrətərɪ] *n* товарищ *или* заместитель министра (*в Англии и США*).

undershirt [ˈʌndəʃəːt] *n* нижняя рубашка.

undersign [ˌʌndəˈsaɪn] *v* подписывать(ся), ставить свою подпись.

undersigned [ˌʌndəˈsaɪnd] *n* (the ~) нижеподписавшийся.

undersized [ˈʌndəˈsaɪzd] *a* 1) недостаточного размера; карликовый; 2) *воен.* низкорослый.

understaffed [ˈʌndəˈstɑːft] *a* неукомплектованный (*штатами*).

understand [ˌʌndəˈstænd] *v* (*past, p. p.* understood) 1) понимать; to give smb. to ~ дать кому́-л. понять; намекнуть; to make oneself understood объясниться; 2) знать основательно; иметь правильное представление; 3) узнавать (*что-л., о чём-л.— that*); 4) предполагать, догадываться; 5) подразумевать; 6) уметь; смыслить, быть знатоком в чём-л.; 7) уславливаться.

understandable [ˌʌndəˈstændəbl] *a* (вполне) понятный, ясный.

understanding I [ˌʌndəˈstændɪŋ] *n* 1) понимание, разумение; a clear ~ of the problem ясное понимание задачи, вопроса; 2) разум, рассудок; способность понять; 3) взаимопонимание, согласие; mutual ~ взаимопонимание; good ~, right ~ доброе, полное согласие; bad ~, ill ~ взаимное непонимание, несогласие; 4) соглашение; on the ~ that при условии, что; предполагая, что; to come to an ~ прийти к соглашению; 5) *pl шутл.* ноги.

understanding II *a* 1) разумный, толковый, способный; 2) чуткий; отзывчивый.

understate [ˈʌndəˈsteɪt] *v* 1) преуменьшать; 2) замалчивать; не высказывать открыто.

understatement [ˈʌndəˈsteɪtmənt] *n* 1) преуменьшение; 2) замалчивание.

understood [ˌʌndəˈstud] *past, p. p. см.* understand.

understrapper [ˈʌndəˌstræpə] *см.* underling.

understudy I [ˈʌndəˌstʌdɪ] *n театр.* дублёр.

understudy II *v театр.* дублировать.

undertake [ˌʌndəˈteɪk] *v* (*past* undertook; *p. p.* undertaken) 1) предпринимать; 2) брать на себя; обязываться; 3) ручаться.

undertaken [ˌʌndəˈteɪkən] *p. p. см.* undertake.

undertaker[a] [ˌʌndəˈteɪkə] *n* предприниматель.

undertaker[b] [ˈʌndəˌteɪkə] *n* содержатель похоронного бюро; гробовщик.

undertaking[a] [ˌʌndəˈteɪkɪŋ] *n* 1) предприятие; 2) обязательство.

undertaking[b] [ˈʌndəˌteɪkɪŋ] *n* 1) похоронное бюро; 2) обслуживание похорон.

under-tenant [ˈʌndəˈtenənt] *n* субарендатор.

undertone [ˈʌndətoun] *n* 1) полутон (*звука, цвета*); to speak (to talk) in ~s говорить (разговаривать) вполголоса; 2) оттенок (*цвета и т. п.*).

undertook [ˌʌndəˈtuk] *past см.* undertake.

undervalue [ˈʌndəˈvæljuː] *v* недооценивать.

underwear [ˈʌndəwɛə] *n* нижнее бельё.

underwent [ˌʌndəˈwent] *past см.* undergo.

underwood [ˈʌndəwud] *n* подлесок; подрост.

underworld [ˈʌndəwəːld] *n* 1) преисподняя; 2) подонки общества; преступный мир.

underwrite [ˈʌndəraɪt] *v* (*past* underwrote; *p. p.* underwritten) 1) подписывать(ся); 2) страховать.

underwriter [ˈʌndəˌraɪtə] *n амер. разг.* страховщик.

underwritten I [ˈʌndəˌrɪtn] *p. p. см.* underwrite.

underwritten II *a* 1) нижеподписавшийся; 2) нижеизложенный.

underwrote [ˈʌndərout] *past см.* underwrite.

underservedly [ˈʌndɪˈzəːvɪdlɪ] *adv* незаслуженно.

undesignedly [ˈʌndɪˈzaɪnɪdlɪ] *adv* неумышленно.

undesirable [ˈʌndɪˈzaɪərəbl] *a* 1) нежелательный; неприятный; 2) неподходящий.

undetermined [ˈʌndɪˈtəːmɪnd] *a* 1) неопределённый; неопределённый; 2) нерешительный.

undeveloped [ˈʌndɪˈveləpt] *a* неразвитой, недоразвитый.

undid [ʌnˈdɪd] *past. см.* undo.

undies [ˈʌndɪz] *n pl разг.* женское бельё.

undisguised [ˈʌndɪsˈgaɪzd] *a* незамаскированный; явный; открытый, откровенный.

undisposed [ˈʌndɪsˈpouzd] *a* 1) нерасположенный (*к — to*); 2) нераспределённый, непроданный (*об имуществе и т. п.*).

undisputed [ˈʌndɪsˈpjuːtɪd] *a* бесспорный, несомненный.

undistinguished [ˈʌndɪsˈtɪŋgwɪʃt] *a* ничем не замечательный, незаметный.

undisturbedly [ˈʌndɪsˈtəːbɪdlɪ] *adv* спокойно; безмятежно.

undo [ʌnˈduː] *v* (*past* undid; *p. p.* undone) 1) расстёгивать, развязывать; раскрывать (*пакет и т. п.*); 2) уничтожать сделанное; аннулировать; расторгать (*договор и т. п.*); what is done cannot be undone сделанного не воротишь; 3) распарывать (*шов*).

undone I [ʌnˈdʌn] *p. p. см.* undo.

undone II *a* 1) несделанный, незаконченный; неготовый; 2) погибший, загубленный; he is ~ он погиб.

undoubted [ʌnˈdautɪd] *a* несомненный, бесспорный.

undreamed-of, undreamt-of [ʌnˈdremtɔv] *a* и во сне не снившийся, неожиданный; невообразимый.

undress I [ˈʌnˈdres] *n* домашний костюм.

undress II *v* раздевать(ся).

undressed [ˈʌnˈdrest] *a* 1) неодетый; 2) невыделанный (*о коже*); 3) неперевязанный (*о ране*).

undue [ˈʌnˈdjuː] *a* 1) неуместный; несвоевременный; 2) чрезмерный.

undulate I [ˈʌndjuleɪt] *a* волнистый; волнообразный.

undulate II v 1) виться (о волосах); 2) быть холмистым (о местности); 3) волноваться, вздыматься.

undulation [ˌʌndjuˈleɪʃən] n 1) волнообразное движение; 2) волнистость; 3) неровность поверхности.

unduly [ʌnˈdjuːlɪ] adv 1) неправильно; 2) чрезмерно, чересчур.

undying [ʌnˈdaɪɪŋ] a бессмертный; вечный, нетленный.

unearned [ˈʌnˈəːnd] a незаработанный; нетрудовой (о доходе).

unearth [ˈʌnˈəːθ] v 1) вырыть, выкопать из земли; перен. раскопать, раскрыть; 2) выгнать из норы (лисицу и т. п.).

unearthly [ʌnˈəːθlɪ] a 1) неземной; сверхъестественный; 2) странный, абсурдный, крайне неподходящий.

uneasiness [ʌnˈiːzɪnɪs] n 1) неловкость; неудобство; 2) стеснённость; 3) беспокойство.

uneasy [ʌnˈiːzɪ] a 1) неловкий; неудобный; 2) смущённый, стеснённый; 3) беспокойный, встревоженный; to feel ~ a) беспокоиться; б) испытывать неловкость.

unemployed I [ˈʌnɪmˈplɔɪd] a 1) безработный; 2) незанятый; 3) неиспользованный.

unemployed II n: the ~ (употр. как pl) безработные.

unemployment [ˈʌnɪmˈplɔɪmənt] n безработица.

unending [ʌnˈendɪŋ] a нескончаемый, непрестанный.

unendurable [ˈʌnɪnˈdjuərəbl] a нестерпимый; невыносимый.

unequal [ˈʌnˈiːkwəl] a 1) неравный (по размеру, качеству и т. п.); неравноценный; 2) несправедливый, неправильный; несоответствующий.

unequalled [ˈʌnˈiːkwəld] a непревзойдённый.

unequivocal [ˈʌnɪˈkwɪvəkəl] a ясный, прямой, недвусмысленный.

unerring [ʌnˈəːrɪŋ] a безошибочный, верный; непогрешимый.

uneven [ˈʌnˈiːvən] a 1) неровный (о поверхности и т. п.); 2) неравный; 3) нечётный.

unexampled [ˌʌnɪgˈzaːmpld] a беспримерный, несравненный.

unexceptionable [ˌʌnɪkˈsepʃnəbl] a 1) безусловный; 2) совершенный.

unexpected [ˈʌnɪksˈpektɪd] a неожиданный; внезапный.

unexperienced [ˈʌnɪksˈpɪərɪənst] a неопытный.

unexploded [ˈʌnɪksˈploudɪd] a неразорвавшийся (о снаряде, бомбе).

unexplored [ˈʌnɪksˈplɔːd] a 1) неисследованный; 2) геол. неразведанный.

unfading [ʌnˈfeɪdɪŋ] a 1) неувядающий, неувядаемый; 2) нелиняющий.

unfailing [ʌnˈfeɪlɪŋ] a неизменный, верный.

unfair [ˈʌnˈfɛə] a несправедливый; нечестный.

unfaithful [ˈʌnˈfeɪθful] a неверный, вероломный; предательский.

unfaltering [ʌnˈfɔːltərɪŋ] a непоколебимый, стойкий.

unfamiliar [ˈʌnfəˈmɪljə] a 1) незнакомый, неведомый; 2) необычный, непривычный; странный; 3) не знающий; не знакомый (с чем-л.).

unfathomable [ʌnˈfæðəməbl] a 1) неизмери-

мый, бездонный; 2) непостижимый; непроницаемый (о тайне и т. п.).

unfavourable [ˈʌnˈfeɪvərəbl] a неблагоприятный; невыгодный; неудобный.

unfeeling [ʌnˈfiːlɪŋ] a 1) бесчувственный, чёрствый; 2) нечувствительный (о нерве и т. п.).

unfeigned [ʌnˈfeɪnd] a непритворный, искренний.

unfit[a] [ˈʌnˈfɪt] a не(при)годный; неподходящий.

unfit[b] [ˈʌnˈfɪt] v делать не(при)годным, портить.

unflagging [ˈʌnˈflægɪŋ] a неослабевающий, неослабный (об интересе, рвении).

unflinching [ʌnˈflɪntʃɪŋ] a непоколебимый, стойкий.

unfold [ˈʌnˈfould] v 1) развёртывать(ся); раскрывать(ся); 2) открывать (секрет, намерения).

unforeseen [ˈʌnfɔːˈsiːn] a непредвиденный.

unforgettable [ˈʌnfəˈgetəbl] a незабываемый; незабвенный.

unforgivable [ˈʌnfəˈgɪvəbl] a непростительный.

unfortunate I [ʌnˈfɔːtʃnɪt] n 1) несчастный человек, горемыка; неудачник; 2) проститутка.

unfortunate II a 1) несчастный, несчастливый; 2) неудачный, неуместный.

unfounded [ˈʌnˈfaundɪd] a неосновательный; необоснованный.

unfriendly I [ˈʌnˈfrendlɪ] a 1) недружелюбный; неприветливый; неприязненный; 2) уст. неблагоприятный.

unfriendly II adv неприязненно; неприветливо.

unfrock [ˈʌnˈfrɔk] v лишать духовного сана.

unfurl [ʌnˈfəːl] v развёртывать.

ungainly [ʌnˈgeɪnlɪ] a неуклюжий, неловкий, нескладный.

un-get-at-able [ˈʌngetˈætəbl] a недоступный.

ungloved [ˈʌnˈglʌvd] a без перчаток.

ungovernable [ʌnˈgʌvənəbl] a неукротимый, неудержимый (о смехе и т. п.).

ungrateful [ʌnˈgreɪtful] a неблагодарный.

ungrounded [ˈʌnˈgraundɪd] a 1) необоснованный, беспочвенный; 2) необученный, неподготовленный.

unguarded [ˈʌnˈgaːdɪd] a 1) незащищённый; 2) неосторожный, беспечный.

unguent [ˈʌŋgwənt] n мазь.

unhand [ʌnˈhænd] v выпускать (из рук).

unhandsome [ˈʌnˈhænsəm] a 1) некрасивый; 2) невежливый, нелюбезный; 3) неблагородный, невеликодушный.

unhandy [ʌnˈhændɪ] a 1) неудобный; 2) неловкий, неповоротливый.

unhappy [ʌnˈhæpɪ] a 1) печальный, грустный; 2) несчастный; 3) неудачный.

unhealthy [ʌnˈhelθɪ] a 1) нездоровый; болезненный; 2) вредный (для здоровья); 3) воен. разг. опасный; обстреливаемый.

unheard [ˈʌnˈhəːd] a 1) неслышный; 2) невыслушанный.

unheard-of [ʌnˈhəːdɔv] a неслыханный.

unhesitatingly [ʌnˈhezɪteɪtɪŋlɪ] adv без колебания; решительно; уверенно.

unhinge [ʌnˈhɪndʒ] v 1) снимать с петель (дверь и т. п.); 2) расстраивать, выбивать из колеи.

unholy [ʌnˈhoulɪ] a 1) нечестивый; 2) разг. безобразный, страшный (о шуме, беспорядке).

unhoused [ʌnˈhauzd] *a* бездо́мный, лишённый кро́ва.

unicorn [ˈjuːnɪkɔːn]. *n* *миф.* единоро́г.

unification [ˌjuːnɪfɪˈkeɪʃən] *n* 1) объедине́ние; 2) унифика́ция.

uniform I [ˈjuːnɪfɔːm] *n* фо́рма, фо́рменная оде́жда.

uniform II *a* 1) единообра́зный; одина́ковый; однообра́зный; 2) равноме́рный; 3) постоя́нный, неизме́нный.

uniform III *v* одева́ть в фо́рму.

uniformed [ˈjuːnɪfɔːmd] *a* оде́тый в фо́рму.

uniformity [ˌjuːnɪˈfɔːmɪtɪ] *n* единообра́зие.

unify [ˈjuːnɪfaɪ] *v* 1) объединя́ть; 2) унифици́ровать.

unilateral [ˈjuːnɪˈlætərəl] *a* односторо́нний.

unimaginable [ˌʌnɪˈmædʒɪnəbl] *a* невообрази́мый.

unimaginative [ˈʌnɪˈmædʒɪnətɪv] *a* лишённый воображе́ния.

unimpaired [ˈʌnɪmˈpɛəd] *a* нетро́нутый; незатро́нутый, непострада́вший.

unimpeachable [ˌʌnɪmˈpiːtʃəbl] *a* 1) несомне́нный; 2) безупре́чный.

unimprovable [ˈʌnɪmˈpruːvəbl] *a* 1) неисправи́мый; 2) безупре́чный, идеа́льный.

unintelligible [ˈʌnɪnˈtelɪdʒəbl] *a* непоня́тный, неразуми́тельный; неразбо́рчивый (*о почерке*).

union [ˈjuːnjən] *n* 1) сою́з; the Soviet Union Сове́тский Сою́з; 2) соедине́ние, объедине́ние; 3) профессиона́льный сою́з (*тж.* trade ~, labour ~); 4) согла́сие, еди́нство; ~ is strength в еди́нении — си́ла; in perfect ~ в по́лном согла́сии; 5) бра́чный сою́з; 6) рабо́тный дом; 7) *тех.* соедини́тельная му́фта.

unionist [ˈjuːnjənɪst] *n* 1) член профсою́за; 2) *ист.* униони́ст.

unique I [juːˈniːk] *n* у́никум.

unique II *a* 1) еди́нственный в своём ро́де; бесподо́бный, несравне́нный; 2) осо́бенный, необы́чный.

unison [ˈjuːnɪzn] *n* 1) согла́сие; in ~ согла́сно, в унисо́н; 2) *муз.* унисо́н.

unit [ˈjuːnɪt] *n* 1) едини́ца; едини́ца измере́ния; thermal ~ едини́ца теплоты́, кало́рия; 2) *воен.* во́инская часть, подразделе́ние; 3) *тех.* агрега́т; компле́кт.

unite [juːˈnaɪt] *v* 1) соединя́ть(ся); 2) объединя́ть(ся).

united [juːˈnaɪtɪd] *a* 1) соединённый; 2) объединённый; 3) дру́жный, сплочённый.

unitedly [juːˈnaɪtɪdlɪ] *adv* все вме́сте, дру́жно, объединёнными уси́лиями.

unity [ˈjuːnɪtɪ] *n* 1) еди́нство; the dramatic unities еди́нство вре́мени, ме́ста и де́йствия (*в дра́ме*); 2) едине́ние, сплочённость; согла́сие; working class ~ еди́нство, солида́рность рабо́чего кла́сса; utmost ~ по́лное еди́нство; 3) *мат.* едини́ца.

universal [ˌjuːnɪˈvəːsəl] *a* 1) всео́бщий; 2) всеми́рный; 3) универса́льный.

universe [ˈjuːnɪvəːs] *n* мир, вселе́нная.

university [ˌjuːnɪˈvəːsɪtɪ] *n* 1) университе́т; 2) *attr* университе́тский.

unjust [ˈʌnˈdʒʌst] *a* несправедли́вый.

unkempt [ˈʌnˈkempt] *a* 1) нечёсаный; 2) неопря́тный, запу́щенный.

unkind [ʌnˈkaɪnd] *a* злой, жесто́кий; недо́брый.

unknown I [ˈʌnˈnoun] *n* (the ~) 1) неизве́стное; неизве́стность; 2) незнако́мец, незнако́мка; 3) *мат.* неизве́стное, неизве́стная величина́.

unknown II *a* неизве́стный; неве́домый; незнако́мый; чу́ждый.

unknown III *adv* та́йно, без ве́дома.

unlace [ˈʌnˈleɪs] *v* расшнуро́вывать.

unlawful [ˈʌnˈlɔːful] *a* незако́нный; противозако́нный, запрещённый.

unlearned [ˈʌnˈləːnɪd] *a* 1) необразо́ванный; неве́жественный; 2) невы́ученный; незау́ченный.

unleash [ˈʌnˈliːʃ] *v* 1) спуска́ть со сво́ры; 2) развяза́ть (*войну́*).

unleavened [ˈʌnˈlevnd] *a* незаква́шенный, пре́сный.

unless [ənˈles] *conj* е́сли не, ра́зве то́лько, без того́ чтобы; I shall not do it ~ absolutely compelled я э́того не сде́лаю, е́сли не (*или* ра́зве то́лько) бу́ду вы́нужден; he never comes ~ called он никогда́ не прихо́дит без зо́ва.

unlettered [ˈʌnˈletəd] *a* 1) необразо́ванный; 2) негра́мотный.

unlike I [ˈʌnˈlaɪk] *a* непохо́жий на; не тако́й, как.

unlike II *prep* в отли́чие от.

unlikely [ʌnˈlaɪklɪ] *a* 1) маловероя́тный, неправдоподо́бный; 2) не обеща́ющий ничего́ хоро́шего.

unlimited [ʌnˈlɪmɪtɪd] *a* безграни́чный, беспреде́льный; неограни́ченный.

unload [ˈʌnˈloud] *v* 1) разгружа́ть(ся), выгружа́ть; 2) *воен.* разряжа́ть; 3) отде́лываться, избавля́ться (*от чего́-л. невы́годного*); спуска́ть (*по дешёвке*).

unlock [ˈʌnˈlɔk] *v* отпира́ть; *перен.* открыва́ть (*ду́шу*).

unlooked-for [ʌnˈluktfɔː] *a* неожи́данный, непредви́денный.

unlucky [ʌnˈlʌkɪ] *a* несчастли́вый; злополу́чный; неуда́чный.

unmanly [ˈʌnˈmænlɪ] *a* не досто́йный мужчи́ны; трусли́вый.

unmanned [ˈʌnˈmænd] *a* 1) непилоти́руемый (*о косми́ческом корабле́*), без челове́ка на борту́; 2) неукомплекто́ванный (*шта́тами*).

unmannerly [ʌnˈmænəlɪ] *a* невоспи́танный, гру́бый.

unmarried [ˈʌnˈmærɪd] *a* холосто́й, нежена́тый; незаму́жняя.

unmask [ˈʌnˈmɑːsk] *v* 1) снима́ть *или* срыва́ть ма́ску; разоблача́ть; 2) *воен.* демаски́ровать.

unmatched [ˈʌnˈmætʃt] *a* не име́ющий себе́ ра́вного, бесподо́бный.

unmeaning [ʌnˈmiːnɪŋ] *a* бессмы́сленный.

unmeant [ʌnˈment] *a* неумы́шленный; ненаме́ренный.

unmeasured [ʌnˈmeʒəd] *a* 1) неизме́ренный; 2) неизмери́мый, безме́рный.

unmindful [ʌnˈmaɪndful] *a* 1) невнима́тельный, беспе́чный; 2) *predic* не обраща́я внима́ния (*на — of*).

unmistakable [ˈʌnmɪsˈteɪkəbl] *a* я́вный, несомне́нный; безоши́бочный.

unmounted [ˈʌnˈmauntɪd] *a* 1) пе́ший; 2) без опра́вы (*о ка́мне*); без ра́мы (*о карти́не*).

unmoved [ʌn'muːvd] *a* 1) неподвижный; 2) равнодушный, бесстрастный; 3) неуязвимый, непоколебимый.

unnatural [ʌn'nætʃrəl] *a* 1) неестественный; 2) чудовищный; противоестественный.

unnavigable [ʌn'nævɪgəbl] *a* несудоходный.

unnecessary [ʌn'nesɪsərɪ] *a* ненужный, излишний.

unnerve [ʌn'nəːv] *v* лишать бодрости, присутствия духа.

unnoticed [ʌn'noutɪst] *a* 1) незамеченный; 2) незаметный; приметный.

unnumbered [ʌn'nʌmbəd] *a* несчитанный; ненумерованный; 2) неисчислимый; несметный; бесчисленный.

unobstructed [ʌnəb'strʌktɪd] *a* беспрепятственный, свободный.

unoccupied [ʌn'ɔkjupaid] *a* 1) незанятый, свободный; 2) праздный, ничем не занятый.

unoffending [ʌnə'fendɪŋ] *a* безобидный, невинный.

unofficial [ʌnə'fɪʃəl] *a* неофициальный.

unpack [ʌn'pæk] *v* распаковывать.

unpaid [ʌn'peɪd] *a* 1) неуплаченный; неоплаченный; ~ for взятый в кредит; 2) неоплатный; 3) не получающий платы.

unparalleled [ʌn'pærəleld] *a* бесподобный, беспримерный.

unpardonable [ʌn'pɑːdnəbl] *a* непростительный.

unpeople [ʌn'piːpl] *v* обезлюдить.

unpleasant [ʌn'pleznt] *a* неприятный.

unpleasantness [ʌn'plezntnɪs] *n* 1) непривлекательность; 2) неприятность; недоразумение.

unpopular [ʌn'pɔpjulə] *a* непопулярный, не пользующийся любовью.

unpractised [ʌn'præktɪst] *a* 1) неопытный, неискусный; 2) не применявшийся.

unprecedented [ʌn'presɪdəntɪd] *a* беспрецедентный, беспримерный.

unprejudiced [ʌn'predʒudɪst] *a* непредубеждённый, без предубеждения; беспристрастный.

unpremeditated [ʌnprɪ'medɪteɪtɪd] *a* непредумышленный; не обдуманный (заранее).

unpretending [ʌnprɪ'tendɪŋ] *a* без претензий, скромный.

unpretentious [ʌnprɪ'tenʃəs] *см.* unpretending.

unprincipled [ʌn'prɪnsəpld] *a* беспринципный; безнравственный.

unprintable [ʌn'prɪntəbl] *a* непечатный, нецензурный.

unprofessional [ʌnprə'feʃənl] *a* 1) непрофессиональный; 2) не имеющий профессии.

unprofitable [ʌn'prɔfɪtəbl] *a* невыгодный; нерентабельный.

unpromising [ʌn'prɔmɪsɪŋ] *a* не обещающий ничего хорошего; неутешительный.

unprovoked [ʌnprə'voukt] *a* ничем не вызванный, неспровоцированный.

unqualified[a] [ʌn'kwɔlɪfaid] *a* 1) не имеющий (соответствующей) квалификации; неподходящий; 2) *разг.* явный; резко выраженный.

unqualified[b] [ʌn'kwɔlɪfaid] *a* 1) неограниченный (условиями и т. п.); 2) безоговорочный; категорический (об отказе).

unquenchable [ʌn'kwentʃəbl] *a* 1) неугасимый; 2) неутолимый.

unquestionable [ʌn'kwestʃənəbl] *a* неоспоримый, несомненный.

unquotable [ʌn'kwoutəbl] *a* нецензурный.

unravel [ʌn'rævəl] *v* 1) распутывать (нитки и т. п.); 2) разгадывать.

unreadable [ʌn'riːdəbl] *a* 1) неразборчивый (о почерке); 2) скучный, неинтересный (для чтения).

unready [ʌn'redɪ] *a* 1) неготовый; 2) неповоротливый; медлительный.

unreal [ʌn'rɪəl] *a* 1) нереальный, воображаемый; 2) ненастоящий.

unrealizable [ʌn'rɪəlaɪzəbl] *a* неосуществимый.

unreasonable [ʌn'riːznəbl] *a* 1) неразумный, неблагоразумный; 2) непомерный; слишком высокий (о цене и т. п.).

unreasoned [ʌn'riːznd] *a* 1) непродуманный; 2) неубеждённый.

unreasoning [ʌn'riːznɪŋ] *a* 1) неразумный, не рассуждающий; 2) беспричинный (о ненависти и т. п.).

unreel [ʌn'riːl] *v* разматывать(ся).

unrelenting [ʌnrɪ'lentɪŋ] *a* безжалостный; немилосердный.

unreliable [ʌnrɪ'laɪəbl] *a* 1) ненадёжный; не заслуживающий доверия; 2) смутный (о представлении).

unremitting [ʌnrɪ'mɪtɪŋ] *a* беспрестанный; неослабный; упорный.

unreserve [ʌnrɪ'zəːv] *n* 1) откровенность; 2) несдержанность.

unreserved [ʌnrɪ'zəːvd] *a* 1) откровенный; 2) несдержанный; 3) не ограниченный (условиями, оговорками).

unrest [ʌn'rest] *n* 1) беспокойство; тревога, смятение; 2) смута; беспорядки.

unriddle [ʌn'rɪdl] *v* разгадать, объяснить.

unrip [ʌn'rɪp] *v* распарывать; разрывать.

unrivalled [ʌn'raɪvəld] *a* не знающий себе равных, бесподобный.

unroll [ʌn'roul] *v* раскрывать, развёртывать.

unruffled [ʌn'rʌfld] *a* 1) гладкий, приглаженный (о волосах и т. п.); 2) спокойный, невозмутимый.

unruly [ʌn'ruːlɪ] *a* непокорный; буйный; распущенный.

unsafe [ʌn'seɪf] *a* ненадёжный, опасный.

unsaid [ʌn'sed] *past, p. p. см.* unsay.

unsavoury [ʌn'seɪvərɪ] *a* 1) безвкусный; 2) невкусный; 3) неприятный; отталкивающий.

unsay [ʌn'seɪ] *v* (*past, p.p.* unsaid) брать обратно (свои слова); отпираться.

unscathed [ʌn'skeɪðd] *a* невредимый.

unschooled [ʌn'skuːld] *a* 1) необученный; неопытный; 2) недисциплинированный.

unscrew [ʌn'skruː] *v* отвинчивать(ся); развинчивать(ся).

unscrupulous [ʌn'skruːpjuləs] *a* 1) неразборчивый в средствах; не слишком щепетильный; 2) беспринципный; бессовестный.

unseal [ʌn'siːl] *v* распечатывать.

unsearchable [ʌn'səːtʃəbl] *a* непостижимый, необъяснимый; таинственный.

unseasoned [ʌn'siːznd] *a* 1) несозревший,

незре́лый; *перен.* нео́пытный; 2) без припра́вы.

unseat [ʌnˈsiːt] *v* 1) сбро́сить (*с седла́*); ссади́ть (*со сту́ла и т. п.*); 2) лиша́ть ме́ста, до́лжности.

unseemly [ʌnˈsiːmlɪ] *a* неподоба́ющий; неприли́чный, непристо́йный.

unseen [ʌnˈsiːn] *a* 1) неви́данный; 2) неви́димый.

unselfish [ʌnˈselfɪʃ] *a* неэгоисти́чный; бескоры́стный.

unsettle [ʌnˈsetl] *v* наруша́ть поря́док, споко́йствие; выбива́ть из коле́й; расстра́ивать.

unsettled [ʌnˈsetld] *a* 1) расстро́енный, не в поря́дке; 2) неустанови́вшийся, неопределённый; неусто́йчивый (*о пого́де*); 3) неопла́ченный (*о счёте и т. п.*); 4) нерешённый; 5) необита́емый, незаселённый; 6) *хим.* неотстоя́вшийся.

unshakable [ʌnˈʃeɪkəbl] *a* непоколеби́мый.

unshaken [ʌnˈʃeɪkən] *a* непоколе́бленный; непоколеби́мый, твёрдый.

unsheathe [ʌnˈʃiːð] *v* вынима́ть из но́жен.

unshod [ʌnˈʃɔd] *a* 1) необу́тый; 2) неподко́ванный.

unsightly [ʌnˈsaɪtlɪ] *a* 1) непригля́дный; невзра́чный; 2) уро́дливый; безобра́зный.

unskilful [ʌnˈskɪlful] *a* 1) неуме́лый, нео́пытный; 2) неуклю́жий, нело́вкий, нескла́дный.

unskilled [ʌnˈskɪld] *a* неквалифици́рованный.

unsleeping [ʌnˈsliːpɪŋ] *a* недре́млющий; бди́тельный.

unsophisticated [ˈʌnsəˈfɪstɪkeɪtɪd] *a* просто́й, безыску́сственный; простоду́шный.

unsound [ʌnˈsaund] *a* 1) нездоро́вый; боле́зненный; 2) ненадёжный; 3) необосно́ванный.

unsparing [ʌnˈspɛərɪŋ] *a* 1) беспоща́дный; 2) ще́дрый; расточи́тельный.

unspeakable [ʌnˈspiːkəbl] *a* 1) невырази́мый, непередава́емый (*слова́ми*); 2) о́чень плохо́й.

unspotted [ʌnˈspɔtɪd] *a* незапя́тнанный, чи́стый.

unstable [ʌnˈsteɪbl] *a* неусто́йчивый; непостоя́нный.

unsteady [ʌnˈstedɪ] *a* 1) неусто́йчивый, нетвёрдый; 2) колеблющийся, ша́ткий; 3) непостоя́нный; ненадёжный.

unstressed [ʌnˈstrest] *a* 1) неподчёркнутый; 2) безуда́рный (*о зву́ке, сло́ге*).

unsuitable [ʌnˈsjuːtəbl] *a* неподходя́щий, неподоба́ющий.

unsuspected [ˈʌnsəsˈpektɪd] *a* 1) незаподо́зренный; 2) непредви́денный; неожи́данно оказа́вшийся (*кем-л., чем-л.*).

untamable [ʌnˈteɪməbl] *a* неукроти́мый, безу́держный.

untapped [ʌnˈtæpt] *a* непоча́тый (*о бочо́нке и т. п.*).

unthinkable [ʌnˈθɪŋkəbl] *a* 1) невообрази́мый; 2) *разг.* неправдоподо́бный.

unthinking [ʌnˈθɪŋkɪŋ] *a* безду́мный, беспе́чный, лекомы́сленный.

untie [ʌnˈtaɪ] *v* развя́зывать, отвя́зывать.

until I [ənˈtɪl] *prep* до; ~ summer до ле́та.

until II *conj* (до тех пор) пока́; he worked ~ he was too tired to do more он рабо́тал (до тех пор), пока́ не уста́л.

untimely I [ʌnˈtaɪmlɪ] *a* несвоевре́менный; безвре́менный.

untimely II *adv* несвоевре́менно, не во́время; безвре́менно.

untiring [ʌnˈtaɪərɪŋ] *a* неутоми́мый.

unto [ˈʌntu] *см.* to I.

untold [ʌnˈtould] *a* 1) нерасска́занный; нераскры́тый (*о секре́те*); 2) бессчётный, несме́тный, неисчисли́мый.

untoward [ʌnˈtouəd] *a* 1) неблагоприя́тный, несчастли́вый; неуда́чный; 2) *уст.* непоко́рный, упря́мый.

untrammelled [ʌnˈtræməld] *a* беспрепя́тственный; неоспори́мый (*о пра́ве и т. п.*).

untranslatable [ˈʌntrænsˈleɪtəbl] *a* непереводи́мый.

untrue [ʌnˈtruː] *a* 1) ло́жный, непра́вильный; 2) неве́рный (*кому́-л.*), нару́шивший ве́рность; 3) несоотве́тствующий (*образцу́, ти́пу*).

untwine [ʌnˈtwaɪn] *v* распу́тывать(ся); расплета́ть(ся).

untwist [ʌnˈtwɪst] *v* раскру́чивать(ся).

unusedᵃ [ʌnˈjuːzd] *a* не употребля́вшийся, не испо́льзованный (*до сих пор*).

unusedᵇ [ʌnˈjuːst] *a* непривы́чный, неприу́ченный (*к чему́-л. — to*).

unusual [ʌnˈjuːʒuəl] *a* 1) необы́чный, ре́дкий; 2) необыча́йный, замеча́тельный.

unutterable [ʌnˈʌtərəbl] *a* невырази́мый.

unvarnished [ʌnˈvɑːnɪʃt] *a* нелакиро́ванный; *перен.* неприкра́шенный.

unveil [ʌnˈveɪl] *v* 1) снима́ть покрыва́ло; раскрыва́ть; 2) торже́ственно открыва́ть (*па́мятник*); 3) открыва́ть (*та́йну*).

unversed [ʌnˈvəːst] *a* несве́дущий, нео́пытный, неиску́сный (*в чём-л. — in*).

unvoiced [ʌnˈvɔɪst] *a* 1) непроизнесённый; 2) *фон.* глухо́й.

unwanted [ʌnˈwɔntɪd] *a* нежела́нный, нежела́тельный; нену́жный, ли́шний.

unwarrantable [ʌnˈwɔrəntəbl] *a* недопусти́мый; ниче́м не опра́вданный.

unwearying [ʌnˈwɪərɪŋ] *a* неутоми́мый.

unwelcome [ʌnˈwelkəm] *a* 1) нежела́нный, нежела́тельный; неприя́тный; 2) непро́шенный.

unwell [ʌnˈwel] *a* нездоро́вый.

unwieldy [ʌnˈwiːldɪ] *a* 1) громо́здкий; 2) нескла́дный.

unwilling [ʌnˈwɪlɪŋ] *a* несклонный, нерасполо́женный.

unwillingly [ʌnˈwɪlɪŋlɪ] *adv* неохо́тно; про́тив во́ли.

unwind [ʌnˈwaɪnd] *v* (*past, p. p.* unwound) разма́тывать(ся).

unwinking [ʌnˈwɪŋkɪŋ] *a* немига́ющий; *перен.* бди́тельный.

unwise [ʌnˈwaɪz] *a* глу́пый, неблагоразу́мный.

unwittingly [ʌnˈwɪtɪŋlɪ] *adv* неча́янно, нево́льно.

unwonted [ʌnˈwountɪd] *a* непривы́чный; необы́чный.

unworldly [ʌnˈwəːldlɪ] *a* 1) духо́вный; 2) не от ми́ра сего́.

unworthy [ʌnˈwəːðɪ] *a* недосто́йный; нестоя́щий.

unwound [ʌnˈwaund] *past, p. p. см.* unwind.

unwritten [ʌnˈrɪtn] *a* непи́саный, незапи́санный; ~ law *юр.* обы́чное пра́во.

unyielding [ʌnˈjiːldɪŋ] *a* неподáтливый; несгибáемый; упóрный; несдаю́щийся.

up I [ʌp] *prep* 1) *указывает на движение вверх* вверх по; up the river вверх по рекé; up the hill в гóру; up the steps вверх по лéстнице; 2) *в сочетании с* to *указывает на:* а) *приближение вплотнýю к другóму предмéту* к, ко; he came up to me он подошёл ко мне; б) *приближение к определённой величинé* до; I counted up to twenty я просчитáл до 20; в) *соответствие какóму-л. кáчеству, стандáрту:* up to the mark на высотé; хорóший, удовлетворительный; not up to the mark не на высотé, неудовлетворительный; not up to his work he соотвéтствует своéй рабóте; up to his income по свои́м дохóдам.

up II *adv* 1) *указывает на движение вверх* вверх; hands up! рýки вверх!; to climb up to the top of the ladder влезть на сáмый верх лéстницы; up and down вверх и вниз; вдоль и поперёк; взад и вперёд; тудá и сюдá; 2) *указывает на бóлее высóкое положéние по сравнéнию с другим предмéтом* наверхý; high up a tree наверхý на дéреве; 3) *в соединéнии с гл. указывает на:* а) *перехóд из горизонтáльного положéния в вертикáльное, из сидя́чего в стоя́чее, из бóлее ни́зкого в бóлее высóкое:* I was up at eight in the morning я встал в 8 часóв утрá; we get up early мы встаём рáно; the patient sat up in bed больнóй сел в постéли; the sun (the moon) is up сóлнце (лунá) взошлó (взошлá); the barometer is up барóметр поднялся; б) *однокрáтный харáктер дéйствия, вы́раженного гл.:* I could not catch him up я не смог догнáть егó; в) *завершéние или результáт дéйствия:* our time is up нáше врéмя истеклó; it is all up with him с ним всё кóнчено; the weather has cleared up погóда проясни́лась.

up III *n* подъём; the ~s and downs of life преврáтности жи́зни.

up IV *a* 1) растýщий; 2) иду́щий вверх; 3) идýщий в центр (*о пóезде*).

up V *v разг.* 1) вставáть; 2) повышáть (*цéны*).

up- [ʌp-] *pref* 1) *с гл., осóбенно в фóрме прич. наст. вр., и с отглагóльными именáми выражáет рост, подъём и т. п.:* upbringing воспитáние; upheaval переворóт (*социáльный*); 2) *с сущ. образýет прил. и наречия со значéнием вверх, квéрху, наверхý;* uphill в гóру; нá гору; upland нагóрный, гори́стый; upstairs вверх по лéстнице, навéрх.

up-and-coming [ˈʌpənˈkʌmɪŋ] *a амер. разг.* 1) энергичный, предприимчивый; напóристый, настóйчивый; 2) осторóжный, осмотрительный.

up-and-down I [ˈʌpənˈdaun] *a* прямóй, откровéнный; я́вный, я́сный.

up-and-down II *adv* 1) прямо, откры́то; 2) там и сям.

upas [ˈjuːpəs] *n* 1) анчáр (*тж.* ~-tree); 2) ядови́тый сок анчáра; *перен.* пáгубное влия́ние.

upbraid [ʌpˈbreɪd] *v* обвиня́ть в чём-л.; брани́ть, упрекáть.

upbringing [ˈʌpˌbrɪŋɪŋ] *n* воспитáние.

upbuilding [ʌpˈbɪldɪŋ] *n* построéние; ~ of communism построéние коммуни́зма.

up-country I [ˈʌpˈkʌntrɪ] *n* внýтренняя часть страны́.

up-country II *a* располóженный внутри́ страны́, удалённый от грани́ц.

up-grade [ˈʌpˌɡreɪd] *n* подъём.

upgrowth [ˈʌpˌɡrouθ] *n* рост, развитие.

upheaval [ʌpˈhiːvəl] *n* 1) сдвиг; 2) *геол.* смещéние пластóв; 3) глубóкие социáльные изменéния; переворóт.

upheave [ʌpˈhiːv] *v* поднимáть; сдвигáть.

upheld [ʌpˈheld] *past, p. p. см.* uphold.

uphill I [ˈʌpˈhɪl] *a* идýщий в гóру; *перен.* трýдный, тяжёлый.

uphill II *adv* в гóру.

uphold [ʌpˈhould] *v* (*past, p. p.* upheld) 1) поддéрживать; окáзывать поддéржку; 2) придéрживаться (*взгля́да и т. п.*).

upholster [ʌpˈhoulstə] *v* 1) обивáть (*мéбель*); 2) меблировáть.

upholsterer [ʌpˈhoulstərə] *n* обóйщик, драпирóвщик.

upholstery [ʌpˈhoulstərɪ] *n* 1) обивочный материáл; 2) ремеслó обóйщика, драпирóвщика.

upkeep [ˈʌpkiːp] *n* 1) содержáние (в испрáвности); ремóнт; 2) стóимость содержáния.

upland I [ˈʌplənd] *n* гори́стая странá; нагóрная часть страны́.

upland II *a* нагóрный, гори́стый.

uplift[a] [ˈʌplɪft] *n* 1) подъём; подня́тие; возвышéние; 2) подъём, воодушевлéние.

uplift[b] [ʌpˈlɪft] *v* поднимáть; возвышáть.

upmost [ˈʌpmoust] *см.* uppermost.

upon [əˈpɔn] *см.* on I.

upper I [ˈʌpə] *a* вéрхний; вы́сший; ◊ the ~ ten (thousand) верхýшка óбщества.

upper II *n* передóк башмакá; ◊ to be (down) on one's ~s остáться без грошá.

upper-cut [ˈʌpəkʌt] *n* апперкóт (*в бóксе*).

uppermost [ˈʌpəmoust] *a* 1) сáмый вéрхний, сáмый вы́сший; 2) сáмый глáвный; преобладáющий, домини́рующий; to be ~ in занимáть глáвное, пéрвое мéсто.

uppish [ˈʌpɪʃ] *a* чвáнный, спеси́вый.

upraise [ʌpˈreɪz] *v* поднимáть; возвышáть.

upright[a] I [ˈʌpraɪt] *n* стóйка; подпóрка.

upright[a] II *a* чéстный, прямóй; справедли́вый.

upright[b] I [ˈʌpˈraɪt] *a* вертикáльный, прямóй.

upright[b] II *adv* прямо, вертикáльно, стоймя́.

uprightness [ˈʌpˌraɪtnɪs] *n* чéстность, прямотá; справедли́вость.

uprise [ʌpˈraɪz] *v* (*past* uprose; *p. p.* uprisen) 1) восставáть; 2) поднимáться.

uprisen [ʌpˈrɪzn] *p. p. см.* uprise.

uprising [ʌpˈraɪzɪŋ] *n* 1) восстáние; 2) вставáние; 3) подъём (*вверх, в гору*).

uproar [ˈʌpˌrɔː] *n* шум, гам, волнéние, суматóха; взрыв (*смéха*).

uproarious [ʌpˈrɔːrɪəs] *a* шýмный, бýйный.

uproot [ʌpˈruːt] *v* вырывáть с кóрнем; *перен. тж.* искореня́ть.

uprose [ʌpˈrouz] *past. см.* uprise.

upset I [ʌpˈset] *n* 1) опроки́дывание; 2) беспоря́док, расстрóйство; 3) ссóра, нелáды; 4) *спорт.* неожи́данный результáт.

upset II *v* (*past, p. p.* upset) 1) опроки́дывать (-ся); 2) расстрáивать (*плáны и т. п.*); 3) нарушáть (*поря́док и т. п.*); 4) выводи́ть из равновéсия, волновáть, огорчáть.

upshot [ˈʌpʃɔt] *n* результáт; развя́зка; заключéние.

upside [ˈʌpsaɪd] *n* ве́рхняя сторона́.

upside-down I [ˈʌpsaɪdˈdaun] *a* 1) перевёрнутый вверх дном; 2) беспоря́дочный, в по́лном беспоря́дке.

upside-down II *adv* вверх дном; вверх нога́ми.

upstairs I [ˈʌpˈstɛəz] *a* в ве́рхнем этаже́; наверху́.

upstairs II *adv* вверх по ле́стнице, наве́рх.

upstanding [ʌpˈstændɪŋ] *a* 1) стоя́чий; вертика́льный; 2) си́льный, здоро́вый.

upstart[a] [ˈʌpˌstɑːt] *n* вы́скочка.

upstart[b] [ʌpˈstɑːt] *v* внеза́пно появи́ться, вы́скочить.

up-stream [ˈʌpˈstriːm] *adv* про́тив тече́ния, вверх по тече́нию.

upsurge [ˈʌpˌsəːdʒ] *n* подъём (*хозя́йства, промы́шленности*); economic ~ бу́рный подъём эконо́мики.

upswing [ˈʌpswɪŋ] *n* подъём, улучше́ние.

uptake [ˈʌpteɪk] *n* 1) подня́тие; 2) *разг.* поня́тливость, сообрази́тельность; quick (slow) in the ~ смышлёный, сообрази́тельный (ме́дленно сообража́ющий).

up-to-date [ˈʌptəˈdeɪt] *a* 1) (вполне́) совреме́нный, нове́йший; 2) сохрани́вшийся до настоя́щего вре́мени.

uptown I [ˈʌpˈtaun] *a* располо́женный *или* находя́щийся в ве́рхней ча́сти го́рода.

uptown II *adv* в ве́рхней ча́сти го́рода.

upturn I [ˈʌpˈtəːn] *n* подъём; улучше́ние.

upturn II *v* перевёртывать.

upward I [ˈʌpwəd] *a* напра́вленный *или* дви́жущийся вверх.

upward II *adv см.* upwards.

upwards [ˈʌpwədz] *adv* 1) вверх; 2) свы́ше, вы́ше; and ~ и бо́лее (того́).

uranium [juəˈreɪnjəm] *n хим.* ура́н.

urban [ˈəːbən] *a* городско́й.

urbane [əːˈbeɪn] *a* 1) ве́жливый, любе́зный; 2) изы́сканный.

urbanity [əːˈbænɪtɪ] *n* 1) ве́жливость, любе́зность; 2) изы́сканность.

urchin [ˈəːtʃɪn] *n* мальчи́шка.

Urdu [əːˈduː] *n* язы́к урду́.

urge I [əːdʒ] *n* побужде́ние, и́мпульс; си́льное жела́ние.

urge II *v* 1) подгоня́ть, торопи́ть; 2) понужда́ть; подстрека́ть; 3) убежда́ть, побужда́ть; наста́ивать.

urgency [ˈəːdʒənsɪ] *n* 1) настоя́тельность, безотлага́тельность; кра́йняя необходи́мость; 2) насто́йчивость, назо́йливость.

urgent [ˈəːdʒənt] *a* 1) настоя́тельный, безотлага́тельный; 2) насто́йчивый, назо́йливый; неотсту́пный.

urinate [ˈjuərɪneɪt] *v* мочи́ться.

urine [ˈjuərɪn] *n* моча́.

urn [əːn] *n* 1) у́рна; 2) кофе́йник, ча́йник.

Ursa [ˈəːsə] *n астр.:* ~ Major Больша́я Медве́дица; ~ Minor Ма́лая Медве́дица.

us [ʌs] *pron pers* (*ко́св. п. от* we) нас, нам; by us на́ми; to us нам; with us с на́ми; of us нас.

usable [ˈjuːzəbl] *a* (при)го́дный к употребле́нию.

usage [ˈjuːzɪdʒ] *n* 1) употребле́ние; 2) обраще́ние, обхожде́ние; rough ~ гру́бое обраще́ние; 3) обы́чай; обыкнове́ние.

use[a] [juːs] *n* 1) употребле́ние, примене́ние, по́льзование; free ~ свобо́дное по́льзование (*без ограниче́ний*); in ~ в употребле́нии, употреби́тельный; in daily ~ в ча́стом употребле́нии; в обихо́де; out of ~ вы́шедший из употребле́ния; to be in ~ быть в употребле́нии; to be (*или* to fall) out of ~ вы́йти из употребле́ния; to make ~ of испо́льзовать, воспо́льзоваться; to have the ~ of по́льзоваться чем-л.; to lose the ~ of потеря́ть спосо́бность по́льзоваться чем-л., не владе́ть чем-л.; to put to ~ испо́льзовать; 2) по́льза; of ~ поле́зный; of no ~ бесполе́зный; there is no ~ бесполе́зно, ни к чему́; is there any ~? сто́ит ли?; 3) обыкнове́ние, привы́чка; обы́чай; ~ and wont установи́вшийся обы́чай; обы́чная пра́ктика; ◊ there is no ~ to cry over spilt milk *посл.* ≅ сде́ланного не воро́тишь.

use[b] [juːz] *v* 1) употребля́ть, по́льзоваться, применя́ть; 2) обраща́ться, обходи́ться с кем-л.; 3) *то́лько past* име́ть обыкнове́ние; it ~d to be said обы́чно говори́ли; he ~d to come at ten o'clock он обыкнове́нно приходи́л в де́сять часо́в; there ~d to be a house здесь стоя́л ра́ньше стоя́л дом; □ to ~ up испо́льзовать; израсхо́довать; истощи́ть; ~d up изнурённый, истощённый.

used[a] [juːst] *a predic* привы́кший; привы́чный; to get ~ привы́кнуть.

used[b] [juːzd] *a амер.* поде́ржанный, ста́рый.

useful [ˈjuːsful] *a* 1) поле́зный; приго́дный; to come in ~ а) появи́ться кста́ти; б) пригоди́ться.

useless [ˈjuːslɪs] *a* бесполе́зный; нену́жный; него́дный.

user [ˈjuːzə] *n* потреби́тель, по́льзующийся.

usher I [ˈʌʃə] *n* 1) швейца́р; привра́тник; 2) капельди́нер; 3) *уст., шутл.* мла́дший учи́тель; репети́тор.

usher II *v* 1) проводи́ть, вводи́ть (*в дом, зал*); 2) докла́дывать (*о ком-л.; тж.* to ~ in).

usual [ˈjuːʒuəl] *a* обыкнове́нный, обы́чный; употреби́тельный (*о сло́ве, выраже́нии*); as ~ как обы́чно, по обыкнове́нию.

usually [ˈjuːʒuəlɪ] *adv* обы́чно, обыкнове́нно.

usurer [ˈjuːʒərə] *n* ростовщи́к.

usurious [juːˈʒuəriəs] *a* ростовщи́ческий.

usurp [juːˈzəːp] *v* захва́тывать незако́нно, завладева́ть, узурпи́ровать.

usurpation [ˌjuːzəːˈpeɪʃən] *n* незако́нный захва́т; узурпа́ция.

usurper [juːˈzəːpə] *n* захва́тчик; узурпа́тор.

usury [ˈjuːʒərɪ] *n* 1) ростовщи́чество; 2) ростовщи́ческий проце́нт; with ~ *перен.* с лихво́й.

utensil [juːˈtensl] *n* 1) у́тварь; kitchen ~s ку́хонная посу́да; 2) принадле́жность; writing ~s пи́сьменные принадле́жности.

uterus [ˈjuːtərəs] *n* 1) *анат.* ма́тка; 2) утро́ба, чре́во.

utilitarian I [ˌjuːtɪlɪˈtɛəriən] *n* утилитари́ст.

utilitarian II *a* утилита́рный.

utility [juːˈtɪlɪtɪ] *n* 1) поле́зность; вы́годность, по́льза; 2): public utilities предприя́тия обще́ственного по́льзования; коммуна́льные предприя́тия; 3) *attr* утилита́рный; сугу́бо практи́ческий.

utility-man [juːˈtɪlɪtɪmæn] *n* 1) *теа́тр. разг.* актёр на выходны́х роля́х; 2) ма́стер на все ру́ки.

utilization [ˌjuːtɪlaɪˈzeɪʃən] *n* испо́льзование.

utilize [ˈjuːtɪlaɪz] *v* испо́льзовать, утилизи́ровать.

utmost I [ˈʌtmoust] *n* вы́сшая сте́пень, са́мое большо́е; всё возмо́жное; to the ~ в вы́сшей сте́пени; как то́лько мо́жно; to do one's ~ сде́лать всё возмо́жное.

utmost II *a* 1) кра́йний; преде́льный; са́мый отдалённый; 2) велича́йший (*о значении, ценности и т. п.*); высоча́йший.

Utopia [juːˈtoupjə] *n* уто́пия.

Utopian I [juːˈtoupjən] *n* утопи́ст.

Utopian II *a* утопи́ческий.

utter[1] [ˈʌtə] *v* 1) издава́ть (*звук, крик*); 2) произноси́ть; выража́ть слова́ми; 3) пуска́ть в обраще́ние, распространя́ть (*фальшивые деньги и т. п.*).

utter[2] *a* 1) по́лный; полне́йший, соверше́нный; абсолю́тный; кра́йний (*об удивлении и т. п.*); 2) отъя́вленный.

utterance [ˈʌtərəns] *n* 1) выраже́ние (*чего-л.*); to give ~ to вы́разить, дать вы́ход (*чувству и т. п.*); разрази́ться (*гневом и т. п.*); 2) произноше́ние; 3) изрече́ние, выска́зывание; public ~ публи́чное заявле́ние.

utterly [ˈʌtəlɪ] *adv* кра́йне, чрезвыча́йно; соверше́нно.

uttermost [ˈʌtəmoust] *a* полне́йший, абсолю́тнейший; са́мый кра́йний.

uvula [ˈjuːvjulə] *n* (*pl* uvulae [ˈjuːvjuliː]) *анат.* язычо́к.

Uzbek I [uzˈbek] *n* 1) узбе́к; узбе́чка; the ~s узбе́ки; 2) узбе́кский язы́к.

Uzbek II *a* узбе́кский.

V

V, v [viː] *n* 22-я бу́ква англ. алфави́та.

vac [væk] *n* разг. кани́кулы.

vacancy [ˈveɪkənsɪ] *n* 1) пустота́; 2) пусто́е, неза́нятое ме́сто, простра́нство; 3) вака́нсия; 4) пра́здность; 5) равноду́шие, безуча́стие; 6) *амер.* помеще́ние, сдаю́щееся внаём.

vacant [ˈveɪkənt] *a* 1) пусто́й, неза́нятый, свобо́дный (*о помещении, месте и т. п.*); 2) вака́нтный (*о должности*); 3) пра́здный (*о жизни*); 4) безуча́стный, отсу́тствующий (*о взгляде*); 5) вы́морочный (*об имуществе, земле*); 6) *тех.* холосто́й (*о ходе*).

vacate [vəˈkeɪt] *v* 1) освобожда́ть (*место, помещение, должность*); 2) упраздня́ть, отменя́ть (*закон, договор и т. п.*).

vacation [vəˈkeɪʃən] *n* 1) кани́кулы; long ~ ле́тние кани́кулы; 2) о́тпуск; 3) освобожде́ние, оставле́ние.

vacationist [vəˈkeɪʃənɪst] *n* амер. отдыха́ющий, отпускни́к.

vaccinate [ˈvæksɪneɪt] *v мед.* де́лать приви́вку.

vaccination [ˌvæksɪˈneɪʃən] *n мед.* приви́вка.

vaccine [ˈvæksiːn] *n мед.* вакци́на.

vacillate [ˈvæsɪleɪt] *v* 1) кача́ться, колыха́ться; 2) колеба́ться, проявля́ть нереши́тельность.

vacillation [ˌvæsɪˈleɪʃən] *n* 1) колеба́ние; 2) нереши́тельность; непостоя́нство.

vacua [ˈvækjuə] *pl см.* vacuum.

vacuity [væˈkjuːɪtɪ] *n* 1) пустота́; 2) отсу́тствие мы́слей, бессодержа́тельность.

vacuous [ˈvækjuəs] *a* 1) пусто́й; 2) бессмы́сленный; невырази́тельный, отсу́тствующий.

vacuum [ˈvækjuəm] *n* (*pl тж.* vacua) 1) безвозду́шное простра́нство; пустота́; ва́куум; 2) *разг.* пылесо́с; 3) *attr* ва́куумный.

vacuum-tube [ˈvækjuəmˈtjuːb] *n радио* 1) электро́нная ла́мпа; 2) *attr* ла́мповый.

vade-mecum [ˈveɪdɪˈmiːkəm] *n* карма́нный спра́вочник.

vagabond I [ˈvægəbənd] *n* 1) бродя́га; бездо́мный; 2) *разг.* безде́льник.

vagabond II *a* бродя́чий; бездо́мный.

vagabond III *v* бродя́жничать, скита́ться.

vagabondage [ˈvægəbəndɪdʒ] *см.* vagabondism.

vagabondism [ˈvægəbəndɪzəm] *n* бродя́жничество.

vagary [ˈveɪgərɪ] *n* 1) бредо́вая иде́я, ди́кая мысль; 2) причу́да, капри́з; 3) чуда́чество.

vagrancy [ˈveɪgrənsɪ] *n* бродя́жничество, скита́ние.

vagrant I [ˈveɪgrənt] *n* бродя́га, скита́лец.

vagrant II *a* 1) бродя́чий, стра́нствующий; кочу́ющий; 2) блужда́ющий.

vague [veɪg] *a* 1) нея́сный, сму́тный, неопределённый; 2) тума́нный (*об ответе, высказывании*); 3) бессмы́сленный, отсу́тствующий (*о взгляде, выражении лица*).

vain [veɪn] *a* 1) тще́тный, напра́сный; in ~ напра́сно, тще́тно; 2) пусто́й (*о мечтах, развлечениях и т. п.*); 3) тщесла́вный; самодово́льный; to be ~ of горди́ться (*чем-л.*).

vainglorious [veɪnˈglɔːrɪəs] *a* тщесла́вный; хвастли́вый.

vainglory [veɪnˈglɔːrɪ] *n* тщесла́вие; хвастли́вость.

valance [ˈvæləns] *n* подзо́р (*у кровати*); ламбреке́н (*над окном, дверью*).

vale[a] [veɪl] *n* 1) *поэт.* доли́на; 2) сто́чная кана́ва.

vale[b] I [ˈveɪlɪ] *n* проща́ние.

vale[b] II *int* проща́йте!

valediction [ˌvælɪˈdɪkʃən] *n* проща́ние; напу́тствие, проща́льное сло́во.

valedictory I [ˌvælɪˈdɪktərɪ] *n* 1) напу́тствие, проща́льное сло́во; 2) *амер.* напу́тственная речь (*при выпуске из учебного заведения*).

valedictory II *a* проща́льный, напу́тственный.

valence [ˈveɪləns] *см.* valency.

valency [ˈveɪlənsɪ] *n хим.* вале́нтность, а́томность.

valentine [ˈvæləntaɪn] *n* 1) возлю́бленный, -ная (*выбирается в шутку в день св. Валенти́на*); 2) посла́ние *или* шу́точные любо́вные стихи́ (*посылаемые в день св. Валенти́на*).

valerian [vəˈlɪərɪən] *n* 1) *бот.* валерья́на; 2) валерья́новые ка́пли.

valet [ˈvælɪt] *n* 1) камерди́нер, лаке́й (*тж.* valet de chambre [vəˈleɪdeˈʃɑːnbr]); 2) *амер.* слу́жащий гости́ницы (*производящий ремонт, чистку и глажение одежды*); 3) *амер.* мастерска́я бытово́го обслу́живания.

valetudinarian I [ˈvælɪˌtjuːdɪˈnɛərɪən] *n* боле́зненный *или* мни́тельный челове́к.

valetudinarian II *a* болезненный; мнительный.

valetudinary I, II [ˌvælɪˈtjuːdɪnərɪ] *см.* valetudinarian I, II.

valiant [ˈvæljənt] *a* храбрый, доблестный, мужественный.

valid [ˈvælɪd] *a* 1) правильный; обоснованный; здравый; 2) действительный, имеющий силу (*о договоре и т. п.*).

validate [ˈvælɪdeɪt] *v* 1) утверждать, ратифицировать; 2) *юр.* объявлять действительным, придавать законную силу.

validation [ˌvælɪˈdeɪʃən] *n* утверждение, ратификация.

validity [vəˈlɪdɪtɪ] *n* 1) основательность, вескость; обоснованность; 2) действительность; законность.

valise [vəˈliːz] *n* 1) дорожная сумка, саквояж; 2) *воен.* перемётная сума.

valley [ˈvælɪ] *n* долина.

valor [ˈvælə] *амер. см.* valour.

valorous [ˈvælərəs] *a* доблестный.

valour [ˈvælə] *n* доблесть, мужество.

valuable [ˈvæljuəbl] *a* 1) ценный; дорогой; 2) ценимый.

valuables [ˈvæljuəblz] *n pl* драгоценности.

valuation [ˌvæljuˈeɪʃən] *n* 1) оценка; 2) цена.

value I [ˈvæljuː] *n* 1) ценность; 2) стоимость, цена; exchange ~, ~ in exchange меновая стоимость; face (relative, surplus) ~ номинальная (относительная, прибавочная) стоимость; surrender ~ сумма, возвращаемая лицу, отказавшемуся от страхового полиса; 3) важность, значительность; 4) значение (*слова*); the precise ~ of a word точное, буквальное значение слова; 5) *мат.* величина; 6) *муз.* длительность (*ноты*); 7) *жив.* соотношение света и тени (*в картине*).

value II *v* 1) оценивать; 2) дорожить, ценить.

valueless [ˈvæljulɪs] *a* ничего не стоящий; бесполезный.

valuer [ˈvæljuə] *n* оценщик.

valve [vælv] *n* 1) *тех., анат.* клапан; 2) створка; 3) *радио* электронная лампа; 4) *attr* ламповый; 5) *attr* клапанный.

vamoose [væˈmuːs] *v амер. сленг* удирать; убираться.

vamose [vəˈmous] *см.* vamoose.

vamp[1] I [væmp] *n* 1) передок (*обуви*); 2) заплата; 3) *муз.* импровизированный аккомпанемент.

vamp[1] II *v* 1) ставить новый передок (*на обувь*); 2) латать, починять, переделывать из старого (*тж.* to ~ up); 3) *муз.* импровизировать аккомпанемент.

vamp[2] I *n разг.* соблазнительница; авантюристка; вымогательница.

vamp[2] II *v разг.* соблазнять, завлекать; вымогать (*деньги*).

vampire [ˈvæmpaɪə] *n* вампир; *перен.* кровопийца; вымогатель(ница).

van[1] [væn] *n* 1) фургон, фура; 2) вагон (*товарный, багажный, служебный*).

van[2] *n* авангард.

vandal I [ˈvændəl] *n* вандал, варвар.

vandal II *a* варварский.

vandalism [ˈvændəlɪzəm] *n* вандализм, варварство.

vane [veɪn] *n* 1) флюгер; 2) крыло (*мельницы, ветряка*); 3) лопасть (*винта*); 4) вентилятор.

vanguard [ˈvænɡɑːd] *n* авангард.

vanilla [vəˈnɪlə] *n* ваниль.

vanish [ˈvænɪʃ] *v* исчезать, пропадать.

vanity [ˈvænɪtɪ] *n* 1) суета, тщета; 2) тщеславие; to tickle smb.'s ~ льстить кому-л.; щекотать чьё-л. самолюбие.

vanquish [ˈvæŋkwɪʃ] *v* побеждать, покорять.

vanquisher [ˈvæŋkwɪʃə] *n* победитель; завоеватель.

vantage [ˈvɑːntɪdʒ] *n редк.* преимущество (*см. тж.* coign).

vantage-ground [ˈvɑːntɪdʒɡraund] *n* удобная, выгодная позиция.

vapid [ˈvæpɪd] *a* безвкусный, пресный; *перен.* бессодержательный, скучный.

vapidity [væˈpɪdɪtɪ] *n* безвкусность, пресность; *перен.* бессодержательность.

vapor I, II [ˈveɪpə] *амер. см.* vapour I, II.

vaporization [ˌveɪpəraɪˈzeɪʃən] *n* испарение; парообразование.

vaporize [ˈveɪpəraɪz] *v* испарять(ся), превращать(ся) в пар.

vaporous [ˈveɪpərəs] *a* 1) парообразный; 2) туманный; насыщенный парами; 3) нереальный.

vapory [ˈveɪpərɪ] *амер. см.* vapoury.

vapour I [ˈveɪpə] *n* 1) пар; 2) испарение; пары; туман; 3) иллюзия, нереальность; 4) *pl уст.* подавленность, угнетённое состояние.

vapour II *v* 1) испаряться; 2) хвастаться.

vapouring [ˈveɪpərɪŋ] *n часто pl* пустое хвастовство.

vapourish [ˈveɪpərɪʃ] *a* 1) хвастливый; 2) угнетённый, подавленный.

vapoury [ˈveɪpərɪ] *a* 1) туманный, затуманенный; 2) унылый; 3) воздушный (*о ткани*).

variability [ˌveərɪəˈbɪlɪtɪ] *n* изменчивость.

variable I [ˈveərɪəbl] *n мат.* переменная величина.

variable II *a* 1) изменчивый, непостоянный; 2) переменный.

variance [ˈveərɪəns] *n* 1) изменение; 2) разногласие, несогласие; размолвка; to set at ~ поссорить; вызвать конфликт; to be at ~ with а) противоречить (*чему-л.*); б) расходиться (*во взглядах и т. п.*); в) быть в ссоре (*с кем-л.*); 3) *юр.* несоответствие, расхождение.

variant I [ˈveərɪənt] *n* вариант.

variant II *a* различный; отличный, иной, другой.

variation [ˌveərɪˈeɪʃən] *n* 1) изменение; 2) отклонение; 3) *мат., муз.* вариация; 4) вариант, разновидность.

varicoloured [ˈveərɪˌkʌləd] *a* разноцветный.

varied [ˈveərɪd] *a* различный; разнообразный.

variegated [ˈveərɪɡeɪtɪd] *a* 1) разноцветный; пёстрый; 2) разнообразный.

variety [vəˈraɪətɪ] *n* 1) разнообразие; 2) множество; ряд; 3) *биол.* разновидность; 4) варьете, эстрада (*тж.* ~ show); 5) *attr* эстрадный.

variform [ˈveərɪfɔːm] *a* различной формы.

various [ˈveərɪəs] *a* 1) различный, разный; 2) разнообразный; разносторонний; 3) (*перед pl*) многие, разные.

varmint [ˈvɑːmɪnt] *n* 1) *разг.* шалопай; 2) (the ~) *охот. сленг* лиса.

varnish I [ˈvɑːnɪʃ] *n* 1) лак; 2) блеск, глянец; 3) внешний лоск; прикрытие, маскировка; 4) глазурь.

varnish II *v* 1) покрывать лаком, глазурью; 2) придавать лоск; 3) прикрывать *(недостатки)*.

varnishing-day [ˈvɑːnɪʃɪŋˈdeɪ] *n* день накануне открытия *(выставки картин)*.

'varsity [ˈvɑːsɪtɪ] *n разг.* университет.

vary [ˈveərɪ] *v* 1) менять(ся), изменять(ся); 2) расходиться, отличаться, разниться; 3) *муз.* исполнять вариации.

vascular [ˈvæskjulə] *a анат.* сосудистый.

vase [vɑːz, *амер.* veɪs] *n* ваза.

vaseline [ˈvæsɪliːn] *n* вазелин.

vassal [ˈvæsəl] *n* 1) вассал; 2) слуга, зависимое лицо; 3) *attr* вассальный.

vassalage [ˈvæsəlɪdʒ] *n* 1) *ист.* вассальная зависимость; 2) полная зависимость.

vast I [vɑːst] *n поэт.* простор.

vast II *a* 1) обширный; безбрежный; 2) *разг.* огромный; безграничный *(о радости, удовольствии)*; 3) многочисленный *(о войсках)*.

vastly [ˈvɑːstlɪ] *adv разг.* очень, чрезвычайно.

vat [væt] *n* 1) чан, бак; цистерна; 2) кадка.

Vatican [ˈvætɪkən] *n* 1) Ватикан; 2) папская власть.

vaudeville [ˈvoudəvɪl] *n театр.* 1) водевиль; 2) *амер.* эстрадное представление, варьете.

vault¹ I [vɔːlt] *n* 1) свод; the ~ of heaven небесный свод; 2) сводчатое помещение; подвал; погреб; 3) склеп; family ~ фамильный склеп; 4) стальная камера *(в банке)*.

vault¹ II *v* покрывать сводом.

vault² I *n* прыжок *(с упором)*.

vault² II *v* перепрыгивать, прыгать *(с упором)*.

vaulted [ˈvɔːltɪd] *a* сводчатый.

vaulting¹ [ˈvɔːltɪŋ] *n* 1) свод, своды; 2) возведение свода.

vaulting² *n* вольтижировка.

vaulting-horse [ˈvɔːltɪŋˈhɔːs] *n* конь *(гимнастический снаряд)*.

vaunt I [vɔːnt] *n* хвастовство.

vaunt II *v* 1) хвастаться, бахвалиться; 2) злорадствовать *(over)*.

've [v] *сокр. разг.* = have.

veal [viːl] *n* 1) телятина; 2) *attr* телячий *(о кушанье)*.

vector I [ˈvektə] *n* 1) *мат.* вектор; 2) переносчик инфекции; 3) *attr* векторный.

vector II *v* направлять, давать направление.

vedette [vɪˈdet] *n* 1) кавалерийский пост *(тж.* ~ post); 2) конный часовой.

veer [vɪə] *v* 1) изменять направление, изменяться *(о ветре)*; *перен.* изменять взгляды; передумать; переменить тему разговора; 2) *мор.* травить *(канат)*.

veering [ˈvɪərɪŋ] *n* поворот.

vegetable I [ˈvedʒɪtəbl] *n* 1) овощ; green ~s зелень; 2) растение.

vegetable II *a* 1) растительный; 2) овощной.

vegetal [ˈvedʒɪtl] *a* растительный.

vegetarian I [ˌvedʒɪˈteərɪən] *n* вегетарианец.

vegetarian II *a* вегетарианский.

vegetate [ˈvedʒɪteɪt] *v* 1) расти, произрастать; 2) прозябать.

vegetation [ˌvedʒɪˈteɪʃən] *n* 1) растительность;

2) произрастание, вегетация; 3) растительная жизнь; прозябание; 4) *attr* вегетационный.

vegetative [ˈvedʒɪtətɪv] *a* 1) растительный; вегетационный; 2) прозябающий.

vehemence [ˈviːɪməns] *n* сила; страстность.

vehement [ˈviːɪmənt] *a* сильный; решительный; страстный, горячий.

vehicle [ˈviːɪkl] *n* 1) экипаж *(любой)*; средство передвижения *или* перевозки; 2) *pl* (авто)транспорт, транспортные средства; 3) *ав.* (летательный) аппарат; unmanned ~ беспилотный летательный аппарат; rocket ~ ракета-носитель; 4) средство выражения, распространения *(идей и т. п.)*; 5) проводник *(звука, света и т. п.)*; 6) *хим.* растворитель.

vehicular [vɪˈhɪkjulə] *a* 1) перевозочный; 2) (авто)гужевой *(о транспорте)*.

veil I [veɪl] *n* 1) вуаль; покрывало; 2) завеса; 3) предлог, прикрытие; ◊ to take the ~ сделаться монахиней.

veil II *v* 1) закрывать вуалью, покрывалом; 2) завуалировать; скрыть.

vein [veɪn] *n* 1) вена; varicose ~s *мед.* варикозное расширение вен; 2) жилка, прожилка; 3) склонность, жилка; 4) *мин.* жила; 5) настроение; to be in the ~ быть в настроении *(что-л. делать; for)*; in the same ~ в том же роде, подобным же образом.

veined [veɪnd] *a* покрытый жилками.

velar I [ˈviːlə] *n фон.* задненёбный звук.

velar II *a фон.* задненёбный.

vellum [ˈveləm] *n* 1) тонкий пергамент; 2) калька; восковка; 3) *attr* веленевый *(о бумаге)*.

velocipede [vɪˈlɔsɪpiːd] *n* 1) *амер.* детский трёхколёсный велосипед; 2) дрезина.

velocity [vɪˈlɔsɪtɪ] *n* 1) скорость; orbital ~ первая космическая скорость; escape ~ вторая космическая скорость; 2) *радио* частота.

velours [veˈluəz] *n* 1) велюр; плюш; 2) велюровая шляпа.

velvet I [ˈvelvɪt] *n* 1) бархат *(тж.* silk ~); cotton ~ бумажный бархат, вельвет; 2) *разг.* выгода, преимущество; to be on ~ а) иметь преимущество; б) процветать; ◊ to prophesy upon ~ предсказывать заранее известные события.

velvet II *a* бархатный.

velvety [ˈvelvɪtɪ] *a* бархатистый.

venal [ˈviːnl] *a* продажный, подкупный.

venality [viːˈnælɪtɪ] *n* продажность.

vend [vend] *v* продавать, торговать.

vendee [venˈdiː] *n юр.* покупатель.

vender [ˈvendə] *n* продавец, торговец.

vendetta [venˈdetə] *n* кровная месть.

vendor [ˈvendɔː] *n* 1) *см.* vender; 2) *юр.* продавец.

veneer I [vəˈnɪə] *n* 1) (однослойная) фанера; 2) тонкий наружный слой; облицовка; глазурь; 3) видимость, налёт *(чего-л.)*; внешний лоск; 4) *attr* фанерный.

veneer II *v* 1) обклеивать, отделывать фанерой; 2) покрывать тонким слоем; облицовывать; 3) придавать видимость *(чего-л.)*; придавать внешний лоск.

venerable [ˈvenərəbl] *a* 1) почтенный; 2) *церк.* преподобный *(титул архидиакона)*.

venerate ['venəreɪt] v благоговеть (*перед кем-л.*); чтить.

veneration [,venə'reɪʃən] n почитание, преклонение, благоговение.

venereal [vɪ'nɪərɪəl] a венерический.

Venetian I [vɪ'niːʃən] n венецианец.

Venetian II a венецианский.

vengeance ['vendʒəns] n месть, мщение; ◊ with a ~ *разг.* здорово, вовсю.

vengeful ['vendʒful] a мстительный.

venial ['viːnjəl] a простительный.

venison ['venzn] n оленина.

venom ['venəm] n яд (*змеи, скорпиона и т. п.*); *перен. тж.* злоба.

venomous ['venəməs] a ядовитый.

venose ['viːnous] a 1) *анат.* венозный; 2) *бот.* жилковатый.

venous ['viːnəs] *см.* venose.

vent I [vent] n 1) входное *или* выходное отверстие; 2) отдушина; 3) выход, выражение (*чувств*); to give ~ дать волю (*чему-л. — to*); 4) клапан (*духового муз. инструмента*).

vent II v 1) выпускать, испускать; 2) давать выход, волю (*чувствам*).

vent-hole ['venthoul] n отдушина.

ventilate ['ventɪleɪt] v 1) вентилировать, проветривать; 2) обсуждать, выяснять (*вопрос и т. п.*).

ventilation [,ventɪ'leɪʃən] n 1) вентиляция, проветривание; 2) обсуждение, выяснение (*вопроса и т. п.*).

ventilator ['ventɪleɪtə] n вентилятор.

ventricle ['ventrɪkl] n *анат.* желудочек.

ventriloquist [ven'trɪləkwɪst] n чревовещатель.

venture I ['ventʃə] n рискованное предприятие; опасная затея; at a ~ наудачу, наугад; 2) спекуляция.

venture II v 1) рисковать; 2) рискнуть; отважиться, осмелиться (*тж.* to ~ on, to ~ upon); ◊ nothing ~, nothing have *посл.* ≅ риск — благородное дело.

venturer ['ventʃərə] n авантюрист.

venturesome ['ventʃəsəm] a 1) рискованный; 2) смелый, предприимчивый; 3) авантюристический.

venturous ['ventʃərəs] *см.* venturesome.

Venus ['viːnəs] n *астр., миф.* Венера.

Venusian [vɪ'njuːsɪən] a относящийся к планете Венера.

veracious [və'reɪʃəs] a 1) правдивый; 2) достоверный, верный.

veracity [və'ræsɪtɪ] n 1) правдивость; 2) достоверность, правда.

veranda(h) [və'rændə] n веранда.

verb [vəːb] n *грам.* глагол; auxiliary (deponent, impersonal, modal) ~ вспомогательный (депонентный, безличный, модальный) глагол; (in)transitive ~ (не)переходный глагол; reflexive ~ возвратный глагол; regular ~ глагол с суффиксацией; irregular ~ глагол с чередованием гласного.

verbal ['vəːbəl] a 1) устный; 2) словесный; 3) буквальный; дословный; 4) *грам.* (от)глагольный; 5) *дип.* вербальный.

verbally ['vəːbəlɪ] adv устно; на словах.

verbatim I [vəː'beɪtɪm] a дословный.

verbatim II adv дословно.

verbose [vəː'bous] a многословный.

verbosity [vəː'bɔsɪtɪ] n многословие.

verdancy ['vəːdənsɪ] n 1) зелень; 2) неискушённость; незрелость; неопытность.

verdant ['vəːdənt] a 1) зелёный, зеленеющий; 2) неискушённый; незрелый.

verdict ['vəːdɪkt] n 1) вердикт, решение присяжных заседателей; to return (*или* to bring in) a ~ of not guilty признать невиновным; 2) суждение, мнение (*о чём-л. — on*).

verdure ['vəːdʒə] n 1) зелень, зелёная трава, листва; 2) свежесть.

verdurous ['vəːdʒərəs] a зеленеющий.

verge I [vəːdʒ] n 1) край; *перен. тж.* грань; on the ~ на грани (*чего-л. — of*); 2) дёрн вокруг клумбы *или* по краям дороги.

verge II v склоняться, опускаться; спускаться; □ to ~ on граничить (*с чем-л.*).

verger ['vəːdʒə] n церковный служитель.

verification [,verɪfɪ'keɪʃən] n 1) проверка; 2) исполнение (*предсказания*); подтверждение (*опасения*).

verify ['verɪfaɪ] v 1) проверять; 2) подтверждать; удостоверять.

verisimilar [,verɪ'sɪmɪlə] a правдоподобный.

verisimilitude [,verɪsɪ'mɪlɪtjuːd] n правдоподобие, вероятность.

veritable ['verɪtəbl] a настоящий, истинный, сущий.

verity ['verɪtɪ] n правда, истина, истинность.

verjuice ['vəːdʒuːs] n кислый сок (*незрелых фруктов*); a look of ~ кислый взгляд, кислое выражение лица.

vermeil ['vəːmeɪl] n 1) позолоченное серебро; 2) киноварь.

vermicelli [,vəːmɪ'selɪ] n вермишель.

vermicide ['vəːmɪsaɪd] n глистогонное (*средство*).

vermifuge ['vəːmɪfjuːdʒ] *см.* vermicide.

vermillion I [və'mɪljən] n 1) киноварь; 2) ярко-красный цвет.

vermillion II a ярко-красный.

vermillion III v красить, окрашивать в ярко-красный цвет.

vermin ['vəːmɪn] n *собир.* вредители; паразиты; *перен.* сброд.

verminous ['vəːmɪnəs] a 1) передаваемый паразитами; 2) заражённый паразитами; 3) вредный.

verm(o)uth ['vəːməθ] n вермут.

vernacular I [və'nækjulə] n 1) родной язык; 2) местный диалект; in the ~ а) на местном диалекте; б) в сильных *или* бранных выражениях; 3) профессиональный язык.

vernacular II a 1) родной (*о языке*); 2) местный (*о диалекте, слове и т. п.*); 3) свойственный данной местности (*о болезни*).

vernal ['vəːnl] a весенний.

versatile ['vəːsətaɪl] a 1) многосторонний, разносторонний (*о таланте, авторе и т. п.*); 2) непостоянный, изменчивый (*о настроении и т. п.*); 3) подвижный.

versatility [,vəːsə'tɪlɪtɪ] n 1) многосторонность, разносторонность; 2) непостоянство, изменчивость.

verse I [vəːs] n 1) стихи; поэзия; 2) стих;

строфа́; blank ~ бе́лый стих; ◊ to give chapter and ~ (for) дать то́чную ссы́лку.

verse II v 1) писа́ть стихи́; 2) выража́ть в стиха́х.

versed [vəːst] a све́дущий; о́пытный.

verse-monger ['vəːsˌmʌŋgə] n рифмоплёт.

versification [ˌvəːsɪfɪ'keɪʃən] n 1) стихосложе́ние; accentual ~ тони́ческое стихосложе́ние; 2) переложе́ние (про́зы) в стихи́.

versifier ['vəːsɪfaɪə] n версифика́тор, стихоплёт.

versify ['vəːsɪfaɪ] v 1) писа́ть, слага́ть стихи́; 2) перелага́ть (про́зу) в стихи́.

version ['vəːʃən] n 1) ве́рсия; вариа́нт; 2) перево́д; 3) текст; the Russian and English ~s of the treaty ру́сский и англи́йский те́ксты догово́ра.

versus ['vəːsəs] prep про́тив.

vertebra ['vəːtɪbrə] n (pl vertebrae ['vəːtɪbriː]) 1) позвоно́к; 2) pl позвоно́чник.

vertebral ['vəːtɪbrəl] a позвоно́чный.

vertebrate I ['vəːtɪbrɪt] n позвоно́чное (живо́тное).

vertebrate II a позвоно́чный.

vertex ['vəːteks] n (pl vertices) 1) верши́на; 2) астр. зени́т.

vertical I ['vəːtɪkəl] n вертика́ль, вертика́льная ли́ния; перпендикуля́р.

vertical II a 1) вертика́льный; перпендикуля́рный; 2) отве́сный.

vertices ['vəːtɪsiːz] pl см. vertex.

vertigo ['vəːtɪgou] n головокруже́ние.

verve [vɛəv] n си́ла, жи́вость, я́ркость (изображе́ния).

very I ['verɪ] a 1) и́стинный, настоя́щий; су́щий; that is the ~ truth э́то и́стинная пра́вда; the veriest scoundrel unhung отъявленне́йший негодя́й; 2) (и́менно) тот са́мый; that is the ~ one э́то тот са́мый; 3) служит для усиления сущ. са́мый, тот са́мый; да́же; at that ~ moment в тот са́мый моме́нт; his ~ look betrayed him да́же его́ взгляд выдава́л ме́ня; the ~ thought frightens me одна́ э́та мысль меня́ пуга́ет; 4) служит для усиления прил.: a ~ little more will do ещё немно́жко, и бу́дет доста́точно.

very II adv 1) о́чень; ~ well о́чень хорошо́, отли́чно; ~ much о́чень; 2) с отрицанием придаёт прил. противоположное значение: not a ~ good bit of work нева́жная рабо́та; I don't sing ~ well я о́чень пло́хо пою́; I am not ~ keen on going there я во́все не хочу́ идти́ туда́; 3) служит для усиления: I did my ~ utmost я сде́лал всё, что мог, всё, что бы́ло в мои́х си́лах; he came the ~ next day он пришёл на сле́дующий же день; the ~ last thing I expected са́мое после́днее, что я мог предположи́ть; to the ~ last drop до после́дней ка́пли; my, his etc ~ own мой, его́ и т. п. со́бственный, дорого́й; you shall have this book for your ~ own вы полу́чите э́ту кни́гу в по́лную со́бственность.

vesicle ['vesɪkl] n анат., биол. пузырёк.

vesper ['vespə] n 1) поэт. ве́чер; 2) (V.) вече́рняя звезда́; 3) вече́рний звон (тж. ~-bell); 4) pl вече́рняя моли́тва или слу́жба; вече́рня.

vespertine ['vespətaɪn] a вече́рний, ночно́й.

vessel ['vesl] n 1) сосу́д (тж. анат.); 2) су́дно, кора́бль; ◊ leaky ~ болту́н, не уме́ющий хра-

ни́ть секре́т; weaker ~ библ., тж. шутл. не́мощнейший сосу́д (т. е. же́нщина).

vest I [vest] n 1) ни́жняя руба́шка или фуфа́йка; 2) жиле́т(ка); 3) церк. облаче́ние.

vest II v 1) церк. облача́ть(ся); 2) облека́ть (вла́стью и т. п.; with); 3) поруча́ть, доверя́ть (кому́-л. — in).

vestal ['vestl] n 1) веста́лка (тж. ~ virgin); 2) чи́стая, непоро́чная же́нщина.

vestee [ves'tiː] n мани́шка, вста́вка (в же́нском пла́тье).

vestibular [ve'stɪbjulə] a анат. вестибуля́рный.

vestige ['vestɪdʒ] n след, при́знак; мале́йший оста́ток.

vestment ['vestmənt] n 1) одея́ние, оде́жда; 2) церк. облаче́ние.

vest-pocket ['vest'pɔkɪt] n 1) жиле́тный карма́н; 2) attr карма́нный (о форма́те).

vestry ['vestrɪ] n 1) церк. ри́зница; 2) помеще́ние для моли́твенных собра́ний; 3) собра́ние прихожа́н.

vet I [vet] n разг. ветерина́р.

vet II v разг. 1) вет. лечи́ть живо́тное (шутл. тж. челове́ка); 2) иссле́довать, проверя́ть; просма́тривать (ру́копись).

vetch [vetʃ] n бот. ви́ка.

veteran ['vetərən] n 1) ветера́н; 2) (бы́вший) уча́стник войны́; 3) быва́лый солда́т; 4) attr о́пытный, ста́рый; 5) attr испы́танный в боя́х.

veterinary I ['vetərɪnərɪ] n ветерина́р.

veterinary II a ветерина́рный.

veto I ['viːtou] n ве́то; пра́во ве́то; to put a ~ on smth. наложи́ть ве́то, запре́т на что-л.

veto II v налага́ть ве́то, запре́т.

vex [veks] v 1) раздража́ть, серди́ть; to be ~ed a) серди́ться (на кого́-л., что-л. — with, at); б) огорча́ться; how ~ing! кака́я доса́да!, как доса́дно!; 2) беспоко́ить, волнова́ть.

vexation [vek'seɪʃən] n 1) раздраже́ние, доса́да; 2) доса́дное обстоя́тельство, неприя́тность.

via ['vaɪə] prep че́рез.

viaduct ['vaɪədʌkt] n виаду́к.

vial ['vaɪəl] n (стекля́нный) пузырёк, буты́лочка.

viands ['vaɪəndz] n pl я́ства.

vibrant ['vaɪbrənt] a 1) вибри́рующий; дрожа́щий; 2) резони́рующий.

vibrate [vaɪ'breɪt] v 1) вибри́ровать; 2) звуча́ть; 3) кача́ть(ся), колеба́ть(ся); 4) трепета́ть, дрожа́ть (от чего́-л. — with).

vibration [vaɪ'breɪʃən] n 1) вибра́ция; 2) колеба́ние.

vicar ['vɪkə] n 1) церк. вика́рий; 2) наме́стник; замести́тель.

vicarious [vaɪ'kɛərɪəs] a 1) замеща́ющий; 2) соверше́нный за друго́го.

vice¹ [vaɪs] n 1) поро́к; 2) недоста́ток (хара́ктера); constitutional ~ физи́ческий недоста́ток; 3) но́ров (у ло́шади).

vice² n тех. тиски́; (as) firm as a ~ ту́го закреплённый, неподви́жный.

vice- [vaɪs-] pref ви́це-.

vice-admiral ['vaɪs'ædmərəl] n ви́це-адмира́л.

vice-like ['vaɪslaɪk] a кре́пкий (о рукопожа́тии).

vice-president ['vaɪs'prezɪdənt] n ви́це-президе́нт.

viceroy ['vaɪsrɔɪ] *n* вице-коро́ль.

vice versa ['vaɪsɪ'vəːsə] *adv* наоборо́т.

vicinity [vɪ'sɪnɪtɪ] *n* 1) окре́стности; 2) сосе́дство, бли́зость; in the ~ (of) побли́зости (от); по сосе́дству (с); in the ~ of sixty о́коло шести́десяти.

vicious ['vɪʃəs] *a* 1) поро́чный; 2) непра́вильный, оши́бочный; 3) зло́бный, ожесточённый; 4) норови́стый (*о лошади*).

vicissitude [vɪ'sɪsɪtjuːd] *n* превра́тность.

victim ['vɪktɪm] *n* же́ртва; ~s of war же́ртвы войны́.

victimize ['vɪktɪmaɪz] *v* 1) де́лать кого́-л. свое́й же́ртвой, му́чить; 2) обма́нывать.

victor ['vɪktə] *n* 1) победи́тель; 2) *attr* победоно́сный.

victoria [vɪk'tɔːrɪə] *n* фаэто́н, викто́рия.

Victorian [vɪk'tɔːrɪən] *a* викториа́нский, эпо́хи короле́вы Викто́рии; *перен.* старомо́дный, устаре́вший.

victorious [vɪk'tɔːrɪəs] *a* победоно́сный.

victory ['vɪktərɪ] *n* побе́да; to gain (*или* to win) the ~ одержа́ть побе́ду (*над кем-л.* — *over*); to secure a ~ обеспе́чить побе́ду; доби́ться побе́ды; to claim the ~ наста́ивать на свое́й побе́де.

victual ['vɪtl] *v* 1) снабжа́ть прови́зией; 2) запаса́ться прови́зией.

victuals ['vɪtlz] *n pl* пи́ща, прови́зия, продово́льствие.

vie [vaɪ] *v* сопе́рничать (*с кем-л.* — *with*; *в чём-л.* — *in*).

Vietnamese I [,vjetnə'miːz] *n* вьетна́мец; вьетна́мка; the ~ (*употр. как pl*) вьетна́мцы.

Vietnamese II *a* вьетна́мский.

view I [vjuː] *n* 1) вид; a glorious ~ вели́чественный, живопи́сный пейза́ж; dissolving ~s тума́нные карти́ны; 2) взгляд, мне́ние; сужде́ние; то́чка зре́ния (*тж.* point of ~); представле́ние; large ~s широ́кие взгля́ды; in my ~ по моему́ мне́нию; in this ~ в э́том отноше́нии, с э́той то́чки зре́ния; to take a dim ~ of *разг.* смотре́ть на что-л. *или* относи́ться к чему́-л. пессимисти́чески; to take long ~s проявля́ть дальнови́дность, предусмотри́тельность; 3) по́ле зре́ния; to be in ~ а) быть ви́димым; б) предви́деться; to come into ~ появи́ться, стать ви́димым; to come in ~ of а) уви́деть что-л.; б) стать ви́димым отку́да-л.; to pass from ~ скры́ться и́з виду; 4) наме́рение, цель, вид; with the ~ of, with a ~ to с це́лью, в це́лях, име́я в виду́, с наме́рением; to bear (*или* to have, to keep) in ~ не теря́ть и́з виду; име́ть в виду́; in ~ of ввиду́, принима́я во внима́ние; 5) осмо́тр; on ~ вы́ставленный для обозре́ния; to the ~ откры́то, откры́тый; private ~ закры́тый просмо́тр (*выставки и т. п.*).

view II *v* 1) осма́тривать; 2) смотре́ть на, рассма́тривать.

viewer ['vjuːə] *n* зри́тель; посети́тель (*в музее, галерее*).

view-finder ['vjuː,faɪndə] *n фото* видоиска́тель.

viewless ['vjuːlɪs] *a* неви́димый.

view-point ['vjuːpɔɪnt] *n* то́чка зре́ния.

vigil ['vɪdʒɪl] *n* бо́дрствование; to keep ~ бо́дрствовать.

vigilance ['vɪdʒɪləns] *n* бди́тельность.

vigilant ['vɪdʒɪlənt] *a* бди́тельный.

vigor ['vɪgə] *амер. см.* vigour.

vigorous ['vɪgərəs] *a* си́льный, энерги́чный, бо́дрый.

vigour ['vɪgə] *n* си́ла, эне́ргия, бо́дрость.

viking ['vaɪkɪŋ] *n ист.* ви́кинг.

vile [vaɪl] *a* 1) по́длый, ни́зкий; 2) *разг.* скве́рный, ме́рзкий; отврати́тельный.

vilify ['vɪlɪfaɪ] *v* поноси́ть, черни́ть (*кого-л.*).

villa ['vɪlə] *n* ви́лла.

village ['vɪlɪdʒ] *n* 1) дере́вня, село́; 2) *attr* дереве́нский, се́льский.

villager ['vɪlɪdʒə] *n* дереве́нский, се́льский жи́тель.

villain ['vɪlən] *n* 1) негодя́й, злоде́й; 2) *шутл.* разбо́йник (*о шаловливом ребёнке*); 3) *ист.* вилла́н.

villainous ['vɪlənəs] *a* 1) по́длый; 2) *разг.* отврати́тельный, ме́рзкий.

villainy ['vɪlənɪ] *n.* 1) по́длость; 2) злоде́йство.

villein ['vɪlɪn] *см.* villain 3).

vim [vɪm] *n разг.* си́ла, эне́ргия.

vindicate ['vɪndɪkeɪt] *v* 1) отста́ивать (*права, дело и т. п.*); подде́рживать; 2) опра́вдывать (*поведение, политику и т. п.*).

vindication [,vɪndɪ'keɪʃən] *n* 1) защи́та; 2) оправда́ние.

vindicative ['vɪndɪkətɪv] *a* 1) защити́тельный; 2) кара́тельный.

vindictive [vɪn'dɪktɪv] *a* мсти́тельный.

vine [vaɪn] *n* 1) виногра́дная лоза́ (*тж.* grape-vine); 2) ползу́чее *или* вью́щееся расте́ние.

vinegar ['vɪnɪgə] *n* у́ксус.

vineyard ['vɪnjəd] *n* виногра́дник.

vinous ['vaɪnəs] *a* ви́нный.

vintage ['vɪntɪdʒ] *n* 1) сбор виногра́да; 2) урожа́й виногра́да; 3) вино́ (*сбора определённого года или определённого сорта винограда*).

viol ['vaɪəl] *n муз.* вио́ла.

viola[a] [vɪ'oulə] *n муз.* альт (*смычковый инструмент*).

viola[b] ['vaɪələ] *n* расте́ние семе́йства фиа́лковых.

violate ['vaɪəleɪt] *v* 1) наси́ловать; применя́ть, соверша́ть наси́лие; 2) (*грубо*) наруша́ть, попира́ть (*закон, права, договор и т. п.*); 3) вторга́ться, врыва́ться; наруша́ть (*тишину и т. п.*); 4) оскверня́ть.

violation [,vaɪə'leɪʃən] *n* 1) наси́лие; 2) (гру́бое) наруше́ние (*закона и т. п.*); 3) оскверне́ние.

violence ['vaɪələns] *n* 1) наси́лие; to do ~ to оскробля́ть, оскверня́ть; наси́ловать; 2) си́ла, неи́стовство.

violent ['vaɪələnt] *a* 1) си́льный; 2) неи́стовый, я́ростный, отча́янный; бу́йный (*о характере*); 3) наси́льственный (*о смерти, мерах*).

violet I ['vaɪəlɪt] *n* 1) фиа́лка; 2) фиоле́товый, лило́вый цвет.

violet II *a* фиоле́товый, лило́вый.

violin [,vaɪə'lɪn] *n* скри́пка.

violinist ['vaɪəlɪnɪst] *n* скрипа́ч(ка).

violoncellist [,vaɪələn'tʃelɪst] *n* виолонче́лист.

violoncello [,vaɪələn'tʃelou] *n* виолонче́ль.

viper ['vaɪpə] *n* 1) гадю́ка (*тж.* common ~);

2) змея, ехидна, вероломный человек; 3) *сленг* курильщик марихуаны.

virago [vɪˈrɑːgou] *n* сварливая женщина, мегера.

virgin I [ˈvəːdʒɪn] *n* дева, девственница; the Virgin богородица.

virgin II *a* 1) девственный; *перен.* чистый; нетронутый; 2) девичий.

virginal [ˈvəːdʒɪnl] *a* девственный, чистый.

virginity [vəːˈdʒɪnɪtɪ] *n* 1) девственность; 2) девичество.

virile [ˈvɪraɪl] *a* 1) сильный, жизнеспособный; мужественный; 2) возмужалый; 3) мужской.

virility [vɪˈrɪlɪtɪ] *n* 1) мужество; 2) возмужалость; 3) половая зрелость.

virtual [ˈvəːtʃuəl] *a* фактический; действительный.

virtually [ˈvəːtʃuəlɪ] *adv* фактически, в сущности.

virtue [ˈvəːtjuː] *n* 1) добродетель; 2) достоинство, хорошее качество; 3) сила, эффективность (*средства и т. п.*); there is little ~ in that medicine мало пользы от этого лекарства; 4) целомудрие; of easy ~ не отличающаяся строгим нравом (*о женщине*); ◇ by ~ of, in ~ of благодаря (*чему-л.*), посредством (*чего-л.*), на основании (*чего-л.*).

virtuous [ˈvəːtjuəs] *a* 1) добродетельный; 2) целомудренный.

virulence [ˈvɪruləns] *n* ядовитость; *перен.* злоба.

virulent [ˈvɪrulənt] *a* 1) ядовитый; *перен.* злобный, оскорбительный; 2) заразный, опасный, смертельный.

virus [ˈvaɪərəs] *n* вирус; *перен.* зараза.

visage [ˈvɪzɪdʒ] *n* лицо; выражение лица.

visard [ˈvɪzəd] *см.* visor.

viscid [ˈvɪsɪd] *см.* viscous.

viscosity [vɪsˈkɔsɪtɪ] *n* 1) вязкость; 2) внутреннее трение.

viscount [ˈvaɪkaunt] *n* виконт.

viscous [ˈvɪskəs] *a* вязкий, липкий.

vise [vaɪs] *см.* vice².

visé I [ˈviːzeɪ] *n* виза.

visé II *v* визировать.

visibility [ˌvɪsɪˈbɪlɪtɪ] *n* видимость.

visible [ˈvɪzəbl] *a* видимый; видный; *перен.* явный, очевидный.

vision [ˈvɪʒən] *n* 1) зрение; beyond our ~ вне нашего поля зрения, вне досягаемости нашего зрения; 2) предвидение; проницательность; 3) видение, мечта.

visional [ˈvɪʒənl] *a* 1) зрительный; 2) воображаемый.

visionary I [ˈvɪʒnərɪ] *n* 1) мечтатель, фантазёр; 2) непрактичный человек; 3) человек, подверженный галлюцинациям.

visionary II *a* 1) мечтательный; 2) непрактичный; 3) призрачный, воображаемый; фантастический.

visit I [ˈvɪsɪt] *n* посещение, визит; to pay (*или* to make) a ~ посетить, навестить; нанести визит; to be on a ~ гостить (*у кого-л.* — to); to come on a ~ приехать в гости; ◇ domiciliary ~ домашний обыск.

visit II *v* посещать; навещать; гостить;

I hope to ~ Leningrad я надеюсь побывать в Ленинграде.

visitant [ˈvɪzɪtənt] *n* 1) посетитель, гость; 2) перелётная птица.

visitation [ˌvɪzɪˈteɪʃən] *n* 1) посещение; визит; 2) инспектирование; осмотр; обыск нейтрального судна (*во время войны*); 3) испытание; кара, наказание.

visitor [ˈvɪzɪtə] *n* 1) гость; посетитель; summer ~ дачник; 2) инспектор.

visor [ˈvaɪzə] *n* 1) козырёк (*фуражки*); 2) *косм.* лицевое стекло (*шлема*); 3) *ист.* забрало.

vista [ˈvɪstə] *n* 1) вид на что-л. (*открывающийся между рядами деревьев и т. п.*); 2) аллея, просека (*с видом на что-л.*); 3) вереница воспоминаний (*о чём-л.* — of).

visual [ˈvɪzuəl] *a* 1) зрительный; оптический; визуальный; 2) наглядный (*о пособиях*).

visualize [ˈvɪzuəlaɪz] *v* воображать, представлять себе; мысленно видеть.

vital [ˈvaɪtl] *a* 1) жизненный; 2) существенный, важный; 3) роковой, смертельный.

vitality [vaɪˈtælɪtɪ] *n* 1) жизнеспособность; жизненность; 2) жизненные силы.

vitals [ˈvaɪtlz] *n pl* 1) жизненно важные органы (*сердце, лёгкие и т. п.*); 2) наиболее важные части (*механизма и т. п.*).

vitamin [ˈvɪtəmɪn] *n* витамин.

vitiate [ˈvɪʃɪeɪt] *v* 1) портить; 2) делать недействительным (*соглашение и т. п.*).

vitreous [ˈvɪtrɪəs] *a* 1) стеклянный; 2) стекловидный.

vitriol [ˈvɪtrɪəl] *n* 1) купорос; blue (*или* copper) ~ медный купорос; green ~ железный купорос; 2) сарказм, язвительность.

vituperate [vɪˈtjuːpəreɪt] *v* бранить, поносить.

vivacious [vɪˈveɪʃəs] *a* весёлый, живой, оживлённый.

vivacity [vɪˈvæsɪtɪ] *n* живость; оживлённость, весёлость.

vivid [ˈvɪvɪd] *a* 1) яркий (*о свете, краске*); 2) живой (*о воспоминании, описании и т. п.*); пылкий (*о воображении*).

vivify [ˈvɪvɪfaɪ] *v* оживлять.

vixen [ˈvɪksn] *n* 1) лисица; 2) сварливая женщина, мегера.

vizi(e)r [vɪˈzɪə] *n* визирь.

vizor [ˈvaɪzə] *см.* visor.

vocable [ˈvoukəbl] *n* слово.

vocabulary [vəˈkæbjulərɪ] *n* 1) словарь (*автора, профессиональный и т. п.*); 2) запас слов; 3) словарный состав (*языка*).

vocal [ˈvoukəl] *a* 1) голосовой; 2) устный; 3) *фон.* звонкий; 4) звучный; 5) вокальный.

vocation [vouˈkeɪʃən] *n* 1) профессия, занятие; 2) призвание.

vocational [vouˈkeɪʃənl] *a* профессиональный.

vocative [ˈvɔkətɪv] *n грам.* звательный падеж.

vociferate [vouˈsɪfəreɪt] *v* кричать, орать.

vociferous [vouˈsɪfərəs] *a* шумный, громогласный.

vogue [voug] *n* мода; популярность; to be in ~ быть в моде; быть популярным; all the ~ последний крик моды.

voice I [vɔɪs] *n* 1) голос; high-pitched ~ высокий голос; to be not in ~ быть не в голосе;

in a loud ~ гро́мко; in a low ~ ти́хо; sweet (*или* soft) ~ не́жный го́лос; to lift up one's ~ возвы́сить го́лос; 2) го́лос (*на вы́борах*); пра́во го́лоса; my ~ is for peace я голосу́ю, выска́зываюсь за мир; with one ~ единогла́сно; negative ~ го́лос про́тив; to have a ~ in име́ть пра́во го́лоса (*в чём-л.*); 3) выраже́ние; to give ~ to выража́ть, дава́ть во́лю; 4) *грам.* зало́г; active (passive, middle) ~ действи́тельный (страда́тельный, сре́дний) зало́г.

voice II *v* 1) выража́ть, выска́зывать; 2) *фон.* произноси́ть зво́нко.

voiced [vɔɪst] *a фон.* зво́нкий.

voiceless ['vɔɪslɪs] *a* 1) безголо́сый; 2) немо́й; 3) *фон.* глухо́й.

void I [vɔɪd] *n* пустота́.

void II *a* 1) пусто́й; незаня́тый; 2) лишённый (*чего-л.— of*), свобо́дный (*от чего-л.— of*); 3) недействи́тельный; to be ~ стать недействи́тельным.

voile [vɔɪl] *n* вуа́ль (*ткань*).

volatile ['vɔlətaɪl] *a* 1) *хим.* лету́чий, испаря́ющийся; 2) непостоя́нный, изме́нчивый.

volatility [,vɔlə'tɪlɪtɪ] *n* 1) *хим.* лету́честь; 2) непостоя́нство, изме́нчивость.

volatilize [vɔ'lætɪlaɪz] *v* улету́чиваться; испаря́ть(ся).

volcanic [vɔl'kænɪk] *a* 1) вулкани́ческий; 2) бу́рный (*о характере и т. п.*).

volcano [vɔl'keɪnou] *n* вулка́н; active (dormant) ~ де́йствующий (безде́йствующий) вулка́н; dead ~, extinct ~ поту́хший вулка́н; mud ~ грязево́й вулка́н.

volition [vou'lɪʃən] *n* 1) жела́ние, хоте́ние; by one's own ~ по со́бственному жела́нию; 2) во́ля.

volley I ['vɔlɪ] *n* 1) залп; *амер.* бе́глый ого́нь; 2) град (*камней, пуль, упрёков и т. п.*); 3) приём мяча́ на лету́ (*в те́ннисе и т. п.*).

volley II *v* 1) стреля́ть за́лпами; *амер.* вести́ бе́глый ого́нь; 2) сы́пать(ся) гра́дом; 3) принима́ть мяч на лету́.

volley-ball ['vɔlɪbɔːl] *n спорт.* волейбо́л.

voltᵃ [voult] *n* 1) *эл.* вольт.

voltᵇ [vɔlt] *n* 1) вольт (*круто́й поворо́т ло́шади*); 2) уклоне́ние от уда́ра (*в фехтова́нии*).

voltage ['voultɪdʒ] *n эл.* напряже́ние то́ка, вольта́ж.

voltaic [vɔl'teɪɪk] *a эл.* 1) гальвани́ческий; 2) во́льтов.

voltameter [vɔl'tæmɪtə] *n эл.* вольта́метр.

volte [vɔltɪ] *см.* voltᵇ.

voltmeter ['voult,miːtə] *n эл.* вольтме́тр.

volubility [,vɔlju'bɪlɪtɪ] *n* говорли́вость; пото́к слов, словоизверже́ние.

voluble ['vɔljubl] *a* многоречи́вый, говорли́вый.

volume ['vɔljum] *n* 1) том, кни́га; 2) вмести́мость, ёмкость; 3) объём; 4) *обыкн. pl* ма́сса; ~s of smoke клубы́ ды́ма; 5) *муз.* полнота́ (*зву́ка*); 6) *ист.* сви́ток (*папируса и т. п.*); ◊ to speak ~s говори́ть красноречи́вее вся́ких слов; говори́ть о мно́гом (*for*).

voluminous [və'ljuːmɪnəs] *a* 1) объёмистый; масси́вный; 2) свобо́дный, просто́рный, широ́кий (*об оде́жде и т. п.*); 3) многото́мный; 4) плодови́тый (*об а́вторе*).

voluntary ['vɔləntərɪ] *a* 1) доброво́льный;

2) доброво́льческий; 3) созна́тельный; умы́шленный; 4) *физиол.* произво́льный.

volunteer I [,vɔlən'tɪə] *n* доброво́лец.

volunteer II *v* 1) поступа́ть доброво́льцем (*на вое́нную слу́жбу*); 2) вызыва́ться (*сде́лать что-л.*).

voluptuous [və'lʌptjuəs] *a* сластолюби́вый, чу́вственный.

voluptuousness [və'lʌptjuəsnɪs] *n* сластолю́бие, чу́вственность.

vomit I ['vɔmɪt] *n* 1) рво́та; 2) рво́тное (сре́дство).

vomit II *v* рвать; *перен.* изверга́ть.

voodoo I ['vuːduː] *n* 1) колдовство́, ведовство́ (*особ. у не́гров*); 2) колду́н (*тж.* ~ doctor, ~ priest).

voodoo II *v* околдо́вывать, заколдо́вывать.

voracious [və'reɪʃəs] *a* прожо́рливый, жа́дный.

vortex ['vɔːteks] *n* (*pl тж.* vortices ['vɔːtɪsiːz]) 1) водоворо́т; вихрь; 2) *attr* вихрево́й.

votaress ['voutərɪs] *n* сторо́нница, защи́тница; почита́тельница.

votarist ['voutərɪst] *см.* votary.

votary ['voutərɪ] *n* сторо́нник, защи́тник; почита́тель.

vote I [vout] *n* 1) голосова́ние; ~ by show of hands голосова́ние подня́тием рук; card ~ голосова́ние манда́тами; roll-call ~ голосова́ние по спи́ску; by closed ~ закры́тым голосова́нием; to put to the ~ ста́вить на голосова́ние; plural ~ голосова́ние одного́ челове́ка в не́скольких места́х; straw ~ неофициа́льный опро́с с це́лью выясне́ния обще́ственного мне́ния; 2) го́лос (*на вы́борах*); the ~ пра́во го́лоса; to cast a ~ подава́ть го́лос, голосова́ть; to lose the ~ лиши́ться пра́ва го́лоса; to split one's ~ голосова́ть за обо́их кандида́тов; 3) голоса́, число́ голосо́в; 4) во́тум; реше́ние, при́нятое голосова́нием; ~ of censure во́тум недове́рия; 5) избира́тельный бюллете́нь.

vote II *v* 1) голосова́ть (*за — for; против —* against); to ~ Democrat (Republican) *амер.* голосова́ть за демокра́тов (республика́нцев); to ~ by short ballot *амер.* голосова́ть за вы́борщиков в це́лом; 2) постановля́ть, присужда́ть большинство́м голосо́в; избира́ть (*куда́-л.; in*); 3) признава́ть; they all ~d the trip a great success все они́ призна́ли прогу́лку о́чень уда́чной; 4) *разг.* предлага́ть; ◊ to ~ **down** провали́ть, отклони́ть (*предложе́ние*); забаллоти́ровать.

voter ['voutə] *n* избира́тель.

voting ['voutɪŋ] *n* голосова́ние, вы́боры; cumulative ~ систе́ма вы́боров, при кото́рой ка́ждый избира́тель располага́ет голоса́ми по числу́ кандида́тов и име́ет пра́во отда́ть их все одному́ кандида́ту.

voting-paper ['voutɪŋ,peɪpə] *n* избира́тельный бюллете́нь.

votive ['voutɪv] *a* испо́лненный по обе́ту.

vouch [vautʃ] *v* руча́ться; поручи́ться.

voucher ['vautʃə] *n* 1) поручи́тель; 2) руча́тельство; поручи́тельство.

vouchsafe [vautʃ'seɪf] *v* удоста́ивать; he ~d no reply он не удосто́ил отве́том, он не снизошёл до отве́та.

vow I [vau] *n* обе́т; to make (*или* to take) a ~ дава́ть обе́т.

vow II *v* 1) дава́ть обе́т; 2) заявля́ть, покля́сться.

vowel ['vauəl] *n* 1) гла́сный звук; open (close) ~ откры́тый (закры́тый) гла́сный; 2) гла́сная бу́ква.

voyage I [vɔɪdʒ] *n* 1) (морско́е) путеше́ствие; 2) полёт, перелёт (*на самолёте*).

voyage II *v* пла́вать, путеше́ствовать (*по мо́рю*); 2) лета́ть (*на самолёте*).

voyager ['vɔɪədʒə] *n* 1) путеше́ственник (*по мо́рю*); 2) морепла́ватель.

vulcanize ['vʌlkənaɪz] *v* вулканизи́ровать (*резину*).

vulgar ['vʌlgə] *a* 1) гру́бый; 2) вульга́рный; 3) простонаро́дный; 4) общераспространённый; 5) просто́й (*о дроби*).

vulgarian [vʌl'gɛərɪən] *n* вульга́рный челове́к.

vulgarity [vʌl'gærɪtɪ] *n* 1) вульга́рность; 2) *pl* вульга́рное поведе́ние; вульга́рные выраже́ния.

vulgarize ['vʌlgəraɪz] *v* 1) вульгаризи́ровать; 2) опошля́ть.

vulnerable ['vʌlnərəbl] *a* уязви́мый.

vulpine ['vʌlpaɪn] *a* хи́трый, лука́вый.

vulture ['vʌltʃə] *n* 1) *зоол.* гриф, стервя́тник; 2) хи́щник.

vulturous ['vʌltʃurəs] *a* хи́щный.

vying ['vaɪɪŋ] *pres. p.* см. vie.

W

W, w ['dʌblju:] *n* 23-я бу́ква англ. алфави́та.

wabble ['wɔbl] см. wobble.

wad I [wɔd] *n* 1) клочо́к чего́-л. мя́гкого, *напр.*, ва́ты, ше́рсти *и т. п.*; 2) пыж; 3) па́чка (*банкно́т, бума́ги*).

wad II *v* 1) прокла́дывать, набива́ть, подбива́ть ва́той; 2) забива́ть пыж; 3) скла́дывать в па́чки.

wadding ['wɔdɪŋ] *n* 1) наби́вка, подби́вка (ва́той); 2) ва́та, шерсть, во́лос *и т. п.* для наби́вки.

waddle I ['wɔdl] *n* перева́ливающаяся похо́дка.

waddle II *v* ходи́ть перева́ливаясь; ковыля́ть.

wade [weɪd] *v* 1) перебира́ться (*вброд, по грязи и т. п.*); 2) набра́сываться на кого́-л., критикова́ть; принима́ться за кого́-л. (in, into); 3) случа́йно наткну́ться, набрести́ (into); □ to ~ **through** одоле́ть, преодоле́ть.

wading ['weɪdɪŋ] *n* 1) перехо́д вброд; 2) *attr* боло́тный (*о птицах*); 3) *attr* пла́вательный.

wafer ['weɪfə] *n* 1) ва́фля; 2) обла́тка.

waffle ['wɔfl] *n* ва́фля.

waft I [wɑːft] *n* 1) взмах; маха́ние; 2) дунове́ние; струя́ (*воздуха, аромата*); 3) *мор.* сигна́л флажко́м.

waft II *v* 1) нести́ (*по воздуху, воде*); 2) рассека́ть (*воду, воздух*).

wag¹ I [wæg] *n* взмах.

wag¹ II *v* 1) маха́ть, разма́хивать; 2) пока́чивать(ся); 3): to ~ one's finger грози́ть па́льцем (*кому-л.*— at); 4) виля́ть (*хвостом*).

wag² *n* 1) шутни́к; 2) *сленг* лентя́й; to play (the) ~ прогуля́ть, не яви́ться (*на работу, в шко́лу*).

wage¹ [weɪdʒ] *n обыкн. pl* 1) жа́лованье, зара-

ботная пла́та; living ~ прожи́точный ми́нимум; dismissal ~ выходно́е посо́бие; to cut (*или* to dock) ~s снижа́ть зарпла́ту; on board ~s на свои́х харча́х; 2) возме́здие.

wage² *v* 1) вести́ (*войну*); 2) вступа́ть (*в конфли́кт и т. п.*).

wage-cut ['weɪdʒˌkʌt] *n* сниже́ние за́работной пла́ты.

wage-freezing ['weɪdʒˌfriːzɪŋ] *n* заморажива́ние за́работной пла́ты.

wager I ['weɪdʒə] *n* пари́, ста́вка.

wager II *v* 1) держа́ть пари́; 2) рискова́ть.

waggery ['wægərɪ] *n* 1) шутли́вость; 2) *pl* ша́лости, шу́тки.

waggle ['wægl] *v разг.* виля́ть, маха́ть (*хвосто́м*).

wag(g)on ['wægən] *n* 1) *ж.-д.* ваго́н-платфо́рма; 2) ваго́нетка; 3) пово́зка, фурго́н; patrol ~ *амер.* тюре́мная каре́та; lunch ~ буфе́т-заку́сочная на колёсах.

wag(g)oner ['wægənə] *n* во́зчик.

wagtail ['wægteɪl] *n* трясогу́зка (*птица*).

waif [weɪf] *n* 1) бездо́мный челове́к; беспризо́рный, бездо́мный ребёнок; ~s and strays беспризо́рные де́ти; 2) бро́шенная вещь; 3) заблуди́вшееся дома́шнее живо́тное.

wail I [weɪl] *n* 1) вопль; вой; 2) причита́ние.

wail II *v* 1) выть, вопи́ть (*от чего-л.*— with); 2) гро́мко опла́кивать кого́-л., причита́ть (*часто* to ~ over).

wain [weɪn] *n* 1) *поэт.* пово́зка; 2): the Wain, Charles's Wain *астр.* Больша́я Медве́дица; the Lesser Wain *астр.* Ма́лая Медве́дица.

wainscot I ['weɪnskət] *n* деревя́нная пане́ль *или* обши́вка.

wainscot II *v* обшива́ть пане́лью.

waist [weɪst] *n* 1) та́лия; slender ~ то́нкая та́лия; 2) лиф, корса́ж; *амер.* ли́фчик.

waist-belt ['weɪstbelt] *n* поясно́й реме́нь.

waistcoat ['weɪskout] *n* жиле́т; strait ~ смири́тельная руба́шка.

waist-deep ['weɪst'diːp] *a* по по́яс.

waist-high ['weɪst'haɪ] см. waist-deep.

wait I [weɪt] *n* 1) ожида́ние; 2) сиде́ние в заса́де; to lay ~, to lie in ~ выжида́ть в заса́де, подстерега́ть (*кого-л.*— for).

wait II *v* 1) ждать, дожида́ться, ожида́ть (for); to keep ~ing заста́вить ждать; 2) прислу́живать, обслу́живать (*тж.* to ~ on, to ~ upon).

waiter ['weɪtə] *n* 1) официа́нт; 2) подно́с.

waiting-room ['weɪtɪŋrum] *n* 1) зал ожида́ния; 2) приёмная.

waitress ['weɪtrɪs] *n* официа́нтка.

waive [weɪv] *v* 1) отка́зываться (*от права, требования*); 2) уклоня́ться, избега́ть.

wake¹ [weɪk] *n*: in the ~ of *мор.* в кильва́тер за; *перен.* сле́дуя; по следа́м, по пята́м.

wake² *v* (*past* woke; *p. p.* woken) 1) (*тж.* to ~ up) просыпа́ться; *перен.* пробужда́ться; 2) (*тж.* to ~ up) буди́ть; *перен.* пробужда́ть, возбужда́ть; 3) бо́дрствовать.

wakeful ['weɪkful] *a* 1) бессо́нный; 2) бо́дрствующий; 3) бди́тельный.

waken ['weɪkən] *v* 1) просыпа́ться; пробужда́ться; 2) буди́ть.

walk I [wɔːk] *n* 1) ходьба́; at the ~ ша́гом;

sharp ~ быстрая ходьба; 2) походка; I know him by his ~ я узнаю его по походке; 3) прогулка (пешком); to go for a ~, to take a ~ идти гулять, прогуляться; 4) аллея, дорожка, тропа (для пешеходов); 5) любимое или обычное место прогулки; 6) обход (своих покупателей); ◊ ~ of life состояние; общественное положение; образ жизни.

walk II v 1) идти, ходить (пешком); обходить; 2) идти, ехать шагом; вести шагом; появляться (о призраке); □ to ~ **about** гулять, прогуливаться; to ~ **along** продвигаться, идти вперёд; to ~ **away** а) уходить; б) уводить; в) легко обгонять (from); г) унести, украсть (with); to ~ **in** входить; to ~ **into** а) входить; б) сленг набрасываться (на); пожирать, уплетать; to ~ **off** а) (внезапно) уходить; б) унести, украсть (with); в): to ~ smb. off his legs утомить ходьбой; to ~ **out** а) амер. (за)бастовать; б) груб. «гулять» с кем-л. (with); to ~ **over** а) перешагнуть; б) легко победить (противника); to ~ **up** подойти к кому-л. (to); ◊ ~ the wards учиться на медицинском факультете, быть студентом-медиком.

walker ['wɔːkə] n ходок; space ~ космонавт, вышедший в открытый космос.

walking I ['wɔːkɪŋ] n ходьба.

walking II a ходячий.

walking-on ['wɔːkɪŋˈɔn] a выходной, без слов (о роли).

walking-out ['wɔːkɪŋˈaut] a воен. выходной (о форме).

walking-papers ['wɔːkɪŋˌpeɪpəz] n pl: to get one's ~ получить увольнение с работы.

walking-stick ['wɔːkɪŋstɪk] n трость, палка для гулянья.

walking-ticket ['wɔːkɪŋˌtɪkɪt] см. walking-papers.

walking-tour ['wɔːkɪŋtuə] n пешеходная экскурсия.

walk-out ['wɔːkˌaut] n 1) выход (из партии, профсоюза и т. п.); 2) амер. забастовка.

walk-over ['wɔːkˌouvə] n лёгкая победа.

wall I [wɔːl] n 1) стена; dead ~, blank ~ глухая стена; 2) стенка (сосуда); ◊ to drive (или to force, to push) to the ~ припереть к стенке, довести до критического состояния; to go to the ~ а) потерпеть неудачу; б) обанкротиться; to give smb. the ~ посторониться, уступить дорогу (или лучшее место); to take the ~ of не уступить дороги (или лучшего места).

wall II v обносить стеной (тж to ~ in); □ to ~ **up** заделать отверстие.

wallet ['wɔlɪt] n 1) бумажник; 2) маленький чемодан, кожаная сумка (для инструментов и т. п.).

wall-eye ['wɔːlaɪ] n бельмо.

wallflower ['wɔːlˌflauə] n 1) бот. желтофиоль; 2) разг. дама, оставшаяся без кавалера (на балу).

wallop I ['wɔləp] n разг. сильный удар.

wallop II v разг. бить, тузить.

wallow ['wɔlou] v 1) валяться, барахтаться; 2) погрязнуть (в чём-л.— in).

wall-painting ['wɔːlˌpeɪntɪŋ] n стенная роспись, фрески.

wallpaper ['wɔːlˌpeɪpə] n обои; to hang ~ оклеивать обоями.

Wall Street ['wɔːlˈstriːt] n Уолл-стрит (улица

в Нью-Йорке, где помещаются биржа и главнейшие банки); перен. американский финансовый капитал.

walnut ['wɔːlnət] n 1) грецкий орех; 2) орех (древесина); 3) attr ореховый.

walrus ['wɔːlrəs] n морж.

waltz I [wɔːls] n вальс.

waltz II v вальсировать.

wan [wɔn] a 1) бледный, измождённый; 2) тусклый, бесцветный; 3) слабый (об улыбке); потухший (о взгляде).

wand [wɔnd] n дирижёрская палочка; жезл.

wander ['wɔndə] v 1) бродить, странствовать (по чему-л.— over); 2) блуждать (о мыслях, глазах и т. п.); 3) заблудиться; 4) бредить; 5) уклоняться (от темы разговора; from).

wanderer ['wɔndərə] n странник.

wanderlust ['wɔndəlʌst] n страсть к путешествиям.

wane I [weɪn] n 1) убывание; to be on the ~ убывать; быть на исходе; the ~ of life закат жизни; 2) ущерб (луны).

wane II v 1) убывать, уменьшаться; лишаться силы, значения; 2) быть на ущербе (о луне).

wangle ['wæŋgl] v сленг 1) суметь добиться, ухитриться получить; 2) представить что-л. в выгодном для себя свете, состряпать (доклад, отчёт и т. п.).

want I [wɔnt] n 1) недостаток (в чём-л.— of); for (или through) ~ of за неимением, из-за недостатка чего-л.; 2) необходимость, нужда (в чём-л.— of); to be in ~ of нуждаться в чём-л.; 3) обыкн. pl потребность; 4) бедность.

want II v 1) желать, хотеть; 2) нуждаться (в чём-л.), требовать (чего-л.); call me if I am ~ed позовите меня, если я буду нужен; he is a little ~ing у него не все дома, он не совсем нормален; 3) недоставать.

wanting I ['wɔntɪŋ] a 1) нуждающийся, имеющий недостаток (в чём-л.— in); 2) недостающий.

wanting II prep без.

wanton I ['wɔntən] n 1) распутница; 2) разг. ракета, отклонившаяся от курса.

wanton II a 1) резвый, живой; 2) капризный, своенравный; 3) буйный (о росте); 4) распутный; 5) бессмысленный.

wanton III v резвиться; проказничать.

wapiti ['wɔpɪtɪ] n канадский олень, вапити.

war I [wɔː] n 1) война; the Great Patriotic War Великая Отечественная война; World War II вторая мировая война; civil ~ гражданская война; cold (push-button) ~ холодная (механизированная, «кнопочная») война; ~ to the death борьба не на жизнь, а на смерть; at ~ в состоянии войны (с кем-л.— with); to wage (или to make) ~ on, to levy ~ against вести войну с; to unleash a ~ развязать войну; to declare (или to proclaim) ~ объявлять войну (кому-л.— on, upon); to go to ~ а) прибегать к оружию; б) пойти на войну, на фронт; 2) борьба; ~ of the elements буря, борьба стихий; стихийное бедствие; 3) attr военный.

war II v уст. воевать; □ to ~ **down** завоевать, покорить.

warble I ['wɔːbl] n трель.

warble II v петь, щебетать (о птицах).

warbler ['wɔːblə] *n* певчая птица.

ward I [wɔːd] *n* 1) опекаемый, подопечный; 2) опёка; 3) больничная палата; 4) тюрёмная камера; 5) административное делёние города.

ward II *v* 1) (*часто* to ~ off) парировать, отражать (*удар, атаку*); отвращать (*опасность, нужду и т. п.*); 2) *уст.* охранять.

warden ['wɔːdn] *n* 1) начальник; 2) директор (*колледжа, госпиталя и т. п.*); 3) *амер.* начальник тюрьмы.

warder ['wɔːdə] *n* 1) тюрёмщик; 2) *уст.* страж, часовой.

wardrobe ['wɔːdroub] *n* гардероб.

ward-room ['wɔːdrum] *n* офицёрская кают-компания.

ware[1] [wɛə] *n* 1) издёлия; brown ~ глиняная посуда; 2) *pl* товар(ы); to push one's ~s рекламировать свой товары.

ware[2] *v* остерегаться; ~! берегись!

warehouse ['wɛəhaus] *n* 1) товарный склад; 2) оптовый магазин.

warfare ['wɔːfɛə] *n* война; приёмы ведёния войны; guerilla ~ партизанская война, действия партизанских отрядов; naval (stationary, germ) ~ морская (позиционная, бактериологическая) война.

warhead ['wɔːhed] *n* боевая головка; боевой заряд.

war-horse ['wɔːhɔːs] *n* 1) *ист.* боевой конь; 2) ветеран; бывалый человек.

warily ['wɛərɪlɪ] *adv* осторожно.

wariness ['wɛərɪnɪs] *n* осторожность.

warlike ['wɔːlaɪk] *a* воённый; войнственный.

warm I [wɔːm] *a* 1) тёплый; it is ~ тепло; I am ~ мне тепло; to make ~ греть, разогревать; to keep ~ держать в теплё; 2) согрётый; жаркий; *перен.* горячий, сердёчный; разгорячённый; to get ~ согревать(ся); *перен.* разгорячиться; рассердиться; ~ with wine разгорячённый вином; 3) горячий, свёжий (*о слёде*); 4) *разг.* богатый, состоятельный; 5) сильный, свёжий (*о запахе*); ◊ to make it ~ for smb. досаждать кому-л.

warm II *n* согревание; теплота; to have a ~ (по)грёться.

warm III *v* греть(ся), согревать(ся), нагревать (-ся), разогревать(ся); *перен.* разгорячить(ся); воодушевлять(ся), оживлять(ся) (*часто* to ~ up).

warm-blooded ['wɔːm,blʌdɪd] *a* 1) *зоол.* теплокровный; 2) горячий (*о темпераменте*).

warm-house ['wɔːmhaus] *n* теплица, оранжерёя.

warming ['wɔːmɪŋ] *n* 1) согревание; 2) *сленг* взбучка, трёпка.

war-monger ['wɔː,mʌŋgə] *n* поджигатель войны.

warmth [wɔːmθ] *n* 1) тепло, теплота; *перен.* сердёчность; 2) горячность; 3) раздражёние.

warn [wɔːn] *v* предостерегать, предупреждать.

warning ['wɔːnɪŋ] *n* 1) предостережёние, предупреждёние; to give ~ сдёлать предупреждёние; предупредить; to take ~ остерегаться; 2) признак; 3) предупреждёние (*об увольнении или уходе с работы*).

warp[1] [wɔːp] *n* основа (*ткани*).

warp[2] I *n* 1) коробление, искривлёние, перекос; *перен.* извращёние, извращённость; 2) (наносный) ил.

warp[2] II *v* 1) коробить(ся), искривлять(ся); *перен.* извращать; 2) удобрять наносным илом.

war-plane ['wɔːpleɪn] *n* воённый самолёт.

warrant I ['wɔrənt] *n* 1) основание; полномочие; ~ of attorney довёренность; 2) ордер, приказ; 3) гарантия, ручательство.

warrant II *v* 1) оправдывать; 2) гарантировать, ручаться.

warren ['wɔrɪn] *n* кроличий садок.

warring ['wɔrɪŋ] *a* непримиримый, противоречивый.

warrior ['wɔrɪə] *n* *поэт.* боёц, войн.

warship ['wɔːʃɪp] *n* воённый корабль.

wart [wɔːt] *n* бородавка.

war-wearied ['wɔː,wɪərɪd] *a* 1) утомлённый войной; 2) износившийся в боях.

war-worn ['wɔːwɔːn] *a* истощённый, опустошённый войной.

wary ['wɛərɪ] *a* осторожный.

was [wɔz (*сильная форма*), wəz, wz (*слабые формы*)] *past sg см.* be.

wash I [wɔʃ] *n* 1) мытьё; to get (*или* to have) a ~ помыться; 2) стирка; бельё (*для или из стирки*); 3) волна (*особ. за кормой парохода*); плеск (*волны*); 4) наносы (*песка, гравия и т. п.*); намытый грунт; 5) овраг, балка; dry ~ высохшее русло; 6) помои (*тж. перен. о жидком чае и т. п.*); 7) тонкий слой; 8) примочка.

wash II *v* 1) мыть(ся), умывать(ся); промывать; 2) стирать (*бельё*); 3) выдёрживать стирку не линяя; *перен.* выдёрживать критику; 4) омывать (*берега*); 5) смывать; размывать; 6) плескаться; 7) наносить тонким слоем; □ to ~ away смывать; to ~ down а) вымывать, смывать; б) *разг.* запивать (*еду*); to ~ off смывать; to ~ out а) смывать, размывать; б) *сленг* лишать (воённого) звания; увольнять; в) *сленг* не считаться; не выполнять (*распоряжений, инструкций*); г): ~ed out застиранный, полинявший; *перен.* утомлённый, вялый, ослабёвший; to ~ up мыть (*посуду*).

washable ['wɔʃəbl] *a* стирающийся, нелиняющий.

washateria [,wɔʃə'tɪərɪə] *n* *амер.* прачечная.

wash-board ['wɔʃbɔːd] *n* стиральная доска.

washer ['wɔʃə] *n* 1) мойщик; 2) мойка; 3) стиральная машина; 4) *тех.* прокладка.

washerwoman ['wɔʃə,wumən] *n* прачка.

wash-hand-stand ['wɔʃhænd,stænd] *n* умывальник.

wash-house ['wɔʃhaus] *n* прачечная.

washing ['wɔʃɪŋ] *n* 1) мытьё; 2) стирка; выстиранное бельё.

washing-up ['wɔʃɪŋ'ʌp] *n* мытьё посуды.

wash-leather ['wɔʃ,leðə] *n* замша.

wash-out ['wɔʃaut] *n* 1) размыв; 2) *сленг* неудача, провал; 3) *сленг* неудачник.

wash-room ['wɔʃrum] *n* *амер.* уборная.

wash-stand ['wɔʃstænd] *n* умывальник.

washwoman ['wɔʃ,wumən] *амер. см.* washerwoman.

washy ['wɔʃɪ] *a* водянистый.

wasn't ['wɔznt] *разг.* = was not.

wasp [wɔsp] *n* 1) оса; 2) *attr* осиный.

waspish ['wɔspɪʃ] *a* раздражительный, злой, язвительный.

wassail I ['wɔseɪl] n уст. 1) пиру́шка, попо́йка; 2) вы́пивка; напи́ток (обыкн. эль с пря́ностями).

wassail II v уст. пирова́ть, выпива́ть.

wastage ['weɪstɪdʒ] n поте́ри, уте́чка.

waste[1] I [weɪst] n 1) отбро́сы, отхо́ды; 2) уще́рб, убы́ток; по́рча; 3) бесполе́зная тра́та (денег, вре́мени, пищи и т. п.); to run to ~ тра́титься по́пусту.

waste[1] II a 1) ли́шний, нену́жный; 2) отрабо́танный, испо́льзованный; него́дный.

waste[1] III v 1) тра́тить, расточа́ть (время, деньги, слова и т.п.); 2) изнуря́ть; 3) истоща́ться; ча́хнуть (тж. to ~ away).

waste[2] I n 1) пусто́е простра́нство, пусты́ня; a ~ of waters морско́й просто́р; 2) пу́стошь.

waste[2] II a пусты́нный, незаселённый; необрабо́танный (о земле); to lay ~ опустоша́ть; to lie ~ быть невозде́ланным или необрабо́танным (о земле).

waste[2] III v опустоша́ть.

waste-basket ['weɪst,bɑːskɪt] см. waste-paper-basket.

waste-bin ['weɪstbɪn] n му́сорный я́щик.

wasteful ['weɪstful] a расточи́тельный.

waste-paper-basket [weɪst'peɪpə,bɑːskɪt] n корзи́на для нену́жных бума́г.

wastrel ['weɪstrəl] n 1) брак(о́ванное изде́лие); 2) беспризо́рный ребёнок; 3) расточи́тельный челове́к; 4) него́дный, никуды́шный челове́к.

watch[1] [wɔtʃ] n часы́ (карманные или ручные); wristlet ~ нару́чные часы́; my ~ is fast, my ~ gains мои́ часы́ иду́т вперёд; my ~ is slow, my ~ loses мои́ часы́ отстаю́т; to set the ~ ста́вить часы́ (по другим — by); by my ~ по мои́м часа́м; на мои́х часа́х; to wind up the ~ завести́ часы́; my ~ has run down мои́ часы́ останови́лись, у мои́х часо́в ко́нчился заво́д.

watch[2] I n 1) бди́тельность, внима́ние; to keep ~ быть начеку́ или насторо́же; to be on the ~ поджида́ть, ожида́ть (for); 2) надзо́р, наблюде́ние; 3) стра́жа, карау́л; to pass as a ~ in the night быть ско́ро забы́тым; 4) мор. ва́хта.

watch[2] II v 1) следи́ть, наблюда́ть; to ~ the train out of sight проводи́ть глаза́ми по́езд; to ~ it быть осторо́жным; 2) сторожи́ть; 3) быть начеку́, бо́дрствовать; □ to ~ for выжида́ть; to ~ out амер. остерега́ться; to ~ over охраня́ть.

watchdog ['wɔtʃdɔg] n сторожево́й пёс.

watcher ['wɔtʃə] n 1) сто́рож; 2) наблюда́тель.

watch-fire ['wɔtʃ,faɪə] n сигна́льный костёр.

watchful ['wɔtʃful] a бди́тельный; осторо́жный.

watch-guard ['wɔtʃgɑːd] n цепо́чка, ремешо́к (для карманных часов).

watch-house ['wɔtʃhaus] n карау́льное помеще́ние.

watch-maker ['wɔtʃ,meɪkə] n часовщи́к.

watchman ['wɔtʃmən] n ночно́й сто́рож.

watch-tower ['wɔtʃ,tauə] n сторожева́я ба́шня.

watchword ['wɔtʃwɜːd] n 1) ло́зунг; 2) паро́ль.

water I ['wɔːtə] n 1) вода́; fresh (или soft) ~ пре́сная вода́; salt (hard, standing) ~ морска́я (жёсткая, стоя́чая) вода́; town ~ вода́ из городско́го водопрово́да; mineral (или table) ~ минера́льная вода́; running ~ водопрово́д; boiling ~ кипято́к; to be (или to get) into hot ~ попа́сть в беду́; cold ~ холо́дная вода́; перен. неодобре́-

ние; to throw cold ~ on перен. обли́ть холо́дной водо́й (кого́-л.); deep ~ больша́я глубина́; in deep ~ в беде́; to hold ~ быть водонепроница́емым; перен. выде́рживать кри́тику; blue ~ мо́ре; the ~s океа́н; by ~ водо́й, во́дным путём; to back ~ грести́ в обра́тном направле́нии; перен. не сдержа́ть своего́ сло́ва; 2) pl (минера́льные) во́ды; to drink the ~s пить (лече́бные) во́ды; 3) прили́в и отли́в; high ~ а) вы́сшая то́чка прили́ва; б) па́водок; low ~ ни́зшая то́чка отли́ва; slack ~ ни́зкая вода́ (при отливе); in low ~ «на мели́», в крити́ческом (фина́нсовом) положе́нии; 4) слёзы; пот; слюна́; моча́; to make (или to pass) ~ мочи́ться; 5) вода́, чистота́ драгоце́нного ка́мня; of the first ~ чи́стой воды́; 6) attr водяно́й; во́дный; ◇ smooth ~ «ти́хая при́стань»; in smooth ~ гла́дко, без затрудне́ний; still ~s run deep погов. ≅ в ти́хом о́муте че́рти во́дятся.

water II v 1) мочи́ть, сма́чивать; 2) полива́ть, сбры́згивать водо́й; 3) разбавля́ть (водо́й; тж. to ~ down); 4) пои́ть живо́тных; 5) ходи́ть на водопо́й; 6) снабжа́ть водо́й (город, район); 7) ороша́ть; 8) слези́ться; пуска́ть слюну́; it makes one's mouth ~ ≅ слю́нки теку́т; □ to ~ down а) обедня́ть (сюжет); б) смягча́ть подро́бности.

water-blister ['wɔːtə,blɪstə] n волды́рь, водяна́я мозо́ль.

water-borne ['wɔːtəbɔːn] a 1) перевози́мый по воде́, по мо́рю; 2) смыва́емый водо́й.

water-bottle ['wɔːtə,bɔtl] n 1) графи́н (для воды); 2) фля́га.

water-colour ['wɔːtə,kʌlə] n 1) акваре́ль(ная кра́ска); 2) акваре́ль (рисунок); 3) attr акваре́льный.

watercourse ['wɔːtəkɔːs] n 1) река́, руче́й; 2) ру́сло.

waterfall ['wɔːtəfɔːl] n водопа́д, каска́д.

waterfowl ['wɔːtəfaul] n 1) водяна́я пти́ца; 2) собир. водяна́я дичь.

water-hole ['wɔːtəhoul] n пруд, водоём; коло́дец.

watering-cart ['wɔːtərɪŋkɑːt] n цисте́рна для поли́вки у́лиц.

watering-place ['wɔːtərɪŋpleɪs] n 1) водопо́й; 2) во́ды, куро́рт для лече́ния минера́льными во́дами; 3) морско́й куро́рт.

watering-pot ['wɔːtərɪŋpɔt] n (садо́вая) ле́йка.

waterless ['wɔːtəlɪs] a безво́дный.

water-lily ['wɔːtə,lɪlɪ] n водяна́я ли́лия, кувши́нка.

water-line ['wɔːtəlaɪn] n мор. ватерли́ния.

waterlogged ['wɔːtəlɔgd] a 1) заболо́ченный; 2) напо́лнившийся водо́й (о судне).

waterman ['wɔːtəmən] n 1) ло́дочник; 2) гребе́ц.

watermark ['wɔːtəmɑːk] n 1) водяно́й знак на бума́ге; 2) отме́тка у́ровня воды́.

water-melon ['wɔːtə,melən] n арбу́з.

water-power ['wɔːtə,pauə] n 1) гидроэне́ргия; во́дная эне́ргия; 2) attr гидроэнергети́ческий, гидроэлектри́ческий.

waterproof I ['wɔːtəpruːf] n 1) непромока́емая ткань; 2) непромока́емый плащ, -мое пальто́; дожде́ви́к.

waterproof II a непромока́емый; водонепроница́емый.

waterproof III *v* дéлать непромокáемым, водонепроницáемым.

water-rate ['wɔːtəreɪt] *n* тарúф водоснабжéния.

watershed ['wɔːtəʃed] *n* водораздéл.

waterside ['wɔːtəsaɪd] *n* береговáя полосá.

waterspout ['wɔːtəspaut] *n* 1) смерч; 2) водостóчная трубá.

watertight ['wɔːtətaɪt] *a* 1) водонепроницáемый; 2) выдéрживающий крúтику.

water-tower ['wɔːtə‚tauə] *n* водонапóрная бáшня.

water-way ['wɔːtəweɪ] *n* (внýтренний) вóдный путь; фарвáтер.

waterworks ['wɔːtəwəːks] *n* водопровóдная стáнция; водопровóдные сооружéния; ◊ to turn on the ~ проливáть слёзы.

water-worn ['wɔːtəwɔːn] *a* размýтый, сглáженный водóй.

watery ['wɔːtərɪ] *a* 1) водянúстый; 2) бесцвéтный, бессодержáтельный; 3) слезýщийся (*о глазах*); слюнýвый; 4) предвещáющий дождь.

watt [wɔt] *n эл.* ватт.

wattle[1] I ['wɔtl] *n* 1) плетéнь; 2) австралúйская акáция.

wattle[1] II *v* 1) дéлать плетéнь; 2) стрóить из плетня.

wattle[2] *n* борóдка, серёжка (*петуха и т. п.*).

wave I [weɪv] *n* 1) волнá, вал; the ~s *поэт.* моря, мóре; tidal ~ огрóмная волнá (*вызванная землетрясением*), цунáми; *перен.* волнá недовóльства, возмущéния, протéста *и т. п.*; brain ~ *разг.* блестýщая мысль; внезáпная мысль; 2) волнúстость; 3) колебáние; 4) махáние, взмах; знак (*рукóй*); 5) завúвка; permanent ~ шестимéсячная завúвка, перманéнт; 6) *воен.* атакýющая цепь; ◊ the tenth ~ девýтый вал.

wave II *v* 1) развевáться, качáться (*на ветру*); волновáться (*о ниве*); 2) махáть, размáхивать; помахáть; сдéлать знак (*рукóй*); to ~ smb. nearer подозвáть когó-л. знáком; 3) завивáть(ся), вúться (*о волосáх*); □ to ~ **aside** отмахнýться (*от когó-л., чегó-л.*); to ~ **away** отослáть, отпустúть когó-л., махнýв рукóй; *перен.* отмахнýться; to ~ **back** махáть в отвéт.

wave-length ['weɪvleŋθ] *n физ.* длинá волнý.

waver ['weɪvə] *v* 1) колыхáться (*о пламени и т. п.*); 2) колебáться, быть в нерешúтельности; 3) дрóгнуть (*о войскáх*).

wavy ['weɪvɪ] *a* 1) волнúстый; 2) бýрный (*о мóре*).

wax[1] I [wæks] *n* 1) воск; mineral ~ озокерúт; 2) céра (*ушнáя; тж.* ear-wax); 3) *attr* восковóй.

wax[1] II *v* вощúть.

wax[2] *v* 1) прибывáть (*о лунé*); 2) *в сочетании с прил.* ознáчает дéлаться, становúться (*обыкн. шутл.*); to ~ old состáриться; to ~ angry рассердúться.

wax[3] *n сленг* прúступ гнéва; to be in a ~ быть в бéшенстве; to put in a ~ привестú в бéшенство; to get into a ~ разгнéваться, рассвирепéть.

waxen ['wæksən] *a* 1) восковóй; 2) мýгкий как воск.

waxy[1] ['wæksɪ] *a* восковóй (*похóжий на воск*).

waxy[2] *a сленг* горýчий, вспýльчивый.

way [weɪ] *n* 1) дорóга, путь; by the ~ a) по дорóге, по путú; б) мéжду прóчим; on the ~ по путú, в путú; на путú; he is on the ~ он в путú; он при-

ближáется; out of the ~ a) не по путú; б) необыкновéнный, из рýда вон выходýщий; в) далёкий, отдалённый; over the ~ напрóтив, чéрез дорóгу; to feel one's ~ идтú ощýпью, нащýпывать дорóгу; *перен.* дéйствовать осторóжно, осмотрúтельно; to find the ~ найтú дорóгу; попáсть (*кудá-л.*); to lose one's (*или* the) ~ заблудúться; to pick one's ~ идтú, выбирáя дорóгу; to show the ~ провестú кудá-л., показáть дорóгу; to get under ~ отправлýться в путь; to get out of smb.'s ~ уйтú с дорóги; to be (*или* to stand) in one's ~ стоýть поперёк дорóги, быть препýтствием; to push one's ~ протáлкиваться; проклáдывать себé путь; to thread one's ~ пробирáться, протúскиваться; to elbow one's ~ протáлкиваться, протúскиваться; to make one's ~ продвигáться, проклáдывать себé дорóгу; to hew one's ~ прорубáть, проклáдывать себé дорóгу; to hammer one's ~ through пробивáться; to make ~ for давáть дорóгу; to pave the ~ for подготóвить пóчву, расчúстить путь; to put out of the ~ *перен.* убрáть с дорóги; 2) расстоýние; a little ~ недалекó; a long ~ (off) далекó; a ~ out в сторонé, неподалёку; 3) движéние, ход; to be under ~ a) быть на ходý, в дéйствии; б) происходúть, имéть мéсто; to gather ~ трóгаться, отправлýться (*о сýдне*); to have ~ on двúгаться вперёд; 4) спóсоб, óбраз дéйствий; which ~ как(úм спóсобом); to go (*или* to take) one's own ~ поступáть самостоýтельно, по-своéму; to have one's own ~ поступáть по-своéму, настоýть на своём; добúться своегó; to see the ~ to do smth. найтú возмóжность сдéлать что-л.; there are no two ~s about it об этом не мóжет быть двух мнéний; one ~ or another так úли инáче; the other ~ инáче; 5) обычай, привýчка, манéра; I don't like the ~ he smiles мне не нрáвится его улýбка; in a family ~ по-дóмашнему, без церемóний; in the family ~ берéменная; 6) óбраз жúзни; занýтие; to pay one's ~ жить по срéдствам; ◊ in a ~ до нéкоторой стéпени; in any ~ во всýком слýчае; in every ~ во всех отношéниях; by ~ of рáди, с цéлью, в вúде, в кáчестве (*когó-л., чегó-л.*); to be in a (great) ~ *разг.* быть взволнóванным, возбуждённым; to give ~ a) подавáться, уступáть; б) поддавáться, предавáться (*отчáянию, гóрю и т. п.*); в) пóртиться, сдавáть (*о механúзме, здорóвье*); г) пáдать в ценé (*об акциях и т. п.*); д) подлáмываться, рýшиться; проломúться (*о льде*); once in a ~ óчень рéдко, в кóи вéки; Milky Way *астр.* Млéчный Путь.

wayfarer ['weɪ‚fɛərə] *n* пýтник; пешехóд.

wayfaring ['weɪ‚fɛərɪŋ] *a* путешéствующий, стрáнствующий.

waylay ['weɪ'leɪ] *v* подстерегáть.

way(-)leave ['weɪliːv] *n* 1) прáво прохóда, проéзда, проклáдки кáбеля и т. п. по чужóй землé; 2) прáво полёта над чужóй территóрией.

wayside ['weɪsaɪd] *n* 1) обóчина дорóги; 2) *attr* придорóжный.

way-station ['weɪ'steɪʃən] *n амер. ж.-д.* полустáнок.

wayward ['weɪwəd] *a* капрúзный, своенрáвный.

we [wiː, wɪ] *pron pers* мы.

weak [wiːk] *a* 1) слáбый; *перен. тж.* нерешúтельный; 2) *грам.* слáбый, с суффиксáцией (*о глагóле*).

weaken ['wiːkən] *v* 1) ослаблýть; 2) слабéть, поддавáться.

weak-eyed [ˈwiːkˌaɪd] *a* со слáбым, с плохи́м зрéнием.

weak-headed [ˈwiːkˈhedɪd] *a* 1) слабоýмный; 2) легкó пьянéющий.

weakling [ˈwiːklɪŋ] *n* слáбый, слабовóльный человéк.

weakly I [ˈwiːklɪ] *a* слáбый, хи́лый.

weakly II *adv* слáбо.

weak-minded [ˈwiːkˈmaɪndɪd] *a* слабоýмный.

weakness [ˈwiːknɪs] *n* 1) слáбость; 2) слáбое мéсто, недостáток.

weal[1] [wiːl] *n*: in ~ and woe в счáстье и несчáстье; for the public (*или* general) ~ для óбщего блáга.

weal[2] *n* полосá, рубéц (*от удара кнутом и т. п.*).

wealth [welθ] *n* 1) богáтство; 2) изоби́лие; 3) богачи́.

wealthy [ˈwelθɪ] *a* богáтый, состоя́тельный.

wean I [wiːn] *n* *шотл.* ребёнок.

wean II *v* 1) отнимáть (*ребёнка*) от груди́; 2) отучáть, отвлекáть (*от чего-л.* — from; *тж.* to ~ away).

weapon [ˈwepən] *n* орýжие; *перен. тж.* срéдство (*борьбы́*); atomic ~s áтомное орýжие; (thermo-) nuclear ~s (термо)я́дерное орýжие; ~ of mass annihilation, ~ of mass destruction орýжие мáссового уничтожéния.

weaponless [ˈwepənlɪs] *a* безорýжный.

wear I [weə] *n* 1) ношéние, нóска (*платья*); out of ~ вы́шло из мóды; не нóсят; for country ~ для зáгорода (*об одежде*); 2) одéжда; изнáшивание, изнóс (*тж.* ~ and tear).

wear II *v* (*past* wore; *p. p.* worn) 1) носи́ть, быть одéтым (*во что-л.*); 2) изнáшивать, протирáть; протáптывать; 3) носи́ться (*о платье*); 4) имéть (*вид, выражение лица*); he ~s well он хорошó сохрани́лся, он прекрáсно вы́глядит; □ to ~ **away** а) стирáть(ся); б) мéдленно тянýться (*о времени*); в) тянýть, проводи́ть (*время*); to ~ away one's life in trifles растрáчивать жизнь на пустяки́; to ~ **down** а) стирáть(ся); изнáшивать(ся); б) изнуря́ть, истощáть, ослабля́ть; в) подави́ть, преодолéть (*сопротивление, оппозицию*); to ~ **off** стирáть(ся); to ~ **on** мéдленно тянýться (*о времени*); to ~ **out** а) изнáшивать(ся); б) истощáть(ся), изнуря́ть(ся).

wearily [ˈwɪərɪlɪ] *adv* 1) утоми́тельно; 2) утомлённо.

weariness [ˈwɪərɪnɪs] *n* 1) устáлость, утомлéние; 2) скýка; утоми́тельность.

wearisome [ˈwɪərɪsəm] *a* 1) утоми́тельный; 2) скýчный, надоéдливый.

weary I [ˈwɪərɪ] *a* 1) устáлый, утомлённый (*чем-л.* — of); I am ~ of it мне э́то надоéло; 2) утоми́тельный, надоéдливый; скýчный.

weary II *v* 1) утомля́ть(ся); 2) тосковáть (*о ком-л.* — for).

wearying [ˈwɪərɪɪŋ] *a* утоми́тельный; изнуря́ющий.

weasel [ˈwiːzl] *n* *зоол.* лáска; to catch a ~ asleep *перен.* застáть врасплóх осторóжного человéка.

weasel-worded [ˈwiːzlwəːdɪd] *a* *амер.* двусмы́сленный, противорéчивый, искажáющий смысл.

weather I [ˈweðə] *n* погóда; fine (fair, settled, foul) ~ хорóшая (я́сная, усто́йчивая, ненáстная) погóда; severe ~ холóдная, вéтреная погóда; fly-

ing ~ *ав.* лётная погóда; ◊ under the ~ *сленг* а) нездорóвый; б) в бедé; to make heavy ~ of smth. находи́ть что-л. трýдным.

weather II *a* *мор.* навéтренный.

weather III *v* 1) вывéтривать(ся); подвергáть(-ся) атмосфéрным влия́ниям; 2) выдéрживать (*бýрю, кри́зис*); 3) *мор.* обходи́ть с навéтренной стороны́.

weather-beaten [ˈweðəˌbiːtn] *a* повреждённый бýрями; *перен.* закалённый (*о человеке*).

weather-bound [ˈweðəbaund] *a* задéржанный непогóдой.

weather-bureau [ˈweðəbjuəˌrou] *n* бюрó погóды.

weathercock [ˈweðəkɔk] *n* флю́гер; *перен.* непостоя́нный человéк.

weather-forecast [ˈweðəˌfɔːkɑːst] *n* прогнóз погóды; a long-range ~ долгосрóчный прогнóз.

weather-stained [ˈweðəsteɪnd] *a* вы́цветший.

weather-station [ˈweðəˌsteɪʃən] *n* метеорологи́ческая стáнция.

weather-vane [ˈweðəveɪn] *см.* weathercock.

weave [wiːv] *v* (*past* wove; *p. p.* woven) 1) ткать; 2) плести́; 3) сочиня́ть.

weaver [ˈwiːvə] *n* ткач, ткачи́ха.

weazen(ed) [ˈwiːzn(d)] *см.* wizen(ed).

web [web] *n* 1) ткань; кусóк, штýка ткáни; *перен.* сплетéние (*лжи и т. п.*); spider's ~ паути́на; to spin a ~ of deceit опýтывать паути́ной лжи; 2) перепóнка (*у водоплáвающих птиц*); 3) перемы́чка; перебóрка; 4) полотнó пилы́.

webbed [webd] *a* перепóнчатый.

web-footed [ˈwebˌfuːtɪd] *a* с перепóнчатыми лáпами.

wed [wed] *v* 1) выдавáть зáмуж; жени́ть; 2) венчáть; 3) *уст.* вступáть в брак; венчáться; 4) соединя́ть.

we'd [wiːd] *разг.* 1) = we had; 2) = we should, we would.

wedding [ˈwedɪŋ] *n* 1) свáдьба; 2) *attr* свáдебный; 3) *attr* обручáльный (*о кольце*).

wedge I [wedʒ] *n* клин.

wedge II *v* 1) закрепля́ть кли́ном; 2) вкли́ниваться; врезáться (*тж.* to ~ in); □ to ~ **away**, to ~ **off** расталкивать.

wedgies [ˈwedʒɪz] *n pl* танкéтки (*обувь*).

wedlock [ˈwedlɔk] *n* супрýжество, брак.

Wednesday [ˈwenzdɪ] *n* средá.

wee [wiː] *a* малю́сенький, крóшечный.

weed I [wiːd] *n* 1) сóрная травá, сорня́к; 2) кля́ча; 3) долговя́зый и тóщий человéк; 4) *разг.* сигáра; ◊ Indian ~ табáк; ill ~s grow apace *посл.* сóрная травá хорошó растёт (*говорится в шýтку детям, выросшим не по возрасту*).

weed II *v* полóть, выпáлывать; □ to ~ **out** удаля́ть.

weeds [wiːdz] *n pl* трáур, трáурная одéжда.

weedy [ˈwiːdɪ] *a* 1) сóрный; заросший сорняками; 2) высóкий и худóй; болéзненный.

week [wiːk] *n* недéля; in a ~ чéрез недéлю; this day ~ недéлю томý назáд; Holy Week *рел.* стрáстная недéля; ◊ a ~ of Sundays óчень дóлго, цéлая вéчность; ~ in, ~ out мнóго недéль подря́д.

week-day [ˈwiːkdeɪ] *n* бýдний день.

week-end I [ˈwiːkˈend] *n* врéмя óтдыха с суббóты до понедéльника, уикэ́нд.

week-end II *v* проводить где-л. время с субботы до понедельника.

week-ender ['wiːkendə] *n* уезжающий отдыхать на время с субботы до понедельника.

weekly I ['wiːklɪ] *n* еженедельник, еженедельное издание.

weekly II *a* 1) еженедельный; 2) недельный.

weekly III *adv* 1) один раз в неделю; 2) еженедельно.

ween [wiːn] *v поэт.* полагать, думать.

weep [wiːp] *v* (*past, p. p.* wept) 1) плакать; оплакивать; 2) покрываться каплями; мокнуть (*об экземе*); ☐ to ~ **away** проплакать; to ~ **out** а) выплакать; to ~ oneself out выплакаться; б) проговорить сквозь слёзы.

weeping ['wiːpɪŋ] *a* плакучий.

weft [weft] *n* 1) *текст.* уток; 2) *разг.* ткань.

weigh [weɪ] *v* 1) взвешивать; 2) весить; *перен.* иметь вес; 3) взвешиваться (*чтобы узнать свой вес*); 4) сравнивать (*against, with*); ☐ to ~ **down** перевешивать; отягощать; *перен.* тяготить; подавлять; to ~ **in** привести (*аргумент, довод и т. п.; with*); to ~ **out** развешивать; отвешивать; to ~ **up** перевешивать; to ~ **upon** тяготить; угнетать; to ~ **with** влиять.

weighing-machine ['weɪŋməʃiːn] *n* весы.

weight I [weɪt] *n* 1) вес; by ~ на вес; atomic ~ атомный вес; unit (*или* specific) ~ удельный вес; short ~ недовес; to give light ~ обвешивать; to put on ~ а) толстеть; б) становиться тяжелее; 2) тяжесть, груз; *перен.* бремя; dead ~ мёртвый груз; 3) важность, значение, влияние; to carry ~ иметь вес, влияние; to lay ~ on, to give ~ to придавать значение; 4) гиря.

weight II *v* 1) нагружать; *перен.* отягощать, обременять; 2) придавать вес, силу.

weightless ['weɪtlɪs] *a* невесомый.

weightlessness ['weɪtlɪsnɪs] *n* невесомость; состояние невесомости.

weighty ['weɪtɪ] *a* 1) тяжёлый; 2) обременительный; 3) веский, важный.

weir [wɪə] *n* плотина, запруда.

weird I [wɪəd] *n* судьба, рок.

weird II *a* 1) таинственный, сверхъестественный; 2) *разг.* странный, чудной; непонятный; 3) роковой, фатальный.

welcome I ['welkəm] *n* 1) приветствие; to bid ~ приветствовать; встречать; 2) гостеприимство, радушный приём; to give a warm (*или* hearty) ~ а) оказать сердечный приём; горячо встретить; б) оказать энергичное сопротивление; to wear out (*или* to outstay) one's ~ злоупотреблять чьим-л. гостеприимством.

welcome II *a* 1) желанный; благоприятный; приятный; to make smb. ~ радостно, радушно встретить кого-л.; ~ as snow in harvest несвоевременный, нежелательный; 2) *predic* охотно разрешаемый; (you are) ~ не стоит благодарности, пожалуйста (*в ответ на благодарность*); you are ~! добро пожаловать!; you are ~ to take what steps you please вы можете предпринять всё, что вам угодно; пожалуйста, действуйте по своему усмотрению.

welcome III *v* 1) приветствовать; 2) радушно, радостно принимать, встречать.

welcome IV *int* добро пожаловать!

weld I [weld] *n тех.* сварка.

weld II *v тех.* сваривать(ся); *перен.* сплачивать, спаивать.

welder ['weldə] *n* сварщик.

welding ['weldɪŋ] *n тех.* сварка; acetylene ~ ацетиленовая сварка; autogenous (*или* oxygen) ~ автогенная сварка.

welfare ['welfɛə] *n* благосостояние, благоденствие; social ~ социальное обеспечение.

well¹ I [wel] *n* 1) колодец; водоём; Artesian (*или* bore) ~ артезианский колодец; 2) родник; *перен.* источник; 3) *горн.* скважина; 4) пролёт (*лестницы*), лестничная клетка.

well¹ II *v* бить ключом (*часто* to ~ forth, out, up).

well² I *adv* (*compar* better; *superl* best) 1) хорошо; very ~ очень хорошо, прекрасно; to come off ~ обойтись хорошо, сойти удачно; ~ enough ничего себе; 2) как следует, основательно; 3) очень, вполне; далеко, значительно; it may ~ be that... вполне возможно, что...; ~ into the night далеко за полночь; ~ advanced in mathematics успевающий по математике, хорошо знающий математику; ~ advanced in years, ~ on in years престарелый, очень пожилой; ◊ as ~ кроме того, вдобавок, к тому же; точно так же; с таким же успехом; as ~ as так же как.

well² II *a* (*compar* better; *superl* best) в прекрасном состоянии; здоровый; I'm perfectly (*или* quite) ~ я совершенно здоров, я прекрасно себя чувствую; he is best in the winter зимой ему лучше, зимой он лучше себя чувствует; to stand ~ быть в хороших отношениях (*с кем-л.— with*).

well² III *n* 1) добро; I wish him ~ я желаю ему добра; 2): the ~ (*употр. как pl*) здоровые.

well² IV *int* служит для выражения удивления, ожидания, согласия, удовлетворения и т. п. ну!; ~, who would have thought it? ну кто бы мог подумать?; ~!, ~ to be sure! ну и ну!, вот так так!; ~, come if you like ну что же, приходите, если хотите; ~ then? ну и что же?, ну и как же?; ~ now! ну что же!, ну!

well- [wel-] *pref указывает на:* а) *хорошее качество выполнения действия, выраженного причастием:* well-preserved хорошо сохранившийся, неиспорченный; well-timed своевременный; б) *доброжелательность:* well-doer благодетель.

we'll [wiːl] *разг.* = we shall, we will.

well-advised ['weləd'vaɪzd] *a* благоразумный.

well-balanced ['wel'bælənst] *a* уравновешенный.

well-being ['wel'biːŋ] *n* благополучие.

well-born ['wel'bɔːn] *a* знатный, родовитый.

well-bred ['wel'bred] *a* 1) (хорошо) воспитанный; 2) чистокровный (*о животном*).

well-disposed ['weldɪs'pouzd] *a* расположенный, благожелательный (*к — to, towards*).

well-favoured ['wel'feɪvəd] *a* красивый.

well-groomed ['wel'gruːmd] *a* ухоженный; выхоленный.

well-judged ['wel'dʒʌdʒd] *a* тактичный; уместный; сделанный вовремя, своевременный.

well-knit ['wel'nɪt] *a* хорошо сложённый; *перен.* хорошо продуманный; хорошо скомпонованный.

well-nigh ['welnaɪ] *adv* почти.

well-off ['wel'ɔːf] *a* зажиточный; обеспеченный (*чем-л.— for*).

well-paid ['wel'peɪd] *a* хорошо́ опла́чиваемый.

well-spring ['welsprɪŋ] *n* исто́чник.

well-timed ['wel'taɪmd] *a* своевре́менный.

well-to-do ['weltə'duː] *a* состоя́тельный, зажи́точный.

well-worn ['wel'wɔːn] *a* поно́шенный; *перен.* изби́тый.

Welsh I [welʃ] *n* 1) жи́тель Уэ́льса, валли́ец; 2) уэ́льский, валли́йский язы́к.

Welsh II *a* уэ́льский, валли́йский.

welsh [welʃ] *v* скры́ться от упла́ты про́игрыша (*о букмекере и т. п.*).

Welshman ['welʃmən] *n* жи́тель Уэ́льса, валли́ец.

welt I [welt] *n* 1) рант (*на обуви*); 2) след, рубе́ц.

welt II *v* 1) шить на ранту́; 2) бить (*кнутом*), полосова́ть.

welter I ['weltə] *n* неразбери́ха, сумбу́р.

welter II *v* бара́хтаться; валя́ться.

welter-weight ['weltəweɪt] *n* спорт. 1) боксёр полусре́днего ве́са; 2) доба́вочный груз (*на ска́чках*).

wen [wen] *n* жирова́я ши́шка; *перен.* перенаселённый го́род; the great ~ Ло́ндон.

wench [wentʃ] *n* 1) *уст., шутл.* де́вушка или молода́я же́нщина (*особ. деревенская*); 2) *уст.* прости́ту́тка.

wend [wend] *v*: .to ~ one's way направля́ть путь.

went [went] *past см.* go I.

wept [wept] *past, p. p. см.* weep.

were [wəː] *past pl см.* be.

we're [wɪə] *разг.* = we are.

weren't [wəːnt] *разг.* = were not.

wer(e)wolf ·['wəːwulf] *n* о́боротень.

west I [west] *n* 1) за́пад; *мор.* вест; to the ~ (of) к за́паду (от); the West За́пад; *амер.* за́падные шта́ты; 2) за́падный ве́тер; *мор.* вест.

west II *a* за́падный.

west III *adv* к за́паду от, на за́пад от; ◊ to go ~ *сленг* а) отпра́виться на тот свет; б) ру́хнуть (*о планах, надеждах*); не уда́ться.

West End ['west'end] *n* Уэ́ст-Э́нд, за́падная (аристократи́ческая) часть Ло́ндона.

West-Ender ['west'endə] *n* жи́тель Уэ́ст-Э́нда, аристокра́т.

westerly I ['westəlɪ] *a* 1) обращённый, напра́вленный к за́паду; 2) ду́ющий с за́пада, за́падный (*о ветре*).

westerly II *adv* 1) к за́паду, на за́пад; 2) с за́пада.

western I ['westən] *n* 1) жи́тель, урожёнец за́пада; 2) *амер.* ковбо́йский фильм, ве́стерн.

western II *a* 1) живу́щий на За́паде; 2) за́падный; 3) обращённый на за́пад.

westerner ['westənə] *n* (*тж.* Westerner) урожёнец За́пада (*обыкн. западных штатов США*).

westernmost ['westənmoust] *a* са́мый за́падный.

Westminster ['westmɪnstə] *n* 1) Вестми́нстер· (*часть Лондона*); 2) англи́йский парла́мент; *перен.* полити́ческая аре́на.

westward I ['westwəd] *n* за́падное направле́ние.

westward II *a* напра́вленный на за́пад, к за́паду.

westward III *adv* к за́паду, на за́пад, в за́падном направле́нии.

westwards ['westwədz] *см.* westward III.

wet I [wet] *n* 1) вла́га, вла́жность; 2) дождли́вая

погода; 3) *сленг* вы́пивка; спиртно́й напи́ток; to have a ~ вы́пить, промочи́ть го́рло.

wet II *a* 1) мо́крый, вла́жный, сыро́й; to get ~ промо́кнуть; ~ to the skin, ~ through промо́кший наскво́зь; 2) дождли́вый; 3) *амер. разг.* «мо́крый» (*разрешающий продажу спиртных напитков*); 4) *сленг* непра́вильный, неле́пый; you're all ~ вы си́льно заблужда́етесь.

wet III *v* мочи́ть, сма́чивать, увлажня́ть.

wet-nurse ['wetnəːs] ·*n* корми́лица.

we've [wiːv] *разг.* = we have.

whack I [wæk] *n* 1) си́льный уда́р; 2) *разг.* до́ля; I have had my ~ of я получи́л свою́ до́лю, я получи́л вдо́воль (*чего-л.*).

whack II *v* ударя́ть, колоти́ть; ~ed to the wide *сленг* изму́ченный вконе́ц.

whale [weɪl] *n* кит; sperm ~ кашало́т; ◊ a ~ of *разг.* ма́сса, мно́жество (*чего-л.*); very like a ~! ≅ так я и пове́рил!

whale-boat ['weɪlbout] *n мор.* вельбо́т.

whalebone ['weɪlboun] *n* кито́вый ус.

whale-oil ['weɪlɔɪl] *n* во́рвань, кито́вый жир.

whaler ['weɪlə] *n* 1) китоло́в, китобо́й; 2) китобо́йное су́дно.

wharf I [wɔːf] *n* (*pl тж.* wharves) при́стань.

wharf II *v* 1) пришварто́вывать (*судно*); 2) скла́дывать груз на при́стани.

wharves [wɔːvz] *pl см.* wharf I.

what [wɔt] *pron* 1) *inter* а) что?; ~ is it? что э́то тако́е?; ~ do you mean? что вы име́ете в виду́?; ~ of it? что из э́того?; and ~ not и так да́лее, и тому́ подо́бное; б) *в ка́честве определения* что, кака́я, како́е; ~ day of the month is it? како́е сего́дня число́?; в) *о профессии* кто?; ~ is your brother? кто ваш брат (*по профессии*)?; 2) *rel.* *demonstr* тот, кото́рый; та, кото́рая; то, кото́рое; те, кото́рые; то, что; I will tell you ~ to say я сообщу́ вам то, что ну́жно сказа́ть; 3) *в восклицательных словосочетаниях* како́й!, что за!; ~ luck! како́е сча́стье!; ~ a pity! кака́я жа́лость!; ~ an idea! а) что за фанта́зия!; б) кака́я мысль!; ◊ he knows what's ~ он себе́ на уме́, он зна́ет что к чему́; ~· for для чего́, для како́й це́ли.

whate'er [wɔt'eə] *поэт.* = whatever.

whatever I [wɔt'evə] *a* како́й бы ни, любо́й.

whatever II *pron* 1) всё что, что бы ни; 2) *после сущ. в отриц. предложениях* никако́й, како́й бы ни; there is no doubt ~ нет никако́го сомне́ния; is there any chance ~? нет ли хоть како́й-нибудь наде́жды, возмо́жности?; I cannot see anyone ~ кто бы э́то ни был — я никого́ не могу́ ви́деть.

what's [wɔts] *разг.* = what is.

whatsoever I, II [,wɔtsou'evə] *см.* whatever I, II.

wheat [wiːt] *n* пшени́ца; Indian ~ кукуру́за; summer (winter) ~ ярова́я (ози́мая) пшени́ца.

wheaten ['wiːtn] *a* пшени́чный.

wheedle ['wiːdl] *v* 1) льстить; прельща́ть, привлека́ть; 2) подольща́ться, подде́лываться (*into*); 3) выма́нивать (*out of*); 4) обойти́ ле́стью.

wheel I [wiːl] *n* 1) колесо́; free ~ свобо́дное колесо́ (*велосипеда*); potter's ~ гонча́рный круг; spur ~ зубча́тое колесо́; 2) *авто* руль, «бара́нка»; *ав., мор.* штурва́л (*тж.* steering-wheel); 3) велосипе́д; 4) круг; оборо́т; 5) колесо́ форту́ны, сча́стье (*тж.* Fortune's ~); ◊ to grease the ~s дать взятку, «подмазать»; to go on ~s идти как по маслу; ~s within ~s сложное взаимодействие; the ~s of State государственная машина.

wheel II *v* 1) катить, двигать (*что-л. на колёсах*); 2) поворачивать(ся); описывать круги; 3) ехать на велосипеде.

wheelbarrow ['wi:l,bærou] *n* тачка.

wheeler ['wi:lə] *n* 1) коренник; 2) колёсный мастер.

wheel-horse ['wi:lhɔ:s] *см.* wheeler 1).

wheelwright ['wi:lrait] *см.* wheeler 2).

wheeze I [wi:z] *n* 1) тяжёлое дыхание; 2) *сленг* шутка; уловка; трюк.

wheeze II *v* 1) тяжело дышать, дышать с хрипом; 2) скрипеть (*о механизме*); □ to ~ **out** прохрипеть.

wheezy ['wi:zɪ] *a* 1) задыхающийся; страдающий одышкой; 2) скрипучий.

whelk [welk] *n* брюхоногий моллюск.

whelm [welm] *v поэт.* поглощать, заливать.

whelp I [welp] *n* щенок (*тж. перен.*); детёныш (*зверя*).

whelp II *v* 1) щениться; 2) замышлять.

when I [wen] *adv* 1) когда?; ~ will you come? когда вы придёте?; 2) когда, в то время как (*тж. в эллиптических оборотах*); it was raining ~ we started шёл дождь, когда мы отправились; we were about to start ~ it began to rain мы были готовы отправиться, когда пошёл дождь; ~ passing проходя мимо; ~ asking спрашивая; say ~ *разг.* скажите, когда (будет) достаточно; 3) после того как; he will go ~ he has had his dinner он пойдёт, после того как пообедает; 4) хотя, несмотря на то, в то время как, тогда как; he keeps on singing ~ he knows it annoys us он продолжает петь, хотя знает, что это нас раздражает.

when II *pron* когда; during the time ~ you were away в то время, когда вы отсутствовали; till ~ до какого времени, до каких пор; since ~ с каких пор; с какого времени.

when III *n*: the ~ and the where когда и где; the ~ and the how когда и как.

whence [wens] *adv* 1) откуда (*обыкн.* from ~); ~ did you come? откуда вы пришли, приехали?; from ~ is he? откуда он (*т. е. из каких мест*)?; 2) как, каким образом; ~ comes it that... как это случилось, что...; 3) туда откуда; go back ~ you came возвращайтесь туда, откуда вы пришли.

whene'er [wen'ɛə] *поэт. см.* whenever.

whenever [wen'evə] *adv* когда бы ни, всякий раз как; как только.

whensoever [,wensou'evə] *см.* whenever.

where I [wɛə] *adv* 1) куда?; ~ are you going? куда вы идёте?; let him go ~ he likes пусть идёт куда хочет; 2) где?; ~ is my hat? где моя шляпа?; he knows ~ they are он знает, где они; ◊ ~ does it concern us? каким образом это нас касается?; ~ will you be if you offend him? в каком положении вы окажетесь, если оскорбите его?; ~ is the use of... какой смысл в том, что...; that's ~ it is *разг.* вот в чём дело.

where II *pron* 1) *inter:* ~ from? откуда?; ~ to? куда?; ~ have you come from? откуда вы пришли?; ~ are you going to? куда вы идёте?; 2) *rel* где; this is ~ I live вот где я живу, здесь я живу;

that is the place ~ he lives вот то место, где он живёт; from ~ откуда; to ~ куда; that's just ~ you're wrong вот тут-то вы и ошибаетесь.

whereaboutsᵃ ['wɛərəbauts] *n* местонахождение, местопребывание.

whereaboutsᵇ ['wɛərə'bauts] *adv* где?

whereas [wɛər'æz] *conj* 1) принимая во внимание; 2) тогда как.

whereat [wɛər'æt] *adv* 1) на это, на что; о чём; 2) затем, после этого.

whereby [wɛə'baɪ] *adv* при помощи, посредством (*чего-л.*); как; чем.

wherefore ['wɛəfɔ:] *adv* почему, по какой причине, из-за чего.

wherein [wɛər'ɪn] *adv* в чём.

whereof [wɛər'ɔv] *adv* 1) из чего, из которого; 2) о чём, о котором.

whereon [wɛər'ɔn] *adv* 1) на чём, на котором; 2) на что.

wheresoever [,wɛəsou'evə] *см.* wherever.

whereto [wɛə'tu:] *adv* для чего.

whereunto [,wɛərʌn'tu:] *см.* whereto.

whereupon [,wɛərə'pɔn] *adv* после чего, тогда, между тем.

wherever [wɛər'evə] *adv* где бы ни, куда бы ни; где бы то ни было; куда бы то ни было.

wherewith [wɛə'wɪθ] *adv уст.* чем.

wherry ['wɛrɪ] *n* лодка, ялик.

whet I [wet] *n* 1) оттачивание; 2) средство, возбуждающее аппетит; глоток спиртного.

whet II *v* 1) точить, оттачивать; 2) возбуждать (*аппетит*).

whether I ['weðə] *conj* ли; ~ or по так или иначе; ~ he is here or not здесь он или нет.

whether II *pron уст.* который из двух.

whetstone ['wetstoun] *n* точильный камень, брусок, оселок.

whew [hwu:] *int* вот тебе на!

whey [weɪ] *n* сыворотка.

which I [wɪtʃ] *a* какой; ~ books did you choose? какие книги вы выбрали?; ~ way shall we go? по какой дороге мы пойдём?

which II *pron* 1) который, какой; ~ is the right road? какая дорога правильна?; ~ of you am I to thank for this? кого из вас должен я благодарить за это?; this is the book ~ I chose это книга, которую я выбрал; 2) что; I lost my way, ~ delayed me considerably я заблудился, что значительно задержало меня; he said he had seen me there ~ was a lie он сказал, что видел меня там, но это была ложь.

whichever [wɪtʃ'evə] *pron* какой бы ни, какой угодно, любой.

whiff I [wɪf] *n* 1) дуновение, струя (*воздуха, аромата*); I want a ~ of fresh air мне нужен глоток свежего воздуха; 2) дымок; 3) затяжка (*сигарой, папиросой*); 4) небольшая сигара; 5) лёгкая лодка, ялик.

whiff II *v* 1) веять (*об аромате, свежести и т. п.*); 2) пускать клубы (*дыма*); попыхивать (*трубкой*).

whiffle ['wɪfl] *v* 1) веять, слегка дуть (*о ветре*); 2) развевать; 3) *амер.* колебаться.

whig [wɪg] *n* 1) *ист.* виг (*член партии вигов*); 2) *амер. ист.* сторонник восстания против английского владычества; 3) *амер.* член республиканской партии.

while I [waıl]′ *n* время, промежуток времени; the ~ в это время; between ~s в промежутках; по временам; a good ~, a great ~ долгое время; for a ~ на время; in a little ~ скоро; once in a ~ время от времени; изредка, редко; in a long ~ ago давным-давно; it is not worth ~, it is not worth my (your *etc*) ~ не стоит того, не стоит труда.

while II *v*: to ~ away the time проводить время.

while III *conj* 1) в то время как, пока; ~ reading во время чтения; 2) несмотря на то, что; тогда как.

whiles [waılz] *conj уст.* пока; в то время как.

whilst [waılst] *conj* в то время как, пока.

whim [wım] *n* каприз, прихоть, увлечение.

whimper I ['wımpə] *n* хныканье.

whimper II *v* хныкать.

whimsical ['wımzıkəl] *a* причудливый, прихотливый, капризный.

whimsy I ['wımzı] *n см.* whim.

whimsy II *a см.* whimsical.

whine I [waın] *n* вой.

whine II *v* выть; скулить; хныкать.

whinny I ['wını] *n* тихое *или* радостное ржание.

whinny II *v* тихо ржать.

whip I [wıp] *n* 1) кнут; 2) кучер; good (poor) ~ хороший (плохой) кучер; 3) *охот.* псарь, доезжачий; 4) парламентский партийный организатор (*в Англии*).

whip II *v* 1) хлестать; 2) подгонять; 3) обматывать; 4) сшивать, обметывать через край; 5) взбивать (*белки*); 6) *разг.* превосходить; □ to ~ **away** а) прогонять, гнать (*кнутом*); б) сбежать; в) схватить, стащить; to ~ **in** сгонять; to ~ **off** а) сбросить, сдёрнуть; б) прогнать; в) убежать, ускользнуть; to ~ **on** подгонять, подстёгивать; to ~ **out** а) выколачивать, выбивать; б) выхватить; в) вырваться, ускользнуть; г) разразиться (*бранью, угрозами*); to ~ **round** а) гонять кругом; б) обматывать; в) быстро повернуться; to ~ **up** а) подгонять, подстёгивать; *перен.* раздувать, разжигать; б) выхватить; подхватить; в) взбежать наверх, быстро подняться; to ~ up and down бегать туда и сюда.

whip-hand ['wıp'hænd] *n*: to have the ~ of (*или* over) держать в руках; держать в полном подчинении (*кого-л.*).

whipper-in ['wıpər'ın] *n охот.* псарь, доезжачий.

whipper-snapper ['wıpə,snæpə] *n* ничтожество, самонадеянный мальчишка.

whippet ['wıpıt] *n* 1) гончая; 2) *воен.* танкетка.

whip-round ['wıpraund] *n* сбор денег экспромтом (*для кого-л.*).

whir I, II [wəː] *см.* whirr I, II.

whirl I [wəːl] *n* 1) вихрь; кружение; вихревое движение; 2) смятение; in a ~ в смятении (*о мыслях*).

whirl II *v* 1) кружить(ся), вертеть(ся); 2) проноситься; 3) быть в смятении; □ to ~ **away**, to ~ **up** уноситься.

whirligig I ['wəːlıgıg] *n* 1) карусель; 2) юла; 3) вихрь, водоворот (*событий и т. п.*); ~ of time превратности судьбы.

whirligig II *a* вихревой.

whirlpool ['wəːlpuːl] *n* водоворот; *перен. тж.* пучина.

whirlwind ['wəːlwınd] *n* 1) вихрь, ураган; смерч; 2) *attr* ураганный; 3) *attr* стремительный.

whirr I [wəː] *n* шум (*крыльев, машин*); рокот (*пропеллера*).

whirr II *v* шуметь; жужжать.

whisk I [wısk] *n* 1) веничек; метёлка; 2) мутовка; 3) взмах, взмахивание, помахивание.

whisk II *v* 1) смахивать (*тж.* to ~ away, to ~ off); 2) умчать(ся); унести(сь) (*тж.* to ~ away, to ~ off); 3) юркнуть, шмыгнуть; 4) помахивать (*хвостом; тросточкой*); 5) взбивать (*белки, сливки*).

whisker ['wıskə] *n обыкн. pl* 1) бакенбарды (*тж.* side ~s); 2) усы (*животного*).

whisky[1] ['wıskı] *n* виски (*водка*).

whisky[2] *n* лёгкая двуколка.

whisper I ['wıspə] *n* 1) шёпот; 2) слух, молва; 3) шорох, журчание; ◊ in a pig's ~ мгновенно, моментально; to give the ~ предостеречь, намекнуть, «шепнуть».

whisper II *v* 1) шептать; говорить шёпотом; 2) нашёптывать; пускать слух, клевету; it is ~ed that ходят слухи, говорят, что; 3) шелестеть; журчать.

whist[1] [wıst] *n* вист (*карточная игра*).

whist[2] *int уст.* тише!

whistle I ['wısl] *n* 1) свист; 2) свисток; ◊ to wet one's ~ *разг.* промочить горло, выпить.

whistle II *v* 1) свистеть; 2) давать свисток; 3) *уст.* ябедничать, доносить.

Whit [wıt] *a*: ~ Sunday *церк.* троицын день; ~ Monday *церк.* духов понедельник.

whit [wıt] *n* чуточка; no ~, not (*или* never) a ~ совсем нет, нисколько.

white I [waıt] *a* 1) белый; *перен.* невинный, чистый; незапятнанный; 2) бледный; to turn ~ побледнеть, побелеть; as ~ as a sheet ≅ белый как полотно; 3) прозрачный (*о воде, воздухе и т. п.*); 4) седой (*о волосах*); 5) бессонный (*о ночи*).

white II *n* 1) белизна; белый цвет; in ~ в белом; 2) белая краска, белила; London ~ свинцовые белила; Chinese (*или* zinc) ~ цинковые белила; 3) белок (*глаза, яйца*); 4) белый человек; ◊ to hit the ~ попасть в точку, оказаться правым.

whitebait ['waıtbeıt] *n* мелкая рыбка.

Whitechapel ['waıt,tʃæpl] *n* Уайтчэпл (*квартал в Лондоне, населённый беднотой*).

whiteguard I ['waıtgɑːd] *n* белогвардеец.

whiteguard II *a* белогвардейский.

Whitehall ['waıt'hɔːl] *n* Уайтхолл (*улица в Лондоне, на которой расположены правительственные учреждения*); *перен.* британское правительство; официальные правящие круги.

white-handed ['waıt'hændıd] *a* 1) честный; 2) невиновный; непричастный.

white-hot ['waıt'hɔt] *a* раскалённый добела.

White House ['waıt'haus] *n* Белый Дом (*официальная резиденция президента США*).

white-livered ['waıt,lıvəd] *a* трусливый.

whiten ['waıtn] *v* 1) белить; 2) белеть; 3) бледнеть.

whitesmith ['waıtsmıθ] *n* 1) жестянщик; 2) лудильщик.

whitethorn ['waıtθɔːn] *n* боярышник.

whitewash I ['waıtwɔʃ] *n* 1) побелка; *перен.* данные, реабилитирующие человека; 2) *амер. спорт. разг.* выигрыш «всухую».

whitewash II *v* 1) белить (*потолок, стены*); *перен.*

реабилити́ровать, пыта́ться обели́ть (кого́-л.); 2) восстана́вливать в права́х (банкро́та); 3) амер. спорт. разг. победи́ть, вы́играть «всуху́ю».

whither ['wɪðə] adv уст. куда́.

Whitsun(day) ['wɪt'sʌn(dɪ)] см. Whit.

whittle ['wɪtl] v строга́ть (ножо́м); □ to ~ away, to ~ down уме́ньшить, свести́ на нёт.

whiz(z) I [wɪz] n свист (рассека́емого во́здуха).

whiz(z) II v свисте́ть, со сви́стом рассека́ть во́здух.

who [huː] pron 1) inter кто?; ~ would have thought it? кто бы мог поду́мать?; 2) rel кото́рый, кто; the man ~ was here челове́к, кото́рый был здесь.

whoa [wou] int стой!, тпру!

whoever [huː'evə] pron кто бы ни, кото́рый бы ни.

whole I [houl] n 1) це́лое; (up)on the ~ в о́бщем, в це́лом; 2) всё; 3) су́мма, ито́г.

whole II a 1) весь, це́лый; по́лный 2) це́лый, невреди́мый (тж. ~ and sound); 3) це́льный (тж. перен.); непоча́тый; 4) непросе́янный (о муке́).

whole-hearted ['houl'hɑːtɪd] a от всего́ се́рдца, и́скренний, чистосерде́чный.

wholeness ['houlnɪs] n це́льность (нату́ры и т. п.).

wholesale I ['houlseɪl] n опто́вая торго́вля; to sell by ~ продава́ть о́птом.

wholesale II a опто́вый; перен. по́лный; огро́мный, в большо́м коли́честве.

wholesale III adv о́птом; перен. по́лностью; в большо́м коли́честве, в кру́пных разме́рах.

wholesome ['houlsəm] a здоро́вый, поле́зный.

wholly ['houlɪ] adv соверше́нно, целико́м.

whom [huːm] pron (косв. п. от who) кого́; кото́рого; кому́; кото́рому; by ~ кем; to ~ кому́, кото́рому; with ~ с кем, с кото́рым; of ~ о ком, о кото́ром.

whoop I [huːp] n 1) крик, ги́канье; 2) коклю́шный ка́шель.

whoop II v 1) ги́кать; 2) зака́тываться ка́шлем.

whoopee ['wuːpiː] n: to make ~ амер. разг. шу́мно весели́ться, гро́мко хохота́ть.

whooping-cough ['huːpɪŋkɔf] n коклю́ш.

whop [wɔp] v разг. 1) бить, колоти́ть; 2) одоле́ть, победи́ть.

whopper ['wɔpə] n на́глая ложь.

whore [hɔː] n проститу́тка.

whortleberry ['wɜːtlberɪ] n черни́ка; bog ~ голуби́ка; red ~ брусни́ка.

whose [huːz] pron poss чей; кото́рого.

whosoever [ˌhuːsou'evə] см. whoever.

why[1] I [waɪ] adv почему́, заче́м; ~ did you do it? почему́ вы э́то сде́лали?

why[1] II n: the ~s of it причи́на э́того, основа́ние для э́того.

why[2] int выража́ет удивле́ние, колеба́ние, проте́ст и т. п.: ~, it's nearly five o'clock! да уж почти́ пять часо́в!; is it true? ~, yes, I think so пра́вда ли э́то? да как сказа́ть? ду́маю, что так; ~, of course, it is so! ну коне́чно, э́то так!; ~, he told me he was only fifty! да он говори́л мне, что ему́ то́лько пятьдеся́т!; ~, what's the harm! ну так что за беда́!; ~, a child could answer that! да́же ребёнок мог бы отве́тить на э́тот вопро́с!

wick [wɪk] n 1) фити́ль; 2) тампо́н.

wicked ['wɪkɪd] a 1) злой; зло́бный; 2) испорчен-

ный, безнра́вственный; поро́чный, вре́дный; 3) со́рный (о тра́вах).

wicker ['wɪkə] n 1) пру́тья для плете́ния; 2) attr плетёный (о корзи́нах, ме́бели и т. п.).

wicker-work ['wɪkəwɜːk] n плетёные изде́лия.

wicket ['wɪkɪt] n 1) кали́тка (в воро́тах или ря́дом с воро́тами); 2) турнике́т; 3) око́шко (ка́ссы); глазо́к (в две́ри); 4) воро́та (в кри́кете).

wide I [waɪd] a 1) широ́кий; 2) тако́й-то ширины́; one metre ~ ширино́й в оди́н метр; 3) большо́й, обши́рный; 4) широко́ откры́тый (о глаза́х); 5) далёкий (от — of).

wide II adv 1) широко́; 2) далеко́; ~ from being... далеко́ не...; 3) повсю́ду (тж. far and ~); 4) ми́мо це́ли; ~ of the mark ми́мо це́ли; невпопа́д; ◊ ~ awake осторо́жный, бди́тельный, осмотри́тельный.

wide III n: broke to the ~ разг. разори́вшийся, прогоре́вший.

wide-awake ['waɪdəweɪk] n 1) мя́гкая фе́тровая шля́па с широ́кими поля́ми; 2) морска́я ла́сточка.

widen ['waɪdn] v расширя́ть(ся).

widespread ['waɪdspred] a широко́ распространённый; широко́ разветвлённый.

widow ['wɪdou] n вдова́; grass ~ соло́менная вдова́.

widowed ['wɪdoud] a овдове́вший.

widower ['wɪdouə] n вдове́ц.

widowhood ['wɪdouhud] n вдовство́.

width [wɪdθ] n 1) ширина́, широта́; in ~ в ширину́; 2) поло́тнище; 3) тех. пролёт.

wield [wiːld] v 1) владе́ть; 2) облада́ть.

wife [waɪf] n (pl wives) жена́.

wig [wɪg] n пари́к; scratch ~ накла́дка из воло́с; ◊ big ~ персо́на, ши́шка.

wigging ['wɪgɪŋ] n разг. брань; нагоня́й.

wight [waɪt] n уст. челове́к, созда́ние.

wigwag ['wɪgwæg] v сигнализи́ровать флажка́ми.

wigwam ['wɪgwæm] n вигва́м.

wild I [waɪld] n обыкн. pl пусты́ня, ди́кая ме́стность.

wild II a 1) ди́кий; to grow (или to run) ~ расти́ на свобо́де, без присмо́тра; 2) пусты́нный; 3) пугли́вый (о живо́тных, пти́цах); 4) бу́рный (о пого́де, восто́рге и т. п.); 5) бу́йный; беспоря́дочный; необу́зданный; 6) поме́шанный, безу́мный; нейстовый, возбуждённый; to be ~ about быть без ума́ от чего́-л.; to drive ~ приводи́ть в бе́шенство, в исступле́ние; it made me ~ to listen to such nonsense меня́ беси́ло, когда́ я слу́шал э́ти глу́пости; 7) необду́манный; сумасбро́дный.

wild III adv как попа́ло, науга́д.

wildcat I ['waɪldkæt] n ди́кая ко́шка.

wildcat II a риско́ванный, фантасти́ческий, несбы́точный.

wilderness ['wɪldənɪs] n 1) пусты́ня; ди́кая ме́стность; 2) запу́щенная часть са́да; 3) ма́сса, мно́жество (of).

wildfire ['waɪldˌfaɪə] n ист. гре́ческий ого́нь; to spread like ~ бы́стро, молниено́сно распространя́ться.

wilding ['waɪldɪŋ] n бот. дичо́к.

wile I [waɪl] n обыкн. pl хи́трость, уло́вка.

wile II v зама́нивать, завлека́ть (away, into).

wilful ['wɪlful] *a* 1) упря́мый, своенра́вный; 2) преднаме́ренный, умы́шленный.

will[1] I [wɪl] *n* 1) во́ля; си́ла во́ли; strong ~ си́льная во́ля; 2) во́ля, жела́ние; free ~ до́брая во́ля; свобо́да во́ли; ill ~ зла́я во́ля; against one's ~ про́тив во́ли; of one's own free ~ по свое́й до́брой во́ле; по со́бственному жела́нию; at one's own sweet ~ науга́д, как (*или* когда́) взду́мается; with a ~ энерги́чно; to work one's ~ сде́лать по-сво́ему; to have one's ~ доби́ться своего́; 3) свобо́да де́йствий; at ~ по усмотре́нию, по жела́нию; 4) завеща́ние; to make a ~ сде́лать завеща́ние.

will[1] II *v* (*past, p. p.* willed) 1) хоте́ть, жела́ть; проявля́ть во́лю, жела́ние; 2) заставля́ть, внуша́ть; 3) завеща́ть.

will[2] *v* (*past* would) 1) *как вспом. гл. испо́льзуется для образова́ния форм бу́дущего вре́мени 2-го и 3-го л.:* he ~ do it он сде́лает э́то; you ~ be there in good time вы бу́дете там во́время; 2) *как модáльный гл. испóльзуется для выраже́ния наме́рения, реши́мости, обеща́ния говоря́щего:* I ~ certainly go and see him я непреме́нно пойду́ и уви́жусь с ним; I shall have to go, whether I ~ or not я до́лжен бу́ду пое́хать, хочу́ я э́того и́ли нет; 3) *выража́ет обы́чное и́ли повто́рное де́йствие в настоя́щем:* now and then a bird ~ call вре́мя от вре́мени раздаётся крик пти́цы; he ~ sit there for hours он сиди́т там часа́ми; 4) *выража́ет заключе́ние, вы́вод, предположе́ние:* this'll be our train, I fancy я полага́ю, что э́то наш по́езд.

willing ['wɪlɪŋ] *a* 1) гото́вый (охо́тно) (*сде́лать что-л.*); 2) доброво́льный; доброво́льно даю́щий *или* выполня́ющий что-л.; 3) стара́тельный; 4) послу́шный (*о лошади*).

willingness ['wɪlɪŋnɪs] *n* гото́вность (*сде́лать что-л.*).

will-o'-the-wisp ['wɪləðwɪsp] *n* 1) блужда́ющий огонёк; 2) не́что обма́нчивое, неулови́мое.

willow ['wɪlou] *n* и́ва; weeping ~ плаку́чая и́ва; 2) бита́ (*для крикета*); to handle the ~ быть игроко́м в кри́кет; ◇ to wear the ~ опла́кивать смерть (*обы́кн. возлю́бленного*).

willowy ['wɪloui] *a* 1) поро́сший ивняко́м; 2) ги́бкий, стро́йный, то́нкий.

willynilly ['wɪlɪ'nɪlɪ] *adv* во́лей-нево́лей.

wilt[1] [wɪlt] *v* 1) вя́нуть, увяда́ть, поника́ть; 2) губи́ть (*цветы*).

wilt[2] *уст. 2-е л. ед. ч. наст. вр. от гл.* will[2]; thou ~ = you will.

wily ['waɪlɪ] *a* кова́рный, хи́трый.

wimble ['wɪmbl] *n* бура́в, сверло́.

win I [wɪn] *n* 1) вы́игрыш; 2) побе́да (*в игре, состяза́нии*).

win II *v* (*past, p. p.* won) 1) выи́грывать; 2) завоёвывать, побежда́ть; оде́рживать побе́ду; 3) достига́ть (с трудо́м), пробива́ться; to ~ clear, to ~ free вы́путаться с трудо́м; 4) располага́ть к себе́; завоева́ть, сниска́ть (*уваже́ние, любо́вь и т. п.*); 5) добыва́ть (*руду́ и т. п.*); 6) *сленг* укра́сть; вы́манить обма́ном; □ to ~ out доби́ться успе́ха; to ~ over склони́ть на свою́ сто́рону; расположи́ть к себе́; to ~ through проби́ться, преодоле́ть (*тру́дности*); to ~ upon постепе́нно завоева́ть (*призна́ние, симпа́тии и т. п.*).

wince I [wɪns] *n* дрожь, содрога́ние.

wince II *v* 1) вздра́гивать; 2) мо́рщиться (*от бо́ли*).

winch [wɪntʃ] *n* 1) лебёдка, во́рот; 2) кривоши́п.

wind[a] I [wɪnd] *n* 1) ве́тер; adverse (*или* contrary, head) ~ проти́вный ве́тер; fair ~ попу́тный ве́тер; wet ~ ве́тер, несу́щий дождь; high ~, strong ~ си́льный ве́тер; against the ~ про́тив ве́тра; down the ~, before the ~ по ве́тру; to sail before the ~ *мор.* идти́ с попу́тным ве́тром; *перен.* процвета́ть; close to the ~, near the ~ *мор.* в круто́й бейдеви́нд; *перен.* на гра́ни прили́чия, поря́дочности; 2) возду́шная струя́, ток во́здуха; 3) дыха́ние; short (*или* bad) ~ оды́шка; second ~ *спорт.* второ́е дыха́ние; to get one's ~ отдыша́ться; to lose ~ задохну́ться, запыха́ться; broken ~ запа́л (*у лошади*); 4) за́пах, дух; *перен.* слух; болтовня́; to get ~ of проню́хать (*о чём-л.*), почу́ять (*кого́-л., что-л.*); to take (*или* to get) ~ распространи́ться; стать изве́стным; 5) (the ~) *муз.* духовы́е инструме́нты; wood (brass) ~ деревя́нные (ме́дные) духовы́е инструме́нты; 6) *мед.* га́зы; ◇ the four ~s четы́ре страны́ све́та; from the four ~s со всех сторо́н; to cast (*или* to fling) to the ~s отбро́сить (благоразу́мие, осторо́жность); to get (*или* to have) the ~ of име́ть преиму́щество, быть в бо́лее благоприя́тном положе́нии; there is smth. in the ~ в во́здухе что́-то но́сится, что́-то до́лжно произойти́; to get the ~ up *сленг* испуга́ться; to put the ~ up *сленг* напуга́ть; to burn the ~ нести́сь во весь опо́р; between ~ and water уязви́мое ме́сто; to raise the ~ *сленг* раздобы́ть де́нег; to sow the ~ and to reap the whirlwind *посл.* посе́ешь ве́тер — пожнёшь бу́рю.

wind[a] II *v* 1) вы́звать оды́шку; заста́вить задохну́ться, запыха́ться; 2) дать перевести́ дух; 3) (по)чу́ять.

wind[b1] I [waɪnd] *n поэ́т. см.* wind[a] I 1).

wind[b1] II *v* труби́ть в рог.

wind[b2] I *n* 1) оборо́т, поворо́т; 2) вито́к.

wind[b2] II *v* (*past, p. p.* wound) 1) ви́ться, извива́ться; 2) нама́тывать(ся), обма́тывать(ся); обвива́ть(ся); 3) заводи́ть (*механи́зм*); 4) повора́чивать; □ to ~ off разма́тывать(ся); to ~ up а) нама́тывать; б) заводи́ть (*часы́, механи́зм*); в) подтя́гивать (*дисципли́ну*); г) конча́ть, ликвиди́ровать.

windbag ['wɪndbæg] *n разг.* пустозво́н, болту́н.

wind-break ['wɪndbreɪk] *n* щит, ветроло́м.

wind-breaker ['wɪnd,breɪkə] *n* ветронепроница́емая ку́ртка (*мехова́я, ко́жаная и т. п.*).

windfall ['wɪndfɔːl] *n* 1) па́данец, плод, сби́тый ве́тром; 2) неожи́данная уда́ча.

winding I ['waɪndɪŋ] *n* 1) изги́б; 2) витки́; 3) *эл.* обмо́тка; 4) нама́тывание.

winding II *a* 1) изви́листый; 2) спира́льный, вито́й.

winding-up ['waɪndɪŋ'ʌp] *n* 1) оконча́ние, коне́ц; 2) ликвида́ция, закры́тие предприя́тия.

wind-instrument ['wɪnd,ɪnstrumənt] *n* духово́й инструме́нт.

wind-jammer ['wɪnd,dʒæmə] *n разг.* 1) торго́вое па́русное су́дно; 2) *воен.* непопуля́рный нача́льник.

windlass ['wɪndləs] *n* лебёдка, во́рот.

windmill ['wɪnmɪl] *n* ветряна́я ме́льница; ветря́к.

window [ˈwɪndou] *n* 1) окно́; blind (*или* blank, dead, dummy, false) ~ ло́жное окно́; gable ~ слуховое окно́; bay ~ окно́ фонарём, э́ркер; bow ~ (полукру́глое) окно́ фонарём; French ~ окно́, доходя́щее до по́ла; wide-view ~ широ́кое окно́ в железнодоро́жном ваго́не; shop ~ витри́на магази́на; to have everything in the shop ~ *перен.* быть пове́рхностным, неглубо́ким; 2) *attr* око́нный.

window-pane [ˈwɪndoupeɪn] *n* (око́нное) стекло́ и ра́ма.

window-sill [ˈwɪndousɪl] *n* подоко́нник.

windpipe [ˈwɪndpaɪp] *n* дыха́тельное го́рло.

wind-screen [ˈwɪndskriːn] *n* пере́днее, ветрово́е стекло́.

wind-shield [ˈwɪndʃiːld] *амер. см.* wind-screen.

wind-up [ˈwɪndˈʌp] *n сленг* страх, не́рвное возбужде́ние; to have (*или* to get) a ~ испуга́ться, испыта́ть страх.

windward I [ˈwɪndwəd] *n* наве́тренная сторона́.

windward II *a* наве́тренный.

windward III *adv* про́тив ве́тра.

windy [ˈwɪndɪ] *a* 1) ве́треный; 2) обдува́емый ве́тром; 3) пусто́й, бессодержа́тельный; 4) *сленг* испу́ганный; трусли́вый.

wine I [waɪn] *n* 1) вино́; green (*или* new) ~ молодо́е вино́; Adam's ~ вода́; in ~ пья́ный, опьяне́вший; 2) *унив.* студе́нческая пиру́шка; 3) *attr* ви́нный; ◊ good ~ needs no bush ≅ хоро́ший това́р сам себя́ хва́лит.

wine II *v* 1) пить вино́; 2) угоща́ть, пои́ть вино́м.

winebibber [ˈwaɪnˌbɪbə] *n* пья́ница.

winecup [ˈwaɪnkʌp] *n* ча́ша.

wineglass [ˈwaɪnɡlɑːs] *n* бока́л; рю́мка.

wine-vault [ˈwaɪnvɔːlt] *n* 1) ви́нный по́греб; 2) ви́нный погребо́к; каба́чок.

wing I [wɪŋ] *n* 1) крыло́; on the ~ на лету́; в полёте; *перен.* в путеше́ствии; гото́вый отпра́виться в путь; to take ~ вспорхну́ть, улете́ть; полете́ть; to take to itself ~s бы́стро исче́знуть, улету́читься; under the ~ of под кры́лышком, под покрови́тельством (*кого́-л.*); to clip smb.'s ~s подре́зать кры́лышки кому́-л.; to singe one's ~s опали́ть себе́ кры́лышки; to lend (*или* to add) ~s ускори́ть; прида́ть кры́лья; 2) крыло́ (*дома*), фли́гель; щит от гря́зи (*у автомаши́ны*); 4) *воен.* фланг; 5) *воен.* авиапо́лк (*в А́нглии*); брига́да (*в США*); 6) *pl театр.* кули́сы.

wing II *v* 1) снабжа́ть кры́льями; 2) окрыля́ть; 3) лете́ть, рассека́ть во́здух, пересека́ть в полёте (*тж.* to ~ the air, to ~ its way through the air, to ~ its flight); 4) ра́нить (*в крыло́, в ру́ку*).

winged [wɪŋd] *a* крыла́тый; *перен. тж.* бы́стрый.

wingless [ˈwɪŋlɪs] *a* бескры́лый.

wing-spread [ˈwɪŋspred] *n* разма́х кры́льев.

wink I [wɪŋk] *n* морга́ние; мига́ние, подми́гивание; to give a ~, to tip smb. the ~ подмигну́ть кому́-л., сде́лать кому́-л. знак украдкой, намекну́ть; 2): not to sleep a ~, not to get a ~ of sleep не засну́ть ни на мину́ту; forty ~s коро́ткий сон.

wink II *v* 1) морга́ть, мига́ть; 2) мерца́ть; □ to ~ at a) подми́гивать (*кому́-л.*); б) смотре́ть сквозь па́льцы, закрыва́ть глаза́ на что-л.

winking [ˈwɪŋkɪŋ] *n*: like ~ *сленг* в мгнове́ние о́ка.

winner [ˈwɪnə] *n* победи́тель (*состяза́ния, игры́*), вы́игравший.

winning [ˈwɪnɪŋ] *a* 1) победи́вший, одержа́вший побе́ду (*в соревнова́нии*); 2) побежда́ющий; реша́ющий (*уда́р, вы́стрел и т. п.*); 3) обая́тельный, чару́ющий (*об улы́бке и т. п.*).

winnings [ˈwɪnɪŋz] *n pl* вы́игрыш, вы́игранные де́ньги.

winnow [ˈwɪnou] *v* 1) ве́ять (*зерно́*); 2) отве́ивать (*мяки́ну; тж.* to ~ away, to ~ out); *перен.* отсе́ивать (*тж.* to ~ away, to ~ out); отбира́ть.

winsome [ˈwɪnsəm] *a* обая́тельный, привлека́тельный.

winter I [ˈwɪntə] *n* 1) зима́; hard (*или* severe) ~ суро́вая зима́; green (*или* mild, open) ~ мя́гкая зима́; it was deep ~ зима́ уже́ вошла́ в свои́ права́, зима́ была́ в разга́ре; 2) *поэт.* год жи́зни; of fifty ~s пяти́десяти лет; 3) *attr* зи́мний; 4) *attr* ози́мый.

winter II *v* 1) проводи́ть зи́му, зимова́ть (*at, in*); 2) пасти́, корми́ть, содержа́ть скот (*во вре́мя зимы́*).

wintering [ˈwɪntərɪŋ] *n* 1) зимо́вка; 2) *attr* зиму́ющий.

wintry [ˈwɪntrɪ] *a* 1) зи́мний, холо́дный; 2) холо́дный, ледяно́й (*об обраще́нии, то́не и т. п.*).

wipe I [waɪp] *n* 1) вытира́ние; to give smth. a ~ вы́тереть что-л.; 2) *сленг* уда́р с разма́ху.

wipe II *v* 1) вытира́ть, утира́ть; осуша́ть; 2) *сленг* замахну́ться на кого́-л., уда́рить с разма́ху кого́-л. (*at*); □ to ~ away, to ~ off стира́ть, вытира́ть; to ~ out а) стира́ть, вытира́ть; смыва́ть (*тж. перен.*); б) разруша́ть, уничтожа́ть, стира́ть с лица́ земли́; to ~ up подтира́ть.

wiper [ˈwaɪpə] *n* 1) полоте́нце; 2) тря́пка для вытира́ния; 3) носово́й плато́к; 4) *авто* «дво́рник».

wire I [ˈwaɪə] *n* 1) про́волока; barbed ~ колю́чая про́волока; 2) *эл.* про́вод; naked ~ неизоли́рованный про́вод; by ~ по телегра́фу, по телефо́ну; 3) *разг.* телегра́мма; ◊ to be on the ~ *сленг* находи́ться в самово́льной отлу́чке; to pull the ~s употреби́ть та́йное влия́ние; нажа́ть та́йные пружи́ны.

wire II *v* 1) телеграфи́ровать; 2) соединя́ть, скрепля́ть про́волокой, провода́ми; 3) де́лать электропрово́дку; □ to ~ in *разг.* энерги́чно вмеша́ться в де́ло; с жа́ром приня́ться за что-л.

wire-haired [ˈwaɪəhɛəd] *a* жесткошёрстный (*о соба́ке*).

wireless I [ˈwaɪəlɪs] *n* 1) ра́дио; беспро́волочный телегра́ф; 2) радиогра́мма.

wireless II *a* беспро́волочный.

wireless III *v* сообща́ть по ра́дио; посыла́ть радиогра́мму.

wirepuller [ˈwaɪəˌpulə] *n* политика́н; полити́ческий интрига́н.

wiring [ˈwaɪərɪŋ] *n* 1) прокла́дка электри́ческих про́водов; 2) *эл.* прово́дка; 3) *воен.* про́волочные загражде́ния.

wiry [ˈwaɪərɪ] *a* 1) похо́жий на про́волоку (*т. е. жёсткий и ги́бкий*); 2) жи́листый, выно́сливый, неутоми́мый.

wisdom [ˈwɪzdəm] *n* му́дрость; благоразу́мие.

wise[1] [waɪz] *a* 1) му́дрый; благоразу́мный; ~ after the event ≅ за́дним умо́м крепо́к; none the ~r ничу́ть не умне́е; 2) осведомлённый, зна́ющий;

to put smb. ~ (to) *амер.* информи́ровать кого́-л. (о чём-л.); раскры́ть кому́-л. глаза́ (на что-л.).

wise² *n уст.* спо́соб; in по ~ нико́им о́бразом; in any ~ каки́м бы то ни́ было о́бразом; in like ~ таки́м же о́бразом.

wiseacre ['waɪzˌeɪkə] *n* всезна́йка.

wisecrack ['waɪzkræk] *n амер. разг.* шутли́вое *или* остроу́мное замеча́ние.

wish I [wɪʃ] *n* 1) жела́ние, пожела́ние; 2) жела́емое.

wish II *v* жела́ть, хоте́ть; пожела́ть; it is to be ~ed that жела́тельно чтобы; could not ~ it better как нельзя́ лу́чше; I ~ it (to be) finished я хочу́, чтобы э́то бы́ло ко́нчено.

wishful ['wɪʃful] *a* жела́ющий, жа́ждущий (*сделать что-л.*).

wishing-bone ['wɪʃɪŋboun] *n* ду́жка (*косточка птицы*).

wishing-cap ['wɪʃɪŋkæp] *n* волше́бная ша́почка (*в сказках*).

wish-wash ['wɪʃwɔʃ] *n* 1) бурда́, помо́и; 2) болтовня́.

wishy-washy ['wɪʃɪˌwɔʃɪ] *a* 1) жи́дкий (*о чае, супе*); 2) сла́бый, вя́лый.

wisp [wɪsp] *n* клок, пучо́к; соло́менный жгут.

wistaria [wɪs'tɛərɪə] *n бот.* глици́ния.

wistful ['wɪstful] *a* тоску́ющий, печа́льный; заду́мчивый (*о взгляде*).

wit¹ [wɪt] *n* 1) *обыкн. pl* ум, ра́зум; mother ~ здра́вый смысл, приро́дный ум; to have a ready (*или* quick) ~ быть нахо́дчивым, сообрази́тельным; to have a slow ~ быть ненахо́дчивым, несообрази́тельным; to have one's ~s about one не теря́ть головы́, сохраня́ть самооблада́ние; быть насторожё; out of one's ~s вне себя́, обезу́мевший; to live by one's ~s кое-ка́к изворáчиваться; 2) остроу́мие; 3) остроу́мный челове́к, остря́к.

wit² *v*: to ~ то есть, а и́менно.

witch I [wɪtʃ] *n* 1) ве́дьма, колду́нья; 2) *разг.* чароде́йка, чаровни́ца.

witch II *v поэт.* околдо́вывать, очаро́вывать.

witchcraft ['wɪtʃkrɑːft] *n* колдовство́.

witchery ['wɪtʃərɪ] *n* 1) *см.* witchcraft; 2) *pl* очарова́ние, ча́ры.

witch-hunt ['wɪtʃhʌnt] *n* 1) *ист.* пресле́дование колду́ний; 2) «охо́та за ве́дьмами», пресле́дование прогресси́вно настро́енных люде́й (*в США*).

with [wɪð] *prep* 1) *выражает совместность, соучастие в одном и том же действии* с; I shall go ~ you я пойду́ с ва́ми; 2) *указывает на лицо или предмет, с которым устанавливается какая-л. связь* с; we talked (argued, sat, dealt) ~ him мы говори́ли (спо́рили, сиде́ли, име́ли де́ло) с ним; 3) *указывает на обладание чем-л., наличие чего-л. у действующего лица, предмета* с, в; a long beard (grey hair, black moustache, a soft hat) с дли́нной бородо́й (седы́ми волоса́ми, чёрными уса́ми, в мя́гкой шля́пе); ~ a stick in his hand с па́лкой в руке́; 4) *указывает на характер производимого действия* с; ~ energy энерги́чно; ~ zeal с рве́нием; ~ all one's heart от всего́ се́рдца, от всей души́; ~ a loud voice гро́мким го́лосом; ~ tears in his eyes со слеза́ми на глаза́х; ~ animation оживлённо; ~ emotion растро́ганно; 5) *выражает причину, вызвавшую данное действие* от (*с род. п.*); to die ~ pneumonia (thirst) умере́ть от воспале́ния лёгких

(от жа́жды); to shiver ~ cold (fear) дрожа́ть от хо́лода (от стра́ха); 6) *указывает на орудие, с помощью которого произведено действие; по-русски переводится тв. п. без предлога*; ~ a spoon, ~ a knife *etc* ло́жкой, ножо́м и т. п.; 7): his coat is covered ~ dust его́ пальто́ покры́то пы́лью.

with- [wɪð] *pref указывает на*: а) *удаление или разделение*: to withdraw уходи́ть, отта́гивать (*войска*); б) *сопротивление*: to withstand сопротивля́ться.

withdraw [wɪð'drɔː] *v* (*past* withdrew; *p. p.* withdrawn) 1) уходи́ть, отходи́ть, отодвига́ться; удаля́ться; ретирова́ться; to ~ from action выходи́ть из бо́я; 2) отдёргивать, отнима́ть, отодвига́ть; удаля́ть; 3) брать наза́д; 4) отзыва́ть; отта́гивать (*войска*); 5) изыма́ть (*из обращения*).

withdrawal [wɪð'drɔːəl] *n* 1) ухо́д, отхо́д, удале́ние; 2) отдёргивание; 3) взя́тие наза́д; 4) отозва́ние; 5) изъя́тие.

withdrawn [wɪð'drɔːn] *p. p. см.* withdraw.

withdrew [wɪð'druː] *past см.* withdraw.

wither ['wɪðə] *v* 1) вя́нуть, со́хнуть; увяда́ть; 2) ослабева́ть, угаса́ть (*о чувствах*); 3) иссуша́ть, лиша́ть све́жести; 4) *шутл.* уничтожа́ть, испепеля́ть (*взглядом*); □ to ~ **away** а) вы́дохнуться; б) увяда́ть, со́хнуть.

withers ['wɪðəz] *n pl* хо́лка; ◊ my ~ are unwrung э́то меня́ не затра́гивает.

withheld [wɪð'held] *past, p. p. см.* withhold.

withhold [wɪð'hould] *v* (*past, p. p.* withheld) 1) отка́зывать (*в чём-л.*); 2) уде́рживать(ся) (*от чего-л. — from*); 3) скрыва́ть, ута́ивать.

within I [wɪ'ðɪn] *prep* 1) внутри́, внутрь; from ~ изнутри́ (*чего-л.*); 2) в преде́лах; ~ hearing в преде́лах слы́шимости, побли́зости; ~ sight of в преде́лах ви́димости; a task well ~ his powers рабо́та по его́ си́лам; 3) не да́лее, не позднее (чем); в тече́ние.

within II *adv* внутри́.

without I [wɪ'ðaut] *prep* 1) без; to do (*или* to go) ~ обходи́ться без чего́-л.; 2) (*перед pres. p. и отглагольными сущ. на* -ing) без того́ чтобы; to come in ~ waking him войти́, не разбуди́в его́; to go away ~ thanking him уйти́, не поблагодари́в его́; 3) вне, за (преде́лами).

without II *adv* снару́жи.

without III *n*: from ~ снару́жи, извне́.

without IV *conj* е́сли не; без того́ чтобы.

withstand [wɪð'stænd] *v* (*past, p. p.* withstood) выде́рживать, противостоя́ть.

withstood [wɪð'stud] *past, p. p. см.* withstand.

witless ['wɪtlɪs] *a* 1) глу́пый; безмо́зглый; 2) бессмы́сленный (*о попытке и т. п.*).

witness I ['wɪtnɪs] *n* 1) свиде́тель (*тж. в суде*); очеви́дец; to call to ~ призыва́ть в свиде́тели, ссыла́ться на; to call in a ~ вы́звать свиде́теля; 2) свиде́тельство, доказа́тельство; to bear ~ свиде́тельствовать, удостоверя́ть (*to, of*); in ~ of в доказа́тельство (*чего-л.*).

witness II *v* 1) быть свиде́телем, очеви́дцем (*чего-л.*); 2) засвиде́тельствовать, заве́рить (*подпись, документ*); 3) дава́ть показа́ния, свиде́тельствовать (*against, for*); 4) свиде́тельствовать о чём-л., служи́ть доказа́тельством.

witticism ['wɪtɪsɪzəm] *n* остроу́мное замеча́ние, остро́та.

wittingly ['wɪtɪŋlɪ] *adv* 1) созна́тельно; 2) умы́шленно, наме́ренно.

witty ['wɪtɪ] *a* остроу́мный.

wives [waɪvz] *pl см.* wife.

wizard ['wɪzəd] *n* колду́н; волше́бник, чароде́й; ◊ ~! *сленг* всё в поря́дке!, отли́чно!

wizen(ed) ['wɪzn(d)] *a* вы́сохший, ссо́хшийся, смо́рщенный.

wo [wou] *int* тпру!

wo-back ['wou'bæk] *int* наза́д!

wobble I ['wɔbl] *n* колеба́ние.

wobble II *v* колеба́ться (*тж. перен.*); шата́ться.

wobbly ['wɔblɪ] *a* ша́ткий, шата́ющийся.

woe [wou] *n поэт., шутл.* го́ре, скорбь; несча́стья; ~ is me! го́ре мне!; ~ be to him!, ~ betide him! будь он про́клят!; to sing ~ сокруша́ться, опла́кивать, горева́ть.

woebegone ['woubɪ,gɔn] *a* удручённый го́рем, мра́чный, пода́вленный.

woeful ['wouful] *a* го́рестный; приско́рбный; жа́лкий.

woke [wouk] *past см.* wake².

woken ['woukən] *p. p. см.* wake².

wold [would] *n* пу́стошь.

wolf I [wulf] *n* (*pl* wolves) 1) волк; 2) обжо́ра; 3) жесто́кий, злой челове́к; ◊ to cry ~ поднима́ть ло́жную трево́гу; to see a ~ онеме́ть, лиши́ться го́лоса (*от страха, изумления и т. п.*); to keep the ~ from the door предотврати́ть го́лод и нищету́; to have a ~ by the ears быть в безвы́ходном положе́нии, не име́ть свобо́ды де́йствий; between dog and ~ су́мерки.

wolf II *v* пожира́ть; есть с жа́дностью (*тж.* to ~ down).

wolf-dog ['wulfdɔg] *n* овча́рка; волкода́в.

wolf-hound ['wulfhaund] *n* волкода́в.

wolfish ['wulfɪʃ] *a* 1) во́лчий; 2) свире́пый.

wolverene ['wulvəriːn] *n зоол.* росома́ха.

wolves [wulvz] *pl см.* wolf I.

woman ['wumən] *n* (*pl* women) 1) же́нщина; kolkhoz ~ колхо́зница; the new ~ передова́я же́нщина; peasant ~ крестья́нка; ~ of the world све́тская же́нщина; single ~ одино́кая, незаму́жняя же́нщина; 2) (the ~) же́нственность; 3) женоподо́бный мужчи́на; 4) *attr* же́нский.

womanhood ['wumənhud] *n* 1) же́нщины, же́нский пол; 2) же́нская зре́лость; 3) же́нственность.

womanish ['wumənɪʃ] *a* же́нский; женоподо́бный.

womankind ['wumən'kaind] *n* же́нщины, же́нский пол; one's ~ же́нская полови́на семьи́.

womanlike ['wumənlaik] *a* же́нский; женоподо́бный.

womanly ['wumənlɪ] *a* же́нственный.

womb [wuːm] *n* 1) *анат.* ма́тка; 2) чре́во.

women ['wɪmɪn] *pl см.* woman.

womenfolk ['wɪmɪnfouk] *pl см.* womankind.

won [wʌn] *past, p. p. см.* win II.

wonder I ['wʌndə] *n* 1) удивле́ние, изумле́ние; I am full of ~ я стра́шно удивлён; no ~ that неудиви́тельно, что; what ~? чему́ удивля́ться?; что удиви́тельного?; for a ~ на удивле́ние; как э́то ни стра́нно; 2) чу́до; to work ~s твори́ть чудеса́; a nine days' ~ злоба́ дня, сенса́ция; гро́мкое, но ско́ро забыва́емое собы́тие.

wonder II *v* 1) удивля́ться (*тж.* to ~ at); 2) хоте́ть знать; I ~ what the time is хоте́л бы я знать, кото́рый час.

wonderful ['wʌndəful] *a* удиви́тельный, замеча́тельный.

wonk(e)y ['wɔŋkɪ] *a сленг* неусто́йчивый, ша́ткий, кача́ющийся.

wont I [wount] *n* привы́чка, обыкнове́ние.

wont II *a predic* име́ющий обыкнове́ние.

won't [wount] *разг.* = will not.

wonted ['wountɪd] *a* обы́чный.

woo [wuː] *v* 1) уха́живать (*за кем-л.*); домога́ться чьей-л. любви́; сва́таться; 2) добива́ться (*богатства, славы и т. п.*).

wood [wud] *n* 1) *часто pl* лес; thick ~ густо́й, дрему́чий лес; 2) де́рево, древеси́на; 3) дрова́; to chop ~ коло́ть дрова́; 4) (the ~) *муз.* деревя́нные духовы́е инструме́нты; 5) изде́лия из де́рева; in the ~ в бочо́нке; from the ~ из бочо́нка (*о вине, пиве*); ◊ to be (*или* to get) out of the ~ быть вне опа́сности; вы́путаться из затрудне́ния; to take to the ~s *амер.* уклоня́ться от исполне́ния обя́занностей (*особ. от голосования*).

woodbine ['wudbain] *n* 1) *бот.* жи́молость; 2) дешёвые папиро́сы; 3) *амер. сленг* англи́йский солда́т.

woodcock ['wudkɔk] *n* ва́льдшнеп.

woodcraft ['wudkrɑːft] *n* зна́ние ле́са и усло́вий охо́ты.

woodcut ['wudkʌt] *n* гравю́ра на де́реве.

woodcutter ['wud,kʌtə] *n* 1) лесору́б, дровосе́к; 2) гравёр, ре́зчик по де́реву.

wooded ['wudɪd] *a* леси́стый.

wooden ['wudn] *a* 1) деревя́нный; 2) вя́лый, безжи́зненный; 3) топо́рный (*о слоге*).

wood-engraver ['wudɪn,greivə] *n* гравёр (по де́реву).

woodland ['wudlənd] *n* леси́стая ме́стность.

woodless ['wudlɪs] *a* безле́сный.

woodman ['wudmən] *n* 1) лесни́к; 2) лесору́б.

woodpecker ['wud,pekə] *n* дя́тел.

wood-wind ['wudwind] *n собир.* деревя́нные духовы́е инструме́нты.

woodwork ['wudwəːk] *n* 1) деревя́нные изде́лия; 2) деревя́нные ча́сти (*рамы, двери и т. п.*); 3) столя́рное иску́сство.

woody ['wudɪ] *a* 1) леси́стый; 2) деревяни́стый.

wooer ['wuːə] *n* возлю́бленный; обожа́тель, уха́жёр.

woof [wuːf] *n текст.* уто́к.

wool [wul] *n* шерсть; (absorbent) cotton ~ (гигроскопи́ческая) ва́та; ◊ to draw (*или* to pull) the ~ over smb.'s eyes втира́ть очки́ кому́-л., вводи́ть кого́-л. в заблужде́ние; to lose one's ~ рассерди́ться.

woolen I, II ['wulɪn] *см.* woollen I, II.

wool-gathering I ['wul,gæðərɪŋ] *n* рассе́янность.

wool-gathering II *a* рассе́янный; вита́ющий в облака́х.

woollen I ['wulɪn] *n pl* шерстяна́я мате́рия; изде́лия из ше́рсти.

woollen II *a* шерстяно́й.

woolly I ['wulɪ] *n* 1) сви́тер; шерстяно́е, вя́заное изде́лие; 2) *pl* тёплая зи́мняя оде́жда; зи́мнее обмундирова́ние.

woolly II *a* 1) шерсти́стый, покры́тый ше́рстью; 2) си́плый (*о голосе*); 3) гру́бый (*о живописи*); напи́санный кру́пными мазка́ми.

word I [wəːd] *n* 1) сло́во; household ~ просто́е, обихо́дное сло́во *или* выраже́ние; знако́мое и́мя; in a ~, in one ~ одни́м сло́вом, коро́тко говоря́; by ~ of mouth у́стно; ~ for сло́во в сло́во, буква́льно; on the ~, with the ~ неме́дленно; in ~ and deed сло́вом и де́лом; to say a good ~ for замо́лвить слове́чко (*за кого́-л.*); to eat one's ~s брать наза́д свои́ слова́; to get a ~ in edgeways вверну́ть, вста́вить слове́чко; 2) *обыкн. pl* речь, разгово́р; soft ~s не́жности; fair (*или* good) ~s а) примири́тельный разгово́р; б) комплиме́нты, лесть; warm (*или* hard, high, sharp, hot) ~s кру́пный разгово́р; брань; big ~s хвастовство́; to bandy ~s перебра́ниваться; to have a ~ with поговори́ть с (*кем-л.*); to have ~s with поссо́риться, кру́пно поговори́ть с (*кем-л.*); to speak the ~ вы́разить жела́ние; to speak ~s of praise хвали́ть, расхва́ливать; 3) обеща́ние; руча́тельство; to give (*или* to pawn) one's ~ дава́ть сло́во; to pass one's ~ руча́ться (*за кого́-л. — for*); to keep (to break) one's ~ держа́ть (наруша́ть) сло́во; to believe smb.'s bare ~ пове́рить кому́-л. на́ слово; upon my ~! че́стное сло́во!; to take smb. at his ~ а) пове́рить кому́-л. на́ слово; б) пойма́ть кого́-л. на́ слове; 4) приказа́ние; ~ of command *воен.* кома́нда; to pass the ~ передава́ть приказа́ние; 5) ве́сти, изве́стие; send me ~ извести́те меня́; to leave ~ оста́вить, переда́ть (*записку, поручение, сообще́ние кому́-л. — for*); 6) *воен.* паро́ль; ◊ weasel ~s слова́, затума́нивающие и́стинный смысл, слова́, соверше́нно искажа́ющие смысл.

word II *v* 1) выража́ть слова́ми; 2) подбира́ть выраже́ния.

word-book ['wəːdbuk] *n* слова́рь.

word-for-word ['wəːdfə,wəːd] *a* досло́вный.

wordiness ['wəːdɪnɪs] *n* многосло́вие.

wording ['wəːdɪŋ] *n* фо́рма выраже́ния; текст; формулиро́вка, реда́кция (*докуме́нта*).

word-perfect ['wəːd'pəːfɪkt] *a* по́мнящий, зна́ющий что-л. наизу́сть.

word-picture ['wəːd,pɪktʃə] *n* о́бразное описа́ние.

word-play ['wəːdpleɪ] *n* 1) игра́ слова́ми; 2) игра́ слов, каламбу́р.

word-splitting ['wəːd,splɪtɪŋ] *n* о́чень то́нкое слове́сное разли́чие.

wordy ['wəːdɪ] *a* 1) многосло́вный; 2) слове́сный.

wore [wɔː] *past см.* wear II.

work I [wəːk] *n* 1) рабо́та; at ~ за рабо́той; in ~ име́ющий рабо́ту; out of ~ безрабо́тный; job ~ сде́льная рабо́та; hard ~ напряжённая, тяжёлая рабо́та; warm ~ опа́сная *или* напряжённая рабо́та; outside ~ рабо́та на во́здухе; welfare ~ мероприя́тия по улучше́нию усло́вий жи́зни рабо́чих; to be hard at ~ рабо́тать напряжённо, не покла́дая рук; to set to ~ принима́ться за рабо́ту; to do poor ~ пло́хо рабо́тать; to knock off ~ прекрати́ть рабо́ту; to strike ~ забастова́ть; to be looking for ~ иска́ть рабо́ту; to give smb. the ~s *амер. сленг* гру́бо обраща́ться с кем-л.; эксплуати́ровать кого́-л.;

≅ взять кого́-л. в оборо́т, в переплёт; 2) де́ло, де́йствие, посту́пок; bloody ~ крова́вое де́ло; to make short ~ of бы́стро разде́латься, спра́виться с чем-л.; 3) произведе́ние, сочине́ние, труд; research ~ иссле́довательская рабо́та; learned ~ нау́чный труд; a beautiful (*или* fine) piece of ~ прекра́сное произведе́ние, прекра́сная вещь; ~ of art произведе́ние иску́сства; complete ~s по́лное собра́ние сочине́ний; 4) *pl* обще́ственные рабо́ты (*по строи́тельству и т. п.; тж.* public ~s); relief ~s обще́ственные рабо́ты для безрабо́тных; 5) *обыкн. pl* сооруже́ние, укрепле́ние; 6) *pl* механи́зм; 7) *attr* рабо́чий; ◊ repetition ~ ма́ссовое произво́дство.

work II *v* 1) рабо́тать (*где́-л. — at; над — on*); to ~ at high (at low) pressure рабо́тать энерги́чно (с прохла́дцей); to ~ to rule проводи́ть италья́нскую забасто́вку; to ~ in distemper (in oils) рабо́тать те́мперой (ма́сляными кра́сками); 2) рабо́тать, быть специали́стом (*в како́й-л. о́бласти*); 3) (*past, p. p. тж.* wrought) обраба́тывать, отде́лывать; 4) де́йствовать; 5) управля́ть; пуска́ть в ход, приводи́ть в движе́ние; заставля́ть рабо́тать; 6) разраба́тывать; эксплуати́ровать; вести́ (*предприя́тие*); 7) пробива́ться; продвига́ться; проника́ть; прокла́дывать себе́ доро́гу; 8) распу́тывать; выпу́тываться, освобожда́ться (*тж.* to ~ loose, to ~ free); 9) причиня́ть, вызыва́ть; 10) вышива́ть; ☐ to ~ **against** де́йствовать про́тив; to ~ **away** продолжа́ть рабо́тать; to ~ **in** а) вставля́ть, вводи́ть; б) соотве́тствовать; to ~ **off** а) распрода́ть, сбыть; б) отде́латься, освободи́ться; в) отрабо́тать (*долг, задо́лженность*); г) вымеща́ть; to ~ off one's bad temper срыва́ть своё плохо́е настрое́ние (*на ком-л. — on*); to ~ **out** а) выража́ться (*в како́й-л. ци́фре*); б) реша́ть (*зада́чу*); в) истоща́ть; г) разраба́тывать (*план, прое́кт*); to ~ **up** (*past, p. p. тж.* wrought) а) разраба́тывать; отде́лывать; б) возбужда́ть.

workable ['wəːkəbl] *a* 1) примени́мый; приго́дный для рабо́ты *или* обрабо́тки; 2) выполни́мый.

workaday ['wəːkədeɪ] *a* бу́дничный, повседне́вный.

workday ['wəːkdeɪ] *n* рабо́чий день.

worker ['wəːkə] *n* 1) рабо́чий; рабо́тник; manual ~ рабо́тник физи́ческого труда́; intellectual (*или* white-collar) ~ рабо́тник у́мственного труда́; ~s by hand and brain рабо́тники физи́ческого и у́мственного труда́; disabled ~ инвали́д труда́; skilled ~ квалифици́рованный рабо́чий; office ~ (канцеля́рский) слу́жащий; shock ~ уда́рник; workers of the world, unite! пролета́рии всех стран, соединя́йтесь!; 2) *attr* рабо́чий; трудово́й.

workhouse ['wəːkhaus] *n* 1) рабо́тный дом; 2) *амер.* исправи́тельный дом.

working I ['wəːkɪŋ] *n* 1) рабо́та; ~ to rule италья́нская забасто́вка; 2) эксплуата́ция, разрабо́тка; произво́дство рабо́т; 3) обрабо́тка (*тж.* working-out); 4) ме́сто разрабо́тки (*ша́хта, карье́р и т. п.*).

working II *a* 1) рабо́чий; трудово́й; 2) приго́дный для рабо́ты; свя́занный с рабо́той.

workman ['wəːkmən] *n* рабо́чий.

workmanlike ['wəːkmənlaik] *a* иску́сный.

workmanship ['wə:kmənʃıp] *n* 1) искусство, мастерство; 2) отделка.

work-out ['wə:k'aut] *n амер. сленг* 1) проверка, испытательный срок; 2) *спорт.* тренировка.

work-people ['wə:k,pi:pl] *n pl* рабочие, трудящиеся.

work-room ['wə:krum] *n* рабочая комната, рабочий кабинет.

works [wə:ks] *n* завод; мастерские.

workshop ['wə:kʃɔp] *n* цех; мастерская.

work-shy I ['wə:kʃaı] *n* лентяй; бездельник.

work-shy II *a* уклоняющийся от работы.

world [wə:ld] *n* 1) мир, свет; вселенная; the outer ~ внешний мир; посторонние; the other ~, the next ~, the ~ to come тот свет, загробный мир; the nether (*или* the lower) ~ ад, преисподняя; to bring into the ~ родить, произвести на свет; to come into the ~ родиться, появиться на свет; to rock the ~ потрясать мир; as the ~ goes с тех пор как существует мир; so goes the ~ такова жизнь, вот как бывает на свете; to tell the ~ *амер.* открыто объявить, рассказать всему свету; 2) общество; мир; the learned ~ научный мир, ученые; the literary ~, the ~ of letters литературный мир; the animal ~ животный мир; to know (*или* to see) the ~ знать жизнь, видеть свет, иметь жизненный опыт; to begin the ~ вступать в жизнь, начинать свою карьеру; to come down in the ~ опуститься, деклассироваться; 3) масса, множество (*чего-л. — of*); a ~ of troubles множество, куча хлопот; a ~ of waters водное пространство; 4) *служит для усиления вопроса:* what in the ~ does it mean? что это наконец значит?; 5) *attr* мировой; всемирный; ◊ a ~ too слишком; ~ without end навсегда, на веки вечные; all the ~ and his wife все без исключения; to the ~ *разг.* совершенно, в высшей степени; for all the ~ like во всех отношениях такой же; · to carry the ~ before one преуспевать, иметь успех.

worldly ['wə:ldlı] *a* 1) земной, мирской; 2) любящий земные блага.

world-wide ['wə:ldwaıd] *a* всемирно известный, мировой; распространённый по всему свету.

worm I [wə:m] *n* 1) червяк, червь; 2) глист(а); 3) жалкий, презренный человек; 4) *тех.* червяк, бесконечный винт; змеевик; ◊ a ~ will turn ≅ всякому терпению приходит конец; the ~ of conscience угрызения совести; I am a ~ today я не в настроении сегодня, я сегодня не в своей тарелке; to satisfy the ~ заморить червячка, поесть.

worm II *v* 1) вползать, проникать (*into, through*); 2) вкрадываться, втираться (*в доверие; into*); 3) выпытать, разузнать (*тж.* to ~ out).

wormwood ['wə:mwud] *n* полынь; *перен.* горечь, источник огорчений.

wormy ['wə:mı] *a* 1) червивый; 2) подлый, низкий.

worn [wɔ:n] *p. p. см.* wear II.

worn-out ['wɔ:n'aut] *a* изношенный; *перен.* истощённый.

worriless ['wʌrılıs] *a* спокойный, не причиняющий беспокойства.

worrisome ['wʌrısəm] *a* беспокойный; доставляющий, причиняющий беспокойство.

worry I ['wʌrı] *n* беспокойство, тревога; заботы.

worry II *v* 1) приставать, надоедать; 2) мучить(ся), терзать(ся), беспокоить(ся); I should ~ *амер. разг.* это меня ничуть не беспокоит; 3) терзать, трепать (*добычу зубами — о собаках*); □ to ~ **along** пробиваться вперёд, невзирая на трудности.

worse I [wə:s] *a* (*compar см.* bad I) худший; he is ~, he is getting ~ ему хуже (*о больном*); to make it ~ и что хуже того, в придачу (*к чему-л. плохому*); not the ~ тем не менее; to grow ~ ухудшаться.

worse II *adv* (*compar см.* badly) хуже; none the ~ ещё лучше, ещё сильнее.

worse III *n* худшее; for the ~ к худшему; the ~ поражение; to have the ~ быть побеждённым; to put to the ~ победить.

worsen ['wə:sn] *v* ухудшать(ся).

worship I ['wə:ʃıp] *n* 1) поклонение, преклонение, почитание; культ; 2) богослужение; divine ~ церковная служба, богослужение; 3) *уст.* почёт; 4): Your Worship ваша милость (*обращение*).

worship II *v* 1) поклоняться, обожать; 2) ходить в церковь.

worst I [wə:st] *a* (*superl см.* bad I) наихудший.

worst II *adv* (*superl см.* badly) хуже всего.

worst III *n* самое худшее, наихудшее; at (the) ~ в худшем случае, в худшем положении; to get the ~ of it быть побеждённым; if the ~ comes to the ~ в худшем случае, на худой конец.

worst IV *v* побеждать, наносить поражение; одержать верх; разбить.

worsted ['wustıd] *a* шерстяной.

worth I [wə:θ] *n* цена, стоимость; ценность; достоинство; of great (little) ~ ценный (малоценный); of no ~ ничего не стоящий; person of ~ достойный, заслуживающий уважения человек; a shilling's ~ (of) стоящий шиллинг, на шиллинг (*чего-л.*).

worth II *a* 1) стоящий; заслуживающий; to be ~ стоить; what is it ~? сколько это стоит?; 2): he is ~ a million у него миллионное состояние; he spent all he was ~ он истратил всё, что имел, всё своё состояние; ◊ for all one is ~ *разг.* изо всех сил, чего бы это ни стоило.

worthily ['wə:ðılı] *adv* достойно; по достоинству; заслуженно.

worthless ['wə:θlıs] *a* ничего не стоящий, никчёмный.

worth-while ['wə:θ'waıl] *a* стоящий; заслуживающий внимания; имеющий смысл.

worthy I ['wə:ðı] *a* 1) достойный, заслуживающий (*of*); ~ of remembrance, ~ to be remembered заслуживающий памяти; 2) (досто)почтенный, достойный (*тж. ирон.*).

worthy II *n* знаменитость (*тж. шутл.*).

would [wud] 1) *past см.* will[2]; 2) *как вспом. гл. употр.:* а) *в форме Subjunctive 2-го и 3-го л. обоих чисел для выражения пожелания:* I wish he ~ know English я хотел бы, чтобы он знал английский язык; б) *в форме Conditional 2-го и 3-го л. обоих чисел для выражения условности:* I should be very glad if you ~ translate this passage я был бы очень рад, если бы вы перевели э́тот отры́вок; в) *в форме Future in the Past 2-го и 3-го л. обоих чисел для выражения буду́щего действия, о котором говорилось в про́шлом:* he ~ come at 9 o'clock он сказа́л, что придёт в 9 часо́в; 3) *как модальный гл. употр. для выражения желания, однако в более слабой степени, чем в форме наст. вр.:* he ~ smoke here, though it was forbidden ему́ хоте́лось кури́ть здесь, хотя́ э́то и бы́ло запрещено́; I ~ rather я предпочёл бы; 4) *употр. для выражения повторности действия в прошлом:* he ~ sit for hours without saying a word он, быва́ло, часа́ми сиде́л, не произноса́ ни сло́ва.

would-be ['wudbiː] *a* 1) изобража́ющий из себя́, вообража́ющий себя́; де́лающий вид; мни́мый; 2) *разг.* «с прете́нзиями».

wouldn't ['wudnt] *разг.* = would not.

woundᵃ I [wuːnd] *n* 1) ра́на; incised (lacerated) ~ ре́заная (рва́ная) ра́на; punctured ~ сквозна́я ра́на; ко́лотая ра́на; vital (*или* mortal) ~ смерте́льная ра́на; to search a ~ зонди́ровать ра́ну; 2) оби́да, оскорбле́ние.

woundᵃ II *v* ра́нить.

woundᵇ [waund] *past, p. p. см.* wind^{b2} II.

wove [wouv] *past см.* weave.

woven ['wouvən] *p. p. см.* weave.

wrack [ræk] *n* 1) во́доросль (*выброшенная морем*); 2): ~ and ruin по́лное разоре́ние, по́лное разруше́ние.

wraith [reɪθ] *n* при́зрак, дух.

wrangle¹ I ['ræŋgl] *n* ссо́ра, пререка́ние; спор.

wrangle¹ II *v* спо́рить, пререка́ться.

wrangle² *v амер.* пасти́ стада́ (верхо́м).

wrangler¹ ['ræŋglə] *n* спо́рщик, крику́н.

wrangler² *n амер.* ковбо́й.

wrap I [ræp] *n* 1) обёртка; 2) шаль, плато́к.

wrap II *v* 1) завёртывать, заку́тывать (*тж.* to ~ up); 2) обёртывать, оку́тывать (*round, about*); □ to ~ up a) ку́таться; б): ~ped up in погружённый в (*работу и т. п.*).

wrapper ['ræpə] *n* 1) обёртка; 2) суперобло́жка (*на книге*); 3) бандеро́ль; 4) наки́дка (*да́мская*); лёгкое широ́кое полупальто́; 5) хала́т, капо́т.

wrath [rɔːθ] *n* гнев, я́рость; to stir one's ~ вы́звать гнев, отвраще́ние.

wrathful ['rɔːθful] *a* гне́вный.

wreak [riːk] *v* дава́ть во́лю, вы́ход (*чу́вствам*).

wreath [riːθ, *pl* riːðz] *n* 1) вено́к; 2) кольцо́ (*ды́ма*).

wreathe [riːð] *v* 1) свива́ть, вить, плести́ (*венки*); 2) озаря́ться (*улы́бкой*); 3) обвива́ть; 4) клуби́ться (*о ды́ме*).

wreck I [rek] *n* 1) ава́рия, круше́ние; to go to ~ разруша́ться, разва́ливаться, приходи́ть в упа́док; 2) обло́мки круше́ния; 3) разва́лина (*тж. перен. о человеке*).

wreck II *v* вы́звать круше́ние, ава́рию; *перен.* разру́шить (*надежды, планы*).

wreckage ['rekɪdʒ] *n* обло́мки круше́ния.

wrecker¹ ['rekə] *n* 1) ремо́нтный рабо́чий; 2) маши́на техни́ческой по́мощи.

wrecker² *n* 1) *полит.* вреди́тель; 2) граби́тель разби́тых судо́в.

wren [ren] *n* крапи́вник, королёк (*птица*).

wrench I [rentʃ] *n* 1) си́льное дёрганье, выкру́-

чивание; to give a ~ at the door-handle си́льно дёрнуть ру́чку две́ри; 2) тоска́, боль (*при разлу́ке*); 3) вы́вих; 4) *тех.* га́ечный ключ.

wrench II *v* 1) с си́лой дёрнуть, сверну́ть, вы́рвать; to ~ open взла́мывать; 2) вы́вихнуть; 3) искажа́ть.

wrest [rest] *v* 1) вырыва́ть (*из рук*); 2) искажа́ть, истолко́вывать в свою́ по́льзу (*закон и т. п.*).

wrestle I ['resl] *n* 1) борьба́ (*спортивная*); 2) упо́рная борьба́, схва́тка.

wrestle II *v* боро́ться.

wrestler ['reslə] *n* боре́ц.

wretch [retʃ] *n* 1) несча́стный, бедня́га; 2) негодя́й; 3) *шутл.* него́дник.

wretched ['retʃɪd] *a* 1) несча́стный, жа́лкий; 2) скве́рный, никуда́ не го́дный.

wriggle I ['rɪgl] *n* изви́в, изги́б.

wriggle II *v* 1) извива́ться, изгиба́ться (*тж.* to ~ oneself); *перен.* увиливать; уклоня́ться; 2) пробира́ться.

wright [raɪt] *n уст.* ма́стер.

wring I [rɪŋ] *n* 1) сжима́ние, сжа́тие; пожа́тие; 2) выжима́ние; to give a ~ выжима́ть.

wring II *v* (*past, p. p.* wrung) 1) скру́чивать; 2) жать, сжима́ть; 3) выжима́ть (*тж.* to ~ out); 4) жать (*об обуви*); 5) терза́ть; 6) вымога́ть, вынужда́ть.

wrinkle¹ I ['rɪŋkl] *n* морщи́на.

wrinkle¹ II *v* мо́рщить(ся).

wrinkle² *n* поле́зный сове́т; to get a ~ of two узна́ть ко́е-что́ (*о предстоящем путешествии, це́нах и т. п.*).

wrist [rɪst] *n* запя́стье.

wristlet ['rɪstlɪt] *n* 1) брасле́т; 2) ремешо́к для часо́в.

wrist-watch ['rɪstwɔtʃ] *n* нару́чные часы́.

writ [rɪt] *n* 1) прика́з, предписа́ние; повестка; 2) *уст.* писа́ние; the Holy Writ свяще́нное писа́ние, би́блия.

write [raɪt] *v* (*past* wrote; *p. p.* written) писа́ть; to ~ large (small) кру́пно (ме́лко) писа́ть; □ to ~ **down** а) запи́сывать; б) пло́хо отзыва́ться в печа́ти (*о ком-л.*); в) опи́сывать, изобража́ть; то ~ **off** а) легко́ и бы́стро (о)писа́ть; б) посла́ть письмо́; в) аннули́ровать; спи́сывать со счёта; to ~ **out** выпи́сывать по́лностью; to ~ oneself out испи́саться, вы́дохнуться (*о писа́теле*); to ~ **up** а) подро́бно опи́сывать; б) зака́нчивать, допи́сывать, доводи́ть до сего́дняшнего дня; в) реклами́ровать, расхва́ливать (*в печати*).

writer ['raɪtə] *n* 1) пи́шущий; present ~ пи́шущий э́ти стро́ки; 2) писа́тель; productive ~ плодови́тый писа́тель; editorial ~ сотру́дник газе́ты, пи́шущий передови́цы; feature ~ фельето́нист; 3) писе́ц, письмоводи́тель.

write-up ['raɪtʌp] *n* 1) газе́тное сообще́ние; 2) хвале́бная статья́ (*в газете*).

writhe [raɪð] *v* 1) ко́рчиться (*от боли*); 2) му́читься (*от злости*); терза́ться.

writing ['raɪtɪŋ] *n* 1) писа́ние; in ~ в пи́сьменной фо́рме; to commit to ~ запи́сать; 2) (*литерату́рное*) произведе́ние; кни́га, статья́; 3) докуме́нт; 4) *attr* пи́счий; для письма́; пи́сьменный.

writing-desk ['raɪtɪŋdesk] *n* конто́рка; па́рта.

writing-materials [ˈraɪtɪŋməˈtɪərɪəlz] *n pl* письменные принадлежности.

writing-paper [ˈraɪtɪŋˌpeɪpə] *n* почтовая бумага; писчая бумага.

writing-table [ˈraɪtɪŋˌteɪbl] *n* письменный стол.

written [ˈrɪtn] *p. p. см.* write.

wrong I [rɔŋ] *n* зло; несправедливость; неправда; you are in the ~ вы ошибаетесь; to put smb. in the ~ сделать кого-л. ответственным за что-л.; свалить вину на кого-л.; to right а ~ исправить зло, несправедливость.

wrong II *a* неправильный, ошибочный; не тот; you are ~ вы неправы, вы ошибаетесь; what is ~? в чём дело?, что случилось?; to go ~ а) сбиться с пути истинного; б) не выйти, не получиться.

wrong III *adv* неверно, неправильно, плохо.

wrong IV *v* быть несправедливым (*к кому-л.*); причинять зло, обижать.

wrongdoer [ˈrɔŋˈduə] *n* 1) обидчик, оскорбитель; 2) преступник; правонарушитель; 3) грешник.

wrongdoing [ˈrɔŋˈdu(ː)ɪŋ] *n* 1) грех, проступок; 2) преступление; правонарушение.

wrongful [ˈrɔŋful] *a* несправедливый; незаконный.

wrong-headed [ˈrɔŋˈhedɪd] *a* упорствующий в заблуждениях.

wrote [rout] *past см.* write.

wroth [rouθ] *a поэт., шутл.* разгневанный.

wrought [rɔːt] *past, p. p. см.* work II, 3.

wrought-iron [ˈrɔːtˈaɪən] *n* кованое железо.

wrung [rʌŋ] *past, p. p. см.* wring II.

wry [raɪ] *a* кривой, перекошенный.

X

X, x [eks] *n* 1) *24-я буква англ. алфавита;* 2) икс, неизвестная величина.

xenophobia [ˌzenəˈfoubɪə] *n* ненависть к иностранцам.

Xmas [ˈkrɪsməs] *см.* Christmas.

X-mitter [ˈeksˈmɪtə] *n разг.* радиопередатчик.

X-ray I [ˈeksˈreɪ] *n обыкн. pl* рентгеновы лучи.

X-ray II *v* просвечивать рентгеновыми лучами.

xylographer [zaɪˈlɔgrəfə] *n* гравёр по дереву, ксилограф.

xylography [zaɪˈlɔgrəfɪ] *n* ксилография; гравирование на дереве.

xylonite [ˈzaɪlənaɪt] *n* целлулоид.

xylophone [ˈzaɪləfoun] *n муз.* ксилофон.

Y

Y, y [waɪ] *n 25-я буква англ. алфавита.*

yacht [jɔt] *n* яхта.

yacht II *v* плавать на яхте.

yacht-club [ˈjɔtklʌb] *n* яхт-клуб.

yachting [ˈjɔtɪŋ] *n* 1) плавание на яхте; 2) управление яхтой.

yachtsman [ˈjɔtsmən] *n* 1) владелец яхты; 2) *спорт.* яхтсмен.

yahoo [jəˈhuː] *n* грубая скотина (*о человеке*).

yak [jæk] *n зоол.* як.

Yank [jæŋk] *n сленг см.* Yankee.

yank I [jæŋk] *n сленг* рывок.

yank II *v сленг* рвануть, дёрнуть; to ~ out выдернуть, выбить.

Yankee [ˈjæŋkɪ] *n* 1) янки, американец; 2) *attr* американский.

yankeefied [ˈjæŋkɪfaɪd] *a* обамериканившийся.

yap I [jæp] *n* пронзительный лай, тявканье.

yap II *v* 1) пронзительно лаять, тявкать; 2) *разг.* болтать.

yard¹ [jɑːd] *n* 1) ярд (*около 91 см*); 2) *мор.* рей.

yard² I *n* 1) двор; 2) *ж.-д.* сортировочная станция, парк (*тж.* railway-yard *u* marshalling yard); 3) склад; ◊ the Yard, Scotland Yard Скотленд-Ярд (*центр уголовной полиции в Лондоне*).

yard² II *v* загонять (*скот*).

yard-man [ˈjɑːdmən] *n ж.-д.* служащий депо.

yard-master [ˈjɑːdˌmɑːstə] *n ж.-д.* 1) начальник парковых путей; 2) составитель поездов.

yarn I [jɑːn] *n* 1) пряжа, нить; 2) *разг.* рассказ (*особ.* неправдоподобный), повествование; анекдот; to spin a ~, to spin ~s рассказывать истории, небылицы; передавать слухи.

yarn II *v* 1) рассказывать истории; 2) болтать.

yataghan [ˈjætəgən] *n* ятаган.

yaw I [jɔː] *n мор., ав.* отклонение от курса.

yaw II *v мор., ав.* отклоняться от курса.

yawl [jɔːl] *n* ялик.

yawn I [jɔːn] *n* зевота; to give a soft (*или а* comfortable) ~ сладко зевнуть.

yawn II *v* 1) зевать; 2) зиять; 3) сказать что-л. зевая.

ye [jiː] *уст. поэт. см.* you.

yea [jeɪ] *adv уст.* да.

year [jɑː] *n* 1) год; light ~ световой год; fiscal ~ бюджетный год; an off ~ неурожайный год; the New Year Новый год; to see the New Year in встречать Новый год; to sing the New Year in встречать с песнями Новый год; to sing the Old Year out провожать с песнями старый год; (I wish you) a happy New Year! с Новым годом!; the ~ of grace год нашей эры; in this ~ of grace *ирон.* в наши дни, в наш век; from ~ to ~, ~ by ~ каждый год; с каждым годом; ~ in ~ out из году в год; once a ~ раз в год; this day ~ ровно год тому назад; all the ~ round весь год, круглый год; in the ~ one в незапамятные времена; school ~ учебный год; 2) *pl* годы, возраст; in ~s пожилой, в летах; he is young for his ~s он молод, не бодр для своих лет.

year-book [ˈjɑːbuk] *n* ежегодник.

yearling I [ˈjɑːlɪŋ] *n* годовалое животное.

yearling II *a* годовалый.

yearlong [ˈjɑːlɔŋ] *a* длящийся год; годичный.

yearly I [ˈjɑːlɪ] *a* ежегодный.

yearly II *adv* ежегодно; раз в год.

yearn [jɑːn] *v* 1) томиться, тосковать (*for, after*); 2) стремиться (*towards, to*).

yeast [jiːst] *n* дрожжи.

yeast-powder [ˈjiːstˈpaudə] *n* сухие дрожжи.

yeasty ['ji:stɪ] *a* пе́нистый; *перен.* пусто́й, бессодержа́тельный.

yelk [jelk] *n* желто́к.

yell I [jel] *n* 1) крик; вопль; 2) *амер.* во́зглас ободре́ния (*на студе́нческих спорт. состяза́ниях; у ка́ждого колле́джа свой во́зглас*).

yell II *v* 1) крича́ть, вопи́ть; 2) выкри́кивать (*тж.* to ~ out); 3) *амер.* хо́ром выкри́кивать во́зглас своего́ колле́джа (*на спорт. состяза́ниях*).

yellow I ['jelou] *a* 1) жёлтый; 2) зави́стливый, ревни́вый; подозри́тельный; 3) *разг.* трусли́вый.

yellow II *n* 1) желтизна́; жёлтый цвет; 2) жёлтая кра́ска; 3) *разг.* тру́сость.

yellow III *v* желте́ть.

yellowback ['jeloubæk] *n* 1) дешёвый бульва́рный рома́н; 2) францу́зский рома́н (*в жёлтой обло́жке*).

yellowish ['jelouɪʃ] *a* желтова́тый.

yellowy ['jelouɪ] *см.* yellowish.

yelp I [jelp] *n* лай, тя́вканье; визг.

yelp II *v* ла́ять, тя́вкать; визжа́ть.

yen [jen] *n* (*pl без измен.*) ие́на (*де́нежная едини́ца Япо́нии*).

yeoman ['joumən] *n* 1) *ист.* ио́мен; 2) фе́рмер; ме́лкий землевладе́лец; ◊ ~ of the guard дворцо́вый страж.

yeomanry ['joumənrɪ] *n ист.* ио́мены.

yes I [jes] *n* утвержде́ние; say ~! согласи́тесь!, да́йте согла́сие!

yes II *part* да; ~? да?, в са́мом де́ле?

yes-man ['jesmæn] *n разг.* всегда́ подда́кивающий челове́к; подхали́м.

yesterday I ['jestədɪ] *n* 1) вчера́шний день; 2) *pl* былы́е времена́, проше́дшее.

yesterday II *adv* вчера́; the day before ~ позавчера́, тре́тьего дня.

yet I [jet] *adv* 1) (всё) ещё; there is ~ time ещё есть вре́мя; much ~ remains to be done всё ещё мно́гое не сде́лано, мно́гое ещё остаётся сде́лать; not ~ ещё не(т); never ~ никогда́ ещё не; 2) ещё, вдоба́вок; more and ~ more бо́льше и ещё бо́льше; he won't listen to me nor ~ to her он не слу́шает ни меня́ ни её; 3) уже́; is he dead ~? он уже́ у́мер?; need you go ~? вам уже́ на́до уходи́ть?; 4) да́же; 5) до тех пор; пока́; as ~ до сих пор; 6) несмотря́ на, тем не ме́нее; всё же, всё-таки; strange and ~ true стра́нно, но тем не ме́нее ве́рно.

yet II *conj* тем не ме́нее, одна́ко, но в то же вре́мя; ~ what is the use of it all? одна́ко что по́льзы во всём э́том?

yeti ['jetɪ] *n* йе́ти, «сне́жный челове́к».

yew [ju:] *n* ти́совое де́рево (*тж.* yew-tree).

yield I [ji:ld] *n* 1) производи́тельность; коли́чество добыва́емого проду́кта; урожа́й.

yield II *v* 1) производи́ть; 2) приноси́ть, дава́ть (*дохо́д, урожа́й и т. п.*); 3) уступа́ть; подава́ться; to ~ to the advice после́довать сове́ту; 4) сдава́ть(ся); to ~ oneself prisoner сда́ться в плен; □ to ~ up отка́зываться (*от чего́-л.*).

yielding ['ji:ldɪŋ] *a* 1) усту́пчивый, покла́дистый; 2) мя́гкий (*о материа́ле*).

yoga ['jougə] *n* уче́ние йо́гов.

yogi ['jougɪ] *n* йог.

yo-heave-ho ['jouhi:v'hou] *см.* yoho.

yoho [jou'hou] *int мор.* ≅ взя́ли!, дру́жно! (*во́зглас при тяжёлой физи́ческой рабо́те*).

yoke I [jouk] *n* 1) ярмо́; *перен. тж.* и́го; у́зы; 2) па́ра воло́в; 3) коромы́сло; 4) коке́тка (*на пла́тье*); 5) *тех.* скоба́, зажи́м.

yoke II *v* 1) впряга́ть в ярмо́; *перен.* соединя́ть; 2) порабоща́ть, угнета́ть; 3) подходи́ть друг к дру́гу.

yokel ['joukəl] *n* дереве́нщина.

yolk [jouk] *n* желто́к.

yonder I ['jɔndə] *a* вон тот.

yonder II *adv* вон там.

yore [jɔ:] *n*: in days of ~ во вре́мя о́но.

York [jɔ:k] *n*: House of ~ *ист.* дина́стия Йо́рков, Бе́лая ро́за.

you [ju:] *pron pers* 1) ты (*тж. ко́св. п.* тебя́, тебе́); by ~ тобо́й; to ~ тебе́; with ~ с тобо́й; 2) вы (*тж. ко́св. п.* вас, вам); by ~ ва́ми; to ~ вам; with ~ с ва́ми; 3) *употр. для усиле́ния восклица́ния, иногда́ не перево́дится:* ~ fool! дура́к!; ~, my friends, listen to me! послу́шайте меня́, друзья́ мои́!; ~, boys, come here! ма́льчики, подойди́ сюда́!; ~ there! эй вы!; 4) *перево́дится безли́чными оборо́тами:* ~ never can tell никогда́ нельзя́ сказа́ть; what are ~ to do with a child like this? ну что (бу́дешь) де́лать с таки́м ребёнком?; 5) *уст. см.* yourself.

young I [jʌŋ] *a* 1) молодо́й, ю́ный; 2) моложа́вый; 3) нео́пытный; 4) неда́вний; 5) ра́нний (*о вре́мени*).

young II *n* детёныш; with ~ сте́льная, супоро́сая *и т. п.*

youngish ['jʌŋɪʃ] *a* моложа́вый.

youngling ['jʌŋlɪŋ] *n поэт.* ребёнок; детёныш.

youngster ['jʌŋstə] *n* ю́ноша, ма́льчик.

your [jɔ:] *pron poss* ваш, твой.

you're [juə] *разг.* = you are.

yours [jɔ:z] *pron poss* 1) *predic* ваш, ва́ша, ва́ше, ва́ши; твой, твоя́, твоё, твои́; some friends of ~ не́сколько ва́ших друзе́й, не́которые из ва́ших друзе́й; 2) *замеща́ет сущ.:* ~ of the 12th ва́ше письмо́ от 12-го; ~ is to hand ва́ше письмо́ полу́чено.

yourself [jɔ:'self] *pron* (*pl* yourselves) 1) *refl* -ся, себя́, себе́, собо́ю; have you hurt ~? вы уши́блись?; dress ~ одева́йтесь; 2) *употр. для усиле́ния* сам, са́ми; you ~ said so, you said so ~ вы са́ми так сказа́ли; by ~ оди́н, в одино́честве; you cannot do it ~ вы не мо́жете э́того сде́лать са́ми; how's ~? *сленг* (а) как вы пожива́ете? (*осо́б. по́сле отве́та на подо́бный же вопро́с*); you are not quite ~ tonight вам сего́дня не по себе́; be ~ *разг.* возьми́те себя́ в ру́ки, успоко́йтесь.

yourselves [jɔ:'selvz] *pl см.* yourself.

youth [ju:θ] *n* 1) мо́лодость, ю́ность; 2) (*pl* youths [ju:ðz]) ю́ноша; 3) *собир.* молодёжь.

youthful ['ju:θful] *a* 1) молодо́й, ю́ный, ю́ношеский; 2) моложа́вый.

you've [ju:v] *разг.* = you have.

yowl I [jaul] *n* вой.

yowl II *v* выть.

yperite ['i:pəraɪt] *n* иприт.

yuft [ju:ft] *n* юфть.

Yugoslav I [ˈjuːgouˈslɑːv] *n* югослав́; югослав́ка; жи́тель (ница) Югославии.

Yugoslav II *a* югослав́ский.

yule [juːl] *n* святки (*тж.* yule-tide).

Z

Z, z [zed, *амер.* ziː] *n* 26-я буква *англ. алфавита.*

zeal [ziːl] *n* усе́рдие, рве́ние.

zealot [ˈzelət] *n* фанати́ческий приве́рженец, фана́тик.

zealous [ˈzeləs] *a* усе́рдный, рья́ный.

zebra [ˈziːbrə] *n* 1) зе́бра; 2) *attr* полоса́тый (как зе́бра).

zebu [ˈziːbuː] *n* *зоол.* зе́бу.

zenith [ˈzeniθ] *n* зени́т.

zenithal [ˈzeniθəl] *a* зени́тный.

zephyr [ˈzefə] *n* 1) за́падный ве́тер; 2) лёгкий ветеро́к, зефи́р; 3) ма́йка, се́тка (*у боксёра, пловца и т. п.*); 4) зефи́р (*ткань*).

zero [ˈziərou] *n* 1) нуль; *перен.* ничто́; to reduce to ~ своди́ть(ся) к нулю́, конча́ться ниче́м; 2) *attr* нача́льный; 3) *attr* нулево́й.

zest [zest] *n* 1) «изю́минка», пика́нтность; 2) интере́с, жар; with ~ с жа́ром, с энтузиа́змом.

zigzag I [ˈzigzæg] *n* зигза́г.

zigzag II *a* зигзагообра́зный.

zigzag III *v* де́лать зигза́ги.

zigzag IV *adv* зигзагообра́зно.

zinc I [ziŋk] *n* 1) цинк; 2) *attr* ци́нковый.

zinc II *v* оцинко́вывать.

zinnia [ˈzinjə] *n* *бот.* ци́нния.

Zionism [ˈzaiənizəm] *n* сиони́зм.

zip I [zip] *n* 1) свист пу́ли; 2) треск разрыва́емой тка́ни; 3) стреми́тельность; жи́вость, эне́ргия, темпера́мент; 4) застёжка «мо́лния».

zip II *v* 1) проноси́ться со сви́стом; 2) бы́стро нести́сь, лете́ть.

zip-fastener [ˈzipˌfɑːsnə] *см.* zip I, 4).

zipper [ˈzipə] *см.* zip I, 4).

zippy [ˈzipi] *a* живо́й, оживлённый, бо́дрый.

zither [ˈziθə] *n* *муз.* ци́тра.

zloty [ˈzlɔti] *n* зло́тый (*денежная единица Польши*).

zodiac [ˈzoudiæk] *n* *астр.* зодиа́к.

zodiacal [zouˈdaiəkəl] *a* *астр.* зодиака́льный.

zonal [ˈzounl] *a* зона́льный.

zone I [zoun] *n* 1) зо́на, по́яс; полоса́, о́бласть; frigid (torrid, temperate) ~ аркти́ческий (тропи́ческий, уме́ренный) по́яс; 2) *attr* зона́льный.

zone II *v* опоя́сывать.

Zoo [zuː] *n* *разг.* зоопа́рк.

zoological [ˌzouəˈlɔdʒikəl] *a* зоологи́ческий.

zoologist [zouˈɔlədʒist] *n* зоо́лог.

zoology [zouˈɔlədʒi] *n* зооло́гия.

zoom I [zuːm] *n* 1) гуде́ние, жужжа́ние; 2) крутой подъём; 3) *ав.* «све́чка», «го́рка».

zoom II *v* 1) гуде́ть, жужжа́ть; 2) кру́то взмыва́ть вверх; 3) *ав.* де́лать «све́чку».

zooman [ˈzuːmən] *n* рабо́тник зоопа́рка.

zounds [zaundz] *int* *уст.* чёрт возьми́.

ГЕОГРАФИЧЕСКИЕ НАЗВАНИЯ *
GEOGRAPHIC NAMES

Abidjan [ˌæbɪ'dʒɑːn] *г.* Абиджа́н.
Abu Dhabi [æ'buː'dɑːbɪ] *г.* Абу́-Да́би. ·
Accra [ɔ'krɑː] *г.* А́ккра.
Addis Ababa ['ædɪs'æbəbə] *г.* Аддис-Абе́ба.
Aden ['eɪdn] *г.* А́ден.
Adriatic Sea [ˌeɪdrɪ'ætɪk...] Адриати́ческое мо́ре.
Aegean Sea [iː'dʒiːən...] Эге́йское мо́ре.
Afghanistan [æf'gænɪstæn] Афганиста́н; **Republic of Afghanistan** [rɪ'pʌblɪkəvæf'gænɪstæn] Респу́блика Афганиста́н.
Africa ['æfrɪkə] А́фрика.
Alabama [ˌælə'bæmə] Алаба́ма.
Alaska [ə'læskə] Аля́ска.
Albania [æl'beɪnjə] Алба́ния; **People's Socialist Republic of Albania** ['piːplz'souʃəlɪstrɪ'pʌblɪkəvæl'beɪnjə] Наро́дная Социалисти́ческая Респу́блика Алба́ния.
Aleutian Isls [ə'luːʃjən...] Але́утские о-ва́.
Algeria [æl'dʒɪərɪə] Алжи́р.
Algiers [æl'dʒɪəz] *г.* Алжи́р.
Al Kuwait [ælku'weɪt] *г.* Эль-Куве́йт.
Alma-Ata ['ɑːlmɑːɑː'tɑː] *г.* Алма́-Ата́.
Alps, the [ælps] А́льпы.
Altai [æl'taɪ] Алта́й.
Amazon ['æməzən] *р.* Амазо́нка.
America [ə'merɪkə] Аме́рика.
Amman [æm'mæn] *г.* Амма́н.
Amsterdam ['æmstə'dæm] *г.* Амстерда́м.
Amur [ə'muːə] *р.* Аму́р.
Andes ['ændiːz] А́нды.
Andorra [æn'dɔrə] Андо́рра.
Angola [æŋ'goulə] Анго́ла; **People's Republic of Angola** ['piːplzrɪ'pʌblɪkəvæn'goulə] Наро́дная Респу́блика Анго́ла.
Ankara ['æŋkərə] *г.* Анкара́.
Antananarivo ['æntəˌnænə'riːvou] *г.* Антананари́ву.
Antarctic Continent [ænt'ɑːktɪk...] Антаркти́да.
Antarctic Regions [ænt'ɑːktɪk...] Анта́рктика.
Antilles [æn'tɪliːz] Анти́льские о-ва́.
Antwerp ['æntwəːp] *г.* Антве́рпен.
Apennines ['æpɪnaɪnz] Апенни́ны.
Arabia [ə'reɪbjə] *п-ов* Ара́вия.
Arabian Sea [ə'reɪbjən...] Арави́йское мо́ре.
Archangel ['ɑːkˌeɪndʒəl] *см.* Arkhangelsk.
Arctic Ocean ['ɑːktɪk...] Се́верный Ледови́тый океа́н.
Arctic Regions ['ɑːktɪk...] А́рктика.
Argentina [ˌɑːdʒən'tiːnə] Аргенти́на.

Arizona [ˌærɪ'zounə] Аризо́на.
Arkansas ['ɑːkənsɔː (штат), ɑː'kænzəs (город)] Арка́нзас.
Arkhangelsk [ɑː'kɑːngəlsk] *г.* Арха́нгельск.
Armenian Soviet Socialist Republic [ɑː'miːnjən'souvɪet'souʃəlɪstrɪ'pʌblɪk] Армя́нская Сове́тская Социалисти́ческая Респу́блика; **Armenia** [ɑː'miːnjə] Арме́ния.
Ashkhabad [ˌɑːʃkɑː'bɑːd] *г.* Ашхаба́д.
Asia ['eɪʃə] А́зия; ~ **Minor** Ма́лая А́зия.
Asuncion [əˌsunsɪ'oun] *г.* Асунсьо́н.
Athens ['æθɪnz] *г.* Афи́ны.
Atlantic Ocean [ət'læntɪk...] Атланти́ческий океа́н.
Australia [ɔs'treɪljə] Австра́лия.
Australia, Commonwealth of ['kɔmənwelθəvɔs'treɪljə] Австрали́йский Сою́з.
Austria ['ɔstrɪə] А́встрия.
Azerbaijan Soviet Socialist Republic ['ɑːzəbaɪ'dʒɑːn'souvɪet'souʃəlɪstrɪ'pʌblɪk] Азербайджа́нская Сове́тская Социалисти́ческая Респу́блика; **Azerbaijan** ['ɑːzəbaɪ'dʒɑːn] Азербайджа́н.
Azores [ə'zɔːz] Азо́рские о-ва́.
Azov ['ɑːzɔv]: **Sea of** ~ Азо́вское мо́ре.

Bag(h)dad ['bægdæd] *г.* Багда́д.
Baikal [baɪ'kɑːl] *оз.* Байка́л.
Baku [bɑː'kuː] *г.* Баку́.
Balkans ['bɔːlkənz] Балка́ны.
Baltic Sea ['bɔːltɪk...] Балти́йское мо́ре.
Bamako [ˌbɑːmɑː'kou] *г.* Бамако́.
Bangkok [bæŋ'kɔk] *г.* Бангко́к.
Bangladesh ['bæŋglə'deʃ] Бангладе́ш.
Bangui [bɑːŋ'giː] *г.* Банги́.
Banjul [bæn'dʒuːl] *г.* Бан(д)жу́л.
Barbados [bɑː'beɪdouz] Барба́дос.
Barents Sea ['bɑːrənts...] Ба́ренцево мо́ре. ·
Beirut [beɪ'ruːt] *см.* Beyrouth.
Belfast ['belfɑːst] *г.* Бе́лфаст.
Belgium ['beldʒəm] Бе́льгия.
Belgrade ['belgreɪd] *г.* Белгра́д.
Bengal [ben'gɔːl]: **Bay of** ~ Бенга́льский зали́в.
Benin [be'nɪn] Бени́н.
Bering ['berɪŋ]: ~ **Sea** Бе́рингово мо́ре; ~ **Strait** Бе́рингов проли́в.
Berlin [bəː'lɪn] *г.* Берли́н.
Bern(e) [bəːn] *г.* Берн.
Beyrouth [beɪ'ruːt] *г.* Бейру́т.
Bhutan [buː'tɑːn] Бута́н.
Birmingham ['bəːmɪŋəm] *г.* Би́рмингем.

---

* Слова Mountain, Mountains, Island, Islands приведены в сокращении Mt., Mts., Isl., Isls и не транскрибированы. Фонетической транскрипцией не снабжены тж. слова, имеющиеся в тексте словаря, как напр.: lake, strait, gulf, а также такие названия, как Black Sea, White Sea, English Channel и др., произношение которых легко установить по тексту словаря.

Biscay ['bɪskeɪ] : Bay of ~ Бискайский залив.
Bissau [bɪ'sau] г. Бисау.
Black Sea Чёрное море.
Bogota [,bougou'tɑ:] г. Богота.
Bolivia [bə'lɪvɪə] Боливия.
Bombay [bɔm'beɪ] г. Бомбей.
Bonn [bɔn] г. Бонн.
Bosporus ['bɔspərəs] Босфор.
Boston ['bɔstən] г. Бостон.
Bothnia ['bɔθnɪɑ:] : Gulf of ~ Ботнический залив.
Botswana [bɔt'swɑ:nə] Ботсвана.
Brahmaputra [,brɑːmə'puːtrə] р. Брахмапутра.
Brasilia [brə'zɪljə] г. Бразилиа.
Brazil [brə'zɪl] Бразилия.
Brazzaville ['bræzəvɪl] г. Браззавиль.
Bridgetown ['brɪdʒtaun] г. Бриджтаун.
Brussels ['brʌslz] г. Брюссель.
Bucharest [,bjuːkə'rest] г. Бухарест.
Budapest ['bjuːdə'pest] г. Будапешт.
Buenos Aires ['bwenəs'aɪərɪz] г. Буэнос-Айрес.
Bujumbura [,buːdʒəm'buərə] г. Бужумбура.
Bulgaria [bʌl'geərɪə] Болгария; People's Republic of Bulgaria ['piːplzrɪ'pʌblɪkəvbʌl'geərɪə] Народная Республика Болгария.
Burkina Faso [bu(r)kɪ'nɑːfʌ'sɔː] Буркина-Фасо.
Burma ['bəːmə] Бирма.
Burundi [bə'ruːndɪ] Бурунди.
Byelorussian Soviet Socialist Republic [,bjelou'rʌʃən'souvɪet'souʃəlɪstrɪ'pʌblɪk] Белорусская Советская Социалистическая Республика; Byelorussia [,bjelou'rʌʃə] Белоруссия.

Cabo Verde ['kʌvuː'vəːdə] Кабо-Верде.
Cairo ['kaɪərou] г. Каир.
Calcutta [kæl'kʌtə] г. Калькутта.
California [,kælɪ'fɔːnjə] Калифорния.
Cambridge ['keɪmbrɪdʒ] г. Кембридж.
Cameroon ['kæməruːn] Камерун.
Canada ['kænədə] Канада.
Canberra ['kænbərə] г. Канберра.
Canterbury ['kæntəbərɪ] г. Кентербери.
Cape Canaveral ['keɪpkə'nævərəl] мыс Канаверал.
Cape Horn ['keɪphɔːn] мыс Горн.
Cape of Good Hope ['keɪpəv'gud'houp] мыс Доброй Надежды.
Capetown, Cape Town ['keɪptaun] г. Кейптаун.
Cape Verde Isls ['keɪp'vəːd...] о-ва Зелёного Мыса.
Caracas [kə'rækəs] г. Каракас.
Caribbean Sea [,kærɪ'biːən...] Карибское море.
Carpathians [kɑː'peɪθɪənz] Карпаты.
Caspian Sea ['kæspɪən...] Каспийское море.
Caucasus, the ['kɔːkəsəs] Кавказ.
Central African Republic Центральноафриканская Республика.
Chad [tʃæd] Чад.
Channel Isls ['tʃænl...] Нормандские о-ва.
Chicago [ʃɪ'kɑːgou] г. Чикаго.
Chile ['tʃɪlɪ] Чили.
China ['tʃaɪnə] Китай; Chinese People's Republic ['tʃaɪ'niːz'piːplzrɪ'pʌblɪk] . Китайская Народная Республика.
Chomolungma ['tʃoumou'luŋmɑ:] Джомолунгма.
Colombia [kə'lɔmbɪə] Колумбия.
Colombo [kə'lʌmbou] г. Коломбо.
Colorado [,kɔlə'rɑːdou] Колорадо.
Columbia [kə'lʌmbɪə] : District of ~ федеральный округ Колумбия (местонахождение столицы США г. Вашингтона).
Conakry ['kɔnəkrɪ] г. Конакри.

Congo ['kɔŋgou] 1) р. Конго; 2) Конго; People's Republic of the Congo ['piːplzrɪ'pʌblɪkəvðə'kɔŋgou] Народная Республика Конго.
Connecticut [kə'nektɪkət] Коннектикут.
Copenhagen [,koupn'heɪgən] г. Копенгаген.
Cordilleras, the [,kɔːdɪ'ljeərəz] Кордильеры.
Corsica ['kɔːsɪkə] о-в Корсика.
Costa Rica ['kɔstə'riːkə] Коста-Рика.
Côte d'Ivoire ['kɔtdɪvuɑː] Кот-д'Ивуар.
Coventry ['kɔventrɪ] г. Ковентри.
Crete [kriːt] о-в Крит.
Crimea, the [kraɪ'mɪə] Крым.
Cuba ['kjuːbə] Куба; Republic of Cuba [rɪ'pʌblɪkəv'kjuːbə] Республика Куба.
Cyprus ['saɪprəs] Кипр.
Czechoslovakia ['tʃekouslou'vækɪə] Чехословакия; Czechoslovak Socialist Republic ['tʃekou'slouvæk'souʃəlɪstrɪ'pʌblɪk] Чехословацкая Социалистическая Республика.

Dacca ['dækə] г. Дакка.
Dakar ['dækə] г. Дакар.
Damascus [də'mɑːskəs] г. Дамаск.
Danube ['dænjuːb] р. Дунай.
Dardanelles [,dɑːdə'nelz] Дарданеллы.
Dar es Salaam ['dɑːressə'lɑːm] г. Дар-эс-Салам.
Dead Sea Мёртвое море.
Delaware ['deləweə] Делавэр.
Delhi ['delɪ] г. Дели.
Denmark ['denmɑːk] Дания.
Djakarta [dʒə'kɑːtə] см. Jakarta.
Djokjakarta [,dʒɔkjə'kɑːtə] см. Jogjakarta.
Dnieper ['dniːpə] р. Днепр.
Dominican Republic [də'mɪnɪkənrɪ'pʌblɪk] Доминиканская Республика.
Dover ['douvə] г. Дувр; Strait of ~ Па-де-Кале.
Dublin ['dʌblɪn] г. Дублин.
Dyushambe [djuː'ʃɑːmbe] г. Душанбе.

Ecuador [,ekwə'dɔː] Эквадор.
Edinburgh ['edɪnbərə] г. Эдинбург.
Egypt ['iːdʒɪpt] Египет; Arab Republic of Egypt ['ærəbrɪ'pʌblɪkəv'iːdʒɪpt] Арабская Республика Египет.
El Salvador [el'sælvədɔː] Сальвадор.
England ['ɪŋglənd] Англия.
English Channel Ла-Манш.
Equatorial Guinea [...'gɪnɪ] Экваториальная Гвинея.
Erie, Lake ['ɪərɪ...] оз. Эри.
Estonian Soviet Socialist Republic [es'tounjən'souvɪet'souʃəlɪstrɪ'pʌblɪk] Эстонская Советская Социалистическая Республика; Estonia [es'tounjə] Эстония.
Ethiopia [,iːθɪ'oupjə] Эфиопия; Socialist Ethiopia ['souʃəlɪst,iːθɪ'oupjə] Социалистическая Эфиопия.
Eton ['iːtn] г. Итон.
Euphrates [juː'freɪtiːz] р. Евфрат.
Europe ['juərəp] Европа.
Everest ['evərɪst] Эверест; см. Chomolungma.

Federal Republic of Germany ['fedərəlrɪ'pʌblɪkəv'dʒəːmənɪ] Федеративная Республика Германия.
Finland ['fɪnlənd] Финляндия.
Florence ['flɔrəns] г. Флоренция.
Florida ['flɔrɪdə] Флорида.
France [frɑːns] Франция.
Freetown ['friːtaun] г. Фритаун.

Frunze ['fru:nze] *г.* Фрунзе.

Gabon [gə'bɔ:n] Габон.
Gaborone [gæbə'rəunə] *г.* Габороне.
Gambia ['gæmbɪə] Гамбия.
Ganges ['gændʒi:z] *р.* Ганг.
Geneva [dʒɪ'ni:və] *г.* Женева.
Georgia ['dʒɔ:dʒjə] Джорджия (*штат в США*).
Georgian Soviet Socialist Republic ['dʒɔ:dʒjən'souviet'souʃəlɪstrɪ'pʌblɪk] Грузинская Советская Социалистическая Республика; **Georgia** ['dʒɔ:dʒjə] Грузия.
German Democratic Republic ['dʒə:mən,demə'krætɪkrɪ'pʌblɪk] Германская Демократическая Республика.
Ghana ['gɑ:nə] Гана.
Gibraltar [dʒɪ'brɔ:ltə] Гибралтар.
Glasgow ['glɑːsgou] *г.* Глазго.
Gobi, the ['goubi:] Гоби (*пустыня*).
Great Britain ['greɪt'brɪtn] Великобритания.
Greece [gri:s] Греция.
Greenland ['gri:nlənd] Гренландия.
Greenwich ['grɪnɪdʒ] *г.* Грин(в)ич.
Guatemala [,gwætɪ'mɑːlə] Гватемала.
Guinea ['gɪnɪ] Гвинея.
Guinea-Bissau ['gɪnɪbɪ'sau] Гвинея-Бисау.
Guyana [gaɪ'ɑːnə] Гайана.

Hague, the [heɪg] *г.* Гаага.
Haiphong ['haɪ'fɔːŋ] *г.* Хайфон.
Haiti ['heɪtɪ] Гаити.
Hamburg ['hæmbə:g] *г.* Гамбург.
Hampshire ['hæmpʃɪə] Гемпшир.
Hanoi [hæ'nɔɪ] *г.* Ханой.
Havana [hə'vænə] *г.* Гавана.
Hawaii [hɑː'waɪi:] Гавайи; **Hawaiian Isls** Гавайские о-ва.
Hebrides ['hebrɪdi:z] Гебридские о-ва.
Hel(i)goland ['hel(ɪ)goulænd] *о-в* Гельголанд.
Helsinki ['helsɪŋkɪ] *г.* Хельсинки.
Himalaya(s), the [,hɪmə'leɪə(z)] Гималаи, Гималайские горы.
Hindu Kush ['hɪndu:'ku:ʃ] Гиндукуш.
Hiroshima [hɪ'rɔʃɪmə] *г.* Хиросима.
Ho-Chi-Minh ['hou,tʃi'mɪn] *г.* Хошимин.
Honduras [hɔn'djuərəs] Гондурас.
Hudson ['hʌdsn] *р.* Гудзон; ~ Вау Гудзонов залив.
Hungary ['hʌŋgərɪ] Венгрия; **Hungarian People's Republic** [hʌŋ'gɛərɪən'pi:plzrɪ'pʌblɪk] Венгерская Народная Республика.
Huron, Lake ['hjuərən...] *оз.* Гурон.
Hwang Ho ['hwæŋ'hou] *р.* Хуанхэ.

Iceland ['aɪslənd] Исландия.
Idaho ['aɪdəhou] Айдахо.
Illinois [,ɪlɪ'nɔɪ(z)] Иллинойс.
India ['ɪndjə] Индия.
Indiana [,ɪndɪ'ænə] Индиана.
Indian Ocean Индийский океан.
Indochina [,ɪndou'tʃaɪnə] *п-ов* Индокитай.
Indonesia [,ɪndou'ni:zjə] Индонезия.
Indus ['ɪndəs] *р.* Инд.
Ionian Sea [aɪ'ounjən...] Ионическое море.
Iowa ['aɪouə] Айова.
Iran [ɪ'rɑːn] Иран.
Iraq [ɪ'rɑːk] Ирак.
Ireland ['aɪələnd] Ирландия.
Islamabad [ɪs'lɑːməbɑːd] *г.* Исламабад.
Israel ['ɪzreɪəl] Израиль.

Istanbul [,ɪstæn'bu:l] *г.* Стамбул.
Italy ['ɪtəlɪ] Италия.

Jakarta [dʒə'kɑːtə] *г.* Джакарта.
Jamaica [dʒə'meɪkə] Ямайка.
Japan [dʒə'pæn] Япония; **Sea of** ~ Японское море.
Java ['dʒɑːvə] *о-в* Ява.
Jerusalem [dʒə'ru:sələm] *г.* Иерусалим.
Jogjakarta [,dʒɔgjə'kɑːtə] *г.* Джокьякарта.
Jordan ['dʒɔːdn] 1) *р.* Иордан; 2) Иордания.

Kabul ['kɔːbl] *г.* Кабул.
Kalimantan [,kɑːlɪ'mɑːntɑːn] *о-в* Калимантан.
Kansas ['kænzəs] Канзас.
Karachi [kə'rɑːtʃɪ] *г.* Карачи.
Kara Sea ['kɑːrɑː...] Карское море.
Kashmir [kæʃ'mɪə] Кашмир.
Katmandu [,kɑːtmɑːn'du:] *г.* Катманду.
Kattegat [,kætɪ'gæt] *пролив* Каттегат.
Kazakh Soviet Socialist Republic [kɑː'zɑːk'souviet'souʃəlɪstrɪ'pʌblɪk] Казахская Советская Социалистическая Республика; **Kazakhstan** [,kɑːzɑːk'stɑːn] Казахстан.

Kentucky [ken'tʌkɪ] Кентукки.
Kenya ['ki:njə, 'kenjə] Кения.
Khart(o)um [kɑː'tu:m] *г.* Хартум.
Kiev ['ki:ev] *г.* Киев.
Kigali [kɪ'gɑːlɪ] *г.* Кигали.
Kingston ['kɪŋstən] *г.* Кингстон.
Kinshasa [kɪn'ʃɑːsɑː] *г.* Киншаса.
Kirghiz Soviet Socialist Republic [kə'gi:z'souviet'souʃəlɪstrɪ'pʌblɪk] Киргизская Советская Социалистическая Республика; **Kirghizia** [kə'gi:zjə] Киргизия.
Kishinev [kɪʃɪ'njɔf] *г.* Кишинёв.
Korea [kə'rɪə] Корея; **Korean People's Democratic Republic** [kə'ri:ən'pi:plz,demə'krætɪkrɪ'pʌblɪk] Корейская Народно-Демократическая Республика.

Kuala Lumpur ['kwɑːlə'lumpuə] *г.* Куала-Лумпур.
Kuril Isls [ku'ri:l...] Курильские о-ва.
Kuwait [ku'weɪt] Кувейт.

Lagos ['leɪgɔs] *г.* Лагос.
Lancashire ['læŋkəʃɪə] Ланкашир.
Laos [lauz] Лаос; **Lao People's Democratic Republic** [lau'pi:plz,demə'krætɪkrɪ'pʌblɪk] Лаосская Народно-Демократическая Республика.
La Paz [lɑː'pæz] *г.* Ла-Пас.
Latvian Soviet Socialist Republic ['lætvɪən'souviet'souʃəlɪstrɪ'pʌblɪk] Латвийская Советская Социалистическая Республика; **Latvia** ['lætvɪə] Латвия.
Lebanon ['lebənən] Ливан.
Leicester(shire) ['lestə(ʃɪə] Лестер(шир).
Leipzig ['laɪpzɪg] *г.* Лейпциг.
Leningrad ['lenɪngrɑːd] *г.* Ленинград.
Lesotho [lə'soutou] Лесото.
Lhasa ['lɑːsə] *г.* Лхаса.
Liberia [laɪ'bɪərɪə] Либерия.
Libia ['lɪbɪə] *см.* Libya.
Libreville [li:brə'vi:l] *г.* Либревиль.
Libya ['lɪbɪə] Ливия.
Liechtenstein ['lɪktənstaɪn] Лихтенштейн.
Lima ['li:mə] *г.* Лима.
Lisbon ['lɪzbən] *г.* Лиссабон.

Lithuanian Soviet Socialist Republic [ˌlɪθjuːˈeɪn-jənˈsouvɪetˈsouʃəlɪstrɪˈrʌblɪk] Литóвская Совéтская Социалисти́ческая Респýблика; **Lithuania** [ˌlɪθjuːˈeɪnjə] Литвá.

Liverpool [ˈlɪvəpuːl] *г.* Ливерпýль.

Lomé [ˌlɔːˈmeɪ] *г.* Ломé.

London [ˈlʌndən] *г.* Лóндон.

Los Angeles [lɔsˈændʒɪliːz] *г.* Лос-Áнджелес.

Louisiana [luːˌɪzɪˈænə] Луизиáна.

Luanda [luːˈændə] *г.* Луáнда.

Lusaka [luːˈsɑːkə] *г.* Лусáка.

Luxemburg [ˈlʌksəmbɜːg] Люксембýрг.

Madagascar [ˌmædəˈgæskə] 1) *о-в* Мадагаскáр; 2) Мадагаскáр; **Democratic Republic of Madagaskar** [ˌdeməˈkrætɪkrɪˈrʌblɪkəvˌmædəˈgæskə] Демократи́ческая Респýблика Мадагаскáр.

Madrid [məˈdrɪd] *г.* Мадри́д.

Magellan [məˈgelən]: Strait of ~ Магеллáнов проли́в.

Maine [meɪn] Мэн.

Malawi [məˈlɑːwɪ] Малáви.

Malaysia [məˈleɪzɪə] Малáйзия.

Maldives [ˈmɔːldɪvz] Мальди́вские о-вá.

Male [ˈmɑːleɪ] *г.* Мáле.

Mali [ˈmɑːlɪ] Мали́.

Malta [ˈmɔːltə] Мáльта.

Managua [məˈnɑːgwə] *г.* Манáгуа.

Manchester [ˈmæntʃɪstə] *г.* Мáнчестер.

Manila [məˈnɪlə] *г.* Мани́ла.

Maputo [məˈpuːtəu] *г.* Мапýту.

Marmora, Sea of [ˈmɑːmərə...] Мрáморное мóре.

Marseilles [mɑːˈseɪlz] *г.* Марсéль.

Maryland [ˈmeərɪlænd] Мэ́риленд.

Maseru [ˈmæzəruː] *г.* Мáсеру.

Massachusetts [ˌmæsəˈtʃuːsets] Массачýсетс.

Mauritania [ˌmɔrɪˈteɪnjə] Мавритáния.

Mauritius [məˈrɪʃəs] Маври́кий.

Mbabane [mbɑːˈbɑːnɪ] *г.* Мбабáне.

Mediterranean Sea [ˌmedɪtəˈreɪnjən...] Средизéмное мóре.

Melbourne [ˈmelbən] *г.* Мéльбурн.

Mexico [ˈmeksɪkou] Мéксика.

Mexico (City) [ˈmeksɪkou(ˈsɪtɪ)] *г.* Мéхико.

Miami [maɪˈæmɪ] *г.* Майáми.

Michigan [ˈmɪʃɪgən] Мичигáн.

Minnesota [ˌmɪnɪˈsoutə] Миннесóта.

Minsk [mɪnsk] *г.* Минск.

Mississippi [ˌmɪsɪˈsɪpɪ] Миссиси́пи.

Missouri [mɪˈzuərɪ] Миссýри.

Mogadishu [ˌmɔgəˈdɪʃuː] *г.* Могади́шо.

Moldavian Soviet Socialist Republic [mɔlˈdeɪvjənˈsouvɪetˈsouʃəlɪstrɪˈrʌblɪk] Молдáвская Совéтская Социалисти́ческая Респýблика; **Moldavia** [mɔlˈdeɪvjə] Молдáвия.

Monaco [ˈmɔnəkou] Монáко.

Mongolia [mɔŋˈgouljə] Монгóлия; **Mongolian People's Republic** [mɔŋˈgouljənˈpiːplzrɪˈrʌblɪk] Монгóльская Нарóдная Респýблика.

Monrovia [mənˈrouvɪə] *г.* Монрóвия.

Montana [mɔnˈtænə] Монтáна.

Montevideo [ˌmɔntɪvɪˈdeɪou] *г.* Монтевидéо.

Montreal [ˌmɔntrɪˈɔːl] *г.* Монреáль.

Morocco [məˈrɔkou] Марóкко.

Moscow [ˈmɔskou] *г.* Москвá.

Mozambique [ˌmouzəmˈbiːk] Мозамби́к.

Munich [ˈmjuːnɪk] *г.* Мю́нхен.

Muscat [ˈmʌskæt] *г.* Мáскат.

Nagasaki [ˌnɑːgəˈsɑːkɪ] *г.* Нагасáки.

Nairobi [naɪˈroubɪ] *г.* Найрóби.

Namibia [nəˈmɪbɪə] Нами́бия.

Nanking [nænˈkɪŋ] *г.* Нанки́н.

Naples [ˈneɪplz] *г.* Неáполь.

N'Djamena [ndʒɑːˈmenə] *г.* Нджамéна.

Nebraska [nɪˈbræskə] Небрáска.

Nepal [nɪˈpɔːl] Непáл.

Netherlands [ˈneðələndz] Нидерлáнды.

Nevada [neˈvɑːdə] Невáда.

Newark [ˈnjuːək] *г.* Нью́арк.

Newcastle [ˈnjuːˌkɑːsl] *г.* Нью́касл.

Newfoundland [ˌnjuːfəndˈlænd] *о-в* Ньюфаунд-лéнд.

New Guinea [ˈnjuːgɪnɪ] *о-в* Нóвая Гвинéя.

New Hebrides [ˈnjuːˈhebrɪdiːz] *о-ва* Нóвые Гебри́ды.

New Jersey [ˈnjuːˈdʒɜːzɪ] Нью-Джéрси.

New Mexico [ˈnjuːˈmeksɪkou] Нью-Мéксико (*штат США*).

New Orleans [ˈnjuːˈɔːlɪənz] *г.* Нóвый Орлеáн.

New South Wales [ˈnjuːsauθˈweɪlz] Нóвый Ю́жный Уэ́льс (*Австралия*).

New York [ˈnjuːˈjɔːk] *г.* Нью-Йóрк.

New Zealand [njuːˈziːlənd] Нóвая Зелáндия.

Niamey [njɑːˈmeɪ] *г.* Ниамéй.

Nicaragua [ˌnɪkəˈrægjuə] Никарáгуа; **Republic of Nicaragua** [rɪˈpʌblɪkəvˌnɪkəˈrægjuə] Респýблика Никарáгуа.

Nicosia [ˌnɪkouˈsiːə] *г.* Никоси́я.

Niemen [ˈniːmən] *р.* Нéман.

Niger [ˈnaɪdʒə] 1) *р.* Ни́гер; 2) Ни́гер (*государство*).

Nigeria [naɪˈdʒɪərɪə] Ниге́рия.

Nile [naɪl] *р.* Нил.

Norfolk [ˈnɔːfək] Нóрфолк.

Normandy [ˈnɔːməndɪ] Нормáндия.

North Carolina [ˈnɔːθˌkærəˈlaɪnə] Сéверная Каролúна.

North Dakota [ˈnɔːθdəˈkoutə] Сéверная Дакóта.

Northern Ireland Сéверная Ирлáндия.

North Sea Сéверное мóре.

Norway [ˈnɔːweɪ] Норвéгия.

Nouakchott [nwɑːkˈʃɔt] *г.* Нуакшóт.

Nuremberg [ˈnjuərəmbɜːg] *см.* Nürnberg.

Nürnberg [ˈnjuːrnberk] *г.* Нюрнбéрг.

Oceania [ˌouʃɪˈeɪnjə] Океáния.

Oder [ˈoudə] *р.* Óдер.

Odessa [ouˈdesə] *г.* Одéсса.

Ohio [ouˈhaɪou] Огáйо.

Okinawa [ˌoukɪˈnɑːwɑː] *о-в* Окинáва.

Oklahoma [ˌoukləˈhoumə] Оклахóма.

Oman [ouˈmɑːn] Омáн.

Ontario, Lake [ɔnˈteərɪou...] *оз.* Онтáрио.

Oregon [ˈɔrɪgən] Орегóн.

Orinoco [ˌɔrɪˈnoukou] *р.* Оринóко.

Oslo [ˈɔzlou] *г.* Осло.

Ottawa [ˈɔtəwə] *г.* Оттáва.

Oxford [ˈɔksfəd] *г.* Óксфорд.

Pacific Ocean [pəˈsɪfɪk...] Ти́хий океáн.

Pakistan [ˌpɑːkɪsˈtɑːn] Пакистáн.

Pamirs, the [pəˈmɪəz] Памир.

Panama [ˌpænəˈmɑː] Панáма; ~ Canal Панáмский канáл.

Paraguay [ˈpærəgwaɪ] Парагвáй.

Paris [ˈpærɪs] *г.* Пари́ж.

Peking [piːˈkɪŋ] *г.* Пеки́н.

Pennsylvania [ˌpensɪlˈveɪnjə] Пенсильвáния.

Persian Gulf [ˈpəːʃən...] Перси́дский зали́в.

Peru [pə'ruː] Перу́.
Philadelphia [ˌfɪlə'delfjə] г. Филаде́льфия.
Philippines, Philippine Isls ['fɪlɪpiːn(z)...] Филип-
пи́нские о-ва́.
Plymouth ['plɪməθ] г. Пли́мут.
Pnompenh, Pnom-Penh [nɔm'pen] г. Пномпе́нь.
Poland ['poulənd] По́льша; Polish People's
Republic ['poulɪʃ'piːplzrɪ'pʌblɪk] По́льская
Наро́дная Респу́блика.
Polynesia [ˌpɔlɪ'niːzjə] Полине́зия.
Port-au-Prince [ˌpɔːtou'prɪns] г. Порт-о-Пре́нс.
Port Louis ['pɔːt'luːɪs] г. Порт-Луи́.
Port-of-Spain ['pɔːtəv'speɪn] г. Порт-оф-Спе́йн.
Porto Novo ['pɔːtou'nouvou] г. По́рто-Но́во.
Port Said [pɔːt'saɪd] г. Порт-Сайд.
Portsmouth ['pɔːtsməθ] г. По́ртсмут.
Portugal ['pɔːtjugəl] Португа́лия.
Prague [prɑːg] г. Пра́га.
Praia ['praɪə] г. Пра́я.
Pretoria [prɪ'touriə] г. Прето́рия.
Puerto Rico ['pwɑːtou'riːkou] Пуэ́рто-Ри́ко.
Pyongyang ['pjɑːŋ'jɑːŋ] г. Пхенья́н.
Pyrenees [ˌpɪrə'niːz] Пирене́и.

Quebec [kwɪ'bek] Квебе́к.
Quito ['kiːtou] г. Ки́то.

Rabat [rə'bɑːt] г. Раба́т.
Red Sea Кра́сное мо́ре.
Republic of South Africa Ю́жно-Африка́нская
Респу́блика.
Reunion [rɪ'juːnjən] о-в Реюньо́н.
Reykjavik ['reɪkjəviːk] г. Ре́йкьявик.
Rhine [raɪn] р. Рейн.
Rhode Island [roud'aɪlənd] Род-А́йленд.
Riga ['riːgə] г. Ри́га.
Rio de Janeiro ['riːoudədʒə'nɪərou] г. Ри́о-де-Жа-
не́йро.
Riyadh [rɪ'jɑːd] г. Эр-Рия́д.
Rockies, the ['rɔkɪz] см. Rocky Mountains.
Rocky Mountains ['rɔkɪ...] Скали́стые го́ры.
Rome [roum] г. Рим.
R(o)umania [ruː'meɪnjə] Румы́ния; Socialist Re-
public of R(o)umania ['souʃəlɪstrɪ'pʌblɪkəv-
ruː'meɪnjə] Социалисти́ческая Респу́блика Ру-
мы́ния.
Ruhr [ruːr] Рур.
Russian Soviet Federative Socialist Republic
['rʌʃən'souviet'fedərətɪv'souʃəlɪstrɪ'pʌblɪk] Рос-
си́йская Сове́тская Федерати́вная Социалисти́-
ческая Респу́блика; Russia ['rʌʃə] Росси́я.
Rwanda [ruː'ændə] Руа́нда.

Sahara [sə'hɑːrə] Саха́ра.
Sakhalin [ˌsækə'liːn] о-в Сахали́н.
Salisbury ['sɔːlzbərɪ] г. Со́лсбери
San'a, Sanaa [sɑː'nɑː] г. Сана́.
San Francisco [ˌsænfrən'sɪskou] г. Сан-Фран-
ци́ско.
San José [sænhou'zeɪ] г. Сан-Хосе́.
San Juan [sæn'hwɑːn] г. Сан-Хуа́н.
San Marino [ˌsænmə'riːnou] Сан-Мари́но.
San Salvador [sæn'sælvədɔː] г. Сан-Сальвадо́р.
Santiago [ˌsæntɪ'ɑːgou] г. Сантья́го.
Santo Domingo ['sæntoudɔ'mɪŋgou] г. Са́нто-До-
ми́нго.
Sardinia [sɑː'dɪnjə] о-в Сарди́ния.
Saudi Arabia ['saudɪə'reɪbjə] Сау́довская Ара́вия.

Scotland ['skɔtlənd] Шотла́ндия.
Seattle [sɪ'ætl] г. Сиэ́тл.
Seine [seɪn] р. Се́на.
Senegal [ˌsenɪ'gɔːl] Сенега́л.
Seoul [soul, seɪ'uːl] г. Сеу́л.
Sevastopol [ˌsevɑːs'tɔpɔl] г. Севасто́поль.
Shanghai [ʃæŋ'haɪ] г. Шанха́й.
Siangan ['sjɑːŋ'gɑːn] Сянга́н.
Siberia [saɪ'bɪərɪə] Сиби́рь.
Sicily ['sɪsɪlɪ] о-в Сици́лия.
Sierra Leone ['sɪərəlɪ'oun] Сье́рра-Лео́не.
Singapore [ˌsɪŋgə'pɔː] Сингапу́р.
Skagerrak ['skægəræk] пролив Скагерра́к.
Sofia ['soufjə] г. Со́фия.
Somalia [sou'mɑːlɪə] Сомали́.
Sound, the [saund] пролив Зунд.
South African Republic ['sauθ'æfrɪkənrɪ'pʌblɪk]
см. Republic of South Africa.
Southampton [sauθ'æmptən] г. Саутге́мптон.
South Carolina ['sauθ,kærə'laɪnə] Ю́жная Каро-
ли́на.
South Dakota ['sauθdə'koutə] Ю́жная Дако́та.
South Korea ['sauθkə'rɪə] Ю́жная Коре́я.
Spain [speɪn] Испа́ния.
Sri Lanka [ˌsrɪ'læŋkə] Шри-Ла́нка.
Stockholm ['stɔkhoum] г. Стокго́льм.
Stratford-on-Avon ['strætfədən'eɪvən] г. Стра́т-
форд-он-Э́йвон.
Sudan [suː'dɑːn] Суда́н.
Suez ['suːɪz] Суэ́ц; ~ Canal Суэ́цкий кана́л.
Suffolk ['sʌfək] Су́ффолк.
Sulawesi [ˌsuːlɑː'weɪsɪ] о-в Сулаве́си.
Sumatra [suː'mɑːtrə] о-в Сума́тра.
Superior, Lake оз. Ве́рхнее.
Sussex ['sʌsɪks] Су́ссекс.
Swaziland ['swɑːzɪˌlænd] Сва́зиленд.
Sweden ['swiːdn] Шве́ция.
Switzerland ['swɪtsələnd] Швейца́рия.
Sydney ['sɪdnɪ] г. Си́дней.
Syria ['sɪrɪə] Си́рия.

Tadjik Soviet Socialist Republic [tɑː'dʒɪk'souviet-
'souʃəlɪstrɪ'pʌblɪk] Таджи́кская Сове́тская
Социалисти́ческая Респу́блика; Tadjikistan
[tɑːˌdʒɪkɪ'stɑːn] Таджикиста́н.
Tahiti [tɑː'hiːtɪ] о-в Таи́ти.
Taiwan [taɪ'wæn] о-в Тайва́нь.
Tallinn ['tɑːlɪn] г. Та́ллинн.
Tanganyika [ˌtæŋgə'njiːkə] оз. Таганьи́ка.
Tanzania [ˌtænzə'nɪə] Танза́ния.
Tashkent [tæʃ'kent] г. Ташке́нт.
Tbilisi [tbɪ'liːsɪ] г. Тби́лиси.
Tegucigalpa [təˌguːsɪ'gɑːlpɑː] г. Тегусига́льпа.
Teh(e)ran [tɪə'rɑːn] г. Тегера́н.
Tel Aviv ['telɑː'viːv] г. Тель-Ави́в.
Tennessee [ˌtenə'siː] Теннесси́.
Texas ['teksəs] Теха́с.
Thailand ['taɪlænd] Таила́нд.
Thames [temz] р. Те́мза.
Thibet [tɪ'bet] см. Tibet.
Thimphu ['θɪmpuː] г. Тхи́мпху.
Tiber ['taɪbə] р. Тибр.
Tibet [tɪ'bet] Тибе́т.
Tien Shan ['tjen'ʃɑːn] Тянь-Ша́нь.
Tierra del Fuego ['tjeradelfuː'eɪgou] о-в Огнен-
ная Земля́.
Tigris ['taɪgrɪs] р. Тигр.
Tirana [tɪ'rɑːnɑː] г. Тира́на.
Togo ['tougou] То́го.

Tokyo ['toukjou] *г.* Токио.

Trinidad and Tobago ['trınıdædəntə'beıgou] Тринидад и Тобаго.

Tsushima ['tsuːʃımə] *о-в* Цусима.

Tunis ['tjuːnıs] *г.* Тунис.

Tunisia [tjuːˈnızıə] Тунис.

Turkey ['təːkı] Турция.

Turkmen Soviet Socialist Republic ['təːkmen'souvıet'souʃəlıstrı'pʌblık] Туркменская Советская Социалистическая Республика; **Turkmenistan** [ˌtəːkmenı'stɑːn] Туркменистан.

Tyrrhenian Sea [tıˈriːnjən...] Тирренское море.

Uganda [juːˈgændə] Уганда.

Ukrainian Soviet Socialist Republic [juːˈkreınjən-ˈsouvıet'souʃəlıstrı'pʌblık] Украинская Советская Социалистическая Республика; **Ukraine** [juːˈkreın] Украина.

Ulan Bator ['uːlɑːn'bɑːtə] *г.* Улан-Батор.

Ulster ['ʌlstə] Ольстер.

Ulyanovsk [ul'jɑːnəvsk] *г.* Ульяновск.

Union of Soviet Socialist Republics Союз Советских Социалистических Республик.

United Arab Emirates [juːˈnaıtıd'ærəbe'mıərıts] Объединённые Арабские Эмираты.

United Kingdom of Great Britain and Northern Ireland Соединённое Королевство Великобритании и Северной Ирландии.

United States of America Соединённые Штаты Америки.

Ural ['juərəl] Урал.

Uruguay ['urugwaı] Уругвай.

USA *см.* United States of America.

U.S.S.R. *см.* Union of Soviet Socialist Republics.

Utah ['juːtɑː] Юта.

Uzbek Soviet Socialist Republic [uz'bek'souvıet-ˈsouʃəlıstrı'pʌblık] Узбекская Советская Социалистическая Республика; **Uzbekistan** [uzˌbekı'stɑːn] Узбекистан.

Vatican ['vætıkən] Ватикан.

Venezuela [ˌvene'zweılə] Венесуэла.

Venice ['venıs] *г.* Венеция.

Versailles [vɛə'saı] *г.* Версаль.

Vienna [vı'enə] *г.* Вена.

Viet Nam ['vjet'næm] Вьетнам; **Socialist Republic of Viet Nam** ['souʃəlıstrı'pʌblıkəv'vjet'næm] Социалистическая Республика Вьетнам.

Vilnius, Vilnyus ['vılnıəs] *г.* Вильнюс.

Virginia [və'dʒınjə] Виргиния; West ~ Западная Виргиния.

Vistula ['vıstjulə] *р.* Висла.

Vladivostok [ˌvlædıvɔ'stɔk] *г.* Владивосток.

Volga ['vɔlgə] *р.* Волга.

Volgograd [ˌvɔlgə'grɑːd] *г.* Волгоград.

Wales [weılz] Уэльс.

Warsaw ['wɔːsɔː] *г.* Варшава.

Washington ['wɔʃıŋtən] Вашингтон.

Wellington ['welıŋtən] *г.* Веллингтон.

West Indies ['west'ındız] Вест-Индия.

White Sea Белое море.

Wight [waıt]: Isle of ~ *о-в* Уайт.

Windhoek ['vınthuːk] *г.* Виндхук.

Wisconsin [wıs'kɔnsın] Висконсин.

Wyoming [waı'oumıŋ] Вайоминг.

Yangtze ['jæŋtsı] *р.* Янцзы.

Yaoundé [jɑːuːn'deı] *г.* Яунде.

Yarmouth ['jɑːməθ] *г.* Ярмут.

Yellow Sea Жёлтое море.

Yemen ['jemən] Йемен; **People's Democratic Republic of Yemen** ['piːplz,demə'krætıkrı'pʌblıkəv'jemən] Народная Демократическая Республика Йемен; **Yemen Arab Republic** ['jemən'ærəbrı'pʌblık] Йеменская Арабская Республика.

Yerevan [ˌjerı'vɑːn] *г.* Ереван.

Yokohama [ˌjoukə'hɑːmə] *г.* Иокогама.

Yorkshire ['jɔːkʃıə] Йоркшир.

Yugoslavia ['jugou'slɑːvjə] Югославия; **Socialist Federal Republic of Yugoslavia** ['souʃəlıst-ˈfedərəlrı'pʌblıkəv'ju:gou'slɑːvjə] Социалистическая Федеративная Республика Югославия.

Yukon ['juːkɔn] *р.* Юкон.

Zaire [zɑː'iːrə] Заир.

Zambia ['zæmbıə] Замбия.

Zimbabwe [zım'bɑːbwı] Зимбабве; **Republic of Zimbabwe** [rı'pʌblıkəvzım'bɑːbwı] Республика Зимбабве.

Zurich ['zjuərık] *г.* Цюрих.

НАИБОЛЕЕ УПОТРЕБИТЕЛЬНЫЕ СОКРАЩЕНИЯ, ПРИНЯТЫЕ В АНГЛИИ И США

ABBREVIATIONS FREQUENTLY USED IN BRITAIN AND THE UNITED STATES

A academy академия.

A.A. anti-aircraft противовоздушный, зенитный.

AAF Army Air Forces объединённые военно-воздушные силы.

A.B. able-bodied годен к военной службе.

abbr., abbrev. 1) abbreviated сокращённый; сокращено; 2) abbreviation сокращение; аббревиатура.

ABC *см. в Словаре.*

abl. ablative творительный падеж.

ABS American Broadcasting System Американская радиовещательная компания.

AC alternating current *эл.* переменный ток.

acc. account счёт.

acc. accusative винительный падеж.

actg acting исполняющий обязанности.

A.D. anno Domini нашей эры.

adj. 1) adjective имя прилагательное; 2) adjourned отложено; 3) adjunct приложение, дополнение; 4) adjutant адъютант.

adv. 1) adverb наречие; 2) advertisement объявление; реклама.

advt advertisement объявление; реклама.

AFL — CIO American Federation of Labour — Congress of Industrial Organizations Американская федерация труда — Конгресс производственных профсоюзов, АФТ — КПП.

A.G. 1) Adjutant-General генеральный адъютант; генерал-адъютант; 2) Attorney General генеральный атторней; министр юстиции (*США*).

Ag August август.

Agcy agency агентство.

Agt agent агент; представитель.

Ala Alabama Алабама (*штат США*).

Alas Alaska Аляска.

Ald. alderman ольдермен, член городского управления.

a.m. ante meridiem до полудня.

amp ampere *эл.* ампер.

amt amount сумма.

anal 1) analogous аналогичный; 2) analogy аналогия.

anal. analysis анализ.

ann. 1) annual годовой; ежегодный; 2) annuity ежегодная рента.

anon. anonymous анонимный.

ans answer ответ.

AP Associated Press информационное агентство «Ассошиэйтед пресс» (*США*).

app. appendix приложение.

approx. approximately приблизительно.

Apr. April апрель.

ar. 1) arrival прибытие; 2) arrives, arrive прибывает, прибывают.

Arch. 1) archbishop архиепископ; 2) archipelago архипелаг.

arch. 1) archaic архаический, устарелый; 2) architecture архитектура.

Ariz. Arizona Аризона (*штат США*).

Ark. Arkansas Арканзас (*штат США*).

AS Anglo-Saxon англосаксонский.

assn association общество, ассоциация.

asst assistant помощник; ассистент.

Aug. August август.

auth. 1) author автор, писатель; 2) authorized авторизованный.

aux. auxiliary вспомогательный.

b. born рождённый; родился.

B.A. 1) Bachelor of Arts бакалавр искусств (*первая учёная степень*); 2) British Academy Британская Академия.

B.Agr(ic) Bachelor of Agriculture бакалавр сельскохозяйственных наук.

BALPA British Airline Pilot's Association Ассоциация пилотов английских авиационных линий.

Bart. baronet баронет.

Bat., batt. 1) battalion батальон; 2) battery батарея.

BBC British Broadcasting Corporation Британская радиовещательная корпорация, «Би-би-си».

B.C. before Christ до нашей эры.

BC British Columbia Британская Колумбия (*провинция Канады*).

B.C.L. Bachelor of Civil Law бакалавр гражданского права.

B.D. Bachelor of Divinity бакалавр богословия.

B.E.A. British European Airways Британская европейская авиакомпания.

B.Ed. Bachelor of Education бакалавр педагогических наук.

bef. before до, перед; ранее.

B.Eng. Bachelor of Engineering бакалавр технических наук (*по гражданскому строительству*).

B.Litt. Bachelor of Letters бакалавр литературы.

B.M. British Museum Британский музей.

Bn. battalion батальон.

BOAC British Overseas Airway Corporation Британская корпорация трансокеанских воздушных сообщений.

B.O.T. Board of Trade министерство торговли; торговая палата (*США*).

Bros brothers братья (*в названиях компаний*).

B.Sc. Bachelor of Science бакалавр физико-математических наук.

bu bushel бушель.

bus business а) дело; занятие; профессия; б) сделка.

C. 1) calorie *физ.* большая калория; 2) cape мыс; 3) catholic католик; 4) centigrade стоградусная температурная шкала (Цельсия).

c. 1) calorie *физ.* малая калория; 2) cent цент; 3) century столетие; век; 4) cubic кубический.

ca circa около, приблизительно.

Cal 1) California Калифорния (*штат США*); 2) calorie *физ.* большая калория.

cal. calorie *физ.* малая калория.

Can Canada Канада.

Cantab. of Cambridge кембриджский.

cap capital, capital letter прописная буква.

capt. captain капитан.

C.B. Companion of the Bath кавалер ордена Бани III степени.

C.C. 1) County Council совет графства; 2) Civil Court гражданский суд.

CCIR International Wireless Communications Advisory Committee Международный консультативный комитет радиосвязи.

cent. 1) central центральный; 2) century столетие, век.

cf. confer сравни, ср.

cg. centigram сантиграмм.

chap. chapter глава.

C.-in-C. Commander-in-Chief (главно)командующий.

C.I.O. Congress of Industrial Organizations Конгресс производственных профсоюзов; КПП; *см. тж.* AFL — CIO.

cit. 1) citation цитата; 2) cited цитируется, цитировано.

cit. citizen гражданин; подданный.

civ. civil гражданский.

CLC Canadian Labour Congress Канадский рабочий конгресс (*объединение профсоюзов*).

cm centimetre сантиметр.

Co 1) company компания (*промышленная, торговая и т. п.*); 2) county графство; округ (*США*).

COD cash on delivery, *амер.* collect on delivery наложенный платёж; уплата при доставке.

Col 1) colonel полковник; 2) Colorado Колорадо (*штат США*).

Coll. college колледж.

colloq. colloquial разговорный.

Colo. Colorado Колорадо (*штат США*).

com. 1) commander командир; начальник; 2) commodore *мор.* коммодор; 3) commission комитет, комиссия.

COMECON, Comecon Council for Mutual Economic Aid Совет экономической взаимопомощи, СЭВ.

conf. confer сравни, ср.

Cong. congress съезд; конгресс.

conj. 1) conjugation спряжение; 2) conjunction *грам.* союз; 3) conjunctive *грам.* сослагательное наклонение.

Conn. Connecticut Коннектикут (*штат США*).

contd. continued продолженный; продолжение следует.

Corp. 1) corporal капрал; 2) corporation корпорация; акционерное общество (*США*).

COSPAR Committee on Space Research Комитет по исследованию космического пространства.

cp. compare сравни, ср.

C.P.G.B. Communist Party of Great Britain Коммунистическая партия Великобритании.

C.P.S.U. Communist Party of the Soviet Union Коммунистическая партия Советского Союза, КПСС.

C.P.U.S.A. Communist Party of the United States of America Коммунистическая партия Соединённых Штатов Америки.

cu., cub cubic кубический.

C.U.P. Cambridge University Press Издательство Кембриджского университета.

cwt hundredweight центнер.

D. 1) December декабрь; 2) democrat демократ (*член демократической партии США*).

d. 1) date дата; 2) daughter дочь; 3) degree а) градус; б) учёная степень; 4) penny пенни, пенс; 5) died скончался.

dbl. double двойной; парный; дублированный.

D.C. District of Columbia федеральный округ Колумбия (*США*).

D.C.L. Doctor of Civil Law доктор гражданского права.

D.D. Doctor of Divinity доктор богословия.

D.D.S. Doctor of Dental Science доктор одонтологии.

Dec. December декабрь.

deg. degree а) градус; б) учёная степень.

Del. Delaware Делавэр (*штат США*).

Dept. 1) department отдел; министерство; департамент; 2) deputy депутат; заместитель.

D.Lit., D. Litt. Doctor of Literature доктор литературы.

D.M. Doctor of Medicine доктор медицины.

D.Mus. Doctor of Music доктор музыковедения.

dol. dollar(s) доллар(ы).

doz. dozen дюжина.

DP displaced person перемещённое лицо.

D.Ph(il). Doctor of Philosophy доктор философии.

Dr 1) doctor доктор; 2) debtor должник; дебитор.

D.Sc. Doctor of Science доктор физико-математических наук.

DSC Distinguished Service Cross «Крест за отличную службу».

D.S.O. Distinguished Service Order орден «За отличную службу».

E. 1) East восток; 2) English английский.

E.B. Encyclopaedia Britannica Британская энциклопедия.

E.C. Executive Committee исполнительный комитет.

Ed editor редактор.

E.E.T.S. Early English Text Society Общество по изучению древних английских текстов.

E.G., e.g. exempli gratia например.

Eng England Англия.

esp. especially особенно, специально.

Esq. esquire эсквайр.

ex. example пример.

exc. except исключая, за исключением, кроме.

exs. examples примеры.

F. 1) Fahrenheit температурная шкала Фаренгейта; 2) Friday пятница; 3) February февраль; 4) fellow член научного общества.

f. feminine женского рода.

F.A.P. first aid post пункт первой медицинской помощи.

F.B.I. Federal Bureau of Investigation Федеральное бюро расследований, ФБР (*США*).

F.C. Football Club футбольный клуб.

Feb. February февраль.

F.H. fire hydrant пожарный гидрант.

Fla Florida Флорида (*штат США*).

F.M. field-marshal фельдма́ршал.

FM frequency modulation *радио* частотная модуля́ция.

FO Foreign Office Министе́рство иностра́нных дел (*Англия до 1968 г.*).

Fr. French францу́зский.

Fri. Friday пя́тница.

F.R.S. Fellow of the Royal Society член Короле́вского (нау́чного) о́бщества.

G. guinea гине́я.

Ga. Georgia Джо́рджия (*штат США*).

gal. gallon галло́н.

G.B. Great Britain Великобрита́ния.

G.B.E. Knight Grand Cross of the Order of the British Empire кавале́р о́рдена Брита́нской импе́рии I сте́пени.

G.C. Grand Cross Большо́й крест (*орден*).

G.C.B. Knight Grand Cross of the Bath кавале́р о́рдена Ба́ни I сте́пени.

Gen. general генера́л.

Ger. German неме́цкий.

GHQ General Headquarters ста́вка, гла́вное кома́ндование.

GI *см. в Словаре.*

Gk Greek гре́ческий.

gm gram(me) грамм.

G-man *см. в Словаре.*

G.M.T. Greenwich mean time сре́днее вре́мя по гри́нвичскому меридиа́ну.

G.O.P. Grand Old Party «Вели́кая ста́рая па́ртия» (*неофициальное название республиканской партии в США*).

Gov. governor губерна́тор; прави́тель.

Govt government прави́тельство.

G.P.O. General Post Office гла́вное почто́вое управле́ние, гла́вный почта́мт.

grm. gram(me) грамм.

G.S. general staff генера́льный штаб.

h. hour час.

h.&.c. hot and cold (water) горя́чая и холо́дная вода́.

HC House of Commons пала́та о́бщин.

HL House of Lords пала́та ло́рдов.

H.M. His (Her) Majesty Его́ (Её) Вели́чество.

H.O. 1) Home Office министе́рство вну́тренних дел; 2) Head Office гла́вная конто́ра; правле́ние.

hon. honorary почётный.

h.p. 1) horsepower лошади́ная си́ла; 2) high pressure *тех.* высо́кое давле́ние.

H.Q. headquarters штаб.

H.R. House of Representatives пала́та представи́телей (*США*).

hr hour час.

I. 1) Idaho Айдахо (*штат США*); 2) Iowa Айова (*штат США*).

Ia Iowa Айова (*штат США*).

IAF International Astronautical Federation Междунаро́дная федера́ция астрона́втики, МФА.

IAU International Astronomical Union Междунаро́дный астрономи́ческий сою́з, МАС.

ib., ibid. ibidem там же.

ICFTU International Confederation of Free Trade Unions Междунаро́дная конфедера́ция свобо́дных профсою́зов, МКСП.

ICSU International Council of Scientific Unions Междунаро́дный сове́т нау́чных сою́зов, МСНС.

ID Intelligence Department разве́дывательное управле́ние.

id. idem то же са́мое.

i.e. id est то́ есть.

Ill. Illinois Иллино́йс (*штат США*).

ILO International Labour Organization Междунаро́дная организа́ция труда́, МОТ.

in. inch дюйм.

Ind. Indiana Индиа́на (*штат США*).

Insp. inspector инспе́ктор.

inst. instant теку́щего ме́сяца.

I.O.M. Isle of Man о-в Мэн.

IOU I owe you долгова́я распи́ска.

Ir. Irish ирла́ндский.

IRW International Rocket Week Междунаро́дная раке́тная неде́ля.

It. Italian италья́нский.

ital. italics курси́в.

IUGG International Union of Geodesy and Geophysics Междунаро́дный сою́з геоде́зии и геофи́зики.

I.W. Isle of Wight о-в Уа́йт.

J. Judge судья́.

Jan. January янва́рь.

J.P. Justice of the Peace мирово́й судья́.

Jr. junior мла́дший.

jun., junr. junior мла́дший.

Kan. Kansas Ка́нзас (*штат США*).

K.C.B. Knight Commander of the Bath кавале́р о́рдена Ба́ни II сте́пени.

K.G. Knight of the Garter кавале́р о́рдена Подвя́зки.

kg. kilogram(me) килогра́мм.

K.K.K. Ku-Klux-Klan ку-клукс-кла́н (*реакцио́нная фаши́стская организа́ция США*).

km. kilometre киломе́тр.

Kt knight а) ры́царь; б) кавале́р о́рдена.

kts knots *мор.* узлы́.

Ky Kentucky Кенту́кки (*штат США*).

L 1) libra фунт (сте́рлингов); 2) lord лорд; член пала́ты ло́рдов; lady ле́ди.

l 1) left ле́вый; 2) litre литр.

La Louisiana Луизиа́на (*штат США*).

Lancs Lancashire Ла́нкашир.

Lat. Latin лати́нский.

lat. latitude широта́.

lb. libra фунт (сте́рлингов).

Ld limited с ограни́ченной отве́тственностью (*о торговой компании*).

lect. lecture ле́кция.

Leics. Leicestershire Ле́стершир.

Lincs. Lincolnshire Ли́нкольншир.

ll. lines стро́ки.

L.L.D. Doctor of Laws до́ктор гражда́нского и канони́ческого пра́ва.

long. longitude долгота́.

L.P. Labour Party лейбори́стская па́ртия.

L.s.d. pounds, shillings, pence фу́нты, ши́ллинги, пе́нсы.

Lt. lieutenant лейтена́нт.

Ltd limited с ограни́ченной отве́тственностью (*о торговой компании*).

M. 1) March март; 2) master маги́стр (*учёное звание*); 3) member член (*общества и т. п.*).

m. 1) masculine мужско́го ро́да; 2) metre метр;

3) mile ми́ля; 4) minute мину́та; 5) month ме́сяц.

Maj. major майо́р.

Mar. March март.

Mass. Massachusetts Массачу́сетс (*штат США*).

MC Member of Congress член конгре́сса.

Md Maryland Мэ́риленд (*штат США*).

M.E. Middle English среднеангли́йский (*язы́к*).

Me Maine Мэн (*штат США*).

mem. memento по́мни.

memo. memorandum мемора́ндум.

mg. milligram(me) миллигра́мм.

M.H.R. Member of the House of Representatives член пала́ты представи́телей (*в США*).

Mich. Michigan Мичига́н (*штат США*).

mil. military вое́нный, во́инский.

Minn. Minnesota Миннесо́та (*штат США*).

Miss. Mississippi Миссиси́пи (*штат США*).

Mlle mademoiselle мадемуазе́ль.

MM Messieurs господа́.

mm millimetre миллиме́тр.

Mme Madame мада́м.

Mmes Mesdames ми́лостивые госуда́рыни.

Mo. Missouri Миссу́ри (*штат США*).

Mods Moderations пе́рвый публи́чный экза́мен на сте́пень бакала́вра (*в Оксфорде*).

Mon. Monday понеде́льник.

Mon. Montana Монта́на (*штат США*).

M.P. 1) Member of Parliament член парла́мента; 2) military police вое́нная поли́ция.

m.p.h. miles per hour (*столько-то*) миль в час.

mr Mister ми́стер, господи́н.

Mrs Mistress ми́ссис, госпожа́.

MS. manuscript ру́копись.

M.Sc. Master of Science маги́стр фи́зико-математи́ческих нау́к.

MSS. manuscripts ру́кописи.

Mt mountain гора́.

mth(s) month(s) ме́сяц(ы).

N. North се́вер.

n. 1) neuter сре́днего ро́да; 2) nominative имени́тельный паде́ж; 3) noun и́мя существи́тельное.

N.A. North America Се́верная Аме́рика.

N.A.T.O. North Atlantic Treaty Organization Организа́ция Североатланти́ческого догово́ра, Североатланти́ческий пакт, Североатланти́ческий сою́з, НАТО.

nav. naval вое́нно-морско́й.

N.B. nota bene обрати́(те) внима́ние, заме́ть(те).

N.C. North Carolina Се́верная Кароли́на (*штат США*).

n.d. no date без да́ты, без числа́.

N.Dak. North Dakota Се́верная Дако́та (*штат США*).

N.E. 1) New England Но́вая А́нглия; 2) North-East се́веро-восто́к.

Neb. Nebraska Небра́ска (*штат США*).

N.E.D. New English Dictionary Но́вый слова́рь англи́йского языка́ (*12 томов*).

Nev. Nevada Нева́да (*штат США*).

N.F. Newfoundland Ньюфаундле́нд.

N.H. New Hampshire Нью-Гэ́мпшир (*штат США*).

NHS National Health Service Национа́льная слу́жба здравоохране́ния (*Англия*).

N.J. New Jersey Нью-Дже́рси (*штат США*).

NLF National Liberation Front (Viet Nam) Национа́льный фронт освобожде́ния Ю́жного Вьетна́ма.

N.Mex. New Mexico Нью-Ме́ксико (*штат США*).

No., no. number но́мер.

Nos., nos numbers номера́.

Notts Nottinghamshire Но́ттингемшир.

Nov. November ноя́брь.

N.S. New Style но́вый стиль.

N.S.W. New South Wales Но́вый Ю́жный Уэ́льс (*Австралия*).

N.Y. New York *г.* Нью-Йо́рк.

N.Z. New Zealand Но́вая Зела́ндия.

O. Ohio Ога́йо (*штат США*).

obs. obsolete устаре́вший.

Oct. October октя́брь.

O.E. Old English древнеангли́йский (*язы́к*).

O.E.D. Oxford English Dictionary Оксфо́рдский слова́рь англи́йского языка́ (*13 томов*).

O.K. all correct *амер.* всё в поря́дке; утверждено́, согласо́вано.

Okla Oklahoma Оклахо́ма (*штат США*).

O.M. Order of Merit о́рден «За заслу́ги».

Ont. Ontario Онта́рио.

o.p. out of print распро́дано.

Oreg. Oregon Орего́н (*штат США*).

O.S. Old Style ста́рый стиль.

O.U. Oxford University Оксфо́рдский университе́т.

O.U.P. Oxford University Press Изда́тельство Оксфо́рдского университе́та.

Oxon. Oxonian Оксфо́рдский.

oz ounce(s) у́нция(-ии).

P. 1) (car-)park стоя́нка (авто)тра́нспорта; 2) pedestrian (crossing) перехо́д (*для пешехо́дов*).

p. page страни́ца.

Pa Pennsylvania Пенсильва́ния (*штат США*).

par. paragraph пара́граф; абза́ц.

Parl. parliament парла́мент.

PAYE pay as you earn упла́та нало́гов при получе́нии за́работной пла́ты.

P.C. 1) postcard почто́вая откры́тка; 2) police constable полице́йский; 3) Privy Council Та́йный сове́т.

p.c. per cent проце́нт.

Penn, Penna Pennsylvania Пенсильва́ния (*штат США*).

per an. per annum ежего́дно, в год.

Ph.B. Bachelor of Philosophy бакала́вр филосо́фии.

Ph.D. Doctor of Philosophy до́ктор филосо́фии.

phr. phrase выраже́ние, оборо́т; словосочета́ние.

P.I. Philippine Islands Филиппи́нские о-ва́.

pl plural *грам.* мно́жественное число́.

P.M. 1) Prime Minister премье́р-мини́стр; 2) postmaster нача́льник почто́вого отделе́ния, почтмей́стер.

p.m. 1) post meridiem по́сле полу́дня; 2) post-mortem а) вскры́тие (*трупа*); б) посме́ртный.

P.O. 1) Post-Office по́чта, почто́вое отделе́ние; 2) postal order де́нежный перево́д по по́чте.

P.O.W. prisoner of war военнопле́нный.

pp. pages страни́цы.

Pref. preface предисло́вие.

Prof. professor профе́ссор.

P.S. postscript постскри́птум.

Pt 1) part часть; 2) port порт.

pt. pint пи́нта.

P.T.O. please, turn over смотри(те) на обороте, см. н/об.

q. question вопрос.

Q.E.D. quod erat demonstrandum что и требовалось доказать.

Que. Quebec Квебек (*провинция Канады*).

quot. quotation цитата.

q.v. quod vide смотри (*там-то*).

R. 1) railway железная дорога; 2) Réaumur температурная шкала Реомюра; 3) river река; 4) road дорога.

r. right правый.

R.A. 1) rear admiral контр-адмирал; 2) Royal Academy Королёвская академия изобразительных искусств.

R.A.D.A. Royal Academy of Dramatic Art Королёвская академия драматического искусства.

R.A.F. Royal Air Force военно-воздушные силы Великобритании.

R.A.M. Royal Academy of Music Королёвская академия музыкального искусства.

R.C. Red Cross Красный Крест.

rd road дорога.

regt regiment полк.

rep. 1) representative а) представитель; делегат; б) член палаты представителей (*в США*); 2) republic республика.

Rev. reverend преподобный (*титул священника*).

R.I. Rhode Island Род-Айленд (*штат США*).

R.N. Royal Navy военно-морские силы Великобритании.

R.S. the Royal Society Королёвское общество.

Rt. Hon. Right Honourable досточтимый (*титул пэра*).

Rus., Russ. Russian русский.

S dollar(s) доллар(ы).

S. 1) saint святой; 2) South юг.

s. 1) second а) второй; б) секунда; 2) singular *грам.* единственное число; 3) shilling шиллинг.

S.A. 1) South Africa Южная Африка; 2) South America Южная Америка.

Sat. Saturday суббота.

S.C. South Carolina Южная Каролина (*штат США*).

S. Dak. South Dakota Южная Дакота (*штат США*).

S.E.A.T.O. South-East Asia Treaty Organization Организация договора Юго-Восточной Азии, СЕАТО.

Sec. secretary а) секретарь; б) министр.

sec. second а) второй; б) секунда.

Sen. 1) senate сенат; 2) senator сенатор.

Sept. September сентябрь.

Sergt sergeant сержант.

sg singular *грам.* единственное число.

sh. shilling шиллинг.

S.O.S. международный радиосигнал бедствия.

S.P.E. Society of Pure English Общество сохранения чистоты английского языка.

Sr. senior старший.

S.S. 1) steamship пароход; 2) Sunday School воскресная школа.

St. 1) saint святой; 2) street улица.

Sta. station железнодорожная станция.

St.Ex. Stock Exchange фондовая биржа.

Su. Sunday воскресенье.

Sub. 1) submarine boat подводная лодка; 2) sub-

altern младший офицер; 3) substitute заменитель; суррогат.

Sun. Sunday воскресенье.

suppl. supplement дополнение, приложение.

surg. surgeon хирург; военный врач.

S.W. South-West юго-запад.

Sw. Swedish шведский.

T. 1) temperature температура; 2) time а) время; б) срок.

t. 1) ton тонна; 2) town город; 3) territory территория.

T.B. 1) torpedo-boat миноносец; торпедный катер; 2) torpedo-bomber бомбардировщик-торпедоносец; 3) tuberculosis туберкулёз.

tech. technical технический.

Tenn Tennessee Теннесси (*штат США*).

Tex Texas Техас (*штат США*).

Th. Thursday четверг.

thr through через, сквозь.

T.O. 1) telegraph office телеграфное отделение; 2) telephone office телефонное отделение; 3) turn over смотри(те) на обороте.

T.U. trade union тред-юнион; профессиональный союз.

T.U.C. Trades Union Congress Конгресс тред-юнионов (*Англия*).

Tues. Tuesday вторник.

TV television телевидение.

U. university университет.

U.K. United Kingdom Соединённое Королевство.

ult. ultimo истёкшего месяца.

U.N. United Nations Объединённые Нации.

U.N.O. United Nations Organization Организация Объединённых Наций, ООН.

U.P.I. United Press International информационное агентство «Юнайтед пресс интернейшнл» (*США*).

U.S. United States Соединённые Штаты.

U.S.A. 1) United States of America Соединённые Штаты Америки, США; 2) United States Army армия США, сухопутные войска США.

U.S.N. United States Navy военно-морские силы США.

U.S.S. 1) United States Senate сенат США; 2) United States Ship корабль военно-морских сил США.

U.S.S.R. Union of Soviet Socialist Republics Союз Советских Социалистических Республик, СССР.

usu. usually обычно, обыкновенно.

Ut. Utah Юта (*штат США*).

v. versus *юр., спорт.* против.

V.A. vice-admiral вице-адмирал.

Va Virginia Виргиния (*штат США*).

V.C. 1) vice-chancellor вице-канцлер; 2) Victoria Cross орден «Крест Виктории».

VD venereal disease венерическая болезнь.

V-Day Victory Day День Победы.

VE-Day Victory in Europe Day День победы в Европе (*над фашистской Германией*).

v.i. verb intransitive непереходный глагол.

v.imp. verb impersonal безличный глагол.

Vis. viscount виконт.

viz videlicet то есть; а именно.

VJ-Day Victory in Japan Day День победы над Японией.

voc. vocative звательный падеж.

vocab. vocabulary словарь.
vol. volume том.
V.P. vice-president вице-президе́нт.
v.p. verb passive глаго́л страда́тельного зало́га.
v.r. verb reflexive возвра́тный глаго́л.
Vt Vermont Вермо́нт (*штат США*).
v.t. verb transitive перехо́дный глаго́л.
vy very о́чень.

W. 1) Wales Уэ́льс; 2) Wednesday среда́; 3) West за́пад.
w. 1) weight вес; 2) watt ватт; 3) with с, вме́сте.
W.A. 1) West Africa За́падная А́фрика; 2) West Australia За́падная Австра́лия.
Wash Washington Вашингто́н (*штат США*).
Wash. D. C. Washington, District of Columbia *г.* Вашингто́н, федера́льный о́круг Колу́мбия.
Wed. Wednesday среда́.
W.F.D.Y. World Federation of Democratic Youth Всеми́рная федера́ция демократи́ческой молодёжи, ВФДМ.
W.F.T.U. World Federation of Trade Unions Всеми́рная федера́ция профессиона́льных сою́зов, ВФП.
W.I. West Indies Вест-И́ндия.
W.I.D.F. Women's International Democratic Federation Междунаро́дная демократи́ческая федера́ция же́нщин, МДФЖ.
Wisc. Wisconsin Виско́нсин (*штат США*).
wk. week неде́ля.
Wks works сочине́ния.
W/L wave length *радио* длина́ волны́.
W.O. Warrant Officer уо́рент-офице́р.
w.o. without без.
Worcs. Worcestershire Ву́стершир.
WPC World Peace Council Всеми́рный Сове́т Ми́ра, ВСМ.
W/T 1) wireless telegraphy радиотелеграфи́я; 2) wireless telephony радиотелефони́я.
wt weight вес.
Wyo Wyoming Вайо́минг (*штат США*).

x extra вы́сшего ка́чества.
Xm., Xmas. Christmas рождество́.

Y.B. year-book ежего́дник.
Y.C.L. Young Communist League Коммунисти́ческий сою́з молодёжи.
yd yard ярд.
Yorks. Yorkshire Йо́ркшир.
yr 1) year год; 2) your ваш.

Z.G. Zoological Garden зоопа́рк.

СПИСОК ИМЕН

LIST OF NAMES

Abel ['eɪbəl] Эйбел; Авель.
Abraham ['eɪbrəhæm] Абрахам; Авраа́м.
Adam ['ædəm] Ада́м.
Adrian ['eɪdrɪən] ‚Адриа́н.
Agatha ['ægəθə] Ага́та.
Agnes ['ægnɪs] Агне́сса.
Albert ['ælbət] ‚Альбе́рт.
Alec(k) ['ælɪk] *уменьш. от* Alexander; А́лек.
Alexander [‚ælɪg'zɑːndə] Алекса́ндр.
Alfred ['ælfrɪd] Альфре́д.
Algernon ['ældʒənən] Элджернон.
Alice ['ælɪs] Э́лис; Али́са.
Allan ['ælən] Алла́н.
Amabel· ['æməbel] А́мабель.
Amelia [ə'miːljə] Аме́лия; Эми́лия.
Amy ['eɪmɪ] *уменьш. от* Amelia; Эми.
Andrew ['ændruː] Э́ндрю; Андре́й.
Andy ['ændɪ] *уменьш. от* Andrew; Э́нди.
Angelica [æn'dʒelɪkə] Анжели́ка.
Ann, Anna [æn,'ænə] Эн, Э́нна; А́нна.
Annabel ['ænəbel] Э́ннабел.
Annie ['ænɪ] *уменьш. от* Ann; Anna; Э́нни.
Anthony ['æntənɪ] Э́нтони; Анто́ний.
Arabella [‚ærə'belə] Арабе́лла.
Archibald ['ɑːtʃɪbəld] А́рчибальд.
Archie ['ɑːtʃɪ] *уменьш. от* Archibald; А́рчи.
Arnold ['ɑːnld] Арно́льд.
Arthur ['ɑːθə] А́ртур.
Aubrey ['ɔːbrɪ] О́бри.
August ['ɔːgʌst] А́вгуст.
Augustus [ɔː'gʌstəs] Оге́стес; А́вгуст.
Aurora [ɔː'rɔːrə] Авро́ра.
Austin ['ɔstɪn] О́стин.

Bab [bæb] *уменьш. от* Barbara; Бэб.
Baldwin ['bɔːldwɪn] Бо́лдуин.
Barbara ['bɑːbərə] Ба́рбара; Варва́ра.
Bart [bɑːt] *уменьш. от* Bartholomew; Барт.
Bartholomew [bɑːˈθɔləmjuː] Варфоломе́й.
Basil ['bæzl] Бе́зил; Васи́лий.
Beatrice, Beatrix ['bɪətrɪs, -ɪks] Беатри́са.
Beck, Becky [bek, 'bekɪ] *уменьш. от* Rebecca; Бек, Бе́кки.
Bel, Bella [bel, 'belə] *уменьш. от* Isabel, Isabella, Annabel *и* Arabella; Бэл, Бэ́лла.
Ben [ben] *уменьш. от* Benjamin; Бен.
Benedict ['benɪdɪkt] Бенеди́кт.
Benjamin ['bendʒəmɪn] Бе́нджамен; Веньями́н.
Benny ['benɪ] *уменьш. от* Benjamin; Бе́нни.
Bernard ['bənəd] Берна́рд.
Bert, Bertie [bət, 'bətɪ] *уменьш. от* Albert, Bertram, Herbert *и* Robert; Берт, Бе́рти.
Bertram ['bətrəm] Бе́ртрам.
Bess, Bessie, Bessy [bes, 'besɪ] *уменьш. от* Elisabeth; Бесс; Бе́сси.

Betsey, Betsy ['betsɪ] *уменьш. от* Elisabeth; Бе́тси.
Betty ['betɪ] *уменьш. от* Elisabeth; Бе́тти.
Bill, Billy [bɪl, 'bɪlɪ] *уменьш. от* William; Бил, Би́лли.
Bob, Bobbie, Bobby [bɔb, 'bɔbɪ] *уменьш. от* Robert; Боб, Бо́бби.
Brian ['braɪən] Бра́йен, Бриан.
Bridget ['brɪdʒɪt] Бри́джит, Бриги́тта.

Carol ['kærəl] Кэ́рол.
Caroline ['kærəlaɪn] Кароли́на.
Carrie ['kærɪ] *уменьш. от* Caroline; Кэ́рри.
Catherine ['kæθərɪn] Кэ́трин; Екатери́на.
Cathie ['kæðɪ] *уменьш. от* Catherine; Кэ́ти.
Cecil ['sesl] Сесл.
Cecilia, Cecily [sɪ'sɪljə, 'sesɪlɪ] Сеси́лия, Цеци́лия.
Charles [tʃɑːlz] Чарл(ь)з; Карл.
Charley, Charlie ['tʃɑːlɪ] *уменьш. от* Charles; Ча́рли.
Chris [krɪs] *уменьш. от* Christian, Christina, Christine *и* Christopher; Крис.
Christian ['krɪstjən] Кри́стиан; Христиа́н.
Christie ['krɪstɪ] *уменьш. от* Christian; Кри́сти.
Christina, Christine [krɪs'tiːnə, 'krɪstiːn, krɪs'tiːn] Кристи́на, Кри́стин.
Christopher ['krɪstəfə] Кри́стофер; Христофо́р.
Clara ['klɛərə] Кла́ра.
Clare [klɛə] Клэр.
Clarence ['klærəns] Кле́ренс, Кла́ренс.
Claud(e) [klɔːd] Клод.
Clem [klem] *уменьш. от* Clement; Клем.
Clement ['klemənt] Кле́мент.
Connie ['kɔnɪ] *уменьш. от* Constance; Ко́нни.
Constance ['kɔnstəns] Ко́нстанс; Конста́нция.
Cora ['kɔːrə] Ко́ра.
Cordelia [kɔː'diːljə] Корде́лия.
Cyril ['sɪrɪl] Си́рил; Кири́лл.
Cyrus ['saɪərəs] Са́йрес; Кир.

Dan [dæn] *уменьш. от* Daniel; Дэн.
Daniel ['dænjəl] Дэ́ниел; Дании́л.
Dannie ['dænɪ] *уменьш. от* Daniel; Дэ́нни.
Dave [deɪv] *уменьш. от* David; Дейв.
David ['deɪvɪd] Дэ́вид; Дави́д.
Davy ['deɪvɪ] *уменьш. от* David; Дэ́ви.
Den(n)is ['denɪs] Де́нис.
Diana [daɪ'ænə] Диа́на.
Dick [dɪk] *уменьш. от* Richard; Дик.
Dickie ['dɪkɪ] *уменьш. от* Richard; Ди́кки.
Dob, Dobbin [dɔb, 'dɔbɪn] *уменьш. от* Robert; Доб, До́бин.
Doll, Dolly [dɔl, 'dɔlɪ] *уменьш. от* Dorothy; Долл, До́лли.
Donald ['dɔnld] До́нальд.

Dora ['dɔːrə] *уменьш.* от Dorothy; Дóра.
Dorian ['dɔːrɪən] Дóриáн.
Doris ['dɔrɪs] Дóрис.
Dorothy ['dɔrəθɪ] Дóроти; Доротéя.
Douglas ['dʌgləs] Дýглас.

Ed [ed] *уменьш.* от Edgar, Edmund, Edward *и* Edwin; Эд.
Eddie, Eddy ['edɪ] *уменьш.* от Edward *и* Edwin; Эдди.
Edgar ['edgə] Эдгáр.
Edith ['iːdɪθ] Эдит.
Edmund ['edmənd] Эдмýнд.
Edward ['edwəd] Эдвард; Эдуáрд.
Edwin ['edwɪn] Эдвин.
Eleanor ['elɪnə] Элинóр; Элеонóра.
Elijah [ɪ'laɪdʒə] Илáйджа; Илия.
Elisabeth, Elizabeth [ɪ'lɪzəbəθ] Элизабет, Елизавéта.
Ellen ['elɪn] *уменьш.* от Eleanor; Элин.
Elmer ['elmə] Элмер.
Elsie ['elsɪ] *уменьш.* от Elisabeth *и* Alice; Элси.
Em [em] *уменьш.* от Emily; Эм.
Emery ['emərɪ] Эмери.
Emilia [ɪ'mɪlɪə] Эмилия.
Emily ['emɪlɪ] Эмили; Эмилия.
Ernest ['əːnɪst] Эрн(é)ст.
Ernie ['əːnɪ] *уменьш.* от Ernest; Эрни.
Essie ['esɪ] *уменьш.* от Esther; Эсси.
Esther ['estə] Эстер; Эсфирь.
Ethel ['eθəl] Этéль.
Eugene ['juːdʒiːn, juːˈdʒiːn] Юджин; Евгéний.
Eustace ['juːstəs] Юстас.
Eva, Eve ['iːvə, iːv] Éва.
Evelina, Eveline, Evelyn [ˌevɪˈliːnə, 'evɪliːn, 'iːvlɪn] Эвелина, Эвелин.

Fanny ['fænɪ] *уменьш.* от Frances; Фáнни.
Felix ['fiːlɪks] Фéликс.
Ferdinand ['fəːdɪnənd] Фердинáнд.
Flo [flou] *уменьш.* от Florence *и* Flora; Фло.
Flora ['flɔːrə] Флóра.
Florence ['flɔrəns] Флóренс.
Flossie ['flɔsɪ] *уменьш.* от Florence; Флóсси.
Floy [flɔɪ] *уменьш.* от Florence; Флой.
Frances ['frɑːnsɪs] Фрáнсис, Франчéска, Франциска.
Francis ['frɑːnsɪs] Фрáнсис; Францисск; Франц.
Frank [fræŋk] *уменьш.* от Francis; Фрэнк.
Fred, Freddie, Freddy [fred, 'fredɪ] *уменьш.* от Frederic(k); Фрэд, Фрэдди.
Frederic(k) ['fredrɪk] Фредерик; Фридрих.

Gabriel ['geɪbrɪəl] Габриéль; Гаврийл.
Geffrey, Geoffrey ['dʒefrɪ] Джéффри, Джóффри; Гóтфрид.
George [dʒɔːdʒ] Джордж; Гéорг(ий).
Gerald ['dʒerəld] Джéрáльд.
Gertie ['gəːtɪ] *уменьш.* от Gertrude; Гéрти.
Gertrude ['gəːtruːd] Гертрýда.
Gideon ['gɪdɪən] Гидеóн.
Gil [gɪl] *уменьш.* от Gilbert; Гил.
Gilbert ['gɪlbət] Гильберт.
Gladys ['glædɪs] Глэдис.
Gloria ['glɔːrɪə] Глóрия.
Godfrey ['gɔdfrɪ] Гóдфри.
Gordon ['gɔdn] Гóрдóн.
Grace [greɪs] Грейс.
Graham ['greɪəm] Грéйем, Грэ́(хе)м.

Gregory ['gregərɪ] Грéгори.
Guy [gaɪ] Гай.
Gwendolen ['gwendəlɪn] Гвéндолин.

Hal [hæl] *уменьш.* от Henry; Хэл.
Harold ['hærəld] Гáрóльд.
Harriet, Harriot ['hærɪət] Генриéтта.
Harry ['hærɪ] Гáрри.
Hatty ['hætɪ] *уменьш.* от Harriet, Harriot; Хэ́тти.
Helen, Helena ['helɪn, 'helɪnə, he'liːnə] Элéн; Елéна.
Henry ['henrɪ] Гéнри; Гéнрих.
Herbert ['həːbət] Гéрберт.
Herman(n) ['həːmən] Гéрман.
Hilary ['hɪlərɪ] Хилари.
Hope [houp] Хóуп.
Horace, Horatio ['hɔrəs, hɔ'reɪʃiou] Гóрас, Горáцио; Горáций.
Howard ['hauəd] Гóвард.
Hubert ['hjuːbəːt] Хьюберт.
Hugh, Hugo [hjuː, 'hjuːgou] Хью, Хьюго.
Humphr(e)y ['hʌmfrɪ] Хáмфри, Гéмфри.

Ida ['aɪdə] Йда.
Ik, Ike [ɪk, aɪk] *уменьш.* от Isaac; Ик, Айк.
Ira ['aɪərə] Áйра.
Irene [aɪ'riːniː, 'aɪriːn] Áйрин, Ирэ́н; Ирина.
Isaac ['aɪzək] Áйзек; Исаáк.
Isabel, Isabella ['ɪzəbel, ˌɪzə'belə] Изабéлла.
Isidore ['ɪzɪdɔː] Исидóра.
Isold(e) [ɪ'zɔld(ə)] Изóльда.

Jack [dʒæk] *уменьш.* от John; Джек.
Jacob ['dʒeɪkəb] Джéкоб; Иáков.
Jake [dʒeɪk] *уменьш.* от Jacob; Джейк.
James [dʒeɪmz] Джемс; Яков; Иáков.
Jane [dʒeɪn] Джейн.
Janet ['dʒænɪt] Джéнет, Жанéт.
Jean [dʒiːn] Джин.
Jeff [dʒef] *уменьш.* от Jeffrey; Джефф.
Jeffrey ['dʒefrɪ] Джéффри.
Jem [dʒem] *уменьш.* от James; Джем.
Jemima [dʒɪ'maɪmə] Джемáйма.
Jen, Jennie [dʒen, 'dʒenɪ] *уменьш.* от Janet; Джен, Джéнни.
Jennifer ['dʒenɪfə] Джéнифер.
Jenny ['dʒenɪ] *уменьш.* от Janet; Джéнни.
Jeremiah [dʒerɪ'maɪə] Джéреми; Иеремия.
Jerome [dʒə'roum, 'dʒerəm] Джерóм.
Jess [dʒes] *уменьш.* от Janet; Джесс.
Jessica ['dʒesɪkə] Джéссика.
Jessie, Jessy ['dʒesɪ] *уменьш.* от Janet; Джéсси.
Jim, Jimmy [dʒɪm, 'dʒɪmɪ] *уменьш.* от James; Джим.
Jo [dʒou] *уменьш.* от Joseph *и* Josephine; Джо.
Joe [dʒou] *уменьш.* от Joseph *и* Josephine; Джо.
John [dʒɔn] Джон; Иоáнн, Ивáн.
Johnny ['dʒɔnɪ] *уменьш.* от John; Джóнни.
Jonathan ['dʒɔnəθən] Джонатáн; Ионафáн.
Joseph ['dʒouzɪf] Джóзеф; Иóсиф.
Josephine ['dʒouzɪfiːn] Джóзефин; Жозефина.
Joshua ['dʒɔʃwə] Джóшуа; Иисýс.
Joy [dʒɔɪ] Джой.
Joyce [dʒɔɪs] Джойс.
Jozy ['dʒouzɪ] *уменьш.* от Josephine; Джóзи.
Judith ['dʒuːdɪθ] Джýдит; Юдифь.
Judy ['dʒuːdɪ] *уменьш.* от Judith; Джýди.
Julia ['dʒuːljə] Джýлия; Юлия.

Juliet ['dʒuːljət] Джульétта; Юлия.
Julius ['dʒuːljəs] Джýлиус; Юлий.

Kate [keɪt] *уменьш.* от Catherine; Кейт.
Kathleen ['kæθliːn] *уменьш.* от Catherine; Кéтлин.
Keith [kiːθ] Кит.
Kenneth ['kenɪθ] Кéннет.
Kit [kɪt] *уменьш.* от Christopher *и* Catherine; Кит.
Kitty ['kɪtɪ] *уменьш.* от Catherine; Кѝтти.

Laurence ['lɔrəns] Лóренс; Лаврéнтий.
Lazarus ['læzərəs] Лáзарь.
Leonard ['lenəd] Леонáрд.
Leonora [,liːə'nɔːrə] Леонóра, Элеонóра.
Lesley, Leslie ['lezlɪ] Лéсли.
Lewis ['luːɪs] Льюис; Людóвик.
Lillian ['lɪlɪən] Лѝллиан; Лилиáна.
Lily ['lɪlɪ] Лѝли.
Lionel ['laɪənl] Лáйонел; Лионéль.
Liz, Liza, Lizzie [lɪz, 'liːzə, 'laɪzə, 'lɪzɪ] *уменьш.* от Elisabeth; Лиз, Лѝза, Лѝззи.
Lucas ['luːkəs] Лýкас.
Lucy ['luːsɪ] Люси.
Luke [luːk] Люк; Лукá.

Mabel ['meɪbəl] Мейбл, Мáбель.
Madeleine ['mædlɪn] Мáделейн; Маделѝна.
Madge [mædʒ] *уменьш.* от Margaret; Мэдж.
Mag [mæg] *уменьш.* от Margaret; Мэг.
Maggie ['mægɪ] *уменьш.* от Margaret; Мэгги.
Malkolm ['mælkəm] Мáлькольм.
Mamie ['meɪmɪ] *уменьш.* от Mary; Мéйми.
Margaret ['mɑːgərɪt] Мáргарет; Маргарѝта.
Margery ['mɑːdʒərɪ] *уменьш.* от Margaret; Мáрджори.
Margie ['mɑːdʒɪ] *уменьш.* от Margaret; Мáрджи.
Maria [mə'raɪə] Марѝя.
Marion ['mɛərɪən] Мариóн.
Mark [mɑːk] Марк.
Martha ['mɑːθə] Мáрта.
Martin ['mɑːtɪn] Мартѝн.
Mary ['mɛərɪ] Мэри; Марѝя.
Mat(h)ilda [mə'tɪldə] Матѝльда.
Matthew, Matthias ['mæθjuː, mə'θaɪɔs] Мэтью, Мáтиас; Матфéй.
Matty ['mætɪ] *уменьш.* от Martha *и* Mat(h)ilda; Мэтти.
Maud(e) [mɔːd] *уменьш.* от Madeleine *и* Mat(h)ilda; Мод.
Maurice ['mɔrɪs] Мóрис.
Max [mæks] Макс.
May [meɪ] *уменьш.* от Mary *и* Margaret; Мэй.
Meg, Meggy [meg, 'megɪ] *уменьш.* от Margaret; Мэг, Мéгги.
Mercy ['mɜːsɪ] Мéрси.
Michael ['maɪkl] Майкл; Михаѝл.
Micky ['mɪkɪ] *уменьш.* от Michael; Мѝки.
Mike [maɪk] *уменьш.* от Michael; Майк.
Mildred ['mɪldrɪd] Мѝлдред.
Mirabel ['mɪrəbel] Мѝрабéль.
Miriam ['mɪrɪəm] Мѝриáм.
Moll, Molly [mɔl, 'mɔlɪ] *уменьш.* от Mary; Молл, Мóлли.
Montagu(e) ['mɔntəgjuː] Мóнтегю.
Monty ['mɔntɪ] *уменьш.* от Montagu(e); Мóнти.
Morgan ['mɔːgən] Мóрган.
Mortimer ['mɔːtɪmə] Мóртимер.

Moses ['mouzɪz] Мóзес; Моисéй.
Muriel ['mjuərɪəl] Мюриéль.

Nance, Nancy [næns, 'nænsɪ] *уменьш.* от Agnes. *и* Ann, Anna; Нэнс, Нэнси.
Nannie, Nanny ['nænɪ] *уменьш.* от Ann, Anna; Нэнни.
Nat [næt] *уменьш.* от Nathan; Нат.
Nathan ['neɪθən] Нáтан.
Ned, Neddie, Neddy [ned, 'nedɪ] *уменьш.* от Edgar, Edmund, Edwin *и* Edward; Нед, Нéдди.
Nell, Nellie, Nelly [nel, 'nelɪ] *уменьш.* от Eleanor *и* Helen, Helena; Нел, Нéлли.
Neville ['nevɪl] Нéвиль.
Nicholas ['nɪkələs] Нѝколас; Николáй.
Nick [nɪk] *уменьш.* от Nicholas; Ник.
Noah ['nouə] Ной.
Noel ['nouəl] Ноэ́ль.
Noll, Nolly [nɔl, 'nɔlɪ] *уменьш.* от Olivia *и* Oliver; Нол, Нóлли.
Nora ['nɔːrə] *уменьш.* от Eleanor *и* Leonora; Нóра.
Norman ['nɔːmən] Нóрман.

Oliver ['ɔlɪvə] Óливер.
Olivia [ɔ'lɪvɪə] Олѝвия.
Ophelia [ɔ'fiːljə] Офéлия.
Oscar ['ɔskə] Оскáр.
Oswald ['ɔzwəld] Óсвальд.
Owen ['ouɪn] Óуэн.

Paddy ['pædɪ] *уменьш.* от Patrick *и* Patricia; Пэдди.
Pat [pæt] *уменьш.* от Patrick, Patricia *и* Martha; Пэт.
Patricia [pə'trɪʃə] Патрѝция.
Patrick ['pætrɪk] Пáтрик.
Patty ['pætɪ] *уменьш.* от Martha *и* Mat(h)ilda; Пэтти.
Paul [pɔːl] Поль.
Peg, Peggy [peg, 'pegɪ] *уменьш.* от Margaret; Пэг, Пéгги.
Pen [pen] *уменьш.* от Penelope; Пен, Пéнни.
Penelope [pɪ'neləpɪ] Пенелóпа.
Percy ['pɜːsɪ] Пéрси.
• **Pete** [piːt] *уменьш.* от Peter; Пит.
Peter ['piːtə] Пѝтер; Пётр.
Phil [fɪl] *уменьш.* от Philip; Фил.
Philip ['fɪlɪp] Фѝлип; Филѝпп.
Pip [pɪp] *уменьш.* от Philip; Пип.
Pol, Polly [pɔl, 'pɔlɪ] *уменьш.* от Mary; Пол, Пóлли.
Portia ['pɔːʃjə] Пóрция.

Rachel ['reɪtʃəl] Рéчел; Рахѝль.
Ralph [rælf, reɪf] Ральф.
Randolph ['rændɔlf] Рáндольф.
Raphael ['ræfeɪəl, 'reɪfl] Рафаэ́ль.
Raymond ['reɪmənd] Раймóнд.
Rebecca [rɪ'bekə] Ребéкка; Ревéкка.
Reg, Reggie ['redʒ, 'redʒɪ] *уменьш.* от Reginald; Редж, Рéджи.
Reginald ['redʒɪnld] Рéджинáльд.
Reynold ['renld] Рейнóльд.
Richard ['rɪtʃəd] Рѝчард.
Rob, Robbie [rɔb, 'rɔbɪ] *уменьш.* от Robert; Роб, Рóбби.
Robert ['rɔbət] Рóберт.
Robin ['rɔbɪn] *уменьш.* от Robert; Рóбин.

Roddy ['rɔdɪ] *уменьш.* от Roderick; Ро́дди.
Roderick ['rɔdərɪk] Ро́дерик.
Roger ['rɔdʒə] Ро́джер.
Roland ['roulənd] Ро́ланд.
Rolf [rɔlf] Рольф.
Romeo ['roumɪou] Роме́о.
Ronald ['rɔnld] Ро́нальд.
Rosa ['rouzə] Ро́за.
Rose [rouz] Ро́уз; Ро́за.
Rosemary ['rouzmərɪ] Розмари́.
Roy [rɔɪ] Рой.
Rudolf, Rudolph ['ru:dɔlf] Рудо́льф.
Rupert ['ru:pət] Ру́перт.
Ruth [ru:θ] Рут.

Sadie ['seɪdɪ] *уменьш.* от Sara(h); Се́йди.
Sal, Sally [sæl, 'sælɪ] *уменьш.* от Sara(h); Сэл, Сэ́лли.
Sam, Sammy [sæm, 'sæmɪ] *уменьш.* от Samuel; Сэм, Сэ́мми.
Sam(p)son ['sæm(p)sn] Сэ́мпсон; Самсо́н.
Samuel ['sæmjuəl] Сэ́мюель; Самуи́л.
Sanders ['sɑːndəz] *уменьш.* от Alexander; Са́ндерс.
Sandy ['sændɪ] *уменьш.* от Alexander; Сэ́нди.
Sara(h) ['sɛərə] Са́ра.
Saul [sɔːl] Сау́л.
Sebastian [sɪ'bæstjən] Себа́стиан.
Sibil, Sibyl, Sibylla ['sɪbɪl, sɪ'bɪlə] Сиби́лла.
Sidney ['sɪdnɪ] Си́дней.
Silas ['saɪləs] Са́йлас.
Silvia ['sɪlvɪə] Си́львия; Си́льва.
Sim [sɪm] *уменьш.* от Simon; Сим.
Simmy ['sɪmɪ] *уменьш.* от Simon; Си́мми.
Simon ['saɪmən] Са́ймон; Си́мон.
Sol, Solly [sɔl, 'sɔlɪ] *уменьш.* от Solomon; Сол, Со́лли.
Solomon ['sɔləmən] Соломо́н.
Sophie, Sophy ['soufɪ] Софи́; Со́фья.
Stanley ['stænlɪ] Стэ́нли.
Stella ['stelə] Сте́лла.

Stephen ['sti:vn] Сти́вн; Стефа́н.
Steve [sti:v] *уменьш.* от Stephen; Стив.
Sue [sju:] *уменьш.* от Susan; Сью.
Susan ['su:zn] Сью́зен; Сюза́нна.
Susie, Susy ['su:zɪ] *уменьш.* от Susan; Сю́зи.

Ted, Teddy [ted, 'tedɪ] Тед, Те́дди.
Theobald ['θɪəbɔːld] Теоба́льд.
T(h)eresa [tə'ri:zə] Тере́за.
Thomas ['tɔməs] То́мас; Фома́.
Tib, Tibbie [tɪb, 'tɪbɪ] *уменьш.* от Isabel, Isabella; Тиб, Ти́бби.
Tim [tɪm] *уменьш.* от Timothy; Тим.
Timothy ['tɪməθɪ] Ти́моти.
Tina ['ti:nə] *уменьш.* от Christina; Ти́на.
Tobias [tə'baɪəs] Тоба́йес.
Toby ['toubɪ] *уменьш.* от Tobias; То́би.
Tom [tɔm] *уменьш.* от Thomas; Том.
Tommy ['tɔmɪ] *уменьш.* от Thomas; То́мми.
Tony ['tounɪ] *уменьш.* от Anthony; То́ни.
Tristan ['trɪstæn] Триста́н.
Tybalt ['tɪbəlt] Тиба́льт.

Victor ['vɪktə] Ви́ктор.
Victoria [vɪk'tɔːrɪə] Викто́рия.
Vincent ['vɪnsənt] Винсе́нт.
Violet ['vaɪəlɪt] Виоле́тта.
Virginia [və'dʒɪnjə] Вирги́ния.
Vivian, Vivien ['vɪvɪən] Ви́вьен.

Wallace ['wɔlɪs] Уо́ллес.
Walt [wɔːlt] *уменьш.* от Walter; Уо́лт.
Walter ['wɔːltə] Уо́лтер; Ва́льтер.
Wilfred, Wilfrid ['wɪlfrɪd] Уи́лфред.
Will [wɪl] *уменьш.* от William; Уи́лл.
William ['wɪljəm] Уи́льям, Ви́льям.
Willy ['wɪlɪ] *уменьш.* от William; Уи́лли, Ви́лли.
Win [wɪn] *уменьш.* от Winifred; Уин.
Winifred ['wɪnɪfrɪd] Уи́нифред.
Winnie ['wɪnɪ] *уменьш.* от Winifred; Уи́нни.

NTC's
New College
RUSSIAN
and
ENGLISH
Dictionary

V. D. Arakin, Z. S. Vigodskaya, N. N. Iljina
A. M. Taube, I. W. Litvinova,
A. D. Miller, R. C. Daglish

Library of Congress Cataloging-in-Publication Data

NTC's new college Russian and English dictionary / V.D. Arakin...[et al.]
     p.   cm.
   ISBN 0-8442-4280-2
   1. Russian language—Dictionaries—English. 2. English language—
Dictionaries—Russian. I. Arakin, Vladimir Dmitrievich.
PG2640.N786 1996   96-33914
491.73'12--dc20   CIP

Contents

PREFACE

The guiding principle in making this dictionary has been to provide in the space available the fullest possible picture of present-day written and spoken Russian rendered correctly and idiomatically into modern English. Dialect words and obsolete expressions have been avoided. On the other hand, the technological revolution has led to the inclusion of many new words and senses that have acquired currency in the newspapers and popular literature.

Although this dictionary is not primarily intended for the reader whose native language is English, the response to its earlier editions has shown that it can be used effectively as a general-purpose Russian-English dictionary by students of either language. The native English speaker will naturally ignore the explanations addressed specifically to the Russian student, but by consulting the list of abbreviations he will be able to draw on all the information supplied concerning the Russian words in the dictionary, such as the gender of nouns, the aspects and government of verbs, stress and stylistic colour. Students of Russian may also become interested in the brief Russian definitions of the different senses of the Russian headwords. These are his signposts to other parts of the dictionary where synonyms and variant expressions may be found. Since these definitions follow those of the above-mentioned Russian dictionaries, and particularly the four-volume **Slovar' russkogo yazyka**, he has at his disposal in the present volume a miniature explanatory dictionary of the Russian language.

A full translation of the article on the structure of the dictionary and the list of abbreviations is provided below.

The present edition has been revised on the basis of the new edition of Ozhegov's **Slovar' russkogo yazyka** (1984) and the **Novyye slova i znacheniya**, edited by N. Z. Kotelova, Moscow, 1984.

STRUCTURE OF THE DICTIONARY

All Russian headwords are entered in alphabetical order. Words with a common root, if they can be arranged alphabetically within the entry, are grouped together. The common part of such words is indicated only once, in the headword, where it is marked off by vertical parallel (|), the swung dash (~) being used to indicate this part in the rest of the entry, e. g.:

горчи́|ца *ж.* mústard. ~чник *м.* mústard pláster; ... ~чница *ж.* mústard-pot. ~чный mústard *attr.*

The swung dash may also be used to denote the whole of the headword, e. g.:

граб|ёж *м.* róbbery; ... ~ на большо́й доро́ге híghway róbbery; ...

Homonyms are given in separate entries, marked with Roman numerals, e. g.:

грана́т I *м. (плод и дерево)* pómegranate.
грана́т II *м. (драгоценный камень)* gárnet.

Different senses of Russian words are set out after Arabic numerals in heavy type (1., 2., *etc.*).

Senses of phraseological combinations and idiomatic expressions are marked off by Arabic numerals enclosed in a single bracket.

The various senses and uses of Russian words are differentiated by brief definitions (italicized in brackets) or by indications of their field of application (medical, technical, *etc.*), and also by reference to stylistic colouring (colloquial, poetic, *etc.*)

Explanatory references to English translations, stylistic, grammatical, and so on, are given in italics after the translation, e. g.: *амер., разг., attr., etc.*

Synonymous or nearly synonymous translations are divided by commas, while more distant synonyms appear after semi-colons, as do the numbered meanings.

Alternative synonyms in English word-combinations are separated by a slanting stroke (/), e. g.:

бензоба́к *м.* pétrol/fuel tank (*read:* pétrol tank *or* fuel tank.).

Alternative synonyms in Russian expressions are separated by commas, e. g.:

выки́дывать, вы́кинуть ...; 2. (*вн.*) *разг.* ...; вы́кинуть но́мер, шту́ку (*read* вы́кинуть но́мер *or* вы́кинуть шту́ку) play a prank/trick.

If the Russian headword is used only in a certain combination, or has no equivalent in English, the combination and its English translation are given after a colon, e. g.:

баклу́ши: бить ~ ídle awáy *one's* time; ≈ twíddle *one's* thumbs.

Phraseological units, and word-combinations that do not correspond to any of the senses given under the headword are placed after a rhombus sign (◇) at the end of the entry.

Nouns are given in the nominative singular, their gender being indicated by the Russian letters *м., ж., с.* (*cf.* list of abbreviations). If the noun has two grammatical genders, both are shown, e. g.:

обжо́ра *м. и ж.* ...

If the noun is used only in the plural, it is given in the plural and marked *мн.,* e. g.:

часы́ *мн.* ...

If the noun is used more commonly, but not exclusively, in the plural, it is given in the plural and marked *мн.,* and its singular form is shown in brackets with an indication of the gender, e. g.:

гало́ши *мн. (ед.* гало́ша *ж.)* ...

In cases when the meanings of the Russian noun have different plural forms, these forms are shown for each meaning, e. g.:

коле́н|о *с.* 1. (*мн.* ~и) knee; ... 3. (*мн.* ~ья, ~а) *тех.* ... ; 4. (*мн.* ~а) ...

If the plural of the noun has a different meaning from the singular, the translations of this meaning are given after those of the singular meaning and marked *мн.*, e. g.:

> деся́ток *м.* 1. ...; ... 3. *мн.* (*мно́жество*) dózens, scores ...

When the English translation is of different grammatical number from that of the Russian, the number is noted in both cases, e. g.:

> бели́ла *мн.* 1. (*кра́ска*) whíting *sg*; ...

The plurals of English nouns of Latin or Greek origin are indicated in brackets, e. g.:

> гипо́теза *ж.* hypóthesis (*pl* -ses).

If a noun is indeclinable its gender is shown and it is marked *нескл.*, e. g.:

> пальто́ *с. нескл.* ...

Collective nouns are marked *собир.*, e. g.:

> беднота́ *ж. собир.* the poor *pl*; ...

Adjectives are normally given in their full form in the nominative singular, masculine. If the masculine form is not in use, the adjective is given in the gender which is in use, e. g.:

> бере́менная prégnant; ...

If the short form of the adjective has an independent meaning, it appears as a headword followed by a reference to the full form, under which its meaning is listed, e. g.:

> вели́к *см.* вели́кий
> вели́кий 1. ...; 2. *тк. кратк. ф.* (*сли́шком большо́й*) (too) big; ...

If an English adjective is used only predicatively or must come after its noun, it is labelled *predic.* or *после сущ.* (*cf.* list of abbreviations), e. g.:

> безынициати́вный ... withóut/lácking initiative *после сущ.*

Substantivized adjectives are marked *в знач. сущ.* and appear as a numbered meaning in the adjective entry, e. g.:

> бе́дный *прил.* 1. ...; ... 6. *в знач. сущ. м.* the poor man*; *мн.* the poor.

If a substantivized adjective is used in the feminine or neuter, this is shown by a gender label after the notation *в знач. сущ.*, e. g.:

> гла́вный *прил.* 1. ...; ... 3. *в знач. сущ. с.* the great/chief thing; ...

Any substantivized adjective that has become a fully independent noun, e. g., столо́вая, мастерска́я, is given as a separate headword with its meaning.

Short-form adjectives that are used predicatively are given in the entry for the corresponding adverb after an Arabic numeral and the notation *в знач. сказ.* or *в знач. сказ. безл.* In many cases short-form adjectives are given as separate entries.

> безопа́сно 1. *нареч.* safely; ... 2. *в знач. сказ.* it is safe...

Verbs which have an imperfective and perfective aspect are presented under the imperfective aspect, which appears as the headword in heavy type and is followed, after a comma, by the perfective aspect in lighter type. The perfective aspect is also given in its alphabetical position with a reference to the corresponding imperfective aspect, e. g.:

> багрове́ть, побагрове́ть...
> побагрове́ть *сов. см.* багрове́ть.

Identical perfective and imperfective aspects are labelled *несов. и сов.*

If there are two or more perfective aspects for an imperfective, all the perfective aspects are appended in ordinary type.

When only one of the perfective aspects may be used for one particular sense of the verb, this aspect is shown under the given meaning and labelled *сов.*, e. g.:

> гла́дить, вы́гладить, погла́дить (*вн.*) 1. *сов.* вы́гладить (*утю́жить*) iron (*smth.*) ...; 2. *сов.* погла́дить (*ласка́ть*) stroke (*smb., smth.*) ...

If in one of its senses the verb is used only in the imperfective aspect, this is indicated after the Arabic numeral by the label *тк. несов.*, e. g.:

> беле́ть, побеле́ть 1. (*станови́ться бе́лым*) turn white; 2. *тк. несов.* (*видне́ться*) show* white.

The English translations offered for verbs usually apply to both imperfective and perfective aspects. However, the label *несов. тж.* denotes a translation that will render only the imperfective aspects, and the label *сов. тж.* a rendering suitable only for the perfective, e. g.:

> выве́дывать, вы́ведать (*вн.*) *разг.* find* (*smth.*) out; *несов. тж.* try to worm (*smth.*) out.
> беси́ться, взбеси́ться... 2. (*неистовствова́ть*) rage; *сов. тж.* fly* into a rage.

If a perfective aspect has its own independent meaning which cannot be combined with the imperfective, the translation of this meaning is given separately, under that perfective aspect.

In cases when there is no common translation for imperfective and perfective aspects, each aspect is treated separately.

Verbs with the ending -ся appear in alphabetical order with their translation. Those that have only a passive meaning are not usually given.

The following devices are used to show how verbs are governed. If the Russian verb and its English equivalent take a direct object, the Russian verb is followed by the label (*вн.*), and the direct object of the English verb is shown by the label (*smb., smth.*), e. g.:

баловáть *несов.* (*вн.*) spoil* (*smb.*); ...

If the Russian verb takes a direct object and the English verb is governed by prepositions, the Russian verb is labelled (*вн.*), and the prepositions are given after the English verb, unitalicized, in brackets, e. g.:

вызывáть, вы́звать 1. (*вн.*) ...; (*посылáть за кем-л.*) send* (for); ...

Where the Russian verb governs a preposition, the preposition is given in brackets unitalicized, followed by the appropriate case in italics, and the English verb is dealt with as in the previous paragraph, e. g.:

глазéть *несов.* (на *вн.*) *разг.* gape (at), stare (at).

In word-combinations within the entry the government of the Russian verb is shown by the indefinite pronoun in the appropriate case in italics without brackets, e. g.:

глáсност|ь *ж.* publicity; ◇ предавáть *что-л.* ~и make* *smth.* públic.

If the Russian verb takes the infinitive, it is labelled (+ *инф.*), while the corresponding English verb is labelled (+ *inf*) or (+ to *inf*), as English usage requires. If the English verb takes the -ing form, this is shown by (+ -ing), e. g.:

начинáть, начáть 1. (*вн.*, + *инф.*) begín* (*smth.*, + to *inf.*, + -ing), start (*smth.*, + -ing); ...

Participial constructions are given in entries under the verb, not as separate vocables.

The pronoun *one* in translations is italicized to show that in practice any personal pronoun may be used. Similarly *one*self stands for the reflexive pronouns myself, yourself, himself, ourselves, yourselves, and themselves;

one's stands for the possessive pronouns my, your, his, her, our and their, which correspond to the forms of the Russian «свой»;

smb. stands for any noun indicating an animate being, and also for the objective forms of the personal pronouns (me, you, him, her, us, them);

smth. stands for any noun indicating an inanimate object, and also for the personal pronouns "it" and "them";

smb.'s stands for any noun in the Saxon genitive, a possessive pronoun, and also the prepositional construction (in the latter case the noun and preposition are given after the noun preceded by *smb.'s*).

Polysyllabic Russian and English words are stressed.

If a monosyllabic headword appears in an entry in an oblique case without any indication of stress, it means that the stress falls on the first syllable, thus:

борт *м.* ...; за ~ом (*read*: за бóртом).

English nouns, adjectives, adverbs and verbs that are irregular in their habits are labelled with an asterisk (*).

In order to save space the authors have tried to avoid duplication of idiomatic phrases. If the required phrase is not to be found under its first component, the other operative words should also be consulted.

ПРЕДИСЛОВИЕ

Настоящий Русско-английский словарь предназначается для широкого круга лиц, занимающихся английским языком, в частности для преподавателей и студентов вузов, а также для учащихся старших классов средней школы. Авторы учитывали также возможность использования словаря зарубежным читателем, изучающим русский язык. Словарь имеет целью помочь читателю при переводе на английский язык русских текстов средней трудности на общественно-политические, литературные и бытовые темы, т. е. текстов, не носящих специального, научного или технического характера.

Особое внимание при составлении словаря уделялось, с одной стороны, такому подбору лексики и фразеологии, который возможно полнее (насколько позволял объем словаря) отразил бы современное состояние русского литературного языка, с другой стороны, семантически, стилистически и идиоматически правильному переводу на английский язык русских слов и выражений.

В основу словника положены новейшие толковые словари русского языка, а также картотека, созданная при расписывании произведений художественной и научно-популярной литературы, газет и журналов. В словарь не вошли узкоспециальные термины, устаревшие и диалектные слова и выражения. Однако, в связи со стремительным развитием науки и техники, в словарь включены новые слова и выражения и новые значения слов, вошедшие в быт и постоянно употребляемые в печати.

В словаре приводятся также словосочетания и идиоматические выражения, представляющие трудности при переводе на английский язык.

В словарных статьях даются грамматические и стилистические пометы, а также указания на сферу употребления русского и, если необходимо, английского слова, что особенно важно для лиц, не владеющих свободно английским языком.

Все замечания и пожелания, касающиеся словаря, редакция просит направлять в издательство «Русский язык» (103012, Москва, Старопанский пер., 1/5).

ЛЕКСИКОГРАФИЧЕСКИЕ ИСТОЧНИКИ

Словарь русского языка тт. I — IV, Академия наук СССР — Институт русского языка, изд-во «Русский язык». Москва, 1981—1984.

Словарь русского языка, составил С. И. О ж е г о в, изд. 16-е, изд-во «Русский язык». Москва, 1984.

Толковый словарь русского языка, тт. I — IV, под ред. проф. Д. Н. У ш а к о в а, Гос. изд-во иностранных и национальных словарей. Москва, 1935 — 1940.

Новые слова и значения. Словарь-справочник по материалам прессы и литературы 60-х годов, Академия наук СССР — Институт русского языка, под ред. Н. З. К о т е л о в о й и Ю. С. С о р о к и н а, изд-во «Советская Энциклопедия». Москва, 1971.

Новые слова и значения. Словарь-справочник по материалам прессы и литературы 70-х годов, Академия наук СССР — Институт русского языка, под ред. Н. З. К о т е л о в о й, изд-во «Русский язык». Москва, 1984.

Англо-русский словарь, составил В. К. М ю л л е р, изд. 17-е, изд-во «Русский язык». Москва, 1978.

Большой англо-русский словарь тт. I — II, под общим руководством доктора филологических наук профессора И. Р. Г а л ь п е р и н а, изд-во «Советская Энциклопедия». Москва, 1972.

Русско-английский словарь, под ред. О. С. А х м а н о в о й и Е. А. М. У и л с о н, изд. 25-е, изд-во «Советская Энциклопедия». Москва, 1973.

The Shorter Oxford English Dictionary, vols. I — II, 3d ed. Oxford, 1973.

The Concise Oxford Dictionary of Current English, Revised by R. E. A l l e n. Oxford, 1990.

Daniel J o n e s. An English Pronouncing Dictionary, 14th ed. London, 1979.

A. S. H o r n b y, E. V. G a t e n b y, H. W a k e f i e l d. The Advanced Learner's Dictionary of Current English. London, 1981.

W e b s t e r's Third New International Dictionary of the English Language. Springfield Mass., 1971.

W e b s t e r's New World Dictionary of the American Language. New York, 1962.

The Oxford Russian-English Dictionary by M a r c u s W h e e l e r, General Editor B.O. Unbegaun. Oxford. At the Clarendon Press, 1972.

О ПОСТРОЕНИИ СЛОВАРЯ

Все заглавные русские слова расположены в алфавитном порядке. Слова с общим корнем, если они следуют друг за другом по алфавиту, объединяются в одно гнездо, в котором общая часть данных слов приводится только один раз в первом слове гнезда, где она отделяется параллелькой (|); в прочих словах того же гнезда она заменяется тильдой (~), напр.:

> горчи́|ца *ж.* mústard. ~чник *м.* mústard pláster; ...~чница *ж.* mústard-pot. ~чный mústard *attr.*

Тильда заменяет в гнезде также все заглавное слово, напр.:

> граб|ёж *м.* róbbery; ... ~ на большо́й доро́ге híghway róbbery; ...

О м о н и м ы даются отдельными статьями и отмечаются светлыми римскими цифрами, напр.:

> грана́т I *м. (плод и дерево)* pómegranate.
> грана́т II *м. (драгоценный камень)* gárnet.

З н а ч е н и я р у с с к и х с л о в выделяются арабскими полужирными цифрами с точкой (1., 2. *и т. д.*), после которых дается пояснение или помета.

З н а ч е н и я ф р а з е о л о г и ч е с к и х с о ч е т а н и й и идиоматических выражений выделяются светлыми цифрами со скобкой.

Различные значения и употребления русского слова дифференцируются либо краткими их пояснениями (курсивом в скобках), либо указанием на область применения слова (медицина, техника *и т. п.*) или на стиль речи (разговорный, поэтический *и т. п.*).

С т и л и с т и ч е с к и е, г р а м м а т и ч е с к и е п о м е т ы и л и п о я с н е н и я к английскому переводу приводятся после соответствующего английского слова курсивом, напр.: *амер., разг., attr., и т. п.*

Б л и з к и е с и н о н и м ы в переводах отделяются друг от друга запятой, далекие синонимы и значения за цифрами — точкой с запятой.

Взаимозаменяемые синонимы в английских сочетаниях разделяются косой чертой (/), напр.:

> бензоба́к *м.* pétrol/fuel tank (*читай:* pétrol tank *или* fuel tank).

Взаимозаменяемые синонимы в русском выражении разделяются запятой, напр.:

> выки́дывать, вы́кинуть...; 2. (*вн.*) *разг.* ... вы́кинуть но́мер, шту́ку (*читай:* вы́кинуть но́мер *или* вы́кинуть шту́ку) play a prank/trick.

Если заглавное русское слово употребляется только в определенном с о ч е т а н и и или не имеет соответствующего эквивалента в английском языке, после него ставится двоеточие, а затем приводится данное сочетание с переводом, напр.:

> баклу́ши: бить ~ ídle awáy *one's* time; ≈ twíddle *one's* thumbs.

В конце словарной статьи за значком ◇ (ромб) даются фразеологические единицы и такие сочетания, которые не подходят ни к одному из данных в словаре значений заглавного слова.

И м е н а с у щ е с т в и т е л ь н ы е даются в именительном падеже единственного числа. При именах существительных дается указание на род: *м., ж., с.* Если существительное имеет два грамматических рода, то указываются оба рода, напр.:

> обжо́ра *м. и ж.* ...

Если существительное употребляется только во множественном числе, оно дается во множественном числе с пометой *мн.,* напр.:

> часы́ *мн.* ...

Если существительное чаще употребляется во множественном числе, оно приводится во множественном числе с пометой *мн.,* а форма единственного числа указывается в скобках с пометой рода, напр.:

> гало́ши *мн. (ед.* гало́ша *ж.)* ...

В тех случаях, когда значения русского существительного имеют различные формы множественного числа, эти формы указываются для каждого значения, напр.:

> коле́н|о *с.* 1. (*мн.* ~и) knee; ... 3. (*мн.* ~ья, ~а) *тех.* ...; 4. (*мн.* ~а) ...

Если слово во множественном числе приобретает другое значение, то переводы этого значения даются после переводов значений единственного числа как новые значения с пометой *мн.*, напр.:

десяток *м.* 1. ...; ... 3. *мн.* (*множество*) dózens, scores; ...

При несовпадении единственного и множественного числа в русском и английском существительном в случае равенства значений при английском переводе дается помета *sg* или *pl*, напр.:

белила *мн.* 1. (*краска*) whiting *sg*; ...

Множественное число английских существительных латинского и греческого происхождения приводится в скобках, напр.:

гипотеза *ж.* hypóthesis (*pl* -ses).

При несклоняемых существительных указывается род и дается помета *нескл.*, напр.:

пальто *с. нескл.* ...

При существительных с собирательным значением дается помета *собир.*, напр.:

беднота *ж. собир.* the poor *pl*; ...

И м е н а п р и л а г а т е л ь н ы е даются в полной форме мужского рода в именительном падеже единственного числа.

Если в мужском роде прилагательное не употребляется, то оно приводится в том роде, в каком употребляется, напр.:

беременная prégnant; ...

Если краткая форма прилагательного имеет самостоятельное значение, она приводится в основном гнезде прилагательного, а на своем месте по алфавиту дается со ссылкой, напр.:

велик *см.* великий.
велик|ий 1. ... ; 2. *тк. кратк. ф.* (*слишком большой*) (too) big; ...

Если английский эквивалент русского прилагательного употребляется только предикативно или должен стоять после существительного, это указывается пометами *predic.* или *после сущ*, стоящими после перевода, напр.:

безынициативный ... without/lácking initiative *после сущ*.

С у б с т а н т и в и р о в а н н ы е п р и л а г а т е л ь н ы е даются в гнезде прилагательного за отдельной цифрой, напр.:

бедный *прил.* 1. ...; ... 6. *в знач. сущ. м.* the poor man*; *мн.* the poor.

Если субстантивированное прилагательное употребляется в женском или среднем роде, то это указывается пометой рода после *в знач. сущ*, напр.:

главн|ый *прил.* 1. ...; ...3. *в знач. сущ. с.* the great/chief thing; ...

Если субстантивированное прилагательное стало полностью самостоятельным существительным, например: столовая, мастерская, то оно дается как отдельное слово-существительное.

Краткие прилагательные, употребляющиеся предикативно, даются в статье соответствующего наречия за отдельной цифрой с пометой *в знач. сказ.* или *в знач. сказ. безл.* В целом ряде случаев предикативное краткое прилагательное дается самостоятельной статьей.

безопасно 1. *нареч.* sáfely; ... 2. *в знач. сказ.* it is safe ...

Г л а г о л ы, имеющие несовершенный и совершенный виды, приводятся под формой несовершенного вида, после которой, через запятую дается форма совершенного вида светлым шрифтом. Совершенный вид дается на своем алфавитном месте со ссылкой на соответствующий глагол несовершенного вида, напр.:

багроветь, побагроветь...
побагроветь *сов. см.* багроветь.

При совпадении формы совершенного и несовершенного вида дается помета *несов. и сов.*

Если к несовершенному виду глагола имеются две или больше форм совершенного вида, то все эти формы даются светлым шрифтом.

При этом в тех случаях, когда в каком-либо значении глагола возможна только одна из этих форм совершенного вида, она указывается при данном значении с пометой *сов.*, напр.:

гладить, выгладить, погладить (*вн.*) 1. *сов.* выгладить (*утюжить*) iron (*smth.*) ...; 2. *сов.* погладить (*ласкать*) stroke (*smb., smth.*); ...

Если в одном из значений глагол употребляется только в несовершенном виде, то после цифры дается помета *тк. несов.*, напр.:

белеть, побелеть 1. (*становиться белым*) turn white; 2. *тк. несов.* (*виднеться*) show* white.

Английский перевод в глагольных статьях, как правило, относится к формам обоих видов. Однако пометой *несов. тж.* вводится такой перевод, который относится только к формам несовершенного вида, пометой *сов. тж.* вводится такой перевод, который относится только к формам совершенного вида, напр.:

вывёдывать, вы́ведать (вн.) разг. find* (smth.) out; несов. тж. try to worm (smth.) out.
беси́ться, взбеси́ться... 2. (неистовствовать) rage; сов. тж. fly* into a rage.

Если глагол совершенного вида имеет свое самостоятельное значение, не соотнесенное с формой несовершенного вида, перевод этого значения дается при совершенном виде.

В тех случаях, когда нет общего перевода для форм совершенного и несовершенного вида, каждая из форм разрабатывается отдельно.

Глаголы на -ся даются на своем месте по алфавиту с переводом. Глаголы на -ся, имеющие значение только страдательного залога, которому в английском языке соответствует пассив, в словаре, как правило, не приводятся.

При глаголах указывается у п р а в л е н и е. Если русский глагол и его соответствие в английском языке управляют прямым дополнением, то при русском глаголе курсивом в скобках дается указание (вн.), а при английском глаголе курсивом в скобках дается прямое дополнение в виде (smb., smth.), напр.:

бáловать несов. (вн.) spoil* (smb.); ...

Если русский глагол управляет прямым дополнением, а английский глагол предлогами, при русском глаголе дается указание (вн.), а при английском глаголе прямым шрифтом в скобках — предлог, напр.:

вызывáть, вы́звать 1. (вн.) ...; (посылать за кем-л.) send* (for); ...

Если русский глагол управляет посредством предлога, то этот предлог приводится прямым шрифтом в скобках и дается указание на падеж (курсивом), а управление английского глагола дано, как указано в предыдущем абзаце, напр.:

глазéть несов. (на вн.) разг. gape (at), stare (at).

В сочетаниях внутри словарной статьи управление русского глагола указывается неопределенно-личным местоимением в соответствующем падеже курсивом без скобок, напр.:

глáсност|ь ж. publícity; ◇ предавáть что-л. ~и make* smth. públic.

Если русский глагол управляет неопределенным наклонением, при нем дается указание в скобках (+ инф.); при английском глаголе, управляющем инфинитивом с to, дается указание (+ to inf); если английский глагол требует инфинитива без to, дается указание (+ inf); если английский глагол управляет формой на -ing, это указывается (+ -ing), напр.:

начинáть, начáть 1. (вн., + инф.) begin* (smth., + to inf, + -ing), start (smth., + to inf, + -ing); ...

Все п р и ч а с т н ы е о б о р о т ы даются не самостоятельными вокабулами, а в статье глагола.

В переводах one означает, что в реальной английской фразе на этом месте должно стоять личное местоимение; oneself заменяет собой возвратные местоимения myself, yourself, himself, ourselves, yourselves, themselves;

one's заменяет собой притяжательные местоимения my, your, his, her, our, their, соответствующие формам русского «свой»;

smb. заменяет собой любое существительное, обозначающее лицо, а также личные местоимения в объектной форме (me, you, him, her, us, them);

smth. заменяет собой любое существительное, обозначающее неодушевленный предмет, а также личные местоимения it, them;

smb.'s заменяет собой любое существительное в форме саксонского родительного падежа, притяжательное местоимение, а также конструкцию с предлогом of (в последнем случае существительное с предлогом of ставится после существительного, перед которым стоит smb.'s).

На многосложных русских и английских словах даны ударения.

Если односложное заглавное слово в статье употребляется в косвенном падеже с соответствующим окончанием без ударения, то в этом случае ударение падает на первый слог, напр.:

борт м. ... ; за ~ом (читай: за бóртом).

Английские существительные, прилагательные, наречия и глаголы, изменяющиеся не по общим правилам, в словаре снабжены звездочкой (*).

СПИСОК
УСЛОВНЫХ СОКРАЩЕНИЙ
LIST OF ABBREVIATIONS

Русские

ав. — авиация — aeronautics
авт. — автомобильное дело — motor transport
амер. — американизм — American
анат. — анатомия — anatomy
архит. — архитектура — architecture
астр. — астрономия — astronomy
бакт. — бактериология — bacteriology
безл. — безличная форма — impersonal form
биол. — биология — biology
биохим. — биохимия — biochemistry
бот. — ботаника — botany
бран. — бранное слово, выражение — abusive
буд. — будущее время — future tense
бухг. — бухгалтерия — book-keeping
вводн. сл. — вводное слово — parenthesis
в знач. вводн. сл. — в значении вводного слова — as parenthesis
в знач. нареч. — в значении наречия — as adverb
в знач. прил. — в значении прилагательного — as adjective
в знач. сказ. — в значении сказуемого — as predicate
в знач. сущ. — в значении существительного — as noun
вн. — винительный (падеж) — accusative (case)
воен. — военное дело, военный термин — military
вопр. — вопросительное (местоимение), вопросительная частица — interrogative
вр. — время — tense
в сложн. — в сложных словах — in compounds
г. — 1) год; 2) город — 1) year; 2) town
гг. — годы — years
геогр. — география — geography
геод. — геодезия — geodesy
геол. — геология — geology
гл. — глагол — verb
горн. — горное дело — mining
грам. — грамматика — grammar
груб. — грубое слово, выражение — vulgar
дет. — детская речь — children's speech
дип. — дипломатический термин — diplomacy
др. — другой, другие — other(s)
дт. — дательный (падеж) — dative (case)
ед. — единственное (число) — singular
ж. — женский (род) — feminine
ж.-д. — железнодорожное дело — railway
знач. — значение — sense
зоол. — зоология — zoology
инф. — инфинитив, неопределенная форма глагола — infinitive
ирон. — в ироническом смысле — ironically
иск. — искусство — art
ист. — относящийся к истории; исторический термин — historical
и т. д. — и так далее — etc., et cetera
и т. п. — и тому подобное — and so on
канц. — канцелярское выражение — officialese
карт. — термин карточной игры — card-playing
кг — килограмм — kilogram

кем-л. — кем-либо — by somebody; as somebody
кино — кинематограф — cinema
км — километр — kilometre
книжн. — книжный стиль — bookish
кратк. ф. — краткая форма — short form
кул. — кулинария — culinary
л. — лицо глагола — person of verb
л — литр — litre
лингв. — лингвистика — linguistics
лит. — литература, литературоведение — literature, literary studies
личн. — личная форма, личное (местоимение) — personal form, personal pronoun
лог. — логика — logic
м. — мужской (род) — masculine
м — метр — metre
мат. — математика — mathematics
мед. — медицина — medicine
межд. — междометие — interjection
мест. — местоимение — pronoun
метеор. — метеорология — meteorology
мин. — минералогия — mineralogy
мн. — множественное (число) — plural
мор. — морское дело, морской термин — maritime
муз. — музыка — music
напр. — например — e. g.
нареч. — наречие — adverb
наст. — настоящее время — present tense
научн. — научный термин — scientific term
нескл. — несклоняемое слово — indeclinable
несов. — несовершенный вид глагола — imperfective aspect
обыкн. — обыкновенно — usually
относ. — относительное (местоимение) — relative pronoun
отриц. — отрицательная частица — negative particle
охот. — охотничий термин — hunting
п. — падеж — case
перен. — в переносном значении — figurative sense
погов. — поговорка — saying
полигр. — полиграфия — printing
полит. — политический термин — political
посл. — пословица — proverb
поэт. — поэтическое слово — poetic
пр. — предложный (падеж) — prepositional case
превосх. ст. — превосходная степень — superlative
пренебр. — пренебрежительно — contemptuous
прил. — имя прилагательное — adjective
притяж. — притяжательное (местоимение) — possessive (pronoun)
прич. — причастие — participle
прош. — прошедшее время — past tense
прям. — в прямом значении — in direct sense
р. — 1) река; 2) род — 1) river; 2) gender
радио — радиотехника — radio
разг. — разговорное слово, выражение — colloquial
рд. — родительный (падеж) — genitive (case)
рел. — религия — religion
рыб. — рыболовство, рыбоводство — fishing
с. — средний (род) — neuter

15

сад. — садоводство — horticulture
сказ. — сказуемое — predicate
скл. — склоняется; склонение — declinable; declension
см. — смотри — see
собир. — собирательное (существительное), собирательно — collective noun, collectively
сов. — совершенный вид глагола — perfective aspect
сокр. — сокращение, сокращенно — abbreviation
сочет. — сочетание — combination
спорт. — физкультура и спорт — physical culture and sport
сравнит. ст. — сравнительная степень — comparative
ст. — степень — degree
стр. — строительное дело — building
сущ. — имя существительное — noun
с.-х. — сельское хозяйство — agriculture
тв. — творительный (падеж) — instrumental (case)
театр. — театроведение, театр — theatre
текст. — текстильное дело — textiles
тех. — техника — technical
тж. — также — also
тк. — только — only
торг. — торговля — trade
употр. — употребляется — used
усил. — усилительная частица — intensifier
уст. — устаревшее слово, выражение — obsolete
утверд. — утвердительная частица — affirmative particle

ф. — форма — form
фарм. — фармацевтический термин — pharmaceutical
физ. — физика — physics
физиол. — физиология — physiology
филос. — философия — philosophy
фин. — финансовый термин — finance
фольк. — фольклор — folklore
фото — фотография — photography
хим. — химия — chemistry
церк. — церковное слово, выражение — ecclesiastical
ч. — число — number
числ. — имя числительное — numeral
шахм. — термин шахматной игры — chess
шутл. — шутливое слово, выражение — jocular
эк. — экономика — economics
эл. — электротехника — electricity
юр. — юридический термин — legal

Английские

attr. attributive атрибутивное употребление
etc. et cetera и так далее
inf infinitive инфинитив, неопределенная форма глагола
pl plural множественное число
predic. predicative предикативное употребление
sg singular единственное число

РУССКИЙ АЛФАВИТ

Аа	Ии	Рр	Шш
Бб	Йй	Сс	Щщ
Вв	Кк	Тт	ъ
Гг	Лл	Уу	ы
Дд	Мм	Фф	ь
Ее, Ёё	Нн	Хх	Ээ
Жж	Оо	Цц	Юю
Зз	Пп	Чч	Яя

А

а I *союз* **1.** (*при сопоставлении, восклицаниях и вопросах*) and; *часто не переводится;* (*при противопоставлении*) but; он инженер, а я врач he's an engineer, (and) I'm a doctor; а вот и он! (and) here he is!; а ты куда? (and) where are you going?; а это кто? and who's that?; я его видел, а он меня нет I saw him, but he didn't see me; не ..., а ... not ... but...; instead of; не 10, а 11 not ten, but eleven; 10, а не 11 ten — not eleven; направо, а налево to the right — not to the left; выплачивать единовременно, а не по частям pay* not by instalments but in a lump sum, pay* in a lump sum instead of by instalments; **2** (*в знач. но, однако*) but; *после предложений с уступительными союзами не переводится*; здесь очень весело, а надо уходить it's very nice here, but I must be going; хотя здесь весело (как здесь ни весело), а надо уходить nice as/though it is here, I must be going; **3.** (*служит для усиления*) but; *обычно не переводится*; а я сам это видел! (but) I saw it with my own eyes!; а я так и сказал ему! I told him!, I did tell him!; поторопись, а (не) то опоздаешь hurry, or (else) you'll be late.

а II *частица разг.* (*при повторном обращении*) **1.** hi!, hi there!; мальчик, а мальчик! hi there, boy!; **2.** *вопр.* eh?

а III *межд.* a!, oh!, ah!

абажур *м.* (lamp-)shade.

аббат *м.* **1.** abbot; **2.** (*во Франции*) abbé. **~ство** *с.* abbey.

аббревиатура *ж.* abbreviation.

аберрация *ж.* aberration.

абзац *м.* **1.** (*отступ в начале строки*) indention; с (нового) ~а indent; (new) paragraph; **2.** (*часть текста*) paragraph.

абитуриент *м.*, ~ка *ж.* university entrant, candidate for university/college admission.

абонемент *м.* season-ticket; межбиблиотечный ~ interlibrary loan system.

абонент *м.* subscriber; (*телефона*) telephone subscriber; (*библиотеки*) reader, borrower.

абориген *м.* aboriginal.

аборт *м.* abortion.

абрикос *м.* **1.** (*плод*) apricot; **2.** (*дерево*) apricot-tree. **~овый** apricot *attr.*

абсолютн|ый absolute; ~ покой complete rest; ~ое невежество complete/utter/abysmal ignorance; ◇ ~ое большинство absolute/overwhelming majority; ~ слух perfect ear, absolute pitch; ~ чемпион absolute/overall champion.

абстрактный abstract.

абстракцион|изм *м.* abstractionism. **~ист** *м.* abstract artist. **~истский** abstractionist.

абстракция *ж.* abstraction.

абсурд *м.* nonsense; довести что-л. до ~а carry smth. to the point of absurdity. **~ность** *ж.* absurdity. **~ный** absurd, ridiculous, nonsensical, ludicrous.

абсцесс *м. мед.* abscess.

абсцисса *ж. мат.* absciss, abscisa (*pl* -sas, -sae).

абхаз|ец *м.*, ~ка *ж.* Abkhazian. **~ский** Abkhazian; ~ский язык Abkhazian, the Abkhazian language.

авангард *м.* van, vanguard; *воен.* advance guard; идти, быть в ~е be* in the forefront/van/vanguard.

авангард|изм *м.* avant-gardism. **~ист** *м.* avant-gardist. **~истский** avant-garde *attr.*

авангардный vanguard *attr.*; (*передовой, ведущий*) leading.

аванс *м.* advance; выдать ~ в размере 10% make* an advance of 10%; выдать кому-л. ~ за месяц advance smb. a month's salary; ~ в счёт зарплаты advance on one's salary; ◇ делать ~ы make* overtures/advances. **~ировать** *несов. и сов.* (*вн.*) make* an advance/prepayment (to), advance money (to); ~ировать завод grant credits to a factory; ~ировать строительство advance money for building. ~ом in advance; платить ~ом pay* in advance.

авансцена *ж.* proscenium.

авантюр|а *ж.* adventure; (*рискованное дело тж.*) hazardous affair, gamble, venture; военная ~ military adventure/gamble. **~изм** *м.* adventurism. **~ист** *м.* adventurer. **~истка** *ж.* adventuress. **~ный 1.** (*рискованный*) risky, hazardous; (*неблаговидный*) shady, doubtful; **2.** (*приключенческий*) adventure *attr.*; ~ный роман novel of adventure; (*литературный жанр*) picaresque novel.

аварийн|ость *ж.* accident rate; breakdowns *pl*; борьба с ~остью accident precautions *pl.* **~ый 1.** emergency *attr.*; ~ый сигнал accident alarm; в ~ом состоянии unsafe; ~ый запас emergency stock; **2.** (*предназначенный для устранения аварии*) breakdown *attr.*; ~ая машина breakdown lorry.

авари|я *ж.* (*порча машины, механизма*) breakdown; (*крушение*) crash; (*несчастный случай*) accident; *перен. разг.* mishap; потерпеть ~ю have* an accident; (*о самолёте*) crash; (*быть повреждённым*) be* damaged.

август *м.* August; в ~е этого года this/in August; в ~е прошлого года last August, last year in August; в ~е будущего года next August. **~овский** August *attr.*

авиа- *в сложн.* air-; aircraft *attr.*

авиа|база *ж.* airbase. **~десант** *м.* airborne landing. **~десантный**: ~десантные войска airborne troops. **~компания** *ж.* airline. **~конструктор** *м.* aircraft designer. **~линия** *ж.* (air-)route. **~моделизм** *м.* aircraft modelling. **~моделист** *м.* model aircraft constructor. **~модель** *ж.* model aircraft. **~носец** *м.* aircraft carrier. **~письмо** *с.* airletter. **~почта** *ж.* airmail; отправлять что-л. ~почтой send* smth. (by) airmail; ~транспорт *м.* air transport. **~транспортный** air(-transport) *attr.* **~трасса** *ж.* air-route; международная ~трасса international air-route.

авиационный aircraft *attr.*; aviation attr. *амер.*; ~ завод aircraft factory/works; ~ мотор aircraft engine; ~ая промышленность aircraft industry; ~ая школа flying school.

авиация *ж.* **1.** (*теория*) aviation; **2.** (*воздушный флот*) aircraft *pl*; военная ~ air force; гражданская ~ civil air fleet; транспортная ~ transport aircraft; сельскохозяйственная ~ agricultural aircraft.

авóсь *разг.* perháps, let's hope; ◇ на ~ on the óff-
-chance.

авóська *ж. разг.* string (shópping) bag.

аврáл *м. мор.* áll-hands evolútion; *перен.* all hands'
job, emérgency job.

аврáльный emérgency *attr.*

австрал│иец *м.,* ~ийка *ж.* Austrálian. ~ийский
Austrálian.

австр│иец *м.,* ~ийка *ж.* Áustrian. ~ийский Áustrian.

áвто- *в сложн.* 1. *(само-, собственный)* áuto-; 2.
(автомобильный) mótor-.

автобáза *ж.* (mótor-)transport dépot; *(место стоянки и ремонта автомобилей)* gárage.

автобиографи́ч│еский, ~ный autobiográphical.

автобиогрáфия *ж.* autobiógraphy.

автоблокирóвка *ж. ж.-д.* automátic block sýstem.

автóбус *м.* (mótor) bus; *(маршрутный, туристский)* coach; éхать на ~e go* by bus.

автовокзáл *м.* bus/coach státion.

автогéнн│ый autogénous; ~ая свáрка autogénous
wélding.

автогóнки *мн.* mótor rácing *sg.*

автогóнщик *м. спорт.* rácing mótorist, ráce-dríver.

автóграф *м.* áutograph.

автодорóжный road tránsport *attr.*

автодрези́на *ж.* (rail) mótor trólley.

автозавóд *м.* mótor works, car fáctory; áutomobile
plant *амер.*

автозапрáвочн│ый: ~ая стáнция pétrol/sérvice/fíl-
ling státion; gas státion *амер.*

автоинспéк│тор *м.* tráffic wárden/policeman; tráffic
cop *разг.* ~ция *ж.* mótor lícencing and inspéction
depártment; *(надзор)* tráffic contról.

автокáр *м.* mótor trólley, mechánical whéelbarrow.

автокормýшка *ж.* (automátic) féeder.

автокрáн *м.* truck crane.

автóл *м.* mótor oil.

автолюби́тель *м.* mótorist, mótoring fan.

автомагистрáль *ж.* trunk road, híghway.

автомáт *м.* 1. *(машина)* automátic machíne; *(действующий при опускании монеты)* slót-machine; ~ для
размéна дéнег cóin-exchange box; 2. *(о человеке)*
áutomaton; róbot; 3. *(оружие)* súbmachine-gun; tómmy-
-gun *разг.*

автоматиз│áция *ж.* automátion. ~и́ровать *несов. и
сов. (вн.)* áutomate (*smth.*).

автомáтика *ж.* 1. *(отрасль науки и техники)*
automátion; 2. *(совокупность механизмов)* automátic
machínery/devíces.

автомати́ческий automátic.

автомáтчик *м. воен.* súbmachíne-gunner.

автомаши́на *ж.* mótor véhicle; *(легковая)* (mótor-)
car; *(грузовая)* lórry; truck *амер.*

автомобилестроéние *с.* automótive/áutomobile
índustry.

автомобил│и́зм *м.* mótoring. ~и́ст *м.* mótorist.

автомоби́л│ь *м. (легковой)* (mótor-)car; áutomobile
амер.; (грузовой) lórry; truck *амер.;* санитáрный ~
ámbulance; ~ технической помощи bréakdown van;
sérvice truck *амер.;* éхать на ~e go* by car; постáвить ~
на стоянку park a car.

автомоби́льн│ый mótor(-car) *attr.;* áutomobile *attr.
амер.;* ~ая дорóга mótor-road; ~ая промышленность
mótor/áutomobile índustry.

автоном│ия *ж.* autónomy. ~ный autónomous; ~ная
респýблика autónomous repúblic; ~ная óбласть
autónomous région.

автопáрк *м.* mótor-véhicle pool; *(легковых автомобилей)* car pool.

автопилóт *м.* automátic/róbot pílot.

автопогрýзчик *м.* automátic lóader, fórk-lift truck.

автопои́лка *ж.* automátic drínker.

автопокры́шка *ж.* (mótor-)tyre.

автопортрéт *м.* self-pórtrait.

автопробéг *м.* mótor-race, mótor rálly.

áвтор *м.* áuthor; *(литературного произведения
тж.)* wríter; *(музыкального произведения)* compóser.

авторáлли *с. нескл.* mótor rálly.

авторемóнтный mótor-repáir *attr.*

авторефе́рáт *м.* (áuthor's) ábstract.

авторизóванный áuthorized.

авторитáрный authoritárian.

авторитéт *м.* authórity; *(влияние тж.)* prestíge;
быть ~ом в чём-л. be* an authórity on *smth.;* пóльзоваться ~ом у кого-л., среди кого-л. have* authórity with
smb.; have*/enjóy prestíge with/amóng *smb.;* завоевáть ~
gain/win* prestíge/authórity. ~ный authóritative; ~ое
мнéние cómpetent/éxpert opínion.

áвторск│ий *прил.* 1. áuthor's; ~ое прáво cópyright;
нарушéние ~ого прáва infríngement of cópyright, píracy;
~ вéчер recítal (of *one's* own works); 2. *в знач. сущ. мн.
разг.* róyalties, áuthor's fees.

áвторство *с.* áuthorship.

авторýчка *ж.* fóuntain-pen.

автосéрвис *м.* sérvice státion, gárage.

автострáда *ж.* mótorway; híghway *амер.*

автотрáкторный mótor-vehicle and tráctor *attr.*

автотрáнспорт *м.* mótor tránsport.

автотрáсса *ж.* mótorway.

автотури́ст *м.* car tóurist.

агáт *м.* ágate.

агглютинати́вн│ый *лингв.* agglútinative; ~ые языки́
agglútinative lánguages.

агглютинáция *ж.* agglutinátion.

агéнт *м.* ágent; *(представитель тж.)*
represéntative; ~ по снабжéнию supply ágent; ~ уголóв-
ного рóзыска police inspéctor; detéctive. ~ство *с.*
ágency.

агентýр│а *ж.* 1. intélligence/sécret sérvice; 2. *собир.
(агенты)* ágents *pl.* ~ный: ~ная развéдка sécret sérvice;
~ные свéдения sécret-service informátion *sg.*

агитáтор *м.* propagándist, ágitator; *(агитирующий
за кандидата)* cánvasser.

агитациóнный propagánda *attr.*

агитáция *ж.* propagánda, agitátion.

агитбригáда *ж.* ágitprop team.

агити́ровать, сагити́ровать 1. *тк. несов. (за вн.)*
campáign (for), ágitate (for), cárry on propagánda (for),
make* propagánda (for); 2. *(вн.) разг. (убеждать в
чём-л.)* urge (*smb.*); *сов. тж.* persuáde (*smb.*).

агитколлекти́в *м.* team of ágitators.

агитмáссов│ый máss-propagánda *attr.;* ~ая рабóта
propagánda work amóng the másses.

агитпýнкт *м.* agitátion céntre; *(во время выборов)*
pólling státion; eléction campáign céntre/óffice.

агóн│ия *ж.* (déath-)agony; déath-throes *pl,* déath-
-pangs *pl;* быть в ~ии be* in *one's* déath-agony.

аграрн│ый agrárian; ~ая рефóрма agrárian refórm.

агрегáт *м.* únit; set, assémbly; убóрочный ~
hárvesting únit; посевнóй ~ sówing únit; силовóй ~ pówer
únit; генерáторный ~ génerating set.

агресси́вный aggréssive.

агрéсс│ия *ж.* aggréssion. ~ор *м.* aggréssor.

агробиолóгия *ж.* agrobiólogy.

агронóм *м.* agrónomist, agricúlturist. ~и́ческий
agronómic(al). ~ия *ж.* agrónomy, agricúltural science.

агротéхн│ик *м.* crop spécialist. ~ика *ж.* agrotéchnics,
agricúltural/fárming práctices *pl,* scientífic fárming. ~и́че-
ский agrotéchnical.

агрохи́мия *ж.* agricúltural chémistry.

ад *м.* hell.

адаптáция *ж.* adaptátion.

адáптер *м.* píck-up.

адапти́ровать *несов. и сов.* (*вн.*) adápt (*smth.*).

адвока́т *м.* láwyer; attórney *амер.*; (*выступающий в суде*) bárrister, ádvocate; (*поверенный*) solícitor; *перен.* ádvocate.

адвокату́р|а *ж.* 1. *собир.* láwyers *pl*, the bar; 2. (*деятельность*) práctice (as a bárrister); занима́ться ~ой práctise at the bar.

адеква́тный equívalent, idéntical, áccurate.

аджа́р|ец *м.*, ~ка *ж.* Adzhár. ~ский Adzhárian.

администрати́вн|ый administrative; ~ аппара́т the administrative staff; ~ое взыска́ние official réprimand; ~ое деле́ние administrative divísion; ◇ в ~ом поря́дке by administrative means.

администр|а́тор *м.* 1. administrator; 2. (*распорядитель*) mánager. ~а́ция *ж.* mánagement, administrátion; вое́нная, гражда́нская, ме́стная ~а́ция mílitary, cívil, lócal authórities *pl*; ~и́рование *с.* high-hánded áction/méasures; го́лое ~и́рование mánagement by decrée.

адмира́л *м.* ádmiral.

адмиралте́йство *с.* the Ádmiralty.

адмира́льский ádmiral's; ~ кора́бль flágship.

а́дрес *м.* addréss; доста́вить письмо́ по ~у delíver a létter at the right addréss; ◇ по его́ ~у abóut him; обрати́ться не по ~у come* to the wrong shop/quárter; э́то по ва́шему ~у that's a dig at you. ~ат *м.* addressée. ~ный: ~ная кни́га diréctory; ~ный стол addréss buréau. ~ова́ть *несов. и сов.* (*вн. дт.*) addréss (*smth.* to). ~ова́ться *несов. и сов.* (*к дт.*, *в вн.*) applý (to).

а́дск|и *разг.* áwfully; ~ий inférnal; héllish; ~ие му́ки tórments of hell; ~ая ску́ка *разг.* intólerable bóredom; ~ий шум *разг.* a hell of a noise, an inférnal din.

адъюта́нт *м.* ádjutant; aide *амер.*; (*генерала*) áide-de-cámp.

ажу́р *м.*: в ~е *разг.* in pérfect órder, típ-tóp.

ажу́рн|ый ópen-work *attr.*; ~ая стро́чка hém-stitch, dráwn-thread work; ~ узо́р lácy desígn/páttern; ◇ ~ая рабо́та filigree work.

аза́рт *м.* excítement; (*увлечение*) férvour; войти́ в ~ get* worked up, get* ínto the swing; в пылу́ ~а in the heat/excítement of the móment; рабо́тать с ~ом work with a will; ~но inténsely, récklessly; ~но игра́ть 1) (*с увлечением*) be* a keen pláyer; 2) (*рискованно*) play récklessly. ~ный réckless, éager, keen; ~ный игро́к 1) (*играющий с увлечением*) keen pláyer; 2) (*рискующий всем*) réckless gámbler; ◇ ~ная игра́ game of chance/házard.

а́збу|ка *ж.* 1. (*алфавит*) álphabet; 2. (*основы*) the ABC; 3. (*букварь*) an ABC(-book); ◇ ~ Мо́рзе Morse code. ~чный: ~чная и́стина trúism.

азербайджа́н|ец *м.*, ~ка *ж.* Azerbaijánian. ~ский Azerbaiján(ian); ~ский язы́к Azerbaijánian, the Azerbaijánian lánguage.

азиа́тский Asian.

а́зимут *м.* ázimuth.

азо́т *м. хим.* nítrogen; о́кись ~а nítric óxide. ~истый *хим.* nítrous.

азотноки́слый *хим.* nítric ácid *attr.*; ~ на́трий sódium nítrate.

азо́тн|ый *хим.* nítric; ~ая кислота́ nítric ácid.

азы́ *мн.* ABC *sg*; rúdiments, élements; начина́ть с азо́в begín* at the véry begínning.

а́ист *м.* stork.

ай *разг.* oh! ◇ ай-ай-а́й! tút-tút!

айв|а́ *ж.* quince; (*дерево тж.*) quínce-tree. ~о́вый quince *attr.*

а́йсберг *м.* íceberg.

акаде́мик *м.* mémber of the Acádemy; Academícian.

академи́ческий acádemic; ~ час téaching périod; э́то представля́ет чи́сто ~ интере́с that is of púrely acádemic válue.

акаде́мия *ж.* 1. Acádemy; Акаде́мия нау́к Acádemy of Sciences; 2. (*учебное заведение*) acádemy, cóllege; вое́нная ~ mílitary cóllege/acádemy.

ака́ция *ж.* acácia; бе́лая ~ black lócust.

аквала́нг *м. спорт.* áqualung. ~и́ст *м.* skín-diver, úriderwater swímmer.

акванавт *м.* áquanaut, úriderwater explórer.

акваре́ль *ж.* 1. (*краски*) wáter-colours *pl*; писа́ть ~ю paint in wáter-colours; 2. (*картина*) wáter-colour (dráwing), aquarélle. ~ный wáter-colour *attr.*; in wáter-colours *после сущ.*; ~ные кра́ски wáter-colours.

аква́риум *м.* aquárium.

акведу́к *м.* áqueduct, cónduit.

акклиматиз|а́ция *ж.* acclimatizátion. ~и́ровать *несов. и сов.* acclímatize (*smb., smth.*). ~и́роваться *несов. и сов.* becóme* acclímatized.

аккомода́ция *ж.* accommodátion, adjústment.

аккомпан|еме́нт *м.* accómpaniment; под ~ чего́-л. to the accómpaniment of *smth.* ~иа́тор *м.* accómpanist. ~и́ровать *несов.* (*дт. на пр.*) accómpany (*smb.* on).

акко́рд *м.* chord; заключи́тельный ~ fínal chord.

аккордео́н *м.* accórdion.

аккордеони́ст *м.* accórdion pláyer.

аккордн|ый: ~ая опла́та труда́ páyment by the piece/job; ~ая рабо́та piecework.

аккредити́в *м. фин.* létter of crédit.

аккредитова́ть *несов. и сов.* (*вн.*) *дип.* accrédit (*smb.*).

аккумуля́тор *м.* báttery, accúmulator.

аккура́тн|о 1. (*опрятно*) néatly; 2. (*тщательно*) thóroughly; он рабо́тает ~ he's a thórough wórker; 3. (*осторожно*) cárefully; 4. (*точно*) áccurately, exáctly; (*о времени и т. п.*) púnctually; он всегда́ прихо́дит ~ he is álways on time; 5. (*регулярно*) régularly. ~ость *ж.* 1. (*опрятность*) néatness; 2. (*тщательность*) thóroughness, atténtion to détail; 3. (*точность*) áccuracy; (*о времени прихода и т. п.*) punctuálity. ~ый 1. (*опрятный*) neat, tídy; 2. (*тщательный*) thórough; 3. (*точный*) áccurate, exáct; (*приходящий вовремя*) púnctual; 4. (*исполнительный*) relíable, consciéntious.

акр *м.* ácre.

акроба́т *м.* ácrobat. ~ика *ж.* acrobátics.

акробати́ческий acrobátic.

акселера́тор *м.* accélerator.

аксио́ма *ж.* áxiom; э́то ~ that's a trúism, that's self-évident.

акт *м.* 1. (*поступок, действие*) act; 2. *театр.* act; коме́дия в трёх ~ах a thrée-áct cómedy; 3. *юр.* deed; обвини́тельный ~ índictment; 4. (*протокол*) státement; соста́вить о чём-л. draw* up a státement on *smth.*; (*о неисправности и т. п.*) draw* up a repórt on *smth.*; 5. (*закон*) Act.

актёр *м.* áctor, pláyer. ~ский áctor's; theátrical; ~ское иску́сство the art of ácting.

акти́в I *м. собир.* the áctivists *pl*, the most áctive mémbers *pl*.

акти́в II *м. фин.* ássets *pl*; в ~е on the crédit side.

активизи́ровать *несов. и сов.* (*вн.*) áctivate (*smb., smth.*); stímulate (*smb., smth.*); ~ рабо́ту speed* up the work. ~ся *несов. и сов.* líven up.

активи́ст *м.* áctive mémber/wórker, áctivist.

акти́вность *ж.* actívity, áction.

акти́вный I áctive.

акти́вный II *фин.*: ~ бала́нс fávourable bálance.

а́ктовый: ~ зал assémbly hall.

актри́са *ж.* áctress.

актуа́льн|ость *ж.* 1. (*насущность*) úrgency; (*злободневность*) topicálity; 2. (*действительное существование*) actuálity. ~ый 1. (*насущный*) úrgent; (*злободневный*) tópical; ~ый вопро́с mátter of cúrrent/tópical ínterest, vítal quéstion; 2. (*существующий в действительности*) áctual.

аку́ла *ж.* shark.

аку́ст|ика ж. acóustics. ~и́ческий acóustic.

акуше́р м. obstetrícian, accouchéur.

акуше́р|ка ж. mídwife*. ~ский obstétric(al). ~ство с. 1. (отдел медицины) obstétrics; 2. (деятельность) mídwifery.

акце́нт м. áccent; (ударение тж.) stress, émphasis; ◇ де́лать ~ на чём-л. stress smth. ~и́ровать несов. и сов. (вн.) stress (smth.); перен. тж. émphasize (smth.).

акционе́р м. sháreholder, stóckholder. ~ный: ~ный капита́л joint stock; ~ное о́бщество jóint-stock cómpany.

а́кци|я I ж. фин. share; привилегиро́ванная ~ preférred share; ~и поднима́ются, па́дают shares are rísing, fálling; ◇ его́ ~и повы́сились his stock stands high; его́ ~и па́дают his stock in góing down.

а́кция II ж. (действие) áction, démarche.

албан|ец м., ~ка ж. Albánian. ~ский Albánian; ~ский язы́к Albánian, the Albánian lánguage.

а́лгебра ж. álgebra. ~и́ческий algebráic(al).

алгори́тм м. álgorithm.

алеба́стр м. álabaster. ~овый álabaster attr.

александри́т м. alexándrite.

але́ть несов. 1. (становиться алым) turn scárlet/red; rédden (о закате) glow; 2. (виднеться) show* red.

алжи́р|ец м., ~ка ж. Algérian. ~ский Algérian.

а́либи с. нескл. юр. álibi; установи́ть чьё-л. ~ estáblish smb.'s álibi; доказа́ть своё ~ prove one's álibi.

алиме́нты мн. álimony sg.

алкало́ид м. хим. álkaloid.

алкоголи́зм м. dipsománia, álcoholism.

алкого́лик м. dipsomániac, alcohólic.

алкого́ль м. álcohol. ~ный alcohólic; ~ные напи́тки alcohólic/strong drinks.

Алла́х м. Állah.

аллегори́ческий allegórical, fígurative.

аллего́рия ж. állegory.

аллерг|е́н м. мед. állergen. ~и́ческий мед. allérgic. ~и́я ж. мед. állergy.

алле́я ж. ávenue; (в парке, саду) path, walk.

аллига́тор м. зоол. álligator.

алло́ hulló!; helló! амер.

аллю́р м. pace.

алма́з м. 1. díamond; 2. (для резки стекла) glázier's díamond. ~ный díamond attr.

ало́э с. нескл. áloe.

алта́йский Altái attr.

алта́рь м. áltar.

алфави́т м. 1. álphabet; по ~у in alphabéticál órder; 2. (перечень чего-л.) alphabéticál list. ~ный alphabéticál; ~ный указа́тель índex (pl -es, índices).

алхи́м|ик м. álchemist. ~ия ж. álchemy.

а́лчн|ость ж. (к дт.) greed (of, for); ~ к деньга́м cupídity. ~ый (к дт.) gréedy (of, for).

а́л|ый red, scárlet; ~ая заря́ crímson sky; ~ стяг scárlet/red bánner; ~ые щёки red/rósy cheeks.

альбо́м м. álbum; (для рисунков) skétch-book; ~ для ма́рок stamp álbum.

альбуми́н м. биохим. álbumen.

альмана́х м. líterary miscéllany.

альпи́йск|ий Álpine; ~ая боле́знь móuntain síckness; ~ая фиа́лка cýclamen; ~ие луга́ Álpine grásslands/méadows.

альпин|и́зм м. móuntain clímbing, mountainéering. ~и́ст м. móuntain clímber, mountainéer. ~и́стский móuntain attr., mountainéer attr.

альт м. 1. (голос, певец) álto; 2. (музыкальный инструмент) vióla.

альтернати́ва ж. altérnative.

альтиме́тр м. ав. áltimeter.

альтру|и́зм м. áltruism, unsélfishness. ~и́ст м. áltruist. ~исти́ческий altruístic, unsélfish.

а́льфа ж. álpha; ◇ ~ и оме́га Álpha and Ómega.

~лучи́ мн. физ. álpha rays. ~-части́ца ж. физ. álpha pártícle.

алюми́н|иевый alumínium attr.; aluminum attr. амер. ~ий м. alumínium; alúminum амер.

аляпова́т|ый 1. (грубо сделанный) crude, tásteless; ~ая бро́шка tásteless/chéap-looking brooch; 2. (грубый, некрасивый) coarse, íll-sháped.

амба́р м. barn, gránary; (для товаров) stórehouse.

амби́ци|я ж. pride, self-respéct; (чванство) vánity; (спесь) árrogance; ◇ уда́риться в ~ю разг. take* offénce, fly* into a huff.

амбразу́ра ж. 1. воен. gún-port; 2. архит. embrásure.

амбулато́р|ия ж. óut-patient/ámbulatory clínic; (при больнице) óut-patient depártment. ~ный: ~ный больно́й óut-patient; ~ное лече́ние óut-patient tréatment.

амёба ж. зоол. amóeba.

америка́н|ец м. Américan. ~ка ж. Américan (wóman). ~ский Américan.

амети́ст м. ámethyst.

аммиа́к м. хим. ammónia.

аммона́л м. ámmonal.

аммо́ний м. хим. ammónium.

амнисти́ровать несов. и сов. (вн.) ámnesty (smb.), grant an ámnesty (to).

амни́сти|я ж. ámnesty; объяви́ть ~ю annóunce an ámnesty.

амора́льный amóral; (безнравственный) immóral.

амортиз|а́тор м. shock absórber. ~а́ция ж. 1. эк. depreciátion; amortizátion; 2. тех. sprínging; (гашение колебаний) dámping.

амо́рфный amórphous.

ампе́р м. физ. ámpere. ~метр м. эл. ámmeter.

ампи́р м. иск. Empire style.

амплиту́да ж. физ. ámplitude.

амплуа́ с. нескл. (special) line; его́ ~ — хара́ктерные ро́ли he spécializes in cháracter parts; э́то не его́ ~ it's not in his line.

а́мпула ж. ámpoule.

ампут|а́ция ж. amputátion. ~и́ровать несов. и сов. (вн.) ámputate (smth.).

амуле́т м. ámulet, charm.

аму́р м. миф. Cúpid.

амфи́бия ж. 1. зоол., бот. amphíbian; 2. (самолёт) flýing boat.

амфибра́хий м. лит. ámphibrach.

амфите́атр м. 1. ámphitheatre; 2. театр. (dréss-) circle.

ана́лиз м. análysis (pl -ses); ~ кро́ви blood test; взять кровь на ~ take* blood counts; сде́лать ~ кро́ви на... ánalyse the blood for...

анализи́ровать несов. и сов. (сов. тж. проанализи́ровать) (вн.) ánalyse (smth.).

анали́т|ик м. ánalyst. ~и́ческий analýtical; ~и́ческий ум analýtical mind; ◇ ~и́ческая геоме́трия analýtic(al) geómetry; ~и́ческая хи́мия analýtical chémistry; ~и́ческие языки́ analýtic lánguages.

аналоги́чн|ый analógous; быть ~ым чему-л. be* análogous to/with smth., be* símilar to smth.; со мной произошёл ~ слу́чай much the same thing háppened to me, I once found mysélf in símilar case.

анало́гия ж. análogy; по ~и by análogy; проводи́ть ~ю с чем-л. draw* a párallel with smth.

анана́с м. (плод и растение) píneapple. ~ный píneapple attr.

ана́пест м. лит. ánapaest.

анарх|и́зм м. ánarchism. ~и́ст м. ánarchist. ~и́стский ánarchist attr. ~и́ческий anárchic. ~и́чный chaótic, disórderly.

ана́рхия ж. ánarchy; (полный беспорядок тж.) cháos.

ана́рхо-синдикали́зм м. anárcho-sýndicalism.

ана́том *м.* anátomist. ~и́ровать *несов. и сов. (вн.)* disséct (*smth.*). ~и́ческий anatómical; ~и́ческий а́тлас hándbook of anatómical charts; ◇ ~и́ческий теа́тр dissécting room.

анато́мия *ж.* anátomy.

анахрони́зм *м.* anáchronism.

ангáр *м.* hángar, áirshed.

а́нгел *м.* ángel.

а́нгельск│ий angélic; ~ая улы́бка angélic smile; ~ое терпе́ние the pátience of an ángel.

ангидри́д *м. хим.* anhýdride.

ангина *ж. мед.* tonsillítis, quínsy.

англи́йск│ий Énglish; (*относящийся к Великобритании*) British; ~ язы́к Énglish, the Énglish lánguage; ~ая делега́ция British delegátion; ◇ ~ая була́вка sáfety pin.

англика́нск│ий Ánglican; ~ая це́рковь the Church of England, the Ánglican Church.

англици́зм *м.* Ánglicism.

англича́н│ин *м.* Énglishman*; *мн. собир.* the Énglish; (*о населении Великобритании тж.*) the British. ~ка *ж.* Énglishwoman*.

а́нгло-америка́нский Ánglo-Américan.

англоса́кс *м.*, ~кий Ánglo-Sáxon.

анго́рск│ий Angóra; ~ая ко́шка Angóra/Pérsian cat; ~ая коза́ Angóra goat.

анекдо́т *м.* stóry, joke; хоро́ший, смешно́й ~ good*, fúnny stóry; остроу́мный ~ amúsing stóry; э́то про́сто ~ it's símply ridículous.

анекдоти́ческий impróbable, extraórdinary; э́то но́сит ~ хара́ктер it seems hárdly sérious. ~и́чный impróbable, cómical; ~и́чный слу́чай incrédible/extraórdinary thing.

анем│и́чный anǽmic. ~и́я *ж.* anǽmia.

анестезио́лог *м.* anaesthesiólogist.

анестез│и́ровать *несов. и сов. (вн.) мед.* anǽsthetize (*smth.*). ~и́я *ж.* anaesthésia; о́бщая ~и́я géneral anaesthésia; ме́стная ~и́я lócal anaesthésia.

анили́н *м. хим.* ániline. ~овый ániline *attr.*; ~овые кра́ски ániline dyes.

ани́с *м.* 1. (*растение*) ánise; 2. (*сорт яблок*) ánise ápple. ~овый: ~овое се́мя ániseed.

а́нкер *м.* 1. *тех.* ánchor, hóldfast; 2. (*в часах*) ánchor escápement.

анке́т│а *ж.* questionnáire, form; заполни́ть ~у fill in/up a form. ~и́рование *с.* survéying, pólling (by questionnáire). ~ный: ~ные да́нные biográphical particulars.

анна́лы *мн.* ánnals, récords.

аннекси́ровать *несов. и сов. (вн.)* annéx (*smth.*).

анне́ксия *ж.* annexátion.

аннот│а́ция *ж.* synópsis. ~и́ровать *несов. и сов. (вн.)* synópsize (*smth.*).

аннули́р│ование *с.* annúlment; (*постановления, решения*) cancellátion; (*отмена*) abrogátion. ~ова́ть *несов. и сов. (вн.)* annúl (*smth.*); (*долг, постановление*) cáncel (*smth.*); (*мандат и т. п.*) núllify (*smth.*); (*отменять*) ábrogate (*smth.*); догово́р ~ован the cóntract is decláred null and void; ~ова́ть бронь cáncel a reservátion.

ано́д *м. физ.* ánode. ~ный *физ.* anódic.

анома́│лия *ж.* anómaly. ~льный anómalous, irrégular.

анони́м *м.* (*автор сочинения*) anónymous áuthor; (*автор письма*) anónymous correspóndent. ~ка *ж. разг. презр.* anónymous létter. ~ный anónymous; ~ное письмо́ anónymous létter. ~щик *м. разг. презр.* anónymous-létter writer.

ано́нс *м.* annóuncement, nótice.

анса́мбль *м.* ensémble; (*певцов и т. п. тж.*) cómpany; (*небольшой*) group; архитекту́рный ~ architéctural ensémble, group of buildings; ~ пе́сни и пля́ски Song and Dance Cómpany.

антагони́зм *м.* antágonism.

антагонисти́ческ│ий antagonístic.

Анта́рктика *ж.* the Antárctic, Antárctica.

антаркти́ческий Antárctic.

анте́нна *ж.* áerial, anténna; передаю́щая ~ transmítting áerial; приёмная ~ recéiving áerial.

анти- *в сложн.* ánti-.

антибио́тики *мн.* (*ед.* антибио́тик *м.*) antibiótics.

антивое́нный ánti-wár, ánti-mílitary.

антиге́н *м. биохим.* ántigen.

антигосуда́рственный (dirécted) agáinst the ínterests of the State *после сущ.*; (*предательский*) tréasonable.

антидемократи́ческий anti-democrátic.

антиистори́ческий unhistórical.

антиква́р *м.* 1. (*продавец*) déaler in antíques, antíque déaler; 2. (*коллекционер*) ántiquary, colléctor of antíques. ~ный antiquárian; ~ная вещь antíque; ~ный магази́н antíque-shop.

антиколониа́льн│ый ánti-colónial.

антиконституцио́нный únconstitútional.

антило́па *ж.* ántelope.

антими́р *м.* antiwórld.

антинаро́дный ánti-nátional, ánti-pópular.

антинау́чный únscientific.

антиобще́ственный antisócial; ~ посту́пок antisócial áction.

антипа́ти│я *ж.* (*к дт.*) antípathy (agáinst, to), avérsion (for, to), dislíke (for, of, to); испы́тывать о́струю ~ю к кому́-л. have* táken a víolent dislíke to *smb.*

антипо́ды *мн.* (*ед.* антипо́д *м.*) antípodes.

антираке́та *ж.* ánti-míssile míssile, ánti-míssile.

антирелигио́зный ánti-relígious.

антисанита́рный insánitary, unsánitary.

антисеми́т *м.* ánti-Sémite. ~и́зм *м.* ánti-Sémitism. ~ский ánti-Semític.

антисепти́ческ│ий antiséptic; ~ое сре́дство antiséptic.

антисове́тский ánti-Sóviet.

антите́за *ж.* antíthesis (*pl* -ses).

антите́ло *с. биохим.* ántibody.

антитокси́н *м.* antitóxin.

антифаши́ст *м.* ánti-fáscist. ~ский ánti-fáscist.

антифри́з *м. ав., авт.* ántifreeze.

антихудо́жественный inartístic; devóid of art *после сущ.*

антицикло́н *м.* anticýclone.

античасти́ца *ж. физ.* ánti-párticle.

анти́чн│ость *ж.* antíquity. ~ый áncient, clássical, Gr(á)eco-Róman; ~ый мир (clássical) antíquity.

антоло́гия *ж.* anthólogy.

анто́ним *м. лингв.* ántonym.

анто́новка *ж.* antónovka ápple.

антра́кт *м.* 1. ínterval; intermíssion *амер.*; 2. (*музыкальное произведение*) éntr'acte, ínterlude.

антраци́т *м.* ánthracite.

антреко́т *м.* rib of beef; entrecôte; steak.

антрепренёр *м.* impresário (*pl* -os), theátrical mánager, diréctor of a theátrical cómpany.

антресо́ли *мн.* 1. áttic *sg*; 2. (*галерея*) gállery *sg*.

антропо́лог *м.* anthropólogist.

антрополо́гия *ж.* anthropólogy.

анфа́с full face; сня́ться ~ be* táken/phótographed full face.

анфила́да *ж.*: ~ ко́мнат suite of rooms.

аншла́г *м.* the "sold out" nótice; пье́са идёт с ~ом the play is dráwing full hóuses.

аню́тин: ~ы гла́зки pánsy *sg*.

ао́рта *ж. анат.* aórta.

апарте́ид *м.* apártheid, rácial segregátion.

апати́т *м. мин.* ápatite. ~овый ápatite *attr.*

апати́чный apathétic; (*равнодушный*) indífferent; (*вялый*) lethárgic, lístless.

апа́тия *ж.* ápathy; (*равнодушие*) indífference.

апелли́ровать *несов. и сов.* 1. *юр.* appéal; ~ в Верхо́вный Суд appéal to the Suprême Court; 2. (*к дт.*; *обращаться за поддержкой и т. п.*) appéal (to); ~ к ма́ссам appéal to the másses.

апелляцио́нн|**ый** appéal *attr.*; ~ая жа́лоба appéal.

апелля́|**ция** *ж.* appéal; пода́ть ~цию send* in an appéal; отклони́ть ~цию dismíss an appéal.

апельси́н *м.* 1. (*плод*) órange; 2. (*дерево*) órange-tree. ~ный, ~овый órange *attr.*; ~овая планта́ция órange-grove; ~ное варе́нье mármalade.

аплоди́ровать *несов.* (*дт.*) appláud (*smb., smth.*), cheer (*smb., smth.*).

аплодисме́нт|**ы** *мн.* appláuse *sg;* clápping *sg;* cheers; продолжи́тельные ~ prolónged appláuse.

апло́мб *м.* assúrance, áplomb, sélf-cónfidence; говори́ть с ~ом speak* glíbly; держа́ться с ~ом be* sélf-assúred; у него́ не хвата́ет ~а he lacks sélf-cónfidence.

апог|**е́й** *м. астр.* ápogee; *перен.* clímax, ácme, zénith; ~ сла́вы height/súmmit/zénith of one's glóry; дости́гнуть своего́ ~е́я reach its clímax.

аполити́чн|**ость** *ж.* political ápathy, indifference to pólitics. ~ый apolítical, kéeping/hólding alóof from pólitics *после сущ.*, indífferent to pólitics *после сущ.*

апологе́т *м.* apólogist, ádvocate.

апоселе́ний *м. астр.* ápolune.

апо́сто|**л** *м.* apóstle. ~льский apostólic.

апостро́ф *м.* apóstrophe.

апофео́з *м.* apotheósis.

аппара́т *м.* 1. apparátus; 2. *физиол.* sýstem; 3. (*совокупность учреждений*) machínery; bódies *pl;* госуда́рственный ~ State machínery, the machínery of State; 4. *собир.* (*штат*) personnél.

аппарату́ра *ж. собир.* apparátus, equípment; (*приборы*) ínstruments *pl.*

аппендици́т *м. мед.* appendicítis.

аппети́т *м.* 1. *тк. ед.* áppetite; дразни́ть чей-л. ~ whet *smb.'s* áppetite, make* *smb.'s* mouth wáter; прия́тного ~a! bon appétit!, I hope you enjóy your bréakfast, lunch, dínner, *etc.;* есть с ~ом eat* with rélish; 2. *обыкн. мн.* (*к дт.*) *разг.* (*желание*) áppetite (for); уме́рить свои́ ~ы curb *one's* áppetite/desíres. ~ный áppetizing.

апплика́ция *ж.* appliqué work.

апре́л|**ь** *м.* Ápril; в э́того го́да this/in Ápril; в ~e про́шлого го́да last Ápril, last year in Ápril; в ~e бу́дущего го́да next Ápril; ◇ пе́рвое ~я All Fools' Day.

апре́льский Ápril *attr.*

априо́р|**и** *adv.* a prióri. ~ный a prióri.

апроби́ровать *несов. и сов.* (*вн.*) (officially), appróve (*smth.*).

апте́к|**а** *ж.* chémist's (shop), phármacy; drúg-store *амер.;* ◇ как в ~ шутл. (right) to a T. ~арский pharmacéutical. ~арь *м.* chémist, phármacist; drúggist *амер.*

апте́ч|**ка** *ж.* first-áid kit; (*ящичек с лекарствами*) médicine chest. ~ный: ~ный за́пах smell of drugs; ~ная посу́да médicine bóttles.

ара́б *м.* Árab.

арабе́ска *ж.* arabésque.

ара́бка *ж.* Árab wóman*.

ара́бск|**ий** Árab; Árabic, Arábian; ~ие стра́ны Árab cóuntries; ~ язы́к Árabic, the Árabic lánguage; ◇ ~ие ци́фры Árabic númerals.

аранжи́р|**овать** *несов. и сов.* (*вн.*) *муз.* arránge (*smth.*). ~о́вка *ж. муз.* arrángement.

ара́хис *м. собир.* ground-nuts *pl,* péanuts *pl.*

арба́ *ж.* wágon; (*на Кавказе*) arbá, búllock cart.

арби́тр *м.* 1. (*посредник в спорах*) árbiter, judge; 2. *спорт.* úmpire.

арбитра́ж *м.* arbitrátion. ~ный arbitrátion *attr.;* ~ный суд court of arbitrátion.

арбу́з *м.* wátermelon.

аргенти́н|**ец** *м.,* ~ка *ж.* Argentínean. ~ский Árgentine.

аргуме́нт *м.* árgument. ~а́ция *ж.* árguments *pl,* réasoning, line of árgument. ~и́ровать *несов. и сов.* (*вн.*) advánce árguments (for); give* réasons (for).

аре́на *ж.* aréna (*тж. перен.*); цирково́вая ~ círcus ring; ~ де́ятельности field/sphere of áction; междунаро́дная ~ internátional scene.

аре́нд|**а** *ж.* 1. (*наём*) lease; (*земли тж.*) ténure; брать что-л. в ~у rent *smth.;* (*на длительное время*) lease *smth.,* take* *smth.* on lease; сдава́ть что-л. в ~у let* *smth.;* (*на длительное время*) lease *smth.,* grant *smth.* on lease; 2. (*плата*) rent. ~а́тор *м.* ténant; lessée, léaseholder. ~ный: ~ный догово́р lease; ~ная пла́та rent. ~ова́ть *несов. и сов.* (*вн.*) rent (*smth.*); lease (*smth.*), have* a lease (on), hold* (*smth.*) on lease.

аре́ст *м.* 1. arrést; взять кого́-л. под ~ put* *smb.* únder arrést; сиде́ть под ~ом be* únder arrést, be* in cústody; 2. *юр.* sequestrátion; наложи́ть ~ на иму́щество seize/sequéster próperty.

аресто́ванный *м.* prísoner.

арестова́ть *несов. и сов.* (*вн.*) arrést (*smb.*).

аристокра́т *м.* áristocrat. ~и́ческий, ~и́чный aristocrátic. ~ия *ж.* aristócracy; фина́нсовая ~ия plutócracy. ~ка *ж.* áristocrat.

аритми́я *ж. мед.* arrhýthmia.

арифме́т|**ика** *ж.* aríthmetic; уче́бник ~ики aríthmetic-book. ~и́ческий aríthmétical; ~и́ческая зада́ча próblem, sum.

арифмо́метр *м.* arithmómeter.

а́рия *ж. муз.* ária, air.

а́рка *ж.* arch.

арка́да *ж. архит.* arcáde.

арка́н *м.* lásso, láriat; лови́ть ~ом lásso.

А́рктика *ж.* the Árctic; Árctic régions *pl.*

аркти́ческий árctic.

арлеки́н *м.* hárlequin.

арма́да *ж.* armáda.

армату́р|**а** *ж. тех.* 1. *собир.* (*приборы*) fíttings *pl;* 2. (*стальной каркас железобетонных сооружений*) steel reinfórcement, steel frámework; reinfórcing bars *pl.* ~щик *м.* steel eréctor; spíderman* *разг.*

арме́йский ármy *attr.*

а́рмия *ж.* ármy; forces *pl;* Сове́тская А́рмия the Sóviet Ármy.

армяни́н *м.* Arménian.

армя́н|**ка** *ж.* Arménian. ~ский Arménian; ~ский язы́к Arménian, the Arménian lánguage.

арома́т *м.* frágrance, pérfume; aróma (*тж. перен.*). ~и́ческий, ~и́чный, ~ный aromátic, frágrant.

арсена́л *м.* ársenal (*тж. перен.*).

арт- в сложн. artíllery.

арта́читься *несов.* 1. (*о лошади*) jib, balk; 2. *разг.* (*упрямиться*) kick; не арта́чься! don't be so stúbborn!

артезиа́нский ~ коло́дец artésian well.

арте́ль *ж.* 1. co-óperative; ~ промысло́вой коопера́ции small prodúcer's co-óperative; сельскохозя́йственная ~ colléctive farm, agricúltural co-óperative; 2. *ист.* artél, work associátion.

артериа́льный *анат.* artérial.

артериосклеро́з *м. мед.* arteriosclerósis, hárdening of the árteries.

арте́рия *ж.* 1. *анат.* ártery; 2. (*путь сообщения*) artérial road; во́дная ~ wáterway.

артилле́р|**ийский** artíllery *attr.;* ~ ого́нь artíllery fire, shéll-fire. ~и́ст *м.* artílleryman*, gúnner.

артилле́рия *ж.* artíllery; (*орудия тж.*) órdnance; тяжёлая ~ héavy artíllery; лёгкая ~ light artíllery; морска́я ~ nával órdnance; самохо́дная ~ sélf-propélled artíllery;

зени́тная ~ ánti-áircraft artíllery; противота́нковая ~ ánti-tánk artíllery; а́томная ~ atómic artíllery.

арти́ст м. 1. (stáge-)ártist, artíste; (драматический) áctor; (концертный исполнитель) perfórmer; (оперный) (бреа-)singer; (балетный) bállet-dancer; заслу́женный ~ Hónoured Ártist; ~ эстра́ды varíety áctor; 2. разг. (мастер своего дела) an ártist in one's own line.

артисти́ческ|ая ж. dréssing-room; (при концертном зале) perfórmers' room. ~ий 1. artístic; 2. (искусный) skílful.

арти́стка ж. artíste; (драматическая) áctress и т. д., ср. арти́ст.

артишо́к м. бот. ártichoke.

артналёт м. artíllery attáck.

артобстре́л м. artíllery bombárdment.

артподгото́вка ж. preparátion fire, sóftening-up.

артри́т м. мед. arthrítis.

а́рф|а ж. harp; ◇ Эо́лова ~ Aeólian harp. ~и́ст м., ~и́стка ж. hárp-player, hárpist.

арха|и́зм м. árchaism. ~и́ческий archáic.

архео́|лог м. archaeólogist. ~логи́ческий archaeológical. ~ло́гия ж. archaeólogy.

архи́в м. 1. (учреждение) Árchives pl, Récord Óffice; (отдел в учреждении) régistry; 2. (письма, документы и т. п.) árchives pl; (личные документы и т. п.) pápers pl; ры́ться в ~ах delve ínto the récords, go* through the files; ◇ сдава́ть что-л. в ~ file smth.; перен. give* smth. up as a bad job. ~ный árchive(s) attr.

архиепи́скоп м. árchbishop.

архиере́й м. bishop.

архипела́г м. archipélago.

архите́кт|ор м. árchitect. ~у́ра ж. árchitecture. ~у́рный architéctural; ~у́рный институ́т acádemy/institute of árchitecture.

арши́н м. уст. archín (=27.95 inches); ◇ ме́рить всех на свой ~ judge/méasure óthers by one's own yárd-stick; сло́вно ~ проглоти́л as stiff as a póker/rámrod.

арык м. irrigátion ditch.

арьерга́рд м. réarguard. ~ный réarguard attr.

ас м. (air) ace; перен. wízard.

асбе́ст м. asbéstos. ~овый asbéstos attr.

асепти́ческий aséptic, stérile.

асимметр|и́ческий, ~и́чный asymmétrical. ~и́я ж. asýmmetry, want/lack of sýmmetry.

аске́т м. ascétic. ~и́зм м. ascéticism. ~и́ческий ascétic.

аскорби́нов|ый: ~ая кислота́ хим. ascórbic ácid.

аспе́кт м. áspect; в э́том ~е regárded in that light; под други́м ~ом from anóther ángle/view-point.

аспира́нт м., ~ка ж. póst-gráduate (stúdent); gráduate stúdent амер. ~у́ра ж. póst-gráduate course.

аспири́н м. áspirin(e).

ассамбле́я ж. assémbly; 20-я се́ссия Генера́льной Ассамбле́и the 20th Géneral Assémbly.

ассенизáция ж. cléaring/émptying of césspools, séwage dispósal.

ассигн|ова́ние с. 1. assignátion, allocátion, appropriátion; 2. мн. (суммы) allocátions. ~ова́ть несов. и сов. (вн. на вн.) assign (smth. to, for); apprópriate (smth. for); (вн. дт.) állocate (smth. to).

ассимил|и́ровать несов. и сов. (вн.) assímilate (smb., smth.). ~и́роваться несов. и сов. (с тв.) becóme* assímilated (to). ~я́ция ж. assimilátion.

ассисте́нт м., ~ка ж. 1. assístant; 2. (преподаватель вуза) assístant lécturer.

ассисти́ровать несов. (дт.) assíst (smb.).

ассортиме́нт м. 1. (подбор) assórtment; хоро́ший ~ това́ров a large seléction of goods; расширя́ть ~ това́ров make* a wíder varíety of goods aváilable; 2. (комплект) set.

ассоциа́ция ж. associátion.

ассоции́р|овать несов. и сов. (вн. с тв.) assóciate (smth. with). ~оваться несов. и сов. (с тв.) assóciate (with); с чем э́то у вас ~уется? what do you assóciate it with?

астеро́ид м. астр. ásteroid.

астигмати́зм м. опт. astígmatism.

а́стма ж. мед. ásthma. ~ти́ческий asthmátic.

а́стра ж. áster.

астра́льный ástral.

астробота́ника ж. astrobótany.

астрогеоло́гия ж. astrogeólogy.

астро́лог м. astróloger.

астроло́гия ж. astrólogy.

астрона́вт м. ástronaut; (космонавт тж.) spáce-man*. ~ика ж. astronáutics.

астроно́м м. astrónomer. ~и́ческий astronómical (тж. перен.); ◇ ~и́ческие ци́фры vast sums, astronómical figures. ~ия ж. astrónomy.

астрофи́зик м. astrophýsicist.

астрофи́зика ж. astrophýsics.

астрофизи́ческ|ий astrophýsical; ~ая обсервато́рия astrophýsical obsérvatory; ~ие наблюде́ния astrophýsical observátions.

асфа́льт м. 1. ásphalt; 2. (дорога) hárd-súrface/métalled road. ~и́ровать несов. и сов. (вн.) ásphalt (smth.). ~овый ásphalt attr.; (покрытый асфальтом) ásphalted, métalled.

атав|и́зм м. átavism. ~исти́ческий atavístic.

ата́к|а ж. attáck; (пехотная, кавалерийская тж.) charge; возду́шная ~ air attáck; идти́ в ~у make* an attáck; charge; перейти́ в ~у switch to the attáck. ~ова́ть несов. и сов. (вн.) attáck (smb., smth.), make* an attáck (on); charge (smb., smth.).

атама́н м. 1. ист. átaman, Cóssack chíeftain; 2. (главарь, предводитель) chief.

ате|и́зм м. átheism. ~и́ст м. átheist. ~исти́ческий atheístic.

ателье́ с. 1. (художника, фотографа) stúdio; 2. (швейная мастерская) táiloring and dréssmaking estáblishment; dréssmaker's; (мужской одежды) táilor's; ~ мод fáshion house; 3.: ~ прока́та réntal/hire sérvice; телевизио́нное ~ télevision sérvice (shop).

атла́с м. 1. (географический) átlas; 2. (собрание рисунков, таблиц, чертежей и т. п.) álbum.

атла́с м. sátin. ~ный 1. (сделанный из атласа) sátin; 2. (похожий на атлас) sátiny.

атле́т м. áthlete. ~ика ж. athlétics; лёгкая ~ика track and field athlétics; тяжёлая ~ика wéightlifting. ~и́ческий 1. athlétic; 2. (свойственный атлету) of an áthlete после сущ.

атмосфе́р|а ж. átmosphere (тж. перен.). ~ный atmosphéric; ~ное давле́ние atmosphéric préssure.

ато́лл м. átoll.

а́том м. átom. ~ник м. разг. núclear spécialist. ~ный atómic, núclear; ~ный вес хим. atómic weight; ~ная бо́мба átom/atómic bomb, Á-bomb; ~ное ору́жие atómic wéapon; ~ная эне́ргия atómic/núclear énergy; ~ное ядро́ atómic núcleus; ~ная электроста́нция atómic/núclear power státion.

атомохо́д м. núclear íce-breaker.

а́томщик м. 1. см. а́томник; 2. átom-bomb wárrior.

атрибу́т м. áttribute. ~и́вный грам. attríbutive.

атроф|и́рованный átrophied. ~и́роваться несов. и сов. átrophy. ~и́я ж. átrophy.

атташе́ м. нескл. attaché.

аттест|а́т м. 1. certíficate; 2. воен. remíttance páper, fámily allótment; ◇ ~ зре́лости schóol-leaving certíficate. ~а́ция ж. 1. (действие) certificátion; 2. (присвоение звания) certificátion (as), promótion (to); 3. (отзыв, характеристика) réference.

аттест|ова́ть несов. и сов. (вн.) 1. (давать отзыв, характеристику) give* (smb.) a réference; 2. (присваивать звание) cértify (smb.) as, promóte (smb.) to; 3.

(*оценивать знания учащихся*) give* (*smb.*) a repórt/mark.

аттракцио́н *м.* 1. (*эффектный номер*) spécial attráction, star turn; 2. (*карусель, тир и т. п.*) síde-show.

аудие́нц|ия *ж.* áudience; дать ~ию кому́-л. give*/grant an áudience to *smb.*; получи́ть ~ию у кого́-л. have* an áudience with *smb.*

аудито́рия *ж.* 1. (*помещение*) lécture-hall, lécture-room; 2. *собир.* (*слушатели*) áudience.

аукцио́н *м.* áuction; продава́ть что́-л. с ~а sell* *smth.* by áuction.

ау́л *м.* aúl, Caucásian víllage.

аутенти́чный authéntic.

афга́н|ец *м.*, ~ка *ж.* Áfghan. ~ский Áfghan.

афе́р|а *ж.* swíndle, fraud; shády transáction. ~и́ст *м.* swíndler; spiv *разг.*

афи́ш|а *ж.* bill, póster; (*небольшая*) nótice; театра́льная ~ pláybill. ~и́ровать *несов. и сов.* (*вн.*) paráde (*smth.*), ádvertise (*smth.*).

афори́зм *м.* áphorism.

африка́н|ец *м.*, ~ка *ж.* Áfrican. ~ский Áfrican.

а́фро-азиа́тский Áfro-Ásian.

ах oh!

а́хать *несов. разг.* sigh, keep* síghing.

ахилле́сов: ~а пята́ weak point, Áchílles' heel.

ахине́|я *ж. разг.* drível, nónsense, rúbbish; нести́ ~ю talk nónsense.

а́хнуть *сов.* gasp; он и ~ не успе́л befóre he could say knife.

ахти́ *разг.:* не ~ како́й! no great shakes!; не ~ како́й актёр, врач *и т. п.* not much of an áctor, dóctor, *etc.*; не ~ как nóthing spécial, not up to much; не ~ что not up to much.

ацетиле́н *м.* acétylene. ~овый acétylene *attr.*

ацето́н *м. хим.* ácetone.

аэро- *в сложн.* aero-, air-.

аэро́бика *ж.* aeróbics.

аэро́бус *м.* áirbus.

аэровокза́л *м.* air términal.

аэродина́м|ика *ж.* aerodynámics. ~и́ческий aerodynámical; ~и́ческая труба́ wind-tunnel.

аэродро́м *м.* áirfield, áerodrome; áirdrome *амер.*

аэрозо́ль *м.* áerosol.

аэроклу́б *м.* ámateur flýing club.

аэро́н *м.* áirsickness táblets *pl.*

аэро|пла́н *м. уст.* áeroplane; áirplane *амер.* ~по́рт *м.* áirport. ~са́ни *мн.* propéller-sleigh *sg.* ~сёв *м.* aerosówing.

аэроста́т *м.* ballóon.

аэроста́тика *ж.* aerostátics.

аэрофотосъёмка *ж.* air/áerial photógraphy, aerosurvéying.

АЭС (*а́томная электроста́нция*) atómic pówer státion.

Б

б *см.* бы.

ба́ба I *ж.* 1. *уст.* (*péasant*) wóman*; 2. *пренебр.* wóman*; (*молодая*) wench; 3. *разг.* (*жена*) wife*, the old wóman*; 4. *ирон.* (*о мужчине*) old wóman*, mílksop, drip; ◇ снéжная ~ snów-man*; ка́менная ~ stone ídol.

ба́ба II *ж. тех.* (*копровая*) ram.

ба́ба III *ж. кул.* (*ромовая*) ~ rum cake/bába.

ба́ба-яга́ *ж.* Bába-Yagá (*a witch in Russian folk tales*), ógress.

ба́б|ий *разг.* wóman's; ◇ ~ье ле́то ≈ Indian súmmer; ~ьи ска́зки old wives' tales/fábles.

ба́бка I *ж.* 1. (*бабушка*) grándmother; 2. *разг.* (*стару́ха*) old wóman*.

ба́бк|а II *ж.* (*надкопытный сустав — у лошади*) pástern; (*у других животных*) knúcklebone.

ба́бочка *ж.* bútterfly; ночна́я ~ moth.

ба́бушка *ж.* grándmother; *ласк.* grándma, gránny; ◇ ~ на́двое сказа́ла we'll see what we'll see.

бага́ж *м.* 1. lúggage; bággage *амер.*; ручно́й ~ hand/small lúggage; сдать ве́щи в ~ в ~ в cláak-room; 2. (*способ отправки вещей*): сдать ве́щи в ~ régister *one's* lúggage; отпра́вить что́-л. ~о́м send* *smth.* on; зал вы́дачи ~а́ bággage claim; ~ интеллектуа́льный ~ intelléctual resóurces *pl*, méntal equípment. ~ник *м.* lúggage compártment, boot; (*на крыше автомашины, в ж.-д. вагоне*) lúggage rack; (*на велосипеде*) cárrier.

баге́т *м.* móulding, béading.

баго́р *м.* hook; (*для лодки*) bóat-hook; (*для рыбной ловли*) gaff.

багрове́ть, побагрове́ть grow*/turn red/crímson/púrple; (*о лице тж.*) flush.

багро́вый crímson; (*с фиолетовым оттенком*) púrple.

бадминто́н *м. спорт.* bádminton.

бадминтони́ст *м.* bádminton pláyer.

бадья́ *ж.* búcket.

ба́з|а *ж.* 1. (*основание, основа чего-л.*) básis, foundátion; экономи́ческая ~ ecónomic básis; материа́льная ~ matérial resóurces *pl*; кормова́я ~ животново́дства fódder/food resóurces for stóck-raising; подвести́ ~у подо что́-л. substántiate *smth.*, give* good grounds for *smth.*, place *smth.* on a sound foundátion/básis; 2. (*опорный пункт*) base; вое́нная ~ mílitary base; вое́нно-морска́я ~ nával base; раке́тная ~ míssile base; 3. (*учреждение по обслуживанию чего-л.*) céntre; тури́стская ~ tóurist hóstel/céntre; 4. (*склад*) dépot.

база́льт *м.* básalt. ~овый básalt *attr.*, basáltic.

база́р *м.* 1. márket; (*восточный*) bazáar; *перен. разг.* béar-garden; 2.: кни́жный ~ book fair/sale. ~ный márket *attr.*; ~ный день márket day; ~ная пло́щадь márket square.

база́дов: ~а боле́знь (exophthálmic) góitre.

бази́ровать *несов.* (*вн. на пр.*) base (*smth.* on, upón), found (*smth.* on, upón), ground (*smth.* on, upón); ~ся *несов.* 1. (*на пр., основываться*) rest (on), be* based/fóunded/gróunded (on); 2. (*размещаться где-л.*) be* based státioned, set* up base, make* *one's* base.

ба́зис *м.* básis (*pl* -ses), foundátion; ~ и надстро́йка básis and súperstructure.

бай-ба́й býe-bye.

байба́к *м.* 1. *зоол.* (steppe) mármot; 2. *разг.* (*ленивый человек*) sléepyhead, lázy-bones.

ба́йк|а I *ж.* flanelétte. ~овый flanelétte *attr.*

ба́йка II *ж. разг.* (*выдумка*) fáble; *мн. тж.* old wives' tales.

бак I *м.* tank; cístern; (*для стирки белья*) bóiler.

бак II *м. мор.* fóre-deck, fórecastle.

бакале́йн|ый grócery *attr.*; ~ая ла́вка grócer's; ~ отде́л grócery depártment.

бакале́я *ж. собир.* gróceries *pl.*

ба́кен *м.* buoy.

бакенба́рды *мн.* (*ед.* бакенба́рда *ж.*) (síde-)whiskers; (*короткие*) sídeburns.

ба́кенщик *м.* buoy kéeper.

баклажа́н *м.* 1. (*плод*) áubergine; 2. (*растение*) égg-plant. ~ный; ~ная икра́ áubergine paste.

баклу́ши: бить ~ idle awáy *one's* time; ≈ twíddle *one's* thumbs.

бактерио́лог *м.* bacteriólogist.

бактериологическ|ий bacteriológical; germ *attr.*; ~ая война germ wárfare.

бактериология ж. bacteriólogy.

бактерия ж. bactérium (*pl* -ia).

бал м. ball; (*небольшой*) dance, dáncing párty.

балаган м. (*зрелище*) show; *перен. разг.* farce, tomfóolery.

балагур м. *разг.* wag, jéster. ~ить *несов. разг.* jest, crack jokes.

балалаечник м. balaláika pláyer.

балалайка ж. balaláika.

баланс м. bálance; годовой ~ ánnual bálance; торговый ~ bálance of trade; мировой топливный ~ world fuel búdget; подвести ~ bálance/square accóunts.

балансир м. 1. *тех.* beam; 2. (*в часах*) bálance.

балансировать *несов.* 1. (*сохранять равновесие*) bálance, keep* one's bálance; 2. (*вн.; приводить в правильное соотношение*) bálance (*smth.*); co-órdinate (*smth.*); 3. (*вн.*) *тех.* bálance (*smth.*).

балансовый bálance *attr.*; ~ отчёт bálance-sheet.

балерина ж. bállet-dancer, ballerína.

балет м. bállet. ~мейстер м. bállet-master. ~ный bállet *attr.*

балка I ж. (*брус*) beam, joist; (*металлическая*) gírder; поперечная ~ cróss-beam.

балка II ж. (*овраг*) ravíne; (*небольшая*) gúlly.

балканский Bálkan.

балкар|ец м., ~ка ж. Balkár. ~ский Balkár; ~ский язык Balkár, the Balkár lánguage.

балкон м. 1. bálcony; 2. *театр.* (*средний ярус*) úpper círcle; (*верхний ярус*) bálcony.

балл м. 1.: ветер в 6 ~ов a fórce-síx wind; землетрясение в 8 ~ов éarthquake of mágnitude eight; 2. (*отметка*) mark; 3. *спорт.* point.

баллада ж. 1. bállad; 2. *муз.* balláde.

балласт м. bállast; *перен.* (*лишнее*) lúmber, dead weight.

баллист|ика ж. ballístics. ~ический ballístic; ~ическая межконтинентальная ракета íntercontinéntal ballístic míssile; ~ические снаряды ballístic míssiles; ~ический снаряд среднего радиуса действия intermédiate-range ballístic míssile.

баллон м. 1. cýlinder; (*резиновая груша*) bulb; газовый ~ gás-container, gás-bag; 2. (*автомобильный*) týre; (*аэростата*) énvelope.

баллотир|овать *несов.* (*кого-л.*) put* (*smb.*) up for eléction; (*что-л.*) put* (*smth.*) to the vote. ~оваться *несов.* (*в вн.*) stand* for eléction (to); stand* for (*smth.*). ~овка ж. vóting, bálloting, pólling.

-балльный 1. (*об отметке*) -mark; пятибалльная система отметок five-márk gráding sýstem; 2. *метеор.*: восьмибалльный шторм fórce-éight gale.

бал-маскарад м. fáncy-dress ball, masked ball, masqueráde.

балованный spoilt, pámpered.

баловать *несов.* (*вн.*) spoil* (*smth.*); (*нежить тж.*) pámper (*smth.*); ~ кого-л. вниманием fávour smb. with atténtion. ~ся *несов.* 1. *разг.* play abóut, play pranks; не балуйся! don't be náughty!, no nónsense!; 2. (*тв.; заниматься чем-л. ради удовольствия*) indúlge (in); dábble (in).

балов|ень м. *разг.* pet; ◇ ~ судьбы mínion of fórtune, fávourite/child* of fórtune. ~ник м. *разг.* míschievous child*, scamp, imp. ~ство с. *разг.* 1. (*потакание*) spóiling; (*потворство*) spóiling; 2. (*шалость*) náughtiness; pranks *pl*, tricks *pl*.

балтийский Báltic.

балык м. balýk (*cured fillet of sturgeon*).

бальзамировать, набальзамировать (*вн.*) embálm (*smth.*).

бальн|ый ball *attr.*; ~ое платье báll-dress; ~ые танцы báll-room dánces.

балюстрада ж. *архит.* bálustrade.

бамбук м. bambóo. ~овый bambóo *attr.*

банальн|ость ж. 1. triviálity, banálity; 2. (*банальная мысль и т. п.*) cómmonplace, plátitude. ~ый cómmonplace, trite; ~ый разговор trívial conversátion, exchánge of plátitudes.

банан м. (*плод и растение*) banána.

банда ж. gang, band.

бандаж м. 1. *мед.* súrgical córset, abdóminal suppórt; (*грыжевый*) truss; 2. (*колёсный*) týre, hoop; *ж.-д.* rim.

бандероль ж. 1. (*бумажная обёртка*) póstal wrápper; 2. (*почтовое отправление*) prínted mátter; посылать что-л. ~ю send* smth. by bóok-post, send* smth. as prínted mátter.

банджо с. *нескл.* bánjo.

бандит м. thug, cút-throat; (*разбойник*) bándit, brígand; gángster *амер.* ~изм м. gángsterism, thúggery. ~ский: ~ский налёт múrderous attáck; ~ская шайка gang of thugs.

банк м. bank; Государственный ~ the State Bank; класть деньги в ~ depósit móney at a bank.

банк|а I ж. 1. (*стеклянная*) jar, pot; (*металлическая, консервная*) tin; can *амер.*; ~ для варенья jám-pot; ~ с вареньем pot of jam; 2. *обыкн. мн. мед.* cúpping glass *sg*, súction cup *sg*; ставить ~и кому-л. cup *smb.*, apply cups to *smb.*

банка II ж. (*сиденье на шлюпке*) thwart.

банка III ж. *мор.* (*отмель*) (sánd-)bank, shoal.

банкет м. bánquet; устраивать ~ give* a bánquet.

банкир м. bánker.

банковский: ~ капитал bánking cápital; ~ служащий bank employée.

банков|ый: ~ое дело bánking; ~ билет bánk-note.

банкрот м. bánkrupt; *перен. тж.* fáilure; объявлять кого-л. ~ом decláre smb. bánkrupt; объявить себя ~ом go* bánkrupt. ~ство с. bánkruptcy; *перен. тж.* fáilure.

банный bath *attr.*

бант м. bow. ~ик м. little bow; ◇ губки ~иком Cúpid's bow.

банту *нескл.* Bántu.

бан|щик м., ~щица ж. báth-attèndant.

бан|я ж. báth-house; коммунальные ~и públic baths; здесь настоящая ~! this place is like a bóiler-house! ◇ задам ему ~ю! I'll give him what for!

бар м. bar.

барабан м. drum. ~ить *несов.* 1. drum, tattóo; (*о дожде*) pátter; ~ить пальцами по стеклу drum on the window-pane; 2. *разг.* (*на рояле*) bang, thump. ~ный: ~ный бой drúmbeat, roll of drums; ~ная палочка drúmstick; ◇ ~ная перепонка *анат.* éar-drum; tympánic mémbrane *научн.* ~щик м. drúmmer.

барак м. hut.

баран м. ram, sheep*; кастрированный ~ wéther. ~ий 1. ram's; (*о меховом изделии*) shéepskin *attr.*; ~ий тулуп shéepskin coat; 2. (*о кушанье*) mútton *attr.*; ~ья котлета mútton chop; ~ий жир mútton fat/dripping; ◇ согнуть кого-л. в ~ий рог make* smb. knúckle únder/down. ~ина ж. mútton; молодая ~ина lamb.

баранка ж. 1. baránka, bágel (*ring-shaped roll*); 2. *разг.* (*руль автомобиля*) the wheel.

барахло с. *собир. разг.* 1. (*старые вещи*) goods and cháttels *pl*; (*старая одежда*) old clothes *pl*; 2. (*хлам*) trash, rúbbish, old íron.

барахтаться *несов. разг.* strúggle, flóunder.

барачн|ый bárrack-like; ~ая постройка témporary building/strúcture; préfab; ~ого типа light-constrúction *attr.*; préfab *attr.*

бараш|ек м. 1. lamb; 2. (*мех*) lámbskin; (*каракуль*) ástrakhan; 3. *тех.* wíng-nut. ~ки *мн.* 1. (*облака*) máckerel sky *sg*, fléecy clouds; 2. (*гребни волн*) white hórses, white caps. ~ковый lámbskin *attr.*; (*каракуле-*

вый) ástrakhan attr.; ~ковая шáпка ástrakhan hat; ~ковый воротни́к ástrakhan cóllar.

барбари́с м. 1. собир. (ягоды) bárberries pl; 2. (об отдельной ягоде) bárberry; 3. (растение) bárberry.

барелье́ф м. bás-relief.

бáржа ж. barge.

бáрий м. хим. bárium.

бáрин м. 1. ист. (помещик) lándowner, squíre; 2. уст. géntleman*; (хозяин) máster; (как обращение) sir; Your Hónour; 3. разг. lord, lóunger; ◇ жить ~ом live a life of ease.

барито́н м. báritone.

бáрка ж. wóoden barge.

бáркас м. 1. (весельный) rówing-boat; рыбáчий ~ fishing-boat; 2. (портовый) launch.

барокáмера ж. préssure chámber.

барóкко с. нескл. иск. baróque; в сти́ле ~ in baróque.

барóметр м. barómeter; ~ пáдает, поднимáется the barómeter is fálling, rísing. ~и́ческий barométric.

баррикáд|а ж. barricáde; стрóить ~ы make*/eréct barricádes. ~и́ровать, забаррикади́ровать (вн.) barricáde (smth.). ~ный barricáde attr.

барс м. зоол. pánther.

бáрск|ий máster's; (высокомерный) lórdly; ~ дом mánsion; (в деревне) mánor(-house); ~ие замáшки háughty/lórdly ways/mánners; ~ая спесь háughtiness; ~ое отношéние к дéлу lórdly/supercílious áttitude to the work.

бáрство с. 1. (изнеженность) efféteness; 2. (высокомерие) lórdliness, árrogance; 3. собир. (помещики) the géntry.

барсу́к м. bádger.

бархáны мн. (ед. бархáн м.) sánd-hills.

бáрхат м. vélvet. ~истый vélvety. ~ный vélvet attr.; (подобный бархату) vélvety; перен. (о голосе) rich, méllow; (о глазах) líquid; soft as a doe's после сущ.; ~ная кóжа sílky skin; ~ный сезóн the méllow séason.

бáрыня ж. 1. ист. (помещица) lánded propríetress; lády of the mánor; (жена помещика) squíre's wife*; 2. уст. lády; (хозяйка) místress; (как обращение) Mádam, Ma'am; (фин.) lády.

бáрыш м. разг. prófit; чи́стый ~ net/clear prófit; дели́ть ~и́ share the prófits; (о воротах и т. п.) divíde the spoil.

бáрышня ж. 1. уст. young lády, girl; (незамужняя женщина) únmárried wóman*; 2. (обращение) Miss.

барье́р м. 1. bárrier; перен. (преграда) bar; тамóженные ~ы táriff walls; 2. спорт. húrdle; брать ~ clear/jump a húrdle.

бас м. 1. (голос, певец) bass; 2. (муз. инструмент) dóuble bass. ~и́стый 1. deep, bass; 2. разг. (обладающий басом) déep-vóiced.

баскетбóл м. básket-ball. ~и́ст м., ~и́стка ж. básket-ball pláyer.

баскетбóльн|ый básket-ball attr.; ~ая комáнда básket-ball team; ~ мяч básket-ball; ~ая площáдка básket-ball court.

баснопи́сец м. fáble-writer, fábulist.

баснослóвный fábulous, incrédible.

бáс|ня ж. 1. fáble; 2. разг. (вымысел, небылица) (old wives') tale, tall stóry; не расскáзывай ~ен! none of your tall stóries!

бассéйн м. 1. (искусственный) pond; закры́тый ~ índoor pool, cóvered pool; откры́тый ~ óutdoor pool, ópen-air pool; 2. (реки) básin; 3. (угольный и т. п.) field.

баст|овáть несов. be* on strike. ~у́ющий прил. 1. stríking; on strike после сущ.; 2. в знач. сущ. м. stríker.

баталист м. жив. páinter of báttle-pieces.

баталь́н|ый báttle attr.; ~ая живопись báttle-painting; ~ая карти́на báttle-piece.

батальóн м. battálion. ~ный battálion attr.; ~ный команди́р battálion commánder.

батарéйка ж. эл. báttery.

батарéя ж. 1. воен. báttery; 2. эл. báttery; ~ аккумуля́торов stórage báttery; сухáя ~ dry báttery; 3. (отопления) rádiator.

бати́ст м. batíste; (льняной) cámbric, lawn. ~овый batíste attr.; cámbric attr., lawn attr.

батóн м. 1. (хлеб) long loaf*; 2. (кондитерское изделие) stick; шоколáдный ~ stick of chócolate.

батрáк м. farm lábourer, fárm-hand.

батрáчить несов. work as a fárm-hand.

баттерфля́й м. (стиль плавания) bútterfly(-stroke).

батýт м. trámpoline.

бáтюшк|а м. 1. уст. (отец) fáther; 2. разг. (священник) priest, párson; (в обращении) (hóly) fáther; ◇ ~и! good héavens!

бáтя м. разг. fáther, dad.

бахвáлиться несов. (тв.) разг. brag (abóut).

бахвáльство с. разг. brágging, bóasting.

бахромá ж. fringe.

бахчá ж. mélon-field.

бахчевóдство с. mélon-grówing.

бахчев|óй: ~ы́е культу́ры gourds; Cucurbitáceae научн.

баци́лла ж. bacíllus (pl -li).

бáшенка ж. túrret.

бáшенный tówer attr.; ~ кран tówer crane.

башкá ж. разг. nóddle, pate; глу́пая ~ blóckhead; у́мная ~ bráiny féllow.

башки́р м., ~ка ж. Bashkír. ~ский Bashkír; ~ский язы́к Bashkír, the Bashkír lánguage.

башмáк м. 1. boot; (не покрывающий щиколотки) shoe; 2. тех. shoe; ◇ быть под ~óм у жены́ be* hénpecked.

бáшня ж. 1. tówer; сторожевáя ~ wátch-tower; 2. (орудийная) (gún-)turret.

баю́кать, убаю́кивать (вн.) lull (smth.); ~ ребёнка lull/sing* a child* to sleep.

баян м. accórdion. ~и́ст м. accórdion pláyer.

бди́тельн|ость ж. vígilance, wátchfulness; проявля́ть ~ displáy vígilance; усыпи́ть чью-л. ~ lull smb.'s vígilance, lull smb. ínto a false sense of secúrity. ~ый vígilant, wátchful.

бег м. 1. run, rúnning; 2. спорт. race; ~ на корóткую дистáнцию sprint; ~ на дли́нную дистáнцию lóng-distance race; состязáние в ~е race; барье́рный ~ húrdle-race, húrdling; ~ на мéсте rúnning on the spot; ◇ в ~áх on the run.

бегá мн. (рысистые испытания) trótting mátches.

бéга|ть несов. 1. run*; (взад и вперёд) run* abóut; 2. (от рд.; избегать) shun (smb., smth.), keep* awáy (from); 3. (сновать) scúrry; (о пальцах) twínkle; (о глазах) shift unéasily; пáльцы её ~ют по клáвишам her fingers twínkle óver the keys; 4. (за тв.) разг. (ухаживать) run* áfter (smb.), chase (smb.).

бегемóт м. hippopótamus (pl -ses, -mi).

беглéц м. fúgitive, rúnaway; (из тюрьмы) escáped cónvict, gáol-breaker.

бéгл|о 1. (о речи) flúently; (об игре на рояле) with facílity; ~ читáть read* quíckly; ~ говори́ть по-англи́йски speak* flúent Énglish; 2. (поверхностно) superficially, cúrsorily; ~ ознакóмиться с чем-л. make* a cúrsory inspéction of smth.; ~ просмотрéть что-л. glance óver/through smth. ~ость ж. (о речи) flúency; (об игре на рояле) facílity. ~ый прил. 1. (о речи) flúent; (об игре на рояле) fácile; ~ое чтéние rápid réading; ~ое исполнéние (на рояле) fácile technique; 2. (поверхностный) cúrsory; ~ый обзóр brief súrvey; ~ое замечáние pássing remárk; 3. (мимолётный) fléeting; ~ый взгляд (pássing) glance; 4. (бежавший) rúnaway, escáped, fúgitive; **5.** *в знач. сущ. м.* fúgitive, rúnaway; ◇ ~ые гла́сные *грам.* "fúgitive" vówels; ~ый ого́нь rápid fire.

бегля́нка *ж.* fúgitive, rúnaway.

бегов|о́й race *attr.*; rúnning; ~а́я доро́жка rúnning track; (*на ипподроме*) rácecourse; ~ы́е коньки́ rácing/speed skates; ~а́я ло́шадь ráce-horse.

бего́м at a run; rúnning; *воен.* at the dóuble; пусти́ться ~ start rúnning, break* into a run; ~! run!; ~ марш! *воен.* (at the) dóuble!; бежа́ть ~ run* hard, run* for dear life.

беготня́ *ж. разг.* bústle, húrry-scúrry, rúnning abóut; у меня́ сего́дня це́лый день ~ I've been on the run all day.

бе́гство *с.* **1.** (*поспешный уход*) flight; обраща́ться в ~ take* to flight; **2.** (*побег*) escápe.

бегу́н *м.* rúnner; ~ на дли́нные диста́нции lóng-distance rúnner; ~ на коро́ткие диста́нции sprínter.

бегуно́к *м.* **1.** *разг.* cléarance sheet; **2.** *тех.* rúnner.

бед|а́ ж. 1. (*несчастье*) misfórtune; (*бедствие*) disáster, calámity; у нас ~ we're in trouble, we've had a misfórtune; быть в ~е́ be* in trouble; оста́вить, покѝнуть *кого-л.* в ~е́ leave* smb. in the lurch; ~е́ there's trouble ahéad!; there's trouble in the óffing!; **2.** *в знач. сказ.* (*плохо; горе, неприятность*): ~ ей с ним she has nóthing but trouble with him, he gives her a lot of trouble; в то́м-то и ~! that's just the trouble!; не ~! it doesn't mátter! ~ (не) в том, что the trouble is (not) that; ◇ вот ~! (*неприятность*) what a núisance!; на ~у́ unlúckily, as luck would have it; как на ~у́ to make mátters worse; что за ~! as though it didn't mátter!; пришла́ ~ — отворя́й воро́та *посл.* misfórtunes néver come síngly; it néver rains but it pours.

бедне́ть, обедне́ть get* póorer, grow*/becóme* poor.

бедн|о́ póorly; (*скудно*) scántily; ~ live póorly; ~ость *ж.* **1.** (*нужда*) póverty, pénury; **2.** (*убожество*) póverty, póorness; ~ость мы́сли want/póverty of íntellect.

беднота́ *ж. собир.* the poor *pl*; дереве́нская ~ the víllage poor; городска́я ~ the úrban poor.

бедн|ый прил. 1. (*неимущий*) poor; ~ челове́к poor man*/pérson; **2.** (*убогий*) wrétched; ~ая обстано́вка scánty fúrniture; ~ое пла́тье cheap attíre; ~ ужин wrétched/méagre súpper; **3.** (*небогатый по содержанию; скудный*) insípid, méagre, jejúne; ~ая фанта́зия féeble imaginátion; **4.** (*тв.; ограниченный*) poor (in), wánting (in), lácking (in), starved (of); **5.** (*несчастный*) poor; ~ челове́к poor man*/chap!; **6.** *в знач. сущ. м.* the poor man*; *мн.* the poor; ~я́га *м. и ж. разг.* poor créature; (*о девушке или девочке тж.*) poor girl; (*о женщине тж.*) poor wóman*; ~я́к *м.* **1.** poor man*; **2.** (*о крестьянине*) poor péasant; ~я́цкий poor péasant's.

бедо́вый *разг.* dáring; (*своевольный*) héadstrong; ~ па́рень a hell of a lad; он у нас ~! he's álways up to sómething!; he's a real dáredevil!

бе́дренн|ый *анат.* fémoral; ~ая кость thígh-bone, fémur.

бедро́ *с.* thigh; (*бок*) hip; ру́ки на бёдра! hips firm!

бе́дственн|ый disástrous, calámitous; ~ое положе́ние disástrous situátion; быть в ~ом положе́нии be* in díre/míserable straits.

бе́дств|ие *с.* disáster, calámity; (*последствие войн, неурожаев и т. п.*) distréss; сигна́л ~ия distréss signal, S.O.S. ~овать *несов.* be* in distréssed/stráitened círcumstances; ~ destítute.

беж beige, fawn; ту́фли цве́та ~ fawn shoes.

бежа́ть *несов.* **1.** run*; (*об облаках*) fly*; ~ ры́сью go* at a trot; ~ мне пора́ ~ I'm afráid I must run; I must fly; **2.** (*о времени*) fly*; ва́ши часы́ бегу́т your watch is fast; **3.** (*течь*) flow, run*; (*при кипении*) boil óver; **4.** *несов. и сов.* (*спасаться бегством*) run* awáy; (*совершать побег*) flee*, take* to flight; (*отступать*) flee*, take* to flight; ~ за грани́цу fly* the country.

бе́жен|ец *м.*, ~ка *ж.* refugée.

без 1. withóut; ~ исключе́ния withóut excéption; ~ меня́ (него́, вас *и т. п.*) (*в отсутствие*) in my (his, your *etc.*) ábsence; ~ движе́ния mótionless; (*о машине и т. п.*) státionary; ~ созна́ния uncónscious; без толку withóut achíeving ánything; ~ уста́ли tírelessly; ~ глу́постей! no nónsense!; и ~ того́ as it is; не ~ того́! a líttle; я́сно, ~ слов it speaks for itsélf; **2.** (*при обозначении часа*) to; ~ пяти́ четы́ре five mínutes to four; ~ че́тверти четы́ре a quárter to four.

безала́бер|о *разг.* háphazardly, cárelessly; они́ живу́т о́чень ~ there is no sýstem in their lives, they're háppy-go-lúcky péople. ~ость *ж. разг.* háphazard ways. ~ый *разг.* háphazard, slápdash; ~ая рабо́та slápdash work.

безалкого́льн|ый nón-alcohólic; ~ые напи́тки álcohol-free/nón-alcohólic béverages; soft drinks *амер.*

безапелляцио́нн|ый 1. (*категорический*) fínal, categórical; сказа́ть *что-л.* ~ым то́ном say* smth. in a perémptory tone; **2.** *юр.* irrévocable; allówing of no appéal *после сущ.*; ~ое реше́ние fínal and irrévocable decísion.

беза́томн|ый núclear-free *attr.*; ~ая зо́на núclear-free zone.

безбе́дн|о: жить ~ live cómfortably, be* fáirly well off. ~ый cómfortable; ~ое существова́ние cómfortable existence/líving.

безбиле́тный withóut a tícket *после сущ.*; ~ пассажи́р fáre-dodger; (*на судне*) stówaway.

безбо́жн|ик *м.* átheist, irrelígious pérson. ~ый **1.** gódless; **2.** *разг.* (*возмутительный*) outrágeous.

безболе́зненн|о páinlessly; *перен. тж.* quíetly, únnóticeably. ~ый páinless; *перен. тж.* smooth.

безбоя́зненный féarless.

безбра́чие *с.* célibacy.

безбре́жный bóundless.

безве́ст|ность *ж.* obscúrity; жить в ~ости live in obscúrity, lead* an obscúre existence. ~ный obscúre; (*неизвестный*) únknówn; ~ный геро́й únknówn héro.

безве́тренн|ый wíndless, still; ~ая пого́да calm wéather.

безве́трие *с.* calm.

безвку́с|ица *ж.* bad/poor taste. ~но in bad/poor taste, vúlgarly, withóut taste; ~но одева́ться wear tásteless clothes, have* no idéa how to dress. ~ный tásteless; (*невкусный, пресный тж.*) insípid.

безвла́стие *с.* ánarchy.

безво́дн|ый 1. árid, wáterless; ~ая степь árid steppe; **2.** *хим.* anhýdrous.

безво́дье *с.* lack of wáter, arídity.

безвозвра́тн|ый 1. (*утраченный навсегда*) irretríevable, irrévocable; **2.** (*не подлежащий возврату*): ~ая ссу́да grant, nón-repáyable súbsidy.

безвозду́шн|ый áir-free; áirless; ~ое простра́нство *физ.* vácuum; (*вне земли*) ímpty) space.

безвозме́здн|о free (of charge), grátis; ~ по́льзоваться *чьими-л.* услу́гами enjóy smb.'s únpaid/gratúitous sérvices. ~ый free; (*невознаграждаемый*) gratúitous, únpaid; переда́ть *что-л.* в ~ое по́льзование *кому-л.* hand óver smth. for the free use of smb.

безво́лие *с.* wéakness of will, lack of will, spínelessness.

безво́льный wéak-willed, flábby, spíneless.

безвре́дный hármless, innócuous; (*о человеке тж.*) inoffénsive.

безвре́менн|о prematúrely; ~ сконча́лся died prematúrely, passed awáy prematúrely. ~ый úntimely, premature.

безвре́менье *с.* **1.** dark days *pl*, tróubled times *pl* **2.** périod of sócial stagnátion.

безвы́ездно cónstantly, úninterrúptedly; withóut quítting the place; он ~ живёт в Москве́ he has lived in Móscow all his life.

безвы́ходн|ый hópeless, désperate; ~ое положе́ние désperate situátion; положе́ние каза́лось мне ~ым I could see no way out.

безголо́вый héadless; *перен. разг.* bráinless; *(забы́вчивый)* scátter-brained, háre-brained.

безголо́сый féeble-vóiced; ~ певе́ц médiocre sínger; он совсе́м ~! he has no voice at all!

безгра́мотн|о 1. *(негра́мотно)* illíterately; *(с оши́бками)* úngrammátically; **2.** *(неве́жественно)* incómpetently, ígnorantly, withóut knówledge. ~ость *ж.* **1.** illíteracy; **2.** *(неве́жество)* incómpetence, ígnorance; полити́ческая ~ость political ígnorance. ~ый **1.** *(негра́мотный)* illíterate; ~ый челове́к an illíterate; **2.** *(неве́жественный)* incómpetent, ígnorant; **3.** *(содержа́щий мно́го оши́бок)* hópelessly ináccurate; full of mistákes *после сущ.*; ~ое сочине́ние éssay full of mistákes; ~ый чертёж bótched-up dráwing.

безграни́чн|ый bóundless, únbounded, ínfinite, límitless; ~ просто́р vast/ínfinite/bóundless expánse; ~ая пусты́ня bóundless désert; ~ая любо́вь bóundless love; ~ая пре́данность ínfinite devótion.

безда́рн|ость *ж.* **1.** lack of tálent, féebleness; **2.** *(о челове́ке)* a mediócrity. ~ый **1.** *(лишённый тала́нта)* dull, médiocre, úngifted; withóut a spark of tálent *после сущ.*; ~ый поэ́т wórthless vérsifier/rhýmer; **2.** *(вы́полненный неталантли́во)* féeble, úninspíred; ~ое произведе́ние work of no signíficance; ~ая карти́на picture útterly devóid of inspirátion.

безде́йств|енный ináctive, ídle. ~ие *с.* ináction, inactívity, inértia.

безде́йствовать *несов.* do* nóthing; fail to take áction; *(о станке́, маши́не и т. п.)* stand* ídle.

безде́лица *ж. разг.* (mere) bagatélle, trífle.

безделу́шка *ж.* knick-knack, trínket, toy; *мн. тж.* bríc-à-brac.

безде́ль|е *с.* ídleness; вы́нужденное ~ станови́лось для него́ невыноси́мым he was begínning to find the enfórced ídleness unbéarable. ~ник *м.*, ~ница *ж.* **1.** *разг.* lóafer, ídler, láyabout; **2.** *бран.* góod-for-nóthing, ne'er-do-well. ~ничать *несов.* do* nóthing, ídle, loaf.

безде́нежн|ый 1.: ~ые расчёты cléaring operátions; **2.** *разг. (не име́ющий де́нег)* pénniless.

безде́нежье *с.* lack of móney.

безде́ти|ость *ж.* chíldlessness. ~ый chíldless.

безде́ятель|ость *ж.* inactívity. ~ый ináctive, pássive, lethárgic.

бе́здна *ж.* **1.** abýss, chasm; **2.** *в знач. сказ. (рд.) разг. (мно́жество)* heaps (of), ány amóunt (of); у него́ ~ дел he is up to his neck in work.

бездоказа́тельн|ый báseless, gróundless, únsubstántiated; ~ые обвине́ния únfóunded accusátions.

бездо́мн|ый hómeless; ~ая соба́ка stray dog.

бездо́нн|ый bóttomless; *перен. тж.* unfáthomable; ~ая про́пасть bóttomless pit.

бездоро́жье *с.* **1.** *(отсу́тствие доро́г)* lack of roads; **2.** *(распу́тица)* impassabílity of roads, bad roads; осе́ннее ~ the múd-locked roads of áutumn.

безду́мный thóughtless.

безду́ш|ие *с.* cállousness, héartlessness. ~но **1.** *(бессерде́чно)* cállously, héartlessly; **2.** *(хо́лодно, без живо́го чу́вства)* hálf-héartedly, indífferently. ~ный **1.** *(бессерде́чный)* cállous, héartless; **2.** *(невырази́тельный, холо́дный)* sóulless, uninspíred.

безды́мный smókeless.

безды́ханный lífeless.

безжа́лостный pítiless, mérciless; *(жесто́кий)* rúthless.

безжи́зненный 1. lífeless; **2.** *(о взгля́де)* dull, spíritless.

беззабо́тн|о líght-héartedly, in a cáre-free mánner; *(беспе́чно)* cárelessly. ~ость *ж.* líght-héartedness; *(беспе́чность)* cárelessness. ~ый cáre-free, líght-héarted;

(беспе́чный) cáreless; ~ый челове́к háppy-go-lúcky pérson; ~ое де́тство cáre-free/úntróubled chíldhood; ~ый смех cáre-free láughter.

беззаве́тн|о devótedly, sélflessly. ~ый devóted, sélfless, whóle-héarted, útter.

беззако́н|ие *с.* **1.** *(отсу́тствие зако́нности)* illegálity, láwlessness; **2.** *(просту́пок)* láwless act. ~ный láwless.

беззасте́нчив|о shámelessly; он ~ лжёт he's a shámeless líar. ~ость *ж.* effróntery; cheek *разг.* ~ый shámeless, brázen; *(о лжи)* báarefaced.

беззащи́тный defénceless, únprotécted.

беззву́чный sóundless, sílent; ~ смех sílent láughter.

безземе́ль|е *с.* lándlessness, lack of land. ~ный lándless.

беззло́бн|о míldly, góod-náturedly; ~ подшу́чивать над кем-л. tease smb. géntly. ~ый kíndly, góod-nátured, ámiable; ~ый смех góod-nátured láughter.

беззу́б|ый tóothless; *перен.* féeble, weak; ~ые остро́ты féeble wítticisms/cracks; ~ая кри́тика féeble/insípid críticism.

безле́сный únwóoded, tréeless.

безли́кий fáceless, féatureless.

безли́чн|ый 1. cháracterless; lácking personálity *после сущ.*; **2.** *грам.* impérsonal; ~ глаго́л impérsonal verb; ~ое предложе́ние impérsonal séntence.

безлю́дн|ый 1. *(малонаселённый)* desérted, úninhábited, thínly pópulated; **2.** *(пусты́нный)* lónely, sólitary; ~ая у́лица quíet/únfrequénted street.

безме́рн|о beyónd méasure *(в конце́ предложе́ния)*. ~ый méasureless, imméasurable.

безмо́зглый *разг.* sílly, bráinless, dim.

безмо́лв|ие *с.* sílence, stíllness. ~ный sílent; *(не вы́раженный в слова́х)* unspóken, mute; ~ное уча́стие mute sýmpathy. ~ствовать *несов.* maintáin sílence, keep* sílent.

безмото́рный éngineless; *(с вы́ключенным мото́ром)* únpówered; ~ полёт glíding.

безмяте́жн|ость *ж.* serénity, tranquíllity, placídity. ~ый seréne, plácid, unrúffled; ~ый поко́й unrúffled serénity, úndistúrbed tranquíllity; ~ый сон tránquil/untróubled slúmber; ~ое сча́стье unrúffled háppiness.

безнадёжный hópeless, désperate; больно́й безнадёжен the case is hópeless.

безнадзо́рный negléected.

безнака́занн|о with impúnity; ему́ э́то не пройдёт ~ he won't get awáy with that. ~ый unpúnished; преступле́ние не оста́лось ~ым the crime did not go unpúnished.

безнали́чн|ый: ~ расчёт *бухг.* páyment by cheque, páyment by wrítten órder; *(ме́жду ба́нками)* cléaring; по ~ому расчёту by wrítten órder.

безнача́лие *с.* ánarchy.

безно́гий légless; *(с одно́й ного́й)* one-légged.

безнра́вственн|ость *ж.* immorálity; *(разврат)* deprávity. ~ый immóral; *(развращённый)* depráved.

безоби́дн|ый ínnocent; *(безвре́дный)* inoffénsive, hármless; ~ая шу́тка ínnocent joke; ~ое существо́ hármless créature.

безо́блачн|ый clóudless; *перен.* únclóuded, seréne; ~ое не́бо clóudless sky; ~ое сча́стье únclóuded háppiness.

безобра́з|ие *с.* **1.** *(уро́дство)* úgliness, hídeousness, defórmity; **2.** *(отврати́тельное явле́ние)* disgráce; там таки́е ~ия творя́тся disgráceful/térrible things are háppening there; **3.** *в знач. сказ. разг.:* ~! outrágeous!, it's a pósitive scándal!; ~, что он опозда́л it's disgráceful that he is late, it's a disgráce/shame that he is late.

безобра́з|ить, обезобра́зить *(вн.; уро́довать)* disfígure *(smb., smth.).* ~ник *м. разг.* lout, míschief-maker; *шутл.* rogue; *(о ребёнке)* (young) víllain/míschief; ~ница *ж. разг.* míschief-maker; *(о ребёнке)* (little) míschief, bad girl. ~ничать *несов. разг.* beháve like a lout, beháve outrágeously/disgrácefully; *(о* *ребёнке*) be* náughty, be* up to míschief. ~ный 1. (*некрасивый*) úgly, hídeous; (*уродливый*) defórmed; ~ая внéшность hídeous appéarance; 2. (*возмутительный*) outrágeous, disgústing; (*постыдный*) disgráceful, shámeful; ~ное поведéние atrócious beháviour; ~ный постýпок disgráceful áction.

безоговóрочн|о úncondítionally, únresérvedly. ~ый úncondítional, únquálified; ~ая капитуляция úncondítional surrénder; ~ое согласие únquálified assént.

безопáсн|о 1. *нареч.* sáfely, in sáfety; 2. *в знач. сказ.* it is safe; э́то совершéнно ~ it is pérfectly safe. ~ость *ж.* sáfety; (*общественная*) secúrity; тут мы бýдем в ~ости we'll be safe here; госудáрственная ~ость nátional/state secúrity; Совéт Безопáсности ООН UN Secúrity Cóuncil. ~ый 1. safe; ~ое мéсто safe place; 2. (*безвредный*) hármless; ~ое срéдство hármless rémedy; ~ая бритва sáfety rázor.

безорýжный únármed; *.перен.* (*беззащитный*) defénceless.

безостанóвочный uncéasing, únintérrupted; nón-stóp.

безотвéтн|ый 1. (*не получающий ответа*) únrecíprocated, únánswered; ~ая любóвь unrequíted love; 2. (*не отвечающий*) sílent, unrespónsive; 3. (*покорный*) meek, submíssive.

безотвéтственн|ость *ж.* irresponsibílity. ~ый 1. irrespónsible; ~ый постýпок irrespónsible áction; 2. (*не несущий ответственности*) únauthóritative; ~ое лицó pérson of no authórity.

безоткáзн|о smóothly, efficiently. ~ый 1. smooth, stéady; 2. *разг.* (*о человеке*) (éver) willing.

безотлагáтельн|о úrgently, without deláy; э́то нáдо сдéлать ~ it is úrgent, it must be done at once. ~ый préssing, úrgent.

безотносительно (к *дт.*) irrespéctive (of).

безотрáдн|ый chéerless, dréary; ~ая картина désolate scene.

безотчётный (*бессознательный*) instínctive, subcónscious, unaccóuntable; ~ страх unaccóuntable fear.

безошибочн|ость *ж.* (*правильность*) corréctness; (*точность*) áccuracy. ~ый unérring, fáultless; (*правильный*) corréct; (*точный*) áccurate, precíse; ~ый расчёт precíse calculátions *pl.*

безрабóт|ица *ж.* unemplóyment. ~ный *прил.* 1. unemplóyed, wórkless, jóbless; быть ~ным be* unemplóyed, be* out of work; 2. *в знач. сущ. м.* unemplóyed; *мн. собир.* the unemplóyed.

безрáдостный jóyless, chéerless, unháppy.

безраздéльн|о úndivídedly. ~ый úndivíded, compléte; ~ое госпóдство úndivíded rule, compléte sway.

безразлич|ие *с.* indífference. ~но 1. *нареч.* with indífference; относиться к *кому-л.* ~но be* indífferent to *smth.*; он отнёсся к э́тому ~но he remáined quite unconcérned; 2. *в знач. сказ.* it's all the same, it makes no difference, it is immatérial; э́то (совершéнно) ~но I don't care (whéther, if), it's a mátter of indífference to me. ~ный 1. (*безучастный*) indífferent, unconcérned; ~ный взгляд indífferent glance; он произнёс э́ти словá ~ным тóном he spoke the words in a tone of indífference; 2. (*не стоящий внимания*) unimpórtant; он мне ~ен he's nóthing to me; я емý совершéнно ~ен he's pérfectly indífferent to me.

безразмéр|ный stretch; ~ые носки stretch socks.

безрассýд|ный reckless, imprúdent; ~ное поведéние réckless cónduct; ~ная смéлость fóolhardiness. ~ство *с.* récklessness, fólly; бы́ло бы ~ством предполагáть... it would be fólly to suppóse.

безрезультáтн|о without resúlt, in vain, to no púrpose/aváil. ~ый inefféctual, fútile; (*безуспешный*) únsuccéssful; ~ая попы́тка abórtive attémpt.

безрóгий hórnless; without horns *после сущ.*; (*об оленях*) without ántlers *после сущ.*

безрóдный 1. (*не имеющий родных*) kíthless; without kith or kin *после сущ.*; 2. (*утративший связь с родиной*) róotless, expátriate.

безрóпотн|о without a múrmur. ~ый uncompláining, únmúrmuring; (*покорный*) meek, resígned.

безрукáвка *ж.* sléeveless jácket; (*из шерсти*) sléeveless cárdigan.

безрýк|ий without arms/hands, ármless; (*с одной рукой*) óne-armed; *перен. разг.* clúmsy, áwkward; онá такáя ~ая her fíngers are all thumbs.

безры́бье *с.*: на ~ и рак ры́ба *погов.* ≈ half a loaf is bétter than no bread; amóng the blind the óne-éyed is king.

безубы́точн|ый óperated/run without loss *после сущ.*; ~ое предприя́тие páying concérn.

безудáрный *лингв.* unstréssed, unaccénted.

безудéрж|ный unrestráined, úncontróllable; (*бурный*) impétuous; ~ое весéлье unrestráined mirth; ~ смех úncontróllable láughter.

безукоризненн|о irrepróachably; ~ чистый spótlessly clean; ~ый (*о произношении, порядке и т. п.*) pérfect, irrepróachable; (*о поведении и т. п. тж.*) unimpéachable, immáculate.

безýм|ец *м.* mádman*. ~ие *с.* 1. (*безрассудство*) mádness, fólly; любить кого-л., что-л. до ~ия mádly, love smb., smth. to distráction; 2. (*сумасшествие*) mádness, insánity; доводить кого-л. до ~ия drive* smb. crázy, drive* smb. to distráction. ~но *разг.* mádly, áwfully; ~но боя́ться кого-л., чего-л. be* térrified of smb., smth., be* áwfully afráid of smb., smth.; ~но увлекáться кем-л., чем-л. be* mad/crázy abóut smb., smth.; ~но увлéчься кем-л., чем-л. be* infátuated with smb.; он ~но любит свою́ мать he símply adóres/ídolizes his móther; я ~но устáл I'm fríghtfully/térribly tíred. ~ный 1. *разг.* (*безрассудный*) réckless; ~ная отвáга réckless dáring; ~ный план réckless plan; 2. *разг.* (*очень сильный*) térrible; ~ная устáлость térrible wéariness; ~ная рóскошь extrávagant lúxury; 3. *уст.* mad, insáne, crázy; ~ные глазá crázy/wíld-lóoking eyes.

безýмство *с.* fólly, mádness. ~вать *несов.* rave, be* in a fúry, be* ráging.

безупрéчн|о irrepróachably. ~ость *ж.* irreproachabílity. ~ый irrepróachable, bláмеless, fáultless; ~ое поведéние irrepróachable beháviour/cónduct; ~ая репутáция unimpéachable/spótless/stáinless reputátion, unblémished récord; ~ая чéстность unimpéachable hónesty/ íntegrity.

безуслóвн|о undóubtedly, cértainly; of course; ~, он чéстен of course, he's hónest; он, ~, придёт he's sure to come. ~ый ábsolute, uncondítional; ~ое повиновéние implícit obédience; ~ый успéх unquálified succéss; ◇ ~ый рефлéкс uncondítioned réflex.

безуспéшн|о únsuccéssfully, in vain, without succéss. ~ый únsuccéssful, unaváiling, inefféctive, abórtive.

безýсый without a moustáche *после сущ.*; *перен. разг.* cállow, green; ~ мальчишка cállow youth, béardless boy.

безутéшный inconsólable.

безýхий éarless; (*с одним ухом*) óne-éared.

безучáст|ие *с.* indífference. ~ный indífferent, lístless, apathétic; ~ное отношéние indífference; detáched áttitude; ~ный зри́тель indífferent ónlooker; ~ный взгляд lístless glance; остáваться ~ным к *чему-л.* show* no ínterest in *smth.*, remáin indífferent towárds *smth.*

безъя́дерн|ый núclear-free; ~ая зóна núclear-free zone.

безыдéйн|ость *ж.* lack of progréssive idéas. ~ый unpríncipled; lácking ideológical cóntent *после сущ.*

безымя́нн|ый námeless; (*анонимный*) anónymous; горá ~ая unnámed peak; ~ труд anónymous work; ◇ ~ пáлец fourth fínger; (*на левой руке тж.*) ríng-fínger.

безынициати́вный unénterprising; withóut/lácking initiative *после сущ.*; ~ рабо́тник stéreotyped mind.

безыску́сный símple.

безыску́сственный ártless, ingénuous, unsophísticated, unaffécted; ~ расска́з ártless tale.

безысхо́дный hópeless; (*нескончаемый*) everlásting, éndless.

бейсбо́л *м. спорт.* báseball.

беко́н *м.* bácon.

белёсый whítish.

беле́ть, побеле́ть 1. (*становиться белым*) turn white; 2. *тк. несов.* (*виднеться*) show* white.

белизна́ *ж.* whíteness.

бели́ла *мн.* 1. (*краска*) whíting *sg*; свинцо́вые ~ white lead *sg*; ци́нковые ~ zinc white *sg*; 2. (*в косметике*) cerúse *sg*.

бели́ть, побели́ть, вы́белить (*вн.*) 1. *сов.* побели́ть (*производить побелку*) whítewash (*smth.*); 2. *сов.* вы́белить (*о ткани*) bleach (*smth.*).

бе́лич|ий squírrel's; squírrel *attr.*; ~ мех squírrel; ~ья шу́ба squírrel coat; шу́ба на ~ьем меху́ squírrel-lined coat.

бе́лка *ж.* squírrel.

белко́в|ый prótein *attr.*, albúminous; ~ое вещество́ albúminous súbstance, prótein.

беллетри́ст *м.* fíction-writer. **~ика** *ж.* fíction.

белово́й: ~ экземпля́р fair cópy.

белогварде́ец *м.* White Guard.

белогварде́йский White Guard *attr.*

бело́к *м.* 1. (*яичный*) white of egg, the white; 2. *биол., хим.* prótein, álbumin, álbumen; 3. (*глаза*) white (of the eye).

белокро́вие *с. мед.* leukáemia.

белоку́р|ый fáir(-háired); blond; ~ая де́вушка blonde (girl).

белору́с *м.*, **~ка** *ж.* Byelorússian. **~ский** Byelorússian; **~ский** язы́к Byelorússian, the Byelorússian lánguage.

белору́чк|а *м. и ж. разг.* shírker; быть ~ой be* afráid of gétting one's hands dírty.

белосне́жн|ый snów-white, snówy; ~ая ска́терть snów-white táblecloth.

белошве́йка *ж.* séamstress.

белу́га *ж.* belúga, white stúrgeon.

бе́л|ый *прил.* 1. white; ~ воротничо́к white cóllar; 2. *в знач. сущ. м.* White (Guard); 3. *в знач. сущ. мн. шахм.* White *sg*; ◇ ~ биле́т mílitary sérvice exémption certíficate; ~ые стихи́ blank verse *sg*; средь ~а дня in broad dáylight; ~ая горя́чка delírium trémens; ~ хлеб white bread; ~ое вино́ 1) white wine; 2) *разг.* vódka; ~ые пя́тна blanks, blank spáces; ~ая воро́на white crow, óutsider.

бельг|и́ец *м.*, **~и́йка** *ж.* Bélgian. **~и́йский** Bélgian.

бельё *с. собир.* línen; (*для стирки, из стирки*) wáshing, láundry; ни́жнее ~ únderwear.

бельево́й línen *attr.*

бельмо́ *с.* wáll-eye; ◇ он у меня́ как ~ на глазу́ ≈ he is a thorn in my flesh, he is an éyesore to me.

бельэта́ж *м.* 1. (*второй этаж*) first floor; 2. *театр.* dress círcle.

бемо́ль *м. муз.* flat.

бенга́л|ец *м.*, **~ка** *ж.* Bengáli.

бенга́льский Bengálese; ~ язы́к Bengáli, the Bengáli lánguage; ◇ ~ ого́нь Bengál light.

бензи́н *м.* pétrol; gásoline, gas *амер.*; очи́щенный ~ benzíne. **~овый** pétrol.

бензоба́к *м.* pétrol/fuel tank.

бензозапра́в|очный fílling. **~щик** *м.* fúelling lórry.

бензоколо́нка *ж.* fílling státion, pétrol státion; gas státion *амер.*

бензопрово́д *м.* fuel pipe/lead.

бензохрани́лище *с.* pétrol store/tank.

бенуа́р *м. театр.* the (gróund-floor) bóxes *pl*; ло́жа ~а (gróund-floor) box.

бе́рег *м.* (*моря, озера*) shore; (*морское побережье*) coast; (*реки, пруда*) bank; ~ мо́ря séashore; (*курорт*) séaside; мы сиде́ли на ~у́ мо́ря we were sítting on the séashore; мы отдыха́ем на ~у́ мо́ря we are stáying at the séaside; ~ реки́ (*прибрежная полоса*) ríverside; на ~у́ ashóre; on shore; сойти́ на ~ go* ashóre.

берегов|о́й wáterside *attr.*; (*при море*) coast *attr.*, cóastal; (*при реке*) ríverside *attr.*; (*при озере*) lákeside *attr.*; ~ ве́тер óff-shore wind, lánd-breeze; ~а́я охра́на cóastguard; ~а́я ли́ния cóastline, shore line.

береди́ть, разбереди́ть (*вн.*) chafe (*smth.*); *перен.* tróuble (*smth.*); ~ ста́рые ра́ны reópen old sores/wounds.

бережли́в|о económically, thríftily; ~ расхо́довать сре́дства húsband one's resóurces. **~ость** *ж.* thrift, économy, húsbandry. **~ый** thrífty, económical; она́ о́чень ~ая хозя́йка she is a véry cáreful hóusewife*.

бе́режн|о (*осторожно*) géntly; (*аккуратно*) cárefully, with care; (*заботливо*) táctfully, with considerátion. **~ый** (*осторожный*) géntle, cáutious; (*аккуратный*) cáreful; (*заботливый*) táctful, considerate; ~ое прикоснове́ние géntle touch; ~ое обраще́ние с кни́гами cáreful hándling of books; ~ое отноше́ние к лю́дям considerátion for péople, táctful áttitude to péople, lóoking áfter péople.

берёз|а *ж.* birch(-tree), ~овый birch *attr.*; ~овая ро́ща birch grove.

бере́менн|ая prégnant; ~ же́нщина prégnant wóman*; expéctant móther. **~ость** *ж.* prégnancy; она́ на четвёртом ме́сяце ~ости she is in her fourth month (of prégnancy).

бере́т *м.* béret.

бере́чь *несов.* (*вн.*) 1. (*хранить*) take* care of *smth.*; keep* (*smth.*); ~ ста́рые пи́сьма keep* old létters; 2. (*не расходовать напрасно*) save (*smth.*), consérve (*smth.*); (*расчётливо тратить тж.*) use (*smth.*) spáringly/cárefully; ~ си́лы save/consérve one's strength/énergy; ~ вре́мя save time; 3. (*заботливо оберегать*) take* (good) care (*of*); ~ здоро́вье take* care of onesélf, take* care of one's health; ~ сы́на look áfter one's son. **~ся** *несов.* take* care of onesélf; береги́сь! take care!, be cáreful!; береги́сь по́езда! bewáre of the trains!

берло́га *ж.* den, lair.

бертоле́тов: ~а соль *хим.* potássium chlórate.

берцо́в|ый: ~ая кость *анат.* tíbia (*pl* -iae), shínbone.

бес *м.* démon; *перен.* urge; како́й ~ в тебя́ всели́лся? what's come óver you?; what's bíting you?; в нём сиди́т како́й-то ~ противоре́чия he seems to have an urge/itch to contradíct éveryone; ◇ ме́лким ~ом рассыпа́ться пе́ред кем-л. lay* onesélf out to please *smb.*

бесе́д|а *ж.* 1. talk, conversátion; chat *разг.*; (*интервью*) ínterview; 2. (*собеседование*) discússion; проводи́ть ~ы среди́ студе́нтов lead*/hold* discússions amóng stúdents; ~ по ра́дио rádio talk.

бесе́дка *ж.* súmmer-house, árbour; bówer *поэт.*

бесе́довать *несов.* (*с тв.*) have* a talk (with); have* a chat (with) *разг.*

бесёнок *м. imp.*, góblin.

беси́ть, взбеси́ть (*вн.*) enráge (*smb.*), mádden (*smb.*). **~ся, взбеси́ться** 1. (*о животных*) go* mad, get* rábies; 2. (*неистовствовать*) rage; *сов. тж.* fly* into a rage.

бескла́ссовый clássless.

бескозы́рка *ж.* péakless cap.

бескомпроми́ссн|о uncómpromisingly, fírmly. **~ость** *ж.* refúsal to cómpromise, uncómpromisingness. **~ый** uncómpromising.

бесконе́чн|о 1. ínfinitely; ~ ма́лый infinitésimal; ~ ма́лая величина́ infinitésimal; 2. (*чрезвычайно длинно*) éndlessly. ~ость *ж.* infinity, infinitude; (*бесконечное пространство*) ínfinite/éndless expánse; ◇ и так дáлее до ~ости and so on, and so on. ~ый 1. (*беспредельный*) ínfinite; 2. (*длинный*) éndless, intérminable; ~ый расскáз intérminable stóry; ~ая дорóга éndless road; 3. (*чрезвычайный по силе проявления*) ínfinite, extréme, éndless; ~ое удовóльствие extréme pléasure; 4. *разг.* (*постоянный, непрекращающийся*) perpétual; ~ые жáлобы perpétual compláints; ◇ ~ая десятúчная дробь *мат.* infinite décimal.

бесконтрóльн|о without contról; (*без надзора*) without supervísion. ~ый uncontrólled; (*безнадзорный*) unsúpervised; ~ое расхóдование дéнег uncontrólled expénditure of móney.

бескорýст|е *с.* disínterestedness. ~ный disínterested; ~ый человéк disínterested pérson; ~ная пóмощь disínterested help/assístance.

бескрúзисный crísis-free.

бескрóвный blóodless.

бесновáться *несов.* rage, rave, storm.

беспáлый fíngerless; (*без пальца*) with one fínger míssing *после сущ.*

беспáмят|ный *разг.* forgétful. ~ство *с.* uncónsciousness; впасть в ~ство lose* cónsciousness.

беспартúйный *прил.* 1. nón-Párty; 2. *в знач. сущ. м.* nón-Párty man*; *мн.* nón-Párty péople.

беспереббóйн|о uninterrúptedly; without a hitch *разг.* ~ый stéady, uninterrúpted; ~ая рабóта мотóра smooth fúnctioning/rúnning of an éngine; ~ое снабжéние régular supplý, contínuous flow of supplíes.

беспересáдочн|ый diréct, through; ~ое сообщéние diréct communicátion.

бесперспектúвн|ость *ж.* lack of próspects, hópelessness. ~ый unpromísing; without prómise/próspects *после сущ.*; hópeless.

беспéчн|о cárelessly, thóughtlessly; (*беззаботно*) light-héartedly; ~ прогýливаться sáunter about in a cárefree mánner; жить ~ have* no wórldly cares; ~ относúться к свойм обязанностям treat one's responsibílities líghtly/cárelessly. ~ость *ж.* cárelessness, irrespónsibility; (*отсутствие забот*) light-héartedness. ~ый cáreless, irrespónsible; (*не обременённый заботами*) cárefree, light-héarted; ~ое отношéние к чему-л. irrespónsible áttitude to smth.; ~ая улыбка light-héarted smile; ~ый харáктер cárefree dispositíon.

беспланóв|ость *ж.* lack of plán(ning), hapházardness. ~ый unplánned, plánless; without a plan *после сущ.*

бесплáтн|о free (of charge), grátis. ~ый free; ~ый билéт free tícket; ~ое приложéние free súpplement; ~ое обучéние free educátion; ~ое медицúнское обслýживание free médical aid/sérvice.

бесплацкáртный únresérved; without resérved seats *после сущ.*

бесплóд|ие *с.* 1. stérility; 2. (*о почве*) infertílity, bárrenness. ~ность *ж.* 1. bárrenness, stérility; 2. (*безуспешность*) futílity, frúitlessness. ~ный 1. stérile, bárren; 2. (*неплодородный — о почве*) bárren; 3. (*безуспешный*) fútile, frúitless, abórtive; ~ные попытки frúitless attémpts.

бесповорóтный irrévocable.

бесподóбный *разг.* inímitable, unrívalled, unéqualled, péerless.

беспозвонóчный invértebrate.

беспокó|ить, обеспокóить (*вн.*) 1. (*нарушать покой, мешать*) distúrb (smb.), tróuble (smb.), bóther (smb.); (*причинять боль*) hurt* (smb.), give* (smb.) tróuble; 2. (*волновать*) wórry (smb.), upsét* (smb.); меня ~úло, что... I was afráid (that)... ~úться, обеспокóиться, побеспокóиться 1. *сов.* обеспокóиться (о *пр.*; *волноваться*) be* ánxious (about), wórry (about), be* unéasy (about); 2. *сов.* побеспокóиться (*утруждать се-*

бя) tróuble, wórry, fret; пожáлуйста, не ~йтесь! please, don't tróuble/bóther!

беспокóйн|о 1. *нареч.* réstlessly; больнóй спал ~ the pátient passed a réstless night; 2. *в знач. сказ. безл.* it is wórrying/distúrbing. ~ый 1. (*тревожный, взволнованный*) réstless, ánxious; ~ый человéк réstless pérson; ~ый вид wórried appéarance/looks; ~ый сон tróubled sleep; ~ые временá tróubled/túrbulent times; 2. (*причиняющий беспокойство*) tróublesome, wórrying, tíresome; ~ая дорóга tíresome/dífficult jóurney; ~ая рабóта wórrying work.

беспокóйство *с.* 1. (*волнение*) anxíety, unéasiness; с ~м ánxiously; испытывать ~ expérience/feel* anxíety; 2. (*хлопоты*) wórry; причинять ~ кому-л. tróuble smb., give* smb. tróuble, put* smb. to tróuble; простúте за ~ I am sórry to tróuble you.

бесполéзн|о 1. *нареч.* úselessly; 2. *в знач. сказ.* it is úseless, it is no good; спóрить ~ it's úseless to árgue, it's no good árguing. ~ый úseless, fútile, vain.

беспóл|ый séxless, aséxual; ~ое размножéние *биол.* parthenogénesis.

беспóмощ|ность *ж.* hélplessness. ~ый 1. hélpless, inefféctual; 2. (*плохой*) féeble.

беспорядок *м.* 1. disórder, confúsion; 2. *мн.* (*волнения*) ríots, distúrbances.

беспорядочн|о in confúsion/disórder; (*непоследовательно*) without sýstem, únsystemátically; ~ читáть read* whatéver comes to one's hand, read* without ány sýstem. ~ость *ж.* disórderliness; (*непоследовательность*) hapházardness, inconsístency. ~ый disórderly; (*непоследовательный*) hapházard, irrégular, únsystemátic; ~ая жизнь irrégular life.

беспосáдочный: ~ перелёт nón-stóp flight.

беспóчвенный únfounded, flímsy.

беспóшлинный dúty-frée; ~ ввоз товáров dúty-frée ímport.

беспощáдный rúthless, mérciless.

беспрáв|ие *с.* ábsence/lack of (légal) rights. ~ный without (légal) rights, háving no (légal) rights *после сущ.*

беспредéльный bóundless, ínfinite.

беспредмéтн|ый áimless, vague; ~ая крúтика íll-defined críticism; ~ спор póintless árgument.

беспрекослóвн|о implícitly, unquéstioningly. ~ый unquéstioning, implícit; ~ое повиновéние implícit obédience, ábsolute submíssion.

беспрепятственн|о without híndrance, fréely. ~ый free, únimpéded.

беспрерывн|о céaselessly, contínuosly, úninterrúptedly; without a break *разг.*; ~ лил дождь it rained without stópping. ~ый céaseless, contínuous, úninterrúpted.

беспрестáнн|о continually, incéssantly; ~ раздавáлись звонкú по телефóну the télephone kept rínging. ~ый incéssant.

беспрецедéнтный unprécedented.

беспрúбыльный unprófitable.

беспризóрн|ик *м.* waif, hómeless child*. ~ость *ж.* hómelessness, destitútion. ~ый *прил.* 1. (*заброшенный*) neglécted, úncared for; 2. (*о детях*) hómeless, déstitute; 3. *в знач. сущ. м. см.* беспризóрник.

беспримéрный unparálleled; unprécedented; ~ пóдвиг unparálleled feat.

беспринцúпн|ость *ж.* ábsence of (guíding) prínciple, unscrúpulousness. ~ый unpríncipled, unscrúpulous.

беспристрáст|ие *с.,* ~ность *ж.* impártiality. ~ный impártial, únbías(s)ed; ~ое мнéние únbías(s)ed opínion; ~ная крúтика únbías(s)ed críticism; ~ный судья impártial judge.

беспричúнн|о for no réason. ~ый gróundless, cáuseless; ~ая грусть inéxplicable sádness.

бесприютный hómeless.

беспробýдн|ый 1. (*очень крепкий*) deep, dead; 2.

разг. (*безудержный*) hópeless; ~ое пья́нство incéssant drínking.

беспрово́лочный wíreless; ~ телегра́ф wíreless (telégraphy).

беспро́игрыш|ый safe; ~ая лотере́я prízes-for-all lóttery; ~ заём repáyable loan; ~ое де́ло sure thing.

беспросве́тн|ый pítch-dárk; *перен.* hópeless, únrelíeved; ~ая тьма útter dárkness; ~ая нужда́ únrelíeved póverty.

беспроце́нтный béaring no ínterest *после сущ.*

беспу́т|ный wáyward, díssolute; (*развра́тный*) díssipated. ~ство *с.* dissipátion.

бессвя́зн|ость *ж.* incohérence. ~ый incohérent, incónsequent, rámbling; ~ый расска́з incohérent stóry/accóunt.

бессеме́йный háving no fámily *после сущ.*

бессерде́ч|ие *с.* héartlessness. ~ный héartless.

бесси́л|ие *с.* 1. (*кра́йняя сла́бость*) féebleness, wéakness, debílity; 2. (*беспо́мощность*) pówerlessness, hélplessness; ímpotence.

бесси́ль|ный 1. (*сла́бый*) weak, féeble, debílitated; 2. (*беспо́мощный*) pówerless, hélpless; ímpotent; ~ гнев ímpotent rage; слова́ ~ны words are inádequate.

бесисте́мн|ость *ж.* lack of sýstem. ~ый únsystemátic.

бессла́вный inglórious, ignomínious; ~ коне́ц inglórious end.

бессле́дн|о withóut (léaving) a trace; он исче́з ~ he disappéared complétely. ~ый léaving no trace *после сущ.*; ~ое исчезнове́ние compléte disappéarance.

бессло́весн|ый 1. (*о живо́тных*) dumb; 2. (*кро́ткий*) meek, únprotésting; ◇ ~ая роль nón-spéaking part.

бессме́нный pérmanent.

бессме́рт|ие *с.* immortálity. ~ник *м.* immortélle. ~ный immórtal; ~ная сла́ва déathless fame, undýing glóry.

бессмы́сленн|о 1. *нареч.* inánely, vácantly; ~ улыба́ться grin vácantly; 2. *в знач. сказ.* it is póintless; ~ говори́ть, идти́, де́лать *и т. п.* it's no use tálking, góing, dóing *etc.* ~ость *ж.* absúrdity. ~ый 1. (*лишённый смы́сла*) absúrd, méaningless; ~ набо́р слов méaningless júmble of words; 2. (*неле́пый*) sénseless, absúrd; ~ый посту́пок sénseless áction; ~ая жесто́кость wánton crúelty; 3. (*неразу́мный*) póintless, fóolish; 4. (*неосмы́сленный*) ináne; ~ый смех ináne láughter; ~ый взгляд vácant look, blank stare; ~ая улы́бка méaningless/vácuous smile.

бессмы́слица *ж. разг.* nónsense; э́то ~! that's absúrd! it dóesn't make sense!

бессне́жный snówless.

бессо́вестный unscrúpulous; shámeless.

бессодержа́тельный émpty, trívial; (*о челове́ке*) shállow, cómmonplace.

бессозна́тельн|ый uncónscious; (*безотчётный тж.*) instínctive; в ~ом состоя́нии uncónscious.

бессо́нн|ица *ж.* sléeplessness, insómnia. ~ый sléepless.

бесспо́рн|о 1. *нареч.* undóubtedly, unquéstionably; 2. *в знач. вводн. сл.* indéed, no doubt. ~ый unquéstionable, incontéstable, indispútable.

бессро́чн|ый pérmanent; ~ о́тпуск indéfinite leave; ~ па́спорт life-passport; ~ая ссу́да loan for an indéfinite term.

бесстра́ст|ие *с.* impássivity. ~но dispássionately. ~ный dispássionate, calm; (*выража́ющий равноду́шие*) impássive; ~ное лицо́ impássive face.

бесстра́ш|ие *с.* féarlessness, intrepídity. ~ный féarless, intrépid.

бессты́д|ник *м. разг.* ímpudent/brázen féllow. ~ница *ж. разг.* shámeless créature; hússy. ~ный shámeless; (*непристо́йный*) indécent. ~ство *с.* shámelessness, immódesty.

беста́ктн|ость *ж.* 1. táctlessness, indélicacy; 2. (*беста́ктный посту́пок*) indiscrétion. ~ый táctless; (*нескро́мный*) indélicate.

бестолко́в|о in a múddled/irrátional mánner; у него́ всё получа́ется ~ he makes a múddle of éverything he puts his hand to. ~ость *ж.* 1. stupídity; 2. (*бессвя́зность*) incohérence. ~ый 1. stúpid, múddle-héaded; 2. (*бессвя́зный*) incohérent; ~ое объясне́ние múddled explanátion.

бесфо́рменный shápeless, fórmless.

бесхара́ктерн|ость *ж.* lack of cháracter, flábbiness. ~ый cháracterless, weak(-willed), spíneless.

бесхво́стый táilless; withóut a tail *после сущ.*

бесхи́тростный ártless, ingénuous.

бесхозя́йственн|ость *ж.* bad mánagement, mismánagement. ~ый unpráctical; (*неэконо́мный*) thríftless, wásteful; ~ое веде́ние дел mismánagement.

бесцве́т|ость *ж.* cólourlessness; *перен. тж.* dúllness, monótony. ~ый cólourless; *перен. тж.* insípid, dull; ~ый газ cólourless gas; ~ые глаза́ cólourless eyes; ~ый расска́з dull/insípid tale.

бесце́льный áimless, púrposeless, póintless.

бесце́нный inváluable, príceless.

бесцено́к *м.*: за ~ *разг.* dírt-chéap, for next to nóthing.

бесцеремо́нн|о hígh-hándedly, cóolly; (*на́гло*) impudently. ~ность *ж.* hígh-hándedness; úndue familiárity; (*на́глость*) ímpudence. ~ый hígh-hánded, cool; (*на́глый*) ímpudent, fórward; ~ое обраще́ние с фа́ктами hígh-handed tréatment of facts.

бесчелове́чн|ость *ж.* inhumánity. ~ый inhúman.

бесче́ст|ить *несов.*, обесче́стить (*вн.*) (*позо́рить*) disgráce (*smb.*); (*поноси́ть*) defáme (*smb.*). ~ный dishónourable.

бесче́стье *с.* dishónour, disgráce.

бесчи́нство *с.* óutrage. ~вать *несов.* commít óutrages, make* hávoc.

бесчи́сленн|ый innúmerable, cóuntless; ~ое коли́чество vast númber/quántity.

бесчу́вственн|ость *ж.* 1. (*неспосо́бность чу́вствовать*) númbness; (*бессерде́чие*) hárshness, lack of féeling/heart. ~ый 1. (*лишённый спосо́бности чу́вствовать*) numb, lífeless; (*бессозна́тельный*) uncónscious; 2. (*бессерде́чный, равноду́шный*) cold, unféeling; (*безжа́лостный*) héartless.

бесчу́встви|е *с.* 1. (*поте́ря созна́ния*) oblívion, loss of cónsciousness; в ~и uncónscious; пьян до ~я dead drunk; 2. (*равноду́шие*) héartlessness.

бесшаба́шный *разг.* réckless, fóolhardy.

бесшу́мный nóiseless, sílent.

бе́та *ж.* béta. ~-лучи́ *мн. физ.* béta rays.

бето́н *м.* cóncrete. ~и́ровать, забетони́ровать (*вн.*) cóncrete (*smth.*). ~ка *ж. разг.* cóncrete road/highway; (*взлётная полоса́*) cóncrete rúnway. ~ный cóncrete.

бечева́ *ж.* tów(ing)-rope.

бечёвка *ж.* string, twine.

бе́шен|ство *с.* 1. (*боле́знь*) hydrophóbia; (*у живо́тных тж.*) rábies; 2. (*неи́стовство*) rage, fúry; приводи́ть кого́-л. в ~ infúriate *smb.*; drive* *smb.* mad; приходи́ть в ~ fall* ínto a pássion. ~ый 1. (*о живо́тных*) mad, rábid; ~ая соба́ка mad dog; 2. (*неи́стовый*, *необу́зданный*) fúrious, víolent; ~ый хара́ктер víolent témper; ~ая страсть víolent pássion; ~ый темп fúrious rate/témpo; ◇ ~ые де́ньги móney to burn.

биатло́н *м.* winter bíathlon. ~и́ст *м.* bíathloner.

библе́йский bíblical.

библио́граф *м.* bibliógrapher.

библиографи́ческий bibliográphical.

библиогра́фия *ж.* bibliógraphy.

библиоте́к|а *ж.* líbrary. ~арь *м.* librárian.

библиоте́ка-чита́льня *ж.* públic líbrary and réading-room.

библиоте́чный líbrary *attr.*

Би́блия ж. Bíble.

би́вень м. tusk.

бигуди́ мн. нескл. cúrlers.

бидо́н м. can; (большой — для молока) mílk-churn.

бие́ние с. béating; (сильное) thróbbing; ~ се́рдца héart-beat; ◇ ~ жи́зни the pulse of life.

бижуте́рия ж. bijóuterie, cóstume jéwellery.

бизо́н м. зоол. bíson; búffalo амер.

биле́т м. 1. (входной, проездной и т. п.) tícket; ~ в теа́тр théatre tícket, tícket to/for the théatre; 2. (членский и т. п.) pass, card; парти́йный ~ Párty (-mémbership) card; студе́нческий ~ stúdent's pass; воѐнный ~ mílitary-sérvice card; 3. (экзаменационный) páper.

билетёр м. tícket colléctor; (в театре, кино) atténdant.

биле́тн|ый tícket attr.; ~ая ка́сса bóoking-office; (в театре, кино) bóx-office.

биллио́н м. thóusand míllion, mílliard; bíllion амер.

билья́рд м. 1. (игра) bílliards pl; 2. (стол) bílliard--table. ~ная ж. bílliard-room. ~ный bílliard.

бино́кль м. binóculars pl; полево́й ~ fíeld-glasses pl; театра́льный ~ ópera-glasses pl.

бино́м м. мат. binómial; ~ Ньюто́на binómial théorem.

бинт м. bándage.

бинтова́ть, забинтова́ть (вн.) bándage (smth.). ~ся, забинтова́ться bándage onesélf.

биогеогра́фия ж. biogeógraphy.

био́граф м. biógrapher. **-и́ческий** biográphic(al).

биогра́фи|я ж. biógraphy; рассказа́ть свою́ ~ю give* a brief accóunt of one's life.

био́лог м. biólogist. ~и́ческий biológical.

биоло́гия ж. biólogy.

био́ника ж. biónics.

биосфе́ра ж. bíosphere.

биото́ки мн. áction cúrrents/poténtial(s).

биофи́зика ж. biophýsics.

биохи́мия ж. biochémistry.

би́рж|а ж. stock exchánge; ◇ ~ труда́ lábour exchánge. **-ево́й**: ~ева́я игра́ stóckjobbing; ~ево́й ма́клер stóckbroker.

би́рка ж. tag.

бирма́н|ец м., ~ка ж. Burmése, Búrman. ~ский Burmése, Búrman; ~ский язы́к Burmése, the Burmése lánguage.

бирю́з|а ж. túrquoise. **-о́вый** 1. túrquoise; ~о́вый ка́мень túrquoise (stone); ~о́вые се́рьги túrquoise éar--rings; 2. (цвета бирюзы) túrquoise; ~о́вое мо́ре túrquoise sea.

бирю́льки мн. (ед. бирю́лька ж.) spíllikins, jáck--straws; ◇ игра́ть в ~ frítter one's time awáy.

бис encóre!; на ~ as an encóre, by way of encóre; исполня́ть что-л. на ~ give* smth. as an encóre.

би́сер м. собир. beads pl; ◇ мета́ть ~ пе́ред свинья́ми cast* pearls before swine; ~ный béaded; ◇ ~ный по́черк fine hand, délicate hándwriting.

биси́ровать несов. и сов. give* an encóre; (вн.) repéat (smth.).

бискви́т м. spónge(-cáke). ~ный: ~ное те́сто sponge pástry; ~ное пиро́жное, пече́нье spónge-cáke.

биссектри́са ж. мат. biséctor.

би́тва ж. báttle.

битко́м: ~ наби́т(ый) crammed, packed, crám-fúll.

бито́к м. ríssole; méat-ball амер.

би́т|ый 1. béaten; 2. (о посуде) bróken (разбитый); cracked (треснувший); ◇ ~ая пти́ца frésh-killed póultry/game; ~ час (for) a sólid hour.

бить, поби́ть, проби́ть, разби́ть 1. тк. несов. (по дт., в вн.; ударять) strike* (smth.), beat* (smth.), hit* (smth.), knock (smth.); конь бьёт копы́том the horse stamps; косо́й дождь бьёт по стёклам the dríving rain

lashed the window-panes; 2. сов. поби́ть (вн.) beat* (smb., smth.); они́ би́ли друг дру́га кулака́ми и нога́ми they punched and kicked éther; 3. тк. несов. (вн.; убивать) kill (smb.); (резать скот) sláughter (smth.); ~ пти́цу kill póultry; ~ ры́бу острого́й spear fish; 4. тк. несов. (стрелять) shoot*; ~ ме́тко shoot* straight; ~ ми́мо це́ли miss one's aim; 5. тк. несов. (на вн.; об оружии) have* an efféctive range (of); револьве́р бьёт на 600 ме́тров the revólver has an efféctive range of six húndred métres; 6. сов. разби́ть (вн.; раздроблять) smash (smth.), break* (smth.); ~ посу́ду break*/smash the cróckery; ~ стёкла break*/smash wíndows; 7. тк. несов. (в вн.) ударами производить звуки) sound (smth.); (глухо) thump (smth.); ~ в ко́локол sound/toll a bell; ~ в бараба́н beat* a drum; 8. тк. несов. (в сочет. с некоторыми сущ.: давать сигнал): ~ зо́рю sound the revéille; ~ трево́гу raise the alárm; 9. сов. проби́ть (о часах) strike*; часы́ бьют по́лночь the clock strikes mídnight; 10. тк. несов. (выбиваться с силой) gush out, spurt out; (о фонтане) play; ~ струёй spurt; ◇ эне́ргия в нём бьёт ключо́м he is búbbling óver with énergy; ~ наверняка́ ónly shoot* once; ~ в одну́ то́чку cóncentrate on one thing; ~ на эффе́кт strain áfter efféct; ~ кого́-л. по карма́ну touch smb. in his, her pócket.

битьё с. 1. (побои) béating; 2. (посуды и т. п.) smáshing, bréaking.

би́ться несов. 1. (с тв.; драться, сражаться) fight* (smb., with); 2. (о вн.; ударяться) knock (agáinst), beat* (agáinst); ~ голово́й об сте́нку knock one's head agáinst a wall; 3. (разбиваться) break*; 4. (о сердце) beat*; 5. (над тв.) sweat (óver); как он ни би́лся... try as he would...; ◇ ~ как ры́ба об лёд strúggle désperately for a líving; ~ об закла́д bet*.

битю́г м. 1. cárt-horse, dráy-horse; 2. перен. strong man.

бифште́кс м. béefsteak.

бич м. whip, lash; перен. scourge. ~ева́ние с. flagellátion; перен. castigátion; ~ева́ть несов. (вн.) flog (smb.), whip (smb.); перен. chástise (smb., smth.), scourge (smb., smth.); ~ева́ть поро́ки cénsure faults, chástise évil.

бла́г|о I с. 1. good, bénefit; о́бщее ~ cómmon good/weal; на ~ челове́чества for the bénefit of mankínd; 2. мн. goods; материа́льные и духо́вные ~а matérial and spíritual goods; произво́дство материа́льных благ prodúction of matérial wealth; ~а жи́зни the things of life, matérial bénefits; ◇ ни за каки́е ~а! not for worlds!; всех благ! good luck!; жела́ю вам вся́ких благ I wish you évery háppiness.

бла́го II союз разг. (тем более, что) (partícularly) since.

благови́дный próper; ~ предло́г pláusible excúse.

благоволи́ть несов. (к дт.) be* well/kíndly dispósed (to).

благовоспи́танный wéll-bréd, well bróught-úp.

благогове́ние с. réverence, venerátion; внуша́ть ~ кому́-л. inspíre smb. with profóund venerátion.

благогове́ть несов. (перед тв.) have* a profóund respéct (for), revére (smb.).

благодар|и́ть, поблагодари́ть (вн.) thank (smb.); ~ю́ вас! thank you!, thanks!

благода́рн|ость ж. 1. grátitude, thánkfulness (for); в ~ за что-л. in acknówledgement/recognítion of smth.; 2. (официальная положительная оценка чьего-л. труда) méssage of thanks/appreciátion; вы́нести кому́-л. ~ за что-л. thank smb. officially for smth.; объяви́ть ~ в прика́зе thank in an órder of the day; получи́ть ~ recéive an official méssage of thanks. ~ый gráteful, thánkful; перен. grátifying, rewárding; ~ая аудито́рия appréciative áudience; ~ый материа́л rewárding matérial; ~ая роль good*/prómising part.

благодаря́ thanks to, ówing to; ◇ ~ тому́, что thanks to the fact that.

благода́тный bléssed; ~ дождь the good/refréshing rain; ~ край land of plénty/abúndance.

благоде́нствовать *несов.* thrive*.

благоде́тельн|ый benefícial.

благодея́ние *с. уст.* boon.

благоду́ш|ие *с.* éuphoria; good húmour. ~ный euphóric; géntle.

благожела́тельн|о fávourably; ~ относи́ться к *кому́-либо* be* wéll-dispósed towárds *smb.* ~ость *ж.* benévolence, góodwill. ~ый wéll-dispósed; kíndly; (*об отзыве и т. п.*) fávourable; ~ый челове́к góod-nátured pérson, fávourably dispósed pérson; ~ое отношéние fávourable áttitude.

благозву́ч|ие *с.*, ~ность *ж.* éuphony, pléasant hármony. ~ный harmónious, euphónious.

благ|о́й I *уст.* good; ~ое де́ло a good job; ~а́я мысль háppy thought; ~ие намéрения good inténtions.

благ|о́й II: крича́ть ~и́м ма́том yell for all *one* is worth, shout at the top of *one's* voice.

благонадёжн|ость *ж. уст.* reliabílity, trústworthiness. ~ый *уст.* relíable, trústworthy.

благообра́зный fíne-lóoking, pérsonable.

благополу́ч|ие *с.* wéll-béing, prospérity; (*счастье*) háppiness. ~но sáfely; all right, well; всё обстои́т ~но éverything is all right, all is well; они́ ~но дое́хали до ме́ста they arríved sáfely at their destinátion. ~ный succéssful, háppy.

благоприобре́тенный acquíred.

благоприя́т|ный fávourable, propítious, ~ момéнт propítious móment; ~ные усло́вия fávourable condítions; ~ное обстоя́тельство propítious círcumstance; ~ фа́ктор condúcive fáctor; ~ отвéт fávourable ánswer; все даю́т о нём ~ные о́тзывы he is véry well spóken of.

благоприя́тствов|ать *несов.* (*дт.*) be* fávourable (to); (*быть полезным*) be* condúctive (to); судьба́ ~ала его́ начина́ниям fate smiled upón his éfforts; кли́мат ~ал его́ выздоровлéнию the clímate was condúcive to his recóvery.

благоразу́м|ие *с.* sense, prúdence, discrétion; образе́ц ~ия a módel of discrétion. ~но sénsibly; ~но умолча́ть о чём-л. maintáin a discréet sílence on *smth.*; он ~но удали́лся *разг.* he had the sense to leave. ~ный réasonable, sénsible, wise; ~ный челове́к réasonable pérson; ~ный совéт sénsible advíce; быть доста́точно ~ным, чтобы... have* the sense to...; са́мое ~ное — э́то уйти́ the wísest course would be to go.

благоро́д|ный nóble; (*великодушный*) génerous (-héarted); ~ поры́в good/génerous ímpulse; ~ посту́пок fine/nóble áction; ~ное де́ло good/nóble cause; ~ная красота́ refíned/nóble béauty; ◇ ~ные мета́ллы précious métals. ~ство *с.* nobílity, nóbleness; (*великодушие*) generósity.

благоскло́нн|о fávourably; ~ вы́слушать *кого-л.* lend* a wílling/fávourable ear to *smth.*; ~ приня́ть *кого-л.* recéive *smb.* kíndly, give* *smb.* a fávourable recéption; относи́ться ~ к *кому-л.* be* fávourably dispósed towárds *smb.* ~ость *ж.* fávour, kíndness; по́льзоваться чьей-л. ~остью be* in *smb.'s* good gráces/books; сниска́ть чью́-либо ~ость find* fávour in *smb.'s* eyes. ~ый fávourable, kíndly; ~ое отношéние góodwill, kíndness; ~ый приём fávourable/córdial recéption; ~ое внима́ние fávourable atténtion; ~ый взгляд kíndly glance.

благослов|и́ть *сов. см.* благословля́ть. ~ля́ть, благослови́ть (*вн.*) **1.** bless (*smb.*); **2.** (*одобрять*) appróve (of), give* *one's* bléssing/appróval (to).

благосостоя́ние *с.* wéll-béing, prospérity; wélfare.

благотвори́тель *м.* philánthropist. ~ность *ж.* chárity, philánthropy. ~ный cháritable, benévolent; chárity *attr.*, philanthrópic; с ~ной це́лью for chárity, with a cháritable/benévolent púrpose.

благотво́рный benefícial, sálutary.

благоустра́ивать, благоустро́ить (*вн.*) províde aménities (for), módernize (*smth.*).

благоустро́|енный cómfortable; with módern convéniences *после сущ.*; with all próper aménities *после сущ.*; (*о квартире, доме тж.*) wéll-appóinted; ~ го́род cíty with all próper aménities. ~ить *сов. см.* благоустра́ивать.

благоустро́йств|о *с.* impróvement, provísion of aménities; ~ го́рода cíty/town impróvement; рабо́та по ~у сéльских посёлков províding hóusing and aménities for rúral séttlements.

благоуха́н|ие *с.* frágrance. ~ный frágrant, swéet-smelling.

благоуха́|ть *несов.* be* frágrant, smell* sweet/nice. ~ющий frágrant, swéet-smelling, swéet-scénted.

блажéн|ный 1. bléssed; (*выражающий блаженство*) blíssful; **2.** *разг.* (*чудаковатый*) dótty. ~ство *с.* bliss.

блажéнствовать *несов.* enjóy onesélf, enjóy/have* a blíssful exístence.

блажь *ж. разг.* whim; на неё нашла́ ~ he was seized with a súdden whim, the fáncy took him.

бланк *м.* form; ~ заявлéния applicátion form; ~ для почто́вого перево́да póstal órder form; телегра́фный ~ télegraph form; запо́лните, пожа́луйста, ~ fill in the form, please.

бледнéть, побледнéть **1.** turn/grow*/becóme* pale; **2.** (*перед тв.; терять свою силу, яркость*) fade/pale ínto insigníficance (before), be* outshóne/overshádowed (by).

бледноли́цый pále(-faced).

блéдн|ость *ж.* **1.** pállor; **2.** (*отсутствие яркости, выразительности*) féebleness, flátness, lack of force/cólour. ~ый **1.** pale, pállid; **2.** (*невыразительный*) cólourless, féeble, insigníficant; ~ый расска́з féeble stóry.

блёк|лый fáded; (*тусклый*) pállid, dim. ~нуть, поблёкнуть fade, wíther; (*тускнеть*) grow* dim.

блеск *м.* glítter; *перен.* brílliance; ~ наря́да spléndour/brílliance of attíre; ~ ума́ brílliance of íntellect; терять ~ lose* its lústre; ◇ во всём ~е in all *one's* spléndour; с ~ом brílliantly.

блесна́ *ж.* spóon-bait.

блес|ну́ть *сов.* flash; *перен.* show* up súddenly; у меня́ ~ну́ла мысль the thought flashed through my mind. ~тéть *несов.* **1.** gleam, glítter; огни́ ~тя́т lights are gléaming; звёзды блéщут stars are shíning/glíttering; **2.** (*о глазах*) shine*; **3.** (*отличаться какими-л. качествами*) shine*; он не блéщет умо́м he has no spécial pówers of íntellect, he's not véry bright.

блёстк|и *мн.* (*ед.* блёстка *ж.*) **1.** (*украшение*) spángles, séquins; в ~ах, укра́шенный ~ами spángled, bespángled; **2.** (*светящиеся точки*) spárkles; *перен.* fláshes; ~ остроу́мия fláshes of wit.

блестя́щ|ий shíning; *перен.* brílliant; ~ метео́р glíttering méteor; ~ие глаза́ shíning eyes; ~ее образова́ние spléndid educátion; ~ лéктор brílliant lécturer; ~ успéх dázzling succéss.

блéять *несов.* bleat.

ближа́йш|ий 1. (*самый близкий*) the néarest; в ~ем бу́дущем in the véry near fúture; в ~ие дни (with)in the next few days; в ~ие же дни as soon as póssible; **2.** (*непосредственный*) immédiate; при ~ем рассмотрéнии on clóser inspéction; при ~ем уча́стии *кого-л.* with the close co-operátion of *smb.*

бли́же (*сравнит. ст. прил.* бли́зкий *и нареч.* бли́зко) néarer; (*об отношениях тж.*) clóser; ~ к дéлу! stick to the point!

бли́зк|ий *прил.* **1.** near; ~яя диста́нция short range; ~им путём by the shórtest route; ~ свет *авт.* dipped héadlights; **2.** *в знач. сущ. м. уст.* *one's* néighbour.

близ near, by, close to.

бли́зиться *несов.* draw* near, appróach.

бли́зкие *мн.* (*родственники*) rélatives, *one's* péople/fámily.

бли́з|**кий 1.** (*на небольшом расстоянии*) near, close; (*близлежащий*) néar-by, néighbouring; на ~ком расстоя́нии от *чего-л.* not far from *smth.*; quite near *smth.*; **2.** (*во времени*) near, impénding; ~кое бу́дущее near fúture; ~ отъе́зд impénding depárture; ~кая смерть appróaching/impénding death; **3.** (к *дт.*; *приближаю-щийся к какому-л. состоянию*) near (to); néarly (+ -ing); ~ к о́бмороку néarly fáinting; **4.** (*связанный род-ством, дружбой*) dear, close, íntimate; ~ ро́дственник near relátion; ~ челове́к íntimate friend, dear one; он мне ~ок I feel véry close to him; ~кие отноше́ния íntimate relátions/terms; **5.** (*сходный*) close, símilar; ~кие взгля́ды reláted/símilar views; ~ к по́длиннику close to the original; ~ перево́д fáithful translátion. ~ко **1.** *нареч.* near, close; ~ко от го́рода quite near the town, not far from the town; ~ко познако́миться 1) (с *чем-л.*) get* well acquáinted (with *smth.*), gain an íntimate knówledge (of *smth.*); **2.** (с *кем-л.*) becóme* close friends (with *smb.*); Это меня́ ~ко каса́ется I am most clósely concérned; **2.** *в знач. сказ.* (*о расстоянии*) it is not far; до го́рода ~ко it is not far to the town, the town is quite close; **3.** *в знач. сказ.* (*о времени*) it is not long; у́тро ~ко mórning is not far off.

близлежа́щий néighbouring, néar-by.

Близнецы́ *мн. астр.* (*созвездие*) Gémini, the Twins.

близнецы́ *мн.* (*ед.* близне́ц *м.*) twins.

близору́к|**ий** néar-síghted, shórt-sighted, myópic; *перен. тж.* púrblind. ~ость *ж.* shórt-sightedness, myópia; *перен. тж.* púrblindness.

бли́зость *ж.* **1.** (*о месте, времени*) néarness, proxímity; ~ сме́рти appróach of death; **2.** (*близкие от-ношения*) íntimacy; **3.** (*сходство*) clóseness, affínity; ~ взгля́дов clóseness of views.

блик *м.* light spot; со́лнечные ~и игра́ли на стене́ the wall was dáppled with súnlight.

блин *м.* páncake; ◇ пе́рвый ~ ко́мом *погов.* ≈ the first try is not álways lúcky, you must spoil befóre you spin well.

блинда́ж *м. воен.* dúg-out.

бли́нчатый páncake *attr.*

бли́нчики *мн.* (*ед.* бли́нчик *м.*) (small) páncakes.

блиста́тельный brílliant.

блиста́ть *несов.* **1.** glow, scíntillate, shine*; **2.** (*тв.*; *ярко проявляться*) spárkle (with), be* rádiant/brílliant (with); ~ красото́й и мо́лодостью be* rádiant with youth and béauty; ~ остроу́мием spárkle with wit; ◇ ~ отсу́т-ствием *ирон.* be* conspícuous by *one's* ábsence.

блицтурни́р *м.* lightning tóurnament.

блок I *м.* (*грузоподъёмное устройство*) púlley, block.

блок II *м.* **1.** (*объединение государств и т. п.*) bloc; **2.** *тех.* block, únit; шлакобето́нные ~и breeze blocks.

блока́д|**а** *ж.* **1.** siege; blockáde (*тж. перен.*); эконо-ми́ческая ~ económic blockáde; **2.** *мед.* blockáde; ново-каи́новая ~ nóvocaine blockáde.

блоки́ровать *несов. и сов.* (*вн.*) **1.** blockáde (*smb., smth.*); *перен.* block (*smb.*); **2.** *ж.-д.* block (*smth.*).

блоки́роваться *несов. и сов.* (*вступать в блок*) form a bloc.

блоко́в|**ка** *ж. ж.-д.* block sýstem. ~очный block *attr.*; ~очная систе́ма block sýstem.

блокно́т *м.* writing-pad.

блонди́н *м.* fáir-háired man*. ~ка *ж.* blonde.

блоха́ *ж.* flea.

бло́чн|**ый** ~ое строи́тельство indústrialized hóusing constrúction, sýstem búilding.

блоши́ный: ~ уку́с fléa-bite.

блу́дный: ~ сын pródigal son.

блужда́ние *с.* róving, wándering, róaming.

блужда́|**ть** *несов.* (*прям. и перен.*) rove, wánder, roam. ~ющий róving, wándering; ~ющий взгляд róving glance; ◇ ~ющие огни́ will-o'-the-wisp *sg*; ~ющая по́ч-ка *мед.* flóating kidney.

блуз *м.* blouse, smock. ~ка *ж.* blouse.

блю́дечко *с. см.* блю́дце.

блю́до *с.* **1.** (*посуда*) dish; **2.** (*кушанье*) dish; (*одно из кушаний в обеде и т. п.*) course; мясно́е ~ meat dish/course; обе́д из трёх блюд thrée-course dínner.

блю́дце *с.* sáucer.

блюсти́, соблюсти́ (*вн.*) keep* (*smth.*), obsérve (*smth.*); ~ поря́док keep*/maintáin órder. ~тель *м.*: ~тель поря́дка custódian of the law.

бля́ха *ж.* badge.

боб *м.* **1.** bean; **2.** *мн.* (*растение*) beans; ◇ оста́ть-ся на ~ах get* nóthing for *one's* pains.

бобёр *м.* (*мех*) béaver.

бобо́в|**ый** *прил.* **1.** bean *attr.*; legúminous *научн.*; ~ стручо́к béan-pod; ~ые культу́ры légumes; **2.** *в знач. сущ. ж. бот.* púlses, légumes.

бобр *м.* béaver. ~о́вый béaver *attr.*

Бог *м.* God; ◇ изба́ви ~!, не дай ~! God forbid; сла́ва ~у! thank God!, thank góodness!; ~ зна́ет кто (что, куда́ *и т. п.*) God/góodness knows who (what, where *etc.*).

богате́ть, разбогате́ть grow* rich, becóme* rich; (*преуспевать*) thrive*.

бога́тство *с.* **1.** (*обилие денег и т. п.*) wealth; ríches *pl*; **2.** (*роскошь, великолепие*) ríchness, respléndence; **3.** *обыкн. мн.* (*совокупность материальных ценностей*) wealth *sg*, resóurces; **4.** (*обилие, многообразие*) wealth; ~ впечатле́ний wealth of impréssions; ~ кра́сок wealth of cólour; ~ языка́ ríchness of lánguage.

бога́т|**ый** *прил.* **1.** rich; (*о людях, странах и т. п. тж.*) wéalthy; ~ урожа́й rich hárvest; ~ о́пыт rich expérience; ~ витами́нами, жира́ми rich in vitamins, fats; край, ~ леса́ми cóuntry abóunding in forests; **2.** *в знач. сущ. м.* the rich man*; *мн.* the rich; ◇ чем ~ы, тем и ра́ды such as it is, you are wélcome to it.

богаты́рск|**ий 1.** (*об эпосе*) heróic; **2.** (*сильный, могучий*) Hercúlean, exúberant; ~ое здоро́вье rude/exúberant health; ~ое телосложе́ние athlétic build; ◇ ~ сон *шутл.* sound sleep.

богаты́рь *м.* **1.** (*эпический*) bogatýr, wárrior; **2.** (*си-лач*) strápping/stálwart féllow.

бога́ч *м.* rich man*; *мн. собир.* the rich.

боге́ма *ж.* Bohémians *pl*; (*образ жизни*) bohémianism.

боги́ня *ж.* góddess.

Богоро́дица *ж.* The Vírgin, Our Lády

богослуже́ние *с.* divíne sérvice.

боготвори́ть *несов.* (*вн.*) wórship (*smb.*), adóre (*smb.*).

бода́ться *несов.* butt.

бодли́вый given to bútting *после сущ.*; bellígerent.

бодр|**и́ть** *несов.* (*вн.*) invígorate (*smb., smth.*), stímulate (*smb., smth.*). ~и́ться *несов.* try to keep *one's* spirits up; как он ни ~и́тся... for all his pluck...

бо́дрость *ж.* vígour; (*бодрое настроение*) chéerfulness; ~ ду́ха pluck, spírit; вселя́ть ~ в кого-л. put* fresh heart into smb.

бо́дрствовать *несов.* be*/stay awáke.

бо́др|**ый** áctive, vígorous; (*весёлый, оживлённый*) chéerful, búoyant; име́ть ~ вид look véry spry; ~ая по-хо́д а jáunty gait; ~ шаг brisk pace; ~ое настрое́ние búoyant spírits *pl*; ~ ду́хом in good spírits, chéerful; на-строе́ние солда́т ~ое the morále of the men is éxcellent.

бодря́щий brácing, invígorating, stímulating.

боеви́к *м.* **1.** (*фильм и т. п.*) hit; **2.** mémber of a fíghting group.

боеви́тый keen, cómbative.

боев|**о́й 1.** fíghting; ~о́е зада́ние cómbat

operátion/míssion; ~áя подготовка cómbat tráining; ~ патрóн live/ball cártridge; в ~ готóвности in fíghting trim, réady for áction; 2. (*воинственный*) fíghting, béllicose; (*воинствующий*) mílitant; ~ дух fíghting spírit; 3. (*решительный, бойкий*) gó-ahead, enérgetic, lívely; 4. (*особо важный*) úrgent, vítal; ~áя задáча vítal task; ~áя тéма impórtant/úrgent tópic.

боеголóвк|**а** ж. (*боевая головка*) wárhead; ракéта с я́дерной ~ой míssile with a núclear wárhead, núclear-tipped míssile.

боеготóвность ж. báttle réadiness/prepáredness.

боеприпáсы мн. ammunítion sg.

боеспосóбн|**ость** ж. fíghting efficiency. ~ый efficient; cápable of fíghting после сущ.

боéц м. 1. (*воин*) fíghter; wárrior поэт.; 2. (*солдат*) (prívate) sóldier, man*; командúры и бойцы́ ófficers and men.

Бóже oh God!; ~ мой! my God!

божéст|**венный** divíne; ~вó с. divínity.

бóж|**ий** God's; ◇ кáждый ~ день évery (bléssed) day; я́сно как ~ день as clear as nóonday. ~и́ться несов. swear*. ~óк м. ídol.

бой м. 1. (*битва, сражение*) báttle, engágement, áction; (*небольшой*) fight, cómbat; бои́ мéстного значéния lócal engágements; по всему́ фрóнту иду́т бои́ fíghting is góing on alóng the whóle front; воздýшный ~ áerial engágement, air báttle; (*небольшой*) air fight; развéдка бóем fíghting recónnaissance; приня́ть ~ fight*, accépt báttle; ввести́ в ~ нóвые си́лы bring* fresh fórces ínto áction; 2. (*борьба, состязание*) fight, fíghting; 3. (*убой*) sláughter; 4. (*разбивание*) bréaking; 5. собир. (*разбитая посуда*) bréakage; 6.: ~ часóв stríking of a clock; the chimes pl; часы́ с бóем a stríking clock; (*карманные*) repéater; ◇ взять что-л. с бóю take* smth. by assáult, перен. have* to fight for smth.; уступи́ть без бóя give* up without a fight; бить кого-л. смéртным бóем beat* smb. within an inch of his, her life.

бóйк|**ий** 1. (*решительный и находчивый*) shrewd, sharp, smart; ~ мáлый a sharp young man*; 2. (*живой, быстрый*) lívely, brisk; ~ ум lívely/réady wit; ~ая речь lívely talk; 3. (*полный движения*) búsy; ~ая ýлица búsy street; ~ая торгóвля brisk trade; ◇ на язы́к glib, glíb-tóngued; ~ое перó у кого-л. he has a lívely pen.

бойкóт м. bóycott. ~и́ровать несов. (вн.) bóycott (smb., smth.); разг. (не общаться) óstracize (smb.).

бойни́ца ж. lóop-hole, slit.

бóйня ж.1. sláughter-house; 2. (*массовое убийство людей*) cárnage, mássacre, bútchery.

бок м. side; спать на прáвом ~ý sleep* on one's right side; у негó боли́т лéвый ~ he has a pain in his left side; по ~áм чего-л. on éither side of smth.; ◇ ~ ó ~ side by side; пóд ~ом near by, just round the córner.

бокáл м. góblet, glass; ◇ поднимáть ~ за кого-л., что-л. give* a toast to smb., smth.

бокóв|**óй** side attr.; láteral научн.; ~ кармáн síde-pocket; ~áя аллéя síde-path.

бóком sídeways; стоя́ть ~ к кому-л. stand* sídeways to smb. ◇ вы́йти ~ turn out bádly.

бокс I м. спорт. bóxing; занимáться ~ом go* in for bóxing.

бокс II м. (*мужская стрижка*) short háircut, crew cut; стри́чься под ~ wear* one's hair clóse-cropped.

бокс III м. (*в лечебных учреждениях*) cúbicle.

боксёр м. bóxer. ~ский bóxer's; ~ские перчáтки bóxing gloves.

бокси́т м. мин. báuxite.

болвáн м. 1. (*деревянная форма*) block, dúmmy; 2. бран. (*дурак*) blóckhead, fool.

болвáнка ж. 1. тех. bíllet, pig; 2. (*заготовка*) blank.

болгáр|**ин** м., ~ка ж. Bulgárian. ~ский Bulgárian; ~ский язы́к Bulgárian, the Bulgárian lánguage.

болев|**óй** páinful; ~óе ощущéние sensátion of pain.

бóлее more; ◇ ~ и́ли мéнее more or less; всё ~ и ~ more and more, incréasingly; не ~ (и) не мéнее как... néither more nor less than...; ~ тогó what is more; тем ~, что... the more so that...

болéзненн|**о:** ~ переживáть, ощущáть feel* kéenly; ~ относи́ться к чему-л. be* véry sénsitive/mórbid abóut smth. ~ый 1. (*нездоровый*) délicate, síckly; ~ый ребёнок délicate child*; 2. (*причиняющий боль*) páinful; 3. (*преувеличенный, чрезмерный*) mórbid; ~ая чувстви́тельность mórbid sensibílity; ~ое самолю́бие pathológical vánity.

болéзн|**ь** ж. diséase, íllness; ~ сéрдца héart-diséase; ◇ ~и рóста grówing pains.

болéльщик м. разг. fan, suppórter; ~ футбóла fóotball fan.

болéть I несов. 1. (*тв.; хворать*) be* ill (with); be* sick (with) амер.; (*перен. переживать*) be* sénsitive (to, abóut), take* (smth.) to heart; ~ гри́ппом, кóрью и т. д. have* influénza, méasles etc.; 2. (*за вн.; о пр.; беспокоиться*) wórry (abóut), feel* (for); get* worked up (abóut) разг.; ~ за успéх дéла have* the succéss of the cause at heart; 3. (*за вн.*) разг. be* a fan (of), suppórt (smth.); он болéет за «Динáмо» he is a Dýnamo fan; ◇ ~ душóй, сéрдцем за кого-л., что-л. wórry abóut smb., smth., take* smth. to heart.

бол|**éть** II несов. (*о какой-л. части тела*) ache, hurt*; у меня́ ~и́т головá I have a héadache, my head aches; у меня́ ~и́т пáлец my finger hurts (me); у меня́ ~я́т зýбы I have a tóothache, у вас ~и́т? what do you compláin of?, where's the pain?; ◇ у меня́ ~и́т душá, сéрдце I'm sick at heart.

болеутоля́ющ|**ий** sédative. ~ее срéдство sédative.

болóнья ж. разг. light nýlon ráincoat.

болóт|**истый** márshy, bóggy; ~истая мéстность márshy área/locálity. ~ный marsh attr.; ~ная водá stágnant wáter; ~ная пти́ца wáder; ◇ ~ный газ marsh gas; méthane научн.

болóто с. marsh, bog; перен. тж. moráss, slough.

болт м. bolt.

болтáнка ж. ав. разг. búmpiness, rough air.

болтáть I несов. 1. (*тв.*) dángle (smth.), let* (smth.) dángle; ~ ногáми let* one's legs dángle; 2. (*вн.*) разг. (*взбалтывать*) shake* (smth.), shake* up (smth.).

болтáть II несов. разг. 1. (*говорить*) chátter; (*о детях*) prate, práttle; (*проговариваться*) blab; ~ глýпости talk nónsense; ~ без ýмолку chátter éndlessly; не нáдо ~ об этом keep* it únder your hat, don't say too much abóut it; 2. (*бегло говорить*) hold* forth; ~ по-англи́йски hold* forth in Énglish.

болтáться несов. разг. 1. dángle, hang* lóosely; 2. (*слоняться*) hang* abóut; ~ без дéла lóiter abóut.

болтли́в|**ость** ж. tálkativeness, garrúlity. ~ый loquácious, gárrulous, vóluble; (*не умеющий хранить тайну*) lóng-tóngued, indiscréet; он стрáшно болтли́в he's a térrible chátterbox.

болтовня́ ж. разг. chátter, twáddle, tittle-táttle.

болтýн I м. разг. chátterbox, práttler.

болтýн II м. (*яйцо*) wind-egg.

боль ж. pain, ache; ревмати́ческая ~ rheumátic pains pl; причиня́ть ~ кому-л. hurt* smb.; душéвная ~ méntal súffering, ánguish (of mind); с ~ю в сéрдце with a héavy/áching heart.

больни́ца ж. hóspital.

больни́чный hóspital attr.; ~ лист dóctor's/médical certíficate.

бóльно I 1. нареч. páinfully; ~ прищеми́ть себé пáлец pinch one's finger bádly; ~ удáрить кого-л. strike* smb. a páinful blow; 2. в знач. сказ. безл. it is páinful; ~! it hurts!; мне ~ it hurts me; мне óчень ~ I am in great pain; ~ ви́деть егó мучéния it's páinful to watch his súfferings; мне ~ ви́деть... it hurts me to see...; ◇ сдéлать ~ *кому-л.* hurt* *smb.*, make* *smb.* súffer.

бóльно II *нареч. разг. (очень);* ~ мнóго ráther a lot; ~ рáно a bit (too) éarly; уж ~ день хорóш! it's such a lóvely day!

больн|óй *прил.* **1.** *(о человеке)* ill, sick; *(о живóтном)* sick; *(о частях тела)* sore, bad; *перен.* sore; он бóлен туберкулёзом he has consúmption; ~áя рукá bad hand; ~óе воображéние mórbid imaginátion; **2.** *в знач. сущ. м.* ínvalid, sick pérson, sick man*; *(пациент)* pátient, case; ◇ ~ вопрóс sore súbject; ~óе мéсто sore/ weak point; свали́ть с ~ головы́ на здорóвую shift the blame on to sómebody else.

бóльше 1. *прил. (сравнит. ст. от большóй) (о размéре)* bígger, lárger; *(о расстоянии, весе)* óver; ~ чем тóнны óver a ton; **2.** *нареч. (сравнит. ст. от мнóго)* more; не ~ чем no more than; как мóжно ~ as much as póssible; в шесть раз ~ (чем) six times as much (as); ~ всегó most of all; э́то мне нрáвится ~ всегó I like this/that the best of all; **3.** *нареч. (с отрицáнием):* ~ не... not... agáin, no lónger, no more; егó ~ нет с нáми he is no lónger in our midst; мы с вáми ~ не уви́димся we shall not meet agáin; он там ~ не рабóтает he no lónger works there, he dóesn't work there ány lónger; я ~ не бýду! I won't do it agáin!, I won't do it ány more!; ◇ ~ тогó moreóver.

большеви́к *м.* Bólshevik. ~и́стский Bólshevik.

большеголóвый with a big head *пóсле сущ.;* macrocéphalous *научн.*

бóльш|ий *(сравнит. ст. прил.* большóй*)* the gréater; ~ая часть the gréater part, most of; ◇ ~ей чáстью, по ~ей чáсти máinly, for the most part; сáмое ~ее at the most/óutside *(в концé предложéния);* ~его я и не жду that's all I ask.

большинств|ó *с.* majórity; *(о людях тж.)* most péople; простóе ~ голосóв majórity vote; ~óм голосóв бы́ло решенó создáть драмкружóк the majórity were in fávour of stárting a dramátics círcle; в ~é слýчаев in most cáses.

больш|óй big, large; *(значи́тельный, вáжный; тж. перен.)* great; ~ гóрод big/large city; ~áя рекá big/great ríver; ~и́е глазá big eyes; ~áя скóрость high/great speed; ~ мáльчик big boy; ~óе big seléction, wide choice; ~ спрос great demánd; ~и́е дéньги a lot of móney; с ~и́ми промежýтками at long íntervals; ~и́е друзья́ great friends; ~áя жизнь full life; ~ успéх great succéss; ~áя пóльза great/much bénefit; получи́ть ~óе удовóльствие от *чего-л.* enjóy *smth.* véry much; ◇ ~áя бýква cápital létter; ~ пáлец *(руки́)* thumb; *(ноги́)* big/great toe; Большóй теáтр the Bolshói Théatre.

боля́чка *ж. разг.* sore, sore place.

бóмба *ж.* bomb; зажигáтельная ~ incéndiary (bomb); фугáсная ~ demolítion bomb.

бомбарди́р *м. разг.* góal-scorer; лýчший ~ сезóна top góal-scorer of the séason.

бомбарди́р|овáть *несов. (вн.) (с вóздуха)* bomb *(smb., smth.); (обстрéливать из орýдий; тж. перен.)* bombárd *(smb., smth.).* ~óвка *ж.* bómbing (attáck), bombárd *(smb., smth.).* ~óвочный bómbing, bombárdment *attr.* ~óвщик *м. ав.* bómber; тяжёлый ~óвщик héavy bómber.

бомб|ёжка *ж. разг.* bómbing. ~и́ть *несов. (вн.) разг.* bomb *(smth.).*

бомбоубéжище *с.* áir-raid shélter.

бондáрь *м.* cóorer.

бор I *м. (лес)* pine fórest; ◇ откýда сыр-~ загорéлся? what stárted all the tróuble?; набрáть с ~у да с сóсенки get* togéther a scratch lot, take* what was, is góing.

бор II *м. хим.* bóron.

бордó I *с. нескл. (винó)* cláret, Bordéaux.

бордó II *прил. (цвет)* cláret-coloured, wine-coloured; плáтье цвéта ~ wine-coloured dress.

бордóвый *см.* бордó II.

бордю́р *м.* bórder.

бор|éц *м.* **1.** fighter, chámpion; ~ за свобóду chámpion of líberty; ~цы́ за мир fighters for peace; **2.** *спорт.* wréstler.

боржóми *м. и с. нескл.* Borzhómi (wáter).

борзáя *ж. (рýсская)* Rússian wólfhound, bórzoi; *(англи́йская)* gréyhound.

бормаши́на *ж.* déntal drill.

бормотáть, пробормотáть *(вн.)* mútter *(smth.).*

бóрн|ый bóric, borácic; ~ая кислотá borácic ácid.

бóров *м.* **1.** boar, hog; **2.** *перен.* obése man.

бородá *ж.* beard.

борóдавка *ж.* wart.

бородáтый béarded.

бородáч *м. разг.* béarded man*.

борóдка *ж.* **1.** small beard; ~ кли́нышком póinted beard; **2.** *(ключá)* (kéy-)bit.

борозд|á *ж.* fúrrow. ~и́ть, изборозди́ть *(вн.)* fúrrow *(smth.),* make* fúrrows (in); морщи́ны ~и́ли егó лоб his fórehead was déeply lined.

борон|á *ж.* hárrow. ~и́ть, заборони́ть *(вн.)* hárrow *(smth.).*

боронов|áние *с.* hárrowing; начáть ~ зя́би start hárrowing land ploughed in áutumn. ~áть *несов. см.* борони́ть.

борóться *несов.* **1.** strúggle, fight*; ~ за свобóду fight* for líberty; ~ за мир strúggle/fight* for peace; ~ с препя́тствиями strúggle agáinst óbstacles/odds; ~ за кáчество продýкции strive* for quálity; **2.** *спорт.* wréstle.

борт *м.* **1.** *(сýдна)* side; ~ ó ~ alóngside (one anóther); за́ ~, за ~ом óverboard; вы́бросить *что-л.* за́ ~ throw* *smth.* óverboard; человéк за ~ом! man* óverboard!; на ~ý on board; брать на ~ take* abóard; **2.** *(одéжды)* (cóat-)breast; **3.** *(билья́рда)* cúshion.

бортжурнáл *м.* lóg(-book).

бортмехáник *м.* flight mechánic.

бортов|óй *attr.; мор. тж.* bróadside *attr.;* журнáл log; ~áя аппаратýра *(искýсственного спýтника)* ón-board equipment.

бортпроводн|и́к *м.* air stéward. ~и́ца *ж.* stéwardess, áir-hostess.

бортради́ст *м.* wíreless/rádio óperator; *(в англи́йской воéнной авиáции)* sígnaller.

борщ *м.* borsch.

борьб|á *ж.* **1.** strúggle; ~ за свобóду и незави́симость strúggle for fréedom and indepéndence; ~ за мир fight/strúggle for peace; ~ с эпидеми́ческими заболевáниями contról of epidémics; ~ нóвого со стáрым strúggle of the new agáinst the old; ~ противополóжностей cónflict of ópposites; **2.** *спорт.* wréstling; класси́ческая ~ Gráeco-Róman (wréstling); вóльная ~ cátch-as-cátch-cán, free style (wréstling).

босикóм *разг.* bárefoot.

бос|óй bárefóot(ed); ~и́е нóги bare feet; ◇ на ~ý нóгу with no stóckings/socks on, bárefóot(ed).

босонóгий bárefóoted, bárefoot; únshód *поэт.*

босонóжки *мн. (ед.* босонóжка *ж.) (обувь)* (ópen-tóe) sándals.

бостóн *м. (ткань)* wóollen súiting.

бося́к *м.* tramp; bum *амер.*

бот *м. (сýдно)* boat.

ботáн|ик *м.* bótanist. ~ика *ж.* bótany. ~и́ческий botánical.

ботвá *ж.* top; *собир.* tops *pl.*

ботви́нья *ж.* botvínnia, cold végetable soup.

бóтики *мн. (ед.* бóтик *м.)* high óvershoes.

боти́нки *мн. (ед.* боти́нок *м.)* boots; high shoes *амер.*

бóты *мн. см.* бóтики.

бóцман *м.* bóatswain, bós'un. ~ский bóatswain's.

бóчка *ж.* **1.** bárrel, cask; **2.** *ав.* (bárrel-)roll.

бочко́м sídeways; пробира́ться ~ sídle.

бочо́нок *м.* keg, small bárrel.

боязли́в│ость *ж.* timídity, apprehénsiveness. ~ый tímid, nérvous, apprehénsive.

боязнь *ж.* fear, dread; ~ простра́нства fear of ópen spáces; agoraphóbia *научн.*

боя́рышник *м.* háwthorn, máy(-bush).

боя́ться *несов.* 1. (*рд.,* + *инф., испытывать страх*) fear (*smb., smth.*); be* afráid (of); ~ тру́дностей shrink* from dífficulties; я бою́сь, что мы опа́здываем I'm afráid we are late; 2. (*рд., не переносить чего-л.*) súffer (from), be* sénsitive (to); ◇ бою́сь вам то́чно сказа́ть I can't say for cértain; не бо́йтесь, он вас прекра́сно по́нял you may be quite sure he knew what you meant.

бра *с. нескл.* wáll-brácket, wall lamp.

брава́да *ж.* bravádo.

брави́ровать *несов.* (*тв.*) defý (*smth.*); (*рисова́ться*) flaunt (*smth.*); ~ опа́сностью brave/defý dánger.

бра́в│о well done!, well played!, brávo! ~урный stírring, inspíriting; ~урная му́зыка bravúra.

бра́вый jáunty, gállant; ~ вид jáunty air.

бразды́ *мн.:* ~ правле́ния the reins of góvernment.

брази́лец *м.* Brazílian.

брази́ль│ский Brazílian. ~янка *ж.* Brazílian.

брак I *м.* márriage; wédlock, mátrimony *юр.;* состоя́ть в ~е с кем-л. be* márried to smb.; расто́ргнуть ~ annúl a márriage; рождённый вне ~a born out of wédlock.

брак II *м.* 1. (*недоброкачественные изделия*) deféctive goods *pl,* réjects *pl,* spóilage; thrów-outs *pl разг.;* 2. (*изъян*) flaw, deféct.

брако́ванный deféctive.

бракова́ть, забракова́ть (*вн.*) scrap (*smth.*), condémn (*smth.*); (*отвергать*) reject (*smth.*).

бракоде́л *м.* slípshod wórker.

браконье́р *м.* póacher. ~ство *с.* póaching.

бракоразво́дн│ый: ~ое де́ло divórce case.

бракосочета́ние *с.* wédding (céremony), mátrimony.

брандспо́йт *м.* nózzle.

брани́ть *несов.* (*вн.*) scold (*smb.*). ~ся *несов.* 1. (*с тв.; ссориться*) quárrel (with); 2. (*ругаться*) scold, swear; ◇ ми́лые браня́тся — то́лько те́шатся the fálling out of fáithful friends renéwal is of love, lóvers' quárrels are quíckly healed.

бра́нн│ый abúsive; ~ое сло́во swéar-word.

брань I *ж.* (*ругательство*) invéctive, abúse, swéaring, bad lánguage.

бран│ь II *ж.:* по́ле ~и field of báttle, strícken field.

брасле́т *м.,* ~ка *ж.* brácelet, bángle.

брасс *м. спорт.* bréast-stroke; плыть ~ом swim*/use the bréast-stroke.

брат *м.* bróther; (*как обращение*) friend, mate, chum, old man*/chap; ◇ ваш ~ писа́тель *разг.* you wríters; по куску́ на ~a a slice each.

брат│а́ние *с.* fraternizátion; ~а́ться, побрата́ться 1. swear* etérnal fríendship; 2. (*на фронте*) fráternize.

бра́т│ец *м.* bróther; (*как обращение*) mate, chum, old chap/féllow; ~цы (my) lads!, boys! ~ишка *м. разг.* little bróther; (*как обращение*) friend, mate, chum.

братоуби́йст│венный fratricídal. ~во *с.* fratrícide.

бра́т│ский fratérnal; brótherly *разг.;* ~ сою́з fratérnal alliance; ~ское сотру́дничество brótherly/fratérnal co-operátion. ~ство *с.* brótherhood, fratérnity; ~ство наро́дов the brótherhood of nátions.

брать, взять 1. (*вн.*) take* (*smb., smth.*); ~ кого́-л. за́ руку take* smb.'s hand; ~ в рот что́-л. put* smth. into one's mouth; ~ те́му для сочине́ния choose* a súbject for an éssay; ~ рабо́ту на́ дом do* work at home; ~ кого́-л., что́-л. с собо́й take*/bring* smb., smth. alóng; ~ ребёнка из шко́лы take* a child* into one's home; ~ что́-л. в долг bórrow smth.; ~ такси́ take* a táxi; ~ биле́ты в теа́тр take*/buy* tíckets for the théatre;

где вы берёте молоко́? where do you get your milk?; 2. (*вн.; взимать, взыскивать*) charge (*smth.*); *перен.* exáct (*smth.*); ~ нало́ги lévy táxes; ~ по́шлины charge dúty; ~ до́рого за что́-л. charge high for smth.; ~ сло́во с кого́-л. exáct a prómise from smb., make* smb. prómise; 3. (*вн.; заимствовать*) bórrow (*smth.*), take* (*smth.*); 4. (*вн.; завладевать, захватывать*) take* (*smth.*), cápture (*smb., smth.*); *перен.* (*овладевать, охватывать*) overcóme* (*smb.*), seize (*smb.*); ~ го́род take*/seize a town; ~ что́-л. при́ступом take*/cárry smth. by storm/assáult; ~ кого́-л. в плен take* smb. prísoner; (меня́) за́висть берёт I am filled with énvy; (меня́) злость берёт it makes me fúrious; 5. (*вн.; преодолевать*) take* (*smth.*); ~ препя́тствие clear an óbstacle; 6. (*тв.; добиваться чего-л.*) succéed (through), get* by (with); он берёт упо́рством it's his óbstinacy does it; ~ наха́льством succéed through sheer árrogance; чем он берёт? what do péople see in him?; 7. (*вн.*) *разг.* (*оказывать действие*) have* an effect (on); хлеб тако́й чёрствый, что его́ нож не берёт the bread's so stale you can't get the knife into it; 8. *разг.* (*направляться*) go*; бери́те леве́е! more to the left!; ~ кру́то в сто́рону turn off shárply; 9. *с некоторыми сущ.:* ~ что́-либо в расчёт take* smth. into accóunt; ~ кого́-л. под защи́ту take* smb. únder one's protéction; ~ что́-л. под сомне́ние quéstion smth., becóme* dóubtful of smth.; ~ курс, направле́ние (на) steer (for), set* course (for); ~ нача́ло originate (in, from); ◇ ~ приме́р с кого́-л. fóllow/take* smb.'s exámple; ~ на себя́ undertáke*; ~ на себя́ отве́тственность за что́-л. assúme responsibílity for smth.; ~ сло́во (на собрании), rise* to speak; take* the floor; ~ себя́ в ру́ки pull onesélf togéther, take* onesélf in hand; на́ша взяла́ our side has won; с чего́ вы э́то взя́ли? what makes you think that?; where did you get that from?

бра́ться, взя́ться 1. (*за вн.; хвататься*) take* (*smth.*); ~ за́ руки take*/join hands; 2. (*за вн.; производить работу каким-л. орудием*) take* (*smth.*), take* up (*smth.*); ~ за руль take* the wheel; ~ за ору́жие take* up arms; 3. (*за вн.; приниматься за что-л.*) set* to work (on); set* abóut (*smth.*), set* abóut (+ -ing); tackle (*smth.*); ~ за де́ло start wórking; вы не так берётесь за де́ло you're not going abóut it in the right way; 4. (+ *инф.; быть в состоянии сделать что-л.*) undertáke* (+ to *inf*); я не беру́сь спо́рить с ним I can't undertáke to árgue with him; 5. (*возникать*) come* (from); отку́да вы взяли́сь? where did you spring from?; ◇ ~ за кого́-л. take* smb. in hand; ~ за ум come* to one's sénses, grow* wíser; отку́да ни возьми́сь súddenly there appéared.

бра́чн│ый márriage *attr.*; cónjugal; ~ сою́з márriage únion; ~ые у́зы cónjugal ties.

бреве́нчатый log *attr.*; made of logs *после сущ.;* ~ дом log house.

бревно́ *с.* log.

бред *м.* 1. delírium; ~ сумасше́дшего the rávings of a mádman*; 2. *разг.* (*бессмыслица*) rúbbish, nónsense, póppycock.

бре́д│ить *несов.* 1. be* delírious, rave; больно́й всю ночь ~ил the pátient spent the night in a state of delírium; 2. (*тв.; увлекаться чем-л.*) be* mad (on); ~ му́зыкой be* mad on músic. ~ни *мн.* nónsense *sg,* móonshine *sg.* ~овой 1. delírious; ~овое состоя́ние delírious state; ~овые виде́ния sick fántasies, hallucinátions; 2. (*нелепый*) nonsénsical, absúrd; ~овая мысль crazy nótion, nonsénsical idéa.

бре́зг│ать, побре́згать (*тв.*) be* squéamish/fastídious (abóut); *перен. тж.* shrink* (from); как вы не ~аете пить из тако́й гря́зной ча́шки? how can you bear to drink from such a dírty cup?; он не ~ает никако́й рабо́той he'll do ánything, no work/job is benéath his dígnity; не ~ никаки́ми сре́дствами stick* at nóthing; have* no scruples. ~ли́вый fastídious, squéamish; ~ли́вый челове́к fastídious pérson; ~ли́вая ми́на fastídious air; вызыва́ть ~ли́вое чу́вство у *кого-л.* make* smb. feel sick, repél smb.

брезе́нт м. tarpáulin. ~овый tarpáulin attr.

бре́зж|**ить** несов. 1. (слабо светиться) gleam fáintly, glímmer; уж ~ит рассве́т day is bréaking; в степи́ чуть ~ит огонёк a light can be seen glímmering fáintly in the steppe; 2. безл. (светать): чуть ~ило it was just grówing light.

брело́к м. charm, trínket.

бре́м|**я** с. búrden; ~ лет the weight of years; ◇ разреши́ться от ~ени be* delívered of a child*.

бре́нн|**ый** уст. tránsitory; ~ые оста́нки mórtal remáins.

бренча́ть несов. 1. jingle; (о саблях и т. п.) clank; (тв.) jingle (smth.); 2. (на пр.) разг. (неискусно играть) strum (on).

брести́ несов. trudge.

брете́льки мн. (ед. брете́лька ж.) shóulder-straps.

брешь ж. breach; проби́ть ~ в чём-л. breach smth.

бре́ющ|**ий**: ~ полёт zéro-áltitude flight; hédge-hopping разг.; лете́ть ~им полётом fly* at zéro áltitude.

брига́д|**а** ж. 1. (производственная группа) team, brigáde; ж.-д. crew; 2. воен. brigáde; ~и́р м. téam-leader.

бри́джи мн. (ríding) bréeches.

бриз м. мор. breeze.

брике́т м. briquétte.

брилья́нт м. díamond, brílliant. ~овый díamond attr.

брита́н|**ец** м. ист. Bríton; разг. Brítisher; мн. the British. ~ский British.

бри́тв|**а** ж. rázor; электри́ческая ~ eléctric rázor/sháver; ~енный sháving; ~енный прибо́р sháving set; ~енные принадле́жности sháving árticles/things.

бри́тый cléan-shaven; (о голове) shaved, sháven.

брить, побри́ть (вн.) shave (smb.).

бритьё с. sháving.

бри́ться, побри́ться shave (onesélf), have* a shave.

бров|**ь** ж. éyebrow; ◇ не в ~, а (пря́мо) в глаз ≈ that hit the mark, that went home; попа́сть не в ~, а в глаз hit* the nail on the head.

брод м. ford; ◇ не зна́я, не спроси́сь ~у, не су́йся в во́ду посл. ≈ look befóre you leap.

броди́ть I несов. roam, rove, rámble; wánder (тж. перен.); ◇ ~ в потёмках be* wándering in the dark, be* at sea.

броди́ть II несов. (подвергаться брожению) fermént.

бродя́га м. tramp, vágrant; hóbo амер.

бродя́жнич|**ать** несов. разг. lead* a vágabond life; (странствовать) rove, roam, be on the road. ~ество с. vágrancy; (постоянные путешествия) róaming, róving.

бродя́ч|**ий** róaming, róving, wándering; ~ая соба́ка stray dog; ~ие музыка́нты itínerant/strólling musícians; ~ о́браз жи́зни únsettled way of life.

броже́ние с. fermentátion; перен. férment; rúmblings pl; ~ умо́в méntal férment.

бром м. 1. хим. brómine; 2. (лекарство) brómide. ~истый хим. brómine; ~истый ка́лий potássium brómide.

бронебо́йный ármour-piercing; ~ снаря́д ármour-piercing shell.

броневи́к м. ármoured car.

броnево́й ármour(ed).

бронено́сный ármoured; ~ кре́йсер ármoured crúiser.

броненосец ármoured train.

бронета́нков|**ый** ármoured; ~ые войска́ ármoured troops.

бронетранспортёр м. ármoured personnél cárrier.

бронз|**а** ж. 1. bronze; 2. собир. (изделия) brónzes pl. ~овый bronze attr.; ◇ ~овый век the Bronze Age.

брони́ровать несов. и сов. (сов. тж. заброни́ро-

вать) (вн.; места и т. п.) resérve (smth.); ~ чью-л. кварти́ру resérve smb.'s flat.

брони́ровать несов. и сов. (вн.; покрывать бронёй) ármour (smth.), protéct (smth.) with ármour.

бронх|**и** мн. (ед. бронх м.) анат. brónchial tubes. ~иа́льный анат. brónchial. ~и́т м. мед. bronchítis.

бро́ня ж. (на места и т. п.) reservátion; (документ тж.) wárrant; (на сотрудника) exémption; железнодоро́жная ~ ráilway wárrant; ~ на жилпло́щадь wárrant for retáining of accommodátion.

броня́ ж. ármour.

брос|**а́ть, бро́сить** 1. (вн., тв.) throw* (smth.); (швырять) fling* (smth.); (опускать) drop (smth.), cast* (smth.); ~ грана́ту throw* a grenáde; ~ снежка́ми в окно́ throw* snowballs at a window; ~ я́корь drop ánchor; перен. тж. find* a háven; 2. обыкн. безл. (сильно качать) throw*, bump; (на море) toss; маши́ну ~а́ло из стороны́ в сто́рону the car was thrown from side to side; 3. (вн.; быстро перемещать) send* (smth., smth.); 4. в сочет. с сущ.: ~ тень cast* a shádow; ~ луч cast* a beam; ~ взгляд на кого-л. cast* a glance at smb.; ~ бы́стрый взгляд на кого-л. dart/shoot* a glance at smb.; 5. (вн.; выки́дывать) throw* awáy (smth.); (класть небрежно) leave* (smth.) in a múddle, leave* (smth.) lýing abóut; 6. (вн.; покидать) leave* (smb., smth.), (в беде и т. п.) abándon (smb., smth.), desért (smb., smth.); 7. (вн., + инф.; прекращать) give* up (smth., + -ing); leave* off (smth., + -ing), stop (smth., + -ing); ~ кури́ть, куре́ние give* up smóking; ~ рабо́ту throw* up a job; quit амер.; брось(те) э́ти глу́пости! stop that nónsense!; 8. безл.: его́ ~а́ло то в жар, то в хо́лод he went hot and cold by turns; его́ бро́сило в жар he felt hot all óver; его́ бро́сило в пот he broke out into a sweat; ◇ ~ грязью в кого-л. fling* mud/dirt at smb.; ~ свет на что-л. throw* light on smth.; ~ ору́жие lay* down one's arms; ~ вы́зов кому-л. chállenge smb.; ~ обвине́ния кому-л. hurl accusátions at smb. ~а́ться, бро́ситься 1. (тв.) throw* (smth.), fling* (smth.); 2. (устремляться) throw* onesélf, rush; (на вн.; нападать) rush (at), dash (at); ~а́ться на по́мощь кому-л. rush to smb.'s help/aid; rush to the réscue; соба́ка ~а́ется на чужи́х the dog will attáck strángers; ~а́ться на коле́ни fall* on one's knees; ~а́ться друг дру́гу в объя́тия rush ínto one anóther's arms; ~а́ться бего́м start rúnning; 3. (прыгать) jump; ~а́ться в во́ду jump ínto the wáter; ~а́ться впла́вь jump in and start swímming; ◇ ~а́ться деньга́ми throw* one's móney abóut/awáy; ~а́ться слова́ми use words líghtly; ~а́ться в глаза́ be* conspícuous/óbvious; leap* to the eye; кровь бро́силась ему́ в лицо́, в го́лову the blood rushed to his face, to his head.

бро́сить(ся) сов. см. броса́ть(ся).

бро́ский разг. stríking.

бросо́в|**ый** разг. tráshy; ◇ ~ э́кспорт dúmping; ~ые зе́мли wásteland sg.

бросо́к м. 1. throw; 2. (стремительное движение) rush; воен. тж. thrust; спорт. sprint; spurt; после́дний ~ final spurt; ~ вперёд fórward rush; перен. leap fórward.

бро́шка ж, брошь ж. brooch.

брошю́ра ж. bóoklet, pámphlet; bróchure.

брошюрова́ть, сброшюрова́ть (вн.) stitch (smth.).

брошюро́в|**ка** ж. stítching. ~щик м., ~щица ж. stítcher.

брус м. 1. beam; (металлический) gírder; 2. мн. спорт. the bars; упражне́ния на бру́сьях éxercises on the bars.

брусни́ка ж. 1. собир. cówberries pl, móuntain cránberries pl; 2. (об отдельной ягоде и растении) cówberry, móuntain cránberry.

брусни́чн|**ый** cówberry attr.; ~ое варе́нье cówberry jam.

брусо́к *м.* 1. (*точильный*) whétstone, hone; 2. (*кусо́к*) bar.

бру́ствер *м. воен.* párapet.

брусча́т|ка *ж.* 1. *собир.* páving (stones *pl*); 2. *разг.* (*мостовая*) paved road. ~ый paved.

бру́тто *неизм. прил. торг.* gross; вес ~ gross weight.

бры́зг|ать, бры́знуть 1. (*тв.*) splash (*smth.*); ~ слюно́й foam at the mouth, sláver; 2. (*разлета́ться*) gush out, spurt; *перен.* spárkle; вода́ ~ала из кра́на wáter spúrted out of the tap; мо́лодость бры́зжет из её глаз her eyes spárkle with youth; 3. (*вн.; опры́скивать*) sprínkle (*smth.*); (*си́льно*) splash (*smth.*); ~ водо́й в лицо́ splash *one's* face with wáter. ~аться *несов.* 1. (*тв.*) splash (*smth.*); 2. (*бры́згать друг на дру́га*) splash each óther.

бры́зги *мн.* spláshes; spray *sg.*

бры́зн|уть *сов.* 1. *см.* бры́згать; 2. (*хлы́нуть*) gush out, spurt out; ~ул дождь it súddenly stárted ráining; слёзы ~ули у неё из глаз tears spúrted from her eyes.

брыка́ть, брыкну́ть (*вн.*) kick (*smb., smth.*). ~ся, брыкну́ться kick.

брыкну́ть(ся) *сов. см.* брыка́ть(ся).

бры́нза *ж.* brýnza, sheep's milk cheese.

брысь shoo!, scat!

брюзг|а́ *м. и ж.* grúmbler. ~ли́вый cantánkerous, bad-témpered.

брюзжа́ть *несов.* grúmble, be* grúmpy.

брю́ква *ж.* swede, rutabága.

брю́ки *мн.* tróusers.

брюне́т *м.* dárk-haired man*. ~ка *ж.* brunétte, dárk(-haired) wóman*, dárk(-haired) girl.

брю́хо *с.* bélly.

брюши́н|а *ж. анат.* peritonéum; воспале́ние ~ы peritonítis.

брюш|ко́ *с.* 1. *разг.* paunch, corporátion, túmmy; нагуля́ть, отрасти́ть себе́ ~ get* (quite) a paunch/túmmy; 2. (*у насеко́мого*) ábdomen. ~но́й abdóminal; ~но́й тиф entéric/týphoid féver.

бря́кать, бря́кнуть *разг.* 1. ráttle, tínkle; (*о металли́ческих веща́х тж.*) jíngle; (*о кру́пных предме́тах*) clank, clang; (*тв.; производи́ть шум*) ráttle (*smth.*), jíngle (*smth.*); 2. (*вн.; с си́лой броса́ть, роня́ть*) bang (*smth.*); бря́кнуть что-л. на пол, на зе́млю put* *smth.* down with a bang; (*урони́ть*) drop *smth.* víolently; 3. (*вн.; необду́манно говори́ть*) blurt out (*smth.*). ~ся, бря́кнуться *разг.* flop (down on).

бря́кнуть(ся) *сов. см.* бря́кать(ся).

бряца́ние *с.* ráttle.

бряца́ть *несов.* 1. ráttle; (*о лёгких металли́ческих веща́х*) jíngle; (*о тяжёлых*) clank, jángle; 2. (*тв.; вызыва́ть звеня́щие зву́ки*) ráttle (*smth.*); (*лёгкими предме́тами*) jíngle (*smth.*); бряца́я шпо́рами with jíngling spurs; ◇ ~ ору́жием ráttle the sábre, brándish *one's* arms.

бу́бен *м.* tambouríne.

бубенцы́ *мн.* bells.

бу́блик *м.* búblik, bréad-ring.

бубни́ть, пробубни́ть *разг.* múmble.

бубно́вый *карт.* of díamonds *после сущ.*

буб|ны́ *мн. карт.* díamonds; шестёрка ~ён six of díamonds.

буго́р *м.* híllock, knoll, rise. ~о́к *м.* 1. (*на земле́*) mound; 2. (*на лёгочной тка́ни*) túbercle, nódule.

бугри́стый únéven.

будд|и́зм *м.* Búddhism. ~и́ст *м.* Búddhist.

бу́дет that'll do!; ~ с меня́! I've had enóugh!; I'm through!; ~ шути́ть! now let's be sérious!

буди́льник *м.* alárm-clóck.

буди́ть, разбуди́ть (*вн.*) wake* (*smb.*), call (*smb.*); *перен.* aróuse (*smth.*); разбуди́те меня́ в 7 часо́в wake me at séven.

бу́дка *ж.* box, cábin; железнодоро́жная ~ línesman's cábin.

бу́дн|и *мн.* 1. wéekdays; *перен.* éveryday life *sg.*; 2. (*однообра́зная жизнь*) drab routíne *sg.* ~ий: ~ий день wéekday. ~ичный 1. wórkaday, wórkday; (*предназна́ченный для бу́дней*) éveryday; ~ичный день wéekday; ~ичное пла́тье éveryday dress; 2. (*ску́чный, однообра́зный*) órdinary, húmdrum.

будора́жить, взбудора́жить (*вн.*) *разг.* excíte (*smb.*), rouse (*smb.*); (*приводи́ть в беспоря́док*) upsét* (*smth.*).

бу́дто 1. *союз* (*как, сло́вно*) as if, as though; он останови́лся, ~ прислу́шиваясь к чему́-то he stopped as though listening to *smth.*; ~ бы, как ~ бы as though, as if; мне послы́шалось, ~ кто́-то меня́ зовёт I thought I heard sómeone cálling me; 2. *союз* (*что — с отте́нком сомне́ния*) *не перево́дится*; он уверя́ет, ~ сам ви́дел he alléges he saw it himsélf; мне сни́лось, ~ я сно́ва в Москве́ I dreamed I was back in Móscow; я слы́шал, ~ он уе́хал I am told he has gone; 3. *частица разг.* (*ка́жется*) it seems; ~ бы for the osténsible púrpose (of); он ~ бы уе́хал he is said to have gone; 4. *частица разг.* (*ра́зве*) indéed?, réally?

бу́дущ|ее *с.* the fúture, time to come. ~ий (*предстоя́щий*) fúture, cóming; (*сле́дующий*) next; ~ее поколе́ние the next/cóming generátion; ~ие поколе́ния fúture generátions; на ~ий год next year; ◇ ~ее вре́мя *грам.* the fúture tense. ~ность *ж.* fúture.

бу́ер *м.* íce-yacht. ~ный íce-yacht *attr.*; ~ный спорт íce-yachting.

буженина́ *ж.* cold boiled pork.

бузина́ *ж.* 1. (*я́года*) élder-berry; 2. (*расте́ние*) élder.

буй *м.* buoy.

бу́йвол *м.* búffalo.

бу́й|ный 1. (*необу́зданный*) wild, víolent, unrúly; (*разгу́льный*) róllicking, rumbústious; (*лихо́й*) bóisterous, impétuous; ~ хара́ктер unrúly cháracter, hárum-scárum; ~ное весе́лье upróarious mirth; 2. (*бу́рный, порыви́стый*) tempéstuous, bóisterous; ~ ве́тер bóisterous wind; 3. (*бы́стро расту́щий*) vígorous; ~ рост vígorous/rápid growth; ~ная расти́тельность lúxúriant/ríotous vegetátion. ~ство *с.* unrúly/disórderly cónduct, bráwling. ~ствовать *несов.* ríot, get* rough; (*о сумасше́дшем*) be* víolent, run* amúck.

бук *м.* beech.

бука́шка *ж.* small ínsect.

бу́кв|а *ж.* létter; прописна́я ~ cápital létter; úpper case *полигр.*; ◇ ~ в ~у líterally, to the létter; ~ зако́на the létter of the law. ~а́льно líterally; я по́нял его́ ~а́льно I took what he said líterally; я ~а́льно не спал I haven't slept a wink. ~а́льный líteral; ~а́льный перево́д líteral traslátion, wórd-for-wórd translátion; в ~а́льном смы́сле сло́ва in the líteral sense of the word.

буква́рь *м.* ABC-book; school prímer.

бу́квенн|ый: ~ое обозначе́ние alphabétical sýmbol.

буквое́д *м. ирон.* pédant.

буке́т *м.* 1. (*цвето́в*) bunch, nósegay, bóuquet; 2. (*совоку́пность вку́совых свойств чего́-л.*) bóuquet.

букини́ст *м.* sécond-hand bóokseller, déaler in sécond-hand books. ~и́ческий sécond-hánd *attr.*; ~и́ческий магази́н sécond-hand bóokshop.

бу́ков|ый beech *attr.*; ~ лес beech wood/fórest; ~ая древеси́на beech (wood); ~ая ме́бель beech-wood fúrniture.

бу́кса *ж. тех.* áxle-box, jóurnal box.

букси́р *м.* 1. (*кана́т*) tow (*line*); 2. (*су́дно*) túg(boat); ◇ брать кого́-л. на ~ take* *smb.* in tow. ~ный tówing *attr.*; ~ный парохо́д *см.* букси́р 2. ~овать *несов.* (*вн.*) tow (*smth.*).

буксова́ть *несов.* skid.

булава́ *ж.* 1. mace; 2. *спорт.* Índian club.

була́в|ка ж. pin; англи́йская ~ка sáfety pin. ~очный pin attr.; ~очный уко́л pínprick; величино́й с ~очную голо́вку the size of a pin's head.

була́ный ísabel, dun.

бу́лка ж. roll; (сдо́бная) bun.

бу́лочн|ая ж. báker's (shop). ~ый: ~ые изде́лия rolls and buns.

бултыха́ться, бултыхну́ться разг. 1. plop, flop; 2. тк. несов. (бара́хтаться) flop about; 3. тк. несов. (пле́скаться о сте́нки сосу́да) slop about.

бултыхну́ться сов. см. бултыха́ться 1.

булы́жн|ик м. cóbble-stone; собир. cóbble-stones pl. ~ый cóbbled; ~ая мостова́я cóbbled road.

бульва́р м. bóulevard. ~ный 1. bóulevard attr.; 2. (по́шлый) low; ~ная пре́сса gútter press; ~ный рома́н tráshy/cheap nóvel.

бульдо́г м. búlldog.

бульдо́зер м. búlldozer.

бульдозери́ст м. búlldozer óperator.

бу́лька|нье с. gúrgle, gúrgling. ~ть несов. gúrgle.

бульо́н м. broth, clear soup; (для больно́го) béef-tea.

бум м. разг. (шуми́ха) boom.

бума́г|а ж. 1. páper; 2. (докуме́нт) dócument; мн. разг. (ли́чные докуме́нты) pápers; 3. мн. (ру́кописи и т. п.) pápers; ◇ оста́ваться на ~e come* to nóthing, remáin ink on páper; це́нные ~и secúrities.

бумагоре́зальн|ый: ~ая маши́на páper-cútting machine.

бума́ж|ка ж. 1. bit of páper, piece of páper; 2. разг. (докуме́нт) páper. ~ник м. wállet.

бума́жн|ый I 1. páper attr.; ~ое произво́дство páper-máking, páper prodúction; ~ые салфе́тки páper nápkins; 2. ~ая волоки́та red tape; 3. (существу́ющий то́лько на бума́ге) fictítious, tóken; ◇ ~ые де́ньги páper cúrrency/móney.

бума́жный II текст. cótton.

бумазе́я ж. fústian.

бу́нкер м. búnker.

бунт м. rebéllion. ~а́рский rebéllious. ~а́рь м. rébel.

бунтов|а́ть несов. rebél. ~щи́к м. rebél.

бур м. тех. drill; (для де́рева, гру́нта) áuger.

бура́ ж. хим. bórax.

бура́в м. gímlet.

бура́вить несов. (вн.) drill (smth.).

бура́н м. blízzard, snów-storm.

бурда́ ж. разг. swill; кака́я ~! hóg-wash!; dísh-water!

бурдю́к м. skin, wíneskin.

бурево́стник м. (stórmy) pétrel.

бурело́м м. собир. fállen wood.

буре́ние с. тех. bóring, drílling; ~ сква́жин drílling (of wells).

буржуази́я с. bourgeoise.

буржуа́зный bóurgeois.

бури́ль|ный bóring attr., drílling attr. ~щик м. dríller.

бури́ть, пробури́ть (вн.) bore (smth.), drill (smth.); ~ нефтяну́ю сква́жину sink*/drill an óil-well.

бу́рка ж. felt cloak.

бу́рки мн. felt boots with léather soles.

бу́ркнуть сов. (вн.) разг. mútter (smth.), say* (smth.) grúffly.

бурла́к м. bárge-hauler.

бурли́ть несов. seethe; перен. тж. buzz with excítement.

бу́рн|ый 1. (о пого́де, мо́ре и т. п.) stórmy, rough, tempéstuous; ночь обеща́ет быть ~ой it looks like béing a rough night; 2. (по́лный собы́тий, волне́ний) evéntful, héctic; 3. (пы́лкий, неи́стовый) wild, enthusiástic; ~ые стра́сти wild/víolent pássions; ~ые аплодисме́нты cheers, tempéstuous appláuse sg, storms of appláuse; ~ая де́ятельность fúrious actívity; 4. (стреми́тельно протека-

ющий, развива́ющийся) rápid, vígorous; ~ рост промы́шленности rápid/vígorous growth of índustry; ~ое тече́ние боле́зни rápid course of the íllness.

буров|о́й bóring; ~а́я сква́жина bóre-hole; ~а́я вы́шка dérrick; rig; ~ молото́к bóre-hámmer.

бурт м. с.-х. clamp.

буру́н м. surf; мн. bréakers.

бурч|а́ть, пробурча́ть 1. (бормота́ть) múmble, mútter; 2. тк. несов. (о бурля́щих зву́ках) rúmble; в животе́ ~и́т my (your etc.) stómach is rúmbling.

бу́рый gréyish-brown; ◇ ~ медве́дь brown bear; ~ у́голь brown coal, lígnite; ~ железня́к límonite, brown íron ore.

бурья́н м. собир. (tall) weeds, scrub.

бу́ря ж. storm, témpest; ~ восто́ргов storm of enthúsiasm; ~ негодова́ния storm of indignátion; ◇ ~ в стака́не воды́ storm in a téa-cup.

буря́т м., ~ка ж. ~ский Búryat; ~ский язы́к Búryat, the Búryat lánguage.

бу́син(к)а ж. bead.

бу́сы мн. beads; béad-necklace sg.

бутафо́р м. próperty-man*; props man* разг. ~ия ж. fake; (в теа́тре) stáge-próperties pl; перен. window-dressing, sham. ~ский próperty attr.; перен. faked.

бутербро́д м. ópen sándwich; ~ с ветчино́й (ópen) ham sándwich.

буто́н м. bud.

бу́тсы мн. (ед. бу́тса ж.) fóotball boots.

буту́з м. разг. chúbby child*.

буты́л|ка ж. bóttle; ~ молока́, кефи́ра bóttle of milk, yóghurt. ~очный bóttle attr., ◇ ~очного цве́та bóttle-green.

буты́ль ж. large bóttle.

бу́фер м. búffer. ~ный búffer attr.

буфе́т м. 1. (ме́бель) sídeboard; 2. (помеще́ние) refréshment room; (небольшо́й) snack bar, búffet. ~чик м. bárman*, bár-tender. ~чица ж. bármaid.

бух разг. bang!, boom!

буха́нка ж. tínned loaf*.

бу́хать, бу́хнуть разг. 1. (издава́ть глухо́й звук) thump, thud; бу́хнул вы́стрел there was a múffled shot; 2. (вн.; роня́ть что-л.) drop (smth.) with a thud; thump (smth.) down. ~ся, бу́хнуться разг. fling* onesélf, throw* onesélf; (в кре́сло и т. п.) flop; бу́хнуться в во́ду throw* oneself ínto the wáter.

бухга́лт|ер м. bóok-keeper, accóuntant; гла́вный ~ chief accóuntant. ~е́рия ж. 1. bóok-keeping, accóuntancy; 2. (отде́л) accóunts depártment; ◇ двойна́я ~е́рия bóok-keeping by dóuble éntry.

бу́хнуть I сов. см. бу́хать.

бу́хнуть II, разбу́хнуть swell*, expánd.

бу́хнуться сов. см. бу́хаться.

бу́хта I ж. (зали́в) bay.

бу́хта II ж. (тро́са) coil.

бу́ч|а ж. разг.: подня́ть ~у raise hell.

бушева́ть несов. rage; перен. тж. storm.

бушла́т м. péa-jacket.

буя́н м. bráwler, rówdy. ~ить несов. get* víolent, go* bersérk.

бы 1. (при выраже́нии жела́ния): он хоте́л бы вас повида́ть he would like to see you; я был бы рад его́ ви́деть I should be glad to see him, I'd love to see him; я хоте́л бы пое́сть I wóuldn't mind a bite of sómething; мне бы тако́й слова́рь if ónly I had a díctionary like that; 2. (при предположе́нии или ве́жливом вопро́се): вам бы отдохну́ть you ought to have a rest; ему́ бы уже́ пора́ быть здесь he should be here by now, he ought to be here by now; не вам бы жа́ловаться it's not for you to compláin, you shóuldn't compláin; 3. (при выраже́нии удивле́ния): кто бы мог подýмать? who could have believed such a thing?; кто бы мог подýмать, что... who could have believed that...; 4. (в усло́вных оборо́тах —

в главных предложениях) would; в придаточных предложениях не переводится; я пришёл бы, éсли бы мог I would have come if I could.

бывáло разг. would (+ inf); used (to); ~, он рабóтал по двенáдцати часóв в сýтки he would work twelve hours a day, he used to work twelve hours a day.

бывáл|**ый** 1. (много видавший) expérienced; ~ вóин, солдáт old campáigner/sóldier, véteran; 2. (привычный) úsual.

быв|**áть** несов. 1. (происходить, случаться) (sómetimes) háppen; (о заседаниях и т. п.) be* held, take* place; со мной э́того никогдá не ~áло such a thing has néver happened to me; с кем э́того не ~áло it's cómmon enóugh; 2. (находиться, быть) be*; не ~ be* néver; по утрáм он не ~áет дóма he is néver at home in the mórning; он ~áет в институ́те с 3-х до 4-х he atténds the ínstitute from three to four; 3. (посещать) go*; я нигдé не ~áю I néver go ánywhere; он у нас чáсто ~áет he óften comes to see us; я там рéдко ~áю I hárdly éver go there; ◇ как ни в чём не ~áло as if nóthing had háppened.

бывш|**ий** fórmer, ex-; ~ие колониáльные стрáны óne-time colónial cóuntries; ◇ ~ие лю́ди háve-beens.

бык I м. bull; здорóв как ~ разг. ≈ as strong as an ox.

бык II м. (моста) pier.

были́на ж. bylína, Rússian épic.

были́нка ж. blade; как ~ as light as air; тóнкая, как ~ wíllowy, véry thin.

были́нный épic.

бы́ло was just góing to, was just on the point of; прекрати́вшийся ~ дождь вдруг снóва поли́л the rain, which had been abóut to stop, súddenly came on éven hárder; он чуть ~ не ушёл he was just on the point of léaving; чуть ~ не вéry néarly; я чуть ~ не забы́л I álmost forgót.

бы́л|**ой** прил. 1. past, bý gone; érstwhile; ~ые временá past times, bý gone days; ~óе счáстье érstwhile háppiness; 2. в знач. сущ. с. the past.

быль ж. true stóry; fact; э́то не скáзка, а ~ it's not just a stóry, it réally háppened; it's a true stóry; сдéлать скáзку ~ю ˉ make* dreams come true.

бы́стри́на ж. rápids pl.

бы́стро quíckly, rápidly, swíftly; ~ соображáть be* quíckwítted, be* quick in the úptake.

быстроглáзый lívely.

быстронóгий fleet, swíft-fóoted.

быстрораствори́мый ínstant; ~ кóфе ínstant cóffee.

быстрорастýщ|**ий** quíck-growing; ~ие потрéбности населéния rápidly grówing requírements of the populátion.

быстрот|**á** ж. speed, rapídity; quíckness; ~ достáвки speed of delívery; с ~óй вéтра like the wind; с ~óй мóлнии as quick as líghtning; ~ отвéта swíftness of one's replý.

быстрохóдный fast.

бы́стр|**ый** rápid, swift; (быстроходный тж.) fast; (проворный, живой тж.) quick; ~ое течéние rápid cúrrent; ~ая лóшадь fast/swift horse; ~ым шáгом at a smart pace; в ~ом тéмпе brískly; муз. in quick time; ~ ум ágile mind; ~ отвéт prompt replý; ~ рост промы́шленности rápid growth of índustry; ~ая речь swift flow of words.

быт м. 1. (уклад жизни) mode/way of life; ~ и нрáвы life and mánners; 2. (повседневная жизнь) éveryday life; домáшний, сéльский ~ doméstic, rúral life.

бытиé с. exístence, béing; ~ определя́ет сознáние béing detérmines cónsciousness; ◇ кни́га Бытия́ Génesis.

бы́тность ж.: в ~ мою́ в Москвé when I was stáying/líving in Móscow, dúring my stay in Móscow; в ~ мою́ студéнтом in my stúdent days.

бытовáть несов. exist.

бытов|**óй**: ~ые удóбства éveryday aménities; ~ое обслýживание sérvice; ~ые услóвия líving condítions; ~ое явлéние éveryday occúrrence; ~áя дрáма play of mánners; ~áя жи́вопись genre páinting.

бытописáтель м. portráyer of órdinary life.

быть 1. (связка и в знач.: находиться, существовáть, присýтствовать) be*; он бýдет у нас в шесть часóв he'll be with us at six; он был рад вас ви́деть he was glad to see you; там, здесь бы́ло мнóго нарóду mány péople were there, here; бы́ло óчень жáрко it was véry hot; будь он здесь if he were here; не будь вас but for you; 2. (иметься) переводится фóрмами гл. have*; у негó бы́ло мнóго друзéй he had mány friends; у негó нé было врéмени he had no time; у негó есть дéти? has he ány chíldren?; 3. (случаться, происходить) háppen; 4. (об одежде и т. п.) be* wéaring, have* on; на нём былá (сéрая) шля́па, он был в (сéрой) шля́пе he had a (grey) hat on; онá былá вся в чёрном she was all in black; онá былá в чёрном плáтье she had a black dress on, she was wéaring a black dress; ◇ ~ бедé! there's tróuble ahéad!; ~ за когó-л., ~ на чьéй-л. сторонé be* on smb.'s side; ~ заодно́ с кéм-л. be* in full agréement with smb.; будь что бýдет come what may, whatéver háppens; былá не былá! (let) come what may!; как ~? what's to be done?; так и ~ véry well, all right; чтобы э́того бóльше нé было! you're not to do that agáin!, don't let it háppen agáin!; что бýдет, то бýдет what is to be will be.

бычáчий, бы́чий bull's; bóvine научн.; ~ язы́к óx-tongue.

бычóк I м. bull-cálf*, young bull.

бычóк II м. (рыба) góby.

бьеф м. reach; вéрхний ~ head wáter; ни́жний ~ tail wáter.

бювáр м. blótting-book, blótter.

бюджéт м. búdget; (личный тж.) fináncial resóurces pl; finánces pl разг.; прéния по ~y debáte on the búdget; ◇ вы́йти из ~а exceéd one's búdget. ~ный búdgetary; ~ная коми́ссия búdget committee; ~ный год búdget year.

бюллетéн|**ь** м. 1. búlletin; ~ погóды wéather repórt; ~ съéзда cóngress búlletin; 2. (избирательный) bállot-paper; 3. (периодическое издание) búlletin; 4. разг. (больничный лист) dóctor's/médical certíficate; быть на ~e be* on sick-leave.

бюрó I с. нескл. 1. (название руководящей части некоторых органов) Buréau; ~ (заседание) méeting of the Buréau; 2. (учреждение) ágency; óffice; ~ путешéствий trável ágency; ~ нахóдок lóst-property óffice.

бюрó II с. нескл. (мебель) buréau.

бюрокрáт м. búreaucrat. ~и́зм м. buréaucratism; red tape. ~и́ческий buréaucratic.

бюрокрáтия ж. buréaucracy.

бюст м. bust.

бюстгáльтер м. brassíère.

бязь ж. únbléached cálico.

В

в 1. (где, в чём) in; (при указании нестоличных городов, местечек, учреждений, заведений и т. п.) at; в СССР, в Москвé, в Лóндоне in the USSR, in Móscow, in Lóndon; в Волгогрáде at Vólgograd; в институ́те, кинó, клýбе, теáтре, универмáге, университéте и т.п. at the ínstitute, cínema, club, théatre, stores, univérsity etc.; в шкóле at school; он гдé-то в здáнии (института и т. п.) he is sómewhere in the búilding; 2. (куда, во что) to; (внутрь) ínto; в СССР, в Москвý to the USSR, to

Móscow; в Волгогра́де to Vólgograd; в институ́т *и т. п.* to the ínstitute *etc.*; в шко́лу to school; отпра́виться в Ки́ев leave* for Kíev; войти́ в дом go* ínto the house, go* indóors; 3. *(когда — о месяце, годе)* in; *(о дне)* on; *(о часе)* at; в январе́ in Jánuary; в 1965 году́ in 1965, in the year 1965; в понеде́льник on Mónday; в после́дний день ме́сяца on the last day of the month; в 2 часа́ at two o'clóck; 4. *(при указании единицы времени)* обы́чно *не переводится;* два ра́за в год, день, ме́сяц, час *и т. п.* twice a year, a day, a month, an hour; 20 оборо́тов в мину́ту twénty revolútions a/per mínute; 5. *(при указании размера и т. п.)* обы́чно *не переводится;* длино́й в три ме́тра three métres long; пье́са в трёх а́ктах play in three acts, thrée-act play; 6. *(при указании расстояния от чего-л.)* at a dístance of... (from); *часто не переводится;* в пяти́ киломе́трах от Москвы́ (at a dístance of) five kílometres from Móscow; 7. *(в течение)* in; он сде́лает э́то в три дня he will do it in three days, it will take him three days; в одно́ мгнове́ние in an ínstant in the twínkling of an eye; 8. *(при указании на вид или форму чего-л.)* in; в чёрном in black; заверну́ть в бума́гу wrap in páper; в фо́рме ша́ра in the form of a sphere; 9. *(покрытый, запачканный чем-л.)* не *переводится;* ру́ки в черни́лах ínk-stained hands; ска́терть в пя́тнах táble-cloth cóvered with stains; лицо́ в прыща́х spótty face; весь в снегу́ cóvered with snow.

вавило́нск|ий: ~ое столпотворе́ние bábel.

ваго́н *м.* 1. *(пассажирский)* (ráilway) cárriage, coach; car *амер.*; *(товарный)* truck; *(закрытый тж.)* (goods) van; (freight) car *амер.*; бага́жный ~ lúggage van; bággage car *амер.*; почто́вый ~ máil-van; máil-car *амер.*; трамва́йный ~ trámcar; stréetcar, trólley *амер.*; 2. *(количество груза)* cárload, trúckload; ~ у́гля trúckload of coal.

вагоне́тка *ж.* truck, trólley.

ваго́нный wágon *attr.*; car *attr.*; ~ парк rólling stock.

вагоновожа́тый *м.* trám-driver.

вагоноремо́нтный: ~ заво́д coach/wágon repáir works.

вагоностроéние *с.* coach/wágon building.

вагонострои́тельный: ~ заво́д coach/wágon-búilding works; cár-building plant *амер.*

ваго́н|-рестора́н *м.* díning-car; díner *разг.* ~-цисте́рна *ж.* tánk-car.

ваго́нчик *м.* *(на полевом стане)* cáravan, tráiler.

ва́жничать *несов. разг.* give* onesélf airs, put* on airs.

ва́жн|о 1. *нареч.* pómpously, with an air of impórtance; 2. *в знач. сказ.* it is impórtant; *(очень)* ~ знать, что ну́жно де́лать it is (extrémely) impórtant to know what to do; э́то не так ~ it dóesn't réally mátter. ~ость *ж.* 1. impórtance; *(значение)* signíficance; большо́й ~ости of great impórtance/signíficance; 2. *(горделивость, надменность)* pompósity; с ~остью pómpously; ◇ не велика́ ~ость! that dóesn't mátter!; э́ка ~ость! what does it mátter?, who cares? ~ый 1. impórtant; *(значительный)* signíficant; ~ое лицо́, ~ая персо́на (véry) impórtant pérson *(сокр.* V. I. P.); ~ая ши́шка *разг.* bigwig, big knob; 2. *(горделивый, надменный)* pómpous; grand; с ~ым ви́дом with an air of (the útmost) impórtance, pómpously.

ва́за *ж.* vase; *(в форме чаши)* bowl; ~ для фру́ктов frúit-stand; ~ для цвето́в flówer-vase, flówer-bowl.

вазели́н *м.* váseline.

вака́нсия *ж.* vácancy.

вака́нтн|ый vácant; ~ое ме́сто vácancy.

ва́куум *м. физ. тех.* vácuum *(pl* -cua, -ums). ~-насо́с *м.* vácuum-pump.

вакхана́лия *ж.* Bacchanália *pl*; *перен.* órgy, révelry.

вакци́н|а *ж. мед.* váccine. ~а́ция *ж. мед.* vaccinátion.

вал I *м.* 1. *(насыпь)* bank, earth wall; *воен.* rámpart; 2. *(волна)* bíllow, róller; ◇ девя́тый ~ the tenth wave, the híghest wave.

вал II *м. тех.* shaft; приводно́й ~ dríving shaft.

вал III *м. эк.* gross; вы́полнить план по ~у fulfíl the plan in the gross.

вале́жник *м. собир.* wíndfallen wood, déadfall.

ва́ленки *мн.* *(ед.* ва́ленок *м.)* felt boots.

вале́нтность *ж. хим.* válency.

валерья́нов|ый valérian; ~ые ка́пли valérian drops; tíncture of valérian *sg.*

вале́т *м. карт.* knave, Jack.

ва́лик *м. тех.* shaft; róller; cýlinder; *(пишущей машинки)* pláten; 2. *(диванный)* bólster.

вали́ть I, повали́ть, свали́ть *(вн.)* 1. *сов.* повали́ть, свали́ть throw* *(smb., smth.)* down, knock *(smb., smth.)* down, bring* *(smb., smth.)* down; *(в борьбе)* throw* *(smb.)*; *(деревья)* fell *(smth.)*; ~ кого́-л. с ног knock *smb.* down; ве́тром повали́ло мно́го дере́вьев the wind blew down mány trees; 2. *сов.* свали́ть *разг.* *(беспоря́дочно складывать)* heap *(smth.)* up, pile *(smth.)* up; 3. *сов.* свали́ть *разг.*: ~ вину́ на кого́-л. blame *smb.*, put* the blame on/upón *smb.*; ◇ ~ всё в одну́ ку́чу lump éverything togéther.

вали́ть II, повали́ть 1. *(двигаться массой)* flock, throng; наро́д ва́лом вали́т (в, из) péople are póuring (into, out of); 2. *(подыматься — о дыме и т. п.)* belch; *(падать — о снеге)* fall* thíckly/héavily, fall* in thick flakes.

вали́ться, повали́ться, свали́ться fall*, drop; ◇ ~ с ног от уста́лости be* drópping with fatígue; у меня́ сего́дня всё ва́лится из рук 1) *(не ладится)* I can't get ánywhere todáy; 2) *(нет сил делать что-л.)* I'm fit for nóthing todáy; у него́ *(вечно)* всё ва́лится из рук his fíngers are all thumbs.

ва́лк|ий unstéady, sháky; *(о корабле)* crank; ◇ ни ша́тко ни ~о fair to míddling.

валов|о́й *эк.* gross; ~ дохо́д gross révenue/íncome; ~а́я при́быль gross prófit; ~а́я проду́кция gross óutput.

валу́н *м.* bóulder.

ва́льдшнеп *м. зоол.* wóodcock.

вальс *м.* waltz; танцева́ть ~ waltz. ~и́ровать *несов.* waltz.

вальц|ева́ть *несов.* *(вн.)* *тех.* roll *(smth.).* ~о́вка *ж. тех.* rólling. ~о́вщик *м.* róller. ~ы́ *мн. тех.* róllers.

валю́т|а *ж.* 1. *(денежная система)* cúrrency; 2. *собир.* *(иностранные деньги)* fóreign cúrrency. ~ный cúrrency *attr.*; ~ная опера́ция cúrrency transáction; ◇ ~ный курс rate of exchánge, exchánge.

валя́ть, сваля́ть, вы́валять 1. *сов.* вы́валять *(вн. в пр.)* roll *(smth.* in); ~ котле́ты в сухаря́х roll cútlets in bréad-crumbs; 2. *тк. несов.* *(вн. по дт.)* *разг.* roll *(smth.* in, on), drag *(smth.)* abóut (on); ~ по́ снегу roll in the snow; ~ по́ полу roll on the floor, drag abóut on the floor; 3. *сов.* сваля́ть *(вн.)* felt *(smth.)*; *(сукно)* full *(smth.)*; ~ ва́ленки make* felt boots; ◇ ~ дурака́ play the fool; валя́й! *разг.* go ahéad!, cárry on!

валя́|ться *несов.* 1. *(кататься)* roll abóut, wállow; ~ в грязи́ wállow in the mud/mire; 2. *разг.* *(лежать)* sprawl, lie*; *(бездельничать)* loll abóut; ~ в посте́ли до 12 часо́в дня lie* in bed till twelve o'clóck; 3. *разг.* *(о вещах)* lie* abóut; всю́ду ~лись кни́ги books were scáttered all óver the place.

вам *(дт. от личн. мест.* вы*)* you; мы к ~ зайдём we'll call on you; мы ~ пока́жем э́ту кни́гу we'll show you the book.

ва́ми *(тв. от личн. мест.* вы*)* by/with you; мы пойдём с ~ we'll go with you; мы за ~ зайдём we'll come to fetch you.

вана́дий *м. хим.* vanádium.

вани́ль *ж.* vanílla. ~ный vanílla *attr.*

ва́нн|а ж. bath; со́лнечная ~ sún-bath. **~ая** ж. báth-room: **~очка** ж.: де́тская ~очка báby's bath.

ва́нька-вста́нька м. tílting doll.

ва́рвар м. barbárian. **~ский** 1. barbárian; 2. (грубый, жестокий) bárbarous, barbáric. **~ство** с. barbárity.

ва́режки мн. (ед. ва́режка ж.) míttens.

варене́ц м. varené́ts (milk baked in an oven and allowed to ferment).

варёный boiled.

варе́нье с. (wholefruit) jam; presérves pl.

вариа́нт м. vérsion; (разночтение тж.) váriant, réading; (шахматный) váriant; ~ прое́кта altérnative desígn.

вариа́ция ж. variátion; биол. тж. modificátion; те́ма с ~ми муз. theme and variátions.

вари́ть, свари́ть (вн.) 1. (отваривать) boil (smth.); (готовить) make* (smth.), cook (smth.); ~ обе́д make*/cook the dínner; ~ варе́нье make* jam/presérves; ~ пи́во brew (beer). 2. (изготовлять путём плавления и т. п.) make* (smth.); ~ мы́ло make* soap; ~ сталь found/make* steel; 3. тех. (сваривать) weld. **~ся, свари́ться** boil; be* bóiling; be* boiled; сов. тж. be* réady; суп уже́ ва́рится the soup is on now; ◇ ~ся в со́бственном соку́ stew in one's own juice.

ва́рка ж. 1. (пищи) cóoking; ~ варе́нья jám-making; 2. (металла) fóunding.

варьете́ с. нескл. varíety show.

варьи́ровать несов. (вн.) váry (smth.). **~ся** несов. váry.

вас (рд., вн., пр. от личн. мест. вы) you; рад ~ ви́деть glad to see you; нет ли у ~ карандаша́? have you a péncil?; мы о ~ вспомина́ли we thought about you.

василёк м. córnflower, báchelor's-bútton.

василько́вый sápphire(-cóloured), róyal blue.

васса́л м. vással; перен. тж. sátellite.

васса́льн|ый vással attr.; **~ая** зави́симость vássalage.

ва́т|а ж. (подкладочная) wádding; (медицинская) cótton wool.

вата́га ж. разг. band, gang.

ватерли́ния ж. мор. wáter-line.

ватерпа́с м. wáter-level.

ватерполи́ст м., **~ка** ж. wáter-polo pláyer.

ватерпо́ло с. нескл. спорт. wáter pólo.

вати́н м. fléecy stóckinet, sheet wádding; пальто́ на ~е wádded coat.

ва́тман м. Whátman (páper).

ва́тник м. разг. wádded jácket.

ва́тн|ый 1. cótton-wool attr.; перен. numb; 2. (на вате) wádded; (стёганый) quílted; **~ое** одея́ло quilt.

ватру́шка ж. chéese-cake, curd tart.

ватт м. эл. watt. **~-мётр** м. эл. wáttmeter.

ва́фельница ж. wáffle-iron.

ва́фля ж. wáfer, wáfer-cake; (из взбитого теста) wáffle.

ва́хт|а ж. 1. мор. watch; стоя́ть ~у, стоя́ть на ~е keep* watch, be* on watch; 2. (исполненная энтузиазма работа) spécial éffort, wórk-effort, wórk-drive; ~ ми́ра wórk-effort for peace.

ва́хтенный прил. 1. watch attr.; ~ команди́р ófficer of the watch; ófficer of the deck амер.; 2. в знач. сущ. м. méssenger (of the watch).

вахтёр м. pórter, dóor-keeper; jánitor амер.

ваш притяж. мест. 1. (перед сущ.) your; (без сущ.) yours; э́то ~а кни́га that is your book; ~у кни́гу я убра́л I put your book awáy; э́то ~? is this yours?; э́та кни́га ~а? is this book yours?; 2. в знач. сущ. мн. (родные) yours; your folks амер.

ва́|ние с. scúlpture. **~тель** м. scúlptor.

вая́ть, извая́ть (вн.) scúlpture (smth.), sculpt (smth.); (высекать) carve (smth.); (лепить) módel (smth.).

вбега́ть, вбежа́ть come* rúnning in, rush in; (в вн.) come* rúnning (ínto), rush (ínto).

вбежа́ть сов. см. вбега́ть.

вбива́ть, вбить (вн.) drive* (smth.) in, knock (smth.) in; (вн. в вн.) drive* (smth. ínto), knock (smth. ínto); он не смог вбить гвоздь he cóuldn't drive the nail in; он вбил гвоздь в сте́ну he knocked the nail ínto the wall; ◇ ~ что-л. кому́-л. в го́лову drive* ínto smb.'s head; вбить себе́ в го́лову get*/take* it ínto one's head.

вбира́ть, вобра́ть (вн.; впитывать) absórb (smth.), soak up (smth.); (вдыхать) inhále (smth.), draw* in (smth.).

вбить сов. см. вбива́ть.

вблизи́ 1. нареч. not far óff/awáy, near/close by; хорошо́, пло́хо ви́деть ~ see* well*, bádly* at a short dístance; он живёт где́-то здесь ~ he lives sómewhere near here; он lives sómewhere in this néighbourhood; 2. предлог (рд.) by, near; ~ от not far from.

вбок разг. to the side.

вброд: переходи́ть ~ cross by fórding; wade acróss; переходи́ть ре́ку ~ ford a ríver, wade acróss a ríver.

вва́ливаться, ввали́ться 1. (становиться впалым) be*/becóme* hóllow/súnken; у него́ глаза́ ввали́лись he has súnken eyes; у него́ щёки ввали́лись he has hóllow cheeks; 2. (в вн.) разг. (входить) burst* (ínto).

вва́лившийся: ~иеся щёки hóllow cheeks; ~иеся глаза́ súnken eyes.

ввали́ться сов. см. вва́ливаться.

введе́ние с. introdúction; ~ в языкозна́ние introdúction to linguístics.

ввезти́ сов. см. ввози́ть.

ввек разг. né́ver; ~ не забу́ду as long as I live I shall né́ver forgét.

вверга́ть, вве́ргнуть (вн. в вн.) plunge (smb. ínto); throw* (smb. ínto); ~ кого́-л. в отча́яние plunge smb. ínto despáir.

вве́ргнуть сов. см. вверга́ть.

вве́рить(ся) сов. см. вверя́ть(ся).

вверну́ть сов. см. вве́ртывать.

вве́ртывать, вверну́ть (вн.) 1. screw (smth.) in; (вн. в вн.) screw (smth. ínto); ~ винт drive*/put* in a screw, insért a screw; ~ ла́мпочку screw/put* a bulb in; 2. разг. put* (smth.) in; вверну́ть слове́чко put* a word in.

вверх up, úpward(s); ~ по ле́стнице úpstáirs; ~ по реке́, ~ по тече́нию úpstréam; ~ нога́ми hang* úpside-dówn; стоя́ть ~ нога́ми stand* on one's head; be* úpside-dówn; ~. дном úpside-dówn; перен. at síxes and sévens, tópsy-túrvy; всё пошло́ ~ дном éverything went tópsy-túrvy.

вверху́ óverhéad, abóve.

вверя́ть, вве́рить (вн. дт.) entrúst (smb. with smth., smth. to smb.); ~ свою́ судьбу́ кому́-л. leave* one's fate in smb.'s hands. **~ся, вве́риться** (дт.) place onesélf in smb.'s hands.

ввести́ сов. см. вводи́ть.

ввиду́ in view of, ówing to; ~ того́, что... in view of the fact that..., considering that...

ввинти́ть сов. см. вви́нчивать.

вви́нчивать, ввинти́ть (вн. в вн.) screw (smth. ínto).

ввод м. 1. (действие) pútting ínto; ~ в де́йствие stárting, pútting ínto operátion; ~ в эксплуата́цию commíssioning, láunching; 2. тех. (устройство) léad-ín.

вводи́ть, ввести́ 1. (вн.) lead* (smb., smth.) in; (вн. в вн.) lead* (smb., smth., ínto); ввести́ кого́-л. в ко́мнату lead* smb. into the room; ~ кого́-л. в семью́ bring* smb. ínto the fámily; ~ войска́ bring* in troops; 2. (вн.; вовлекать, ввергать): ~ кого́-л. в расхо́ды put* smb. to expénse; 3. (вн.; учреждать, внедрять) introdúce (smth.); 4.: ~ в де́йствие но́вую ша́хту put* a new mine ínto operátion, ópen a new mine; ~ что-л. в употребле́ние introdúce smth., start úsing smth.; ~ войска́ в бой engáge one's troops; ~ что-л. в мо́ду bring* smth. ínto fáshion; ◇ ~ кого-л. в курс (дéла) put* *smb.* in the way of things; show* *smb.* the ropes *разг.*

ввóдн|ый **1.** introdúctory; **2.** *грам.* parenthétic(al); ~ое предложéние parénthesis (*pl* -ses), parenthétic clause; ~ое слóво parénthesis.

ввоз *м.* **1.** (*дéйствие*) importátion; предмéт ~a ímport; **2.** (*общее количество ввозимых товаров*) ímports *pl*, impórted goods *pl.* ~ить, ввезти (*вн.*) bring* (*smth.*); in; (*импортировать*) impórt (*smth.*).

ввóзн|ый impórted; ~ая пóшлина import dúty.

вволю *разг.* to one's heart's contént.

ввысь high ínto the air.

ввязáться *сов. см.* ввязываться.

ввязываться, ввязáться (в *вн.*) *разг.* get* invólved (in), get* mixed up (in).

вглубь deep ínto.

вглядéться *сов. см.* вглядываться.

вглядываться, вглядéться (в *вн.*) peer (ínto); (*рассматривать*) take* a good look (at); пристáльно ~ во что-л. gaze stéadily at *smth.*

вгонять, вогнáть (*вн.* в *вн.*) drive* (*smth.* ínto); (*молотком тж.*) knock (*smth.* ínto); ◇ вогнáть кого-л. в крáску make* *smb.* blush.

вдавáться, вдáться (в *вн.*) project (ínto); jut out (ínto); ~ клином form a wedge in; мóре глубокó вдаётся в бéрег the sea forms a deep ínlet; ◇ ~ в крáйности go* to extрéмes; ~ в подрóбности go* ínto détails; ~ в тóнкости split* hairs.

вдавить *сов. см.* вдáвливать.

вдáвливать, вдавить (*вн.* в *вн.*) press (*smth.* ínto), force (*smth.* ínto), squeeze (*smth.* ínto).

вдáлбливать, вдолбить (*вн.*) *разг.* hámmer (*smth.*) in, ram (*smth.*) in.

вдалекé, вдали **1.** *нареч.* in the distance; исчéзнуть ~ disappéar from sight, disappéar out of sight; disappéar ínto the distance; **2.** *предлог:* ~ от a long way from, far from, remóte from.

вдаль ínto the distance.

вдáться *сов. см.* вдавáться.

вдвигáть, вдвинуть (*вн.*) push (*smth.*) in.

вдвинуть *сов. см.* вдвигáть.

вдвóе **1.** twice, dóuble; (*с прил.*) twice as; (*с сущ.*) twice/dóuble the; ~ бóльше twice as much; ~ мéньше half as much; ~ выше twice as high/tall, twice the height; much higher/táller; ~ ниже half the height; much lówer/shórter; ~ дорóже twice as expénsive, dóuble the price; much déarer, much more expénsive; ~ дешéвле twice as cheap, half the price; much chéaper; ~ ближе much néarer; ~ дáльше twice as far, twice the distance; much fúrther; ~ дóльше twice as long; much lónger; я ~ стáрше вас I'm twice your age; он ~ молóже вас he's half your age; he's (éver so) much yóunger than you; увеличить ~ dóuble; уменьшить ~ halve; **2.** (*пополам*) in half; сложить ~ fold in two/half.

вдвоём the two of them (us, you); ~ веселéе it's more fun together; he's ~ alóne together.

вдвойнé dóuble; dóubly; платить кому-л. ~ pay* *smb.* dóuble; ~ дóрог dóubly dear.

вдевáть, вдеть (*вн.*) thread (*smth.*); (*всовывать*) put* (*smth.*); ~ нитку в игóлку thread a néedle.

вдеть *сов. см.* вдевáть.

вдобáвок *разг.* besídes; (к *дт.*) in addítion (to).

вдовá *ж.* widow.

вдовéц *м.* widower.

вдóвий widow's.

вдóволь **1.** *нареч.* (*вволю*) to one's heart's contént; есть, пить ~ eat*, drink* one's fill; мы ~ поéли фрýктов we had as much fruit as we could eat; наговориться ~ talk to one's heart's contént; **2.** *в знач. сказ.* (*много*) in plénty; у нас всегó ~ we have plénty of éverything, we have all we need.

вдóвый widowed.

вдогóнку *разг.* áfter; пуститься ~ за кем-л. run* áfter *smb.*; кричáть ~ кому-л. call áfter *smb.*; послáть кого-л. ~ за кем-л. send* *smb.* áfter *smb.*

вдолбить *сов. см.* вдáлбливать.

вдоль **1.** *нареч.* léngthwise; **2.** *предлог* (*рд.*) alóng; ◇ ~ и поперёк **1)** (*во всех направлениях*) far and wide; **2.** (*основательно*) thóroughly; изъéздить странý ~ и поперёк trável the length and breadth of a cóuntry.

вдох *м.* inhalátion; сдéлать глубóкий ~ take* a deep breath; ~! (*команда*) breathe in!

вдохновéн|ие *с.* inspirátion; прилив ~ия a rush of inspirátion. ~но in an inspíred mánner, with inspirátion; with enthúsiasm, enthusiástically; ~но трудиться work with enthúsiasm. ~ный inspíred.

вдохнов|итель *м.* inspírer, inspirátion, móving spírit. ~ить(ся) *сов. см.* вдохновлять(ся).

вдохновлять, вдохновить **1.** (*вн.*) inspíre (*smth.*); успéх вдохновил егó he was encóuraged by succéss; succéss lent him wings; **2.** (*вн.* на *вн.*) inspíre (*smb.* to); вдохновить кого-л. на пóдвиг inspíre *smb.* to héroism. ~ся, вдохновиться (*тв.*) be* inspíred/encóuraged (by); be* filled with inspirátion (by).

вдохнýть *сов.* **1.** *см.* вдыхáть; **2.** (*вн.* в *вн.*; *внушить*) breathe (*smth.* ínto), instíl (ínto); ~ жизнь в кого-л. breathe new life ínto *smb.*; ~ силы, мýжество в кого-л. put*/instíl fresh strength, cóurage ínto *smb.*; inspíre *smb.* with fresh strength, cóurage.

вдрéбезги **1.** to smitheréens, to píeces; разбить что-либо ~ smash *smth.* to smitheréens; разбиться ~ be* smashed to smitheréens; **2.** *разг.:* пьян ~ dead/blind drunk.

вдруг **1.** (*неожиданно*) súddenly, unexpéctedly; (*внезапно тж.*) all of a súdden, all at once; ~ кóмната погрузилась во мрак all of a súdden the room was plunged in dárkness; **2.** (*одновременно*) togéther; все ~ all togéther; не все ~! one at a time!; **3.** *разг.* (*а если*) suppóse; a ~ у негó нет дéнег? suppóse he hasn't any móney?

вдýматься *сов. см.* вдýмываться.

вдýмчив|о thóughtfully; ~ относиться к чему-л. take* a thóughtful áttitude to *smth.* ~ый thóughtful, sérious; (*о взгляде*) pénsive; ~ый человéк thóughtful pérson; ~ое отношéние к чему-л. sérious áttitude towárds *smth.*

вдýмываться, вдýматься (в *вн.*) consíder (*smth.*), think* óver (*smth.*), go* ínto (*smth.*); вдýматься в смысл пóвести consíder the méaning of the stóry.

вдыхáние *с.* inhalátion.

вдыхáть, вдохнýть (*вн.*) breathe in (*smth.*), inhále (*smth.*).

вегетариáнский vegetárian.

вегетативн|ый *биол.* végetative; ◇ ~ая нéрвная система végetative nérvous sýstem.

вегетациóнный *бот.* végetative.

вед|áть *несов.* **1.** (*тв.; заведовать*) be* in charge (of); mánage (*smth.*); **2.** (*вн.*) *уст.* (*знать*) know* (*smth.*); не знáю, не ~аю I háven't the fáintest idéa.

вéдени|е *с.* authórity, contról; находиться в ~и кого-л. be* únder the authórity of *smb.*; не в моём ~и not withín my cómpetence.

ведéние *с.* (*рд.*) cónduct (of); ~ бухгáлтерских книг bóok-keeping; ~ хозяйства hóusekeeping; ~ собрáния condúct(ing) of a méeting; ~ протокóла kéeping of the mínutes.

вéдома: с, без *чего-л.* ~ with, withóut the knówledge of *smth.*; без моегó ~ withóut my knówledge.

вéдомость *ж.* list, régister.

вéдомственн|ый departméntal; ~ые барьéры bureaucrátic/departméntal bárriers.

вéдомство *с.* (góvernment) depártment.

вéдомый: ~ самолёт suppórting áircraft, No 2 (of a flight).

ведр|ó с. pail, búcket; пóлное ~ *чего-л.* a búcketful of *smth.*; ◇ дождь льёт как из ~á it's ráining cats and dogs, it's símply póuring/pélting.

ведущ|ий *прил.* 1. léading; ~ая óтрасль промышленности a léading branch of índustry; игрáть ~ую роль play the chief/léading role; ~ее положéние в мировóй наýке léading place in world science; 2. *тех.* dríving; 3. *в знач. сущ. м. ав.* léader.

ведь 1. *частица (всё-таки)* áfter all; you see; (*но*) but; ~ он ваш брат! áfter all, he is your bróther; он ~ не ребёнок! he isn't a child*, áfter all!; ~ я вам сказáл! but I told you!; да ~ ... why...; да ~ э́то товáрищ Ивáнов! Why, it's Cómrade Ivanóv!; он ~ болéл he's been ill, you know; ~ он ваш брат? he is your bróther; он ~ не придёт? he isn't cóming, is he?; ~ вы егó вѝдели? you saw him, dídn't you?; 3. *союз не перевóдится*; ~ я сам вѝдел I saw it with my own eyes!

ведьма ж. 1. *фольк.* witch; 2. *бран.* witch, hárridan, víxen; стáрая ~ old hag.

вéер м. fan.

вéжлив|ость ж. políteness, civílity; (*любезность*) cóurtesy; элементáрная ~ órdinary cóurtesy. ~ый políte, cívil; (*любезный*) cóurteous.

вездé éverywhere; ~ и всюду here, there and éverywhere.

вездесýщий ubíquitous.

вездехóд м. cróss-cóuntry véhicle, lánd-róver. ~ный cróss-cóuntry *attr.*, róugh-cóuntry *attr.*

везтѝ, повезтѝ 1. *тк. несов. см.* возѝть; 2. *безл. разг.*: емý везёт he's lúcky, he's in luck.

век м. 1. (*столетие*) céntury; двадцáтый ~ the twéntieth céntury; освящённый ~ами tíme-honoured; 2. (*эпоха*) age; кáменный ~ the Stone Age; 3. (*жизнь*) (span of) life; доживáть свой ~ live out *one's* remáining days; на наш ~ хвáтит it will last our time; на своём ~ý in the course of *one's* life; ~ живѝ — ~ учѝсь! live and learn!; 4. *разг.* (*очень долгое время*): цéлый ~ не видáлись háven't seen one anóther for ages; ◇ во ~и ~óв for éver and éver; до сконцáния ~а till the end of time; в кóи ~и once in a blue moon; на ~и вéчные for éver.

вéко с. éyelid.

вековéчный everlásting, etérnal.

веков|óй áncient; áge-óld; ~ые чáяния нарóда the lóng-cherished desíres of the péople; ~áя отстáлость áge-long báckwardness.

вéксель м. (*простóй*) prómissory note; (*перевóдный*) bill of exchánge. ~ный: ~ный курс rate of exchánge.

велéние с. díctates *pl.*

вел|éть *несов. и сов.* tell*, órder; ~ѝте емý уйтѝ tell him to go; я ~ю убрáть э́то I will have it remóved; дéлайте, как вам вéлено! do as you're told!; дóктор не ~ел мне выходѝть the dóctor won't let me go out.

велѝк см. велѝкий.

великáн м. gíant.

велѝк|ий 1. great; (*при сóбственных именах*) the Great; Велѝкая Октя́брьская социалистѝческая револю́ция the Great Octóber Sócialist Revolútion; ~ие держáвы the Great Pówers, the súperpowers; ~ учёный great scíentist; Пётр Велѝкий Péter the Great; 2. *тк. кратк. ф.* (*слишком большóй*) (too) big; э́ти ботѝнки мне ~ѝ these boots are (too) big for me; ◇ от мáла до ~a young and old.

великовозрастный overgrówn.

великодержáвный Great Pówer *attr.*; ~ шовинѝзм Great Pówer cháuvinism.

великодýш|ие с. generósity, magnanímity. ~ный génerous, bíg-héarted, magnánimous.

великолéп|о: ~! that's spléndid! ~ый 1. (*роскошный*) magníficent, spléndid; 2. *разг.* (*отлѝчный*) fine, spléndid.

величáвый státely, majéstic.

велѝчественн|о majéstically. ~ый státely, majéstic, impósing; ~ое здáние státely búilding; ~ая осáнка majéstic cárriage/béaring; ~ое зрéлище impósing spéctacle.

велѝчество с. Májesty; вáше ~ Your Májesty.

велѝчи|е с. grándeur; ~ дýха gréatness (of soul); ◇ во всём (своём) ~и in all its grándeur; с высоты своегó ~я from the peak of *one's* éminence.

величин|á ж. 1. (*размер*) size; звездá пéрвой ~ы a star of the first mágnitude; 2. *мат.* quántity, válue; 3. (*выдающийся человек*) great fígure.

велогóн|ка ж. (bí)cycle-race. ~щик м. rácing cýclist.

велопробéг м. cýcle-race.

велосипéд м. bícycle; cýcle; bike *разг.* ~ѝст м. cýclist. ~ный: ~ный спорт cýcle-racing; ~ная ездá cýcling.

велотрéк м. cýcle-track.

вельвéт м. *текст.* velvetéen. ~овый *текст.* velvetéen *attr.*

вельмóжа м. 1. *уст.* great nóble; grandée; 2. *ирон.* grandée.

вéна ж. *анат.* vein.

венгéрец м. см. венгр.

венгéрка I ж. Hungárian (wóman*).

венгéрка II ж. (*танец*) Hungárian dance.

венгéрский Hungárian; ~ язы́к Hungárian, the Hungárian lánguage.

венгр м. Hungárian.

венесуэ́л|ец м. Venezuélan. ~ка ж. Venezuélan wóman*.

венесуэ́льский Venezuélan.

венéц м. 1. (*корона*) crown; *перен. тж.* crówning point, consummátion; 2. *астр.* coróna, hálo; ◇ тернóвый ~ crown of thorns; конéц — дéлу ~ *посл.* the end crowns all.

вéнзель м. mónogram.

вéник м. (straw) bésom; (*в бане*) switch of green birch twigs.

венóзный vénous, venóse.

венóк м. wreath; gárland.

вентилѝровать, провентилѝровать (*вн.*) véntilate (*smth.*), air (*smth.*).

вéнтиль м. *тех.* valve.

вентиля|тор м. véntilator; (*с вращающимися крыльями*) fan. ~циóнный ventilátion *attr.* ~ция ж. ventilátion.

венчáльный wédding *attr.*, márriage *attr.*, núptial; ~ наря́д wédding-dress; ~ обря́д márriage/núptial rites *pl.*

венчáние с. (*свадьба*) wédding.

венч|áть, повенчáть, увенчáть (*вн.*) 1. *сов.* повенчáть (*соединять брáком*) márry (*smb.*); 2. *сов.* увенчáть (*на цáрство*) crown (*smb.*); 3. *сов.* увенчáть (*завершáть*) crown (*smth.*); 4. *сов.* увенчáть *архит.* top (*smth.*). ~áться, повенчáться be* márried (in church).

вéр|а ж. 1. (*убеждённость, уверенность*) faith, belief; ~ в успéх дéла cónfidence; ~ в человéка belief/faith in man/humánity; 2. (*религия*) faith; 3 *разг.* (*доверие*) cónfidence, trust; ◇ принять что-л. на ~у take* smth. on trust.

верáнда ж. veránda(h).

вéрб|а ж. (pússy-)willow. ~ный: ~ное воскресéнье *рел.* Palm Súnday.

вербáльн|ый vérbal; ◇ ~ая нóта *дип.* vérbal note.

верблю́|д м. cámel; навью́ченный как ~ lóaded like a páck-mule. ~жий cámel's; ~жья шерсть cámel's hair.

верб|овáть, завербовáть (*вн.*) recrúit (*smb.*), enlíst (*smb.*). ~óвка ж. recrúiting, enlístment. ~óвщик м. lábour contráctor; hírer of lábour.

верёв|ка ж. горе; (*тóнкая*) string, cord; (*для белья*) clóthes-line. ~очка ж. bit of string. ~очный string *attr.*; ~очная лéстница rópe-ladder.

верени́ц|а *ж.* file, string; ~ автомоби́лей string/stream of cars; дви́гаться ~ей file; проноси́ться несконча́емой ~ей pass in néver-énding succéssion.

веретено́ *с.* spíndle.

верзи́ла *м. разг.* lánky féllow; gángling féllow.

вери́тельн|ый: ~ые гра́моты *дип.* credéntials; вруча́ть (свои́) ~ые гра́моты *дип.* presént one's credéntials.

вер|ить *несов.* 1. (в *вн.;* быть убеждённым в чём--либо) belíeve (in), have* faith (in); мы ~им в успе́х борьбы́ we belíeve we shall succéed in our éfforts; ~ в правоту́ своего́ де́ла belíeve in the jústice of one's cause; 2. (быть религио́зным) belíeve (in God); 3. (в *вн.; дт.;* принима́ть за и́стину) belíeve (in); е́сли мо́жно ~ слу́хам if what is said is true; хоти́те ве́рьте, хоти́те нет belíeve it or not; 4. (дт.; доверя́ть) belíeve (smb.), trust (smb.); я вам и так ~ю I'll take your word for it. ~иться *несов. безл.:* мне не ~ится I can't belíeve; ~ится с трудо́м it is hard to belíeve; it is scárcely crédible.

вермише́ль *ж.* vermicélli.

верне́е 1. *сравнит. ст. прил.* ве́рный *и нареч.* ве́рно; 2. *в знач. вводн. сл.* or ráther, at least; вчера́ но́чью, ~, сего́дня ра́но у́тром late last night, or ráther, éarly this mórning; мы рабо́тали, ~, я рабо́тал, а он смотре́л we worked — at least, I worked, and he looked on.

верниса́ж *м.* ópening day; (предвари́тельный просмо́тр) préview.

верн|о 1. *нареч.* (преданно) fáithfully, lóyally; 2. *нареч.* (правильно) corréctly; right; ~ петь sing* in tune; 3. *в знач. сказ. безл.:* э́то ~! that's true; ~! quite right; 4. *в знач. вводн. сл.* (вероятно) próbably; он, ~, не придёт próbably he's not cóming, it looks as if he's not cóming. ~ость *ж.* 1. (преданность) fáithfulness, lóyalty; ~ость прися́ге lóyalty to one's oath; ~ость до́лгу devótion to dúty; 2. (правильность) truth, corréctness, áccuracy; (о перево́де тж.) fáithfulness.

верну́ть *сов.* (вн.) 1. (отда́ть обра́тно) retúrn (smth.), give* (smth.) back, bring* (smth.) back; (поте́рянное кем-л.) restóre (smth.); ~ кни́гу retúrn a book; ~ долг repáy a debt; 2. (вновь обрести́) recóver (smth.); ~ зре́ние, здоро́вье restóre one's sight, health; 3. (заста́вить возврати́ться) make* (smb.) come back. ~ся *сов.* 1. come* back, go* back; retúrn; be* back; ~ся домо́й come*/go* back/home; верну́лся ли он? is he back?; когда́ он вернётся? when will he be back?; оди́н самолёт не верну́лся one áircraft is míssing; 2. (к дт.; восстанови́ться): нему́ верну́лось самооблада́ние he regáined/recóvered his sélf-contról.

ве́рн|ый 1. (преданный) fáithful, true, lóyal; ~ друг fáithful friend; ~ сторо́нник lóyal suppórter/adhérent; ~ свои́м убежде́ниям true to one's prínciples; 2. (надёжный) relíable, safe; ~ спо́соб the best way; э́то де́ло ~ое it's a sure thing; 3. (точный, правильный) corréct, right, áccurate; э́то ~ые часы́ this watch/clock keeps véry good time; ~ое изображе́ние, описа́ние fáithful descríption; ~ перево́д fáithful translátion; ~ глаз true eye; у него́ ~ взгляд на ве́щи he sees things in their próper light; 4. (неизбежный) sure, cértain; ~ая ги́бель, смерть cértain ruin, death; идти́ на ~ую смерть go* to one's death.

ве́рова|ние *с.* belief. ~ть *несов.* (в *вн.*) belíeve (in).

вероиспове́дание *с.* faith, religión, creed.

веролом|ный tréacherous, perfídious. ~ство *с.* tréachery.

веротерпи́мость *ж. рел.* tolerátion.

вероя́тн|о próbably; в пять часо́в я, ~, бу́ду до́ма I expéct to be home at five o'clóck. ~ость *ж.* probabílity, líkelihood; ~ость safe; ~ости in all probabílity, véry líkely; тео́рия ~остей *мат.* théory of probabílity. ~ый próbable, líkely.

ве́рсия *ж.* vérsion.

верст|а́ *ж. уст.* verst (= *3,500 feet*); ◇ его́ за́ ~у ви́дно you can't miss him — he tówers óver éverybody; его́ за́ ~у слы́шно you can hear him a mile off.

верста́к *м.* jóiner's/cárpenter's bench.

верста́ть, сверста́ть (вн.) *полигр.* make* (smth.) up in páges, make* (smth.) into páges, impóse (smth.).

вёрстка *ж. полигр.* 1. (действие) máke-up; 2. (корректурный оттиск) páge-proofs.

ве́ртел *м.* spit; осетри́на на ~е grílled stúrgeon.

верте́ть *несов.* 1. (вн.) turn (smth.); (быстро враща́ть) spin* (smth.), twirl (smth.); ~ в рука́х что-л. fidget with smth., play with smth.; 2. (тв.) *разг.* (распоряжа́ться) lord it óver (smb., smth.); twist (smb.) round one's líttle finger; ~ всем до́мом rule the roost. ~ся *несов.* 1. turn, go* round, revólve; (быстро враща́ться) spin*; ~ся волчко́м spin* (like a top); ~ся перед зе́ркалом twist and turn before the mírror; разгово́р верти́тся вокру́г одного́ предме́та the conversátion turns upón the same súbject; 2. *разг.* (постоянно находи́ться): ~ся среди́ кого́-л. be* álways with smb.; ~ся о́коло кого́-л. be* álways at smb.'s side; он всё вре́мя верти́тся среди́ взро́слых he's álways with grówn-ups; 3. *разг.* (увиливать) hedge, beat* abóut the bush; ◇ ~ся под нога́ми keep* gétting in the way; назва́ние верти́тся на языке́ the name is on the tip of my tongue; как ни верти́сь, а придётся согласи́ться there's nóthing for it but to consént; ничего́ не выхо́дит, как тут ни верти́сь it won't work, whatéver you do.

вертика́ль *ж.* 1. vértical line; 2. *шахм.* file. ~ный vértical.

вертля́вый *разг.* fidgety.

вертолёт *м.* hélicopter.

верту́шка *ж. разг.* 1. (враща́ющаяся этаже́рка) revólving bóokcase; (враща́ющаяся дверь) revólving door; (телефонный диск) dial; 2. (легкомысленная женщина) flighty créature.

ве́рующий *м.* belíever, religious pérson.

верфь *ж.* shípyard, dóckyard.

верх *м.* 1. (ве́рхняя часть) top, úpper part; 2. (ве́рхний эта́ж) top floor; top stórey; 3. (экипа́жа) hood; 4. (оде́жды) óutside, coat; э́то на подкла́дку, а э́то для ~а this is for the líning, and this is for the coat/óutside; 5. (рд.; высшая степень) the height (of); (в положит. смысле тж.) the ácme (of); ~ соверше́нства the height/ácme of perféction; ~ неприли́чия the height of bad mánners; ~ блаже́нства the height/ácme of bliss; ◇ быть на ~у́ блаже́нства be* in the séventh héaven; взять ~ над кем-л. gain the úpper hand of smb.; его́ мне́ние одержа́ло ~ his opínion preváiled.

верх|и́ *мн.* 1. (общества) the úpper stráta; 2. (руководи́тели) léaders; совеща́ние в ~а́х súmmit cónference, tóp-level cónference; 3. (высокие ноты) high notes; 4.: нахвата́ться ~о́в have* a mere smáttering of the súbject; скользи́ть по ~а́м skim the súrface.

верхн|ий top; úpper; ~ие слои́ атмосфе́ры úpper láyers/stráta of the átmosphere; ~яя по́лка top shelf*; ~ эта́ж top floor/stórey; ~яя че́люсть úpper jaw; ~ее пла́тье (óver)coats pl; ~ее тече́ние úpper wáters pl; ~ее тече́ние Во́лги the Úpper Vólga; ~ реги́стр *муз.* úpper régister.

верхо́вн|ый supréme; ~ая власть supréme/sóvereign pówer; Верхо́вный Суд Росси́йской Федера́ции Supréme Court of the Rússian Federátion.

верхово́д *м. разг.* ríngleader. ~ить *несов.* (тв.) *разг.* be* the léading spírit (amóng).

верхов|о́й 1. *прил.:* ~а́я езда́ hórse-ríding; ~а́я ло́шадь sáddle-horse; иску́сство ~о́й езды́ hórsemanship, equéstrian skill; 2. *в знач. сущ. м.* ríder.

верхо́вье *с.* úpper wáters pl; ~ Во́лги 1) the Úpper Vólga; 2) (о ме́стности) the úpper réaches of the Vólga.

верхогля́д м. разг. superfícial pérson, trífler. **~ство** с. разг. superficiálity.

верхола́з м. stéeplejack; spíderman* разг.

ве́рхом (по верху) alóng the top; пойти́ ~ take* the úpper path.

верхо́м (на лошади) on hórseback; (на осле) on a dónkey; сесть ~ на стул sit* astríde a chair; е́здить ~ (на ло́шади) ride* (on hórseback).

верху́ш|ка ж. 1. (верхняя часть) top; ~ де́рева top of a tree; ~ки дере́вьев trée-tops; ~ лёгкого ápex of a lung; 2. разг. (руководящая часть общества, организации) úpper crust; bósses; пра́вящая ~ rúling clíque.

верши́н|а ж. 1. top, súmmit; (остроконечная) peak; на са́мой ~е at the véry top; 2. (рд.; высшая степень) the height (of), ápex (of); ◇ ~ угла́ мат. vértex (pl -tices).

верши́ть несов. (вн.; решать) decíde (smth.); (тв.; распоряжаться) diréct (smth.); ~ чью-л. судьбу́ decíde smb.'s fate; ~ все́ми дела́ми be* at the head of affáirs; boss the show разг.; (в доме) rule the roost.

вес I м. weight; перен. weight, ínfluence; его́ ~ 65 килогра́ммов he weighs síxty-five kílograms; ~ом в 65 килогра́ммов wéighing síxty-five kílograms; на ~ by weight, by the pound; име́ть ~ cárry weight; ◇ цени́ться на ~ зо́лота be* worth its weight in gold.

вес II м.: держа́ть что-л. на ~у́ hold* smth. súspended (in mid-air); держа́ть винто́вку на ~у́ cárry one's rífle at the trail.

весели́ть несов. (вн.; радовать) cheer (smb.) up; (забавлять) amúse (smb.). **~ся** несов. have* a good time, enjóy onesélf; как вы весели́тесь? have you had a good time?

ве́село 1. нареч. gáily, mérrily; ~ проводи́ть вре́мя enjóy onesélf, have* a good time; как бы́ло ~! wásn't it fun/jólly?, háven't we had a good time?; смотре́ть на жизнь веселе́е take* a bríghter view (of things); веселе́е! 1) (бодрее) cheer up!; 2) (быстрее) look alíve!; 2. в знач. сказ. безл.: мне ~ I'm enjóying mysélf; мне ~ смотре́ть на них it makes me glad to look at them.

весёл|ость ж. gáiety, mérriness, chéerfulness. **~ый** 1. (жизнерадостный) mérry, lívely, jólly; (бодрый) chéerful, light-héarted; ~ое лицо́ mérry face; ~ая компа́ния mérry párty/band, jólly cómpany; ~ое настрое́ние high/blíthe spírits pl, mérry mood; ~ый хара́ктер jólly/jóvial disposítion; он всегда́ ве́сел he's álways in good spírits; 2. (забавный) amúsing, entertáining; ~ая шу́тка good joke; 3. (приятный для взора) chéerful, pléasing; ~ая расцве́тка chéerful páttern.

весе́ль|е с. 1. (жизнерадостность) high spírits pl; 2. (развлечение) mérriment, mérry-making; fun. **~ча́к** м. разг. bright spark.

весе́нний spring attr., spríngtime attr.; vérnal книжн.

ве́с|ить несов. weigh; ско́лько он ~ит? what is his weight?, what does he weigh? **~кий** wéighty; ~кий до́вод wéighty/fórmidable árgument. **~ко**: ~ко говори́ть speak* with authórity; ~ко возража́ть raise sérious objéctions.

весло́ с. oar; (парное тж.) scull.

весн|а́ ж. spring, spríngtime. **~о́й** in (the) spring.

весну́ш|ка ж. fréckle. **~чатый** fréckled.

весо́в|о́й weight attr.; ~а́я едини́ца weight únit, únit of weight; ~ това́р goods sold by weight; ~а́я ги́ря weight. **~щи́к** м. wéigher.

весо́м|ость ж. weight; перен. pónderability. **~ый** wéighable; перен. wéighty, pónderable.

вест м. мор. 1. (направление) west; 2. (ветер) west wind.

вести́ несов. 1. (вн.) take* (smb.), lead* (smb.); condúct (smth.) книжн.; ~ на прогу́лку take* the children out for a walk; ~ слепо́го lead* a blind man*; ~ аресто́ванного escórt a prísoner; 2. (вн.; автомобиль, поезд, трамвай) drive* (smth.); (судно) steer (smth.); (самолёт) fly* (smth.). 3. (вн.; руководить занятия-

ми, делом и т. п.) condúct (smth.), run* (smth.); ~ семина́р condúct a séminar; ~ больно́го (о лечащем враче) be* in charge of a pátient; ~ хозя́йство do* the hóusekeeping, run* the house; 4. (тв. по дт.) см. води́ть 3; 5. (к дт.; о дороге, двери и т. п.) lead* (to); э́та тропи́нка ведёт к ле́су this path leads to the fórest; 6. (приводить) lead*; не пойму́, к чему́ он ведёт! I can't think what he's dríving at!; 7. (вн.): ~ протоко́л keep* the mínutes; ~ расска́з tell* a stóry; ~ счета́ keep* accóunts; ~ дневни́к keep* a díary; ~ перегово́ры condúct negotiátions, cárry on negotiátions; ~ ми́рные перегово́ры condúct peace negotiátions, negótiate for peace; ~ войну́ wage war; ~ бой be* in áction; ~ ого́нь (по) fire (on); ~ своё нача́ло (от) have* its órigin (in); ~ свой род от кого-л. trace one's áncestry/líneage back to smb.; ~ себя́ beháve; веди́ себя́ прили́чно! beháve yoursélf!

вестибуля́рный vestíbular; ~ аппара́т vestíbular apparátus.

вестибю́ль м. (в театре, гостинице и т. п.) lóbby, vestíbule, fóyer; (в жилых домах, учреждениях) (éntrance-)hall.

вести́сь несов.: так уж ведётся such is the cústom; так уж у нас ведётся! it's our way!, that's how we do things!; летосчисле́ние ведётся с... time is réckoned from...

ве́стник м. 1. méssenger, hérald; hárbinger поэт.; 2. (в названиях журналов) bulletin.

вестово́й м. rúnner, órderly.

ве́сточк|а ж. news; я получи́л ~у из дому I have heard from home; да́йте о себе́ ~у let us hear from you.

вест|ь I ж. news; tídings pl поэт.; ◇ пропа́сть без ~и disappéar, go*/be* míssing; он пропа́л без ~и he has been repórted míssing.

весть II разг.: бог ~ góodness knows; э́то не бог ~ что тако́е it's nóthing spécial.

весы́ мн. scales; (для больших тяжестей тж.) wéighing-machine sg.

весь, вся, всё, все мест. 1. all, the entíre, the whole (of); ~ день all day (long); ~ о́пыт all the expérience; все на́ши ресу́рсы the whole of our resóurces; все кни́ги all the books; вся, всю жизнь all one's life, one's whole life; всё населе́ние the entíre populátion; все остальны́е all the óthers; вся шко́ла the whole/entíre school; по всему́ го́роду all óver the town; во всём ми́ре in the whole world, throughóut the world; 2. (целиком) вся в бе́лом all in white; ~ в цвета́х (о саде и т. п.) full of flówers; (украшенный) decked with flówers; ◇ он ~ в отца́ he takes áfter his fáther; мир во всём ми́ре world peace, peace acróss the world.

весьма́ extrémely, híghly; ~ удовлетвори́тельно híghly satisfáctory.

ветви́стый bránchy, búshy.

ветвь ж. 1. branch, limb, bough; 2. (отрасль чего-либо) branch.

ве́тер м. wind; ~ стих the wind dropped; подня́лся ~ the wind sprang up, the wind stárted to blow; ◇ броса́ть слова́ на ~ use words líghtly; идти́, куда́ ~ ду́ет be* a wéathercock; держа́ть нос по ве́тру trim one's sails to the wind.

ветера́н м. véteran; ~ войны́ war-véteran.

ветерина́р м. véterinary (súrgeon); vet разг. **~ия** ж. véterinary scíence. **~ный** véterinary; ~ный институ́т véterinary cóllege.

ветеро́к м. breeze.

ве́тка ж. 1. branch; (цветущая) spray; 2. ж.-д. bránch-line.

ветла́ ж. wíllow.

ве́то с. нескл. véto; пра́во ~ right of véto; наложи́ть ~ на что-л. véto smth., place/put* a véto on smth.

ве́тошь ж. rags pl.

ве́трен|о 1. нареч. разг. frívolously; 2. в знач. сказ.

безл. it is wíndy. ~ый 1. wíndy; ~ая погóда wíndy wéather; 2. *разг. (легкомысленный)* frívolous; ~ое повéдение fíckle cónduct.

ветров|óй wind *attr.*; ~óe стеклó windscreen.

ветря́нка *ж. разг.* chícken-pox.

ветря́н|óй wind *attr.*; ~ двигатель wind wheel; ~áя мéльница windmill.

вéтх|ий 1. dilápidated, ríckety; *(о здании тж.)* rámshackle; *(об одежде тж.)* thréadbare; 2. *(о человеке)* decrépit, infírm. ~ость *ж.* dilápidated state; прийти́ в ~ость fall* into disrepáir.

ветчина́ *ж.* ham.

ветша́ть, обветша́ть fall* into decáy.

вéха *ж.* 1. stake; *мор.* spár-buoy; 2. *обыкн. мн. (основной этап в развитии чего-л.)* lándmark *sg*, mílestone *sg*.

вéчер *м.* 1. évening; под ~, к ~у towárds évening; 2. *(собрание)* párty, évening; ~, посвящённый па́мяти Пу́шкина Púshkin memórial gáthering; ~ áнгло-совéтской дру́жбы Brítish-Sóviet fríendship párty.

вечер|éть *несов. обыкн. безл.:* ~éет dusk is fálling, night is cóming on.

вечери́нк|а *ж.* (évening) párty; устра́ивать ~у hold*/give* a párty.

вечéрн|ий évening *attr.*; ~яя заря́ súnset glow; ~ee нéбо évening sky; ~яя газéта évening páper; ~ee пла́тье évening dress.

вечéрня *ж. рел.* véspers.

вéчером in the évening; сегóдня ~ this évening, toníght; сегóдня ~ мы идём в теа́тр we're góing to the théatre toníght; вчера́ ~ yésterday évening, last night; за́втра ~ tomórrow évening/night; пóздно ~ late in the évening.

вéчеря *ж. рел.* súpper; тáйная ~ the Last Súpper.

вéчн|о 1. for éver, etérnally; жить ~ live for éver; 2. *разг. (постоянно)* álways, perpétually; он ~ опа́здывает he is álways late. ~ость *ж.* etérnity; ◇ кáнуть в ~ость go*/disappéar for éver, sink* into oblívion; мы не вида́лись *(цéлую)* ~ость *разг.* we háven't met for áges!; мне пришло́сь ждать цéлую ~ость *разг.* I had to wait for an etérnity. ~ый 1. etérnal, everlásting; *(непрерывный)* perpétual; ~ое владéние perpétual posséssion; ~ое пóльзование use in perpetúity; 2. *разг. (постоянный)* perpétual, éndless; ~ые ссóры éndless quárrelling *sg*; ~ые приди́рки incéssant fáultfinding; ◇ ~ое перó fóuntain-pen.

вечóрка *ж. разг.* évening páper.

вéшалка *ж.* 1. *(для верхнего платья и головных уборов)* hát-and-coat-stánd; hát-and-coat-ráck *(на стене)*; *(крючок)* peg; 2. *(плечики)* hánger; 3. *(у платья)* hánger, tab; *разг. (помещение)* clóak-room.

вéшать I, повéсить *(вн.)* 1. hang* *(smth.)*, hang* up *(smth.)*; ~ карти́ну put* up a pícture; hang* a pícture; ~ бельё hang* up/out the wáshing; ~ тру́бку *(телефонную)* hang* up the recéiver, put* down the recéiver; 2. *(казнить)* hang *(smb.)*; ◇ ~ гóлову hang* one's head; не нáдо ~ гóлову! chin up!, keep smíling!, néver say die!

вéшать II, свéшать *(вн.)* weigh *(smth.)*

вéшаться, повéситься *(кончать с собой)* hang onesélf; ◇ ~ на шéю кому́-л. throw* onesélf at *smb.'s* head.

веща́ть *несов. радио* be* on the air.

вещевóй: ~ мешóк pack, knápsack; ~ склад wárehouse; stores *pl*.

вещéственн|ый matérial; ~ые доказáтельства *юр.* matérial évidence *sg*.

вещество́ *с.* súbstance.

вéщий wise, prophétic.

вещи́ца *ж.* ●*(безделушка)* knick-knack, trífle; *(драгоценность)* bíjou (*pl* -oux).

вещ|ь *ж.* 1. thing; 2. *мн. (имущество и т. п.)*

things, belóngings; из всех ~ей я привёз тóлько... the ónly thing I brought was...; 3. *(о пьесе, книге и т. п.)* piece, thing; чья э́то ~? who is it by?; э́то егó лу́чшая ~ it's the best thing he éver did, wrote *etc.*; 4. *(факт, дéло)* thing, mátter, affáir; хочу́ сказáть вам одну́ ~ I have sómething to tell you.

вéяние *с.* 1. *(ветра)* bréathing, blówing; 2. *(направление)* trend, téndency; ~ врéмени the spírit of the age; 3. *с.-х.* wínnowing.

вéять *несов.* 1. *(о ветре)* blow* sóftly, breathe; 2. *обыкн. безл.:* вéет прохлáдой there is a gráteful cóolness in the air; вéет весной the air has a breath of spring in it; 3. *(развеваться — о знамёнах)* flútter; 4. *(вн.) с.-х.* wínnow *(smth.)*.

вжива́ться, вжи́ться *разг.* get* used (to); ~ в óбраз *театр.* get* the feel of one's part.

вжив|и́ть *сов. см.* вживля́ть. ~лéние *с.* implantátion. ~ля́ть, вживи́ть *(вн.)* implánt *(smth.)*.

вжи́ться *сов. см.* вжива́ться.

взад *разг.:* ~ и вперёд up and down; to and fro; back and forth; ходи́ть ~ и вперёд по кóмнате walk up and down the room; walk to and fro acróss the room; ни ~ ни вперёд at a stándstill, at a déadlock, déadlocked.

взаи́мн|ость *ж.* recíprocity; любóвь без ~ости únrequited love; доби́ться ~ости win* *smb.'s* afféction. ~ый mútual; *(ответный)* recíprocal; ~ая пóмощь mútual aid; ~ое уважéние mútual respéct; ~ые обвинéния recriminátions; ~ое соглáсие mútual consént; ◇ ~ый глагóл *грам.* recíprocal verb.

взаимовы́годн|ый mútually benefícial/advantágeous; ~ые экономи́ческие отношéния mútually advantágeous económic relátions.

взаимодéйств|ие *с.* 1. *(взаимное влияние)* interáction; ~ сил прирóды the interáction of nátural fórces; 2. *(согласованность действий)* co-operátion. ~овать *несов.* interáct; *(действовать согласованно)* co-óperate.

взаимозаменя́ем|ость *ж.* ínterchangeabílity. ~ый interchángeable.

взаимоотношéние *с.* relátion; interrelátion.

взаимопóмощ|ь *ж.* mútual aid, mútual assístance; договóр о ~и agréement/tréaty of mútual assístance.

взаимопонима́ние *с.* cómmon/mútual understánding.

взаимосвя́занн|ый ínterconnécted; ~ые телевизиóнные стáнции línk-up sýstem of télevision státions.

взаимосвя́зь *ж.* (ínter)communicátion.

взаймы́: давáть ~ lend*; брать ~ bórrow.

взамéн 1. *нареч. (вместо)* instéad; *(в обмен)* in exchánge; 2. *предлог (рд.)* instéad (of); in exchánge (for); предложи́ть нóвое пальтó ~ стáрого óffer a new coat in exchánge for an old one.

взаперти́ 1. *(под замкóм)* únder lock and key; locked up; держáть когó-л. ~ keep* *smb.* shut up; keep* *smb.* únder lock and key; 2. *(в уединéнии)* in seclúsion; жить ~ live in seclúsion; keep* onesélf to onesélf.

взápуски *разг.:* бéгать ~ run* ráces, chase each other.

взбалмóшный *разг.* únbálanced, eccéntric, cránky.

взбáлтывать, взболтáть *(вн.)* shake* *(smth.)*; перед употреблéнием ~ shake well befóre táking.

взбегáть, взбежáть run* up; взбежáть на пя́тый эта́ж run* up to the fourth floor; ~ по лéстнице run* úpstairs.

взбежáть *сов. см.* взбегáть.

взбеси́ть(ся) *сов. см.* беси́ть(ся).

взбешённый fúrious, enráged.

взбивáть, взбить *(вн.)* 1. *(делать пышным)* puff up *(smth.)*; взбить поду́шки shake* up the pillows; 2. *(вспénивать)* churn up *(smth.)*; взбить белки́ beat* up the whites of eggs; взбить сли́вки whip cream.

взбирáться, взобрáться *(на вн. по дт.)* go* up *(smth.,* ínto, on to, to), climb (up) *(smth.,* ínto, on to, to); *сов. тж.* reach/gain (the top of), get* (to the top of); (*влезать, вставать*) get* (on to); ~ по лéстнице go* up the stairs, ascénd the stairs; (*по приставной*) climb/go* up the ládder; взобрáться нá гору climb (up) the móuntain; взобрáться на вéрхний этáж reach the top floor; взобрáться на крышу climb (up) on to the roof; взобрáться на дéрево climb (up) a tree; взобрáться на стол, подокóнник get* on to the táble, windowsill.

взбить *сов. см.* взбивáть.

взболтáть *сов. см.* взбáлтывать.

взбре|сти *сов.*: емý ~лá в гóлову, на ум глýпая мысль he was seized by a fóolish idéa; емý ~лó в гóлову, на ум... he took it ínto his head...; что это вам ~лó на ум? what posséssed you?

взбудорáживать, взбудорáжить (*вн.*) tróuble (*smb., smth.*), distúrb (*smb., smth.*), upsét* (*smb., smth.*).

взбудорáжить *сов. см.* взбудорáживать *и* будорáжить.

взбунтовáться *сов.* revólt, rise* in revólt.

взбýчка *ж. разг.* híding, thráshing; (*нагоняй тж.*) wígging.

взвáливать, взвалить (*вн. на вн.*) 1. hoist (*smth.* on to), heave* (*smth.* on to); ~ мешóк себé нá спину shóulder a sack; 2. *разг.* (*обременять кого-л.*); ~ всю рабóту на *кого-л.* sáddle *smb.* with all the work; ~ винý на *кого-л.* throw* the blame on *smb.*, make* *smb.* to blame.

взвалить *сов. см.* взвáливать.

взвéсить(ся) *сов. см.* взвéшивать(ся).

взвести *сов. см.* взводить.

взвéшивать, взвéсить (*вн.; прям. и перен.*) weigh (*smth.*); (*давать взвесить*) get*/have* (*smth.*) weighed; взвéсить свои возмóжности assess* stock of one's resóurces; взвéсив все обстоятельства... áfter due considerátion... ~ся, взвéситься weigh onesélf.

взвивáться, взвиться 1. (*о птице*) soar úpwards; 2. (*о флаге*) go* up, be* raised.

взвизгивать, взвизгнуть squeal; *сов. тж.* give* a shriek; (*о собаке*) yelp.

взвизгнуть *сов. см.* взвизгивать.

взвинтить *сов. см.* взвинчивать.

взвинченн|ый: ~ые цéны infláted prices; он вéчно взвинчен he is in a contínual state of excítement/nerves.

взвинчивать, взвинтить (*вн.*) *разг.* excíte (*smb., smth.*); ~ себé нéрвы get* térribly worked up; ◇ ~ цéны jack up prices.

взвиться *сов. см.* взвивáться.

взвод I *м. воен.* platóon.

взвод II *м.* cócking notch; на боевóм ~e cocked, at full cock; на предохранительном ~e at half cock; ◇ на ~e 1) keyed up; 2) (*слегка пьян*) líght-héaded.

взводить, взвести (*вн.*): ~ курóк cock a gun; ~ клеветý на *кого-л.* slánder *smb.*; ~ обвинéние на *кого-л.* accúse *smb.* fálsely; put* the blame on *smb.*

взволнóванн|о with emótion. ~ый ágitated, excíted; (*растроганный*) moved *predic.*; у негó ~ый вид he looks wórried/pertúrbed.

взволновáть *сов. см.* волновáть. ~ся *сов. см.* волновáться 1, 2.

взвыть *сов.* howl.

взгляд *м.* 1. glance, look; прикóвывать ~ы attráct all eyes; все ~ы были устремлены на негó all eyes were fixed upón him; чувствовать на себé чей-л. ~ have* a féeling that *smb.* is lóoking at you; 2. (*выражение глаз*) look, expréssion; ýмный ~ intélligent expréssion; тяжёлый, неприятный ~ unpléasant look in one's eyes; 3. (*точка зрения*) view, opínion; у негó прáвильный (непрáвильный) ~ на вéщи he takes the right (a false) view of things; разделять чьи-л. ~ы share *smb.'s* views; ~ на жизнь óutlook on life; ◇ на мой ~ in my view/opínion; my view is that...; на пéрвый ~ at first sight; с одногó ~а at a glance; с пéрвого ~а видно было, что... it was

50

óbvious from the first that...; он мне понрáвился с пéрвого ~а I liked him the móment I set eyes on him.

взглядывать, взглянуть (*на вн.*) look (at), glance (at) (*тж. перен.*); *несов. тж.* cast* glánces (at); *сов. тж.* have*/take* a look (at) (*тж. перен.*); взглянуть на часы take* a look at the time.

взглянуть *сов. см.* взглядывать.

взгромождáть, взгромоздить (*вн.*) *разг.* hoist (*smth.*). ~ся, взгромоздиться (на *вн.*) *разг.* hoist onesélf (on to), clámber (upón).

взгромоздить(ся) *сов. см.* взгромождáть(ся).

взгрустну|ться *сов. безл. разг.*: мне ~лось my spírits have gone down, I feel sad all of a súdden.

вздёрнутый: ~ нос snub nose.

вздор *м. разг.* nónsense, rúbbish; ~! stúff-and--nónsense!, what nónsense!; чистéйший ~ útter nónsense. ~ный *разг.* 1. absúrd, ridículous; 2. (*сварливый*) quárrelsome.

вздорож|áние *с.* rise in prices; (*чего-л.*) rise in the price (of); ~ жизни íncrease in the cost of líving; ~áть *сов. см.* дорожáть.

вздох *м.* sigh; ~ облегчéния sigh of relíef; ◇ испустить послéдний ~ breathe one's last.

вздохнуть *сов.* 1. *см.* вздыхáть 1; 2. *разг.* (*отдохнуть*) rest, take* a bréather; он мне ~ не даёт he hárdly gives me time to breathe; ~ свобóдно breathe fréely.

вздрáгивать, вздрóгнуть start, give* a start; (*от боли*) flinch, wince; (*от ужаса*) shúdder; *несов. тж.* trémble, quíver.

вздремнýть *сов. разг.* doze, have*/take* a nap.

вздрóгнуть *сов. см.* вздрáгивать.

вздувáть, вздуть (*вн.*) 1. (*поднимать — о ветре*) raise (*smth.*); 2. *разг.* (*о ценах*) infláte (*smth.*). ~ся, вздýться swell*; (*о ценах*) jump, soar.

вздýм|ать *сов.* (+ *инф.*) *разг.* take* it ínto one's head (+ to *inf.*); что (это) вы вдруг ~али отказáться? what made you súddenly decíde to refúse?; ◇ и не ~айте! and don't you dare!; ~аться *сов. безл. разг.*: емý ~алось... he took it ínto his head...; как ~ается at one's own sweet will; поступáть как ~ается fóllow one's fáncy.

вздуть I *сов. см.* вздувáть.

вздуть II *сов.* (*вн.*) *разг.* (*отколотить*) thrash (*smb.*), give* (*smb.*) a híding/lícking.

вздýться *сов. см.* вздувáться.

вздымáться *несов. рise*; (*о волнах, груди*) heave*.

вздыхáть, вздохнуть 1. sigh; (*переводить дыхание*) draw* breath; вздохнуть пóлной грýдью breathe déeply, fill one's lungs; 2. *тк. несов.* (о, по *пр.*; *московать*) sigh (for), yearn (for).

взимáть *несов.* (*вн.*) lévy (*smth.*); ~ налóги lévy táxes; ~ плáту colléct páyment; ~ штраф impóse a fine.

взирáть *несов.* (на *вн.*) *уст.* gaze (at).

взлáмывать, взломáть (*вн.*) break* (*smth.*) ópen; (*сейф, замок*) force (*smth.*).

взлёт *м.* 1. (*птицы*) flight; (*самолёта*) táke-óff; 2.: ~ мысли elevátion of thought, flight of inspirátion.

взлетáть, взлетéть 1. (*о птице*) take* wing; (*о самолёте*) take* off; 2. *разг.* (*стремительно подниматься*) run* up; взлетéть по лéстнице rush up the stairs; ◇ взлетéть на вóздух blow* up, be* blown sky-hígh; *перен.* collápse.

взлетéть *сов. см.* взлетáть.

взлётно-посáдочн|ый: ~ая полосá (táke-off and lánding) rúnway.

взлёт|ый táke-óff *attr.*; ~ая дорóжка (táke-off) rúnway.

взлом *м.* bréaking ópen; bréaking in.

взломáть *сов. см.* взлáмывать.

взлóмщик *м.* búrglar.

взлохмáтить *сов. см.* взлохмáчивать.

взлохмáченный dishévelled.

взлохма́чивать, **взлохма́тить** *(вн.)* tóusle *(smth.)*, rúffle *(smth.)*.

взмах *м.* *(весла, косы, руки пловца и т. п.)* stroke, sweep; *(руки)* wave, móvement; *(крыльев)* sweep, flap.

взма́хивать, **взмахну́ть** *(тв.)* *(крыльями)* flap *(smth.)*; *(рукой, флажком)* wave *(smth.)*; *(веслом, косой и т. п.)* strike* (with); make* strokes (with).

взмахну́ть *сов. см.* **взма́хивать**.

взметну́ться *сов.* fly up, soar.

взмоли́ться *сов.* *(о пр.)* beg (for), implóre (for); ~ о поща́де cry quárter, beg/cry for mércy.

взмо́рье *с.* (séa-)shóre; *(только суша)* beach.

взмыва́ть, **взмыть** soar.

взмы́ленный fóaming, fóam-flecked; in a láther *после сущ.*

взмыть *сов. см.* **взмыва́ть**.

взнос *м.* 1. *(платёж)* páyment; очередно́й ~ instálment; 2. *(внесённые деньги)* fee; dues *pl.*

взнузда́ть *сов. см.* **взну́здывать**.

взну́здывать, **взнузда́ть** *(вн.)* brídle *(smth.)*, curb *(smth.)*.

взобра́ться *сов. см.* **взбира́ться**.

взойти́ *сов. см.* **всходи́ть** *и* **восходи́ть** 1.

взор *м.* gaze, glance; устреми́ть ~ *(на вн.)* fix one's eyes (on).

взорв|а́ть *сов.* 1. *см.* **взрыва́ть** 1; 2. *разг.* *(возмути́ть)* его́ ~а́ло he exploded; э́то меня́ ~а́ло it infúriated/exásperated me; it made my blood boil. **~а́ться** *сов.* 1. *см.* **взрыва́ться**; 2. *разг.* *(возмути́ться, рассерди́ться)* blow* up.

взро́слый *прил.* 1. ádult; grówn-up *разг.*; 2. *в знач. сущ. м.* an ádult, a grówn-up.

взрыв *м.* 1. explósion; ~ снаря́да shéll-burst; 2. *(разрушение)* blówing up; ~ моста́ blówing up of a bridge; 3. *(внезапное, бурное проявление чего-л.)* *(out)*burst; ~ негодова́ния burst of indignátion, óutburst of wrath.

взрыва́тель *м.* *mex.* fuse.

взрыва́ть I, **взорва́ть** *(вн.)* blow* up *(smth.)*; *(мину, заряд)* explóde *(smth.)*, détonate *(smth.)*, fire *(smth.)*; set* off *(smth.)*; *(горную породу)* blast *(smth.)*.

взрыва́ть II, **взрыть** *(вн.)* dig* up *(smth.)*, plough *(smth.)*.

взрыва́ться, **взорва́ться** be* blown up; *(о заряде и т. п.)* explóde.

взрывн|о́й 1. explósive; ~а́я волна́ blast; ~ы́е рабо́ты blásting *sg*; 2. лингв.: ~ звук stop; explósive/stopped sound.

взрывча́тка *ж. разг.* demolítion explósive/chárge(s).

взры́вчат|ый explósive; ~ое вещество́ explósive *(súbstance)*.

взрыть *сов. см.* **взрыва́ть** II.

взрыхли́ть *сов. см.* **взрыхля́ть**.

взрыхля́ть, **взрыхли́ть** *(вн.)* lóosen *(smth.)*; *(мотыгой)* hoe *(smth.)*.

взъеро́шенный dishévelled, tóusled.

взъеро́шить *сов. см.* **еро́шить**.

взыва́ть *несов.* *(к дт., о пр.)* appéal (to *smb.*, *smth.*; for *smth.*); ~ к чьей-л. со́вести appéal to *smb.'s* cónscience; ~ о по́мощи call for help, appéal for aid; ~ к справедли́вости demánd jústice.

взыска́н|ие *с.* 1. *(долга и т. п.)* recóvery; пода́ть на *кого-л.* ко ~ию procéed agáinst *smb.*; 2. *(наказание)* pénalty; наложи́ть ~ на *кого-л.* pénalize *smb.*; подве́ргнуться ~ию incúr a pénalty.

взыска́тельн|ость *ж.* high stándards *pl*; strictness. **~ый** exácting, strict; быть ~ым к себе́ set* onesélf high stándards.

взыска́ть *сов. см.* **взыскивать**.

взы́скивать, **взыска́ть** 1. *(вн. с рд.)* exáct *(smth. from)*; взыска́ть штраф с *кого-л.* exáct a fine from *smb.*; ~ долг с *кого-л.* recóver a debt from *smb.*; 2. *(с рд.; под-*

верга́ть наказа́нию) pénalize *(smb.)*; ◇ не взыщи́те! it's the best I can do!; don't expéct too much!

взя́тие *с.* séizure, táking; ~ кре́пости cápture/táking of a fórtress.

взя́тка *ж.* 1. *(подкуп)* bribe; 2. *(в картах)* trick; ◇ с него́ ~и гла́дки you won't get ánything out of him.

взя́точни|к *м.* bríbe-taker. **~чество** *с.* táking of bribes; graft.

взя́ть(ся) *сов. см.* **брать(ся)**.

виаду́к *м.* víaduct.

вибра́ция *ж.* vibrátion.

вибри́ровать *несов.* vibráte.

виго́нь *ж.* vicúna (wool).

вид I *м.* 1. *(наружность)* appéarance, look; *(выражение)* air; вну́тренний ~ intérior; нару́жный ~ extérior; гро́зный ~ fórmidable áspect; скро́мный ~ módest appéarance; с са́мым неви́нным, равноду́шным ~ом with an air of the útmost ínnocence, indífference; име́ть тако́й ~, бу́дто... look as if...; у вас больно́й ~ you don't look well; 2. *(состояние)* state, condítion; в испра́вном ~е in wórking órder; в неиспра́вном ~е out of órder; в пья́ном ~е in a state of intoxicátion; drunk; 3. *(пейзаж, перспектива)* view; ~ на мо́ре view of the sea; ~ сбо́ку side view; ~ спе́реди front view; ко́мната с ~ на Во́лгу, на пло́щадь a room overlóoking the Vólga, the square; 4. *(поле зрения)* sight; скры́ться из ~у disappéar from view/sight; на ~у́ in sight of *smth.*; 5. *мн.* *(намерения, предположения)* próspect(s); óutlook *sg.*; ~ы на урожа́й próspect for the hárvest; ~ы на успе́х chánces of success; ◇ ему́ на ~ (мо́жно дать) лет 40, ему́ с ~у 40 лет he looks about fórty; с ~у он совсе́м ю́ноша he looks a mere youth; нельзя́ суди́ть о лю́дях по вне́шнему ~у néver judge by appéarances; он ви́дывал ~ы he has seen a lot of life, he has seen a good deal of the world; под ~ом *чего-л.* únder/on the prétext of *smth.*; ни под каки́м ~ом on no accóunt; не показа́ть ~у show*/give* no sign (of); име́ть ~ы на *кого-л.* have* one's eye on *smb.*; име́ть ~ы на *что-л.* count on *smth.*; быть на ~у́ be* conspícuous; у всех на ~у́ in front of éverybody; нака́зывать, хвали́ть *и т. п.* для ~а make* a show of púnishing, práising *etc.*; име́ть в ~у́ 1) *(подразумевать)* mean*, imply*; 2) *(помнить)* bear*/have* in mind; поста́вить на ~ *кому-л.* reprimánd *smb.*; не теря́ть из ~у not lose sight of.

вид II *м.* 1. *(разновидность)* form; *mex.* type, class; но́вый ~ обще́ственных отноше́ний new form of sócial relátions; 2. *биол.* spécies; 3. *лингв.* áspect; несоверше́нный ~ imperféctive áspect; соверше́нный ~ perféctive áspect.

ви́данн|ый: ~ое ли э́то де́ло? did you éver hear such a thing?

ви́даться *несов. см.* **ви́деться**.

ви́дение *с.* sight; ~ на расстоя́нии long sight.

виде́ние *с.* vísion; *(привидение тж.)* apparítion.

видеоза́пись *ж.* vídeotape recórding.

видеомагнитофо́н *м.* vídeo (recórder). **~ный** vídeo, vídeotáped.

видеотелефо́н *м.* vídeotélephone. **~ный** vídeotélephone *attr.*

ви́деть, **уви́деть** *(вн.)* see* *(smb., smth.)*; хорошо́ ~ see* well; я ви́жу его́ как живо́го I can see him before me now; уви́деть свет see* the light; что я ви́жу! what's this?, what have we here?; ~ го́род вдали́ see* a town in the dístance; я вчера́ ви́дел его́ два ра́за I saw him twice yésterday; я мно́гое ви́дел на своём веку́ I have seen much in my time; ~ сон dream*, have* a dream; ~ *что-л.* во сне dream* of/about *smth.*; ~ то́лько его́ и ви́дели he disappéared as súddenly as he appéared, he was off agáin at once; ~ *кого-л.* наскво́зь see* through *smb.*; ~ его́ не могу́ I can't bear the sight of him; как ви́дно *в знач. вводн. сл.* you see; вот уви́дите, он придёт he'll come — see if he dóesn't!; рад ~ (вас) glad to see you;

поживём — уви́дим! we shall see what we shall see! ~ся, уви́деться see* each óther; ~ся с кем-л. see* smb.

ви́димо appárently.

ви́димо-неви́димо разг. lots, véry mány; наро́ду бы́ло ~ there was a huge crowd; you néver saw such crowds!

ви́дим|**ость** ж. 1. visibílity; 2. (подобие) sémblance, appéarance; э́то одна́ ~ it ónly seems so; ◇ по всей ~ости to all (óutward) appéarances; для ~ости púrely for the sake of appéarance, just for show. ~ый 1. vísible; 2. (явный) appárent, mánifest; без вся́кой ~ой причи́ны without appárent cause; 3. разг. (кажущийся) appárent, séeming; ~ая весёлость appárent chéerfulness.

видне́|**ться** несов. be* discérnible/vísible; чуть ~ be* bárely discérnible; вдали́ ~ется мо́ре the sea can be discérned in the dístance.

ви́дно 1. в знач. сказ. безл. one can see; отсю́да хорошо́ ~ one can, see béautifully from here; отсю́да не ~ до́ма you can't see the house from here; по́езда не ~ (ещё не показался) the train isn't yet in sight; (уже скрылся) the train is out of sight; никого́ не ~ there's no one to be seen; (вне помещения тж.) there's no one in sight; ничего́ не ~ one can't see a thing; конца́ не ~ one can see no end to it; по всему́ ~ all the facts go to prove; éverything points to the fact; éverything índicates; 2. в знач. вводн. сл. разг. apparently, évidently; ~, мне придётся пойти́ самому́ it looks as if I shall have to go mysélf.

вид|**ный** 1. (видимый) vísible; (заметный) conspícuous; чуть ~ scárcely discérnible; на са́мом ме́сте in the mоşt conspícuous place; (о вещах) conspícuously displáyed; по́езд уже́ ~ен the train is alréady in sight; дом ~ен отсю́да you can see the house from here; конца́ уже́ ~ен the end is in sight; 2. (выдающийся) próminent; 3. разг. (представительный) impréssive; ~ мужчи́на fine-looking man*, man* of hándsome présence.

видо|**во́й** I: ~а́я кинокарти́на trável film.

видово́й II биол. specífic.

видоизмен|**е́ние** с. 1. modificátion; 2. (разновидность) type; (вариант) váriant. ~и́ть(ся) сов. см. видоизменя́ть(ся).

видоизменя́ть, видоизмени́ть (вн.) módify (smth.), álter (smth.). ~ся, видоизмени́ться change, álter.

видоиска́тель м. фото, кино víewfinder.

ви́з|**а** ж. (разрешение и пометка) vísa; наложи́ть ~у на что-л. vísa smth.; отказа́ть кому́-л. в ~е refúse (to grant) smb. a vísa.

визави́ 1. нареч. vis-à-vis, ópposite, fácing each óther; 2. м. и ж. нескл. vis-à-vis, pártner, ópposite númber.

визг м. squeal; (многоголосый) squéaling. ~ли́вый shrill; (резкий) strídent; squéaky; ~ли́вый го́лос shrill voice.

визжа́ть несов. squeal, screech.

визи́ровать несов. и сов. (сов. тж. завизи́ровать) (вн.) vísa (smth.); ~ па́спорт stamp/vísa a pássport.

визи́т м. (официальный) vísit; (частный тж.) call; прибы́ть с ~ом arríve on a state vísit. ~ка ж. разг. vísiting card. ~ный vísiting; ~ная ка́рточка (vísiting-)card.

ви́ка ж. бот. vetch.

викторина ж. quízzing game, quiz.

ви́лка ж. 1. fork; 2. тех.: штепсельная ~ plug.

вило́к м. разг. head of cábbage.

ви́л|**ы** мн. pítchfork sg; ◇ э́то ещё ~ами на воде́ пи́сано ≈ it may or may not come off; it's all in the air still.

вильну́ть сов. см. виля́ть.

виля́ть, вильну́ть 1. (тв.) wag (smth.); ~ хвосто́м wag its tail; 2. (двигаться по извилистой линии) weave*, dodge; 3. разг. (лукавить) hedge, be* evásive.

вин|**а́** ж. 1. fault, blame; э́то моя́, ва́ша ~ it's my, your fault; я признаю́ свою́ ~у́ I know I'm to blame; все-

му́ ~о́й его́ небре́жность it's all ówing to his négligence/cárelessness; по ~е́ кого-л. becáuse of smb.; не по мое́й, его́ ~е́ through no fault of mine, his; поста́вить что-л. в ~у́ кому́-л. repróach smb. with smth.; 2. (виновность) guilt; его́ ~ была́ дока́зана his guilt was estáblished.

винегре́т м. 1. (кушанье) Rússian sálad (chopped beetroot, gherkins etc., dressed with oil and vinegar); 2. разг. (смесь разнородных предметов, понятий) júmble, hótchpotch.

вини́тельный: ~ паде́ж грам. accúsative (case).

вин|**и́ть** несов. (вн.) blame (smb.); во всём ~и́те са́мого себя́ you have ónly yoursélf to blame.

ви́нн|**ый** wine attr.; ~ по́греб wíne-cellar; ~ спирт spírits of wine; ◇ ~ ка́мень tártar; ~ая я́года fig.

вино́ с. 1. (виноградное) wine; 2. разг. (водка) vódka.

винова́т|**ый** 1. (виновный) guílty; я не винова́т it's not my fault, кто винова́т? whose fault is it?; никто́ не винова́т it's nóbody's fault, no one is to blame; 2. (выражающий сознание вины) guílty, apologétic; у него́ ~ вид he looks guílty; ~ взгляд apologétic glance; ~ым то́ном apologétically; ◇ винова́т! (как извинение) sórry!, I beg your párdon!; (что помешал) excúse me!

вино́в|**ник** м. 1. the guílty pérson; (обвиняемый) cúlprit; ~ происше́ствия cúlprit; 2. (тот, кто является причиной чего-л.) cause; ~ торжества́ héro of the day/occásion. ~ность ж. guilt, culpabílity; ~ный (в пр.) guílty (of); он ни в чём не ~ he is complétely ínnocent; признаёте ли вы себя́ ~ным? do you admít your guilt?; призна́ть обвиня́емого ~ным bring* a vérdict of guílty agáinst the accúsed.

виногра́д м. 1. собир. (плоды) grapes pl; 2. (растение) vine; ◇ зе́лен ~! the grapes are sour!, sour grapes!

виногра́д|**арство** с. víne-growing, vitículture. ~арь м. víne-grower, vitículturist. ~ник м. víneyard. ~ный vine attr.; ~ное вино́ wine; ~ная ко́сточка grápe-stone, pip; ~ная лоза́ vine; ~ный са́хар grápe-sugar.

винт м. screw; (самолёта) áirscrew, propéller.

ви́нтик м. small screw; ◇ у него́ (в голове́) ~а не хвата́ет he has a screw loose.

винто́вка ж. rifle.

винтов|**о́й** 1. (спиральный) spíral; тех. screw attr., hélical; ~а́я ле́стница spíral stáircase; ~а́я наре́зка thread (of screw); 2. (приводимый в движение винтом) screw attr.; (о самолёте) propéller-driven; prop attr. разг.

виолончели́ст м. violoncéllist, 'céllist.

виолонче́ль ж. violoncéllo (pl -os), 'céllo (pl -os).

вира́ж I м. 1. (поворот) turn; 2. спорт. bank, banked turn.

вира́ж II м. фото tóning solútion.

вира́ж-фикса́ж м. фото fíxer.

виртуо́з м. virtuóso (pl -sos, -si); 2. (знаток своего дела) éxpert (at, in), past máster (in). ~ность ж. 1. virtuósity; 2. (высокое мастерство в каком-л. деле) skill, dextérity. ~ный brílliant, másterly.

ви́рус м. vírus. ~ный vírus attr., víral; ~ные заболева́ния vírus diséases.

вирусоло́гия ж. virólogy.

ви́селица ж. gállows pl.

висе́ть несов. hang*, be* suspénded; ◇ ~ в во́здухе be* all in the air.

виско́за ж. 1. víscose; 2. (искусственный шёлк) víscose ráyon. ~ный víscose; ~ный шёлк víscose ráyon, viscose silk.

ви́снуть, пови́снуть 1. (свисать) hang* down; 2. (на пр.) hang* (on).

висо́к м. témple.

високо́сный: ~ год léap-year.

висо́чный témporal.

вися́ч|**ий** hánging; péndent; ~ замо́к pádlock; ~ мост suspénsion bridge; в ~ем положéнии hánging, suspénded.

витамúн *м.* vítamin.

витаминизúрованный vítaminized.

витамúнный vítamin *attr.*

витáть *несов.* hóver; ◇ ~ в облакáх have* one's head in the clouds.

витиевáтый ornáte, flówery, flórid.

вит|óй twísted; *архит.* cónvoluted; ~ая лéстница wínding stáirway.

витóк *м.* 1. (*оборот спирали*) spíral, spíre, turn; 2. (*моток, свитый спиралью*) coil, wínding; 3. (*вокруг Земли*) círcuit.

витрáж *м.* stáined-glass wíndow.

витрúна *ж.* 1. (*окно магазина*) shop wíndow, shów-window; 2. (*для показа музейных экспонатов*) shówcase.

вить, свить (*вн.*) twine (*smth.*), twist (*smth.*); weave* (*smth.*); ~ венкú make* wreaths; ~ верёвку lay* rope; ~ гнездó build*/make* a nest; ◇ ~ верёвки из *кого-л.* twist *smb.* round one's little finger.

вúться *несов.* 1. (*о растениях*) climb, twine; 2. (*о волосах*) curl; 3. (*о дороге, реке*) wind*; 4. (*о пыли, дыме и т. п.*) éddy; 5. (*о птицах, насекомых*) círcle; 6. (*о змее*) writhe, úndulate; 7. (*развеваться*) flútter.

вих|óр *м.* 1. tuft; 2. *мн. разг.* rebéllious locks; отодрáть *кого-л.* за ~рь pull *smb.'s* hair; приглáдить ~ры smooth down one's hair. ~рáстый *разг.* shóck-headed; with rebéllious hair *после сущ.*

вúхрем like a whírlwind; летéть ~ run* like the wind; влетéть ~ burst*/come* in like a whírlwind.

вихрь *м.* whírlwind; *перен.* vórtex (*pl* -xes, -tices); снéжный ~ éddy of snow.

вице- *в сложн.* více-.

вице-президéнт *м.* více-président.

вишнёв|ка *ж.* chérry brándy. ~ый 1. chérry; ~ый сад chérry órchard; 2. (*о цвете*) dárk-red.

вúшня *ж.* 1. (*плод*) chérry; 2. (*дерево*) chérry-tree.

вкатúть(ся) *сов. см.* вкáтывать(ся).

вкáтывать, вкатúть (*вн.*) roll (*smth.*). ~ся, вкатúться (в *вн.*) come* rólling (ínto); *перен. разг.* (*вбегать*) burst* (ínto).

вклад *м.* (*в банк, сберкассу*) depósit; *перен.* contribútion; срóчный ~ depósit accóunt; бессрóчный ~ cúrrent accóunt; сдéлать цéнный ~ в наýку make* a váluable contribútion to science.

вклáдка *ж. полигр.* ínset; (*в журнале и т. п. тж.*) súpplement; (*вложенная репродукция*) plate.

вклáдчик *м.* depósitor.

вклáдывать, вложúть (*вн. в вн.*) 1. put* (*smth.* ínto); ~ меч в нóжны sheathe a sword; ~ мнóго трудá во *что-л.* put* a lot of work ínto *smth.*; 2. (*капитал*) invést (*smth.* in).

вклéивать, вклéить (*вн.*) paste (*smth.*) in, stick* (*smth.*) in; (*вн. в вн.*) paste (*smth.* ínto), stick* (*smth.* ínto).

вклéить *сов. см.* вклéивать.

вклéйка *ж.* 1. (*действие*) pásting in; 2. (*что-л. вклеенное*) ínset.

вклúниваться, вклúниться (в *вн.*) be* wedged in; (*вторгаться*) force one's way (ínto); дорóга вклúнилась в лес the road cut ínto the fórest.

вклúниться *сов. см.* вклúниваться.

включáть, включúть (*вн.*) 1. *тк. несов.* (*охватывать*) inclúde (*smth.*); 2. (*вн. в вн.; вводить, вносить куда-л.*) put* (*smth.* ínto), take* (*smth.* ínto); ~ *кого-л.* в кружóк take* *smb.* into the group; ~ *что-л.* в прогрáмму put*/inclúde *smth.* in the prógramme; 3. (*ток, мотор и т. п.*) switch (*smth.*) on, turn (*smth.*) on; ~ газ, свет turn on the gas, light; ~ рáдио switch on the rádio. ~ся, включúться 1. (в *вн.*) join in (*smth.*), take* part

(in), partícipate (in); 2. (*начинать действовать*) begín* óperating, start.

включáя *предлог* inclúding; inclúded *после сущ.*

включúтельно inclúsive; от пéрвой до четвёртой главы́ ~ chápters one to four inclúsive.

включúть *сов. см.* включáть 2, 3. ~ся *сов. см.* включáться.

вкóлачивать, вколотúть (*вн.*) *разг.* drive* (*smth.*) in, hámmer (*smth.*) in.

вколотúть *сов. см.* вкóлачивать.

вконéц *разг.* quite, altogéther, tótally, útterly; ~ отчáявшись... útterly despóndent..., háving lost all hope...

вкóпанный: как ~ as if róoted to the ground; он остановúлся как ~ he stopped dead.

вкось diágonally, aslánt; ◇ вкривь и ~ in all diréctions.

вкрáдчив|ость *ж.* insinuáting ways *pl,* súbtle fláttery. ~ый ingrátiating, insínuating.

вкрáдываться, вкрáсться 1. (в *вн.*) creep* (ínto); в текст вкрáлась опечáтка a mísprint has crept ínto text; 2. (*о мыслях, чувствах*) aríse*; вкрáлось подозрéние a suspícion aróse; ◇ вкрáсться в *чьё-л.* довéрие worm onesélf ínto *smb.'s* cónfidence, trick *smb.* ínto trústing one.

вкрáпленный embédded.

вкрáсться *сов. см.* вкрáдываться.

вкрáтце in brief, bríefly.

вкривь *разг.:* ~ и вкось *см.* вкось.

вкрутýю: яйцó ~ hard-bóiled egg; сварúть яйцó ~ boil/do* an egg hard.

вкус *м.* taste; быть прия́тным на ~ have* a pléasant taste; в моём ~е to my taste; имéть ~ к *чему-л.* have* a taste for *smth.*; положúте сáхару, сóли по ~у add súgar, salt to taste; ~ вхóдишь во ~ begín* to enjóy; на ~ и цвет товáрищей нет there's no accóunting for tastes.

вкусúть *сов. см.* вкушáть.

вкýсн|о: ~ готóвить cook well, be* a good* cook; ~ есть eat* well, live on good* food; ~ поéсть have* a good* meal. ~ый nice, good*, delícious, pálatable; ~ый кусóк tásty mórsel.

вкусов|óй gústatory; ~ое ощущéние sense of taste. ~щúна *ж. разг. неодобр.* týranny of taste.

вкушáть, вкусúть (*вн., рд.*) taste (*smth.*); ~ рáдость taste joy.

влáга *ж.* móisture.

влагáлище *с. анат. бот.* vagína (*pl* -ae, -as).

влагозадержáние *с.* móisture-reténtion.

владé|лец *м.* ówner, posséssor; (*недвижимости тж.*) propríetor. ~ние *с.* 1. (*обладание*) posséssion; (*недвижимостью тж.*) propríetorship; 2. (*собственность*) próperty; (*земельное*) domáin, estáte; 3. *мн.* (*территория*) posséssions.

владéть *несов.* (*тв.*) 1. (*иметь*) have* (*smth.*), posséss (*smth.*) (*тж. перен.*); own (*smth.*); 2. (*держать в своей власти*) hold* (*smth.*); *перен.* contról (*smth., smth.*); ~ умáми sway the minds; ~ чýвствами contról one's féelings; 3. (*о мыслях, чувствах*) posséss (*smb.*); 4. (*уметь обращаться с чем-л., хорошо знать*) be* able to use (*smth.*); ~ орýжием hándle a wéapon with skill; ~ рýсским, англúйским языкóм have* a compléte commánd of Rússian, Énglish; 5.: (не) ~ рукáми, ногáми have* (lost) the use of one's arms, legs; ◇ ~ перóм write* well; умéть хорошó ~ собóй have* plénty of sélf-contról; не ~ собóй have* no sélf-contról, be* lácking in sélf-contról.

влады́|ка *м.* 1. sóvereign, rúler; 2. *рел.* mémber of hígher órders of clérgy. ~чество *с.* domínion.

влáжн|ость *ж.* dámpness, humídity. ~ый damp, moist; (*о климате, воздухе тж.*) húmid; ~ое бельё damp línen/wáshing; ~ые глазá líquid eyes; (*от слёз*) téar-filled eyes.

влáмываться, вломúться (в *вн.*) burst* (ínto); ~ в

комнату burst* ínto a room; ~ к *кому-л.* burst* in on *smb.*

вла́ствовать *несов.* (*тв.,* над *тв.*) rule (óver), hold* sway (óver).

властели́н *м.* rúler, pótentate.

власти́тель *м. уст. см.* властели́н; ◇ ~ дум acknówledged léader, inspírer.

власт|ный 1. (*имеющий власть*) pówerful, strong; я над ним не ~ен I have no authórity óver him; он не ~ен измени́ть положе́ние he has no pówer to álter the situátion; 2. (*склонный повелевать; повелительный*) impérious, másterful; commánding; ~ная рука́ hand of íron; ~ тон perémptory tone.

власто|люби́вый másterful, dominéering; он о́чень ~люби́в he is véry fond of pówer. ~лю́бие *с.* love of pówer.

власт|ь *ж.* 1. pówer; находи́ться у ~и be* in pówer; прийти́ к ~и come* to pówer; 2. (*образ правления*) form of góvernment; сове́тская ~ Sóviet pówer; the Sóviets *pl разг.*; 3. *обыкн. мн.* (*должностные лица, администрация*) the authórities; ~ на места́х lócal authórities *pl*; вое́нные ~ mílitary authórities; 4. (*право распоряжаться*) authórity; роди́тельская ~ paréntal authórity; ◇ быть во ~и *кого-л.* be* in *smb.'s* pówer; быть во ~и *чего-л.* be* in the grip of *smth.*; име́ть ~ над *кем-л.* have* pówer over *smb.*; have* *smb.* in *one's* pówer.

влачи́ть *несов.* (*вн.*) *уст.* drag (*smth.*); ◇ ~ жа́лкое существова́ние drag out a wrétched/míserable existence. ~ся *несов. уст.* drag (alóng); (*о человеке тж.*) línger.

вле́во to the left; ~ от on the left of; сверну́ть ~ turn to the left.

влеза́ть, влезть 1. get* in; (*в вн.*) get* (into); ~ в окно́ get*/climb in through the window; 2. (*на вн.; наверх*) climb (*smth.*), scale (*smth.*); ◇ влезть в ду́шу *кому-л.* worm *onesélf* into *smb.'s* cónfidence; ~ в долги́ get* ínto debt.

влезть *сов. см.* влеза́ть.

влет|а́ть, влете́ть 1. (*в вн.*) fly* ín(to), come* flýing ín(to); в окно́ влете́ла пти́ца a bird flew in through the window; 2. (*в вн.*) *разг.* (*быстро войти, вбежать*) burst* (ínto), dash (ínto); он влете́л в ко́мнату he burst ínto the room; 3. *безл.* (*дт.*) *разг.:* ему́ здо́рово влете́ло he got it hot.

влете́ть *сов. см.* влета́ть.

влече́ние *с.* (к *дт.*) bent (for), inclinátion (for); чу́вствовать ~ к *кому-л.* feel* *smb.'s* attráction; feel* attrácted to *smb.*; ~ к му́зыке, иску́сству bent for músic, art; име́ть ~ к литерату́ре have* líterary léanings; име́ть ~ к нау́ке be* of a scientífic turn of mind.

вле|чь *несов.* (*вн.*) 1. (*тащить*) draw* (*smb., smth.*); 2. (*привлекать*) attráct (*smb.*); ◇ ~ за собо́й *что-л.* bring* *smth.* in its train, entáil *smth.*

влива́ние *с.* infúsion, injéction; ~ глюко́зы glúcose injéction; внутриве́нное ~ intravénous infúsion.

влива́ть, влить 1. (*вн., рд.*) pour (*smth.*) in; *перен.* instíl (*smth.*), infúse (*smth.*); ~ *что-л.* по ка́пле pour *smth.* a drop at a time, instíl *smth.*; ~ бо́дрость instíl cóurage; 2. (*вн.; включать*) amálgamate (*smth.*) with, merge (*smth.*) with, make* (*smth.*) part of; отря́д был влит в брига́ду the detáchment was made part of a brigáde. ~ся, вли́ться 1. flow in, stream in; (*в вн.*) flow (ínto), stream (ínto); 2. join.

влипа́ть, вли́пнуть (*в вн.*) 1. get* ínto (smth.); 2. *разг.:* вли́пнуть в исто́рию get* ínto a prétty mess.

вли́пнуть *сов. см.* влипа́ть.

влить(ся) *сов. см.* влива́ть(ся).

влия́ние *с.* ínfluence; находи́ться под ~м *кого-л.* be* únder the ínfluence of *smb.*; по́льзоваться ~м be* influéntial.

влия́тельный influéntial.

влия́ть, повлия́ть (на *вн.*) ínfluence (*smb., smth.*), have* an ínfluence (on); (*более конкретно или быст-*

ро) afféct (*smb., smth.*); ~ на свои́х това́рищей ínfluence *one's* friends/cómrades; э́то повлия́ло на их здоро́вье it affécted their health.

влож|е́ние *с.* 1. (*капитала*) invéstment; 2. (*в письмо, пакет*) enclósure. ~и́ть *сов. см.* вкла́дывать.

вломи́ться *сов. см.* вла́мываться.

влюби́ться *сов. см.* влюбля́ться.

влюблённ|ый *прил.* 1. in love *после сущ.*; enámoured, lóve-sick *поэт.*; ~ взгляд ámorous glance; быть ~ым в *кого-л.* be* in love with *smb.*; 2. *в знач. сущ. мн.* lóvers, lóving cóuple.

влюбля́ться, влюби́ться (в *вн.*) fall* in love (with).

влюбчив|ость *ж.* susceptibílity; ámorous dispositíon *книжн.* ~ый of an ámorous dispositíon *после сущ.*

вменить *сов. см.* вменя́ть.

вменя́ем|ость *ж.* responsibílity. ~ый respónsible.

вменя́ть, вмени́ть: ~ *что-л.* в вину́ *кому-л.* impúte *smth.* to *smb.*; ~ *что-л.* в обя́занность *кому-л.* make* *smb.* respónsible for *smth.*, make* it *smb.'s* dúty to do *smth.*

вме́сте togéther; ~ с togéther with; все ~ all togéther; всё ~ взя́тое éverything (put togéther); ◇ ~ с тем at the same time.

вмести́|лище *с.* recéptacle. ~мость *ж.* capácity. ~тельный (*о сосуде, карманах и т. п.*) capácious; (*о помещении*) large, spácious, róomy.

вмести́ть *сов. см.* вмеща́ть 1, 3. ~ся *сов. см.* вмеща́ться.

вме́сто (*рд.*) instéad (of); ~ меня́, вас instéad of me, you; ~ э́того instéad of this); ~ того́, что́бы пойти́, отве́тить *и т. п.* instéad of góing, ánswering *etc.*; рабо́тать ~ *кого-л.* do* *smb.'s* work.

вмеша́тельство *с.* 1. (*в чужие дела*) interférence; (*в дела другого государства*) intervéntion; вооружённое ~ armed intervéntion; 2.: хирурги́ческое ~ súrgical intervéntion.

вмеша́ться *сов. см.* вме́шиваться.

вме́шиваться, вмеша́ться 1. (*в вн.*) (*в чужие дела*) interfére (with), méddle (in), intervéne (in); ~ не в своё де́ло méddle in óther péople's búsiness; он ве́чно во всё вме́шивается he's for éver interféring; 2. (*для пресечения нежелательных действий*) step in, intervéne; вме́шаться, что́бы предотврати́ть кровопроли́тие step/go* in to prevént blóodshed.

вмеща́ть, вмести́ть (*вн.*) 1. (*заключать в себе*) contáin (*smth.*), hold* (*smth.*); (*о помещении*) accómmodate (*smb., smth.*), seat (*smb., smth.*), hold* (*smb., smth.*); 2. *тк. несов.* (*иметь ёмкость*) contáin (*smth.*), hold* (*smth.*); 3. (*в вн.; помещать внутри*) get* (ínto). ~ся, вмести́ться (*в вн.*) go* (ínto).

вмиг in a flash, in the twínkling of an eye, at the drop of a hat.

вмя́тина *ж.* dent.

внаём, внаймы́: брать ~ híre; отдава́ть ~ (*помещение*) let*; (*машину и т. п.*) híre out, let* out on híre.

внаки́дку: наде́ть пальто́ ~ fling*/drape *one's* coat óver *one's* shóulders.

внакла́де *разг.:* оста́ться ~ be* the lóser; не оста́ться ~ be* none the worse off.

внакла́дку *разг.:* пить чай ~ drink* tea with súgar in it.

внача́ле at first, at the begínning, at the óutset.

вне 1. outsíde; out of; ~ до́ма awáy from home; ~ го́рода outsíde the town; ~ опа́сности out of dánger; 2. (*помимо*) in addítion (to); ~ пла́на óver and abóve the plan; 3. (*минуя что-л.*) out of, beyónd; ~ о́череди out of turn; ~ ко́нкурса not compéting; out of competítion; ◇ ~ игры́ offsíde; ~ вся́кого сомне́ния beyónd all mánner of doubt; ~ подозре́ний abóve/beyónd suspícion; быть ~ себя́ от *чего-л.* be* besíde *onesélf* with *smth.*; объяви́ть *кого-л.* ~ зако́на óutlaw *smb.*

внебра́чный: ~ ребёнок nátural child*, child* born out of wédlock.

внедре́ние с. inculcátion, adóption; ~ передово́го о́пыта introdúction of advánced knów-how; ~ но́вой те́хники inculcátion of new techníques; ~ в произво́дство достиже́ний нау́ки adóption of scientífic achíevements in índustry.

внедри́ть(ся) сов. см. внедря́ть(ся).

внедря́ть, внедри́ть (вн. в вн.) ínculcate (smth. in, on); instíl (smth. in, ínto); (технику и т. п.) introdúce (smth. in, ínto). ~ся, внедри́ться take* (deep) root.

внеза́пн|о súddenly, all of a súdden; ~ замолча́ть, ~ останови́ться stop short. ~ость ж. súddenness. ~ый súdden; (об атаке и т. п.) surprise attr.

внекла́ссн|ый óut-of-cláss; ~ые заня́тия óut-of-cláss work sg; ~ое чте́ние home réading.

внекла́ссовый nón-class.

внеко́нкурсный out-of-competítion.

внема́точн|ый: ~ая бере́менность мед. extra-úterine prégnancy.

внеочередн|о́й out of turn после сущ.; (вне устано́вленного сро́ка) extraórdinary; ~а́я се́ссия extraórdinary séssion.

внепарла́ментск|ий óutside párliament после сущ.

внепла́нов|ый éxtra; óver and abóve the plan после сущ.; ~ое зада́ние task not stípulated in the plan, addítional task; ~ расхо́д unforeséen expénses pl.

внесе́ние с. introdúction, insértion; ~ в протоко́л insértion in the mínutes; pútting on récord; ~ в спи́сок insértion in the list.

внести́ сов. см. вноси́ть.

внешко́льн|ый óut-of-schóol; ~ая рабо́та óut-of-schóol work.

вне́шне óutwardly.

внешнеполити́ческ|ий fóreign-pólicy attr., of fóreign pólicy после сущ.; ~ курс fóreign pólicy; ~ие пробле́мы próblems of fóreign pólicy.

внешнеторго́вый of fóreign trade после сущ.

внешнеэкономи́ческий extérnal económic.

вне́шн|ий 1. óutward, extérnal; (поверхностный) supérficial; súrface attr.; ~ вид (óutward) appéarance; ~ мир the óutside world; ~ее оформле́ние extérnal decorátion; (книги) cóver design; ~ при́знак óutward sign; ~ее схо́дство (между людьми) supérficial resémblance; (на портрете) supérficial líkeness; ~ее споко́йствие óutward calm; ~ лоск (mere) súrface pólish, thin venéer; ~ у́гол мат. extérior ángle; 2. (относящийся к сношениям с другими государствами) fóreign; ~яя торго́вля fóreign trade; ~яя поли́тика fóreign pólicy.

вне́шность ж. extérior, appéarance; looks pl разг.; внуши́тельная ~ impósing appéarance/présence; непривлека́тельная ~ únprepossésing appéarance/extérior.

внешта́тный non-stáff, non-sálaried; supernúmerary; ~ сотру́дник, рабо́тник non-sálaried mémber of the staff; frée-lance.

вниз down; dównwards; спуска́ться ~ descénd; ~ голово́й 1) (падать, прыгать в воду) head first; 2) (висеть) úpside-dówn; ~ по ле́стнице downstáirs; ~ по Во́лге down the Vólga; ~ по тече́нию downstréam.

внизу́ 1. нареч. belów; (в нижнем этаже) downstáirs; 2. в знач. предлога (рд.) (в нижней части) at the foot/bóttom (of), undernéath; (здания) in the lówer part (of).

**вн

ика́ть,** вни́кнуть (в вн.) go* (ínto), look deep (ínto); ~ в суть де́ла get* to the heart of the mátter.

вни́кнуть сов. см. вника́ть.

внима́ни|е с. 1. atténtion; слу́шать с ~ем lísten atténtively/clósely; 2. (забота) atténtion, considerátion; относи́ться с больши́м ~ем к кому́-л. be* véry atténtive to smb.; ◇ ~! atténtion!; обраща́ть чьё-л. ~ на кого́-л., что-л. draw*/call smb.'s atténtion to smb., smth.; обра-

ща́ть ~ на кого́-л., что-л. pay* atténtion to smb., smth.; обрати́ть на себя́ ~ attráct smb.'s atténtion; оста́вить что-л. без ~я pay* no atténtion to smth., take* no nótice of smth., ignóre smth.; быть в це́нтре ~я be* the céntre of atténtion; удели́ть чему́-л. (осо́бое) ~ pay* (spécial) atténtion to smth.

внима́тельн|о 1. atténtively, kéenly, clósely; ~ следи́ть, ~ наблюда́ть за чем-л. fóllow smth. clósely; 2.: ~ относи́ться к кому́-л. be* consíderate to smb. ~ость ж. 1. atténtiveness; 2. (к дт.; заботливость) considerátion (towárds), kíndness (towárds); (любезность) cóurtesy (towárds). ~ый 1. atténtive; ~ый учени́к atténtive púpil; ~ый взгляд intént gaze; 2. (к дт.; заботливый) consíderate (to); (любезный) políte (to), cóurteous (to).

внима́ть, внять (дт.) поэт. heed (smb., smth.); ~ го́лосу рассу́дка lísten to the voice of réason; ~ мольба́м heed smb.'s práyers.

вничью́: зако́нчиться ~ end in a draw; они́ сыгра́ли ~ their game énded in a draw.

вновь 1. (снова) once agáin, once more; 2. (недавно) néwly, recéntly.

внос|и́ть, внести́ 1. (вн. в вн.; внутрь) take* (smth. ínto), bring* (smb., smth. ínto), cárry (smb., smth. ínto); он внёс чемода́н в ваго́н he took the súitcase ínto the cárriage; он внёс её в ко́мнату (на рука́х) he cárried her ínto the room (in his arms); 2. (вн.; платить, делать взнос) pay* (smth.); 3. (вн.; включать, вписывать) put* (smb., smth.) in; внести́ попра́вку в текст insert a corréction in the text/aménd the text; ~ кого́-л. в спи́сок énter smb.'s name on the list; ~ но́вые усло́вия в догово́р insert new condítions in a tréaty; 4. (вн.; представлять, предлагать) submit (smth.); ~ законопрое́кт introdúce a bill; ~ что-л. на рассмотре́ние кого́-л. submit smth. for (the) considerátion of smb.; ~ предложе́ние submit a propósal; (на собрании) move a propósal; 5. (вн. в вн.; вызывать, приносить с собой) introdúce (smth. ínto); ~ не́что но́вое во что-л. introdúce a fresh note into smth.; внести́ свой вклад во что-л. make* one's contribútion to smth.; do* one's bit for smth. разг.; ~ ра́дость bring* háppiness; ~ разложе́ние demóralize; ~ смяте́ние spread* confúsion.

внук м. grándson, grándchild*.

вну́тренне ínwardly; ~ почу́вствовать feel* intúitively.

вну́тренн|ий 1. (находящийся внутри) ínner, intérior, intérnal, inside; перен. ínner, ínward; (присущий) intrínsic, inhérent; ~ двор ínner court; ~яя сторона́ the ínside; ~яя дверь, стена́ ínside door, wall; ~яя пове́рхность ínner súrface; ~ее оформле́ние intérior decorátions pl; ~ее мо́ре ínland sea; ~ие о́бласти страны́ the intérior; ~ие резе́рвы intérnal resóurces; (финансовые) ínner resérves; ~ смысл, мир ínner méaning, life; ~ее чутьё intuítion; ~ подъём ínward elátion, spontáneous urge; ~ие причи́ны intrínsic cáuses; 2. (внутригосударственный) home, doméstic, intérnal; ~ие во́дные пути́ ínland wáterways; ~ заём doméstic/intérnal loan; ~ ры́нок home márket; ~яя торго́вля intérnal/home trade; ~яя поли́тика home/doméstic pólicy; ~ие дела́ intérnal affáirs; ◇ ~ие боле́зни intérnal diséases. ~ость ж. 1. intérior, the ínside; 2. мн. intérnal órgans; guts разг.

внутри́ 1. нареч. ínside; 2. предлог (рд.) withín.

внутриве́нный intravénous.

внутрипарти́йн|ый withín the párty после сущ.

внутриполити́ческ|ий intérnal polítical; ~ая обстано́вка intérnal polítical situátion.

внутриэкономи́ческ|ий intérnal económic; ~ое положе́ние intérnal económic situátion.

внутригосуда́рственный intranúclear.

внутрь 1. нареч. in(síde); intérnally; принима́ть лека́рство ~ take* a médicine intérnally; 2. предлог (рд.) in(to), inside; ~ страны́ ínland.

внуча́та мн. grándchildren.

вну́чка *ж.* gránddaughter, grándchild*.

внуш|а́ть, внуши́ть (*вн. дт.*) inspíre (*smb.* with); ~, что... try to suggést that...; ~ уваже́ние *кому-л.* command *smb.'s* respéct, inspíre *smb.* with respéct; ~ кому́-л. опасе́ния, подозре́ние *smb.'s* apprehénsion, suspísion; ~ кому́-л. мысль (+ *инф.*) put* it ínto *smb.'s* head (+ to *inf.*); внуши́ть себе́ get* it ínto *one's* head.

внуше́ни|е *с.* 1. (*воздействие*) instílling; для ~я стра́ха *кому-л.* to instíl fear ínto *smb.*; 2. (*гипноз*) (hypnótic) suggéstion; лечи́ть ~ем treat by hypnósis; 3. (*выговор*) admonítion, réprimand; сде́лать *кому-л.* ~ admónish/réprimand *smb.*

внуши́тельный impósing, impréssive.

внуши́ть *сов. см.* внуша́ть.

вня́тный 1. (*отчётливый*) distínct; ~ го́лос clear voice; 2. (*понятный*) intélligible.

внять *сов. см.* внима́ть.

во *см.* в; во вре́мя dúring, in; во вре́мя войны́, револю́ции dúring the war, revolútion; во что бы то ни ста́ло at all costs, at ány price.

во́бла *ж.* vóbla, Cáspian roach.

вобра́ть *сов. см.* вбира́ть.

вове́к(и) 1. for éver; 2. (*при гл. с отрицанием; никогда*) néver.

вовлека́ть, вовле́чь (*вн. в вн.*) draw* (*smb.* ínto), invólve (*smb.* in); ~ кого́-л. в разгово́р draw* *smb.* ínto conversátion.

вовлече́ние *с.* dráwing ínto.

вовле́чь *сов. см.* вовлека́ть.

во́время at the right móment; in time; ~ ска́занное сло́во a word in séason; не ~ inópportunely; прийти́ не ~ come* just at the wrong móment, arríve inópportunely.

во́все *разг.*: ~ не not a bit, not at all; ~ э́то ~ не он! it ísn't him!; я э́того ~ не говори́л I néver said that; ~ нет! nóthing of the sort!

вовсю́ *разг.* to the útmost, with might and main; гнать ло́шадь ~ drive* the hórses as fast as they will go.

во-вторы́х sécondly, in the sécond place.

вогна́ть *сов. см.* вгоня́ть.

во́гнутый concáve.

вод|а́ *ж.* 1. wáter; морска́я ~ séa-water; пре́сная ~ fresh wáter; 2. *см.* во́ды; ◇ чи́стой, чисте́йшей ~ы́ (*о драгоценном камне; тж. перен.*) of the first wáter; толо́чь во́ду в сту́пе, решето́м во́ду носи́ть ≈ beat* the air, mill the wind, cárry wáter in a sieve; вы́йти сухи́м из ~ы́ get* out of it; как в во́ду опу́щенный créstfallen; как (бу́дто) в во́ду гляде́л! he must have sécond sight!; с ви́ду он ~ы́ не замути́т *разг.* ≈ he looks as if bútter wóuldn't melt in his mouth.

водвори́ть(ся) *сов. см.* водворя́ть(ся).

водворя́ть, водвори́ть (*вн.*) 1. séttle (*smb.*), instáll (*smb.*); (*возвращать на прежнее место*) put* (*smth.*) back; send* (*smb., smth.*) back; (*устанавливать*) estáblish (*smth.*). ~ся, водвори́ться 1. instáll *oneself*, estáblish *onesélf*, séttle; 2. (*устанавливаться*) be* estáblished; наконе́ц водвори́лся поря́док órder was at last (re-)estáblished; водвори́лась тишина́ sílence fell.

водеви́ль *м.* vaudeville, músic-hall sketch.

води́тель *м.* dríver. ~ский dríver's; ~ские права́ dríver's licence *sg.*

води́ть *несов.* 1. (*вн.*) lead* (*smb., smth.*), take* (*smb., smth.*); ~ слепо́го lead* a blind man*; ~ сы́на в шко́лу take* *one's* son to school; ~ ребёнка гуля́ть take* a child* out for a walk; ~ в ата́ку lead* in the attáck; 2. (*вн.; управлять автомобилем и т. п.*) drive* (*smth.*); (*самолёт*) fly* (*smth.*). 3. (*тв. по дт.; проводить*) draw* (*smth.* óver), pass (*smth.* óver); ~ смычко́м по стру́нам draw* the bow óver the strings; ~ руко́й по лицу́ pass *one's* hand óver *one's* face; 4. (*вн.; поддерживать знакомство и т. п.*) keep* (*smth.*); keep* up (*smth.*); ~ компа́нию с кем-л. go* abóut with *smb.*; ~ дру́жбу с кем-л. be* friends with *smb.*, keep* up a

friendship with *smb.*; ◇ ~ кого́-л. за́ нос make* a fool of *smb.*, fool *smb.*

води́ться *несов.* 1. (*иметься*) be* found, be*; здесь во́дятся медве́ди there are bears in these parts, bears are to be found here; 2. (с *тв.*) *разг.* (*дружить*) assóciate (with); (*о детях*) play (with); 3. (за *тв.*; *наблюдаться*): за ним во́дится ма́ленькая сла́бость he has one small wéakness; за ним э́то во́дится that's what you may expéct from him; ◇ как во́дится as úsual.

во́дка *ж.* vódka.

во́дник *м.* wáter-transport wórker.

воднолы́жн|ик *м. спорт.* wáter-skíer. ~ый wáter-ski *attr.*; ~ спорт wáter-skíing.

во́дн|ый 1. wáter *attr.*; ~ая прегра́да wáter óbstacle; ~ое простра́нство expánse of wáter; ~ рубе́ж wáter-line; ~ тра́нспорт wáter tránsport; ~ спорт aquátic/wáter sports *pl*; ~ по́ло wáter pólo; ~ая ста́нция wáter-sports céntre; ~ые лы́жи wáter skis; 2. *хим.* áqueous, hýdrous; ~ раство́р áqueous solútion.

водобо́язнь *ж.* hydrophóbia; (*у животных*) rábies.

водово́з *м.* wáter-carrier.

водоворо́т *м.* whírlpool; (*речной, мелкий*) éddy; *перен.* vórtex (*pl* -xes, -tices), máelstrom.

водоём *м.* wáter bódy, réservoir.

водоизмеще́ние *с.* displácement, tónnage; ~м в 800 тонн of eight húndred tons displácement.

водока́чка *ж.* pump-house.

водола́з *м.* 1. díver; 2. (*собака*) Newfóundland (dog). ~ный díving; ~ный костю́м díving suit/dress.

Водоле́й *м.* (*созвездие*) Aquárius, the Wáter-carrier.

водолече́бница *ж.* hydropáthic (estáblishment).

водолече́ние *с.* hydrópathy.

водонапо́рн|ый: ~ая ба́шня wáter-tower.

водонепроница́емый wátertight.

водоотво́д *м.* dráinage sýstem. ~ный drain *attr.*, dráinage *attr.*; ~ный кана́л dráinage caná́l.

водоотта́лкивающ|ий wáter-repéllent; ~ая ткань wáter-repellent fábric.

водопа́д *м.* wáterfall; (*небольшой*) cascáde; cátaract *поэт.*; (*с названием*) falls *pl*, the falls of...

водопла́вающ|ий: ~ая пти́ца aquátic bird; *собир.* aquátic birds *pl*, wáterfowl.

водопо́й *м.* 1. (*место*) wátering-place; 2. (*действие*) wátering.

водопрово́д *м.* wáter-supply; (*в доме*) plúmbing. ~ный: ~ный кран wáter-tap; ~ная магистра́ль wáter-main; ~ная сеть wáter sýstem; ~ная труба́ wáter-pipe. ~чик *м.* plúmber.

водоразде́л *м.* wátershed; divide *амер.*

водоро́д *м. хим.* hýdrogen. ~ный *хим.* hydrógenous; hýdrogen *attr.*; ~ная бо́мба hýdrogen bomb, H-bomb.

во́доросль *ж.* aquátic plant; (*морская*) séaweed; álga (*pl* -ae) *научн.*

водоснабже́ние *с.* wáter-supply.

водосто́к *м.* drain; (*жёлоб*) gútter. ~чный drain *attr.*; ~чная труба́ dráin-pipe.

водохрани́лище *с.* réservoir; (*небольшое*) tank.

водружа́ть, водрузи́ть (*вн.*) eréct (*smth.*); ~ флаг set* up a flag.

водрузи́ть *сов. см.* водружа́ть.

во́ды *мн.* 1. (*водные пространства*) rívers and lakes; 2. (*минеральные*) wáters; пить ~ take* the wáters; 3. (*курорт*) wátering-place *sg*, spa *sg*.

водяни́стый 1. wátery; 2. (*бесцветный*) cólourless, wíshy-wáshy.

водя́нка *ж.* drópsy; hýdropsy *научн.*

водян|о́й I *прил.* wáter *attr.*; (*живущий в воде*) aquátic; ~о́е расте́ние aquátic plant; ~а́я турби́на hydráulic/wáter túrbine; ~о́й знак wátermark; ~о́е отопле́ние hot-wáter héating, céntral héating.

водяно́й II *м. фольк.* wáter-sprite, píxy.

воева́ть *несов.* (с *тв.*) 1. make*/wage war (on), be*

at war (with); 2. *разг.* (*стараться одолеть кого-л.,* *что-л.*) fight* (*smb., smth.*).

воедино togéther; собрáть ~ colléct, gáther up.

военачáльник *м.* mílitary léader, commánder.

вениз|áция *ж.* militarizátion. ~**ировать** *несов. и* *сов.* (*вн.*) mílitarize (*smth.*).

военкомáт *м.* (*военный комиссариáт*) recrúiting--óffice.

воённо-воздýшн|ый áir-force *attr.*; ~**ые сúлы** the Air Fórce(s).

воённо-морск|óй nával; ~**ие сúлы** nával fórces; ~ **флот** Návy.

военнообязанный *м.* pérson líable to mílitary sérvice; (*состоящий в запасе*) resérvist.

военноплённый *м.* prísoner of war.

воённо-полевóй field *attr.*; ~ **суд** court mártial.

военнослýжащий *м.* mílitary man*; sérviceman*.

воённо-экономúческий mílitary and económic; ~ **потенциáл** mílitary and económic poténtial.

воённ|ый *прил.* 1. (*относящийся к войне*) war *attr.*, mártial; ~**ое искýсство** art of war; ~**ое положéние** mártial law; ~**ое врéмя** time of war; ~**ого врéмени** wár--time *attr.*; ~ **завóд** munítion(s) fáctory; ~ **корáбль** mán--of-wár (*pl* men-), wárship; 2. (*относящийся к армии,* *к военнослýжащему*) mílitary; ~**ая слýжба** mílitary sérvice, sérvice in the armed fórces; ~**ое учúлище** mílitary tráining estáblishment; ~ **врач** ármy (áir-force, nával) dóctor, médical ófficer; ~**ая выправка** mílitary/sóldierly béaring; 3. *в знач. сущ. м.* mílitary man*, sérviceman*; ◇ **Воéнный совéт** 1) Mílitary Cóuncil; 2) (*совещание*) cóuncil of war; ~ **коммунúзм** war cómmunism.

воéнщина *ж. собир. презр.* mílitary clíque.

вожáк *м.* 1. léader; (*проводник, поводырь тж.*) guide; 2. (*животное, птица*) léader.

вожáтый *м.* 1. (*пионéрского отряда*) Young Pionéer léader; 2. *разг.* (*вагоновожáтый*) trám-dríver.

вожделéние *с.* lónging, cráving; **смотрéть с ~м на** *кого-л., что-л.* gaze lóngingly at *smb., smth.*

вождь *м.* 1. léader; 2. (*предводитель племени*) chief.

вóжжи *мн.* (*ед.* вожжá *ж.*) rein(s).

воз *м.* 1. cart; 2. (*рд.; количество*) cárt-load (of) (*тж. перен.*); wágon-load (of); ◇ **а ~ и ныне там ≈** things háven't budged an inch; **что с ~у упáло, то пропáло ≈** it's no use crýing óver spilt milk.

возбрáн|яться *несов. уст.* be* forbídden, be* prohíbited; **никомý не ~яется... éveryone is allówed...**

возбудúмость *ж.* excitabílity. ~**ый** éxcitable.

возбудú|тель *м.* 1. cause, stímulus (*pl* -li), stímulant; 2. *биол.* ágent; ~ **болéзни** ágent of a diséase; 3. *тех.* excíter. ~**ть(ся)** *сов. см.* возбуждáть(ся).

возбужд|áть, возбудúть 1. (*вн.; вызывать*) aróuse (*smth.*), stímulate (*smth.*); ~ **аппетúт** stímulate the áppetite; ~ **жáлость, негодовáние** *и т. п.* aróuse compássion, indignátion *etc.*; ~ **любопытство, подозрéние, suspícion; ~ в ком-л. интерéс к** *чему-л.* stímulate *smb.'s* interest in *smth.*; ~ **страсть в** *ком-л.* inspíre *smb.* with pássion; 2. (*вн.; предлагать на* *обсуждéние*) raise (*smth.*); ~ **вопрóс** raise the quéstion; ~ **дéло, иск прóтив** *кого-л.* ínstitute procéedings agáinst *smb.*; ~ **ходáтайство** make* an applicátion; 3. (*вн.; вол-* *новáть*) excíte (*smth.*); 4. (*вн. прóтив рд.; восстанáв-* *ливать*) stir up (*smb.* agáinst), try to put (*smb.* agáinst). ~**áться**, возбудúться 1. awáken, be* aróused; 2. (*волно-* *вáться*) get* excíted. ~**áющий** excíting; ~**áющее срéдст-** **во** stímulant. ~**éние** *с.* 1. (*состояние*) excítement; **в** ~**éнии** in a state of excítement; 2. (*дéйствие*) excitátion; stimulátion; ~**éние дéятельности сéрдца** stimulátion of the áction of the heart.

возбуждённ|ый excíted; ~ **вид** excíted appéarance; ~**ые голосá** excíted vóices; **в** ~**ом состоянии** in a state of excítement, híghly excíted.

возведéние *с.* 1. (*сооружéние*) eréction; 2. *мат.* ráising; ~ **в стéпень** involútion; ~ **в трéтью, пятую стé-** **пень** ráising to the third, fifth pówer.

возвелúчивать, возвелúчить (*вн.*) exált (*smb.,* *smth.*), glórify (*smb., smth.*).

возвелúчить *сов. см.* возвелúчивать.

возвестú *сов. см.* возводúть.

возвестúть *сов. см.* возвещáть.

возвещ|áть, возвестúть (*вн., о пр.*) annóunce (*smth.*), procláim (*smth.*).

возводúть, возвестú (*вн.*) 1. (*сооружáть*) eréct (*smth.*); 2. (*возвышáть*) élevate/promóte (*smb.*) (to the rank of); ~ **кого-л. на престóл** enthróne *smb.*; 3. *мат.* raise (*smth.*); ~ **что-л. в квадрáт** square *smth.*; ~ **что-** **-либо в куб** cube *smth.*; ~ **в четвёртую стéпень** raise to the fourth pówer; 4.: ~ **клеветý на** *кого-л.* calúmniate *smb.*; ~ **обвинéние на** *кого-л.* accúse *smb.*

возврáт *м.* retúrn; (*издержек*) reimbúrsement; *юр.* restitútion; **к прóшлому нет ~а** there's no brínging back the past. ~**úть(ся)** *сов. см.* возвращáть(ся).

возврáт|ный 1. *грам.* refléxive; ~ **глагóл** refléxive verb; ~**ое местоимéние** refléxive prónoun. 2. (*о болéзни*) recúrrent; 3. (*о деньгáх*) repáyable; ~**ая ссýда** loan.

возвращ|áть, возвратúть (*вн.*) 1. (*отдавáть*) retúrn (*smth.*), give* (*smth.*) back; 2. (*вновь обретáть*) recóver (*smth.*); **возвратúть здорóвье** recóver *one's* health; **возвратúть сúлы** regáin *one's* strength; 3. (*спо-* *сóбствовать возвращéнию*) bring* (*smb., smth.*) back, recáll (*smb., smth.*), call (*smb.*) back; ~ **кого-** *-л.* **к жúзни** restóre *smb.* to life. ~**áться**, возвратúться 1. go* back; come* back, retúrn (*тж. перен.*); *сов. тж.* be* back; 2. (*к дт.; к прéжнему, к мысли и т. п.*) go* back (to), retúrn (to), revért (to). ~**éние** *с.* retúrn; ~**éние** **домóй** retúrn (home), hóme-coming.

возвысить *сов. см.* возвышáть 1, 2. ~**ся** *сов. см.* возвышáться.

возвыш|áть, возвысить (*вн.*) 1. raise (*smth.*); (*зна-* *чéние, положéние тж.*) élevate (*smth.*); 2. (*усиливать*) raise (*smth.*); ~ **гóлос** raise *one's* voice; 3. *тк. несов.* (*облагорáживать*) uplíft (*smth.*), élevate (*smth.*). ~**áться,** **возвыситься** 1. *тк. несов.* (*над тв.*) tówer (abóve, óver), rise* high (abóve); *перен.* be* (abóve); 2. (*усили-* *ваться*) rise*; ◇ ~**áться в чьём-л. мнéнии** rise* in *smb.'s* estéem, go* up in *smb.'s* estimátion. ~**éние** *с.* 1. (*дéйствие*) elevátion, éminence, rise; 3. (*сооружéние*) plátform, dáis.

возвышенн|ость *ж.* 1. height, hill; **Валдáйская ~** Váldai Hills *pl*; 2. (*благорóдство*) sublímity; ~ **мыслей,** **чувств** elevátion of thought, féeling. ~**ый** 1. high, élevated; 2. (*о мыслях, чýвствах*) sublíme, lófty, exálted.

возглáвить *сов.* (*вн.*) take* óver the léadership (of), becóme* the léader (of), head (*smth.*); **вы должны ~ это** **дéло** you must take the lead in this mátter, you must take charge.

возглавл|ять *несов.* (*вн.*) lead* (*smth.*), head (*smth.*); ~ **борьбý** lead* the strúggle; ~ **делегáцию** be* the léader of the delegátion, head a delegátion; ~ **учреж-** **дéние** be* at the head of a depártment; ~ **экспедúцию** lead* an expedítion.

вóзглас *м.* cry, exclamátion.

возгорáться, возгорéться kíndle.

возгордúться *сов.* (*тв.*) be* proud (of), grow* proud (of); **get* a swelled head** (óver) *разг.*

возгорéться *сов. см.* возгорáться.

воздавáть, воздáть (*вн.*) rénder (*smth.*); ~ **дóлжное** *кому-л.* give* *smb.* his (her, their) due.

воздáть *сов. см.* воздавáть.

воздвигáть, воздвúгнуть (*вн.*) set* up (*smth.*), put* up (*smth.*), eréct (*smth.*), raise (*smth.*).

воздвúгнуть *сов. см.* воздвигáть.

воздéйствие *с.* ínfluence; **физúческое ~** force,

coércion; оказывать моральное ~ на *кого-л.* bring* móral préssure to bear upón *smb.*

воздействовать *несов. и сов.* (на *вн.*) ínfluence (*smb., smth.*); bring* préssure to bear (upón); ~ на *кого-л.* лаской mánage *smb.* by kíndness; ~ на *кого-л.* силой use force to ínfluence *smb.*; ~ на ход событий ínfluence the course of evénts.

возделать *сов. см.* возделывать.

возделывать, **возделать** (*вн.*) 1. cúltivate (*smth.*), till (*smth.*); 2. (*выращивать*) grow* (*smth.*), cúltivate (*smth.*).

воздержавш|ийся *м.* (*от голосования*): при четырёх ~ихся with four absténtions.

воздержание *с.* (от *рд.*) absténtion (from); ~ от пищи ábstinence.

воздержанн|ость *ж.* abstémiousness, moderátion. ~ый abstémious, témperate.

воздержаться *сов. см.* воздерживаться.

воздерживаться, **воздержаться** (от *рд.*) refráin (from); (*от голосования*) abstáin (from); воздержаться от суждения resérve *one's* júdgement; я советую вам воздержаться от поездки I advíse you to refráin from máking this journey.

воздух *м.* air; в ~е in the air; подышать свежим ~ом get* a breath of (fresh) air; ◇ на (вольном, открытом) ~е in the ópen, out of doors; выйти на ~ go* out for a breath of air.

воздухоплав|ание *с.* aerostátics, ballóoning. ~атель *м.* áeronaut, ballóonist.

воздушно-десантн|ый: ~ые войска áirborne troops; (*парашютисты*) páratroops.

воздушн|ый 1. air *attr.*, áerial; ~ое пространство air space; ~ поток áir cúrrent; ~ое сообщение air sérvice; ~ая трасса áir-route; ~ая яма áir-pocket; 2. (*лёгкий*) aethéreal; ~ое платье aethéreal/góssamery dress; ~ая походка búoyant stride/gait; ~ пирог meríngue; ◇ ~ шар ballóon; ~ые замки cástles in the air; посылать ~ поцелуй blow* a kiss, kiss *one's* hand to.

воззвание *с.* appéal; proclamátion.

воззрение *с.* view; *мн.* views, opínions.

возить *несов.* 1. (*вн.; перевозить*) convéy (*smb., smth.*), transpórt (*smb., smth.*), cárry (*smb., smth.*); (*с указанием места назначения*) take* (*smb., smth.*); (*толкая*) push (*smth.*); (*людей в автомобиле и т. п.*) drive* (*smb.*); 2. (*привозить*) bring* (*smb., smth.*).

возиться *несов.* 1. (*беспокойно ворочаться*) stir réstlessly; (*копошиться — о котёнке и т. п.*) scámper abóut; (*о птице*) hop abóut, flútter abóut; 2. (*шуметь, резвиться*) play, romp; 3. (*с тв.; заниматься*) be* búsy (óver, with); bóther (with), take* tróuble (with); мне некогда с вами ~ I have no time to bóther with you; 4. (*медленно делать что-л.*) fíddle abóut; что ты там так долго возишься? what are you dóing there all this time?

возлагать, **возложить** (*вн.* на *вн.*) 1. lay* (*smth.* on), place (*smth.* on); возложить венок на могилу lay* a wreath on a grave; 2. (*поручать*) charge (*smb.* with); ~ задачу на *кого-л.* assign a míssion/task to *smb.*, entrúst *smb.* with a task/míssion; ~ на *кого-л.* обязанность place a dúty on *smb.*; ◇ ~ надежды на *кого-л.*, на *что-л.* set*/pin *one's* hopes on *smb., smth.*; ~ ответственность на *кого-л.* make* *smb.* respónsible.

возле 1. *нареч.* close, near by; 2. *предлог* (*рд.*) by, near, besíde, next to; ~ меня besíde me, next to me.

возложить *сов. см.* возлагать.

возлюбленная *ж.* belóved, swéetheart; *разг.* (*любовница*) místress.

возлюбленный I *прил.* belóved.

возлюбленный II *м.* belóved, swéetheart; *разг.* (*любовник*) lóver.

возмездие *с.* retribútion; получить ~ get* *one's* desérts, get* what *one* desérves.

возместить *сов. см.* возмещать.

возмещ|ать, **возместить** (*вн. дт.*) cómpensate (*smb.* for); récompense (*smb.* for); ~ *кому-л.* издержки reimbúrse *smb.*, refúnd *smb.'s* expénses; ~ *кому-л.* убытки cómpensate *smb.* for lósses incúrred; ~ потерянное время make* up for lost time. ~ение *с.* compensátion; ~ение издержек reimbúrsement of expénses; ~ение убытков compensátion for lósses; *юр.* dámages *pl.*

возможно 1. *нареч.* (*с нареч. в сравнит. ст.*) as... as póssible; (*с прил. в превосх. ст.*) the... póssible; ~ больше, меньше, лучше *и т. п.* as much, little, well, *etc.*, as póssible; ~ больший, меньший, лучший *и т. п.* the gréatest/lárgest, least/smállest, best, *etc.*, póssible; 2. *в знач. сказ. безл.* it is póssible, it may be; (*очень*) ~! véry líkely!; насколько ~ as far as póssible; если ~ if póssible; 3. *в знач. вводн. сл.* (*вероятно*) póssibly, perháps; он, ~, придёт he may come.

возможное *с.*: сделать всё ~ do* all *one* can; do* éverything in *one's* pówer; сделать всё ~ и невозможное move héaven and earth; leave* no stone untúrned.

возможн|ость *ж.* 1. possibílity; 2. (*удобный случай*) opportúnity, chance; давать, предоставлять *кому-л.* ~ сделать *что-л.* enáble *smb.* to do *smth.*, give* *smb.* a chance to do *smth.*; иметь ~ сделать *что-л.* be* áble to do *smth.*; be* in a posítion to do *smth.*; не иметь ~ости сделать *что-л.* be* únable to do *smth.*; если предстáвится ~ should an opportúnity aríse; предоставляется ~ an opportúnity presénts itsélf; 3. *мн.* (*внутренние силы, ресурсы*) means, resóurces; poténtial *sg.*; материáльные ~ости means; ◇ нет никакой ~ости there is not the fáintest chance; по ~ости, по мере ~ости as far as póssible; при первой ~ости at the first opportúnity. ~ый 1. (*вероятный, допустимый*) póssible, líkely; 2. (*осуществимый*) póssible, féasible; ~ый случай a líkely occásion.

возмужал|ость *ж.* matúrity, mánhood. ~ый matúre, grówn-up.

возмуж|ать *сов.* grow* ínto a man*; он очень ~ал he looks quite grówn-up.

возмутительн|о 1. *нареч.* disgrácefully, outrágeously; ~ вести себя act/behave outrágeously; 2. *в знач. сказ. безл.* it is a scándal, it is scándalous; это ~! disgráceful!, outrágeous!; it's a disgráce!, it's a pérfect scándal! ~ый disgráceful, outrágeous; ~ая несправедливость shócking injústice; ~ое поведение disgráceful/outrágeous behaviour; ~ый случай disgráceful íncident.

возмутить(ся) *сов. см.* возмущать(ся).

возмущ|ать, **возмутить** (*вн.*) rouse *smb.'s* indignátion, óutrage (*smth.*). ~áться, возмутиться be* indignant, be* óutraged. ~ение *с.* indignátion; с ~ением indignantly. ~ённый indígnant.

вознаградить *сов. см.* вознаграждать.

вознагражд|ать, **вознаградить** (*вн.* за *вн.*) rewárd (*smb.* for); ~ *кого-л.* за его услуги rewárd *smb.* for his sérvices. ~ение *с.* rewárd; (*оплата*) remunerátion; денежное ~ение móney rewárd; за небольшое ~ение for a small considerátion.

возненавидеть *сов.* (*вн.*) concéive a hátred (for), begín* to detést (*smb.*).

вознес|ение *с.* 1. ascént; 2. *рел.* Ascénsion (Day). ~тись *сов. см.* возноситься.

возника|ть, **возникнуть** spring* up; (*зарождаться*) aríse*; ~ют новые города new towns are sprínging up; ~ет вопрос the quéstion aríses; у меня возникла мысль (+ *инф.*) I got the idéa (of + -ing), it occúrred to me (+ to *inf*).

возникновение *с.* órigin, rise, beginning(s).

возникнуть *сов. см.* возникать.

возница *м.* dríver.

возноситься, **вознестись** 1. rise; ascénd; 2. *разг.* becóme concéited.

возня *ж. разг.* 1. fuss, a great to-dó; детская ~

children's rómping; ~ мышéй под пóлом the scúffling of mice únder the floor; **2.** (*хлопоты*) tróuble; **3.** *разг.* (*скрытная деятельность, интриги*) machinátions *pl*, pétty intrígue.

возобновить *сов. см.* возобновлять.

возобновлéние *с.* renéwal; (*после перерыва*) recomméncement, resúmption; (*театральной постановки*) revíval; ~ подписки renéwal of subscríption; ~ догóвора renéwal of an agréement/cóntract.

возобновлять, возобновить (*вн.*) renéw (*smth.*); (*после перерыва*) resúme (*smth.*); take* up (*smth.*) *разг.*; (*театральную постановку*) revíve (*smth.*); ~ подписку renéw one's subscríption; ~ договóр renéw an agréement; ~ рабóту resúme work; ~ отношéния resúme relátions.

возомнить *сов.*: ~ о себé have* a high opínion of oneself, think* a lot of oneself; get* a swelled head *разг.*

возраж|áть, возразить (*дт.*) objéct (to), raise objéctions (to); (*докладчику*) replý (to), disagrée (with); éсли вы не ~áете if you have no objéctions; я не ~áю I have no objéctions, I don't mind, I don't objéct (to). **~éние** *с.* objéction; (*ответ*) retórt; без ~éний! no árguing!

возразить *сов. см.* возражáть.

вóзраст *м.* age; одногó ~a the same age; предéльный ~ áge-limit; ◇ выйти из ~a be* óver age.

возрастáние *с.* growth, íncrease.

возрастáть, возрасти grow*, incréase; (*о ценах тж.*) rise.

возрасти *сов. см.* возрастáть.

возрастнóй age *attr.*; ~ состáв age strúcture.

возродить(ся) *сов. см.* возрождáть(ся).

возрожд|áть, возродить (*вн.*) revíve (*smb., smth.*), regénerate (*smb., smth.*); ~ когó-л. к жизни restóre smb. to life, breathe new life ínto smb. **~áться,** возроди́ться revíve, be* regénerated; (*чувствовать прилив новой силы*) be* born agáin *разг.* **~áющийся** revíving, renáscent.

Возрождéние *с.* Renáissance.

возрождéние *с.* regenerátion, rebírth, revíval.

вóзчик *м.* cárter.

возыметь *сов.*: ~ дéйствие work, prodúce the desíred efféct; ~ желáние concéive a desíre; ~ сíлу come* ínto force, take* efféct.

вóин *м.* sóldier, fighting man*; wárrior *поэт.* **~ский** mílitary; ~ский долг the dúty of a sóldier; всеóбщая ~ская обязанность univérsal mílitary sérvice; ~ский устáв ármy regulátions *pl.*

войнственн|ый wárlike, mártial; (*связанный с войной*) aggréssive; bellícose (*тж. перен.*); ~ые племенá wárlike/mártial tribes; ~ое настроéние aggréssive mood; bellícose mood *книжн.*; иметь ~ вид look aggréssive.

войнствующий mílitant.

вой *м.* **1.** howl, hówling, wáiling; ~ вéтра the hówling of the wind; жáлобный ~ píteous wáiling; **2.** *разг.* (*плач*) wáiling, kéening.

вóйл|ок *м.* felt. **~очный** felt *attr.*, félted.

войн|á *ж.* war; (*приёмы ведения войны*) wárfare; манёвренная ~ war of móvement; позициóнная ~ trench wárfare; на ~é in/at the war.

войскá *мн.* (*ед.* вóйско *с.*) troops; (*military*) force *sg.*

войсковóй troop *attr.*

войти *сов. см.* входить.

вокáльн|ый vócal; ~ая пáртия voice (part).

вокзáл *м.* (ráilway) státion; речнóй ~ ríver-boat términal; морскóй ~ sea términal.

вокрýг 1. *нареч.* round, aróund; abóut; ~ всё бы́ло тíхо all aróund was sílence; **2.** *предлог* (*рд.*) (a)róund (*smb.*), aróund (*smth.*); ~ себя́ (all) róund one; ~ гóрода round/aróund the town; ◇ ходить ~ да óколо *погов.* ≈ beat* abóut the bush.

вол *м.* ox*, búllock; ◇ рабóтать как ~ ≈ work like a horse.

волáн 1. (*на платье*) flounce; **2.** (*мячик для игры в бадминтон*) shúttlecock.

волды́рь *м.* (*пузырь*) blíster; (*шишка*) bump, swélling.

волев|óй 1. volítional; of the will *после сущ.*; **2.** (*решительный*) stróng-willed, résolute, detérmined; ~ человéк stróng-willed indivídual; ~ командир detérmined léader; ~óе лицó résolute face.

волейбóл *м.* vólley-ball.

волейболист *м.*, ~ка *ж.* vólley-ball pláyer.

вóлей-невóлей whéther *one* likes it or not, willy-nílly.

волк *м.* wolf*; ◇ морскóй ~ séa-dog; ~ в овéчьей шкýре a wolf* in sheep's clóthing; ~ов боя́ться — в лес не ходить *посл.* ≈ nóthing vénture, nóthing have!; с ~áми жить — по-вóлчьи выть *погов.* ≈ when in Rome do as the Rómans do, who keeps cómpany with the wolf, shall learn to howl.

волкодáв *м.* wólf-hound.

волнá *ж.* wave (*тж. перен.*); (*бурун*) bréaker; нóвая ~ атакýющих fresh wave of attáckers; ~ протéста wave of prótest.

волнéние *с.* **1.** (*движение волн*) rough wáter(s); (*на море*) rough sea; сильное ~ héavy seas *pl*; на Вóлге бывáет сильное ~ the Vólga can be véry rough at times; **2.** (*нервное возбуждение*) (*душевное*) emótion; я слýшал её расскáз с ~м I was moved by her stóry; **3.** *мн.* (*народные*) únrest *sg*, distúrbances.

волнист|ый wávy; (*о ландшафте*) úndulating, rólling; ~ые вóлосы wávy hair *sg*; ~ое желéзо córrugated íron; ~ая линия wávy/úndulating line; ~ая мéстность rólling cóuntry.

волн|овáть, взволновáть (*вн.*) **1.** (*водную повéрхность*) rúffle (*smth.*); **2.** (*беспокоить, тревожить*) upsét* (*smb.*), wórry (*smth.*); ágitate (*smth.*); всё это меня́ óчень ~ýет the whole thing wórries me, I'm áwfully upsét abóut it all. **~овáться, взволновáться 1.** (*о море, озере и т. п.*) be* rough; surge; **2.** (*нервничать*) be*/get* upsét; be*/becóme ágitated; (*о пр.*) *беспокóиться*) be* unéasy (abóut); не ~ýйтесь don't get excíted!, keep calm!, don't you wórry!; онá óчень ~ýется she is térribly wórried, she's áwfully upsét; **3.** *тк. несов.* (*о народных массах*) be* in a férment; нарóд ~ýется there is tróuble bréwing amóng the péople.

волнообрáзн|ый wávy, úndulating; ~ое движéние undulátion.

волнорéз *м.* bréakwater.

волнýющий stírring, excíting; thrílling *разг.*; (*тревожный*) pertúrbing, distúrbing; (*трогательный*) móving.

волокита I *ж.* (*канцелярская*) red tape; bureaucrátic deláys *pl.*

волокита II *м. уст. разг.* (*любитель ухаживать*) ládies' man*.

волокнистый fíbrous; filaméntous.

волокнó *с.* fibre; filament; льнянóе ~ flax fibre/filament; нéрвные волóкна nerve fíbres.

вóлос *м.* hair; *мн. собир.* hair *sg*; белокýрые ~ы fair hair *sg*; шáпка волóс a shock of hair; кóнский ~ hórsehair; ◇ ни на ~ not at all; (*косматый*) shággy; ~нóй capíllary; ~нáя трéщина háirline crack. **~óк** *м.* **1.** hair; **2.** (*пружина*) háirspring; **3.** (*в лампочке*) filament; ◇ быть на ~óк от гибели escápe death by a háirbreadth; на ~óк от смéрти within a háirbreadth of death; висéть на ~кé hang* by a thread. **~янóй** hair *attr.*

волочить *несов.* (*вн.*) **1.** drag (*smth.*); **2.** *тех.* draw* (*smth.*); ◇ он éле волочит нóги he can scárcely put one foot áfter the óther. **~ся** *несов.* **1.** drag, trail; ~ся по землé trail alóng the ground; **2.** (*медленно идти*) drag onesélf alóng; 3. (за тв.) уст. разг. (ухаживать) run* (áfter).

волч|ий wólfish; ~ья стáя pack of wolves; ◇ ~ аппетит vorácious áppetite; ~ья ягода mezéreon.

волчица ж. shé-wolf*.

волчóк м. 1. (игрушка) top; (за)пускáть ~ spin* a top; 2. физ. gýroscope; 3. сад. (побег) súcker.

волчóнок м. wólf-cub.

волшéбн|ик м. magícian, wízard; (колдун) sórcerer. ~ица ж. enchántress; (колдунья) sórceress. ~ый 1. mágic; ~ая пáлочка mágic wand; ~ая скáзка fáiry-tale; ~ое цáрство fáiry-land; 2. (чарующий) mágical, enchánting, bewítching.

волшебств|ó с. 1. mágic, wízardry; как по ~ý as if by mágic; 2. (очарование) mágic, charm, enchántment.

волы́нк|а ж. 1. муз. bágpipes pl; 2. разг. (канитель) (a lot of) bóther; завести ~у cause deláys; тянýть ~у keep* on pútting things off.

вольгóтный разг. free.

вольéр м., вольéра ж. enclósure.

вóльничать несов. разг. take* líberties.

вóльно 1. fréely; ~ обращáться с фáктами take* líberties with the facts; stretch the facts; 2.: ~! (команда) (stand) at ease!; rest! амер.

вольнолюби́вый fréedom-loving.

вольномы́слие с. frée-thought.

вольнонаёмный civílian; ~ врач cóntract súrgeon; ~ служащий civílian employée; ~ состáв emplóyed personnél, enrólled civílian personnél.

вóльн|ость ж. 1. (несдержанность) familiárity, líberty; позволя́ть себé ~ости take* líberties; 2. (отступление от общих правил) líberty; поэти́ческая ~ poétic lícence. ~ый 1. free; 2. тк. кратк. ф. free, at líberty; он вóлен поступи́ть, как ему́ хóчется let him do as he pléases!; 3. (фамильярный) familiar; ~ое поведéние úndúe familiárity; ◇ он ~ая пти́ца he is his own máster; ~ый гóрод free cíty; ~ый перевóд free translátion.

вольт м. эл. volt.

вольтмéтр м. эл. vóltmeter.

вольфрáм м. хим. túngsten.

вóл|я ж. 1. will; воспитáние ~и cultivátion of will-power; исполнить чью-л. ~ю obéy smb.'s will, do* as smb. wíshes; по своéй дóброй ~е of one's free will; сдéлать по своéй ~е do* vóluntarily; не по своéй ~е not of one's own will; прóтив ~и когó-л. agáinst the will of smb.; 2. (свобода) fréedom; líberty; выпускáть когó-л. на ~ю set* smb. free; ◇ давáть ~ю комý-л. let* smb. loose; давáть ~ю воображéнию give* (free) rein to one's fáncy; дать ~ю слезáм let* one's tears flow; давáть ~ю рукáм use one's fists; рукáм ~и не давáй! keep your hands to yoursélf!; ~ вáша just as you please.

вон I нареч. разг. 1. (прочь) out; вы́гнать когó-л. ~ turn smb. out (of); вы́йти ~ leave* (с из в знач. межд.: ~ отсю́да! get out!; ◇ ~ из рук (плóхо) it cóuldn't be worse, (совсéм) из умá ~ clean forgótten.

вон II частица разг. 1. (там) there, óver there; ~ он идёт! that's him!, there he comes!; 2.: ~ вы какóй ýмный! so you're as cléver as all that! ◇ вóн (онó) что! so that's it!

вонзáть, вонзи́ть (вн. в вн.) thrust* (smth. into), plunge (smth. into). ~ся, вонзи́ться go* into, pierce.

вонзи́ть(ся) сов. см. вонзáть(ся).

вон|ь ж. разг. stench, stink. ~ю́чий разг. smélly; stínking груб. ~я́ть несов. (тв.) разг. stink* (of), smell* (of).

воображáем|ый imáginary, imágined, fáncied; ~ая опáсность imáginary dánger.

вообража́|ть, вообрази́ть (вн.) imágine (smth.); ◇ ~ о себé think* a lot of onesélf; вообрази́те (себé)! just fáncy!, ónly fáncy!, try and imágine! ~ение с. imaginátion; э́то однó ~ение! (it's) pure imaginátion!

вообрази́ть сов. см. воображáть.

вообщé 1. in géneral; 2. (совсем) at all; он ~ не пришёл he dídn't come at all, he néver came; ◇ ~ говоря́ génerally spéaking.

воодушев|и́ть(ся) сов. см. воодушевля́ть(ся). ~лéние с. inspirátion; enthúsiasm; без вся́кого ~лéния in a half-héarted way, without enthúsiasm. ~лённый férvent; (вдохновенный) inspíred.

воодушевля́ть, воодушеви́ть (вн.) fill (smb.) with enthúsiasm; (вн. тв.) inspíre (smb. with); ~ когó-л. на пóдвиг inspíre smb. to héroism. ~ся, воодушеви́ться be* inspíred/filled with enthúsiasm.

вооружáть, вооружи́ть 1. (вн.) arm (smb., smth.); 2. (вн. тв.; снабжáть) equíp (smb. with) (тж. перен.); ~ промы́шленность нóвой тéхникой equíp índustry with new machínery; ~ когó-л. знáниями arm/equíp smb. with knówledge; 3. (вн. прóтив рд.; восстанáвливать) set* (smb. agáinst). ~ся, вооружи́ться arm (onesélf) (тж. перен.).

вооружéни|е с. 1. (действие) ármament, árming; 2. (оружие) ármaments pl, arms pl; wéaponry; принимáть, брать чтó-л. на ~ adópt smth. (amóng one's wéapons), add smth. to one's ármoury (тж. перен.); ~й редукция arms; сокращéние ~й redúction of arms; 3. (принадлежности какого-л. устройства) táckle; (парусное) rig.

вооружённ|ый armed; ~ые си́лы armed fórces; ~ отря́д armed detáchment; force; ~ое нападéние armed attáck.

вооружи́ть(ся) сов. см. вооружáть(ся).

вóочию with one's own eyes; (нагля́дно) in reálity; убеди́ться в чём-л. see* smth. for onesélf; see* smth. with one's own eyes; ~ предстáвить себé чтó-л. imágine smth. in reálity.

во-пéрвых first, in the first place.

вопи́ть несов. разг. howl, cry out; (плáкать) wail.

вопию́щ|ий flágrant, gross, crýing; ~ее безобрáзие a disgráce; ~ая несправедли́вость crýing/flágrant/gross injústice; ~ая a crýing shame разг.

воплоти́ть(ся) сов. см. воплощáть(ся).

воплощ|áть, воплоти́ть (вн.) embódy (smth.), incárnate (smth.); ◇ ~ чтó-л. в жизнь put* smth. into práctice; ~ в себé чтó-л. be* the personifi-cátion/embódiment of smth. ~áться, воплоти́ться (в пр.) be* embódied (in), be* incárnated (in). ~éние с. embódi-ment, incarnátion; (олицетворение) personificátion; ~éние в жизнь чего-л. (áctual) realizátion of smth.; он ~éние здорóвья he is the incarnátion/picture of health.

воплощённ|ый incárnate после сущ., persónified после сущ.; ~ое великодýшие the véry soul of magnáimity; он ~ая чéстность he is hónesty itsélf, he is the véry soul of hónesty.

вопль м. howl; (скорбный) wail.

вопреки́ in spite of, despíte; ~ моемý желáнию in defiance of my wish; ~ ожидáниям cóntrary to expectátions; ~ рассýдку in defiance of réason.

вопрóс м. 1. quéstion; 2. (проблема) próblem, íssue; (дело) point, mátter; ~ы языкознáния próblems of linguístics; ~ большóй госудáрственной вáжности a mátter of the útmost impórtance to the State; ~ состои́т в том... the quéstion is...; вот в чём ~ that is the quéstion; э́то ещё ~ it remáins to be seen; ~ы, стоя́щие на повéстке дня points on the agénda; 3. (чего-л.) mátter, point; ~ вréмени mátter of time; ~ чéсти point of hónour; ◇ под (больши́м) ~ом súbject to doubt, problemátic; стáвить чтó-л. под ~ quéstion the necéssity/validity of smth.; ~ жи́зни и́ли смéрти a mátter of life and death.

вопроси́тельн|ый inquíring, interrógative; ~ взгляд inquíring glance; ~ знак quéstion-mark, note of interrogátion; ~ое предложéние грам. quéstion.

вопрóсник м. questionnáire.

вор м. thief*; кармáнный ~ píckpocket.

ворва́ться *сов. см.* врыва́ться.

вори́шка *м.* pílferer, pétty thief*.

воркова́|нье *с.* cóoing. ~ть *несов.* coo; *перен.* bill and coo.

воркотня́ *ж. разг.* grúmbling.

воробе́й *м.* spárrow; ◇ стре́ляный ~ a knówing old bird; ста́рого воробья́ на мяки́не не проведёшь *посл.* an old bird is not to be caught with chaff.

воробьи́ный spárrow's.

воро́в|анный stólen. ~а́тый 1. thíevish, light--fingered; 2. (*опасливый*) fúrtive.

ворова́ть *несов.* steal*.

воро́в|ка́ *ж.* thief*. ~ски́ thíevishly, dishónestly; (*опасливо*) fúrtively; like a thief*. ~ско́й thieves'; ~ско́й язы́к, жарго́н thieves' cant. ~ство́ *с.* stéaling.

во́рон *м.* ráven.

воро́на *ж.* 1. crow; 2. *перен.* gáper, lóafer; Jóhnny--head-in-áir; ◇ ~ в павли́ньих пе́рьях jáckdaw in péacock's féathers; счита́ть воро́н *разг.* gape.

воронёный búrnished.

воро́ний crow's.

воро́нка *ж.* 1. (*для наливания*) fúnnel; 2. (*от взры-ва*) cráter; (*от снаряда тж.*) shéll-hole.

во́ронов ráven's.

вороно́й *прил.* 1. black; 2. *в знач. сущ. м.* black horse.

во́рот I *м.* (*воротник*) cóllar; (*рубашки тж.*) néckband; схвати́ть за́ ~ take* by the scruff of the neck.

во́рот II *м. тех.* windlass.

воро́та *мн.* 1. gate *sg*; в ~х in the gáteway; 2. *спорт.* goal *sg*.

вороти́ла *м. разг.* mágnate, big-búsiness man*; big shot *амер.*

вороти́ть *сов.* (*вн.*) *разг.* call (*smb., smth.*) back, bring* (*smb., smth.*) back; сде́ланного не воро́тишь what's done can't be úndone. ~ся *сов. разг.* come* back.

вороти́|к *м.*, ~чо́к *м.* cóllar.

во́рох *м.* (*прям. и перен.*) heap; ~ новосте́й batch of news.

вороча́ть *несов.* 1. (*вн.; сдвигать*) move (*smth.*), shift (*smth.*); 2. (*перевёртывать*) turn (*smth.*) round; 3. (*тв.*) *разг.* (*управлять*) run* (*smth.*), hándle (*smth.*); ~ дела́ми boss the show. ~ся *несов. разг.* turn; (*в постели*) toss and turn.

вороши́ть, развороши́ть (*вн.*) stir (*smth.*); ~ се́но toss the hay.

ворс *м.* (*ковра, бархата*) pile; (*сукна*) nap.

ворси́нка *ж.* fibre.

ворч|а́ние *с.* (*собаки и т. п.*) gŕowling; 2. *разг.* (*брюзжание*) grúmbling. ~а́ть *несов.* 1. (*о собаке и т. п.*) growl; 2. (*на вн.*) *разг.* (*брюзжать*) grúmble (at, abóut); ~ли́вый quérulous, grúmbling; grúmpy *разг.*; ~ли́вый стари́к quérulous old man*; ~ли́вый тон péevish tone.

ворчу́н *м.*, ворчу́нья *ж.* grúmbler.

восво́яси *разг.:* отпра́виться ~ go* home, take* the hómeward road.

восемнадцатиле́тний 1. ·(*о сроке*) eightéen-year *attr.*; of eightéen years *после сущ*; 2. (*о возрасте*) eighteen-year-óld; of eighteen *после сущ.*

восемна́дца|тый eighténth. ~ть eighteen.

во́семь eight. ~деся́т éighty. ~со́т eight húndred.

воск *м.* wax; ◇ го́рный ~ míneral wax, ozócerite.

воскли́кнуть *сов. см.* восклица́ть.

восклица́|ние *с.* exclamátion. ~тельный excláma-tory; ~тельный знак exclamátion mark/point.

восклица́ть, воскли́кнуть excláim.

воско́вка *ж.* wax(ed)-páper.

воско́в|ой *ж.* wax *attr.*; perfen. wáxen; ~ая бле́дность wáxen pállor; ~ое лицо́ wáxen compléxion/féatures; ◇ ~ая спе́лость, зре́лость gold/wax rípeness.

воскреса́ть, воскре́снуть 1. *рел.* rise*, from the dead,

come* back to life; *перен.* revíve, retúrn to life; 2. (*о чув-ствах и т. п.*) be* revíved; воскре́сли воспомина́ния mémories were revíved.

воскресе́ние *с. рел.* Resurréction; *перен. тж.* revíval.

воскресе́нье *с.* (*день*) Súnday.

воскреси́ть *сов. см.* воскреша́ть.

воскре́снуть *сов. см.* воскреса́ть.

воскре́сный Súnday *attr.*

воскреша́ть, воскреси́ть (*вн.*) 1. *рел.* resurréct (*smb.*), raise (*smb.*) from the dead; bring* (*smb.*) back to life, restóre (*smb.*) to life (*тж. перен.*); 2. (*восстанав-ливать в памяти*) revíve (*smth.*).

воспал|е́ние *с.* inflammátion; ~ брюши́ны peritonítis; ~ кишо́к enterítis; ~ лёгких pneumónia; ~ по́чек nephrítis. ~ённый 1. inflámed; 2. (*разгорячённый*) févered, féverish.

воспаля́ть, воспали́ть *процесс* inflámmatory; inflámmatory prócess. ~и́ться *сов. см.* воспаля́ться.

воспаля́ться, воспали́ться becóme* inflámed.

воспева́ть, воспе́ть (*вн.*) praise (*smb., smth.*), praise (*smb., smth.*) in song; sing* (*smth.*) *поэт.*

воспе́ть *сов. см.* воспева́ть.

воспита́ние *с.* 1. (*действие*) brínging up; (*образова-ние*) educátion; (*подготовка*) tráining; ~ дете́й brínging up children; 2. (*воспитанность*) bréeding, úpbringing.

воспи́танн|ик *м.*, ~ица *ж.* 1. púpil; 2. (*приёмыш*) adópted child*; 3. (*школы*) púpil, stúdent; (*окончивший институт*) gráduate.

воспи́танн|ость *ж.* bréeding. ~ый well-bréd, well bróught-úp (*о мужчине тж.*) géntlemanly; пло́хо ~ый ill-bréd, bádly bróught-úp.

воспита́тель *м.* éducator, tútor. ~ница *ж.* éducator, tútoress; (*в детском саду*) kíndergarten/núrsery-school téacher. ~ный well educátional, éducative; име́ть огро́мное ~ное значе́ние be* of vast educátional impórtance.

воспита́ть(ся) *сов. см.* воспи́тывать(ся).

воспи́тывать, воспита́ть (*вн.*) 1. bring* up (*smb.*), rear (*smb.*); (*давать образование*) éducate (*smb.*); 2. (*формировать чей-л. характер*) train (*smb.*); воспи-та́ть хоро́шего бойца́ train *smb.* to be a good sóldier; 3. (*прививать, внушать какие-л. чувства*) cúltivate (*smth.*); ~ся, воспита́ться be* bróught up.

воспламен|е́ние *с.* 1. cátching fíre, combústion; 2. (*зажигание*) ignítion, sétting fíre (to); температу́ра, то́ч-ка ~е́ния ignítion point. ~и́ть(ся) *сов. см.* воспламе-ня́ть(ся). ~я́емость *ж.* inflammabílity, ~я́емый inflámmable.

воспламеня́ть, воспламени́ть (*вн.*) set* (*smth.*) on fire; *тех.* igníte (*smth.*); *перен.* fíre (*smth.*). ~ся, воспла-мени́ться 1. take/catch* fire; 2. (*тв.; увлекаться ка-кой-л. мыслью и т. п.*) be* fíred with a pássion (for); be* fíred with zeal (for).

воспо́лнить *сов. см.* восполня́ть.

восполня́ть, воспо́лнить (*вн.*) make* good (*smth.*), make* up (for); ~ пробе́л в зна́ниях fill a gap in *one's* knówledge, make* good *one's* knówledge.

воспо́льзоваться *сов.* (*тв.*) 1. (*употребить в свою пользу*) aváil onesélf (of), prófit (by), take* advántage (of); ~ чьей-л. нео́пытностью take* advántage of *smb.'s* inexpérience; ~ чьим-л. приглаше́нием aváil onesélf of *smb.'s* invitátion; (*удобным*) слу́чаем size the opportúnity, aváil onesélf of the opportúnity; 2. (*употре-бить для какой-л. цели*) make* use (of).

воспомина́ние *с.* 1. mémory, recolléction; оста́лось одно́ ~ nóthing but the mémory remáins; 2. *мн.* (*запи-ски*) mémoirs, reminíscences.

воспрети́ть *сов. см.* воспреща́ть.

воспрещ|а́ть, воспрети́ть (*вн.*) prohíbit (*smth.*), forbíd* (*smth.*). ~а́ться *несов.* be* prohíbited; вход ~а́ет-ся no éntrance; кури́ть ~а́ется! no smóking! ~е́ние *с.* prohibítion.

восприи́мчив|ость *ж.* receptívity; (*к впечатлениям,*

болезням) susceptibílity. ~ый recéptive; (*к впечатлени- ям, болезням*) susceptibílity. ~ый recéptive; (*к впечат- лениям, болезням*) suscéptible; ~ый ум recéptive mind.

воспринимáть, **восприня́ть** (*вн.*) percéive (*smth.*), apprehénd (*smth.*), take* (*smth.*), be recéptive (to).

восприня́ть *сов. см.* воспринимáть.

восприя́тие *с.* percéption, apprehénsion.

воспроизведéние *с.* reprodúction.

воспроизвести́ *сов. см.* воспроизводи́ть.

воспроизводи́ть, **воспроизвести́** (*вн.*) reprodúce (*smth.*).

воспроизвóдство *с. эк.* reprodúction; простóе ~ simple reprodúction; расши́ренное ~ exténded reprodúction.

воспроти́виться *сов. см.* проти́виться.

воспря́нуть *сов.* aróuse *oneself*, bestír *onesélf*; ◇ ~ ду́хом take* fresh heart, cheer up.

воссоедин|éние *с.* reúnion. ~и́ть(ся) *сов. см.* воссо- единя́ть(ся).

воссоединя́ть, **воссоедини́ть** (*вн.*) reuníte (*smth.*). ~ся, воссоедини́ться reuníte.

воссоздавáть, **воссоздáть** (*вн.*) re-creáte (*smth.*), recónstitute (*smth.*); ~ о́бразы про́шлого reconstrúct the past.

воссоздáть *сов. см.* воссоздавáть.

восставáть, **восстáть** 1. rise*; revólt; ~ с ору́жием в рукáх rise* in arms; 2. (*про́тив рд.; проти́виться*) revólt (agáinst), oppóse (*smth.*).

восстáвший insúrgent; ~ нарóд insúrgent péople.

восстанáвливать, **восстанови́ть** 1. (*вн.; приводи́ть в прéжнее состоя́ние*) restóre (*smth.*), reconstrúct (*smth.*), rehabílitate (*smth.*); (*постро́йку*) rebuíld* (*smth.*); *перен.* reconstrúct (*smth.*); ~ промы́шленность, хозя́йство restóre/rehabílitate índustry, the ecónomy; ~ первоначáльный текст restóre the origínal text; ~ поло- жéние retríeve the situátion; ~ здорóвье, си́лы recóver *one's* health, strength; ~ дипломати́ческие отношéния resúme diplomátic relátions; reconstrúct the past; ~ кого́-л. в правáх restóre smb. to his, her rights, rehabílitate *smb.*; восстанови́ть кого́-л. в дóлжности réinstate *smb.*; 3. (*вн. про́тив рд.; враж- дéбно настрáивать*) set* (*smb.* agáinst); ~ кого́-л. про́- тив себя́ antágonize *smb.*, álienate *smb.'s* sýmpathies, set* *smb.* agáinst *one*; он всех восстанови́л про́тив себя́ he set éveryone agáinst him. ~ся, восстанови́ться 1. (*прихо- ди́ть в прéжнее состоя́ние*) recóver, be* restóred; (*возо- бновля́ться*) be* resúmed, contínue as befóre; 2. (*в пá- мяти*) recúr, come* back; 3. (*в пр.; в прéжнем общé- ственном положéнии*) be* reinstáted (in).

восстáние *с.* úprising, rísing, rebéllion, insurréction.

восстанови́тельн|ый: ~ перио́д périod of reconstrúction; ~ые рабо́ты restorátion work *sg.*

восстанови́ть(ся) *сов. см.* восстанáвливать(ся).

восстановлéн|ие *с.* restorátion, reconstrúction, rehabilitátion; recóvery; (*постро́йки*) rebuílding; про- грáмма ~ия recóvery prógramme, rehabilitátion plan; ра- бо́ты по ~ию restorátion/rehabilitátion work *sg.*

восстáть *сов. см.* восставáть.

востóк *м.* 1. (*странá свéта*) the east; к ~у (от) east (of); на ~ éastward(s); выходи́ть на ~ look east; на ~е in the east; 2. (В.) (*восто́чные стрáны*) the East; the Órient *книжн.:* Бли́жний Востóк the Míddle East; Дáль- ний Востóк the Far East; Срéдний Востóк the Míddle East.

востоковéд *м.* orientálist. ~éние *с.* oriéntal stúdies/reséarch. ~ческий of oriéntal stúdies *после сущ.,* oriéntal.

востóрг *м.* enthúsiasm; (*восхищéние*) delíght; смот- рéть на кого́-л. с ~ом gaze rápturously at *smb.*; быть в

~е от чего́-л. be* in ráptures óver *smth.*, be* enthusiástic abóut *smth.*, be* delíghted with *smth.*; приводи́ть кого́-л. в ~ delíght *smb.*; приходи́ть в ~ от чего́-л. be* delíghted with *smth.*, be* enthusiástic abóut *smth.*; ~ам нé было концá the enthúsiasm was bóundless. ~áть *несов.* (*вн.*) delíght (*smb.*). ~áться *несов.* (*тв.*) be* enthusiástic (abóut), be* delíghted (with), be* enráptured (with.).

восто́рженн|ость *ж.* 1. (*состоя́ние восто́рга*) enthúsiasm, exaltátion; 2. (*скло́нность к восто́ргу*) effúsiveness, excitabílity. ~ый 1. enthusiástic; ~ая встрéча enthusiástic recéption; 2. (*скло́нный к восто́ргу*) effúsive, exálted; ~ая натýра exálted dispositíon; 3. (*вы- ражáющий восто́рг*) rápturous; ~ая речь effúsive talk, impássioned addréss; ~ый взгляд rápturous glance.

восторжествовáть *сов.* tríumph.

восто́чн|ый 1. éastern*, east; ~ая грани́ца éastern fróntier; ~ вéтер east wind; 2. (*о странах Восто́ка*) oriéntal; ~ые нарóды oriéntal péoples; ~ые обы́чаи oriéntal cústoms; ~ые языки́ oriéntal lánguages; Восто́ч- ная Еврóпа Éastern Éurope.

вострéбован|ие *с.:* до ~ия (*на пи́сьмах*) póste réstante, to be cálled for.

востро́: держáть ýхо ~ be* on the alért, keep* a sharp lóok-óut (for).

восхвали́ть *сов. см.* восхваля́ть.

восхваля́ть, **восхвали́ть** (*вн.*) extól (*smb.*), laud (*smb.*), éulogize (*smb.*).

восхити́|тельный éxquisite, delíghtful. ~ть(ся) *сов. см.* восхищáть(ся).

восхищ|áть, **восхити́ть** (*вн.*) delíght (*smb.*), charm (*smb.*), enrápture (*smb.*). ~áться, восхити́ться (*тв.*) admíre (*smb., smth.*), be* delíghted (with); be* in ráptures (óver). ~éние *с.* admirátion; в ~éнии от чего́-л. in ráptures óver *smth.*; с ~éнием with admirátion.

восхóд *м.* 1. rise, rísing; ~ сóлнца súnrise; ~ луны́ móonrise; 2. (*восхождéние на вéршину горы́*) ascént. ~и́ть, взойти́ 1. rise*, ascénd; 2. *тк. несов.* (к *дт.*; имéть свои́м начáлом) go* back (to). ~я́щий rísing, ascénding; ◇ ~я́щее свети́ло rísing star/génius.

восхождéние *с.* (на *вн.*) ascént (of), scáling (of).

восьмёрка *ж.* 1. (*ци́фра*) an eight; 2. (*фигýра*) fígure-of-éight; 3. (*кáрта*) the eight (of); 4. (*шлю́пка*) éight(-oar boat); 5. *ав.* flight of eight áircraft.

во́сьмеро eight (pérsons); нас ~ there are eight of us.

восьмигрáнн|ик *м.* óctahédron. ~ый óctahédral.

восьмидесяти|лéт|ие *с.* 1. (*перио́д*) éighty years *pl.*; 2. (*годовщи́на*) éightieth annivérsary. ~ний 1. (*о сро́ке*) éighty-year *attr.*; of éighty years *после сущ.*; 2. (*о воз- расте*) éighty-year-óld; of éighty *после сущ.*

восьмидеся́т|ый éightieth; ~ые гóды the éighties.

восьмиклáсс|ник *м.* boy in his éighth year at school, éighth-form boy. ~ица *ж.* girl in her éighth year at school, éighth-form girl.

восьмикрáтный éightfold.

восьмилéтний 1. (*о сро́ке*) éight-year *attr.*; of eight years *после сущ.*; 2. (*о во́зрасте*) éight-year-óld; of eight *после сущ.*; ~ ребёнок child* of eight.

восьмимéсячный 1. (*о сро́ке*) eight months'; éight- -month *attr.*; 2. (*о во́зрасте*) éight-month-óld; of eight months *после сущ.*

восьмисóтый éight-húndredth.

восьмиугóльн|ик *м.* óctagon. ~ый octágonal.

восьмичасовóй 1. éight-hour *attr.*; ~ рабóчий день éight-hour wórking day; 2. *разг.* (*о пóезде, парохóде*) éight-o'clock *attr.*

восьмóй éighth.

вот 1. (*здесь*) here; (*там*) there; *иногда не перево- дится;* ~ вам!, ~, возьми́те! here you are!; ~ вам билéт here's your ticket; ~ и я! here I am!; а ~ и он! and here he is!; ~ они́! here they are!; ~ типи́чный пример... here is a týpical exámple...; 2. (*с мест. и нареч.*) this is, that's; *иногда не перево́дится;* ~ как он живёт that's how he lives; ~ где мы живём this is where we live; ~ чего он хотёл that's what he wánted; ◇ ~ и всё (and) that's all; ~ как? réally?; ~ тáк! and that's that!; вóт (онó) что! so that's it!; ~ так истóрия! what a mess!; ~ так тáк!, ~ тебé páз! well, well!; my, my! *амер.;* ~ ещё! I like that!

вот-вóт *разг.* aný móment; он ~ придёт he'll be here ány mínute now.

воткнýть *сов. см.* втыкáть.

вóтум *м.* vote; ~ довéрия vote of cónfidence; ~ недовéрия vote of no cónfidence, vote of cénsure.

воцарúться *сов. см.* воцаря́ться.

воцар|**я́ться**, воцарúться 1. *(наступать)* reign; воцарúлось молчáние sílence reigned; 2. *уст. (вступать на престол)* ascénd the throne.

вошь *ж.* louse*.

воюющ|**ий** belligerent; ~ие стóроны the belligerents.

воя́ка *м.* fighter; храбрый ~ *ирон.* some sóldier/fighter; ну какóй он ~? he's no sóldier!

впадáть, впасть 1. *тк. несов. (о реке)* flow into; 2. *(становиться впалым)* be* súnken, becóme* hággard; егó глазá, щёки впáли his eyes, cheeks are súnken; 3. *(в вн.)*: доходúть до какого-л. состояния sink* (into), lapse (into); ~ в отчáяние sink* ínto despáir; ◇ ~ в противорéчие invólve onesélf in contradíctions, contradíct onesélf.

впáдина *ж. (в земле)* hóllow, depréssion; *(в стене)* cávity; ◇ глазнáя ~ éyehole, éye-socket.

впáл|**ый** hóllow, súnken; ~ая грудь hóllow/púny chest; ~ые щёки hóllow cheeks; с ~ыми щекáми hóllow-cheeked.

впасть *сов. см.* впадáть 2, 3.

впервы́е for the first time, first.

впереáлку *разг.*: ходúть ~ wáddle.

вперегонки́ *разг.*: бéгать ~ race one anóther.

вперёд *нареч.* 1. fórward; ahéad, ón(ward), шагнýть ~ step fórward; смотрéть ~ look ahéad; put* one's hand out; движéние ~ héadway, advánce, prógress; 2. *разг. (впредь)* in fúture; ~ э́того не дéлай! don't do it agáin!; 3. *(в счёт будущего)* in advánce; заплатúть ~ pay* in advánce; 4.: часы́ идýт ~ the watch is fast; 5. *в знач. межд.* on!; ~ к побéде! ónward to víctory!

впередú 1. *нареч.* in front; ~ шёл оркéстр a band led the way; there was a band in front; 2. *нареч. (в будущем)* у нас ~ мнóго врéмени there's plénty of time; у вас ещё цéлая жизнь ~ all your life is befóre you; 3. *предлог (рд.)* in front of.

вперемéжку altérnately; дубы́ стоя́ли тут ~ с ёлями here oaks álternated with firtrees.

вперемéшку mixed up, in a júmble; кни́ги лежáли на столé ~ с тетрáдями téxtbooks and éxercise-books lay mixed up on the táble.

вперя́ть *сов. см.* вперя́ть.

вперя́ть, вперúть *(вн.)* fix *(smth.)*; ~ взóр(ы) во *что-л.* fix one's gaze on *smth.*

впечатлéние *с.* impréssion; под сúльным ~м чего-л. déeply impréssed by *smth.*; находúться под ~м *чего-л.* be* únable to forgét *smth.*, be* háunted by *smth.*; э́то произвелó на меня́ глубóкое ~ I was déeply impréssed by it; под ~м всегó вúденного únder the ínfluence of what one has seen.

впечатлúтельн|**ость** *ж.* impressionability. ~ый impréssionable.

впивáться, впúться: ~ зубáми во *что-л.* sink* one's teeth ínto *smth.*; ~ кóгтями во *что-л.* dig* its claws ínto *smth.*; колючка впилáсь емý в рýку the thorn had sunk deep ínto his hand; ~ глазáми в *кого-л.* fix one's eyes on *smb.*

вписáть(ся) *сов. см.* впúсывать(ся).

впúсывать, вписáть *(вн.)* 1. insért *(smth.)*, add *(smth.)*; вписáть прóпущенное слóво insért the omítted word; 2. *(делать запись)* énter *(smth.)*; inscríbe *(smth.)*

книжн.; вписáть слáвную страни́цу в истóрию войны́ add a glórious chápter to the hístory of the war; 3. *мат.* inscríbe *(smth.)*. ~ся, вписáться (в *вн.*) blend (with).

впитáть(ся) *сов. см.* впúтывать(ся).

впúтывать, впитáть *(вн.)* absórb *(smth.)*, soak *(smth.)* up; imbíbe *(smth.)* *(тж. перен.)*. ~ся, впитáться soak in.

впúться *сов. см.* впивáться.

впúхивать, впихнýть *(вн.)* *разг.* cram *(smb., smth.)* in, shove *(smb., smth.)* in, push *(smb., smth.)* in.

впихнýть *сов. см.* впúхивать.

вплавь: ~ переправля́ться чéрез рéку swim* acróss a ríver.

вплести́ *сов. см.* вплетáть.

вплетáть, вплести́ *(вн. в вн.)* entwíne *(smth. in)*, thread *(smth. through)*; plait *(smth., ínto)*.

вплотнýю close, clósely; in immédiate cóntact (with); *перен.* in éarnest; подойтú ~ к *кому-л.* come* right up to *smb.*; подойтú ~ к протúвнику *воен.* come* to close quárters with the énemy; подойтú ~ к решéнию вопрóса be* on the verge of sólving a próblem.

вплоть: ~ до right until, up to; *(включая)* éven; ~ до настоя́щей минýты up to this véry mínute.

вповáлку *разг.* side by side; лежáть ~ lie* side by side.

вполгóлоса in an úndertone, in a low voice.

вползáть, вползти́ crawl in, creep* in.

вползти́ *сов. см.* вползáть.

вполнакáла at half préssure; *перен.* half-héartedly.

вполнé pérfectly, quite, fúlly; ~ довóльный pérfectly cóntent; ~ достáточно quite enóugh; ~ заслужúть fúlly/ríchly desérve; ~ заслýженный well-desérved; ~ подхóдит и quite well; не ~ not ábsolutely.

вполоборóта half-túrned; *(о портрете)* half-fáce.

вполови́ну *разг.* half; ~ дешéвле half the price.

вполси́лы half-héartedly.

впопáд *разг.* to the point; отвечáть ~ ánswer véry much to the point.

впопыхáх *(наскоро)* in a húrry, hástily; *(в спешке)* in one's haste; ~ он забы́л кни́гу in his haste he forgót his book.

впорý 1. *нареч. (надлежащего размера)*: быть ~ fit; как раз ~ (it's) an exáct fit; пальтó емý ~ the coat is just the right size for him; 2. *в знач. сказ.* (+ *инф.*) the ónly thing to do is (+ *inf*).

впослéдствии láter; *(с гл. в прош. вр. тж.)* súbsequently.

впотьмáх in the dark.

впрáве: быть ~ (+ *инф.*) have* the right (+ to *inf*); он ~ трéбовать э́то he has a right to demánd it.

впрáвить *сов. см.* вправля́ть.

вправля́ть, впрáвить *(вн.)* set* *(smth.)*.

впрáво to the right; ~ от on the right of; сверну́ть ~ turn to the right.

впредь from now on, in the fúture; hénceforth *книжн.*; ◇ ~ до until, pénding *книжн.*

вприкýску *разг.*: пить чай ~ drink* tea with a small piece of súgar in one's mouth.

вприпры́жку with a hop, skip and a jump; бежáть ~ skip alóng.

вприся́дку squátting.

впритык *разг.* edge to edge; flush.

впрóголодь half-stárved, half-stárving; жить ~ be* half-stárved.

впрок 1. *нареч. (про запас)* in store; заготовля́ть *что-л.* ~ lay* smth. in store; *(о продуктах)* presérve *smth.*, cure *smth.*; 2. *в знач. сказ. (быть в пользу)* be* good (for); емý всё ~ he turns éverything to accóunt; all is grist that comes to his mill; ◇ идти́, пойти́ *кому-л.* ~ bénefit *smb.*, do* *smb.* good.

впросáк *разг.*: попáсть ~ ≈ put* one's foot in it.

впро́чем 1. *союз* but, howéver; **2.** *в знач. вводн. сл.* incidéntally.

впры́скив|ание *с.* injéction. **~ать, впры́снуть** (*вн.*) injéct (*smth.*), give* an injéction (of); впры́снуть больно́му мо́рфий give* the pátient (an injéction of) mórphia.

впры́снуть *сов. см.* впры́скивать.

впряга́ть, впрячь (*вн.*) hárness (*smth.*); ~ ло́шадь hárness a horse; ◇ ~ кого́-л. в рабо́ту *разг.* set* smb. to work. **~ся, впря́чься** hárness onesélf; ◇ ~ся в рабо́ту get* to work.

впрямь *разг.* réally.

впрячь(ся) *сов. см.* впряга́ть(ся).

впуск *м.* admíssion; *тех. тж.* íntake, ínlet. **~а́ть, впусти́ть** (*вн.*) let* (*smb., smth.*) in(to), admít (*smb., smth.*) to/into; не ~а́ть кого́-л. keep* smb. out. **~но́й:** ~но́й кла́пан íntake/ínlet valve; ~на́я труба́ íntake/feed pipe.

впусти́ть *сов. см.* впуска́ть.

впусту́ю in vain, to no púrpose; рабо́тать ~ plough the sand, lábour in vain.

впу́тать(ся) *сов. см.* впу́тывать(ся).

впу́тывать, впу́тать (*вн. в вн.*)- *разг.* invólve (*smb.* in); он впу́тал меня́ в э́то де́ло he got me ínto this mess. **~ся, впу́таться** (*в вн.*) *разг.* be*/becóme* invólved (in); get* mixed up (in); (*вмешиваться*) méddle (in); впу́таться в неприя́тную исто́рию get* mixed up in an unpléasant afáir.

впя́теро five times; ~ бо́льше five times as much; ~ ме́ньше one fifth.

впятеро́м the five of them (us, you); они́ рабо́тали ~ the five of them worked in a group.

в-пя́тых in the fifth place.

враг *м.* énemy; foe *поэт.*

вражд|а́ *ж.* hostílity, énmity; (*личного характера*) animósity; (*длительная*) feud; пита́ть ~у́ к кому́-л. feel* animósity against smb.; они́ пита́ют ~у́ друг к дру́гу there is animósity betwéen them.

враждéбн|ость *ж.* énmity, hostílity; (*личная*) animósity. **~ый** hóstile, inímical; ~ые де́йствия hóstile acts; быть в ~ых отноше́ниях с кем-л. be* on hóstile/bad terms with smb.; ~ый прогре́ссу inímical to prógress.

враждова́ть *несов.* (*с тв.*) have* a feud (with); ~ ме́жду собо́й be* at dággers drawn.

вра́жеский énemy('s), hóstile.

вразби́вку *разг.* at rándom; спра́шивать кого́-л. ~ quéstion smb. at rándom, ask smb. spot quéstions; спра́шивать что́-л. ~ put* quéstions at rándom on smth.

вразбро́д *разг.* hapházardly; (*недружно, несогласованно*) without co-ordinátion, rággedly.

вразва́лку *разг.:* ходи́ть ~ wáddle.

вразре́з cóunter to; идти́ ~ с чем-л. run* cóunter to smth.

вразуми́тельный clear, intélligible.

вразуми́ть *сов. см.* вразумля́ть.

вразумля́ть, вразуми́ть (*вн.*) put* sense (into), make* (*smth.*) lísten to réason.

вра́ки *мн. разг.* (*вздор*) nónsense *sg*, rúbbish *sg*; (*ложь*) lies; a pack of lies *sg*.

враньё *с. разг.* **1.** (*действие*) lýing; **2.** (*ложь*) lies *pl*, a pack of lies.

врасплóх unawáres, by surpríse; заста́ть кого́-л. ~ take* smb. unawáres, take* smb. by surpríse.

врассыпну́ю hélter-skélter; пусти́ться ~ run* hélter-skélter, make* off in different diréctions.

враста́ние *с.* g.rówing in.

враста́ть, врасти́ (*в вн.*) grow* (into); (*оседать*) becóme* embédded (in).

врасти́ *сов. см.* враста́ть.

врастя́жку *разг.* **1.** at full length; **2.:** говори́ть ~ drawl.

врата́рь *м. спорт.* góalkeeper.

врать, совра́ть *разг.* **1.** lie, tell* lies; ври, да знай ме́ру!, ври, да не завира́йся! ≈ you don't expéct me to believe that, do you?; **2.** (*быть неточным*) be* wrong; мои́ часы́ врут my watch is wrong; **3.** (*фальшивить в пении и т. п.*) make* a mistáke, be* out of tune.

врач *м.* dóctor; physícian *книжн.*

враче́бный médical.

враща́тельный rótary, rotátory, gýratory.

враща́|ть *несов.* (*вн.*) revólve (*smth.*), rotáte (*smth.*), turn (*smth.*); ◇ ~ глаза́ми roll one's eyes. **~ся** *несов.* **1.** revólve, rotáte, turn; **2.** (*бывать в обществе*) move, mix; ~ться среди́ молодёжи mix with young péople. **~ние** *с.* rotátion, revolútion, gyrátion.

вред *м.* harm, ínjury; таки́е посту́пки прино́сят большо́й ~ such áctions do great harm; без ~а́ для кого́-либо without détriment/ínjury to smb.; во ~ кому́-л., чему́-л. hármful to smb., smth., to the détriment of smb., smth.; и от э́того не бу́дет ни́какого harm won't do ány harm.

вреди́тель *м.* **1.** *с.-х.* pest; **2.** (*человек*) sabotéur, wrécker. **~ский** sábotaging, wrécking; ~ская де́ятельность sábotage. **~ство** *с.* sábotage, wrécking.

вреди́ть, повреди́ть (*дт.*) harm (*smb., smth.*), ínjure (*smb.*), hurt* (*smb.*), dámage (*smth.*); ~ де́лу harm the cause; ~ здоро́вью dámage the health, be* injúrious to the health; э́то вам не повреди́т it won't hurt you, it will do you no harm.

вре́дн|о 1. *нареч.* injúriously; (*неблагоприятно*) unfávourably; ~ отража́ться на чём-л. reáct unfávourably upón smth., have* a bad* efféct on smth.; **2.** *в знач. сказ.* it is bad*/hármful/injúrious; ~ для здоро́вья bad* for one, bad* for one's health; ему́ ~ кури́ть it is bad* for him to smoke. **~ость** *ж.* harm, hármfulness, injúriousness; ~ость произво́дства unhéalthy condítions of work, work injúrious to the health. **~ый** hármful, injúrious, bad*; deletérious *книжн.*; (*нездоровый*) unhéalthy; ~ый кли́мат unhéalthy clímate; ~ая привы́чка bad* hábit; ~ое произво́дство dángerous trade/índustry; ~ый для здоро́вья bad* for the health.

вре́зать *сов. см.* вреза́ть.

вреза́ть, вре́зать (*вн.*) fit (*smth.*) in.

вре́заться *сов. см.* вреза́ться.

вреза́ться, вре́заться (*в вн.*) **1.** cut* (into), run* (into); ло́дка вре́залась в бе́рег the boat ran ínto the bank, the boat ran up the beach; **2.** (*врываться*) cut* (into), plunge (into); маши́на вре́залась в толпу́ the car tore ínto the crowd; **3.** (*запечатлеваться*) be* imprínted (on), be* engráved (on).

вре́менн|о témporarily, provísionally; ~ исполня́ющий обя́занности дире́ктора ácting diréctor. **~ый** témporary, provísional; ~ая постро́йка témporary strúcture; ~ое прави́тельство provísional góvernment.

вре́м|я *с.* **1.** time; со́лнечное ~ sólar time; промежу́ток ~ени ínterval; ~ лети́т time flies; ~ идёт time goes by, time is pássing; простра́нство и ~ space and time; до настоя́щего ~ени up to the présent; до после́днего ~ени till quite récently; на бу́дущее ~ in fúture, hencefórth; с того́ ~ени since then; в свобо́дное ~ at one's leisure, in one's spare time; у меня́ есть ~ чита́ть I have time to read; в э́то ~ at that time; (*между тем*) méanwhile; in the méanwhile; а в э́то ~ ... méanwhile...; во ~ dúring; во ~ рабо́ты while wórking; за э́то ~ in this périod, since then; за коро́ткое ~ in a véry short time; в то ~ at that/ the time; **2.** (*пора*) time; (*года тж.*) séason; лу́чшее ~ су́ток the best time of the day; вече́рнее ~ évening hours *pl*; у́треннее ~ mórning hours *pl*; ~ жа́твы hárvest time; дождли́вое ~ the ráiny séason; нена́стное ~ bad spell of wéather; **3.** (*эпоха*) time(s), age; дух ~ени the spírit of the age/ times; в на́ше ~ (*о прошлом*) in our day; (*о настоящем*) nówadays, in this day and age; бы́ло ~ когда́... the time was when..., there was a time when...; во ~ена́ Екатери́ны in the days of Cátherine; в те ~ена́ in those days; **4.** *грам.* tense; ◇ в после́днее ~, за послѐднее ~ látely, of late; (в) пѐрвое ~ at first, in the begínning; ~ от ~ени from time to time; в своё ~ 1) (когда-то) at one time; 2) (в извѐстный перио́д жи́зни) in one's day; 3) (своеврѐменно) in due time, when the time comes; всё в своё ~ all in good time; всему́ своё ~ there's a time for éverything; (тепѐрь) ~ this is not the момент; не ~ шути́ть no time for jóking; (тепѐрь) сáмое ~ it's the véry móment, it's just the time; в то же ~ at the same time; со ~енем in due course, in time; всё ~ all the time; во ~ óно at one time; во все ~енá at all times.

времяпрепровождён|ие с. pástime; рáди ~ия to kill time, to pass the time awáy.

вро́вень (с тв.) lével (with), flush (with); ~ с края́ми up to the brim.

вро́де 1. (предлог (рд.) in the náture (of), not únlike; 2. частица разг. sómehow; kind of, sort of; он ~ постарѐл he seems to have aged, he looks ólder sómehow; 3. частица (перед перечислѐнием) such as, like.

врождён|ый innáte, inbórn, congénital, inhérent; ~ая скро́мность inhérent módesty; ~ талáнт inbórn/nátural tálent.

врозь apárt, séparately.

врукопáшную hánd-to-hánd; би́ться, сражáться ~ engáge in hánd-to-hánd fighting.

врун м., **врýнья** ж. разг. fíbber, líar.

вруч|áть, вручи́ть (вн.) hand in (smth.), delíver (smth.); (вн. дт.) hand (smth. to· smb.), delíver (smth. to smb.); (ордена и т. п.) presént (smth. with); юр. serve (smth. on smb.); ~ перен. entrúst (smth. to smb., smb. to smth.); ~ кому́-л. повѐстку в суд serve a súmmons on smb.; ~ прави́тельственные нагрáды presént góvernment awárds; ~ свою́ судьбу́ кому́-л. entrúst one's déstiny to smb. **~ѐние** с. delívery; (ордена) presentátion. **~и́ть** сов. см. вручáть.

вручну́ю by hand.

врывáть, врыть: врыть столбы́ в зѐмлю fix posts in the ground.

врыв|áться, ворвáться (куда-л.) burst* ín(to); вѐтер ~áется в ко́мнату the wind bursts ínto the room.

врыть сов. см. врывáть.

вряд ли it's unlíkely; он ~ придёт he's not líkely to come; он ~ знáет I don't suppóse he knows.

всади́ть сов. см. всáживать.

всáдник м. rider; ло́шадь без ~а ríderless horse.

всáживать, всади́ть (вн.) thrust* (smth.), stick* (smth.); всади́ть пу́лю (в) put* a búllet (in, ínto); всади́ть нож в спи́ну кому́-л. stick* a knife* ínto smb.'s back.

всáсыв|ание с. súction; (впи́тывание) absórption. **~ать, всосáть** (вн.) soak (smth.) up, absórb (smth.); ◇ всосáть что́-л. с молоко́м мáтери imbíbe smth. with one's mother's milk.

все мест. 1. см. весь; 2. в знач. сущ. мн. éveryone sg; éverybody sg; all; все егó знáют éverybody knows him; все соглáсны, что... all are agréed that...; он всех знáет he knows éverybody.

всё I мест. 1. см. весь; 2. в знач. сущ. с. all the, éverything; всё необходи́мое all that is néeded, all the nécessaries/réquisites; всё про́чее all the rest, éverything else; всё, что нáдо all that is required; ~ э́то нам давно́ извѐстно we have known all that for a long time; всё в поря́дке! éverything is all right!; всё! (конец) that's all!; и всё такóе and all that; он всё знáет he knows éverything; э́то ещё не всё and that's not all, there's more to come.

всё II нареч. разг. 1. (всегда, постоянно) álways, all the time; а он всё говори́л да говори́л he went on tálking and tálking; 2. (до сих пор) still; 3. (только, исключи́тельно): э́то всё вы винова́ты it is all your fault, you are the one to blame; 4. в знач. усил. частицы: всё бо́лее и бо́лее more and more; всё ещё still; всё лу́чше

и лу́чше bétter and bétter; всё увели́чиваться be* on the íncrease; он всё стоя́л и смотрѐл he stood there gázing; я всё ду́маю I keep thínking; всё же still; а всё же but all the same.

всевозмо́жн|ый all kinds/sorts of, évery póssible, évery descríption of; ~ые догáдки, предположѐния the most váried speculátions, conjéctures; ~ых цветóв of évery póssible cólour.

всегдá álways; ~ готóв! álways réady!; как ~ as úsual, as éver.

всегдáшний úsual, cústomary.

всего́ 1. нареч. (итого) in all; altogéther; 2. в знач. усил. частицы (лишь) ónly, in all, altogéther; all told; ~ тóлько ónly; ◇ ~-нáвсего ónly, nóthing but; тóлько и ~ and that's all.

всезнáйка м. и ж. разг. know-all.

вселѐние с. installátion; (въезд в квартиру) móving-in.

вселённая ж. úniverse, world.

всели́ть(ся) сов. см. вселя́ть(ся).

вселя́ть, всели́ть (вн. в вн.) 1. (поселять) move (smth. ínto), instáll (smth. in); ~ к себѐ жильцá take* in a lódger; 2. (внушать) inspíre (smb. with); ~ надѐжду instíl hope; ~ подозрѐния, тревóгу aróuse suspícions, alárm; ~ увѐренность instíl cónfidence. **~ся, всели́ться** (в вн.) move (ínto); перен. take* root; в меня́ всели́лось подозрѐние I was assáiled by suspícion.

всемѐри|о in évery póssible way. **~ый** évery kind of, áll-róund; comprehénsive; ~ое содѐйствие évery kind of assístance.

всеми́рно-истори́ческ|ий world-históric; э́то бы́ло ~ое собы́тие it was an evént in world hístory.

всеми́рн|ый world attr., wórld-wíde; ~ое движѐние сторо́нников ми́ра the world peace móvement; ~ конгрѐсс world cóngress.

всемогу́щий áll-pówerful, omnípotent.

всенаро́дн|ый nátional, nátion-wíde; ~ое голосовáние (nátion-wíde) reféréndum; ~ прáздник nátional hóliday.

всѐнощная ж. рел. night sérvice.

всеóбщ|ий univérsal, géneral; ~ая истóрия univérsal/world hístory; ~ая забастóвка, стáчка géneral strike; ~ее избирáтельное прáво univérsal súffrage.

всеобъѐмлющий comprehénsive, áll-embrácing, acróss the board.

всеору́жи|е с.: во ~и wéll-ármed, wéll-prepáred, fúlly equípped; во ~и знáний primed with knówledge.

всепобеждáющий áll-cónquering, éver-victórious.

всеросс│йский Áll-Rússia attr.

всерьёз разг. in éarnest; вы э́то ~? do you réally mean it?; принимáть что́-л. ~ take* smth. sériously.

всеси́льный omnípotent, áll-pówerful.

всесою́зный Áll-Únion attr.

всесторо́нн|е thóroughly, in detáil; comprehénsively; ~ развиты́е лю́ди harmóniously devéloped péople. **~ий** thórough, detáiled; comprehénsive; ~ие знáния comprehénsive knówledge sg; ~ее обсуждѐние thórough/detáiled considerátion.

всё-таки 1. союз for all that, still, nevertheléss, all the same; ~ он мне понрáвился I liked him all the same; 2. частица обычно не переводится; где же ~ я ви́дел э́того человѐка? now where have I seen that man* before?

всеуслы́шание с.: во ~ públicly, for all to hear, from the house-tops.

всецѐло entírely, complétely, whólly; ~ поглощён чем-л. complétely wrapped up in smth.; я был ~ предостáвлен самому́ себѐ I was left entírely to my own devíces; я на егó сторонѐ I thóroughly agrée with him.

всея́дный omnívorous.

вскáкивать, вскочи́ть 1.: вскочи́ть в вагóн leap* ínto the cárriage; ~ на подно́жку swing* on to the fóotboard;

2. (*быстро вставать*) jump up; ~ нá ноги, ~ с мéста jump/spring* to one's feet; ~ с постéли jump out of bed; **3.** *разг.* (*о прыщике и т. п.*) break* out, come* up; у негó на лбу вскочи́ла ши́шка a bump came up on his fórehead.

вскáпывать, вскопáть (*вн.*) dig* (*smth.*).

вскарáбкаться *сов.* (на *вн.*) *разг.* climb (*smth.*); clámber (on to).

вскáрмливать, вскорми́ть (*вн.*) (*животных, птиц*) rear (*smth.*), raise (*smth.*); (*детей*) bring* up (*smb.*), rear (*smb.*), raise (*smb.*).

вскачь at a gállop; пусти́ться ~ break* into a gállop; нести́сь ~ gállop/charge alóng.

вски́дывать, вски́нуть 1. (*вн.* на *вн.*) heave* (*smth.* on to); вски́нуть мешóк нá спину heave* a sack on to one's back; **2.** (*вн.; быстро поднимать*) throw* up (*smth.*); ~ ружьё raise one's gun; ~ гóлову throw* up one's head; ◇ ~ глазá на *кого-л.* look up súddenly at smb.

вски́нуть *сов. см.* вски́дывать.

вскипáть, вскипéть 1. come* to the boil; молокó вскипéло the milk has boiled; **2.** (*о чувстве негодования и т. п.*) flare up; ~ гнéвом fly* into a rage.

вскипéть *сов. см.* вскипáть.

вскипяти́ть *сов. см.* кипяти́ть. ~ся *сов. разг.* flare up.

всклокóченн|ый dishévelled; ~ая бородá mátted beard.

всколыхнýть *сов.* (*вн.*) stir (*smth.*); *перен.* rouse (*smb., smth.*); stímulate (*smb.*) to áction. ~ся *сов.* stir; *перен. тж.* be* aróused.

вскользь cásually; замéтить ~ remárk cásually; коснýться вопрóса ~ touch upón a quéstion in pássing.

вскопáть *сов. см.* вскáпывать.

вскóре soon, shórtly; befóre long.

вскорми́ть *сов. см.* вскáрмливать.

вскочи́ть *сов. см.* вскáкивать.

вскри́кивать, вскри́кнуть scream, shriek; *сов. тж.* give*/útter a cry; вскри́кнуть от стрáха give* a scream of térror, cry out in fright.

вскри́кнуть *сов. см.* вскри́кивать.

вскруж|и́ть *сов.:* ~ *кому-л.* гóлову turn smb.'s head; успéх ~и́л емý гóлову succéss went to his head.

вскрывáть, вскрыть (*вн.*) **1.** ópen (*smth.*); ~ конвéрт, письмó ópen an énvelope, létter; **2.** (*выявлять*) expóse (*smth.*); úncover (*smth.*), revéal (*smth.*); ~ злоупотреблéния expóse abúses; ~ и́стинный харáктер *чего-л.* disclóse the true náture of smth.; **3.** (*анатомировать*) disséct (*smth.*); ~ труп disséct a corpse; **4.** (*разрезать*) lance (*smth.*); ~ нары́в lance an ábscess. ~ся, вскры́ться **1.** (*обнаруживаться*) be* expósed/discóvered; **2.:** рекá вскры́лась the ice is bréaking up on the ríver; **3.** (*о нарыве*) burst*.

вскры́ти|е *с.* **1.** ópening; **2.** (*разоблачение*) expósure; **3.** (*реки*) bréak-up; ждать ~я реки́ wait for the ríver to break up, wait for the ríver to move; **4.** (*трупа*) áutopsy, póst-mórtem (examinátion); **5.** (*нарыва и т. п.*) láncing.

вскры́ть(ся) *сов. см.* вскрывáть(ся).

вслáсть *разг.* to one's heart's contént.

вслед 1. *нареч.* áfter; **2.** *предлог* (*дт.*) behínd; in the wake of; смотрéть ~ *кому-л.* watch smb. go, fóllow smb. with one's eyes; ~ емý раздали́сь угрóзы he was pursúed by threats, threats fóllowed in his wake; ◇ ~ за тем áfter this, next.

вслéдствие (*по причине*) ówing to, on accóunt of; (*в результате*) in cónsequence.

вслепýю *разг.* blíndly; печáтать на маши́нке ~ tóuch-type; дéйствовать ~ move in the dark; игрáть в шáхм. play withóut lóoking at the board.

вслух alóud.

вслýшаться *сов. см.* вслýшиваться.

вслýшиваться, вслýшаться (в *вн.*) lísten (atténtively) (to); ~ в кáждое слóво lísten to évery word, drink* in the words.

всмáтриваться, всмотрéться (в *вн.*) peer (into), scrútinize (*smth.*); *сов. тж.* take* a good look (at); при́стально ~ (*вблизи*) look clósely (at); (*вдаль*) peer (into), gaze (into).

всмотрéться *сов. см.* всмáтриваться.

всмя́тку: яйцó ~ soft-bóiled egg; свари́ть яйцó ~ boil an egg líghtly.

всóвывать, всýнуть (*вн.* в *вн.*) thrust* (*smth.* into), shove (*smth.* into); slip (*smth.* into).

всосáть *сов. см.* всáсывать.

вспáивать, вспои́ть (*вн.*) (*животных, птиц*) rear (*smth.*), raise (*smth.*); (*детей*) bring* up (*smb.*), rear (*smb.*), raise (*smb.*); вспои́ть, вскорми́ть *кого-л. разг.* bring* up smb. with évery care, nurse smb.

вспахáть *сов. см.* вспáхивать.

вспáхивать, вспахáть (*вн.*) plough (*smth.*).

вспáшка *ж.* plóughing.

всплакнýть *сов. разг.* shed* a tear, have* a little weep.

всплеск *м.* splash.

всплёскивать, всплеснýть splash; ◇ всплеснýть рукáми fling* up one's hands.

всплеснýть *сов. см.* всплёскивать.

всплывáть, всплыть come*/rise* to the súrface, emérge; (*о подводной лодке*) súrface; *перен.* (*обнаруживаться*) aríse*, come* up, emérge; come* to light.

всплыть *сов. см.* всплывáть.

вспои́ть *сов. см.* вспáивать.

всполоши́ть *сов.* (*вн.*) *разг.* stártle (*smb., smth.*), rouse (*smb., smth.*). ~ся *сов. разг.* be* stártled, take* alárm.

вспомин|áть, вспóмнить (*вн., о пр.*) remémber (*smb., smth.*), recáll (*smb., smth.*); я дóлго ~áл, но никáк не мог вспóмнить I thought and thought, but I cóuldn't remémber. ~áться, вспóмниться (*дт.*) come* back (to); мне ~áется дéтство my childhood comes back to me.

вспóмнить(ся) *сов. см.* вспоминáть(ся).

вспомогáтельный auxíliary; (*второстепенный*) subsídiary, ancíllary; ◇ ~ глагóл *грам.* auxíliary verb.

вспорхнýть *сов.* take* wing.

вспотéть *сов. см.* потéть 1.

вспры́с|кивать, вспры́снуть (*вн.*) **1.** sprínkle (*smth.*); **2.** *разг.* (*лекарство*) injéct (*smth.*); **3.** *разг.* (*ознаменовывать что-л. выпивкой*) célebrate (*smth.*); вспры́снуть сдéлку wet the bárgain/deal. ~нуть *сов. см.* вспры́скивать.

вспýгивать, вспугнýть (*вн.*) scare (*smb., smth.*) awáy; (*птиц тж.*) flush (*smth.*).

вспугнýть *сов. см.* вспýгивать.

вспыли́ть *сов. разг.* fly* into a témper, flare up.

вспы́льчив|ость *ж.* hot témper, irascibílity; егó всем извéстна he is notórious for his témper. ~ый hót-témpered, iráscible.

вспых|ивать, вспы́хнуть 1. (*быстро загораться*) blaze up; (*о пламени*) flare up; (*о свете*) flash; ~ плáменем burst* into flames; **2.** (*краснеть*) flush; лицó её мгновéнно вспы́хнуло her face grew súddenly pink; **3.** (*внезапно возникать*) break* out; вспы́хнула ссóра a quárrel broke out; a quárrel flared up; **4.** (*раздражаться*) grow* ángry, flare up. ~нуть *сов. см.* вспы́хивать.

вспы́шк|а *ж.* **1.** (*огня*) flash; температýра ~и *тех.* flásh-point; **2.** (*проявление чего-л.*) óutburst; (*эпидемии*) óutbreak; ~ гнéва ángry óutburst, burst of ánger.

вспять báckwards; нельзя́ повернýть колесó истóрии ~ the course of history cánnot be revérsed.

вставáние *с.* rísing; рáннее ~ éarly rísing; почти́ть пáмять ~м stand* in mémory, hónour the decéased by rísing.

вставать, встать 1. (*подниматься*) get* up; rise*; aríse* *поэт.*; ~ из-за стола rise* from the table; ~ с постели get* up; не ~ с постели (*о больном*) be* bédridden; порá ~! time to get up!; 2. (*ногами*) step on to; ~ на ковёр step on to the cárpet; 3. (*о солнце, луне*) rise*; солнце уже встало the sun is up; 4. (*на борьбу и т. п.*) rise*; aríse* *поэт.*; ~ на защиту отечества spring*/rise* to the defénce of one's cóuntry; 5. (*возникать*) arise*, come* up; ~ перед глазами come* into sight; (*о прошлом*) come* back; встал вопрос о деньгах the quéstion of móney came up; 6. *разг.* (*останавливаться*) stop; ◇ ~ на путь *чего-л.* énter the path of smth.; встать на чью-л. стóрону take* smb.'s side, side with smb.; встать поперёк доróги *кому-л.* balk smb., stand* in smb.'s way; не вставая without a break.

вставить *сов. см.* вставлять.

встáвка *ж.* 1. insértion; móunting; 2. (*у платья*) ínset.

вставлять, вставить (*вн.*) put* (smth.) in(to); *тех.* insért (smth.); (*вделывать*) fit (smth.); ~ стёкла put* in window-panes; ~ что-л. в опрáву mount smth., set* smth.; ~ что-л. в раму frame smth.; ~ зуб get* a false tooth* made; ~ замечáние put* in a remárk.

встав|ой detáchable; (*о зубах*) false, artificial; ~ые рамы dóuble window-frames, storm windows.

встарь in the old days, in ólden days/times.

встать *сов. см.* вставáть.

встревóженный alármed, distúrbed.

встревóжить *сов. см.* тревóжить 1. ~ся *сов. см.* тревóжиться.

встрёпанный dishévelled, tóusled; ◇ вскочить как ~ ≈ jump like a shot.

встрепенýться *сов.* 1. start; (*о птице*) ópen/spread* its wings; 2. (*оживиться*) rouse onesélf; 3. (*о сердце*) begín* to throb.

встрéтить(ся) *сов. см.* встречáть(ся).

встрéч|а *ж.* 1. méeting; (*на фестивале и т. п.*) gét-together; 2. (*приём*) wélcome, recéption; устрóить торжéственную ~у arránge a grand recéption; 3. *спорт.* match; (*по лёгкой атлéтике тж.*) méeting; meet *амер.*; ~ Нóвого гóда New-Yéar('s) párty.

встреч|áть, встрéтить (*вн.*) 1. (*прям. и перен.*) meet* (smb., smth.), encóunter (smb., smth.); случáйно встрéтить *кого-л.* come* acróss smb., háppen to meet smb.; встрéтить поддéржку recéive suppórt; встрéтить отпóр encóunter stiff resístance; 2. (*принимáть*) recéive (smb.); (*приветствовать*) greet (smb.), wélcome (smb.); ~ гостéй recéive/greet one's guests; ~ делегáцию recéive/greet/wélcome a delegátion; ~ аплодисмéнтами greet with appláuse; ◇ ~ Нóвый год see* the New Year in, célebrate the New Year. ~áться, встрéтиться 1. meet*; рéдко ~áться с *кем-л.* meet* smb. séldom; чáсто ~áться с *кем-л.* meet* smb. fréquently; 2. (*попадáться*) be* found; turn up, occúr; такúе ошибки чáсто ~áются that kind of mistáke óften occúrs.

встрéчн|ый *прил.* 1. appróaching, óncoming; ~ пóезд train trávelling in the ópposite diréction, appróaching/óncoming train; ~ вéтер cóntrary wind, head wind; 2. (*ответный*) recíprocal; ~ое обязáтельство recíprocal undertáking; ~ план supplementary plan (propósed by the wórkers themsélves); ~ бой encóunter báttle; ~ое обвинéние *юр.* cóunter-charge; 3. *в знач. сущ. м.:* кáждый ~ и попéречный ánybody and éverybody; the firstcomer.

встрáска *ж. разг.* sháke-up, sháking; это былá хорóшая ~ it was a héalthy jolt/shock.

встрáхивать, встряхнýть (*вн.*) shake* (smth.); jolt (smth.); *перен.* shake* (smth.) up; встряхнýть кудрями shake* one's curls; нас сúльно встряхнýло we got a sevére jolt. ~ся, встряхнýться shake* onesélf; встряхнúсь!, встряхнúтесь! cheer up!, pull yoursélf togéther!; вам нýжно встряхнýться what you need is a change.

встряхнýть(ся) *сов. см.* встрáхивать(ся).

вступáть, вступить (в *вн.*) 1. énter (smth.); ~ в гóрод énter a town; 2. (*поступáть, зачисляться*) join (smth.); ~ в пáртию, в профсоюз join the Párty, a trade únion; 3. (*начинáть*) énter (into), begín*; ~ в борьбý take* up the strúggle; ~ в переговóры énter into/upón negotiátions; ~ в разговóр énter into conversátion; ~ в спор take* up an árgument; ~ в бой с *кем-л.* engáge in báttle with smb.; ~ в дрáку start fighting; ~ в соглашéние, союз énter into an agréement, alliance; ~ во владéние come* into posséssion; ◇ ~ на престóл ascénd the throne; вступить в брак márry; вступить в свой правá come* into one's own; зимá вступила в свой правá winter came into its own; ~ на путь *чего-л.* take* the road of smth., embárk on smth. ~ся, вступиться (за *вн.*) intercéde (for), take* smb.'s part; stand*/stick* up (for) *разг.*

вступúтельн|ый 1. (*вводный*) introdúctory, ópening; ~ое слóво ópening addréss; 2. (*связанный с поступлéнием куда-л.*) éntrance *attr.*; ~ взнос éntrance fee; ~ экзáмен éntrance examinátion.

вступúть(ся) *сов. см.* вступáть(ся).

вступлéние *с.* 1. (*действие*) éntry; ~ войск в гóрод éntry of troops into a town; ~ в пáртию jóining the Párty; 2. (*введéние*) introdúction; *муз. тж.* prélude; (*увертюра*) óverture; ~ к поэме introdúction to the póem.

всýнуть *сов. см.* всóвывать.

всухомятку *разг.:* питáться ~ live on snacks, live on dry rátions.

всухýю without scóring a point; сыгрáть ~ make* no score; score a duck *разг.*

всучить *сов.* (*вн. дт.*) *разг.* foist (smth. on), fob off (smth. on), palm off (smth. on).

всхлúп|нуть *сов.* give* a sob. ~ывание *с.* sóbbing.

всхлúпывать *несов.* sob.

всходить, взойти 1. (*на вн.*) climb (smth.), mount (smth.), ascénd (smth.); 2. (*о солнце, луне*) rise*; 3. (*о семенах*) sprout, come* up.

всхóды *мн.* shoots; дрýжные ~ vígorous young growth *sg*; зазеленéли ~ the corn is green.

всхóжесть *ж. с.-х.* gérminating pówer.

всыпáть *сов.* 1. *см.* всыпáть; 2. (*дт.*) *разг.* make* it hot (for), warm (smb.).

всыпáть, всыпать (*вн., рд. в вн.*) pour (smth. into).

всюду éverywhere; (*где угóдно*) ánywhere.

вся *мест. см.* весь.

всяк|ий *мест.* 1. (*любой*) ány; (*каждый*) évery, each; ~ раз, как whenéver; во ~ое врéмя at ány time; 2. (*разный*) all sorts of; ~е люди all sorts of péople; ~е товáры all sorts of things; 3. (*какой-л.*) ány; без ~ого сожалéния without ány regrét, with no regrét whatsoéver; 4. *в знач. сущ. м.* (*любой*) ányone; (*каждый*) éveryone; ◇ во ~ом слýчае in ány case, whatéver háppens; at ány rate; на ~ слýчай in case; to be on the safe side; as a sáfeguard.

всячеcк|и *разг.* in évery way. ~ий *разг.* all sorts of.

всячина *ж.:* всякая ~ all sorts of odds and ends, all sorts of things.

втáйне in sécret, sécretly.

втáлкивать, втолкнýть (*вн.*) push (smth.) in, shove (smth.) in; (*вн. в вн.*) push (smth. into), shove (smth. into).

втáптывать, втоптáть (*вн. в вн.*) trámple (smth. into); ◇ втоптáть *кого-л.* в грязь trámple smb. underfóot, ride* roughshod óver smb.

втáскивать, втащить 1. (*вн.*) pull (smth.) in, drag (smth.) in; (*вн. в вн.*) pull (smth. into), drag (smth. into); 2. (*вн. наверх*) pull (smth., smth.) up, drag (smth., smth.) up; втащить чемодáн на трéтий этáж drag a case up to the sécond floor.

втащить *сов. см.* втáскивать.

втерéть(ся) *сов. см.* втирáть(ся).

втира́ть, втере́ть (*вн.*) rub (*smth.*) in; (*вн. в вн.*) rub (*smth.* ínto); ◇ ~ очки́ кому́-л. ≈ throw* dust in *smb.'s* eyes. ~ся, втере́ться 1. (*впитываться*) rub in, pénetrate; 2. (*в вн.*) *разг.* (*протискиваться*) make* *one's* way (ínto); *перен.* worm onesélf (ínto); ~ся в компа́нию insínuate onesélf, get* onesélf accépted; ~ся в дове́рие к кому́-л. worm onesélf ínto *smb.'s* cónfidence.

вти́скивать, вти́снуть (*вн. в вн.*) squeeze (*smth.* ínto). ~ся, вти́снуться (*в вн.*) squeeze onesélf (ínto).

вти́снуть(ся) *сов. см.* вти́скивать(ся).

втихомо́лку *разг.* on the quíet, on the sly.

втолкну́ть *сов. см.* вта́лкивать.

втолкова́ть *сов. см.* втолко́вывать.

втолко́вывать, втолкова́ть (*вн. дт.*) *разг.* make* (*smb.*) understánd (*smth.*); ника́к э́того ему́ не втолку́ешь you símply can't get it ínto his head.

втопта́ть *сов. см.* вта́птывать.

вторга́ться, вто́ргнуться (*в вн.*) inváde (*smth.*); *перен.* intrúde (upón, ínto); ~ в страну́ inváde a cóuntry; ~ в чужи́е дела́ intrúde into *smb.'s* affáirs; ~ в чужу́ю о́бласть, сфе́ру tréspass upón sómebody élse's ground.

вто́ргнуться *сов. см.* вторга́ться.

вторже́ние *с.* (*в вн.*) invásion (of); encróachment (upón); *перен.* intrúsion (upón, ínto).

вто́рить *несов.* 1. (*дт.; повторять*) écho (*smb.*, *smth.*); ~ кому́-л., ~ чьи́м-л. слова́м écho *smb.'s* words; 2. *муз.* take* the sécond part.

вто́ричн|о agáin, a sécond time. ~ый 1. (*повторный*) sécond; ~ое напомина́ние sécond remínder; 2. (*производный*) sécondary; ~ый проду́кт bý-product; ~ые го́рные поро́ды Mesozóic/sécondary rocks.

вто́рник *м.* Túesday.

второго́дник *м.* púpil remáining in the same class for anóther year.

втор|о́й *прил.* 1. sécond; (*после имени*) the sécond; 2. (*второстепенный*) sécondary; (*хуже по качеству*) sécond; на ~о́м пла́не in the báckground; ~ сорт sécond grade/quálity; каю́та ~о́го кла́сса sécond-class cábin; ~ соста́в *театр.* únderstudies *pl*; 3. *в знач. сущ. ж.*: одна́ ~а́я one half, a half; 4. *в знач. сущ. с.* (*блюдо*) sécond course; ◇ ~а́я мо́лодость sécond youth; из ~ы́х рук at sécond hand.

второку́рсни|к *м.*, ~ца *ж.* sécond-year stúdent; sóphomore *амер.*

второпя́х hástily; ~ я забы́л... in my húrry I forgót...

второразря́дный sécond-gráde; of the sécond grade *после сущ.*; *разг.* (*посредственный*) sécond-ráte.

второсо́ртн|ый sécond-gráde; of the sécond grade *после сущ.*; *разг.* (*посредственный*) sécond-ráte; ~ая мука́ sécond-grade flour.

второстепе́нн|ый sécondary; of mínor impórtance *после сущ.*; ◇ ~ые чле́ны предложе́ния *грам.* sécondary parts of a séntence.

в-тре́тьих in the third place, thírdly.

втри́дорога *разг.*: плати́ть ~ pay* through the nose.

втро́е three times, thréefold; ~ бо́льше three times as much; ~ ме́ньше a third of; сложи́ть ~ fold in three; увели́чить ~ incréase thréefold; уме́ньшить ~ redúce to a third.

втроём the three of them (us, you); они́ сде́лали э́то ~ the three of them did/made it togéther.

втро́йне three times as much.

вту́лка *ж.* 1. bush, búshing, sleeve; 2. (*пробка*) bung, plug, stópper.

втыка́ть, воткну́ть (*вн. в вн.*) thrust* (*smth.* ínto), drive* (*smth.* ínto); (*булавку и т. п.*) stick* (*smth.* ínto).

втя́гивать, втяну́ть 1. (*вн.*) draw* (*smb.*, *smth.*) in; (*поднимать*) draw* / pull (*smth.*) up; 2. (*вн.; вбирать в себя*) breathe (*smth.*) in, take* in, draw* in, inhále; 3. (*вн. в вн.*) *разг.* (*привлекать к участию*) draw* (*smb.* ínto), get* (*smb.*) invólved (in), invólve (*smb.* in); втяну́ть кого́-л. в разгово́р draw* *smb.* ínto

conversátion; втяну́ть кого́-л. в рабо́ту get* *smb.* to join in the work; втяну́ть кого́-л. в войну́ invólve *smb.* in war. ~ся, втяну́ться 1. (*в вн.; постепенно входить куда-л.*) drift (ínto); 2. (*в вн.*) becóme* invólved (in), be* drawn (ínto); (*привыкать*) get* used to (*smth.*); (*в рабо́ту*) get* ínto *one's* stride; 3.: его́ щёки втяну́лись his cheeks are drawn in, he looks hóllow-chéeked.

втяну́ть(ся) *сов. см.* втя́гивать(ся).

вуа́ль *ж.* 1. veil; 2. *фото* fog, haze.

вуз *м.* (*высшее учебное заведе́ние*) institútion of hígher educátion/léarning, hígher school, cóllege.

ву́зовск|ий cóllege *attr.*; ~ая програ́мма cóllege sýllabus/prógramme.

вулка́н *м.* volcáno.

вулканизи́ровать *несов. и сов.* (*вн.*) *тех.* vúlcanize (*smth.*).

вулкани́ческ|ий volcánic; ~ого происхожде́ния of volcánic órigin, ígneous.

вульгариз|а́тор *м.* vúlgarizer. ~а́ция *ж.* óver-simplificátion, vulgarizátion.

вульгаризи́ровать *несов. и сов.* (*вн.*) vúlgarize (*smth.*), óver-símplify (*smth.*).

вульга́рн|ость *ж.* vulgárity. ~ый vúlgar.

вундерки́нд *м.* ínfant pródigy.

вход *м.* 1. (*вступле́ние, вхожде́ние*) éntry; ~ беспла́тный admíssion free; ~а нет no éntrance; 2. (*дверь, воро́та*) éntrance, way in.

входи́ть, войти́ 1. go* in, come* in, énter, get* in; (*в вн.*) go* (ínto), come* (ínto), énter (*smth.*), get* (ínto); он вошёл he came in; войди́те! come in!; ~ в порт steam/sail ínto port; ~ в ваго́н get* ínto a cárriage; 2. (*в соста́в, в до́лю и т. п.*) be* in; войти́ в спи́сок be* on the list; войти́ в соста́в прави́тельства be* in the góvernment, becóme* a mémber of the góvernment; 3. (*быть составно́й ча́стью чего-л.*) be* included in; расска́зы, воше́дшие в э́тот том the stóries inclúded in this vólume; 4. (*вмеща́ться*) go* in; э́то сюда́ не войдёт it won't go in here; 5. (*вника́ть*) get* to the bóttom of; войти́ в суть де́ла get* to the heart of the mátter; ◇ ~ в мо́ду come* ínto fáshion; войти́ в исто́рию go* down in history, make* history; ~ в положе́ние understánd* the position; ~ в погово́рку becóme* a býword; ~ в привы́чку (у) becóme* a hábit (with); (*про́чно*) ~ в произво́дственную пра́ктику becóme* an íntegral part of indústrial techníque.

входн|о́й éntrance *attr.*; ~а́я дверь éntrance; ~ биле́т éntrance tícket/card; ~а́я пла́та admíssion (fee), charge for admíttance.

входя́щая *ж.* (*бума́га*) íncoming mail.

вхо́жий *разг.* accépted; он вхож к ним, он вхож в их дом he is an accépted guest in their fámily.

вцепи́ться *сов. см.* вцепля́ться.

вцепля́ться, вцепи́ться (*вн.*) seize (*smth.*), clutch (*smth.*); ~ в во́лосы кому́-л. seize *smb.* by the hair.

вчера́ *нареч.* 1. yésterday; ~ ве́чером last night, yésterday évening; ~ но́чью last night; ~ у́тром yésterday mórning; 2. *в знач. сущ. с. нескл.* yésterday. ~шний yésterday's; ~шний день yésterday; жить ~шним днём live on yésterdays, live in the past.

вчерне́ in (the) rough; ~ зако́нчить *что-л.* fínish the rough draft of *smth.*; гото́вый ~ básically compléte.

вче́тверо four times, fóurfold; ~ бо́льше four times as much; ~ ме́ньше a quárter, redúced to a quárter; увели́чить ~ incréase fóurfold; уме́ньшить ~ quárter, redúce to a quárter.

вчетверо́м the four of them (us, you).

в-четвёртых in the fourth place, fóurthly.

вчи́тываться, вчита́ться (*в вн.*) read* (*smth.*) cárefully; (*осва́иваться с чем-л.*) make* onesélf thóroughly famíliar (with).

вчита́ться *сов. см.* вчи́тываться.

вшива́ть, вшить (*вн.*) sew* (*smth.*) in.

вширь in breadth.

вшить *сов. см.* вшивать.

въедаться, въесться (в *вн.*) 1. (*вонзаться*) bite* (into); 2. (*впитываться*) eat* (into).

въезд *м.* 1. (*действие*) entry; ~ запрещён no entry; 2. (*место*) entrance; (*дорога*) drive(way). ~ной: ~ная виза entry visa; ~ные ворота entrance gate *sg.*

въезжать, въехать 1. drive* in, enter; (*в квартиру*) move in; (*в вн.*) drive* (into), enter (smth.); (*в квартиру и т. п.*) move (into); ~ в дом, квартиру move into a house, flat; 2. (*на вн.*) drive* up (smth.); ~ на гору drive* up a hill.

въесться *сов. см.* въедаться.

въехать *сов. см.* въезжать.

вы *личн. мест.* (*рд.* вас, *дт.* вам, *вн.* вас, *тв.* вами, *пр.* о вас) you.

выбалтывать, выболтать (*вн.*) *разг.* blurt out (smth.); ~ секрет let*/blurt out a secret; let* the cat out of the bag *идиом.*

выбегать, выбежать run* out, come* running out; ~ навстречу кому-л. run* out to meet *smth.*; ~ из дома run* out of the house.

выбежать *сов. см.* выбегать.

выбелить *сов. см.* белить 2.

выбивать, выбить (*вн.*) 1. knock (smb., smth.) out; (*противника тж.*) dislodge (smb.); 2. (*штампом*) stamp (smth.); 3. *разг.* (*ударяя, очищая*) beat* (smth.); ~ ковёр beat* a carpet; ~ трубку knock out one's pipe; 4. (*уничтожать градом*) beat* (smth.) down; 5. (*молотком придавать новую форму*) hammer (smth.) out; ◇ выбить дорогу break* up a road, knock a road to pieces; ~ дурь из кого-л. *разг.* knock the nonsense out of smb. ~ся, выбиться; ~ся из сил strain every nerve/muscle; выбиться из сил be* at the end of one's tether; be* dead-beat; ~ся на дорогу get* on one's feet; make* good; её волосы выбились из-под шляпы, косынки her hair was showing from under her hat, kerchief.

выбир|ать, выбрать (*вн.*) 1. choose* (smth.), select (smth.), pick (smth.); (*отбирать*) sort (smth.); *сов. тж.* make* one's choice; ~айте по вкусу choose what you like; 2. (*голосованием*) elect (smth.); 3.: ~ снасть take*/haul in the nets; ~ якорь weigh anchor; 4. *разг.* (*освобождать для чего-л.*) find* (smth.); ~ время find* time; выбрать удобную минуту choose* a favourable opportunity.

выбир|аться, выбраться *разг.* 1. (*из рд.*) find* one's way out (of); мы долго ~ались из леса it took us a long time to find our way out of the forest; мы наконец выбрались из леса at last we got/were out of the forest; 2. (*выселяться*): ~ из квартиры move out of a flat; 3. (*отыскиваться — о времени*) be* available/free; если выберется свободный час, приезжайте к нам come and see us if you have an hour to spare; я не могу выбраться в театр I have no time to go out to the theatre.

выбить(ся) *сов. см.* выбивать(ся).

выбоин|а *ж.* hole, scar; (*на дороге*) pot-hole; здание было всё в ~ах the building was badly scarred.

выболтать *сов. см.* выбалтывать.

выбор *м.* choice; (*ассортимент тж.*) selection; (*право замены*) option; сделать хороший ~ make* a good* choice; нет никакого ~а there is no choice; нет другого ~а there is no choice/alternative; остановить свой ~ на чём-л. choose* smth., select smth.; ◇ предложить на ~ offer the choice; без ~а indiscriminately.

выборка *ж.* 1. (*сети и т. п.*) raising; (*цитат*) excerpting; 2. *обыкн. мн.* (*из рд.; выписки из чего-л.*) excerpts (from), extracts (from), selections (from).

выборн|ость *ж.* electiveness. ~ый *прил.* 1. elective; ~ая должность elective office; ~ый судья elected judge; 2. (*относящийся к выборам*) election *attr.*, electoral; 3. *в знач. сущ. м.* delegate.

выборочн|ый selective; ~ая рубка леса selective felling.

выборщик *м.* elector.

выборы *мн.* election *sg*; всеобщие ~ general election; дополнительные ~ by-election *sg.*

выбрасывать, выбросить (*вн.*) 1. throw* (smth.) away; (*одежду тж.*) discard (smth.); *перен. разг.* (*выпускать, исключать*) omit (smth.), leave* (smth.) out, exclude (smth.); (*тратить попусту*) throw* away (smth.), waste (smth.); выбросить на берег cast* ashore; 2. (*выдвигать резким движением*) throw* out (smth.), fling* out (smth.), make* a lunge (with); выбросить флаг hoist a flag; *мор.* break* a flag; 3. (*высылать вперёд*) send* (smth., smb.) out ahead; ◇ выбросить что-л. из головы get* smth. out of one's head; выбросить лозунг put* out a slogan; ~ кого-л. на улицу (*выгонять*) turn smb. out into the street, make* smb. homeless; выбросить с работы fire smb., throw* smb. out of work; ~ что-л. на рынок release smth. for sale, put* smth. on the market. ~ся, выброситься 1. throw* oneself out; (*с парашютом*) bale out; 2. (*о дыме, пламени и т. п.*) gush out.

выбрать *сов. см.* выбирать.

выбраться *сов. см.* выбираться.

выбривать, выбрить (*вн.*) shave* (smth.); выбрить себе голову have* one's head shaved. ~ся, выбриться shave*; чисто выбриться have* a close shave.

выбрить(ся) *сов. см.* выбривать(ся).

выбросить(ся) *сов. см.* выбрасывать(ся).

выброшенн|ый wasted; ~ые деньги money wasted; money down the drain *разг.*

выбывать, выбыть leave*; выбыть из школы leave* school; выбыть из игры retire, leave* the field; ◇ выбыть из строя be* put out of action.

выбыть *сов. см.* выбывать.

вываливать, вывалить (*вн.*) *разг.* dump (smth.), shoot* (smth.); ~ уголь из тачки empty/shoot* coal out of a barrow. ~ся, вывалиться (*из рд.*) *разг.* fall* out (of), tumble out (of).

вывалить(ся) *сов. см.* вываливать(ся).

вывалять(ся) *сов. см.* валять 1.

вываривать, выварить (*вн.*) 1. (*лишать вкусовых или питательных свойств*) boil (smth.) to nothing; 2. (*извлекать*) boil (smth.) out, extract (smth.) by boiling, decoct (smth.); ~ соль produce salt by evaporation; ~ жир render fat. ~ся, вывариться be* boiled to pulp.

выварить(ся) *сов. см.* вываривать(ся).

выведать, выведать (*вн.*) *разг.* find* (smth.) out; *несов. тж.* try to worm (smth.) out; ~ тайну у кого-л. pump/worm a secret out of smb.

вывезти *сов. см.* вывозить 1, 2, 3.

вывер|ить *сов. см.* выверять. ~ка *ж.* adjustment, regulation; (*хронометра*) rating; (*списка*) verification, checking.

вывернуть(ся) *сов. см.* вывёртывать(ся).

вывёртыва|ть, вывернуть (*вн.*) 1. (*вывинчивать*) unscrew (smth.); 2. (*руку, ногу*) wrench (smth.), twist (smth.); 3. (*наизнанку*) turn (smth.) inside out. ~ться, вывернуться 1. (*вывинчиваться*) come* unscrewed; винт легко ~ается the screw turns quite easily; 2. (*выскальзывать, высвобождаться*) slip away; 3. *разг.* (*из затруднительного положения*) wriggle out, extricate oneself.

выверять, выверить (*вн.*) regulate (smth.), adjust (smth.), set* (smth.); (*хронометр*) rate (smth.); (*список*) check (smth.); verify (smth.).

вывесить I, II *сов. см.* вывешивать I, II.

вывеска *ж.* sign, signboard; *перен.* mask.

вывести(сь) *сов. см.* выводить(ся).

выветривание *с.* 1. ventilation, airing; 2. *геол.* weathering, (wind) erosion.

выве́тривать, вы́ветрить (вн.) 1. air (smth.), ventílate (smth.); ~ за́пах нафтали́на air a room to remóve the smell of náphthalene; 2. геол. wéather (smth.), eróde (smth.). ~ся, вы́ветриться 1. (о запахе) eváporate; перен. fade; вы́ветриться из головы́, из па́мяти be* effáced from the mémory; 2. геол. be* wéathered/eróded.

вы́ветрить(ся) сов. см. выве́тривать(ся).

выве́шивать I, вы́весить (вн.) 1. hang* out (smth.); ~ фла́ги hoist flags; ~ бельё (для просушки) hang* out the wáshing; 2. (помещать для обозрения) displáy (smth.), post (up) (smth.); ~ объявле́ние displáy a nótice, post (up) a nótice.

выве́шивать II, вы́весить (вн.) (определять вес) test the weight (of).

вы́винтить(ся) сов. см. выви́нчивать(ся).

выви́нчивать, вы́винтить (вн.) únscréw (smth.). ~ся, вы́винтиться come* únscréwed.

вы́вих м. dislocátion. ~нуть сов. (вн.) díslocate (smth.); ~нуть себе́ но́гу (в лодыжке) díslocate one's ánkle; (в колене) díslocate one's knee.

вы́вод м. 1. (увод; удаление) remóval; 2. (умозаключение) conclúsion, ínference; прийти́ к ~у come* to a conclúsion; 3. (выращивание) réaring, bréeding; 4. (высиживание) hátching; 5. (истребление) extermination.

выводи́ть, вы́вести 1. (вн.; удалять за пределы чего-л.) bring* (smb.) out, remóve (smb.), send* (smb.) out, take* (smb.) out; (войска) withdráw* (smth.); 2. (вн.; ведя, направлять куда-л.) lead* (smb., smth.) out; take* (smb., smth.) out; ~ дете́й в сад take* the chíldren out ínto the gárden; ~ ло́шадь из коню́шни lead* the horse out of the stáble; вы́вести спу́тник на орби́ту put* a spútnik ínto órbit; 3. (вн. из рд.; исключать) remóve (smb. from); вы́вести кого́-л. из соста́ва прези́диума remóve smb. from the presídium; вы́вести кого́-л. из игры́ disquálify smb.; 4. (вн. из рд.): ~ кого́-л. из состоя́ния поко́я distúrb smb.'s compósure; ~ цех из прорыва get* the shop/depártment out of difficulties; вы́вести самолёт из пике́ pull a plane out of a dive; 5. (вн.; делать вывод) draw* (smth.), arríve (at); ~ фо́рмулу deríve a fórmula; 6. (вн.; высиживать — о птицах) hatch (smth.); вы́вести цыпля́т hatch chíckens; 7. (вн.; выращивать) breed* (smth.), raise (smth.), ~ но́вую поро́ду скота́ breed* a new strain of cáttle; ~ засухоусто́йчивую пшени́цу breed* dróught-resistant wheat; 8. (вн.; сооружать) put* up (smth.); 9. (вн.; уничтожать) extérminate (smth.); ~ пятно́ take* out a spot; 10. (вн.; старательно писать, рисовать и т. п.) trace out (smth.); ~ бу́квы trace out the létters; ◇ ~ отме́тку define the áverage mark; вы́вести что́-л. нару́жу bring* smth. out ínto the ópen; вы́вести кого́-л. в лю́ди give* smb. a start in life, introdúce smb. to the world; вы́вести кого́-л. из себя́ infúriate smth., drive* smth. to distráction; вы́вести кого́-л. из равнове́сия distúrb smb.'s bálance/equilíbrium, upsét* smth.; get* smb. ráttled разг.; вы́вести кого́-л. на чи́стую во́ду show* smb. up in his true cólours. ~ся, вы́вестись 1. (переставать существовать) die out, becóme* extínct; 2. (выходить из употребления) go* out of use; (об обычаях) die out; go* out; 3. (исчезать) disappéar; (о пятнах тж.) come* out; 4. (появляться на свет — о птенцах) hatch out.

вы́водок м. brood.

вы́воз м. 1. (действие) convéyance; 2. эк. éxport.

вывози́ть, вы́везти (вн.) move (smb., smth.) out/awáy; (мусор и т. п.) take* (smth.) awáy, remóve (smth.); 2. (доставлять куда-л.) take* (smth.); ~ това́ры на ры́нок take* goods to márket; 3. (привозить с собой откуда-л.) bring* (back) (smth.); 4. тк. несов. эк. expórt (smth.).

вы́воз|ка ж. remóval. ~но́й эк. éxport attr.; ~ы́е по́шлины éxport dúty sg.

выволáкивать, вы́волочь (вн) разг. drag (smth.) out of.

вы́волочь сов. см. выволáкивать.

вы́гадать сов. см. выга́дывать.

выга́дывать, вы́гадать (вн.) (получать выгоду) gain (smth.); (сберегать) save (smth.), económize (smth.); вы вы́гадали you've done well for yoursélf; вы́гадать вре́мя save time.

вы́гиб м. bend, curve.

выгибáть, вы́гнуть (вн.) bend* (smth.), curve (smth.); ~ спи́ну arch one's back. ~ся, вы́гнуться bend*.

вы́гладить сов. см. гла́дить 1.

выгляде́ть несов. look; ~ моло́же свои́х лет look young for one's age; она́ вы́глядит моло́же свои́х лет she does not look her age; ~ ста́рше свои́х лет look ólder than one réally is; хорошо́ ~ look well; пло́хо ~ look ill.

выгля́дывать, вы́глянуть 1. (смотреть откуда-л.) look out; (украдкой) peep out; 2. (показываться, появляться) appéar, show*; со́лнце вы́глянуло из-за туч the sun appéared from behínd the clouds.

вы́глянуть сов. см. выгля́дывать.

вы́гнать сов. см. выгоня́ть.

вы́гнутый bent.

вы́гнуть(ся) сов. см. выгибáть(ся).

выгова́ривать, вы́говорить 1. (вн.) say* (smth.); (произносить) pronóunce (smth.); он не мог вы́говорить ни сло́ва he could not útter a word; 2. (вн.) разг. (обусловливать) stípulate (smth.); он вы́говорил себе́ льго́тные усло́вия he obtáined fávourable terms for himsélf; 3. тк. несов. (дт.) разг. (делать замечание) scold (smb.), repróve (smb.). ~ся, вы́говориться разг. unbúrden onesélf, unbúrden one's féelings, get* it off one's chest.

вы́говор м. 1. (произношение) áccent, pronunciátion; 2. (порицание) réprimand; объяви́ть кому́-л. ~ give* smb. an official réprimand.

вы́говорить сов. см. выгова́ривать 1, 2. ~ся сов. см. выгова́риваться.

вы́год|а ж. 1. (прибыль) prófit, gain; ра́ди ~ы for the sake of prófit; 2. (польза) bénefit, advántage; извлекáть ~у из чего́-л. deríve advántage from smth.; без вся́кой ~ы для себя́ without the slíghtest bénefit to onesélf. ~но 1. нареч. fávourably; ~но отличáться от compáre fávourably with; 2. в знач. сказ. (прибыльно) be* prófitable; (полезно) be* advantágeous; кому́ э́то ~но? who stands to gain?; (ожидая отрицательного ответ) what use is it to ányone? ~ный 1. (доходный) prófitable, páying; 2. (благоприятный) fávourable, advantágeous.

вы́гон м. pásture, méadow.

выгоня́ть, вы́гнать (вн.) 1. turn (smb.) out; ~ кого́-л. из до́му turn smb. out; 2. разг. (исключать) expél (smb.); (увольнять) give* (smb.) the sack; fire (smb.) амер.; ~ скот drive* cáttle to pásture.

выгорáживать, вы́городить (вн.) 1. (отделять огра́дой) fence (smth.) off; 2. разг. (оправдывать) shield (smb.), protéct (smb.); вы́городить прия́теля exónerate one's friend.

выгорáть I, вы́гореть 1. (сгорать) be* burnt down; (о траве) be* burnt up; ~ дотлá be* burnt to the ground; 2. (выцветать) fade.

выгорáть II, вы́гореть разг. (удаваться) come* off; де́ло вы́горело it came off; де́ло не вы́горело it fell through.

вы́гореть I, II сов. см. выгорáть I, II.

вы́городить сов. см. выгорáживать.

вы́греб|áть, вы́грести 1. (вн.; удалять) clean (smth.) out; (из печки) rake (smth.) out; 2. (вёслами) row, pull. ~но́й: ~ная я́ма césspool.

вы́грести сов. см. выгребáть.

выгружáть, вы́грузить (вн.) únlóad (smth.); (груз с корабля́) dischárge (smth.); (войска с судна) disembárk (smb.). ~ся, вы́грузиться get* off (with one's lúggage); (с судна) disembárk, bring* one's lúggage/equípment off the ship; (из вагона) detráin.

вы́груз|и́ть(ся) сов. см. выгружа́ть(ся). ~ка ж. únlóading; (с судов) disembarkátion; (из вагона) detráining.

выдава́ть, вы́дать 1. (вн.) íssue (smth.), give* out (smth.); ~ удостовере́ние íssue a certíficate; ~ зарпла́ту кому́-л. pay* smb. his, her wáges; 2. (вн.; обнаружи-вать; разоблача́ть) give* (smb., smth.) awáy, betráy (smb., smth.); ~ секре́т give* awáy a sécret, betráy a sécret; улы́бка вы́дала его́ his smile gave him awáy; 3. (вн.; возвраща́ть кого́-л. про́тив его́ во́ли) hand óver (smth.); (друго́му госуда́рству) extradíte (smth.); вы́дать перебе́жчика hand óver a desérter; вы́дать престу́пника extradíte a críminal; 4. (вн. за вн.; непра́вильно пред-ставля́ть) pass (smb.) off as (smth.); он вы́дал меня́ за своего́ учи́теля he preténded I was his téacher; он выда-ёт себя́ за худо́жника he póses as an ártist, he gives himsélf out to be an ártist; 5. (вн.; добыва́ть, выпу-ска́ть) turn out (smth.), prodúce (smth.); вы́дать у́голь на-гора́ prodúce coal; 6. разг. (сообща́ть что-л. при-меча́тельное) come* out with (smth.); 7. разг. (руга́ть) give* it (to); ◇ вы́дать себя́ give* onesélf awáy.

выдава́ться, вы́даться 1. (выступа́ть) jut out, projéct; 2. (отлича́ться) be* distínguished; он ниче́м осо́бенным не выдаётся he is in no way remárkable; there is nóthing spécial abóut him; 3. разг. (случа́ться): сего́дня вы́дался хоро́ший денёк the day has turned out fine.

вы́давить сов. см. выда́вливать.

выда́вливать, вы́давить (вн.) 1. (выжима́ть) squeeze (smth.) out, force (smth.) out (тж. перен.); 2. (прода́вливать) break* (smth.); вы́давить стекло́ break* a window-pane; 3. (выти́снять) embóss (smth.), stamp (smth.).

выда́лбливать, вы́долбить (вн.) gouge (out) (smth.), hóllow out (smth.).

вы́дать сов. см. выдава́ть.

вы́даться сов. см. выдава́ться.

вы́дача ж. íssue, gíving out; ~ де́нег páyment; ~ зар-пла́ты páyment of sálary/wáges.

выдаю́щийся outstánding, distínguished; remárkable; ниче́м не ~ in no way remárkable; ~ успе́х sígnal succéss; ~ актёр distínguished áctor.

выдвига́ть, вы́двинуть (вн.) 1. push (smth.) fórward; pull (smth.) out; ~ я́щик стола́ ópen a drawer; 2. (пред-лага́ть для обсужде́ния) bring* up (smth.), put* (smth.) fórward; ~ предложе́ние bring* up a propósal; ~ тео́рию propóund a théory; ~ чью́-л. кандидату́ру propóse/nóminate smb. as a cándidate; 3. (на бо́лее от-ве́тственную рабо́ту) recomménd (smb.) for promótion. ~ся, вы́двинуться 1. (вперёд) advánce, move fórward; 2. тк. несов. (быть выдвижны́м) slide*/pull out; я́щик легко́ выдвига́ется the drawer ópens smóothly; 3. (по рабо́те) rise*, get* promóted.

выдвиже́ние с. 1. móving fórward; 2. (для обсужде́-ния) brínging up; ~ кандида́тов nominátion of cándidates; 3. (по рабо́те) promótion.

выдвижно́й slíding; (об анте́нне и т. п.) telescópic; ~ я́щик drawer.

вы́двинуть сов. см. выдвига́ть. ~ся сов. см. выдви-га́ться 1, 3.

вы́делать сов. см. выде́лывать 1, 2.

выделе́ние с. 1. (организацио́нное) síngling out; ~ в осо́бый райо́н formátion ínto a séparate dístrict; 2. (средств) allocátion; 3. физ., физиол. dischárge; физи-ол. тж. secrétion; ~ гно́я suppurátion; 4. мн. физиол. excrétions.

вы́делить(ся) сов. см. выделя́ть(ся).

вы́делк|а ж. 1. (изготовле́ние) manufácture; ~ ко́-жи dréssing of léather; 2. (ка́чество) quálity; fínish;

осо́бо про́чной ~и of éxtra-stróng quálity; 3. (рельéфный рису́нок на тка́ни) embóssing.

выде́лывать, вы́делать (вн.) 1. make* (smth.), fáshion (smth.); 2. (подвергáть специáльной обрабо́т-ке) treat (smth.), dress (smth.); ~ ко́жу под за́мшу give* a suéde fínish to a piece of léather; 3. тк. несов. (производи́ть) manufácture (smth.); 4. тк. несов. разг. (совершáть что-л. необы́чное) do* (smth.), perfórm (smth.).

выдел|я́ть, вы́делить (вн.) 1. (отбира́ть, обособ-ля́ть) seléct (smb., smth.), pick out (smb., smth.), síngle out (smb., smth.); ~ в отде́льный райо́н make* ínto a séparate dístrict; 2. (отлича́ть) distínguish (smb., smth.); give* próminence (to); э́то ~я́ет его́ среди́ дру-ги́х it distínguishes him from the rest; ~ что́-л. курси́вом put* smth. in itálics; 3. (предназначáть для какой-л. це́ли) állocate (smth.), éarmark (smth.); ~ сре́дства set* asíde funds, állocate funds; 4. (часть иму́щества) appórtion (smth.); 5. физиол. (отрабо́танное веще́ст-во) excréte (smth.); (гной) dischárge (smth.); (пот) exúde (smth.); ~ мокро́ту cough up phlegm. ~я́ться, вы́-делиться 1. (тв.; отлича́ться) be* distínguished (by, for), stand* out (for); ~я́ться на фо́не чего́-л. stand* out agáinst smth.; 2. (обособля́ться) emérge; ~я́ться в са-мостоя́тельное учрежде́ние be* reórganized as a séparate institútion; 3. физиол. be* dischárged, exúde; 4. (о па́ре, га́зе и т. п.) be* gíven off, escápe.

выдёргивать, вы́дернуть (вн.) pull out (smth.), pluck (smth.); ~ зуб extráct a tooth*; вы́дернуть себе́ зуб have* a tooth* out.

вы́держанный 1. (о хара́ктере, челове́ке) self--contrólled; 2. (после́довательный) sustáined, consístent; ~ стиль úniform style; 3. (о лесоматериáле) séasoned; (о сы́ре, табаке́) ripe; (о вине́) old, matúre.

вы́держать сов. см. выде́рживать.

выде́ржив|ать, вы́держать 1. (вн.; не поддава́ться) bear* (smth.), stand* (smth.), sustáin (smth.); мост ~ает тя́жесть в 30 тонн the bridge can bear a weight of thírty tons; 2. (вн.; терпе́ть, сто́йко переноси́ть) bear* (smth.), endúre (smth.), stand* (smth.), sustáin (smth.); вы́держать оса́ду withstánd* a siege; вы́держать пы́тку endúre tórture; я не могу́ э́того вы́держать I can't stand it; 3. разг. (проявля́ть вы́держку) hold* out, bear* it; она́ не вы́держала, что́бы не подразни́ть его́ she cóuldn't help/resíst téasing him; 4. (вн.; удовлетворя́ть тре́бованиям) pass (smth.); вы́держать экза́мен pass an examinátion; 5. (вн.; сохраня́ть) maintáin (smth.), sustáin (smth.), keep* up (smth.); ~ ско́рость maintáin the speed; ~ те́мпы keep* up the pace; ~ направле́ние (о журна́ле и т. п.) adhére to its line; 6. (вн.; для улуч-ше́ния ка́чества) séason (smth.); вы́держать вино́ matúre wine; ◇ вы́держать не́сколько изда́ний go* through séveral edítions; вы́держать па́узу keep* up a pause, maintáin a pause; вы́держать хара́ктер stand* firm; stick* to one's guns.

вы́держка I ж. 1. (самооблада́ние) self-contról; (вы-носливость) endúrance; (сде́ржанность) resérve, restráint; 2. фо́то expósure; больша́я ~ long expósure.

вы́держка II ж. (отры́вок) éxtract, éxcerpt.

вы́дернуть сов. см. выдёргивать.

выдира́ть, вы́драть (вн.) разг. tear* (smth.) out.

вы́долбить сов. см. выда́лбливать.

вы́дох м. exhalátion; ~! breathe out! ~нуть(ся) сов. см. выдыха́ть(ся).

вы́дра ж. (живо́тное и мех) ótter.

вы́драть I сов. см. выдира́ть.

вы́драть II сов. см. драть 3.

выдрессирова́ть сов. см. дрессирова́ть.

выдува́ть, вы́дуть (вн.) blow* (smth.); всё тепло́ вы́-дует all the heat will escápe.

вы́дум|анный fictítious. ~ать сов. см. выду́мывать. ~ка ж. 1. (вы́мысел) fíction, invéntion; чи́стая ~ка pure invéntion, trúmped-úp stóry; **2.** *разг.* (*изобретатель-ность*) invéntiveness, invéntion, imaginátion; **3.** (*изобре-тение, затея*) invéntion. ~**щик** *м.* *разг.* **1.** man* of idéas; **2.** (*клеветник*) táttler, góssip.

выду́мыв|ать, вы́думать (*вн.*) **1.** (*изобретать*) invént (*smth.*); think* (*smth.*) up *разг.*; **2.** (*создавать воображением*) make* (*smth.*) up, invént (*smth.*); что ты ~аешь? what have you got ínto your head?; ◇ он по́роха не вы́думает he's no génius.

вы́дуть *сов. см.* выдува́ть.

выдыха́ть, вы́дохнуть (*вн.*) exhále (*smth.*), breathe out (*smth.*). ~**ся, вы́дохнуться 1.** lose* its pówer/strength; (*о пиве*) becóme* flat; **2.** *разг.* (*терять силу*) péter out; наступле́ние вы́дохлось the attáck came to a stándstill; **3.** *разг.* (*утомляться*) get* tíred/exháusted, be* played out.

выеда́ть, вы́есть (*вн.*) **1.** eat* out (*smth.*), peck out (*smth.*); **2.** (*кислотой и т. п.*) corróde (*smth.*), eat* (*smth.*) away.

вы́езд *м.* **1.** (*отъезд*) depárture; **2.** (*место, через которое выезжают*) éxit road, way out; **3.** (*экипаж и лошади*) túrn-óut.

вы́езд|ить *сов. см.* выезжа́ть II. ~**ка** *ж.* (*лошадей*) tráining, bréaking in.

выездн|о́й: ~**а́я ви́за** éxit vísa; ~**а́я се́ссия суда́** assízes *pl.*

выезжа́ть I, вы́ехать 1. (*уезжать*) go* awáy, leave*; (*с квартиры*) move, leave*; **2.** (*из ворот, на прогулку и т. п.*) drive* out; **3.** (*появляться*) come* out; вы́ехать на шоссе́ come* out on to the main road.

выезжа́ть II, вы́ездить (*вн.; лошадь*) train (*smth.*).

вы́емка *ж.* **1.** (*действие*) táking out, excavátion; (*писем*) colléction; **2.** (*углубление*) depréssion, hóllow; (*на железной дороге*) cútting; **3.** (*вырез*) ópening.

вы́есть *сов. см.* выеда́ть.

вы́ехать *сов. см.* выезжа́ть I.

вы́жать *сов. см.* выжима́ть.

вы́ждать *сов. см.* выжида́ть.

вы́жечь *сов. см.* выжига́ть.

выжива́ние *с.* survíval.

выжива́ть I, вы́жить (*оставаться в живых*) survíve, live; (*о больном тж.*) pull through *разг.*; он вряд ли вы́живет he is unlíkely to recóver, I don't suppóse he'll live; ◇ вы́жить из ума́ becóme* féeble-mínded.

выжива́ть II, вы́жить (*вн.*) *разг.* (*выгонять откуда-л.*) get* rid (of); ~ кого́-л. из дому force smb. to leave the house.

выжига́ние *с.* búrning; ~ **по де́реву** póker-work.

выжига́ть, вы́жечь (*вн.*) **1.** (*уничтожать огнём*) burn* (*smth.*), raze (*smth.*); со́лнцем вы́жгло посе́вы the young crops wíthered in the sun; вы́жженная со́лнцем земля́ the sún-scórched earth; **2.** (*какие-л. узоры, знаки*) burn* (*smth.*), burn* (*smth.*) out; ~ клеймо́ на чём-л. brand (*smth.*); ~ **по де́реву** do* póker-work.

выжида́ние *с.* témporizing; expéctancy.

выжида́тельн|ый expéctant; ~**ая поли́тика** témporizing pólicy, wáit-and-sée pólicy.

выжида́ть, вы́ждать (*вн.*) wait (for), témporize (until); ~ удо́бный слу́чай bide* *one's* time; вы́ждать вре́мя wait till the time is ripe.

выжима́ть, вы́жать (*вн.*) **1.** wring* out (*smth.*); squeeze out (*smth.*); *перен.* squeeze (*smth.*) out of, extráct (*smth.*) from; ~ бельё wring* out clothes; ~ лимо́н squeeze a lémon; ~ сок из плодо́в squeeze the juice out of fruit; **2.** *спорт.* lift (*smth.*); вы́жать ги́рю lift a dúmb-bell; вы́жать со́рок килогра́ммов lift fórty kílograms.

вы́жить I, II *сов. см.* выжива́ть I, II.

вы́звать(ся) *сов. см.* вызыва́ть(ся).

вы́зволить *сов. см.* вызволя́ть.

вызволя́ть, вы́зволить (*вн.*) *разг.* help (*smb.*) out.

выздора́влив|ать, вы́здороветь get* bétter, get* well, recóver; он ~**ает**, но ещё не вы́здоровел he's gétting bétter, but he's not well yet. ~**ающий** *м.* convaléscent.

выздоров|еть *сов. см.* выздора́вливать. ~**ле́ние** *с.* recóvery.

вы́зов *м.* **1.** call; ~ **ско́рой по́мощи** emérgency call, call for first aid; ~ **по телефо́ну** télephone-call; ~ **на бис** encóre; **выходи́ть на ~ы** come* befóre the cúrtain; **2.** (*требование явиться*) súmmons; **получи́ть ~ в суд** recéive a súmmons; **3.** (*на соревнование, борьбу*) chállenge; **приня́ть ~** take* up a chállenge, accépt a chállenge; **4.** (*дт.; предложение вступить в борьбу*) chállenge, defíance; **с ~ом сказа́ть, посмотре́ть** say, look chállengingly/defíantly.

вы́зубрить *сов.* (*вн.*) *разг.* cram (*smth.*), swot up (*smth.*).

вызыв|а́ть, вы́звать 1. (*вн.*) call (*smb.*); (*посылать за кем-л.*) send* (for); (*предлагать явиться*) súmmon (*smb.*); ~ **врача́** call a dóctor, send* for the dóctor; ~ **ско́рую по́мощь** phone an ámbulance, send* for an ámbulance; **вы меня́ ~а́ли?** did you want to see me?; ~ **кого́-л. в суд** subpóena smb., súmmon(s) smb.; ~ **кого́-л. к доске́** call smb. to the bláckboard; ~ **по спи́ску** call péople by name; ~ **актёра** recáll an áctor; **2.** (*вн. на вн., вн. + инф.; на состязание*) chállenge (smb. to, smb. to inf.); **3.** (*вн. на вн., вн. + инф.; побуждать*) prompt (smb. + to inf.); **вы́звать кого́-л. на открове́нность** indúce smb. to be frank, draw* smb. out; **вы́звать кого́-л. на разгово́р** get* smb. to talk; **4.** (*вн.; быть причиной*) cause (*smth.*), bring* (*smth.*) about; (*о мыслях, чувствах и т. п.*) aróuse (*smth.*), evóke (*smth.*); ~ **аппети́т** stímulate the áppetite; ~ **кровотече́ние, рво́ту** cause bléeding, vómiting; ~ **смех** provóke láughter; ~ **улы́бку** evóke a smile; ~ **гнев** rouse smb.'s íre; ~ **воспомина́ния** evóke/aróuse mémories; ~ **сомне́ния** give* rise to doubts; ~ **представле́ние о чём-л.** suggést smth.; ~ **большо́й интере́с** evóke/rouse great ínterest; ~**а́ться, вы́зваться** (*+ инф.*) voluntéer (for, + to inf.); **э́то не ~а́ется необходи́мостью** there's no need for it. ~**а́ющий** provócative; ~**а́ющий взгляд** provócative glance; ~**а́ющее поведе́ние** defíant behávìour.

вы́играть *сов. см.* выи́грывать.

выи́грывать, вы́играть 1. (*вн.*) win* (*smth.*); вы́играть сто рубле́й win* a húndred róubles; ~ **в ка́рты** win* at cards; **вы́играть па́ртию в ша́хматы** win* a game of chess; **вы́играть сраже́ние** win* a báttle; **2.** (*вн.; получать выгоду*) gain (*smth.*), acquíre (*smth.*); населе́ние вы́играло от сниже́ния цен the públic has gained by the price redúction; **3.** (*в пр.; преуспевать*) gain (in); вы́играть в чьём-л. мне́нии rise* in smb.'s opínion; ◇ вы́играть вре́мя gain time; стара́ться вы́играть вре́мя play for time.

вы́игрыш *м.* **1.** (*то, что выиграно*) prize; (*в ка́рты и т. п.*) wínnings *pl*; **2.** (*выгода*) gain, advántage; ~ **во вре́мени** sáving of time; **3.** (*победа в чём-л.*) succéss, víctory; ◇ **быть в ~е 1)** have* won some móney; **2)** (*извлечь выгоду*) be* the gáiner. ~**ный 1.** (*о займе и т. п.*) lóttery *attr.*; **2.** (*выгодный*) advántageous; (*способствующий успеху*) wínning; ~**ная роль** rewárding part; ~**ный ход** good move; ~**ное положе́ние** wínning/strong posítion.

вы́искать(ся) *сов. см.* выи́скивать(ся).

выи́скивать, вы́искать (*вн.*) *разг.* look for (*smth.*); *сов. тж.* find* (*smth.*) out. ~**ся, вы́искаться** *разг.* turn up; како́й у́мник вы́искался! what a cléver pérson we have found!

вы́йти *сов. см.* выходи́ть 1, 2, 3, 4, 5, 7, 8, 9.

вы́казать *сов. см.* выка́зывать.

выка́зывать, вы́казать (*вн.*) *разг.* displáy (*smth.*), show* (*smth.*); ~ **хра́брость** displáy cóurage.

выка́лывать, вы́колоть (*вн.*) prick out (*smth.*);

(*глаз*) put* out (*smth.*); ◇ (*темно́*) хоть глаз вы́коли it is pítch-dárk.

выка́пывать, вы́копать (*вн.*) 1. dig* (*smth.*); выкопать я́му dig* a pit; вы́копать пруд dig* a pond; 2. (*извлека́ть из земли́*) dig* (*smth.*) up; exhúme (*smth.*) *книжн.*; 3. *разг.* (*оты́скивать*) dig* (*smth.*) up; отку́да вы э́то вы́копали? where on earth did you get that from?

выкара́бкаться *сов. см.* выкара́бкиваться.

выкара́бкиваться, вы́карабкаться *разг.* scrámble out; *перен.* get* out, éxtricate onesélf.

выка́рмливать, вы́кормить (*вн.*) bring* (*smb., smth.*) up; raise (*smb., smth.*) *амер.*

вы́катить(ся) *сов. см.* выка́тывать(ся).

выка́тывать, вы́катить (*вн.*) roll (*smth.*) out; (*о коля́ске, велосипе́де и т. п.*) wheel (*smth.*) out; ◇ глаза́ *разг.* ópen one's eyes wide; stare góggle-eyed. ~**ся,** вы́катиться roll out.

вы́качать *сов. см.* выка́чивать.

выка́чивать, вы́качать (*вн.; прям. и перен.*) pump (*smth.*) out.

выки́дывать, вы́кинуть 1. *см.* выбра́сывать; 2. (*вн.*) *разг.* play (*smth.*); вы́кинуть но́мер, шту́ку play a prank/trick; 3. *разг.* (*о бере́менной*) have* a miscárriage.

вы́кидыш *м.* 1. miscárriage; 2. (*плод*) prémature báby.

вы́кинуть *сов. см.* выки́дывать.

выкипа́ть, вы́кипеть boil awáy.

вы́кипеть *сов. см.* выкипа́ть.

вы́кладк|а *ж.* 1. обы́кн. *мн.* (*расчёты, вычисле́ния*) computátion *sg*; 2. *воен.* kit, equípment; с по́лной ~ой in full equípment/kit; 3. *разг.* (*кирпичо́м, плита́ми*) fácing (*снару́жи*); líning (*изнутри́*).

выкла́дыв|ать, вы́ложить 1. (*вн.*) put* (*smth.*) out; ~ ве́щи из чемода́на take* one's things out of one's súitcase; 2. (*вн.*) *разг.* (*выска́зывать, сообща́ть*) make* a clean breast of it; ~ но́вости give* the látest news; ~ай! out with it!; 3. (*вн. тв.; обкла́дывать*) face (*smth.* with) (*снару́жи*); line (*smth.* with) (*изнутри́*); ~ что́-л. дёрном turf *smth.*; ~ двор ка́мнем pave a cóurtyard.

выкла́дываться, вы́ложиться *разг.* give* all *one* has got.

вы́клевать *сов. см.* выклёвывать.

выклёвывать, вы́клевать (*вн.*) 1. (*вырыва́ть клю́вом*) peck (*smth.*) out; 2. (*склёвывать*) peck (*smth.*) up.

выклика́ть, вы́кликнуть (*вн.*) call (*smb.*) out; ~ по спи́ску call the roll.

вы́кликнуть *сов. см.* выклика́ть.

выключа́тель *м.* switch; автомати́ческий ~ cút-out.

выключа́ть, вы́ключить (*вн.*) turn (*smth.*) off, switch (*smth.*) off; (*всю сеть*) cut* (*smth.*) off; ~ свет turn out the light; ~ ра́дио switch off the rádio; ~ сцепле́ние disengáge the clutch.

вы́ключить *сов. см.* выключа́ть.

выкля́нчивать, вы́клянчить (*вн. у рд.*) *разг.* cadge (*smth.* off), whéedle (*smth.* out of).

вы́клянчить *сов. см.* выкля́нчивать.

вы́ковать *сов. см.* выко́вывать.

выко́вывать, вы́ковать (*вн.; прям. и перен.*) forge (*smth.*); *перен. тж.* devélop (*smth.*).

выкови́ривать, вы́ковырять (*вн.*) *разг.* pick (*smth.*) out.

вы́ковырять *сов. см.* выкови́ривать.

выкола́чивать, вы́колотить (*вн.*) beat* (*smth.*) out, knock out (*smth.*); (*ковры́ и т. п.*) beat* (*smth.*); ~ пыль из *чего́-л.* beat* the dust out of *smth.*

вы́колотить *сов. см.* выкола́чивать.

вы́колоть *сов. см.* выка́лывать.

вы́копать *сов. см.* выка́пывать.

вы́кормить *сов. см.* выка́рмливать.

вы́корчевать *сов. см.* выкорчёвывать.

выкорчёвывать, вы́корчевать (*вн.*) grub up (*smth.*); upróot (*smth.*), root (*smth.*) out; *перен.* erádicate (*smth.*), root (*smth.*) out.

выкра́ивать, вы́кроить (*вн.*) cut* (*smth.*) out; *перен. разг.* find* (*smth.*); ~ вре́мя make*/find* time; ~ де́ньги на *что́-л.* make* one's móney run to smth.

вы́крашивать, вы́красить (*вн.*) paint (*smth.*); (*о мате́рии, во́лосах*) dye (*smth.*). ~**ся** *сов.* dye.

вы́красть *сов.* (*вн.*) steal* (*smth.*).

вы́крик *м.* cry, shout.

выкри́кивать, вы́крикнуть (*вн.*) shout (*smth.*).

вы́крикнуть *сов. см.* выкри́кивать.

вы́кроить *сов. см.* выкра́ивать.

вы́кройк|а *ж.* páttern; альбо́м вы́кроек páttern-book; шить *что́-л.* по ~e make* *smth.* from a páttern.

вы́крутить(ся) *сов. см.* выкру́чивать(ся).

выкру́чивать, вы́крутить (*вн.*) *разг.* 1. (*выви́нчивать*) unscréw (*smth.*); 2.: ~ ру́ку twist one's arm. ~**ся,** вы́крутиться *разг.* come* unscréwed; *перен.* wríggle out.

вы́куп *м.* 1. (*де́йствие*) ránsom, redémption; (*зало́женных веще́й*) búying back, repúrchase; 2. (*пла́та*) ránsom.

выкупа́ть, вы́купить (*вн.*) 1. redéem (*smth.*), buy* (*smth.*) back, repúrchase (*smth.*); 2. (*пле́нного*) ránsom (*smb.*), pay the ránsom (for).

вы́купаться *сов. см.* купа́ться.

вы́купить *сов. см.* выкупа́ть.

выку́ривать, вы́курить (*вн.*) 1. (*папиро́су и т. п.*) smoke (*smth.*); 2. (*выгоня́ть ды́мом*) smoke (*smb.*) out; *перен. разг.* get* rid (of).

вы́курить *сов. см.* выку́ривать.

выла́вливать, вы́ловить (*вн.*) fish (*smth.*) out; вы́ловить бревно́ из воды́ fish a log out of the wáter.

вы́лазк|а *ж.* 1. *воен.* sórtie; sálly (*тж. перен.*); сде́лать ~у make* a sórtie; враждёбная ~ hóstile sálly; 2. (*прогу́лка*) excúrsion, óuting; лы́жная ~ ski-trip.

выла́мывать, вы́ломать, вы́ломить (*вн.*) out; вы́ломать дверь break* ópen a door; вы́ломать замо́к wrench out a lock.

вы́лежать *сов.* stay in bed (until *one* is bétter). ~**ся** *сов.* 1. *разг.* have* a spell in bed, have* a complete rest; 2. (*о фру́ктах и т. п.*) rípen/matúre in stórage.

вылеза́ть, вы́лезти, вы́лезть 1. get* out, climb out; 2. (*о волоса́х*) fall* out.

вы́лезти, вы́лезть *сов. см.* вылеза́ть.

вы́лепить *сов. см.* лепи́ть 1.

вы́лет *м.* 1. táke-off; вре́мя ~a time of depárture/táke-off, plane depárture; 2. (*полёт*) flight; боево́й ~ sórtie, operátion; operátional flight.

вылета́ть, вы́лететь 1. fly* out; (*о самолёте*) leave*, take* off; (*на самолёте*) leave* (by air); (*о про́бке*) pop out; *перен. разг.* fly* out, go* flýing, be* flung out; вы́лететь из седла́ be* flung out of the sáddle; 2. (*стреми́тельно выезжа́ть, выбега́ть*) dash out, charge out, rush out; (*о маши́не и т. п.*) shoot* out; ◇ у меня́ э́то вы́летело из головы́ it went right out of my head.

вы́лететь *сов. см.* вылета́ть.

выле́чивать, вы́лечить (*вн.; прям. и перен.*) cure (*smb.*). ~**ся,** вы́лечиться (*прям. и перен.*) be* cured, recóver; get* bétter *разг.*

вы́лечить(ся) *сов. см.* выле́чивать(ся).

вылива́ть, вы́лить (*вн.*) 1. pour (*smth.*) out; (*опора́жнивать*) émpty (*smth.*); *перен.* pour (*smth.*) out, vent (*smth.*); вы́лить во́ду из ведра́ pour the wáter out of the pail; он вы́лил на них всё своё негодова́ние he vénted his indignátion on them; 2. (*изготовля́ть литьём*) cast* (*smth.*). ~**ся,** вы́литься 1. flow out, run* out; 2. (*в вн.; принима́ть каку́ю-л. фо́рму*) take* the shape (of), devélop (ínto).

вы́лизать *сов. см.* выли́зывать.

вылизывать, вылизать (вн.) lick (smth.) clean; перен. разг. make* (smth.) spótless.

вылинять сов. 1. fade; 2. (о животных) moult.

вылитый: ~ отец the image of one's father.

вылить(ся) сов. см. выливать(ся).

выловить сов. см. вылавливать.

выложить сов. см. выкладывать.

выложиться сов. см. выкладываться.

выломать сов. см. выламывать.

выломить сов. разг. см. выламывать.

вылупиться сов. см. вылупляться.

вылупляться, вылупиться hatch out.

вымаз|ать сов. (вн. тв.) smear (smth. with), cóver (smth. with); ~ что-л. дёгтем tar smth.; ~ что-л. салом grease smth.; ~анный в грязи all múddy; all dírty. ~аться сов. разг. (be) smear onesélf; get* dírty; ~аться в чернилах be* cóvered with ink.

вымаливать, вымолить (вн.) implóre (smth.); сов. тж. get* (smth.) by pléading; ~ прощение implóre forgíveness; он вымолил себе прощение his plea for párdon was gránted.

выманивать, выманить разг. 1. (вн.; побуждать выйти) lure (smth.) out/awáy; 2. (вн. у рд.; добывать лестью) coax (smth. out of); (обманом) defráud (smb. of), cheat (smb. out of).

выманить сов. см. выманивать.

вымарать сов. см. вымарывать.

вымарывать, вымарать (вн.) разг. 1. (пачкать) dírty (smth.); 2. (вычёркивать) strike* (smth.) out, smudge (smth.) out.

вымачивать, вымочить (вн.) 1. (промачивать) drench (smb., smth.); 2. (в чём-л.) soak (smth.), steep (smth.); mex. ret (smth.).

выменивать, выменять (вн. на вн.) bárter (smth. for).

выменять сов. см. выменивать.

вымереть сов. см. вымирать.

вымерзать, вымерзнуть 1. (гибнуть от мороза) be* destróyed by frost; 2. (обращаться в лёд) freeze* sólid.

вымерзнуть сов. см. вымерзать.

вымерший extínct; dead.

вымести сов. см. выметать.

выместить сов. см. вымещать.

выметать, вымести (вн.) sweep* (smth.); вымести пол sweep* the floor; вымести сор sweep* up/out the litter.

вымещать, выместить 1. (вн.; отплачивать) avénge (smth.); ~ обиду avénge an ínsult; 2. (вн. на пр.; удовлетворять чувство злобы) take* (it) out (on); ~ (свою) злобу на ком-л. wreak/vent one's ánger on smb.

вымирать, вымереть 1. die out; (о роде, виде тж.) becóme* extínct; 2. (о селении, городе и т. п.) pérish, die; улицы словно вымерли the streets seemed to be dead, there was not a líving soul to be seen in the streets.

вымогатель м. extórtioner. ~ство с. extórtion.

вымогать несов. (вн.) extórt (smth.).

вымокать, вымокнуть 1. (промокать) be* wet through; 2. (в жидкости) be* soaked, be* steeped; 3. (погибать от обилия влаги) becóme* sódden, rot.

вымокнуть сов. см. вымокать.

вымолвить сов. (вн.) разг. útter (smth.).

вымолить сов. см. вымаливать.

вымочить сов. см. вымачивать.

вымпел м. 1. stréamer; мор. pénnant, péndant; 2. ав. méssage bag.

вымученный разг. (о стиле, рифме и т. п.) láboured; (об улыбке) forced.

вымывать, вымыть (вн.) 1. (мыть) wash (smth.); 2. (размывать) hóllow out (smth.); 3. (смывать) wash awáy (smth.).

вымысел м. fíction, fígment of the imaginátion; (ложь) lie, fabricátion; сплошной ~ pure invéntion.

вымыть сов. см. вымывать и мыть. ~ся сов. см. мыться.

вымышленный imáginary, fictítious.

вымя с. údder.

вынашивать, выносить (вн.); ~ ребёнка be* prégnant; cárry a child*; ~ мысль let* an idéa rípen in one's mind.

вынести сов. см. выносить.

вынимать, вынуть (вн. из рд.) take* (smth.) out (of); ~ что-л. из ящика take* smth. out of a drawer; ~ револьвер pull out a revólver; ~ шпагу из ножен unshéathe one's sword; draw* one's sword; ◇ вынь да положь prodúce it on the spot; as if it were one's for the ásking.

вынос м. cárrying out; ~ тела назначен на 12 часов the fúneral cortège will start at twelve.

выносить сов. см. вынашивать.

выносить, вынести (вн.) 1. take* (smth.) out, cárry (smth.) out, remóve (smth.); вынести мебель из комнаты cárry fúrniture out of a room; 2. разг. (доставлять куда-л.) bring* (smth.); ~ что-л. на рынок bring* smth. to márket; 3. (ставить на обсуждение) submit (smth. for); 4. (выбрасывать течением) cárry (smth.) out, sweep* (smth.) out; лодку вынесло на берег the boat was swept up on the shore; 5. (выдерживать, переносить) stand* (smth.), bear* (smth.), endúre (smth.); ~ тяжёлые испытания stand* a sevére test; он не вынес этого удара he néver recóvered from the blow; не ~ постороннего вмешательства brook no interférence; 6.: ~ приговор give*/pronóunce júdgement; ~ решение make*/give* a decísion/rúling; ~ резолюцию pass a resolútion; ◇ вынести всю тяжесть чего-л. на своих плечах bear* the búrden of smth.; ~ за скобки put* óutside the bráckets; я не выношу его I can't stand him.

вынослив|ость ж. endúrance, stáying power; (растений) hárdiness. ~ый tough, wíry; hárdy (тж. о растениях).

вынудить сов. см. вынуждать.

вынуждать, вынудить (вн.; вн. + инф.) force (smth.; smb. + to inf.), compél (smth.; smb. + to inf.); вынудить обещание у кого-л. extráct a prómise from smb.

вынужденн|ый forced; ~ое признание únwilling admíssion; ~ая посадка ав. forced lánding.

вынуть сов. см. вынимать.

вынырнуть сов. emérge 1. (тж. перен.); come* to the súrface; 2. перен. разг. turn up.

вынянчить сов. (вн.) разг. bring* up (smb.), nurse (smb.).

выпад м. 1. спорт. lunge, thrust; (в фехтовании тж.) pass, passáde, passádo; 2. (враждебное выступление) attáck; сделать ~ против кого-л. make* an attáck on smb.; 3. физ. fáll-out.

выпад|ать, выпасть 1. fall* out; (о волосах тж.) come* out; у него ~ают зубы he's lósing his teeth; 2.: ~ из памяти, поля зрения slip one's mind, one's mémory; 3. (об осадках) fall*; 4. (дт.; доставаться) fall* (to); ему выпало счастье he had the good fórtune; 5. (случаться) háppen to be; ночь выпала тёмная it háppened to be a dark night, the night háppened to be a dark one; ◇ ~ кому-л. на долю fall* to smb.'s lot. ~ение с. 1. fall; (зубов, волос) loss; 2. мед. prólapsus.

выпалить сов. разг. 1. fíre; ~ из ружья fire off a gun; 2. (вн.; сказать) come* out (with), blurt (smth.) out.

выпаривать, выпарить (вн.) 1. eváporate (smth.); 2. (очищать паром) steam (smth.).

выпарить сов. см. выпаривать.

выпарывать, выпороть (вн.) rip out (smth.).

выпасть сов. см. выпадать.

вы́пачк|ать *сов.* (вн.) *разг.* get*/make* (*smth.*) dirty; ~ па́льцы черни́лами get* ink on *one's* fingers; я ~ала пла́тье I got my dress dirty; ~аться *сов. разг.* get* dirty; smudge *oneself*; ~аться в са́же make* *oneself* sooty.

выпека́ть, вы́печь (вн.) bake (*smth.*). ~ся, вы́печься bake; *сов. тж.* be* baked.

вы́печка *ж.* baking.

вы́печь(ся) *сов. см.* выпека́ть(ся).

выпив|а́ть, вы́пить 1. (вн.) drink* (*smth.*); (о *спиртном тж.*) have* a drop (of); вы́пить стака́н ча́ю, ко́фе *и т. п.* have* a glass of tea, coffee *etc.*; вы́пить до дна drink* up; drain *one's* glass; вы́пить за́лпом gulp/toss down; 2. *тк. несов. разг.* (*иметь склонность к спиртным напиткам*) drink*, go* in for drinking; он иногда́ ~а́ет he has a few drinks occásionally.

вы́пивка *ж. разг.* 1. (*попойка*) drinking session, drinking-bout; 2. (*напитки*) drinks *pl.*

вы́пиливание *с.* fretwork.

выпи́ливать, вы́пилить (вн.) 1. (*вырезать отверстие*) saw* (*smth.*); 2. (*изготовлять что-л. пилкой*) cut* out (*smth.*); вы́пилить ра́мку cut* out a frame.

вы́пилить *сов. см.* выпи́ливать.

выпира́ть *несов. разг.* bulge, protrúde; *перен.* be* óbvious.

вы́писать(ся) *сов. см.* выпи́сывать(ся).

вы́писка *ж.* 1. (*извлечение из книги и т. п.*) extract; éxcerpt; ~ из протоко́ла extract from the minutes; 2. (*газет и т. п.*) subscription (to); 3. (*из больницы*) dischárge.

выпи́сывать, вы́писать (вн.) 1. (*делать выписки*) extráct (*smth.*), cópy out (*smth.*); ~ отры́вки из кни́ги extráct pássages from a book, cópy out pássages from a book; 2. (*тщательно писать*) write* (*smth.*) out; ~ ка́ждую бу́кву form each létter cárefully; 3. (*квитанцию, ордер и т. п.*) make* out (*smth.*); 4. (*заказывать*) órder (*smth.*); 5. (*газету, журнал и т. п.*) take* (*smth.*), subscríbe (to); 6. (*вызывать письмом и т. п.*) write* for (*smb.*) to come; 7. (*исключать из списка*) dischárge (*smb.*); ~ кого́-л. из больни́цы dischárge *smb.* from hóspital; ~ся, вы́писаться check out; ~ся из больни́цы be* dischárged from hóspital.

вы́пить *сов. см.* пить 1, 3 *и* выпива́ть 1.

выпи́хивать, вы́пихнуть (вн.) *разг.* push (*smb.*) out, shove (*smb.*) out.

вы́пихнуть *сов. см.* выпи́хивать.

вы́плавить *сов. см.* выплавля́ть.

вы́плавк|а *ж.* 1. (*действие*) smelting; ~ чугуна́ production of pig-iron; 2. (*количество выплавленного металла*) melt, óutput; увели́чить су́точную ~у incréase the dáily melt.

выплавля́ть, вы́плавить (вн.) smelt (*smth.*), make* (*smth.*); ~ сталь make* steel.

вы́плакать *сов.*: ~ го́ре sob out *one's* grief; ~ все глаза́ cry *one's* eyes out. ~ся *сов.* have* a good cry, cry *one's* heart out.

вы́плат|а *ж.* páyment. ~ить *сов. см.* выпла́чивать.

выпла́чива|ть, вы́платить (вн.) pay* (*smth.*); (*полностью*) pay* (*smth.*) off, pay* (*smth.*) in full; ~ в рассро́чку pay* by instálments, pay* on the instálment plan.

выплёвывать, вы́плюнуть (вн.) spit* (*smth.*) out.

выплёскивать, вы́плеснуть (вн.) tip (*smth.*) out.

вы́плеснуть *сов. см.* выплёскивать.

выплыва́ть, вы́плыть 1. (*подниматься на поверхность воды*) come* up, break* súrface; (*выбираться на берег*) swim* ashóre; 2. (*возникать — о вопросе и т. п.*) emérge, come* up; 3. (*плывя, появляться*) swim* out, emérge; (*на парусах*) sail out (*тж. перен.*); луна́ вы́плыла из-за туч the moon sailed out from behind the clouds.

вы́плыть *сов. см.* выплыва́ть.

вы́плюнуть *сов. см.* выплёвывать.

выпола́скивать, вы́полоскать (вн.) rinse (out) (*smth.*).

выполза́ть, вы́ползти creep* out, crawl out.

вы́ползти *сов. см.* выполза́ть.

выполн|е́ние *с.* (*плана*) fulfilment, cárrying-out, execútion; (*обязанностей*) dischárge, performance. ~и́мый féasible; cápable of execútion *после сущ.*

вы́полнить *сов. см.* выполня́ть.

выполня́ть, вы́полнить (вн.) 1. (*осуществлять*) fulfíl (*smth.*), cárry out (*smth.*), éxecute (*smth.*); (*обязанности*) perfórm (*smth.*), dischárge (*smth.*); ~ свой долг do*/perfórm *one's* dúty; ~ своё обеща́ние keep* *one's* prómise; ~ обяза́тельство fulfíl/implement an obligátion; ~ план на 110% excéed the plan by ten per cent; ~ прика́з cárry out *one's* órders; не ~ прика́за fail to comply; 2. (*создавать*) do* (*smth.*), make* (*smth.*), éxecute (*smth.*).

выполня́ться *несов.* be* fulfílled, be* cárried out.

вы́полоскать *сов. см.* выпола́скивать.

вы́полоть *сов.* (вн.) pull (*smth.*) out; (*грядки и т. п.*) weed (*smth.*).

вы́пороть I *сов. см.* выпа́рывать.

вы́пороть II *сов. см.* пороть II.

вы́порхнуть *сов.* flútter out, flit out.

вы́потрошить *сов. см.* потроши́ть.

вы́править(ся) *сов. см.* выправля́ть(ся).

вы́правка *ж.* (*осанка*) béaring, cárriage.

выправля́ть, вы́править (вн.) 1. (*выпрямлять*) stráighten out (*smth.*); 2. (*исправлять*) corréct (*smth.*); (*ошибку*) réctify (*smth.*); 3. (*улучшать*) put* (*smth.*) right. ~ся, вы́правиться 1. (*выпрямляться*) stráighten out; 2. *разг.* (*исправляться*) impróve.

выпра́шивать, вы́просить (вн. у рд.) cadge (*smth.* off), wheedle (*smth.* out of); *несов. тж.* try to wheedle (*smth.* out of).

выпрова́живать, вы́проводить (вн.) *разг.* send* (*smb.*) about his, her búsiness, send* (*smb.*) pácking.

вы́проводить *сов. см.* выпрова́живать.

вы́просить *сов. см.* выпра́шивать.

выпры́гивать, вы́прыгнуть jump out (of); ~ в окно́ jump out of a window; ~ из маши́ны jump out of a car.

вы́прыгнуть *сов. см.* выпры́гивать.

выпряга́ть, вы́прячь (вн.) únhárness (*smth.*), únhítch (*smth.*).

выпрями́тель *м. эл.* réctifier.

выпрям|и́ть(ся) *сов. см.* выпрямля́ть(ся). ~ле́ние *с.* stráightening out; ~ле́ние то́ка *эл.* rectificátion.

выпрямля́ть, вы́прямить (вн.) 1. stráighten (*smth.*); ~ ток *эл.* réctify the cúrrent. ~ся, вы́прямиться stráighten *one's* back; ~ся во весь рост draw* *oneself* up to *one's* full height.

вы́прячь *сов. см.* выпряга́ть.

вы́пукло in relíef; *перен.* (*выразительно*) vívidly.

вы́пукло-во́гнутый cónvéxo-cóncáve.

вы́пукл|ость *ж.* 1. (*свойство*) convéxity; 2. (*выпуклое место*) bulge; protúberance. ~ый 1. cónvéx; 2. (*выдающийся вперёд*) protúberant; (*о глазах, лбе*) búlging; *перен.* (*выразительный*) vívid, clear, distínct; ~ый о́браз vívid pícture.

вы́пуск *м.* 1. (*денег, акций и т. п.*) íssue; (*книг, газет*) publicátion; (*в продажу, на экран*) reléase; (*пара, воды и т. п.*) dischárge; (*из учебного заведения*) graduátion; 2. *уст.* (*сокращение, исключение*) cut; 3. (*номер журнала*) númber, íssue; (*часть издания*) instálment; 4. (*количество выпущенной продукции*) óutput; 5. (*количество окончивших вуз*) (the númber of) gráduates; (*количество окончивших среднюю школу*) (the númber of) léavers; ~ про́шлого го́да last year's léavers.

выпуск|а́ть, вы́пустить (вн.) 1. let* (*smb., smth.*) out; не ~ кого́-л. и́з дому not let *smb.* out of the house; вы́пустить что́-л. из рук let* *smth.* go, relínquish *one's* hold on *smth.*; **2.** (*дым, воду и т. п.*) dischárge (*smth.*); ~ пары́ blow* off steam; **3.** (*освобождать*) reléase (*smb., smth.*); вы́пустить кого́-л. на свобо́ду set* *smb.* at líberty; **4.** (*из учебного заведения*) prepáre (*smb.*), train (*smb.*); институ́т ~ает в э́том году́ 150 студе́нтов the húndred-and-fífty stúdents will gráduate from the ínstitute this year; институ́т ~ает матема́тиков и фи́зиков the ínstitute prepáres/trains mathematícians and phýsicists; **5.** (*изделия, товары и т. п.*) prodúce (*smth.*), turn out (*smth.*); ~ проду́кцию сверх пла́на excéed *one's* prodúction tárget; ~ что-л. в прода́жу reléase *smth.* for sale; ~ что-л. на ры́нок put* *smth.* on the márket; **6.** (*книги и т. п.*) públish (*smth.*); (*фильм*) reléase (*smth.*); **7.** (*пускать в обращение*) íssue (*smth.*); ~ заём íssue a loan; ~ ма́рки íssue stamps; **8.** (*исключать, выкидывать*) omít (*smth.*), cut* (*smth.*); вы́пустить стро́чку omít/miss a line; **9.** (*выставлять наружу*) shoot* out (*smth.*), thrust* out (*smth.*); ~ ко́гти show* its claws; ◇ вы́пустить снаря́д ejéct a shell; вы́пустить в свет públish, íssue.

выпускн|и́к *м.* fínal-year stúdent; (*школьник тж.*) léaver. ~о́й: ~о́й класс léavers' class; graduátion-class; ~о́й курс fínal-year stúdents *pl*; ~о́й экза́мен fínal/pássing-out examinátion; finals *pl*; ~о́е отве́рстие óutlet; ~о́й кла́пан exháust-valve.

вы́пустить *сов. см.* выпуска́ть.

вы́путаться *сов. см.* выпу́тываться.

вы́путываться, вы́путаться éxtricate onesélf, disentángle onesélf.

вы́пучить *сов.*: ~ глаза́ *разг.* góggle.

вы́пытать *сов. см.* выпы́тывать.

выпы́тывать, вы́пытать (*вн. у рд.*) *разг.* drag (*smth.* out of), pump (*smth.* out of); *несов. тж.* try to elícit (*smth.* from).

вы́пятить(ся) *сов. см.* выпя́чивать(ся).

выпя́чивать, вы́пятить (*вн.*) *разг.* thrust* out (*smth.*); *перен.* (*особо подчёркивать*) play up (*smth.*); émphasize (*smth.*), lay* stress (upón). ~ся, вы́пятиться *разг.* protrúde; stick* out (*тж. перен.*).

выраба́тывать, вы́работать (*вн.*) **1.** (*производить*) manufácture (*smth.*), prodúce (*smth.*). **2.** (*план и т. п.*) work (*smth.*) out; **3.** (*воспитывать*) devélop (*smth.*); ~ в себе́ си́лу во́ли devélop *one's* will; **4.** (*зарабатывать*) earn (*smth.*), make* (*smth.*); ~ся рабо́тается form, devélop; у него́ вы́работалась привы́чка ра́но встава́ть he has devéloped the hábit of gétting up éarly.

вы́работать(ся) *сов. см.* выраба́тывать(ся).

вы́работк|а *ж.* **1.** (*производство*) manufácture; тка́ни ручно́й ~и handmáde fábrics; **2.** (*количество выработанного*) óutput, prodúction; (*средняя*) ~ на одного́ рабо́чего (áverage) indivídual óutput; **3.** *разг.* (*качество*) quálity; гру́бая ~ coarse quálity; **4.** *обыкн. мн.* (*место добычи*) wórkings.

выра́внивать, вы́ровнять (*вн.*) **1.** (*делать ровным, гладким*) smooth (*smth.*), lével (*smth.*); ~ доро́гу lével a road, give* a road a lével súrface; **2.** (*выпрямлять*) steer/fly* (*smth.*) straight; (*в горизонтальной плоскости*) fly* (*smth.*) lével; **3.** (*располагать в ряд*) align (*smth.*); *воен.* dress (*smth.*); ◇ вы́ровнять шаг keep* in step. ~ся, вы́ровняться **1.** (*выпрямляться*) stráighten out; (*горизонтально*) flátten out; (*располагаться в ряд*) line up; *воен.* dress; **3.** (*выправляться*) impróve.

выраж|а́ть, вы́разить (*вн.*) **1.** expréss (*smth.*); ~ благода́рность кому́-л. expréss *one's* thanks to smb.; ~ что-л. слова́ми put* *smth.* into words; **2.** *тк. несов.* (*обозначать*) denóte (*smth.*), expréss (*smth.*); **3.** (*обозначать в каких-л. единицах*) expréss (*smth.*). ~а́ться, вы́разиться **1.** (в *пр.*) (*проявляться*) find* expréssion (in), mánifest itsélf (in); (*принимать форму*) take* the form (of); ~а́ться в том, что... expréss itsélf in the fact that...; **2.** (*высказываться*) expréss onesélf; ◇ мя́гко ~а́ясь to put it mildly. ~е́ние *с.* expréssion; ~е́ние лица́

expréssion; си́льные ~е́ния strong lánguage *sg*; ◇ чита́ть без ~е́ния read* monótonously, read* withóut ány expréssion; с ~е́нием with expréssion.

вы́раженн|ый: я́рко, ре́зко ~ pronóunced, marked; сла́бо ~ slight; я́рко ~ая фо́рма боле́зни an acúte form of a diséase.

вырази́тель *м.* spókesman*, móuthpiece.

вырази́тельн|ость *ж.* expréssiveness. ~ый **1.** expréssive; ~ые глаза́ éloquent eyes; **2.** *разг.* (*многозначительный*) méaningful, signíficant.

вы́разить *сов. см.* выража́ть 1, 3. ~ся *сов. см.* выража́ться.

выраста́ть, вы́расти **1.** (*становиться больше*) grow*; как вы вы́росли! how you have grown!; де́рево вы́росло до огро́мных разме́ров the tree grew to an enórmous size; ~ из оде́жды grow* out of *one's* clothes; **2.** (*достигать зрелого возраста*) grow* up; он совсе́м вы́рос he is quite grówn-up now; **3.** (в *вн.*) (*становиться кем-л.*) becóme (*smb.*), devélop (ínto); он вы́рос в кру́пного учёного he becáme a great scíentist; **4.** (*увеличиваться*) incréase, grow*; **5.** (*появляться*) appéar, come* into sight; ◇ вы́расти в чьих-л. глаза́х grow*/impróve in *smb.'s* opínion, go* up in *smb.'s* estimátion.

вы́расти *сов. см.* выраста́ть.

вы́растить *сов. см.* выра́щивать.

выра́щивать, вы́растить (*вн.*) (*растения*) grow* (*smth.*), raise (*smth.*), cúltivate (*smth.*); (*животных*) rear (*smth.*), breed* (*smth.*); (*детей*) bring* up (*smth.*); *перен.* (*кадры*) train (*smth.*).

вы́рвать I *сов. см.* вырыва́ть I.

вы́рва|ть II *сов. безл. разг.:* его́ ~ло he was sick, he was ill.

вы́рваться *сов. см.* вырыва́ться 2, 3, 4.

вы́рез *м.* cut, slit; блу́зка с треуго́льным ~ом blouse with a V-neck; пла́тье с ни́зким ~ом lów-necked dress.

вы́резать *сов. см.* выреза́ть и ре́зать 4.

выреза́ть, вы́резать (*вн.*) **1.** cut* out; (*удалять*) remóve (*smth.*); **2.** (*гравировать*) carve (*smth.*) (*на дереве*) engráve (*smth.*) (*на металле*); **3.** (*истреблять*) sláughter (*smb., smth.*).

вы́резка *ж.* **1.** (*действие*) cútting out; **2.** (*вырезанное место*) cut; газе́тная ~ press cútting; press clípping; **3.** (*часть туши*) fíllet, sírloin.

вы́рисовать(ся) *сов. см.* вырисо́вывать(ся).

вырисо́вывать, вы́рисовать (*вн.*) trace (*smth.*) out; (*тщательно писать*) inscríbe (*smth.*). ~ся, вы́рисоваться be* óutlined, come* into view.

вы́ровнять(ся) *сов. см.* выра́внивать(ся).

вы́родиться *сов. см.* вырожда́ться.

вы́родок *м. разг.* degénerate.

вырожд|а́ться, вы́родиться degénerate. ~е́ние *с.* degéneracy.

вы́ронить *сов.* (*вн.*) drop (*smth.*), let* (*smth.*) fall; ~ что-л. из рук drop *smth.*

выруба́ть, вы́рубить (*вн.*) **1.** (*срубать*) cut* (*smth.*) down; (*о деревьях тж.*) fell (*smth.*); **2.** (*извлекать, рубя*) cut* (*smth.*) out; (*топором*) hack (*smth.*) out; **3.** (*высекать*) cut* (*smth.*) out; carve (*smth.*); **4.** *горн.* cut* (*smth.*), dig* (*smth.*).

вы́рубить *сов. см.* выруба́ть.

вы́рубка *ж.* **1.** (*действие*) cútting; **2.** (*вырубленное место в лесу*) cléaring.

вы́ругать *сов. см.* руга́ть. ~ся *сов.* swear*.

выруча́ть, вы́ручить (*вн.*) *разг.* **1.** (*помогать*) réscue (*smb.*), help (*smb.*) out; ~ кого́-л. из беды́ help *smb.* out of a dífficulty; **2.** (*получать за проданное*) recéive (*smth.*) (in cash).

вы́ручить *сов. см.* выруча́ть.

вы́ручк|а *ж.* **1.** *разг.* (*помощь*) aid; прийти́ на ~у кому́-л. come* to the assístance/réscue of *smb.*; **2.** (*деньги*) tákings *pl.*

вырыва́ть I, **вы́рвать** (*вн.*) pull (*smth.*) out; (*с большой силой*) wrench (*smth.*) out; (*о растении*) pull (*smth.*) up, tear* (*smth.*) up; *перен.* force (*smth.*); ~ что-л. из рук snatch *smth.* out of *smb.'s* hands; ~ зуб extract a tooth*, take* out a tooth*; ~ страни́цу tear* out a page; вы́рвать согла́сие у *кого-л.* wring* consént from *smb.*; вы́рвать призна́ние у *кого-л.* force an admission from *smb.*

вырыва́ть II, **вы́рыть** (*вн.*) 1. (*яму и т. п.*) dig* (*smth.*); 2. (*извлека́ть*) dig* up (*smth.*).

вырыва́ться, вы́рваться 1. *тк. несов.* (*пыта́ться освободи́ться*) strúggle to get free, try to break awáy; 2. (*высвобожда́ться*) break* awáy; break* loose, get* awáy (from); вы́рваться на свобо́ду escápe, free onesélf; вы́рваться из окруже́ния escápe from encírclement; 3. (*стреми́тельно появля́ться*) escápe, burst* out, break* through; (*о пла́мени, дыме тж.*) gush out; у меня́ нево́льно вы́рвалось это сло́во I didn't mean to use that word; 4. (*уходи́ть вперёд*) break* awáy, forge ahéad.

вы́рыть *сов. см.* **вырыва́ть** II.

выряди́ться *сов. разг.* get*/dress onesélf up; (*о же́нщинах тж.*) put* on *one's* best bib and túcker.

выса́д|ить(ся) *сов. см.* **выса́живать(ся).** ~ка *ж.* 1. (*с су́дна*) disembarkátion, debarkátion, lánding; (*с по́езда*) detráinment; ~ка (*возду́шного*) деса́нта (áirborne) lánding; 2. (*расте́ний*) bédding out, transplánting.

выса́живать, вы́садить (*вн.*) 1. put* (*smb., smth.*) down; (*принуди́тельно*) put* (*smb.*) off; (*на бе́рег*) put* (*smb.*) ashóre, disembárk (*smb.*), land (*smb.*); 2. (*расте́ния*) bed (*smth.*) out; transplánt (*smth.*). ~ся, вы́садиться land; (*из рд.*) get* out (of), get* off (*smth.*), alight (from); (*с су́дна*) disembárk (from).

выса́сывать, вы́сосать (*вн.*) suck (*smth.*) out; ◇ ~ из па́льца что-л. make* *smth.* up, concóct *smth.*

вы́свободить(ся) *сов. см.* **высвобожда́ть(ся).**

высвобожда́ть, вы́свободить (*вн.*) 1. free (*smth.*), liberate (*smth.*); ~ но́гу из стре́мени take* *one's* foot* out of the stírrup; 2. (*сре́дства, люде́й*) make* (*smth.*) aváilable, reléase (*smb., smth.*). ~ся, вы́свободиться 1. free onesélf, reléase onesélf; 2. (*о сре́дствах и т. п.*) becóme* aváilable.

высева́ть, вы́сеять (*вн.*) sow* (*smth.*).

высека́ть, вы́сечь 1. (*вн. на, в пр.; выруба́ть*) cut* (*smth.* on, out of), hew* (*smth.* out of); 2. (*ваять*) carve (*smth.* out of); вы́сеченный из ка́мня carved out of stone, hewn from stone; ◇ ~ ого́нь strike* fire, strike* a spark.

выселе́ние *с.* evíction.

вы́селить(ся) *сов. см.* **выселя́ть(ся).**

выселя́ть, вы́селить (*вн.*) evíct (*smb.*). ~ся, вы́селиться move.

вы́сечь I *сов. см.* **высека́ть.**

вы́сечь II *сов. см.* **сечь** I.

вы́сеять *сов. см.* **высева́ть.**

вы́сидеть *сов. см.* **высиживать.**

высиживать, вы́сидеть 1. *разг.* (*остава́ться*) remáin, stay; я не мог вы́сидеть до конца́ I simply cóuldn't sit it out; 2. (*вн.; птенцо́в*) hatch out (*smth.*).

вы́ситься *несов.* (*над тв.*) tówer (abóve).

выска́бливать, вы́скоблить (*вн.*) 1. (*пове́рхность*) scrape (*smth.*); 2. (*удаля́ть скобле́нием*) scrape (*smth.*) off; (*напи́санное*) scrape (*smth.*) out; 3. *мед.* curétte (*smth.*).

выска́зать(ся) *сов. см.* **выска́зывать(ся).**

выска́зывание *с.* státement.

выска́зывать, вы́сказать (*вн.*) state (*smth.*), expréss (*smth.*), voice (*smth.*); (*вн. дт.*) tell* (*smb. smth.*); ~ предположе́ние voice a supposítion; вы́сказать *кому-л.* всю пра́вду в глаза́ tell* *smb.* the truth to his, her face; вы́сказать сомне́ние expréss doubt. ~ся, вы́сказаться 1. speak* (out), expréss/state *one's* opinion; да́йте ему́ вы́сказаться! let him have his say!; ~ся в по́льзу *кого-л.*

чего-л. speak* up for *smb., smth.*; предложи́ть *кому-л.* вы́сказаться invíte *smb.* to state his, her opínion; 2. (*за вн., про́тив рд.*) speak* (for, agáinst), come* out (in fávour of, agáinst).

выска́кивать, вы́скочить 1. jump out, leap* out; вы́скочить из окна́ jump/leap* out of a window; 2. *разг.* (*поспе́шно выбега́ть и т. п.*) pop out; вы́скочить вперёд get* in front, forge ahéad; 3. *разг.* (*с тв.; ра́ньше други́х вя́зываться в како́е-л. де́ло*) be* in a húrry (with, + to *inf.*); ~ с замеча́ниями be* in a húrry to make remárks; 4. *разг.* (*па́дать отку́да-л.*) come* out; вы́скочить из рук slip out of *one's* hands; ◇ вы́скочить из головы́, из па́мяти go* right out of *one's* head, slip *one's* mémory.

выска́льзывать, вы́скользнуть slip out.

вы́скоблить *сов. см.* **выска́бливать.**

вы́скользнуть *сов. см.* **выска́льзывать.**

вы́скоч|ить *сов. см.* **выска́кивать.** ~ка *м. и ж. разг.* úpstart.

вы́слать *сов. см.* **высыла́ть.**

вы́следить *сов. см.* **выслёживать.**

выслёживать, вы́следить (*вн.*) track (*smb.*); trail (*smb.*); trace (*smb.*); *сов. тж.* track (*smb.*) down, run* (*smb.*) to earth.

вы́слуг|а *ж.*: за ~у лет for length of sérvice.

выслу́живаться, вы́служиться (*перед тв.*) *разг.* cúrry fávour (with); ingrátiate onesélf (with).

вы́служиться *сов. см.* **выслу́живаться.**

вы́слушать *сов. см.* **выслу́шивать.**

выслу́шивание *с. мед.* auscultátion.

выслу́шивать, вы́слушать (*вн.*) 1. listen (to); (*до конца́*) listen to the whole (of); вы́слушать *кого-л.* listen to what *smb.* has to say; hear* *smb.* out; я не вы́слушал ле́кции до конца́ I didn't stay to the end of the lécture; вы́слушать о́бе сторо́ны listen to both sides of the stóry; 2. *мед.* examine (*smb., smth.*); (*лёгкие*) sound (*smth.*).

высма́тривать, вы́смотреть (*вн.*) 1. (*находи́ть, замеча́ть*) spot (*smb., smth.*), detéct (*smb., smth.*); 2. (*разгля́дывать*) obsérve (*smth.*); *сов. тж.* spot (*smth.*); ◇ вы́смотреть глаза́ tíre *one's* eyes out.

высме́ивать, вы́смеять (*вн.*) scoff (at), make* fun (of), rídicule (*smb.*), deríde (*smb.*).

вы́смеять *сов. см.* **высме́ивать.**

вы́сморкать *сов.*: ~ нос blow* *one's* nose. ~ся *сов. см.* **сморка́ться.**

вы́смотреть *сов. см.* **высма́тривать.**

высо́вывать, вы́сунуть (*вн.*) put* out (*smth.*), thrust* out (*smth.*); ~ язы́к put*/stick* out *one's* tongue. ~ся, вы́сунуться lean* out; (*торча́ть*) stick* out, show*; ~ся из окна́ lean*/put* *one's* head out of the window.

высо́к|ий 1. high; (*о челове́ке, живо́тном*) tall; ~ ма́льчик tall boy; ~ дом tall/high búilding; ~ая ме́стность high locálity, high ground; ко́мната с ~им потолко́м room with a high céiling; ~ая вода́ high wáter; (*при прили́ве*) high tide; 2. (*большо́й, значи́тельный*) high; ~ урожа́й high yield, big crop, búmper crop/hárvest; ~ая производи́тельность труда́ high productívity of lábour; 3. (*отли́чный, хоро́ший*) great; ~ое мастерство́ great skill; ~ая оце́нка high appreciátion/asséssment; 4. (*почётный, ва́жный*) high; ~ая награ́да high awárd; ~ая честь great hónour; ~ гость hónoured guest; 5. (*возвы́шенный*) élevated, lófty; ~ поры́в lófty urge/impulse; 6. (*о зву́ках*) high, high-pítched; ◇ Высо́кие Догова́ривающиеся Сто́роны the High Contrácting Párties; ~ая грудь high breast; ~ лоб high fórehead; lófty brow; ~ая та́лия short waist; быть ~ого мне́ния о *ком-л.* have* a high opínion of *smb.*, think* híghly of *smb.*

высо́ко 1. *нареч.* high, high up, ~ в не́бе high (up) in the sky; (*о свети́лах тж.*) high in the héavens; ~ над голово́й far abóve *one's* head; ~ подня́ться climb high; ~ держа́ть го́лову hold* *one's* head high; ~ цени́ть *кого-л.* válue *smb.* híghly, hold* *smb.* in high estéem; 2. *в знач.*

сказ. it is too high; до вершины горы ещё ~ it is still a long way to the top of the móuntain.

высоково́льтн|ый *эл.* high vóltage *attr.*, high-ténsion *attr.*; ~ые се́ти high-ténsion lines.

высокого́рный high-móuntain *attr.*, high-áltitude *attr.*, Álpine.

высокоиде́йный high-príncipled.

высокока́чественный high-quálity *attr.*, high-gráde *attr.*

высококвалифици́рованный híghly skilled.

высококульту́рный: ~ челове́к véry cúltivated/cúltured pérson.

высокоме́р|ие *с.* háughtiness, supercíliousness, árrogance. ~ный háughty, supercílious, árrogant.

высокомолекуля́рный high-molécular.

высокоодарённый véry tálented; híghly endówed; gífted.

высокопа́рный high-flówn, grandíloquent.

высокопоста́вленный high-ránking.

высокопродукти́вн|ый híghly prodúctive; ~ая о́трасль се́льского хозя́йства híghly prodúctive branch of ágriculture.

высокопроизводи́тельн|ый híghly efficient, híghly prodúctive; ~ые станки́ híghly efficient machínes; ~ые ме́тоды труда́ híghly prodúctive (work) méthods.

высокора́звит|ый híghly devéloped; ~ая страна́ híghly devéloped cóuntry.

высокосо́ртный high-quálity *attr.*

высокоурожа́йн|ый high-yíeld *attr.*; ~ые культу́ры high-yíeld crops.

высокочасто́тный high fréquency *attr.*

вы́сосать *сов. см.* выса́сывать.

высот|а́ *ж.* **1.** height; *ав.*, *геогр.*, *астр. тж.* áltitude; **2.** (*возвышенность, холм*) elevátion; height; **3.** (*звука*) pitch; ◇ быть на ~е́ положе́ния rise* to the occásion; не на ~е́ not at one's best.

высо́тник *м.* **1.** (*строитель*) spíderman*; **2.** (*о лётчике*) high-áltitude pílot; (*об альпинисте*) high-áltitude clímber.

высо́тн|ый 1. high-áltitude *attr.*; **2.** (*о здании*) tall; ~ дом high-rise(r).

вы́сох|нуть *сов. см.* высыха́ть. ~ший dry; (*о листьях и т. п.*) shrívelled, wíthered; *перен.* (*о человеке*) wízened, dríed-up.

вы́спаться *сов. см.* высыпа́ться II.

выспра́шивать, вы́спросить (*вн. у рд.*) *разг.* pump (*smth.* out of).

вы́спросить *сов. см.* выспра́шивать.

вы́став|ить(ся) *сов. см.* выставля́ть(ся). ~ка *ж.* exhibítion, show; exposítion *амер.*; ~ка в витри́не магази́на window-display; ~ка карти́н exhibítion of páintings; ~ка соба́к dóg-show; всеми́рная ~ка world fair; Вы́ставка достиже́ний наро́дного хозя́йства Exhibítion of Nátional Económic Achíevement.

выставля́ть, вы́ставить (*вн.*) **1.** (*вынимать вставленное*) take* (*smth.*) out, remóve (*smth.*); ~ ра́му remóve the window-frame; **2.** (*наружу*) put* (*smth.*) out; *перен. разг.* (*выгонять*) turn (*smb.*) out; ~ на свет expóse to the light; ~ кого́-л. за дверь turn *smb.* out of doors, turn *smb.* out of the house; **3.** (*выдвигать вперёд*) put* (*smth.*) fórward; stick* out (*smth.*); ~ кула́к put* up one's fist; ~ но́гу stick* out one's foot; **4.** (*для обсуждения*) propóse (*smth.*); bring* (*smth.*) up; ~ чью́-л. кандидату́ру propóse *smb.'s* candidature; **5.** (*охрану и т. п.*) mount (*smth.*); post (*smb.*, *smth.*), set* (*smb.*, *smth.*); ~ карау́л mount/post the guard; ~ охране́ние place/man the óutposts; ~ часово́го post a séntry; set* a séntinel *амер.*; **6.** (*помещать для обозрения*) displáy (*smth.*); exhíbit (*smth.*), show* (*smth.*); **7.** *разг.* (*представлять, изображать*) presént (*smth.*, *smth.*); ~ что́-л. в хоро́шем све́те put* *smth.* in a fávourable light; ~ кого́-л. на осмея́ние make* a

láughing-stock of *smb.* ~ся, вы́ставиться **1.** (*помещать свои работы на выставке*) exhíbit; **2.** *разг.* (*показывать свои достоинства*) show* off; **3.** *разг.* (*высовываться*) show* onesélf, lean* out, emérge.

вы́ставочный exhibítion *attr.*; ~ комите́т exhibítion committee; (*выставки картин*) hánging committee; ~ зал shów-room.

выста́ивать, вы́стоять 1. stand*; ~ часа́ми в о́череди queue for hours; **2.** (*удерживаться*) stand*; *перен.* hold* out; э́то зда́ние вы́стоит ещё мно́го лет that building will stand for years. ~ся, вы́стояться **1.** (*о вине и т. п.*) matúre; **2.** (*о лошади*) rest.

выстила́ть, вы́стлать (*вн. тв.*) (*пол, землю*) cóver (*smth.* with); (*изнутри*) line (*smth.* with); (*мостить*) pave (*smth.* with).

вы́стирать *сов. см.* стира́ть II.

вы́стлать *сов. см.* выстила́ть.

вы́стоять(ся) *сов. см.* выста́ивать(ся).

вы́страд|ать *сов.* (*вн.*) **1.** súffer (*smth.*), endúre (*smth.*); он мно́го ~ал he has been through a lot; **2.** (*добиться ценой страданий*) achíeve (*smth.*) through súffering, concéive (*smth.*) in súffering; learn* (*smth.*) the hard way *разг.*; ~ своё сча́стье achíeve háppiness through súffering.

выстра́ивать, вы́строить (*вн.*) **1.** build* (*smth.*), put* up (*smth.*); **2.** (*располагать*) draw* up (*smb.*), form up (*smb.*). ~ся, вы́строиться form up, line up.

вы́стрел *м.* shot; (*звук*) repórt; произвести́ ~ fire a shot; ◇ без еди́ного ~а withóut firing a shot; ~ within shóoting distance; не подпуска́ть кого́-л. на расстоя́ние пу́шечного ~а от чего́-л. not let* *smb.* get ánywhere near *smth.* ~ить *сов.* fire (a shot); (*об оружии*) go* off; ~ить из ружья́ fire a gun; ~ить в кого́-л., во что́-л. fire at/on *smb.*, *smth.*; ~ить в кого́-л. из револьве́ра fire a revólver at *smb.*

вы́строить *сов. см.* выстра́ивать. ~ся *сов.* **1.** *см.* выстра́иваться; **2.** (*возникнуть*) spring* up.

вы́стукать *сов. см.* высту́кивать.

высту́кивать, вы́стукать (*вн.*) **1.** tap out (*smth.*); ~ сообще́ния tap out méssages; **2.** *мед.* percúss (*smth.*), tap (*smth.*); sound (*smb.*, *smth.*) by percússion/tápping.

вы́ступ *м.* projéction; (*стены тж.*) búttress; (*горизонтальный*) ledge.

выступа́ть, вы́ступить 1. (*выходить вперёд*) step out, come* fórward; emérge (*тж. перен.*); **2.** (*отправляться в путь и т. п.*) march out; ~ из ла́геря leave* camp; ~ в похо́д take* the field; **3.** *тк. несов.* (*важно шагать*) strut; **4.** *тк. несов.* (*выдаваться*) jut out, project; (*нависать*) óverháng; **5.** ~ из берего́в overflów its banks; **6.** (*появляться, проступать*) appéar, come* out; на лбу у него́ вы́ступил пот the sweat stood out on his fórehead; сыпь вы́ступила по всему́ те́лу a rash broke out all óver one's bódy; слёзы вы́ступили у неё на глаза́х tears came/rose/stárted to her eyes; **7.** (*публично*) speak*; (*на сцене*) appéar; ~ на собра́нии addréss a méeting; ~ с докла́дом make* a repórt; (*с научным*) give* a lécture; ~ в защи́ту свои́х прав stand* up for one's rights; ~ в защи́ту кого́-л. stand* up for *smb.*, speak* in defénce of *smb.*; ~ в печа́ти с письмо́м, со статьёй have* a létter, an árticle in the press; ~ с манифе́стом íssue a manifésto/státement; зате́м вы́ступил Ивано́в the next to speak was Ivanóv; (*об артисте*) next perfórmer was Ivanóv.

вы́ступить *сов. см.* выступа́ть 1, 2, 5, 6, 7.

выступле́ние *с.* **1.** (*на сцене*) appéarance; (*исполнение*) perfórmance; (*речь*) speech; (*в печати*) státement; **2.** (*отправление*) depárture.

вы́сунуть(ся) *сов. см.* высо́вывать(ся).

высу́шивать, вы́сушить (*вн.*) dry (*smth.*); *перен.* drain (*smth.*), exháust (*smth.*). ~ся, вы́сушиться dry.

вы́сушить *сов. см.* высу́шивать и суши́ть. ~ся *сов. см.* высу́шиваться и суши́ться.

вы́считать *сов. см.* высчи́тывать.

высчи́тывать, **вы́считать** *(вн.)* cálculate *(smth.)*; compúte *(smth.)*, réckon *(smth.)*.

вы́сш|ий 1. *(превосх. ст. прил. высокий 3, 4)* the highest; *(о качестве и т. п.)* supérior; ~ая то́чка clímax, ~его ка́чества of supérior/éxcellent quálity; tóp-quality; **2.** *(самый главный, руководящий)* supréme; ~ие о́рганы госуда́рственной вла́сти the supréme órgans of State pówer; ~ая суде́бная инста́нция the supréme/híghest judícial lével; **3.** *(совершенный)* the highest, pérfect; ~ая фо́рма организа́ции the highest form of organizátion; ~ пило́таж aerobátics; **4.**: ~ее образова́ние hígher educátion, educátion at univérsity lével; ~ие уче́бные заведе́ния hígher educátional institútions, hígher schools; **5.** *(более развитой, сложный)* hígher; ~ие млекопита́ющие hígher mámmals; ~ая матема́тика hígher mathemátics, cálculus; ◇ ~ая ме́ра наказа́ния death/supréme pénalty.

высыла́ть, **вы́слать** *(вн.)* **1.** *(отправлять)* send* *(smth.)*; dispátch *(smth.)*; **2.** *(изгонять)* éxile *(smb.)*; *(из страны)* depórt *(smb.)*.

вы́сылка *ж.* **1.** *(посылка)* dispátch; **2.** *(административная)* éxile; *(из страны)* deportátion.

высыпа́ть *сов. см.* высыпа́ть.

высыпа́ть, **вы́сыпать 1.** pour *(smth.)* out; *(нечаянно)* spill* *(smth.)*; **2.** *разг.* *(выходить, выбегать)* pour out; они́ вы́сыпали на у́лицу they poured out into the street; **3.** *(о сыпи)* break* out.

вы́сыпаться *сов. см.* высыпа́ться I.

высыпа́ться I, **вы́сыпаться** fall* out, spill* out.

высып|а́ться II, **вы́спаться** have* a good/próper sleep; *(ночью)* have* a good night's rest; он всё это вре́мя не ~а́ется he still isn't sléeping próperly.

высыха́ть, **вы́сохнуть 1.** dry (up); **2.** *(увядать)* wíther; **3.** *(худеть — о человеке)* waste awáy.

высь *ж.* height; *мн.* the heights, the lóftiest régions.

выта́лкивать, **вы́толкнуть** *(вн.)* push *(smb.)* out, hústle *(smb.)* out.

выта́птывать, **вы́топтать** *(вн.)* *(портить)* trámple *(smth.)* down; *(протаптывать)* tread* *(smth.)*; вы́топтать тропи́нку в снегу́ tread* a path in the snow.

вы́таращить *сов. см.* тара́щить.

выта́скивать, **вы́тащить** *(вн.)* **1.** drag *(smth.)* out; *(вынимать, выдёргивать)* pull *(smth.)* out; *перен. разг.* get* *(smth.)* out; вы́тащить кого́-л. гуля́ть get* smb. to come/go out for a walk; **2.** *разг.* *(красть, похищать)* steal* *(smth.)*, take* *(smth.)*.

вы́тащить *сов. см.* выта́скивать.

вытек|а́ть, **вы́течь 1.** *(откуда-л.)* run* out; **2.** *тк. несов.* *(из рд.; брать начало — о реке и т. п.)* rise* (from), take* its source (from); **3.** *тк. несов.* *(являться следствием)* fóllow; отсю́да ~а́ет сле́дующее заключе́ние from this may be drawn the fóllowing conclúsion; отсю́да ~а́ет, что... it fóllows that...; со все́ми ~а́ющими отсю́да после́дствиями with all the cónsequences ensúing therefróm.

вы́тереть(ся) *сов. см.* вытира́ть(ся).

вы́терп|еть *сов. (вн.)* endúre *(smth.)*, go* through *(smth.)*; *разг.* stand* it; он не ~ел и посмотре́л he could not resíst táking a look; не ~ев бо́ли, он закрича́л unáble to bear the pain ány lónger, he cried out.

вы́тертый *разг. (поношенный)* thréadbare.

вытесне́ние *с.* óusting, supersé́ding.

вы́теснить *сов. см.* вытесня́ть.

вытесня́ть, **вы́теснить** *(вн.)* **1.** force *(smth.)* out; *(противника тж.)* dislódge *(smb.)*; **2.** *(заменять собой)* oust *(smth.)*, supersé́de *(smth.)*; *физ.* displáce *(smth.)*; но́вые маши́ны вы́теснили ста́рые the old machínes were supersé́ded by new ones.

вы́течь *сов. см.* вытека́ть 1.

вытир|а́ть, **вы́тереть** *(вн.)* wipe *(smth.)*; *(мокрое*

тж.) dry *(smth.)*; ~ лоб mop/wipe one's brow; ~ пыль dust; ~ что́-л. до́суха wipe smth. dry; ~а́йте но́ги! please, wipe your feet! ~ться, вы́тереться dry onesélf; ~ться до́суха rub onesélf (quite) dry.

вы́толкнуть *сов. см.* выта́лкивать.

вы́топтать *сов. см.* выта́птывать.

вы́требовать *сов. (вн.)* **1.** get* *(smth.)*, obtáin *(smth.)*; **2.** *(заставлять явиться)* súmmon *(smb.)*; send* (for).

вытряса́ть, **вы́трясти** *(вн.)* shake* *(smth.)* out.

вы́трясти *сов. см.* вытряса́ть.

вытря́хивать, **вы́тряхнуть** *(вн.)* shake* *(smth.)* out.

вы́тряхнуть *сов. см.* вытря́хивать.

выть *несов.* howl, *(о ветре тж.)* wail, moan.

вытя́гивать, **вы́тянуть** *(вн.)* **1.** stretch *(smth.)*; ~ ше́ю crane one's neck; **2.** *разг.* *(вытаскивать)* pull *(smth.)* out; extráct *(smth.)*; *перен.* get* *(smth.)* out, extráct *(smth.)*; из него́ слова́ не вы́тянешь you can't get a word out of him; **3.** *(удалять тягой)* draw* *(smth.)* out; дым вы́тянуло the smoke has escáped; ◇ ~ ду́шу, все жи́лы у кого́-л. tíre smb. out, tíre smb. to death. ~ся, вы́тянуться **1.** *(растягиваться)* stretch; *разг.* *(вырастать)* grow*; он о́чень вы́тянулся he has grown enórmously; **2.** *(выпрямляться)* stand* up straight, draw* onesélf up; **4.** *(ложиться)* stretch onesélf, throw* onesélf down at full length; лежа́ть вы́тянувшись lie* stretched out; ◇ у него́ вы́тянулось лицо́ his face fell.

вытяжн|о́й: ~ вентиля́тор exháust-fán; ~ шкаф exháust-hóod; ~а́я труба́ exháust-pípe; ~о́е кольцо́ у парашю́та rip-córd.

вы́тянуть(ся) *сов. см.* вытя́гивать(ся).

вы́удить *сов. см.* выу́живать.

выу́живать, **вы́удить** *(вн.) разг.* fish *(smth.)* out; *перен. соах* *(smth.)* out; ~ де́ньги у кого́-л. coax móney out of smb.

выу́чивать, **вы́учить 1.** *(что-л.)* learn* *(smth.)*; **2.** *(кого-л.)* teach* *(smb.)*. ~ся, вы́учиться **1.** *(дт., + инф.)* learn* *(smth., + to inf)*; **2.** *(заканчивать учёбу)* finish one's educátion.

вы́учить(ся) *сов. см.* выу́чивать(ся).

вы́учка *ж.* **1.** *(действие)* tráining; **2.** *(умение)* trained skill/ability; боева́я ~ fíghting expérience, the skill of a trained and expérienced sóldier.

выха́живать, **вы́ходить** *(вн.) разг.* **1.** *(больного)* nurse/pull *(smb.)* through an íllness; nurse *(smb.)* back to health; **2.** *(выращивать)* bring* up *(smb.)*.

вы́хватить *сов. см.* выхва́тывать.

выхва́тывать, **вы́хватить 1.** *(вн. из, у рд.)* snatch *(smth. from)*; ~ что́-л. из рук snatch smth. out of smb.'s hands; **2.** *(вн.; вынимать)* whip out *(smth.)*; ~ ша́шку whip out one's sword; ~ цита́ты quote out of cóntext, dig* up irrélevant quotátions.

вы́хлопотать *сов. (вн.) разг.* mánage to get *(smth.)*, succéed in gétting *(smth.)*, obtáin *(smth.)*.

вы́ход *м.* **1.** *(действие)* góing out; *(из какой-л. организации)* withdráwal; *(на сцену)* éntrance; э́то был мой пе́рвый ~ по́сле боле́зни it was the first time I had been out (of doors) since my íllness; ~ на орби́ту góing into órbit; **2.** *(место выхода)* éxit, way out; *(выходное отверстие)* óutlet; в э́том до́ме не́сколько ~ов the house has séveral éxits; стоя́ть у ~а stand* at the door; ~ к мо́рю an óutlet to the sea; **3.** *(из затруднения и т. п.)* way out; друго́го ~а нет there's no altérnative; найти́ ~ find* a solútion; из вся́кого положе́ния есть ~ there's a way out of évery difficulty; **4.** *(журнала)* publicátion, íssue; *(книги тж.)* appéarance; **5.** *(продукции)* yield, óutput; ~ зерна́ с ка́ждого гекта́ра óutput per héctare; **6.** *геол. (жилы, пласта)* óutcrop; ~ слоя́ на пове́рхность óutcropping (of a strátum); ◇ дать ~ чу́вству give* vent to one's féelings; знать все ходы и ~ы know* all the ins and outs.

выход|ец *м.*: его родители ~цы из... his parents were natives of..., his parents came from...

выходит *в знач. вводн. сл. разг.* so; it turns out; ~, (что) я был прав I was right, after all.

выходить *сов. см.* выхаживать.

выход|ить, выйти 1. go* out, leave*; (*появляться*) come* out, emérge; (*выбывать из состава*) withdráw*, leave*; (*на поверхность — о жиле, пласте*) crop out, come* to the súrface; ~ из комнаты leave* the room; ~ на улицу go* out into the street; go* óutside; ~ из вагона, машины get* out of the cárriage, car; ~ из-за стола get* up, rise* from the táble; ~ из-за туч come* out from behind the clouds; ~ в море put* (out) to sea; ~ со станции (*о поезде*) pull out; ~ на сцену step on to the stage; appéar (on the stage); make* one's entry; ~ в тыл противнику gain the énemy's rear; ~ из боя *воен.* withdráw* from áction; ~ из войны withdráw* from the war; выйти на первое (второе) место move up into first (sécond) place; **2.** (*издаваться*) appéar, come* out; выйти из печати be* públished, come* off the press; **3.** (*становиться, делаться кем-л.*) be*, make*; из него выйдет хороший врач *и т. п.* he will make a good dóctor *etc.*; он вышел победителем в этом соревновании he was the winner of the competítion/match; **4.** (*удаваться*) come* off; (*о задаче, фотоснимке*) come* out; **5.** (*получаться, случаться*): вышло так, что... (as) it turned out...; у него никогда ничего не выйдет he'll néver amount to ánything; из этого ничего хорошего не выйдет no good will come of it; как бы чего не вышло something may háppen; ничего не выходит it's no use; что из этого выйдет? what will be the good of that?; **6.** *тк. несов.* (на, в *вн.*; *быть обращённым*) look (on to), face (*smth.*); комната выходит окнами на улицу the room fáces/overlóoks the street; окна выходят на юг the windows face south; **7.**: ~ замуж за кого-л. márry *smb.*; **8.** (*происходить*) come*, be*; он вышел из крестьян he comes of péasant stock; **9.** (*расходоваться*): у нас выходит много дров we use a lot of wood; у нас вышел весь бензин, сахар *и т. п.* we have run out of pétrol, súgar *etc.*; ◇ выйти в люди make* one's mark in life, achíeve a posítion in life; ~ на пéнсию retíre on one's pénsion; ~ в отставку resígn; (*по возрасту*) retíre; ~ из берегов overflów its banks; ~ из себя lose* one's témper, lose* contról of onesélf; fly* off the hándle *разг.*; ~ из затруднительного положения get* out of a tight córner, get* out of a difficulty; ~ из доверия lose* one's position of trust, becóme* distrústed; ~ из моды go* out of fáshion; ~ из повиновения get*/go* out of contról, get* out of hand; ~ из употребления fall* into disúse, go* out of use; ~ наружу come* out, come* to light.

выходка *ж.* trick, prank, escapáde.

выходн|ой: ~ день day off; free day, rést-day; ~ое отверстие óutlet; ~ое платье best clothes *pl*, one's best; ~ое пособие dischárge pay; ~ые данные públisher's/prínter's ímprint *sg*.

выхолащивать, выхолостить (*вн.*) geld (*smth.*), castráte (*smth.*); *перен.* emásculate (*smth.*), dilúte (*smth.*); выхолостить содержание чего-л. destróy the súbstance of *smth.*

выхоленный well-gróomed; well cáred-for.

выхолостить *сов. см.* выхолащивать.

выхухоль *ж.* **1.** (*животное*) músk-rat; **2.** (*мех*) músquash.

выцарапать *сов. см.* выцарапывать.

выцарапывать, выцарапать (*вн.*) **1.** scratch (*smth.*) out; **2.** *разг.* (*добывать с трудом*) squeeze (*smth.*) out of *smb.*; **3.** (*царапая, написать что-л.*) scratch (*smth.*).

выцвести *сов. см.* выцветать.

выцветать, выцвести fade, lose* cólour.

вычёркивать, вычеркнуть (*вн.*) cross (*smth.*) out, strike* (*smth.*) out, deléte (*smth.*); (*часть текста тж.*) expúnge (*smth.*); ◇ ~ из своей жизни кого-л. strike* *smb.* out of one's life; ~ кого-л. из памяти eráse *smb.* from one's mémory.

вычеркнуть *сов. см.* вычёркивать.

вычерпать *сов. см.* вычёрпывать.

вычёрпывать, вычерпать (*вн.*) scoop out (*smth.*); (*из лодки*) bail (out) (*smth.*).

вычёсывать, вычесать (*вн.*) comb out (*smth.*).

вычесть *сов. см.* вычитать.

вычет *м.* dedúction; ◇ за ~ом (*рд.*) exclúsive (of), mínus (*smth.*), allówing (for).

вычисление *с.* calculátion, computátion.

вычислитель|ный compúting; compúter *attr.*; ~ные машины compúters; ~ный центр compúter céntre; ~ная техника compúter technólogy.

вычислить *сов. см.* вычислять.

вычислять, вычислить (*вн.*) cálculate (*smth.*); compúte (*smth.*); réckon (*smth.*), éstimate (*smth.*).

вычистить *сов. см.* вычищать.

вычита|емое *с. мат.* súbtrahend. ~ние *с. мат.* subtráction; знак ~ния subtráction mark.

вычитать *сов. см.* вычитывать.

вычитать, вычесть (*вн.*) **1.** *мат.* subtráct (*smth.*); вычесть семь из десяти subtráct séven from ten, take* séven awáy from ten; **2.** (*удерживать*) dedúct (*smth.*).

вычитывать, вычитать (*вн.*) **1.** (*рукопись и т. п.*) read* (*smth.*) for the press; **2.** *разг.* (*узнавать, читая*) read* (*smth.*); вычитать из книги, что... read* in a book that...; где вы это вычитали? where did you get that from?

вычищать, вычистить (*вн.*) clean (*smth.*); вычистить что-л. щёткой brush *smth.*

вычурный preténtious.

вышвыривать, вышвырнуть (*вн.*) *разг.* throw* (*smth.*) out, chuck (*smth.*) out.

вышвырнуть *сов. см.* вышвыривать.

выше 1. (*сравнит. ст. прил.* высокий *и нареч.* высоко́) hígher; (*ростом*) táller; **2.** *нареч.* (*вверх от чего-л., сверх чего-л.*) óver, abóve; этажом ~ on the floor abóve, on the next floor; дети от пяти лет и ~ children of five and óver; **3.** *предлог* (*рд.*; *вне чего-л.*) beyónd, abóve; это ~ моих сил it is beyónd me; это ~ моего понимания it pásses my comprehénsion; it beats me *разг.*; **4.** *нареч.* (*на той же странице*) abóve; (*на предыдущей*) on a prévious page; как сказано ~ as státed abóve.

вышеизложенн|ый: всё ~ое the abóve, the fóregoing (státement).

вышеприведённый the above-méntioned, the afóresaid.

вышестоящий hígher; ~ орган hígher bódy, hígher authórity.

вышеуказанный *см.* вышеприведённый.

вышивание *с.* embróidery.

вышивать, вышить (*вн.*) embróider (*smth.*); ~ шёлком *и т.п.* embróider in silk *etc.*

вышивка *ж.* embróidery.

вышин|а *ж.* height; в ~é high up, alóft; (*в небе тж.*) in the sky.

вышитый embróidered.

вышить *сов. см.* вышивать.

вышка *ж.* tówer; (*для прыжков в воду*) díving-board; наблюдательная ~ watch / observátion tówer.

вышкол|енный *разг.* schooled, well-tráined, disciplined. ~ить *сов.* (*вн.*) *разг.* train (*smb.*), discipline (*smb.*).

выщипать *сов. см.* выщипывать.

выщипывать, выщипать (*вн.*) pull (*smth.*) out.

вы́яв|ить(ся) *сов. см.* выявля́ть(ся). ~ле́ние *с.* 1. discóvery; 2. (*разоблачение*) expósure.

выявля́ть, вы́явить (*вн.*) 1. revéal (*smth.*), bring* (*smth.*) to light; 2. (*разоблачать*) expóse (*smth.*), show* (*smth.*), lay* bare (*smth.*). ~ся, вы́явиться come* to light, be* revéaled.

выясне́ние *с.* elucidátion, clarificátion; ~ отноше́ний héart-to-héart talk; shów-down *разг.*

вы́ясн|ить(ся) *сов. см.* выясня́ть(ся).

выясн|я́ть, вы́яснить (*вн.*) elúcidate (*smth.*); (*устанавливать*) ascertáin (*smth.*); *несов. тж.* look (ínto), inquíre (ínto); *сов. тж.* find* out (*smth.*); вы́яснить вопро́с sort the mátter out, clear the mátter up. ~я́ться, вы́ясниться turn out; тепе́рь ~я́ется, что..., как тепе́рь вы́яснилось ... it now appéars that...

вьетнам|ец *м.,* ~ка *ж.* Vietnamése. ~ский Vietnám *attr.,* Vietnamése; ~ский язы́к Vietnamése, the Vietnamése lánguage.

вью́га *ж.* snów-storm.

вьюк *м.* pack, páck-load.

вьюн *м.* 1. (*рыба*) loach; 2. (*о человеке*) eel, slíppery féllow; ◇ ви́ться ~о́м о́коло кого́-л. dance atténdance on *smb.*

вьюно́к *м. бот.* bíndweed, convólvulus; mórning glóry *амер.*

вью́чн|ый pack *attr.;* ~ое живо́тное pack ánimal, beast of búrden; ~ая тропа́ brídle-path.

вью́шка *ж.* 1. (*печная*) dámper; 2. *тех.* (*для наматывания*) reel.

вью́щ|ийся: ~иеся во́лосы cúrly hair *sg;* ~ееся расте́ние créeper, clímbing-plant.

вя́жущий astríngent; ~ вкус astríngent taste.

вяз *м. бот.* elm.

вяза́льн|ый knítting; ~ая спи́ца knítting-needle; ~ крючо́к crochét-hook.

вяза́льщ|ик *м.,* ~ица *ж.* 1. knítter; 2. (*снопов*) bínder.

вяза́ние *с.* 1. (*связывание*) bínding; ~ снопо́в bínding of sheaves; ~ сете́й máking of nets; 2. (*спицами*) knítting; (*крючком*) crochét-work.

вяза́нка *ж.* (*дров и т. п.*) fággot; (*соломы, сена*) búndle, truss.

вяза́нье *с.* (*вещь, которая вяжется или связана*) knítting (*спицами*); crochét-work (*крючком*).

вяза́ть, связа́ть 1. (*вн.; связывать*) bind* (*smb., smth.*), tie (*smb., smth.*) up; bind* (*smth.*) togéther; ~ снопы́ bind* sheaves; 2. (*вн.; на спицах*) knit* (*smth.*); (*крючком*) crochét (*smth.*); 3. *тк. несов.* (*быть вяжущим*) be* astríngent; вя́жет во рту it draws the mouth.

вяза́ться *несов.* (*с тв.*) (*соответствовать*) fit in (with), tálly (with), be* compátible (with); э́то (ка́к-то) не вя́жется с... it (sómehow) doesn't seem compátible with..., it doesn't seem to fit in with...

вя́зка *ж.* 1. bínding, týing; 2. (*спицами*) knítting; (*крючком*) crochét-work; 3. *разг.* (*связка чего-л.*) búndle.

вя́зк|ий 1. (*липкий*) stícky, víscous; 2. (*топкий*) míry, spóngy, sóggy; (*о почве тж.*) swámpy. ~ость *ж.* 1. stíckiness, viscósity; 2. (*о почве*) swámpiness.

вя́знуть *несов.* stick*, get* stuck; ~ в грязи́ get* stuck in the mud.

вя́лен|ый sún-cured, dried; ~ое мя́со jerked meat; ~ая ры́ба dried fish.

вя́лить, провя́лить (*вн.*) dry (*smth.*); (*мясо*) cure (*smth.*), jerk (*smth.*).

вя́л|ость *ж.* slúggishness; (*мускулов*) flábbiness. ~ый 1. (*о растении*) fáded, dróoping; 2. (*о коже, мускулах*) flábby; (*о движениях, настроении*) slúggish; ~ая рука́ limp hand; 3. (*лишённый бодрости*) lánguid, spíritless; half-héarted; (*бессильный*) nérveless; 4. (*о рынке, торговле*) slack.

вя́н|уть, завя́нуть wilt, droop, fade, wíther; (*о деревьях*) turn; *перен.* (*о человеке*) fade, declíne, lose* heart; ◇ у́ши ~ут I am sick and tíred of héaring it.

Г

га *м.* héctare.

габарди́н *м.* gábardine. ~овый gábardine *attr.*

габари́т *м.* 1. cléarance, gabarít; (*размер*) diménsions *pl,* size; ~ы станко́в óverall machíne diménsions; 2. *ж.-д.* cléarance gauge.

га́вань *ж.* hárbour; háven *поэт.;* входи́ть в ~ énter hárbour.

га́га *ж. зоол.* éider(-duck).

гага́р|а *ж. зоол.* loon. ~ка *ж. зоол.* auk.

гага́чий: ~ пух éiderdown.

гад *м.* 1. *обыкн. мн. зоол.* réptile *sg;* 2. *бран.* skunk, réptile.

гада́|лка *ж.* fórtune-teller. ~ние *с.* 1. (*предсказывание*) divinátion; fórtune-telling; 2. (*предположение*) guéssing, guéss-work. ~тельный conjéctural; (*сомнительный*) problemátic, dóubtful.

гад|а́ть 1. погада́ть 1. tell* fórtunes; (*дт.*) tell* (*smb.*) his, her fórtune; 2. *тк. несов.* о *пр., строить дога́дки*) guess (at), surmíse (*smth.*), conjécture (*smth.*); ~ о бу́дущем spéculate abóut the future; ◇ ~ на кофе́йной гу́ще ≈ read* the téa-leaves, tell* fórtunes in a téacup; не ду́мал, не ~ал who would have thought it.

га́дина *ж.* 1. *разг.* réptile; 2. *бран.* swine, beast.

га́дк|ий násty; fílthy; ~ая пого́да násty/foul wéather; ~ посту́пок vile act, foul deed; ~ ребёнок náughty child*, hórrid líttle thing; он мне га́док I find him repúlsive; ◇ ~ утёнок úgly dúckling.

гадли́в|ость *ж.* disgúst, lóathing. ~ый disgústed; э́то вызыва́ет ~ое чу́вство it's lóathsome/disgústing, it's enóugh to make *one* sick.

га́дост|ь *ж. разг.* 1. filth; 2. (*подлость*) dírty trick; сде́лать ~ кому́-л. play *smb.* a dírty trick, play a dírty trick on *smb.;* кака́я ~! what a násty thing to do!; 3.: говори́ть ~и о ком-л. say* fílthy/násty things abóut *smb.*

гадю́ка *ж.* ádder; víper (*тж. перен.*).

га́ечн|ый nut *attr.;* ~ ключ spánner, wrench; ~ая резьба́ fémale thread.

газ I *м.* 1. gas; веселя́щий ~ láughing gas; слезоточи́вый ~ téar gas; приро́дный ~ nátural gas; 2. *мн.* (*в кишечнике*) flátulence *sg;* wind *sg разг.;* ◇ дать ~ *разг.* press down the accélerator; step on the gas *амер.;* сба́вить ~ *разг.* slow down; на по́лном ~у́ *разг.* at full speed.

газ II *м.* (*ткань*) gauze.

газго́льдер *м.* gásholder, gasómeter.

газе́т|а *ж.* néwspaper; páper *разг.;* ◇ стенна́я ~ wall néwspaper. ~ный néwspaper *attr.;* ~ная бума́га néwsprint; ~ный стиль journalése; ~ный кио́ск néwsstand. ~чик *м.* 1. *разг.* (*сотрудник газеты*) jóurnalist, préssman, néws-writer; 2. (*продавец*) néws-vendor, néwspaper-boy, néws-boy.

газиро́ванн|ый áerated; ~ая вода́ áerated wáter; ≈ sóda-water; ~ напи́ток effervéscent béverage, fízzy/spárkling drink.

газифи|ка́ция *ж.* 1. (*превращение в газ*) gasificátion; 2. (*снабжение газовой энергией*) installátion of gas; ~ городо́в и сёл installátion of gas in towns and víllages. ~ци́ровать *несов. и сов.* (*вн.*) 1. (*превращать в газ*) gásify (*smth.*); génerate gas (from); 2. (*проводить газ*) instáll gas (in), lay* gás-mains; го́род ~ци́рован the cíty is supplíed with gas.

газоаппарату́ра ж. gás-fittings *pl.*

газобалло́н *м.* gás-cylinder.

газовщи́к *м.* (*слесарь*) gás-fitter; (*контролёр и т. п.*) gásman*.

га́зов|ый I gas *attr.*; ~ заво́д gásworks; ~ая коло́нка géyser; ~ая плита́ gas stove/cóoker; ~ счётчик gás-meter; ~ая магистра́ль gas pípe-line; ◇ ~ая гангре́на gas gángrene; ~ая ре́зка gas cútting; ~ая сва́рка acétylene/gas wélding.

га́зовый II *текст.* gauze *attr.*; ~ шарф (fine) silk scarf.

газоли́н *м. тех.* gásolene.

газо́н *м.* lawn; по ~ам не ходи́ть ≈ keep off the grass.

газонепроница́емый (*о ткани*) gás-proof; (*о соединении*) gás-tight.

газоно́сный gás-bearing.

газообра́зный gáseous, gásiform.

газопрово́д *м.* gás-main, gás-pipe.

газоснабже́ние *с.* gas supplý.

газохрани́лище *с.* gasómeter.

га́йка ж. nut.

гак *м. разг.*: с ~ом and óver, or móre.

гала́ктика ж. *астр.* gálaxy.

галантере́йный: ~ магази́н háberdasher's (shop), háberdashery; dry goods store *амер.*

галантере́я ж. háberdashery; fáncy goods *pl*; dry goods *pl амер.*

гала́нт|ость ж. gállantry; ~ый gállant; cóurtly, cívil.

галдёж *м. разг.* húbbub of vóices, din; подня́ть ~ raise a din.

галде́ть *несов. разг.* chátter lóudly; make* a húbbub.

галере́я ж. gállery; карти́нная ~ pícture-gallery.

галёрка ж. *театр. разг.* 1. gállery; 2. (*публика*) the gods *pl.*

гале́та ж. bíscuit, ship's bíscuit.

галима́|я́ *м. разг.* rúbbish, rígmarole; нести́ ~ю make* up a rígmarole; Э́то сплошна́я ~ this is sheer nónsense.

галифе́ *мн. нескл.* ríding-breeches.

га́лка ж. (jáck)daw.

га́ллий *м. хим.* gállium.

галлюцин|а́ция ж. hallucinátion. ~и́ровать *несов.* súffer from hallucinátions; see* things *разг.*

галоге́н *м. хим.* hálogen.

галои́д *м. хим.* háloid.

гало́п *м.* 1. gállop; 2. (*танец*) gálop. ~и́ровать *несов.* gállop. ~ом at a gállop; скака́ть ~ом gállop.

гало́чк|а ж. *разг.* (*значок*) tick; ста́вить ~у на чём--л. tick (off) *smth.*

гало́ш|и *мн.* (*ед.* гало́ша ж.) galóshes; óver-shoes *разг.*; rúbbers *амер.*

галс *м. мор.* tack; пра́вым ~ом on the stárboard tack; ле́вым ~ом on the port tack.

га́лстук *м.* (néck)tie.

галу́н *м.* (gold, sílver) lace.

гальваниз|а́ция ж. *физ.* galvanizátion. ~и́ровать *несов. и сов.* (*вн.*) *физ.* gálvanize (*smth.*); *тех. тж.* eléctroplate (*smth.*).

гальвани́ческий *физ.* galvánic; ~ элеме́нт galvánic cell; ~ ток galvánic/díríct cúrrent.

га́льк|а ж. pébble; *собир.* pébbles *pl*; shíngle; морско́й бе́рег был усы́пан ~ой the beach was strewn with shíngle.

гам *м. разг.* húbbub, úproar; шум и ~ a terrific rácket/din.

гама́к *м.* hámmock.

гама́ши *мн.* (*ед.* гама́ша ж.) gáiters.

гамби́т *м. шахм.* gámbit.

га́мм|а I ж. *муз.* scale; *перен.* gámut; ~ до мажо́р scale of C májor; игра́ть ~ы play/práctise scales; ~ цвето́в range of cólours.

га́мма II ж. (*греческая буква*) gámma. ~-лучи́ *мн. физ.* gámma rays.

гангре́н|а ж. *мед.* gángrene. ~озный *мед.* gángrenous; ~озный проце́сс mortificátion.

га́нгстер *м.* gángster.

гандбо́л *м. спорт.* hándball.

гандика́п *м. спорт.* hándicap.

гантéль ж. *спорт.* dúmb-bell.

гара́ж *м.* gárage.

гара́нт *м. юр.* guarantór.

гаранти́йн|ый guarantée *attr.*; ~ срок guarantée (períod); ~ое письмо́ létter of guarantée/indémnity.

гаранти́рованн|ый guaranteéd; ~ая опла́та труда́ guaranteéd íncome/wáges.

гаранти́р|овать *несов. и сов.* 1. (*вн.; ручаться*) guarantée (*smth.*); wárrant (*smth.*); я ~ую вам успе́х I'll ánswer for your succéss; 2. (*вн. от рд.; защищать*) ensúre (*smth.* against), sáfeguard (*smth.* against).

гаранти|я ж. guarantée; ~ безопа́сности guarantée of secúrity; служи́ть ~ей успе́ха ensúre succéss; ~ на́ год a year's guarantée; с ~ей на́ два го́да guaranteéd for two years.

гардеро́б *м.* 1. (*шкаф*) wárdrobe; 2. (*помещение*) clóakroom; 3. (*одежда*) wárdrobe. ~щик *м.*, ~щица ж. clóakroom atténdant.

гарди́на ж. cúrtain.

га́рев|ый: ~ая доро́жка *спорт.* cínder track, cínder--path.

гаре́м *м.* hárem.

га́ркать, **га́ркнуть** (на *вн.*) *разг.* bark (at), shout (at).

га́ркнуть *сов. см.* га́ркать.

гармонизи́ровать *несов. и сов.* (*вн.*) *муз.* hármonize (*smth.*).

гармо́ника ж. accórdion; (*концертино*) concertína; ◇ губна́я ~ móuth-organ.

гармони́ровать *несов.* (с *тв.*) be* in hármony (with); (*о цвете*) go* (with).

гармони́ст *м.* accórdion pláyer.

гармони́ч|еский harmónic; (*гармоничный*) harmónious; ~ ряд harmónic séries. ~ность ж. harmóniousness, hármony. ~ный 1. (*благозвучный*) harmónious, concórdant; wéll-attúned; 2. (*соразмерный*) harmónious.

гармо́ния ж. hármony; *перен. тж.* cóncord.

гармо́нь ж. *разг. см.* гармо́ника.

гарнизо́н *м.* gárrison; нача́льник ~а gárrison/post commánder. ~ный gárrison *attr.*; ~ная слу́жба gárrison dúty.

гарни́р *м.* gárnish; trímmings *pl. разг.*; (*овощной*) végetables *pl*; с ~ом из чего́-л. (gárnished) with *smth.*

гарниту́р *м.* set; ~ ме́бели suíte; спа́льный ~ bédroom suíte; ~ белья́ set of únderwear.

гарпу́н *м.* harpóon; бить ~ом harpóon.

гарт *м. полигр.* týpe-metal.

га́рус *м.* wórsted (yarn). ~ный wórsted.

гарцева́ть *несов.* prance, prance alóng.

гарь ж. 1. fumes *pl*; па́хнет ~ю there's a smell of búrning; 2. (*остатки сгоревшего вещества*) cínder, ash, dross.

гаси́ть, **погаси́ть** (*вн.*) 1. put* out (*smth.*), extínguish (*smth.*); (*электричество тж.*) switch (*smth.*) off, turn (*smth.*) off; 2. *тех.* redúce (*smth.*); (*колебания*) damp (*smth.*); 3. (*погашать*) cáncel (*smth.*); 4. *спорт.*: ~ мяч kill the ball; ◇ ~ и́звесть slake lime.

га́сну|ть, **пога́снуть** fade; *перен.* (*терять силы*) wéaken, fade awáy; sink*. ~щий: ~щий свет dýing/fáding light.

гастролёр *м.* guést-performer; áctor on tour; *перен. разг.* bird of pássage. ~и́ровать *несов.* tour, be* on tour.

гастро́л|и *мн.* tour *sg*; на ~ях on tour. ~ьный:

~льная поéздка tour; ~льный спектáкль guést-
-perfórmance.

гастронóм *м.* 1. (*знаток пищи*) góurmet; 2. (*магазин*) food store(s). ~и́ческий gastronómical; ~и́ческий
магази́н food store(s); delicatéssen (store) *амер.* ~ия *ж.*
1. gastrónomy; 2. (*продукты*) gróceries and provísions
pl; delicatéssen *pl амер.*

гать *ж.* (*бревенчатая*) córduroy road, lóg-path; (*из
хвороста*) brúshwood-road.

гáубица *ж. воен.* hówitzer.

гауптвáхта *ж. воен.* guárdhouse.

гашён|ый: ~ая и́звесть slaked lime.

гашётк|а *ж. воен.* trígger; нажáть на ~y pull the
trígger.

гвалт *м. разг.* húbbub, row; поднимáть ~ raise a
hullaballóo/úproar.

гвард|éец *м.* guárdsman*. ~éйский Guards *attr.*;
~éйское знáмя Guards bánner; ~éйская диви́зия Guards
division, division of Guards.

гвáрди|я *ж.* Guards *pl*; ~и майóр, капитáн, лейте-
нáнт, рядовóй májor, cáptain, lieuténant, prívate/sóldier
of the Guards; ◇ стáрая ~ the old guard.

гвозди́ка I *ж.* (*цветок*) pink; махрóвая ~ carnátion;
туре́цкая ~ swéet-william.

гвозди́ка II *ж.* (*пряность*) clove.

гвозди́чн|ый: ~ое мáсло oil of cloves.

гвозд|ь *м.* nail; прибивáть ~я́ми nail.

где where; ~ бы ни, ~ бы (то) ни́ бы́ло wheréver; ◇
~ ему́...! he'll néver...! ~ уж нам! how can we?

где́|-либо, ~-нибудь, ~-то sómewhere; (*в вопр.
предложениях*) ánywhere; ~ в другóм мéсте sómewhere
else.

гегемóн *м.* predóminant force/pówer, léader. ~ия *ж.*
hegémony.

гéйзер *м.* géyser, hot spring.

гектáр *м.* héctare.

гекто- *в сложн.* hecto-.

гектовáтт *м. эл.* héctowatt.

гектóграф *м.* héctograph.

гéлий *м. хим.* hélium.

гелиоэнергéтика *ж.* sólar pówer enginéering.

гематолóгия *ж.* haematólogy.

гемоглоби́н *м. физиол.* haemoglóbin.

геморрóй *м. мед.* h(á)emorrhoid(s); piles *pl разг.*

ген *м. биол.* gene.

генеалоги́ческ|ий genealógical; ~ое дéрево fámily-
-tree.

генеалóгия *ж.* genealógy.

гéнезис *м.* génesis, órigin.

генерáл *м.* géneral; ~ áрмии Géneral of the Ármy.

генерáл-губернáтор *м.* góvernor géneral.

генерали́ссимус *м.* Generalíssimo (*pl* -os).

генералитéт *м. собир.* the génerals *pl.*

генерáл|-лейтенáнт *м.* lieuténant-géneral. ~-майóр
м. májor-géneral. ~-полкóвник *м.* cólonel-géneral.

генерáльн|ый géneral; (*основной тж.*) básic; ~
кóнсул cónsul-géneral; ~ секретáрь géneral sécretary; ~
секретáрь ООН UN Sécretary-géneral; ~ штаб
Géneral Staff; Генерáльная Ассамблéя Géneral
Assémbly; ~ая репети́ция *театр.* dress rehéarsal; ~ое
сражéние géneral engágement.

генерáльский géneral's.

генерáтор *м.* génerator; ~ постоя́нного тóка diréct-
-cúrrent génerator; ~ переме́нного тóка álternator. ~ный
génerator *attr.*

генéти|к *м.* genéticist. ~ка *ж.* genétics.

генети́ческий genétic.

гениáльн|ость *ж.* génius; gréatness, brílliance. ~ый
of génius *после сущ.*, great, brílliant; ~ый полковóдец
brílliant géneral, military génius; ~ый худóжник great
ártist; ~ое предви́дение brílliant fóresight; ~ое произведéние work of génius.

гéний *м.* génius; (*о человеке тж.*) man* of génius;
◇ дóбрый (злой) ~ good (évil) génius.

геноци́д *м.* génocide.

генштáб *м.* (*генерáльный штаб*) *см.* генерáльный.

геóграф *м.* geógrapher. ~и́ческий geográphic(al);
~и́ческая кáрта geográphical map.

геогрáфия *ж.* geógraphy.

геодез|и́ст *м.* geódesist. ~и́ческий geodétical.

геодéзия *ж.* geódesy.

геóлог *м.* geólogist. ~и́ческий geológical.

геолóгия *ж.* geólogy.

геологорáзвéд|ка *ж.* geológical explorátion/pro-
spécting. ~очный (geológical) prospécting *attr.*; ~очная
экспеди́ция prospécting expedítion.

геометри́ческий geométrical.

геомéтрия *ж.* geómetry.

георги́н *м. бот.* dáhlia.

геофи́зика *ж.* geophýsics.

геофизи́ческий geophýsical; ~ год geophýsical year.

геохи́мия *ж.* geochémistry.

герáнь *ж. бот.* geránium.

герб *м.* coat of arms, armórial béarings *pl*; госудáрственный ~ State Émblem, Nátional Émblem; королéвский
~ róyal crest.

гербáрий *м.* herbárium.

гербици́ды *мн.* (*ед.* гербици́д *м.*) *хим.* hérbicides,
wéed-killers.

гéрбов|ый: ~ая бумáга officially stámped/héaded
páper; ~ая мáрка révenue stamp.

гериатри́я *ж.* geriátrics.

геркулéс *м.* 1. (*силач*) Hércules; 2. (*крупа*) rolled
oats *pl*, pórridge oats *pl.* ~ов: ~овы столпы́ the Píllars of
Hércules.

гермáний *м. хим.* germánium.

гермáнск|ий 1. *ист., лингв.* Germánic, Teutónic;
~ие языки́ Germánic lánguages; 2. (*немецкий*) Gérman.

гермети́ческ|и hermétically; ~ закýпоренный
hermétically sealed. ~ий hermétic, áir-tight, léak-tight;
~ая каби́на *ав.* préssure cábin.

герои́зм *м.* héroism; (*в бою тж.*) válour.

герóика *ж.* heróic spírit; ~ нáших дней heróic spirit
of our time.

герои́н *м.* héroin.

герóй|ня *ж.* héroine. ~ческий heróic, váliant.

герóй *м.* 1. héro; 2. (*действующее лицо*) cháracter;
~ ромáна cháracter of a nóvel; ◇ Герóй Совéтского
Сою́за Héro of the Sóviet Únion. ~ский heróic. ~ство *с.*
héroism.

геронтолóгия *ж.* gerontólogy.

герýндий *м. грам.* gérund.

герц *м. эл.* cýcle per sécond.

гéрцог *м.* duke. ~и́ня *ж.* dúchess. ~ский dúcal.
~ство *с.* dúchy.

рестáпо *с. нескл.* gestápo. ~вец *м.* gestápo
políceman*.

гетерогéнный héterogéneous.

гéтры *мн.* (*длинные*) gáiters, léggings; (*короткие*)
spats.

гéтто *с. нескл.* ghétto.

гиаци́нт *м. бот.* hýacinth.

гиббóн *м. зоол.* gíbbon.

ги́бель *ж.* 1. (*полное разрушение*) destrúction, ruin;
(*падение чего-л.*) dównfall; (*смерть*) death, destrúction;
~ сýдна the loss/wreck of a ship; э́то грози́т емý ~ю that
may ruin him, that may be the end of him; приводи́ть
кого-л. к ги́бели bring* smb. to ruin; он обречён на ~
he is doomed (to destrúction); ~ надéжд the wreck/ruin
of *one's* hopes; 2. *в знач. сказ.* (*рд.*) *разг.* (*множество*)
heaps (of); (*о людях*) crowds (of); (*о насекомых и
т.п.*) swarms (of); ~ вся́ких дел heaps of things to do.
~ный (*бедственный*) disástrous; (*вредный*) pernícious;
~ные послéдствия fátal cónsequences.

ги́бк|ий 1. (*упругий*) fléxible, súpple; (*о движениях*) súpple, plíable, lithe; ~ая ве́тка súpple twig; ~ие па́льцы súpple fíngers; ~ое те́ло súpple bódy/fígure; ~ие движе́ния súpple/lithe móvements; **2.** (*применяющийся к обстоятельствам*) fléxible; (*уступчивый*) plíable; ~ ум vérsatile mind; ~ хара́ктер fléxible/plíable/adáptable cháracter; ~ое руково́дство adáptable léadership; ~ое реше́ние elástic decísion. **~ость** *ж.* flexibílity, súppleness, pliabílity, plíancy; ~ость хара́ктера flexibílity/pliabílity of cháracter; ~ость ума́ méntal flexibílity.

ги́бл|ый *разг.*: ~ое де́ло bad job, lost cause; ~ое ме́сто gód-forsaken spot, wrétched hole.

ги́бн|уть, поги́бнуть (от *рд.*; *от боле́зней, нужды́*) die (of), pérish (from); (*от засухи, мороза*) be* killed (by); (*о государстве, цивилизации*) fall* to píeces, be* góing to rack and ruin; (*о судах*) be* lost; кора́бль ~ет the ship is sínking.

гибри́д *м.* hýbrid. **~иза́ция** *ж.* hybridizátion, cróss- -fertilizátion.

гига́нт *м.* gíant; промы́шленный ~ gíant fáctory, vast indústrial plant. **~ский** gigántic; ~ские масшта́бы gigántic scale *sg;* ◇ ~ские шаги́ *спорт.* gíant stride *sg;* дви́гаться вперёд ~скими шага́ми advánce with gíant strides; make* treméndous prógress.

гигие́н|а *ж.* hýgiene; ли́чная ~ pérsonal hýgiene. **~и́ческий, ~и́чный** hygíenic; (*о мерах и т. п.*) sánitary.

гигро́граф *м.* *физ.* hýgrograph.

гигро́метр *м.* *физ.* hygrómeter.

гигроско́п *м.* *физ.* hýgroscope. **~и́ческий** *физ.* hygroscópic; ~и́ческая ва́та absórbent cótton wool.

гид *м.* guide.

гидра́вл|ика *ж.* hydráulics. **~и́ческий** hydráulic; ~и́ческий то́рмоз hydráulic brake; ~и́ческий пресс hydráulic press; ~и́ческий спо́соб добы́чи угля́ hydráulic cóal-mining.

гидра́т *м.* *хим.* hýdrate.

гидри́д *м.* *хим.* hýdride.

гидро- *в сложн.* hýdro.

гидробиоло́гия *ж.* hýdrobiólogy.

гидро́|граф *м.* hydrógrapher. **~графи́ческий** hydrográphic(al); ~графи́ческое су́дно súrvey-vessel. **~гра́фия** *ж.* hydrógraphy.

гидродина́мика *ж.* hýdrodynámics.

гидро́лиз *м.* hydrólysis (*pl* -ses). **~ный** hydrolýtic.

гидро́|лог *м.* hydrólogist. **~логи́ческий** hydrológical. **~ло́гия** *ж.* hydrólogy.

гидромеханиза́ция *ж.* hydráulic míning.

гидромеха́ника *ж.* hýdromechánics.

гидромонито́р *м.* hydráulic mónitor.

гидропо́ника *ж.* hydropónics.

гидросамолёт *м.* séaplane; (*летающая лодка*) flýing-boat.

гидроста́нция *ж.* hydroeléctric (pówer) státion.

гидротерапи́я *ж.* *мед.* hydrópathy, hýdrothérapy, hýdrotherapéutics.

гидроте́хн|ик *м.* hydráulic enginéer. **~ика** *ж.* hydráulic enginéering. **~и́ческий** hydrotéchnical.

гидротурби́на *ж.* wáter-túrbine, hydráulic túrbine.

гидроу́зел *м.* hydroeléctric pówer devélopment.

гидроэлектроста́нция *ж.* hydroeléctric (pówer) státion.

гидроэнергети́ческий wáter-power *attr.*; (*об установках*) wáter-driven.

гидроэнергоресу́рсы *мн.* wáter-power resóurces.

гие́на *ж.* *зоол.* hyéna.

ги́к|ать, ги́кнуть *разг.* whoop. **~нуть** *сов. см.* ги́кать.

ги́льд|ия *ж.* *ист.* guild; пе́рвой ~ии of the first guild.

ги́льза *ж.* **1.** (*патронная*) cártridge)case; (*орудийного патрона*) shéll-case; **2.** (*папиросная*) (cigarétte-) sheath.

гимн *м.* **1.** ánthem; госуда́рственный ~ Nátional Ánthem; **2.** (*прославление*) hymn (of praise).

гимнази́ст *м.* grámmar-school boy, hígh-school boy. **~ка** *ж.* grámmar-school girl, hígh-school girl.

гимна́зия *ж.* grámmar school, high school, gymnásium.

гимна́ст *м.* gýmnast; выступле́ния ~ов gymnástic displáy.

гимнастёрка *ж.* hígh-collared túnic.

гимна́ст|ика *ж.* gymnástics; спорти́вная ~ compétitive gymnástics; худо́жественная ~ free callisthénics; занима́ться ~икой go* in for gymnástics. **~и́ческий** gymnástic; ~и́ческий зал gymnásium (*pl* -siums, -sia); gym *разг.*; ~и́ческие упражне́ния gymnástic éxercises, gymnástics; ~и́ческие снаря́ды gymnástics apparátus *sg.* **~ка** *ж.* gýmnast.

гинеко́лог *м.* gynaecólogist.

гинекологи́ческий gynaecológical.

гинеколо́гия *ж.* gynaecólogy.

гипе́рбол|а *ж.* **1.** *мат.* hypérbola; **2.** *лит.* hypérbole; *перен.* exaggerátion. **~и́ческий 1.** *мат.* hyperbólic; **2.** *лит.* hyperbólical.

гипертони́я *ж.* *мед.* hyperténsion, high blood préssure.

гипертроф|и́рованный hypértrophied. **~и́я** *ж.* hypértrophy.

гипно́з *м.* **1.** (*состояние*) hypnósis; **2.** (*сила внушения*) hýpnotism; быть под ~ом be* in a hypnótic trance; *перен.* be* hýpnotized.

гипно́т|изёр *м.* hýpnotist, mésmerist. **~изи́ровать,** загипнотизи́ровать (*вн.*) hýpnotize (*smb.*). **~и́зм** *м.* hýpnotism, mésmerism. **~и́ческий** hypnótic; ~и́ческий сон hypnótic trance.

гипосульфи́т *м.* *хим.* hyposúlphite.

гипо́тез|а *ж.* hypóthesis (*pl* -ses); рабо́чая ~ wórking hypóthesis; стро́ить ~ы frame/form hypótheses.

гипотену́за *ж.* *мат.* hypótenuse.

гипотони́я *ж.* *мед.* hypoténsion, low blood préssure.

гиппопота́м *м.* *зоол.* hippopótamus (*pl* -ses, -mi).

гипс *м.* **1.** *мин.* gýpsum; **2.** (*употр. в скульптуре и хирургии*) pláster (of Páris); наложи́ть ~ на что-л. put* *smth.* in pláster; **3.** (*скульптура*) pláster cast. **~ова́ть** *несов.* (*вн.*) **1.** *мед.* pláster (*smth.*); **2.** *с.-х.* gýpsum (*smth.*) apply gýpsum (to).

ги́псовый 1. gýps(e)ous; **2.** (*сделанный из гипса*) pláster(-of-Páris) *attr.*; ~ сле́пок pláster cast.

гипю́р *м.* guipúre.

гиреви́к *м.* *спорт.* wéight-lifter.

гирля́нда *ж.* gárland, festóon; украша́ть что-л. ~ми festóon *smth.*, deck *smth.* with gárlands.

гироко́мпас *м.* gyroscópic cómpass, gýrocompass.

гироско́п *м.* gýroscope, **~и́ческий** gyroscópic.

ги́ря *ж.* weight.

гисто́лог *м.* histólogist.

гистоло́гия *ж.* histólogy.

гита́р|а *ж.* guitár; гава́йская ~ ukuléle. **~и́ст** *м.* guitár pláyer.

ги́чка *ж.* *мор., спорт.* gig.

глав- *в сложн.* **1.** (*главный*) chief; **2** (*главное управление*) céntral board.

глав|а́ I 1. *м. и ж.* (*главное лицо*) head; chief *разг.*; ~ семьи́ head of the fámily; ~ прави́тельства head of the góvernment, prémier; ~ госуда́рства Head of State; **2.** *ж.* (*купол*) cúpola; ◇ во ~е́ чего-л. at the head of *smth.*; во ~е́ с кем-л. héaded/led by; ста́вить что-л. во ~у́ угла́ make* *smth.* the córner-stone of *smth.*

глава́ II *ж.* (*в книге и т. п.*) chápter.

глава́рь *м.* léader; (*зачинщик*) ríngleader.

гла́венств|овать *с.* suprémacy. ~ **вать** *несов.* (в *пр.*) be* predóminant (in); (над *тв.*) have* suprémacy (óver), dóminate (*smth.*), contról (*smth.*).

главнокома́ндующий *м.* Commánder-in-Chief; Верхо́вный Главнокома́ндующий Suprême Commánder-in--Chíef.

гла́вн|ый *прил.* **1.** chief, main, príncipal; ~ го́род príncipal town; (*столица*) cápital; ~ая у́лица main street; ~ уда́р *воен.* main attáck/blow; ~ые си́лы *воен.* main bódy/fórces; **2.** (*старший по положению*) head *attr.*, chief *attr.*; ~ врач head physícian; (*в армии*) chief médical ófficer; ~ хиру́рг head súrgeon; ~ инжене́р chief engíneer; ~ бухга́лтер chief accóuntant; **3.** *в знач. с.* the great/chief thing; what réally mátters; са́мое ~ое — не опа́здывать the great thing is not to be late; whatéver you do, don't be late!, abóve all, don't be late!; са́мого ~ого вы и не сказа́ли you have left out the most impórtant part; он не ви́дит са́мого ~ого he misses the point; ◇ ~ым о́бразом máinly, in the main; ~ая кни́га *бухг.* lédger; ~ое предложе́ние *грам.* príncipal/main clause.

-гла́вый *в сложн.* **1.** (*о головах*) -héaded; двугла́вый орёл double éagle; **2.** (*о куполах*) with... domes; трёхгла́вая це́рковь church with three domes.

глаго́|л *м. грам.* verb. ~**льный** vérbal.

глади́ль|ный íroning *attr.*, smóothing *attr.*; ~ная доска́ íroning-board.

гладио́лус *м. бот.* gladiólus (*pl* -li, -luses).

гла́дить, вы́гладить, погла́дить (*вн.*) **1.** *сов.* вы́гладить (*утюжить*) íron (*smth.*); (*верхнее платье*) press (*smth.*); **2.** *сов.* погла́дить (*ласкать*) stroke (*smb., smth.*); ~ кого́-л. по голове́ stroke *smb.'s* hair, pat *smb.* on the head; ◇ ~ кого́-л. про́тив ше́рсти stroke/rub *smb.* the wrong way; *перен.* put* *smb.'s* back up, rub *smb.* up the wrong way; ~ кого́-л. по голо́вке ≈ pat *smb.* on the back.

гла́д|кий 1. (*ровный*) smooth; ~кая доро́га smooth road; ~кая причёска símple háir-style; **2.** (*плавный*) fácile; (*о речи*) flúent; ~ стиль éasy style; **3.** (*без рисунка — о ткани*) plain; **4.** *разг.* (*холёный*) sleek. ~ко (*прям. и перен.*) smóothly; (*без задержки*) withóut a hitch; ~ко вы́бритый clean-sháven; ~ко причёсываться wear* *one's* hair straight, do* *one's* hair símply; ~ко говори́ть be* a glib tálker; be* smóoth-spóken; (*об ораторе*) be* a flúent/persuásive spéaker; ~ко писа́ть have* an éasy style; проходи́ть, сходи́ть ~ко go* off smóothly, go* withóut a hitch. ~кость *ж.* smóothness; ~кость сти́ля éasy style, ease of style.

гладь I *ж.* (*водной поверхности*) smooth/mírror-like súrface.

гладь II *ж.* (*вышивка*) sátin-stitch.

гла́женье *с.* íroning.

глаз *м.* **1.** eye; (*взгляд, взор*) glance, look; голубы́е ~а́ blue eyes; отвести́ ~а́ look awáy; подня́ть ~а́ look up, raise/lift *one's* eyes; оки́нуть что́-л. ~а́ми look *smth.* óver; **2.** (*зрение*) sight; плохи́е (хоро́шие) ~а́ poor (éxcellent) éyesight; по́ртить себе́ ~а́ spoil* *one's* eyes, ruin *one's* éyesight; **3.** *тк. ед.* (*особая способность видения*) eye; *перен. разг.* (*присмотр*) wátching; ве́рный ~ good eye; за ним ну́жен ~ да ~ you can't take your eyes off him for a móment; ◇ в мои́х ~а́х to my eye, in my opínion; за ~а́ **1)** (*в отсутствие*) in *smb.'s* ábsence; withóut háving seen *smb.*; withóut *smb.'s* knówledge; **2)** (*за спиной*) behínd *smb.'s* back; **3)** (*в избытке*) ámply, quite enóugh; за ~а́ доста́точно enóugh and to spare; на ~ by eye; на ~а́х у кого́-л. in front of *smb.*, únder *smb.'s* véry eyes; он ~а́ми у нас на ~а́х we watched him grow up; ра́ди прекра́сных глаз for love, for *smb.'s* (sweet) sake; с ~у на ~ in prívate, alóne; бесе́да с ~у на ~ confidéntial/prívate talk; идти́ куда́ ~а́ гляди́т wánder áimlessly; смея́ться в ~а́ ко-му́-л. laugh in *smb.'s* face; смотре́ть во все ~а́ на кого́-л., что́-л. gaze inténtly at *smb., smth.*; смотре́ть пра́вде в ~а́ face the truth; face it *разг.*; хозя́йским ~ом with a thrífty eye; смотре́ть больши́ми ~а́ми на кого́-л., что́-л. stare wíde-éyed at *smb.*,

smth.; сде́лать больши́е ~а́ ≈ raise *one's* éyebrows; с глаз доло́й — из се́рдца вон *посл.* out of sight, out of mind; вон, доло́й с глаз мои́х! get out of my sight!

глаза́стый *разг.* **1.** (*большеглазый*) róund-éyed, lárge-éyed; **2.** (*зоркий*) shárp-éyed, quíck-síghted.

глазе́ть *несов.* (*на вн.*) *разг.* gape (at), stare (at).

глазиро́ванн|ый 1. (*о посуде*) glazed; **2.** (*о фруктах и т.п.*) glacé, cándied; ~ые чере́шни glacé chérries; ~ экле́р iced éclair; **3.** (*о бумаге*) glóssy; gloss *attr.*

глазирова́ть *несов. и сов.* (*вн.*) **1.** (*посуду*) glaze (*smth.*); **2.** (*фрукты*) cándy (*smth.*); (*кондитерские изделия*) ice (*smth.*); **3.** (*бумагу*) give* a glóssy fínish (to).

глазни́к *м. разг.* éye-doctor.

глазни́ца *ж. анат.* éye-socket.

глазн|о́й eye *attr.*; ~ые боле́зни diséases of the eye; ~ нерв óptic nerve; ~ врач óculist, éye-specialist; ~а́я больни́ца éye-hospital; ◇ ~ые зу́бы éye-teeth, cánine teeth.

глаз|о́к *м.* **1.** eye; **2.** (*отверстие*) péephole; ◇ одни́м ~ко́м with half an eye; на ~ róughly, at a guess; стро́ить гла́зки кому́-л. make* eyes at *smb.*

глазоме́р *м.* eye (for distance); плохо́й ~ fáulty eye.

глазу́нья *ж.* (*яичница*) fried eggs *pl.*

глазу́рь *ж.* (*на посуде*) glaze; (*сахарная*) ícing; покрыва́ть что́-л. ~ю (*посуду*) glaze *smth.*; (*печенье и т.п.*) ice *smth.*

гла́нды *мн. анат.* (*ед.* гла́нда *ж.*) tónsils; удали́ть ~ have* *one's* tónsils out.

глас *м. уст. поэт.* voice; ◇ ~ вопию́щего в пусты́не the voice (of one crýing) in the wilderness.

глас|и́ть *несов.* state; зако́н ~и́т the law reads; письмо́ ~и́т the létter runs; как ~и́т посло́вица as the próverb has it, as the próverb says.

гла́сност|ь *ж.* publicity; glásnost ◇ предава́ть что́--л. ~и make* *smth.* públic.

гла́сный I (*открытый, публичный*) públic, ópen.

гла́сн|ый II *прил. лингв.* **1.** vowel *attr.*; **2.** *в знач. сущ. м.* vówel; ~ые пере́днего ря́да front vówels.

гла́уберов: ~а соль Gláuber's salts *pl*; só́dium súlphate *хим.*

глаша́тай *м.* tówn-crier, hérald; *перен.* procláimer, spókesman*; ~ и́стины procláimer of the truth.

глин|а́ *ж.* clay; (*гончарная*) árgil, pótter's clay; бе́лая ~, фарфо́ровая ~ káolin; огнеупо́рная ~ fire-clay. ~истый clay *attr.*, cláyey; ~истая по́чва clay soil; ~истый сла́нец shale.

глиноби́т|ный adóbe; ~ая постро́йка adóbe building; ~ая стена́ adóbe wall, múd-wall.

глинозём *м.* alúmina.

глинтве́йн *м.* múlled wine.

гли́нян|ый clay *attr.*, éarthen; ~ горшо́к éarthenware pot; ~ая посу́да *собир.* éarthenware, póttery; ~ая тру́бка clay pipe.

гли́ссер *м.* hýdroplane.

глист *м.* (*intéstinal*) worm, hélminth.

глистого́н|ный vermífugal; ~ое сре́дство vérmifuge.

глицери́н *м.* glycerín(e). ~**овый** glycéric.

глици́ния *ж. бот.* wistária.

глоба́ль|ный adj глóbal.

гло́бус *м.* globe.

глода́ть *несов.* (*вн.; прям. и перен.*) gnaw (*smb., smth.*); его́ гло́жет за́висть he is consúmed with énvy.

глосса́рий *м. лингв.* glóssary.

глота́ть *несов.* (*вн.*) swállow (*smth.*); (*быстро*) bolt (*smth.*), gulp (*smth.*) down; *перен.* devóur (*smth.*); ~ кни́ги devóur books; ◇ ~ во́здух gulp air ínto *one's* lungs; ~ слёзы choke/gulp down *one's* tears; ~ слова́ swállow half *one's* words, múmble.

глотк|а *ж.* **1.** *анат.* gúllet; **2.** *разг.* (*горло*) throat; ◇

заткну́ть *кому-л.* ~у gag *smb.*, shut* *smb.* up; не лезть в ~у stick* in *one's* throat; ора́ть во всю ~у yell.

глотну́ть *сов.* take* a sip.

глот|о́к *м.* 1. *(действие)* gulp; сде́лать ~ take* a sip; одни́м ~ко́м at a draught/gulp; 2. *(количество)* drop; drink; *(маленький)* sip, mouthful; ~ воды́ a drink/sip of water; пить больши́ми ~ка́ми gulp; пить ма́ленькими ~ка́ми sip.

гло́хнуть, огло́хнуть, загло́хнуть 1. *сов.* огло́хнуть *(терять слух)* go* deaf, grow* deaf, become* deaf; 2. *сов.* загло́хнуть *(затихать)* die away; 3. *сов.* загло́х-нуть *(постепенно исчезать)* dwindle; *(о слухах)* die down; 4. *сов.* загло́хнуть *(зарастать)* run* wild, be* overgrown; 5. *сов.* загло́хнуть *(о моторе)* stall.

глу́бже *(сравнит. ст. прил.* глубо́кий *и нареч.* глубо́ко*)* deeper.

глубин|а́ *ж.* depth; *перен. тж.* profundity, intensity; на ~е трёх ме́тров at a depth of three metres; два метра в ~у two metres deep; измеря́ть ~у *чего-л.* sound (the depth) of *smth.*; *(лином)* plumb *smth.*; в ~е ко́мнаты at the back of the room, in the interior of the room; ~ мы́сли profundity of thought; ~ чувств depth/intensity of feeling; deep/intense feelings; ◇ в ~е души́ at heart, in *one's* heart of hearts; до ~ы́ души́ to the bottom of *one's* heart; из ~ы́ души́ *one's* innermost soul, from the bottom of *one's* soul/heart; в ~е веко́в in ancient days, in the remote past.

глубинн|ый 1. deep; *(на глубине реки)* deep-water *attr.*; *(на глубине моря)* deep-sea *attr.*; ~ая бо́мба depth-charge; 2. *геол.* abyssal; 3. *(отдалённый)* remote, out-of-the-way; ~ райо́н remote district.

глубо́к|ий 1. deep; *перен. тж.* profound; ~ая ша́хта deep mine/shaft; ~ая вспа́шка deep ploughing; ~ая таре́лка soup-plate; ~ие морщи́ны deep wrinkles; ~ие ко́рни deep roots; ~ая ра́на deep wound; ~ая оборо́на defence in depth; в ~ом тылу́ deep in the rear, far behind the lines; ~ая разве́дка deep reconnaissance; ~ая дре́вность remote past; ~ие зна́ния deep knowledge *sg;* ~ мысли́тель deep thinker; ~ая мысль deep/profound thought; ~ие противоре́чия deep contradictions; ~ое неве́жество profound/utter ignorance; ~ тра́ур deep mourning; ~ сон deep/profound sleep; 2. *(поздний)* late; ~ая о́сень late autumn; late fall *амер.*; ~ая ночь the dead of night; the small hours *pl;* ~ой но́чью at the dead of night; до ~ой но́чи far/deep into the night; ~ая ста́рость extreme old age, venerable age; до ~ой ста́рости till a great age.

глубоко́ 1. *нареч.* deeply; *перен. тж.* profoundly; in depth; ~ заду́маться fall* into deep thought; 2. *в знач. сказ.* deep.

глубоково́дн|ый deep-water *attr.;* ~ая река́ deep river; ~ые иссле́дования deep-water research *sg;* ~ые ры́бы deep-sea fish *sg.*

глубокомы́сл|енный profound, grave; ~енное выска́зывание profound statement; с ~енным ви́дом with a thoughtful air; *ирон.* with an air of profound wisdom; looking (very) wise. ~ие *с.* depth of thought, profundity of thought.

глубокоуважа́емый deeply respected, highly respected; *(в обращении)* honoured.

глубь *ж.* the depths *pl,* the heart; в ~ ле́са into the heart of the forest; в ~ страны́ inland, towards the interior.

глум|и́ться *(над тв.)* mock *(smb.),* jeer (at); commit an outrage (upon, against). ~ле́ние *с. (над тв.)* mockery (of), outrage (upon, against). ~ли́вый 1. *(издеватель-ский)* mocking, jeering; 2. *(склонный к глумлению)* derisive; ~ли́вый челове́к scoffer, mocker.

глуп|е́ть, поглупе́ть get*/become* stupid. ~е́ц *м.* blockhead. ~и́ть, сглупи́ть *разг.* be* foolish/silly, commit follies; не ~и́! don't be foolish/silly!

глупова́тый dull, not very bright; ~ па́рень dull fellow; у него́ ~ вид he doesn't look very bright.

глу́пост|ь *ж.* 1. stupidity, foolishness; 2. *разг. (по-ступок, слова)* foolish/silly thing; наде́лать ~ей do* a lot of foolish/silly things; 3. *(чепуха)* rubbish, nonsense; брось э́ти ~и! stop that nonsense!; ~и! nonsense!, rubbish!

глу́п|ый stupid, silly; *(о поступке и т.п.)* foolish; он ещё глуп *(о ребёнке)* ≈ he's too little to understand; он от приро́ды глуп he was born stupid; он не так глуп, что́бы... he has more sense than to...; ~ вид foolish appearance; ~ая зате́я silly idea; ~ое положе́ние embarrassing/awkward situation.

глупы́ш I *м. разг.* silly little thing, goose*.

глупы́ш II *м. (птица)* fulmar.

глуха́рь *м. зоол.* capercailzie, wood-grouse.

глу́хо 1. *нареч. (тихо, неясно)* quietly, softly, indistinctly; 2. *в знач. сказ. безл.* there is a hush.

глух|о́й *прил.* 1. deaf *(тж. перен.);* ~ на о́ба у́ха deaf in both ears; ~ на одно́ у́хо deaf in one ear; он соверше́нно глух he is stone-deaf; 2. *(о голосе)* toneless; *(о звуке)* dull, hollow, indistinct, muffled; ~ согла́сный *лингв.* voiceless consonant; 3. *(смутный, скрытый)* suppressed; ~ое недово́льство suppressed/inarticulate discontent; ~а́я молва́ vague rumours *pl;* 4. *(отдалён-ный)* remote; *(безлюдный)* lonely; ~ое ме́сто remote/out-of-the-way place; ~а́я у́лица lonely/solitary street; 5. *(заросший)* wild, overgrown; ~ лес dense forest; 6. *(сплошной, без отверстий)* blind; ~а́я стена́ blank wall; ~ая *в знач. сущ. м.* deaf man*, deaf boy; *ж.* deaf woman*, deaf girl; *мн. собир.* the deaf; ◇ ~ но́чью at the dead of night; ~о́е вре́мя a time of darkness and stagnation.

глухома́нь *ж. разг.* remote place/corner; out-of-the--way place/corner.

глухонемо́й *прил.* 1. deaf-and-dumb; 2. *в знач. сущ. м.* deaf-mute; *ж.* deaf-mute; *мн. собир.* the deaf-and--dumb.

глухота́ *ж.* deafness.

глуши́тель *м. тех.* silencer.

глуши́ть *несов. (вн.)* 1. *(звук)* muffle *(smth.),* deaden *(smth.);* ~ радиопереда́чи jam broadcasts; 2. *(мотор)* throttle down *(smth.);* 3. *(не давать расти)* choke *(smth.); перен. (подавлять)* stifle *(smth.);* ~ кри́тику stifle criticism; 4. *разг. (оглушать)* stun *(smb.);* ◇ ~ ры́бу stun fish.

глуш|ь *ж.* remote place; *(дикие места)* the wilds *pl;* жить в ~и́ live miles from anywhere; лесна́я ~ remote woodlands/forest; the backwoods *pl.*

глы́ба *ж.* great lump, block; ~ земли́ clod; ~ у́гля great lump of coal; ка́менная ~ boulder, block of stone.

глюко́за *ж.* glucose, dextrose, grape-sugar.

гляд|е́ть, погляде́ть 1. look; *(на вн.)* look (at); 2. *(за тв.) разг. (присматривать)* look (after); ~ за поря́дком see*/attend to order; 3. *тк. несов. (на вн.)* *(вы-ходить на)* face *(smth.),* look (on); *(об окнах)* give* (on); ◇ ~ в о́ба be* on the alert, be* on *one's* guard; ~ не́ на что it's hardly worth mentioning; того́ и ~и it's more than likely; на́ ночь гля́дя when it's nearly dark, at this time of night.

гляде́ться, погляде́ться *(в вн.)* look at oneself (in); ~ в зе́ркало look at oneself in the glass/mirror.

гля́нец *м.* gloss; *(на материи и т.п.)* lustre; *(на де́реве, коже)* polish.

гля́нуть *сов. (на вн.) разг.* glance (at); cast* a glance (at); куда́ ни глянь wherever one looks.

гля́нцев|ый glossy, lustrous; ~ая бума́га glossy paper.

гм ahem!, h'm!

гнать *несов. (вн.)* 1. drive* *(smth.);* ~ ста́до drive* a herd; 2. *(погонять; вести на большой скорости)* urge *(smth.)* on, drive* *(smth.)* on; ~ ло́шадь urge on a horse; ~ маши́ну *разг.* drive* hard, belt alóng; **3.** (*быстро ехать*): ~ во весь дух drive* at full speed; (*верхом*) ride* at full speed; **4.** (*преследовать зверя*) chase (*smth.*); *перен.* hound (*smth.*); **5.** (*выгонять*) drive* (*smb.*) awáy; ~ кого-л. и́з дому turn smb. out of the house; ~ кого-л. прочь drive* smb. awáy; (*добывать перегонкой*) distíl (*smth.*). ~ся *несов.* (за *тв.*) **1.** (*преследовать*) chase (*smb.*), pursúe (*smb.*); **2.** *разг.* (*стремиться*) strive* (for), strain (áfter), be* out (for).

гнев *м.* ánger; wrath *поэт.*; припа́док ~a fit of ánger; в ~e in (a fit of) ánger. ~ный ángry; wráthful *поэт.*

гнедо́й bay.

гнезди́ться *несов.* **1.** nest, make* its nest; *перен.* (*ютиться*) have* one's dwélling, lodge, put* up; **2.** (*корениться*) have* its seat, be* implánted.

гнездо́ *с.* **1.** nest (*тж. перен.*); вить ~ build* a nest; **2.** (*выводок, семья*) brood; **3.** (*скопление, группа*) clúster; ~ грузде́й a clúster of milk múshrooms; **4.** (*тайное пристанище*) den; воровско́е ~ den of thieves; **5.** *тех.* seat; sócket; (*для шипа*) mórtise; кла́панное ~ valve séat(ing); штепсельное ~ sócket; **6.** *лингв.* fámily; ◇ свить (себе́) ~ build* one's nest. ~ва́ние *с. зоол.* nidificátion, nésting. ~во́й: ~во́й посе́в *с.-х.* clúster sówing.

гнёздышко *с.* nest; свить себе́ тёплое ~ féather one's nest.

гнейс *м. геол.* gneiss.

гне|сти́ *несов.* (*вн.*) oppréss (*smb.*); меня́ ~тёт тоска́ my heart is héavy with distréss/grief, I am sick at heart.

гнёт *м.* (*бремя, угнетение*) oppréssion, yoke; под ~ом чего-л. únder the yoke of smth.

гнету́щ|ий oppréssive, depréssing; ~ие забо́ты cárking cares; ~ая мысль oppréssive nótion, ágonizing thought; ~ая тоска́ ánguish.

гни́да *ж.* nit.

гние́ние *с.* decáy, rótting.

гнил|о́й **1.** rótten, decáyed, pútrid; ~ое де́рево rótting tree; (*о древесине*) rótten wood; ~ зуб decáyed tooth*; **2.** (*сырой*) foul, damp; ~ая пого́да damp wéather; **3.** (*порочный*) corrúpt; ~ая тео́рия corrúpt théory.

гни́л|остный **1.** (*вызываемый гниением*) pútrefying; **2.** (*вызывающий гниение*) putrefáctive, séptic. ~ость *ж.* róttenness, putrídity.

гнилу́шка *ж.* piece of rótten wood; *разг.* (*кусок чего-л.*) rótten scrap.

гниль *ж.* **1.** rot; **2.** (*плесень*) mould.

гнить, сгнить (*прям. и перен.*) rot, decáy; ~ на корню́ rot on the stalk.

гнои́ть, сгнои́ть (*вн.*) rot (*smth.*), let* (*smth.*) rot; ~ наво́з ferment manúre; ~ кого-л. в тюрьме́ leave* smb. to rot in gaol. ~ся *несов.* súppurate; (*о ране*) féster; dischárge pus.

гной *м.* pus; mátter *разг.* ~ни́к *м.* gáthering, ábscess; вскрыть ~ни́к ópen/lance/drain an ábscess.

гно́йн|ый púrulent; ~ая ра́на féstering/súppurative wound; ~ аппендици́т súppurative appendicítis.

гном *м. миф.* gnome, góblin, elf*.

гносеологи́ческий epistemológical, gnosiológical.

гносеоло́гия *ж.* epistemólogy, gnosiólogy, théory of knówledge.

гну *м. и ж. нескл. зоол.* gnu.

гнус *м. собир.* (*мошкара*) mídges *pl.*

гнуса́в|ить *несов.* speak*/talk with a twang/snúffle. ~о with a násal twang. ~ый násal, snúffling.

гну́сн|ый base, vile; (*о человеке*) villáinous; ~ое зре́лище hídeous spéctacle; ~ая клевета́ scúrrilous líbel; ~ое преда́тельство base tréachery; ~ое преступле́ние héinous/atrócious crime.

гну́т|ый curved; bent; ~ая ме́бель bént-wood fúrniture.

гнуть *несов.* **1.** (*вн.*) bend* (*smth.*); (*наклонять*) bow (*smth.*); *перен.* (*подчинять своей воле*) force (*smb.*); **2.** (*к дт.*) *разг.* (*клонить к чему-л.*) be* dríving (at); я понима́ю, куда́ он гнёт I see what he is dríving at; ◇ ~ спи́ну toil, lábour hard; ~ спи́ну, ше́ю перед кем-л. cringe to/before smb.; ~ свою́ ли́нию go* one's own way. ~ся *несов.* bend*; *перен. тж.* give* way, wáver.

гнуша́ться *несов.* (*тв.*; *пренебрегать*) disdáin (*smth.*); (*брезгать*) have*/feel* an avérsion (for, to); не ~ ниче́м stop at nóthing; не ~ никаки́ми сре́дствами be* complétely unscrúpulous.

гобеле́н *м.* Góbelin (tápestry).

гобои́ст *м.* óboe pláyer, óboist.

гобо́й *м. муз.* óboe.

го́вор *м.* **1.** sound of tálking/vóices; *перен.* sound, múrmur(ing); ~ волн múrmur of the waves; **2.** (*манера говорить*) mánner of speech/spéaking; **3.** (*местный диалект*) díalect.

говори́льня *ж. разг. пренебр.* tálking-shop.

говор|и́ть, сказа́ть **1.** *тк. несов.* (*владеть устной речью*) speak*, talk; ребёнок ещё не говори́т the child* dóesn't talk yet; ~и́те (по)гро́мче! speak (a little) lóuder; speak up!; ~ на не́скольких языка́х speak* séveral lánguages; ~ по-ру́сски, по-англи́йски *и т. п.* speak* Rússian, English *etc.*; **2.** (*вн.*; *выражать в устной речи, сообщать*) speak* (*smth.*); не ~я́ ни сло́ва without sáying a word; ~ перед аудито́рией speak* to an áudience; ~ пра́вду speak*/tell* the truth; ~ комплиме́нты pay* cómpliments; ~ с уве́ренностью speak*/talk cónfidently; **3.** *тк. несов.* (*дт.*; *вызывать какие-л. чувства*) appéal (to); **4.** *тк. несов.* (*разговаривать*) talk; ~ с кем-л. speak* to/with smb.; кто ~и́т? who's spéaking?; нам ~я́т we are told; об э́том все ~я́т éverybody is tálking about it; об э́том мно́го ~я́т it is widely discússed; **5.** *тк. несов. безл.*: ~я́т (so) they say; ~я́т, (что) they say; it is said; ~я́т, что он в Москве́ he is said to be in Móscow; ~я́т, что они́ уе́хали they are believed/said to have left; **6.** *тк. несов.* (*вн.*; *свидетельствовать о чём-л.*) show* (*smth.*), revéal (*smth.*); ~ (не) в по́льзу кого-л., чего-л. (not) do* smb., smth. crédit, (not) speak* well for smb., smth.; фа́кты ~я́т не в ва́шу по́льзу the facts are not in your fávour; всё э́то ~и́т о том, что... éverything points to the fact that...; **7.** *тк. несов.* (*в пр.*; *проявляться*) come* out (in); в нём ~и́т со́бственник the próperty-owner is cóming out in him; ◇ ~и́т Москва́ *радио* this is rádio Móscow; что вы ~и́те? oh, réally?; is that so?; само́ за себя́ ~и́т it speaks for itsélf; что и ~ of course, it goes without sáying; что (*или* как) ни ~и́... say what you like...; на ра́зных языка́х not speak the same lánguage; что я вам ~и́л! I told you so!; вам хорошо́ ~! it's all véry well for you!; вообще́ ~я́ génerally spéaking; не ~я́ (уже́) о apárt from, not to méntion, to say nóthing of; ина́че ~я́ in óther words; открове́нно ~я́ fránkly spéaking; по пра́вде ~я́ to tell the truth; со́бственно ~я́ as a mátter of fact; стро́го ~я́ strictly spéaking. ~и́ться *несов.* be* said; как э́то ~и́тся? how do you say it?; ◇ как ~и́тся as the sáying goes; as the phrase is.

говорли́в|ость *ж.* tálkativeness, gárrulousness, loquácity. ~ый tálkative, loquácious; (*о ручейке*) bábbling.

говору́н *м. разг.* great tálker, chátterbox.

говя́|дина *ж.* beef. ~жий beef *attr.*

го́гол|ь *м. зоол.* gólden-eye; ◇ ходи́ть ~ем strut (like a túrkey-cock).

го́голь-мо́голь *м.* gógol-mógol (*yolk of egg and sugar beaten up together*).

го́гот *м.*, ~анье *с.* **1.** (*гусей*) cáckling; **2.** *разг.* (*хохот*) loud láughter; roars of láughter *pl.* ~а́ть *несов.* **1.**

(*о гусях*) cáckle; **2.** *разг.* (*хохотать*) roar with láughter, guffáw.

год *м.* **1.** year; текущий ~ cúrrent year; астрономический ~ astronómic year; сóлнечный ~ sólar year; урожáйный ~ good year, búmper-crop year; в будущем ~ý next year; в прóшлом ~ý last year; в 1941 ~ý in (the year) 1941; (*в устной речи*) in ninetéen fórty-óne; в тот ~ that year; в этом ~ý this year; два рáза в ~ý twice a year; ему 22 ~a he's twénty-twó (years old); зá ~ dúring the year, in (the course of) a year; ~ до a year befóre; за этот ~ in the course of the year; на одúн ~ for one year; раз в два ~a évery two years; спустя три гóда three yéars láter; **2.** *мн.* (*возраст*) age *sg*; в егó ~ы at his age, at his time of life; рáзница в ~áx dispárity in years, age gap; **3.** *мн.*: шестидесятые, девянóстые ~ы the síxties, níneties; ◇ Нóвый ~ New Year; с Нóвым ~ом! háppy New Year!; из ~a в ~ from year to year, year áfter year; в ~áx (*о возрасте*) gétting on (in years), advánced in years; с ~áми in the course of time, as the years go by; бéз ~y недéля a véry short time, but a few days; не по ~áм beyónd *one's* years; не по ~áм серьёзный too sérious for *one's* age, sérious beyónd *one's* years; ~ нá ~ не прихóдится next year is álways dífferent from this; there are no two years alíke; ~ от ~a évery year; ~ за ~ом year áfter year.

годáми for years (on end).

гóден *см.* **гóдный.**

годúн|а *ж.* time, year; в ~y бéдствий in the year of great disásters; тяжёлая ~ hard times *pl*.

годú|ться *несов.* (на *вн.*) be* fit (for), do* (for); (*о человеке*) be* fítted/súitable (for), be* fit (+ to *inf*); (*быть впору*) fit; это никудá не ~тся! that won't do at all!, that is no good at all!; так дéлать не ~тся you shóuldn't do that; так поступáть не ~тся that's not the way to beháve.

годúч|ный 1. (*продолжающийся в течение года*) a year's; of a year *после сущ.*; в ~ срок within a year/twélvemonth; **2.** (*бывающий раз в год*) ánnual; ◇ ~ое кольцó (*дéрева*) ánnual ring (of a tree).

гóдн|ость *ж.* suitabílity, fítness; (*о билете и т. п.*) valídity. ~ый súitable, fit (for); (*о билете и т. п.*) válid; ~ый для питья fit for drínking, fit to drink, drínkable; билéт гóден на зáвтра the tícket is válid for tomórrow; ни к чему́ не ~ый wórthless, good for nóthing; никудá не ~ый útterly wórthless.

годовáл|ый óne-year-óld; ~ младéнец twélve-months child*, yéar-old báby/child*; ~ое живóтное yéarling.

годовóй ánnual, yéarly; ~ дохóд ánnual íncome; (*государственный*) ánnual révenue; ~ отчёт ánnual repórt.

годовщúна *ж.* annivérsary.

гол *м.* *спорт.* goal; забúть ~ score a goal.

голáвль *м.* *зоол.* chub.

голгóфа *ж.* Cálvary *тж. перен.*

голенáстые *мн.* *зоол.* wáding birds, wáders.

голенúще *с.* bóot-top.

гóлень *ж.* shin, shank.

голлáнд|ец *м.* Dútchman*; *мн. собир.* the Dutch. ~ка *ж.* Dútchwoman*. ~ский Dutch; ◇ ~ское отоплéние stove héating; ~ская печь tiled stove; ~ское полотнó hólland; ~ская черепúца pántile.

голов|á *ж.* **1.** head (*в знач. единицы счёта скота pl* head); *перен.* (*ум*) mind; (*умственные способности*) brains *pl*; у меня болúт ~ my head aches, I have a héadache; над ~óй óverhéad; ~óй вперёд head first; он ушёл в вóду с ~óй the wáter came óver his head; свéтлая ~ clear/lúcid mind; тупáя ~ dull brain; не выходúть из ~ы́ not go out of *one's* mind; рабóтать ~óй use *one's* brains; у негó ~ хорошó рабóтает he has a good head on his shóulders; his head is screwed on the right way *разг.*; это мне и в гóлову бы не пришлó it would néver have éntered my head, it would néver have occúrred to me; 100 голóв скотá a húndred head of cáttle; **2.** (*саха-*

ру) súgar-loaf*; **3.**: городскóй ~ *ист.* máyor; ◇ он человéк с ~óй he is a man* of brains, he has brains; ~ в гóлову (*о лошадях на скáчках*) néck-and-néck; с ~ы́ до ног from head to foot, from top to toe; в пéрвую гóлову first and fóremost; сдéлать *что-л.* на свою гóлову bring* *smth.* upón *one*sélf; дел — вы́ше ~ы́ up to the ears in work; (*мчáться*) слóмя гóлову (go*) at bréakneck speed; бежáть слóмя гóлову rush; run* héadlong; отвечáть, ручáться ~óй за *что-л.* take* full responsibílity for *smth.*; вы́дать себя с ~óй give* *one*sélf awáy; очертя гóлову héadlong.

головáстик *м.* *зоол.* tádpole.

головéшка *ж.* fire-brand; потýхшая ~ charred brand.

головúзна *ж.* jowl (of stúrgeon *etc.*).

головка *ж.* **1.** head; **2.** (*гвоздя, винта, булавки*) head; (*снаряда*) nóse-cap, tip, point; **3.** *разг.* (*руководúтели*) those at the head, those on top; the léaders *pl*; big shots; **4.** *мн.* (*обуви*) vamp *sg*; **5.** (*лука, чеснока*) bulb.

головн|óй *прил.* **1.** head *attr.*; ~áя боль héadache; ~ мозг brain; cérebrum (*pl* -ra) *научн.*; **2.** (*находящийся впередú, ведущий*) léading; ~ отряд vánguard; ~ые вагóны the front of the train, the front cárriages; **3.** *в знач. сущ. м.* léader.

головня *ж.* **1.** *см.* головéшка; **2.** *бот.* (*болезнь злаков*) smut.

головокруж|éние *с.* dízziness, gíddiness; испытывать ~ feel*/get* dízzy/giddy, have* fits of giddiness/dízziness; он почувствовал ~ his head swam; ◇ ~ от успéхов intoxicátion with succéss. ~ительный (*прям. и перен.*) dízzy; ~ительный успéх intóxicating succéss; с ~ительной быстротóй at a giddying/dízzy speed.

головолóм|ка *ж.* púzzle, téaser. ~ный púzzling; ~ная загáдка púzzle, póser, bráin-twister.

головомóйк|а *ж.* *разг.* dréssing down; задáть *кому-л.* ~y give* *smb.* a good dréssing down; bawl *smb.* out *амер.*

головорéз *м.* *разг.* **1.** (*сорвиголова*) dáre-devil; **2.** (*бандит*) cútthroat; (*хулиган*) rúffian.

головотяп *м.* *разг.* múddler. ~ство *с.* *разг.* múddling, (*stúpid*) búngling.

гóлод *м.* **1.** húnger; (*голодание*) starvátion; испытывать, чувствовать ~ be* húngry; умирáть с ~a die of starvátion, starve to death; я умирáю от ~a I'm símply stárving; **2.** (*бéдствие*) fámine; **3.** (*недостаток*) shórtage, fámine; книжный ~ book shórtage. ~áние *с.* starvátion. ~áть *несов.* **1.** starve, go* húngry; **2.** (*воздéрживаться от пищи*) fast. ~áющий **1.** *прич.* stárving; **2.** *в знач. сущ. м.* stárving/húngry pérson; (*объявивший голодóвку*) húnger-striker.

голóд|ный *прил.* **1.** (*чувствующий голод*) húngry; быть ~ным be* húngry; feel* émpty *разг.*; на ~ желýдок on an émpty stómach; **2.** (*вызванный голодом*) húnger *attr.*; ~ая смерть death from starvátion; **3.** (*неурожайный*) bárren; ~ край bárren région; ~ год year of fámine; **4** *разг.* (*скудный*) húnger *attr.*; scánty; ~ обéд scánty meal; на ~ом пайкé on short/húnger rátions; **5.** *в знач. сущ. м.* húngry pérson; ◇ ~ как волк ▪ húngry as a húnter.

голодóвк|а *ж.* **1.** *разг.* (*голод*) starvátion; **2.** (*в тюрьмé*) húnger-strike; объявúть ~y go* on húnger-strike.

гололёд *м.* *см.* гололéдица.

гололéдица *ж.* black ice, íce-crusted ground; (*о погóде*) glazed frost, ícing; сегóдня стрáшная ~ it's áwfully slíppery todáy.

гóлос *м.* **1.** voice; поднять ~ raise *one's* voice; **2.** (*при голосовании*) vote; ~ за vote for, and the noes; отдáть свой ~ за *кого-л.* vote for *smth.*, give* *one's* vote for *smb.*; прáво ~a the (right to) vote; решáющий ~ (*при разделении голосóв*) cásting vote; с прáвом решáющего ~a with the right to vote; с пра́вом совеща́тельного ~a with a voice but no vote; 3. *муз.* part; пе́сня на два ~a two-part song; для ~a и хо́ра for sólo voice and chórus; 4. (*мнение*) voice, opínion; ~ масс the voice of the másses; 5.: ~ рассу́дка the voice of réason; ~ со́вести the voice/appéal of cónscience; ◇ во весь ~ at the top of *one's* voice; быть в ~e be* in voice; зау́чивать *что-л.* с ~a pick up *smth.* from héaring it; в оди́н ~ in one voice, unánimously; хвали́ть в оди́н ~ uníte in práising; с чужо́го ~a говори́ть écho sómebody else, écho óther péople.

голоси́стый loud-vóiced; (*звонкий*) rínging.

голоси́ть *несов.* wail; ~ по поко́йнику keen.

голосло́вн|**о** withóut the slíghtest proof, on *one's* bare word, blánkly. ~**ый** unfóunded, gróundless, próofless; ~**ое** обвине́ние unfóunded accusátion; ~**ое** утвержде́ние mere allegátion; чтобы не быть ~ым by way of proof.

голосова́ни|**е** *с.* vóting; (*во время выборов*) poll; поимённое ~ róll-call vote; поста́вить предложе́ние на ~ put* the mótion to the vote; провести́ ~ по *чему-л.* take* a vote on *smth.*; результа́ты ~**ия** resúlts of the vóting/vote; (*в англ. парламенте*) division fígures; каби́на для ~**ия** pólling booth; ◇ маши́на ~**ия** vóting machine.

голосова́ть, проголосова́ть 1. (*за вн.; участвовать в голосовании*) vote (for); ~ подня́тием руки́ vote by (a) show of hands; ~ за (про́тив) предложе́ния vote in fávour of (agáinst) the mótion; 2. (*вн.; ставить на голосование*) put* (*smth.*) to the vote, take* a vote (on); (*чью-л. кандидату́ру*) vote (for); 3. *разг.* (*останавливать машину*) thumb a lift, (try to) hitch a lift.

голосов|**ой** vócal; ~**ые** свя́зки *анат.* vócal chords; ~**а́я** щель *анат.* glóttis.

голубе́|**ть** *несов.* 1. (*становиться голубым*) becóme*/turn blue; 2. (*виднеться*) show* blue; вдали́ ~**ло** мо́ре the sea showed blue in the dístance.

голубизна́ *ж.* ázure, the blue.

голуби́ка *ж.* 1. *собир.* bog whórtleberries *pl*, great bílberries *pl*; 2. (*об отдельной ягоде и растении*) bog whórtleberry, great bílberry.

голуби́н|**ый** pígeon *attr.*; ~**ая** по́чта pígeon-post.

голу́бка *ж.* 1. fémale dove/pígeon; 2. *ласк.* dear, dárling.

голубогла́зый blúe-eyed.

голуб|**о́й** 1. light-blúe, sky-blúe; 2. (*идеализированный*) idéalized; ◇ ~ экра́н TV, télevision.

голу́бушка *ж. ласк.* dear, dárling.

голубцы́ *мн. кул.* (*ед.* голубе́ц *м.*) stuffed cábbage-rolls.

голу́бчик *м. ласк.* old man*/féllow, my dear man*.

го́луб|**ь** *м.* pígeon, dove; ~ свя́зи, почто́вый ~ cárrier-pigeon, hóming pígeon; гоня́ть ~**ей** go in for pígeon-fáncying, race pígeons; ◇ ~ ми́ра the dove of peáce.

голубя́т|**ник** *м.* 1. (*любитель*) pígeon-fáncier, pígeon-flyer; 2. (*ястреб*) pígeon-hawk. ~**ня** *ж.* dóve-cot(e), pígeon-loft, pígeon-house.

го́л|**ый** 1. náked, nude (*обыкн. о человеке*); (*ничем не покрытый*) bare; (*лишённый растительности*) bald, bare; ~**ое** те́ло náked bódy; ~ пол báre/úncarpeted floor; ~**ые** дере́вья bare trees; ~**ые** сте́ны bare walls; спать на ~**ой** земле́ sleep* on the bare ground; 2. (*без прикрас*) náked, bare; ~**ая** и́стина the náked truth; ~**ые** фа́кты the bare facts; ◇ ~**ыми** рука́ми ≈ without firing a shot; ~**ое** администри́рование púrely bureaucrátic méthods *pl.*

голы́ш *м.* 1. *разг.* (*о ребёнке*) náked child*/boy*; (*о кукле*) náked báby doll; 2. (*камень*) pébble, shíngle; ~**о́м** *разг.* náked, with nóthing on.

голь *ж. собир.*: ~ на вы́думки хитра́ ≈ necéssity is the móther of invéntion.

гольф *м. спорт.* golf; игра́ть в ~ play golf, golf.

го́льфы *мн.* (knée-)bréeches; (*чулки*) gólf-stóckings.

гомеопа́т *м.* hómoeopath, homoeópathist. ~**и́ческий** homoeopáthic; в ~**и́ческих** до́зах in mínute quántities. ~**ия** *ж.* homoeópathy.

гоме́рический Homéric; ~ хо́хот Homéric láughter.

го́мон *м. разг.* húbbub; ~ толпы́ the hum of the crowd.

гонг *м.* gong; уда́рить в ~ strike*/sound the gong.

гондо́|**ла** *ж.* 1. (*лодка*) góndola; 2. (*дирижабля*) car. ~**лье́р** *м.* gondolíer.

гоне́н|**ие** *с.* persecútion; подверга́ться ~**иям** be* pérsecuted; (*об отдельных людях тж.*) be* víctimized.

гоне́ц *м.* méssenger.

го́нк|**а** *ж.* 1. *тк. ед. разг.* (*спешка*) húrry; 2. *тк. ед.* (*сплав плотов*) ráfting; 3. *мн.* ráces; (*лодочные*) regátta *sg*; бо́ат-race *sg*; па́русные ~ sáiling regátta *sg*; ~ вооруже́ний ármaments/arms race drive.

го́нор *м. разг.* árrogance; с ~**ом** árrogant.

гонора́р *м.* fee; а́вторский ~ áuthor's fee; áuthor's emóluments *pl*; (*с тиража*) róyalties *pl.*

го́ночный rácing; ~ автомоби́ль rácing car; ~ велосипе́д rácing bícycle; rácing bike *разг.*

гонча́р *м.* pótter. ~**ный** pótter's; ~**ные** изде́лия éarthenware *sg*, póttery *sg*; ~**ный** круг pótter's wheel.

го́нчая *ж.* hound.

го́нщик *м. спорт.* rácer; rácing dríver.

гоня́ть *несов.* (*вн.*) 1. drive* (*smb., smth.*); drive* (*smb.*) awáy; ~ кого́-л. с ме́ста make* smb. run all óver the place; ≈ drive* smb. from píllar to post; 2. *разг.* (*с поручениями*) send* (*smb.*) (on érrands); 3. (*по дт.*) *разг.* (*спрашивать — о преподавателе*) make* smb. go through smth., grill smb. on smth. ~**ся** *несов.* (*за тв.*) chase (*smb., smth.*); pursúe (*smb., smth.*); (*искать*) seek* (*smth.*).

гоп hóop-la!; ◇ не говори́ ~, пока́ не перепры́гнешь ≈ don't halló till you're out of the wood, don't speak too soon.

гор- в сложн. cíty *attr.*; (*о небольшом городе*) town *attr.*

гор|**а́** *ж.* móuntain; (*невысокая*) hill, *перен.* (*множество*) heap (of); снегов́ы́е го́ры snów-capped móuntains; америка́нские го́ры (*для катания в вагонетках*) switchback *sg*; ката́ться с гор (*на санках*) tobóggan; в го́ру úphill; под ~у dównhill; ~ бума́г heap of páper; ◇ идти́ в го́ру go* up in the world; стоя́ть ~**о́й** за кого́-л., что́-л. stand* firm for smb., smth.; be* sólidly behínd smb.; stick* up for smb., smth. *разг.*; сули́ть золоты́е го́ры prómise a fórtune; ~ с плеч (свали́лась) (it's) a load off *one's* mind; не за ~**а́ми** not far off.

горазд *в знач. сказ. разг.*: кто во что ~ each in his own fáshion and as hard as he can; он на э́то ~ he's a dab at that, that's just what he's good at.

гора́здо much, far; в ~ бо́льшей сте́пени to a far gréater extént.

горб *м.* hump; ◇ свои́м ~**о́м** ≈ by the sweat of *one's* brow. ~**а́тый** *прил.* 1. (*с горбом*) hunched, humped; 2. (*изогнутый, с горбинкой*): ~**а́тый** нос áquiline nose; ~**а́тый** мост húmpback bridge; 3. *в знач. сущ. м.* húnchback; ◇ ~**а́того** моги́ла испра́вит *погов.* ≈ can the léopard change his spots?

горб|**и́ть**, сго́рбить: ~ спи́ну bend* *one's* back. ~**ться**, сго́рбиться stoop; не ~**сь!** don't stoop!

горбоно́сый with an áquiline nose *после сущ.*; hóok-nósed.

горб|**у́н** *м.*, ~**у́нья** *ж.* húnchback, húmpback.

горбу́ша *ж.* gorbúsha, húmpbacked sálmon.

горбу́шка *ж.* crust/óutside (of a loaf*).

гордел́ивый proud.

го́рдиев: ~ у́зел Górdian knot.

горди́ться *несов.* 1. (*тв.; испытывать гордость*) be* proud (of), take* pride (in), pride onesélf (on); 2.

разг. (*быть высокомерным*) show* pride, have* a high opinion of one*self.

горд|ость *ж.* pride. **~ый** proud.

гор|е *с.* 1. (*глубокая печаль*) grief, sórrow; в ~ sórrow-stricken, in great grief, gríeving (óver); поседéть от ~я turn grey with sórrow; причинять кому-л. мнóго ~я cause *smb.* much distréss; причинять кому-л. ~ cause *smb.* pain; 2.: ~ емý! woe betíde him!; ~ мне! woe is me!; ~ мне с тобóй! you are the bane of my exístence/life!; 3. (*беда, несчастье*) tróuble, misfórtune; её постúгло ~ a sad thing háppened to her; какóе ~! what a misfórtune!; э́то для нас большóе ~ it is a great sórrow to us; ◇ емý и ~я мáло what does he care!

горе- *в сложн.* sórry; **~поэт** poetáster, apólogy for a póet.

горевáть *несов.* (*о пр.*) mourn (fór), grieve (óver).

горéлка *ж.* búrner; гáзовая ~ gás-burner.

горéлки *мн.* (*игра*) catch *sg*; игрáть в ~ play catch.

горéлый burnt.

горельéф *м.* high relíef.

горемы́|ка *м. и ж. разг.* hápless créature. **~чный** *разг.* wrétched, hápless.

горéние *с.* combústion, búrning; жизнь егó былá непрерúвным ~м his whole life was an unquénchable flame.

гóрестный sad, gríevous, sórrowful.

горест|ь ж. 1. (*печаль, скорбь*) grief, distréss; с ~ью sórrowfully; 2. *мн.* (*несчастья*) sórrows; пережúть мнóго ~ей know* much sórrow.

гор|éть, сгорéть 1. burn* (*тж. перен.*); (*о пожаре*) be* on fire; ~ я́рким плáменем burn* with a clear flame; ~úм! fire!; ~ нетерпéнием burn* with impátience; ~ желáнием burn* with desíre; в огнé не ~úт и в водé не тóнет it pásses únscáthed through fire and flood; 2. *тк. несов.* (*давать свет, пламя*) be* búrning, be* on; свет ~úт the light is (switched) on; 3. *тк. несов.* (*быть в лихорадке*) burn*; be* féverish; головá у меня́ ~úт my head is búrning/féverish; 4. *тк. несов.* (*сверкать*) flash, blaze; глазá ~éли я́ростью the eyes blazed with ánger; гóрод ~úт огня́ми the town is abláze with light; ◇ рабóта ~úт в егó рукáх he works like lightning; земля́ ~úт под ногáми the place is gétting too hot for *one*.

гóрец *м.* móuntain-dwéller, híghlander.

гóречь ж. 1. (*вкус*) bítter taste; 2. (*что-л. горькое*) bítter stuff; 3. (*горькое чувство*) bítterness.

горизóнт *м.* 1. horízon (*тж. перен.*); (*линия горизонта*) skýline; скрúться за ~ом disappéar from the horízon; (*о солнце*) sink* belów the horízon; 2. *мн.* (*круг действий, возможностей*) horízons; открúть нóвые ~ы в наýке ópen up new térritory/horízons in science; перед нáми раскрывáются широкие ~ы vast perspéctives lie before us.

горизонтáль *ж.* horizóntal line; (*на карте*) cóntour line; (*на шахматной доске*) rank. **~ный** horizóntal.

горúлла *ж. зоол.* gorílla.

гориспóлкóм *м.* (*исполнительный комитет городского Совета депутатов*) Exécutive (Committee) of the City/Town Sóviet (of Péople's Députies); City/Town Exécutive *разг.*

горúстый móuntainous.

горихвóстка *ж. зоол.* rédstart.

горицвéт *м. бот.* lýchnis.

гóрка ж. 1. hill; 2. (*шкафчик*) cábinet; 3. *ав.* vértical climb.

гóркнуть, прогóркнуть go* bad, spoil*; (*о масле*) turn (ráncid).

горкóм *м.* (*городскóй комитéт*) City/Town Committee.

горлá|нить *несов. разг.* bawl. **~стый** *разг.* lóud-vóiced.

гóрл|инка ж., **~ица ж.** *зоол.* túrtle-dove.

гóрл|о *с.* throat; лáрупх *анат.*; у негó болúт ~ he

has a sore throat; ◇ дыхáтельное ~ wíndpipe; быть сúтым по ~ be* full; *перен.* be* fed up; have* had enóugh; кричáть во всё ~ shout lústily, shout at the top of *one's* voice; (как) с ножóм к ~у пристáть к кому-л. péster *smb.*, bádger *smb.*; стать поперёк ~а кому-л. make* *smb.* sick, be* a thorn in *smb.'s* flesh; промочúть ~ have* a drink.

горловóй 1. throat *attr.*; of the throat *после сущ.*; 2. (*о голосе*) gúttural, thróaty.

гóрлышк|о *с.* neck; пить из ~а drink* straight from the bóttle.

гормóн *м. физиол.* hórmone.

горн I *м. тех.* 1. fúrnace; кузнéчный ~ forge; 2. (*нижняя часть доменной печи*) hearth.

горн II *м.* (*сигнальный*) búgle.

горнúло *с.* crúcible (*тж. перен.*).

горнúст *м.* búgler.

гóрничная *ж.* hóusemaid; (*в гостинице*) chámbermaid; (*на пароходе*) stéwardess.

горнодобывáющий míning.

горнозавóдский míning and metallúrgical; ~ райóн míning and smélting área.

горнолы́жный: ~ спорт móuntain skíing.

горнопромы́шленный míning *attr.*; ~ райóн míning área.

горнопрохóдческ|ий: ~ие рабóты drífting; wórking a mine.

горнорабóчий *м.* míner.

горноспасáтельный (míne-)réscue *attr.*

горностáй *м.* 1. (*животное*) stoat; 2. (*мех*) érmine.

гóрн|ый 1. móuntain *attr.*; (*гористый*) móuntainous; ~ хребéт móuntain chain/range; ~ая рéчка móuntain stream; ~ая странá híghlands *pl*; 2. (*добываемый из недр земли*) míneral; ~ая порóда rock; 3. (*относящийся к разработке земных недр*) míning; ~ое дéло míning; ~ая промы́шленность míning índustry; ~ инженéр míning engíneer; ~ институ́т míning ínstitute; ◇ ~ая болéзнь móuntain síckness; ~ хрустáль róck-crystal; ~ лён *мин.* móuntain flax, amiánthus.

горн|я́к *м. разг.* (*рабочий*) míner; (*инженер*) míning engíneer; **~я́цкий** *разг. разг.* míners', míning.

гóрод *м.* town; (*крупный центр*) city; ~ Москвá the city of Móscow; столúчный ~ cápital (city); провинциáльный ~ províncial town; зá ~ out of town, to the cóuntry; зá ~ом out of town, in the cóuntry; ~ и дерéвня town and cóuntry; в ~áх и посёлках in (large and small) úrban commúnities.

гóрод-герóй *м.* Héro City.

городúть *несов. разг.*: ~ вздор talk (a lot of) nónsense; не стóит огорóд ~ ≈ it's nóthing to make a song and dance abóut.

городúще *с. археол.* site of áncient town/séttlement.

городкú *мн.* gorodkí (*a kind of skittles*); игрáть в ~ play gorodki.

городóк *м.* 1. (small) town, tównship; 2.: студéнческий ~ stúdents' hóstels *pl*; университéтский ~ cámpus; воéнный ~ cantónment.

городск|óй town *attr.*, city *attr.*, úrban; municipal; ~ жúтель tówn-dweller; tównsman* (*pl* tównspeople, tównsfolk); ~óе населéние úrban populátion; ~ сад the municipal gárdens *pl*; ~ Совéт нарóдных депутáтов City/Town Sóviet (of Péople's Députies); ~ трáнспорт úrban/municipal tránsport (sýstem); ~óе строúтельство town building, úrban devélopment; (*раздел архитектуры*) town plánning; ~óе хозя́йство municipal facílities and sérvices *pl*.

горожáнин *м.* tówn-dweller, tównsman* (*pl* tównspeople, tównsfolk).

горонó *м. нескл. ист.* (*городскóй отдéл нарóдного образовáния*) City/Town Board of Educátion.

горóх *м.* 1. (*растение*) pea; 2. *собир.* (*семена*) peas *pl*; лущёный ~ split peas; ◇ при царé Горóхе ≈ in the year dot/one, áges agó; как об стену ~ you might as well talk to a brick wall. ~овый 1. pea attr.; ~овое поле field of peas; ~овый суп pea soup; 2. (о цвете) pea--green; ◇ шут ~овый, чучело ~овое clown, buffóon.

горош|ек м. 1. бот. vetch, tare; 2. (крапинки на ткани) spots pl; ситец в ~ spótted cótton stuff; ◇ зелёный ~ green peas pl. ~ина ж. pea; с ~ину no bígger than a pea.

горсовет м. (городской Совет народных депутатов) City/Town Sóviet (of Péople's Députies).

горстка ж. hándful; ~ людей a (mere) hándful of péople.

горсть ж. 1. (руки) one's cupped hand, the cup of one's hand; 2. (количество) hándful (тж. перен.).

гортанный gúttural.

гортань ж. анат. lárynx.

гортензия ж. бот. hydrángea.

горчить несов. taste bitter, have* a bítter taste.

горчи|ца ж. mústard. ~чник м. mústard pláster; поставить ~чники кому-л. use mústard plásters on smb. ~чница ж. mústard-pot. ~чный mústard attr.

горшок m. pot.

горь|кий 1. bítter; ~ как полынь bítter as wórmwood; 2. (горестный, тягостный) sad, bítter; ~кая доля sad/bítter fate; ◇ ~кая истина the bítter truth; ~кие слёзы bítter tears; ~ пьяница hópeless drúnkard. ~ко 1. нареч. bítterly; ~ плакать cry bítterly, shed* bítter tears; 2. в знач. сказ. безл. ~ко во рту a bítter/bad taste in one's mouth; ~ко слышать такие слова it pains one to hear such words.

горючее с. fuel; (бензин тж.) pétrol; gásoline, gas амер.

горючий I combústible; (легко воспламеняющийся) inflámmable.

горючий II: ~ие слёзы scálding tears.

горяч|ий 1. hot; ~ие угли live coals; 2. (пылкий) fíery, keen, éager; (выражающий глубину чувства) árdent, férvent; ~ие головы hótheads; ~ее сердце warm heart; ~ая любовь pássionate love; ~ее желание árdent desíre; ~ спор héated debáte; ~ приём enthusiástic wélcome; встретить ~ую поддержку recéive whole-héarted suppórt; 3. (вспыльчивый) hot-témpered; (резвый — о лошади) fíery, spírited; 4. (при высоких температурах) heat attr.; ~ая обработка металлов heat tréatment of métals; 5. (напряжённый) búsy; ~ее время búsy séason; crówded days pl; ◇ ~ая кровь férvent náture; по ~им следам while the scent is hot; попасть под ~ую руку run* into a squall.

горячить, разгорячить (вн.) excite (smb.). ~ся, разгорячиться be*/becóme* excíted; (раздражаться) be*/becóme* ángry, be* in a témper.

горячк|а ж. разг. 1. féver; 2. (азарт) rush; биржевая ~ a rush on the stóck-market; 3. (спешка) rush (and tear), hot haste; ◇ пороть ~у do* things in a rush.

горячность ж. 1. (увлечение) zeal, férvour, éagerness; 2. (вспыльчивость) hot témper.

горячо 1. нареч. férvently, éagerly, pássionately; ~ говорить speak* with férvour; ~ приняться за дело set* to enthusiástically; ~ любить кого-л. love smb. déarly; 2. в знач. сказ. безл.: мне ~ it is too hot for me.

гос- в сложн. State.

госбанк м. (Государственный банк) the State Bank.

госбезопасност|ь ж.: органы ~и (State) secúrity órgans.

госбюджет м. the State Búdget.

госпитализация ж. hospitalizátion.

госпиталь м. (mílitary) hóspital.

господа мн. 1. géntlemen; (в обращении) géntlemen! (при наличии мужчин и женщин) ládies and géntlemen!; (в присутствии одной женщины) Mádam!, Géntlemen!; 2. (при фамилии или звании) Messrs.

['mesəz]; 3. (хозяева) másters; слуга двух господ the sérvant of two másters.

господин м. 1. géntleman*; (в обращении) sir! 2. (при фамилии или звании) Mr. ['mɪstə]; (в официальной речи — о французах) Monsieur [mə'sjə :] (сокр. M.); (об итальянцах) Signor ['si:njɔ:]; (о немцах) Herr [hɛə] — председатель! Mr. Cháirman!; ~ президент! Mr. Président!; 3. (хозяин) máster; ◇ сам себе ~ one's own máster.

господств|о с. 1. (власть) dominátion; 2. (преобладание) suprémacy; мировое ~ world dominátion; ~ в воздухе air suprémacy. ~овать несов. 1. (над тв.; властвовать) dóminate (óver); 2. (преобладать) preváil; 3. (над тв.; возвышаться) command (smth.), dóminate (smth.). ~ующий 1. (находящийся у власти) rúling; ~ующий класс rúling class, the class in pówer; 2. (преобладающий) preváiling, dóminant; ~ующие взгляды preváiling views/opínions.

госпож|а ж. 1. lády; 2. (при фамилии) Mrs. ['mɪsɪz]; (о незамужней женщине) Miss; (в официальной речи — о француженках, часто русских и др.) Mádam (сокр. Mme.), Mademoisélle [mædəm'zel] (сокр. Mlle); (об итальянках) Signóra [sɪ'njɔ:rə], Signorína [sɪnjo'ri:nə]; (о немках) Frau [frau], Fräulein ['frɔɪlaɪn]; 3. (без фамилии) Mádam; 4. (хозяйка) místress.

гостев|ой: ~ билет invitátion card; ~ые места на трибуне pláces for vísitors.

гостеприим|ный hóspitable. ~ство с. hospitálity; оказывать ~ство кому-л. show* hospitálity to smb.; be* host to smb.

гостиная ж. 1. dráwing-room; (в небольшой квартире) sítting-room; 2. (в гостиницах и т.п.) lounge; 3. (мебель) dráwing-room suite.

гостиниц|а ж. hotél; остановиться в ~e put* up at a hotél, stay/stop at a hotél.

гостить несов. (у рд.) stay (with).

гост|ь м. guest, vísitor; незваный ~ uninvited guest; редкий ~ infréquent vísitor; у нас ~и we have vísitors; ◇ быть в ~ях у кого-л. be* on a vísit to smb.; идти в ~и к кому-л. go* to see smb.; прийти в ~и к кому-л. come* to see smb.; в ~ях хорошо, а дома лучше погов. ≈ East or West, home is best.

государственно-монополистический státe-monópoly.

государственн|ость ж. political sýstem; (государственный суверенитет) státehood. ~ый State attr.; (национальный) nátional; ~ый строй political/State sýstem; ~ое устройство political organizátion, form of góvernment; ~ая власть State pówer; ~ый флаг nátional flag; ~ая граница State fróntier; ~ый язык official lánguage (of the State); ~ый деятель státesman*; ~ый долг nátional debt; ~ые доходы (públic) révenues; ~ая служба públic sérvice; ~ый переворот coup-d'état; ~ый преступник State críminal, political offénder; дело ~ой важности affáir of nátional impórtance; ~ые закупки State púrchases; ◇ ~ое право юр. constitútional law.

государств|о с. State; (страна) cóuntry, nátion; ~а--участники member States/nátions; содружество государств the commonwealth of states.

государыня ж. уст. 1. (царица) sóvereign; 2. (в обращении) Your Májesty, Mádam.

государ|ь м. уст. 1. (царь) sóvereign; 2. (в обращении) Your Májesty, Sir; ◇ милостивый ~ Dear Sir; милостивые ~и Géntlemen.

гот|ика ж. Góthic. ~ический Góthic; ~ический стиль Góthic style; ~ический шрифт Góthic (type), black létter.

готовальня ж. set/case of dráwing instruments.

готовить несов. (вн.) 1. prepáre (smth.); ~ торжественную встречу órganize an official recéption; 2. (обучать) train (smb.); ~ кадры train wórkers/personnél; 3. (стряпать) cook (smth.), make* (smth.); ~ обед make* dínner, get* dínner réady; хорошо ~ be* a good cook; уме́ть ~ know* how to cook. ~ся *несов.* 1. (к *дт.*) prepáre (for), make* réady (for); ~ся к бою stand* by for áction; ~ся к отъе́зду make* preparátions for depárture; ~ся к экза́мену prepáre/stúdy for an examinátion; ~ся к зачёту по геогра́фии revíse *one's* geógraphy; get*/read* up *one's* geógraphy *разг.*; 2. (*на-двига́ться, назрева́ть*) appróach, be* in the óffing.

гото́вность *ж.* réadiness; (*согласие тж.*) wíllingness; выража́ть ~ expréss *one's* réadiness/wíllingness.

гото́в|ый 1. (к *дт.*) réady (for); (*подготовленный*) prepáred (for); ~о! réady!; 2. (*на вн.,* + *инф. соглас-ный*) wílling (+ to *inf*), réady (for, + to *inf*), prepáred (for, + to *inf*); мы ~ы вести́ переговоры we are prepáred to negótiate; он для вас готов на всё he'd do ánything for you; я был уже́ готов согласи́ться, когда́... I was on the point of agréeing, when...; 3. (*сделанный, закончен-ный*) fínished; (*об одежде*) réady-máde; ~о блюдо dish réady to serve; ~ое изде́лие fínished 'próduct/árticle; manufáctured goods *pl*; ~ое пла́тье réady-máde clothes; 4. (*заранее обдуманный*) cút-and-dríed; ◇ всегда́ го-то́в! (*девиз пионеров*) éver réady!

го́тский Góthic; ~ язы́к Góthic, the Góthic lánguage.

гофриро́ванный crimped; (*о платье*) góffered; (*о металле*) córrugated.

гофрирова́ть *несов.* (*вн.*) crimp (*smth.*); (*платье*) góffer (*smth.*); (*металл*) córrugate (*smth.*).

граб *м. бот.* hórnbeam.

граб|ёж *м.* róbbery; (*вооружённый*) armed róbbery; hóld-up *разг.*; ~ на большо́й доро́ге híghway róbbery; занима́ться ~ежом rob, plúnder; ~и́тель *м.* róbber. ~и́тельский rapácious, prédatory; ~и́тельская поли́тика expánsionist pólicy; ~и́тельские во́йны prédatory wars; ~и́тельские це́ны exórbitant príces.

гра́бить *несов.* (*вн.*) rob (*smb., smth.*) (*тж. перен.*); plúnder (*smb., smth.*).

гра́бли *мн.* rake *sg*; ко́нные ~ hórse-rake *sg.*

гравёр *м.* engráver; (*офортист*) étcher; ~ по де́ре-ву wóodcutter, wóod-engraver; ~ по ка́мню lápidary.

гра́ви|й *м.* grável; посыпа́ть *что-л.* ~ем grável *smth.*

гравиро́в|а́льный engráver's, engráving; (*для офор-та*) étcher's, étching. ~а́ть *несов.* engráve; (*травлени-ем*) etch.

гравю́ра *ж.* engráving, print; (*офорт*) étching; ~ на де́реве wóodcut.

град I *м.* hail; *перен. тж.* vólley; ~ идёт it is háiling, hail is fálling; ~ пуль hail of búllets; ~ руга́тельств vólley of oaths.

град II *м. уст. поэт. см.* го́род.

града́ция *ж.* gradátion(s).

гра́дина *ж.* háilstone.

гради́рня *ж.* 1. (*в производстве соли*) sált-pan, sált-pond; 2. (*охладитель*) cóoling tówer.

гра́дом thick and fast; слёзы ка́тятся ~ tears are rólling down *one's* cheeks; пот с него́ льётся ~ the sweat is póuring off him; уда́ры сы́пались ~ the blows fell thick and fast.

градостро|е́ние, ~и́тельство *с.* town plánning, town building, úrban devélopment.

градуи́ровать *несов. и сов.* (*вн.*) *тех.* gráduate (*smth.*).

гра́дус *м.* degrée; пять ~ов вы́ше, ни́же нуля́ five degrées abóve, belów zéro; пять ~ов моро́за, тепла́ five degrées of frost, abóve zéro; ско́лько сего́дня ~ов? what is the témperature todáy?; у́гол в 45 ~ов an ángle of fórty-five degrées. ~ник *м. разг.* thermómeter; поста́вить ~ник *кому-л.* take* *smb.'s* témperature.

гражд|ани́н *м.*, ~а́нка *ж.* cítizen.

гражда́нск|ий 1. cívil; ~ое пра́во cívil law; ~ иск *юр.* civil áction/suit; ~ ко́декс cívil code; 2. (*свойственный гражданину*) cívic; ~ долг dúty as a cítizen; cívic dúty;

cívic obligátions *pl*; ~ое му́жество cívic vírtue; 3. (*невоен-ный*) civílian; ~ое пла́тье civílian clothes *pl*; ~ возду́ш-ный флот cívil air fleet; ◇ ~ая война́ cívil war; ~ая па-нихи́да fúneral méeting; ~ брак cívil márriage.

гражда́нств|о *с.* cítizenship; получи́ть права́ ~а be* admítted to cítizenship; *перен.* win* recognítion, win* an acknówledged place; приня́ть росси́йское ~ becóme* a Rússian cítizen, be* náturalized as a Rússian cítizen.

грамза́пис|ь *ж.* (grámophone) recórding; му́зыка в ~и músic on grámophone recórds, recórded músic.

грамм *м.* gram(me).

грамм|а́тика *ж.* grámmar; (*книга*) grámmar(-book). ~и́ст *м.* grammárian. ~и́ческий grammátical; де́лать ~и́ческие оши́бки speak*, write* úngrammátically/ illíterately, make* grámmar mistákes; он де́лает мно́го ~и́ческих оши́бок his grámmar is bad; производи́ть ~и́ческий разбо́р *чего-л.* parse *smth.*

грамм|-а́том *м. физ., хим.* gram(me) átom. ~-моле́-кула *ж. физ., хим.* gram(me) mólecule.

граммофо́н *м.* grámophone.

гра́мот|а *ж.* 1. réading and wríting; учи́ться ~е learn* to read and write; 2. (*документ*) deed; почётная ~ (*honorary*) diplóma; ◇ фи́лькина ~ *ирон.* (*о доку-менте*) a scrap of páper. ~но 1. grammátically; писа́ть ~но write* grammátically; 2. (*умело*) cómpetently, skílfully. ~ность *ж.* 1. líteracy; 2. (*осведомлённость*) cómpetence, skílfulness; полити́ческая ~ность political knówledge. ~ный 1. (*умеющий читать и писать*) líterate; 2. (*не содержащий грамматических ошибок*) grammátical; 3. (*умелый, осведомлённый*) cómpetent, skilled, knówledgeable.

грампласти́нка *ж.* (grámophone) récord, disc.

грана́т I *м.* (*плод и дерево*) pómegranate.

грана́т II *м.* (*драгоценный камень*) gárnet.

грана́т|а *ж. воен.* grenáde; (*артиллерийская*) high--explósive shell; ручна́я ~ hánd-grenade; противота́нко-вая ~ anti-tánk grenáde.

грана́тов|ый I pómegranate *attr.*; ~ое де́рево pómegranate(-tree).

грана́товый II 1. (*о драгоценном камне*) gárnet *attr.*; ~ брасле́т gárnet brácelet; 2. (*о цвете*) gárnet-red.

грандио́зн|ый (*огромный*) vast, huge, treméndous, colóssal; (*внушительный*) grándiose, impósing; ~ая де-монстра́ция huge demonstrátion; ~ое строи́тельство treméndous work of constrúction; ~ое зда́ние huge building; ~ое зре́лище impósing spéctacle; ~ план gigántic/huge plan; ~ые масшта́бы colóssal scale *sg.*

гранён|ый cut; (*о драгоценном камне*) fáceted; ~ое стекло́ cut glass; ~ графи́н cút-glass decánter; ~ стака́н thick glass túmbler.

грани́т *м.* gránite. ~ный gránite *attr.*

грани́ть *несов.* (*вн.*) cut* (*smth.*); (*драгоценный ка-мень тж.*) fácet (*smth.*).

грани́ц|а *ж.* 1. bórder; (*естественная*) bóundary; (*государственная*) frontíer; переходи́ть ~у cross the frontíer; 2. *обыкн. мн.* (*предел*) límit *sg*, bound *sg*, end *sg*; не знать грани́ц know* no bounds; переходи́ть ~ы go* beyónd all bounds; э́то перехо́дит все ~ы! that's the límit!; э́то pásses the bounds!; ◇ за ~у, за ~ей abróad; из-за ~ы from abróad.

грани́чить *несов.* (*с тв.*) bórder (on, upón), be* contíguous (to), adjóin (*smth.*); *перен.* verge (on), bórder (on); ~ с безу́мием verge on lúnacy/insánity.

гра́нка *ж. полигр.* (gálley)proof.

гран|ь *ж.* 1. (*граница*) bórder, brink, verge; на ~и войны́ on the brink of war; 2. (*плоскость*) side, edge; (*драгоценного камня*) fácet.

граф *м.* count; (*английский*) earl.

графа́ *ж.* 1. (*колонка*) cólumn; 2. (*раздел*) séction, héading.

гра́фик I *м.* 1. (*чертёж*) chart, graph; ~ движе́ния поездо́в ráilway tíme-table; 2. (*план работ*) schédule, (tíme-)table; ~ рабо́т óperating schédule; по ~у accórding to schédule.

гра́фик II *м.* (*художник*) péncil ártist, black-and-white ártist.

гра́фик|а *ж.* 1. dráwing; black-and-white art; 2. *собир.* dráwings *pl*; вы́ставка ~и an exhibítion of dráwings.

графи́н *м.* (*для воды*) wáter-bottle, caráfe; (*для вина*) decánter.

графи́ня *ж.* cóuntess.

графи́т *м.* plumbágo, black lead.

графи́ть *несов.* (*вн.*) rule (*smth.*) (*make lines*).

графи́ческ|и in díagram form. ~ий gráphic.

графлёный ruled.

графома́н *м.* graphomániac, compúlsive scríbbler.

графств|о *с.* (*административный район в Англии, Ирландии*) cóunty, shíre; центра́льные ~a the Mídlands.

грацио́зный gráceful.

гра́ци|я *ж.* 1. grácefulness, grace; 2. *миф.* три Гра́ции the Gráces; 3. (*корсет*) córset.

грач *м. зоол.* rook.

гребёнк|а *ж* comb; стричь *кого-л.* под ~y crop *smb.'s* hair (close); ◇ стричь всех под одну́ ~у redúce éveryone to the same lével.

гре́бень *м.* 1. comb; 2. (*у птицы*) comb; crest; петуши́ный ~ cock's comb; 3. (*волны*) crest; (*горы*) ridge; 4. *mex.* comb; *текст.* card; (*для льна и т. п.*) háckle, hátchel.

гребе́ц *м.* óarsman*, rówer; он хоро́ший ~ he pulls a good oar.

гребешо́к *м.* 1. small comb; 2. (*у птиц*) comb.

гре́бля *ж.* rówing; академи́ческая ~ *спорт.* bóat-racing; наро́дная ~ *спорт.* dínghy rácing.

гребн|о́й: ~ спорт rówing, bóating; ~а́я шлю́пка rówing-boat; ~ винт scréw-propeller; ~о́е колесо́ páddle-wheel.

гребо́к *м.* 1. (*взмах весла*) stroke; 2. (*весло, лопасть*) páddle.

грёза *ж.* dream, dáy-dream, réverie.

гре́зить dream*; ~ наяву́ dáy-dream*.

гре́йдер *м.* 1. *mex.* gráder; 2. *разг.* (*дорога*) dirt road. ~ный gráder *attr.*; ~ная доро́га dirt road.

грейпфру́т *м.* 1. (*плод*) grápe-fruit; 2. (*дерево*) grápefruit-tree.

грек *м.* Greek.

грёлка *ж.* hot-wáter bóttle; электри́ческая ~ héating pad.

грем|е́ть, прогреме́ть thúnder; (*звенеть*) ráttle, clank; (*о ключах*) jíngle; *перен.* resóund; гром ~и́т thúnder roars/cráshes; ~ посу́дой ráttle díshes; его́ сла́ва ~и́т по всему́ ми́ру his fame resóunds/revérberates throughóut the world.

гремуч|ий ráttling; ◇ ~ газ fíre-damp; ~ая змея́ ráttlesnake.

гренки́ *мн.* (*ед.* грено́к *м.*) *кул.* toast *sg*; (*для супа*) síppets.

грести́ *несов.* 1. (*вёслами*) row; pull; (*парными вёслами*) scull; (*гребком*) páddle; 2. (*вн.*; *граблями*) rake (*smth.*).

гре|ть *несов.* 1. (*излучать тепло*) give* warmth/heat, be* warm; (*сохранять тепло — об одежде*) keep* warm; со́лнце ~ет the sun is warm; печь ~ет ко́мнату the stove heats the room; моя́ шу́ба хорошо́ ~ет my fúr-coat keeps me nice and warm; 2. (*вн.; нагревать*) warm (*smth.*) up, heat (*smth.*) up; ~ во́ду heat wáter. ~ться *несов.* warm onesélf; ~ться на со́лнце bask in the sun.

грех *м.* 1. *рел.* sin; 2. (*предосудительный поступок*) offénce; мой ~! my fault!; 3. *в знач. сказ. разг.* it's wrong; ◇ от ~а́ подáльше out of harm's way; вы́держать экза́мен с ~о́м попола́м scrape through an examinátion; сде́лать *что-л.* с ~о́м попола́м make* a

rough/poor job of *smth.*; что (*или* нéчего) ~á тáить let's tell the whole stóry, let's face it.

гре́цкий: ~ оре́х wálnut.

греча́нка *ж.* Greek wóman*.

гре́ческий Greek; (*о стиле*) Grécian; ~ язы́к Greek, the Greek lánguage.

гречи́ха *ж. бот.* búckwheat.

гре́чнев|ый búckwheat *attr.*; ~ая кáша búckwheat pórridge; ~ая крупá búckwheat.

греши́ть, согреши́ть, погреши́ть 1. *сов.* согреши́ть sin, transgréss; 2. *сов.* погреши́ть (*против рд., допускать ошибки*) err (from); (*тв.; иметь недостаток*) err (in the diréction of), err (towárds); ~ про́тив и́стины err from the truth, sin against the truth.

греш|ник *м.*, ~ница *ж.* sínner. ~нó *в знач. сказ.* (+ *инф.*) *разг.* it is a sin (+ to *inf*); ~нó так говори́ть it's a shame to talk like that. ~ный sínful; (*о мыслях*) guílty, cúlpable; ◇ ~ным де́лом sad to say.

гриб *м.* fúngus (*pl* -gi, -ses); (*съедобный*) múshroom; (*несъедобный*) tóadstool; собирáть ~ы́ go* múshroom-picking; бéлый ~ bolétus édulis. ~ни́ца *ж. бот.* múshroom spawn; mycélium; ~но́й múshroom *attr.*; ~но́е мéсто a good spot for múshrooms; ~но́й суп múshroom soup; ◇ ~но́й дождь shówer of fine warm rain, rain dúring súnshine. ~о́к *м.* 1. *биол.* fúngus (*pl* -gi); 2. (*укрытие*) (wóoden) umbrélla.

гри́ва *ж.* mane.

гри́венник *м. разг.* tén-cópeck piece/coin.

грим *м.* 1. máke-up; 2. (*краски*) gréase-paint.

грима́с|а *ж.* grimáce; стро́ить ~ы make*/pull fáces. ~ничать *несов.* grimáce.

гримёр *м.* máke-up ártist/man*. ~ша *ж. разг.* máke-up ártist/wóman*.

гримировáть, нагримировáть, загримировáть 1. *сов.* нагримировáть (*вн.*) make* (*smb.*) up; 2. *сов.* загримировáть (*вн. тв.*) make* (*smth.*) up (as *smb.*). ~ся, нагримировáться, загримировáться make* (onesélf) up; загримировáться под *кого-л.* make* (onesélf) up as *smb.*

Гри́нвич *м.:* 15 ч. 30 м. по ~у three thírty (3.30) p.m. Gréenwich (mean) time (*сокр.* G.M.T.).

грипп *м.* grippe, influénza; flu(e) *разг.* ~овáть *несов. разг.* have* the flu(e). ~о́зный influénzal.

гриф I *м.* 1. *миф.* gríffin; 2. (*птица*) gríffon (-vulture).

гриф II *м. муз.* neck, fínger-board.

гриф III *м.* (*печать*) stamp.

гри́фель *м.* sláte-pencil. ~ный: ~ная доскá slate.

грифо́н *м.* 1. *миф!* gríffin; 2. (*собака*) gríffon-térrier.

гроб *м.* cóffin; идти́ за ~ом *кого-л.* fóllow *smb.'s* remáins; ◇ до ~а all one's life, to the day of one's death, till one's dýing day; вогнáть *кого-л.* в ~ drive* *smb.* to his, her grave; по ~ жи́зни to the end of one's life; одно́й ного́й в ~у one foot in the grave. ~ни́ца *ж.* tomb, sépulchre.

гробов|о́й cóffin *attr.*; ◇ ~ го́лос sepúlchral voice; ~о́е молчáние dead sílence; встречáть *кого-л., что-л.* ~ы́м молчáнием receíve *smb., smth.* in dead sílence; meet* *smb., smth.* with dead sílence; до ~о́й доски́ to the end of one's days/life. ~щи́к *м.* cóffin-máker.

грозá *ж.* 1. thúnderstorm; *перен.* storm; 2. (*опасность*) dánger; 3. (*кто-л. или что-л., внушающее страх*) térror.

гроздь *ж.* clúster; ~ виногрáда bunch of grapes.

грози́|ть, погрози́ть 1. *тк. несов.* (*дт.*) thréaten (*smb.*); ему́ ~т опáсность he is in grave dánger; ~ катастро́фой thréaten to cause disáster; 2. (*дт. тв.*; *делать угрожающий жест*) make* threatening géstures (at); ~ кому́-л. кулако́м, пáльцем shake* one's fist, finger at *smb.* ~ться *несов.* (+ *инф.*) *разг.* thréaten (+ to *inf*).

грозн|ый 1. (*угрожающий*) ménacing, thréatening; ~ая по́за intímidating áttitude; ~ взгляд féarsome gaze; 2. (*внушающий страх*) fórmidable; ~ое ору́жие fórmidable wéapon; ~ проти́вник fórmidable ádversary/oppónent; ◇ Ива́н Гро́зный Ivan the Térrible.

грозов|о́й thúndery; ~áя атмосфе́ра thúnder in the air; ~ое о́блако, ~áя ту́ча thúnder-cloud, stórm-cloud.

гром м. thúnder; ~ пу́шек the roar/thúnder of the guns; ~ аплодисме́нтов storm/thúnder of appláuse; ◇ ~ побе́ды the thúnders of víctory; как ~ом поражённый thúnderstruck; ~ среди́ я́сного не́ба a bolt from the blue; мета́ть ~ы и мо́лнии fúlminate, rage, storm.

грома́д|а ж. mass, bulk; enórmous thing; се́рые ~ы незако́нченных постро́ек the huge grey shapes of únfinished buíldings. ~ный huge, enórmous, vast, imménse; ~ое зда́ние enórmous buílding; ~ое значе́ние imménse sígnificance.

громи́ла м. разг. 1. (вор-взло́мщик) hóuse-breaker; 2. (погро́мщик) thug.

громи́ть, разгроми́ть (вн.) 1. (разруша́ть, разоря́ть) break* (smth.) up, smash (smth.) up, wreck (smth.), ránsack (smth.); 2. (разбива́ть врага́) rout (smb., smth.), deféat (smb., smth.), smash (smb., smth.); 3. разг. (облича́ть) flay (smb.), belábour (smb.), make* a slá́shing attáck (on); (тео́рию и т. п.) anníhilate (smth.).

гро́мк|ий 1. loud; ~им го́лосом in a loud voice; 2. (изве́стный) notórious, fámous; ~ое де́ло notórious case; ~ое и́мя fámous name; ~ая побе́да resóunding víctory; 3. (высокопа́рный) high-flown, grandíloquent; ~ие слова́, фра́зы high-sounding phráses; ирон. big words.

гро́мко loud, lóudly; ~ болта́ть chátter lóudly; ~ крича́ть shout; ~ sing* at the top of one's voice; ~ разгова́ривать talk loud; ~ смея́ться laugh alóud.

громкоговори́тель м. lóudspeaker.

громов|о́й thúnder attr.; перен. thúnderous; ~ые раска́ты peals of thúnder; ~ го́лос voice of thúnder, stentórian voice.

громогла́сн|о lóudly. ~ый 1. (о го́лосе, пе́нии и т. п.) loud, thúnderous; 2. (о челове́ке) lóud-vóiced.

громозд|и́ть несов. (вн.) heap (up) (smth.), pile (up) (smth.). ~и́ться несов. 1. tówer; го́ры ~я́тся одна́ за друго́ю the peaks rise in majéstic succéssion; 2. (на вн.) разг. (влеза́ть) clámber (on to).

громо́здкий cúmbersome, búlky, unwíeldy; ~ бага́ж búlky lúggage.

громоотво́д м. líghtning-conductor; (в аппара́те) líghtning-arrester.

гро́мче (сравнит. ст. прил. гро́мкий и нареч. гро́мко) lóuder.

громыха́ть несов. разг. rúmble.

гроссме́йстер м. шахм. grándmaster.

грот I м. (пеще́ра) grótto (pl -oes, -os).

грот II м. (па́рус) máinsail.

гроте́ск м. the grotésque. ~ный grotésque.

грот-ма́чта ж. мор. máin-mast.

гро́хнуться сов. разг. fall* with a bang, come* crashing down.

гро́хот I м. thúnder.

гро́хот II м. (решето́) screen, ríddle.

грохота́ть, загрохота́ть rúmble.

грош м. 1. уст. hálf-copeck piece; 2. обыкн. мн. (ма́ленькая су́мма де́нег) pénny sg, fárthing sg; за ~и́ for a song; ◇ ~á ло́маного, ме́дного не сто́ит ≈ not worth a rap/scrap; без ~á (в карма́не) pénniless; оста́ться без ~á be* pénniless, be* stóny-broke, be* broke to the world: не име́ть ни ~á за душо́й have* not a pénny to bless oneself with; ни в ~ не ста́вить кого́-л., что́-л. not give*/care túppence/a fig for smb., smth. ~о́вый разг. cheap, twópenny-hálfpenny.

грубе́ть, огрубе́ть cóarsen; перен. get* coarse.

груби́ть, нагруби́ть (дт.) be* rude (to); (о ребёнке) ánswer back.

грубия́н м. разг. rude féllow, boor.

гру́б|о rúdely, róughly; ~ обходи́ться с кем-л.

treat/hándle smb. róughly, be* rough to smb.; ~ отвеча́ть ánswer rúdely; ◇ ~ говоря́ róughly spéaking. ~ость ж. rúdeness; (о лице́, мате́рии, пи́ще) cóarseness; гово́ри́ть ~ости be* rude; отве́тить ~остью ánswer rúdely; допусти́ть ~ость спорт. play rough.

грубошёрстный (о сукне́) coarse; (о костю́ме и т. п.) of coarse cloth по́сле сущ.

гру́б|ый 1. (недоста́точно отде́ланный; приблизи́тельный) rough; перен. crude, gross; ~ая рабо́та rough work; ~ подсчёт rough éstimate; ~ая лесть gross fláttery; 2. (жёсткий, шерохова́тый) rough, coarse; ~ые ру́ки hórny/cálloused hands; 3. (ре́зкий — о го́лосе, сме́хе) harsh, rough, gruff; 4. (малокульту́рный) rude; (об обраще́нии тж.) rough; ~ое сло́во bad word, swéar-word; 5. (недопусти́мый) gross, gláring; ~ое искаже́ние фа́ктов gross distórtion of the facts; ~ое наруше́ние догово́ра gross/flágrant violátion of a tréaty; ~ая оши́бка bad*/grave mistáke.

гру́да ж. pile, heap; ~ камне́й heap of stones; ~ обло́мков pile of wréckage; ~ книг pile of books.

груди́нка ж. breast, brísket; (копчёная свини́на) bácon; теля́чья ~ breast of veal.

грудни́ца ж. mastítis.

грудн|о́й 1. chest attr.; péctoral нау́чн.; ~а́я железа́ анат. milk gland; ма́мма нау́чн.; 2.: ~ младе́нец báby, ínfant in arms; ◇ ~ го́лос deep voice, résonant voice.

грудь ж. 1. chest; поэт. breast, bósom; 2. (же́нская) breast; корми́ть ~ю give* the breast, nurse; 3. (ве́рхняя часть руба́шки) shirt-front; ◇ встать ~ю за кого́-л. stand* up for smb., smth.

ружёный lóaded; мор. láden.

груз м. 1. тк. ед. (тя́жесть) load; поле́зный ~ páy-load; мёртвый ~ dead weight; с тяжёлым ~ом héavily lóaded; мор. héavily láden; 2. (това́ры) goods pl; (судово́й) cárgo, freight.

груздь м. milk múshroom, péppery milk cap; ◇ назва́лся ~ем, полеза́й в ку́зов ≈ you can't back out now that you've begun.

грузи́ло с. рыб. plúmmet, sínker.

грузи́н м., ~ка ж. Geórgian. ~ский Geórgian; ~ский язы́к Geórgian, the Geórgian lánguage.

грузи́ть, нагрузи́ть 1. сов. нагрузи́ть (вн. тв.; наполня́ть что-л. гру́зом) load (smth. with); 2. сов. погрузи́ть (вн.; скла́дывать груз куда́-л.) load (smth.); (люде́й на суда́) embárk (smb.); (в по́езд) entráin (smb.). ~ся, погрузи́ться 1. load; (о парохо́де тж.) take* on cárgo; ~ся углём coal; 2. (о лю́дях — на суда́) embárk; (в ваго́ны) entráin.

гру́зный héavy; (о челове́ке тж.) córpulent, thíck-sét; (о похо́дке) pónderous.

грузови́к м. lórry; truck амер.

грузов|о́й cárgo attr., freight attr.; ~а́я маши́на lórry; truck амер.; ~о́е движе́ние goods tráffic; ~о́е су́дно fréighter, cárgo-boat; cárgo-vessel.

грузооборо́т м. freight túrnover/tráffic; ~ речно́го, морско́го тра́нспорта ríver-borne, séa-borne freight.

грузоотправи́тель м. consígner (of goods).

грузоподъёмность ж. cárrying capácity.

грузополуча́тель м. consígnee.

грузопото́к м. goods/freight tráffic; мо́щность ~ов vólume/amóunt of goods tráffic.

гру́зчик м. freight hándler; (портово́й) dócker, stévedore; lóngshoreman* амер.; (на лесоскла́де) tímber hándler.

грунт м. 1. (по́чва) soil; (дно) bed, ground; песча́ный ~ sándy soil; 2. жив. príming; (пе́рвый слой кра́ски тж.) prímer, first coat (of paint). ~ова́ть несов. (вн.) жив. prime (smth.). ~о́вка ж. жив. príming. ~ово́й: ~овы́е во́ды súbsoil wáters; ~ова́я доро́га unmétalled road; dirt road амер.

гру́ппа ж. group; ~ дере́вьев clump/clúster of trees; деса́нтная ~ lánding párty; ~ кро́ви биол. blood group.

группирова́ть, сгруппирова́ть (вн.) group (smth., smth.); (классифицировать) clássify (smth.). ~ся, сгруппирова́ться group; ~ся вокру́г кого-л., чего-л. form a group round smb., smth.

группиро́вк|а ж. 1. (действие) grouping; 2. (группа) group, gróuping, alígnment; полити́ческие ~и political groups; вое́нные ~и troop concentrátions.

группово́|й group attr.; ~ые заня́тия group stúdy sg; ~ косми́ческий полёт group space flight; ~ые интере́сы ínterests of a ná́rrow group/set, fáctional ínterests.

грусти́ть несов. grieve, be* sad; ~ по кому-л. miss smb.; (по умершем) mourn for the loss of smb.

гру́стн|о 1. нареч. sádly, só́rrowfully; 2. в знач. сказ. безл. (дт.): мне ~ I am sad. ~ый sad, só́rrowful, mélancholy; ~ая пе́сня sad/mó́urnful song; ~ое настрое́ние mélancholy mood; ~ая карти́на mélancholy/sad spéctacle; име́ть ~ый вид look só́rry for oneself.

грусть ж. grief, só́rrow.

гру́ша ж. 1. (плод) pear; 2. (дерево) péar-tree; 3. (резиновая) bulb; ◇ земляна́я ~ Jerúsalem ártichoke.

грушеви́дный péar-shaped, pýriform.

гры́жа ж. rúpture; hérnia научн.; ущемлённая ~ strángulated hérnia.

грызня́ ж. разг. 1. (драка между животными) fight; 2. (перебранка, мелочный спор) squá́bbling, bíckering.

грыз|ть несов. (вн.) 1. (раскусывать) gnaw (smth.); (откусывать понемногу) níbble (smth.); ~ оре́хи eat* nuts; ~ пече́нье níbble (at) a bíscuit; ~ себе́ но́гти bite* one's nails; ~ се́мечки eat* súnflower seeds; 2. разг. (докучать придирками) nag (smth.); 3. (терзать) tó́rture (smth.), tormént (smth.); его́ ~ёт раска́яние he is torménted by remó́rse; его́ ~ёт тоска́ he is éating his heart out. ~ться несов. 1. (о собаках) fight*; 2. разг. (постоянно ссориться) bícker, squá́bble, wrá́ngle.

грызу́н м. зоол. ró́dent.

гряда́ ж. 1. (садовая) (fló́wer)bed; (огородная) (végetable) bed; 2. (гор) range; 3. (ряд однородных предметов) bank, ridge.

гря́дк|а ж. см. гряда́ 1; копа́ть ~и dig* beds.

гряду́щ|ее с. the fúture, the time/days to come. ~ий có́ming; to come после сущ.; ◇ на сон ~ий before góing to sleep; чита́ть на сон ~ий read* in bed, read* oneself to sleep.

грязев|о́й mud attr.; ~а́я ва́нна mú́d-bath.

грязе|лече́бница ж. mú́d-baths pl. ~лече́ние с. mú́d-cure, mú́d-treatment.

грязни́ть, загрязни́ть (вн.) soil (smth.), make* (smth.) dírty/só́iled. ~ся, загрязни́ться becó́me*/get* dírty/só́iled.

гря́зно 1. нареч. dírtily; э́то ~ напи́сано it is untídily wrítten; 2. в знач. сказ. безл. it is dírty; на у́лице ~ it is mú́ddy óutside.

грязну́|ля м. и ж., ~ха м. и ж. разг. dírty créature; (о мужчине тж.) dírty féllow; (о женщине тж.) slut; (о ребёнке) dírty líttle thing, líttle pig.

гря́зн|ый 1. (покрытый грязью) dírty; (о дороге, земле тж.) mú́ddy, slúshy; ~ая у́лица mú́ddy street; 2. (запачканный) soiled, dírty; (о детях) untídy, grúbby; ~ое бельё soiled línen; 3. (непристойный) dírty, só́rdid, fílthy; ~ая исто́рия разг. unpléasant affáir, násty búsiness; ~ые мы́сли unclé́an thoughts; ~ые разгово́ры fílthy talk sg, smut sg.

грязь|ж. 1. тк. ед. (нечистота, сор) dirt; filth (тж. перен.); въе́вшаяся ~ grime; 2. тк. ед. (размокшая земля) mud; (слякоть) slush; ми́ре поэт.; весь в ~и́ all mú́ddy; 3. мн. (лечебное средство) mud sg; лечи́ть кого-л. ~ями bathe smb. in mud; ◇ меси́ть ~ squelch through the mud; забра́сывать кого-л. ~ью fling*/throw* mud at smb.; не уда́рить лицо́м в ~ not disgrá́ce oneself.

гря́ну|ть сов. 1.: ~л вы́стрел a shot rang out; ~ла

му́зыка the músic blared/pealed out; ~л гром there was a clap of thúnder; 2. (разразиться) break* out.

губа́ I ж. lip; ◇ у него́ губа́ не ду́ра he knows a good thing when he sees it, he knows what's good for him.

губа́ II ж. геогр. bay.

губерна́тор м. gó́vernor. ~ский gó́vernor's, gubernató́rial.

губе́рн|ия ж. ист. próvince. ~ский ист. províncial; ~ский го́род principal town of a próvince.

губи́тельный destrúctive, disá́strous; ~ ого́нь múrderous/withering fire.

губи́ть, погуби́ть, сгуби́ть (вн.) ruin (smb., smth.); (портить) spoil* (smb., smth.); (разрушать) destró́y (smth.).

гу́бк|а ж. 1. sponge; вытира́ть ~ой sponge; 2. (на дереве) fúngus (pl -gi, -ses).

губн|о́й 1. lip attr.; ~а́я пома́да lípstick; 2. лингв. (о звуке) lábial.

гу́бчат|ый spó́ngy; ~ая рези́на foam rúbber.

гугу́: ни ~! разг. mum's the word!; он (сиди́т и) ни ~ he is ké́eping mum.

гуде́ние с. hum; (громкое) roar; (глухое) drone, dró́ning; (ветра) mó́aning.

гуде́ть, прогуде́ть 1. hum, buzz; (о низком звуке) drone; 2. (давать сигнал) hoot; (об автомобиле тж.) honk.

гуд|о́к м. (автомобильный) horn; (пароходный) síren; (паровозный) whístle; (фабричный) síren, hó́oter; дава́ть ~ки hoot; (об автомобиле) toot/honk the horn.

гудро́н м. тех. tar, petró́leum á́sphalt. ~и́рованный: ~и́рованное шоссе́ tá́rmac road. ~и́ровать несов. и сов. (вн.) тех. tar (smth.); (о дорогах тж.) tár macá́damize (smth.).

гуж м. (в упряжи) tug, trace; ◇ взя́вшись за ~, не говори́, что не дюж посл. ≈ néver give up once you've stá́rted. ~ево́й á́nimal-drawn; ~ево́й тра́нспорт cá́rting; cá́rtage; на ~ево́й тя́ге á́nimal-drawn. ~о́м (конной тя́гой) by á́nimal-drawn tránsport.

гул м. drone, dró́ning; (машины тж.) hum; ~ голосо́в hum of vó́ices.

гу́лкий 1. (имеющий сильный резонанс) resó́unding, hó́llow, échoing; 2. (громкий) loud.

гуля́ка м. и ж. réveller, rake.

гуля́нье с. 1. wá́lking, tá́king a walk; 2. (празднество) ó́pen-air pá́rty, gá́rden fête/féstival; наро́дное ~ féstival.

гуля́|ть 1. (совершать прогулку) have*/take* a walk; (быть не дома) be* out (for a walk); (о детях) be* óut-of-dóors; води́ть кого-л. ~ take* smb. out, take* smb. for a walk; (о детях) take* smb. óut-of-dóors; идти́ ~ go* for a walk; в па́рке ~ет мно́го наро́ду the park is full of stróllers; 2. разг. (быть свободным от рабо́ты) have* time-off, have* free time; 3. (веселиться, развлекаться) enjó́y oneself; be* on the spree разг.

гуля́ш м. кул. gó́ulash, stew.

гума́н|изм м. húmanism. ~и́ст м. húmanist.

гуманита́рн|ый humanístic, humá́ne; ~ые нау́ки the humá́nities; the Arts.

гума́нн|ость ж. húmaneness, humá́nity. ~ый humá́ne.

гуммиараби́к м. gum, glue.

гумно́ с. с.-х. thré́shing-floor.

гу́мус м. с.-х. húmus.

гурт м. herd, drove, ~овщи́к м. dró́ver. ~о́м разг. 1. (оптом) en bloc; 2. (всей компанией) in a bunch.

гурьб|а́ ж. crowd. ~о́й in a crowd.

гуса́к м. gá́nder, тж. перен.

гу́сени|ца ж. 1. зоол. cá́terpillar; 2. тех. track, cá́terpillar track. ~чный cá́terpillar attr., trá́ck-laying attr.; ~чный тра́ктор cá́terpillar/crá́wler tráctor; на ~чном ходу́ cá́terpillar attr., trá́ck-laying attr.

гусёнок м. gó́sling.

гуси́н|ый goose *attr.*; ~ое са́ло góose-fat; ◇ ~ая ко́жа góose-flesh, góose-skin; ~ое перо́ quill pen.

гу́сл|и *мн. муз.* psáltery *sg.* ~áр *м.* psáltery pláyer.

густе́ть *несов.* thícken, get*/grow* thícker.

гу́сто thíckly, dénsely; (*изобильно*) in abúndance; ~ покрасне́ть flush crímson.

густ|о́й 1. thick; (*плотный*) dense; ~ые бро́ви búshy éyebrows; ~ые во́лосы thick hair *sg*; ~ лес dense/thick fórest; ~ суп thick soup; ~ дым dense smoke; ~ое населе́ние dense populátion; ~ая толпа́ dense crowd; 2. (*о голосе, цвете*) deep, rich; ~ бас deep bass.

густоли́ственный with thick fóliage *после сущ.*

густонаселённый pópulous, dénsely pópulated.

густота́ *ж.* thíckness, dénsity.

гу́сыня *ж.* goose*.

гусь *м.* goose*; ◇ ~ ла́пчатый sly rogue; как с гу́ся вода́ ≈ like wáter off a duck's back; хоро́ш ~! he's a queer cústomer.

гусько́м in síngle file.

гуся́тина *ж.* góose(-flesh).

гуся́тница *ж.* póultry cásserole.

гутали́н *м.* bóot-polish, shóe-polish.

гуттапе́рч|а *ж.* gutta-pércha. ~евый gutta-pércha *attr.*

гу́щ|а *ж.* 1. (*осадок*) dregs *pl*; 2. в са́мой ~е чего́-л. in the thick of *smth.*

гу́ще (*сравнит. ст. прил.* густо́й *и нареч.* гу́сто) thícker.

гю́йс *м. мор.* (stém-)jack.

Д

да I *частица* 1. *утверд.* yes; *переводится тж. вспомогательным гл. в утверд. предложении* yes, I do!; yes, he is!; yes, they will!; (*в утверждении отрицания*) no; вам э́то не нра́вится? — Да, не нра́вится don't you like it? No, I don't; 2. *вопрос. переводится вспомогательным гл. в вопрос. предложении* do you?; is he?; will they?; can('t) she?; have you?; он ушёл — Да? he's gone. — Has he?; 3. *усил. обычно не переводится*; да вот и он! here he is/comes!; да что вы говори́те! you don't say so!; réally?; 4. (*пусть*): да бу́дет вам изве́стно, что... allów me to infórm you that..; да здра́вствует..! long live..!

да II *союз* 1. *соед.* and; он да я he and I; то́лько сосна́ да оси́на ónly píne-trees and a few áspens; 2. *противит.* (*в условных оборотах*) but; я бы пошёл, да он не хо́чет I would like to go, but he dóesn't want to; ◇ да и 1) (*а кроме того*) besídes; 2) (*и наконец*) and (at last); ду́мал, ду́мал, да и наду́мал I thought and thought, and at last I made up my mind.

дава́ть, дать (*вн.*) 1. give* (*smth.*); дать кому́-л. кни́гу give* smb. a book; give* smb. a book; ~ кому́-л. чей-л. а́дрес, телефо́н give* smb.'s address, télephone númber to smb.; ~ кому́-л. зада́ние give* smb. an assignment, set* smb. a task; ~ кому́-л. взя́тку bribe smb.; 2. (*наносить удар*) give* (*smth.*); ~ кому́-л. пощёчину slap/smack smb.'s face, box smb.'s ears; 3. (*устраивать*) give* (*smth.*); ~ обе́д give* a dínner; ~ конце́рт give* a cóncert; 4. (*приносить как результат*) yield (*smth.*); ~ урожа́й yield a hárvest; ~ плоды́ bear*/yield fruit; ~ дохо́д be* prófitable; 5. *в сочет. с некоторыми сущ* (*производить, делать*): ~ сигна́л give* a signal; ~ звоно́к ring*; ~ отбо́й 1) (*по телефону*) ring* off; 2) (*тревоги*) sound the all-cléar; ~ залп fire a vólley; 6. *в сочет. с рядом сущ. имеет знач. действия*: ~ распоряже́ние кому́-л. give* instructions to

smb., instrúct smb.; ~ обеща́ние give* a prómise, prómise; ~ отсро́чку grant a deláy; 7. (*дт. + инф; предоставлять возможность*) let* (*smb. + inf*); не ~ спать кому́-л. not let* smb. sleep; да́йте мне поду́мать let me think; ~ кому́-л. говори́ть let* smb. speak; дать кому́-л. вы́сказаться let* smb. have his, her say; 8. *тк. несов. повел.*: дава́й(те) (*пойдём, сделаем и т. п.*) let's (+ *inf*) (*начинайте, действуйте*) go ahéad!; дава́йте я вам помогу́ let me help you; 9. *разг.* (*определять возраст по внешнему виду*) give* (*smth.*); ему́ нельзя́ дать бо́льше 30 лет he dóesn't look a year óver thírty; ◇ дать знак кому́-л. let* smb. know; дать себя́ знать make* itself felt; го́ды даю́т себя́ знать the years are begínning to tell; ~ нача́ло чему́-л. give* a start to smth.; дать себе́ труд tróuble, take* the tróuble; он не дал себе́ труда́ поду́мать he did not tróuble to think; ~ кому́-л. поня́ть give* smb. to understánd; ~ сло́во 1) (*обещать*) give* one's word; 2) (*оратору*) give* smb. the floor; ~ себе́ во́лю not to..; ~ показа́ния bear* witness; give* évidence. ~ся, да́ться *разг.* 1.: ~ся в ру́ки кому́-л. (*увёртываться*) dodge smb.; 2. (*дт.; легко усваиваться*) come* éasy (to); э́то ему́ легко́ даётся it comes éasy/náturally to him; э́то мне нелегко́ даётся it's not éasy for me; I find it véry difficult.

дави́ть *несов.* 1. (*вн.; на вн.; нажимать*) press (*smth.*); (*тяжестью*) weigh (*smth.*) down, weigh down (on), weigh héavily (on); *перен.* (*угнетать*) oppréss (*smb.*); 2. (*вн.; разминать, выжимая сок*) squeeze (*smth.*), crush (*smth.*); ~ лимо́н squeeze a lémon; 3. (*вн.; сбивая с ног, убивать*) run* (*smb.*) óver, kill (*smb.*); 4. (*стискивать, сжимать*) be* (too) tight; pinch; пра́вый боти́нок мне да́вит the right shoe pínches. ~ся *несов.* 1. (*тв.*) be* choked (by); ~ся ко́стью get* a bone in one's throat; 2. (*от рд.*) choke (with); ~ся от сме́ха choke with láughter.

да́вка *ж. разг.* throng, press, crush.

давле́ние *с.* (*прям. и перен.*) préssure; высо́кое ~ high préssure; кровяно́е ~ blood préssure.

да́вн|ий old, áncient; (*существующий с давних пор*) of long stánding *после сущ*; с ~их пор for a long time, for áges.

давни́шн|ий *см.* да́вний; ~ знако́мый old acquáintance; ~яя ссо́ра áncient feud, quárrel of long stánding.

давно́ 1. (*много времени тому назад*) long agó, a long time agó; не так ~ not so long agó; 2. (*долго*) for a long time, for áges; я (так) ~ не ви́дел I háven't seen you for áges; it's áges since we met; ◇ ~ бы так!, ~ пора́! and high time it is!

давнопроше́дш|ий: ~ее вре́мя *грам.* past perfect.

да́вность *ж.* 1. (*отдалённость по времени совершения*) remóteness (in time), antíquity; э́то де́ло име́ет большу́ю ~ it's a véry old affáir; 2. (*длительность существования*) long durátion/stánding; двадцатиле́тней ~и of twénty years' stánding; 3. *юр.* prescríption; искова́я ~ limitátion; де́ло бы́ло прекращено́ за ~ью the case was dismíssed únder the státute of limitátions; потеря́ть си́лу за ~ью becóme* void by prescríption.

давны́м-давно́ *разг.* éver so long agó, áges agó.

дагеста́н|ец *м.*, ~ка *ж.* Daghestán. ~ский Daghestán.

да́же éven; (*при усилении тж.*) áctually; он ~ не попроща́лся he didn't éven say good-býe; э́то ~ хорошо́ it's áctually a good thing; е́сли ~ éven if.

дактилоскопи́я *ж.* dactýloscopy.

да́лее fúrther; и так ~ and so on, et cétera (*сокр.* etc.); и так ~, и так ~ and so on, and so forth; не ~ как вчера́ ónly yésterday.

далёк|ий 1. distant; (*имеющий большое протяжение*) long; ~ бе́рег distant shore; ~ друг distant friend; ~ое путеше́ствие long jóurney; ~ое расстоя́ние long distance; 2. (*отдалённый большим промежутком вре-*

мени) dístant, remóte; ~ое прóшлое, бýдущее dístant/remóte past, fúture; **3.** (_имеющий мало общего с кем-л._) dissímilar; with líttle in cómmon _после сущ._; **4.** (_от рд._; _не думающий делать что-л._) far (from), by no means inclíned (to); он далёк от и́стины he has no ínkling of the truth; он не óчень далёк от и́стины he's not far wrong; ~ от действи́тельности far from reálity; я далёк от тогó, чтóбы... I am far from...; он далёк от подозрéний he has not the fáintest suspícion.

далекó 1. _нареч._ far*; (_о расстоянии_ тж.) a long way; он живёт (óчень) ~ he lives a long way off/awáy; он уéхал ~ he has gone awáy (on a long jóurney), he's gone far awáy; оставля́ть _кого-л._ ~ позади́ leave* _smb._ far behínd; **2.** _в знач. сказ._ it's a long way; дó дóму ещё ~ it's still far to home, home is a long way off; **3.** _в знач. сказ._ (_о времени_) it is a long time (to); ◇ ~ за... 1): ~ зá полдень, зá полночь far/well ínto the áfternóon, night; 2): ~ за 40 he is well óver fórty; ~ не far from...; by no means...; я ~ не увéрен в э́том I'm by no means sure of that; зайти́ сли́шком ~ go* too far; ~ ходи́ть за примéром не ну́жно one does not have to look far for an exámple; он ~ пойдёт he will go far.

даль _ж._ expánse, dístance; голубáя ~ the blue dístance; зелёная ~ полéй the green expánse of the fields; ◇ такáя ~ such a long way off!; кудá нам éхать в такýю ~! how can we go so far awáy!

дальневостóчный Fár-Éastern.

дальнéйш|ий fúrther, súbsequent; ◇ в ~ем 1) (_в будущем_) in the fúture, súbsequently; 2) (_ниже в тексте_) hénceforth, hereáfter; belów; в ~ем именýемый... (_в документе_) hereináfter reférred to as...

дáльн|ий 1. (_о расстоянии_) dístant; fár-óff; (_имеющий большое протяжение_) long; ~ие райóны dístant/fár-off régions; ~его дéйствия lóng-ránge; ~яя дорóга long jóurney; ~ее плáвание long vóyage, ócean cruise; **2.**: ~ рóдственник dístant rélative; **3.**: ~ свет _авт._ undípped héadlights; ◇ поли́тика ~его прицéла fár-réaching pólicy.

дальнобóйн|ый lóng-range; ~ая артилле́рия lóng-range artíllery.

дальнови́дн|ость _ж._ fóresight. ~ый farséeing, farsíghted.

дальнозóрк|ий longsíghted, farsíghted. ~ость _ж._ long sight, longsíghtedness.

дальномéр _м._ ránge-finder.

дáльность _ж._ dístance; (_действия, стрельбы_) range; ~ плáвания, полёта (crúising-)ránge.

дальтони́зм _м._ dáltonism, cólour-blindness; страдáть ~ом be* cólour-blind.

дáльше 1. (_сравнит. ст. прил._ далёкий _и нареч._ далекó) fárther; **2.** _нареч._ (_затем, потом_) then; а ~ что?, а что же ~? well, what next?, and then (what)?; **3.** _нареч._ (_продолжая начатое_) fúrther; tell* fúrther, go* on with _one's_ stóry; он продолжáл читáть ~ he went on réading fúrther; ~! (_продолжайте_) go on!; ◇ не ви́деть ~ своегó нóса not see beyónd _one's_ nose; ~ — бóльше it gets worse and worse; ~ — кáк..., не — чем... ónly; не ~ как на дня́х no more than a few days agó; ~ нéкуда that's the límit.

дáма _ж._ **1.** lády; **2.** (_в танцах_) pártner; **3.** _карт._ queen.

дáмба _ж._ dam; (_защитная_) dike.

дáмк|а _ж._ (_в шашках_) king; провести́ (шáшку) в ~и crown a (dráughts)man*.

дáмский wóman's, lády's; ~ портнóй ládies' táilor; ~ парикмáхер (ládies') háirdresser.

дáнн|ые _мн._ **1.** dáta, facts; informátion _sg_; цифровы́е ~ figures; по всем (имéющимся) ~ым accórding to informátion (aváilable); мы имéем ~, что... we are in posséssion of informátion shówing that...; ~ разве́дки sécret informátion; **2.** (_свойства, способности_) mákings; (_качества_) quálities; внéшние ~ appéarance _sg_; у негó

все ~, чтóбы стать хорóшим инженéром he has the mákings of a first-rate engínéer; у негó отсýтствуют необходи́мые ~ he lacks the nécessary quálities. ~ый gíven; (_настоящий_) présent; ~ый вопрóс the quéstion befóre us, the quéstion únder considerátion; в ~ую минýту, в ~ое врéмя, в ~ый момéнт at présent; в ~ом слýчае in the présent ínstance; ◇ ~ая величинá _мат._ gíven quántity.

дань _ж._ **1.** _ист._ tríbute; облагáть _кого-л._ ~ю lay* _smb._ únder contribútion; **2.** (_должное_) tríbute, hómage; ◇ отдáть, заплати́ть ~ _кому-л._, _чему-л._ pay* tríbute to _smb._, _smth._, acknówledge _smb._, _smth._

дар _м._ **1.** (_подарок_) gift; **2.** (_способность, талант_) gift, pówer; ~ красноречи́я gift of éloquence; ◇ ~ рéчи, ~ слóва pówer of speech; потеря́ть ~ рéчи lose* the pówer of speech, be* spéechless.

дарвини́зм _м._ Dárwinism.

дарён|ый _разг._ gift _attr._; ◇ ~ому коню́ в зýбы не смóтрят _посл._ don't look a gift horse in the mouth.

дари́ _ж. нескл._ Dári.

дари́ть, подари́ть (_вн._ _дт._) give* (_smb. smth._), presént (_smb._ with).

дармоéд _м._ _разг._ spónger, drone.

дарова́ни|е _с._ gift, tálent; приро́дное ~ nátural abílity; рéдкое ~ unúsual tálent; ю́ные ~я gífted young péople.

дарова́ть _несов. и сов._ (_вн._) _уст._ grant (_smth._); ◇ ~ _кому-л._ жизнь, свобо́ду grant _smb._ his, her life, líberty.

дарови́т|ость _ж._ tálent. ~ый gífted, tálented.

даров|óй free (of charge); ~óе зрéлище free entertáinment; ~ы́е биле́ты на спектáкль free tíckets to a perfórmance.

дáром 1. (_бесплатно_) free of charge, grátis, for nóthing; отдáть _что-л._ ~ give* _smth._ awáy; достáться ~ cost* nóthing; емý э́то не ~ далóсь he dídn't get it for nóthing; **2.** _разг._ (_очень дёшево_) for next to nóthing, for a trífle, for a song; он купи́л э́то совсéм ~ he paid next to nóthing for it; **3.** (_напрасно_) all for nóthing, in vain; ~ трáтить врéмя waste _one's_ time; все нáши труды́ пропáли ~ all our work went for nóthing; ◇ э́то емý ~ не пройдёт he'll pay for that, he won't get awáy with that.

дáрственн|ый dónative; ~ акт grant; ~ая зáпись deed, séttlement; ~ая нáдпись dédicatory inscríption.

дáт|а _ж._ date; без ~ы úndáted; постáвить ~у на чём-л. date _smth._

дáтельный: ~ падéж _грам._ the dátive (case).

дати́ровать _несов. и сов._ (_вн._) date (_smth._); ~ письмó пя́тым мáя date the létter the fifth of May; ~ _что-л._ бóлее пóздним числóм postdáte _smth._; ~ _что-л._ бóлее рáнним числóм ántedate _smth._; невéрно ~ _что-л._ misdáte _smth._

дáт|ский Dánish; ~ язы́к Dánish, the Dánish lánguage. ~чáнин _м._, ~чáнка _ж._ Dane.

дáтчик _м._ _эл._ dáta únit, sénsing élement, sénsor, transmítter.

дать _сов. см._ давáть 1, 2, 3, 4, 5, 6, 7, 9. ~ся _сов. см._ давáться.

дáч|а I _ж._ **1.** (_загородный дом_) cóuntry house, house in the cóuntry; (_небольшая_) cóuntry cóttage; **2.** (_загородная местность_) the cóuntry; на ~e in the cóuntry, out of town; éхать на ~у go* to the cóuntry; go* out of town; жить на ~e live out of town.

дáча II _ж._ (_действие_) gíving; ~ показáний deposítion.

дáчник _м._ súmmer résident.

дáчн|ый cóuntry _attr._; ~ая мéстность óut-of-tówn resórt.

два two; в двух словáх to cut a long stóry short; расскажи́те мне в двух словáх tell me bríefly; в двух шагáх (_от_) within a few steps (of); ◇ в ~ счётá _разг._ in (less than) no time, in a tick; ни ~ ни полторá ≈ néither one thing, nor anóther.

двадцатилёт|ие с. 1. (период) twénty years pl, score of years; 2. (годовщина) twéntieth annivérsary. ~ний 1. (о сроке) twénty-year attr.; of twénty years после сущ.; 2. (о возрасте) twénty-year-óld; of twénty после сущ.

двадцат|ый twéntieth; ~ые гóды the twénties; ~ нómep twénty; емý ~ год he is in his twéntieth year.

двадца|ть twénty; a score (два десятка); ~ одúн twénty-óne; ~ пéрвый twénty-first; емý окóло ~тú лет he is about twénty.

дважды twice; ~ два — четы́ре twice two is four; ~ Герóй Совéтского Сою́за twice Héro of the Sóviet Únion; ◇ как ~ два четы́ре ≈ as plain as a píkestaff, as plain as the nose on your face.

двенадцатилéтний 1. (о сроке) twélve-year attr.; of twélve years после сущ.; 2. (о возрасте) twélve-year-óld; of twélve после сущ.

двенадцат|атый the twélfth. ~ать twélve.

двéрца ж. door.

двер|ь ж. door; (дверной проём) dóorway; стоя́ть в ~я́х stand* in the dóorway; ◇ при закры́тых ~я́х behínd closed doors, in prívate; при откры́тых ~я́х in públic (séssion); ломи́ться в откры́тую ~ force an ópen door, knock at an ópen door; поли́тика откры́тых ~éй ópen-dóor pólicy; показáть комý-л. на ~ show* smb the door.

двéсти two húndred.

дви́гатель м. mótor, éngine; ~ внýтреннего сгорáния intérnal-combústion éngine; ракéтный ~ jet éngine. ~ный mótive; ~ный нерв mótor (nerve); ~ная сúла mótive pówer/force.

дви́гать, дви́нуть 1. (вн.; перемещáть, толкáть) move (smth.); ~ мéбель move fúrniture; 2. (тв.; шевелúть) move (smth.); ~ ногóй, рукóй move one's foot*, hand; 3. (вн.; развивáть, совершéнствовать) promóte (smth.); ~ вперёд наýку и тéхнику advánce science and technólogy. ~ся, дви́нуться 1. (перемещáться, идти́ вперёд) move; врéмя дви́жется вперёд time moves on; дéло не дви́жется things are not móving; 2. (дéлать движéния, шевелúться) stir; не ~ся с мéста not budge; 3. разг. (трóгаться с мéста) start, move; порá ~ся! it's time to go!; ~ся в путь start on one's way, set* out; ◇ ~ся по слýжбе rise* stéadily in one's caréer.

движéн|ие с. 1. (перемещéние) mótion, móvement; (дéйствие какóго-л. механúзма тж.) wórking, fúnctioning; вращáтельное ~ rótary mótion; ~ии in mótion; без ~ия mótionless; лежáть без ~ия lie* mótionless; приводúть в ~ set*/put* in mótion, get* góing; приходúть в ~ start móving, begín* to move, get* únder way; (оживля́ться) come* to life; ~ войск troop móvement; 2. (изменéние положéния тéла) móvement; ~ головы́ móvement of the head; ~ рукú gésture; 3. (общéственное) móvement; всенарóдное ~ nátional/nátion-wide móvement; ~ в защи́ту ми́ра peace móvement; 4. (дéйствие трáнспорта) tráffic; (ходьбá) cóming and góing; большóе ~ héavy tráffic; ~ поездóв rail tráffic; train sérvices pl; 5. (внýтреннее побуждéние) ímpulse; душéвные ~ия emótions; 6. филос. mótion.

движи́м|ость ж. móvables pl, móvable próperty; pérsonal belóngings pl; cháttels pl. ~ый móvable; ~ое имýщество см. движи́мость.

движóк м. 1. (движущаяся детáль в механúзмах) slide; 2. разг. (небольшóй двúгатель) mótor.

дви́жущ|ий mótive; ~ая сúла mótive pówer; перен. dríving/mótive force; ~ие сúлы истóрии the dríving fórces of hístory.

дви́нуть(ся) сов. см. дви́гать(ся).

двó|е two (péople); нас ~ there are two of us; ◇ на свóих (на) ~úх ≈ on Shanks's mare/póny.

двоебóрье с. (в тяжёлой атлéтике) snatch, clean and jerk combinátion; (лы́жное) Nórdic/Wínter combinátion; Álpine combinátion; bíathlon.

двоевлáстие с. díarchy.

двоетóчие с. cólon.

двой|ться несов. 1. (раздвáиваться) fork; 2. (казáться двóйным) go* out of fócus; becóme* blurred; в глазáх ~тся I am séeing dóuble, éverything is out of fócus.

двóйк|а ж. 1. (цифра) a two; 2. (отмéтка) two, "poor"; он получи́л ~у по áлгебре he got two for álgebra; у негó ~ по истóрии he has a "poor" for hístory; 3. (кáрта) the two (of); 4. спорт (распашнáя) páir(-oar boat); (пáрная) dóuble sculls.

двойни́к м. dóuble.

двойн|óй 1. dóuble; ~ые рáмы dóuble glázing, storm windows; 2. (удвóенный) dóuble, twófold; ~ая плáта dóuble pay; э́то ~ая трáта врéмени it takes dóuble the time; в ~óм размéре twice as much; 3. (двóйственный) twó-fáced, dóuble; вестú ~ýю игрý play a dóuble game; ◇ ~ая бухгалéрия bóok-keeping by dóuble éntry; перен. dóuble-déaling.

двóйня ж. twins pl.

двóйственн|ый 1. (противоречи́вый) ambívalent; ~ харáктер ambívalent chárácter; 2. (двулúчный) dóuble-fáced; 3. (касáющийся двух) dúal; bilátеral; ~ое соглашéние bilátеral/bipártite agréement.

двор I м. 1. (при дóме) yard, cóurtyárd; во ~é in the yard; 2. (крестья́нское хозя́йство) hómestead; ◇ на ~é (вне дóма) óut-of-doors, outdóors, out; на ~é темнó it's dark outsíde; на ~é непогóда it's a véry bad day; веснá на ~é spring has come; быть, прийти́сь ко ~ý fit in well; быть не ко ~ý not fit in; remáin an óutsíder.

двор II м. (короля́ и т. п.) court; при ~é at court; при ~é когó-л. at the court of smb.

дворéц м. 1. pálace; 2.: ~ культýры Pálace of Cúlture, commúnity céntre; ~ бракосочетáний Márriage Pálace.

двóр|ник м. 1. (рабóтник) yárd-keeper, cáretaker; jánitor амер.; 2. разг. (на автомашúне) windscreen wíper.

дворня́|га ж., ~жка ж. móngrel.

дворóв|ый прил. 1. yard attr.; ~ пёс wátch-dog; ~ые пострóйки óutbuildings; 2. в знач. сущ. м. ист. hóuse-serf.

дворцóвый pálace attr.; ◇ ~ переворóт pálace revolútion; coup d'état, coup.

дворяни́н м. nóbleman*, nóble.

дворя́н|ка ж. nóblewoman*. ~ский nóbleman's, nóble. ~ство с. 1. (сослóвие) nobílity; (звáние) nóble rank; 2. собир. (дворя́не) nóbles pl; (мéлкое и срéднее) géntry.

двою́родн|ый: ~ брат, ~ая сестрá (first) cóusin.

двоя́|кий dóuble. ~ко in two ways.

двоя́ко|вóгнутый concávo-concáve. ~вы́пуклый convéxo-convéx.

двубóртный dóuble-bréasted; ~ пиджáк dóuble-bréasted coat.

двугóрбый: ~ верблю́д Báctrian cámel.

двугри́венный м. разг. twénty-copeck piece.

двузнáчн|ый: ~ое числó twó-digit nómber.

двукóлка ж. twó-whéeled cart, twó-whéeler.

двукрáт|ный twó-fold; (произведённый два рáза) réiterated, twíce(-repéated); в ~ом размéре dóuble the amóunt; ~ чемпиóн twíce chámpion; пóсле ~ого предупреждéния áfter the sécond wárning.

двули́ч|ие с., ~ность ж. duplícity. ~ный twó-fáced, dóuble-fáced; быть ~ным be* twó-fáced.

двунóгий twó-légged; bíped научн.

двуóкись ж. хим. dióxide.

двуру́шни|к м. dóuble-déaler. ~ческий dóuble-déaling. ~чество с. dóuble-déaling.

двускáт|ный: ~ая крыша gábled/rídged roof.

двуслóжный лингв. twó-sýllable, disýllábic.

двусмы́сленн|ость ж. 1. ambigúity; 2. (непристóйность) innuéndo, dóuble enténdre. ~ый 1. ambíguous, equívocal; 2. (*непристойный*) dúbious; ~ая шýтка dúbious joke.

двуспáльн|ый: ~ая кровáть dóuble bed.

двуствóлка ж. dóuble-barrelled gun.

двустворчат|ый: ~ая дверь dóuble-doors *pl*.

двустúшие *с.* cóuplet.

двусторóнн|ий 1. dóuble; ~ее воспалéние лёгких dóuble pneumónia; ~ее ýличное движéние twó-way tráffic; ~ драп dóuble-síded cloth; 2. (*обоюдный*) bipártite, biláteral; ~ее соглашéние bipártite/biláteral agréement; 3.: ~яя радиосвязь twó-way rádio communicátion.

двухвéсельн|ый: ~ая шлюпка, лóдка páir(-oar boat).

двухгóд|ичный twó-year *attr.*; ~ичное плáвание twó-year vóyage. ~овáлый twó-year-óld; of two *после сущ.*

двухднéвный twó-day *attr*.

двухзáльный twó-screen *attr.*; ~ кинотеáтр twó-screen cínema.

двухколéйн|ый: ~ая желéзная дорóга dóuble-track ráilway/ráilroad.

двухколёсный twó-whéel(ed).

двухкóмнатн|ый twó-room *attr.*; ~ая квартúра twó-room flat.

двухлéтн|ий 1. (*о сроке*) twó-year *attr.*; of two years *после сущ.*; 2. (*о возрасте*) twó-year-óld; of two *после сущ.*; 3. *бот.* biénnial; ~ее растéние biénnial.

двухмéстн|ый: ~ое купé twó-berth compártment; ~ая машúна twó-séater.

двухмéсячный 1. (*о сроке*) two months'; twó-month *attr.*; 2. (*о возрасте*) twó-month-óld; of two months *после сущ.*; 3. (*об издании*) públished évery two months *после сущ.*; bí-mónthly.

двухмотóрный twó-engine *attr.*, twó-éngined.

двухнедéльный 1. (*о сроке*) twó-week *attr.*; two weeks'; 2. (*о возрасте*) twó-week-óld; of two weeks *после сущ.*; 3. (*об издании*) fórtnightly; ~ журнáл fórtnightly (magazine).

двухпалáтный twó-chamber *attr*.

двухсмéнный twó-shift *attr*.

двухсóтый twó-húndredth.

двухцвéтный twó-cólour *attr.*, dichromátic.

двухчасовóй 1. (*продолжающийся два часа*) twó-hour *attr.*; 2. (*назначенный на два часа*) two o'clóck *attr*.

двухэтáжный twó-storey *attr.*; ~ автóбус double-décker (bus).

двучлéн *м. мат.* binómial.

двуязычный bilíngual.

дебатúровать *несов.* (*вн., о пр.*) debáte (*smth.*)

дебáты *мн.* debáte *sg.*

дéбет *м. бухг.* débit.

дебúт *м. тех.* dischárge.

дебитóр *м. бухг.* débtor.

дебóш *м.* row.

дебошúрить *несов.* make* an úproar, kick up a row.

дéбри *мн.* júngle *sg*, thíckets; *перен.* maze *sg*, lábyrinth *sg*.

дебют *м.* 1. début; 2. *шахм.* ópening. ~áнт *м.* débutant. ~áнтка *ж.* débutante. ~úровать *несов. и сов.* make* one's début, make* one's first appéarance.

дéва *ж. поэт.* máiden; ◇ стáрая ~ old maid, spínster.

девальвáция ж. devaluátion.

девá|ть, деть (*вн.*) *разг.* put* (*smth.*); кудá вы дéли кнúгу? where on earth did you put the book? ◇ не знáть, кудá глазá деть not know where to hide onesélf; не знать, кудá деть себя not know what to do with onesélf. ~ться, дéться *разг.* go*, get*; кудá ~лось письмó? where on earth is the létter?, where has that létter got to?; кудá он ~лся? what's becóme of him?; ◇ не

знать, кудá ~ться (*от смущения и т. п.*) feel* útterly at a loss, wish the earth would ópen and swállow *one* up; никудá не дéнешься (*от чего-л.*) there is no gétting awáy from it.

дéверь *м.* húsband's bróther, bróther-in-law (*pl* brothers-).

девиáция ж. deviátion.

девúз *м.* mótto.

девúца *ж.* girl; *поэт.* dámsel.

девúческий *см.* дéвичий.

дéвич|ий gírlish; ~ья фамúлия máiden name.

дéвочка ж. (little) girl.

дéвственн|ик *м.*, ~ица *ж.* vírgin. ~ость *ж.* virgínity. ~ый vírgin, vírginal; ~ый лес vírgin/primével fórest.

дéв|ушка ж. girl; lass, lássie *разг.* ~чáта *мн. разг.* girls, lásses. ~чóнка ж. *разг.* girl; kid *разг.*

девянóсто nínety.

девяностолéт|ие *с.* 1. (*период*) nínety years *pl*; 2. (*годовщина*) nínetieth annivérsary. ~ний 1. (*о сроке*) nínety-year *attr.*; of nínety years *после сущ.*; 2. (*о возрасте*) nínety-year-óld; of nínety years *после сущ.*

девянóст|ый nínetieth; ~ые гóды the níneties.

девятилéтний 1. (*о сроке*) níne-year *attr.*; of nine years *после сущ.*; 2. (*о возрасте*) níne-year-óld; of nine *после сущ.*

девятисóтый níne-húndredth.

девятка ж. 1. (*цифра*) a nine; 2. *карт.* the nine (of).

девятнадцатилéтний 1. (*о сроке*) ninetéen-year *attr.*; of ninetéen years *после сущ.*; 2. (*о возрасте*) ninetéen-year-óld; of ninetéen *после сущ.*

девятнáдца|тый ninetéenth. ~ть ninetéen.

девятый the ninth.

дéвять nine.

девятьсóт nine húndred.

дегаз|áция *ж.* decontaminátion. ~úровать *несов. и сов.* (*вн.*) decontáminate (*smth.*)

дегенерáт *м.* degénerate.

дéготь *м.* tar; древéсный ~ wóod-tar; каменноугóльный ~ cóal-tar; ◇ лóжка дёгтя в бóчке мёда ≈ a fly in the óintment.

деград|áция *ж.* degradátion. ~úровать *несов. и сов.* becóme* degráded.

дегтярный tar *attr*.

дегустá|тор *м.* táster. ~ция *ж.* tásting.

дед *м.* 1. grándfather; 2. *разг.* (*старик*) old man*; 3. *мн.* (*предки*) fórefathers; ◇ ~-морóз Jack Frost; (*на ёлке*) Fáther Christmas, Sánta Claus.

дéдовский grándfather's.

дéдушка *м.* grándfather; (*обращение тж.*) grándad, grándpa.

деепричáстие *с. грам.* advérbial párticiple.

дееспосóбн|ость *ж.* 1. ability, efficiency; 2. *юр.* cómpetence. ~ый 1. áble, efficient; 2. *юр.* cómpetent; ~ый гражданúн cómpetent cítizen.

дежýр|ить *несов.* 1. be* on dúty; 2. (*неотлучно находиться где-л.*) watch; ~ у постéли больнóго watch by a síck-bed. ~ный *прил.* 1. (*о людях*) on dúty *после сущ.*; ~ный администрáтор (*гостиницы*) recéptionist; ~ный офицéр ófficer of the day, dúty ófficer; órderly ófficer *амер.*; 2. (*об учреждении*): ~ный магазúн shop with exténded búsiness hours; 3. (*заранее приготовленный*): ~ное блюдо stánding dish, plat du jour; 4. *неодобр.* (*постоянно употребляемый*) rún-of-the-míll; 5. *в знач. сущ. м.* official on dúty, man* on dúty; (*в школе*) mónitor; ~ный по стáнции *ж.-д.* assistant státion-master on dúty. ~ство *с.* dúty; ночнóе ~ство night dúty/watch.

дезертúр *м.* desérter; *перен.* shírker, quítter. ~овать *несов. и сов.* desért; *перен.* shirk, quit. ~ство *с.* desértion; *перен.* shírking, quítting.

дезинфекциóнн|ый disinféction *attr.*; ~ая кáмера disinféction chámber.

дезинфе́кция ж. disinféction.

дезинфици́р|овать *несов. и сов.* (*вн.*) disinféct (*smth.*). ~ующий disinféctant; (*для ран и т. п.*) antiséptic; ~ующее сре́дство disinféctant.

дезинформа́ция *ж.* misinfórming, misléading; bráinwashing.

дезинформи́ровать *несов. и сов.* (*вн.*) misinfórm (*smb.*), misléad* (*smb.*); bráinwash (*smb.*).

дезорганиза́тор *м.* disórganizer.

дезорганиз|а́ция *ж.* disorganizátion; вноси́ть ~а́цию cause disorganizátion; (*намеренно тж.*) spread* confúsion. ~ова́ть *несов. и сов.* (*вн.*) disórganize (*smth.*).

дезориент|а́ция *ж.* disorientátion. ~и́ровать *несов. и сов.* (*вн.*) confúse (*smb.*).

де́йственн|ость *ж.* éfficacy, efféctiveness. ~ый efféctive, efficácious.

де́йстви|е *с.* 1. áction; (*деятельность тж.*) actívity; actívities *pl*; руково́дство к ~ю a guide to áction; план ~й plan of áction; самово́льные ~я árbitrary áction(s); 2. (*о работе механизма и т. п.*) operátion, fúnctioning; в ~и in operátion; вступа́ть в ~ (*о заводе и т. п.*) come* into operátion; ~ введён be* commissioned; приходи́ть в ~ come* into operátion; ~ кише́чника móvement of the bówels; 3. (*применение на практике*) efféct; ввести́ зако́н в ~ put* the law into efféct; 4. (*воздействие*) efféct; под ~ем únder the influence; 5. (*события*) áction; ~ происхо́дит в Москве́ the scene is laid in Móscow; 6. *театр.* act; пье́са в пяти́ ~ях five-act play; 7. *мат.* operátion, prócess; четы́ре ~я арифме́тики the four rules of aríthmetic; ◇ вое́нные ~я hostílities; (*mílitary*) operátions.

действи́тельн|о 1. *нареч.* réally, áctually; э́то ~ случи́лось it áctually háppened; 2. *в знач. вводн. сл.* indéed; ~, вы пра́вы indéed, you are right. ~ость *ж.* reálity; совреме́нная ~ость módern conditions *pl*, módern life; ◇ в ~ости in reálity; в ~ости произошло́ то, что... what áctually háppened was that... ~ый 1. (*реальный*) real, áctual; (*истинный*) true, génuine; ~ая жизнь real life; ~ый факт áctual fact; ~ое происше́ствие true stóry, real-life íncident/occúrrence; 2. (*имеющий законную силу*) válid; биле́т действи́телен на два ме́сяца the tícket is válid for two months; 3. *грам.:* ~ый зало́г áctive voice; ◇ ~ая вое́нная слу́жба áctive sérvice, sérvice with the cólours; ~ый член Акаде́мии нау́к (full) Mémber of the Acádemy of Sciences.

де́йств|овать, поде́йствовать 1. *тк. несов.* (*совершать что-л.*) act; (*о войсках*) be* in áction, óperate; ~ реши́тельно take* áction, act résolutely; ~ нереши́тельно hésitate to take áction, act irrésolutely; ~уй(те)! go ahéad!; 2. *тк. несов.* (*функционировать*) work, fúnction; (*о машине тж.*) run*; ~ безотка́зно work/run* pérfectly; прибо́р не ~ует the ínstrument is out of órder, the ínstrument does not work; 3. *тк. несов.* (*иметь силу — о законах и т. п.*) be* in force, be* válid; 4. *тк. несов.* (*тв.*) *разг.* (*двигать, управлять*) use (*smth.*); ~ вёслами use one's oars, row; ~ лопа́той use a spade; 5. (*на вн.; влиять*) work (on), have* an efféct (on), efféct (*smth.*); не ~ have* no efféct; ~ благотво́рно have* a good/fávourable efféct; сре́дство не ~ует the rémedy dóesn't work; э́то лека́рство хорошо́ ~ует this medicine is efféctive; на меня́ э́то (ниско́лько) не ~ует it dóest't efféct me (in the least); на него́ никаки́е угово́ры не ~уют he is not to be preváiled upón, nóthing will sway him.

действующ|ий: ~ вулка́н áctive volcáno; ~ая а́рмия Ármy in the Field; Field Fórces *pl амер.*; ~ее лицо́ *театр., лит.* cháracter.

дейте́рий *м. хим.* deutérium, héavy hýdrogen.

де́ка *ж. муз.* sóunding-board.

декабри́ст *м. ист.* Decémbrist.

декабр|ь *м.* Decémber; в ~е́ э́того го́да this/in

Decémber; в ~е́ про́шлого го́да last Decémber, last year in Decémber; в ~е́ бу́дущего го́да next Decémber.

дека́брьский Decémber *attr.*

дека́да *ж.* 1. ten days; 2.: ~ литерату́ры и иску́сства Ten-day Féstival of Literature and the Arts.

декаде́нт *м.* décadent. ~ский décadent. ~ство *с.* décadence.

дека́н *м.* dean. ~а́т *м.* dean's óffice.

деквалифици́роваться *несов. и сов.* lose* one's skill.

деклам|а́тор *м.* reciter. ~ацио́нный declámatory. ~а́ция *ж.* recitátion; *перен.* (*напыщенная речь*) harángue. ~и́ровать, продеклами́ровать 1. (*вн.*) recíte (*smth.*); 2. *тк. несов.* (*говорить напыщенно*) decláim.

деклар|ати́вный declárative. ~а́ция *ж.* declarátion; прави́тельственная ~а́ция góvernment státement. ~и́ровать *несов. и сов.* (*вн.*) decláre (*smth.*).

деклассиро́в|анный déclassé.

декольт|é *с. нескл.* 1. low neck; 2. *в знач. неизм. прил.* low-nécked. ~и́рованный 1. (*о платье*) low-nécked; 2. (*о женщине*) in a low-nécked dress *после сущ.*

декорати́вно-прикладн|о́й: ~ое иску́сство décorative and applied art; arts and crafts *pl.*

декорати́вн|ый décorative; (*служащий для украшения и т. п.*) ornaméntal; ~ое иску́сство décorative art; ~ое расте́ние ornaméntal plant.

декор|а́тор *м.* 1. (*театральный*) scéne-painter; 2. (*помещений*) intérior décorator. ~а́ция *ж.* set, stage set; *мн.* scénery *sg; перен.* show; trímmings *pl*; всё э́то одна́ ~а́ция it's all for show; переме́на ~а́ций change of scene. ~и́ровать *несов. и сов.* (*вн.*) décorate (*smth.*).

декре́т *м.* decrée; ~ о ми́ре the Decrée on Peace. ~ный: ~ный о́тпуск matérnity leave.

де́ланн|ость *ж.* afféctation. ~ый affécted; ~ая улы́бка forced smile.

де́л|ать, сде́лать (*вн.*) do* (*smth.*); (*изготовлять, совершать*) make* (*smth.*); ~ поле́зное де́ло do* úseful work; ~ что-л. по-сво́ему do* smth. in one's own way; ~ 100 оборо́тов в мину́ту do* one húndred revolútions per mínute; по́езд ~ает 60 киломе́тров в час the train does sixty kílometres an hour; ~ упражне́ния do* éxercises; ~ прыжо́к jump; ~ уро́ки do* one's léssons; ~ кого́-л. свои́м помо́щником make* smb. one's assistant; ~ кого́-л. счастли́вым make* smb. háppy; ~ оши́бки make* mistákes; ~ вы́воды draw* conclúsions; ~ наблюде́ния make* observátions; ~ вы́говор кому́-л. réprimand smb.; ~ попы́тки make* attémpts; ~ всё для того́, что́бы... do* éverything to...; ◇ ~ вид preténd; он ~ает вид, что сли́шком испуга́н, что спит he preténds to be afráid, to be asléep; ~ честь кому́-л. 1) (*оказывать уважение*) do* smb. an hónour; 2) (*являться заслугой*) do* smb. crédit; э́то ~ает ему́ честь it does him crédit; э́то не ~ает ему́ че́сти it is not to his crédit; ~ не́чего it can't be helped, nóthing can be done abóut it; от не́чего ~ for want/lack of ánything bétter to do, out of sheer ídleness. ~аться, сде́латься 1. (*становиться*) becóme*, get*; 2. (*происходить*) be* góing on, háppen; не зна́ю, что со мной ~ается I don't know what's háppening to me; что там ~ается? what's góing on there?; ◇ что ему́ сде́лается! he'll be all right!

делега́т *м.*, ~ка *ж.* délegate. ~ский délegate *attr.*

делега́ция *ж.* delegation.

делеги́ровать *несов. и сов.* (*вн.*) send* (*smth.*) as a délegate.

делёж *м.*, ~ка *ж. разг.* sháring.

деле́ни|е *с.* 1. division (*тж. мат.*); ~ о́бщества на кла́ссы the division of society into clásses; 2. *биол.* físsion; 3. (*на шкале*) point, division; ртуть в термо́метре подняла́сь на одно́ ~ (the mércury in) the thermómeter went up a point; наноси́ть ~я subdivide, gráduate.

деле́ц *м.* búsiness man*; óperator *разг.*

деликате́с *м.* dáinty, délicacy, títbit.

деликáт|ичать *несов. разг.* treat too géntly; ~ с *кем-л.* stand* on céremony with *smb.* **~ость** *ж.* délicacy, tact. **~ый 1.** (*вежливый, предупредительный*) considerate, táctful; **2.** *разг.* (*щекотливый*) délicate, tícklish; **~ый вопрóс** délicate próblem/mátter.

дели́м|ое *с. мат.* dividend. **~ость** *ж.* divisibílity; **~ость клéтки** cell divísion; при́знаки **~ости** *мат.* dividing sign *sg.* **~ый** divísible.

дели́тель *м. мат.* divísor, denóminator; óбщий наибóльший ~ the gréatest cómmon divísor.

дели́ть *несов.* **1.** (*вн.; на части*) divíde (*smth.*); ~ *что-л.* на три чáсти divíde *smth.* into three parts; ~ *что-л.* пополáм divíde *smth.* in half, halve *smth.*; ~ *что-л.* порóвну share/divíde équally; **2.** (*вн. на вн.*) *мат.* divíde (*smth.* by); **3.** (*вн. с тв.*) share (*smth.* with); ~ дéньги с *кем-л.* share the móney with *smb.*; ~ с *кем-л.* и рáдость и гóре share *one's* joys and sórrows with *smb.*; ◇ нам ~ нéчего we have nóthing to quárrel óver; ~ шкýру неубúтого медвéдя ≈ count *one's* chíckens before they are hatched. **~ся** *несов.* **1.** (*на вн.*) divíde (ínto); **2.** (*тв. с тв.*) share (*smth.* with) (*тж. перен.*); **~ся с кем-л.** кускóм хлéба share a crust with *smb.*; **~ся впечатлéниями** compáre notes; **~ся новостя́ми** exchánge news; **~ся óпытом рабóты** share/pool *one's* knów-how; **3.** (*разделять имущество*) divíde the próperty; **4.** (*на вн.*) *мат.* be* divísible (by).

дéл|о *с.* **1.** afffáir; (*занятие*) work, búsiness; (*чего-л.*) mátter (of); ~ спóрится the work goes with a swing; у меня́ мнóго дел I have a lot to do; сидéть без **~а 1**) be dóing nóthing; **2.** (*быть без работы*) have* nóthing to do; по **~у** on búsiness; ~ привы́чки, вкýса a mátter of hábit, taste; как (*ваши*) **~á**? how are you?, how's éverything?; вмéшиваться не в своё ~ interfére in óther péople's affáirs; не суйся не в своё **~!** mind your own búsiness!; **2.** (*поступок, деяние*) deed, act, áction; и на словáх и на **~е** in word and deed; **3.** (*специальность*) búsiness; (*круг знаний*) science; воéнное ~ mílitary science; mílitary skills *pl*; **4.** (*цель, интересы*) cause; служи́ть **~у** ми́ра serve the cause of peace; **5.** (*предприятие*) búsiness, откры́ть своё ~ start *one's* own búsiness, start up on *one's* own; **6.** *юр.* case; **7.** *канц.* file; подши́ть *что-л.* к **~у** file *smth.*; ◇ в чём ~? what's the mátter?; э́то (*совсéм*) другóе **~!** that's quite anóther thing!; that's different!; какóе мне **~?** what do I care?; в сáмом **~е** réally, indéed; мéжду **~ом** at odd móments; он занимáется э́тим мéжду **~ом** he does this in bits as a sídeline; ~ за вáми it depénds on you; it is up to you; ~ за материáлом *и т. n.* it's now ónly a mátter of materíal, *etc.*; за нáми ~ не стáнет there will be no híndrance from our side, there will be no lack of co-operátion on our part; имéть ~ с *кем-л.* have* to deal with *smb.*; на ~е in práctice; на сáмом **~е** as a mátter of fact, in reálity; пéрвым **~ом** first of all; то и ~ incéssantly, perpétually; он то и ~ смотрéл в окнó he kept lóoking out of the wíndow; то ли ~ but it is quite a different mátter; ~ не в том, что it isn't that; ~ в том, что the point is that; не в э́том ~ that's not the point; я ~ говорю́ I am tálking sense.

делови́т|ость *ж.* práctical náture, búsiness ability. **~ый** búsiness-like.

делов|óй 1. (*связанный с работой*) búsiness *attr.*; **~óе письмó** búsiness létter; **~ы́е связи** búsiness connéctions; **~ы́е кáчества** proféssional quálities; **2.** (*касающийся существа*) práctical, realístic; **~ая кри́тика** práctical críticism; **~óе обсуждéние** realístic discússion; ~ подхóд realístic/práctical appróach; **3.** (*деловитый*) búsiness-like, práctical; ~ тон búsiness-like tone; **4.** (*занятый коммерческой деятельностью*) búsiness *attr.*; ~ человéк búsiness man*; **~ы́е круги́** búsiness círcles.

делопроизвóдство *с.* óffice-work.

дéльно *to* the point. **~ый 1.** (*способный, деловой*) áble, effícient; **~ый человéк** áble pérson; **2.** (*заслуживающий внимания*) práctical, sénsible; **~ая мысль** sénsible idéa; **~ое предложéние** sénsible propósal; **~ый совéт** sénsible/práctical advíce.

дéльта I *ж.* (*реки*) délta.

дéльта II *ж.* (*греческая буква*) délta. **~-лучи́** *мн. физ.* délta rays.

дельфи́н *м.* dólphin.

деля́че|ский: ~ подхóд *см.* деля́чество. **~ство** *с.* utilitárian appróach.

демагóг *м.* démagogue. **~и́ческий** demagógic. **~ия** *ж.* démagogy.

демаркацио́нн|ый demarcátion *attr.*; **~ая ли́ния** line of demarcátion.

демáрш *м. дип.* démarche.

демилитариз|áция *ж.* demilitarizátion. **~óванный** demílitarized.

демилитаризовáть *несов. и сов.* (*вн.*) demílitarize (*smth.*).

демисезóнн|ый: ~ое пальтó óvercoat.

демобилиз|áция *ж.* demobilizátion. **~óванный** *прич.* **1.** demóbilized; demóbbed *разг.*; **2.** *в знач. сущ. м.* éx-sérviceman*.

демобилизовáть *несов. и сов.* (*вн.*) demóbilize (*smth.*); demób (*smth.*) *разг.* **~ся** *несов. и сов.* be* demóbilized.

демóграф *м.* demógrapher.

демогрáфия *ж.* demógraphy.

демокрáт *м.* démocrat. **~изи́ровать** *несов. и сов.* (*вн.*) démocratize (*smth.*). **~и́ческий** democrátic. **~ия** *ж.* demócracy.

дéмон *м.* démon. **~и́ческий** demónic, demoníacal.

демонстрáнт *м.* démonstrator, márcher.

демонстрати́вн|о póintedly, ostentátiously; ~ покúнуть зал leave* the hall as a sign of prótest. **~ый 1.** (*нарочито подчёркнутый*) póinted, ostentátious; **~ый откáз** póinted refúsal/rejéction; **~ый ухóд** wálk-out in prótest; **2.** (*основанный на показе чего-л.*) demonstrátion *attr.*

демонстр|ацио́нный: ~ зал lécture-hall; (*для показа изделий и т. n.*) shów-room. **~áция** *ж.* **1.** demonstrátion; устрóить **~áцию** make* a demonstrátion; **2.** (*показ*) displáy, show; (*фильма*) shówing; состои́тся **~áция** нóвого фи́льма a new film will be shown. **~и́ровать 1.** démonstrate; **2.** *сов. тж.* (*вн.; показывать*) displáy (*smth.*); **~и́ровать фильм** show* a film.

демонт|áж *м. тех.* dismántling; ~ предприя́тий dismántling of indústrial plants. **~и́ровать** *несов. и сов.* (*вн.*) *тех.* dismántle (*smth.*).

деморализ|áция *ж.* demoralizátion. **~óванный** demóralized, dispírited. **~овáть** *несов. и сов.* (*вн.*) demóralize (*smb., smth.*).

дéмпинг *м. эк.* dúmping.

денатурáт *м.* denátured álcohol; méthylated spírits *pl.*

дендрáрий *м.* arborétum.

дéнежно-креди́тн|ый: ~ая систéма mónetary and crédit sýstem.

дéнежн|ый 1. mónetary; (*выражающийся в деньгах*) móney *attr.*; **~ое обращéние** *эк.* móney circulátion; **~ые срéдства** fináncial/móney resóurces; в **~ом** выражéнии in terms of móney; **~ая рефóрма** mónetary/cúrrency refórm; ~ перевóд móney órder; ~ знак cúrrency note; **~ые затруднéния** pecúniary difficulties; **~ая пóмощь** fináncial aid; ~ гóлод shórtage of móney; **2.** *разг.* (*богатый*) móneyed, wéll-to-dó; ~ человéк móneyed man*; ◇ ~ мешóк móney-bag.

дéнно: ~ и нóщно day and night.

день *м.* day; прáздничный ~ hóliday; ~ вы́дачи зарплáты páy-day; ~ óтдыха rést-day; День Побéды Víctory Day; в ~ a day, per day; он зарабáтывает дéсять рублéй в ~ he makes ten róubles a day; в оди́н ~ in the course of one day; в оди́н и тот же ~ the same day; в э́тот, тот ~ that day; какóй сегóдня ~? what day is it todáy?; зá ~ (*в продолжение дня*) dúring the day; зá ~

до (того) the day befóre; по сей ~ still; to this day; с
кáждым днём évery day; ◇ ~ за днём, изо дня в ~ day
áfter day; со дня нá ~ 1) from one day to the next; 2) (*в
ближáйшее врéмя*) ány day; отклáдывать *что-л.* со
дня нá ~ keep* pútting *smth.* off till anóther day; мы
ждём егó со дня нá ~ we are expécting him ány day
now; ~ ото дня (with) évery (pássing) day, from day to
day; на чёрный ~ for/agáinst a ráiny day; *чьи-л.* дни
сочтены́ *smb.'s* days are númbered; (и) ~ и ночь day
and night; в одúн прекрáсный ~ one fine day; не по
дням, а по часáм évery day, évery hour; мáльчик растёт не по дням, а по часáм the boy is shóoting up like a
béanstalk; средú бéла дня in broad dáylight; на днях 1)
(*о предстоя́щем*) in a day or two, one of these days; 2)
(*о прошлом*) a few days agó, the óther day.

дéньг|и *мн.* móney *sg*; мéлкие ~ (small) change *sg*;
налúчные ~ cash; ◇ ни за какúе ~ ≈ not for (all the
móney in) the world; э́того не достáть ни за какúе ~
you can't get it for love or móney; быть при ~áx have*
móney; быть не при ~áx be* short of cash/móney.

деньскóй: день-~ all day long; the lívelong day *поэт.*

департáмент *м.* depártment.

депó *с. нескл.* dépot; пожáрное ~ fire-station.

депрéссия *ж.* 1. *мед.* depréssion; 2. *эк.* depréssion,
recéssion, declíne; (*большáя*) slump.

депут|áт *м.* députy. ~áтский députy *attr.*, députy's.
~áция *ж.* depután.

дёрг|ать, дёрнуть 1. (*вн.*) pull (*smth.*), jerk (*smth.*);
(*за вн.*) tug (at); ~ вóжжи jerk the reins; ~ *кого-л.* зá
волосы, за рукáв pull *smb.'s* hair, sleeve; 2. *тк. несов.*
(*вн.*) *разг.* (*выдёргивать*) pull (*smth.*) out; ~ гвóзди
pull out nails; ~ зуб pull out a tooth*; 3. (*тв.; рéзко
двúгать какой-л. чáстью тéла*) jerk (*smth.*); 4. *безл.*:
егó всегó ~ает he is twítching all óver; 5. *тк. несов.*
(*вн.; надоедáть*) hárass (*smb.*), péster (*smb.*). ~аться,
дёрнуться twitch; у негó ~алась бровь one of his
éyebrows kept twítching.

дерáч *м.* (*птица*) córn-crake, lándrail.

деревéнский víllage *attr.*; (*харáктерный для дерéв-
ни*) cóuntry *attr.*, rúral, rústic; ~ жúтель cóuntryman*,
cóuntry dwéller.

дерéвн|я *ж.* 1. (*селéние*) víllage; жúтель ~и víllager;
2. (*сéльская мéстность*) the cóuntry; 3. (*сéльское насе-
лéние*) cóuntry folk/péople, rúral populátion.

дéрево *с.* 1. tree; 2. *тк. ед.* (*материáл*) wood;
крáсное ~ mahógany; чёрное ~ ébony.

деревообдéлочн|ик *м.* wóod-worker. ~ый
wóodworking.

деревообрабáтывающ|ий: ~ая промы́шленность
tímber índustry.

деревýшка *ж.* hámlet.

деревя́нн|ый wóoden (*тж. перен.*); ~ гóлос tóneless
voice; ~ое лицó wóoden cóuntenance/face; ~ая похóдка
stiff stride.

деревя́шка *ж.* chunk/piece/bit of wood.

держáв|а *ж.* State, Power. ~ный sóvereign; *перен.*
majéstic.

держáтель *м.* hólder.

держáть *несов.* 1. (*вн.; не выпускáть, не отдá-
вать*) hold* (*smth.*); ~ *что-л.* в рукáх hold* *smth.* (in
one's hands); ~ *что-л.* в зубáх hold* *smth.* betwéen one's
teeth; ~ рубéж hold* the line; 2. (*вн.; поддéрживать*)
suppórt (*smth.*), hold* (*smth.*), hold* (*smth.*) up; (*сдéрживать напор*) stop (*smth.*), hold* back (*smth.*); бáлка
дéржит кры́шу the beam suppórts the roof; 3. (*вн., за-
стáвлять находúться где-л.*) keep* (*smb.*), hold*
(*smb.*); ~ *кого-л.* в плену́ hold*/keep* smb. prísoner; ~
кого-л. дóма keep* *smb.* at home, keep* smb. índoors; 4.
(*вн.; хранúть где-л.*) keep* (*smth.*); ~ дéньги в сбер-
бáнке keep* móney in the sávings-bank; 5. (*вн.; владéть*) keep* (*smth.*); ~ собáку keep* a dog; 6. (*дви-

гáться в определённом направлéнии*) steer; ~ на зáпад
steer west; ◇ ~ слóво keep* one's word; be* true to one's
word; не ~ слóва break* one's word; ~ речь
make*/deliver a speech; ~ связь maintáin communicátion,
keep* in touch; ~ экзáмен go* in for an examinátion, sit*
for an examinátion; ~ себя́ (*вести себя́*) beháve; ~ себя́
в рукáх keep* onesélf in hand; ~ *кого-л.* в рукáх keep*/
have* smb. well in hand; ~ *кого-л.* в кýрсе *чего-л.* keep*
smb. infórmed of *smth.*, keep* smb. advised/pósted on
smth.; ~ под контрóлем maintáin in hand upón; ~ *что-л.*
про себя́ keep* smth. to onesélf; ~ у́хо востро́ be* on
one's guard, keep* one's wéather eye ópen; ~ курс (на)
set* one's course (for), steer (for); ~ курс на зáпад steer
a wésterly course; ~ путь (на) head (for), be* héaded
(for). ~ся *несов.* 1. (*за вн.*) hold* on (to); cling* (to)
(*тж. перен.*); ~ся рукáми за перúла hold* on to the
rail; 2. (*быть укреплённым*) stay in place, stay on,
keep* on; мост дéржится на бы́ках the bridge is
suppórted/cárried by piers; пýговица дéржится на однóй нúточке the bútton is hánging by a thread; дéржится? will it hold?; 3. (*в каком-л. положéнии*) stay; ~ся
на водé stay aflóat, float; 4. (*занимáть какое-л. мéсто, положéние*) keep*, stay; ~ся вмéсте keep* togéther;
~ся в сторонé, на расстоя́нии keep* awáy; *перен.* hold*
onesélf alóof; 5. (*сохраня́ть определённое положéние
тéла*) hold* onesélf; ~ся пря́мо hold* onesélf straight/
eréct, stand* straight; 6. (*вести себя́*) beháve; ~ся прóсто be* straightfórward in one's mánner; 7. (*сохраня́ть-
ся, удéрживаться*) last; нéсколько дней держáлась хорóшая погóда the fine wéather held for séveral days; ~
(*не сдавáться*) hold* out; ~ся из послéдних сил be*
just hólding out, be* at the end of one's téther; 9. (*придéрживаться определённого направлéния*) keep*; ~ся
прáвой стороны́ keep* to the right; 10. (*рд.; слéдовать
чему-л.*) adhére (to), stick* (to); ~ся прéжнего мнéния
adhére to one's fórmer opínion; упóрно ~ся *чего-л.* stick*
to *smth.*; ◇ едвá ~ся на ногáх be* scárcely áble to
stand.

дерз|áние *с.* dáring, énterprise; *мн.* dáring attémpts.
~áть, дерзнýть dare.

дерзúть, надерзúть *разг.* be* ínsolent, talk back.

дéрзк|ий 1. (*грýбый, вызывáющий*) ínsolent,
impértinent, ímpudent; ~ мальчúшка rude boy; с ~им
вúдом with an ínsolent air; ~ отвéт impértinent ánswer; 2.
(*смéлый*) dáring, bold, audácious.

дерзнýть сов. *см.* дерзáть.

дéрзост|ь *ж.* 1. ínsolence, impértinence, ímpudence;
2. (*дéрзкий постýпок, выскáзывание*) impértinence; говорúть ~и be* rude, be* ínsolent, talk back; 3. (*смéлость*) dáring, audácity.

дерматúн *м.* leatherétte.

дерматолóгия *ж.* dermatólogy.

дёрн *м.* turf.

дёрн|уть сов. 1. *см.* дёргать 1, 3, 4; 2. (*трóнуться
с мéста*) start off; лóшади ~ули the hórses stárted off.
~уться сов. 1. *см.* дёргаться; 2. *см.* дёрнуть 2; 3. (*рéзко подáться куда-л.*) start with a jerk, jerk ínto mótion.

дерю́га *ж.* búrlap, sácking.

десáнт *м.* *воен.* 1. (*войскá*) expedítionary force; (*небольшóй*) lánding/ráiding párty; воздýшный ~ áirborne
force; вы́садка ~а lánding of troops; 2. (*вы́садка войск*)
lánding, lánding operátion. ~ник *м.* commándo (*pl -os,
-oes*). ~ный lánding *attr.*

десéрт *м.* dessért. ~ный dessért *attr.*; ~ная лóжка ~ное винó dessért/áfter-dínner
wine.

деснá *ж.* gum.

déспот *м.* déspot. ~úзм *м.* déspotism. ~úческий
despótic.

десятибóрье *с.* *спорт.* decáthlon.

десятиднéвный tén-day *attr.*

десятиклассн|ик *м.* ténth-form boy. ~ица *ж.* ténth--form girl.

десятикрáтн|ый ténfold; в ~ом размére ten times the amóunt.

десятилéт|ие *с.* 1. (*период*) décade; 2. (*годовщина*) tenth annivérsary. ~ка *ж.* (*школа*) (tén-year) sécondary school. ~ний 1. (*о сроке*) tén-year attr.; of ten years *после сущ.*; 2. (*о возрасте*) tén-year-óld; of ten *после сущ.*

десяти́чн|ый décimal; ~ая дробь décimal (fráction).

десятка *ж.* 1. (*цифра*) a ten; 2. *разг.* tén-rouble note; 3. *карт.* the ten (of).

десятник *м.* fóreman*.

десят|ый 1. ten, half a score; ~ яйц ten eggs; 2.: ему уже седьмóй ~ he is past síxty, he is in his séventies; 3. *мн.* (*множество*) dózens, scores; ~ки киломéтров болóтных земéль mile áfter mile of bógland; ~ки людéй dózens/scores of péople; ◇ он не рóбкого ~ка he is no cóward.

десят|ый the tenth; ◇ рассказывать *что-л.* с пя́того на ~ое give* a disjóinted accóunt of *smth.*; это дело ~ое *разг.* that's a small mátter.

десять ten.

детализáция *ж.* détailed elaborátion.

детализи́ровать *несов. и сов.* (*вн.*) work (*smth.*) out in détail, work out détails (of); ~ план строи́тельства work out the détails of a búilding prógramme.

детáль *ж.* 1. détail; 2. (*механизма*) part.

детáльн|о in détail. ~ый détailed, élaborate.

детворá *ж. собир. разг.* children *pl*, kids *pl*, kíddies *pl.*

детдóм *м.* (дéтский дом) children's home.

детекти́в *м.* 1. (*сыщик*) detéctive; 2. (*произведение*) detéctive stóry/nóvel. ~ный detéctive.

детéктор *м.* detéctor. ~ный: ~ный приёмник crýstal recéiver.

детёныш *м.* báby(-ánimal); (*крупного хищника*) cub; *мн. собир.* the young.

дéт|и *мн.* children; кни́га для ~éй children's book; они́ ~ своегó вéка they are children of the age they live in.

дети́на *м. разг.* stúrdy/húsky féllow.

дети́шки *мн.* children; kíddies *разг.*

дéтище *с.* child*, óffspring; *перен.* (*творение*) creátion; bráin-child *разг.*

детон|áтор *м.* détonator. ~ация *ж.* detonátion.

детони́ровать I *несов. тех.* détonate.

детони́ровать II *несов. муз.* be* off pitch, be* out of tune.

деторождéние *с.* child-birth, child-bearing.

детоуби́й|ство *с.* infánticide. ~ца *м. и ж.* infánticide, báby-killer.

детсáд *м.* (дéтский сад) núrsery school, kíndergarten. ~овский kíndergarten *attr.*

дéтск|ий 1. children's, child's; ~ крик the cry of a child; ~ие и́гры children's games; ~ие болéзни children's diséases; ~ая смéртность ínfant mortálity; ~ие гóды childhood *sg*; ~ая игру́шка pláything, toy; ~ая кни́га book for children, children's book; ~ая кли́ника children's clínic; 2. (*свойственный детям*) child's, childlike; *перен.* (*ребяческий, незрелый*) childish; неви́нная ~ая улы́бка ínnocent, childlike smile; ~ пóчерк childish hánd(wríting); ◇ ~ дом children's home; ~ сад núrsery school, kíndergarten; ~ие я́сли núrsery, crèche.

дéтств|о *с.* childhood; с ~a from childhood; ◇ впасть в ~ énter *one's* sécond childhood, grow* childish, be* in *one's* dótage.

дéть(ся) *сов. см.* девáть(ся).

де-фáкто de fácto; признáние ~ de fácto recognítion.

дефéкт *м.* deféct. ~ивный deféctive. ~ный impérfect.

дефини́ция *ж.* definítion.

дефи́с *м.* hýphen.

дефици́т *м.* 1. (*бюджетный*) déficit; покры́ть ~ make* good the déficit; 2. (*товаров*) shórtage; ~ в тóпливе shórtage of fuel, fuel shórtage. ~ный 1. (*убыточный*) unprófitable; rúnning at a loss *после сущ.*; ~ное предприя́тие énterprise sustáining lósses; 2. (*не имею-щийся в достаточном количестве*) scarce; ~ный товáр scarce commódity; быть ~ным be* in short supplý.

дефóрм|ация *ж.* distórtion, deformátion. ~и́ровать *несов. и сов.* (*вн.*) change the shape (of). ~и́роваться *несов. и сов.* lose* shape.

децентрализ|ация *ж.* decentralizátion. ~овáть *несов. и сов.* (*вн.*) décentralize (*smth.*).

деци- *в сложн.* déci-.

дешев|éть, подешевéть becóme* chéaper, fall* in price. ~и́зна *ж.* low prices *pl.*

дешёвк|а *ж. разг.* 1. low price, bárgain; купи́ть что-л. по ~е buy* *smth.* dirt-chéap, get* *smth.* for a song; 2. (*нечто безвкусное*) trash, cheap stuff.

дёшево cheap; ~ купи́ть *что-л.* get* *smth.* cheap; ◇ ~ отдéлаться come*/get* off lightly.

дешёв|ый (*прям. и перен.*) cheap; ~ая электро-энéргия cheap electrícity; купи́ть *что-л.* по ~ой ценé buy* *smth.* cheap; ~ успéх cheap/éasy succéss; ~ая остро́та cheap witticism.

де-ю́ре de júre.

деяние *с.* deed, act.

дéятель *м.* figure; ~ искýсства ártist; ~ наýки scientist, man* of science. ~ность *ж.* 1. (*занятия, труд*) actívities *pl*, work; общéственная ~ность públic/sócial actívities; врачéбная ~ность médical práctice; 2. (*о работе каких-л. органов, о действии сил природы*) actívity, áction; ~ность сéрдца áction/fúnctioning of the heart; вы́сшая нéрвная ~ность higher nérvous actívity; ~ность вéтра и воды́ the áction of wind and wáter. ~ный áctive; принимáть ~ное учáстие в чём-л. take* an áctive part in *smth.*

джаз *м.* 1. (*оркестр*) jazz band; 2. (*музыка*) jazz.

джем *м.* jam.

джéмпер *м* júmper; (*мужской*) púll-over.

джентльмéн *м.* géntleman*. ~ский géntlemanly; ◇ ~ское соглашéние géntleman's agréement.

джéрси *с нескл. и неизм. прил.* jérsey; костю́м ~ jérsey suit.

джи́нсы *мн.* (blue) jeans.

джóуль *с. физ.* joule.

джу́нгли *мн.* júngle *sg*.

джут *м.* jute.

дзот *м. воен.* pillbox.

дзюдó *с. нескл. спорт.* júdo.

дзюдóист *м.* júdoka.

диабéт *м. мед.* diabétes. ~ик *м.* diabétic. ~и́ческий diabétic.

диáгноз *м.* diagnósis (*pl* -oses); постáвить ~ give* a diagnósis.

диагонá|ль *ж.* 1. diágonal; 2. (*материя*) diágonal (cloth); ◇ по ~ли diágonally. ~льный diágonal.

диагрáмма *ж.* diagram, chart, graph.

диакрити́ческий: ~ знак *лингв.* diacrítical mark/sign.

диалéкт *м.* díalect.

диалéктика *ж.* dialéctics; материалисти́ческая ~ matérialist dialéctics; ~ собы́тий the dialéctics of évents.

диалекти́ческий dialéctical.

диалéктный dialéctal.

диалóг *м.* dialogue; в фóрме ~a in díalogue.

диáметр *м.* diámeter.

диаметрáльн|о diamétrically; ~ противополóжный diamétrically oppósed. ~ый diamétrical; ~ая плóскость diámetral plane; ~ая противополóжность diamétrical ópposite.

диапазóн *м.* range, scope; (*голоса, инструмента тж.*) cómpass; ~ частóт *радио* fréquency range; ~ знаний intelléctual scope; актёр большо́го ~a híghly vérsatile áctor.

диапозити́в *м. фото* slide. ~ный slide *attr.*; ~ный фильм slide film.

диатони́ческий *муз.* diatónic.

диафи́льм *ж.* slide film.

диафра́гма *ж.* díaphragm.

дива́н *м.* sófa, couch.

дива́н-крова́ть *м.* diván(-bed).

диверс|а́нт *м.* sabotéur, wrécker. ~ио́нный wrécking; ~ио́нный акт act of sábotage.

диве́рсия *ж.* 1. *воен.* (*тактическая*) divérsion; 2. (*вредительская*) sábotage.

дивиде́нд *м. эк.* dividend.

дивизио́н *м.* (*артиллерийский*) báttery; (artíllery) battálion *амер.* ~ный báttery *attr.*; battálion *attr. амер.*

диви́зия *ж.* division.

диви́ться *несов.* (*дт.*) márvel (at), wónder (at).

ди́вн|ый márvellous, wónderful; ~ая пого́да glórious wéather; ~ день glórious/fine day.

ди́в|о *с.* márvel; ◇ не ~ (it is) no wónder; ~у даёшься one can but márvel (at); на ~ márvellously.

дидакти́ческий didáctic.

дие́з *м. муз.* sharp.

дие́т|а *ж.* díet; быть на ~e be* on a díet; посади́ть кого́-л. на ~у put* *smb.* on a díet.

диетвра́ч *м.* dietícian.

диети́ческий dietétic, díetary.

диетоло́г *м.* dietícian.

дизайнер *м.* (art) desígner.

ди́зель *м. тех.* díesel éngine.

ди́зель-мото́р *м.* díesel éngine.

ди́зельный díesel *attr.*; ~ тра́ктор díesel tráctor.

ди́зель-электрохо́д *м.* díesel-eléctric ship.

дизентер|и́йный *мед.* dysentéric. ~и́я *ж. мед.* dýsentery.

дика́р|ка *ж.* sávage; *перен. разг.* shy girl, shy wóman*. ~ский sávage.

дика́рь *м.* 1. sávage; *перен. разг.* shy boy, shy man*; 2. *разг.* hóliday-maker with no advánce bóoking.

ди́к|ий 1. wild; ~ зверь wild ánimal/beast; ~ виногра́д wild grapes; ~ие, угрю́мые го́ры wild and sómbre móuntains; 2. (*первобытный*) sávage; ~ие племена́ sávage tribes; 3. (*необузданный*) wild; ~ нрав wild témperament; с ~им ви́дом wíldly; 4. (*невероятный*) wild; прийти́ в ~ восто́рг becóme* wíldly enthusiástic; ~ая зло́ба frénzied ánger; ~ая боль ágonizing pain; 5. (*странный, нелепый*) absúrd; ~ая мысль mónstrous idéa; (*застенчивый, нелюдимый*) shy, unsóciable; 7. *разг.* (*действующий самостоятельно*) indepéndent; ◇ ~ое мя́со proud flesh; ~ ка́мень rock.

дикобра́з *м. зоол.* pórcupine.

дико́вин|(к)а *ж. разг.* márvel; ◇ э́то ему́ в ~(к)у he has néver seen ánything like it; э́то ему́ не в ~(к)у he sees nóthing óut-of-the-wáy in it. ~ный *разг.* odd, bizárre.

дикорасту́щий wild; in its native state *после сущ.*

ди́кость *ж.* 1. (*некультурность*) wildness, uncívilized state; ~ нра́вов uncivilized/barbáric ways; 2. (*нелюдимость*) shýness, unsociability; 3. *разг.* (*нелепость*) absúrdity.

дикта́нт *м.* dictátion.

дикта́т *м.* díctates *pl*; diktát; поли́тика ~a pólicy of dictátion/diktát. ~ор *м.* dictátor. ~орский dictatórial.

диктату́ра *ж.* dictátorship.

диктова́ть, продиктова́ть (*вн.*) dictáte (*smth.*).

дикто́в|ка *ж.* dictátion; писа́ть под ~ку кого́-л. take* down from *smb.'s* dictátion; ◇ под чью-л. ~ку at *smb.'s* bídding, just becáuse *one* is told by *smb.*

ди́ктор *м.* annóuncer.

диктофо́н *м.* díctophone, dictáting machine.

ди́кция *ж.* enunciátion, díction.

диле́мма *ж.* dilémma.

дилета́нт *м.* ámateur; *неодобр.* dilettánte, dábbler. ~и́зм *м.* amatéurishness. ~ский amatéurish. ~ство *с.* amatéurishness.

динами́зм *м.* dýnamism, dynámic pówer.

дина́мик *м. радио* loud spéaker.

дина́мика *ж.* 1. (*наука*) dynámics *sg*; 2. (*состояние движения, ход развития чего-л.*) the dynámics *pl*; 3. (*движение, действие*) móvement, áction.

динами́т *м.* dýnamite; подрыва́ть что́-л. ~ом dýnamite *smth.*

динами́ч|еский, ~ный dynámic.

дина́стия *ж.* dýnasty.

диора́ма *ж.* dioráma.

дипкурье́р *м.* (*дипломатический курьер*) diplomátic cóurier; (*английский*) Queen's méssenger.

дипло́м *м.* 1. diplóma; (*университетский*) first degrée; ~ с отли́чием first-cláss diplóma; 2. *разг.* (*работа*) graduátion work.

диплома́т *м.* díplomat, díplomatist. ~и́ческий (*прям. и перен.*) diplomátic; ~и́ческие отноше́ния diplomátic relátions; ~и́ческий ко́рпус diplomátic corps*; ~и́ческий отве́т diplomátic ánswer. ~и́чный diplomátic, táctful. ~ия *ж.* díplomacy.

дипломи́рованный gráduate *attr.*

дипло́мн|ик *м.*, ~ица *ж.* stúdent engáged on degrée thésis.

дипло́мн|ый ~ прое́кт graduátion work; ~ая рабо́та graduátion éssay/work.

директи́в|а *ж.* diréctive. ~ный diréctive; ~ное письмо́ létter of instrúctions; ~ные указа́ния diréctions, instrúctions.

дире́ктор *м.* diréctor, mánager; ~ шко́лы diréctor of a school; school príncipal; (*мужчина тж.*) head máster; (*женщина тж.*) head místress. ~ский diréctor's, managérial.

дире́кция *ж.* 1. the mánagement; 2. (*помещение*) diréctor's/mánager's óffice, mánagement óffice.

дирижа́бль *м.* dírigible, áirship.

дирижёр *м.* condúctor; ~ хо́ра chóir-master. ~ский: ~ская па́лочка condúctor's báton; ~ский пульт condúctor's desk/stand.

дирижи́ровать *несов.* (*тв.*) condúct (*smth.*).

дисгармони́ровать *несов.* be* out of hármony; (с *тв.*) *перен.* clash (with), be* out of kéeping (with).

дисгармо́ния *ж.* dishármony, discórdance.

диск *м.* 1. disk, disc; 2. *спорт.* díscus.

ди́скант *м.* tréble.

дисквалифи|ка́ция *ж.* disqualificátion. ~ци́ровать *несов. и сов.* (*вн.*) disquálify (*smb.*). ~ци́роваться *несов. и сов.* lose* *one's* proféssional qualificátion/skill.

дискобо́л *м.* díscus thrówer.

дискреди́т|ация *ж.* discréditing. ~и́ровать *несов. и сов.* (*вн.*) bring* discrédit (on), discrédit (*smb.*), cómpromise (*smb.*).

дискрими|на́ция *ж.* discriminátion. ~и́ровать *несов. и сов.* (*вн.*) discríminate (agáinst).

дискуссио́нн|ый debátable; в ~ом поря́дке as a básis for discússion.

диску́ссия *ж.* discússion, debáte.

дискути́ровать *несов.* (*вн., о пр.*) discúss (*smth.*), debáte (*smth.*)

дислока́ци|я *ж.* 1. *мед.* dislocátion; *геол. тж.* shífting; 2. *воен.* distribútion (of troops); в райо́не ~и диви́зии in the área where the division is locáted.

дислоци́ровать *несов. и сов.* (*вн.*) *воен.* státion (*smth.*). ~ся *несов. и сов.* be* statióned.

диспансе́р *м.* prophyláctic céntre. ~иза́ция *ж.* prophyláctic sýstem. ~ный: ~ое наблюде́ние régular médical chéck-up.

диспе́тчер *м.* contróller; (*на железной дороге*)

dispátcher. ~ская ж. contróller's óffice; ав. contról tówer. ~ский contról attr.; ~ский пункт contróller's óffice.

дисплéй м. displáy.

диспропóрция ж. dispropórtion.

діспут м. disputátion, debáte.

диссертá|нт м. áuthor of a thésis/dissertátion. ~ция ж. thésis (pl -ses), dissertátion; кандидáтская ~ция máster's thésis.

диссон|áнс м. муз. díscord, díssonance; discórdant note (тж. перен.). ~íровать несов. муз. be* díssonant.

дистанциóнн|ый remóte; ~ое управлéние remóte contról; ~ая трýбка (tíme-)fuse.

дистáнц|ия ж. 1. dístance; 2. воен. range; 3. ж.-д. (ráilway) divísion; ◇ сойтú с ~ии спорт. fall* out of the race.

дистилл|íрованный distílled; ~ированная водá distílled wáter. ~íровать несов. и сов. (вн.) distíl (smth.). ~ция ж. distillátion.

дисциплíна I ж. тк. ед. (установленный порядок) díscipline.

дисциплíна II ж. (отрасль науки) díscipline, branch (of knówledge); súbject.

дисциплин|áрный dísciplinary; ~áрное взыскáние súmmary púnishment. ~íрованный dísciplined. ~íровать несов. и сов. (вн.) díscipline (smb.).

дитя́ с. child*.

дифирáмб м. díthyramb; петь ~ы кому-л. sing* the práises of smb., laud smb. to the skies.

дифтерíт м. мед. diphthéria. ~ный мед. diphthéria attr.

дифтóнг м. лингв. díphthong.

диффамáция ж. юр. defamátion.

дифференци|áл м. мат. differéntial. ~áльный differéntial; ~áльное исчислéние мат. differéntial cálculus; ~áльный тариф differéntial dúties pl.

дифференциáция ж. differentiátion.

дифференцúрованный differéntiated; ~ подхóд indivídual appróach/tréatment.

дифференцúровать несов. и сов. (вн.) differéntiate (smth.).

диффýзия ж. физ. diffúsion.

дич|áть, одичáть 1. (о растениях) run* wild; (о животных) becóme*/grow* wild; 2. (о людях) becóme* shy/unsóciable; онá совсéм одичáла she has becóme a pérfect sávage. ~иться несов. (рд.) разг. be* shy (of). ~óк м. бот. wílding.

дичь ж. тк. ед. 1. собир. game; крýпная ~ big game; 2. (мясо дичи как пища) game; 3. разг. (чепуха) nónsense; порóть ~ talk rot/rúbbish.

длин|á ж. тк. ед. length; мéры ~ы́ méasures of length; ~ окрýжности circúmference; в ~ý léngthwise; имéть в ~ý 15 мéтров be* fiftéen métres long; ~ волны́ rádio wáve-length; наибóльшая ~ mex. óverall length.

длинно|волóсый long-háired. ~нóгий long-légged. ~нóсый long-nósed. ~рýкий with long arms после сущ.

длиннóты мн. prolíxities.

длинно|хвóстый long-táiled. ~шёрст(н)ый long-háired.

длúнн|ый long; ◇ ~ язык long tongue; гнáться за ~ым рублём be* áfter a big páy-packet.

длítельн|ость ж. durátion. ~ый protrácted, prolónged, long.

длúться, продлúться last, go* on, contínue.

для 1. for; он это сдéлает ~ неё he will do it for her; 2. (по отношению к) to, for; полéзно ~ детéй good* for children; ~ негó это типично that's týpical of him; 3. (с целью) for, for the púrpose of (+ -ing); ~ изучéния for the púrpose of stúdying; не ~ (б)тогó that's not what... for; я не ~ этого пришёл сюдá that's not what I've come for; ~ тогó, чтóбы (перед инф.) (in órder) to; (перед подлежащим или дополнением) in órder that, so that; ~ тогó, чтóбы мы пóняли это in órder that we

should understánd it, to make us understánd it; ~ чегó? why?, what for?; ~ чегó это? what's it for?

дневáльный воен. man* on dúty.

дневáть несов.: ~ и ночевáть разг. spend* all one's time.

дневнúк м. 1. díary; ~ боевых дéйствий war díary; вестú ~ keep* a díary; 2. (ученический) púpil's mark book.

дневн|óй 1. day attr.; diúrnal астр., поэт.; ~бе врéмя dáy-time; ~ свет dáylight, the light of day; ~ спектáкль matinée; ~я смéна dáy-shift; 2. (приходящийся на один день) dáily, day's; ~ зáработок dáily éarnings pl.

днём by day, in the dáy-time; (после полудня) in the áfternóon; сегóдня ~ this áfternóon; ◇ ~ с огнём не найтú it's nówhere to be found.

днúще с. bóttom; (судна тж.) bilge.

дно с. bóttom; (моря, реки тж.) bed; на дне at the bóttom; пить до дна drain the cup; drink* to the dregs; ◇ вверх дном úpside-dówn; tópsy-túrvy; идтú ко дну go* to the bóttom, fóunder; золотóе ~ góld-mine.

до I нескл. муз. do, C.

до II предлог 1. (указывает предел распространения действия) to, up to, down to; as far as; до вершú-ны далекó it's a long way to the top; проводúть когó-л. до углá see* smb. to the córner; до Лóндона 100 киломéтров it is one húndred kílometres to Lóndon; от Москвы́ до Калýги from Móscow to Kalúga; 2. (указывает временнóй предел действия) till, untíl, up to, to; до послéдней минýты to the véry last; нáдо ждать до обéда we must wait till dínner-time; с утрá до вéчера from mórning till night; 3. (раньше чего-л.) before; он встал до рассвéта he got up befóre dawn; 4. (указывает стéпень действия) to, to the point of; (целиком, полностью) to; онú дошлú до дрáки they came to blows; промёрзнуть до костéй be* frózen to the bone; мóкрый до нúтки wet to the skin; выпить что-л. до послéдней кáпли drink* smth. to the last drop; 5. (указывает колúчественный предел) as much as; (не больше) up to; (приблизительно) abóut; зарабáтывать до ста рублéй earn as much as one húndred róubles; на собрáнии было до пятидесяти человéк there must have been about fifty péople at the méeting; дéти до шестнáдцати лет chíldren únder sixtéen; 6. (указывает предмет, лицо, к которому относится действие): до нас дошлú слýхи rúmours have reached us; ◇ до тех пор, покá till, untíl; до тогó, что till; до сих пор 1) (по времени) up to now, to this day; (пока) so far; 2) (по месту) up to here; мне не до тогó I have no time for that, I am in no mood for that.

добáвить сов. см. добавлять.

добáв|ка ж. разг. addítion; (при еде) anóther hélping. ~лéние с. addítion; в ~лéние ко всемý on top of éverything; он сдéлал нéкоторые ~лéния к статьé he made some addítions to the árticle.

добавлять, добáвить (вн.) add (smth.).

добáвочный additional, éxtra.

добегáть, добежáть (до рд.) reach (smth.), run* (to).

добéг|аться сов. разг.: ~ался! now he's in tróuble!

добежáть сов. см. добегáть.

добелá to a white heat; раскалённый ~ white-hót; раскалúть что-л. ~ make* smth. white-hót.

добивáть, добúть (вн.) 1. kill (smb., smth.), finish (smb., smth.) off; (вражескую áрмию) compléte the destrúction (of); 2. (разбивать) break* (smth.), finish (smth.) off.

добивá|ться несов. (рд.) strive* (for, + tυ inf); try/strive* to get (smth.), seek* (smth.); ~ встрéчи с кем-л. try to meet smb.; seek* out smb.; он всегдá ~лся своегó he álways got what he wánted; ~ признáния strive* for recognítion; ◇ ~ реше́ния seek* a decísion, try to get a decísion; ~ сла́вы seek* fame.

добира́|ться, добра́ться arríve, get* there; (до рд.) reach (smth.), arríve (at, in), get* (to) (тж. перен.); ~ до бе́рега мо́ря reach the sea-shore; мы до́лго ~лись до́ дому it took us a long time to get home; добра́ться до гор get* to the móuntains, reach the móuntains; не добра́ться fail to get there; (до рд.) fail to get (to); fail to reach (smth.); ~ до и́стины get*/arríve at the truth; ◇ я ещё до него́ доберу́сь wait till I have a go at him.

доби́ть сов. см. добива́ть.

доби́ться сов. (рд.) obtáin (smth.), achíeve (smth.), succéed in gétting (smth.); он доби́лся встре́чи с ним he succéeded in gétting an ínterview with him; ~ отве́та succéed in gétting an ánswer; я не доби́лся отве́та I cóuldn't get an ánswer, I failed to get an ánswer; ~ (по́лного) успе́ха succéed; achíeve (compléte) succéss; ~ реше́ния obtáin a decísion; ~ своего́ succéed in gétting one's own way, get* one's own way; achíeve/attáin one's óbject; не ~ чего́-л. fail to get smth., fail to achíeve smth.; ничего́ не ~ gain nóthing, get* nóthing for one's pains; ~ попада́ний воен. get* on tárget.

до́блестный váliant; ~ труд váliant lábour.

до́блесть ж. válour, cóurage.

добра́сывать, добро́сить (вн.) throw* (smth.) so far; (вн. до рд.) throw* (smth. as far as); не добро́сить not throw far enóugh; (до рд.) throw* short (of).

добра́ться сов. см. добира́ться.

добре́ть, подобре́ть becóme kínder; ~ к кому́-л. sóften towárds smb.

добр|о́ I с. тк. ед. 1. (the) good; де́лать ~ do* good; жела́ть ~а́ кому́-л. wish smb. well; э́то до ~а́ не доведёт nóthing good will come of it; от ~а́ ~а́ не и́щут посл. one ought to know when one is well off; 2. разг. (имущество, пожитки) things pl, posséssions pl, próperty; помина́ть кого́-л. ~о́м разг. recáll smb.'s good points; speak* well of smb.; э́то не к ~у́ that's a bad ómen/sign; дать (получи́ть) ~ на что́-л. give* (get*) the go-ahéad for smth.

добро́ II нареч. разг. 1. в знач. сказ. безл. all right!; 2.: ~ бы it would be a dífferent mátter; ~ бы но́чью, а то средь бе́ла дня it would have been a dífferent mátter at night but this was in broad dáylight; ◇ ~ пожа́ловать! (you are) wélcome!

доброво́лец м. voluntéer.

доброво́льн|о vóluntarily; of one's own free will. ~ость ж. vóluntary náture, ábsence of compúlsion. ~ый vóluntary; на ~ых нача́лах on a vóluntary básis.

доброво́льческий voluntéer attr., vóluntary; ~ батальо́н voluntéer battálion.

доброде́тель ж. vírtue. ~ный vírtuous.

добро́душ|ие с. good náture. ~ный good-nátured, kíndly; с са́мым ~ным ви́дом with an air of the útmost good húmour.

доброжела́тель м. well-wisher. ~ность ж. benévolence. ~ный (желающий добра) well-méaning, benévolent; (выражающий расположение) fríendly, well-dispósed; ~ная улы́бка fríendly smile. ~ство с. goodwíll.

доброка́чественн|ость ж. sound/good quálity; sóundness. ~ый 1. good-quálity attr.; of good quálity после сущ.; 2. мед. benígn, non-malígnant.

добро́м разг. of one's own accórd.

добросерде́ч|ие с., ~ность ж. kind-héartedness. ~ный kind-héarted.

добро́сить сов. см. добра́сывать.

добросо́вестн|ость ж. consciéntiousness. ~ый consciéntious; (старательный) páinstaking.

добрососе́дск|ий good-néighbour, néighbourly; ~ие отноше́ния fríendly relátions, good-néighbour relátions.

доброта́ ж. kíndness, góodness.

добро́тн|ость ж. sóundness, (good) quálity. ~ый (good) sound, dúrable; ~ая ткань good sound matérial.

до́бр|ый 1. good*, kind; ~ое се́рдце kind heart; ~ые лю́ди kíndly souls; ~ые наме́рения good inténtions; ~ые дела́ kind deeds; ~ое и́мя good name/reputátion; ~ая сла́ва good fame; 2. разг.: ~ых два (три) часа́ a full two (three) hours; ~ час a sólid hour; ~ая полови́на a good half; ◇ ~ ма́лый разг. a good sort; бу́дьте ~ы would you mind (+ -ing), be so kind (as + to inf); в ~ час! good luck!; всего́ ~ого! goodbýe!; ~ ве́чер! good évening!; ~ день! good mórning!; (после полудня) good afternóon!; ~ой но́чи! good night!; по ~ой во́ле of one's own accórd; визи́т ~ой во́ли goodwíll vísit; чего́ ~ого I'm afráid; пойдём скоре́е, а то, чего́ ~ого, дождь пойдёт húrry up! I'm afráid it's góing to rain; наде́ньте пальто́, а то, чего́ ~ого, просту́дитесь put on your coat if you don't want to catch cold; бюро́ ~ых услу́г pérsonal sérvices buréau.

добря́к м. разг. good/kíndly soul, good-nátured pérson.

добуди́ться сов. (рд.) разг. succéed in róusing/wáking (smb.).

добыв|а́ние с. 1. gáining, obtáining; 2. (из недр и т. п.) extráction. ~а́ть, добы́ть (вн.) 1. mánage to get* (smth.), obtáin (smth.), gain (smth.); ~а́ть све́дения obtáin/elícit informátion; ~а́ть сре́дства к существова́нию earn one's líving/bread; 2. (извлекать) extráct (smth.); (в рудниках) mine (smth.); (в карьерах) quárry (smth.). ~а́ющий: ~а́ющая промы́шленность extráctive índustry.

добы́ть сов. см. добыва́ть.

добы́ч|а ж. 1. (действие) gétting; (угля и т. п. тж.) extráction; вы́йти на ~у (о зверях) go* húnting, go* out in search of prey; 2. (добытое из недр земли) óutput; 3. (захваченное) bóoty, plúnder, loot; 4. (хищника) bag; quárry.

дова́ривать, довари́ть (вн.) fínish bóiling (smth.); (суп) fínish máking (smth.). ~ся, довари́ться fínish bóiling; (о супе) be* bóiled enóugh.

довари́ть(ся) сов. см. дова́ривать(ся).

довезти́ сов. см. довози́ть.

дове́ренн|ость ж. létter/power of attórney; по ~ости únder a power of attórney. ~ый прил. 1. confidéntial; ~ое лицо́ (confidéntial) ágent, accrédited represéntative; 2. в знач. сущ. м. próxy, ágent.

дове́р|ие с. cónfidence, trust, faith; пита́ть ~ к кому́-л. have* faith/cónfidence in smb.; оказа́ть ~ кому́-л. put* cónfidence in smb.; отсу́тствие ~ия credibílity gap.

дове́рить сов. см. доверя́ть 2. ~ся сов. см. доверя́ться.

до́верху to the top.

дове́рчив|ость ж. trústfulness; (наивная) credúlity. ~ый trústing, trústful, confíding; (наивный) crédulous.

доверш|а́ть, доверши́ть (вн.) compléte (smth.). ~éние с. complétion; ◇ в ~éние всего́ to crown all. ~и́ть сов. см. доверша́ть.

доверя́ть, дове́рить 1. тк. несов. (дт.; верить) trust (smb., smth.), have* cónfidence/faith (in smb., smth.); не ~ кому́-л., чему́-л. not trust smb., smth., have* no cónfidence/faith in smb., smth.; místrust smb., smth., distrúst smb., smth.; 2. (вн. дт.; поручать) entrúst (smb. with, smb., smth. to); (сообщать тж.) confíde (smth. to); ~ кому́-л. своего́ ребёнка entrúst one's child* to smb.'s care; ~ кому́-л. та́йну confíde a sécret to smb. ~ся, дове́риться (дт.) trust (in), put* one's trust (in).

дове́сок м. mákeweight.

довести́ сов. см. доводи́ть. ~сь сов. см. доводи́ться 1.

до́вод м. árgument, réason; ~ы за и про́тив the pros and cons; приводи́ть ~ы advánce/addúce réasons.

доводи́ть, довести́ (вн.) 1. (вн. до: ведя, доставляя) bring* (smb. to), take* (smb. to); ~ кого́-л. до угла́ take* smb. to the córner; go* as far as the córner with smb.; 2. (*достигать какого-л. предела*) bring* (*smth.*); ~ что-л. до совершéнства bring* *smth.* to perféction, perféct *smth.*; ~ что-л. до концá see* *smth.* through, go* through with *smth.*; ~ что-л. до тóчки кипéния bring* *smth.* to bóiling-point; ~ что-л. до мúнимума redúce *smth.* to the mínimum; 3. (*приводить в какое-л. состояние*) redúce (*smb.*), drive* (*smb.*); ~ когó-л. до отчáяния drive* *smb.* to despáir; ~ себя до чего-л. work one*sélf* into *smth.*; 4. (*сообщать, передавать*) get* (*smth.*); ~ что-л. до потребúтеля get* *smth.* to the consúmer; ~ до свéдения когó-л., что... bring* it to *smb.'s* nótice that..., infórm *smb.* that... ~ся, довестúсь 1. *безл.* (+ *инф.*) *разг.*: мне не доводúлось, не довелóсь там нáм I have néver been there; вот кáк нам довелóсь встрéтиться! this is how we meet!; мне не доводúлось егó вúдеть I néver had occásion to meet him; 2. *тк. несов.* (*дт. тв.*; *о родстве*) be* (*smth.* of); он доводится мне брáтом he's my bróther.

довоéнный pre-wár.

довозúть, довезтú (*вн.*) take* (*smb., smth.*) there.

довóльн|о 1. *нареч.* (*с удовольствием*) conténtedly, with satisfáction; ~ *нареч.* (*достаточно*) enóugh; с нас ~ we've had enóugh; (*надоело тж.*) we're fed up; 3. *в знач. сказ. безл.* it is enóugh; (*как восклицание*) enóugh!; enóugh (of it)!; that'll do!; 4. *нареч.* (*порядочно*) ráther, fáirly, quíte; ~ далекó a good way off/awáy; ~ далекó от чего-л. a fair dístance from *smth.*, ráther a long way from *smth.*; ~ дóлго ráther a long time; ~ хорошó not bad, quíte/fáirly good; чувствовать себя ~ хорошó feel* prétty well. ~ый 1. (*тв.*) pleased (with); (*удовлетворённый*) content (with), sátisfied (with); он всем довóлен he's éasily pleased; 2. (*выражающий довольство*) conténted; ~ое лицó conténted face, the look of pléasure on one's face; ~ый вид sátisfied/pleased expréssion.

довóльств|ие *с. воен.* allówance; allówances *pl*; вещевóе ~ clóthing allówance; дéнежное ~ móney allówances *pl*; принимáть когó-л. на ~ put* *smb.* down for allówances; снимáть когó-л. с ~ия depríve *smb.* of his allówances.

довóльство *с.* 1. (*удовлетворение*) conténtment, content; 2. *разг.* (*достаток*) ease, prósperity.

довóльствоваться *несов.* 1. (*тв.*; *удовлетворяться*) be* content (with); ~ мáлым be* content with véry little, be* éasily sátisfied; 2. *воен.* draw* allówances; (*получать питание*) mess.

дог *м.* Great Dane.

догадáться *сов. см.* догáдываться.

догáд|ка *ж.* súrmise, conjécture, guess; *мн. тж.* guéss-work sg; стрóить ~ки conjécture, make* conjéctures. ~ливость *ж.* chréwdness, shárpness. ~ливый shrewd, quick-wítted, sharp.

догáд|ываться, догадáться guess, form a prétty good idéa; (+ *инф.*) have* the sense (+ to *inf*); вы не ~áетесь? can't you guess?; я ~аюсь о егó намéрениях I think I know what he's up to; я не знáю, но ~аюсь I don't know but I can guess; он догадáлся выключить вóду he had the sense to turn off the wáter.

доглядéть *сов. разг.* (*вн.*; *до конца*) stay to the end (of); see* the end (of).

догм|а *ж.* dógma. ~атúзм *м.* dógmatism. ~áтик *м.* dógmatist. ~атúческий dogmátic.

догнáть *сов. см.* догонять.

догнивáть, догнúть rot, decáy.

догнúть *сов. см.* догнивáть.

догговáрив|ать, договорúть 1. finish télling; не договорúть break* off, stop short; 2. (*вносить ясность*) speak* out; ~ай (же)! out with it!; не ~ чего-л. keep* *smth.* back. ~аться, договорúться 1. (с *тв.* о *пр.*) make* arrángements (with *smb.* abóut *smth.*); *сов.* come* to an agréement/understánding (with *smb.* abóut *smth.*); договорúлись? is it séttled?; 2. (*вести переговоры*)

negótiate; 3. (до *рд.*) go* as far as to say (*smth.*); он договорúлся до абсýрда his árguments lánded him in absúrdity.

договóр *м.* agréement; *юр.* cóntract; (*между государствами*) tréaty, pact; ~ на постáвку лéса cóntract for the delívery of timber; ~ о дрýжбе и взаúмной пóмощи tréaty of fríendship/ámity and mútual assístance; ~ о ненападéнии non-aggréssion pact.

договорённость *ж.* understánding.

договорúть(ся) *сов. см.* договáривать(ся).

договóрн|ый contráctual; (*о договоре между государствами*) tréaty *attr.*; ~ая ценá agréed price; ~ые обязáтельства contrácted commítments; tréaty obligátions; на ~ых начáлах on a contráctual básis.

доголá: раздéть(ся) ~ strip to the skin, strip náked.

догон|я́ть, догнáть (*вн.*) overtáke* (*smb., smth.*), catch* up (with) (*тж. перен.*); *несов. тж.* gain on (*smb., smth.*); ~áй егó! catch him!

догорáть, догорéть burn* out, burn* down; (*гаснуть*) go* out; дровá догорéли the logs had burnt out.

догорéть *сов. см.* догорáть.

додавáть, додáть (*вн.*) give* (*smth.*) to make up the amóunt, add on (*smth.*).

додáть *сов. см.* додавáть.

додéлать *сов. см.* додéлывать.

додéлывать, додéлать (*вн.*) finish (*smth.*), put* the finishing touch (to).

додýма|ться *сов.* (до *рд.*) hit* upón (the idéa of), arríve (at); он дóлго дýмал, но (так) ни до чегó (и) не ~лся he racked his brains but could arríve at no conclúsion.

доедáть, доéсть (*вн.*) eat* (*smth.*) up, finish (*smth.*) up.

доезжá|ть, доéхать (до *рд.*) arríve (at); (*до какого-л. пункта тж.*) reach (*smth.*); не ~я до... befóre you get to...; не ~я трёх киломéтров до гóрода within three kílometres of the town.

доéсть *сов. см.* доедáть.

доéхать *сов. см.* доезжáть.

дожáривать, дожáрить (*вн.*) finish frýing (*smth.*); (*до готовности*) do* (*smth.*) to a turn. ~ся, дожáриться be* próperly fried.

дожáрить(ся) *сов. см.* дожáривать(ся).

дожáть *сов.* (*вн.*; *кончить жатву*) reap (*smth.*), finish réaping (*smth.*).

дожд|áться *сов.* (*рд.*) 1. wait till (*smb., smth.*); ~ дóктора wait till the dóctor comes; ~ наступлéния темнотý wait till nightfall; он не ~áлся нас he left before we came; я дóлго ждал (егó), но так и не ~áлся I wáited (for him) till I could wait no lónger; I wáited (for him) in vain; он вас ждёт не ~ётся he's dýing to see you; наконéц мы егó ~áлись at long last he came; 2.: ты у меня ~ёшься! you'll catch it one day!

дождевáльн|ый; ~ая устанóвка sprínkler.

дождевúк *м.* 1. *разг.* (*плащ*) ráincoat, wáterproof; 2. (*гриб*) púff-ball.

дождев|óй rain *attr.*; ~áя кáпля ráindrop; ~áя водá ráin-water.

дождемéр *м.* ráin-gauge.

дóждик *м.*, дóждичек *м. см.* дождь; ◇ пóсле дóждичка в четвéрг one fine day when it's ráining.

дождлúв|ый ráiny; ~ая погóда ráiny/wet wéather.

дождь *м.* rain (*тж. перен.*); проливнóй ~ dównpour; ~ идёт it rains, it is ráining; идёт сúльный ~ it is ráining héavily; в ~, под дождём in the rain; перестáл ~ the rain has stopped, it has stopped ráining; золотóй ~ искр a gólden rain of sparks.

доживáть, дожúть 1. live; дожúть до глубóкой стáрости live to a ripe old age; ~ до седых волóс be* góing grey (with age), live till one is gréy-héaded; не дожúть (*не дождаться*) not live to see; емý не дожúть до э́того дня he won't live as long as that; **2.** *тк. несов.*: ~ свою́ жизнь live out the remáinder of *one's* days.

дожид|а́ться *несов.* (*рд.*) *разг.* wait (*smb.*, *smth.*), be* wáiting (for); awáit (*smb.*); он уже́ давно́ (вас) ~а́ется he has been wáiting (for you) a long time.

дожи́ть *сов. см.* **дожива́ть 1.**

до́за *ж.* dose; *перен. тж.* share; сли́шком больша́я ~ óverdose; небольши́ми ~ми in small dóses.

дозва́ться *сов.* (*вн.*) *разг.*: наконе́ц я его́ дозва́лся at last he respónded to my repéated calls; его́ ника́к не дозовёшься I símply can't get him; he néver comes when he's called.

дозво́ленн|ый *прил.* **1.** permíssible; **2.** *в знач. сущ. с.* the allówable; переходи́ть грани́цы ~ого overstép the bounds of décency.

дозвон|и́ться *сов.* (*у две́ри*) go* on rínging till the door is ópened; (*к дт.; по телефо́ну*) get* (*smb.*) on the phone; не ~ get* no ánswer to *one's* rínging; к нему́ ника́к не ~и́шься (*по телефо́ну*) you símply can't get him on the phone.

дознава́ться, дозна́ться find* out, ascertáin.

дозна́ние *с. юр.* prelíminary investigátion; (*в слу́чае внеза́пной сме́рти*) ínquest; производи́ть ~ hold* an ínquest (on).

дозна́ться *сов. см.* **дознава́ться.**

дозо́р *м.* patról; уходи́ть в ~ go* out on patról; ◇ быть, находи́ться в ~e be* (out) on patról. **~ный** *прил.* **1.** patról *attr.*; ~ное су́дно patról boat; **2.** *в знач. сущ. м.* scout.

дозрева́ние *с.* matúring, rípening.

дозрев|а́ть, дозре́ть rípen; *сов. тж.* be* ripe; я́блоки ~а́ют the ápples are néarly ripe.

дозре́ть *сов. см.* **дозрева́ть.**

доигр|а́ть *см.* **дои́грывать. ~а́ться** *сов.* (*до рд.*) play (untíl); *перен.* get* ínto tróuble; ~а́лся! now he's in tróuble!, now he's done it!

дои́грыв|ать, доигра́ть (*вн.*) fínish (pláying) (*smth.*); (*конча́ть ту́ры игр*) play off (*smth.*); вчера́ они́ ~а́ли па́ртию в тече́ние трёх часо́в it took them three hours to fínish their game yésterday; за́втра мы бу́дем ~ остальны́е ма́тчи we'll play off the remáining mátches tomórrow.

дои́льн|ый mílking *attr.*; ~ая маши́на mílking machíne, mílker.

доиска́ться *сов.* (*рд.*) *разг.* **1.** (*найти́, отыска́ть*) find* (*smth.*); **2.** (*разузна́ть о чём-л.*) find* out (*smth.*), get* at (*smth.*), seek* out (*smth.*); ~ пра́вды get* at the truth.

дои́скиваться *несов.* (*рд.*) *разг.* try to find out (*smth.*).

доистори́ческий prehistóric.

дои́ть, подои́ть (*вн.*) milk (*smth.*). **~ся** *несов.* yield milk; хорошо́ ~ся be* a good* mílker.

до́йн|ый milch; ~ корóва mílking cow, mílker; (*перен.*) milch cow.

дойти́ *сов. см.* **доходи́ть.**

док *м.* dock; вводи́ть кора́бль в ~ dock a ship; стоя́ть в ~e be* docked.

доказа́тель|ный demónstrative, conclúsive. **~ство** *с.* **1.** proof; (*подтвержде́ние*) évidence; в ви́де ~ства by way of proof/évidence; в ~ство чего́... in proof of which...; приводи́ть ~ства fúrnish proofs; служи́ть ~ством чего́-л. be* évidence of *smth.*, serve as évidence of *smth.*; я́ркое ~ство чего́-л. stríking évidence of *smth.*; **2.** *лог., мат.* demonstrátion.

доказа́ть *сов. см.* **дока́зывать.**

дока́зывать, доказа́ть (*вн.*) prove (*smth.*), démonstrate (*smth.*); *несов. тж.* árgue (*smth.*), seek* to prove (*smth.*); ~ что-л. на пра́ктике prove *smth.* in práctice; что и тре́бовалось доказа́ть which was to be démonstrate; *мат.* Q.E.D.

дока́нчивать, доко́нчить (*вн.*) fínish (*smth.*); *несов. тж.* be* fínishing (*smth.*).

докапиталисти́ческий pre-cápitalist.

дока́пываться *несов.* (*до рд.*) dig* down (to); *перен.* try to find out (*smth.*), try to worm out (*smth.*).

докати́ться *сов.* (*до рд.*) **1.** reach (*smth.*); (*о мяче́ и т. п.*) roll as far as (*smth.*); **2.** *разг.* (*опусти́ться*) sink* (to, ínto).

до́кер *м.* dócker.

докла́д *м.* **1.** (*у́стный*) lécture; (*пи́сьменный*) pа́рer; де́лать ~ о чём-л. speak* on *smth.*, addréss the méeting on *smth.*, lécture on *smth.*, give* a lécture on *smth.*; read* a pа́рer on *smth.*; **2.** (*официа́льное сообще́ние руководи́телю*) repórt; **3.**: входи́ть без ~а énter unannóunced. **~но́й**: ~ная запи́ска repórt, memorándum (*pl* -da). **~чик** *м.* spéaker, lécturer; (*на конфере́нциях и т. п.*) rapportéur.

докла́дывать I, доложи́ть 1. (*вн., о пр.; сообща́ть*) repórt (on *smth.*); (*вн.*) repórt on a situátion; **2.** (*о пр.; о посети́теле*) annóunce (*smb.*).

докла́дывать II, доложи́ть (*вн., рд.; добавля́ть*) add (*smth.*).

докла́ссовый pre-cláss; befóre the formátion of clásses *по́сле сущ.*

докон|а́ть *сов.* (*вн.*) *разг.* fínish (*smb.*, *smth.*); э́то его́ ~а́ло that finished him, that did for him.

доко́нчить *сов. см.* **дока́нчивать.**

докопа́ться *сов.* (*до рд.*) **1.** dig* down (to); **2.** *разг.* (*разузна́ть*) find* out (*smth.*); ~ до су́ти де́ла get* to the root of the mа́tter.

докрасна́ to rédness; раскалённый ~ red-hót; раскали́ть что́-л. ~ make* *smth.* red-hót.

докрич|а́ться *сов.* **1.** (*рд.*) *разг.* make* (*smb.*) hear, make* *one's* shouts heard; никого́ не ~и́шься you can't make ányone hear; **2.**: ~ до хрипоты́ shout onesélf hoarse.

до́ктор *м.* **1.** (*учёная сте́пень*) dóctor; ~ филологи́ческих нау́к Dóctor of Philólogy; **2.** (*врач*) physícian, dóctor. **~ант** *м.* áspirant/cándidate for a dóctor's degrée. **~ский** dóctor's, dóctoral; ~ская диссерта́ция thésis for a dóctor's degrée, dóctor's/dóctoral thésis.

доктри́на *ж.* dóctrine.

доктринёр *м.* doctrináire, doctrinárian. **~ский** doctrináire. **~ство** *с.* doctrináirism.

докуме́нт *м.* dócument; *юр.* deed; *мн. тж.* pа́рers, credéntials; ва́ши ~ы! show your pа́рers (please)!; прове́рка ~ов examinátion of pа́рers. **~а́льный** documéntary; ◇ ~а́льный фильм documéntary (film). **~а́ция** *ж.* documentátion.

документи́ровать *несов. и сов.* (*вн.*) dócument (*smth.*).

доку́ривать, докури́ть (*вн.*) fínish smóking (*smth.*); ~ папиро́су fínish *one's* cigarétte.

докури́ть *сов. см.* **доку́ривать.**

долби́ть *несов.* **1.** (*вн.; пробива́ть отве́рстие*) gouge (*smth.*), hóllow out (*smth.*); **2.** (*вн.; ударя́ть*) thump (*smth.*); *перен.* hа́mmer (*smth.*); **3.** (*вн., дт.*) *разг.* (*повторя́ть*) tell* (*smb., smth.*) agа́in and agа́in, hа́mmer it ínto *smb.*; ~ одно́ и то́ же keep* repéating the same thing.

долг *м.* **1.** *тк. ед.* (*обя́занность*) dúty; **2.** (*взя́тое взаймы́*) debt; наде́лать ~ов incúr debts; обременённый ~а́ми dept-lа́den; héavily in debt; ◇ дава́ть в ~ lend*; быть в ~у́ пе́ред ке́м-л. be* indébted to *smb.*; быть в ~у́ у кого́-л. be* in *smb.'s* debt; влезть в ~и́ get*/run* into debt; не оста́ться в ~у́ пе́ред ке́м-л. give* as good as one gets; по ~у слу́жбы officially, in *one's* official capа́city; отда́ть после́дний ~ кому́-л. pay* the last hónours to *smb.*

дол|гий long; по́сле ~ой разлу́ки áfter béing apа́rt for a long time; ◇ откла́дывать что́-л. в ~ я́щик keep*

pútting *smth.* off, procrástinate óver *smth.*, shelve *smth.*

долговечн|ость ж. 1. longévity; 2. (*прочность*) durabílity. **~ый** 1. long-líved; 2. (*прочный*) lásting, dúrable.

долговрéменный 1. prolónged; 2. *воен.* (*о сооружениях*) pérmanent.

долговязый *разг.* lánky, léggy; gángling *амер.*

долгождáнный long-awáited, long-expécted.

долгоигрáющ|ий: **~ая** пластинка ˈlong-pláying récord, lóng-pláyer.

долголет|ие *с.* longévity. **~ний** long; of mány years *после сущ.*, of long stánding *после сущ.*

долгонóсик *м. зоол.* wéevil.

долгосрóчный long-térm; **~** кредит long-térm crédit; **~** óтпуск long leave.

долготá ж. 1. (*продолжительность*) length; 2. *геогр.* lóngitude.

долезáть, долéзть (до *рд.*) climb up (to), reach (*smth.*).

долéзть *сов. см.* долезáть.

долетáть, долетéть 1. (*о камне, снаряде и т. п.*) reach its mark; (*о самолёте тж.*) reach its destinátion, compléte its flight; (до *рд.*) reach (*smth.*) fly* as far as (*smth.*); не долетéть до *чего-л.* fail to reach *smth.*; (*о камне, снаряде и т. п.*) fall* short of *smth.*; 2. (*доноситься — о звуках и т. п.*) reach.

долетéть *сов. см.* долетáть.

долечить *сов.* (*вн.*) finish tréating (*smb.*). **~ся** *сов.* finish one's tréatment; он вышел из больницы не долечившись he came out of hóspital withóut finishing his tréatment.

долж|ен *в знач. сказ.* 1. (+ *инф.*; *обязан*) must (+ *inf*), ought (+ to *inf*), have (+ to *inf*); ты **~** кончить эту рабóту you must finish this work; так **~**бó было быть it had to be, it was to be; этого не **~**но быть that ought not to be, that's wrong; он не **~** был говорить, делать этого he should not have said, done it; he ought not to have said, done it; 2. (+ *инф.*; *для выражения возможности, вероятности*) should (+ *inf*), ought (+ to *inf*); он **~** скóро вернуться he should be back soon; это **~**но емý понравиться that ought to please him; это не **~**но служить препятствием it shóuldn't be an impédiment; 3. (*дт.*; *задолжал*) owe (*smb.*), owes (*smb.*); он **~** мне 20 рублéй he owes me twénty róubles; я **~** емý him...; ◇ **~**но быть (*вероятно*) próbably, I dare say; ought to; should (+ *inf*), must (+ *inf*); вы, **~**но быть, встречáли егó you must have met him; он, **~**но быть, дóма he's próbably at home, he ought to be at home, he should/must be at home.

должник *м.* débtor.

должностн|óй: **~óе** лицó official, fúnctionary; **~óе** преступлéние breach of trust.

дóлжность ж. post, posítion; занимáть **~** hold* a post; он занимáет отвéтственную **~** he occupies a major post.

дóлжн|ый *прил.* 1. due, próper; **~ым** óбразом próperly, dúly; относиться к *чему-л.* с **~ым** внимáнием give* due atténtion to *smth.*; 2. *в знач. сущ. с.* due.

доливáть, долить (*вн.*, *рд.*) top up (*smth.*), fill up (*smth.*); долить молокá в стакáн fill up a glass with milk; долить чáйник fill up a kéttle.

долина ж. válley.

долить *сов. см.* доливáть.

дóллар *м.* dóllar.

доложить I, II *сов. см.* доклáдывать I, II.

долóй *разг.* down with; с глаз моих **~**! out of my sight!; **~** войнý! down with war!

долотó *с.* chísel.

дóлька ж. (*чеснока*) clove; (*апельсина*) ségment, quárter.

дóльше (*сравнит. ст. прил.* дóлгий *и нареч.* дóлго) lónger.

дóл|я ж. 1. (*часть*) share, part, quóta; делить *что-л.* на рáвные **~и** divide *smth.* into équal parts; книга в четвёртую **~ю** листá quárto; 4to; вносить свою **~ю** contríbute *one's* quóta/share; в этом есть **~** прáвды there's grain of truth in it; в егó словáх нé было и **~и** истины there was not a párticle of truth in what he said; 2. (*судьба*) fate, lot; выпасть *кому-л.* на **~ю** fall* to *smb.'s* lot; ◇ войти в **~ю** с *кем-л.* go* shares with *smb.*

дом *м.* 1. (*здание*) búilding; house; жилóй **~** (dwélling-)house; дойти до **~а** reach the búilding; 2. (*домáшний очáг*) home; в роднóм **~е** in *one's* own home; выйти из **~у** leave* the house, go* out; дойти до **~у** get*/reach home; 3. (*семья*) house, home; мы знакóмы **~ами** our fámilies are acquáinted; 4. (*хозяйство однóй семьи*) house, hóusehold; онá ведёт весь **~** she runs the house; 5. (*учреждéние*): **~** культýры cúltural céntre, House of Cúlture; **~** óтдыха guésthouse, rest home; **~** твóрчества писáтелей, худóжников *и т. п.* guésthouse for writers, ártists *etc.*; **~** ребёнка ínfant's home; ◇ на **~ý** at *one's* own house; пóмощь на **~ý** óut-relief, home médical atténdance; урóки на **~ý** prívate léssons; брать рабóту нá **~** take* work home.

дóма at home; **~** ли он? is he in?, is he at home?; егó нет **~** he's not at home; ◇ быть как **~** make* onesélf at home; у негó не все **~** he's not quite all there.

домáшн|ие *мн.* (*семья*) *one's* péople. **~ий** 1. home; **~ий** áдрес home addréss; **~ий** телефóн home (télephone) númber; 2. (*об одежде, обуви*) house *attr.*; **~ий** костюм house clothes *pl*; 3. (*относящийся к хозяйству семьи*) doméstic; hóusehold *attr.*; **~ее** имýщество hóusehold goods *pl*; **~ие** делá doméstic affáirs; **~ие** расхóды hóusehold/hóusekeeping expénses; **~ее** хозяйство hóusekeeping; 4. (*приготовленный дома*) home; **~** обéд home-cóoked dínner; 5. (*семейный, частный*) home, prívate; по **~им** обстоятельствам for doméstic réasons; 6. (*прирученный, не дикий*) doméstic; **~яя** птица *собир.* póultry; ◇ **~ий** арéст house arrést; *воен.* arrést in quárters.

дóмен|ный: **~ная** печь blást-fúrnace. **~щик** *м.* blást-fúrnace wórker/óperative.

доминиóн *м.* domínion.

доминир|овать *несов.* 1. (*преобладáть*) predóminate, preváil, be* úppermost; 2. (*над тв.*; *возвышаться*) commánd (*smth.*), dóminate (*smth.*). **~ующий** dóminant, prévalent; **~ующее** положéние léading posítion; игрáть **~ующую** роль play a léading part, be* an impórtant fáctor.

доминó I *с. нескл.* (*костюм*) dómino.

доминó II *с. нескл.* (*игрá*) dóminoes *pl*.

домкрáт *м. тех.* (lífting) jack; поднимáть *что-л.* **~ом** jack *smth.* up.

дóмна ж. *тех.* blást-furnace.

домовит|ый thrífty, cáreful; **~ая** хозяйка good hóusewife*.

домовладéл|ец *м.*, **~ица** ж. hóuseholder, propríetor.

домовóдств|о *с.* hóusekeeping; hóusecraft; курс **~а** hóusecraft/doméstic science course.

домовóй *м. фольк.* hóbgoblin, góblin.

домóв|ый: **~ая** книга house-régister.

домогá|тельство *с.* solicitátions *pl*, importúnity. **~ться** *несов.* (*рд.*) solícit (*smth.*), raise an óutcry (for); **~ться** *чего-л.* у *кого-л.* press/péster/impórtune *smb.* for *smth.*

домóй home; (*в сторону дома тж.*) hómewards; емý порá **~** it's time for him to go home.

доморóщенный 1. hóme-bréd; 2. *ирон.* ámateur *attr.*

домосéд *м.*, **~ка** ж. stáy-at-hóme.

домостроéние *с.* hóuse-búilding.

домостроитель|ный (hóuse-)búilding *attr.* **~ство** *с.* house-búilding, hóusing constrúction.

домострóй *м. ист.* doméstic týranny.

домотка́ный hómespun.

домоуправле́ние *с.* house mánagement; (*помещение*) hóuse-management óffice.

домохозя́|ин *м.* hóuseholder, lándlord. ~йка *ж.* 1. (*домовладелица*) hóuseholder, lándlady; 2. (*ведущая хозяйство*) hóusewife*.

домоча́дцы *мн.* hóusehold *sg.*

до́мра *ж. муз.* dómra (*Russian mandoline-type instrument*).

домрабо́тница *ж.* dáily help.

домча́ть *сов.* (*вн.* куда́-л.) *разг.* take* (*smb. sómewhere*) in no time. ~ся *сов.* (куда́-л.) *разг.* get*/be* (*sómewhere*) in no time.

домыва́ть, домы́ть (*вн.*) fínish wáshing (*smth.*).

до́мысел *м.* conjécture, invéntion.

домы́ть *сов. см.* домыва́ть.

донага́ stark náked.

дона́шивать, доноси́ть (*вн.*) 1. (*одежду*) wear* (*smth.*) out; 2. (*ребёнка*) give* nórmal birth (to). ~ся, доноси́ться be* worn out.

Донба́сс *м.* (Доне́цкий у́гольный бассе́йн) Donéts cóal-field(s).

доне́льзя *разг.* útterly, as can be; он ~ уста́л he was tíred as could be.

донесе́ние *с.* repórt; (*письменное*) dispátch.

донести́ I, II *сов. см.* доноси́ть I, II.

донести́сь *сов. см.* доноси́ться II.

до́низу to the bóttom; све́рху ~ from top to bóttom.

донима́ть, доня́ть (*вн.*) *разг.* péster (*smb.*), wear* (*smb.*) out, annóy (*smb.*).

донкихо́тство *с.* quíxotry.

до́нор *м.* dónor.

доно́с *м.* denunciátion, repórt to the authórities.

доноси́ть I, донести́ (*вн.*; *приносить*) bring* (*smth.*), cárry (*smth.*); донести́ бага́ж до ваго́на take* the lúggage as far as the cárriage.

доноси́ть II, донести́ 1. (*о пр.*; *сообщать*) repórt (*smth.*); 2. (*на вн.*; *делать донос*) infórm (agáinst), denóunce (*smb.*).

доноси́ть III *сов. см.* дона́шивать.

доноси́ться I *сов. см.* дона́шиваться.

доноси́ться II, донести́сь (*о звуке и т. п.*) be* heard; (*до рд.*) reach (*smb., smth.*).

доно́сч|ик *м.*, ~ица *ж.* infórmer.

доны́не to this day.

доня́ть *сов. см.* донима́ть.

допека́ть, допе́чь (*вн.*) 1. bake (*smth.*) to a turn; 2. *разг. см.* донима́ть. ~ся, допе́чься be* well báked, be* báked to a turn.

допе́ть *сов.* (*вн.*) fínish (sínging) (*smth.*), sing* the rest (of).

допеча́тать *сов. см.* допеча́тывать.

допеча́тывать, допеча́тать (*вн.*) 1. (*докончить печатание*) fínish prínting (*smth.*), print the rest (of); (*на машинке*) fínish týping (*smth.*), type the rest (of); вы должны́ бы́ли допеча́тать де́сять страни́ц you should have typed the remáining ten páges; 2. (*дополнительно*) print addítional cópies (of).

допе́чь(ся) *сов. см.* допека́ть(ся).

допива́ть, допи́ть (*вн.*) drink* (*smth.*) up, fínish (*smth.*) up. ~ся, допи́ться (*до рд.*) *разг.* drink* onesélf ínto a state (of), get* *smth.* from drínking.

дописа́ть *сов. см.* допи́сывать.

допи́сыв|ать, дописа́ть (*вн.*) 1. fínish wríting (*smth.*); он ~ал письмо́, статью́ he was fínishing a létter, an árticle; он дописа́л письмо́, статью́ he (has, had) fínished a létter, an árticle; 2. (*писать дополнительно*) add (*smth.*); дописа́ть не́сколько строк к письму́ add a few lines to a létter.

допи́ть(ся) *сов. см.* допива́ть(ся).

допла́т|а *ж.* addítional charge; (*за билет*) excéss fare; (*за письмо*) excéss póstage. ~и́ть *сов. см.* допла́чивать. ~ной: ~но́е письмо́ unstámped létter.

допла́чивать, доплати́ть (*вносить остающуюся часть платы*) pay* the rest/remáinder; (*уплачивать всё до конца*) pay* in full; (*вносить дополнительную плату*) pay* the éxtra/excéss; доплати́ть два рубля́ pay* the remáining two róubles.

доплыва́ть, доплы́ть make* the dístance; get* there, make* it *разг.*; (*о пловце*) swim* so far; (*до рд.*) reach (*smth.*); (*о пловце*) swim* to *smth.*, as far as *smth.*).

доплы́ть *сов. см.* доплыва́ть.

допо́длинн|о *разг.* for cértain; мне э́то ~ изве́стно I know it for cértain. ~ый *разг.* authéntic, real.

допо́лзать, доползти́ crawl so far, creep* so far; get* there *разг.*; (*до рд.*) crawl (to, as far as), creep* (to, as far as).

доползти́ *сов. см.* допо́лзать.

дополне́ние *с.* 1. addítion; (*приложение*) súpplement; 2. *грам.* óbject; ко́свенное ~ indiréct óbject; прямо́е ~ diréct óbject; ◇ ~ к чему́-л. in addítion to *smth.*

дополни́тельн|о in addítion; ~ый 1. addítional; (*дополняющий*) supplementáry; ~ый о́тпуск éxtra leave, exténsion of leave; ~ое разъясне́ние fúrther explanátions *pl*; ~ый у́гол *мат.* (*до 90°*) cómplement; (*до 180°*) súpplement; ~ые цвета́ *физ.* complementáry cólours; 2. *грам.*: ~ое прида́точное предложе́ние óbject clause.

дополни́ть *сов. см.* дополня́ть.

дополня́ть, допо́лнить (*вн.*) súpplement (*smth.*); ~ слова́рь expánd a díctionary; ◇ ~ друг дру́га be* the cómplement of one anóther.

дополуча́ть, дополучи́ть (*вн.*) recéive (*smth.*), get* (*smth.*); дополучи́ть недостаю́щую су́мму recéive the remáinder.

дополучи́ть *сов. см.* дополуча́ть.

допото́пный antedilúvian; (*старомодный тж.*) ántiquated.

допра́шивать, допроси́ть (*вн.*) intérrogate (*smth.*), quéstion (*smth.*), exámine (*smth.*); ~ пле́нного, свиде́теля intérrogate/quéstion a prísoner, a wítness.

допризы́вн|ик *м.* pre-conscríption tráinee. ~ый pre--conscríption *attr.*

допро́с *м.* interrogátion, examinátion; ~ свиде́теля interrogátion/examinátion of a wítness.

допроси́ть *сов. см.* допра́шивать.

допроси́ться (*рд.*; *рд. + инф.*) *разг.* persuáde/get* (*smth.*) out of *smb.*; persuáde (*smb. + to inf*), get* (*smb. + to inf*); мы е́ле допроси́лись обе́да we had to ask a long time befóre we got a meal; его́ не допро́сишься дверь закры́ть no amóunt of ásking will indúce him to shut the door.

до́пуск *м.* 1. (*право входа*) admíssion, admíttance; áccess; 2. *тех.* tólerance.

допуск|а́ть, допусти́ть 1. (*вн.* до *рд.*; *вн.* к *дт.*) admít (*smb. to*); ~ кого́-л. к кому́-л. admít *smb.* to *smb.'s* présence; ~ кого́-л. до экза́менов admít *smb.* to the examinátions; ~ кого́-л. к ко́нкурсу allów *smb.* to énter a competítion; не ~ (до) keep* (from); 2. (*вн.*; *позволять*) allów (*smth.*), permít (*smth.*); (*терпеть*) tólerate (*smth.*); 3. (*вн.*; *предполагать*) assúme (*smth.*); ~а́ю, что... I can well believe that...; допу́стим, что... let us assúme that...; не ~ мы́сли о чём-л. refúse to admít the possibílity of *smth.*; ◇ ~ оши́бку make* a mistáke, go* wrong; здесь была́ допу́щена оши́бка a mistáke has crept in here.

допусти́мый admíssible, permíssible.

допусти́ть *сов. см.* допуска́ть.

допуще́ние *с.* assúmption.

допыта́ться *сов. разг.* find* out.

допы́тываться *несов. разг.* try to find*/worm out.

допьяна́ *разг.*: напи́ться ~ drink* onesélf stúpid; напои́ть кого́-л. ~ make* *smb.* rólling drunk.

дораба́тывать, дорабо́тать (вн.) finish (smth.), put* the finishing touches (to), polish up (smth.).

дорабо́тать сов. см. дораба́тывать.

дораста́ть, дорасти́ 1. grow* as high as; 2. (достигать какого-л. возраста) reach (the age of); перен. attain; не дорасти до чего-л. fail to come up to smth.

дорасти́ сов. см. дораста́ть.

дорва́ться сов. (до рд.) разг. get* (to), fall* greedily (upon).

дореволюцио́нный pre-revolutionary.

дорисова́ть сов. см. дорисо́вывать.

дорисо́вывать, дорисова́ть (вн.) finish (drawing) (smth.); complete (smth.); пусть ва́ше воображе́ние дорису́ет остально́е I leave the rest to your imagination.

дори́ческий иск. Doric.

доро́г|а ж. 1. road; way; больша́я, шоссе́йная ~ main/high road, highway; ~ шла ле́сом the road passed through a forest, the road was wooded; при ~е by the roadside; 2. (место прохода или проезда) way, path; стул стоя́л на са́мой ~е the chair was just in the way; 3. (путешествие) journey; в ~е on the way; на ~у for the journey; отдохну́ть с ~и have* a rest after one's journey; уста́ть с ~и be* tired from the journey, be* travel-weary; ◇ желе́зная ~ см. желе́зный; идти́ свое́й ~ой go* one's own way; по ~е 1) on the way; 2): нам с ва́ми по ~е we are going the same way; нам с ва́ми не по ~е we are going different ways; перен. тж. your way is not our way; быть на хоро́шей ~е have* made a good start; станови́ться кому́-л. поперёк ~и stand* in smb.'s path; туда́ ему́ и ~! it serves him right!; дать кому́-л. ~у make* way for smb.; перен. give* smb. a free hand.

до́рого dear; перен. тж. dearly; ~ заплати́ть pay* dear, pay* a lot; э́то ему́ ~ обойдётся it will cost him dear; ◇ он ~ бы дал, заплати́л would give a lot, he would pay a lot; ~ отда́ть свою́ жизнь sell* one's life dearly.

дороговизна́ ж. high prices pl; (чего-л.) high price (of); ~ жи́зни high cost of living.

дорого́й on the way.

дорог|о́й прил. 1. dear, expensive; (ценный) costly; ~и́е кни́ги expensive books; ~и́е ка́мни costly jewels; по ~ цене́ at a high price; 2. (который дорожат) precious; ему́ до́рог ваш сове́т he values your advice; 3. (милый) dear; ~ друг! (my) dear friend!; 4. в знач. сущ. м. dear, darling.

дорогосто́ящий expensive.

доро́дный burly, beefy; (полный) portly, corpulent.

дорож|а́ть, вздорожа́ть rise* (in price); жизнь ~а́ет the cost of living is going up.

доро́же сравнит. ст. прил. дорого́й и нареч. до́рого.

дорожи́ть несов. (тв.) 1. (ценить) value (smb., smth.), prize (smb., smth.); 2. (беречь) cherish (smb., smth.), treasure (smb., smth.); take* care (of); ~ ка́ждой мину́той treasure every minute; не ~ чем-л. not care for smth., care nothing for smth.; не ~ жи́знью place no value on one's life.

доро́жка ж. 1. path; (в саду тж.) walk; 2. спорт. track; 3. (половик) strip of carpet; (скатерть) runner; ◇ во́дная ~ lane; лётная ~ runway.

доро́жный 1. (относящийся к дороге) road attr.; of the road после сущ.; ~ знак road-sign; 2. (для путеше́ствия) travelling attr.; ~ костю́м travelling clothes pl.

ДОСА́АФ м. (Доброво́льное о́бщество соде́йствия а́рмии, авиа́ции и фло́ту) ист. Voluntary Association/ Society for Assisting Army, Air Force and Navy.

доса́д|а ж. vexation, annoyance; кака́я ~! how annoying!, what a nuisance!; с ~ы out of annoyance, from annoyance. ~ить сов. см. досажда́ть. ~но в знач. сказ. безл. it is regrettable; как ~но! what a nuisance!, what a bore!; мне ~но, что... I deeply regret (that)... ~ный regrettable; (раздражающий) annoying; ~ный слу́чай

regrettable incident; ~ная опеча́тка regrettable mistake; ~ное чу́вство annoying feeling.

доса́довать несов. (на кого́-л.) be* annoyed/vexed (with smb.); (на что́-л.) be* annoyed/vexed (about smth.), be* irritated (by smth.).

досажда́ть, досади́ть (дт.) annoy (smb.), vex (smb.).

досиде́ть сов. см. доси́живать.

доси́живать, досиде́ть (до рд.) stay (till); ~ до конца́ stay till the end; sit* it out разг.; не ~ (до конца́) leave* before the end.

доск|а́ ж. board; (строи́тельная тж.) plank; ~ объявле́ний notice-board, bulletin-board; ме́дная ~ brass plate; мра́морная ~ marble plaque; откидна́я ~ flap; ◇ ~ почёта roll of honour; от ~и́ до ~и́ from cover to cover; ста́вить на одну́ до́ску с кем-л. put* on a level with smb.

досказа́ть сов. (вн.) tell* (smth.) as far as, get* (to); (око́нчить) finish (smth.); тепе́рь он доска́жет свою́ исто́рию now he will tell the rest of his story; ~ ска́зку до середи́ны get* to the middle of the tale.

доскона́льн|о thoroughly; мне всё ~ изве́стно I know everything about it. ~ый thorough.

досла́ть сов. см. досыла́ть.

досло́вн|о word for word; (о перево́де тж.) literally. ~ый literal, verbatim; ~ый перево́д literal translation; ~ая переда́ча verbatim report.

дослужи́ться сов. (до рд.) rise* to the rank (of).

дослу́ш|ать сов. (вн.) listen (to smth.) to the end; я не ~ал докла́да I didn't stay to the end of the lecture; он не ~ал меня́ he didn't listen to the rest (of what I was saying).

досма́тривать, досмотре́ть (вн.) 1. тк. несов. (осма́тривать) examine (smth.); 2. (до конца́) stay to the end (of), sit* (smth.) out; (о кни́ге, журна́ле и т. п.) look through (smth.) to the end, look all the way through (smth.).

досмо́тр м. examination.

досмотре́ть сов. см. досма́тривать 2.

досмо́трщик м. (на тамо́жне) examiner, customs official.

досо́хнуть сов. dry up.

доспа́ть сов. см. досыпа́ть I.

доспе́хи мн. armour sg.

досро́чн|о ahead of schedule/time; ~ вы́полнить план fulfil the plan ahead of schedule. ~ый advance attr.; ahead of schedule после сущ.; ~ое выполне́ние пла́на completion of the plan/programme ahead of schedule/time.

достав|а́ть, доста́ть 1. (до рд.) reach (smth.), touch (smth.); он достаёт руко́й до потолка́ he can touch the ceiling with his hand; 2. (вн. из, с рд.; брать, извлека́ть что-л.) get* (smth. out of), take* (smth. out of), produce (smth. from); (снима́ть) get* (smth. from); 3. (вн., рд.; приобрета́ть, получа́ть) get* (smth.), obtain (smth.). ~а́ться, доста́ться (дт.) 1. (поступа́ть в чью́-л. со́бственность) fall* to smb.'s share; ему́ доста́лась в насле́дство ты́сяча рубле́й he came into a thousand roubles; 2. безл. разг. (о наказа́нии): ему́ доста́лось he caught it; и доста́лось же ему́! what a hiding/beating he got!

доста́в|ить сов. см. доставля́ть. ~ка ж. delivery; (на большо́е расстоя́ние) carriage; ~ка на́ дом delivery; с ~кой на́ дом (о цене́) including delivery; carriage paid.

доставля́ть, доста́вить (вн.) 1. (привози́ть, приноси́ть) deliver (smb., smth.); ~ что-л. на́ дом deliver smth.; ~ кого́-л. домо́й на маши́не take* smb. home in a car; ~ све́дения furnish information; 2. (причиня́ть) give* (smth.), cause (smth.); ~ кому́-л. беспоко́йство give*/cause smb. trouble; 3. (предоставля́ть) give* (smth.), afford (smth.); ~ кому́-л. удово́льствие afford/give* smb. the pleasure.

достат|ок *м.* 1. prospérity; жить в ~ке be* in éasy círcumstances, be* cómfortably off; 2. *разг.* (*достаточное количество чего-л.*) sufficiency; 3. *мн. разг.* (*доходы*) íncome sg.

достаточн|о 1. *нареч.* enóugh *после прил.*; sufficiently; (*порядочно*) ráther, fáirly; он ~ сильный he is ráther strong; 2. *в знач. сказ. безл.* it's enóugh; этого (будет) ~ that will do, that will be enóugh; этого было ~, чтобы... no more was required to..., that sufficed to...; у нас всего ~ we have enóugh of éverything; ~ сказáть suffice it to say. **~ый** sufficient; быть ~ым suffice, be* enóugh.

достать(ся) *сов. см.* доставáть(ся).

достиг|áть, достигнуть, достичь (*рд.*) 1. reach (*smth.*); никто не ~áл вершины (этой горы) nóbody has éver reached the top (of that móuntain); достигнуть совершеннолétия attáin *one's* majórity, come* of age; достигнуть стáрости reach old age; достигнуть высшего предéла reach its clímax; достигнуть соглашéния reach an understánding; 2. (*успеха, цели и т. п.*) achíeve (*smth.*), attáin (*smth.*); не достигнуть *чего-л.* fail to achíeve *smth.*; этим вы ничегó не достигнете you won't get ánywhere by dóing that, that won't get you ánywhere.

достиж|éние *с.* 1. (*действие*): для ~éния своéй цéли to achíeve *one's* óbject; по ~éнии *чего-л.* on réaching *smth.*; 2. (*успех*) achíevement; ~éния наýки и тéхники scientífic and téchnical achíevement(s). **~имый** attáinable; within the bounds of possibílity *после сущ.*

достичь *сов. см.* достигáть.

достовéрн|о for cértain, for sure; мне (это) ~ извéстно I know (it) for a fact. **~ость** *ж.* authentícity, reliabílity. **~ый** authéntic, relíable; trústworthy; из ~ых истóчников from relíable sóurces; нам сообщáют из ~ых истóчников we are crédibly infórmed, we have it on the best authórity.

достоинств|о *с.* 1. *тк. ед.* dígnity; ниже своегó ~а benéath *one's* dígnity; 2. (*хорошее качество*) mérit; 3. (*стоимость, ценность*) válue, worth; облигáция ~ом в 25 рублéй 25-rouble bond; ◇ оценить *кого-л., что-л.* по ~у appréciate *smb., smth.*

достойн|о in a fítting mánner, (be)fíttingly; ~ отмéтить *что-л.* célebrate *smth.* in a fítting mánner. **~ый** 1. (*рд.; заслуживающий, стоящий*) wórthy (of), desérving (*smth.*); быть ~ым *чего-л.* be* wórthy of *smth.*; desérve *smth.*, mérit *smth.*; ~ый внимáния nóteworthy; ~ый похвалы práiseworthy; 2. (*заслуженный*) mérited, wéll-desérved; ~ая награда wéll-desérved rewárd; 3. (*почтенный*) wórthy.

достопримечáтельн|ость *ж.* one of the sights; осмáтривать ~ости гóрода see* the sights of the town. **~ый** *уст.* nóteworthy, remárkable; ~ый слýчай remárkable íncident; ~ый факт nóteworthy fact.

достоя́ни|е *с. тк. ед.* próperty; *перен. тж.* bírthright; обществéнное ~ públic próperty; сдéлать *что-л.* ~ем *кого-л.* make* *smth.* accéssible to *smb.*

дострáивать, дострóить (*вн.*) compléte (*smth.*), fínish búilding (*smth.*).

дострóить *сов. см.* дострáивать.

достýп *м.* áccess; открыть *кому-л.* ~ к *чему-л.* make* *smth.* accéssible to *smb.*; получить ~ (на, в *вн.*) gain áccess (to *smth.*).

достýпн|ость *ж.* 1. accessibílity; 2. (*простота*) simplícity, intelligibílity; 3. (*внимательность к другим*) approachabílity, affabílity. **~ый** 1. (*по которому можно пройти*) negótiable; (*к которому можно подойти*) accéssible, get-át-able; тропá, ~ая тóлько для пешехóдов fóotpath ónly; 2. (*подходящий для всех*) aváilable; ~ые цéны réasonable/pópular príces; 3. (*соответствующий силам, возможностям*) within the capácity (of), within reach (of); 4. (*лёгкий для понимания*) símple, intélligible; изложить свою мысль в ~ой фóрме find* a símple form of expréssion for *one's* idéa; 5. (*о человеке*) appróachable, áffable.

достýч|áться *сов.* knock till *one* is heard; ~ у двéри knock till the door is ópened; ~ýсь ли я? will they hear my knócking?; не ~ knock in vain.

досý|г *м.* 1. léisure; часы ~га léisure (hours); на ~ге at léisure; 2. *в знач. сказ. (дт.) разг. one* has the time. **~жий** *разг.* ídle.

дóсуха thóroughly dry; ~ вытереть рýки dry *one's* hands thóroughly; ~ вытереться ~ wipe *oneself* dry, dry *oneself* thóroughly.

досчитáть *сов.* fínish cóunting; (*до рд.*) count (to).

досылáть, дослáть (*вн.*) send* the remáining (*smth.*); (*дополнительно*) send* (*smth.*) addítionally; дослáть недостáющий том словаря send* the remáining vólume of the díctionary; ~ 10 рублéй send* the ten róubles due.

досыпáть *сов. см.* досыпáть II.

досыпáть I, доспáть *разг.* sleep*.

досыпáть II, досыпать (*вн., рд.*) (*добавлять*) add (*smth.*) to; (*доверху*) fill (*smth.*) up.

дóсыта to *one's* heart's contént; есть, наéсться ~ eat* *one's* fill; ~ наговориться talk to *one's* heart's contént.

досьé *с. нескл.* dóssier, file.

досюда *разг.* up to here.

досягáем|ость *ж.* reach; *воен.* range; в предéлах ~ости within reach; вне предéлов, за предéлами ~ости beyónd reach, out of reach; *воен.* out of range.

дотáция *ж.* súbsidy.

дотáщ|ить *сов.* (*вн.*) drag (*smth.*); он éле ~ил мешóк he bárely mánaged to drag the sack there. **~иться** *сов. разг.* drag *oneself*.

дотлá: сгорéть ~ be* burned to the ground; сжечь *что-л.* ~ redúce *smth.* to áshes.

дотóшный *разг.* keen, metículous; (*пытливый*) inquísitive; ~ человéк a stíckler for détail; какóй вы ~! what a stíckler you are!

дотрáгиваться, дотрóнуться (*до рд.*) touch (*smb., smth.*).

дотрóнуться *сов. см.* дотрáгиваться.

дотýда *разг.* up to there.

дотя́гивать, дотянуть 1. (*вн. до рд.; таща, доставлять*) drag (*smth.* to, as far as); 2. (*вн.*) *разг.* (*доставлять машину, самолёт и т. п.*) mánage to bring (*smth.*); он дотянýл повреждённую машину до аэродрóма he mánaged to fly the dámaged áircraft to the áerodrome; 3. *разг.* (*с трудом доезжать и т. п.*) make*; мы не дотянýли до Москвы we dídn't make Móscow; 4. (*вн. до рд.; протягивать*) stretch (*smth.* to); они дотянýли верёвку до столбá they stretched the rope to the post; 5. *разг.* (*до какого-л. времени*) last out, hold* out; дотянýть до весны live to see the spring; дотянýть до утрá last/hold* out till mórning, last out the night; 6. (*вн. до рд.*) *разг.* (*медлить с чем-л.*) spin* (*smth.*) out (till). **~ся**, дотянýться (*до рд.*) 1. (*доставать*) reach (*smth.*); *несов. тж.* try to reach (*smth.*); 2. *разг.* (*простираться*) stretch (to, as far as *smth.*); 3. *разг.* (*доходить*) make* *one's* way (to), get* as far as (*smth.*).

дотянýть(ся) *сов. см.* дотя́гивать(ся).

доýчивать, доучить 1. (*кого-л.*) round off *smb.'s* tráining/educátion; 2. (*что-л.*) learn (*smth.*); (*до конца*) fínish léarning (*smth.*); вы доучили стихотворéние? have you fínished léarning the póem? **~ся**, доучиться 1. (*кончать учиться*) compléte *one's* stúdies; 2. (*до рд.; до какого-л. срока*) contínue *one's* stúdies (till); доучиться до седьмóго клáсса go* through six clásses, leave* at the end of *one's* sixth year.

доучить(ся) *сов. см.* доýчивать(ся).

дохá *ж.* fúr-cóat.

дóхлый 1. (*о животном*) dead; 2. *разг.* (*слабый, больной — о человеке*) púny, síckly, áiling.

до́хнуть *несов.* die; ~ с го́лоду die of húnger.

дохну́ть *сов.* breathe; ◇ ~ не́когда there ísn't time to breathe; боя́ться ~ be* afráid to breathe.

дохо́д *м.* íncome; (*государственный тж.*) révenue; чи́стый ~ net prófit.

дохо́д|и́ть, дойти́ 1. (*до рд.*) reach (*smb., smth.*), go*/get* as far as (*smth.*); (*о письмах и т. п.*) arríve (at); они́ дошли́ до ста́нции за 15 мину́т they reached the státion in fiftéen mínutes; не ~я́ this side of, just before you get to; 2. (*до рд.; достига́ть — о звуках, известиях и т. п.*) reach (*smb., smth.*); 3. (*до рд.*) *разг.* (*становиться понятным*) come* acróss (to); э́то до меня́ не дохо́дит; не дошло́ I don't see the point, I didn't get it; му́зыка не дохо́дит до слу́шателей the músic dóesn't come acróss to the áudience; 4. (*до рд.; о преданиях и т. п.*) come* down (to); 5. (*до рд.; достига́ть какого-л. предела*) reach (*smth.*), come* up (to); ~ до коле́н reach to the knee; 6. (*до рд.*) *разг.* (*доду́мываться*) reach (*smth.*), arríve (at); до всего́ сам дошёл it is all his own achíevement; дойти́ до э́того свои́м умо́м think* it out *oneself*, reach this conclúsion unáided; 7. (*до рд.; приходить в какое-л. состояние, положение*) be* redúced (to); ~ до отча́яния be* redúced to despáir; ~ до дра́ки come* to blows; до чего́ он дошёл! look what he's come to!, how low he has fállen!; 8. *безл.* ~ до... it came to...; дойти́ до того́, что... reach a point where...; 9. *разг.* (*ослабевать, обессилевать*) be* on *one's* last legs; ◇ ~ до абсу́рда run* into absúrdity; у меня́ не дохо́дят ру́ки до э́того I have no time for that.

дохо́дн|ость *ж.* prófit-making capácity, prófit-ableness; ~ предприя́тия the capácity of an énterprise to make a prófit. ~ый 1. crédit *attr.*; ~ая статья́ бюдже́та révenue ítem; 2. (*прибыльный*) prófit-yíelding, prófitable, páying, remúnerative; ~ая о́трасль хозя́йства prófitable branch of the ecónomy.

дохо́дчивый understándable, éasily understóod.

доце́нт *м.* (univérsity) réader; assístant proféssor *амер.*

доче́рний 1. dáughter's, fílial; 2. (*о предприятиях и т. п.*) branch *attr.*; 3. биол. dáughter *attr.*

до́чиста clean; вы́мыть что-л. ~ clean *smth.* pérfectly, leave* *smth.* spéckless; ~ огра́бить кого-л. clean *smb.* out, rob *smb.* of éverything.

дочи́т|ывать, дочита́ть (*вн.*) read* (*smth.*) through; *несов. тж.* be* fínishing (*smth.*); (*вн. до рд.*) read* (*smth.* as far as); дочита́ть кни́гу, письмо́ fínish a book, a létter, come* to the end of a book, a létter; ~ до второ́й главы́ read* as far as the sécond chápter; не дочита́ть not fínish. ~ся, дочита́ться *разг.*: дочита́ться до головно́й бо́ли give* *oneself* a héadache from réading.

дочь *ж.* dáughter.

дошко́льн|ик *м.*, ~ица *ж.* child* únder school age. ~ый pre-schóol; де́ти ~ого во́зраста children únder school age; ~ые учрежде́ния pre-schóol institútions.

доща́тый board *attr.*, plank *attr.*; ~ мо́стик plank bridge.

дои́ярка *ж.* mílkmaid.

дра́га *ж.* *тех.* dredge.

драгоце́нн|ость *ж.* 1. jéwel; *мн.* jéwels; jéwelry *sg*; 2. (*то, что дорого*) précious thing/object; précious posséssion. ~ый précious (*тж. перен.*); ~ый ка́мень précious stone; (*гранёный*) gem, jéwel.

дразни́ть *несов.* (*вн.*) 1. tease (*smb., smth.*); (*животное тж.*) bait (*smth.*); 2. (*возбуждать*) whet (*smth.*); ~ чей-л. аппети́т whet *smb.'s* áppetite.

дра́ить *несов.* (*вн.*) *мор.* scrub (*smth.*).

дра́ка *ж.* fight, brawl.

драко́н *м.* dragon. ~овский Dracónian, Dracónic; ~овские зако́ны rígorous laws.

дра́м|а *ж.* dráma; *перен. тж.* trágedy; теа́тр ~ы théatre; семе́йная ~ doméstic trágedy.

драмат|и́зм *м.* 1. *лит.* dramátic efféct/ténsion; 2. (*напряжённость чего-л.*) dráma; ~ положе́ния the dráma of the situátion. ~и́ческий dramátic; ~и́ческое произведе́ние dramátic work; ~и́ческие же́сты dramátic gestures; ~и́ческий слу́чай dramátic íncident.

драмату́рг *м.* pláywright, drámatist. ~ия *ж.* 1. (*искусство*) dramátic art; 2. *собир.* (*совокупность драматических произведений*) plays *pl*; сове́тская ~ия Sóviet plays; ~ия Го́голя the plays of Gógol.

драмкружо́к *м.* (*драматический кружо́к*) dramátic círcle.

дра́нка *ж.* 1. *тк. ед. собир.* (*штукатурная*) laths *pl*; (*кровельная*) shíngles *pl*; 2. (*одна дощечка*) shingle.

дра́н|ый *разг.* rágged; с ~ыми локтя́ми óut-at--élbows; ходи́ть с ~ыми локтя́ми be* óut-at-élbows.

драп *м.* héavy wóollen cloth.

дра́пир|ова́ть *несов.* (*вн.*) drape (*smth.*). ~о́вка *ж.* dráperies *pl.*, hángings *pl.* ~о́вщик *м.* uphólsterer.

дра́пов|ый (made) of héavy wóollen cloth *после сущ.*; ~ое пальто́ héavy óvercoat.

дра́тва *ж.* *тк. ед.* wáx-end, waxed thread.

драть, вы́драть (*вн.*) *разг.* 1. *тк. несов.* (*рвать*) tear* (*smth.*); 2. *тк. несов.* (*отрывать, снимать*) strip (*smth.*); 3. (*сечь*) thrash (*smb.*), give* (*smth.*) a thráshing/whípping; ~ кого-л. за во́лосы pull *smb.'s* hair; ~ кого-л. за́ уши tweak *smb.'s* ears; ◇ ~ втри́дорога charge exórbitant príces, charge the earth; ~ гло́тку yell, bawl; от э́того моро́з по ко́же дерёт it makes *one's* flesh creep.

дра́ться, подра́ться 1. fight*; come* to blows, have* a fight; я с ним подра́лся we had a fight; ма́льчи́шки ка́ждый день деру́тся друг с дру́гом the boys fight every day; ~ на кула́чках have* a fist fight; 2. *тк. несов.* (*сражаться*) fight*; ~ на дуэ́ли fight* a dúel; 3. *тк. несов.* (*за вн.; бороться за что-л.*) fight* (for).

драч|ли́вый *разг.* pugnácious. ~у́н *м. разг.* fighter, pugnácious féllow; он большо́й ~у́н he loves fighting, he's álways réady for a fight.

дребезж|а́ть *несов.* jíngle, ráttle. ~а́щий: ~а́щий го́лос trémulous voice.

древеси́на *ж. тк. ед.* 1. wood; 2. *собир.* (*лесоматериалы*) tímber.

древе́сн|ый wood *attr.*; ~ая ма́сса wóod-pulp; ~ спирт wood spírit.

дре́вко *с.* shaft; (*знамени*) staff.

древнеангли́йский Old Énglish; ~ язы́к Old Énglish.

древнегре́ческий (áncient) Greek; (*об архитекту́ре*) Grécian; ~ язы́к áncient Greek.

древнееврейский Hébrew.

древнеру́сский Old Rússian.

дре́вние *мн.* the áncients.

дре́вн|ий 1. áncient; 2. (*очень старый*) áged, véry old; ~ стари́к áged man*. ~ость *ж.* 1. antíquity; (*вещь*) antique; 2. *мн.* antíquities.

древонасажде́ние *с.* plánting of trees.

дрези́на *ж. ж.-д.* trólley; (*railroad*) hánd-car *амер.*

дрейф *м. мор.* 1. drift; 2. (*действие*) drífting; 3.: лечь в ~ lie* to. ~ова́ть *несов.* drift. ~у́ющий drífting; ~у́ющая ста́нция drífting státion.

дрель *ж.* drill.

дрем|а́ть *несов.* doze; nod; *перен.* slúmber; ◇ не ~ be* on the alért, keep* *one's* wits abóut one. ~о́та *ж.* drówsiness, sómnolence. ~о́тный drówsy, sómnolent.

дремучий dense, thick.

дрен|а́ж *м.* 1. *мед., тех.* dráinage; 2. *мед.* (*трубка*) drain. ~и́ровать *несов. и сов.* (*вн.*) drain (*smth.*).

дрессиро́в|анный trained; (*для цирка*) perfórming. ~а́ть, вы́дрессировать (*вн.*) train (*smth.*). ~ка *ж.* tráining. ~щик *м.*, ~щица *ж.* ánimal-trainer.

дроб|и́ть, раздроби́ть (*вн.*) 1. (*размельчать*) crush (*smth.*), pound (*smth.*); 2. (*делить*) divíde (*smth.*) up, split* (*smth.*) up; ~ си́лы dismémber/scátter *one's* fórces.

~**и́ться**, раздроби́ться 1. (*размельчаться*) be* crushed/púlverized; (*раскалываться*) splínter; (*о волна́х*) break*; 2. (*делиться*) divíde up, split* up. ~**лёный** crushed.

дробн|ый 1. (*расчленённый*) séparate; 2. (*частый — о зву́ках, шага́х и т. п.*) rhýthmic; ~ стук дождя́ stéady pátter of rain; ~ цо́кот копы́т drúmming of hoofs; ме́лким ~ым ша́гом with short quick steps; 3. *мат.* fráctional; ~ое число́ fráctional númber.

дробь *ж.* 1. *мат.* fráction; проста́я ~ vúlgar fráction; пра́вильная (непра́вильная) ~ próper (impróper) fráction; 2. *собир. охот.* shot; кру́пная ~ búck-shot; ме́лкая ~ small shot, bird-shot; 3. (*частые преры́вистые зву́ки*) táp(ping); ча́стая ~ каблуко́в a drúmming of heels; бараба́нщики отбива́ли суро́вую, ме́рную ~ the drúmmers beat out a grim tattóo.

дрова́ *мн.* fírewood *sg*; берёзовые ~ birch logs.

дровосе́к *м. уст.* wóodcutter.

дровян|о́й wood *attr.*; ~ сара́й wóodshed; ~ склад wóod-store; ~о́е отопле́ние wood fíring.

дро́ги *мн.* dray cart *sg*; похоро́нные ~ hearse *sg*.

дро́гнуть I *несов.* (*мёрзнуть*) shíver; полчаса́ он дрог на моро́зе he shívered in the cold for half an hour.

дро́гн|уть II *сов.* 1. (*вздро́гнуть*) trémble, quíver; ни оди́н му́скул не ~ул на его́ лице́ not a múscle in his face moved; се́рдце у него́ ~уло his heart missed a beat; his heart gave a shúdder; 2. (*поколеба́ться*) wáver, flinch, fálter; не ~ néver flinch, stand* *one's* ground; неприя́тель ~ул the énemy wávered; ◇ рука́ не ~ет without a qualm.

дрожа́ние *с.* trémbling; (*вибра́ция*) vibrátion.

дрожа́|ть *несов.* 1. (*трясти́сь*) trémble, shake*, quíver; (*о го́лосе тж.*) break*; ~ от хо́лода shake*/shíver with cold; ~ ме́лкой дро́жью trémble all óver; be* in a trémor; ~ от возбужде́ния shake*/trémble with excítement; 2. (*боя́ться*) trémble, shúdder; (*перед тв.*) live in fear (of); ~ от стра́ха shake*/shúdder/trémble with fear; 3. (*за вн.*) obeper`áть) trémble (for); 4. (*над тв.*) watch ánxiously (óver), fuss (óver); ~ над ка́ждой копе́йкой grudge évery cópeck. ~**щий** trémbling; trémulous; ~**щим го́лосом** in a trémulous voice; ~**щими рука́ми** with sháking/trémbling hands.

дро́жжи *мн.* yeast *sg*; пивны́е ~ bréwer's yeast.

дро́жки *мн.* dróshky *sg*; бегов́ые ~ rácing súlky *sg*.

дрожь *ж.* trémbling; shívering; (*не́рвная*) trémor; с ~ю в го́лосе (with) a trémor in *one's* voice; его́ броса́ет в ~ при (одно́й) мы́сли об э́том he shúdders at the (mere) thought of it, it gives him the shúdders (mérely) to think of it.

дрозд *м.* thrush; певчий ~ sóng-thrush; чёрный ~ bláckbird; ◇ дать ~а́ кому́-л. *разг.* give* *smb.* a wígging.

дрок *м. бот.* genísta, broom.

дро́ссель *м. тех.* thróttle, choke; *эл.* chóking coil. ~**ный** thróttling; ~**ная засло́нка** bútterfly valve.

дрофа́ *ж. зоол.* great bústard.

друг I *м.* friend; ~ де́тства chíldhood friend, pláyfellow; ◇ ста́рый ~ лу́чше но́вых двух *посл.* an old friend is bétter than two new ones.

друг II: ~а each óther, one anóther; ~ без ~а without each óther; ~ за ~ом one áfter the óther; ~ про́тив ~а ópposite one anóther, vis-à-vis.

друг|о́й *прил.* 1. (*не э́тот*) óther, anóther; (*не тако́й*) dífferent; (*ещё оди́н*) anóther; кто́-то ~ sómeone else; никто́ ~ не... nóne óther than..., who but...; оди́н за ~и́м one áfter the óther; соверше́нно ~а́я те́ма a whólly dífferent súbject/tópic; быть ~и́м челове́ком be* a changed man*; 2. (*сле́дующий, второ́й*) next; на ~ день the next day, the day áfter; в ~ раз anóther time; на ~ год for another year; 3. *в знач. сущ. м.* anóther pérson, a different pérson; (*из двух*) the óther; 4. *в знач. сущ. с.* anóther thing; 5. *в знач. сущ. мн.* óther people; (*ос-*

та́льные) the rest, the óthers; ◇ ~и́ми слова́ми in óther words; смотре́ть ~и́ми глаза́ми на что́-л. look dífferently upón *smth.*, take* a dífferent view of *smth.*; ни тот ни ~ néither; и тот и ~ both; с ~ стороны́ on the óther hand; с одно́й стороны́..., с ~ стороны́ on the one hand..., on the óther hand.

дру́жб|а *ж.* fríendship; быть в ~е с кем-л. be* friends with *smb.*

дружелю́б|ие *с.* fríendliness, fríendly/ámicable spírit. ~**ный** fríendly, ámicable.

дру́жеск|и in a fríendly way, ámicably, ~**ий** fríendly, ámicable; ~**ий тон** ámicable/fríendly tone; ~**ое уча́стие** the sýmpathy of a friend; оказа́ть ~**ую услу́гу** do* a fríendly sérvice.

дру́жественн|ый fríendly, ámicable; ~**ые стра́ны** fríendly cóuntries.

дружи́на *ж.* 1. (*гру́ппа, отря́д*) squad, group; пожа́рная ~ vólunteer fíre-fíghting squad; наро́дная ~ vólunteer públic órder squad; 2. *ист.* bódyguard; fíghting men *pl.*

дружи́нник *м.* 1. vólunteer; наро́дные ~и públic órder vólunteers; 2. *ист.* bódyguard, fíghting man*, man* at arms.

дружи́ть *несов.* (с тв.) be* friends (with).

дру́жище *м. разг.* old chap.

дру́жн|о 1. (*в согла́сии*) ámicably, in a fríendly way/mánner; жить ~ live in hármony; live in cóncord, get* on well; 2. (*одновреме́нно*) in únison, (all) togéther; ~ принима́ться за де́ло set* to work all togéther; раз-два ~! altogéther — heave!. ~**ый** 1. (*свя́занный дру́жбой*) harmónious, fríendly; ~**ая семья́** united fámily; они́ о́чень ~**ы** they're great friends; ~**ый коллекти́в** harmónious group; 2. (*согласо́ванный*) concérted; (*с уча́стием всех*) géneral; ~**ый смех** géneral láughter; ~**ая рабо́та** (pérfect) téamwork; ~**ыми уси́лиями** by *one's* united/concérted éfforts; 3. (*бы́стро возника́ющий, протека́ющий*) súdden; ны́нче ожида́ется ~**ая весна́** spring is expécted to come with a rush this year; на поля́х появи́лись ~**ые всхо́ды** the fields were súddenly green with young shoots.

дружо́к *м.* pal; мой ~! (*обраще́ние*) my dear!

дры́гать *несов.* (тв.) *разг.* jerk (*smth.*); ~ нога́ми kick.

дря́бл|ость *ж.* flábbiness, flaccídity. ~**ый** flábby, fláccid.

дря́зги *мн. разг.* squábbles.

дрянн|о́й *разг.* wórthless; rótten; (*о материа́ле*) shóddy; ~ челове́к wórthless féllow; ~**а́я пого́да** rótten wéather.

дрянь *ж. разг.* 1. *собир.* trash, rúbbish; 2. (*о челове́ке*) skunk, a bad lot; 3. *в знач. сказ.*: де́ло ~ things are lóoking bad.

дряхле́ть, одряхле́ть becóme* sénile, grow* decrépit.

дряхл|ость *ж.* decrépitude, senílity. ~**ый** decrépit, sénile.

дуали́зм *м.* dúalism.

дуб *м.* 1. (*де́рево*) óak(-tree); 2. *тк. ед.* (*древеси́на*) oak; 3. *разг.* (*о челове́ке*) block of wood; square; ◇ дать ~а kick it.

дуба́сить, отдуба́сить *разг.* 1. (*вн.*) clóbber (*smb.*); ~ друг дру́га púmmel each óther; 2. *тк. несов.* (по дт.; в вн.) sílsón stúchать) knock víolently (at); ~ в дверь hámmer/thump on the door.

дуби́н|а *ж.* 1. cúdgel; 2. *разг.* (*о ту́пом челове́ке*) blóckhead. ~**ка** *ж.* cúdgel, club.

дублён|ый tanned; ~**ые ко́жи** tanned léathers; ~ полушу́бок shéepskin (coat).

дублёр *м.* 1. dúplicate, cóunterpart; ópposite númber *разг.*; (*о космона́вте*) báckup (man*); заво́д-~ dúplicate fáctory, fáctory óperating in párallel with another; 2. *теа́тр.* únderstudy; 3. *кино́* dúbbing áctor, voice; (*актёр для отде́льных эпизо́дов*) stánd-in.

дублёт *м.* 1. dúplicate; 2. (*два выстрела*) dóublet.

дубликат *м.* dúplicate, réplica.

дублированный dubbed; ~ фильм dubbed film.

дублировать *несов.* (*вн.*) 1. dúplicate (*smth.*); ~ работу другого предприятия dúplicate the work of another énterprise; 2. *театр.* únderstudy (*smb.*); 3. *кино* dub (*smth.*); ~ фильм dub a film.

дубль *м.* 1. *кино* take; 2. *спорт.* dóuble (víctory); 3. *спорт. разг.* (*второй состав команды*) resérves *pl.*

дубняк *м.* óak wood.

дуб|овый 1. oak *attr.*; of oak *после сущ.*; ~óвая роща grove of óak-trees; ~ стол oak táble; 2. *разг.* (*грубый, тяжеловесный*) wóoden; ~ стиль wóoden style. ~óк *м.* óak-sapling.

дубрава *ж.* 1. oak fórest/wood; 2. (*лиственная роща*) léafy grove.

дуг|а *ж.* 1. (*часть конской упряжи*) sháft-bow; 2. (*часть окружности*) arc; описать циркулем ~ý draw* an arc with cómpasses; брови ~óй arched brows; изогнуться ~óй arch *one's* back; ~ реки bend/curve of a ríver; ◇ электрическая ~ *физ.* eléctric arc. ~овóй arc *attr.*; ~овáя печь arc fúrnace; ~овáя электрическая лáмпа arc lamp.

дугообразный arched, curved.

дудеть *несов. разг.* pipe.

дудк|а *ж.* pipe; ◇ плясáть под чью-л. ~y dance to *smb.'s* tune.

дужка *ж.* hoop.

дуло *с.* bárrel; (*выходное отверстие*) múzzle; под ~м пистолéта at pístol point.

дум|а *ж.* 1. (*мысль*) thought; 2. *лит.* élegy, bállad; 3. *ист.* cóuncil, dúma; городскáя ~ city/town cóuncil, municipal cóuncil; Государственная ~ State Dúma.

дум|ать, подумать 1. (*над тв.*, *о пр.*; *размышлять*) think* (abóut, of), consíder (*smth.*), refléct (upón); pónder (*smth.*); ~ над проблéмой think* abóut a próblem; о ком вы ~али? who were you thinking of?; об этом следует подумать that is worth thinking abóut; я подумаю об этом I'll think it óver; дáйте мне врéмя подýмать give me time to think it óver; 2. *тк. несов.* (*полагáть, считáть*) think*; вы так ~аете? do you think so?; вы как ~аете? what do you think?, what's your opínion?; 3. *тк. несов.* (+ *инф.*; *намереваться сдéлать что-л.*) think* of (+ -ing), inténd (+ to *inf,* + -ing); когдá вы ~аете éхать в дерéвню? when are you thinking of góing to the cóuntry?; 4. (*о пр.*; *заботиться, беспокоиться*) think* (of), be* concérned (abóut); он ~ает тóлько о себé he thinks ónly of himsélf; 5. (*на вн.*) *разг.* (*подозревáть*) suspéct (*smb.*); напрáсно вы на негó ~али you were quite wrong to suspéct him; ◇ я ~аю! (*конечно*) I should think so!; не ~аю! (*едвá ли*) I don't think so!, hárdly!; и не ~аю! (*вовсе нет*) nóthing of the kind; не знáю, что об этом и ~ I don't know what to make of it; мнóго о себé ~ *разг.* have* a high opínion of onesélf, think* a lot of onesélf; не дóлго ~ая without stópping to think. ~аться *несов. безл.* seem; мне ~ается it seems to me.

думпкар *м. тех.* dúmp-car.

дуновéние *с.* puff, breath.

дýнуть *сов.* blow*.

дуплистый hóllow.

дуплó *с.* hóllow.

дур|а *ж.*, ~áк *м. разг.* fool; ◇ остáвить когó-л. в ~акáх fool *smb.*; остáться в ~акáх be* duped, be* a fool for *one's* pains; не ~áк (+ *инф.*) *шутл.* be* a great one for (+ -ing); без ~акóв without any nónsense, on the lével. ~áцкий *разг.* idiótic; ~áцкое положéние idiótic situátion; ~áцкая привычка fóolish hábit. ~áчество *с. разг.* tomfóolery. ~áчить, одурáчить (*вн.*) *разг.* fool (*smth.*). ~áчиться *несов. разг.* play the fool. ~ачóк *м. разг.* 1. goose*; 2. (*слабоумный*) hálf-wit. ~áшливый *разг.* fóolish; (*шаловливый*) pláyful.

дурéть, одурéть *разг.* 1. becóme* stúpid; go* crázy; 2. (*одурмáниваться*) grow* bemúsed.

дур|йть *несов. разг.* fool abóut; не ~й! stop fóoling!

дурмáн *м. бот.* thórnapple, stramónium; *перен.* fúddle. ~ить, одурмáнить (*вн.*) intóxicate (*smb.*, *smth.*), stúpefy (*smb.*), fúddle (*smb.*); ~ить голову комý-л. make* *smb.'s* head swim. ~ящий intóxicating, héady.

дурнéть, подурнéть lose* *one's* (good) looks, go* off; онá óчень подурнéла she is not néarly so góod-looking.

дýрно 1. *нареч.* bádly, bad*, ill*; ~ вести себя misbeháve, beháve bádly; ~ говорить, отзывáться о комý-л. speak ill of *smb.*; ~ обращáться с кем-л. treat *smb.* bádly; 2. *в знач. сказ. безл.*: ей ~ she feels faint; почýвствовать себя ~ feel* faint/ill.

дурн|óй 1. (*плохóй*) bad*; (*нрáвственно*) wícked, évil*; ~ поступок wícked áction/act, piece of wíckedness; ~óе поведéние misbeháviour, bad* beháviour; ~óе воспитáние bad* úpbringing; ~áя слáва bad* reputátion; о нём идёт ~áя слáва he is held in bad* repúte, he has a bad* reputátion; 2. (*некрасивый*) plain; hómely *амер.*; ◇ ~óй глаз évil eye.

дурнотá *ж. разг.* fáintness, gíddiness; почýвствовать ~ý feel* faint.

дурнýшка *ж. разг.* plain girl; hómely girl *амер.*

дýрочка *ж. разг.* 1. sílly (young) créature, goose*; 2. (*слабоумная*) hálf-wit.

дуршлáг *м.* cólander.

дурь *ж. разг.* nónsense; ◇ выбить ~ из когó-л. knock the nónsense out of *smb.*; выкинь эту ~ из головы! get rid of those nonsénsical idéas!

дýт|ый 1. (*о стекле, метáлле*) blown*; ~ые шины pneumátic týres; 2. (*преувеличенный*) exággerated; ~ые цифры exággerated figures; ~ые цéны inflated príces.

дуть, подуть blow*; дýет вéтер a big wind is blówing, it's blówing hard; как здесь дýет! what a draught!; от окнá (*сильно*) дýет there's a térrible draught cóming from the window; ◇ ~ гýбы pout, sulk; и в ус себé не ~ not turn a hair, not give a damn.

дутьё *с. тех.* blast; горячее ~ hot blast.

дýться *несов.* (*на вн.*) sulk (at), be* súlky (with).

дух *м.* 1. *тк. ед.* spírit; морáльно ~ morále; пасть ~ом lose* heart, be* dejécted, becóme* dówn-héarted; поднимáть ~ raise morále; в том же ~е on the same lines; чтó-то в этом ~е words to that effect; 2. (*сознáние, мышлéние*) mind; 3. *тк. ед.* (*дыхáние*) breath; перевести ~ get* *one's* breath; не переводя ~а without stópping to rest; 4. (*сверхъестéственное существо*) spírit, ghost; святóй ~ the Hóly Ghost; злой ~ évil spírit; ◇ быть в ~е be* in high spírits; быть не в ~е be* in low spírits, be* depréssed; во весь ~, что есть ~y with all *one's* might; одним ~ом in a flash; ни слýху ни дýху о ком-л. not a sound from *smb.*

духи *мн.* pérfume *sg*, scent *sg*.

духовéнство *с. тк. ед. собир.* clérgy.

духóвн|ый 1. spíritual; ~ óблик spíritual máke-up, soul; ~ая близость commúnity of féeling, spíritual affínity; ~ мир ínner devélopment; 2. (*церкóвный*) ecclesiástical; ~ая мýзыка sácred músic; ~ое лицó clérgyman*, cléric.

духов|óй: ~ инструмéнт wínd-instrument; деревянные ~ые инструмéнты the wóod-wind *sg*; ~ оркéстр brass band; ~ое ружьё áir-gun.

духотá *ж.* sweltering heat; (*в помещéнии*) stúffiness; какáя ~! how stúffy!; how hot it is!

душ *м.* shówer; принимáть ~ have*/take* a shówer.

душ|á *ж.* 1. soul; дóбрая ~ kíndly soul; низкая ~ low/mean créature; с ~óй (*игрáть, петь*) with féeling; говорить от ~и speak* straight from the heart; ~ óбщества the life and soul of the párty; 2. *разг.* (*человéк*) pérson; на дýшу each; на дýшу населéния per head of the populátion; производство на дýшу населéния per cápita prodúction; ◇ ни ~и not a soul; семья из семи душ a fámily of séven; ◇ ~ в дýшу in pérfect hármony; ~й не чáять в ком-л. ídolize *smb.*, dote *(upón)*; ~óй и тéлом heart and soul; в ~é in *one's* heart; всей ~óй, от всей ~й with all *one's* heart; разговóр по ~áм héart-to-héart talk; скóлько ~é угóдно to *one's* heart's contént.

душевáя *ж.* shówer-room.

душевнобольнóй *прил.* 1. insáne; 2. *в знач. сущ. м.* insáne; *мн.* the insáne *sg.*

душéвн|ый 1. emótional; ~ое состоя́ние state of mind; ~ая бóдрость fórtitude; ~ое потрясéние emótional shock; ~ подъём elátion, elevátion of spírits; 2. *(искренний)* sincére; *(прочувствованный)* héartfelt; ~ человéк wárm-héarted pérson; ~ое отношéние consíderate/córdial áttitude; ~ая болéзнь méntal disórder, insánity.

душегýбка *ж.* 1. *(для умерщвления людей газом)* móbile gás-chamber; 2. *(лодка)* canóe.

душераздирáющий héart-rending; ~ крик blóod-curdling shriek.

душúстый frágrant; ◇ ~ горóшек *бот.* sweet peas *pl.*

душ|úть I, задушúть *(вн.)* 1. *(убивать)* strángle *(smb., smth.)*, thróttle *(smb., smth.)*; 2. *(подавлять)* strángle *(smth.)*, crush *(smth.)*, suppréss *(smth.)*; ~ свобóду strángle fréedom; 3. *тк. несов. (затруднять дыхание; тж. перен.)* choke *(smb.)*, súffocate *(smb.)*; егó дýшит кáшель his cough is chóking him; егó дýшит смех he is chóking with láughter; злóба ~и́ла егó he choked with ánger; ◇ ~ в объя́тиях hug.

душúть II, надушúть *(вн.; духами)* put* scent/pérfume (on), scent *(smb., smth.)*. ~ся, надушúться use scent/pérfume, scent onesélf.

дýшн|о *в знач. сказ.* 1. *безл.:* здесь ~ it's stúffy here; 2. *(дт.):* мне ~ I can hárdly breathe. ~ый close, stúffy; ~ый день close/oppréssive day; ~ая кóмната stúffy room.

душ|óк *м. разг.* bad smell; *перен. тж.* taint, tinge; э́то мя́со с ~кóм the meat is high/táinted.

душóнка *ж. пренебр.:* ни́зкая, пóдлая ~ mean soul, base créature.

дуэ́ль *ж.* dúel.

дуэ́т *м. (спортивный)* pair. ~ом: спеть что-л. ~ом sing* *smth.* as a duét; петь ~ом sing* a duét.

ды́бом: вóлосы встáли ~ *one's* hair stood on end.

ды́бы: станови́ться на ~ rear; *перен.* bristle up, kick.

ды́лда *м. и ж. разг.* spíndle-shanks; great húlking féllow/girl.

дым *м.* smoke; ◇ ~ коромы́слом *разг.* hullaballóo; нет ~а без огня́ *погов.* there's no smoke without fire. ~ся *несов.* smoke; плитá ~и́т the stove is smóking; ~и́ть папирóсой puff awáy at *one's* cigarétte; ~и́ться *несов.* 1. smoke; 2. *(испускать пар)* steam; 3. *(о тумане и т. п.)* rise*, roll.

ды́мка *ж.* haze.

ды́мный smóky.

дымов|óй smoke *attr.*; ~áя трубá chímney; *(паровозная, судовая)* fúnnel, smóke-stack.

дымóк *м.* tin cólumn of smoke; *(от папиросы)* wisp/thread of smoke.

дымохóд *м.* flue, smóke-duct.

ды́мчат|ый smóky, grey; ~ая кóшка grey cat; ~ые очки́ tínted glásses.

ды́ня *ж.* mélon.

дырá *ж.* hole.

ды́рка *ж. разг.* hole.

дыря́в|ый torn; full of holes *после сущ.*; ~ая кастрю́ля a sáucepan with a hole in it.

дыхáни|е *с.* bréathing, respirátion; *(воздух при выходе)* breath *(тж. перен.)*; удéрживать ~ hold* *one's* breath; ~ весны́ breath of spring; ~ вторóе ~ sécond wind; до послéднего ~я to the last móment of *one's* life.

дыхáтельн|ый respíratory; ~ые пути́ respíratory ducts; болéзнь ~ых путéй respíratory diséase.

дыш|áть *несов.* 1. breathe; *(тв.) перен.* be* frágrant (with), émanate *(smth.)*; тяжелó ~ breathe hard, pant; чуть ~á hárdly dáring to breathe; 2. *(на вн.; дуть)* blow* (on); 3. *(тв.; выражать что-л.)* rádiate *(smth.)*, breathe *(smth.)*; ~ довóльством breathe contéentment; ◇ ~ на лáдан be* at death's door, have* one foot in the grave, be* on *one's* last legs; не ~á with báted breath.

ды́шло *с.* pole.

дья́вол *м.* dévil. ~ёнок *м. разг.* imp.

дьявольск|и dévilish(ly); ~ трýдно dévilish hard. ~ий dévilish, diabólical.

дья́кон *м. церк.* déacon.

дю́жий *разг.* strápping.

дю́жина *ж.* dózen; ◇ чёртова ~ báker's dózen.

дюйм *м.* inch.

-дю́ймовый *в сложн.* -inch; трёхдюймóвый thrée-inch *attr.*

дю́на *ж.* dune.

дюралюми́ний *м.* duralumínium; dúralumin *амер.*

дя́дя *м.* úncle.

дя́тел *м. зоол.* wóodpecker.

Е

Евáнгел|ие *с.* the Góspel; *перен. ирон.* góspel. ~и́ческий evangélical.

éвнух *м.* éunuch.

еврéй *м.* Jew. ~ка *ж.* Jéwish wóman*; *(девушка)* Jéwish girl. ~ский Jéwish; *(древнееврейский)* Hébrew.

европ|éец *м.* Européan. ~éйский Européan.

éгерь *м.* 1. húntsman*; 2. *воен.* chasséur.

еги́петский Egýptian.

египтя́н|ин *м.*, ~ка *ж.* Egýptian.

егó 1. *(рд., вн. от личн. мест.* он *и* онó) *(о мужчинах, самцах)* him; *(о младенцах, животных тж.)* it; *(о неодушевлённых предметах)* it; *(о судах)* it, her; ~ здесь нет he's not here; ~ нет he's out; *(уехал надолго)* he's awáy; 2. *в знач. притяж. мест. (о мужчинах, самцах)* his; *(о младенцах, животных тж.)* its; *(о неодушевлённых предметах)* its; *(о судах)* its, hers.

егоз|á *м. и ж. разг.* fidget. ~и́ть *несов. разг.* fidget.

едá *ж.* 1. *(принятие пищи)* meal; во врéмя еды́ dúring a meal, while éating; 2. *разг. (пища)* food.

едвá 1. *нареч. (с трудом)* hárdly, scárcely; я ~ разыскáл егó I could hárdly/scárcely find him; я ~ дышý *(от усталости)* I can hárdly/scárcely move; 2. *нареч. (чуть)* bárely; ~ замéтный bárely nóticeable/percéptible, scárcely visible; ~ избежáть чего-л. bárely escápe *smth.*; 3. *нареч. (только что)* ónly just; hárdly, scárcely; 4. *союз* по sóoner... than, scárcely/bárely... when; ~ встáло сóлнце, как... hárdly/scárcely had the sun rísen when...; no sóoner had the sun rísen than...; ~ ~ не... álmost...; ~~ hárdly; ~ ли it's unlíkely; он ~ ли придёт he's not líkely to come; он ~ ли знáет, хóчет *и т. д.* I don't suppóse he knows, wants to *etc.*; ~ ли э́то возмóжно it's hárdly póssible; ~ ли не *(с превосх. ст.)* próbably; ~ ли не лýчший шахмати́ст в странé próbably the best chéss-player in the cóuntry.

единéние *с.* únity.

едини́ц|а *ж.* 1. únit; ~ измерéния únit of méasurement; 2. *(цифра)* one; 3. *(плохая отметка)* bad mark; 4. *мн. (немногие)* indivíduals; тóлько ~ы only a few.

едини́ч|ный 1. *(единственный)* síngle; ~ слýчай síngle/sólitary ínstance; э́тот слýчай не ~ен this case is not the ónly one; 2. *(отдельный)* ísolated, indivídual; ~ные фáкты ísolated facts.

единобо́рство *с.* síngle cómbat; вступа́ть в ~ engáge in síngle cómbat.

единобра́чие *с.* monógamy.

единовла́ст|**ие** *с.* autocrátic pówer. ~ный autocrátic; ~ное правле́ние autocrátic rule.

единовре́менн|**о** (*один раз*) once; (*сразу*) in a lump, all at once; уплати́ть *что-л.* ~ pay* *smth.* in a lump sum. ~ый lúmp-sum *attr.*; ~ое посо́бие síngle--páyment grant, lúmp-sum grant.

единогла́с|**ие** *с.* unanímity. ~но unánimously; при́нято ~но passed unánimously. ~ный unánimous.

единоду́ш|**ие** *с.* accórd, unanímity. ~ный unánimous.

единокро́вн|**ый** *несов.* 1. consanguíneous; ~ брат hálf--brother; ~ая сестра́ hálf-sister.

единоли́чн|**ик** *м. ист.* indivídual péasant; fármer. ~ый 1. *ист.* indivídual péasant *attr.*; 2. (*осуществля́емый одним лицо́м*) indivídual; ~ое реше́ние indivídual decísion.

единомы́|**слие** *с.* agréement. ~шленник *м.* 1. like--mínded pérson, sýmpathizer; 2. (*соо́бщник*) álly.

единонача́лие *с.* one-mán mánagement, undivíded authórity.

единообра́з|**ие** *с.* unifórmity. ~ный úniform.

единоплеме́нник *м.* féllow-tríbesman*; (*принадлежа́щий к той же наро́дности*) féllow-cóuntryman*.

единоутро́бн|**ый** *уст.* úterine; ~ брат hálf-brother; ~ая сестра́ hálf-sister.

еди́нственн|**о** ónly; ~ возмо́жное реше́ние the ónly póssible solútion; ~, о чём говоря́т... the sole súbject of discússion is...; ~, о чём я прошу́ all I ask; ~, что я могу́ сказа́ть all I can say is. ~ый *прил.* 1. ónly, sole; ~ый ребёнок ónly child*; ~ в своём ро́де unique; ~ая наде́жда sole hope; 2. *в знач. сущ. с.* the ónly thing; ~ое, что остаётся де́лать, э́то... the ónly thing left is to...; ◇ ~ое число́ *грам.* síngular.

еди́нство *с.* únity; ~ взгля́дов únity of opínion/views.

еди́н|**ый** 1. (*один, еди́нственный*) a síngle; там не́ было ни ~ой души́ there wásn't a soul in the place; он не произнёс ни ~ого сло́ва he dídn't útter a (síngle) word; 2. (*объединённый, це́льный*) united; ~ое це́лое united/íntegral whole; ~ фронт united front; ~ технологи́ческий проце́сс únified/íntegrated technológical prócess; 3. (*о́бщий, одина́ковый*) cómmon; ~ое мне́ние cómmon opínion; ~ все до ~ого éveryone without excéption; они́ яви́лись все до ~ого they turned up to a man; ~ (прое́здной) биле́т bús-trám-and-túbe tícket.

е́дк|**ий** 1. *хим.* corrósive, cáustic; 2. (*раздража́ющий*) púngent, ácrid; ~ дым ácrid smoke; 3. (*ко́лкий, язви́тельный*) cáustic, cútting, bíting; ~ое замеча́ние cáustic/cútting remárk; ~ая иро́ния bíting írony. ~ость *ж.* 1. *хим.* corrósiveness, caustícity; 2. (*ко́лкость*) ácrimony.

едо́к *м.* 1. (*потреби́тель*) consúmer; (*в семье́*) a mouth to feed; коли́чество проду́ктов на ~á food per pérson/consúmer; семья́ из трёх ~о́в fámily of three (péople); 2. *разг.* éater; плохо́й ~ poor éater.

её 1. (*рд., вн. от личн. мест.* она́) (*о же́нщинах, са́мках*) her; (*о младе́нцах, живо́тных тж.*) it; (*о неодушевлённых предме́тах*) it; её здесь нет she's not here; 2. *в знач. притяж. мест.* (*перед сущ.*) (*о же́нщинах, са́мках*) her; (*о младе́нцах, живо́тных тж.*) its; (*о неодушевлённых предме́тах*) its; (*без сущ.*) hers, its.

ёж *м.* hédgehog; ◇ морско́й ~ séa-úrchin.

ежеви́ка *ж.* 1. *собир.* bláckberries *pl*; 2. (*об отде́льной я́годе*) bláckberry; 3. (*расте́ние*) bláckberry-bush, brámble.

ежего́дник *м.* yéar-book, ánnual.

ежего́дн|**о** yéarly, évery year. ~ый yéarly, ánnual.

ежедне́вн|**о** dáily, évery day. ~ый dáily; ~ая газе́та dáily (páper); ~ые забо́ты dáily/éveryday cares.

ежеме́сяч|**ник** *м.* mónthly (magazíne). ~но mónthly,

évery month. ~ный mónthly; ~ный отчёт mónthly repórt; ~ный журна́л mónthly (magazíne).

ежемину́тн|**о** 1. évery mínute; 2. (*постоянно*) perpétually. ~ый 1. at óne-minute íntervals *по́сле сущ.*; occúrring évery mínute *по́сле сущ.*; 2. (*непреры́вный*) cónstant, perpétual; мне надое́ли эти ~ые звонки́ по телефо́ну I'm sick of these everlásting télephone-calls.

еженеде́льн|**ик** *м.* wéekly (magazíne). ~ый wéekly, évery week.

ежесеку́ндно 1. évery sécond; 2. (*постоянно*) incéssantly, cónstantly.

ежеча́сн|**о** hóurly. ~ый hóurly.

ёжиться *несов.* 1. shíver (with); 2. *разг.* (*стесня́ться*) be* shy; (*колеба́ться*) hésitate, wáver.

ежо́в|**ый**: держа́ть *кого-л.* в ~ых рукави́цах rule *smb.* with a rod of íron.

езд|**а́** *ж.* 1. (*в маши́не*) dríving; (*верхова́я, на велосипе́де*) ríding; (*по желе́зной доро́ге, водо́й*) trávelling; до́лгая ~ в маши́не утоми́ла его́ the long drive tíred him; 2.: в двух часа́х ~ы́ от *чего-л.* two hours jóurney from *smth.*

езд|**ить** *несов.* go*; (*в маши́не, экипа́же*) drive*; (*верхо́м, на велосипе́де*) ride*; (*на пр.*) go* (by); (*по желе́зной доро́ге*) trável (by); он ка́ждый день ~ит в го́род he goes to town évery day; ~ на трамва́е go* by tram; ~ на оле́нях ride* in a réindeer sledge. ~ка́ *ж. разг.* jóurney; run.

ездов|**о́й** *прил.* draught; ~ые соба́ки draught/sledge dogs.

ездо́к *м.* (*верхо́м*) ríder, hórseman*; (*на велосипе́де*) cýclist; (*на мотоцикле*) mótor-cyclist; хоро́ший ~ good* ríder; плохо́й ~ bad* ríder; ◇ туда́ я бо́льше не ~ you don't catch me góing there ány more.

ей (*дт. от личн. мест.* она́) (*о же́нщинах, са́мках*) (to) her; (*о младе́нцах, живо́тных тж.*) (to) it; *в безл. выраже́ниях обы́чно* she; ей хо́лодно she is cold; ей всё равно́ she dóesn't care; it's all the same to her.

ей-бо́гу *разг.* réally.

ёкать, ёкнуть *разг.* miss a beat.

ёкнуть *сов. см.* ёкать.

е́ле hárdly, scárcely; ~ слы́шный звук hárdly áudible sound; я ~ дошёл сюда́ I could hárdly drag mysélf here; ◇ он ~ ды́шит he's half dead.

е́ле-е́ле hárdly.

еле́йн|**ый** únctuous, sanctimónious; ~ым го́лосом únctuously, sanctimóniously.

ёлка *ж.* 1. fir(-tree); 2. (*нового́дняя*) Néw-Yéar's tree; (*рожде́ственская*) Chrístmas-tree; 3. (*пра́зднество*) (chíldren's) Néw-Yéar's párty.

ело́в|**ый** fir *attr.*, spruce *attr.*; ~ая ши́шка fír-cone.

ёлочка *ж.* fir(-tree).

ёлочн|**ый**: ~ые украше́ния Néw-Yéar's tree decorátions; Chrístmas-tree decorátions.

ель *ж.* spruce, fir(-tree). ~ник *м.* 1. (*лес*) fir-grove; 2. (*ве́тки*) twigs/bránches of fir *pl.*

ёмк|**ий** capácious. ~ость *ж.* capácity.

ему́ (*дт. от личн. мест.* он) (*о мужчи́нах, са́мцах*) (to) him; (*о младе́нцах, живо́тных тж.*) (to) it; *в безл. выраже́ниях обы́чно* he; ~ хо́лодно he is cold; ~ всё равно́ he dóesn't care; it's all the same to him.

ено́т *м.* 1. (*зверь*) ra(c)cóon; 2. (*мех*) ra(c)cóon fur, cóon-skin. ~овый ra(c)cóon *attr.*, cóon-skin *attr.*

епи́скоп *м.* bíshop.

ерала́ш *м. разг.* múddle, mess.

е́ресь *ж.* héresy; *перен. разг.* (*чушь*) rúbbish, rot.

ёрзать *несов. разг.* fidget.

еро́шить, взъеро́шить (*вн.*) *разг.* rúffle (*smth.*), rúmple (*smth.*), dishével (*smth.*). ~ся *несов. разг.* brístle up.

ерунд|**а́** *ж. разг.* 1. (*чепуха́*) rúbbish, (stuff and) nónsense; говори́ть ~у́ talk nónsense; 2. (*пустя́к*) trífle; ~! néver mind that!

ёрш *м.* **1.** *(рыба)* ruff; **2.** *(щётка)* см. ёршик. **~ик** *м.* *(проволочный)* wire brush; *(щетинный)* bristle-scourer.

ерши́ться *несов. разг.* bristle up; *перен. тж.* get* into a témper.

е́сли 1. if; ~ вы за́няты, приходи́те за́втра if you are búsy come tomórrow; ~ не хоти́те, не приходи́те don't come if you don't want to, don't come unléss you want to; ~ бы if; ~ бы он был свобо́ден, он пришёл бы сего́дня he would have come todáy if he had been free; о ~ бы..! if ónly..!; что, ~ бы... what if...; ~ не if... not, unléss; ~ бы не кто-л., что-л. but for *smb., smth.*; ~ он и был там, я его́ не ви́дел éven if he was there I dídn't see him; **2.** *(при сопоставлении)* обычно *не переводится*; ~ до войны́ здесь бы́ло де́сять школ, то сейча́с их уже́ два́дцать befóre the war there were ten schools here, now there are twénty.

есте́ственн|о 1. *нареч.*, náturally; **2.** *в знач. вводн. сл.* náturally, of course. **~ость** *ж.* náturalness, simplícity. **~ый** nátural; *(непринуждённый тж.)* unaffécted; **~ые** бога́тства страны́ the cóuntry's nátural resóurces; **~ые** нау́ки nátural scíences; **~ая** смерть nátural death; **~ый** цвет лица́ nátural compléxion.

естествозна́ние *с.* scíence; nátural scíences *pl.*

естествоиспыта́тель *м.* náturalist.

есть I, **съесть** *(вн.)* **1.** *(питаться)* eat* *(smth.);* мне хо́чется ~ I am húngry; не ~ мя́са eat* no meat; **2.** *тк. несов.* *(разъедать)* corróde *(smth.)*, eat* *(into)*; **3.** *тк. несов.* *(раздражать — о дыме и т. п.)* sting* *(smth.);* ~ глаза́ кому́-л. make* *smb.'s* eyes smart; **4.** *разг.* *(попрекать)* nag *(smb.);* ◇ ~ кого́-л. глаза́ми devóur *smb.* with *one's* eyes; ~ чужо́й хлеб sponge, live on óther péople.

есть II *(наст. вр. гл. быть)* **1.** is; ~ о чём говори́ть! it's not worth méntioning!; **2.** *в знач. сказ.* *(имеется)* there is, there's; there are *мн.*; *переводится также ли́чными фо́рмами глаго́ла* have*; у меня́ (него́ и т. п.) ~ мно́го книг I have (he has *etc.*) mány books; ~ ли? is there?; are there? *мн.*; ~ ли у кого́-л. каранда́ш? has ányone got a péncil?; ◇ так и ~! and there you are!

есть III *межд.* *(ответ на команду)* véry good!

ефре́йтор *м.* córporal.

е́хать *несов.* **1.** см. е́здить; он е́дет в Москву́ he's góing to Móscow; ~ бы́ло о́чень ве́село we had a véry pléasant jóurney; **2.** *(уезжать)* go* off; сейча́с е́ду! I'm off; **3.** *разг.* *(сдвигаться, скользить)* slip, slide*; ◇ да́льше ~ не́куда! it's the límit!

ехи́дна *ж.* **1.** *(животное)* echídna, pórcupine ánt-eater; **2.** *разг.* *(о злом, язви́тельном человеке)* víper, spíteful/vénomous créature.

ехи́дн|ичать, **съехи́дничать** *разг.* be* spíteful, be* sarcástic. **~ый** spíteful, malícious; **~ый** челове́к malícious pérson; **~ое** замеча́ние malícious remárk.

ехи́дство *с.* spite, málice, malévolence.

ещё 1. *нареч.* *(дополнительно, больше)* (some) more, anóther; ~ хле́ба some more bread; ~ ча́шку ча́ю anóther cup of tea; хоти́те ~? will you have some more?; ~ немно́го a líttle more; подожди́те ~ немно́го wait a little lónger; ~ оди́н just one more; ~ оди́н! yet anóther!; ~ полчаса́ anóther half-hóur; ~ раз once more; ~ раз! *(сделайте)* (do it) agáin!; *(скажите)* say it agáin!; остаётся ~ мно́го сде́лать much yet remáins to be done; **2.** *нареч.* *(до сих пор, пока)* still; ~ есть вре́мя there's still time; вре́мени ~ доста́точно there's plénty of time; ~ не по́здно it's not too late; он ~ мо́лод he's still young; ~ не not yet; ~ не вре́мя the time is not ripe, the time has not yet come; он ~ не пришёл he hásn't come yet; **3.** *нареч.* *(уже)*: в 1917 году́ as far back as 1917; as long agó as 1917; он уе́хал ~ на про́шлой неде́ле, a year agó he left néarly a week, a year agó; **4.** *нареч.* *(при сравнит. ст.)* still, éven; ~ бо́льше, лу́чше *и т. п.* still more, bétter *etc.*; **5.** *усил. частица*; како́й ~..! what a..!;

э́то ~ ничего́! that's not so bad!; ◇ ~ бы!, да ~ как! I should think/say so!; and how! *амер.* ~ бы он отказа́лся! as if he would refúse!; ~ и ~ more and more, incréasingly; всё ~ still.

е́ю *(тв. от личн. мест. она́)* by her; *(о неодушевлённых предметах)* by it; э́та рабо́та сде́лана ~ this work was done by her; он ~ дово́лен he is pleased with her; он ~ кома́ндует she is ruled by him.

Ж

ж I, II см. же I, II.

жа́ба *ж.* toad.

жабо́ *с. нескл.* jábot.

жа́бры *мн.* gills.

жа́воронок *м. зоол.* lark, skýlark.

жа́дничать, **пожа́дничать** *разг.* be* gréedy; *(скупиться)* be* mean/stíngy.

жа́дн|о gréedily; *перен. (с интересом)* éagerly; ~ есть eat* gréedily; ~ слу́шать lísten éagerly. **~ость** *ж.* **1.** *(к дт., на вн., до рд.)* greed (for, of), ávarice (for); cupídity (for); **2.** *(прожорливость)* gréediness; **3.** *(скупость)* méanness, stínginess. **~ый 1.** *(на вн., до рд., к дт.; страстно желающий чего-л.)* gréedy (for); húngry (for); **2.** *(жаждущий удовлетворения)* ávid, éager; **~ое** любопы́тство éager curiósity; **3.** *(прожорливый)* gréedy, vorácious; **4.** *(выражающий жадность)* yéarning, húngry; grásping, avarícious.

жа́жд|а *ж.* *(прям. и перен.)* thirst; испы́тывать ~у be* thírsty; ~ зна́ний thirst for knówledge. **~ать** *несов.* *(рд.)* thirst (for), húnger (for), crave (for).

жаке́т *м.*, **~ка** *ж.* jácket.

жале́|ть, **пожале́ть 1.** *(вн.; чувствовать жалость)* píty *(smb.);* be* sórry (for), feel* sórry (for); **2.** *(о пр., что; сожалеть)* regrét *(smth.),* be* sórry (abóut); *(о несделанном)* wish *one* had, be* sórry *one* didn't; *(о сделанном)* wish *one* hádn't, be* sórry *one* did; **3.** *(вн., рд., беречь)* spare *(smth.);* *(скупиться)* grudge *(smth.);* не ~ уси́лий (чтобы) spare no pains (+ to *inf*); не ~ затра́т spare no expénse; не ~я затра́т regárdless of expénse; **4.** *разг. (любить)* be* kind/good (to), care ténderly (for).

жа́лить, **ужа́лить** *(вн.)* sting* *(smb., smth.);* *(о змее)* bite* *(smb., smth.).*

жа́лк|ий 1. *(вызывающий жалость)* pítiful, pítiable; *(страдальческий)* pathétic; **~ое** зре́лище sórry/pítiful sight; её лицо́ вдруг ста́ло ста́рым и ~им she súddenly looked old and pathétic; *(невзрачный, бедный)* wrétched, míserable; *(ничтожно малый тж.)* páltry; ~ вид wrétched appéarance; име́ть ~ вид look wrétched; ~ие оста́тки pítiful remáins/rémnants; ~ая су́мма páltry sum; **3.** *(презренный, мелкий)* míserable; ~ая попы́тка pítiful attémpt; игра́ть ~ую роль play a sórry part; ~ трус míserable cóward.

жа́лко см. жаль.

жа́ло *с.* sting.

жа́лоб|а *ж.* compláint; приноси́ть ~у lodge/make* a compláint; рассмотре́ть ~у consíder a compláint. **~ный 1.** pláintive; dóleful; **~ный** го́лос pláintive voice; **2.** *(о жалобой на кого-л.)* compláints *attr.;* ~ная кни́га compláints book. **~щик** *м. юр.* pláintiff.

жа́лованье *с.* sálary; *(рабочих)* wáges *pl.*

жа́л|овать, **пожа́ловать 1.** *(вн. тв., дт. тв.)* уст. *(давать)* grant *(smb. smth., smth. to smb.);* **2.** *тк. несов.* *(вн.)* разг. *(уважать)* like *(smb.),* care (for);

про́сим люби́ть да ~ we relý on your good óffices; он вас не ~уeт you're not amóng his fávourites.

жа́л|оваться, пожа́ловаться (на *вн.*) compláin (of); на что вы ~уeтесь? what's your compláint?, what's the mátter?; where does it hurt you?

жа́лостливый *разг.* **1.** soft-héarted, compássionate; (*выражающий сострада́ние*) sympathétic; **2.** (*печа́льный*) sad, mótrnful.

жа́лостный *разг.* **1.** pítiful, pláintive; **2.** (*сострада́тельный*) sympathétic.

жа́лост|ь ж. píty, compássion, sýmpathy; из ~и к кому́-л. out of compássion for *smb.*; ◇ кака́я ~! what a píty!

жаль **1.** *в знач. сказ. безл.:* как ~! what a píty!; мне вас ~ I'm sórry for you; мне не ~ про́шлого I have no regréts for the past; ~, что... it's a píty...; what a píty...; ~ потеря́нного вре́мени a píty so much time has been wásted; **2.** *в знач. сказ. безл. (рд., + инф.: о нежела́нии лиша́ться чего́-л.)* grudge (*smth.*, + -ing); мне ~ отдава́ть де́ньги I grudge the móney; **3.** *в знач. вводн. сл.* unfórtunately.

жалюзи́ *с. нескл.* Venétian blinds *pl.*

жанр *м.* **1.** genre; **2.** *иск.* genre-páinting; **3.** (*мане́ра*) style, mánner.

жа́нров|ый: ~ая жи́вопись genre-páinting; ~ая карти́на conversátion (piece).

жар *м.* **1.** heat; **2.** *разг. (горя́чие у́гли)* live coals *pl*, émbers *pl*; **3.** (*повы́шенная температу́ра*) (high) témperature; в ~ý in a high féver; у него́ ~ he has a témperature; **4.** (*лихора́дочное состоя́ние*) féver of excítement; броса́ет в ~ и в хо́лод it makes *one* go hot and cold; **5.** (*рве́ние*) árdour, férvour; (*горя́чность*) warmth; ~ говори́ть с ~ом speak* with animátion/heat; с ~ом приня́ться за де́ло set* to work with enthúsiasm; зада́ть ~у кому́-л. give* it *smb.* hot; чужи́ми рука́ми ~ загреба́ть ≅ make* óthers do the dírty work for one.

жар|á ж. heat; в са́мую ~ý at the hóttest time of the day, in the heat of the day.

жа́рен|ый (*на сковороде́*) fried; (*на пла́мени*) grilled; (*в духо́вке*) roast; ~ая ры́ба fried fish; ~ая карто́шка fried potátoes *pl*, chips *pl*.

жа́р|ить *несов.* **1.** (*вн.*) (*на сковороде́*) fry (*smth.*); (*на пла́мени*) grill (*smth.*); (*в духо́вке*) roast (*smth.*); **2.** *разг.* (*обжига́ть луча́ми*) scorch; нещáдно ~ит со́лнце the sun is fierce. ~иться *несов.* **1.** (*на сковороде́*) fry; (*в духо́вке*) roast; **2.** *разг.:* ~иться на со́лнце roast in the sun.

жа́рк|ий **1.** hot; ~ день hot day; ~ие стра́ны hot/trópical cóuntries; ~ пояс *геогр.* tórrid zone; **2.** (*пы́лкий, стра́стный*) árdent; **3.** (*бу́рный*) héated; ~ спор héated árgument; **4.** (*си́льный, интенси́вный*) fierce; inténse; ~ие бои́ fierce fíghting.

жа́рко **1.** *нареч.:* ~ нато́пленная печь hot stove; **2.** *в знач. сказ. безл.* it is hot; **3.** *в знач. сказ. (дт.):* мне ~ I'm hot.

жарко́е *с.* roast, roast meat.

жаро́вня *ж.* brázier.

жаропонижа́ющее *с.* fébrifuge, cóoling médicine.

жароупо́рный héatproof, héat-resístant.

жар-пти́ца *ж. фольк.* fire-bird.

жасми́н *м.* jásmin(e), jéssamin(e).

жа́тв|а ж. **1.** (*де́йствие*) réaping; **2.** (*вре́мя убо́рки хле́бных зла́ков*) hárvest-time; **3.** (*урожа́й*) hárvest. ~енный hárvesting.

жа́тка *ж. с.-х.* hárvester; réaper.

жать I *несов.* **1.** (*вн.; дави́ть*) press (*smth.*), squeeze (*smth.*); ~ кому́-л. ру́ку press *smb.'s* hand; **2.** (*быть те́сным*) be* tight; (*об о́буви*) pinch.

жать II, сжать (*вн.*) *с.-х.* reap (*smth.*).

жа́ться *несов.* **1.** húddle up; (*тесни́ться*) be*

húddled togéther; ~ от хо́лода stand* húddled up in the cold; **2.** (*к дт.; льнуть*) press (agáinst), cling* (to); ~ к ма́тери cling* to *one's* móther; ~ в у́гол cówer in the córner; **3.** *разг.* (*проявля́ть нерешительность*) díther, hésitate; **4.** *разг.* (*скупиться*) skimp, scrimp.

жбан *м.* jug.

жва́ч|ка ж. **1.** cud; жева́ть ~ку chew the cud; rúminate; *перен.* grind* the órgan; **2.** *разг.* chéwing gum; búbble gum. ~ный: ~ное живо́тное rúminating ánimal, rúminant.

жгут *м.* rope; соло́менный ~ twist of straw; сверну́ть что́-л. ~о́м twist *smth.* into a rope.

жгу́ч|ий búrning; ~ee со́лнце scórching/báking sun; ~ая крапи́ва stínging néttles *pl*; ~ стыд búrning shame; ~ие слёзы scálding tears; ◇ ~ брюне́т ráven-head; ~ вопро́с búrning quéstion.

ждать *несов.* **1.** (*вн., рд.*) wait (for); awáit (*smb., smth.*); ~ по́езда wait for a train; **2.** (*вн., рд.; рассчи́тывать на что-л.*) expéct (*smb., smth.*); ~ пи́сем от кого́-л. expéct létters from *smb.*; а мы вас и не жда́ли we wéren't expécting (to see) you; **3.** (*вн.; предстоя́ть*) be* in store (for), awáit (*smb.*); что ждёт его́ в жи́зни? what has life in store for him?; ◇ ~ не дожда́ться *кого́-л., чего́-л.* just can't wait for *smb., smth.* to come; не заста́вить себя́ ~ be* not long in cóming.

же I *союз* **1.** (*при противоположе́нии*) but, and; в не́которых же слу́чаях in some cáses, indéed; е́сли же... if, howéver...; и́ли же... or (perháps)...; **2.** (*ведь*): э́то же совсе́м друго́е де́ло (but) that's quite different; я же вам сказа́л but I told you; я же вам говори́л I told you so.

же II *частица усил.*: он тогда́ же посла́л письмо́ he sent the létter at once; приходи́те же! do come!; сего́дня же todáy.

жёваный chewed; *перен. разг.* crúmpled.

жева́ть *несов.* (*вн.*) chew (*smth.*), másticate (*smth.*); (*о жва́чных тж.*) rúminate (*smth.*); *перен. разг.* jaw (abóut).

жезл *м.* báton.

жела́ем|ый: принима́ть, выдава́ть ~ое за действи́тельное mistáke* the wish for the reálity; indúlge in wíshful thínking.

жела́н|ие *с.* wish, desíre; (*си́льное*) lónging (for); по ~ию at will; про́тив ~ия agáinst *one's* will; по ~ию пу́блики at the requést/desíre of the públic; по со́бственному ~ию at *one's* own requést; при всём моём ~ии much as I should like to; горе́ть ~ем be* búrsting with a desíre. ~ный *прил.* **1.** lónged-for, wélcome; ~ный гость wélcome guest; **2.** (*ми́лый, дорого́й*) dárling; déarest; **3.** *в знач. сущ. м. разг.* dárling; мой ~ный my best belóved.

жела́тельн|о *в знач. сказ. безл.* it is desírable; it is to be hoped; préferably; ~, что́бы вы уе́хали it might be as well for you to leave. ~ый desírable; (*необходи́мый*) desíred.

желати́н *м.* gelátine.

жел|а́ть, пожела́ть **1.** (*вн., рд., + инф.*) wish (*smth.*), desíre (*smth.*); (*стра́стно*) long (for); **2.** (*дт. рд.*) wish (*smb. smth.*); ~а́ю вам всего́ хоро́шего I wish you luck, good luck to you; не ~ зла *кому́-л.* not wish *smb.* any harm.

жела́ющ|ие *мн.* those who wish; ányone who wishes *sg*; откры́то для всех ~их ópen to all.

желе́ *с. нескл.* jélly.

железа́ *ж. анат.* gland; же́лезы вну́тренней секре́ции éndocrine glands.

желе́зистый I *хим.* férrous.

желе́зистый II *анат.* glándular.

желе́зка *ж. разг.* piece of iron, iron bar.

железнодоро́жн|ик *м.* ráilwayman*; ráilman*; ráilroader *амер.* ~ый ráilway *attr.*; ráilroad *attr. амер.*;

~ый путь track; rails *pl*, pérmanent way; ~ое движéние rail tráffic; ~ый ýзел rail júnction.

желéзн|ый íron (*тж. перен.*); *хим.* férrous; ~ая рудá íron-ore; ~ая стрýжка íron sháving; ~ купорóс green vítriol, súlphate of íron; ~ая крýша métal roof; ~ая бáнка tin; can *амер.*; ~ая вóля will of íron, íron will; ~ человéк íron-willed pérson; ~ая вýдержка íron sélf--contról; ~ая лóгика cást-iron lógic; ◇ ~ая дорóга ráilway; ráilroad *амер.*; по ~ой дорóге by rail, by train.

железнЯк *м.* íron-stone; крáсный ~ h(á)ematite.

желéзо *с.* (*металл, тж. лекарство*) íron; *собир.* (*изделия*) íronmongery, hárdware; листовóе ~ sheet íron; свáрочное ~ wrought íron.

железобетóн *м.* reinfórced cóncrete, ferrocóncrete. ~ный reinfórced-cóncrete *attr.*, ferrocóncrete *attr.*

железопрокáтный: ~ завóд rólling mill.

жёлоб *м.* chute, shoot, trough; (*на крыше*) gútter.

желт|éть, пожелтéть 1. (*становиться жёлтым*) yéllow, turn yéllow; 2. *тк. несов.* (*виднеться*) show* yéllow. ~изнá *ж.* yéllow hue, yéllowness.

желтóк *м.* yolk.

желторóтый yéllow-beaked; *перен. разг.* cállow; ~ птенéц cállow fledg(e)ling.

жёлт|ый yéllow (*тж. перен.*); ~ая прéсса yéllow press.

желýд|ок *м.* stómach; на голóдный ~ on an émpty stómach/bélly. ~очек *м. анат.* véntricle. ~очный gástric; ~очный сок gástric juice.

жёлудь *м.* ácorn.

жёлч|ный bílious, jáundiced; *перен.* jáundiced, bítter; ~ пузýрь gáll-bladder; ~ человéк bítter/acrimónious pérson.

жёлч|ь *ж.* 1. bile; (*животных*) gall; у негó разлилáсь ~ he has a bílious attáck; 2. (*раздражение*) spleen, bile, bítterness; пóлный ~и embíttered; излúть ~ на когó-л. vent one's spleen on smb.

жемáн|иться *несов. разг.* mince, símper. ~ный míncing, símpering. ~ство *с.* airs and gráces *pl.*

жéмч|уг *м.* pearls *pl.* ~ýжина *ж.* (*прям. и перен.*) pearl. ~ýжный 1. (*из жемчуга*) pearl *attr.*; 2. (*напоминающий жемчуг*) péarly.

женá *ж.* wife*. ~тый márried.

жéнин one's wife's.

жени|ть *несов. и сов.* (*вн.*) márry off (*smb.*); (*вн. на пр.*) márry (*smb. to*). ~ба *ж.* márriage. ~ся *несов. и сов.* márry; (*на пр.*) márry (*smb.*), get* márried (to).

женúх *м.* fiancé; (*в день свадьбы*) brídegroom.

женоподóбный efféminate.

жéнск|ий 1. wóman's, fémale; ~ пол the fémale sex; ~ие болéзни gynaecológical diséases; Междунарóдный ~ день Internátional Wómen's Day; 2. (*свойственный женщине*) a wóman's, wómanly, féminine; ~ая лóгика a wóman's lógic; ◇ ~ род *грам.* féminine génder.

жéнственн|ость *ж.* feminínity, femínity, wómanliness. ~ый féminine, wómanly.

жéнщина *ж.* wóman*.

женьшéнь *м. бот.* gínseng.

жёрдочка *ж.* perch.

жердь *ж.* pole; длúнный как ~ lánky.

жеребёнок in foal *после сущ.*

жереб|ёнок *м.* foal. ~éц *м.* stállion; (*до 4-х лет*) colt. ~úться, ожеребúться foal.

жеребьёвка *ж.* cásting of lots.

жерлó *с.* mouth; (*дуло тж.*) múzzle.

жёрнов *м.* míllstone.

жéртв|а *ж.* 1. sácrifice; ценóй больш́их жертв at great sácrifice; 2. (*пострадавший*) víctim; ~ы войны́ víctims of war; быть ~ой чегó-л. be* the víctim of smth. ◇ приносúть ~у чемý-л. make* a sácrifice to smth.; приносúть что-л. в ~у sácrifice smth.; пасть ~ой чегó--л. fall* a prey to smth. ~енник *м.* áltar. ~енный sacríficial.

жéртвовать, пожéртвовать 1. (*вн.; дарить*) give* (*smth.*), donáte (*smth.*); 2. (*тв.*) sácrifice (*smb., smth.*); ~ собóй sácrifice onesélf; ~ жúзнью sácrifice one's life.

жертвоприношéние *с.* sácrifice, óffering.

жест *м.* gésture; крас́ивый ~ fine gésture.

жестикул|úровать *несов.* gesticuláte. ~Яция *ж.* gesticulátion.

жёстк|ий 1. hard; (*о материи*) harsh; (*о волосах*) coarse; (*об органической ткани, пище*) tough; ~ матрáц hard máttress; ~ая кóжа tough skin; 2. (*суровый, резкий*) hard; ~ харáктер hard náture; дул холóдный ~ вéтер the wind blew cold and hard; 3. (*строгий*) rígid, strict; ~ грáфик rígid tíme-table; ~ие срóки strict tíme-limits; ~ое прáвило rígid rule, hard and fast rule; ~ие услóвия hard terms; ◇ ~ вагóн cárriage with úncushioned seats; éхать ~им trável 2nd class, trável «hard»; ~ая водá hard wáter.

жестóк|ий 1. cruel; (*грубый*) brútal; ~ человéк cruel pérson; ~ие нрáвы cruel cústoms; учинúть ~ую распрáву над кем-л. deal* brútally with smb.; 2. (*очень сильный*) fierce, víolent; ~ удáр crúshing/sávage blow; ~ое сопротивлéние fierce resístance; ~ое поражéние púnishing/crúshing deféat; ~ие страдáния térrible súfferings; ~ое разочаровáние bítter/cruel disappóintment; ~ морóз cruel/sevére frost; ◇ ~ая необходúмость díre necéssity. ~ость *ж.* 1. crúelty, inhumánity; 2. (*жестокий поступок*) crúelty, brutálity; cruel act/deed, act of crúelty; 3. (*суровость, резкость*) sevérity.

жест|ь *ж.* tin(-plate). ~Янка *ж.* tin, can. ~янóй tin (-plate) *attr.* ~Янщик *м.* whítesmith, tínsmith.

жетóн *м.* cóunter.

жечь *несов.* 1. (*вн.*) burn* (*smth.*); (*здания*) burn* down (*smth.*); 2. (*припекать — о солнце*) be* fierce; 3. (*причинять боль*) burn*, sear; (*о крапиве и т. п.*) sting*. ~ся *несов. разг.* 1. get* hot; (*о крапиве и т. п.*) sting*; 2. (*обжигаться*) burn* onesélf, get* burned; (*обжигать язык*) burn* one's tongue.

жжéние *с.* búrning sensátion.

жжёный burnt.

живúтельный invígorating; (*о воздухе тж.*) brácing.

жúвность *ж. собир. разг.* líving créatures, life; (*домашняя птица, мелкий скот*) líve-stock.

жúво 1. (*ярко*) vívidly; ~ описáть что-л. give* a vívid descríption of smth.; 2. (*сильно, остро*) kéenly, stróngly; э́то всех ~ заинтересовáло it aróused keen ínterest; 3. (*оживлённо*) ánimatedly, spíritedly; 4. *разг.* (*быстро*) quíckly; ~! quick!, look alíve!

жив|óй 1. líving, live; alíve *predic.*; ~ое существó líving béing, ánimated béing. ~ая рýба fresh fish; остáться в ~ых remáin alíve, survíve; он как ~ (*на портрете, фотокарточке и т. п.*) it's the líving ímage of him; 2. (*органический*) líving, ánimate; nátural; ~ая прирóда ánimate náture; ~ органúзм líving órganism; ~ая úзгородь hedge; ~ые цветы́ real/nátural flówers; 3. (*полный жизненных сил*) lívely; (*подвижный*) ágile, sprítely; (*о чертах лица*) móbile; ~ нрав, харáктер lívely disposítion; ~ая бесéда ánimated discússion/discóurse; ~ые talk/conversátion; ~ обмéн мнéниями lívely/ánimated exchánge of opínion; ~ ребёнок lívely child*; ~ые глазá bright eyes; ~ое лицó lívely/móbile face; 4. (*подлинный, реальный*) líving, real; ~ая действúтельность real life; 5. (*жизненный, насýщный*) vítal; 6. (*интенсивно проявляющийся*) lívely; (*остро переживаемый*) inténse; ~ воображéние lívely/vívid imaginátion; проявúть ~ интерéс к чемý-л. show* a lívely/keen ínterest in smth.; ~ óтклик на что-л. lívely respónse to smth.; 7. (*яркий, выразительный*) vívid; ~ое воспоминáние vívid mémory; ◇ ~ вес live weight; ~ая сúла líving force; ~ ум quick mind; quick wits *pl*; ~ язы́к líving lánguage; ~áя páна óрen wound; ни жив ни мёртв páralysed with fear; ~ портре́т spéaking líkeness; заде́ть *кого-л.* за ~бе sting* *smb.* to the quick; ~ уголо́к pets' córner.

живопи́сец *м.* páinter, ártist.

живопи́сный picturésque.

жи́вопис|**ь** *ж.* 1. páinting; 2. *собир.* *(картины)* páinting(s), píctures *pl*; вы́ставка ~и exhibítion of páinting(s).

живородя́щий *зоол.* vivíparous.

жи́вость *ж.* 1. *(подвижность)* líveliness, agílity; ~ умá méntal agílity/alértness; 2. *(оживлённый)* animátion, móvement; 3. *(острота, сила)* inténsity; *(яркость)* vívidness; ~ чувств inténsity of féeling.

живо́т *м.* bélly, stómach; ábdomen *книжн.*

животво́рный invígorating.

животново́д *м.* stóck-breeder. ~ство *с.* stóck-breeding, ánimal húsbandry. ~ческий stóck-breeding *attr.*

живо́тное *с.* ánimal; *перен. тж.* brute.

живо́тный 1. ánimal; ~ мир the ánimal kíngdom; 2. *(низменный, грубый)* béstial; ~ страх ánimal fear.

животрепе́щущий 1. *(живой)* líving; quívering with life *после сущ.*; *(зыбкий)* quívering; 2. *(злободневный)* vítal; ~ вопро́с vítal íssue, búrning quéstion.

живу́ч|**есть** *ж.* vitálity, pówer of survíval; *(выносливость)* hárdiness. ~ий hárdy; *перен.* endúring; ~ee расте́ние hárdy plant; ста́рые привы́чки ~и old hábits die hard; ◇ живу́ч как ко́шка *погов.* he has as mány lives as a cat.

живьём *разг.* alíve; взять *кого-л.* ~ take *smb., smth.* alíve.

жи́дк|**ий** 1. líquid; *(текучий)* flúid; ~ое то́пливо líquid fuel, oil fuel; 2. *(негустой)* thin; *(водянистый)* wátery, weak; ~ая ка́ша tin gruel; ~ суп wátery soup; ~ чай weak tea; 3. *(редкий)* thin, scánty; ~ие во́лосы thin/sparse hair; ~ лес thínly scáttered wood. ~ость *ж.* líquid, flúid.

жи́жа *ж.* mess; гря́зная ~ líquid mud.

жизнедея́тельн|**ость** *ж.* *биол.* vítal fúnctions *pl*; *перен.* vítal actívity. ~ый *биол.* cápable of life *после сущ.*, víable; *перен.* áctive, vígorous.

жи́зненн|**ость** *ж.* 1. *см.* жизнеспосо́бность; 2. *(близость к действительности)* néarness to life. ~ый 1. *после сущ.* life; ~ый путь path/road in life; ~ый о́пыт expérience of life; *(высокий)* ~ый у́ровень (high) stándard of líving; 2. *(близкий к действительности)* lifelike; 3. *(общественно необходимый)* vítal; ~ые интере́сы vítal ínterests.

жизнеописа́ние *с.* bíography.

жизнера́достн|**ость** *ж.* búoyancy, chéerfulness, abílity to enjóy life. ~ый búoyant, chéerful; ~ый хара́ктер bright disposítion; ~ый челове́к optimístic pérson, búoyant personálity.

жизнеспосо́бн|**ость** *ж.* viabílity, vitálity; ~ семя́н gérminating pówer of seed. ~ый víable; ~ый органи́зм víable órganism; ~ый коллекти́в víable colléctive; ~ое предприя́тие góing concérn.

жизнеутвержда́ющ|**ий** life-assérting; ~ие иде́и life-assérting idéas.

жизн|**ь** *ж.* life*; возникнове́ние ~и на Земле́ the órigin of life on Earth; ~ ме́дленно возвраща́лась к нему́ life slówly retúrned to his bódy; при ~и dúring *one's* lífetime; нача́ть но́вую ~ start a new life; борьба́ за ~ fight for life; в тече́ние всей ~и in all *one's* life/days; на всю ~ for life; о́браз ~и way of life; вести́ бродя́чую ~ lead* a nomádic exístence; по́лный ~и full of life; ◇ никогда́ в ~и néver in *one's* life; *(ни за что на свете)* not on your life!; ме́жду ~ью и сме́ртью within an inch of death; не на ~, а на смерть for dear life.

жи́ла *ж.* 1. vein; *(сухожилие)* téndon, sínew; 2. *горн.* vein, seam.

жиле́т *м.*, ~ка *ж.* wáistcoat, vest; вя́заный ~ cárdigan.

жиле́ц *м.* lódger, ténant; ◇ он не ~ (на бе́лом све́те) he has not long to live.

жи́лист|**ый** stríngy; *(мускулистый)* sínewy; ~oe мя́со stríngy meat; ~ые ру́ки sínewy arms.

жили́чка *ж.* *разг.* lódger, ténant.

жили́щ|**е** *с.* home, dwélling. ~ный hóusing; ~ный вопро́с hóusing próblem; ~ное строи́тельство hóuse-building, constrúction of hóuses; ~ные усло́вия líving condítions; ~ный отде́л hóusing depártment.

жи́лка *ж.* vein; *перен.* flair, bent; романти́ческая ~ romántic streak.

жил|**о́й** dwélling *attr.*; *(обитаемый)* hábitable; ~ масси́в hóusing estáte; ~о́е зда́ние dwélling house; ко́мната име́ет ~ вид the room looks líved-in.

жилпло́щадь *ж.* *(жилая площадь)* líving-space.

жиль|**ё** *с.* 1. *(жилое место)* inhábited place; приго́дный для ~я́ fit for habitátion; 2. *разг.* *(жилище)* home, dwélling.

жим *м.* *спорт.* the press.

жи́молость *ж.* *бот.* hóneysuckle, wóodbine.

жир *м.* fat, grease; *(от жаренья)* drípping; расти́тельный ~ végetable oil; живо́тный ~ ánimal fat.

жира́ф *м.*, ~а *ж.* giráffe.

жире́ть, разжире́ть get*/grow* fat.

жи́рн|**ый** 1. *(содержащий много жира)* fat; *(о пище)* rich; ~ое мя́со fat/fátty meat; ~ суп rich soup; 2. *(сальный)* gréasy; *(лоснящийся)* shíny; ~oe пятно́ grease spot/stain; 3. *(толстый, тучный)* fat, fléshy; 4. *(насыщенный)* rich; ~ая земля́ rich soil; 5. *(толстый — о линии, черте)*: ~ шрифт bold/héavy type; ~ым шри́фтом in bold type, bóldly prínted.

жиро́вка *ж.* *разг.* rent bill.

жиров|**о́й** fátty; ~а́я ткань ádipose tíssue.

жите́йск|**ий** wórldly; éveryday; ~ая му́дрость wórldly wísdom.

жи́тель *м.* inhábitant, dwéller, résident. ~ство *с.* résidence; ме́сто постоя́нного ~ства place of résidence, pérmanent addréss; вид на ~ство résidence permít.

жи́тница *ж.* gránary.

жить *несов.* live; *(быть в живых)* be* alíve; ~ ску́ченно live in crówded condítions; ~ ве́село lead* a gay life; ~ по́лной жи́знью live a full life; ~ свои́м трудо́м keep* onesélf, live on *one's* own éarnings; ~ воспомина́ниями live on *one's* mémories; ◇ ~ свои́м умо́м live as *one* thinks fit.

жить|**ё** *с.* *разг.* (way of) life, exístence; ◇ ~я́ от него́ нет he makes life intólerable.

житьё-бытьё *с.* *разг.* the way *one* lives.

жи́ться *безл. разг.*: ему́ живётся непло́хо he is well off; как вам живётся? how are things with you?; how are you gétting on?; ему́ не живётся на одно́м ме́сте he is néver content to stay in one place.

жму́рить *несов.*: ~ глаза́ *см.* жму́риться. ~ся *несов.* screw up *one's* eyes; *(от солнца, яркого света)* blink.

жму́рки *мн.* blind-man's-buff *sg.*

жмых *м. обыкн. мн.* óilcake.

жне́йка *ж.* *с.-х.* réaper, hárvester.

жнец *м.* réaper.

жнивь|**ё** *с.* 1. *(поле с остатками соломы на корню)* stúbble-field; 2. *(солома)* stúbble.

жни́ца *ж.* réaper.

жоке́й *м.* jóckey.

жонгл|**ёр** *м.* júggler. ~ёрство *с.* júgglery, sléight-of-hánd. ~и́ровать *несов.* *(тв.; прям. и перен.)* júggle *(smth., with)*; ~и́ровать фа́ктами júggle with facts.

жрать, сожра́ть *(вн.)* 1. *(о животных)* góbble up *(smth.)*, devóur *(smth.)*; 2. *груб.* *(о человеке)* gúzzle *(smth.)*, hog *(smth.)*.

жре́бий *м.* lot, ticket; *перен.* *(судьба)* fate, lot; броса́ть ~ cast* lots; ◇ ~ бро́шен the die is cast.

жрец *м.* priest; ◇ ~ы́ иску́сства árt-pundits; ~ы́ нау́ки the high priests of science.

жри́ца *ж.* príestess.

жу́желица *ж. зоол.* gróund-beetle.

жужж|а́ние *с.* hum, buzz. ~а́ть *несов.* hum, buzz.

жук *м.* 1. béetle; bug *амер.* 2. *разг.* rógue.

жу́лик *м. (вор)* thief*; *(мошенник)* swíndler, cheat; *разг.* crook, tríckster.

жуликова́тый *разг.* shády, cróoked.

жу́льнич|ать *несов. разг.* cheat, swíndle. ~еский *разг.* únderhand. ~ество *с. разг.* swíndling, chéating, swíndle.

жу́пел *м.* búgaboo, búgbear.

журавлёнок *м.* young crane.

журавли́н|ый crane *attr.*; *перен.* cráne-like; ~ая ста́я flock of cranes; ~ые но́ги spíndly legs.

жура́вль *м.* 1. *(птица)* crane; 2. *(у колодца)* wéll-sweep.

жури́ть *несов. (вн.) разг.* chide* *(smb.)*, repróve *(smb.)*.

журна́л *м.* 1. magazíne, jóurnal, periódical; *(трёхмесячный)* quárterly; ~ мод fáshion-magazíne; 2. *(книга для записи)* díary; кла́ссный ~ class régister; ~ боевы́х де́йствий wár-diary; ~ заседа́ний mínutes; ва́хтенный ~ lóg-book.

журнали́ст *м.* jóurnalist, néwspaperman*. ~ика *ж.* 1. jóurnalism; 2. *собир. (периодические издания)* periódicals *pl.*

журна́льный magazíne *attr.*

журча́ние *с.* múrmur, bábbling.

журча́ть *несов.* múrmur, bábble.

жу́ткий ghásty, hórrible, térrible.

жу́тко *в знач. сказ. безл.:* нам бы́ло ~ we were fríghtened/térrified.

жуть *ж. разг.* hórror.

жу́х|лый wíthered; *(о краске)* fáded. ~нуть *несов.* wíther; *(о красках)* fade.

жюри́ *с. нескл. собир.* júry.

З

за 1. *(по ту сторону)* beyónd, the óther side of; *(через)* acróss, óver; *(позади)* behínd; жить за реко́й live the óther side of the ríver; уе́хать за́ реку go* awáy acróss the ríver; вы́йти за дверь go* óutside the door; поста́вить *что-л.* за шкаф put* *smth.* behínd the wárdrobe; стоя́ть за шка́фом stand* behínd the wárdrobe; за кули́сами behínd the scenes; 2. *(около, у)* at, to; сесть за стол sit* down to/at táble; сиде́ть за столо́м sit* at the táble; за роя́лем at the piáno; 3. *(указывает на направление действия)* for; боро́ться за свобо́ду fight* for fréedom; беспоко́иться за дете́й be* wórried abóut the chíldren; наблюда́ть за детьми́ watch the chíldren; 4. *(по причине, вследствие)* for, on accóunt of; цени́ть *кого-л.* за ум válue *smb.* for *his* intélligence; за отсу́тствием вре́мени for lack of time; 5. *(употребляется при указании лица, предмета, до которого дотрагиваются)* by; *(при обозначении действия, которое начинают)* to; взять *кого-л.* за́ руку take* *smb.'s* hand; вести́ *кого-л.* за́ руку lead* *smb.* by the hand; держа́ться за пери́ла hold* the rail; приня́ться за рабо́ту set* to work; 6. *(свыше какого-л. предела)* óver; ему́ уже́ за 30 he is alréady óver thírty; 7. *(на расстоянии)* at a dístance of или не перево́дится; за пять киломе́тров отсю́да five kílometres from here; 8. *(до какого-л. временно́го предела)* не перево́дится; за де́сять дней до сро́ка ten

days befóre schédule; 9. *(в течение)* dúring, in; *иногда не переводится*; мно́гое сде́лано за после́дний год much has been done dúring the past year; за после́днее вре́мя in récent times, of late; э́то мо́жно сде́лать за час it can be done in an hour; 10. *(вместо кого-л.)* for; *(в качестве кого-л.)* as; я за тебя́ всё сде́лаю I will do éverything for you; рабо́тать за секретаря́ work as a sécretary; 11. *(в возмещение, в обмен)* for; плати́ть за рабо́ту pay* for the work; купи́ть *что-л.* за де́сять рубле́й buy* *smth.* for ten róubles; 12. *(ради, в пользу, во имя)* for; сража́ться за Ро́дину fight* for *one's* cóuntry; голосова́ть за предложе́ние vote for the propósal; 13. *(одно вслед за другим; преследуя)* áfter; год за го́дом year áfter year; чита́ть кни́гу за кни́гой read* book áfter book; бежа́ть, гна́ться за кем-л. run* áfter *smb.*, chase *smb.*; 14. *(во время чего-л.)* at; поговори́ть за обе́дом have* a talk at dínner; 15. *(с целью получить, достать что-л.)* for; посла́ть за до́ктором send* for a dóctor; пойти́ за биле́тами go* for the tíckets; 16.: кни́га чи́слится за мной the book is régistered in my name; за тобо́й долг you have a debt to pay; де́ло за деньга́ми it's a quéstion of móney; за по́дписью *(о документе)* signed by.

заале́ть *сов.* gleam red/scárlet.

заатланти́ческий transatlántic.

заба́ва *ж.* amúsement, pástime; э́то для него́ де́тская ~ it is child's play to him.

забавля́ть *несов. (вн.)* amúse *(smb.)*, entertáin *(smb.)*. ~ся *несов.* amúse onesélf.

заба́вн|о 1. *нареч.* amúsingly, fúnnily, in a fúnny má́nner; 2. *в знач. сказ. (дт.):* мне ~ I find it fun, I enjóy it. ~ый amúsing, fúnny.

забаллоти́ровать *сов. (вн.)* rejéct *(smb.)*.

забаррикади́ровать *сов. см.* баррикади́ровать.

забастова́ть *сов.* go* on strike, strike*; come* out *разг.*

забасто́в|ка *ж.* strike; объяви́ть ~ку decláre a strike. ~очный strike *attr.*; ~очный комите́т strike committee; ~очное движе́ние strike móvement. ~щик *м.* stríker.

забве́ни|е *с. уст.* 1. *(утрата воспоминаний)* oblívion, forgétfulness; 2. *(невнимание к чему-л.)* negléct; ~ до́лга derelíction of dúty; ◇ преда́ть *что-л.* ~ю consign *smth.* to oblívion, búry *smth.* in oblívion.

забе́г *м. спорт.* heat; предвари́тельный ~ tríal; ~ на 100 ме́тров húndred-metre race, the 100 mètres.

забе́гать *сов.* begín* to bústle (abóut), begín* to scúrry; *(о глазах)* becóme* shífty, assúme a shíffy expréssion.

забега́ть *сов.*, **забежа́ть** 1. *(бегом входить)* run*; 2. *разг. (заходить)* drop in; забежа́ть к кому́-л. drop in to see *smb.*; 3. *(убегать далеко)* run* off; ◇ ~ вперёд 1) go* too fast, run* ahéad; 2) *(опережать кого-л. в чём-л.)* anticipate *smb.*, forestáll *smb.*; beat* *smb.* to it *разг.*

забега́ться *сов. разг.* be* run off *one's* legs.

забежа́ть *сов. см.* забега́ть.

забере́менеть *сов.* becóme* prégnant.

забето́ни́ровать *сов. см.* бетони́ровать.

забива́ть *несов.*, **заби́ть** *(вн.)* 1. *(вбивать)* drive* *(smth.)* in; *(молотком)* hámmer *(smth.)* in; ~ сва́и sink* píles; ~ гво́зди в сте́ну knock nails into a wall; 2. *(закрывать наглухо)* nail up/down *(smth.)*; ~ я́щик гвоздя́ми nail up/down a box; ~ о́кна доска́ми board up the wíndows; 3. *(заполнять)* block up *(smth.)*; *(засорять тж.)* choke *(smth.)*, choke up *(smth.)*; все прохо́ды бы́ли заби́ты *(толпой)* all the aisles/gángways were blocked/thrónged; 4. *спорт.* drive* in *(smth.)*, score *(smth.)*; ~ мяч в воро́та score a goal; 5. *разг. (превосходить в чём-л.)* outdó* *(smth.)*; он нас всех заби́л he outdíd us all; ◇ ~ кому́-л. го́лову чем-л. wórry *smb.'s* head with *smth.*

забива́ться, **заби́ться** *разг.* 1.: ~ в у́гол húddle in a córner; 2. *(засоряться)* becóme* obstrúcted, get* blocked up; 3. (*проникать, попадать — о снеге, пыли*) cake, clog, lodge.

забинтова́ть(ся) *сов. см.* бинтова́ть(ся).

забира́ть, забра́ть 1. (*вн.*) take* (*smth.*); 2. (*вн.; арестовывать*) arrést (*smb.*), take* (*smb.*); 3. (*отклоняться от прямого направления*) bear*; забра́ть впра́во bear* (to the) right; 4. (*уменьшать*) gáther; ~ в шов gáther at the seam; ◇ забра́ть себе́ что-л. в го́лову take* *smth.* ínto *one's* head.

забира́ться, забра́ться 1. (*залезать, карабкаться*) get*; (*наверх*) climb (on); (*внутрь*) creep*; ~ на де́рево climb (up) a tree; ~ под одея́ло creep* únder the béd-clothes; 2. (*в вн.; проникать куда-л.*) get* (ínto), pénetrate (ínto); в дом забрали́сь во́ры thieves broke ínto the house; 3. (*уходить, уезжать далеко*) go* awáy/off; (*прятаться*) hide*.

заби́тый (*запуганный*) dówntrodden; ~ вид hángdog expréssion; ~ челове́к dówntrodden indivídual.

заби́ть I *сов. см.* забива́ть.

заби́ть II *сов.* (*начать бить*) begín* to strike; (*о фонтане*) gush forth.

заби́ться I *сов. см.* забива́ться.

заби́ться II *сов.* (*начать биться*) begín* to beat.

забия́ка *м. и ж. разг.* fighter, gáme-cock; (*задира*) tease.

заблаговре́менно in good time; (*заранее*) beforehand; in advánce.

заблагорассу́ди|ться *сов. безл.* seem fit; как ему́ ~тся as he thinks fit; ско́лько ему́ ~тся as much as he likes/chooses.

заблесте́|ть *сов.* 1. (*выделяться своим блеском*) show* up bríghtly, gleam; 2. (*стать блестящим*) shine*, begín* to shine; его́ глаза́ ~ли his eyes shone; *~.*: глаза́ ~ли слеза́ми *one's* eyes grew bright with tears.

заблуди́ться *сов.* lose* *one's* way, get* lost, go* astráy.

заблу́дш|ий stray; ◇ ~ая овца́ lost sheep*.

заблужд|а́ться *несов.* err, be* mistáken, be* únder a misapprehénsion. ~а́ющийся misgúided. ~е́ние *с.* érror, fállacy, delúsion, misconcéption; вводи́ть кого́-л. в ~е́ние mislead* (*smb.*); вы́вести кого́-л. из ~е́ния undecéive *smb.*, disillúsion *smb.*; находи́ться в ~е́нии be* únder a misapprehénsion/delúsion, be* in érror.

забод|а́ть *сов.* (*вн.*) gore (*smb.*); его́ ~а́л бык he was gored by a bull.

забо́й *м. горн.* face; (*угольный*) cóal-face. ~ный *горн.* cóal-face *attr.*, face *attr.* ~щик *м.* cóal-cútter, fáce-worker.

забола́чивать, заболо́тить (*вн.*) make* (*smth.*) bóggy. ~ся, заболо́титься becóme* bóggy.

заболев|а́емость *ж.* morbídity, sick rate; ~ ра́ком cáncer rate. ~а́ние *с.* diséase, íllness. ~а́ть, заболе́ть fall* ill/sick, be* táken ill; заболе́ть гри́ппом catch*/get* the flu(e).

заболе́ть I *сов. см.* заболева́ть.

заболе́|ть II *сов.* (*начать болеть; о какой-л. части тела*) begín* to hurt/ache, ache; у него́ ~ла голова́ he has a héadache.

за́болонь *ж.* sáp-wood.

заболо́тить(ся) *сов. см.* забола́чивать(ся).

заболо́ченный márshy, bóggy; wáterlogged; ~ луг wáterlogged méadow.

заболт|а́ть *сов. разг.* (*увлечься болтовнёй*) have* a long chat; ну и ~а́лись! what a talk we've had!

забо́р *м.* fence.

заборони́ть *сов. см.* борони́ть.

забо́т|а *ж.* 1. (*тревога*) anxíety, wórry; 2. (*о пр.; увлечение, хлопоты*) care (for); concérn (for); ~ о челове́ке concérn for the indivídual; ~ о лю́дях concérn for péople's wellbéing; ◇ э́то уже́ ва́ша ~ that's your lóokout. ~ить *несов.* (*вн.*) wórry (*smb.*). ~иться, позабо́титься (*о пр.*) 1. (*тревожиться*) be*

wórried/ánxious (abóut); он ни о чём не ~ится he shows no concérn for ánything, he takes no ínterest in ánything; ~иться о том, чтобы... see* to it that...; 2. (*окружать заботой*) look áfter (*smb.*), take* care (of); ~иться о де́тях take* care of children. ~ливый (*внимательный*) consíderate, solícitous, thóughtful; (*старательный*) cáreful; ~ливое отноше́ние к де́лу cáreful áttitude to *one's* work.

забракова́ть *сов. см.* бракова́ть.

забра́ло *с.* vísor.

забра́сывать I, заброса́ть (*вн. тв.; осыпать, покрывать*) cóver (*smth.* with), throw* (*smth.* óver); (*закидывать*) pelt (*smb., smth.* with); *перен.* bombárd (*smb.* with); ~ ров землёй fill a ditch with earth; ~ кого́-л. вопро́сами ply/bombárd *smb.* with quéstions.

забра́сывать II, забро́сить (*вн.*) 1. (*бросать далеко*) throw* (*smth.*), fling* (*smth.*), toss (*smth.*); *перен.* take* (*smth.*); судьба́ забро́сила его́ на се́вер fate took/brought him to the north; 2. (*оставлять без внимания*) negléct (*smb., smth.*); (*переставать заниматься*) give* up (*smth.*), abándon (*smth.*); 3. *разг.* (*доставлять*) delíver (*smth.*); (*по дороге*) drop (*smb., smth.*).

забра́ть *сов. см.* забира́ть.

забра́ться *сов. см.* забира́ться.

забре́зжить *сов.* begín* to grow light.

забрести́ *сов. разг.* 1. (*сбившись с пути*) stray, wánder, drift; 2. (*зайти мимоходом*) drop in; ~ к кому́-л. drop in at *smb.'s* house.

заброни́ровать *сов.* (*вн.*) resérve (*smth.*).

заброса́ть *сов. см.* забра́сывать I.

забро́сить *сов. см.* забра́сывать II.

забро́шенн|ый neglécted; ~ая ша́хта dérelict mine.

забры́згать *сов.* (*вн.*) splash (*smb., smth.*); (*мелкими брызгами*) sprínkle (*smb., smth.*); ~ водо́й sprínkle with wáter; ~ что-л. гря́зью splash/bespátter *smth.* with mud.

забыва́|ть, забы́ть 1. (*вн., о пр.*) forgét* (*smb., smth.*); (*упускать*) overlóok (*smth.*); ~ оби́ду forgíve* an ínjury; forgíve* and forgét*; нельзя́ ~ о том, что... we must not overlóok the fact that...; 2. (*вн.; оставлять где-л.*) leave* (*smth.*); я забы́ла у вас су́мку I left my bag at your house; ◇ об э́том и ду́май забу́дь! get that right out of your head!; забу́дь туда́ доро́гу! néver go there agáin! ~ться, забы́ться 1. (*не удерживаться в памяти*) be* forgótten, pass; 2. (*засыпать*) doze off; ~ться трево́жным сном fall* ínto an unéasy sleep; 3.: ~ться в мечта́х lose* onesélf in dreams; 4. (*терять самообладание*) forgét* onesélf.

забы́вчив|ость *ж.* absent-míndedness, forgétfulness. ~ый absent-mínded, forgétful.

забы́тый 1. forgótten; 2. (*заброшенный*) neglécted; 3. (*оставленный где-л.*) lost.

забы́ть *сов. см.* забыва́ть.

забытьё *с.* 1. (*неполная потеря сознания*) (state of) semi-cónsciousness; 2. (*полусон*) trance, drówsiness; 3. (*глубокая задумчивость*) réverie, muse, (fit of) abstráction; 4. (*сильное возбуждение*) tránsport.

забы́ться *сов. см.* забыва́ться.

зава́л *м.* obstrúction; снёжный ~ snów-drift.

зава́ливать, завали́ть (*вн.*) 1. (*засыпать*) cóver (*smth.*); (*наполнять*) fill up (*smth.*); (*упав, засыпать*) búry (*smth.*); (*загромождать*) block up (*smth.*); доро́гу завали́ло сне́гом the road is snów-bound; платфо́рма зава́лена чемода́нами the plátform is piled high with cáses; 2. *разг.* (*снабжать в изобилии*) flood (*smth.*); магази́ны зава́лены това́рами the shops are overflówing with goods; 3. *разг.* (*обременять*) overlóad (*smth.*); он зава́лен рабо́той he is up to the eyes in work; 4. *разг.* (*обрушивать*) pull down; 5. *разг.* (*проваливать*) spoil* (*smth.*), wreck (*smth.*); make* a mess of (*smth.*). ~ся, завали́ться 1. (*падать за что-л.*)

fall* behínd, slip behínd; be* misláid; 2. *разг.* (*запрокидываться*) drop, slip to one side; (*всем телом*) slump; 3. (*обрушиваться, падать*) collápse, túmble down; 4. *разг.* (*ложиться*) flop down; завали́ться спать flop ínto bed; 5. *разг.* (*терпеть неудачу*) collápse, fall* through.

завали́ть(ся) *сов. см.* зава́ливать(ся).

заваля́|ться *сов. разг.* be* misláid; (*остаться непроданным*) remáin unsóld; письмо́ ~лось на по́чте the létter got misláid in the post; кни́га где́-то ~лась the book must be misláid sómewhere. ~щий *разг.* old, rúbbishy, unwánted; (*об одежде*) discárded.

зава́ривать, завари́ть 1. (*вн., рд.; чай, кофе*) make* (*smth.*); (*обдавать кипятком*) pour bóiling wáter (óver); 2. (*вн.*) *тех.* weld (*smth.*); ◇ сам завари́л ка́шу, сам и расхлёбывай! you got yoursélf ínto the mess, so get yoursélf out of it!, you made the broth, now sup it! ~ся, завари́ться: чай завари́лся the tea is made/réady; ~лось де́ло! *разг.* now the fat is in the fire!; now we are in for it!

завари́ть(ся) *сов. см.* зава́ривать(ся).

зава́рк|а *ж. разг.* brew; ча́ю оста́лось на одну́ ~у there is ónly enóugh tea for one more brew/pot.

заведе́ние *с.* estáblishment, institútion.

заве́довать *несов.* (*тв.*) mánage (*smth.*), be* in charge (of).

заве́дом|о (*явно*) óbviously; (*известно*) known to be *после сущ.*; дава́ть ~ ло́жные показа́ния give* évidence known to be false, give* delíberately fálsified évidence. ~ый (*явный*) óbvious; (*известный*) notórious; ~ая ло́жь óbvious lie; ~ый лжец notórious líar.

заве́дующий *м.* mánager, diréctor; ~ уче́бной ча́стью diréctor of stúdies; ~ магази́ном shop mánager.

завезти́ *сов. см.* завози́ть.

завербова́ть *сов. см.* вербова́ть.

завере́ние *с.* assúrance.

заве́|ренн|ый *cértified; ~ая ко́пия cértified cópy.

заве́рить *сов. см.* заверя́ть.

заверну́ть(ся) *сов. см.* завёртывать(ся).

заверте́ть I *сов. (вн.) разг.* (*увлечь*) turn *smb.'s* head.

заверте́ть II *сов.* (*вн.; начать вертеть*) set* (*smth.*) spínning, set* (*smth.*) in rotátion.

заверте́ться I *сов. разг.* (*захлопотаться*) be* in a spin/whirl, be* véry búsy.

заверте́ться II *сов.* (*начать вертеться*) begín* to rotáte/spin.

завёртывать, заверну́ть 1. (*вн.; обёртывать*) wrap (*smth.*), wrap up (*smth.*); ~ кого́-л. в одея́ло wrap a blánket round smb., roll smb. up in a blánket; ~ 'паке́т wrap up a párcel; 2. (*поворачивать*) turn; ~ за́ угол turn a córner; 3. (*к дт.*) *разг.* (*заходить*) drop in (at *smb.'s* house/place); 4. (*вн.*) *завинчивать*) screw up (*smth.*); ~ кран turn off the tap; ~ кры́шку screw on the cap/top. ~ся, заверну́ться 1. (*закутываться*) wrap onesélf up; ~ся в плато́к wrap *one's* shawl round *one*; 2. (*загибаться*) turn up, get* turned up.

заверш|а́ть, заверши́ть compléte (*smth.*), accómplish (*smth.*). ~а́ться *несов.* be* near complétion; ~а́ться чем-л. end with smth. ~а́ющий fínishing, fínal, crówning; ~а́ющий уда́р fínishing stroke; coup de grâce. ~е́ние *с.* consummátion, complétion.

заверши́ть *сов. см.* заверша́ть. ~ся *сов.* be* compléted.

заверя́ть, заве́рить 1. (*вн. в пр.; уверять*) assúre (*smb.* of); 2. (*вн.; удостоверять подлинность чего-л.*) cértify (*smth.*), authénticate (*smth.*); ~ по́дпись wítness a signature.

заве́с|а *ж.* 1. screen, cúrtain; 2. (*то, что скрывает собой*) veil; ды́мовая ~ veil of snow; smóke-screen; огнева́я ~ fire-curtain; приподня́ть ~у lift the veil. ~ить *сов. см:* заве́шивать I.

завести́(сь) *сов. см.* заводи́ть(ся).

заве́т *м.* 1. precépt; behést; 2. *рел.* Ве́тхий, Но́вый ~ the Old, the New Téstament.

заве́тн|ый 1. (*сокровенный*) chérished, fóndest; ~ые жела́ния chérished aspirátions; ~ая мечта́ fóndest dream; ~ая цель chérished goal; 2. (*связанный с обещанием, тайным условием*) sécret, pledged.

заве́шать *сов. см.* заве́шивать II.

заве́шивать I, заве́сить (*вн.*) veil (*smth.*), cúrtain (*smth.*), cóver (*smth.*); ~ карти́ну cóver up a picture; ~ окно́ cúrtain a window.

заве́шивать II, заве́шать (*вн. тв.; вешать повсюду*) hang* (*smth.* with); сте́ны бы́ли заве́шаны чертежа́ми the walls were cóvered with dráwings.

завеща́|ние *с.* will; сде́лать ~ make* one's will; умере́ть, не оста́вив ~ия die intéstate.

завеща́ть *несов. и сов.* 1. (*вн. дт.; имущество*) leave* (*smb. smth.*) in one's will, bequéath (*smth.* to); 2. (*дт. + инф.; выражать предсмертную волю*) adjúre (*smb.* + to *inf*).

завзя́тый *разг.* invéterate; ~ кури́льщик invéterate smóker.

завива́ть, зави́ть (*вн.*) 1. (*волосы*) wave (*smth.*); (*локонами*) curl (*smth.*); ~ себе́ во́лосы wave/curl *one's* hair; 2. (*закручивать*) twist (*smth.*), coil (*smth.*). ~ся, зави́ться 1. (*о волосах*) wave, curl; 2. (*делать завивку*) wave/curl *one's* hair; (*у парикмахера*) have* *one's* hair waved/curled.

зави́вка *ж.* 1. (*действие*) wáving; (*локонами*) cúrling; 2. (*причёска*) háir-do; холо́дная ~ wáter/fínger wave; шестимеся́чная ~ pérmanent wave.

завиде́ть *сов. (вн.)* catch* sight (of).

зави́дно 1. *нареч.* énviably; 2. *в знач. сказ. безл. (дт.):* мне ~ I am énvious; ему́ да́же ~ ста́ло he felt quite énvious.

зави́дный énviable.

зави́д|овать, позави́довать (*дт.*) énvy (*smb.; smth.*); ~ую его́ здоро́вью I énvy his health; я не ~ую его́ успе́ху I don't grudge him his success.

завизжа́ть *сов.* (*начать визжать*) begín* to scream/squall.

завизи́ровать *сов. (вн.)* vísa (*smth.*), give* a vísa (to).

завинти́ть *сов. см.* зави́нчивать.

зави́нчивать, завинти́ть (*вн.*) screw/tíghten up (*smth.*).

зави́с|еть *несов.* (*от рд.*) depénd (on); он ни от кого́ не ~ит he is not depéndent on ányone; мы сде́лали всё, что от нас ~ело we have done éverything in our pówer; э́то не ~ит от нас it dóesn't depénd upón them.

зави́сим|ость *ж.* depéndence; находи́ться в ~ости от кого́-л. be* depéndent on/upón smb.; ◇ в ~ости от обстоя́тельств depénding on circumstances. ~ый depéndent.

зави́стлив|о énviously, with énvy. ~ый énvious, cóvetous.

за́висть *ж.* énvy; возбужда́ть ~ в ком-л. aróuse énvy in smb., aróuse smb.'s énvy.

зави́т|ой 1. curled, waved; with *one's* hair curled/waved *после сущ.*; 2. (*закрученный*) twísted. ~о́к *м.* 1. (*локон*) rínglet; 2. (*у растения*) téndril; 3. (*украшение*) scroll, flóurish; *архит.* volúte; 4. (*росчерк*) flóurish.

зави́ть(ся) *сов. см.* завива́ть(ся).

завихре́ние *с.* 1. (*образование вихрей*) éddying, eddy; 2. *разг. (мозгов)* fáncy, odd nótion, wild idéa.

завко́м *м.* (*заводско́й комите́т*) fáctory (tráde-union) committee.

завладе́|вать, завладе́ть (*тв.*) 1. take* posséssion (of), seize (*smb., smth.*); *воен. тж.* cápture (*smb., smth.*); про́чно завладе́ть чем-л. get* a firm hold of smth., get* a firm grip on smth.; 2. (*сильно увлекать*) grip (smth.); завладе́ть чъим-л. внима́нием compél smb.'s atténtion; завладе́ть ума́ми sway the minds; 3. (подчинять себе) take* posséssion (of), cáptivate (smth.), grip (smth.).

завладе́ть сов. см. завладева́ть.

завлека́ть, завле́чь (вн.) 1. entíce (smb.), lure (smb.), témpt (smth.); 2. (пленять) cáptivate (smb.), enthráll (smb.), cárry (smb.) awáy.

завле́чь сов. см. завлека́ть.

заво́д I м. 1. works, fáctory, plant, mill; машинострои́тельный ~ enginéering works/plant; чугунолите́йный ~ íron-works; маслобо́йный ~ créamery, bútter-factory; 2.: ко́нный ~ stúd-farm.

заво́д II м. (механизм) wínding méchanism; ~ ко́нчился (у часо́в) the watch has run down.

заводи́ть, завести́ (вн.) 1. (вводить куда-л.) bring* (smb., smth.), take* (smb., smth.), lead* (smb., smth.); 2. разг. (отводить куда-л. мимоходом) take* (smb.) somewhere on one's way, drop (smb.) somewhere; 3. (уводить далеко) take* (smb.) far awáy; перен. lead* (smb.) far astráy; куда́ ты нас завёл? where on earth have you brought us?; объясне́ние причи́н далеко́ бы завело́ меня́ it would lead me far from the point to expláin all the cáuses; 4. (приобретать) get* (smth.), acquíre (smth.); ~ но́вое обору́дование instáll new equipment; ~ соба́ку get* onesélf a dog; 5. (вводить) introdúce (smth.); ~ но́вые поря́дки introdúce/estáblish new procédure; lay* down new rules; 6. (начинать) start (smth.); ~ знако́мство с кем-л. strike* up an acquáintance with smb., get* to know smb.; ~ разгово́р с кем-л. get* tálking to smb.; 7. (приводить в действие) wind* up (smth.); ~ маши́ну start a car; 8. разг. (будоражить) get* (smb.) worked up; ◇ завести́ кого́-л. в тупи́к put* smb. in an impóssible position. ~ся, завести́сь 1. (появляться): у него́ завели́сь де́ньги he has got hold of some móney; у него́ завели́сь но́вые знако́мства he has got to know new péople; 2. разг. (устанавливаться) be* estáblished; завели́сь но́вые поря́дки a new sýstem came into béing; 3. (о мото́ре) start; (о часа́х и т. п.) be* wound (up); мото́р не заво́дится the éngine won't start; 4. разг. (приходить в возбуждение) get* worked up.

заводн|о́й 1. mechánical; ~а́я игру́шка clóckwork/mechánical toy; 2. (служащий для завода) wínding, cránking, stárting; ~ механи́зм wínding méchanism; ~а́я рукоя́тка stárting-handle; 3. разг. (легко возбудимый) lively.

заводоуправле́ние с. fáctory/works mánagement.

заводск|и́й, заводско́й fáctory attr.; ~и́е корпуса́ fáctory buildings.

за́водь ж. creek, báckwater; ти́хая ~ quíet báckwater.

завоева́ние с. 1. cónquest; 2. обыкн. мн. (достижения) achíevements, gains.

завоева́тель м. cónqueror.

завоева́тельный expánsionist.

завоева́ть сов. см. завоёвывать.

завоёвывать, завоева́ть (вн.) cónquer (smth.); перен. win* (smth.); несов. тж. try to get (smth.); ~ побе́ду attáin a víctory; завоева́ть пе́рвое ме́сто спорт. take*/gain first place, come* first; завоева́ть чье́-л. расположе́ние win*/gain smb.'s sýmpathies; завоева́ть всео́бщее уваже́ние win* univérsal respéct.

заво́з м. разг. delívery; ~ сырья́ delívery of raw matérials.

завози́ть, завезти́ (вн.) 1. (привозить по пути) delíver (smth.) en route, drop (smb.) on the way; 2. (отвозить далеко) take* (smb.) miles awáy; 3. разг. (доставлять что-л. куда-л.) delíver (smth.).

завола́кивать, заволо́чь (вн.) cloud (smth.); не́бо заволокло́ ту́чами the sky becáme a mass of clouds; слёзы заволокли́ её глаза́ her eyes were clóuded with

tears. ~ся, заволо́чься be*/becóme* shróuded (in), cloud óver.

заволнова́ться сов. (встревожиться) get* wórried/upsét; (прийти в возбуждение) get* excíted; (о мо́ре) get*/becóme* rough.

заволо́чь(ся) сов. см. завола́кивать(ся).

заворо́живать, заворожи́ть (вн.) cast* a spell (óver), charm (smb.).

заворож|ённый spéllbound, enchánted. ~и́ть сов. см. заворо́живать.

заворо́т м.: ~ кишо́к мед. vólvulus.

заворо́чаться сов. разг. begín* to toss and turn, stir réstlessly.

заворча́ть сов. begín* to grúmble.

завсегда́тай м. frequénter (of), habitué (of).

за́втра нареч. 1. tomórrow; 2. в знач. сущ. с нескл. tomórrow; откла́дывать на ~ put* off till tomórrow; ◇ до ~! goodbýe till tomórrow!, see you tomórrow!

за́втрак м. (первый) bréakfast; (второй) lúnch(eon); вку́сный ~ a nice/tásty bréakfast/lunch; взять с собо́й ~ take* one's bréakfast/lunch with one, take* a packed lunch. ~ать, поза́втракать (утром) bréakfast, have* bréakfast; (днём) lunch, have* lunch.

за́втрашн|ий the next day's, tomórrow's; ~ее число́ tomórrow's date; ~ день tomórrow; начина́я с ~его дня begínning from tomórrow.

завуали́ровать сов. (вн.) veil (smth.); перен. disguíse (smth.); ~ фа́кты disguíse the facts.

за́вуч м. разг. diréctor of stúdies.

завхо́з м. разг. supplý mánager.

завши́веть сов. becóme* inféstеd with lice.

завыва́ние с. hówling, wáiling.

завыва́ть несов. howl, wail, make* a wáiling sound.

завы́сить сов. см. завыша́ть.

завы́ть сов. start hówling, howl.

завыш|а́ть, завы́сить (вн.) overstáte (smth.), set* (smth.) too high; ~ но́рмы set* the quótas too high. ~е́ние с. overstátement, sétting too high.

завы́шенн|ый overstáted; ~ые но́рмы excéssive quótas; ~ые оце́нки marks that are too high.

завяза́ть(ся) сов. см. завя́зывать(ся).

завя́зка ж. 1. (тесёмка) tape; (лента) ríbbon; 2. (литературного произведения) plot, build-up; 3. (начало) start, óutset; ~ бо́я initial fighting.

завя́знуть сов. (прям. и перен.) get* stuck; ~ в долга́х sink* into debt.

завя́зывать, завяза́ть (вн.) 1. tie (smth.); (пакет, шнурок) do* up (smth.), tie up (smth.); ~ га́лстук knot a (néck-)tie; ~ глаза́ кому́-л. blíndfold smb.; ~ что-л. узло́м knot smth.; 2. (начинать) start (smth.); ~ бой start fíghting, engáge in a fight; завяза́ть знако́мство с кем-л. strike* up an acquáintance with smb.; ~ отноше́ния с кем-л. énter into relátions with smb.; завяза́ть разгово́р с кем-л. énter into conversátion with smb.; start a conversátion with smb. ~ся, завяза́ться (начинаться) start; (о дружбе, знакомстве) spring* up.

за́вязь ж. 1. бот. óvary; 2. (образование плода) frúiting.

завя́нуть сов. см. вя́нуть.

загада́ть сов. см. зага́дывать.

зага́дить сов. (вн.) foul (smth.), befóul (smth.); перен. besmírch (smth.).

зага́д|ка ж. ríddle; перен. тж. enígma, mýstery. ~очный enigmátic, mystérious; (о выражении лица тж.) inscrútable; (о словах) mystérious, crýptic; ~очный слу́чай mystérious íncident/case.

зага́дывать, загада́ть 1.: ~ зага́дку set* a ríddle; 2. (вн.) задумывать что-л.) think* (of); 3. разг. (предполагать что-л. сделать) think* ahéad.

загазо́ванный (загрязнённый газами) gas-pollúted, smógged-up; thick with fumes после сущ.

загáр *м.* tan, súnburn, brown.

загвóздка *ж. разг.* snag; вот в чём ~! that's the snag!, that's just it!

загерметизи́ровать *сов. (вн.)* seal (*smth.*) hermétically.

заги́б *м.* 1. (*поворот*) bend, curve; *перен.* deviátion; 2. (*загнувшееся место*) crease.

загибáть, загну́ть 1. (*вн.*) (*вверх*) turn up (*smth.*); (*вниз*) turn down (*smth.*); ~ страни́цу turn down the page; ~ пáльцы (*для счёта*) tick off on *one's* fingers; 2. *разг.* (*высказывать что-л. нелепое*) go* a bit too far. ~ся, загну́ться curl, turn up.

загипнотизи́ровать *сов. см.* гипнотизи́ровать.

заглáв|ие *с.* títle. ~ный: ~ный лист títle-page; ~ная бýква cápital létter.

заглáдить *сов. см.* заглáживать.

заглáживать, заглáдить (*вн.*) 1. (*делать гладким*) smooth out (*smth.*); (*утюгом*) íron out (*smth.*); ~ склáдки íron out the créases; 2. (*смягчать*) sóften (*smth.*); (*искупать*) atóne (for); make* up (for); ~ свою́ вину́ atóne for *one's* offénce.

заглóхнуть *сов. см.* глóхнуть 2, 3, 4, 5.

заглóхший (*запущенный*) neglécted, overgrówn.

заглушáть, заглуши́ть (*вн.*) 1. (*звук*) déaden (*smth.*), múffle (*smth.*), smóther (*smth.*); (*более громким звуком*) drown (*smth.*); шум вéтра заглуши́л егó словá the noise of the wind drowned his words; 2. (*ослаблять какое-л. чувство, ощущение*) déaden (*smth.*); ~ боль déaden pain; 3. (*растения*) choke (*smth.*); 4. (*подавлять*) stífle (*smth.*); ~ гóлос сóвести stífle the voice of cónscience.

заглуши́ть *сов. см.* заглушáть.

заглядéнье *с. разг.* lóvely sight; feast for the eyes *идиом.*; онá прóсто ~! she's simply lóvely!

заглядéться *сов. см.* заглядываться.

заглядывать, заглянýть 1. (*смотреть*) look; (*незаметно*) peep, peer; заглянýть кому́-л. в лицó peer/look into *smb.'s* face; ~ в словáрь look in a dictionary; 2. (*бегло прочитывать*) take* a look/glance (at), glance through; 3.: ~ в дýшу человéка seek* an insight into a pérson's heart, try to pénetrate a pérson's ínnermost féelings; 4. *разг.* (*заходить куда-л.*) look in (at), drop in (at); ◇ ~ вперёд look ahéad; ~ в бýдущее get* a glimpse of the fúture.

заглядываться, заглядéться (на *вн.*) be* lost in contemplátion (of); (*любоваться*) be* lost in admirátion (of).

заглянýть *сов. см.* заглядывать.

зáгнанный 1. (*о лошади*) overwórked, exháusted; (*затравленный*) húnted; ~ зверь hunted ánimal; 2. (*запуганный, забитый*) pérsecuted, dówntrodden.

загнáть *сов.* 1. *см.* загонять I; 2. (*вн.; утомить быстрой ездой*) óverdrive* (*smth.*); ~ лóшадь óverdrive* a horse; (*до смерти*) ride* a horse to death.

загнив|áть, загни́ть rot; decáy (*тж. перен.*). ~áющий decáying.

загни́ть *сов. см.* загнивáть.

загнýть(ся) *сов. см.* загибáть(ся).

заговáривать I *несов.* (*вступать в разговор*) ópen the conversátion; addréss (*smb.*) first.

заговáривать II, заговори́ть (*вн.*) 1. (*утомлять разговором*) talk *smb.'s* head off, talk (*smb.*) silly *разг.*; 2. (*действовать заговором*) bewítch (*smb.*); ~ зýбы кому́-л. tell* *smb.* the tale, talk *smb.* round.

заговáриваться, заговори́ться *разг.* 1. *тк. несов.* (*говорить бессвязно*) wánder (in *one's* speech), becóme* incohérent; 2. (*завираться*) let* *one's* tongue run awáy with *one*; говори́, да не заговáривайся! don't let your tongue run awáy with you!

зáговор I *м.* (*тайный сговор*) plot, conspíracy; быть в ~е be* in a conspíracy/plot; состáвить ~ make* a plot, plot, conspíre; ◇ ~ молчáния conspíracy of sílence.

зáговор II *м.* (*заклинание*) charm.

заговори́ть I *сов. см.* заговáривать II.

заговори́ть II *сов.* 1. (*начать говорить*) speak*, begín* to speak; 2. (*овладеть речью*) begín* to talk.

заговори́ться *сов.* 1. forgét* the time in conversátion, talk too long; 2. *см.* заговáриваться 2.

заговóрщик *м.* conspírator.

заголóвок *м.* héading, héadline.

загóн *м.* 1. (*действие*) driving; 2. (*для крупного скота*) enclósure, pen; (*для овец*) shéep-fold; ◇ быть в ~е be* neglécted.

загоня́ть I, загнáть (*вн.*) 1. drive* (*smth.*); (*скот тж.*) round up (*smth.*); загнáть корóву в сарáй drive* a cow into a shed; 2. (*заставлять уйти, уехать очень далеко*) send* (*smb.*) far awáy; 3. *разг.* (*вбивать что-л. с силой*) drive* (*smth.*), knock (*smth.*); 4. *разг.* (*продавать*) flog (*smth.*).

загоня́ть II *сов.* (*вн.*) *разг.* (*утомить работой и т. п.*) off his, her feet.

загорáжив|ать, загороди́ть (*вн.*) 1. (*обносить оградой*) fence in (*smth.*); ~ двор забóром enclóse a yard, fence in a yard; 2. (*преграждать*) block (*smth.*), obstrúct (*smth.*), bar (*smth.*); ~ кому́-л. дорóгу block *smb.'s* way; 3. (*заслонять*) shield (*smth.*); ~ кому́-л. свет be* in *smb.'s* light; не ~áйте мне свет would you mind kéeping out of my light. ~аться, загороди́ться 1. fence *onesélf* off, shut* *onesélf* off; 2. (*заслоняться*) screen *onesélf*, shield *onesélf*.

загор|áть, загорéть get* súnburnt; *несов. тж.* súnbathe, bask in the sun; кáждое ýтро мы ~áем на сóлнце we súnbathe every mórning; как он загорéл! how brown/brónzed he is!

загорáться, загорéться 1. catch* fire, take* fire; на чердакé загорéлось the áttic's on fire; 2. (*зажигаться*) glow*, shine* forth; в óкнах загорéлись огни́ lights came on in the windows; 3. (*появляться, излучая свет*) begín* to glow; загорéлись пéрвые звёздочки the first stars came out; 4. (*тв.; о глазах*) light* up (with); 5. (*тв., от рд.; покрываться румянцем*) flush (with), burn* (with); на егó щекáх загорéлся румя́нец a flush appéared in his cheeks; 6. (*тв.; быть охваченным каким-л. чувством*) concéive (*smth.*), be* consúmed (with); загорéться желáнием сдéлать что-л. concéive a desíre to do *smth.*; 7. *безл.* (*дт. + инф.*) *разг.* (*сильно захотеться*) have* a víolent urge (+ to *inf*); мне вдруг загорéлось уви́деть егó I súddenly had a víolent urge to see him; 8. (*о споре и т. п.*) break* out, flare up.

загорди́ться *сов. разг.* get* a swelled head, start swánking, get*/be* stúck-up.

загорéлый súnburnt, tanned, brown.

загорéть *сов. см.* загорáть.

загорéться *сов. см.* загорáться.

загороди́ть(ся) *сов. см.* загорáживать(ся).

загорóдка *ж.* fence, ráiling; (*внутри помещения*) partítion.

зáгородн|ый óut-of-tówn *attr.*, cóuntry *attr.*; ~ дом house in the cóuntry; ~ая прогýлка trip to the cóuntry, trip out of town.

загости́ться *сов. разг.* stay too long, overstáy *one's* time.

заготáвливать, заготóвить *см.* заготовля́ть.

заготови́тель *м.* purvéyor; official in charge of State púrchases. ~ный: ~ная организáция púrchasing organizátion; ~ный пункт purvéying céntre; ~ная ценá púrchase price.

заготóвить *сов. см.* заготовля́ть и заготáвливать.

заготóвка *ж.* 1. (*действие*) láying in, stócking up; (*закупка*) púrchasing/purvéyance; 2. (*полуфабрикат*) intermédiate próduct; (*сапожная*) úpper.

заготовля́ть, заготóвить (*вн.*) 1. (*приготовлять заранее*) prepáre (*smth.*) in advánce, have* (*smth.*) réady; 2. (*запасать*) lay* in (*smth.*), store up (*smth.*);

build* up stocks (of); ~ дрова́ на́ зиму lay* in firewood for the winter.

загради́тельный féncing *attr.*; *воен.* defénsive, cóvering; ~ аэроста́т bárrage ballóon; ~ ого́нь bárrage.

загради́ть *сов. см.* заграж||да́ть.

заграж||да́ть, загради́ть *(вн.)* block *(smth.)*. ~е́ние *с.* bárrier, block, obstrúction; *воен. тж.* bárrage; возду́шное ~е́ние ballóon-bárrage; ми́нное ~е́ние mínefield.

заграни́ца *ж. разг.* fóreign cóuntries *pl*, abróad.

заграни́чный fóreign; ~ па́спорт pássport for trávelling abróad; ~ това́р fóreign goods *pl*.

загреба́ть, загрести́ *(вн.) разг.* rake up *(smth.)*; *перен.* rake in *(smth.)*; ~ се́но rake up hay; ~ жар bank (up) the fire; ~ де́ньги make* heaps of móney, rake in the móney.

загребн||о́й *прил. мор.* 1. stroke *attr.*; ~о́е весло́ stróke-oar; 2. *в знач. сущ., м.* stroke; быть ~ы́м be* at stroke.

загреме́||ть I *сов. (начать греметь)* roar, rúmble; ~л гром the thúnder roared; ~ посу́дой make* a clátter with the dishes; его́ го́лос ~л на весь зал his voice resóunded through the hall.

загреме́ть II *сов. разг. (упасть)* fall* with a crash, come* down with a crash, crash to the floor.

загрести́ *сов. см.* загреба́ть.

загри́вок *м.* 1. *(у лошади)* withers *pl*; 2. *разг. (у человека)* nape of the neck.

загримирова́ть *сов. см.* гримирова́ть 2. ~ся *сов. см.* гримирова́ться.

загриппова́ть *сов. разг.* catch* the flu(e).

загробн||ый: ~ая жизнь life beyónd the grave; ~ мир the next world; ~ го́лос sepúlchral voice.

загроможда́ть, загромозди́ть *(вн.)* clútter up *(smth.)*; *перен.* overlóad *(smth.)*; ~ ко́мнату ме́белью clútter up a room with fúrniture; ~ что́-л. нену́жными подро́бностями búrden *smth.* with unnécessary détail.

загромозди́ть *сов. см.* загроможда́ть.

загрохота́ть *сов.* 1. *см.* грохота́ть; 2. *(начать грохотать)* begín* to ráttle/rúmble.

загрубе́л||ый 1. *(жёсткий)* cóarsened, cálloused; ~ые ру́ки cálloused/hórny hands; 2. *(ставший грубым)* rough; *(ставший чёрствым)* cállous, coarse.

загрубе́ть *сов.* cóarsen, becóme* cóarsened.

загружа́ть, загрузи́ть *(вн.)* 1. load *(smth.)*; по́лностью ~ что́-л. load *smth.* to capácity; ~ печь charge a fúrnace; 2. *разг. (обеспечивать работой)* keep* *(smb.)* búsy; ~ преподава́телей give* téachers a full prógramme; ~ рабо́чий день fill up *one's* day; он загру́жен рабо́той he has plénty of work, he has plénty to do.

загрузи́ть *сов. см.* загружа́ть.

загру́зк||а *ж.* 1. *(действие)* lóading, fílling; *(печи)* chárging; 2. *разг. (загруженность)* wórk-load; *(машин и т. п.)* charge, load; заво́д име́ет по́лную ~у the fáctory is wórking to full capácity.

загрунто́ванный: ~ холст prímed cánvas.

загрусти́ть *сов.* grow* sad; *(о пр.)* miss *(smb.)*.

загры́з||ть *сов. (вн.)* kill *(smth.)*; tear* *(smth.)* (to píeces); *перен. разг.* make* *smb.'s* life a hell; его́ ~ла тоска́ he is éating his heart out.

загрязн||е́ние *с.* sóiling; *(воды)* pollútion, contaminátion. ~и́ть(ся) *сов. см.* загрязня́ть(ся) *и* грязни́ть(ся).

загрязня́ть, загрязни́ть *(вн.)* soil *(smth.)*, make* *(smth.)* dirty; *(воду)* pollúte *(smth.)*, contáminate *(smth.)*. ~ся, загрязни́ться get* dírty, make* onesélf dírty.

ЗАГС *м.* (отде́л за́писи а́ктов гражда́нского состоя́ния) régistry óffice.

загуби́ть *сов. (вн.)* 1. *(погубить)* ruin *(smb.,*

smth.); 2. *разг. (истратить напрасно)* waste *(smth.)*; ◇ ~ чью́-л. жизнь ruin *smb.'s* life.

загуде́ть *сов. begín* to hoot.

загуля́ть *сов. разг.* go* on the spree.

загуля́ться *сов. разг. (долго гулять)* stay out wálking, stay out late.

загусте́ть *сов.* thícken.

зад *м.* 1. *(задняя часть)* back; rear; бить ~ом *(о лошади)* kick; поверну́ться к кому́-л. ~ом turn *one's* back on *smth.*; 2. *(седалище)* behínd, báckside; *(у животного)* rump; hind quárters *pl*.

задабривать, задо́брить *(вн.)* get* round *(smb.)*; *(уговаривать)* cajóle *(smb.)*, coax *(smb.)*.

задава́ть, зада́ть *(вн.)* give* *(smth.)*, set* *(smth.)*; ~ уро́к set* hómework; ~ зада́чу set* a próblem; что за́дано? what is the hómework?; ~ рабо́ту assign work; ~ пир give* a bánquet; ~ корм give* fódder; ◇ ~ вопро́с ask/put* a quéstion; я тебе́ зада́м! I'll give it to you! ~ся, зада́ться: ~ся це́лью сде́лать что́-л. set* onesélf the task of dóing *smth.*

задави́ть *сов. (вн.)* kill *(smb., smth.)*; *(автомобилем и т. п.)* run* *(smb., smth.)* óver, knock *(smb., smth.)* down.

зада́н||ие *с.* task, assígnment; *(плановое)* tárget; *(упражнение, урок)* task; рабо́тать по чьему́-л. ~ию work únder *smb.'s* órders; дома́шнее ~ hómework.

зада́ривать, задари́ть *(вн.)* 1. *(подносить много подарков)* lávish/heap gifts (upón); 2. *(подкупать)* bribe *(smb.)* with gifts.

задари́ть *сов. см.* зада́ривать.

зада́ром *разг. см.* да́ром.

зада́тки *мн.* ínborn quálities, ínstincts, potentiálities; у него́ хоро́шие ~ there's good stuff in him, he has the mákings.

зада́ток *м.* depósit; down páyment; дать ~ leave* a depósit.

зада́ть(ся) *сов. см.* задава́ть(ся).

зада́ч||а *ж.* 1. task; *(цель)* goal; боева́я ~ táctical task; cómbat míssion *амер.*; вы́полнить ~у cárry out a task, accómplish a task/míssion; поста́вить ~у set* a task; ста́вить ~у перед кем-л. brief *smb.*; поста́вить перед собо́й ~у (+ инф.) make* it *one's* aim (+ to inf), set* onesélf the task of (+ -ing); 2. *(упражнение)* próblem; *(арифметическая тж.)* sum; реша́ть ~у work on a próblem; реша́ть ~и do* sums; реши́ть ~у solve a próblem. ~ник *м.* book of (mathemátical) próblems.

задвига́ть *сов. begín* to move.

задвига́ть, задви́нуть *(вн.)* push 'smth.); *(о дверях, я́щиках)* close *(smth.)*.

задви́гаться *сов. begín* to move.

задви́ж||ка *ж.* bolt; *(маленькая)* catch; *mex.* slíde-valve; закры́ть дверь на ~ку bolt a door, put* a door on the catch. ~но́й slíding, slídable.

задви́нуть *сов. см.* задвига́ть.

задво́рк||и *мн.* báckyards, backs; *перен.* the back of beyónd; ◇ на ~ах in the báckground.

задева́ть I, заде́ть *(вн., за вн.)* *(касаться)* brush (agáinst); *(цепляться)* catch* *(smth.)*; пу́ля заде́ла кость the búllet grazed the bone; заде́ть за гвоздь catch* on a nail; заде́ть ного́й за ковёр catch* *one's* foot* in the cárpet, trip óver the cárpet; 2. *(волновать)* afféct *(smb.)*; *(обижать)* sting* *(smb.)*, wound *(smb.)*.

задева́ть II *сов. (вн.) разг. (затерять)* mislá́y* *(smth.)*.

заде́л *м.* 1. *(начатая работа)* start; 2. *(запас)* resérve, márgin.

заде́лать *сов. см.* заде́лывать.

заде́лка *ж.* pátching up, stópping up, séaling.

заде́лывать, заде́лать *(вн.)* patch up *(smth.)*, stop up *(smth.)*, seal *(smth.)*; ~ дверь wall up a door; ~ что́-л. доска́ми board up *smth.*; ~ что́-л. кирпичо́м brick up *smth.*; ~ пробо́ину fill up a hole, seal a hole.

задёргать I *сов.* (*вн.*) *разг.* (*измучить, утомить*) wear* (*smb.*) out, nag (*smb.*) to death.

задёргать II *сов.* (*начать дёргать*) begín* to pull; (*заболеть*) begín* to throb.

задёргивать, задёрнуть 1. (*вн.*) draw* (*smth.*); ~ занавéску draw* the cúrtain; 2. (*вн. тв.*; *закрывать чем-л.*) cóver (*smth.* with); mask (*smth.* with). ~ся, задёрнуться draw*, be* drawn.

задеревенéлый *разг.* numbed, stiff.

задеревенéть *сов. разг.* becóme* numb/stiff.

задержáние *с.* reténtion; *юр.* deténtion; ~ престýпника deténtion of a críminal.

задержáть(ся) *сов. см.* задéрживать(ся).

задéрживать, задержáть (*вн.*) 1. (*воспрепятствовать*) detáin (*smb.*), deláy (*smb., smth.*); impéde (*smth.*), check (*smth.*); *перен.* (*мешать чему-л.*) hold* up (*smth.*); меня задержáли I was deláyed/detáined; я вас дóлго не задержý I won't keep you long; ~ достáвку *чего-л.* hold* up (the) delívery of *smth.*; ~ протívника *воен.* deláy the énemy; 2. (*замедлять что-л.*) slow (*smth.*) down, retárd (*smth.*); ~ шагú slow one's steps/pace; ~ дыхáние hold* one's breath; 3. (*не выдавать вовремя*) withhóld* (*smth.*), deláy (*smth.*), keep* (*smth.*) back; ~ зарплáту fail to pay out sálaries/wáges on time, withhóld* sálaries/wáges; ~ уплáту дóлга get* ínto arréars; 4. (*арестовывать*) arrést (*smb.*), take* (*smb.*) in charge. ~ся, задержáться 1. be* deláyed, be* kept; (*намеренно*) línger; дóлго не задéрживайтесь! don't be long!; 2. (*затягиваться, откладываться*) lag, be* late.

задéржка *ж.* deláy; (*помеха*) sétback, hitch.

задёрнуть(ся) *сов. см.* задёргивать(ся).

задéть *сов. см.* задевáть I.

задúра *м. и ж. разг.* tease, búlly; tróuble-maker.

задирáть, задрáть (*вн.*) 1. *разг.* (*поднимать кверху*) lift (*smth.*), stick* up (*smth.*); ~ гóлову crane one's neck; 2. (*кожу, ноготь и т. п.*) scratch (*smth.*), tear* (*smth.*) off; 3. *тк. несов. разг.* (*дразнить*) tease (*smb.*); ◇ задрáть нос put* on airs.

задне|нёбный *лингв.* vélar. ~прохóдный *анат.* ánal. ~язы́чный *лингв.* vélar, back.

задн|ий back, rear; (*о конечностях*) hind; ~ee колесó rear wheel; ~яя ногá hind leg; ~ кармáн híp--pocket; ~ ход revérse; báckward móvement; идтú ~им хóдом back; move báckwards; (*о судне*) go* astérn; ~ прохóд *анат.* ánus; ~ ~яя мысль ultérior mótive; это бы́ло скáзано не без ~ей мы́сли that was not said withóut a púrpose; без ~их ног réady/fit to drop; ~им умóм крéпок wise áfter the evént; ~им числóм áfter the evént, in rétrospect; подписáть что-л. ~им числóм ántedáte *smth.*

задник *м.* 1. (*обуви*) back; 2. *театр.* báckdrop, báckcloth.

задóбрить *сов. см.* задáбривать.

задóлго long befóre; (*заранее*) well in advánce (of).

задолж|áть *сов.* be* in debt, get* ínto debt; он ~áл мне 100 рублéй he owes me a húndred róubles.

задóлженность *ж.* debts *pl*, indébtedness; (*по взносам и т. п.*) arréars *pl*; (*по выполнению заказов*) bácklog; академúческая ~ fáilure to take examinátions/tést-papers at the requíred time.

задóлжник *м. разг.* defáulter.

зáдом (*о движении*) báckwards; идтú ~ walk báckwards; ◇ ~ наперёд back to front.

задóр *м.* árdour, vígour, zeal; молодóй ~ yóuthful árdour. ~ный bold, lívely; (*бойкий*) pérky; ~ный мотúв lívely/róusing tune.

задохнýться *сов. см.* задыхáться.

задрáивать, задрáить (*вн.*) *мор.* bátten down (*smth.*).

задрáить *сов. см.* задрáивать.

задрáть *сов.* 1. *см.* задирáть 1, 2; 2. (*вн.*) (*растерзать*) kill (*smb., smth.*).

задремáть *сов.* doze off, fall* ínto a doze.

задрожáть *сов.* begín* to trémble; (*от холода*) begín* to shíver.

задувáть I, **задýть** (*вн.*; *гасить*) blow* out (*smth.*), extínguish (*smth.*), put* out (*smth.*).

задувáть II, **задýть** (*вн.*) *тех.* blow* in (*smth.*); задýть дóмну blow* in a blást-fúrnace.

задувáть III *несов.* 1. (*о ветре*) blow*; 2. (*проникать*) get* in, blow* in, cause a draught; 3. (*вн.*; *заносить дуновением*) blow* (*smth.*) in.

задýмать(ся) *сов. см.* задýмывать(ся).

задýмчив|ость *ж.* thóughtfulness, pénsiveness; в глубóкой ~ости in deep thought, in a réverie. ~ый thóughtful, pénsive; с ~ым вúдом with a thóughtful-/pénsive air.

задýмыв|ать, задýмать 1. (*вн.*, + *инф.*) think* (of, + -ing), plan (+ to *inf*), concéive (*smth.*); 2. (*вн.*; *мысленно выбирать что-л.*) think* of (*smth.*); задýмайте какóе-нибудь числó think of a númber. ~ться, задýматься 1. (*над тв. и пр.*) pónder (óver), brood (óver); о чём вы задýмались? what are you so thóughtful about?; 2. (*впадать в задýмчивость*) becóme* thóughtful, grow* pénsive, plunge ínto a réverie, be* drowned in thought; 3. (*колебаться*) hésitate; отвéтить не ~ясь ánswer without a móment's hesitátion.

задýть I, II *сов. см.* задувáть I, II.

задýть III *сов. разг.* (*начать дуть*) begín* to blow.

задушéвн|ость *ж.* sincérity, soul, féeling. ~ый (*о людях*) kind, génuine, sincére; (*о чувствах*) héartfelt; (*сокровенный*) íntimate; ~ый разговóр héart-to-héart talk.

задушúть *сов. см.* душúть I 1, 2.

зад|ы́ *мн.* 1. (*дворов*) the back (of the hóuses) *sg*; пробирáться ~áми go* round the back way; 2.: повторя́ть ~ go* óver old ground.

задымúть I *сов.* (*начать дымить*) begín* to smoke, begín* to emít/dischárge smoke, start bélching smoke.

задымúть II *сов.* (*вн.*; *закоптить дымом*) blácken (*smth.*) with soot; (*заполнять дымом*) fill (*smth.*) with smoke.

задымлённый smóky.

задыхáться, задохнýться (*от рд.*) choke (with); be* súffocated (by); (*от утомления*) be* out of breath; ~ от смéха choke with láughter.

заедáть, заéсть (*вн.*; *загрызать*) kill (*smb., smth.*); (*мучить укусами*) plague (*smb.*); нас заéли комары́ we were plagued by mosquítoes; 2. (*вн. тв.*; *закусывать*) eat* (*smth.* with) to take awáy the taste; 3. (*вн.*) *разг.* (*изводить*) get* (*smb.*) down; 4. (*вн.*; *пагубно влиять*) drag (*smb.*) down, corrúpt (*smb.*), demorálize (*smb.*); егó заéла средá he was corrúpted by his envíronment; 5. *обыкн. безл. разг.* (*застревать*) stick*, jam; 6. *обыкн. безл. разг.* (*задевать самолюбие*) get* on one's nerves.

заéзд *м.* 1. vísit; без ~a (в) without cálling/stópping (at); с ~ом (в) cálling/stópping (at); 2. *спорт.* heat; полуфинáльный ~ the semifínal; 3. (*приезд отдыхающих*) arríval.

заéздить *сов.* (*вн.*) *разг.* (*лошадь*) óverdrive* (*smth.*); *перен.* (*человека*) overwórk (*smb.*), óverdrive* (*smb.*).

заезжáть, заéхать 1. (*останавливаться по пути*) stop (at), break* one's jóurney (at); (*к дт.*; *посещать*) drop in (at smb.'s), look in (at smb.'s); 2. (*за тв.*) come* and fetch (*smb.*); 3. (*уезжать далеко или не туда, куда следует*) stray ínto; 4. (*подъезжать со стороны*) appróach; он заéхал с лéвой стороны́ he appróached from the left, he rode in from the left.

заéзженный *разг.* (*о лошади*) overwórked, óverdriven; *перен.* (*банальный*) háckneyed.

заёзжий *прил.* 1. vísiting; 2. *в знач. сущ. м.* pássing tráveller, pérson pássing through.

заём *м.* loan; вы́игрышный ~ lóttery loan; вне́шний ~ fóreign loan.

зае́сть *сов. см.* заеда́ть.

зае́хать *сов. см.* заезжа́ть.

зажа́ривать, зажа́рить (*вн.*) roast (*smth.*); (*на сковороде*) fry (*smth.*). ~ся, зажа́риться be* róasted; (*на сковороде*) be* fried.

зажа́рить(ся) *сов. см.* зажа́ривать(ся).

зажа́ть *сов. см.* зажима́ть.

зажд|а́ться *сов.* (*рд.*) *разг.* be* wáiting impátiently (for); мы вас ~али́сь! ≈ you've come at last!

заже́чь(ся) *сов. см.* зажига́ть(ся).

зажива́ть, зажи́ть heal.

зажива́ться, зажи́ться *разг.* live too long, live beyónd one's time.

заживи́ть *сов. см.* заживля́ть.

заживля́ть, заживи́ть (*вн.*) *разг.* heal (*smth.*).

за́живо alíve; ~ погребённый búried alíve.

зажига́|лка *ж.* (*для сигарет*) (cigarétte) líghter. ~ние *с.* 1. (*действие*) líghting; 2. *тех.* ignítion. ~тельный 1. igníting *attr.*; (*о снаряде, бомбе*) incéndiary; 2. (*возбуждающий*) róusing, stírring.

зажиг|а́ть, заже́чь (*вн.*) 1. light* (*smth.*); ~ свет (*электрический*) turn on the light; ~ спи́чку strike* a match; 2. (*вызвать подъём энергии и т. п.*) stir (*smb.*), fire (*smb.*), rouse (*smb.*). ~а́ться, заже́чься 1. light* up, be* lit; когда́ ~а́ются огни́ when the lights go on, when the lights are turned on; зажгла́сь спи́чка a match flared; 2. (*появляться*) come* out; зажгла́сь пе́рвая звезда́ the first star came out; 3. (*о глазах*) flare (with), blaze (with); её глаза́ зажгли́сь не́навистью hátred glíttered in her eyes; 4. (*возникать — о чувствах и т. п.*) blaze up, flame up; в его́ душе́ зажгло́сь вдохнове́ние he was fired with inspirátion.

зажи́м *м.* 1. (*приспособление*) clip; (*большой*) clamp; 2. (*стеснение, подавление*) restríction; ~ кри́тики restríction/suppréssion of críticism. ~а́ть, зажа́ть (*вн.*) 1. (*стискивать*) squeeze (*smth.*); grip (*smth.*), hold* (*smth.*) tight; ~а́ть что-л. в руке́ clasp *smth.* tíghtly in one's hand; 2. (*затыкать*) stop (*smth.*); ~а́ть нос hold* one's nose; ~а́ть у́ши stop one's ears; ~а́ть кому́-л. рот руко́й put* one's hand óver *smb.'s* mouth; *разг.* (*стеснять, подавлять*) restríct (*smth.*), suppréss (*smth.*), hámper (*smth.*); ~а́ть инициати́ву restríct initiative; ◇ зажа́ть рот *кому́-л.* sílence *smb.*, gag *smb.*

зажи́точн|ость *ж.* prospérity. ~ый wéll-to-dó, prósperous; ~ая жизнь prospérity.

зажи́ть I *сов. см.* зажива́ть.

зажи́ть II *сов.* (*начать жить*) begín* to live; ~ но́вой жи́знью begín* a new life.

зажи́ться *сов. см.* зажива́ться.

зажму́рить *сов.:* ~ глаза́ *см.* зажму́риться. ~ся *сов.* screw up one's eyes.

зажужжа́ть *сов.* begín* to buzz.

зазва́ть *сов. см.* зазыва́ть.

зазвене́ть *сов.* begín* to tínkle.

зазвон|и́ть *сов.* begín* to ring; (*о будильнике*) go* off; ~и́л телефо́н the télephone rang.

заздра́вный: ~ тост toast.

зазева́ться *сов.* (*на вн.*) *разг.* gape (at).

зазелене́ть *сов.* 1. (*стать зелёным*) turn green; 2. (*показаться — о чём-л. зелёном*) show* green.

заземл|е́ние *с.* 1. (*действие*) éarthing; 2. (*приспособление*) earth. ~и́ть *сов. см.* заземля́ть.

заземля́ть, заземли́ть (*вн.*) earth (*smth.*), ground (*smth.*).

зазнава́ться, зазна́ться *разг.* get* a swelled head, get* concéited, give* onesélf airs.

зазна́йство *с. разг.* concéit.

зазна́ться *сов. см.* зазнава́ться.

зазо́р *м. тех.* cléarance.

зазре́н|ие *с.:* без ~я (со́вести) shámelessly, without compúnction, without ány scrúples.

зазу́бренный I (*имеющий зазубрины*) notched.

зазу́бренный II *разг.* (*заученный*) párroted, mugged up.

зазу́бривать I, зазубри́ть (*вн.; делать зазубрины*) notch (*smth.*).

зазу́бривать II, зазубри́ть (*вн.*) *разг.* (*заучивать*) learn* (*smth.*) mechánically/párrot-fáshion, mug up (*smth.*).

зазу́брина *ж.* notch; с ~ми notched.

зазубри́ть I, II *сов. см.* зазу́бривать I, II.

зазыва́ть, зазва́ть (*вн.*) *разг.* press (*smb.*) to come.

заигра́нн|ый 1. (*ставший негодным*) worn, defáced; ~ая пласти́нка worn récord; 2. (*избитый*) háckneyed.

заигра́ть I *сов. см.* заи́грывать I.

заигра́ть II *сов.* (*начать играть*) begín* to play; (*об оркестре*) strike* up.

заигра́ться *сов. см.* заи́грываться.

заи́грывание *с. разг.* flírting, flirtátion.

заи́грывать I, заигра́ть (*вн.*) 1. (*приводить в негодность*) wear* out (*smth.*), deface (*smth.*); заигра́ть пласти́нку wear* out a récord, 2. (*опошлять*) make* (*smth.*) háckneyed, play (*smth.*) to death.

заи́грывать II *несов.* (*с тв.*) *разг.* 1. (*кокетничать*) make* advánces (to), flirt (with); 2. (*заискивать*) make* up (to).

заи́грываться, заигра́ться be* cárried awáy with one's game.

за́йка *м. и ж.* stámmerer, stútterer.

заик|а́ние *с.* stámmer(ing), stútter(ing). ~а́ться, заикну́ться 1. *тк. несов.* stámmer, stútter; си́льно ~а́ться have* a bad stámmer; 2. *разг.* (*запинаться на полуслове*) stop short; 3. (*о пр.*) *разг.* (*намекать*) breathe/útter a word (abóut), hint (at); он да́же не заикну́лся об э́том he did not so much as hint at it.

заикну́ться *сов. см.* заика́ться 2, 3.

заимообра́зно as a loan; брать что-л. ~ bórrow *smth.*

займствов|а́ние *с.* 1. adóption, bórrowing; 2. *лингв.* (*слово*) lóan-word. ~ать *несов. и сов.* (*вн.*) bórrow (*smth.*), adópt (*smth.*); ~ать о́пыт передовико́в bórrow from the expérience of advánced wórkers.

заиндеве́|вший ríme-covered, frósted; cóvered with hóarfrost *после сущ.* ~ть *сов.* be* cóvered with rime/hóarfrost.

заинтересо́ванн|ость *ж.* ínterest; материа́льная ~ matérial ínterest/incéntive. ~ый ínterested; ~ые ли́ца péople with ínterests at stake; ~ые сто́роны the párties concérned; быть ~ым в чём-л. have* an ínterest/stake in *smth.*

заинтересова́ть *сов.* (*вн. тв.*) ínterest (*smb.* in); ~ кого́-л. расска́зом win*/gain *smb.'s* atténtion with a stóry. ~ся *сов.* (*тв.*) becóme/get* ínterested (in), take* an ínterest (in).

заинтригова́ть *сов. см.* интригова́ть 2.

заи́скив|ать (*перед тв.*) try to ingrátiate onesélf (with), cúrry fávour (with). ~ающий ingrátiating.

заи́скриться *сов.* begín* to spárkle.

зайти́ *сов. см.* заходи́ть.

за́йч|иха *ж.* dóe-hare. ~о́нок *м.* young hare.

закаба́л|е́ние *с.* enslávement. ~и́ть(ся) *сов. см.* закабаля́ть(ся).

закабаля́ть, закабали́ть (*вн.*) ensláve (*smb.*). ~ся, закаба́литься tie onesélf down.

закавка́зский Tráns-Caucásian.

закады́чный *разг.:* ~ друг, прия́тель bósom friend.

зака́з *м.* 1. órder; отде́л ~ов delívery-órder depártment; 2. *разг.* (*заказанная вещь*) órder, job; ваш

~ ужé готóв your órder is réady; ◇ на ~ to órder; по ~y to órder; custom-made; не могý писáть по ~y I can't write to órder.

заказáть *сов. см.* закáзывать.

заказн|óй régistered; послáть письмó ~ым send* a létter by régistered post, régister a létter.

заказч|ик *м.*, ~ица *ж.* cústomer.

закáзывать, заказáть (*вн.*) órder (*smth.*), book (*smth.*); ~ билéт book a tícket.

закалённый 1. hárdened; 2. (*обладающий выдержкой*) séasoned, tóughened, wéll-tríed; 3. (*крепкий, выносливый*) trained; in good tráining *после сущ.*

закáливать(ся) *несов. см.* закалять(ся).

закалить(ся) *сов. см.* закалять(ся).

закáл|ка *ж.* 1. hárdening, témpering; 2. (*физическая*) tráining; получáть ~ку get* ínto good tráining, get* fit; 3. (*выдержка, стойкость*) trained endúrance, acquíred tóughness.

закáлывать, заколóть (*вн.*) 1. (*убивать*) stab (*smb.*); (*животных*) sláughter (*smth.*); 2. (*закреплять*) pin up (*smth.*), fásten (*smth.*) with a pin; ~ вóлосы pin up *one's* hair.

закалять, закалить (*вн.*) 1. (*путём нагрева*) hárden (*smth.*), témper (*smth.*); ~ сталь témper/hárden steel; 2. (*делать выносливым*) steel (*smb., smth.*); ~ вóлю steel *one's* will; закалённый в бою́ báttle-hárdened, steeled in báttle; 3. (*делать физически крепким*) train (*smb.*). ~ся, закалиться 1. (*о стали*) be* hárdened/témpered; 2. (*делаться выносливым*) make* oneself fit, impróve *one's* endúrance; *сов. тж.* get* fit.

закáнчивать, закóнчить (*вн.*) end (*smth.*), fínish (*smth.*); (*завершать*) compléte (*smth.*); (*отделывать*) put* the fínishing tóuches (to), round off (*smth.*); ~ речь, письмó conclúde a speech, a létter. ~ся, закóнчиться 1. come* to its close; 2. *тк. несов.* (*тв.*) end (in, with), términate (in).

закáпать I *сов.* (*вн.*) 1. (*забрызгать*) spot (*smth.*); ~ стол черни́лами spot the táble with ink; 2. *разг.* (*лекарство и т. п.*) put* (a few) drops (of).

закáп|ать II *сов.* (*начать капать*) begín* to drip; слёзы ~али из глаз the tears begán to flow.

закáпывать, закопáть (*вн.*) 1. búry (*smb., smth.*); (*прятать*) hide* (*smth.*); 2. (*заполнять землёй*) fill in (*smth.*); ~ яму fill in a hole/pit. ~ся, закопáться búry oneself; (*о войсках*) entrénch oneself, dig* oneself in.

закáрмливать, закормить (*вн.*) óverféed* (*smb., smth.*), stuff (*smb., smth.*).

закáт *м.* (*солнца*) súnset; *перен.* declíne; ◇ на ~е дней in the évening of life.

закáтать *сов. см.* закáтывать II.

закатить *сов. см.* закáтывать I.

закатиться *сов. см.* закáтываться.

закáтывать I, закатить (*вн.*) 1. roll (*smth.*); 2. *разг.* (*устраивать*): ~ скандáл make* a scene; ◇ закатить глазá roll *one's* eyes.

закáтывать II, закатáть (*вн. в вн.; обёртывать, обматывать*) roll up (*smth.* in); wrap up (*smth.* in); ~ рукавá roll up *one's* sleeves.

закáтываться, закатиться 1. roll; 2. (*о солнце*) set*, go* down.

закáч|ать I *сов.* (*вн.*) 1. rock (*smb.*) to sleep; 2. (*вызвать головокружение*) make* (*smb.*) sick; егó ~áло the rócking has made him sick.

закачáть II *сов.* (*начать качать*) begín* to rock/sway.

закáшл|ять *сов.* begín* to cough. ~яться *сов.* have* a fit of cóughing; я ~ялся от ды́ма the smoke made me cough.

заквáска *ж.* léaven; *перен.* strain, stock; (*плохая тж.*) taint, streak.

заквáшивать(ся) *несов. см.* квáсить(ся).

закидáть *сов. см.* закидывать I.

закидывать I, закидáть (*вн. тв.*) *разг.* scátter (*smb., smth.* with), strew* (*smb., smth.* with); (*снегом, грязью и т. п.*) pláster (*smb., smth.* with), bespátter (*smb., smth.* with); pelt (*smb., smth.* with); *перен.* bombárd (*smb.* with), shówer (*smb.* with); закидáть вопрóсами bombárd with quéstions.

закидывать II, закинуть 1. *см.* забрáсывать II; 2.: ~ гóлову throw* back *one's* head; ~ нóгу нá ногу put* *one's* leg óver *one's* knee; ~ рýки зá голову put* *one's* hands behínd *one's* head; ◇ ~ ýдочку cast* a line; *перен.* put* out a féeler.

закинуть *сов. см.* закидывать II.

закипáть, закипéть begín* to boil; boil; *перен.* seethe; водá закипéла the wáter is bóiling; рабóта закипéла work is in full swing, the job got únder way.

закипéть *сов. см.* закипáть.

зáкись *ж. хим.* protóxide.

заклáдка *ж.* 1. (*действие*) láying; ~ гóрода fóunding of a city; ~ кораблá láying of a ship's keel; ~ силоса fílling of a sílo; ~ сáда máking of a gárden; 2. (*в книге*) bóok-mark.

закладнáя *ж. юр.* mórtgage.

заклáдывать, заложить 1. (*вн.; засовывать, класть*) put* (*smth.*); (*терять*) misláy* (*smth.*); (*помещать куда-л. с какой-л. целью*) lay* (*smth.*), set* (*smth.*); ~ мины lay* mines; 2. (*вн.; основывать*) lay* (*smth.*); ~ фундáмент lay* the foundátions; ~ корáбль lay* a ship's keel; заложить нóвый гóрод found a new town/city; 3. (*вн. тв.; заполнять чем-л.*) stop (*smth.* with), block up (*smth.* with); заложить дымохóды кирпичóм brick up the chímneys; заложить стол книгами pile a táble with books; 4.: ~ лошадéй hárness hórses; 5. (*вн.; отдавать в залог — вещи*) pawn (*smth.*); (*недвижимость*) mórtgage (*smth.*); ~ заложить осно́ву чего-л. lay* the foundátion of *smth.*

заклевáть I *сов.* (*вн.*) peck (*smb., smth.*) to death; *перен. разг.* pérsecute (*smb.*), búlly the life out (of).

заклевáть II *сов.* (*начать клевать*) begín* to peck.

заклéивать, заклéить (*вн.*) stick* (*smth.*); (*запечатывать*) seal (*smth.*); ~ конвéрт stick* down an énvelope, seal an énvelope; ~ окóнные рáмы seal the window-frames; ~ся, заклéиться stick*.

заклéить(ся) *сов. см.* заклéивать(ся).

заклеймить *сов. см.* клеймить.

заклепáть *сов. см.* заклёпывать.

заклёпка *ж.* 1. (*действие*) ríveting; 2. (*металлический стержень*) rívet.

заклёпывать, заклепáть (*вн.*) rívet (*smth.*).

заклин|áние *с.* 1. charm, spell; (*слова тж.*) incantátion; 2. (*мольба, просьба*) conjurátion, entréaty. ~áть *несов.* 1. (*вн.; заколдовывать*) charm (*smb., smth.*), bewítch (*smb., smth.*); 2. (*вн. + инф.; умолять, просить*) entréat (*smb.* + to *inf*), implóre (*smb.* + to *inf.*).

заклинивать, заклинить (*вн.*) 1. (*вбивать клин*) drive*/fix a wedge (ínto); 2. (*повреждать*) jam.

заклинить *сов. см.* заклинивать.

заключáть, заключить 1. *тк. несов.* (*вн.; содержать*) contáin (*smth.*); 2. (*вн.; лишать свободы*) lock up (*smb.*), confíne (*smb.*); ~ когó-л. в тюрьмý imprison (*smb.*), gaol (*smb.*); 3. (*вн. в вн.; помещать*) put* (*smth.* in), enclóse (*smth.* in); ~ что-л. в скóбки put* *smth.* in bráckets; 4. (*вн. тв.; заканчивать*) conclúde (*smth.* with), end (*smth.* with); 5. (*делать вывод*) conclúde, dedúce; 6. (*вн.; вступать в соглашение*) conclúde (*smth.*); заключить мир make* peace; заключить сою́з form an alliance; ~ соглашéние, договóр conclúde an agréement, a tréaty; ~ся *несов.* 1. (*в пр.; находиться*) be* (in), be* contáined (in); 2. (в *пр.; содержаться*) be* (in); lie* (in), consíst (in); **3.** (*тв.; заканчиваться*) end (in); conclúde (with, in).

заключéни|е *с.* **1.** (*соглашения и т. п.*) conclúsion; ~ договóра the conclúsion of a tréaty; ~ сою́за the fórming of an allíance; ~ мира conclúsion of peace, sígning a peace tréaty; **2.** (*лишение свободы*) confínement; одинóчное ~ sólitary confínement; находи́ться в ~и be* in prison; **3.** (*вывод*) conclúsion, dedúction, ínference; **4.** (*конец чего-л.*) conclúsion, end; ◇ в ~ in conclúsion.

заключённый *м.* prísoner; (*осуждённый*) cónvict.

заключи́тельн|ый clósing, fínal; ~ое слóво conclúding speech, súmming up; ~ая часть рéчи perorátion; ~ая сцéна *театр.* last/fínal scene.

заключи́ть *сов. см.* заключáть 2, 3, 4, 5, 6.

закля́тый irréconcilable; ~ враг sworn énemy.

заковáть *сов. см.* закóвывать.

закóвывать, заковáть (*вн.*) chain (smb.), scháckle (smb.), fétter (smb.); *перен.* lock (smth.) fast, hold* (smth.) fast, imprison (smth.); ~ когó-л. в кандалы́ scháckle smb.; chain smb., put* smb. in írons.

закоди́рованный códed, encóded.

заколáчивать, заколоти́ть (*вн.*) *разг.* **1.** nail down (smth.); ~ дом board up the windows and doors of a house; **2.** (*избивать*) beat* (smth.).

заколдóванный charmed, enchánted; ◇ ~ круг vícious círcle.

заколдовáть *сов. см.* заколдóвывать.

заколдóвывать, заколдовáть (*вн.*) cast* a spell (óver).

закóлка *ж. разг.* kírby-grip, slide.

заколоти́ть I *сов. см.* заколáчивать.

заколот|и́ть II *сов.* (в *вн.; начать колотить*) start knócking (at); в дверь ~и́ли there was/came a sharp knócking at the door.

заколóть I *сов. см.* закáлывать.

заколó|ть II *сов. безл.* (*начать колоть*): у меня ~ло в боку́ I have the stitch.

закóн *м.* law; дéйствующие ~ы the law(s) in force; объяви́ть, постáвить *когó-л.* вне ~а óutlaw smb.; ~ сохранéния энéргии the law of the conservátion of énergy.

закóнн|ость *ж.* **1.** legálity; láwfulness, legítimacy; ~ докумéнта legálity of a dócument; **2.** (*общественная деятельность в соответствии с законами*) legálity, rule of law; укрепля́ть ~ stréngthen legálity. ~ый **1.** légal, láwful, legítimate; ~ый докумéнт légal dócument; ~ый владéлец láwful ówner; **2.** (*справедливый, обоснованный*) legítimate, nátural; ~ое трéбование legítimate demánd; ~ое возмущéние nátural indignátion; ◇ ~ый брак láwful wédlock.

законовéд *м.* júrist. ~ение *с.* júrisprudence.

законодáтель *м.* législator, láwgiver, láwmaker; *перен.* árbiter; ~ мод árbiter of fáshion; ~ный láwmaking, législative; ~ная власть législative pówer. ~ство *с.* legislátion.

закономéрн|о nórmally; развивáться ~ devélop in confórmity to/with cértain laws. ~ость *ж.* láw-góverned náture, (objéctive) regulárity; law; ~ость развития óбщества the láw-góverned náture of sócial devélopment; ~ости поведéния behávioural pátterns. ~ый láw-góverned; (*естественный*) nátural, régular, nórmal; ~ое явлéние natural phenómenon; истóрия как ~ый процéсс history as a prócess góverned by cértain laws; э́то вполнé ~о that's quite in the order of things, that's quite nórmal.

законопáтить *сов. см.* законопáчивать.

законопáчивать, законопáтить (*вн.*) caulk (smth.).

законопроéкт *м.* bill, draft law.

законсерви́ровать *сов.* (*вн.*) **1.** (*продукт*) presérve (smth.); (*в жестяных банках*) tin (smth.); can (smth.) *амер.* **2.** (*предприятие и т. п.*) lay* up (smth.).

законспекти́ровать *сов.* (*вн.*) make* a synópsis (of).

законтрактовáть *сов.* (*вн.*) make*/have* a cóntract (for). ~ся *сов.* contráct, put* onesélf únder cóntract.

закóнч|енный **1.** compléted, compléte; **2.** (*достигший совершенства*) cónsummate, accómplished. ~ить *сов. см.* закáнчивать. ~иться *сов. см.* закáнчиваться I.

закопáть(ся) *сов. см.* закáпывать(ся).

закоптéлый sóot-covered, sóoty, smóke-blackened.

закопти́ть I *сов.* (*вн.*) **1.** (*покрыть копотью*) blácken (smth.) with soot; **2.** (*приготовить копчением*) smoke (smth.).

закопти́ть II *сов.* (*начать коптить*) begín* to smoke.

закопти́ться *сов.* **1.** (*покрыться копотью*) be* cóvered/thick with soot; **2.** (*о рыбе, мясе*) be* well smoked.

закопчённый sóoty; thick with soot *после сущ.*

закоренéлый 1. (*укоренившийся*) invéterate, deep-séated, deep-róoted; **2.** (*упорный, неисправимый*) hárdened, invéterate, confírmed.

закоренéть *сов.* **1.** (*укорениться*) becóme* deep-séated, take* deep root; **2.** (в *пр.; стать упорным*) be*/becóme* confírmed (in); ~ в предрассу́дках be* steeped in préjudice.

закóрк|и *разг.* shóulders; на ~ах on one's shóulders.

закорми́ть *сов. см.* закáрмливать.

закорю́чка *ж. разг.* **1.** (*почерка*) flóurish, hook; **2.** (*трудность*) snag.

закоснéл|ый 1. (*застарелый*) invéterate; ~ое невéжество rank ígnorance; **2.** (*неисправимый*) hárdened, invéterate.

закоу́лок *м.* **1.** (*глухой переулок*) back street; **2.** (*потайной уголок*) nook, cránny.

закоченéлый numb (with cold), frózen stiff.

закоченéть *сов. см.* коченéть.

закрáдываться, закрáсться steal*; в егó ду́шу закрáлось подозрéние a suspícion crept ínto his mind.

закрáшивать *сов. см.* закрáшивать.

закрáсться *сов. см.* закрáдываться.

закрáшивать, закрáсить (*вн.*) paint (smth.), cóver (smth.) with paint, paint (smth.) óver.

закрепи́тель *м. фото* fíxing ágent.

закрепи́ть(ся) *сов. см.* закрепля́ть(ся).

закрéпка *ж.* clip, fástener.

закрепля́ть, закрепи́ть 1. (*вн.*) secúre (smth.), fásten (smth.), fix (smth.); **2.** (*вн.* за *тв.; обеспечивать права на когó-л., что-л.*) attách (smb. to); assign (smth. to); **3.** (*вн.; упрочивать*) consólidate (smth.); *воен. тж.* reinfórce (smth.); ~ побéду consólidate a víctory; ~ успéх consólidate a succéss; fóllow up a succéss; **4.** (*вн.*) *фото* fix (smth.); **5.** (*вн.; желудок*) stéady (smth.), bind* (smth.). ~ся, закрепи́ться **1.** (*принимать устойчивое положение*) hold* firm; **2.** (*упрочиваться*) take* root; **3.** *воен.* mount defénces, dig* in; ~ся на захвáченной пози́ции consólidate the position.

закрепости́ть *сов. см.* закрепощáть.

закрепощáть, закрепости́ть (*вн.*) ensláve (smb.).

закричáть *сов.* **1.** (*издать крик*) cry out, shout; give* a cry; **2.** (*начать кричать*) begín* to shout.

закрóйщ|ик *м.*, ~**ица** *ж.* cútter.

закрóм *м.* bin, córn-bin.

закругл|éние *с.* **1.** (*действие*) róunding off; **2.** (*изгиб*) curve. ~ённый róunded. ~и́ть(ся) *сов. см.* закругля́ть(ся).

закругля́ть, закругли́ть (*вн.*) make* (smth.) round; round (smth.); *перен.* round off (smth.). ~ся, закругли́ться becóme*/grow* round; (*о пути*) curve.

закружи́ть I *сов.* (*вн.*) whirl (smb.); ~ когó-л. в тáнце make* smb. dízzy with dáncing.

закружи́ть II *сов.* (*начать кружить*) begín* to whirl/spin.

закружи́ться I *сов.* whirl round; *перен. разг.* be* in a whirl, be* in a spin.

закруж|и́ться II *сов.* (*начать кружиться*) begin* to whirl, begin* to spin; у меня́ ~и́лась голова́ my head is going round, I'm dizzy.

закрути́ть *сов. см.* закру́чивать.

закру́чивать, закрути́ть (*вн.*) 1. twist (*smth.*); закрути́ть ус twirl *one's* moustáche; 2. *разг.* (*завинчивать*) tíghten (*smth.*) up, make* (*smth.*) tight.

закрыва́ть, закры́ть (*вн.*) 1. (*делать недоступным*) shut* (*smth.*), close (*smth.*); ~ шкаф close a cúpboard; ~ дверь close/shut* a door; ~ грани́цу close the fróntier; ~ путь bar the way; 2. (*покрывать*) cóver (*smb., smth.*); shield (*smth.*); ~ что-л. кры́шкой put* the lid on *smth.*; ~ что-л. от со́лнца shield *smth.* from the sun; 3. (*складывать, смыкать*) close (*smth.*), shut* (*smth.*); ~ глаза́ close *one's* eyes; ~ зо́нтик let* down *one's* umbrélla; 4. (*запирать*) lock (*smb., smth.*) in; shut* (*smb.*) in; ~ дете́й в ко́мнате shut* children in a room; 5. (*прекращать действие*) turn (*smth.*) off, shut* (*smth.*) off; ~ газ turn off the gas; 6. (*прерывать деятельность*) close down (*smth.*); ~ заво́д close down a fáctory; ~ собра́ние decláre a méeting closed; ◇ ~ глаза́ на что-л. shut* *one's* eyes to *smth.*, blink at *smth.*; ~ счёт close an accóunt; закры́ть рот кому́-л. stop *smb.'s* mouth. ~ся, закры́ться 1. shut*, close; (*о сезоне*) come* to an end, come* to its close; 2. (*тж.; укрываться, накрываться*) wrap/cóver onesélf up (in); (*от рд.; защищаться*) protéct/shield onesélf (*from*); 3. (*оставаться в помещении*) shut* onesélf up in; 4. (*прекращать деятельность*) close down; (*о собрании*) end, come* to an end.

закры́т|ие *с.* clósing, close; ~ театра́льного сезо́на the close/end of the théatre séason; вре́мя ~ия магази́нов shop clósing-time. ~ый closed; ~ое пла́тье high-nécked dress; ~ое заседа́ние closed méeting; (*съезда и т. п.*) closed/private/sécret séssion; ~ое уче́бное заведе́ние private school; ~ый просмо́тр private view; ~ое голосова́ние sécret bállot; в ~ом помеще́нии indóors; ~ое мо́ре ínland sea.

закры́ть(ся) *сов. см.* закрыва́ть(ся).

закули́сн|ый báckstage *attr.; перен.* báckstáirs, clándestine; ~ые перегово́ры clándestine negotiátions.

закупа́ть, закупи́ть (*вн.*) buy* a stock (of).

закупи́ть *сов. см.* закупа́ть.

заку́пка *ж.* búying a stock, bulk púrchase.

заку́пор|ивать, заку́порить (*вн.*) stópper up (*smth.*); (*пробкой*) cork (*smth.*). ~ить *сов. см.* заку́поривать. ~ка *ж.* 1. córking, plúgging; 2. *мед.* obstrúction; ~ка вен vénous thrombósis.

заку́п|очный púrchasing; ~очная цена́ (Státe) púrchase price. ~щик *м.* whólesale púrchaser/búyer.

закури́в|ать, закури́ть (*вн.*) light* up (*smth.*); ~ папиро́су, тру́бку light* a cigarétte, a pipe; закури́м! shall we light up?, let's have a smoke!; разреши́те закури́ть? do you mind if I smoke? ~а́ться, закури́ться light*; папиро́са не ~а́ется the cigarétte won't light.

закури́ть *сов.* 1. *см.* закури́вать; 2. (*начать курить*) begin* to smoke. ~ся *сов.* 1. *см.* закури́ваться; 2. (*начать куриться*) begin* to smoke.

закуса́ть *сов.* (*вн.*) *разг.* maul (*smb.*), bite* (*smth.*) to death.

закуси́ть I, II *сов. см.* заку́сывать I, II.

заку́с|ка *ж.* sávouries *pl*, snacks *pl*; (*перед обедом*) hors d'oeuvres *pl*, áppetizers *pl*, stárters *pl*; ◇ на ~ку as a (final) tídbit. ~очная *ж.* lunch cóunter, snack bar.

заку́сывать I, **закуси́ть** 1. (*есть немного, наскоро*) have* a snack, have* a bite; закуси́ть на ско́рую ру́ку have* a quick snack; 2. (*вн. тж.; заедать*) eat* (*smth.* with); 3. *разг.* (*перед обедом*) have* the hors d'oeuvres.

заку́сывать II, **закуси́ть** (*вн.*) (*захватывать зубами*) bite* (*smth.*); ~ гу́бу bite* *one's* lip; ◇ закуси́ть удила́ take* the bit betwéen *one's* teeth; *перен. тж.* be* well awáy; прикуси́ть язы́к stop short.

заку́танный múffled.

заку́тать(ся) *сов. см.* заку́тывать(ся).

заку́ток *м. разг.* nook, córner.

заку́тывать, заку́тать (*вн.*) wrap up (*smb., smth.*), múffle (*smb., smth.*). ~ся, заку́таться wrap onesélf up, múffle onesélf up.

зал *м.* 1. (*помещение*) hall; (*танцевальный*) báll-room; ~ заседа́ний суда́ cóurt-room; ~ ожида́ния wáiting-room; 2. (*в частном доме*) dráwing-room.

залá́д|ить *сов. разг.* 1. (*повторять одно и то же*) repéat the same thing óver and óver agáin; 2. (+ *инф.; делать одно и то же*) take* to (+ -ing); он ~ил ка́ждый день ходи́ть в кино́ he took to góing to the cínema évery day.

залáмывать, заломи́ть (*вн.*) *разг.* charge up (*smth.*); ~ це́ну jack up the price; ◇ ~ ша́пку cock *one's* hat; заломи́ть ру́ки wring* *one's* hands; заломи́ть ру́ки за спи́ну twist *one's* arms behínd *one's* back.

заласка́ть *сов.* (*вн.*) *разг.* smóther (*smb.*) with carésses.

залата́ть *сов. см.* лата́ть.

заля́ть *сов.* begin* to bark.

залег|а́ние *с. геол.* occúrrence. ~а́ть *несов. геол.* lie*; пласт ~а́ет на глубине́ 25 ме́тров the seam lies 25 métres down.

заледене́лый 1. (*покрывшийся льдом*) íced-up; 2. (*холодный*) ícy.

заледене́ть *сов.* 1. (*покрыться льдом*) be* cóvered with ice; 2. (*закоченеть*) freeze*.

залежа́лый *разг.* lóng-képt; stale; ~ това́р old stock; (*о продуктах питания*) stale goods *pl*.

залежа́ться *сов. см.* зале́живаться.

зале́живаться, залежа́ться be* kept a long time, lie* a long time; пи́сьма залежа́лись на по́чте the létters got deláyed in the post; э́тот това́р не залежи́тся these goods won't lie long on the shelves.

за́лежн|ый long-fállow; ~ые зе́мли long-fállow land *sg.*

за́лежь *ж.* 1. (*месторождение*) depósit; 2. *мн.* (*завал*) accumulátions; 3. *с.-х.* long-fállow land, abándoned land.

залеза́ть, зале́зть 1. (*на вн.; взбираться*) climb (on to); (*на дерево и т. п.*) climb (*smth.*); зале́зть на кры́шу climb on to the roof; 2. (*в вн.; прятаться*) creep* (ínto); зале́зть в кана́ву creep* ínto a ditch; 3. (*в вн.; проникать куда-л.*) get* (ínto); во́ры зале́зли в дом thieves got ínto the house; 4. (*в вн.; забираться рукой*) put* *one's* hand (ínto); ~ кому́-л. в карма́н put*/slip *one's* hand into *smb.'s* pócket; ◇ зале́зть кому́-л. в ду́шу intrúde on *smb.'s* féelings.

зале́зть *сов. см.* залеза́ть.

залепи́ть *сов. см.* залепля́ть.

залепля́ть, залепи́ть (*вн. тв.*) 1. (*заделывать*) paste up (*smth.* with), stick* up (*smth.* with), plug (*smth.* with); 2. (*облеплять*) pláster (*smth.* with); ~ сте́ну объявле́ниями stick* nótices all óver the wall.

залета́ть, залете́ть 1. (*в вн.; влетать куда-л.*) get* (ínto), fly* (ínto); (*о брошенном*) fall* (ínto); 2. (*подниматься высоко*) soar, fly* high.

залете́ть *сов. см.* залета́ть.

залётн|ый ~ая пти́ца bird of pássage.

залечи́вать, залечи́ть (*вн.*) 1. heal (*smth.*); 2. *разг.* dóctor (*smb.*) to death. ~ся, залечи́ться heal.

залечи́ть(ся) *сов. см.* залечи́вать(ся).

зале́чь *сов.* 1. lie* down; ~ в берло́гу take* to its den; 2. *воен.* drop flat, take* cóver; (*занимать позицию*) take* up *one's* position.

зали́в *м.* (*глубоко вдающийся*) gulf; (*открытый*) bay.

залива́ть, зали́ть 1. (*вн., затоплять, покрывать*) flood (*smth.*) (*тж. перен.*); overflów (*smth.*); (*судно и т. п.*) swamp (*smth.*); ~ све́том flood with light; ко́мната была́ залита́ со́лнцем the room was bathed in súnlight; кра́ска залила́ её лицо́ the cólour flew ínto her cheeks; лицо́ её бы́ло за́лито слеза́ми her face was wet with tears; **2.** (*вн. тв.; обливать*) pour (*smth. óver*); (*нечаянно*) spill* (*smth.* on); ~ что-л. со́усом pour sauce óver *smth.*; **3.** (*вн.; тушить*) put* out (*smth.*); extínguish (*smth.*); ~ пожа́р put* out a fire; **4.** (*вн. тв.; покрывать чем-л. жидким*) cóat (*smth.* with); ~ что-л. асфа́льтом ásphalt *smth.*

залив|а́ться I, зали́ться 1. (*тв.; покрываться водой*) be* flóoded (with); **2.** (*проникать*) tríckle; вода́ ~а́ется за воротни́к wáter is trickling down one's neck.

залива́ться II, зали́ться: зали́ться ла́ем (begin* to) bark víolently; ~ сме́хом rock with láughter; зали́ться пе́сней burst* ínto song; зали́ться пла́чем, сме́хом burst* out crýing, laughing.

заливно́е *с. кул.* jélly.

заливн|о́й 1.: ~ луг wáter-meadow; **2.** (*о кушанье*) jéllied.

зали́занный sleek, sléeked-down.

зализа́ть *сов. см.* зали́зывать.

зали́зывать, зализа́ть (*вн.*) **1.** (*лизаньем очищать*) lick (*smth.*) clean; **2.** *разг.* (*гладко причёсывать*) sleek down (*smth.*).

зали́ть *сов. см.* залива́ть.

зали́ться I, II *сов. см.* залива́ться I, II.

залихва́тск|ий *разг.* bóisterous, róllicking; ~ вид dévil-may-cáre appéarance; jáunty air; ~ая пе́сня róllicking song.

зало́г I *м.* **1.** (*вещей*) páwning; (*недвижимости*) mórtgaging; под ~ чего́-л. on the secúrity of *smth.*; **2.** (*заложенная вещь*) guarantée, secúrity; **3.** (*свидетельство чего-л.*) guarantée, pledge, wárrant; ~ дру́жбы pledge of fríendship.

зало́г II *м. грам.* voice.

заложи́ть *сов. см.* закла́дывать.

заложн|ик *м.*, ~ица *ж.* hóstage.

заломи́ть *сов. см.* зала́мывать.

залп *м.* vólley; (*орудийный*) sálvo; дать ~ fire a vólley.

за́лпом 1. in a vólley; вы́стрелить ~ fire a vólley; **2.** *разг.:* вы́пить что-л. ~ drink* *smth.* at a gulp; сказа́ть всё ~ blurt out éverything.

залуча́ть, залучи́ть (*вн.*) *разг.* entíce (*smb., smth.*); залучи́ть кого́-л. в го́сти entíce *smb.* to pay one a vísit.

залучи́ть *сов. см.* залуча́ть.

залюбова́ться (*тв.*) gaze with admirátion (at); be* lost in admirátion (of); éю мо́жно ~ one could look at her for éver.

зама́зать(ся) *сов. см.* зама́зывать(ся).

зама́зка *ж.* pútty.

зама́зывать, зама́зать (*вн.*) **1.** (*краской и т. п.*) paint (*smth.*) out; **2.** *разг.* (*умышленно скрывать*) gloss (*smth.*) óver, cóver up (*smth.*); ~ недоста́тки cóver up defécts; **3.** (*залеплять*) seal (*smth.*), fill up (*smth.*); ~ о́кна seal wíndows; ~ щель fill up a crévice; **4.** (*пачкать*) dírty (*smth.*), get* (*smth.*) dírty; make* a mess (of). ~ся, зама́заться get* onesélf dírty.

зама́лчивать, замолча́ть (*вн.*) *разг.* hush up (*smth.*), gloss óver (*smth.*).

зама́нивать, замани́ть (*вн.*) lure (*smth.*); (*противника*) draw* (*smb.*) on; замани́ть кого́-л. в лову́шку entráp *smb.*

замани́ть *сов. см.* зама́нивать.

зама́нчивый témpting, allúring.

замара́ть *сов. см.* мара́ть 1. ~ся *сов. см.* мара́ться.

замара́шка *м. и ж. разг.* slóven; (*о детях*) dírty little píggy.

замаринова́ть *сов. см.* маринова́ть.

замаскиро́ванный disguísed, cámouflaged.

замаскирова́ть(ся) *сов. см.* маскирова́ть(ся).

зама́сленный gréase-stained, gréasy.

зама́тывать, замота́ть (*вн.*) *разг.* wind* (*smth.*). ~ся, замота́ться **1.** be* wound up; **2.** *разг.* (*уставать*) be* worn out.

замаха́ть *сов.* begín* to wave.

зама́хиваться, замахну́ться (*на вн.*) make* as if to stríke (*smb.*); ~ кулако́м draw* back one's fist; ~ па́лкой на кого́-л. brándish a stick at *smb.*

замахну́ться *сов. см.* зама́хиваться.

зама́чивать, замочи́ть (*вн.*) **1.** wet (*smb., smth.*); не замочи́в ног without gétting one's feet wet; **2.** (*опускать в жидкость*) steep (*smth.*), soak (*smth.*).

зама́шки *мн. разг.* ways.

замедле́ни|е *с.* **1.** (*хода*) slówing down, decelerátion; *физ.* moderátion; **2.** *уст.* (*задержка*) del

замедле́нн|ый slówed-up; бо́мба ~ого де́йствия delúy(ed)-action bomb; ~ая съёмка slów-motion shot.

заме́длить(ся) *сов. см.* замедля́ть(ся).

замедля́ть, заме́длить 1. (*вн.*) slow down (*smth.*); *физ.* móderate (*smth.*); ~ ход slow down, decélerate; коло́нна заме́длила ход the cólumn slowed its pace; **2.** (*вн.; задерживать*) deláy (*smth.*), hold* up (*smth.*), slow up (*smth.*); **3.** (*с тв., + инф.; запаздывать*) be* slow (with, + to inf); заме́длить с отве́том be* slow in replýing; слу́чай не заме́длил предста́виться it was not long before an opportúnity presénted itsélf. ~ся, заме́длиться **1.** slow down; **2.** (*задерживаться*) be* deláyed.

заме́на *ж.* **1.** (*действие*) substitútion, replácement; ~ спекта́кля change of prógramme; **2.** (*заменяющее лицо или предмет*) substitute.

замени́мый repláceable.

замени́тель *м.* substitute; ~ ко́жи substitute for léather.

замени́ть *сов. см.* заменя́ть.

заменя́ть, замени́ть 1. (*вн. тв.; сменять*) substitute (*smth.* for), change (*smth.* for), repláce (*smth.* by/with); ~ мета́лл пластма́ссой substitute plástics for métals, repláce métals by/with plástics; **2.** (*вн.; замещать*) repláce (*smb., smth.*), take* the place (of); (*о вещах*) do* dúty as (*smth.*); serve as (*smth.*); она́ замени́ла сиро́там мать she becáme a móther to the órphans.

замере́ть *сов. см.* замира́ть 1, 2.

замерза́ни|е *с.* fréezing; ◇ то́чка ~я fréezing-point; на то́чке ~я at a stándstill.

замерза́ть, замёрзнуть 1. (*превращаться в лёд*) freeze*; (*покрываться льдом*) be* frózen óver, be* cóvered with ice; вода́ замёрзла the wáter froze; окно́ замёрзло the window is all frósted up; **2.** (*погибать от мороза*) freeze* to death; (*о растениях*) be* killed by frost, die in the frost; **3.** (*сильно зябнуть*) get*/be* frózen; я совсе́м замёрз! I am frózen!

замёрзнуть *сов. см.* замерза́ть.

за́мертво as if dead; он упа́л ~ he fell down in a dead faint.

замеси́ть *сов. см.* заме́шивать II.

замести́ *сов. см.* замета́ть I.

замести́тель *м.*, ~ница *ж.* **1.** (*могущий заменить*) substitute; **2.** (*должность*) députy; ~ нача́льника, дире́ктора députy chief, diréctor.

замести́ть *сов. см.* замеща́ть 1.

замета́ть I, замести́ (*вн.*) **1.** (*подметать*) sweep* (*smth.*); **2.** (*засыпать — снегом, песком*) cóver up (*smth.*); сне́гом замело́ все доро́ги all the roads are deep in snow; ◇ ~ следы́ cóver up one's tracks; замести́ следы́ преступле́ния concéal all tráces of a crime.

замета́ть II *сов. см.* замётывать.

замета́ться *сов.* get* ínto flúrry; ~ по ко́мнате start rúshing abóut the room; ~ в постéли begín* to toss abóut in bed; ~ в отчáянии ≈ be* frántic with despáir.

замéтить *сов. см.* замечáть.

замéтк|а *ж.* 1. (*знак*) mark; 2. (*запись*) note; 3. (*в газете*) páragraph; ◇ взять *что-л.* на ~у make* a note of *smth.*

замéтн|о 1. *нареч.* percéptibly, appréciably, nóticeably; он ~ вы́рос he has grown appréciably; 2. *в знач. сказ. безл.* it is nóticeable, it is seen, one can see. ~ый 1. (*видимый*) vísible, nóticeable; (*ощутительный*) percéptible, appréciable; 2. (*видный, известный*) nótable, nóted, conspícuous.

замётывать, **заметáть** (*вн.*) baste (*smth.*), sew* up (*smth.*).

замечáн|ие *с.* 1. (*высказывание*) remárk, observátion; cómment; 2. (*выговор*) repróof; дéлать ~ *кому-л.* repróve *smb.*; tell* *smb.* off *разг.*; он не выно́сит никаки́х ~ий he can't stand a word of críticism.

замечáтельн|о spléndid, fine. ~ый 1. spléndid; (*исключительный*) remárkable; *разг.* (*очень хороший*) fine; ~ая побéда spléndid/sígnal víctory; 2. (*примечательный*) nóteworthy.

замечáть, **заметить** 1. (*вн.; видеть*) nótice (*smb., smth.*), percéive (*smb., smth.*); be* cónscious (of); *сов. тж.* catch* sight (of); он замéтил две ло́дки в бу́хте he nóticed two boats in the bay; не ~ *кого-л., чего-л.* fail to nótice *smb., smth.*; (*намеренно*) ignóre (*smb., smth.*); 2. (*вн.; обращать внимание*) obsérve (*smth.*), note (*smth.*); 3. (*вн.; запоминать*) take* note (of), make* a note (of), mark (*smth.*); замéтьте mind (you); 4. (*делать замечание*) remárk, nóte.

замечáться *сов.* be* lost in dreams/réverie.

замéшанный mixed up, invólved, ímplicated.

замешáтельство *с.* confúsion; (*растерянность тж.*) consternátion, dismáy; привести́ *кого-л.* в ~ disconcért *smb.*, throw* *smb.* into confúsion; прийти́ в ~ be* disconcérted, be* put off.

замешáть *сов. см.* замéшивать I.

замешáться *сов. см.* замéшиваться.

замéшивать I, **замешáть** (*вн.; вовлекать в какое-л. дело*) ímplicate (*smb.*).

замéшивать II, **замеси́ть** (*вн.*) mix (*smth.*); ~ тéсто knead dough.

замéшиваться, **замешáться** (*в пр.; быть причастным к чему-л.*) be* ímplicated (in), becóme* ímplicated (in), get* invólved (in).

замéшкаться *сов. разг.* línger, hang* abóut.

замещ|áть, **замести́ть** 1. (*вн. тв.*) súbstitute (*smth.* for), repláce (*smb., smth.* with); 2. *тк. несов.* (*вн.; собою*) take* the place (of); 3. *тк. несов.* (*вн.; временно исполнять обязанности*) act (for). ~éние *с.* substitútion.

зами́нк|а *ж. разг.* (*задержка*) hitch; произнести́ с ~ой say* hésitantly.

замирáние *с.* dýing awáy; *радио* fáding; ◇ с ~м сéрдца with *one's* heart in *one's* mouth.

замир|áть, **замерéть** 1. (*становиться неподвижным*) stand* still; (*о сердце*) sink*; он зáмер от у́жаса he froze with hórror; замерéть на мéсте stop short/dead, stand* róoted to the spot; 2. (*прекращаться*) stop, come* to a stándstill; (*о звуках*) die awáy, fade; 3. *тк. несов.* (*прерываться*) fálter; ~а́ющим го́лосом in a fáltering voice.

зáмкнут|ый 1. (*обособленный*) exclúsive; seclúded; ~ кружо́к exclúsive círcle; вести́ ~ую жизнь lead* a seclúded life; 2. (*необщительный*) réticent, resérved, unsóciable; 3. (*смыкающийся*) closed; ~ нáкоротко short-círcuited; ~ая электри́ческая цепь closed círcuit.

замкну́ть(ся) *сов. см.* замыка́ть(ся).

замоги́льн|ый *разг.:* ~ым го́лосом in sepúlchral tones.

зáмок *м.* cástle.

зам|о́к *м.* lock; вися́чий ~ pádlock; заперéть дверь на ~ lock the door; на ~ке́ locked; под ~ко́м únder lock and key; ◇ за семью́ ~ка́ми sealed and guárded.

замо́лвить *сов. разг.:* ~ сло́во, словéчко за *кого-л.* put* in a word for *smb.*

замо́лк|ать, **замо́лкнуть** fall* sílent; (*о звуках*) cease, be* hushed; пти́цы замо́лкли the birds fell sílent; the birds stopped sínging; разгово́р не ~а́л ни на мину́ту the conversátion néver flagged for a móment; шаги́ на лéстнице замо́лкли the fóotsteps died awáy on the stáircase.

замо́лкнуть *сов. см.* замолка́ть.

замолча́ть I *сов.* stop (tálking, crýing, sínging *etc.*); (*во время разговора*) lapse ínto sílence; (*о пушках и т. п.*) stop fíring; заста́вить *кого-л.* ~ sílence *smb.*

замолча́ть II *сов. см.* зама́лчивать.

замора́живан|ие *с.* fréezing; ~ пищевы́х проду́ктов fóod-freezing; ◇ ~ зáработной пла́ты *эк.* wáge-freezing, wáge-freeze; не допуска́ть ~ия материáльных ресу́рсов not allów matérial resóurces to lie ídle.

замора́живать, **заморо́зить** (*вн.*) 1. (*давать замёрзнуть*) freeze* (*smth.*); (*вино*) chill (*smth.*); 2. *разг.* (*давать озябнуть*) get* (*smb., smth.*) frózen, make* (*smb., smth.*) numb with cold; 3. (*оставлять неиспользованным*) keep* (*smth.*) ídle; заморо́зить срéдства keep* funds ídle.

замори́ть *сов.* (*вн.*) *разг.* 1. (*плохо кормить*) starve (*smb., smth.*), underféed* (*smb., smth.*); 2. (*изнурить*) overwórk (*smb., smth.*); ◇ ~ червячка́ stay the pangs of húnger.

заморо́женн|ый: ~ напи́ток iced drink; ~ые фру́кты chilled/quick-frozen fruit *sg*; ~ое мя́со chilled/refrígerated meat.

заморо́зить *сов. см.* замора́живать.

заморо́зки *мн.* frost(s); осéнние ~ éarly frosts; весéнние ~ late frosts; ~ на по́чве ground frost(s).

замо́рыш *м. разг.* stárveling.

замота́ть(ся) *сов. см.* зама́тывать(ся).

замочи́ть *сов. см.* зама́чивать.

замо́чн|ый lock *attr.*; ~ая сква́жина kéyhole.

зáмуж: вы́дать *кого-л.* ~ за *кого-л.* give* *smb.* in márriage to *smb.*; consént to *smb.'s* márrying *smb.* ~ем márried; быть ~ем за *кем-л.* be* márried to *smb.*

зáмуж|ество *с.* márriage, márried life. ~няя márried.

замурова́ть *сов. см.* замуро́вывать.

замуро́вывать, **замурова́ть** (*вн.*) wall (*smb., smth.*) up.

замусо́лить *сов.* (*вн.*) *разг.* soil (*smth.*), besméar (*smth.*).

замути́ть(ся) *сов. см.* мути́ть(ся) 1.

заму́ч|ить *сов.* (*вн.*) 1. (*до смерти*) tórture (*smb., smth.*) to death; 2. (*заставить страдать*) tórture (*smb.*), tormént (*smth.*); (*изнурить*) wear* (*smb.*) out, péster (*smb.*) to death; боле́знь ~ила ребёнка the diséase sapped all the child's strength. ~иться *сов.* have* a bad/térrible time.

зáмш|а *ж.* suède, dóe-skin, chámois-leather; (*для вытирания*) wásh-leather. ~евый suède *attr.*

замыва́ть, **замы́ть** (*вн.*) wash out (*smth.*).

замыка́ние *с.:* коро́ткое ~ *эл.* short círcuit.

замыка́ть, **замкну́ть** (*вн.*) 1. *разг.* lock (*smb., smth.*); 2. (*смыкать*) close (*smth.*); ~ цепь close the círcuit; 3.: ~ коло́нну bring* up the rear; 4. (*окружать*) surróund (*smth.*), ring (*smth.*) round, encírcle (*smth.*). ~ся, замкну́ться 1. (*в вн., в пр.; обособляться*) withdráw* (ínto); ~ся в своём кругу́ immérse onesélf in fámily afáirs; 2. (*смыкаться*) close; ◇ ~ся в себé retíre ínto onesélf.

зáмысел *м.* 1. (*намерение*) inténtion, scheme, design; вели́чественный ~ grándly concéived plan; стратеги́ческий ~ strátegic idéa; ~ опера́ции cóncept of an operátion, téntative plan of an operátion; 2.

(*художественного произведения*) idéa, concéption; ~ пьéсы the main/underlýing idéa of a play; худóжественный ~ artístic concéption.

замы́слить *сов. см.* замышля́ть.

замыслова́т|ый íntricate, ingénious; ~ые ре́чи róund-abóut talk *sg.*

замы́ть *сов. см.* замыва́ть.

замышля́ть, замы́слить (*вн.*, + *инф.*) cóntemplate (*smth.*, + -ing).

замя́ть *сов.* (*вн.*) *разг.* hush up (*smth.*), suppréss (*smth.*), smóther (*smth.*); ~ де́ло hush up an affáir.

замя́ться *сов. разг.* 1. (*смутиться*) becóme* confúsed; 2. (*остановиться, подыскивая нужное слово*) stúmble.

за́навес *м.* cúrtain; ◇ под ~ at the last móment.

занаве́с|ить *сов. см.* занаве́шивать. ~ка *ж.* cúrtain.

занаве́шивать, занаве́сить (*вн.*) drape (*smth.*), cúrtain (*smth.*).

зана́шивать, заноси́ть (*вн.*) wear* out (*smth.*); ~ что-л. до дыр wear* *smth.* into holes.

занемо́чь *сов.* be* тáken ill, fall* ill.

занести́ *сов. см.* заноси́ть I.

занести́сь *сов. см.* заноси́ться.

занижа́ть, зани́зить (*вн.*) understáte (*smth.*), set* (*smth.*) too low; ~ нóрму understáte the quóta.

зани́женный understáted, artificially lówered.

зани́зить *сов. см.* занижа́ть.

занима́тельный entertáining, ínteresting.

заним|а́ть I, заня́ть (*вн.*) 1. (*пространство*) take* up (*smth.*), óccupy (*smth.*); ~ мнóго мéста take* up a lot of room/space; ~ кóмнату have* a room; я ~áю э́ту кóмнату this is my room; заня́ть мéсто для когó-л. keep* a place for *smb.*; ~áйте свои́ местá! take your seats!; 2. (*должность, положение*) hold* (*smth.*); ~ высóкий пост hold* a high post; ~ пéрвое мéсто head the list, be* first; ~ вторóе мéсто be* sécond, take* sécond place; 3. (*овладевать территорией и т. п.*) óccupy (*smth.*); ~ гóрод óccupy a town; 4. (*время*) take* (*smth.*), take* up (*smth.*); 5. (*давать работу*) emplóy (*smb.*); 6. (*развлекать*) entertáin (*smb.*); ~ детéй keep* the children amúsed; ~ когó-л. разговóром keep* *smb.* engáged in conversátion; ◇ ~ оборóну *воен.* hold* a defénsive position/line; ~ пози́цию *воен.* hold* a position, be* in position; какýю пози́цию он ~áет в э́том вопрóсе? what is his áttitude to this quéstion?; егó ~áет мысль (о) he is táken up with the idéa (of + -ing), he is cóntemplating (+ -ing).

занима́ть II, заня́ть (*вн.* у *рд.*; *брать взаймы*) bórrow (*smth.* from).

заним|а́ться I, заня́ться 1. (*тв.*; *быть занятым чем-л.*) do* (*smth.*), be* óccupied/búsy (with); чем он сейчáс ~áется? what is he dóing now?; ~ дéлом do* some work; ~ упакóвкой вещéй do* the pácking, be* búsy with the pácking; 2. (*тв.*; *выполнять какую-л. работу*) be* engáged (in), be* óccupied (in), have* to do (with); (*посвящать себя чему-л.*) devóte onesélf (to), take* up (*smth.*), go* in (for); ~ поли́тикой be* engáged in pólitics; ~ иску́сством be* concérned with art; он реши́л ~ медици́ной he decíded to go in for médicine; вы должны́ ~ спóртом you ought to take up sport; 3. *тк. несов.* (*учиться*) stúdy, learn*; (у *рд.*) take* léssons (from); ~ англи́йским языкóм learn* Énglish; не мешáйте емý ~ let him get on with his work; 4. (с *тв.*; *учить*) teach* (*smb.*), give* léssons (to); ~ с отстаю́щими ученикáми give* spécial atténtion to báckward púpils; 5. (*тв.*; *заботиться*) look (áfter); ~ покупáтелем atténd to a cústomer.

заним|а́ться II, заня́ться 1. (*загораться*) catch* fire; занялся́ хвóрост, и вскóре костёр разгорéлся the twigs caught and soon a fire was blázing; 2. (*наступать*) begín*; ~áется день day is bréaking; ◇ дух ~áется it takes *one's* breath awáy.

за́ново all óver agáin; (*по-новому*) afrésh, anéw; передéлывать что-л. ~ do* *smth.* all óver agáin, recást* *smth.*; написáть что-л. ~ rewríte* *smth.*; отдéлывать что-л. ~ rénovate *smth.*

зано́з|а 1. *ж.* splínter; 2. *м. и ж. разг.* (*о человеке*) príckly cháracter, thorn in the flesh. ~истый *разг.* rough, jagged; *перен.* príckly; ~и́ть *сов.* (*вн.*) get* a splínter (in).

зано́с *м.* drift; снéжные ~ы snów-drifts.

заноси́ть I, занести́ (*вн.*) 1. (*приносить*) bring* (*smth.*); ~ зарáзу bring*/cárry (the) inféction; 2. (*доставлять по пути*) drop in with (*smth.*), drop (*smth.*) in; товáрищ занёс мне кни́гу a friend dropped in with a book for me; 3. *разг.*: каки́м вéтром вас занеслó сюдá? what brings you here?; кудá вас занеслá судьбá! look where fate has lánded us!; 4. (*записывать*) énter (*smth.*) in; ~ что-л. в протокóл énter *smth.* in the mínutes; ~ что-л. в спи́сок put* *smth.* down on the list; 5. (*поднимать или отводить в сторону*) lift (*smth.*); ~ рýку для удáра raise *one's* hand to strike; ~ нóгу в стрéмя swing* *one's* foot* into the stírrup; ~ конéц бревнá slew the end of the log round; 6. *безл.:* маши́ну всё врéмя занóсит the car keeps skídding; 7. (*засыпать, заметать чем-л.*): дорóгу занеслó снéгом the road is blócked with snow.

заноси́ть II *сов. см.* зана́шивать.

заноси́ться *сов.* занести́сь *разг.* 1. (*далеко заходить в мыслях*) be* cárried awáy; 2. (*гордиться*) get* stúck-up.

зано́счив|ость *ж.* árrogance. ~ый árrogant, proud.

заночевáть *сов.* spend* the night, stay the night.

заношенный worn out, thréadbare.

заня́т|ие *с.* 1. (*дело, труд, работа*) proféssion, trade, occupátion; (*в учреждении и т. п.*) work; практи́ческие ~ия по чемý-л. práctical work in *smth.*; род ~ий occupátion; вы́брать себé ~ по вкýсу choose* the proféssion *one* preférs; 2. *мн.* (*учебные*) léssons, stúdies; начáло ~ий 1-го сентября́ the term begins on the first of Septémber; начáло ~ий в 9 часóв léssons begín at nine; опоздáть к начáлу ~ий be* late for school; часы́ ~ий school hours; 3. (*города, страны и т. п.*) occupátion; 4. *разг.* (*времяпрепровождение*) pástime.

заня́тный *разг.* amúsing, ínteresting.

занятóй búsy.

за́нятость *ж.* 1. emplóyment; 2. (*перегруженность работой*) préssure of work.

за́нят|ый (*несвободный*) engáged; (*делами*) búsy; я за́нят I'm búsy; э́то мéсто ~о 1) this seat is táken; 2) (*о должности*) this post is alréady filled; телефóн у них всегдá за́нят their númber is álways engáged; 2. (*войсками*) óccupied; ◇ быть ~ым тóлько собóй be* ínterested ónly in onesélf, be* self-céntred.

заня́ть I, II *сов. см.* занимáть I, II.

заня́ться *сов. см.* занимáться I 1, 2, 4, 5; 2. (*тв.*; *приступить*) start (*smth.*), set* to work (on); take* up (*smth.*); ~ подготóвкой к конферéнции start prepáring for the cónference.

заня́ться II *сов. см.* занимáться II.

заóблачн|ый ethéreal; ~ая высь régions beyónd the clouds; ~ые мечты́ ethéreal dreams.

заоднó *нареч.* 1. togéther, in cóncert; дéйствовать ~ с кéм-л. act in cóncert with *smth.*; 2. *в знач. сказ.:* мы с ним ~ we understánd each óther; 3. *разг.* (*кстати, попутно*) at the same time.

заокеáнский 1. ovérseas, transoceánic; 2. (*американский*) transatlántic.

заострённый (*sharp-*)póinted; (*суживающийся к концу*) tápering.

заостри́ть(ся) *сов. см.* заостря́ть(ся).

заостря́ть, заостри́ть (*вн.*) shárpen (*smth.*); *перен.* (*подчёркивать*) accéntuate (*smth.*); (*обострять*) cóncentrate (*smth.*); заостри́ть чьё-л. внимáние на чём-

-либо draw* smb.'s spécial atténtion to smth.; заострить вопрóс accéntuate the impórtance of a quéstion. ~ся, заостри́ться nárrow to a point, becóme* póinted; táper; перен. becóme* acúte.

заóчн|ик м., ~ица ж. correspóndence/extramúral stúdent.

заóчн|о 1. (в отсутствие) in smb.'s ábsence; суди́ть когó-л. ~ try smb. in his, her ábsence; суди́ться ~ be* tried in one's ábsence; 2. (об обучении) by correspóndence; ~ окóнчить институ́т take* an extérnal degrée. ~ый: ~ый пригово́р júdgement by defáult; ~ые ку́рсы correspóndence course; ~ое обучéние tuítion by correspóndence.

за́пад м. 1. the west; находи́ться к ~у от чего-л. be* west of smth.; с ~a from the west; 2. (3.) (Западная Европа) the West.

запада́ть, запа́сть 1. stick* (inside); кла́виши запада́ют the keys are sticking; 2. (становиться впалым) becóme* súnken; её щёки запа́ли her cheeks were súnken/hóllow; 3. (в вн.; запечатлеваться) make* a deep impréssion (on), sink* (into); запа́сть в ду́шу sink* into one's heart.

западно|германский Wést-Gérman. ~европейский Wést-Européan.

за́падн|ый 1. wéstern; ~ая грани́ца wéstern fróntier; в ~ом направлéнии wéstward(s), in a wésterly diréction; ~ ве́тер west wind; 2. (о странах Запада) Wéstern; За́падная Евро́па Wéstern Éurope.

западн|я́ ж. (прям. и перен.) trap; пойма́ть когó-л. в ~ю́ trap smb.

запа́здывать, запозда́ть 1. be* late; 2. (с тв., + инф.) be* late (with; in + -ing).

запа́ивать, запая́ть (вн.) sólder (smth.).

запакова́ть сов. см. запакóвывать.

запакóвывать, запакова́ть (вн.) pack (smth.).

запа́л I м. 1. fuse, prímer; 2. разг. (горячность) the heat of the móment.

запа́л II м. (одышка у животных) bróken wind; the heaves pl.

запалённый (о лошади) bróken-winded.

запа́льчив|ость ж. irascibílity, quick témper; (задор) véhemence. ~ый iráscible, hásty, quick-témpered; (задорный) fiery.

запанибра́та разг.: быть ~ с кем-л. be* on équal terms with smb., be* frée-and-éasy with smb.

запа́с м. 1. resérve, stock; (о сырье тж.) stóckpile; ~ горю́чего, тóплива fuel resérves/stocks pl; ~ боеприпа́сов stock of ammunítion; дéлать ~ы lay* in supplies; ~ безопа́сности, прóчности тех. márgin of sáfety; ~ слов vocábulary; имéть большо́й ~ слов have* a rich vocábulary; ~ впечатлéний store of impréssions; рассчита́ть с ~ом leave* a wide márgin; 2. разг. (излишек ткани за швом) hem; 3. воен. resérve; ◇ в ~е in resérve; у нас ещё два часá в ~е we still have two hours to spare; про ~ as a resérve; оставля́ть что́-л. про ~ keep* smth. for fúture use.

запаса́ть, запасти́ (вн., рд.) store (smth.), lay* in (smth.); (сырьё и т. п.) stóckpile (smth.). ~ся, запасти́сь (тв.) store (smth.), build* up resérves (of), lay* in (smth.), lay* in a stock/supply (of); ◇ ~ся терпéнием be* pátient; posséss one's soul in pátience.

запа́сливый thrífty, próvident.

запа́сник м. 1. resérvist; 2. (хранилище в музее) resérve (stock).

запасн|óй прил. 1. см. запа́сный; ~ игрóк resérve; ~а́я покры́шка spare (týre); ~ые ча́сти spare parts, spares; 2. воен. resérve attr.; 3. в знач. сущ. м. воен. resérvist.

запа́сный spare; ~ вы́ход emérgency éxit; ~ путь ж.-д. síding, shúnting-track; переводи́ть на ~ путь síde-track, shunt.

запасти́(сь) сов. см. запаса́ть(ся).

запа́сть сов. см. запада́ть.

за́пах м. smell; ódour книжн.

запаха́ть сов. см. запа́хивать I.

запа́хивать I, запаха́ть (вн.) 1. (вспахивать) plough (smth.); 2. (заваливать землёй при вспашке) plough (smth.) in.

запа́хивать II, запахну́ть ~ шу́бу wrap one's coat clóser round one. ~ся, запахну́ться: ~ся в шу́бу wrap/húddle onesélf up in one's coat.

запахну́ть сов. см. запа́хивать II. ~ся сов. см. запа́хиваться.

запа́чкать сов. (вн.) dírty (smth.), make* (smth.) dírty; перен. stain (smth.). ~ся сов. get* onesélf dírty.

запа́шка ж. с.-х. 1. (вспашка) plóughing; 2. (количество запаханного) ploughed área, tíllage.

запая́ть сов. см. запа́ивать.

запева́ла м. и ж. léading sínger, sóloist; перен. léading spírit.

запев|а́ть несов. lead* the sínging/chórus, strike* up the first notes; ~а́ет Петрóв sólo-part by Petróv.

запека́нка ж. 1. (кушанье) baked púdding; картóфельная ~ shépherd's pie; 2. (наливка) zapekánka (kind of brandy).

запека́ть, запéчь (вн.) bake (smth.). ~ся, запéчься 1. bake; 2. (о губах) parch; 3. (о крови) clot, coágulate.

запёкш|ийся: ~иеся гу́бы parched lips; ~аяся кровь clótted blood.

запелена́ть сов. (вн.) swáddle (smth.).

запере́ть(ся) сов. см. запира́ть(ся).

запéть сов. begín* to sing.

запеча́тать сов. см. запеча́тывать.

запечатлева́ть, запечатлéть: запечатлéть собы́тие на карти́не commémorate an evént on cánvas; ~ что́-л. в па́мяти fix smth. in one's mémory. ~ся, запечатлéться (в пр.) impréss itsélf (on).

запечатлéть(ся) сов. см. запечатлева́ть(ся).

запеча́тывать, запеча́тать (вн.) seal (smth.).

запéчь(ся) сов. см. запека́ть(ся).

запива́ть, запи́ть (вн. тв.) take* (smth. with), drink* (smth. with); wash down (smth. with) разг.; запи́ть лека́рство водóй take* medicine with wáter.

запина́|ться, запну́ться hésitate; stúmble in one's speech; сов. тж. stop short; говори́ть ~ясь fálter.

запи́нк|а ж.: без ~и glíbly.

запира́тельство с. denial, refúsal to conféss.

запир|а́ть, запере́ть (вн.) 1. (на замок) lock (smth.), lock up (smth.); (засовом) bolt (smth.); ~ дверь lock the door; ~ дом lock up a house; ~ замóк turn the key in the lock; 2. (где-л.) lock in (smb., smth.); 3. (прекращать доступ, лишать выхода): ~ проли́вы block the straits; ~ флот проти́вника blockáde the énemy fleet. ~а́ться, запере́ться 1. (в помещении) lock onesélf up; запере́ться в своéй кóмнате lock onesélf in one's room; 2.: замóк не ~ется the lock dóesn't work; я́щик ~ется на замóк the box has a lock; the box can be locked; 3. разг. (не сознаваться) dený one's guilt, persíst in one's denial.

записа́ть(ся) сов. см. запи́сывать(ся).

запи́ск|а ж. 1. note; любóвная ~ lóve-letter, bíllet-dóux; 2. (официальное сообщение о чём-л.) memorándum (pl -da); подáть доклáдную ~у submít a repórt; 3. мн. notes; (воспоминания) mémoirs; учёные ~и (издание) transáctions, procéedings; читáть лéкцию по ~ам lécture from notes.

записн|óй I: ~áя кни́жка nótebook.

записнóй II разг. (рьяный) óut-and-óut, thórough-góing.

запи́сывать, записа́ть (вн.) 1. write* (smb., smth.) down, put* (smb., smth.) down, recórd (smth.); (поспешно) jot (smth.) down; (со слов) take* (smth.) down; (систематически) keep* a record (of); записáть áдрес take* down an address; 2. (на пластинку, на плёнку) recórd (smth.). ~ся, записа́ться (на вн.) put* one's name down (for); put* oneself down (for); ~ся доброво́льцем enlíst as a voluntéer, voluntéer; ~ся к врачу́ make* an appóintment at the dóctor's; ~ся в библиоте́ку join a líbrary.

за́пис|ь ж. 1. (де́йствие) registrátion; (на пласти́нку) recórding; 2. (запи́санное) éntry; (системати́ческая) récord; мн. notes; ◇ в литерату́рной ~и кого́-л. as told to smb.

запи́ть I сов. см. запива́ть.

запи́ть II сов. разг. (запья́нствовать) take* to drink, go* on the bóttle.

запиха́ть сов. см. запи́хивать.

запи́хивать, запиха́ть, запихну́ть (вн.) разг. thrust* (smth.), cram (smth.), stuff (smth.).

запихну́ть сов. см. запи́хивать.

запла́канн|ый: ~ые глаза́ eyes red with wéeping; с ~ыми глаза́ми réd-éyed; ~ое лицо́ téar-stained face.

запла́кать сов. begín* to cry.

заплани́ровать сов. см. плани́ровать I.

запла́т|а ж. patch; поста́вить ~у на что́-л. patch smth., put* a patch on smth.

заплати́ть сов. 1. (вн. за вн.) pay* (smth. for); 2. (тв.; отплати́ть) repáy* (with).

заплева́ть сов. (вн.) soil (smth.) with spíttle; ~ (весь) пол spit* all óver the floor.

заплесневе́лый móuldy, míldewed.

заплесневе́ть сов. см. пле́сневеть.

заплести́ сов. см. заплета́ть.

заплет|а́ть, заплести́ (вн.) 1. plait (smth.), braid (smth.); ~ ко́су plait one's hair; 2. (оплета́ть) weave* round (smth.). ~а́ться несов. stúmble; у него́ но́ги ~а́ются he is stággering, he can't walk straight; у него́ язы́к ~а́ется he can ónly múmble, his speech is slurred.

запломбирова́ть сов. см. пломбирова́ть.

заплыв м. спорт. race; (часть состяза́ния) heat.

заплыва́ть I, заплы́ть swim*; (о суда́х) sail; (о веща́х) float.

заплыва́ть II, заплы́ть (тв.) 1.: его́ глаза́ заплы́ли his eyes were mere slits (amid thick folds of fat); 2. swell* (with), becóme* blóated (with); ~ жи́ром becóme* blóated.

заплы́вший (отёкший) swóllen; (жи́ром) blóated.

заплы́ть I, II сов. см. заплыва́ть I, II.

запляса́ть сов. begín to dance.

запну́ться сов. см. запина́ться.

запове́дн|ик м. resérve, presérve; (пти́чий) sánctuary. ~ый 1. (охраня́емый зако́ном) protécted; ~ый лес protécted fórest, fórest resérve; 2. (сокрове́нный) sécret; 3. (заве́тный) chérished.

за́поведь ж. commándment; перен. тж. précept.

заподо́зрить сов. 1. (вн. в пр.; счита́ть кого́-л. вино́вным в чём-л.) suspéct (smb. of); ~ кого́-л. в кра́же suspéct smb. of stéaling; 2. (вн.; предположи́ть) suspéct (smth.); ~ обма́н suspéct tríckery.

запое́м разг. non-stóp; чита́ть ~ read* ávidly, be* an ávid réader; пить ~ have* fits of drínking.

запозда́лый belated.

запозда́ние с.: с ~м на три мину́ты three mínutes late.

запозда́ть сов. см. запа́здывать.

запо́|й м. fit of drínking; страда́ть ~ем be* gíven to drink, drink* héavily.

заполза́ть, заползти́ (в, под вн.) creep* (into, únder).

заползти́ сов. см. заполза́ть.

запо́лнить(ся) сов. см. заполня́ть(ся).

заполня́ть, запо́лнить (вн.) 1. (наполня́ть) fill (smth.), fill up (smth.); зри́тели запо́лнили зал spectátors filled the hall, the hall was filled with spectátors; ~ вре́мя fill in the time; 2. (впи́сывать) fill in (smth.); ~ бланк make* out a form, fill in a form. ~ся,

запо́лниться fill, fill up; пло́щадь запо́лнилась наро́дом the square filled with péople.

заполя́рный pólar.

запомин|а́ть, запо́мнить (вн.) remémber (smb., smth.); твёрдо запо́мнить что́-л. fix smth. in one's mind. ~а́ться, запо́мниться (дт.) remáin in smb.'s mémory; мне э́то хорошо́ запо́мнилось it has remáined fírmly in my mémory; тру́дно ~а́ться be* hard to remémber. ~а́ющий: ~а́ющее устро́йство mémory, mémory device.

запо́мнить(ся) сов. см. запомина́ть(ся).

за́понка ж. (для воротника́) stud; (для манже́ты) cúff-link.

запо́р I м. bolt; (замо́к) lock; дверь на ~e the door is bólted.

запо́р II м. мед. constipátion.

запороши́|ть сов. (вн.) pówder (smth.), dust (smth.); доро́гу ~ло сне́гом the road was pówdered with snow.

запот|ева́ть, запоте́ть becóme* damp; (о стекле́ и т. п.) cloud óver, mist óver. ~е́вший, ~е́лый: ~е́вшее стекло́ místed glass.

запоте́ть сов. см. запотева́ть и поте́ть 2.

заправи́ла м. разг. ríngleader, boss.

запра́вить сов. см. заправля́ть 1, 2, 3. ~ся сов. см. заправля́ться.

запра́вка ж. 1. (ку́шанья) séasoning; 2. (автомаши́ны) refúelling, filling (-up).

заправля́ть, запра́вить 1. (вн.; засо́вывать) tuck (smth.) in; 2. (вн. тв.; класть припра́ву) séason (smth. with), flávour (smth.); ~ сала́т dress a sálad; 3. (вн.; автомаши́ну) refúel (smth.), fill up (smth.); 4. тк. несов. (тв.) разг. (быть заправи́лой) run*/boss the show; ◇ запра́вить ко́йку make* a bed. ~ся, запра́виться разг. 1. (горю́чим) fill up; 2. (есть до́сыта) eat*, have* a square meal.

запра́вочный filling attr.; ~ пункт filling státion.

запра́вский разг. régular; ~ игро́к confirmed gámbler.

запра́шивать, запроси́ть 1. (вн. о пр.; осведомля́ться) send* an inquíry (to smb. about smth.); 2. (вн.; называ́ть высо́кую це́ну) ask the exórbitant sum (of); запроси́ть вдво́е ask dóuble the price.

запре́т м. prohibítion, ban; (на вы́воз) embárgo; наложи́ть ~ на что́-л. véto smth.; ◇ быть, находи́ться под ~ом be* strictly prohíbited; держа́ть ~ под ~ом maintáin a ban on smth. ~и́тельный prohíbitive. ~и́ть сов. см. запреща́ть. ~ный forbídden, prohíbited, banned; ~ная зо́на restrícted área; ◇ ~ный плод forbídden fruit.

запрещ|а́ть, запрети́ть (вн.) forbíd* (smth.); (ча́ще зако́ном и т. п.) ban (smth.). ~е́ние с. prohibítion, ban; ~е́ние я́дерного ору́жия prohibítion/bánning of núclear wéapons. ~ённый forbídden; (зако́ном тж.) banned, prohíbited; ~ённый приём спорт. foul; (в борьбе́) barred hold.

заприхо́довать сов. см. приходовать.

запрограмми́ров|анный prógrammed. ~ать сов. см. программи́ровать.

запроекти́ровать сов. (вн.) design (smth.); (наме́тить) plan (smth.).

запроки́дывать, запроки́нуть (вн.) разг.: ~ го́лову throw* one's head back. ~ся, запроки́нуться разг. fall* back.

запроки́нуть(ся) сов. см. запроки́дывать(ся).

запропа́ст|и́ться сов. разг. get* lost, disappéar; куда́ он ~и́лся? what can have becóme of him?

запро́с м. 1. (вопро́с) inquíry; обрати́ться куда́-л. с ~ом make* an inquíry at; 2. обыкн. мн. (спрос) demánds, requírements; expectátions; ~ы потреби́телей requírements of the consúmer; 3. обыкн. мн. (стремле́ния) aspirátions; име́ть больши́е ~ы have* great aspirátions; **4.** *разг.* (*о цене*) overchárging; цена́ без ~a réasonable price. ~и́ть *сов. см.* запра́шивать.

за́просто *разг.* without fuss/adó, quite infórmally.

запру́да *ж.* **1.** (*плотина*) weir, dam; **2.** (*запруженный водоём*) pond, réservoir; ме́льничная ~ míll-pond.

запруди́ть *сов. см.* запру́живать.

запру́живать, **запруди́ть** (*вн.*) **1.** (*воду*) dam up (*smth.*); **2.** *разг.* (*заполнять*) throng (*smth.*), block (*smth.*); толпа́ запруди́ла у́лицы crowds thronged the streets.

запры́гать *сов.* begín* to jump.

запряга́ть, **запря́чь** (*вн.*) **1.** (*лошадь, собак и т. п.*) hárness (*smth.*); (*повозку и т. п.*) put* the hórses (to); **2.** *разг.* (*нагружать тяжёлой работой*) make* (*smb.*) work. ~ся, запря́чься *разг.* get* down to; ~ся в рабо́ту get* down to work.

запря́жка *ж.* **1.** (*действие*) hárnessing; **2.** (*сбруя, упряжь*) hárness.

запря́тать *сов.* (*вн.*) hide* (*smth.*) awáy. ~ся *сов.* hide* onesélf.

запря́чь(ся) *сов. см.* запряга́ть(ся).

запу́ганный cowed, brówbeaten.

запуга́ть *сов. см.* запу́гивать.

запу́гивать, **запуга́ть** (*вн.*) intímidate (*smb.*), cow (*smb.*), brówbeat* (*smb.*).

за́пуск *м.* (*мотора*) stárting; (*ракеты*) láunching; ~ косми́ческого корабля́ láunching of a spáceship, space láunching.

запуска́ть I, **запусти́ть 1.** (*вн. в вн., тв. в вн.; бросать*) hurl (*smth.* at); **2.** (*вн.; заставлять взлетать*) send* up (*smth.*); ~ змей fly* a kite; запусти́ть иску́сственный спу́тник Земли́ launch an artíficial Earth sátellite; **3.** (*вн.; приводить в действие*) start (*smth.*); ~ мото́р start an éngine; **4.** (*вн. в вн.*) *разг.* (*засовывать, вонзать*) plunge (*smth.* into); ~ ко́гти dig* its claws in.

запуска́ть II, **запусти́ть** (*вн.; доводить до состояния упадка, разрушения*) negléct (*smth.*), not look áfter (*smth.*), let* (*smth.*) slide.

запусте́ни|е *с.* desolátion; (*заброшенность*) state of negléct/dísrepáir; дом в ~и the house has gone to rack and ruin; прийти́ в ~ fall* into a state of negléct.

запусти́ть I, II *сов. см.* запуска́ть I, II.

запу́танн|ость *ж.* confúsion. ~ый tángled; *перен.* íntricate, invólved; ~ый вопро́с knótty quéstion; оказа́ться ~ым в чём-л. becóme* invólved in *smth.*

запу́тать(ся) *сов. см.* запу́тывать(ся).

запу́тывать, **запу́тать** (*вн.*) **1.** tángle (*smth.*), entángle (*smth.*); *перен.* confúse (*smth.*), múddle (*smth.*); запу́тать ни́тки tángle the threads; запу́тать де́ло confúse the íssue, búngle the affáir, múddle mátters; **2.** *разг.* (*сбивать с толку*) confúse (*smb.*); **3.** *разг.* (*впутывать*) invólve (*smb.*), ímplicate (*smb.*). ~ся, запу́таться **1.** get* into a tángle; *перен.* (*усложняться*) becóme* confúsed/cómplicated; верёвка запу́талась the rope got tángled; де́ло запу́талось complicátions aróse; **2.** (*в пр.; оказываться опутанным чем-л.*) get* tángled up (in), get* caught (in); **3.** *разг.* (*сбиваться с толку*) get* mixed up (in), запу́таться в отве́тах give* conflícting ánswers, contradíct onesélf.

запу́щенн|ый neglécted, uncáred-for; ~ сад neglécted gárden; ~ая боле́знь neglécted íllness.

запыла́ть *сов.* blaze up, flare up.

запыли́ть *сов.* (*вн.*) make* (*smth.*) dústy. ~ся *сов.* becóme* dústy.

запыха́ться *сов. разг.* be* out of breath.

запя́стье *с. анат.* wrist.

запята́я *ж.* cómma.

запятна́ть *сов. см.* пятна́ть.

зараба́тывать, **зарабо́тать** (*вн.*) earn (*smth.*); дать

кому́-л. зарабо́тать give* smb. a chance to earn some móney; ~ на жизнь earn/make* one's líving.

зарабо́тать I *сов. см.* зараба́тывать.

зарабо́тать II *сов.* (*начать работать*) start (wórking), begín* to work.

зарабо́т|аться *сов. разг.* be* overwórked, overwórk onesélf; мы ~ались до по́здней но́чи we worked far ínto the night; он совсе́м ~ался he is térribly overwórked.

зарабо́тн|ый: ~ая пла́та wáges *pl*; (*служащих*) sálary; реа́льная ~ая пла́та real wáges.

за́работок *м.* éarnings *pl.*

зара́внивать, **заровня́ть** (*вн.*) lével (*smth.*).

заража́|ть, **зарази́ть** (*вн. тв.*) inféct (*smth.* with); (*тж. перен.*); (*воздух и т. п. тж.*) contáminate (*smth.* with); зарази́ть кого́-л. скарлати́ной inféct smb. with scárlet féver; ~ кого́-л. свои́м приме́ром inféct smb. by one's exámple. ~ться, зарази́ться (*тв.*) be* infécted (with) (*тж. перен.*); catch* (*smth.*); зарази́ться гри́ппом от кого́-л. catch* the flu from smb.; зарази́ться о́бщим весе́льем be* infécted with the géneral mérriment, enjóy the fun. ~е́ние *с.* inféction; (*воздуха и т. п.*) contaminátion; ~е́ние кро́ви blóod-poisoning; ~е́ние ме́стности contaminátion of the locálity.

зара́з|а *ж.* inféction; (*через прикосновение*) contágion. ~и́тельный inféctious; ~и́тельный смех inféctious láughter. ~и́ть(ся) *сов. см.* заража́ть(ся). ~ный inféctious; (*передающийся через прикосновение*) contágious; ~ный больно́й inféctious pátient.

зара́нее in advánce, befórehand; ~ обду́мать что-л. consider smth. befórehand.

зарапортова́ться *сов. разг.* let* one's tongue run awáy with one, talk through one's hat.

зараста́ть, **зарасти́ 1.** (*тв.*) be* overgrówn (with); ~ сорняка́ми be* choked/overrún with weeds; **2.** *разг.* (*заживать*) heal.

зарасти́ *сов. см.* зараста́ть.

зарва́ться *сов. см.* зарыва́ться II.

зарде́ться *сов.* be* flushed, rédden, grow* red; (*румянцем*) flush.

зареве́ть *сов.* **1.** (begín* to) roar; (*о быке*) (begín* to) béllow; **2.** *разг.* (*начать плакать*) burst out crýing.

за́рево *с.* glow; (*заката*) áfterglow.

зарегистри́ровать *сов.* (*вн.*) régister (smb., smth.). ~ся *сов.* **1.** régister onesélf; **2.** (*оформить брак*) get* márried (at a régistry óffice); régister one's márriage.

заре́з *м. разг.*: мне до ~у ну́жно вас ви́деть! I must see you!, I've símply got to see you!

заре́зать *сов. см.* ре́зать 3. ~ся *сов. разг.* cut* one's throat.

зарека́ться, **заре́чься** (+ *инф.*) vow not (+ to *inf*), pledge onesélf not (+ to *inf*); ~ кури́ть vow not to smoke ány more.

зарекомендова́ть *сов.*: ~ себя́ с хоро́шей, плохо́й стороны́ make* a good, bad shówing; ~ себя́ хоро́шим рабо́тником show* onesélf to be a good wórker.

заре́чься *сов. см.* зарека́ться.

заржа́в|еть *сов. см.* ржа́веть. ~ленный rústy.

заржа́ть *сов.* (begín* to) neigh.

зарис|ова́ть *сов. см.* зарисо́вывать. ~о́вка *ж.* **1.** (*действие*) skétching; **2.** (*рисунок*) sketch.

зарисо́вывать, **зарисова́ть** (*вн.*) sketch (*smth.*).

зарни́ца *ж.* súmmer lightning.

заровня́ть *сов. см.* зара́внивать.

зароди́ться *сов. см.* зарожда́ться.

заро́дыш *м.* émbryo (*pl* -os); *бот.* germ; ◇ в ~е in émbryo; подави́ть что-л. в ~e nip smth. in the bud. ~евый embryónic.

зарожд|а́ться, **зароди́ться** oríginate; ~а́ется но́вая жизнь a new life is dáwning; у него́ зароди́лась мысль he concéived the idéa; э́то у него́ зароди́лась така́я мысль it was he who oríginated the idéa.

зарóк *м.* pledge, vow; взять ~ с *кого-л.* make* *smb.* prómise; дать ~ не курйть pledge *oneself* néver to smoke.

заросл|ь *ж.* growth; (*чаща*) thícket; ~и кустáрника dense búshes *pl.*

заро́сший overgrówn.

зарпла́та *ж. разг.* wáges *pl*; (*служащих*) sálary.

заруб|áть, зарубить (*вн.*) **1.** (*убивать*) slash/sábre (*smb.*) to death; (*топором*) kill (*smb.*) with an axe; **2.** (*делать зарубку*) notch (*smth.*), nick (*smth.*); ◇ ~й себé на носý bear it/that in mind, put that in your pipe and smoke it.

зарубéжн|ый fóreign; ~ая делегáция fóreign delegátion, delegátion from abróad.

зарубить *сов. см.* зарубáть.

зарубка *ж.* (*метка*) notch, nick.

зарубцевáться *сов. см.* зарубцо́вываться.

зарубцо́вываться, зарубцевáться cícatrize, form a scar; (*заживать*) heal.

зарумя́нить *сов. см.* румя́нить 1, 3. ~ся *сов. см.* румя́ниться 1, 3, 4.

заруча́ться, заручи́ться (*тв.*) secúre (*smth.*); заручи́ться поддéржкой *кого-л.* enlist *smb.'s* aid.

заручи́ться *сов. см.* заруча́ться.

зарыва́ть, зары́ть (*вн.*) búry (*smth.*).

зарыва́ться, зары́ться (в *вн.*) búry *oneself* (in), búrrow (into); (*прятать лицо, голову*) búry *one's* face (in).

зарыва́ться II, зарва́ться *разг.* go* too far, overdó* things; зарва́ться в свои́х трéбованиях get* more and more exácting, lose* all sense of moderátion.

зарыда́ть *сов.* begín* to sob. .

зары́ть *сов. см.* зарыва́ть. ~ся *сов. см.* зарыва́ться I.

зар|я́ *ж.* **1.** (*утренняя*) dawn; (*вечерняя*) áfterglow; вставáть с ~ёй rise* with the dawn; на ~é at dawn; **2.** (*начало, зарождение*) dawn; ~ нóвой жи́зни the dawn of a new life; **3.** *воен.* (*сигнал*) retréat; игрáть зóрю sound the retréat; ◇ от ~и́ до ~и́ (*с вечера до утра*) from dusk to dawn; (*с утра до вечера*) from dawn to dusk.

заря́д *м.* charge; *перен.* fund, supplý, store; ~ энéргии store of énergy.

заряди́ть I *сов. см.* заряжа́ть.

заря́д|ить II *сов. разг.:* ~ однó и тó же keep* hárping on the same string; дождь ~и́л надóлго the rain had set in for a long time.

заря́дка *ж.* **1.** (*аккумулятора*) chárging; **2.** *спорт.* (*setting-úp*) éxercises.

заря́дный: ~ я́щик *воен.* ammunítion wágon; cáisson *амер.*

заряжа́ние *с.* lóading.

заряжа́ть, заряди́ть (*вн.*) **1.** (*оружие, фотоаппарат и т. п.*) load (*smth.*); **2.** (*электричеством*) charge (*smth.*).

заса́д|а *ж.* ámbush, сидéть в ~e líe* in ámbush; устрóить ~y lay* an ámbush.

засади́ть *сов. см.* заса́живать.

заса́живать, засади́ть **1.** (*вн. тв.*; *растениями*) plant (*smth.* with); **2.** (*вн.*) *разг.* (*подвергать заключению*) shut* up (*smb.*); засади́ть *кого-л.* в тюрьмý clap *smb.* in gaol; **3.** (*вн. за вн., вн. + инф.*) *разг.* (*заставлять делать что-л.*) make* (*smb.*) get down (to *smth.*); засади́ть *кого-л.* за кни́ги make* *smb.* stúdy; **4.** (*вн. в вн.*) *разг.* (*вонзать*) stick* (*smth.* in).

заса́ленный *разг.* gréasy.

заса́ливать I, заса́лить (*вн.*) make* (*smth.*) gréasy.

заса́ливать II, засоли́ть (*вн.*) salt (*smth.*); (*мясо*) corn (*smth.*).

заса́ливаться, заса́литься becóme* gréasy.

заса́лить *сов. см.* заса́ливать I. ~ся *сов. см.* заса́ливаться.

заса́сывать, засосáть (*вн.*) suck in (*smth.*); *перен.* swállow up (*smb., smth.*).

заса́харенн|ый cándied, crýstallized

заса́хар|ивать, заса́харить (*вн.*) cándy (*smth.*). ~иваться, заса́хариться: варéнье заса́харилось the jam has súgared/crýstallized. ~ить(ся) *сов. см.* заса́харивать(ся).

засвети́ть I *сов.* (*вн.*) light* (*smth.*).

засвети́ть II *сов. см.* засвéчивать.

засвети́ться I *сов.* light* up.

засвети́ться II *сов. см.* засвéчиваться.

за́светло dúring dáylight; befóre dark, befóre níghtfall.

засвéчивать, засвети́ть (*вн.*) *фото* expóse (*smth.*), let* the light (into). ~ся, засвети́ться *фото* get* expósed.

засвидéтельствовать *сов.* (*вн.*) téstify (*smth.*); (*документ*) cértify (*smth.*), witness (*smth.*).

засевáть, засéять (*вн.*) sow* (*smth.*).

заседáни|е *с.* cónference, méeting; (*суда, парламента и т. п.*) séssion, sítting; ~ Верхóвного Совéта séssion/sítting of the Supréme Sóviet; на ýтреннем ~и at the mórning séssion.

заседáтель *м.* asséssor; ◇ нарóдный ~ Péople's asséssor.

заседáть *несов.* sit*, be* in cónference/séssion.

засекáть I, засéчь (*вн.*) **1.** (*делать засечки*) notch (*smth.*), nick (*smth.*); **2.** (*установив местоположение, нанести на план, на карту*) plot (*smth.*); map (*smth.*); ◇ засéчь врéмя note the time.

засекáть II, засéчь (*вн.*) (*до смерти*) flog (*smb.*) to death.

засекрé|тить *сов. см.* засекрéчивать. ~ченный sécret; húsh-hush *разг.*

засекрéчивать, засекрéтить (*вн.*) **1.** (*сведения, документы*) restríct (*smth.*), make* (*smth.*) sécret; **2.** *разг.* (*работника*) give* (*smb.*) áccess to sécret dócuments, entrúst (*smb.*) with sécret work.

заселéние *с.* (*края, области*) séttling; (*дома*) pútting ténants in; ~ нóвого дóма начнётся в декабрé péople will start móving ínto the house in Decémber, the ténants will take óver the house in Decémber; ~ нóвых земéль séttling of new térritory.

засели́ть *сов. см.* заселя́ть.

заселя́ть, засели́ть (*вн.*) (*область, край*) séttle (*smth.*); (*дом*) put* ténants (ínto), óccupy (*smth.*), ténant (*smth.*).

засéсть *сов. разг.* **1.** (*усесться где-л.*) sit* down; **2.** (*за вн., + инф.*) (*приняться за что-л.*) séttle down (to, + to *inf*) ~ за рабóту séttle down to *one's* work; ~ писáть séttle down to write; **3.** (*надолго расположиться где-л.*) búry/hide* *oneself*; ~ дóма búry *oneself* indóors, stay at home; **4.** *воен.* take* up a posítion, dig in; **5.** (*застрять*) lodge.

засéчь I, II *сов. см.* засекáть I, II.

засéять *сов. см.* засевáть.

засидéться *сов. см.* заси́живаться.

заси́живаться, засидéться stay late; ~ за рабóтой sit* long óver *one's* work; (*ночью*) sit* up wórking.

заси́лье *с.* dominátion, prepónderance, dóminating ínfluence.

заси|я́ть *сов.* **1.** shine*; *перен.* becóme* rádiant; **2.** (*показаться*) gleam; вдали́ ~я́л кýпол цéркви the gléaming dome of a church rose in the dístance.

заскирдовáть *сов. см.* скирдовáть.

заскóк *м. разг.* whim, méntal block.

заскорýзл|ый hárdened, hórny; ~ые рýки cálloused hands.

заскрежетáть *сов.:* ~ зубáми grind*/gnash *one's* teeth.

заскучáть *сов.* feel* míserable, get* depréssed.

заслáть *сов. см.* засылáть.

заслон *м.* 1. (*преграда*) bárrier; снéжный ~ snow wall; 2. *воен.* cóvering force.

заслони́ть(ся) *сов. см.* заслоня́ть(ся).

заслонка *ж.* 1. (*печи*) door; 2. (*щит в шлюзах*) gate.

заслоня́ть, заслони́ть (*вн.*) shield (*smb., smth.*), screen (*smb., smth.*); *перен.* overshádow (*smth.*); ~ свет be* in the light. ~ся, заслони́ться: ~ся от свéта shield *one's* eyes from the light.

заслуг|**а** *ж.* sérvice; ~и перед Рódиной sérvices to *one's* cóuntry; ~и в óбласти науки sérvices to science; это ва́ша ~ it's all thanks to you; ◇ по ~ам accórding to *one's* desérts.

заслуженн|**ый** 1. well-desérved, well-éarned; (*справедливый*) desérved; ~ая награда well-desérved rewárd; ~ упрёк desérved/mérited repróach; 2. (*имеющий заслуги*) célebrated, distínguished; ~ человéк distínguished pérson, man* of mérit; 3. (*в составе звания*) Hónoured; ~ арти́ст респу́блики Hónoured Ártist of the Repúblic.

заслу́живать, заслужи́ть 1. (*вн.; какого-л. отношения*) desérve (*smth.*); заслужи́ть любовь desérve love; заслужи́ть награ́ду desérve a rewárd; заслужи́ть всеобщее довéрие win* univérsal cónfidence; 2. *тк. несов.* (*рд.; быть достойным чего-л.*) mérit (*smth.*), desérve (*smth.*); ~ довéрия be* perfectly crédible; 3. (*вн.*) *разг.* (*зарабатывать*) earn (*smth.*).

заслужи́ть *сов. см.* заслу́живать 1, 3.

заслу́шать(ся) *сов. см.* заслу́шивать(ся).

заслу́шивать, заслу́шать (*вн.*) hear* (*smth.*); заслу́шать отчёт hear* a repórt. ~ся, заслу́шаться (*рд.*) listen to (*smb., smth.*) with delight.

заслы́ш|**ать** *сов.* (*вн.*) catch* the sound (of); я и́здали ~ал их голоса́ I could hear their vóices in the distance.

засма́триваться, засмотрéться (на *вн.*) be* lost in contemplátion (of), be* unáble to take *one's* eyes off (*smb., smth.*).

засмея́ть *сов.* (*вн.*) *разг.* hold* (*smb.*) up to rídicule, scoff (at).

засмея́ться *сов.* laugh, begín* to laugh.

засмотрéться *сов. см.* засма́триваться.

засне́женный snów-cóvered.

засну́ть *сов. см.* засыпа́ть I.

засня́ть *сов.* (*вн.*) *разг.* take* a phótograph (of); (*в кино*) shoot* (*smb., smth.*).

засо́в *м.* bolt.

засо́вывать, засу́нуть (*вн.*) thrust* (*smth.*); я куда́-то засу́нул егó письмо́ I put his létter awáy sómewhere.

засо́л *м.* 1. (*действие*) sálting; píckling; 2.: вку́сный ~ tásty píckle.

засоли́ть *сов. см.* заса́ливать II.

засорéние *с.* clógging, obstrúction; (*сорными травами*) chóking; ~ рек и водоёмов clógging of rívers and réservoirs; ◇ ~ желу́дка clógging (of the bówels).

засори́ть(ся) *сов. см.* засоря́ть(ся).

засоря́ть, засори́ть (*вн.*) 1. (*загрязнять*) lítter (*smth.*); 2. (*повреждать чем-л.*) clog (*smth.*); ~ желу́док clog (the bówels); засори́ть себé глаз get* sómething in *one's* eye; 3. (*заполнять собой — о сорных травах*) choke (*smth.*) with weeds; 4. (*заполнять чем-л. ненужным*) clútter up (*smth.*); ~ язы́к clútter up the lánguage. ~ся, засори́ться be* clogged.

засоса́ть I *сов. см.* заса́сывать.

засос|**а́ть** II *сов. разг.* (*начать сосать*) suck; у меня́ ~а́ло под ло́жечкой I have a sínking sensátion in the pit of my stómach.

засо́хнуть *сов. см.* засыха́ть.

за́спанн|**ый** sléepy; héavy with sleep *после сущ.*; у негó ~ вид he looks half-aslées; ~ые глаза́ sléepy eyes.

заспа́ться *сов. разг.* oversléep (*onesélf*).

заста́ва *ж. воен.* pícket; пограни́чная ~ fróntier post.

заста́вать, заста́ть (*вн., smth.*); (*застигать*) catch* (*smb.*); не заста́ть кого-л. дома not find *smb.* at home.

заста́вить I, II *сов. см.* заставля́ть I, II.

заста́вка *ж.* héad-piece, vignétte.

заставля́ть I, **заста́вить** (*вн. + инф.; принуждать*) make* (*smb. + inf.*), force (*smb. + to inf.*); не могу́ заста́вить себя́ прочита́ть эту кни́гу I can't bring mysélf to read that book; ~ кого-л. замолча́ть sílence *smb.*; ~ долго ждать себя́ be* a long time (cóming), keep* *one* waiting; ~ долго проси́ть себя́ be* hard to persuáde.

заставля́ть II, **заста́вить** (*вн.*) 1. (*загораживать*) block (*smth.*); ~ дверь шка́фом block a dóorway with a cúpboard/wárdrobe; 2. (*загромождать*) clútter (*smth.*); заста́вить ко́мнату мéбелью clútter a room with fúrniture, overfúrnish a room.

застава́ться, застоя́ться 1. (*о лошади*) becóme* réstive; 2. (*о воде, воздухе*) becóme* stale/stágnant.

застарéлый invéterate; (*о болезни*) chrónic.

заста́ть *сов. см.* застава́ть.

застёгивать, застегну́ть (*вн.*) fásten (*smth.*), do* up (*smth.*); (*на пуговицы тж.*) bútton up (*smth.*); (*на крючки тж.*) hook up (*smth.*). ~ся, застегну́ться 1. (*застёгивать на себе одежду*) do* *one's* coat up; do* onesélf up *разг.*; застегну́ться на все пу́говицы bútton *one's* coat up tight; 2. (*о пуговицах и т. п.*) fásten, do* up.

застегну́ть(ся) *сов. см.* застёгивать(ся).

застёжка *ж.* fástener; frog.

застекли́ть *сов. см.* застекля́ть.

застекля́ть, застекли́ть (*вн.*) glaze (*smth.*), put* glass (in).

засте́нок *м.* tórture-chamber.

засте́нчив|**ость** *ж.* shýness, timídity. ~ый shy, tímid.

застига́ть, засти́гнуть, засти́чь (*вн.*) catch* (*smth.*), overtáke (*smth.*); засти́чь кого-л. враспло́х catch* *smb.* únawáres; засти́чь кого-л. на мéсте преступлéния catch* *smb.* in the act, catch* *smb.* red-hánded; гроза́ засти́гла нас в лесу́ we were in the woods when the storm overtóok/caught us.

засти́гнуть *сов. см.* застига́ть.

застила́ть, застла́ть (*вн.*) 1. (*покрывать*) spread* (*smth.*); ~ стол ска́тертью put*/spread* a táblecloth on the táble; 2. (*о тумане*) veil (*smth.*); (*о слезах*) dim (*smth.*). ~ся, застла́ться (*туманом*) be* veiled; (*слезами*) becóme* dim.

застира́ть *сов. см.* засти́рывать.

засти́рывать, застира́ть (*вн.*) 1. (*отмывать*) wash (*smth.*) out; застира́ть пя́тна на ска́терти wash the spots out of a táblecloth; 2. (*портить плохой стиркой*) spoil* (*smth.*) in the wash; ~ бельё spoil* the línen in the wash.

засти́чь *сов. см.* застига́ть.

застла́ть(ся) *сов. см.* застила́ть(ся).

засто́й *м.* immobílity, stánding still; *перен.* stándstill, stagnátion; ~ в промы́шленности stagnátion/stándstill in índustry.

застона́ть *сов.* begín* to moan/groan.

засто́поривать, засто́порить (*вн.*) stop (*smth.*). ~ся, засто́пориться stop, come* to a stándstill.

засто́порить(ся) *сов. см.* засто́поривать(ся).

застоя́ться *сов. см.* застава́ться.

застра́ивать, застро́ить (*вн.*) put* up búildings (on, all óver), devélop (*smth.*), build* (on). ~ся, застро́иться be* built óver, be* devéloped.

застрахова́ть *сов. см.* страхова́ть 1. ~ся *сов. см.* страхова́ться.

застра́чивать, застрочи́ть (*вн.*) seam (*smth.*), stitch (*smth.*).

застрева́ть, застря́ть 1. stick* (fast); 2. *разг.*

(*задерживаться где-л.*) be* held up; ◇ застрять в го́рле stick* in *one's* throat.

застрели́ть *сов.* (*вн.*) shoot (*smb.*, *smth.*). ~ся *сов.* shoot* *oneself*.

застре́льщ|ик *м.*, ~ица *ж.* ínitiator, pionéer.

застро́|енный búilt-up, devéloped. ~ить(ся) *сов. см.* застра́ивать(ся).

застро́й|ка *ж.* búilding; пра́во ~ки the right to build. ~щик *м.* pérson building his own house.

застрочи́ть I *сов. см.* застра́чивать.

застрочи́ть II *сов. разг.* (*о пулемёте*) (begín* to) chátter.

застря́ть *сов. см.* застрева́ть.

застуди́ть(ся) *сов. см.* засту́живать(ся).

засту́живать, застуди́ть (*вн.*) chill (*smth.*), make* (*smb.*, *smth.*) cold; застуди́ть лёгкие catch* a chill on one's chest. ~ся, застуди́ться catch* a chill.

за́ступ *м.* spade.

заступа́ться, заступи́ться (за *вн.*) intercéde (for), take* the part (of), stand* up (for).

заступи́ться *сов. см.* заступа́ться.

засту́пн|ик *м.*, ~ица *ж.* intercéssor, protéctor. ~ичество *с.* intercéssion.

застыва́ть, засты́ть 1. (*сгущаться*) thícken, congéal; *кул.* jélly; 2. (*замерзать*) freeze*, be* cold, be* frózen; 3. (*оставаться без изменения*) freeze*, stíffen; на его́ лице́ засты́ла улы́бка his face set in a fixed smile; ~ на ме́сте be* róoted to the spot, stop dead.

застыди́ться *сов.* be* embárrassed.

засты́ть *сов. см.* застыва́ть.

засу́нуть *сов. см.* засо́вывать.

за́суха *ж.* drought.

засухоусто́йчивый dróught-resistant.

засу́чивать, засучи́ть (*вн.*) roll up (*smth.*); засучи́ть рукава́ roll up *one's* sleeves.

засучи́ть *сов. см.* засу́чивать.

засу́шивать, засуши́ть (*вн.*) 1. dry (*smth.*); (*цветы*) press (*smth.*); 2. *разг.* (*кушанье*) overdó* (*smth.*).

засуши́ть *сов. см.* засу́шивать.

засу́шлив|ый dróughty, dry; ~ые райо́ны árid/wáterless dístricts; ~ год dry year.

засчита́ть *сов. см.* засчи́тывать.

засчи́тывать, засчита́ть (*вн.*) count (*smth.*); ~ в упла́ту до́лга 50 рубле́й count fífty róubles towárds páyment of a debt.

засыла́ть, засла́ть (*вн.*) *разг.* send* (*smb.*, *smth.*).

засы́пать *сов. см.* засыпа́ть II.

засыпа́ть I, засну́ть go* to sleep, fall* asléep.

засыпа́ть II, засы́пать (*вн.*) 1. (*заполнять*) fill in (*smth.*), fill up (*smth.*); 2. (*покрывать*) cóver (*smth.*), heap (*smth.*); 3. (*вн., рд.*) *разг.* (*насыпать*) pour (*smth.*); ~ крупу́ в суп stir a céreal ínto the soup; засы́пать овса́ ло́шади give* a horse some oats; 4.: ~ кого́-л. пода́рками shówer *smb.* with gifts; ~ кого́-л. вопро́сами bombárd/pelt *smb.* with quéstions.

засы́паться I *сов. см.* засыпа́ться I, II.

засыпа́ться I, засы́паться 1. trickle; песо́к засы́пался за воротни́к sand tríckled down *one's* neck; 2. (*тв.*; *покрываться*) be* cóvered/sprínkled óver (with).

засыпа́ться II, засы́паться *разг.* 1. (*попадаться*) be* caught; 2. (*проваливаться на экзамене*) fail, flunk.

засыха́ть, засо́хнуть 1. dry, get* dry; (*о грязи*) cake; 2. (*о растениях*) wíther.

зата́ённый sécret; (*сдерживаемый*) suppréssed.

затаи́ть *сов.* (*вн.*) 1. (*утаить что-л.*) keep* (*smth.*) for *oneself*; 2. (*чувство, мысль*) hárbour (*smth.*); ~ оби́ду hárbour a gríevance, nurse a grudge; ◇ ~ дыха́ние hold* *one's* breath.

зата́лкивать, затолкну́ть (*вн.*) push (*smb.*, *smth.*), shove (*smb.*, *smth.*).

зата́пливать, затопи́ть (*вн.*) light* (*smth.*).

зата́птывать, затопта́ть (*вн.*) 1. stamp (*smth.*),

tread* down (*smth.*); 2. *разг.* (*оставлять следы*) leave* dirty fóotmarks (on); ◇ затопта́ть кого́-л. в грязь drag *smb.* in/through the mud.

зата́сканный *разг.* (*изношенный*) shábby, worn out; *перен.* (*избитый, опошленный*) stale, háck-neyed.

затаска́ть *сов. см.* зата́скивать I.

зата́скивать I, затаска́ть (*вн.*) *разг.* (*занашивать*) wear* out (*smth.*); *перен.* overwórk (*smth.*), make* (*smth.*) háckneyed.

зата́скивать II, затащи́ть (*вн.*) (*уносить куда-л.*) cárry (*smth.*) off.

затащи́ть *сов. см.* зата́скивать II.

затвердева́ть, затверде́ть hárden; (*о жидкости*) solídify.

затверде́|лый hard, sólid. ~ние *с.* (hard) lump.

затверде́ть *сов. см.* затвердева́ть.

затверди́ть I *сов.* (*вн.*) (*заучить*) get* (*smth.*) by heart.

затверди́ть II *сов.* (*вн.*) *разг.* (*начать твердить*): ~ одно́ и то́ же keep* on repéating the same thing.

затво́р *м.* 1. *разг.* (*засов*) bolt; 2. (*фотоаппарата*) shútter; (*винтовки*) bolt; (*орудия*) bréech-block.

затвори́ть(ся) *сов. см.* затворя́ть(ся).

затворя́ть, затвори́ть (*вн.*) shut* (*smth.*). ~ся, затвори́ться 1. (*о двери и т. п.*) shut*; 2. (*о человеке*) shut* *oneself* up.

затева́ть, зате́ять (*вн.*, + *инф.*) *разг.* start (*smth.*, + -ing), undertáke* (*smth.*, + to *inf.*); ~ возню́ start scúffling abóut, start máking a noise; ~ игру́ start a game; ~ спор start an árgument.

зате́й|ливый (*замысловатый*) eláborate; (*лишённый простоты*) íntricate, ingénious; ~ рису́нок eláborate páttern. ~ник *м.* 1. entertáining féllow; 2. (*руководитель массовых развлечений*) amúsements órganizer.

затека́ть, зате́чь 1. (*попадать, проникать*) leak, tríckle; вода́ затекла́ в подва́л the wáter leaked through ínto the céllar; 2. (*распухать*) swell*; 3. (*неметь*) grow* numb; у меня́ затекла́ нога́ my leg has gone dead/numb.

зате́м 1. (*потом*) then; 2. (*для того*): я ~ и пришёл that's what I've come for; ◇ ~, чтобы to.

затемн|е́ние *с.* 1. dárkening; 2. (*маскировка света*) bláck-out; 3. (*затемнённое место*) dark patch/spot. ~и́ть *сов. см.* затемня́ть.

за́темно *разг.* 1. (*до рассвета*) befóre dawn; 2. (*когда стемнеет*) áfter dark.

затемня́ть, затемни́ть (*вн.*) 1. dárken (*smth.*); *перен.* obscúre (*smth.*); 2. (*маскировать свет*) black out (*smth.*).

затени́ть *сов. см.* затеня́ть.

затеня́ть, затени́ть (*вн.*) shade (*smth.*).

затере́ть *сов. см.* затира́ть.

затеря́вшийся lost; ~ в лесу́ до́мик a hut búried in the heart of the fórest.

затеря́нный lost.

затеря́ть *сов.* (*вн.*) *разг.* lose* (*smth.*), misláy* (*smth.*). ~ся *сов. разг.* 1. (*потеряться*) be* lost, go* astráy; 2. (*скрыться, пропасть из виду*) vánish, disappéar; 3. (*оказаться неприметным среди кого-л., чего-л.*) be* lost, be* dwarfed to insígnificance.

зате́чь *сов. см.* затека́ть.

зате́|я *ж.* 1. (*замысел*) idéa, inténtion; (*предприятие*) vénture; но́вая, очередна́я ~ látest whim, new fad; 2. (*забава*) game, amúsement; ребя́чьи ~и chíldish tricks; ◇ по́просту, без ~й quite infórmally/símply.

зате́ять *сов. см.* затева́ть.

затира́ть, затере́ть (*вн.*) 1. (*стирать*) rub (*smth.*) out, effáce (*smth.*); 2. (*теснить*) hold* (*smb.*, *smth.*) fast, trap (*smb.*, *smth.*); затёртый льда́ми stuck in the ice, íce-bound; **3.** *разг.* (*не давать хода*) push (*smb.*) ínto the báckground, keep* (*smb.*) down, upstáge (*smb.*).

затиха́ть, затихнуть **1.** grow* quíet, quíeten down; (*переставать слышаться*) die awáy; го́род опусте́л и зати́х the cíty becáme desérted and quíet; шаги́ зати́хли the steps died awáy; **2.** (*прекращаться*) die down, abáte; бу́ря зати́хла the storm abáted.

зати́хнуть *сов. см.* затиха́ть.

зати́шье *с.* **1.** (*безветрие*) calm, lull; **2.** (*тишина*) hush; **3.** (*тихое место*) shéltered spot; **4.** (*приостановка, ослабление*) lull.

заткну́ть *сов. см.* затыка́ть.

затмева́ть, затми́ть (*вн.*) dárken (*smth.*), eclípse (*smth.*); *перен.* put* (*smb.*) in the óther hand.

затме́ние *с.* **1.** eclípse; по́лное ~ tótal eclípse; **2.** *разг.:* на него́ нашло́ ~ his mind went blank.

затми́ть *сов. см.* затмева́ть.

зато́ but; no ~ but, on the óther hand.

затова́р|ивание *с.* óverstócking. **~ивать,** затова́рить (*вн.*) stock too much (of). **~ить** *сов. см.* затова́ривать.

затолка́ть *сов.* (*вн.*) **1.** (*толчками замучить*) jóstle (*smb.*); **2.** (*толкая, заставить войти, въехать куда-либо*) push (*smb., smth.*).

затолкну́ть *сов. см.* зата́лкивать.

зато́н *м.* báckwater.

затону́ть *сов.* sink*, go* down; (*о корабле тж.*) fóunder.

затопи́ть I *сов. см.* зата́пливать.

затопи́ть II *сов. см.* затопля́ть.

затопле́ние *с.* flóoding.

затопля́ть, затопи́ть (*вн.*) **1.** (*заливать*) flood (*smth.*), ínundate (*smth.*); **2.** (*пускать ко дну*) sink* (*smth.*), scúttle (*smth.*).

затопта́ть *сов. см.* зата́птывать.

зато́р *м.* block, congéstion; (*при сплаве леса*) lóg-jam; ~ в у́личном движе́нии tráffic-jam.

затормо́з|и́ть *сов.* (*вн.*) **1.** brake (*smth.*), put* on the brake(s); води́тель ре́зко ~и́л the dríver braked shárply; **2.** *разг.* (*задержать развитие*) slow down (*smth.*), check (*smth.*), hold* up (*smth.*).

заторопи́ться *сов.* begín* to bústle abóut.

зато́ч|а́ть, заточи́ть (*вн.*) *уст.* incárcerate (*smb.*), confíne (*smb.*); ~е́ние *с. уст.* incarcerátion, confínement.

заточи́ть I *сов. см.* заточа́ть.

заточи́ть II *сов.* (*вн.*) *разг.* shárpen (*smth.*).

затошн|и́ть *сов. безл.:* его́ ~и́ло he begán to feel sick.

затрави́ть *сов.* (*вн.*) hunt down (*smth.*); *перен.* hound (*smb.*), pérsecute (*smb.*).

затра́гивать, затро́нуть (*вн.*) **1.** (*касаться*) touch (*smb., smth.*); *перен. тж.* afféct (*smb., smth.*); пу́ля затро́нула кость the búllet touched the bone; ~ чьи́-л. интере́сы afféct smb.'s ínterests; ~ чье́-л. самолю́бие wound smb.'s vánity; **2.** (*касаться чего-л. в разговоре и т. п.*) touch (upón).

затра́|та *ж.* expénditure; *мн.* óutlay *sg*; не щадя́ ~т regárdless of expénse, spáring no cost; ~ труда́ expénditure of lábour. **~тить** *сов. см.* затра́чивать.

затра́чивать, затра́тить (*вн. на вн.*) expénd (*smth.* on), spend* (*smth.* on).

затре́бовать *сов.* (*вн.*) demánd (*smth.*); ~ что-л. по телефо́ну órder *smth.* by télephone; ~ све́дения demánd informátion.

затру́живать *сов. см.* затра́гивать.

затрудн|е́ние *с.* difficulty; (*препятствие*) impédiment; материа́льные ~е́ния móney/fináncial difficulties; быть в ~е́нии be* in difficulty. **~ённый** lábonred, impéded; (*содержащий трудности*) difficult, áwkward; ~и́тельный difficult, embárrassing; ~и́тельное положе́ние áwkward predícament, embárrassing situátion.

затрудн|и́ть(ся) *сов. см.* затрудня́ть(ся). **~я́ть,** затрудни́ть **1.** (что-л.) make* (*smth.*) difficult; **2.** (*кого-*

-*л.*) bóther (*smb.*), tróuble (*smb.*); ◇ е́сли вас не затрудни́т if it's not too much tróuble. **~я́ться,** затрудни́ться find* it difficult; я ~я́юсь сказа́ть I hárdly know what to say.

затума́н|ивать, затума́нить (*вн.*) veil (*smth.*) in mist, mist (*smth.*); (*слезами*) dim (*smth.*); *перен.* fúddle (*smth.*). **~иваться,** затума́ниться be* veiled in mist; (*о стекле*) be* místed óver; *перен.* be* fúddled; её глаза́ затума́нились her eyes grew místy. **~ить(ся)** *сов. см.* затума́нивать(ся).

затупи́ть *сов.* (*вн.*) *разг.* blunt (*smth.*). **~ся** *сов. разг.* get* blunt.

затух|а́ние *с.* (*о радиоволнах и т. п.*) fade, fáding. **~а́ть,** затухнуть **1.** *разг.* (*переставать гореть*) go* out; ~а́ть от дождя́ be* put out by the rain; **2.** (*о радиоволнах и т. п.*) subsíde, fade.

зату́хнуть *сов. см.* затуха́ть.

затушева́ть *сов. см.* затушёвывать.

затушёвывать, затушева́ть (*вн.*) **1.** (*покрывать тушёвкой*) shade (*smth.*) in; **2.** (*сглаживать*) veil (*smth.*), gloss (*smth.*) óver; ~ социа́льные противоре́чия veil sócial contradíctions.

затуши́ть *сов.* (*вн.*) *разг.* put* out (*smth.*), extínguish (*smth.*).

за́тхлый músty, fústy; ~ во́здух stale air.

затыка́ть, заткну́ть (*вн.*) **1.** (*закрывать*) stop up (*smth.*); (*пробкой*) cork (*smth.*); **2.** *разг.* (*засовывать*) thrust* (*smth.*); ◇ заткну́ть за́ пояс кого́-л. eclípse smb., outshíne* smb.; ~ рот кому́-л. stop smb.'s mouth, gag smb.

заты́лок *м.* back of the head; почеса́ть ~ scratch one's head; сдви́нуть ша́пку на ~ push one's hat on to the back of one's head, tilt one's hat báckwards.

заты́чка *ж. разг.* plug; *перен.* stópgap.

затя́гивать I, затяну́ть **1.** (*вн.; натягивать, стягивать концы*) tíghten (*smth.*); **2.** (*вн. тв.; покрывать*) cóver (*smth.* with); **3.:** ра́ну затяну́ло the wound has heáled óver; **4.** (*вн.; засасывать*) draw* in (*smb., smth.*); **5.** (*вн.; задерживать*) drag out (*smth.*).

затя́гивать II, затяну́ть (*вн.*) *разг.* strike* up (*smth.*); ~ пе́сню start sínging, strike* up a song.

затя́гив|аться, затяну́ться **1.** (*стягиваться*) belt onesélf, búckle one's belt; он ту́го затяну́лся ремешко́м he drew his belt tight; **2.** (*тв.; покрываться*) be* cóvered (by); не́бо ~а́ется ту́чами the sky is clóuding óver; **3.:** ра́на ~а́ется the wound is heáling óver; **4.** (*задерживаться*) drag on; собра́ние затяну́лось the méeting drágged on; **5.** (*при курении*) inhále; ~ папиро́сой inhále the smoke of a cigarétte.

затя́ж|ка *ж.* **1.** (*промедление*) deláy; **2.** (*при курении*) inhalátion, draw; он сде́лал не́сколько ~ек he took a few puffs/drags.

затяжн|о́й protrácted; ~а́я боле́знь língering íllness; ◇ ~ прыжо́к *спорт.* free-fáll jump, deláyed jump.

затяну́ть I, II *сов. см.* затя́гивать I, II.

затяну́ться *сов. см.* затя́гиваться.

зау́мный abstrúse.

зауны́вн|ый móurnful; ~ая пе́сня móurnful song.

заупря́миться *сов.* be* óbstinate; (*о человеке тж.*) dig* one's heels in *идиом.*

заура́дный órdinary, medíocre.

заусе́н|ец *м.,* ~ица *ж.* **1.** (*у ногтя*) hángnail; **2.** (*на металле*) burr.

зау́ченный stúdied, mechánical; ~ жест stúdied gésture.

зау́чивать, заучи́ть (*вн.*) mémorize (*smth.*); ~ что-л. наизу́сть learn* *smth.* by heart. **~ся,** заучи́ться *разг.* stúdy too hard.

заучи́ть(ся) *сов. см.* зау́чивать(ся).

зафикси́ровать *сов.* (*вн.*) fix (*smth.*).

заха́живать *несов. разг.* drop in.

захва́ливать, **захвали́ть** (вн.) разг. overpráise (smb.), give* (smb.) too big an idéa of himsélf.

захвали́ть сов. см. захва́ливать.

захва́т м. séizure, cápture; (территории тж.) annexátion.

захва́т|анный разг. soiled; (о книге) múch-thúmbed. **-ать** сов. см. захва́тывать I.

захвати́ть сов. см. захва́тывать II.

захва́тническ|ий prédatory, rapácious, expánsionist; **-ие** войны wars of cónquest.

захва́тчик м. inváder, aggréssor; (власти) usúrper.

захва́тывать I, **захвата́ть** (вн.) разг. soil (smth.), leave* dírty fínger-marks (on).

захва́т|ывать II, **захвати́ть** (вн.) 1. (брать какое-л. количество чего-л.) take* (smth.), seize (smth.); (крепко зажимать) grasp (smth.), get* hold (of); 2. (брать с собой) bring* (smth.) (приходя); take* (smth.) (уходя); 3. (завладевать) seize (smth.), cápture (smth.); (территории тж.) annéx (smth.); захвати́ть власть seize pówer; захвати́ть инициати́ву cápture the initiative; 4. (увлекать) engróss (smb.); рабо́та захвати́ла его́ целико́м he is complétely engróssed in his work; 5. разг. (вовремя принять меры): во́время захвати́ть боле́знь check an íllness in time; ◇ захвати́ть кого́-л. враспло́х take* smb. unawáres, take* smb. by surprise; дух **-ывает** it takes one's breath awáy.

захва́тывающ|ий absórbing, thrílling; с **-им** интере́сом with absórbing ínterest; **-ая** сце́на thrílling scene.

захвора́ть сов. разг. fall* ill; (тв.) be* down (with), have* (smth.).

захире́ть сов. см. хире́ть.

захлебну́ться сов. см. захлёбываться.

захлёбыв|аться, **захлебну́ться** 1. choke; захлебну́ться кро́вью choke in one's own blood; он захлебну́лся и утону́л his lungs filled with wáter and he drowned; 2. (от рд.; испытывать затруднение в дыхании) choke (with); **-** от волне́ния splútter with excítement, be* álmost chóking with excítement; говори́ть **-аясь** splútter; 3. (прекращаться) stop, péter out; 4. разг. (о моторе) stall.

захлестну́ть сов. см. захлёстывать.

захлёстывать, **захлестну́ть** 1. (вн. тв.; верёвкой и т. п.) fling* (smth. óver, round); (обвивать) wind* (smth. round); 2. (вн.; обдавать — о воде) sweep* óver (smb.); (заливать) swamp (smth.).

захло́пать сов. begín* to clap, start clápping; **-** в ладо́ши clap.

захло́пнуть(ся) сов. см. захло́пывать(ся).

захлопота́ться сов. разг. be* run off one's legs.

захло́пывать, **захло́пнуть** (вн.) bang (smth.), slam (smth.); захло́пнуть дверь bang the door to; **-** кры́шку bang the lid down. **-ся**, захло́пнуться bang shut, slam to.

захо́д м. 1.: **-** со́лнца súnset; 2. (в вн.; куда-л.) stop (at); **-** в порт pútting in to a port; без **-а** (в) without stópping; **-** на цель ав. run óver the tárget.

заход|и́ть, **зайти́** 1. (в вн.) call (at), drop in (at); (к дт.) call (on smb.), look in (at smb.'s), call in (at smb.'s); **-и́** домо́й without góing home first; 3а (тв.) call (for), come* (for), call round (for); **-и́(те)** за мной call for me, come and fetch me; **-и́(те)** за кни́гами call round for the books; 3. (подходить со стороны) go* round (to the óther side), appróach from the óther side; зайти́ сза́ди go* round to the óther side of the car; зайти́ в тыл проти́внику take* the énemy in the rear; 4. (за вн.; скрываться) go* (behínd); со́лнце зашло́ за ту́чу the sun went behínd a cloud; 5. (попадать, оказываться) get*, find* onesélf; куда́ мы зашли́? where have we got to?; **-** сли́шком далеко́ go* too far (тж. перен.); 6. (о небесных светилах) set*; 7.:

разгово́р зашёл о нём the conversátion touched on him; ◇ де́ло зашло́ далеко́ the mátter has gone too far.

захолу́стный out-of-the-wáy, províncial.

захолу́стье с. óut-of-the-wáy place.

захоте́ть(ся) сов. см. хоте́ть(ся).

захохота́ть сов. begín* to laugh, burst* out láughing.

захрипе́ть сов. разг. begín* to croak.

захрома́ть сов. разг. begín* to limp; (о лошади) go* lame.

захуда́лый (незначительный) insigníficant, shábby; уст. (обедневший) impóverished.

зацвести́ I сов. burst* into blóssom, blóssom.

зацвести́ II сов. см. зацвета́ть.

зацвета́ть, **зацвести́** 1. (о стоячей воде) turn green; 2. разг. (покрываться плесенью) becóme* cóvered with míldew.

зацелова́ть сов. (вн.) разг. smóther (smb.) with kísses.

зацепи́ть(ся) сов. см. зацепля́ть(ся).

заце́пка ж. разг. 1. (крючок) catch, hook; 2. (предлог) prétext.

зацепля́ть, **зацепи́ть** 1. (вн., за вн.) get* hold (of); 2. (за вн.; задевать) catch* (on). **-ся**, зацепи́ться 1. get* caught; (за вн.) catch* (on); зацепи́ться ного́й за ковёр catch* one's foot in the cárpet; 2. (за вн.) разг. (ухватиться) get* hold (of).

зачасти́ть сов. разг. 1. (стать более частым) becóme* more fréquent; 2. (заговорить быстро) ráttle on, speed* on; 3. (к дт.) becóme* a fréquent vísitor (at smb.'s house).

зачасту́ю разг. óften, fréquently.

зача́тие с. concéption.

зача́т|ок м. 1. émbryo (pl -os); 2. обыкн. мн. (начало чего-л.) rúdiments. **-очный** rudiméntary; в **-очном** состоя́нии in an embryónic state.

зача́хнуть сов. см. ча́хнуть.

зачём what... for, why; **-** вы пришли́? what did you come for?; what made you come?; вот **-** он пришёл! so that's why he came! **-то** for some púrpose.

зачерви́веть сов. becóme* wórm-eaten.

зачёркивать, **зачеркну́ть** (вн.) deléte (smth.), cross out (smth.), strike* out (smth.).

зачеркну́ть сов. см. зачёркивать.

зачерпну́ть сов. см. зачёрпывать.

зачёрпывать, **зачерпну́ть** (вн.) scoop up (smth.).

зачерстве́лый stale; перен. hard, crábbed.

зачерстве́ть сов. см. черстве́ть I.

зачеса́ть сов. см. зачёсывать.

зачеса́ться сов. begín* to itch.

зачесть сов. см. зачи́тывать I. **-ся** сов. см. зачи́тываться I.

зачёсывать, **зачеса́ть** (вн.) comb (smth.).

зачёт м. test; поста́вить **-** кому́-л. pass smb.; сдава́ть **-** по матема́тике take* a test in mathemátics; сдать, получи́ть **-** pass a test. **-ный**: **-ная** кни́жка stúdent's récord book; **-ная** рабо́та páper; **-ная** стрельба́ воен. classificátion shoot.

зачина́тель м. initiator.

зачи́нщ|ик м., **-ица** ж. instigator.

зачи́слить сов. см. зачисля́ть.

зачисля́ть, **зачи́слить** (вн.) énter (smb.); **-** кого́-л. на рабо́ту take* smb. on; **-** кого́-л. на до́лжность секретаря́ take* smb. on as sécretary; **-** кого́-л. в штат take* smb. on the staff; **-** кого́-л. в спи́ски énter smb. on the list; воен. take* smb. on the strength.

зачита́ть сов. см. зачи́тывать II. **-ся** сов. см. зачи́тываться II.

зачи́тывать I, **зачесть** (вн.) 1. (учитывать) count (smth.); э́та су́мма должна́ быть зачтена́ в упла́ту до́лга this sum must be cóunted as páyment of the debt; 2. (признавать выполненным) accépt (smth.), pass (smth.).

зачи́тывать II, зачита́ть (*вн.*) 1. (*оглашать*) read* out (*smth.*); 2. *разг.* (*читая, истрепать*) read* a book to tátters; 3. *разг.* (*не возвращать*); зачита́ть кни́гу néver retúrn a book, apprópriate a book.

зачи́тываться I, зач́сться be* cóunted; (*дт.*) be* put/placed to smb.'s crédit.

зачи́тываться II, зачита́ться *разг.* (*увлекаться чтением*) be* absórbed in *one's* réading; (*тв.*) be* an enthusiástic réader (of); зачита́ться до утра́ read* the whole night through.

зашага́ть *сов.* step out.

зашата́ться *сов.* sway, stágger, begín* to stágger.

зашевели́ть *сов.* (*тв.*) stir (*smth.*), begín* to stir (*smth.*). ~ся *сов.* stir.

зашива́ть, заши́ть (*вн.*) 1. (*чинить*) mend (*smth.*), stitch up (*smth.*); ~ ра́ну put* stítches in a wound; 2. (*упаковывать*) sew* up (*smth.*).

заши́ть *сов. см.* зашива́ть.

зашифрова́ть *сов. см.* зашифро́вывать.

зашифро́вывать, зашифрова́ть (*вн.*) cípher (*smth.*), code (*smth.*).

зашнурова́ть *сов. см.* зашнуро́вывать.

зашнуро́вывать, зашнурова́ть (*вн.*) lace up (*smth.*).

зашпи́л|ивать, зашпи́лить (*вн.*) fásten (*smth.*) with a pin, pin up (*smth.*); ~ во́лосы pin up *one's* hair. ~ить *сов. см.* зашпи́ливать.

зашто́панный darned.

зашто́пать *сов.* (*вн.*) darn (*smth.*).

заштрихова́ть *сов. см.* штрихова́ть.

зашуме́ть *сов.* begín* to make a noise.

защёлка *ж.* latch.

защёлкивать, защёлкнуть (*вн.*) snap (*smth.*); click (*smth.*) to. ~ся, защёлкнуться close with a snap, snap shut.

защёлкнуть(ся) *сов. см.* защёлкивать(ся).

защеми́ть I *сов. см.* защемля́ть.

защем|и́ть II *сов. безл.*: у него́ се́рдце ~и́ло he felt a twinge at heart, his heart ached.

защемля́ть, защеми́ть (*вн.*) squeeze (*smth.*), pinch (*smth.*), crush (*smth.*).

защи́т|а *ж.* 1. protéction; defénce; ~ ми́ра defénce of peace; будь(те) мое́й ~ой be my protéctor; иска́ть ~ы у кого́-л. seek* smb.'s protéction; 2. *собир. юр., спорт.* defénce; ◊ брать кого́-л. под ~у take* smb. under *one's* protéction, protéct smb.; ~ диплóмных прое́ктов defénce of graduátion work.

защи́ти́тельн|ый defénsive; ~ая речь speech for the defénce.

защити́ть *сов. см.* защища́ть 1, 2. ~ся *сов. см.* защища́ться.

защи́тник *м.* 1. protéctor, defénder; (*теории, мероприятия*) ádvocate; 2. *юр.* cóunsel for the defénce; колле́гия ~ов Board of Cóunsels; 3. *спорт.* back.

защи́тн|ый 1. protéctive; ~ые очки́ protéctive góggles; ~ экра́н реа́ктора protéctive screen of a reáctor; ~ скафа́ндр protéctive suit; ~ шлем crash hélmet; 2. *разг.* (*о цвете*) kháki; ◊ цвет khák; ~ая окра́ска *зоол.* protéctive cólouring.

защища́ть, защити́ть (*вн.*) 1. (*от нападения и т. п.*) defénd (*smth., smth.*); (*отстаивать тж.*) uphóld* (*smth.*), maintáin (*smth.*); 2. (*предохранять от чего-либо*) protéct (*smth., smth.*); ~ от хо́лода keep* the cold out; 3. *тк. несов. юр.* plead (for); ~ подсуди́мого defénd the accúsed, be* cóunsel for the defénce; ~ диссерта́цию defénd *one's* thésis/dissertátion. ~ся, защити́ться 1. (*от нападения*) defénd onesélf; 2. (*предохранять себя от чего-л.*) protéct onesélf; 3. *разг.* (*публично защищать диссертацию и т. п.*) defénd *one's* thésis/dissertátion.

заяви́ть *сов. см.* заявля́ть.

зая́в|ка *ж.* 1. (*заявление о правах*) claim; ~ на изобрете́ние claim/application for invéntion rights; 2. (на

вн.; *требование, заказ*) applicátion (for), órder (for); сде́лать ~ку на что-л. place an órder for smth. ~ле́ние с. 1. státement; сде́лать ~ле́ние make* a státement; 2. (*письменная просьба*) requést application; пода́ть ~ле́ние submit an application.

заявля́ть, заяви́ть (*вн. о пр.*) state (*smth.*), decláre (*smth.*); ~ о своём жела́нии make* *one's* wishes known; ~ о свое́й реши́мости procláim *one's* determinátion; ~ о своём согла́сии sígnify *one's* consént; ~ прете́нзию lodge/make* a compláint; ~ проте́ст énter/file a prótest.

за́й́длый *разг.* confirmed.

за́я|ц *м.* hare. ~чий hare's; ~чий мех rábbit-skin; ◊ ~чья губа́ *мед.* hárelip; ~чья капу́ста *бот.* stónecrop.

зва́ние с. rank; (*почётное*) títle; учёное ~ académic rank; во́инское ~ mílitary rank.

зва́ный invíted; ~ гость invíted guest; ~ обе́д fórmal dínner-party.

зва́тельный: ~ паде́ж *грам.* vócative (case).

звать, позва́ть 1. (*вн.*) call (*smb.*); ~ на по́мощь call for help; ~ кого́-л. на по́мощь súmmon smb. to *one's* aid; 2. (*приглашать*) ask (*smb.*), invíte (*smb.*); 3. *тк. несов.* (*тв.; называть*): его́ зову́т Петро́м his name is Péter; как вас зову́т? what's your name? ~ся *несов.* be* called.

звезда́ *ж.* star; о́рден Кра́сной Звезды́ Órder of the Red Star; ◊ морска́я ~ stár-fish; он звёзд с не́ба не хвата́ет he's no génius.

звёздн|ый 1. star *attr.*; sidéreal *научн.*; ~ая ка́рта star map, astronómical chart; ~ год *астр.* sidéreal year; 2. (*покрытый звёздами*) stárry; ~ое не́бо 1) stárry sky; stárry firmament *поэт.*; 2) *астр.* the night sky; ~ая ночь stárry/stárlit night; 3. *спорт.* convérging; ~ пробе́г convérging race; ~ час hour of tríumph; ~ая боле́знь *шутл.* star féver, big-héadedness.

звездолёт *м.* spáceship, spácecraft.

звездо|лётчик *м.*, ~пла́ватель *м.* spáceman*, ástronaut.

звёздочк|а *ж.* 1. star; 2. *полигр.* ásterisk; отмеча́ть что-л. ~ой ásterisk smth.

звене́ть *несов.* (*о голосе, звонке*) ring*; (*тв.*) clink (*smth.*), jingle (*smth.*); ~ моне́тами jíngle coins.

звено́ с. 1. (*цепи; тж. перен.*) link; (*конструкции*) séction; ~ моста́ bridge séction; 2. (*группа*) séction; ~ самолётов flight of áircraft.

звеньев|а́я *ж.*, ~о́й *м.* séction-leader.

зверёк *м.* líttle ánimal/beast.

звере́ть, озвере́ть becóme* like an ánimal, lose* húman shape; (*приходить в ярость*) fly* into a rage.

звери́нец *м.* menágerie.

звери́н|ый ánimal *attr.*; (*свойственный зверю*) brútish; *перен.* (*жестокий*) ferócious; (*очень сильный*) ~ая шку́ра ánimal skin, pelt; ~ая не́нависть ferócious hátred.

зверобо́й I *м.* séa-hunter.

зверобо́й II *м.* (*трава*) St. John's wort.

зверобо́йный: ~ про́мысел séa-hunting índustry.

зверово́дство с. fúr-fárming.

зверолóв *м.* trápper.

звероподо́бный ánimal-like, brútish.

зве́рск|ий ferócious; ~ посту́пок inhúman act; ~ое уби́йство atrócious/brútal múrder.

зве́рство с. 1. (*жестокость*) ferócity; 2. *обыкн. мн.* (*крайне жестокие поступки*) atrócities.

звер|ь *м.* 1. (wild) beast, (wild) ánimal; пушно́й ~ fúr-bearing ánimal; 2. (*жестокий человек*) beast, brute; ◊ смотре́ть ~ем have* a báleful/ferócious look in *one's* eye.

зверьё с. *собир. разг.* wild ánimals *pl.*

звон *м.* (*металла*) ring, rínging; (*мелких колоколов, монет*) jíngling; (*посуды*) cláttering; ~ колоколо́в sound of bells; (*монотонный*) tólling of bells;

~ бока́лов clink of glásses; ◇ ~ в уша́х rínging in *one's* ears.

звони́ть, позвони́ть 1. ring*; (*о колоколе тж.*) toll; ~ в ко́локол ring*/toll a bell; 2. (*дт.; по телефону*) ring* (*smb.*) up, call (*smb.*) up.

звон|кий rínging, clear; (*издающий громкие звуки*) sonórous, resóunding; ◇ ~ согла́сный *лингв.* voiced cónsonant; ~ая фра́за resóunding phrase; ~ая моне́та hard cash.

звон|о́к *м.* 1. (*прибор*) bell; дверно́й ~ dóorbell; 2. (*звук*) ring; вызыва́ть кого́-л. ~ко́м ring* for *smb.*; два ~ка́ ring twice; по ~ку́ when the bell rings; встава́ть по ~ку́ be* roused by a bell; разда́лся ~ a bell rang; ~ по телефо́ну télephone call.

звук *м.* 1. sound; ~ вы́стрела sound of a shot; repórt; под ~и орке́стра to the strains of a band; 2. *лингв.*: гла́сный ~ vówel; согла́сный ~ cónsonant; ◇ ни ~а not a sound; пусто́й ~ méaningless/émpty phrase.

звуков|о́й sound *attr.*; *физ. тж.* sónic; ~а́я волна́ *физ.* sóund-wave; ~о́е кино́ tálking píctures *pl*; tálkies *pl разг.*; ~а́я доро́жка *кино* sóundtrack; ~ фильм tálking film; ~ сигна́л sónic sígnal, áudible sígnal; ~ые зако́ны *лингв.* rules of phonétics.

звукоза́пись *ж.* (sóund-)recórding.

звуконепроница́емый sóundproof.

звукоопера́тор *м.* sóund-prodúcer, sóund-technícian.

звукоподража́|ние *с.* onomatopóeia. ~тельный onomatopóeic.

звукопрово́д|ность *ж.* sóund-transmíssion, sóund-conductívity. ~ящий sóund-transmítting, sóund-condúcting.

звукоснима́тель *м.* pick-up.

звукоула́вливатель *м.* sóund-locátor.

звуч|а́ть, прозвуча́ть 1. ring*; sound (*тж. перен.*); ~ убеди́тельно ring* true; в его́ го́лосе ~а́ла трево́га his voice sóunded ánxious; 2. (*раздаваться, быть слышным*) be* heard; ~а́ла пе́сня a song was heard.

звучн|ость *ж.* 1. sonórity; (*отчётливость*) clárity; 2. (*музыкальных инструментов и т. п.*) résonance, fine tone. ~ый 1. sonórous; (*отчётливый*) clear, rínging; 2. (*издающий звонкий звук*) résonant; (*о музыкальных инструментах тж.*) fine-tóned.

звя́кать, звя́кнуть jíngle, clink; (*о цепях и т. п.*) clank; звя́кнуть шпо́рами jíngle *one's* spurs.

звя́кнуть *сов. см.* звя́кать.

зги: ни зги не ви́дно it is pitch-dárk.

зда́ние *с.* búilding; édifice.

здесь 1. (*в этом месте*) here; (*о стране тж.*) in this cóuntry; есть ~ кто́-нибудь? is there ánybody here?; ~ нико́го нет there's nóbody here; 2. (*в этом случае*) at this point; ~ на́до сказа́ть... at this point it should be méntioned...; ~ нет ничего́ предосуди́тельного I see nóthing wrong in this.

зде́шний *разг.* of this place *после сущ.*, lócal; ~ жи́тель lócal résident; он ~ жи́тель he lives here.

здоро́в|аться, поздоро́ваться (*с тв.*) greet (*smb.*); (*взаимно*) greet one anóther; exchánge gréetings; ~ за́ руку shake* hands; он никогда́ не ~ается he néver says good mórning.

здорове́ть, поздорове́ть *разг.* grow* strong and héalthy.

здо́рово *разг.* 1. (*хорошо, ловко*) fine; вот э́то ~! that's fine!; 2. (*сильно, очень*): сего́дня ~ хо́лодно it's áwfully cold today; ему́ ~ попа́ло he got a terrífic blast; мы ~ уста́ли we're áwfully tíred.

здоро́в|ый 1. héalthy, sound; *перен.* sound, whólesome; ~ое се́рдце sound/strong heart; ~ые лёгкие good lungs; ~ вид róbust appéarance; ~ая атмосфе́ра héalthy átmosphere; ~ая кри́тика sound críticism; 2. (*полезный*) héalthy; (*о пище*) whólesome; 3. *разг.* (*крепкий, сильный*) strápping, húsky; ~ па́рень big lad;

◇ бу́дьте ~ы! (*до свидания*) chéerio!; (*при чихании*) bless you!

здоро́вье *с.* health; кре́пкое ~ spléndid health; сла́бое ~ poor health; как ва́ше ~? how are you?, how are you kéeping?; ◇ (за) ва́ше ~! your health!; пить (за) ~ кого́-л. drink* *smb.'s* health; на ~! you're wélcome!

здорова́к *м. разг.* héalthy pérson, strápping féllow.

здра́виц|а *ж.* toast; провозгласи́ть ~у procláim a toast.

здра́вница *ж.* sanatórium (*pl* -ria), resórt.

здра́во sénsibly, rátionally; ~ рассужда́ть have* sound víews; ~ суди́ть о чём-л. take* a sane view of *smth.*; поступа́ть ~ act/beháve sénsibly.

здравомы́слящий sane, réasonable.

здравоохране́ни|е *с.* protéction of health; health sérvices *pl*; Министе́рство ~я Ministry of Health.

здра́вств|овать *несов.* be* in good health; ◇ да ~ует..! long live..!; ~уй(те)! good mórning/afternóon/évening!; (*при первом знакомстве*) how do you do!

здра́в|ый sound; ~ая мысль sound idéa; ~ смысл cómmon sense; ~ ум sound mind; быть в ~ом уме́ be* of sound mind; здрав и невреди́м safe and sound.

зе́бра *ж.* zébra.

зев *м. анат.* phárynx.

зева́ка *м. и ж. разг.* ídler, ídle ónlooker.

зев|а́ть, зевну́ть, прозева́ть 1. *сов.* зевну́ть yawn; сла́дко зевну́ть luxúriously yawn; 2. *тк. несов. разг.* (*глазеть*) gape; 3. *сов.* прозева́ть *разг.* (*упускать, не замечать*) miss *one's* chance; (*вн.*) overlóok (*smth.*); не ~а́й! look alíve!, keep your eyes ópen!

зевну́ть *сов. см.* зева́ть 1.

зев|о́к *м.* yawn. ~о́та *ж.* yáwning.

зелене́|ть, позелене́ть 1. *тк. несов.* (*покрываться зеленью*) turn green; 2. (*становиться зелёным*) becóme* green; 3. *тк. несов.* (*виднеться*) show* green; вдали́ ~ла ро́ща a cóppice showed green in the dístance. ~ющий vérdant.

зеле́нщик *м.* gréengrocer.

зелён|ый green; ~ые насажде́ния trees and shrubs; ~ые щи (*из шпината*) spínach soup; (*из щавеля*) sórrel broth; ◇ ~ая молодёжь cállow youth; дать ~ую у́лицу give* the green light.

зе́лень *ж. собир.* 1. (*растительность*) gréenery, green; vérdure *поэт.*; 2. (*овощи*) green végetables *pl*; greens *pl разг.*

зе́лье *с. уст.* (*яд*) póison; (*напиток*) póison draught, póisonous concóction.

земе́льн|ый 1. land *attr.*; of land *после сущ.*; ~ уча́сток plot of land; 2. (*относящийся к землевладению*) agrárian; ~ая рефо́рма agrárian refórm; ~ая со́бственность lánded próperty.

землевладе́|лец *м.* lándowner; кру́пный ~ big lándowner; ме́лкий ~ pétty lándowner, smállholder. ~льческий lándowners'. ~ние *с.* ównership of land.

земледе́|лец *м.* fármer, cróp-grower. ~лие *с.* cróp-growing; ágriculture. ~льческий agricúltural.

землеко́п *м.* návvy.

землеме́р *м.* lánd-survéyor.

землепо́льзование *с.* land use.

землепрохо́дец *м.* explórer.

землеро́йн|ый dígging *attr.*, éxcavating *attr.*; ~ая маши́на éxcavator, mechánical shóvel.

землесо́с *м.* súction drédger.

землетрясе́ние *с.* éarthquake.

землеустро́йство *с.* sýstem of land use/utilizátion.

землечерпа́лка *ж.* drédge(r).

земли́стый éarthy; ~ цвет лица́ sállow compléxion.

земл|я́ *ж.* 1. earth; на ~е in this world; мир на ~е́ peace on earth; 2. (З.) (*планета*) the Earth; 3. (*суша, страна, владения*) land; больша́я ~ the máinland;

чужи́е зе́мли foreign lands; 4. (почва) soil; плодоро́дная ~ rich/fértile soil; 5. (поверхность земли) ground; сиде́ть на ~é sit* on the ground; ◇ сло́вно из ~й, из-под ~й вы́расти appéar from nówhere; ~й под собо́й не слы́шать be* wálking on air.

земля́к м. (féllow-)cóuntryman*; мы с ним ~и́ we come from the same part of the cóuntry.

земляни́|ка ж. 1. собир. (садовая) stráwberries pl; (лесная) wild stráwberries pl; 2. (об отдельной ягоде) (wild) stráwberry, 3. (куст) (wild) stráwberry plant. ~чный stráwberry attr.

земля́нка ж. dúg-out.

земля́н|о́й earth attr., éarthen; ~ пол éarthen floor; ~ые рабо́ты éarthwork sg; ~ое укрепле́ние éarthworks pl; ~ оре́х gróund-nut.

земля́чка ж. cóuntrywoman*.

земново́дн|ые мн. зоол. amphíbia. ~ый amphíbian; ~ое живо́тное amphíbian.

земн|о́й 1. terréstrial; of the earth после сущ.; ~а́я ось the earth's áxis; 2. (относящийся к земле как месту жизни) éarthly, перен. éarthy, dówn-to-éarth; ~ые бла́га éarthly bléssings.

земснаря́д м. (súction) drédger.

зени́т м. (прям. и перен.) zénith; в ~е сла́вы at the height of one's fame.

зени́т|ка ж. разг. anti-áircraft gun. ~ный 1. астр. zénithal; 2. воен. anti-áircraft. ~чик м. anti-áircraft gúnner.

зени́ц|а ж.: бере́чь кого́-л., что́-л. как ~у о́ка guard smb., smth. like the ápple of one's eye.

зе́ркал|о с. lóoking-glass; mírror (тж. перен.); ~ прожёктора refléctor; как в ~е as in a mírror/glass.

зерка́льн|ый mírror attr.; перен. smooth, unrúffled; ~ое стекло́ pláte-glass; ~ шкаф wárdrobe with a mírror; ~ая гладь unrúffled súrface; ◇ ~ карп mírror carp.

зерни́ст|ый gránular; ◇ ~ая икра́ soft/gránulated cáviar.

зерн|о́ с. grain; перен. тж. kérnel, core; хлеб в ~é grain; семенно́е ~ seed grain; ко́фе в зёрнах cóffee-béans; ~ и́стины a grain/átom of truth; рациона́льное ~ филос. rátional kérnel.

зернобобо́в|ый: ~ые культу́ры legúminous crops.

зернов|о́й прил. 1. grain attr.; ~о́е хозя́йство gráin (-growing) farm; ~ые культу́ры gráin-crops; 2. в знач. сущ. мн. gráin-crops.

зерно|дроби́лка ж. córnmill, mill. ~суши́лка ж. grain drýer. ~храни́лище с. gránary.

зёрнышко с. grain.

зефи́р м. 1. уст. поэт. (ветерок) zéphyr; 2. (ткань) zéphyr; 3. (род пастилы) márshmallow.

зигза́г м. zigzag.

зигзагообра́зный zígzag attr.

зи́ждиться несов. (на пр.) be* based (on), be* fóunded (on), rest on.

зим|á ж. winter; всю зи́му the whole winter; к ~é by the winter; (для зимы) for the winter; на́ зиму for the winter.

зи́мн|ий winter attr.; ~ ве́чер winter évening; ~яя оде́жда winter clóthing.

зимова́ть, прозимова́ть spend* the winter; (о животных) hibernate.

зимо́вк|а ж. 1. wintering; подгото́виться к ~е prepáre to stay the winter; 2. (место, помещение) winter camp; winter quárters pl.

зимо́вщик м. winterer.

зимо́вье с. 1. winter quárters pl; 2. (животных) wintering place.

зимо́й in (the) winter.

зимосто́йкий winter-hárdy.

зия́ние с. лингв. hiátus.

зия́ть несов. gape.

злак м.: хле́бные ~и céreals. ~овый céreal.

злейший: ~ враг one's worst énemy.

злить, обозли́ть (вн.) make* (smb., smth.) cross; ánger (smb., smth.). ~ся, обози́ться (на вн.) be* cross (with), get* annóyed (with); что ты зли́шься? what makes you so cross?

зло I с. 1. тк. ед. (всё дурное) évil; не по́мнить зла bear* no ill-will; причиня́ть зло кому́-л. harm smb.; причини́ть мно́го зла кому́-л. do* smb. great harm; 2. (несчастье, неприятность) évil, harm, ill; из двух зол выбира́ть ме́ньшее choose* the lésser of two évils; 3. разг. (досада) spite; зло берёт it makes one fúrious; сде́лать что́-л. со зла do* smth. out of spite.

зло II нареч. malíciously; ~ подшути́ть над кем-л. play smb. a mean trick; ~ посме́иваться chúckle malíciously.

зло́б|а ж. málice, spite; (гнев) ánger, fúry, бесси́льная ~ ímpotent rage; пита́ть ~у к кому́-л. bear* smb. ill-will; ◇ ~ дня the tópic of the day; на ~у дня on a tópical súbject. ~ный malícious; ~ный взгляд malígnant glance; ~ный враг vícious énemy.

злободне́вный tópical; ~ вопро́с búrning quéstion.

злове́щий óminous, sínister.

зловон|ие с. stench. ~ный fétid.

зловре́дный malícious, vícious, spíteful.

злоде́й м., ~ка ж. víllain, scóundrel. ~ский scóundrelly, ráscally; ~ское уби́йство foul múrder. ~ство с. 1. víllainy; 2. (злодейский поступок) évil deed, évil act.

злодея́ние с. crime.

злой 1. cruel, wícked, vícious; (о людях тж.) ill-nátured; ~ челове́к ill-nátured/vícious pérson; 2. (выражающий злобу) spíteful, malícious; злы́е глаза́ malícious eyes; зла́я улы́бка sarcástic/násty smile; у него́ ~ вид he looks cross; 3. тк. кратк. ф. в знач. сказ. cross, ángry, bad-témpered; он зол на вас he's cross with you; как вы сего́дня злы! how bítter/násty you are todáy!; 4. (вызванный злобой) spíteful, malícious; ~ у́мысел malícious inténtion; зла́я шу́тка mean trick; зла́я во́ля évil intent; пита́ть зло́е чу́вство к кому́-л. hárbour ill féelings agáinst smb.; 5. (свирепый — о животных) sávage, fierce; 6. (приносящий беду) évil; злы́е времена́ évil days pl, time of évil; зла́я судьба́ cruel fate; 7. (приносящий боль) páinful, ágonizing; ~ неду́г cruel síckness; 8. разг. (едкий, острый) перен. (язвительный) bíting, sávage; зла́я горчи́ца hot/strong mústard; зла́я иро́ния sávage írony; зла́я насме́шка cruel jest; зла́я сати́ра bíting sátire; ~ язы́к wícked tongue; ◇ злы́е языки́ évil tongues.

злока́чественн|ый мед. malígnant; ~ая о́пухоль malígnant túmour.

злоключе́ние с. misadvénture, míshap; мн. тж. tribulátions.

злонаме́ренный ill-inténtioned, malévolent, malícious; ~ посту́пок malícious act.

злопа́мят|ный unforgíving. ~ство с. unforgívingness.

злополу́чный ill-fáted; (о человеке тж.) ill-stárred, hápless.

злопыха́тель м. malígnant pérson, fáultfinder. ~ский snáppish; ~ская кри́тика cárping/préjudiced críticism. ~ство с. spite, fáultfinding.

злора́д|ный spíteful; glóating attr. ~ство с. fíendish pléasure/delíght. ~ствовать несов. gloat (óver).

злосло́в|ие с. scándal. ~ить несов. talk scándal.

злостн|ый 1. malícious; ~ клевета́ scúrrilous líbel; ~ клеветни́к slánderer; ~ые наме́рения evil inténtions; 2. (сознательно недобросовестный) delíberate; ~ непла́тельщик persístent/delíberate defáulter; ~ наруши́тель дисципли́ны persístent offénder.

злость ж. málice, ráncour; fúry; меня́ ~ берёт it makes me fúrious; говори́ть со ~ю о ком-л. speak* ángrily abóut smb.

злосча́стный ill-stárred, ill-fáted.

злоупотреб|и́ть *сов. см.* злоупотребля́ть. ~ле́ние *с.* (*тв.*) abúse (of); (*пищей и т. п.*) óver-indúlgence (in).

злоупотребля́ть, злоупотреби́ть (*тв.*) abúse (*smth.*); (*пищей и т. п.*) óver-indúlge (in); ~ чьим-л. дове́рием abúse· *smb.'s* cónfidence; ~ чьим-л. гостеприи́мством abúse *smth.'s* hospitálity; ~ чьей-л. добротой impóse upón *smb.'s* kíndness; ~ вла́стью abúse of pówer/authórity.

злю́|ка *м. и ж.*, ~чка *м. и ж. разг.* spítfire.

змееви́дный sérpentine.

змееви́к *м.* 1 *тех.* coil (pipe); 2. *мин.* sérpentine.

змеи́н|ый snake *attr.*, snake's; reptílian *зоол.*; *перен.* cúnning, sínister; ~ая ко́жа snákeskin; ~ая улы́бка sínister smile.

зме|и́ться *несов.* wind*; на губа́х его́ ~лась презри́тельная улы́бка his lips curved in a contémptuous smile.

змей *м.* 1. *фольк.* drágon; 2. (*бумажный*) kite.

змея́ *ж.* snake, sérpent; ◇ ~ подколо́дная *разг.* víper, snáke-in-the-grâss.

знава́ть *несов.* use to know.

знак *м.* 1. sign, mark; (*условное обозначение*) sýmbol; ~ ра́венства équal-sign; фабри́чный ~ trade mark; ~ внима́ния mark of esté em/respéct; дурно́й *разг.* bad sign; 2. (*сигнал*) sign, sígnal; ~ руко́й a sign with *one's* hand; подава́ть ~и make* signs; 3. (*след*) mark; ~и вре́мени marks of time; 4. (*значок*) badge; ◇ ~и препина́ния punctuátion marks; под ~ом *чего-л.* guíded by *smth.*; в ~ *чего-л.* to sígnify *smth.*; в ~ дру́жбы as a tóken/sign of friéndship; в ~ призна́тельности as a mark of grátitude; в ~ согла́сия as a sign of assént/consént.

знако́мить, познако́мить 1. (*вн. с кем-либо*) introdúce (*smb.* to); меня́ познако́мили с ним I was introdúced to him; 2. (*вн. с чем-л.*) acquáint (*smb.* with), tell* (*smb.* abóut). ~ся, познако́миться 1. (с кем-либо) get* to know (*smb.*); 2. (с чем-л.; *получать сведения*) acquáint *oneself* (with), make* *oneself* familiar (with), get* to know (*smth.*); ~ся с го́родом see* the sights, have* a look at the town; ~ся с обстано́вкой make* *oneself* familiar with the círcumstances/situâtion.

знако́мств|о *с.* 1. acquáintance; пе́рвое ~ с кем-л. introdúction to *smth.*; 2. (*круг знакомых*) acquáintances *pl*; больши́е ~а númerous acquáintances, wide círcle of friends; 3. (*наличие знаний*) knówledge; ~ с исто́рией, матема́тикой *и т. п.* knówledge of hístory, mathemátics *etc.*

знако́м|ый *прил.* 1. (*известный*) familiar; ~ по́черк familiar hándwriting; 2. (с *тв.*; *дт.*; *испытавший, знающий что-л.*) acquáinted (with), familiar (with); всё э́то нам давно́ ~о we have known all about that for a long time; я знако́м со всей литерату́рой по э́тому вопро́су I am familiar with all the literature on the súbject; I know all the literature on the subject; 3. (с *тв.*; *состоящий в знакомстве с кем-л.*) acquáinted (with); быть ~ым с *кем-л.* be* acquáinted with *smb.*; мы с ним давно́ ~ы we've known each óther for some time; 4. *в знач. сущ. м.* acquáintance; он мой ~ he's a friend of mine.

знамена́тел|ь *м. мат.* denóminator; приводи́ть к о́бщему ~ю redúce to a cómmon denóminator.

знамена́тельный great, mémorable; (*значительный*) signíficant.

зна́мение *с. уст.* sign; (*предзнаменование*) ómen; ◇ ~ вре́мени sign(s) of the times.

знамени́т|ость *ж.* celébrity; стать ~остью becóme* fámous, becóme* a celébrity. ~ый fámous, nótable, célebrated; ~ый учёный fámous scíentist.

знаменова́ть *несов.* mark (*smth.*).

знамено́сец *м.* stándard-bearer.

зна́м|я *с.* bánner; ◇ высоко́ держа́ть ~ *чего-л.* raise high the bánner of *smth.*; под ~енем *чего-л.* únder the bánner of *smth.*

зна́ни|е *с.* 1. *тк. ед.* knówledge; ~ де́ла skill; руководи́ть чем-л. со ~ем де́ла diréct/mánage *smth.* with skill, be* a skílful/cápable órganizer; о́бласть ~я field of knówledge; 2. *мн.* knówledge *sg*; обши́рные ~я exténsive knówledge *sg*; облада́ть ~ями be* wéll- -infórmed; приобрести́ ~я acquire knówledge.

зна́тн|ый 1. (*выдающийся*) distínguished, out- stánding, nóted, ~ые лю́ди на́шей страны́ the distínguished men and wómen of our cóuntry; ~ шахтёр nóted míner; 2. *ист.* (*принадлежащий к знати*) high- -born (*о человеке*); nóble (*о роде*).

знато́к *м.* connoisséur; он ~ своего́ де́ла he knows his job.

знать I *несов.* (*вн.*) know* (*smb.*, *smth.*); ~ англи́йский язы́к know* Énglish; ~ мно́го люде́й know* mány péople; ◇ ~ ме́ру know* when to stop; во всём на́до ~ ме́ру the great thing is moderátion; ~ что к чему́ know* what's what; кто его́ зна́ет? who knows?; ~ толк в чём-л. know* what *smth.* is about; ~ це́ну кому-л., чему-л. know* what *smb.*, *smth.* is worth.

знать II *ж.* nobílity.

зна́ться *несов.* (с *тв.*) *разг.* assóciate (with), have* to do (with).

значе́ни|е *с.* 1. (*смысл*) méaning, sense, signíficance; в буква́льном ~и сло́ва in the literal sense of the word; 2. (*важность*) impórtance, signíficance; имéть (большо́е) ~ be* of great signíficance/impórtance; не имéть (никако́го) ~я be* of no impórtance, not mátter (in the least); придава́ть большо́е ~ чему-л. attách great impórtance to *smth.*; не прида́ть ~я чему-л. attách no impórtance to *smth.*; приобрета́ть большо́е ~ acquire great signíficance.

зна́чим|ость *ж.* signíficance. ~ый significant.

зна́чит *разг.* so, then; ~, вы ничего́ не ви́дели! so you saw nóthing!; ~, он придёт so/then he's cóming.

значи́тельн|ость *ж.* impórtance, signíficance. ~ый 1. (*большой*) considerable; в ~ой сте́пени to a great extént; 2. (*важный*) impórtant, signíficant.

знач|и́ть *несов.* mean*, sígnify; что э́то ~ит? what does it/this mean?; what is the méaning of this?; what's all this about?; э́то не ~ит, что... it doesn't mean that..., this is not to say that...; ма́ло, мно́го ~ be* of little, great impórtance. ~иться *несов.* be* listed (as); он ~ится в о́тпуске he is listed as on leave; он нигде́ не ~ится he isn't listed/régistered ánywhere.

значо́к *м.* 1. (*носимый на одежде*) badge; 2. (*пометка*) mark.

зна́ющ|ий áble, cómpetent; ~ие лю́ди well-infórmed péople.

зноб|и́ть *несов. безл.*: меня́ (си́льно) ~и́т I feel féverish/shívery.

зной *м.* scórching/inténse heat. ~ный búrning, súltry; ~ное ле́то súltry súmmer.

зоб *м.* 1. (*у птицы*) crop; 2. (*болезнь*) góitre.

зов *м.* 1. appéal; 2. *разг.* (*приглашение*) call; прийти́ по пе́рвому ~у come* at the first call.

зодиа́к *м. астр.* Zódiac.

зо́дч|ество *с.* árchitecture. ~ий *м.* árchitect.

зола́ *ж.* ash(es).

золо́вка *ж.* húsband's síster, síster-in-law (*pl* sísters-).

золоти́стый gólden.

золоти́ть, позолоти́ть (*вн.*) gild* (*smth.*).

золотни́к *м. тех.* valve, slide.

зо́лото *с.* gold; листово́е ~ góldleaf; ◇ не всё то ~, что блести́т *посл.* all is not gold that glítters.

золотоиска́тель *м.* góld-prospéctor.

золот|о́й *прил.* 1. gold; (*похожий на золото*) gólden (*тж. перен.*); ~ сли́ток gold búllion; ~ые ро́ссыпи plácer *sg*; ~ые часы́ gold watch *sg*; ~а́я валю́та gold cúrrency; ~ые ку́дри gólden curls/locks; ~ое се́рдце heart of gold; ~ рабо́тник inváluable wórker; 2. *в знач. сущ. м.* gold coin, gold piece; ◇ ~ станда́рт the gold stándard; ~ое содержáние валю́ты gold cóntent of a cúrrency, extént to which a cúrrency is backed by gold; ~ запáс gold resérve(s); ~ых дел мáстер *уст.* góldsmith; ~ век the Gólden Age; ~ая óсень gólden áutumn; ~áя порá gólden days; ~ая середи́на the gólden mean; ~ые ру́ки a wónderful pair of hands; y негó ~ые ру́ки he is a wízard with his hands/fíngers.

золотонóсный auríferous, góld-bearing; ~ песóк góld-bearing grável.

золотопромы́шленн|ик *м.* 1. (*работник*) wórker in the góld-mining índustry; 2. (*владелец золотых приисков*) ówner of a góldmine. ~ость *ж.* góld-mining.

золоту́|ха *ж. уст. разг.* scrófula. ~шный *разг.* scrófulous.

золочёный gilt, gílded.

Зóлушка *ж. фольк.* Cinderélla.

зóльник *м. тех.* ásh-pit.

зóна *ж.* zone.

зонáльн|ый zónal; ~ое совещáние zónal cónference.

зонд *м.* probe. ~и́ровать *несов.* (*вн.; прям. и перен.*) sound (*smth.*); *мед.* probe (*smth.*); ◇ ~и́ровать пóчву find* out the lie of the land, find* out how things stand.

зонт *м.* 1. *см.* зóнтик; 2. (*навес*) áwning. ~ик *м.* (*от дождя*) umbrélla; (*от солнца*) súnshade.

зоóлог *м.* zoólogist. ~и́ческий zoológical.

зоолóгия *ж.* zoólogy.

зоомагази́н *м.* pet shop.

зоопáрк *м.* zoológical gárdens *pl*; the Zoo *разг.*

зоотéхни|к *м.* lívestock éxpert, stóck-breeder. ~ка *ж.* zootéchnics.

зóркий 1. (*о глазах*) sharp, keen; (*о человеке*) sharp-éyed, lynx-éyed; 2. (*проницательный*) far-séeing, clear-sighted, percéptive.

зрачóк *м.* púpil.

зрéлищ|е *с.* 1. spéctacle, sight; печáльное ~ pathétic/móurnful sight; 2. (*представление*) show, perfórmance. ~ный entertáinment *attr.*; ~ные предприя́тия shows, entertáinments.

зрéл|ость *ж.* 1. (*спелость*) rípeness; 2. (*полное развитие организма*) matúrity (*тж. перен.*). ~ый 1. (*спелый*) ripe; 2. (*достигший полного развития*) matúre (*тж. перен.*); ~ый вóзраст matúre age; ~ое решéние decísion táken áfter matúre deliberátion; ~ый ум matúre mind, well-devéloped mind.

зрéни|е *с.* sight, éyesight; лиши́ться ~я lose* one's sight; ◇ пóле ~я sight, field of vísion; *перен.* scope; тóчка ~я point of view, stándpoint; с тóчки ~я from the point of view (of), from the stándpoint (of), as regárds.

зреть *несов.* 1. (*стать спелым*) ripen; 2. (*достигать полного развития*) matúre (*тж. перен.*).

зри́тель *м.* 1. ónlooker, spectátor; 2. (*в театре, кино*) mémber of the áudience; *собир.* áudiences *pl; мн.* áudience *sg.* ~ный 1. vísual, óptic(al); ~ный нерв óptic nerve; ~ная пáмять vísual mémory; ~ный сигнáл vísual sígnal; 2.: ~ный зал auditórium; ~ная трубá télescope.

зря *разг.* for nóthing, in vain; ~ трáтить *что-л.* waste *smth.*; вы э́то ~! there you're wrong!

зря́чий síghted.

зуб *м.* 1. (*мн.* зу́бы) tooth*; молóчный ~ first-tooth*, milk-tooth*; ~ный ~ы have* déntal tréatment; в ~áх between one's teeth; 2. (*мн.* зу́бья) tooth*; (*шестерни тж.*) cog; ◇ не по ~áм too hard for one, a hard nut to crack; имéть ~ прóтив *кого-л.* bear* a grudge agáinst *smb.*; класть ~ы на пóлку ≈ tíghten one's belt; y меня́ ~ нá ~ не попадáет my teeth are cháttering; ни в ~ (ногóй) not know a thing abóut it.

зубáстый *разг.* sharp-tóothed; *перен.* sharp-tóngued.

зубéц *м.* 1. (*грабель*) tooth*; (*колеса*) tooth*, cog; (*вил, вилки*) prong; (*пилы*) (sáw-)tooth*; 2. *обыкн. мн.* (*на стене башни*) báttlement.

зуби́ло *с. тех.* chísel, póint-tool.

зубн|óй 1. tooth *attr.*, déntal; ~ нерв the nerve of a tooth; ~ая боль tóothache; ~ врач déntist; ~ протéз déntal plate; déntures *pl амер.*; ~ая щётка tóoth-brush; ~ порошóк tóoth-powder; 2. *лингв.* déntal; ~ соглáсный déntal cónsonant.

зубоврачéбный déntal; ~ кабинéт déntal súrgery.

зубоскá|л *м. разг.* scóffer. ~лить *несов. разг.* scoff. ~льство *с.* scóffing, derísion.

зубочи́стка *ж.* tóothpick.

зубр *м.* 1. *зоол.* Européan bíson; 2. (*о крайнем реакционере*) díe-hard, báckwoodsman*; 3. *разг.* (*об опытном специалисте*) púndit.

зубрёжка *ж. разг.* crámming. ~и́ть *несов.* (*вн.*) *разг.* cram (*smth.*), grind* (*smth.*); ~и́ть урóки grind* awáy at one's stúdies.

зубчá́т|ый toothed; ~ое колесó cóg-wheel; ~ая шестерня́ pínion, géar-wheel.

зуд *м.* (*прям. и перен.*) itch; писáтельский ~ the líterary urge, the itch to write.

зуд|éть *несов.* itch; ру́ки ~я́т (+ *инф.*) one is ítching (+ to *inf*); y негó язы́к ~éл сообщи́ть об э́том he was ítching to tell abóut it.

зы́бк|ий unstéady; únstable; ~ая пóчва shífting soil.

зыбь *ж.* lop; (*после бури*) swell; лёгкая ~ rípples *pl.*

зы́чный stentórian.

зюйд *м. мор.* 1. South; 2. (*ветер*) south (wind).

зюйд|-вéст *м. мор.* 1. south-wést; 2. (*ветер*) south-wést wind, southwéster. ~вéстка *ж. разг.* (*шапка*) sou'wéster.

зюйд-óст *м. мор.* 1. south-éast; 2. (*ветер*) south-éast wind, southéaster.

зя́бкий *разг.* chílly.

зя́блев|ый: ~ая вспáшка áutumn plóughing.

зя́блик *м. зоол.* cháffinch.

зя́бнуть *несов.* 1. feel* the cold, be* chílled; 2. (*о растениях*) súffer from frost.

зябь *ж. с.-х.* 1. áutumn plóughing; 2. (*поле*) land plóughed in áutumn.

зять *м.* (*муж дочери*) són-in-law (*pl* sóns-); (*муж сестры*) bróther-in-law (*pl* bróthers-).

И

и I *союз* 1. (*соединительный*) and; гóрод и дерéвня town and cóuntry; дождь шёл сильнéе и сильнéе it was ráining fáster and fáster; стáрые и мáлые young and old; 2. (*перечислительный*) and; и на мóре, и на землé, и в вóздухе at sea, on land and in the air; я́блоки, гру́ши и апельси́ны ápples, pears and óranges; и то и другóе both (the one and the óther); 3. (*усилительный*) не перевóдится; и как он бежáл! how he ran!; и как вы егó не ви́дели? I just don't know how you could have missed him; 4. (*уступительный в знач. хотя́*) though; чáсто не перевóдится; и хóчется пойти́ в кинó, да нéкогда I want to go to the cínema, but I have no time; и мой ты сын, а не пойму́ я тебя́ I can't understánd you, though you are my son; 5. (*именно*) that is...; так он и сдéлал that is what he did; вот об э́том я и говори́л that is what I was tálking abóut.

и II *частица* 1. (*употр. для усиления*) не перевóдится; и какóй ты счастли́вый! how lúcky you are!; 2. (*тоже, также*) too; (*при отрицании*) éither; он и к нам зашёл he came to see us too; он и тудá не пошёл he did not go there éither; 3. (*даже*) éven; он и не попрощáлся he didn't éven say goodbýe.

и́бо for, becáuse.

и́ва *ж.* willow.

ива́н-да-ма́рья *ж. бот.* со́w-wheat.

ива́н-ча́й *м. бот.* willow-herb, rose-bay.

ивня́к *м.* 1. (*заросли ивы*) willow-bed, ósier-bed; 2. *собир.* (*ивовые прутья*) willow(-branches).

и́вовый willow *attr.*

и́волга *ж.* óriole.

игла́ *ж.* 1. néedle (*тж. хвойных деревьев*); (*у животных*) quill; spine *научн.*; вяза́льная ~ knítting-needle; хирурги́ческая ~ súture néedle; 2. (*остроконечный предмет*) spíre.

иглоука́лывание *с.* acupúncture.

игнори́ровать *несов. и сов.* (*вн.*) ignóre (smb., smth.); (*не обращать внимания*) disregárd (smb., smth.); (*пренебрегать*) defý (smb., smth.); ~ чьи-л. распоряже́ния defý smb.'s órders; ~ фа́кты ignóre the facts.

и́го *с.* yoke.

иго́л|**ка** *ж.* néedle; ~ сиде́ть как на ~ках be* on ténterhooks. **~очка** *ж.* néedle; ◇ с ~очки brand-néw; костю́м с ~очки brand-néw suit; оде́т с ~очки dressed up to the nines.

иго́льн|**ый** néedle *attr.*; ~ое ушко́ the eye of a néedle.

иго́рный gámbling; ~ дом gámbling/gáming house.

игр|**а́** *ж.* 1. play; 2. (*вид игры, тж. спорт. — партия*) game; 3. (*исполнение*) ácting; perfórmance; (*на муз. инструменте тж.*) pláying; слу́шать ~у́ на роя́ле, скри́пке lísten to the piáno, violín; 4. (*интриги*) íntrigue, tríckery; ultérior mótives; *pl*; ◇ ~ воображе́ния the work of smb.'s imaginátion; биржева́я ~ stóck-exchánge gámbling; ~ на бега́х, на ска́чках ráce-bétting; ~ приро́ды freak of náture; ~ слов play on words, pun; ~ с огнём pláying with fíre; ~ судьбы́ a trick of fáte; ~ не сто́ит свеч the game is not worth the cándle.

игра́льн|**ый**: ~ые ка́рты (pláying-)cards; ~ые ко́сти dice.

игр|**а́ть**, сыгра́ть 1. *тк. несов.* (*забавляться*) play; де́ти ~а́ют в саду́ children are pláying in the gárden; 2. (*в вн.; в какую-л. игру*) play (smth.); ~ в ша́хматы play chess; ~ в футбо́л play fóotball; ~ в ка́рты на де́ньги play cards for móney; 3. (*вн., на пр.; исполнять музыкальное произведение*) play (smth.); (*на пр.*) перен. play (on); ~ вальс play a waltz; ~ на роя́ле play the piáno; ~ на чьих-л. сла́бостях play on smb.'s wéaknesses; 4. (*вн.*) *театр* act (smb., smth.), perfórm (smth.), play (smth.); ~ роль кого́-л. play/take* the part of smb.; 5. *тк. несов.* (*тв.*) play (with); (*вертеть в руках*) toy (with); он стоя́л, ~я́ плётью he stood tóying with his whip; 6. *тк. несов.* (*искриться*) spárkle; ◇ ~ пе́рвую скри́пку play first fíddle; ~ большу́ю роль play an impórtant part; э́то не ~а́ет (никако́й) ро́ли! it dóesn't mátter (in the least)!; ~ на́ руку кому́-л. play ínto smb.'s hands; ~ свое́й жи́знью take* one's life in one's hands; ~ на не́рвах у кого́-л. get*/play on smb.'s nerves.

игра́ючи *разг.* without éffort, éffortlessly; он де́лает э́то ~ it's child's play to him.

игри́в|**ый** pláyful; ~ котёнок frísky/pláyful kítten; ~ое настрое́ние pláyful mood.

игри́стый spárkling.

игрово́й: ~ фильм fíction film/pícture.

игро́к *м.* pláyer; (*в азартные игры*) gámbler.

игроте́ка *ж.* colléction of children's games.

игру́шечный toy *attr.*; перен. (*маленький*) tíny; ~ парово́з toy lócomotive; ~ до́мик doll's house.

игру́ш|**ка** *ж.* toy; pláything (*тж. перен.*); магази́н ~ек tóyshop.

идеа́л *м.* idéal. **~иза́ция** *ж.* idealizátion. **~изи́ровать** *несов. и сов.* (*вн.*) idéalize (smb., smth.).

идеал|**и́зм** *м.* idéalism. **~и́ст** *м.* idéalist. **~исти́ческий** 1. idéalist; ~исти́ческая филосо́фия

idéalist philósophy; 2. *разг.* (*свойственный идеалисту*) idealístic.

идеа́льный idéal; (*превосходный тж.*) pérfect.

иде́йн|**ость** *ж.* móral súbstance/fíbre, high-mindedness. **~ый** 1. (*идеологический*) ideológical; ~ая борьба́ ideológical strúggle; 2. (*выражающий основную мысль*): ~ое содержа́ние пье́сы the méssage of the play; 3. (*о человеке*) high-mínded.

иденти́чн|**ость** *ж.* idéntity. **~ый** idéntical.

идеогра́|мма *ж. лингв.* ídeograph, ídeogram. **~фи́ческий** *лингв.* ideográphic(al). **~фия** *ж. лингв.* ideógraphy.

иде́о|лог *м.* ideólogist. **~логи́ческий** ideológical. **~ло́гия** *ж.* ideólogy.

иде́|я *ж.* idéa; (*понятие*) concéption, cóncept, nótion; ~ добра́ concéption of good; передовы́е ~и progréssive/advánced idéas; полити́ческие ~и polítical cóncepts; ~ рома́на underlýing idéa/theme of a nóvel; счастли́вая ~ háppy thought; что за ~! what an idéa!

идилли́ческий idýllic.

иди́ллия *ж.* idýll.

идио́м *м.*, ~а *ж. лингв.* ídiom.

идиома́тика *ж. лингв.* 1. (*учение*) stúdy of ídiom; 2. (*совокупность идиом*) ídioms *pl*.

идиомати́ческ|**ий** *лингв.* idiomátic; ~ое выраже́ние idiomátic expréssion.

идио́т *м.* ídiot. **~и́зм** *м.* ídiocy. **~ка** *ж.* ídiot. **~ский** idiótic. **~ство** *с. разг.* ídiocy, imbecílity.

и́дол *м.* ídol.

идолопокло́н|**ник** *м.* idólater. **~ство** *с.* ídolatry.

идти́, пойти́ 1. *тк. несов.* go*; он шёл по у́лице he was góing down/up/alóng the street; она́ шла по мосту́ she was góing acróss the bridge, she was cróssing the bridge; ему́ пришло́сь ~ пешко́м he had to walk, he had to go on foot; ло́шадь идёт ры́сью, гало́пом the horse is trótting, gálloping; 2. *тк. несов.* (*двигаться, перемещаться*) move, go*, trável; по́езд идёт бы́стро the train is góing/trávelling at high speed; та́нки иду́т пря́мо на нас the tanks are cóming/móving straight towárds us; самолёты шли на восто́к the planes were flýing east; флот шёл на всех паруса́х the fleet was in full sail; по не́бу ме́дленно иду́т облака́ the clouds are móving/drífting slówly acróss the sky; лёд идёт по реке́ the ice is góing down the ríver; 3. *тк. несов.* (*о моменте отправления поезда и т. п.*) go*, leave*; по́езд идёт в 12 часо́в но́чи the train goes/leaves at mídnight; 4. *тк. несов.* (*доставляться*) come*; пи́сьма до́лго иду́т the mail is véry slow, létters take a long time to arríve; 5. *тк. несов.* (*приближаться, появляться*) come*; перен. тж. appróach; по́езд идёт! the train is cóming; весна́ идёт spring is on the way; 6. *тк. несов.* (*в вн., + инф.; направляться с какой-л. целью*) go* (to, + to inf, + -ing); ~ гуля́ть go* for a walk; ~ в шко́лу go* to school; ~ на охо́ту go* húnting; 7. (*на вн.; нападать*) march (on), advance (on); перен. attáck (on); враг идёт на Москву́ the énemy is adváncing on Móscow; 8. (*в, на вн.; вступать, поступать куда-л.*) join (smth.), énter (smth.); ~ на биологи́ческий факульте́т énter the bíology fáculty; ~ в а́рмию join the ármy; 9. *тк. несов.* (*развиваться*) progréss, head; (*действовать тем или иным образом*) march, go*; ~ по пути́ техни́ческого прогре́сса take* the path of téchnical prógress; всё идёт к лу́чшему éverything is for the best; 10. *тк. несов.* (*за тв.; следовать*) fóllow (smb., smth.); ~ за толпо́й fóllow the crowd; 11. *тк. несов.* (*от, из рд.; распространяться, исходить*) come* (from); (*о слухах, вестях*) go* (a)róund; из трубы́ идёт дым there is smoke cóming from the chímney; идёт слух, что... a rúmour is going round that...; 12. *тк. несов.* (*поступать, подаваться*) be* on, flow; ток идёт the cúrrent is on; 13. *разг.* (*находить сбыт*) sell*; э́тот това́р хорошо́ идёт these goods are in demánd; **14.** *тк. несов.* (*простира́ться, пролега́ть*) run*, stretch; доро́га идёт по́лем the road runs acróss the field; го́рная гряда́ идёт с се́вера на юг the móuntain range strétches from north to south; **15.** *тк. несов.* (*находи́ться в де́йствии*) work; часы́ иду́т то́чно the watch keeps exáct time; **16.** *тк. несов.* (*об оса́дках*) fall*; дождь, снег идёт it is ráining, snówing; **17.** *тк. несов.* (*протека́ть, проходи́ть*) go* by, pass; шли неде́ли the weeks went by; **18.** *тк. несов.* (*дли́ться, продолжа́ться*) be*; идёт 1965 год it is the year níneteen (húndred and) síxty-five; **19.** *тк. несов.* (*име́ть ме́сто, происходи́ть*) be* in prógress, procéed; (*ста́виться — о пье́се и т. п.*) go*; иду́т экза́мены the examinátions are in prógress; идёт но́вый фильм there is a new film on; **20.** (*на вн.; соглаша́ться*) agrée (to); пойти́ на предло́женные усло́вия agrée to the terms óffered; **21.** (*в, на вн.; предназнача́ться, испо́льзоваться*) be* used (for); лучи́на идёт на расто́пку the sticks are used for fuel; **22.** (*на вн.; расхо́доваться*) be* spent (on); go* (on); мно́го де́нег идёт на кни́ги a lot of móney goes on books; на костю́м пойдёт три ме́тра тка́ни it takes three métres of matérial to make a suit; **23.** (*дт.; подходи́ть*) suit (*smb., smth.*); пиджа́к ему́ не идёт the jácket dóesn't suit him; **24.** *разг.* (*получа́ться, ла́диться*) go* right; рабо́та не шла the work wóuldn't go right; **25.** (*тв., с рд.; де́лать ход в игре́*) play (*smth.*); (*в ша́хматах*) move (*smth.*); тепе́рь ~ вам now it's your move, now it's your turn/go; ~ с туза́ play the ace; ◇ ~ на сме́ну кому́-л., чему́-л. take* the place of *smb., smth.*, repláce *smb., smth.*; не ~ да́льше *чего́-л.* not go fúrther than; речь идёт о том, что... the point is that...

иезуи́т *м.* Jésuit. **~ский** Jesuítical.

иера́рхи́ческий hierárchic(al).

иера́рхия *ж.* híerarchy.

иеро́глиф *м.* **1.** híeroglyph; *мн.* hieroglýphics, cháracters; **2.** *обыкн. мн.* (*о непоня́тном письме́*) scrawl *sg.* **~и́ческий** hieroglýphic; **~и́ческое письмо́** hieroglýphic wríting.

иждиве́|ец *м.* depéndant. **~ие** *с.*: состоя́ть на **~ии** у кого́-л. be* depéndent on *smb.*

из, изо 1. (*отку́да*) from; (*изнутри́*) out of; прие́хать из Волгогра́да come from Vólgograd; вы́йходить из до́му come out of the house; цита́та из газе́ты a quotátion from a néwspaper; **2.** (*при указа́нии материа́ла, соста́ва*) of; (*о сырье́*) from; э́ти боти́нки сде́ланы из ко́жи these shoes are made of léather; из одного́ куска́ де́рева made from a síngle piece of wood; ма́сло де́лается из молока́ bútter is made from milk; буке́т, вено́к из роз bunch, wreath of róses; аппара́т состои́т из двух часте́й the machine is in two parts; обе́д из двух блюд two-cóurse dínner; **3.** (*по́сле сравни́т. или превосх. ст.*) of; лу́чший из всех the best of all; мла́дший из бра́тьев (*двух*) the younger of the two; **4.** (*по причи́не*) out of, for; из уваже́ния (к) out of respéct (for); из любопы́тства out of curiósity; из стра́ха перед кем-л., чем-л. féaring *smb., smth.*, for fear of *smb., smth.*; из любви́ ко мне for me, for my sake; ◇ одно́ из двух one or the óther; оди́н из ты́сячи one in a thóusand; изо всех сил with all *one's* might, with might and main.

изба́ *ж.* izbá, péasant's house/cóttage, log cábin.

избави́тель *м.*, **~ница** *ж.* delíverer, sáviour.

избав|и́ть(ся) *сов. см.* избавля́ть(ся). **~ле́ние** *с.* delíverance (from).

избавля́ть, изба́вить (*вн. от рд.*) save (*smb.* from); ~ кого́-л. от сме́рти, опа́сности save *smb.* from death, dánger; ~ кого́-л. от необходи́мости де́лать что́-л. save *smb.* the tróuble of dóing *smth.*; ~ кого́-л. от хлопо́т save *smb.* tróuble; изба́вьте меня́ от него́! can't you get rid of him for me?; изба́вьте меня́! spare me that, please!;

изба́вьте меня́ от своего́ прису́тствия! kíndly take yoursélf off! **~ся, изба́виться** (от *рд.*) get* rid (of), shake* off (*smb., smth.*); изба́виться от неприя́тностей rid* onesélf of tróuble; изба́виться от просту́ды shake* off a cold.

избало́ванный spoilt.

избалова́ть *сов.* (*вн. тв.*) spoil* (*smb.* by, with). **~ся** *сов.* becóme/get* spoilt.

избега́ть, избе́гнуть, избежа́ть (*рд.*) **1.** (*уклоня́ться*) avóid (*smb., smth.*), shun (*smb., smth.*); ~ чьего́-л. взгля́да avóid *smb.'s* eye; ~ о́бщества кого́-л. shun the society of *smb.*; ~ просту́ды try not to catch cold; ~ встре́чи с кем-л. keep* out of *smb.'s* way; избежа́ть неприя́тного разгово́ра avóid an unpléasant ínterview; **2.** (*спаса́ться, избавля́ться*) escápe (*smth.*), eváde (*smth.*), elúde (*smth.*); избежа́ть ги́бели be* saved; (*о лю́дях тж.*) escápe death.

избе́гнуть *сов. см.* избега́ть.

избеж|а́ние *с.*: во ~ чего́-л. to prevént *smth.*; во ~ недоразуме́ния in órder to prevént a misunderstánding; so that there should be no misunderstánding; во ~ нарека́ний to avóid críticism. **~а́ть** *сов. см.* избега́ть.

изби|ва́ть, изби́ть (*вн.*) beat* (*smb.*), give* (*smb.*) a térrible béating; beat* up (*smb.*) *разг.* **~е́ние** *с.* béating; béating-up *разг.*

избира́тель *м.* eléctor, vóter; *мн. собир.* the eléctorate *sg.* **~ный** eléctoral; eléction *attr.*; **~ный** бюллете́нь bállot-paper, vóting-paper; **~ная** кампа́ния eléction campáign; **~ная** коми́ссия eléction committee; **~ный** о́круг eléctoral district, constítuency; **~ный** уча́сток 1) pólling-district; 2) (*помеще́ние*) pólling-station; **~ное** пра́во súffrage, right to vote; **~ный** зако́н eléctoral law; **~ная** систе́ма eléctoral sýstem, eléction sýstem; **~ная** у́рна, **~ный** я́щик bállot-box.

избира́ть, избра́ть (*вн.*) **1.** (*выбира́ть*) seléct (*smb., smth.*), choose* (*smb., smth.*); **2.** (*на вы́борах*) eléct (*smb., smth.*).

изби́т|ый 1. (*проторённый*) béaten, famíliar; **~ая** доро́га the béaten track; **2.** (*опо́шленный*) trite, stale, háckneyed; ~ сюже́т óutworn theme.

изби́ть *сов. см.* избива́ть.

изборозди́ть *сов. см.* борозди́ть.

избра́н|ие *с.* eléction. **~ник** *м.* chosen one; *мн.* the eléct *sg*; наро́дный **~ник** chósen represéntative of the péople.

и́збранн|ый *прил.* **1.** seléct; ~ круг люде́й a seléct circle; **~ые** произведе́ния selécted works; **2.** *в знач. сущ. мн.* the chósen ones; для **~ых** for the élite.

избра́ть *сов. см.* избира́ть.

избу́шка *ж.* hut, log cábin.

избы́т|ок *м.* **1.** (*изли́шек*) súrplus; ~ хле́ба grain súrplus; **2.** (*оби́лие, полнота́*) abúndance; ~ усе́рдия excéss of zeal; ~ка чувств out of the fúl(l)ness of *one's* heart; ◇ в ~ке, с ~ком in abúndance. **~очный** súrplus *attr.*, excéss *attr.*

изва́яние *с.* státue.

изва́ять *сов. см.* вая́ть.

изве́дать *сов.* (*вн.*) expérience (*smth.*), know* (*smth.*); ~ сча́стье know* háppiness, taste of háppiness.

и́зверг *м.* fiend, mónster.

изверга́ть, изве́ргнуть (*вн.*) **1.** erúpt (*smth.*), spout (*smth.*), eject (*smth.*); (*о пи́ще*) vómit (*smth.*); **2.** (*изгоня́ть*) expél (*smth.*). **~ся** *несов.* erúpt.

изве́ргнуть *сов. см.* изверга́ть.

изверже́ние *с.* erúption.

изве́риться *сов.* (*в пр.*) lose* faith (in).

изверну́ться *сов. см.* извора́чиваться.

извести́ *сов. см.* изводи́ть.

изве́стие *с.* **1.** news; tídings *pl книжн.*; прия́тное ~ good* news; **2.** *мн.* (*периоди́ческое изда́ние*) Procéedings.

извести́сь *сов. см.* изводи́ться.

извести́ть *сов. см.* извеща́ть.

извёстка *ж. разг.* lime; (*для побелки стен*) whitewash.

известко́вый lime *attr.*; ~ раство́р solútion of lime, slaked lime.

изве́стно *в знач. сказ. безл.* it is known; хорошо́ ~ it is well·known, it is cómmon knówledge; всему́ ми́ру ~ the whole world knows.

изве́стн|ость *ж.* populárity; (*слава*) fame, renówn; по́льзоваться ~остью be* well-knówn, be* pópular; ◇ поста́вить *кого-л.* в ~ inform *smb.*, nótify *smb.* ~ый 1. (*знакомый*) known; ~ый факт known fact; ~ый свои́м ма́стерством known for *one's* skill; ~ый как хоро́ший учи́тель known as a good téacher; 2. (*знаменитый*) well-knówn, pópular, fámous; (*с плохой стороны*) notórious; ~ый писа́тель well-known wríter; ~ый моше́нник notórious swíndler; 3. (*определённый*) cértain; при ~ых усло́виях únder cértain condítions.

известня́к *м.* límestone.

и́звесть *ж.* lime.

изве́чн|ый perénnial; ~ые скотово́ды cáttle-bréeders since éarliest times.

извеща́ть, извести́ть (*вн. о пр.*) inform (*smb.* of, abóut), nótify (*smb.* of, abóut); (*дать знать*) let* (*smb.*) know (of, abóut). ~éние *c.* nótice, notificátion.

изви́в *м.* bend, twist. ~а́ться *несов.* wríggle; (*о реке, дороге*) wind*, méander.

изви́ли|на *ж.* bend; convolútion *научн.*; ~ны мо́зга convolútions of the brain. ~стый wínding, méandering; ~стые у́лицы wínding streets; ~стая ре́чка méandering/wínding stream.

извине́ни|е *c.* apólogy; приноси́ть (свой) ~я за *что-л.* óffer (*one's*) apólogies for *smth.*; проси́ть ~я у *кого-л.* beg *smb.'s* párdon; 2. (*оправдание*) excúse.

извини́тельный párdonable.

извин|и́ть(ся) *сов. см.* извиня́ть(ся). ~я́ть, извиня́ть (*вн.*) excúse (*smb.*, *smth.*), párdon (*smb.*, *smth.*); ~и́те! (I'm) sórry!, excúse me!, I beg your párdon! ~я́ться, извини́ться (*пе́ред тв.*) apólogize (to); я извини́лся I said I was sórry.

извлека́ть, извле́чь (*вн. из рд.*) extráct (*smth.* from); *перен.* derive (from); ~ пу́лю из ра́ны extráct a búllet from a wound; ~ по́льзу из *чего-л.* derive bénefit from *smth.*; ~ удово́льствие derive/extráct pléasure; ◇ ~ ко́рень *мат.* extráct the root.

извлече́ние *c.* 1. extráction; 2. (*выдержка*) éxtract; ◇ ~ ко́рня *мат.* extráction of the root.

извле́чь *сов. см.* извлека́ть.

извне́ from óutside; без по́мощи ~ withóut óutside help.

изводи́ть, извести́ (*вн.*) 1. (*тратить*) waste (*smth.*), spend* (*smth.*); 2. (*мучить*) tormént (*smb.*), wórry (*smb.*) to death. ~ся, извести́сь tíre onesélf out, exháust onesélf.

изво́зчик *м.* 1. (*кучер*) cábman*; cábby *разг.*; 2. (*экипаж*) cab; взять ~а take* a cab; éхать на ~е go* by cab.

извора́чиваться, изверну́ться twist and turn; *перен.* wríggle, shift, dodge.

изворо́тливый 1. (*увёртливый*) slíppery, nímble, ágile; 2. (*находчивый, ловкий*) resóurceful.

извраща́ть *сов. см.* извраща́ть.

извращ|а́ть, изврати́ть (*вн.*) distórt (*smth.*), pervért (*smth.*); ~ фа́кты distórt/twist the facts. ~е́ние *c.* 1. (*искажение*) distórtion; 2. (*болезненное отклонение от нормы*) pervérsion.

извращённ|ость *ж.* pervérsity. ~ый 1. (*искажён-ный*) distórted; 2. (*противоестественный*) pervérted, pervérse; ~ый вкус deprável taste.

изги́б *м.* bend, curve.

изгиба́ть, изогну́ть (*вн.*) bend* (*smth.*), curve (*smth.*); ~ спи́ну arch *one's* back. ~ся, изогну́ться bend*, curve.

изгла́дить(ся) *сов. см.* изгла́живать(ся).

изгла́живать, изгла́дить (*вн.*) effáce (*smth.*), oblíterate (*smth.*), blot (*smth.*) out; ◇ изгла́дить *что-л.* из па́мяти oblíterate *smth.* from *one's* mémory. ~ся, изгла́диться disappéar, effáce onesélf, becóme* oblíterated, be* blótted out; ◇ изгла́диться из па́мяти fade from mémory.

изгна́н|ие *c.* 1. (*действие*) expúlsion, bánishment; 2. (*ссылка*) éxile, bánishment. ~ник *м.*, ~ница *ж.* éxile.

изгна́ть *сов. см.* изгоня́ть.

изго́й *м.* sócial óutcast.

изголо́вь|е *c.* head of the bed; сиде́ть у ~я sit* at the bédside.

изголода́ться *сов.* 1. be* stárving; 2. (*по дт.*) be* yéarning/lónging (for).

изгоня́ть, изгна́ть (*вн.*) 1. drive* (*smb.*, *smth.*) out; (*ссылать*) éxile (*smb.*), bánish (*smb.*); 2. (*искоренять*) do* awáy (with).

и́згородь *ж.* fence.

изгота́вливать *несов. см.* изготовля́ть.

изгото́вить *сов. см.* изготовля́ть.

изготовл|е́ние *c.* manufácture. ~я́ть, изгото́вить (*вн.*) manufácture (*smth.*), make* (*smth.*).

издава́ть I, изда́ть (*вн.*) 1. (*выпускать в свет*) públish (*smth.*); bring* out, íssue (*smth.*); 2. (*обнародовать*) íssue (*smth.*), prómulgate (*smth.*); ~ прика́з íssue an órder; ~ зако́н prómulgate a law.

издава́ть II, изда́ть (*вн.*) (*звук*) emít (*smth.*), útter (*smth.*); (*запах*) give* (*smth.*) off, exhále (*smth.*); он не изда́л ни зву́ка he did not útter a word.

и́здавна long, long since; from time immemórial, long since; знать *кого-л.* have* known *smb.* for a long time; ~ знать (что) have* long known (that); ~ установи́вшийся long--estáblished.

издалека́ from afár; (*издали тж.*) from a distance; ~ докати́лся гро́хот ору́дий from afár came the rúmble of artíllery; он уви́дел его́ ~ he saw him from a distance; прие́хать ~ come* from far awáy; го́сти ~ guests from afár, guests from distant parts; ◇ нача́ть (разгово́р) ~ take* a róundabout appróach to the súbject.

и́здали from a distance, from afár.

изда́ние *c.* 1. (*действие*) publicátion, públishing; (*закон*) íssue, promulgátion, íssuing; 2. (*печатное произведение*) publicátion; 3. (*род издания*) edítion; дешёвое ~ cheap edítion; второ́е ~ 2nd edítion.

изда́тель *м.* públisher. ~ский públishing; ~ское де́ло the públishing trade. ~ство *c.* públishing house.

изда́ть I, II *сов. см.* издава́ть I, II.

издева́тель|ский jéering, derísive; (*оскорби-тельный*) insúlting; ~ское отноше́ние derísive áttitude; ~ тон tone of derísion/rídicule. ~ство *c.* 1. (*действие*) (vícious) móckery; jéering, derísion; 2. (*злая насмешка*) malícious insult; ~ство над людьми́ violátion of húman dígnity.

издева́ться *несов.* (*над тв.*) treat (*smb.*, *smth.*) with contémpt; jeer (at), mock (*smb.*, *smth.*), taunt (*smb.*).

издёвк|а *ж. разг.* gibe, taunt; посмотре́ть с ~ой на *кого-л.* look táuntingly at *smb.*

изде́ли|е *c.* 1. (*выделка*) make; часы́ ме́стного ~я watch of lócal make, lócally made watch; 2. (*предмет, вещь*) árticle, próduct; goods *pl*; промы́шленное ~ indústrial próduct; желе́зные ~я hárdware *sg*, íronmongery *sg*.

издёрганн|ый *разг.* hárried, hárassed; ~ые не́рвы overtáxed nerves.

издёргать *сов.* (*вн.*) *разг.* hárass (*smb.*). ~ся *сов. разг.* get* into a bad state of nerves.

издержа́ть *сов.* (*вн.*) spend* (*smth.*), expénd (*smth.*). ~ся *сов.* have* spent all *one's* móney.

издёржки *мн.* óutlay *sg*; ~ произвóдства prodúction costs.

издóхнуть *сов. см.* издыхáть.

издыхáть, издóхнуть die.

изжáрить *сов.* (*вн.*) (*на сковороде*) fry (*smth.*); (*в духовке, на вертеле*) roast (*smth.*). ~ся *сов.* be* réady.

изживáть, изжи́ть (*вн.*) get* rid (of), elíminate (*smth.*); ◇ изжи́ть себя́ becóme* óbsolete.

изжи́ть *сов. см.* изживáть.

изжóга *ж.* héartburn.

из-за 1. (*откуда*) from, from behínd; ~ мóря from acróss the sea, from overséas; ~ двере́й from the óther side of the door; встать ~ столá rise* from the táble, get* up; ~ углá вы́ехала маши́на a car came round the córner; ~ óблака вы́плыла лунá the moon came out from behínd a cloud; 2. (*по причине*) becáuse of, ówing to; (*по вине*) through; ~ вас (all) becáuse of you; ~ дождя́ on accóunt of the rain.

иззя́бнуть *сов. разг.* be* frózen stiff, be* chilled to the bone.

излагáть, изложи́ть (*вн.*) expóund (*smth.*), state (*smth.*), set* (*smth.*) forth; ~ своё дéло state *one's* case; ~ прóсьбу frame a requést; ~ что-л. в пи́сьменной фóрме state/put* *smth.* in wríting; ~ что-л. свои́ми словáми put* *smth.* in *one's* own words, páraphrase *smth.*

излени́ться *сов. разг.* get* lázy.

излёт *м.*: пу́ля на ~е spent búllet.

излéчени|е *с.* 1. (*лечение*) tréatment, cure; находи́ться на ~и be* únder médical tréatment; 2. (*выздоровление*) recóvery.

излéчивать, излечи́ть (*вн.*) cure (*smb., smth.*). ~ся, излечи́ться 1. (*от рд.*) be* cured (of); 2. *тк. несов.* (*поддаваться лечению*) respónd to tréatment.

излечи́мый cúrable. ~и́ть *сов. см.* излéчивать. ~и́ться *сов. см.* излéчиваться 1.

изливáть, изли́ть (*вн.*) pour (*smth.*) out/forth, effúse (*smth.*); ~ гнев на когó-л. vent *one's* ánger on *smb.*, pour out (the víals of) *one's* wrath upón *smb.*; ~ комý-л. свои́ чу́вства pour out *one's* féelings to *smb.* ~ся, изли́ться relíeve *one's* féelings; ~ся в выраже́ниях благодáрности pour out *one's* grátitude/thanks, be* profúse in *one's* thanks.

изли́ть(ся) *сов. см.* изливáть(ся).

изли́ш|ек *м.* 1. (*то, что остаётся*) súrplus; ~ки хлéба súrplus grain; 2. (*чрезмерное количество*) excéss; ◇ э́того хвáтит с ~ком thát'll be enóugh and to spare. ~ество *с.* excéss, óver-indúlgence; архитекту́рные ~ества architéctural extrávagances. ~ний 1. (*чрезмерный*) supérfluous, excéssive; ~ние подрóбности supérfluous détail *sg*; 2. (*ненужный*) unnécessary; ~няя предосторóжность únwárranted precáution.

излия́ния *мн.* óutpourings; ~ чувств effúsions.

излови́ть *сов.* (*вн.*) *разг.* catch* (*smb., smth.*), get* (*smb., smth.*).

изловчи́ться *сов.* (+ *инф.*) *разг.* mánage (+ to *inf*), contríve (+ to *inf*).

изложе́ни|е *с.* 1. exposítion, interpretátion; 2. (*пересказ*) páraphrase, réndering in *one's* own words. ~ть *сов. см.* излагáть.

излóм *м.* 1. (*место разлома*) crack, break; 2. (*болезненный надрыв*) bréakdown; душе́вный ~ psychológical collápse.

излóманн|ый 1. (*сломанный*) bróken; *тех.* fráctured; 2. (*непрямой*) zígzag *attr.*; ~ почерк ángular/unéven hand (wríting); ~ая ли́ния zígzag line; 3. (*неестественный*) affécted; (*изуродованный*) defórmed; (*о языке*) bróken.

излóмать *сов.* (*вн.*) 1. (*сломать*) break* (*smth.*), break* up (*smth.*), smash (*smth.*) to píeces; 2. *разг.* (*сделать неестественным*) defórm (*smb., smth.*), warp (*smb., smth.*); ~ человéку жизнь warp a pérson's life. ~ся *сов.* break* up.

излучáть несов. (*вн.*) emít (*smth.*), rádiate (*smth.*), erádiate (*smth.*). ~áться несов. rádiate, émanate. ~éние *с.* radiátion, eradiátion.

излу́чина *ж.* bend.

излю́бленн|ый fávourite; ~ое выраже́ние pet expréssion.

измáзать *сов.* (*вн.*) smear (*smb., smth.*), dírty (*smb., smth.*); ~ плáтье dírty *one's* dress, mess up *one's* dress; ~ ру́ки dírty *one's* hands; ~ себé лицó get* *one's* face all óver onesélf; ~ся *сов.* get* dírty; ~ся черни́лами get* ink all óver onesélf; ~ся крáсками get* onesélf cóvered with paint.

измáтывать, измотáть (*вн.*) *разг.* exháust (*smb., smth.*), wear* (*smb., smth.*) out. ~ся, измотáться *разг.* be* worn out.

измельчáть I *сов. см.* мельчáть.

измельчáть II, измельчи́ть (*вн.*) redúce (*smth.*) to frágments; (*рубить*) chop (*smth.*) fine; (*толочь*) pound (*smth.*); измельчи́ть что-л. в порошóк grind* *smth.* to a pówder, púlverize *smth.*

измельчи́ть *сов. см.* измельчáть II.

измéна *ж.* 1. (*предательство*) tréason; государственная ~ high tréason; 2. (*отказ от чего-л.*) betráyal; 3. (*нарушение верности в любви*) unfáithfulness; супру́жеская ~ adúltery.

изменéни|е *с.* 1. (*действие*) chánging, alterátion; ~ плáна change of the plan, alterátion in the plan; ~ направлéния change in/of diréction; 2. (*поправка*) change, alterátion, améndment; без ~я unchánged; вноси́ть ~я в констру́кцию самолётов módify the desígn of áircraft.

измени́ть I, II *сов. см.* изменя́ть I, II.

измени́ться *сов. см.* изменя́ться.

измéнни|к *м.* tráitor; ~ рóдины tráitor to *one's* cóuntry. ~ческий tráitorous, tréacherous.

изме́нчив|ость *ж.* changeabílity, incónstancy. ~ый chángeable, incónstant; (*о человеке тж.*) fíckle, unstáble.

изменя́ть I, измени́ть (*вн.*) álter (*smth.*), change (*smth.*); (*видоизменять*) módify (*smth.*); измени́ть курс álter (the) course; ~ óбраз жи́зни change *one's* mode of líving; измени́ть своё мнéние о ком-л., чём-л. change *one's* opínion abóut *smth., smth.*; несколько измени́ть своё отношéние к комý-л. módify *one's* áttitude towárds *smb.*; ~ ход собы́тий álter the course of evénts.

изменя́ть II, измени́ть (*дт.*) 1. (*предавать*) betráy (*smb., smth.*); измени́ть рóдине betráy *one's* cóuntry; 2. (*нарушать верность чему-л.*) betráy (*smth.*); ~ прися́ге break* *one's* oath; измени́ть своемý дóлгу fail in *one's* dúty; 3. (*нарушать верность в любви*) be* unfáithful (to); 4. (*переставать действовать*) fail (*smb.*); éсли пáмять мне не ~ет if my mémory does not decéive me, if my mémory serves me well; пáмять емý ~ет his mémory is fáiling; си́лы измени́ли емý his strength fáiled him.

изменя́ться, измени́ться change; измени́ться к лу́чшему change for the bétter; ◇ измени́ться в лицé change cóuntenance.

измерéние *с.* 1. (*действие*) méasuring; (*землемерное*) súrvey; (*глубины*) sóunding; (*температуры*) táking; 2. *мат.* (*измеряемая величина*) diménsion.

измери́тель *м.* gauge, méasure. ~ный méasuring.

измéрить *сов. см.* измеря́ть.

измеря́ть, измéрить (*вн.*) méasure (*smth.*); (*землю*) survéy (*smth.*); (*глубину*) sound (*smth.*), fáthom (*smth.*); (*температуру*) take* (*smth.*). ~я́ться несов. be* méasured; врéмя ~я́лось тепéрь секу́ндами évery sécond cóunted now; запáсы ~я́ются тóннами supplíes may be éstimated by the ton.

измождённый emáciated, hággard.

измока́ть, измо́кнуть *разг.* be* wet through, be* sódden.

измо́кнуть *сов. см.* измока́ть.

измо́р *м.:* брать, взять *кого-л.* ~ом starve *smb.* ínto surrénder; *перен.* wear* down *smb.'s* resístance.

и́зморозь *ж.* (*иней*) hóarfrost, rime.

и́зморось *ж.* drízzle.

измота́ть(ся) *сов. см.* изма́тывать(ся).

изму́ченный worn-óut, exháusted; у него́ ~ вид he looks worn-óut, he looks played out.

изму́чить *сов.* (*вн.*) break* (*smb.*) by tórture; (*утомить*) wear* (*smb.*) out. ~ся *сов.* be* tíred out, be* worn out.

измыва́ться *сов.* (*над тв.*) *разг.* jeer (at), poke fun (at).

изму́слить *сов. см.* измышля́ть.

измышл|е́ние *с.* invéntion, fabricátion; (*ложь*) lie, fálsehood. **~я́ть**, измы́слить (*вн.*) invént (*smth.*), fábricate (*smth.*); (*придумывать*) think* up (*smth.*), invént (*smth.*).

измя́тый crúmpled, creased; (*с вмятинами*) dénted, báttered.

измя́ть *сов.* (*вн.*) 1. crúmple (*smth.*); (*постель*) rúmple (*smth.*); (*покрыть вмятинами*) dent (*smth.*), bátter (*smth.*); 2. (*придавить; прям. и перен.*) crush (*smb., smth.*). ~ся *сов.* be* crúmpled/creased.

изна́нк|а *ж.* wrong side; séamy side (*тж. перен.*); ◇ с ~и on the inside, on the únderside.

изнаси́лов|ание *с.* rape, violátion. **~ать** *сов. см.* наси́ловать 1.

изна́шивать, износи́ть (*вн.*) wear* (*smth.*) out. **~ся**, износи́ться be* worn out.

изне́женн|ость *ж.* délicacy, sóftness; (*о мужчине тж.*) efféminacy. **~ый** délicate, soft, códdled; (*о мужчине тж.*) efféminate.

изне́живать, изне́жить (*вн.*) códdle (*smb.*), make* (*smb.*) soft. **~ся**, изне́житься grow* soft.

изне́жить(ся) *сов. см.* изне́живать(ся).

изнемога́ть, изнемо́чь be* exháusted; *сов. тж.* break* down; ~ от уста́лости be* faint with exháustion/fatígue, be* tíred out, drop with exháustion.

изнеможе́ние *с.* exháustion, prostrátion.

изнемо́чь *сов. см.* изнемога́ть.

изне́рвнича|ться *сов.* wreck *one's* nerves; она́ совсе́м ~лась her nerves are all to píeces, she is a nérvous wreck.

изно́с *м.* 1. (*изношенность*) wear, wear and tear, depreciátion; 2. (*изнашиваемость*) wear; э́той мате́рии нет ~а this stuff can néver wear out, this stuff will stand ány amóunt of wear.

износи́ть(ся) *сов. см.* изна́шивать(ся).

изно́шенный worn-óut; (*о ткани тж.*) thréadbare.

изнур|е́ние *с.* exháustion. **~ённый** exháusted, enféebled, énervated, worn-óut.

изнури́тельн|ый exháusting, grúelling; ~ая жара́ énervating heat.

изнури́ть *сов. см.* изнуря́ть.

изнуря́ть, изнури́ть (*вн.*) exháust (*smb., smth.*), énervate (*smb.*), wear* (*smb., smth.*) out.

изнутри́ from (the) inside; (*с внутренней стороны*) on the inside; дверь заперта́ ~ the door is locked on the inside.

изныва́ть *несов.* lánguish, droop; ~ от жары́ be* lánguishing in the heat; be* dýing of heat; ~ от ску́ки be* dýing of bóredom; ~ от тоски́ pine with grief.

изо *см.* из.

изоба́ра *ж. геогр., физ.* ísobar.

изоби́л|ие *с.* abúndance, plénty; в ~ии in abúndance, in plénty. **~овать** *несов.* (*тв.*) abóund (in, with).

изоби́льный abúndant, pléntiful.

изоблич|а́ть, изобличи́ть (*вн.*) 1. (*уличать в чём-либо*) expóse (*smb., smth.*); unmásk (*smb.*); изобли-

чи́ть *кого-л.* во лжи catch* *smb.* out in a lie, prove *smb.* a líar; 2. *тк. несов.* (*ясно показывать*) revéal (*smth., smth.*); то́лько меч ~а́л в нём во́ина ónly the sword revéaled him as a wárrior. **~е́ние** *с.* expósure. **~и́ть** *сов. см.* изобличáть 1.

изображ|а́ть, изобрази́ть (*вн.*) 1. portráy (*smth., smth.*); (*графически тж.*) represént (*smb., smth.*); (*в литературе тж.*) delíneate (*smb., smth.*), depíct (*smb., smth.*); 2. (*на сцене*) act/play the part (of); 3. (*выражать*) show* (*smth.*); его́ лицо́ изобрази́ло трево́гу his face displáyed anxíety; 4. *тк. несов.* (*быть изображением*) represént (*smth., smth.*); ◇ ~ из себя́ give* one*self*; ~а́ться, изобрази́ться: на его́ лице́ изобрази́лось кра́йнее изумле́ние his face/féatures expréssed extréme astónishment. **~е́ние** *с.* portráyal, representátion, delineátion; (*то, что изображено тж.*) pícture; (*оптическое*) ímage.

изобрази́тельн|ый representátional; ◇ ~ые иску́сства the fine arts.

изобрази́ть *сов. см.* изображáть 1, 2, 3. **~ся** *сов. см.* изображáться.

изобрести́ *сов. см.* изобретáть.

изобрета́тель *м.* invéntor. **~ность** *ж.* invéntiveness. **~ный** invéntive. **~ство** *с.* invéntion.

изобрет|а́ть, изобрести́ (*вн.*) invént (*smth.*). **~е́ние** *с.* invéntion.

изогну́ть(ся) *сов. см.* изгибáть(ся).

изойти́ *сов. см.* исходи́ть III.

изолга́ться *сов.* becóme* an incórrigible líar.

изоли́рованный 1. (*обособленный*) ísolated; 2. *тех.* ínsulated, sealed; ~ про́вод ínsulated wíre.

изоли́ровать *несов. и сов.* 1. (*обособлять*) ísolate (*smb., smth.*); 2. *тех.* ínsulate (*smth.*), seal (*smth.*).

изоля́|тор *м.* 1. *эл.* ínsulator; 2. (*больничный*) isolátion ward. **~цио́нный** ínsulating *attr.* **~ция** *ж.* 1. isolátion; 2. *эл.* insulátion.

изорва́ть *сов.* (*вн.*) tear* up (*smth.*). **~ся** *сов.* get* torn, come* to píeces.

изоте́рм|а *ж. геогр., физ.* ísotherm. **~и́ческий** isothérmal.

изото́п *м.* ísotope.

изощрённ|ость *ж.* súbtlety, refínement. **~ый** acúte, súbtle; ~ый слух acúte ear; ~ый ум súbtle/percéptive mind.

изощри́ть(ся) *сов. см.* изощря́ть(ся).

изощря́ть, изощри́ть (*вн.*) perféct (*smth.*), refíne (*smth.*); ~ свой вкус, ум train *one's* taste, mind. ~ся, изощри́ться: ~ся в остроу́мии éxercise *one's* wits, strain *one's* ingenúity; (*стараться быть остроумным*) try to be wítty.

из-под 1. (*откуда*) from únder, from benéath; вы́лезти ~ стола́ crawl out from únder the táble; 2.: буты́лка ~ молока́ mílk-bottle; коро́бка ~ конфе́т swéet-box; 3. (*из района, города, деревни*) from sómewhere near; ~ Ку́рска from sómewhere near Kursk.

израз|е́ц *м.* tile. **~цо́вый** tiled.

изра́ильский Isráeli.

израильтя́н|ин *м.*, **~ка** *ж.* Isráeli.

изра́ненный lácerated; cóvered with wounds *после сущ.*

израсхо́довать *сов. см.* расхо́довать.

и́зредка 1. (*иногда*) évery now and then, from time to time; 2. (*местами*) here and there.

изре́занный (*о береге и т. п.*) indénted, jagged.

изре́з|ать *сов.* (*вн.*) 1. (*на куски*) cut* (*smth.*) up; 2. (*сделать много порезов*) gash (*smth.*), slash (*smth.*); (*стол, доску и т. п.*) hack (*smth.*) about; 3. (*пересечь*) cut* (*smth.*) acróss, incíse (*smth.*); ме́стность ~ана овра́гами the cóuntry is scarred with ravínes.

изре|ка́ть, изре́чь (*вн.*) pronóunce (*smth.*), útter (*smth.*); ~ и́стину útter a truth. **~че́ние** *с.* díctum (*pl*

-ums, -ta), sáying; ~чёния велиќих людёй the útter- ances/sáyings of great men.

изрéчь *сов. см.* изрекáть.

изрешети́ть *сов. (вн.)* riddle (*smb.*, *smth.*).

изрисовáть *сов. (вн.)* cóver (*smth.*) with dráwings.

изруби́ть *сов. (вн.)* 1. chop (*smth.*); мéлко ~ *что-л.* cut*/chop *smth.* up (into little bits), mince *smth.*; 2. (*шашками*) put* (*smb.*, *smth.*) to the sword; cut* down (*smb.*, *smth.*) with one's sword.

изругáть *сов. (вн.)* heap abúse (on), revíle (*smb.*).

изры|áть, изрыгну́ть *(вн.)* 1. belch (*smth.*) out; *перен.* spout (*smth.*); 2. (*произносить, выкрикивать*) mouth (*smth.*). ~ну́ть *сов. см.* изрыгáть.

изры́тый churned up; ~ óспой pitted with smállpox scars *после сущ.*; póck-marked.

изры́ть *сов. (вн.)* churn (*smth.*) up, tear* (*smth.*) up.

изря́дн|о *разг.* consíderably, ráther, much. ~ый *разг.* quite a; ~ое расстоя́ние quite a dístance, ~ая су́мма дéнег quite a sum, quite a lot of móney.

изувéр *м.* fanátic, mónster; фаши́стские ~ы fáscist mónsters. ~ский fanátical, fanátically cruel. ~ство *с.* fanáticism, fanátical cruélty.

изувéчить *сов. (вн.)* maim (*smb.*, *smth.*), mútilate (*smb.*, *smth.*).

изуми́тельный (*удивительный*) amázing, astóund- ing; (*замечательный*) márvellous, wónderful.

изум|и́ть(ся) *сов. см.* изумля́ть(ся). ~лéние *с.* amázement; (*неприятное*) consternátion, dismáy. ~лённый amázed, astóunded; быть (неприя́тно) ~лённым be* dismáyed. ~ля́ть, изуми́ть *(вн.)* amáze (*smb.*), astóund (*smb.*). ~ля́ться, изуми́ться be* amázed/astóunded.

изумру́д *м.* émerald. ~ный émerald *attr.*

изурóдованный disfígured.

изурóдовать *сов. см.* урóдовать.

изуч|áть, изучи́ть *(вн.)* stúdy (*smb.*, *smth.*); (*исследовать тж.*) invéstigate (*smth.*); ~ вопрóс go* into the quéstion. ~éние *с.* stúdy; внимáтельное ~éние scrútiny. ~и́ть *сов. см.* изучáть.

изъéденный eaten; (*кислотой, ржавчиной*) corróded; ~ мóлью móth-eaten; ~ мыша́ми níbbled by mice *после сущ.*

изъéздить *сов. (вн.) разг.* trável all óver (*smth.*).

изъяви́тельн|ый: ~ое наклонéние *грам.* indícative (mood).

изъяв|и́ть *сов. см.* изъявля́ть. ~лéние *с.* expréssion.

изъявля́ть, изъяви́ть *(вн.)* expréss (*smth.*), decláre (*smth.*); ~ желáние expréss a wish; ~ соглáсие give* one's consént, consént (to).

изъя́н *м.* flaw, deféct; без ~а fláwless; товáр с ~ом deféctive árticle.

изъясня́ться *несов.* speak*, make* onesélf under- stóod.

изъя́ти|е *с.* 1. (*действие*) withdráwal; (*конфиска- ция*) confiscátion; ~ чего-л. из употреблéния, обращé- ния withdráwal of (*smth.*); 2. (*исключение*) excéption; все без ~я éveryone withóut excéption.

изъя́ть *сов. см.* изымáть.

изымáть, изъя́ть *(вн.)* withdráw* (*smth.*); (*конфисковать*) cónfiscate (*smth.*); изъя́ть что-л. из обращéния withdráw* *smth.* from circulátion.

изыскáние *с.* 1. (*действие*) fínding, procúring; ~ срéдств fínding/procúring of funds; 2. *обыкн. мн.* (*научные исследования*) reséarch *sg*, investigátion *sg*; 3. *обыкн. мн.* (*исследование местных условий*) survéying *sg*; (*геологические*) prospécting *sg*.

изы́сканный éxquisite, súbtle, refíned.

изыскáть *сов. (вн.)* (*деньги, средства*) obtáin (*smth.*); (*способ, средство*) find* (*smth.*), discóver (*smth.*).

изы́скивать *несов. (вн.)* seek* (*smth.*), look for (*smth.*).

изю́бр *м.* Manchúrian deer.

изю́м *м.* ráisins *pl.* ~ина *ж.* ráisin. ~инка *ж.* 1. *см.* изю́мина; 2. (*своеобразие*) píquancy; (*у человека*) spark; в ней есть ~инка she has a spark.

изя́щ|ество *с.* élegance; (*движений*) grace; (*стиля, манеры и т. п.*) pólish. ~ный élegant; (*о движениях*) gráceful; ~ное плáтье smart dress; ~ная фигу́ра gráceful figure.

икáть, икну́ть híccough.

икну́ть *сов. см.* икáть.

икóна *ж.* ícon.

иконопи́сец *м.* ícon-painter.

икóт|а *ж.* híccoughs *pl*; припáдок ~ы fit/attáck of híccoughs.

икрá I *ж.* 1. roe; 2. (*кушанье*) cáviare.

икрá II *ж.* (*ноги*) calf*.

икрометáние *с.* spáwning.

ил *м.* silt.

и́ли or; ~... or~... éither... or...

и́листый sílty.

иллю́з|ия *ж.* illúsion. ~óрный illúsory.

иллюминáтор *м. мор.* pórthole; *ав.* window.

иллюмин|áция *ж.* illuminátions *pl*; прáздничная ~ féstive illuminátions. ~и́ровать, ~овáть *несов. и сов.* (*вн.*) illúminate (*smth.*).

иллюстр|ати́вный íllustrative; ~ матери́áл illustrative matérial. ~áтор *м.* íllustrator. ~áция *ж.* illustrátion. ~и́ровать *несов. и сов. (сов. тж.* проиллюстри́ровать) (*вн.; прям. и перен.*) íllustrate (*smth.*).

им 1. (*тв. от личн. мест.* он) by him; 2. (*дт. от личн. мест.* они́) (to) them.

имби́рный gínger *attr.*

имби́рь *м.* gínger.

имéние *с.* estáte, (lánded) próperty.

имени́н|ник *м.*, ~ица *ж.* pérson célebrating his, her náme-day; *перен.* héro of the day; он ~ it's his náme- -day; *перен.* he is the héro of the day.

имени́ны *мн.* náme-day *sg.*

имени́тельный: ~ падéж *грам.* nóminative (case).

имени́тый éminent.

и́менно 1. (*как раз*) precísely, exáctly, just; ~ он э́то сказáл it was he who said it, he was the one who said it; ~ э́то он сказáл that's precísely/exáctly/just what he said; вы ~ тот, когó я хотéл ви́деть you're the véry pérson I wánted to see; ~ вас пошлю́т it'll be you they'll send; ~ потому́, что... it is (precísely) becáuse...; ~ так и слéдует понимáть that's just what it means; 2. (*при перечислении*) námely (*сокр.* viz.); три цвéта, а ~: крáсный, си́ний и жёлтый three cólours, námely: red, blue and yéllow; я получи́л при́я́тное извéстие, а ~, что мой проéкт при́нят I have had good news — my design has been accépted; 3.: кто, что ~? who, what, may I ask?; скóлько ~? how mány, much may I ask?; вот ~! exáctly!, that's right!, that's just the point!

именн|óй 1. inscríbed; (*о металлических вещах*) engráved; ~ые часы́ watch with the ówner's name engráved on it; ~ билéт, прóпуск ticket, pass made out in *smb.'s* name; ~ые áкции inscríbed stock *sg*; 2. *грам.* nóminal; ◇ ~ спи́сок nóminal list.

именóванн|ый: ~ое число́ *мат.* cóncrete númber.

именовáть *несов. (вн.)* name (*smb.*). ~ся *несов.* be* called, bear* the name.

имéть *несов. (вн.)* have* (*smth.*); ◇ ~ мéсто take* place; ~ цéлью have* as its aim (+ *noun*), be* aimed at (+ -ing); ничегó не ~ прóтив *чего-л.* have* nóthing agáinst *smth.*, have* no objéction to *smth.* ~ся *несов.* перевóдится действи́тельными фóрмами *гл.* have или оборóтами there is, there are; у меня́, у вас имéется I, you have; имéются в продáже (are) on sale; в продáже имéются нóвые радиоприёмники new rádio-

-sets are on sale; имéется в чьём-л. распоряжéнии is at smb.'s dispósal; éсли таковы́е имéются if aváilable; здесь имéется в виду́... the réference is to..., by this is meant...

имéющ|ийся aváilable; ~иеся фáкты подтверждáют the aváilable facts prove; кни́ги, ~иеся налицó the books aváilable.

и́ми (тв. от личн. мест. они́) by them.

имит|áтор м. ímitator. ~áция ж. imitátion. ~и́ровать несов. (вн.) ímitate (smb., smth.).

иммигр|áнт м., ~áнтка ж. ímmigrant. ~áция ж. 1. (дéйствие) immigrátion; 2. собир. (имми́гранты) ímmigrants pl. ~и́ровать несов. и сов. ímmigrate.

иммуниз|áция ж. immunizátion. ~и́ровать несов. и сов. (вн.) мед., юр. rénder (smb.) immúne, ímmunize (smb.).

иммунитéт м. мед., юр. immúnity; пóльзоваться ~ом enjóy immúnity; имéть ~ к óспе be* immúne agáinst/to smállpox.

императ|ор м. émperor. ~орский impérial. ~ри́ца ж. émpress.

империал|и́зм м. impérialism. ~и́ст м. impérialist. ~исти́ческий, ~и́стский imperialístic, impérialist.

импéр|ия ж. émpire. ~ский impérial.

импозáнт|ый ímposing; у негó ~ая фигýра he is a pérson of impósing appéarance.

импони́ровать несов. (дт.) impréss (smb.), inspíre smb.'s respéct.

и́мпорт м. ímport. ~ёр м. impórter. ~и́ровать несов. и сов. (вн.) impórt (smth.). ~ный impórted; import attr.

импотéнция ж. мед. ímpotence.

импрессион|и́зм м. impréssionism. ~и́ст м. impréssionist. ~и́стский impressionístic.

импровиз|áтор м. improvisátor, ímproviser. ~áция ж. improvisátion. ~и́рованный ímprovised, extémpore. ~и́ровать несов. и сов. (вн.) ímprovise (smth.).

и́мпульс м. 1. ímpulse, ímpetus; 2. физ. pulse; ◇ нéрвный ~ nérvous impulse; электри́ческий ~ eléctric pulse/impulse. ~и́вный impúlsive. ~ный pulsed; ~ный реáктор pulsed reáctor; ~ная фотолáмпа phótoflash lamp.

иму́щественный próperty attr.; ~ ценз próperty qualificátion.

иму́щество с. próperty.

иму́щ|ий propértied; ◇ власть ~ие those in pówer, the pówers that be.

и́м|я с. 1. name; (в отличие от фами́лии тж.) first name; gíven name амер.; по ~ени Ивáн named Iván; извéстный под ~енем Ивáнова known as Ivanóv; 2. (извéстность, популя́рность) name, reputátion; учёный с мировы́м ~енем world-fámous scíentist; 3. грам.: ~ существи́тельное noun; ~ прилагáтельное ádjective; ~ числи́тельное númeral; ~ завóд ~ени Ки́рова the Kírov works/plant; (адресóванный) на ~ addréssed to; остáвить что-л. на чьё-л. ~ leave* smth. for; перевести́, положи́ть дéньги на ~ когó-л. crédit móney to smb.'s accóunt; во ~ чегó-л. in the name of smth.; во ~ ми́ра во всём ми́ре in the name of world peace; от ~ени когó-л. on behálf of smb.; называ́ть вéщи свои́ми ~енáми call things by their próper names; call a spade a spade идиом.

инáче 1. нареч. dífferently, in a dífferent way, ótherwise; дýмать, поступáть ~ think*, act ótherwise; ~ обстои́т дéло с... quite dífferent is the case of...; 2. в знач. союза разг. ótherwise, or else; ◇ так и́ли ~ in ány case, ányhow; так и́ли ~, приходи́те! you come, ányhow!

инвали́д м. ínvalid, disábled man; ~ войны́ disábled sóldier; ~ трудá disábled wórker. ~ность ж. disáblement; disabílity; пéнсия по ~ности disabílity pénsion. ~ный ínvalid's; ~ный дом home for invalids.

инвентариз|áция ж. táking stock; про(из)води́ть ~áцию чегó-л. draw* up an ínventory of smth.;

(проверя́ть) take* stock of smth. ~овáть несов. и сов. (вн.) draw* up an ínventory (of); (проверя́ть) take* stock (of).

инвентáрн|ый: ~ая кни́га ínventory; ~ нóмер ínventory númber.

инвентáрь м. 1. (предмéты) ínventory, stock; 2. (о́пись) ínventory; ◇ живóй ~ lívestock; мёртвый ~ ímplements pl.

инвéрсия ж. лингв. invérsion.

инвести́ровать несов. и сов. (вн.) эк. invést (smth.).

ингаля|тор м. inháler. ~ция ж. мед. inhalátion.

индéец м. Américan Índian.

индéйка ж. túrkey(-hen).

индéйский (Américan) Índian; ◇ ~ петýх túrkey (-cock).

и́ндекс м. índex (pl -es; эк., мат. índices); ~ цен price índex.

индиáнка I ж. Índian wóman*.

индиáнка II ж. (Américan) Índian wóman*.

индивидуал|изи́ровать несов. и сов. (вн.) individualize (smb., smth.). ~и́зм м. indivídualism. ~и́ст м. indivídualist.

индивидуáльн|ость ж. 1. individuálity; 2. (человéк) pérson, indivídual. ~ый indivídual; ~ые осóбенности indivídual peculiárities; ~ое хозя́йство indivídual/private farm/hólding; ~ое жили́щное строи́тельство indivídual/ prívate búilding; ~ый подхóд indivídual appróach.

индиви́дуум м. indivídual.

инди́го с. нескл. índigo.

инди́ец м. Índian.

инди́йский Índian.

индикáтор м. тех., хим. índicator, márker. ~ный тех. índicator attr.; índicated; ~ная бумáга índicator/test páper.

индифферéнтн|ость ж. indífference. ~ый indífferent.

индоевропéйск|ий Índo-Européan; ~ие языки́ Índo-Européan lánguages.

индонез|и́ец м., ~и́йка ж. Indonésian. ~и́йский Indonésian; ~и́йский язы́к Indonésian, the Indonésian lánguage.

индукти́вный indúctive.

индукцио́н|ный indúction attr.; ~ная катýшка indúction coil.

инду́кция ж. indúction.

инду́с м., ~ка ж., ~ский Hindú.

индустриализ|áция ж. industrializátion. ~и́ровать несов. и сов. (вн.) indústrialize (smth.).

индустриáльный indústrial.

инду́стрия ж. índustry.

индю́|к м. túrkey(-cock). ~шка ж. túrkey(-hen). ~шóнок м. túrkey-poult.

и́ней м. hóarfrost, rime.

инéртн|ость ж. inértia, inértness, sláckness, slúggishness. ~ый 1. физ. inért; 2. (бездéятельный) slúggish, slóthful.

инéрци|я ж. 1. физ. inértia; (движущегося тела) moméntum; момéнт ~ moment of inértia; по ~и by one's own moméntum; перен. mechánically; 2. (бездéятельность) slúggishness, inértia.

инженéр м. enginéer; ~-механик mechánical enginéer; ~-строи́тель cívil enginéer; ~-электрик electrical enginéer. ~ный enginéering; ~ные войскá enginéer troops, enginéers; sáppers разг.; ~ная психолóгия indústrial psychology.

инжи́р м. 1. (плод) fig; 2. (дерево) fig(-tree).

инициáлы мн. inítials.

инициати́в|а ж. initiative; по ~е когó-л. on the initiative of smb.; прояви́ть ~y show* initiative; взять ~y в свои́ ру́ки take* the initiative; творческая ~ creative initiative. ~ный resóurceful; ~ный человéк pérson with initiative.

инициа́тор *м.* ínitiator; быть ~ом *чего-л.* take* the lead in *smth.*

инквизи́|тор *м.* inquísitor. ~торский inquisitórial. ~ция *ж.* inquisítion.

инко́гнито *с. нескл. и нареч.* incógnito.

инкримини́ровать *несов. и сов. (вн. дт.)* accúse (*smb.* of), charge (*smb.* with).

инкруст|а́ция *ж.* ínlay, ínláid work. ~и́ровать *несов. и сов. (вн.)* ínláy* (*smth.*).

инкуба́|тор *м.* íncubator. ~торный íncubator *attr.*

инкубацио́нный incubátion *attr.*; ~ пери́од (*болезни*) incubátion (périod), látency.

инкуба́ция *ж.* incubátion.

иногда́ sómetimes.

иногоро́дн|ий 1. (*живущий в другом городе*) líving in anóther town *после сущ.*; 2. (*о корреспонденции*): ~ее письмо́ non-lócal létter.

иноземе́|ец *м.*, ~ка *ж. уст.* fóreigner. ~ный *уст.* fóreign.

ин|о́й *прил.* 1. (*другой, не такой*) óther, anóther; ~ы́ми слова́ми in óther words; 2. (*некоторый*) some (*с сущ. во мн. ч.*); 3. *в знач. сущ. м.* some (péople) *pl*; ~о́му э́то мо́жет не понра́виться some péople may not like it; ◇ совсе́м ~о́е де́ло quite anóther thing, quite different; не кто ~, как none óther than; не что ~ое, как nóthing but; ~ раз sómetimes.

инопланет́ный of anóther plánet *после сущ.*

инопланет́янин *м.* pérson from anóther plánet.

иноро́дн|ый heterogéneous; ◇ ~ое те́ло fóreign body.

иносказа́|ние *с.* állegory. ~тельный allegórical.

иностра́н|ец *м.*, ~ка *ж.* fóreigner. ~ный fóreign.

иноходе́ц *м.* pácer, ámbler.

и́ноходь *ж.* ámble; идти́ ~ю ámble.

иноязы́чн|ый 1. (*о населении*) spéaking anóther lánguage *после сущ.*; 2. (*о выражении, обороте*) belónging to anóther lánguage *после сущ.*; ~ое заи́мствование fóreign bórrowing.

инсину|а́ция *ж.* insinuátion. ~и́ровать *несов. и сов.* insínuate.

инспекти́ровать *несов. (вн.)* inspéct (*smb., smth.*).

инспе́к|тор *м.* inspéctor. ~торский inspéctor's. ~цио́нный inspéction *attr.*; ~цио́нная пое́здка tour of inspéction; ~цио́нные о́рганы inspéction bódies. ~ция *ж.* 1. inspéction; 2. (*учреждение*) inspéction board.

инспири́ровать *несов. и сов. (вн.)* inspíre (*smth.*).

инста́нц|ия *ж.* ínstance; depártment; *воен.* échelon; вы́сшая ~ hígher authórity; переда́ть де́ло в вы́сшую ~ию *юр.* refér the mátter to hígher authórity; по ~иям through all the stáges.

инсти́нкт *м.* ínstinct. ~и́вный instínctive.

институ́т *м.* 1. (*учреждение, учебное заведение*) ínstitute; 2. *юр.* institútion.

инструкт|а́ж *м. разг.* 1. (*действие*) instrúction, instrúcting; 2. (*руководящие указания*) instrúctions *pl.* ~и́вный instrúctional.

инструкти́ровать *несов. и сов. (сов. тж.* проинструкти́ровать) *(вн.)* instrúct (*smb.*), give* (*smb.*) instrúctions.

инстру́к|тор *м.* instrúctor. ~торский instrúctor's. ~ция *ж.* instrúctions *pl*, diréctions *pl.*

инструме́нт *м.* ínstrument; *собир.* ínstruments *pl*, tóol-kit; хирурги́ческие ~ы súrgical ínstruments; ~ музыка́льный músical ínstrument. ~а́льный 1. *тех.* tool *attr.*, ínstrument *attr.*; 2. *муз.* instruméntal. ~а́льщик *м.* tóolmaker. ~а́рий *м. тех.* set of tools, ínstrument set.

инструментова́ть *несов. и сов. (вн.) муз.* ínstrument (*smth.*); (*для оркестра*) órchestrate (*smth.*).

инструменто́вка *ж. муз.* instrumentátion; (*для оркестра*) orchestrátion.

инсули́н *м. мед.* ínsulin.

инсу́льт *м. мед.* cérebral thrombósis; stroke *разг.*

инсцени́ровать *несов. и сов. (вн.)* 1. (*переделывать в пьесу*) drámatize (*smth.*), prodúce (*smth.*) for the stage; ~ рома́н drámatize a nóvel; 2. (*притворно изображать что-л.*) feign (*smth.*); ~ боле́знь feign íllness; ~ суде́бный проце́сс rig a tríal.

инсцениро́вка *ж.* 1. (*переделка в пьесу*) dramatizátion; 2. (*симуляция*) preténce, act; ~ суде́бного проце́сса fráme-up; 3. (*инсценированное произведение*) stage vérsion.

интегра́л *м. мат.* íntegral.

интегра́льн|ый *мат.* íntegral; ~ое исчисле́ние íntegral cálculus.

интегри́ровать *несов. и сов. (вн.) мат.* íntegrate (*smth.*).

интелле́кт *м.* íntellect. ~уа́л *м.* intelléctual. ~уа́льный intelléctual.

интеллиге́нт *м.* an intelléctual, cúltivated pérson. ~ность *ж.* cúltural lével. ~ный intelléctual; (*культурный тж.*) cúltured, cúltivated.

интеллиге́нция *ж.* the intelligéntsia; intelléctuals *pl.*

интенда́нт *м.* quártermaster. ~ский quártermaster's; sérvice corps *attr.* ~ство *с.* sérvice corps*.

интенси́вн|ость *ж.* inténsity; ~ зву́ка inténsity of sound; ~ све́та inténsity of light; ~ труда́ inténsiveness of lábour, lábour inténsity. ~ый inténsive.

интерва́л *м.* ínterval, space; с ~ом в пять мину́т at five-mínute íntervals.

интерве́н|т *м.* intervéntionist. ~ция *ж.* intervéntion.

интерви́дение *с.* Intervísion.

интервью́ *с. нескл.* ínterview; дать *кому-л.* ~ grant *smb.* an ínterview. ~и́ровать *несов. и сов. (сов. тж.* проинтервью́и́ровать) *(вн.)* ínterview (*smth.*).

интере́с *м.* ínterest; ~ к иску́сству ínterest in art; в ~ах де́ла for the good of the cause; в *чьих-л.* ~ах in *smb.'s* ínterests; э́то в ва́ших ~ах it is to/in your ínterest; представля́ть большо́й ~ be* of the útmost ínterest, be* of great ínterest.

интере́сн|о 1. *нареч.* in an ínteresting mánner; ~ расска́зывает be* a good tálker; ~ расска́зывать о *чём-либо* give* an ínteresting descríption of *smth.*; 2. *в знач. сказ. безл.* it is ínteresting; э́то не ~ there's no point in it. ~ый 1. ínteresting; как ~о! how ínteresting!; 2. *разг.* (*красивый*) attráctive, good-lóoking; ~ая же́нщина attráctive wóman*.

интере́с|ова́ть *несов. (вн.)* ínterest (*smth.*); э́то меня́ ~ует it ínterests me, I am ínterested in it, I take an ínterest in it; э́то меня́ не ~ует! I'm afráid that dóesn't ínterest me!; не э́то меня́ ~ует that's not what ínterests me; меня́ не ~ует их мне́ние! I don't care what they think abóut it! ~ова́ться *несов. (тв.)* be* ínterested (in), take* an ínterest (in); жи́во ~ова́ться *чем-л.* take* a lívely ínterest in *smth.*

интерме́дия *ж. театр.* ínterlude.

интерна́т *м.* 1. (*школа*) bóarding-school; 2. (*общежитие при школе*) (schóol-)hóstel.

Интернациона́л *м.* 1. Internatiónal; 2. (*пролетарский гимн*) the Internatiónale.

интернационал|изи́ровать *несов. и сов. (вн.)* internatiónalize (*smth.*). ~изм *м.* internátionalism. ~и́ст *м.* internátionalist. ~и́стский internátionalist *attr.*

интернациона́льный 1. internátional; 2. (*соответствующий принципам интернационализма*) internátionalist *attr.*; ~ долг internátionalist dúty.

интерни́ров|ание *с.* intérnment. ~ать *несов. и сов. (вн.)* intérn (*smb., smth.*).

интерпрет|а́ция *ж.* interpretátion. ~и́ровать *несов. и сов. (вн.)* ínterpret (*smth.*).

интерье́р *м.* intérior.

инти́мн|ость *ж.* íntimacy. ~ый íntimate; ~ый разгово́р íntimate conversátion; ~ая те́ма íntimate súbject; ~ая обстано́вка íntimate surróundings *pl.*

интоксика́ция *ж. мед.* intoxicátion.

интона́ция ж. 1. (в речи) intonátion; (модуляция) infléction; 2. муз. intonátion.

интри́г|а ж. 1. intrígue; plot; вести́ ~у про́тив кого́--либо plot/intrígue against smb.; 2. (в пьесе, книге) plot.

интрига́н м., ~ка ж. schémer, intríguer. ~ство с. plótting, schéming, intrígue.

интригова́ть, заинтригова́ть 1. тк. несов. (про́тив рд.) plot (against), scheme (against), intrígue (against); 2. (вн.; возбуждать любопытство) rouse the curiósity (of).

интроду́кция ж. муз. introdúction.

инту|ити́вный intuítive. ~иция ж. intuítion; по ~иции by intuition, intuítively.

интури́ст м. fóreign tóurist, tóurist/vísitor from abróad.

инфанти́льный infantíle.

инфа́ркт м. мед. infárction; heart attáck разг.

инфекцио́нн|ый мед. inféctious; (передающийся через прикосновение) contágious; ~ое заболева́ние inféctious disease.

инфе́кция ж. мед. inféction.

инфинити́в м. грам. infinitive.

инфици́рование с. infécting.

инфля́ция ж. эк. inflátion.

информа́тор м. infórmant.

информацио́нн|ый informátion attr.; ~ое сообще́ние búlletin.

информа́ция ж. informátion; (сообщение) repórt.

информи́рованн|ый well-infórmed; ~ые круги́ well--infórmed círcles.

информи́ровать несов. и сов. (сов. тж. проинформи́ровать) (вн.) infórm (smb.), keep* (smb.) infórmed.

инфракра́сн|ый infraréd; ~ые лучи́ infraréd rays.

инфузо́рия ж. зоол. infusórian (pl -ria).

инциде́нт м. íncident.

инъе́кци|я ж. мед. injéction; сде́лать ~ю give* an injéction.

ио́н м. физ. íon. ~иза́ция ж. физ. ionizátion. ~ный физ. iónic; íon attr.

ионосфе́ра ж. íonosphere.

ипоте́|ка ж. эк. mórtgage. ~чный эк. mórtgage attr.

ипохо́ндрия ж. hypochóndria.

ипподро́м м. rácecourse.

ипри́т м. mústard gas, ýperite.

ира́кский Iráqi, Iráquian.

ира́н|ец м., ~ка ж. Iránian. ~ский Iránian.

и́рис м. бот. íris.

ирла́нд|ец м. Írishman*. ~ка ж. Írishwoman*. ~ский Írish.

иро́н|изи́ровать несов. (над тв.) speak* irónically (of), be* sarcástic (abóut). ~и́ческий irónical; quízzical.

иро́ния ж. írony; ◇ ~ судьбы́ the írony of fate.

иррациона́льн|ый irrátional; ~ое число́ мат. irrátional númber.

иррегуля́рный irrégular.

ирригацио́нный irrigátion attr.

иррига́ция ж. irrigátion.

иск м. claim, áction; suit; предъявля́ть ~ кому́-л. sue smb., lodge a claim agáinst smb.; bring* an áction agáinst smb.; ◇ встре́чный ~ cóunter-claim, cóuntercharge, cróss-action.

искаж|а́ть, искази́ть (вн.) 1. (сильно изменять) distórt (smth.); боле́знь искази́ла то́нкие черты́ его́ лица́ his fine féatures had been déeply changed by illness; 2. (извращать) distórt (smth.), gárble (smth.), twist (smth.); ~ фа́кты twist facts. ~а́ться, искази́ться becóme* distórted; (о лице тж.) twist. ~е́ние с. 1. (действие) distórtion; misrepresentátion; 2. (неправильность, ошибка) distórtion. ~ённый 1. (о лице, наружности) distórted; 2. (неправильный, извращённый) gárbled, misrepreseńted.

искази́ть(ся) сов. см. искажа́ть(ся).

искале́ченный maimed, críppled; перен. rúined.

искале́чить сов. (вн.) maim (smb., smth.), crípple (smb.); перен. ruin (smb.).

иска́ния мн. search (áfter) sg, quest (for) sg.

иска́тель м., ~ница ж. séeker (áfter); ~ жёмчуга péarl-diver; ◇ ~ приключе́ний advénturer.

иска́ть несов. 1. (вн.) look (for), search (for); 2. (рд.; добиваться чего-л., стремиться) seek* (smth.); ~ сове́та seek* advíce; ~ по́вода seek* an excúse/prétext.

исключ|а́ть, исключи́ть 1. (вн. из рд.) exclúde (smb., smth. from); (удалять из состава) expél (smb. from); ~ кого́-л. из спи́сков strike* smb.'s name off the lists; исключи́ть кого́-л. из шко́лы expél smb. from school; 2. тк. несов. (вн.; устранять, не допускать) elíminate (smth.); rule out (smth.); ~ возмо́жность чего́--либо rule out the possibility of smth. ~а́ться несов.: взаи́мно ~а́ться be* mútually exclúsive. ~а́я except, with the excéption of, bárring; не ~а́я not excépting. ~е́ние с. 1. (удаление) expúlsion, exclúsion; 2. (отступление) excéption; ~е́ние из пра́вила excéption to the rule; нет пра́вила без ~е́ния there is álways an excéption to the rule; в ви́де ~е́ния as an excéption; все без ~е́ния éveryone without excéption; ◇ за ~е́нием кого́-л., чего́--либо except smb., smth., with the excéption of smb., smth.

исключи́тельн|о 1. (лишь, только) exclúsively; nóthing but; 2. (особенно) excéptionally; он ~ тала́нтлив he's excéptionally gífted. ~ость ж. 1. (особенность) excéptional náture, exceptionálity; 2. (обособленность) exclúsiveness. ~ый 1. (особенный, необыкновенный) excéptional; ~ый слу́чай excéptional case; 2. (единственный) sole, exclúsive; ~ое пра́во the sole/exclúsive right.

исключ|и́ть сов. 1. см. исключа́ть 1; 2.: не ~ена́ возмо́жность it's quite póssible; э́та возмо́жность ~ена́ ány such contíngency may be dismíssed (as impóssible); э́то ~ено́ it's out of the quéstion.

исковерканн|ый 1. (изломанный) misshápen, twísted; 2. (нравственно изуродованный) corrúpted; rúined; ~ая жизнь rúined life; 3. (неправильный) distórted; на ~ом англи́йском языке́ in bróken Énglish.

искове́ркать сов. см. кове́ркать.

исколеси́ть сов. (вн.) разг. trável all óver (smth.).

исколот|и́ть сов. (вн.) разг. 1. beat* (smb.) up, rain blows (on); его́ ~и́ли he was béaten up; 2. (вколачивая, испортить) chip and dent (smth.) all óver; вся дверь была́ исколо́чена the door was chipped and dénted all óver.

исколо́ть сов. (вн.) 1. (изранить) prick and scratch (smb., smth.) all óver; 2. stud (smth.); ка́рта была́ исколо́та флажка́ми the map was dótted/stúdded with flags.

иско́м|ое с. мат. an unknówn (quántity). ~ый 1. sóught-for; 2. мат. sought после сущ., to be found после сущ.

искони́ уст. from time immemórial.

иско́нный long-stánding, tíme-honoured.

ископа́ем|ый прил. 1. (добываемый) míneral; ~ое сырьё míneral raw matérials; 2. в знач. сущ. мн.: поле́зные ~ые (económic) mínerals; 3. (о животном, растении) fóssil; 4. в знач. сущ. с. (о человеке) fóssil, old fóssil; 5. шутл. (допотопный) fóssilized.

ископа́ть сов. (вн.) dig* up (smth.).

искорёженный twísted; (о дереве) warped.

искорене́ние с. eradicátion, extirpátion.

искорени́ть сов. см. искореня́ть.

искореня́ть, искорени́ть (вн.) root out (smth.), erádicate (smth.), éxtirpate (smth.); ~ зло root out an évil; ~ предрассу́дки erádicate préjudices.

и́скоса sídeways, askánce; ~ посмотре́ть на кого́-л. look askánce at smb.

и́скр|а ж. spark; ~ надéжды gleam/glímmer of hope; ◇ у меня́ ~ы из глаз посы́пались I saw stars.

и́скренн|е sincérely, cándidly. ~ий sincére. ~ость ж. sincérity.

искриви́ть(ся) сов. см. искривля́ть(ся).

искривлéние с. twist, cúrvature; distórtion (тж. перен.); ~ позвонóчника cúrvature of the spine; ~ политúческой лúнии distórtion of the political line.

искривля́ть, искриви́ть (вн.) (дéлать кривы́м) twist (smth.), bend* (smth.); (о чертáх лицá) distórt (smth.). ~ся, искриви́ться becóme* twísted, twist; becóme* distórted; егó лицó искриви́лось от бóли his face twísted with pain.

и́скристый spárkling.

и́скри́ться несов. spárkle.

искрогаси́тель м. тех. spárk-arrester.

искромса́ть сов. см. кромса́ть.

искроши́ть сов. (вн.) crúmble (smth.), púlverize (smth.); перен. разг. slash (smb., smth.) to píeces. ~ся сов. crúmble, fall* to píeces.

искря́щийся spárkling.

искупа́ть I, искупи́ть (вн.) 1. redéem (smth.), éxpiate (smth.); atóne (for); ~ свою́ вину́ atóne for one's guilt; 2. (возмещáть) make* up (for), make* aménds (for), cómpensate (for).

искупа́ть II сов. (вн.) разг. (вы́купать) give* (smb.) a bath.

искупа́ться I, искупи́ться 1. be* redéemed (by), be* atóned (by); 2. (возмещáться) be* made up for (by), be* cómpensated (by).

искупа́ться.II сов. разг. have* a bath.

искупи́тельн|ый éxpiatory; ~ая жéртва péace-offering.

искупи́ть сов. см. искупа́ть I. ~ся сов. см. искупа́ться I.

искуплéние с. redémption, expiátion, atónement.

искуса́|ть сов. (вн.) bite* (smb.) (bádly); комары́ меня́ ~ли I've been bítten all óver by mosquítoes.

искус|и́тель м. témpter. ~и́ть сов. см. искуша́ть.

искýсн|ик м., ~ица ж. разг. past máster, éxpert.

искýсный skílful; ~ стрелóк skilled márksman*.

искýсственн|ость ж. artificiálity. ~ый 1. artificial; тех. тж. synthétic; ~ое орошéние artificial irrigátion; ~ое питáние artificial féeding; ~ые цветы́ artificial flówers; ~ое волокнó synthétic/mán-made fibre; 2. (притвóрный) afféted, artificial; ~ая улы́бка afféted smile; ◇ ~ый спýтник Землú artificial Earth sátellite, spútnik.

искýсств|о с. 1. art; произведéние ~a a work of art; драматúческое ~ dramátics; 2. (умéние, мастерствó) skill, art; владéть ~ом шáхматной игры́ be* proficient at chess.

искусствовéд м. árt-critic. ~ение с. árt-criticism. ~ческий art attr.

искуш|áть, искуси́ть (вн.) tempt (smb., smth.); ◇ ~ судьбý tempt fate. ~éние с. temptátion.

искушённый expérienced; ◇ ~ óпытом well-tríed.

ислáм м. Íslam.

исланд|ец м., ~ка ж. Ícelander. ~ский Íceland attr.; Icelándic; ~ский язы́к Icelándic, the Icelándic language.

испáн|ец м. Spániard. ~ка ж. Spánish wóman*; онá ~ка she's Spánish. ~ский Spánish; ~ский язы́к Spánish, the Spánish lánguage.

испарéни|е с. 1. (дéйствие) evaporátion; 2. обыкн. мн. (испаря́ющееся веществó) fume, vápour; врéдные ~я hármful/nótious fumes.

испáрина ж. perspirátion.

испари́ть(ся) сов. см. испаря́ть(ся).

испаря́ть, испари́ть (вн.) eváporate (smth.). ~ся, испари́ться eváporate.

испáчкать сов. (вн.) make* (smb., smth.) dírty. ~ся сов. make* onesélf dírty.

испепели́ть сов. см. испепеля́ть.

испепел|я́ть, испепели́ть (вн.) redúce (smb., smth.) to áshes; lay* (smth.) waste. ~я́ющий: ~я́ющий взгляд wíthering glance.

испéчь сов. см. печь II 1. ~ся сов. см. пéчься I 1.

испещри́ть сов. см. испещря́ть.

испещр|я́ть, испещри́ть (вн. тв.) spot (smth. with), dot (smth. with), cóver (smth. with).

исписáть(ся) сов. см. испи́сывать(ся).

испи́сывать, исписáть (вн.) 1. fill up (smth.), cóver (smth.) with wríting; он исписáл три тетрáди he fílled up three nótebooks; 2. разг. (израсхóдовать) use up (smth.); онá исписáла послéдний карандáш she has used up her last péncil. ~ся, исписáться 1. (расхóдоваться) be* used up; карандáш исписáлся the péncil is worn to a stump; 2. (о писáтеле) exháust one's pówers/inspirátion, write* onesélf out.

испитóй разг. hággard, emáciated.

испи́ть сов. (вн.) drain (smth.); ~ гóрькую чáшу страдáний drain the cup of woe.

исповéдовать несов. и сов. (вн.) 1. тк. несов. (слéдовать учéнию) proféss (smth.); 2. церк. hear* smb.'s conféssion; перен. (расспрáшивать) quéstion (smb.) clósely. ~ся несов. и сов. церк. conféss; перен. unbósom onesélf.

и́споведь ж. conféssion.

и́сподволь разг. líttle by líttle, grádually, at one's léisure; ~ готóвиться к чему́-л. prepáre well in advánce for smth.

исподлóбья: смотрéть ~ на когó-л., чтó-л. scowl at smb., smth., lour at smb., smth.

исподтишкá разг. stéalthily, surreptítiously.

испокóн: ~ векóв, ~ вéку from time immemórial, since time begán.

исполúн м. gíant. ~ский huge, gigántic; человéк ~ского рóста huge man*.

исполкóм м. (исполнúтельный комитéт) exécutive committee.

исполнéни|е с. 1. (выполнéние) execútion, fulfílment, perfórmance; ~ приказáния execútion of an órder; ~ дóлга fulfílment of dúty; ~ желáния, обещáния fulfílment of a wish, prómise; при ~и служéбных обя́занностей in the perfórmance of one's dúties, in line of dúty; не при ~и служéбных обя́занностей when off dúty; 2. (передáча худóжественного произведéния) perfórmance, réndering; тéхника ~я execútion; ~ ромáнса réndering of a song; вúдеть пьéсу в хорóшем (плохóм) ~и see* a good* (bad*) perfórmance of a play; в ~и когó-л. perfórmed by smb.

исполненн|ый (рд.) full (of); ~ желáния filled with the desíre; глазá, ~ые печáли sórrowful eyes, sórrowing eyes.

исполнúм|ый féasible; вáше желáние вполнé ~о your wish can éasily be grátified; это вполнé ~о! that's pérfectly féasible!

исполнúтель м. 1. dóer, exécutor; ~ послéдней вóли exécutor; 2. (артúст) perfórmer; ◇ судéбный ~ báiliff, officer of the law. ~ница ж. 1. exécutrix (pl -ixes, -ices); 2. (артúстка) perfórmer.

исполнúтельн|ый 1. exécutive; ~ая власть the exécutive (pówer); ~ комитéт exécutive committee; 2. (о человéке) efficient, consciéntious; ◇ ~ лист court órder, writ, wárrant.

исполнúтельск|ий: ~ое мастерствó téchnical skill/brílliance; mástery.

исполни́ть сов. см. исполня́ть. ~ся сов. см. исполня́ться 1, 3, 4.

исполн|я́ть, испóлнить (вн.) 1. (осуществля́ть) execute (smth.), fulfíl (smth.); (обя́занность) dischárge (smth.), atténd (to), perfórm (smth.); ~ чьё-л. желáние fulfíl/meet* smb.'s wish; ~ долг dischárge one's dúty; ~ приказáние cárry out an órder, éxecute an órder; 2.

(*пьесу, музыкальное произведение*) perfórm (*smth.*); (*о пении тж.*) sing* (*smth.*); ~ роль take* the part; *перен.* play the role. ~*яться*, исполниться 1. (*осуществляться*) be* fulfilled; 2. *тк. несов.* (*о пьесе, музыкальном произведении*) be* perfórmed; ~*яется впервые* perfórmed for the first time; 3. (*о времени, сроке*) be*; исполнилось 30 лет со дня окончáния войны thírty years have passed since the end of war; 4. *безл.* (*о возрасте*): емý тóлько что исполнилось 18 лет he is just eightéen; зáвтра емý исполняется 18 лет he will be eightéen tomórrow.

исполня́ющий: ~ обязанности директора ácting diréctor.

использование *с.* utilizátion, emplóyment; ~ всех возможных средств the emplóyment of all póssible means.

использовать *несов. и сов.* (*вн.*) use (*smth.*), útilize (*smth.*), make* use (of), emplóy (*smth.*); ~ слýчай, возмóжность take* the opportúnity; ~ своё влияние use one's ínfluence; ~ отхóды произвóдства útilize waste материáls; ~ резéрвы make* use of (*one's*) resérves; ~ своё преимýщество explóit one's advántage; ~ специалистов make* use of éxperts; ~ все средства emplóy all means; пóлностью ~ что-л. make* full use of smth.

испóртить(ся) *сов. см.* пóртить(ся).

испóрченный 1. spoilt; (*о зубе*) decáyed; (*о продуктах*) táinted; ~ замóк bróken lock; 2. (*распущенный*) depráved; ~ ребёнок spoilt child*.

исправим|ый remédiable, réctifiable; (*о человеке*) córrigible; это ~о that can be set right.

исправительно-трудовóй corréctive-lábour.

исправительн|ый corréctive; ~ая колóния refórmatory, appróved school; ~ые меры corréctive méasures.

испра́вить(ся) *сов. см.* исправля́ть(ся).

исправлéни|е *с.* 1. (*действие*) corréction, corrécting; (*починка*) repáir; 2. (*поправка*) corréction; вносить ~я make* corréctions.

исправля́ть, исправить (*вн.*) 1. (*чинить*) repáir (*smth.*); ~ радиоприёмник repáir a rádio; 2. (*устранять недостатки*) corréct (*smth.*), put* (*smth.*) right; ~ ошибку corréct a mistáke; исправленное и дополненное revísed and enlárged edition; 3. (*улучшать*) refórm (*smth.*); испрáвить харáктер refórm one's cháracter. ~ся, исправиться impróve, refórm, mend one's ways; он совсéм исправился he is quite a refórmed cháracter.

испра́вн|ость *ж.*: в ~ости in wórking órder; (*в хорошем состоянии*) in good condition. ~ый 1. (*в порядке*) in wórking órder *после сущ.*, in good repáir *после сущ.*; эта машина ~а this machíne is in good wórking órder; 2. (*старательный*) consciéntious.

испражнéни|е *мн.* éxcrements. ~*ться*, испражниться evácuate the bówels, défecate.

испрóбовать *сов.* (*вн.*) 1. (*проверить качество, годность*) test (*smth.*); 2. *разг.* (*на вкус*) taste (*smth.*); 3. (*испытать*) try (*smth.*).

испýг *м.* fright; в ~e in a fright; с ~y in one's fright.

испýганн|о in fright; (*робко*) tímidly. ~ый frightened, scared, térrified.

испугáть(ся) *сов. см.* пугáть(ся).

испускáть, испустить (*вн.*) give* off (*smth.*); ~ зáпах give* off an ódour; испустить крик útter a cry; ◇ испустить дух expíre.

испустить *сов. см.* испускáть.

испытáни|е *с.* 1. test, tríal; производить ~ чего-л. test *smth.*; ~ я́дерного орýжия núclear wéapon test; проводить ~я condúct tests; выдержать ~ врéменем stand* the test of time; (*экзамен*) examinátion; 3. (*тягостное переживание*) ordéal, tríal.

испы́танн|ый tried; ~ое срéдство well-tríed rémedy; ~ друг tried friend; ~ в боях tried in báttle, báttle-tésted.

испытáтельный test *attr.*, tríal *attr.*; ~ полигóн próving ground; ~ срок périod of probátion; ~ рейс tríal run.

испыт|áть *сов. см.* испытывать 1, 2. ~ýющий séarching, scrútinizing; ~ýющий взгляд séarching look.

испы́тывать, испытáть (*вн.*) 1. (*проверять*) try (*smth.*), test (*smb., smth.*); ~ мотóр test an éngine; ~ чьё-л. терпéние try *smb.'s* pátience; 2. (*узнавать на собственном опыте*) feel* (*smth.*), expérience (*smth.*), undergó* (*smth.*); ~ испытáть что-л. на себé have* pérsonal expérience of *smth.*; ~ лишéния expérience/know* hárdship; 3. *тк. несов.* expérience; ~ недостáток в чём-л. be* short of *smth.*

исслéдова|ние *с.* 1. (*действие*) reséarch (into); investigátion (of); (*страны*) explorátion (of); *хим.* análysis (of); ~ больнóго médical examinátion; ~ния в óбласти использования я́дерной энéргии reséarch into the úses of núclear énergy; ~ космического прострáнства space explorátion; 2. (*научный труд*) work (on), stúdy (of). ~тель *м.* reséarcher; scientist, éxpert; (*страны*) explórer. ~тельский reséarch *attr.*

исслéдовать *несов. и сов.* (*вн.*) invéstigate (*smth.*); (*изучать*) stúdy (*smth.*); (*территорию*) explóre (*smth.*); *хим.* anályse (*smth.*); ~ больнóго exámine a pátient.

исстари since ólden days; так ~ ведётся it's an áncient cústom.

исстрадáться *сов.* súffer bítterly, be* worn out with súffering.

исступл|éние *с.* frénzy; в ~éнии in a frénzy; приходить в ~ fly* into a rage. ~ённый frénzied, frántic, frenétic.

иссуш|áть, иссушить (*вн.*) dry up (*smth.*); (*о растении*) wíther (*smth.*); *перен.* consúme (*smb.*); гóре иссушило её she is wásted with grief. ~ить *сов. см.* иссушáть.

иссякáть, иссякнуть 1. (*об источнике, воде*) dry up; 2. (*кончаться*) run* out; (*о терпении и т. п.*) give* out, be* exháusted; егó сúлы иссякли his strength gave out.

иссякнуть *сов. см.* иссякáть.

истáптывать, истоптáть (*вн.*) 1. (*мять*) trámple (*smth.*); 2. *разг.* (*пачкать*): истоптáть пол leave* fóotmarks on the floor; 3. *разг.* (*об обуви*) wear* out (*smth.*).

истекáть, истéчь 1. (*кончаться, проходить*) expíre, elápse; врéмя истеклó time is up; 2.: ~ крóвью be* bléeding to death; *перен.* pour out one's life-blood.

истéкш|ий past; за ~ год (*о сроке*) for the past year; (*о периоде*) dúring/in the past year; цифры за ~ год the fígures for the past year, last year's fígures; за ~ год мнóго сдéлано much has been done dúring the past year; 20-го числá ~его мéсяца on the 20th últ(imo).

истéрзанный (*израненный*) lácerated, gashed; (*о чувствах, нервах*) lácerated; (*измученный*) worn out, torménted; (*изуродованный*) torn, twísted; (*растрёпанный*) bedrággled.

истерзáть *сов.* 1. (*изранить*) tear* (*smb.*) to píeces; 2. (*измучить*) wear* (*smb.*) out, tormént (*smb.*).

истéр|ик *м.* hystériac. ~ика *ж.* fit of hystéria; быть в ~ике be* in hystérics; ◇ впадáть в ~ику, закáтывать ~ику go* into hystérics, make* a hystérical scene. ~ический hystérical. ~ичка *ж.* hystérical wóman*; онá ~ичка she gets hystérical. ~ичный hystérical.

истерия *ж.* hystéria.

истéц *м. юр.* pláintiff.

истечéни|е *с.* 1. flow; 2. (*окончание*) terminátion, expirátion; по ~и двух часóв áfter two hours, two hours láter; по ~и извéстного врéмени áfter a cértain lapse of time.

истéчь *сов. см.* истекáть.

йстин|а *ж.* truth; в э́том есть до́ля ~ы there is a grain of truth in that; ◇ святáя ~ góspel truth.

йстинн|о trúly, véritably. ~ый true; ~ая прáвда the truth; ~ый друг true friend; ~ое сóлнечное врéмя *астр.* appárent sólar time; э́тот ребёнок — ~ое наказáние! the child's a véritable inflíction!

истлевáть, истлéть 1. (*гнить*) rot; 2. (*сгорать*) be* redúced to áshes; у́гли истлéли the coals had burned to áshes.

истлéть *сов. см.* истлевáть.

истóк *м.* 1. source; 2. *обыкн. мн.* (*начало чего-л.*) source, root.

истолков|áние *с.* interpretátion. ~áть *сов. см.* истолкóвывать.

истолкóвывать, истолковáть (*вн.*) intérpret (*smth.*); непрáвильно истолковáть *что-л.* misintérpret *smth.*, misréad* *smth.*, put* a wrong constrúction on *smth.*

истолóчь *сов.* (*вн.*) pound (*smth.*), grind* (*smth.*).

истóма *ж.* lánguor, lássitude.

истомúть *сов.* (*вн.*) wéary (*smb.*), exháust (*smb.*). ~ся *сов.* be* wéaried.

истопúть *сов.* (*вн.*) (*печь*) heat (*smth.*).

истопнúк *м.* stóker; bóiler-man*.

истоптáть *сов. см.* истáптывать.

истóрик *м.* histórian.

историóграф *м.* historiógrapher.

историогрáфия *ж.* historiógraphy.

истори́ческ|ий 1. histórical; ~ая наýка the science of history; ~ факт histórical fact; ~ая эпóха histórical périod/époch; ~ ромáн histórical nóvel; ~ подхóд к изучáемым явлéниям histórical appróach to *one's* súbject; ~ая геогрáфия histórical geógraphy; 2. (*значительный*) históric, époch-making; ~ая речь históric speech; ~ое решéние époch-making decísion.

истóри|я *ж.* 1. history; закóны ~и laws of history; ~ срéдних векóв history of the Míddle Áges, mediéval history; ~ искýсства history of art; ~ э́того дéла таковá the truth about this affáir is as fóllows; 2. (*повествование*) stóry; 3. *разг.* (*происшествие*) event, thing; épisode; попáсть в неприя́тную ~ю run* into tróuble; ◇ ~ болéзни case history; вéчная ~! álways the same old stóry!; вот так ~! what a núisance!

истосковáться *сов.* grow* sick with lónging; (*по дт.*) miss (*smb., smth.*); ~ по рóдине, по семьé yearn for home, be* hómesick.

источáть *несов.* (*вн.*) shed* (*smth.*), yield (*smth.*).

истóчник *м.* 1. (*родник*) spring; горя́чий ~ hot spring; нефтянóй ~ óil-well; 2. (*то, что даёт начало чему-л.*) órigin, source; ~ сырья́ sóurces of raw matérials; ~ повышéния дохóдов means of increásing íncome, source of increásed íncome; 3. (*письменный памятник*) source, sóurce-book.

истóшн|ый *разг.* blóod-curdling; закричáть ~ым гóлосом give* a blóod-curdling shriek.

истощ|áть, истощи́ть (*вн.*) exháust (*smb., smth.*); ~ пóчву impóverish the soil; ~ запáсы exháust stocks; ~ си́лы drain/sap énergy. ~áться, истощи́ться 1. (*ослабевать*) wéaken, dwíndle; (*о почве*) be* impóverished/exháusted; 2. (*приходить к концу*) be* exháusted, get* low, run* out; (*о залежах, ископаемых*) run* thin; моё терпéние истощи́лось my pátience is exháusted, my pátience is at an end. ~éние *с.* 1. (*изнурение*) exháustion; (*о почве тж.*) impóverishment; нéрвное ~éние nérvous exháustion; 2. (*уменьшение*) deplétion; ~éние месторождéния желéзной руды́ deplétion of íron depósits.

истощ|ённый 1. exháusted; 2. (*ослабевший*) emáciated. ~и́ть(ся) *сов. см.* истощáть(ся).

истрати́ть(ся) *сов. см.* трáтить(ся).

истреби́тель *м.* 1. destróyer; 2. (*самолёт*) fighter (áircraft). ~ный 1. destrúctive; ~ная войнá war of

exterminátion/annihilátion; 2. *ав.* fighter *attr.*; ~ная авиáция fighter áircraft; fighter fórce.

истреби́ть *сов. см.* истреблять.

истребл|éние *с.* destrúction, exterminátion; ~ лесóв whólesale destrúction of fórests. ~я́ть, истреби́ть (*вн.*) destróy (*smb., smth.*), extérminate (*smb., smth.*).

истрёпанный *разг.* dilápidated, táttered; véry much the worse for wear *после сущ., идиом.*; *перен.* worn, jáded.

истрепáть *сов.* (*вн.*) *разг.* (*об одежде и т. п.*) wear* (*smth.*) to rags; (*о книгах и т. п.*) spoil* (*smth.*), wear* (*smth.*) out; ◇ ~ нéрвы fray *one's* nerves. ~ся *сов. разг.* 1. get* worn out; 2. (*измучиться*) wear* onesélf out, wear* onesélf to a shádow.

истукáн *м.* idol; ◇ стоя́ть ~ом 1) (*неподвижно*) stand* stock-still; 2) (*ничего не понимая*) stand* like a dúmmy.

йстый true.

истяз|áние *с.* tórture. ~áтель *м.* tórturer. ~áть *несов.* (*вн.*) tórture (*smb.*).

исхóд *м.* 1. (*способ разрешить затруднение*) way out, solútion; э́то для меня́ еди́нственный ~! it's my ónly way out!; 2. (*завершение*) end, close; (*результат*) óutcome, íssue, culminátion; смертéльный ~ fátal óutcome; ◇ день на ~е the day is dráwing to its close; на ~е дня towárds évening; съестны́е запáсы бы́ли на ~е food supplíes were rúnning out.

исходи́ть I *сов.* (*вн.; обойти*) go* all óver (*smth.*).

исходи́ть II *несов.* 1. (*от, из рд.; происходить*) come* (from); (*о слухе*) originate (with, from); 2. (*из рд.; основываться*) procéed (from); ~ из предположéния... procéed from the supposítion..., start with the assúmption...

исходи́ть III, изойти́: ~ слезáми be* in floods of tears; sob *one's* heart out; изойти́ крóвью bleed* to death.

исхóдн|ый stárting; ~ момéнт, ~ пункт stárting-point; ~ые дáнные inítial dáta; ~ое положéние 1) point of depárture; (*в гимнастике*) stárting position; ~ рубéж stárting line, stárting-point.

исхуд|áлый wásted, emáciated, hággard. ~áть *сов.* becóme* emáciated.

исцарáпанный lácerated, bádly scratched.

исцарáпать *сов.* (*вн.*) scratch (*smb., smth.*); ~ рýки scratch *one's* hands bádly. ~ся *сов. разг.* scratch onesélf, get* scratched all óver.

исцел|éние *с.* 1. cure; héaling; 2. (*выздоровление*) recóvery. ~и́тель *м.* héaler. ~и́ть(ся) *сов. см.* исцеля́ть(ся).

исцеля́ть, исцели́ть (*вн.*) cure (*smb.*), heal (*smb.*). ~ся, исцели́ться (*от рд.*) be* cured (of), be* healed (of), recóver (from).

исчáдие *с.:* ~ áда dévil incárnate.

исчáхнуть *сов.* waste awáy.

исчез|áть, исчéзнуть disappéar, vánish; боль исчéзла the pain disappéared; кудá вы исчéзли? where did you disappéar to? ~новéние *с.* disappéarance.

исчéзнуть *сов. см.* исчезáть.

исчéрпать *сов. см.* исчéрпывать.

исчéрп|ывать, исчéрпать (*вн.*) 1. exháust (*smth.*), drain (*smth.*); 2. (*доводить до конца*) compléte (*smth.*); вопрóс исчéрпан the mátter is séttled; ◇ ~ себя́ reach the límit of *one's* resóurces. ~аться *несов.:* э́тим дéло не ~áется the mátter will not rest here; э́тим не ~áется значéние егó трудá his work has impórtance beyónd this. ~ающий exháustive; ~ающий отвéт exháustive/comprehénsive ánswer; ~ающее объяснéние exháustive explanátion.

исчерти́ть *сов. см.* исчéрчивать.

исчéрчивать, исчерти́ть (*вн.*) cóver (*smth.*) (with lines).

исчисле́ние с. 1. (*вычисление*) calculátion, computátion; 2. *мат.* cálculus.

исчисля́ть *сов. см.* исчисля́ть.

исчисля́ть, исчи́слить (*вн.*) éstimate (*smth.*), cálculate (*smth.*); compúte (*smth.*); ~ расхо́ды éstimate/cálculate expénses.

исчисл|я́ться *несов.* (в *пр.*) come* (to), amóunt (to); сто́имость ~я́ется в 500 рубле́й the cost is cálculated/éstimated at five húndred róubles.

ита́к so, thus; ~, вопро́с решён so the quéstion is séttled.

италья́н|ец *м.*, ~ка *ж.* Itálian. ~ский Itálian; ~ский язы́к Itálian, the Itálian lánguage; ◇ ~ская забасто́вка sit-down strike.

и т. д. (и так да́лее) and so on; etc.

ито́г *м.* 1. (*сумма*) tótal; о́бщий ~ grand tótal; подвести́ ~ sum up; 2. (*результат*) resúlt; ~и разви́тия наро́дного хозя́йства the géneral resúlt of the devélopment of the nátional ecónomy; ◇ в ~е as a resúlt; в коне́чном ~е in the long run, in the end.

ито́го in all; súm-total *бухг.*

итого́в|ый 1. tótal; ~ая су́мма tótal amóunt; 2. (*заключающий*) final; ~ые заня́тия final léssons/stúdies.

и т. п. (и тому́ подо́бное) and the like, and so on (and so forth).

их 1. (*рд., вн. от личн. мест.* они́) them; 2. *в знач. притяж. мест.* (*при сущ.*) their; (*без сущ.*) theirs.

ихтиоза́вр *м.* ichthyosáurus.

ихтиоло́гия *ж.* ichthýology.

иша́к *м.* dónkey, ass, *тж. перен.*

и́шиас *м. мед.* sciática.

ишь *разг.:* ~ ты! fáncy that!; ~ ты како́й! what a one you are!

ище́йка *ж.* blóodhound, trácker dog.

ию́л|ь *м.* Julý; в ~е э́того го́да this/in Julý; в ~е про́шлого го́да last Julý, last year in Julý; в ~е бу́дущего го́да next Julý.

ию́льский Julý *attr.*; ~ день day in Julý, Julý day.

ию́н|ь June; в ~е э́того го́да this/in June; в ~е про́шлого го́да last June, last year in June; в ~е бу́дущего го́да next June.

ию́ньский June *attr.*; ~ день day in June, June day.

Й

йог *м.* yógi.

йо́га *ж.* yóga.

йогу́рт *м.* yóghurt.

йод *м.* íodine. ~истый íodic. ~ный: ~ная насто́йка tíncture of íodine.

йодофо́рм *м. фарм.* íodoform.

йот *м. лингв.* létter J.

йо́т|а *ж.* íota, jot; ◇ де́ло ни на ~у не сдви́нулось things háven't budged (an inch); положе́ние ни на ~у не измени́лось the situátion hásn't changed a bit; он ни на ~у не усту́пит he will not yield one íota/an inch.

К

к 1. (*указывает на направление движения*) to; (*при подчёркивании направления*) towards; спуска́ться к реке́ go* to the ríver; плыть к бе́регу swim* to the shore; е́хать к сестре́ go* to see one's síster; поверну́ться к окну́ turn towárds the wíndow; наклони́ться к ребёнку bend* down to the child*; на пути́ к on the way to; обраще́ние к молодёжи an appéal to young péople; ходи́ть от до́ма к до́му go* from house to house; 2. (*для обозначения лица, предмета, с которым соприкасается кто-л., что-л. или к которому присоединяется что-л.*) to; прислони́вшись к стене́ léaning against the wall; парохо́д приста́л к бе́регу the ship came in to the shore; припа́сть к земле́ stoop to the ground; лицо́м к лицу́ face to face; к двум приба́вить три add two and three togéther; ко всем про́чим неудо́бствам in addítion to óther inconvéniences; 3. (*при указании на срок совершения или завершения действия*) by; towárds; к утру́ бред прошёл the delírium passed off by the mórning; к ве́черу жара́ спа́ла towárds évening the heat subsíded; вам ну́жно прийти́ к трём часа́м you must be here by three o'clóck; он яви́лся к отхо́ду по́езда he arríved in time for the train's depárture; 4. (*для обозначения побуждения, мотива, при указании на назначение действия или предмета*) for; гото́виться к се́ву, к экза́менам prepáre for the sówing, the examinátions; приучи́ть кого́-л. к поря́дку teach* smb. régular hábits; пода́рок ко дню рожде́ния présent for smb.'s bírthday; предисло́вие к кни́ге introdúction/préface to a book; 5. (*при обозначении предмета, лица, с которыми связано какое-л. действие, признак, отношение*) for, towárds; любо́вь к ро́дине love for one's cóuntry; гото́вность к бою réadiness for báttle/áction; приго́дный к употребле́нию fit for use; 6. (*в заглавиях*) towárds; *часто не переводится*; «К кри́тике Го́тской програ́ммы» A Contribútion to the Critique of the Gótha Prógramme; 7. (*в призывах*) to; вперёд, к побе́де! fórward, to the víctory!; 8. *с некоторыми сущ.:* к сча́стью fórtunately; к несча́стью unfórtunately; к сло́ву (сказа́ть) by the way; ◇ к чему́ э́то? what use is that?; э́то ни к чему́ that's no use/good; к тому́ же moreóver, besídes, furthermóre; всё к лу́чшему it's all for the best.

-ка 1. (*при повел.*) come on; *часто не переводится*; доста́нь-ка кни́гу с по́лки! come on, fetch the book; ну́-ка, покажи́! let's see it!; спо́й-ка! do sing!, give us a song!; 2. (*при будущем времени*): напишу́-ка я ему́ what if I write to him.

каба́к *м. уст.* públic house, pub, távern; *перен. разг.* béargarden, pígsty.

кабал|а́ *ж.* bóndage, sérvitude; быть в ~е́ у кого́-л. be* in bóndage to smb.; пойти́ в ~у́ к кому́-л. sell* onesélf into bóndage to smb.

каба́льн|ый ensláving, féttering; ~ая зави́симость forced depéndence (on), bóndage; ~ые усло́вия ensláving/crippling terms.

каба́н *м.* 1. (*дикий*) wild boar; 2. (*самец домашней свиньи*) boar.

кабарди́н|ец *м.*, ~ка *ж.* Kabárdian. ~ский Kabárdian; ~ский язы́к Kabárdian, the Kabárdian lánguage.

кабаре́ с. *нескл.* cábaret.

кабачо́к I *м.* (*овощ*) végetable márrow.

кабачо́к II *м.* small réstaurant.

ка́бель *м.* cáble.

ка́бельтов *м. мор.* 1. (*мера*) cáble('s) length; 2. (*трос*) cáble.

каби́на *ж.* booth, box, cúbicle; (*на самолёте*) cábin; (*открытая*) cóckpit; ~ води́теля dríver's cab; купа́льная ~ báthing-hut, dréssing cúbicle; душева́я ~ shówer cúbicle; ~ ли́фта lift car.

кабине́т *м.* 1. (*в учреждении*) (prívate) óffice; (*дома*) stúdy; ~ дире́ктора the diréctor's óffice; 2. (*специальный*) room; ~ врача́ dóctor's consúlting room; зубоврче́бный ~ déntal súrgery; физи́ческий ~ phýsics labóratory; 3. (*правительство*) cábinet; ~ мини́стров the Cábinet; **4.** *разг.* *(мебель)* (óffice, stúdy) suite. ~ный: ~ный рояль báby-gránd; ~ный стратéг ármchair strátegist; ~ный учёный mere theoretícian; ◇ ~ный портрéт cábinet phótograph.

каблогрáмма *ж.* cáblegram, cáble.

каблýк *м.* heel; тýфли на высóких ~áx high-heeled shoes; ◇ быть под ~óм у кого-л. be* únder smb.'s thumb.

каботáж *м.* *мор.* cóasting-trade, cábotage. ~ный cóasting; ~ное сýдно cóasting véssel, cóaster; ~ное плáвание cóasting navigátion.

кáбы *разг.* **1.** *(если)* if; **2.** *(если бы только)* if ónly; ◇ éсли бы да ~ if ifs and ans were pots and páns.

кавалéр I *м.* **1.** *(в танцах)* pártner; **2.** *разг.* *(поклонник)* admírer.

кавалéр II *м.* *(награждённый орденом)* hólder, knight.

кавалер|и́йский cávalry *attr.* ~и́ст *м.* cávalryman*.

кавалéрия *ж.* cávalry.

кавардáк *м.* *разг.* mess, múddle.

кавéрз|а *ж.* intrígue; *(злая шалость)* mean trick; устрóить ~у кому-л. play a mean trick on *smb.* ~ный trícky; ~ный вопрóс trícky quéstion; ~ный человéк schémer.

кавéрна *ж.* cávity.

кавкáз|ец *м.*, ~ский Caucásian.

кавы́чк|и *мн.* *(ед.* кавы́чка *ж.)* quotátion marks, invérted cómmas; откры́ть (закры́ть) ~ ópen (close) the quotátion marks; ◇ учёный в ~ах so-cálled scíentist; pséudoscientist.

кадéнция *ж.* *муз.* **1.** *(гармонический оборот)* cádence; **2.** *(сольная вставка в концерте с оркестром)* cadénza.

кадéт I *м.* *ист.* *(воспитанник кадетского корпуса)* cadét.

кадéт II *м.* *ист.* *(член конституционно-демократической партии)* Constitútional Démocrat.

кадéтский: ~ кóрпус *ист.* mílitary school/cóllege.

кади́ло *с.* *церк.* cénser, thúrible.

кади́ть *несов.* cense, burn* íncense; *(дт.)* *перен.* *разг.* flátter *(smb.).*

кáдка *ж.* tub.

кáдмий *м.* cádmium.

кадр *м.* *кино* **1.** frame; за кáдром off screen; **2.** *(отдельная сцена)* séquence; *(фотография кадра)* still.

кáдровый 1. trained; ~ рабóчий trained wórker; **2.** *воен.* régular; ~ офицéр régular ófficer.

кáдр|ы *мн.* **1.** (trained) personnél; подбирáть ~ seléct personnél; воспи́тывать ~ train personnél; молоды́е (стáрые) ~ young (old) personnél; **2.** *воен.* régulars, cádres; cádre *sg*; ◇ отдéл ~ов personnél depártment; начáльник отдéла ~ов personnél/staff mánager.

кады́к *м.* Ádam's ápple.

каёмка *ж.* édging, bórder.

каждоднéвный dáily, éveryday.

кáжд|ый *мест.* **1.** each, évery; ~ из each of; ~ день, с ~ым днём évery day; **2.** *в знач. сущ. м.* éveryone, éverybody; ~ дóлжен знать éveryone must know.

кáжется 1. *см.* казáться; **2.** *в знач. ввод. сл.* it seems; ~, хóлодно it seems to be cold; он, ~, прав he seems to be right.

кáжущийся appárent.

казáк *м.* Cóssack.

казáлось 1. *см.* казáться; **2.** *в знач. вводн. сл.* it seemed; ~ бы it would seem.

казáрм|а *ж.* bárrack; *мн. воен.* bárracks. ~енный bárrack *attr.*

казáть *несов.* *разг.:* он к нам не кáжет глаз he néver comes near us.

казáться, показáться 1. seem, appéar; *(выглядеть)* look; ~ стáрше свои́х лет look ólder than *one* is, be* old for *one's* age; он мне показáлся óчень стáрым he

---

seemed véry old to me; **2.** *безл.* *(дт.)*: мне кáжется, что... it seems to me (that)...; **3.** *обыкн.* *безл.* *(чудиться, мерещиться)* seem; мне всё казáлось, что кто́-то стучи́т в ворóта I kept imágining sómeone was knócking at the gate; вам показáлось! it's your imaginátion!

казáх *м.* Kazákh. ~ский Kazákh; ~ский язы́к Kazákh, the Kazákh lánguage.

казáцкий Cóssack *attr.*

казáч|ество *с.* the Cóssacks *pl.* ~ий Cóssack *attr.*

казáшка *ж.* Kazákh wóman*.

казён|ный 1. *(государственный)* góvernment *attr.*; за ~ счёт at góvernment expénse; ~ные дéньги públic funds; **2.** *(бюрократический, формальный)* bureaucrátic; ~ язы́к official járgon; officialése; ~ ~ная часть *(оружия)* breech. ~щина *ж.* *разг.* réd-tápe.

казначéй *м.* tréasurer. ~ский tréasury *attr.*; ~ский билéт tréasury note. ~ство *с.* tréasury.

казни́ть *несов. и сов.* *(вн.)* éxecute *(smb.)*; *перен.* tórture *(smb.)*, tormént *(smb.).* ~ся *несов.* tormént onesélf.

казнокрáд *м.* embézzler of públic funds.

казн|ь *ж.* execútion; смéртная ~ cápital púnishment; приговори́ть кого-л. к смéртной ~и séntence *smb.* to death.

кáзус *м.* *разг.* íncident; неприя́тный ~ áwkward íncident.

каймá *ж.* edge, bórder.

как 1. *нареч.* how; ~ э́то случи́лось? how did it háppen?; я забы́л, ~ э́то дéлается I have forgótten how to do it; ~ давнó э́то бы́ло? how long agó was it?; ~ я рад! how glad I am!; **2.** *частица* *(для выражения удивления, негодования)* what!; **3.** *союз* *(сравнительный)* as; бéлый ~ sneг white as snow; **4.** *союз* *(в качестве)* as; совéтую вам э́то ~ друг I advíse you as a friend; **5.** *союз* *(всякий раз, когда)* when, évery time; *(с того времени, когда)* since; **6.** *союз* *(кроме, только)* but, excépt; комý ~ не тебé who else but you; **7.** *союз* *(присоединяет дополнительные придаточные предложения)* не переводится; он не замéтил, ~ вы вошли́ he did not nótice you come in; ◇ ~ бýдто 1) *(как если бы)* as if, as though; 2) *(кажется)* it looks as if; ~ бы as if, as though; ~ бы то ни́ было at all evénts, at ány rate; ~ вдруг when all of a súdden; ~ же of course; когдá ~ it depénds; пиши́ ~ мóжно чáще write as óften as póssible; ~ нельзя́ лýчше extrémely well; ~ ни though, no mátter how.

какáо *с. нескл.* **1.** *(растение)* cacáo; **2.** *(порошок, напиток)* cócoa.

кáк-либо sómehow (or óther).

кáк-нибудь 1. *(так или иначе)* sómehow (or óther); **2.** *разг.* *(кое-как)* ányhow; **3.** *разг.* *(когда-нибудь в будущем)* some day/time; ~ вечеркóм one évening; ~ в другóй раз some óther time.

какóв *мест.* **1.** *вопр.* what?; ~ он собóй? what's he like to look at?; **2.** *относ.* *(присоединяет придаточные определительные)* as; *(присоединяет придаточные дополнительные)* what (kind of); мы вы́яснили, ~ы нáши ресýрсы we éstimated what resóurces we had; ~..., такóв... like... like; ◇ он-то ~! he's a fine one!; ~ поп, такóв и прихóд ≈ like máster, like man.

каковó: ~! well!; ~ емý тепéрь! what must his féelings be now!; ~ нам э́то слýшать! to think we should have to lísten to this!

как|óй 1. *(в вопросах; что за)* what sort of *(какого рода)*; what *(о названии, назначении)*; ~ýю мýзыку вы лю́бите? what sort of músic do you like?; ~óe э́то здáние? what is that búilding?; ~áя сегóдня погóда? what's the wéather like todáy?; ~ сегóдня день? what's todáy?; ~óe сегóдня числó? what's the date?; **2.** *(который из многих)* what; *(из двух)* which; **3.** *(в восклицании)* what (a); *(при прил. и при отвлечённом* *сущ.*) how; ~ человéк! what a man!; ~áя (чýдная) погóда! what (lóvely) wéather!; ~ он дóбрый! how kind he is!; ~áя рáдость! how lóvely; ~ ýжас! how áwful!; ~áя прéлесть! how sweet!; (*о живом существе*) what a dárling/pet!; 4. (*в риторическом вопросе*): ~ же он учёный? call him a scíentist?; ~ э́то парк? is that what you call a park?; ~ я инженéр? what kind of an enginéer would I make!; ◇ ~ ни на есть just ány; ~ угóдно ány... you like; ~ бы то ни бы́ло ány... whatsoéver; ~ бы whatéver; ~у бы оши́бку он ни соверши́л whatéver mistáke he might commít, whatéver mistáke he has committed.

какóй-либо some; (*в отрицательных или условных предложениях*) ány.

как|óй-нибудь 1. (*тот или иной*) *см.* какóй-либо; **2.** *разг.* (*с числ.*) ónly abóut, not more than; остáлось ~их-нибудь два киломéтра there's ónly abóut two kílometres more to go.

как|óй-то 1. some... or óther; a/some sort of; ~ человéк вас спрáшивал sómebody has been ásking for you; он сегóдня ~ стрáнный he's in a queer mood todáy; он сегóдня ~ устáлый, несчáстный *и т. п.* he seems to be tíred, unháppy, *etc.* todáy; иногдá они́ выражáют ~ протéст sómetimes they make a sort of prótest; **2.** (*в вопрос. употреблении*) what kind/sort of?; лéто бы́ло дождли́вое, ~áя-то бýдет óсень? we had a wet súmmer, what sort of áutumn are we góing to have?

какофóния *ж.* cacóphony.

кáк-то (*каким-то образом, необъяснимо*) sómehow; емý ~ удалóсь вы́рваться he sómehow mánaged to escápe; здесь ~ неую́тно sómehow it's not véry cósy here; он ведёт себя́ ~ стрáнно there's sómething strange in his beháviour; **2.** (*однажды*) once; ~ вéчером one évening; ~ раз one day; я ~ был у негó I háppened to be at his place; **3.** *разг.* (*а именно*) námely; *часто не переводится*; **4.** (*риторический вопрос*) I wónder how...; how... I wónder!; ~ они́ живýт там без нас? how are they gétting on there all by themsélves, I wónder!

кáктус *м.* cáctus.

кал *м. тк. ед.* éxcrements *pl.*

каламбýр *м.* pun.

каланчá *ж.* (fíreman's) wátch-tower; *перен. разг.* (*о высоком человеке*) lámp-post.

калáч *м.* kalátch (*small white loaf shaped like a padlock*); ◇ тёртый ~ tough cústomer; меня́ тудá ~óм не замáнишь! I wóuldn't go there for ánything!, nóthing would make me go there! ~иком: сверну́ться ~иком curl up in a ball.

калейдоскóп *м.* kaléidoscope.

калéка *м. и ж.* crípple.

календáрный cálendar *attr.*

календáрь *м.* cálendar.

калéни|е *с.* (*окраска раскалённого металла*) incandéscence; бéлое ~ white heat, incandéscence; крáсное ~ red heat; ◇ довести́ когó-л. до бéлого ~я make* *smb.* frántic (with rage).

калён|ый 1. (*раскалённый*) réd-hót; **2.** (*поджаренный*) róasted; ~ые орéхи róasted nuts; ◇ вы́жечь что-л. ~ым желéзом ≈ root out *smth.* mércilessly, éxtirpate *smth.*

калéчить *несов.* (*вн.*) crípple (*smb.*), disáble (*smb.*), maim (*smb.*); *перен.* (*портить*) ruin (*smb., smth.*).

калибр *м.* **1.** (*оружия*) cálibre, bore; **2.** *тех.* gauge, stándard. ~овáть *несов.* (*вн.*) *тех.* cálibrate (*smth.*).

кáлий *м.* potássium; хлóристый ~ potássium chlóride.

калийн|ый potássium *attr.*, pótash *attr.*, potássic; ~ые удобрéния pótash fértilizers.

кали́на *ж.* (*куст*) guélder-rose, snówball-tree.

кали́тка *ж.* wícket(-gate), wícket-door.

кали́ф *м.* cáliph; ◇ ~ на час ≈ king for a day.

каллиграфи́ческий calligráphic; ~ пóчерк cópy-book hand.

каллигрáфия *ж.* calligraphy.

калмы́|к *м.* Kálmyk. ~цкий Kálmyk; ~цкий язы́к Kálmyk, the Kálmyk lánguage. ~чка *ж.* Kálmyk.

калори́йн|ость *ж.* calorífic válue. ~ый hígh-calorie *attr.*; ~ая пи́ща food rich in cálories; ~ое тóпливо hígh--calorie fuel.

калори́фер *м.* rádiator, héater.

калóрия *ж.* cálorie.

калóш|и *мн.* (*ед.* калóша *ж.*) *см.* галóши; ◇ сесть в ~у make* a fool of onesélf.

кáльк|а *ж.* **1.** (*чертёж*) trácing; **2.**: бумáжная ~ trácing-paper; полотня́ная ~ trácing-cloth; **3.** *лингв.* loan translátion, calque. ~и́ровать *несов. и сов.* (*вн.*) **1.** trace (*smth.*), make* a trácing (of); **2.** *лингв.* make* a loan translátion (of).

калькул|и́ровать *несов.* (*вн.*) cálculate (*smth.*), compúte (*smth.*). ~я́тор *м.* cálculator. ~я́ция *ж.* calculátion, éstimate.

кальсóны *мн.* drawers, pants.

кáльций *м. хим.* cálcium.

кáмбала *ж.* plaice, flát-fish.

кáмбуз *м.* gálley, cabóose.

камвóльный *текст.* wórsted.

камéдь *ж.* gum.

камелёк *м. уст.* **1.** (*камин*) small fire-place; **2.** (*небольшой очаг*) hearth.

камéлия *ж.* camélia.

каменéть *несов.* **1.** pétrify, turn to stone; **2.** (*становиться неподвижным*) be* pétrified, stíffen; **3.** (*становиться бесчувственным*) hárden, becóme* hard/cállous.

камени́стый stóny; (*с большими камнями*) rócky.

каменноýгольн|ый coal *attr.*; ~ая промы́шленность coal índustry, cóal-mining índustry; ~ бассéйн cóal-field, cóal-mining dístrict; ~ые кóпи cóal-mines.

кáменн|ый 1. (*из камня*) stone *attr.*; (*из кирпича*) brick *attr.*; ~ые пли́ты flágstones, páving stones; **2.** (*неподвижный*) set; **3.** (*бесчувственный*) hard, cállous, stóny; ~ое сéрдце heart of stone/flint; ◇ ~ ýголь coal.

каменолóмня *ж.* quárry.

каменотёс *м.* stóne-cutter.

кáменщик *м.* (stóne-)mason, brícklayer.

кáм|ень *м.* **1.** *тк. ед.* (*порода*) stone, rock; **2.** (*отдельный кусок*) stone; **3.** (*гнетущее чувство*) load; у меня́ на сéрдце ~ my heart is héavy; сéрдце не ~ one ísn't made of stone, one has a heart; **4.** *мн. мед.* gáll--stones; ~ни в пéчени stones in the líver; ◇ ~ня на ~не не остáвить raze it to the ground; (*раскритиковать*) tear* it to shreds.

кáмера *ж.* **1.** chámber; тюрéмная ~ cell; ~ хранéния багажá clóakroom; left-lúggage óffice; check room *амер.*; **2.** (*шины*) ínner tube; (*мяча*) bládder; **3.** *фото* cámera; скры́тая ~ hídden/concéaled cámera.

кáмерн|ый chámber *attr.*; ~ая мýзыка chámber músic.

камертóн *м.* túning fork.

камéя *ж.* cámeo.

ками́н *м.* fire-place; (*горящий*) fire; ◇ электри́ческий ~ eléctric fire.

камóрка *ж.* tíny room, clóset.

кампáния *ж.* campáign; (*общественная тж.*) drive.

камуфля́ж *м. воен.* cámouflage.

камф|арá *ж.* cámphor. ~áрный cámphor *attr.*; ~áрный спирт spirits of cámphor; ◇ ~áрное мáсло cámphorated oil.

камчáт(н)ый dámasked.

камы́ш *м.* rush, reed.

канáва *ж.* ditch, trench.

канавокопáтель *м.* dítcher.

канáд|ец *м.*, ~ка *ж.*, ~ский Canádian.

кана́л *м.* 1. canál; 2. *тех.* chánnel; 3. *анат.* canál, duct; 4. *мн.* (*пути, способы к достижению чего-л.*) chánnels; дипломати́ческие ~ы diplomátic chánnels.

канализ|ацио́нный séwage *attr.* ~а́ция *ж.* séwage sýstem; sanitátion *разг.*

канаре́йка *ж.* canáry.

кана́т *м.* горе; (*якорный*) cáble. ~ный горе *attr.*, cáble *attr.*; ◇ ~ная доро́га cábleway.

канатохо́дец *м.* rópe-walker.

канва́ *ж.* (*для вышивания*) cánvas; *перен.* gróundwork, sketch, óutline, skéleton.

кандалы́ *мн.* fétters, írons; ручны́е ~ hándcuffs, mánacles; закова́ть *кого-л.* в ~ fétter *smb.*, put* *smb.* in fétters/írons.

кандида́т *м.* 1. (*намеченный к избранию*) cándidate; ~ в депута́ты городско́го Сове́та cándidate for eléction to the town Sóviet; 2. (*учёная степень*) Cándidate (*roughly equivalent to Master*); ~ нау́к Cándidate of Science (*сокр.* Cand. Sc.). ~ский Cándidate's ◇ ~ский ми́нимум mínimum requírements for a Cándidate's degrée. ~ура *ж.* 1. cándidature; снять свою́ ~уру withdráw* *one's* cándidature; 2. (*кандидат*) cándidate; подходя́щая ~ура súitable cándidate.

кани́кул|ы *мн.* hólidays; vacátion *sg.* ~я́рный hóliday *attr.*, vacátion *attr.*

канители́ться *несов. разг.* fiddle abóut; dáwdle.

канитéль *ж.* 1. purl; золота́я ~ gold purl; 2. *перен. разг.* lóng-drawn-óut procéedings *pl*; разводи́ть, тяну́ть ~ dáwdle; spin out; procrastináte. ~ный *разг.* lóng-drawn-óut; tédious, tíresome; ~ное де́ло long/tédious búsiness.

канифо́ль *ж.* rósin.

кано́н *м.* cánon.

канона́да *ж.* cannonáde.

канони́ческий canónical.

кант *м.* 1. (*на одежде*) píping; 2. (*окантовка*) binding.

канта́та *ж.* cantáta.

кану́н *м.* eve; ~ Но́вого го́да New-Year's eve; в ~ *чего-л.* on the eve of *smth.*

ка́нуть *сов.* sink*; ◇ как в во́ду ~ ≈ vánish ínto thin air.

канцеля́р|ия *ж.* óffice; (*в посольстве и т. п.*) cháncellery. ~ский óffice *attr.*; ~ские принадле́жности státionery *sg*; ~ский слу́жащий clerk; ~ский слог bureaucrátic style; ~ский стиль руково́дства bureaucrátic style of léadership/mánagement. ~щина *ж.* red tape.

канцероге́н *м.* carcínogen. ~ный carcinogénic.

ка́нцлер *м.* cháncellor.

каоли́н *м. мин.* káolin, chína-clay.

ка́п|ать, ка́пнуть 1. (*падать каплями*) be* drípping (from); (*о слезах*) fall*; с крыш ~ает wáter is drípping from the roofs; 2. (*вн.; тв.; лить по капле*) pour (*smth.*) out drop by drop; ~ лека́рство в стака́н pour a few drops of médicine ínto a glass; 3. (*вн., тв.; проливать*) spill* (*smth.*), drip (*smth.*); не ~ай на ска́терть don't make spots on the táblecloth; 4. (*на вн.*) *разг.* (*доносить*) tell* tales (abóut); ◇ над на́ми не ~лет there's plénty of time; there's no húrry.

капéль *ж.* dripping of mélted snow/ice.

ка́пельк|а *ж.* 1. dróplet; 2. *разг.* (*маленькое количество*) grain, little bit; ◇ ни ~и not the least (bit).

капельме́йстер *м.* condúctor; (*духового оркестра*) bándmaster.

капилля́р *м.* capíllary. ~ный capíllary *attr.*

капита́л *м.* cápital; кру́пный ~ big búsiness.

капитал|и́зм *м.* cápitalism. ~и́ст *м.* cápitalist. ~исти́ческий cápitalist *attr.*, capitalístic; ~исти́ческое хозя́йство cápitalist ecónomy.

капиталовложе́ния *мн.* (*ед.* капиталовложе́ние *с.*) invéstments.

капита́льн|ый cápital; ~ труд fundaméntal work; ◇ ~ая стена́ main wall; ~ое строи́тельство cápital constrúction; ~ ремо́нт májor repáirs *pl.*; (*машины, механизма*) overhául; ~ые вложе́ния cápital invéstments.

капита́н *м.* cáptain; (*торгового судна*) máster; skípper *разг.* ~ский cáptain's.

капите́ль *ж.* 1. *архит.* cápital; 2. (*шрифт*) small cápitals *pl.*

капитул|и́ровать *несов. и сов.* capítulate, surrénder. ~я́нт *м.* deféatist, capítulator. ~я́ция *ж.* capitulátion, surrénder.

капка́н *м.* trap.

ка́пл|я *ж.* 1. drop; по ~е a drop at a time; 2. *тк., ед.* (*рд.*) *разг.* (*малое количество чего-л.*) grain (of); ни ~и благоразу́мия not a grain of sense; 3. *мн.* (*лекарство*) drops; ◇ ~ в мо́ре a drop in the ócean; ~, перепо́лнившая ча́шу the last drop which overflówed the cup; после́дняя ~ ≈ the last straw; би́ться до после́дней ~и кро́ви fight* to the last; ~ за ~ей drop by drop; ни ~и not in the least; как две ~и воды́ ≈ like two peas (in a pod).

ка́пнуть *сов. см.* ка́пать.

ка́пор *м.* bónnet.

капо́т *м.* 1. *уст.* (*одежда*) dréssing-gown; 2. *тех.* bónnet, hood.

капра́л *м.* córporal.

капри́з *м.* whim; capríce (*тж. перен.*). ~ничать *несов.* be* wáyward, be* frétful. ~ный caprícious, fíckle, frétful; *перен.* (*неустойчивый*) uncértain.

капро́н *м.* kápron. ~овый kápron *attr.*; ~овое волокно́ kápron fíbre.

ка́псула *ж.* cápsule.

ка́псюль *м.* cap; prímer.

капу́ста *ж.* cábbage; ки́слая ~ sáuerkraut; ◇ брюссе́льская ~ Brússels sprouts *pl*; морска́я ~ (édible) séaweed.

капу́стник *м.* (*самодеятельное представление*) (ámateur) cóncert párty.

капу́стница *ж.* (*бабочка*) cábbage bútterfly.

капу́стный cábbage *attr.*

капу́т *м. нескл. разг.* kapút; ему́ (пришёл) ~ he's done for.

капюшо́н *м.* hood.

ка́ра *ж.* púnishment, pénalty; (*возмездие*) retribútion.

караби́н *м.* cárbine.

кара́бкаться *несов.* (*на вн.*) clámber (up).

карава́й *м.* round loaf*.

карава́н *м.* 1. caraván; 2. *мор.* cónvoy.

кара́им *м.*, ~ка *ж.* Káraite. ~ский Káraite.

каракалпа́к *м.* Karakalpák. ~ский Karakalpák; ~ский язы́к Karakalpák, the Karakalpák lánguage.

каракалпа́чка *ж.* Karakalpák wóman*.

карака́тица *ж.* (*моллюск*) cúttlefish.

кара́кулевый astrakhán *attr.*

кара́куль *м.* astrakhán.

кара́кул|я *ж.* scrawl; scríbble.

караме́ль *ж.* 1. *собир.* (*конфеты*) cáramels *pl*; 2. (*жжёный сахар*) cáramel, burnt súgar.

каранда́ш *м.* péncil; ◇ в ~é in péncil. ~ный péncil *attr.*

каранти́н *м.* 1. quárantine; 2. (*санитарный пункт*) quárantine státion.

карапу́з *м. разг.* little tot, tóddler.

кара́сь *м.* crúcian.

кара́т *м.* cárat.

кара́тель *м.* mémber of a púnitive expedition. ~ный púnitive; ~ная экспеди́ция púnitive expedition.

кара́ть, покара́ть (*вн.*) púnish (*smb.*), chastíse (*smb.*).

карау́л *м.* 1. *воен.* guard; быть в ~е be* on guard dúty; нести́ ~ be* on guard (dúty); смени́ть ~ relíeve the guard; 2. *в знач. межд.* (*помогите!*) help!; ◇ почётный ~ guard of hónour; стоять в почётном ~e be* in the guard of hónour; (брать) на ~ presént arms; просто хоть ~ кричи! it's simply unbéarable! ~ить *несов.* (*вн.*) 1. (*охранять*) guard (*smb.*, *smth.*); 2. *разг.* (*подстерегать*) be* on the watch/lóokout (for).

карау́л|ный *прил.* 1. guard *attr.*; ~ное помещение guárdroom; ~ная служба guard dúty; 2. *в знач. сущ. м. воен.* séntry. ~щик *м. разг.* wátchman*.

карбюра́тор *м.* carburéttor.

карга́ *ж. разг.* hag.

кардина́л *м.* cárdinal.

кардина́льный cárdinal.

кардио|гра́мма *ж.* cárdiogram. ~хирурги́я *ж.* heart/cárdiac súrgery.

каре́л *м.*, ~ка *ж.* Karélian.

каре́льский Karélian.

каре́т|а *ж.* coach; ◇ ~ скорой помощи ámbulance. ~ка *ж. тех.* cárrier, cárriage.

ка́рий brown.

карикату́р|а *ж.* caricatúre; (*политическая тж.*) cartóon; *перен.* párody; нарисовать ~у на кого-л. make* a caricatúre of *smb.* ~и́ст *м.* caricatúrist; cartóonist. ~ный grotésque, lúdicrous.

ка́рканье *с.* 1. cáwing; 2. *разг.* (*зловещее предсказание*) cróaking.

карка́с *м.* fráme(work), shell; железобетонный ~ strúctural frame of reinfórced cóncrete. ~ный frame *attr.*; ~ная конструкция frame constrúction.

ка́ркать, **ка́ркнуть** 1. caw; 2. *тк. несов. разг.* (*предсказывать неприятности*) croak, cast gloom.

ка́ркнуть *сов. см.* ка́ркать 1.

ка́рлик *м.* dwarf; (*о незначительном человеке*) pígmy. ~овый dwárfish, dwárf-like; (*очень маленький*) dwarf *attr.*; ~овый рост dwárf-like/dimínutive státure; ~овая пальма dwarf palm.

карма́н *м.* pócket; ◇ не по ~у beyónd *one's* means, too dear for *one*; мне это не по ~у I can't afford it, it's beyónd my means, it's too dear for me; держи ~ (ши́ре)! no hope!; not a hope! ~ник *м. разг.* píckpocket. ~ный pócket *attr.*; ~ные часы (pócket-)watch *sg*; ~ный словарь pócket díctionary; ~ные деньги pócket móney.

карми́н *м.* cármine, crímson.

карми́нный cármine, crímson.

карнава́|л *м.* cárnival. ~льный cárnival.

карни́з *м. архит.* córnice.

карп *м.* carp.

ка́рт|а *ж.* 1. (*географическая*) map; (*морская*) chart; 2. (*игральная*) card; ◇ поставить всё на ~у stake éverything, stake *one's* all; раскрыть свои ~ы show* *one's* hand/cards.

карта́в|ить *несов.* burr. ~ость *ж.* burr. ~ый 1. (*о человеке*) búrring; with a burr in *one's* voice *после сущ.*; 2. (*о произношении*) burred.

картёжн|ик *м.*, ~ица *ж.* cárd-player.

карте́ль *м. эк.* cartél.

карте́чь *ж. воен.* cáse-shot; 2. (*дробь*) búck-shot.

карти́н|а *ж.* 1. (*художника*) páinting, pícture; ~ы Репина the páintings of Répin; 2. (*изображение, зрелище*) pícture, scene; ~ быта scene from life; 3. (*часть действия*) scene; 4. *разг.* (*кинофильм*) film, pícture. ~ка *ж.* (*иллюстрация в книге*) pícture; книга с ~ками pícture-book. ~ный 1. pícture *attr.*; 2. (*живописный*) picturésque.

карто́граф *м.* cartógrapher, máp-máker. ~и́ческий cartográphic(al).

картогра́фия *ж.* cartógraphy, máp-máking.

карто́н *м.* cárdboard; (*толстый*) míllboard. ~ажный cárdboard *attr.* ~ка *ж.* cárton, cárdboard box; (*фанерная*) plýwood box. ~ный cárdboard *attr.*; в ~ном переплёте with a stiff bínding, bound in boards.

картоте́к|а *ж.* card índex; библиотечная ~ cárd-catalogue; составлять ~у compíle a cárd-index; составление ~и cárd-indexing.

картофелесажа́лка *ж.* potáto plánter.

картофелеубо́рочный: ~ комбайн potáto hárvester.

картофели́на *ж. разг.* potáto, spud.

карто́фель *м.* potátoes *pl*; хрустящий ~ potáto crisps/chips *pl*. ~ный potáto *attr.*; ◇ ~ная мука potáto flour.

ка́рточка *ж.* 1. card; 2. (*фотографическая*) phóto(graph).

ка́рточный card *attr.*; ~ каталог cárd-catalogue.

карто́шк|а *ж. разг.* 1. *собир.* (*картофель*) potátoes *pl*; сажать ~у plant potátoes; 2. (*отдельная картофелина*) potáto.

карту́з *м.* cap.

карусе́ль *ж.* mérry-go-round, róundabout, whírligig.

ка́рцер *м.* púnishment cell.

карье́р I *м.* (*ход лошади*) chárging pace; ~ом at a chárging pace; ◇ с места в ~ straight awáy.

карье́р II *м.* (*каменоломня*) quárry; песчаный ~ sánd-pit.

карье́р|а *ж.* caréer; сделать ~у make* *one's* caréer; get* to the top *разг.* ~и́зм *м.* caréerism. ~и́ст *м.*, ~и́стка *ж.* caréerist, clímber, self-séeker.

каса́ни|е *с.* cóntact; ◇ точка ~я *мат.* point of cóntact.

каса́тельная *ж. мат.* tángent.

каса́тельств|о *с.* relátion, connéction; не иметь никакого ~a к чему-л. have* nóthing to do with *smth.*

кас|а́ться, **косну́ться** (*рд.*) 1. (*дотрагиваться*) touch (*smb.*, *smth.*); ~ дна touch bóttom; 2. (*упоминать*) touch (upón); ~ вопроса о чём-л. touch upón the próblem of *smth.*; 3. (*иметь отношение*) concérn (*smb.*); это вас не ~ается 1) (*не затрагивает*) it dóesn't refér to you; 2) (*не ваше дело*) it's no concérn of yours, it is not your búsiness; ◇ что ~ается as to/for; что ~ается меня as for me, for my part, as far as I am concérned.

ка́ска *ж.* hélmet.

каска́д *м.* cascáde; ◇ ~ гидроэлектростанций séries of hýdroeléctric státions.

ка́сс|а *ж.* 1. (*в учреждении*) cashíer's óffice; (*в магазине*) cásh-desk; (*железнодорожная*) bóoking-office; (*театральная*) bóx-office; tícket-office *амер.*; 2. (*кассовый аппарат*) cásh-register; 3. (*учреждение*): сберегательная ~ sávings-bank; 4. (*деньги*) cash; 5. *полигр.* case; ◇ ~ взаимопомощи mútual assístance fund.

кассацио́нн|ый *юр.*: ~ая жалоба appéal; ~ суд Court of Appéal/Cassátion.

кассаци|я *ж.* cassátion; подать ~ю *разг.* appéal.

кассе́та *ж. фото* (*для плёнки*) casséte, drum; (*для пластинок*) pláte-holder, dark slide.

касси́р *м.* cashíer; (*в банке тж.*) téller; (*продающий билеты*) bóoking-clerk; (*в театре*) bóx-office clerk.

ка́ссов|ый cash *attr.*; ~ая книга cásh-book.

ка́ста *ж.* caste.

кастеля́нша *ж.* línen místress.

ка́стовый caste *attr.*

ка́стор|ка *ж. разг.* cástor oil. ~овый: ~овое масло cástor oil.

кастр|а́ция *ж.* castrátion. ~и́ровать *несов. и сов.* (*вн.*) castráte (*smb.*, *smth.*); (*животное тж.*) geld (*smth.*).

кастрю́ля *ж.* sáucepan, pan.

катако́мбы *мн.* (*ед.* катакомба *ж.*) cátacombs.

ката́лиз *м. хим.* catálysis. ~а́тор *м. хим.* cátalyst.

катало́г *м.* cátalogue. ~изи́ровать *несов. и сов.* (*вн.*) cátalogue (*smth.*).

катамара́н *м.* catamarán.

ката́ние *с.* 1. rólling; 2.: ~ в экипаже dríving; ~

верхо́м ~ ríding; ~ на ло́дке bóating; (*под парусами*) sáiling; ~ на саня́х sléighing; ~ на конька́х skáting.

катапу́льт|а *ж.* cátapult; взлёт самолёта с ~ы cátapult start/láunching.

катапульти́ровать *несов. и сов.* (*вн.*) cátapult (*smb.*). ~ся *несов. и сов.* cátapult.

катапульти́рующ|ий: ~ее устро́йство cátapult (device).

ката́р *м. мед.* catárrh; ~ желу́дка gastrítis, gástric catárrh.

катара́кта *ж. мед.* cátaract.

катара́льный *мед.* catárrhal.

катастро́ф|а *ж.* disáster, catástrophe; железнодоро́жная ~ ráilway áccident. ~ный disástrous.

ката́ть *несов.* (*вн.*) 1. roll (*smth.*); ~ мяч roll a ball; ~ те́сто roll pástry/dough; ~ мета́лл roll métal; 2. (*возить*) drive* (*smb.*); take* (*smb.*) out; ~ кого́-л. на маши́не take* *smb.* for a drive. ~ся *несов.* 1. roll, roll abóut; 2. (*ездить*) drive*; (*верхом*) ride*, ~ся на велосипе́де go* for a cýcle ride; ~ся на конька́х skate; ~ся на маши́не go* for a car ride; ~ся на ло́дке go* out in a boat, go* bóating; ◇ ~ся со́ смеху rock with láughter.

катафа́лк *м.* cátafalque; (*погребальная колесница*) hearse.

категори́ческ|и categórically, flátly; ~ возража́ть stróngly objéct; ~ запреща́ть ábsolutely forbíd*. ~ий categórical, explícit, ~ий отве́т categórical/explícit ánswer; ~ий отка́з· categórical/flat refúsal; ~ое возраже́ние únqualified objéction.

катего́рия *ж.* cátegory, class.

ка́тер *м.* launch; (*парусно-гребной*) cútter; мото́рный ~ mótor boat; сторожево́й ~ patról boat.

ка́тет *м. мат.* leg/side of a triangle.

кати́ть *несов.* 1. (*вн.*) roll (*smth.*); (*на колёсах*) push (*smth.*); (*обруч*) bowl (*smth.*); 2. *разг.* (*ехать*) drive*. ~ся *несов.* 1. roll; (*скользить*) slide*; 2. (*ехать — об автомобиле и т. п.*) move*; 3. (*разноситься — о звуках*) roll, écho; гро́хот кати́лся по ущелью the roar échoed through the raví́ne; 4. (*течь, струиться*) roll; пот кати́лся у него́ со лба the sweat was rólling down his fórehead.

като́д *м. физ.* cáthode. ~ный *физ.* cáthode *attr.*; ~ные лучи́ cáthode rays.

като́к *м.* 1. (*ледяная площадка*) skáting-rink; 2. (*машина*) róller; (*для белья*) mángle.

като́л|ик *м.* cátholic, Róman Cátholic. ~ици́зм *м. см.* католи́чество. ~и́ческий Róman Cátholic. ~и́чество *с.* cathólicism.

ка́тор|га *ж.* pénal sérvitude, hard lábour; (*место*) pénal/cónvict cólony; отбыва́ть ~гу serve a pénal séntence, do* hard lábour. ~жа́нин *м.* (*обычно политический*) State cónvict; éx-convict. ~жник *м.* cónvict. ~жный: ~жные рабо́ты pénal sérvitude *sg*, hard lábour *sg*; ~жная жизнь *перен.* unbéarable life; ~жный труд *перен.* kílling work, drúdgery.

кату́шка *ж.* bóbbin, reel; *эл.* coil.

катю́ша *ж. воен. разг.* Katyúsha, múltiple rócket projéctor/láuncher.

ка́урый light-chéstnut.

ка́уст|ик *м.* cáustic sóda. ~и́ческий cáustic.

каучу́к *м.* rúbber. ~овый rúbber *attr.*

каучуконо́сы *мн.* (*ед.* каучуконо́с *м.*) rúbber--bearing plants.

кафе́ *с. нескл.* café.

ка́федр|а *ж.* 1. (*возвышение*) réading-desk, róstrum (*pl* -ra, -rums); говори́ть с ~ы speak* from the róstrum; 2. (*научная отрасль как предмет преподавания в вузе, объединение учёных одной специальности*) chair, depártment; ~ органи́ческой хи́мии chair of orgánic chémistry; получи́ть ~y get the chair; заве́довать ~ой

hold the chair; заве́дующий ~ой head of the chair; заседа́ние ~ы fáculty méeting. ~а́льный: ~а́льный собо́р cathédral.

ка́фель *м.* tile. ~ный tiled.

кафе́-моло́чная *с.* milk-bar.

кафете́рий *м.* cafetéria.

кафта́н *м.* cáftan.

кача́лка *ж.* rócking-chair.

кача́ние *с.* 1. swáying, swínging; 2. (*воды насосом*) púmping; 3. (*колебание маятника и т. п.*) swing.

кач|а́ть *несов.* 1. (*вн., тв.*) sway (*smth.*), rock (*smth.*), swing* (*smth.*); ~ ного́й swing* one's foot*; ~ колыбе́ль rock a crádle; ве́тер ~а́ет верху́шки дере́вьев the wind is swáying the trée-tops; the tree-tops are swáying in the wind; 2. *безл.*: его́ ~а́ет во все сто́роны he stággers from side to side; ло́дку, су́дно ~а́ет the boat, ship is rólling and pítching; си́льно ~а́ет (*на море*) the sea is véry rough; совсе́м не ~а́ет it's quite calm; 3. (*вн.; подбрасывать*) toss (*smth.*); 4. (*вн.; убаюкивать*) dándle (*smb.*); 5. (*вн.; воду и т. п. насосом*) pump (*smth.*); ◇ ~ голово́й shake* one's head. ~ся *несов.* 1. sway, rock; (*на качалке*) rock onesélf; (*на качелях*) swing* onesélf; ~ся на волна́х rock on the waves; 2. (*пошатываться*) sway, stágger.

каче́ли *мн.* swing *sg*.

ка́чественный 1. quálitative; 2. (*высокого качества*) high-quality *attr.*, high-grade *attr.*; ~ ана́лиз *хим.* quálitative análysis.

ка́честв|о *с.* quálity; неотъе́млемое ~ esséntial quálity; ~ проду́кции the quálity of the próduct; ◇ в ~e as; в ~e доказа́тельства by way of évidence; в ~e сове́тника as an adviser, in an advísory capácity.

ка́чка *ж.* mótion; бортова́я ~ *мор.* rólling; килева́я ~ *мор.* pítching.

качну́ть *сов.* (*вн.*) give* (*smth.*) a push. ~ся *сов.* lurch, give* a lurch.

ка́ш|а *ж.* 1. pórridge; (*жидкая*) pap, gruel; вари́ть ~у make* pórridge; 2. (*полужидкая масса*) sóggy mass; 3. (*путаница*) múddle, hódgepodge; hótchpotch *амер.*; ◇ сапоги́ ~и про́сят *smb.'s* boots are gáping; с ним ~и не сва́ришь you won't get ánywhere with him; завари́ть ~y get* into a mess, start sómething.

кашало́т *м.* cáchalot, spérm-whale.

кашева́р *м.* cook.

ка́ш|ель *м.* cóughing; (*болезнь*) cough; сухо́й, хри́плый ~ dry, hoarse cóughing.

ка́шлянуть *сов.* cough, give* a (slight) cough.

ка́шлять *несов.* cough.

кашне́ *с. нескл.* scarf*, múffler.

кашпо́ *с. нескл.* cáche-pot, ornaméntal pot.

кашта́н *м.* chéstnut; (*дерево тж.*) chéstnut-tree. ~овый 1. chéstnut *attr.*; 2. (*каштанового цвета*) chéstnut(-cóloured); ~овые во́лосы áuburn hair.

каю́та *ж.* cábin, státe-room.

каю́т-компа́ния *ж. мор.* (*на военном корабле*) wárdroom; (*на пассажирском судне*) salóon.

ка́яться, пока́яться 1. repént; 2. (*в пр.; сознаваться*) conféss (*smth.*); 3.: ка́юсь, винова́т! sórry, my fault!

квадра́т *м.* square.

квадра́тно-гнездово́й squáre-clúster *attr.*

квадра́т|ный square; ~ное уравне́ние quadrátic equátion; ко́рень ~ (*из*) square root (of). ~у́ра: ~у́ра кру́га squáring the circle.

квак|анье *с.* cróaking. ~ать *несов.* croak. ~нуть *сов.* give* a croak.

квалификацио́нн|ый: ~ая коми́ссия board of éxperts.

квалифика́ц|ия *ж.* qualificátion(s); (*навык*) skill; приобрести́ ~ию becóme* quálified (in a proféssion/trade); повы́сить ~ию impróve one's qualificátions.

квалифици́ров|анный skilled, quálified; ~ рабо́тник skilled wórker; ~ труд skilled lábour. **~ать** *несов. и сов.* (*вн.*) **1.** (*определять степень чего-л.*) quálify (*smth.*); **2.** (*выяснять квалификацию*) test/detérmine *smth.'s* qualificátions.

квант *м. физ.* quántum (*pl* -ta).

ква́нтовый quántum *attr.*; ~ генера́тор máser.

кварта́л *м.* **1.** (*четверть года*) quárter; **2.** (*часть города*) dístrict, néighbourhood; *разг.* (*часть улицы между двумя перекрёстками*) block.

кварта́льный quárterly.

кварте́т *м.* quartétte.

кварти́р|а *ж.* **1.** (*часть жилого дома*) flat; apártment *амер.*; lódgings *pl* (*нанимаемое помещение*); сдава́ть ~у let* a flat; жить на ~е live in lódgings; ~ из трёх ко́мнат thrée-room flat; **2.** *мн. воен.* bíllets; ◇ коммуна́льная ~ "cómmunal" flat; гла́вная ~ *воен. уст.* Géneral Héadquárters. **~а́нт** *м.* lódger. **~ный:** ~ная пла́та rent; ~ные усло́вия hóusing condítions; ~ный вопро́с housing próblem. **~ова́ть** *несов.* (*у рд., в пр.*) **1.** *разг.* (*жить на квартире*) lodge (with, in); **2.** *воен.* be* bílleted (on, at).

квартиросъёмщик *м.* ténant.

квартпла́та *ж.* rent.

кварц *м.* quartz. **~евый** quartz *attr.*; ◇ ~евая ла́мпа quartz lamp.

квас *м.* kvass.

ква́сить *несов.* (*вн.*) fermént (*smth.*); (*о тесте*) léaven (*smth.*); ~ капу́сту píckle cábbage. **~ся** *несов.* fermént.

квасцы́ *мн.* álum *sg.*

ква́шен|ый: ~ая капу́ста sáuerkraut.

квашня́ *ж.* dóugh-trough.

кве́рху up, úpward(s); подня́ть глаза́ ~ raise *one's* eyes.

кви́нта *ж. муз.* fifth.

квинте́т *м. муз.* quintét(te).

квинтэссе́нция *ж.* quintéssence.

квита́нци|я *ж.* recéipt; бага́жная ~ lúggage recéipt; вы́дать кому́-л. ~ю give* *smb.* a recéipt.

кви́ты *в знач. сказ. разг.:* тепе́рь мы ~ now we are quits.

кво́рум *м.* quórum.

кво́та *ж. эк.* quóta.

кегельба́н *м.* bówling-alley.

ке́гли *мн.* (*ед.* ке́гля *ж.*) skíttles.

кегль *м. полигр.* point.

кедр *м.* cédar. **~овый** cédar *attr.*; ~овый оре́х cédar nut.

ке́ды *мн. спорт.* rúbber-soled sports boots.

кекс *м.* plúm-cake.

келе́йн|о in sécrecy. **~ый** sécret; ~ая жизнь hérmit's existence.

кельт *м.* Celt. **~ский** Céltic; ~ские языки́ the Céltic lánguages.

ке́лья *ж.* cell.

кем (*тв. от мест.* кто) by whom, who by.

ке́мпинг *м.* cámping-site.

кенгуру́ *м. нескл. зоол.* kangaróo.

ке́пка *ж. разг.* cap.

кера́мика *ж. собир.* cerámics *pl.*

керами́ческий cerámic.

кероси́н *м.* kérosene; páraffin *разг.* ~ка *ж.* oil-stove. **~овый** kérosene *attr.*

кессо́н *м.* cáisson. **~ный:** ~ная боле́знь *мед.* cáisson diséase; the bends *pl разг.*

кет|а *ж.* Sibérian/chum sálmon. **~овый:** ~овая икра́ red́ cáviare.

кефа́ль *ж.* grey múllet.

кефи́р *м.* kefir (*kind of yoghurt*).

киберне́тик *м.* cybernéticist, cybernetícian.

киберне́тика *ж.* cybernétics.

кива́ть, кивну́ть **1.** nod; ~ голово́й nod; **2.** (*на вн.*; *указывать кивком*) nod in the diréction (of); *перен. разг.* hint (at).

кивну́ть *сов. см.* кива́ть.

кивок *м.* nod.

кид|а́ть, ки́нуть **1.** (*вн., тв.*; *бросать*) throw* (*smth.*) (*тж. перен.*); fling* (*smth.*), cast* (*smth.*); ~ ка́мешки в во́ду throw* pébbles ínto the wáter; ~ не́вод cast* a net; **2.** *обыкн. безл.* (*сильно качать*) toss; су́дно ~а́ло из стороны́ в сто́рону the ship was tossed from side to side; **3.** (*вн.*; *направлять, устремлять*) cast* (*smth.*), throw* (*smth.*); ~ тень cast* a shádow; ~ взгляд throw* a glance; **4.** (*вн.*; *небрежно класть*) fling* (*smth.*), toss (*smth.*); **5.** *безл. в сочет. с сущ.:* меня́ в сон ~а́ет I keep drópping off to sleep; его́ ~а́ло в дрожь he felt sháky all of a súdden. **~а́ться, ки́нуться** **1.** *тк. несов.* (*тв.*; *бросаться*) throw* (*smth.*) at one anóther; *перен. разг.* (*не дорожить*) treat (*smth., smth.*) líghtly, trífle (with); **2.** (*устремляться*) rush, fling*/throw* onesélf; ~а́ться на ше́ю кому́-л. rush to embráce *smb.*; **3.** (*метаться*) dart abóut, prance abóut; ◇ ~а́ться в го́лову (*о вине*) go* to *one's* head; кровь ки́нулась в го́лову the blood rushed to *one's* head.

кизи́л(ь) *м.* (*ягода и растение*) cornélian chérry.

кий *м.* (*billiard*) cue.

кило́ *с. нескл. разг.* kílo(gram).

килова́тт *м. эл.* kílowatt. **~-час** *м. эл.* kílowatt-hour.

килогра́мм *м.* kílogram.

киломе́тр *м.* kílometre.

киль *м.* **1.** *мор.* keel; **2.** *ав.* fin.

кильва́тер *м. мор.* wake; идти́ в ~е, в ~ fóllow in the wake of; строй ~ line ahéad; cólumn *амер.*

ки́лька *ж.* sprat.

кинема́тика *ж. физ.* kinemátics.

кинема́то́граф *м.* **1.** cinemátograph; **2.** (*киноискус- ство*) the cínema. **~и́чный** cinemátic.

кинематогра́фия *ж.* cinematógraphy, the cínema.

кинеско́п *м.* télevision tube.

кине́т|ика *ж.* kinétics. **~и́ческий** kinétic; ~и́ческая эне́ргия kinétic énergy.

кинжа́л *м.* dágger.

кино́ *с. нескл.* **1.** (*искусство*) cinematógraphy, the cínema; films; the móvies *амер.*; **2.** *разг.* (*фильм*) film; **3.** *разг.* (*кинотеатр*) cínema; ходи́ть в ~ go* to the cínema/píctures; go* to the móvies *амер.*

кино|актёр *м.* film áctor. **~актри́са** *ж.* film áctress. **~аппара́т** *м.* cinecámera. **~аппарату́ра** *ж.* mótion-picture equipment. **~боеви́к** *м.* film hit, smásh-hit.

ки́новарь *ж.* cínnabar.

кино|докуме́нт *м.* documéntary (film). **~журна́л** *м.* film magazíne. **~звезда́** *ж.* film/móvie star. **~зри́тель** *м.* filmgoer, cínemagoer, móvie-goer *амер.* **~иску́сство** *с.* the art (of film) cínema, cinemátic art. **~ка́мера** *ж.* mótion- -picture cámera, (móvie-)cámera. **~карти́на** *ж.* film, picture; móvie *амер.* **~коме́дия** *ж.* cómedy film. **~кри́тика** *ж.* film críticism. **~ле́нта** *ж.* (cínema) film. **~люби́тель** *м.* amateur film-máker. **~ма́ния** *ж.* cínema operátor. **~опера́тор** *м.* cámeraman*. **~панора́ма** *ж.* cineráma; кругова́я ~панора́ма círclorama. **~передви́жка** *ж.* pórtable film projéctor. **~плёнка** *ж.* film. **~прока́т** *м.* film distribútion. **~промы́шленность** *ж.* film índustry. **~режиссёр** *м.* (film) diréctor. **~сеа́нс** *м.* (cínema) perfórmance. **~сту́дия** *ж.* film stúdio. **~сцена́рий** *м.* film script, scréenplay. **~съёмка** *ж.* shóoting, fílming. **~теа́тр** *м.* cínema. **~фестива́ль** *м.* film féstival.

кинофика́ция *ж.* provísion of film shows.

кинофи́льм *м.* film, pícture; móvie *амер.*

кинофици́ровать *несов. и сов.* (*вн.*) bring* the cínema (to).

кино|хро́ника *ж.* néwsreel. **~экра́н** *м.* (cínema) screen. **~эпопе́я** *ж.* film épic.

ки́нуть *сов. см.* кида́ть. **~ся** *сов. см.* кида́ться 2, 3.

киóск *м.* kiósk, booth; газéтный ~ néwsstand, néws-stall; книжный ~ bóokstall.

киоскёр *м.* néwsagent; néwsdealer *амер.*

кипа *ж.* 1. (*пачка, связка*) búndle; (*груда*) pile, heap; ~ книг búndle of books; ~ бумáг sheaf* of pápers; 2. (*упаковочная мера*) bale; ~ хлóпка bale of cótton.

кипарúс *м.* cýpress. ~овый cýpress *attr.*

кипéние *с.* bóiling.

кипé|ть *несов.* boil, seethe; (*о работе*) be* in full swing; досáда так и ~ла в нём he was séething with annóyance.

кипýч|ий séething; *перен. тж.* ebúllient; ~ая дéятельность ebúllient/tíreless actívity; ~ая натýра impétuous cháracter.

кипят|úть, вскипятúть (*вн.*) boil (*smth.*); bring* (*smth.*) to the boil. ~úться *несов.* 1. (*нагреваться*) be* bóiling; 2. *разг.* (*волноваться, горячиться*) be* worked up, get* worked up. ~óк *м.* bóiling wáter.

кипяч|éние *с.* bóiling. ~ёный boiled; ~ёная водá boiled wáter.

кирг|úз *м.*, ~ка *ж.* Kirghíz. ~ский Kirghíz; ~ский язык Kirghíz, the Kirghíz lánguage.

киркá *ж.* pick(-axe).

кирпúч *м.* brick; облицóвочный ~ fácing bricks *pl*; класть ~й lay* bricks. ~ный 1. brick *attr.*; ~ный завóд bríckyard, bríckfield; 2. (*о цвете*) brick-réd, rúddy; ◇ ~ный чай brick-tea.

кисéйн|ый múslin *attr.*; ◇ ~ая бáрышня ≈ bréad-and-bútter miss.

кисел|ь *м.* 1. kíssel (*fruit juice, milk etc. thickened with potato flour*); 2. *разг.* (*о человеке*) wet rag; он такóй ~ he's so spíneless; ◇ седьмáя водá на ~е sécond cóusin twice remóved.

кисéт *м.* tobácco-pouch.

кисéя *ж.* múslin.

кислорóд *м. хим.* óxygen. ~ный óxygen *attr.*, oxýgenous; ~ное голодáние óxygen starvátion; ◇ ~ная подýшка óxygen/bréathing bag.

кúсло-слáдкий sóur-sweet.

кислотá *ж.* 1. (*свойство*) acídity; 2. *хим.* ácid.

кислóтн|ость *ж.* acídity. ~ый ácid.

кúсл|ый 1. (*прям. и перен.*) sour; ~ые яблоки sóur/tart ápples; ~ое молокó sour milk; ~ое тéсто léavened dough; ~ая улыбка ácid smile; дéлать ~ое лицó make* a sour face; 2. *хим.* ácid; ◇ ~ые щи sáuerkraut soup. ~ятина *ж. разг.* sour stuff.

кúснуть *несов.* turn sour; (*о молоке тж.*) turn, go* off; *перен. разг.* mope.

кистá *ж. мед.* cyst.

кист|ь *ж.* 1. (*часть руки*) hand; тóнкая ~ slénder hand; 2. (*гроздь*) bunch, clúster; 3. (*украшение*) tássel; с ~ями tásselled; 4. (*для краски, клея и т. п.*) brush; ~ для бритья sháving-brush; 5. (*искусство живописи*) the brush (of the ártist).

кит *м.* whale.

китáец *м.* Chínése.

китáйский Chínése; ~ язык Chínése, the Chínése lánguage.

китаянка *ж.* Chínése wóman*.

кúтель *м.* hígh-nécked túnic.

китобóец *м.* wháler, whále-boat, wháling ship.

китобóй *м.* 1. (*занимающийся китобойным промыслом*) wháler; 2. (*судно*) см. китобóец.

китобóйн|ый wháling; ~ое сýдно whále-boat, wháling ship; ~ промысел wháling, wháling índustry.

китóвый whale *attr.*; ~ жир blúbber; ◇ ~ ус whálebone.

китолóвный см. китобóйный.

кичúться *несов.* (*тв.*) boast (of), pride onesélf (on).

кичлú́в|ость *ж.* concéit. ~ый vain, concéited, búmptious.

киш|éть *несов.* (*тв.*) swarm (with), teem (with); (*паразитами*) be* infésted (with).

кишéчн|ик *м.* bówels *pl*, intéstines *pl.* ~ый intéstinal.

кишкá *ж.* 1. *анат.* intéstine, gut; двенадцатипéрстная ~ duodénum; прямáя ~ réctum (*pl* -ta); 2. *разг.* (*резиновая трубка*) rúbber tube; (*шланг*) hose; пожáрная ~ fire-hose.

кишлáк *м.* kishlák (*village in Central Asia*).

кишмя: ~ кишéть кем-л., чем-л. be* téeming with *smb., smth.*

клавиатýра *ж.* kéyboard.

клáвиш *м.*, ~а *ж.* key.

клад *м.* hídden tréasure; *перен.* tréasure.

клáдб|ище *с.* cémetery, gráveyard. ~ищенский cémetery *attr.*

клáдезь *м.*: ~ премýдрости *шутл.* fóuntain of wísdom.

клáдка *ж.* láying; кáменная ~ másonry; кирпúчная ~ bricklaying, bríckwork.

кладов|áя *ж.* stóre-room; (*для продуктов тж.*) lárder. ~щúк *м.* stórekeeper.

кладь *ж. собир.* load; ручнáя ~ hand lúggage.

клáняться, поклонúться 1. (*дт.; делать поклон*) bow (to); не ~ с кем-л. not be* on spéaking terms with *smb.*; низко ~ кому-л. bow low to *smb.*; 2. (*дт.; посылать привет*) send* gréetings (to); клáняйтесь им от меня remémber me kíndly to them; он просúл вам ~ he sends you his regárds/gréetings; 3. (*дт., перед тв.; просить*) beg (of).

клáпан *м.* 1. valve; выхлопнóй ~ exháust valve; 2. *анат.*: сердéчный ~ cárdiac valve; 3. (*на одежде и т. п.*) flap.

кларнéт *м. муз.* clarinét. ~úст *м.* clarinéttist.

класс I *м.* (*социальная группа*) class.

класс II *м.* 1. (*группа, разряд; тж. биол.*) class; 2. (*в школе*) class, form; grade *амер.*; 3. (*комната*) cláss-room.

клáссик *м.* 1. clássic, clássic(al) áuthor; 2. clássical schólar.

классифи|кáтор *м.* clássifier. ~кáция *ж.* classificátion, gróuping. ~цúровать *несов. и сов.* (*вн.*) clássify (*smth.*), group (*smth.*).

классицúзм *м.* clássicism.

классúческ|ий 1. clássical; ~ая рýсская литератýра the clássics of Rússian literature, the great works of Rússian literature; ~ая мýзыка clássical músic; ~ие языкú the clássical lánguages; ~ие черты лицá clássical féatures; 2. (*типичный, характерный*) clássic; ~ образéц clássic exámple.

клáссн|ый 1. (*учебный*) class *attr.*; ~ руководúтель form máster; ~ая доскá bláckboard; 2. *спорт.* (*квалифицированный*) tóp-level; clássy *амер.*

клáссов|ый class *attr.*; ~ая борьбá class strúggle, class war; ~ые противорéчия contradíctions betwéen clásses; ~ые разлúчия class dífferences.

класть, положúть, сложúть (*вн.*) 1. *сов.* положúть put* (*smb., smth.*), lay* (*smb., smth.*), place (*smb., smth.*); ~ дéньги в кармáн put* móney in one's pócket; ~ кого-л. в больнúцу put* *smb.* in hóspital; ~ рáненого на стол lay* an ínjured man* on a táble; ~ крáски на холст put* paint on a cánvas, applý paint to a cánvas; ~ печáть на что-л. rúbber-stamp *smth.*; *перен.* leave* its mark on *smth.*; ~ сáхар в чай put* súgar in one's tea; ~ нóгу нá ногу cross one's legs; 2. *сов.* сложúть (*строить*) build* (*smth.*), make* (*smth.*); ~ печь build*/make* a stove; ~ стéну build* a wall; ~ фундáмент lay* a foundátion; ~ яйца lay* eggs; положúть словá на мýзыку put*/set* words to músic; положúть жизнь за рóдину lay* down one's life for one's cóuntry.

клёв *м.* bíting, báit-taking; вечéрний ~ the évening rise.

клевáть, клюнуть 1. (*вн.; о птицах*) peck (*smth.*);

2. (*о рыбе*) bite*; ◇ ~ носом nod, be* nódding, be* drówsy.

клевер *м.* clóver.

клевет|**á** *ж.* slánder, cálumny; (*в печати тж.*) líbel. ~**áть** *несов.* (*на вн.*) slánder (*smb.*), calúmniate (*smb.*); (*в печати тж.*) líbel (*smb.*). ~**ни́к** *м.* slánderer. ~**ни́ческий** slánderous, líbellous.

клеев|**óй** glue *attr.*; ~**áя кра́ска** non-wáshable distémper, cólour-wash.

клеён|**ка** *ж.* (*скатерть*) óilcloth; (*для компресса и т. п.*) óilskin. ~**чатый** óilcloth *attr.*; (*из тонкой клеёнки*) óilskin attr.

клé|**ить** *несов.* (*вн.*) glue (*smth.*); (*клейстером*) paste (*smth.*); (*растительным клеем*) gum (*smth.*). ~**иться** *несов.* 1. stick*; 2. *разг.*: де́ло не ~**ится** it ísn't wórking out; разгово́р не ~**и́лся** the conversátion flagged.

клей *м.* glue.

клéйк|**ий** sticky. ~**ость** *ж.* stíckiness.

клейм|**ёный** bránded. ~**и́ть**, заклейми́ть (*вн.*) brand (*smth.*); *перен. тж.* stígmatize (*smb., smth.*); ~**и́ть кого́--л.** позо́ром hold* smb. up to shame/ígnominy, brand smb. with ínfamy.

клеймó *с.* (*знак*) stamp; (*выжженное*) brand (*тж. перен.*); ~ позо́ра the brand of shame, stígma.

клéйстер *м.* paste.

клён *м.* máple.

клепáть *несов.* (*вн.*) *тех.* rívet (*smth.*).

клёпка *ж.* 1. *тех.* ríveting; 2. (*бочечная*) stave.

клéтк|**а** *ж.* 1. cage; посади́ть кого́-л. в ~**у** put* smth. in a cage, cage smth.; 2. (*рисунок*) square; (*на материи*) check, в ~**у** checked; 3. *биол.* cell; ◇ грудна́я ~ chest; thórax *анат.*

клéточный 1. cage attr.; 2. *биол.* céllular.

клетýшка *ж. разг.* cúbby-hole.

клетчáтка *ж.* céllulose.

клéтчатый 1. (*в клетку*) checked; 2. *биол.* céllular.

клеть *ж.* (*в шахте*) cage.

клёцки *мн. кул.* (*ед.* клёцка *ж.*) dúmplings.

клёш: брю́ки ~ béll-bottomed tróusers; ю́бка ~ clóche-skirt.

клешня́ *ж.* claw, nípper.

клещ *м. зоол.* mite; (*крупный*) tick.

клещеви́на *ж. бот.* cástor-oil plant.

клéщи́ *мн.* píncers, níppers.

клиéнт *м.* clíent; (*покупатель тж.*) cústomer. ~**ýра** *ж.* clientéle.

кли́зм|**а** *ж.* énema; поста́вить кому́-л. ~**у** give* smb. an énema.

кли́ка *ж. неодоб.* clique, (tight) set, bunch.

кли́мат *м.* clímate. ~**и́ческий** climátic.

клин *м.* 1. wedge; вбить ~ во что́-л. drive* a wedge ínto smth.; 2. (*участок*) field; ози́мый ~ área únder winter crops; яровой ~ área únder spring crops; 3. (*материи*) gússet; ◇ ~ ~**ом** вышиба́ют *погов.* like cures like.

кли́н|**ика** *ж.* clínic. ~**и́ческий** clínical.

клиновидн|**ый** wédge-shaped; ~**ые** письмена́ cúneiform cháracters.

клинóк *м.* blade.

кли́ном: борода́ ~ wédge-shaped/póinted beard.

кли́нопись *ж.* cúneiform.

кли́псы *мн.* (*ед.* клипс *м.*) éarclips, éar-rings.

клич *м.* call, appéal; ◇ кли́кнуть ~ íssue an appéal.

кли́чка *ж.* 1. (*животного*) name; 2. (*прозвище человека*) níckname; конспирати́вная ~ assúmed name, álias.

клише́ *с нескл. полигр.* cliché.

клок *м.* 1. (*волос*) wisp, tuft; (*шерсти*) tuft, flock; ~ се́на wisp of hay; 2. (*обрывок*) shred; (*о бумаге*) scrap; *перен.* clúster; разорва́ть что́-л. в кло́чья tear* smth. to shreds.

клокот|**áть** *несов.* 1. (*о жидкости*) splútter, búbble;

2. *безл.*: в груди́ ра́неного ~**áло** a gúrgling sound rose from the chest of the wóunded man*; 3. (*бурно проявляться*) seethe, boil; (*о радости*) búbble; в нём клокóчет гнев he is séething with ánger; ра́дость ~**áла** в нём he was búbbling with joy.

клон|**и́ть** *несов.*: ве́тер клóнит дере́вья the trees bow/bend befóre the wind; к чему́ он клóнит? what's he dríving at?; меня́ клóнит ко сну I feel sléepy/drówsy. ~**и́ться** *несов.* 1.: де́рево клóнится от ве́тра the tree is bénding in the wind; со́лнце ~**и́лось** к зака́ту the sun was góing down; 2. (*к дт.; приближаться*) near (*smth.*); день ~**и́лся** к ве́черу the day was wáning/declíning; 3. (*к дт.; иметь своей целью*) lead* up (to); я ви́жу, к чему́ э́то клóнится I can see what that's léading up to; де́ло клóнится к развя́зке mátters are cóming to a head.

клоп *м.* 1. bug; (*постельный*) béd-bug; 2. *разг.* (*малыш*) mite.

клóун *м.* clown.

клохтáть *несов.* cluck.

клоч|**óк** *м.* 1. *см.* клок; 2.: ~ земли́ bit of land; разорва́ть что́-л. в ~**ки́** tear* smth. into líttle píeces.

клуб I *м.* 1. (*общественная организация*) club; 2. (*здание*) clúb-house.

клуб II *м.* (*дыма, пара и т. п.*) cloud, mass, éddy; (*небольшой*) puff.

клýбень *м. бот.* túber.

клуби́ться *несов.* swirl, éddy; (*о дыме тж.*) curl.

клубни́|**ка** *ж.* 1. *собир.* stráwberries *pl*; 2. (*об отдельной ягоде*) stráwberry; 3. (*куст*) stráwberry plant. ~**чный** stráwberry attr.; ~**чное** варе́нье stráwberry jam.

клуб|**óк** *м.* ball; *перен.* tángle; ◇ сверну́ться ~**ком** roll onesélf up ínto a ball; ~ в гóрле a lump in the throat.

клýмба *ж.* (flówer-)bed.

клык *м.* 1. (*у животного*) fang; (*бивень*) tusk; 2. (*у человека*) cánine (tooth*).

клюв *м.* beak, bill.

клю́кв|**а** *ж.* 1. *собир.* cránberries *pl*; 2. (*об отдельной ягоде*) cránberry; 3. (*куст*) cránberry (shrub). ~**енный** cránberry attr.

клю́нуть *сов. см.* клева́ть.

ключ I *м.* 1. key; *перен. тж.* clue; запере́ть что́-л. на ~ lock smth.; ~ к зада́чнику solútions *pl*, ánswers *pl*; ~ к реше́нию пробле́мы the key to the próblem; 2. *муз.* clef.

ключ II *м.* (*родник*) spring; ◇ жизнь бьёт ~**óм** things are góing with a swing, the place is thróbbing with life; жизнь в нём бьёт ~**óм** he's brímming óver with life.

ключев|**óй** *аи* ~**áя** пози́ция key posítion; ~**áя** óтрасль промы́шленности key (branch of) índustry; 2. *муз.*: ~ знак clef.

ключев|**óй II**: ~**áя** вода́ spring-water.

ключи́ца *ж. анат.* cóllar-bone.

клю́шка *ж. спорт.* íce-hóckey stick; (*для гольфа*) club.

кля́кс|**а** *ж.* blot; посади́ть ~**у** make* a blot.

кля́нчить *несов. разг.* beg; (*вн. у рд.*) péster (*smb.* for).

кляп *м.* gag.

клясть *несов.* (*вн.*) curse (*smb., smth.*). ~**ся**, покля́сться (*вн.*) vow *книжн.*; ~**ся** в ве́чной дру́жбе swear* etérnal fríendship.

кля́тв|**а** *ж.* oath, vow; взять ~**у** с кого́-л. make* smb. swear; дать ~**у** swear*, make*/take* an oath; нару́шить ~**у** break* one's oath. ~**енный**: ~**енное** обеща́ние sólemn oath; дать ~**енное** обеща́ние give* a sólemn oath/prómise, swear*.

кля́уз|**а** *ж. разг.* smear, false repórt. ~**ник** *м. разг.* báckbiter, múck-raker, sneak. ~**ничать** *несов. разг.* smear, múck-rake, speak* évil. ~**ный** *разг.*: ~**ное** де́ло dúbious affáir, dirty búsiness.

кля́ча ж. jade, nag, hack.

кни́г|а ж. 1. book; 2.: бухга́лтерская ~ lédger; ~ за́писей а́ктов гражда́нского состоя́ния régister; ◇ ему́ и ~и в ру́ки he knows best, he ought to know; ~ за семью́ печа́тями a sealed book.

книгове́дение с. bibliólogy, bibliógraphy.

книгоизда́тель|ский: ~ское де́ло book públishing. ~ство с. públishing house.

книгоно́ша м. и ж. 1. (продаве́ц) bóok-vendor; 2. (библиоте́карь) móbile-líbrary assístant.

книгообме́н м. book exchánge.

книгопеча́тание с. (bóok-)prínting.

книготорго́вля ж. book trade.

книгохрани́лище с. 1. book depósitory; 2. (библиоте́ка) líbrary.

кни́жк|а ж. book; чле́нская ~ mémbership card; положи́ть де́ньги на ~у (в сберба́нк) put* móney in the sávings-bank.

кни́жник м. connoisséur of books, bóoklover; ирон. bóokish pérson, bóokworm.

кни́жн|ый 1. book attr.; ~ая торго́вля book trade; ~ шкаф bóokcase; ~ магази́н bóokshop; 2. (отвлечённый, далёкий от жи́зни) bóokish; ~ые выраже́ния bóokish expréssions; ~ стиль, язы́к bóokish style; ◇ Кни́жная пала́та Céntral Ínstitute of Bibliógraphy.

кни́зу down, dównwards; опусти́ть ~ lówer.

кно́пк|а ж. 1. (канцеля́рская) dráwing-pin; 2. (нажимна́я) (púsh-)bútton; (звонка́) béll-push; нажа́ть ~y press the bútton; 3. (застёжка) dréss-stud, dréss-fastener.

кнут м. knout; поли́тика ~а́ и пря́ника pólicy of threats and bríbery, pólicy of stick and cárrot.

кнутови́ще с. whíp-handle.

княги́ня ж. princéss; вели́кая ~ ист. Grand Dúchess.

кня́жес|кий prínce's. ~тво с. principálity.

княжна́ ж. princéss.

князь м. prince; вели́кий ~ ист. Grand Duke.

ко см. к.

коалицио́нн|ый coalítion attr.; ~ое прави́тельство coalítion góvernment.

коали́ц|ия ж. coalítion; заключа́ть ~ию form a coalítion.

ко́бальт м. 1. хим. cóbalt; 2. (кра́ска) cóbalt blue.

кобе́ль м. (male) dog.

кобура́ ж. hólster.

кобы́л|а ж. 1. (ста́рше 4 лет) mare; (до 4 лет) filly; 2. спорт. váulting-horse. ~ка ж. 1. (молода́я ло́шадь) filly; 2. (у стру́нного инструме́нта) bridge.

ко́ваный 1. (сде́ланный посре́дством ко́вки) forged; 2. (оби́тый желе́зом) íron-bound.

кова́р|ный tréacherous; (тая́щий в себе́ опа́сность и т. п.) insídious; ~ враг tréacherous énemy; ~ная улы́бка insídious smile. ~ство с. 1. guile, decéit; 2. (посту́пок) tréachery.

кова́ть несов. (вн.) 1. forge (smth.) (тж. перен.); 2. (подко́вывать) shoe (smth.); ◇ куй желе́зо, пока́ горячо́ посл. strike while the íron is hot.

ковбо́й м.ców-boy.

ковбо́йка ж. разг. checked sports shirt.

ковёр м. cárpet (тж. перен.); (небольшо́й) rug.

ковёркать, исковёркать (вн.) defórm (smth.), distórt (smth.); перен. spoil* (smb., smth.); (неве́рно произноси́ть) mispronóunce (smth.); ~ язы́к bútcher the lánguage.

ко́вк|а ж. 1. fórging; 2. (лошаде́й) shóeing. ~ий málleable. ~ость ж. malleabílity.

коври́|га ж. large round loaf*. ~жка ж. gíngerbread; ◇ ни за каки́е ~жки ≈ not for the world.

ко́врик м. rug, mat; (у две́ри) dóor-mat.

ковро́в|щица ж. cárpet-maker. ~ый cárpet attr.

ковш м. scoop; (экскава́тора тж.) búcket; лите́йный ~ ládle.

ковы́ль м. féather-grass.

ковыля́ть несов. разг. limp, hóbble; (о ребёнке) tóddle.

ковыря́ть несов. (вн.) разг. pick (at); (тв. в пр.) pick (smth. with); ~ ры́бу pick at a piece of fish; ~ в зуба́х зубочи́сткой pick one's teeth with a tóothpick. ~ся (в пр.) разг. (ры́ться) rúmmage (in).

когда́ I нареч. 1. when; ~ он придёт? when will he come?; он не зна́ет, ~ э́то бы́ло he dóesn't know when it was; в (тот) день, ~ мы... the day we...; 2.: ~... ~... разг. sómetimes... sómetimes; он рабо́тает ~ у́тром, ве́чером sómetimes he works in the mórning, sómetimes in the évening; 3.: ~ бы ни whenéver; no mátter when; ~ бы вы ни пришли́ whenéver you come; ◇ есть ~! there's no time!; ре́дко ~ véry rárely.

когда́ II союз when; (в то вре́мя как) while; (с проше́дшим вре́менем тж.) as; ~ б(ы) if; ~ б я знал if I had ónly known; он уе́дет, ~ ко́нчит рабо́ту he will leave when he has fínished his work.

когда́|-либо, ~-нибудь (в бу́дущем) one day; (в вопрос. и усло́вных предложе́ниях) éver.

когда́-то 1. (в про́шлом) at one time; я ~ встреча́лся с ним I used to meet him; я ~ чита́л э́ту кни́гу I did read that book once; 2. (в бу́дущем): ~ мы опя́ть уви́димся! who knows when we shall meet agáin!; ~ он придёт! will he éver come!

кого́ (рд., вн. от мест. кто) whom, who.

ко́г|оть м. claw; ◇ держа́ть кого́-л. в ~тя́х have* smb. in one's clútches; показа́ть свои́ ~ти ≈ show* one's claws.

код м. code.

ко́декс м. code; мора́льный ~ móral code.

коди́ровать несов. и сов. (вн.) encóde (smth.).

кодифици́ровать несов. и сов. (вн.) códify (smth.).

кое-где́ here and there.

кое-ка́к 1. (как-нибудь) sómehow or óther; (небре́жно) just ányhow; 2. (с трудо́м, еле-еле) sómehow.

кое-како́й some.

кое-когда́ sómetimes.

кое-кто́ some péople pl; sómebody.

кое-куда́ sómewhere.

кое-что́ sómething.

ко́ж|а ж. 1. skin; (кру́пного живо́тного тж.) hide; 2. (материа́л) léather; теля́чья ~ calf*, cálfskin; ◇ из ~и вон лезть lay* onesélf out, do* one's útmost.

ко́жанка ж. разг. léather-coat; (ку́ртка) léather-jacket.

ко́жаный léather attr.

кожгалантере́я ж. собир. háberdashery and léather goods pl.

коже́венн|ый léather-prócessing; ~ая промы́шленность léather índustry; ~ заво́д tánnery; ~ това́р léather-ware.

ко́жица ж. skin; (у ногте́й) cúticle.

ко́жн|ый skin attr.; cutáneous научн.; ~ покро́в skin; ~ые боле́зни skin diséases.

кожура́ ж. peel, skin; (апельси́на, лимо́на тж.) rind.

кожу́х м. 1. (тулу́п) léather coat; 2. mex. hóusing, cásing.

коза́ ж. (shé-)goat, (nánny-)goat.

козёл м. (hé-)goat; ◇ ~ отпуще́ния scápegoat.

ко́з|ий goat's. ~лёнок м. kid. ~линый goat's; ~линая боро́дка goatée.

ко́злы мн. 1. (экипа́жа) box sg; 2. (подста́вка) tréstle sg; 3. (для пи́лки дров) sáw-horse sg.

ко́зни мн. machinátions; стро́ить ~ кому́-л., про́тив кого́-л. plot agáinst smb.

козырёк *м.* peak (of a cap); vízor *амер.*, ◇ взять под ~ salúte.

козыр|ьбо́й trump *attr.*; ~я ка́рта trump card. ~у́ть I, II *сов. см.* козыря́ть I, II.

козы́рный *см.* козырно́й.

ко́зыр|ь *м.* (*прям. и перен.*) trump, trump card; бить, крыть ~ем take* with a trump, trump.

козыря́ть I, козырну́ть 1. *карт.* trump; 2. (*тв.; хвастаться*) show* off (*smth.*); ~ свои́ми зна́ниями air one's knówledge.

козыря́ть II, козырну́ть *разг.* (*отдавать честь*) salúte.

козя́вка *ж. разг.* small ínsect.

ко́йка *ж.* 1. (*кровать*) bed; пала́та на пять ко́ек ward contáining five beds; 2. (*подвесная*) hámmock.

кок *м.* (ship's) cook.

ко́ка-ко́ла *ж.* Coca-Cóla; coke *разг.*

кока́рда *ж.* cáp-badge.

коке́т|ка *ж.* 1. coquétte; 2. (*верхняя часть платья*) yoke. ~ливый 1. coquéttish, arch; ~ливая де́вушка flirtátious/coquéttish girl; ~ливая улы́бка wínsome smile; 2. (*имеющий нарядный вид*) attráctive, smart; ~ливый наря́д fétching gét-up/attíre. ~ничать *несов.* 1. (с *тв.*) flirt (with); 2. (*тв.; рисоваться*) paráde (*smth.*), flaunt (*smth.*). ~ство *с.* cóquetry.

коклю́ш *м. мед.* whóoping-cough.

ко́кон *м.* cocóon.

коко́с *м.* 1. cóco; 2. (*плод*) cóconut. ~овый cóconut *attr.*; ~овый оре́х cóconut; ~овое ма́сло cóconut oil; ~овый трос cóir-rope; ◇ ~овая па́льма cóconut palm, cóco-tree.

коко́шник *м.* kokóshnik (*woman's head-dress in old Russia*).

кокс *м.* coke.

кокс|ова́ние *с. mex.* cóking. ~ова́ть *несов.* (*вн.*) *mex.* coke (*smth.*). ~ова́ться *несов. mex.* coke. ~у́ющийся: ~у́ющийся у́голь cóking coal.

кокте́йль *м.* cócktail.

кол I *м.* pícket, stake; ◇ хоть ~ на голове́ теши́ *кому-л.* you can't knock it into *smb.'s* head.

кол II *м.*: ни ~а́ ни двора́ néither house, nor home, not a pénny to bless onesélf.

ко́лба *ж.* retórt.

колбаса́ *ж.* sáusage.

колба́сный sáusage *attr.*

колго́тки *мн.* tights; pánty hóse *амер.*

колдов|а́ть *несов.* práctise wítchcraft; *перен.* be* mystériously búsy/engáged. ~ство́ *с.* sórcery, wítchcraft.

колду́|н *м.* sórcerer. ~нья *ж.* sórceress.

колеба́|ние *с.* 1. (*качание*) oscillátion; (*вибрация*) vibrátion; 2. (*неустойчивость*) fluctuátion; 3. (*нерешительность*) hesitátion. ~тельный óscillatory; (*вибрирующий*) víbratory.

колеба́ть, поколеба́ть (*вн.*) shake* (*smth.*), rock (*smth.*), sway (*smth.*); *перен.* shake* (*smb.*, *smth.*). ~ся, поколеба́ться 1. *тк. несов.* (*покачиваться*) sway; óscillate; (*раскачиваться*) swing*; (*вибрировать*) vibráte; 2. (*терять прежнее значение*) tótter; 3. *тк. несов.* (*меняться*) flúctuate; 4. (*не решаться*) wáver, hésitate; díther *разг.*

коленко́р *м.* cálico.

коле́нный knee *attr.*

коле́н|о *с.* 1. (*мн.* ~и) knee; встать на ~и kneel* down; стоя́ть на ~ях kneel*; 2. *мн.* (~и) (*сидящего*) knees; lap *sg*; посади́ть кого́-л. к себе́ на ~и take* smb. on one's knees/lap; 3. (*мн.* ~ья, ~а) *mex.* (*отрезок*) length, séction; (*изгиб*) élbow; 4. (*мн.* ~а) (*поколение*) generátion; 5. (*мн.* ~а) *муз.* phrase; (*фигура в танце*) figure; ◇ ему́ мо́ре по ~ he cóuldn't care less, he's ábsolutely réckless.

коле́нчатый *mex.*: ~ вал cránkshaft.

колеси́ть *несов. разг.* 1. (*ехать непрямым путём*) zigzag; 2. (*много ездить*) rove abóut.

колесни́ца *ж.* cháriot.

колёсн|ый wheel *attr.*, wheeled; ~ая мазь cárt-grease; ~ ма́стер wheelwright.

колес|о́ *с.* wheel; рулево́е ~ stéering-wheel; веду́щее ~ dríving-wheel; ◇ как бе́лка в ~é верте́ться be* cónstantly on the go; грудь ~о́м búlging chest.

коле|я́ *ж.* 1. (*наезженная*) rut; 2. *ж.-д.* track; ◇ войти́ в ~ю́ resúme one's nátural course, get* back into one's routíne; вы́бить кого́-л. из ~и́ unséttle *smb.*, upsét* *smb.'s* routíne; вы́биться из ~и́ be* unséttled, have* one's routíne upsét.

ко́ли *уст.*, *разг.* if; (*уж*) ~ на то пошло́ for that mátter, if that is the case.

коли́бри *м. и ж. нескл.* húmming-bird.

ко́лики *мн.* (*ед.* ко́лика *ж.*) cólics.

коли́т *м. мед.* colítis.

коли́чественный quántitative; ◇ ~ ана́лиз *хим.* quántitative análysis.

коли́честв|о *с.* quántity; (*число*) númber; большо́е ~ наро́да a great mány people; перехо́д ~а в ка́чество the transformátion of quántity into quálity.

ко́лкий I 1. (*колючий*) príckly; 2. (*язвительный*) cáustic, bíting.

ко́лкий II *разг.* (*легко раскалывающийся*) éasily split.

ко́лкост|ь *ж.* cáustic remárk; говори́ть ~и make* cáustic remárks.

колле́га *м. и ж.* cólleague.

коллегиа́льн|о colléctively, jóintly. ~ость *ж.* collegiálity; (*руководства*) colléctive léadership. ~ый colléctive, joint, collégial; ~ое реше́ние colléctive decísion.

колле́гия *ж.* board, collégium.

колле́дж *м.* cóllege.

коллекти́в *м.* colléctive (bódy), group; нау́чный ~ bódy/team of scíentists, scientífic bódy; ~ заво́да the fáctory's wórk-force; рабо́чий ~ work colléctive, bódy of wórkers.

коллективиз|а́ция *ж.* collectivizátion. ~и́ровать *несов. и сов.* (*вн.*) cóllectivize (*smth.*).

коллективи́зм *м.* colléctivism.

коллекти́вн|ость *ж.* colléctive náture. ~ый colléctive; ~ое хозя́йство colléctive farm, kolkhóz; ~ое руково́дство colléctive léadership; систе́ма ~ой безопа́сности sýstem of colléctive secúrity; ◇ ~ый догово́р colléctive agréement.

колле́ктор *м.* 1. (*учреждение*) distribútion céntre; библиоте́чный ~ céntral óffice for the distribútion of books to líbraries; 2. *mex.* colléctor.

коллекцион|е́р *м.* colléctor. ~и́ровать *несов.* (*вн.*) colléct (*smth.*).

колле́кция *ж.* colléction.

колли́зия *ж.* clash.

колло́дий *м.* collódium.

колло́ид *м. хим.* cólloid. ~а́льный, ~ный *хим.* collóidal.

колло́квиум *м.* tutórial.

коло́д|а I *ж.* 1. (*лежачее бревно*) log; *перен.* (*о неповоротливом человеке*) (great) lump; 2. (*обрубок бревна*) block; ◇ че́рез пень ~у half-héartedly, in a slípshod mánner.

коло́да II *ж.* (*комплект карт*) pack; deck *амер.*

коло́дец *м.* well.

коло́дка *ж.* 1. block; 2. (*тормоза*) shoe; 3. (*сапожная*) last; (*для сохранения обуви*) bóot-tree; 4. (*орденская*) médal-holder; *разг.* (*планка, носимая вместо ордена, медали*) médal ríbbon(s).

ко́локол *м.* bell.

колоко́ль|ный: ~ звон rínging of bells; (*монотонный*) tólling of bells. ~ня *ж.* church tówer, bell tówer; ◇ смотре́ть на всё со свое́й ~ни see* о́nly one's own point of view. ~чик м. 1. bell; 2. (цветок) blúebell.

колониали́зм м. colónialism.

колониа́льн|ый colónial.

колониз|а́тор м. cólonizer. ~а́ция ж. colonizátion. ~и́ровать несов. и сов. (вн.) 1. (превращать в колонию) make* a cólony (of); turn (smth.) ínto a cólony; 2. (заселять) cólonize (smth.)

колони́ст м. séttler, cólonist.

коло́ния ж. 1. cólony; 2. (исправительная) refórmatory.

коло́нка ж. 1. (столбец) cólumn; 2. (для нагрева воды) géyser; 3. (водопроводное устройство) pump; ◇ запра́вочная ~ fílling státion.

коло́нн|а ж. cólumn; архит. тж. píllar; с ~ами cólumned; похо́дная ~ márching cólumn; ~ демонстра́нтов cólumn of démonstrators. ~а́да ж. colonnáde. ~ный cólumned; ~ый зал hall of cólumns.

колонти́тул м. полигр. rúnning títle.

колорату́р|а ж. муз. coloratúra. ~ный муз. coloratúra attr.; ◇ ~ное сопра́но coloratúra sopráno.

колори́т м. cólour (тж. перен.); ~ эпо́хи histórical átmosphere; ме́стный ~ lócal cólour. ~ный cólourful.

ко́лос м. ear, spike; ~ пшени́цы ear/spike of wheat. ~и́стый full-éared. ~и́ться несов. be* fórming ears/spikes.

колосники́ мн. (ед. колосни́к м.) 1. тех. fire-bars; 2. театр. flies; grídiron sg.

колоснико́в|ый: ~ая решётка тех. fire-grate.

колосовы́е мн. бот. héaded grains.

коло́сс м. colóssus (pl -si), giant. ~а́льный colóssal, huge, enórmous.

колоти́ть несов. 1: (по дт., в вн.; ударять) thump (smth.), bang (at); 2. (вн.) разг. (бить) hit* (smth.), thrash (smb.), give* (smb.) a drúbbing/hiding; 3. (вн.) разг. (разбивать) break* (smth.), smash (smth.). ~ся несов. разг. 1. (о сердце) thump; 2. (ударяться): ~ся головой обо что-л. bang one's head on smth.

ко́лот|ый I (проколотый) pérforated; ~ая ра́на stab*(-wound).

ко́лотый II (разбитый на куски) bróken; ~ са́хар lúmp-sugar.

коло́ть I, кольну́ть (вн.) 1. (остриём) prick (smth.); 2. тк. несов. (пронзать оружием) stab (smb.); 3. (задевать язвительными замечаниями) taunt (smb.), gibe (at); 4. тк. несов. (убивать скот) sláughter (smth.); 5. безл.: у меня́ ко́лет в боку́ I have a stitch in my side; ◇ пра́вда глаза́ ко́лет посл. the truth hurts.

коло́ть II несов. (вн.; дробить) split* (smth.); ~ дрова́ split*/chop wood; ~ оре́хи crack nuts; ~ са́хар break* súgar ínto lumps.

коло́ться I несов. (вызывать ощущение укола) prick; (о растении) be* príckly.

коло́ться II несов. (поддаваться колке) split*.

колпа́к м. 1. cap; 2. (абажур) lamp-shade; 3. тех. cowl; (защитный) hood; стекля́нный ~ glass cóver; ◇ держа́ть кого́-л. под (стекля́нным) ~о́м ≈ keep* smb. in cótton wool.

колумба́рий м. columbárium (pl -ia).

колу́н м. wóod-chopper, axe.

колхо́з м. colléctive farm, kolkhóz. ~ник м., ~ница ж. colléctive fármer, mémber of a colléctive farm. ~ный colléctive-farm attr., kolkhóz attr.

колча́н м. ист. quíver.

колчеда́н м. мин. pyríites.

колыбе́ль ж. crádle. ~ный: ~ная (пе́сня) lúllaby, crádle-song.

колыха́ть, колыхну́ть (вн.) (листья и т. п. — о ветре) sway (smth.); (покачивать) rock (smth.). ~ся,

колыхну́ться sway; (о флаге) flútter, wave; (о лодке) rock; (о груди) heave*; (о пламени) leap*, blaze.

колыхну́ть(ся) сов. см. колыха́ть(ся).

ко́лышек м. peg.

коль см. ко́ли; ◇ ~ ско́ро (если) if; (как только) as soon as.

колье́ с. нескл. nécklace.

кольну́ть сов. см. коло́ть I 1, 3, 5.

кольцев|а́ние с. rínging. ~а́ть несов. (вн.) ring (smth.). ~о́й círcular.

кольцо́ с. 1. ring; ~ для ключе́й kéy-ring; обруча́льное ~ wédding ring; 2. мн. (гимнастический снаряд) the rings; 3. (маршрут метро, автобуса) círcular route; circle; 4. (кольцевая дорога) ring road.

кольчу́га ж. ист. chain mail.

колю́ч|ий 1. (с колючками) príckly, thórny; ~ая про́волока barbed wíre; 2. (колющийся) príckly; ~ая пыль stínging dust; 3. (язвительный, злой) cáustic, bíting; ~ взгляд sávage look. ~ка ж. thorn, príckle.

коля́ск|а ж. 1. (экипаж) cárriage; 2. (детская) perámbulator, pram; báby-carriage амер.; 3.: мотоци́кл с ~ой mótorcycle and síde-car.

ком I м. lump; снежный ~ lump of snow.

ком II (пр. от мест. кто) abóut whom, who abóut.

кома́нд|а ж. 1. (приказание) commánd; по ~е at the commánd; 2. (начальствование) commánd; под ~ой кого́-л. únder the commánd of smb., únder smb.; приня́ть ~у над кем-л. take* commánd of smb.; 3. (воинская часть) párty; 4. (группа лиц, выполняющих определённое задание) squad, team; 5. (экипаж судна) crew, ship's cómpany; 6. (спортивный коллектив) team; ◇ как по ~е as if at a commánd, as one man; пода́ть ра́порт по ~е воен. repórt to one's supérior ófficer.

команди́р м. 1. воен. commánder, commánding ófficer; ~ полка́ régiment commánder; 2. мор.: ~ корабля́ cáptain of the ship, ship's cáptain; ~ подво́дной ло́дки submárine cáptain; 3. (руководитель) léader.

командиро́ванный м. pérson on búsiness, búsiness tráveller.

командир|ова́ть несов. и сов. (вн.) send* (smb.) (on a míssion). ~о́вка ж. míssion, búsiness trip; нау́чная ~о́вка stúdy tour; в ~о́вке, в ~о́вку on a míssion, on a búsiness trip; получи́ть ~о́вку be* sent on a míssion. ~о́вочный: ~о́вочные де́ньги trávelling allówance sg; ~о́вочное удостовере́ние credéntials pl, trávelling pápers pl.

команди́рский ófficer's, commánder's.

кома́ндн|ый: ~ая высота́ commánding height/position; ~ пункт commánd post; ~ соста́в the ófficers; ~ приз спорт. team prize.

кома́ндование с. 1. (действие) commánd; приня́ть ~ take* commánd; сдать ~ relínquish commánd; под ~м кого́-л. únder smb., únder smb.'s commánd; 2. собир. commánd; héadquárters pl (сокр. H.Q.); гла́вное ~ High Commánd, Géneral Héadquárters.

кома́ндовать несов. 1. give* órders; воен. commánd; 2. (тв.) commánd (smth.), be* in commánd (of); ~ полко́м commánd a régiment; 3. (тв., над тв.) разг. give* órders (to), mánage (smb.).

командо́р м. 1. ист. (Knight) Commánder; 2. (яхт-клуба) Cómmodore.

кома́ндующий прил. 1. commánding; 2. в знач. сущ. м. géneral ófficer commánding (сокр. G.O.C.); ~ а́рмией ármy commánder.

кома́р м. mosquíto; gnat; ◇ ~ но́су не подто́чит погов. there's not a weak spot ánywhere.

комба́йн м. cómbine. ~ер м. cómbine-óperator.

комба́т м. 1. (командир батальо́на) battálion commánder; 2. (командир батаре́и) báttery commánder.

комбико́рм м. (комбини́рованный корм) mixed feed.

комбина́т *м.* 1. (*промышленный*) íntegrated plant; cómplex; cómbine; целлюлóзно-бума́жный ~ íntegrated púlp-and-páper mill; мя́со-моло́чный ~ íntegrated méat--and-dáiry próducts plant; 2. (*учебный*) tráining céntre; ◇ ~ бытового обслу́живания sérvice shop.

комбина́тор *м. разг.* maní pulator, schémer.

комбина́ция *ж.* 1. combinátion; *перен.* scheme; 2. (*белье́*) slip; 3. *спорт.* (*в шахматах*) combinátion; (*в футболе и т. п.*) móvement, manóeuvre.

комбинезо́н *м.* óveralls *pl.*

комбини́рованн|ый combíned; ~ уда́р combíned attáck; ~ое пла́тье twó-colour dress.

комбини́ровать, скомбини́ровать 1. (*вн.*) combíne (*smth.*); 2. *разг.* (*строить комбинации*) maní pulate, scheme.

комеди́йный cómedy *attr.*

коме́ди|я *ж.* cómedy; *перен. тж.* farce; музыка́льная ~ músical cómedy; ◇ разы́грывать ~ю put* on an act; брось лома́ть ~ю! stop pláy-acting!

команда́нт *м.* 1. *воен.* commandánt; ~ го́рода town májor; ~ кре́пости commandánt, góvernor of a fórtress; 2. (*здания, общежития*) superinténdent, wárden.

команда́нтский: ~ час cúrfew.

команда́тура *ж. воен.* commandánt's óffice/héadquárters *pl.*

коме́та *ж.* cómet.

ко́ми *нескл.* Kómi; язы́к ~ Kómi, the Kómi lánguage.

коми́зм *м.* cómic(al) side.

ко́мик *м.* (*актёр*) cómic áctor; *перен. разг.* húmorist, wit.

ко́микс *м.* cómic (páper); (*серия рисунков*) cómic strip.

комисса́р *м.* 1. commissár; вое́нный ~ enlístment ófficer; 2. (*за границей*) commíssioner. ~иа́т *м.* commissáriat; вое́нный ~иа́т mílitary registrátion and enlístment óffice.

комиссионе́р *м.* commíssion-ágent.

комиссио́нн|ый *прил.* 1. commíssion *attr.*; ~ое вознагражде́ние commíssion; ~ магази́н sécond-hand shop; 2. *в знач. сущ. мн.* commíssion *sg.*

коми́сси|я *ж.* 1. (*орган*) commíttee; (*временная*) commíssion; парла́ментская ~ parliaméntary commíttee; прави́тельственная ~ góvernment commíssion; экзаменацио́нная ~ board of exáminers; 2. (*поручение*) commíssion; брать на ~ю *что-л.* accépt *smth.* for sale on a commíssion básis, táke on commíssion.

комите́т *м.* commíttee; исполни́тельный ~ exécutive commíttee.

коми́ческий cómic; ◇ ~ актёр cómic áctor, comédian.

коми́чный cómical.

ко́мкать, ско́мкать (*вн.*) (*мять*) crúmple (*smth.*); *перен. разг.* húrry/rush through (with), cut* (*smth.*) short.

коммент|а́рий *м.* 1. cómmentary, explánatory note; 2. *мн.* (*рассуждения*) cómments; ◇ ~а́рии изли́шни it speaks for itsélf, no cómment néeded. ~а́тор *м.* cómmentator. ~и́ровать *несов. и сов.* (*сов. тж.* прокоммент́ровать) (*вн.*) 1. (*текст, книгу*) ánnotate (*smth.*); 2. (*толковать*) cómment (on).

коммерса́нт *м.* mérchant, búsiness man*.

комме́р|ция *ж.* cómmerce, trade. ~ческий commércial; ◇ ~ческий дире́ктор finánсial/commércial mánager.

комму́на *ж.* cómmune; ◇ Пари́жская ~ the Páris Cómmune.

коммуна́льн|ый 1. (*общественный*) cómmunal; 2. (*связанный с городским хозяйством*) muní cipal; ~ые услу́ги públic utílities; ~ое хозя́йство muní cipal sérvices *pl.*

коммуна́р *м. ист.* Cómmunard.

коммуни́зм *м.* cómmunism.

коммуника́бельн|ость *ж.* appróachability, sociabílity. ~ый appróachable, sóciable.

коммуникацио́нн|ый: ~ая ли́ния line of communicátion.

коммуника́ция *ж.* communicátion; *воен. тж.* line of communicátion.

коммуни́ст *м.* cómmunist.

коммунисти́ческ|ий cómmunist; ~ая па́ртия Cómmunist Párty.

коммута́тор *м.* 1. (*телефонный*) swítchboard; 2. (*переключатель тока*) cómmutator.

коммюнике́ *с. нескл.* communiqué.

ко́мнат|а *ж.* room; кварти́ра из трёх ко́мнат thrée-room flat; ◇ ~ ма́тери и ребёнка mothers' room. ~ный: ~ное расте́ние índoor plant; ~ная соба́ка láp-dog; ~ная температу́ра room témperature.

комо́д *м.* chest of drawers.

комо́к *м.* lump; ◇ ~ не́рвов a búndle of nerves; ~ в го́рле a lump in one's throat.

компа́ктдиск *м.* (*компа́ктный диск*) compáct disc.

компа́ктн|ость *ж.* compáctness. ~ый compáct.

компане́йский *разг.* sóciable, companionable.

компа́ни|я *ж.* 1. (*о людях*) cómpany, párty; соста́вьте нам ~ю won't you join us?; keep us cómpany; не ~ кому́-л. по cómpany for *smb.*; 2. (*торговое или промышленное товарищество*) cómpany, corporátion; ◇ за ~ю to be sóciable; for cómpany('s) sake; води́ть ~ю с кем-л. assóciate with *smb.*; поддержа́ть ~ю join in.

компаньо́н *м.* 1. (*сотоварищ*) compánion; 2. (*член торговой или промышленной компании*) pártner.

компа́ртия *ж.* Cómmunist Párty.

ко́мпас *м.* cómpass.

компенс|а́ция *ж.* compensátion. ~и́ровать *несов. и сов.* (*вн.*) cómpensate (*smth.*)

компете́нтн|ость *ж.* cómpetence, authórity. ~ый cómpetent, authóritative.

компете́нци|я *ж.* cómpetence; (*круг полномочий тж.*) jurisdíction; входи́ть в чью-л. ~ю be* within *smb.'s* cómpetence; вне (*сферы*) чьей-л. ~и óutside *smb.'s* cómpetence; вне ~и суда́ beyónd the court's jurisdíction.

компил|и́ровать *несов.* (*вн.*) compíle (*smth.*). ~я́ция *ж.* compilátion.

ко́мплекс *м.* cómplex, group; архитекту́рный ~ architéctural cómplex. ~ный íntegrated, cómposite; ~ная механиза́ция íntegrated mechanizátion; ~ная экспеди́ция cómposite/combíned expedítion; ~ная брига́да combíned team; ~ное соглаше́ние páckage deal; ~ый обе́д set meal.

компле́кт *м.* 1. (*набор предметов*) set; ~ белья́ set of únderwear; ~ инструме́нтов set of tools, tóol-kit; 2. (*предельное число лиц*) full cómplement; сверх ~а éxtra. ~ный compléte.

комплекто́в|а́ние *с.* 1. collécting, máking up ínto sets; 2. (*дополнение до комплекта*) máking up, compléting; (*кадров и т. п.*) brínging up to strength. ~а́ть *несов.* (*вн.*) 1. make* (*smth.*) up ínto sets; 2. (*дополнять до комплекта*) make* up (*smth.*), compléte (*smth.*); (*кадры и т. п.*) make* (*smth.*) up to strength; ~а́ть библиоте́ку colléct a library; make* up (the míssing vólumes in) a líbrary; ~а́ть полк bring* a régiment up to strength.

компле́кция *ж.* build, constitútion.

комплиме́нт *м.* cómpliment; сказа́ть ~ pay* a cómpliment; напра́шиваться на ~ fish for cómpliments.

компо́зер *м.* compóser.

композ́тор *м.* compóser.

композ|ицио́нный compositíonal. ~и́ция *ж.* composítion.

компоне́нт *м.* compónent.

компон|ова́ть, скомпонова́ть (*вн.*) make* up (*smth.*). ~о́вка *ж.* arrángement; (*способ, метод тж.*) máke-up.

компо́ст *м. с.-х.* cómpost.

компости́ровать, прокомпости́ровать (*вн.*) date (*smth.*); ~ биле́т date/punch a ticket.

компо́т *м.* (*из варёных фруктов*) stewed fruit; (*из консерви́рованных фруктов*) fruit salad.

компре́сс *м.* cómpress.

компре́ссор *м.* compréssor, blówer. ~ный compréssor *attr.*

компромети́ровать, скомпромети́ровать (*вн.*) cómpromise (*smb.*).

компроми́сс *м.* cómpromise; пойти́ на ~ make* a cómpromise. ~ный cómpromise *attr.*; ~ное реше́ние, соглаше́ние cómpromise agréement.

компью́тер *м.* compúter; персона́льный ~ pérsonal compúter. ~иза́ция *ж.* computerizátion.

комсомо́л *м.* the Kómsomol, the Young Cómmunist League. ~ец *м.*, ~ка *ж.* mémber of the Kómsomol, mémber of the Young Cómmunist League, YCLer. ~ьский Kómsomol *attr.*

комсо́рг *м.* (*комсомо́льский организа́тор*) Kómsomol órganizer.

кому́ (*дт. от мест.* кто) to whom, who to.

комфо́рт *м.* cómfort.

комфорта́бельн|ый cómfortable; ~ое кре́сло cósy ármchair; ~ая кварти́ра cómfortable flat, well-appóinted flat.

конве́йер *м.* convéyor; ~ом, по ~у by convéyor, on the convéyor belt. ~ный convéyor *attr.*; ~ная систе́ма convéyor sýstem.

конве́нци|я *ж.* convéntion; подписа́ть ~ю sign a convéntion.

конве́рсия *ж.* фин. convérsion.

конве́рт *м.* énvelope, cóver.

конверти́р|овать *несов. и сов.фин.* convért. ~уемый convértible; ~уемая валю́та convértible/hard cúrrency.

конво́ир *м.* éscort. ~овать *несов.* (*вн.*) escórt (*smb., smth.*); (*о корабля́х и т. п. тж.*) cónvoy (*smth.*).

конво́й *м.* éscort. ~ный *прил.* 1. éscort *attr.*; ~ное су́дно éscort ship; 2. *в знач. сущ. м.* éscort.

конвульси́вный convúlsive.

конву́льсия *ж.* convúlsion.

конгре́сс *м.* 1. cóngress; Всеми́рный ~ сторо́нников ми́ра World Peace Cóngress; 2. (*законода́тельный о́рган в США*) Cóngress.

конгрессме́н *м.* Cóngressman*.

конденс|а́тор *м.* condénser. ~а́ция *ж.* condensа́tion. ~и́ровать *несов. и сов.* (*вн.*) condénse (*smth.*).

конди́тер *м.* conféctioner. ~ская *ж.* conféctioner's (shop). ~ский: ~ские изде́лия conféctionery *sg*; ~ская фа́брика conféctionery.

кондиционе́р *м.* áir-conditioner.

кондициони́ров|ание *с.:* ~ание во́здуха áir-conditioning. ~ать *несов. и сов.* (*вн.*) condítion (*smth.*).

конду́ктор *м.* ж.-д. guard; (*в городско́м тра́нспорте*) condúctor's.

коневóд *м.* hórse-breeder. ~ство *с.* hórse-breeding. ~ческий hórse-breeding *attr.*; ~ческая фе́рма stud farm.

конёк I *м.* 1. (*излюбленный предмет разговоров*) pet súbject, hóbby-horse; 2. (*крыши*) ridge; ◇ сесть на своего́ конька́ be*/get* on one's pet súbject.

конёк II *м. см.* коньки́.

кон|е́ц *м.* 1. end; подходи́ть к ~цу́ draw* to its close, come* to an end; день бли́зится к ~цу́ the day is dráwing* to its close; в ~це сороковы́х и т. п. годо́в in the late fórties *etc.*; 2. (*смерть, кончина*) end; ему́ прихо́дит ~ his end is appróaching; 3. (*расстояние*) way; в о́ба ~ца́ there and back; де́лать больши́е ~цы́ cóver great dístances; 4. *мор.* rope's end; ◇ до ~ца́ to the end/last; без ~ца́ éndlessly; говори́ть без ~ца́ speak* without stópping; по ~ца́ towards the end; в ~це́ ~цо́в áfter all; всё равно́ оди́н ~! it all comes to the same thing in the end; взя́ться не с того́ ~ца́ have* got the wrong end of the stick, begín*/start at the wrong end; не знать, с

какого́ ~ца́ нача́ть not know where to begín; со всех ~цо́в from évery quárter; из ~ца́ в ~ from one end to the óther; во все ~цы́ in all diréctions; и ~цы́ в во́ду and nóbody was (will be) a pénny the wíser; ~ца́-кра́ю нет there is no end to it; па́лка о двух ~ца́х sómething that cuts both ways, a dóuble-édged wéapon.

коне́чно 1. *вводн. сл.* of course, náturally; он, ~, прав he is right, of course; 2. *утверд.* of course; cértainly; мо́жно мне войти́? — ~! may I come in? Why, of course!

коне́чности *мн.* (*ед.* коне́чность *ж.*) limbs, extrémities; ни́жние (ве́рхние) ~ lówer (úpper) limbs.

коне́чн|ый 1. (*находя́щийся в конце́*) end *attr.*, last; ~ая остано́вка the last stop; ~ая ста́нция términus; 2. (*оконча́тельный, заверша́ющий*) final, últimate; ~ая цель últimate aim, final goal; ◇ ~ая величина́ *мат.* finite quántity.

кони́на *ж.* hórse-flesh.

кони́ческий cónic(al).

конкретизи́ровать *несов. и сов.* (*вн.*) cóncretize (*smth.*), rénder (*smth.*) cóncrete.

конкре́тн|ость *ж.* cóncreteness, solídity, súbstance; ~ руково́дства efféctive léadership. ~ый cóncrete, specífic; ~ая цель specífic aim; ~ое предложе́ние cóncrete propósal.

конкуре́н|т *м.* compétitor, rival. ~ция *ж.* (márket) competítion; ◇ вне ~ции beyónd compáre, unrívalled.

конкури́ровать *несов.* (*с тв. в пр.*) compéte (with *smb.* in).

ко́нкурс *м.* competítion; ~ на лу́чшую пье́су competítion for the best play; быть при́нятым в университе́т по ~у be* admítted to the univérsity by compétitive examinátion; замеща́ть до́лжность по ~у fill a post by о́pen competítion. ~ный compétitive; ~ный экза́мен compétitive examinátion.

ко́нн|ик *м.* cávalryman*. ~ица *ж.* cávalry.

ко́нн|ый 1. horse *attr.*; ~ая тя́га horse tráction; 2. (*состоя́щий из вса́дников*) móunted; ~ая мили́ция móunted milítia; ◇ ~ый заво́д stud (farm).

ко́новязь *ж.* 1. téthering post/rail; 2. (*верёвка для спутывания лошади*) hóbble.

конокра́д *м.* hórse-thief*, hórse-stealer. ~ство *с.* hórse-stealing.

конопа́тить *несов.* (*вн.*) caulk (*smth.*)

конопля́ *ж.* hemp.

конопля́нка *ж. зоол.* línnet.

конопля́н|ый: ~ое ма́сло hémp-seed oil.

коносаме́нт *м. торг.* bill of láding.

консерват|и́вный consérvative. ~и́зм *м.* consérvatism.

консерва́тор *м.* 1. consérvative; 2. (*член па́ртии консерва́торов*) tóry, consérvative.

консервато́рия *ж.* conservatóire, consérvatory.

консерви́рованный tinned, préserved.

консерви́ровать *несов. и сов.* (*вн.*) 1. presérve (*smth.*); 2. (*предприя́тие и т. п.*) témporarily close (*smth.*); móth-ball (*smth.*).

консе́рвн|ый: ~ая ба́нка tin; can *амер.*; ~ нож tín-opener; can píercer *амер.*; ~ая фа́брика cánnery.

консе́рвы *мн.* tinned foods; canned foods *амер.*; мясны́е, овощны́е, ры́бные ~ tinned/canned meat, végetables, fish.

конси́лиум *м.* consultátion.

консисте́нция *ж.* consístency.

ко́нский horse *attr.*

консолид|а́ция *ж.* consolidátion. ~и́ровать *несов. и сов.* (*вн.*) consólidate (*smth.*).

консо́ль 1. *ж. архит.* córbel; cónsole; 2. *ж. эл.* cónsole, contról pánel; 3. *м. тех.* cántilever.

конспе́кт *м.* synópsis (*pl* -ses), précis, ábstract. ~и́вный concíse, brief. ~и́ровать, проконспекти́ровать (*вн.*) súmmarize (*smth.*), make* a súmmary/ábstract (of).

конспир|ати́вный sécret; ~ати́вная кварти́ра sécret addréss. ~а́тор м. conspírator. ~а́ция ж. sécrecy.

конста́нта ж. мат., физ. cónstant.

констат|а́ция ж. státement. ~и́ровать несов. и сов. (вн.) estáblish (smth.), ascertáin (smth.); (отмечать) note (smth.); ~и́ровать смерть cértify death; ~и́ровать факт estáblish/ascertáin a fact.

конституцио́нный constitútional.

конститу́ция ж. 1. (основной закон) constitútion; 2. (строение организма) constitútion, phýsical máke-up.

констру́и́ровать, сконстру́и́ровать (вн.) 1. (проектировать) design (smth.); 2. (учреждать) órganize (smth.), form (smth.).

констру́кти́вн|ый constrúctive; ~ое предложе́ние constrúctive suggéstion.

констру́ктор м. 1. desígner; 2. (детская игра) meccáno. ~ский: ~ское бюро́ desígners' óffice.

констру́кция ж. 1. (взаимное расположение частей сооружения и т. п.) desígn; 2. (сооружение) strúcture; 3. грам. constrúction.

ко́нсул м. cónsul.

ко́нсуль|ский cónsular; ~ская конве́нция the Cónsular Convéntion. ~ство с. cónsulate; генера́льное ~ство cónsulate-géneral.

консульт|а́нт м. consúltant; (врач тж.) consúlting physician. ~а́ция ж. 1. (совет специалиста) éxpert opínion. 2. (помощь преподавателя учащимся) pérsonal tuítion; 3. (учреждение): де́тская ~а́ция ínfant wélfare céntre; же́нская ~а́ция matérnity advíce buréau. ~и́ровать, проконсульти́ровать (вн.; давать советы) advíse (smb.), give* (smb.) advíce. ~и́роваться, проконсульти́роваться (с тв.) consúlt (smb.), ask smb.'s advíce.

конта́кт м. 1. cóntact; вступа́ть в ~ с кем-л. come* ínto cóntact with smb., get* in touch with smb.; устана́вливать ~ с кем-л. estáblish cóntact with smb.; ли́чные ~ы pérsonal cóntacts; 2. тех. cóntact.

конте́йнер м. contáiner.

конте́кст м. cóntext; ◇ вы́рвать что-л. из ~а wrench smth. out of its cóntext.

континге́нт м. 1. (группа, категория) contíngent, batch; 2. (определённое количество) quóta.

контине́нт м. cóntinent. ~а́льный continéntal; ◇ ~а́льный кли́мат continéntal clímate.

конто́р|а ж. óffice. ~ский óffice attr.; ~ское помеще́ние óffice prémises pl.

контраба́нд|а ж. 1. (занятие) smúggling; занима́ться ~ой smúggle; 2. собир. (предметы) cóntraband. ~и́ст м. smúggler, cóntrabandist. ~и́стский smúggler's. ~ный cóntraband attr.; перен. illégal; ~ный ввоз illégal ímport; ~ные това́ры cóntraband, smúggled goods.

контраба́с м. муз. double-báss.

контраге́нт м. contráctor.

контр-адмира́л м. rear ádmiral.

контра́кт м. cóntract; заключа́ть ~ sign a cóntract, énter ínto a contract. ~а́ция ж. contrácting. ~ова́ть несов. (вн.) contráct (for).

контра́льто с. нескл. contrálto.

контрама́рка ж. free pass, compliméntary tícket.

контра́ст м. cóntrast. ~и́ровать несов. (с тв.) contrást (with). ~ный 1. contrásting; 2. фото cóntrast attr.

контрата́к|а ж. cóunter-attack; предприня́ть, произвести́ ~у deliver a cóunter-attack. ~ова́ть несов. и сов. (вн.) cóunter-attack (smb., smth.).

контргайка ж. тех. lóck-nut.

контрибу́ци|я ж. 1. (по мирному договору) indémnity; 2. (принудительный побор с населения) contribútion; наложи́ть ~ю impóse/lévy a contribútion.

контрнаступле́ние с. воен. cóunter-offensive; перейти́ в ~ launch a cóunter-offensive.

контролёр м. 1. (на производстве) exáminer, inspéctor; фина́нсовый ~ áuditor; 2. (билетный) tícket-colléctor, inspéctor.

контроли́ровать, проконтроли́ровать (вн.) check (smb., smth.); ~ чью-л. рабо́ту check smb.'s work; ~ отчётность check accóunts.

контро́л|ь м. 1. contról, chécking; взять что-л. под ~ set* up contról óver smth., put* smth. únder contról; ~ рублём contról by the róuble, fináncial contról; 2. (учреждение) Contról; госуда́рственный ~ State Contról; отде́л техни́ческого ~я chécking/exámining depártment; 3. собир. (контролёры) inspéctors pl.

контро́льн|ый 1. (осуществляющий контроль) contról attr.; inspéction attr.; 2. (служащий для контроля) test attr.; check attr.; ◇ ~ые ци́фры éstimated/schéduled fígures.

контрразве́д|ка ж. cóunter-intelligence, cóunter-espionage; secúrity sérvice. ~чик м. cóunter-intelligence ágent; secúrity man*.

контрреволюц|ионе́р м. cóunter-revolutionary. ~ио́нный cóunter-revolutionary.

контрреволю́ция ж. cóunter-revolution.

контруда́р м. cóunter-stroke.

конту́женный contúsed; (при разрыве снаряда) shéll-shocked.

конту́з|ить сов. (вн.) contúse (smth.); (при разрыве снаряда) shéll-shock (smth.). ~ия ж. contúsion; (при разрыве снаряда) shéll-shock; (сотрясение) concússion.

конту́р м. 1. óutline; мн. тж. cóntours; 2. эл. círcuit, loop. ~ный óutline attr., cóntour attr.; ◇ ~ная ка́рта óutline-map, skéleton-map.

конура́ ж. kénnel (тж. перен.); dóg-house амер.

ко́нус м. cone.

конфедерати́вный conféderative.

конфедера́ция ж. confederátion.

конферансье́ м. нескл. máster of céremonies, compère.

конфере́нц-зал м. cónference hall.

конфере́нция ж. cónference; ми́рная ~ peace cónference.

конфе́т|а ж. sweet; cándy амер. ~ный sweet attr.; cándy attr. амер.; перен. (слащавый) chócolate-box attr.

конфетти́ с. нескл. confétti.

конфигура́ция ж. configurátion; ~ ме́стности configurátion of the ground.

конфиденциа́льн|о in cónfidence, confidéntially. ~ый confidéntial.

конфиск|а́ция ж. confiscátion. ~ова́ть несов. и сов. (вн.) cónfiscate.

конфли́кт м. cónflict. ~ный: ~ная коми́ссия dísputes committee. ~ова́ть несов. и сов. разг. (с тв.) clash (with).

конфо́рка ж. (cóoking-)ring; га́зовая ~ gás-ring.

конформи́зм м. confórmism.

конфронта́ция ж. confrontátion.

конфу́з м. embárrassment; како́й ~! how embárrassing! ~ить, сконфу́зить (вн.) embárrass (smb.). ~иться, сконфу́зиться be* embárrassed; (рд.) be* shy (of). ~ливый shy.

концентра́т м. 1. cóncentrated próduct; пищевы́е ~ы food cóncentrates; 2. с.-х. cóncentrate; кормовы́е ~ы cóncentrated feed/fódder sg.

концентрацио́нный: ~ ла́герь concentrátion camp.

концентр|а́ция ж. 1. concentrátion; ~ произво́дства concentrátion of industry; 2. хим. strength. ~и́ровать, сконцентри́ровать (вн.) cóncentrate (smth.). ~и́роваться, сконцентри́роваться cóncentrate.

концентр|и́ческий, ~и́чный concéntric.

конце́пция ж. concéption.

конце́рн м. эк. combinátion.

конце́рт м. 1. cóncert; (одного исполнителя тж.) recítal; 2. (музыкальное произведение) concérto.

концерт|и́ровать *несов.* give* cóncerts. **~ме́йстер** *м.* 1. (*руководитель группы исполнителей в оркестре*) léader; 2. (*аккомпаниатор на репетиции*) accómpanist.

конце́ртный cóncert *attr.*; ~ зал cóncert hall; ◇ ~ роя́ль cóncert grand.

концесси|оне́р *м.* concessionnáire, concéssion-holder. **~о́нный** concéssion *attr.*

конце́ссия *ж.* concéssion.

концо́вка *ж.* 1. *полигр.* (*украшение в книге*) táil-piece; 2. (*заключительная часть*) énding.

конча́ть, ко́нчить 1. (*вн., с тв., + инф.*) fínish (*smth.*, + -ing); ко́нчить ремо́нт fínish the repáir(s); ко́нчить писа́ть, чита́ть кни́гу fínish (wríting, réading) a book; 2. (*вн., тв., на пр.*; *завершать чем-л.*) end (*smth.*, with, by + -ing), conclúde (*smth.*, with, by + -ing); ~ речь призы́вом end *one's* speech with an appéal; 3. (*вн.; высшее учебное заведение*) gráduate (from, at); (*школу, курс и т. п.*) fínish (*smth.*); (*тв.; получать какую-л. квалификацию*) quálify (as); ко́нчить Моско́вский университе́т gráduate from Móscow Univérsity; 4. (*вн., с тв.; прекращать что-л.*) stop (*smth.*); ~ рабо́ту по гудку́ stop wórking at the sound of the hóoter; ◇ ~ самоуби́йством commít súicide. **~ся, ко́нчиться** 1. (*приходить к концу*) come* to an end; be* óver; 2. (*тв.; завершаться*) end (in), resúlt (in); 3. (*умирать*) die.

ко́нчен|о *в знач. сказ. безл.* 1. (*обыкн. с тв.*) *разг.*: бою́сь, что с на́ми ~ I fear it is all up with us; 2. (*довольно, достаточно*) that'll do!; ◇ всё ~! it's all óver! **~ый** *разг.* fínished; ◇ ~ый челове́к fáilure, álso-ran, nó-good.

ко́нчик *м.* tip; (*острие*) point; ~и па́льцев finger-tips; ~ языка́ tip of *one's* tongue.

кончи́на *ж.* death, pássing, decéase.

ко́нчить(ся) *сов. см.* конча́ть(ся).

конъюнктиви́т *м. мед.* conjunctivítis.

конъюнкту́р|а *ж.* situátion; *эк. тж.* conjúncture, state of the márket. **~ный** marketéering; **~ные** це́ны prices at a gíven móment; принципиа́льная поли́тика вме́сто ~ных реше́ний a príncipled pólicy instéad of ad hoc decísions. **~щик** *м. разг.* trímmer, ópportunist.

кон|ь *м.* 1. horse; *поэт.* steed, chárger; 2. (*в шахматах*) knight; 3. *спорт.* (*váulting*) horse; ◇ не в ~я́ корм wásted éffort.

коньки́ *мн.* (*ед.* конёк *м.*) skates; ро́ликовые ~ róller-skates.

конькобе́ж|ец *м.* skáter. **~ный** skáting; **~ный** спорт skáting.

конья́к *м.* cógnac, brándy.

ко́нюх *м.* groom, stábleman*.

коню́шня *ж.* stáble.

коoperatíв *м.* 1. co-óperative, co-óperative society; жили́щный ~ housing co-óperative; 2. *разг.* (*магазин*) co-óperative store. **~ный** co-óperative.

коопер|а́тор *м.* co-óperative official; employée of a co-óperative. **~а́ция** *ж.* 1. (*форма организации труда*) co-operátion; 2. (*производственное, торговое и т. п. объединение*) co-óperative; потреби́тельская ~а́ция consúmers' co-óperative; сельскохозя́йственная ~а́ция agricúltural co-óperative organizánions *pl.*

коопери́ров|ать *несов. и сов.* (*вн.*) draw* (*smth.*) into co-óperative organizátions. **~аться** *несов. и сов.* co-óperate, form a co-óperative.

коопт|а́ция *ж.* co-optátion. **~и́ровать** *несов. и сов.* (*вн.*) co-ópt (*smth.*).

координа́тный co-órdinate.

координа́ты *мн.* 1. (*ед.* координа́та *ж.*) co-órdinates; 2. *разг.* (*местонахождение*) whéreabouts.

координ|а́ция *ж.* co-ordinátion. **~и́ровать** *несов. и сов.* (*вн.*) co-órdinate (*smth.*).

копа́ть *несов.* (*вн.*) 1. dig* (*smth.*); ~ зе́млю dig* the earth/ground; 2. (*выкапывать*) dig* up (*smth.*); ~

карто́фель dig* up potátoes. **~ся** *несов.* 1. (*в пр.*): ры́ться) dig* (*smth.*); *перен.* (*ворошить*) rúmmage (in); 2. (*тщательно разбираться*) probe (into); ~ в душе́ ánalyse *one's* féelings, indúlge in sélf-análysis; 3. *разг.* (*мешкать*) dáwdle; ве́чно он копа́ется! he's such a dáwdler!; что ты там копа́ешься? what are you dáwdling óver?

копе́еч|ка *ж.*: стать, обойти́сь в ~ку cost* one a prétty pénny. **~ный** cópeck *attr.*; (*недорогой*) cheap; *перен.* pétty; **~ный** расхо́д trífling expénse; **~ые** счёты pétty calculátions.

копе́йк|а *ж.* 1. cópeck; 2. *собир. разг.* (*денежные средства*) funds *pl*, purse; бере́чь наро́дную ~у guard the públic purse; ◇ ~ в ~у exáctly; до (*после́дней*) ~и to the last fárthing; без ~и pénniless; дрожа́ть над ка́ждой ~ой grudge évery pénny.

ко́пи *мн.* (*ед.* копь *ж.*) mines; соляны́е ~ (róck-)salt mines.

копи́лка *ж.* móney-box.

копи́рк|а *ж. разг.* cárbon-paper; писа́ть под ~у make* cárbon cópies.

копирова́льн|ый cópying; ~ аппара́т cópying device/machine, dúplicator; **~ая** бума́га cárbon-paper.

копи́ровать, скопи́ровать (*вн.*) cópy (*smth.*); (*подражать тж.*) ímitate (*smb., smth.*)

копиро́в|ка *ж. разг.* cópying. **~щик** *м.* cópyist.

копи́ть *несов.* (*вн.*) save up (*smth.*), accúmulate (*smth.*); *перен.* build* up (*smth.*); ~ де́ньги save up; ~ си́лы build* up *one's* strength.

ко́пи|я *ж.* 1. cópy; снима́ть ~ю с чего-л. make*/take* a cópy of *smth.*; 2. *разг.* (*о ком-л. похожем*) the ímage; он то́чная ~ своего́ отца́ he's the (líving/spítting) ímage of his fáther.

копн|а́ *ж.*: ~ се́на háycock; ~ снопо́в shock; ◇ ~ воло́с shock of hair. **~и́тель** *м. с.-х.* shócker. **~и́ть** *несов.* (*вн.*) *с.-х.* shock (*smth.*).

ко́поть *ж.* soot.

копоши́ться *несов.* 1. stir; (*о насекомых*) crawl abóut; 2. *разг.* (*возиться*) pótter abóut.

копте́ть *несов.* smoke.

копти́лка *ж.* wick light.

копти́льная *ж.* smóke-house, cúring-house.

копти́ть *несов.* 1. (*испускать копоть*) smoke; 2. (*вн.; покрывать копотью*) make* (*smth.*) black/smóky; 3. (*вн.; рыбу и т. п.*) smoke (*smth.*), cure (*smth.*).

копче́ние *с.* smóking, cúring.

копчён|ости *мн.* (*ед.* копчёность *ж.*) smoked próducts. **~ый** smoked; **~ая** сельдь smoked hérring.

ко́пчик *м. анат.* cóccyx.

копы́тный *прил.* 1. hoof *attr.*; 2. *в знач. сущ. мн. зоол.* hoofed ánimals, úngulates.

копы́то *с.* hoof*.

копьё *с.* spear; ◇ не сто́ит из-за э́того копья́ лома́ть it's not worth máking an issue out of it.

кора́ *ж.* 1. (*древесная*) bark; 2. (*корка*) crust; ◇ ~ головно́го мо́зга córtex; земна́я ~ *геол.* the earth's crust.

корабе́л *м.* shípbuilder.

корабе́льн|ый ship *attr.*, ship's; **~ая** верфь shípyard; ◇ ~ лес shíp-timber.

корабле|вожде́ние *с.* navigátion. **~круше́ние** *с.* shípwreck. **~строе́ние** *с.* shípbuilding. **~строи́тель** *с.* shípbuilder; (*конструктор тж.*) nával árchitect. **~строи́тельный** shípbuilding *attr.*

корабл|ь *м.* 1. ship; на ~е on board (ship); лине́йный ~ báttleship; вое́нный ~ wárship; ~ на подво́дных кры́льях (*pássenger-cárrying*) hýdroplane; 2. (*летательный аппарат*) ship, véhicle; косми́ческий ~ spácecraft, spáceship.

кора́бль-спу́тник *м.* órbital spácecraft.

кора́лл *м.* córal. **~овый** córal *attr.*; **~овый** риф córal reef.

Кора́н *м. рел.* the Kóran.

корвёт *м.* *мор.* corvétte.

кордебалёт *м.* *театр.* corps de ballét.

кордóн *м.* 1. (*заградительный отряд*) córdon; 2. (*местопребывание охраны*) (guárd-)post, cómpound; 3. (*граница*) bórder.

корéец *м.* Koréan.

корéйский Koréan; ~ язы́к Koréan, the Koréan lánguage.

коренáстый thicksét, stócky.

корени́ться *несов.* (в *пр.*) be* róoted (in).

коренн|óй 1. (*основной*, *постоянный*) nátive; indígenous; ~ москви́ч nátive of Móscow; ~óе населéние the nátive populátion; 2. (*существенный*) fundaméntal, rádical; ~ вопрóс fundaméntal próblem; ~ые вопрóсы совремéнности fundaméntal íssues of the présent day; ◇ ~ зуб mólar (tooth*); ~ая лóшадь sháft-horse; ~ы́м óбразом rádically.

кор|éнь *м.* root; ◇ вырывáть *что-л.* с ~нем erádicate *smth.*, root out *smth.*; в ~не пресéчь *что-л.* nip *smth.* in the bud; пусти́ть (глубóкие) ~ни strike*/take* (deep) root; измени́ть *что-л.* в ~не change *smth.* rádically; смотрéть в ~ look belów the súrface, get* to the root of things; хлеб на ~ню́ stánding crops *pl.*

корéнья *мн.* *кул.* cúlinary roots.

корешóк *м.* 1. (*корень*) róotlet; 2. (*переплёта*) back; 3. (*квитанции*) cóunterfoil.

кореянка *ж.* Koréan wóman*.

кóржик *м.* shórtbread.

корзи́на *ж.* básket; (*с крышкой*) hámper; бельевáя ~ línen/láundry básket; ~ для бумáги wáste-paper básket; wáste-basket *амер.*

коридóр *м.* córridor, pássage. ~ный *прил.* 1. córridor *attr.*; 2. *в знач. сущ.* *м.* flóor-attendant.

кори́нка *ж.* cúrrants *pl.*

кори́ть *несов.* (*вн.* за *вн.*) *разг.* (*упрекать*) repróach (*smb.* for).

корифéй *м.* lúminary, léading light; ~ нау́ки lúminary of science.

кори́ца *ж.* cínnamon.

кори́чневый brown.

кóрк|а *ж.* 1. (*твёрдый слой*) crust; ~ хлéба crust of bread; ~ сы́ра chéese-rind; 2. (*плода*) rind, peel; апельси́нная ~ órange peel; арбу́зная ~ wáter-melon rind; ◇ от ~и до ~и from cóver to cóver.

корм *м.* feed; (*сухой*) fódder; грубы́е ~á roughage *sg;* сóчные ~á súcculent fódder *sg.*

кормá *ж.* *мор.* stern.

кормёжка *ж.* *разг.* féeding.

корми́л|ец *м.* (*семьи*) bréad-winner. ~ица *ж.* 1. (*няня*) wét-nurse; fóster-mother; 2. (*семьи*) bréad--winner.

корми́л|о *с.:* стоя́ть у ~а влáсти, правлéния be* at the helm (of State).

корми́ть, **накорми́ть** (*вн.*) 1. feed* (*smb.*, *smth.*); 2. (*ребёнка*, *детёныша своим молоком*) súckle (*smb.*, *smth.*); (*ребёнка тж.*) nurse (*smb.*); 3. *тк.* *несов.* (*содержать*) keep* (*smb.*, *smth.*); ~ обещáниями keep* prómising. ~ся *несов.* 1. feed*, eat*; (*пастись*) graze; 2. (*тв.*) live (on); ~ся свои́м трудóм keep* onesélf, live by one's work.

кормлéние *с.* 1. féeding; 2. (*своим молоком*) suckling; núrsing.

кормов|óй I fódder *attr.*; ~ые трáвы fódder grass *sg;* ◇ ~áя бáза fódder supply.

кормов|óй II *мор.* stern *attr.*, áfter; ~óе веслó steering oar; ~áя часть áfter-body.

корму́шка *ж.* féeding trough; (*для сена*) mánger; (*для птицы*) séed-can.

кóрмчий *м.* hélmsman*.

корневи́ще *с.* róotstock, rhízome.

корневóй root *attr.*

корнеплóды *мн.* (*ед.* корнеплóд *м.*) édible roots, root crops.

корнишóн *м.* ghérkin.

кóроб *м.* básket, hámper; ◇ цéлый ~ новостéй a búdget of news; наговори́ть с три ~а talk ninetéen to the dózen.

корóб|ить, **покорóбить** (*вн.*) warp (*smth.*); *перен.* grate (on); меня́ ~ит егó неи́скренность, меня́ ~ит от егó неи́скренности his insincérity grates on me. ~иться, покорóбиться 1. warp; 2. (*об одежде и т. п.*) curl.

корóбка *ж.* 1. box; 2. (*остов здания*) frame; 3.: двернáя ~ dóor-frame; ◇ ~ передáч, скоростéй *тех.* géar-box.

коробóк *м.* box; ~ спи́чек box of mátches.

корóва *ж.* cow.

корóв|ий cow *attr.*, cow's; ~ье мáсло bútter. ~ка *ж.:* бóжья ~ка ládybird. ~ник *м.* ców-house, býre.

королéв|а *ж.* queen. ~ский róyal. ~ство *с.* kíngdom.

королёк *м.* 1. (*птица*) kínglet, gólden-crested wren; 2. (*апельсин*) blood órange.

корóль *м.* king.

коромы́сло *с.* 1. (*для вёдер*) yoke; 2. (*весов*) beam; 3. *тех.* rócker.

корóн|а *ж.* 1. crown; 2. *астр.* coróna; сóлнечная ~ coróna. ~áция *ж.* coronátion.

корóнк|а *ж.* 1. (*зуба*) crown; постáвить ~у crown a tooth*; 2. (*бура*) bit.

коронн|ый crown *attr.*; ◇ ~ нóмер star turn/perfórmance; ~ая роль best part.

коронов|áние *с.* *см.* коронáция. ~áть *несов. и сов.* (*вн.*) crown (*smth.*). ~áться *несов. и сов.* be* crowned.

коростéль *м.* lándrail, córn-crake.

коротáть *несов.* coróntáть: ~ врéмя while awáy the time.

корóтк|ий 1. short; (*непродолжительный тж.*) brief; 2. (*близкий*, *дружественный*) íntimate; ~ое знакóмство íntimate fríendship; 3. (*быстрый*, *решительный*) quick, sharp; ~ая распрáва short shrift; у негó распрáва ~á he will show no mércy; ◇ ~ая волнá short wave; ~ая пáмять short/bad mémory; быть на ~ой ногé с кем-л. be* on íntimate/good terms with *smb.*; ру́ки корóтки у кого-л. *smb.* hásn't got the pówer.

корóтко 1. short; ~ остри́женный close-crópped; 2. (*вкратце*) bríefly; ~ говоря́ to put it bríefly; ~ и я́сно! pláinly; withóut mákíng ány bones abóut it; 3. (*близко*) íntimately.

коротковолнóвый *радио* shórt-wave *attr.*; ~ передáтчик shórt-wave transmítter.

короткометрáжный short; ~ фильм short (film).

коротконóгий short-légged, stúmpy.

короткохвóстый short-táiled.

короткошёрст(н)ый short-háired.

корóче (*сравнит. ст. прил.* корóткий *и нареч.* корóтко) shórter; говори́те ~ be as brief as póssible; ◇ ~ говоря́ to be brief, in short.

корпéть *несов.* (*над тв.*) *разг.* drudge (at), plod awáy (at).

корпорáция *ж.* corporátion.

кóрпус *м.* 1. (*мн.* ~ы) (*туловище*) trunk, tórso; держи́те ~ прямо! the trunk úpright!; подáться всем ~ом вперёд lean forward; прийти́ к фи́нишу на два ~а вперёд (*о лошади*) win* by two lengths; 2. (*мн.* ~á) (*оболочка механизмов*, *приборов и т. п.*) bódy, móunting, frame; 3. (*мн.* ~á) (*судна*, *танка*) hull; 4. (*мн.* ~á) (*здание*) block; глáвный ~ the main building; 5. (*мн.* ~á) *воен.* corps*; 6. *тк. ед.* (*совокупность лиц одной профессии и т. п.*) corps*; корреспондéнтский ~ press corps*.

корректи́в *м.* corréction, améndment; внести́ ~ы во *что-л.* aménd *smth.*

корректи́ров|ание *с.* 1. corréction; ~ стрельбы́ adjústment of fire, spótting; 2. (*исправление ошибок в корректуре*) próof-reading. ~ать, прокорректи́ровать (*вн.*) 1. corréct (*smth.*); ~ать стрельбу́ adjúst the fire, spot for the guns; 2. (*исправлять ошибки в корректуре*) read* the proofs.

корре́ктн|ость *ж.* corréctness, propríety. ~ый corréct, próper.

корре́кт|ор *м.* próof-reader. ~у́ра *ж.* 1. (*исправление ошибок*) corréction; 2. (*гранки*) proofs *pl.*

корреспонд|е́нт *м.* correspóndent; (*журналист тж.*) néwspaper man*, repórter; специа́льный ~ spécial correspóndent; ◇ член-корреспонде́нт correspónding mémber. ~е́нтский *attr.*, correspóndent's; ~е́нтское удостовере́ние press card. ~е́нция *ж.* 1. (*переписка*) correspóndence; 2. *собир.* (*почта*) létters *pl*, mail; 3. (*сообщение в газете*) repórt, néws-item.

корро́зия *ж.* corrósion.

коррумпи́рованный corrupt.

корру́пция *ж.* corrúption.

корса́ж *м.* bódice.

корсе́т *м.* 1. stays *pl*, córsets *pl*; 2. (*лечебный*) córset, súrgical bándage.

корт *м. спорт.* (ténnis-)court.

корте́ж *м.* procéssion; (*автомобилей*) mótorcade.

ко́ртик *с.* dirk.

ко́рточк|и *мн.*: присе́сть на ~, сиде́ть на ~ах squat (down).

корчева́ть *несов.* (*вн.*) stub up (*smth.*), grub up (*smth.*)

ко́рчить, ско́рчить 1. *безл.*: его́ ко́рчит от бо́ли he is writhing with pain; 2. *тк. несов.* (*вн; прикидываться кем-л.*) pose as (*smth.*); ~ из себя́ кого́-л. give* onesélf airs. ~ся, ско́рчиться (от *рд.*) writhe (with).

ко́ршун *м.* kite.

коры́стн|ый sélfish; ~ые побужде́ния mércenary/sórdid mótives; ~ челове́к mércenary/sélfish pérson.

корыстолюби́вый mércenary, cóvetous, avarícious.

корыстолю́бие *с.* mércenary spírit, love of gain, cupídity.

коры́сть *ж.* 1. (*выгода*) advántage, prófit; кака́я мне в э́том ~? what good would it do me?, what would I gain by it?; 2. *см.* корыстолю́бие.

коры́т|о *с.* tub; (*как кормушка*) trough; ◇ оста́ться у разби́того ~а be* no bétter off than when *one* stárted, be* back where *one* stárted.

корь *ж. мед.* méasles *pl.*

корю́шка *ж.* (*рыба*) smelt.

коря́вый 1. (*неровный, уродливый — о растениях*) gnarled, twisted, rúgged; 2. (*загрубевший, узловатый — о руках, пальцах*) gnarled; 3. *разг.* (*неумелый, неискусный*) clúmsy; (*о почерке*) crabbed.

коря́га *ж.* snag.

коса́ I *ж.* (*волос*) plait, braid.

коса́ II *ж.* (*с.-х. орудие*) scythe.

коса́ III *ж.* (*мыс*) spit (of land).

коса́рь I *м.* (*косец*) mówer.

коса́рь II *м.* (*нож*) chópper.

ко́свенн|ый indirect; ~ые ули́ки circumstántial/indirect évidence *sg*; ◇ ~ паде́ж *грам.* oblique case; ~ая речь *грам.* indirect/oblique speech.

косе́канс *м. мат.* cosécant.

коси́лка *ж. с.-х.* mówer.

ко́синус *м. мат.* cósine.

коси́ть I, скоси́ть (*вн.; траву*) mow (*smth.*); *перен.* mow down (*smb., smth.*).

коси́ть II, скоси́ть 1. (*вн.; кривить*) twist (*smth.*); ~ рот make* a wry face; 2.: ~ глаза́, глаза́ми squint; 3. (*быть косым*) squint. ~ся, покоси́ться (на *вн.*) 1. squint (at); cast* a sídelong glance (at); 2. *тк. несов. разг.* (*относиться неодобрительно*) take* a dim view (of).

косма́тый shággy.

космет|ика *ж.* 1. (*мероприятия*) béauty tréatment;

2. *собир.* (*средства*) cosmétics *pl.* ~и́ческий cosmétic; ~и́ческое сре́дство cosmétic.

косми́ческ|ий 1. space *attr.*, cósmic; ~ое простра́нство óuter space; ~ полёт space flight; ~ аппара́т space véhicle; ~ие лучи́ cósmic rays; ~ая радиа́ция cósmic radiátion; пе́рвая ~ая ско́рость órbital velócity; втора́я ~ая ско́рость escápe velócity; 2. (*грандиозный*) cósmic, vast.

космого́ния *ж.* cosmógony.

космодро́м *м.* spácedrome, láunching site.

космона́вт *м.* cósmonaut, ástronaut, spáceman*.

космона́втика *ж.* astronáutics, space explorátion.

космона́втка *ж.* spácewoman*.

космополи́т *м.* cosmópolitan, cosmópolite. ~и́зм *м.* cosmópolitanism. ~и́ческий cosmopólitan.

космопсихоло́гия *ж.* space psychólogy.

ко́смос *м.* (óuter) space, the cósmos; покоре́ние, освое́ние ~a space explorátion.

ко́смо|фи́зика *ж.* space phýsics. ≃ хи́мия *ж.* space chémistry, cosmochémistry.

космоце́нтр *м.* space céntre.

ко́смы *мн. разг.* dishévelled locks.

косне́ть *несов.* 1. (*пребывать в состоянии застоя*) stágnate (in); ~ в неве́жестве wállow in ignorance; 2. (*терять гибкость, подвижность*) stíffen.

ко́сность *ж.* inértness, slúggishness, bígotry; (*застой*) stagnátion.

коснояз|ы́ч|ие *с.* inartículateness. ~ный tóngue-tied; (*невнятный — о речи*) inartículate.

косну́ться *сов. см.* каса́ться.

ко́сный inért, slúggish; ~ ум slow/slúggish mind; ~ челове́к bígot.

ко́со oblíquely; смотре́ть ~ look askánce.

косо́бокий lop-síded.

коси́вица *ж.* 1. (*косьба*) mówing; 2. (*время косьбы*) mówing(-time).

косоворо́тка *ж.* blouse (with side cóllar fástening).

косогла́з|ие *с.* squint; strabísmus *научн.* ~ый cróss-éyed.

косого́р *м.* slope.

кос|о́й 1. (*расположенный наклонно*) slánting, oblíque; ~ая черта́ oblíque stroke; ~ дождь driving/slánting rain; ~ по́черк slóping hándwriting; 2. (*искривлённый*) cróoked; ~ плете́нь cróoked fence; ~ пробо́р side párting; 3. (*косоглазый*) cróss-éyed; (*косящий — о глазах*) squínting; он ~ he squints; y него́ ~ глаз he has a squint in one eye; 4. (*недоверчивый, недружелюбный*) scówling; ~ взгляд scowl; ◇ ~ па́рус fóre-and-áft sail; ~ у́гол *мат.* oblíque ángle; ~ая са́жень в плеча́х broad-shóuldered.

косола́пый pígeon-toed, ín-toed; *перен. разг.* (*неуклюжий*) áwkward, clúmsy; ~ медве́дь lúmbering bear.

косоуго́льный *мат.* oblíque-ángled; ~ треуго́льник oblíque tríangle.

костене́ть, окостене́ть 1. (*о трупе*) stíffen; 2. (от *рд.; терять чувствительность*) grow* numb (with); *перен.* be* pétrified (with).

костёр *м.* (cámp-)fire; (*большой*) bónfire.

кост|и́стый, ~ля́вый bóny.

ко́стный ósseous; ~ туберкулёз tubercúlosis of the bones; ◇ ~ мозг *анат.* bone márrow.

ко́сточк|а *ж.* 1. bone; 2. (*плода*) stone; (*мелкая*) pip; ◇ перемыва́ть ~и кому́-л. pick *smb.* to pieces; по ~ам разбира́ть кого́-л., что́-л. dissect *smb., smth.*

косты́л|ь *м.* 1. crutch; ходи́ть на ~я́х go*/walk on crútches; 2. (*гвоздь*) spike.

кост|ь *ж.* 1. bone; 2. *собир.* (*бивни, клыки*) tusks *pl*; слоно́вая ~ ívory; 3. *мн.* (*игральные*) dice, bones; 4. (*шарик на счётах*) bead; ◇ ко́жа да ~и, одни́ ~и nóthing but skin and bones; лечь костьми́ 1) be* killed, lay* down *one's* life; 2) *обыкн. шутл.* kill *oneself*; ~ей не собрáть you'll néver come out alíve!

костю́м *м.* 1. (*одежда*) dress; вечéрний ~ dress suit; космúческий ~ space suit; 2. (*вид одежды*) suit; (*женский тж.*) cóstume.

костюмéр *м.*, ~ша *ж. театр.* costúmier.

костюмирóванный in fáncy dress *после сущ.*; ~ бал fáncy-dress ball.

костя́к *м.* 1. *анат.* skéleton; 2. (*рд.; основа, опора*) báckbone (of), main bódy (of).

костяно́й bone *attr.*; ~ клей bone glue.

костя́шка *ж.* 1. (*на пальцах*) knúckle; 2. (*шарик на счётах*) bead, ball.

косу́ля *ж.* roe deer*.

косы́нка *ж.* (thrée-cornered) scarf, kérchief.

косьба́ *ж.* mówing.

косяк I *м.* (*двери, окна*) jamb; (*двери тж.*) dóor-post.

косяк II *м.* 1. (*лошадей*) herd; 2. (*рыб*) shoal, school; 3. (*птиц*) flock.

кот *м.* tómcat; ◇ не всё ~у́ мáсленица! life ísn't all beer and skíttles!, you can't álways be lúcky!; купúть ~а в мешкé ≈ buy* a pig in a poke.

котáнгенс *м. мат.* cotángent.

кот|ёл *м.* 1. (*кухонный*) large sáucepan, bóiler; (*большой*) cáuldron; из óбщего ~лá from the same pot; 2. *тех.* bóiler; áтомный ~ núclear reáctor; 3. *воен.* (*окружение*) pócket.

котелóк *м.* 1. pot, sáucepan; 2. (*походный*) méss-tin; 3. (*шляпа*) bówler (-hat).

котéль|ная *ж.* bóiler-room. ~ный bóiler *attr.*; ~ный завóд bóiler works; ~ное желéзо bóiler-plate.

котёнок *м.* kítten.

кóтик *м.* 1. *ласк.* (*кот*) pússy; 2. *зоол.* fúr-seal; 3. (*мех*) séalskin. ~овый séalskin *attr.*

котúровать *несов. и сов.* (*вн.*) *фин.* quote (*smth.*). ~ся *несов. фин.* 1. (*оцениваться*) be* quóted; *перен.* be* regárded; 2. (*иметь хождение*) be* in demánd.

котирóвка *ж. фин.* quotátion.

котúться, окотúться give* birth; (*о кошке*) have* kíttens.

котлéта *ж.* (*отбивная*) cútlet, chop; (*рубленая*) ríssole, méat-ball; hámburger *амер.*; свинáя ~ pórk-chop; теля́чья ~ veal cútlet.

котловáн *м.* foundátion pit.

котловúна *ж.* hóllow.

котóмка *ж.* knápsack.

котóр|ый 1. *вопр.* (*по порядку, при выборе*) which; (*какой*) what; ~ час? what's the time?; 2. *относит.* (*о неодушевл.*) which, that; (*об одушевл.*) who; *часто не переводится*; та кнúга, ~ая стои́т на пóлке the book (that is) on the shelf*; мой брат, ~ живёт в Ленингрáде my bróther, who lives in Léningrad; тот человéк, ~... the man* who...; ~ого вы вúдели вчерá the man* (whom) you saw yésterday; пьéса, о ~ой вы мне говорúли the play (which) you told me abóut; (та) гостúница, ~ая нахóдится напрóтив вокзáла the hotél (that is) ópposite the ráilway státion; лýчшая в гóроде гостúница, ~ая нахóдится на глáвной плóщади the best hotél in the town, which is in the main square; ◇ ~ раз я тебé говорю́? how mány times have I told you?; уж ~ раз э́то с ним случáется it's álways háppening to him.

коттéдж *ж.* (subúrban) vílla.

кóфе *м. нескл.* cóffee; чёрный ~ black cóffee; ~ в зёрнах cóffee beans.

кофевáрка *ж.* cóffee machine; esprésso; percólator; cóffee máker *амер.*

кофеúн *м.* cáffeine.

кофéйн|ик *м.* cóffee-pot. ~ица *ж.* 1. (*ручная мельница*) cóffee-mill; 2. (*банка*) cóffee jar/tin. ~ый 1. cóffee *attr.*: ~ая гýща cóffee-grounds *pl*; ~ая мéльница cóffee-mill; 2. (*о цвете*) cóffee-cóloured.

кофемóлка *ж.* (eléctric) cóffee-mill.

кóфт|а *ж.*, ~очка *ж.* blouse; (*вязаная*) púllover, swéater.

кочáн *м.*: ~ капýсты head of cábbage.

кочевáть *несов.* 1. roam, wánder; (*о птицах и т. п.*) migráte; 2. *разг.* (*часто менять местожительство*) be* álways on the road/move.

кочéв|ник *м.* nómad. ~ой nomádic.

кочéвье *с.* 1. (*действие*) migrátion; 2. (*стоянка*) nómad camp; 3. (*местность*) nómad área/térritory.

кочегáр *м.* stóker, fíreman*. ~ка *ж.* stóke-hold; fíre-room *амер.*

кочéнеть, закочéнеть, окочéнеть 1. (*замерзать*) becóme*/get* stiff, grow* numb (with cold); 2. *сов.* закочéнеть (*о трупе*) stíffen.

кочергá *ж.* póker.

кочеры́жка *ж.* stump of cábbage.

кóчк|а *ж.* húmmock, tússock. ~овáтый húmmocky, tússocky.

кошáчий cat's; féline *научн.*; (*свойственный кошке*) cátlike.

кошелёк *м.* purse.

кóшечка *ж.* cat, pússy.

кóшк|а *ж.* 1. cat; 2. *тех.* grápnel; ◇ жить как ~ с собáкой live a cát-and-dóg life; мéжду нúми пробежáла чёрная ~ they have fállen out; у негó на сéрдце ~и скребýт he is sick at heart.

кóшки-мы́шки: игрáть в ~ play cát-and-móuse; *перен.* play híde-and-séek.

кошмáр *м.* nightmare. ~ный ghástly; nightmare *attr*; hórrible, áwful.

кощýнственный sacrilégious, blásphemous.

кощýнство *с.* sácrilege, blásphemy. ~вать *несов.* blasphéme, commít a sácrilege.

коэффициéнт *м.* coefficient, rátio, fáctor; ~ полéзного дéйствия efficiency.

краб *м.* crab.

крáги *мн.* 1. (*на ноги*) léggings; 2. (*у перчаток*) gáuntlets.

крáден|ое *с. собир.* stólen goods *pl.* ~ый stólen.

крáдучись stéalthily; идтú ~ creep*.

краевéд *м.* régional ethnógrapher. ~ение *с.* régional stúdies/ethnography. ~ческий: ~ческий музéй muséum of régional stúdies/ethnógraphy.

краевóй régional.

краеугóльный básic; ◇ ~ кáмень córner-stone.

крáеш|ек *м. разг.* edge; слы́шать *что-л.* ~ком ýха *разг.* chance to hear *smth.*

крáжа *ж.* theft; ~ со взлóмом búrglary; мéлкая ~ pílfering, pétty lárceny.

кра|й *м.* 1. edge, bórder. (*обрыва, пропасти*) brink; (*сосуда*) brim; ~ дорóги wáyside, róadside; лéвый, прáвый ~ left, right edge; пóлный до ~ёв full to the brim, brím-full; 2. (*страна, местность*) land, région; в э́тих ~я́х in these parts; роднóй ~, роднáя ~я́ one's own cóuntry; в чужúх ~я́х in fóreign parts; 3. (*административно-территориальная единица*) krai, térritory; Краснодáрский ~ Krásnodar Krai/Térritory; ◇ с ~ю from the end; чéрез ~ in plénty; ~ем ýха слы́шать *что-л.* chance to hear *smth.*; на ~ю́ гúбели on the brink/verge of ruin; на ~ю́ свéта at the world's end.

край|испóлком *м.* (исполнúтельный комитéт краевóго Совéта нарóдных депутáтов) Exécutive (Committee) of the Krai/Térritory Sóviet (of Péople's Députies). ~кóм *м.* (краевóй комитéт) Krai/Térritory Committee.

крáйне extrémely; ~ необходúмый ábsolutely esséntial.

крáйн|ий 1. extréme; ~яя лéвая, прáвая *полит.* the extréme left, right; ~яя нужда́ díre need; extréme póverty; ~ срок the last/látest date; ~яя ценá the lówest price; на Крáйнем Сéвере in the Far North; 2 *спорт.*

óutside; wing *attr.*; ~ нападáющий óutside fórward; ◇ ~ие мéры extréme méasures; в ~ем слýчае in the last resórt, if the worst comes to the worst; по ~ей мéре at ány rate. ~ость *ж.* 1. extréme; 2. (*опасное положение*) extrémity; ◇ до ~ости excéssively; впадáть в ~ость go* to extrémes.

кран I *м.* (*водопроводный и т. п.*) tap, cock; fáucet *амер.*; ~ с горя́чей водóй hót-water tap.

кран II *м.* (*подъёмный*) crane.

крановщ|и́к *м.*, ~и́ца *ж.* crane óperator.

крапи́в|а *ж.* (stínging-)nettle(s). ~ница *ж.* néttle--rash; urticária *мед.* ~ный néttle *attr.*

крáпинк|а *ж.* dot, spot; си́тец в ~у dótted cótton.

крас|á *ж.* 1. *поэт. уст.* (*красота*) béauty; *мн.* (*прелести*) charms; 2. (*украшение*) órnament; ~ и гóрдость the pride and joy; ◇ во всей своéй ~é 1) in all *one's* béauty; 2) *ирон.* in all *one's* glóry.

красáв|ец *м.* 1. góod-looking/hándsome féllow; 2.: ~-гóрод a béautiful cíty. ~ица *ж.* 1. béauty; 2.: ~ица--лóшадь spléndid horse, fine spécimen of a horse.

краси́в|о béautifully. ~ый 1. béautiful, lóvely; (*о женщине и ребёнке тж.*) prétty; (*о мужчине*) góod--looking, hándsome; он ~ый? is he góod-looking?; онá ~ая? is she prétty/béautiful?; 2. (*хороший в нравственном отношении*) fine; ~ый постýпок fine áction; 3. (*эффектный*) fine; ~ые словá fine words.

краси́ль|ный dye *attr.*; ~ завóд dýe-works. ~ня *ж.* dýe-house. ~щик *м.* dýer.

краси́|тель *м.* dýe-stuff.

крас|и́ть, покрáсить (*вн.*) 1. (*покрывать краской*) paint (*smth.*); (*волосы, материю*) dye (*smth.*); (*щёки*) paint (*smth.*), rouge (*smth.*); ~ гýбы put* on lípstick, paint *one's* lips; 2. *тк. несов.* (*украшать*) impróve (*smb., smth.*); э́то плáтье её óчень ~ит this dress shows her to great advántage. ~иться *несов.* 1.: матéрия хорошó ~ится the stuff takes the dye well; 2. (*красить лицо, губы*) use/wear* máke-up; (*красить волосы*) dye *one's* hair; 3. *разг.* (*пачкать краской*) run*, stain.

крáск|а I *ж.* 1. (*вещество*) cólour, paint, pígment; (*для тканей, волос*) dye; писáть ~ами paint; ~ для шéрсти wool dye; 2. (*цвет*) cólour; *мн.* cólouring *sg*, tints; 3. *мн.* (*выразительные средства*) cólours; не жалéя крáсок láying it on thick; опи́сывать чтó-л. в я́рких (мрáчных) ~ах paint *smth.* in bright (dark) cólours; 4. (*румянец*) flush; (*стыда, смущения*) blúsh(es); ~ удовóльствия a flush of pleasure.

крáск|а II *ж. разг.* (*окрашивание*) dýeing; отдáть чтó-л. в ~у have* *smth.* dyed.

красне́|ть, покраснéть 1. (*становиться красным*) rédden, grow*/turn red; (*от прилива крови к коже*) rédden; (*о лице*) flush; (*от смущения, стыда тж.*) blush; рýки ~ют от хóлода *one's* hands grow red with cold; 3. *тк. несов.* (*стыдиться*) be* ashámed; мне за тебя́ прихóдится ~ you make me ashámed of you; 4. *тк. несов.* (*виднеться*) show* red.

красноарм|éец *м. ист.* Red Ármy man*. ~éйский Red Ármy *attr.*

красногвардéец *м. ист.* Red Guard.

краснодерéвщик *м.* cábinet-maker.

краснознамённый Red Bánner *attr.*; awárded the Órder of the Red Bánner; ~ полк Red Bánner régiment.

краснолéсье *с.* cónifers *pl.*

красноречи́вый éloquent; ~ орáтор éloquent spéaker; ~ взгляд éloquent look.

краснорéчие *с.* éloquence.

краснотá *ж.* rédness.

краснофлóтец *м. ист.* Red Návy man*, Red sáilor.

краснощёкий réd-cheeked, ápple-chéeked.

краснýха *ж. мед.* Gérman méasles *pl.*

крáсн|ый red; (*о лице тж.*) rúddy, rúbicund; ~ое знáмя Red Bánner; ◇ Óбщество Крáсного Крестá и Крáсного Полумéсяца Red Cross and Red Créscent

Socíety; Крáсная плóщадь Red Square; Крáсная Áрмия *ист.* Red Ármy; ~ая ры́ба stúrgeons *pl*; ~ая икрá red cáviar; ря́ди ~ого словцá for the sake of a wítty remárk; ~ая строкá new páragraph; (э́тому) ~ая ценá ámple/fair price (for that); проходи́ть ~ой ни́тью be* the kéy-note; ~ая дéвица fair/lóvely máiden; ~ое сóлнышко the gólden/bright sun.

красовáться *несов.* 1. stand* out béautifully, stand* out in all its béauty; 2. (*рисоваться*) show* off.

крас|отá *ж.* béauty; ~óты приро́ды the béauties of náture.

красóтка *ж. разг.* béauty.

крáсочн|ый 1. paint *attr.*, dye *attr.*; ~ое произвóдство dýestuffs índustry; 2. (*исполненный красками*) cóloured; 3. (*яркий*) cólourful, picturésque; ~ое описáние cólourful descríption.

красть, укрáсть 1. (*вн.*) steal* (*smth.*); 2. *тк. несов.* (*заниматься кражами*) be* a thief*. ~ся *несов.* steal*, prowl; ~ся вслед за *кем-л.* creep* up behínd *smb.*, stalk *smb.*

крáсящ|ий: ~ее вещество́ cólouring mátter.

крат: во сто ~ a/one húndredfold.

крáтк|ий 1. (*непродолжительный по времени*) short, brief; ~ая встрéча brief mééting; 2. *лингв.* short; ~ие глáсные short vówels; 3. (*недлинный — о дороге*) short; ~ путь the short way/route; 4. (*изложенный коротко*) brief, concíse, short; ~ое изложéние concíse/brief súmmary; в ~их словáх in a few words; ◇ ~ое прилагáтельное *грам.* the short form of the ádjective.

крáтко bríefly, with brévity.

кратковрéменн|ый short, brief, shórt-lived; of short durátion *после сущ.*; ~ое пребывáние short stay; ~ успéх shórt-lived success.

краткосрóчн|ый shórt-térm, shórt-dáted; ~ óтпуск short leave (of ábsence); ~ая ссýда shórt-térm loan; ~ вéксель shórt-dáted bill.

крáткость *ж.* brévity.

крáтн|ое *с. мат.* múltiple; óбщее наимéньшее ~ least cómmon múltiple. ~ый *мат.* múltiple.

крах *м.* crash, fáilure, bánkruptcy; *перен.* fáilure, collápse; ~ бáнка fáilure of a bank; потерпéть пóлный ~ fail útterly.

крахмáл *м.* starch. ~ить, накрахмáлить (*вн.*) starch (*smth.*)

крахмáльный 1. starch *attr.*; 2. (*накрахмаленный*) starched; ~ воротничóк stiff cóllar.

крáшеный páinted; (*о материи, волосах*) dyed.

краю́ха *ж. разг.* ~ хлéба hunch/hunk of bread.

крéдит *м. бухг.* crédit.

креди́т *м.* 1. crédit; предостáвить ~ *кому-л.* give* *smb.* crédit; 2. *мн.* (*ассигнования*) allocátion *sg*, appropriátion *sg*; ◇ госудáрственный ~ эк. State loan sýstem; в ~ on crédit; ~ный crédit *attr.*

кредит|овáть *несов. и сов.* (*вн.*) 1. (*давать в долг*) crédit (*smth.*), give* (*smth.*) crédit; ~ когó-л. большóй сýммой crédit a large sum to smb., crédit smb. with a large sum; 2. *фин.* finánce (*smth.*), grant crédits (to); ~ строи́тельство finánce búilding. ~óр *м.* créditor.

кредитоспосóб|ность *ж.* sólvency. ~ный sólvent.

крéдо *с. нескл.* crédo.

крéйсер *м.* crúiser. ~ский crúising *attr.* ~ство *с.* cruise.

крейси́ровать *несов.* cruise.

крéкер *м.* crácker; (*картофельный*) crisp.

крем *м.* cream; сапóжный ~ shóe-cream, bóot-polish.

крем|атóрий *м.* cremató rium (*pl* -ms, -ia). ~áция *ж.* cremátion.

кремéнь *м.* 1. flint; 2. *разг.* (*о человеке с твёрдым характером*) man* of íron; (*о скупом человеке*) skínflint; не человéк, а ~ he has a heart of flint.

кремль *м.* Krémlin; (*в Москве*) the Krémlin.

крéмний *м. хим.* sílicon.

кремнúстый I (*каменистый*) stóny; *перен.* (*непреклонный*) hard.

кремнúстый II *хим.* silíceous.

крéмовый 1. cream *attr.*; 2. (*о цвете*) créam-coloured.

крен *м.* list; (*при качке*) heel; парохóд идёт с сúльным ~ом the ship is lísting héavily.

крéндель *м.* twist of bread.

кренú|ть, накренúть (*вн.*) give* (*smth.*) a list; (*при качке*) make* (*smth.*) heel óver; парохóд сúльно ~ло the ship was lísting héavily. ~ться, накренúться list, heel óver.

креозóт *м. хим.* créosote.

креóл *м.*, ~ка *ж.* Creóle.

креп *м.* 1. (*ткань*) crêpe; 2. (*траурный*) crape.

крепдешúн *м.* crêpe de Chine.

креп|úть *несов.* 1. (*вн.; укреплять*) fix (*smth.*), fásten (*smth.*); 2. (*вн.*) *горн.* shore up (*smth.*) (with pit props); 3. (*вн.*) *мор.* (*привязывать*) lash (*smth.*) down; 4. (*вн.; делать прочным, усиливать*) stréngthen (*smth.*); ~ оборóну stréngthen the defénce(s); 5. (*о желудке*) cónstipate, make* one cónstipated; егó ~úт he is cónstipated. ~úться *несов.* (*сдерживаться*) hold* out; ~úтесь! keep your chin up!, bear up!

крéпк|ий 1. strong; (*твёрдый*) tough, hard; ~ орéх tough nut; ~ая верёвка strong/stout rope; 2. (*неизношенный*) sound; ~ие сапогú sound boots; 3. (*здоровый, выносливый*) hárdy, strong; ~ органúзм strong constitútion; 4. (*стойкий, непоколебимый*) firm; 5. (*надёжный*) relíable; (*неизменный, глубокий*) lásting, endúring; ~ая любóвь endúring love; 6. (*насыщенный*) strong; ~ чай strong tea; ~ табáк strong tobácco; ~ сон sound sleep; ~ое словцó swéar-word, strong lánguage.

крéпко fírmly; ~ сложённый stúrdily built; ~ выражáться use strong lánguage; ~ полюбúть *кого-л.* becóme* véry fond of *smb.*; ~ спать (*в данный момент*) be* fast asléep; (*вообще*) sleep* sóundly, be* a sound/héavy sléeper; ~ целовáть *кого-л.* give* *smb.* a big/real kiss; ~ (*вас*) целую (*в письме*) love and kísses!

креплéние *с.* 1. (*действие*) fástening; *мор.* láshing; 2. *горн.* tímbering, cásing; 3. (*у лыж*) bínding.

крéпнуть, окрéпнуть be*/grow* strong, get* strónger, grow*/incréase in strength; (*после болезни*) recóver *one's* strength.

крепостнúчество *с.* sérfdom.

крепостн|óй I *прил.* serf *attr.*, féudal; based on sérfdom *после сущ.*; ~ая завúсимость sérfdom, bóndage; ~ое прáво sérfdom; ~ труд serf lábour; ~ое хозяйство ecónomy based on sérfdom, féudal ecónomy; 2. *в знач. сущ. м.* serf.

крепостнóй II *воен.* fórtress *attr.*

крéпость I *ж.* (*прочность, сила*) strength.

крéпость II *ж. воен.* fórtress; *перен.* búlwark, cítadel.

крепчáть *несов.* (*о морозе*) incréase in sevérity, tíghten its grip; (*о ветре*) blow* hárder.

крепы́ш *м. разг.* stúrdy féllow.

крепь *ж. горн.* tímbering.

крéсло *с.* ármchair, éasy chair; lóunger *амер.* (*в театре*) stall.

крéсло-кровáть *с.* béd-chair; cháir-bed *амер.*

крест *м.* cross; ◇ постáвить ~ на чём-л. give* *smth.* up (as a bad job, as a hópeless case).

крестéц *м. анат.* sácrum (*pl* -rums, -ra).

крестúны *мн.* 1. (*обряд*) chrístening *sg*; 2. (*празднество*) chrístening-party *sg*.

крестúть, окрестúть, перекрестúть (*вн.*) 1. *сов.* окрестúть baptíze (*smb.*), chrísten (*smb.*); 2. *тк. несов.* (*быть крёстным у кого-л.*) stand* gódfather to *smb.'s* child*; 3. *сов.* перекрестúть (*делать знак креста*)

make* the sign of the cross (óver). ~ся, окрестúться, перекрестúться 1. *сов.* окрестúться (*принимать христианство*) be* baptízed; 2. *сов.* перекрестúться (*делать знак креста*) cross onesélf.

крест-нáкрест crósswise.

крёстная *ж. разг.* gódmother.

крéстн|ик *м.* gódchild*, gódson. ~ица *ж.* gódchild*, góddaughter.

крéстн|ый *прил.* 1.: ~ая мать gódmother; ~ отéц gódfather; 2. *в знач. сущ. м.* gódfather.

крестовúна *ж.* 1. cróss-piece; 2. *ж.-д.* frog.

крестóвый: ~ похóд *ист.* crusáde.

крестонóсец *м. ист.* crusáder.

крестообрáзн|о crósswise. ~ый cróss-shaped, crúciform.

крестцóв|ый: ~ая кость *анат.* sácral bone.

крестья́н|ин *м.* péasant. ~ка *ж.* péasant wóman*. ~ский *attr.* ~ство *с.* péasantry.

кретúн *м.* 1. crétin; 2. *разг.* nítwit, ímbecile.

крéчет *м.* gérfalcon.

крещéние *с.* 1. *рел.* (*обряд*) báptism; 2. *церк.* (*праздник*) twélfth-day, Epíphany; ◇ боевóе ~ báptism of fire, first time únder fire.

крещёный baptízed.

кривáя *ж.* curve; ~ температýры témperature curve; ◇ ~ вы́везет we might be lúcky.

кривизнá *ж.* cúrvature.

кривúть, скривúть, покривúть (*вн.*) twist (*smth.*); ◇ ~ душóй play the hýpocrite, dissémble (*one's* féelings); ~ рот, гýбы twist *one's* mouth, curl *one's* lip, make* a wry face. ~ся, скривúться go* out of shape, lose* its shape; (*о лице, рте, губах*) twist.

кривл|я́ка *м. и ж. разг.* affécted pérson; онá такáя ~ she's full of airs and gráces, she's so affécted. ~я́нье *с.* afféctation. ~я́ться *несов.* be* affécted; не ~я́йся! don't be so affécted!; none of your airs and gráces!

кривобóкий lop-síded.

крив|óй 1. (*изогнутый*) curved; (*перекошенный*) cróoked, léaning óver; ~ая лúния curve; ~ые нóги bándy legs; 2. *разг.* (*слепой на один глаз*) óne-eyed; blind in one eye *после сущ.*; ◇ ~ая улы́бка wry/irónic smile; ~ое зéркало distórting mirror.

кривонóгий bándy-legged, bów-legged.

кривотóлки *мн.* false rúmours.

кривошúп *м. тех.* crank.

крúзис *м.* crísis (*pl* -ses); *эк. тж.* depréssion; ◇ прáвительственный ~ cábinet crísis; политúческий ~ polítical crísis.

крик *м.* 1. сгу; (*громкий*) shout; (*пронзительный*) scream, shriek, yell; (*шум голосов*) shóuting, clámour; 2. (*животных, птиц*) cry; ◇ ~ душú cri de coeur; послéдний ~ мóды the látest fáshion/style, the látest thing out.

криклúвый 1. nóisy; 2. (*о голосе*) shrill; (*о птицах и т. п.*) ránting, lóud-voiced; 3. (*вычурный*) gárish; ~ наря́д fláshy/gárish attíre.

крúк|нуть *сов.* give* a cry/shout; cry out. ~ýн *м.*, ~ýнья *ж. разг.* nóisy pérson; ребёнок у вас ~ýн! how your báby cries!

криминалúст *м.* críminalist. ~ика *ж.* criminalístics.

криминáльный críminal.

криминолóгия *ж.* criminólogy.

крúнка *ж. см.* кры́нка.

кристáлл *м.* crýstal; *эл. тж.* chip. ~изáция *ж.* crystallizátion. ~изовáться *несов. и сов.* crýstallize. ~úческий crýstalline.

кристáльн|ый crýstal, crýstal-clear; ~ая душá pure soul; ~ой чистоты́ человéк a man* of pérfect intégrity.

критéрий *м.* critérion (*pl* -ia).

крúтик *м.* crític; стрóгий ~ sevére crític; театрáльный ~ dramátic crític.

крúтик|а *ж.* 1. críticism; (*исследование тж.*)

critíque; ~ тéкста téxtual críticism; **2.** *собир.* *(критики)* the crítics *pl*; ◇ это не выдéрживает ~и ≈ it is wide ópen to críticism; it dóesn't hold wáter; эта тeóрия не выдéрживает ~и the théory dóesn't hold wáter; нúже всякой ~и benéath contémpt. **~áн** *м.* críticizer, fáultfinder, críticaster. **~áнство** *с.* cárping/íll-nátured críticism. **~овáть** *несов.* *(вн.)* críticize *(smb., smth.)*.

критицúзм *м.* críticism.

критúческ|ий I *(содержащий критику)* crítical; **~ая** статья críticism, critíque; **~ие** замечáния crítical remárks; **~ ум** crítical mind.

критúческ|ий II 1. *(переломный)* crítical, decísive; **~** вóзраст crítical age; **2.** *(трудный, опасный)* crítical; **~** момéнт crítical/crúcial móment; ◇ **~ая** температýра *физ.* crítical témperature.

крич|áть *несов.* **1.** сгу; *(громко)* shout, bawl; *(пронзительно)* cry out, scream, shriek, yell; *(об осле)* bray; **~** от бóли shriek with pain; **2.** *(на вн.; бранить)* shout (at); **3.** *(вн.; звать)* call *(smb.)*; **4.** *(бросаться в глаза)* stick* out; *(о пр.; быть ярким свидетельством чего-л.)* proclaím *(smth.)*; **5.** *(о пр.) разг.* *(обсуждать)* shout (abóut), raise a clámour (abóut). **~áщий** gláring, loud; **~áщие** цветá loud/gláring cólours; **~áщий** нарáд gáwdy attíre.

кров *м.* shélter, roof; остáться без **~а** be* hómeless, be* left without a roof óver *one's* head.

кровáв|ый 1. blóody; *(окровавленный тж.)* blóod-stained; *(кровопролитный тж.)* múrderous; **~ая** рáна blóody/bléeding wound; **~ое** пятнó blood stain; **~ая** бúтва, **~** бой blóody báttle; **2.** *(ярко-красный)* blóod-réd; ◇ **~ые** слёзы bítter tears; **~ая** бáня blóod-bath.

кровáтка *ж.* cot.

кровáть *ж.* bed; *(остов)* bédstead.

кровéль|ный róofing *attr.*; **~** материáл róofing. **~щик** *м.* *(по настилу железных крыш)* róofer; *(по настилу черепичных крыш)* tíler.

кровенóсн|ый: ~ сосýд blóod-vessel; **~ая** систéма círculatory sýstem.

кровúнк|а *ж.*: ни **~и** в лицé déathly pale; not a drop of blood in *one's* face.

крóвл|я *ж.* róofing; *(черепичная)* tíling; жить под однóй **~ей** live únder the same roof.

крóвн|о: ~ связанный bound by ties of blood/kínship; **~** заинтересóванный vítally ínterested; **~** обúйеду когó-л. mórtally offénd/wound *smb.* **~ый 1.** *(родственный)* blood *attr.*; **~** родствó blood relátionship; **2.** *(чистокровный, породистый)* púrebred, thóroughbred; **3.** *(насущный)* vítal; **~ый** интерéс vítal ínterest; **~ое** дéло immédiate concérn; **4.** *разг.* *(добытый тяжёлым трудом)* hárd-earned; **~ые** дéньги hárd-earned móney; ◇ **~ая** обúда mórtal/gríevous offénce; **~ый** враг déadly énemy; **~ая** месть blood feud, vendétta.

кровожáдн|ость *ж.* blóod-thirstiness. **~ый** blóod-thirsty.

кровоизлиянние *с.* háemorrhage; **~** в мозг cérebral háemorrhage.

кровообращéние *с.* circulátion (of the blood).

кровоостанáвливающ|ий stýptic; **~ее** срéдство stýptic.

кровопúйца *м. и ж.* blóod-sucker.

кровоподтёк *м.* intérnal bruise/contúsion.

кровопролúт|ие *с.* blóodshed. **~ный** blóody; **~ные** вóйны blóody/múrderous wars.

кровопускáние *с.* blóod-letting, bléeding.

кровотечéние *с.* bléeding; háemorrhage *научн.*; **~** из носу nóse-bleed; bléeding at the nose; у меня **~** из носу my nose is bléeding.

кровоточ|áщий bléeding. **~úть** *несов.* bleed*.

кровохáрканье *с.* spitting of blood.

кров|ь *ж.* **1.** blood; gore *поэт.*; останови́ть **~** stop the blood, stop a wound; налитóй **~ю** blóodshot; **2.** *(порода животных)* breed, strain; бульдóг чúстых **~ей**

thóroughbred búlldog; **3.** *(о происхождении людей)* descént; по **~и** by descént; **4.** *(кровопролитие)* blóodshed, blood; ◇ это у негó в **~и** it runs in his blood; пóртить себé **~** upsét* onesélf, wórry unnécessarily; пóртить **~** кому-л. upsét* *smb.*; **~** с молокóм blóoming; in the pink of health; сéрдце **~ю** обливáется *one's* heart bleeds, it makes *one's* heart bleed; **~** стúнет в жúлах *one's* blood freezes, it's enóugh to make *one's* blood freeze; **~** игрáет the blood is fresh in *one's* veins, *one* has plénty of good red blood in *one*; бифштéкс с **~ю** rare steak. **~яной** blood *attr.*; **~яное** давлéние blood préssure.

кроúть, скроúть *(вн.)* cut* out *(smth.)*.

крóйк|а *ж.* cútting(-out); кýрсы **~и** и шитья dréss-making school.

крокéт *м.* cróquet.

крокодúл *м.* crócodile. **~ов: ~овы** слёзы crócodile tears. **~овый** crócodile *attr.*

крóкус *м. бот.* crócus.

крóлик *м.* rábbit.

кроликовóд *м.* rábbit-breeder. **~ство** *с.* rábbit-breeding. **~ческий** rábbit *attr.*; **~ческая** фéрма rábbit-farm.

крóлич|ий rábbit *attr.*; **~** мех rábbit-skin; **~ья** норá rábbit-hole, rábbit-burrow; **~** садóк rábbit-warren.

крол|ь *м. спорт.* crawl; плáвать **~ем** swim* the crawl.

крольч|áтник *м.* rábbit-hutch. **~úха** *ж.* dóe-rabbit, móther-rábbit; *(в сказках)* búnny-rabbit.

крóме 1. *(исключая)* excépt(ing); **2.** *(вдобавок)* besídes; ◇ **~** тогó besídes, moreóver, what is more; **~** шýток jóking apárt.

кромéшн|ый: ~ ад pérfect hell; a régular inférno; тьма **~ая** pítch-dárkness.

крóмка *ж.* **1.** *(материи)* sélvage, sélvedge; **2.** *(металла и т. п.)* edge; **3.** *(край чего-л.)* edge; **~** льда the edge of the ice.

кромсáть, искромсáть *(вн.) разг.* hack *(smth.)*; cut* *(smth.)* jággedly.

крóна I *ж.* *(верхушка дерева)* crown, top.

крóна II *ж.* *(монета)* crown.

кронцúркуль *м.* cállipers *pl.*

кроннштéйн *м.* brácket, hólder.

кропúть *несов.* *(вн. тв.)* sprínkle *(smth. with)*.

кропотлúв|ый labórious; *(о человеке)* páinstaking, díligent; **~ая** рабóта close/íntricate work.

кросс *м.* cróss-cóuntry race; *(бег тж.)* stéeplechase; лыжный **~** cróss-cóuntry ski-race.

кроссвóрд *м.* cróssword (púzzle).

кроссóвки *мн.* *(ед.* кроссóвка *ж.)* tráining/sports shoes, tráiners.

крот *м.* **1.** *(животное)* mole; **2.** *(мех)* móleskin.

крóткий meek, géntle.

кротóв|ый 1. mole *attr.*; **~** мех móleskin; **~ая** нóрка mole's búrrow; **2.** *(сделанный из меха крота)* móleskin *attr.*

крóтость *ж.* méekness, géntleness.

крохобóрство *с.* **1.** *(скупость)* pétty méanness; **2.** *(мелочность)* háir-splitting.

крóхотный *разг.* tíny.

крóшечный tíny.

крошúть *несов.* **1.** *(вн.)* chop up *(smth.)*, chop *(smth.)* fine; *(хлеб)* crúmble *(smth.)*; **~** картóшку в суп chop up potátoes and put* them in the soup; **2.** *(вн.) разг. (ломать)* smash *(smth.)* up; *перен.* cut* *(smb.)* to píeces; **3.** *(сорить)* make*/drop a lot of crumbs. **~ся** *несов.* crúmble.

крóшк|а 1. *ж.* crumb; **~** хлéба (bréad-)crumb; **2.** *м. и ж. разг. (о ребёнке)* líttle one, mite; ◇ ни **~и** not a mórsel/scrap.

круг *м.* **1.** circle; вы́числить плóщадь **~а** cálculate the área of the circle; дéлать, опúсывать **~(и)** *(в воздухе)* circle; **2.** *(сомкнутая цепочка людей)* ring;

стать в ~ form a ring; **3.** (*предмет, имеющий форму круга*) ring; round; ~ колбасы́ ring of sáusage; спаса́тельный ~ life-buoy; **4.** (*цепь де́йствий, собы́тий*) round, course; **5.** (*пе́речень чего-л.*) list; ~ вопро́сов class of próblems; **6.** (*сфе́ра де́ятельности*) sphere; ~ де́ятельности sphere/scope/range of actívity; **7.** (*гру́ппа люде́й*) circle; прави́тельственные ~и́ góvernment circles; в ~у́ семьи́ in the fámily circle; в те́сном ~у́ among íntimates; ◇ ~и́ под глаза́ми rings round *one's* eyes; ~и́ перед глаза́ми плыву́т *one* feels dízzy; голова́ идёт кру́гом *one's* head is spínning; сде́лать ~ make* a détour, go* a róundabout way; на ~ on the/an áverage; ~ почёта lap of hónour.

кру́гленьк|ий 1. round; **2.** (*то́лстенький*) plump; ◇ ~ая су́мма big sum of móney.

кругле́ть *несов.* becóme* round.

круглоли́цый róund-faced.

круглосу́точн|ый róund-the-clock *attr.*; dáy-and-níght *attr.*

кру́гл|ый 1. round; **2.** (*то́лстый*) plump; **3.:** ~ год all the year round; ~ые су́тки all day and night, round the clock; **4.:** ~ дура́к útter fool; ~ неве́жда compléte ignorámus; ◇ конфере́нция ~ого стола́ róund-table cónference; ~ сирота́ órphan; ~ отли́чник púpil/stúdent with distínctions in évery súbject; учи́ться на ~ые пятёрки have* éxcellent marks in évery súbject; ~ые ско́бки round bráckets; ~ая су́мма round sum; ~ым счётом, для ~ого счёта in round fígures; де́лать ~ые глаза́ ópen *one's* eyes wide, góggle.

кругов|о́й círcular; ◇ ~а́я пору́ка 1) (*коллекти́вная отве́тственность*) colléctive responsibílity; 2) (*взаи́мное укрыва́тельство*) mútual protéction.

кругово́рот *м.* rotátion; cýcle; ~ собы́тий the cónstant flow of evénts.

кругозо́р *м.* óutlook, range of vísion; челове́к с широ́ким (у́зким) ~ом pérson of broad (nárrow) views, pérson with a broad (nárrow) óutlook.

круго́м 1. *нареч.* (*вокру́г*) (all) aróund; ~ леса́, ~ мно́го лесо́в all aróund there are fórests; ~ всё ти́хо all aróund is quiet; посмотре́ть ~ look a(róund); поверну́ться ~ turn (right) round; *воен.* turn abóut; ~! abóut turn!; **2.** *нареч. разг.* (*по́лностью*): вы винова́ты it's all your fault; он ~ до́лжен he's in debt all round; он ~ обма́нут he has been thróroughly táken in, he has been thóroughly fooled; **3.** *предлог* (*рд.*) aróund.

кругооборо́т *м.* circulátion.

кругосве́тн|ый róund-the-world *attr.*; ~ое путеше́ствие vóyage/tour aróund the world, world tour.

кружев|а́ *мн. см.* кру́жево. ~но́й lace *attr.*; *перен.* láсу, láce-like.

кру́жево *с.* lace.

кружи́ть *несов.* **1.** (*вн.; верте́ть*) whirl (*smb., smth.*), spin* (*smb., smth.*); ~ кого́-л. в та́нце dance round with *smb.*; **2.** (*о пти́це, самолёте*) circle; **3.** (*блужда́ть*) wánder aróund; ~ кому́-л. го́лову turn *smb.'s* head. ~ся *несов.* **1.** go* round; (*бы́стро враща́ться, нести́сь*) whirl, spin*; *перен. разг.* hang* abóut; **2.** (*о пти́це, самолёте*) circle; ◇ у меня́ голова́ кру́жится my head is góing round; I'm dízzy (*тж. перен.*).

кру́жка *ж.* mug; (*металли́ческая*) tánkard.

кружн|ый: е́хать ~ым путём make* a détour, go* round; узна́ть ~ым путём get* to know in a róundabout fáshion.

кружо́к *м.* **1.** (small) círcle; деревя́нный ~ wóoden disc, círcular piece of wood; **2.** (*гру́ппа люде́й*) group, circle; дру́жеский ~ the circle of *one's* friends; литерату́рный ~ líterary círcle/group; ◇ стри́чься в ~ have* *one's* hair bobbed.

круи́з *м.* cruise.

круп I *м.* (*ло́шади*) crúpper, croup.

круп II *м.* (*боле́знь*) croupe.

круп|а́ *ж.* **1.** céreals *pl*; **2.** (*снег*) tíny péllets of snow. ~и́нка *ж.* grain; ~и́нка песка́ grain of sand; ни ~и́нки пра́вды not a grain of truth.

крупи́ца *ж. см.* крупи́нка.

кру́пно: ~ наре́зать *что-л.* cut* *smth.* in large píeces; ~ писа́ть write* large; ◇ ~ поговори́ть, поспо́рить с *кем-л.* have* (high) words with *smb.*

крупнобло́чн|ый lárge-block *attr.*; ~ое строи́тельство lárge-block constrúction.

крупнокали́берный lárge-calibre *attr.*

крупнопане́ль|ый lárge-panel *attr.*; ~ое строи́тельство lárge-panel constrúction.

кру́пн|ый 1. cóarse(-grained); ~ песо́к coarse sand; **2.** (*большо́й*) big, large; (*ро́слый тж.*) héavily built, strápping, mássive; ~ые черты́ лица́ mássive féatures; **3.** (*многочи́сленный*) large, strong; ~ отря́д large detáchment; **4.** (*большо́го масшта́ба*) lárge-scale *attr.*; ~ая промы́шленность lárge-scale índustry; ~ая буржуази́я úpper bourgeoísie; **5.** (*значи́тельный*) impórtant, próminent; ~ учёный próminent/distínguished scíentist; **6.** (*ва́жный, суще́ственный*) great, mássive; ~ая побе́да great víctory; ~ успе́х great/huge succéss; ~ое достиже́ние great/mássive achíevement; ~ые де́ньги large móney/notes; ~ая су́мма large sum (of móney); ~ разгово́р high words *pl*; show-down *разг.*; ~ рога́тый скот horned cáttle; вести́ ~ую игру́ play high, play for high stakes; снима́ть кого́-л. ~ым пла́ном take* a clóse-up of *smb.*

крупо́зн|ый: ~ое воспале́ние лёгких cróupous/lóbar pneumónia.

крупору́шка *ж.* húlling-mill.

крутизна́ *ж.* stéepness; (*круто́й спуск*) steep (slope).

крути́ть *несов.* **1.** (*вн.; враща́ть, верте́ть*) turn (*smth.*), whirl (*smth.*), twirl (*smth.*); **2.** (*вн.; скру́чивать*) twist (*smth.*); ~ папиро́су roll a cigaré́tte; **3.** (*вн.; вздыма́я, кружи́ть*) whip up (*smth.*), swirl (*smth.*); **4.** (*тв.*) *разг.* (*распоряжа́ться*) órder (*smth.*) abóut, have* *one's* way (with); ~ кому́-л. ру́ки twist *smb.'s* arms; (*свя́зывать*) tie *smb.'s* hands behínd *his* back. ~ся *несов.* **1.** (*верте́ться*) twirl round; **2.** (*скру́чиваться*) spin*; **3.** (*вздыма́ясь, кружи́ться*) whirl, swirl.

крут|о́ 1. (*внеза́пно*) súddenly; ~ останови́ться pull up short; ~ поверну́ть make* a sharp turn; **2.** (*ту́го*) tíghtly, fírmly. ~о́й **1.** (*отве́сный*) steep; **2.** (*ре́зкий, внеза́пный*) sharp, súdden, abrúpt; ~о́й поворо́т sharp/abrúpt turn; ~о́й перело́м abrúpt/súdden change; **3.** (*суро́вый*): ~о́й нрав, ~о́й хара́ктер infléxible/harsh témper, cháracter; ~ые ме́ры drástic méasures; ~о́й ве́тер high wind; ~о́й моро́з sharp frost; **4.** (*густо́й*) thick; ~ое те́сто héavy dough; ~о́е яйцо́ hárd-boiled egg; ◇ ~о́й кипято́к fást-boiling wáter. ~ость *ж.* **1.** (*отве́сность*) slope; **2.** (*хара́ктера*) hárshness.

круча *ж.* steep slope, cliff.

кручён|ый twisted; ~ая ни́тка lisle thread.

круше́ние *с.* crash; (*судна́*) loss; *перен.* dównfall, collápse; ~ по́езда train crash, ráilway áccident.

крыжо́вник *м.* **1.** *собир.* (*я́годы*) góoseberries *pl*; **2.** (*об отде́льной я́годе*) góoseberry; **3.** (*куст*) góoseberry-bush.

крыла́т|ый winged; ◇ ~ые слова́ winged words.

крыло́ *с.* **1.** wing; взма́хивать кры́льями flap its wings; ~ до́ма wing of a house; ~ самолёта áircraft wing; **2.** (*ветряно́й ме́льницы*) arm, sail; **3.** (*автомаши́ны, велосипе́да и т. п.*) múdguard; ◇ подре́зать кры́лья кому́-л. clip *smb.'s* wings; опусти́ть кры́лья мо́ре.

крыльц|о́ *с.* the steps *pl*; (*с наве́сом*) porch; стоя́ть на ~е́ stand* on the steps, stand* in the porch.

кры́нка *ж.* éarthenware jar.

крыс|а *ж.* rat. ~и́ный rat's; rat *attr.*; ~и́ная нора́ rát-hole.

крысоло́вка ж. 1. (*ловушка*) rát-trap; 2. (*собака*) rátter.

кры́тый cóvered; ~ ры́нок cóvered márket.

крыть, покры́ть (*вн.*) cóver (*smth.*); (*крышу*) roof (*smth.*); ~ кры́шу желе́зом roof the house with shéet-iron; ◇ ~ не́чем one has not a leg to stand on. ~ся *несов.*: причи́на кро́ется в... the cause lies in...; здесь кро́ется недоразуме́ние there is some misunderstánding here; здесь что́-то кро́ется there's sómething behind this.

кры́ш|а ж. roof; соло́менная ~ thátched roof; черепи́чная ~ tiled roof; ◇ под одно́й ~ей únder the same roof.

кры́шка ж. 1. lid; (*верхняя часть*) top; 2. *в знач. сказ. разг.*: ему́ ~ he's done for!, it's all up with him!, he's had it!

крюк м. 1. hook; 2. *разг.* (*окольный путь*) détour; сде́лать большо́й ~ make* a big détour, go* a long way round.

крюч|ить, скрючить *обыкн. безл. разг.*: его́ ~ит от бо́ли he is racked with pain; его́ скрючило от бо́ли he is/was dóubled up with pain. ~иться, скрючиться *разг.* be* dóubled up; он весь скрючился he is all dóubled up.

крючкова́тый hooked.

крючкотво́р м. *уст.* péttifogger. ~ство с. *уст.* péttifoggery; юриди́ческое ~ство chicánery.

крючо́к м. hook; (*дверной тж.*) catch; (*в механизме*) claw.

крюшо́н м. cold frúit-punch; (*с вином*) hóck-cup.

кряж м. 1. (*горный*) ridge; 2. (*бревно*) stump.

кря́жистый thicksét.

кря́канье с. 1. (*утки*) quácking; 2. (*человека*) grúnting.

кря́кать, кря́кнуть 1. (*об утках*) quack; 2. *разг.* (*о человеке*) grunt.

кря́кнуть *сов. см.* кря́кать.

кряхте́ть *несов. разг.* groan.

ксилогра́фия ж. wood engráving.

кста́ти *нареч.* 1. (*уместно*) to the point; о́чень ~ véry much to the point; э́то о́чень ~! that is just what was wánted!; it'll come in véry hándy!; э́то случи́лось о́чень ~ it came in the véry nick of time; 2. (*заодно*) while one is abóut it; когда́ пойдёте гуля́ть, ~ зайди́те к нему́ while you're táking your walk, you might as well drop in and see him; 3. *в знач. вводн. сл.* (*между прочим*) by the by, by the way; incidéntally; ~, где он сейча́с? by the way, where is he?

кто *мест.* (*рд., вн.* кого́, *дт.* кому́, *тв.* кем, *пр.* о ком) 1. *вопр., относ.* who; ~ тако́й? who's that?; ма́ло ~ зна́ет few péople know; 2. *неопр.* ánybody, ányone; ~ чита́л, ~ писа́л пи́сьма some read, some wrote létters; кому́ что нра́вится éveryone to his taste; ◇ ~~, а он не мог сде́лать э́того óthers might have done it, but not he; ~~, а он знал, что тако́е аркти́ческая зима́ he knew, if ányone did, what an Árctic winter was like; кому́-кому́, а вам на́до бы знать you ought to know if ányone does; они́ разбежа́лись ~ куда́ they scáttered in all diréctions; ~ где some here; some there; ~ как in várious ways; что whatéver ányone; ~ кого́ who beats who; ~ ни, ~ бы ни whoéver; ~ бы то ни был whoéver it may be; ~ ни есть ányone.

кто́|-либо sómebody, sómeone; (*в вопросе и при отрицании*) ányone, ánybody.

куб I м. 1. *мат.* cube; ~ двух ра́вен восьми́ the cube of two is eight, two cubed makes eight; 2. *разг.* (*кубический метр*) cúbic métre.

куб II м. (*котёл*) bóiler; перего́нный ~ still.

куба́рем *разг.*: кати́ться ~ roll head óver heels.

кубату́ра ж. cúbic capácity.

ку́бик м. 1. cube; 2. *разг.* (*кубический сантиметр*) cúbic céntimetre; 3. *мн.* (*детская игрушка*) bricks.

куби́н|ец м. Cúban. ~ка ж. Cúban wóman*. ~ский Cúban.

куби́ческ|ий cúbic; ~ ко́рень *мат.* cúbe-root, cúbic root; ◇ ~ие ме́ры cúbic méasures.

кубо́к м. 1. góblet; 2. (*как приз*) cup; переходя́щий ~ chállenge cup.

кубоме́тр м. cúbic métre.

ку́брик м. *мор.* mess deck; crew's quárters *pl.*

кубы́шк|а ж. 1. (*копилка*) móney-box; держа́ть де́ньги в ~е hoard one's money; 2. *разг.* (*толстушка*) plump girl, whópper.

кувши́н м. jug, pítcher, éwer.

кувши́нка ж. wáter-lily.

кувырк|а́ться *несов.* turn sómersaults, turn héad-over-héels. ~ну́ться *сов.* turn a sómersault. ~о́м *разг.* héad-over-héels.

куда́ *нареч.* 1. *вопр., относ.* where; whither *поэт.*; 2. *неопр. разг.* sómewhere; 3. *в знач. частицы разг.* (*гораздо*) much, far; ~ лу́чше much/far bétter; ◇ ~ бы ни wheréver; ~ бы то ни́ было ánywhere.

куда́-либо sómewhere. ~-то sómewhere or óther. ~-то sómewhere.

куда́хтанье с. cáckle.

куда́хтать *несов.* cáckle.

ку́др|и *мн.* locks, curls. ~я́вый 1. cúrly; ~я́вые во́лосы cúrly hair; 2. (*о человеке*) cúrly-héaded; ~я́вый ма́льчик cúrly-héaded boy.

кузне́ц м. blácksmith.

кузне́чик м. grásshopper.

кузне́чный blácksmith's.

ку́зница ж. smíthy, forge.

ку́зов м. 1. (*лукошко*) básket; 2. (*автомашины*) back, bódy.

кукаре́кать *несов.* crow.

кукареку́ cóck-a-doodle-dóo.

ку́кла ж. doll; (*театральная*) púppet (*тж. перен.*).

кукова́ть *несов.* cúckoo.

ку́колка ж. 1. dólly; 2. (*насекомого*) chrýsalis (*pl* -ices, -ides), púpa (*pl* -ae).

ку́кольный doll's; (*похожий на куклу*) dóll-like; *перен.* tíny; ~ теа́тр púppet-show.

ку́кситься *несов. разг.* be* in the dumps.

кукуру́з|а ж. maize; corn *амер.*; возду́шная ~ pópcorn. ~ный maize *attr.*; corn *attr. амер.*; ~ный си́лос maize sílage; ~ные хло́пья córnflakes.

куку́шка ж. 1. cúckoo; 2. *разг.* (*небольшой паровоз*) shúnting éngine.

кула́к I м. 1. (*руки*) fist; 2. (*войска, сосредоточенные в одном месте*) stríking force; брониро́ванный ~ the mailed fist; ◇ держа́ть кого́-л. в ~é keep* smb. únder one's thumb.

кула́к II м. *ист.* kúlak.

кула́чн|ый ~ бой físt-fighting; físticuffs *pl*; ~ое пра́во club law.

кулачо́к м. 1. small fist; 2. *тех.* cam, táppet.

кулебя́ка ж. *кул.* kulebyáka, sávoury pátty (*with meat, fish or cabbage filling*).

кулёк м bag.

кули́к м. *зоол.* sándpiper.

кулина́р м spécialist in cóokery.

кулина́р|ия ж. 1. cóokery, the cúlinary art; 2. *собир.* (*кушанья*) cuisíne, cóoking; магази́н ~ии delicatéssen shop, prepáred-food shop. ~ный cúlinary; ~ное иску́сство the art of cóoking; ~ная кни́га cóokery-book.

кули́с|а ж. *обыкн. мн. театр.* wings; ◇ за ~ами, за ~ы behínd the scenes.

кули́ч м. kulích, Éaster cake.

кули́чк|и *мн.*: у чёрта на ~ах *разг.* on the óther side of the world, in the back of beyónd; к чёрту на ~ *разг.* to the óther side/end of the world.

кулуа́рн|ый únofficial; behínd-the-scénes *attr.*; ~ые интри́ги wíre-pulling (in the lóbby).

кулуа́ры *мн.* lóbby *sg.*

куль м. sack.

культminацио́нный cúlminating; ~ пункт clímax, culminátion, cúlminating point.

культминáция ж. culminátion.

культ м. cult, wórship; ~ ли́чности personálity cult, cult of personálity.

культивáтор м. с.-х. cúltivator.

культиви́ровать *несов.* (*вн.*) 1. с.-х. cúltivate (*smth.*); 2. (*разводить растения*) grow* (*smth.*); 3. (*развивать, совершенствовать*) cúltivate (*smth.*), encóurage (*smth.*), fóster (*smth.*).

культмáссов|ый: ~ая рабóта cúltural work amóng the másses.

культпохóд м. (cúltural) óuting/excúrsion.

культрабóтник м. cúltural órganizer.

культтовáры мн. recreátional goods.

культу́р|а ж. 1. cúlture; ~ дре́вних гре́ков the cúlture of Áncient Greece; челове́к высóкой ~ы man* of cúlture; 2. (*уровень, степень развития чего-л.*): ~ земледе́лия efficiency in ágriculture; ~ производства prodúction stándards/efficiency; ~ ре́чи speech hábits *pl;* ~ труда́ wórkmanship; ~ бы́та cúlture in éveryday life; 3. (*разведение растений*) cultivátion, grówing; (*обработка земли*) cultivátion, tílling; 4. (*растение*) crop; техни́ческие ~ы indústrial crops; 5. *бакт.* cúlture.

культу́рно in a cúltured/cívilized mánner.

культу́рно-бытов|óй: ~óе обслу́живание provísion of cúltural and pérsonal sérvices.

культу́рно-воспитáтельн|ый cúltural and educátional; ~ая рабóта cúltural and educátional work.

культу́рно-мáссовый for spréading cúlture amóng the másses *после сущ.*

культу́рно-просвети́тельный cúltural and educátional.

культу́рн|ость ж. cúlture; высóкая ~ high lével of cúlture. ~ый 1. (*относящийся к культуре*) cúltural; ~ый у́ровень cúltural lével; ~ые запрóсы intelléctual interest *sg;* ~ые свя́зи cúltural relátions; 2. (*образованный*) cúltured; ~ый челове́к man* (wóman*) of cúlture, cúltivated/cúltured pérson; ~ый óтдых hóliday/recreátion with cúltural opportúnities; 3. с.-х. cúltivated; ~ые расте́ния cúltivated plants.

культя́ ж. stump.

кум м. gódfather of *one's* child*. ~á ж. gódmother of *one's* child*.

кумáч м. red cótton.

куми́р м. ídol.

кумовствó с. *разг.* népotism.

ку́мушка ж. (*сплетница*) góssip.

кумы́с м. kóumiss.

кунжу́т м. *бот.* sésame. ~ный: ~ное мáсло sésame oil.

куни́ца ж. (*животное и мех*) márten.

купáль|ный báthing *attr.;* ~ костю́м báthing-suit. ~ня ж. báth-house. ~щик м. báther.

купáни|е с. báthing; морски́е ~я séa-bathing *sg.*

купáть, вы́купать (*вн.*) give* (*smb.*) a bath, bath (*smb.*). ~ся, вы́купаться bathe, have* a bath.

купé с. *нескл.* compártment.

купé|ц м. mérchant. ~ческий mérchant's. ~чество с. 1. (*сословие*) mérchantry; 2. собир. (*купцы*) the mérchants *pl.*

купи́рованный compártment *attr.;* ~ вагóн compártment cárriage.

купи́ть *сов. см.* покупáть.

куплéт м. cóuplet.

ку́пля ж. púrchase; ◇ ~-продáжа sale and púrchase.

ку́пол м. cúpola; dome (*тж. перен.*); ~ парашю́та cánopy.

купóн м. cóupon.

купорóс м. vítriol; мéдный ~ blue/cópper vítriol.

купю́ра I ж. (*сокращение*) cut, excísion.

купю́ра II ж. *фин.* bond.

курагá ж. *собир.* dried ápricots.

курáнты *мн.* chime *sg.*

кургáн м. búrial-mound.

курдю́|к м. fat tail. ~чный: ~чные óвцы fát-tailed sheep.

куре́ние с. 1. (*действие*) smóking; 2. (*благовоние*) íncense.

кури́льщик м. smóker.

кури́н|ый hen's; ~ бульóн chícken-broth; ~ое яйцó (hen's) egg; ◇ ~ая грудь chícken-breast, pígeon-breast; ~ая слепотá 1) (*болезнь глаз*) night-blíndness; 2) (*название цветка*) chickweed.

кури́тельный smóking *attr.*

кури́ть *несов.* (*вн.*) 1. smoke (*smth.*); 2. (*добывать перегонкой*) distíl (*smth.*). ~ся *несов.* 1. smoke; 2. (*тв.; выделять испарения, туман, пар*) give* off (*smth.*); 3. (*носиться в воздухе — о дыме, тумане и т. п.*) swirl, roll.

ку́рица ж. hen, fowl; *кул.* chícken; холóдная ~ cold chícken; ◇ мóкрая ~ 1) bedrággled créature; 2) (*бесхарактерный человек*) wéakling, spíneless créature; у негó дéнег ку́ры не клюю́т ≈ he is rólling in móney; ку́рам нá смех ≈ it's enóugh to make a cat laugh.

курлы́кать *несов.* call (*of cranes*).

курнóсый *разг.* 1. (*о носе*) túrned-up; 2. (*о человеке*) snúb-nosed.

курóк м. cock, hámmer; (*винтовки*) cócking-piece; спусти́ть ~ pull the trígger; взвести́ ~ cock the gun.

куропáтка ж. pártridge; бéлая ~ white grouse, ptármigan.

курóрт м. health resórt. ~ник м. *разг.* vísitor at/to a health resórt. ~ный: ~ное лече́ние tréatment at a health resort; ~ный сезóн hóliday séason.

курс м. 1. (*направление движения*) course; *перен.* pólicy; взять ~ на чтó-л. set* *one's* course for *smth.*, steer for *smth.*; взять ~ на сéвер steer/set* a nórtherly course, steer north; 2. (*год обучения*) year; на пéрвом (вторóм *и т. д.*) ~е in *one's* first (sécond *etc.*) year; 3. (*учебник*) hándbook, mánual; 4.: ~ лече́ния course of tréatment; cure; 5. (*денежный*) rate of exchánge, exchánge; ~ рубля́ rate of exchánge of the róuble; ◇ быть в ~е know* all abóut it; быть в ~е поли́тики be* well infórmed abóut pólitics; держáть когó-л. в ~е keep* *smb.* infórmed (as to).

курсáнт м. stúdent.

курси́в м. itálics *pl;* вы́делить слóво ~ом put* a word in itálics. ~ный itálic.

курси́ровать *несов.* run*, ply.

курсóвка ж. entítlement to tréatment and board at a sanatórium and óutside accommodátion.

курсов|óй: ~áя рабóта undergráduate's thésis (*pl* -ses).

ку́рсы *мн.* school *sg,* cóllege *sg;* ~ заóчного обуче́ния correspóndence cóllege.

ку́ртка ж. jácket; (*спортивная с капюшоном*) ánorak; párka *амер.;* кóжаная ~ léather jácket.

курчáвый 1. (*о волосах*) cúrly; 2. (*о человеке*) cúrly-héaded.

курьёз м. strange/queer thing. ~ный strange, queer; (*о вещах тж.*) cúrious.

курьéр м. méssenger, cóurier. ~ский: ~ский пóезд expréss train; как на ~ских at top speed, póst-háste.

куря́т|ина ж. chícken. ~ник м. fówl-house, hén-coop.

куря́щ|ий м. smóker; вагóн для ~их smóking-carriage; smóker *разг.*

кусáть *несов.* (*вн.*) 1. bite* (*smb., smth.*); (*ранить жалом тж.*) sting* (*smb., smth.*); (*ранить клювом*) peck (*smb., smth.*); ~ себé гу́бы bite* *one's* lip; 2. *разг.* (*о крапиве*) sting* (*smb.*); (*о морозе*) nip (*smb.*); (*о шерсти*) irritate (*smb.*), tíckle (*smb.*). ~ся *несов.* 1. bite*; 2. (*кусать друг друга*) bite* each óther.

кусково́й lump *attr.*; ~ cа́хар lump súgar.

кусо́к *м.* **1.** piece, bit; (*пищи*) mórsel; ~ льда chunk of íce; ~ мы́ла cake of soap; ~ cа́хара lump of súgar; **2.** (*часть чего-л.*) part; ◇ ~ хлеба (*заработок*) bread, lívelihood; зараба́тывать на ~ хле́ба make* one's bread, earn one's lívelihood; ~ в го́рло не идёт *one* can't eat a mórsel.

кусо́чек *м.* bit.

куст *м.* bush, shrub; ◇ спря́таться в ~ы́ back out. ~а́рник *м. собир.* búshes *pl*, úndergrowth.

куста́рн|ый **1.** hóme-máde; ~ые изде́лия hándicraft wares; ~ про́мысел hóme-índustry, cóttage craft; **2.** (*примитивный*) crude, amatéurish.

куста́рщина *ж. разг.* crude/amatéurish work.

куста́рь *м.* hándicraftsman*, ártisan.

ку́тать *несов.* (*вн.*) múffle (*smb.*, *smth.*), wrap (*smb.*, *smth.*); (*одевать слишком тепло*) múffle (*smb.*) up. ~ся *несов.* **1.** (*в вн.*) wrap *oneself* (in); ~ся в платок wrap one's shawl round *one*, wrap oneself up in one's shawl; **2.** (*одеваться слишком тепло*) múffle onesélf up, dress too wármly.

кутёж *м.* drínking(-bout), caróusing.

кутерьма́ *ж. разг.* fuss, confúsion.

кут|и́ла *ж. разг.* rake, fast líver. ~и́ть *несов.* drink*, caróuse; booze; *шутл.* be* on the spree.

кухáрка *ж.* cook.

ку́х|ня *ж.* **1.** kítchen; **2.** (*подбор кушаний*) cuisíne. ~онный kítchen *attr.*; ~онные принадле́жности kítchen uténsils, pots and pans.

ку́цый **1.** (*о хвосте*) short, docked; **2.** (*о живо́тных, птицах*) stúmpy-tailed; **3.** (*об одежде*) short, skímpy; **4.** *ирон.* (*ограниченный*) curtáiled.

ку́ча *ж.* **1.** heap; **2.** *разг.* (*множество*) a lot (of), heaps (of).

ку́чев|о́й: ~ые облака́ cúmulus cloud *sg.*

ку́чер *м.* cóachman*; (*возница*) dríver, cárter.

ку́чка *ж.* **1.** heap; **2.** (*небольшая группа*) bunch; ~ люде́й hándful of péople, собира́ться ~ми gáther in small groups.

кушáк *м.* sash, gírdle.

ку́ш|анье *с.* food; (*блюдо*) dish. ~ать *несов.* (*вн.*) eat* (*smth.*), take* (*smth.*), have* (*smth.*).

кушéтка *ж.* (stúdio) couch, sófa.

кювéт *м.* ditch.

Л

лабиáльный *лингв.* lábial.

лабири́нт *м.* maze, lábyrinth.

лабора́нт *м.*, ~ка *ж.* labóratory assístant.

лаборато́р|ия *ж.* labóratory (*тж. перен.*). ~ный labóratory *attr.*; ~ные о́пыты labóratory expériments; ~ная рабо́та labóratory reséarch.

лáва I *ж.* (*вулкана*) láva; *перен.* flood, ávalanche.

лáва II *ж. горн.* drift, drive.

лави́н|а *ж.* (*прям. и перен.*) ávalanche. ~ой in an ávalanche.

лави́ровать *несов. мор.* tack; *перен.* manóeuvre.

лáвка I *ж.* (*скамья*) bench, seat.

лáвка II *ж.* (*магазин*) shop; store *амер.*

лáвочка I *ж.* (*скамейка*) bench, seat.

лáвочк|а II *ж.* **1.** (*небольшой магазин*) shop; **2.** *разг.* (*нечестное предприятие*) rácket; ◇ закры́ть ~у shut* up shop.

лáвочник *м. уст.* shópkeeper; stórekeeper *амер.*

лавр *м.* **1.** láurel; **2.** (*дерево тж.*) báy-tree; ◇ почи́ть на ~ах rest on one's láurels.

ла́вро́вый láurel *attr.*, bay *attr.*; лáвровая ро́ща láurels *pl*, láurel grove; ◇ лавро́вый вено́к wreath of láurels; лавро́вый лист báy-leaf*.

лавсáн *м.* lávsan (*man-made fabric*). ~овый lávsan *attr.*; ~овое волокно́ lávsan fíbre.

лáгерный camp *attr.*

лáгер|ь *м.* camp (*тж. перен.*); раски́нуть ~ pitch a camp; снять ~ break* (up) camp, strike* tents; стать ~ем camp; стоя́ть ~ем be* encámped; ◇ пионе́рский ~ Young Pioneer camp.

лагу́на *ж.* lagóon.

лад *м.* **1.** *разг.* (*гармония, согласие*) hármony; быть не в ~áх not get on, get* on véry bádly; он с ней не в ~áх they don't get on; **2.** (*способ, манера*) way; на свой ~ in one's own way; повторя́ть одно́ и то́ же на все ~ы́ be* álways hárping on the same string/note; **3.** *муз.* (*тональность*) mode, key; мажо́рный ~ májor key; **4.** *обыкн. мн.* (*на струнных инструментах*) stop *sg*, fret *sg*; **5.** *обыкн. мн.* (*клавиши гармоники и т. п.*) keys; перебира́ть ~ы́ run* one's fingers óver the keys; ◇ петь в ~ sing* in tune; петь не в ~ sing* out of tune; де́ло идёт на ~ things are lóoking up; де́ло не идёт на ~ things are not góing well.

лáдан *м.* íncense; кури́ть ~ом burn* íncense.

лáд|ить *несов.* (*с тв.*) get* on (with); мы с ним ~им we get on véry well; они́ (совсе́м) не ~ят they don't get on (at all); как вы с ним ~ите? how do you get on? ~иться *несов.* succéed, go* well; де́ло не ~ится nóthing goes right.

лáдно *разг.* all right!; okáy!, O.K. *амер.*

лáдный *разг.* **1.** (*хорошо сложённый, сделанный*) wéll-built; **2.** (*дельный*) smart, sharp; **3.** (*ловкий*) ágile, light-fóoted; **4.** (*согласованный, согласный*) harmónious.

лáдо|нь *ж.* palm (of the hand); ◇ ви́дно как на ~ни pláinly/cléarly vísible, plain to see. ~ши *мн.*: бить, хло́пать в ~ши clap one's hands.

ладья́ *ж. шахм.* cástle.

лаз *м.* **1.** *разг.* hole; **2.** *тех.* mánhole.

лазаре́т *м.* infírmary; sick quárters *pl*; (*полевой*) field-ambulance; *мор.* síck-bay.

лáзать *несов. см.* лáзить.

лазéйк|а *ж.* hole; *перен.* lóop-hole; оста́вить себе́ ~у leave* onesélf a lóop-hole.

лáзер *м.* láser. ~ный láser *attr.*

лáз|ить *несов.* climb; (*неуклюже*) clámber; (*на вн.*; *на стену, возвышенность*) climb (*smth.*), climb up (*smth.*), scale (*smth.*); ~ по дере́вьям climb trees; ~ в окно́ get* in by the window; он ~ил на голубя́тню he climbed up to the pígeon-loft.

лазо́ревый, лазу́рный ázure.

лазу́рь *ж.* ázure.

лазу́тчик *м. уст.* spy.

лай *м.* bárk(ing); бросáться с лáем на *кого-л.* rush at *smb.* bárking.

лáйка I *ж.* (*собака*) Éskimo dog, húsky.

лáйк|а II *ж.* (*кожа*) kid. ~овый kid *attr.*; ~овые перчáтки kíd-gloves.

лáйнер *м.* líner; (*многоместный самолёт*) air líner.

лак *м.* várnish, lácquer; покрывáть *что-л.* ~ом lácquer *smth.*, várnish *smth.*; ~ для ногте́й nail várnish/pólish.

лакáть *несов.* (*вн.*) lap (*smth.*).

лаке́й *м.* fóotman*, mán-servant; *перен.* láckey, flúnkey. ~ский fóotman's, mán-servant's; *перен.* sérvile.

лакиро́ванн|ый várnished, lácquered; *перен.* lústrous, dázzling; ~ая ко́жа pátent léather; ~ые ту́фли pátent-léather shoes.

лакирова́ть *несов.* (*вн.*) várnish (*smth.*); *перен. тж.* embéllish (*smth.*), touch up (*smth.*); ~ действи́тельность put* a glóssy appeárance on things.

лакиро́в|ка *ж.* **1.** (*действие*) várnishing; *перен. тж.*

embéllishment, tóuching-up; **2.** (*слой лака*) várnish. ~щик *м.* várnisher; *перен.* embéllisher, whítewasher.

ла́кмус *м.* lítmus. ~овый: ~овая бума́га lítmus-paper.

ла́ковый 1. várnish *attr.*; **2.** (*покрытый лаком*) várnished, lácquered; **3.** (*о кожаных изделиях*) pátent-léather *attr.*

ла́комиться, пола́комиться (*тв.*) enjóy (*smth.*), regále onesélf (on).

ла́комк|а *м. и ж.* góurmand, lóver of food; быть ~ой have* a sweet tooth*.

ла́ком|ство *с.* **1.** *обыкн. мн.* (*сласти*) swéetmeats, sweets; **2.** (*вкусная пища*) dáinty, délicacy. ~ый **1.** (*очень вкусный*) tásty, témpting; **2.** (*до рд.; падкий на что-л.*) fond (of); ◇ ~ый кусо́чек títbit.

лакон|и́зм *м.* térseness, concíseness. ~и́ческий terse, concíse; (*о речи тж.*) lacónic. ~и́чно lacónically. ~и́чность *ж.* térseness. ~и́чный *см.* лакони́ческий; ~и́чный стиль concíse style.

лакто́за *ж.* láctose.

ла́ма I *ж.* (*животное*) lláma.

ла́ма II *м.* (*буддийский монах*) láma.

ла́мпа *ж.* lamp; *радио* valve, tube; электри́ческая ~ eléctric bulb; ~ дневно́го све́та fluoréscent lamp/bulb; ~ нака́ливания incandéscent bulb.

лампа́д|а *ж.*, ~ка *ж.* ícon lamp.

лампа́с *м.* stripe.

ламп|овый lamp *attr.*; *радио* valve *attr.*; ~овое стекло́ (lamp-)chímney; ~ приёмник valve recéiver. ~очка *ж.* bulb.

ланге́т *м.* (long) flank steak.

ландша́фт *м.* **1.** (*вид местности*) view, lándscape; scénery; **2.** (*картина*) lándscape; **3.** *геогр.* lándscape.

ла́ндыш *м.* líly of the válley.

ланце́т *м.* láncet.

лань *ж.* **1.** (*порода оленей*) fállow-deer*; **2.** (*самка*) doe (of fállow-deer*).

ла́п|а *ж.* **1.** paw, foot*; (*лисицы, зайца тж.*) pad; **2.** (*ветвь хвойного дерева*) branch; **3.** *тех.* claw; ~ я́коря ánchor-fluke; попа́сть в ~ы к кому́-л. fall* ínto smb.'s clútches; быть в ~ах у кого́-л. be* in smb.'s clútches; наложи́ть свою́ ~у на что-л. get* one's paws on smth.

лапида́рный lápidary, terse; ~ стиль terse style.

ла́п|ка *ж.*; ◇ ходи́ть на за́дних ~ах перед кем-л. dance atténdance on smb.

ла́пник *м. разг.* fir bránches *pl.*

ла́поть *м.* bást-shoe.

лапта́ *ж.* **1.** (*игра*) laptá (*a game similar to rounders*); **2.** (*бита*) bat.

ла́пчатый pálmate; (*имеющий лапы с перепонками тж.*) wéb-footed; ◇ гусь ~ sly féllow.

лапша́ *ж.* **1.** nóodles *pl*; **2.** (*суп*) nóodle soup.

лапше́вник *м.* nóodle púdding.

ларёк *м.* stall.

ларе́ц *м.* cásket.

ларинги́т *м. мед.* laryngítis.

ларинго́лог *м.* laryngólogist.

лариноло́гия *ж.* laryngólogy.

ларингоско́п *м.* láryngoscope.

ларингофо́н *м.* láryngophone.

ла́рчик *м.* cásket; ◇ а ~ про́сто открыва́лся ≈ the explanátion was quite símple.

ларь *м.* bin.

ла́ска I *ж.* **1.** caréss; **2.** (*ласковое отношение*) kíndness, afféction.

ла́ска II *ж. зоол.* wéasel.

ласка́тельн|ый 1. (*нежный*) afféctionate; ~ое сло́во term of afféction; **2.** *грам.* dimínutive.

ласк|а́ть *несов.* (*вн.*) caréss (*smb., smth.*), fóndle (*smb., smth.*); *перен.* please (*smb., smth.*), soothe (*smb., smth.*); ~ слух soothe the ear. ~а́ться *несов.* (к *дт.*) make* up (to); (*о собаке*) fawn (upón). ~а́ющий sóothing.

ла́сковый 1. (*о человеке*) afféctionate; (*о голосе, взгляде и т. п.*) ténder; ~ ребёнок afféctionate child*; ~ приём córdial recéption; **2.** (*ласкающий*) géntle, caréssing; ~ ветеро́к géntle breeze.

ласт *м.* **1.** flípper; **2.** *мн. спорт.* flíppers, fins.

ла́сточк|а *ж.* swállow; ◇ пе́рвая ~ the first signs/pórtent; одна́ ~ ещё не де́лает весны́ *посл.* ≈ one swállow does not make a súmmer. ~ин swállow's.

лата́ть, залата́ть (*вн.*) *разг.* patch (*smth.*), patch up (*smth.*).

латви́йский Látvian.

латини́ст *м.* Látin schólar; (*преподаватель*) Látin téacher.

латиноамерика́нск|ий: ~ие стра́ны Látin-Américan cóuntries, cóuntries of Látin América.

лати́нский Látin; ~ алфави́т Róman álphabet; ~ язы́к Látin.

лату́к *м. бот.* léttuce.

лату́нный brass *attr.*

лату́нь *ж.* brass.

ла́ты *мн.* ármour *sg*, cuiráss *sg.*

латы́нь *ж. разг.* Látin.

латы́ш *м.*, ~ка *ж.* Lett. ~ский Léttish; ~ский язы́к Léttish, the Léttish lánguage.

лауреа́т *м.* príze-winner, láureate.

лафе́т *м.* gún-carriage.

ла́цкан *м.* lapél.

лачу́га *ж.* hóvel, shánty, shack.

ла́ять *несов.* bark.

лганьё *с.* **1.** (*действие*) lýing; **2.** (*ложь*) lies *pl*, fálsehood.

лгать, солга́ть lie, tell* lies.

лгун *м.* líar.

лебеда́ *ж.* góose-foot.

лебеди́н|ый swan *attr.*; ~ая ста́я flock of swans; **2.** (*напоминающий лебедя*) swánlike, swan's; ~ая ше́я swánlike neck; ~ая по́ступь gráceful walk; ◇ ~ая пе́сня swan song.

лебёдка *ж. тех.* winch.

ле́бедь *м.* swan; (*самец*) cob; (*молодой*) cýgnet.

лебези́ть *несов.* (перед *тв.*) *разг.* fawn (on), kowtów (to).

лебя́жий swan *attr.*, swan's; *перен. тж.* swánlike; ~ пух swan's down.

лев *м.* líon.

лев|е́ть *несов.* go* left. ~изна́ *ж.* rádicalism.

левко́й *м. бот.* stock.

левобере́жный léft-bank *attr.*

левша́ *м. и ж.* léft-hánded pérson; léft-hánder; он ~ he's léft-hánded.

ле́в|ый прил. **1.** (*о стороне, направлении*) left; léft-hand *attr.*; *мор.* port *attr.*; в ~ом углу́, я́щике in the léft-hand córner, drawer; ~ая сторона́ left side; ~ карма́н léft-hand pócket; ~ борт *мор.* port side; ~ фланг left flank/wing, the left; **2.** *полит.* léft-wing *attr.*; **3.** *разг.* (*о работе, заработке*) unofficial; on the side *после сущ.*; **4.** *в знач. сущ. м. полит.* léft-winger; *мн. собир.* the Left, léft-wingers.

лега́в|ый: ~ая соба́ка (*длинношёрстная*) sétter; (*короткошёрстная*) póinter.

легализ|и́ровать *несов. и сов.* (*вн.*) légalize (*smb., ...*). ~и́роваться *несов. и сов.* becóme* légal. ~ова́ть(ся) *несов. и сов. см.* легализи́ровать(ся).

лега́льн|ость *ж.* legálity. ~ый légal.

леге́нд|а *ж.* **1.** légend; **2.** (*вымысел*) fáiry-tale; **3.** (*разведчика*) stóry, légend. ~а́рный **1.** légendary; *перен. тж.* fábulous; **2.** (*породивший легенду*) renówned, célebrated; ~а́рный го́род city of renówn; **3.** (*вымышленный*) fictítious.

легио́н *м.* légion.

леги́рованн|ый allóy(ed); ~ая сталь allóy steel.

легитим|и́зм *м.* legitimism. ~и́ст *м.* legítimist.

лёгк|ий 1. (*по весу*) light; боре́ц ~ого ве́са líght-weight; 2. (*ло́вкий, изя́щный*) light, líght-fóoted, gráceful; (*бы́стрый*) fléet-fóoted; ~ие шаги́ light fóotsteps; 3. (*нетру́дный*) éasy; (*развлека́тельный*) light; ~ уро́к éasy lésson; ~ая му́зыка light músic; ~ое чте́ние light líterature/réading; ~ успе́х éasy succéss; ~ слог éasy style; ~ая жизнь life of ease, éasy life; 4. (*незначи́тельный, сла́бый*) light, slight; ~ моро́з light frost; ~ое наказа́ние light púnishment; ~ая боль slight pain; ~ на́сморк slight cold; ~ое заболева́ние mild case; ~ таба́к mild tobácco; 5. (*пове́рхностный, несерьёзный*) light, líght-minded, frívolous; ~ие нра́вы éasy/loose mórals; 6. (*покла́дистый*) nice, éasy-góing; ~ хара́ктер sweet/nice disposítion; ◇ ~ая промы́шленность light índustry; у него́ ~ая рука́ he brings luck; с ~им се́рдцем, с ~ой душо́й with a light héart; лёгок на поми́не! talk of the dévil (and he is sure to appéar).

легко́ 1. *нареч.* líghtly; (*без труда́*) éasily; (*беззабо́тно*) áirily; (*немно́жко, слегка́*) slíghtly; ~ ра́нен slíghtly wóunded; 2. *в знач. сказ. безл.* it is éasy; ◇ ~ сказа́ть it's all véry well (to talk), it's éasier said than done.

легкоатле́т *м.* track and field áthlete. ~и́ческий track and field *attr.*

легкове́р|ие *с.* credúlity. ~ный crédulous.

легкове́с *м. спорт.* light-weight. ~ный líght-weight *attr.*; light; *перен.* flímsy, trívial; ~ный до́вод flímsy árgument.

легков|о́й: ~ автомоби́ль, ~а́я маши́на (pássenger-)car.

лёгк|ое *с.* 1. lung; боле́знь ~их púlmonary diséase, lúng-diséase; 2. *тк. ед.* (*как ку́шанье*) lights *pl.*

легкомы́сленн|ый frívolous, líght-minded, thóughtless; ~ челове́к líght-minded pérson; ~ое отноше́ние к де́лу irrespónsibility; ~ посту́пок thóughtless áction.

легкомы́слие *с.* frivólity, frívolousness, líght-mindedness, lévity.

легкопла́вкий fúsible.

лёгкость *ж.* 1. líghtness; 2. (*рабо́ты, зада́чи и т. п.*) ease, facílity; с ~ю with ease; 3. (*подви́жность*) nímbleness.

лёгочный púlmonary; ~ больно́й lúng-pátient.

легча́ть, полегча́ть *разг.* 1. abáte; мне полегча́ло I begán to feel bétter.

ле́гче 1. (*сравни́т. ст. прил. лёгкий и нареч.* легко́) (*по весу*) líghter; (*по тру́дности*) éasier; 2. *в знач. сказ. безл.*: ему́ ~ he is féeling bétter; больно́му ~ the pátient is féeling bétter; ◇ мне от э́того не ~ it's no cómfort to me; час о́т часу не ~ things are góing from bad to worse; ~! (*осторо́жнее*) not so fast!; ~ на поворо́тах! watch your step!

лёд *м.* ice; ~ идёт the ice has begún to move; затёртый льда́ми caught in the ice; ◇ слома́ть ~ break* the ice, start the ball rólling; ~ тро́нулся things are móving.

леден|е́ть *несов.* 1. turn to ice; 2. (*замерза́ть, коченеть*) be* chilled to the bone; ру́ки ~е́ют my hands are fréezing; 3. (*цепене́ть*) freeze*; ~ от у́жаса freeze* with hórror.

ледене́ц *м.* frúit-drop.

леден|и́ть *несов.* (*вн.*) freeze* (*smth.*) (*тж. перен.*); turn (*smth.*) to ice. ~я́щий ícy (*тж. перен.*); fréezing, chílling; ~я́щее дыха́ние ве́тра ícy blast of wind; его́ охвати́л ~я́щий у́жас he was chilled with hórror; ~я́щий взгляд ícy look.

ле́ди *ж. нескл.* lády.

ле́дник *м.* íce-house; (*ко́мнатный*) refrígerator; íce-box *амер.*

ледни́к *м.* glácier.

леднико́вый glácial; ~ пери́од glácial périod, íce-age.

ледо́в|ый 1. ice *attr.*; ~ покро́в ice cóver; 2.: ~ые

пла́вания Árctic vóyages; ◇ ~ая разве́дка ice recónnaissance; ~ая обстано́вка ice condítions *pl.*

ледоко́л *м.* íce-breaker.

ледоре́з *м.* 1. (*сооруже́ние*) stárling; 2. (*су́дно*) íce-breaker.

ледору́б *м.* íce-axe.

ледоста́в *м.* fréeze-up.

ледохо́д *м.* drífting of the ice; начался́ ~ the ice has begún to move.

леды́шк|а *ж. разг.* lump of ice; у него́ ру́ки как ~и his hands are like ice.

ледян|о́й 1. ice *attr.*; 2. (*холо́дный*) (*тж. перен.*) ícy; ~ ве́тер ícy wind; ~а́я вода́ íce-cold wáter; ~ взгляд ícy/chilling look.

лежа́к *м.* plank bed; chaise-lóngue, deck chair.

лежа́лый stale.

леж|а́ть *несов.* lie*; ~ в лихора́дке be* down with féver; ~ в посте́ли be* in bed; (*о больно́м*) keep* one's bed; ~ в больни́це be* in hóspital; кни́га ~и́т на столе́ the book is on the táble; ~ без употребле́ния lie* ídle; на нас ~и́т отве́тственность за э́то it is our responsibílity; ◇ ~ в разва́линах lie* in rúins; у меня́ душа́ не ~и́т к э́тому my heart ísn't in it; ~ под сукно́м lie* on the shelf. ~а́чий *прил.* 1. recúmbent; ~а́чий больно́й bed-pátient. 2. *в знач. сущ. м.*: ~а́чего не бьют don't hit a man* when he's down; ◇ в ~а́чем положе́нии lýing, in a lýing posítion.

ле́жбище *с.* 1. (*морски́х живо́тных*) róokery; bréeding ground; 2. *охот.* bed.

лежебо́ка *м. и ж. разг.* lázy-bones.

ле́звие *с.* blade.

лезги́н *м.* Lezghín.

лезги́нка I *ж.* Lezghín wóman*.

лезги́нка II *ж.* (*та́нец*) lezghínka.

лезги́нский Lezghín.

лезть *несов.* 1. *см.* ла́зить; 2. (*внутрь*) get* in; ~ в окно́ get* in by/through the wíndow; 3. (*в вн.*) *разг.* (*проника́ть руко́й внутрь чего́-л.*) put* one's hand (into); 4. *разг.* (*насто́йчиво идти́, продвига́ться*) push; ~ вперёд push fórward; 5. (*к дт.*) *разг.* (*надоеда́ть, вме́шиваться*) butt in (on); ~ в чужи́е дела́ poke one's nose ínto óther péople's affáirs; 6. (*выпада́ть — о волоса́х и т. п.*) come* out, fall* out; (*располза́ться — о мате́рии*) wear* thin; 7. (*быть впору*) go* on; сапо́г не ле́зет the boot won't go on, I can't get the boot on; ◇ ~ в дра́ку be* lóoking for a fight; в го́лову ле́зут ра́зные мы́сли all sorts of thoughts pass through one's mind; ~ на глаза́ push onesélf forward; не ~ за сло́вом в карма́н have* a réady tongue; ~ на́ стену от чего́-л. be* frántic with smth., be* beside onesélf with smth.

лейбори́ст *м.* mémber of the Lábour Párty. ~ский Lábour *attr.*; ~ская па́ртия the Lábour Párty.

ле́йденск|ий: ~ая ба́нка Léyden jar.

ле́йка *ж.* 1. (*для поли́вки*) wátering-can; 2. *разг.* (*воро́нка*) fúnnel; 3. *мор.* (*черпа́к*) scoop.

лейкоци́т *м.* физиол. léucocyte, white blood córpuscle.

лейтена́нт *м.* lieuténant; ста́рший ~ sénior lieuténant; (*в англи́йской армии*) first lieuténant; мла́дший ~ júnior lieuténant; (*в англи́йской армии*) sécond lieuténant.

лейтмоти́в *м. муз.* léit-motif; *перен.* búrden, theme.

лека́ло *с.* (*для черче́ния*) curve.

лека́рственн|ый medícinal; ~ые тра́вы medícinal herbs.

лека́рство *с.* médicine; дава́ть ~ give*/adminíster médicine; принима́ть ~ take* one's médicine.

ле́карь *м. уст.* dóctor.

ле́ксика *ж.* vocábulary.

лексико́|граф *м.* lexicógrapher. ~графи́ческий lexicográphical. ~гра́фия *ж.* lexicógraphy. ~лог *м.* lexicólogist. ~ло́гия *ж.* lexicólogy.

лексикóн м. 1. уст. (словарь) léxicon; 2. (запас слов) vocábulary.

лексúческий léxical.

лéктор м. lécturer.

лектóрий м. 1. lécturing buréau (pl -éaux, -éaus); 2. (помещение) lécture-hall.

лéкторский lécturing; ~ óпыт lécturing expérience.

лекциóнно-демонстрациóнный: ~ зал lécture-hall (equípped with demonstrátion apparátus).

лекциóнн|ый lécture attr.; ~ые часы́ lécture hours/times; ~ зал lécture-hall, lécture-room.

лéкци|я ж. lécture; ~ по языкознáнию lécture on linguístics; посещáть ~и atténd léctures; прочéсть ~ю give*/déliver a lécture; читáть ~и lécture.

лелéять несов. (вн.; прям. и перен.) chérish (smb., smth.); ~ мечту́ chérish the hope.

лéмéх м. с.-х. plóughshare.

лён м. flax.

ленúв|ец м. 1. (лентяй) ídler, lázy féllow; lázy-bones разг.; 2. (животное) sloth. ~ый 1. (избегающий труда) lázy, ídle; ~ый ученúк lázy púpil; 2. (выражающий лень) índolent; ~ая пóза índolent áttitude; 3. (медлительный) slúggish; slow (тж. перен.); ~ая похóдка sáunter, sáuntering gait.

ленингрáд|ец м. inhábitant of Léningrad. ~ский Léningrad attr.

лен|úться несов. be* lázy; не ~úсь! don't be so lázy!; ~ рабóтать be* too lázy to work.

лéность ж. láziness, sloth.

лéнта ж. 1. ríbbon (тж. перен.); ~ на шля́пе hát-band; 2. тех. tape; измерúтельная ~ tápe-measure; изоляцóнная ~ ínsulating tape; конвéйерная ~ convéyor belt; 3. (кинофильм) film; ◇ пулемётная ~ machíne-gun belt.

лéнточка ж. ríbbon.

лéнточн|ый 1. ríbbon attr.; 2. (в форме ленты): ~ые чéрви tápeworms; 3.: ~ая пилá bánd-saw; ~ая подáча belt feed.

лентя́й м., ~ка ж. разг. slácker, slúggard, lázy-bones; он ~ he's lázy. ~ничать несов. разг. loaf, ídle, slack.

лен|á ж. разг.: с ~óй ráther lázy; рабóтать с ~óй work half-héartedly, slack.

лень ж. 1. láziness, índolence, sloth; 2. в знач. сказ. разг.: ему́ (ей) ~ (+ инф.) he (she) is too lázy (+ to inf); ◇ (все) комý не ~ ányone who feels like it, ányone who will take the tróuble.

леопáрд м. léopard.

лепестóк м. pétal; ~ рóзы róse-leaf*.

лéпет м. (ребёнка) prátling; (нежный; тж. перен.) múrmuring; ◇ дéтский ~ prátle, drível. ~áть несов. bábble; (о ребёнке) prátle; (нежно говорúть; тж. перен.) múrmur.

лепёшка ж.1. (из теста) scone; 2. (лекарство, конфета) lózenge; 3. (что-л. плоское и круглое) clot; ~ грязи clot of mud.

лепúть, вы́лепить, слепúть (вн.) 1. сов. вы́лепить módel (smth.); ~ бюст make*/módel a bust; 2. сов. слепúть build* (smth.); ~ гнёзда build* nests; ~ из глúны módel in clay. ~ся несов. (к дт.) cling* (to); дóмики лéпятся по склóну горы́ the hóuses hug the slope.

лéп|ка ж. módelling. ~нóй: ~ны́е рабóты pláster work sg; ~ны́е украшéния stúcco móulding sg; ~нóй потолóк móulded céiling.

лéпт|а ж. mite, contribútion; внестú свою́ ~у во что-л. make* one's contribútion to smth.

лес м. 1. wood; (обширный) fórest; прогу́лка в ~у́ a walk in the woods; 2. тк. ед. (материал) tímber; lúmber амер.; ◇ как в ~у́ ● all at sea; кто в ~, кто по дровá погов. ● at síxes and sévens.

лесá I мн. (строительные) scáffolding sg, stáging sg; (в шахте) pit props.

лесá II ж. (для рыбной ловли) físhing-line.

лесúст|ый wóoded; ~ая мéстность wóoded locálity, wóodland.

лéска ж. см. лесá II.

лесн|úк м. fórest guard; fórest ránger амер. ~чество с. fórestry. ~чий м. fórester, fórest wárden.

лесн|óй fórest attr., wóodland attr.; ~ жúтель fórest-dwéller; ~ пейзáж wóodland scénery/lándscape; ~ы́е богáтства tímber resóurces; ~áя тропá fórest/wóodland path; ~áя земляника wild stráwberries pl; ~ пúтомник fórest núrsery, trée-nursery; ~áя промы́шленность tímber índustry; lúmber índustry амер.

лесовóд м. fórestry éxpert. ~ство с. fórestry. ~ческий fórestry attr.

лесозавóд м. tímber mill.

лесозагото́вки мн. (ед. лесозаготóвка ж.) lógging sg; lúmbering sg амер.

лесозащúтный fórest-protéction attr.

лесоматериáл|ы мн. (ед. лесоматериáл м.) tímber sg; склад ~ов tímber-yard.

лесонасаждéн|ие с. 1. (действие) afforestátion; 2. обыкн. мн. (посаженные деревья) plantátion sg; полезащúтные ~ия shélter-belts; protéctive afforestátion sg.

лесопáрк м. fórest park. ~овый fórest-park attr.

лесо|пúлка ж. разг. sáwmill. ~пúльный wóod-sawing; ~пúльный завóд sáwmill.

лесопúтомник м. fórest núrsery, trée-nursery.

лесополосá ж. wóodland belt, fórest belt.

лесопосáдочн|ый: ~ые материáлы sáplings; ~ые маши́ны trée-plánting machínes.

лесопромы́шленн|ость ж. tímber índustry. ~ый of the tímber índustry после сущ.

лесоразрабóтки мн. (ед. лесоразрабóтка ж.) lógging sg; (место) lógging área.

лесору́б м. lógger, wóodcutter; lúmberjack амер.

лесо|сéка ж. félling área. ~сплáв м. ráfting.

лесо|степнóй ~степны́е райóны pártially-wóoded steppe dístricts. ~степь ж. pártially-wóoded steppe. ~ту́ндра ж. wóoded tú́ndra, fórest tú́ndra.

лёсс м. lóess.

лéстн|ица ж. 1. (постоянная) stairs pl, stáircase; (переносная) ládder; steps pl; 2. (последовательное расположение) ládder, órder; обще́ственная ~ the sócial ládder. ~чный: ~чная клéтка stáircase.

**лéстн|о 1. нареч. fláteringly; (одобрительно) appróvingly, in compliméntary terms; 2. в знач. сказ. безл.: мне óчень ~ слы́шать... I have been déeply grátified to hear... ~ый 1. fláttering; 2. (одобрительный) compliméntary, grátifying.

лесть ж. fláttery; (превозношéние) adulátion.

лёт м.: на летý on the wing; хватáть что-л. на летý take* smth. in one's stride, grasp smth. at once.

летá мн. 1. (годы) years; 2. (возраст) age sg; скóлько вам лет? how old are you?; мне 30 лет I'm thírty; мне бы́ло 20 лет, когдá... I was twénty (years old) when...; с дéтских лет from chíldhood; егó ~ не позволя́ют э́того he's too old for that at his age; ◇ в ~х élderly; он ужé в ~х he's gétting on in years; на стáрости лет in one's old age; по мóлодости лет on accóunt of one's youth; по развúтию не по ~м he's véry intélligent for his age; he's a little precócious.

летáрг|úческий lethárgic; ~ сон lethárgic sleep. ~úя ж. léthargy.

летáтельный flýing; ~ аппарáт flýing machíne; ~ аппарáт лéгче вóздуха líghter-than-áir craft; ~ аппарáт тяжелéе вóздуха héavier-than-áir craft.

летáть несов. fly*.

летéть несов. 1. см. летáть; 2. (мчаться) fly* alóng; 3. разг. (падать) go* flýing, fall*; 4. (о времени) fly* (by).

лéтний súmmer attr.

лётн|ый flýing *attr*.; ~ая погóда flýing wéather; ~ костюм flýing suit; ~ая шкóла flýing school; ◇ ~ое пóле áirfield.

лéто *c*. súmmer; ◇ скóлько лет, скóлько зим! fáncy méeting you áfter all this time!, it's áges since we met!

лéтом in (the) súmmer; ~ 1965 гóда in the súmmer of 1965.

летопи́сец *m*. chrónicler.

лéтопись *ж*. chrónicle; ánnals *pl*.

летосчислéние *c*. (sýstem of) chronólogy.

летýн *m. разг*. flýer; *перен*. rólling-stone.

летýч|есть *ж*. volatílity. ~ий 1. flýing (*тж. перен.*); ~ий отрáд flýing cólumn; 2. (*легко испаряющийся*) vólatile; 3. (*мимолётный*) fléeting; ◇ ~ая мышь 1) bat; 2) (*фонарь*) storm lántern; ~ий ми́тинг ón-the-spót méeting; ~ий ревмати́зм shífting rhéumatism. ~ка *ж. разг*. (*краткое собрание*) quick bríefing.

лётчик *m*. áirman*, pílot, flýer, flýing man*. ~-испытáтель *m*. test pílot. ~-истреби́тель *m*. fíghter pílot. ~-космонáвт *m*. space pílot. ~-наблюдáтель *m*. áir-obsérver.

лётчица *ж*. áirwoman*, wóman* pílot/flýer.

лéчащий: ~ врач dóctor in charge of the case.

лечéбн|ица *ж*. (spécial) hóspital. ~ый (*врачебный*) médical; (*целебный*) medícinal; ~ое заведéние médical estáblishment; ~ые трáвы medícinal herbs; ~ая физкультýра therapéutic phýsical tráining.

лечéние *c*. tréatment.

лечи́ть *несов*. (*вн*.) treat (*smb., smth.*); (*вн. от рд.*) treat (*smb.* for); кто вас лéчит? who's your dóctor?; ~ сéрдце treat the heart; ~ туберкулёз treat tuberculósis. ~ся *несов*. take* a cure; (*от рд.*) undergó* tréatment (for), be* tréated (for); он лечи́лся у дóктора N he was Dr. N's pátient; у когó вы лéчитесь? who's your dóctor?

лечь *сов. см*. ложи́ться.

лéший *m. фольк*. góblin (of the woods).

лещ *m*. bream.

лженау́|ка *ж*. pséudo-science. ~чный pséudo-scientífic.

лжесвидéтель *m*. pérjurer, pérjured witness. ~ство *c*. false witness, pérjury. ~ствовать *несов*. commít pérjury.

лжетеóрия *ж*. false théory.

лже|учéние *c*. false dóctrine. ~учёный *m*. pséudo-scientist.

лжец *m*. líar.

лжи́в|ость *ж*. mendácity. ~ый mendácious; (*о человеке тж*.) untrúthful; ~ые рéчи false words; ~ый язык lýing tongue.

ли 1. *частица* (*в прямом вопросе выражается обычной вопр. формой*): нрáвится ли вам áто? do you like it?; плати́л ли он? has he paid?; придёт ли он? is he cóming?; 2. *союз* if, whéther; (*после отрицания*) whéther; посмотри́, пришёл ли он go and see if/whéther he's come; я не знáю, пришёл ли он I don't know whéther he's come.

лиáна *ж. бот*. liána.

либерáл *m*. líberal. ~изм *m*. líberalism.

либерáльн|ичать *несов. разг*. be* óver-tólerant. ~ость *ж*. líberalism; líberal views *pl*. ~ый líberal.

ли́бо or; ~..., ~... éither... or...

либрéтто *c. нескл*. librétto, book; (*краткое изложение оперы и т. п.*) stóry.

ли́вень *m*. dównpour; (*кратковременный*) héavy shówer; *перен*. hail.

ли́вер *m*. pluck. ~ный pluck *attr*.

ливрéйный lívery *attr*.

ливрé|я *ж*. lívery; в ~e líveried.

ли́га *ж*. league.

лигатýра *ж*. 1. (*примесь*) allóy; 2. *лингв., мед*. lígature.

лигни́т *m*. lígnite.

ли́дер *m*. léader. ~ство *c*. 1. léadership; 2. (*первенство*) the lead.

лиди́ровать *несов. и сов*. be* in the lead.

лизáть, лизну́ть (*вн*.) lick (*smth.*). ~ся *несов*. 1. lick onesélf; 2. (*лизать друг друга*) lick one anóther.

лизну́ть *сов. см*. лизáть.

лик I *m. уст*. cóuntenance; (*на иконах*) ímage; *перен*. face.

лик II *m. уст.* (*сонм, собрание*) commúnion, причи́слить когó-л. к ~у святы́х cánonize *smb.*

ликвид|áтор *m*. líquidator. ~áция *ж*. 1. (*прекращение деятельности чего-л.*) liquidátion; 2. (*уничтожение*) abolítion. ~и́ровать *несов. и сов.* (*вн.*) 1. (*прекращать деятельность чего-л.*) líquidate (*smth.*), wind* up (*smth.*); 2. (*уничтожать*) abólish (*smth.*), elíminate (*smth.*), wipe out (*smth.*); ~и́ровать задóлженность wipe out a debt; ~и́ровать безгрáмотность put* an end to illíteracy, do* awáy with illíteracy. ~и́роваться *несов. и сов.* be* liquidated, be* wound up.

ликёр *m*. liquéur.

ликов|áние *c*. rejóicing, jubilátion. ~áть *несов*. rejóice, exúlt, tríumph.

лику́ющий júbilant, exúltant.

лилипýт *m*. Lillipútian, dwarf.

ли́лия *ж*. líly; ◇ водянáя ~ wáter-lily.

лилóвый púrple, mauve.

лимáн *m*. lagóon.

лимб *m. тех*. limb, gráduated circle.

лими́т *m*. límit. ~и́ровать *несов. и сов.* (*вн.*) límit (*smth.*).

лимóн *m.* (*плод и дерево*) lémon. ~áд *m*. lemonáde. ~ный 1. lémon *attr*.; 2. (*цвета лимона*) lémon-cóloured; ◇ ~ная кислотá cítric ácid.

ли́мфа *ж. физиол*. lymph. ~ти́ческий *физиол*. lymphátic.

лингафóн *m*. línguaphone.

лингви́ст *m*. línguist. ~ика *ж*. linguístics. ~и́ческий linguístic.

линéй|ка *ж*. 1. (*линия*) line; тетрáдь в ~ку lined nótebook; 2. (*чертёжная*) rúler; 3. (*строй в одну шеренгу*) line; paráde; выстрáиваться в ~ку form up in line, go* on paráde; ~ (*сбор пионеров, военных*) paráde; вечéрняя ~ évening paráde; торжéственная ~ ceremónial paráde.

линéйн|ый *прил*. 1. línear; 2. *в знач. сущ. m. воен*. márker; ~ые мéры línear méasures.

ли́нза *ж*. lens.

ли́ни|я *ж*. line; провести́ ~ю draw* a line; ~ желéзной дорóги ráilway-line; ráilroad-track *амер*.; ~ поведéния line of áction; pólicy; ~ прицéливания line of sight; ◇ вести́ свою́ ~ю pursúe one's own pólicy; по ~и наимéньшего сопротивлéния alóng the line of least resístance.

линкóр *m*. báttleship.

линóванный ruled, lined.

линовáть, налиновáть (*вн*.) rule (*smth.*), line (*smth.*).

линогравю́ра *ж*. línocut.

линóлеум *m*. linóleum.

линоти́п *m. полигр*. línotype.

линчевá|ние *c*. lýnching. ~ть *несов. и сов.* (*вн.*) lynch (*smb.*).

линь I *m.* (*рыба*) tench.

линь II *m. мор*. line.

ли́нька *ж*. móulting.

лин|ю́чий *разг*. fáding; ~ю́чая матéрия matérial that runs (in the wash). ~я́лый *разг*. fáded, discóloured. ~я́ть, полиня́ть 1. moult; (*о животных тж*.) lose* its fur/coat; 2. (*терять окраску*) fade, lose* cólour; (*при стирке*) run*.

ли́па *ж*. lime(-tree), línden.

ли́п|кий stícky; adhésive *тех*.; ~ плáстырь

sticking/adhésive pláster. ~нуть *несов.* (к *дт.*) stick* (to), cling* (to); *перен. разг.* fásten (on to), cling* (to).

ли́повый lime *attr.*; ◇ ~ цвет (dried) líme-blossom.

ли́ра *ж.* lýre.

ли́рик *м.* lýric póet.

ли́рик|а *ж.* 1. lýricism; 2. (*стихи*) lýric póetry; 3. *разг.* (*чувствительность*) séntiment; пуска́ться в ~у indúlge in séntiment.

лири́ч|еский 1. (*о поэзии*) lýric; 2. (*чувствительный*) lýrical; ~еское отступле́ние lýrical digréssion. ~ность *ж.* lýricism.

лис|а́ *ж.* fox. ~ёнок *м.* fóx-cub.

ли́сий fox *attr.*; ~ след fox tracks *pl*; ли́сьи но́ры fox holes; ли́сья шу́ба coat lined with fóx-skin.

лиси́|ца *ж.* fox; (*самка*) víxen. ~чка *ж.* 1. fox; 2. (*гриб*) chanterélle.

лист *м.* 1. (*мн.* ли́стья *и* листы́) (*растения*) leaf*; 2. (*мн.* листы́) (*бумаги, металла*) sheet*; 3. (*мн. листы́*) (*документ*): похва́льный ~ testimónial; 4. (*мн. листы́*) *полигр.* (*16 страниц*) sheet (*containing sixteen pages*); све́рстанные ~ы́ páge-proofs; ◇ а́вторский ~ signature (*containing 40,000 characters*); петь, игра́ть с ~а́ sing*, play at sight. ~а́ж *м.* númber of sheets (in a book).

листа́ть *несов.* (*вн.*) *разг.* go* through the páges (of), turn the páges (of).

листва́ *ж. собир.* fóliage; leaves *pl.*

ли́ственн|ица *ж.* larch. ~ый decíduous, bróad-léaved; ~ый лес decíduous/bróad-léaved fórest.

ли́стик *м.* leaf*

листо́вка *ж.* léaflet.

листов|о́й 1. leaf *attr.*; 2. sheet *attr.*; ~а́я лату́нь léaf-brass; ~а́я сталь steel plate; sheet steel; ◇ ~ таба́к leaf tobácco.

листо́к *м.* 1. leaf*; 2. (*бумаги*) sheet (of páper).

листопа́д *м.* fall of the leaf, turn of the year.

литавр|ы *мн.* (*ед.* лита́вра *ж.*) *муз.* kéttle-drum *sg.*

лите́й|ный fóundry *attr.*; ~ заво́д fóundry; ◇ ~ двор cásting bed. ~щик *м.* fóunder, fóundryman*.

ли́тер *м. разг.* trávelling wárrant.

ли́тера *ж.* 1. *полигр.* type; 2. *уст.* (*буква*) létter.

литера́тор *м.* man* of létters, líterary man*.

литерату́р|а *ж.* literature; техни́ческая ~ téchnical publicátions *pl.* ~ный líterary; ~ный ве́чер líterary gáthering; ~ное насле́дство líterary légacy; ~ная переда́ча (*по радио*) literary/book prógramme; ◇ ~ный язы́к líterary lánguage.

литературове́д *м.* literary schólar. ~ение *с.* history and críticism of literature; literary stúdies *pl.* ~ческий líterature *attr.*

ли́терный (*обозначенный буквой*) léttered.

ли́тий *м. хим.* líthium.

лито́в|ец *м.* ~ка *ж.* Lithuánian. ~ский Lithuánian; ~ский язы́к Lithuánian, the Lithuánian lánguage.

лито́граф *м.* lithógrapher. ~и́ровать *несов. и сов.* (*вн.*) líthograph (*smth.*).

литогра́ф|ия *ж.* 1. (*печатание*) lithógraphy; 2. (*оттиск*) líthograph; 3. (*предприятие*) lithográphical works. ~ский lithográphic.

лит|о́й cast; ~о́е желе́зо íngot iron.

литр *м.* litre; ~ *амер.* ~о́вый litre *attr.*; ~о́вая буты́лка óne-litre bóttle.

литурги́я *ж. церк.* líturgy.

лить *несов.* 1. (*вн.*; *жидкость*) pour (*smth.*); *перен.* shed* (*smth.*), cast* (*smth.*); ~ во́ду в стака́н pour wáter ínto a glass; 2. (*течь*) pour; вода́ льёт из кра́на wáter is póuring out of the tap; 3. (*вн.*) *тех.* cast* (*smth.*); ◇ ~ слёзы shed* tears.

литьё *с. тех.* 1. (*действие*) cásting; 2. *собир.* (*изделия*) cástings *pl.*

ли́ться *несов.* flow, stream, pour.

лиф *м.* bódice.

лифт *м.* lift; élevator *амер.*

лифтёр *м.* líftboy, líftman; élevator boy *амер.* ~ша *ж. разг.* lift-girl; élevator girl *амер.*

ли́фчик *м.* (*детский*) bódice; (*бюстгальтер*) brassiére; bra *разг.*

лиха́ч *м.* 1. (*храбрый человек*) dáre-devil; 2. (*на автомобиле*) réckless dríver; road hog *разг.*

лиха́чество *с.* récklessness.

лихв|а́ *ж.*: с ~о́й with ínterest.

лих|о́ I *с разг.* évil; ◇ не помина́й(те) ~ом! don't think bádly of me!; узна́ть, почём фунт ~а have* a taste of misfórtune.

ли́хо II *нареч. разг.* 1. (*смело, храбро*) dáringly, dáshingly, with dash; 2. (*быстро*) at a spánking pace; 3. (*бойко*) jáuntily; 4. (*ловко*) smártly, déftly.

лих|о́й I *разг.* (*плохой*) évil; ◇ ~а́ беда́ нача́ло it's the first step that counts.

лихо́й II *разг.* 1. (*удалой*) dáring, dáshing; 2. (*быстрый*) fast; (*о лошадях*) spírited; 3. (*бойкий*) jáunty; 4. (*ловкий*) smart, deft.

лихора́д|ить *несов. безл.*: меня́ ~ит I am féverish. ~ка *ж.* féver. ~очность *ж.* féverishness; *перен. тж.* féverish excítement. ~очный féverish; ~очная поспе́шность féverish haste.

ли́хость *ж.* 1. (*смелость*) dáring, dash; 2. (*быстрота*) speed; 3. (*бойкость*) jáuntiness; 4. (*ловкость*) déftness.

лицев|о́й 1. fácial; 2. (*наружный, верхний*): ~а́я сторона́ the right side; (*монеты, медали*) óbverse; 3. *фин.*: ~ счёт pérsonal accóunt.

лицезре́ть *несов.* (*вн.*) *ирон.* behóld* (*smb., smth.*).

лицеме́р *м.* hýpocrite. ~ие *с.* hypócrisy. ~ить *несов.* be* hypocrítical, be* a hýpocrite; dissémble *книжн.* ~ный hypocrítical; ~ный челове́к hypocrítical pérson; ~ная улы́бка hypocrítical smile.

лице́нзия *ж. эк.* lícence.

лиц|о́ *с.* 1. (*часть головы*) face; 2. (*отличительные черты*) cháracter; не име́ть своего́ ~а́ have* no cháracter; сохрани́ть своё ~ presérve one's idéntity/image; 3. (*человек*) pérson; гражда́нское ~ civílian; физи́ческое ~ *юр.* nátural pérson; 4. (*лицевая сторона*) right side; 5. *грам.* pérson; ◇ быть к ~у́ кому́-л. suit smb., be* becóming to smb.; э́та шля́па ей не к ~у́ that hat suits her; быть не к ~у́ кому́-л. not suit smb., be* unbecóming to smb.; вам не к ~у́ осужда́ть, жа́ловаться it is not for you to críticize, to compláin; на нём ~á нет he looks térrible/áwful; перед ~о́м кого́-л., чего́-л. in the face of smb., smth.; в ~ кому́-л. to smb.'s face; в ~ кого́-л. in the pérson of smb.; от ~á кого́-л. on behálf of smb.; ~о́м к кому́-л., чему́-л. fácing smb., smth.; ~о́м к ~у́ face to face; поверну́ться ~о́м к чему́-л. turn to face smth.; показа́ть това́р ~о́м make* the best of what one has; не уда́рить в грязь ~о́м not disgráce onesélf; знать кого́-л. в ~ know* smb. by sight; смотре́ть в ~ чему́-л. face smth.

ли́чико *с.* (little) face.

личи́н|а *ж.* mask; под ~ой дру́жбы únder the guise of friéndship.

личи́нка *ж. зоол.* grub; lárva (*pl* -vae).

ли́чно pérsonally; ~ ознако́миться с чем-л. get* a first-hand view of smth.; see* smth. for onesélf; быть ~ заинтересо́ванным в чём-л. have* a pérsonal stake in smth.

личн|о́й face *attr.*; ~о́е полоте́нце fáce-towel.

ли́чн|ость *ж.* 1. (*индивидуальность*) personálity; (*в сочетании с определением*) pérson, cháracter; зага́дочная ~ mystérious pérson; 2. (*индивидуум*) indivídual; роль ~ости в исто́рии the role of the indivídual in hístory. ~ый pérsonal; (*принадлежащий толькс данному лицу тж.*) prívate; ~ая со́бственность pérsonal próperty; ~ый секрета́рь prívate sécretary; ~ое мне́ние pérsonal opínion; ~ое клеймо́ (*рабочего*) pérsonal stamp;

◇ ~ый соста́в personnél; mémbers pl; ~ое де́ло pérsonal records/dócuments pl; dóssier.

лиша́й м. 1. мед. hérpes; стригу́щий ~ ríngworm; 2. бот. líchen.

лиш|а́ть, лиши́ть (вн. рд.) 1. deprive (smb. of); dený (smb., smth.); ~ кого́-л. насле́дства deprive smb. of his, her inhéritance; лиши́ть кого́-л. свобо́ды imprison smb.; лиши́ть кого́-л. сло́ва deprive smb. of the right to speak; ~ себя́ удово́льствия foregó* the pléasure; ~ённый избира́тельных прав disfránchised; 2.: он ~ён вообра́же́ния he is unimáginative, he has no imaginátion; он ~ён ю́мора he has no sense of húmour; ~ённый (вся́кого) смы́сла (whólly) void of sense; ◇ ~ кого́-л. жи́зни take* awáy smb.'s life; ~ себя́ жи́зни commit súicide. ~а́ться, лиши́ться (рд.) lose* (smth.); лиши́ться иму́щества have* one's próperty cónfiscated; ~а́ться зре́ния lose* one's sight; ~а́ться да́ра ре́чи lose* the pówer of speech; ~а́ться созна́ния lose* cónsciousness, faint; ~ лиши́ться рассу́дка lose* one's réason, go* out of one's mind.

ли́ш|ек м. разг.: с ~ком or more; со́рок киломе́тров с ~ком fórty kilométres or more.

лише́ни|е с. 1. (де́йствие) deprivátion; ~ избира́тельных прав disfránchisement; ~ свобо́ды imprísonment; 2. мн. (нужда́) privátion sg, privátions; hárdships; терпе́ть ~я súffer hárdship.

лиши́ть(ся) сов. см. лиша́ть(ся).

ли́шн|ий прил. 1. supérfluous; ~ие де́ньги supérfluous cash, móney to spare; 2. (нену́жный) unnécessary; ~ие расхо́ды unnécessary expénse sg; э́то соверше́нно ~ее that's quite unnécessary; 3. (доба́вочный, дополни́тельный) éxtra; ~ раз once more; 4. в знач. сущ. с. more than nécessary; вы́пить ~ее have* had a drop too much; э́то ~ее not come amíss; позво́лить себе́ ~ее go* too far; не позволя́ть себе́ ~его not go too far; не говори́те ~его! be* cáreful what you say!; сказа́ть ~ее let* one's tongue run awáy with one; с ~им more than; 300 рубле́й с ~им more than three húndred róubles; ему́ 50 с ~им лет he is óver fifty; ~ие лю́ди supérfluous/unwánted péople.

лишь 1. части́ца (то́лько) ónly; всего́ ~ раз ónly once; я ~ косну́лся э́того I ónly/just touched it; ~ бы if ónly; ~ бы отде́латься от simply/just to get rid of; 2. сою́з (едва́, как то́лько) as soon as; ~ то́лько as soon as.

лоб м. fórehead; brow разг.; це́литься пря́мо в ~ кому́-л. aim straight at smb.'s face; ◇ атакова́ть в ~ attáck fróntally; пусти́ть себе́ пу́лю в ~ blow* one's brains out.

лобзик м. frét-saw.

лобн|ый анат. fróntal; ~ая кость fróntal/corónal bone; ◇ ~ое ме́сто ист. place of execútion.

лобов|о́й fróntal; ~ая ата́ка воен. fróntal attáck; ~о́е сопротивле́ние ав. drag.

лобогре́йка ж. с.-х. réaper.

лов м. cátching.

лов|е́ц м. húnter; (рыба́к) fisherman*; ◇ на ~ца́ и зверь бежи́т посл. just what I, he, she, etc., was áfter.

лови́ть, пойма́ть (вн.) 1. catch* (smb., smth.); несов. тж. try to catch (smb., smth.); ~ ры́бу fish; 2. (изоблича́ть) catch* (smb.) out; ◇ ~ ка́ждое сло́во hang* on smb.'s lips; ~ кого́-л. на сло́ве 1) take* smb. at his, her word; 2) (придира́ться) twist smb.'s remárk; ~ чей-л. взгляд catch* smb.'s eye; ~ на себе́ чей-л. взгляд nótice smb.'s glance; ~ волну́, ста́нцию pick up a wáve-length, a státion; в му́тной воде́ ры́бу ~ fish in tróubled wáters.

ловка́ч м. разг. sharp féllow.

ло́вк|ий 1. (иску́сный) déxterous, deft, adróit; 2. разг. (сообрази́тельный) sharp(-witted), smart; (изворо́тливый) cráfty, slíppery.

ло́вк|о 1. нареч. néatly; ~ вы́вернуться из чего́-л. wríggle adróitly out of smth.; ~ пойма́ть кого́-л. catch*

smb. néatly; 2. в знач. межд. разг.: вот э́то ~! well done!, véry neat! ~ость ж. 1. dextérity, déftness, adróitness; 2. разг. (изворо́тливость) cúnning, slípperiness; ◇ ~ость рук sleight of hand.

ло́вля ж. cátching; ры́бная ~ fishing.

лову́шк|а ж. trap, pítfall; попа́сть(ся) в ~у fall* into a trap.

лог м. ravíne.

логари́фм м. мат. lógarithm; табли́ца ~ов táble of lógarithms; ~и́ческий мат. logaríthmic; ~и́ческая лине́йка slíde-rule.

ло́гика ж. lógic; ~ веще́й the lógic of things; ~ собы́тий the lógic of evénts; у него́ своя́ ~ he acts accórding to a lógic of his own.

логи́ч|еский lógical; ~ вы́вод lógical conclúsion. ~ность ж. lógic. ~ный lógical.

ло́гов|ище с., ~о с. (прям. и перен.) lair, den.

ло́джия ж. lóggia.

ло́дка ж. boat.

ло́дочка ж. 1. small boat; 2. мн. (ту́фли) pumps.

ло́дочн|ик м. bóatman*; ~ый boat attr.; ~ые го́нки bóat-races; ~ая ста́нция bóat-house.

лоды́жка ж. ánkle.

ло́дырничать несов. разг. loaf, idle awáy one's time.

ло́дырь м. разг. shírker, slácker.

ло́жа I ж. (театра́льная) box.

ло́жа II ж. и ло́же с. (руже́йные) stock.

ложби́на ж. depréssion, hóllow.

ло́же с. bed.

ло́жечк|а ж. 1. small spoon; 2.: под ~ой in the pit of the stómach; у меня́ сосёт под ~ой I have a sínking sensátion.

ложи́ться, лечь 1. lie* down; ~ спать go* to bed; 2. (покрыва́ть собо́й что-л.) fall* (on), spread* óver; 3. (о морщи́нах, зага́ре) form; 4. (располага́ться тем или ины́м о́бразом) set* (in); во́лосы легли́ волна́ми the hair set in waves, the hair turned wávy; 5. (брать направле́ние — о самолётах и т. п.) get*; ~ на курс get* on course; ~ на но́вый курс change course; 6. (на вн.; об отве́тственности и т. п.) rest (with), fall* (on); ◇ ~ тяжёлым бре́менем на кого́-л. be* a héavy búrden to smb.

ло́жк|а ж. 1. spoon; разлива́тельная ~ ládle; 2. (как ме́ра) spóonful; ◇ че́рез час по ча́йной ~е погов. in microscópic dóses.

ло́жн|ость ж. fálsity. ~ый false; (оши́бочный) mistáken, erróneous; ~ая скро́мность false módesty; ~ые показа́ния юр. false téstimony sg; ~ые вы́воды erróneous árguments; ~ое обвине́ние false/spúrious chárges; ~ое со́лнце móck-sun, parhélion; ~ое положе́ние false/ambíguous position; ~ый шаг false step; представля́ть что-л. в ~ом све́те presént smth. in a false light, distórt smth.; идти́ по ~ому пути́ fóllow a mistáken path.

ложь ж. fálsehood; (вы́мысел) tale.

лоз|а́ ж. 1. (и́ва) wíllow(s); 2. (то́нкий сте́бель) switch; ве́рбная ~ wíllow switch; виногра́дная ~ vine. ~ня́к м. wíllows pl, ósiers pl.

ло́зунг м. 1. (при́зыв) slógan, wátchword; 2. (плака́т) slógan.

локализ|а́ция ж. localizátion. ~и́ровать(ся) несов. и сов. см. локализова́ть(ся).

локализова́ть несов. и сов. (вн.) lócalize (smth.). ~ся несов. и сов. becóme* lócalized.

лока́льный lócal.

лока́тор м. rádar.

лока́ут м. lóck-out.

локомоти́в м. lócomotive, éngine.

ло́кон м. lock, curl.

ло́к|оть м. élbow; ◇ чу́вство ~тя воен. touch, cóntact; перен. ésprit de corps, cómradeship. ~тево́й cúbital; ~тева́я кость úlna; fúnny-bone разг.

лом I м. (ору́дие) crów-bar.

лом II *м. собир.* frágments *pl*, scrap; желéзный ~ scráp-iron.

ломáка *м. и ж. разг.* símpering/afféoted pérson, símperer.

лóман│ый 1. bróken; ~ое крéсло bróken ármchair; говорúть на ~ом англúйском, францýзском *и т. п.* языкé speak* bróken Énglish, French *etc.*; 2. *(изогнутый под углом)* cróoked; ◇ ~ая лúния *мат.* bróken line.

ломáнье *с.* afféoted airs *pl*, affectátion, símpering, pósing.

ломáть, сломáть *(вн.)* 1. break* *(smth.)*; *(на куски)* break* up *(smth.)*; *(сносить постройку)* pull *(smth.)* down, demólish *(smth.)*; 2. *тк. несов. (добывать камень и т. п.)* quárry *(smth.)*, break* *(smth.)*; 3. *(уничтожать)* sweep* awáy *(smth.)*, do* awáy (with), destróy *(smth.)*; ~ традúции destróy tradítions; ~ стáрые обычаи sweep* awáy old cústoms; 4. *(резко, круто изменять)* transfórm *(smth.)*, álter *(smth.)*; force *(smth.)* ínto a new mould; ~ харáктер álter the charácter; 5. *(изменять в худшую сторону)* wreck *(smth.)*; ~ свою жизнь wreck one's life; ◇ ~ себé рýки wring* one's hands; ~ гóлову над *чем-л.* rack/cúdgel one's brains óver *smth.*

лом│áться, сломáться 1. break*; get* bróken; игрýшки чáсто ~áются у детéй old get bróken; 2. *тк. несов. (быть ломким, хрупким)* break*, be* bréakable; 3. *(уничтожаться)* be* swept awáy, crúmble, tótter, disappéar; ~áлся стáрый вековóй обычай the old cústoms were swept awáy; 4. *(резко, круто изменяться)* undergó* a súdden change, be* transfórmed; 5. *(меняться в худшую сторону)* collápse, be* rúined; 6. *тк. несов. (о голосе)* break*; 7. *тк. несов. (кривляться)* make* fáces, símper, pose; 8. *тк. несов. (заставлять себя просить)* preténd, make* a fuss, play hárd-to-gét.

ломбáрд *м.* páwnshop. **~ный** pawn *attr.*; **~ная квитáнция** páwn-ticket.

ломúть *несов. разг.* 1. break*; 2. *безл. (болеть)* ache; у меня лóмит пояснúцу I have pains in the small of my back. **~ся** *несов.* 1. *(от рд.)* be* weighed down (with); сундукú лóмятся от вещéй the trunks are búrsting with things; 2. *разг. (стараться проникнуть)* try to force; ◇ ~ся в открытую дверь knock at an ópen door.

лóмка *ж.* bréaking; bréak-up; destrúction; ~ старого быта the bréak-up of the old ways; ~ харáктера change of charácter.

лóмкий bríttle, frágile.

ломов│óй *прил.* 1. dray; ~ извóзчик cárter, dráyman*; **~áя лóшадь** cárt-horse, dráy-horse; 2. *в знач. сущ. м.* cárter.

ломóта *ж.* aches and pains *pl.*

ломóть *м.* chunk, hunk.

лóмтик *м.* slice.

лóн│о *с.* lap; ◇ на ~е прирóды out in the cóuntry, alóne with náture, in the ópen air.

лóпасть *ж.* blade; *(гребного колеса)* páddle.

лопáт│а *ж.* spade; *(совковая)* shóvel. **~ка** *ж.* 1. *см.* лопáта; ~ка штукатýра trówel; 2. *анат.* shóulder-blade; ◇ положúть *кого-л.* на óбе ~ки 1) *(в борьбе)* pin *smb.* down, pin *smb.* to the floor; 2) *(одержать полную победу над кем-л.)* beat* *smb.*; положúл он тебя на óбе ~ки! he's got you beat! во все ~ки at full speed.

лоп│áться, лóпнуть 1. burst*; *(о нарыве тж.)* break*; *(о веревке, струне и т. п.)* snap, break*; 2. *разг. (терпеть неудачу)* go* phut, collápse; ◇ ~ от смéха split* one's sides with láughter; моё терпéние лóпнуло I can't stand ány more, my pátience is exháusted. **~нуть** *сов. см.* лóпаться.

лопотáть *несов. разг.* jábber, gábble; *перен.* múrmur, whisper.

лопýх *м.* 1. *бот.* dock, búrdock; 2. *разг. (простак, глупый человек)* nóddy, goof, boob.

лорд *м.* lord.

лорнéт *м.* lorgnétte.

лосúн│а *ж.* 1. *(кожа)* élk-skin, búckskin, chámois léather; 2. *(мясо)* elk meat, vénison. **~ый** elk *attr.*; *(из кожи лося)* búckskin *attr.*; **~ые порá** elk ántlers.

лоск *м. (прям. и перен.)* gloss.

лоскýт *м.* rag, shred, scrap.

лоснúться *несов.* shine*, glísten; ~ от жúра be* shíny with grease, shine* with grease.

лоснящийся shíny, glístening.

лососёвый sálmon *attr.*

лососúна *ж.* sálmon.

лосóсь *м.* sálmon.

лось *м.* elk.

лосьóн *м.* face lótion.

лот *м. мор.* lead, plúmmet; бросáть ~ cast* the lead.

лотерéйный lóttery *attr.*; ~ билéт lóttery tícket.

лотерéя *ж.* lóttery; *(на вечере и т. п.)* ráffle.

лотó *с. нескл.* lótto.

лотóк *м.* 1. *(разносчика)* (stréet-vendor's) tray; 2. *(прилавок)* (stréet-)stall; 3. *(жёлоб)* chute, shoot.

лóтос *м. бот.* lótus.

лотóчник *м.* háwker, pédlar, stréet-vendor.

лохáн│ка *ж. см.* лохáнь; ◇ пóчечная ~ *анат.* rénal pélvis; воспалéние пóчечных ~ок pyelítis.

лохáнь *ж.* (wásh-)tub.

лохмáтый 1. shággy; ~ пёс shággy dog; 2. *(непричёсанный)* dishévelled, tóusled.

лохмóтья *мн.* rags, tátters; в ~х in rags.

лóц│ия *ж. мор.* sáiling diréctions *pl.* **~ман** *м.* pílot. **~манский** pílot's. **~манство** *с.* pílotage.

лошадú│ный 1. horse *attr.*; ~ое лицó équine féatures *pl*; ◇ ~ая сúла *физ.* hórse-power *(сокр. h. p.)*; ~ая дóза huge dose.

лошáдник *м. разг.* 1. hórse-fancier; 2. *(торговец)* hórse-dealer.

лóшад│ь *ж.* horse; на ~и on hórseback, móunted.

лошáк *м.* hínny.

лощёный glóssy; *перен.* pólished.

лощúна *ж.* dell, hóllow.

лоя́льн│ость *ж.* lóyalty. **~ый** lóyal.

луб *м.* bast.

луб│óк *м.* 1. *мед.* splint(s); накладывать ~ на *что-л.* splint *smth.*, put* in splints; 2. *(доска)* wóod-block; 3. *(картинка)* pópular print. **~óчный:** ~óчная картúнка pópular print; ~óчная литератýра cheap líterature.

луг *м.* méadow, grássland. **~овóй** méadow *attr.*, grássland *attr.*

луд│úльщик *м.* tínner. **~úть** *несов.* tin.

лýж│а *ж.* púddle, pool; ◇ сесть в ~у get* ínto a mess.

лужáйка *ж.* méadow; *(перед домом)* grass, lawn; sward *поэт.*

луж│éние *с.* tínning. **~ёный** tinned.

лужóк *м.* gráss-plot.

лýза *ж.* pócket.

лук I *м.* 1. *(растение)* ónion; 2. *собир.* ónions *pl*; зелёный ~ spring ónions *pl.*

лук II *м. (оружие)* bow.

лукá *ж.* 1. *(реки, дороги)* bend; 2. *(седла)*: зáдняя ~ cántle; передняя ~ pómmel.

лукáв│ить, слукáвить be* sly, be* cúnning; *(притворяться)* dissémble. **~ство** *с.* 1. *(коварство, хитрость)* árchness, slýness; 2. *(задор)* róguishness. **~ый** 1. *(коварный, хитрый)* arch, cúnning; 2. *(задорный)* róguish.

лýков│ица *ж.* 1. bulb; 2. *(головка лука)* ónion. **~ичный** búlbous; ~ичные растéния búlbous plants. **~ый** ónion *attr.*; of ónions *после сущ.*

лукóшко с. bast básket.

лунá ж. moon; полёт на Луну flight to the Moon.

лунáтик м. sléep-walker; мед. somnámbulist.

лýнка ж. 1. (углубление) hóllow; (отверстие) hole; 2. анат. álveole.

лýнник м. разг. lúnik, Moon rócket.

лýнн|ый moon attr.; lúnar научн.; ~ свет móonlight; ~oe затмéние lúnar eclípse; ~ая ночь móonlit night; ~ мéсяц lúnar month; ~ая повéрхность lúnar/moon's súrface; ◇ ~ кáмень móonstone.

лунохóд м. Lunokhód, Móoncar.

лунь м. зоол. hárrier; ◇ седóй как ~ white-háired.

лýпа ж. mágnifying glass.

лупúть, облупúть, отлупúть (вн.) 1. сов. облупúть (очищать от шелухи, сдирать) peel (smth.); 2. сов. отлупúть разг. (бить) thrash (smb., smth.). ~ся несов. разг. (шелушиться) peel; (о краске, штукатурке и т. п. тж.) peel off, flake off, come* off; у негó лупúтся лицó his face is péeling.

лупоглáзый разг. póp-eyed, góggle-eyed.

луч м. 1. ray, beam; перен. ray; ~ свéта shaft of light; ~ надéжды ray of hope; 2. мн. физ. rays; ◇ расхóдиться ~áми rádiate. ~евóй 1. физ. radiátion attr.; 2. (расходящийся лучами) rádial; ◇ ~евáя кость анат. rádius (pl -dii); ~евáя болéзнь radiátion síckness.

лучезáрный rádiant.

лучúна ж. splínter.

лучúст|ый 1. lámbent, sóftly rádiant; ~ые глазá sóftly rádiant eyes; 2. физ. rádiant; ~ая энéргия rádiant énergy.

лýчник м. árcher.

лýчше 1. (сравнит. ст. прил. хороший и нареч. хорошо) bétter; ~ всегó best of all; ~ в знач. сказ. безл. it is bétter; больнóму сегóдня ~ the pátient is bétter todáy; 3. в знач. частицы: вам ~ подождáть you'd bétter wait; вам бы ~ уйтú you'd bétter go; ~ не спрáшивай! bétter not ask!; ◇ тем ~ all the bétter; тем ~ для негó so much the bétter for him; как мóжно ~ as well as póssible; как нельзя ~ to perféction.

лýчш|ий прил. 1. (сравнит. ст. от хороший) bétter; ~ из двух the bétter of the two; 2. (превосх. ст. от хороший) the best; 3. в знач. сущ. с. sómething bétter; я хотéл ~его I wánted sómething bétter; за неимéнием ~его for want of ánything bétter; ◇ в ~ем слýчае at the best; всегó ~его! goodbýe!; всё к ~ему it's all for the best.

лущúть несов. (вн.) (очищать от скорлупы и т. п.) shell (smth.); (семечки) husk (smth.).

лыж|и мн. (ед. лыжа ж.) skis; ходúть на ~ax ski; 2. разг. (вид спорта) skíing; ◇ вóдные ~ wáter skis. ~ник м., ~ница ж. skíer. ~ный ski attr.; ~ный спорт skíing; ~ный костюм skí-suit; ~ная мазь skí-wax; ~ные креплéния skí-bindings; ~ная бáза skíing lodge/céntre. ~ня ж. skí-track.

лык|о с. bast; ◇ не всякое ~ в стрóку погов. you mústn't be too exácting/fínicky; он ~а не вяжет прост. he's dead drunk; он не ~ом шит прост. he's no fool.

лысéть, облысéть, полысéть go* bald, grow* bald, bald.

лыс|ина ж. bald patch/spot. ~ый bald; báld-héaded.

льв|ёнок м. líon-cub. ~íный líon's; ◇ ~íная дóля the líon's share; ~íный зев бот. snápdragon, antirrhínum. ~íца ж. líoness.

льгóт|а ж. prívilege. ~ный spécial; fávourable; ~ный срок spécial tíme-límit; ~ные услóвия fávourable condítions; на ~ных услóвиях on fávourable terms, at redúced rates.

льдúна ж. íce-floe, block of ice.

льновóд м. fláx-grówer. ~ство с. fláx-grówing. ~ческий fláx-grówing attr.; ~ческий райóн fláx-grówing dístrict.

льнопряд|éние с. fláx-spínning. ~úльный fláx-spínning attr.

льноубóрочн|ый fláx-púlling attr.; ~ые машúны fláx-púlling machínes, fláx-púllers.

льнуть, прильнýть (к дт.) 1. cling* (to), snúggle up (to); 2. тк. несов. разг. (испытывать влечение) feel* drawn (to), make* up (to).

льнян|óй 1. flax attr.; (о холсте и т. п.) línen; ~oe мáсло línseed oil; 2. (о цвете волос) fláxen.

льст|ец м. flátterer. ~úвый fláttering; ~úвый человéк flátterer, sýcophant; ~úвые рéчи fláttering spéeches.

льстить, польстúть (дт.) 1. flátter (smb.); 2. (быть приятным) flátter (smb., smth.); ~ самолюбию flátter one's vánity; ◇ ~ себя надéждой flátter onesélf with the hope.

любéзн|ичать несов. (с тв.) разг. pay* cómpliments (to), make* up (to). ~ость ж. 1. cóurtesy, amiabílity; 2. обыкн. мн. (комплименты) cómpliments; 3. (одолжение) fávour, kíndness; окажúте ~ость, не откажúте в ~ости be so kind (as to). ~ый cóurteous, ámiable, génial; ◇ бýдьте ~ы please; be so kind (as to).

любúм|ец м., ~ица ж. fávourite. ~чик м. разг. pet. ~ый прил. 1. déarly loved; 2. (предпочитаемый) fávourite; ~oe занятие hóbby; 3. в знач. сущ. м. swéetheart, déarest, dárling; belóved поэт.

любúтель м. lóver; ~ мýзыки músic-lover; быть большúм любúтелем чего-л. be* véry fond of smth.; (непрофессионал) ámateur. ~ский ámateur; ~ский спектáкль ámateur perfórmance.

любúть несов. (вн.) 1. love (smb., smth.); ~ своúх детéй love one's children; ~ свою рóдину love one's cóuntry; 2. (чувствовать склонность к чему-л.) be* fond (of); like (smth.); ~ читáть be* fond of réading; ~ мýзыку like músic; 3. (быть довольным чем-л.) like; он не любит, чтóбы емý возражáли he does not like béing contradícted.

любо в знач. сказ. безл. разг.: ~ смотрéть на когó-л., что-л. it's a pléasure to look at smb., smth.

любовáться, полюбовáться (тв., на вн.) admíre (smb., smth.); полюбýйтесь на негó! just look at him!

любóвн|ик м. lóver. ~ица ж. místress. ~ый 1. ámorous; love attr.; ~oe письмó love létter; ~ая песнь love song; ~ый взгляд ámorous glance; 2. (заботливый, бережный) lóving; ~oe отношéние lóving care.

люб|óвь ж. love; ~ к рóдине love of/for one's cóuntry; ~ к дéтям love of/for children; ~ с пéрвого взгляда love at first sight; ~ к мýзыке love of músic; женúться по ~ú márry for love.

любознáтельн|ость ж. love of knówledge, intelléctual curiósity. ~ый cúrious; with a taste for knówledge после сущ.; быть ~ым be* of an inquíring turn of mind, have* a love of knówledge.

любóй прил. 1. ány; в ~ день ány day; 2. в знач. сущ. м. ányone; ~ из вас ány(one) of you.

любопы́т|но 1. нареч. (интересно) ínterestingly; (странно) cúriously, strángely; 2. в знач. сказ. безл. it is cúrious/strange; óddly enóugh; ~, что никтó не замéтил егó óddly enóugh, no one nóticed him. ~ный прил. 1. (нескромный) inquísitive; (интересующийся) cúrious; 2. (интересный) ínteresting; ~ное событие cúrious íncident; он человéк ~ный he's an ínteresting/unúsual man*; в знач. сущ. м. cúrious pérson. ~ство с. curiósity. ~ствовать несов. be* cúrious/inquísitive.

любящий lóving.

люд м. собир. разг. péople, folk.

люд|и мн. péople; воен. уст. тж. men; ◇ ~ дóброй вóли péople of good will; выбиться (выйти) в ~ make* one's way (in life). ~ный 1. (с большим населением) pópulous; 2. (многолюдный) crówded.

людоéд м. cánnibal. ~ство с. cánnibalism.

людскóй human; род ~ the húman race, mankínd.

люк _м._ 1. hatch; (_на улице_) mánhole; 2. (_для орудия_) gún-port.

люкс _м. переводится через прил._ de luxe; каюта ~ de luxe cábin.

люлька _ж._ crádle.

люпин _м. бот._ lúpin.

люрекс _м._ lúrex.

люстра _ж._ chandelíer, candelábrum (_pl_ -ra).

лютик _м. бот._ búttercup, crówfoot.

лютня _ж._ lute.

лют|ость _ж._ ferócity. ~ый 1. ferócious; ~ый враг rúthless/vícious énemy; 2. (_мучительный_) excrúciating; (_тяжкий_) inténse; 3. (_сильный_) sevére; ~ый мороз sevére/wíthering frost.

люцерна _ж. бот._ alfálfa.

ля _с. нескл. муз._ la, A.

ляг|áть, лягнуть (_вн._) kick (_smb., smth._). ~áться _несов._ kick; эта лошадь ~áется this horse kicks. ~нуть _сов. см._ лягáть.

лягушáтник _м. разг._ (_бассейн для начинающих_) páddle pool.

лягушáчий, лягушечий frog's.

лягушка _ж._ frog.

ляжка _ж._ thigh.

лязг _м._ clánging, clánking. ~ать, лязгнуть clang, clank; (_зубами_) chátter.

лязгнуть _сов. см._ лязгать.

лямк|а _ж._ strap; ◇ тянуть ~y drudge, bear* the búrden.

ляпать, ляпнуть (_вн._) _разг._ blurt (_smth._) out.

ляпис _м._ sílver nítrate, lúnar cáustic.

ляпис-лазурь _ж. мин._ lápis lázuli.

ляпнуть _сов. см._ ляпать.

ляпсус _м._ blúnder.

M

мавзолей _м._ mausoléum.

мавр _м._ Moor. ~итанский Móorish.

маг _м._ (_волшебник_) magícian, wízard.

магазин _м._ 1. (_лавка_) shop; store _амер._; универсáльный ~ depártment store; 2. (_в оруж..и_) magazine; 3. _тех._: ~ сопротивлéния resístance box.

магазин|ный 1. shop _attr._; 2. (_об оружии_) magazine _attr._; ~ая коробка magazine.

магистр _м._ Máster.

магистрáль _ж._ 1. (_дорожная_) main road, artérial road; железнодорóжная ~ main line, trúnk-line; вóдная ~ main wáterway; 2. (_водопроводная и т. п._) main; нефтянáя ~ oil pípeline. ~ный artérial, main.

магический mágic; _перен._ mágical.

магия _ж._ mágic; ◇ чёрная ~ black mágic.

магма _ж._ mágma.

магнáт _м._ mágnate.

магнезия _ж._ magnésia.

магнетизм _м._ mágnetism; ◇ земнóй ~ terréstrial mágnetism.

магнетит _м._ mágnetite, magnétic íron ore.

магнето _с. нескл._ magnéto.

магниевый magnésian.

магний _м. хим._ magnésium.

магнит _м._ mágnet. ~ный magnétic; ◇ ~ная аномáлия mágnetic anómaly; lócal attráction; ~ная буря magnétic storm; ~ный железняк magnétic íron ore, mágnetite; ~ный меридиáн magnétic merídian; ~ное пóле magnétic field; ~ный пóлюс magnétic pole; ~ное наклонéние ángle of dip/inclinátion.

магнитофóн _м._ tápe-recorder. ~ный tápe(-recorder) _attr._; ~ная зáпись tápe(-recording); ~ная лéнта recórding tape.

магнóлия _ж. бот._ magnólia.

магометáн|ин _м._, ~ка _ж._ Mohámmedan. ~ский Mohámmedan. ~ство _с._ Mohámmedanism, the Mohámmedan creed.

мадéра _ж._ madéira.

мадригáл _м._ mádrigal.

мадьяр _м._, ~ка _ж._ Mágyar. ~ский Mágyar.

мажóр _м._ 1. _муз._ májor key; гáмма ля ~ the scale of A-májor; 2. _разг._ (_весёлое настроение_) good spírits/mood; быть в ~e be* in good form. ~ный _муз._ májor.

мáзанка _ж._ cláy-walled cóttage/house.

мáзаный 1. _разг._ (_грязный_) grúbby; 2. (_сделанный из глины_) cláy-walled, adóbe.

мáзать, помáзать (_вн._) 1. (_чем-л. жидким, жирным_) spread* (_smth._) on; (_стену и т. п. красками_) paint (_smth._); ~ хлеб мáслом bútter _one's_ bread; 2. _тк. несов._ (_пачкать_) dírty (_smth._); (_вн._) smear (_smth._ with), stain (_smth._ with). ~ся, помáзаться 1. (_мазью и т. п._) smear onesélf; 2. _тк. несов. разг._ (_пачкаться_) get* onesélf dírty; 3. _разг._ (_краситься_) put* on máke-up.

мáзер _м._ máser.

мазня _ж._ 1. (_о картине_) daub; (_о плохой работе_) bótching, botched/pátchy work; 2. (_неумелая игра_) fúmbling.

мазóк _м._ 1. (_кистью_) dab, stroke, touch; 2. _мед._ smear.

мазурка _ж._ mazúrka.

мазут _м._ black oil, mazút. ~ный black oil _attr._, mazút _attr._

маз|ь _ж._ óintment; сапóжная ~ blácking; ◇ дéло на ~й éverything is góing smóothly.

майс _м._ maize, Índian corn. ~овый maize _attr._

май _м._ May; в мáе этого гóда this/in May; в мáе прóшлого гóда last May; last year in May; в мáе будущего гóда next May; ◇ Пéрвое мáя the first of May, May Day.

мáйка _ж._ (_sléeveless_) vest; (_спортивная тж._) fóotball shirt; spórts-shirt _амер._

майóлика _ж._ majólica.

майонéз _м. кул._ mayonnáise.

майóр _м._ májor.

мáйский May _attr._; ~ день day in May; ◇ ~ жук cóckchafer.

мак _м._ 1. (_цветок_) póppy; 2. (_семена_) póppy-seeds _pl._

макáка _ж._ macáque.

макарóны _мн._ macaróni _sg._

макáть _несов._ (_вн._) dip (_smth._).

макéт _м._ módel, móck-up.

мáклер _м._ bróker. ~ство _с._ brókerage, bróking.

мáков: как ~ цвет póppy-red; красный как ~ цвет red as a rose.

мáков|ка _ж._ 1. (_плод мака_) póppy-head; 2. (_купол_) cúpola; 3. _разг._ (_головы_) crown, pate. ~ый póppy _attr._

макрокóсм _м._ mácrocosm.

макромир _м._ the great world, mácrocosm.

мáкси- _в сложн._ máxi-.

максимáльный máximum _attr._, máximal; gréatest; top _attr._

мáксимум _м._ 1. máximum; 2. _в знач. нареч._ at most; ~, что я могу сдéлать the most I can do.

макулатура _ж._ 1. (_негодная бумага_) spóilage, wáste-paper; 2. _разг._ (_бездарное литературное произведение_) rúbbish, pulp.

макушка _ж._ 1. top; 2. (_головы_) crown, pate.

мал _см._ мáлый I.

малá|ец _м._, ~йка _ж._ Maláyan.

малайский Maláyan.

малахи́т *м. мин.* málachite. **~овый** málachite *attr.*

малева́ть, намалева́ть 1. *(вн.)* paint *(smb., smth.)*; **2.** *разг. (плохо рисовать)* daub.

малейш|ий *(превосх. ст. прил. ма́лый)* the slightest, the faintest; **ни ~ей** опа́сности not the slightest danger; **ни ~его** поня́тия not the faintest idea.

ма́леньк|ий *прил.* **1.** little*; *(обычно только о размере)* small; *(низкорослый тж.)* short; **2.** *(незначительный)* slight, little*; **~ие** моро́зы light frosts; **~ая** неприя́тность slight unpléasantness, spot of tróuble; **3.:** **~ие** лю́ди péople of no impórtance; **4.** *(малолетний)* little*; **5.** *в знач. сущ. м.* child*, little one.

мали́н|а *ж.* **1.** *собир. (ягоды)* ráspberries *pl*; **2.** *(об отдельной ягоде)* ráspberry; **3.** *(растение)* ráspberry (-cane). **~ник** *м.* patch of ráspberries.

мали́новка *ж. зоол.* róbin.

мали́нов|ый 1. ráspberry *attr.*; **~ое** варе́нье ráspberry jam; **2.** *(о цвете)* crímson.

ма́ло *нареч.* **1.** *(немного)* little*; **он говори́л ~** he said little*, he had little* to say; **он ~ чита́ет** he dóesn't read much; **2.** *(недостаточно)* not enóugh; **~!** that's not enóugh!; **ра́зве э́того ~?** isn't that enóugh?; **пяти́ дней бу́дет ~** five days won't be enóugh; **~ сказа́ть — на́до показа́ть** it's not enóugh to expláin — you must show how it's done; **3.** *в знач. числ.* not much; not mány, *(only* a) few *(с сущ. во мн. ч.)*; **~ де́нег** not much móney; **~ книг, наро́да** not mány books, péople; **~ посети́телей** ónly a few vísitors; **о́чень ~** véry little *(с сущ. в ед. ч.)*; véry few *(с сущ. во мн. ч.)*; **о́чень ~ книг** véry few books; **о́чень ~ наро́да** véry few péople; **4.** *с мест. и нареч.*: **~ кто** hárdly ánybody, few (péople); **~ что** hárdly ánything; **~ где** hárdly ánywhere; **~ когда́** hárdly éver; **~ ли чего́ челове́к не наговори́т** a pérson may say ánything; **~ ли кто придёт** ányone may come; **~ ли что мо́жет случи́ться** ánything might háppen; **◇ ~ того́** and what's more; **~ того́ что...** not ónly...; **~ ли что!** what of it?, that dóesn't mean ánything!

малоавторите́тный insufficiently authóritative.

малова́жный insigníficant, unimpórtant.

малове́р *м.* scéptic.

малове́роятный impróbable, scárcely próbable.

малово́дный 1. *(о реке и т. п.)* shállow; **2.** *(о местности)* árid.

малогабари́тн|ый compáct, small; **~ приёмник** small rádio set; **~ая** ме́бель compáct fúrniture, fúrniture of convénient size.

малогра́мотн|ость *ж.* semi-líteracy. **~ый 1.** semi-líterate, half-éducated; **2.** *(сделанный без достаточных знаний)* unskílled; **~ый** чертёж unskílled dráwing.

малоду́ш|ие *с.* faint-héartedness, cráven spírit. **~ный** faint-héarted, cráven, púsillánimous; *(о поступке)* cówardly.

малозаме́тный 1. unobtrúsive; **2.** *(мало себя проявляющий)* insigníficant, undistínguished.

малозе́мель|е *с.* land shórtage, land-hunger; **~ный** land-starved, land-hungry.

малознако́мый unfamíliar.

малозначи́тельный insigníficant.

малоизве́стный little-knówn.

малоиму́щий néedy, poor.

малоинтере́сный uninteresting.

малокали́берный small-bore *attr.*

малокро́в|ие *с.* anáemia. **~ный** anáemic.

малоле́т|ний *прил.* **1.** young, underáge; **2.** *в знач. сущ. м.* júvenile. **~ство** *с. разг.* childhood.

малолитра́жный: ~ автомоби́ль small(-displácement) car.

малолю́дный *(о крае)* thínly pópulated; *(об улице)* émpty, desérted; *(о собрании)* póorly atténded.

мало-ма́льски *разг.* a little bit, in the slightest

degrée; **~ культу́рный челове́к** ányone with the slightest preténsions to cúlture.

маломо́щн|ый 1. *(физически слабый)* féeble; **2.** *(бедный)* small; **~ое** крестья́нское хозя́йство small péasant farm; **3.** *(небольшой мощности)* low-pówered.

малонаселённый spársely/thínly pópulated.

малоосво́енный little-devéloped; **~ райо́н** little-devéloped área.

малоподви́жный slow, ináctive; slúggish; **~ суста́в** stiff joint.

ма́ло-пома́лу *разг.* little by little.

малопоня́тный not véry comprehénsible, obscúre.

малопродукти́вн|ый 1. unprodúctive; **~ая** рабо́та unprodúctive work; **2.** *с.-х.* low-yield; **~ скот** póor-yielding/low-yield cáttle.

малопроизводи́тельный unprodúctive; **~ труд** unprodúctive mánual lábour.

малоразви́тый 1. *(физически)* undevéloped, half-grówn; **2.** *(недостаточно развитый)* underdevéloped; **3.** *(недостаточно образованный)* half-éducated, uncúltivated.

малоро́слый undersized, stúnted.

малосеме́йный with a small fámily *после сущ.*

малоси́льный 1. weak; **2.** *(о машине и т. п.)* low-pówered.

малосодержа́тельный émpty, unsubstántial, uninteresting.

малосо́льный míldly sálted.

малосостоя́тельный 1. *(небогатый)* not véry prósperous; **2.** *(неубедительный)* not véry convíncing.

ма́лость *ж. разг.* **1.** trífle; **са́мая ~ оста́лась** there's hárdly ány left; **2.** *в знач. нареч.* a bit, a little.

малотира́жный small-circulátion *attr.*

малоубеди́тельный not véry convíncing.

малоупотреби́тельный rárely-used.

малоурожа́йн|ый low-yield; **~ые** культу́ры low-yield crops.

малоутеши́тельный not véry consóling/cómforting.

малоце́нный of little worth *после сущ.*, of little válue *после сущ.*

малочи́сленный small, not númerous.

малоэффекти́вный inefféctive.

мал|ый I *прил.* **1.** *(по величине, возрасту)* small; **~ые** де́ти small chíldren; **2.** *(незначительный)* slight, light; **3.** *тк. кратк. ф. (не впору, тесный)* (too) small; **пальто́ ~о** the coat is too small; **4.** *в знач. сущ. с.* a little; **дово́льствоваться ~ым** be* sátisfied with a little; **◇ ~ая** ско́рость *ж.-д.* low speed; **~ ход** *мор.* slow speed; **~ые** фо́рмы *театр.* short plays; **с ~ых лет** from childhood, éver since *one* was a child; *(с младенчества)* from ínfancy; **са́мое ~ое** at least; **без ~ого** néarly, álmost; **за ~ым де́ло ста́ло** one thing is míssing; **мал ~а́** ме́ньше one smáller than the óther.

ма́лый II *м. разг. (парень)* féllow, boy, lad; kid *амер.*

малы́ш *м. разг.* **1.** kíddy, little one; **2.** *(о человеке маленького роста)* little man*, short féllow.

ма́льва *ж. бот.* mállow; *(садовая)* hóllyhock.

ма́льчик *м.* boy; **◇ ~ с па́льчик** hóp-o'-my-thúmb.

мальчи́ш|еский bóyish; *(ребяческий)* chíldish. **~ество** *с.* chíldishness; *(шалость)* childish prank. **~ка** *м. разг.* boy; **вести́ себя́ как ~ка** beháve like a boy.

мальчуга́н *м. разг.* little chap, little féllow.

малю́сенький *разг.* tíny, wee.

малю́тка *м. и ж.* báby.

маля́р *м.* **1.** (house-)páinter; **2.** *(о плохом художнике)* dáubster.

маляри́|йный malárial. **~я** *ж. мед.* malária.

маля́рн|ый: ~ые рабо́ты páinting *sg*; **~ая** кисть páintbrush.

мам|а *ж.* múmmy. **~аша** *ж. разг.* móther. **~енькин**

разг. mother's; ◇ ~енькин сынок mother's darling, milksop.

ма́монт *м.* mámmoth.

мандари́н *м.* 1. (*плод*) tangeríne; 2. (*дерево*) tangeríne-tree.

мандари́новый tangeríne *attr.*

манда́т *м.* mándate; (*на съезд и т. п.*) credéntials *pl.* ~ный mándate *attr.*; ~ная коми́ссия Credéntials Commission.

мандоли́н|**а** *ж.* mándoline. ~и́ст *м.* mándoline pláyer.

манёвр *м.* 1. *воен.* manóeuvre; *перен. тж.* devíce, wile; 2. *мн. воен.* (*тактические занятия*) manóeuvres; 3. *мн. ж.-д.* shúnting *sg.*

манёвренный 1. manóeuvrable; 2. *воен.* manóeuvre *attr.*

маневри́ровать *несов.* 1. manóeuvre; *перен.* (*хитрить*) dodge; 2. *ж.-д.* shunt.

манёж *м.* 1. (*для верховой езды*) ríding-school; (*крытый тж.*) ríding-hall; 2. (*в цирке*) ring; 3. (*для детей*) play pen. ~ить *несов.* (*вн.*) *разг.* keep* pútting (*smb.*) off, keep* (*smb.*) hánging abóut.

манеке́н *м.* dúmmy.

манеке́нщ|**ик** *м.*, ~**ица** *ж.* módel, mánnequin.

мане́р *м. разг.* way, mánner; на ~ чего́-л. like *smth.*; на свой ~ in one's own mánner.

мане́ра *ж.* 1. mánner; (*привычка, способ*) way; ~ держа́ть себя́ behaviour, béaring; 2. *мн.* (*внешние формы поведения*) mánners; 3. (*особенности творчества, исполнения*) mánner, style.

манже́та *ж.* cuff.

маниака́льный maníacal.

маникю́р *м.* mánicure. ~ша *ж.* mánicurist.

манипули́ровать *несов.* (*тв.*) manípulate (*smth.*). ~**я́тор** *м.* manípulator. ~**я́ция** *ж.* manipulátion.

мани́ть, помани́ть (*вн.*) 1. (*звать*) sígnal (*smb.*, to); (*пальцем*) béckon (*smb.*); 2. *тк. несов.* (*привлекать*) attráct (*smth.*), have* an attráction (for); мо́ре ма́нит меня́ the sea draws me.

манифе́ст *м.* manifésto.

манифеста́ция *ж.* demonstrátion.

мани́шка *ж.* shirt-front; (*пристёгивающаяся*) dícky.

ма́ния *ж.* mánia; ~ вели́чия megalománia; ~ пресле́дования persecútion mánia.

манки́ровать *несов. и сов.* 1. (*тв.*; *пренебрегать*) negléct (*smth.*); ~ свои́ми обя́занностями negléct one's dúties; ~ заня́тиями negléct one's stúdies; 2. *уст.* (*не посещать*) fail to atténd; be* irrégular in one's atténdance; (*о школьниках*) play trúant.

ма́нн|**ый**: ~ая крупа́ semolína; ~ая ка́ша cooked semolína.

мано́метр *м.* manómeter, préssure-gauge.

манса́рда *ж.* áttic(-room).

манти́лья *ж.* mantílla.

ма́нтия *ж.* cloak.

манто́ *с. нескл.* coat.

мануфакту́р|**а** *ж. тк. ед.* (*ткани*) téxtiles *pl*; ~ный téxtile; (*магазин*) drápers'; dry-goods store *амер.*; ~ные изде́лия téxtiles.

маньчжу́р *м.*, ~**ка** *ж.* Manchúrian. ~ский Manchúrian.

манья́к *м.* mániac.

мара́зм *м.* debílity, marásmus; ста́рческий ~ sénile debílity.

мара́ть, замара́ть, намара́ть (*вн.*) *разг.* 1. *сов.* замара́ть dírty (*smth.*), make* (*smth.*) dírty; *перен.* soil (*smth.*), cast* a slur (on); ~ репута́цию soil one's reputátion; 2. *сов.* намара́ть (*неряшливо писать, рисовать*) scríbble (*smth.*), scrawl (*smth.*); ◇ бума́гу waste páper, scríbble; ~ ру́ки об кого́-л., обо что́-л. soil one's hands on *smb.*, *smth.* ~ся, замара́ться get* onesélf dírty, dírty onesélf.

марафо́н|**ец** *м.* Márathon rúnner. ~ский: ~ бег *спорт.* Márathon race.

марга́н|**ец** *м. хим.* manganése. ~цевый manganésian; manganése *attr.*

маргари́н *м.* margaríne. ~овый margaríne *attr.*

маргари́тка *ж. бот.* dáisy.

ма́рево *с.* 1. mírage; 2. (*дымка, туман*) haze.

мари́ *м. и ж. нескл. см.* мари́ец, мари́йка.

мар|**и́ец** *м.*, ~**и́йка** *ж.* Mári. ~и́йский Mári; ~и́йский язы́к Mári, the Mári lánguage.

марина́д *м.* 1. marináde; 2. обыкн. мн. (*маринованный продукт*) marináde *sg*; (*овощи*) píckles *pl.*

марини́ст *м.* painter of séa-scapes.

марин|**о́ванный** marináted, píckled. ~**ова́ть**, замарино́вать (*вн.*) 1. marináte (*smth.*), píckle (*smth.*); 2. *разг.* (*задерживать исполнение чего-л.*) shelve (*smth.*); (*заставлять ждать*) keep* (*smb.*) wáiting; ~ова́ть де́ло put* things off.

марионе́т|**ка** *ж.* marionétte; púppet (*тж. перен.*). ~**очный** púppet *attr.*; ~очное прави́тельство púppet góvernment.

марихуа́на *ж.* marijuána; pot *разг.*

ма́рк|**а** *ж.* 1. (*почтовая*) (póstage-)stamp; 2. (*клеймо*) mark; brand; 3. (*сорт, тип изделия, товара*) make; ◇ вы́сшей ~и of the first wáter; под ~ой чего́-л. únder the guise of *smth.*; держа́ть ~у maintáin one's reputátion (for).

маркизе́т *м.* marquisétte.

ма́ркий éasily soiled; э́то ~ материа́л this stuff shows the dirt.

маркси́зм *м.* Márxism.

маркси́ст *м.* Márxist. ~ский Márxist, Márxian.

маркше́йдер *м.* míne-survéyor.

ма́рля *ж.* gauze; (*для процеживания*) chéese-cloth.

мармела́д *м.* fruit jéllies *pl.*

мародёр *м.* lóoter, maráuder. ~ство *с.* lóoting. ~ствовать *несов.* loot.

марсиа́нин *м.* Mártian.

март *м.* March; в ~е э́того го́да this/in March; в ~е про́шлого го́да last March; last year in March; в ~е бу́дущего го́да next March.

марте́н *м.* ópen-hearth fúrnace.

мартёновск|**ий** ópen-hearth; ~ая печь *см.* марте́н; ~ проце́сс ópen-hearth prócess; ~ая сталь ópen-hearth steel.

ма́ртовский March *attr.*

марты́шка *ж.* mármoset.

марш I *м.* 1. march (*тж. муз.*); 2. (*лестницы*) flight (of steps).

марш II *межд.*: ша́гом ~! quick march!; ~ отсю́да! off with you!

ма́ршал *м.* márshal; ~ Сове́тского Сою́за Márshal of the Sóviet Únion.

ма́ршальский márshal's.

марши́р|**овать** *несов.* march. ~**о́вка** *ж.* márching, fóot-drill.

маршру́т *м.* itínerary, route. ~ный: ~ный по́езд *ж.-д.* through goods train; ~ное такси́ route táxi.

ма́ск|**а** *ж.* mask; посме́ртная ~ déath-mask; ◇ наде́ть (на себя́) ~у put* on a mask, mask onesélf; сбро́сить (с себя́) ~у throw* off the mask; сорва́ть ~у с кого́-л. unmásk *smb.*, expóse *smb.*

маскара́д *м.* 1. (*бал*) fáncy-dress ball, cóstume-ball, masqueráde; 2. (*необычный костюм*) fáncy dress; *перен.* pláy-acting. ~ный fáncy-dress *attr.*; ~ный костю́м fáncy dress.

маскир|**ова́ть**, замаскирова́ть (*вн.*) 1. mask (*smb.*), disguíse (*smb.*); 2. (*закрывать, прикрывать*) cámouflage (*smth.*); conceál (*smth.*) (*тж. перен.*). ~**ова́ться**, замаскирова́ться 1. put* on a mask; (*тв.*) dress up (as); 2. (*закрывать, прикрываться*) cámouflage onesélf; *перен.* bluff. ~**о́вка** *ж.* 1. (*действие*) concéalment; 2. (*то, чем маскируют*) cámouflage. ~овочный cámouflage *attr.*

масленица *ж.* Shróvetide; ◇ не житьё, а ~ this is the life!

маслёнка *ж.* 1. (*посуда*) bútter-dish; 2. *тех.* lúbricator; (*ручная*) óilcan.

маслёнок *м.* (*гриб*) Bolétus lúteus.

масленый búttered, rich; (*запачканный маслом*) óily, gréasy.

масли|на *ж.* 1. (*плод*) ólive; 2. (*дерево*) ólive(-tree).

масли́чный óil-bearing; oleáginous *научн.*; ~ые культу́ры óil-producing crops.

масли́чный ólive.

масл|о *с.* 1. (*растительное*) oil; (*коровье*) bútter; 2. *жив.* oil; писа́ть ~ом paint in oils; ◇ как по ~у swímmingly.

масло|бойка *ж.* churn. ~бо́йня *ж.* óil-mill. ~де́лие *с.* bútter-making. ~де́льный bútter-making *attr.*; ~де́льный заво́д bútter-factory, créamery.

масляни́стый 1. óily; 2. (*лоснящийся*) gréasy-looking.

масля́н|ый óily, gréasy; ~ое пятно́ grease spot; ◇ ~ая кра́ска óil-paint; oils *pl.*

ма́сс|а *ж.* 1. mass; 2. (*тестообразное вещество*) mass; dough, pulp, súbstance; 3. (*большинство*) the bulk; (*скопление*) mass; основна́я ~ чего-л. the bulk of *smth.*; в ~е as a whole, the majórity (of); мураве́й густо́й ~ой копоши́лись в траве́ the grass was a séething mass of ants; 4. (*рд.*) *разг.* (*множество*) a lot (of); heaps (of) *pl.*

масса́ж *м.* mássage. ~и́ст *м.* masséur. ~и́стка *ж.* masséuse.

масси́в *м.* 1. (*горный*) mássif, móuntain mass; 2. (*большое пространство*) tract; лесно́й ~ tract of fórest, large fórest área; торфяно́й ~ péat-bog.

масси́вный mássive.

масси́рованный mass *attr.*, massed.

масси́ровать I *несов. и сов.* (*вн.*; *делать массаж*) mássage (*smb.*, *smth.*).

масси́ровать II *несов. и сов.* (*вн.*) *воен.* (*сосредоточивать*) mass (*smth.*), cóncentrate (*smth.*).

массови́к *м.* *разг.* órganizer of mass cúltural and sports actívities.

ма́ссов|ость *ж.* mass cháracter. ~ый mass *attr.*; (*общедоступный*) pópular; ~ая демонстра́ция mass demonstrátion; ~ые и́гры pópular games; ~ое произво́дство lárge-scale prodúction; ~ые сре́дства информа́ции mass média; ~ый чита́тель the géneral réader; това́ры ~ого потребле́ния consúmer goods; ~ые сце́ны crowd scenes.

ма́ссы *мн.* the másses.

ма́стер *м.* 1. skilled cráftsman*; máker; сапо́жный ~ shóemaker; 2. (*большой специалист своего дела*) máster, éxpert; ~ худо́жественного сло́ва skilled recíter; ~ своего́ де́ла éxpert, a great máster in *one's* line; 3. (*на вн.*) *разг.* (*искусный человек*) good hand (at); он ~ на вы́думки he's véry invéntive; 4. (*цеха и т. п.*) fóreman*; сме́нный ~ shift fóreman*; 5. (*звание*): ~ спо́рта Máster of Sport, Spórt-Master; ◇ ~ на все ру́ки vérsatile wórker, jáck-of-all-trádes; де́ло ~a бои́тся you've ónly got to know how, cléver hands make light work.

мастер|и́ть, смастери́ть (*вн.*) *разг.* make* (*smth.*), contríve (*smth.*). ~ска́я *ж.* 1. wórkshop; ремо́нтная ~ска́я repáir shop; 2. (*на заводе*) shop; 3. *мн.* wórkshops; железнодоро́жные ~ские ráilway wórkshops; 4. (*художника, скульптора*) stúdio (*pl* -os).

мастер|ско́й másterly. ~ство́ *с.* 1. (*ремесло*) hándicraft, trade; 2. (*искусство, умение*) skill, mástery.

масти́ка *ж.* 1. mástic; 2. (*для натирания полов*) flóor-polish.

масти́тый vénerable.

мастодо́нт *м.* mástodon.

масть *ж.* 1. (*животного*) coat; 2. (*в картах*) suit; ходи́ть в ~ fóllow suit.

масшта́б *м.* scale; в большо́м ~е on a large scale; в междунаро́дном ~е on an internátional scale.

мат *м.* *шахм.* chéckmate.

матема́тик *м.* mathematícian.

матема́т|ика *ж.* mathemátics. ~и́ческий mathemátical.

материа́л *м.* matérial; (*ткань тж.*) stuff, fábric.

материал|и́зм *м.* matérialism; истори́ческий ~ histórical matérialism; диалекти́ческий ~ dialéctical matérialism. ~и́ст *м.* matérialist. ~исти́ческий matérialist. ~исти́чный materialístic.

материа́льность *ж.* materiálity.

материа́льно-техни́ческ|ий matérial and téchnical; ~ая ба́за the matérial and téchnical básis.

материа́льн|ый matérial; (*денежный тж.*) fináncial, pecúniary; ~ мир matérial úniverse; ~ые ресу́рсы matérial resóurces; ~ое положе́ние fináncial posítion; затрудни́тельное ~ое положе́ние pecúniary embárrassment; быть в хоро́шем ~ом положе́нии be well-óff; ~ая заинтересо́ванность matérial incéntives *pl*; ~ые це́нности matérial válues; ~ая отве́тственность fináncial responsibílity; ~ые и духо́вные потре́бности matérial and intelléctual/spíritual needs; ◇ ~ая часть matériel, equípment.

матери́к *м.* cóntinent; (*в отличие от острова*) máinland.

матери́нский 1. (*принадлежащий матери*) móther's; 2. (*свойственный матери*) matérnal, mótherly.

матери́нство *с.* matérnity, mótherhood.

матери́|я *ж.* 1. mátter; строе́ние ~и strúcture of mátter; 2. (*ткань*) fábric, stuff; 3. *разг.* (*тема, разговор*) súbject.

матеро́й: ~ волк adúlt/fúll-grown wolf*; ~ дуб áncient oak.

матёрчатый *разг.* fábric *attr.*

матёрый 1. *см.* матеро́й; 2. *разг.* (*опытный*) véteran, expérienced; 3. (*закоренелый*) invéterate; ~ враг invéterate énemy.

ма́тка *ж.* 1. (*самка*) fémale; (*пчелиная*) quéen (-bee); 2. *анат.* womb; úterus *мед.*

ма́товый 1. (*тусклый*) lústreless, dull; (*о цвете лица*) mat; 2. (*о стекле*) frósted.

ма́точный úterine.

матра́с *м.*, **матра́ц** *м.* máttress.

ма́трица *ж.* mátrix (*pl* -ices, -ixes).

матро́с *м.* séaman*; sáilor *разг.* ~ка *ж.* (*блуза*) sáilor's blouse. ~ский sáilor *attr.*; sáilor's; ~ский костю́м sáilor-suit.

ма́тушка *ж.* móther.

матч *м.* *спорт.* match; ~ на пе́рвенство ми́ра по футбо́лу match for the World Fóotball Chámpionship, the World Cup match.

матч-турни́р *м.* tóurnament.

мать *ж.* móther.

мать-и-ма́чеха *ж.* *бот.* cóltsfoot.

ма́фия *ж.* Máfia.

мах *м.* stroke; (*колеса*) turn; ◇ одни́м ~ом at one stroke; at a síngle bound (*прыжком*); с ~у ráshly; дать ~у fail, make* a blúnder.

маха́ть, махну́ть (*тв.*) wave (*smth.*); (*крыльями*) flap (*smth.*), flútter (*smth.*); ~ руко́й кому-л. wave (*one's* hand) to smb.; ~ хвосто́м swish its tail; (*о собаке*) wag its tail.

махина́ция *ж.* trick, machinátion; *мн. тж.* machinátions.

махну́ть *сов.* 1. *см.* маха́ть; 2. *разг.* (*прыгнуть*) leap*; 3. *разг* (*поехать*) go*; (*в другой город*) dash óver (to); ◇ ~ руко́й на кого-л., что-л. give* smb., smth. up (as hópeless, as a bad job).

махов|и́к *м. тех.* flý-wheel. **~о́й: ~о́е колесо́** *см.* махови́к.

махро́в|ый 1. (*о цветах*) double; **2.** (*отъявленный*) diehard *attr.;* **~ реакционе́р** diehard reáctionary; **3.** *текст.* térry; **~ое полоте́нце** térry tówel.

ма́чеха *ж.* stépmother.

ма́чт|а *ж.* mast; (*высотная конструкция для антенн и т. п. тж.*) tówer. **~овый** mast *attr.;* **~овый лес** ship-timber.

машбюро́ *с.* (*машинописное бюро*) týping pool.

маши́н|а *ж.* **1.** machíne; (*двигатель*) éngine; *мн. собир.* machínery *sg;* *перен.* (*организация*) machíne; **вое́нная ~** war machíne; **2.** (*автомобиль*) (mótor) car; (*грузовик*) lórry; **е́хать на ~е** drive*, go* by car.

машина́льный mechánical.

машини́ст *м.* **1.** óperator, machínist; **~ экскава́тора** éxcavator óperator; **2.** *ж.-д.* éngine-driver; engineer *амер.*

машини́стка *ж.* týpist.

маши́нк|а *ж.* **1.** machíne; **2.** (*для стрижки*) clíppers *pl;* **3.** *разг.* (*пишущая*) týpewriter; **печа́тать на ~е** type.

маши́нн|ый machíne *attr.;* **~ое произво́дство** méchanized prodúction; **~ое отделе́ние** machíne-room, éngine-room; **~ое ма́сло** machíne/lúbricating oil.

машинопи́сный: ~ текст týpewritten text.

машинопись *ж.* týpewriting.

машиностро|е́ние *с.* mechánical engineering. **~и́тельный** machíne-building.

машиносчётный compúter *attr.*

мая́к *м.* líghthouse; béacon (*тж. перен.*).

ма́ятник *м.* péndulum; (*ручных часов*) bálance.

ма́яться *несов. разг.* **1.** (*заниматься утомительной работой*) sweat; (*переносить лишения*) rough it; **2.** (*мучиться, томиться*) súffer.

мая́чить *несов. разг.* loom.

мгл|а *ж.* **1.** (*пелена тумана и т. п.*) haze; **2.** (*сумрак*) gloom, dárkness. **~и́стый** házy.

мгнове́ни|е *с.* ínstant; **<> в одно́ ~** ínstantly; **в ~ о́ка** in the twínkling of an eye. **~но** ínstantly, in a trice. **~ный** instantáneous; (*быстро проходящий*) mómentary.

ме́бель *ж. собир.* fúrniture. **~ный** fúrniture *attr.;* **~ный магази́н** fúrniture shop.

меблиро́ванный fúrnished.

меблирова́ть *несов. и сов.* (*вн.*) fúrnish (*smth.*).

меблиро́вка *ж.* **1.** (*действие*) fúrnishing; **2.** *собир.* (*мебель*) fúrniture.

мегафо́н *м.* mégaphone.

меге́ра *ж.* térmagant.

мёд *м.* **1.** hóney; **2.** (*напиток*) mead; **<> ва́шими бы уста́ми да ~ пить** *погов.* if ónly it were true!, would it were so!

медали́ст *м.,* **~ка** *ж.* médallist.

меда́л|ь *ж.* médal; **золота́я ~** gold médal; **<> оборо́тная сторона́ ~** the revérse side of the médal.

медальо́н *м.* medállion, lócket.

медве́дица *ж.* she-bear; **<> Больша́я Медве́дица** *астр.* the Great Bear; **Ма́лая Медве́дица** *астр.* the Líttle Bear.

медве́|дь *м.* bear; **бе́лый ~** white/pólar bear. **~жий 1.** bear *attr.;* úrsine *научн.;* **2.** (*похожий на медведя*) béar-like; **<> оказа́ть ~жью услу́гу кому́-л.** confér a dúbious bénefit upón *smb.* **~жо́нок** *м.* (béar-)cub.

медеплави́льный: ~ заво́д cópper works.

ме́дик *м.* médical man*.

медикаме́нты *мн.* médicaments, drugs.

медици́на *ж.* médicine. **~ский** médical; **~ский пункт** first-áid státion, médical room; **~ский институ́т** médical ínstitute; **<> ~ская сестра́** (tráined) nurse; (*в больнице*) hóspital nurse.

ме́дленный slow.

медли́тельн|ый slúggish, slow; (*неторопливый*) léisurely; **~ ум** slúggish brain; **~ челове́к** slów-moving pérson; **~ые движе́ния** léisurely móvements.

ме́длить *несов.* línger; (*откладывать*) deláy; **~ с отве́том** deláy one's ánswer, be* slow in ánswering.

ме́дно-кра́сный cópper-coloured.

ме́дн|ый 1. cópper *attr.;* (*из жёлтой меди*) brass *attr.;* **~ сли́ток** cópper bar; **~ая руда́** cópper ore; **~ колчеда́н** cópper pyrítes; **~ые де́ньги** cópper (coin/móney); **~ые пу́говицы** brass búttons; **2.** (*о цвете*) cóppery; **3.** (*о звуке*) metállic; (*о голосе*) brássy; **<> ~ век** the áge of Cópper; **~ лоб** blóckhead.

медо́в|ый hóney *attr.;* *перен.* hóneyed; **~ые со́ты** hóneycomb *sg;* **~ пря́ник** hóney-cake; **~ые ре́чи** hóneyed words; **<> ~ ме́сяц** hóneymoon.

медоно́сн|ый hóney-bearing; **~ые пчёлы** hóney-bees.

медосмо́тр *м.* médical examinátion.

медпу́нкт *м.* first-áid státion, médical room.

меду́за *ж. зоол.* jélly-fish.

мед|ь *ж.* **1.** cópper; **жёлтая ~** brass; **кра́сная ~** red cópper; **2.** *собир. разг.* (*медные деньги*) cóppers *pl.* **~я́к** *м. разг.* cópper (coin).

медя́нка *ж.* **1.** (*змея*) gráss-snake; (*гадюка*) víper; **2.** (*краска*) vérdigris.

межа́ *ж.* bóundary(-line); (*нераспаханная полоса*) balk.

междоме́тие *с. грам.* interjéction.

междоусо́б|ица *ж.* internécine war. **~ный** internécine.

ме́жду 1. betwéen; **2.** (*среди*) amóng; **<> ~ на́ми (говоря́)** betwéen you and me, betwéen oursélves; **~ тем** méanwhile; **~ тем как** while, whereás; **~ про́чим 1)** *нареч.* in pássing; **2)** *вводн. сл.* by the way, incidéntally; **~ де́лом** while *one* is about it, in odd móments.

междуве́домствен|ый interdepartméntal; **~ая коми́ссия** joint commíttee; **~ая перепи́ска** correspóndence betwéen depártments.

междугоро́дный interúrban; **~ телефо́н** trúnk-line; **~ разгово́р** trunk-call, lóng-distance call.

междунаро́дн|ый internátional; **Междунаро́дная демократи́ческая федера́ция же́нщин** Internátional Federátion of Democrátic Wómen; **~ое пра́во** internátional law, law of nátions.

междуря́дный *с.-х.* interrów; between rows *после сущ.*

междуца́рствие *с.* interrégnum.

меж|ева́ние *с.* fíxing of bóundaries, lánd-survéying. **~ева́ть** *несов.* (*вн.*) set*/fix bóundaries (to). **~ево́й: ~ево́й знак** lándmark, bóundary-mark; **~ево́й столб** bóundary-post.

межзвёздн|ый: ~ое простра́нство interstéllar space.

межколхо́зный sérving séveral colléctive farms *после сущ.*

межконтинента́льный intercontinent(al).

межплане́тн|ый interplánetary; **~ полёт** interplánetary flight; **~ое простра́нство** interplánetary space; **~ая ста́нция** interplánetary státion.

межреспублика́нск|ий interrepúblic; **~ие хозя́йственные о́рганы** interrepúblic económic órgans.

межсезо́нье *с.* óff-season.

мезозо́йский *геол.* mesozóic.

мезони́н *м.* mézzanine.

мексика́н|ец *м.,* **~ка** *ж.* Méxican. **~ский** Méxican.

мел *м.* chalk; (*для побелки*) whítewash; **писа́ть ~ом** write* in chalk.

меланхо́л|ик *м.* mélancholy pérson. **~и́ческий** mélancholy. **~ия** *ж.* mélancholy, depréssion.

меле́ть, обмеле́ть becóme* shállow.

мелиор|ати́вный reclamátion *attr.* **~а́ция** *ж.* reclamátion, impróvement.

ме́лк|ий 1. (*состоящий из малых частиц*) small, fine; **~ дождь** fine rain, drízzle; **~ песо́к** fine sand; **2.** (*небольшой*) small; **~ие оре́хи** small nuts; **~ие черты́ лица́** small féatures; **~ скот** sheep and goats; **3.** (*экономически маломощный*) small(-scale), pétty; **~ие едино-**

ли́чные хозя́йства small indivídual farms, small hóldings; ~ое хозя́йство small fárming; ~ со́бственник small/pétty proprίetor; ~ая буржуазίя pétty bourgeoisίe; 4. (незначи́тельный) pétty; ~ие расхо́ды minor expénses; ~ая кра́жа pétty theft/lárceny, pίlfering; 5. (неглубо́кий) shállow; ~ая река́ shállow rίver; ~ая таре́лка (méat-) plate; 6. (низме́нный, по́шлый) nárrow, líttle, méan--spírited; ~ая душо́нка mean soul; ◇ ~ой ры́сью at a géntle trot; ~ие де́ньги (small) change sg; ~ая со́шка pίp-squeak.

ме́лко 1. (некру́пно) fine, small; ~ моло́ть grind* fine/small; ~ писа́ть write* a fine/small hand; 2. (неглубо́ко) shállow.

мелкобуржуа́зн|ый pétty-bóurgeois; ~ые взгля́ды nárrow views/opίnions.

мелково́дный shállow.

мелково́дье с. shoal-water; shállows pl.

мелкокали́берный small-bore attr.

мелколе́сье с. small fórest.

мелкосо́бственнический small próperty-owner attr.

мелкота́ ж. собир. разг. small fry.

мелкотова́рн|ый эк. smáll-scale; ~ое хозя́йство pétty ecónomy.

мелов|о́й chalk attr.; ~ые го́ры chalk hills; ◇ ~а́я бума́га art páper; ~ пери́од геол. the Cretáceous périod.

мелодеклама́ция ж. recitátion to músic.

мело́дика ж. melódics.

мелод|и́ческий 1. (относя́щийся к мело́дии) melódic; 2. (благозву́чный) melódious, túneful. ~ήчный см. мелоди́ческий 2.

мело́дия ж. mélody, tune.

мелодра́ма ж. mélodrama.

мелодрамати́ческий melodramátic.

мелочн|о́й 1. pétty; ~а́я торго́вля pétty tráding; pédlary; 2. см. ме́лочный.

ме́лочн|ость ж. péttiness. ~ый 1. pétty; ~ые интере́сы pétty ínterests; ~ые приди́рки pétty objéctions; 2. (о челове́ке) smáll-mínded.

ме́лоч|ь ж. 1. small árticles pl, small things pl; (о ры́бе) small fry; вся́кая ~ all sorts of odds and ends pl; 2. собир. (ме́лкие де́ньги) change; 3. (пустя́к) trίfle; ◇ по ~а́м on trίfles; разме́ниваться на ~и frίtter awáy one's énergy.

мел|ь ж. shoal; на ~и́ stránded, high and dry (тж. перен.); снять с ~и́ set* aflóat, float; посади́ть на ~ ground.

мелька́ние с. fláshing.

мелька́ть, мелькну́ть 1. (пока́зываться) show* (up); (попада́ться) turn up; перен. come*; у него́ мелькну́ла мысль the thought flashed through his mind; 2. (бы́стро сле́довать) flash, 3. (мерца́ть) glίmmer, gleam.

мелькну́ть сов. см. мелька́ть.

ме́льком: ви́деть кого́-л., что́-л. ~ see* smb., smth. for a móment; заме́тить, уви́деть кого́-л., что́-л. ~ catch* a glimpse of smb., smth.; взгляну́ть ~ на кого́-л., что́-л. cast* a perfúnctory/héedless glance at smb., smth.; слы́шать что́-л. ~ hear* smth. méntioned.

ме́льни|к м. mίller. ~ца ж. mill; ◇ лить во́ду на чью-л. ~цу bring* grist to smb.'s mill.

мельча́йш|ий (превосх. ст. прил. ме́лкий) the smállest; до ~их подро́бностей down to the minútest détails.

мельча́ть, измельча́ть 1. (станови́ться ме́льче по величине́) get* small; перен. detériorate, go* off; 2. (о реке́ и т. п.) grow* shállow.

ме́льче (сравнит. ст. прил. ме́лкий и нареч. ме́лко) 1. (по величине́) smáller; 2. (о реке́ и т. п.) shállower.

мельчи́ть несов. (вн.; дроби́ть) crush (smth.).

мелюзга́ ж. собир. разг. small fry; tíny créatures pl.

мембра́на ж. díaphragm.

мемора́ндум м. memorándum (pl -da).

мемориа́л м. 1. (соревнова́ния) memórial match; 2. (архитекту́рный анса́мбль) memórial.

мемориа́льн|ый memórial; ~ая доска́ táblet, memórial táble.

мемуа́рн|ый: ~ая литерату́ра mémoirs pl; ~ стиль style of pérsonal reminίscence.

мемуа́ры мн. mémoirs.

ме́на ж. bárter, exchánge (in kind).

ме́нее нареч.; ◇ тем не ~ none the less, nevertheléss.

мензу́рка ж. méasuring-glass.

менинги́т м. мед. meningítis.

менов|о́й exchánge attr., bárter attr.; ~а́я сто́имость exchánge válue; ~а́я торго́вля exchánge in kind, bárter.

менструа́ция ж. menstruátion.

менто́л м. ménthol.

ме́нтор м. méntor. ~ский édifying, didáctic; ~ским то́ном in édifying tones.

ме́ньше 1. (сравнит. ст. прил. ма́ленький, ма́лый) smáller; 2. (сравнит. ст. нареч. ма́ло) less; немно́го ~ 50-ти лет (о во́зрасте) a little únder 50, a little short of 50; как мо́жно ~ движе́ний as little móvement as póssible; как мо́жно ~ дви́гаться move as little as póssible; ◇ ~ всего́ least of all.

меньшев|и́зм м. ист. Ménshevism. ~и́к м. Ménshevik. ~и́стский Ménshevik attr., Ménshevist.

ме́ньш|ий 1. (сравнит. ст. прил. ма́лый, ма́ленький) lésser; 2. (превосх. ст. прил. ма́лый, ма́ленький) the least; 3. разг. (мла́дший) yóunger; ◇ по ~ей ме́ре to say the least of it; са́мое ~ее at least; not less than.

меньшинств|о́ с. minórity; оказа́ться в ~е́ be* outnúmbered; (при голосова́нии) be* outvóted.

меню́ с. нескл. ménu, bill of fare.

меня́ (рд., вн. от личн. мест. я) me.

меня́ть несов. (вн.) change (smth.); ~ свою́ вне́шность change one's appéarance. ~ся несов. 1. (тв.; обме́ниваться) exchánge (smth.); 2. (изменя́ться) change; 3. (замеща́ть друг дру́га) relίeve one anóther, be* changed; ◇ ~ся в лице́ change cóuntenance.

ме́р|а ж. 1. méasure; ~ы пло́щади square méasures; ~ы жи́дкости líquid méasures; 2. (мероприя́тие) méasure, step; принима́ть ~ы take* áction; приня́ть все ~ы take* all due méasures; ~ы взыска́ния disciplinary méasure; 3. (преде́л, грани́ца чего́-л.) límit; всему́ есть ~ éverything has a límit; сохраня́ть чу́вство ~ы retáin a sense of propórtion; ◇ по ~е того́ как as; по ~е возмо́жности as far as póssible; по ~е необходи́мости as the necéssity aríses, if nécessary; в значи́тельной ~е to a considerable extént; в изве́стной ~е to a cértain extént; в ~у (сто́лько, ско́лько ну́жно) móderately; (сообразу́ясь с чем-л.) in accórdance with; всё в ~у éverything in moderátion; не в ~у beyónd méasure, inórdinately; в по́лной ~е complétely; в той ~е, в како́й... to the extént that...

мере́жка ж. dráwn-work.

мере́щ|иться, помере́щиться (дт.) разг. seem (to); ему́ ~ся, что... he fáncies (that)..., it seems to him (that)...

мерза́в|ец м., ~ка ж. разг. scóundrel, ráscal.

ме́рзкий 1. (вызыва́ющий отвраще́ние) lóathsome, disgústing, filthy; ~ посту́пок vile act; 2. разг. (о́чень плохо́й) áwful, foul.

ме́рзко 1. нареч. disgústingly, revóltingly, in a vile mánner; 2. в знач. сказ. безл.: ему́ ста́ло ~ he felt disgústed/revólted.

мерзлота́ ж.: ве́чная ~ pérmafrost, etérnal frost.

мёрз|лый frózen. ~нуть несов. freeze*.

ме́рзость ж. 1. víleness; 2. (то, что вызыва́ет отвраще́ние) abominátion, lóathsome/abóminable thing; ~ запусте́ния abominátion of desolátion.

меридиа́н м. merídian.

мери́ло с. critérion.

ме́рин *м.* gélding.

мерино́с *м.* 1. (*порода овец*) meríno (sheep); 2. (*шерсть*) meríno (wool). ~овый meríno *attr.*

ме́рить, сме́рить (*вн.*) 1. méasure (*smth.*) (*тж. перен.*); ~ кому́-л. температу́ру take* smb.'s témperature; ~ глубину́ sound the depth; 2. тк. несов. (*примерять*) try on (*smth.*); ~ ту́фли try on a pair of shoes. ~ся, поме́риться: ~ся си́лами с кем-л. try their (our, your) strength on each óther, engáge in a trial of strength.

ме́рк|а *ж.* 1. méasurements *pl;* снять ~у с кого́-либо take* smb.'s méasurements (*предмет для измерения*) méasure (*тж. перен.*); ме́рить кого́-л. свое́й ~ой judge *smb.* by one's own stándard/yárdstick.

мерканти́льн|ый mércantile; *перен. тж.* mércenary; ~ая систе́ма mércantile sýstem; ~ дух mércenary spírit.

ме́ркнуть, поме́ркнуть fade, grow* dim.

мерлу́шк|а *ж.* lámbskin. ~овый lámbskin *attr.*

ме́рн|ый méasured; ~ая по́ступь méasured steps *pl;* ~ая речь méasured words *pl,* róunded périods *pl.*

мероприя́тие *с.* méasure.

ме́ртвенно-бле́дный déathly pale.

ме́ртвенный lífeless; *перен.* déathly.

мертв|е́ть, омертве́ть, поме́ртветь 1. сов. омертве́ть (*о клетках, тканях*) die; (*неметь*) grow*/be* numb; ру́ки ~е́ют от хо́лода one's hands grow numb with cold; 2. сов. поме́ртветь (*приходить в оцепенение*) be* páralysed; помертве́ть от у́жаса be* páralysed with térror.

мертве́ц *м.* corpse, dead man*; мн. the dead. ~ки: ~ки пьян *разг.* dead drunk.

мертворождённый (*прям. и перен.*) still-born.

мёртв|ый *прил.* 1. dead; *перен.* (*безжизненный*) lífeless; ~ая тишина́ déathly sílence; 2. в знач. сущ. м. dead man*/pérson; мн. the dead; ~ спать ~ым сном sleep* like the dead; ~ая голова́ death's head; ~ая зыбь gróundswell; ~ капита́л dead stock; ~ язы́к dead lánguage; ~ая петля́ *ав.* loop; де́лать ~ую петлю́ *ав.* loop the loop; на ~ой то́чке at dead céntre; сдви́нуть что-л. с ~ой то́чки get* smth. móving; ~ое простра́нство *воен.* dead ground.

мерц|а́ние *с.* twinkling, shímmering, flíckering, scintillátion. ~а́ть несов. twinkle, shímmer, flícker.

ме́сиво *с. разг.* 1. mess; (*грязь*) míre; 2. (*корм для скота*) mash.

меси́ть, смеси́ть (*вн.*) (*тесто*) mix (*smth.*), knead (*smth.*); (*глину*) púddle (*smth.*); ◇ ~ грязь plough through mud.

ме́сса *ж.* mass.

месте́чко I *с.* place; ◇ тёплое ~ cúshy/snug job.

месте́чко II *с.* (*селение*) tównship.

мести́ *несов.* (*вн.*) 1. sweep* (*smth.*); ~ cop sweep* up/awáy the rúbbish; ~ пол sweep* the floor; 2. (*гнать*) sweep* (*smth.*), drive* (*smth.*); 3. безл.: метёт (*о метели*) the wind is dríving the snow.

месткóм *м.* (*местный комитет профсоюза*) lócal tráde-union commíttee.

ме́стн|ость *ж.* 1. locálity, cóuntry; гори́стая ~ hílly cóuntry; 2. (*край, район*) dístrict, région. ~ый lócal; ~ый жи́тель lócal inhábitant; ~ый уроже́нец nátive; ~ый го́вор lócal díalect; ~ое сырьё lócal raw matérials *pl;* ~ые óрганы вла́сти lócal authórities; ◇ ~ое вре́мя lócal time; ~ый колори́т lócal cólour; ~ая промы́шленность lócal índustry; ~ый паде́ж *грам.* lócative (case).

ме́ст|о *с.* 1. (*пространство*) place, spot; (*свободное пространство*) room; (*для постройки, сада и т. п.*) site; (*действия, происшествия*) scene; ~ преступле́ния scene of the crime; быть на ~е be* on the spot, be* présent; 2. (*сиденье, кресло*) seat; зри́тельный зал на 500 мест séating five húndred; заня́ть ~ take* one's seat; 3. обыкн. мн. (*местность*) locálity *sg,* área *sg;* знако́мые ~á familiar locálity; 4. мн. (*периферия*) the próvinces; províncial organizátions; на ~áx in the próvinces; 5. (*часть, отрывок книги и т. п.*) part (of), place (in); 6. (*положение*) position; (*в спорте*) place; 7. (*должность*) post, place, work; 8. (*отдельный предмет багажа*) piece, bag; сдать в бага́ж пять мест régister five píeces of lúggage; ◇ я бы на ва́шем ~е... in your place I would...; стоя́ть, остава́ться на ~е stand* still; уби́ть кого́-л. на ~е kill smb. on the spot; заста́ть, пойма́ть кого́-л. на ~е преступле́ния catch* smb. in the act, catch* smb. réd-hánded; де́тское ~ placénta; ~á о́бщего по́льзования (públic) convéniences; не находи́ть себе́ ~а not know what to do with onesélf; к ~у súitable for/to the occásion; знать своё ~ know* one's place; поста́вить кого́-л. на ~ put* smb. in his, her place; нет ~а, не должно́ быть ~а кому́-л., чему́-л. there should be no place for smth., smth.; о́бщее ~ plátitude, cómmonplace; на (своём) ~е dóing what one should be dóing; не на (своём) ~е be* a mísfit, be* a square peg (in a round hole); не к ~у out of place, irrélevant; не ~ 1) (кому́-л.) this is no place (for smb.); 2) (чему́-л., + инф.) this is no place (for + -ing), this isn't the place (for); ни с ~а 1) stay where you are!; 2) (*в том же положении*) not a scrap of prógress.

местожи́тельство *с.* place of résidence.

местоиме́н|ие *с. грам.* prónoun. ~ный *грам.* pronóminal.

местонахожде́ние *с.* locátion; whéreabouts *разг.*

местоположе́ние *с.* situátion, site; locátion *амер.*

местопребыва́ние *с.* résidence, abóde, seat; ~ прави́тельства the seat of Góvernment.

месторожде́ние *с. геол.* depósit.

месть *ж.* revénge.

ме́сяц *м.* 1. (*календарный*) month; янва́рь, февра́ль и т. п. ~ the month of Jánuary, Fébruary *etc.;* 2. (*луна*) moon; ~ на уще́рбе the moon is on the wane; молодо́й ~ new moon.

ме́сячник *м.* month; ~ безопа́сности движе́ния róad-sáfety month.

ме́сяч|ный month's; (*ежемесячный*) mónthly; ~ о́тпуск a month's leave; ~ план a month's plan, plan for the month; ~ая зарпла́та mónthly sálary/wáges.

мета́лл *м.* métal.

металли́ст *м.* métal-worker.

металли́ческ|ий métal *attr.; перен.* metállic; ~ие изде́лия métal goods; ~ го́лос metállic voice.

металлоло́м *м.* scrap métal.

металлообраба́тывающ|ий métal-working *attr.;* ~ая промы́шленность métal-working índustry.

металлопла́вильн|ый smélting; ~ая печь smélting fúrnace; ~ заво́д fóundry.

металлопрока́тный métal-rolling *attr.;* ~ цех rólling depártment/shop.

металлоре́жущий métal-cutting *attr.*

металлу́рг *м.* metállurgist.

металлу́рг|и́ческий metallúrgical; ~ заво́д metallúrgical works/plant. ~ия *ж.* metállurgy.

метаморфо́за *ж.* metamórphosis (*pl* -ses), transformátion.

мета́ние *с.* 1. thrówing; ~ ди́ска *спорт.* díscus-thrówing; 2.: ~ икры́ spáwning.

метаста́з *м. мед.* metástasis (*pl* -ses).

мета́тельный míssile; ~ снаря́д míssile.

мета́ть I, метну́ть (*вн.*) 1. (*бросать*) throw* (*smth.*), cast* (*smth.*), fling* (*smth.*); ~ диск throw* the díscus; ~ копьё throw*/fling* the jávelin; 2. тк. несов.: ~ икру́ spawn; ◇ ~ банк keep* the bank; рвать и ~ be* in a flýing rage.

мета́ть II, смета́ть (*вн.; шить*) baste (*smth.*), tack (*smth.*); ◇ ~ пе́тли make* búttonholes.

мета́ться *несов.* rush abóut; (*в постели*) toss and turn; ~ по ко́мнате fling* onesélf abóut the room.

метафи́з|**ик** *м.* metaphysícian. ~**ика** *ж.* metaphýsics. ~**и́ческий** metaphýsical.

метафóр|**а** *ж. лит.* métaphor. ~**и́ческий** *лит.* metaphórical.

метёлка *ж.* 1. whisk, broom; 2. *бот.* ear, pánicle.

метéль *ж.* snów-storm, dríving snow.

метеóр *м.* méteor, shóoting star.

метеори́т *м.* méteorite.

метеорóлог *м.* meteorólogist. ~**и́ческий** meteorológical.

метеоролóгия *ж.* meteorólogy.

метео|**слýжба** *ж.* meteorológical/wéather sérvice. ~**спýтник** *м.* wéather sátellite.

мети́с *м.* 1. hálf-breed; 2. (*в антропологии*) métis.

мéтить I *несов.* (*вн.; ставить знак, метку*) mark (*smth.*); (*скот*) brand (*smth.*).

мéтить II *несов.* 1. (*в вн.; целиться*) aim (at); 2. (*на вн.*) *разг.* (*намекать*) hint (at); 3. (*в вн.*) *разг.* (*стремиться*) aspíre (to).

мéтк|**а** *ж.* 1. (*действие*) márking; 2. (*знак*) mark; без ~**и** únmárked.

мéтк|**ий** 1. áccurate; (*о пуле, ударе и т. п.*) well-áimed; ~ **стрелóк** good shot; márksman*; ~**ая стрельбá** áccurate fire; ~ **глаз** true/keen eye; 2. (*выразительный*) keen, intélligent; ~**ое замечáние** apt remárk. ~**ость** *ж.* 1. (*стрелкá*) márksmanship; (*стрельбы*) áccuracy; 2. (*выразительность*) kéenness, intélligence.

метлá *ж.* broom; ◇ **нóвая ~ чи́сто метёт** *посл.* a new broom sweeps clean.

метнýть *сов. см.* метáть I 1.

мéтод *м.* méthod.

метóд|**ика** *ж.* 1. (*наука о методах преподавания*) methódics; 2. (*совокупность методов выполнения чего-л.*) méthods *pl.* ~**и́ст** *м.*, ~**и́стка** *ж.* spécialist in educátional méthods.

методи́ческ|**ий** 1. methódics *attr.*; ~ **кабинéт** methódics depártment; ~**ое пособие** téxtbook of methódics; 2. (*последовательный*) methódical.

методи́чный *см.* методи́ческий 2.

методол|**оги́ческий** methodológical. ~**óгия** *ж.* methodólogy.

метоними́мия *ж. лит.* metónymу.

метр I *м.* 1. (*единица длины*) métre; 2. (*линейка*) métre méasure/rule.

метр II *м. лит.* métre.

метрáж *м.* 1. (*длина чего-л. в метрах*) length (in métres); ~ **фи́льма** length of film, fóotage; 2. (*площадь чего-л. в кв. метрах*) méasurements *pl.,* (métric) área.

метрдотéль *м.* head wáiter.

мéтрика I *ж. лит.* métre.

мéтрика II *ж.* (*документ*) birth-certíficate.

метри́ческ|**ий** I métric; ~**ая систéма мер** the métric sýstem.

метри́ческ|**ий** II *лит.* métrical; ~**ое стихосложéние** métrical versificátion.

метри́ческ|**ий** III: ~**ая кни́га** régister of births, deaths and márriages; ~**ое свидéтельство** birth-certíficate.

метрó *с. нескл. см.* метрополитéн.

метрóном *м.* métronome.

метрополитéн *м.* the únderground; the Métro; súbway *амер.*

метрополия *ж.* párent state, móther cóuntry.

мех I *м.* 1. (*шкура*) fur; **на ~ý, подби́тый ~ом** fúr-lined; 2. (*для вина*) skin.

мех II *м. см.* мехи́.

механизáтор *м.* 1. mechanizer, mechanizátion éxpert; 2. (*в сельском хозяйстве*) machíne óperator. ~**ский** óperating *attr.*

механиз|**áция** *ж.* mechanizátion. ~**и́рованный** méchanized. ~**и́ровать** *несов. и сов.* (*вн.*) méchanize (*smth.*).

механи́зм *м.* méchanism; **часовóй ~** clóckwork

(devíce); **дви́жущий ~** dríving-gear; **госудáрственный ~** machínery of State.

механик *м.* 1. mechánical enginéer; 2. (*тот, кто обслуживает машины*) mechánic.

механ|**ика** *ж.* (*прям. и перен.*) mechánics. ~**и́ческий** mechánical; ~**и́ческая обрабóтка** machíning.

мехи́ *мн.* (*ед.* мех *м.*) béllows.

мехов|**óй** fur *attr.*; ~**áя шýба** fur coat; ~**áя промышленность** fur índustry.

меценáт *м.* Maecénas, pátron of the arts. ~**ство** *с.* pátronage (of the arts).

мéццо-сопрáно *с. нескл.* mézzo-sopráno.

меч *м.* sword; **blade** *поэт.*; ◇ **вложи́ть ~ в нóжны** sheathe the sword; **обнажи́ть ~, подня́ть ~** take* up one's sword; **Дамóклов ~** the sword of Dámocles; **предáть ~ý** put* to the sword; **скрести́ть ~и** cross/méasure swords (with).

мéчен|**ый** marked; ◇ ~**ые áтомы** tagged átoms.

мечéть *ж.* mosque.

мечтá *ж.* 1. dream; **несбы́точная ~** vain dream; 2. (*предмет сильного желания*) ambítion; **егó ~ стать капитáном корабля́** his ambítion is to becóme a ship's cáptain; 3. *в знач. сказ. разг.*: **это не плáтье, а ~!** it's a dream of a dress! ~**ние** *с.* 1. dreams *pl,* dréamings *pl,* réverie; 2. (*мечта*) dream. ~**тель** *м.,* ~**тельница** *ж.* dréamer. ~**тельность** *ж.* 1. dréaminess; 2. (*мечтание*) dreams *pl,* dréamings *pl,* réverie.

мечтáтельн|**ый** 1. dréamy; ~ **человéк** dréamy/imáginative pérson; ~**ое выражéние** dréamy expréssion; 2. (*созданный мечтой*) dream *attr.*; (*несбыточный*) fantástic.

мечтáть *несов.* dream*.

мешани́на *ж. разг.* hótchpot(ch), hódge-podge; (*в голове*) múddle.

меш|**áть** I, помешáть (*дт.*) (*препятствовать*) prevént (*smb.*), interfére (with), hínder (*smb.*); (*беспокоить*) be* in the way (of); ~ **кому-л.** be* in *smb.'s* way; **не ~áй!** leave me, him, *etc.* alóne! don't interrúpt!; **не ~áйте мне рабóтать!** let me work!; ◇ **не ~áло бы..., не ~áет...** there would be no harm in...

меш|**áть** II, помешáть (*вн.*) 1. (*размешивать*) stir (*smth.*); 2. *тк. несов.* (*соединять в одно*) mix (*smth.*); ~ **крáски** mix cólours.

меш|**áться** I *несов. разг.* 1. (*быть помехой*) get* in the way; ~ **под ногáми** be* in the way; 2. (*вмешиваться*) interfére, meddle.

меш|**áться** II *несов.* 1. (*с тв.; соединяться*) míngle (with); 2. (*сливаться в одну массу*) be* blurred, blur; 3. (*путаться*) becóme* confúsed.

мéш|**ать** *несов.* lóiter, línger; (*медлить*) be* slow (+ to *inf*); **не ~áй!** húrry up!; **он ~ал с отвéтом** he del áyed his replý, he was slow to replý.

мешковáтый 1. (*об одежде*) bággy; 2. (*о человеке*) clúmsy.

мешкови́на *ж.* sácking, sáckcloth.

меш|**óк** *м.* 1. bag; (*из мешковины*) sack; 2. (*как мера*) sack of, sáckful; 3. (*окружение*) pócket, encírclement; **попáсть в ~** get* caught in a pócket; **огневóй ~** fire pócket; ◇ **сидéть ~óм** hang* lóosely on one's limbs; be* bággy; **костю́м сиди́т на нём ~óм** the suit is far too loose for him, the suit is bággy; ~**и́ под глазáми** bags únder the eyes.

мещ|**ани́н** *м.* 1. pétty bóurgeois, míddle-class pérson; 2. (*обыватель*) Phílistine, vulgárian. ~**áнский** nárrow-mínded, vúlgar. ~**áнство** *с.* 1. (*сословие*) míddle clásses *pl*; 2. (*обывательщина*) míddle-class conventionálity.

ми *с. нескл. муз.* mi, E.

миг *м.* móment, ínstant; ◇ **в оди́н ~** in a trice; **в тот же ~** in the same ínstant.

мигáть, мигнýть 1. (*непроизвольно*) blink; 2. (*дт.; подавать знак*) wink (at); 3. (*мерцать*) twínkle, blink, glímmer.

мигну́ть *сов. см.* мига́ть.

ми́гом *разг.* in a trice/flash.

мигра́ция *ж.* migrátion.

мигре́нь *ж.* mígraine.

мигри́ровать *несов.* migráte.

мизансце́на *ж. театр.* stage sétting, set.

мизантро́п *м.* mísanthrope. **~и́ческий** misanthrópic. **~ия** *ж.* misánthropy.

мизе́рный wrétched, scánty, pítiful.

мизи́нец *ж.* (*на руке*) little fínger; (*на ноге*) little toe.

микроавто́бус *м.* mínibus.

микро́б *м.* mícrobe.

микробиоло́гия *ж.* microbiólogy.

микроволно́вый: ~ радиотелефо́н mícrowave rádio télephone.

микрокли́мат *м.* microclímate.

микроко́см *м.* mícrocosm.

микро́метр *м.* micrómeter. **~и́ческий** micrométrical.

микроми́р *м. см.* микрокосм.

микро́н *м.* mícron.

микроорганизм *м. биол.* microórganism.

микропо́ристый microcéllular.

микрорайо́н *м.* mícro-dístrict.

микроско́п *м.* mícroscope. **~и́ческий** microscópic.

микрофо́н *бот.* mícrophone; the mike *разг.*

ми́ксер *м.* míxer.

миксту́ра *ж.* míxture; ~ от ка́шля cough míxture.

ми́лая *ж.* (*возлюбленная*) swéetheart, dárling.

ми́ленький *прил. разг.* 1. (*хорошенький*) sweet líttle, nice líttle; 2. (*родной, любимый*) dear, sweet; 3. *в знач. сущ. м.* dárling.

милитариз|а́ция *ж.* militarizátion. **~и́ровать** *несов. и сов.* (*вн.*) mílitarize (*smth.*).

милитар|и́зм *м.* mílitarism. **~и́ст** *м.* mílitarist. **~исти́ческий** militarístic.

милице́йск|ий milítia *attr.*; **~ая фо́рма** milítia úniform.

милиционе́р *м.* milítiaman*.

мили́ция *ж.* 1. milítia; 2. *собир. разг.* (*работники милиции*) the milítia; 3. (*милиционная армия*) territórial ármy.

миллиа́рд mílliard; bíllion *амер.*; два ~а рубле́й two mílliard róubles, two thóusand míllion róubles.

миллиарде́р *м.* multimíllionáire.

миллиа́рдный 1. *числ.* mílliardth; bíllionth *амер.*; 2. *прил.* (*исчисляемый миллиардами*) rúnning ínto mílliards/bíllions *после сущ.*

миллигра́мм *м.* mílligramme.

миллиме́тр *м.* míllimetre.

миллио́н 1. míllion; 2. *обыкн. мн.* (*большое количество*) míllions.

миллионе́р *м.* 1. millionáire; 2. (*о колхозе*) millionáire colléctive farm (in terms of ánnual íncome).

миллио́н|ый 1. *числ.* míllionth; 2. *прил.* (*оцениваемый, исчисляемый миллионами*) worth a míllion *после сущ.*; rúnning ínto míllions *после сущ.*; 3. *прил.* (*о большом количестве*) míllions-strong; cóunting míllions of men *после сущ.*; **~ые а́рмии** míllions-strong ármies.

ми́ло 1. *нареч.* (*хорошо*) nícely; (*приятно, приветливо*) swéetly; 2. *в знач. сказ. безл.*: о́чень ~ с ва́шей стороны́ that's véry kind of you; о́чень ~! véry nice!; как ~! how sweet!

милови́дный prétty.

милосе́рд|ие *с.* mércy; ◇ сестра́ **~ия** *уст.* síster of mércy, hóspital nurse. **~ный** mérciful.

ми́лостивый *уст.* mérciful; (*выражающий снисходительность*) kind.

ми́лост|ня *ж.* alms; проси́ть **~ю** beg alms; подава́ть **~ю** give* alms.

ми́лост|ь *ж.* 1. (*хорошее отношение*) kíndness, góodness; (*сострадание, снисхождение*) fávour; сде́лать

кому-л. ~ do* *smb.* a fávour; 2. (*пощада, помилование*) mércy; 3. (*доброе дело, благодеяние*) chárity; из ~и out of chárity; 4. *разг.* (*полное доверие, расположение*) fávour; быть в **~и** у кого́-л. be* in *smb.'s* good gráces; втере́ться в ~ к кому́-л. worm onesélf ínto *smb.'s* fávour; ◇ сда́ться на ~ победи́теля give* onesélf up to the ténder mércies of the énemy; **~и про́сим!** *разг.* I'll, we'll be delíghted to see you!, wélcome to my house!, you are wélcome!; скажи́те на **~!** (*выражение удивления*) well, I néver!, would you belíeve it!; по чьей-л. **~и** thanks to *smb.*

ми́лый I *прил.* 1. sweet, nice; 2. (*дорогой, люби́мый, тж. как обращение*) dear.

ми́лый II *м.* swéetheart, dárling.

ми́ля *ж.* mile.

ми́мика *ж.* expréssion (of *smb.'s* face); бога́тая ~ móbile féatures *pl.*

ми́мо 1. *нареч.* past, by; прое́хать, пройти́ ~ go* past, pass by; бить ~ miss; **~!** missed!, a miss!; 2. *предлог* (*рд.*) past, by; ~ це́ли besíde the mark, wide of the mark; ◇ пропусти́ть что-л. ~ уше́й pay* no atténtion to *smth.*, turn a deaf ear to *smth.*; пройти́ ~ кого́-л., чего́-л. 1) miss *smb., smth.*, fail to nótice *smb., smth.*; 2) (*обходить молчанием*) pass óver *smth.*

мимое́здом *разг.* on the way.

мимо́за *ж. бот.* mimósa.

мимолёт|ный fléeting, ephémeral, tránsient; **~ое впечатле́ние** hásty impréssion; ~ взгляд hásty glance; **~ое знако́мство** fléeting acquáintance.

мимохо́дом 1. on the way, in pássing; 2. (*между прочим*) in pássing.

мин|а I *ж. воен.* 1. (*для установки в земле, воде*) mine; 2. (*для стрельбы*) mórtar bomb; ◇ подложи́ть **~у** кому́-л. undermíne *smb.'s* reputátion.

мин|а II *ж.* (*выражение лица*) expréssion; сде́лать ки́слую **~у** pull a wry face; ◇ де́лать весёлую, хоро́шую **~у** при плохо́й игре́ put* a good face on the mátter.

минаре́т *м.* mínaret.

миндалеви́дн|ый álmond-shaped; **~ая железа́** tónsil.

минда́лина *ж.* 1. álmond; 2. *анат.* tónsil.

минда́ль *м.* 1. *собир.* (*плоды*) álmonds *pl*; 2. (*дерево*) álmond-tree. **~ный** álmond *attr.*; **~ные оре́хи** álmonds; **~ное ма́сло** álmond oil; **~ное молоко́** milk of álmonds.

мине́р *м.* 1. míner, sápper; 2. (*на корабле*) torpédo-man*.

минера́л *м.* míneral.

минерало́гия *ж.* minerálogy.

минера́льный míneral.

ми́ни- *в сложн.* míni-.

миниатю́р|а *ж.* míniature; ◇ в **~е** in míniature; сде́лать ~е моде́ль чего́-л. make* a smáll-scale módel of *smth.* **~ный** 1. míniature; 2. (*очень маленький*) tíny.

минима́льный mínimum *attr.*

ми́нимум *м.* 1. mínimum; прожи́точный ~ subsístence/líving wage; доводи́ть что-л. до ~ redúce *smth.* to a mínimum; 2. (*совокупность знаний и т. п.*) mínimum requírements *pl*, mínimum qualificátion; 3. *в знач. нареч.* at least, at the mínimum.

мини́ровать *несов. и сов.* (*вн.*) mine (*smth.*).

министе́рский ministérial.

министе́рство *с.* mínistry, óffice; depártment *амер.*; Министе́рство вну́тренних дел Mínistry for Intérnal Affáirs; Home Óffice (*в Англии*); Depártment of the Intérior (*в США*); Министе́рство иностра́нных дел Mínistry for Fóreign Affáirs; Fóreign Óffice (*в Англии*); Depártment of State, State Depártment (*в США*); Министе́рство торго́вли Mínistry of Trade; Board of Trade (*в Англии*).

мини́стр *м.* mínister; Sécretary (*в США*); ~ иностра́нных дел Mínister for Fóreign Affáirs; Fóreign

Sécretary (*в Англии*); Secretary of State (*в США*); ◇ ~ без портфе́ля mínister without portfólio.

ми́ни-ю́бка *ж.* míniskirt.

ми́нный mine *attr.*

мин|ова́ть *сов.* 1. (*вн.; проехать, пройти мимо*) pass (*smth.*); 2. с отрица́нием (*рд.; не избежать*) escápe (*smth.*); ему́ э́того не ~ he can't escápe it; 3. (*окончиться*) be* óver, be* past; опа́сность ~ова́ла the dánger is óver/past; зима́ ~ова́ла the winter is óver; ◇ ~у́я подро́бности omítting détails; двум смертя́м не быва́ть, а одно́й не ~ *посл.* you can ónly die once.

минога *ж. зоол.* lámprey.

миномёт *м. воен.* mórtar. ~**ный** *воен.* mórtar *attr.* ~**чик** *м.* mórtar man*, mórtar gúnner.

миноно́сец *м.* torpédo-boat; эска́дренный ~ destróyer.

мино́р *м.* 1. *муз.* mínor key; га́мма соль ~ the scale of G-mínor; 2. *разг.* (*грустное настроение*) mélancholy/sad mood. ~**ный** 1. *муз.* mínor; 2. *разг.* (*грустный*) sad.

ми́нус *м.* 1. *мат.* mínus; пять ~ четы́ре равно́ одному́ four from five leaves one; 2. (*о температуре*): сего́дня ~ 20 it is twénty belów todáy; 3. *разг.* (*недостаток*) deféct, dráwback.

мину́т|а *ж.* 1. mínute; без 10-и мину́т семь ten mínutes to séven; 20 мину́т пя́того twénty mínutes past four; 2. (*мгновение*) móment; подожди́те ~у! wait a mínute!; я ни ~ы не спал I háven't closed an eye, I háven't slept a wink; ◇ в одну́ ~у in no time; ~ в ~ on the dot; с ~ы на ~у at ány mínute; сию́ ~у! (*как ответ*) in a mínute!; (*как приказ*) at once!; одну́ ~у just a mínute. ~**ный** 1. mínute's; of a mínute *после сущ.*; ~**ная** стре́лка mínute-hand; 2. (*длящийся минуту*) mínute's; (*кратковременный*) shórt-líved, mómentary, tránsient; ~**ная** па́уза a pause of a mínute; ~**ная** заба́ва shórt-líved amúsement; ◇ ~**ное** де́ло the work of a mínute, it won't take a mínute.

мину́ть *сов.* 1. (*пройти*) pass; уже́ пять лет ми́нуло с тех пор, как... five years have passed since...; 2. (*о возрасте*): ему́ ми́нуло три́дцать лет he is óver thírty.

мир I *м.* world, úniverse; происхожде́ние ~а the órigin of the úniverse; со всего́ ~а from all óver the world; окружа́ющий ~ the óutside world; органи́ческий ~ the orgánic world; ◇ не от ~а сего́ unwórldly; ходи́ть по́ ~у live by bégging.

мир II *м.* (*отсутствие вражды, войны*) peace; в ~е at peace; де́ло ~а the cause of peace; угро́за ~у a ménace to peace; защи́та ~а defénce of peace.

мирабе́ль *ж.* 1. *собир.* (*плоды*) mirabélle plum; 2. (*дерево*) mirabélle plúm-tree.

мира́ж *м.* (*прям. и перен.*) mírage.

мири́ть, помири́ть (*вн.*) réconcile (*smb.*). ~**ся**, помири́ться, примири́ться 1. *сов.* помири́ться (*взаимно*) be*/becóme* réconciled; make* it up; дава́й ~ся! let's make it up!; 2. *сов.* примири́ться (с *тв.; терпимо относиться к чему-л.*) resign onesélf (to); réconcile onesélf (to).

ми́рн|ый 1. (*миролюбивый*) péaceable, péaceful, péace-lóving; ~ челове́к man* of peace; ~ разгово́р péaceable conversátion; 2. (*невоенный*) peace *attr.*; ~ое вре́мя time of peace, péace-time; в ~ых усло́виях únder péace-time condítions; ~ое населе́ние civílians *pl*; ~ая поли́тика pólicy of peace; ~ догово́р peace tréaty; 3. (*спокойный*) péaceful, péaceable.

миров|а́я *ж. разг.* ámicable séttlement; пойти́ на ~у́ю séttle the mátter ámicably.

мировоззре́ние *с.* world óutlook, world view.

миров|о́й I world *attr.*; ~о́е простра́нство óuter

space; ~ ры́нок world márket; ~**ая** война́ world war; ~**ая** реко́рд world récord.

мирово́й II (*примирительный*): ~ судья́ Jústice of the Peace.

миролюби́в|ый péace-lóving; ~**ые** наро́ды péace-lóving péoples; ~**ая** поли́тика péaceful pólicy.

миролю́бие *с.* péaceableness, péacefulness.

мироощуще́ние *с.* áttitude to the world.

миропонима́ние *с.* interpretátion of the world/úniverse.

миротво́рец *м.* péacemaker.

ми́ска *ж.* bowl; (*большая*) básin.

миссионе́р *м.* míssionary.

ми́ссия *ж.* 1. míssion; ~ до́брой во́ли góodwill míssion; 2. (*дипломатическое представительство*) legátion; 3. (*делегация*) delegátion, míssion; торго́вая ~ trade delegátion; вое́нная ~ mílitary míssion.

мисте́рия *ж.* mýstery, míracle play.

ми́стик *м.* mýstic.

ми́стика *ж.* mýsticism.

мистифи|ка́тор *м.* mýstifier, hóaxer. ~**ка́ция** *ж.* mystificátion, hoax; práctical joke. ~**ци́ровать** *несов. и сов.* mýstify.

мист|ици́зм *м.* mýsticism. ~**и́ческий** mýstical.

ми́тинг *м.* méeting.

митингова́ть *несов. разг.* hold* a méeting; *перен.* condúct éndless discússions.

митрополи́т *м. церк.* Metropólitan.

миф *м.* (*прям. и перен.*) myth. ~**и́ческий** (*прям. и перен.*) mýthical.

мифо|логи́ческий mytholόgical. ~**ло́гия** *ж.* mythόlogy.

ми́чман *м.* wárrant ófficer.

мише́нь *ж.* (*прям. и перен.*) tárget; служи́ть кому́--л. ~ю для насме́шек be* the butt of *smb.*

миш|ура́ *ж.* tínsel; *перен.* trúmpery. ~**у́рный** tínsel; *перен.* táwdry, trúmpery.

младе́н|ец *м.* ínfant, báby. ~**ческий** ínfantile. ~**чество** *с.* ínfancy.

мла́дший 1. (*по возрасту*) the yόunger; (*самый младший*) the yόungest; 2. (*по службе*) júnior; ~ нау́чный сотру́дник júnior reséarch wórker; ~ кома́ндный соста́в júnior ófficers; ~ партнёр júnior pártner.

млекопита́ющие *мн.* (*ед.* млекопита́ющее *с.*) *зоол.* mámmals.

млеть *несов.* 1. (*томиться*) melt, lánguish, go* limp; (*быть расслабленным*) reláx, nod; 2. *разг.* (*становиться нечувствительным*) go* numb.

мле́чный: Мле́чный Путь *астр.* the Mílky Way.

мне 1. (*дт. от личн. мест. я*) (to) me; *в безл. выражениях обычно* I; ~ хо́лодно, жа́рко *и т. п.* I am cold, hot etc.; 2. (*пр. от личн. мест. я*) (abóut, of) me.

мне́ни|е *с.* opínion; быть хоро́шего, плохо́го ~я о ком-л. have* a high, low opínion of *smb.*; по моему́ ~ю in my opínion, as I see it.

мни́мый 1. (*воображаемый*) imáginary, illúsory; 2. (*притворный, ложный*) feigned, affécted.

мни́тельн|ость *ж.* hypochóndria; (*подозрительность*) suspíciousness. ~**ый** hypochóndriac, héalth--cónscious; (*подозрительный*) suspícious, mistrústful.

мнить *несов. уст.* think*, imágine; ~ себя́ кем-л., чем-л. imágine onesélf to be *smb.*, *smth.*; сли́шком мно́го о себе́ think* a lot of onesélf.

мно́гие *прил. мн.* 1. mány; 2. *в знач. сущ.* mány (péople); ~ сочу́вствовали на́шему де́лу there were mány who sýmpathized with our cause; ~ ду́мают, что... mány péople consíder that...

мно́го *нареч.* 1. (*в большом количестве*; с гл.) a lot; (*пр. и нареч.*) much; он ~ рабо́тает he works a lot; сли́шком ~ too much; too mány (*с сущ. во мн. ч.*) он сли́шком ~ рабо́тает he works too much; о́чень ~ a great deal of; a great mány, lots of (*с сущ. во мн. ч.*);

так ~ so much; so mány, such a lot of (*с сущ. во мн. ч.*); 2. (*больше, чем нужно*) too much; 3. *в знач. числ.* much; mány (*с сущ. во мн. ч.*); plénty of (*с собир. сущ. и с сущ. во мн. ч.*); lots of, a lot of *разг.*; у меня ~ свободного времени I have plénty/lots of time; у вас (ещё) ~ работы? have you got much work (to do)?; ~ бумаги, карандашей much páper, mány péncils; было ~ народу there were a great mány péople présent, a lot of péople were there; ~ раз mány times; во ~ раз much, a great deal; 4.: ~ ли вам надо? do you need much?; 5. (*не больше, чем*) no more than; пройдёт год, ~ два a year or two will pass, not more; ◇ ни ~ ни мало as much as.

многобо́рец *м.* áll-róund compétitor.

многобо́рье *с. спорт.* áll-róund evént(s).

многовеково́й áncient, cénturies-óld.

многово́дн|ый 1. fúll-flówing; ~ые ре́ки deep/fúll-flówing rívers; 2. (*хорошо орошаемый*) wéll-wátered.

многоголо́в|ый mány-héaded; ~ое чудо́вище hýdra-héaded mónster.

многоголо́сый 1. of (mány) vóices *после сущ.*; (*исполняемый многими голосами*) sung by mány vóices *после сущ.*; ~ гул roar of vóices; 2. *муз.* polyphónic.

многогра́нн|ик *м. мат.* polyhédron. ~ый 1. polyhédral; 2. (*разносторонний*) many-síded, vérsatile.

многоде́тн|ый ~ая mother of a large fámily.

мно́го|е *с.* much; a lot *разг.*; во ~м in mány respécts; он ~то не зна́ет ещё there is much of which he is still ígnorant.

многоземе́льный lánd-rich; rich in land *после сущ.*

многозначи́тельн|о méaningly, significantly. ~ый méaning, significant.

многозна́чн|ость *ж. лингв.* polýsemy. ~ый 1. *мат.* multicíphered; ~ое число́ multidígit númber; 2. *лингв.* polysemántic.

многокана́льный múlti-chánnel.

многокра́сочн|ый *полигр.* polychromátic, polychrómic; ~ая улы́бка prómising smile.

многокра́тн|о repéatedly. ~ый repéated, fréquent; ~ый о́пыт repéated expérience; ◇ ~ый глаго́л frequéntative verb.

многола́мповый *радио* multiválve.

многоле́т|ий 1. of long stánding *после сущ.*; ~яя безупре́чная рабо́та long and distínguished sérvice; 2. *бот.* perénnial.

многолю́дн|ый pópulous, crówded; ~ое собра́ние well-atténded méeting; crówded méeting; ~ го́род pópulous city.

многоме́стный with exténsive séating capácity *после сущ.*

многомиллио́нный of mány míllions *после сущ.*

многонациона́льн|ый multinátional; ~ое госуда́рство multinátional State.

многообеща́ющ|ий prómising; ~ хиру́рг prómising súrgeon; ~ая улы́бка prómising smile.

многообра́з|ие *с.* varíety, divérsity. ~ный váried, divérse.

многоотрасле́в|ой vérsatile; ~ое се́льское хозя́йство divérsified ágriculture.

многопрогра́ммный multiprógramme *attr.*; (*об аппарате, выполняющем много заданий тж.*) vérsatile.

многоречи́вый gárrulous, loquácious.

многосеме́йный with a large fámily *после сущ.*

многосери́йный sérial; ~ телефи́льм TV sérial.

многосло́в|ие *с.* verbósity. ~ный verbóse.

многосло́жн|ый polysyllábic; ~ое сло́во polysýllable.

многостано́чник *м.* wórker óperating séveral machínes simultáneously.

многосторо́нн|ий 1. *мат.* polýgonal; 2. (*о договоре и т. n.*) multiláteral; ~ее соглаше́ние multiláteral agréement; 3. (*разнообразный*) vérsatile, mány-síded; ~ая де́ятельность vérsatile actívity.

многострада́льный long-súffering.

многоступе́нчат|ый: ~ая раке́та multistáge rócket.

многотира́жка *ж. разг.* fáctory néwspaper.

многотира́жн|ый lárge-circulátion *attr.*; ~ая газе́та lárge-circulátion néwspaper.

многото́мный múlti-vólume; in mány vólumes *после сущ.*

многото́чие *с.* dots *pl.*

многоуважа́емый déeply respécted; (*в письме*) dear.

многоуго́льник *м. мат.* pólygon. ~ый *мат.* polýgonal.

многофа́зный multipháse; ~ электри́ческий ток multipháse cúrrent.

многоцве́тный 1. multicólour(ed); 2. *полигр.* polychromátic, polychrómic; 3. *бот.* multiflórous.

многочи́сленн|ость *ж.* large númber, great size; ~ áрмии the great size of the ármy; ~ о́пытов the large númber of expériments. ~ый 1. (*состоящий из большого числа кого-л., чего-л.*) large; ~ая толпа́ large crowd; 2. (*имеющийся в большом количестве*) númerous.

многочле́н *м. мат.* multinómial, polynómial.

многоэта́жный múlti-stórey, mány-stóreyed; ~ дом tall búilding.

многоязы́чный pólyglot.

мно́жественн|ый plúral; ~ое число́ *грам.* the plúral.

мно́жество *с.* large númber, host, múltitude, any amóunt.

мно́жи|мое *с. мат.* multiplicánd. ~тель *м. мат.* fáctor.

мнóжительный múltiplying; ~ аппара́т (print) dúplicator, dúplicating machíne.

мно́жить, помно́жить, умно́жить (*вн.*) 1. *мат.* múltiply (smth.); 2. *сов.* умно́жить (*увеличивать*) incréase (smth.). ~ся *несов.* (*увеличиваться*) incréase, grow*, múltiply.

мной, мно́ю (*тв. от личн. мест.* я) by me.

мобилиз|ацио́нный mobilizátion *attr.* ~а́ция *ж.* mobilizátion. ~ованный *м.* enlísted man*.

мобилизова́ть *несов. и сов.* 1. (*вн.*) móbilize (smth., smb.); 2. (*вн. на вн.; поднимать, воодушевлять*) rálly (smb. to). ~ся *несов. и сов.* (*на вн.*) móbilize onesélf (for), brace onesélf (for).

моги́л|а *ж.* grave; ◇ бра́тская ~ cómmon grave; найти́ (себе́) ~у pérish; рыть ~у кому́-л. dig* a pit/grave for smb.; ~ Неизве́стного солда́та grave/tomb of the Únknówn Sóldier.

моги́ль|ный 1. grave *attr.*; ~ холм grave mound; ~ная плита́ grávestone, tómbstone; 2. (*напоминающий могилу*) sepúlchral; ~ная тишина́ the sílence of the grave, tómb-like sílence. ~щик *м.* gráve-digger.

могу́чий pówerful; míghty *поэт.*

могу́щест|венный pówerful; míghty *поэт.* ~во *с.* might, pówer.

мо́д|а *ж.* fáshion; vogue; быть в ~e be* in fáshion; по ~e fáshionable, fáshionably; не по ~e unfáshionable, unfáshionably; по после́дней ~e in the látest fáshion; вводи́ть ~у set* the fáshion (for); ◇ э́то что ещё за ~? now what have you táken ínto your head?

модели́ровать *несов. и сов.* (*сов. тж.* смодели́ровать) (*вн.*) 1. (*изготовлять образец*) design (smth.), módel (smth.); ~ пла́тье design a dress; 2. (*представлять в виде модели*) símulate (smth.). ~ся *несов. и сов.* be* símulated, be* repróduced.

модели́рующ|ий: ~ее устро́йство símulator.

моде́ль *ж.* módel.

моде́льн|ый quality *attr.*, fáshion *attr.*; ~ая о́бувь fáshion shoes *pl.*

моде́рн *м.* módernist style; the módern.

модерниз|а́ция *ж.* modernizátion; ~ обору́дования modernizátion of equipment. ~и́ровать *несов. и сов.* (*вн.*) módernize (smth.).

модерни́стск|ий modernístic; ~ое иску́сство modernístic art.

модѐрновый, модѐрный módern; úp-to-the-mínute *attr.*

мо́дн|ый fáshionable; ~ое пла́тье fáshionable dress; ~ое увлечѐние the látest craze; ~ журна́л fáshion-magazíne.

модул|и́ровать *несов.* 1. *муз.* change key; 2. *(вн.) физ.* módulate *(smth.).* ~яция *ж.* modulátion.

моё *притяж. мест. с. см.* мой.

мо́жет *3 л. ед. см.* мочь I.

можжевѐльник *м.* júniper.

мо́жно *в знач. сказ. безл.* 1. *(возможно)* one/you can, it can be; всё, что ~ éverything that is póssible, all in *one's* pówer; 2. *(позволительно)* one/you may; *(в вопросах)* may one?, may I?; здесь ~ кури́ть one/you may smoke here; здесь ~ кури́ть? may one smoke here?; окно́ ~ откры́ть you may/can ópen the window; ~ откры́ть окно́? may I ópen the window?; ѐсли ~ так вы́разиться if one may say so; ~ (мне войти́)? may I come in?; ◇ как ~ бо́льше as much as póssible; как ~ лу́чше as well as póssible; как ~ ра́ньше as éarly as póssible; как ~ скорѐе as soon as póssible; как ~! incrédible!; you don't say so!

моза́ика *ж.* mosáic, ínlay.

моза́ичный mosáic *attr.*, téssellated, ínlaid.

мозг *м.* 1. brain *(тж. перен.);* спинно́й ~ spínal cord; 2. *(костный)* márrow; 3. *мн. (кушанье)* brains; ◇ до ~а костѐй to *one's* véry márrow; продро́гнуть до ~а костѐй be* chilled to the bone/márrow; шевели́ть ~а́ми use *one's* brains.

мозгов|о́й *анат.* cérebral; brain *attr. (тж. перен.);* ~ое заболева́ние cérebral diséase, diséase of the brain; ~а́я рабо́та bráin-work.

мозжечо́к *м. анат.* líttle brain, cerebéllum.

мозо́листый cálloused, hórny.

мозо́лить, намозо́лить: ~ глаза́ кому́-л. *разг.* be* an éyesore to *smb.*

мозо́ль *ж.* corn; ◇ наступи́ть кому́-л. на люби́мую ~ tread* on *smb.'s* pet corn.

мой *притяж. мест.* 1. *(перед сущ.)* my; *(без сущ.)* mine; по моему́ мнѐнию in my opínion; 2. *в знач. сущ. мн. (родные)* my péople.

мо́йка *ж.* 1. wáshing; 2. *(устройство)* wásher.

мо́йщик *м.* wásher.

мокаси́ны *мн. (ед.* мокаси́н *м.)* móccasins.

мо́кнуть *несов.* 1. get* wet; ~ под дождём be* out in the rain; 2. *(быть погружённым в жидкость)* soak.

мокри́ца *ж. зоол.* wóod-louse*.

мо́кро 1. *нареч.* wétly; 2. *в знач. сказ. безл. разг.* it is wet.

мокро́та *ж.* phlegm.

мокрота́ *ж. разг.* 1. *(сырость)* damp, wet; 2. *(мелкий дождь, мокрый снег)* drízzle, sleet.

мо́кр|ый wet; ◇ у неё глаза́ на ~ом мѐсте she's álways réady to cry; she's a crý-baby.

мол I *м.* bréakwater, pier; *(небольшой)* jétty.

мол II *частица разг.:* он, ~, не винова́т he says it's not his fault.

молва́ *ж.* rúmour; дурна́я ~ bad reputátion.

молдава́н|ин *м.,* ~ка *ж.* Moldávian. ~ский Moldávian.

молда́вский Moldávian; ~ язы́к Moldávian, the Moldávian lánguage.

молѐбен *м.* sérvice; públic prayers *pl;* отслужи́ть ~ hold* a sérvice.

молѐкул|а *ж.* mólecule. ~я́рный molécular; ~я́рный вес molécular weight.

моли́тв|а *ж.* prayer; *(перед едой и после еды)* grace. ~енник *м.* práyer-book.

моли́ть *несов. (вн.)* beg *(smb.),* entrèat *(smb.),* implóre *(smb.);* ~ о поща́де cry (for) mércy, implóre párdon; cry quárter *идиом.* ~ся, помоли́ться 1. *(дт.)*

pray (to); 2. *тк. несов. (на вн.; боготворить)* ídolize *(smb., smth.).*

моллю́ск *м.* móllusc.

молниено́сн|о ínstantly, at líghtning speed. ~ый líghtning *attr.;* с ~ой быстрото́й at líghtning speed; ~ая война́ blítzkrieg.

молниеотво́д *м.* líghtning-condúctor, líghtning-rod.

мо́лни|я *ж.* 1. líghtning; 2. *(телеграмма)* expréss télegram; 3. *(застёжка)* zípper, zíp-fastener; slíde-fastener *амер.;* 4. *(стенная газета)* néws-flash; ◇ с быстрото́й ~и at líghtning speed; распространя́ться с быстрото́й ~и spread* like wildfire.

молодёжный youth *attr.;* téen-age *attr.; (состоящий из молодёжи тж.)* young péople's.

молодёжь *ж. собир.* youth; young péople *pl;* the young (ones *pl);* уча́щаяся ~ the stúdents *pl.*

молодѐть, помолодѐть get* yóunger and yóunger.

молод|ѐц *м.* 1. young stálwart; 2. *в знач. сказ. разг.:* ~! well done!, good lad!; ◇ ~ к ~цу́ fine féllows to a man, évery one of them a stálwart.

молодѐчество *с. (удаль)* dáring; *(ухарство)* fóolhardiness, récklessness, bravádo.

молоди́ть *несов. (вн.)* make* *(smb.)* look yóunger. ~ся *несов.* try to look yóunger than *one* is, put* on yóuthful airs.

молодня́к *м.* 1. *(лес)* sáplings *pl;* 2. *собир. (молодые животные)* young ánimals *pl;* cubs *pl (льва́та, тигря́та, медвежа́та и т. п.);* calves *(теля́та, слоня́та и т. п.);* yéarlings *(жеребя́та, ягня́та и т. п.);* 3. *собир. (птицы)* young birds *pl;* 4. *собир. разг. (молодёжь)* the yóunger generátion.

молодожёны *мн.* young cóuple *sg,* néwly-weds.

молодо́й *прил.* 1. young; *(юный)* yóuthful; *(о неодушевлённых предметах)* new; *(свежий)* fresh; ~ карто́фель new potátoes; 2. *в знач. сущ. мн.* young péople, the young; 3. *в знач. сказ. разг.* too young; вы ещё мо́лоды, чтобы так разгова́ривать you are too young to talk like that.

мо́лодост|ь *ж.* youth; ◇ не пѐрвой ~и past *one's* prime.

молодцева́тый dáshing.

молодцо́м *разг.:* вести́ себя́ ~ beháve magníficently.

молодчик *м. разг.* tough, thug.

молодчи́на *м. и ж. разг.* brick, trump.

молоды́е *мн. (супруги)* the young cóuple *sg.*

моложа́в|о: ~ вы́глядеть be* véry yóung-looking. ~ый yóung-looking; имѐть ~ый вид look young for *one's* age.

моло́ки *мн.* soft roe *sg,* milt *sg.*

молоко́ *с.* milk; ◇ у негó ~ на губа́х не обсо́хло ≈ he is véry green.

молоково́з *м.* milk lórry.

молокосо́с *м. разг. ирон.* strípling, a raw youth; *бран.* young púppy.

моло́т *м.* hámmer; парово́й ~ stéam-hammer; кузнѐчный ~ slédge-hammer.

молоти́|лка *ж.* thréshing-machine.

молоти́ть, смолоти́ть *(вн.)* thresh *(smth.).*

молотобо́ец *м.* hámmerer; hámmerman*, hammer-smith.

молот|о́к *м.* hámmer; ◇ прода́ть с ~ка́ sell* by áuction; пойти́ с ~ка́ come* únder the hámmer.

мо́лотый ground; ~ ко́фе ground cóffee.

моло́ть, смоло́ть *(вн.)* grind* *(smth.);* ◇ ~ вздор talk nónsense, drível, talk drível.

молотьба́ *ж.* 1. *(действие)* thréshing; 2. *(время, пора)* thréshing-time.

молочн|ая *ж.* dáiry. ~ик *м.* 1. *(посуда)* mílk-jug; 2. *(продавец)* mílkman*. ~ица *ж.* mílkwoman*, mílkmaid.

моло́чно-воско́в|ой: ~а́я спѐлость milk-wax rípeness.

моло́чн|ый 1. *(дающий, производящий молоко)* dáiry *attr.;* ~ скот dáiry cáttle; ~ая коро́ва mílking cow;

~ое хозяйство dáiry farm; ~ая промышленность dáiry índustry; 2.: ~ поросёнок súcking pig; 3. (*приготовленный из молока*) milk *attr.*; ~ые продукты dáiry/milk próduce *sg*; ~ая каша milk púdding; ~ая диéта milk díet; 4. (*похожий на молоко*) mílky; 5. *хим.* láctic; ~ая кислота láctic ácid; ◇ ~ брат fóster-brother; ~ые зубы mílk-teeth.

молча sílently, withóut a word; *перен.* in sílence, unprotéstingly.

молчали́в|**ый** 1. (*неразговорчивый*) táciturn, shórt-spóken, réticent; sílent (*тж. перен.*); 2. (*понимаемый без слов*) tácit; ~ое согласие tácit consént.

молчáние *c.* sílence; хранить (упóрное) ~ maintáin a (stúbborn) sílence; обойти что-л. ~м pass *smth.* óver in sílence; ~ — знак согласия sílence gives consént.

молчáть *несов.* 1. be* sílent; ~! hold your tongue!; 2. (*скрывать*) say* nóthing, keep* sílent; 3. (*безропотно терпеть что-л.*) make* no compláint.

молчóк *в знач. сказ. разг.*: об этом ~! not a word!, keep it únder your hat!

моль *ж.* moth.

мольб|**á** *ж.* prayer, entréaty; внять ~é hear* one's prayer.

мольбéрт *м.* éasel.

момéнт *м.* 1. (*о времени*) móment; удóбный ~ opportúnity, súitable móment; в тот ~, когда just when; 2. (*отдельная сторона какого-л. явления*) féature; ◇ в (один) ~ in a móment; в данный ~ at the (gíven) móment; в любóй ~ at any móment.

момента́льн|**о** immédiately. ~**ый** instantáneous; ~ый снимок snápshot.

монáрх *м.* mónarch. ~**изм** *м.* mónarchism. ~**ист** *м.* mónarchist. ~**и́ческий** monárchical.

монáрхия *ж.* mónarchy.

монасты́рский monastérial; (*о женском монастыре*) convéntual.

монасты́рь *м.* mónastery; (*женский*) núnnery, cónvent; ◇ в чужóй ~ со своим устáвом не хóдят ≈ when you go to Rome, do as Rome does; подвести когó-л. под ~ get* *smth.* ínto tróuble.

монáх *м.* monk; постричься в ~и take* monástic vows. ~**иня** *ж.* nun; постричься в ~ини take* the veil.

монáшеский monástic, mónkish.

монгóл *м.*, ~**ка** *ж.* Mongól(ian).

монгóльский Mongólian; ~ язык Mongólian, the Mongólian lánguage.

монéт|**а** *ж.* coin; мéлкая ~ small coin; ◇ отплатить комý-л. той же ~ой pay* *smb.* in his, her own coin. ~**ный** mónetary; ◇ ~ный двор the mint.

монеторазмéнник *м.* cóin (-exchánge) box.

моногáмия *ж.* monógamy.

монограмма *ж.* mónogram.

монография *ж.* mónograph, stúdy.

монóкль *м.* mónocle.

монолит|**ость** *ж.* monolíthic cháracter. ~**ый** 1. monolíthic; 2. (*сплочённый*) mássive, united.

монолóг *м.* mónologue, solíloquy.

моноплáн *м.* mónoplane.

монополиз|**áция** *ж.* monopolizátion. ~**и́ровать** *несов. и сов.* (*вн.*) monópolize (*smth.*).

монополи́ст *м.* monópolist. ~**и́ческий** monopolístic; ~и́ческий капитáл monópoly cápital.

монопóлия *ж.* monópoly; ~ внéшней торгóвли fóreign-trade monópoly.

монопóльн|**ый** monópoly *attr.*, exclúsive; ~ое прáво exclúsive right.

монорéльсов|**ый** mónorail *attr.*; ~ая дорóга mónorail.

моноти́п *м. полигр.* mónotype. ~**ный** *полигр.* mónotype *attr.*

монотóнн|**ость** *ж.* monótony. ~**ый** monótonous; ~ый гóлос expréssionless voice; ~ая жизнь unevéntful life.

монтáж *м.* 1. *тех.* assémbly; (*установка*) installátion; ~ электростáнции assémbly of a pówer-státion; 2. (*фильма, литературного произведения и т. п.*) éditing; 3. (*о фильме, произведении и т. п.*) montáge, arrángement; литератýрный ~ book prógramme.

монтáжник *м.* assémbly wórker, fitter.

монтёр *м.* 1. (*монтажник*) fitter; 2. (*электромонтёр*) electrícian.

монти́ровать, смонти́ровать (*вн.*) 1. *тех.* assémble (*smth.*); (*устанавливать*) instáll (*smth.*); ~ машину instáll/assémble a machine; 2. (*о фильме*) édit (*smth.*).

монумéнт *м.* mónument. ~**áльный** monuméntal; ~áльное здáние building on the grand scale; ~áльная фигýра monuméntal fígure; ~áльный труд monuméntal work.

мопéд *м.* móped.

морá|**ль** *ж.* 1. (*нравственность*) mórals *pl*, morálity; при́нципы ~и móral précepts; 2. (*вывод*) móral; 3. *разг.* (*нравоучение*) móral instrúction; читáть ~ комý-л. preach to *smb.*; ◇ прописнáя ~ cópy-book máxims/morálity.

морáльно mórally.

морáльн|**ый** móral; (*духовный тж.*) spíritual; ~ое состоя́ние méntal state, morále; ◇ ~ износ (*машины и т. п.*) эк. obsoléscence.

моратóрий *м. фин., полит.* moratórium; объяви́ть ~ grant a moratórium.

морг *м.* morgue.

моргáть, моргнýть 1. blink; 2. (*дт.; подавать знак*) wink (at); 3. (*мерцать*) glímmer, wink, blink; ◇ глáзом не моргнýть withóut bátting an éyelid.

моргнýть *сов. см.* моргáть.

мóрда *ж.* 1. múzzle; (*кошачья*) face; 2. *груб.* (*о лице*) mug.

мордви́н *м.*, ~**ка** *ж.* Mordví́nian.

мордóвский Mordví́nian; ~ язы́к Mordví́nian, the Mordví́nian lánguage.

мóр|**е** *c.* sea; *перен.* (*большое количество*) ócean; вы́йти в ~ put* to sea; в откры́том ~ on the ópen sea, on the high seas; у ~я at the séaside; ◇ ждать у ~я погóды indúlge in vain hopes.

морепла́в|**ание** *c.* navigátion, hígh-seas navigátion. ~**атель** *м.* návigator.

морехóд|**ность** *ж.* séaworthiness. ~**ный** séaworthy. ~**ство** *c.* navigátion.

морж *м.* 1. wálrus; 2. *разг.* (*купальщик*) winter báther.

мори́ть *несов.* (*вн.*) 1. (*истреблять*) extérminate (*smth.*); ~ таракáнов extérminate cóckroaches; 2. *разг.* (*изнурять*) wear* down (*smth.*); ~ гóлодом когó-л. starve *smb.*

морко́вный 1. cárrot *attr.*; ~ сок cárrot juice; 2. (*цвета моркови*) cárroty.

морко́вь *ж.* 1. cárrot; 2. *собир.* cárrots *pl*.

моро́жен|**ое** *c.* íce-créam; шокола́дное ~ chócolate íce-créam; ~**щик** *м.* íce-créam véndor. ~**ый** frózen; ~ое мя́со frózen meat.

моро́з *м.* frost; си́льный ~ hard/bítter frost; 20 грáдусов ~a twénty degrées of frost, twénty belów zéro; ◇ по кóже подирáет ≈ it's enóugh to make one's flesh creep; ~**ить** *несов.* 1. (*вн.*) freeze* (*smth.*); (*об овощах и т. п.*) put* (*smth.*) in cold stórage; 2. *безл.*: ~ит it is fréezing, there is a frost. ~**но** *в знач. сказ. безл.* there's a frost. ~**ный** frósty.

морозосто́йк|**ий** fróst-resistant, fróst-hardy; ~ая ози́мая пшени́ца fróst-resistant winter wheat.

морос|**и́ть** *несов.* 1. drízzle; 2. *безл.*: ~и́т it is drízzling.

моро́шка *ж.* 1. *собир.* clóudberries *pl*; 2. (*об отдельной ягоде и растении*) clóudberry.

морс *м.* frúit-drink.

морск|**óй** 1. sea *attr.*; (*живущий, растущий в море* *тж.*) maríne; ~ая вода́ séa-water; ~ая ка́рта chart; sea map; ~ бе́рег séashore; ~ие живо́тные maríne ánimals; ~ие расте́ния maríne plants; ~ая держа́ва séa-power; 2. (*связанный с военным флотом*) nával; ~ флот návy; ~ офице́р nával ófficer; ~ая пехо́та marínes *pl*; ~ бой nával engágement; ~бе учи́лище nával cóllege/school; ◇ ~ая боле́знь séasickness; страда́ть ~ боле́знью be* séasick; ~ кли́мат máritime clímate.

морти́ра *ж. воен.* mórtar.

морфе́ма *ж. лингв.* mórpheme.

морфо|логи́ческий morphológical. ~ло́гия *ж.* 1. (*наука о строении организмов*) morphólogy; 2. *лингв.* morphólogy, áccidence.

морщи́н|а *ж.* wrínkle; (*на ткани и т. п. тж.*) crease; ~ы у глаз crów's-feet. ~истый wrínkled; (*о лице тж.*) lined.

мо́рщить, намо́рщить, смо́рщить (*вн.*) 1. *сов.* намо́рщить wrínkle (up) (*smth.*); ~ лоб wrínkle *one's* fórehead; 2. *сов.* смо́рщить wrínkle (*smth.*); ~ нос wrínkle *one's* nose; ~ гу́бы purse *one's* lips; 3. *сов.* смо́рщить (*образовывать рябь на воде*) rípple (*smth.*). ~ся, намо́рщиться, смо́рщиться 1. *сов.* намо́рщиться wrínkle, break* ínto wrínkles; 2. *сов.* смо́рщиться (*делать гримасы*) frown, make*/pull fáces; *сов. тж.* make*/pull a face; 3. *сов.* смо́рщиться (*об одежде*) crease, crúmple; (*о водной поверхности*) rípple, be* rúffled.

моря́к *м.* séaman*; sáilor *разг.*

москате́льн|ый chándlery *attr.*, chándler's; ~ые това́ры chándlery *sg*; ~ая ла́вка chándlery-shop, chándler's.

москви́ч *м.*, ~ка *ж.* Múscovite, inhábitant of Móscow.

моски́т *м.* mosquíto.

моско́вский Móscow *attr.*

мост *м.* 1. bridge; вре́менный ~ témporary bridge; разводно́й ~ dráwbridge; 2. (*для зубов*) plate; 3. *тех.* end; за́дний ~ rear end.

мо́стик *м.* 1. small bridge, fóot-bridge; 2.: капита́нский ~ the cáptain's bridge.

мости́ть *несов.* (*вн.*) pave (*smth.*).

мостки́ *мн.* bóard-walk *sg*; (*на судне*) gángway *sg*.

мостова́я *ж.* road, róadway.

мота́ть *несов.* 1. (*вн.; нитки и т. п.*) wind* (*smth.*); reel (*smth.*); 2. (*тв.*) *разг.* (*качать, махать*) shake* (*smth.*); ~ хвосто́м wag its tail; ◇ ~ (себе́) на ус *что-л.* make* a méntal note of *smth.*, get* *smth.* ínto *one's* head.

моте́ль *м.* motél.

моти́в *м.* 1. (*причина*) mótive; 2. (*довод*) réason; 3. (*тема*) theme; 4. (*мелодия*) tune.

мотиви́р|овать *несов. и сов.* (*вн.*) expláin (*smth.*), give* réasons (for); find* a mótive (for). ~о́вка *ж.* réasons *pl*, explanátion.

мотого́н|ки *мн.* mótor-cycle ráces; (*на стадионе*) spéedway ráces. ~щик *м.* rácing mótor-cyclist.

мото́к *м.* ball.

мотоклу́б *м.* mótor-cycle club.

мотокро́сс *м.* cróss-country mótor-cycle race.

мотопехо́та *ж.* mótorized ínfantry.

мотопробе́г *м.* mótor-cycle rálly.

мото́р *м.* éngine, mótor; останови́ть ~ stop the éngine.

мотора́лли *с.* mótor-cycle rálly.

моторизо́ванный mótorized.

мото́рн|ый mótor *attr.*; ~ ваго́н frónt-car; ~ая ло́дка mótor boat.

моторо́ллер *м.* (mótor) scóoter.

моторосбо́рочный éngine-assembly *attr.*

моторострои́тельный éngine-building; ~ заво́д éngine-building works.

мотоци́кл *м.* mótor-cycle. ~и́ст *м.* mótor-cyclist.

мотыга *ж.* hoe, máttock.

мотылёк *м.* bútterfly; ночно́й ~ moth.

мох *м.* moss; заро́сший мхом móss-grown; ◇ ~ом обрасти́ ≈ run*/go* to seed.

мохе́р *м.* móhair. ~овый móhair *attr.*

мохна́т|ый 1. (*обросший шерстью*) shággy, háiry, fúrry; 2. (*из густых прядей волос, шерсти*) búshy, shággy (*тж. перен.*); ~ые бро́ви shággy/búshy éyebrows; 3. (*с густым ворсом*) rough, flúffy; (*о ковре*) thíck-pile *attr.*; 4.: ~ое полоте́нце Túrkish tówel.

моцио́н *м.* éxercise, constitútional.

моча́ *ж.* úrine.

моча́лка *ж.* bast, wásh-rag.

мочев|о́й úrinary; ~ пузы́рь (úrinary-)bládder; ◇ ~а́я кислота́ úric ácid.

мочего́нн|ый: ~ое сре́дство diurétic.

мочеиспуска́|ние *с.* urinátion. ~тельный: ~тельный кана́л *анат.* uréthra.

мочён|ый soused; ~ые я́блоки soused ápples.

мочеполово́й urinogénital.

моче́точник *м. анат.* uréter.

мочи́ть *несов.* (*вн.*) 1. wet (*smb., smth.*), make* (*smb., smth.*) wet; 2. (*вымачивать*) soak (*smth.*), steep (*smth.*); ~ лён ret flax. ~ся *несов.* (*испускать мочу*) úrinate, make* wáter.

мо́чка *ж.* (*часть уха*) lobe.

мочь I, смочь be* áble; мо́жет ли он пойти́ туда́? (*возможно ли это?*) can he go there?; (*позволено ли это?*) may he go there?; я не могу́ прийти́ сего́дня I shall not be able to come todáy; мо́жете ли вы э́то сде́лать? can you do that?; е́сли (с)могу́ if I can, if I am áble (to); ◇ мо́жет быть, быть мо́жет perháps; не мо́жет быть! not réally!; как живёте-мо́жете? how are you?, how are you gétting alóng?

моч|ь II *ж. разг.* pówer, might; во всю ~ with all *one's* might, with might and main; ◇ ~и никако́й нет! it's unbéarable!

моше́нн|ик *м.* swíndler. ~ичать, смоше́нничать cheat, swíndle. ~ичество *с.* swíndle.

мо́шка *ж.* midge. ~ра́ *ж. собир.* midges *pl*.

мощёный paved; ~ бу́лыжником cóbbled.

мо́щи *мн.* rélic *sg*; ◇ живы́е ~ wálking skéleton *sg*.

мо́щн|ость *ж.* 1. pówer; 2. *физ., тех.*, capácity; (*производительность*) óutput; фа́брика рабо́тает на по́лную ~ the fáctory is wórking at full capácity; 3. (*толщина жилы, пласта*) depth, thíckness; 4. *мн.* (*производственные объекты*) capácities. ~ый 1. pówerful; (*о физической силе тж.*) strong; 2. (*о жиле, пласте и т. п.*) thick, mássive.

мощь *ж.* pówer, might.

мо́ющ|ий: ~ие сре́дства detérgents.

моя́ *притяж. мест. ж. см.* мой.

мрак *м.* gloom, dárkness, obscúrity; ◇ покры́тый ~ом неизве́стности wrapped in mýstery.

мракобе́с *м.* obscurántist. ~ие *с.* obscurántism.

мра́мор *м.* márble. ~ный márble *attr.*

мрачне́ть, помрачне́ть becóme* glóomier; (*о лице*) dárken.

мра́чн|ый glóomy, sómbre, dísmal; (*о человеке тж.*) moróse; име́ть ~ хара́ктер be* of a moróse dispositión; име́ть ~ вид look glum; ~ое настрое́ние sómbre mood.

мсти́тель *м.* avénger. ~ность *ж.* vindíctiveness, revéngefulness. ~ный vindíctive, revéngeful.

мстить, отомсти́ть (*дт.*) revénge onesélf (on), take*/have* revénge (on), pay* (*smb.*) back; я отомщу́ за него́ I will avénge him.

мудрено́ *в знач. сказ. безл.* (+ *инф.*) it is hard/difficult (+ to *inf*); ~ поня́ть его́ he's hard to understánd; ◇ не ~, что... no wónder...; ~ ли? is it ány wónder?

мудр|ёный *разг.* 1. (*трудный для понимания*) íntricate; 2. (*трудный для выполнения*) all but impóssible; 3. (*странный*) queer; (*о вещах*) outlándish; ◇ в э́том ничего́ ~ёного нет it's pérfectly símple; у́тро ве́чера ~ене́е *посл.* an hour in the mórning is worth two in the évening; ≈ bétter sleep on it!

мудре́ц *м.* sage; ◇ на вся́кого ~á дово́льно просто-ты́ ≈ éveryone has a fool in his sleeve.

мудр|и́ть *несов. разг.* be* óver-súbtle, súbtilize; не ~и́те! don't try to be súbtle!, don't make a púzzle of it!, don't split hairs!

му́дрост|ь *ж.* wísdom; наро́дная ~ folk wísdom; ◇ зуб ~и wísdom tooth*.

му́дрств|овать *несов. разг.* philósophize; ◇ не ~уя лука́во without fúrther adó.

му́др|ый wise; ~ челове́к wise man*; ~ое реше́ние wise decísion; ~ сове́т sage cóunsel.

муж *м.* húsband.

мужа́ть *несов.* matúre.

мужа́ться *несов.* take* heart/cóurage.

му́жественн|ый brave, courágeous; váliant; ~ наро́д courágeous péople, ~ая же́нщина brave wóman*; ~ хара́ктер brave cháracter; ~ая фигу́ра mánly fígure; ~ая пе́сня váliant song.

му́жество *с.* cóurage; (*стойкость*) fórtitude.

мужи́к *м.* 1. *уст.* (*крестьянин*) péasant; 2. *разг.* (*мужчина*) man*; 3. *уст. разг.* (*муж*) húsband.

мужско́й másculine; (*мужского пола*) male; (*предназначенный для мужчин*) men's; в ~ компа́нии in the cómpany of men, in male cómpany.

мужчи́на *м.* man*.

му́за *ж.* muse.

музе́й *м.* muséum. ~ный muséum *attr.*; ◇ ~ная ре́дкость rare/príceless óbject; сде́латься ~ной ре́дкостью becóme* a rárity.

музе́й-уса́дьба *ж.* cóuntry-house muséum, memórial está te.

му́зык|а *ж.* músic; положи́ть что́-л. на ~у set* *smth.* to músic; занима́ться ~ой learn* músic, have* músic léssons; танцева́ть под ~у dance to músic; люби́ть ~у be* fond of músic; люби́тель ~и músic-lover.

музыка́льн|ость *ж.* musicálity; (*талант тж.*) gift for músic. ~ый músical; (*имеющий отношение к нотам*) músic *attr.*; ~ое сопровожде́ние accómpaniment; ~ый челове́к músical pérson; ~ая шко́ла músic school; ~ый магази́н músic shop; ~ый слух an ear for músic.

музыка́нт *м.* musícian.

му́к|а *ж.* 1. tórment, tórture; *мн.* pangs; ~и го́лода pangs of húnger; ~и тво́рчества throes of compositíon; 2. *в знач. сказ.* it is (sheer) tórture; одна́ ~ nóthing but tróuble; ◇ хожде́ние по ~ам the road of sórrows.

мука́ *ж.* flour.

мукомо́льн|ый: ~ое произво́дство flóur-mílling.

мул *м.* mule.

мула́т *м.*, ~ка *ж.* mulátto.

мультипликацио́нн|ый: ~ фильм ánimated cartóon; ~ая съёмка animátion/cartóon work.

мультиплика́ция *ж. кино* (máking of an) ánimated cartóon.

му́мия *ж.* múmmy.

мунди́р *м.* (*full-dress*) úniform; ◇ карто́фель в ~е potátoes cooked in their jáckets.

мундштук *м.* 1. (*твёрдая часть папиросной гиль-зы*) móuth-piece; 2. (*для сигар*) cigár-holder; (*для сигаре́т*) cigarétte-holder; 3. (*духового инструмента*) móuth-piece; 4. (*для лошадей*) curb.

муниципа́льный municipal.

мураве́й *м.* ant. ~ник *м.* ánt-hill.

мурави́н|ый ant *attr.*; ◇ ~ая кислота́ *хим.* fórmic ácid.

мура́шк|а *ж.*: ~и бе́гают по спине́ it makes *one's* flesh creep, it's enóugh to give *one* the shívers/creeps.

мурлы́к|анье *с.* púrring. ~ать *несов.* 1. purr; 2. *разг.* (*напевать*) hum.

муска́т *м.* 1. (*орех*) nútmeg; 2. (*виноград*) múscat; 3. (*вино*) múscat wine. ~ный múscat *attr.*, nútmeg *attr.*; ◇ ~ный оре́х nútmeg; ~ный цвет mace.

му́скул *м.* múscle. ~ату́ра *ж.* múscles *pl.* ~истый múscular.

му́скус *м.* musk.

му́сор *м.* dust, rúbbish, réfuse, gárbage; строи́тель-ный ~ búilders' réfuse. ~ный: ~ный я́щик dúst-bin; gárbage-can *амер.*; ~ная я́ма rúbbish-heap.

мусоропрово́д *м.* rúbbish chute.

мусс *м. кул.* mousse.

мусси́ровать *несов.* (*вн.*) exággerate (*smth.*); ~ слу́-хи exággerate/spread* rúmours.

муссо́н *м.* monsóon.

мусульма́н|ин *м.* Móslem, Mússulman. ~ский Móslem, Mússulman. ~ство *с.* Móslemism, Mohámmedanism, Íslam.

мута́нт *м.* mútant. ~ный mútant *attr.*

мута́ция *ж.* mutátion.

мут|и́ть, замути́ть 1. (*вн.; делать мутным*) stir up (*smth.*), múddy (*smth.*); 2. *тк. несов. безл.*: меня́ ~и́т I feel sick/queer; ◇ ~ во́ду stir up tróuble. ~и́ться, замути́ться, помути́ться 1. *сов.* замути́ться grow* múddy/túrbulent; 2. *сов.* помути́ться grow* dull; его́ созна́ние помути́лось his brain went dull; ◇ у меня́ в голове́, глаза́х ~и́тся I feel dízzy.

мутне́ть, помутне́ть (*о жидкости*) becóme* túrbid; (*о стекле*) becóme* dim, mist óver, be* místed.

му́тн|ый 1. (*непрозрачный*) túrbid; múddy; 2. (*потускневший*) dim, dull; о́кна, ~ые от дождя́ ráin-dimmed windows; 3. (*неясный, окутанный туманом*) místy, bléary.

му́фта *ж.* 1. muff; 2. *тех.* cóupling, connéction.

му́х|а *ж.* fly; ◇ де́лать из ~и слона́ ≈ make* móuntains out of mólehills; слы́шно, как ~ пролети́т you could hear a pin drop.

мухомо́р *м.* flý-agaric.

муче́ние *с.* tórture, tórment; (*мне*) с ним одно́ ~ I have nóthing but tróuble with him.

му́чен|ик *м.*, ~ица *ж.* mártyr. ~ический mártyr's. ~ичество *с.* mártyrdom.

мучи́тель *м.* torméntor. ~ный excrúciating, rácking, ágonizing; ~ная боль excrúciating pain; ~ная зубна́я боль rácking tóothache; ~ный ка́шель excrúciating cough; ~ное ожида́ние ágonizing suspénse; ~ные сомне́-ния ágonizing doubts; ~ная процеду́ра (*лечение*) páinful tréatment.

му́ч|ить *несов.* (*вн.*) tormént (*smb., smth.*), tórture (*smb., smth.*); (*дразнить*) tease (*smb., smth.*); (*беспо-коить*) wórry (*smb.*); меня́ ~ит со́весть I am cónscience--stricken; меня́ ~ит неизве́стность I can't bear the suspénse. ~иться *несов.* 1. súffer, be* in ágony; ~иться перед сме́ртью die in ágony; 2. (*тв.; томиться*) be* tórtured (by), be* wórried (by); ~иться сомне́ниями be* tórtured by doubts, be* a prey to doubt; ~иться угрызе́-ниями со́вести be* racked/tórtured by remórse; 3. (*с, над тв.*) *разг.* (*испытывать затруднения*) have* a hard time (with).

мучни́стый méaly, flóury, farináceous; ~ карто́фель méaly/flóury potáto.

му́шк|а I *ж.* (*на оружии*) bead; взять кого́-л. на ~у aim at *smth.*, draw* a bead on *smth.*

му́шка II *ж.* (*на лице*) béauty spot.

муштр|а́ *ж.* drill. ~ова́ть *несов.* (*вн.*) drill (*smb.*), díscipline (*smb.*). ~о́вка *ж.* drill.

мчать *несов.* (*вн.*) rush (*smb., smth.*); (*уносить бы-стрым движением*) sweep* (*smb., smth.*) alóng; по́езд мчал меня́ на юг the train rushed me to the south; ве́тер мчит облака́ the wind is dríving the clouds. ~ся *несов.* rush, race; ~ся по у́лице race down the street.

мще́ние *с.* véngeance.

мы *личн. мест. (рд. вн.* нас, *дт.* нам, *тв.* на́ми, *пр.* о нас) we; мы все we all, all of us; we are all; мы уста́ли we are all tíred; мы с бра́том my bróther and I; мы с ва́ми you and I; мы с ним he and I.

мы́л|ить, намы́лить *(вн.)* soap *(smb., smth.).* ~ся, намы́литься 1. soap oneself; 2. *тк. несов. (о мыле)* láther.

мы́лкий soft, dissólvent.

мы́л|о *с.* 1. soap; туале́тное ~ tóilet soap; ~ для бритья́ sháving-soap; 2. *тк. ед. (пот у лошади)* foam, láther; ло́шадь вся в ~е the horse is in a láther.

мылова́рение *с.* sóap-boiling.

мылова́рен|ый soap *attr.*; ~ заво́д sóap-works; ~ая промы́шленность soap índustry.

мы́льн|ица *ж.* sóap-dish. ~ый 1. soap *attr.*; ~ая пе́на láther; sóap-suds *pl*; ~ый пузы́рь sóap-bubble; пуска́ть ~ые пузыри́ blow* sóap-bubbles; 2. *(намыленный)* sóapy; ~ые ру́ки sóapy hands.

мыс *м.* cape, héadland.

мы́сленн|о in one's thoughts/mind, méntally. ~ый 1. *(воображаемый)* imáginary; 2. *(существующий в мыслях)* méntal.

мы́слим|ый concéivable, póssible; ◇ ~ое ли э́то де́ло? ~о ли э́то? can one think of such things?, is such a thing póssible?, did you éver hear of such a thing?

мысли́тель *м.* thínker.

мы́слит|ь *несов.* think*; как вы ~е себе́ э́то? what are your idéas abóut it?

мысл|ь *ж.* thought; *(размышление)* cogitátion; *(идея)* idéa; *(мнение)* view; интере́сная ~ ínteresting idéa; основна́я *(произведения)* underlýing/fundaméntal idéa; счастли́вая, уда́чная ~ good idéa, háppy thought; прийти́ к ~и arríve at the idéa; погрузи́ться в свои́ ~и becóme* lost in thought; give* oneself up to one's thoughts; ◇ о́браз ~ей óutlook, way of thínking; не допуска́ть да́же ~и о чём-л. not éven admit the thought of *smth.*; there can be no quéstion of *smth.*; у меня́ э́того и в ~ях не́ было I dídn't mean that for a móment, it néver crossed my mind.

мы́слящий thínking.

мыта́рить *несов. (вн.) разг.* tormént *(smb.)*, make* *(smb.)* súffer. ~ся *несов. разг.* have* a rough time; go* through the mill *идиом.*

мыта́рств|о *с.* trial, trýing expérience, ordéal; пройти́ че́рез все ~а endúre évery ordéal.

мыть, вы́мыть, помы́ть *(вн.)* wash *(smth.)*; ~ посу́ду wash up the (díshes); ◇ ~ зо́лото wash gold; рука́ ру́ку мо́ет *погов.* ≈ you scratch my back and I'll scratch yours.

мытьё *с.* wáshing; ~ головы́ shampóo; ~ посу́ды wáshing-úp; ◇ не ~м, так ка́таньем by hook or by crook.

мы́ться, вы́мыться, помы́ться wash (onesélf); *(в ванне)* have* a bath.

мыч|а́ние *с.* 1. lówing; móoing *разг.*; *(быка)* béllowing; 2. *разг. (неясные звуки)* múmbling. ~а́ть *несов.* 1. low; moo *разг.*; *(о быке)* béllow; 2. *разг. (издавать неясные звуки)* múmble.

мышело́вка *ж.* móuse-trap.

мы́шечн|ый múscular; ~ые тка́ни múscular tíssues.

мыши́н|ый 1. mouse *attr.*; of mice *после сущ.*; ~ писк squéaking of mice; 2. *(напоминающий мышь)* móuse-like; 3. *(серый)* grey; ◇ ~ая возня́ fuss abóut nóthing; подня́ть ~ую возню́ вокру́г чего́-л. make* a great fuss abóut *smth.*

мы́шк|а *ж.*: под ~ой, под ~у únder one's/the arm; пла́тье порвало́сь под ~ой the dress has torn únder the arm; он взял ша́пку под ~у he put his cap únder his arm.

мышле́ние *с.* 1. thought, mentálity; 2. *(действие)* thínking.

мы́шца *ж.* múscle.

мышь *ж.* mouse*; полева́я ~ field-mouse*.

мышья́к *м.* arsénic. ~ови́стый arsénious. ~о́вый arsénic(al).

мю́зикл *м.* músical.

мя́гк|ий 1. soft; *(о металлах)* málleable; ~ие во́лосы sg; 2. *(свежий, нечёрствый)* fresh; ~ хлеб fresh bread; 3. *(приятный для глаз, слуха, плавный)* géntle, méllow; ~ го́лос géntle voice; ~ свет géntle light; ~ая похо́дка géntle tread; light fóotsteps *pl*; 4. *(о чувствах, настроениях)* mild; 5. *(с неопределёнными чертами, границами)* géntle; ~ие черты́ лица́ géntle féatures; 6. *(кроткий, уступчивый)* plíable, adáptable; ~ челове́к géntle pérson; ~ хара́ктер plíable cháracter; 7. *(сердечный, отзывчивый)* kind, respónsive; 8. *(нестрогий)* mild, lénient; ~ пригово́р mild séntence; ~ое наказа́ние mild púnishment; ~ое обраще́ние lénient tréatment; 9. *(вежливый)* mild; ~ упрёк mild repróach; 10. *(о погоде, климате)* mild, clément; ~ ваго́н uphólstered cárriage, first-cláss cárriage; ~ое кре́сло éasy chair; ~ая ме́бель uphólstered fúrniture; ~ая вода́ soft wáter; ~ знак soft sigh; ~ие согла́сные зву́ки soft cónsonants.

мя́гко sóftly; ~ выража́ясь to put it míldly.

мягкосерде́ч|ие *с.* sóft-héartedness. ~ный sóft-héarted.

мя́гкость *ж.* sóftness; *перен.* géntleness.

мягкоте́лый flábby, spíneless.

мяки́на *ж.* chaff.

мя́киш *м.* the crumb.

мя́кнуть *несов. разг.* get* soft; *перен.* droop, go* limp.

мя́коть *ж.* 1. flesh; 2. *разг. (мясо без костей)* meat; 3. *(фруктов, ягод)* pulp.

мя́млить, промя́млить *разг.* 1. *(вяло говорить)* múmble; 2. *тк. несов. (действовать медлительно)* díther.

мя́мля *м. и ж. разг.* múmbler; *(нерешительный человек)* dítherer.

мяси́ст|ый 1. *(с большим количеством мяса)* fléshy, méaty; ~ая белу́га fléshy stúrgeon; 2. *разг. (о частях тела)* fléshy; ~ нос fléshy nose.

мясни́к *м.* bútcher.

мясн|о́й *прил.* 1. meat *attr.*; ~а́я ла́вка bútcher's shop; ~а́я пи́ща méaty food; ~ бульо́н méat-broth, beef tea; 2. *в знач. сущ. с.* meat, sómething with meat in it.

мя́с|о *с.* flesh; *(как еда)* meat; бе́лое *(чёрное)* ~ white (brown) meat; ◇ вы́рвать с ~ом *(пуговицу и т. п.)* tear* off with the cloth.

мясозагото́вки *мн. (ед.* мясозагото́вка *ж.)* meat purvéyance.

мясокомбина́т *м.* méat-packing fáctory.

мясопоста́вки *мн. (ед.* мясопоста́вка *ж.)* delíveries of meat.

мясору́бка *ж. (прям. и перен.)* míncing-machine; meat grínder *амер.*

мя́та *ж.* mint.

мяте́ж *м.* mútiny, rebéllion. ~ник *м.* mutinéer, rébel. ~ный 1. *(причастный к мятежу)* rébel *attr.*, mútinous, rebéllious; 2. *(бурный)* rebéllious, tempéstuous; ~ный хара́ктер rebéllious náture.

мя́т|ый mint *attr.*; ~ые пря́ники péppermint cakes.

мя́т|ый *(негладкий)* crúmpled, rúmpled; ~ая бума́га crúmpled páper; ~ая посте́ль rúmpled béd-clothes *pl*; ~ая трава́ trámpled grass; 2. *(раздавленный)* crushed, smashed; *(слегка)* bruised; ~ая я́года crushed bérries *pl*.

мять *несов. (вн.)* 1. *(делать неровным)* crush *(smth.)* crúmple *(smth.)*, rúmple *(smth.)*; ~ бума́гу crúmple páper; ~ посте́ль rúmple the béd-clothes; ~ траву́ trámple down the grass; 2. *(давить, размягчая)* smash *(smth.)*; *(слегка)* bruise *(smth.)*; ~ гли́ну knead clay. ~ся *несов.* 1. get* rúmpled/crúmpled/crushed; э́тот

intímidate *smb.*; ~ тоску́ evóke despáir; **4.** (*вн.; оружие, приборы*) point (*smth.*), aim (*smth.*); **5.**: ~ мост че́рез ре́ку build*/throw* a bridge óver/acróss a ríver; **6.** (*вн.; покрыва́ть, кра́сить*) put* (*smth.*); ~ гля́нец, лоск на что-л. pólish *smth.*; ◇ ~ спра́вки make* inquíries; ~ поря́док put* things in órder. stráighten things out; ~ красоту́ make* onesélf béautiful.

наво́дк|а ж. **1.** (*моста*) búilding; **2.** воен. láying; прямо́й ~ой póint-blánk, at póint-blánk range.

наводн|е́ние с. flood, inundátion. ~**и́ть** сов. см. наводня́ть.

наводня́ть, наводни́ть (*вн. тв.*) flood (*smth.* with), ínundate (*smth.* with); наводни́ть ры́нок това́рами flood the márket with goods.

наво́дчик м. **1.** (*ору́дия*) gún-layer; **2.** (*пособник воровско́й ша́йки*) spótter.

наводя́щий: ~ вопро́с léading quéstion.

наво́з м. manúre, dung. ~**ить** несов. (*вн.*) manúre (*smth.*), dung (*smth.*).

навози́ть сов. (*вн., рд.*) bring* in (a supply of) (*smth.*); ~ дров на́ зиму bring* in (a supply of) wood for the winter; ~ се́на bring* in a lot of hay.

наво́зн|ый manúre attr., dung attr.; ~**ая** ку́ча manúre-heap, dúng-heap; ~ жук dúng-beetle.

на́волочка ж. pillow-case.

наворова́ть сов. (*вн., рд.*) steal* (a lot of) (*smth.*).

навостри́ть сов. разг.: ~ у́ши prick up one's ears; ~ лы́жи ≈ pack up one's traps.

навра́ть сов. разг. **1.** (*налга́ть*) (tell* a) lie, tell* a pack of lies; **2.** (*в пр.; сде́лать оши́бку*) make* a mistáke (in); **3.** (*на вн.; наклевета́ть*) tell* lies (abóut), make* up a lot of rúbbish (abóut).

навреди́ть сов. (*дт.*) разг. cause (*smb., smth.*) a lot of harm.

навря́д ли разг. hárdly, it's not líkely.

навсегда́ for éver, for good; уе́хать ~ go* for good; ◇ раз (и) ~ once (and) for all.

навстре́чу to meet, towárds; идти́ ~ кому́-л. go* towárds *smb.*; перен. meet* *smb.* hálf-wáy; идти́ ~ опа́сности go* to meet dánger; идти́ ~ чьим-л. пожела́ниям respónd to *smb.'s* wishes.

на́вык м. skill; *мн.* práctical knówledge *sg*; приобрета́ть но́вые ~и acquíre new skills; трудовы́е ~и skills.

навы́кат(е): глаза́ ~ próminent/protúberant eyes.

навы́лет right through; ра́нен в грудь ~ shot right through the chest.

навы́пуск outside (one's boots, tróusers, skirt *etc.*).

навы́тяжку: стоя́ть ~ stand* at atténtion.

навью́чивать, навью́чить (*вн. тв.*) load (*smth., smth.* with).

навью́чить сов. см. навью́чивать.

навяза́ть I сов. см. навя́зывать.

навяза́ть II, **навя́знуть** clog; гли́на навя́зла на колёсах the wheels are clogged with clay; ◇ э́то у всех навя́зло в зуба́х éveryone is sick and tíred of it.

навяза́ться сов. см. навя́зываться.

навя́знуть сов. см. навяза́ть II.

навя́зчив|ый 1. tíresome; (*назойливый*) impórtunate; ~ челове́к a tíresome pérson, a núisance; **2.** (*неотступный*) obséssive, háunting; ~ моти́в háunting mélody; ~**ая** иде́я obséssion, fíxed idéa.

навя́зывать, навяза́ть 1. (*вн. на вн.; прикрепля́ть*) fásten (*smth.* on); (*завя́зывать*) tie (*smth.* on); **2.** (*вн., рд.; наготовить вязаных изделий*) knit* (a lot. of) (*smth.*); **3.** (*вн. дт.; заставля́ть приня́ть*) impóse (*smth.* upón); ~ свои́ взгля́ды кому́-л. force one's idéas upón *smb.* ~**ся**, навяза́ться разг. impóse (onesélf); ~**ся** в го́сти get* onesélf invíted, fish for an invitátion.

нага́йка ж. whip, lash.

нага́н м. revólver.

нага́р м. scale, (cárbon) depósit; (*на свече́*) snuff.

нагиба́ть, нагну́ть (*вн.*) bend* (*smth.*). ~**ся**, нагну́ться stoop, bend* down.

нагишо́м разг. stárk-náked.

нагле́ть, обнагле́ть becóme* more and more ínsolent.

нагле́ц м. ímpudent/ínsolent féllow.

на́глость ж. ínsolence, ímpudence; cheek разг.; име́ть ~ сказа́ть ... have* the cheek to say...

наглота́ться сов. (*рд.*) swállow (*smth.*); ~ пы́ли get* a móuthful of dust.

на́глухо 1. (*очень плотно*) fírmly; ~ заби́ть дверь nail up a door; **2.** (*на все пуговицы и т. п.*) tíghtly; ~ застегну́ться bútton onesélf up tíghtly, do* up all one's búttons.

на́гл|ый ínsolent, ímpudent; ~**ая** ложь báre-fáced lie.

нагляде́ться сов. (на вн.) see* enóugh (of); я не могу́ ~ на него́ I can't take my eyes off him; ну и нагляде́лся я у́жасов и т. д. I have seen enóugh hórrors *etc.*

нагля́дн|о cléarly. ~**ый 1.** (*основанный на показе*) vísual; ~**ое** обуче́ние demonstrátion, vísual téaching méthods; ~**ые** посо́бия vísual aids; ~**ый** уро́к object--lesson; **2.** (*убедительный*) óbvious, gráphic, clear; ~**ый** приме́р gráphic exámple; ~**ое** доказа́тельство clear proof.

нагна́ть сов. см. нагоня́ть.

нагнести́ сов. см. нагнета́ть.

нагнета́ть, нагнести́ (*вн.*) force (*smth.*), pump (*smth.*).

нагное́ние с. suppurátion, féstering.

нагну́ть(ся) сов. см. нагиба́ть(ся).

нагова́ривать, наговори́ть 1. (на вн.) разг. slánder (*smb.*); ~ на кого́-л., что он взял, сде́лал и т. д. say* *smb.* took, did *etc.*; **2.**: ~ пласти́нку recórd one's voice.

наговор м. разг. slánder, múck-raking, títtle-tattle.

наговор|и́ть сов. **1.** см. нагова́ривать; **2.** (*вн., рд.; сказа́ть мно́го чего-л.*) talk (a lot of) (*smth.*); ~ глу́постей talk a lot of nónsense; ~ де́рзостей say* a lot of rude things. ~**и́ться** сов. have* a good talk; они́ ника́к не ~**ятся** they can't stop tálking.

наго́й náked, nude; (*без растительности тж.*) bare.

на́голо bare; остри́чься ~ have* one's head shaved.

наголо́ bared; с ша́шками ~ with bared swords.

на́голову: разби́ть ~ wipe out, útterly deféat, rout.

нагоня́й м. разг. ráting, tícking-óff; дать кому́-л. ~ rate *smb.*; получи́ть ~ get* a good tícking-óff.

нагоня́ть, нагна́ть 1. (*вн.; догоня́ть*) overtáke* (*smb., smth.*); catch* (*smb., smth.*) up (*тж. перен.*); **2.** (*вн.; навёрстывать*) make* up (for); нагна́ть упу́щенное вре́мя make* up for lost time; **3.** (*вн., рд.; сосредоточивать в одно́м ме́сте*) bring* up (*smb., smth.*); ве́тер нагна́л ту́чи the wind brought up stórm-clouds; **4.** (*вн., рд. на вн.*) разг. (*внуша́ть какое-л. чу́вство*) put* (*smth.* ínto); нагна́ть сон на кого́-л. make* *smb.* sléepy; нагна́ть на кого́-л. стра́ху put* the fear of God ínto *smb.*, scare *smb.* stiff; ~ тоску́ bore to death.

на-гора́ горн. to the súrface; вы́дать у́голь ~ hoist coal.

нагора́ть, нагоре́ть 1. (*дать нага́р*) begín* to splútter; **2.** безл. (*израсхо́доваться — об электри́честве и т. п.*) be* burned/consúmed; **3.** безл. разг. (*достава́ться за что-л.*): нагори́т тебе́ за э́то you'll get* ínto hot wáter for it, you'll catch* it for this.

нагоре́ть сов. см. нагора́ть.

наго́рный 1. (*гори́стый*) móuntainous, high; ~ бе́рег móuntainous coast; **2.** (*располо́женный на горах*) úpland, híghland.

наго́рье с. platéau, úpland.

нагот|а́ ж. núdity, nákedness; ◇ во всей (свое́й) ~**е́** náked and unadórned.

нагото́ве in réadiness.

нагото́вить сов. (*вн., рд.*) **1.** (*запасти́*) lay* in (*smth.*); ~ проду́ктов lay* in provísions; **2.** (*настря*-

пать) cook (a lot of) (*smth.*); смотри́те, ско́лько я наготóвила! look what a lot I've cooked!

награб|и́ть *сов.* (*вн., рд.*) steal* (a lot of) (*smth.*). **~ленный** stólen.

награ́д|а *ж.* rewárd; (*в школе*) prize; (*знак отличия*) decorátion; **в ~у** as a rewárd; **дéнежная ~** gratúity. **наградúть** *сов. см.* **награжда́ть.**

награжда́ть, наградúть (*вн.*) rewárd (*smth.*); (*вн. тв.*) confér (*smth.* on); *перен.* endów (*smb.* with), bestów (*smth.* upón); ~ *кого-л.* óрденом confér an órder on *smb.*; приро́да наградúла его́ необыкновéнной си́лой náture had endówed him with remárkable strength.

награждéние *с.* rewárding.

нагревáние *с.* héating, wárming.

нагревáтельн|ый héating *attr.*; ~ые прибóры héating applíances.

нагревáть, нагрéть (*вн.*) heat (*smth.*), warm (*smth.*); сóлнце нагрéло песóк the sand was warm from the heat of the sun; ◇ **нагрéть рýки** line one's pócket. **~ся**, нагрéться get* warm, warm up; get* hot.

нагрéть(ся) *сов. см.* **нагревáть(ся).**

нагримировáть *сов. см.* **гримировáть** 1. **~ся** *сов. см.* **гримировáться.**

нагромождáть, нагромоздúть (*вн., рд.*) pile up (*smth.*). **~éние** *с.* 1. (*дéйствие*) píling up; 2. (*грýда*) conglomerátion.

нагромоздúть *сов. см.* **нагромождáть.**

нагрубúть *сов. см.* **грубúть.**

нагрýдн|ик *м.* 1. (*дéтский*) bib; 2. (*в латах*) bréastplate; 3. (*прóбковый*) lífebelt. **~ый** chest *attr.*, breast *attr.*; ~ый знак (chest) badge.

нагружáть, нагрузúть (*вн. тв.*) 1. load (*smth.* with); 2. *разг.* (*рабóтой, поручéниями*) keep* (*smb.*) búsy (with).

нагрузúть *сов. см.* **нагружáть** *и* **грузúть** 1.

нагрýзка *ж.* 1. (*дéйствие*) lóading; 2. (*груз*) load; 3. (*стéпень зáнятости*) amóunt of work to be done; у меня́ больша́я ~ I have a lot of work to do; 4. *тех.* load.

нагрязнúть *сов.* make* a mess.

нагря́нуть *сов.* descénd out of the blue; (*к дт.*) descénd upón), turn up (at).

нагýливать, нагуля́ть 1. (*вн., рд.*; *прибавля́ть в вéсе*) put* on (*smth.*); 2. (*вн.*) *разг.* (*гуля́я, приобрести*) walk up (*smth.*); нагуля́ть аппетúт, румя́нец walk up an áppetite, a cólour.

нагуля́ть *сов. см.* **нагýливать.**

нагуля́ться *сов.* have* enóugh wálking.

над óver; (*выше*) abóve; ля́мпа висúт ~ столóм there is a lamp óver the táble; ~ гóродом пролетéл самолёт an áircraft flew óver the town; имéть власть ~ *кем-л.* have* pówer óver *smb.*; заснýть ~ кнúгой fall* asléep óver a book; возвышáться ~ *чем-л.* rise* abóve *smth.*; (*о гóре, бáшне и т. п.*) tówer óver *smth.*; ~ ýровнем мóря abóve séa-level; рабóтать ~ проéктом work on a plan; смея́ться ~ *кем-л.* laugh at *smb.*

надавúть *сов. см.* **надáвливать.**

надáвливать, надавúть (*вн., на вн.*) press (*smth.*).

надбáв|ить *сов. см.* **надбавля́ть. ~ка** *ж.* addítion; ~ка к зарплáте rise in wáges.

надбавля́ть, надбáвить (*вн.*) incréase (*smth.*).

надвúг|áть, надвúнуть: надвúнуть шля́пу *one's* hat óver *one's* eyes. **~áться,** надвúнуться appróach; *перен. тж.* be* impénding, be* ímminent; тýчи надвúнулись clouds have gáthered; ночь ~áлась night was appróaching.

надвúнуть(ся) *сов. см.* **надвигáть(ся).**

надвóдный súrface *attr.*

нáдвое in two; доро́га раздели́лась ~ the road forked; ◇ **бáбушка ~ сказáла** *погов.* you néver can tell.

надвяза́ть *сов. см.* **надвя́зывать.**

надвя́зывать, надвяза́ть (*вн.*) 1. (*увеличивать, до-*

вя́зывая) add (to) by knítting; (*чулки тж.*) refóot (*smth.*); 2. (*верёвку и т. п.*) add a piece (to).

надгрóбн|ый: ~ая нáдпись inscríption on a tómbstone, épitaph; ~ая плитá tómbstone; ~ памятник tómbstone, mónument; ~ая речь gráveside speech, fúneral orátion.

надевáть, надéть (*вн.*) put* (*smth.*) on; ~ ботúнки put* on one's shoes; ~ очкú put* on one's spéctacles.

надéжд|а *ж.* hópe; ◇ подавáть большúе ~ы be* véry prómising, show* great prómise; в ~е на *что-л.* in the hope of *smth.*; питáть ~у chérish the hope.

надёжн|ый 1. (*внушающий довéрие*) relíable, depéndable; ~ друг relíable friend; 2. (*крéпкий, прóчный*) firm; ~ фундáмент firm/relíable foundátion; 3. (*вéрный*) sure, efféctive; ~ое срéдство efféctive rémedy.

надéл|ать *сов.* (*вн., рд.*) 1. make* (a lot of) (*smth.*); ~ игрýшек make* a lot of toys; 2. (*достáвить, причинúть*) do* (a lot of) (*smth.*), cause (a lot of) (*smth.*); ~ ошúбок make* a lot of mistákes; ~ мнóго шýма make* a stir; что ты ~ал! look what you've done!; ~ глýпостей do* a lot of sílly things.

наделúть *сов. см.* **наделя́ть.**

наделя́ть, наделúть (*вн. тв.*) (*предоставля́ть как дóлю*) allót (*smth.* to); (*дáрить*) províde (*smb.* with); *перен.* (*одаря́ть*) endów (*smb.* with); приро́да щéдро наделúла его́ талáнтами náture has shówered gifts on him.

надёргать *сов.* (*вн., рд.*) 1. pull (*smth.*); 2. *разг.* (*набрáть произвóльно, неумéло*) wrench (*smth.*); ~ цитáт drag in quotátions.

надерзúть *сов. см.* **дерзúть.**

надéть *сов. см.* **надевáть.**

надé|яться *несов.* 1. (*на вн., + инф; рассчúтывать на что-л.*) expéct (*smth.*, + to *inf*); hope (for, + to *inf*); ~ на лýчшее hope for the best; ~ на возвращéние hope to retúrn; я не ~я́лся егó увúдеть I did not expéct to see him; 2. (*на вн.; полагáться*) relý (on).

надзéмн|ый óverhead; abóve (the) ground *пócле сущ.*; (*над повéрхностью земли́*) óverhead; ~ая желéзная дорóга óverhead/élevated ráilway.

надзирáтель *м.* óverseer, súpervisor.

надзирáть *несов.* (*за тв.*) súpervise (*smb., smth.*).

надзóр *м.* 1. supervísion; (*слéжка*) surveíllance; быть под ~ом be* únder surveíllance/supervísion; установúть ~ за *кем-л.* put*/keep* *smb.* únder serveíllance/supervísion; 2.: санитáрный ~ sánitary inspéction; (*грýппа людéй*) sánitary inspéctors *pl*; прокурóрский ~ procuratórial supervísion, supervísion by the públic prósecutor.

надивúться *сов. разг.:* не могý ~ на *кого-л., что-л.* (*удивля́юсь*) I am amázed at *smb., smth.*; (*восхищáюсь*) I am lost in admirátion for *smb., smth.*

надклáссов|ый indepéndent of class *пócле сущ.*; stánding abóve clásses *пócле сущ.*; ~ая идеолóгия ideólogy indepéndent of class.

надкóстниц|а *ж. анат.* periósteum; воспалéние ~ы periostítis.

надкусúть *сов. см.* **надкýсывать.**

надкýсывать, надкусúть (*вн.*) bite* (*smth.*); (*откýсывать*) bite* a piece (out of); надкусúть я́блоко bite* a piece out of an ápple.

надлáмывать, надломúть (*вн.*) pártly break* (*smth.*), crack (*smth.*); (*о кóсти тж.*) frácture (*smth.*); *перен.* (*сúлы*) overtáx (*smth.*); (*здорóвье*) ruin (*smth.*), crípple (*smth.*). **~ся**, надломúться crack; *перен.* collápse, have* a bréak-down; crack up *разг.*

надлеж|áть *безл.:* рабóту ~úт сдать в двухнедéльный срок the work must be réady in two weeks. **~ащий** próper, fítting; (*надлежáщие мéры*) apprópriate méasures; **в ~ащем поря́дке** in good órder; **~ащим óбразом** próperly, thóroughly, súitably; **в ~ащий срок** in due course, at the appóinted time.

надлóм *м.* break, crack; (*кости*) gréenstick frácture; *перен.* collápse, bréak-down.

надломи́ть(ся) *сов. см.* надлáмывать(ся).

надлóмленный bróken; *перен. тж.* enféebled, stém-bróken.

надмéнн|ость *ж.* háughtiness, árrogance, superciliousness. **~ый** háughty, árrogant, supercílious.

нáдо I *в знач. сказ. безл.* 1. (*следует*) it is nécessary; one must; *переводится тж. личными формами гл.* have* (+ to *inf*); ~ учи́ться, слу́шаться *и т. п.* you must stúdy, obéy *etc.*; it is nécessary to stúdy, obéy *etc.*; ~ бы́ло всё стрóить зáново éverything had to be rebuílt from the foundátions; мне, емý *и т. д.* ~ I, he, *etc.* must; I have, he has, *etc.* to; не ~! don't (do that)!; 2. (*о потребности*): мне *и т. д.* ~... I, *etc.* want...; что вам ~? what do you want?; ◇ так емý и ~! it serves him right!; óчень мне ~! what do I care!, why should I?; ~ ду́мать, ~ полагáть 1) it must be assúmed; 2) (*как ответ*) próbably.

нáдо II *предлог см.* над.

нáдобност|ь *ж.* necéssity, need; в слу́чае ~и if nécessary; без ~и unnécessarily; по мéре ~и as required.

надоед|áть, надоéсть 1. (*дт.*) bóther (*smb.*), péster (*smb.*); bore (*smb.*); ~ комý-л. прóсьбами péster *smb.* with requésts; он всем надоéл éveryone is sick of him; 2. *безл.* ~áет бездéльничать *one* gets sick of dóing nóthing; мне ~áет напоминáть емý I'm sick of reminding him.

надоéдливый tíresome, impórtunate; ~ человéк, собесéдник bore.

надоéсть *сов. см.* надоедáть.

надои́ть *сов.* (*вн.*) receíve a milk yield (of).

надóй *м. с.-х.* milk yield.

надóлго for long, for a long time.

надóмн|ик *м.*, **~ица** *ж.* pérson wórking at home, hóme-worker.

надорвáть *сов. см.* надрывáть. **~ся** *сов.* 1. *см.* надрывáться 1; 2. *разг.* (*повредить себе внутренние органы*) overstráin *onesélf*; 3. (*измучиться нравственно*) break* down; crack up *разг.*

надоýм|ить *сов.* (*вн.*) *разг.* suggést (to), put* in into *smb.'s* head; он ~ил меня обрати́ться к... he suggésted to me that I applý to...

надписáть *сов. см.* надпи́сывать.

надпи́сывать, надписáть (*вн.*) write* on (*smth.*); (*снабжать своей надписью*) put* *one's* áutograph (*smth.*); ~ тетрáдь put* *one's* name on an éxercise-book; ~ фотогрáфию write* an inscríption on a phótograph.

нáдпись *ж.* inscríption, superscríption.

надрáть *сов.:* ~ у́ши комý-л. *разг.* pull *smb.'s* ears.

надрéз *м.* incísion, notch. **~ать** *сов. см.* надрезáть.

надрезáть, надрéзать (*вн.*) make* an incísion (in), notch (*smth.*).

надругáтельство *с.* (*над тв.*) óutrage (of, upón).

надругáться *сов.* (*над тв.*) óutrage (*smb., smth.*), commít an óutrage (upón).

надры́в *м.* 1. tear; 2. (*чрезмерное усилие*) (great) éffort; с ~ом with a great éffort; 3. (*резкое ослабление сил*) collápse; (*подавленное состояние*) depréssion.

надрыв|áть, надорвáть (*вн.*) 1. tear* (*smth.*) slíghtly, make* a tear (in); 2. (*повреждать*) strain (*smth.*), overstráin (*smth.*); ~ си́лы overtáx *one's* strength; ~ здорóвье undermíne *one's* health; ~ ду́шу, сéрдце комý-л. break* *smb.'s* heart. **~áться, надорвáться** 1. have* a tear in it, be* torn slíghtly; пакéт надорвáлся the pácket was slíghtly torn; 2. *тк. несов.* (*делать что-л. с большим напряжением сил*) lábour; ~áясь, он тащи́л рáненого в окóп he strúggled to drag the wóunded man* into the trench; 3. *тк. несов.* (*кричать*) yell; 4. *тк. несов.* (*от рд.; страдать*) súffer (*smth.*); ◇ сéрдце, душá ~áется *one's* heart is bréaking.

надсмóтр *м.* supervísion. **~щик** *м.* óverseer, súpervisor.

надстрáивать, надстрóить (*вн.*) incréase the height (of), add (a súperstructure) (to); ~ этáж add a stórey to a house.

надстрóить *сов. см.* надстрáивать.

надстрóйка *ж.* 1. (*действие*) búilding on; 2. (*надстроенная часть чего-л.*) súperstructure (*тж. филос.*).

надтрéснутый cracked (*тж. перен.*).

надувáтельство *с. разг.* tríckery, chéating, swíndling.

надувáть, надýть (*вн.*) 1. (*наполнять воздухом, газом*) infláte (*smth.*); blow* up (*smth.*); (*напрягивать действием ветра*) fill (*smth.*); 2. *разг.* (*обманывать*) dupe (*smb.*), cheat (*smb.*); swíndle (*smb.*); ◇ надýть гу́бы *разг.* pout; надýть щёки puff up *one's* cheeks. **~ся, надýться** 1. becóme* infláted; (*о парусе*) fill; (*раздувать щёки*) puff up *one's* cheeks; 2. (*набухать*) swell*.

надувн|óй inflátable; **~áя лóдка** rúbber inflátable boat; **~áя подýшка** áir-cushion.

надýманный forced; (*об образах, сравнениях и т. п.*) fár-fétched.

надýмать *сов.* (+ *инф.*) *разг.* make* up *one's* mind (+ to *inf*); (*придумать*) take* it into *one's* head (+ to *inf*).

надýтый 1. (*набухший*) swóllen; 2. (*надменный*) puffed up; 3. (*обиженный*) súlky.

надý|ть *сов.* 1. *см.* надувáть; 2. *безл.:* емý ~ло в у́хо the draught gave him éar-ache. **~ться** *сов.* 1. *см.* надувáться; 2. (*обидеться*) make* a súlky face, sulk; 3. *разг.* (*принять важный вид*) put* *one's* nose in the air.

надýш|енный scénted, perfúmed. **~и́ть II. ~и́ться** *сов. см.* души́ться.

надши́ть *сов. см.* надшивáть.

надшивáть, надши́ть (*вн.*) 1. sew* a piece on (to); 2. (*делать длиннее*) léngthen (*smth.*).

надши́ть *сов. см.* надшивáть.

надыми́ть *сов.* smoke, make* a lot of smoke.

надышáть *сов.* make* it warm with *one's* breath; (*сделать душным*) make* it stúffy. **~ся** *сов.* (*тв.*) breathe *one's* fill (of); ◇ не ~ся на *кого-л.* dote on *smb.*

наедáться, наéсться 1. (*досыта*) eat* enóugh, have* *one's* fill; я наéлся I've had enóugh; 2. (*тв., рд.; есть что-л. в большом количестве*) eat* plénty (of); gorge (*onesélf*) (on); наéсться слáдкого gorge on sweets.

наединé alóne; (*без свидетелей*) in prívate, prívately.

наéздн|ик *м.* ríder, hórseman*; прекрáсный ~ spléndid hórseman*; циркóвой ~ círcus ríder. **~ица** *ж.* hórsewoman*.

наéздом on a flýing vísit; бывáть ~ pay* flýing vísits.

наезжáть, наéхать 1. (*на вн.; наталкиваться*) run* (into); (*на неодушевлённый предмет тж.*) collíde (with); (*встречать кого-л., что-л. во время езды*) come* upón (*smb., smth.*); 2. *разг.* (*приезжать в каком-л. количестве*) come*, arríve; наéхало мнóго гостéй a lot of guests arríved; 3. *тк. несов. разг.* (*бывать наездом*) pay* flýing vísits (to).

наéзженн|ый whéel-worn; **~ая дорóга** whéel-worn track; (*зимняя*) smooth/firm sléigh-road.

наём *м.* 1. (*рабочих*) híring; рабóтать по нáйму work for wáges/hire; 2. (*помещения*) rénting. **~ник** *м.* híreling. **~ный** 1. híred; ~ный труд wage/híred lábour; 2. (*подкупленный*) mércenary; ~ные войскá mércenaries, híred troops; ~ный уби́йца híred assássin.

наéсться *сов. см.* наедáться.

наéхать *сов. см.* наезжáть.

нажáрить *сов.* (*вн., рд.*) fry (a lot of) (*smth.*). roast (a lot of) (*smth.*). **~ся** *сов. разг.* roast *onesélf*; ~ся на сóлнце roast (*onesélf*) in the sun.

нажáть I *сов. см.* нажимáть.

нажáть II *сов.* (*вн., рд.; сжать какое-л. количество*) reap (a lot of) (*smth.*), hárvest (a lot of) (*smth.*).

наждá|к *м.* émery. **~чный** émery *attr.*

нажи́в|а I *ж. разг.* acquisítion; gain, prófit; погóня за ~ой greed for gold/gain; лёгкая ~ éasy móney.

нажи́ва II *ж. см.* нажи́вка.

нажива́ть, нажи́ть 1. (*вн.; приобретать постепенно*) get* (*smth.*), acquíre (*smth.*); (*получать прибыль и т. п.*) make* (*smth.*), amáss (*smth.*); ~ состоя́ние amáss/make* a fórtune; 2. (*вн., рд.; получать что-л. неприятное*): нажи́ть боле́знь contráct a diséase; нажи́ть враго́в make* énemies; нажи́ть себé хлопо́т let* onesélf in for a lot of tróuble. ~ся, нажи́ться get* rich, make* a fórtune.

нажи́вка *ж.* (líve-)bait.

нажи́м *м.* 1. préssure; 2.: писа́ть с ~ом press on one's pen.

нажима́ть, нажа́ть 1. (*вн., на вн.; надавливать*) press (*smth.*); (*ногой тж.*) tread* (on); ~ на акселера́тор press the accélerator; 2. (*на вн.*) *разг.* (*оказывать воздействие*) put* préssure (on), bring* préssure to bear (on); 3. (*на вн.*) *разг.* (*энергично приниматься за что-л.*) exért onesélf (óver), put* one's back ínto (*smth.*).

нажи́ть(ся) *сов. см.* нажива́ть(ся).

наза́втра *разг.* the next day.

наза́д 1. (*в противоположном направлении*) báckward(s); шаг ~ a step báckward; 2. (*в обратную сторону*) back; огляну́ться ~ look back; заложи́ть ру́ки ~ put* one's hands behínd one's back; 3. (*обратно*) back; взять ~ своё обеща́ние withdráw one's prómise; отда́ть что-л. ~ give* smth. back; 4. (*тж.* тому́ ~) agó.

назади́ *разг.* behínd.

назва́ние *с.* name; (*книги тж.*) títle.

назва́ть I *сов. см.* называ́ть.

назва́ть II *сов.* (*вн., рд.; пригласить многих*) invíte (a lot of) (*smth.*).

назва́ться I *сов. см.* называ́ться I 2, 3.

назва́ться II *сов. см.* называ́ться II.

назе́мн|ый (*существующий, действующий на земле, суше*) land *attr.*; (*невоздушный*) ground *attr.*; ~ые войска́ land/ground fórces; ~ая желе́зная доро́га súrface ráilway.

на́земь to the ground.

назида́|ние *с.* edificátion; *мн.* sérmons; сказа́ть что-л. в ~ кому́-л. say* smth. for smb.'s edificátion. ~тельный édifying, didáctic; ~тельный тон didáctic tone of voice.

назло́ out of spite; как ~ as ill luck would have it; ~ кому́-л. to spite smb.; они́ сде́лали э́то ~ мне they did it just to spite me.

назнач|а́ть, назна́чить (*вн.*) 1. (*заранее намечать*) fix (*smth.*); назна́чить день отъе́зда fix the day of depárture; назна́чить свида́ние make* a date; 2. (*устанавливать, определять*) allót (*smth.*), állocate (*smth.*), assígn (*smth.*); ~ пе́нсию, посо́бие grant a pénsion, súbsidy; ~ це́ну fix/name a price; (*на должность*) appóint (*smb.*); 4. *разг.* (*предписывать*) prescríbe (*smth.*), órder (*smth.*). ~éние *с.* 1. (*пособия и т. п.*) assignment, allocátion; 2. (*на должность*) appóintment; 3. (*функция*) fúnction, púrpose; отвеча́ть своему́ ~éнию ánswer/serve its púrpose; испо́льзовать что-л. по ~éнию use smth. próperly, use smth. for its próper púrpose; 4. (*лечебное*) prescríption; по ~éнию врача́ on dóctor's órders; ◊ ме́сто ~éния destinátion.

назна́чить *сов. см.* назнача́ть.

назо́йлив|ость *ж.* importúnity. ~ый impórtunate; (*о человеке*) tíresome, púshing; ~ая мысль intrúsive thought; ~ая мело́дия háunting tune.

назрева́ть, назре́ть 1. (*становиться неизбежным*) becóme* ímminent; come* to a head; кри́зис назре́л the crísis is ímminent; 2. *разг.* (*о нарыве*) gáther.

назре́вш|ий úrgent, préssing; ~ие вопро́сы úrgent quéstions.

назре́ть *сов. см.* назрева́ть.

назубо́к *разг.*: знать что-л. ~ have* smth. at one's fingertips, be* wórd-pérfect in smth.; знать роль ~ be* wórd-pérfect.

называ́емый: так ~ 1) (*как обычно называют*) what is known as; 2) *ирон.* the so-cálled.

называ́ть, назва́ть (*вн.*) 1 (*давать имя*) name (*smb.*); (*определять каким-л. словом*) call (*smth.*); 2. (*произносить имя, название*) give* the name (of); ~ себя́ give* one's name, say* who one is; он не назва́л себя́ he did not revéal his name; 3. (*объявлять*) name (*smth.*), state (*smth.*); ~ день name a day.

называ́ться I, **назва́ться** 1. *тк. несов.* (*иметь название*) be* called; как э́то называ́ется? what is it called? 2. (*присваивать себе какое-л. название*) call onesélf; 3. (*сообщать своё имя и т. п.*) give* one's name, say* who one is.

называ́ться II, **назва́ться** *разг.* (*напрашиваться*) invíte onesélf; (*предлагать своё участие в чём-л.*) voluntéer; take* it upón onesélf.

наибо́лее the most.

наибо́льший the lárgest, the gréatest.

наи́вн|ость *ж.* naïveté, naívety; crédulousness; (*безыскусственность*) ártlessness. ~ый naïve, crédulous; (*безыскусственно-простой*) ingénuous, ártless, unsophísticated; ~ый ребёнок crédulous child*; ~ая улы́бка ártless/ingénuous smile; ~ый вопро́с naïve question.

наивы́сший the gréatest.

найгранн|ый affécted, assúmed; ~ жест affécted gésture; ~ая весёлость assúmed gáiety.

найгра́ть *сов. см.* найгрывать 2, 3. ~ся *сов.* play to one's heart's contént.

найгрывать, найгра́ть 1. *тк. несов.* (*играть тихо*) play sóftly; 2. (*вн.*) *разг.* (*передавать основную мелодию*) run* through (*smth.*); найгра́ть моти́в run* through a tune; 3. (*вн.; для звукозаписи*): найгра́ть пласти́нку make* a recórding.

наизна́нку inside out.

наизу́сть by heart.

наилу́чший the best.

наиме́нее the least.

наименова́ние *с.* 1. appellátion, name; 2. (*вид*) denominátion, type.

наиме́ньш|ий the least, the shórtest; ~ее расстоя́ние ме́жду двумя́ то́чками the shórtest dístance betwéen two points.

наискосо́к *разг. см.* на́искось.

на́искось oblíquely.

наиху́дший the worst.

найми́т *м. презр.* híreling.

найти́ I, II *сов. см.* находи́ть I, II.

найти́сь *сов.* 1. *см.* находи́ться I 1, 2; 2. (*не растеряться*) néver be* at a loss (for); он бы́стро нашёлся he reácted quíckly to the situátion, he rose to the occásion; он не нашёлся, что отве́тить he was at a loss.

нака́з *м.* mándate; ~ избира́телей депута́ту députy's mándate from his eléctors/constituents.

наказа́ние *с.* púnishment; ◊ ~ мне с тобо́й! you'll drive me mad!; не ребёнок, а су́щее ~! the child* is a pérfect núisance!

наказ|а́ть *сов. см.* нака́зывать. ~уемый *юр.* púnishable.

нака́зывать, наказа́ть (*вн.*) púnish (*smb.*); он сам себя́ наказа́л it was himsélf he hurt.

нака́л *м.* 1. incandéscence; бе́лый, кра́сный ~ white, red heat; ла́мпочка гори́т в не по́лный ~ the bulb is úsing dimínished cúrrent; 2. (*состояние крайнего напряжения*) ténsion.

накалённ|ый 1. overhéated; ~ая земля́ the báking/róasted earth; ~ песо́к the scórching sand; 2. (*напряжённый, неспокойный*) tense; ~ая атмосфе́ра strained/tense átmosphere.

нака́ливать, накали́ть (*вн.*) heat (*smth.*), incandésce (*smth.*), bring* (*smth.*) to a high témperature; *перен.* strain (*smb., smth.*), make* (*smth.*) strained/tense; накали́ть что-л. до́красна́ make* *smth.* red-hót. ~ся, накали́ться get* véry hot; *перен.* becóme* héated.

накали́ть(ся) *сов. см.* нака́ливать(ся).

нака́лывать, наколо́ть 1. (*вн.; повреждать*) prick (*smth.*); 2. (*вн. на вн.; прикреплять*) pin (*smth.* to). ~ся, наколо́ться prick onesélf.

накали́ть(ся) *несов. см.* нака́ливать(ся).

накану́не 1 *нареч.* the day befóre; 2. *предлог* (*рд.*) on the eve (of).

нака́пать *сов.* 1. (*вн., рд.*) pour drops (of); méasure (*smth.*) out in drops; 2. (*вн., тв.; пролить*) spill* (*smth.*).

нака́пливать, накопи́ть (*вн.*) accúmulate (*smth.*); *перен. тж.* gain (*smth.*); (*о деньгах*) save up (*smth.*), amáss (*smth.*); ~ о́пыт gain expérience. ~ся, накопи́ться accúmulate, pile up.

накача́ть *сов. см.* нака́чивать.

нака́чивать, накача́ть (*вн.*) pump up (*smth.*); ~ ши́ну pump up a týre; накача́ть бо́чку воды́ fill a bárrel (at a pump); накача́ть воды́ pump up wáter.

накида́ть *сов.* (*вн.; кидая, наполнить что-л.*) fill (*smth.*); (*вн., рд.; набросать*) throw* (*smth.*), heap (up) (*smth.*).

наки́дка ж. 1. (*одежда*) cape; (*длинная*) cloak; 2. (*покрывало*) pillow cóver; 3. *разг.* (*надбавка к цене*) súrcharge.

наки́дывать, наки́нуть (*вн.*) 1. throw* on (*smth.*); он наки́нул пальто́ и вы́шел he threw on his coat and walked out; 2. *разг.* (*набавлять*) put* on (*smth.*). ~ся, наки́нуться (на *вн.*) pounce on (*smb., smth.*), attáck (*smb., smth.*).

наки́нуть(ся) *сов. см.* наки́дывать(ся).

накипа́ть, накипе́ть form a scum; *перен.* rise*, ferment; в душе́ у него́ накипе́ло he was séething with reséntment.

накипе́ть *сов. см.* накипа́ть.

на́кипь ж. 1. (*пена*) scum; 2. (*в котле*) fur, scale.

накла́дка ж. 1. (*искусственные волосы*) háir-piece; 2. *разг.* (*ошибка*) blúnder.

накладна́я ж. ínvoice; (*корабельного груза*) bill of láding.

накладн|о́й superimpósed, addítional; ~ сере́бро́ pláted sílver; ◇ ~ые расхо́ды óverhead expénses, óverheads.

накла́дывать, наложи́ть (*вн.*) 1. put* (*smth.*); ~ себе́ на таре́лку что-л. help onesélf to *smth.*; 2. *мед.* apply (*smth.*); ~ повя́зку кому́-л. bándage *smb.*; ~ швы put* in stítches; 3.: ~ резолю́цию appénd one's decision.

накле́ивать, накле́ить (*вн.*) stick* (*smth.*) on; ~ ма́рку put* a stamp on, stamp a létter/énvelope; ~ афи́ши paste up nótices.

накле́ить *сов. см.* накле́ивать.

накле́йка ж. 1. (*действие*) stícking on; 2. (*ярлычок*) (stícky) lábel.

накло́н м. 1. (*действие*) sídeways mótion; móvement sídeways; 2. (*наклонное положение*) slope.

наклоне́ние с. *грам.* mood.

наклони́ть(ся) *сов. см.* наклоня́ть(ся).

накло́н|ность ж. téndency, inclinátion, bent, propénsity. ~ный slánting, inclíned; ~ная пло́скость inclíned plane; ◇ кати́ться по ~ной пло́скости go* dównhill, rápidly detériorate.

наклоня́ть, наклони́ть (*вн.*) bend* (*smth.*), inclíne (*smth.*), lean* (*smth.*). ~ся, наклони́ться bend*, lean*; она́ наклони́лась ко мне she bent/léaned óver me.

накова́льн|я ж. ánvil; ◇ ме́жду мо́лотом и ~ей ≈ betwéen the dévil and the deep sea.

наколо́ть I *сов. см.* нака́лывать.

наколо́ть II *сов.* (*вн., рд.*) (*дров*) chop (a lot of) (*smth.*); (*сахару*) break* (a lot of) (*smth.*).

наколо́ться *сов. см.* нака́лываться.

наконе́ц 1. *нареч.* at last, evéntually; (*в заключение*) finally; 2. *вводн. сл.* at last; (*при перечислении*) finally; 3. *вводн. сл.:* да уходи́те же, ~! oh, go awáy, do!; ◇ ~-то! at (long) last!

наконе́чник м. tip; (*карандаша*) top.

накопа́ть *сов.* (*вн., рд.*) 1. (*копая, сделать углубления*) dig* (a lot of) (*smth.*); 2. (*выкопать*) dig* up (a lot of) (*smth.*).

накопи́ть(ся) *сов. см.* нака́пливать(ся).

накопле́ние с. 1. (*действие*) accumulátion; 2. *мн.* (*сбережения*) accumulátion *sg.*

накопля́ть(ся) *несов. см.* нака́пливать(ся).

накорми́ть *сов. см.* корми́ть 1, 2.

накра́пыв|ать *несов.* sprinkle down; ~ает дождь ráin-drops begin to fall; it is spitting *разг.*

накра́сить *сов.* 1. (*вн.*) make* up (*smth.*); 2. (*вн., рд.; выкрасить в каком-л. количестве*) paint (a lot of) (*smth.*). ~ся *сов. разг.* make* up.

накрахма́л|енный starched. ~ить *сов. см.* крахма́лить.

накрени́ть(ся) *сов. см.* накреня́ть(ся) *и* крени́ть(ся).

накреня́ть, накрени́ть 1. (*вн.*) make* (*smth.*) lean óver; (*корабль*) give* a list (to); 2. *безл.:* ло́дку накрени́ло the boat heeled óver; дом накрени́ло the house is léaning óver on one side. ~ся, накрени́ться (*о корабле*) heel óver, take* a list; (*о стене, здании*) lean*.

на́крепко 1. fast, firmly; 2. *разг.* (*решительно*) strictly.

на́крест crósswise.

накрича́ть *сов.* shout; (*на вн.; выругать*) scold (*smb.*); go* for (*smb.*) *разг.*

накроши́ть *сов.* 1. (*вн., рд.*) crúmble (*smth.*); ~ таре́лку мя́са chop up a plate of meat; 2. (*насорить*) make* a lot of crumbs; ~ на столе́ cóver the táble with crumbs.

накрыва́ть, накры́ть (*вн.*) 1. cóver (*smb., smth.*); 2. *разг.* (*захватить врасплох*) catch* (*smb.*) in the act, catch* (*smb.*) réd-handed; 3. *воен.* hit* (*smth.*), knock out (*smth.*); ◇ ~ на стол lay* the táble. ~ся, накры́ться (*тв.*) cóver onesélf (with).

накры́ть(ся) *сов. см.* накрыва́ть(ся).

накупи́ть *сов.* (*вн., рд.*) buy* (a lot of) (*smth.*).

наку́рен|ный smóky; full of smoke *после сущ.*; как тут ~о! how smóky it is here!

накури́ть *сов.* make* (a room) smóky. ~ся *сов.* smoke to one's heart's contént, smoke as much as one likes.

налага́ть, наложи́ть (*вн.*) impóse (*smth.*); ~ наказа́ние inflíct a pénalty/púnishment; наложи́ть аре́ст на иму́щество seize/sequéster próperty.

нала́дить(ся) *сов. см.* нала́живать(ся).

нала́дчик м. adjúster.

нала́жив|ать, нала́дить (*вн.*) 1. (*исправлять, делать пригодным*) put* (*smth.*) in órder; (*регулировать*) adjúst (*smth.*); нала́дить маши́ну adjúst a machíne; 2. (*создавать, организовывать*) órganize (*smth.*); нала́дить произво́дство маши́н órganize the prodúction of machínery. ~аться, нала́диться come* right; всё нала́дится éverything will come right; рабо́та ещё не нала́дилась the work has not got góing próperly yet; дела́ постепе́нно ~аются things are gradually beginning to take shape.

налга́ть *сов.* 1. (*наговорить лжи*) tell* a pack of lies; 2. (*на вн.; наклеветать*) tell* lies (abóut), slánder (*smb.*).

нале́во 1. to the left; ~ от чего-л. on the left of *smth.*; ~ от меня́ to/on my left; ~! (*команда*) left turn!; 2. *разг. неодобр.* (*незаконно используя служебные возможности*) on the side.

налега́ть, нале́чь (на *вн.*) 1. (*с силой опираться*) lean* (on); (*придавливать*) press (on); 2. (*с силой нажимать на что-л.*) push (*smth.*) hard, pull (*smth.*) hard; ~ на вёсла ply the oars with a will; 3. *разг.* (*приниматься за что-л.*) get* down (to); нале́чь на рабо́ту get* down to work.

налегке́ 1. (*без багажа*) without lúggage; путеше́ствовать ~ trável light; 2. (*в лёгкой одежде*) lightly clad.

налёт *м.* 1. (*нападение*) raid; (*с целью грабежа тж.*) búrglary; возду́шный ~ air attáck/raid; 2. (*тонкий слой чего-л.*) film; ~ пы́ли film of dust; 3. (*оттенок*) tinge; 4. *мед.*: ~ в го́рле patch; ~ на языке́ fur; ◇ с ~a, с ~y at full speed; *перен.* in a flash.

налета́ть, налете́ть 1. (на *вн.*) swoop (on); *перен. разг.* (*наскакивать*) run* into (*smb., smth.*); 2. (на *вн.*) *разг.* (*обрушиваться с обвинениями и т. п.*) jump on (*smb.*); 3. (*внезапно начинаться*) blow* up; налете́л ве́тер there was a súdden gust of wind.

налете́ть *сов. см.* налета́ть.

налётчик *м.* róbber.

нале́чь *сов. см.* налега́ть.

налива́ть, нали́ть 1. (*вн.; наполнять*) fill (*smth.*); нали́ть ведро́ воды́ fill a pail with wáter; 2. (*вн., рд.; вливать во что-л.*) pour (*smth.*); нали́ть во́ду в стака́н pour some wáter into a glass; 3. (*вн., рд.; разливать*) spill* (*smth.*); нали́ть воды́ на́ пол spill* wáter óver the floor. ~ся, нали́ться 1. (в *вн.; натекать во что-л.*) flow (into); вода́ сра́зу налила́сь ему́ в рот, в нос, в у́ши he got his mouth, nose, ears full of wáter at once; 2. (*наполняться*) fill; её глаза́ налили́сь слеза́ми her eyes filled with tears; 3. (*созревать*) rípen; *несов. тж.* swell*; ◇ нали́ться кро́вью becóme* blóodshot.

нали́вка *ж.* córdial, liqúeur.

наливн|о́й: ~о́е я́блоко júicy ápple; ~о́е су́дно tánker; ~ груз líquid cárgo/freight.

нали́м *м.* búrbot, éel-pout.

налинова́ть *сов. см.* линова́ть.

нали́ть(ся) *сов. см.* налива́ть(ся).

налицо́ aváilable, to hand; ули́ки ~ there is ámple proof, there's no gétting awáy from it; все ~ éverybody is here; преступле́ние ~ it is clear that a crime has been committed.

нали́чи|е *с.* availability; (*существование*) exístence; при ~и кво́рума if there is a quórum; при ~и де́нег if *one* has the móney; ~ бы́ть в ~е be* aváilable.

нали́чн|ость *ж.* 1. amóunt aváilable; 2. (*о деньгах*) cash; 3. *см.* нали́чие; все маши́ны в ~ости all aváilable véhicles. ~ый *прил.* 1. aváilable; ~ые де́ньги réady móney, cash; 2. *в знач. сущ. мн.:* плати́ть ~ыми pay* (in) cash; ◇ ~ый расчёт cásh-páyment; за ~ый расчёт for cash (down).

налови́ть *сов.* (*вн., рд.*) catch* (a lot of) (*smth.*).

наловчи́ться *сов.* (в *пр.*, + *инф.*) *разг.* becóme* proficient (at), get* the knack (of + *ing*).

нало́г *м.* tax; прямо́й ~ diréct tax; ко́свенный ~ indiréct tax; взима́ть ~и colléct táxes; обложе́ние ~ом taxátion; сниже́ние ~а a redúction of tax.

нало́гов|ый tax *attr.*, taxátion *attr.*; ~ая систе́ма sýstem of taxátion.

налогоплате́льщик *м.* táxpayer.

наложе́нн|ый: ~ый платёж C. O. D., cash on delivery; отпра́вить груз ~ым платежо́м send* a consígnment cash on delivery.

наложи́ть *сов. см.* накла́дывать *и* налага́ть.

налома́ть *сов.* (*вн., рд.*) 1. break* off (a lot of) (*smth.*); 2. (*ломая, привести в негодность*) break* (a lot of) (*smth.*); ◇ ~ дров make* a real mess of things.

нало́паться *сов. разг.* gorge onesélf.

нам (*дт. от личн. мест.* мы) to us; ~ бы́ло ска́зано we were told.

нама́зать *сов.* 1. (*вн., тв.; покрыть слоем чего-л.*) put* (*smth.* on); spread* (*smth.* on); ~ хлеб ма́слом

bútter bread, put* bútter on *one's* bread; 2. (*вн.*) *разг.* (*накрасить*) make* up (*smth.*); ~ гу́бы use lípstick; 3. *разг.* (*напачкать*) make* a mess; 4. *разг.* (*небрежно нарисовать*) daub, botch up. ~ся *сов.* 1. (*тв.*) smear onesélf (with); 2. *разг.* (*накраситься*) make* (*onesélf*) up.

намалева́ть *сов. см.* малева́ть.

намара́ть *сов. см.* мара́ть 2.

намарина́ть *сов.* (*вн., рд.*) píckle (a lot of) (*smth.*); ~ грибо́в píckle some múshrooms.

нама́тывать, намота́ть (*вн.*) wind* (*smth.*), spool (*smth.*), reel (*smth.*); намота́ть не́сколько клубко́в ше́рсти wind* a few balls of wool; ~ ни́тки на кату́шку wind* cótton on a reel.

намёк *м.* hint; поня́ть ~ take* a hint; сде́лать ~ give*/drop a hint; нея́сные ~и vague/cóvert hints.

намек|а́ть, намекну́ть (на *вн.*) hint (at); *сов. тж.* drop a hint (at); на что вы ~а́ете? what are you dríving at? ~ну́ть *сов. см.* намека́ть.

намерева́ться *несов.* (+ *инф.*) inténd (+ -ing, + to *inf.*)

наме́рен *в знач. сказ.:* он ~ (+ *инф.*) he inténds (+ to *inf,* + -ing); он ~ уе́хать сего́дня he inténds to leave tóday.

наме́рени|е *с.* inténtion; ◇ с ~ем inténtionally; без ~я úninténtionally.

наме́ренный inténtional, delíberate.

намести́ *сов. см.* намета́ть.

намета́ть, намести́ 1. (*вн., рд.*) sweep* togéther (*smth.*); 2. (*вн.; наносить ветром*) drift (*smth.*); намело́ це́лые сугро́бы сне́га the snow was packed in huge drifts, great drifts of snow had formed.

наме́тить I, II *сов. см.* намеча́ть I, II.

наме́титься *сов. см.* намеча́ться.

наме́тка *ж.* (*предварительный план*) óutline.

намеча́ть I, наме́тить (*вн.*) 1. (*обозначать метками*) mark (*smth.*); наме́тить доро́гу ве́шками mark a road with posts; 2. (*обозначать штрихами*) óutline (*smth.*) (*тж. перен.*); ~ пути́ подъёма се́льского хозя́йства óutline ways of adváncing ágriculture.

намеча́ть II, наме́тить (*вн.; заранее назначать*) plan (*smth.*); наме́тить день отъе́зда fix *one's* day of depárture.

намеча́ться I, наме́титься (*обозначаться*) show*; *перен.* be* óutlined, emérge, form, take* shape.

намеча́ться II *несов.* (*предполагаться*) be* planned.

на́ми (*тв. от личн. мест.* мы) by us; с ~ with us; он пойдёт за ~ he'll fóllow us.

намно́го much, far; стать ~ сильне́е becóme* much strónger.

намозо́лить *сов. см.* мозо́лить.

намока́ть, намо́кнуть get* wet, be* soaked.

намо́кнуть *сов. см.* намока́ть.

намола́чивать, намолоти́ть (*вн., рд.*) thresh (*smth.*); намолоти́ть мешо́к ржи thresh a sáckful of rye.

намоло́т *м. с.-х.* amóunt of threshed grain.

намолоти́ть *сов. см.* намола́чивать.

намоло́ть *сов.* (*вн., рд.*) (*размолоть какое-л. количество*) grind* (*smth.*); ~ ко́фе grind* some cóffee.

намо́рдник *м.* múzzle; наде́ть ~ на соба́ку múzzle a dog.

намо́рщить *сов. см.* мо́рщить 1. ~ся *сов. см.* мо́рщиться 1.

намота́ть *сов. см.* нама́тывать.

намочи́ть *сов.* 1. (*вн.; пропитать водой*) soak (*smth.*); 2. (*наплескать*) splash, make* the place wet.

намучиться *сов. разг.* have* an áwful lot of tróuble, have* a hell of a time.

намыва́ть, намы́ть (*вн.*) 1. (*наносить течением*) depósit (*smth.*); 2. (*добывать*) pan out (*smth.*); намы́ть золото́го песку́ pan out góld-bearing grável.

намы́ливать, намы́лить (*вн.*) soap (*smth.*); ◇ на-

мы́лить *кому́-л.* го́лову rap *smb.* óver the knúckles, give* it (to) *smb.* hot. ~ся, намы́литься soap onesélf.

намы́лить *сов. см.* намы́ливать *и* мы́лить. ~ся *сов. см.* намы́ливаться *и* мы́литься 1.

намы́ть *сов. см.* намыва́ть.

нанести́ *сов.* 1. *см.* наноси́ть II; 2. *(вн., рд.; принести́ много чего́-л.)* bring* (a lot of) *(smth.)*; 3. *(вн., рд.; снести́ много яи́ц — о пти́цах)* lay* (a lot of) *(smth.)*.

наниза́ть *сов. см.* нани́зывать.

нани́зывать, наниза́ть *(вн., рд.)* thread *(smth.)*.

нанима́тель *м.* 1. *(рабо́чего)* emplóyer; 2. *(кварти́ры)* ténant.

нанима́ть, наня́ть *(вн.)* 1. *(на рабо́ту)* hire *(smb.)*, emplóy *(smb.)*, engáge *(smb.)*; 2. *(автомоби́ль, экипа́ж и т. п.)* hire *(smth.)*; *(помеще́ние)* rent *(smth.)*. ~ся, наня́ться take* a job; *несов. тж.* apply for a job.

нано́с *м.* allúvium *(pl* -ums, -ia), depósit.

наноси́ть I *сов.* *(вн., рд.)* bring* (a lot of) *(smth.)*; ~ бо́чку воды́ fill a bárrel with wáter pail by pail; ~ гру́ду камне́й pile up a heap of stones.

наноси́ть II, нанести́ 1. *(вн.; нагроможда́ть)* pile up *(smth.)*; *(о сне́ге, песке́)* pile up *(smth.)* into drifts; вода́ нанесла́ на бе́рег мно́го во́дорослей the wáter piled up a lot of séa-weed on the shore; 2. *безл.:* нанесло́ мно́го сне́га there are héavy drifts of snow éverywhere; 3. *(вн.; обознача́ть, отмеча́ть)* trace *(smth.)*, óutline *(smth.)*; ~ что-л. на ка́рту mark/trace *smth.* on the map; 4. *(вн.; причиня́ть)* inflíct *(smth.)*; ~ оскорбле́ние кому́-л. insúlt *smb.*; ~ ра́ну inflíct a wound (on); ~ уще́рб cause dámage; ~ вред *кому́-л., чему́-л.* cause harm to *smb., smth.*, dámage *smb., smth.*, ínjure *smb., smth.*; ◇ нанести́ визи́т кому́-л. pay* a vísit to *smb.*, vísit *smb.*, call on *smb.*

нано́с|ый 1. allúvial; 2. *(не сво́йственный кому́-л., чему́-л., привнесённый со стороны́)* extráneous; superfícial; ~ое влия́ние extráneous ínfluence.

наня́ть(ся) *сов. см.* нанима́ть(ся).

наобеща́ть *сов. (вн., рд.) разг.* prómise (a lot of) *(smth.)*.

наоборо́т *нареч.* 1. *(соверше́нно ина́че)* the wrong way, the óther way round; как раз ~ just the óther way abóut; де́лать ~ do* just the ópposite; он всё понима́ет ~ he puts a wrong constrúction on éverything; 2. *в знач. вво́дн. сл.* on the cóntrary, quite the revérse.

наобу́м *разг.* at rándom.

наотма́шь with the full swing of *one's* arm; уда́рить кого́-л. ~ deal* *smb.* a swíngeing/smáshing blow.

наотре́з flátly; отказа́ть ~ refúse point-blánk, flátly refúse.

напа́д|ать *сов.:* ~ало мно́го сне́га a lot of snow has fállen.

напада́ть, напа́сть *(на вн.)* 1. attáck *(smb., smth.)* assáult *(smb., smth.)*; 2. *(натáлкиваться)* come* across *(smb., smth.)*, come* upón *(smb., smth.)*; 3. *(овладева́ть)* come* óver *(smb.)*; на него́ напа́л страх he was seized with fear; 4. *разг. (обру́шиваться с упрёками и т. п.)* jump on *(smb.)*.

напада́ющий *м.* fórward.

нападе́ни|е *с.* 1. attáck, assáult; 2. *спорт.* the fórwards *pl*, the fórward line; центр ~я céntre fórward.

нападки *мн.* attácks.

напа́ивать, напая́ть *(вн.)* sólder *(smth.)*.

напа́сть I *сов. см.* напада́ть.

напа́сть II *ж. разг.* misfórtune, disáster.

напа́хивать *сов. см.* напа́ивать.

напе́в *м.* tune, mélody.

напева́ть, напе́ть 1. *тк. несов. (петь вполго́лоса)* hum, croon; 2. *(вн.) разг. (мело́дию и т. п.)* sing* *(smth.)*; напе́ть моти́в sing* a tune; 3. *(для звукоза́писи)* recórd *(smth.)*; напе́ть а́рию на пласти́нку recórd an ária.

напе́вный melódious, túneful.

наперебо́й *разг.:* говори́ть ~ interrúpt one anóther; расска́зывать что́-л. ~ vie with each óther in télling *smth.*

наперегонки́: бе́гать ~ race one anóther, chase each óther.

напереко́р 1. *нареч.* contrárily; идти́ ~ be* contráry; 2. *предло́г:* ~ чему́-л. in defíance of *smth.*; ~ кому́-л. to spite *smb.*

наперере́з: идти́ кому́-л. ~ cut* acróss *smb.'s* path; бежа́ть ~ cut* acróss.

наперечёт 1. *нареч.:* знать всех ~ know* évery síngle one; 2. *в знач. сказ.* few; таки́е, как он, ~ there are not many like him.

наперсток *м.* thímble.

напе́ть *сов. см.* напева́ть 2, 3.

напеча́тать *сов. см.* печа́тать.

напе́чь *сов. (вн., рд.)* bake (a lot of) *(smth.)*.

напива́ться, напи́ться *разг.* 1. drink* *one's* fill, quench *one's* thirst; 2. *(допьяна́)* get* drunk.

напили́ть *сов. (вн., рд.)* saw* *(smth.)*; ~ тёсу, дров saw* some boards, firewood.

напи́льник *м.* file.

напира́ть *несов. разг.* 1. *(тесни́ть)* press hard; 2. *(на вн.; де́лать упо́р)* come* down (on); *(подчёркивать)* put* the émphasis (on); stress *(smth.)*.

напис|а́ние *с.* spélling. ~а́ть *сов. см.* писа́ть 1, 2, 6.

напи́ток *м.* drink; béverage *книжн.*

напи́ться *сов. см.* напива́ться.

напиха́ть *сов. см.* напи́хивать.

напи́хивать, напиха́ть *разг.* 1. *(вн., рд. в вн.)* cram *(smth.* into); напиха́ть веще́й в чемода́н cram things into a case; 2. *(вн. тв.)* stuff *(smth.* with); напиха́ть шкаф бельём stuff a wárdrobe with línen.

напи́чкать *сов. см.* пи́чкать.

напла́каться *сов.* 1. *(вдо́воль попла́кать)* have* a good cry; 2. *(с тв.) разг. (получи́ть мно́го неприя́тностей)* have* tróuble (with).

напластова́ние *с.* stratificátion.

наплева́тельск|ий *разг.;* ~ое отноше́ние slápdash áttitude, cóuldn't-care-léss áttitude.

наплева́ть *сов.* 1. spit*; 2. *разг.* ему́ ~ he dóesn't care; ему́ ~ на всё he dóesn't give a damn for ánything.

наплести́ *сов. (вн., рд.)* 1. *(изгото́вить плете́нием)* weave* (a lot of) *(smth.)*; 2. *разг. (наговори́ть взд́ора)* talk (a lot of) nónsense.

наплы́в *м.* 1. *(большо́е коли́чество)* flow, wave; *(прие́зжих)* ínflux; 2. *бот. (наро́ст на дере́вьях)* excréscence; 3. *кино́* dissólve.

наповал: уби́ть кого́-л. ~ kill *smb.* outríght.

наподо́бие like, resémbling.

напои́ть *сов. (вн.)* 1. *(дать пить)* give* *(smb.)* a drink; *(скот)* wáter *(smth.)*; ~ кого́-л. ча́ем, молоко́м и *т. п.* give* *smb.* some tea, milk *etc.*; 2. *(спиртны́м)* make* *(smb.)* drunk; 3. *(напо́лнить, насы́тить чем-л.)* fill *(smth.)*.

напока́з 1. on show; выставля́ть това́ры ~ put* goods on show; 2. *(для ви́ду)* for show; де́лать что́-л. ~ do* *smth.* for show.

напо́лнить(ся) *сов. см.* наполня́ть(ся).

наполня́ть, напо́лнить *(вн.)* fill *(smth.)*; ~ корзи́ну гриба́ми fill a básket with múshrooms. ~ся, напо́лниться fill, be* filled.

наполови́ну half; сде́лано то́лько ~ ónly half done.

напомин|а́ние *с.* 1. *(де́йствие)* méntion; *(при одно́м ~а́нии о...* at the mere méntion of...; 2. *(извеще́ние)* remínder. ~а́ть, напо́мнить 1. *(дт. вн., о пр.)* remind *(smb.* of, abóut); не забу́дь напо́мнить мне об э́том don't forget to remind me abóut it; письмо́ напо́мнило про́шлое the létter brought back the past; 2. *тк. несов. (вн., быть похо́жим)* look like *(smb., smth.)*; resémble (*smb.*, *smth.*); он ~áет мне моегó брáта he reminds me of my bróther.

напóмнить *сов. см.* напоминáть 1.

напóр *м.* 1. (*давление*) préssure, thrust; ~ воды the préssure of the wáter; 2. (*решительное действие*) préssure; под ~ом врагá únder énemy préssure; 3. *разг.* (*настойчивость*) énergy, drive; со свóйственным емý ~ом with his cústomary énergy.

напóрист|ость *ж.* drive, énergy, assértiveness; ~ харáктера fórceful cháracter. ~ый fórceful, vígorous, energétic; ~ый человéк gó-ahead pérson.

напослéдок *разг.* (*под конец*) towárds the end; (*на прощание*) by way of fárewéll.

напрáвить(ся) *сов. см.* направлять(ся).

направлéн|ие *с.* 1. diréction (*тж. перен.*); по всем ~иям in all diréctions; по ~ию к in the diréction of; ~ полúтики diréction of pólicy; 2. (*течение*) trend; ~ мыслей the trend of *one's* thoughts; ~ умá turn of mind; литератýрное ~ líterary school; 3. (*документ*) órder, permít; получúть ~ на завóд be* assígned to a fáctory, be* dirécted to work at a fáctory; 4. (*участок фронта*) séctor; line of advánce.

напрáвлен|ость *ж.* púrposefulness, sense of púrpose; идéйная ~ sense of ideológical púrpose. ~ый púrposeful.

направлять, напрáвить (*вн.*) 1. diréct (*smb.*, *smth.*); (*устремлять*) turn (*smth.*); (*оружие*) aim (*smth.*); level (*smth.*); ~ свои сúлы на что-л. diréct *one's* énergies to *smth.*; ~ удáр прóтив когó-л., чегó-л. aim/diréct a blow at *smb.*, *smth.*; ~ струю на что-л. turn a jet of wáter upón *smth.*; 2. (*посылать*) send* (*smb.*, *smth.*); ~ когó-л. к врачý send* *smb.* to a dóctor. ~ся, напрáвиться set* off (for); ~ся к двéри move towárds the door, move in the diréction of the door.

напрáво to the right; ~ от чегó-л. on the right of *smth.*; ~ от меня on my right hand; ~! (*команда*) right turn!; ~ и налéво right and left.

напрактиковáться *сов. см.* практиковáться 1.

напрáсн|о 1. *нареч.* (*зря*) without réason; ~ вы емý рассказáли you shóuldn't have told him; ~! you shóuldn't have (done that)!; 2. *в знач. сказ.* (*тщетно, бесполезно*) in vain; всё было ~ it was no use/good. ~ый 1. (*тщетный*) vain; 2. (*ненужный*) unwárranted, unnécessary; 3. *уст.* (*несправедливый*) unjúst.

напрáшив|аться, напросúться 1. (*добиваться*) ask for; ~ в гóсти fish for an invitátion; 2. (*на вн.; вызывать что-л.*) ask (for); ~ на неприятности ask for tróuble; ~ на оскорблéние ask for a snub; 3. *тк. несов.* (*о мысли и т. п.*) suggést itsélf; вывод ~ается сам собóй the conclúsion is forced upón one; невóльно ~ается сравнéние a compárison suggésts itsélf.

напримéр for exámple, for ínstance (*сокр.* e.g.).

напрокáзить *сов. см.* прокáзить.

напрокáзничать *сов. см.* прокáзничать.

напрокáт: брать что-л. ~ híre *smth.*; (от)давáть что-л. ~ híre out *smth.*, let* *smth.* out on híre.

напролёт *разг.:* весь день ~ all day long; the whole day; просúживать нóчи ~ sit* up night áfter night.

напролóм *разг.* straight through/ahéad; идтú ~ go* straight ahéad, break* through.

напропалýю *разг.* récklessly.

напрорóчить *сов. см.* прорóчить.

напросúться *сов. см.* напрáшиваться 1, 2.

напрóтив 1. *нареч.* ópposite; (*на противоположной стороне улицы*) acróss the street, óver the way; он сидéл ~ he sat ópposite; 2. *нареч.* (*наоборот*) on the cóntrary; 3. *предлог* (*рд.*) ópposite, fácing.

напрягáть, напрячь (*вн.*) 1. (*делать упругим*) brace (*smth.*), táuten (*smth.*); ~ мýскулы brace/táuten the múscles; 2. (*повышать степень проявления чего-л.*) brace (*smth.*), exért (*smth.*), strain (*smth.*); ~ все усúлия strain évery nerve; use/exért évery éffort, do*

one's útmost; ~ слух strain *one's* ears; ~ зрéние strain *one's* eyes. ~ся, напрячься 1. (*становиться упругим*) táuten, becóme* taut, tíghten; 2. (*собрать все свои силы*) brace onesélf, exért onesélf; 3. (*усиливаться в своём проявлении*) be* inténsified.

напряжéние *с.* 1. (*усилие*) éffort, strain, exértion; слýшать с ~м lísten with strained atténtion; 2. (*трудное положение*) préssure, strain; ~ на трáнспорте в часы пик strain on tránsport dúring the rush hours; 3. *тех.* stress; 4. *эл.* ténsion, vóltage; высóкое ~ high ténsion/vóltage.

напряжённ|ость *ж.* 1. inténsity; 2. (*натянутость*) ténsion; ~ый 1. (*неослабевающий*) inténse, tense; (*интенсивный*) strénuous, inténsive; ~ое внимáние strained atténtion; ~ая рабóта hard/strénuous work; 2. (*затруднительный, натянутый*) strained, tense; ~ая атмосфéра tense átmosphere; ~ые отношéния strained relátions; 3. (*принуждённый, неестественный*) forced, strained.

напрямúк *разг.* 1. by the diréct way; идтú ~ take* a short cut; (*за городом*) go* acróss cóuntry; ~ бýдет два киломéтра it's two kílometres as the crow flies; 2. (*откровенно*) straight (out), point-blánk; сказáть комý-л. ~ tell* *smb.* point-blánk, tell* *smb.* straight.

напрячь(ся) *сов. см.* напрягáть(ся).

напýганный fríghtened, scared.

напугáть *сов.* (*вн.*) fríghten (*smb.*), térrify (*smb.*). ~ся *сов.* be* fríghtened, be* térrified.

напýдрить(ся) *сов. см.* пýдрить(ся).

напускáть, напустúть 1. (*вн., рд.*) admít (*smb., smth.*) let* in (*smb., smth.*); (*о воде, дыме и т. п.*) let* (*smth.*); напустúть жильцóв в дом take* in a lot of lódgers; напустúть пóлную вáнну воды fill a bath with wáter; напустúть дыма в кóмнату let* a lot of smoke ínto the room; 2. *разг.:* ~ на себя вáжность put* on airs; 3. (*вн. на вн.*) *разг.* (*натравливать*) set* (*smth.* on). ~ся, напустúться (*на вн.*) *разг.* pitch ínto (*smb.*).

напуски|óй assúmed, affécted; ~óе равнодýшие stúdied indífference.

напустúть(ся) *сов. см.* напускáть(ся).

напýт|ать *сов.* (*вн.*) *разг.* múddle (*smth.*); ~ в áдресе get* the addréss wrong; ~ в вычислéниях make* mistákes in calculátion; здесь чтó-то ~ано there's some mistáke here; он всё ~ал he has múddled éverything up.

напýтственн|ый: ~ое слóво ~ напýтствие.

напýтствие *с.* párting words/injúnctions *pl.*

напýтствовать *несов. и сов.* say* in párting.

напыхáться *сов. см.* пыхáться.

напыщенный 1. pómpous; 2. (*о речи, стиле*) bombástic, híghflown, grandíloquent.

нарабóтать *сов.* (*вн., рд.*) *разг.* 1. (*произвести*) make* (a lot of) (*smth.*): 2. (*заработать*) earn (*smth.*). ~ся *сов. разг.* work enóugh.

наравнé 1. (*на одном уровне*) on the same lével (as), lével (with); 2. (*на равных правах*) on équal terms.

нараспáшку *разг.* unbúttoned; он нóсит пальтó ~ he wears his coat unbúttoned, he does not bútton his coat; ◇ у негó душá ~ he is open-héarted.

нараспéв in a síngsong, síngingly.

нарастáние *с.* íncrease, growth; ~ революциóнного движéния the móunting actívity of the revolútionary móvement; ~ тéмпов accelerátion, spéeding-up.

нарастáть, нарастú 1. (*вырастать на чём-л.*) grow*, form; 2. *тк. несов.* (*увеличиваться*) íncrease, grow*; (*о звуке*) swell*; 3. (*накапливаться — о процентах и т. п.*) accúmulate.

нарастú *сов. см.* нарастáть 1, 3.

нарасхвáт: билéты берýт ~ the tíckets are sélling like hot cakes; эту кнúгу покупáют, берýт ~ this book is in great demánd.

наращéние *с.* growth, íncrease, augmentátion.

нара́щивание с. íncrease; ~ те́мпов произво́дства sté́pping up the rate of prodúction.

нарва́ть I *сов. см.* нарыва́ть.

нарва́ть II *сов. (вн., рд.)* 1. *(цветов, плодов и т. п.)* pick (a lot of) *(smth.)*; 2. *(разорвать на куски)* tear* up *(smth.)*.

нарва́ться *сов. см.* нарыва́ться.

наре́зать *сов.* 1. *см.* нареза́ть; 2. *(вн., рд.; какое-л. количество)* cut* (a lot of) *(smth.)*; ~ таре́лку ветчины́ cut* a plate of ham.

нареза́ть, наре́зать *(вн.)* 1. cut* *(smth.)*; *(хлеб)* slice *(smth.)*, cut* *(smth.)* ínto slices; *(мясо за столом)* carve *(smth.)*; 2. *(винт)* thread *(smth.)*; *(ствол оружия)* rífle *(smth.)*; 3. *(участки земли)* allót *(smth.)*.

наре́зка ж. *тех.* thread; *(в канале ствола)* rífling.

нарека́ни|е с. repróach, repróof; вы́звать ~я evóke únfávourable críticism.

наре́чие I с. *лингв.* díalect.

наре́ч|ие II с. *грам.* ádverb. ~ный *грам.* advérbial.

нарисова́ть *сов. см.* рисова́ть.

нарица́тельн|ый: и́мя ~ое *грам.* cómmon noun; ~ая сто́имость эк. nóminal value.

нарко́з м. 1. *мед.* narcósis, anaesthésia; под ~ом únder (an) anaesthétic; 2. *разг. (средство)* anaesthétic, narcótic.

наркома́н м. drug áddict. ~ия ж. drug addíction. ~ка ж. drug áddict.

нарко́т|ик м. (narcótic) drug; злоупотребле́ние ~иками drug abúse. ~и́ческий narcótic.

наро́д м. 1. *(население государства)* the péople; ру́сский ~ the Rússian péople; 2. *(нация)* a péople; все ~ы ми́ра all péoples/nátions; 3. *тк. ед. (люди)* péople; мно́го ~у a great mány péople; 4: *тк. ед. (основная, трудовая масса населения)* the péople; ◇ просто́й ~ the cómmon péople; на ~е in públic.

наро́дность ж. 1. natiónality; 2. *тк. ед. (национальная, народная самобытность)* nátional cháracter; nátional roots *pl;* kínship with the péople; ~ в поэ́зии Пу́шкина the nátional cháracter of Púshkin's póetry.

народнохозя́йственный nátional ecónomic.

наро́дн|ый of the péople *после сущ.,* péople's; *(принадлежащий народу, стране тж.)* nátional; *(о песнях, обычаях и т. п.)* folk *attr.;* ~ые ма́ссы the péople; ~ое хозя́йство nátional ecónomy; ~ое достоя́ние próperty of the péople; ~ое тво́рчество pópular/folk art; ~ая пе́сня fólk-song; ~ суд Péople's Court; ~ арти́ст Péople's Ártist; ~ое ополче́ние nátional voluntéers; ~ фронт pópular front; ~ университе́т культу́ры públic lécture céntre.

народонаселе́ние с. populátion.

наро́ст м. 1. excréscence; 2. *(опухоль)* growth.

наро́читый delíberate; *(показной)* affécted.

наро́чно 1. *(сознательно)* on púrpose; *(специально)* púrposely; 2. *разг. (в шутку)* for fun; ◇ как ~ of course, it had to háppen.

наро́чн|ый м. cóurier; с ~ым (by) spécial delívery.

на́рт|а ж., ~ы *мн.* sledge; *(для езды на собаках)* dóg-sledge.

наруби́ть *сов. (вн., рд.)* *(срубить в каком-л. количестве)* fell (a lot of) *(smth.)*, cut* down (a lot of) *(smth.)*; *(рубя, приготовить)* chop/cut* (a lot of) *(smth.)*.

нару́жн|ость ж. 1. appéarance; looks *pl;* прия́тной ~ости of pléasant appéarance; 2. *(внешний вид чего-л.)* extérior. ~ый 1. extérior, extérnal; *(обращённый наружу тж.)* óutside; *(производимый снаружи)* from óutside; 2. *(показной)* óutward; ~ое споко́йствие óutward calm/compósure; 3. *(о лекарстве)* for extérnal use ónly.

нару́жу out, óutside; on the óutside; *перен.* ín(to) the ópen; ◇ весь ~ compléte ópen; всё ~ éverything in the ópen.

нарука́вники *мн. (ед.* нарука́вник *м.)* óversleeves.

наруми́нить *сов. см.* румя́нить 2. ~ся *сов. см.* румя́ниться 2.

нару́чники *мн. (ед.* нару́чник *м.)* hándcuffs, mánacles.

наруш|а́ть, нару́шить *(вн.)* 1. *(не соблюдать)* break* *(smth.)*, víolate *(smth.)*; *(закон, договор и т. п. тж.)* infrínge *(smth.)*; ~ дисципли́ну víolate díscipline; ~ госуда́рственную грани́цу víolate the State fróntier; 2. *(мешать, прерывать)* distúrb *(smth.)*; ~ тишину́ break*/distúrb the stíllness. ~е́ние с. 1. breach, violátion; *(договора и т. п.)* infríngement; ~е́ние обще́ственного поря́дка breach of the peace; ~е́ние грани́цы illégal cróssing of the fróntier, bórder violátion; 2. *(покоя)* distúrbance. ~и́тель м. offénder; ~и́тель грани́цы fróntier intrúder/víolator; ~и́тель обще́ственного поря́дка distúrber of the peace.

нару́шить *сов. см.* наруша́ть.

нарци́сс м. *бот.* narcíssus *(pl* -ssi); жёлтый ~ dáffodil.

на́ры *мн.* plank bed *sg.*

нары́в м. boil; *(внутренний)* ábscess; gáthering *разг.*

нарыв|а́ть, нарва́ть féster; gáther *разг.;* у меня́ па́лец ~а́ет my finger is begínning to féster.

нарыва́ться, нарва́ться *(на вн.) разг.* run* (ínto).

наря́д I м. *(одежда)* attíre, appárel; *мн.* clothes.

наря́д II м. 1. *(документ)* órder; *(на получение товаров)* wárrant; 2. *воен. (задание)* dúty; ~ вне о́череди éxtra dúty; 3. *(группа лиц)* (spécial-duty) squad; detáil.

наряди́ть I, II *сов. см.* наряжа́ть I, II.

наряди́ться *сов. см.* наряжа́ться.

наря́дн|ый smart, wéll-dréssed; *(празднично убранный)* gáily décorated, féstive; ~ое пла́тье smart dress; ~ая де́вушка wéll-dréssed girl.

наряду́: ~ с on a lével with; *(на одинаковых правах)* togéther with; ~ со все́ми like éveryone else; ◇ ~ с э́тим at the same time.

наряжа́ть I, наряди́ть *(вн.; одевать)* dress *(smb.)* up.

наряжа́ть II, наряди́ть *(вн.)* 1. *(давать наряд)* assign *(smb.)*; send* *(smb.)*; 2. *(назначать в наряд)* detáil *(smb.)*.

наряжа́ться, наряди́ться dress up.

нас *(рд., вн. от личн. мест.* мы) us; ~ дво́е (тро́е и т. д.) there are two (three *etc.)* of us.

насади́ть *сов. (вн.)* 1. *(растения)* plant *(smth.)*; 2. *(плотно надеть что-л.)* fix *(smth.)*; 3. *см.* насажда́ть.

насажд|а́ть, насади́ть *(вн.; распространять)* spread* *(smth.)*; ~ нау́ку spread* knówledge. ~е́ние с. 1. *(растений)* plánting; 2. *(распространение)* spréading, propagátion; 3. *обыкн. мн. (посаженные деревья и т. п.)* plantátions.

насви́стывать *несов.* 1. pipe; 2. *(о птицах)* pipe, twitter.

наседа́ть, насе́сть 1. *(о пыли)* séttle (on); 2. *(на вн.) разг. (наваливаться)* fall* on *(smth.)*; *перен. (требовать)* press *(smth.)*; *сов. тж.* pounce on *(smth.)*; 3. *тк. несов. (на вн.) разг. (теснить)* press *(smth.)* hard.

насе́дка ж. bróody (hen).

насеко́мое с. ínsect.

населе́ние с. populátion; inhabitants *pl.*

населён|ость ж. dénsity of populátion. ~ый 1. *(тв.)* pópulated (with); inhábited (by); 2. *(имеющий много жителей)* pópulous; *(о квартире)* crówded; ◇ ~ый пункт pópulated área/locálity.

насели́ть *сов. см.* населя́ть 1.

населя́ть, насели́ть *(вн.)* 1. *(заселять)* pópulate *(smth.)*, put* péople (ínto); ~ но́вый дом put* péople/ténants ínto a new house; 2. *тк. несов. (составлять население)* inhábit *(smth.)*, pópulate *(smth.)*.

насе́ст м. roost, perch.

насе́сть *сов. см.* наседа́ть 1, 2.

насе́чка *ж.* 1. (*действие*) incising; 2. (*украшение на металле*) ínlay, damascéne.

наси́женн|ый: ~ое ме́сто cómfortable perch.

наси́л|ие *с.* víolence; (*принуждение*) coércion. ~овать, изнаси́ловать (*вн.*) 1. (*женщину*) rape (*smb.*); 2. *тк. несов.* (*принуждать*) coérce (*smb., smth.*); force; ~овать чью-л. во́лю coérce *smb.*; ~овать себя́ force onesélf.

наси́лу *разг.* ónly just, hárdly; я ~ добра́лся (до) I thought I should néver get (here, there, home *etc.*); ~ я вас дожда́лся I thought you would néver come.

наси́ль|ник *м.* týrant, oppréssor. ~но by force, agáinst *one's* will; ~но мил не бу́дешь *погов.* love cánnot be forced.

наси́льственн|ый fórcible, víolent; ◇ ~ая смерть death by víolence, víolent death; умере́ть ~ой сме́ртью come* to a víolent end.

наска́кивать, наскочи́ть (на *вн.*) 1. (*натыкаться*) run* (ínto) (*тж. перен.*); наскочи́ть на ми́ну strike* a mine; 2. (*набрасываться, нападать*) pounce on (*smb.*); 3. *разг.* (*накидываться с упрёками*) jump at (smb.), fly* at (smb.).

наска́льн|ый rock *attr.;* ~ые изображе́ния rock cárvings.

наскандалить *сов. см.* скандалить.

наскво́зь 1. through; ~ прогни́вший *презр.* rótten to the core; 2. (*через всё протяжение чего-л.*) from end to end; овра́г ~ простре́ливался проти́вником the whole ravíne, from one end to the óther, was expósed to énemy fíre; 3. *разг.* (*полностью*) complétely, throughóut.

наско́лько as far as; (*в вопросах, восклицаниях*) how much; ~ мне изве́стно as far as I know; ~ второ́е изда́ние лу́чше пе́рвого! how much bétter the sécond edítion is than the first one!

на́скоро *разг.* hástily, húrriedly; (*о работе тж.*) in a slápdash mánner; ~ пообе́дав... áfter a húrried dínner...

наскочи́ть *сов. см.* наска́кивать.

наскрести́ *сов.* (*вн.; прям. и перен.*) scrape (*smth.*) up/togéther, scratch (*smth.*) up/togéther.

наску́ч|ить *сов.* (*дт.*) tire (*smb.*), wéary (*smb.*); мне э́то ~ило I am tíred of it.

наслади́ться *сов. см.* наслажда́ться.

наслажд|а́ться, наслади́ться (*тв.*) enjóy (*smth.*), rével (in). ~е́ние *с.* delíght, pléasure, enjóyment.

насла́ивать, насло́иться form láyers *перен.* accúmulate, accréte.

насле́дие *с.* légacy.

насле́дить *сов. см.* следи́ть II.

насле́д|ник *м.* 1. heir; 2. (*преемник*) succéssor. ~ница *ж.* héiress. ~ование *с.* inhéritance.

насле́довать *несов. и сов.* 1. (*вн.; получать в наследство*) inhérit (*smth.*); 2. (*дт.*) be* heir (to), succéed (to).

насле́дственн|ость *ж.* herédity. ~ый heréditary.

насле́дств|о *с.* 1. inhéritance; (*по завещанию*) légacy; лиша́ть кого-л. ~а disínherit *smb.*; 2. (*наследие*) légacy.

насло|е́ние *с.* *геол.* stratificátion, láyer; *перен.* accrétion. ~и́ться *сов. см.* насла́иваться.

наслу́шаться *сов.* (*рд.*) 1. (*услышать много чего-л.*) hear* (a lot of) (*smth.*); 2. (*вдоволь послушать*) hear* enóugh (of, *smth.*).

наслы́шаться *сов.* (о *пр.*) *разг.* hear* enóugh (abóut).

насма́рку *разг.:* идти́ ~ come* to nóthing.

на́смерть mórtally; *перен.* to the last; разби́ться ~ be* killed (in a crash); have* a fátal áccident; стоя́ть ~ make* one's last stand.

насмеха́ться *несов.* (над *тв.*) mock (*smb., smth.*), jeer (at), taunt (*smb.*), gíbe at.

насмеши́ть *сов.* (*вн.*) make* (*smb.*) laugh.

насме́ш|ка *ж.* gibe, sneer, taunt; *мн. тж.* móckery *sg*, derísion *sg*; в ~ку derísively. ~ливый 1. (*склонный к насмешкам*) sarcástic, sardónic; ~ливый челове́к sarcástic pérson; 2. (*выражающий насмешку*) derísive, mócking; ~ливый тон derísive tone. ~ник *м. разг.* scóffer, mócker.

на́сморк *м.* cold (in the head).

насмотре́ться *сов.* 1. (на *вн.*) (*вдоволь посмотреть на*) gaze *one's* fill (upón), gaze long enóugh (at); 2. (*рд.; увидеть много чего-л.*) see* (plénty of) (*smth.*).

насол|и́ть *сов.* 1. (*вн., рд.*) salt (a lot of) (*smth.*), píckle (a lot of) (*smth.*); ~ грибо́в на́ зиму píckle a good supply of múshrooms for the winter; 2. (*вн.*) *разг.* (*сильно посолить*) oversált (*smth.*); 3. (*дт.*) *разг.* (*сделать неприятность*) make* tróuble (for); он э́то сде́лал, что́бы ~ мне he did it to spite me; он мне поря́дком ~и́л he did me a lot of harm.

насори́ть *сов.* lítter; ~ на́ пол lítter the floor with rúbbish.

насо́с *м.* pump.

на́спех in a húrry.

насплётничать *сов. см.* сплётничать.

наст *м.* frózen snow, íce-encrústed snow.

настава́ть, наста́ть come*; наста́ла ночь night has fállen; вре́мя ещё не наста́ло the time has not yet come.

настави́тельный didáctic; ~ тон didáctic tone.

наста́вить I *сов. см.* наставля́ть I; 2. (*вн., рд.; поставить в большом количестве*) put* (a lot of) (*smth.*).

наста́вить II *сов. см.* наставля́ть II.

наставле́ние *с.* 1. injúnction; 2. (*руководство, инструкция*) diréctions *pl.*

наставля́ть I, наста́вить (*вн., удлинять*) léngthen (*smth.*); ~ не́сколько сантиме́тров add a few céntimetres.

наставля́ть II, наста́вить (*вн.; поучать*) admónish (*smb.*); ◇ ~ кого-л. на путь и́стинный set* *smb.* in the right way.

наста́вник *м.* téacher, instrúctor; tútor.

наста́ивать I, настоя́ть (на *пр.*) insíst (on); настоя́ть на своём get* *one's* way.

наста́ивать II, настоя́ть (*вн.; приготавливать настой чего-л.*) make* an infúsion (of).

наста́иваться, настоя́ться draw*; (*о чае*) brew.

наста́ть *сов. см.* настава́ть.

на́стежь wide ópen; окно́ бы́ло (о́ткрыто) ~ the window was wide ópen.

настига́ть, насти́гнуть, насти́чь (*вн.*) overtáke* (*smb.*), catch* up (with).

насти́гнуть *сов. см.* настига́ть.

насти́л *м.* flóoring; (*из досок*) plánking.

настила́ть, настла́ть (*вн., рд.*) 1. (*расстилать*) spread* (*smth.*); 2. (*плотно укладывать*) lay* (*smth.*); ~ пол lay* a floor.

насти́лка *ж.:* ~ поло́в láying floors.

насти́чь *сов. см.* настига́ть.

настла́ть *сов. см.* настила́ть и стлать 2.

насто́й *м.* infúsion; (*лекарственный*) éxtract.

насто́йка *ж.* 1. (*спиртной напиток*) liquéur; 2. (*раствор*) tíncture.

насто́йчив|ость *ж.* persevérance, persístence. ~ый 1. (*о человеке*) persevéring, persístent, dógged; 2. (*выражающий настойчивость*) insístent; ~ые про́сьбы insístent/préssing requests.

насто́лько so; не ~ умён, силён *и т. д.* not cléver, strong, *etc.* enóugh.

насто́льн|ый 1. desk *attr.;* ~ая ла́мпа desk lamp; (*на ночном столике*) réading-lamp; 2.: ~ая кни́га hándbook; (*любимая*) fávourite book, béd-side book, desk compánion.

насторо́живать, насторожи́ть (*вн.*) put* (*smb.*) on his, her guard. ~ся, насторожи́ться be* alérted.

насторожё on the alért; быть ~ be* on the alért.

насторожённый tense, wátchful; ~ взгляд guárded look.

насторожить(ся) *сов. см.* настора́живать(ся).

настоя́н|ие *с.* insistence; по ~ию *кого-л.* on smb.'s insistence; по ~ию врача́ on dóctor's órders.

настоя́тель *м.* 1. (*монастыря́*) ábbot, príor; 2. (*старший свяще́нник собо́ра*) dean.

настоя́тельн|ый 1. (*настойчивый*) insistent; (*упо́рный*) persístent; ~ое тре́бование préssing demánd; 2. (*насущный*) úrgent, préssing; ~ая необходи́мость úrgent necéssity.

настоя́ть I, II *сов. см.* наста́ивать I, II.

настоя́ться *сов. см.* наста́иваться.

настоя́щ|ее *с.* the présent. ~ий 1. (*тепе́решний*) présent; в ~ее время at présent; (*в наши дни*) todáy; 2. (*подлинный*) real, true; (*истинный тж.*) génuine; régular *разг.*; (*натуральный*) real; ~ий ко́фе real cóffee; ~ее зо́лото real gold; 3. (*этот, да́нный*) the présent; ~ая кни́га the présent book, this book; ◇ ~ее время *грам.* présent (tense).

настра́ивать, **настро́ить** (*вн.*) 1. (*музыка́льный инструме́нт*) tune (*smth.*); 2. (*нала́живать стано́к и т. п.*) adjúst (*smth.*); 3. (*радиоприёмник*) tune in (*smth.*); 4. (*в по́льзу кого́-л.*) influence (*smb.*) in smb.'s fávour; (*про́тив кого́-л.*) set* (*smb.*) agáinst; 5. (*приводи́ть в како́е-л. настрое́ние*): ~ кого́-л. на гру́стный лад put* smb. in a mélancholy frame of mind. ~ся, настро́иться 1. (*испытывать како́е-л. чу́вство по отноше́нию к кому́-л.*) feel* dispósed; он сра́зу настро́ился про́тив воше́дшего he took an immédiate dislike to the néwcomer; 2. (*на вн.*, + *инф.*; *намерева́ться*) be* just góing (+ to inf), inténd (+ to inf); get* into the mood (for).

на́строго *разг.* strictly.

настрое́ни|е *с.* mood; frame of mind; (*дух*) spírits *pl*; у меня́ нет ~я игра́ть I am not in the mood for pláying, I am in no mood to play; испо́ртить ~ кому́-л. put* smb. out of húmour; в дурно́м (хоро́шем) ~и in low (high) spírits; ◇ быть не в ~и be* off form; челове́к ~я pérson/man* of moods, pérson of chángeable disposítion.

настро́ить I *сов.* (*вн.*, *рд.*) build* (a lot of) (*smth.*).

настро́ить II *сов. см.* настра́ивать. ~ся *сов. см.* настра́иваться.

настро́й|ка *ж.* 1. (*музыка́льного инструме́нта*) túning; 2. (*радиоприёмника*) túning (in). ~щик *м.* 1. (*роя́лей*) piáno-túner; 2. (*станко́в*) adjúster.

настрочи́ть *сов. см.* строчи́ть 2.

наступа́тельн|ый offénsive; ~ бой offénsive; ~ая война́ war of offénce; ~ая поли́тика vígorous/áctive pólicy.

наступа́ть I, **наступи́ть** 1. (*на вн.*; *ного́й*) tread* (on); 2. *тк. несов. воен.* advánce, attáck; undertáke*/launch an offénsive (*тж. перен.*); на пусты́ню launch an offénsive agáinst the désert; 3. *тк. несов.* (*на вн.*; *подступа́ть с про́сьбами и т. п.*) péster (*smb.*), nag (*smb.*); 4. *тк. несов.* (*на вн.*; *вплотну́ю подходи́ть к чему́-л.*) begín* to encróach (on).

наступа́ть II, **наступи́ть** (*начина́ться, настава́ть*) come*, set* in; (*о ве́чере, тишине́*) fall*; наступи́ло ле́то súmmer has come.

наступи́ть I *сов. см.* наступа́ть I 1.

наступи́ть II *сов. см.* наступа́ть II.

наступле́ние I *с. воен.* offénsive, advánce, attáck.

наступле́ни|е II *с.* (*нача́ло*) cóming; (*приближе́ние*) appróach; с ~ем но́чи when night came; с ~ем темноты́ with the cóming of dárkness; до ~я зимы́ before winter sets in.

настурция *ж. бот.* nastúrtium.

насу́п|ить *сов.*: ~ бро́ви frown, knit* one's brows. ~ся *сов.* 1. (*приня́ть суро́вый вид*) scowl; 2. (*сдви́нуться — о бровя́х*) draw* togéther, contráct, knit*.

на́сухо dry; вы́тереть *что-л.* ~ wipe *smth.* dry.

насуши́ть *сов.* (*вн.*, *рд.*) dry (a lot of) (*smth.*).

насу́щн|ый vítal, esséntial; ~ вопро́с quéstion of vítal impórtance, vítal íssue; ~ые потре́бности vítal/esséntial needs.

насчёт *разг.* abóut, as regárds; concérning; ~ э́того on that score.

насчита́ть *сов. см.* насчи́тывать 1.

насчи́тыва|ть, **насчита́ть** (*вн.*) 1. count (*smth.*); ско́лько страни́ц вы насчита́ли? how mány páges do you make it?; 2. *тк. несов.* (*содержа́ть*) númber (*smth.*); го́род ~ает три́дцать ты́сяч жи́телей the town has thírty thóusand inhábitants. ~аться *несов.* númber.

насыпа́ть *сов. см.* насыпа́ть.

насыпа́ть, **насы́пать** 1. (*вн.*; *наполня́ть*) fill (*smth.*); насы́пать мешо́к ро́жью fill a sack with rye; 2. (*вн. рд.*; *всыпа́ть в како́м-л. коли́честве*) pour (*smth.*); насы́пать мешо́к муки́ pour a sáckful of flour; 3. (*вн.*; *наброса́ть*) strew* (a lot of) (*smth.*); 4. (*вн.*; *возводи́ть*) make* (*smth.*), eréct (*smth.*); ~ плоти́ну make* a dam.

на́сыпь *ж.* embánkment.

насы́пать(ся) *сов. см.* насыща́ть(ся).

насыщ|а́ть, **насы́тить** (*вн.*) 1. (*пи́щей*) fill (*smb.*); sátiate (*smb.*, *smth.*) (*тж. перен.*) 2. *хим.* sáturate (*smth.*). ~а́ться, насы́титься 1. (*пи́щей*) have* had enóugh, be* sátisfied; 2. *хим.* sáturate. ~е́ние *с.* 1. (*едо́й*) satiátion, satíety; 2. *хим.* saturátion.

насы́щенный 1. *хим.* sáturated; 2. (*о́чень содержа́тельный*) méaningful, cóncentrated.

ната́лкивать, **натолкну́ть** (*вн. на вн.*) incíte (*smb.* to); натолкну́ть кого́-л. на мысль give* *smb.* the idéa, suggést the idéa to *smb.* ~ся, натолкну́ться (*на вн.*) 1. knock (agáinst), run* (into); strike* (*smth.*), *перен.* come* up (agáinst); 2. (*неожи́данно находи́ть, обнару́живать*) come* acróss (*smb.*, *smth.*).

натаска́ть *сов.* (*вн.*, *рд.*) fetch/bring* (a lot of) (*smth.*).

натвор|и́ть *сов.* (*вн.*, *рд.*) *разг.* do* (*smth.*), be* up to (*smth.*); что вы ~и́ли? look what you've done!

натере́ть *сов.* 1. *см.* натира́ть; 2. (*вн.*, *рд.*; *измельчи́ть*) grate (*smth.*); ~ морко́вь grate some cárrots.

натерпе́ться *сов.* (*рд.*) *разг.* have* súffered a great deal (of); ~ стра́ху have* a térrible fright.

натира́ть, **натере́ть** (*вн.*) 1. rub (*smth.*); ~ грудь скипида́ром rub one's chest with túrpentine; 2. (*раздража́ть, поврежда́ть*) rub (*smth.*) sore, make* (*smth.*) sore; натере́ть себе́ мозо́ль get* a corn; хому́т натёр ше́ю ло́шади the hórse's neck has been galled by the cóllar; 3. (*начища́ть*) pólish (*smth.*), wax (*smth.*).

на́тиск *м.* ónslaught, ónset.

наткну́ться *сов. см.* натыка́ться.

натолкну́ть(ся) *сов. см.* ната́лкивать(ся).

натоло́чь *сов.* (*вн.*, *рд.*) crush (a lot of) (*smth.*), pound (a lot of) (*smth.*), pówder (a lot of) (*smth.*).

натопи́ть *сов.* (*вн.*) heat (*smth.*) (well, thóroughly).

натопта́ть *сов. разг.* (*насле́дить*) leave* fóot-marks.

наточи́ть *сов. см.* точи́ть 1.

натоща́к on an émpty stómach.

натрави́ть *сов. см.* натра́вливать.

натра́вливать, **натрави́ть** (*вн. на вн.*) set* (*smth.* on); *перен.* set* (*smb.* agáinst).

натренирова́ть(ся) *сов. см.* тренирова́ть(ся).

на́трий *м. хим.* sódium, nátrium; углеки́слый ~ sódium cárbonate; хло́ристый ~ sódium chlóride.

нату́р|а *ж.* 1. (*хара́ктер*) disposítion, náture; 2. *иск.* real life; рисова́ть с ~ы paint/draw* from life; 3. (*нату́рщик*) (ártist's) módel; 4. *кино* locátion; на ~е on locátion; 5.: плати́ть ~ой pay* in kind; ◇ привы́чка — втора́я ~ hábit is sécond náture.

натура́л|иза́ция *ж.* naturalizátion. ~и́зм *м.* náturalism. ~и́ст *м.* 1. (*естествоиспыта́тель*) náturalist; юный ~ист young náturalist; 2. (последователь натурализма) expónent of náturalism. ~истический naturalístic.

натурáльн|ый 1. (настоящий) real; ~ шёлк real silk; ~ мёд pure hóney; 2. (соответствующий действительности) nátural, true; ~ цвет nátural cólour; в ~ую величину life-size attr.; 3. (естественный, искренний) nátural; 4. (оплачиваемый натурой) in kind после сущ.; ~ налóг tax in kind; ◇ ~ое хозяйство subsístence ecónomy.

натýрн|ый: выехать на ~ые съёмки go* on locátion.

натýрщ|ик м., ~ица ж. (ártist's) módel.

натыкáться, наткнýться (на вн.) 1. run* (into); наткнýться на гвоздь catch* oneself on a nail; наткнýться на засáду run* into an ámbush; 2. разг. (неожиданно найти, встретить) come* across (smb., smth.).

натюрмóрт м. still life.

натя́гивать, натянýть 1. (вн.) tíghten (smth.); tãuten (smth.); (прикреплять) put* (smth.) on/up; ~ верёвку для белья put* up a clóthes-line; ~ нóвую струну на скрипке put* a new string on a violin; натянýть вóжжи tíghten/pull the reins; ~ холст на рáмку stretch a cánvas on a frame; 2. (вн. на вн.) pull (smth. óver), draw* (smth. óver); ~ на себя одеяло pull up the béd-clothes; 3. (вн.; надевать) pull on (smth.); ~ чулки, сапоги pull* on one's stóckings, boots. ~ся, натянýться tíghten, tãuten.

натя́жк|а ж. irregulárity; (в толковании) strained interpretátion; это ~! that would be to stretch a point!; с ~ой by strétching a point, at a pinch.

натя́нут|ый taut; перен. strained; ~ая улыбка forced/embárrassed smile; ~ые отношения strained relátions.

натянýть(ся) сов. см. натя́гивать(ся).

наугáд at rándom.

наудáчу on the óff-chance.

наýк|а ж. 1. science; 2. (как профессия) stúdy, léarning; посвятить себя ~е devóte oneself to stúdy/léarning; 3. (навыки, знания) knówledge; 4. (нечто поучительное) lésson; это вам ~! let that be a lésson to you!

наукообрáзный scientífic-looking.

наýскать, сов. см. наýскивать.

наýскивать, наýскать (вн.) разг. set* (smth.) on; перен. egg (smb.) on.

наутёк разг. in flight, on the run; пуститься ~ take* to one's heels.

наýтро the next mórning.

научить сов. 1. (вн. дт., вн. + инф.) teach* (smb. smth.), teach* (smb. + to inf); 2. (вн.) разг. (подговорить сделать что-л.) put* (smth.) up to it, give* (smb.) the hint; 3. (вн.; убедить в чём-л.) teach* (smth.). ~ся сов. (дт., + инф.) learn* (+ to inf).

научно-исследовательск|ий (scientífic) reséarch; ~ институт reséarch institute; ~ая рабóта reséarch work; занимáться ~ой рабóтой be* engáged in reséarch.

научно-популя́рн|ый pópular-science attr.; ~ая литератýра pópular-science líterature; ~ые фильмы pópular-science films.

научно-техническ|ий scientífic and téchnical; ~ая литератýра scientífic and téchnical líterature; ~ая интеллигéнция scientists and enginéers; ~ая револю́ция scientífic and technológical revolútion.

научно-фантастический science-fiction attr.; ~ ромáн science-fiction nóvel.

наýчн|ый scientífic; ~ая рабóта scientífic work; ~ рабóтник scientífic/reséarch wórker, scientist; ~ труд ·scientífic work; (в области литературы и т. п.) work of schólarship, stúdy; ~ое обоснование scientífic básis/substantiátion; ~ые учреждéния scientífic institútions.

наýшники мн. (ед. наýшник м.) 1. (на шапке) éar-flaps; 2. (телефона, радио) éar-phones, héad-phones.

нафталин м. náphthalene; (в шариках) móth-balls pl.

нахáл м. ímpudent/ínsolent féllow. ~ка ж. ímpudent wóman*.

нахáль|ный ímpudent, impértinent, ínsolent; ~ человéк ímpudent pérson; ~ постýпок impértinent áction; ~ вид ímpudent appéarance. ~ство с. ímpudence, impértinence, ínsolence; cheek разг.

нахимов|ец м. púpil of the Nakhímov Nával Cóllege. ~ский Nakhímov; ~ское учи́лище Nakhímov Nával Cóllege.

нахлéбник м. hánger-ón (pl hángers-), spónger.

нахлобýчивать, нахлобýчить (вн.) разг. cram (smth.) on; нахлобýчить шáпку pull one's cap óver one's eyes.

нахлобýчить сов. см. нахлобýчивать.

нахлы́н|уть сов. surge; перен. тж. assáil; к нему ~ула молодёжь he was assáiled on all sides by young péople; на негó ~ули воспоминáния mémories of his past life came súrging into his mind.

нахмýренн|ый 1. frówning; ~ое лицó glóomy face; 2. (суровый) grim.

нахмýрить(ся) сов. см. хмýрить(ся).

нахо|дить I, найти (вн.) 1. find* (smb., smth.); (обнаруживать тж.) discóver (smb., smth.); ~ применéние find* application, be* used; я не ~жý слов, чтобы... I can find no words to...; 2. (полагать, считать, что) find* (smth., that), consíder (smth., that); егó нахóдят глýпым he is considered stúpid; ◇ найти свою смерть meet* one's end/death.

находить II, найти (на вн.) 1. (надвигаться) cóver (smth.); нахóдят тýчи héavy clouds are gáthering; 2. разг. (овладевать) overcóme* (smth.); на меня нахóдит тоскá I am overcóme by mélancholy/depréssion.

находиться I, найтись 1. (обнаруживаться в результате поисков) be* found/discóvered, turn up; 2. (оказываться налицо) be*, be* found; не найдётся ли у вас..? do you háppen to have..?; у вас, навéрное, найдётся... you próbably have...; 3. тк. несов. (быть) be*; он нахóдится сейчáс в Москвé he is now in Móscow.

находиться II сов. (много ходить) do* a lot of wálking, walk a long way.

нахóдка ж. 1. a find; 2. (о ком-л., о чём-л. удачно найденном) discóvery, a (háppy) find.

нахóдчив|ость ж. ingenúity, resóurcefulness. ~ый ingénious, resóurceful; ~ый человéк resóurceful pérson; быть ~ым be* réady-witted; ~ый отвéт resóurceful ánswer, smart replý.

нацéнка ж. éxtra charge.

нацепить сов. см. нацеплять.

нацеплять, нацепить (вн.) 1. fásten (smth.); 2. разг. (надевать что-л., приколов, пристегнув) pin (smth.) on; stick* (smth.) on.

национализ|áзия ж. nationalizátion. ~и́ровать несов. и сов. (вн.) nátionalize (smth.).

национал|и́зм м. nátionalism. ~и́ст м. nátionalist. ~исти́ческий nationalístic.

национáльно-освободи́тельн|ый nátional-liberátion attr.; ~ое движéние nátional-liberátion móvement, móvement for nátional liberátion.

национáльност|ь ж. nationálity; какóй он ~и? what's his nationálity?; он рýсский по ~и he is of Rússian nationálity.

национáльн|ый 1. nátional; ~ вопрóс the próblem of nationálities; ~ое движéние nátional móvement; ~ая культýра nátional cúlture; ~ óкруг nátional área; 2. (государственный) nátional; State attr.; ~ суверенитéт nátional sóvereignty; ~ гимн nátional ánthem; ~ дохóд nátional íncome; ◇ ~ое меньшинствó nátional minórity.

нáция ж. nátion.

начадить *сов. см.* чадить.

начал|о *с.* 1. beginning; óutset, start; положить ~ чему-л. mark the beginning of *smth.*; ~ концерта в 8 часов the cóncert begíns at eight o'clóck; с самого ~a right from the start/óutset; в ~e сороковых *и т. п.* годов in the éarly fórties *etc.*; 2. (*источник*) órigin, source; река берёт ~ в... the ríver ríses in...; 3. (*основа чего-л.*) source, élement; организующее ~ órganizing élement; 4. *мн.* (*принципы*) prínciples; 5. *мн.* (*способы, методы*) lines; básis *sg*; ◇ под ~ом у кого-л. únder *smb.'s* authórity.

начальник *м.* chief, head; *воен.* commánder; ~ станции státion-máster; ~ цеха shop superintendent.

начальн|ый 1. (*находящийся в начале чего-л.*) first, inítial; 2. (*первоначальный*) prímary, eleméntary; ~ое образование prímary education.

начальственный authóritative, dictatórial; ~ тон perémptory tone.

начальство *с.* 1. *собир.* (*начальники*) the authórities *pl*; 2. *разг.* (*начальник*) chief; 3. (*власть начальника*) commánd, authórity.

начальствующ|ий: ~ие лица commánders, péople in charge/authórity.

начатки *мн.* rúdiments, élements.

начать *сов. см.* начинать. ~ся *сов. см.* начинаться 1.

начеку on the alért.

начерно róughly; написать что-л. ~ make* a rough draft/cópy of smth.

начерта|ние *с.* óutline; (*внешняя форма*) óutward shape. ~тельный: ~тельная геометрия descríptive geómetry.

начертить *сов.* 1. *см.* чертить; 2. (*вн., рд., какое-л. количество*) draw* (a lot of) (*smth.*).

начёс *м.* 1. (*причёска*) báck-combing; 2. *текст.* nap.

начётчик *м.* pédant, dógmatist.

начинание *с.* undertáking, próject, inítiative.

начинательный: ~ глагол ínchoative/incéptive verb.

начинать, начать 1. (*вн., + инф.*) begín* (*smth.*, + to *inf*, + -*ing*), start (*smth.*, + to *inf*, + -*ing*), comménce (+ -*ing*); ~ работу begín* work, begín* to work, begín* wórking; ~ лекцию begín* *one's* lécture; ~ кампанию ópen/start/launch a campáign; ~ новую жизнь make* a fresh start; turn óver a new leaf*; ~ всё сначала begín*/do* *smth.* all óver agáin; 2. (*вн., тв., с рд.*) begín* (with), start (with); ~ с того, что... in the first place..., to begín with... ~ся, начаться 1. begín*, start; (*тв., с рд.*) begín* (with), start (with); лекция началась в 9 часов the lécture begán at nine; 2. *тк. несов.* begín*; река начинается в болотах the ríver ríses in the marshes.

начинающий *прил.* 1. begínner *attr.*; ~ писатель begínner wríter; 2. *в знач. сущ. м.* begínner.

начиная: ~ с (beginning) from; ~ с сегодняшнего дня from todáy, from this day forth.

начинить *сов. см.* начинять.

начинк|а *ж.* stúffing; (*сладкая*) filling; пирог с мясной ~ой méat-pie.

начинять, начинить (*вн.*) stuff (*smth.*), fill (*smth.*).

начислить *сов. см.* начислять.

начислять, начислить (*вн.*) *бухг.* 1. (*проценты и т. п.*) add (*smth.*); 2.: начислить трудодни кому-л. crédit *smb.* with wórk-day únits.

начисто 1. clean, cléanly; переписать что-л. ~ make* a clean/fair cópy of *smth.*; 2. *разг.* (*полностью*) complétely; ограбить кого-л. ~ clean *smb.* out.

начистоту fránkly, ópenly; поговорить ~ speak* *one's* mind.

начитанн|ость *ж.* erudítion. ~ый well-réad; он человек ~ый he is well-réad, he is a man* of some erudítion.

начитаться *сов.* read* enóugh; ~ романов have* *one's* head full of nóvels.

наш *притяж. мест.* 1. (*перед сущ.*) our; (*без сущ.*) ours; это ~а половина that's our half; это ~е! that's ours!; эта половина ~а that half is ours; по ~ему мнению in our opínion; 2. *в знач. сущ. с. разг.* what is ours; 3. *в знач. сущ. мн.*: ~и ещё не приехали our péople/lot háven't come yet; ◇ ~а взяла! our side won!; он и ~им и вашим he runs with the hare and hunts with the hounds; ~е дело that's our búsiness; не ~е дело that's none of our búsiness, that's nóthing to do with us.

нашатырный: ~ спирт (líquid) ammónia.

нашатырь *м.* sal ammóniac.

нашептать *сов. см.* нашёптывать.

нашёптывать, нашептать (*вн., рд.*) whisper (*smth.*) in *smb.'s* ear.

нашествие *с.* invásion.

нашивать, нашить (*вн.*) sew* on (*smth.*).

нашивка *ж.* badge; (*полоса*) stripe.

нашить *сов.* 1. *см.* нашивать; 2. (*вн., рд.; сшить в каком-л. количестве*) get* (a lot of) (*smth.*) made; ~ себе много платьев get* a lot of drésses made.

нашумевш|ий sensátional, much tálked-of; ~ее дело much tálked-of case; ~ая история notórious affáir, affáir that caused a great stir.

нашуметь *сов.* 1. (*произвести шум*) make* a noise; 2. (*вызвать много толков*) make* a sensátion, cause a stir.

нащуп|ать *сов.* (*вн.*) 1. (*отыскать ощупью*) grope (for) and find (*smth.*); он ~ал камень his gróping hand touched a stone; 2. (*обнаружить в результате поисков*) find* (*smth.*), sniff out (*smth.*); ◇ ~ почву judge the lie of the land.

наэлектризовать *сов.* (*вн.; прям. и перен.*) eléctrify (*smb., smth.*); ~ зрителей eléctrify the áudience. ~ся *сов.* (*прям. и перен.*) be* eléctrified.

наяву when awáke; это сон ~ it is like a dream; видеть не во сне, а ~ see* with *one's* own eyes; áctually see*.

не I *частица* 1. (*сообщает слову значение полного отрицания*) not; (*при сравнит. ст.*) no, not... ány; (*при именном сказ.*) no; (*при деепричастии*) without (+ -*ing*); он не знает he does not know; he dóesn't know *разг.*; он не пойдёт he will not go; he won't go *разг.*; мы не придём we shall not come; we shan't come *разг.*; разве вы не знаете? do you not know?; don't you know? *разг.*; ей не хуже she is no worse, she is not ány worse; нам от этого не легче that makes it ány éasier for us; он не гений he is no génius; не долетев до цели without réaching the tárget; он ничего не сказал he said nóthing, he did not say ánything; 2. (*придаёт значение неполного отрицания*) (*в положении между повторяющимися сущ.*) perháps not (*опускается первое сущ.*); (*между повторяющимися гл.*) whether... or not; счастье не счастье, а что-то очень похожее perháps not háppiness, but sómething véry much like it; хочешь не хочешь, а придётся сделать whether you like it or not, you'll have to do it; 3. (+ *инф.; в значении невозможности*) will néver; ему этого не сделать he'll néver (be áble to) do it; ему не уйти he won't escápe; его не узнать you would néver know him; 4. (*придаёт выражению утвердительное значение*) *обыкн.* не переводится; какие тут цветы не растут! there are so mány flówers grówing here!; как не радоваться! how can one help béing pleased!, one cánnot help béing pleased!; кто не любит поесть! éveryone likes a good meal!, who dóesn't enjóy a good meal!; 5. (*с предлогом без придаёт значение ограниченного утверждения*) not; *часто* передаётся утвердительным оборотом; не без трудностей not without difficulty, with some difficulty; не без сожаления not without regrét, with some regrét.

не II *в сочетании с предлогами является отделяемой частью местоимений* некого, нечего; не с кем поговорить there is nóbody to talk to; выбрать было не из чего there was nóthing to choose from, there was no choice.

неаккура́тн|ость ж. 1. (*неточность*) unpunctuálity; 2. (*небрежность*) cárelessness; 3. (*неопря́тность*) untídiness. **~ый** 1. (*неточный*) unpúnctual; 2. (*небре́жный*) cáreless; 3. (*неопря́тный*) untídy.

неантагонисти́ческий non-antagonístic.

неаппети́тный unáppetizing.

небезопа́сный ráther dángerous.

небезоснова́тельный not entírely unfóunded; not withóut foundátion/ground *после сущ.*

небезразли́чный not indífferent, ráther ínterested.

небезрезульта́тный not entírely frúitless; not withóut resúlt *после сущ.*

небезупре́чный not entírely blámeless.

небезызве́стн|о: ~, что... it is no sécret that...; вам, вероя́тно, ~, что... you are próbably awáre that..., you can scárcely be unawáre that... **~ый** well-knówn.

небезынтере́сный ráther ínteresting.

небеса́ *мн. см.* небо.

небе́сн|ый celéstial, héavenly; **~ая сфе́ра** celéstial sphere; **~ свод** fírmament, sky; héavens *pl*; ◇ **~ цвет** sky-blúe (cólour).

небесполе́зный ráther úseful; of some use *после сущ.*

неблагови́дный unséemly.

неблагода́рн|ость ж. ingrátitude. **~ый** ungráteful; *перен.* thánkless; unrewárding; **~ый труд** thánkless task.

неблагозву́ч|ие *с.* dishármony, discórdance. **~ный** inharmónious, dishármonious, discórdant; **~ный акко́рд** túneless chord.

неблагонадёжный *уст.* 1. (*ненадёжный*) unreliable, untrústworthy; 2. (*политически*) súspect, politically unreliable.

неблагополу́чие *с.* tróubles *pl.*

неблагополу́чн|о 1. *нареч.* bádly; 2. *в знач. сказ. безл.:* у нас ~ things are not well with us. **~ый** unháppy, unfórtunate, unlúcky; **~ый год** unfórtunate year.

неблагоприя́тн|ый unfávourable; **~ая пого́да** unfávourable wéather; **~ отве́т** unfávourable reply.

неблагоразу́м|ие *с.* imprúdence. **~ый** imprúdent, unwíse.

неблагоро́дн|ый ignóble, base; **~ посту́пок** ignóble áction; ◇ **~ые мета́ллы** base métals.

неблагоустро́енный ill-províded; lácking aménities *после сущ.*; withóut módern convéniences *после сущ.*

нёбн|ый 1. *анат.* pálatine; 2. *лингв.* pálatal; **~ые согла́сные** pálatal cónsonants.

не́б|о *с.* the sky; (*небеса*) the héavens *pl*; **на ~е in** the sky; ◇ **попа́сть па́льцем в ~** ≈ get* the wrong sow by the ear, miss the point by a mile; **с ~а свали́ться** drop from the clouds; **превозноси́ть кого́-л. до небе́с** laud/praise *smb.* to the skies.

нёбо *с. анат.* pálate; **мя́гкое ~** soft pálate; **твёрдое ~** hard pálate.

небога́тый 1. of módest means *после сущ.*; 2. (*скромный*) módest, unpreténtious; 3. (*скудный*) poor, limited.

небольш|о́й 1. (*по величине, размерам*) (ráther) small; (*о расстоянии*) (ráther) short; **~а́я ко́мната** room of módest size; **~а́я глубина́** comparátive shállowness; **~а́я высота́** low áltitude; **~а́я су́мма де́нег** móderate/small sum of móney; **~ тира́ж** small/límited circulátion; 2. (*непродолжительный по времени*) brief, short; 3. (*незначительный*) small; у меня́ к вам **~а́я про́сьба** I have a small requést to make of you; 4. (*не имеющий веса в обществе*) mínor; of no great impórtance *после сущ.*; 5.: я ~ люби́тель ша́хмат I don't care much for chess, I'm not particularly keen on chess; ◇ **с ~и́м** a little óver; odd; ему́ бы́ло лет 20 **с ~и́м** he was a little óver twénty.

небосво́д *м.* fírmament, sky.

небоскло́н *м.* horízon.

небоскрёб *м.* sky-scraper.

небо́сь *разг.* próbably, súrely.

небре́жн|ость ж. cárelessness; (*халатность тж.*) négligence; (*пренебрежительность*) alóofness; допусти́ть оши́бку по **~ости** make* a mistáke through cárelessness/négligence; ~ то́на cásual tone; преступ́ная ~ críminal négligence. **~ый** cáreless; (*халатный тж.*) négligent; slípshod *разг.*; (*пренебрежительный*) alóof, cásual; **~ая причёска** cárelessly done hair, untídy hair; **~ая рабо́та** slípshod work; **~ый тон** cásual tone.

небри́тый unsháven.

небыва́лый unprécedented, unhéard of, prodígious.

небыли́ца ж. 1. (*выдумка*) cóck-and-búll stóry; 2. (*фантастический рассказ*) (tale of) fántasy.

небью́щийся unbréakable; *тех.* shátterproof.

неважн|о 1. *нареч.* not véry well; он себя́ ~ чу́вствует he dóesn't feel véry well; 2. *в знач. сказ.* (*несущественно*) it dóesn't mátter! **~ый** 1. (*несущественный*) insigníficant, unimpórtant; **~ый вопро́с** unimpórtant mátter; 2. *разг.* (*посредственный*) poor; **~ое здоро́вье** poor health.

невдалеке́ not far off.

невдомёк *разг.*: мне ~ it néver occúrred to me.

неве́дени|е *с.* ígnorance; по **~ю** out of ígnorance, through ígnorance; пребыва́ть в **~и** know* nóthing abóut it.

неве́дом|о *разг.*: ~ зачём no one knows/knew why; ~ откýда there is/was no knówing where from, no one knows/knew where from. **~ый** unknówn; (*таинственный*) mystérious; по **~ой причи́не** for some unknówn réason.

неве́жа *м. и ж.* boor.

неве́жда *м. и ж.* ignorámus.

неве́жественный ígnorant.

неве́жество *с.* 1. ígnorance; 2. *разг.* (*невежливый поступок*) impolíteness.

неве́жлив|ость ж. impolíteness, incivílity. **~ый** rude, impolíte, discóurteous; **~ый челове́к** rude pérson; **~ый отве́т** rude/impolíte ánswer.

невезе́ние *с. разг.* bad luck.

невели́к|ий *обыкн. кратк. ф.* 1. (*небольшой*) no great; невели́к ро́стом not véry tall, ráther short; 2. (*пустяковый*) insigníficant; **~á беда́**! it dóesn't mátter!, no harm done!

неве́рие *с.* lack of faith (in).

неве́рн|о 1. *нареч.* incorréctly, wrong; 2. *в знач. сказ. безл.* it is not true. **~ость** ж. 1. (*ошибочность*) incorréctness; 2. (*измена*) infidélity, unfáithfulness. **~ый** 1. (*ошибочный*) incorréct, wrong, erróneous; 2. (*вероломный*) unfáithful; fáithless *книжн.*; 3. (*подверженный ошибкам*) errátic; **~ый глаз** errátic eye; 4. (*нетвёрдый*) unstéady; **~ая рука́** unstéady hand.

невероя́тн|ость ж. incredibílity; ◇ **до ~ости** unbelíevably. **~ый** incrédible.

неве́рующий *прил.* 1. unbelíeving; 2. *в знач. сущ. м.* disbelíever, átheist.

неве́сел|о 1. *нареч.* not véry chéerfully, chéerlessly, glóomily; 2. *в знач. сказ. безл.* it is glóomy, it is not véry chéerful.

невесёл|ый 1. chéerless, jóyless; ~ смех mírthless láughter; **~ые мы́сли** chéerless thoughts; **~ое положе́ние** unháppy situátion; **~ое заня́тие** chéerless occupátion; что́-то ты сего́дня ~ you seem ráther lów-spírited todáy; 2. (*мрачный, безрадостный*) glóomy, dréary, glum.

невесо́м|ость ж. wéightlessness; состоя́ние **~ости** (state of) wéightlessness. **~ый** wéightless.

неве́ста ж. fiancée; (*незадолго до дня свадьбы*) bride.

неве́стка ж. (*жена сына*) dáughter-in-law (*pl* dáughters-*); (*жена брата*) síster-in-law (*pl* sísters-*).

невеще́ственный immatérial.

невзго́да ж. advérsity, misfórtune, affliction.

невзирая: ~ **на** in spite of, nótwithstánding, regárdless of; ~ **на ли́ца** withóut respéct of pérsons.

невзлюби́ть *сов. (вн.)* take* a dislíke (to).

невзнача́й *разг.* by chance, uninténtionally.

невзра́чный unattráctive, plain; (*о предметах*) unsíghtly.

невзыска́тельный lax, éasy-going, undemánding.

не́видаль *ж. разг.* wónder, pródigy; э́ка ~! a pródigy indéed!

неви́данный prodígious, unprécedented; (*таинственный*) mystérious; ~ **урожа́й** búmper hárvest.

невиди́мк|а 1. *м. и ж.* invísible pérson, invísible béing; **стать** ~**ой** becóme* invísible; **челове́к-**~ the invísible man*; 2. *ж.* (*шпилька*) invísible háirpin.

неви́димый invísible.

неви́дный 1. (*невидимый*) invísible; 2. *разг.* (*незначительный*) insígnificant; 3. *разг.* (*некрасивый*) unimpósing, unimpréssive.

неви́дящ|ий unséeing; (*слепой*) síghtless; **он смотре́л** ~**им взо́ром** he stared with unséeing eyes.

неви́нн|ость *ж.* 1. ínnocence; 2. (*целомудрие*) virgínity. ~**ый** 1. ínnocent; (*безвредный*) hármless, innócuous; 2. (*целомудренный*) vírgin.

невино́вн|ость *ж.* ínnocence. ~**ый** ínnocent, not gúilty.

невку́сн|о: ко́рмят ~ the food is unpálatable, the food is bad. ~**ый** tásteless, unpléasant.

невменя́ем|ость *ж.* irrespónsibílity; **быть в состоя́нии** ~**ости** not be respónsible for *one's* áctions. ~**ый** 1. irrespónsible; 2. (*раздражённый*) besíde *oneself predic.*

невмеша́тельств|о *с.* non-interférence, non-intervéntion; **поли́тика** ~**а** pólicy of non-interférence; ~ **во вну́тренние дела́** (*какой-л. страны*) non-interférence in intérnàl affáirs.

невнима́ние *с.* 1. (*рассеянность*) inatténtion; 2. (*равнодушие, пренебрежение*) lack of considerátion, negléct.

невнима́тельн|ость *ж.* 1. (*рассеянность*) inatténtiveness; 2. (*равнодушное отношение*) inconsíderateness, lack of considerátion. ~**ый** 1. (*рассеянный*) inatténtive; (*небрежный тж.*) cáreless; 2. (*равнодушный, нелюбезный*) inconsíderate.

невня́тный indistínct, inartículate.

не́вод *м.* seine, swéep-net.

невозвра́тн|ый irretríevable; ~**ая поте́ря** irretríevable loss; ~**ые го́ды** years that will néver retúrn.

невозде́ланный untílled, uncúltivated.

невозде́ржанн|ость *ж.* lack of self-restráint, intémperance. ~**ый** intémperate, immóderate, unrestráined; **он невозде́ржан на язы́к** he is intémperate in his speech.

невозде́ржный *см.* невозде́ржанный.

невозмо́жн|о 1. *нареч.* impóssibly; *разг.* (*чрезвычайно*) véry; 2. *в знач. сказ. безл.* it is impóssible. ~**ость** *ж.* impossibílity; **в слу́чае** ~**ости** should it be found impóssible. ~**ый** 1. (*неосуществимый*) impóssible; 2. *разг.* (*невыносимый*) intólerable; ~**ая боль** intólerable pain.

невозмути́м|ость *ж.* cóolness, imperturbabílity. ~**ый** 1. (*спокойный*) cool, impertúrbable, unrúffled; ~**ый челове́к** self-posséssed pérson/indivídual; cool cústomer *разг.*; ~**ый тон** nónchalant tone; ~**ый взгляд** impássive gaze; 2. (*ничем не нарушаемый*) undistúrbed; ~**ая тишина́** undistúrbed tranquíllity; ~**ое споко́йствие** pérfect/undistúrbed calm, unrúffled compósure.

невознагради́м|ый 1. (*непоправимый*) irréparable; 2. (*очень значительный*) irrépayable.

нево́лить *несов. (вн.) разг.* compél (*smb.*), force (*smb.*).

нево́льн|ик *м.,* ~**ица** *ж.* slave. ~**ичество** *с.* slávery, bóndage.

нево́льн|о 1. (*неумышленно*) uninténtionally,
unwíttingly, accidéntally; 2. (*непроизвольно*) invóluntarily, automátically. ~**ый** 1. (*неумышленный*) uninténtional, unwítting; ~**ая ложь** uninténtional lie; 2. (*непроизвольный*) invóluntary; ~**ая улы́бка** invóluntary smile; 3. (*принуждённый*) forced, unwílling.

нево́л|я *ж.* 1. (*рабство*) slávery, bóndage; (*плен*) captívity; 2. *разг.* (*необходимость, нужда*) need; **охо́та пу́ще** ~**и** *посл.* ≈ desíre is strónger than compúlsion.

невообрази́мый unimáginable, incónceivable; ~ **беспоря́док** incrédible disórder.

невооружённ|ый unármed; ◇ ~**ым гла́зом** with the náked eye.

невоспи́танн|ость *ж.* ill bréeding. ~**ый** ill-bréd.

невосприи́мчивый 1. (*плохо усваивающий*) dull, slów(-wítted); 2. (*к болезни*) not suscéptible *после сущ.*

невостре́бованн|ый unclaímed; ~**ое письмо́** unclaímed létter.

невпопа́д at the wrong móment; out of turn, quite inapprópriately.

невразуми́тельный unintélligible, obscúre; ~ **отве́т** unintélligible replý.

невралги́ческий *мед.* neurálgic.

невралги́я *ж. мед.* neurálgia.

неврасте́н|ик *м.* neurótic. ~**и́ческий** neurótic. ~**и́я** *ж. мед.* neurasthénia.

невреди́мый unhármed; (*целый*) intáct.

невре́дн|о *в знач. сказ. разг.* it does no harm (+ to *inf*); **вам бы́ло бы** ~ **погуля́ть иногда́** it would do you no harm to go out for a walk occásionally. ~**ый** hármless.

невро́з *м. мед.* neurósis (*pl* -ses).

невропато́лог *м.* neurólogist, nérve-spécialist.

невы́года *ж.* disadvántage.

невы́годн|о 1. *нареч.* at a loss; **он** ~ **про́дал маши́ну** he sold the car at a loss; 2. *в знач. сказ.* (*не даёт прибыли*) it is not prófitable, it does not pay; 3. *в знач. сказ.* (*не даёт преимуществ*) it is not good, it is no good; **э́то вам бу́дет** ~ it will do you no good. ~**ый** 1. (*не приносящий прибыли*) unremúnerative, unprófitable; ~**ая сде́лка** unprófitable deal/transáction; 2. (*неблагоприятный*) unfávourable, disadvantágeous; ~**ые усло́вия** unfávourable terms; 3. (*непривлекательный*) unattráctive; **показа́ть себя́ с** ~**ой стороны́** show* *oneself* at a disadvántage, show* *oneself* in an unfávourable light; ◇ **в** ~**ом све́те** in an unfávourable light.

невы́держанн|ость *ж.* 1. lack of self-contról; 2. (*о стиле и т. п.*) inconsístency, shórt-wíndedness. ~**ый** 1. (*не владеющий собой*) unrestráined; 2. (*непоследовательный*) inconsístent, unéven, shórt-wínded; ~**ый стиль** unéven style; 3. (*не совсем готовый*) new; ~**ое вино́** new wine.

невыноси́м|о 1. *нареч.* unbéarably, intólerably; 2. *в знач. сказ. безл.* it is unbéarable/intólerable/impóssible. ~**ый** intólerable, unbéarable; (*о боли тж.*) excrúciating.

невыполн|е́ние *с.* non-fulfílment, failure to fulfíl. ~**и́мый** imprácticable; ~**и́мое жела́ние** impóssible desíre.

невырази́мый inexpréssible; ~ **у́жас** unspéakable hórror.

невырази́тельн|ость *ж.* inexpréssiveness, flátness, vapídity. ~**ый** inexpréssive, flat, insípid, féeble.

невысо́к|ий low; (*о росте*) short; **быть** ~**ого мне́ния о чём-л.** have* a low opínion of *smth.*; ~**ое ка́чество** poor quálity; ~**ая пла́та** móderate price; ~**ая оце́нка** low ráting.

негармони́чный inharmónious.

негати́в *м.* négative.

негашён|ый: ~**ая и́звесть** quícklime.

не́где nówhere; ~ **поверну́ться** there's scárcely room to turn round; **ему́** ~ **жить** he has nówhere to live.

неги́бкий infléxible; *перен. тж.* rígid.

негигиени́ч|еский, ~**ный** unhygíenic, insánitary.

негла́сный prívate; sécret.

неглубо́к|ий 1. shállow; 2. (*поверхностный*)

superficial; ~ие знания superficial knówledge *sg*; ~ сон light slúmber.

неглу́пый 1. (*довольно умный*) sénsible, quite intélligent; ~ человéк quite an intélligent pérson; **2.** (*о содержании*) sound; ~ совéт a sound piece of advíce.

него́ 1. (*рд., вн. от личн. мест.* он) him; **2.** (*рд., вн. от личн. мест.* оно́) it.

него́дн│ость *ж.* unfítness; прийти́ в ~ becóme* úseless, be* unfit for use; (*износиться*) fall* ínto disrepáir, wear* out. **~ый 1.** (к, для) unfit (for), not fit (for); ~ый к военной службе inéligible/unfit for mílitary sérvice; **2.** *разг.* (*плохой*) wórthless; (*о человеке тж.*) góod-for-nóthing.

негодова́ние *с.* indignátion; привести́ кого́-л. в ~ infúriate *smb.*; с ~м indígnantly.

него́д│ова́ть *несов.* (на что-л., про́тив чего́-л.) be* índignant (at), rail (at); (на, про́тив кого́-л.) be* índignant (with). **~ующий** indígnant, óutraged.

негодя́й *м.* scóundrel, bláckguard.

негостеприи́мный inhóspitable.

негр *м.* Négro.

негра́мотн│ость *ж.* **1.** illíteracy; *перен.* (*отсутствие знаний в какой-л. области*) ignorance; ликвида́ция ~ости abolition of illíteracy; техни́ческая ~ téchnical ígnorance; **2.** (*наличие грамматических ошибок*) grammátical ígnorance; *перен.* (*несоответствие основным требованиям*) incómpetence; ~ сочинéния the grammátical ígnorance displáyed in the éssay; ~ чертежа́ the téchnical incómpetence displáyed in the dráwing. **~ый** *прил.* **1.** illíterate; *перен.* (*малоопытный, неумелый*) ignorant (of); **2.** (*содержащий ошибки*) ungrammátical; *перен.* (*выполненный без знания дела*) ináccurate, incómpetent; ~ая речь ungrammátical/unéducated speech; **3.** *в знач. сущ. м.* an illíterate.

негритёнок *м.* Négro child*, Négro báby.

негритя́н│ка *ж.* Négro wóman*. **~ский** Négro *attr.*; of the Négroes *после сущ.*

негро́мк│ий low; ~им го́лосом in a low voice.

неда́вн│ий récent; ~ие собы́тия evénts of récent date; с ~его вре́мени quite récently; до ~его вре́мени until quite récently; ~ее знакóмство récent acquáintance.

неда́вно récently, not long agó; ~ прибы́вший récently arríved.

недалёк│ий 1. not dístant, néar-by; (*о путешествии, расстоянии и т. п.*) short; **2.** (*близкий по времени*) the not véry dístant; в ~ом бу́дущем in the not véry dístant fúture; в ~ом про́шлом quite récently, not so long agó; недалёк тот день, когда́... the day/time is not far off, when...; **3.** (*неумный*) límited; он ~ человéк he is a ráther límited pérson.

недалеко́, недалёко 1. *нареч.* not far; им ~ идти́ they háven't got far to go; **2.** *в знач. сказ. безл.* it is not far; недалекó то вре́мя... the time is not fár-dístant...

недальнови́дн│ость *ж.* lack of fóresight. **~ый** shórt-sighted; ~ый человéк shórt-sighted pérson, pérson of no fóresight; ~ая поли́тика shórt-sighted pólicy.

неда́ром 1. (*не без оснований*) not for nóthing, without réason; он ~ так говори́л he had a réason for spéaking as he did; **2.** (*не без цели, не без умысла*) for some púrpose/réason; он ~ сюда́ приезжа́л he came here for some réason; **3.** (*не напрасно, небесполезно*) not for nóthing, not in vain; он ~ рабóтал his work was not in vain, his work was not wásted.

недви́жим│ость *ж.* real estáte; immóvables *pl.* **~ый:** ~ое иму́щество real estáte; immóvables *pl.*

недви́жимый (*неподвижный*) mótionless; (*неспособный двигаться*) immóbile.

недвусмы́сленн│о in no uncértain terms. **~ый** unequívocal; unambíguous, unmistákable; ~ый отвéт unequívocal/unambíguous ánswer; ~ый намёк unmistákable hint; ~ая угрóза unmistákable/óbvious threat.

недееспосо́бн│ость *ж.* **1.** (*неспособность к действию*) inefféctiveness; **2.** *юр.* incapácity. **~ый 1.** (*неспособный к действию*) inefféctive; **2.** *юр.* incápable.

недействи́тельный inválid, null, void.

неделика́тн│ость *ж.* indélicacy; (*нетактичность*) táctlessness; ~ обраще́ния inconsíderate tréatment. **~ый** indélicate; (*нетактичный*) táctless.

недели́м│ость *ж.* indivisibílity. **~ый** indivísible; ~ые чи́сла prime númbers; ◇ ~ый фонд non-distríbutable fund.

неде́льный week's; ~ срок a week; ~ óтпуск a week's leave/hóliday.

неде́л│я *ж.* week; две ~и two weeks, a fórtnight; чéрез ~ю in a week, in a week's time; на э́той ~е this week.

недержа́ние *с.* incóntinence.

недёшево not cheap, ráther dear/expénsive; *перен.* at no líttle cost, at great cost.

недисциплини́рованный undísciplined; ~ учени́к undísciplined púpil.

недоброжела́тель│ный unfriéndly; hóstile, ill-dispósed. **~ство** *с.* ill-will.

недоброка́чественн│ый inférior, poor; ~ая рабóта inférior piece of work; ~ые товáры inférior/shóddy goods; ~ материáл poor matérial.

недобросо́вестн│о unconsciéntiously; (*нечестно*) unscrúpulously; (*небрежно*) cárelessly; négligently. **~ость** *ж.* lack of consciéntiousness; (*нечестность*) unscrúpulousness; lack of íntegrity; (*небрежность*) cárelessness, négligence. **~ый** unconsciéntious; (*нечестный, непорядочный*) unscrúpulous; (*небрежный*) cáreless.

недо́бр│ый 1. (*злой*) unkínd; (*выражающий неприязнь*) hóstile; питáть ~ые чу́вства к кому́-л. bear* *smb.* ill-will; ~ые намéрения hóstile/évil inténtions; ~ взгляд hóstile glance; **2.** (*плохой*) évil, bad; ~ая весть bad/óminous news; в ~ая порá unfávourable/unpropítious time; ~ая слáва évil reputátion.

недова́ривать, недовари́ть (*вн.*) not cook (*smth.*) próperly. **~ся, недовари́ться** not cook próperly.

недовари́ть(ся) *сов. см.* недовáривать(ся).

недове́р│ие *с.* (к *дт.*) distrúst (of), mistrúst (of), lack of cónfidence (in); питáть ~ к кому́-л. feel* no cónfidence in *smb.*; вы́разить ~ expréss distrúst; отнести́сь с ~ем treat with distrúst, distrúst. ~**чиво** distrústfully; относи́ться ~чиво к кому́-л. feel* distrústful of *smb.* **~чивость** *ж.* distrúst, lack of cónfidence (in). **~чивый** distrústful, mistrústful; (*о человеке тж.*) untrústing.

недове́с *м.* short weight. **~ить** *сов. см.* недовéшивать.

недове́шивать, недове́сить (*вн., рд.*) give* short weight (of).

недово́ль│но disconténtedly. **~ный** disconténted; (*тв.*) dissátisfied (with); displéased (with); он был недово́лен тем, что... he was displéased that... **~ство** *с.* dissatisfáction, discontént; ~ство собóй dissatisfáction with onesélf.

недовыполне́ние *с.* fáilure to fulfíl; shórtfall.

недовы́полнить *сов.* (*вн.*) not quite fulfíl (*smth.*), fail to fulfíl (*smth.*), fall* short of fulfílling (*smth.*).

недога́длив│ость *ж.* lack of percéption, impercípience. **~ый** slów(-witted), unobsérvant, uncercéptive; dense, thick *разг.*

недогляде́ть *сов. разг.* **1.** (*вн., рд.; пропустить*) overlóok (*smth.*); **2.** (за *тв.; не уберечь*) fail to look áfter (*smth.*), fail to keep an eye on (*smb.*).

недогова́ривать, недоговори́ть (*вн., рд.*) hold* (*smth.*) back, leave* (*smth.*) unsáid.

недоговорённость *ж.* **1.** (*несогласованность*) fáilure to come to an agréement; **2.** (*умалчивание*) réticence.

недоговори́ть *сов. см.* недоговáривать.

недодавать, недода́ть 1. (дт. вн., рд.) fail to supplý (smb. with), fail to delíver (smth. to); (недоплачивать) pay* (smb. smth.); 2. (вн., рд.; изготовлять меньше, чем требуется) fail to prodúce (smth.), fall* short of prodúcing (smth.).

недода́ть сов. см. недодава́ть.

недоде́л|анный unfínished. ~ать сов. (вн., рд.) not fínish (smth.) off. ~ка ж. 1. unfínished (item of) work; 2. (упущение) deféct; bug разг.

недоеда́ние с. malnutrítion; undernóurishment.

недоеда́ть, недое́сть 1. тк. несов. (не иметь достаточного питания) be* undernóurished; not get enóugh to eat; 2. (есть не досыта) not eat enóugh.

недое́сть сов. см. недоеда́ть 2.

недозре́лый unrípe, green; перен. тж. immatúre.

недока́занн|ый unpróved; ~ое обвине́ние unpróved accusátion.

недо́лгий brief, short.

недо́лго 1. нареч.: я бу́ду там ~ I won't be there long; он жил ~ he did not live long; ~ ду́мая withóut páusing to think; 2. в знач. сказ. разг. (легко, нетрудно) ónly too éasy; ~ и утону́ть it's ónly too éasy to get drowned.

недолгове́чный short-líved; (непрочный) mákeshift.

недолю́бливать несов. (вн.) be* not véry fond (of), have* líttle líking (for).

недомога́ние с. indispositíon; чу́вствовать ~ feel* out of sorts, be* indispósed.

недомога́ть несов. feel* unwéll; feel* off cólour разг.

недомо́лвка ж. réticence.

недомы́слие с. lack/want of understánding, thóughtlessness.

недоно́|сок м. prematúre báby. ~шенный prematúre.

недооце́нивать, недооцени́ть (вн., рд.) underéstimate (smb., smth.), underráte (smb., smth.).

недооцени́ть сов. см. недооце́нивать.

недооце́нка ж. underestimátion.

недопусти́м|ый inadmíssible, impermíssible; ~ое поведе́ние impóssible beháviour.

недорабо́танн|ый ónly half fínished/compléted; ~ые пье́сы plays that are ónly half compléted.

недорабо́тка ж. см. недоде́лка.

недора́звитый underdevéloped; (умственно отсталый) báckward, retárded.

недоразуме́ние с. misunderstánding.

недо́рого (quite) cheap, for a réasonable price.

недорого́й cheap (тж. перен.); inexpénsive.

недо́росль м. young ignorámus.

недослы́шать сов. (вн.) not (quite) hear; 2. разг. (быть глуховатым) be* a líttle hard of héaring.

недосмо́тр м. óversight; по ~у by an óversight.

недосмотре́ть сов. (вн., рд.) overlóok (smth.); (за тв.) negléct (smb., smth.).

недоспа́ть сов. см. недосыпа́ть.

недоста|ва́ть несов. безл. 1. (не хватать) lack (smth.); be* lácking, be* míssing; ему́ ~ёт терпе́ния he lacks pátience; чего́ вам ~ёт? what do you need?, what háven't you got?; чего́-то ~ёт there is sómething lácking; 2. (быть необходимым) miss (smb., smth.); be* much néeded; нам о́чень ~ва́ло вас we missed you véry much; ◇ э́того ещё ~ва́ло! I call that the límit!, if that ísn't the límit!

недоста́т|ок м. 1. (нехватка) defíciency; lack, shórtage; за ~ком чего́-л. for lack/want of smth.; он ни в чём не испы́тывал ~ка he wánted for nóthing; 2. (изъян) deféct; defíciency; мн. тж. shórtcomings; 3. обыкн. мн. разг. (нужда) want sg, póverty sg.

недоста́точн|о 1. нареч. insufficiently; (слабо, не очень хорошо) not... well enóugh; not fúlly, inádequately; 2. в знач. сказ. безл. there is not enóugh; ~ то́плива there is not enóugh fuel. ~ость ж.

insufficiency; серде́чная ~ость cárdiac insufficiency. ~ый insufficient; (слабый, малый) inádequate; ~ые запа́сы чего́-л. inádequate supplíes of smth.; ~ый о́пыт insufficient expérience, lack of expérience; ~ые све́дения inádequate informátioin sg; ~ая причи́на для огорче́ния insufficient cause for disappóintment; ~ый глаго́л грам. deféctive verb.

недоста́ча ж. разг. 1. shórtage; 2. (обнаруженная при проверке) déficit.

недостаю́щий míssing.

недостижи́мый unattáinable, unachíevable.

недостове́рный unrelíable, dóubtful.

недосто́йно 1. нареч. bádly, unwórthily; 2. в знач. сказ. безл. (рд.) it is unwórthy (of).

недосто́йный 1. (рд.) unwórthy (of); 2. (не заслуживающий уважения) wórthless, unwórthy, déspicable.

недостро́енный unfínished, half-fínished.

недосту́п|ный 1. inaccéssible; 2. (превышающий чьи-л. возможности) unattáinable (for), beyónd the pówers (of); (в денежном отношении) beyónd the means (of); 3. (трудный для понимания) too dífficult (for), incomprehénsible (to), beyónd the comprehénsion (of); э́то ~о моему́ понима́нию that's beyónd me, that's beyónd my understánding; 4. (о человеке) unappróachable, alóof.

недосу́г: мне ~ I have no time.

недосчита́ться сов. см. недосчи́тываться.

недосчи́тываться, недосчита́ться (рд.) be* short (of); недосчита́лись трои́х three were (found to be) míssing; он недосчита́лся трёх рубле́й he (found he) was three róubles short, he was short of three róubles.

недосыпа́ть, недоспа́ть not get enóugh sleep; я недоспа́л I háven't had enóugh sleep.

недосяга́емый unattáinable; (недоступный) inaccéssible.

недотро́га м. и ж. tóuchy pérson; она́ така́я ~ she is such a tóuch-me-nót.

недоумев|а́ть несов. be* bewíldered, be* púzzled, wónder. ~а́ющий bewíldered, púzzled.

недоуме́н|ие с. bewílderment; (озадаченность) perpléxity; останови́ться в ~ии halt/stop in bewílderment. ~ный perpléxed, púzzled; ~ный вопро́с púzzled quéstion.

недоу́чка м. и ж. разг. half-táught pérson, half-tráined pérson.

недочёт м. 1. (недостача) déficit; 2. обыкн. мн. (недостаток) deficiency sg, shórtcoming sg.

не́дра мн. 1. depths; ~ земли́ bówels of the earth; 2. (внутренняя часть чего-л.) heart; déepest recésses pl; в ~х души́ in the ínmost recésses of one's soul; в ~х ста́рого о́бщества in the womb of the old society.

недре́млющий vígilant, wátchful.

не́друг м. énemy.

недружелю́б|ие с. unfríendliness. ~ный unfríendly.

неду́г м. íllness.

неду́рно 1. нареч. fáirly well; 2. в знач. сказ. безл. it is not bad; ~! that's not bad!, I like that!; 3. в знач. сказ. безл. (+ инф.) it's not a bad idéa/thing (+ to inf); ~ бы... it wóuldn't be a bad idéa...

недурно́й 1. not bad*; 2. обыкн. кратк. ф. (о наружности) quite prétty, not bád-lóoking.

недю́жинный unúsual, uncómmon; ~ ум uncómmon intélligence.

неё (вн., рд. от личн. мест. она́) her.

неесте́ственн|ый unnátural; (деланный тж.) affécted; ~ая улы́бка affécted/unnátural smile.

нежда́нный unexpécted.

нежела́ние с. unwíllingness, relúctance, disinclinátion.

нежела́тельн|ый undesírable.

не́жели than.

нежена́тый unmárried, síngle.

нёженка *м. и ж. разг.* mólly-coddle, móther's dárling.

неживой 1. (*мёртый*) dead, lífeless; **2.** (*неорганический*) inánimate; **3.** (*вялый*) lífeless, dull.

нежизненный 1. (*нереальный*) imprácticable; **2.** (*неправдоподобный*) unlífelike, unréal.

нежизнеспособный (*прям. и перен.*) unvíable.

нежилой 1. (*в котором не живут*) that is not líved-in *после сущ.*; (*неуютный*) unlíved-in; **2.** (*необитаемый*) uninhábited; **3.** (*негодный для жилья*) uninhábitable.

нёжить *несов.* (*вн.*) pámper (*smb.*), códdle (*smb.*). ~**ся** *несов.* enjóy one's/the cómfort, luxúriate; ~**ся на солнце** bask in the sun.

нёжн|ость *ж.* **1.** ténderness; **2.** *мн. разг.* (*ласковые слова, поступки*) endéarments. ~**ый 1.** (*ласковый*) géntle, ténder-héarted; **2.** (*мягкий*) ténder; ~**ая кожа** ténder skin; **3.** (*приятный*) géntle, pléasant; ~**ый аромат** délicate frágrance; ~**ый голос** géntle/caréssing voice; **4.** (*слабый, хрупкий*) frail.

незабвённый néver-to-be-forgótten.

незабудка *ж. бот.* forgét-me-not.

незабываемый unforgéttable.

незавидн|ый unénviable; ~**ое положение** unénviable position.

независим|о indepéndently; **держать себя** ~ beháve indepéndently; ◇ ~ **от чего-л.** regárdless of *smth.*, irréspective of *smth.* ~**ость** *ж.* indepéndence. ~**ый** indepéndent; ~**ые страны** indepéndent cóuntries; ~**ый вид** indepéndent/cásual air; air of detáchment.

независящ|ий indepéndent (of); **по** ~**им от меня обстоятельствам** ówing to círcumstances beyónd my contról.

незадач|а *ж. разг.* bad luck. ~**ливый** *разг.* únlúcky; hápless.

незадолго shórtly befóre, not long befóre.

незаинтересованный 1. (*не проявляющий интереса*) indífferent, unínterested; **2.** (*бескорыстный*) dísinterested.

незаконный illégal, unláwful; (*юридически не оформленный*) illegítimate.

незаконченный incompléte, unfínished.

незаменимый irrepláceable; (*очень нужный тж.*) indispénsable.

незаметн|о 1. *нареч.* impercéptibly; (*неприметно*) inconspícuously, quíetly; **время прошло** ~ the time passed unnóticed; **2.** *в знач. сказ. безл.* it is not nóticeable; ~ **для себя** withóut nóticing it. ~**ый 1.** impercéptible; (*неприметный*) inconspícuous; **2.** (*незначительный*) insigníficant; ~**ый человек** insigníficant pérson.

незамеченный unnóticed.

незамужняя unmárried, síngle.

незамысловатый símple, uncómplicated; ~ **узор** símple páttern.

незанятый unóccupied; (*свободный*) free.

незапамятн|ый: с ~**ых времён** from time immemórial.

незапятнанный unblémished, unsúllied.

незаразн|ый non-inféctious; ~**ая болезнь** non-inféctious diséase; ~ **больной** non-inféctious pátient.

незаслуженн|о undesérvedly. ~**ый** undesérved, unmérited; ~**ый упрёк** undesérved repróach.

незатейливый símple, unpreténtious.

незаурядн|ый outstánding; ~**ые способности** outstánding ability *sg.*

нёзачем *разг.* there's no need; there's no point; **мне** ~ **идти туда** there's no need for me to go there.

незащищённый (*от рд.*) unprotécted (from); expósed (to).

незваный uninvíted, unbídden.

нездёшний *разг.* álien, strange; **я** ~ I am a stránger here.

нездоров|иться *несов. безл.* (*дт.*): **мне** ~**ится** I

don't feel well. ~**ый** unhéalthy; (*о пище, климате тж.*) unwhólesome; **он нездоров** he's not well.

нездоровье *с.* ill health; (*недомогание*) indisposítion, íllness.

незлой not unkíndly.

незлопамятный forgíving.

незнаком|ец *м.* stránger. ~**ый 1.** unfamíliar; ~**ые места** unfamíliar locálity *sg*; **2.** (*о людях*) strange; (**с** *тв.*) unacquáinted (with); ~**ые человек** stránger; **быть** ~**ым с кем-л.** not know *smb.*, be* unacquáinted with *smb.*

незнание *с.* ígnorance.

незначительный insigníficant; (*небольшой*) small, slight; (*маловажный*) trívial.

незрёл|ый 1. (*неспелый*) únrípe; ~ **виноград** únrípe grapes; **2.** (*не достигший полного развития*) immatúre (*тж. перен.*); ~ **юноша** immatúre young man*, raw youth; ~**ая мысль** immatúre idéa; ~**ое произведёние** immatúre work.

незримый invísible.

незыблемый firm, unshák(e)able, stáble.

неизбёжн|о inévitably. ~**ость** *ж.* inevitabílity. ~**ый** inévitable.

неизвёдан|ный (*незнакомый*) unknówn; (*неизученный*) únexplóred; (*неприметный*) nóvel; ~**ное чувство** nóvel féeling.

неизвёстн|о *в знач. сказ. безл.* it is not knówn; **ему** ~ **he** dóesn't know; (*никому*) ~! nóbody knows!; ~ **почему** for some unknówn réason; ~ **где** no one knows where. ~**ость** *ж.* **1.** uncértainty; **2.** (*скромное, незаметное существование*) obscúrity; **жить в** ~**ости** live in obscúrity. ~**ый** *прил.* **1.** unknówn; **2.** *в знач. сущ. м.* stránger; **3.** *в знач. сущ. с. мат.* unknówn quántity.

неизгладимый ineffáceable, indélible.

неизданный unpúblished.

неизлечимый incúrable.

неизмённый 1. (*постоянный*) inváriable, immútable, fixed, firm; **2.** (*всегдашний*) cústomary; **3.** (*преданный*) cónstant, unfáiling.

неизменяемый immútable.

неизмерим|о ínfinitely, éver so much. ~**ый** imméasurable; **в** ~**ых глубинах** in the unfáthomable/fáthomless depths.

неизрасходованный unexpénded.

неимёние *с.*: **за** ~**м чего-л.** for lack of *smth.*; **за** ~**м** лучшего in defáult of ánything bétter.

неимовёрный incrédible.

неимущий *прил.* **1.** índigent, poor, néedy; **2.** *в знач. сущ. мн.* the poor.

неинтерёсный 1. unínteresting, dull; ~ **рассказ** féeble tale; **2.** *разг.* (*некрасивый*) unattráctive; **он совсём** ~ he is nóthing to look at.

неискоренимый inerádicable.

нейскренн|ий insincére. ~**ость** *ж.* insincérity.

неискушённый unsophísticated; (*неопытный*) inexpérienced.

неисполнёние *с.* non-perfórmance; fáilure to cárry out; (*о правилах и т. п.*) non-obsérvance.

неисполним|ый imprácticable; ~**ое желáние** impóssible desíre.

неисполнительный inefficient, slack, cáreless.

неиспользован|ный unúsed; ~**ные мощности** ídle capácities.

неиспорченный unspóilt, pure, fresh.

неисправимый incórrigible, hópeless.

неисправн|ость *ж.* disrepáir. ~**ый 1.** (*повреждённый*) fáulty; out of órder *predic.*; ~**ые механизмы** fáulty méchanisms; **маши́на** ~**а** the car is out of órder; **2.** (*неаккуратный*) cáreless, slóvenly.

неиспытанный 1. (*непроверенный*) úntríed; **2.** (*непережитый*) nóvel.

неисслёдованный únexplóred.

неиссякаем|ый inexháustible; ~ родни́к unfáiling source; ~ые бога́тства inexháustible wealth sg.

нейств|о frántically. ~ство с. 1. fúry, rage, frénzy; прийти́ в ~ство fly* ínto a rage; 2. (жестокость) atrócity. ~ствовать несов. rage, storm. ~ый frántic; ~ый гнев tówering/frénzied rage; ~ые аплодисме́нты frénzied appláuse sg.

неистощи́мый inexháustible; он неистощи́м на вы́думки he has an inexháustible fund of invéntiveness.

неисчерпа́емый inexháustible, ínfinite.

неисчисли́мый innúmerable, númberless, cóuntless.

ней 1. (дт. от личн. мест. она́) to her; 2. (тв. от личн. мест. она́) by her; 3. (пр. от личн. мест. она́) about her.

нейло́н м. nýlon. ~овый nýlon attr.

нейрохиру́рг м. néuro-súrgeon.

нейрохирурги́я ж. néuro-súrgery.

нейтрализа́ция ж. neutralizátion.

нейтрализова́ть несов. и сов. (вн.) néutralize (smth.).

нейтралите́т м. neutrálity.

нейтра́льн|ость ж. neutrálity. ~ый néutral.

нейтри́но с. нескл. физ. neutríno.

нейтро́н м. физ. néutron. ~ный физ. néutron attr.; ~ная бо́мба néutron bomb.

неказ́истый разг. plain, hómely, unpreposséssing.

некапиталисти́ческий non-cápitalist.

нека́чественн|ый lów-quálity attr.; ~ые изде́лия lów-quálity árticles.

неквалифици́рованный unskilled, unquálified; ~ рабо́чий géneral/unskilled wórker; ~ труд unskilled work/lábour.

не́кем мест. тв. см. не́кого.

не́кий мест. a cértain.

не́когда I в знач. сказ. there is no time; мне ~ I have no time.

не́когда II нареч. (когда-то) once, at one time, in fórmer times.

не́кого мест. (дт. не́кому, тв. не́кем, пр. не́ о ком) (+ инф.) there is no one (+ to inf).

некомпете́нт|ость ж. incómpetence. ~ый not cómpetent, incómpetent.

не́кому мест. дт. см. не́кого.

некорре́ктный táctless.

не́котор|ый мест. 1. a cértain; мн. some; ~ое вре́мя, с ~ых пор for some time, в ~ой сте́пени, ме́ре to a cértain extént. ~ым о́бразом in some way; 2. в знач. сущ. мн. some (péople).

некраси́в|ый 1. úgly; (о человеке тж.) unattráctive, plain; 2. разг. (о поступке, поведении) unséemly, impróper; (подлый) low; э́то ~о that's not nice.

некре́пкий 1. (непрочный) weak, frail; (о ткани) thin; (шаткий) unstéady; 2. (нездоровый) frail, délicate.

некрити́ческий uncrítical.

некроло́г м. obítuary (nótice).

некста́ти at the wrong móment, inópportunely, irrélevant; ~ ска́зано quite irrélevant; замеча́ние бы́ло ~ the remárk was most untímely; вот ~!, как ~! what a núisance!

не́кто мест. sómeone; ~ Смирно́в one Smirnóv, a cértain Smirnóv; ~ в се́ром a pérson in a grey coat.

не́куда there is nówhere; ему́ ~ де́ваться, пойти́ he has nówhere to go; ~ де́ваться (от) there's no escápe (from).

некульту́рн|о in an uncúltured/uncívilized way. ~ость ж. lack of cúlture, cúltural báckwardness, low lével of cúlture; ~ость поведе́ния uncúltured beháviour. ~ый 1. uncúltured, uncívilized, uncúltivated; ~ый челове́к an uncúltured pérson, a boor; ~ое поведе́ние uncívilized/uncúltured beháviour; 2. (о растениях) uncúltivated.

некуря́щ|ий прил. 1. who does not smoke после сущ.; я ~ I don't smoke; 2. в знач. сущ. м. non-smóker; ваго́н для ~их non smóking cárriage, non-smóker.

нела́дн|о 1. нареч. bádly, in a poor way; я дела́ ~ повёл I made a poor job of things; 2. в знач. сказ.: что́-то ~ there's sómething wrong/amíss. ~ый 1. bad; wrong, amíss predic.; 2. (неуклюжий) clúmsy, áwkward.

нела́ды мн. разг.: у них ~ they don't get on, they have fállen out.

нелега́льный illégal.

нелёгк|ий 1. (тяжёлый) héavy; 2. (трудный) hard, not éasy; ~ая зада́ча no éasy task, task of some difficulty.

неле́п|ость ж. absúrdity. ~ый absúrd, ridículous.

неле́стн|ый unfláttering; быть ~ого мне́ния о ком-л. have*/hold* an unfláttering opínion of smb.

нелётный non-flýing; unfit for flýing после сущ.

нели́шн|е в знач. сказ. (+ инф.) it does no harm (+ to inf); ~ бы́ло бы ещё раз посмотре́ть one had bétter have anóther look at it. ~ий úseful, nécessary.

нело́вк|ий 1. (неуклюжий) clúmsy, áwkward; он о́чень нело́вок he is véry clúmsy/áwkward; сде́лать ~ое движе́ние make* an áwkward móvement; 2. (неприятный) áwkward, uncómfortable; поста́вить кого-л. в ~ое положе́ние put* smb. in an áwkward posítion.

нело́вк|о 1. нареч. áwkwardly; чу́вствовать себя́ ~ feel* áwkward; 2. в знач. сказ. безл. it is uncómfortable; о́чень ~ сиде́ть на э́том сту́ле this chair is uncómfortable to sit on; 3. в знач. сказ. безл. (дт.; о чувстве стесне́ния, стыда́) it is áwkward/embárrassing (for); мне ~ говори́ть об э́том I hardly like to méntion it. ~ость ж. áwkwardness; (неловкий поступок) blúnder; почу́вствовать ~ость feel* áwkward.

нелоги́чный illógical.

нелоя́льный dislóyal.

нельзя́ в знач. сказ. (обыкн. + инф.) 1. (невозмо́жно) it is impóssible (+ to inf); ~ теря́ть ни мину́ты there's not a mínute to lose; ина́че ~ it's the ónly way; ~ бы́ло предполага́ть... no one could have suppósed...; 2. (запрещено) it is not allówed; здесь ~ кури́ть smóking is not allówed here; ему́ ~ кури́ть he is not allówed to smoke; ~ тро́гать! don't touch!; ~ входи́ть! you can't come in!; ◇ ~ не согласи́ться, призна́ться и т. п. it must be agréed, admítted etc.; ~ сказа́ть, что мне э́то нра́вится I can't say I like it; ~ сказа́ть, что он умён nóbody could call him cléver; ~ ли поти́ше? cóuldn't you be a líttle quíeter?; как ~ лу́чше spléndidly.

нелюбе́зный ungrácious, alóof.

нелюби́мый that one does not love/like после сущ.; ~ ребёнок unlóved child*.

нелюбо́вь ж. dislíke.

нелюди́м м. unsóciable pérson, bad míxer; он тако́й ~ he's véry unsóciable. ~ый unsóciable.

нём 1. (пр. от личн. мест. он) about/of him; 2. (пр. от личн. мест. оно́) about/of it.

нема́ло 1. (довольно много) much, a good deal (of), quite a númber/lot (of); (вполне достаточно) plénty (of); 2. (очень, довольно сильно) considerably, to quite an extént.

немалова́жный not unimpórtant, by no means unimpórtant.

нема́лый considerable.

нема́ркий that does not show the dirt после сущ.

неме́дленн|о immédiately, at once; (тут же) then and there, on the spot; fórthwith книжн. ~ый immédiate.

неме́ркнущий unfáding, immórtal.

немета́лл м. хим. non-métal, metallóid.

неме́ть, оне́меть 1. becóme* dumb; (перен. be* spéechless, be* struck dumb; онеме́ть от изумле́ния be* dumbfóunded; 2. (цепенеть, коченеть) grow* numb.

не́мец м. Gérman.

неме́цкий Gérman; ~ язы́к Gérman, the Gérman lánguage.

неми́лост|ь *ж.* disfávour, disgráce; быть в ~и у *кого́-л.* be* out of fávour with *smb.*

немину́емый inévitable.

не́мка *ж.* Gérman (wóman*).

немно́г|ие *мн.* (véry) few péople; ~им изве́стно few péople are awáre; ~им дано́... it is gíven to few.

немно́г|ий: в ~их слова́х in a few words; ~им бо́льше a líttle more; ~им ме́ньше a líttle less.

немно́го 1. a líttle; ónly a líttle, not much; few, not mány (*с сущ. во мн. ч.*); **2.** (*слегка*) ráther, slíghtly, sómewhat, a líttle.

немно́гое *с.* the líttle.

немногосло́вный 1. (*краткий*) lacónic; terse; **2.** (*о человеке*) táciturn; of few words *после сущ.*

немногочи́сленн|ый 1. small; ~ая семья́ small fámily; ~ые замеча́ния a few remárks; **2.** *мн.* the few; ~ые пассажи́ры дрема́ли the few pássengers were dózing.

немну́щ|ийся uncrúshable; ~иеся тка́ни uncrúshable fábrics.

нем|о́й *прил.* **1.** dumb; *перен.* mute; **2.** *в знач. сущ. м.* dumb pérson; *мн.* the dumb; ◇ ~ фильм sílent pícture/film; ~а́я а́збука sígn-lánguage; ~а́я ка́рта óutline/skéleton map; ~а́я сце́на dumb show.

немолодо́й élderly; gétting on in years *после сущ.*

немота́ *ж.* dúmbness.

не́мощный féeble.

нему́ 1. (*дт. от личн. мест.* он) to him; **2.** (*дт. от личн. мест.* оно́) to it.

немудрено́ *в знач. сказ.* no wónder; ~, что no wónder (that).

немудрёный *разг.* símple, éasy.

немы́слим|ый unthínkable, impóssible; э́то ~о! that's impóssible!

ненави́деть *несов.* (*вн.*) hate (*smb., smth.*), detést (*smb., smth.*).

ненави́стный 1. (*вызывающий ненависть*) háted, háteful; **2.** (*выражающий ненависть*) háte-filled; fill of hate *после сущ.*

не́нависть *ж.* hátred; hate *поэт.*; ~ к кому́-л. hátred of *smb.*

ненагля́дный dárling, belóved.

ненадёжный unrelíable; (*о человеке тж.*) untrústworthy.

ненадо́бность *ж.*: за ~ю as supérfluous; вы́бросить что-л. за ~ю throw* *smth.* awáy as béing of no fúrther use.

ненадо́лго for a short while/time, not for long.

ненаме́ренный uninténtional.

ненападе́ни|е *с.* non-aggréssion; пакт о ~и non-aggréssion pact.

нена́стный wet, ráiny, bad*.

нена́стье *с.* wet/ráiny wéather.

ненасы́тный insátiable (*тж. перен.*).

ненатура́льный 1. (*искусственный*) artifícial; **2.** (*неестественный*) unnátural.

ненау́чный unscientífic.

не́нец *м.* Nénets. ~кий Nénets; ~кий язы́к Nénets, the Nénets lánguage.

не́нка *ж.* Nénets wóman*.

ненорма́льн|ость *ж.* abnormálity. ~ый **1.** abnórmal; **2.** *разг.* (*психически больной*) mad.

ненорми́рованный: ~ труд work with no fíxed hours; ~ рабо́чий день irrégular wórking hours *pl.*

нену́жный unnécessary; (*о человеке тж.*) únwanted.

необду́манн|ый rash, uncónsidered; ~ посту́пок unconsídered áction; ~ое реше́ние rash decísion.

необеспе́ченн|ость *ж.* insecúrity, lack of means; ~ существова́ния ill-próvided exístence. ~ый without means *после сущ.*; он челове́к ~ый he has no régular lívelihood.

необита́емый uninhábited; ~ о́стров désert ísland.

необозри́м|ый bóundless, vast; ~ые да́ли bóundless expánse *sg.*

необосно́ванный gróundless, báseless, unfóunded; ~ вы́вод unfóunded conclúsion; ~ упрёк unjustífied repróach.

необрабо́танный 1. (*о земле*) uncúltivated, untílled; **2.** (*не подвергшийся обработке*) crude, unwróught; **3.** (*о произведении*) rough, unfínished.

необразо́ванн|ость *ж.* lack of educátion, ígnorance. ~ый unéducated, ígnorant.

необстоя́тельный superfícial.

необстре́лянный that has néver been únder fíre *после сущ.*; untésted, inexpérienced.

необу́зданный unbrídled, ungóvernable.

необходи́м|о *в знач. сказ.* (+ *инф.*) it is nécessary/esséntial (+ to *inf*), one must (+ *inf*). ~ость *ж.* necéssity, need; по ~ости from necéssity, out of necéssity; по ме́ре ~ости as requíred. ~ый **1.** (*очень нужный*) nécessary, esséntial; that *one* needs *после сущ.*; **2.** (*неизбежный*) nécessary, inévitable.

необщи́тельный unsóciable.

необъекти́вн|ый bías(s)ed; ~ая оце́нка bías(s)ed júdgement/asséssment.

необъясни́мый inéxplicable, unaccóuntable.

необъя́тный bóundless.

необыкнове́нн|ый extraórdinary, uncómmon; (*странный*) strange; в э́том нет ничего́ ~ого there's nóthing spécial/unúsual in that.

необыча́йный extraórdinary, remárkable.

необы́чн|ость *ж.* **1.** (*особенность*) singulárity; **2.** (*непривычность*) unfamiliárity, stràngeness. ~ый **1.** (*особенный*) unúsual; **2.** (*непривычный*) unfamíliar, strange, odd.

необяза́тельный 1. not esséntial *predic.*; (*не подлежащий обязательному изучению*) óptional; **2.** (*о человеке*) unreliable.

неограни́ченн|ый unlímited, unrestrícted; (*о власти*) ábsolute; ~ое коли́чество unlímited quántity; ~ые полномо́чия unrestrícted pówers.

неодина́ков|ый (*неравный*) unéqual; (*разный*) différent; они́ ~ы they are not the same.

неоднокра́тн|о more than once, repéatedly. ~ый repéated.

неодноро́дный 1. (*несходный*) dissímilar; **2.** (*разнородный по составу*) heterogéneous.

неодобре́ние *с.* disappróval, disapprobátion.

неодобри́тельн|о disappróvingly. ~ый disappróving.

неодоли́мый irrepréssible; irresístible; (*непобедимый*) invíncible.

неодушевлённый inánimate.

неожи́данн|о unexpéctedly; (*вдруг*) súddenly; ~ для самого́ себя́ to *one's* own surprise. ~ость *ж.* **1.** unexpéctedness; (*внезапность*) súddenness; **2.** (*события и т. п.*) surprise; больша́я ~ость great surprise; вздро́гнуть от ~ости give* a start of surprise. ~ый **1.** unexpécted; (*внезапный*) súdden; ~ая ра́дость unlóoked-for pléasure.

неоколониал|и́зм *м.* néo-colónialism. ~и́стский néo-colónialist.

неоконча́тельный inconclúsive, not final, téntative.

неоконче́нный unfínished.

неологи́зм *м. лингв.* néologism, new word.

нео́н *м.* **1.** *хим.* néon; **2.** (*свет*) néon light.

неонац|и́зм *м.* néonázism. ~и́стский néonázi.

нео́нов|ый néon *attr.*; ~ свет néon líghting; ◇ ~ая ла́мпа néon tube.

неопа́сн|о 1. *нареч.* sáfely, without dánger, **2.** *в знач. сказ.* it is quite safe. ~ый safe; ~ое путеше́ствие safe jóurney; ~ый проти́вник safe oppónent; ра́на была́ ~ая the wound was not dángerous.

неопера́бельный inóperable.

неопери́вшийся unfle̊dged; ~ птене́ц fle̊dg(e)ling.

неопису́емый indescri̊bable; *перен. тж.* unspe̊akable.

неопла́тный unpåyable; ~ долг unpåyable debt.

неопла́ченный unpåid.

неопо́знанный uniden̊tified.

неопра́вданн|ый unwårranted, unjůstified; ~ое обвине̊ние unwårranted accusåtion.

неопределённ|ость *ж.* 1. (*нея́сность*) vågueness; 2. (*неопределённое положе́ние*) unce̊rtainty; ~ му́чит меня́ the suspe̊nse is ki̊lling me. ~ый 1. inde̊finite, inde̊terminate; идти́ в ~ом направле́нии go̊ no̊where in parti̊cular; челове́к ~ых заня́тий pe̊rson of no de̊finite occupåtion; он уе́хал на ~ое вре́мя he has gone awåy for an inde̊finite pe̊riod; 2. (*сму́тный, нея́сный*) vague; 3. (*ничего́ не выража́ющий*) våcant; ◇ ~ые местоиме́ния *грам.* inde̊finite pro̊nouns; ~ая фо́рма глаго́ла *грам.* the infi̊nitive; ~ый арти́кль inde̊finite årticle.

неопроверж́им|ый i̊ncontrove̊rtible, irre̊futable; ~ые доказа́тельства i̊ncontrove̊rtible proof(s).

неопря́тн|ость *ж.* slo̊venliness, unti̊diness. ~ый slo̊venly, unti̊dy; fro̊wzy *разг.*; (*о же́нщинах*) slåtternly; ~ый вид unke̊mpt/slo̊venly appe̊arance; ~ый костю́м shåbby suit; ~ый ребёнок unti̊dy child*.

неопублико́ванный unpůblished.

неопы́тн|ость *ж.* inexpe̊rience. ~ый inexpe̊rienced; ~ый челове́к inexpe̊rienced pe̊rson; (*новичо́к*) no̊vice.

неорганизо́ванн|ость *ж.* lack of organizåtion. ~ый uno̊rganized.

неоргани́ческ|ий inorgånic; ◇ ~ая хи́мия inorgånic che̊mistry.

неореали́зм *м.* ne̊oreålism.

неосведомлённость *ж.* i̊gnorance, lack of informåtion.

неосведомлённый bådly info̊rmed, ill-info̊rmed.

неосла́бн|ый unremi̊tting, assi̊duous; ~ое внима́ние unremi̊tting atte̊ntion.

неосмотри́тельн|ость *ж.* imprůdence. ~ый imprůdent; ~ый челове́к imprůdent pe̊rson; ~ый посту́пок imprůdent åction.

неоснова́тельный 1. unfo̊unded, te̊nuous, fli̊msy; 2. *разг.* (*легкомы́сленный*) håppy-go-lůcky.

неоспори́мый inconte̊stable, i̊ndispůtable.

неосторо́жн|ость *ж.* cårelessness; (*неблагоразу́мие*) imprůdence; ~ый cåreless; (*неблагоразу́мный*) imprůdent, incåutious.

неосуществи́мый unfe̊asible, impråcticable.

неосяза́емый intångible, impålpable.

неотврати́мый ine̊vitable.

неотвя́з|ный håunting; någging; ~чивый persi̊stent, någging.

неотдели́мый ~ от *чего-л.* inse̊parable from *smth.*

неотёсанный rough; *перен. разг.* unco̊uth.

неотзы́вчивый not respo̊nsive *predic.*, unrespo̊nsive.

нео́ткуда there is no̊where; ~ ждать по́мощи there is no̊where to expe̊ct help from; ~ ему́ знать э́то he co̊uldn't know that, there was no way he could know that.

неотло́жка *ж. разг.* åmbulance (se̊rvice).

неотло́жн|ый ůrgent, pre̊ssing; ~ое де́ло ůrgent måtter; ~ая по́мощь first aid.

неотрази́мый irresi̊stible; ~ уда́р crůshing/irresi̊stible blow; ~ до́вод irresi̊stible årgument.

неотсту́пн|ый insi̊stent, impo̊rtunate; ~ое пресле́дование rele̊ntless pursůit; ~ая мысль inescåpable thought.

неотъе́млем|ый inålienable; ~ая часть i̊ntegral part.

неофаш́|и́зм *м.* ne̊ofåscism. ~и́ст *м.* ne̊ofåscist. ~и́стский ne̊ofåscist.

неофициа́льный unoffi̊cial.

неохо́т|а *ж.*1. (*нежела́ние*) relůctance, unwi̊llingness; 2. *в знач. сказ. (дт., + инф.) разг.:* ~ мне говори́ть с ним I don't feel like speaking to him. ~но with relůctance, unwi̊llingly; ~ный relůctant, unwi̊lling.

неоцени́мый invåluable, ine̊stimable.

неощути́мый intångible; (*незначи́тельный*) inappre̊ciable.

непа́рный odd; that does, do not match *после сущ.*

непарти́йн|ый (*не состоя́щий в па́ртии*) non-pårty.

непереводи́мый untranslåtable.

непередава́емый inexpre̊ssible, unůtterable.

непереходный ~ глаго́л *грам.* intrånsitive verb.

неперспекти́вный låcking in pro̊spects *после сущ.*; unpro̊mising.

непи́саный unwri̊tten; ~ зако́н unwri̊tten law.

неплатёж *м.* fåilure to pay, non-påyment, defåult.

неплатёжеспосо́бн|ость *ж.* inso̊lvency. ~ый inso̊lvent.

неплате́льщик *м.* defåulter.

неплодоро́дный bårren, infe̊rtile.

непло́тно: ~ закры́тый half-clo̊sed; ~ закрыва́ть(ся) not shut pro̊perly.

непло́хо 1. *нареч.* not bådly, quite well; 2. *в знач. сказ. безл.* it is not bad.

неплохо́й quite a good.

непобеди́м|ость *ж.* invincibi̊lity. ~ый invi̊ncible, unco̊nquerable.

непови́нный i̊nnocent.

неповинове́ние *с.* disobe̊dience, refůsal to obe̊y.

неповоро́тливый (*нело́вкий*) clůmsy; (*медли́тельный*) slow, slůggish.

неповтори́мый ini̊mitable, uni̊que.

непого́да *ж.* bad we̊ather.

непогреши́м|ость *ж.* infallibi̊lity. ~ый infållible.

неподалёку not far off; ~ от *чего-л.* not far from *smth.*

непода́тливый unyi̊elding.

неподви́жн|о mo̊tionless, still. ~ый mo̊tionless, still; (*медли́тельный*) immo̊bile, slůggish; ~ое лицо́ sto̊ny face; ~ый взгля́д fixed stare; ~ый челове́к slůggish/sto̊lid pe̊rson.

неподде́льн|ый 1. (*по́длинный*) ge̊nuine, authe̊ntic; ~ые докуме́нты authe̊ntic påpers; 2. (*и́скренний*) since̊re, unfe̊igned; ~ая ра́дость since̊re joy.

неподку́пный incorrůptible.

неподходя́щ|ий impro̊per, unbeco̊ming; (*неприли́чный*) unse̊emly, inde̊corous; ~им о́бразом impro̊perly, unbeco̊mingly, in an impro̊per månner.

неподража́емый ini̊mitable.

неподходя́щий unsůitable; (*некста́ти*) inappro̊priate.

неподчине́ние *с.* insubordinåtion.

непозволи́тельный impermi̊ssible.

непоколеби́мый unshåkeable, ste̊adfast.

непоко́рный unrůly, rebe̊llious.

непокры́т|ый unco̊vered; с ~ой голово́й båre-headed; (*без шля́пы*) håtless.

непола́дки *мн.* (*ед.* непола́дка *ж.*) 1. defe̊cts; trouble *sg*; so̊mething wrong; организацио́нные ~ organizåtional difficulties; 2. *разг.* (*ссо́ры, нела́ды*) trouble *sg.*

неполнопра́вный underpri̊vileged; not enjo̊ying full rights *после сущ.*

неполнота́ *ж.* incomple̊teness; ~ све́дений insufficient informåtion.

неполноце́нн|ость *ж.* defe̊ctiveness; ко́мплекс ~ости *психол.* inferio̊rity co̊mplex. ~ый defe̊ctive.

непо́лн|ый 1. (*за́нятый чем-л. не до краёв*) that is not full *после сущ.*; ~ое ведро́ a pail that is not full; 2. (*не дости́гший определённого разме́ра, преде́ла и т. п.*) incomple̊te; ~ пе́речень *чего-л.* incomple̊te list of *smth.*; по ~ым да́нным accoording to incomple̊te dåta; ~ вес short weight; ~ая рабо́чая неде́ля short week.

непоме́рный exce̊ssive; (*о цене́*) exo̊rbitant.

непонима́ние *с.* incomprehe̊nsion, inabi̊lity/fåilure to understánd; взаймное ~ lack of understánding, inabílity to understánd one anóther.

непоня́тливый slów-wítted; dense *разг.*

непоня́тн|**о** 1. *нареч.* incomprehénsibly, unintélligibly; 2. *в знач. сказ. безл.:* ~, что он хо́чет сказа́ть it's not quite clear what he means; мне ~ I don't understánd. **~ый** unintélligible, incomprehénsible.

непоправи́м|**ый** irretríevable, irréparable, irremédiable; ~ шаг irretríevable step; **~ая** оши́бка fátal mistáke.

непоро́чный ínnocent, pure.

непоря́док *м.* disórder.

непоря́дочный dishónourable.

непосвящённый uninítiated.

непосе́д|**а** *м. и ж. разг.* fidget, réstless pérson. **~ли́вый** fidgety, réstless.

непоси́льн|**ый** exháusting, báck-breaking; **~ая** рабо́та work beyónd *one's* strength, work that is too much for *one.*

непосле́довательн|**ость** *ж.* inconsístency. **~ый** inconsístent.

непослуша́ние *с.* disobédience.

непослу́шн|**ый** disobédient; *перен.* unrúly; **~ые** ку́дри unrúly curls.

непосре́дственн|**ость** *ж.* (*непринуждённость*) spontanéity; (*простота*) ingénuousness, náturalness. **~ый** 1. diréct, immédiate; **~ый** нача́льник immédiate supérior; 2. (*непринуждённый, естественный*) spontáneous; (*простой*) ingénuous, nátural.

непостижи́м|**ый** incomprehénsible, inconcéivable, unfáthomable; ◇ уму́ ~o beyónd húman understánding.

непостоя́н|**ный** chángeable; (*о человеке тж.*) unstáble, fíckle; **~ная** пого́да chángeable wéather. **~ство** *с.* changeabílity; instabílity; incónstancy.

непохо́жий unlíke, dífferent.

непоча́т|**ый** untóuched; *перен.* untápped, abúndant; **~ая** буты́лка unópened bóttle; ◇ ~ край abúndance; рабо́ты — ~ край there's no end of work to be done.

непочте́ние *с.* disrespéct.

непочти́тельн|**ость** *ж.* disrespéct. **~ый** disrespéctful.

непра́вда *ж.* 1. untrúth, lie; э́то ~! it's a lie!, it's not true!; 2. (*обман, мошенничество*) decéption.

неправдоподо́б|**ие** *с.* improbabílity. **~ный** unlíkely, impróbable.

непра́вильн|**о** 1. wrong, incorréctly; ~ отвеча́ть ánswer wrong; ~ написа́ть а́дрес на конве́рте addréss the létter incorréctly, put* the wrong addréss on the létter; ~ указа́ть но́мер, фами́лию *и т. п.* give* the wrong númber, name *etc.*; 2. *в сочетании с гл.* информи́ровать, истолко́вывать, понима́ть, представля́ть, суди́ть, цити́ровать, произноси́ть *переводится приста́вкой* mis-, *напр.:* misinfórm, mispronóunce *etc.*; ~ указа́ть доро́гу *кому-л.* misdiréct *smb.* **~ый** 1. (*отклоняющийся от обычных норм*) abnórmal; (*непропорциональный*) irrégular; *разг.* (*не соблюдающий правил морали*) wáyward; 2. (*ошибочный*) wrong, incorréct, false; 3. (*несправедливый*) unjúst, unfáir; ◇ **~ые** глаго́лы *грам.* irrégular verbs; **~ая** дробь *мат.* impróper fráction.

неправоме́рный illegítimate.

неправомо́чный incómpetent; withóut authórity *после сущ.*

непра́в|**ый** 1. *обыкн. кратк. ф.* wrong; вы **~ы** you are wrong; 2. (*несправедливый*) unjúst.

непракти́чный unprácticaI.

непревзойдённ|**ый** unsurpássed, mátchless; sécond to none *predic.*; ~ ма́стер unsurpássed máster; **~ая** глу́пость mátchless stupídity.

непредви́денный unforeséen; ~ расхо́д unforeséen expénse.

непредпреднаме́ренн|**ый** uninténtional; *юр.* unpremédi-tated; **~ое** оскорбле́ние uninténtional ínsult.

непредубеждённый unbíás(s)ed, unpréjudiced.

непредусмо́тренный unprovíded for, unenvísaged; not províded for *после сущ.*

непредусмотри́тельн|**ость** *ж.* imprόvidence. **~ый** imprόvident.

непреклόнн|**ость** *ж.* inexorabílity, determinátion. **~ый** inéxorable, indόmitable, unyíelding; **~ая** во́ля infléxible will; **~ый** в достиже́нии свои́х це́лей indόmitable in the pursúit of *one's* aims.

непрекраща́ющийся incéssant.

непрело́жн|**ый** immútable; (*неоспоримый*) indispútable, incontéstable; ~ зако́н indeféasible law; **~ая** и́стина incontéstable truth.

непреме́нн|**о** cértainly, súrely; withóut fail; он ~ придёт he is sure to come. **~ый** indispénsable; **~ое** усло́вие indispénsable condítion, a síne qua nón.

непреодоли́м|**ый** insúperable, insurmóuntable; **~ое** жела́ние overmástering desíre; **~ая** си́ла irresístible force; **~ое** препя́тствие insurmóuntable bárrier/óbstacle.

непререка́емый indispútable.

непреры́вн|**о** contínuously, uninterrúptedly. **~ость** *ж.* continúity. **~ый** contínuous, uninterrúpted; **~ая** цепь собы́тий unbróken chain/succéssion of evénts; **~ый** рост произво́дства uninterrúpted growth of prodúction.

непреста́нн|**о** incéssantly. **~ый** incéssant, céaseless.

неприве́тлив|**ый** 1. ungrácious, unfríendly; ~ челове́к ungrácious pérson; ~ взгляд unwélcoming glance; 2. (*мрачный, угрюмый*) unhóspitable, uninvíting; **~ая** ме́стность unhóspitable locálity.

непривлека́тельный unattráctive.

непривы́чк|**а** *ж. разг.* lack of hábit; с **~и** béing unaccústomed (to), not béing used (to); э́то с **~и** it's becáuse *one* is not used to it.

непривы́чн|**о** *в знач. сказ. безл.* it seems strange; ~ ему́ на но́вом ме́сте he feels strange in his new surróundings. **~ый** 1. (*новый, чуждый для кого-л.*) strange, unaccústomed; **~ая** обстано́вка unaccústomed círcumstances/situátion; 2. (*о человеке*) of líttle expérience *после сущ.*

непригля́дный unattráctive, unpreposséssing.

неприго́дный úseless; ~ к *чему-л.* unfit for *smth.*

неприе́млем|**ый** 1. unaccéptable; **~ые** усло́вия unaccéptable terms; 2. (*недопустимый*) inadmíssible.

непри́знанный unrécognized, unacknówledged.

неприкоснове́нн|**ость** *ж.* inviolabílity; (*дипломати́ческая*) immúnity; ~ ли́чности inviolabílity of pérson; ~ жили́ща the sánctity/inviolabílity of the home. **~ый** 1. untóuchable; **~ый** запа́с untóuchable resérve; (*продово́льствия*) emérgency/íron rátion; 2. (*находящийся под защитой закона*) invíolable; **~ое** лицо́ protécted pérson.

неприкра́шенн|**ый** unvárnished; **~ая** и́стина unvárnished/unadúlterated truth.

неприкры́т|**ый** 1. (*неплотно закрытый*) slíghtly ópen; оста́вить дверь **~ой** leave* the door ajár; 2. (*не покрытый сверху*) bare, uncóvered; (*оставленный без защиты*) unprotécted, undefénded; 3. (*явный*) ópen, unconcéaled; **~ая** пра́вда the náked truth.

неприли́ч|**ие** *с.* impropríety; (*непристойность*) indécency; груб до ~ия scándalously rude. **~но** impróperly, not próperly; **~но** вести́ себя́ beháve impróperly/shóckingly. **~ный** impróper; (*непристойный*) indécent.

непримени́мый inápplicable.

неприме́тн|**ый** 1. (*незаметный*) impercéptible; **~ая** ра́зница impercéptible dífference; 2. (*непримечательный*) inconspícuous.

непримири́м|**ый** irréconcilable; ~ враг irréconcilable/sworn énemy; **~ые** противоре́чия irréconcilable contradíctions.

непринуждённ|**ость** *ж.* éasiness, fréedom; ~ обстано́вки córdial átmosphere. **~ый** nátural, éasy; **~ый** тон nátural tone; **~ая** по́за éasy pósture/áttitude.

непpисоединение *с.* non-alignment.

непpисоединивш|ийся: ~иеся госудáрства the non-aligned cóuntries.

непpиспособленный unpráctical.

непpистóйн|ость *ж.* 1. indécensy; ~ поведéния indécent/báwdy beháviour; 2. (*поступок, речь и т. п.*) obscénity; говоpить ~ости make* indécent remárks. ~ый indécent, obscéne, lewd.

непpистýпный 1. unassáilable, imprégnable; ~ая высотá unassáilable peak; 2. (*о человеке*) unappróachable, alóof.

непpитвóрный unafféctted, unféigned, undisguísed.

непpитязáтельный undemánding; (*простóй*) unassúming, módest.

непpихотлив|ый 1. (*нетребовательный*) not hard to please *после сущ.*, unfastídious; (*о растениях*) hárdy; 2. (*простóй, незатéйливый*) plain, símple; ~ рисýнок símple dráwing; ~ая пи́ща plain food.

непpиязненный unfríendly, hóstile.

непpиязнь *ж.* dislíke; hostílity.

непpиятель *м. собир.* énemy; ~ский énemy *attr.*

непpиятн|о 1. *нареч.* unpléasantly; 2. *в знач. сказ. безл. (дт.)* it is unpléasant (for); емý бы́ло ~ слýшать э́то he found it unpléasant to lísten; э́то бýдет вам ~ it will be unpléasant for you. ~ость *ж.* míshap; *мн.* (*огорчéния*) tróuble *sg*, unpléasantness *sg*; какáя ~ость! how unpléasant! ~ый unpléasant, disagréeable; ~ый пáрень unpléasant féllow; ~ый разговóр unpléasant conversátion.

непpобивáемый impénetrable *тж. перен.*

непpобýдн|ый 1. wákeless; ~ сон deep sleep; *перен.* (*смерть*) the etérnal sleep; спать ~ым сном be* fast asléep; *перен.* sleep* the sleep of death; 2. (*о пьянице*) invéterate.

непpоводник *м. физ.* non-condúctor.

непpоглядн|ый impénetrable; (*тёмный*) pitch-dárk; ~ая ночь impénetrable night.

непpодолжи́тельн|ый short, brief; в течéние ~ого вpéмени for a short time.

непpодукти́вн|ый unprodúctive (*тж. лингв.*); ~ труд unprodúctive work; ~ая трáта вpéмени waste of time; ~ые сýффиксы unprodúctive súffixes.

непpодýманный ill-consídered.

непpоéзжий impássable; (*затруднительный для езды́*) difficult.

непpозрáчный opáque.

непpоизводи́тельн|ость *ж.* unprodúctiveness. ~ый unprodúctive; ~ый труд unprodúctive lábour; ~ая трáта вpéмени waste of time; ~ые расхóды unprodúctive expénditure.

непpоизвóльный invóluntary.

непpолáзн|ый *разг.* impássable; по дорóгам былá ~ая грязь the roads were a sea of mud.

непpомокáемый wáterproof; ~ плащ wáterproof máckintosh.

непpоницáем|ость *ж.* impenetrabílity. ~ый 1. impénetrable; (*для воды́, гáзов тж.*) impérvious; ~ый для звýка sóund-proof; ~ый мрак impénetrable dárkness; 2. (*скры́тный*) enigmátic.

непpопоpционáльн|ость *ж.* dispropórtion. ~ый dispropórtionate.

непpосвещённый unenlíghtened.

непpости́тельн|о unforgíveably. ~ый unpárdonable, inexcúsable.

непpотивлéние *с.* non-resístance.

непpоторённ|ый unexplóred, unúsual; пойти́ по ~ому пути́ *перен.* take* an unexplóred path.

непpофессионáл *м.* nonproféssional, ámateur.

непpоходи́м|ый 1. impássable; ~ лес impénetrable fórest; 2. *разг.* (*совершéнный, пóлный*) útter, rank; ~ дурáк útter fool; ~ая глýпость rank stupídity.

непpóчный 1. flímsy; (*о сооружéниях*) unstáble, insecúre; 2. (*о чýвствах*) fléeting, precárious.

непpóшен|ый uninvíted; (*нежелательный*) unásked-for; (*невóльный*) unbídden, invóluntary; ~ гость uninvíted guest; ~ совéт unásked-for advíce; ~ые мы́сли unbídden thoughts.

непpямóй 1. indiréct; 2. (*неоткровенный*) not stráightforward; ~ отвéт evásive ánswer.

неpаботоспосóбный incapácitated, disábled; unáble to work *predic.*

неpабóч|ий 1.: ~ее происхождéние non-wórking-cláss órigin; ~ая одéжда léisure clothes; 2. (*о скóте*) non-wórking; 3. (*о вpéмени*) non-wórking, off; ~ день non-wórking day, off day; 4. (*не располагáющий к работе*) distrácting; ~ая обстанóвка not the right átmosphere for work.

неpáвенство *с.* inequálity.

неpавнодýшный (*к дт.*) not indífferent (to).

неpавномéрн|ость *ж.* unévenness; ~ развития unévenness of devélopment, unéven devélopment. ~ый unéven; ~ое развитие unéven devélopment.

неpавнопрáв|ие *с.* (*sócial*) inequálity. ~ный unéqual; posséssing unéqual rights *после сущ.*

неpáвн|ый unéqual; ~ые си́лы unéqual fórces; пасть в ~ом бою́ die fíghting against odds; ~ брак misallíance.

неpади́в|ый slack, half-héarted; (*небрéжный*) cáreless; ~ое отношéние к занятиям half-héarted áttitude to *one's* stúdies; ~ учени́к, рабóтник slack púpil, wórkman*.

неpазбери́ха *ж. разг.* múddle.

неpазбóрчивый 1. (*о пóчерке*) illégible; (*невнятный*) incomprehénsible; 2. (*невзыскательный*) undiscríminating; 3. (*беспринци́пный*) unscrúpulous; ~ в срéдствах unscrúpulous.

неpазвитóй undevéloped; (*ýмственно*) báckward.

неpазгáданный unsólved; (*нерасшифрóванный*) undecíphered.

неpазговóрчив|ость *ж.* tacitúrnity. ~ый táciturn, sílent; ~ый человéк man* of few words.

неpаздéльный indivísible.

неpазличи́мый indistínguishable.

неpазлýчн|ый inséparable; ~ые друзья́ inséparable friends.

неpазреш|ённый 1. (*запрещённый*) prohíbited, forbídden; 2. (*нерешённый*) unsólved; ~ вопрóс unsólved próblem. ~и́мый insóluble.

неpазруши́мый indestrúctible.

неpазры́вн|ый indissóluble, inséparable; ~ая связь indissóluble ties *pl*; ~ая дрýжба indissóluble fríendship.

неpазýмный unréasonable, unwíse, irrátional; ~ человéк irrátional/unréasonable pérson; ~ поступóк unwíse áction.

неpасположéние (*к дт.*) dislíke (of, for).

неpаспоряди́тельн|ость *ж.* inefficiency. ~ый ineffícient.

неpаспространéние *с.* non-proliferátion. ~ я́дерного орýжия non-proliferátion of núclear wéapons.

неpассуди́тельный irrátional, unréasonable; ~ человéк irrátional pérson; ~ поступóк irrátional/unréasonable áction.

неpасторóпный slow, lánguid.

неpасчётливый impróvident; (*в денéжном отношéнии тж.*) thríftless, extrávagant.

неpационáльный irrátional.

нерв *м.* nerve; крéпкие ~ы strong nerves; ◇ дéйствовать комý-либо на ~ы get* on *smb.'s* nerves.

нерви́ровать *несов.* (*вн.*) make* (*smb.*) nérvous.

нéрвничать *несов.* be* nérvous, feel* nérvous, be* excíted; (*волновáться*) wórry.

нервнобольнóй *м.* nérve-patient, neurótic.

нéрвн|ость *ж.* nérvousness. ~ый nérvous; ~ая систéма nérvous sýstem; ~ый припáдок fit of nerves; ~ый человéк nérvous pérson; ~ое состоя́ние nérvous state of mind; ~ая рабóта trýing/hárassing work.

нерво́зн|ость ж. (nérvous) ténsion; ~ый nérvy, híghly strung; jíttery разг.

нереа́льн|ость ж. 1. unreálity; 2. (невыполни́мость) impracticabílity. ~ый 1. (фантасти́ческий) unréal;·2. (невыполни́мый) imprácticable, unrealístic.

нерегуля́рн|ость ж. irregulárity. ~ый irrégular.

нере́дк|ий not infréquent; (обы́чный) not unúsual. ~о not infréquently; quite óften.

нерента́бельный unprófitable.

не́рест м. spáwning.

нереши́тельн|о hésitantly. ~ость ж. indecísion; быть в ~ости be* hésitating, be* in doubt, vácillate. ~ый indecísive, irrésolute, hésitant; ~ый челове́к irrésolute pérson; ~ый тон hésitant tone.

нержаве́ющ|ий rústproof; ~ая сталь stáinless steel.

неритми́чн|ый unrhýthmical; ~ые движе́ния unrhýthmical/errátic móvements; ~ая рабо́та unstéady work, wórking in fits and starts.

неро́бк|ий brave, féarless.

неро́вн|ый 1. (негла́дкий) unéven, rough; ~ая ме́стность rough/rúgged cóuntry; 2. (криво́й) cróoked, not straight; ~ая ли́ния cróoked line; 3. разг. (неодина́ковый) unéqual; 4. (неравноме́рный, преры́вистый) unéven, unstéady; ~ пульс unstéady pulse; ~ое дыха́ние unéven bréathing; 5. (неусто́йчивый) errátic, eccéntric; ~ хара́ктер errátic témper.

не́рпа ж. зоол. ringed seal.

неру́сский non-Rússian; (не сво́йственный ру́сским) not Rússian predic., un-Rússian.

неруши́мый invíolable, indestrúctible.

неря́|ха м. и ж. slóven; (о же́нщине тж.) sláttern, slut. ~шество с., ~шливость ж. slóvenliness. ~шливый 1. (неопря́тный) slóvenly; ~шливый челове́к slóvenly pérson; ~шливый вид slóvenly appéarance; 2. (небре́жный) cáreless, slípshod; ~шливая рабо́та cáreless/slípshod work.

несамостоя́тельн|ый 1. lácking in inítiative по́сле сущ., cháracterless; (материа́льно зави́симый) not self-supporting, depéndent; ~ челове́к pérson lácking in inítiative; 2. (о труде́, произведе́нии) unoríginal, ímitative.

несбы́точн|ый unrealízable; ~ые мечты́ cástles in the air; ~ые наде́жды unfóunded hopes.

несваре́ние с.: ~ желу́дка indigéstion.

несве́дущий uninfórmed, ill-infórmed; (в пр.) ígnorant (of), unconvérsant (with).

несве́ж|ий 1. (испо́рченный) stale; ~ее мя́со meat that is not fresh, táinted meat; 2. (лишённый све́жести) not fresh predic.; име́ть ~ вид look tíred; 3. разг. (уста́релый) old; ~ но́мер газе́ты back númber; 4. (нечи́стый) soiled.

несвоевре́менн|ый unpúnctual, irrégular; (неуме́стный) inópportune, ill-tímed; ~ая я́вка на рабо́ту unpúnctual/irrégular atténdance (at work).

несвя́зный incohérent, disconnécted.

несгиба́емый infléxible; перен. тж. unbénding.

несгово́рчивый intráctable, óbstinate.

несгора́емый incombústible; fíreproof; ~ шкаф safe.

несде́ржан|ность ж. lack of restráint. ~ный 1. (об обеща́нии и т. п.) unfulfílled; 2. (о хара́ктере) uncontrólled; (ре́зкий) unrestráined, víolent; ~ный челове́к excítable/impétuous pérson; ~ный тон víolent tone.

несдоброва́ть сов. ему́ ~ he is héading for tróuble.

несерьёзн|ый 1. (легкомы́сленный) líght-mínded, trívial, supérficial, shállow; ~ые лю́ди shállow/trívial péople; ~ вид frívolous appéarance; ~ое отноше́ние к де́лу líght-mínded/supérficial áttitude to the mátter; 2. (незначи́тельный) unimpórtant, trívial; ~ое де́ло trívial mátter, trífle; ~ая ра́на slight wound.

несессе́р м. dréssing-case.

несимметри́чный asýmmetric(al).

несказа́нный inexpréssible.

нескла́дн|ый 1. (неуклю́жий) ungáinly, áwkward; ~ая фигу́ра bad/áwkward figure; 2. (неуда́чно вы́раженный) clúmsy, disjóinted; ~ое предложе́ние clúmsy séntence; 3. (неуда́чный) fútile.

несклоня́емый грам. indeclínable.

не́скольк|о I числ. séveral; (немно́го) a few; ~ раз séveral times; в ~их места́х in séveral pláces; сказа́ть ~ слов say* a few words; ◇ в ~их слова́х in a few words. не́сколько II нареч. slíghtly, sómewhat, a little.

несконча́емый intérminable, éndless, perpétual.

нескро́мный 1. immódest, presúmptuous; 2. (бесцеремо́нный, нетакти́чный) indiscréet, rude; 3. (неприли́чный) indécent, impróper, immódest.

нескрыва́емый unconcéaled, undisguísed.

несло́жн|ый símple; ~ механи́зм símple méchanism; ~ая нату́ра símple/uncómplicated náture; ~ вопро́с símple/éasy quéstion.

неслы́ханн|ый prodígious, unhéard-of; ~ая уда́ча prodígious succéss.

неслы́шный ináudible.

несме́лый tímid.

несме́т|ный cóuntless, vast; ~ое бога́тство vast wealth; ~ые сокро́вища cóuntless tréasures.

несмолка́емый céaseless, uncéasing.

несмотря́: ~ на in spite of, despíte, notwithstánding; ~ на то, что... despíte the fact that...; ◇ ~ ни на что in spite of all.

несмыва́емый indélible.

несно́сный intólerable, unbéarable; (о челове́ке) insúfferable.

несоблюде́ние с. non-obsérvance; (наруше́ние) infríngement.

несовершенноле́т|ие с. minórity. ~ний прил. 1. únder age по́сле сущ.; 2. в знач. сущ. м. mínor.

несоверше́нный I impérfect.

несоверше́нный II: ~ вид грам. imperféctive áspect.

несоверше́нство с. imperféction.

несовмести́м|ость ж. incompatibílity; ~ тка́ней мед. incompatibílity of tíssues. ~ый incompátible; ~ые поня́тия incompátible idéas.

несогла́с|ие с. 1. disagréement, dífference of opínion; 2. (разла́д, ссо́ра) disagréement; 3. (отка́з) refúsal, dissént. ~ный 1.: быть ~ным not agrée, disagrée; 2. (несогласо́ванный) únco-órdinated; (о пе́нии) discórdant.

несогласо́ванн|ость ж. lack of co-ordinátion. ~ый únco-órdinated; ~ые де́йствия únco-órdinated áctions.

несозву́чный díssonant; ~ эпо́хе not in the spírit of the times.

несозна́тельн|ость ж. 1. thóughtlessness, méntal immatúrity; 2. (полити́ческая отста́лость) polítical unawáreness/ígnorance; 3. (безотве́тственность) irresponsibílity. ~ый 1. thóughtless; (неосозна́нный) uncónscious; ~ый ребёнок thóughtless child*; 2. (полити́чески отста́лый) polítically ígnorant; ~ые ма́ссы polítically ígnorant másses; 3. (безотве́тственный) irrespónsible; ~ое отноше́ние к де́лу irrespónsible áttitude.

несоизмери́м|ый incomménsurable; перен. incompátible; ~ые величи́ны incomménsurable quántities; ~ые поня́тия incompátible idéas.

несокруши́м|ый invíncible; ~ая во́ля uncónquerable will.

несо́лоно: уйти́ ~ хлеба́вши разг. get* nóthing for one's pains.

несомне́нн|о undóubtedly, indispútably; он ~ придёт he's sure to come. ~ость ж. cértainty. ~ый undóubted, unmistákable, indispútable; ~ый успе́х an indispútable/indúbitable succéss.

несообрази́тельный slow(-witted); dense разг.

несообра́зн|ость ж. incongrúity; (неле́пость) absúrdity. ~ый incóngruous; (неле́пый) absúrd, prepósterous.

несоотве́тствие *с.* dispárity (between), discrépancy (between); ~ хара́ктеров incompatibílity (of témperament).

несоразме́рный dispropórtionate.

несорто́в|о́й: ~ые семена́ lów-grade seeds.

несостоя́тельн|ость *ж.* 1. insólvency; объяви́ть о ~ости declа́re onesélf insólvent/bа́nkrupt; 2. (*необоснованность*) unsóundness, flímsiness. ~ый 1. insólvent, bа́nkrupt; ~ый должни́к insólvent; 2. (*небогатый*) of módest means *после сущ.*; 3. (*необоснованный*) unsóund; ~ая тео́рия unsóund/bа́nkrupt théory.

неспе́лый unrípe.

неспоко́й|о 1. *нареч.* réstlessly, а́nxiously; 2. *в знач. сказ. безл.* it is distúrbing/wórrying; на се́рдце у меня́ бы́ло ~ I felt distúrbed/unéasy; 3. *в знач. сказ. безл.* (*о нарушении спокойствия где-л.*): в до́ках ~ the а́tmosphere at the docks is tense. ~ый réstless, а́nxious, tróubled.

неспосо́бн|ость *ж.* inability. ~ый incа́pable; (*к учению*) dull; not cléver *predic.*, not bright *predic.*; ~ый ма́льчик dull/bа́ckward boy; ~ый к рисова́нию with no abílity to draw; ~ый на же́ртвы incа́pable of sа́crifice.

несправедли́в|ость *ж.* injústice. ~ый unjúst, unfа́ir.

неспроста́ *разг.* with a définite púrpose, with an últimáte aim; э́то ~! there's more in this than meets the eye!; он ~ заговори́л об э́том there was something behínd what he said.

неспряга́емый *грам.* that does not cónjugate *после сущ.*

несравне́нн|о 1. (*замечательно*) supérbly; 2. (*гораздо*) much, far. ~ый incómparable, mа́tchless.

несравни́мый 1. (*очень хороший*) incómparable; 2. (*различный, непохожий*) that cа́nnot be compа́red *после сущ.*

нестанда́ртный unstа́ndardized, non-stа́ndard.

нестерпи́мый intólerable, unbéarable.

нести́ I, понести́ (*вн.*) 1. (*перемещать на себе*) cа́rry (*smb., smth.*); *перен.* bring* (*smth.*); ~ мешо́к на спине́ cа́rry a sack on one's back; ~ культу́ру в ма́ссы bring* cúlture to the mа́sses; ~ мир наро́дам bring* peace to the world; 2. (*быстро передвигать, мчать*) cа́rry (*smb., smth.*) swíftly, bear* (*smb., smth.*) swíftly; (*о ветре, течении тж.*) sweep* (*smth.*) (alóng), drive* (*smth.*); (*о лошади*) bolt; ве́тер несёт ту́чи the wind drives the clouds; тече́ние несёт ло́дку the cúrrent bears/sweeps the boat alóng; 3. *безл.* (*тв.*): с мо́ря несло́ сыры́м во́здухом damp air drífted in from the sea; от него́ несёт табако́м he reeks of tobа́cco; 4. *тк. несов.* (*выполнять*) perfórm (*smth.*); ~ обя́занности perfórm the dúties; ~ слу́жбу *воен.* serve; 5. (*терпеть что-л.*) bear* (*smth.*); ~ поте́ри bear*/sustа́in lósses; ~ расхо́ды bear* the expénse; ~ убы́тки lose* móney; ~ наказа́ние undergó* púnishment; 6. *разг.* (*говорить что-л. неразумное*) búrble (*smth.*); что ты несёшь? what are you drívelling abóut?; ~ вздор, чепуху́ talk nónsense; ◇ ~ отве́тственность bear* the responsibílity; высоко́ ~ го́лову hold* one's head high.

нести́ II, снести́: ~ я́йца lay* eggs.

нести́сь I, понести́сь 1. (*мчаться*) rush (alóng), tear* alóng; по́езд нёсся с необыкнове́нной быстрото́й the train rushed alóng at terrífic speed; ту́чи несу́тся по не́бу clouds are scúdding acróss the sky; 2. *разг.* (*быстро бежать*) rush, tear*.

нести́сь II, снести́сь (*о птицах*) lay* (*eggs*).

несто́йк|ий unstа́ble; ~ие духи́ weak pérfume *sg.*

несто́ящ|ий trívial; э́то ~ee де́ло it's not worth while; ~ челове́к wórthless féllow.

нестроево́й I *прил. воен.* 1. non-cómbatant; 2. *в знач. сущ. м.* non-cómbatant.

нестроево́й II (*не годный для постройки*) that is not fit for búilding *после сущ.*

нестро́йн|о discórdantly. ~ый 1. (*лишённый строй-*

ности) ill-propórtioned; 2. (*беспорядочно расположенный*) disórderly; ~ые ряды́ disórderly ranks; 3. (*неслаженный*) discórdant.

несудохо́дный unnа́vigable.

несура́зн|ый *разг.* 1. (*нелепый, бессмысленный*) absúrd; ~ разгово́р absúrd conversа́tion; 2. (*неуклюжий*) clúmsy, а́wkward.

несуще́ственный unimpórtant, unessе́ntial.

несхо́дство *с.* dissimilа́rity.

несчастли́вый unhа́ppy; (*неудачный*) unlúcky.

несча́стн|ый *прил.* 1. unhа́ppy, unfórtunate, míserable; сде́лать кого́-л. ~ым make* smb.'s life míserable; 2. *разг.* (*злополучный*) ill-stа́rred; 3. *разг.* (*жалкий*) wrе́tched; 4. *в знач. сущ. м.* wretch, unfórtunate pérson.

несча́сть|е *с.* misfórtune; (*бедствие*) calа́mity, disа́ster; ◇ к ~ю unfórtunately; я име́л ~ (+ *инф.*) I had the bad luck (+ to *inf.*)

несчётный innúmerable.

несъедо́бн|ый inédible; (*невкусный*) unéatable; ~ые грибы́ inédible fúngi.

нет I *отриц. частица* 1. (*при ответе*) no; (*как опровержение отрицательного предположения*) yes; вы согла́сны пое́хать туда́? — Нет (*не согла́сен*) do you agrée to go there? — No (I do not); пойдёшь в кино́? — Нет (*не пойду́*) will you go to the cínema? — No (I won't); он не́ был сего́дня в шко́ле? — Нет, был he wа́sn't at school todа́y, was he? — Yes, he was; 2. (*в начале реплики*, *с оттенком возражения, удивления*) but; ~, вы его́ не ви́дели but you didn't see him; 3. (= *не + данное сказ. — при том же подлежащем*) not; (*в безл. предложении после союза или тж.*) no; (*при другом подлежащем*) передаётся через сокращённое *сказ.* + not; ку́пит он кни́гу и́ли ~? will he buy the book or not?; совсе́м ~, во́все ~ not at all, not in the least; ещё ~, ~ ещё тот; почему́ ~? why not?; хорошо́ и́ли ~, но э́то так good or no/not, it is so; я чита́л э́ту кни́гу, а он ~ I have read this book, but he hа́sn't; он мо́жет э́то сде́лать, а она́ ~ he can do it, but she can't; ◇ ~~ да и... once in a while...; ни да ни ~ néither yes, nor no; свести́ на ~ bring* to nought; сойти́, свести́сь на ~ come* to nought/nóthing.

нет II *в знач. сказ. безл.* 1. (*не имеется*) there is/are no...; ~ оши́бок there is no..., у меня́ ничего́ ~... I have, he has no...; 2. (*отсутствует — о местонахождении человека*) is/are not; ва́шего бра́та здесь ~ your bróther is not here; никого́ ~ до́ма there is nóbody at home; ◇ ~ и ~, ~ да ~ still no sign, not a sign; ~ как ~ nówhere to be seen; чего́ (*только*) ~! the amóunt of stuff there!

нетакти́чн|ость *ж.* tа́ctlessness. ~ый tа́ctless; ~ый вопро́с tа́ctless/indiscréet quéstion.

нетала́нтливый untа́lented, médiocre.

нетвёрд|о: ~ знать *что-л.* not know *smth.* próperly; ~ стоя́ть на нога́х be* unstéady/shа́ky on one's legs. ~ый 1. (*мягкий*) soft; 2. (*неустойчивый*) unstéady, shа́ky; ~ая похо́дка unstéady gait; ~ый по́черк a shа́ky hand; 3. (*нерешительный, неуверенный*) írrésolute; ~ый хара́ктер írrésolute chа́racter; он нетвёрд в матема́тике his mathemа́tics are shа́ky.

нетерпели́в|ость *ж.* impа́tience. ~ый impа́tient.

нетерпе́ние *с.* impа́tience; ждать с ~м кого́-л., чего́-л. wait impа́tiently for *smb., smth.*; (*о чём-л. приятном*) look fórward to *smth.*; выража́ть ~ expréss impа́tience.

нетерпи́м|ость *ж.* intólerance. ~ый 1. (*недопустимый*) intólerable; ~ое положе́ние intólerable situа́tion; 2. (*о человеке*) intólerant.

нетова́рищеск|ий uncómradely, unfríendly; ~ое отноше́ние uncómradely а́ttitude.

нетороплив|о unhúrriedly, tа́king one's time; он ~ откры́л я́щик he took his time ópening the box. ~ость *ж.*

léisureliness, unhúrried mánner. ~ый léisured, delíberate; (*медлительный*) unhúrried, slow; ~ые шагú méasured tread *sg*.

нетóчн|ость ж. ináccuracy; (*ошибка тж.*) érror. ~ый ináccurate, inexáct.

нетрéбовательный 1. (*не предъявляющий больших требований*) unexácting, lax; ~ учúтель unexácting téacher; 2. (*неприхотливый*) undemánding; éasy to please *predic*.

нетрéзв|ый drunk, intóxicated; в ~ом вúде drunk, in a state of intoxicátion.

нетрóнутый untóuched; *перен*. fresh, unsúllied.

нетрýдн|ый not dífficult, quite éasy; это ~ая задáча it is not a dífficult task.

нетрудов|óй 1. non-wórking; ~ элемéнт non-wórking élements *pl*; 2. (*получаемый не от своего труда*) unéarned; ~ые дохóды unéarned íncome *sg*.

нетрудоспосóбн|ость ж. disáblement, incapácity for work; пóлная (частúчная) ~ pérmanent (pártial) disáblement. ~ый disábled; быть ~ым be* unáble to work.

нéтто *прил. неизм. торг.* net; вес ~ net weight.

неубедúтельный unconvíncing.

неýбранн|ый: ~ая кóмната untídied room; ~ая постéль unmáde bed; ~ урожáй ungáthered hárvest; ~ые поля unréaped fields.

неувáж|éние *с.* disrespéct, lack of respéct. ~úтельный 1. (*недостаточно основательный*) inádequate; ~úтельная причúна insufficient/inádequate excúse; 2. *разг.* (*непочтительный*) disrespéctful; ~úтельный тон disrespéctful tone.

неувéренн|ость ж. lack of cónfidence; (в *пр.*) uncértainty (as to); ~ в себé díffidence. ~ый uncértain, hésitant; ~ый в себé díffident, not sure of onesélf.

неувядáем|ый unfáding, undýing; ~ая слáва undýing fame.

неувя́зка ж. *разг.* hitch; ~ в рабóте hitch.

неугасúмый inextínguishable; *перен. тж.* unquénchable.

неугомóнный *разг.* réstless; (*подвижный, шумливый*) bóisterous; (*непрекращающийся*) céaseless, uncéasing.

неудáч|а ж. fáilure, revérse; потерпéть ~у súffer a revérse; (*о плане и т. п.*) fail, miscárry. ~ник *м.* a fáilure. ~ный 1. unsuccéssful; 2. (*неудовлетворительный*) poor, unsuccéssful; ~ный перевóд unháppy translátion; ~ный фотоснúмок poor phótograph.

неудержúмый irrepréssible, irresístible.

неудивúтельно в знач. сказ. it is not surprísing.

неудóбн|о 1. нареч. áwkwardly; uncómfortably; 2. в знач. сказ. безл. (об ощущении неудобства) it is uncómfortable; сидéть бы́ло ~ it was an uncómfortable seat; 3. в знач. сказ. безл. (о чувстве смущения): мне ~ I feel áwkward/embárrassed; мне бы́ло ~ за негó his beháviour embárrassed me, I found his beháviour embárrassing; 4. в знач. сказ. безл. (+ инф.) (о сознании неуместности чего-л.) it is áwkward (+ to inf); ~ начинáть такóй разговóр в машúне a car is not the place for a conversátion of that kind. ~ый 1. uncómfortable, inconvénient; 2. (*неловкий*) áwkward; 3. (*неприятный, затруднительный*) áwkward, embárrassing.

неудобочитáемый unréadable.

неудóбство *с.* 1. inconvénience; *мн.* discómforts; 2. (*смущение, неловкость*) embárrassment.

неудовлетворённ|ость ж. dissatisfáction. ~ый unsátisfied; (*недовольный*) dissátisfied; ~ое любопы́тство unsátisfied curiósity.

неудовлетворúтельн|о нареч. 1. unsatisfáctorily; 2. в знач. сущ. с. нескл. unsatisfáctory mark. ~ый unsatisfáctory.

неудовóльствие *с.* displéasure.

неужéли réally; ~ он хóчет пойтú тудá? does he réally want to go there?, súrely he dóesn't want to go there; ~ это прáвда? is it réally true?, do you réally mean it?; ~! réally?, you don't mean it!

неужúвчивый unsóciable, dífficult; ~ человéк dífficult pérson; ~ харáктер unsóciable cháracter.

неузнавáем|ость ж.: до ~ости beyónd recognítion. ~ый unrecógnizable; он стал совсéм неузнавáем you wóuldn't know him.

неуклóнн|о stéadily, unswérvingly; (*непрерывно*) uninterrúptedly, stéadily. ~ый stéady; (*непоколебимый*) stéadfast, unswérving.

неуклю́жий clúmsy, áwkward.

неукротúмый indómitable; (о животных) untámable; ~ гнев ungóvernable ánger.

неуловúмый 1. elúsive; он неуловúм he is dífficult to catch; 2. (*незаметный*) bárely percéptible, súbtle; ~ звук bárely áudible sound.

неумé|лый unskílful; (*сделанный неумело*) clúmsy. ~ние *с.* inability, lack of skill.

неумéренн|ость ж. lack of moderátion, immoderátion; (*в еде, питье*) intémperance, excéss. ~ый 1. (*о человеке*) intémperate, immóderate; 2. (*чрезмерный*) immóderate, excéssive; ~ый аппетúт immóderate áppetite.

неумéстн|ый inapprópriate; out of place *predic.*; ~ое замечáние irrélevant remárk.

неýмн|ый not cléver, unintélligent, misguíded; ~ человéк unintélligent pérson; ~ые рéчи misguíded talk *sg*.

неумолúмый reléntless, inéxorable.

неумолкáемый incéssant, céaseless.

неумы́шленный unintentional.

неуплáт|а ж. fáilure to pay; non-páyment; в слýчае ~ы fáiling páyment.

неупорядоченный unsystemátic, unrégulated.

неупотребúтельн|ый unúsual, uncómmon; not in use *predic.*; ~ые выражéния expréssions not in cómmon use, little-úsed expréssions.

неуправля́емый out of contról *после сущ.*, uncontróllable; uncontrólled.

неуравновéшенн|ость ж. instabílity, lack of bálance; ~ харáктера unbálanced cháracter. ~ый unbálanced.

неурожáй *м.* cróp-failure, bad hárvest; ~ пшенúцы bad wheat hárvest, wheat cróp-failure. ~ный lów-yield *attr.*; ~ный год a year of poor crops, bad year.

неурóчн|ый unúsual; в ~ое врéмя at an unúsual hour.

неуря́дица ж. разг. 1. múddle, confúsion; 2. обыкн. мн. (ссоры) squábbling *sg*.

неусúдчивый unpersevéring; (*подвижный*) réstless; ~ ребёнок réstless child*.

неуспевáемость ж. poor prógress, lágging behínd.

неуспевáющий прил. 1. báckward, lágging; ~ студéнт báckward stúdent; 2. в знач. сущ. м. báckward púpil/stúdent.

неуспéх *м.* fáilure, lack of succéss.

неустáнный indefátigable, untíring, tíreless.

неустóйка ж. fórfeit.

неустóйчив|ый 1. (*шаткий*) unstéady, unstáble; 2. (*непостоянный*) chángeable, unséttled; ~ая погóда unséttled wéather; 3. (*колеблющийся*) unstáble, wávering; ~ харáктер wávering cháracter; ◇ ~ое равновéсие *физ.* unstáble equilíbrium.

неустранúм|ый inerádicable; ~ые противорéчия inerádicable/inhérent contradíctions; ~ое препя́тствие unavóidable/insúperable óbstacle.

неустрашúмый féarless, intrépid.

неустрóенный ill-províded; (*плохо устроенный*) póorly órganized; ~ человéк a pérson with no estáblished posítion; lame duck *разг.*

неустрóйство *с.* múddle, disórder.

неусту́пчивый unyíelding, óbstinate; ~ челове́к óbstinate pérson; ~ хара́ктер unyíelding cháracter.

неутеши́тельный unconsóling, not véry cómforting.

неуте́шный inconsólable.

неутоли́мый unquénchable; *перен.* reléntless.

неутоми́м|ый indefátigable, untíring, tíreless; ~ая де́ятельность tíreless actívity; ~ иссле́дователь indefátigable explórer.

нѐуч *м. разг.* ignorámus.

неучти́в|ость *ж.* impolíteness, discóurtesy. ~ый impolíte, discóurteous.

неую́тн|о *в знач. сказ. безл.* 1. it is uninvíting; в кварти́ре ~ the flat was uninvíting; 2. (*дт.; о неприя́тном чу́встве*) it is not véry agréeable (for). ~ый uncómfortable, bleak, uninvíting.

неуязви́мый invúlnerable.

нефтега́зовый oil and gas *attr.*

нефтедобыва́ющ|ий óil-extrácting; ~ая промы́шленность óil-extrácting índustry.

нефтедобы́ча *ж.* oil extráction.

нефтенали́в|ой; ~ое су́дно (óil-)tánker.

нефтено́сн|ый óil-bearing; ~ые пласты́ óil-bearing stráta.

нефтеперего́нн|ый; ~ заво́д oil refínery; ~ая аппарату́ра óil-refíning equípment.

нефтеперераба́тывающ|ий óil-prócessing; ~ие заво́ды oil refíneries.

нефтепрово́д *м.* oil pípeline.

нефтепроду́кты *мн.* (*ед.* нефтепроду́кт *м.*) oil próducts.

нефтепро́мысел *м.* óil-extrácting énterprise, óil-field.

нефтепромы́шленн|ость *ж.* oil índustry. ~ый óil-prodúcing *attr.*

нефтехими́ческий pétrochémical.

нефтехи́мия *ж.* pétrochémistry.

нефтехрани́лище *с.* óil-tank.

нефть *ж.* oil, petróleum (-oil).

нефтя́ник *м.* óil-industry wórker, óilman*.

нефтян|о́й oil *attr.*, petróleum *attr.*; ~ фонта́н óil-gusher; ~а́я вы́шка dérrick, rig.

нехва́тка *ж. разг.* shórtage.

нехи́трый 1. (*о челове́ке*) guíleless, ártless; 2. *разг.* (*просто́й, незате́йливый*) símple.

нехоро́ший bad*.

нехорошо́ 1. *нареч.* bádly; 2. *в знач. сказ. безл.* it is bad, it is wrong; ~! that's not right!; ~ так поступа́ть it's wrong to do that; 3. *в знач. сказ. безл.* (*о самочу́вствии*) ~ мне I feel ill/rótten.

нехотя́ 1. (*неохо́тно*) relúctantly; 2. (*нево́льно*) willy-nílly.

нецелесообра́зн|ый inexpédient, póintless; ~ая тра́та вре́мени waste of time.

неча́янн|о by áccident, by mistáke, inadvértently. ~ый 1. (*неожи́данный*) únexpécted; chance *attr.*; ~ая встре́ча chance encóunter; 2. (*случа́йный*) accidéntal; chance *attr.*

не́чего I *мест.* (*дт.* не́чему, *тв.* не́чем, *пр.* не́ не́ чем) (+ *инф.*) there is nóthing (+ to *inf*); там ~ смотре́ть there's nóthing to be seen there; there's nóthing worth séeing there; мне ~ сказа́ть I have nóthing to say; мне ~ сказа́ть вам I have nóthing to tell you; мне ~ скрыва́ть (от вас) I have nóthing to concéal (from you); нам не́чем похва́статься we have nóthing to boast of; мне не́чем похва́статься I have nóthing to write with; не́чему ра́доваться! it's nóthing to rejóice abóut!; тут не́чему удивля́ться! there's nóthing surprising in it!; ◇ де́лать ~! it can't be helped!; ~ де́лать, де́лать ~, придётся... there's nóthing for it but (+ to *inf*); ~ и говори́ть cértainly, of course; ~ сказа́ть, прия́тное положе́ние! a fine mess, I must say!; от ~ де́лать háving nóthing bétter to do; for want of sómething to do; to while awáy the time.

не́чего II *в знач. сказ.* (+ *инф.*; *незаче́м*) it's no use/good (+ -ing); (*нет надо́бности*) there is no need (+ to *inf*); ~ беспоко́иться there's nóthing to wórry abóut; вам ~ беспоко́иться you have nóthing to wórry abóut; ~ спеши́ть there's no húrry; ~ рассужда́ть! it's no use arguing!; об э́том и ду́мать ~ that's out of the quéstion.

нечелове́ческ|ий 1. (*не сво́йственный челове́ку*) inhúman; 2. (*о́чень си́льный*) superhúman; ~ие уси́лия superhúman éfforts.

не́чем *мест. тв. см.* не́чего I.

не́чему *мест. дт. см.* не́чего II.

нечёсаный unkémpt.

нечестн|ость *ж.* dishónesty. ~ый dishónest.

нечётк|ий indistínct, vague; (*о по́черке*) illégible; ~ая рабо́та cáreless/slípshod work; ~ое изложе́ние чего-л. vague/uncléar expositíon of *smth.*

нечётный odd.

нечистокро́вный half-bréd.

нечистопло́тный dírty; *перен.* unscrúpulous, shády.

нечисто́ты *мн.* séwage *sg.*

нечи́ст|ый 1. dírty, uncléan; 2. (*с при́месью*) adúlterated; 3. (*непра́вильный, нето́чный*) fáulty; ~ое произноше́ние fáulty articulátion; 4. (*нече́стный*) dishónourable; ~ая со́весть soiled/guílty cónscience; ◇ он на́ руку нечи́ст he's a bit of a thief.

нечленоразде́льный inartículate.

не́что *мест.* sómething; ~ вро́де sómething like, a kind of.

нечувстви́тельный insénsitive.

нечу́ткий insénsitive; (*неотзы́вчивый тж.*) hard, unféeling.

неширо́кий ráther nárrow.

нешу́точн|ый *разг.* fórmidable, sérious; де́ло ~ое! it's no láughing mátter!, it's no joke!

неща́дн|о rúthlessly, mércilessly. ~ый rúthless, mérciless.

неэконо́мн|ый unconómical; ~ая хозя́йка poor/bad hóusekeeper; ~ое расхо́дование средств uneconómical use of resóurces.

неэти́чн|ый unéthical; ~ посту́пок unéthical act; ~ое поведе́ние impróper cónduct.

не́ю (*тв. от личн. мест.* она́) by her.

нея́вка *ж.* ábsence, fáilure to appéar.

нея́рк|ий faint, dim; subdúed (*тж. перен.*); ~ие цвета́ subdúed cólours.

нея́сн|о 1. *нареч.* dímly, fáintly, indistínctly; 2. *в знач. сказ. безл.* it is not clear. ~ый 1. (*ту́склый*) indistínct, dim; 2. (*неразбо́рчивый*) múffled, faint; 3. (*неопределённый*) vague, indéfinite.

ни I 1. *союз:* ни... ни néither... nor (*отрица́ние не не перево́дится*); ни он, ни его́ брат не пришли́ néither he nor his bróther came; он не говори́т ни по-францу́зски, ни по-неме́цки he speaks néither French nor Gérman; 2. *частица* (*перед сущ. в ед. числе, перед сло́вом оди́н или одна́*) not a (*отрица́ние не не перево́дится*); не упа́ло ни (одно́й) ка́пли not a (síngle) drop fell; ни сло́ва нé было ска́зано not a word was úttered; ни зву́ка! not anóther sound!; ни с ме́ста! don't stir!; 3. *частица:* ни оди́н, ни одна́, ни одно́... не (*да́же оди́н... не*) not a; (*никако́й... не*) no; не... ни одного́, ни одно́й *передаётся через отрица́ние при глаго́ле* + a síngle; ни оди́н челове́к не пошевели́лся not a pérson stirred; ни оди́н челове́к не мо́жет сде́лать э́того no man can do that; он не сказа́л ни одного́ сло́ва he did not útter a word; ◇ ни в мале́йшей сте́пени не... not in the least...; не име́ть ни мале́йшего представле́ния have* not the slíghtest idéa; ни то ни друго́е! néither!; ни то ни сё néither one thing nor the óther; ни с того́ ни с сего́ all of a súdden, for no appárent réason; ни взад ни вперёд it won't move éither way; э́то ни к селу́ ни к го́роду that is néither here nor there.

ни II (*в сочетании с предлогами является отделяемой частью местоимений* никто, ничто, никакой, ничей, никой): ни... какого, ни... какой *и т. д.* не по (... whatéver); *или передаётся через отрицание при гл.* + *any* (... whatéver); ни... кого, ни... кому *и т. д.* не nóbody; *или передаётся через отрицание при гл.* + *anybody*; ни... чего, ни... чему *и т. д.* не nóthing; *или передаётся через отрицание при гл.* + *anything*; это ни к чему не приведёт no good will come of it; ◇ ни за что! not for the world!; я ни за что туда не пойду! nóthing will indúce me to go there!; I wóuldn't go there for the world!; я бы ни за что туда не пошёл I would néver have gone there.

ни́ва *ж.* córnfield; *перен.* field, sphere.

нивели́р *м.* lével ~овать *несов. и сов.* (*вн.*) *тж. перен.* lével (*smth.*). ~бвка *ж.* lévelling.

нигде́ nówhere; (*при гл. с отрицанием тж.*) not... ánywhere; он ~ не мог найти их he could find them nówhere, he could not find them ánywhere; его ~ нет he is nówhere to be found.

нидерла́нд|ец *м.*, ~ка *ж.* Nétherlander. ~ский Nétherlands *attr.*; ~ский язык Dutch, the Dutch lánguage.

ни́же 1. (*сравнит. ст. прил.* ни́зкий *и нареч.* ни́зко) lówer; 2. *нареч.* (*вниз от чего-л.*) lówer, belów; этажом ~ on the floor belów; октáвой ~ an óctave lówer; 3. *нареч.* (*далее, позже*) belów, fúrther on; смотри об этом ~ see belów; 4. *в знач. предлога* (*рд.*) belów; ~ нуля́ belów zéro; 5. *предлог* (*рд.*; *вниз по течению реки*) dównstréam (from); belów; ◇ ~ чьего-л. достóинства benéath *smb.'s* dígnity.

нижеподписа́вшийся the undersigned.

нижеслéдующий the fóllowing.

нижестоя́щий lówer-ránking.

ни́жн|ий lówer; ~ие нóты low notes; ~ее бельё únderclothes *pl*, únderwear; ~яя юбка pétticoat, únder-skirt; ~яя полка bóttom shelf*; ~яя ступéнька bóttom step; ~ этáж lówer floor.

низ *м.* lówer part; (*дно*) bóttom.

низа́ть *несов.* (*вн.*) thread (*smth.*).

низвергáть, низвергнуть (*вн.*) overthrów* (*smb., smth.*); ~ся, низвéргнуться come* rúshing down, húrtle down.

низвéргнуть(ся) *сов. см.* низвергáть(ся).

низвержéние *с.* óverthrow.

низвести́ *сов. см.* низводи́ть.

низводи́ть, низвести́ (*вн. до рд.*) redúce (*smb., smth.* to).

низи́на *ж.* low ground, depréssion, bóttom.

ни́зк|ий 1. low; ~ дом lów-built house; ~ забóр low fence; ~ каблу́к low heel; ~ бéрег low bank; ~ая температу́ра low témperature; ~ое давлéние low préssure; ~ лоб low fórehead; ~ая производи́тельность трудá low productívity of lábour; ~ое кáчество poor quálity; ~ сорт inférior grade; ~ая культу́ра low lével of cúlture; ~ го́лос deep voice; 2. (*подлый*) base, mean; ~ посту́пок mean áction; ~ поклóн low bow.

ни́зко 1. low; 2. (*подло*) méanly, básely.

низковóльтный *эл.* lów-tension *attr.*

низкоопла́чиваемый lów-paid.

низкопоклóн|ство *с.* servility (towárds), self-abásement (befóre); grôvelling (befóre).

низкопрóбный lów-grade; *перен.* sécond-ráte.

низкорóслый undersized, dwárfish; (*о растениях*) stúnted.

низкосóртный lów-grade.

низлагáть, низложи́ть (*вн.*) overthrów* (*smb., smth.*), depóse (*smb.*).

низложéние *с.* óverthrow. ~и́ть *сов. см.* низлагáть.

ни́зменн|ость *ж.* 1. lówland; 2. (*бесчестность*) báseness. ~ый 1. lów-lying; 2. (*бесчестный*) base, vile; 3. (*животный*).

низов|óй (*периферийный*) lócal; ~áя печáть lócal press.

низóвье *с.* the lówer réaches *pl*; ~ Вóлги the Lówer Vólga.

ни́зом low, by the lówer path.

ни́зость *ж.* báseness, méanness; это ~ it is mean.

ни́зш|ий 1. (*превосх. ст. прил.* ни́зкий) the lówest; 2. (*подчинённый*) júnior; ~ая инстáнция júnior depártment; 3. (*простейший*) lówest; ~ие органи́змы the lówest órganisms; 4. (*начальный*) prímary.

низы́ *мн.* 1. (*непривилегированные круги общества*) the másses; 2. (*нижние ноты*) low notes.

никáк I *нареч.* símply, just; ~ не (*никаким образом не*) símply (+ *гл. в отрицательной форме*); ~ не могу́ I símply can't; он ~ не мог открыть ящик he símply cóuldn't ópen the box; это ~ не подойдёт that won't do at all; ~ нельзя́ допусти́ть it cánnot be allówed.

никáк II *частица разг.* (*как будто*): ~ он просну́лся! look — he's awáke!

никáк|ой *мест.* 1. no; нет ~ого сомнéния there can be no doubt; нет ~ надéжды there is no hope; ~ого беспокóйства it's no tróuble; это ~ое не + *сущ.* no; я ~ не социóлог I am no sociólogist; 3. *в знач. прил. разг.* (*плохой*) no good at all; дóктор он ~ he's no good at all as a dóctor.

никелирóванный níckel *attr.*, níckel-pláted.

никелировáть *несов. и сов.* (*вн.*) plate (*smth.*) with níckel.

ни́кель *м.* níckel.

никéм *мест. тв. см.* никтó.

никогдá néver; (*при отрицательном подлежащем*) éver; ~ в жи́зни (*в будущем*) néver; (*в прошлом*) néver in *one's* life; как ~ в жи́зни as néver befóre; никтó ~ не ви́дел егó no one has éver seen him.

никогó *мест. рд., вн. см.* никтó.

ник|óй: ~óим óбразом on no accóunt, néver, by no means.

никому́ *мест. дт. см.* никтó.

никоти́н *м.* nícotine.

никтó *мест.* (*рд., вн.* никогó, *дт.* никому́, *тв.* никéм, *пр.* ни о ком) 1. no one, nóbody; никтó, никéм не *передаётся тж. через отрицание при гл.* + *anybody*; ~ этому не повéрит no one will éver believe that; он никогó там не ви́дел he didn't see ánybody there; 2. *в знач. сущ. м. разг.* (*ничтожная личность*) a nóbody; 3. *в знач. сущ. м. нескл.* (*дт.*) *разг.* (*о рóдственных отношениях*) nóbody (to), no one (to).

никудá nówhere; ~ не nówhere; *или передаётся через отрицание при гл.* + *anywhere*; мы сегóдня ~ не идём we are góing nówhere todáy, we are not góing ánywhere todáy; ◇ это ~ не годи́тся! this won't do!; ~ негóдный pérfectly úseless; wórthless.

никчёмный *разг.* úseless.

ним 1. (*тв. от личн. мест.* он) by him; 2. (*дт. от личн. мест.* они́) to them.

нимáло not a bit, not in the least; ◇ ~ he not in the least, not at all.

ни́ми (*тв. от личн. мест.* они́) by them.

ниоткýда: ~ не not from ánywhere; я ~ письмá не ожидáл I was not expécting a létter from ánywhere.

нипочём *разг.*: ему́ всё ~ it's nóthing to him, he's not afráid of ánything; ему́ ~ хóлод he dóesn't mind cold; ему́ ~ солгáть he thinks nóthing of télling a lie.

нискóлько not in the least, not a bit; ~ не not in the least, not a bit; *передаётся тж. через отрицание при гл.* + at all, a bit, in the least; я ~ не устáл I'm not a bit tíred; я ~ не удивля́юсь I'm not a bit surprísed; ему́ сегóдня ~ не лýчше he is not ány bétter todáy.

ниспадáть *несов.* fall*.

ниспровергáть, ниспровéргнуть (*вн.*) overthrów* (*smb., smth.*).

ниспровéргнуть *сов. см.* ниспровергáть.

ниспровержёние *с.* óverthrow.

нисходя́щ|**ий** descénding; в ~ем поря́дке in descénding órder; (*о числах*) in decréasing/descénding séries.

ни́тк|**а** *ж.* 1. cótton; (*толстая*) thread; 2. (*бус, жемчуга*) string; ◇ на живу́ю ~у róughly; промо́кнуть до ~и be* wet through, be* drípping wet; обобра́ть кого́--л. до ~и clean *smb.* out; бе́лыми ~ами ши́то transpárent, óbvious.

ни́точк|**а** *ж.* (bit of) thread; ◇ висе́ть на ~е hang* by a thread; ходи́ть (как) по ~е be* as quíet as a mouse, go* abóut on típ-toe.

нит|**ь** *ж.* 1. thread; 2. (*то, что похоже на нитку*) thread, fílament; ~ ла́мпы накáливания bulb fílament; нéрвные ~и nerve fíbres; 3. (*то, что соединяет одно с другим*) thread; потеря́ть ~ разгово́ра lose* the thread of the conversátion.

них 1. (*рд., вн. от личн. мест.* они́) them; 2. (*пр. от личн. мест.* они́) abóut/of them.

ниц: (у)па́сть ~ prostráte onesélf.

ничего́ I *мест. рд. см.* ничто́.

ничего́ II *разг.* 1. *нареч.* (*довольно хорошо*) not bádly, so-so; ~ себе́ not bad; 2. *в знач. сказ.* (*не имеет значения*) it dóesn't mátter; ~! néver mind!, it dóesn't mátter!

ничей *мест.* 1. nóbody's; ничья́ земля́ no man's land; 2. (*любой, всякий*) ánybody's; не ну́жно вам ничьи́х сове́тов you need no advíce from ányone.

ничéйн|**ый** 1. *разг.* nóbody's; 2. *спорт.* drawn; ~ результа́т draw.

ничéм *мест. тв. см.* ничто́.

ничему́ *мест. дт. см.* ничто́.

ничко́м *мест.* próstrate; лежа́щий ~ prone; упа́сть ~ fall* face dównwards; лежа́ть ~ lie* prone, lie* face dównwards.

ничто́ *мест.* (*рд.* ничего́, *дт.* ничему́, *тв.* ничéм, *пр.* ни о чём) nóthing; ничего́, ничему́, ничéм не *передаётся тж. через отрицание при гл.* + ánything; ~ не могло́ помо́чь nóthing could (have) help(ed); он ничего́ не зна́ет 1) (*вообще*) he dóesn't know a thing; 2) (*не осведомлён*) he knows nóthing abóut it; 3) (*ещё не узна́л*) he knows nóthing, he has heard nóthing; я ничего́ подо́бного не ви́дел I néver saw ánything like it; э́то ничего́ не зна́чит that's nóthing; он ничéм не отлича́ется от други́х he is no dífferent from ányone else; я ничéм не мог вам помо́чь there is nóthing I can do for you; его́ ничéм не удиви́шь there's no surprísing him; его́ ничéм не проймёшь nóthing makes ány impréssion on him; он никогда́ ничéм не быва́ет дово́лен he's néver sátisfied; ◇ ничего́ подо́бного! nóthing of the sort!

ничто́ж|**ество** *с.* (*о человеке*) nonéntity, a nóbody. ~ный 1. (*очень маленький*) infinitésimal, trífling; ~ная до́ля расхо́да an infinitésimal part of the íncome; ~ное меньшинство́ tíny minórity; 2. (*незначительный*) trívial, contémptible; ~ная роль trívial role; 3. (*о человеке*) wórthless.

ничу́ть *разг.* not a bit, not in the least; ◇ ~ не быва́ло! nóthing of the sort!

ничь|**я́** *ж. спорт.* a draw, drawn game; они́ сде́лали ~ю it was a draw.

ни́ша *ж.* niche, recéss.

нища́ть, обнища́ть becóme* impóverished/déstitute, be* redúced to póverty.

ни́щая *ж.* béggar(-wóman*).

ни́щен|**ский** béggarly; *перен. тж.* wrétched; ~ская пла́та píttance; ~ство *с.* 1. bégging; 2. (*крайняя бедность*) béggary, destitútion. ~ствовать *несов.* 1. beg; 2. (*жить в крайней бедности*) be* déstitute, pass a béggarly existence.

нищета́ *ж.* 1. destitútion, extréme póverty; *перен.* póverty; душе́вная ~ spíritual póverty; 2. *собир. разг.* (*нищие люди*) the béggars *pl.*

ни́щий I *прил.* póverty-stricken, déstitute; *перен.* mean; ~ ду́хом méan-spírited.

ни́щий II *м.* béggar.

но I *союз* but; *в главном предложении после уступительного придаточного с* хотя́*, как ни и т. п. не переводится*; как ни тру́дно, но на́до сде́лать hard though it may be, it must be done.

но II *межд.* 1. gée-úp!; 2. (*предостережение*) now then!, now, now!

нова́тор *м.* ínnovator; ~ы произво́дства ínnovators in índustry, prodúction ínnovators. ~ский innovátory; ~ские ме́тоды new/innovátory méthods. ~ство *с.* innovátion.

нове́йш|**ий** the látest; (*современный*) récent; ~ая исто́рия récent hístory.

нове́лла *ж.* short stóry.

новелли́ст *м.* short-story wríter.

но́венький *прил.* 1. new; 2. *в знач. сущ. м.* néw-cómer; (*в университете*) fréshman*; (*в школе*) new boy.

новизна́ *ж.* nóvelty.

нови́нк|**а** *ж.* sómething new; ~и литерату́ры récent publicátions; ~и мо́ды the látest fáshions; ◇ в ~у sómething new, a nóvelty.

новичо́к *м.* 1. nóvice, begínner; 2. (*о школьнике*) new boy.

новобра́нец *м.* recrúit.

новобра́чн|**ая** *ж.* the bride. ~ые *мн.* néwly márried cóuple *sg.* ~ый *м.* the young húsband.

нововведе́ние *с.* innovátion.

нового́дний New-Yéar('s).

новолу́ние *с.* new moon.

новообразова́ние *с.* new growth; new formátion; néoplasm *науч.*

новоприбы́вший *прил.* 1. néwly-arríved; 2. *в знач. сущ. м.* néwcomer, new arríval.

новорождённый *прил.* 1. néwborn; 2. *в знач. сущ. м.* néwborn child*, the new báby.

новосёл *м.* new séttler; (*в доме*) new ténant.

новосе́лье *с.* 1. (*новое жилище*) new home/dwélling; 2. (*празднование*) hóuse-wárming.

новостро́йк|**а** *ж.* 1. (*новое здание*) new búilding; жить в ~е live in a new búilding; шко́ла-~ néwly-built school; 2. (*строительство*) new búilding; búilding devélopment/próject.

но́вост|**ь** *ж.* 1. (*известие*) news; э́то для меня́ (не) ~! that's (no) news to me!; 2. (*что-л. ранее неизвестное*) discóvery, nóvelty; ~и нау́ки и те́хники discóveries in science and enginéering; ◇ э́то что ещё за ~и!, вот ещё ~и! what's all this abóut?

но́вшество *с.* innovátion, nóvelty.

но́в|**ый** *прил.* 1. new; ~ костю́м new suit; ~ые знако́мые new friends; ~ое изобрете́ние new invéntion; ~ое для кого́-л. де́ло new work to *smb.*; нача́ть ~ую жизнь begín* a new life; ~ урожа́й new hárvest; ~ карто́фель new potátoes *pl*; 2. (*современный*) módern, ~ая исто́рия módern hístory; 3. *в знач. сущ. с.* the new, what is new; (*новость*) news; чу́вство ~ого sense of what is new, féeling for the new; борьба́ ста́рого с ~ым the cóntest between old and new; что ~ого? what's the news?; что у вас ~ого? what's your news?; ◇ ~ стиль New Style.

новь *ж.* vírgin soil.

ног|**а́** *ж.* leg; (*ступня*) foot*; положи́ть но́гу на́ ногу cross *one's* legs; ◇ на ~áх on *one's* feet; перенести́ боле́знь на ~áх have* an íllness without lýing up; в ~áх at the foot; идти́ в но́гу keep* in step; (*не отставать от кого-л., чего-л.*) keep* pace with; идти́ в но́гу с жи́знью, со вре́менем be* in step with life, with the times; со всех ног as fast as *one* can; сбить кого́-л. с ног knock *smb.* down; быть без (за́дних) ног (*от усталости*) be* déad-béat; подня́ть всех на́ ~и raise the alárm; поста́вить кого́-л. на́ ~и set* *smb.* on his, her feet; стать на́ ~и 1) (*оправиться после болезни и т. п.*) get* on one's feet agáin; 2) *(стать самостоятельным)* find* one's feet, becóme* indepéndent; жить на широкую нóгу live in (grand) style; вверх ~áми úpside-dówn; стоя́ть однóй ~óй в могúле have* one foot in the grave; встать с лéвой ~ú get* out of bed on the wrong side; не чýвствовать под собóй ног *(от радости)* be* wálking on air; наступи́ть *кому-л.* нá ногу tread* on *smb.'s* foot; *(сделать кому-л. неприятное)* do* smb. harm; он éле волочи́т нóги he can hárdly drag himsélf alóng; с тех пор я тудá ни ~óй I've néver set foot there since then.

нóготь *м.* nail; *(на руке тж.)* fínger-nail; *(большого пальца)* thúmb-nail; *(на ноге)* tóe-nail; куса́ть нóгти bite* one's nails.

нож *м.* knife*; ◇ ~ в спи́ну a stab in the back; быть на ~áх с *кем-л.* be* at dággers drawn with *smb.*; как ~óм пó сердцу like a stab in the heart; ~ óстрый *кому-л.* ≈ it is death to *smb.*

ножев|óй knife *attr.*; ~áя páна knife wound.

нóжик *м.* knife*.

нóжк|а *ж.* 1. lítle leg; *(ступня)* ти́пу foot*; корóтенькие ~и short legs; ма́ленькие ~и ти́пу feet; 2. *(у мебели)* leg; *(у рюмки)* stem; ~ сту́ла chair leg; 3. *(гриба, стебель растений)* stem.

нóжницы *мн.* 1. scíssors; a pair of scíssors *sg.*; *(садовые, для стрижки животных)* shears; дáйте мне ~ pass me the scíssors; купи́ть ~ buy* a pair of scíssors; 2. *тех.* cútters, clíppers; 3. *(резкое расхождение)* sharp divérgence, discrépancy.

ножн|óй foot *attr.*; ~áя вáнна fóot-bath; ~áя *(швейная)* маши́на tréadle-machíne.

нóжны *мн.* scábbard *sg.*, sheath *sg.*

ножóвка *ж.* hándsaw; *(узкая)* cómpass saw.

ноздревáтый pórous.

ноздря́ *ж.* nóstril.

нокáут *м. спорт.* knóck-out.

нокаути́ровать *несов. и сов. (вн.) спорт.* knock *(smb.)* out.

нокдáун *м. спорт.* knóck-down.

ноктю́рн *м.* nócturne.

нолевóй *см.* нулевóй.

ноль *м.* 1. *см.* нуль; 2. *спорт.* nil; счёт ноль — ноль there is no score; они́ вы́играли со счётом три — ноль they won three nil; ◇ ~~: он придёт в пять ~~ he will arríve at 05.00 ['ou'faɪv'ou'ou].

номенклату́р|а *ж.* nomenclátural; ~ный спи́сок noménclature; ~ный рабóтник top official (appóinted by hígher authórity).

нóмер *м.* 1. númber; ~ телефóна télephone númber; автóбус ~ 17 bus númber séventéen, númber séventéen bus; 2. *(ярлычок, планка)* check; ~ маши́ны car númber-plate; 3. *(размер)* size; 4. *(газеты и т. п.)* issue, númber; 5. *(в гостинице)* room; 6. *(часть концерта и т. п.)* item, piece; *(выход)* turn; объяви́ть слéдующий ~ прогрáммы annóunce the next item on the prógramme; 7. *разг. (неожиданный, странный поступок)* trick; ◇ э́тот ~ не пройдёт! that won't do!, that won't wash!

номерóванный *см.* нумерóванный.

номерóк *м.* check.

номинáл *м. фин.* nóminal price, face válue; по ~у at face válue, at par.

номинáльн|ый *фин.* nóminal; ~ая ценá nóminal price; ~ая стóимость nóminal válue.

нонпарéль *ж. полигр.* nónpareil.

норá *ж.* búrrow, hole; *(крупного зверя)* lair, den.

норвéж|ец *м.*, ~ка *ж.* Norwégian; ~ский Norwégian; ~ский язы́к Norwégian, the Norwégian lánguage.

норд *м. мор.* 1. *(направление)* North; 2. *(ветер)* north (wind).

норд-вéст *м. мор.* 1. *(направление)* north-wést; 2. *(ветер)* north-wést wind, northwéster.

норд-óст *м. мор.* 1. *(направление)* north-éast; 2. *(ветер)* north-éast wind, northéaster.

нóрк|а *ж. (животное и мех)* mink. ~овый: ~овый мех mink.

нóрм|а *ж.* 1. stándard; norm; ~ поведéния rule of cónduct; ~ы литератýрного языкá líterary stándards; ~ы междунарóдного прáва the stándards/rúles of internátional law; 2. *(размер чего-л.)* quóta, rate; сверх ~ы abóve quóta; ~ вы́работки óutput quóta; выполня́ть ~у fulfíl one's quóta; ◇ войти́ в ~у get* back to nórmal.

нормализáция *ж.* normalizátion; ~ междунарóдной обстанóвки normalizátion of the internátional situátion.

нормализовáть *несов. и сов. (вн.)* nórmalize *(smth.).* ~ся *несов. и сов.* becóme* nórmal, retúrn to nórmal.

нормáльн|ый 1. nórmal; ~ая температýра nórmal témperature; ~ рост nórmal height; 2. *(психически здоровый)* sane, nórmal.

нормати́в *м.* stándard. ~ный nórmative.

нормировáние *с.* standardizátion, rate sétting; *(снабжения)* rátioning.

нормирóванный: ~ рабóчий день fixed wórking hours *pl.*

нормировáть *несов. и сов. (вн.)* stándardize *(smth.)*, set* the rate/quóta (of); *(снабжение)* rátion *(smth.).*

норов|и́ть *несов. разг.* contríve; так и ~и́т (+ инф.) álways contríves (+ to *inf*)

нос *м.* 1. nose; у негó кровь идёт и́з ~у his nose is bléeding; 2. *(клюв птицы)* beak; 3. *(судна)* bows *pl*, bow; *(самолёта)* nose; на ~ý in the bows; ◇ говори́ть в ~ speak* through one's nose, speak* with a twang; показа́ть ~ *кому-л.* make* a long nose at *smb.*; thumb one's nose at *smb.*; дáльше своегó ~а не ви́деть not see an inch beyónd one's nose; из-под сáмого ~а from únder one's véry nose; остáться с ~ом be* left in the lurch, be* made a fool; совáть свой ~ в чужи́е делá poke one's nose ínto óther péople's búsiness; закрывáть дверь перед сáмым ~ом shut* the door in *smb.'s* face; зимá на ~ý wínter is just round the córner.

носáтый *разг.* lóng-nósed.

нóсик *м.* 1. lítle nose; 2. *(у чайника)* spout; *(у кувшина)* lip.

носи́лки *мн.* strétcher *sg.*; *(для песка и т. п.)* tray *sg.*

носи́льщик *м.* pórter.

носи́тель *м.* 1. béarer, véhicle; *(инфекции)* (gérm-)cárrier; ~ языкá nátive spéaker (of the lánguage); 2. *вчт.* médium; ~ дáнных dáta médium.

носи́|ть *несов. (вн.)* 1. cárry *(smb., smth.)*; *перен.* bear* *(smth.)*; ~ ребёнка на рукáх cárry a child* in one's arms; ~ мешки́ cárry sacks; 2. *(гнать — о ветре, течении)* bear* *(smth.)* alóng, drive* *(smth.)*; ветерóк ~л по вóздуху семенá the seeds were borne alóng on the breeze; 3. *(иметь на себе)* wear* *(smth.)*, have* *(smth.)* on; ~ плáтье, шля́пу, кольцó wear* a dress, hat, ring; ~ очки́ wear* spéctacles/glásses; ~ часы́ have* a watch on; ~ корóткую причёску wear* one's hair short; ~ усы́ have* a moustáche; 4.: ~ фами́лию мýжа use one's húsband's name, go* únder one's húsband's name; 5. *(характеризоваться чем-л.)* bear* *(smth.)*, have* *(smth.)*; ~ харáктер *чего-л.* be* in the náture of *smth.*; ~ слéды *чего-л.* bear* the tráces of *smth.*; ◇ ~ орýжие bear*/cárry arms; ~ *кого-л.* на рукáх make* much of *smb.*; он нóсит её на рукáх he makes much of her, he can't do enóugh for her.

носи́ться *несов.* 1. *(быстро двигаться)* rush abóut; rush up and down; *(скакать)* gállop abóut; gállop up and down; *(по воздуху, воде)* float, drift; в вóздухе нóсятся снежи́нки snówflakes are flýing abóut; 2. *(об одежде и т. п.)* wear*; э́то плáтье хорошó нóсится this dress wears well; 3. *(с тв.) разг. (уделять много вни-*

мания) make* a great fuss (óver), make* too much (of); ~ с теóрией péddle a théory.

носки́ *мн.* (*ед.* носóк *м.*) socks.

носк|и́й 1. *разг.* (*прóчный*) hárd-wéaring; 2. (*о птицах*) fértile, prolífic; ~ая ку́рица good láyer.

носов|о́й 1. ~ы́е зву́ки násal sounds; 2. (*на носу́ судна*) fórward; ~áя пáлуба the fórward deck; ◇ ~ платóк (pócket) hándkerchief.

носоглóтка *ж. анат.* násophárynx.

нос|óк *м.* 1. (*пере́дняя часть ступни́, тж. обуви, чулка́*) toe; на ~кáх on one's toes; 2. *см.* носки́.

носорóг *м.* rhinóceros.

нóт|а I *ж.* 1. note (*тж. перен.*); взять ~у sound a note; 2. *мн.* (*музыка́льный текст*) músic *sg*; игрáть, петь по ~ам play, sing* from the músic; ◇ как по ~ам разыгрáть *что-л.* perfórm *smth.* with clóck-work precísion; на однóй ~е álways on the same string.

нóта II *ж. дип.* note; ~ протéста note of prótest; обмéн ~ми exchánge of notes.

нотариáльн|ый nótary's, notárial; ~ая контóра nótary's óffice.

нотáриус *м.* nótary (públic).

нотáци|я I *ж.* (*нравоуче́ние*) réprimand, lécture; читáть ~и *кому́-л.* lécture *smb.*

нотáция II *ж.* (*систе́ма обозначе́ний*) notátion.

нóтка *ж.* note; ~ недовéрия note of distrúst.

нóтн|ый músic *attr.*; ~ магази́н músic shop; ~ая тетрáдь músic book; ~ая бумáга músic-paper.

ночевáть *несов. и сов.* stay the night, stay overníght, put* up (for the night); ~ под откры́тым нéбом spend* the night in the ópen; ~ на сеновáле sleep* in a háyloft.

ночёвк|а *ж.* spénding the night; остáться на ~у stay the night.

ночлéг *м.* 1. a place to sleep; искáть ~a seek* shélter for the night; 2. (*ночёвка*) spénding the night; останови́ться на ~ (*в доме*) put* up for the night; (*в лесу́ и т. п.*) halt for the night.

ночни́к *м.* níght-light.

ночнóе *с.* níght-watch (*over horses at grass*).

ночн|óй night *attr.*; nóctúrnal; of the night *после сущ.*; в ~óе врéмя at night; пусты́нная ~áя у́лица dark desérted street; ~ стóлик béd-table; ~áя рабóта night work; ~ стóрож night wátchman*; ~ пóезд night train.

ноч|ь *ж.* night; по ~áм at night, in the night; до пóздней ~и till late at night, late ínto the night; ◇ бéлые ~и the mídnight sun; Варфоломéевская ~ night of térror; нá ~ befóre (góing to) bed, at bédtime.

нóчью at night, by night; днём и ~ day and night.

нóша *ж.* búrden, load.

ноющ|ий: ~ гóлос whíning voice; ~ая боль dull pain.

ноябр|ь *м.* Novémber; в ~é э́того гóда this/in Novémber; в ~é прóшлого гóда last Novémber; last year in Novémber; в ~é бу́дущего гóда next Novémber.

ноя́брьский Novémber *attr.*

нрав *м.* 1. (*хара́ктер*) dispositíon; 2. *обыкн. мн.* (*обы́чаи, уклад жи́зни*) ways; the mánners and cústoms; ◇ э́то ему́ не по ~у it's not to his líking; it goes agáinst the grain with him.

нрáв|иться, понрáвиться (*дт.*) please (*smb.*); мне (нам и т. д.) ~ится I (we *etc.*) like; мне (нам и т. д.) не ~ится I (we *etc.*) don't like; он мне óчень не ~ится I dislíke him inténsely; как вам ~ится..? how do you like..?, what do you think of..?; вам э́то понрáвится you'll like it; мне здесь не ~ится I like it here; мне ~ится его́ смéлость I admíre his cóurage; карти́на ему́ не понрáвилась he did not like the pícture; вы ему́ óчень понрáвились he is gréatly táken with you.

нравоучéни|е *с.* préaching; читáть ~я *кому́-л.* read* *smb.* a lécture, preach *smb.*

нравоучи́тельный móralizing; ~ ромáн móral tale.

нрáвственн|ость *ж.* 1. morálity; 2. (*мора́льные ка́чества*) mórals *pl.* ~ый móral.

ну why, well; ну хорошó! véry well, then!; ну, скорéе! do come on!; ну, так что же! well, what abóut it!; ну, не серди́сь! don't be cross now!; ну так вот as I was sáying; ну вот ещё! come now!; ну да! yes, indéed!; (*с недовéрием*) tell me anóther!; go on!; ну конéчно! why, cértainly!; да ну? you don't say so!; да ну тебя́! stop that!; а ну егó! to hell with him!; ну, погоди́ же! just you wait!

ну́дн|о *разг.* 1. *нареч.* monótonously, tíresomely; 2. *в знач. сказ. безл.* it is bóring/tédious. ~ый *разг.* bóring, tédious; какóй он ~ый! what a bore he is!

нужд|á *ж.* 1. *тк. ед.* (*бе́дность*) need, want; жить в ~é live in póverty; терпéть ~у́ endúre póverty; 2. (*надо́бность*) need, necéssity; испы́тывать ~у́ в чём-л. feel* the need of *smth.*; без ~ы́ néedlessly; нет ~ы́ it is unnécessary, there is no need; в слу́чае ~ы́ in case of need; ◇ ~ы́ нет néver mind; ~ы́ мáло кому́-л. smb. dóesn't care.

нужд|áться *несов.* 1. (*находи́ться в бе́дности*) be* poor; он óчень ~áется he is extrémely poor; 2. (*в пр.*) need (*smb., smth.*), require (*smth.*), be* in need (of); óчень ~ в деньгáх be* in great need of móney; он ~áется в пóмощи he needs assístance; он перестáл в нём ~ he no lónger had any need of him.

ну́жн|о *в знач. сказ. безл. см.* нáдо I. ~ый nécessary; ~ая кни́га indispénsable book; сон ну́жен для здорóвья sleep is esséntial for health; он здесь ну́жен he is wánted here; как раз то, что ~o the véry thing; всё, что ~o éverything nécessary; ~o ли э́то? is it réally nécessary?

ну́-ка *разг.* come on!

нулев|óй zéro *attr.*; ~áя температу́ра zéro témperature.

нул|ь *м.* 1. zéro, nought; (*при обозначе́нии телефо́нного но́мера*) o [ou]; ни́же ~я́ belów zéro; своди́ть что-л. к ~ю́ bring* smth. to nought; 2. (*о ничто́жном челове́ке*) a nóbody, a nonéntity.

нумер|áция *ж.* númbering. ~óванный númbered; ~óванное мéсто resérved seat. ~овáть, пронумеровáть (*вн.*) númber (*smth.*); ~овáть страни́цы númber the pàges.

нумизмáтика *ж.* numismátics.

ну-ну́ *разг.* 1. now then!; 2. (*выража́ет негодова́ние*) well!; 3. (*выража́ет согла́сие*) now.

ну́трия *ж.* 1. (*водяна́я кры́са*) cóypu (rat); 2. (*мех*) nútria.

нутр|ó *с. разг.* ínside(s); *перен.* éssence, core; чу́вствовать всем ~óм feel* instínctively; ◇ э́то ему́ не по ~у́ it goes agáinst the grain with him.

ны́не now, at présent.

ны́нешн|ий *разг.* présent; ~ год this year; в ~ие временá nówadays; ~яя молодёжь the young péople of todáy.

ны́нче 1. *разг.* nówadays; 2. *уст.* (*сего́дня*) todáy; ◇ не ~ — зáвтра any day now.

нырну́ть *сов. см.* ныря́ть.

ныря́ть, нырну́ть 1. dive, plunge; 2. (*о ло́дке, самолёте*) pitch.

ны́тик *м. разг.* whíner, móaner.

ныть *несов.* 1. (*жа́ловаться*) whine, whímper; 2. *разг.* (*издава́ть жа́лобные зву́ки*) whine; 3. (*боле́ть*) ache.

нытьё *с.* 1. (*надое́дливые жа́лобы*) móaning; 2. (*жа́лобные зву́ки*) whíning; 3. (*тупа́я боль*) dull pain, ache.

нэп *м.* (*но́вая экономи́ческая поли́тика*) *ист.* NEP (the New Económic Pólicy).

нюáнс *м.* nuánce, shade, sútbtle dífference.

нюх *м.* scent; *перен.* flair; ◇ собáчий ~ extraórdinary nose (for); имéть ~ have* a nose (for).

ню́хать, поню́хать (*вн.*) smell* (*smth.*); ~ табáк take* snuff.

ня́нчить *несов.* *(вн.)* nurse *(smb.)*. ~**ся** *несов.* (с *тв.)* nurse *(smb.)*; *разг. (возиться)* fuss *(óver)*.

ня́н|ька *ж. разг. (прям. и перен.)* núrse-maid; ◇ у семи́ ~ек дитя́ без гла́зу *посл.* ≈ too mány cooks spoil the broth.

ня́ня *ж.* 1. nurse; 2. *разг. (в больни́це)* núrse's assístant.

О

о I, об, обо *предлог* 1. *(относительно)* abóut, of; *(на тему тж.)* on; о чём вы говори́ли? what were you tálking abóut?; поду́мать, вспо́мнить о чём-л. think* of *smth.*; ле́кция о диалекти́ческом материали́зме a lécture on dialéctical matérialism; кни́га о живо́тных a book abóut/on ánimals; заботиться о ком-л. have* considerátion for *smb.*; пла́кать о поги́бших weep* for the fállen; 2. *(указывает на соприкосновение и т. п.)* against, on; опере́ться о стол lean* against the táble; споткну́ться о ка́мень stúmble on/óver a stone.

о II *межд.* oh!; *поэт.* o!

оа́зис *м.* oásis *(pl* oáses).

об *см.* о I.

о́ба, о́бе both, the two; ~ бра́та both bróthers, the two bróthers; мы, вы, они́ ~ both of us, you, them; ухвати́ться за что-л. обе́ими рука́ми seize *smth.* with both hands; *перен.* jump at *smth.*

обагрённый crímsoned, réd-stáined; stained/dyed red *после сущ.*; ~ кро́вью crímsoned with blood, blóod-stáined.

обагри́ть(ся) *сов. см.* обагря́ть(ся).

обагря́ть, обагри́ть *(вн.)* crímson *(smth.)*; stain *(smth.)* red; обагри́ть ру́ки в крови́ stain *one's* hands with/in blood. ~**ся**, обагри́ться turn crímson/red.

обанкро́титься *сов.* go* bánkrupt, fail; *перен.* be* discrédited.

оба́яние *с.* charm; *(чего-л. тж.)* appéal, attráction.

обая́тельн|ость *ж.* charm. ~**ый** chárming.

обва́л *м.* 1. *(падение)* collápse; зда́ние грози́т ~ом the whole building may collápse; 2. *(груда камней и т. п., обрушившаяся с гор)* lándslide; *(лавина снега)* snówslide, snówslip.

обва́ливаться, обвали́ться collápse, fall*, cave in; *(осыпаться)* break* off, come* off.

обвали́ться *сов. см.* обва́ливаться.

обва́ривать, обвари́ть *(вн.)* scald *(smb., smth.)*. ~**ся**, обвари́ться scald onesélf.

обвари́ть(ся) *сов. см.* обва́ривать(ся).

обвева́ть, обвея́ть *(вн. тв.; воздухом, ветром)* fan *(smb. with, by)*; *перен.* infúse *(smth. with)*.

обве́ивать, обве́ять *(вн.) с.-х.* wínnow *(smth.)*, fan *(smth.)*, sift *(smth.)*.

обвенча́ть *сов. (вн. с тв.)* márry *(smb. to)*. ~**ся** *сов.* (с *тв.)* be* márried (to).

обверну́ть *сов. см.* обвёртывать.

обвёртывать, оберну́ть *(вн.)* wrap *(smth.)*, wrap *(smth.)* up.

обве́сить I, II *сов. см.* обве́шивать I, II.

обвести́ *сов. см.* обводи́ть.

обве́тр|енный 1. wéathered, wínd-eróded; 2. *(огрубевший)* chapped; *(о лице тж.)* wéather-béaten. ~**иться** *сов.* 1. be* eróded by the wind; 2. *(огрубеть от ветра)* get* chapped, get* rough, wéather-béaten.

обветша́лый dilápidated; rámshackle *(тж. перен.)*.

обветша́ть *сов.* becóme* dilápidated, go* to pieces.

обве́шать *сов. см.* обве́шивать I.

обве́шивать I, обве́шать, обве́сить *(вн. тв.)* hang* *(smth.)* all óver *(smth.)*, load *(smth.* with); он обве́шал все сте́ны карти́нами he hung píctures all óver the walls.

обве́шивать II, обве́сить *(вн.; недовешивать)* give* *(smb.)* short weight, cheat *(smb.)*.

обвея́ть *сов. см.* обвева́ть и обве́ивать.

обвива́ть, обви́ть *(вн. тв.; smth. round)*, twine *(smth. round)*, wind* *(smth. round)*; *(о растениях)* entwíne *(smth. with)*, wreathe *(smth. with)*; обви́ть ше́ю рука́ми put* *one's* arms round *smb.'s* neck, twine/wind* *one's* arms round *smb.'s* neck. ~**ся**, обви́ться wind*/wrap itsélf round; *(обхватывать — о руках)* encírcle.

обвине́ни|е *с.* 1. *(в пр.)* accusátion (of), charge (of); по ~ю в уби́йстве on a charge of múrder; бро́сить ~ кому́-л. hurl an accusátion at *smb.*; 2. *(приговор)* vérdict of guílty; вы́нести ~ pass a vérdict of guílty; 3. *тк. ед. юр. (обвиняющая сторона на суде)* prosecútion.

обвини́тель *м.* accúser; *юр.* prósecutor. ~**ный** accúsatory; ~**ный** пригово́р vérdict of guílty; ~**ное** заключе́ние indíctment; ~**ная** речь denunciátion; *юр.* speech for the prosecútion.

обвини́ть *сов.* 1. *см.* обвиня́ть 1, 2, 3; 2. *(вн.; осуди́ть)* decláre *(smb.)* guílty, condémn *(smb.)*.

обвиня́емый *м.* the deféndant, the accúsed.

обвиня́ть, обвини́ть 1. *(вн. в пр.; считать виновным)* consider *(smb.)* to blame (for); 2. *(вн. в пр.; привлекать к судебному разбирательству)* charge *(smb. with)*; bring* a charge (against); 3. *(вн. в пр.; упрекать)* accúse *(smb. of)*; 4. *тк. несов. юр. (выступать обвини́телем)* condúct the case for the prosecútion, represént the prosecútion.

обвиса́ть, обви́снуть droop, flop; *(под тяжестью чего-л.)* sag; *(о подоле)* hang* down; *(о щеках и т. п.)* becóme* péndulous, sag.

обви́слый *разг.* dróoping, ságging; *(о щеках тж.)* péndulous.

обви́снуть *сов. см.* обвиса́ть.

обви́ть(ся) *сов. см.* обвива́ть(ся).

обводи́ть, обвести́ 1. *(вн.; вокруг чего-л.)* take* *(smb.)* round; lead* *(smb.)* round; обвести́ кого́-л. вокру́г са́да take* *smb.* round the gárden; 2. *(вн.; в футбо́ле, хоккее)* dodge *(smb.)*, síde-step *(smb.)*; 3. *(вн. тв.; делать круговое движение)* pass *(smth.)* round *(smth.)*; ~ что-л. руко́й pass *one's* hand round *smth.*; ~ что-л. взгля́дом cast* a look round *smth.*, survéy *smth.*, look round *smth.*; 4. *(вн. тв.; окаймлять)* ring *(smth.* with); 5. *(вн.; по намеченным контурам)* go* óver *(smth.)*, trace *(smth.)* out; *(чернилами, тушью)* ink *(smth.)* in; ~ чертёж ту́шью ink in a dráwing; ◇ обвести́ кого́-л. вокру́г па́льца ~ pull the wool óver *smb.'s* eyes.

обводн|е́ние *с.* irrigátion. ~**и́тельный** irrigátion *attr.*; ~**и́тельная** систе́ма irrigátion sýstem. ~**и́ть** *сов. см.* обводня́ть.

обводня́ть, обводни́ть *(вн.)* írrigate *(smth.)*.

обволáкивать, обволо́чь *(вн.)* envélop *(smth.)*; ту́чи обволокли́ не́бо héavy clouds envéloped the sky. ~**ся**, обволо́чься be*/becóme* envéloped (in), be*/becóme* cóvered (with).

обволо́чь(ся) *сов. см.* обволáкивать(ся).

обворова́ть *сов. см.* обворо́вывать.

обворо́вывать, обворова́ть *(вн.) разг.* rob *(smb., smth.)*.

обворожи́тельн|ый entráncing, enchánting, bewítching; ~**ая** улы́бка enchánting smile.

обворожи́ть *сов. (вн.)* enchánt *(smb.)*, bewítch *(smb.)*.

обвяза́ть(ся) *сов. см.* обвя́зывать(ся).

обвя́зывать, обвяза́ть 1. *(вн. тв.; обматывать)* tie *(smth. with)*, bind* *(smth. round)*; ~ что-л. верёвкой tie a rope round *smth.*; ~ го́лову платко́м tie/bind* a kérchief round *one's* head; 2. *(вн.; спицами, крючком)* edge (*smth.*), bind* (*smth.*). ~ся, обвязáться (*тв.*): ~ся верёвкой tie a rope round *one's* waist.

обглáдывать, обглодáть (*вн.*) pick (*smth.*); (*о животных*) gnaw (*smth.*).

обглодáть *сов. см.* обглáдывать.

обгóн *м.* pássing, overtáking; идти на ~ overtáke; ~ запрещён! do not overtáke!, no pássing!

обгонять, обогнáть (*вн.*) pass (*smb.*), outdístance (*smb.*); перен. surpáss (*smb.*), outstríp (*smb.*); посмóтрим, кто когó обгóнит! let's see who gets there first!

обгорáть, обгорéть 1. be* pártly burnt down; be* scorched/bláckened with fire; 2. *разг.* (*на солнце*) get* burnt by the sun.

обгорéлый 1. charred; 2. *разг.* (*обожжённый солнцем*) súnburnt.

обгорéть *сов. см.* обгорáть.

обгрызáть, обгрызть (*вн.*) níbble/bite* round the edge (of); ~ нóгти bite* *one's* nails.

обгрызть *сов. см.* обгрызáть.

обдавáть, обдáть (*вн.*) sweep* óver (*smb., smth.*); (*вн. тв.*) splash (*smb., smth.* with), douche (*smb.* with); ~ что-л. кипяткóм pour hot wáter óver *smth.*; ~ когó-л. грязью splash/bespátter *smb.* with mud; splash/spátter mud on/óver *smb.*; ~ зáпахом чегó-л. envélop in the scent/smell of *smth.*; ◇ обдáть когó-л. хóлодом snub *smb.*, give* *smb.* the cold shóulder.

обдáть *сов. см.* обдавáть.

обделáть *сов. см.* обдéлывать.

обделять, обделить (*вн. тв.*) cheat/depríve (*smb.*) (of his, her láwful share); перен. deprive (*smb.* of); он не был обделён умóм he was not wánting in intélligence.

обдирáть, ободрáть (*вн.*) 1. strip (*smth.*); (*тушу*) skin (*smth.*), flay (*smth.*); 2. *разг.* (*царапать*) graze (*smth.*); ободрáть лицó graze *one's* face; 3. *разг.* (*обирать, брать непомерную цену*) rook (*smb.*), fleece (*smb.*); ободрáть когó-л. как лúпку strip *smb.* of his, her belóngings. ~ся, ободрáться rub off, be* scratched.

обдувáть, обдуть (*вн.*) blow* on (*smth.*); (*сдувая, очищать*) blow* (*smth.*) off.

обдýманн|о delíberately. ~ый considered, delíberate; ~ое решéние considered decision; с зарáнее ~ым намéрением with delíberate intént.

обдýмывать, обдýмать (*вн.*) think* (*smth.*) óver, consider (*smth.*); зарáнее обдýмать что-л. think* *smth.* out in advánce.

обдýть *сов. см.* обдувáть.

óбе *см.* óба.

обегáть *сов. см.* обегáть I.

обегáть I, обéгать (*вн.*) make* a quick round (of).

обегáть II, обежáть run* (round); обежáть вокрýг дóма run* round a house; ◇ обежáть когó-л., что-л. глазáми, взглядом run* *one's* eyes óver *smb., smth.*, scan *smb., smth.*

обéд *м.* dínner; вкýсный ~ good* dínner; пригласить когó-л. на ~ invite *smb.* to dínner; за ~ом at/óver dínner; пóсле ~a áfter dínner; (*после полудня*) in the afternóon; до ~a before dínner; приéхать в сáмый ~ come* just at dínner-time; ◇ ~ы нá дом táke-hóme meals.

обéд|ать, пообéдать have* (*one's*) dínner, dine; остáться ~ stay to dínner. ~енный dínner *attr.*; ~енный стол dínner táble; ~енный перерыв lunch break.

обеднé|вший impóverished. ~ние *с.* impóverishment.

обеднéть *сов. см.* беднéть.

обéдня *ж. церк.* mass.

обежáть *сов. см.* обегáть II.

обезбóлив|ать, обезбóлить (*вн.*) anáesthetize (*smth.*); (*роды и т. п.*) relíeve the pain (of). ~ающий anaesthétic; ~ающее срéдство anaesthétic; páinkiller.

обезбóлить *сов. см.* обезбóливать.

обезвóдеть *сов.* becóme* wáterless/árid.

обезвóдить *сов. см.* обезвóживать.

обезвóживать, обезвóдить (*вн.*) depríve (*smth.*) of wáter; (*продукты и т. п.*) dehýdrate (*smth.*).

обезврéдить *сов. см.* обезврéживать.

обезврéживать, обезврéдить (*вн.*) rénder (*smb., smth.*) hármless.

обезглáвить *сов.* (*вн.*) behéad (*smth.*), decápitate (*smth.*); перен. destróy the bráin-centre (of).

обездóленный déstitute, índigent.

обездóливать, обездóлить (*вн.*) make* (*smb.*) déstitute.

обездóлить *сов. см.* обездóливать.

обезлéс|ение *с.* deforestátion. ~ить *сов.* (*вн.*) defórest (*smth.*).

обезлúчивать, обезлúчить (*вн.*) 1. (*лишать индивидуальных особенностей*) take* awáy *smb.'s* individuálity, depérsonalize (*smth.*); 2. (*работу и т. п.*) elíminate pérsonal responsibílity (in).

обезлúч|ить *сов. см.* обезлúчивать.

обезлюдеть *сов.* be*/becóme* depópulated.

обезобрáживать, обезобрáзить (*вн.*) disfigure (*smb., smth.*).

обезобрáзить *сов. см.* обезобрáживать и безобрáзить.

обезопáсить *сов.* (*вн.*) protéct (*smb., smth.*), make* (*smb., smth.*) safe, make* (*smth.*) secúre. ~ся *сов.* make* onesélf safe.

обезорýживать, обезорýжить (*вн.; прям. и перен.*) disárm (*smb.*).

обезорýжить *сов. см.* обезорýживать.

обезýмевш|ий (*от рд.*) máddened (with); смотрéть на что-л. ~ими глазáми stare wíld-éyed at *smth.*

обезýметь *сов.* (*от рд.*) be* mad (with), be* crazed (with).

обезьян|а *ж.* mónkey; (*человекообразная*) ape. ~ий mónkey *attr.*, ápe-like. ~ничать, собезьянничать 1. (*вн.*) *разг.* cópy (*smth.*); 2. *тк. несов.* ape.

обелúск *м.* óbelisk.

обелúть *сов. см.* обелять.

обелять, обелúть (*вн.*) whitewash (*smb.*), víndicate (*smb.*), jústify (*smb.*).

оберегáть *несов.* (*вн. от рд.*) protéct (*smb., smth.* from, against), guard (*smb., smth.* from, against), shield (*smb., smth.* from, against). ~ся *несов.* (*от рд.*) shield/protéct onesélf (from).

обернýть(ся) *сов. см.* обёртывать(ся) и оборáчивать(ся).

обёртка *ж.* wrápper, cóver.

обёрточн|ый wrápping; ~ая бумáга wrápping-paper; (*неотбелённая*) brown páper.

обёртывать, обернýть (*вн.*) 1. (*завёртывать*) wrap (*smth.*) up; 2. (*обвивать*) wind* (*smth.*) round, wrap (*smth.*) round; обернýть шарф вокрýг шéи wrap a scarf round *one's* neck; 3. (*поворачивать*) turn (*smth.*) (*тж. перен.*); обернýть дéло в свою пóльзу turn mátters in *one's* fávour; ◇ обернýть когó-л. вокрýг пáльца twist *smb.* round *one's* little finger. ~ся, обернýться 1. (*повёртываться*) turn round, look round; 2. (*о делах, событиях и т. п.*) turn out; неизвéстно, как обернётся дéло who knows what turn mátters will take, who knows how things will turn out; 3. (*ехать и возвращаться обратно*) get* there and back (again).

обескрóвить *сов.* (*вн.*) 1. bleed* (*smb., smth.*) white; 2. перен. wéaken *smb.*; emásculate (*smth.*).

обескурáженный discóuraged.

обескурáживать, обескурáжить (*вн.*) discóurage (*smb.*).

обескурáжить *сов. см.* обескурáживать.

обеспéчен|ие *с.* 1. (*действие*) ensúring; (*чем-л.*) provísion; ~ промышленности ýглем kéeping índustry supplíed with coal; материáльно-технúческое ~ áрмии ármy's logístical suppórt; 2. (*материальные средства к жизни*) secúrity; прáво на материáльное ~ в стáрости the right to matérial secúrity in old age; 3. (*гарантия*) guarantée, secúrity. ~ность ж. 1. (*степень обеспечения*) provísion; Это зави́сит от ~ности школ кни́гами it depénds on how well the schools are províded with books; 2. (*достаток*) secúrity. ~ный (*зажиточный*) wéll-to--dó, cómfortably off.

обеспе́чивать, обеспе́чить 1. (*вн.; гарантировать*) secúre (*smth.*), ensúre (*smth.*); ~ безопа́сность движе́ния achíeve sáfety on the roads, ensúre road sáfety; ~ успе́х ensúre succéss; обеспе́чить дальне́йший подъём эконо́мики ensúre fúrther económic prógress; 2. (*вн. тв.; снабжать*) províde (*smb., smth.* with); ~ кого́-л. всем необходи́мым províde *smb.* with éverything he needs; 3. (*вн.; материально*) províde for (*smb., smth.*). ~ся, обеспе́читься (*тв.*) províde onesélf (with).

обеспе́чить(ся) сов. см. обеспе́чивать(ся).

обеспоко́ить сов. см. беспоко́ить. ~ся сов. см. беспоко́иться.

обесси́леть сов. becóme* weak/enféebled.

обессла́вить сов. (*вн.*) defáme (*smb., smth.*), disgráce (*smb., smth.*).

обессме́ртить сов. (*вн.*) immórtalize (*smth.*).

обесцве́тить сов. см. обесцве́чивать.

обесцве́чивать, обесцве́тить (*вн.*) take* the colour out (of).

обесце́н|ение с. depreciátion. ~ивать, обесце́нить (*вн.*) depréciate (*smth.*). ~иваться, обесце́ниться depréciate.

обесце́нить(ся) сов. см. обесце́нивать(ся).

обесче́стить сов. см. бесче́стить.

обе́т м. vow; дава́ть ~ prómise, vow; дава́ть ~ молча́ния take* a vow of sílence.

обеща́ние с. prómise.

обещ|а́ть несов. и сов. (+ инф., вн.) 1. (*сов. тж.* пообеща́ть) prómise (+ to *inf, smth.*); он ~а́л прийти́ во́время he prómised to be púnctual; 2. *тк. несов.* (*подавать надежды*) prómise (+ to *inf, smth.*); день ~а́ет быть я́сным the day looks like béing fine.

обжа́ловани|е с. *юр.* appéal (against); пригово́р ~ю не подлежи́т the séntence cárries no right of appéal.

обжа́ловать сов. (*вн.*) appéal (against).

обжа́ривать, обжа́рить (*вн.*) fry (*smth.*) (on both sides). ~ся, обжа́риться be* fried on both sides.

обжа́рить(ся) сов. см. обжа́ривать(ся).

обже́чь(ся) сов. см. обжига́ть(ся).

обжига́ть, обже́чь (*вн.*) 1. burn* (*smth.*), sear (*smth.*); 2. (*повреждать огнём*) burn* (*smb., smth.*); (*вызывать ощущение жжения*) sting* (*smth.*); *перен.* sear (*smb., smth.*); 3. (*кирпич*) bake* (*smth.*). ~ся, обже́чься burn* onesélf; (*напитком*) burn* one's tongue/mouth; (*крапивой и т. п.*) get* stung; *перен.* burn* one's fingers.

обжито́й that has been lived in *после сущ.*; (*уютный*) hómelike; име́ть ~ вид look hómelike, have* a lived-in appéarance.

обжо́р|а м. и ж. *разг.* glútton. ~ство с. *разг.* glúttony.

обзавести́сь сов. см. обзаводи́ться.

обзаводи́ться, обзавести́сь (*тв.*) *разг.* províde onesélf (with); ~ хозя́йством set* up house; обзавести́сь семе́йством start a fámily; обзавести́сь знако́мыми acquíre friends.

обзо́р м. 1. (*действие*) observátion, obsérving; 2. (*возможность обозреть*) view, field of vísion; 3. (*сжатое сообщение*) revíew, súrvey, róund-up. ~ный 1. (*содержащий обзор*) súmmarizing; ~ная ле́кция súmmarizing lécture; 2. (*позволяющий обозревать*) observátion *attr.*; look-out; ~ная пози́ция look-out post.

обзыв|а́ть, обозва́ть (*вн. тв.*) call (*smb. smth.*); его́ по-вся́кому ~а́ют they call him all sorts of names.

обива́ть, оби́ть (*вн. тв.*) cóver (*smth.* with); (*мебель*

тж.) uphólster (*smth.* with); ~ что-л. желе́зом sheet (*smth.*) with íron; ◇ ~ поро́ги camp on the dóorstep.

оби́вка ж. 1. (*действие*) uphólstering; 2. (*материал*) uphólstery.

оби́д|а ж. ínjury, wrong, ínsult; (*чувство досады*) reséntment; (*горестное чувство*) sense of ínjury; wóunded féelings *pl*, gríevance; нанести́ ~у кому́-л. give* offénce to *smb.*; ◇ не дава́ться в ~у not allów onesélf to be put upón; be* quite áble to stand/stick up for onesélf; не дать кого́-л. в ~у see* that no harm comes to *smb.*, take* care of *smth.*; быть в ~е на кого́-л. have* a grudge agáinst *smb.*; не в ~у бу́дет ска́зано no offénce meant.

оби́деть(ся) сов. см. обижа́ть(ся).

оби́дн|о 1. *нареч.* offénsively, insúltingly; 2. *в знач. сказ. безл.* (*дт.*): мне, ему́ *и т. д.* ~ it offénds me, him *etc.*, it hurts me, him *etc.*; мне ~ слу́шать I am páined to hear; мне ~ за него́ I feel (véry) sórry on his accóunt; ~, что... it is a píty that...; ~, что вы не могли́ прийти́! what a shame you cóuldn't be there! ~ый 1. (*оскорбительный*) offénsive, slíghting, wóunding; ~ое замеча́ние slíghting remárk; сказа́ть что-л. в ~ой фо́рме say* smth. in an offénsive way; 2. *разг.* (*досадный*) annóying, regréttable; ~ая опеча́тка regréttable mísprint.

оби́дчив|ость ж. tóuchiness, susceptibílity. ~ый tóuchy.

обижа́ть, оби́деть 1. (*вн.; нанести обиду*) offénd (*smb.*); hurt*/wound *smb.'s* féelings; 2. (*вн.*) *разг.* (*наносить ущерб кому-л.*) do* (*smb.*) down; 3. (*вн. тв.*) *разг.* (*лишать чего-л.*): приро́да не оби́дела его́ си́лой he was no wéakling, he had plénty of strength. ~ся, оби́деться take* offénce; (*на вн.*) be* hurt/offénded (with); be*/get* húffy (with).

оби́женн|о offéndedly; húffily *разг.*; (*недовольно*) reséntfully. ~ый 1. (*на вн.; обидевшийся*) offénded (with); он на вас оби́жен he's offénded with you; он оби́жен тем, что... he is offénded that...; 2. (*выражающий обиду*) offénded, reséntful, hurt; ~ым го́лосом reséntfully, in reséntful/ínjured tones; с ~ым ви́дом with an air of reséntment.

оби́лие с. 1. (*большое количество*) abúndance; ~ ди́чи an abúndance of game; 2. (*достаток*) plénty.

оби́льн|о lávishly. ~ый 1. (*отличающийся обилием*) abúndant, pléntiful; (*щедрый, роскошный*) lávish; ~ый урожа́й abúndant hárvest; ~ый у́жин lávish súpper; 2. (*тв.*) (*изобилующий чем-л.*) rich (in), abúndant (in), ríchly/génerously endówed (with); (*о дичи и т. п.*) téeming (with).

обиня́к м.: говори́ть ~а́ми beat* about the bush; сказа́ть что-л. без ~о́в tell* smth. pláinly; not mince mátters.

обира́ть, обобра́ть (*вн.*) *разг.* fleece (*smb.*), clean (*smb.*) out.

обита́емый inhábited.

обита́тел|ь м. inhábitant; ~и до́ма the óccupants of the house.

обита́ть несов. dwell*, live.

оби́ть сов. см. обива́ть.

обихо́д м. course, way of life; (*употребление*) use, úsage; войти́ в ~ come* into géneral use; вы́йти из ~а go* out of use; дома́шний ~ doméstic use; предме́ты ~а árticles of (dáily) use. ~ный éveryday; ~ное выраже́ние cómmon/éveryday expréssion.

обката́ть сов. см. обка́тывать.

обка́тка ж. 1. (*дороги*) rólling; 2. (*автомашины и т. п.*) rún-in.

обка́тывать, обката́ть (*вн.*) 1. (*дорогу*) roll (*smth.*) (smooth); 2. (*автомашину и т. п.*) run* (*smth.*) in.

обкла́дывать, обложи́ть 1. (*вн. тв.; окружать чем--л.*) surróund (*smth.*); обложи́ть больно́го поду́шками put* píllows únder a sick man's back; ~ дёрном turf; 2. (*вн.; обволакивать*) cóver (*smth.*); всё не́бо обложи́ли ту́чи the whole sky was banked with clouds; 3.

безл.: всё нёбо обложи́ло the sky is óvercast; язы́к обло-жи́ло the tongue is furred; **4.** (*вн. тв.; облицо́вывать*) face (*smth.* with); ~ сте́ны мра́мором face walls with márble. ~ся, обложи́ться (*тв.*) surróund onesélf (with); обложи́ться кни́гами surróund onesélf with books.

обко́м *м.* (областно́й комите́т) Régional Committee.

обкра́дывать, обокра́сть (*вн.*) rob (*smb., smth.*).

обкуса́ть *сов. см.* обку́сывать.

обку́сывать, обкуса́ть (*вн.*) níbble (*smth.*), bite* (*smth.*) (round the édges).

обла́ва *ж.* **1.** róund-up; полице́йская ~ police swoop/raid; **2.** *охот.* róund-up, drive; (*цепь загонщи-ков*) ring of béaters.

облага́ть, обложи́ть: ~ *кого-л.* нало́гами tax *smb.*, impóse táxes on *smb.*

облагора́живать, облагоро́дить (*вн.*) **1.** exért an élevating/ennóbling ínfluence (on); **2.** (*улучшать породу животных, качество растений*) impróve (*smth.*). ~ся, облагоро́диться **1.** be* ennóbled; **2.** (*о животных, рас-тениях*) impróve.

облагоро́дить(ся) *сов.* см. облагора́живать(ся).

облада́|ние *с.* posséssion. ~тель *м.* posséssor, ówner; (*кубка, титула*) hólder.

облада́ть *несов.* (*тв.*) have* (*smth.*), posséss (*smth.*). ~ больши́м тала́нтом have* great tálent; ~ хо-ро́шим здоро́вьем enjóy good* health; ~ исто́чником сырья́ posséss sóurces of raw matérials.

о́блак|о *с.* cloud; под ~а́ми just benéath the clouds.

обла́мывать, обломо́ть, обломи́ть (*вн.*) **1.** break* off (*smth.*); **2.** *сов.* обломо́ть (*уговаривать*) break* *smb.'s* resístance/will. ~ся, обломо́ться, обломи́ться break* off.

обласка́ть *сов.* (*вн.*) show* kíndness (to), be* nice (to).

областн|о́й 1. régional; ~ центр régional céntre; **2.** (*диалектный*) díalect *attr.*, dialéctal; ~о́е сло́во díalect word.

о́бласть *ж.* **1.** (*часть страны*) région, área; **2.** (*ад-министративно-территориальная единица*) óblast, région; Моско́вская ~ the Móscow Région; **3.** (*отрасль знаний, деятельности*) sphere, field, próvince; но́вая ~ зна́ний new field of knówledge; э́то не моя́ ~ that is not (withín) my próvince; **4.** *анат.* région; ране́ние в ~ се́рд-ца wound in the région of the heart.

о́блачн|ость *ж.* clóudiness; сплошна́я ~ tén-ténths cloud; ни́зкая ~ low cloud. ~ый clóudy; ~ый день clóudy day.

обла́ять *сов.* (*вн.*) **1.** bark (at); **2.** *разг.* (*обругать*) swear* (at).

облег|а́ть *несов.* fit clósely; (*о пальто и т. п.*) fit snúgly; пла́тье пло́тно ~а́ет фигу́ру the dress is clóse--fítting, the dress óutlines the fígure.

облегч|а́ть, облегчи́ть (*вн.*) **1.** (*уменьшать вес че-го-л.*) líghten (*smth.*), redúce the weight (of), make* (*smth.*) líghter; **2.** (*упрощать*) símplify (*smth.*); **3.** (*де-лать менее трудным*) facílitate (*smth.*), make* (*smth.*) éasy; облегчи́ть усло́вия труда́ impróve wórking condítions; ~ реше́ние зада́чи facílitate the solútion of a próblem; **4.** (*смягчать, ослаблять*) relíeve (*smth.*), ease (*smth.*); облегчи́ть боль ease the pain; **5.** (*успокаи-вать*) relíeve (*smb., smth.*); облегчи́ть ду́шу relíeve one's féelings. ~е́ние *с.* **1.** (*действие*) máking líghter; simplificátion; ~е́ние ве́са redúction of weight; **2.** (*чувст-во успокоения*) (sense of) relíef; вздохну́ть с ~е́нием draw*/heave* a sigh of relíef.

облегчи́ть|о: ~ вздохну́ть draw* a sigh of relíef. ~ый **1.** (*более лёгкий*) light-wéight *attr.*; **2.** (*упрощён-ный*) símplified; постро́йка ~ого ти́па líghtly built strúcture, líghtly constrúcted búilding; **3.** (*выражающий облегчение*) ~ый вздох sigh of relíef.

облегчи́ть *сов. см.* облегча́ть.

обледене́|лый íce-cóated. ~ние *с.* ícing(-up).

обледене́ть *сов.* ice up, be* cóated with ice.

облеза́ть, облезть *разг.* **1.** (*лишаться волос, шер-*

сти и т. п.) moult, lose* *one's* hair, fur *etc.*; **2.** (*о кра-ске, лаке и т. п.*) come*/peel off; (*о стенах*) peel.

обле́зть *сов. см.* облеза́ть.

облека́ть, обле́чь 1. (*вн. тв.; окружать чем-л.*) envélop (*smth.* in); ~ *что-л.* та́йной envélop *smth.* in mýstery; **2.** (*вн.; выражать, воплощать*) clothe (*smth.*); ~ мы́сли слова́ми, в слова́ clothe thoughts in words, put* thoughts ínto words; **3.** (*вн. тв.; наделять*) (in)vést (*smb.* with), fúrnish (*smb.* with); ~ кого́-л. пол-номо́чиями (in)vést *smb.* with pówers; ◇ обле́чь кого́-л. дове́рием place trust in *smb.* ~ся, обле́чься (в *вн.*) be* embódied (in), be* clothed (in).

облени́ться *сов.* get* lázy/slack.

облепи́ть *сов. см.* облепля́ть.

облепи́ха *ж. бот.* séa-búckthorn.

облепля́ть, облепи́ть 1. (*вн.; прилипать со всех сторон*) stick* all óver (*smth.*); боти́нки облепи́ла грязь the shoes were plástered with mud; **2.** (*вн. тв.; покры-вать со всех сторон*) cóver (*smth.* with); **3.** (*вн.) разг.* (*окружать*) cling* (to); (*о мухах и т. п.*) swarm all óver (*smth.*).

облесе́ние *с.* afforestátion.

облета́ть I, облете́ть 1. (*вн.; вокруг*) fly* round (*smth.*); **2.** (*вн.; пролетать стороной*) skirt (*smth.*), pass óver (*smth.*); **3.** (*вн.; распространяться*) spread* (through); облете́ть го́род с быстрото́й мо́лнии spread* through the town like wíldfire; **4.** (*опадать — о листь-ях*) fall*; (*оставаться без листьев*) becóme* bare, lose*/shed* its leaves.

облет|а́ть II *сов.* (*вн.*) **1.** (*летая, побывать всюду*) fly* all óver (*smth.*); ~ всю страну́ fly* all óver the cóuntry; **2.** *разг.:* я ~а́л все магази́ны I've been all round the shops; **3.** *ав.* (*испытать самолёт и т. п.*) put* (*smth.*) through its tríals.

облете́ть *сов. см.* облета́ть I.

обле́чь(ся) *сов. см.* облека́ть(ся).

обливо́ние *с.* dóusing, slúicing; ~ холо́дной водо́й dóusing with cold wáter, cold shówer.

облива́ть, обли́ть (*вн. тв.*) **1.** pour (*smth.* óver); об-ли́ть кого́-л. водо́й pour wáter óver *smb.*, douse *smb.* with wáter; **2.** (*покрывать собой — о росе, слезах и т. п.*) drench (*smth.* with, in); **3.** (*проливать что-л.*) spill* (*smth.* óver); обли́ть ска́терть черни́лами spill*/pour ink all óver the táblecloth; ◇ обли́ть кого́-л. гря́зью, помо́ями fling* mud at *smb.* ~ся, обли́ться (*тв.*) pour (*smth.*) óver onesélf; (*покрываться чем-л.*) be* cóvered (with); обли́ться холо́дной водо́й take* a shówer-bath, sluice onesélf down with cold wáter; ~ся по́-том be* drenched in sweat; ~ся слеза́ми be* drowned in tears; ~ся кро́вью bleed* profúsely.

облига́ция *ж.* bond.

облиза́ть *сов. см.* обли́зывать. ~ся *сов. см.* обли́зы-ваться 2.

обли́зывать, облиза́ть (*вн.*) lick (*smth.*); ◇ па́льчи-ки обли́жешь it'll make you long for more. ~ся, обли-за́ться **1.** *тк. несов.* (*о человеке*) lick *one's* lips; (*на вн.*) *перен.* eye (*smth.*) húngrily; **2.** (*о животных*) lick itsélf.

о́блик *м.* appéarance; (*характер*) cháracter, máke--up; *перен.* face, appéarance; нра́вственный ~ móral cháracter; ~ го́рода the face of a cíty.

облисполко́м *м.* (исполни́тельный комите́т област-но́го Сове́та наро́дных депута́тов) Exécutive (Committee) of the Óblast/Régional Sóviet (of Péople's Députies).

обли́ть(ся) *сов. см.* облива́ть(ся).

облицева́ть *сов. см.* облицо́вывать.

облицо́вка *ж.* fácing; (*кафелем*) tíling; (*деревом*) pánelling.

облицо́вочный fácing; ~ кирпи́ч áshlar brick.

облицо́вывать, облицева́ть (*вн. тв.*) face (*smth.* with); (*кафелем*) tile (*smth.* with); (*деревом*) pánel (*smth.* with).

облич|а́ть *несов.* (*вн.*) 1. (*разоблачать*) expóse (*smth.*); 2. (*показывать*) revéal (*smb., smth.*). ~е́ние *с.* expósure. ~и́тель *м.* denóuncer. ~и́тельный accúsatory; full of denunciátion *после сущ.*

обложе́ние *с.* impositíon; (*налогами*) taxátion.

обложи́ть *сов. см.* обкла́дывать *и* облага́ть. ~ся *сов. см.* обкла́дываться.

обло́жка *ж.* 1. cóver; 2. (*для документа*) case; 3. *разг.* (book) jácket.

обложно́й *разг.:* ~ дождь stéady dównpour.

облока́чиваться, облокоти́ться (*на вн.*) put*/lean* *one's* élbows (on), lean* (on).

облокоти́ться *сов. см.* облока́чиваться.

обломи́ть *сов. см.* обла́мывать(ся).

обломи́ть *сов. см.* обла́мывать 1. ~ся *сов. см.* обла́мываться.

обло́мок *м.* 1. frágment; *мн.* débris *sg*, wréckage *sg*, rúbble *sg*; 2. (*остаток чего-л. исчезнувшего*) véstige, frágment.

облупи́ть *сов. см.* лупи́ть 1.

облуч|а́ть, облучи́ть (*вн.*) irrádiate (*smth.*), expóse (*smb., smth.*) to rays; ~ ква́рцем treat with ultravíolet light. ~а́ться, облучи́ться be* expósed to radiátion. ~е́ние *с.* irradiátion, expósure to rays; (*лечебное*) radiátion tréatment. ~и́ть(ся) *сов. см.* облуча́ть(ся).

облы́сеть *сов. см.* лысе́ть.

облюбова́ть *сов.* (*вн.*) take* a fáncy (to).

обма́зать(ся) *сов. см.* обма́зывать(ся).

обма́зывать, обма́зать (*вн. тв.*) 1. cóver (*smth.* with); coat (*smth.* with); 2. *разг.* (*пачкать*) dírty (*smth.* with). ~ся, обма́заться *разг.* get*/make* *one*sélf dírty.

обма́кивать, обмакну́ть (*вн.*) dip (*smth.*).

обмакну́ть *сов. см.* обма́кивать.

обма́н *м.* 1. (*действия, поступки*) decéption, tríckery, fraud; (*ложь*) lies *pl*; доби́ться *чего-л.* ~ом gain/achíeve *smth.* by decéption, acquíre *smth.* fráudulently; 2. (*заблуждение, ошибка*) delúsion, illúsion; вводи́ть *кого-л.* в ~ decéive *smb.*; ~ зре́ния óptical illúsion; ~ чувств hallucinátion. ~ный fráudulent; ~ным путём fráudulently, by fraud.

обману́ть(ся) *сов. см.* обма́нывать(ся).

обма́нчив|ый decéptive; (*мнимый*) illúsory; нару́жность ~а appéarances are decéptive.

обма́нщик decéiver.

обма́ныв|ать, обману́ть (*вн.*) 1. (*вводить в заблуждение*) decéive (*smb.*); (*не выполнять обещание*) let* (*smb.*) down; (*поступать нечестно по отношению к кому-л.*) cheat (*smb.*); *перен.* betráy (*smb.*), disappóint (*smb.*); обману́ть чью-л. бди́тельность throw* *smb.* off his, her guard; ~ чьи-л. наде́жды disappóint *smb.'s* hopes; е́сли па́мять меня́ не ~ает if my mémory does not decéive me; 2. (*изменять мужу, жене*) decéive (*smb.*); 3. (*соблазнять*) sedúce (*smb.*). ~ся, обману́ться be* delúded, be* mistáken; ~аться в *ком-л.* be* mistáken in *smb.*; я в нём о́чень обману́лся I was gréatly mistáken in him; ~аться в *чём-л.* be* decéived in *smth.*, be* disappóinted in *smth.*

обма́тывать, обмота́ть (*вн. тв.*) wind* (*smth.* aróund); (*окутывать*) wrap (*smth.* round). ~ся, обмота́ться (*тв.*) *разг.* wrap *one*sélf (in).

обма́хивать *несов.* (*вн.*) fan (*smth.*); ~ лицо́ ве́ером fan *one's* face. ~ся *несов.* fan *one*sélf.

обмеле́ть *сов. см.* меле́ть.

обме́н *м.* 1. exchánge; ~ докуме́нтов renéwal of pápers; ~ о́пытом exchánge/sháring/póoling of (*one's*) expérience; ~ мне́ниями exchánge/interchánge of views; ~ информа́цией exchánge of informátion; в ~ на... in exchánge for...; by way of exchánge; 2. *эк.* exchánge; ◇ ~ веще́ств metábolism.

обме́нивать, обменя́ть (*вн. на вн.*) exchánge (*smth.* for). ~ся, обменя́ться (*тв.*) exchánge (*smth.*) (*тж. перен.*); ~ся с *кем-л.* фотогра́фиями exchánge phótographs with *smb.*, give* *smb.* *one's* phótograph in exchánge for *his*; ~ся шу́тками bándy jokes; ~ся впечатле́ниями compáre notes.

обменя́ть(ся) *сов. см.* обме́нивать(ся), меня́ть(ся).

обмере́ть *сов. см.* обмира́ть.

обме́ривать, обме́рить (*вн.*) (*измерять*) méasure (*smth.*).

обме́рить *сов. см.* обме́ривать.

обмеря́ть *несов. см.* обме́ривать.

обмести́ *сов. см.* обмета́ть.

обмета́ть, обмести́ (*вн.*) (*очищать что-л. от пыли и т. п.*) brush (*smth.*); (*удалять пыль и т. п. с чего-л.*) brush (*smth.*) off/awáy; ~ пыль do* some dústing.

обмира́ть, обмере́ть *разг.:* ~ от стра́ха *и т. п.* be* páralyzed with fear *etc.*

обмола́чивать, обмолоти́ть (*вн.*) *с.-х.* thresh (*smth.*).

обмолв|иться *сов.* 1. (*оговориться*) use the wrong word; я ~ился it was a slip of the tongue (on my part); 2. (*проговориться*) let* (it) out; ◇ не ~ (ни еди́ным) сло́вом, что... not say a word abóut the fact that..., not give the slíghtest intimátion that... ~ка *ж.* slip of the tongue, chance remárk.

обмоло́т *м. с.-х.* 1. (*действие*) thréshing; 2. (*обмолоченное зерно*) threshed grain.

обмолоти́ть *сов. см.* обмола́чивать.

обмора́живать, обморо́зить: обморо́зить себе́ лицо́ *и т. п.* get* *one's* face, *etc.* fróst-bitten. ~ся, обморо́зиться get* fróst-bitten.

обморо́женный fróst-bitten.

обморо́зить(ся) *сов. см.* обмора́живать(ся).

о́бморок *м.* faint, fáinting-fit; глубо́кий ~ dead faint; па́дать в ~ faint, fall* down in a faint.

обморочн|ый: ~ое состоя́ние faint, state of uncónsciousness.

обмота́ть(ся) *сов. см.* обма́тывать(ся).

обмо́тка *ж.* 1. *эл.* wínding; 2. *мн.* (*для ног*) púttees.

обмундирова́ние *с.* 1. (*действие*) recéiving úniform(s), kítting up; 2. (*комплект одежды*) úniform, óutfit, kit.

обмундирова́ть *сов.* (*вн.*) clothe (*smb., smth.*), fit (*smb., smth.*) out, kit (*smb., smth.*) up. ~ся *сов.* get* fítted out, get* kítted up.

обмыва́ть, обмы́ть (*вн.*) wash (*smth.*), bathe (*smth.*). ~ся, обмы́ться 1. have* a wash all óver; 2. (*о предметах*) be* washed clean.

обмы́ть(ся) *сов. см.* обмыва́ть(ся).

обмя́кнуть *сов. разг.* go* limp; *перен.* sóften.

обнагле́ть *сов. см.* нагле́ть.

обнадёживать, обнадёжить (*вн.*) raise *smb.'s* hopes.

обнадёжить *сов. см.* обнадёживать.

обнаж|а́ть, обнажи́ть (*вн.*) 1. (*оголять*) bare (*smth.*), uncóver (*smth.*); обнажи́ть го́лову bare *one's* head; 2. (*лишать листвы*) bare (*smth.*), denúde (*smth.*); 3. (*освобождать от покрова*) lay* (*smth.*) bare, expóse (*smth.*) (*тж. перен.*); 4. (*вынимать из ножен*) bare (*smth.*), unshéathe (*smth.*); 5. (*открыть правду*) expóse (*smth.*), revéal (*smth.*). ~а́ться, обнажи́ться 1. (*обнажать своё тело*) strip náked; 2. (*о какой-л. части тела*) be* expósed, be* uncóvered; 3. (*лишаться листвы, хвои*) becóme* bare; (*оказываться ничем не прикрытым*) be* expósed, be* laid bare; *перен.* (*обнаруживаться*) revéal itsélf. ~ённый 1. (*о теле*) náked; (*о частях тела*) bare; ~ённая спина́ bare back; с ~ённой голово́й baréheaded; 2. (*лишённый листвы, растительности*) bare, náked; 3. (*ничем не прикрытый*) expósed; *перен.* undisguísed, bárefaced.

обнажи́ть(ся) *сов. см.* обнажа́ть(ся).

обнаро́дов|ание *с.* publicátion; (*закона*) promulgátion. ~ать *сов.* (*вн.*) públish (*smth.*); (*закон*) prómulgate (*smth.*).

обнару́живать, обнару́жить (*вн.*) 1. (*находить*)

discóver (*smb.*, *smth.*); (*раскрывать*) detéct (*smth.*); обнару́жить проти́вника spot/find* the énemy; 2. (*открывать взору*; *проявлять*) displáy (*smth.*). ~ся, обнару́житься 1. (*отыскиваться*) be* found, be* discóvered; come* to light; turn up *разг.*; 2. (*проявляться*) revéal itself, come* out; 3. (*становиться видимым*) be* reveáled.

обнару́жить(ся) *сов. см.* обнару́живать(ся).

обнести́ *сов. см.* обноси́ть.

обнима́ть, обня́ть (*вн.*) 1. (*заключать в объятия*) embráce (*smb.*, *smth.*), give* (*smb.*) a hug; (*обхватывать руками что-л.*) put* one's arm(s) (about, round); 2. (*охватывать взглядом*) take* in (*smth.*); не обня́ть глáзом fárther than the eye can see; 3. (*захватывать — о чувствах*) overcóme* (*smth.*); 4. (*охватывать*) take* in (*smth.*), embráce (*smth.*). ~ся, обня́ться embráce.

обнищ|áлый impóverished; (*о человеке тж.*) déstitute. ~áние impóverishment; (*о человеке тж.*) destitútion; pauperizátion.

обнища́ть *сов. см.* нища́ть.

обнови́ть(ся) *сов. см.* обновля́ть(ся).

обнóвка *ж. разг.* sómething new, new óutfit, new posséssion.

обновле́ние *с.* 1. (*восстановление первоначального вида*) renovátion, restorátion; *перен.* (*возрождение*) regenerátion; 2. (*замена новым*) renéwal.

обновля́ть, обнови́ть (*вн.*) 1. (*восстанавливать первоначальный вид*) rénovate (*smth.*); *перен.* (*возрождать*) regénerate (*smth.*); ~ свои́ зна́ния refrésh one's knówledge; 2. (*заменять, пополнять новым*) renéw (*smth.*); replénish (*smth.*); ~ репертуа́р renéw one's répertoire; 3. *разг.* (*впервые употреблять новую вещь*) put* on (*smth.*) for the first time; обнови́ть пла́тье put* on a new dress for the first time; обнови́ть лы́жи try out one's new skis. ~ся, обнови́ться 1. be* rebórn, be* born anéw; 2. (*становиться новым по составу*) be* renéwed, be* replénished.

обнос|и́ть, обнести́ 1. (*вн. тв.*; *окружать*) enclóse (*smth.* with); ~ что-л. забóром fence *smth.* in/round; ~ что-л. стенóй put* a wall round *smth.*; 2. (*вн. тв.*; *угощать всех*) serve (*smb.* with); их ~и́ли фру́ктами the fruit was served round; 3. (*вн.*; *пропускать при угощении*) pass óver; (*вн. тв.*) not serve (*smb.* with).

обнос|и́ться *сов. разг.* 1. (*изнашивать одежду, обувь*) wear* out one's clothes; я совсéм ~и́лся I have ábsolutely nóthing to wear; 2. (*истрепаться — об одежде, обуви*) be* worn out.

обню́хать *сов. см.* обню́хивать.

обню́хивать, обню́хать (*вн.*) sniff (at).

обня́ть(ся) *сов. см.* обнима́ть(ся).

обо *см. о* I.

обобра́ть *сов. см.* обира́ть.

обобщ|а́ть, обобщи́ть (*вн.*) 1. (*объединять*) uníte (*smth.*), make* (*smth.*) into a whole; 2. (*делать общее в отдельных явлениях и т. п.*) draw* a géneral conclúsion (from), géneralize (from). ~е́ние *с.* generalizátion; смéлые ~е́ния bold generalizátions. ~ённый géneralized; (*не затрагивающий деталей*) súmmarized, géneral.

обобществ|и́ть *сов. см.* обобществля́ть. ~ле́ние *с.* socializátion; ~лéние средств произвóдства socializátion of the means of prodúction; ~лённый sócialized; ~лённый труд sócialized lábour.

обобществля́ть, обобществи́ть (*вн.*) sócialize (*smth.*).

обобщи́ть *сов. см.* обобща́ть.

обогати́ть(ся) *сов. см.* обогаща́ть(ся).

обогащ|а́ть, обогати́ть (*вн.*) 1. (*прям. и перен.*) enrích (*smb.*, *smth.*); 2. (*повышать полезные качества чего-л.*) dress (*smth.*); (*о рудах тж.*) cóncentrate (*smth.*); ~ пóчву азóтом dress soil with nítrogen; ~ руду́

cóncentrate ore. ~а́ться, обогати́ться 1. (*прям. и перен.*) get*/grow* rícher; (*тв.*) be* enríched (by); ~а́ться за счёт *кого-л.* enrich oneself at *smb.'s* expénse; 2. (*о почве*) be* enríched; (*о руде и т. п.*) be* cóncentrated. ~éние *с.* 1. (*прям. и перен.*) enríchment; 2. (*почвы, руды и т. п.*) dréssing; (*руды тж.*) concentrátion.

обогна́ть *сов. см.* обгоня́ть.

обогну́ть *сов. см.* огиба́ть.

обогрéв *м.*, ~áние *с.* wárming, héating.

обогрева́ть, обогрéть (*вн.*) *разг.* heat (*smth.*). ~ся, обогрéться *разг.* warm oneself; (*о помещении*) get* wármer.

обогрéть(ся) *сов. см.* обогрева́ть(ся).

óбод *м.*, ~óк *м.* rim.

ободрáнн|ый *разг.* rágged; (*о человеке тж.*) in rags *после сущ.*; ~ые обóи torn wállpaper.

ободра́ть *сов. см.* обдира́ть(ся).

ободрéние *с.* encóuragement.

ободри́ть(ся) *сов. см.* ободря́ть(ся).

ободр|я́ть, ободри́ть (*вн.*) encóurage (*smb.*), put* heart (in). ~я́ться, ободри́ться take* heart. ~я́ющий encóuraging.

обожа́ние *с.* adorátion, wórship.

обожа́ть *несов.* (*вн.*) adóre (*smb.*, *smth.*), wórship (*smb.*, *smth.*).

обожда́ть *сов.* (*вн.*) *разг.* wait (for).

обожеств|и́ть *сов. см.* обожествля́ть. ~лéние *с.* déifying, ídolizing.

обожествля́ть, обожестви́ть (*вн.*) déify (*smb.*, *smth.*), ídolize (*smb.*, *smth.*).

обóз *м.* wággon train, string of carts, slédges *etc.*

обозва́ть *сов. см.* обзыва́ть.

обозли́ть(ся) *сов. см.* зли́ть(ся).

обознава́ться, обозна́ться *разг.* take* (*smb.*) for sómebody else; прости́те, я обозна́лся! excúse me, I took you for sómebody else!

обозна́ться *сов. см.* обознава́ться.

обознач|а́ть, обозна́чить (*вн.*) 1. (*помечать*) mark (*smth.*), denóte (*smth.*), désignate (*smth.*); 2. (*указывать, называть*) índicate (*smth.*); 3. *тк. несов.* (*значить*) mean* (*smth.*), sígnify (*smth.*); 4. (*делать заметным*) delíneate (*smth.*), émphasize (*smth.*), bring* out (*smth.*). ~а́ться, обозна́читься 1. (*намечаться, делаться видимым*) take* shape, come* into view, appéar; 2. (*становиться ощутимым*) be* felt, make* itsélf felt. ~éние *с.* designátion; услóвное ~éние convéntional sign.

обозна́чить *сов. см.* обознача́ть 1, 2, 4. ~ся *сов. см.* обознача́ться.

обозрева́тель *м.* cómmentator, obsérver; спорти́вный ~ sports cómmentator.

обозрева́ть, обозрéть (*вн.*) survéy (*smth.*).

обозре́ние *с.* 1. (*действие*) víewing, lóoking óver; 2. (*в газете, по радио и т. п.*) revíew, cómmentary; спорти́вное ~ sports róundup; кни́жное ~ review of books; 3. (*эстрадное представление*) revúe.

обозрéть *сов. см.* обозрева́ть.

обóи *мн.* wállpaper *sg*; окле́ить кóмнату обо́ями páper the room.

обóйма *ж.* hólder; (*патронная*) clip, chárger; *перен.* range.

обойти́ *сов. см.* обходи́ть.

обойти́сь *сов. см.* обходи́ться.

обóйщик *м.* uphólsterer.

обокра́сть *сов. см.* обкра́дывать.

оболга́ть *сов.* (*вн.*) slánder (*smb.*), calúmniate (*smb.*).

оболóчка *ж.* 1. énvelope, óuter skin, shell; *биол.* cápsule; *перен.* (*outward*) form, appéarance; 2. *анат.*: ра́дужная ~ íris; роговáя ~ córnea; сéтчатая ~ rétina; сли́зистая ~ múcous mémbrane.

обольсти́ть *сов. см.* обольща́ть. ~ся *сов. см.* обольща́ться 2.

обольща́ть, обольсти́ть (*вн.*) tempt (*smb.*); (*соблазнять*) sedúce (*smb.*). ~ся, обольсти́ться (*тв.*) 1. *тк. несов.* delúde onesélf (with); flátter onesélf (that); 2. (*поддаваться соблазну*) be* carried awáy (by); ~ся надéждами delúde onesélf with hopes; ~ся успéхами have* one's head turned by succéss.

обольщéние *с.* temptátion, charm.

обоня́|ние *с.* sense of smell; то́нкое ~ a keen sense of smell, a good nose; о́рганы ~ния olfáctory órgans.

обора́чиваемость *ж.* túrnover; (*судов и т. п.*) túrn-round; ~ оборо́тных средств túrnover of cápital.

обора́чивать, оберну́ть (*вн.*) turn (*smth.*); *перен. тж.* give* (*smth.*) a turn/twist. ~ся, оберну́ться 1. turn round (*делать круг вращения*) revólve; 2. (*принимать тот или иной характер*) turn out; 3. (*тв.; выливаться во что-л.*) end (in), resúlt (in), entáil (*smth.*); 4. *разг.* (*съездив, сходив куда-л., возвращаться назад*) go* there and back; 5. *разг.* (*справляться с чем-л.*) mánage; 6. (*тв.; превращаться — в сказках*) turn (ínto).

оборва́нец *м. разг.* rágamuffin.

обо́рванный 1. rágged; 2. (*незаконченный*) frágmentary, scáttered.

оборва́ть(ся) *сов. см.* обрыва́ть(ся).

обо́рка *ж.* frill; (*широкая*) flounce.

оборо́н|а *ж.* 1. (*действие*) defénce; перейти́ от ~ы к нападéнию switch from defénce to attáck; 2. (*совокупность оборонительных средств*) defénce(s); 3. (*линия оборонительных сооружений*) кругова́я ~ áll-róund defénce; держа́ть ~у hold* the line; прорва́ть ~у проти́вника breach/pierce the énemy's defénces.

оборони́ть(ся) *сов. см.* обороня́ть(ся).

оборо́нный defénce *attr.*

обороноспосо́бность *ж.* defénce(s), defénce cápacity/poténtial.

обороня́ть, оборони́ть (*вн.*) defénd (*smth.*). ~ся, оборони́ться 1. hold* the line; 2. *разг.* (*защищать себя*) defénd onesélf.

оборо́т *м.* 1. (*вращение*) turn, revolútion; коли́чество ~ов в мину́ту númber of revolútions per minute, R. P. M.; 2. (*цикл*) rotátion; túrnover; (*совокупность работ, операций*) cýcle of operátions; ~ капита́ла túrnover of cápital; 3. (*коммерческая операция*) operátion; пусти́ть дéньги в ~ put* móney ínto operátion; 4. (*денежные суммы как итог коммерческих операций*) túrnover; годово́й ~ ánnual túrnover; 5. (*употребление, использование*) use; 6. (*поворот*) bend; 7. (*новое направление в ходе, развитии чего-л.*) turn, stage; дéло при́няло дурно́й ~ things have táken a turn for the worse; 8. (*обратная сторона*) the back; на ~e on the óther side, on the back; смотри́ на ~e *пишется* P. T. O. (*т. е.* please turn óver); 9. (*словесное выражение*) expréssion, constrúction; ~ рéчи turn of speech; ◇ брать кого-л. в ~ — take* *smb.* in hand.

оборо́тн|ый 1. (*находящийся в обращении*) círculating; ~ые срéдства círculating/wórking ássets/cápital; 2. (*являющийся не лицевой стороной*) revérse, wrong; ~ая сторона́ листа́ the back of the page.

обору́дов|ание *с.* 1. (*действие*) equípping; зако́нчить ~ заво́да finish equípping a fáctory; 2. (*предметы*) equípment, plant; обнови́ть ~ цéха ré-equíp a depártment/shop. ~ать *несов. и сов.* (*вн.*) equíp (*smth.*), fit out (*smth.*); ~ать мастерску́ю equíp a wórkshop; ~ать площа́дку для игр fit out a pláyground.

обоснова́ние *с.* 1. (*действие*) substantiátion; 2. (*довод*) grounds *pl,* réasons *pl.*

обосно́в|анный wéll-fóunded; (*доказанный*) válid, substántiated; ~ вы́вод wéll-fóunded conclúsion. ~а́ть *сов. см.* обосно́вывать.

обоснова́ться *сов. см.* обосно́вываться.

обосно́вывать, обоснова́ть (*вн.*) substántiate (*smth.*),

give* proof (of); обоснова́ть своё предложéние substántiate/mótivate one's propósal.

обосно́вываться, обоснова́ться (в *пр.*) *разг.* (*поселяться*) séttle down (in).

обосо́бленный ísolated; (*замкнутый тж.*) exclúsive.

обострéние *с.* 1. (*чувств, ощущений*) intensificátion, shárpening; 2. (*ухудшение*) wórsening; ~ болéзни acúte attack of a diséase; 3. (*отношений и т. п.*) aggravátion; ~ противорéчий shárpening/aggravátion of contradíctions.

обострённ|ый 1. (*о чертах лица*) sharp, tápering, póinted; 2. (*об ощущении, восприятии и т. п.*) héightened, enhánced; ~ слух stráining ears; ~ое внима́ние héightened atténtion; 3. (*враждебно напряжённый*) tense, ággravated; ~ые отношéния strained/tense relátions.

обостри́ть(ся) *сов. см.* обостря́ть(ся).

обостря́ть, обостри́ть (*вн.*) 1. (*о чувстве, ощущении*) intensify (*smth.*), héighten (*smth.*); (*о слухе, зрении и т. п.*) shárpen (*smth.*); 2. (*ухудшать*) wórsen (*smth.*); 3. (*делать более напряжённым*) ággravate (*smth.*), exácerbate (*smth.*), shárpen (*smth.*); ~ отношéния strain relátions. ~ся, обостри́ться 1. (*о чертах лица*) becóme* sharp/ángular; 2. (*о чувстве, ощущении*) be* inténsified, becóme* more acúte; (*о слухе, зрении и т. п.*) becóme* kéener/shárper; 3. (*о болезни*) get*/becóme* worse; 4. (*становиться более напряжённым*) becóme* more acúte, be* ággravated; отношéния обостри́лись до предéла relátions were strained to bréaking-point.

обою́дный mútual.

обоюдоо́стр|ый (*прям. и перен.*) dóuble-édged; ~ое ору́жие dóuble-édged wéapon.

обраба́тыв|ать, обрабо́тать (*вн.*) 1. prócess (*smth.*), (*на станке*) machíne (*smth.*); обрабо́тать дета́ль machíne a part; 2. (*возделывать*) till (*smth.*), cúltivate (*smth.*); 3. (*придавать законченный вид*) work up (*smth.*), pólish (*smth.*); ~ материа́лы для статьи́ work up (the matérials for) an árticle, put* an árticle togéther. ~ающий: ~ающая промы́шленность manufácturing índustry.

обрабо́т|ать *сов. см.* обраба́тывать. ~ка *ж.* 1. prócessing; (*на станке*) machíning; ~ка информа́ции informátion prócessing; 2. (*земли*) tílling, cultivátion; 3. (*статьи и т. п.*) pútting ínto shape, éditing; ~ка стати́стических да́нных statístical análysis; ◇ взять кого-л. в ~ку get* to work on *smb.*

обра́довать(ся) *сов. см.* ра́довать(ся).

о́браз *м.* 1. *тк. ед.* (*внешний вид, облик кого-л.*) áspect, appéarance; 2. *обыкн. мн.* (*живое представлéние о ком-л., чём-л.*) image, concéption; свéтлые ~ы бу́дущего the bright óutlines of the fúture; 3. (*тип, характер в художественном произведении*) cháracter, type; 4. (*характер, склад*) mode, way; ~ дéйствия mode of áction; ~ жи́зни mode/way of life; ~ мы́слей áttitude of mind, way of thínking; ~ правлéния form of góvernment; ◇ каки́м ~ом? how?; таки́м ~ом (*так*) and so, thus; никаки́м ~ом by no means; ра́вным ~ом équally; нéкоторым ~ом in some way.

образ|éц *м.* 1. spécimen, sámple; ~цы́ но́вых издéлий sámples (of new próducts); ~цы́ бума́ги spécimen sheets (of páper); 2. (*рд.; пример*) módel (of); ~ добродéтели a módel/páttern of vírtue; ~ му́жества módel of bravery; 3. *тех.* módel, páttern.

о́бразн|ость *ж.* imagery; (*яркость*) cólour, vívidness. ~ый cólourful, gráphic, evócative; ~ое выражéние gráphic phrase; (*метафора*) figure of speech.

образова́ни|е I *с.* 1. (*действие*) formátion; ~ водяны́х паро́в formátion of steam; ~ госуда́рства formátion of a State; 2. (*то, что образовано*) formátion; го́рные ~я hill formátions.

образова́ние II *с.* (*просвещение*) educátion; пра́во

на ~ right to educátion; специáльное ~ spécialized educátion; всеóбщее обязáтельное срéднее ~ univérsal compúlsory sécondary educátion; дать ~ *кому-л.* give* *smb.* an educátion, éducate *smb.*; получи́ть ~ be* éducated.

образóванность *ж.* erudítion.

образóванный éducated.

образовáтельный educátional; ◇ ~ ценз educátional qualificátion.

образовáть *несов. и сов. (вн.)* 1. *(создать)* form *(smth.)*; 2. *(организовать)* órganize *(smth.)*; ~ комúссию set* up a commíttee.

образовáться *несов. и сов.* 1. *(получаться)* form, be* formed; *(возникать)* come* ínto béing; из водьí образу́ется пар steam is génerated from wáter; 2. *(организоваться)* be* órganized, be* set up; 3. *разг. (улаживаться)* come* right, turn out right.

образу́мить *сов. (вн.) разг.* bring* *(smb.)* to réason, bring* *(smb.)* to his, her sénses, sóber down. ~ся *сов. разг.* come* to *one's* sénses, sóber down.

образцóв|ый módel *attr.; (отличный тж.)* exémplary; ~ порáдок pérfect órder; ~ая типогрáфия módel prínting works; ~ое поведéние exémplary cónduct.

обра́зчик *м. (прям. и перен.)* sámple, spécimen.

обрамлéние *с.* 1. *(действие)* fráming, móunting; 2. *(то, что обрамляет что-л.)* frame, frámework, surróund.

обрамля́ть *несов. (вн.)* frame *(smth.)*, mount *(smth.)*, set* *(smth.)* (in a frámework of), surróund *(smth.)*.

обрастáть, **обрасти́** *(тв.)* 1. *(зарастать)* be*/becóme* overgrówn (with); кáмень обрóс мóхом the rock becáme overgrówn with moss; 2. *разг. (покрываться волосами, шерстью)*: ~ бородóй let* *one's* beard grow; 3. *разг. (покрываться слоем чего-л.)* be*/becóme* cóvered (with); ~ жúром put* on fat; ~ грáзью be* encrústed with mud.

обрасти́ *сов. см.* обрастáть.

обрати́ть *сов. см.* обращáть. ~ся *сов. см.* обращáться 1, 2.

обрáтн|о 1. back; повернýть ~ turn back; получи́ть что-л. ~ get* *smth.* back; 2. *разг. (наоборот)* the óther way round; 3.: ~ пропорционáльный *чему-л.* in ínverse rátio to *smth.* ~ый 1.: в ~ом направлéнии in the ópposite diréction; ~ый ход revérse mótion; ~ый путь way back, retúrn jóurney; ~ый поезд a train back; 2. *(противоположный)* ópposite; ~ый смысл ópposite sense; в ~ом поря́дке in revérse órder; 3. *(оборотный)* revérse; ~ая сторонá the back; 4. *мат.* ínverse; ~ая пропóрция invérse propórtion; ◇ ~ áдрес retúrn addréss; ~ый билéт retúrn tícket; ~ая си́ла закóна retrospéctive áction of a law; ~ая связь féedback.

обращáть, **обрати́ть** 1. *(вн.)* turn *(smth.)*; обрати́ть взгляд на *кого-л., что-л.* turn *one's* eyes on *smb., smth.*; ~ взóры (на) look (to); 2. *(вн. в вн.; превращать)* turn *(smth.* into); ~ что-л. в шýтку turn *smth.* into a joke; ◇ ~ *кого-л.* в бéгство put* *smb.* to flight. ~ся, обрати́ться 1. *(к дт.) (заговаривать)* addréss *(smb.)*; ~ся к *кому-л.* с прóсьбой appéal to *smb.*, addréss a requést to *smb.*; ~ся к *кому-л.* за пóмощью appéal to *smb.* for aid; ~ся к *кому-л.* за совéтом ask *smb.'s* advíce, come* for advíce; ~ся к врачý see* a dóctor; ~ся к *кому-л.* с письмóм write* a létter to *smb.*; 2. *(в вн.; превращаться)* turn (ínto); 3. *тк. несов. (с тв.; обходиться с кем-л.)* treat *(smb.)*; плóхо ~ся с *кем-л.* ill-tréat *smb.*; 4. *тк. несов. (с тв.; пользоваться чем-л.)* use *(smth.)*; умéть ~ся с инструмéнтом know* how to hándle tools; осторóжно обращáйтесь с огнём! take no risks with fire!; 5. *тк. несов. (находиться в употреблении)* círculate.

обращéни|е *с. (к дт.; призыв)* appéal (to); addréss (to); *(в письме)* form of addréss; 2. *(с тв.; по-*

стýпки по отношéнию к *кому-л.)* tréatment (of); плохóe ~ с *кем-л.* ill-tréatment of *smb.*; жестóкое ~ с *кем-л.* crúelty to *smb.*; 3. *(с тв.; пользование чем-л.)* hándling (of); неосторóжное ~ с огнём cárelessness with fire, cáreless hándling of fire; 4. *(употребление)* use; circulátion *(тж. эк.)*; изъя́ть что-л. из ~я prohíbit the use of *smth.*; товáрное ~ commódity circulátion; 5. *грам.* form of addréss.

обрéз *м.* 1. *(у книги)* edge; с золоты́м ~ом gílt-édged; 2. *(оружие)* sáwn-óff rifle; ◇ в ~ véry short; дéнег в ~ móney is véry short; врéмени в ~ time is véry short.

обрезáть, **обрéзать** *(вн.)* 1. cut* *(smth.)*, clip *(smth.)*; *(деревья)* prune *(smth.)*, trim *(smth.)*; 2. *(ранить)* cut* *(smth.)*; обрéзать пáлец cut* *one's* finger; л. *разг. (обрывать кого-л.)* cut* *(smb.)* short; ◇ обрéзать кры́лья *кому-л.* clip *smb.'s* wings.

обрéзаться *сов. разг.* cut* onesélf; ~ оскóлком стеклá cut* onesélf on a piece of glass.

обрекáть, **обрéчь** *(вн. на вн.)* doom *(smb., smth.* to), condémn *(smb., smth.* to); обрéчь что-л. на провáл doom *smth.* to failure.

обремен|ённый *(тв.)* lóaded (with), búrdened (with); *перен. тж.* encúmbered (with). ~ительный ónerous, búrdensome.

обременéть *сов. см.* обременя́ть.

обременя́ть, **обремени́ть** *(вн. тв.)* búrden *(smb.* with); чрезмéрно ~ *кого-л.* overbúrden *smb.*

обрести́ *сов. см.* обретáть.

обретáть, **обрести́** *(вн.)* find* *(smth.)*; обрести́ счáстье find* háppiness.

обречённ|ость *ж.*: чýвство ~ости sense of doom. ~ый doomed; он был ~ым человéком he was a doomed man*.

обрéчь *сов. см.* обрекáть.

обрисовáть(ся) *сов. см.* обрисóвывать(ся).

обрисóвывать, **обрисовáть** *(вн.)* 1. *(очерчивать)* péncil in *(smth.)*; *(чернилами)* ink in *(smth.)*; 2. *(облегать — об одежде)* fit *(smth.)*; плáтье хорошó обрисóвывает её фигýру the dress gives her a good figure; 3. *(описывать, характеризовать)* óutline *(smth.)*, descríbe *(smth.)*; ~ своё положéние descríbe the position *one* is in. ~ся, обрисовáться 1. be* óutlined, take* shape; вдали́ обрисовáлись гóры the óutlines of móuntains could be seen in the dístance; 2. *(выявляться)* becóme* clear, take* clear shape; я́сно обрисовáлись задáчи поéздки the aims of the jóurney took clear shape.

обри́ть *сов. (вн.)* shave* *(smth.)* off. ~ся *сов.* have* *one's* head shaved.

оброни́ть *сов. (вн.)* 1. drop (and lose*) *(smth.)*; 2. *(сказать небрежно)* let* fall *(smth.)*; ~ замечáние let* fall a remárk.

обрубáть, **обруби́ть** *(вн.)* chop the end off *(smth.)*, lop (off) *(smth.)*; ~ сýчья lop off the bránches.

обруби́ть *сов. см.* обрубáть.

обрýбок *м.* 1. *(отрубленная часть чего-л.)* log; 2. *(обрубленный кусок чего-л.)* stump.

обругáть *сов. (вн.)* swear* (at); call *(smb.)* names; *(раскритиковать в печати)* críticize *(smth., smth.)*, attáck *(smb., smth.)*.

обрусé|вший *прил.* Rússified.

обрусéть *сов.* becóme* Rússified.

óбруч *м.* hoop; *(для волос)* band.

обручáльн|ый wédding *attr.*; ~ое кольцó wédding-ring.

обруч|áть, **обручи́ть** *(вн.)* betróth *(smb.)*. ~áться, обручи́ться *(с тв.)* be* engáged/betróthed (to). ~éние *с.* betróthal. ~и́ть(ся) *сов. см.* обручáть(ся).

обрýш|ивать, **обрýшить** 1. *(вн.)* bring* *(smth.)* down; 2. *вн. на вн.; с силой направлять)* hurl *(smth.* at); ~ удáр на врагá bring* crúshing force to bear on the énemy. ~иться *сов.* 1. fall* in, collápse; (*тяжело упасть*) crash down; *перен.* (*о несчастье*) descénd on; дом ~ился the house collápsed; 2. (на *вн.*; *стремительно напасть*) fall* (up)ón (*smb.*), swoop on (*smb.*); (*наброситься с упрёками и т. п.*) attáck (*smb.*), set* (upón).

обры́в *м.* précipice; (*на берегу*) bluff, cliff.

обрыва́ть, **оборва́ть** (*вн.*) 1. tear* (*smth.*) off; (*верёвку и т. п.*) break* (*smth.*); (*цветы, плоды*) pick (*smth.*); 2. (*резко прекращать*) break* off (*smth.*); оборва́ть разгово́р на полусло́ве break* off in the míddle of *one's* séntence; 3. *разг.* (*заставлять замолчать*) cut* (*smb.*) short. ~ся, оборва́ться 1. (*о верёвке и т. п.*) break* (*smth.*); 2. (*внезапно прекращаться*) break* off; разгово́р оборва́лся the convérsation came súddenly to an end; 3. (*падать откуда-л.*) lose* one's grip.

обры́вистый 1. (*крутой, отвесный*) steep, precípitous, abrúpt; 2. (*прерывающийся*) disjóinted, disconnécted.

обры́в|ок *м.* scrap; (*материи тж.*) shred; ~ верёвки bit/end of string; ~ки фраз scraps of convérsation; bróken phráses; ~ки мы́слей stray thoughts; ~ки пе́сни snátches of song; ~ки све́дений scraps of knówledge.

обры́вочный disjóinted, scráppy.

обры́згать(ся) *сов. см.* обры́згивать(ся).

обры́згивать, **обры́згать** (*вн. тв.*) splash (*smth.* óver); обры́згать что-л. духа́ми sprínkle scent óver *smth.*, обры́згаться (*тв.*) get* splashed (with).

обрю́зг|лый flábby, fláccid, blóated. ~нуть *сов.* get* flábby. ~ший *см.* обрю́зглый.

обря́д *м.* rite, rítual.

обсади́ть *сов. см.* обса́живать.

обса́живать, **обсади́ть** (*вн. тв.*) plant (*smth.* with).

обса́сывать, **обсоса́ть** (*вн.*) suck (*smth.*).

обсервато́рия *ж.* obsérvatory.

обскака́ть *сов.* (*вн.*) 1. (*кругом*) gállop round (*smth.*); 2. (*обогнать*) pass (*smb.*) at a gállop; *перен.* outdó* (*smb.*).

обсле́дование *с.* inspéction; investigátion; ~ путём опро́са opínion pólling; лечь в больни́цу на ~ go* ínto hóspital for a chéck-up.

обсле́довать *несов. и сов.* (*вн.*) inspéct (*smb.*, *smth.*); (*исследовать*) invéstigate (*smth.*), inquíre (ínto).

обслу́живани|е *с.* sérvice, atténdance; техни́ческое ~ sérvicing; медици́нское ~ населе́ния públic médical/health sérvice; médical atténdance for the populátion.

обслу́жив|ать, **обслужи́ть** (*вн.*) 1. serve (*smb.*); (*за столом тж.*) wait on (*smb.*); ~ покупа́теля serve a cústomer, atténd to a cústomer; 2. (*машину, станок*) óperate (*smth.*), hándle (*smth.*), tend (*smth.*); ~ одновре́менно не́сколько станко́в óperate séveral lathes simultáneously. ~ающий óperating; ~ающий персона́л (óperating) staff.

обслужи́ть *сов. см.* обслу́живать.

обсоса́ть *сов. см.* обса́сывать.

обсо́хнуть *сов. см.* обсыха́ть.

обста́вить(ся) *сов. см.* обставля́ть(ся).

обставля́ть, **обста́вить** 1. (*вн. тв.*; *окружать*) surróund (*smth.* with), encírcle (*smth.* with); 2. (*вн.*; *меблировать*) fúrnish (*smth.*); обста́вить кварти́ру fúrnish a flat; 3. (*вн.*; *устраивать*) arránge (*smth.*); 4. (*вн.*) *разг.* (*обманывать*) cheat (*smb.*); 5. (*вн.*) *разг.* (*обгонять*) get* ahéad (of). ~ся, обста́виться *разг.* 1. (*тв.*; *окружать себя*) be* surróunded (by); 2. (*обставлять жилище мебелью*) fit *one*sélf out; он о́чень хорошо́ обста́вился he's made his place very nice.

обстано́вк|а *ж.* 1. (*комнаты и т. п.*) fúrniture; *театр.* set, sétting; 2. (*положение*) situátion, átmosphere; sét-up *разг.*; де́ти живу́т в здоро́вой ~е the chíldren live in a héalthy átmosphere; междунаро́дная ~ internátional situátion; торже́ственная ~ impréssive átmosphere/sétting.

обстоя́тельный 1. (*подробный*) détailed, circumstántial; ~ отве́т détailed replý; 2. *разг.* (*о человеке*) thórough.

обстоя́тельств|о *с.* 1. (*событие, факт*) círcumstance; все ~а де́ла all the facts of the case; вы́яснить все ~а де́ла find* out all abóut a case; то ~, что... the fact that...; 2. *мн.* (*условия, обстановка*) círcumstances; при таки́х ~ах únder the círcumstances; при други́х ~ах únder any óther círcumstances; при всех ~ах all things consídered; ни при каки́х ~ах я не приду́ únder no círcumstances will I come; по незави́сящим от кого-л. ~ствам ówing to círcumstances óutside *one's* contról; 3. *грам.* advérbial módifier; ~ вре́мени, ме́ста, о́браза де́йствия advérbial módifier of time, place, mánner; ◇ смотря́ по ~ам accórding to círcumstances; (*как ответ*) it all depénds.

обсто|я́ть *несов.*: как ~и́т де́ло? how are things góing?; всё ~и́т благополу́чно all's well, éverything is all right; де́ло ~и́т так... it's like this...

обстра́иваться, **обстро́иться** *разг.* 1. (*строить для себя жильё*) build* a house for *one*sélf; 2. (*застраиваться*) acquíre new búildings.

обстре́л *м.* fire; артиллери́йский ~ artíllery bombárdment; попа́сть под ~ (*прям. и перен.*) come* únder fire.

обстре́ливать, **обстреля́ть** (*вн.*) fire (on); (*из орудий тж.*) shell (*smb.*, *smth.*); ~ кого-л. из пулемётов machine-gun *smb.*

обстре́лянный báttle-hárdened; ~ солда́т báttle-hárdened sóldier; ~ полк régiment with expérience of báttle.

обстреля́ть *сов. см.* обстре́ливать.

обстрога́ть *сов.* (*вн.*) plane (*smth.*); (*заострить*) whittle (*smth.*).

обстро́иться *сов. см.* обстра́иваться.

обстру́кц|ия *ж.* obstrúction; *полит. тж.* fílibuster; устро́ить кому-л. ~ию obstrúct *smb.*

обступа́ть, **обступи́ть** (*вн.*) crowd round (*smb.*, *smth.*), clúster round (*smb.*, *smth.*).

обступи́ть *сов. см.* обступа́ть.

обсуди́ть *сов. см.* обсужда́ть.

обсужд|а́ть, **обсуди́ть** (*вн.*) discúss (*smth.*), debáte (*smth.*). ~е́ние *с.* discússion; предложи́ть что-л. на ~е́ние put* *smth.* fórward for discússion; приня́ть уча́стие в ~е́нии take* part in a discússion.

обсуши́ть *сов.* (*вн.*) dry (*smth.*). ~ся *сов.* get* dry.

обсчита́ть(ся) *сов. см.* обсчи́тывать(ся).

обсчи́тывать, **обсчита́ть** (*вн.*) cheat (*smb.*). ~ся, обсчита́ться make* a mistáke in calculátion.

обсы́пать *сов. см.* обсыпа́ть.

обсыпа́ть, **обсы́пать** (*вн. тв.*) sprínkle (*smth.* with), pówder (*smth.* with), dust (*smth.* with).

обсыха́ть, **обсо́хнуть** dry off.

обта́чивать, **обточи́ть** (*вн.*) (*на токарном станке*) turn (*smth.*); (*на точильном камне*) grind* (*smth.*), smooth.

обтека́ем|ый stréamlined; *ав. тж.* aerodynámic(al); *перен. разг.* evásive, glib; придава́ть чему-л. ~ую фо́рму stréamline *smth.*; ~ отве́т evásive replý.

обтека́ть, **обте́чь** (*вн.*) flow round (*smth.*); *перен.* býpass (*smth.*).

обтере́ть(ся) *сов. см.* обтира́ть(ся).

обтеса́ть *сов. см.* обтёсывать.

обтёсывать, **обтеса́ть** (*вн.*) trim (*smth.*), róugh-héw (*smth.*); *перен.* lick (*smb.*) ínto shape.

обте́чь *сов. см.* обтека́ть.

обтира́ни|е *с.* rúbdown, spónge-down; холо́дные ~я cold sponge bath.

обтира́ть, **обтере́ть** (*вн.*) wipe (*smth.*), wipe (*smth.*) dry. ~ся, обтере́ться (*вытираться*) rub *one*sélf down; ~ся холо́дной водо́й have* a cold spónge-down/sponge bath.

обточи́ть *сов. см.* обта́чивать.

обто́чка *ж.* túrning, grínding.

обтрёпанный shábby; (*о человеке тж.*) shábbily dressed.

обтрепа́ть *сов.* (*вн.*) wear* (*smth.*) out; ~ рукава́ fray *one's* sleeves. ~ся *сов.* fray, be* frayed, rável.

обтя́гивать, обтяну́ть (*вн.*) 1. cóver (*smth.*); 2. (*прилегать — об одежде*) sheathe (*smth.*). ~ся, обтяну́ться 1. (*покрываться чем-л.*) becóme* cóvered/cóated/sheathed; 2. (*о лице*) becóme* drawn.

обтя́жк|а *ж.:* пла́тье в ~у skín-tight/clóse-fitting dress.

обтяну́ть(ся) *сов. см.* обтя́гивать(ся).

обув|а́ть, обу́ть (*вн.*) 1. put* *smth.'s* shoes on (for him, her); обу́ть ребёнка put* a child's shoes on for him; 2. *разг.* (*снабжать обувью*) províde (*smb.*) with shoes/boots. ~а́ться, обу́ться put* *one's* boots/shoes on. ~но́й shoe *attr.;* ~но́й магази́н shoe shop; ~на́я промы́шленность shóe-manufacturing (índustry).

о́бувь *ж.* fóotwear; boots and shoes *pl;* ко́жаная ~ léather fóotwear; ле́тняя ~ súmmer shoes; изя́щная ~ élegant shoes; спорти́вная ~ sports fóotwear; носи́ть хоро́шую ~ wear* good shoes.

обу́гленный charred.

обу́гливаться, обу́глиться char, becóme* charred.

обу́глиться *сов. см.* обу́гливаться.

обу́живать, обу́зить (*вн.*) make* (*smth.*) too tight; обу́зить пла́тье make* a dress too tight.

обу́з|а *ж.* búrden, encúmbrance; быть ~ой для кого́-л. be* a búrden on/to *smb.*

обу́здать *сов. см.* обу́здывать.

обу́здывать, обузда́ть (*вн.; прям. и перен.*) curb (*smb., smth.*); обузда́ть агре́ссоров curb the aggréssors.

обу́зить *сов. см.* обу́живать.

обусло́вить(ся) *сов. см.* обусло́вливать(ся).

обусло́вливать, обусло́вить 1. (*вн. тв.; ограничивать каким-л. условием*) make* (*smth.*) depéndent (on), límit (*smth.* by), stípulate (*smth.* in, by); 2. (*вн.; вызывать что-л.*) bring* abóut (*smth.*), cause (*smth.*). ~ся, обусло́виться (*тв.*) be* condítioned (by), depénd (on).

обу́тый with (*one's*) shoes on *после сущ.;* (*обеспеченный обувью*) províded with shoes *после сущ.*

обу́ть(ся) *сов. см.* обува́ть(ся).

о́бух *м.* blunt side, butt; ◇ как ~ом по голове́ ≈ like a bolt from the blue.

обуч|а́ть, обучи́ть (*вн. дт.*) teach* (*smb. smth.*), instrúct (*smb.* in). ~а́ться, обучи́ться 1. (*дт., + инф.*) learn* (*smth., + to inf*); ~а́ться стрельбе́ be* léarning to shoot; 2. *тк. несов.* (*получать образование где-л.*) stúdy, be* éducated. ~е́ние *с.* instrúction, educátion; ~е́ние гра́моте instrúction in réading and wríting.

обучи́ть *сов. см.* обуча́ть. ~ся *сов. см.* обуча́ться 1.

обуя́|ть *сов.* (*вн.*) seize (*smb.*); его́ ~л страх he was seized with térror.

обха́живать *несов.* (*вн.*) *разг.* make* up (to); cúltivate (*smb.*).

обхва́т *м.* full stretch (of the arms); (*толщина ствола дерева*) girth, circúmference; де́рево в три ~а tree of great girth.

обхвати́ть *сов. см.* обхва́тывать.

обхва́тывать, обхвати́ть (*вн.*) clasp (*smb., smth.*), put* *one's* arm(s) round (*smb., smth.*).

обхо́д *м.* 1. (*для осмотра*) rounds *pl;* соверша́ть ~ go*/make* *one's* rounds; 2. (*кружный путь*) détour; 3. *воен.* túrning móvement, wide envélopment; ◇ в ~ 1) (*обходя стороной*) skírting; 2) (*уклоняясь от соблюдения чего-л.*) by evásion.

обходи́тельный cóurteous, áffable, urbáne.

обходи́ть, обойти́ (*вн.*) 1. (*проходить вокруг чего́-л.*) go* round (*smth.*), walk round (*smth.*); он обошёл дом he walked round the house; 2. *воен.* outflánk (*smb.,*

smth.); обойти́ проти́вника с фла́нга turn the énemy's flank; 3. (*проходить стороной, огибать*) avóid (*smth.*), go* round (*smth.*), skirt (*smth.*); *перен.* (*не затрагивать кого-л.*) pass óver (*smb.*); обойти́ лу́жу go* round a púddle; сча́стье вас не обойдёт háppiness will not pass you by; 4. (*избегать*) avóid (*smth.*); get* round (*smth.*); pass (*smth.*) óver; обойти́ вопро́с pass óver a quéstion, eváde the íssue; 5. (*уклоняться от исполнения чего-л.*) eváde (*smth.*); 6. (*оставлять без повышения*) pass (*smb.*) óver; 7. (*проходить по всему простра́нству*) go* all óver (*smth.*), go* all round (*smth.*); обойти́ весь сад go* all round the gárden; обойти́ все ко́мнаты go* into évery room, go* from room to room; 8. *разг.* (*обгонять*) pass (*smb., smth.*), outpáce (*smb., smth.*); *перен.* outdó* (*smb.*); 9. *разг.* (*обманывать*) take* (*smb.*) in, diddle (*smb.*).

обходи́ться, обойти́сь 1. (*с тв.; обращаться с*) treat (*smb.*); 2. *разг.* (*стоить*) cost*, come* to; ~ недо́рого not cost much; ~ сли́шком до́рого be* too expénsive; во ско́лько э́то обойдётся? how much will it come to?; э́то до́рого вам обойдётся that will cost you a lot of móney; *перен.* you'll pay déarly for that; 3. (*тв.*) *разг.* (*удовлетворяться чем-л.*) mánage (with); (*без рд.; довольствоваться*) do* withóut (*smth.*); отли́чно ~ без чего́-л. do* véry well withóut *smth.*; ~ без чье́й-л. по́мощи, услу́г dispénse with *smb.'s* assístance, sérvices; 4. (*благополучно заканчиваться*): всё обошло́сь благополу́чно éverything turned out all right; ка́к-нибудь обойдётся one way or anóther things will séttle themsélves.

обходно́й, обхо́дный 1. (*кружный*) róundabout (*тж. перен.*); обхо́дный путь róundabout way; 2. *воен.* túrning, outflánking; ◇ обходно́й лист cléarance chit.

обхожде́ние *с.* (*с тв.*) tréatment (of).

обша́ривать, обша́рить (*вн.*) *разг.* ránsack (*smth.*).

обша́рить *сов. см.* обша́ривать.

обшива́ть, обши́ть 1. (*вн. тв.; отделывать*) trim (*smth, with*); (*зашивать во что-л.*) sew* (*smth.*) up (in); обши́ть воротни́к ка́нтом bind* a cóllar; обши́ть посы́лку холсто́м sew* up a párcel in cánvas; 2. (*вн. тв.; покрывать, обтягивать*) cóver (*smth.* with), case (*smth.* in); ~ что-л. доска́ми lag *smth.* with boards; 3. (*вн.*) *разг.* (*шить одежду для кого-л.*) make* clothes (for); она́ обшива́ет всю семью́ she makes clothes for the whole fámily.

обши́вка *ж.* 1. (*отделка*) trímmings *pl;* 2. (*покрытие*) cásing, shéathing; (*досками, войлоком*) lágging.

обши́рн|ый vast, enórmous; ~ое простра́нство enórmous área; ~ые знако́мства vast círcle of acquáintances; ~ые зна́ния vast knówledge *sg.*

обши́тый 1. (*отделанный*) trimmed; 2. (*покрытый*) cased, encásed; ~ бронёй ármour-plated; ~ асбе́стом asbéstos-sheathed; ~ ме́дью cópper-sheathed.

обши́ть *сов. см.* обшива́ть.

обшла́г *м.* cuff.

обща́ться *несов.* (*с тв.*) assóciate (with), be* assóciated (with).

общегородско́й town *attr.;* city *attr.*

общегосуда́рственн|ый nátion-wide, nátional; ~ые интере́сы interests of the whole country, interests of the country at large.

общедосту́пн|ый 1. génerally aváilable; (*недорогой*) móderate, pópular; по ~ым це́нам at pópular príces; 2. (*понятный*) pópular, génerally comprehénsible.

общежи́т|ие *с.* 1. (*помещение*) hóstel; жить в ~ии live in a hóstel; 2. (*общественный быт*) society; commúnity/sócial life; (*повседневная жизнь*) éveryday life.

общеизве́стный well-knówn; of cómmon/públic knówledge.

общенаро́дн|ый nátional; of the whole péople *после сущ.;* ~ое достоя́ние the próperty of the whole péople.

общенациона́льн|ый nátional; ~ые зада́чи nátional próblems, tasks invólving the whole nátion.

обще́ние с. íntercourse; déalings pl, cóntacts pl; ~ с людьми́ cóntact/míxing with péople.

.общеобразова́тельн|ый of géneral educátion после сущ.; ~ые предме́ты géneral súbjects.

общепи́т м. (обще́ственное пита́ние) públic cátering.

общепри́знанный génerally acknówledged, univérsally récognized.

общепри́нят|ый (génerally) accépted; в ~ом смы́сле сло́ва in the accépted sense of the term.

обще́ственник м. sócially áctive pérson.

обще́ственност|ь ж. собир. 1. (передовая часть общества) the públic; мне́ние ~и públic opínion; театра́льная ~ the theátrical world; нау́чная ~ the scientífic world; 2. (общественные организации) sócial organizátions pl, sócially áctive mémbers pl.

обще́ственн|ый 1. (относящийся к обществу) sócial; of society после сущ.; (протекающий, возникающий в обществе тж.) públic; ~ строй sócial órder/sýstem; зако́ны ~ого разви́тия laws of sócial devélopment; ~ые отноше́ния sócial relátions; ~ая жизнь sócial/públic life; (в философии и т. п.) the life of society; ~ые интере́сы sócial ínterests; ~ долг públic dúty, dúty to the commúnity; ~ое положе́ние sócial státus; опро́с ~ого мне́ния públic opínion poll; ~ые нау́ки sócial sciences; ~ де́ятель públic fígure, cívic léader; 2. (связанный с обслуживанием нужд коллектива) sócial; vóluntary; for the commúnity после сущ.; ~ые организа́ции sócial organizátions; вести́ ~ую рабо́ту do* work for the commúnity; ~ое поруче́ние sócial assígnment; 3. (принадлежащий обществу) públic, sócialized; ~ые фо́нды públic funds; ~ая со́бственность públic ównership; ~ое иму́щество públic próperty; 4. разг. (любящий общество) sóciable, gregárious; ◇ ~ обвини́тель prósecutor (representing a trade union organization, etc.); ~ое порица́ние públic réprimand; на ~ых нача́лах as a sócial/públic sérvice; ~ое пита́ние públic cátering.

обществ|о с. 1. society; интере́сы ~a the ínterests of society; 2. (окружение) sócial círcle(s); 3. (компания) cómpany; в ~е свои́х друзе́й in the cómpany of one's friends; 4. (организация) society; cómpany; спорти́вное ~ sports society; ~ с ограни́ченной отве́тственностью límited liabílity cómpany (Ltd).

обществове́дение с. sócial science.

общеупотреби́тельный in géneral use predic., wídely used.

общечелове́ческий húman; cómmon to humánity после сущ.

о́бщ|ий 1. géneral; ~ее пра́вило géneral rule; ~ вид géneral view; в ~их слова́х in óutline, in géneral terms; в ~их черта́х in broad óutline; ~ее впечатле́ние géneral impréssion; ~ее мне́ние géneral opínion; ~ее бла́го géneral good; 2. (совместный; сходный) cómmon; in cómmon после сущ.; ~ие интере́сы ínterests in cómmon; ~ее де́ло cómmon cause; ~ими си́лами, ~ими уси́лиями by combíned éfforts; ~ие знако́мые friends in cómmon; оди́н из на́ших ~их знако́мых a friend of ours; наш ~ друг our mútual friend; 3. (весь, целый) tótal, óverall, ággregate; ~ая су́мма sum tótal, tótal (amount); ◇ ~ее собра́ние géneral méeting; в ~ей сло́жности altogéther; ~ее ме́сто cómmonplace, plátitude; в ~ем, в ~ем и це́лом on the whole; мно́го ~его much in cómmon; э́то не име́ет ничего́ ~его с кем-л., чем-л. it has no connéction with smb., smth.; найти́ ~ язы́к learn* to understánd one anóther, find* cómmon ground; на ~их основа́ниях on the same básis as éveryone else, in accórdance with the géneral práctice.

общи́на ж. commúnity, cómmune.

общи́нный cómmon, commúnal.

общипа́ть сов. см. общи́пывать.

общи́пывать, общипа́ть (вн.) pluck (smth.); общипа́ть гу́ся pluck a goose*.

общи́тельн|ость ж. sociabílity. ~ый sóciable; ~ый челове́к sóciable pérson.

о́бщность ж. commúnity, communálity; ~ интере́сов commúnity of ínterests; ~ взгля́дов cómmon óutlook; ~ зада́ч commúnity of aim.

объеда́ть, объе́сть (вн.) разг. (быть в тягость) eat* (smb.) out of house and home. ~ся, объе́сться overéat* (onesélf); eat* too much; ~ся чем-л. have* one's fill of smth.

объедин|е́ние с. 1. (действие) unificátion, consolidátion; (ресурсов и т. п.) póoling; 2. (союз) associátion; ~ предпринима́телей emplóyers' association. ~ённый 1. uníted, amálgamated; 2. (совместный) joint; ~ённое заседа́ние joint séssion. ~и́ть(ся) сов. см. объединя́ть(ся).

объединя́ть, объедини́ть (вн.) uníte (smb., smth.); (предприятия и т. п.) amálgamate (smth.); объедини́ть си́лы ми́ра uníte/consólidate the fórces of peace. ~ся, объедини́ться uníte, be* consólidated; (о предприятиях и т. п.) be* amálgamated.

объе́дки мн. (ед. объе́док м.) разг. léavings, léft-overs, scraps.

объе́зд м. 1. (действие) góing/ríding/dríving round; détour (с целью посещения, доставки) round; 2. (место) divérsion.

объе́зд|ить сов. см. объезжа́ть 1, 3. ~но́й 1. (окольный) róundabout attr.; 2. (для охраны) patról(ling). ~чик м. 1. fórest ránger; 2. (лошадей) hórse-breaker.

объезжа́ть, объе́здить, объе́хать (вн.) 1. go* round (smth.), drive* round (smth.); (с целью посещения, доставки) make* the round (of); (путешествуя) tour (smth.), trável all óver (smth.); (верхом) ride* round (smth.); объе́хать всё побере́жье tour the whole coast; 2. сов. объе́хать (проехать стороной) skirt (smth.), go* round (smth.); объе́хать боло́то skirt a bog; 3. сов. объе́здить (лошадь) break* in (smth.).

объе́кт м. 1. óbject; воен. objéctive; ~ изуче́ния óbject of stúdy; 2. (предприятие, стройка и т. п.) installátion, próject.

объекти́в м. lens, objéctive; (в телескопе) óbject-lens.

объективи́зм м. objéctivism.

объекти́вн|ость ж. 1. objéctive náture, objectívity; ~ вне́шнего ми́ра the objéctive náture of the extérnal world; 2. (беспристрастность) impartiálity; ~ сужде́ний impártial réasoning. ~ый 1. objéctive; ~ая действи́тельность objéctive reálity; ~ые причи́ны objéctive cáuses; 2. (беспристрастный) impártial, fair, objéctive; ~ая оце́нка fair/impártial asséssment; ~ый отве́т impártial/únbías(ed) replý.

объём м. vólume; (ёмкость) cúbic capácity; перен. amóunt, scope; ~ ко́мнаты áir-space of a room; ~ рабо́т amóunt/scope of the work. ~истый volúminous, capácious; (большой) búlky. ~ный 1. volumétric; ~ное измере́ние volumétric méasurement; 2. (связанный с передачей трёхмерности предмета) thrée-diménsional, 3-D, stéreo; ~ное изображе́ние thrée-diménsional projéction; 3. текст. high-búlk; ~ная пря́жа high-bulk yarn.

объе́сть(ся) сов. см. объеда́ть(ся).

объе́хать сов. см. объезжа́ть 1, 2.

объяв|и́ть(ся) сов. см. объявля́ть(ся). ~ле́ние с. 1. (действие) declarátion; ~ле́ние войны́ declarátion of war; ~ле́ние реше́ния суда́ pronóuncement of a vérdict; ~ле́ние благода́рности в прика́зе públic acknówledgement (of smb.'s sérvices) in órders of the day; 2. (извещение) annóuncement; (о спросе и предложении, рекламное) advértisement, ad; ádvert; дать ~ле́-

ние в газе́ту put* an ad/advértisement in the páper; переда́ча ~ле́ний по ра́дио bróadcasting of annóuncements/ádverts.

объявля́ть, объяви́ть 1. (вн.; *о пр.; заявля́ть*) decláre (*smth.*); объяви́ть кому́-л. о своём реше́нии tell* *smb.* of *one's* decision; **2.** (вн.; *оглаша́ть*) annóunce (*smth.*); объяви́ть пригово́р pronóunce a vérdict; объяви́ть прика́з íssue an órder; **3.** (вн.; *официа́льно устана́вливать, заявля́ть*) decláre (*smth.*); ~ войну́ кому́-л. decláre war on *smb.*; ~ подпи́ску на газе́ты annóunce néwspaper subscríption dates; **4.** (вн. тв.; *официа́льно признава́ть кем-л., чем-л.*) decláre (*smb. smth., smth. smth.*); объяви́ть собра́ние закры́тым decláre a méeting closed; ~ кого́-л. кем-л. procláim *one*sélf *smb.* ~ся, объяви́ться *разг.* show* up.

объясне́ние с. explanátion; (*разгово́р*) discússion; háving things out; ◇ ~ в любви́ declarátion of love.

объясни́мый éxplicable.

объясни́тельный explánatory; ~ая запи́ска explánatory note, note of explanátion.

объясн|я́ть, объясни́ть 1. (вн.) expláin (*smth.*), make* (*smth.*) clear; объясни́ть кому́-л. зада́ние expláin a task/job to *smb.*; **2.** (вн. тв.; *устана́вливать причи́ну*) attríbute (to); put* (down to) *разг.*; чем вы ~я́ете то, что... how do you accóunt for (the fact that)..?; как объясни́ть его́ поведе́ние? what is the explanátion of his beháviour? ~я́ться, объясни́ться **1.** (с тв.; *ула́живать недоразуме́ния*) have* it out (with); **2.** (*выясня́ться*) becóme* clear, be* accóunted for; **3.** тк. несов. (*разгова́ривать, бесе́довать*) convérse; ~я́ться по-англи́йски и т. п. make* *one*sélf understóod in Énglish, *etc.*; **4.** тк. несов. (тв.; *находи́ть себе́ объясне́ние в чём-л.*) be* due (to); ◇ объясни́ться кому́-л. в любви́ decláre *one's* love to *smb.*

объя́ти|е с. embráce; заключи́ть кого́-л. в свои́ ~я throw* *one's* arms round *smb.*, hug *smb.*; ◇ приня́ть, встре́тить кого́-л. с распростёртыми ~ями recéive *smb.* with ópen arms.

объя́ть сов. (вн.) **1.** seize (*smth.*); **2.** (*поня́ть*) grasp (*smth.*).

обыва́тель м. Phílistine. ~ский Phílistine, pétty, nárrow; ~ское рассужде́ние nárrow-mínded árguments *pl*; ~ская то́чка зре́ния nárrow óutlook.

обыгра́ть сов. см. обы́грывать.

обы́грывать, обыгра́ть (вн.) **1.** (*одержа́ть верх в игре́*) beat* (*smth.*); обыгра́ть кого́-л. в ша́хматы beat* *smb.* at chess; обыгра́ть кого́-л. на кру́пную су́мму win* a large sum of móney from *smb.*; **2.** *теа́тр.* use (*smth.*) to the best effect; **3.** *разг.* (*испо́льзовать в свои́х це́лях*) take* advántage (of), play up (*smth.*).

обы́денн|ый éveryday; ~ое явле́ние éveryday occúrrence.

обыкнове́н|ие с. hábit, cústom; име́ть ~ де́лать что-л. be* in the hábit of dóing *smth.*; be* wont to do *smth.*; ◇ по ~ию, по своему́ ~ию as úsual; про́тив ~ия cóntrary to cústom.

обыкнове́нн|о úsually; как ~ as úsual. ~ый **1.** (*постоя́нно встреча́ющийся*) úsual; **2.** (*ниче́м не примеча́тельный*) órdinary.

обы́ск м. search; произвести́ ~ make* a search.

обыска́ть сов. см. обы́скивать.

обы́скивать, обыска́ть (вн.) search (*smb., smth.*); (*помеще́ние, предме́ты тж.*) go* through (*smth.*); (*тк. помеще́ние*) raid (*smth.*).

обы́чай м. cústom; (*привы́чка тж.*) hábit.

обы́чн|о úsually. ~ый **1.** (*постоя́нный, привы́чный*) úsual, cústomary; **2.** (*ниче́м не примеча́тельный*) órdinary; ~ое явле́ние órdinary/úsual thing; ◇ ~ые вооруже́ния convéntional ármaments *pl*.

обя́занн|ость ж. **1.** dúty, responsibílity; счита́ть

своей ~остью... consíder it *one's* dúty/responsibílity...; **2.** *мн.* dúties; work *sg*; исполня́ть ~ости кого́-л. **1)** work as *smb.*, do* the work of *smb.*; **2)** (*заменя́ть*) act for *smb.*; исполня́ющий ~ости дире́ктора ácting diréctor.

обя́зан|ный 1. (+ *инф.*) oblíged (+ to *inf*); bound (+ to *inf*); вы ~ы сде́лать э́то you are bound to do it; **2.** (*дт.*) indébted (to); я мно́гим ему́ обя́зан I am much indébted to him; э́тим я обя́зан вам I have you to thank for this.

обяза́тельн|о withóut fail; приходи́те ~! be sure to come!; он ~ придёт he will come withóut fail; не ~ not nécessarily. ~ый **1.** compúlsory, oblígatory; (*неизме́нный*) inévitable; ~ое усло́вие oblígatory condítion; ~ое обуче́ние compúlsory educátion; в ~ом поря́дке withóut fail; **2.** (*услу́жливый*) oblíging.

обяза́тельство с. **1.** obligátion, undertáking; commítment; дать ~ give* an undertáking; взять на себя́ ~ сде́лать что-л. undertáke* to do *smth.*, commít *one*sélf to do *smth.*; вы́полнить своё ~ meet* *one's* obligátion/commítments, fulfíl *one's* pledge; **2.** эк. liabílity.

обяза́ть сов. см. обя́зывать 1, 3. ~ся сов. см. обя́зываться 1.

обя́зыв|ать, обяза́ть (вн.) **1.** (*заставля́ть*) charge (*smb.*), make* (*smb.*); **2.** тк. несов. (*налага́ть изве́стные обя́занности*) bind* (*smb.*), make* it incúmbent (upón); положе́ние ~ает noblésse oblíge; э́то вас ни к чему́ не ~ает this does not bind you in any way; его́ дове́рие нас ко мно́гому ~ает his cónfidence impóses a deep obligátion upón us; **3.** (*ока́зывать услу́гу*) oblíge (*smb.*); вы меня́ о́чень обя́жете you will gréatly oblíge me. ~я́ться, обяза́ться **1.** (+ *инф.*) undertáke* (+ to *inf*); commít *one*sélf (+ to *inf*); **2.** тк. несов. (*дт., пе́ред*; *станови́ться обя́занным кому́-л.*) be* behólden (to).

обя́зывающ|ий письма, слова́ и т. п., ни к чему́ его́ не ~ие létters, words, *etc.* that commít him to nóthing, non-commítal létters, words, *etc.*

ова́л óval; ~ лица́ shape of the face.

ова́льный óval.

ова́ц|ия ж. ovátion; устро́ить ~ию кому́-л. give* *smb.* an ovátion; до́лго не смолка́ющая ~ prolónged appláuse.

овдове́вший wídowed.

овдове́ть сов. (*о мужчи́не*) becóme* a wídower; (*о же́нщине*) becóme* a wídow, be* left a wídow.

овёс м. oats *pl*.

ове́ч|ий sheep's. ~ка ж. lamb.

овеществи́ть сов. см. овеществля́ть.

овеществля́ть, овеществи́ть книжн. (вн.) matérialize (*smth.*), réify (*smth.*).

овладева́ть, овладе́ть (тв.) **1.** (*захва́тывать*) seize (*smth.*), cápture (*smth.*), take* (*smth.*); овладе́ть го́родом cápture a town; **2.** (*подчиня́ть себе́*) seize (*smb., smth.*), grip (*smb., smth.*), take* hold (of); овладе́ть внима́нием слу́шателей take* hold of the áudience; овладе́ть разгово́ром take* óver the conversátion; **3.** (*о мы́слях, чу́вствах*) seize (*smb.*), overcóme* (*smb.*); мно́ю овладе́л страх I was overcóme with térror, fear grípped me; им овладе́ло беспоко́йство he was overcóme with anxíety; **4.** (*усва́ивать*) máster (*smth.*); овладе́ть зна́ниями acquíre knówledge; овладе́ть но́вой профе́ссией máster a new trade; ◇ овладе́ть собо́й contról *one*sélf, éxercise self-contról.

овладе́ние с. **1.** (*захва́т*) séizure, cápture; **2.** (*усвое́ние*) mástering; ~ зна́ниями acquíring knówledge.

овладе́ть сов. см. овладева́ть.

о́вод м. gád-fly.

овощево́д м. végetable grówer. ~ство с. végetable grówing. ~ческий végetable-grówing.

овощехрани́лище с. végetable-stórage céllar/shed.

о́вощ|и *мн.* (*ед.* о́вощ м.) végetables. ~но́й végetable; ~ны́е культу́ры végetable crops; ~но́й магази́н gréengrocer's/végetable shop; ~ные консéрвы tinned végetables.

овра́г *м.* ravíne, gúlly.

овся́нка I *ж.* 1. (*крупа*) óatmeal; 2. (*каша*) (óatmeal) pórridge.

овся́нка II *ж.* (*птица*) búnting.

овся́н|**ой** *attr.* ~ое по́ле óatfield.

овся́н|**ый** óatmeal *attr.*; ~ая ка́ша (óatmeal) pórridge; ~ая крупа́ óatmeal.

овца́ *ж.* sheep*.

овцево́д *м.* shéep-breeder. ~ство *с.* shéep-breeding. ~ческий sheep *attr.*, shéep-breeding *attr.*

овча́рка *ж.* shéep-dog; неме́цкая, восточноевропе́йская ~ Alsátian.

овча́рня *ж.* shéep-fold.

овчи́н|**а** *ж.* shéepskin. ~ка: ~ка вы́делки не стóит ≈ the game is not worth the cándle; нéбо с ~ку показа́лось *кому́-л.* smb. saw stars. ~ный shéepskin *attr.*; ~ный тулу́п shéepskin coat.

ога́рок *м.* cándle-end.

огиба́ть, обогну́ть (*вн.*) go* round (*smth.*), skirt (*smth.*); *мор.* dóuble (*smth.*).

оглавле́ние *с.* (table of) cóntents.

огласи́ть(**ся**) *сов. см.* оглаша́ть(ся).

огла́ск|**а** *ж.* publícity; де́ло получи́ло ~у the mátter was made públic; преда́ть *что-л.* ~е make* smth. públic.

оглаша́ть, огласи́ть 1. (*вн.*) (*объявлять*) procláim (*smth.*), annóunce (*smth.*); ~ телегра́мму read* a télegram; огласи́ть прика́з read* out an órder; 2. (*вн. тв.; наполнять звуками*) make* (*smth.*) resóund/ring (with). ~ся, огласи́ться (*тв.*) resóund (with), ring* (with).

оглаше́ни|**е** *с.* proclamátion; ~ пригово́ра pronóuncement of a vérdict; не подлежи́т ~ю not for publicátion/circulátion.

огло́бл|**я** *ж.* shaft; в ~ях in/betwéen the shafts; ◇ поверну́ть ~и ≈ go* awáy (émpty-hánded).

оглохну́ть *сов. см.* глóхнуть 1.

оглуша́ть, оглуши́ть (*вн.*) 1. (*звуком*) déafen (*smb.*); 2. (*ударом и т. п.*) stun (*smb.*); *перен. тж.* stágger (*smb.*).

оглуши́тельный déafening.

оглуши́ть *сов. см.* оглуша́ть.

огляде́ть *сов. см.* огля́дывать. ~ся *сов.* 1. *см.* огля́дываться 2; 2. (*освоиться*) get* one's bearings, séttle down.

огля́дк|**а** *ж.*: с ~ой with cáution; без ~и récklessly; бежа́ть без ~и run* for one's life, bolt.

огля́дывать, огляде́ть, огляну́ть (*вн.*) survéy (*smb., smth.*), glance óver (*smb., smth.*), look óver (*smb., smth.*); glance round (*smth.*), look round (*smth.*); ~ кого́-л. с головы́ до ног exámine smb. from head to foot; огляде́ть мéстность survéy the surróunding cóuntry; огля́деть дом look óver the búilding; огляде́ть кóмнату glance round the room. ~ся, огляде́ться, огляну́ться 1. *сов.* огляну́ться look round; 2. *сов.* огляде́ться look aróund/abóut, take* a glance round one; ◇ не успе́ешь огляну́ться как... before you know where you are...

огляну́ть *сов. см.* огля́дывать. ~ся *сов. см.* огля́дываться 1.

огнев|**о́й** *воен.* fire *attr.*; ~а́я завéса cúrtain fire; ~а́я тóчка wéapon emplácement; ~а́я пози́ция firing position.

огнемёт *м.* fláme-thrower.

о́гненн|**ый** fíery; *перен. тж.* árdent; ~ые глаза́ búrning eyes; ~ взгляд fíery glance; ~ое слóво árdent words *pl.*

огнеопа́сный inflámmable.

огнесто́йкий fire-resístant.

огнестрéльн|**ый**: ~ое ору́жие fire-arm(s); ~ая ра́на gúnshot wound.

огнетуши́тель *м.* fire extínguisher.

огнеупóрн|**ый** fíreproof, refráctory; ~ая гли́на fíre-clay; ~ кирпи́ч fire-brick(s).

огова́ривать, оговори́ть (*вн.*) 1. (*обусловливать*) spécify (*smth.*), stípulate (*smth.*); 2. *разг.* (*клеветать*) slánder (*smb.*). ~ся, оговори́ться 1. (*делать оговорку*) spécify; 2. (*ошибаться*): я оговори́лся ≈ it was a slip of the tongue.

огово́р *м. разг.* slánder. ~и́ть(ся) *сов. см.* огова́ривать(ся).

огово́рк|**а** *ж.* 1. (*условие*) reservátion, províso (*pl* -os, -oes); дéлать ~у make* a províso; 2. (*обмолвка*) slip of the tongue.

оголённый bare.

оголи́ть(**ся**) *сов. см.* оголя́ть(ся).

оголя́ть, оголи́ть (*вн.*) 1. (*обнажать*) bare (*smth.*), uncóver (*smth.*); 2. (*лишать покрывающего слоя*) strip (*smth.*); (*лишать листвы тж.*) denúde (*smth.*); оголи́ть прóвод strip the wíre; 3. (*делать беззащитным*) expóse (*smth.*). ~ся, оголи́ться 1. *разг.* strip; 2. (*о какой-л. части тела*) be* expósed, be* bared; 3. (*лишаться листвы*) be* stripped, be* bare; 4. (*становиться видимым*) be* expósed (to view).

огонёк *м.* 1. little flame, flícker; *перен.* (*увлечение, задор*) spark/touch of inspirátion; 2. (*свет*) (gleam/glímmer of) light; *перен.* (*блеск глаз*) gleam; у негó в глаза́х загорéлись весёлые огоньки́ sparks of amúsement/mérriment glowed in his eyes; ◇ зайти́ на ~ drop in for a chat (and a song).

огóнь *м.* 1. *тк. ед.* fire (*тж. перен.*); (*о человеке*) fire-brand, live wíre; развести́ ~ make* a fire; сгорéть в огнé go* up in flames, be* burnt in a fire; грéться у огня́ warm onesélf at/by a fire; 2. (*свет*) light; *перен.* (*блеск глаз*) gleam; заже́чь ~ light* a lamp; (*об электричестве*) put*/switch on the light; погаси́ть ~ put* out the light; в дома́х ужé засвети́лись огни́ lights were alréady búrning in the windows; горéть огнём (*о глазах*) glow; 3. *тк. ед.* (*стрельба, обстрел*) fire; (*из тяжёлых ору́дий*) gun-fire; откры́ть ~ ópen fire; вести́ ~ fire; под нём únder fire; ◇ в огнé 1) (*в жару*) in a féver; 2) (*в бою́*) únder fire; в ~ и в вóду за *кого́-л.* would go through fire and wáter for smb.'s sake; из огня́ да в пóлымя out of the frýing-pan into the fire; мéжду двух огнéй betwéen two fires; огнём и мечóм пройти́ rávage with fire and sword; боя́ться *кого́-л.* как огня́ be* scared to death of smb.; пройти́ ~ и вóду have* been through the mill; игра́ть с огнём play with fire.

огора́живать, огороди́ть (*вн.*) fence (*smth.*) in, enclóse (*smth.*).

огорóд *м.* (*при доме*) kitchen gárden; (*большой*) márket gárden *амер.*; truck gárden *амер.*

огороди́ть *сов. см.* огора́живать.

огорóдн|**ик** *м.* márket-gardener; truck gárdener *амер.* ~ичество *с.* márket-gardening; truck gárdening *амер.* ~ый márket-garden *attr.*; ~ый учáсток végetable allótment; ~ые растéния végetables.

огорóшивать, огорóшить (*вн.*) *разг.* bowl (*smb.*) óver.

огорóшить *сов. см.* огорóшивать.

огорч|**а́ть, огорчи́ть** (*вн.*) distréss (*smb.*), grieve (*smb.*), disappóint (*smb.*). ~а́ться, огорчи́ться (*тв.*) be* distréssed (abóut); grieve (óver); не ~а́йтесь! don't take it to heart! ~éние *с.* grief, distréss, afflíction; к моему́ вели́кому ~éнию much to my regrét. ~ённый aggríeved, disappóinted; ~ённый вид the disappóintment on smb.'s face. ~и́ть(ся) *сов. см.* огорча́ть(ся).

огра́бить *сов.* (*вн.*) rob (*smb.*); *перен. тж.* fleece (*smb., smth.*), plúnder (*smth.*).

ограбле́ние *с.* róbbery; *перен. тж.* fléecing, plúnder.

огра́да *ж.* fence, enclósure.

огради́ть *сов. см.* огражда́ть.

огражд|**а́ть, огради́ть** 1. (*вн.*; *отгораживать*) fence off (*smth.*); 2. (*вн. от рд.*; *защищать*) protéct (*smb.*, *smth.* agáinst); shield (*smb.*, *smth.* from); огради́ть кого́-л. от напа́док shield *smb.* from attáck. **~éние** *c.* 1. bárrier; 2. (*защита*) protéction.

ограничéни|е *c.* restríction, limitátion; без ~й without restríction, unrestríctedly.

ограни́ченн|ость *ж.* 1. (*средств и т. п.*) insufficiency; 2. (*узость*) nárrow-míndedness, nárrowness. **~ый** 1. (*небольшой, незначи́тельный*) límited; в ~ом коли́честве in límited quántities; ~ые возмо́жности límited opportúnities; 2. (*недалёкий*) nárrow, bígoted; ~ый ум nárrow mind; ~ый челове́к nárrow-mínded pérson.

ограни́чивать, ограни́чить (*вн.*) límit (*smb.*, *smth.*), restríct (*smb.*, *smth.*); ~ себя́ в чём-л. stint onesélf of smth.; ~ ора́тора вре́менем give* the spéaker a tíme-límit. **~ся, ограни́читься** (*тв.*) 1. (*довольствоваться чем-л.*) confíne onesélf (to); do* no more than (+ *inf*); ограни́читься то́лько рукопожа́тием confíne onesélf to a brief hándshake; 2. (*сводиться к чему-л. незначи́тельному*) amóunt to nóthing more than, be* confíned (to); boil down (to) *разг.*; де́ло ограни́чилось тем, что... the mátter énded in...

ограничи́тельный restríctive.

ограни́чить(ся) *сов. см.* ограни́чивать(ся).

огро́мн|ый enórmous, huge, imménse; (*обширный*) vast; ~ зверь enórmous beast; челове́к ~ого ро́ста enórmous man*; ~ое простра́нство vast expánse; ~ая ра́зница huge/enórmous dífference; ~ успе́х enórmous/huge success; ~ое сча́стье imménse háppiness.

огрубéлый 1. (*о коже*) cálloused, rough; 2. (*о челове́ке*) cóarsened.

огрубéть *сов. см.* грубе́ть.

огрыза́ться, огрызну́ться snarl; *перен. тж.* snap.

огрызну́ться *сов. см.* огрыза́ться.

огры́зок *м.* 1. (*недоеденный кусок*) gnawed bit; ~ я́блока gnawed ápple; 2. *разг.* (*остаток предмета*) stump; ~ каранда́ша péncil stub.

огу́льн|о indiscríminately. **~ый** 1. *разг.* (*касающийся всех, всего*) indiscríminate; 2. (*не имеющий основа́ния*) swéeping; ~ое обвине́ние swéeping/unfóunded accusátion.

огуре́ц *м.* cúcumber; (*небольшой*) ghérkin.

огуре́чный cúcumber *attr.*

о́да *ж. лит.* ode.

одарённ|ость *ж.* tálents *pl*, gíftedness; endówments *pl.* **~ый** gífted, tálented.

ода́ривать *несов. см.* одаря́ть 1.

одари́ть *сов. см.* одаря́ть.

одаря́ть, одари́ть 1. (*вн.*; *дарить*) give* présents (to); (*вн. тв.*) présent (*smb.* with); 2. (*вн. тв.*; *наделя́ть*) endów (*smb.* with).

одева́ть, оде́ть (*вн.*) 1. dress (*smb.*); (*вн. тв.*; *наряжа́ть кем-л.*) dress up (*smb.* as); оде́ть ребёнка dress a child*; 2. *разг.* (*обеспечивать одеждой*) clothe (*smb.*), províde (*smb.*) with clóthing; оде́ть всю семью́ províde clothes for the whole fámily; 3. (*покрывать*) cóver (*smth.*), clothe (*smth.*); 4. *тк. несов.* (*обеспечивать одеждой того или иного качества*) dress (*smb.*); ~ ребёнка со вку́сом dress a child* próperly. **~ся, оде́ться** 1. dress (onesélf); (в *вн.*) put* on (*smth.*); (*тв.*; *наряжа́ться кем-л.*) dress up (as *smb.*); 2. (*приобретать необходимую одежду*) fit onesélf out (with clothes); 3. (*покрываться*) be* clothed, be* clad; дере́вья оде́лись листво́й the trees were clothed in fóliage; 4. *тк. несов.* (*носить одежду*) dress; хорошо́ ~ся dress well; про́сто ~ся dress pláinly, wear* símple clothes.

оде́жда *ж.* clothes *pl*; ве́рхняя ~ stréet-clothes *pl*, óuterwear; фо́рменная ~ úniform.

одёж|ка *ж. разг.*: по ~е протя́гивай но́жки cut one's coat accórding to one's cloth.

одеколо́н *м.* éau-de-Cológne.

одели́ть *сов. см.* оделя́ть.

оделя́ть, одели́ть (*вн. тв.*) présent (*smb.* with).

одёргивать, одёрнуть (*вн.*) 1. (*поправлять платье и т. п.*) pull (*smth.*) straight; 2. *разг.* (*заставлять замолча́ть*) check (*smb.*), pull (*smb.*) up.

одеревенéлый 1. hárdened; 2. (*онемелый*) numb; 3. (*безучастный*) numb, apathétic.

одеревенéть *сов.* 1. becóme* hard, hárden; *перен. тж.* stíffen; 2. (*онеметь*) go* numb; (*оцепенеть*) freeze*; 3. (*стать безразличным*) lose* interest, dry up.

одержа́ть *сов. см.* оде́рживать.

оде́рживать, одержа́ть: одержа́ть верх gain the úpper hand; одержа́ть побе́ду win* a víctory.

одержи́мый *прил.* 1. (*тв.*) posséssed (by); 2. в *знач. сущ. м.* one posséssed.

одёрнуть *сов. см.* одёргивать.

оде́тый 1. dressed; (*в одежде, не голый*) clothed; with one's clothes on *после сущ.*; я ещё не оде́т I have no clothes on; хорошо́ ~ smártly dressed; 2. (*обеспеченный одеждой*) háving clothes to wear *после сущ.*; 3. (*покрытый, окутанный*) clad, cóvered; ~ сне́гом, листво́й snów-clad, léaf-clad; ~ и́неем ríme-covered.

оде́ть *сов. см.* одева́ть 1, 2, 3. **~ся** *сов. см.* одева́ться 1, 2, 3.

оде́яло *c.* blánket.

оде́яние *c.* attíre, ráiment, garb.

оди́н (*одна́, одно́, мн.* одни́) *числ.* 1. one (*тж. цифра*); ~-два one or two; ~ еди́нственный раз just once; 2. в *знач. прил.* (*какой-то*) а, an; одна́ кни́га, кото́рая мне понра́вилась a book (which) I liked; я ви́дел одного́ челове́ка, кото́рый... I met a man* who...; ~ писа́тель сказа́л... a cértain wríter once said...; it was a wríter who once said...; 3. в *знач. прил.* (*наедине, сам*) alóne; by onesélf; вы одни́? are you alóne?; совсе́м ~ all by onesélf, quite alóne; 4. в *знач. прил.* (*тот же самый*) the same; одного́ го́да рожде́ния born in the same year; одного́ разме́ра the same size; 5. в *знач. прил.* (*никто другой, ничто другое*) no one but, nóbody but (*о человеке*); nóthing but (*о животных, предметах*); ónly; alóne (*обыкн. употребляется перед гл.*); там бы́ли одни́ де́ти there was no one but children there; круго́м бы́ли одни́ ка́мни there was nóthing but stones all aróund; он рабо́тает с одно́й молодёжью he works ónly with young péople; (*только*) он ~ мо́жет, зна́ет *и т. п.* he alóne can, knows, *etc.*; 6. в *знач. сущ. м.* one, *мн.* some péople; ~ из ста, ты́сячи *и т. п.* one in a húndred, thóusand, *etc.*; ~ из них (нас *и т. п.*) one of them (us *etc.*); по одному́ one at a time; ко́мната на одного́ single room; ни ~ one, nóbody; одни́ хотя́т идти́ в теа́тр, други́е не хотя́т some want to go to the théatre, some don't; 7. в *знач. сущ. c.* one thing; одно́ и то же the same thing; одно́ мне изве́стно one thing I do know; ◇ ~ на ~ (*наедине*) quite alóne; face to face; сража́ться ~ на ~ meet* in single cómbat; все до одного́ to a man; все как ~ like one man; одно́ из двух one thing or the óther (you can't have both); одно́ вре́мя at one time; одни́м сло́вом in a word; ~-одинёшенек all alóne.

одина́ков|о équally; относи́ться ко всем ~ treat éveryone équally. **~ый** the same; équal; в ~ой ме́ре équally.

одина́рный single.

одиннадцатилéтний 1. (*о сроке*) eléven-year; of eléven years *после сущ.*; 2. (*о возрасте*) eléven-year-óld; of eléven *после сущ.*

оди́ннадц|атый eléventh; ~ год eléventh year. **~ать** éleven.

одино́к|ий *прил.* 1. sólitary, lónely; lone *поэт.*; 2. (*бессемейный*) single, unmárried; ~ая мать unmárried móther; 3. в *знач. сущ. м.* (*бессемейный*) single/unmárried man*, báchelor. **~о**: жить ~о lead* a sólitary life; ~о стоя́щий дом sólitary house.

одино́чество *c.* sólitude; (*чувство*) lóneliness.

одиночк|а *м. и ж.* 1. pérson by himsélf, pérson on his, her own; *(действующий один)* indivídual; запоздáвшие ~и lone strágglers; 2. *(человек, живущий без семьи)* síngle man*; 3. *ж. разг. (тюремная камера)* sólitary confinement cell; 4. *ж. (лодка)* síngle sculls *pl*; ◇ в ~у 1) *(по одному)* síngly, indivídually; 2) *(своими силами)* síngle-hánded.

одиночн|ый 1. *(о насекомых, животных)* lone, síngle; 2. *(отдельный, случайный)* sólitary, ísolated; ~ые вы́стрелы sólitary/síngle shots; 3. *(совершаемый силами одного)* síngle-hánded, síngle, indivídual; ~ бой síngle cómbat; 4. *(предназначенный для одного человека)* síngle; *(о камере, заключении)* sólitary.

одио́зный ódious, offénsive.

одича́|лый half-wíld; that has (been allówed to) run wild *после сущ.*; ~лая ко́шка stray cat, half-wíld cat. ~ние *с.* becóming/rúnning wild, retúrn to its nátive state; *перен.* degenerátion.

одича́ть *сов. см.* дича́ть.

одна́ *см.* оди́н.

одна́жды 1. *(один раз)* once; 2. *(как-то раз)* once, one day.

одна́ко *(часто ~ же, ~ ж)* 1. *союз* howéver; but *(тк. в начале фразы)*; though *(тк. в конце фразы)*; ~ он не пришёл howéver, he did not come; but he did not come; he did not come, though; вы, ~, не забу́дьте обéщанного but don't forgét what you prómised; 2. *в знач. межд.* indéed!, is that so!, oh, is it!, oh, does it!

одни́ *см.* оди́н.

одно́ *см.* оди́н.

одно- *в сложн.* one-.

одноа́кт|ый óne-act *attr.*; ~ая пьéса óne-act play.

однобо́кий lop-síded; *перен.* one-síded.

однобо́ртный síngle-bréasted; ~ пиджа́к síngle-bréasted jácket.

одновремéнн|о simultáneously, at the same time. ~ый simultáneous.

одногла́зый óne-eyed; with ónly one eye *после сущ.*

одногоди́чный óne-year *attr.*

одного́рбый ~ верблю́д óne-húmped/Arábian cámel, drómedary.

одноднéвный óne-day *attr.*; ~ дом о́тдыха óne-day/wéek-end gúest-house.

однозву́чный monótonous.

однозна́чн|ый 1. synónymous; ~ые выраже́ния synónymous expréssions; 2. *(имеющий только одно значение)* monosemántic, unequívocal; 3. *мат.* símple; ~ое число́ dígit.

одноимённ|ый of the same name *после сущ.*; по ~ому рома́ну áfter the nóvel of the same name.

однока́шник *м. разг.* schóol-fellow, schóol-mate; *(о студентах)* féllow stúdent.

однокла́ссн|ик *м.*, ~ица *ж.* clássmate, fórm-mate.

однокле́точный *биол.* unicéllular.

одноклу́бник *м. разг.* pláyer of the same club; вы́играть у свои́х ~ов beat* a team from *one's* own club.

одноковшо́вый *тех.* síngle-bucket *attr.*, síngle-scoop *attr.*

одноколéйный *ж.-д.* síngle-track *attr.*

однокóмнатн|ый óne-room *attr.*; ~ая кварти́ра óne-room flat.

однокýрсн|ик *м.*, ~ица *ж.* cóurse-mate; pérson in the same year (at univérsity).

однолéтний 1. yéar-óld; 2. *(о растении)* ánnual.

однолéт|ок *м.*: они́ ~ки they're just of the same age.

одномéстн|ый síngle-séater *attr.*; ~ая каю́та síngle cábin.

одномото́рный síngle-éngine(d); ~ самолёт síngle-éngined áircraft.

одноно́гий one-légged; with ónly one leg *после сущ.*

однообра́з|ие *с.* monótony. ~ный monótonous.

однопала́тн|ый síngle-chámber *attr.*; ~ая парла́ментская систéма síngle-chámber parliaméntary sýstem.

однопалу́бн|ый síngle-decked; ~ое су́дно síngle-decked ship.

однополча́н|ин *м.* regiméntal cómrade, bróther-sóldier; *(офицер)* bróther-ófficer; мы с ним ~е we served in the same régiment; we were sóldiers togéther.

однопо́лый *бот.* uniséxual.

однородн|ость *ж.* 1. homogenéity; 2. *(сходство)* similárity, unifórmity. ~ый 1. *(одинаковый во всех своих частях)* homogéneous; ~ое тéло homogéneous bódy; 2. *(сходный)* símilar, úniform, of the same kind *после сущ.*; ~ые явлéния phenómena of the same kind; ~ая стати́стика úniform statístics; ◇ ~ые члéны предложéния *грам.* símilar parts of a séntence.

однору́кий one-ármed; with one arm *после сущ.*; with ónly one hand *после сущ.*

односельча́н|ин *м.* man* from the same víllage. ~ка *ж.* wóman* from the same víllage.

односло́жн|о cúrtly; отвеча́ть ~ give* monosyllábic replíes. ~ый monosyllábic; *перен. тж.* brief; ~ое сло́во monosýllable.

односпа́льн|ый síngle; ~ая крова́ть síngle bed.

односторо́нн|ий 1. one-síded; ~ее движéние тра́нспорта one-wáy tráffic; ~ее воспалéние лёгких síngle pneumónia; ~ее развитие lop-síded devélopment; ~ее воспита́ние one-síded educátion; ~яя ткань irrevérsible fábric; ~ ум óne-track mind; ~ее мышлéние one-síded thínking; 2. *(совершаемый одной стороной, одним лицом)* uniláteral; ~ее прекраще́ние воéнных дéйствий uniláteral cessátion of mílitary operátions.

одноти́пн|ый of the same type/módel *после сущ.*; ~ые маши́ны machínes of the same type.

однотóмн|ик *м. разг.* óne-vólume edítion. ~ый óne-vólume *attr.*

однофами́л|ец *м.*, ~ица *ж.* pérson of the same name, námesake.

одноцвéтн|ый óne-cólour *attr.*; unicólour(ed) *научн.*; ~ая ткань óne-colour fábric; plain fábric.

одночлéн *м. мат.* monómial.

одноэта́жный óne-stórey(ed).

одобрéние *с.* appróval.

одобри́тельн|о appróvingly, with appróval. ~ый appróving; ~ый о́тзыв fávourable respónse; ~ый взгляд glance of appróval.

одо́брить *сов. см.* одобря́ть.

одобря́ть, одо́брить *(вн.)* appróve (of); не ~ disappróve (of), not appróve (of).

одолева́ть, одолéть *(вн.)* 1. *(побеждать)* overpówer *(smb., smth.)*; одолéть проти́вника overpówer *one's* oppónent; 2. *разг. (овладевать чем-л.)* máster *(smth.)*; get* through *(smth.)*; одолéть курс фи́зики get* through a course of phýsics; 3. *(о каком-л. состоянии)* overcóme* *(smb.)*; его́ одолéла лень láziness got the bétter of him; 4. *разг. (лишать покоя)* try *(smb.'s)* pátience, get* smb. down; меня́ комары́ одолéли I'm sick of these mosquítoes.

одолéть *сов. см.* одолева́ть.

одолж|а́ть, одолжи́ть *(вн., рд.)* lend* *(smth.)*. ~éние *с.* fávour; проси́ть кого́-л. об ~éнии ask smb. a fávour; ◇ сдéлайте ~éние! 1) *(просьба)* would you mind (+ -ing); 2) *(ответ)* of course (you may)!; please, do!

одолжи́ть *сов. см.* одолжа́ть.

одр *м.*: на смéртном ~е on *one's* déath-bed.

одряхлéние *с.* decrépitude, flágging strength.

одряхлéть *сов. см.* дряхлéть.

одува́нчик *м. бот.* dándelion.

оду́маться *сов.* 1. *(изменить свои намерения)* think* bétter of it, change *one's* mind; ~ в послéднюю мину́ту change *one's* mind at the last mínute; 2. *разг. (опомниться)* come* to *one's* sénses.

одура́чивание *с.* fóoling.

одура́чивать, одура́чить (вн.) разг. fool (smb.), bamboozle (smb.), dupe (smb.).

одура́чить сов. см. одура́чивать и дура́чить.

одуре́|лый разг. dazed. ~ние с. разг. stúpor; до ~ния till one is blue in the face.

одуре́ть сов. см. дуре́ть.

одурма́нивать, одурма́нить (вн.) intóxicate (smb.), stúpefy (smb.).

одурма́нить сов. см. одурма́нивать и дурма́нить.

одуря́ющий stúpefying, overpówering.

одутлова́т|ость ж. púffiness. ~ый púffy.

одухотворённ|ость ж. spirituálity. ~ый exálted, inspíred; ~ое лицо́ exálted face.

одушев|и́ть(ся) сов. см. одушевля́ть(ся). ~ле́ние с. animátion. ~лённый ánimated.

одушевля́ть, одушеви́ть (вн.) ánimate (smb., smth.). ~ся, одушеви́ться be*/becóme* ánimated.

оды́шк|а ж. shórtness/lack of breath; страда́ть ~ой have* difficulty in bréathing.

ожереби́ться сов. см. жереби́ться.

ожере́лье с. nécklace.

ожесточ|а́ть, ожесточи́ть (вн.) embítter (smb.), hárden smb.'s heart. ~а́ться, ожесточи́ться (озлобля́ться) becóme* embíttered; (черстветь) grow* hard; (становиться жестоким) becóme* víolent/cruel. ~е́ние с. 1. (озлобление) bítterness; (очерствение) hárdness; 2. (упорство, рьяность) frántic zeal; де́лать что-л. с ~е́нием do* smth. with demónic énergy, go* at smth. tooth and nail. ~ённый 1. (безжалостный, суровый) embíttered; 2. (исполненный упорства, напряжения) fierce, frántic; ~ённый бой fierce fight; ~ённый спор frántic árgument.

ожесточи́ть(ся) сов. см. ожесточа́ть(ся).

ожива́ть, ожи́ть revíve, come* back to life.

ожив|и́ть(ся) сов. см. оживля́ть(ся). ~ле́ние с. 1. (действие) resuscitátion, reanimátion; ~ле́ние органи́зма reanimátion of the órganism; 2. (весёлость, живость) líveliness, excítement, jóllity; 3. (движение, суета) animátion, excítement, cóming and góing; на у́лицах цари́ло большо́е ~ле́ние there was great excítement in the streets. ~лённый 1. (весёлый, возбуждённый) excíted, bright, lívely; pérky разг.; ~лённый вид lívely appéarance; ~лённая бесе́да excíted conversátion; 2. (исполненный жизни, движения) ánimated, búsy; ~лённые у́лицы búsy streets.

оживля́ть, ожива́ть (вн.) 1. (возвращать к жизни) resúscitate (smb.), reánimate (smb.); 2. (восстанавливать физические и душевные силы) revíve (smb., smth.), перен.); 3. (лицо, глаза) ánimate (smth.); 4. (наполнять жизнью, движением) bring* life (to); 5. (делать более активным, ярким) enlíven (smth.), bríghten up (smth.); give* (smth.) a lift разг. ~ся, оживи́ться becóme* ánimated, líven up, come* to life; (становиться более весёлым тж.) bríghten up.

ожида́ни|е с. 1. wáiting; по́сле до́лгого ~я áfter a long périod of wáiting; в ~и чего́-л. pénding smth.; в ~и перегово́ров pénding the negotiátions; в ~и while wáiting for the train; 2. обыкн. мн. (предположение, надежда) expectátions; про́тив ~й cóntrary to expectátions; сверх (вся́ких) ~й beyónd all expectátions; обману́ть чьи-л. ~я disappóint/dash smb.'s expectátions/hopes.

ожида́ть несов. 1. (вн., рд.) wait (for); с нетерпе́нием ~ чего́-л. look fórward éagerly to smth.; 2. (рд.; надеяться, предполагать) expéct (smth.); от него́ э́того мо́жно бы́ло ~ it's just what was to be expécted of him; 3. (вн.; предстоять кому-л.) be* in store (for), awáit (smb.).

ожире́ние с. obésity; ~ се́рдца ádipose/fátty heart, fátty deteriorátion of the heart.

ожире́ть сов. run* to fat.

ожи́ть сов. см. ожива́ть.

ожо́г м. burn; (кипящей жидкостью тж.) scald.

озабо́тить сов. (вн.) give* (smb.) sómething to wórry abóut.

озабо́титься сов. (о пр.) take* care (of); (тв.) atténd (to), see* (to); ~, что́бы... see* to it that...

озабо́ченн|ость ж. anxíety. ~ый wórried, ánxious; ~ый вид ánxious looks pl.

озагла́вить сов. см. озагла́вливать.

озагла́вливать, озагла́вить (вн.) províde (smth.) with a títle; (главу тж.) entítle (smth.), head (smth.).

озада́чивать, озада́чить (вн.) perpléx (smb.), bewílder (smb.).

озада́чить сов. см. озада́чивать.

озари́ть(ся) сов. см. озаря́ть(ся).

озаря́ть, озари́ть (вн.) 1. illúminate (smb., smth.), light* up (smth.); перен. тж. bríghten (up) (smb., smth.); 2. (приходить в голову) strike* (smb.), dawn (upón); его́ озари́ла мысль, дога́дка it súddenly dawned upón him (that). ~ся, озари́ться (прям. и перен.) be* illúminated, light* up.

озвере́|вший, ~лый brútal, ferócious.

озвере́ть сов. см. звере́ть.

озву́ченный: ~ фильм sound film.

озву́чивать, озву́чить: ~ фильм make* the sound track for a film.

озву́чить сов. см. озву́чивать.

оздорови́тельн|ый héalth-impróvement attr.; sánitary; ~ые мероприя́тия sánitary méasures; ~ые лагеря́ для дете́й health camps for children.

оздоров|и́ть сов. см. оздоровля́ть. ~ле́ние с. máking héalthier, impróvement of sánitary condítions; перен. impróvement, normalizátion.

оздоровля́ть, оздорови́ть (вн.) make* (smb., smth.) héalthier; перен. (улучшать) impróve (smth.), nórmalize (smth.).

озелене́ние с. plánting trees and shrubs; ~ городо́в plánting trees and shrubs in towns.

озелени́ть сов. см. озеленя́ть.

озеленя́ть, озелени́ть (вн.) plant trees and shrubs (in).

озёрный lake attr.

о́зеро с. lake.

ози́м|ый прил. 1. winter attr.; ~ые культу́ры winter crops; ~ая пшени́ца winter wheat; ~ое по́ле field of winter crops; 2. в знач. сущ. мн. winter crops.

о́зимь ж. (young) winter crop(s).

озира́ться несов. look round; ~ по сторона́м look from side to side.

озло́б|ить(ся) сов. см. озлобля́ть(ся). ~ле́ние с. bítterness; (против рд.) animósity (agáinst); (злость) rage. ~ленный embíttered, hárdened.

озлобля́ть, озло́бить (вн.) embítter (smb.). ~ся, озло́биться 1. becóme* embíttered; 2. разг. (раздражаться) fly* into a témper.

ознако́мить(ся) сов. см. ознакомля́ть(ся).

ознакомля́ть, ознако́мить (вн. с тв.) acquáint (smb. with). ~ся, ознако́миться (с тв.) acquáint/famíliarize onesélf (with); ознако́миться с резолю́цией acquáint oneself with a resolútion.

ознаменов|а́ние с.: в ~ чего́-л. on the occásion of smth.; to célebrate smth.; (в память) in commemorátion of smth. ~а́ть сов. (вн.) 1. (вн.; явиться свидетельством чего-л.) mark (smth.); 2. (вн. тв.; сделать памятным) mark (smth. by); (отметить) célebrate (smth. with). ~а́ться сов. (тв.) be* marked (by).

означа́ть несов. (вн.) mean* (smth.), sígnify (smth.).

озно́б м. fit of shívering; the shívers pl разг.; почу́вствовать си́льный ~ expérience a sevére fit of shívering.

озо́н м. ózone.

озорн|и́к м. разг. 1. (о ребёнке) míschievous child*; 2. (буян, скандалист) gay dog. ~ича́ть несов. be* up to some míschief or óther. ~о́й míschievous, náughty; (буйный) wild.

озорств|о́ *с. разг.* 1. míschief, skýlarking; tricks *pl*; из ~а́ out of míschief; 2. (*бесчинство*) víolence, wild cónduct.

озя́бнуть *сов. разг.* be* chílly.

ой oh; ой-ой-о́й! oh, dear!

оказа́ни|е *с.* réndering; ~ медици́нской по́мощи réndering of médical aid; для ~я по́мощи to rénder assístance.

оказа́ть *сов. см.* ока́зывать.

оказа́ться *сов. см.* ока́зываться 1, 2, 3, 4.

оказѝ|я *ж.:* посла́ть письмо́ с ~ей find* *smb.* to take a létter; что за ~! what an odd thing!

ока́зывать, оказа́ть (*вн.*) rénder (*smth.*), show* (*smth.*); ~ влия́ние на *кого-л.* exércise ínfluence on *smb.*; ~ внима́ние *кому-л.* show* *smb.* atténtion; ~ давле́ние на *кого-л., что-л.* exért préssure upón *smb., smth.*; bring* préssure to bear upón *smb., smth.*; ~ де́йствие на *кого-л., что-л.* have* an efféct on *smb., smth.*; ~ содействие, по́мощь *кому-л.* rénder *smb.* assístance, help; ~ подде́ржку give* one's suppórt; ~ предпочте́ние *кому-л.* show* (a) préference for *smb.*; ~ сопротивле́ние óffer resístance; ~ упо́рное, отча́янное сопротивле́ние put* up a désperate fight; ~ услу́гу *кому-л.* rénder *smb.* a sérvice; ~ честь *кому-л.* do* *smb.* the hónour; ~ по́чести *кому-л.* recéive *smb.* with hónour.

ока́зыв|аться, оказа́ться 1. (*быть налицо*) be*; turn out to be; в гости́нице не оказа́лось свобо́дных номеро́в there turned out to be no room in the hotel; кни́га оказа́лась на ме́сте the book was in its place (all the time); спи́чек у него́ не оказа́лось he had no mátches; 2. (*очути́ться где-л., в каком-л. состоя́нии*) find* onesélf; оказа́ться в опа́сности find* onesélf in dánger; магази́н оказа́лся закры́тым the shop was shut; 3. (*явля́ться на де́ле кем-л., чем-л.*) prove to be; он оказа́лся о́чень ми́лым челове́ком he turned out to be a véry nice man*; мои́ опасе́ния оказа́лись напра́сными my fears proved gróundless; 4. *безл.* (*выясня́ться*) it turns out, it transpíres; как оказа́лось as things turned out; 5. *тк. несов.:* ~ается в знач. вводн. сл. it turns out; ~ается, что... it appéars that...

окайми́ть *сов. см.* окаймля́ть.

окаймля́ть, окайми́ть (*вн. тв.*) bórder (*smth.* with), edge (*smth.* with).

ока́лина *ж. тех.* scale.

окамене́л|ость *ж.* fóssil. ~ый 1. pétrified; *перен.* (*твёрдый, чёрствый — о пище*) róck-hard, íron-hard; 2. (*безучастный*) wóoden, fixed; (*суровый*) stóny; ~ое се́рдце stóny heart.

окамене́ть *сов.* 1. turn ínto stone, be* turned ínto stone; *перен.* (*стать чёрствым — о хлебе и т. п.*) becóme* as hard as a rock; 2. (*от рд.; засты́ть, оцепене́ть*) be* pétrified (with); 3. (*стать безуча́стным*) be* númbed; 4. (*ожесточи́ться*) hárden, becóme* hard.

ока́нчив|ать, око́нчить (*вн.*) fínish (*smth.*), end (*smth.*), compléte (*smth.*), round off (*smth.*); око́нчить рабо́ту round off one's work; око́нчить заседа́ние end a mée ting; око́нчить шко́лу fínish school; око́нчить университе́т gráduate (from/at the univérsity). ~а́ться, око́нчиться 1. fínish, end, be* óver; 2. *тк. несов.* (*тв.; иметь свои́м оконча́нием*) end (with, in); сло́во ~ается на гла́сную the word ends in a vówel.

ока́пывать, окопа́ть (*вн.*) 1. dig*/trench round (*smth.*); ~ де́рево trench round a tree; 2. *воен.* entrénch (*smth.*). ~ся, окопа́ться dig* in; entrénch onesélf (*тж. перен.*).

окати́ть(ся) *сов. см.* ока́чивать(ся).

ока́чивать, окати́ть (*вн.*) douse (*smb., smth.*); окати́ть *кого-л.* холо́дной водо́й throw* cold wáter óver *smb.*; *перен.* discóurage *smb.* ~ся, окати́ться (*тв.*) douse onesélf (with).

океа́н *м.* ócean.

океана́вт *м.* déep-sea/ócean explórer.

океани́ческ|ий oceánic; ócean *attr.*; ~ая ры́ба oceánic/salt-wáter fish.

океанографи́ческий oceanográphic(al).

океаногра́фия *ж.* oceanógraphy.

океаноло́гия *ж. см.* океаногра́фия.

океа́нский ócean *attr.*; ~ ла́йнер ócean líner.

оки́дывать, оки́нуть: оки́нуть *кого-л.* взгля́дом cast* a glance at *smb.*

оки́нуть *сов. см.* оки́дывать.

о́кисел *м. хим.* óxide.

окисле́ние *с. хим.* oxidátion.

окисли́тель *м. хим.* óxidizing ágent, óxidizer.

окисли́ть(ся) *сов. см.* окисля́ть(ся).

окисля́ть, окисли́ть (*вн.*) *хим.* óxidize (*smth.*). ~ся, окисли́ться *хим.* óxidize.

о́кись *ж. хим.* óxide; ~ углеро́да cárbon (mon)-óxide.

оккуп|а́нт *м.* inváder; *мн.* occupátion troops. ~аци́онный occupátion *attr.* ~а́ция *ж.* occupátion. ~и́ровать *несов. и сов.* (*вн.*) óccupy (*smth.*).

окла́д I *м.* (*размер заработной платы*) (rate of) wáges/sálary; pay.

окла́д II *м.* (*металлическое покрытие на иконе*) sétting, móunting.

оклевета́ть *сов.* (*вн.*) slánder (*smth.*); calúmniate (*smth.*), defáme (*smth.*); smear (*smth.*) *разг.*

окле́ивать, окле́ить (*вн.*) paste (*smth.*) all óver; ~ ко́мнату обо́ями páper a room.

окле́ить *сов. см.* окле́ивать.

о́клик *м.* hail, call; ~ часово́го séntry's chállenge.

оклика́ть, окли́кнуть (*вн.*) hail (*smth.*), call (to); (*о часовом*) chállenge (*smth.*).

окли́кнуть *сов. см.* оклика́ть.

окн|о́ *с.* 1. wíndow; ко́мната в три ~а́ room with three wíndows; откры́ть ~ ópen a wíndow; без о́кон wíndowless; стоя́ть под ~о́м stand* únder a wíndow; вы́бросить что-л. в ~ throw* *smth.* out of the wíndow; 2. *разг.* (*подоконник*) wíndowsill; положи́ть что-л. на ~ put* *smth.* on the wíndowsill; цветы́ на о́кнах flówers on wíndowsills; 3. (*просвет, отверстие*) gap, ópening; 4. *разг.* (*промежуток времени между уроками, лекциями*) break.

о́ко *с. поэт.* eye; ◇ ~ за ~, зуб за́ зуб an eye for an eye, and a tooth for a tooth.

окова́ть *сов. см.* око́вывать.

око́вы *мн.* (*прям. и перен.*) sháckles, fétters, chains.

око́вывать, окова́ть (*вн.*) bind* (*smth.*); *перен. тж.* seal (*smth.*).

околдова́ть *сов. см.* околдо́вывать.

околдо́вывать, околдова́ть (*вн.*) bewítch (*smb.*), cast* a spell (upón).

околева́ть, околе́ть die, pérish.

околе́сиц|а *ж. разг.* rúbbish; нести́ ~у talk a lot of rúbbish.

околе́ть *сов. см.* околева́ть.

око́лица *ж.* 1. (*изгородь*) víllage fence; (*ворота*) víllage gate; 2. (*окраина селения*) edge/óutskirts of the víllage.

о́коло 1. *предлог* (*рд.*) (*возле*) close to, besíde; (*недалеко от*) not far from; (*рядом*) next to, besíde, by; 2. *предлог* (*рд.*) (*приблизительно*) abóut; сейча́с ~ двух часо́в it's abóut two; ~ того́ thereabóuts; 3. *нареч.* close by; quite near.

околозе́мн|ый néar-Earth; ~ое простра́нство néar-Earth space.

око́лыш *м.* cáp-band.

око́льн|ый róundabout; ~ путь róundabout way; ~ыми путя́ми in a róundabout way.

око́нн|ый wíndow *attr.*; ~ая ра́ма wíndow-frame; ~ое стекло́ (*в раме*) wíndow-pane; (*не вставленное в ра́му*) wíndow-glass.

оконча́ни|е *с.* 1. (*завершение*) complétion; по ~и

шко́лы on léaving school; по ~и университе́та on gráduating from/at the univérsity; 2. (коне́ц) end; ~ в сле́дующем но́мере final instálment in (our) next íssue; 3. грам. énding.

оконча́тельн|о definitively; (совсе́м) finally; ~ доде́лать что-л. put* the final/finishing tóuches to smth.; ~ убеди́ться в чём-л. be* finally persuáded of smth. ~ый final; (по́лный) compléte; ~ый вы́вод final conclúsion; ~ый отве́т definitive/final ánswer.

око́нчить сов. см. ока́нчивать. ~ся сов. см. ока́нчиваться 1.

око́п м. trench, entrénchment; рыть ~ы dig* trénches.

окопа́ть(ся) сов. см. ока́пывать(ся).

о́корок м. (ветчины) ham; (теля́тины) leg of veal; (бара́нины) leg of mútton.

окостене́лый 1. óssified (тж. перен.); ~ ум óssified mind; 2. (утра́тивший ги́бкость) stiff.

окостене́ть сов. см. костене́ть.

око́т м. (об о́вцах, ко́зах) lámbing; (о ко́шках) háving kíttens.

окоти́ться сов. см. коти́ться.

окочене́лый stiff, numb.

окочене́ть сов. см. кочене́ть 1.

око́шко с. window.

окра́ин|а ж. 1. (населённого пу́нкта) the óutskirts pl; 2. (страны́) bórderlands pl; óutlying dístricts pl; далёкая ~ remóte part of the cóuntry. ~ный on the edge of town по́сле сущ. on the óutskirts по́сле сущ.; (перифери́йный) bórderland attr.

окра́сить(ся) сов. см. окра́шивать(ся).

окра́ск|а ж. 1. (де́йствие) páinting, cólouring; (мате́рии, воло́с) dýeing; 2. (цвет, кра́ска) cólour; colorátion, cólouring науч.; перен. compléxion; придава́ть совсе́м другу́ю ~у чему́-л. put* a véry different compléxion on smth.; принима́ть совсе́м другу́ю ~у assúme a véry different compléxion.

окра́шивать, окра́сить (вн.) páint (smth.); cólour (smth.) (тж. перен.); (мате́рию, во́лосы) dye (smth.); ~ что-л. в кра́сный цвет paint/cólour smth. red. ~ся, окра́ситься take* paint; (о мате́рии, волоса́х) dye; (принима́ть како́й-л. цвет) be* tinged; верши́ны гор окра́сились в ро́зовый цвет the móuntain-tops were tinged pink.

окре́п|нуть сов. см. кре́пнуть. ~ший much strónger, fórtified in health.

окрести́ть сов. 1. см. крести́ть 1; 2. (вн. тв.) разг. (дать про́звище) níckname (smb. smth.). ~ся сов. см. крести́ться 1.

окре́стн|ость ж. 1. (прилега́ющая к чему́-л. ме́стность) néighbourhood; (го́рода) environs pl; 2. (окружа́ющее простра́нство) locálity. ~ый 1. (располо́женный в окре́стности) néighbouring; ~ые дере́вни néighbouring víllages; ~ые леса́ surróunding fórests; 2. (живу́щий в сосе́дней ме́стности) lócal; ~ые жи́тели lócal inhábitants.

о́крик м 1. (о́клик) hail, call; 2. (гру́бый) thréatening shout, bawled órder.

окрова́вленный blóodstained.

окро́шка ж. 1. okróshka (soup made of kvass, greenstuff and meat and served cold); 2. разг. (смесь) médley, mix-up.

о́круг м. dístrict; вое́нный ~ military district.

окру́га ж. разг. the néighbourhood.

округли́ть(ся) сов. см. округля́ть(ся).

округля́ть, округли́ть (вн.) 1. (де́лать кру́глым) make* (smth.) round; перен. разг. (придава́ть зако́нченную фо́рму фра́зе и т. п.) round off (smth.), compléte (smth.); ~ глаза́ stare wíde-éyed; 2. (выража́ть в кру́глых ци́фрах) expréss (smth.) as a whole númber; округли́ть деся́тичную дробь round off the décimal, cárry óver the décimal to the néarest whole númber. ~ся, округли́ться 1. (приобрета́ть кру́глую

фо́рму) grow* round; (станови́ться по́лным) fill out; перен. разг. (о ре́чи, мы́слях и т. п.) take* final shape; 2. разг. (увели́чиваться) mount up.

окруж|а́ть, окружи́ть 1. тк. несов. (вн., прям. и перен.) surróund (smb., smth.); пруд ~а́ли дере́вья the pond was surróunded by trees, there were trees all round the pond; его́ ~а́ло всео́бщее уваже́ние he was the óbject of univérsal respéct; 2. (вн.; располага́ться вокру́г кого́-л., чего́-л.) gáther round (smb., smth.); окружи́ть расска́зчика gáther round a stóryteller; 3. (вн. тв.; обноси́ть, обводи́ть чем-л.) encírcle (smth. with); ~ что-л. рвом encírcle smth. with a moat; 4. (вн.) воен. encírcle (smb., smth.); окружи́ть и уничто́жить проти́вника encírcle and destróy the énemy; 5. (вн. тв.; создава́ть каку́ю-л. обстано́вку) surróund (smb. with); его́ окружи́ли внима́нием и забо́той he had évery care and atténtion; 6. тк. несов. (вн.; составля́ть чьё-л. о́бщество): его́ ~а́ли то́лько и́збранные his círcle was confíned to the élite; нас ~а́ли хоро́шие лю́ди we were in good* cómpany. ~а́ющий прил. 1. surróunding; ~а́ющая среда́ envíronment; surróundings pl; 2. в знач. сущ. мн. the péople of one's círcle/acquáintance; 3. в знач. сущ. с. one's surróundings pl; всё ~а́ющее éverything aróund one.

окруже́ни|е с. 1. (среда́, обстано́вка) envíronment; 2. воен. encírclement; вы́йти из ~я break* out of encírclement; попа́сть в ~ be* encírcled, be* hemmed in on all sides; ◇ в ~и кого́-л. accómpanied by smb.

окружи́ть сов. см. окружа́ть 2, 3, 4, 5.

окружн|о́й 1. district attr.; ~а́я избира́тельная коми́ссия district eléctoral committee; ~ центр district céntre; 2. (окружа́ющий) círcular; ~а́я желе́зная доро́га círcular ráilway.

окру́жност|ь ж. circúmference; име́ть 10 ме́тров в ~и have* a circúmference of ten métres, be* ten métres round; на 10 киломе́тров в ~и within a tén-kílometre rádius.

окрылённый eláted; inspíred; ~ наде́ждой búoyant with hope.

окрыли́ть(ся) сов. см. окрыля́ть(ся).

окрыл|я́ть, окрыли́ть (вн.) eláte (smb.), inspírit (smb.); его́ ~я́ла наде́жда hope lent him wings. ~я́ться, окрыли́ться acquíre wings; перен. тж. be* uplífted.

окта́ва ж. 1. муз., лит. óctave; 2. (разнови́дность ба́са) deep bass.

октя́бр|ь м. Octóber; в ~é э́того го́да this/in Octóber; в ~é про́шлого го́да last Octóber; last year in Octóber; в ~é бу́дущего го́да next Octóber.

октя́брьский Octóber attr.

октября́та мн. (ед. октябрёнок м.) Octóbrians (schoolchildren aged 7 — 10).

окули́ст м. óculist; éye-doctor разг.

окуля́р м. éyepiece, éye-lens; ~ периско́па éye-piece of a périscope.

окуна́ть, окуну́ть (вн.) dip (smb., smth.). ~ся, окуну́ться dip; перен. plunge, be* plunged.

окуну́ть(ся) сов. см. окуна́ть(ся).

о́кунь м. perch.

окупа́емость ж. recóupment; ~ вкла́да в уста́вный фонд recóupment of contribútions to the áuthorized fund.

окупа́ть, окупи́ть (вн.) pay* (smth.), cóver (smth.); ~ расхо́ды cóver the expénse. ~ся, окупи́ться pay* for itsélf, repáy*/recóup the invéstment; перен. be* repáid/rewárded.

окупи́ть(ся) сов. см. окупа́ть(ся).

оку́ривать, окури́ть (вн.) fúmigate (smth.).

окури́ть сов. см. оку́ривать.

оку́рок м. (cigarétte-)butt, stub, fag end.

окута́ть(ся) сов. см. оку́тывать(ся).

оку́тывать, оку́тать (вн.) wrap (smth.); перен. тж. shroud (smth.); оку́тать ше́ю ша́рфом wrap a scarf* round one's neck. ~ся, оку́таться wrap onesélf up.

окучивание *с. с.-х.* éarthing.

окучивать, **окучить** (*вн.*) *с.-х.* earth (*smth.*) up, bank (*smth.*).

окучить *сов. см.* окучивать.

оладья *ж.* thick páncake; ~ с яблоками ápple frítter.

оленевод *м.* déer-breeder. ~ство *с.* déer-breeding. ~ческий déer-breeding *attr.*

олен|ий deer's; ~ьи пора ántlers; ~ьи пимы déerskin boots. ~ина *ж.* vénison. ~уха *ж.* doe, hind.

олень *м.* deer*; (*самец*) buck, hart; (*крупных пород*) stag; (*самка*) doe, hind; северный ~ réindeer*.

олив|а *ж.* 1. (*плод*) ólive; 2. (*дерево*) ólive-tree. ~ка *ж.* ólive. ~ковый 1. ólive *attr.*; ~ковая роща ólive grove; 2. (*о цвете*) ólive-green.

олигархия *ж.* óligarchy.

олимпиада *ж.* 1. (*Олимпийские игры*) the Olýmpic Games, the Olýmpics; 2. (*соревнование, смотр*) cóntest, review.

олимпийск|ий Olýmpian; Olýmpic; ◇ Олимпийские игры the Olýmpic Games, the Olýmpics; ~ая деревня Olýmpic víllage; ~ое спокойствие Olýmpian calm.

олифа *ж.* drýing oil.

олицетвор|ение *с.* personificátion, embódiment. ~ённый personified *после сущ.*; он ~ённая доброта, любезность *и т. п.* he is kindness, políteness, *etc.* itsélf; he is the soul of kíndness, políteness, *etc.* ~ить *сов. см.* олицетворять 1, 2.

олицетворять, **олицетворить** (*вн.*) 1. (*представлять в образе живого существа*) pérsonify (*smth.*), embódy (*smth.*); 2. (*воплощать в каком-л. образе*) portráy (*smth.*), creáte (*smth.*); 3. *тк. несов.* (*являться совершенным образцом чего-л.*) pérsonify (*smth.*); ~ собой что-л. be* the embódiment/personificátion of *smth.*

олово *с.* tin.

оловянный tin *attr.*

олух *м. разг.* oaf.

ольх|а *ж.* álder. ~овый álder *attr.*

ольшаник *м.* álder thícket(s).

ом *м. эл.* ohm.

омар *м.* lóbster.

омега *ж.* ómega.

омерз|ение *с.* lóathing. ~ительный lóathsome, revólting; síckening.

омертвелый 1. dead; *мед.* necrótic; 2. (*неподвижный*) fixed, stiff; 3. (*опустевший*) (déathly) still.

омертветь *сов. см.* мертветь 1.

омлет *м.* omelét(te).

омолаживать, **омолодить** (*вн.*) rejúvenate (*smb., smth.*). ~ся, омолодиться rejúvenate.

омолодить(ся) *сов. см.* омолаживать(ся).

омоложение *с. биол.* rejuvenátion.

омоним *м. лингв.* hómonym.

омонимия *ж. лингв.* homónymy.

омрачать, **омрачить** (*вн.*) dárken (*smth.*), cloud (*smth.*); ~ праздничный день cast* gloom óver the festívities. ~ся, омрачиться.

омрачённый glóomy; ничем не ~ unclóuded.

омрачить(ся) *сов. см.* омрачать(ся).

омут *м.* pool; (*водоворот*) whírlpool; *перен.* slough; ◇ в тихом ~е черти водятся *посл.* ≅ still wáters run deep.

омывать, **омыть** (*вн.*) 1. wash (*smth.*); 2. *тк. несов.* (*о реках, морях*) wash (*smth.*), surróund (*smth.*). ~ся *несов.* (*тв.*) be* washed (by).

омыть *сов. см.* омывать 1.

он *личн. мест.* (*рд., вн.* его, него, *дт.* ему, нему, *тв.* им, ним, *пр.* о нём) (*о мужчинах, самцах*) he; (*о младенцах, животных*) it; (*о неодушевлённых предметах*) it; (*о месяце*) it; she *поэт.* (*о судах*) she.

она *личн. мест.* (*рд., вн.* её, неё, *дт.* ей, ней, *тв.* ею, ей, нею, ней, *пр.* о ней) (*о женщинах*) she; (*о жи-*

вотных тж.) it; (*о неодушевлённых предметах*) it; (*о странах*) she, it; (*о луне*) it; she *поэт.*

ондатра *ж.* músk-rat; (*мех*) músquash.

онемелый *разг.* numb(ed).

онеметь *сов. см.* неметь.

они *личн. мест.* (*рд., вн.* их, них, *дт.* им, ним, *тв.* ими, ними, *пр.* о них) they.

онкологический oncológical.

онкология *ж.* oncólogy.

оно *личн. мест.* (*рд., вн.* его, него, *дт.* ему, нему, *тв.* им, ним, *пр.* о нём) it.

опадать, **опасть** 1. fall*; 2. (*уменьшаться в объёме*) subside, go* down; 3. *разг.* (*худеть, вваливаться*) shrink*.

опаздывать, **опоздать** 1. (*на вн.; прибывать позже, чем нужно*) be* late (for); он опоздал на урок he was late for the lésson; ~ на полчаса be* half an hour late; он опоздал на поезд he missed the train; поезд опоздал на два часа the train was two hours late/óverdúe; 2. (*с тв., + инф.; не делать своевременно*) be* late (with); опоздать с отчётом be* late with *one's* repórt.

опаивать, **опоить** (*вн.*) give* (*smb., smth.*) too much to drink; (*чем-л. хмельным тж.*) make* (*smb.*) drunk.

опал *м.* ópal.

опал|а *ж.* disgráce; быть в ~е be* in disgráce.

опаливать, **опалить** (*вн.*) singe (*smth.*).

опалить *сов. см.* опаливать, опалять и палить I 1.

опальный disgráced.

опалять, **опалить** (*вн.*) sear (*smth.*), scorch (*smth.*).

опара *ж.* léavened dough.

опаршиветь *сов. см.* паршиветь.

опас|аться *несов.* (*рд.*) 1. (*бояться*) fear (*smb., smth.*); 2. (*остерегаться*) be* cáreful (of); вам надо ~ простуды be cáreful not to catch cold. ~ение *с.* apprehénsion, misgíving; есть ~ение, что... it is feared that...; вызывать ~ения cause misgívings.

опаск|а *ж. разг.*: с ~ой nérvously, cáutiously; без ~и withóut any misgívings.

опасн|о 1. *нареч.* dángerously; 2. *в знач. сказ.* it is dángerous. ~ость *ж.* dánger; в ~ости in dánger/péril; с ~остью для жизни at the risk of *one's* life; отвратить ~ость avért a dánger, ward off a dánger. ~ый dángerous; (*о путешествии и т. п. тж.*) périlous; ~ый участок пути dángerous séction of the road; ~ая переправа périlous cróssing; ~ый преступник dángerous críminal; ~ое заболевание dángerous íllness.

опасть *сов. см.* опадать.

опека *ж.* 1. guárdianship, wárdship; (*над имуществом*) trustéeship; 2. *собир.* (*опекуны*) guárdians *pl*, Board of guárdians; 3. (*забота*) care; survéillance; tútelage.

опекать *несов.* (*вн.*) 1. be* the guárdian (of); 2. (*заботиться*) watch (óver), take* care (of).

опекун *м.* guárdian.

опёнок *м.* hóney ágaric.

опера *ж.* ópera.

оперативн|о: действовать ~ act prómptly. ~ость *ж.* efféctiveness, prómptitude. ~ый 1. (*хирургический*) óperative; ~ое вмешательство súrgical intervéntion; 2. *воен.* operátional; operátion(s) *attr.*; ~ое искусство strátegy, campáign táctics; ~ая сводка operátions súmmary; 3. (*гибкий, действенный*) efféctive, prompt, efficient; 4. (*практически осуществляющий что-л.*) operátions *attr.*; ~ый отдел operátions séction; ~ая группа (*штаба*) operátions group; (*тактическая*) task force.

оператор *м.* óperator; (*в кино тж.*) cámeraman*.

операционн|ая *ж.* óperating-room, óperating-theatre. ~ый стол óperating-table.

операци|я *ж.* operátion; *воен.* (stratégic) operátion; сделать ~ю perfórm an operátion; десантная ~ lánding operátion; финáнсовые ~и fináncial operátions.

опереди́ть *сов. см.* опережа́ть.

опережа́|ть, опереди́ть (*вн.*) 1. (*обгонять*) overtáke* (*smb., smth.*), leave* (*smb., smth.*) behínd; 2. (*делать что-л. раньше другого*) forestáll (*smb.*), antícipate (*smb.*); get* one's blow in first *разг.*; 3. (*превосходить*) surpáss (*smb., smth.*), excél (*smb., smth.*).

опере́ние *с.* plúmage; ◇ хвостово́е ~ самолёта tail únit.

опере́т|ка *ж. разг. см.* опере́тта. ~очный músical--cómedy *attr.*; ~очный актёр músical-cómedy áctor.

опере́тта *ж.* operétta; músical, músical cómedy.

опере́ться *сов. см.* опира́ться.

опери́ровать *несов.* 1. *тж. сов.* (*вн.*) óperate (on); ~ больно́го óperate on a pátient; ~ желу́док óperate on the stómach; 2. (*тв.; пользоваться чем-л.*) use (*smth.*); ~ фа́ктами use facts; ~ ци́фрами use fígures.

опери́ться *сов. см.* опера́ться.

о́перн|ый о́пера *attr.*, operátic; ~ая а́рия ária, song from ópera; ~ певе́ц ópera-singer; ~ теа́тр ópera-house; ~ая сце́на operátic stage.

опери́ться, опери́ться (*тв.*) feather, be* full-flédged; *перен.* matúre, find* one's feet.

опеча́л|енный sad, despóndent; (*тв.*) distréssed (by). ~ить(ся) *сов. см.* печа́лить(ся).

опеча́тать *сов. см.* опеча́тывать.

опеча́т|ка *ж.* mísprint; спи́сок ~ок (list of) erráta.

опеча́тывать, опеча́тать (*вн.*) seal (*smth.*).

опе́шить *сов. разг.* be* táken abáck.

опива́ться, опи́ться (*тв.*) drink*/have* too much (*smth.*).

опи́лки *мн.* sáwdust *sg*; (*металлические*) fílings.

опира́ться, опере́ться (на *вн.*) 1. lean* (on); ~ на чью́-л. ру́ку lean* on *smb.'s* arm; 2. (*находить себе поддержку в ком-л.*) relý (on); (*брать что-л. за осно́ву своих рассуждений*) base onesélf (on); ~ на ма́ссы relý upón the másses; ~ на фа́кты base onesélf on facts.

описа́ние *с.* descríption.

опи́санный *мат.* círcumscribed.

описа́тельный descríptive.

описа́ть *сов. см.* опи́сывать. ~ся *сов.* make* a slip in wríting.

опи́ска *ж.* slip (of the pen), mistáke in wríting.

опи́сывать, описа́ть (*вн.*) 1. descríbe (*smth.*); (*литературно тж.*) depíct (*smth.*); 2. *мат.* círcumscribe (*smth.*); 3. (*составлять перечень чего-л.*) make* an invéntory (of); 4. (*имущество*) arrést (*smth.*), seize (*smth.*); 5. (*совершать движение по кривой*) descríbe (*smth.*); ~ круг descríbe a círcle.

о́пись *ж.* 1. (*действие*) séizure; ~ имущества (*за долги*) séizure; 2. (*перечень вещей, бумаг и т. п.*) invéntory.

опи́ться *сов. см.* опива́ться.

о́пиум *м.* ópium.

опла́кать *сов. см.* опла́кивать.

опла́кивать, опла́кать (*вн.*) mourn (for, óver), weep* (for), bewáil the loss (of).

опла́т|а *ж.* páyment. ~ить *сов. см.* опла́чивать.

опла́ченн|ый paid for *после сущ.*; телегра́мма с ~ым отве́том replý-paid télegram.

опла́чиваемый paid; ~ о́тпуск paid hóliday, hóliday with pay.

опла́чивать, оплати́ть (*вн.*) pay* (*smb., smth.*); ~ чьи́-л. услу́ги pay* *smb.* for his, her sérvices; ~ счёт pay* a bill; оплати́ть расхо́ды по командиро́вке pay* trávelling expénses.

оплеу́ха *ж. разг.* box on the ear; *перен.* slap in the face.

оплеши́веть *сов. см.* плеши́веть.

оплодотвор|е́ние *с.* fertilizátion. ~и́ть *сов. см.* оплодотворя́ть.

оплодотворя́ть, оплодотвори́ть (*вн.*) fértilize (*smth.*).

оплóт *м.* strónghold, búlwark.

опло́ш|а́ть *сов. разг.* make* a blúnder; смотри́, не ~а́й! mind you don't slip up!

опло́шност|ь *ж.* cárelessness, slip, inadvértence; допусти́ть ~ make* a slip; по ~и out of cárelessness.

оповести́ть *сов. см.* оповеща́ть.

оповещ|а́ть, оповести́ть (*вн.*) nótify (*smb.*), infórm (*smb.*). ~е́ние *с.* notificátion.

опозда́ни|е *с.* láteness, béing late; *мн.* únpunctuálity *sg*; без ~я púnctually; on time; пóезд идёт без ~я the train is on time; с ~ем на 10 мину́т ten mínutes late; идти́, прийти́ с (больши́м) ~ем be* (véry) late; уйти́ с (больши́м) ~ем start (véry) late.

опозда́ть *сов. см.* опа́здывать.

опознава́тельн|ый: ~ые огни́ recognítion/identificátion lights; ~ знак márking.

опозн|ава́ть, опозна́ть (*вн.*) idéntify (*smb., smth.*). ~а́ние *с.* identificátion.

опозна́ть *сов. см.* опознава́ть.

опозо́рить(ся) *сов. см.* позо́рить(ся).

опо́йть *сов. см.* опа́ивать.

опола́скивать, ополосну́ть (*вн.*) rinse (*smth.*). ~ся, ополосну́ться *разг.* have* a (bit of a) wash.

ополза́ть, оползти́ (*оседать*) slip.

о́ползень *м.* lándslip, lándslide.

оползти́ *сов. см.* ополза́ть.

ополосну́ть(ся) *сов. см.* опола́скивать(ся).

ополча́ться, ополчи́ться (на *вн.*, про́тив *рд.*) be* up in arms (agáinst).

ополче́н|ец *м.* mémber of the emérgency voluntéer corps. ~ие *с.* emérgency voluntéer corps.

ополчи́ться *сов. см.* ополча́ться.

опо́мниться *сов.* 1. (*прийти в сознание*) come* to one's sénses; (*прийти в себя*) recóver/gáther one's wits; 2. (*одуматься*) come* to one's sénses; опо́мнитесь! think!

опо́р *м.*: мча́ться во весь ~ gállop at top speed.

опо́р|а *ж.* suppórt; (*моста*) pier; *перен.* (*поддержка, помощь*) stánd-by; тóчка ~ы (*рычага*) fúlcrum; *перен.* básis, firm ground, fóothold.

опора́жнивать, опоро́жни́ть (*вн.*) émpty (*smth.*), drain (*smth.*).

опо́рн|ый suppórting, béaring; ~ая плита́ báse-plate; ~ая пове́рхность béaring área/súrface; ~ пункт *воен.* strong point.

опоро́жн|и́ть *сов. см.* опора́жнивать. ~я́ть *несов. см.* опора́жнивать.

опоро́с *м. с.-х.* fárrow. ~и́ться *сов. см.* пороси́ться.

опоро́чить *сов. см.* поро́чить.

опо́ссум *м. зоол.* opóssum, póssum *амер.*

опохмели́ться *сов. см.* опохмеля́ться.

опохмеля́ться, опохмели́ться *разг.* take* a drink to cure a háng-over; take* a hair of the dog that bit you *идиом.*

опо́шлить(ся) *сов. см.* опошля́ть(ся).

опошл|я́ть, опо́шлить (*вн.*) 1. (*делать пошлым*) vúlgarize (*smth., smb.*), trívialize (*smth., smb.*), chéapen (*smth., smb.*); 2. (*делать избитым*) make* (*smth.*) trite, deface (*smth.*) by óveruse, debáse (*smth.*). ~ся, опо́шлиться 1. becóme* vúlgar/cheap; 2. (*становиться избитым*) becóme* trite.

опоя́сать(ся) *сов. см.* опоя́сывать(ся).

опоя́сывать, опоя́сать (*вн.*) 1. (*надевать на кого-л. пояс*) belt (*smb.*), gírdle (*smb.*); 2. (*окружать собой*) encírcle (*smth.*), engírdle (*smth.*). ~ся, опоя́саться (*тв.*) 1. gird* onesélf (with); опоя́саться ремнём put* on one's belt; 2. (*окружать себя чем-л.*) acquíre a círcle (of), be* círcled (by).

оппозицио́нн|ый opposítion *attr.*; ~ая па́ртия opposítion párty; ~ые настрое́ния mood of opposítion *sg*, hóstile áttitudes.

оппози́ци|я ж. opposítion; быть в ~и к кому-л., чему-л. be* oppósed to smb., smth.

оппоне́нт м. oppónent.

оппортун|и́зм м. tíme-serving, ópportunism. ~и́ст м. tíme-server, ópportunist. ~исти́ческий ópportunist attr.

опра́в|а ж. móunting, sétting; (очков) frame; rims pl; тех. hólder; вставля́ть что-л. в ~у mount smth.; в золото́й ~e set in gold; (об очках) góld-rimmed.

оправда́|ние с. 1. justificátion; 2. юр. acquíttal; 3. (объяснение, извинение) excúse; что вы мо́жете сказа́ть в своё ~? what have you to say for yoursélf? ~тельный: ~тельный пригово́р vérdict of nót-guílty; ~тельный докуме́нт cóvering vóucher.

оправда́ть сов. см. опра́вдывать. ~ся сов. см. опра́вдываться 1, 2, 4.

опра́вдыв|ать, оправда́ть (вн.) 1. (доказывать чью-л. правоту) jústify (smth.); (подсудимого) acquít (smth.), judge (smth.) not guílty; 2. (извинять что-л.) excúse (smth.); jústify (smth.); 3. (быть достойным чего-л.) wárrant (smth.); оправда́ть свою́ репута́цию live up to one's reputátion; оправда́ть чьи-л. наде́жды come* up to smb.'s expectátions; не оправда́ть чьих-л. наде́жд fall* short of smb.'s expectátions; ~ чьё-л. дове́рие jústify smb.'s cónfidence; 4. (возмещать) cóver (smth.); оправда́ть расхо́ды cóver expénses. ~аться, оправда́ться 1. clear onesélf; 2. (подтверждаться на деле) prove to be corréct; (сбываться) come* true; 3. тк. несов. (объяснять свои поступки) defénd onesélf; (ссылаться) make* excúses; он ~ался тем, что по́езд опозда́л he excúsed himsélf by sáying the train was late; 4. (окупаться) be* wárranted.

опра́вить I, II сов. см. оправля́ть I, II.

опра́виться сов. см. оправля́ться.

оправля́ть I, опра́вить (вн.) (платье) adjúst (smth.), smooth (smth.); (постель) make* (smth.).

оправля́ть II, опра́вить (вн.) set* (smth.), mount (smth.); ~ драгоце́нный ка́мень set* a jéwel.

оправля́ться, опра́виться 1. (приводить в порядок свой туалет, причёску) make* onesélf tidy; 2. (после болезни) recóver.

опра́шивать, опроси́ть (вн.) quéstion (smb.); (население) poll (smb.).

определе́ние с. 1. (установление чего-л.) determinátion; 2. (формулировка) definítion; 3. грам. áttribute; 4. юр. rúling, decísion.

определённо| definitely; он ~ придёт he is sure to come; я ~ зна́ю I know for a fact. ~ость ж. clárity; définiteness. ~ый 1. (установленный) appóinted; в ~ое вре́мя at the appóinted time; 2. (отчётливый, ясный) définite; 3. (некоторый) cértain; при ~ых усло́виях únder cértain condítions; 4. разг. (несомненный) undóubted.

определи́ть(ся) сов. см. определя́ть(ся).

определя́ть, определи́ть (вн.) 1. (устанавливать, обусловливать) detérmine (smth.); ~ направле́ние ве́тра detérmine/tell* the diréction of the wind; ~ боле́знь give* a diagnósis; ~ расстоя́ние на глаз judge the distance; 2. (давать определение) defíne (smth.); 3. (назначать) appóint (smb., smth.), fix (smth.). ~ся, определи́ться 1. (выявляться) be* cléarly defíned; (о характере тж.) form, take* shape; 2. (определять местонахождение) find* one's posítion.

опресни́ть сов. см. опресня́ть.

опресня́ть, опресни́ть (вн.) distíl (smth.).

опробовать сов. (вн.) test (smth.).

опроверга́ть, опрове́ргнуть (вн.) refúte (smth.).

опрове́ргнуть сов. см. опроверга́ть.

опроверже́ние с. refutátion; (отрицание) deníal, disclаimer; помести́ть ~ в газе́те públish a deníal.

опроки́дывать, опроки́нуть (вн.) 1. upsét* (smth.), overtúrn (smth.); (судно) capsíze (smth.); (сбивать с ног) knock (smb.) óver; 2. (заставлять беспорядочно

отступать) rout (smth.), knock out (smth.); 3. (лишать прежнего значения) overthrów* (smth.), do* awáy with (smth.), explóde (smth.). ~ся, опроки́нуться overtúrn; (о судне) capsíze; (падать) fall* óver báckwards.

опроки́нуть(ся) сов. см. опроки́дывать(ся).

опроме́тчив|ость ж. 1. (необдуманность) hástiness, impúlsiveness; 2. (опрометчивый поступок) blúnder. ~ый hásty, impúlsive, rash, precípitate, ill-consídered.

о́прометью héadlong.

опро́с м. quéstioning; ~ свиде́телей quéstioning of wítnesses; ~ населе́ния opínion poll.

опроси́ть сов. см. опра́шивать.

опро́сный: ~ лист questionnáire.

опротестова́ть сов. см. опротесто́вывать.

опротесто́вывать, опротестова́ть (вн.) 1. юр. appéal (agáinst); опротестова́ть реше́ние суда́ appéal agáinst a court decísion; 2. торг. protést (smth.); опротестова́ть ве́ксель protést a bill.

опроти́в|еть сов. (дт.) becóme* distásteful (to), pall (on); мне э́то ~ело I'm sick of it.

опры́скать сов. см. опры́скивать.

опры́скивать, опры́скать (вн.) (be)sprínkle (smth.), spray (smth.); ~ фрукто́вые дере́вья spray frúit-trees.

опря́тн|ость ж. tídiness, néatness. ~ый tídy, neat, clean.

о́птик м. optícian.

о́птика ж. 1. (отдел физики) óptics; 2. собир. (приборы и т. п.) óptical apparátus.

оптима́льный óptimum attr., óptimal.

оптим|и́зм м. óptimism. ~и́ст м. óptimist. ~исти́ческий optimístic.

опти́ческий óptical.

о́пт|овый whólesale; ~ая торго́вля whólesale trade; ~ые це́ны whólesale príces.

о́птом whólesale; ~ и в ро́зницу whólesale and retáil.

опубликов|а́ние с. publicátion; (закона) promulgátion. ~а́ть сов. см. опублико́вывать и публикова́ть.

опублико́вывать, опубликова́ть (вн.) públish (smth.); (закон) prómulgate (smth.).

опуска́ть, опусти́ть 1. (вн.) lówer (smth.); (ставить) put* (smth.) down; ~ глаза́ lówer/drop one's eyes; опусти́в глаза́ with dówncast eyes; ~ го́лову hang* one's head; опусти́в го́лову with one's head down; ~ што́ру pull down the blind; ~ (вн. в; погружать) put* (smth. into), lówer (smth. into); ~ письмо́ в почто́вый я́щик drop/put* a létter into the box; ~ гроб в моги́лу lówer a cóffin into a grave; 3. (вн.; пропускать) omít (smth.), leave* out (smth.). ~ся, опусти́ться 1. go* down; (о голове) sink*; перен. fall*, descénd; ~ся на коле́ни kneel*, go* down on one's knees; 2. (перемещаться сверху вниз) drop, come* down; 3. (морально) let* onesélf go/slíde; go* to seed.

опусте́лый desérted.

опусте́ть сов. см. пусте́ть.

опусти́вшийся degráded.

опусти́ть(ся) сов. см. опуска́ть(ся).

опусто́ш|а́ть, опустоши́ть (вн.) 1. (разорять) dévastate (smth.), rávage (smth.), lay* (smth.) waste; 2. разг. (опорожнять) émpty (smth.); 3. (нравственно) drain smb.'s spírit. ~е́ние с. devastátion; мн. rávages. ~ённость ж. émptiness; вну́тренняя ~ённость spíritual émptiness. ~ённый bróken, dispírited. ~и́тельный dévastating.

опустоши́ть сов. см. опустоша́ть.

опу́тать сов. см. опу́тывать.

опу́тывать, опу́тать (вн.) entángle (smth.); перен. тж. ensnáre (smb.).

опуха́ть, опу́хнуть swell*.

опу́хнуть сов. см. опуха́ть.

о́пухоль ж. swélling; (внутренняя) túmour.

опушённый trimmed; ~ мéхом fúr-trimmed; ~ снéгом pówdered with snow.

опýшка I ж. (*леса*) edge (of the fórest).

опýшка II ж. (*отдéлка*) trímming.

опущéние с. 1. (*прóпуск*) omíssion; 2. мед. prolápsus.

опыл|éние с. бот. pollinátion. ~йть сов. см. опылять.

опылять, опылйть (вн.) бот. póllinate (*smth.*).

óпыт м. 1. expérience; (*знáние дéла*) knów-how; житéйский ~ knówledge of the world; убедйться на сóбственном ~e learn* from *one's* own expérience; ~ новáторов произвóдства the knów-how of wórker ínnovators; чýвственный ~ филос. sénsory/sénsual expérience; 2. (*эксперимéнт*) expériment; 3. (*попытка*) attémpt, try.

óпыт|ость ж. expérience. ~ый 1. (*имéющий óпыт*) expérienced; 2. (*служáщий для óпыта, оснóванный на óпыте*) experiméntal; (*прóбный*) test attr.; trial attr.; pílot attr.; доказáть что-л. ~ым путём prove *smth.* by means of expériment; ~ый учáсток experiméntal plot.

опьянéние с. intoxicátion.

опьянéть сов. см. пьянéть.

опьянйть сов. см. опьянять и пьянйть.

опьянять, опьянйть (вн.) intóxicate (*smb.*); перен. тж. exhílarate (*smb.*).

опять agáin; ◊ ~ двáдцать пять! the same old thing!

орáва ж. разг. mob, gang, horde.

орáкул м. óracle.

орангутáнг м. orangután(g).

орáнжевый órange(-cóloured).

оранжерéйн|ый hóthouse attr.; ~ые растéния hóthouse plants.

оранжерéя ж. consérvatory, hóthouse, gréenhouse.

орáтор м. spéaker; órator; предыдýщий ~ the prévious/last spéaker.

оратóрия ж. муз. oratório (pl -os).

орáторск|ий oratórical; ~ое искýсство the art of públic-spéaking; ~ талáнт gift of óratory.

орáторствовать несов. разг. ирон. hold* forth, oráte; ~ перед кем-л. harángue smb.

орáть несов. разг. 1. yell, bawl; (*от бóли тж.*) scream; (*о птйцах*) shriek; (*о живóтных*) roar, snort; (*ревéть — о ребёнке*) squawl, yell; (*говорйть слйшком грóмко*) shout; ~ во всё гóрло shout at the top of *one's* voice; 2. (*на вн.; ругáть когó-л.*) shout (at).

орбйт|а ж. órbit; на ~e in órbit; вывести корáбль на ~y put* a spáceship into órbit. ~áльный órbital; ~áльная стáнция órbital státion.

орг- в слож. organizátional, órganizing.

óрган м. 1. órgan; ~ы слýха órgans of héaring; ~ы кровообращéния círculatory órgans; 2. (*учреждéние*) bódy; ágency амер.; ~ы влáсти, руководящие ~ы the authórities; исполнйтельный ~ exécutive bódy; ~ы слéдствия invéstigating bódies/ágencies; 3. (*печáтное издáние*) órgan, publicátion.

оргáн м. муз. órgan.

организáтор м. órganizer; (*инициáтор тж.*) spónsor. ~ский órganizing; ~ский талáнт gift for órganizing; ~ские спосóбности órganizing ability sg.

организацióнн|ый órganizing; ~ комитéт órganizing committee; ~ перйод organizátion périod; ~ые вопрóсы próblems of organizátion, organizátional mátters.

организáция ж. organizátion; Организáция Объединённых Нáций United Nátions Organizátion.

организм м. órganism; (*человéка тж.*) constitútion.

организóванн|о in an órganized fáshion/mánner, on a planned básis; ~ проводйть óтдых have* a well--órganized hóliday, órganize *one's* léisure. ~ость ж. good organizátion; ~ый órganized; ~ые дéйствия órganized áction sg; ~ый человéк efficient/well-órganized pérson.

организов|áть несов. и сов. (вн.) órganize (*smb.*, *smth.*); ~ спортйвное óбщество órganize a sports society.

~áться несов. и сов. 1. (*возникáть*) be* órganized; 2. (*объединяться*) órganize (*onesélf*), get* órganized.

организм м. órganist.

органйчески orgánically; ~ неспосóбный к чемý-л. constitútionally incápable of *smth.*

органйческ|ий I (*живóй*) orgánic; ~ мир the orgánic world; ~ие удобрéния orgánic fértilizers; ◊ ~ая хймия orgánic chémistry.

органйческ|ий II (*касáющийся внýтреннего стрóения óрганов человéка*) orgánic; перен. тж. fundaméntal; ~ порóк сéрдца orgánic deféct of the heart.

óргия ж. órgy.

орграбóта ж. (организацióнная рабóта) organizátional work.

ордá ж. horde.

óрден м. 1. (*мн. орденá*) (*знак отлйчия*) órder, decorátion; ~ Крáсного Знáмени Órder of the Red Bánner; наградйть когó-л. ~ом dec.órate *smb.*; представить когó-л. к ~y recommend *smb.* for a decorátion; 2. (*мн. óрдены и орденá*) (*организáция*) órder; ~ иезуйтов the Órder of Jésuits.

óрденонóс|ец м. hólder of an Órder; ~ный hólding an Órder/decorátion пóсле сущ.

óрденск|ий médal attr.; ~ая лéнта médal ríbbon.

óрдер м. (*докумéнт*) wárrant, vóucher; ~ на жилплóщадь wárrant for living accommodátion; прихóдный ~ recéipt vóucher; crédit slip разг.; расхóдный ~ expénditure vóucher; débit slip разг.

ординáрец м. воен. órderly.

ординáрный órdinary.

ординáта ж. мат. órdinate.

орёл м. éagle; ◊ ~ йли рéшка ≈ heads or tails.

орeóл м. hálo; перен. áura.

орéх м. 1. (*плод*) nut; (*грéцкий*) wálnut; 2. тк. ед. (*дéрево*) nút-tree; 3. тк. ед. (*древесйна*) wálnut; ◊ емý достáлось на ~и he got it hot.

орéхов|ый 1. nut attr.; ~ая рóща wálnut grove; ~ торт wálnut cake; 2. (*из орéхового дéрева*) wálnut attr.; ~ая мéбель wálnut fúrniture.

оригинáл м. 1. oríginal; 2. разг. (*чудáк*) crank, eccéntric.

оригинáль|ничать несов. разг. try to be oríginal. ~ный 1. oríginal; 2. (*пóдлинный*) génuine.

ориентáция ж. orientátion.

ориентйр м. lándmark, réference point. ~ный: ~ная кáрта sketch map.

ориентйровать несов. и сов. 1. (вн.) tell* (*smb.*) his, her position/whéreabouts; (*прáвильно направлять прибóр*) órientate (*smth.*); 2. (вн.; помогáть разобрáться) órientate (*smb.*), put* (*smb.*) on the right track, help (*smb.*) to find his, her béarings; 3. (вн. на вн.; нацéливать) órientate (*smb.* towárds + -ing), give* (*smb.*) a lead (towárds + -ing); ~ когó-л. на испóльзование мéстных ресýрсов órientate smb. towárds úsing lócal resóurces. ~ся несов. и сов. 1. find* *one's* way; get* *one's* béarings; (*тж. перен.*); хорошó ~ся в лесý be* good at finding *one's* way in a fórest; 2. (*на вн.; определять направлéние свéей дéятельности*) be* órientated (towárds), lean* (towárds); ~ся на мáссового читáтеля aim at the broad réading públic.

ориентирóвка ж. gétting *one's* béarings.

ориентирóвочн|о as a géneral guide; (*приблизйтельно*) appróximately. ~ый 1. réference attr.; ~ый пункт réference point; 2. (*приблизйтельный*) téntative; ~ые срóки téntative tíme-limits.

оркéстр м. (*симфонйческий*) órchestra; (*духовóй, джаз*) band.

оркéстр|áнт м. mémber of an órchestra, orchéstral pl'áyer. ~овáть несов. и сов. (вн.) órchestrate (*smth.*). ~óвка ж. orchestrátion.

орлёнок _м._ éaglet.

орли́н|ый éagle's; _перен._ éagle _attr._; ~ое гнездо́ éagle's nest, éyrie; ~ взгляд éagle eye; ◇ ~ нос áquiline nose.

орли́ца _ж._ fémale éagle.

орна́мент _м._ órnament.

орнито́з _м. мед._ ornithósis (_pl_ -ses).

орнито́лог _м._ ornithólogist.

орнитоло́гия _ж._ ornithólogy.

оробе́ть _сов._ get* shy, feel* intímidated.

ороси́тель|ый irrigátion _attr._, irrigátory; ~ые рабо́ты irrigátion work _sg_; ~ кана́л irrigátion canál; ~ая систе́ма irrigátion sýstem.

ороси́ть _сов. см._ ороша́ть.

орош|а́ть, ороси́ть (_вн._) 1. sprínkle (_smth._); 2. (_почву_) wáter (_smth._), írrigate (_smth._). ~е́ние _с._ wátering, irrigátion.

ортодокса́льный órthodox.

ортопеди́ческ|ий orthopáedic; ~ая о́бувь orthopáedic fóotwear.

ору́ди|е _с._ 1. (_труда_) tool, ínstrument (_тж. перен._); сельскохозя́йственные ~я agricúltural ímplements/ equípment; ~я произво́дства ínstruments of prodúction; послу́шное ~ в рука́х кого́-л. convénient tool/ínstrument in the hands of _smb._; 2. (_артиллери́йское_) gun, piece (for órdnance).

оруди́йный gun _attr._; ~ залп sálvo; ~ расчёт gun crew.

ору́д|овать _несов. разг._ 1. (_тв._) use (_smth._); (_распоряжа́ться_) boss (_smth._); ~ топоро́м use/wield an axe; 2. (_де́йствовать_) be* at work; здесь ~овал о́пытный жу́лик an expérienced thief has been at work here.

оруже́йник _м._ gúnsmith.

ору́жи|е _с._ wéapon; _собир._ arms _pl_, wéapons _pl_; _перен._ wéapon, ínstrument; ~ ма́ссового уничтоже́ния wéapons of mass destrúction/exterminátion; к ~ю! to arms!; бить проти́вника его́ же ~ем beat*/fight* the énemy with his own wéapons.

орфографи́ческ|ий spélling _attr._; ~ая оши́бка spélling mistáke.

орфогра́фия _ж._ spélling.

орфоэпи́ческий orthoépic; ~ слова́рь pronóuncing díctionary.

орфоэ́пия _ж._ orthóepy.

орхиде́я _ж._ órchid.

оса́ _ж._ wasp.

оса́да _ж._ siege.

осади́ть I _сов. см._ осажда́ть I.

осади́ть II _сов. см._ осажда́ть II.

осади́ть III _сов. см._ оса́живать.

оса́дк|а _ж._ 1. (_почвы, сооруже́ния_) subsídence; дать ~у subsíde; 2. _мор._ draught; име́ть ~у 3 ме́тра draw* ten feet.

оса́дки _мн._ precipitátion _sg_; ожида́ются ~ в ви́де дождя́ и сне́га rain and some snow are expécted.

оса́дн|ый siege _attr._; ~ое положе́ние state of siege.

оса́док _м._ sédiment, depósit; _перен._ (áfter)taste; у меня́ оста́лся неприя́тный ~ от на́шего разгово́ра our talk left an unpléasant áftertaste.

оса́дочный sediméntary.

осажда́ть I, осади́ть (_вн.; подверга́ть оса́де_) besíege (_smth._); lay* siege (to); _перен._ besíege (_smb., smth._); ~ го́род besíege a town.

осажда́ть II, осади́ть (_вн._) _хим._ precípitate (_smth._). ~ся _несов. хим._ séttle, be* depósited.

осажд|а́ющий _м._ besíeger. ~ённый beléaguered; besíeged (_тж. перен._).

оса́живать, осади́ть 1. (_вн._) rein in (_smth._), check (_smth._); 2. (_ре́зко останови́ться — о ло́шади, зве́ре_) stop; 3. (_вн.; заста́вить попяти́ться наза́д_) force (_smb., smth._) back; 4. (_вн.; одёргивать кого́-л._) rebúff (_smb._), snub (_smb._); put* (_smb._) in his, her place.

оса́н|истый impósing, státely. ~ка _ж._ cárriage, béaring.

осва́ивать, осво́ить (_вн._) 1. máster (_smth._); ~ о́пыт кого́-л. prófit by the expérience of _smb._; ~ но́вые ме́тоды произво́дства máster new méthods of prodúction; 2. (_обжива́ть_) devélop (_smth._), pionéer (_smth._), séttle (_smth._); ~ цели́нные зе́мли devélop the vírgin lands, bring* the vírgin lands ínto cultivátion. ~ся, осво́иться séttle down; (с _тв._) get* used (to); (_постига́ть_) have* (_smth._) at one's fíngertips/fínger-ends.

осведоми́тель _м._ infórmer. ~ный infórmative.

осве́домить(ся) _сов. см._ осведомля́ть(ся).

осведомл|е́ние _с._ informátion, notificátion. ~ённый (well-)infórmed; пло́хо ~ённый ill-infórmed.

осведомл|я́ть, осве́домить (_вн. о пр._) infórm (_smb._ of), nótify (_smb._ of). ~ся, осве́домиться (о _пр._) inquíre (abóut), make* inquíries (abóut).

освеж|а́ть, освежи́ть (_вн._) 1. refrésh (_smb., smth._); fréshen (_smth._); дождь освежи́л во́здух the rain has fréshened the air; бы́страя езда́ освежи́ла его́ the fast ride cleared his head; ~ в па́мяти что́-л. refrésh one's mémory of _smth._; освежи́ть свои́ зна́ния rub/brush up one's knówledge; 2. (_подновля́ть_) touch up (_smth._). ~ся, освежи́ться 1. be* refréshed; 2. (_о челове́ке_) refrésh onesélf.

освежева́ть _сов. см._ свежева́ть.

освежи́ть(ся) _сов. см._ освежа́ть(ся).

освети́тель|ый illúminating, líghting; ~ прибо́р illúminator, líghting applíance; ~ые раке́ты flares.

освети́ть(ся) _сов. см._ освеща́ть(ся).

освещ|а́ть, освети́ть (_вн._) 1. light* up (_smth._), illúminate (_smth._), illúmine (_smth._); _перен._ (_оживля́ть_) bríghten (_smth._); взошло́ со́лнце и я́рко освети́ло сад the rísing sun bathed the gárden in light; освети́ть часы́ спи́чкой light* a match to look at one's watch; ~ у́лицы электри́чеством províde eléctric stréet-lighting; улы́бка освети́ла её лицо́ her face bríghtened with a smile; 2. (_излага́ть, истолко́вывать_) elúcidate (_smth._), illúminate (_smth._), intérpret (_smth._); по-но́вому ~ вопро́с cast* a new light on a próblem. ~а́ться, освети́ть(ся) be* líghted, be* illúmined; (_о лице́_) light* up. ~е́ние _с._ 1. (_де́йствие_) líghting; вече́рнее ~ние the évening light; иску́сственное ~ние artifícial líghting; 3. (_объясне́ние, толкова́ние_) presentátion, interpretátion; 4. (_обору́дование_) líghting; электри́ческое ~ние eléctric light(ing).

освиде́тельствов|ание _с._ examinátion. ~ать _сов._ (_вн._) exámine (_smb._).

освиста́ть _сов. см._ освистывать.

осви́стывать, освиста́ть (_вн._) hiss (_smb._); ~ актёра hiss an áctor.

освободи́тель _м._ líberator. ~ный líberating; liberátion _attr._; ~ное движе́ние liberátion móvement; ~ная война́ war of liberátion.

освободи́ть(ся) _сов. см._ освобожда́ть(ся).

освобожд|а́ть, освободи́ть 1. (_вн.; предоставля́ть свобо́ду_) free (_smb., smth._), líberate (_smb., smth._), set* (_smb., smth._) free, set* (_smb._) at líberty; (_от ра́бства_) emáncipate (_smb._); (_из тюрьмы́_) dischárge (_smb._); ~ военнопле́нных líberate/free prísoners of war; 2. (_вн.; высвобожда́ть_) reléase (_smb., smth._); _перен. тж._ give* (_smb._) his, her fréedom; освободи́ть зве́ря из капка́на reléase an ánimal from a trap; 3. (_вн. от рд.; избавля́ть_) exémpt (_smb._ from), reléase (_smb._ from); освободи́ть кого́-л. от наказа́ния exémpt _smb._ from púnishment; 4. (_вн.; отстраня́ть_) reléase (_smb._); 5. (_вн.; очища́ть, опорожня́ть_) clear (_smth._); освободи́ть кни́жный шкаф clear a bóokcase; освободи́ть помеще́ние от посторо́нних clear the prémises (of all unáuthorized pérsons); 6. (_вн.; покида́ть что́-л._) vacáte (_smth._), leave* (_smth._); ~ ко́мнату vacáte one's room; 7. (_вн.; вре́мя для чего́-л._) set* aside (_smth._). ~а́ться, освободи́ться 1. free one*sélf, líberate one*sélf; освободи́ться из плёна be* reléased; 2. (от *рд.*; *избавля́ться*) free one*sélf (from); 3. (*станови́ться пусты́м*) be* émpty; (*о помеще́нии тж.*) be* vácant; (*очища́ться от чего́-л.*) clear, be* cleared; не́бо освободи́лось от туч the sky cleared; 4. (*располага́ть вре́менем*) be* free; я сейча́с освобожу́сь I'll be free in a mínute. ~е́ние *с.* liberátion; (*от гнёта, эксплуата́ции тж.*) emancipátion; (*из тюрьмы́*) reléase, dischárge.

освое́ни|е *с.* 1. mástering, assimilátion; ~ совреме́нных маши́н mástering the use of úp-to-dáte machínery; пери́од ~я bréaking-in périod; 2. (*обжива́ние*) devélopment, pionéering, séttling; ~ пусты́ни reclamátion of the désert.

осво́ить(ся) *сов. см.* осва́ивать(ся).

освяти́ть *сов. см.* освяща́ть.

освяща́ть, освяти́ть (*вн.*) sánctify (*smth.*), hállow (*smth.*).

оседа́ть, осе́сть séttle; (*о гру́нте*) subsíde.

оседла́ть *сов. см.* осёдлывать *и* седла́ть.

осёдлость *ж.* séttled way of life.

осёдлывать, оседла́ть (*вн.*) sáddle (*smth.*); *разг.* (*надева́ть очки́*) put* (*smth.*) on, fix (*smth.*) on; *разг.* (*сади́ться верхо́м на что́-л.*) stráddle (*smth.*); *перен. разг.* (*подчиня́ть себе́*) dóminate (*smth.*), sáddle (*smth.*).

осёдл|ый séttled; вести́ ~ о́браз жи́зни lead* a séttled life; ~ые племена́ tribes that have séttled.

осека́ться, осе́чься stop short; (*о го́лосе*) fail, break* off.

осёл *м.* dónkey; ass (*тж. бран.*).

осело́к *м.* 1. (*точи́льный*) whétstone, hone; 2. (*ка́мень для испыта́ния драгоце́нных мета́ллов*) tóuchstone (*тж. перен.*).

осени́ть *сов. см.* осеня́ть.

осе́нний áutumn *attr.*; autúmnal *поэт.*

о́сень *ж.* áutumn; fall *амер.* ~ю in the áutumn; in the fall *амер.*

осеня́ть, осени́ть (*вн.*) 1. (*покрыва́ть*) shade (*smb., smth.*); *перен.* shield (*smb., smth.*); 2. (*приходи́ть в го́лову*) strike* (*smb.*), occúr (to); меня́ осени́ла мысль it dawned on me (that); меня́ осени́ло I had an inspirátion.

осе́сть *сов. см.* оседа́ть.

осети́н *м.*, ~ка *ж.* Ósset(e). ~ский Ossétic; ~ский язы́к Ossétic, the Ossétic lánguage.

осётр *м.* stúrgeon.

осетри́на *ж.* stúrgeon (flesh).

осе́чк|а *ж.* mísfire, fáilure to fire; дать ~у miss fire, fail to fire.

осе́чься *сов. см.* осека́ться.

оси́ливать, оси́лить (*вн.*) *разг.* 1. overpówer (*smb.*); *перен.* máster (*smth.*), overcóme (*smth.*); 2. (*справля́ться с чем́-л.*) mánage (*smth.*), cope (with); оси́лить кни́гу get* through a book.

оси́лить *сов. см.* оси́ливать.

оси́н|а *ж.* áspen. ~овый áspen.

оси́н|ый wasp's; ◇ ~ое гнездо́ hórnets' nest.

осироте́|вший, ~лый órphaned; (*лиши́вшийся бли́зкого челове́ка*) beréaved; *перен.* (*опусте́вший*) forsáken.

осироте́ть *сов.* be* órphaned, becóme* an órphan; (*потеря́ть бли́зкого челове́ка*) be* beréaved; *перен.* (*опусте́ть*) becóme* désolate.

оска́л *м.:* ~ зубо́в bared teeth. ~ить *сов.:* ~ить зу́бы bare/show* one's teeth. ~иться *сов.* bare/show* one's teeth.

оскандáлиться *сов. разг.* disgráce one*sélf, look sílly.

оскверн|éние *с.* desecrátion. ~и́ть *сов. см.* оскверня́ть.

оскверня́ть, оскверни́ть (*вн.*) 1. *рел.* désecrate (*smth.*); 2. (*оскорбля́ть чу́вства и т. п.*) defíle (*smth.*).

осклáбиться *сов. разг.* grin.

оско́л|ок *м.* splínter, frágment; ~ снаря́да shéll--splinter. ~очный *attr.*; (*поража́ющий оско́лками*) fragmentátion *attr.*; ~очная ра́на shrápnel wound; ~очная бóмба fragmentátion bomb.

оско́мина *ж.* dráwing/sóreness of the mouth.

оскопи́ть *сов. см.* оскопля́ть.

оскопля́ть, оскопи́ть (*вн.*) castráte (*smth.*).

оскорби́тель *м.* insúlter. ~ный insúlting; ~ный тон insúlting tone.

оскорб|и́ть(ся) *сов. см.* оскорбля́ть(ся). ~ле́ние *с.* 1. (*де́йствие*) insúlting; 2. (*оскорби́тельное сло́во, поведе́ние и т. п.*) insúlt. ~лённый insúlted; (*оби́женный*) offénded, ínjured, wóunded; ~лённое достоинство wóunded dígnity; ~лённая неви́нность ínjured ínnocence.

оскорбля́ть, оскорби́ть (*вн.*) insúlt (*smb.*); (*обижа́ть*) offénd (*smb.*), wound (*smb.*), ínjure (*smb.*); ~ кого́-л. в лу́чших чу́вствах óutrage smb.'s féelings; ◇ ~ чей-л. слух offénd smb.'s ears; оскорби́ть кого́-л. де́йствием phýsically insúlt smb. ~ся, оскорби́ться take* offénce, feel* insúlted.

оскудева́ть, оскуде́ть fall* ínto declíne, be* depléted/impóverished.

оскуде́|лый declíning, depléted. ~ние *с.* declíne, deplétion.

оскуде́ть *сов. см.* оскудева́ть.

ослабева́ть, ослабе́ть 1. (*станови́ться физи́чески сла́бым*) wéaken, becóme* wéaker, be*/becóme*/grow* weak; 2. (*уменьша́ться в сте́пени проявле́ния*) reláx, slácken, ease; (*о шу́ме, ве́тре*) abáte, subsíde; 3. (*станови́ться ме́нее туги́м*) lóosen, becóme* lóoser.

ослабе́ть *сов. см.* ослабева́ть.

осла́б|ить *сов. см.* ослабля́ть. ~ле́ние *с.* 1. wéakening, wéakness; 2. (*уменьше́ние сте́пени проявле́ния чего́-л.*) relaxátion, sláckening, éasing; (*шу́ма, ве́тра*) abátement; ~ле́ние внима́ния loss of atténtion; ~ле́ние у́мственных спосо́бностей wéakening of the íntellect; ~ле́ние напряжённости в междунаро́дных отноше́ниях détente.

ослабля́ть, осла́бить (*вн.*) 1. wéaken (*smb., smth.*); make* (*smb., smth.*) wéak(er); 2. (*уменьша́ть си́лу, сте́пень чего́-л.*) reláx (*smth.*), ease (*smth.*), redúce (*smth.*); ~ внима́ние reláx one's atténtion; 3. (*де́лать ме́нее туги́м*) lóosen (*smth.*).

осла́вить *сов.* (*вн.*) *разг.* drag smb.'s name in the mud; (*вн. тв.*) give* (*smb.*) a name (as; for + -ing). ~ся *сов. разг.* get* a bad name.

ослёнок *м.* young/líttle dónkey.

ослепи́тель|ный blínding; dázzling (*тж. перен.*); ~ая красота́ dázzling béauty.

ослеп|и́ть *сов. см.* ослепля́ть. ~ле́ние *с.* blínding; *перен.* blíndness; (*от любви́ тж.*) infatuátion. ~лённый blínded; (*любо́вью и т. п.*) infátuated.

ослепля́ть, ослепи́ть (*вн.*) blind (*smb.*) (*тж. перен.*); (*лиша́ть на вре́мя спосо́бности ви́деть*) dázzle (*smb.*); ~ красото́й blind/dázzle with béauty; ~ я́ркими луча́ми dázzle with bright rays.

ослёпнуть *сов. см.* слёпнуть.

осли́н|ый asses'; *перен.* múlish, ásinine; ~ое упря́мство múlish óbstinacy.

осли́ца *ж.* shé-ass.

осложн|е́ние *с.* 1. complicátion; 2. (*по́сле боле́зни*) complicátions *pl*, áftereffects *pl*; ~ по́сле гри́ппа áftereffects of inflúenza. ~и́ть(ся) *сов. см.* осложня́ть(ся).

осложня́ть, осложни́ть (*вн.*) 1. cómplicate (*smth.*), bedévil (*smth.*); 2. (*боле́знь*) ággravate (*smth.*), cómplicate (*smth.*). ~ся, осложни́ться 1. becóme* cómplicated; 2. (*тв.*) be* ággravated (by), be* cómplicated (by); боле́знь осложни́лась complicátions have set in.

ослу́шаться *сов. разг.* (*чего́-л.*) disregárd (*smth.*);

(кого́-л.) disobéy (smb.); disregárd smb.'s órders/commánd.

ослы́шаться сов. mishéar*, not hear próperly.

осма́тривать, осмотре́ть (вн.) exámine (smb., smth.); look (smb.) óver; (обходя́, ознако́миться) see* (smth.), vísit (smth.), inspéct (smth.), look round (smth.); ~ кого́-л. с головы́ до ног look smb. óver from top to toe; ~ больно́го exámine a pátient; ~ го́род have* a look at the town; ~ достопримеча́тельности go* síghtseeing; ~ вы́ставку go* to an exhibítion; ~ музе́й vísit a muséum. ~ся, осмотре́ться look round; take* a look round (тж. перен.); ~ся по сторона́м look all round; я уже́ осмотре́лся now I know the lie of the land.

осме́ивать, осмея́ть (вн.) rídicule (smb., smth.), deríde (smb., smth.).

осмеле́вший embóldened, plúcking up cóurage.

осмеле́ть сов. см. смеле́ть.

осме́ливаться, осме́литься dare; осме́люсь сказа́ть I vénture to say.

осме́литься сов. см. осме́ливаться.

осмея́ние с. rídicule.

осмея́ть сов. см. осме́ивать.

осмо́тр м. súrvey, examinátion; (учрежде́ния и т. п.) inspéction; (музе́я, вы́ставки) vísit; ~ достоприме-ча́тельностей síghtseeing; ~ больно́го examinátion of a pátient.

осмотре́ть(ся) сов. см. осма́тривать(ся).

осмотри́тельн|ость ж. wáriness, circumspéction. ~ый wáry, círcumspect.

осмысле́ние с. comprehénsion; ~ происходя́щих собы́тий comprehénsion of what is háppening.

осмы́сленный intélligent.

осмы́сл|ивать, осмы́слить (вн.) grasp the idéa (of), comprehénd (smth.). ~ить сов. см. осмы́сливать, ~ять несов. см. осмы́сливать.

оснасти́ть сов. см. оснаща́ть.

осна́стка ж. мор. (де́йствие) equípping, fitting out.

оснащ|а́ть, оснасти́ть (вн.) 1. equíp (smth.); 2. (су́дно) rig (smth.). ~е́ние с. 1. (де́йствие) equípping; 2. (совоку́пность техни́ческих средств) equípment.

осно́в|а ж. 1. (карка́с, осто́в) base, fráme(work); перен. core; 2. (гла́вное, на чём зи́ждется что-л.) ба́sis (pl -ses); мн. prínciples, foundátions; 3. мн. (исхо́дные положе́ния како́й-л. нау́ки) fundaméntals, prínciples; 4. текст. warp; 5. грам. stem; ◇ брать что́-л. за ~у, положи́ть что́-л. в ~у take* smth. as a básis, base smth. upón; лежа́ть в ~е чего́-л. form the básis of smth.; ~ осно́в bédrock.

основа́ни|е с. 1. (де́йствие) foundátion, fóunding; 2. (фунда́мент) foundátion; (ни́жняя часть чего́-л.) base, foot, bóttom; перен. (гла́вное) básis (pl -ses); 3. (оправда́ние, причи́на) réason; grounds pl; без вся́ких ~й without the slíghtest grounds; лишённый вся́ких ~й unfóunded; с по́лным ~ем with good réason; на како́м ~и? on what grounds?; есть ~я ду́мать there are réasons to belíeve; нет никаки́х ~й there are no réasons whatsoéver, there are not the slíghtest grounds; 4. мат., хим. base; ◇ на ~и чего́-л. on the strength of smth.; разру́шить что́-л. до ~я raze smth. to the ground; потрясённый до ~я be* sháken to the core.

основа́тель м. fóunder.

основа́тельн|о thóroughly; ~ закуси́ть have* a good meal. ~ый 1. (обосно́ванный) well-fóunded; ~ые причи́ны good réasons; 2. (соли́дный, про́чный) sólid; 3. (тща́тельный) thórough.

основа́ть сов. см. осно́вывать. ~ся сов. см. осно́вываться 2, 3.

осно́вн|о́е с. the esséntial/main thing; ◇ в ~о́м on the whole.

основн|о́й básic, fundaméntal; (гла́вный) main, príncipal; ~ зако́н fundaméntal law; ~а́я зада́ча key/príncipal task; ◇ ~ капита́л básic/fixed cápital; ~ые фо́нды fixed ássets.

основополо́жник м. fóunder.

осно́вывать, основа́ть 1. (вн.; создава́ть, учрежда́ть) found (smth.); 2. (вн. на пр.; обоснова́ть) base (smth. on). ~ся, основа́ться 1. тк. несов. (на пр.) base one's árguments/théories (upón); (име́ть что-л. свое́й осно́вой) be* based (on); осно́вываясь на... táking as a básis...; 2. (возника́ть) aríse*, be* fóunded; 3. (поселя́ться) séttle down.

осо́б|а ж. pérson; ирон. persónage.

осо́бенн|о 1. particularly, in partícular; spécially разг.; ~ люби́ть что-л. be* particularly fond of smth.; 2. (необы́чно) in a spécial way; ◇ не ~ not spécially/véry. ~ость ж. spécial féature, peculiárity; ~ость кни́ги состои́т в том... what puts the book in a class by itself is that...; ◇ в ~ости espécially. ~ый 1. partícular, spécial; espécial кни́жн.; 2. (своеобра́зный) pecúliar, unúsual; ◇ ничего́ ~ого nóthing spécial.

особня́к м. (prívate) house/mánsion.

особняко́м apárt; жить, держа́ться ~ hold* onesélf alóof; стоя́ть ~ stand* by itself.

осо́бый spécial; (осо́бенный) partícular.

о́собь ж. spécimen.

осознава́ть, осозна́ть (вн.) réalize (smth.), becóme* awáre (of).

осозна́ть сов. см. осознава́ть.

осо́ка ж. бот. sedge.

осоко́рь м. бот. black póplar.

о́сп|а ж. smállpox; изры́тый ~ой póck-marked, pítted; привива́ть ~у кому́-л. váccinate smb.

оспа́ривать, оспо́рить (вн.) 1. contést (smth.), dispúte (smth.); ~ чьи-л. права́ contést smb.'s rights; 2. тк. несов. (добива́ться) conténd (for); ~ зва́ние чемпио́на conténd for the chámpionship, make* a bid for the chámpionship.

о́спина ж. póck-mark.

оспопривива́ние с. vaccinátion.

оспо́рить сов. см. оспа́ривать 1.

осрами́ть сов. см. срами́ть 1. ~ся сов. см. срами́ться.

оста|ва́ться, оста́ться 1. remáin; (заде́рживаться) stay; ~ ночева́ть stay (for) the night; ~ на второ́й год (в шко́ле) not get one's remóve, stay down; 2. (быть в нали́чии) be* left; ~ётся 5 мину́т до отхо́да по́езда (закры́тия магази́на, нача́ла спекта́кля и т. п.) there are five mínutes left befóre the train goes (the shop clóses, the cúrtain ríses, etc.); 3. (не переставать быть каким-л., находи́ться в како́м-л. состоя́нии) remáin; ~ сиде́ть keep* one's seat, remáin sítting; ~ в си́ле remáin in force, hold* good; ~ при своём мне́нии remáin of the same mind; 4. (ока́зываться в како́м-л. состоя́нии, положе́нии) be*; (без рд.) be* left (without); ~ без рабо́ты be* out of work; ~ одному́ be* (left) alóne; оста́вшись оди́н... when alóne...; оста́ться дово́льным be* pleased/delíghted; оста́ться ни с чем be* left déstitute, be* left with nóthing; 5. безл. (+ инф.; сле́дует лишь) it ónly remáins (+ to inf); нам оста́лось дочита́ть всего́ три страни́цы we have ónly three páges left to read; ничего́ не ~ётся как there is nóthing for it but (+ to inf); не ~ётся друго́го вы́бора, как..., не ~ётся ничего́ друго́го, как... the ónly altérnative is...; ◇ ~ до́лжным кому́-л. owe smb.; за ним оста́лось 20 рубле́й he still had twénty róubles to pay; оста́ться ни при чём achíeve nóthing; счастли́во ~! goodbýe and good luck!

оста́вить сов. см. оставля́ть.

остав|ля́ть, оста́вить (вн.) 1. leave* (smb., smth.); (покида́ть тж.) abándon (smb., smth.); оста́вить по себе́ хоро́шую па́мять leave* pléasant mémories of onesélf; оста́вить наде́жду give* up hope; э́та мысль не ~ля́ла его́ this thought néver left him; 2. (сохраня́ть) keep* (smth.), retáin (smth.); оста́вить ме́сто для кого́-

-л., чего-л. keep* a place for *smb., smth.*; 3. *(задерживать кого-л.)* keep* *(smb.)*; оставить кого-л. на второй год keep* *smb.* down, not give *smb.* his, her remove; 4. *(переставать заниматься чем-л.)* give* up *(smth.)* *(тж. перен.)*, leave* *(smth.)*; *(откладывать в сторону)* put* down *(smth.)*, lay* down *(smth.)*; оставь (же)! stop that!; оставить в покое leave* alóne, leave* in peace; оставить за собой что-л. keep* *smth.*; это ~ля́ет жела́ть лу́чшего it leaves much to be desired.

остальн|о́й *прил.* 1. the remáining, the rest of the óther; 2. *в знач. сущ. с.* the rest; всё ~о́е éverything else; в ~о́м in óther respécts; 3. *в знач. сущ. мн.* the rest *sg*, the óthers, все ~ы́е all the óthers.

остана́вливать, останови́ть 1. *(вн.)* stop *(smb., smth.)*; make* *(smb.)* stop; *(машину, лошадей тж.)* pull up *(smth.)*; останови́ть прохо́жего stop a pásser-by; он ре́зко останови́л маши́ну he pulled up shárply; ~ стано́к stop a lathe; ~ кровотече́ние stop the bléeding; 2. *(вн.; удерживать от чего-л.)* check *(smb.)*, restráin *(smb.)*; 3. *(вн. на пр.; задерживать взор, внимание и т. п.)* fix *(smth.* on*)*; ~ взгляд на ком-л., чём-л. let* one's glance rest upón *smb.*, *smth.*; останови́ть своё внима́ние на чём-л. pay* atténtion to *smth.* ~ся, останови́ться 1. stop, come* to a stop/stándstill; *(о машине)* pull up; 2. *(временно поселиться где-л.)* put* up (at), stay (at); *(у друзей, знакомых)* stay (with); 3. *(на пр.; задерживаться)* rest (upón); fall* (upón); его́ вы́бор останови́лся на... his choice fell upón...; 4. *(на пр.; задерживать своё внимание)* dwell* (upón); ~ся на вопро́се dwell* upon the quéstion, take* up the point; на чём мы останови́лись? where were we?, where did we stop?; ◇ ни пе́ред чем не ~ся stop at nóthing.

оста́нки *мн.* remáins.

останови́ть(ся) *сов. см.* остана́вливать(ся).

остано́вк|а *ж.* 1. *(действие)* stópping, stop; 2. *(перерыв, пауза)* pause; без ~и without (a) pause, without stópping; 3. *(временное пребывание где-л.)* stop-off, stay; 4. *(пункт, место)* stópping-place, stop; *(расстояние между пунктами)* stop, stage; ~ авто́буса bús-stop; ◇ ~ то́лько за ни́ми it's ónly they who are hólding us up.

оста́т|ок *м.* 1. the remáinder, the rest; the remáins *pl*; *(материи)* rémnant; 2. *обыкн. мн. (то, что уцелело от разрушения, гибели и т. п.)* the remáins; *(следы чего-л. минувшего)* véstiges, tráces; 3. *тк. ед. (последняя часть чего-л.)* the rest, the remáinder; ~ пути́ the rest of the jóurney; ~ до́лга the remáinder of a debt; 4. *мат.* remáinder, resídual; дели́ться без ~ка divíde exáctly; ◇ всё без ~ка absolútely éverything (one has).

оста́точный 1. remáining, resídual; 2. *физ.* resídual; ~ магнети́зм resídual mágnetism.

оста́ться *сов. см.* остава́ться.

остекленёть *сов.* glaze.

остекле́ние *с.* glázing.

остекли́ть *сов. см.* остекля́ть.

остекля́ть, остекли́ть *(вн.)* glaze *(smth.)*, glass *(smth.)*.

остепени́ться *сов.* sóber/séttle down; *(о молодом мужчине)* have* sown one's wild oats.

остервене́|лый frénzied. ~ние *с.* frénzy; прийти́ в ~ние fall* into a frénzy; ◇ с ~нием with compléte abándon, like a maníac.

остерега́ться, остере́чься *(рд.)* be* cáreful (of); *(опасаться кого-л.)* bewáre (of).

остере́чься *сов. см.* остерега́ться.

о́стов *м.* fráme(work) *(тж. перен.)*; *(скелет)* skéleton.

остолбене́ть *сов.* be* dumbfóunded.

осторо́жн|о *cárefully; (осмотрительно)* cáutiously; ~! take care!, be cáreful!, look out! ~ость *ж.* care, cárefulness; *(осмотрительность)* cáution; с ~остью with care; забы́ть о вся́кой ~ости throw* cáution to the

winds. ~ый cáreful; *(осмотрительный)* cáutious; ~ый отве́т cáutious/gúarded replý.

остра́стк|а *ж. разг.* a taste of what might háppen; для ~и as a wárning; дать ~у кому́-л. show* *smb.* what to expéct.

острига́ть, остри́чь *(вн.)* cut* *(smth.)*; *(ребёнка)* cut* *smb.'s* hair; *(овец и т. п.)* shear* *(smth.)*. ~ся, остри́чься cut* one's hair; *(в парикмахерской)* have* one's hair cut.

остриё *с.* 1. *(кончик)* point; 2. *(режущий край)* edge; *перен. (критики, сатиры)* sharp edge; быть напра́вленным свои́м ~м на что-л. be* spéarheaded agáinst *smth.*

остри́ть I *несов. (вн.; точить)* shárpen *(smth.)*.

остр|и́ть II, остри́ть be* witty, make* jokes; *(об игре слов)* make* a pun; ~ на чей-л. счёт be* witty at *smb.'s* expénse; не ~и́те! don't try to be fúnny!; неуда́чно ~ make* féeble jokes.

остри́чь(ся) *сов. см.* острига́ть(ся).

о́стров *м.* ísland; *(в географических названиях и поэт. тж.)* isle (of).

островерхий rídge-róofed.

островитя́н|ин *м.*, ~ка *ж.* íslander.

остров|но́й ísland *attr.* ~о́к *м.* íslet.

острог| *м. ж.* harpóon; бить ры́бу ~о́й harpóon a fish.

острокoне́чный póinted.

остросовреме́нный híghly contémporary, úp-to-the--minute.

остро́та *ж.* witticism, quip, sálly; wísecrack *амер.*; зла́я ~ malícious joke.

острота́ *ж.* 1. shárpness; *(ощущения)* píquancy, kéenness; *(положения)* acúteness; ~ го́ря póignancy of one's grief; ~ впечатле́ний fréshness of impréssions; ~ зре́ния kéenness of sight; ~ кри́зиса acúteness of a crísis; 2. *(пищи)* high séasoning, sávouriness, hot flávour.

остроуго́льный acúte-ángled; ~ треуго́льник acúte--ángled tríangle.

остроу́м|ие *с.* wit. ~ный witty, sharp.

о́стр|ый sharp *(тж. перен.)*; *(о чувствах)* póignant, acúte, keen; *(о вкусе, запахе)* púngent, strong; ~ клино́к keen/sharp blade; ~ая боль acúte/sharp pain; ~ое ощуще́ние, жела́ние víolent sensátion, desíre; люби́тели ~ых ощуще́ний advénture-séekers; ~ое зре́ние keen éyesight; ~ со́ус púngent sauce; ~ сыр strong cheese; ~ое блю́до híghly séasoned dish, púngent dish; ~ недоста́ток в чём-л. acúte shórtage of *smth.*; ~ кри́зис acúte crísis; ◇ ~ у́гол *мат.* acúte ángle; ~ое словцо́ witticism; ~ язы́к у кого́-л. *smb.* has a sharp tongue.

остря́к *м.* wit.

остуди́ть *сов. см.* остужа́ть и студи́ть.

остужа́ть, остуди́ть *(вн.)* cool *(smth.)*, chill *(smth.)*.

оступа́ться, оступи́ться stúmble; *(на лестнице)* miss a step; *перен.* trip up.

оступи́ться *сов. см.* оступа́ться.

остыва́ть, осты́ть cool off, get* cool/cold; *перен.* cool (down); суп осты́л the soup is cold; интере́с осты́л ínterest has waned.

осты́ть *сов. см.* остыва́ть.

осуди́ть *сов. см.* осужда́ть.

осужд|а́ть, осуди́ть 1. *(вн.; приговаривать)* convíct *(smb.)*; *(вн. на вн. тж.)* condémn *(smb. to)*, séntence *(smb. to)*; осуди́ть кого́-л. за уби́йство convíct *smb.* of múrder; осуди́ть кого́-л. на два го́да séntence *smb.* to two years; 2. *(вн. за вн.; порицать)* blame *(smb. for)*; 3. *(вн. на вн.; обрекать на что-л.)* condémn *(smb., smth.* to*)*, doom *(smb., smth.* to*)*. ~е́ние *с.* 1. convíction; 2. *(порицание)* blame, cénsure. ~ённый *м.* convícted pérson, cónvict.

осу́нуться *сов.* look drawn/hággard, becóme* hóllow--chéeked.

осуш|а́ть, осуши́ть *(вн.)* 1. dry *(smth.)*; *(отводить воду)* drain *(smth.)*; ~ боло́то drain a marsh; 2. *(выпи-*

вать содержимое чего-л.) drain (smth.), émpty (smth.); ~ бокáл drain/émpty a glass. ~éние с. dráining; dráinage; ~éние и освоéние болóт recláiming of márshes. ~úтельный dráinage attr.; ~úтельный канáл dráinage canál.

осуши́ть сов. см. осушáть.

осу́шка ж. dráinage.

осуществи́м|ость ж. feasibílity, practicabílity. ~ый féasible, prácticable; практи́чески ~ый prácticable.

осуществ|и́ть(ся) сов. см. осуществля́ть(ся). ~лéние с. realizátion; (выполнение тж.) fulfílment; ~лéние проéкта the realizátion of a plan.

осуществля́ть, осуществи́ть (вн.) cárry out (smth.), réalize (smth.), put* (smth.) ínto efféct/práctice; ~ план cárry out a plan; ~ за́мыселربло́т an idéa ínto práctice; ~ своё намéрение put* one's inténtion ínto efféct. ~ся, осуществи́ться be* fulfílled, be* réalized; (о планах, мечтах тж.) come* true, matérialize; (о проекте) be* put ínto efféct.

осцилло́граф м. oscíllograph.

осчастли́вить сов. (вн.) make* (smb.) háppy, grátify (smb.).

осы́пать сов. см. осыпáть.

осыпáть, осы́пать (вн. тв.) 1. cóver (smb., smth. with), strew* (smb., smth. with); перен. shówer (smb. with); ~ кого-л. подáрками, похвалáми shówer gifts, práises upón smb.; ~ кого-л. удáрами rain blows upón smb.; 2. (терять листву) shed* (smth.); 3. (разваливать) scátter; ~ песóк scátter sand.

осыпáться сов. см. осыпáться.

осыпáться, осы́паться 1. (обваливаться) fall*, peel off; (о земле) crúmble, crúmble awáy; 2. (опадать — о листьях, зерне) fall*; 3. (покрываться множеством чего-л.) be* strewn/scáttered/spáttered (with).

ось ж. áxis (pl áxes); (машины, механизма) áxle; перен. hub; ~ вращéния áxis of revolútion; опти́ческая ~ áxis of vísion; ~ собы́тий hub of evénts.

осьмино́г м. óctopus.

осяза́|емый tángible, pálpable. ~ние с. sense of touch. ~тельный 1. (об органе) táctile; 2. (ощутимый) tángible, percéptible.

осяза́ть несов. (вн.) feel* (smth.); перен. percéive (smth.), be* pálpably awáre (of).

от 1. (указывает на исходную точку чего-л.) from, awáy from; отъéхать от гóрода drive* awáy from the town; от гóрода до стáнции from the town to the station; 2. (при обозначении стороны) of; с лéвой стороны́ от чего-л. on the left of smth. 3. (указывает на источник чего-л.) from; узнáть что-л. от дрýга hear* smth. from a friend; ребёнок от пéрвого брáка a child* by one's first húsband. 4. (указывает на связь с чем-л.) of; рабóчий от станкá the man* at the bench; 5. (указывает на целое, которому принадлежит часть) of, off; ключ от замкá key of the lock; пýговица от пальтó bútton off an óvercoat, óvercoat bútton; крышка от корóбки the lid of a box; (отделившаяся) the lid off the box; 6. (указывает на что-л., подлежащее устранению, прекращению и т. п.) from, for; срéдство от зубнóй бóли rémedy for tóothache; укры́тие от дождя́ shélter from the rain; 7. (указывает на причину, основание чего-л.) for, from, with; петь от рáдости sing* for joy; глазá, крáсные от слёз eyes red from wéeping; почернéвший от врéмени black with age; 8. (указывает на другой предмет, который противопоставляется первому) from; отлича́ть добро́ от зла know* good from évil; 9. (употр. при обозначении даты документа) of; письмо́ от пéрвого октября́ one's létter of Octóber 1; 10.: врéмя от врéмени from time to time; день ото дня with évery (pássing) day.

отáва ж. с.-х. áfter-grass, áftermath.

отáпливать, отопи́ть (вн.) heat (smth.).

отáра ж. flock (of sheep).

отбáвить сов. см. отбавля́ть.

отбав|ля́ть, отбáвить (вн. рд.; отнимать, вынимать) take* out a little (smth.); (отливать, отсыпать) pour out a little (smth.); ◇ хоть ~ля́й galóre, enóugh and to spáre; more than enóugh.

отбегáть, отбежáть run* awáy; ~ в стóрону run* a few steps off.

отбежáть сов. см. отбегáть.

отбéливать, отбели́ть (вн.) bleach (smth.).

отбели́ть сов. см. отбéливать.

отбéлка ж. bléaching.

отбивáть, отби́ть 1. (вн.; отламывать) break* (smth.) off; ~ молоткóм hámmer (smth.) off; 2. (вн.; отражать) beat* off, repúlse (smb., smth.); ~ мяч retúrn a ball; ~ удáр párry a blow; отби́ть нападéние beat* off an attáck; 3. (вн.; отнимать силой) take* (smth.) awáy; (брать обратно) get* (smth.) back, recápture (smth.); 4. (вн.; ушибать) ~ себé рýку, нóгу hurt* one's arm, foot*; 5. (вн. у рд.) разг. (привлекать к себе) win* (smb., smth.) awáy (from), snatch (smb., smth. from); 6. (вн.; выстукивать, выбивать) beat* (smth.); ~ такт beat* time; ~ побýдку sound the revéille; 7. (вн.) разг. (делать незаметным) take* awáy (smth.); ~ вкус, зáпах take* awáy the taste, smell. ~ся, отби́ться 1. (отламываться) be* bróken off; 2. (отражать удары, атаки) resist; repél (smb., smth.); 3. (отставать от кого-л.) stray; корóва отби́лась от стáда a cow has strayed from the herd; 4. (от рд.) разг. (переставать заниматься чем-л.) give* up (smth.), get* out of the way (of); ◇ отби́ться от рук get* (quite) out of hand.

отбивнáя ж. cútlet; (с косточкой) chop; свинáя ~ pork chop.

отбирáть, отобрáть 1. (вн. у рд.; отнимать) take* (smth.) awáy (from), cónfiscate (smth. from); (билеты) colléct (smth. from); 2. (вн.; выбирать) seléct (smth.), pick (smth.).

отби́ть(ся) сов. см. отбивáть(ся).

отблагодари́ть сов. (вн.; вознаградить) repáy* smb.'s kíndness; (вн. за) show* (smb.) one's appreciátion (of).

óтблеск м. refléction, gleam.

отбó|й м. (после воздушной тревоги) the all-cléar (sígnal); (к отступлению или в конце дня) the retréat; ◇ бить ~ beat* the retréat; перен. beat* a retréat, back out; ~ю нет от кого-л., чего-л. there is no end to smb., smth., there is no gétting rid of smb., smth.; ~ю нет от покупáтелей the shop is besíeged by cústomers.

отбóйный: ~ молотóк pick, píckhammer.

отбóр м. seléction; ~ый 1. (отличный, первосортный) seléct(ed); choice; picked; ~ые семенá selécted seeds; ~ые войскá picked/crack troops; 2. разг. (непристойный): в сáмых ~ых выражéниях in the chóicest lánguage; ~ная рýгань the vílest abúse.

отбóрочн|ый seléction attr.; ~ая коми́ссия seléction commíttee; ~ые соревновáния tríals.

отбрáсывать, отбрóсить (вн.) 1. (назад) throw*/fling* (smb., smth.) back; (в сторону) throw*/fling* (smb., smth.) aside; перен. (отвергать) cast* (smth.) aside, reject (smth.), discárd (smth.); ~ сомнéния throw* aside one's doubts; отбрóсить мысль cast* aside the thought; ~ невéрную теóрию rejéct a false théory; 2. (врага) repúlse (smb., smth.), throw* back (smb., smth.); 3.: ~ тень cast* a shádow.

отбрóсить сов. см. отбрáсывать.

отбрóсы мн. (ед. отбрóс м.) réfuse sg; пищевы́е ~ gárbage sg, óffal sg.

отбывáть, отбы́ть 1. (уезжать) leave* (for); ~ из Москвы́ в Волгогрáд leave* Móscow for Vólgograd; 2.: ~ наказáние serve a séntence; отбы́ть наказáние compléte one's term.

отбы́т|ие *с.* 1. (*отъезд*) depárture; 2.: по ~ии нака-
зáния on complétion of *one's* term.

отбы́ть *сов. см.* отбывáть.

отвáга *ж.* gállantry; (*смелость*) audácity; pluck
разг.

отвáдить *сов. см.* отвáживать.

отвáживать, отвáдить (*вн.*) *разг.* (*от дома*) choke
(*smb.*) off; (*от привычки*) break* (*smb.*) of the hábit
(of).

отвáж|иваться, отвáжиться dare, vénture. ~иться
сов. см. отвáживаться. ~ный gállant; (*смелый*)
audácious; plúcky *разг.*

отвáл *м.* 1. *мор.* (*отплытие*) sáiling; 2. (*плуга*)
móuld-board; ◇ наéсться до ~а stuff onesélf; накормúть
кого́-л. до ~а stuff *smb.* to búrsting point.

отвáливать, отвалúть 1. (*вн.*; *отодвигать в сторону*) throw* (*smth.*) asíde; 2. (*вн.*) *разг.* (*расщедрив-
шись, одаривать*) hand out (*smth.*); 3. *мор.* (*отчали-
вать*) cast* off. ~ся, отвалúться 1. fall* off, peel off; 2.
разг. (*откидывать назад корпус*) lean* back.

отвалúть(ся) *сов. см.* отвáливать(ся).

отвáр *м.* brew; мяснóй ~ (meat) broth; рúсовый ~
ríce-water.

отвáривать, отварúть (*вн.*) boil (*smth.*).

отварúть *сов. см.* отвáривать.

отварн|óй boiled; ~áя рыба boiled fish.

отвéдать *сов. см.* отвéдывать.

отвéдывать, отвéдать (*вн., рд.*) *разг.* 1. (*пробовать*) try (*smth.*), taste (*smth.*); 2. (*узнавать что-л.,
испытывать*) taste (*smth.*), know* what (*smth.*) feels
like.

отвезти́ *сов. см.* отвозúть.

отвергáть, отвéргнуть (*вн.*) 1. rejéct (*smb., smth.*);
refúse (*smth.*); turn (*smth.*) down *разг.*; 2. *тк. несов.*
(*отрицать*) repúdiate (*smth.*).

отвéргнуть *сов. см.* отвергáть 1.

отверд|евáть, отвердéть becóme* firm; (*о жидко-
сти*) solídify. ~éлый firm; (*о почве тж.*) caked.

отвердéть *сов. см.* отвердевáть.

отвéрженный *прил.* 1. óutcast; 2. *в знач. сущ. м.*
óutcast.

отвернýть(ся) *сов. см.* отвёртывать(ся).

отвéрстие *с.* ópening, áperture; órifice *научн.*; (*дыра*) gap, hole.

отвёртка *ж.* scréw-driver.

отвёртывать, отвернýть (*вн.*) 1. (*отвинчивать*)
screw (*smth.*) off; (*винт*) unscréw (*smth.*); 2. (*кран и
т. п.*) turn on (*smth.*); 3. (*отгибать*) fold back
(*smth.*), turn back (*smth.*); 4. (*повёртывать в сторону*) turn (*smth.*) awáy. ~ся, отвернýться 1. (*отвинчи-
ваться*) come* unscréwed, unscréw; 2. (*отгибаться*)
fold back; 3. (*в сторону*) turn awáy, look awáy, avért
one's face; (*от рд.*) *перен.* turn awáy (from); все отвер-
нýлись от негó everyone turned awáy from him.

отвéс *м.* 1. plumb, plúmb-line, plúmmet; 2. (*склон*)
sheer/vértical face, précipice.

отвéсить *сов. см.* отвéшивать.

отвéсный sheer, vértical.

отвести́ *сов. см.* отводúть.

отвéт *м.* 1. ánswer, replý; (*к арифметической задаче*) ánswer; дать ~ кому́-л. на что́-л. give* *smb.* an
ánswer to *smth.*; 2. (*ответное чувство*) respónse,
ánswer; 3. (*ответственность*) responsibílity; призвáть
кого́-л. к ~у call *smb.* to accóunt; за это мóжно вас
призвáть к ~у you can be made ánswer for that; ◇ в
~ на что́-л. in ánswer/replý to *smth.*; in respónse to
smth.; улыбнýться в ~ smile back; быть в ~е за что́-л.
be* respónsible for *smth.*, ánswer for *smth.*; семь бед —
одúн ~! *погов.* ≅ you might as well be hung for a sheep
as for a lamb; in for a pénny, in for a póund.

отвéтв|úться *сов. см.* ответвля́ться. ~лéние *с.*
branch, óffshoot, ramificátion.

ответвля́ться, ответвúться branch off.

отвéт|ить *сов.* 1. *см.* отвечáть 1; 2. (*за вн.*; *поне-
сти наказание*) pay* (for); ты за это ~ишь you'll pay
for that; ~ головóй за что́-л. ánswer with *one's* life for
smth. ~ный: ~ный визúт retúrn vísit; ~ное письмó létter
in replý; ~ная речь ánswering speech; ~ное чýвство
respónse, recíprocal féeling.

ответственн|ость *ж.* responsibílity; на свою ~ on
one's own responsibílity. ~ый respónsible; ~ый перед
кем-л. за что́-л. respónsible/accóuntable/ánswerable to
smb. for *smth.*; ~ый момéнт crúcial móment; ~ая рабóта
respónsible work; ~ое поручéние impórtant assígnment;
~ый рабóтник sénior official; ~ый съёмщик квартúры
respónsible ténant.

отвéтч|ик *м.*, ~ица *ж. юр.* deféndant.

отвечáть, отвéтить 1. (*дт.*) ánswer (*smb.*), replý
(to); (*отзываться*) respónd (to); ~ на вопрóс replý to a
quéstion; ~ на письмó ánswer/acknówledge a létter; ~ на
огóнь протúвника retúrn the énemy's fíre; ~ кому-л.
взаúмностью, ~ на чьи-л. чýвства recíprocate *smb.'s*
féelings; ~ отказом на прóсьбу refúse a requést; ~ урóк
ánswer the téacher's quéstions, give* an accóunt of what
one has learned; 2. *тк. несов.* (*за вн.*; *быть ответственным*) ánswer (for); be* respónsible (for); ~ за кáчество be* respónsible for quálity; вы бýдете ~ за это you
will be held accóuntable for it; 3. *тк. несов.* (*дт.*; *соответствовать*) ánswer (to), correspónd (to); ~ трéбованиям ánswer the requírements.

отвéшивать, отвéсить (*вн., рд.*) weigh out (*smth.*);
◇ ~ поклóн bow, make* a bow; ~ поклóны bow; отвéсить пощёчину кому-л. *разг.* give* *smb.* a good slap on
the face.

отвúливать, отвильнýть (*от рд.*) *разг.* dodge
(*smth.*); *несов. тж.* try to wríggle out (of); ~ от отвéта
hedge.

отвильнýть *сов. см.* отвúливать.

отвинтúть(ся) *сов. см.* отвúнчивать(ся).

отвúнчивать, отвинтúть (*вн.*) unscréw (*smth.*). ~ся,
отвинтúться unscréw, come* unscréwed.

отвисáть, отвúснуть hang* down, droop.

отвисéться *сов. разг. тж.* lose* its créases on the hánger.

отвúсл|ый ságging, dróoping; с ~ыми ушáми lóp-
-eared.

отвúснуть *сов. см.* отвисáть.

отвлекáть, отвлéчь (*вн.*) 1. (*отрывать от чего-л.*)
divért (*smb., smth.*), distráct (*smb., smth.*); ~ внимáние
divért atténtion; ~ кого́-л. от дел distráct *smb.* from his,
her work, take* *smb.'s* mind off his, her work; ~ кого́-л.
от мы́слей divért *smb.*, províde *smb.* with a
divérsion/distráction; 2. (*заставлять изменить направление*) divért (*smb., smth.*); ~ резéрвы протúвника
на себя draw* the énemy's resérvers. ~ся, отвлéчься
divért *one's* atténtion; (*при рассказе, изложении*)
digréss.

отвлечéни|е *с.* distráction; divérsion; для ~я внимá-
ния to divért atténtion.

отвлечённ|ый ábstract; ~ое понятие ábstract
concéption; ~ые идéи ábstract idéas; ◇ ~ое ímя сущест-
вúтельное *грам.* ábstract noun; ~ое числó *мат.* ábstract
númber.

отвлéчь(ся) *сов. см.* отвлекáть(ся).

отвóд *м.* 1. (*воды*) divérsion; 2. (*участка земли и
т. п.*) allótment, grant; 3. (*свидетеля, кандидата*)
rejéction; objéction; заявúть ~ свидéтелю chállenge a
witness; 4. (*войск*) withdráwal; 5. *тех.* bránch-pipe; 6.
эл. tap, tápping; ◇ для ~а глаз to distráct atténtion; as a
blind *разг.*

отводúть, отвестú (*вн.*) 1. (*доставлять куда-л.*)
take* (*smb.*), condúct (*smb.*); отвестú ребёнка в дéтский сад take* a child* to a núrsery school; 2. (*уводить откуда-л.*) lead* (*smb.*) awáy, bring* (*smb.*)
awáy, take* (*smb.*) awáy; ~ кого́-л. от окнá bring* *smb.*

awáy from the wíndow; полк отвелú в тыл the régiment was withdráwn to the rear; 3. (*направлять в сторону om*) divért (*smth.*); draw* (*smth.*) aside; перен. avért (*smth.*), ward off (*smth.*); ~ вéтви draw* aside the bránches; отвестú бедý ward off disáster; отвестú удáр defléct a blow; 4. (*отвергать*) rejéct (*smb., smth.*); ~ кандидатýру rejéct smb.'s cándidature; 5. (*предназначать для чего-л.*) allót (*smth.*), assign (*smth.*); ~ учáсток под сад set* aside a gárden plot; ~ врéмя на *что-л.* allów time for *smth.*; ◇ ~ дýшу unbósom onesélf, unlóad one's heart.

отводнóй, отвóдный: ~ канáл drain, dráinage canál.

отвоевáть сов. 1. см. отвоёвывать; 2. разг. (*кончить воевать*) finish fighting; 3. разг. (*провоевать*) fight*; ~ две войнý go* through two wars.

отвоевáться сов. разг. have* done (*one's*) fighting, one's fighting days are óver.

отвоёвывать, отвоевáть (*вн. у рд.; прям. и перен.*) win* (back) (*smth. from.*)

отвозúть, отвезтú (*вн.*) take* (*smth.*); (*человека тж.*) drive* (*smb.*).

отворáчивать, отворотúть (*вн.*) разг. 1. (*вороча, отодвигать*) pull (*smth.*) aside, heave* (*smth.*) aside; ~ кáмень heave* aside a rock; 2. (*в сторону*) turn (*smth.*) awáy; ~ нос turn up one's nose; 3. (*отгибать*) fold (*smth.*) back. ~ся, отворотúться разг. turn awáy.

отворúть(ся) сов. см. отворáть(ся).

отворóт м. (*одежды*) lapél; (*рукава*) cuff; (*на брюках*) túrn-up.

отворáть, отворúть (*вн.*) óрen (*smth.*). ~ся, отворúться óрen, come* óрen.

отвратúтельн|о disgústingly, abóminably; ~ пáхнуть smell* disgústing; ~ себя́ чýвствовать feel* áwful; ~ вы́глядеть look áwful. ~ый disgústing; (*отталкивающий*) repúlsive, lóathsome; (*плохой*) abóminable; ~ая погóда foul wéather; ~ое поведéние abóminable beháviour.

отвратúть сов. см. отвращáть.

отвращ|áть, отвратúть (*вн.*) avért (*smth.*), ward off (*smth.*). ~éние с. disgúst, repúgnance, lóathing, avérsion; питáть ~éние к *кому-л.* feel* an avérsion for *smb.*

отвыкáть, отвы́кнуть (*от рд.*) 1. (*отучаться*) lose* the hábit (of); get* out of the way (of); несов. тж. try to give up (+ -ing); try to break onesélf (of + -ing); 2. (*забывать кого-л., что-л.*) lose* one's attáchment (to); (*людей тж.*) becóme* estránged (from).

отвы́кнуть сов. см. отвыкáть.

отвязáть(ся) сов. см. отвя́зывать(ся).

отвя́зывать, отвязáть (*вн.*) untie (*smth.*), unfásten (*smth.*). ~ся, отвязáться 1. come* untied/unfástened; 2. (*от рд.*) разг. (*отделываться*) get* rid (of), shake* (*smb.*) off; 3. (*от рд.*) разг. (*оставлять в покое*) leave* (*smb.*) alóne.

отгадáть сов. см. отгáдывать.

отгáдка ж. ánswer, solútion.

отгáдывать, отгадáть (*вн.*) guess (*smth.*); (*загадку*) solve (*smth.*).

отгибáть, отогнýть (*вн.*) 1. (*распрямлять*) straighten out (*smth.*), unbénd* (*smth.*); 2. (*завёртывать край чего-л.*) turn back (*smth.*), bend* back (*smth.*); ~ рукавá turn back the sleeves.

отглагóльн|ый грам. vérbal; ~ое существúтельное vérbal noun.

отглáдить(ся) сов. см. отглáживать(ся).

отглáживать, отглáдить (*вн.*) press (*smth.*); (*небольшие вещи*) íron (*smth.*). ~ся, отглáдиться press, íron.

отговáривать, отговорúть (*вн. от рд.*) dissuáde (*smb.* from), talk (*smb.*) out of it; несов. тж. try to talk (*smb.*) out of it; отговорúть кого-л. от поéздки talk *smb.* out of góing. ~ся, отговорúться (*тв.*) plead (*smth.*), use

(*smth.*) as an excúse; ~ся незнáнием, болéзнью *и т. п.* plead ígnorance, íllness *etc.*

отговорúть(ся) сов. см. отговáривать(ся).

отговóр|ка ж. excúse; без ~ок! no excúses!

отголóсок м. (*прям. и перен.*) écho, reverberátion.

отгоня́ть, отогнáть (*вн.*) 1. drive* (*smb., smth.*) awáy; 2.: ~ мысль dismíss the thought, shake* off the thought.

отторáживать, отгородúть (*вн.*) rail (*smth.*) off; (*верёвкой*) rope (*smth.*) off; (*перегородкой*) partítion (*smth.*) off; (*земельный участок*) enclóse (*smth.*), shut* (*smth.*) in; (*вн. от рд.*) перен. shut* (*smth.*) off (from), keep* (*smb.*) awáy (from). ~ся, отгородúться be* fenced/railed off; (*ширмой*) be* screened off; перен. (*отстраняться*) hold* onesélf alóof.

отгородúть(ся) сов. см. отгорáживать(ся).

отгребáть, отгрестú 1. (*вн.; граблями и т. п.*) rake (*smth.*) awáy/aside; 2. (*вёслами*) row awáy.

отгремéть сов. (thúnder and) die awáy.

отгрестú сов. см. отгребáть.

отгружáть, отгрузúть (*вн.*) dispátch (*smth.*), ship (*smth.*).

отгрузúть сов. см. отгружáть.

отгрýзка ж. dispátch, shípping.

отгрызáть, отгры́зть (*вн.*) bite* (*smth.*) off, gnaw (*smth.*) off.

отгры́зть сов. см. отгрызáть.

отгýл м. compénsatory leave / hóliday.

отгýл|я́ть сов.: я ~я́л свой óтпуск I've had my hóliday; ~ два дня за ночнóе дежýрство take*/have* two days off to make up for night dúty.

отдавáть, отдáть 1. (*вн.; возвращать*) give* (*smth.*) back, retúrn (*smth.*); ~ кому-л. долг pay* smb. a debt; 2. (*вн.; давать*) give* (*smth.*); ~ up (*smth.*), перен. (*посвящать чему-л.*) devóte (*smth.*); ~ зéмлю в арéнду rent land; ~ тýфли в ремóнт take* one's shoes to be repáired; отдáть статью́ на рецéнзию submít an árticle for revíew; ~ жизнь за кого-л., что-л. give* one's life for *smb., smth.*; 3. (*вн.; отправлять куда-л. учиться*) put* (*smb.*), send* (*smth.*); ~ детéй в шкóлу send* the children to school; 4. *тк. несов.* (*тв.*) (*иметь привкус*) taste (of); (*иметь запах*) smell* (of); перен. разг. sávour (of), smack (of); 5. (*вн. за вн.; выдавать зáмуж*) márry (*smb.* to), give* (*smb.*) in márriage (to); 6.: ~ прикáз íssue an órder; ~ распоряжéние give* instrúctions; ~ предпочтéние give* préference; ~ кого-л. под суд take* *smb.* to court; 7. (*вн. за вн.*) разг. (*продавать*) let* (*smth.*) go (for); ~ за бесцéнок let* it go for next to nóthing; 8. (*об оружии*) kick, recóil; 9. (*вн.*) мор. cast* (*smth.*); ~ концы́ cast* off*; ~ я́корь cast*/ drop ánchor; ◇ не ~ себé отчёта в чём-л. fail to réalize *smth.*; ~ дóлжное кому-л. give* smb. his, her due. ~ся, отдáться 1. (*дт.*) give* onesélf up (to), abándon onesélf (to); 2. (*дт.; посвящать себя*) devóte onesélf (to); 3. (*раздаваться*) écho, ring*, revérberate.

отдавúть сов.: ~ кому-л. нóгу tread* on smb.'s foot*.

отдалéни|е с. (*отчуждение*) estrángement; ◇ в ~и in the dístance; ~ я́ от чего-л. remóte from *smth.*

отдалённ|ый remóte; dístant; (*имеющий большое протяжение тж.*) long; ~ райóн remóte área; ~ое схóдство distant/faint líkeness; ~ые прéдки remóte áncestors; в ~ые временá in fár-óff days; ~ое бýдущее the dístant fúture.

отдалúть(ся) сов. см. отдаля́ть(ся).

отдаля́ть, отдалúть 1. (*вн. от рд.*) hold* (*smth.*) awáy (from); 2. (*вн.; отсрочивать*) postpóne (*smth.*), put* (*smth.*) off; 3. (*вн.; вызывать отчуждение*) estránge (*smb.*). ~ся, отдалúться (*от рд.*) 1. move awáy (from); бéрег отдаля́лся the shore recéded; 2. (*перестáвать общаться с кем-л.*) shun (*smb.*).

отдáть сов. см. отдавáть 1, 2, 3, 5, 6, 7, 8, 9. ~ся сов. см. отдавáться.

отда́ч|а ж. 1. giving; ~ внаём létting; 2. (возвраще́ние) retúrn; 3. (ору́жия) recóil, kick; ◇ без ~и with no inténtion of repáying/retúrning; с по́лной ~ей to full efféct.

отде́л м. 1. (в кни́ге и т. п.) séction; 2. (нау́ки) branch; 3. (учрежде́ния) depártment; ~ ка́дров personnél depártment; спра́вочный ~ informátion buréau; ~ здравоохране́ния Board of Health.

отде́лать(ся) сов. см. отде́лывать(ся).

отделе́ние с. 1. (де́йствие) separátion; 2. (учрежде́ния) séction; (отде́л) depártment; (филиа́л) branch; ~ мили́ции branch óffice of the milítia; 3. (помеще́ния) compártment, séction; (пи́сьменного стола́) pigeon-hole; (я́щика) partítion; 4. (конце́рта и т. п.) part; 5. воен. séction; squad амер.

отдели́мый detáchable.

отдели́ть сов. см. отделя́ть 1, 2, 4. ~ся сов. см. отделя́ться.

отде́лк|а ж. 1. (де́йствие) finishing off; (кварти́ры) décorating, decorátion; (пла́тья) trímming; он за́нят оконча́тельной ~ой свое́й рабо́ты he is pútting the finishing tóuches to his work; 2. (украше́ние — на пла́тье) trímmings pl; (помеще́ния) decorátions pl; (пове́рхности материа́ла) finish; вну́тренняя ~ intérior decorátion.

отде́лочн|ый finishing; ~ые рабо́ты páinting and décorating.

отде́лывать, отде́лать (вн.) 1. (придава́ть зако́нченный вид чему́-л.) perféct (smth.), bring* (smth.) to perféction; 2. (украша́ть) décorate (smth.); (оде́жду) trim (smth.); (пове́рхность чего́-л.) put* a finish (on). ~ся, отде́латься разг. 1. (от рд.; освобожда́ться, зако́нчив что-л.) finish (smth.), be* through (smth.); 2. (от рд.; избавля́ться) get* rid (of), shake* (smth.) off; 3. (тв.; испы́тывать что-л. незначи́тельное) get* off (with); отде́латься испу́гом, просту́дой get* off with nóthing more than a fright, a cold; легко́ отде́латься get* off líghtly; 4.: отде́латься отгово́рками avóid gíving a diréct ánswer.

отде́льн|о séparately; (в одино́чку) indivídually, síngly; жить ~ от кого́-л. live apárt from smb.; ~ стоя́щий detáched. ~ость ж.: ка́ждый в ~ости each séparately; взя́тый в ~ости táken séparately. ~ый séparate; ~ая кварти́ра a flat to onesélf; sélf-contáined flat; ~ый ход prívate éntrance; ~ые ли́ца some indivíduals; в ка́ждом ~ом слу́чае in each indivídual case.

отделя́ть, отдели́ть (вн.) 1. séparate (smb., smth.); (изоли́ровать) remóve (smb.) from cóntact (with); (разъединя́ть) cut off (smth.); ~ что-л. перегоро́дкой partítion smth. off; ~ что-л. занаве́ской cúrtain smth. off; 2. (отлича́ть) distínguish (smth.); ~ пра́вду от лжи distínguish truth from fálsehood; 3. тк. несов. (служи́ть грани́цей чего́-л.) divíde (smth.), séparate (smth.); 4. (выделя́ть) allót (smth.). ~ся, отдели́ться (от рд.) 1. (отпада́ть от чего́-л.) come* off (smth.), part (from), detách itsélf (from), come* awáy (from); кора́ отдели́лась от ствола́ the bark came/peeled off the trunk; 2. (отходи́ть, удаля́ться) leave* (smth.), move awáy (from), detách onesélf (from).

отдёргивать, отдёрнуть (вн.) draw* (smth.) back; (ре́зко) jerk (smth.) back; (занаве́ску) draw* (smth.) aside.

отдёрнуть сов. см. отдёргивать.

отдира́ть, отодра́ть (вн.) tear* (smth.) off, rip (smth.) off.

отдохну́ть сов. см. отдыха́ть.

отдуба́сить сов. см. дубаси́ть I.

отдува́ться несов. 1. blow*, pant; 2. разг. (нести́ отве́тственность за каки́е-л. оши́бки) take* the rap (for); мне прихо́дится ~ за всех éverything is left to me, I have to stand the rácket.

отду́шина ж. vent; перен. тж. sáfety-valve.

о́тдых м. rest; (в тече́ние не́скольких дней тж.) hóliday; (развлече́ние) recreátion, relaxátion; нужда́ться в ~e need rest; пра́во на ~ the right to rest; ◇ без ~a incéssantly; не дава́ть кому́-л. ни ~у ни сро́ку néver give* smb. a móment's peace.

отдыха́ть, отдохну́ть (have* a) rest; (брать о́тпуск) take* a hóliday; вам на́до отдохну́ть you need a rest.

отдыха́ющий м. hóliday-maker; (в до́ме о́тдыха) guest.

отдыша́ться сов. recóver one's breath, get* one's breath back.

отёк м. (дро́псикал) swélling; ~ лёгких oedéma of the lungs; ~и под глаза́ми púffiness únder the eyes.

отека́ть, оте́чь 1. swell*; (о лице́) becóme* púffy; (неме́ть) becóme* numb; 2. (о свече́) drip.

отёл м. cálving.

отели́ться сов. см. тели́ться.

оте́ль м. hotél.

отепли́ть сов. см. отепля́ть.

отепля́ть, отепли́ть (вн.) make* (smth.) winterproof, winterize (smth.).

оте́ц м. fáther.

оте́ческ|ий patérnal, fátherly; ~ая ла́ска patérnal afféction, a fáther's kíndness; ~ая забо́та о ком-л. patérnal care for smb.

оте́чественн|ый doméstic, home; ~ая нау́ка the science of our cóuntry; това́ры ~ого произво́дства home-próduced goods; ◇ ~ая война́ patriótic war.

оте́чество с. nátive land, fátherland.

отёчный drópsical.

отéчь сов. см. отека́ть.

отжа́ть сов. см. отжима́ть.

отжива́ть несов. 1. pass the rest of one's life; 2. (устарева́ть) be* fálling into disúse, be* becóming a thing of the past, be* obsoléscent.

отжи́вший 1. who has had his, her day по́сле сущ.; 2. (устаре́лый) óbsolete, óut-of-dáte.

отжима́ть, отжа́ть (вн.) wring* (smth.) out; ~ бельё wring* (out) the wáshing; ~ во́ду из чего́-л. wring* the wáter out of smth.

отжи́ть сов. 1. have* had one's life; перен. pass, die awáy; ~ свой век have* had one's day; 2. (устаре́ть) becóme* óbsolete, fall* into disúse, be* óut-of-dáte.

отзвене́ть сов. finish rínging.

отзвони́ть сов. 1. (вн.; о часа́х) strike* (smth.); 2. (переста́ть звони́ть) finish rínging; (о часа́х) finish stríking.

о́тзвук м. 1. écho; (доноси́щийся издалека́ звук) reverberátion; 2. (отве́тное чу́вство) respónse; 3. (отраже́ние, сле́дствие чего́-л.) reverberátion.

отзвуча́ть сов. sound, die awáy.

о́тзыв м. 1. (мне́ние) repórt, opínion; (характери́стика) testimónial; (реце́нзия) críticism, revíew; кни́га получи́ла благоприя́тные ~ы the book had a good press; 2. воен. repl̀y (to the pássword).

отзы́в м. (отзва́ние) recáll; ~ посла́ recáll of an ambássador.

отзыва́ть I, отозва́ть (вн.) 1. (позва́в, заставля́я отойти́ отку́да-л.) take* (smb.) aside; (соба́ку) call of (smth.); отозва́ть кого́-л. в сто́рону take* smb. aside; 2. (заставля́ть поки́нуть како́й-л. пост) recáll (smb.); отозва́ть посла́ recáll an ambássador.

отзыва́ть II несов. (тв.) разг. (име́ть при́вкус, за́пах) taste (of); smell* fáintly (of).

отзыва́ться, отозва́ться 1. (откли́каться) respónd; никто́ не отозва́лся there was no respónse; 2. (о пр.; выска́зывать своё мне́ние) speak* (of); пло́хо ~ о ком-л. speak* well* of smb.; пло́хо ~ о ком-л. give* a bad repórt of smb.; как он о нём отзыва́ется? what does he say abóut him?; what repórt does he give of him?; 3. (на пр.; отража́ться) afféct (smb.).

отзывн|о́й *дип.* recáll *attr.*; ~ые гра́моты létters of recáll.

отзы́вчив|ость *ж.* sýmpathy; respónsiveness. ~ый 1. sympathétic; ~ый челове́к sympathétic pérson; 2. (*живо реаги́рующий на что-л.*) respónsive.

отка́з *м.* refúsal; (*отрече́ние*) rejéction, repudiátion; ~ в про́сьбе refúsal of *one's* requést; получи́ть ~ meet* with a refúsal; не знать ни в чём ~a néver have* had a síngle wish refúsed; ◇ де́йствовать, рабо́тать без ~a work fáultlessly/pérfectly; до ~a to capácity.

отказа́ть(ся) *сов. см.* отка́зывать(ся).

отка́зывать, отказа́ть 1. (*дт. в пр.; отвеча́ть отрица́тельно на про́сьбу и т. п.*) refúse (smb. smth.), dený (smb. smth.); отказа́ть кому́-л. в по́мощи refúse/dený smb. assistance, refúse to help smb.; ~ кому́-л. в деньга́х refúse smb.'s requést for móney; 2. (*дт. в пр.; лиша́ть чего́-л.*) dený (smb. smth.), depríve (smb. of); отказа́ть себе́ в са́мом необходи́мом dený onesélf the bárest necéssities; не ~ себе́ ни в чём dený onesélf nóthing; 3. (*дт. в пр.; не признава́ть нали́чия чего́-л. у кого́-л.*): ему́ нельзя́ отказа́ть в тала́нте there's no denýing he has tálent; ему́ нельзя́ отказа́ть в остроу́мии it cánnot be denied that he is witty; 4. *разг.* (*переставать де́йствовать*) fail, go* phut, pack up; мото́р отказа́л the éngine packed up; ◇ не откажи́те в любе́зности... be so kind as to... ~ся, отказа́ться 1. (*от рд., + инф.; не соглаша́ться на что-л.*) declíne (+ to inf); 2. (*от рд.; не принима́ть что-л., отверга́ть*) rejéct (smth.), declíne (smth.), give* up (smth.); ~ся от свои́х прав renóunce/relínquish one's rights; 3. (*от рд.; отрека́ться от кого́-л.*) disówn (smb.), renóunce (smb.), repúdiate (smb.); 4. (*от рд., + инф.; не признава́ть свои́м*) renóunce (smth.); ~ся от свои́х слов renóunce/withdráw* one's words; ~ся от свое́й по́дписи refúse to acknówledge one's signature; 5. (*от рд.; отступа́ться от чего́-л.*) give* up (smth.); ~ся от· мы́сли give* up the idéa; ~ся от свои́х убежде́ний recánt; 6. (*переставать де́йствовать, повинова́ться*) fail, refúse to obéy one; (*о механи́змах*) fail; ◇ не откажу́сь, не отказа́лся бы (+ инф.) I wóuldn't mind at all; I wóuldn't mind (+ -ing); не откажу́сь от ча́шки ча́ю I wóuldn't mind a cup of tea.

отка́лывать I, отколо́ть (*вн.; отруба́ть*) chop (smth.) off; отколо́ть кусо́к са́хару break* off a lump of súgar.

отка́лывать II, отколо́ть (*вн.; отшпи́ливать*) unpín (smth.); отколо́ть бант unpín a ríbbon.

отка́лываться I, отколо́ться break* off; break* awáy (*тж. перен.*).

отка́лываться II, отколо́ться (*о чём-л. приколо́том*) come* unpínned/unfástened; бант отколо́лся the ríbbon came unpínned.

отка́пывать, откопа́ть (*вн.*) dig* (smth.) up; (*те́ло*) exhúme (smth.); *перен. разг.* dig* up (smth.); где вы э́то откопа́ли? where on earth did you get it?

отка́рмливать, откорми́ть (*вн.*) fátten (smth.) (up); ~ свинью́ на убо́й fátten a pig for sláughter.

отка́т *м.* (*ору́дия*) recóil.

откати́ть(ся) *сов. см.* отка́тывать(ся).

отка́тка *ж. горн.* háulage, háuling.

отка́тчик *м.* háuler.

отка́тывать, откати́ть (*вн.*) roll (smth.) awáy; (*в сто́рону*) roll (smth.) asíde; (*у́голь*) truck (smth.); откати́ть бревно́ roll a log asíde. ~ся, откати́ться 1. roll awáy; (*в сто́рону*) roll asíde; (*об ору́дии*) recóil; (*на конька́х*) skate awáy; (*о войска́х*) roll back.

откача́ть *сов. см.* отка́чивать.

отка́чивать, откача́ть (*вн.*) 1. (*насо́сом*) pump (smth.) out; 2. (*утопле́нника*) give* (smb.) artifícial respirátion.

откачну́ться *сов.* swing* back; (*о челове́ке*) reel back.

отка́шливаться, отка́шляться clear one's throat.

отка́шляться *сов. см.* отка́шливаться.

откидн|о́й fólding; ~ борт flap; ~о́е сиде́нье hinged seat; ~ верх fólding hood.

отки́дывать, отки́нуть (*вн.*) 1. (*отбра́сывать*) throw* (smb., smth.), fling* (smb., smth.), throw*/fling* (smb., smth.) asíde; *перен.* cast* (smth.) asíde, bánish (smth.); ре́зкий толчо́к отки́нул его́ наза́д the sharp jolt threw him back; отки́нуть ка́мень с доро́ги throw* a stone off the road; отки́нь все свои́ сомне́ния cast aside all your doubts; 2. (*отогну́в, откры́ть*) raise (smth.), lówer (smth.); отки́нуть кры́шку роя́ля raise the lid of a piáno; отки́нуть борт грузовика́ lówer the side of a lórry; 3. *разг.* (*заставля́ть отступи́ть*) throw* back (smb., smth.). ~ся, отки́нуться lean* back.

отки́нуть(ся) *сов. см.* отки́дывать(ся).

откла́дывать, отложи́ть (*вн.*) 1. (*в сто́рону*) lay* (smth.) asíde, put* (smth.) asíde; (*про запа́с*) lay* (smth.) up/by, put* (smth.) by; ~ де́ньги save móney, save up; 2. (*отсро́чивать*) put* (smth.) off, postpóne (smth.), adjóurn (smth.), shelve (smth.); ~ па́ртию *шахм.* adjóurn the game.

откла́няться *сов. уст.* take* one's leave.

откле́ивать, откле́ить (*вн.*) unstíck (smth.), unglúe (smth.). ~ся, откле́иться come* off, come* unstúck.

откле́ить(ся) *сов. см.* откле́ивать(ся).

о́тклик *м.* 1. (*отве́т*) respónse (*тж. перен.*); (*о́тзвук, э́хо*) écho, reverberátion; 2. *обыкн. мн.* (*о́тзывы*) cómment(s); reáction *sg*; ~и в печа́ти press cómments; ~и на статью́ reáction to an árticle.

откли́каться, откли́кнуться (на *вн.*) respónd (to); откли́кнуться на собы́тия show* an ínterest in what is góing on; на э́ту про́сьбу откли́кнулись все éveryone respónded (to this requést).

откли́кнуться *сов. см.* откли́каться.

отклон|е́ние *с.* 1. (*в сто́рону*) defléction, deviátion; ~ стре́лки defléction of the néedle; 2. (*предложе́ния и т. п.*) rejéction; (*про́сьбы*) refúsal, deníal; ~ ва refúsal of an applicátion; 3. (*от рд.; отступле́ние от чего́-л.*) depárture (from), deviátion (from); ~ от те́мы digréssion; ~ от но́рмы depárture from the norm. ~и́ть(ся) *сов. см.* отклоня́ть(ся).

отклоня́ть, отклони́ть (*вн.*) 1. (*в сто́рону*) defléct (smth.); 2. (*предложе́ние и т. п.*) rejéct (smth.), turn (smth.) down; (*про́сьбу*) refúse (smth.), dený (smth.). ~ся, отклони́ться 1. déviate; стре́лка отклони́лась впра́во the néedle swung to the right; 2. (*от рд.; уклоня́ться от первонача́льного направле́ния*) déviate (from); *перен.* (*отвлека́ться*) digréss (from); кора́бль отклони́лся от взя́того ку́рса the ship deviated from its course; отклони́ться от те́мы digréss; stray from the súbject.

отключа́ть, отключи́ть (*вн.*) disconnéct (smth.). ~ся, отключи́ться becóme* disconnécted.

отключи́ть(ся) *сов. см.* отключа́ть(ся).

отко́зыря́ть *сов.* (*дт.*) *разг.* salúte (smb.).

отколоти́ть *сов.* (*вн.*) *разг.* (*изби́ть*) beat* (smb.) up, give* (smb.) a béating/híding.

отколо́ть I, II *сов. см.* отка́лывать I, II.

отколо́ться I, II *сов. см.* отка́лываться I, II.

откомандирова́ть *сов.* (*вн.*) send* (smth.).

откопа́ть *сов. см.* отка́пывать.

отко́рм *м. с.-х.* fáttening.

откорми́ть *сов. см.* отка́рмливать.

отко́рмленный well-nóurished; (*для убо́я*) fáttened.

отко́с *м.* slope; ◇ пусти́ть по́езд под ~ deráil a train.

открепи́тельный tránsfer *attr.*

открепи́ть(ся) *сов. см.* открепля́ть(ся).

открепля́ть, открепи́ть (*вн.*) 1. unfásten (smth.); 2. (*снима́ть с учёта*) strike* (smb.) off the list. ~ся, открепи́ться 1. come* unfástened; 2. (*снима́ться с учёта*) be* struck off the list.

открове́ние *с.* revelátion.

откровéнничать *несов.* (с *тв.*) *разг.* confide (in), speak* of prívate mátters (to); ópen one's heart (to).

откровéнн|ость ж. fránkness. **~ый 1.** (*чистосердéчный, искренний*) frank, outspóken; **~**ый человéк outspóken pérson; **~**ое признáние frank avówal; **2.** (*нескрывáемый, явный*) undisguísed, ópen; в егó глазáх вспыхнуло **~**ое презрéние a gleam of undisguísed contémpt came into his eyes.

открутить *сов. см.* **откручивать.**

откручивать, открутить (*вн.*; *отвинчивать*) unscréw (*smth.*).

открывáть, открыть (*вн.*) **1.** ópen (*smth.*); **~** ящик (столá) (pull) ópen a drawer; открыть роя́ль ópen the piáno; открыть кастрюлю take* the lid off a sáucepan; открыть границу ópen the fróntier; открыть зóнтик ópen one's umbrélla; открыть нóвую школу ópen a new school; **2.** (*освобождáть от чего-л. покрывáющего*) uncóver (*smth.*); (*дéлать видимым*) disclóse (*smth.*), revéal (*smth.*); show* (*smth.*); **~** лицó, гóлову uncóver one's face, head; **~** пáмятник unvéil a státue/mónument; **3.** *разг.* (*вводить в дéйствие*) turn on (*smth.*); **~** кран turn on the tap; **4.** (*начинáть что-л.*) start (*smth.*), launch (*smth.*); открыть собрáние ópen a méeting; открыть сезóн launch the séason; **5.** (*тáйну и т. п.*) revéal (*smth.*); **6.** (*находить, выявля́ть*) discóver (*smth.*); открыть нóвую планéту discóver a new plánet; открыть нефть strike* oil; ◇ **~** комý-л. глазá на что-л. ópen smb.'s eyes to smth.; открыть счёт 1) *бухг.* ópen an accóunt; 2) *спорт.* ópen the score. **~ся, открыться 1.** ópen; *перен.* ópen up; чемодáн открылся the case ópened; зóнтик открылся the umbrélla ópened; **2.** (*покáзываться, представáть взóру*) be* revéaled (to), ópen up (beföre); **3.** (*становиться поня́тным*) be* revéaled, come* clear; **4.** (*становиться извéстным*) come* to light, come* out; **5.** (*об учреждéниях и т. п.*) ópen; (*начинáться*) begín*; **6.** (*признавáться в чём-л.*) confíde; **~ся** во всём комý-л. tell* smb. éverything; ◇ у меня́ открылись глазá my eyes were ópened.

открыт|ие *с.* **1.** ópening; день **~я** ópening-day; **2.** (*то, что устанóвлено в результáте изыскáний и т. п.*) discóvery; *перен.* (*откровéние*) revelátion.

открытка ж. póstcard; (*с худóжественным изображéнием*) pícture póstcard.

открыт|о ópenly; (*откровéнно*) fránkly. **~ый 1.** (*доступный взóру*) ópen, únrestrícted; **~ая** мéстность ópen cóuntry; **2.** (*без навéса, покрытия*) ópen; **~ая** платфóрма ópen plátform; **3.** (*доступный для нападéния*) expósed; **~ые** флáнги expósed flanks; **4.** (*обнажённый*) bare; (*глубокó вырезанный — о плáтье*) lów-nécked; **5.** (*доступный для всех*) ópen; **6.** (*искренний*) ópen, cándid; **~ый** взгляд frank expréssion; **7.** (*нескрывáемый, явный*) ópen, undisguísed; **8.** *горн.* ópen, ópencast; **~ая** разрабóтка месторождéний ópencast wórking/míning of depósits; ◇ **~ая** рáна ópen wound; **~ый** вопрóс ópen quéstion; **~ое** мóре ópen sea; **~ое** письмó (*для публикуемое в газéте*) ópen létter; **~ое** голосовáние vóting by show of hands, ópen vote; объявля́ть заседáние **~ым** decláre the méeting ópen; под **~ым** нéбом óut-of-dóors, in the ópen air; **~ым** тéкстом in so many words.

открыть(ся) *сов. см.* **открывáть(ся).**

откýда 1. *вопр.* where... from; **~** вы? where are you góing from?; (*о происхождéнии тж.*) where do you come from?; вы (э́то) знáете? how d'you know?; **2.** *отнóс.* from which; гóрод, **~** он приéхал, óчень большóй the cíty he has come from is a véry big one; **~** слéдует, что... from which it fóllows that...; hence; ◇ **~** ни возьмись súddenly, out of the blue.

откýда|-либо, ~-нибудь from sómewhere or óther.

откýда-то from sómewhere.

откýпоривать, откýпорить (*вн.*) (*бутылку*) ópen (*smth.*); (*бóчку*) tap (*smth.*), broach (*smth.*).

откýпорить *сов. см.* **откýпоривать.**

откусить *сов. см.* **откýсывать.**

откýсывать, откусить (*вн.*, *рд.*) **1.** bite* (*smth.*) off; откусить хлéба bite* off a piece of bread, take* a bite of bread; **2.** (*клещáми, кусáчками*) cut* off (*smth.*), nip off (*smth.*).

отлагáтельство *с.* deláy, procrastinátion.

отлагáть, отложить 1. *см.* **откладывать 2; 2.** (*вн.*) *геол.* depósit (*smth.*).

отлáмывать, отломáть, отломить (*вн.*) break* (*smth.*) off; отломáть рýчку двéри pull/break* the hándle off a door; отломить кусóк хлéба break* off a piece of bread. **~ся, отломáться, отломиться** break* off.

отлежáть *сов.*: **~** себé бок get* stiff from lýing.

отлежáться *сов. см.* **отлёживаться I.**

отлёживаться, отлежáться *разг.* **1.** have* a thórough rest; **2.** *тк. несов.* (*лежáть, пережидáя что-л.*) lie* low.

отлёт *м.* depárture; **~** птиц на юг начинáется в сентябрé the birds begín to leave for the South in Septémber; ◇ дом стоит на **~е** the house is in a véry lónely situátion; жить на **~е** live far awáy from éverywhere, live in a lónely spot.

отлетáть, отлетéть 1. (*улетáть*) fly* awáy, fly* off; **2.** (*отскáкивать*) reel back; (*о мячé*) rebóund.

отлетéть *сов. см.* **отлетáть.**

отлé|чь *сов.*: у меня́ **~**лó от сéрдца I felt véry much relíeved, it was a weight off my mind.

отлив *м.* **1.** ebb, fálling tide; *перен.* fálling off, withdráwal; **2.** (*оттéнок*) tinge; с золотистым **~ом** shot with gold.

отливáть, отлить 1. (*вн.*, *рд.*; *выливáть*) pour (*smth.*) out; отлéйте немнóго молокá pour a little milk out; **2.** (*вн.*; *откáчивать*) pump (*smth.*) out; отлить вóду из трюма pump wáter out of the hold; **3.** (*вн.*; *изготовля́ть литьём*) cast* (*smth.*); **4.** *тк. несов.* (*тв.*; *о матéри тж.*) be* shot (with).

отливка ж. *тех.* cásting.

отлить *сов. см.* **отливáть 1, 2, 3.**

отлич|áть, отличить (*вн.*) **1.** (*различáть*) distínguish (*smb., smth.*), tell* (*smb., smth.*) from; я не **~**áю их друг от дрýга I can't tell one from the óther; **2.** (*отмечáть нагрáдой*) hónour (*smb.*); **3.** *тк. несов.* (*быть характéрной осóбенностью*) distínguish (*smb., smth.*). **~áться, отличиться 1.** *тк. несов.* (*от рд.*; *быть непохóжим на других*) díffer (from); чем **~**áется... от...? what's the difference betwéen... and...?; **2.** *тк. несов.* (*тв.*; *характеризовáться*) be* remárkable (for); не **~**áться умóм, тáктом и т. п. be* in no way conspícuous for íntellect, tact etc.; **3.** (*выделя́ться чем-л.*) distínguish onesélf; отличиться в бою distínguish onesélf in áction; **4.** *разг.* (*дéлать что-л., вызывáющее удивлéние*) cause a stir.

отличи|е *с.* **1.** distínguishing féature, dífference; внéшние **~я** extérnal dífferences; незначительные **~я** mínor dífferences; **2.** (*нагрáда, óрден*) distínction; диплóм с **~ем** hónours diplóma; знак **~я** decorátion; ◇ в **~** от чего-л. unlíke smth., as distínct from smth., in contradistínction to smth.

отличительн|ый distínctive; **~** признак distínction; **~ая** чертá distínctive féature; **~ая** осóбенность peculiárity.

отличить *сов. см.* **отличáть 1, 2. ~ся** *сов. см.* **отличáться 3, 4.**

отличн|ик *м.*, **~ица** ж. **1.** (*учащийся*) éxcellent púpil, stúdent; **2.** (*отлично выполня́ющий свои обя́занности*) outstánding / éxcellent wórker.

отличн|о 1. *нареч.* véry well; spléndidly; он **~** знáет he knows pérfectly well; **~** знать своё дéло be* véry good at one's job; **~** нести службу give* spléndid sérvice; **2.** *в знач. сказ.* it is fine/spléndid; здесь мне **~** I'm dóing véry well here; **3.** *в знач. сущ. с нескл.* (*отмéтка*) an éxcellent; учи́ться на ~ be* an éxcellent stúdent; получи́ть ~ по исто́рии get*/gain an éxcellent mark for/in history; сдать все экза́мены на ~ get* top/éxcellent marks in all subjects. ~ый 1. (*превосходный*) éxcellent, spléndid; ~ая игра́ актёров spléndid ácting; проду́кция ~ого ка́чества tóp-quality prodúction; ~ое обслу́живание éxcellent sérvice; 2. (*отличающийся от кого-л., чего-л.*) different, unlíke, dissímilar.

отло́гий slóping.

отложе́ние *с. геол., мед.* depósit, sedimentátion.

отложи́ть *сов. см.* откла́дывать *и* отлага́ть.

отложно́й: ~ воротни́к túrn-down cóllar.

отлома́ть(ся) *сов. см.* отла́мывать(ся).

отломи́ть(ся) *сов. см.* отла́мывать(ся).

отлупи́ть *сов. см.* лупи́ть 2.

отлуча́ться, отлучи́ться go* awáy; отлучи́ться и́з дому leave* the house, go* out; отлучи́ться на час be* awáy for an hour.

отлучи́ться *сов. см.* отлуча́ться.

отлу́чк|а *ж.* ábsence; быть, находи́ться в ~е be* awáy.

отлы́нивать *несов.* (от *рд.*) *разг.* shirk (*smth.*); ~ от рабо́ты shirk (*one's* work); ~ от заня́тий slack; shirk *one's* stúdies.

отма́лчиваться, отмолча́ться maintáin sílence.

отма́тывать, отмота́ть (*вн., рд.*) wind* off (*smth.*); отмота́ть мото́к шѐрсти wind* off a ball of wool.

отма́хиваться, отмахну́ться 1. (от *рд.*) wave (*smth.*) awáy; *перен. разг.* brush/wave the mátter asíde; отмахну́ться от реше́ния вопро́са turn *one's* back on a próblem; 2. (*махать рукой, отвергая что-л.*) make* a négative gésture, dismíss the mátter with a wave of the hand.

отмахну́ться *сов. см.* отма́хиваться.

отма́чивать, отмочи́ть (*вн.*) soak (*smth.*) off.

отмежева́ться *сов. см.* отмежёвываться.

отмежёвываться, отмежева́ться (от *рд.*) dissóciate onesélf (from).

о́тмель *ж.* sándbank, shállow.

отме́на *ж.* abolítion; (*закона*) abrogátion, repéal; (*постановления, приказа*) cancellátion; (*приговора*) repéal.

отмени́ть *сов. см.* отменя́ть.

отме́нный (*превосходный*) spléndid; (*исключительный, необыкновенный*) excéptional.

отменя́ть, отмени́ть (*вн.*) abólish (*smth.*); (*закон*) ábrogate (*smth.*), repéal (*smth.*); (*приказ, постановление*) rescínd (*smth.*), cáncel (*smth.*); (*приговор*) repéal (*smth.*).

отмира́ть *сов. см.* отмира́ть.

отме́рить *сов. см.* отмеря́ть.

отмеря́ть, отме́рить (*вн.*) méasure off (*smth.*).

отмести́ *сов. см.* отмета́ть.

отме́стк|а *ж. разг.*: в ~у за *что-л.* in revénge for *smth.*; в ~у он... he retáliated by (+ -ing).

отмета́ть, отмести́ (*вн.*) rejéct (*smth.*).

отме́тить(ся) *сов. см.* отмеча́ть(ся).

отме́тк|а *ж.* 1. mark; (*запись в документе*) note; (*штамп*) stamp; (*оценка знаний*) mark; получи́ть хоро́шую ~у get* a good* mark.

отмеча́ть, отме́тить (*вн.*) 1. (*обозначать какой-л. меткой*) mark (*smth.*); отме́тить ну́жное ме́сто в кни́ге mark the place in a book; 2. (*записывать с целью учѐта*) recórd (*smth.*); отме́тить отсу́тствующих в спи́ске tick off the absentées on the list; 3. (*обращать внима́ние*) note (*smb., smth.*), take* note (of); 4. (*указывать на что-л.*) draw* atténtion (to); ~ досто́инства и недоста́тки рабо́ты draw* atténtion to the mérits and demérits of the work; 5. (*удостаивать похвалы, награды*) comménd (*smb., smth.*); ~ чьи-л. достиже́ния comménd *smb.'s* achievements; 6. (*праздновать*) célebrate (*smth.*), mark (*smth.*). ~ся, отме́титься régister, get* onesélf régistered.

отмира́ние *с.*: ~ госуда́рства wíthering awáy of the State.

отмира́ть, отмере́ть 1. (*утрачивать жизнеспособность*) die; (*о конечностях*) becóme* átrophied; 2. (*исчезать*) die out, disappéar.

отмолча́ться *сов. см.* отма́лчиваться.

отморо́женный fróst-bitten.

отморо́зить *сов.* (*вн.*): ~ себе́ нос, щѐку get* *one's* nose, cheek fróst-bitten.

отмота́ть *сов. см.* отма́тывать.

отмочи́ть *сов. см.* отма́чивать.

отмыв|а́ть, отмы́ть (*вн.*) (*пятна и т. п.*) wash off (*smth.*); (*что-л. от грязи, пятен*) wash (*smth.*); ~ грязь wash off the dirt; ~ ру́ки wash *one's* hands. ~а́ться, отмы́ться (*о грязи, пятнах и т. п.*) wash out, come* out, wash off, come* off; (*становиться чистым*) wash clean, come* clean; пятно́ не ~а́ется, не отмо́ешь, не отмы́ть the spot won't wash/come out; кра́ска отмы́лась the paint washed off, the paint came off in the wash; ру́ки отмы́лись my hands came clean, I washed my hands clean.

отмы́ть(ся) *сов. см.* отмыва́ть(ся).

отмы́чка *ж.* skéleton-key, máster-key.

отнекив|а́ться *несов. разг.* protést, refúse; (*отказываться*) refúse; не ~а́йся! don't shake your head at me!, come on, no excúses!

отнести́ *сов. см.* относи́ться 4.

отнима́ть, отня́ть (*вн.*) 1. take* awáy (*smth.*); (*вн. у рд.; лишать*) depríve (*smb.* of) rob (*smb.* of) (*тж. перен.*); отня́ть у *кого-л.* де́ньги rob *smb.* of his, her móney; отня́ть у *кого-л.* наде́жду depríve *smb.* of hope; 2. (*заставлять потратить время, энергию*) take* (*smth.*); ~ у *кого-л.* мно́го вре́мени take* *smb.* a lot of time; э́то о́тняло у нас три часа́ it took us three hours (to do that); я не хочу́ ~ у вас вре́мя I don't like to take up your time; 3. *разг.* (*ампутировать*) ámputate (*smth.*); 4. *разг.* (*вычитать*) subtráct (*smth.*), take* (*smth.*); от пяти́ отня́ть четы́ре остаѐтся оди́н four from five leaves one; ◇ отня́ть от груди́ wean; нельзя́ отня́ть *чего-л.* у *кого-л.* it cánnot be deníed that *smb.* has merit. ~ся, отня́ться be* páralysed; *разг.* (*неметь*) go* numb; у него́ отня́ли́сь но́ги his legs were páralysed; от смуще́ния у него́ отня́лся язы́к he was spéechless with embárrassment.

относи́тельн|о 1. *нареч.* rélatively, compáratively; день прошѐл ~ споко́йно the day passed fáirly quíetly; 2. *предлог* (*рд.*) about, of, concérning, in regárd/respéct to; (*что касается*) as to. ~ость *ж.* relatívity, rélative náture. ~ый 1. rélative; ~ая и́стина rélative truth; 2. (*некоторый*) compárative; ~ый успе́х compárative/fair succéss; 3. *грам.* rélative; ~ое местоиме́ние rélative prónoun.

относи́ть, отнести́ 1. (*вн.; уносить*) take* (*smth.*); отнести́ письмо́ на по́чту take* a létter to the post; ~ что-л. на ме́сто put* smth. in its place; 2. (*вн.; перемеща́ть*) cárry (*smth.*) awáy; drive* (*smth.*) (to, from); нас относи́т ве́тром we are béing dríven off course by the wind; 3. (*вн. к дт.; приписывать*) attríbute (*smth.* to), ascríbe (*smth.* to); (*причислять*) clássify (*smth.* as, únder); учѐные отно́сят э́ти разва́лины к 12-му ве́ку scientists belíeve these ruins date from the 12th céntury; ◇ отнести́ что-л. на счѐт *кого-л., чего-л.* attríbute/ascríbe smth. to smb., smth.; put* smth. down to smb., smth.

относи́ться, отнести́сь 1. *тк. несов.* (к *дт.; иметь отношение*) be* reláted (to), have* to do (with), applý (to); не ~ к де́лу beside the point, be* néither here, nor there; э́то отно́сится к вам that applíes to you; э́то ко мне не отно́сится that's nóthing to do with me; 2. *тк. несов. мат.* be*; ~ как 3 к 5 be* as three to five; 3. *тк. несов.* (к *дт.; принадлежать*) belóng (to); (к году, *эпохе*) date (from); ~ к такóму-то клáссу, категóрии fall* únder the cátegory (of), be* clássified (as); 4. (к *дт.*; проявлять какое-л. отношение к кому-л., чему-л.) be* dispósed (to), treat (*smb., smth.*); скепти́чески ~ к чему́-л. be* scéptical abóut *smth.*; ~ к комý-л. с довéрием герóse/put* one's trust in *smb.*; ~ к комý-л. с сочýвствием be* in sýmpathy with *smb.*; хорошó (плóхо) ~ к комý-л. be* well (ill) dispósed to *smb.*, treat *smb.* well (bádly); как он к ней отнóсится? how does he feel abóut her?, is he nice to her?

относя́щийся: не ~ к дéлу irrélevant.

отношéни|е *с.* 1. (к *дт.*; взгляд, образ действия) áttitude (to); (обращение тж.) tréatment (of), care (of); добросóвестное ~ к дéлу consciéntious áttitude to one's work; 2. (связь с чем-л.) relátion; relátionship; имéть ~ к чему́-л. concérn *smth.*; э́то не имéет никакóго ~я к дéлу that has nóthing to do with the case; 3. *мн.* relátions; мы (с ним) в óчень хорóших ~ях we are on the best of terms; we get on spléndidly; в каки́х вы (с ним) ~ях? how do you (and he) get on?; быть в бли́зких ~ях с кéм-л. be* on íntimate terms with *smb.*; 4. (документ) memorándum (*pl* -da); 5. *мат.* rátio; ◇ в ~и когó-л., чегó-л. по ~ю к комý-л., чему́-л. as regárds *smb., smth.*, regárding *smb., smth.*, in respéct of *smb., smth.*; в э́том ~и in this respéct; в нéкотором ~и in a (cértain) sense, in a way; во всех ~ях in évery respéct.

отны́не héncefórth, from now on.

отню́дь (обыкн. с отрицанием не) by no means; ánything but.

отня́ть(ся) *сов. см.* отнима́ть(ся).

отображ|а́ть, отобрази́ть (*вн.*) refléct (*smth.*); (изображать) depíct (*smth.*). ~éние *с.* refléction; (описание) pícture.

отобрази́ть *сов. см.* отобража́ть.

отобра́ть *сов. см.* отбира́ть.

отовсю́ду from éverywhere, from all parts.

отогна́ть *сов. см.* оттоня́ть.

отогну́ть *сов. см.* отгиба́ть.

отогрева́ть, отогрéть (*вн.*) warm (*smb., smth.*); ◇ отогрéть змею́ на своéй груди́ chérish a sérpent in one's bósom. ~ся, отогрéться get* warm, warm onesélf.

отогрéть(ся) *сов. см.* отогрева́ть(ся).

отодвига́ть, отодви́нуть (*вн.*) 1. push (*smth.*); (в сторону) push (*smth.*) awáy / asíde; ~ засóв unbólt a door/gate; ~ что́-л. на зáдний план rélegate *smth.* to the báckground; 2. *разг.* (о сроке и m. n.) put* (*smth.*) off, postpóne (*smth.*). ~ся, отодви́нуться 1. (назад) draw* back; (в сторону) move asíde, draw* asíde; 2. *разг.* (о сроке) be* postpóned.

отодви́нуть(ся) *сов. см.* отодвига́ть(ся).

отодра́ть *сов.* 1. *см.* отдира́ть; 2. (*вн.*) *разг.* (побить) give* (*smb.*) a (good) thráshing; ~ когó-л. зá волосы pull *smb.'s* hair; ~ когó-л. зá уши tweak *smb.'s* ears.

отождестви́ть *сов. см.* отождествля́ть.

отождествл|éние *с.* identificátion. ~я́ть, отождестви́ть (*вн.*) idéntify (*smth.*).

отождеств|и́ть, ~лéние, ~ля́ть *см.* отождестви́ть, отождествлéние, отождествля́ть.

отозва́ние *с.* recáll; ~ депутáта recáll of a députy.

отозва́ть *сов. см.* отзыва́ть I. ~ся *сов. см.* отзыва́ться.

отойти́ *сов. см.* отходи́ть I.

отомсти́ть *сов. см.* мсти́ть.

отопи́тельный héating; ~ прибóр héater, héating appliance.

отопи́ть *сов. см.* отáпливать.

отоплéние *с.* héating.

отóрванн|ость *ж.* isolátion. ~ый (от *рд.*) torn (from); *перен.* cut off (from); ~ый от жи́зни remóte from real life.

оторва́ть *сов. см.* отрыва́ть I. ~ся *сов. см.* отрыва́ться.

оторопéть *сов. разг.* be* struck dumb.

отосла́ть *сов. см.* отсыла́ть.

отоспа́ться *сов. см.* отсыпа́ться.

отоща́ть *сов. см.* тоща́ть.

отпад|а́ть, отпа́сть 1. (отделяться) come* off, peel off; 2. (терять смысл, силу) lose* validity; (исчезать) pass, disappéar; вопрóс ~áет the quéstion no lónger aríses; необходи́мость в э́том ~áет there is no lónger any necéssity for this; желáние отпáло the desíre disappéared.

отпари́ровать *сов.* (*вн.*; прям. и перен.) párry (*smth.*); ~ удáр párry a blow.

отпáрывать, отпорóть (*вн.*) unpíck (*smth.*); ~ рукáв unpíck a sleeve. ~ся, отпорóться come* unstítched; воротни́к отпорóлся the cóllar has come unstítched.

отпа́сть *сов. см.* отпадáть.

отперéть(ся) *сов. см.* отпирáть(ся).

отпéтый *разг.* invéterate.

отпеча́т|ать *сов.* (*вн.*) 1. print (*smth.*); (на пишущей машинке) type (*smth.*); 2. фото print (*smth.*); 3. (сняв печать, открыть) unséal (*smth.*). ~ся *сов.* leave* an impréssion; (запечатлеться тж.) make* an impréssion.

отпеча́ток *м.* (прям. и перен.) ímprint; ~ пáльца finger-print; наложи́ть на что-л. ~ грýсти leave* a mark of sórrow upón *smth.*

отпива́ть, отпи́ть (*вн.*, *рд.*) sip (*smth.*); отпи́ть глотóк чáю take* a sip of tea.

отпи́ливать, отпили́ть (*вн.*) saw* off (*smth.*).

отпили́ть *сов. см.* отпи́ливать.

отпира́тельство *с.* (stúbborn) deníal, disavówal.

отпира́ть, отперéть (*вн.*) unlóck (*smth.*); (открывать) ópen (*smth.*). ~ся, отперéться 1. unlóck; дверь отперлáсь the door unlócked, the door came unlócked; 2. (от *рд.*) *разг.* (не сознаваться в чём-л.) dený (*smth.*), go* back (on).

отписа́ться *сов. см.* отпи́сываться.

отпи́ска *ж.* fórmal/non-committal replý.

отпи́сываться, отписа́ться *разг.* send* a fórmal/non-committal replý.

отпи́ть *сов. см.* отпивáть.

отпи́хивать, отпихнýть (*вн.*) *разг.* (назад) push (*smb., smth.*) back; (в сторону) shove (*smb., smth.*) out of the way. ~ся, отпихнýться *разг.* push off.

отпихнýть(ся) *сов. см.* отпи́хивать(ся).

отпла́та *ж.* repáyment.

отпла́тить *сов. см.* отплáчивать.

отпла́чивать, отплати́ть (*дт. тв.*) repáy* (*smb.* with); (*дт.*; мстить) pay* (*smb.*) back; отплати́ть добрóм за зло retúrn good for évil.

отплёвываться *несов. разг.* spit* in disgúst.

отплыва́ть, отплы́ть (о судах) sail; (о людях, животных) swim* awáy; отплы́ть от бéрега swim* awáy from the shore.

отплы́тие *с.* sáiling, depárture.

отплы́ть *сов. см.* отплывáть.

отпля́сывать *несов. разг.* dance awáy.

óтповедь *ж.* repróof, rebúke.

отполза́ть, отползти́ crawl awáy.

отползти́ *сов. см.* отползáть.

отполирова́ть *сов. см.* полировáть.

отпóр *м.* repúlse; перен. rebúff; давáть ~ комý-л. rebúff *smb.*, repúlse *smb.*; получи́ть реши́тельный ~ be* decísively repúlsed.

отпорóть(ся) *сов. см.* отпáрывать(ся).

отпочкова́ться *сов.* gemmáte; перен. detách onesélf, hive off.

отправи́тель *м.* sénder.

отправ|ить *сов. см.* отправля́ть. ~иться *сов. см.* отправля́ться 1, 2. ~ка *ж.* разг. dispátch; (товаров тж.) shipping.

отправлени|е I с. 1. (отсылка) dispátch; 2. (поезда) depárture; (судна) sáiling; 3. (отправляемое по почте) (item of) mail; ◇ тóчка ~я point of depárture.

отправлени|е II с.: ~я органи́зма bódily fúnctions.

отправля́ть, отпра́вить (вн.) 1. (отсылать) send* (smth.); dispátch (smth.); отпра́вить письмо́, посы́лку send* a létter, párcel; 2. (снаряжать в дорогу) send* (smb.) off, get* (smb.) réady for a jóurney; 3. (давать распоряжение к отходу) send* (smth.) off; несов. тж. súpervise the depárture (of); отпра́вить пóезд send* off a train; (парохо́д súpervise a ship's depárture; ◇ отпра́вить кого́-л. на тот свет do* awáy with smb.; send* smb. to kíngdom-come шутл. ~ся, отпра́виться 1. leave* (for); ~ся в путь set* off; ~ся домой пешко́м set* off for home on foot, walk home; 2. (отходить от станции) leave*; пóезд отправля́ется в 9 часо́в утра́ the train leaves at nine a.m.; 3. тк. несов. (от рд.; основываться на чём-л.) procéed (from).

отправн|о́й 1. (откуда отправляют что-л.) dispátch attr.; ~ пункт place of dispátch; 2. (исходный) initial; ~а́я тóчка point of depárture, stárting-point.

отпра́здновать сов. см. пра́здновать.

отпра́шиваться, отпроси́ться get* permíssion to absént oneself; он отпроси́лся на два часа́ he got two hours off.

отпроси́ться сов. см. отпра́шиваться.

о́трыск м. shoot, óffshoot; перен. óffspring, scíon.

отпря́нуть сов. recóil.

отпу́гивать, отпугну́ть (вн.) scare (smb., smth.) off.

отпугну́ть сов. см. отпу́гивать.

о́тпуск м. 1. hóliday, leave (of ábsence); vacátion амер.; ~ по боле́зни sick-leave; ~ с сохране́нием содержа́ния hóliday with pay; ~ без сохране́ния содержа́ния hóliday withóut pay; в ~е on leave; on one's hólidays/vacátion; е́хать в ~ go* for a hóliday; когда́ вы идёте в ~? when do you go on hóliday?; 2. (выдача) íssue; sélling.

отпуска́ть, отпусти́ть (вн.) 1. (разрешать уйти, уехать) let* (smb.) go; отпусти́ть дете́й гуля́ть let* the children go for a walk; 2. (освобождать) reléase (smb., smth.), let* (smb., smth.) go; отпусти́ть пти́цу из кле́тки let* a bird out of its cage; ~ кого́-л. на во́лю set* smb. free, reléase smb.; 3. (выпускать из рук) let* go (of); ~ верёвку let* go of a rope; 4. (ослаблять) lóosen (smth.); ~ по́вод slácken the rein(s); отпусти́ть реме́нь lóosen one's belt; 5. разг. (о боли) let* up for a bit, get* off; 6. (отращивать) grow* (smth.), let* (smth.) grow; ~ бóроду grow* a beard, let* one's beard grow; 7. (выдавать, ассигновывать) grant (smth.); allót (smth.), assign (smth.); отпусти́ть сре́дства на строи́тельство grant funds for búilding; 8. (продавать) sell* (smth.); отпусти́ть товáр sell* goods; 9. разг. (обслуживать) serve (smb.); deal* (with); отпусти́ть клие́нта deal* with a client; 10. разг. (говорить что-л. неуместное) come* out with (smth.); ~ шу́тки crack jokes; ~ комплиме́нты óffer cómpliments.

отпускн|и́к м. pérson on leave. ~о́й: ~ые де́ньги hóliday pay; ~а́я цена́ эк. sale price.

отпусти́ть сов. см. отпуска́ть.

отраба́тывать, отрабо́тать (вн.) 1. (возмещать долг работой) work (smth.) off; 2. разг. (совершенствовать) polish (smth.), perféct (smth.); work out (smth.) to the last détail; 3. (упражняясь, добиваться искусного выполнения чего-л.) perféct (smth.).

отрабо́танн|ый: ~ые га́зы exháust fumes; ~ое ма́сло used/waste oil.

отрабо́тать сов. 1. см. отраба́тывать; 2. (вн.; проработать какой-л. срок) have* worked (smth.); 3. разг. (кончить работу) finish wórk(ing).

отра́ва ж. póison (тж. перен.).

отра́вить(ся) сов. см. отравля́ть(ся).

отравле́ние с. póisoning; ~ свинцо́м léad-poisoning.

отравля́ть, отрави́ть (вн.) póison (smb., smth.); ~ кому́-л. существова́ние be* the bane of smb.'s existence; всё удово́льствие бы́ло отра́влено all pléasure was gone, it killed all the pléasure. ~ся, отрави́ться 1. (принимать яд) take* póison; 2. (случайно) súffer from póisoning; get* póisoned; отрави́ться несве́жими проду́ктами get* fóod-poisoning.

отравля́ющ|ий: ~ее вещество́ tóxic ágent; (газ) póison gas.

отра́д|а ж. delight. ~ный grátifying, encóuraging, cheerful; ~ное изве́стие encóuraging news; ~ное чу́вство feeling of delight.

отража́тель м. refléctor.

отраж|а́ть, отрази́ть (вн.) 1. (отбивать) repúlse (smth.), repél (smth.); перен. rebúff (smth.); ~ нападе́ние repúlse an attáck; ~ уда́р párry a blow; ~ чьи́-л. нападки rebúff smb.'s attácks; 2. (свет, звук) refléct (smth.); refléct back (smth.); 3. (воспроизводить) refléct (smth.); зе́ркало отрази́ло его́ улыба́ющееся лицо́ he saw his smíling face reflécted in the glass; 4. (выражать) refléct (smth.); отрази́ть жизнь в иску́сстве refléct life in art. ~ться, отрази́ться 1. (в пр.) be* reflécted (in); 2. (проявляться) show*, be* reflécted; на лице́ его́ отрази́лось то, что он ду́мал his face reflécted what he was thínking; 3. (на пр.; влиять) afféct (smb., smth.); хорошо́ ~ться на здоро́вье be* good* for the health; ду́рно ~ться на здоро́вье be* detriméntal to health. ~е́ние с. 1. refléction; 2. (нападения) repúlse, dríving back.

отражённ|ый reflécted; ~ свет reflécted light; ~ые радиово́лны reflécted rádio waves.

отрази́ть(ся) сов. см. отража́ть(ся).

отрапортова́ть сов. repórt.

отраслев|о́й sectoral.

о́трасль ж. branch.

отраста́ть, отрасти́ grow*.

отрасти́ сов. см. отраста́ть.

отрасти́ть сов. см. отра́щивать.

отра́щивать, отрасти́ть (вн.) grow* (smth.).

отреаги́ровать сов. (на вн.) reáct (to).

отре́бье с. собир. rábble.

отрегули́ровать сов. (вн.) régulate (smth.).

отредакти́ровать сов. (вн.) édit (smth.).

отре́з м. (материи) length (of stuff); ~ на костю́м suit length.

отре́занность ж. (от рд.) isolátion (from).

отре́зать сов. см. отреза́ть.

отреза́ть, отре́зать 1. (вн.) cut* (smth.), cut* off (smth.); 2. (вн.; разъединять) cut* off (smb., smth.); отреза́ть кого́-л. от гла́вных сил cut* smb. off from the main fórces; 3. (вн.; доступ и т. п.) cut* (smth.); все пути́ отре́заны all escápe routes are cut; 4. разг. (резко отвечать) say* cúrtly, bark, snap out.

отрезве́ть сов. см. трезве́ть.

отрезви́ть сов. см. отрезвля́ть.

отрезвля́ть, отрезви́ть (вн.) sóber (smb.); перен. тж. bring* (smb.) down to earth.

отрезвля́юще: де́йствовать ~ на кого́-л. have* a sóbering influence upón smb.

отрезн|о́й 1. (такой, который отрезается) detáchable; 2.: ~о́е пла́тье dress with a bódice.

отре́зок м. 1. (небольшой кусок чего-л.) length, piece; 2. (ограниченная часть чего-л.) stretch, length, séction; после́дний ~ пути́ the last stretch of the jóurney; ~ ли́нии séction of a line.

отрека́ться, отре́чься (от рд.) renóunce (smb., smth.), disavów (smb., smth.), repúdiate (smb., smth.); ~ от свои́х слов dený one's words; ~ от свое́й пóдписи disavów one's sígnature; ~ от свои́х убежде́ний recánt; give* up one's beliefs; ◇ ~ от престо́ла ábdicate.

отрекомендова́ться сов. introdúce oneself.

отремонти́ровать сов. см. ремонти́ровать.

отречёние с. (от рд.) renunciátion (of), disavówal (of), repudiátion (of); ◇ ~ от престóла abdicátion.

отрéчься сов. см. отрекáться.

отрешáться, отреши́ться (от рд.) renóunce (smth.), give* up (smth.).

отрешённ|ость ж. isolátion, alóofness, detáchment. ~ый alóof, remóte.

отреши́ться сов. см. отрешáться.

отрицáние с. 1. deniál; (отказ от чего-л.) rejéction, repudiátion; 2. филос. negátion; 3. грам. négative.

отрицáтельн|о: дéйствовать ~ на когó-л., что-л. have* a bad efféct on smb., smth.; ~ относи́ться к комý-л., чемý-л. disappróve of smb., smth.; ~ покачáть головóй shake* one's head; отвéтить ~ replý in the négative. ~ый négative; (неблагоприятный) unfávourable; ~ый жест négative gésture; ~ое дéйствие на что-л. unfávourable efféct on smth.; ~ое отношéние к чемý-л. disappróval of smth.; ~ое отношéние к ромáну unfávourable áttitude to the nóvel; ~ые чертьí харáктера négative traits in smb.'s cháracter.

отрицáть несов. (вн.) dený (smth.).

отрóг м. spur.

óтроду разг.: ~ не néver in one's life.

отрóдье с. презр. spawn.

отрóсток м. 1. shoot, branch; 2. (ответвление) branch; ~ слепóй кишки́ appéndix.

óтроче|ский adoléscent; ~ вóзраст adoléscence; teens. ~ство с. adoléscence.

отрубáть, отруби́ть (вн.) chop off (smth.).

óтруби мн. bran sg.

отруби́ть сов. 1. см. отрубáть; 2. разг. (ответить резко) bark, say* cúrtly.

отрул|и́ть сов. ав. táxi asíde; самолёт ~и́л в стóрону the plane táxied asíde.

отрыв м.: ~ от земли́ ав. táke-of; (ракеты) lift-off; ◇ без ~а от произвóдства without gíving up one's work; в ~е от чего-л. in isolátion from smth.; критиковáть когó-л. за ~ от действи́тельности accúse smb. of béing cut off from reálity.

отрывáть I, оторвáть 1. (вн.) pull off (smth.), break* off (smth.), tear* off (smth.); оторвáть пýговицу pull/tear* off a bútton; оторвáть ни́тку break* off a thread; 2. обыкн. безл.: снарядом емý оторвалó рýку his arm was torn off by a shell; 3. (вн. от рд.: отнимать, отстранять) tear* (smth., smb. from); перен. tear* (smb., smth.) awáy (from); я не мог оторвáть глаз от карти́ны I could not tear mysélf awáy from the pícture; 4. (вн. от рд.: разлучать) séparate (smb. from), tear* (smb.) awáy (from); ~ когó-л. от семьи́ tear* smb. awáy from (the bósom of) his, her fámily; 5. (вн. от рд.: отвлекать) interrúpt (smb. at), distúrb (smb. at), take* (smb.) awáy (from); ~ когó-л. от рабóты distúrb smb. at his, her work; ◇ оторвáть от себя́ что-л. depríve onesélf of smth.; с рукáми оторвáть что-л. разг. jump at smth.

отрывáть II, отрьíть (вн.) 1. (откапывать) dig* up (smth.); 2. воен. dig* (smth.); ~ окóпы dig* trénches.

отрывáться, оторвáться (от рд.) 1. (отделяться) come* off (smth.); break* awáy (from); пýговица оторвалáсь a bútton has come off; ~ от привязи break* loose; 2. (отходить, удаляться) eváde (smb., smth.), break* awáy (from); емý удалóсь оторвáться от проти́вника he mánaged to give the énemy the slip; 3. (о летательном аппарате) leave* (smth.); самолёт оторвáлся от земли́ the plane left the ground; 4. (утрачивать связь с кем-л., чем-л.) lose* touch/cóntact (with); оторвáться от масс lose* cóntact with the másses; оторвáться от жи́зни live alóof from the world, lose* touch with éveryone; 5. (переставать делать что-л.) tear* onesélf awáy (from); рабóтать не отрывáясь work withóut stópping; смотрéть не отрывáясь néver take*

one's eyes off; он не мог оторвáться от кни́ги he cóuldn't tear himsélf awáy from the book.

отрьíвист|ый abrúpt; ~ые замечáния disjóinted remárks; ~ смех staccáto láughter.

отрывнóй detáchable; ~ календáрь téar-off cálendar, blóck-cálendar.

отрьíвок м. frágment, pássage; (рассказа, оперы и т. п.) éxcerpt.

отрьíвочн|ый 1. (мало связанный) frágmentary; ~ые свéдения scánty informátion sg; 2. (прерываемый паузами) disjóinted.

отрьíжка ж. belch; перен. hángover.

отрьíть сов. см. отрывáть II.

отря́д м. 1. воен. detáchment, (detáched) force; 2. (группа людей) group, contíngent; 3. зоол. órder.

отряди́ть сов. см. отряжáть.

отряжáть, отряди́ть (вн.) détail (smb.); отряди́ть когó-л. за кем-л. détail smb. to fetch smb.

отря́хивать, отряхнýть (вн.) shake* (smth.) off. ~ся, отряхнýться shake* onesélf.

отряхнýть(ся) сов. см. отря́хивать(ся).

отсади́ть сов. см. отсáживать.

отсáживать, отсади́ть (вн.) 1. (сажать отдельно) seat (smb.) apárt; 2. (о животных) séparate (smth.); 3. (о растениях) transplánt (smth.).

отсáсывать, отсосáть (вн.) draw* off (smth.); (воду тж.) drain (smth.).

óтсвет м. refléction; glímmer (тж. перен.).

отсвéчивать несов. 1. (давать отблеск) refléct the light; ~ розовáтым блéском glow pink; 2. (отражаться) be* reflécted.

отсебя́тина ж. разг. concóction of one's own; (слова тж.) words of one's own, invéntion; (поступки) góing it alóne.

отсéв м. 1. sífting out; перен. тж. eliminátion; 2. (то, что отсеяно) síftings pl; перен. thrów-outs pl.

отсéивать, отсéять (вн.) sift out (smth., smb.); перен. тж. elíminate (smb.). ~ся, отсéяться be* sífted out; перен. тж. be* elíminated, drop out.

отсéк м. compártment; (космического корабля) módule.

отсекáть, отсéчь (вн.) cut* (smth.) off, chop (smth.) off.

отсечéние с. cútting off; ◇ даю́ гóлову на ~ I'd stake my life on it.

отсéчь сов. см. отсекáть.

отсéять(ся) сов. см. отсéивать(ся).

отсидéть(ся) сов. см. отси́живать(ся).

отси́живать, отсидéть 1. (вн.): отсидéть себé нóгу get* pins and néedles in one's leg (from sítting); 2. разг. (сидеть где-л. в течение какого-л. времени) sit* it out; отсидéть два áкта sit* out two acts; отсидéть весь спектáкль sit* through the whole play; 3. (отбывать наказание) serve one's time/term. ~ся, отсидéться разг. shélter; (скрываться) lie* low.

отскáбливать, отскоби́ть (вн.) scrape (smth.) off.

отскáкивать, отскочи́ть 1. (назад) jump back, leap* back; (в сторону) jump asíde, leap* asíde; 2. (от рд.: ударившись, отлетать обратно) rebóund (off); мяч отскочи́л от стеньí the ball bounced back off the wall; 3. разг. (отделяться) come* off; пýговица отскочи́ла a bútton came off.

отскоби́ть сов. см. отскáбливать.

отскочи́ть сов. см. отскáкивать.

отслужи́ть сов. serve (smth.); ~ свой срок (о вещах) have* outlíved its úsefulness.

отсовéтов|ать сов. (дт. + инф.) dissuáde (smb. from + -ing); persuáde (smb.) not (+ to inf); talk (smb. out of + -ing) разг.; емý ~али уезжáть he was persuáded not to leave.

отсосáть сов. см. отсáсывать.

отсóхнуть сов. см. отсыхáть.

отсро́чивать, отсро́чить (вн.) 1. (переносить на более поздний срок) postpóne (smth.), put* (smth.) off; отсро́чить платёж defér páyment; 2. разг. (продлевать срок действия документа) exténd (smth.).

отсро́ч|ить сов. см. отсро́чивать. ~ка ж. 1. postpónement; (платежа) deférment; 2. разг. (продление срока действия документа) exténsion.

отстава́ние с. lágging behínd, lag; ликвиди́ровать ~ catch* up arréars, get* rid of the báck-log.

отстава́ть, отста́ть 1. (от рд.; быть позади) fall*/lag behínd (smb.); (в учениш, работе) lag behínd (smb., smth.); не ~ от кого-л. keep* pace with smb., keep* up with smb.; вы отста́ли! you're behínd the times!; отста́ть от по́езда get* left behínd by one's train; ~ от кла́сса lag behínd the rest of the class; ~ в разви́тии be* báckward; ~ на 10 лет be* ten years behínd; 2. (о часах) be* slow; ~ на четы́ре мину́ты be* four mínutes slow; ~ на две мину́ты в су́тки lose* two mínutes a day; 3. (отделяться) come* off; 4. (от рд.; оставлять в покое) leave* (smb.) alóne.

отста́вить сов. 1. см. отставля́ть; 2.: ~! (команда) as you were!; recóver! амер.

отста́вк|а ж. retirement; в ~е retíred; подава́ть в ~у apply for retírement, send* in one's pápers; ◇ ~ прави́тельства resignátion of the góvernment.

отставля́ть, отста́вить (вн.) move (smth.) aside, move (smth.) to one side; отста́вить стул move a chair to one side; отста́вить мизи́нец raise one's little finger.

отставно́й retíred.

отста́ивать, отстоя́ть (вн.) defénd (smb., smth.), fight* (for); (не давать в обиду) stand* up (for); ~ свою́ незави́симость fight* for one's indepéndence; сов. тж. win* one's indepéndence; ~ свои́ права́ assért one's rights; ~ своё мне́ние maintáin/uphóld one's opinion.

отста́иваться, отстоя́ться (осаждаться) séttle.

отста́л|ость ж. báckwardness. ~ый báckward; (устарелый) old-fáshioned; ~ый челове́к báckward pérson; ~ая страна́ báckward cóuntry; ~ая те́хника old--fáshioned/outmóded techníques/equipment; ~ый взгляд outdáted view.

отста́ть сов. см. отстава́ть.

отстаю́щий báckward.

отстёгивать, отстегну́ть (вн.) unfásten (smth.), undó* (smth.). ~ся, отстегну́ться come* undóne.

отстегну́ть(ся) сов. см. отстёгивать(ся).

отстира́ть(ся) сов. см. отстира́ть(ся).

отсти́рывать, отстира́ть (вн.) wash (smth.) off. ~ся, отстира́ться come* out (in the wash).

отстоя́ть I сов. см. отста́ивать.

отстоя́ть II (вн.; простоять) stand* through (smth.); ~ ва́хту keep*/fínish one's watch.

отсто|я́ть III несов. (от рд.; быть на расстоянии): ~ на 25 киломе́тров от... be* twénty-five kílometres (awáy) from; ~ друг от дру́га на 10 шаго́в be* ten páces apárt; дере́вня ~и́т от ста́нции на де́сять киломе́тров the víllage is ten kílometres awáy from the státion.

отстоя́ться сов. см. отста́иваться.

отстран|е́ние с. remóval. ~и́ть(ся) сов. см. отстраня́ть(ся).

отстраня́ть, отстрани́ть (вн.) 1. (отодвигать от себя в сторону) push (smb., smth.) awáy (a little); 2. (освобождать от исполнения обязанностей) remóve (smb.); ~ кого-л. от до́лжности remóve smb. from his, her post. ~ся, отстрани́ться 1. (отодвигаться) move aside, make* way; 2. (от рд.; уклоняться от какого-л. дела) hold* alóof (from), keep* awáy (from); отстрани́ться от уча́стия в чём-л. not partícipate in smth.

отстре́ливаться, отстреля́ться fire back, retúrn the fire; (отходить) shoot* one's way out.

отстреля́ться сов. см. отстре́ливаться.

о́тступ м. indéntion, space.

отступ|а́ть, отступи́ть 1. (отодвигаться) step back; перен. recéde; отступи́ть на не́сколько шаго́в step back a pace or two; го́ры постепе́нно ~а́ли the móuntains grádually recéded into the distance; 2. воен. retréat (тж. перен.); fall* back; ~ пе́ред тру́дностями retréat in the face of difficulties; отступи́ть пе́ред опа́сностью balk at dánger; 3. (от рд.; изменять чему-л.) abándon (smth.), déviate (from); ~ от свои́х взгля́дов abándon one's views. ~ся, отступи́ться (от рд.) give* up (smth., smb.); я не отступлю́сь! I won't give it up!

отступи́ть(ся) сов. см. отступа́ть(ся).

отступле́ние с. 1. retréat; 2. (отказ от чего-л.) deviátion; ~ от пра́вил deviátion from the rules; 3. (отклонение от основной темы) digréssion.

отсту́пник м. apóstate, recánter.

отсту́пничество с. apóstasy, recánting.

отступя́ awáy, off; ~ два-три шага́ a few páces awáy; немно́го ~ a little way off.

отсу́тстви|е с. ábsence; (недостаток тж.) lack; быть в ~и be* ábsent; (в отъезде) be* awáy; ~ вку́са lack/ábsence of taste; ◇ в чьё-л. ~ in smb.'s ábsence.

отсу́тствовать несов. 1. (не присутствовать) be* ábsent, fail to atténd; ~ на ле́кции be* ábsent from a lécture; 2. (не иметься) be* lácking/wánting; отсу́тствует аппети́т one has no áppetite.

отсу́тствующ|ий прил. 1. ábsent; ~ взгляд vácant glance; 2. в знач. сущ. м. absentée; мн. those ábsent; спи́сок ~их list of absentées.

отсчёт м. márking off; cóunting out; (по прибору) réading; обра́тный ~ вре́мени cóunt-down.

отсчита́ть сов. см. отсчи́тывать.

отсчи́тывать, отсчита́ть (вн.) mark (smth.) off, count (smth.) off; (деньги) count (smth.) out; отсчита́ть 10 шаго́в mark off ten páces.

отсыла́ть, отосла́ть 1. (вн.; посылать) send* (smth.) awáy/off; ~ что-л. обра́тно send* smth. back; 2. (вн.; велеть выйти, уйти) send* (smb.) awáy; 3. (вн. к дт.; к источнику и т. п.) refér (smb. to).

отсы́лка ж. 1. dispátch; 2. (к источнику и т. п.) réference.

отсыпа́ть сов. см. отсыпа́ть.

отсыпа́ть, отсы́пать (вн., рд.) pour out (smth.); (отмерять) méasure out (smth.); отсы́пать зерна́ из мешка́ pour some grain out of a sack; отсы́пать два стака́на я́год méasure out two glásses of bérries.

отсыпа́ться, отоспа́ться have* a good sleep; have* a lie-in разг.; ~ по́сле чего-л. sleep* off smth.; я отосплю́сь I'll sleep it off.

отсыре́ть сов. см. сыре́ть.

отсыха́ть, отсо́хнуть wíther.

отсю́да 1. (из этого места) from here; вон ~! get out (of here)!; 2. (вследствие этого) hence; ~ сле́дует hence it fóllows.

отта́ивать, отта́ять thaw.

отта́лкивание с. физ. repúlsion.

отта́лкивать, оттолкну́ть (вн.) 1. (отодвигать толчком — назад) push (smb., smth.) back, thrust* (smb., smth.) back; (в сторону) push (smb., smth.) aside, thrust* (smb., smth.) aside; перен. (отказываться от чего-л.) rejéct (smth.); оттолкну́ть ло́дку от бе́рега push the boat off; 2. (отдалять кого-л. от себя) rejéct (smb.); 3. (внушать кому-л. неприязнь к себе) repél (smb.); оттолкну́ть от себя́ друзе́й repél one's friends. ~ся, оттолкну́ться 1. (от рд.) push off (from); перен. depárt (from), make* a start (from); оттолкну́ться от земли́ spring*; оттолкну́ться от бе́рега push off; 2. тк. несов. физ. be* repélled.

отта́лкивающий repúlsive, disgústing; ~ вид repúlsive appéarance.

отта́скивать, оттащи́ть 1. (вн.; в сторону) drag (smb., smth.) to one side; 2. (вн. от рд.) разг. pull (smb.) awáy (from).

отта́чивать, отточи́ть (вн.) shárpen (smth.); перен.

turn (*smth.*), mould (*smth.*), pólish (*smth.*); ~ ка́ждый стих pólish évery verse; его́ слова́ бы́ли отто́чены his words were pérfectly phrased.

оттащи́ть *сов. см.* отта́скивать.

оттая́вш|ий thawed; сквозь ~ее окно́ through the window, now entírely free of frost.

отта́ять *сов. см.* отта́ивать.

оттени́ть *сов. см.* оттеня́ть.

оттен|ок *м.* 1. shade, tinge; (*о красках тж.*) tint, hue; с розова́тым ~ком tinged with pink; 2. (*разновидность чего-л.*) súbtlety, núance; ~ значе́ния shade of méaning; 3. (*рд.; слабое проявление*) shade (of), hint (of), trace (of); без ~ка смуще́ния withóut a trace of embárrassment; с ~ком раздраже́ния with a shade/tinge/hint of irritátion.

оттеня́ть, оттени́ть (*вн.*) shade (*smth.*), shade in (*smth.*); *перен.* émphasize (*smth.*), set* (*smth.*) off.

о́ттепель *ж.* thaw.

оттере́ть *сов. см.* оттира́ть.

оттесни́ть *сов. см.* оттесня́ть.

оттесня́ть, оттесни́ть (*вн.*) press (*smb.*) back, drive* (*smb.*) back; *перен.* oust (*smb., smth.*), supplánt (*smb., smth.*).

оттира́ть, оттере́ть (*вн.*) 1. (*удалять*) rub (*smth.*) off; оттере́ть пятно́ rub off a spot; 2. (*возвращать чувствительность*) rub warmth back (into); оттере́ть замёрзшие ру́ки сне́гом rub warmth back into one's hands with snow; 3. *разг.* (*оттеснять*) push (*smb.*) aside; *перен.* oust (*smb.*).

о́ттиск *м.* 1. (*отпечаток, след чего-л.*) ímprint, mark; ~ па́льца fínger-print; 2. (*отпечаток текста, рисунка*) print, impréssions; (*гравюры*) proof; 3. (*отдельно сброшюрованная статья*) óffprint.

оттого́ that's why; ~ что becáuse.

оттолкну́ть *сов. см.* отта́лкивать. ~**ся** *сов. см.* отта́лкиваться 1.

оттопы́ренн|ый protrúding; ~ые у́ши próminent ears, jug ears; у него́ ~ые у́ши his ears stick out.

оттопы́риваться, оттопы́риться *разг.* (*об ушах*) stick* out; (*о кармане*) bulge.

оттопы́рить *сов. см.* оттопы́ривать.

оттопы́риться *сов. см.* оттопы́риваться.

отторга́ть, отто́ргнуть (*вн.*) seize (*smth.*).

отто́ргнуть *сов. см.* отторга́ть.

отторже́ние *с.* séizure.

отто́ченный sharp; *перен.* pólished; о́стро ~ нож sharp knife*; ~ стиль pólished/fínished style.

отточи́ть *сов. см.* отта́чивать.

отту́да from there.

оття́гивать, оттяну́ть (*вн.*) 1. draw* (*smth.*) back, retráct (*smth.*); 2. *разг.* (*уводить силой*) pull (*smb., smth.*) back; 3. (*отвлекать*) divért (*smb., smth.*); оттяну́ть войска́ draw* off troops, divért fórces; 4. (*тяжестью*) weigh (*smth.*) down; make* (*smth.*) sag; оттяну́ть карма́ны make* the póckets sag; вёдра оттяну́ли ру́ки one's hands were áching with the weight of the pails; 5. (*затягивать; откладывать*) deláy (*smth.*), put* off (*smth.*), drag (*smth.*) out; ~ реше́ние keep* pútting off a decision; ◇ ~ вре́мя play for time.

оття́жка *ж.* 1. (*отсрочка*) deláy; 2. (*трос, проволока*) stay.

оттяну́ть *сов. см.* оття́гивать.

отупе́ние *с.* stúpor.

отупе́ть *сов.* grow* dull.

отутю́жить *сов. см.* утю́жить.

отуча́ть, отучи́ть (*вн. от рд., вн. + инф.*) break* (*smb.*) of the hábit (of + -ing), train (*smb.*) not (+ to *inf.*). ~**ся, отучи́ться** (*от рд., + инф.*) break* onesélf of the hábit (of + -ing); grow* unúsed (to + -ing).

отучи́ть(ся) *сов. см.* отуча́ть(ся).

отха́ркивать, отха́ркнуть (*вн.*) expéctorate (*smth.*), cough up (*smth.*). ~**ся, отха́ркнуться** expéctorate.

отха́ркнуть(ся) *сов. см.* отха́ркива,(ся).

отхлебну́ть *сов. см.* отхлёбывать.

отхлёбывать, отхлебну́ть (*вн., рд.*) *разг.* take* a gulp (of).

отхлеста́ть *сов.* (*вн.*) *разг.* give* (*smb., smth.*) a good whípping.

отхлы́нуть *сов.* surge back, fall* back.

отхо́д *м.* 1. (*отправление*) depárture; (*судна тж.*) sáiling; до ~а по́езда оста́лось 5 мину́т there are five mínutes to go befóre the train leaves; 2. *воен.* withdráwal.

отходи́ть I, отойти́ 1. (*от рд.*) move awáy (from); (*в сторону*) move asíde (from); отойти́ от окна́ move awáy from the window; не ~ от телефо́на hold* the line; 2. (*отбывать — о средствах передвижения*) leave*; по́езд отхо́дит в 7 утра́ the train leaves at 7 a. m., the train leaves at séven in the mórning; по́езд отхо́дит от ста́нции the train is púlling out of the státion; 3. *воен.* withdráw*, fall* back; 4. (*от рд., отклоняться*) depárt (from); (*от темы*) digréss (from); ~ от оригина́ла depárt from the oríginal; 5. (*отделяться, отставать*) come* off; (*об обоях и т. п.*) peel off; 6. (*приходить в обычное состояние*) recóver; 7. (*переставать сердиться*) calm down; ◇ отойти́ в о́бласть преда́ния be* consígned to légend.

отходи́ть II *сов.* (*вн.*) *разг.* (*добиться выздоровле́ния кого-л.*) nurse (*smb.*) back to health; ~ больно́го nurse a sick man* back to health.

отхо́дчивый forgíving *attr.*; он отхо́дчив(ый) челове́к) he has a forgíving náture, he soon gets óver it.

отхо́ды *мн.* waste *sg*; пищевы́е ~ gárbage *sg*, scraps; промы́шленные ~ indústrial waste *sg*.

отцвести́ *сов. см.* отцвета́ть.

отцвета́ть, отцвести́ (*о цветах*) finish blóoming, fade; (*о деревьях*) shed* its blóssom; *перен.* lose* one's bloom, fade.

отцепи́ть(ся) *сов. см.* отцепля́ть(ся).

отцепля́ть, отцепи́ть (*вн.*) unhóok (*smth.*); *ж.-д.* uncóuple (*smth.*). ~**ся, отцепи́ться** come* unhóoked.

отцо́в|ский patérnal; ~ дом one's fáther's house. ~**ство** *с.* patérnity, fátherhood.

отча́иваться, отча́яться be* in despáir; (+ *инф., в пр.*) despáir (of + -ing); отча́яться спасти́ чью-л. жизнь despáir of *smb.'s* life; я уже́ отча́ялся вас уви́деть I had given up hope of séeing you.

отча́ливать, отча́лить cast* off; парохо́д отча́лил от при́стани the ship cast off from the wharf.

отча́лить *сов. см.* отча́ливать.

отча́сти pártly; to some extént.

отча́яни|е *с.* despáir; в ~и in despáir, in desperátion; я в ~и I am at my wits' end.

отча́янн|о 1. désperately; 2. *разг.* (*очень*) áwfully. ~**ый** 1. (*проникнутый отчаянием*) désperate; ~ый шаг désperate step; ~ое положе́ние désperate situátion; 2. *разг.* (*безрассудно смелый*) réckless, fóolhardy; ~ый посту́пок réckless act; 3. *разг.* (*увлекающийся каким-л. занятием*) mádly keen; ~ый танцо́р mádly dáncer; 4. *разг.* (*неисправимый*) áwful; ~ый лгун áwful líar.

отча́яться *сов. см.* отча́иваться.

отчего́ why; ~ твой друг переста́л быва́ть у нас? why has your friend stopped cóming to see us?; ~ же? why not?; не зна́ю, ~ он не пришёл I don't know why he didn't come; он засмея́лся, ~ лицо́ его́ ста́ло гора́здо прия́тнее he laughed and this máde his face far more pléasant.

отчего́|-либо, ~-нибудь, ~-то for some réason.

отчека́нивать, отчека́нить (*вн.*) 1. (*изготовлять чеканкой*) coin (*smth.*); 2. (*произносить чётко и раздельно*) rap out (*smth.*).

отчека́нить *сов. см.* отчека́нивать.

отчёркивать, отчеркну́ть (*вн.*) mark (*smth.*), mark round (*smth.*).

отчеркну́ть *сов. см.* отчёркивать.

о́тчество *с.* patroný́mic.

отчёт м. 1. (о работе и т. п.) repórt; ~ о научной работе report on scientific work; финансовый ~ fináncial repórt; 2. (объяснение) accóunt, repórt; отдавать кому--л. ~ в чём-л. give* smb. an accóunt of smth.; требовать ~a demánd an explanátion; ◇ брать что-л. под ~ take* smth. that has to be accóunted for; отдавать себе ~ в чём-л. réalize smth.; не отдавая себе ~a not réalizing.

отчётлив|ый clear, well-defined, distínct; ~ое произношение clear díction; ~ые движения well-defined/crisp móvements; ~ое изображение well-defined ímage/picture.

отчётно-выборн|ый: ~ое собрание eléction méeting; méeting to hear a repórt on the work of the organizátion and elect new exécutives.

отчётность ж. 1. repórting, accóunting; accountabílity; 2. (документация) repórts pl, accóunts pl.

отчётный: ~ период the périod únder revíew/súrvey; ~ год the year únder revíew; (финансовый) fináncial year; ~ доклад (súmmary) repórt.

отчизна ж. nátive land.

отчим м. stépfather.

отчисление с. 1. (вычет) dedúction; 2. обыкн. мн. (ассигнование) allocátions; 3. (исключение) dischárge.

отчислять, отчислить (вн.) 1. (вычитать) dedúct (smth.); 2. (ассигновать) állocate (smth.); 3. (исключать) dischárge (smb.).

отчистить(ся) сов. см. отчищать(ся).

отчитать сов. см. отчитывать.

отчитаться сов. см. отчитываться.

отчитывать, отчитать (вн.) разг. give* (smb.) a good tálking to, tell* (smb.) off.

отчитываться, отчитаться (перед тв.) repórt back (to); ~ перед избирателями repórt back to one's constítuents.

отчищать, отчистить (вн.) clean (smth.); take* (smth.) out; (щёткой) brush (smth.) clean; отчистить пятно бензином take* out a spot with pétrol. ~ся, отчиститься come* off.

отчужд|ать несов. (вн.) 1. estránge (smb.); 2. юр. (собственность) álienate (smth.). ~аться несов. 1. becóme* estránged; 2. юр. (о собственности) be* álienated, becóme* álienated. ~ение с. 1. estrángement; 2. юр. (собственности) alienátion.

отчуждённ|ость ж. estrángement. ~ый 1. estránged; (выражающий отчуждение) forbídding, unwélcoming; 2. юр. (о собственности) álienated.

отшатнуться сов. см. отшатываться.

отшатываться, отшатнуться stágger back; (от рд.) recóil (from); перен. разг. тж. turn awáy (from), turn one's back (on); все от него отшатнулись éveryone gave him the cold shóulder.

отшвыривать, отшвырнуть (вн.) разг. fling* (smth.) awáy; (назад) fling* (smth.) back.

отшвырнуть сов. см. отшвыривать.

отшельник м. hérmit; перен. reclúse; жить ~ом lead* a secluded life.

отшиб м.: жить на ~е live on the óutskirts.

отшлёпать сов. (вн.) разг. spank (smb.).

отшлифовать сов. см. отшлифовывать.

отшлифовывать, отшлифовать (вн.; прям. и перен.) pólish (smth.).

отшутиться сов. см. отшучиваться.

отшучиваться, отшутиться turn it all ínto a joke, come* back with a joke.

отщепенец м. (ренегат) rénegade; (изгнанник) óutcast.

отщепить(ся) сов. см. отщеплять(ся).

отщеплять, отщепить (вн.) split* (smth.) off, chip (smth.) off. ~ся, отщепиться be* chipped off.

отщипнуть сов. см. отщипывать.

отщипывать, отщипнуть (вн.) nip (smth.) off, pinch (smth.) off.

отъедаться, отъесться (после голода) get* one's weight back; (поправляться) grow* sleek.

отъезд м. depárture; ◇ быть в ~e be* awáy.

отъезж|ать, отъехать drive* off/awáy; отъехать на восемь километров от чего-л. get* eight kílometres awáy from smth. ~ающий м. one who is léaving.

отъесться сов. см. отъедаться.

отъехать сов. см. отъезжать.

отъявленный árrant; ~ плут régular scóundrel.

отыграть(ся) сов. см. отыгрывать(ся).

отыгрывать, отыграть (вн.) win* (smth.) back. ~ся, отыграться 1. win* it all back; get* one's revénge; 2. разг. (выходить из затруднительного положения) make* up for it (by).

отыскать(ся) сов. см. отыскивать(ся).

отыскивать, отыскать (вн.) seek* out (smth.), find* (smth.), discóver (smth.). ~ся, отыскаться be* found, be* discóvered.

отягчать, отягчить (вн.) ággravate (smth.).

отягчить сов. см. отягчать.

отяжелеть сов. becóme*/grow* héavy.

офицер м. ófficer; ~ запаса resérve ófficer; ~ связи liáison ófficer; ~ флота nával ófficer. ~ский ófficer's; ófficers'; ~ское звание commíssioned rank.

официальн|ый official; (с соблюдением формальностей тж.) fórmal; ~ое сообщение official communicátion; по ~ым данным accórding to official dáta/figures/statístics; ~ое лицо official; ~ язык official lánguage; ~ое приглашение fórmal invitátion; ~ тон fórmal tone.

официант м. wáiter. ~ка ж. wáitress. ~ский wáiter's; wáitress's.

официоз м. semiofficial órgan/publicátion. ~ный semiofficial; (о статье) inspíred.

оформитель м. desígner; (сцены) stage desígner.

оформ|ить(ся) сов. см. оформлять(ся). ~ление с. 1. (выполнение формальностей) official registrátion; ~ление на работу official registrátion as a mémber of the staff; ~ление документов official registrátion of pápers, stámping of dócuments; 2. (внешний вид чего-л.) desígn; (газеты тж.) láy-out; (спектакля) décor; sets pl; музыкальное ~ músical sétting; художественное ~ artístic arrángement.

оформлять, оформить (вн.) 1. (придавать чему-л. законченную внешнюю форму) desígn (smth.), arránge (smth.); ~ книгу desígn a book; ~ спектакль desígn the sets/décor for a play; 2. (придавать чему-л. законную силу) put* (smth.) in órder; légalize (smth.); ~ документы put* smb.'s pápers in órder; ~ соглашение make* an agréement légal; ~ отношения légalize relátions; 3. (зачислять куда-л.) put* (smb.) on the staff. ~ся, оформиться 1. (принимать форму) take* shape; 2. (поступать куда-л.) be* táken on the staff.

офорт м. étching.

ох oh, dear!

охаивать, охаять (вн.) разг. run* (smth.) down, speak* ill (of).

охапк|а ж. ármful; ~ дров ármful of wood; ◇ взять, схватить в ~у gáther up.

охарактеризовать сов. (вн.) cháracterize (smb., smth.), descríbe (smb., smth.).

охать, охнуть moan, sigh; сов. тж. gasp.

охаять сов. см. охаивать.

охватить сов. см. охватывать.

охватывать, охватить (вн.) 1. (обнимать) put* one's arms round (smb., smth.), embráce (smb., smth.); 2. (окутывать) envélop (smth.); пламя охватило здание flames envéloped the búilding; 3. (о чувствах) seize (smb.), overcóme* (smb.); он охвачен радостью he is full of joy; 4. (распространяться на) spread* all óver (smth.); 5. (воспринимать многое) take* in (smth.), embráce (smth.); 6. разг. (вовлекать) draw* (smb., smth.) in; охвати́ть всех подпи́ской на газе́ты give* éveryone the opportúnity of subscríbing to the néwspapers; ◇ охвати́ть взгля́дом что-л. survéy smth., cast* a glance round smth.

о́хи мн. разг.: ~ и а́хи moans and sighs, gasps and groans.

охладева́ть, охладе́ть (к дт.) cool (towárds), grow* cold (towárds); охладе́ть к пре́жним друзья́м cool towárds one's fórmer friends.

охладе́ть сов. см. охладева́ть.

охлади́ть(ся) сов. см. охлажда́ть(ся).

охлажд|а́ть, охлади́ть (вн.) cool (smth.), chill (smth.); перен. defláte (smb., smth.), dámpen (smth.). ~а́ться, охлади́ться get* cool, cool. ~е́ние с. 1. cóoling; с водяны́м ~е́нием wáter-cooled; с возду́шным ~е́нием áir-cooled; 2. (о чу́вствах) cóolness.

о́хнуть сов. см. о́хать.

охо́т|а I ж. hunting; (с ружьём тж.) shóoting; ~ на волко́в wólf-hunting; ~ на у́ток dúck-shooting; ходи́ть на ~у go* shóoting.

охо́т|а II ж. 1. (жела́ние) desire, fáncy; по свое́й ~е of one's own free will; с большо́й ~ой with the útmost pléasure; 2. в знач. сказ. безл. (дт. + инф.): ему́ ~ чита́ть he feels like réading; ◇ что вам за ~?, ~ вам (+ инф.) why should you bóther (+ to inf); ~ тебе́ спо́рить с ним! why árgue with him!

охо́титься несов. (на вн., за тв.) hunt (smth.); (с ружьём) go* shóoting (smth.), shoot* (smth.); (за тв.) перен. look (for), hunt (for); ~ на медве́дя hunt bears, go* béar-shooting; ~ за перепела́ми shoot* quails.

охо́тник I м. húnter; (непрофессиона́л) spórtsman*.

охо́тник II м. 1. (жела́ющий) voluntéer; найти́ ~а (+ инф.) find* sómebody keen (+ to inf); найти́ ~а на э́то find* sómebody who wants to do it; 2. (до рд., + инф.; люби́тель чего-л.): быть больши́м ~ом до чего-л. be* véry fond of smth.

охо́тни|чий húnting, spórting; ~ до́мик shóoting-box, húnting-box; ~чье ружьё spórting gun; (для ме́лкой дро́би) fówling-piece; ~чья соба́ка húnting-dog, gúndog; (го́нчая) hound.

охо́тно gládly, willingly, réadily; ~! with pléasure!

о́хра ж. óchre.

охра́н|а ж. 1. (защи́та) protéction; ~ здоро́вья health protéction; ~ здоро́вья ма́тери и ребёнка móther-and-child health institútions pl; ~ поря́дка preservátion of law and órder; под ~ой кого-л. guárded by smb.; 2. (стра́жа) guard; guards pl; ли́чная ~ bódyguard; пограни́чная ~ fróntier guards pl. ~е́ние с. protéction; боево́е ~е́ние báttle óutposts pl; похо́дное ~е́ние protéction on the move.

охра́н|ый secúrity attr.; ◇ ~ая гра́мота, ~ лист safe cónduct.

охраня́ть несов. (вн.) guard (smb., smth.), protéct (smb., smth.); (интере́сы и т. п.) sáfeguard (smth.); ~ зда́ние guard a búilding; ~ интере́сы трудя́щихся sáfeguard the interests of the wórking péople.

охри́п|нуть сов. grow*/ becóme* hoarse. ~ший hoarse, húsky.

охроме́ть сов. разг. go* lame, be* lame.

оцара́пать сов. (вн.) scratch (smth.). ~ся сов. scratch onesélf.

оце́нивать, оцени́ть 1. (вн. в вн.) válue (smth. at); оцени́ть кни́гу в 2 рубля́ válue a book at two róubles; 2. (вн.; составля́ть представле́ние, сужде́ние) appréciate (smth., smth.), appráise (smth., smth.); пра́вильно оцени́ть созда́вшееся положе́ние form a corréct éstimate of the situation.

оцени́ть сов. см. оце́нивать.

оце́нк|а ж. 1. (де́йствие) váluing, valuátion; ~ това́ров váluing of goods; ~ иму́щества valuation of próperty; 2. (мне́ние, сужде́ние о ком-л., чём-л.) appráisal, appreciátion; дава́ть ~у произведе́нию иску́сства give*

an appreciátion of a work of art; дава́ть высо́кую ~у кому́-л. expréss a high opínion of smb.; 3. (экзаменацио́нная отме́тка) mark(s); получи́ть хоро́шую ~у за сочине́ние recéive good* marks for compositíon.

оце́нщик м. váluer.

оцепене́л|ый stunned, stúpefied; ~ое состоя́ние stupefáction.

оцепене́ние с. stúpor.

оцепене́ть сов. см. цепене́ть.

оцепи́ть сов. см. оцепля́ть.

оцепля́ть, оцепи́ть (вн.) surróund (smb., smth.); córdon (smth.) off.

оча́г м. 1. hearth; дома́шний ~ the home; 2. (центр) céntre, seat; ~ культу́ры cúltural céntre; ~ инфе́кции céntre of inféction; ~ войны́ hótbed/seat of war; ~ пожа́ра seat of the fire.

очарова́ние с. charm, fascinátion.

очаро́ванный charmed, fáscinated.

очарова́тельный chárming, fáscinating.

очарова́ть сов. см. очаро́вывать.

очаро́вывать, очарова́ть (вн.) charm (smb.), fáscinate (smb.).

очеви́дец м. éyewitness.

очеви́дн|о 1. нареч. óbviously; 2. в знач. сказ. безл. it is óbvious/évident; бы́ло ~, что он э́того не знал he óbviously did not know it; э́то соверше́нно ~! that's (pérfectly) óbvious!; 3. в знач. вводн. сл. évidently; (по-ви́димому) appárently; он, ~, не придёт he is évidently not cóming; вы, ~, счита́ете... you apparently consíder..., you seem to think...; ~ый óbvious; ~ая вы́года óbvious advántage; ~ый факт óbvious fact.

о́чень (при прил. и нареч.) véry; (при гл.) véry much; ~ мно́го (с сущ. в ед. ч.) lots of, a lot of; (с сущ. во мн. ч.) a great mány; с ~ дово́льным ви́дом lóoking véry pleased; мне э́то ~ нра́вится I like it véry much; he ~ not véry; not much; ему́ э́то не ~ нра́вится he's not véry pleased abóut it; он был ~ удивлён he was gréat/much surprísed; он был ~ заинтересо́ван he was much ínterested.

очередн|о́й 1. (ближа́йший) next, immédiate; ~а́я зада́ча the task at hand, immédiate task; ~ые дела́ immédiate affáirs; 2. (сле́дующий по поря́дку) régular, órdinary; ~ о́тпуск one's (régular) leave; ~ съезд (órdinary) cóngress; 3. (повторя́ющийся) recúrrent; just anóther; ~ сканда́л recúrrent row, just anóther row.

очерёдность ж. próper séquence, órder of priórity.

о́черед|ь ж. 1. (поря́док) turn; соблюда́ть ~ wait one's turn; в поря́дке ~и in órder of priórity; ~ за ва́ми it is your turn; 2. (гру́ппа люде́й, ожида́ющих чего-л.) queue; line амер.; ~ за биле́тами tícket-queue; ~ за хле́бом bréad-queue, bréad-line амер.; стоя́ть в ~и queue, stand* in a queue; stand* in line амер.; станови́ться в ~ за кем-л. queue up behínd smb., line up behínd smb.; 3. воен.: пулемётная ~ burst of machine-gun fire; ◇ на ~и next (in turn); по ~и 1) in turns; 2) (сменя́ясь) by turns, in rotátion; в свою́ ~ in one's turn; в пе́рвую ~ in the first place.

о́черк м. (расска́з) (féature) árticle, stóry; (литера́турно-крити́ческий) éssay; ~ о жи́зни и тво́рчестве Пу́шкина an éssay on the life and wrítings of Púshkin; вое́нный ~ árticle abóut ármy life. ~и́ст м. éssayist, éssay-writer.

очерни́ть сов. см. черни́ть.

очерстве́лый hard, cállous.

очерстве́ть сов. см. черстве́ть 2.

очерстви́ть сов. (вн.) hárden (smb., smth.), depríve (smb., smth.) of féeling.

очерта́ния мн. (ед. очерта́ние с.) óutlines, cóntours.

очёски мн. cómbings.

очини́ть сов. см. чини́ть I 2.

очисти́тельный cléansing.

очи́стить(ся) сов. см. очища́ть(ся).

очи́стк|а ж. cléaning, cléaring; purificátion, refíning; ◇ для ~и со́вести to set *one's* mind at ease.

очи́стки *мн.* péelings.

очища́ть, очи́стить (*вн.*) 1. cleaп (*smth.*), clear (*smth.*); *перен.* purge (*smb., smth.*), cleanse (*smth.*); ~ пруд clean a pond; ~ дно реки́ dredge a river; 2. (*освобожда́ть от при́месей*) púrify (*smth.*); *хим. тж.* refine (*smth.*); очи́стить спирт púrify / refine spírit; 3. (*удаля́ть ве́рхний покро́в, оболо́чку*) peel (*smth.*), skin (*smth.*); очи́стить карто́фель peel potátoes; очи́стить яйцо́ shell an egg; очи́стить ры́бу clean a fish; 4. (*освобожда́ть от прису́тствия*) clear (*smth.*); (*освобожда́ть от своего́ прису́тствия*) vacáte (*smth.*); очи́стить помеще́ние clear prémises. ~ся, очи́ститься 1. becóme* clean; becóme* púrified; (*о во́здухе*) becóme* clear/fresh; *перен.* be* purged; 2. (*освобожда́ться*) clear, becóme* free; не́бо очи́стилось the sky cleared; река́ очи́стилась ото льда́ the river becáme free of ice.

очи́щенный 1. *хим.* refined; 2. (*от кожи*) skinned; (*от кожуры*) peeled.

очки́ *мн.* (pair of) spéctacles; glásses; защи́тные ~ góggles.

очк|о́ *с.* 1. (*на ка́ртах, костя́х*) pip; 2. (*в счёте*) point; набра́ть де́сять ~о́в score ten points; 3. (*отве́рстие*) hole; (*глазо́к*) péephole; ◇ он мо́жет дать вам не́сколько ~о́в вперёд he can give you points; втира́ть ~и́ кому́-л. throw* dust in *smb.'s* eyes.

очковтира́тель *м.* fáker, húmbug, blúffer. ~ство *с.* éyewash, bluff.

очко́в|ый: ~ая змея́ cóbra.

очну́ться *сов.* 1. (*просну́ться*) awáken; 2. (*прийти́ в чу́вство*) come* to onesélf, recóver/regáin cónsciousness.

о́чн|ый: ~ая ста́вка *юр.* confrontátion; ~ое обуче́ние full-time instrúction.

очути́ться *сов.* find* onesélf, come* to be; как он здесь ~и́лся? how did he get here?

ошара́шить *сов.* (*вн.*) *разг.* dumbfóund (*smb.*), flábbergast (*smb.*).

оше́йник *м.* cóllar.

ошеломи́ть *сов. см.* ошеломля́ть.

ошеломля́ть, ошеломи́ть (*вн.*) stun (*smb.*), stúpefy (*smb.*).

ошельмова́ть *сов. см.* шельмова́ть.

ошиб|а́ться, ошиби́ться be* mistáken, be* wrong; make* mistákes; *сов. тж.* make* a mistáke; ~ в ком-л. be* mistáken in *smb.*; ~ в чём-л. be* wrong abóut *smth.*; вы ~а́етесь! you're quite mistáken!; е́сли не ~а́юсь if I am not mistáken; мо́жет быть, я ~а́юсь I may be mistáken; не ошибу́сь, е́сли скажу́ I shan't be far out in sáying; смотри́, не ошиби́сь! mind you don't make a mistáke!

ошиби́ться *сов. см.* ошиба́ться.

оши́бк|а ж. mistáke; (*заблужде́ние*) érror; по ~e by mistáke.

оши́бочн|о (*непра́вильно*) wróngly, mistákenly; (*по оши́бке*) by mistáke. ~ый erróneous, mistáken; ~ое представле́ние erróneous idéa, misconcéption.

ошпа́ривать, ошпа́рить (*вн.*) *разг.* scald (*smth., smth.*). ~ся, ошпа́риться scald onesélf.

ошпа́рить(ся) *сов. см.* ошпа́ривать(ся).

оштрафова́ть *сов. см.* штрафова́ть.

оштукату́рить *сов. см.* штукату́рить.

още́ниться *сов. см.* щени́ться.

ощети́ниться *сов. см.* щети́ниться.

ощипа́ть *сов. см.* ощи́пывать.

ощи́пывать, ощипа́ть (*вн.*) pluck (*smth.*).

ощу́пать *сов. см.* ощу́пывать.

ощу́пывать, ощу́пать (*вн.*) feel* (*smb., smth.*) (all óver).

о́щупь ж.: на ~ to the touch, by touch.

о́щупью: иска́ть *что-л.* ~ grope for *smth.*; ~ выби-

ра́ться из grope *one's* way out of; пробира́ться ~ grope *one's* way.

ощути́|мый percéptible, pálpable; (*значи́тельный*) appréciable; ~мая ра́зница appréciable dífference.

ощути́ть *сов. см.* ощуща́ть.

ощущ|а́ть, ощути́ть (*вн.*) sense (*smth.*), feel* (*smth.*); becóme* awáre (of); ~ о́строе жела́ние expérience a keen desíre. ~а́ться *несов.* make* itself felt, be* felt; во всём ~а́лось, что у́тро бли́зко éverything seemed to suggést that mórning was near. ~е́ние *с.* sensátion; у меня́ тако́е ~е́ние, сло́вно... I feel as if...

П

па *с. нескл.* step.

па́ва ж. *зоол.* péahen.

павильо́н *м.* 1. pavílion; 2. (*для киносъёмок*) stúdio (*pl* -os).

павли́н *м.* *зоол.* péacock.

па́водок *м.* fréshet, flood; весе́нний ~ spring floods *pl.*

па́вшие *мн.* the fállen.

па́года ж. pagóda.

па́губ|а ж. *уст.* ruin. ~но: ~но влия́ть, де́йствовать *и т. п.* на кого́-л., что-л. have* a disástrous ínfluence/efféct on *smth.*, *smth.* ~ный (*губи́тельный*) disástrous; (*вре́дный*) pernícious, hármful; ~ное влия́ние hármful ínfluence.

па́даль ж. *обыкн. собир.* cárrion.

пад|а́ть, пасть, упа́сть 1. fall*, drop; ~ на коле́ни go* down on *one's* knees, fall* on *one's* knees; упа́сть на зе́млю fall*/drop to the ground; он упа́л he fell óver; упа́сть со стола́, с кры́ши *и т. п.* fall* off a táble, roof *etc.*; упа́сть с большо́й высоты́ fall* from a great height; 2. *тк. несов.* (*об атмосфе́рных оса́дках*) fall*; ~а́ет снег snow is fálling; 3. *сов.* пасть (*ни́зко опуска́ться*) fall*; его́ голова́ ~а́ла на грудь his head begán to nod; 4. *тк. несов.* (*свиса́ть, ниспада́ть*) fall*; с волоса́ми, ~а́вшими до плеч with hair down to *one's* shóulders; 5. *сов.* пасть (*о росе́, тума́не*) fall*; 6. (*на вн.; о све́те, те́ни*) fall*, be* cast; (*распространя́ться*) fall*; от поле́й шля́пы ~а́ла тень на её лицо́ the brim of the hat cast a shádow on her face; 7. *сов.* пасть (*на вн.; приходи́ться кому́-л., чему́-л.*) fall* (on); жре́бий ~а́ет на меня́ the choice is upón me; 8. *тк. несов.* (*на вн.*) fall* (on); ударе́ние ~а́ет на после́дний слог the stress falls on the last sýllable; 9. *тк. несов. разг.* (*о волоса́х, зуба́х*) come* out, fall* out; 10. (*уменьша́ться, ослабева́ть*) fall*, drop; давле́ние ~а́ет the préssure is fálling; 11. *сов.* пасть (*станови́ться слабе́е, ничто́жнее*) decline, wane, be* on the decline; *перен.* (*по́ртиться*) detériorate; влия́ние его́ ~а́ет his ínfluence is declíning; настрое́ние больно́го ~а́ет the pátient's morále is detériorating; 12. *сов.* пасть (*до́хнуть — о ско́те*) die off, pérish; ◇ ~ в о́бморок faint (awáy); ~ от уста́лости be* réady to drop (with fatígue); се́рдце ~а́ет *one's* heart sinks; упа́сть в чьих-л. глаза́х fall*/sink* in *smb.'s* estimátion.

па́дающий fálling; (*ослабева́ющий*) declíning, wáning.

паде́ж *м. грам.* case.

падёж *м.* cáttle-plague.

падёжн|ый *грам.* case *attr.*; ~ые оконча́ния cáse-éndings.

паде́ни|е *с.* 1. fall; ~ температу́ры fall in témperature; ~ цен drop/fall in príces; у́гол ~я angle of íncidence; 2. (*мора́льное*) degradátion, dównfall.

па́дк|ий (на *вн.*, до *рд.*) ávid (for, of), gréedy (for, of); быть ~им до сла́дкого have* a sweet tooth.

па́дчерица *ж.* stépdaughter.

паёк *м.* rátion.

паз *м.* 1. chink; 2. *тех.* slot; (*жёлоб*) groove.

па́зух|а *ж.* 1. bósom; положи́ть что-л. за ~у slip *smth.* into one's bósom; (*о мужчине*) slip *smth.* únder one's shirt; 2. *анат.* sínus; ло́бные ~и fróntal sínuses; ◇ держа́ть ка́мень за ~ой hárbour thoughts of revénge.

пай *м.* share; ◇ на пая́х on a sháring/co-óperative básis.

па́йка *ж. тех.* sóldering.

па́йщик *м.* sháreholder.

пакга́уз *м.* wárehouse.

паке́т *м.* 1. (small) párcel, pácket; (*для продуктов*) páper-bag; (*упаковка*) pack; 2. (*официальное письмо*) létter; 3. (*комплект, совокупность*) páckage (*тж. перен.*); ◇ индивидуа́льный перевя́зочный ~ *воен.* field dréssing. ~ик *м.* bag; чай в ~иках tea bags. ~и́рование *с.* páck-aging.

пакиста́н|ец *м.*, ~ка *ж.* Pakistáni. ~ский Pakistáni.

па́кля *ж.* tow, fíbre pácking; (*из рассученных верёвок*) óakum.

пакова́ть, упакова́ть (*вн.*) pack (*smth.*).

па́костить *несов. разг.* 1. (*вн.; грязнить*) dírty (*smth.*); (*о животных*) make* a mess; 2. (*вн.; портить*) spoil* (*smth.*); 3. (*дт.; делать неприятности*) do* the dírty (on).

па́костный *разг.* 1. (*отвратительный*) disgústing, filthy; 2. (*делающий пакости*) abóminable.

па́кость *ж. разг.* 1. filth, muck; 2. (*гадкий поступок*) filthy/dírty trick; 3. (*непристойное выражение*) obscénity.

пакт *м.* pact.

пала́т|а *ж.* 1. (*в больнице*) ward; 2. (*высшее законодательное учреждение*) house, chámber; ~ы Верхо́вного Сове́та РФ the Chámbers of the Supréme Sóviet of the RF; ве́рхняя ~ Úpper House; Úpper Chámber *амер.*; ни́жняя ~ Lówer House; Lówer Chámber *амер.*; ~ ло́рдов (*в Англии*) the House of Lords; ~ о́бщин (*в Англии*) the House of Cómmons; ~ представи́телей (*в США*) the House of Represéntatives; ~ депута́тов (*во Франции*) the Chámber of Députies; 3. (*учреждение*) chámber, óffice; торго́вая ~ Chámber of Cómmerce; ~ мер и весо́в Board of Weights and Méasures; 4. *мн.* (*хоромы*) pálace *sg.*; ◇ Оруже́йная ~ the Armoury (*in the Kremlin*); Грано́витая ~ the Hall of Fácets (*in the Kremlin*); у него́ ума́ ~ he has a wónderful brain.

пала́тка *ж.* 1. tent; 2. (*ларёк*) stall, booth.

пала́точн|ый 1. tent *attr.*; ~ая жизнь life únder cánvas; ~ городо́к encámpment; 2. (*ларёчный*) stall *attr.*

пала́ч *м.* execútioner, hángman*; *перен.* bútcher.

па́левый stráw-coloured.

палёный scorched; (*о шерсти, волосах и т. п.*) singed.

па́лец *м.* 1. (*на руке*) fínger; (*на ноге*) toe; ди́гит *науч.*; сре́дний ~ míddle/sécond fínger; 2. *тех.* pin, cam; ◇ ~ о ~ не уда́рить not stir/lift a fínger; смотре́ть, гляде́ть на что-л. сквозь па́льцы turn a blind eye to *smth.*; wink/conníve at *smth.*; знать как свои́ пять па́льцев know* *smth.* báckwards.

палиса́дник *м.* 1. (*небольшой садик*) front gárden; 2. (*сквозной забор*) (stake) fence.

пали́тра *ж.* pálette; *перен. тж.* range of expréssion.

пали́ть I, опали́ть, спали́ть (*вн.*) 1. *сов.* опали́ть (*обжигать*) singe (*smth.*); ~ гу́ся singe a goose*; 2. *тк. несов.* (*обдавать жаром, зноем*) scorch (*smth.*); со́лнце пали́т the sun is béating down; 3. *сов.* спали́ть *разг.* (*жечь*) burn* (*smth.*), scorch (*smth.*).

пали́ть II *несов. разг.* (*стрелять*) shoot*, fire.

па́лк|а *ж.* stick; (*для прогулок тж.*) wálking-stick; (*посох*) staff; ◇ вставля́ть кому́-л. ~и в колёса put* a

---

spoke in *smb.'s* wheel; де́лать что-л. из-под ~и do* *smth.* únder compúlsion; как из-под ~и as if one were forced, as if únder the lash

паллиати́в *м.* pálliative.

пало́мни|к *м.* pílgrim; ~чество *с.* pílgrimage (*тж. перен.*).

па́лочка *ж.* 1. small stick; (*дирижёрская*) báton; 2. (*предмет в виде маленького бруска*) stick; ~ ме́ла stick of chalk; 3. *бакт.* bacíllus (*pl* -li); туберкулёзная ~ túbercle bacíllus; 4. *мн. анат.* rods.

па́луб|а *ж.* deck; ве́рхняя ~ úpper deck; сре́дняя ~ míddle deck; ни́жняя ~ lówer deck; вы́йти на ~у go* on deck. ~ный deck *attr.*

пальба́ *ж. разг.* fíring; (*пушечная*) cannonáde.

па́льм|а *ж.* ~ pálm-tree; ◇ ~ пе́рвенства the palm. ~овый palm *attr.*; ~овая ветвь pálm-branch.

пальто́ *с. нескл.* coat, óvercoat.

паля́щий búrning, scórching.

па́мпасы *мн.* pámpas.

памфле́т *м.* lampóon. ~и́ст *м.* lampóoner.

па́мятка *ж.* memorándum (*pl* -da); (*свод правил*) (list of) instrúctions; (*книжка*) hándbook.

па́мятник *м.* 1. mónument, memórial (*тж. перен.*); ~ Пу́шкину the Púshkin mónument; 2. (*на кладбище*) tómbstone, tomb; 3. (*произведение древней культуры, письменности*) mónument; литерату́рный ~ literary mónument; ~и старины́ mónuments to the past.

па́мятн|ый 1. mémorable; ~ день mémorable day; 2. (*служащий для напоминания*): ~ая кни́жка nótebook, memorándum-book; ◇ ~ая запи́ска memorándum (*pl* -da).

па́мят|ь *ж.* mémory; хоро́шая ~ good*/reténtive mémory; плоха́я ~ bad* mémory; свежо́ в ~и fresh in one's mémory; лиши́ться ~и lose* one's mémory; вре́заться в ~ be* engráved on the mémory, stick* in one's mémory; в ~ кого́-л. in mémory of *smb.*; ◇ на чьей-л. ~и within the mémory of *smb.*; прийти́ на ~ кому́-л. come* to *smb.'s* mind; игра́ть на ~ play from mémory; выпада́ть из ~и escápe/slip one's mémory; подари́ть что-л. на ~ give* *smth.* as a kéepsake/sóuvenir; без ~и 1) (*без сознания*): быть без ~и be* uncónscious; 2): люби́ть кого́-л. без ~и be* mádly in love with *smb.*; 3): быть без ~и от кого́-л. adóre *smb.*, be* pássionately fond of *smb.*

пана́м|а *ж.* sún-hat; (*из тонкой соломы*) panamá. ~ка *ж.* sún-hat.

панаце́я *ж.* panacéa.

пане́ль *ж.* 1. (*тротуар*) pávement, fóotway; sídewalk *амер.*; 2. (*деревянная обшивка стен*) pánelling, wáinscot(ing); 3. *стр.* pánel. ~ный pánel-constrúction *attr.*

панибра́т|ский *разг.* famíliar, báck-slapping, háil-fellow-wéll-mét *attr.* ~ство *с. разг.* familiárity.

па́ник|а *ж.* pánic, scare; быть в ~е be* pánic-stricken; наводи́ть ~у create/cause a pánic.

паникёр *м.* pánic-monger, alármist. ~ский alármist *attr.* ~ство *с.* pánic-mongering.

панихи́да *ж. церк.* the last óffices *pl*, fúneral sérvice.

пани́ческ|ий 1. (*проникнутый паникой*) pánic-stricken, pánic-struck; pánic *attr.*; (*вызывающий панику*) alármist *attr.*; ~ое настрое́ние pánicky mood; ~ страх pánic fear; 2. *разг.* (*легко поддающийся панике*) pánicky, tímorous.

панно́ *с. нескл.* pánel.

панора́м|а *ж.* 1. (*вид*) view; 2. (*картина*) panoráma. ~ный panorámic; ~ная съёмка cineráma; ~ный кинотеа́тр cineráma théatre.

пансио́н *м.* 1. (*учебное заведение*) bóarding school; 2. (*гостиница*) bóarding house; 3. (*полное содержание*) board and lódging.

пансиона́т *м.* hóliday hotél.

пантало́ны *мн.* 1. *уст.* (*брюки*) tróusers; 2. (*женские*) kníckers, pants.

панталы́к *м. разг.*: сби́ться с ~у get* ínto a múddle, go* wrong; сбить *кого-л.* с ~у put* smb. off his, her stroke, put* smb. out of his, her stride.

пантео́н *м.* pántheon.

панте́ра *ж. зоол.* pánther; *(самка)* pántheress.

пантоми́ма *ж.* pántomime; *(жесты, мимика как средство общения)* dumb show.

па́нцирный 1. *(о доспехах)* cháin-mail attr.; **2.** *(о животных)* testácean, testáceous.

па́нцирь *м.* **1.** *(доспех)* coat of mail, cuiráss; **2.** *(животных)* shell.

па́па I *м. разг.* dád(dy).

па́па II *м. (римский)* Pópe.

папа́ха *ж.* papákha *(tall astrakhan hat)*.

па́паша *м. разг.* fáther.

па́перть *ж.* chúrch-porch.

папиро́с|**а** *ж.* cigarétte (with a cárdboard hólder). ~ный cigarétte attr.; ◇ ~ная бума́га tíssue-páper.

папи́рус *м.* papýrus *(pl -ri).*

па́пка *ж.* **1.** *(для бумаг)* fólder; file; **2.** *(род портфеля)* under-árm (dócument) case.

па́поротник *м.* fern, brácken; зоро́сший ~ом férny. ~овый fern attr.

па́п|**ский** pápal. ~ство *с.* pápacy.

папуа́с *м.*, ~ка *ж.* Pápuan. ~ский Pápuan.

папье́-маше́ *с. нескл.* papier-mâché.

пар I *м.* **1.** steam; разводи́ть ~ы́ get* up steam, raise steam; **2.** *мн. (испарения)* vápour *sg;* ◇ под ~ами únder steam; на всех ~áx at full steam, at full speed.

пар II *м. с.-х.* fállow; земля́ под ~ом fállow ground; лежа́ть под ~ом lie* fállow.

па́р|**а** *ж.* **1.** pair; ~ чуло́к pair of stóckings; **2.** *(мужской костюм)* suit (of clothes); **3.** *(запряжка в две лошади)* two hórses; **4.** *(двое)* cóuple; танцу́ющие ~ы dáncing cóuples; влюблённая ~ two lóvers, pair of lóvers; **5.** *разг. (две штуки чего-л.)* two, a cóuple; **6.** *разг. (немного, несколько)* a few; **7.** *в знач. сказ. (дт.) разг.* match (for); она́ ему́ не ~ she's not good enóugh for him; ◇ постро́иться, встать в ~ы form up in pairs; в ~е togéther, as a pair; ~ пустяко́в *разг.* piece of cake; два canopá ~ ≈ birds of a féather.

парабе́ллум *м.* automátic (pístol).

пара́бола *ж. мат.* parábola.

пара́граф *м.* páragraph.

пара́д *м.* paráde; *воен. тж.* revíew; принима́ть ~ *воен.* revíew the troops; ◇ в по́лном ~е in full dress.

паради́гма *ж. грам.* páradigm.

пара́дн|**ое** *с.* front door. ~ость *ж.* magníficence; *(показная)* ostentátion. ~ый **1.** ceremónial; ~ая фо́рма ceremónial dress, full dress; **2.** *(праздничный)* smart, féstive; *(показной)* ostentátious, shówy; ~ое пла́тье best/Súnday clothes; ~ый спекта́кль gála perfórmance; **3.** *(главный)* main; ~ая дверь front door; ~ый подъе́зд main éntrance.

парадо́кс *м.* páradox. ~а́льный paradóxical.

парази́т *м.* párasite; *перен. тж.* drone.

парази́т|**и́зм** *м.* párasitism. ~и́ровать *несов.* live parasítically, párasitize. ~и́ческий parasític(al).

парализо́ванный páralysed.

парализова́ть *несов. и сов. (вн.)* páralyse *(smb., smth.)* *(тж. перен.)*; у него́ парализо́ваны о́бе но́ги he is páralysed in both legs. ~ся *несов. и сов.* be* páralysed.

парали́тик *м. разг.* paralýtic.

паралити́ческий paralýtic.

парали́ч *м.* parálysis *(pl -ses)* *(тж. перен.)*; прогресси́рующий ~ créeping parálysis; разби́т ~о́м strícken with parálysis. ~ный paralýtic.

параллелепи́пед *м. мат.* parallelépiped.

параллели́зм *м.* párallelism; *(дублирование)* duplicátion.

параллелогра́мм *м. мат.* parallélogram.

паралле́ль *ж.* párallel; провести́ ~ draw* a párallel. ~ный párallel; ◇ ~ные бру́сья *спорт.* the párallel bars; ~ное соедине́ние *эл.* connéction in párallel.

пара́метр *м.* parámeter.

паранджа́ *ж.* páranja, hórsehair veil.

парапе́т *м.* párapet.

парафи́н *м.* páraffin (wax). ~овый páraffin attr.; ~овое ма́сло páraffin oil.

парафи́ровать *несов. и сов. (вн.) дип.* initial *(smth.)*; ~ соглаше́ние, догово́р inítial an agréement, a tréaty.

парафра́з|**а** *ж. лит., муз.* páraphrase. ~и́ровать *несов. и сов. (вн.) лит., муз.* páraphrase *(smth.).*

парашю́т *м.* párachute; прыжо́к с ~ом párachute jump; спасти́сь, вы́бросившись с ~ом párachute to sáfety; вы́броситься с ~ом bale out. ~и́зм *м.* párachute-jumping. ~и́ст *м.* párachutist, párachute-jumper; *(спортсмен тж.)* ský-diver.

парашю́тн|**ый** párachute attr.; ~ая вы́шка párachute tówer; ~ деса́нт **1)** *(войска)* párachute troops *pl;* **2)** *(высадка)* párachute drop, lánding of párachute troops.

паре́ние *с.* sóaring.

па́рен|**ый** steamed; ◇ деше́вле ~ой ре́пы ≈ dírt-chéap.

па́рень *м. разг.* féllow, lad, chap; guy *амер.*

пари́ *с. нескл.* bet, wáger; ◇ держа́ть ~ bet*, lay* a bet.

пари́жск|**ий** Parísian; ~ая зе́лень Páris green; ~ая лазу́рь Páris blue.

пари́к *м.* wig.

парикма́хер *м.* háirdressser; *(мужской)* bárber. ~ская *ж.* háirdresser's (shop); *(мужская)* bárber's (shop); в ~ской at the háirdresser's/bárber's.

пари́лка *ж. (в бане)* swéating room.

пари́ровать *несов. и сов. (вн.)* **1.** *(отбивать)* párry *(smth.)*, ward off *(smth.)*; ~ уда́р ward off a blow; **2.** *(опровергать)* párry *(smth.)*, cóunter *(smth.)*; ~ до́вод párry an árgument.

парите́т *м.* **1.** *юр.* párity, equálity; **2.** *эк.* par, párity. ~ный *юр.* párity attr., équal; на ~ных нача́лах on a párity básis.

па́р|**ить** *несов.* **1.** *(вн.; варить на пару)* steam *(smth.)*; **2.** *(вн.; подвергать действию пара)* scald *(smth.)*; *(прогревать паром)* soak *(smth.)* in hot wáter; **3.** *обыкн. безл.* ~ит it is súltry; **4.** *(выделять пар)* steam, give* off vápour.

пари́ть *несов.* soar; *(о птицах тж.)* float, sail; ~ в облака́х *перен.* be*/live in the clouds.

па́риться *несов.* **1.** *(вариться на пару)* steam; **2.** *(в бане)* beat* onesélf with birch twigs in a steam bath; **3.** *разг. (изнемогать от жары)* be* boiled, swélter.

па́рия *м. и ж.* páriah, óutcast.

парк *м.* **1.** park; ~ культу́ры и о́тдыха recreátion park; разби́ть ~ lay* out a park; **2.** *(место стоянки подвижного состава)* dépot; *(автомашин тж.)* gárage; **3.** *(совокупность средств передвижения, механизмов и т. п.)* stock; *(автомашин тж.)* fleet; ~ подвижно́го соста́ва rólling stock.

парке́т *м.* **1.** *собир.* párquetry; **2.** *(пол)* párquet (floor), inláid floor. ~ный: ~ный пол см. парке́т 2.

парла́мент *м.* párliament. ~ари́зм *м.* parliamentárianism, parliaméntary sýstem. ~а́рий *м.* mémber of párliament, M. P. ~а́рный parliaméntary.

парламентёр *м.* truce énvoy. ~ский truce attr.; ~ский флаг flag of truce.

парла́ментск|**ий** parliaméntary; ~ие вы́боры parliaméntary eléctions.

парни́к *м.* hótbed, fórcing frame. ~о́вый hótbed attr.; ~о́вые ра́мы fórcing frames; ~о́вые о́вощи forced végetables; ~о́вое огоро́дничество ráising végetables únder glass.

парн|**о́й** **1.** fresh; ~о́е молоко́ fresh milk, milk fresh from the cow; ~ое мя́со fresh-killed meat; 2. *разг.* (*душный*) súltry, stúffy, stícky.

па́рн|ый 1. (*составляющий пару*) twin; pair *attr.*; (*о листьях*) cónjugate; 2. (*об экипаже, санях*) for two hórses *после сущ.*; 3. (*производимый парой*) pair *attr.*; ~ая игра́ в те́ннис dóubles; ~ое ката́ние на конька́х pair figure-skáting.

парово́з *м.* (steam) lócomotive. ~ный (steam) lócomotive *attr.*

паро́в|о́й I steam *attr.*; ~ коте́л stéam-boiler; ~ дви́гатель stéam-engine; ~ое отопле́ние stéam-heating.

паро́в|о́й II *с.-х.* (*находящийся под паром*) fállow; ~ое по́ле fállow land.

паро́дийн|ый burlésque *attr.*; ~ая пье́са burlésque.

пароди́ровать *несов. и сов.* (*вн.*) párody (*smb., smth.*), trávesty (*smb., smth.*), burlésque (*smb., smth.*); (*представить в смешном виде*) take* (*smb., smth.*) off.

паро́дия *ж.* párody, trávesty, burlésque; ~ на справедли́вость trávesty of jústice.

парокси́зм *м.* paroxysm.

паро́ль *м.* pássword.

паро́м *м.* férry(-boat); перепра́виться на ~е férry acróss/óver the ríver; перепра́ва на ~е férrying acróss.

паро́мщик *м.* férryman*.

парообра́зный váporous.

парообразова́ние *с.* generátion of steam, vaporizátion.

пароотво́дн|ый: ~ая труба́ *тех.* exháust/stéam-escape pipe.

парохо́д *м.* stéamer; (*речной, небольшой*) stéamboat; (*морской*) stéamship. ~ный stéamship *attr.* ~ство *с.* stéamship line; Во́лжское ~ство the Vólga stéamship line.

па́рочка *ж.* pair, cóuple.

парт- *в сложн.* Párty *attr.*

па́рт|а *ж.* (school) desk; за одно́й ~ой с кем-л. share the same desk (at school) with *smb.*

партбиле́т *м.* Párty(-mémbership) card. ~бюро́ *с. нескл.* Párty buréau. ~взно́сы *мн.* Párty dues.

парте́р *м. театр.* (*передние ряды*) the stalls *pl*; (*задние ряды*) the pit; ме́сто в ~е seat in the stalls.

парти́ец *м. разг.* Párty man*/pérson.

партиза́н *м.* partisán, guerrílla (fighter). ~ить *несов. разг.* fight* as a partisán. ~ка *ж. см.* партиза́нка. ~ский partisán *attr.*; guerrílla *attr.*; ~ская война́ guerrílla war/wárfare; ~ский отря́д partisán/guerrílla detáchment.

парти́йн|ость *ж.* (*принадлежность к партии*) Párty-mémbership; ~ый Párty *attr.*; ~ый рабо́тник Párty official; ~ое руково́дство Párty léaders *pl.*

партиту́ра *ж. муз.* score.

па́ртия *ж.* 1. (*политическая организация*) párty; 2. (*группа лиц*) group, párty; (*пленных и т. п.*) batch; поиско́вая ~ prospécting párty; 3. (*количество каких-л. предметов*) consígnment, shípment; batch; ~ това́ра consígnment of goods; ~ гру́за shípment of freight; о́пытная ~ initial lot; 4. (*часть музыкального произведения*) part; 5. (*игра*) game; ~ в ша́хматы, ша́шки a game of chess, draughts.

партко́м *м.* (парти́йный комите́т) Párty Commíttee.

партконфере́нция *ж.* Párty Cónference.

партнёр *м.*, ~ша *ж.* pártner; (*компаньон*) compánion; (*противник в игре*) oppónent; делово́й ~ búsiness pártner.

парт|собра́ние *с.* Párty méeting. ~съезд *м.* Párty Cóngress.

па́рус *м.* sail; подня́ть ~ hoist the sail; спусти́ть ~ lówer the sail; убра́ть ~ take* in sail; идти́ под ~а́ми procéed únder sail; нести́сь на всех ~а́х be* únder full sail, have* all sails set; *перен.* go* full speed.

паруси́н|а *ж.* cánvas; (*для парусов тж.*) sáil-cloth; ~овый cánvas *attr.*

па́русн|ик *м.* sáiling-ship. ~ый sáiling *attr.*; ~ая ло́дка sáiling-boat; ~ый спорт sáiling yáchting.

парфюме́р|ия *ж. собир.* pérfume and cosmétics *pl*; perfúmery. ~ный perfúmery *attr.*; ~ный магази́н pérfume and cosmétics shop.

парч|а́ *ж.* brocáde. ~о́вый brocáde *attr.*, brocáded.

парш|а́ *ж.* mange, scab. ~и́веть, опарши́веть *разг.* get* the mange. ~и́вый 1. (*больной паршой*) scábby, mángy; 2. *разг.* (*плохой, дрянной*) rótten; (*о человеке, поступке тж.*) mean, shábby; ~и́вая пого́да rótten wéather; ~и́вое настрое́ние rótten mood.

пас I 1. *межд.* pass, no bid; 2. *в знач. сказ.*: я ~ count me out.

пас II *м. спорт.* pass; то́чный ~ в центр áccurate pass to the céntre.

па́сека *ж.* ápiary.

па́сечник *м.* bée-keeper.

па́сквил|ь *м.* lampóon, squib; писа́ть ~и на кого́-л. write* lampóons agáinst/abóut *smb.* ~я́нт *м.* lampóoner, lampóonist.

па́смурн|о 1. *нареч.* clóudy, dull; 2. *в знач. сказ. безл.* it is clóudy, it is dull; *перен.* it is glóomy; сего́дня ~ it is clóudy todáy; на душе́ у него́ станови́лось ~ he felt glóomy. ~ый clóudy, óvercast; *перен.* (*о человеке*) glóomy; ~ая пого́да dull / óvercast wéather; ~ый вид glóomy appéarance; ~ое настрое́ние despóndent mood.

пасова́ть I, спасова́ть 1. (*в картах*) pass; 2. (*перед тв.*; *сдаваться*) give* in (to), yield (to); спасова́ть пе́ред кем-л. be* unáble to hold *one's* ground agáinst *smb.*; спасова́ть перед тру́дностями shrink* from dífficulties, dodge dífficulties.

пасова́ть II *несов. спорт.* pass.

пасо́вка *ж. спорт.* pássing.

паспарту́ *с. нескл.* pásse-partout.

па́спорт *м.* 1. (*удостоверение личности*) pássport; 2. (*регистрационное свидетельство оборудования и т. п.*) registrátion certíficate. ~ный pássport *attr.*; ~ная систе́ма pássport sýstem.

пасса́ж *м.* 1. arcáde; 2. *муз.* pássage.

пассажи́р *м.* pássenger; зал для ~ов wáiting-room. ~ский pássenger *attr.*; ~ский по́езд pássenger train; ~ский ваго́н pássenger cárriage; pássenger car *амер.*; ~ское движе́ние pássenger tráffic.

пасса́т *м.* trade wind.

пасси́в *м.* 1. *фин.* liabílities *pl*; 2. *грам.* pássive voice.

пасси́вн|ость *ж.* inértia, passívity, slúggishness. ~ый pássive; ~ые зри́тели unrespónsive áudience *sg.*; ~ое выжида́ние pássive expectátion; ~ый бала́нс вне́шней торго́вли *эк.* unfávourable trade bálance; ~ая констру́кция *грам.* pássive constrúction.

па́ста *ж.* paste; зубна́я ~ tóoth-paste.

па́стбищ|е *с.* pásture, pásture-ground, grázing-ground; (*для овец тж.*) shéep-walk, shéep-run; выгоня́ть скот на ~ take* cáttle out to pásture, drive* cáttle to pásture. ~ный pásture *attr.*

пасте́ль *ж.* pastél; рисова́ть ~ю draw* in pastél. ~ный pastél *attr.*; ~ная жи́вопись pastél (dráwing); ~ные тона́ pastél shades.

пастеризо́ванный pásteurized.

пастеризова́ть *несов. и сов.* (*вн.*) pásteurize (*smth.*).

пастерна́к *м. бот.* pársnip.

пасти́ *несов.* (*вн.*) graze (*smth.*); (*птиц*) feed* (*smth.*).

пастила́ *ж.* pastilá, fruit fudge.

пасти́сь *несов.* graze, pásture; (*о птицах*) feed*.

пастора́ль *ж.* 1. *лит.* pástoral; 2. *муз.* pastorále (*pl* -li, -s).

пасту́|х *м.* hérdsman*; (*пасущий овец*) shépherd. ~шеский hérdsman's; shépherd *attr.* ~ший shépherd's; ~ший рожо́к shépherd's horn.

пастушо́к *м.* shépherd boy.

па́стырь *м. рел.* pástor.

пасть I *сов.* 1. *см.* па́дать 1, 3, 5, 6, 7, 10, 11, 12; 2. *(погибнуть на поле боя)* fall*; 3. *(быть свергнутым)* fall*, collápse; 4. *(сдаться)* fall*.

пасть II *ж.* *(рот)* jaws *pl*, maw.

па́сха *ж.* 1. *рел.* *(христианская)* Éaster; *(еврейская)* the Pássover; 2. *(кушанье)* páskha *(rich mixture of sweetened curds, butter and raisins eaten at Easter)*.

пасха́льный Éaster *attr.*

па́сынок *м.* stépson.

пат *м.* *шахм.* stálemate.

пате́нт *м.* pátent; *перен.* title; получи́ть ~ на изобре́тение take* out a pátent for an invéntion.

патенто́ванн|ый pátent *attr.*; ~ое сре́дство pátent médicine.

патентова́ть *несов. и сов.* *(вн.)* pátent *(smth.)*, take* out a pátent (for, on); ~ изобрете́ние pátent an invéntion.

патети́ческий férvent, pássionate.

патефо́н *м.* *уст.* grámophone; заводи́ть ~ play the grámophone. ~ный grámophone *attr.*; ~ная пласти́нка grámophone récord.

па́тока *ж.* tréacle; *(очищенная)* sýrup; *(чёрная)* molásses.

патологи́ческий pathológical.

патоло́гия *ж.* pathólogy.

патриа́рх *м.* pátriarch. ~а́льный patriárchal; *(устарелый тж.)* ántiquated; ~а́льные взгля́ды ántiquated nótions. ~а́т *м.* 1. *(строй)* pátriarchy; 2. *церк.* pátriarchate.

патрио́т *м.* 1. pátriot; 2. *(преданный какому-л. делу человек)* devotée. ~и́зм *м.* pátriotism. ~и́ческий patriótic; ~и́ческие чу́вства patriótic séntiments. ~ка *ж.* pátriot.

патро́н I *м.* 1. *воен.* cártridge; охо́тничий ~ spórting cártridge; 2. *тех.* chuck; 3. *эл.* lámp-socket.

патро́н II *м.* 1. *(покровитель)* pátron; 2. *(хозяин, начальник)* boss.

патрона́ж *м.* home núrsing. ~ный hóme-núrsing *attr.*; ~ная сестра́ vísiting nurse.

патро́нник *м.* *воен.* (cártrige-)chámber.

патро́нн|ый cártridge *attr.*; ~ая су́мка cártridge-pouch.

патронта́ш *м.* cártridge-belt, bándolier.

патрули́ровать *несов.* be* on patról; *(вн.)* patról *(smth.)*.

патру́ль *м.* patról; ко́нный ~ móunted patról; милице́йский ~ police patról; нача́льник патруля́ patról léader; зелёный ~ fórest patról. ~ный *прил.* 1. patról *attr.*; 2. *в знач. сущ. м.* patrólman*.

па́уз|а *ж.* pause *(тж. муз.)*; де́лать ~у pause; наступи́ла ~ в разгово́ре there was a pause in the conversátion.

пау́к *м.* spíder.

паукообра́зный spíderlike, spídery.

паути́на *ж.* cóbweb, spíder's web; *(осенняя)* góssamer; *перен.* web; ~ лжи web of lies.

па́фос *м.* 1. férvour, pássion, inspirátion, fire; *(излишняя приподнятость тона)* effúsiveness, gush; говори́ть с ~ом speak* with inspirátion; 2. *(воодушевление)* enthúsiasm; *(источник воодушевления)* (source of) inspirátion.

пах *м.* groin.

па́хан|ый ploughed; ~ая земля́ ploughed land.

па́харь *м.* plóughman*;

паха́ть *несов.* *(вн.)* plough *(smth.)*, till *(smth.)*; ~ зе́млю plough/till the soil.

пахн|у́ть *несов.* *(тв.)* smell* (of); *перен. тж.* smack (of); си́льно ~ smell* strong; хорошо́ (пло́хо) ~ smell* nice (násty); ро́зы прия́тно ~ут róses smell sweet, róses have a sweet smell; ~ет бедо́й there is trouble in store; э́то ~ет больши́ми убы́тками this may mean héavy lósses; ◇ ~ет по́рохом war is in the air, war is bréwing.

пахн|у́ть *сов.*: в ко́мнату ~у́ло арома́том цветов the

fragrance of flówers was wáfted into the room; в лицо́ ему́ ~у́ло све́жестью he felt a puff of fresh air in his face; от реки́ ~у́ло хо́лодом a cold air drífted up from the river.

пахово́й groin *attr.*

па́хот|а *ж.* 1. *(действие)* plóughing; 2. *(вспаханное поле)* plóugh-land, ploughed field. ~ный árable; ~ная земля́ árable land.

па́хтать *несов.* *(вн.)* churn *(smth.)*.

паху́ч|есть *ж.* frágrance; aróma. ~ий frágrant, ódorous, aromátic.

пацие́нт *м.*, ~ка *ж.* pátient.

пациф|и́зм *м.* pácifism. ~и́ст *м.* pácifist. ~и́стский pácifist.

па́че *уст.*: ~ ча́яния cóntrary to all expectátions; тем ~! all the more!, the more so!

па́чка *ж.* búndle; *(в упаковке)* pácket, páckage; ~ де́нег wad of notes; ~ газе́т búndle of néwspapers; ~ папиро́с pácket of cigaréttes. ~ми in bátches.

па́чк|ать *несов.* *(вн.)* 1. dírty *(smth.)*, soil *(smth.)*; *(чернилами)* blot *(smth.)*; *(делать пятна)* stain *(smth.)*; 2. *разг.* *(плохо рисовать, писать)* scrawl *(smth.)*; *(краской)* daub *(smth.)*; ◇ ~ чьё-л. до́брое и́мя súlly/tárnish/blémish smb.'s good name. ~аться *несов.* get* dírty; бе́лые ту́фли бы́стро ~аются white shoes éasily get dírty, white shoes show the dirt.

пачкотня́ *ж.* *разг.* *(плохо написанная картина)* daub; *(грязно написанное)* scrawl.

пачку́н *м.* *разг.* 1. slóven; 2. *пренебр.* *(плохой худо́жник)* dáuber.

па́шня *ж.* plóugh-land, ploughed field.

паште́т *м.* paste; *(гусиный, из дичи)* pâté.

па́юсн|ый: ~ая икра́ pressed cáviar(e).

па́йл|ник *м.* sóldering-iron. ~ный sóldering *attr.*; ~ная ла́мпа sóldering lamp, blówlamp.

пая́сничать *несов.* *разг.* clown, fool abóut, act like an ídiot.

пая́ть *несов.* *(вн.)* sólder *(smth.)*.

пая́ц *м.* buffóon, clown.

пев|е́ц *м.* sínger; *перен.* bard. ~и́ца *ж.* sínger.

певу́н *м.* *разг.* sóngster.

певу́нья *ж.* *разг.* sóngstress.

певу́ч|есть *ж.* melódiousness, lilt. ~ий 1. *(мелодичный)* melódious, lílting; 2. *разг.* *(любящий петь)* sóngful; given to song *после сущ.*; ~ий наро́д a péople given to song.

пе́вч|ий *прил.* 1. sínging; ~ие пти́цы sóng-birds; 2. *в знач. сущ. м.* chórister; chóir-boy.

пе́гий skéwbald, píebald.

педаго́г *м.* téacher. ~и́ка *ж.* pedagógics.

педагоги́ческ|ий pedagógical; ~ сове́т másters'/téacher's méeting; ~ тала́нт gift for téaching; ~ие спосо́бности téaching abílity; ~ институ́т téacher-training cóllege, pedagógical ínstitute; ~ое учи́лище prímary-school téachers' course; ~ие ка́дры téachers; ~ая пра́ктика téaching práctice, stúdent téaching; ~ая литерату́ра líterature on educátion; ~ое образова́ние pedagógical tráining; с ~ой то́чки зре́ния from the educátional point of view.

педагоги́чный corréct from the stándpoint of pedagógics, educátionally/pedagógically corréct.

педа́ль *ж.* pédal; *(на швейной машине и т. п.)* tréadle; нажа́ть ~ press the pédal; отпусти́ть ~ reléase the pédal. ~ный pédal *attr.*; ~ная переда́ча pédal gear.

педа́нт *м.* pédant. ~и́зм *м.* pédantry, háir-splitting. ~и́чность *ж.* pédantry. ~и́чный pedántic, hypercrítical, fastídious.

педиа́тр *м.* children's dóctor, pediatrícian. ~и́я *ж.* pediátrics.

педикю́р *м.* pédicure, chirópody.

пейза́ж *м.* 1. *(вид местности)* lándscape, scénery; 2. *(картина)* lándscape. ~и́ст *м.* lándscape páinter.

~ный lándscape *attr*.; ~ная жи́вопись lándscape páinting.

пека́рня *ж*. bákery.

пе́карь *м*. báker.

пёкл|о *с. разг.* scórching heat; *перен.* hell; в са́мом ~е бо́я in the thick of the fighting.

пелена́ *ж*. blánket; ◇ сло́вно ~ с глаз упа́ла the scales fell from *one's* eyes.

пелена́ть, спелена́ть (*вн.*) swáddle (*smb.*).

пе́ленг *м*. béaring.

пеленга́тор *м*. diréction finder.

пеленгова́ть *несов. и сов.* (*сов. тж.* запеленгова́ть) (*вн.*) take* béarings (on); ~ радиоста́нцию take* béarings on a rádio státion.

пелён|ка *ж*. wrap; *мн.* swáddling clothes; ◇ с ~ок from the crádle; вы́йти из ~ок be* out of swáddling clothes.

пелери́на *ж*. (*женская*) pélerine, mántle; (*мужская*) short hóoded cape.

пелика́н *м*. pélican.

пельме́ни *мн.* (*ед.* пельме́нь *м.*) meat dúmplings.

пе́мза *ж*. púmice(-stone).

пён|а *ж*. 1. foam; (*в бокале вина, пива*) froth; (*на лошади*) láther; 2. (*мыльная*) láther; (soap-)suds *pl*; ◇ с ~ой у рта in a great heat, véhemently.

пена́л *м*. péncil-box.

пена́льти *м. и с. нескл. спорт.* pénalty.

пенёк *м*. stump.

пе́ни|е *с*. sínging; (*петуха*) crówing; учи́тель ~я sínging téacher; учи́ться ~ю stúdy sínging; уро́ки ~я sínging léssons.

пе́нист|ый fóamy, fóaming, fróthy; ~ые во́лны fóaming waves; ~ое мы́ло soap that makes a lot of foam/suds.

пе́нить *несов.* (*вн.*) make* (*smth.*) foam/froth. ~ся *несов.* foam, froth.

пеницилли́н *м*. penicíllin(e).

пе́нк|а *ж*. cóating, film, skin; (*накипь*) scum; ◇ снима́ть ~и skim the cream.

пенопла́ст *м*. (rígid) foam plástic. ~овый foam plástic *attr*.

пенсионе́р *м*., ~ка *ж*. pénsioner.

пенсио́нн|ый pénsion *attr*.; ~ое обеспе́чение provísion of pénsions; ~ во́зраст pénsion/pénsionable age; ~ая кни́жка pénsion-book.

пе́нсия *ж*. pénsion.

пенсне́ *с. нескл.* pince-néz.

пень *м*. stump, stub; *перен.* blóckhead; корчева́ть пни stub up trée-stumps; ◇ стоя́ть как ~ stand* (there) like a stuffed dúmmy.

пенька́ *ж*. hemp. ~о́вый hemp *attr*.

пе́ня *ж*. fine.

пен|я́ть, попеня́ть (на *вн.*) *разг.* blame (*smb.*); ◇ ~я́й на себя́! you have ónly yoursélf to blame!

пе́пел *м*. áshes *pl*; ◇ обраща́ть *что-л.* в ~ redúce/burn* *smth.* to áshes; подня́ть *что-л.* из пе́пла retríeve *smth.* from áshes, build* *smth.* anéw. ~ище *с. уст.* 1. the site/scene of a fire; 2. (*родной дом*) home; верну́ться на ста́рое ~ище retúrn to *one's* old home.

пе́пельница *ж*. áshtray.

пе́пельн|ый ásh-coloured, áshen; ~ые ко́сы ásh-blond trésses.

пе́рвен|ец *м*. first-born; *перен.* fírstling. ~ство *с*. the first place; *спорт.* chámpionship; завоева́ть ~ство win* the first place; ~ство ми́ра по футбо́лу world fóotball chámpionship.

пе́рвенствовать *несов.* (над *тв.*, среди́ *рд.*) take* first place (amóng); rule the roost идио́м.

перви́чн|ый 1. (*первоначальный*) prímary; inítial; ~ая обрабо́тка мета́лла inítial prócess in the tréatment of métal; ~ые поро́ды *геол.* prímary rocks; ~ пери́од боле́зни inítial stage of a diséase; 2. (*низовой*) prímary.

первобытнообщи́нный: ~ строй prímitive commúnal sýstem.

первобы́тн|ый 1. prímitive; ~ челове́к prímitive man*; ~ые времена́ prehistóric times; ~ое о́бщество prímitive socíety; ~ коммуни́зм tríbal cómmunism; 2. (*нетронутый, невозде́ланный*) primévat; ~ лес primévat fórest; 3. (*некультурный*) sávage; ~ые нра́вы sávage cústoms; 4. (*вымерший*) fóssil; ~ые живо́тные fóssil ánimals.

первоисто́чник *м*. oríginal work/source; рабо́тать с ~ами stúdy the oríginal works; че́рпать све́дения из ~а get* *one's* informátion at first hand.

первокла́сс|ик *м*. first-form boy. ~ица *ж*. first-form girl.

первокла́сс|ый first-ráte; ~ая те́хника first-ráte machínery.

первоку́рсн|ик *м*. first-year man*/stúdent; fréshman*. ~ица *ж*. first-year stúdent/girl.

Первома́й *м*. Máy Day.

первома́йск|ий Máy Day *attr*.; ~ая демонстра́ция Máy Day demonstrátion.

первонача́льн|о oríginally, in the first place. ~ый 1. (*исходный*) oríginal, inítial; ~ый план oríginal plan; ~ые устано́вки inítial arrángements/sét-up; 2. (*являющийся первым этапом чего-л.*) prímary; ~ое обуче́ние prímary tráining/educátion; ~ое накопле́ние капита́ла prímary accumulátion of cápital; 3. (*элементарный*) eleméntary; ~ые све́дения из грамма́тики first élements of grámmar.

первообра́з *м*. prótotype.

первооткрыва́тель *м*. discóverer.

первоочередн|о́й úrgent; ~а́я зада́ча úrgent task.

первопеча́тн|ый *м*. pioneer of prínting. ~ый 1. éarly prínted; ~ые кни́ги éarly prínted books; 2. (*изданный впервые*) first prínted.

первопрохо́дец *м*. explórer, pioneer, tráil-blázer.

первопу́ток *м. разг.* first sledge road of winter.

перворазря́дн|ик *м*. first-grade spórtsman*/pláyer. ~ица *ж*. first-grade spórtswoman*/pláyer.

первосо́ртный first-ráte, éxcellent.

первостепе́нн|ый páramount; ~ой ва́жности of páramount impórtance.

первоцве́т *м*. prímrose.

пе́рв|ый *прил.* 1. first, the first; ~ое (*число месяца*) the first (day) of the month; ~ое января́ the first of Jánuary, Néw-Year's day; в ~ых чи́слах сентября́ éarly in Septémber; полови́на ~ого half past twelve; 2. (*при перечислении — первый из двух*) the fórmer; из э́тих двух ме́тодов я предпочита́ю ~ of the two méthods I prefér the fórmer; 3. (*впервые совершённый, произнесённый и т. п.*) máiden; ~ая речь máiden speech; ~ полёт máiden flight; 4. (*начальный, вступительный*) ópening; ~ ход ópening; 5. (*находящийся впереди*) front; ~ ряд the first/front row; быть в ~ых ряда́х take* the lead; быть в ~ых ряда́х движе́ния сторо́нников ми́ра be in the vánguard of the peace móvement; 6. *в знач. сущ. с.* (*блюдо*) first course; ◇ при ~ой возмо́жности at the first opportúnity; вы́двинуть *что-л.* на ~ план bring* *smth.* to the fóre(ground); из ~ых рук at first hand; быть ~ым в кла́ссе be* at the top of the class/form; ~ая по́мощь first aid.

перга́мент *м*. 1. (*кожа*) párchment; 2. (*рукопись*) párchment mánuscript; 3. (*бумага*) gréase-proof páper. ~ный párchment *attr*.; ~ая бума́га gréase-proof páper.

переадресова́ть *сов.* переадресо́вывать.

переадресо́вывать, переадресова́ть (*вн.*) readdréss (*smth.*), fórward (*smth.*); ~ письмо́ fórward a létter.

перебази́ровать *сов.* (*вн.*) transfér (*smth.*), move (*smth.*). ~ся *сов.* move/transfér *one's* base.

переба́рщивать, переборщи́ть *разг.* go* too far, overdó* it.

перебега́ть, перебежа́ть 1. (*вн., через вн.*) run*

acróss (*smth.*); ~ чéрез дорóгу, ýлицу run* acróss the road, street; ~ мост run* acróss the bridge; 2. (*бегом миновáть что-л.*) run* acróss; ~ с мéста на мéсто keep* rúnning from one place to anóther; ~ на другóе мéсто run* acróss to anóther place; 3. (*переходить на сторону противника*) desért; go* óver to the énemy; 4. *тк. несов.* (*быстро передвигáться — о свете, тени, взгляде*) dart, flit; ◇ ~ комý-л. дорóгу cross *smb.*, thwart *smb.*

перебежáть *сов. см.* перебегáть 1, 2, 3.

перебéж|ка *ж.* dash, short run. ~чик *м. воен.* desérter; *перен.* deféctor, túrncoat.

перебеси́ться *сов.* 1. go* mad; 2. *разг.* (*остепениться*) stéady down, have* sown *one's* wild oats.

перебивáть, переби́ть (*вн.*) 1. (*прерывáть*) interrúpt (*smb.*); 2. (*нарушáть*) spoil* (*smth.*), kill (*smth.*); ~ аппети́т spoil* *one's* áppetite. ~ся, переби́ться *разг.* mánage.

перебирáть, перебрáть (*вн.*) 1. (*сортировáть*) sort (*smth.*); ~ картóфель sort potátoes; 2. (*пересмáтривать*) exámine (*smth.*), go* through (*smth.*); ~ пи́сьма go* through the létters; 3. (*мысленно воспроизводи́ть*) go* óver (*smth.*); ~ что-л. в пáмяти go* óver *smth.* in *one's* mind; 4. (*касáться пáльцами всего, многого*) run* *one's* fingers (óver); ~ стрýны гитáры run* *one's* fingers óver the strings of a guitár; 5. (*тв.; дéлать чáстые движéния чем-л.*) stir (*smth.*) réstlessly. 6. *полигр.* (*дéлать новый нáбор*) resét* (*smth.*). ~ся, перебрáться *разг.* (*переправляться*) get* acróss, pass óver; ~ся чéрез рéку get* acróss a river; 2. (*переселяться*) move; ~ся на нóвую кварти́ру move (to a new flat).

переби́ть *сов. см.* перебивáть 1. (*вн.*); 2. (*вн.; убить многих*) kill (a lot of); 3. (*вн.; разби́ть всё*) break* (*smth.*); ~ всю посýду break* all *one's* cróckery/chína. ~ся *сов. см.* перебивáться.

перебó|й *м.* 1. (*неравномéрность биéния сéрдца*) irregulárity; пульс с ~ями irrégular pulse; ~и сéрдца irrégular héartbeat *sg*; 2. (*в рабóте механи́зма*) misfire; мотóр рабóтает с ~ями the éngine keeps misfiring/báckfiring; маши́ны рабóтают без ~ев work smóothly; 3. (*в рабóте и т. п.*) stóppage, irregulárity.

перебол|éть *сов.* (*тв.*) 1. (*перенести́ каку́ю-л. болéзнь*) have* been ill (with); have* (*smth.*); go* through (*smth.*) (*тж. перен.*); он тóлько что ~éл воспалéнием лёгких he has just had pneumónia; 2. (*перенести́ много болéзней*) have* évery (concéivable) íllness; 3. (*перенести́ каку́ю-л. болéзнь — о многих*): все дéти ~éли кóрью all the children have had méasles.

перебóрка *ж.* 1. (*дéйствие*) sórting; ~ картóфеля sórting potátoes; 2. (*перегорóдка*) partítion; (*на корáбле*) búlkhead.

переборóть *сов.* (*вн.*) overcóme* (*smb.*, *smth.*) (*тж. перен.*); get* the bétter (of); ~ себя́ take* a grip on onesélf; ~ страх overcóme* fear.

переборщи́ть *сов. см.* перебáрщивать.

перебрáсывать, перебрóсить (*вн.*) 1. throw* (*smth.*) óver; fling* (*smth.*) óver; ~ что-л. чéрез плечó fling* *smth.* óver *one's* shóulder; 2.: ~ мост чéрез рéку build* a bridge óver/acróss a river; 3. (*переводи́ть куда-л.*) send* (*smb.*), transfér (*smb.*); (*доставлять что-л.*) transpórt (*smth.*). ~ся, перебрóситься 1. spring* acróss; rush acróss; 2. (*распространяться*) spread*; огóнь перебрóсился на сосéдний дом the fire spread to the next house; 3. (*тв.; бросáть друг другу*) toss *smth.*; *перен.* (*обмéниваться*) exchánge (*smth.*); ~ся мячóм throw* a ball to one anóther; ~ся словáми exchánge a few words; ~ся шýтками bándy jokes.

перебрáть(ся) *сов. см.* перебирáть(ся).

переброди́ть *сов.* fermént.

перебрóсить(ся) *сов. см.* перебрáсывать(ся).

перебрóска *ж.* (*перемещéние куда-л.*) tránsfer, tránsference; (*достáвка*) transportátion.

перебыв|áть *сов.* make* the round (of); ~ у всех знакóмых make* the round of *one's* friends; он ~áл у всех врачéй he has consúlted all the dóctors.

перевáл 1. (*дéйствие*) cróssing; ~ чéрез гóры прошёл успéшно we (they *etc.*) crossed the móuntains succéssfully; 2. (*горный*) (móuntain) pass.

перевáливать, перевали́ть 1. (*вн.; с трудóм перемещáть что-л.*) heave* (*smth.*); 2. (*вн., чéрез вн.; перемещáться*) cross (*smth.*), top (*smth.*); перевали́ть чéрез гóры cross the móuntains; 3. *разг.* (*переходи́ть какие-л. предéлы*) pass, top; *безл.* be* past; сýмма на текýщем счетý перевали́ла за 5000 рублéй the accóunt came to more than 5,000 róubles; перевали́ло зá полночь it is past mídnight; 4. *безл.* (*дт., о вóзрасте*) be* past; емý перевали́ло зá сóрок he is past fórty. ~ся, перевали́ться 1. heave* onesélf óver, roll óver; 2. *тк. несов.* (*о похóдке*) wáddle.

перевали́ть *сов. см.* перевáливать. ~ся *сов. см.* перевáливаться 1.

перевáрив|ать, перевари́ть (*вн.*) 1. (*по́ртить*) overdó* (*smth.*); перевари́ть óвощи overdó* the végetables; 2. (*усвáивать*) digést (*smth.*) (*тж. перен.*); ~ прочи́танное digést what *one* has read; 3. *разг.* (*переноси́ть*): я егó не ~аю I can't stand him. ~áться, перевари́ться 1. be* overdóne; 2. (*усвáиваться в процéссе пищеварéния*) be* digésted.

перевари́ть(ся) *сов. см.* перевáривать(ся).

перевезти́ *сов. см.* перевози́ть.

перевернýть(ся) *сов. см.* перевёртывать(ся).

перевёртывать, переверну́ть (*вн.*) 1. (*с одной стороны на другу́ю*) turn (*smb.*, *smth.*) óver; (*вверх дном*) turn (*smth.*) upside-dówn; (*опроки́дывать*) overtúrn (*smth.*); *разг.* (*перелицóвывать*) turn (*smth.*); переверну́ть страни́цу turn a page; переверну́ть всё вверх дном turn éverything upside-dówn; 2. *разг.* (*прерывáть всё, многое*) turn (*smth.*) upside-dówn; 3. *разг.* (*дéлать совершéнно другим*) make* a great change (in). ~ся, переверну́ться turn; (*опроки́дываться*) overtúrn.

перевéс *м.* 1. (*изли́шек в вéсе*) óverweight; 2. (*превосхóдство*) superiórity, prepónderance; чи́сленный ~ numérical superiórity; имéть чи́сленный ~ над врагóм be* numérically supérior to the énemy; ~ сил prepónderance of fórces.

перевéсить(ся) *сов. см.* перевéшивать(ся).

перевести́(сь) *сов. см.* переводи́ть(ся).

перевéшивать, перевéсить (*вн.*) 1. (*на другóе мéсто*) rearránge (*smth.*), reháng* (*smth.*); 2. (*превосходи́ть вéсом*) outwéigh (*smth.*) (*тж. перен.*). ~ся, перевéситься (*чéрез вн.*) hang* (óver).

перевирáть, перевра́ть (*вн.*) mix up (*smth.*); misquóte (*smth.*); перевра́ть фами́лии mix up péople's names; ~ чьи-л. словá misquóte *smb.*; перевра́ть цитáту misquóte a pássage, distórt a quotátion.

перевóд 1. (*перемещéние*) móving, tránsfer; ~ на другу́ю рабóту tránsfer to óther work; 2. (*на другóй язык*) translátion; (*устный*) óral translátion; 3. (*изменéние, превращéние*) convérsion; 4. (*денéжное отправлéние*) remíttance; почтóвый ~ (*докумéнт*) póstal órder; 5. *разг.* (*бесполéзная трáта*): пустóй ~ дéнег sheer waste of móney.

переводи́ть, перевести́ 1. (*вн. чéрез вн.*) take* (*smb.*, *smth.* acróss); перевести́ когó-л. чéрез у́лицу take* *smb.* acróss a street; 2. (*вн.; перемещáть*) transfér (*smb.*, *smth.*), move (*smb.*, *smth.*); ~ когó-л. на другу́ю рабóту transfér/move *smb.* to anóther post/job; ~ шкóлу в нóвое здáние move the school to new prémises; ~ пóезд на другóй путь shunt the train to anóther track; ~ часы́ вперёд (назáд) put* a watch, clock on/fórward (back); ~ когó-л. в слéдующий класс move *smb.* up a class; 3. (*вн. с рд. на вн.; на другóй язык*) transláte (*smth.*, from... ínto); (*устно*) intérpret (*smth.* from... ínto); ~ с английского языка́ на ру́сский transláte from Énglish ínto Rússian; ~ статью́ transláte an árticle; ~ чьи-л. выступле́ния (*устно*) intérpret for *smb.*; **4.** (*вн.; ставить в другие условия*) transfér (*smth.*), put* (*smth.*); перевести́ предприя́тие на семичасово́й рабо́чий день put* the énterprise on a séven-hour day; **5.** (*вн.; деньги и т. п.*) remít (*smth.*), transmít (*smth.*); **6.** (*вн. в вн.; выражать в других величинах*) convért (*smth.* to); **7.** (*вн.*) *разг.* (*истреблять*) extérminate (*smth.*); **8.** (*вн.*) *разг.* (*попусту тратить*) waste (*smth.*); зря ~ де́ньги waste móney; **9.** (*вн.; рисунок*) transfér (*smth.*); ◇ перевести́ дыха́ние get* one's breath back; не переводя́ дыха́ния withóut páusing for breath. ~ся, *перевестись* **1.** (*в другое учреждение, другой город и т. п.*) be* transférred, be* moved; **2.** *разг.* (*исчезать*) disappéar; у него́ де́ньги никогда́ не перево́дятся he is néver short of móney.

перево́дн|ой I: ~а́я карти́нка tránsfer.

перево́дн|о́й II *и* перево́дн|ый **1.** (*переведённый с какого-л. языка*) transláted; ~а́я литерату́ра transláted líterature. **2.:** ~ бланк móney-order form.

перево́дческий translátor's; ~ труд the work of a translátor, translátion work.

перево́дч|ик *м.*, ~ица *ж.* translátor; (*устный*) intérpreter.

перево́з *м.* **1.** (*действие*) transportátion, convéyance; **2.** (*место переправы*) férry.

перевози́ть, перевезти́ **1.** (*вн.; из одного места в другое*) cárry (*smb., smth.*), convéy (*smb., smth.*), transpórt (*smb., smth.*); (*на другую квартиру*) move (*smb., smth.*); (*мебель*) remóve (*smth.*); **2.** (*вн. через вн.; через какое-л. пространство*) transpórt (*smb., smth.* acróss), take* (*smb., smth.* acróss); перевезти́ кого́-л. че́рез ре́ку férry *smb.* acróss a ríver.

перево́з|ка *ж.* convéyance, transportátion. ~чик *м.* férryman*.

переволнова́ться *сов. разг.* get* worked up, get* overexcíted.

перевооруж|а́ть, перевооружи́ть (*вн.*) **1.** (*снабжать новым вооружением*) reárm (*smth.*); **2.** (*снабжать новыми орудиями труда*) re-equíp (*smth.*); техни́чески ~ промы́шленность equíp índustry with new plant. ~а́ться, перевооружи́ться **1.** (*заменять старое вооружение новым*) reárm; **2.** (*тв.; оснащаться новыми орудиями труда*) renéw one's plant/equípment. ~е́ние *с.* **1.** (*снабжение новым вооружением*) reármament; **2.** (*снабжение новыми орудиями труда*) re-equípment.

перевооружи́ть(ся) *сов. см.* перевооружа́ть(ся).

перевоплоти́ть(ся) *сов. см.* перевоплоща́ть(ся).

перевоплощ|а́ть, перевоплоти́ть (*вн.*) embódy (*smth.*), expréss (*smth.*). ~а́ться, перевоплоти́ться transfórm onesélf, be* transfórmed. ~е́ние *с.* transformátion; дар ~е́ния the pówer to change onesélf complétely.

перевора́чивать(ся) *несов.см.* переверты́вать(Ься).

переворо́т *м.* **1.** (*перелом*) rádical change; ~ в нау́ке revolútion in scíence; техни́ческий ~ téchnical revolútion; **2.** (*изменение общественно-политической системы*) revolútion, uphéaval; социа́льный ~ sócial uphéaval.

переворош|и́ть *сов.* (*вн.*) *разг.* **1.** (*сено*) ted (*smth.*), toss (*smth.*); **2.** (*в памяти*) go* óver (*smth.*) in one's mind; **3.** (*приводить в беспорядок*) disarránge (*smth.*).

перевоспита́ть(ся) *сов. см.* перевоспи́тывать(ся).

перевоспи́тывать, перевоспита́ть (*вн.*) re-éducate (*smb.*); (*исправлять*) refórm (*smb.*). ~ся, перевоспи́тываться refórm, be* refórmed.

перевра́ть *сов. см.* перевира́ть.

перевы́борн|ый eléction *attr.*; ~ая кампа́ния eléction (éering) campáign; ~ое собра́ние eléction méeting.

перевы́боры *мн.* **1.** (*выборы*) eléction *sg*; **2.** (*повторные выборы*) re-eléction *sg*.

перевыполне́ние *с.* óverfulfilment.

перевы́полнить *сов. см.* перевыполня́ть.

перевыполня́ть, перевы́полнить (*вн.*) óverfulfil (*smth.*), excéed (*smth.*); ~ план на 15 проце́нтов excéed the plan (by) fiftéen per cent.

перевяза́ть(ся) *сов. см.* перевя́зывать(ся).

перевя́зк|а *ж.* bándaging; сде́лать ~у applý a dréssing, dress a wound.

перевя́зочный dréssing *attr.*; ~ пункт dréssing státion; ~ материа́л bándaging matérial.

перевя́зывать, перевяза́ть (*вн.*) **1.** (*перебинтовывать*) bándage (*smb., smth.*); (*рану*) dress (*smth.*); **2.** (*обвязывать*) bind* (*smth.*), tie up (*smth.*); перевяза́ть чемода́н tie up a case; **3.** (*заново завязывать*) tie (*smth.*) up agáin; **4.** (*заново вязать спицами*) reknít (*smth.*). ~ся, перевяза́ться **1.** bándage onesélf, bándage/dress one's wound; **2.** (*тв.*) *разг.* (*обвязываться кругом*) tie (*smth.*) round onesélf.

перевя́зь *ж.* **1.** shóulder-belt; **2.** (*для больной руки*) sling.

переги́б *м.* bend; (*складка*) fold; *перен.* (*крайность*) excéss, exaggerátion, extréme; допуска́ть ~ в чём-л. cárry *smth.* too far, cárry *smth.* to extrémes; не допуска́ть ~ов avóid extrémes/excésses; э́то ~ that's góing too far.

перегиба́ть, перегну́ть (*вн.*) bend* (*smth.*); (*вдвое*) fold (*smth.*); *перен.* go* to extrémes, go* too far; ◇ перегну́ть па́лку overshóot* the mark, go* too far. ~ся, перегну́ться bend* óver, lean óver; ~ся попола́м bend* dóuble.

перегласо́вка *ж.* *лингв.* vówel mutátion.

перегля́дываться, перегляну́ться exchánge glánces.

перегляну́ться *сов. см.* перегля́дываться.

перегна́ть *сов. см.* перегоня́ть.

перегно́й *м.* (*végetable-*)mould, húmus, cómpost. ~ный: ~ная по́чва húmus, végetable-mould; ~ные горшо́чки cómpost pots/bricks.

перегну́ть(ся) *сов. см.* перегиба́ть(ся).

перегова́ривать(ся) *несов.* exchánge remárks, talk.

переговори́ть *сов.* **1.** talk, have* a talk; ~ по телефо́ну speak* óver the télephone; ~ о де́ле talk things óver; **2.** (*вн.*) *разг.* (*поговорить обо всём*) talk (*smth.*) óver, discúss (*smth.*); **3.** (*вн.*) *разг.* (*заставить других замолчать*) out-tálk (*smb.*).

переговорн|ый: ~ пункт call óffice; ~ая бу́дка télephone box.

переговор|ы *мн.* negotiátions, talks; ~ на высо́ком у́ровне high-lével talks/negotiátions; ~ на у́ровне мини́стров talks/negotiátions at ministérial lével; вести́ ~ о заключе́нии догово́ра negótiate a tréaty; де́ло нахо́дится в ста́дии ~ов the mátter is únder negotiátion.

перего́н *м.* (*участок пути между двумя станциями*) stage (between státions), run.

перего́н|ка *ж.* *хим., тех.* distillátion; ~ не́фти distillátion of oil. ~ный distillátion *attr.*, distílling *attr.*; ~ный заво́д distíllery; ~ный куб still.

перегоня́ть, перегна́ть (*вн.*) **1.** (*обгонять*) outdístance (*smb., smth.*); (*в беге тж.*) outrún* (*smb.*); *перен.* (*превосходить в чём-л.*) outstríp (*smb., smth.*), leave* (*smb., smth.*) behínd; **2.** (*на другое место*) drive* (*smth.*); (*самолёты*) férry (*smth.*); **3.** *хим., тех.* distíl (*smth.*).

перегора́живать, перегороди́ть (*вн.*) divíde (*smth.*) with a partítion; ~ ко́мнату divíde a room with a partítion, partítion off part of a room.

перегора́ть, перегоре́ть **1.** (*портиться от длительного горения*) burn* out; ла́мпочка перегоре́ла the bulb has burnt out; про́бка перегоре́ла the fuse has blown; **2.** (*сгорать*) burn* down; *перен.* die down; **3.** (*гнить*) rot, decompóse.

перегоре́ть *сов. см.* перегора́ть.

перегороди́ть *сов. см.* перегора́живать.

перегоро́дка *ж.* partítion; *перен.* bárrier.

перегре́в *м.*, ~а́ние *с.* overhéating; *(пара и т. п.)* superhéating.

перегрева́ть, перегре́ть *(вн.)* 1. overhéat *(smth.)*; 2. *тех.* superhéat *(smth.)*. ~ся, перегре́ться becóme* overhéated; *(о людях тж.)* make* onesélf too hot.

перегре́ть(ся) *сов. см.* перегрева́ть(ся).

перегружа́ть, перегрузи́ть *(вн.)* 1. *(чрезмерно нагружать)* overlóad *(smth.)*, overbúrden *(smth.)*; *перен.* overbúrden *(smb., smth.)*; *(работой тж.)* overwórk *(smb.)*; кни́га перегру́жена цита́тами the book is overbúrdened with quotátions; 2. *(перекладывать что-л. с одного места на другое)* transfér *(smth.)*, move *(smth.)*, load *(smth.)*. ~ся, перегрузи́ться 1. becóme*/be* overlóaded; 2. *(перемещать груз)* transfér one's load/cárgo.

перегру́женность *ж.* *(судна, вагона и т. п.)* overlóading; *перен.* overbúrdening.

перегру́зка *ж.* 1. óverload, overlóading; *(двигателя тж.)* strain (on); *перен.* overbúrdening; *(работой тж.)* overwórk; 2. *(перемещение груза)* tránsfer of cárgo.

перегруппирова́ть(ся) *сов. см.* перегруппиро́вывать(ся).

перегруппиро́вка *ж.* regróuping.

перегруппиро́вывать, перегруппирова́ть *(вн.)* regróup *(smb., smth.)*. ~ся, перегруппирова́ться regróup.

перегрыза́ть, перегры́зть *(вн.)* gnaw *(smth.)*, bite* *(smth.)*; *(надвое)* bite* *(smth.)* in two, bite* through *(smth.)*.

перегры́зть *сов. см.* перегрыза́ть. ~ся *сов. разг. (о животных)* fight*; snap at óther *(тж. перен.)*.

перед, передо 1. *(о времени и т. п.)* befóre; *(о месте тж.)* in front of; ~ сном befóre góing to bed; ~ обе́дом befóre dínner; ~ тем как befóre (+ -ing); ~ до́мом in front of the house; ~ гостя́ми, посторо́нними befóre visitors, strángers, in front of vísitors, strángers; ~ но́сом únder one's véry nose; ~ ва́ми Кремль you see befóre you the Krémlin; предста́ть ~ судо́м appéar befóre the court; 2. *(по сравнению с кем-л., чем-л.)* compáred (with, to); что он ~ тобо́й? he can't compáre with you; 3. *(по отношению к)*: ~ лицо́м опа́сности in the face of dánger; не отступа́ть ~ тру́дностями not shrink from difficulties.

перёд *м.* front.

передава́ть, переда́ть *(вн.)* 1. pass *(smth.)*; *(вручать)* hand *(smth.)*; *(сидящему рядом)* pass *(smth.)* on; он переда́л ей письмо́ he hánded her a létter; ~ поруче́ние delíver the instrúctions; прочти́те э́то и переда́йте друго́му read this and pass *smth.* on; 2. *(предоставлять, отдавать в распоряжение)* hand óver *(smth.)*, turn óver *(smth.)*; ~ зе́млю крестья́нам turn óver the land to the péasants; ~ кого́-л. в ру́ки правосу́дия hand *smb.* over to jústice; 3. *(сообщать)* repórt *(smth.)*; *(рассказывать)* tell* *(smth.)*, give* *(smth.)*; *(излагать)* convéy *(smth.)*; ~ мысль а́втора convéy the áuthor's idéa; ~ кому́-л. ва́жное изве́стие tell* *smb.* an ímportant piece of news; ~ кому́-л. приве́т give* *smb.'s* kind regárds to *smb.*; ~ что́-л. по телегра́фу transmít *smth.* by télegraph; ~ что́-л. по ра́дио bróadcast *smth.*; *тех.* transmít *smth.*; ~ что́-л. по телеви́дению télevise *smth.*, show* *smth.* on télevision; ~ конце́рт по ра́дио bróadcast a cóncert; 4. *(на рассмотрение)* submit *(smth.)*, refér *(smth.)*; ~ де́ло в суд submít the case to the court, take* the mátter to court; ~ де́ло на реше́ние кому́-л. refér the quéstion to *smb.'s* decísion; 5. *(уступать)* hand óver *(smth.)*, transfér *(smth.)*; ~ свои́ права́ кому́-л. transfér one's rights to *smb.*; ~ свои́ полномо́чия délegate one's authórity; 6. *(распространять)*

spread* *(smth.)*, pass on *(smth.)*; ~ инфе́кцию spread* inféction; 7. *(воспроизводить, изображать)* reprodúce *(smth.)*, portráy *(smth.)*, convéy *(smth.)*; 8. *(переплачивать)* overpáy* *(smth.)*, pay* *(smth.)* too much. ~ся, переда́ться *(дт.)* commúnicate itsélf (to); ~ся по насле́дству be* heréditary.

переда́точн|ый 1. transmíssion *attr.*; ~ механи́зм dríving gear, drive; ~ вал transmíssion shaft; 2. ~ая на́дпись *(на векселе, чеке)* endórsement.

переда́тчик *м.* transmítter.

переда́ть(ся) *сов. см.* передава́ть(ся).

переда́ча *ж.* 1. *(вручение)* pássing; hánding; *(прав)* tránsfer; *(тепла, света и т. п.)* transmíssion; ~ электроэне́ргии transmíssion of pówer; 2. *(то, что передаётся по радио)* bróadcast, transmíssion; *(то, что передаётся по телевидению)* télecast; 3. *(образа, выразительности речи и т. п.)* réndering; 4. *(в больницу и т. п.)* párcel; 5. *тех.* transmíssion, gear, drive.

передвиг|а́ть, передви́нуть *(вн.)* 1. move *(smth.)*, shift *(smth.)*; ~ ме́бель move/shift fúrniture; ~ войска́ move troops; он е́ле но́ги ~а́ет he can scárcely drag his feet; 2. *разг. (переносить на другое время)* transfér *(smth.)*, shift *(smth.)*; передви́нуть сро́ки экза́менов shift the examinátion dates. ~а́ться, передви́нуться 1. move, shift; 2. *разг. (о сроке)* change; 3. *тк. несов.* move; больно́й с трудо́м ~а́ется the pátient finds it dífficult to move abóut.

передвиже́ние *с.* móvement.

передви́ж|ка *ж. разг.* 1. *(действие)* móving, shífting; 2.: библиоте́ка-~ móbile líbrary. ~ник *м.* Peredvízhnik *(painter of 19-th century Russian realist school with democratic tendencies)*. ~но́й 1. móvable, adjústable; *(портативный)* pórtable; 2. *(о выставке и т. п.)* trávelling *attr.*, móbile.

передви́нуть *сов. см.* передвига́ть. ~ся *сов. см.* передвига́ться 1, 2.

переде́л *м.* redistribútion, repartítion.

переде́л|ать *сов.* 1. *см.* переде́лывать; 2. *(вн.; сделать всё, многое)* do* *(smth.)*; всех дел не ~аешь you can't do éverything. ~ка *ж.* 1. alterátion; *(полная)* convérsion; *(литературного произведения)* adaptátion; *(в пьесу)* dramatizátion; отда́ть костю́м в ~ку have* a suit áltered; 2. *(затруднительное положение)* áwkward situátion; попа́сть в ~ку get* into a mess/spot/jam.

переде́лывать, переде́лать *(вн.)* álter *(smth.)*, remáke* *(smth.)*; *перен.* change *(smb., smth.)*; ~ пальто́ álter a coat; ~ столо́вую в кабине́т make* the díning-room into a stúdy; ~ свой хара́ктер, себя́ change one's náture.

передёргивать, передёрнуть 1. *(тв.)* twitch *(smth.)*; 2. *безл.* wince, writhe; его́ передёрнуло от бо́ли he winced/writhed with pain; меня́ передёрнуло it made me wince/writhe; 3. *(вн.) разг. (подтасовывать)* distórt *(smth.)*, twist *(smth.)*; ~ фа́кты distórt facts, júggle with the facts. ~ся, передёрнуться shúdder, shiver; *(о лице)* convúlse.

передержа́ть *сов. см.* переде́рживать.

передерж|ивать, передержа́ть *(вн.)* keep* *(smth.)* in too long; *(фотоплёнку)* overexpóse *(smth.)*; ~ка *ж. (фотоплёнки)* overexpósure.

передёрнуть(ся) *сов. см.* передёргивать(ся).

пере́дн|ий front; ~яя часть fórepart, front séction; ~ие но́ги живо́тного fórelegs; ~ее колесо́ front wheel; ◇ ~ край front line.

пере́дник *м.* ápron; *(детский)* pínafore.

пере́дняя *ж.* hall, lóbby; ánteroom.

передо́ *см.* перед.

передова́я *ж.* 1. léader, léading árticle, editórial; 2. *воен.* front line.

передови́к *м.* advánced wórker, léading wórker; top-nótch wórker *разг.*

передови́ца *ж. разг. см.* передова́я 1.

передов|о́й 1. (движущийся, идущий впереди) léading, fóremost; (расположенный впереди чего-л.) fóremost; in front после сущ.; ~ отря́д advánced guard, vánguard; 2. (превосходящий других в чём-л.) advánced; (прогрессивный тж.) progréssive; ~ые спо́собы произво́дства advánced prodúction méthods; ~ о́пыт advánced expérience/knów-how; ~ая мы́сль advánced/progréssive thínking; ~ые иде́и, взгля́ды progréssive idéas, views; ~ые лю́ди progréssive péople; ◇ ~ая статья́ léading árticle, editórial, léader; ~ая пози́ция воен. fórward position; ~ая ли́ния воен. front line.

передохну́ть сов. 1. (перевести дух) take* a breath, breathe in; 2. разг. (немного отдохнуть) get*/recóver one's breath, take* a rest.

передра́знивать, передразни́ть (вн.) mímic (smb.), ímitate (smb.), take* (smb.) off.

передразни́ть сов. см. передра́знивать.

передра́ться сов. разг. have* a fight, have* a frée-for-áll, come* to blows.

переду́мать сов. 1. (изменить решение) change one's mind; 2. (о пр.) разг. (обдумать всё, многое) think* (abóut, óver), méditate (upón).

переды́шк|а ж. rest, bréathing-space; без ~и 1) (без отдыха) without a réspite, unremíttingly; 2) (непреры́вно) uncéasingly.

перееда́ть, перее́сть (есть лишнее) overéat*, have* too much to eat.

перее́зд м. 1. (передвижение) jóurney; (по воде) pássage, cróssing; 2. (на другую квартиру, в другой го́род) move, remóval; 3. (место, где можно переехать) cróssing; железнодоро́жный ~ lével cróssing.

переезжа́ть, перее́хать 1. (вн., че́рез вн.) cross (smth.); 2. (переселяться) move; ~ в го́род move ínto town.

перее́сть сов. см. перееда́ть.

перее́ха|ть сов. 1. см. переезжа́ть; 2. (вн.; задавить) run* óver (smb., smth.); его́ ~ла маши́на he was run óver by a car.

пережа́рить сов. (вн.) 1. (испортить) overdó* (smth.); 2. (изжарить многое) fry plénty (of).

пережда́ть сов. см. пережида́ть.

пережева́ть сов. см. пережёвывать 1.

пережёвывать, пережева́ть (вн.) 1. chew (smth.), másticate (smth.); 2. тк. несов. (надоедливо говорить одно и то же) assért (smth.) at great length, drum (smth.) in; ~ всем изве́стные и́стины grind* out plátitudes.

переже́чь сов. см. пережига́ть.

пережива́ние с. expérience; (волнение) emótion, excítement, emótional expérience.

пережива́ть, пережи́ть (вн.) 1. (жить дольше кого-л., чего-л.) outlíve (smb., smth.), survíve (smb., smth.); пережи́ть свою́ сла́ву outlíve one's reputátion; 2. (выживать) survíve (smth.); (терпеть, выносить что-л.) endúre (smth.); он не переживёт э́того уда́ра he will néver survíve the blow; я э́того не переживу́ it will kill me; му́жественно пережи́ть несча́стье endúre misfórtune brávely; 3. (испытывать) expérience (smth.); go* through (smth.); (огорчения, страдания) undergó* (smth.); (остро чувствовать) feel* (smth.) kéenly, take* to heart.

пережига́ть, переже́чь (вн.) burn* (smth.); переже́чь ко́фе roast cóffee too long; переже́чь ла́мпочку burn* out a bulb.

пережида́ть, пережда́ть wait; (вн.) wait for (smth.) to pass; sit* (smth.) out; ~ грозу́ wait for the storm to pass.

пережито́е с. what one went through; one's expériences pl.

пережи́ток м. survíval, véstige; ~ про́шлого survíval of the past.

пережи́|ть сов. 1. см. пережива́ть; 2. (вн.; прожить како́е-л. время) live through (smth.), last (smth.), survíve (smth.); больно́й не ~ивёт э́ту ночь the pátient will not last/survíve the night.

перезаключа́ть, перезаключи́ть (вн.) renéw (smth.); ~ догово́р renéw a cóntract/tréaty.

перезаключи́ть сов. см. перезаключа́ть.

перезаряди́ть сов. см. перезаряжа́ть.

перезаря́дка ж. 1. (оружия, фотоаппарата) relóading; 2.: ~ аккумуля́тора báttery rechárge.

перезаряжа́ть, перезаряди́ть (вн.) rechárge (smth.); (оружие) relóad (smth.).

перезво́н м. chíming.

перезимова́ть сов. 1. (провести зиму где-л.) wínter, pass the wínter; 2. (выдержать зимние холода) survíve the wínter/cold.

перезрева́ть, перезре́ть becóme* overrípe; перен. be* past one's prime.

перезре́|лый overrípe. ~ть сов. см. перезрева́ть.

переигра́ть сов. 1. см. переи́грывать; 2. (вн.; сыгра́ть всё, многое) play (smth.); ~ все сона́ты play all the sonátas.

переи́грывать, переигра́ть 1. (вн.; играть повто́рно) play (smth.) agáin; потре́бовать переигра́ть матч demánd a réplay; 2. театр. (играть роль ненатура́льно) overáct.

переизбира́ть, переизбра́ть (вн.) re-eléct (smb., smth.).

переизбр|а́ние с. re-eléction. ~а́ть сов. см. переизбира́ть.

переиздава́ть, переизда́ть (вн.) repúblish (smth.), reíssue (smth.).

переизд|а́ние с. 1. (действие) republicátion, reíssue; 2. (книга) reíssue. ~а́ть сов. см. переиздава́ть.

переименов|а́ние с. renáming. ~а́ть сов. (вн.) renáme (smth.).

перейти́ сов. см. переходи́ть.

переко́пывать, перекопа́ть (вн.) 1. (вскапывать всё, многое) dig* up (smth.); 2. (вскапывать заново) dig* (smth.) agáin.

переко́рмливать, перекорми́ть (вн.) overféed* (smb., smth.).

перека́т м. 1. (на реке) shoal; shállows pl; 2. мн. (продолжительный гул) rúmblings; rúmble sg.

перекати́-по́ле с. бот. túmble-weed.

перека́ти́ть(ся) сов. см. перека́тывать(ся).

перека́тывать, перекати́ть (вн.) roll (smth.), move (smth.). ~ся, перекати́ться roll.

перекача́ть сов. см. перека́чивать.

перека́чивать, перекача́ть (вн.) pump. (smth.).

перека́шивать, перекоси́ть (вн.; делать кривым) put* (smth.) out of shape, put* (smth.) awrý/askéw; ра́му перекоси́ло the frame was all askéw; 2. обыкн. безл. (искажать) distórt; (надолго) defórm; рот перекоси́ло the mouth was defórmed/misshápen; его́ перекоси́ло his face was distórted. ~ся, перекоси́ться 1. (о предметах) get* out of shape; 2. (о лице и т. п.) be* distórted; (надолго) be* defórmed.

переквалифи|ка́ция ж. tráining for a new trade/proféssion, retráining. ~ци́ровать несов. и сов. (вн.) train (smb.) for a new trade/proféssion, retráin (smb.). ~ци́роваться несов. и сов. acquíre a new trade/proféssion, requálify.

перекида́ть сов. см. переки́дывать 1.

переки́дывать, перекида́ть, переки́нуть (вн.) 1. сов. перекида́ть (бросать одно за другим) throw* (smth.); перекида́ть зе́млю move earth; 2. сов. переки́нуть throw* (smth.) óver; переки́нуть мяч че́рез забо́р throw*/toss a ball óver a fence; переки́нуть полоте́нце че́рез плечо́ throw* a tówel óver one's shóulder. ~ся, переки́нуться 1. (на вн.; распространяться) spread* (to); ого́нь переки́нулся на сосе́дние постро́йки the fire spread to the néighbouring buíldings; 2. (тв.; кидать друг дру́гу) throw*/toss (*smth.*) to one anóther; *перен.* (*словами и т. п.*) exchánge (*smth.*).

переки́нуть *сов. см.* переки́дывать 2. ~ся *сов. см.* переки́дываться.

пе́рекись *ж. хим.* peróxide; ~ водоро́да hýdrogen peróxide; ~ ма́рганца mangánése peróxide.

переклади́на *ж.* 1. cróss-bar, cróss-beam; (*лестни́цы*) rung; 2. *спорт.* the horizóntal bar.

переклады́вать, переложи́ть 1. (*вн.; перемеща́ть*) shift (*smth.*); ~ что-л. с ме́ста на ме́сто shift *smth.* from place to place; 2. (*вн. на вн.; рабо́ту, вину́ и т. п.*) throw* (*smth.* on to), shift (*smth.* on to); переложи́ть отве́тственность на кого́-л. throw*/shift the responsibílity on to *smb.*; 3. (*вн.; тв.; прокла́дкой*) pack (*smth.* in, with); ~ я́блоки стру́жкой pack the ápples in shávings; 4. (*вн.; переде́лывать*) remáke* (*smth.*), rebúild* (*smth.*); ~ печь resét* a stove; 5. (*вн.; укла́дывать за́ново*) repáck (*smth.*), rearránge (*smth.*); 6. (*вн.; излага́ть в ино́й фо́рме*) rearránge (*smth.*), transpóse (*smth.*); ~ переложи́ть что-л. на му́зыку set* *smth.* to músic; 7. (*вн., рд.*) *разг.* (*класть сли́шком мно́го*) put* too much (*smth.*) in.

переклика́ться *несов.* call to one anóther; (*с тв.*) *перен.* have* sómething in cómmon (with).

перекли́чк|а *ж.* róll-call, cáll-over; де́лать ~у call the roll.

переключа́тель *м. тех.* switch; ~ скоросте́й gear léver/shift.

переключа́ть, переключи́ть (*вн.*) 1. (*изменя́ть направле́ние, си́лу*) rediréct (*smth.*), switch (*smth.*); ~ свет (*на автомаши́не*) dip one's lights; ~ телефо́н change the line; ~ что-л. на обра́тный ход put* *smth.* ínto revérse; 2. (*переводи́ть на ины́е фо́рмы рабо́ты*) transfér (*smth., smth.*), switch (*smth.*), *перен.* change (*smth.*); ~ цех на произво́дство холоди́льников switch the shop to refrígerator prodúction; переключи́ть разгово́р на другу́ю те́му change for the súbject, switch the conversátion on to a new súbject. ~ся, переключи́ться (на вн.) go* óver (to), be* put (on); *перен.* turn (to), switch (to); заво́д переключи́лся на произво́дство турби́н the fáctory has gone óver to prodúcing túrbines.

переключе́ние *с.* switching (óver); (*перехо́д*) chánge-over.

переключи́ть(ся) *сов. см.* переключа́ть(ся).

перекова́ть *сов. см.* переко́вывать.

переко́вывать, перекова́ть (*вн.*) 1. refórge (*smth.*); *перен.* re-éducate (*smb.*), remóuld (*smb.*); перекова́ть мечи́ на ора́ла beat*/hámmer swords ínto plóughshares; 2. (*ло́шадь*) re-shóe (*smth.*).

переконстру́ировать *несов. и сов.* (*вн.*) redesígn (*smth.*).

перекопа́ть *сов. см.* перека́пывать.

перекорми́ть *сов. см.* перека́рмливать.

переко́сить(ся) *сов. см.* перека́шивать(ся).

переко́шенный twísted; askéw *predic.*; (*о лице́*) distórted, contórted, twísted.

перекра́ивать, перекро́ить (*вн.*) cut* (*smth.*) agáin, refáshion (*smth.*); *перен.* (*переде́лывать*) reshápe (*smth.*), recást* (*smth.*).

перекра́сить(ся) *сов. см.* перекра́шивать(ся).

перекра́шивать, перекра́сить (*вн.*) (*масляно́й кра́ской*) repáint (*smth.*); (*о тка́ни*) redýe (*smth.*) agáin. ~ся, перекра́сить change cólour; *перен.* sail únder false cólours.

перекрести́ть *сов. см.* крести́ть 3 *и* перекре́щивать. ~ся *сов. см.* крести́ться 2 *и* перекре́щиваться.

перекре́стн|ый cross *attr.*; ~ допро́с cróss-examinátion; ~ ого́нь *воен.* cróss-fire; ~ое опыле́ние *бот.* cróss-pollinátion.

перекрёст|ок *м.* cróss-roads *pl*; cróssing; ◇ крича́ть о чём-л. на всех ~ках procláim/cry *smth.* from the hóuse-tops, raise a hue and cry abóut *smth.*

перекре́щивать, перекрести́ть (*вн.*) (*о ли́ниях и т. п.*) cross (*smth.*). ~ся, перекрести́ться cross.

перекрича́ть *сов.* (*вн.*) shout (*smb.*) down, outvóice (*smb.*).

перекро́йть *сов. см.* перекра́ивать.

перекрути́ть *сов. см.* перекру́чивать.

перекру́чивать, перекрути́ть (*вн.*) *разг.* 1. (*по́ртить*) overwínd* (*smth.*); перекрути́ть заво́д у часо́в overwínd* a watch/clock; 2. (*скру́чивать*) fásten up (*smth.*).

перекрыва́ть, перекры́ть (*вн.*) 1. (*крыть за́ново*) re-cóver (*smth.*); ~ кры́шу make* a new roof; 2. (*превыша́ть*) excéed (*smth.*); *разг.* (*превосходи́ть в чём-л.*) break* (*smth.*), beat* (*smth.*); ~ ста́рые но́рмы вы́работки excéed the old rate of óutput; ~ пре́жний реко́рд beat* the old récord; 3. (*де́лать прегра́ду в чём-л.*) stop up (*smth.*), block (*smth.*); (*выключа́ть*) cut* off (*smth.*); перекры́ть во́ду cut* off the wáter; перекры́ть ру́сло реки́ dam a ríver; перекры́ть доро́ги block the roads, set* up róad-blocks.

перекры́тие *с.* céiling; (*междуэта́жное*) floor.

перекры́ть *сов. см.* перекрыва́ть.

перекуви́ркиваться, перекувырну́ться *разг.* tópple óver; (*о во́здухе*) turn a sómersault.

перекувырну́ться *сов. см.* перекуви́ркиваться.

перекупа́ть I, перекупи́ть (*вн.*) *разг.* buy* (*smth.*) first, buy* (*smth.*) befóre ányone else.

перекупа́ть II *сов.* (*вн.*) *разг.* 1. (*до́лго продержа́ть в воде́*) bath (*smb.*) too long, keep* (*smb.*) in the bath too long; ~ ребёнка keep* a báby in the bath too long; 2. (*вы́купать всех, мно́гих*) bath (*smb.*); ~ всех дете́й bath all the children. ~ся *сов. разг.* bathe too much/long, stay/be* in the wáter too long.

перекупи́ть *сов. см.* перекупа́ть I.

переку́пщик *м.* míddleman*, déaler.

переку́р *м. разг.* (smoke) break.

перекуси́ть *сов.* 1. (*вн.; прокуси́ть*) bite* (*smth.*) in two; (*куса́чками*) cut* (*smth.*); ~ ни́тку bite* a thread in two; 2. *разг.* (*закуси́ть*) take* a quick bite, have* a snack.

перелага́ть *несов. см.* переклады́вать 2, 6.

перела́мывать, переломи́ть (*вн.*) break* (*smth.*) in two; (*поврежда́ть при паде́нии, уда́ре*) break* (*smth.*); fráctúre (*smth.*) *научн.*; *перен.* (*преодолева́ть*) cónquer (*smth.*); переломи́ть па́лку break* a stick in two; переломи́ть свой хара́ктер cónquer one's témper; ◇ переломи́ть себя́ 1) (*стать ины́м*) change onesélf; 2) (*преодоле́ть како́е-л. чу́вство*) máster/contról one's féelings. ~ся, переломи́ться break* (in two).

перелеза́ть, переле́зть 1. climb óver; 2. (*вн.; че́рез вн.*) climb óver (*smth.*).

переле́зть *сов. см.* перелеза́ть.

перелесо́к *м.* cóppice, copse.

перелёт *м.* 1. flight; (*переселе́ние птиц*) migrátion; 2. (*снаря́да*) overshót.

перелета́ть, перелете́ть 1. (*вн., че́рез вн.*) fly* (acróss); *перен. тж.* spring* (óver); ~ че́рез океа́н fly* across the ócean; ~ че́рез забо́р spring* over a fence; 2. (*перемеща́ться*) fly*; ~ с де́рева на де́рево fly*/flit from tree to tree; 3. (*о снаря́де и т. п.*) trável too far, overshóot*.

переле́теть *сов. см.* перелета́ть.

перелётн|ый mígratory; ~ая пти́ца bird of pássage.

перелива́ние *с.* póuring; ~ вина́ в графи́н decantátion of wine; ~ кро́ви blood transfúsion.

перелива́ть, перели́ть 1. (*вн.; из одного́ ме́ста в друго́е*) pour (*smth.*); ~ вино́ в графи́н decánt the wine; ~ во́ду из ведра́ в бак pour wáter from a pail ínto a tank; ~ кому́-л. кровь give* *smb.* a blood transfúsion; 2. (*вн.; налива́ть бо́льше, чем ну́жно*) pour (*smth.*) too much; 3. (*вн.; переде́лывать литьём*) remélt (*smth.*), recást* (*smth.*); 4. *тк. несов.* (*блесте́ть*) gleam, glísten. ~ся, перели́ться 1. (*через край*) overflów, run* óver; 2. *тк. несов.* (*о красках*) gleam, glísten; (*о звуках*) rise* and fall*, módulate; ~ся всéми цветáми рáдуги shine* with all the cólours of the ráinbow.

перели́вы *мн.* (*красок*) play *sg;* (*звуков*) modulátion *sg,* rise and fall.

перелистáть *сов. см.* перели́стывать.

перели́стывать, перелистáть (*вн.*) 1. turn óver the páges (of); 2. (*бегло прочитывать*) glance through (*smth.*), skim through (*smth.*); ~ ромáн skim/leaf through a nóvel.

перели́ть *сов. см.* переливáть 1, 2, 3. ~ся *сов. см.* переливáться 1.

перелицевáть *сов. см.* перелицóвывать.

перелицóванный turned.

перелицóвывать, перелицевáть (*вн.*) turn (*smth.*).

переложéние *с. муз.* arrángement.

перекладывать *сов. см.* перекла́дывать.

перелóм *м.* 1. break; 2. (*кости*) frácture; 3. (*крутой поворот в развитии*) change; cróss-roads *pl;* túrning-point; (*в болезни*) crísis (*pl* -ses); вели́кий ~ great change; нрáвственный ~ móral túrning-point.

перелом|áть *сов.* (*вн.*) break* (*smth.*) (to bits); ~ все игрýшки break* all the toys. ~áться *сов. разг.* be* bróken (to bits); все карандаши́ ~áлись all the péncils are bróken.

переломи́ть(ся) *сов. см.* перела́мывать(ся).

перелóмный crítical; ~ момéнт crítical/crúcial móment, túrning-point.

перемáзать *сов.* (*вн.*) *разг.* (*перепачкать*) smear (*smth.*), dírty (*smth.*); ~ пáльцы черни́лами dírty one's fíngers with ink, make* one's fíngers ínky. ~ся *сов. разг.* get* dírty.

перема́лывать, перемолóть (*вн.*) mill (*smth.*), grind* (*smth.*). ~ся, перемолóться be* milled, be* ground; ◇ перемéлется — мукá бýдет *посл.* it will all come right in the end.

перема́нивать, перемани́ть (*вн.*) entíce (*smb.*), tempt (*smb.*) óver to one's side; *несов. тж.* try to win (*smb.*) óver.

перемани́ть *сов. см.* перема́нивать.

перема́тывать, перемотáть (*вн.*) rewínd (*smth.*).

перемеж|áть *несов.* (*вн. тв.*) álternate (*smth.* with); ~ рабóту óтдыхом álternate work with rest. ~áться *несов.* be* intermíttent; (*с тв.*) álternate (with); ~áющийся intermíttent; ~áющаяся лихорáдка intermíttent féver.

перемéна *ж.* 1. change; ~ обстанóвки change in the situátion; ~ клímата change of clímate; ~ вéтра change in the wind; с ним произошлá большáя ~ a great change has come óver him; 2. *разг.* (*комплект белья*) change of únderwear; (*постельного*) change of béd-linen; 3. (*перерыв между уроками*) break, ínterval; большáя (*ма́ленькая*) ~ long (short) break.

перемен|и́ть *сов.* (*вн.*) change (*smth.*); ~ тéму разговóра change the súbject; ~ тон change one's tune. ~и́ться *сов.* change; вéтер ~и́лся the wind changed; он ~и́лся ко мне he has changed towárds me, his áttitude towárds me has changed.

перемéнн|ый chángeable, váriable; ~ая погóда, ~ вéтер chángeable/váriable wéather, wind; ◇ ~ая величинá *мат.* váriable quántity; ~ капитáл *эк.* váriable cápital; ~ ток álternating cúrrent; с ~ым успéхом with várying succéss.

перемéнчивый *разг.* chángeable.

перемести́ть(ся) *сов. см.* перемещáть(ся).

перемёт *м.* seine.

переметнýться *сов. разг.:* ~ на стóрону врагá go* óver to the énemy, sneak off.

перемётн|ый: ~ая сумá sáddle-bag; ◇ сумá ~ая wéathercock.

перемешáть(ся) *сов. см.* переме́шивать(ся).

переме́шивать, перемешáть (*вн.*) 1. (*смешивать*)

(*inter*)mix (*smth.*); ~ цемéнт с пескóм mix cemént with sand; 2. (*перемещать*) mix (*smth.*) togéther, stir (*smth.*); перемешáть ýгли в пéчке poke the fire; 3. (*приводить в беспорядок*) confúse (*smth.*), mix (*smth.*) up; перемешáть бумáги mix up the pápers. ~ся, перемешáться 1. (*смешиваться*) be* mixed up; 2. (*перепутываться*) be* confúsed, get* ínto a múddle; всё перемешáлось éverything is in confúsion, éverything is in a múddle.

перемещ|áть, перемести́ть (*вн.*) 1. move (*smb., smth.*); 2. (*по службе*) tránsfer (*smb.*). ~áться, перемести́ться move, shift. ~éние *с.* 1. tránsference, mótion, shíft(ing); (*перемена должности*) tránsfer; 2. *геол.* dislocátion.

перемещённ|ый: ~ые лíца displáced pérsons.

перемíгиваться, перемигнýться (с *тв.*) exchánge winks (with).

перемигнýться *сов. см.* перемíгиваться.

переминáться *несов.:* ~ с ногí нá ногу shift one's feet.

перемíрие *с.* ármistice; (*короткое*) truce; заключи́ть ~ conclúde/sign an ármistice, make* a truce.

перемножáть, перемнóжить (*вн.*) múltiply (*smth.*).

перемнóжить *сов. см.* перемножáть.

перемогáть *несов.* (*вн.*) *разг.* fight* off (*smth.*); ~ болéзнь fight* off an íllness. ~ся *несов. разг.* brace onesélf, try to keep góing.

перемóлвить *сов. разг.:* ~ слóво с кем-л. exhánge a word with *smb.;* ~ словéчка не́ с кем there's not a soul to talk to. ~ся *сов. разг.:* ~ся слóвом с кем-л. have* a word with *smb.*

перемолóть(ся) *сов. см.* перема́лывать(ся).

перемотáть *сов. см.* перема́тывать.

перемы́чка *ж.* 1. cróss-piece; (*оконной рамы*) líntel; 2. (*водонепроницаемая*) dam.

перенапрягáть, перенапрячь (*вн.*) overstráin (*smth.*). ~ся, перенапря́чься overstráin onesélf.

перенапряжéние *с.* 1. overstráin, overexértion; 2. *эл.* overvóltage.

перенапря́чь(ся) *сов. см.* перенапрягáть(ся).

перенаселéние *с.* overpopulátion.

перенаселённ|ость *ж.* overcrówding; overpopulátion; ~ гóрода overcrówding in the city. ~ый overcrówded; (*о городе и т. п. тж.*) overpópulated; ~ая странá overpópulated cóuntry; ~ый дом overcrówded house.

перенаселённость *сов. см.* перенаселять.

перенаселя́ть, перенасели́ть (*вн.*) overcrówd (*smth.*); (*город и т. п. тж.*) overpópulate (*smth.*).

перенесéние *с.* tránsference, remóval; ~ собрáния postpónement of a méeting.

перенести́(сь) *сов. см.* переноси́ть(ся).

перенимáть, переня́ть (*вн.*) take* (*smth.*), adópt (*smth.*); ~ привы́чку take*/catch* the hábit; ~ манéру, манéры cópy the style, mánners; ~ мéтод adópt a méthod.

перенóс *м.* 1. cárrying; (*перемещение*) tránsference, móving; 2. (*на другую страницу*) cárrying óver; ~ слóва division of a word; 3. *разг.* (*знак переноса*) hýphen.

переноси́ть, перенести́ (*вн.*) 1. cárry (*smb., smth.*); (*перемещать*) tránsfer (*smth.*); перенести́ ребёнка чéрез ручéй cárry a child* acróss a stream; перенести́ столи́цу tránsfer the cápital; 2. (*откладывать*) put* off (*smth.*), postpóne (*smth.*); ~ заседáние (на) postpóne the méeting (to); 3. (*на другую строку, страницу*) cárry (*smth.*) óver; 4. (*выдерживать*) endúre (*smth.*), bear* (*smth.*); ~ боль endúre pain; ~ скарлатíну get* óver scárlet féver; перенести́ операцию come* through an operátion; ◇ не ~ кого-л., чего-л. be* unáble to stand/bear *smb., smth.;* find* *smth.* unendúrable. ~ся, перенести́сь 1. *разг.* (*стремительно двигаться*) rush; fly* (*тж. перен.*); 2. (*мысленно*) tránsfer onesélf, turn one's mind.

перено́сица ж. bridge of the nose.

переносн|ый 1. (*портативный*) pórtable; 2. (*иносказательный*) metaphórical, fígurative; ~ое значе́ние fígurative méaning; в ~ом значе́нии in the fígurative sense, fíguratively.

перено́счик м. cárrier; ~ боле́зни cárrier (of a disease).

переночева́ть сов. spend* the night.

перенумерова́ть сов. (*вн.*) 1. (*пронумеровать заново*) renúmber (*smth.*); 2. (*всё, многое*) númber (*smth.*).

переня́ть сов. см. перенима́ть.

переобору́дование с. re-equípment.

переобору́довать несов. и сов. (*вн.*) re-equíp (*smth.*), re-tóol (*smth.*), rejíg (*smth.*).

переобува́ть, **переобу́ть** (*кого-л.*) change smb.'s shoes, boots; (*что-л.*) change (*smth.*); переобу́ть дете́й change the chíldren's shoes; переобу́ть боти́нки change one's shoes, boots. ~ся, переобу́ться change one's shoes, boots.

переобу́ть(ся) сов. см. переобува́ть(ся).

переодева́ть, **переоде́ть** 1. (*кого-л.*) change smb.'s clothes; (*что-л.*) change (*smth.*); переоде́ть ребёнка change the báby's clothes; переоде́ть пла́тье change (*one's dress*); 2. (*вн. тв., в вн.*; *с целью маскировки*) dress (*smb.*) up (as), disguíse (*smb.* as). ~ся, переоде́ться 1. change (*one's clothes*); переоде́ться в но́вое пла́тье change into a new dress; 2. (*тв.*; *для маскировки*) dress up (as), disguíse onesélf (as).

переоде́тый (*тв.*) dressed (up) (as), disguísed (as).

переоде́ть(ся) сов. см. переодева́ть(ся).

переосвиде́тельствование с. мед. re-examinátion.

переосвиде́тельствовать несов. и сов. (*вн.*) мед. re-exámine (*smth.*).

переохлади́ть(ся) сов. см. переохлажда́ть(ся).

переохлажд|а́ть, **переохлади́ть** (*вн.*) make* (*smth.*) too cold. ~а́ться, переохлади́ться becóme* too cold. ~е́ние с. 1. becóming too cold; 2. физ. supercóoling.

переоце́нивать, **переоцени́ть** (*вн.*) 1. (*оценивать заново*) reválue (*smth.*), álter the price (of); переоцени́ть това́ры álter commódity príces; 2. (*давать слишком высокую оценку*) overéstimate (*smb., smth.*), overráte (*smb., smth.*); переоцени́ть свои́ си́лы overráte one's strength.

переоцени́ть сов. см. переоце́нивать.

переоце́нка ж. 1. (*заново*) revaluátion, reappráisal; ~ це́нностей revaluátion/reappráisal of válues; 2. (*слишком высокая оценка*) overestimátion, overráting.

перепад|а́ть, **перепа́сть** 1. (*изредка выпадать*); ~ют дожди́ it rains now and then; 2. чаще безл. разг. (*доставаться на чью-л. долю*): ему́ немно́го перепа́ло he got/recéived véry líttle, véry líttle came his way.

перепа́лка ж. разг. héated árgument, wrángle.

перепа́сть сов. см. перепада́ть.

перепаха́ть сов. см. перепа́хивать.

перепа́хивать, **перепаха́ть** (*вн.*) 1. (*вспахивать заново*) plough (*smth.*) again; 2. (*вспахивать целиком*) plough (*smth.*).

перепа́шка ж. разг. sécond plóughing.

перепе́в м. 1. (*действие*) repetítion; 2. (*то, что является повторением чего-л.*) réhash, écho.

перепева́ть несов. (*вн.*) rehásh (*smth.*), écho (*smth.*).

пе́репел м. quail.

перепёлка ж. (hen-)quail.

перепеча́т|ать сов. см. перепеча́тывать. ~ка ж. 1. (*действие*) (re)prínting; (*на пишущей машинке*) (re-)týping; 2. (*перепечатанное*) réprint.

перепеча́тывать, **перепеча́тать** (*вн.*) 1. (*печатать с печатного текста*) reprínt (*smth.*), reprodúce (*smth.*); 2. (*переписывать на пишущей машинке*) type (*smth.*); (*вторично*) retýpe (*smth.*).

перепи́ливать, **перепили́ть** (*вн.*; *пополам*) saw* (*smth.*) in two, saw* through smth.

перепили́ть сов. см. перепи́ливать; 2.: ~ все дрова́ saw* up all the fírewood.

переписа́ть сов. см. перепи́сывать.

перепи́с|ка ж. 1. (*действие*) cópying; (*на пишущей машинке*) týping; 2. (*обмен письмами*) correspóndence, exchánge of létters; состоя́ть в ~ке с кем-л. correspónd with smb.; 3. (*собрание писем*) correspóndence. ~чик м., ~чица ж. cópyist.

перепи́сывать, **переписа́ть** (*вн.*) 1. (*списывать*) cópy (*smth.*) out; (*на пишущей машинке*) type (*smth.*); ~ ру́копись на́бело make* a fair cópy of a mánuscript; 2. (*писать заново, иначе*) rewríte* (*smth.*), write* anéw; 3. (*делать список*) make* out a list (of), draw* up a list (of); (*имущество*) take* an invéntory (of), draw* up an invéntory (of); ~ прису́тствующих take* down the names of those présent. ~ся несов. (с тв.) correspónd (with), keep* up a correspóndence (with).

пе́репись ж. 1. (*массовый учёт кого-л., чего-л.*) enumerátion, lísting; 2. (*населения*) cénsus; производи́ть ~ населе́ния take* a cénsus (of the populátion).

перепи́ть сов. разг. have* too much to drink.

перепла́вить I, II сов. см. переплавля́ть I, II.

перепла́вка ж. remélting, melting down.

переплавля́ть I, **перепла́вить** (*вн.*) 1. (*металл*) remélt (*smth.*), recást* (*smth.*); (*руду*) smelt (*smth.*); 2. (*всё, многое*) melt (*smth.*).

переплавля́ть II, **перепла́вить** (*вн.*; *лес*) float (*smth.*).

переплани́ровать сов. (*вн.*) replán (*smth.*).

переплани́ровка ж. replánning; ~ городо́в replánning of towns.

переплати́ть сов. см. перепла́чивать.

перепла́чивать, **переплати́ть** (*вн. дт.*) overpáy* (*smb., smth.*); (*дт. вн. за вн.*) pay* (*smb., smth.*) too much (for); pay* through the nose (for) разг.

переплести́(сь) сов. см. переплета́ть(ся).

переплёт м. 1. (*действие*) bínding; отда́ть кни́гу в ~ have* a book bound; 2. (*крышка книги, тетради*) bínding, cóver; в ~е with a hard cóver; 3. (*оконный*) sash; ◇ попа́сть в ~ get* ínto a tight córner/spot.

переплета́ть, **переплести́** (*вн.*) 1. (*книги*) bind* (*smth.*); переплести́ два то́ма в оди́н make* two vólumes ínto one; 2. (*сплетать*) weave* (*smth.*) togéther; (*о пальцах и т. п.*) interlóck (*smth.*); 3. (*заплетая, перевить чем-л.*) twine (*smth.*), weave* (*smth.*); ~ ко́сы ле́нтами weave* ríbbons ínto one's plaits. ~ся, переплести́сь (*прям. и перен.*) interláce, intertwíne, be* interwóven.

переплете́ние с. 1. (*действие*) interwéaving, interlácing; 2. (*то, что сплетено между собой*) web, tángle; ~ обстоя́тельств tángle of círcumstances; 3. текст. weave.

переплёт|ный bóokbinding attr.; ~ное де́ло bóokbinding; ~ цех bínding depártment. ~чик м. bóokbinder.

переплыва́ть, **переплы́ть** (*вн., через вн.*) cross (*smth.*); (*вплавь тж.*) swim* (acróss); (*на вёслах тж.*) row (acróss).

переплы́ть сов. см. переплыва́ть.

переподгота́вливать, **переподгото́вить** (*вн.*) give* (*smb.*) a refrésher course, give* (*smb.*) fúrther tráining.

переподгото́в|ить сов. см. переподгота́вливать. ~ка ж. fúrther tráining, refrésher course; ~ка ка́дров fúrther tráining of staff; ~ка учителе́й téacher's refrésher course.

переполза́ть, **переползти́** 1. (*вн., через вн.*) creep* (acróss), crawl (acróss); ~ че́рез доро́гу creep* acróss a road; 2. (*перемещаться куда-л.*) creep*, crawl.

переползти́ сов. см. переполза́ть.

переполнéние *с.* overcrówding; (*сосуда*) overfílling.

переполн|енный filled to overflówing *после сущ.;* crámmed; (*людьми тж.*) crówded; ~ зал crówded hall; ~ сундýк crámmed trunk; зал ~ен the hall is filled to overflówing; сéрдце ~ено рáдостью *one's* heart is overflówing with joy. ~ить(ся) *сов. см.* переполнять(ся).

переполнять, переполнить (*вн.*) fill (*smth.*) to overflówing; *перен. тж.* overwhélm (*smth.*). ~ся, переполниться be* filled to overflówing; сéрдце переполнилось рáдостью *one's* heart overflówed with joy.

переполóх *м.* pánic, commótion; вызвать ~ cause a pánic/commótion; в дóме поднялся ~ the house was in a state of commótion.

переполошить *сов.* (*вн.*) *разг.* throw* (*smth.*) into a pánic. ~ся *сов. разг.* be* thrown into a pánic.

перепóн|ка *ж.* mémbrane; (*у утки, лебедя и т. п.*) web. ~чатый membráneous; (*об утках и т. п.*) webbed, wéb-fóoted.

перепоручáть, перепоручить (*вн. дт.*) entrúst (*smth.* to); ~ дéло другóму лицý the mátter to anóther pérson.

перепоручить *сов. см.* перепоручáть.

переправа *ж.* 1. (*действие*) cróssing; 2. (*место*) cróssing(-place); (*брод*) ford; (*временная*) témporary/flóating bridge.

переправить(ся) *сов. см.* переправлять(ся).

переправлять, переправить 1. (*вн. через вн.*) take* (*smb.* across, óver), convéy (*smb.* across, óver); ~ когó-л. чéрез рéку на пароме férry *smb.* óver/across the ríver; 2. (*вн.; пересылать*) fórward (*smth.*); 3. (*вн.*) *разг.* (*исправлять*) put* (*smth.*) to rights. ~ся, переправиться (*через вн.*) cross (*smth.*), get* across (*smth.*); ~ся чéрез рéку на пароме, лóдке cross the ríver by férry, boat; ~ся вплавь swim* (*across*) the ríver.

перепрéлый rótten, decáyed.

перепрóбовать *сов.* (*вн.*) try (*smth.*).

перепрод|авáть, перепродáть (*вн.*) reséll* (*smth.*). ~áжа *ж.* resále. ~áть *сов. см.* перепродавáть.

перепроизвóдство *с.* overprodúction.

перепрыгивать, перепрыгнуть 1. (*вн., через вн.*) jump (óver, across); ~ чéрез канáву jump óver a ditch; ~ чéрез забóр jump óver a fence; 2. (*перемещаться прыжками*) jump across, jump; ~ с кáмня на кáмень jump from stone to stone.

перепрыгнуть *сов. см.* перепрыгивать.

перепýг *м. разг.*: с ~у он заболéл the fright made him ill; с ~у он забыл нóмер телефóна in his fright he forgót the télephone númber. ~анный fríghtened; ~анное лицó fríghtened/scared face.

перепугáть *сов.* (*вн.*) fríghten (*smb.*), scare (*smb.*). ~ся *сов.* be* fríghtened/scared (to death).

перепýтанный tángled; (*о бумагах и т. п.*) mixed up; in confúsion predíc.

перепýтать *сов.* (*вн.*) 1. tángle (*smth.*); ~ нитки tángle the threads; 2. (*привести в беспорядок*) múddle (*smth.*) (up); *перен.* confúse (*smth.*); ~ делá múddle things up; 3. (*спутать с чем-л.*) mix (*smth.*) up; ~ адресá mix up the addrésses. ~ся *сов.* 1. (*о нитках и т. п.*) get* tángled; 2. (*приходить в беспорядок*) be* mixed up; *перен. тж.* confúse; всё перепýталось éverything is mixed up.

перепýтье *с.* cróssroads *pl;* ◇ на ~ at the cróssroads.

перерабáтывать, переработать 1. (*вн.; сырьё*) prócess (*smth.*), treat (*smth.*); ~ нефть refíne oil; 2. (*вн.; делать пригодным для усвоения*) digést (*smth.*), take* in (*smth.*); 3. (*вн.; переделывать*) revíse (*smth.*) thóroughly; make* rádical chánges (in); ~ книгу для юношества adápt the book for young péople; 4. (*работать дольше положенного времени*) work/do* óvertime.

переработать *сов. см.* перерабáтывать.

переработка *ж.* 1. (*выделка*) convérsion (into); ~ хлóпка в пряжу the convérsion of cótton into yarn; ~ нéфти oil refíning; 2. (*переделка*) thórough revísion; 3. *разг.* (*работа сверх нормы*) óvertime (work).

перераспредел|éние *с.* redistribútion. ~ить *сов. см.* перераспределять.

перераспределять, перераспределить (*вн.*) redístribute (*smth.*).

перерастáние *с.* 1. outgrówing; 2. (*в вн.; превращение*) devélopment (into).

перерастáть, перерасти 1. (*вн.; стать выше ростом*) grow*/be* táller than (*smth.*); *перен.* outgrów* (*smb., smth.*), surpáss (*smb., smth.*); произведéние перерослó первоначáльный зáмысел áвтора the work devéloped beyónd the áuthor's original concéption; 2. (*по возрасту*) be* óver age, pass the age límit; 3. (*в вн.; превращаться*) devélop (into).

перерасти *сов. см.* перерастáть.

перерасхóд *м.* 1. (*действие*) overexpénditure; ~ электричества overconsúmption of electrícity; 2. (*сумма*) óverdraft. ~овать *несов. и сов.* (*вн.*) use too much (*smth.*); (*о деньгах*) overspénd* (*smth.*), spend* too much (*smth.*); ~овать электрúчество use/consúme too much electrícity; ~овать крéдиты overdráw (on *one's* crédit).

перерасчёт *м.* re-calculátion; сдéлать ~ revíse an accóunt.

перервáть *сов. см.* перерывáть I. ~ся *сов. см.* перерывáться.

перерегистрáция *ж.* re-registrátion.

перерегистрúровать *несов. и сов.* (*вн.*) re-régister (*smb., smth.*). ~ся *несов. и сов.* re-régister.

перерéзать *сов.* 1. *см.* перерезáть; 2. (*вн.*) *разг.* (*убить всех, многих*) kill (*smb., smth.*), sláughter (*smb., smth.*).

перерезáть, перерéзать 1. (*вн.; разрезать надвое*) cut* (*smth.*), séver (*smth.*); перерéзать канáт cut*/séver a rope; 2. (*вн.; пересекать что-л. в каком-л. направлении*) travérse (*smth.*), score (*smth.*); 3. (*вн. дт.; преграждать*) bar (*smth.* to), block (*smth.* for); перерéзать путь протúвнику block the énemy's path.

перерéзаться *сов. см.* перерезáться; 2. *разг.* (*зарезаться*) kill onesélf, stab onesélf; (*в драке*) start knifing each óther, knife each óther.

перерезáться, перерéзаться part (únder the knife*).

перереш|áть *сов.* 1. *разг.* (*менять решение*) change *one's* mind; 2. (*вн.; решать иначе*) revíse (*smth.*); перерешить задáчу solve a próblem in anóther way.

перерешáть II *сов.* (*вн.*) *разг.* (*решить всё, многое*) solve (*smth.*); ~ все задáчи solve all the próblems.

перерешить *сов. см.* перерешáть I.

перерисовáть *сов. см.* перерисóвывать.

перерисóвка *ж.* cópying.

перерисóвывать, перерисовáть (*вн.*) 1. (*срисовывать*) cópy (*smth.*); 2. (*рисовать заново*) draw* (*smb., smth.*) afrésh/anéw.

перерод|úть(ся) *сов. см.* перерождáть(ся).

перерождáть, переродúть (*вн.*) make* a new man*, wóman* (of). ~ся, переродúться 1. becóme* a new man*, wóman*, be* (complétely) regénerated; 2. (*вырождаться*) degénerate.

перерождéние *с.* 1. (*преображение*) regenerátion; 2. (*вырождение*) degenerátion.

перербсток *м.* overáge child*; ученúк-~ overáge púpil.

перерубáть, перерубúть (*вн.*) cut* (*smth.*) in/into two, chop (*smth.*) in/into two.

перерубúть *сов.* 1. *см.* перерубáть; 2. (*вн.*) *разг.* (*изрубить, срубить всё, многое*) cut* down (*smth.*).

переругáться *сов.* (*с тв.*) *разг.* quárrel, fall* out (with); fall* foul (of).

переру́гиваться *несов. разг.* call one anóther names.

переры́в *м.* break; (*временное прекращение чего-л. тж.*) ínterval, adjóurnment; рабóтать без ~a work withóut an intermíssion, work uninterrúptedly; ~ на обéд lúnch--hour/lúnch-time/lúnch-break.

перерыва́ть I, перерва́ть (*вн.; разрывать*) tear* (*smth.*), tear* (*smth.*) apárt.

перерыва́ть II, переры́ть (*вн.*) 1. (*перекапывать*) dig* up (*smth.*); turn óver (*smth.*); 2. *разг.* (*в поисках чего-л.*) ránsack (*smth.*), rúmmage through (*smth.*); он перерýл всё в кóмнате he ránsacked the room.

перерыва́ться, перерва́ться come* apárt, break*.

переры́ть *сов. см.* перерыва́ть II.

пересади́ть *сов. см.* переса́живать.

переса́дк|а *ж.* 1. (*растений*) transplánting; (*ткани тж.*) gráfting; ~ сéрдца heart tránsplant; 2. (*на железной дороге и т. п.*) change; без ~и withóut chánging, straight through.

переса́живать, пересади́ть (*вн.*) 1. (*кого-л. на другое место*) give* (*smb.*) anóther seat, move (*smb.*); пересади́ть ученика́ на другýю па́рту move a púpil to anóther desk; ~ пассажи́ров в другóй вагóн move pássengers to anóther cárriage; 2. (*растения*) transplánt (*smth.*); (*комнатные растения*) repót (*smth.*); ~ огурцы́ из парника́ на гря́дки plant out cúcumbers; 3. *мед.* transplánt (*smth.*); пересади́ть рогови́цу гла́за transplánt the córnea. ~ся, пересéсть 1. (*на другое место*) change one's seat; 2. (*с одного транспорта на другой*) change; ~ся на другóй пóезд change trains.

переса́ливать, пересоли́ть (*вн.*) put* too much salt (in), oversált (*smth.*); *перен.* go* too far, overdó* it.

пересдава́ть, пересда́ть (*вн.*) 1. (*помещение*) sublét (*smth.*); 2.: ~ экза́мен resít* an examinátion.

пересда́ть *сов. см.* пересдава́ть.

пересека́ть, пересéчь 1. (*вн.; переходить, переезжать поперёк*) cross (*smth.*); 2. (*вн.; проходить по поверхности*) run* acróss (*smth.*), travérse (*smth.*); 3. (*вн. дт.; преграждать путь*) bar (*smth.* to); ~ путь неприя́телю bar the énemy's path. ~ся, пересéчься cross, interséct.

переселéнец *м.* séttler.

переселéн|ие *с.* migrátion; (*устройство на новых землях*) reséttlement; (*на новую квартиру*) move, remóval; ◇ Вели́кое ~ нарóдов the great transmigrátion of péoples. ~ческий reséttlement *attr.*; (*относящийся к переселенцам*) séttlers'.

переселя́ть(ся) *сов. см.* переселя́ть(ся).

переселя́ть, пересели́ть (*вн.*) move (*smth.*); (*на новые земли тж.*) reséttle (*smb.*). ~ся, пересели́ться move; (*на новые земли*) migráte.

пересéсть *сов. см.* переса́живаться.

пересечéни|е *с.* cróssing, interséction; тóчка ~я point of interséction.

пересечéнн|ый: ~ая мéстность bróken ground/country.

пересéчь(ся) *сов. см.* пересека́ть(ся).

пересидéть *сов. см.* переси́живать.

переси́живать, пересидéть *разг.* 1. (*вн.; сидеть где-л. дольше кого-л.*) outstáy (*smb.*); 2. (*просидеть дольше, чем следует*) stay too long; (*в гостях тж.*) outstáy one's wélcome; 3. (*в ожидании конца чего-л.*) sit* it out.

переси́ливать, переси́лить (*вн.*) overpówer (*smb.*); *перен.* overcóme* (*smth.*); ~ себя́ force onesélf.

переси́лить *сов. см.* переси́ливать.

пересказ *м.* 1. (*действие*) retélling; 2. (*изложение*) páraphrase, réndering. ~а́ть *сов. см.* переска́зывать.

переска́зывать, пересказа́ть (*вн.*) retéll* (*smth.*); páraphrase (*smth.*); пересказа́ть что-л. свои́ми слова́ми put* smth. into one's own words.

переска́кивать, перескочи́ть 1. (*вн., через вн.*) jump (*smth., óver*), leap* (*smth., óver*); ~ чéрез забóр jump óver a fence; 2. (*скачком перемещаться*) jump, leap*; перескочи́ть с ка́мня на ка́мень leap* from rock to rock; 3. *разг.* (*не кончив одного, переключаться на другое*) skip; ~ с однóй тéмы на другýю skip from one súbject to anóther; перескочи́ть чéрез две гла́вы skip (óver) two chápters.

перескочи́ть *сов. см.* переска́кивать.

пересла́ть *сов. см.* пересыла́ть.

пересма́тривать, пересмотрéть (*вн.*) 1. (*заново просма́тривать*) revíse (*smth.*), go* óver (*smth.*) agáin; 2. (*заново обсуждать*) revíse (*smth.*), reconsíder (*smth.*), revíew (*smth.*); ~ пригово́р revíew a séntence; ~ решéние revíse a decísion; ~ нóрмы вы́работки revíse óutput quótas.

пересмéиваться *несов. разг.* glance at each óther and chúckle/útter, exchánge smiles.

пересмóтр *м.* revísion, revíew, reconsiderátion.

пересмотрéть *сов.* 1. *см.* пересма́тривать; 2. (*вн.; всё, многое*) see* (*smth.*); мнóго карти́н я пересмотрéл на своём векý I have seen a lot of píctures in my time.

переснима́ть, перенсня́ть (*вн.*) 1. (*снимать что-л. заново фотоаппаратом и т. п.*) retáke* (*smth.*), take* (*smth.*) agáin; (*кинонаппаратом тж.*) reshóot* (*smth.*), shoot* (*smth.*) agáin; 2. (*делать новый снимок с уже имеющегося*) cópy (*smth.*), make* a photográphic cópy (of); 3. (*делать новую съёмку чего-л.*) remáke* (*smth.*); ~ план дорóги resurvéy a road. ~ся, перенсня́ться *разг.* have* one's phótograph táken agáin; (*в кино*) do*/make* a rétake.

перенсня́ть(ся) *сов. см.* переснима́ть(ся).

пересоли́ть *сов. см.* переса́ливать.

пересортирова́ть *сов.* (*вн.*) 1. (*заново*) re-sórt (*smth.*); 2. (*рассортировать всё, многое*) sort (*smth.*).

пересóхнуть *сов. см.* пересыха́ть.

переспа́ть *сов. разг.* 1. (*проспать долго*) oversléep (*onesélf*); 2. (*переночевать*) spend the night.

переспéлый overrípe.

переспéть *сов.* be* overrípe.

переспóр|ить *сов.* beat* (*smb.*) in árgument, out-árgue (*smb.*); егó не ~ишь ≈ it's no use árguing with him.

переспра́шивать, переспроси́ть (*вн.*) (*повторять вопрос*) ask (*smth.*) agáin; (*просить повторить*) ask (*smb.*) to repéat what he, she said.

переспроси́ть *сов. см.* переспра́шивать.

пересcóрить *сов.* (*вн.*) set* (*smb.*) at lóggerheads, cause (*smb.*) to quárrel (*smb.*), fall* out. ~ся *сов.* quárrel (with éverybody), fall* out.

перестава́ть, переста́ть stop; cease; они́ переста́ли встреча́ться they don't meet ány more; дождь переста́л the rain has stopped; переста́нь шумéть! stop that noise!; переста́ньте болта́ть! stop tálking/cháttering!

переста́вить *сов. см.* переставля́ть 1, 2.

переставля́ть, переста́вить (*вн.*) 1. move (*smth.*); переста́вить стол к окнý move the táble to the window; 2. (*изменять порядок*) rearránge (*smth.*); ~ мéбель move the fúrniture abóut; rearránge the fúrniture; ~ слова́ во фра́зе transpóse the words in a séntence; 3. *тк. несов.* ёле нóги ~ plod alóng.

переста́ивать, перестоя́ть 1. (*вн.; пережидать*) wait until (*smth.*) pásses, wait for (*smth.*) to pass; перестоя́ть бýрю в портý wait in hárbour till the storm pásses; 2. (*портиться от долгого стояния*) stand* too long.

перестанóвка *ж.* 1. rearrángement; (*слов в предложении*) transposítion; в кóмнате пóлная ~ the room has been complétely rearránged; 2. *мат.* permutátion.

перестара́ться *сов. разг.* overdó* it, try too hard, be* overzéalous.

переста́ть *сов. см.* перестава́ть.

перести́лать, перестла́ть (*вн.*) ~ постéль make* a bed agáin; ~ пол lay* a new floor; ~ пол в кóмнате re-flóor a room.

перестла́ть *сов. см.* перестила́ть.

перестоя́ть *сов. см.* переста́ивать.

перестрада́ть *сов.* (*вн.*) live through (*smth.*), súffer (*smth.*); (*вытерпеть*) bear* (*smth.*); (*понять*) come* to understánd (*smth.*) through súffering.

перестра́ивать, перестро́ить (*вн.*) 1. (*о постройке, сооружении*) rebuíld* (*smth.*), reconstrúct (*smth.*); 2. (*переделывать*) change (*smth.*); перестро́ить всё на свой лад change éverything to suit *one's* own idéas; перестро́ить расписа́ние поездо́в change/revíse the train tíme-table; перестро́ить фра́зу recást* a séntence; 3. (*реорганизовывать*) reórganize (*smth.*); ~ систе́му управле́ния reórganize a sýstem of mánagement; ~ рабо́ту це́ха reórganize the work of a depártment; 4. (*менять строй чего-л.*) refórm (*smth.*); перестро́ить ро́ту refórm a cómpany; 5. (*о рояле, приёмнике и т. п.*) retúne (*smth.*). ~ся, перестро́иться 1. (*изменять свои взгляды*) adópt a new áttitude/appróach; (*в работе тж.*) change *one's* méthods; 2. (*располагаться в строю по-иному*) (re)fórm; перестро́иться в одну́ шере́нгу (re)fórm ínto síngle file; 3. (*настраиваться на новую радиоволну*) change the wávelength.

перестрах|ова́ть(ся) *сов. см.* перестрахо́вывать(ся). ~о́вка *ж.* 1. reinsúrance; 2. *разг.* (*чрезмерная осторожность*) dóuble insúrance; для ~о́вки to be on the safe side. ~о́вщик *м. разг.* overcáutious pérson, sáfety-first man*.

перестрахо́вывать, перестрахова́ть (*вн.*) reinsúre (*smth.*). ~ся, перестрахова́ться 1. (*страховаться снова*) reinsúre; 2. *разг.* (*проявлять чрезмерную осторожность*) play safe, make* *one*sélf safe.

перестре́л|иваться *несов.* exchánge shots/fire. ~ка *ж.* shóoting, fíring, exchánge of shots/fire.

перестреля́ть *сов.* (*вн.*) 1. (*убить всех, многих*) kill (*smb., smth.*), shoot* down (*smb., smth.*); 2. *разг.* (*израсходовать стрельбой*) use up (*smth.*); ~ все патро́ны use up all the cártridges.

перестро́ить(ся) *сов. см.* перестра́ивать(ся).

перестро́йка *ж.* 1. (*взглядов, направления де́ятельности*) perestróyka, reformátion; reorientátion; chánging *one's* áttitude/appróach; (*в работе*) chánging *one's* méthods; 2. (*реорганизация*) reorganizátion; resháping (*prócess*); ~ хозя́йства reorganizátion of the ecónomy; 3. (*здания и т. п.*) rebuílding, reconstrúction; 4. (*переделка*) remóulding, recásting, revísion; 5. (*приёмника, рояля*) retúning.

пересту́киваться *несов.* 1. knock, tap; 2. (*о заключённых*) commúnicate by rápping/tápping.

переступа́ть, переступи́ть 1. (*вн.; через вн.; перешагивать*) step (óver), cross (*smth.*); ~ поро́г cross the thréshold/dóorstep; 2. (*перемещаться*) step; ~ с ноги́ на́ ногу shift from one foot to anóther; 3. *тк. несов.* (*идти, двигаться*) walk, step; 4. (*вн.; нарушать*) overstép (*smth.*), transgréss (*smth.*); ~ грани́цы прили́чия overstép the bounds of décency.

переступи́ть *сов. см.* переступа́ть 1, 2, 4.

пересу́ды *мн. разг.* góssip *sg.*

пересчи́тывать *сов. см.* пересчи́тывать.

пересчи́тывать, пересчита́ть (*вн.*) 1. (*считать вторично*) count (*smth.*) again; recóunt (*smth.*); 2. (*считать всё одно за другим*) count all (*smth.*).

пересыла́ть, пересла́ть (*вн.*) send* (*smth.*); (*переадресовывать*) fórward (*smth.*), send* on (*smth.*).

пересы́лк|а *ж.* sénding; (*переадресовка*) fórwarding; уплати́ть за ~у pay* the póstage.

пересы́пать *сов. см.* пересыпа́ть.

пересыпа́ть, пересы́пать 1. (*вн.; в другое место*) pour (*smth.*); ~ зерно́ в мешо́к pour grain ínto a sack; 2. (*вн.; насыпать слишком много*) put* in (*smth.*) too much; 3. (*вн. тв.; обсыпать*) sprínkle (*smth.* with); *перен. тж.* interspérse (*smth.* with); ~ вещи нафтали́ном

sprínkle clothes with náphthalene; ~ речь остро́тами sprínkle/interspérse *one's* speech with witticisms.

пересыха́ть, пересо́хнуть 1. (*становиться суше, чем нужно*) get* too dry (*о языке, губах и т. п.*) be* parched, be* dry; у меня́ в го́рле пересо́хло my throat is dry/parched; 2. (*иссякать*) dry up, run* dry; коло́дец пересо́х the well has dried up.

перета́скивать, перетащи́ть 1. (*вн., через вн.*) drag (*smb., smth.* acróss); 2. (*вн.*) cárry (*smth.*) awáy, move (*smth.*); ~ дива́н в сосе́днюю ко́мнату move the sófa ínto the next room.

перетасова́ть *сов. см.* перетасо́вывать.

перетасо́вывать, перетасова́ть (*вн.*) reshúffle (*smth.*).

перетащи́ть *сов. см:* перета́скивать.

перетере́ть *сов.* 1. *см.* перетира́ть; 2. (*вн.; вытереть всё, многое*) wipe (*smth.*); ~ всю посу́ду wipe all the díshes. ~ся *сов. см.* перетира́ться.

перетерпе́ть *сов.* (*вн.*) 1. (*вытерпеть многое*) súffer much (*smth.*); 2. (*терпя, преодолеть*) endúre (*smth.*), overcóme.

перетира́ть, перетере́ть (*вн.*) 1. (*растирать*) grate (*smth.*); ~ минда́ль grate álmonds; 2. (*трением разорвать*) fray (*smth.*) through. ~ся, перетере́ться break*, fray through.

перетолков|а́ть *сов.* 1. (*вн.*) misintérpret (*smth.*); он ~а́л мои́ слова́ по-своему he put his own interpretátion on my words; 2. *разг.* (*поговорить*) talk things óver; (*с тв.*) discúss (with smb.).

перетру́сить *сов. разг.* get* fríghtened.

перетя́гивать, перетяну́ть 1. (*вн.; перетаскивать*) drag (*smth.*); (*машину и т. п.*) coax (*smth.*); *перен. разг.* (*переманивать*) entíce (*smb.*); перетяну́ть кого́-л. на свою́ сто́рону win* óver to *one's* side; 2. (*вн. тв.; туго перевязывать*) bind* (*smth.*) tíghtly (with), fásten (*smth.* with); ~ та́лию по́ясом fásten* a belt tíghtly round *one's* waist; 3. (*вн.; перевешивать*) outwéigh (*smth.*); tip the bálance; 4. (*вн.; натягивая заново*) fásten (*smth.*) agáin, tíghten up (*smth.*). ~ся, перетяну́ться lace *one*sélf too tight.

перетяну́ть(ся) *сов. см.* перетя́гивать(ся).

переубеди́ть(ся) *сов. см.* переубежда́ть(ся).

переубежда́ть, переубеди́ть (*вн.*) make* (*smb.*) change his, her mind. ~ся, переубеди́ться change *one's* mind.

переу́л|ок *м.* síde-street; (*узкий*) lane; (*с названием*) Lane; ходи́ть ~ками cut* through the síde-streets.

переустра́ивать, переустро́ить (*вн.*) reórganize (*smth.*), reconstrúct (*smth.*).

переустро́ить *сов. см.* переустра́ивать.

переустро́йство *с.* reorganizátion, reconstrúction.

переутом|и́ть(ся) *сов. см.* переутомля́ть(ся). ~ле́ние *с.* exháustion, overstráin. ~лённый exháusted, overtíred; у вас ~лённый вид you look exháusted/overtíred.

переутомля́ть, переутоми́ть (*вн.*) exháust (*smb.*), overtíre (*smb.*). ~ся, переутоми́ться be* exháusted, be* overtíred.

переу́чивать, переучи́ть 1. (*что-л.; учить снова*) learn* (*smth.*) all óver agáin; 2. (*кого-л.; обучать заново*) teach* (*smb.*) all óver agáin, retráin (*smb.*). ~ся, переу́читься learn* the job/súbject all óver agáin, retráin *one*sélf.

переучи́ть(ся) *сов. см.* переу́чивать(ся).

перефрази́ровать *несов. и сов.* (*вн.*) páraphrase (*smth.*).

перехва́ливать, перехвали́ть (*вн.*) overpráise (*smb.*).

перехвали́ть *сов. см.* перехва́ливать.

перехва́тывать, перехвати́ть (*вн.*) 1. (*задерживать*) catch* (*smb., smth.*); (*выйдя навстречу, натолкнуться*) intercépt (*smb., smth.*); он перехвати́л его́ по доро́-

ге на рабо́ту he intercépted/caught him on the way to work; **2.** (*запи́ску и т. п.*) intercépt (*smth.*), get* hold of (*smth.*) first; *перен.* (*взгляд и т. п.*) catch* (*smth.*), intercépt (*smth.*); перехвати́ть письмо́ intercépt a létter; **3.** (*схва́тывать друго́й руко́й*) take* (*smth.*) in one's óther hand; **4.** (*перевя́зывать поперёк*) tie (*smth.*) round; *перен.* (*прегражда́ть чем-л.*) travérse (*smth.*); **5.** (*вы́звав спазм, приостана́вливать*) check (*smth.*) mómentarily; ра́дость перехвати́ла ей дыха́ние she súddenly felt she ·could scárcely breathe for joy; **6.** *разг.* (*наско́ро заку́сывать*) have* a snack.

перехитри́ть *сов.* (*вн.*) outwít (*smb.*), be* too smart (for), get* the bétter (of).

перехо́д *м.* **1.** (*через что-л.*) cróssing, góing acróss; при ~е у́лицы... when cróssing the street...; ~ че́рез грани́цу cróssing a fróntier; **2.** (*переме́на ме́ста и́ли ро́да заня́тий*) tránsfer; (*в сле́дующий класс*) remóve; ~ на другу́ю рабо́ту chánging one's place of work; **3.** (*из одного́ ла́геря в друго́й*) góing óver; **4.** (*переме́на вероиспове́дания*) convérsion; ~ в католи́чество convérsion to Cathólicism; **5.** (*из одного́ состоя́ния в друго́е*) transítion; ~ на семичасово́й рабо́чий день the change to a séven-hour day; ~ в наступле́ние tá́king the offénsive; **6.** (*расстоя́ние*) march; **7.** (*ме́сто*) cróssing; подзе́мный ~ súbway, únderground pedéstrian cróssing; **8.** (*коридо́р*) pássage, gállery.

переходи́ть, перейти́ **1.** (*вн., через вн.; переправля́ться*) cross (*smth.*); ~ че́рез мост cross a bridge; ~ у́лицу cross a street; **2.** (*в друго́е ме́сто*) move, pass; ~ с ме́ста на ме́сто move/shift from place to place; **3.** (*меня́ть ме́сто и́ли род заня́тий*) transfér; ~ на другу́ю рабо́ту take* up óther work; **4.** (*на сле́дующий курс, в сле́дующий класс*) move up; перейти́ в пя́тый класс move up to the fifth form; **5.** (*в друго́й ла́герь*) go* óver; **6.** (*дт.; поступа́ть в со́бственность, распоряже́ние кого́-л.*) pass ínto the hands (of); (*передава́ться кому́-л.*) be* passed on (to); ~ из рук в ру́ки pass from hand to hand; **7.** (*ко́нчив одно́, приступа́ть к друго́му*) move on, procéed; ~ к друго́й те́ме move on to anóther súbject; перейти́ к заключи́тельной ча́сти докла́да procéed to the final séction of a repórt; разгово́р перешёл от археоло́гии к семе́йной жи́зни the conversátion drifted from archéology to fámily life; **8.** (*меня́ть о́браз де́йствий*) change/go* óver (to); adópt; перейти́ на передовы́е ме́тоды рабо́ты go* óver to advánced méthods; ~ в наступле́ние take* the offénsive; **9.** (*в вн.; постепе́нно превраща́ться во что-л. друго́е*) turn (ínto), devélop (into); (*о цве́те, зву́ке*) merge (into); ◊ перейти́ от слов к де́лу stop tálking and get* down to búsiness.

перехо́дный **1.** (*служа́щий для перехо́да*): ~ тонне́ль pedéstrian túnnel; **2.** (*промежу́точный*) transítion(al); ~ пери́од transítion périod; ~ во́зраст transítional age; **3.** *грам.* tránsitive; ~ глаго́л tránsitive verb.

переходя́щ|ий **1.** (*вруча́емый но́вому победи́телю в соревнова́нии, состяза́нии*) challenge *attr.*; ~ ку́бок challenge cup; **2.** *фин.* cárried óver после *сущ.*

пе́рец *м.* pépper; чёрный, кра́сный ~ black, red pépper; ◊ зада́ть пе́рцу кому́-л. give* it *smb.* hot.

пе́речень *м.* (*перечисле́ние*) enumerátion; (*спи́сок*) list; ~ това́ров invéntory.

перечёркивать, перечеркну́ть (*вн.*) cross out (*smth.*), strike* out (*smth.*); (*при редакти́ровании*) blúe-péncil (*smth.*).

перечеркну́ть *сов. см.* перечёркивать.

перечерти́ть *сов. см.* перечё́рчивать.

перечё́рчивать, перечерти́ть (*вн.*) **1.** (*черти́ть за́ново*) draw* (*smth.*) agáin; **2.** (*снима́ть ко́пию с чертежа́*) make*/take* a trácing (of).

перечисле́ние *с.* **1.** enumerátion; **2.** *бухг.* tránsfer; **3.** (*пе́речень*) list.

перечи́слить *сов. см.* перечисля́ть.

перечисля́ть, перечи́слить (*вн.*) **1.** enúmerate (*smth.*); (*люде́й*) méntion (*smb.*); **2.** *бухг.* transfér (*smth.*).

перечита́ть *сов.* **1.** *см.* перечи́тывать; **2.** (*вн.; всё, мно́гое*) read* (*smth.*); ~ все кни́ги read* all the books.

перечи́тывать, перечита́ть (*вн.*) re-réad* (*smth.*).

пере́чить *несов.* (*дт.*) *разг.* contradíct (*smb.*).

пе́речница *ж.* pépper-pot.

перечу́вствовать *сов.* (*вн.*) go* through (*smth.*), feel* (*smth.*).

переша́гивать, перешагну́ть **1.** (*вн., через вн.*) step (óver); *перен.* (*не поддава́ться како́му-л. чу́вству*) overcóme* (*smth.*), get* óver (*smth.*); **2.** (*вн., за вн.; перехо́дит за како́й-л. преде́л*) be* past (*smth.*); перешагну́ть за со́рок be* past fórty.

перешагну́ть *сов. см.* переша́гивать.

переше́ек *м.* ísthmus.

перешёптываться *несов.* whisper (to one anóther).

перешива́ть, переши́ть (*вн.*) álter (*smth.*); ~ пла́тье álter a dress; (*отдава́я в переде́лку*) have* one's dress áltered.

переши́ть *сов. см.* перешива́ть.

перещеголя́ть *сов.* (*вн.*) *разг.* outdó* (*smb.*).

переэкзаменова́ть *сов.* (*вн.*) re-exámine (*smb.*).

переэкзамено́вка *ж.* re-examinátion.

периге́й *м. астр.* périgee.

периге́лий *м. астр.* perihélion.

пери́ла *мн.* ráil(ings), balustráde *sg*; (*ле́стницы внутри́ до́ма*) bánisters.

пери́метр *м. мат.* perímeter.

пери́на *ж.* féather-bed.

пери́од *м.* périod; в ~ чего́-л. dúring *smth.*; в тече́ние дли́тельного ~а óver a long périod (of time); дли́тельный ~ дожде́й, хоро́шей пого́ды long spell of rain, of fine wéather.

периодиза́ция *ж.* divísion ínto périods, periodizátion.

периоди́ка *ж. собир.* periódical press; periódicals *pl*.

периоди́ческ|ий **1.** periódically; ~ий periódic(al); ~ие дожди́ intermíttent rain *sg*; ~ое изда́ние periódical; ~ая печа́ть periódical press; ◊ ~ая дробь *мат.* repéating décimal; ~ая систе́ма элеме́нтов *хим.* periódic sýstem (of élements).

периоди́чность *ж.* periodícity, regulárity.

периселе́ний *м. астр.* périlune.

периско́п *м.* périscope.

пе́ристо-ку́чев|ой: ~ые облака́ círrocúmulus *sg*, máckerel sky *sg*.

пе́рист|ый: ~ые облака́ círrus *sg*.

перифери́йный óutlying; in an óutlying área/district после *сущ.*; ~ рабо́тник official in an óutlying área/district.

перифери́ческий perípheral.

перифери́|я *ж.* óutlying área/district; (*ме́стные организа́ции*) óutlying/lócal organizátions; жить, рабо́тать на ~и live, work in an óutlying área; live, work in the próvinces; прие́хать с ~и come* from an óutlying área, come* up from an óutlying área, come* up from the próvinces.

перифра́з *м.*, ~а *ж. лит.* períphrasis (*pl* -ses), circumlocútion. ~и́ровать *несов. и сов.* (*вн.*) *лит.* périphrase (*smth.*).

перице́нтр *м. астр.* péricentre.

перл *м.* gem, pearl.

перламу́тр *м.* móther-of-péarl. ~овый móther-of--péarl *attr.*

перло́в|ый: ~ая крупа́ péarl-bárley; ~ суп péarl--bárley soup; ~ая ка́ша péarl-bárley pórridge.

перма́нент *м. разг.* (*зави́вка*) pérmanent wave.

перма́нентный pérmanent.

перна́т|ый *прил.* **1.** féathered; ~ое ца́рство the féathered tribe; **2.** *в знач. сущ. мн.* birds.

перо́ *с.* **1.** (*пти́чье*) féather; (*для украше́ния*)

plume; 2. (*писчее*) pen, nib; 3. (*зелёный лист чеснока, лука*) leaf*; ◇ взя́ться за ~ put*/set* pen to páper.

перочи́нный: ~ нóж(ик) pén-knife.

перпендикуля́р *м.* perpendícular; опусти́ть ~ drop a perpendícular. ~ный perpendícular; ~ная ли́ния perpendícular line.

перрóн *м.* plátform. ~ный plátform *attr.*

перс *м.* Pérsian.

перси́дский Pérsian; ~ язы́к Pérsian, the Pérsian lánguage.

пе́рсик *м.* 1. (*плод*) peach; 2. (*дерево*) péach-tree. ~овый peach *attr.*; ~ового цве́та péach-coloured.

перси́янка *ж.* Pérsian (wóman*).

персóн|а *ж.* pérson; (*важная особа*) pérson of distínction, high pérsonage; серви́з на шесть персóн set for six; два рубля́ с ~ы two róubles per pérson; ◇ cóбственной ~ой in pérson; ~ нон гра́та *дип.* persóna non gráta; ~ гра́та *дип.* persóna gráta.

персона́ж *м.* cháracter.

персона́л *м.* personnél, staff.

персона́льн|ый pérsonal; ~ая пéнсия spécial/mérit pénsion; ~ пенсионéр pérson recípient of a spécial/mérit pénsion.

перспекти́в|а *ж.* 1. perspéctive; 2. (*открывающийся вид*) vísta; 3. обыкн. *мн.* (*виды на будущее*) próspects; óutlook *sg*; ~ы на урожáй отли́чные the óutlook for the hárvest is good, there is every próspect of an éxcellent hárvest; ◇ в ~е in próspect. ~ный 1. (*отражающий перспективу*) perspéctive; gíving an impréssion of depth *после сущ.*; ~ное изображéние perspéctive dráwing; 2. (*предусматривающий будущее развитие*) lóng-térm; for the fúture *после сущ.*; 3. (*имеющий перспективы*) with good próspects *после сущ.*, wórth-while; ~ная рабóта wórth-while work.

перст *м. уст.* fínger; ◇ оди́н как ~ ≈ all alóne in the world.

пе́рстень *м.* ring.

перуа́н|ец *м.*, ~ка *ж.* Perúvian. ~ский Perúvian.

перфока́рта *ж.* punched card.

перфоле́нта *ж.* punched tape.

перфора́|тор *м.* 1. pérforator, punch; 2. (*машина для бурения*) drill, bóring machíne. ~ция *ж.* perforátion, púnching.

пéрхоть *ж.* dándruff; scurf *разг.*

перча́тк|а *ж.* glove; надéть ~и put* on *one's* gloves; ◇ брóсить ~у комý-л. throw* down the gáuntlet to *smb.*; подня́ть ~у take* up the gáuntlet, accépt the chállenge.

пéрчить, попéрчить (*вн.*) pépper (*smth.*).

перш|и́ть *несов. безл. разг.*: у меня́ ~и́т в гóрле I feel a tíckle in my throat, I have a dry throat.

пéрышко *с.* féather; лёгкий как ~ light as a féather.

пёс *м.* dog.

пéсен|ка *ж.* ditty; ◇ егó ~ спéта he's done for, it's all up with him. ~ник *м.* 1. (*певец*) sínger, chórister; 2. (*автор песен*) sóng-wríter; 3. (*сборник песен*) sóng-book; colléction of songs.

песéц *м.* 1. (*животное*) Árctic fox; голубóй ~ blue fox; 2. (*мех*) blue fox.

пескáрь *м.* gúdgeon.

пéсн|я *ж.* song; ◇ тянýть всё тý же ~ю harp on the same string; э́то стáрая ~ it's the same old stóry.

пес|óк *м.* 1. sand; золотóй ~ góld-dúst; 2. *мн.* sands; ◇ сáхарный ~ gránulated súgar; стрóить на ~é build* on sand.

песóчн|ый 1. sand *attr.*; ~ые часы́ sánd-glass *sg*; 2. *разг.* (*о цвете*) sánd-coloured; 3. (*о тесте*) short; ~ торт fáncy shórtcake; ~ое печéнье shórtcake bíscuits *pl.*

пессим|и́зм *м.* péssimism. ~и́ст *м.* péssimist. ~исти́ческий pessimístic.

пéстик *м. бот.* pístil.

пестр|éть I *несов.* 1. (*виднеться*) show* up cólourfully; вдали́ ~éли цветы́ the flówers showed up

cólourfully in the dístance, the flówers made a splash of cólour in the dístance; 2. (*тв.*; *быть пёстрым от чего-л.*) be* bright (with), be* spángled (with); 3. (*становиться пёстрым*) becóme* múlticoloured.

пестр|éть II *несов.* 1. (*тв.*; *изобиловать чем-л.*) be* dótted (with); *перен.* be* interspérsed (with), be* lárded (with); речь ~и́т цитáтами the speech is interspérsed/lárded with quotátions; 2. *разг.* (*быть слишком пёстрым*) be* gáudy.

пестр|и́ть *несов. безл.*: у меня́ ~и́т в глазáх I am dázzled.

пестрот|á *ж.* varíety of cólours; *перен.* varíety, divérsity; толпá отличáлась ~óй it was a véry mixed crowd.

пёстр|ый párticoloured, váriegated; *перен.* mixed, divérse; ~ые крáски gay cólours.

песцóвый white-fox *attr.*; blúe-fox *attr.*

песчáн|ик *м.* sándstone. ~ый sándy; ~ая пóчва sándy soil.

песчи́нка *ж.* grain of sand.

петáрда *ж. ж.-д.* détonator.

пети́т *м. полигр.* brevíer.

пети́ция *ж.* petítion.

петли́ца *ж.* 1. búttonhole; 2. (*на форменной одежде*) tab.

пéтл|я *ж.* 1. loop; 2. (*в вязании*) stitch; 3. (*круговое движение*) meánder; дорóга ~ями шла по склóну the road snaked/meándered down the slope; 4. *ав.* loop; дéлать ~ю loop the loop; 5. *спорт.* sómersault in míd-áir); 6. *мн. охот.* (*следы зверя*) wínding/meándering track *sg*; 7. (*для пуговицы*) búttonhole; (*для крючка*) eye; 8. (*дверей, окон*) hinge; дверь соскочи́ла с пéтель the door is off its hínges; ◇ влезть в ~ю put* *one's* head in the noose; хоть в ~ю лезь it's enóugh to drive *one* mad.

петрýшка I *ж. бот.* pársley.

петрýшка II 1. *м.* (*кукла*) Petrúshka; Punch; 2. *ж.* (*кукольный театр*) púppet-show.

петýх *м.* 1. cock, cóckerel; róoster *разг.*; 2. *мн.* (*пение петухов*) cóck-crow *sg*; вставáть с ~áми rise* at cóck-crow; сидéть до ~óв sit* up till cóck-crow; ◇ пусти́ть комý-л. крáсного ~á set* fire to *smb.'s* home.

петýш|ий, ~и́ный cock *attr.*; ~ грéбень cock's comb; ~и́ный бой cóck-fight, cóck-fighting. ~и́ться *несов. разг.* get* on *one's* high horse, ride* the high horse.

петушóк *м.* cock, cóckerel.

петь, спеть, пропéть 1. (*вн.*) sing* (*smth.*); ~ ромáнс sing* a song; ~ пáртию Лéнского sing* the part of Lénsky; 2. *тк. несов.* (*иметь голос*) sing*; (*профессионально заниматься пением тж.*) be* a sínger; ~ бáсом sing* bass; ~ в óпере be* an ópera sínger; 3. (*издавать мелодичные звуки*) hum; (*о муз. инструментах*) play/sound swéetly; слýшать, как поют скри́пки lísten to the sweet sound of violíns; 4. *сов.* пропéть (*о птицах*) sing*; (*о петухе*) crow*; 5. *тк. несов.* (*вн.*) (*воспевать*) praise (*smth.*), sing* (*smth.*).

пехóт|а *ж.* ínfantry. ~и́нец *м.* ínfantryman*, foot sóldier. ~ный ínfantry *attr.*; ~ный полк ínfantry régiment.

печáлить, опечáлить (*вн.*) grieve (*smb.*), distréss (*smb.*). ~ся, опечáлиться be* sad, be* grieved/distréssed.

печáль *ж.* 1. grief, sádness, sórrow; 2. *разг.* (*забота*) care, wórry. ~ный 1. sad, sórrowful, sórrowing; ~ный человéк sórrowful pérson; ~ный взгляд sórrowful/sad glance; 2. (*вызывающий печаль*) sómbre, sad; ~ные пусты́ни sómbre déserts; 3. (*достойный сожаления*) regréttable, lámentable, deplórable, sórry; ~ная слáва lámentable/sórry reputátion.

печáтание *с.* prínting; (*на машинке*) týping.

печáтать, напечáтать (*вн.*) 1. print (*smth.*); (*на машинке*) type (*smth.*); 2. (*публиковать*) públish (*smth.*). ~ся *несов.* 1. be* prínted; (*издаваться*) be* públished;

2. (*помещать свои произведения в печати*) have* one's works públished; начáть ~ся get* ínto print.

печáтн|ик *м.* prínter. ~ый **1.** prínting; ~ый цех prínting shop; ~ая машúна prínting machíne; **2.** (*напечатанный*) prínted; ~ая продýкция prínted mátter; **3.** (*опубликованный*) públished; **4.** (*имеющий форму напечатанного*): ~ые бýквы block létters; писáть ~ыми бýквами write* in block létters; ◇ ~ый лист sígnature, prínter's sheet; (*сфальцованный*) quíre.

печáт|ь *ж.* **1.** seal; stamp (*тж. перен.*); запечáтать письмó ~ью seal (up) a létter; постáвить ~ на что-л. put*/set*/affíx a seal to *smth.*; наложúть свою ~ на что-л. leave* an ímpress upón *smth.*; носúть ~ чего-л. bear* the stamp of *smth.*; **2.** (*печатание*) prínt(ing), press; кнúга нахóдится в ~и the book is in the press; кнúга готóвится к ~и the book is béing prepáred for the press; вы́йти из ~и, появúться в ~и appéar in print, come* out, come* off the press; **3.** (*отрасль производства*) prínting; высóкая ~ létterpress/relíef prínting; глубóкая ~ intáglio prínting; плóская ~ súrface/planográphic prínting; цветнáя ~ cólour prínting; **4.** (*внешний вид отпечатанного*) type, print; крýпная ~ large type; мéлкая ~ small type; **5.** (*пресса*) the press; кнúга вы́звала благоприя́тные óтзывы в ~и the book had/recéived a good press.

печéние *с.* báking.

печёнка *ж.* líver.

печёный baked; ~ картóфель baked potáto(es).

печен|ь *ж.* líver; болéзнь ~и líver diséase/compláint.

печéнье *с.* bíscuits *pl*; cráckers *pl*, cóokies *pl амер.*

печ|кá *ж.* stove; ◇ танцевáть от ~ки begín* at the begínning. ~ник *м.* stóve-máker, stóve-sétter. ~нóй stove *attr.*; ~нáя трубá chímney; ~нóе отоплéние stove héating.

печь I *ж.* stove; (*духовка*) óven; *тех.* fúrnace; ~ для óбжига kiln; кремациóнная ~ incínerator.

печь II, **испéчь 1.** (*вн.*) bake (*smth.*); ~ пирогú bake pies; **2.** *тк. несов.* (*обдавать жаром*) beat* down (on), scorch; сóлнце печёт the sun is scórching; сегóдня сúльно печёт it's scórching/blázing hot todáy.

печься I, **испéчься 1.** bake; **2.** *тк. несов. разг.* (*греться на солнце*) bask in the sun.

печься II *несов.* (о *пр.*) take* care (of), look áfter (*smb.*, *smth.*), wórry abóut (*smb.*, *smth.*).

пешехóд *м.* pedéstrian; тропá для ~ов fóotpath. ~ный **1.** (*для ходьбы пешком*) pedéstrian; foot *attr.*; ~ный перехóд pedéstrian cróssing; **2.** (*совершаемый пешком*) wálking *attr.*; on foot *после сущ.*; ~ная прогýлка walk.

пéш|ий 1. foot *attr.*; on foot *после сущ.*; ~ие путешéственники trávellers on foot; **2.** *воен.* unmóunted.

пéшка *ж. шахм.* pawn; *перен. разг.* a mere pawn.

пешкóм on foot; ходúть ~ walk, go* on foot.

пещéр|а *ж.* cave, cávern; (*грот*) grótto (*pl* -oes, -os). ~ный *attr.*; ~ный человéк cáve-dweller, cáve-man*; ~ное óзеро subterránean lake.

пианúно *с. нескл.* (úpright) piáno; игрáть на ~ play the piáno.

пианúст *м.*, ~ка *ж.* piánist.

пивн|áя *ж.* pub *разг.*; bár-room *амер.* ~óй beer *attr.*; ~óй завóд bréwery; ~áя крýжка beer mug.

пúво *с.* beer; варúть ~ brew beer. ~вáр *м.* bréwer. ~варéние *с.* bréwing.

пивовáренный bréwing *attr.*; ~ завóд bréwery.

пигмéй *м.* pygmy (*тж. перен.*).

пигмéнт *м.* pigment. ~áция *ж.* pigmentátion.

пиджáк *м.* coat, jácket.

пижáма *ж.* pyjámas *pl*; pajámas *pl амер.*

пижóн *м. разг. неодобр.* (young) fop. ~ство *с. разг. неодобр.* fóppishness.

пик *м.* (móuntain) peak; ◇ часы́ ~ rush hours.

пúка I *ж.* (*оружие*) lance; (*пехотная*) pike.

пúк|а II *ж. разг.*: в ~у комý-л. to spite *smb.*

пикáнтн|ость *ж.* píquancy, sávour; *перен.* spice; (*соблазнительность*) fascinátion. ~ый píquant, sávoury; *перен.* spícy; (*соблазнительный*) fáscinating, fétching.

пикáп *м.* (light) van, píck-up.

пикé I *с. нескл. ав.* dive.

пикé II *с. нескл.* (*ткань*) piqué.

пикéйн|ый piqué *attr.*; ~ая рубáшка piqué shirt.

пикéт *м.* pícket; ~ стáчечный ~ strike pícket.

пикетúровать *несов.* (*вн.*) pícket (*smth.*); ~ завóд pícket a fáctory.

пúки *мн. карт.* spades.

пикúрование *с. ав.* dive, díving.

пикúровать *несов. и сов. ав.* dive.

пикúроваться *несов.* (с *тв.*) bícker óver/abóut (with).

пикирóвка *ж.* (*перебранка*) bíckering.

пикирóвщик *м. разг.* díve-bómber.

пикнúк *м.* pícnic.

пúкнуть *сов.* útter a sound; он и ~ не успéл, как... before he could ópen his mouth..., before he could say knife...; попрóбуй тóлько ~ don't you dare say a word, one squeak out of you and...

пúков|ый of spades *после сущ.*; ~ая дáма queen of spades; ◇ ~ое положéние prétty mess; остáться при ~ом интерéсе have* all the tróuble for nóthing, get* nóthing for *one's* pains.

пúкули *мн. кул.* píckles.

пилá *ж.* saw; *перен.* nágger; крýглая ~ círcular saw.

пилёный sawn; ~ лес sawn tímber.

пилúть *несов.* (*вн.*) saw* (*smth.*); *перен.* (*изводить*) nag (at); ~ дровá saw* wood.

пúлка I *ж.* (*действие*) sáwing.

пúлка II *ж.* **1.** (*ручная пила*) small hánd-saw; **2.** (*напильник*) file; ~ для ногтéй náil-file.

пилóт *м.* pílot. ~áж *м.* píloting, flýing.

пилотúровать *несов.* (*вн.*) pílot (*smth.*).

пилóтка *ж.* field cap, fórage cap.

пúльщик *м.* sáwyer.

пилю́л|я *ж.* pill; ◇ гóрькая ~ bítter pill; подсластúть ~ю swéeten/súgar the pill; проглотúть ~ю swállow the pill.

пинáть, **пнуть** (*вн.*) *разг.* kick (*smb.*, *smth.*).

пингвúн *м.* pénguin.

пинóк *м. разг.* kick.

пинцéт *м.* twéezers *pl*, píncers *pl*.

пиóн *м. бот.* péony.

пионéр I *м.* (*зачинатель чего-л.*) pionéer.

пионéр II *м.* (*член детской организации*) Young Pionéer. ~вожáтый *м.* Young Pionéer léader.

пипéтка *ж.* pipétte, drópper.

пир *м.* feast, bánquet; ◇ ~ горóй súmptuous feast.

пирамúда *ж.* **1.** pýramid; **2.** *воен.* (rifle) stack.

пирамидáльный pyrámidal, pýramid-shaped; ~ тóполь Lómbardy póplar.

пирáт *м. ист.* pírate. ~ский *ист.* pírate *attr.* ~ство *с. ист.* píracy.

пирúт *м.* pyríte.

пировáть *несов.* feast; (*в гостях*) bánquet; (*шумно*) caróuse.

пирóг *м.* pie, pásty; (*сладкий открытый*) tart; ~ с мя́сом méat-pie, méat-pásty; ~ с ры́бой fish-pie, físh-pásty; ~ с я́блоками ápple-pie; (*открытый*) ápple-tárt.

пирóжное *с.* (fáncy) cake, pástry; слóёное ~ púff-pástry.

пирож|óк *м.* pátty; ~кú с мя́сом meat pátties.

пироксилúн *м.* pyróxylin, sóluble gún-cotton.

пиротéхника *ж.* pyrotéchnics.

пирс *м. мор.* pier, jétty.

писá|ка *м. и ж. разг.* scríbbler; продáжный ~ hack. ~ние *с.* wríting.

пúсан|ый 1. hánd-written; **2.** (*разукрашенный*)

páinted; ◇ ~ая краса́вица béauty; говори́ть как по ~о́-му speak* as from the book.

писа́тель *м.* wríter, áuthor, man* of létters. **~ница** *ж.* wríter, áuthoress. **~ский:** ~ский труд wríting, the work of a wríter; ~ский тала́нт tálent for wríting.

писа́ть, написа́ть 1. (*вн.*) write* (*smth.*); ~ бу́квы write* létters; ~ карандашо́м write* in péncil; ~ кру́пно, ме́лко write* large, small; ~ на маши́нке type; ~ расска́-зы write* stóries; 2. (*дт.; письмо*) write* (to); он ей ча́сто пи́шет he óften writes to her; 3. *тк. несов.* (*быть писа́телем*) write*, be* a wríter; он давно́ пи́шет he has been a wríter for some time; 4. *тк. несов.* (в *пр.*; *сотрудничать в периодическом издании*) write* (for); ~ в газе́тах write* for the pápers; 5. *тк. несов.* (*быть годным для письма*) write*; 6. (*вн.*; *создавать произведения живописи*) paint (*smth.*); ~ портре́т ма́слом paint a pórtrait in oils; ~ акваре́лью paint in wáter-colours; ◇ зако́н не пи́сан кому́-л. *smb.* is a law únto himself; пиши́ пропа́ло you can say good-býe to it, it is as good as lost. **~ся** *несов.* 1. be* wrítten; (*о правописании*) be* spelt; как пи́шется э́то сло́во? how is that word spelt?; 2. *безл. разг.*: мне сего́дня не пи́шется my wríting goes véry bádly todáy.

писк *м.* squéak(ing); (*птенцов*) péep(ing), chéep(ing), ~ли́вый 1. (*о голосе*) squéaky, high-pítched; 2. (*обладающий тонким, высоким голосом*) squéaky-vóiced; 3. (*о предметах*) squéaky, scrátchy; ~ли́вая скри́пка scrátchy violín; 4. (*плаксивый*) squéaling, whíning.

пи́скнуть *сов.* give* a squeak.

пистоле́т *м.* pístol. **~ный** pístol *attr.*

писто́н *м.* 1. cap; 2. (*металлическая оправа*) éyelet; 3. *муз.* valve, píston.

писчебума́жн|ый státionery *attr.*; ~ магази́н státioner's shop; ~ые принадле́жности státionery *sg.*

пи́сч|ий wríting *attr.*; ~ая бума́га wríting páper.

письмена́ *мн.* cháracters, létters.

письменн|ость *ж.* in wrítten form. **~ость** *ж.* 1. (*система графических знаков*) wríting; cháracters *pl*, álphabet; 2. (*совокупность письменных памятников*) líterature. **~ый** 1. (*написанный*) wrítten; ~ая рабо́та wrítten work; в ~ом ви́де in wríting, in wrítten form; 2. (*служащий для письма*) wríting *attr.*; ~ый стол desk, wríting-table; ~ый прибо́р desk set, wríting-set.

письм|о́ *с.* 1. (*послание*) létter; заказно́е ~ régistered létter; 2. *тк. ед.* (*умение писать*) wríting; иску́сство ~á callígraphy; 3. *тк. ед.* (*система графических знаков*) wríting, script; cháracters *pl*; разви́тие ~á the evolútion of wríting; готи́ческое ~ Góthic script; 4. *тк. ед. иск., лит.* mánner.

письмоно́сец *м.* póstman*.

пита́ние *с.* 1. (*действие*) féeding; (*снабжение*) supplýing; *перен.* nóurishing; 2. (*пища*) food, nóurishment, díet; недоста́точное ~ underféeding; 3. (*горючее*) fuel supplý; (*рации*) power supplý.

пита́тельн|ость *ж.* food-value, nutrítiousness. **~ый** 1. nutrítious, nóurishing; ~ое вещество́ nútritive; 2. *тех.* feed *attr.*; supplý *attr.*; ◇ ~ая среда́ *биол.* cúlture médium.

пита́ть *несов.* (*вн.*) 1. feed* (*smb.*); 2. (*снабжать чем-л. необходимым*) supplý (*smth.*), keep* (*smth.*) supplíed, *перен.* nóurish (*smth.*); ~ го́род электроэне́ргией supplý a cíty with power; ~ воображе́ние nóurish/feed* the imaginátion; 3. (*испытывать*) feel* (*smth.*); chérish (*smth.*), entertáin (*smth.*); ~ отвраще́ние к кому́-л. feel*/have* an avérsion for *smb.*; ~ не́нависть nurse/nóurish hátred. **~ся** *несов.* (*тв.*) 1. (*есть*) eat* (*smth.*), live (on), feed* (on); хорошо́ ~ся be* well-féd, eat* well; пло́хо ~ся be* underféd; ~ся мя́сом, фру́ктами live/feed* on meat, fruit; 2. (*получать что-л. необходимое*) be* fed (by); *перен.* be* nóurished

(by), draw* (on); ~ся ме́стным у́глем work on lócal coal.

пито́м|ец *м.* púpil. **~ник** *м.* núrsery.

пить, вы́пить 1. (*вн.*) drink* (*smth.*); (*лекарство, чай, кофе и т. п. тж.*) take* (*smth.*), have* (*smth.*); ~ ма́ленькими глотка́ми sip; ~ минера́льные во́ды take*/drink* the wáters; 2. *тк. несов.* (*пьянствовать*) drink*; 3. (*за вн.*) drink* (to); ◇ как ~ дать as sure as fate.

пить|ё *с.* 1. (*действие*) drínking; 2. (*напиток*) drink, béverage. **~ево́й** drínking; ~ева́я вода́ drínking wáter; ~ева́я со́да bicárbonate of sóda, báking/cóoking sóda.

пиха́ть, пихну́ть (*вн.*) *разг.* 1. (*толкать*) push (*smb., smth.*), shove (*smb., smth.*); (*локтями*) élbow (*smb.*); 2. (*засовывать*) thrust* (*smth.*) in.

пихну́ть *сов. см.* пиха́ть.

пи́хта *ж.* fir.

пи́чкать, напи́чкать (*вн. тв.*) *разг.* (*прям. и перен.*) cram (*smb.* with), stuff (*smb.* with); (*лекарствами*) dose (*smb.* with).

пи́шущ|ий wríting; ~ая маши́нка týpewriter.

пищ|а *ж.* food (*тж. перен.*), nóurishment; ~ для ума́ food for the thought; ◇ дава́ть ~у чему́-л. províde food for *smth.*

пища́ть, пропища́ть squeak; (*о ребёнке*) squeal; (*о птенцах*) cheep, peep.

пищеваре́ни|е *с.* digéstion; расстро́йство ~я indigéstion; плохо́е ~ bad*/poor digéstion.

пищевари́тельн|ый digéstive; ~ые о́рганы digéstive órgans.

пищево́д *м.* gúllet; oesóphagus (*pl* -gi, -es) *научн.*

пищев|о́й food *attr.*; ~ы́е проду́кты fóodstuffs; ~а́я промы́шленность food índustry.

пия́вк|а *ж.* leech; ста́вить ~и applý léeches; приста-ва́ть как ~ *разг.* stick* like a leech.

пла́вани|е *с.* 1. swímming; ~ на ло́дках bóating; 2. (*путешествие на судне*) vóyage, cruise; кругосве́тное ~ vóyage round the world; быть в ~и be* at sea; отправ-ля́ться в ~ set* out on a vóyage; ◇ большо́му кораблю́ большо́е (и) ~ *посл.* great ships need deep wáters.

пла́вательн|ый swímming *attr.*; nátatory *научн.*; ~ бассе́йн swímming pool; ~ пузы́рь swímming-bladder, áir-bladder; ~ая перепо́нка (*у птиц*) web.

пла́вать *несов.* 1. (*о человеке и животном*) swim*; (*о предметах; об облаках*) float, drift; (*о судне*) sail; (*о пароходе*) steam; 2. (*держаться на поверхности жидкости*) float; 3. (*на судне и т. п.*) sail, cruise, návigate; ~ на плоту́ float on a raft, raft; ~ на парохо́де по Байка́лу make* a bóat-trip on Lake Baikál; 4. *разг.* (*служить на судне*) serve, sail; 5. *разг.* (*отвечать сбивчиво и путано*) be* all at sea, be* out of *one's* depth.

плавба́за *ж.* flóating fish-factory.

плави́льн|ый smélting; ~ое произво́дство métal prodúction; ~ая печь smélting fúrnace.

пла́в|ить *несов.* (*вн.*) melt (*smth.*); (*получать металл из руды*) smelt (*smth.*). **~иться** *несов.* melt; smelt. **~ка** *ж.* 1. (*процесс*) smélting; 2. (*один производственный цикл процесса плавления*) melt; скоростна́я ~ка high-speed mélt(ing); 3. (*продукт*) melt.

пла́вки *мн.* swímming trunks.

пла́вк|ий méltable, fúsible. **~ость** *ж.* fusibílity.

плавле́ние *с.* mélting, fúsion.

пла́вленый: ~ сыр prócessed cheese.

плавни́к *м.* fin; (*у тюленя, кита*) flípper.

пла́вн|ость *ж.* ease; (*речи*) flúency. **~ый** éasy, smooth; (*о речи*) flúent; ~ая похо́дка gráceful/fine cárriage; ◇ ~ые согла́сные *лингв.* líquid cónsonants.

плаву́ч|есть *ж.* búoyancy. **~ий** 1. flóating; ~ий рыбообраба́тывающий заво́д flóating fish-factory; ~ая льди́на ice-floe; 2. (*способный держаться на поверхности*) buóyant.

плагиа́т *м.* plágiarism. ~ор *м.* plágiarist.

пла́зма *ж.* plásma.

плака́т *м.* póster.

плак|ать *несов.* 1. cry; weep* *поэт.*; го́рько ~ cry bítterly; ~ от ра́дости weep* for joy; 2. (о *пр.*) weep* (for, óver), cry (for, óver); ◇ ~али на́ши де́нежки it was good-býe to our móney. ~аться *несов.* (на *вн.*) *разг.* moan (abóut), whímper (abóut).

пла́кс|а *м. и ж.* crý-baby; sníveller. ~ивый téarful; ~ивый ребёнок child* who is álways crýing, crý-baby; ~ивый го́лос whíning/téarful voice.

плаку́ч|ий wéeping; ~ая и́ва wéeping wíllow.

пламене́ть *несов.* blaze, flame.

пла́менный fíery; *перен. тж.* árdent; ~ взгляд fíery glance; ~ приве́т héartfelt/wármest gréeting.

пла́м|я *с.* (*прям. и перен.*) flame(s); вспы́хнуть ~енем burst*/break* ínto fláme(s); go* up in flame(s); из и́скры возгори́тся ~ the spark will becóme a flame; ~ гне́ва the flames of ánger/wrath.

план *м.* 1. plan; произво́дственный ~ prodúction plan/prógramme; разраба́тывать ~ draw* up a plan; выполня́ть ~ fulfil the plan; стро́ить ~ы на бу́дущее plan for the fúture; снять ~ ме́стности survéy a district; 2. (*расположение предмета в перспективе*): пере́дний ~ fóreground; за́дний ~ báckground; кру́пный ~ *кино* clóse-up; о́бщий ~ *кино* long shot; ◇ отойти́ на за́дний ~ be* rélegated to the báckground; здоро́вье у него́ на после́днем ~е he takes no care of his health; вопро́с обсужда́лся в теорети́ческом, о́бщем ~е the quéstion was discússed on a theorétical, géneral plane.

планёр *м.* glíder; (*спортивный тж.*) sáil-plane.

планер|и́зм *м.* glíding. ~и́ст *м.*, ~и́стка *ж.* glíder-pílot.

плане́т|а *ж.* plánet; больши́е ~ы májor plánets; ма́лые ~ы mínor plánets, ásteroids.

планета́рий *м.* planetárium (*pl* -ria).

плане́тный plánetary.

планиме́трия *ж.* planímetry, plane geómetry.

плани́рование I *с.* plánning; ~ городо́в tówn-plánning.

плани́рование II *с. ав.* glíding.

плани́ровать I, заплани́ровать, сплани́ровать (*вн.*) plan (*smth.*).

плани́ровать II, сплани́ровать *ав.* glide.

планиро́в|ка *ж.* plánning; (*расположение чего-л.*) láy-out. ~щик *м.* plánner.

планисфе́ра *ж. астр.* plánisphere.

пла́нка *ж.* plank, lath; (*металлическая*) métal strip, plate.

планкто́н *м. биол.* planktón.

планови́к *м.* (prodúction) plánner.

планов|ость *ж.* planned náture. ~ый 1. planned; ~ая рабо́та planned work; 2. (*занимающийся составлением планов*) plánning *attr.*; ~ый отде́л plánning depártment.

планоме́рн|ость *ж.* planned/systemátic cháracter, regulárity. ~ый planned, systemátic, accórding to plan *после сущ.*

планта́|тор *м.* plánter. ~ция *ж.* plantátion.

планше́т *м.* 1. *геод.* plane táble, dráwing board; 2. (*полевая сумка*) map case.

пласт *м.* 1. (*плотный слой чего-л.*) láyer; 2. (*слой горной породы*) bed, strátum (*pl* -ta); (*угля*) seam; ◇ лежа́ть ~о́м lie* próstrate, be* flat on one's back.

пла́стика *ж.* 1. (*искусство ваяния*) plástic art; 2. (*пластичность*) plastícity; 3. (*искусство ритмических движений*) sense of rhythm.

пла́стики *мн.* (*ед.* пла́стик *м.*) plástics.

пла́стиков|ый plástic; ~ая бо́мба plástic bomb.

пластили́н *м.* plásticine.

пласти́нка *ж.* 1. plate, strip of métal, táblet; 2. (*патефонная*) récord, recórding; disc *разг.*; 3. *фото* plate; 4. *бот.* blade, lámina; (*гриба*) gill.

пласти́ческ|ий plástic; ~ие движе́ния rhýthmic/plástic móvements; ~ая хирурги́я plástic súrgery; ◇ ~ая ма́сса plástic.

пласти́чн|ость *ж.* plastícity. ~ый plástic.

пластма́сс|а *ж.* plástic. ~овый plástic.

пла́стырь *м.* pláster; вытяжно́й ~ blístering pláster; ли́пкий ~ stícking/adhésive pláster.

пла́т|а *ж.* 1. (*вознаграждение за труд*) pay, páyment; поштучная ~ páyment by the piece; 2. (*возмещение*) charge (for), cost (of); вноси́ть ~у за *что-л.* pay* for *smth.*; вноси́ть ~у за кварти́ру pay* the rent; ~ за прое́зд fare.

платёж *м.* páyment; кру́пные платежи́ large páyments; ◇ долг платежо́м кра́сен *посл.* ≈ one good turn desérves anóther.

платёжеспосо́бн|ость *ж. фин.* sólvency, páying capácity; ~ ба́нка the capácity of a bank to meet its liabílities. ~ый *фин.* sólvent.

платёжн|ый pay *attr.*; ~ день páy-day; ~ая ве́домость páy-sheet, páy-roll; ~ бала́нс bálance of páyments.

пла́тина *ж. фин.* plátinum.

плати́ть *несов.* 1. pay*; ~ нали́чными pay* in cash; ~ за кварти́ру pay* the rent; ~ за прое́зд pay* the fare; ~ по счёту pay* the bill; ~ в рассро́чку pay* in/by instálments; ~ долги́ pay* one's debts; 2. (*тв.* за *вн.*; *делать что-л. в ответ на чей-л. поступок*) repáy* (*smth.* with); ~ добро́м за добро́ repáy*/retúrn (a) kindness; ~ кому́-л. взаи́мностью retúrn smb.'s love. ~ся, поплати́ться pay*; он поплати́лся жи́знью за свою́ неосторо́жность his carelessness cost him his life.

пла́тн|ый 1. (*подлежащий оплате*) that is charged for *после сущ.*, paid; ~ вход paid admíssion; 2. (*оплачиваемый*) paid; ~ рабо́тник wáge-lábourer; 3. (*оплачивающий*) páying.

плато́ *с. нескл. геогр.* pláteau.

плато́к *м.* shawl; (*головной*) kérchief; носово́й ~ (pócket) hándkerchief.

платфо́рма *ж.* 1. (*перрон*) plátform; 2. (*товарный вагон*) ópen truck, plátform car; 3. (*программа действий*) plátform, prógramme.

пла́ть|е *с.* 1. *собир.* (*одежда*) clothes *pl*, clóthing; магази́н гото́вого ~я réady-máde shop; 2. (*женское*) dress, frock, gown.

пла́тян|о́й: ~ шкаф wárdrobe; ~а́я щётка clóthes-brush.

плафо́н *м.* 1. (*расписной или лепной потоло́к*) décorated céiling; 2. (*абажур*) lamp/bowl shade.

плацда́рм *м.* base (*тж. перен.*); spring-board, júmping-off place; (*предмостное укрепление*) brídge-head.

плацка́рт|а *ж.* resérved-seat tícket; взять биле́т с ~ой resérve/book a seat, make* a reservátion/bóoking; вы хоти́те биле́т с ~ой? do you wish to resérve/book your seat? ~ный: ~ный ваго́н cárriage/car with resérved seats; ~ное ме́сто resérved seat.

плач *м.* wéeping, wáiling.

плаче́вн|ый 1. (*скорбный*) laménting, wáiling; 2. (*бедственный*) deplórable, lámentable; (*ничтожный*) pítiful; ~ое состоя́ние deplórable condition/state; результа́ты бы́ли ~ые the resúlts were lámentable/pítiful.

пла́чущий téarful; whíning; ~ го́лос téarful voice.

плашко́ут *м. мор.* pontóon. ~ный *мор.* pontóon *attr.*; ~ный мост pontóon bridge.

плашмя́ flat; упа́сть ~ fall* flat on the ground; уда́рить кого́-л. ша́шкой ~ strike* smb. with the flat of one's sword.

плащ *м.* 1. ráincoat, máckintosh, wáterproof; 2. (*без рукавов*) cloak, mántle.

плащ-палáтка *ж.* (tént-)cape.

плебисци́т *м.* plébiscite.

плевá *ж.* mémbrane, film.

плевáтельница *ж.* spittóon; cúspidor *амер.*

плевáть, плю́нуть spit*; (*на вн.*) *перен. разг.* shrug off (*smth.*); ~ мне на него́ I don't care a damn/hang for him; ему́ ~ на всё he dóesn't care a fig for ánything; ◇ ~ в потоло́к ≈ sit* twíddling *one's* thumbs. **~ся** *несов. разг.* spit*; (*брызгать слюною*) splútter.

плево́к *м.* spíttle; (*мокрота*) spútum (*pl* -ta).

плéвра *ж. анат.* pléura (*pl* -ae).

плеври́т *м. мед.* pléurisy.

плед *м.* plaid, (trávelling-)rug.

плексиглáс *м.* pérspex. **~овый** pérspex *attr.*

племенн|о́й 1. (*о племени*) tríbal; 2. (*породистый*) pédigree, thóroughbred; ~бык pédigree bull; **~ое** живо́тноводство púre-strain/pédigree stóck-breeding.

плéм|я *с.* 1. tribe; кочевы́е ~енá nómad tribes; 2. *тк. ед.* (*поколение, современники*) generátion; ◇ на плéмя *с.-х.* for bréeding púrposes.

племя́нн|ик *м.* néphew. **~ица** *ж.* niece.

плен *м.* captívity; *перен.* spell; находи́ться в ~у́ be* in captívity; быть в ~у́ у кого́-л. *перен.* be* únder *smb.'s* spell; быть в ~у́ предрассу́дков be* a slave to préjudice.

пленáрн|ый plénary, **~ое** заседáние plénary séssion, full assémbly.

плени́тельный chárming, cáptivating, fáscinating.

плени́ть(ся) *сов. см.* пленя́ть(ся).

плёнк|а *ж.* 1. film; ~ льда film of ice; 2. (*фотографическая*) film; засня́ть кого́-л. на ~у take* *smb.'s* picture; 3. (*магнитофонная*) tape; записáть что́-л. на ~у recórd *smth.*

плённ|ик *м.*, **~ица** *ж.* cáptive; prísoner (*тж. перен.*).

плённ|ый *прил.* 1. cáptured, cáptive; 2. *в знач. сущ. м.* prísoner; брать ~ых take* prísoners.

плéнум *м.* plénum.

пленя́ть, плени́ть (*вн.*) cáptivate (*smb.*), fáscinate (*smth.*). **~ся, плени́ться** (*тв.*) be* cáptivated (by), be* fáscinated (by).

плёс *м.* reach, stretch of ópen wáter.

плéсень *ж.* mould; místiness (*тж. перен.*); (*о людях*) scum; покры́ться ~ю be* móuldy.

плеск *м.* splash; (*волн о берег*) lápping.

плескáть, плесну́ть 1. (*о волнах, море*) lap; 2. (*брызгать водой*) splash. **~ся** *несов.* 1. splash; 2. (*переливаться через край*) splash óver.

плéсневеть, заплéсневеть grow*/get* móuldy.

плесну́ть *сов. см.* плескáть.

плести́ *несов.* (*вн.*) 1. weave* (*smth.*) (*тж. перен.*); (*косу*) plait (*smth.*); braid (*smth.*) *поэт.*; (*паутину*) spin* (*smth.*); ~ сéти make* nets; ~ корзи́ну weave*/make* a básket; ~ интри́гу weave* a plot; 2. *разг.* (*сочинять*) make* up (*smth.*), spin* (*smth.*); ~ вздор talk nónsense/rot.

плести́сь *несов. разг.* trudge alóng; ~ в хвостé lag/drag behínd, be at the táil-end.

плетён|ый wícker *attr.*; ~ стул wícker chair; ~ые изде́лия wícker-work *sg.*

плетéнь *м.* wáttle-fence.

плётка *ж.*, **плеть** *ж.* lash.

плечев|о́й shóulder *attr.*; húmeral *научн.*; ~áя кость *анат.* húmerus (*pl* -ri).

плéчики *мн.* (*вешалка для платья*) cóat-hanger *sg.*, clóthes-hanger *sg.*

плечи́стый broad-shóuldered.

плеч|о́ *с.* 1. shóulder; 2. *анат.* húmerus (*pl* -ri); 3. *тех.* arm; ◇ ~о́м к ~у́ shóulder to shóulder; име́ть го́лову на ~áх have* a head on *one's* shóulders; с плеч доло́й that's done, that's off my mind; это ему́ не по ~у́ it's

---

beyónd his pówers, he's not up to it; с чего́-л. ~á passed on to *one* by *smb.*, inhérited from *smb.*; с чужо́го ~á cást-off; у него́ за ~áми 40 лет трудово́й жи́зни fórty years of toil lie behínd him.

плеши́в|еть, оплеши́веть get*/grow* bald. **~ость** *ж.* báldness. **~ый** bálding *attr.*, half-báld; (*лысый*) bald.

плешь *ж.* bald spot/patch.

плея́да *ж.* gálaxy.

пли́нтус *м.* 1. (*планка*) skírting(-board); 2. *архит.* plinth.

плитá *ж.* 1. (*плоский кусок камня, металла и т. п.*) plate, slab; (*для мощения*) flágstone, páving-stone; мрáморная ~ márble slab; 2. (*кухонная*) (kitchen-)range, stove; электри́ческая ~ eléctric cóoker.

пли́тка *ж.* 1. (*облицовочная*) tile; 2. (*шоколада и т. п.*) bar; 3. (*электрическая*) hot plate.

пли́точный: ~ пол tiled floor; ~ чай brick-tea; ~ шоколáд sláb-chocolate.

пловéц *м.* swimmer.

плод *м.* 1. fruit; приноси́ть ~ы́ bear* fruit; 2. *биол.* fóetus; 3. (*результат чего-л.*) fruit(s); ~ы́ нáших трудо́в the fruit(s) of our lábours.

плоди́ть *несов.* (*вн.*) breed* (*smth.*), bring* forth (*smth.*); *перен.* breed* (*smb., smth.*). **~ся** *несов. разг.* (*прям. и перен.*) breed*, múltiply.

плодови́т|ость *ж.* fertílity; *перен.* productívity. **~ый** fértile; *перен.* prolífic; productíve; **~ый** писáтель prolífic wríter.

плодово́д *м.* frúit-grower, frúit-farmer. **~ство** *с.* frúit-growing, frúit-farming. **~ческий** frúit-growing *attr.*

плодо́в|ый fruit *attr.*; ~ые дере́вья frúit-trees; ~ сад órchard.

плодоконсéрвный: ~ завóд frúit-tínning fáctory, fruit cánnery.

плодоноси́ть *несов.* bear* fruit.

плодоно́сный frúit-béaring.

плодоово́щной gréengrocery *attr.*; frúit-and-végetable *attr.*

плодоро́д|ие *с.* fertílity. **~ный** fértile; **~ная** по́чва fértile soil.

плодотво́рн|о frúitfully, productívely. **~ый** frúitful; **~ая** рабо́та frúitful work.

пломб|á *ж.* 1. (*свинцовая*) (lead) seal; 2. (*зубная*) stópping, filling; постáвить серéбряную ~у stop/fill a tooth* with silver.

пломби́р *м.* cream ice.

пломбировáть, запломбировáть (*вн.*) 1. (*запечатывать*) seal (*smth.*), seal up (*smth.*); 2. (*зубы*) stop (*smth.*), fill (*smth.*).

пло́ск|ий 1. (*с ровной поверхностью*) flat; *мат.* plane; 2. (*неглубокий*) shállow, flat; ~ я́щик shállow box; 3. (*банальный*) féeble; ~ая шу́тка féeble/sílly joke; ◇ ~ая стопá flat foot.

плоского́рье *с.* pláteau, táble-land.

плоскогу́бцы *мн.* plíers.

плоскодо́н|ка *ж.* flat-bóttomed boat. **~ный** flat-bóttomed.

плоскосто́пие *с.* flat-fóotedness; у него́ ~ he is flat-fóoted.

пло́скост|ь *ж.* 1. flátness; 2. (*поверхность*) plane; 3. (*сфера каких-л. явлений, отношений*) sphere, plane; рассмотре́ть вопрóс в разли́чных ~áх examíne a próblem from várious ángles; 4. (*плоское замечание*) plátitude; говори́ть ~и platitúdinize.

плот *м.* raft.

плотвá *ж.* roach.

плоти́на *ж.* dam.

плóтни|к *м.* cárpenter. **~чать** *несов.* cárpenter, do* (a bit of) cárpentry.

плóтнич|ий, ~ный cárpenter's.

плóтн|о 1. clóse(ly), tíghtly; ~ облегáть (*о платье*) fit close (to), fit snúgly (on); ~ закры́ть дверь close the door fírmly; ~ прижа́ть(ся) к чему́-л. press close up to/agáinst smth.; 2. разг.: ~ пое́сть, пообе́дать и т. п. have* a héarty meal. ~ость ж. 1. solídity, hárdness; 2. (непроница́емость) dénsity; 3. (тка́ни) thíckness, clóseness of téxture; 4. (про́чность) strength; ◇ ~ость населе́ния dénsity of the populátion. ~ый 1. sólid, compáct, firm; 2. (густо́й, непроница́емый) dense, thick; ~ые слои́ атмосфе́ры dénser láyers of the átmosphere; 3. (о тка́ни) thick, clóse-wóven; 4. (кре́пкий, про́чный) thick, strong; ~ая бума́га strong páper; 5. (упи́танный, кре́пко сло́женный) thickset; 6. разг. (сы́тный) substántial, héarty; ~ый обе́д héarty dínner/meal.

плотоя́дный carnívorous; перен. sénsual, lascívious.

плот|ь ж. flesh; ◇ во ~и́ in the flesh; ~ и кровь чья́-л. one's own flesh and blood; войти́ в ~ и кровь incarnáte, embódy in flesh; обле́чься в ~ и кровь becóme* a reálity; обле́чь в ~ и кровь свою́ иде́ю embódy one's idéa.

пло́хо 1. нареч. bádly, not well; ~ себя́ чу́вствовать feel* unwéll; ~ себя́ вести́ beháve bádly; ~ обраща́ться с кем-л. treat smb. bádly; ill-tréat smb.; ~ отно́ситься к кому́-л. dislíke smb., ~ па́хнуть smell* bad*; ~ вы́глядеть look ill*/bad*; ~ ко́нчить come* to a bad end; ~ ко́нчиться end bádly; ~ знать язы́к not know the lánguage well, have* a poor commánd of the lánguage; 2. в знач. сказ. безл. that's bad; одно́ ~ there is ónly one thing wrong; с деньга́ми бы́ло ~ móney was short; 3. в знач. сказ. безл. (дт.; о тяжёлом состоя́нии): ему́ о́чень ~ he is véry ill; 4. в знач. сущ. с. нескл. (отме́тка) bad mark.

плох|о́й bad*, poor; ~ обе́д poor/tásteless meal, rótten dínner; ~а́я пого́да bad*/násty wéather; ~а́я па́мять poor mémory; ~ урожа́й poor hárvest; ~и́е ве́сти bad* news; ~ при́знак bad* sign; ~а́я привы́чка bad* hábit; ~о́е утеше́ние poor consolátion; ~ актёр bad* áctor; ~а́я репута́ция bad* name/reputátion; ~о́е настрое́ние low spírits pl; у него́ ~ хара́ктер he is a dífficult pérson (to get on with); пло́хо твоё де́ло! things look bad for you!; на него́ ~а́я наде́жда it's no good relýing on him; его́ дела́ пло́хи he's in a bad way; ◇ с ним шу́тки пло́хи he's not a man* to be trífled with, he's a tough cústomer.

площа́дка ж. 1. ground; те́ннисная ~ ténnis-court; 2. (ле́стничная) lánding; 3. (ваго́на) plátform.

пло́щадь ж. 1. (простра́нство; тж. мат.) área; ~ треуго́льника área of a tríangle; 2. (в го́роде и т. п.) square; база́рная ~ márket-place; 3. (помеще́ние) space/accommodátion; жила́я ~ líving space/accommodátion; ◇ производ́ственная ~ próductive área/space.

плуг м. plough; ◇ снегово́й ~ snow plough.

плут м. 1. cheat, swíndler; 2. разг. (хитре́ц) rogue.

плута́ть несов. разг. be* lost, stray, wánder.

плути́шка м. разг. líttle rogue/imp.

плутова́тый 1. cúnning, ártful; 2. (выража́ющий плутовство́) róguish.

плутова́ть, сплутова́ть разг. cheat, swíndle.

плуто́вка ж. cheat, swíndler; 2. разг. (лука́вая же́нщина) rogue.

плутов|ско́й 1. swíndling; ~ски́е приёмы únderhand méthods/tricks; 2. разг. (выража́ющий хи́трость) róguish; ~ско́е лицо́ róguish face. ~ство́ с. 1. (обма́н) tríckery; (в игре́) chéating; 2. разг. (хи́трость, лука́вство) ártfulness.

плыть несов. см. пла́вать; ~ по не́бу float/drift acróss the sky; ◇ ~ по тече́нию drift; ~ про́тив тече́ния go* against the stream, conténd with the tide.

плюга́вый разг. mean, shábby; úndersized.

плю́нуть сов. см. плева́ть.

плюс м. 1. plus; 2. разг. (преиму́щество) advántage.

плюх|а́ться, плю́хнуться разг. flop (down); плю́хнуться в кре́сло flop ínto a chair. ~нуться сов. см. плю́хаться.

плюш м. plush. ~евый plush attr.

плю́шка ж. bun.

плющ м. ívy.

пляж м. beach. ~ный beach attr.

пляс м. разг. dance; пуска́ться в ~ fling* onesélf into a dance.

пляса́ть, спляса́ть разг. dance, do* folk dáncing.

пля́с|ка ж. cóuntry/folk dance. ~ово́й прил. 1. cóuntry dáncing attr.; 2. в знач. сущ. ж. cóuntry dance (-tune). ~у́н м., ~у́нья ж. разг. (folk) dáncer.

пневма́т|ика ж. pneumátic tools/apparátus. ~и́ческий pneumátic.

пнуть сов. см. пина́ть.

по 1. (на пове́рхности) on, óver; (в преде́лах чего́-л.) through, abóut; (вдоль) alóng, down; идти́ по ковру́ walk on the cárpet; идти́ по у́лице walk down/alóng the street; ходи́ть по у́лицам walk the streets; ходи́ть по го́роду walk through the town; ходи́ть по ко́мнате walk abóut the room; pace up and down the room; броди́ть по све́ту wánder abóut the world; по́лзать по́ полу crawl abóut the floor; кни́ги разбро́саны по всему́ столу́ the books are scáttered all óver the táble; 2. (посре́дством чего́-л.) by, óver; по желе́зной доро́ге by rail; по во́здуху by air; по су́ше by land; по телефо́ну, ра́дио óver the télephone, the rádio; посла́ть что́-л. по по́чте send* smth. by post; 3. (согла́сно) accórding to, by; по пра́ву by right; по мои́м часа́м by my watch; по его́ жела́нию accórding to his wish; по прика́зу by órder (of); по ми́рному догово́ру únder the peace tréaty; по пла́ну accórding to plan; по со́бственному вы́бору of one's own choice; 4. (всле́дствие чего́-л.) due to, ówing to; по боле́зни due/ówing to íllness; по любви́ for love; по рассе́янности through ábsent-míndedness, in a móment of ábsent-míndedness; 5. (при обозначе́нии вре́мени) in, on; (в тече́ние) during; по воскресе́ньям on Súndays; по вечера́м in the évening; не писа́ть по меся́цам not write for months; 6. (в о́бласти чего́-л., в сфе́ре чего́-л.) in, on; специализи́роваться по фи́зике spécialize in phýsics; кни́га по матема́тике a book on mathemátics; рабо́тать по до́му do* hóusework; матч, встре́ча по те́ннису ténnis match; 7. (на основа́нии каки́х-л. при́знаков) by, in; дру́жеский по хара́ктеру kind by náture; сапо́жник по профе́ссии shóemaker by trade; челове́к по и́мени Алекса́ндр a man* by the name of Alexánder; крестья́нин по происхожде́нию a péasant by órigin; пе́рвый по величине́ first in size; отли́чный по ка́честву of éxcellent quálity; 8. (в сочета́нии с числи́тельными) in, by; по́ два in twos; по́ двое in twos, two by two, two and two; по́ три in/by threes; по де́сять in tens; 9. (ука́зывает на коли́чество чего́-л. при распределе́нии, обозначе́нии цены́ и т. п.): по десяти́ рубле́й шту́ка ten róubles each; дать де́тям по конфе́те give* the children a sweet each, give* each child* a sweet; 10. (вплоть до, up to, inclúsive; по по́яс up to the waist; с деся́того по двадца́тое ма́я from the tenth to the twéntieth of May inclúsive; 11. (по́сле чего́-л.) on; по прибы́тии on arríval; ◇ по мне as for me, as far as I am concérned.

по-англи́йски in Énglish; (в англи́йском сти́ле) in the Énglish way; говори́ть ~ speak* Énglish.

побагрове́ть сов. см. багрове́ть.

поба́иваться несов. (рд., + инф.) be* ráther afráid (of).

поба́ливать несов. разг. ache, hurt/ache a bit.

побе́г I м. (бе́гство) flight, escápe; соверши́ть ~ make* an/one's escápe.

побе́г II м. (росто́к) shoot, sprout.

побе́гать сов. run* a líttle, have* a run.

побегу́шк|и мн.: быть на ~ах у кого́-л. be* smb.'s érrand-boy; перен. тж. be* at smb.'s beck and call.

побе́да ж. víctory; (торжество тж.) tríumph.

победи́тель м., ~ница ж. cónqueror; (в состязаниях) winner, víctor.

победи́ть сов. см. побежда́ть.

побе́дн|ый 1. víctory attr.; ~ клич víctory cry; 2. (победоносный) tríumphant, victórious; ◇ до ~ого конца́ till final víctory.

победоно́сный victórious; перен. тж. tríumphant.

побежа́ть сов. run*, start rúnning, break* into a run.

побежда́ть, победи́ть 1. (наносить поражение) win*; (вн.) deféat (smb., smth.); победи́ть кого́-л. в бою́ deféat smb. in báttle; 2. (вн.; преодолевать) cónquer (smth.), overcóme* (smth.); 3. (в состязаниях) win*; победи́ть в бе́ге win* the rúnning events.

побеле́ть сов. см. беле́ть 1.

побели́ть сов. см. бели́ть 1.

побе́лка ж. whitewashing.

побере́жье с. coast, cóastline, séaboard, líttoral.

побере́чь сов. (вн.) 1. (сохранить) keep* (smth.); 2. (проявить заботливость) take* care (of). ~ся сов. take* care of onesélf.

побесе́довать сов. (с тв.) have* a talk (with).

побеспоко́ить сов. (вн.) distúrb (smb.). ~ся сов. см. беспоко́иться 2.

побира́ться несов. разг. beg, ask for alms.

поб|и́ть сов. (вн.) 1. см. бить 2; 2. (нанести поражение) beat* (smb., smth.), deféat (smb., smth.); 3. (убить всех, многих) kill (smb., smth.), sláughter (smb., smth.); 4. (повредить посевы и т. п.) beat* down (smth.), knock (smth.) flat; гра́дом ~и́ло хлеб the grain was béaten down by hail; 5. разг. (разбить всё, многое) smash (smth.); ~ всю посу́ду smash all the dishes; ◇ ~ реко́рд beat*/break* the récord. ~и́ться сов. 1. (оказаться повреждённым) be* bruised/dámaged; 2. разг. (о посуде) get* smashed/bróken.

поблагодари́ть сов. см. благодари́ть.

побла́жк|а ж. разг. allówance, indúlgence; дава́ть ~у кому́-л. show* indúlgence towárds smb.; без вся́ких побла́жек кому́-л. máking no allówances for smb., withóut any féather-bedding.

побледне́ть сов. см. бледне́ть.

поблёклый fáded.

поблёкнуть сов. см. блёкнуть.

вблизи́ close by; héreabouts; ~ от... close to...

побо́и мн. thráshing sg, béating sg; (удары) blows.

побо́ище с. 1. уст. (сражение) báttle, sláughter; 2. разг. (драка) brawl.

побо́рн|ик м., ~ица ж. chámpion.

поборо́ть сов. (вн.) 1. (одержать верх) beat* (smb.), deféat (smth.); (на войне тж.) cónquer (smth.); ~ проти́вника deféat/beat* one's ádversary; 2. (преодолеть, превозмочь что-л.) overcóme* (smth.), surmóunt (smth.), get* óver (smth.); ~ чу́вство стра́ха overcóme*/cónquer one's fear; ~ тоску́ overcóme* one's depréssion; ~ боле́знь fight* a diséase, get* the bétter of a diséase.

побо́ры мн. (ед. побо́р м.) exáctions, extórtions.

побо́чн|ый sécondary, subórdinate; side attr.; ~ые явле́ния side effécts; игра́ть ~ую роль play a subórdinate/mínor part; ~ проду́кт bý-product.

побоя́ться сов. (рд., + инф.) be* afráid (of, + to inf), not dare (+ to inf).

побра́таться сов. см. брата́ться.

побрати́м м. sworn friend/bróther; города́-~ы twín-cíties.

побре́згать сов. см. бре́згать.

побрести́ сов. wánder off, plod.

побри́ть сов. см. брить. ~ся сов. см. бри́ться.

поброди́ть сов. разг. (походить некоторое время) stroll, roam, wánder, rove; ~ по у́лицам roam (through)

the streets; ~ по го́роду roam through the town; ~ по све́ту wánder/rove abóut the world.

поброса́ть сов. (вн.) 1. (бросить в беспорядке) throw* down (smth.); 2. (оставить) abándon (smb., smth.).

побры́зг|ать сов. spray a little, sprínkle a little; дождь ~ал и переста́л there was ónly a sprínkle of rain. ~аться сов. splash one anóther.

побря́кивать несов. разг. ráttle.

побряку́шка ж. разг. (безделушка) trínket, báuble, géwgaw; (погремушка) ráttle.

побуди́ть сов. см. побужда́ть.

побужд|а́ть, побуди́ть (вн. к дт., вн. + инф.) prompt (smb. + to inf), indúce (smb. + to inf), impél (smb. + to inf). ~е́ние с. urge, mótive, stímulus (pl -li), indúcement.

побыв|а́ть сов. 1. be*; он ~а́л в И́ндии he has been to Índia; 2. разг. (посетить) look in, vísit.

побы́вк|а ж. разг. short stay/vísit; воен. short leave; он прие́хал на ~у he has come on a short stay/vísit.

побы́ть сов. stay (for a while); он побы́л у нас три дня he stayed with us for three days.

повад|иться сов. (+ инф.) разг. 1. get* ínto the hábit (of + -ing); 2. (часто ходить куда-л.) make* a hábit of góing/cóming. ~ка ж. разг. hábit, way; (потворство) chance, excúse.

пова́дно разг.: чтобы не́ было ~ кому́-л. to put smb. off, to break smb. of the hábit (of dóing smth.).

повали́ть I сов. см. вали́ть I 1.

повали́ть II сов. см. вали́ть II.

повали́ться сов. см. вали́ться.

пова́льн|ый géneral; mass attr.; ~ое увлече́ние чем-л. géneral/mass enthúsiasm for smth.; ~ о́быск géneral search.

поваля́ть сов. (вн.) roll (smth.); ~ в сухаря́х roll in bréadcrumbs. ~ся сов. 1. roll; ~ся в снегу́ roll in the snow; ~ся на траве́ lie* in/on the grass; 2. разг. (в постели) have* a lie-ín, stay in bed.

по́вар м. cook.

пова́ренн|ый cóokery attr., cooking attr.; ~ая кни́га cóokery book; ~ое иску́сство art of cóoking; cúlinary arts pl; ◇ ~ая соль cómmon/táble salt.

по́вар|иха ж. cook. ~ско́й cook's.

по-ва́шему 1. (по вашему мнению) to your mind, in your opínion; 2. (по вашему желанию) as you wish; пусть бу́дет ~ have it your way.

поведе́н|ие с. behaviour, cónduct; ли́ния ~ия line of cónduct. ~ческий behaviour attr., cónduct attr.; ~ческие стереоти́пы behaviour stereotypes.

повезти́ сов. см. везти́ 2.

повелев|а́ть несов. 1. (тв.; править) rule (smb.); 2. (дт. + инф.; приказывать) bid* (smb. + to inf); мой долг ~ мне сде́лать э́то I am in dúty bound to do it.

повели́тельн|ый imperative, peremptory, commánding; ~ го́лос commánding voice; ~ тон peremptory tone; ◇ ~ое наклоне́ние грам. imperative mood.

повенча́ть сов. см. венча́ть 1. ~ся сов. см. венча́ться.

пове́ренный м. 1. attórney; 2. cónfidant; ◇ ~ в дела́х дип. chargé d'afáires.

пове́р|ить сов. 1. (дт.) believe (smb., smth.); 2. см. поверя́ть. ~ка ж. 1. check, test; ~ка вре́мени time check; 2. (перекличка) róll-call; ◇ на ~ку when it came to the test/point.

поверну́ть(ся) сов. см. повёртывать(ся) и повора́чивать(ся).

поверте́ть сов. (вн.) turn (smth.); (тв.; повернуть несколько раз в разные стороны) turn (smth.) this way and that; ~ что-л. в рука́х fiddle with smth. ~ся сов. 1. turn, make* a few turns; (покружиться в танце) dance a little; 2. разг. (поворачиваться из стороны в сторону) turn this way and that; ~ся пе́ред зе́ркалом pose in front of the (lóoking-)glass; 3. *разг.* (*пробыть где-л.*) hang* abóut for a while.

повёртывать, повернуть 1. (*вн.*) turn (*smth.*) (*тж. перен.*); ~ ключ в замке́ turn the key in the lock; поверну́ть разгово́р change the súbject; 2. (*менять направление*) turn; ~ наза́д turn back; ~ напра́во turn right; доро́га кру́то поверну́ла нале́во the road turned shárply to the left. ~ся,. поверну́ться turn; *перен.* turn out; де́ло поверну́лось не так, как он предполага́л things did not turn out as he inténded; у меня́ язы́к не повернётся сказа́ть ему́ I can't bring mysélf to tell him.

пове́рх óver.

пове́рхностн|о superfícially. ~ый 1. (*лежащий на поверхности*) súrface *attr.*; ~ый слой по́чвы súrface-soil; ~ый сев súrface plánting; ~ая ра́на superfícial wound; 2. (*несерьёзный, неглубокий*) superfícial; (*о человеке тж.*) shállow, unpercéptive; ~ые зна́ния superfícial knówledge *sg.*

пове́рхност|ь *ж.* súrface; ~ земно́го ша́ра the earth's súrface; ◇ скользи́ть по ~и néver go* belów the súrface; всплы́ть на ~ come* to the súrface.

пове́рху *разг.* on the top; *перен.* on the súrface.

пове́рье *с.* pópular belíef; superstítion.

поверя́ть, пове́рить 1. (*вн. дт.; доверять*) confíde (*smth.* to); ~ та́йну кому́-л. confíde a sécret to *smb.*; 2. (*вн.; проверять*) check (*smth.*), test (*smth.*).

повеселе́ть *сов.* cheer up.

повесели́ться *сов.* enjóy onesélf, have* a good time.

по-весе́ннему as in spring; пого́да была́ ~ тёплая the wéather was warm and springlike.

пове́сить *сов. см.* ве́шать I. ~ся *сов. см.* ве́шаться.

повествова́|ние *с.* narrátion, nárrative. ~тельный nárrative.

повествова́ть *несов.* (*о пр.*) descríbe (*smth.*), tell* (of), reláte (*smth.*).

повести́ *сов.* 1. (*вн.*) lead* (*smb., smth.*), take* (*smb., smth.*); 2. *см.* поводи́ть II.

повести́сь *сов.* 1. (*войти в обычай*) becóme* the cústom; 2. (*с тв.*) *разг.* (*начать дружить*) make* friends (with); ◇ с кем поведёшься, от того́ и наберёшься *посл.* tell me whom you live with and I will tell you who you are.

пове́стк|а *ж.* nótice, notificátion; (*в суд*) súmmons, subpóena; (*в армию и т. п.*) cáll-up pápers *pl*; ◇ ~ дня agénda; на ~е дня on the agénda.

по́весть *ж.* tale, stóry, novélla.

пове́шен|ие *с.* (death by) hánging. ~ный *м.* the hanged man*, the hanged; ◇ в до́ме ~ного о верёвке не говоря́т ≈ name not a rope in the house of him that hanged himsélf.

пове́|ять *сов.* (*подуть*) begin to blow*; 2. *обыкн. безл.* (*тв.*): ~яло прохла́дой it becáme/grew a little cóoler; от реки́ ~яло прохла́дой cool air drífted up from the ríver.

повзросле́ть *сов.* matúre, becóme* matúre.

повида́ть *сов.* (*вн.*) *разг.* see* (*smb., smth.*); мно́го ~ на своём веку́ see* a lot in *one's* lifetime; ~ друзе́й see* *one's* friends. ~ся *сов.* (*с тв.*) *разг.* see* (*smb.*); see*/meet* each óther.

по-ви́димому appárently, évidently, próbably.

пови́дло *с.* jam.

пови́нн|ость *ж.* sérvice; *перен.* dúty, obligátion. ~ый guílty; ни в чём не ~ые лю́ди complétely ínnocent péople; он ни в чём не пови́нен he is perfectly ínnocent; ◇ прийти́ с ~ой (голово́й) confess *one's* guilt; (*явиться*) give* onesélf up; ~ую го́лову меч не сечёт *посл.* a fault conféssed is half redréssed.

повинова́|ться (*дт.*) obéy (*smb., smth.*); ~ распоряже́ниям obéy órders. ~ние *с.* obédience, submíssion.

повиса́ть, повиснуть 1. hang*, dángle, be* suspénded; (*на пр.; хвататься*) cling* (to); пови́снуть на ше́е у кого́-л. hang* on *smb's* neck, cling* to *smb.*; 2.

(*свешиваться*) droop; (*обвисать*) sag; 3. (*представляться взору неподвижным*) hóver, be* poised; ◇ пови́снуть в во́здухе remáin poised in mid-air; *перен.* be* all in the air as yet, be* hánging in the air.

повисе́ть *сов.* hang* for a while.

пови́снуть *сов. см.* повиса́ть.

повле́чь *сов.* cause (*smth.*), invólve (*smth.*), entáil (*smth.*); ~ за собо́й неприя́тности invólve/entáil tróuble; ~ за собо́й пожа́р cause a fire.

повлия́ть *сов. см.* влия́ть.

по́вод I *м.* (*у лошади*) brídle-rein; отда́ть пово́дья give* a horse the brídle, give* a horse its head; ◇ быть на ~у́ у кого́-л. be* únder *smb's* thumb.

по́вод II *м.* (*обстоятельство*) occásion, ground, réason; (*предлог*) prétext, excúse; без вся́кого ~a for no réason at all; for no éarthly réason *разг.*; по любо́му ~у at the slíghtest prétext; ◇ ~ к войне́ cásus bélli; дать ~ для ссо́ры give* rise to disséntion; по ~у чего́-л. with regárd to *smth.*, in connéction with *smth.*, ápropos of *smth.*; по э́тому ~у in this connéction.

поводи́ть I *сов.* 1. (*вн.; походить с кем-л.*) walk (*smb.*); ~ кого́-л. по ко́мнате walk *smb.* round the room; 2. (*тв. по дт.*) draw* (*smth.* óver), pass (*smth.* óver).

поводи́ть II, повести́ (*тв.*) move (*smth.*); ~ бровя́ми move *one's* éyebrows; ~ глаза́ми pass/cast* *one's* eyes (óver); ◇ он и бро́вью не повёл he didn't éven bat an éyelid.

поводо́к *м.* 1. rein; 2. (*для собак*) lead.

поводы́рь *м.* guíde.

пово́з|ить *сов.* (*вн.*) give* (*smb.*) a ride; (*в коляске, на машине*) take* (*smb.*) for a drive; (*вещи*) cart (*smth.*), do* some cárting. ~и́ться *сов.* 1. (*поворочаться*) stir réstlessly; 2. (*с тв.*) *разг.* (*потратить время на что-л.*) spend* time/éffort (on), have* tróuble (with); мне пришло́сь с ним мно́го ~и́ться he gave me a lot of tróuble, I had my hands full with him.

пово́зка *ж.* horse-drawn véhicle; wággon, cart.

поволнова́ться *сов.* be* wórried/unéasy.

повора́чивать(ся) *несов. см.* повёртывать(ся).

поворо́т *м.* 1. (*действие*) turn; 2. (*место*) turn, túrning; (*изгиб*) bend; пе́рвый ~ напра́во first túrning on the right; 3. (*изменение, перелом в чём-л.*) change, turn, túrning-point; круто́й ~ в поли́тике a rádical/sharp change in pólicy; ◇ ле́гче на ~ах! watch your step!

поворо́тлив|ость *ж.* 1. agílity, nímbleness; 2. (*о машинах, самолётах и т. п.*) manoeuvrabílity. ~ый 1. ágile, nímble, quick; 2. (*о машинах, самолётах*) manóeuvrable.

поворо́тн|ый 1. rotáting, túrning; swível *attr.*, swing *attr.*; ~ые механи́змы rotáting mechanisms; ~ круг túrn-table; 2. (*переломный*) túrning, crúcial; ~ пункт túrning-point.

поворча́ть *сов.* grúmble (a bit); (*о собаке*) give* a growl.

повреди́ть *сов. см.* поврежда́ть *и* вреди́ть.

поврежд|а́ть, повреди́ть 1. (*вн.; портить*) dámage (*smth.*), spoil* (*smth.*); повреди́ть замо́к dámage the lock; 2. (*вн.; ранить*) ínjure (*smth.*), hurt* (*smth.*); он повреди́л себе́ но́гу при паде́нии he hurt his foot* in fálling. ~е́ние *с.* 1. (*действие*) dámaging; 2. (*изъян, поломка и т. п. sg*) dámage (*mk. sg*); ~е́ние телефо́нного ка́беля fault in a télephone cáble.

повремени́ть *сов. разг.* 1. (*с тв., + инф.*) (*помедлить*) wait a bit (befóre + -ing); 2. (*подождать*) wait.

повремён|ный ~ая рабо́та time-work; ~ая опла́та páyment by the hour (day, week *etc.*).

повседне́вн|ый dáily, éveryday; ~ые ну́жды dáily needs; ~ая жизнь éveryday life.

повсеме́стн|о éverywhere. ~ый géneral; in all áreas *после сущ.*; ~ые за́морозки frosts in all áreas.

повста́н|ец *м.* insúrgent, rébel. ~ческий insúrgent; rébel *attr.*; ~ческая а́рмия insúrgent ármy.

повстречать *сов.* (*вн.*) *разг.* meet* (*smb.*), run* ínto (*smb.*). ~**ся** *сов.* (*дт.*, с *тв.*) *разг.* meet* (*smb.*).

повсюду éverywhere, far and wide.

повтор|éние *с.* repetítion; (*многократное*) reiterátion. ~**ить(ся)** *сов. см.* повторять(ся).

повторн|ый repéated, sécond; ~ анáлиз reanálysis; ~**ые** требования repéated requésts.

повторять, повторить (*вн.*) 1. repéat (*smth.*); (*многократно*) reíterate (*smth.*); ~ одно́ и тó же go* on repéating the same thing; 2. (*ранее заученное*) revíse (*smth.*), go* óver (*smth.*); 3. (*воспроизводить*) cópy (*smth.*). ~**ся**, повторúться 1. recúr, be* repéated; 2. (*о людях*) repéat onesélf; он нáчал ~**ся** he is repéating himsélf.

повысить(ся) *сов. см.* повышать(ся).

повышать, повысить (*вн.*) 1. (*делать более высоким*) raise (*smth.*); 2. (*увеличивать, усиливать*) raise (*smth.*), incréase (*smth.*); повысить продуктивность скотá make* cáttle/herds more prodúctive; повысить требовательность к своéй рабóте raise the stándard of one's work, adópt a more exácting áttitude to one's (own) work; повысить цены raise príces, put* príces up; ~ зарплáту raise/incréase wáges; 3. (*по службе*) promóte (*smb.*); повысить кого-л. в чúне promóte *smb.*; 4. (*усовершенствовать, улучшать*) impróve (*smth.*); ◇ повысить гóлос raise one's voice. ~**ся**, повыситься rise*; (*увеличиваться тж.*) incréase; у́ровень воды́ повы́сился the wáter has rísen; дохóды повысились íncome has incréased; повы́ситься в чьём-л. мнéнии rise* in *smb.'s* estéem; ~**ся** по слу́жбе be* promóted.

повышéние *с.* 1. (*действие*) rise; (*по службе*) promótion; ~ жизненного у́ровня rise/impróvement in the stándard of living; ~ зарплáты rise in wáges; ~ квалификáции impróvement of one's qualificátions; 2. (*высокое место*) elevátion.

повы́шенн|ый: ~**ая** температýра (slight) témperature; ~**ые** цены incréased príces; ~**ые** требования incréased demánds/requírements; ~ интерéс к *чему-л.* héightened/incréased ínterest in *smth.*; говорúть в ~**ом** тóне raise one's voice, talk lóud(ly).

повязать(ся) *сов. см.* повязывать(ся).

повязка *ж.* 1. (*бинт*) bándage; 2. (*нарукавная*) ármlet, ármband; (*на голову*) héadband, fíllet.

повязывать, повязать (*вн.*) tie (*smth.*); ~ гáлстук tie one's nécktie; ~ гóлову cóver one's head. ~**ся**, повязáться (*тв.*) put* (*smth.*) on, tie (*smth.*) on; ~**ся** платкóм put* on one's kérchief.

погадáть *сов. см.* гадáть 1.

поганка *ж.* (*гриб*) tóadstool.

погáн|ый 1. (*о грибах*) póisonous; 2. *разг.* (*предназначенный для отбросов*) slop *attr.*, rúbbish *attr.*; ~**ое** ведрó slop pail; 3. *разг.* (*неприятный*) foul, násty; rótten; ~ вкус во рту́ a bad/rótten taste in the mouth.

погасáть, погаснуть 1. go*/burn* out; (*о глазах, взоре*) fade, grow* dim; 2. (*о чувствах и т. п.*) die, fade; 3. (*чахнуть*) die, fade awáy.

погасúть *сов. см.* погашáть *и* гасúть.

погаснуть *сов. см.* гáснуть *и* погасáть.

погаш|áть, погасúть (*вн.*) (*долги*) líquidate (*smth.*), redéem (*smth.*), pay* off (*smth.*); (*марки*) cáncel (*smth.*). ~**éние** *с.* (*долгов*) liquidátion, redémption, páying off; (*марок*) cancellátion; тирáж ~**éния** final draw.

погáшенн|ый cáncelled; ~**ые** мáрки used stamps.

погектáрный per-héctare *attr.*

погибáть, погúбнуть be* lost, pérish; (*о людях тж.*) be* killed; погúбнуть на войнé be* killed in the war.

погúбель I *ж. уст.* death, ruin, doom.

погúбел|ь II *ж.*: согну́ться в три ~**и** bend* dóuble; согну́ть кого-л. в три ~**и** get* *smb.* únder one's thumb.

погúб|нуть *сов. см.* погибáть *и* гúбнуть. ~**ший** ruined, lost.

погладить *сов. см.* глáдить 2.

поглáживать *несов.* (*вн.*) stroke (*smth.*, *smth.*).

поглотúть *сов. см.* поглощáть.

поглощ|áть, поглотúть (*вн.*) 1. absórb (*smth.*), soak up (*smth.*); *перен.* (*усваивать многое*) absórb (*smth.*); он ~**áет** кнúгу за кнúгой he devóurs book áfter book; 2. (*скрывать в своих недрах*) swállow up (*smb.*, *smth.*); 3. (*всецело захватывать*) absórb (*smb.*), engróss (*smb.*); он весь поглощён наýкой he is complétely engróssed/absórbed in science; 4. (*требовать много затрат, времени и т. п.*) use up (*smth.*), consúme (*smth.*); печь ~**áет** мнóго тóплива the stove eats up fuel; рабóта ~**áет** у негó мнóго врéмени his work takes up much of his time. ~**éние** *с.* absórption. ~**ённый** absórbed, engróssed.

поглупéть *сов. см.* глупéть.

поглядéть *сов. см.* глядéть 1, 2. ~**ся** *сов. см.* глядéться.

погля́дывать *несов.* 1. (*на вн.*) cast* a glance (at), look (at); 2. (*за тв.*) *разг.* (*присматривать*) look* (áfter), keep* an eye (on).

погнáть *сов.* (*вн.*) 1. (*заставить двигаться*) drive* (*smth.*); set*/get* *smth.* móving; ~ стáдо в пóле drive* the cáttle to pásture; 2. (*лошадь*) whip up (*smth.*); ~ лóшадь вскачь put* a horse ínto a gállop. ~**ся** *сов.* (*за тв.*) run* (áfter), pursúe (*smb.*, *smth.*), chase (*smb.*, *smth.*); ◇ ~**ся** за двумя́ зáйцами try to do two things at once.

погнúть *сов. разг.* rot, decáy.

погну́ть *сов.* (*вн.*) bend* (*smth.*). ~**ся** *сов.* be* bent.

погова́рив|ать *несов.* (о *пр.*) *разг.* talk (of); ~**ают** о егó возвращéнии there is some talk of his retúrning.

поговор|úть *сов.* 1. talk; он любит ~ he loves to talk; 2. (о *пр.*; *обсудить*) talk óver (*smth.*), discúss (*smth.*); мы ~**úли** о вáшем дéле we have discússed your case.

поговóрка *ж.* provérbial phrase, sáying.

погóда *ж.* wéather.

погод|úть *сов. разг.* wait; ~**úте!** you wait!; ◇ немнóго ~**я́** a líttle láter (on).

погóжий fine; ~ день a fine day.

поголóвн|ый (*о ком-л.*) to a man. ~**ый** géneral.

поголóвье *с.* tótal númber; кóнское ~ tótal stock/númber of hórses; ~ крýпного рогáтого скотá tótal númber/head of cáttle; ~ скотá и птúцы the cáttle and póultry populátion.

погóн *м.* shóulder-strap.

погóнщик *м.* dríver; (*скота*) dróver.

погóн|я *ж.* 1. (*действие*) pursúit; chase; 2. (*группа преследующих*) pursúers *pl*; 3. (*за тв.*; *усиленное стремление к чему-л.*) pursúit of; в ~**е** за счáстьем in pursúit of háppiness.

погоня́ть *несов.* (*вн.*) whip up (*smth.*); *перен.* urge on (*smb.*); ~ лошадéй кнутóм whip up the hórses.

погорéлец *м.* hómeless fire víctim.

погорéть *сов.* lose* éverything in a fire; (*о здании и вещах*) be* burnt; *перен. разг.* slip up.

погорячи́ться *сов.* lose* one's témper, get* excíted.

погóст *м.* víllage/cóuntry chúrchyard.

погостúть *сов.* be* on a short vísit.

погранзастáва *ж.* (*пограничная застава*) fróntier post.

погранúчн|ик *м.* bórder/fróntier-guard. ~**ый** bórder *attr.*, fróntier *attr.*; ~**ый** райóн fróntier área; ~**ый** столб fróntier post; ~**ые** войскá bórder/fróntier troops.

пóгреб *м.* céllar; пороховóй ~ pówder-magazine; *перен.* gúnpowder.

погреб|áльный fúneral; ~ звон tólling of the fúneral bell. ~**áть**, погрестú (*вн.*) búry (*smth.*). ~**éние** *с.* búrial.

погремýшка *ж.* ráttle.

погрестú *сов. см.* погребáть.

погрéть *сов.* (*вн.*) warm (*smth.*) for a while, give* (*smth.*) a wárming; (*о солнце*) be* warm for a while. ~ся *сов.* warm oneself for a while, get* warm (for a bit).

погрешить *сов. см.* грешить 2.

погрешность|ь *ж.* érror; ~и в вычислéнии érrors of calculátion; ~и в мотóре deféects in an éngine.

погрозить *сов. см.* грозить 2.

погром *м.* mássacre, pógrom. ~ный 1. (*призывающий к погрому*) rábble-róusing *attr.*; 2. *разг.* (*содержащий резкие выпады*) dévastating, sláshing; ~ная статья dévastating árticle. ~щик *м.* pógrom-maker, thug.

погруж|áть, погрузить (*вн. в вн.*) dip (*smth.* into), immérse (*smth.* in); plunge (*smb., smth.* into) (*тж. перен.*). ~áться, погрузиться sink*, plunge; be* immérsed (*тж. перен.*); (*о подводной лодке*) submérge; dive; ~áться в рабóту, размышлéния be* deep/immérsed in *one's* work, thought; ~áться в чтéние be* immérsed in *one's* réading; ~áться в глубóкий сон sink* into a deep sleep. ~éние *с.* immérsion, dípping; (*подводной лодки*) submérgence.

погрузить *сов. см.* погружáть *и* грузить 2. ~ся *сов. см.* погружáться *и* грузиться.

погрузка *ж.* lóading.

погрузочно-разгрузочн|ый: ~ые рабóты lóading and unlóading operátions.

погрузочный lóading *attr.*

погрузчик *м.* mechánical lóader.

погряз|áть, погрязнуть (*в пр.*) stick* (in); *перен.* be* steeped (in), wállow (in); погрязнуть в невéжестве be* steeped in ígnorance; погрязнуть в разврáте wállow in vice; погрязнуть в долгáх be* up to the eyes/ears in debt.

погрязнуть *сов. см.* погрязáть.

погубить *сов. см.* губить.

погуливать *несов.* 1. stroll; 2. (*веселиться*) go* on the spree now and then.

погулять *сов.* go* for a stroll/walk.

под, подо 1. (*ниже чего-л.*) únder, underneáth; стоя́ть под дéревом stand* únder a tree; постáвить чемодáн под кровáть put* a case únder a bed; под водóй únder wáter; рабóтать под землёй work undergróund; пóд гóру downhíll; 2. (*около, в непосрéдственной блúзости*) near, close to; жить под Москвóй live near Móscow; бúтва под Полтáвой the Báttle of/at Poltáva. 3. (*в зóне дéйствия чего-л.*) únder; под огнём протúвника únder énemy fire; гулять под дождём walk in the rain; 4. (*указывает на состояние, положéние*) únder; под рукóводством únder the léadership of, под наблюдéнием врачá únder the dóctor; под комáндой кого-л. únder (the) commánd of *smb.*; под замкóм únder lock and key; заключáть под стрáжу put* únder arrést, take* into cústody; быть под угрóзой be* únder (a) threat; взять под свою защúту take* únder *one's* protéction; под влия́нием under the ínfluence; отдáть кого-л. под суд bring* *smb.* to tríal, put* *smb.* on tríal; 5. (*для какой-л. цéли*) for, as; э́тот сарáй зáнят под сéно this barn is for hay; 6. (*о врéмени*) towárds; (*о вóзрасте тж.*) close on; (*накануне*) on the eve of; под вéчер towárds évening; в ночь под Нóвый год on Néw-Year's Eve; емý под шестьдесят he is close on síxty, he is néarly síxty, he is not far off síxty; 7. (*похóжий на*) in imitátion of; под крáсное дéрево in imitátion of mahógany; 8. (*в обмен на какое-л. ручáтельство*) on; под залóг on secúrity; под распúску gíving a recéipt; получúть что-л. под чéстное слóво take* *smth.* on *one's* word of hónour (to retúrn it); 9. (*в сопровождéнии чего-л. звучáщего*) with, to; под аккомпанемéнт роя́ля with a piáno accómpaniment; танцевáть под мýзыку dance to the músic; 10. (*при налúчии прúзнака, свóйства*) with; дом под желéзной крышей house with an iron roof; 11. (*при указáнии прúзнака, выделяющего лицó, предмéт, понятие*) únder, by; писáть под псевдонúмом write* únder an assúmed name.

подавáльщица *ж.* wáitress.

подавáть, подáть 1. (*вн. дт.*) give* (*smb. smth.*); подáть кому-л. портфéль hand *smb.* his bríefcase; подáть кому-л. стул give*/bring* *smb.* a chair; ~ кому-л. пальтó help *smb.* on with his, her coat; 2. (*вн.; стáвить на стол*) serve (*smth.*); ~ обéд serve dínner; кóфе был пóдан в кабинéт cóffee was served in the stúdy; 3. (*давáть мúлостыню*) give* alms; подáть нúщему give* alms to a béggar; 4. (*вн.; подводить для посáдки, погрýзки*) drive* (*smth.*) up; машúну пóдали к подъéзду the car was sent up to the door; пóезд пóдан на трéтью платфóрму the train comes in at plátform three; 5. (*вн.; в пúсьменном вúде*) make* (*smth.*), file (*smth.*); ~ заявлéние file an applicátion; ~ жáлобу на кого-л. make*/lodge a compláint agáinst *smb.*; ~ на кого-л. bring* an áction agáinst *smb.*; 6. (*вн.*) *спорт.* serve (*smth.*); ~ мяч serve (the ball); ◇ подáть совéт give* advíce; подáть пóмощь rénder assístance; подáть гóлос 1) make* *one's* présence known; 2) (*за вн.; проголосовáть*) vote (for); ~ знак make* a sign, give* a sígnal; подáть мысль suggést an idéa; подáть примéр give*/set* an exámple; ~ рýку кому-л. 1) (*протя́гивать*) hold* out *one's* hand to *smb.*; 2) (*чтобы вести под рýку*) óffer *one's* arm to *smb.*; подáть друг дрýгу рýку shake* hands; подáть рýку пóмощи кому-л. give* *smb.* a hélping hand; ~ прúзнаки жúзни show* signs of life. ~ся, подáться yield (*тж. перен.*); (*изменять положéние*) move, shift; lean*; дверь подалáсь под напóром door yíelded to a push; толпá подалáсь назáд the crowd fell back; ~ся тýловищем назáд lean* back; ◇ подáться нéкуда there is no way out.

подавúть *сов. см.* подавля́ть.

подавúться *сов.* choke; ~ кóстью get* a bone in *one's* throat.

подавлéние *с.* suppréssion.

подавлéни|ость *ж.* depréssion, despóndency. ~ый 1. (*угнетённый, мрáчный*) depréssed, despóndent; ~ое настроéние low spírits *pl*, dejéction; 2. (*приглушённый*) suppréssed.

подавл|я́ть, подавúть 1. (*вн.; сúлой прекращáть что-л.*) suppréss (*smth.*), put* down (*smth.*), quell (*smth.*); *перен.* suppréss (*smth.*); подавúть мятéж put* down a rebéllion; подавúть улыбку suppréss/hide* a smile; 2. (*вн.; получáть перевéс над кем-л., чем-л.*) overpówer (*smb., smth.*), overwhélm (*smb., smth.*); 3. (*вн. тв.; производúть сúльное впечатлéние*) overáwe (*smb.* with, by), overpówer (*smb.* with); ~ свойм авторитéтом overáwe with *one's* authórity; 4. (*вн.; приводúть в угнетённое состояние*) depréss (*smb.*). ~я́ющий 1. (*превосходя́щий*) overwhélming; ~я́ющим большинствóм голосóв by an overwhélming majórity; 2. (*гнетýщий*) depréssing.

подáвно *разг.* all the more, so much the more.

подáгр|а *ж.* gout. ~úческий góuty; ~úческая боль góuty pain.

подáльше *разг.* a little fúrther (awáy).

подарúть *сов. см.* дарúть.

подáрок *м.* présent; gift; сдéлать ~ кому-л. give*/make* *smb.* a présent.

подáтель *м.*, ~ница *ж.* (*письмá*) béarer; (*заявлéния*) petútioner.

подáтлив|ость *ж.* 1. málleableness, sóftness; (*воздéйствию*) plíancy; 2. (*устýпчивость, сговóрчивость*) plíancy, compláisance. ~ый 1. málleable, soft; (*легко поддающийся воздéйствию*) plíable, plíant; 2. (*устýпчивый, сговóрчивый*) plíable, compláisant; ~ый харáктер plíant cháracter.

подáть *ж. ист.* tax, dúty.

подáть(ся) *сов. см.* подавáть(ся).

подáч|а *ж.* 1. (*дéйствие*) ~ заявлéния presénting of an applicátion; ~ вагóнов márshalling of trucks; ~ тóплива fuel supplý; 2. *спорт.* sérvice, serve.

подáчка *ж. разг.* scrap; sop (*тж. перен.*).

подая́ние *с.* alms; проси́ть ~ ask for alms.

подба́вить *сов. см.* подбавля́ть.

подбавля́ть, подба́вить (*вн., рд.*) add (*smth.*); подба́вить са́хару в чай put* some more súgar in *one's* tea.

подба́дривать, подбодри́ть (*вн.*) cheer up (*smb.*). ~ся, подбодри́ться cheer up, feel* more chéerful.

подбега́ть, подбежа́ть come* rúnning up, run* up.

подбежа́ть *сов. см.* подбега́ть.

подберёзовик *м.* (*гриб*) brówn-cap bolétus.

подбива́ть, подби́ть 1. (*вн.; прибивать подмётку и т. п.*) nail (*smth.*) on, fix (*smth.*) on; подби́ть каблуки́ tip the heels; 2. (*вн. тв.*) *разг.* (*подшивать с изнанки*) line (*smth.* with); ~ шу́бу ме́хом line a coat with fur; 3. (*вн. на, вн. + инф.*) *разг.* (*подстрекать*) egg (*smb.*) on (+ to *inf*), incite (*smb.* + to *inf*); 4. (*вн.*) *разг.* (*сбивать ударом снизу*) trip (*smb.*) (up), knock (*smth.*) óver; (*повреждать*) dámage (*smth.*); подби́ть глаз кому́-л. give* *smb.* a black eye, black *smb.'s* eye; подби́ть танк crípple/dámage a tank; подби́ть у́тку wing a duck.

подбира́ть, подобра́ть (*вн.*) 1. (*поднимать*) pick up (*smb., smth.*), gáther (*smth.*); ~ ра́неных с по́ля сраже́ния bring* in the wóunded (from the báttle-field); ~ ко́лосья glean; 2. (*выбирать, отбирать*) choose* (*smb., smth.*), seléct (*smb., smth.*); ~ ключ к замку́ find* a key to fit the lock; ~ люде́й seléct/choose* péople; ~ кни́ги collect books; ~ недоста́ющие номера́ журна́ла make* up the missing númbers of a magazine; ~ цвета́ match cólours; ~ себе́ костю́м choose* onesélf a suit; 3. (*убирать, прятать подо что-л.*) tuck up (*smth.*), do* up (*smth.*); (*поджимать*) purse (*smth.*), pull in (*smth.*), (*делать туже*) tíghten (*smth.*); ~ подо́л ю́бки tuck up *one's* skirt; ~ гу́бы purse *one's* lips. ~ся, подобра́ться 1. (*составляться*) be* selécted; подобра́лась хоро́шая компа́ния the cómpany was well selécted; 2. *разг.* (*подкрадываться*) steal* up; 3. *разг.* (*принимать более строгий вид*) brace onesélf, draw* onesélf up.

подби́ть *сов. см.* подбива́ть.

подбодри́ть(ся) *сов. см.* подба́дривать(ся).

подбодря́ть(ся) *см.* подба́дривать(ся).

подбо́р *м.* seléction; (*сочетание*) combinátion; ~ книг seléction of books; ~ ка́дров seléction of personnél; ◇ как на ~ choice *attr.*; well-mátched; (*о людях*) to a man; гру́ши как на ~ choice pears; брига́да вся как на ~ the team is the pick of the bunch; в ~ *полигр.* run on.

подбо́рка *ж.* 1. (*действие*) seléction; 2. (*в газете*) box, séction.

подборо́док *м.* chin.

подбоче́ниться *сов. разг.*: стоя́ть подбоче́нившись stand* with *one's* hands on *one's* hips.

подбра́сыв|ать, подбро́сить 1. (*вн.; кидать вверх*) throw* (*smb., smth.*) up, toss (*smb., smth.*) (up); ~ мяч toss a ball into the air; 2. *обыкн. безл.* (*сильно трясти во время движения*) jolt, shake*; маши́ну си́льно ~ало the car jólted víolently; 3. (*вн., рд.; добавлять*) add (*smth.*); ~ дров в пе́чку put* some more wood in the stove; 4. (*тайком подкладывать, подкидывать*) plant (*smth.*); (*ребёнка*) abándon (*smb.*); ~ докуме́нты plant dócuments (on).

подбро́сить *сов. см.* подбра́сывать.

подва́л *м.* 1. básement; (*погреб*) céllar; 2. (*в газете*) lówer half of the page; (*статья*) árticle cóvering the whole lówer half of the page.

подва́льный básement *attr.*; ~ эта́ж básement (floor).

подвезти́ *сов. см.* подвози́ть.

подверга́ть, подве́ргнуть (*вн. дт.*) subject (*smb., smth.* to); ~ что-л. кри́тике críticize *smth.*, subject *smth.* to críticism; ~ что-л. обсужде́нию discúss *smth.*; ~ кого́-л. наказа́нию inflict a púnishment on *smb.*; ~ кого́-л. опа́сности expóse *smb.* to dánger; ~ что-л. сомне́нию call/bring* *smth.* in quéstion. ~ся, подве́ргнуться (*дт.*) be* subjécted (to), be* expósed (to); ~ся обсужде́нию be* discússed; подве́ргнуться (серьёзной) кри́тике be*

(sevérely) críticized; ~ся опа́сности be* expósed to dánger; ~ся опера́ции undergó* an operátion.

подве́р|гнуть(ся) *сов. см.* подверга́ть(ся). ~женный (*дт.*) súbject (to), líable (to), prone (to); ~женный ревмати́зму líable/prone to rhéumatism; он ~жен просту́де he cátches cold éasily.

подверну́ть(ся) *сов. см.* подвёртывать(ся).

подвёртывать, подверну́ть (*вн.*) 1. (*завинчивать*) screw (*smth.*); ~ га́йку screw (up) a nut; 2. (*засучивать*) turn up (*smth.*), roll up (*smth.*); ~ брю́ки roll up *one's* тро́users; 3. (*подгибать края*) tuck in (*smth.*); ~ одея́ло tuck in the blánket; 4. (*повреждать*) sprain (*smth.*), twist (*smth.*); подверну́ть себе́ но́гу sprain/twist *one's* ankle. ~ся, подверну́ться 1. (*о рукавах, брюках*) be* rolled up; 2. (*о ноге*) get* twisted; 3. *разг.* (*случайно попадаться на глаза*) turn up.

подве́с|ить *сов. см.* подве́шивать. ~ка *ж.* 1. (*действие*) hánging, hánging up; 2. (*устройство для подвешивания*) brácket; (*автомашины*) suspénsion; (*украшение*) péndant. ~но́й 1. (*висящий*) hánging, suspénded; ~на́я ко́йка hámmock; 2. (*устроенный для передвижения*) suspénsion *attr.*, óverhead; ~но́й мост suspénsion bridge; ~но́й конве́йер óverhead convéyor; ~на́я доро́га óverhead trólley, cábleway.

подвести́ *сов. см.* подводи́ть.

подве́тренн|ый lee *attr.*; léeward; ~ая сторона́ lee side.

подве́шивать, подве́сить (*вн.*) suspénd (*smth.*), hang* (*smth.*); подве́сить ла́мпу к потолку́ hang* a lamp from the céiling.

по́двиг *м.* feat, achíevement; (*связанный с большим риском*) éxploit; трудово́й ~ feat of lábour; геройче́ский ~ heróic deed; боево́й ~ feat of arms.

подвига́ть, подви́нуть (*вн.*) 1. (*перемещать*) move (*smth.*); подви́ньте стул move up your chair; 2. *разг.* (*содействовать развитию чего-л.*) advánce (*smth.*), make* prógress (in); make* héadway (in); подви́нуть свою́ рабо́ту make* prógress in *one's* work. ~ся, подви́нуться 1. (*перемещаться*) move; 2. (*двигаться вперёд в каком-л. отношении*) advánce, make* prógress; перегово́ры подви́нулись вперёд the negotiátions have made some prógress.

подви́д *м. биол.* súbspecies.

подви́жн|ик *м.*, ~ица *ж. церк.* ascétic, hérmit; *перен.* enthúsiast. ~ический self-sácrificing. ~ичество *с.* héroism, self-sácrifice.

подвижн|о́й (*двигающийся*) trávelling, móbile; ~ госпиталь móbile hóspital; ◇ ~ые и́гры óutdoor games.

подвижн|ость *ж.* 1. mobílity; ~ лица́ fácial mobílity; 2. (*о человеке*) líveliness; отлича́ться ~остью be* véry energétic/lívely. ~ый (*отличающийся живостью*) lívely, quick; ~ый ребёнок lívely child*; ~ое лицо́ móbile féatures *pl*; ~ый ум quick/nímble mind.

подвинти́ть *сов. см.* подви́нчивать.

подви́нуть(ся) *сов. см.* подвига́ть(ся).

подви́нчивать, подвинти́ть 1. (*вн.*) tíghten up (*smth.*); 2. (*вн. к дт.; привинчивать*) screw (*smth.* on).

подвла́стный (*дт.*) depéndent (on), in the pówer (of).

подво́да *ж.* cart, dray.

подводи́ть, подвести́ (*вн.*) 1. (*приближать*) lead* (*smb., smth.*); (*доставлять*) bring* up (*smb., smth.*); ему́ подвели́ друго́го коня́ they brought him anóther horse; подвести́ резе́рвы bring* up *one's* resérves; 2. (*доводить до какого-л. места*) exténd (*smth.*), take* (*smth.*) as far as; ~ доро́гу к бе́регу exténd the road to the shore; 3. (*подкладывать подо что-л., устраивать под чем-л.*) put* (*smth.*); *перен.* furnish (*smth.*); ~ фунда́мент под зда́ние underpin a búilding; ~ ми́ну под укрепле́ния (under)mine fortificátions; 4. *разг.* (*ставить в затрудни́тельное положе́ние*) let* (*smth.*) down; ◇

подвести черту под *чем-л.* round off *smth.*; подвести часы́ álter *one's* watch; ~ ито́ги sum up; живо́т подвело́ feel* émpty, feel* hóllow inside.

подво́дн|ик *м.* 1. súbmariner; 2. (*водолаз*) díver. ~ый súbmarine; ~ая ло́дка súbmarine; ~ые расте́ния súbmarine plants; ~ое тече́ние úndercurrent; ◇ ~ый ка́мень snag, hídden reef/rock.

подвоз *м.* supplý, delívery. ~и́ть, подвезти́ 1. (*вн.*; *привозить куда-л.*) take* (*smb., smth.*); (*попутно*) give* (*smb.*) a lift; подвезти́ *кого-л.* до дере́вни take* *smb.* to the víllage; мы тебя́ подвезём we'll give you a lift; 2. (*вн., рд.*; *доставлять, снабжать*) bring* in (*smth.*), delíver (*smth.*); (*дополнительно*) supplý éxtra (*smth.*); подвезти́ дров bring* in wood.

подворотничо́к *м.* ínside cóllar (*sewn in under the collar of a tunic*).

подворо́тня *ж.* 1. (*щель*) space únder a gate; 2. (*доска*) únderboard (of a gate); 3. (*проём в стене дома*) gáteway.

подво́х *м. разг.* trick.

подвяза́ть(ся) *сов. см.* подвя́зывать(ся).

подвя́зка *ж.* 1. (*действие*) týing up; 2. (*резинка*) gárter (*женская*); suspénder (*мужская*).

подвя́зывать, подвяза́ть (*вн.*) tie (*smth.*); (*повязывать*) tie up (*smth.*). ~ся, подвяза́ться tie *smth.* round one.

подгиба́ть, подогну́ть (*вн.*) 1. (*загибать края чего--л.*) turn (*smth.*) up; 2. (*сгибать*) tuck (*smth.*) únder; (*слегка сгибать в коленях*) bend* (*smth.*); подогну́ть под себя́ но́ги tuck *one's* legs únder one. ~ся, подогну́ться 1. be* tucked in; 2.: у него́ но́ги подогну́лись his legs are gíving way.

подгляде́ть *сов.* 1. *см.* подгля́дывать; 2. (*вн.*; *случайно заметить*) nótice (*smth.*), spot (*smth.*).

подгля́дывать, подгляде́ть peep at; ~ в замо́чную сква́жину peep through the kéyhole; ~ за *кем-л.* spy on *smb.*

подгова́ривать, подговори́ть (*вн. на вн., вн. + инф.*) instigate (*smb.* + to *inf*), indúce (*smb.* + to *inf*), put* (*smb.*) up to (*smth.*).

подговори́ть *сов. см.* подгова́ривать.

подголо́сок *м.* suppórting/sécond voice; *перен. презр.* yés-man*.

подгоня́ть, подогна́ть (*вн.*) 1. (*пригонять*) drive* (*smth.*); подогна́ть плот к бе́регу steer a raft to the bank; 2. (*торопить*) urge (*smb., smth.*) on, drive* (*smb., smth.*) on; ~ ло́шадь urge a horse fórward; 3. (*прилаживать*) adjúst (*smth.*), fit (*smth.*), make* (*smth.*) fit; ~ ключ к замку́ make* the key fit the lock.

подгор|а́ть, подгоре́ть 1. (*о пище*) get* burnt; 2. (*гореть у основания*) burn* through (underneáth). ~е́лый burnt.

подгоре́ть *сов. см.* подгора́ть.

подгота́вливать, подгото́вить (*вн.*) prepáre (*smb., smth.*), get*/make* (*smb.*) réady; (*обучать*) train (*smth.*); ~ по́чву для перегово́ров prepáre the way for negotiátions; ~ *кого-л.* к экза́мену prepáre *smb.* for an examinátion; ~ враче́й train dóctors; ~ сце́ну для спекта́кля get* the stage réady for the perfórmance. ~ся, подгото́виться (к *дт.*) prepáre (for), make* onesélf réady (for).

подготови́тельн|ый prepáratory; ~ пери́од prepáratory périod; ~ая рабо́та spade work; ~ая ста́дия prelíminary stage; ~ые мероприя́тия prelíminaries; ~ые ку́рсы prelíminary cóurse(s).

подгото́в|ить(ся) *сов. см.* подгота́вливать(ся). ~ка *ж.* 1. preparátion; (*обучение*) tráining; вое́нная ~ка mílitary tráining; ~ка ка́дров tráining of spécialists; без ~ки (*экспромтом*) withóut preparátion, extémpore; 2. (*запас знаний*) schóoling, educátion, gróunding; у него́ хоро́шая ~ка he has a good gróunding; у него́ сла́бая

~ка he lacks tráining; ◇ артиллери́йская ~ка preparátion fire, sóftening-up.

подгото́вленн|ость *ж.* (degrée of) tráining; всё зави́сит от ~ости на́ших ка́дров éverything depénds on how well our personnél are trained. ~ый prepáred.

подготовля́ть(ся) *несов. см.* подгота́вливать(ся).

подгру́ппа *ж.* súbgroup.

подгу́зник *м.* náppy; díaper *амер.*

поддава́ть, подда́ть 1. (*вн. тв.*; *подбрасывать ударом, снизу*) knock (*smth.*) up; ~ мяч раке́ткой lob the ball, play a lób-shot; подда́ть мяч ного́й kick the ball in the air, punt the ball; 2. (*вн.*) *разг.* (*шашку, карту и т. п.*) give* (*smth.*) awáy; ◇ подда́ть жа́ру, па́ру *разг.* put* on steam. ~ся, подда́ться (*дт.*) 1. give* way (to), yield (to); ~ся де́йствию огня́ yield to the flames, catch* fire; подда́ться искуше́нию give* way to temptátion; он легко́ поддаётся угово́рам he is éasily persuáded; мы не поддаёмся угро́зам we do not surrénder to threats; 2. *тк. несов.* respónd (to); материа́л поддаётся обрабо́тке the matérial is good to work on; ◇ не ~ся описа́нию defý/béggar descríption; не ~ся никако́му сравне́нию defý (all) compárison.

подда́кивать, подда́кнуть (*дт.*) *разг.* signify assént (to), écho (*smb.*); *перен.* play up to (*smb.*).

подда́кнуть *сов. см.* подда́кивать.

по́ддан|ная *ж.*, ~ный *м.* súbject, cítizen; англи́йский ~ный British súbject. ~ство *с.* cítizenship; приня́ть ~ство take* out cítizenship.

подда́ть *сов. см.* поддава́ть. ~ся *сов. см.* поддава́ться 1.

поддева́ть, подде́ть (*вн.*) 1. léver (*smth.*) up; 2. *разг.* (*говорить колкости*) bait, tease, have* a dig (at); ло́вко я его́ подде́л I got in a nice dig at him.

подде́л|ать(ся) *сов. см.* подде́лывать(ся). ~ка *ж.* 1. (*действие*) fórging, fórgery; 2. (*подделанная вещь, имитация*) imitátion; fake; (*документ и т. п.*) fórgery, cóunterfeit.

подде́лывать, подде́лать (*вн.*) forge (*smth.*), cóunterfeit (*smth.*); ~ чужу́ю по́дпись forge *smb.'s* signature. ~ся, подде́латься 1. (под, подо *вн.*; *подражать*) imitate (*smb., smth.*); 2. (к *дт.*) *разг.* (*искать расположения*) play up to (*smb.*), ingrátiate onesélf (with), get* ínto *smb.'s* good books.

подде́льный 1. (*фальшивый*) false; fake *attr.*; faked; 2. (*искусственный*) artificial; imitátion *attr.*

подде́ржание *с.* máintenance; ~ поря́дка máintenance of órder.

поддержа́ть *сов. см.* подде́рживать 1, 2, 3, 4.

подде́рж|ивать, поддержа́ть (*вн.*) 1. (*не давать упасть*) suppórt (*smb., smth.*); ~ *кого-л.* под руку hold* *smb.'s* arm; 2. (*оказывать помощь*) suppórt (*smb., smth.*), back (*smb., smth.*) up; поддержа́ть наступле́ние артиллери́йским огнём give* an offénsive artíllery suppórt; 3. (*выражать своё согласие*) suppórt (*smb., smth.*), sécond (*smb., smth.*); back (*smb., smth.*) *разг.*; поддержа́ть чью-л. кандидату́ру suppórt *smb.'s* cándidature; ~ чье-л. предложе́ние suppórt/sécond *smb.'s* propósal; (*на собрании*) suppórt a mótion; 4. (*не давать прекратиться*) keep* up (*smth.*), maintáin (*smth.*); ~ перепи́ску keep* up a correspóndence; ~ дисципли́ну keep*/uphóld* discipline; ~ ого́нь keep* up a fire; ~ отноше́ния keep in touch; ~ разгово́р keep* up the conversátion; ~ поря́док maintáin órder; ~ диплома́ти́ческие отноше́ния maintáin diplomátic relátions; 5. *тк. несов.* (*служить опорой*) keep* up (*smth.*), hold* (*smth.*), suppórt (*smth.*); коло́нны ~ивают кры́шу the cólumns suppórt the roof. ~ка *ж.* 1. (*помощь, одобрение*) suppórt, bácking; материа́льная ~ка fináncial suppórt; 2. (*опора*) suppórt, prop.

подде́ть *сов. см.* поддева́ть.

поддра́знивать, поддразни́ть (*вн.*) tease (*smb.*), chaff (*smb.*), taunt (*smb.*).

поддразни́ть *сов. см.* поддра́знивать.

поддува́ло *с.* (*в печке*) ásh-pan; (*в топке*) ásh-box.

поддув|а́ть, подду́ть 1. *разг.* blow*; creáte a draught; 2. *тк. несов. безл.*: ~áет it's ráther dráughty, there is a slight draught.

подду́ть *сов. см.* поддува́ть 1.

поде́йствовать *сов. см.* де́йствовать 5.

поде́лать *сов.* (*вн.*) *разг.* 1. (*заняться чем-л. в течение некоторого времени*) do* a bit (of); 2. (*сделать что-л.*) make* (*smth.*); ◇ ничего́ не могу́ с ним ~ he is difficult to mánage, I don't know how to mánage him; ничего́ не поде́лаешь! it can't be helped!, no one can do ánything about it; no way!

подел|и́ть *сов.* 1. (*вн.*) divíde (*smth.*), share (*smth.*); они́ чего́-то не ~и́ли they have fállen out, they have had a quárrel; 2. (*вн. с тв.*) share (*smth.* with). ~и́ться *сов.* (*тв. с тв.*) 1. (*уделить*) share (*smth.* with); ~и́ться кни́гами с кем-л. share one's books with *smth.*; 2. (*сообщить*) tell* (*smb. smth.*), share (*smth.* with); ~и́ться с кем-л. свои́ми впечатле́ниями tell* *smb.* one's impréssions; ~и́ться о́пытом с кем-л. impárt one's knówledge to *smb.*, share one's expérience with *smb.*

поде́лка *ж.* hand-máde árticle.

поде́лом *разг.*: ~ ему́ (ей, вам *и т. д.*) it serves him (her, you, *etc.*) right.

поде́лыв|ать *несов. разг.*: что ~аете? how are you gétting alóng/on?; how are you dóing?

подён|но by the day; плати́ть ~ pay* by the day. ~ный by the day *после сущ.*; ~ная рабо́та tíme-work, dáy-labour; ~ная опла́та páyment by the day; ~ный рабо́чий dáy-labourer, tíme-worker. **~щик** *м.*, **~щица** *ж.* dáy-labourer, tíme-worker.

подёргивание *с.* jerk, twitch, twítching.

подёргив|ать *несов.* 1. (*тв.*) twitch (*smth.*); 2. *безл.*: гу́бы его́ ~ало his lips were twítching; его́ всего́ ~ает he is twítching all óver. **~аться** *несов.* twitch.

подёржанн|ый sécond-hand; ~ое пла́тье sécond-hand clothes *pl.*

подержа́ть *сов.* (*вн.*) keep* (*smth.*) for a time. **~ся** *сов.* 1. (*за вн.*) hold* on (to); 2. (*находиться в определённом положении*) stay for a while; 3. (*сохраняться*) last for a while; 4. (*не сдаваться*) hold* out for a while.

подёрн|уть *сов.* (*вн.*) cloud (*smth.*), cóver (*smth.*); о́зеро бы́ло ~уто льдом the lake was cóvered with a thin film of ice. **~уться** *сов.* be* clóuded, be* cóvered; её глаза́ ~улись слеза́ми her eyes are clóuded with tears.

подешеве́ть *сов. см.* дешеве́ть.

поджа́ривать, поджа́рить (*вн.*) (*на сковороде*) fry (*smth.*); (*на пламени*) grill (*smth.*), broil (*smth.*); (*хлеб*) toast (*smth.*); (*в духовке*) roast (*smth.*); (*обжаривать поверхность*) brown (*smth.*). **~ся**, поджа́риться be* róasted, be* fried, be* tóasted.

поджа́ристый nice and brown.

поджа́рить(ся) *сов. см.* поджа́ривать(ся).

поджа́ть *сов. см.* поджима́ть.

поджелу́дочн|ый: ~ая железа́ *анат.* páncreas.

поджа́ть *сов. см.* поджига́ть.

поджига́тель *м.* ársonist, incéndiary; *перен.* instigator.

поджига́ть, подже́чь (*вн.*) set* (*smth.*) on fire, set* fire (to); подже́чь дом set* a house on fire.

поджида́ть *несов.* (*вн., рд.*) wait (for).

поджи́лки *мн. разг.*: ~ трясу́тся у кого́-л. *smb.* is sháking at the knees.

поджима́ть, поджа́ть: ~ гу́бы purse one's lips; ~ но́ги cross one's legs; сиде́ть, поджа́в но́ги sit* cross-légged, sit* with one's legs tucked únder one; поджа́ть хвост put* its tail betwéen its legs; *перен.* sing* small; соба́ка убежа́ла, поджа́в хвост the dog ran off with its tail betwéen its legs.

поджо́г *м.* árson.

подзаголо́вок *м.* súbtitle, súbheading.

подзадо́ривать, подзадо́рить (*вн.*) *разг.* encóurage (*smb.*); (*подстрекать*) egg (*smb.*) on, incíte (*smb.*).

подзадо́рить *сов. см.* подзадо́ривать.

подзаты́льник *м. разг.* cuff, clip (on the back of the head).

подзащи́тн|ая *ж.*, **~ый** *м. юр.* clíent.

подземе́лье *с.* vault; (*пещера*) cave; (*темница*) dúngeon.

подзе́мн|ый únderground; subterránean *книжн.*; ~ ход únderground pássage; ~ взрыв únderground explósion; ~ые испыта́ния únderground tests.

подзо́рн|ый: ~ая труба́ télescope, spýglass.

подзыва́ть, подозва́ть (*вн.*) call (*smb.*), call up (to); (*жестом*) béckon (to).

подка́лывать, подколо́ть (*вн.*) pin (*smth.*) to, pin up (*smth.*); *перен. разг.* tease (*smb.*), have* a dig (at); (*о документе*) attách.

подка́пывать, подкопа́ть (*вн.*) undermíne (*smth.*), sap (*smth.*). **~ся**, подкопа́ться (под *вн.*) dig* únder (*smth.*), undermíne (*smth.*); *воен.* sap (*smth.*); *перен.* intrígue (agáinst).

подкара́уливать, подкара́улить (*вн.*) *разг.* be* on the lóokout (for), watch (for); (*находиться в засаде*) lie* in wait (for).

подкара́улить *сов. см.* подкара́уливать.

подка́рмливать, подкорми́ть (*вн.*) 1. feed* (*smb.*, *smth.*) up; 2. *с.-х.* apply/give* (*smth.*) a tóp-dréssing, give* (*smth.*) éxtra fértilizer. **~ся**, подкорми́ться *разг.* feed* onesélf up.

подкати́ть(ся) *сов. см.* подка́тывать(ся).

подка́тывать, подкати́ть (*вн.*; *катя, приближать к чему-л.*) push (*smth.*) up; (*помещать подо что-л.*) push (*smth.*) únder, roll (*smth.*) únder; 2. *разг.* (*подъезжать*) roll up, drive* up; маши́на подкати́ла к подъе́зду the car drove up to the éntrance; 3. (*к дт.*) *разг.* rise* (in); у него́ подкати́ло к го́рлу he felt a lump in his throat. **~ся**, подкати́ться 1. (*к дт.*, под *вн.*) roll (to, únder); 2. *разг.* (*приближаться — о поезде и т. п.*) run*.

подка́шивать, подкоси́ть (*вн.*) 1. cut* (*smth.*); 2. (*сваливать с ног*) cut* (*smth.*) down; 3. (*лишать силы, бодрости*) sap/undermíne *smb.'s* spírits/vígour; боле́знь подкоси́ла его́ illness sapped his spirits. **~ся**, подкоси́ться give* way; bend*; у него́ но́ги подка́шиваются (от уста́лости) he is réady to drop.

подки́дывать, подки́нуть *см.* подбра́сывать 1, 3, 4.

подки́дыш *м.* fóundling.

подки́нуть *сов. см.* подки́дывать.

подкла́дка *ж.* 1. líning; 2. (*основа чего-л.*) foundátion; кака́я тут ~? what is behínd all this?

подкла́дочный líning *attr.*

подкла́дывать, подложи́ть (*вн.*) 1. put* (*smth.*) únder; 2. *разг.* (*подшивать подкладку*) line (*smth.*); ~ шёлк под пальто́ have* a coat lined with silk; 3. (*вн., рд.*; *добавлять*) add (*smth.*); put* out some more (*smth.*), refill *smb.'s* plate; 4. (*тайно*) plant (*smth.*); ему́ подложи́ли докуме́нты the dócuments were plánted on him; ◇ подложи́ть свинью́ кому́-л. play *smb.* a mean trick, do* the dírty on *smb.*

подкла́сс *м. биол.* súbclass.

подкле́ивать, подкле́ить (*вн.*) paste up (*smth.*), glue up (*smth.*).

подкле́ить *сов. см.* подкле́ивать.

подключа́ть, подключи́ть (*вн.*) put* (*smth.*) in; (*вн. к дт.*) connéct up (*smth.* to). **~ся**, подключи́ться be* connécted up.

подключи́ть(ся) *сов. см.* подключа́ть(ся).

подко́ва *ж.* hórseshoe.

подкова́ть *сов. см.* подко́вывать.

подко́вывать, подкова́ть (*вн.*) shoe (*smth.*); *перен. разг.* train (*smb.*), prepáre (*smb.*); быть подко́ванным в

чём-л. be* well up in *smth.*; он хорошо подкован по математике he is well up in mathematics.

подкожн|ый hypodérmic; ~ое впры́скивание hypodérmic injéction.

подколо́ть *сов. см.* подка́лывать.

подкомиссия *ж.* súbcommittee.

подконтро́льный únder the contról (of) *после сущ.*

подко́п *м.* 1. (*действие*) undermíning; 2. (*подземный ход*) túnnel; 3. *обыкн. мн. разг.* (*происки, козни*) intrígues. ~а́ть(ся) *сов. см.* подка́пывать(ся).

подко́рм *м. с.-х.* éxtra feed.

подкорми́ть(ся) *сов. см.* подка́рмливать(ся).

подко́рмка *ж. с.-х.* tóp-dréssing.

подкоси́ть(ся) *сов. см.* подка́шивать(ся).

подко́шенный: он упа́л как ~ he went down like a nínepin.

подкра́дываться, подкра́сться steal* up, sneak up; stéalthily appróach (*тж. перен.*).

подкра́сить(ся) *сов. см.* подкра́шивать(ся).

подкра́сться *сов. см.* подкра́дываться.

подкра́шивать, подкра́сить (*вн.*) 1. touch up (*smth.*) (*тж. перен.*); (*жидкость*) cólour (*smth.*); ~ гу́бы touch up *one's* lips; ~ щёки put* on a little rouge; 2. (*подновля́ть окра́ску*) touch up (*smth.*), renéw the páint-work (of); подкра́сить око́нные ра́мы touch up the window-frames. ~ся, подкра́ситься *разг.* put* on a little máke-up.

подкреп|и́ть(ся) *сов. см.* подкрепля́ть(ся). ~ле́ние *с.* 1. (*действие*) suppórt; (*пищей*) refréshing, refréshment; (*здоро́вья*) fórtifying; 2. *воен.* reinfórcement.

подкрепля́ть, подкрепи́ть (*вн.*) 1. (*придава́ть про́чность*) prop (*smth.*), underpín (*smth.*); suppórt (*smth.*) (*тж. перен.*); 2. (*подде́рживать*) suppórt (*smth., smth.*); (*пищей и т. п.*) refrésh (*smth.*). ~ся, подкрепи́ться refrésh onesélf, have* a snack.

подкрути́ть *сов. см.* подкру́чивать.

подкру́чивать, подкрути́ть (*вн.*) *разг.* screw (up) (*smth.*) tight; ~ га́йку screw (up) a nut tight.

по́дкуп *м.* bríbery, graft.

подкуп|а́ть, подкупи́ть 1. (*вн.*) bribe (*smb.*), buy* (*smb.*); *перен.* appéal (to), cáptivate (*smb.*); ~а́ет его́ и́скренность his appéal lies in his sincérity; 2. (*вн.; рд.; покупа́ть дополни́тельно*) buy* some more (*smth.*), buy* éxtra (*smth.*). ~а́ющий appéaling, cáptivating, attráctive; ~а́ющая улы́бка winning smile.

подку́пи́ть *сов. см.* подкупа́ть.

подла́мывать, подломи́ть (*вн.*) break* (*smth.*) undernéath; *перен.* take* all the heart out of (*smb.*). ~ся, подломи́ться crack; (*о нога́х, коле́нях*) give* way.

по́дле 1. *нареч.* near, close by; 2. *предлог* (*рд.*) near, by the side of; он сиде́л ~ меня́ he was sítting by my side.

подлёдный únder the ice *после сущ.*; ~ релье́ф subglácial relief; ~ лов ры́бы ice fishing.

подлеж|а́ть *несов.* (*дт.*) be* súbject (to); ~ обложе́нию нало́гами be* súbject to taxátion; не ~и́т оглаше́нию not to be made públic; ◇ это не ~и́т сомне́нию it is not to be dóubted, it is beyónd doubt, it is indispútable.

подлежа́щее *с. грам.* súbject.

подлеза́ть, подле́зть crawl/creep únder.

подле́зть *сов. см.* подлеза́ть.

подле́сок *м.* únderwood, únderbrush, úndergrowth.

подлета́ть, подлете́ть 1. fly* up; 2. *разг.* (*быстро приближа́ться*) run* up.

подлете́ть *сов. см.* подлета́ть.

подле́ц *м.* scóundrel, víllain.

подле́чивать, подлечи́ть (*вн.*) *разг.* give* some tréatment (to), cure (*smb.*) témporarily. ~ся, подлечи́ться get* some tréatment.

подлечи́ть(ся) *сов. см.* подле́чивать(ся).

подлива́ть, подли́ть (*рд.*) add (*smth.*); ◇ подли́ть

ма́сла в ого́нь add fuel to the flame/fire, pour oil on the flame.

подли́вка *ж.* sauce; (*мясна́я*) grávy.

подли́за *м. и ж. разг.* tóady, whéedler.

подлиза́ть(ся) *сов. см.* подли́зывать(ся).

подли́зывать, подлиза́ть (*вн.*) lick (*smth.*) up. ~ся, подлиза́ться (к *дт.*) *разг.* tóady (to), make* up (to), fawn (on); lick *smb.'s* foot.

по́длинник *м.* originál; предста́вить докуме́нты в ~ах prodúce the originál dócuments; чита́ть кла́ссиков в ~ax read* the clássics in the originál.

по́длинн|ость *ж.* authentícity, truth. ~ый 1. (*явля́ющийся оригина́лом*) authéntic, génuine, originál; ~ый докуме́нт originál dócument; ~ое письмо́ authéntic létter; 2. (*и́стинный*) real, true, génuine; ~ый худо́жник real/true ártist; ~ый геро́изм real héroism; ◇ с ~ым ве́рно cértified true cópy.

подли́ть *сов. см.* подлива́ть.

подлича́ть *несов.* act méanly.

подло́г *м.* fórgery.

подложи́ть *сов. см.* подкла́дывать.

подло́жный forged, cóunterfeit; fake *разг.*

подломи́ть(ся) *сов. см.* подла́мывать(ся).

подл|ость *ж.* 1. méanness, báseness; 2. (*по́длый посту́пок*) mean/vile/low áction, foul thing; сде́лать ~ do* a foul thing; кака́я ~! what a foul thing to do! ~ый mean, foul, vile, únderhand; ~ый посту́пок mean/low trick.

подма́зать(ся) *сов. см.* подма́зывать(ся).

подма́зывать, подма́зать (*вн.*) apply a little more (*smth.*); (*жи́ром, ма́слом*) grease (*smth.*). ~ся, подма́заться *разг.* 1. (*подкра́шивать гу́бы*) put* on a little máke-up; 2. (к *дт.*) (try to) get* into *smb.'s* fávour.

подманда́тный mandáted.

подмасте́рье *м.* appréntice.

подма́чивать, подмочи́ть (*вн.*) wet (*smth.*) slightly, móisten (*smth.*), damp (*smth.*); (*дава́ть подмо́кнуть*) get* (*smth.*) wet/damp.

подме́н|а *ж.* súbstitute, substitútion. ~и́ть *сов. см.* подменя́ть.

подменя́ть, подмени́ть (*вн.*) 1. (*незаме́тно заменя́ть что-л.*) quíetly súbstitute (*smth.*), change (*smth.*) on the quíet; 2. (*вре́менно заменя́ть кого́-л.*) repláce (*smb.*), stand* in for (*smb.*).

подмерза́ть, подмёрзнуть freeze* slightly, tíghten up (in the frost).

подмёрзнуть *сов. см.* подмерза́ть.

подмести́ *сов. см.* подмета́ть.

подмета́льщ|ик *м.*, ~ица *ж.* swéeper.

подмета́ть, подмести́ (*вн.*) sweep* (*smth.*).

подме́тить *сов. см.* подмеча́ть.

подмётк|а *ж.* sole; подбива́ть ~и (*о сапо́жнике*) resóle boots; (*о зака́зчике*) have* *one's* boots resóled; ◇ в ~и не годи́ться кому́-л. be* not fit to hold a cándle to *smb.*, be* not a patch on *smb.*

подмеча́ть, подме́тить (*вн.*) nótice (*smth.*), obsérve (*smth.*).

подми́гивать, подмигну́ть (*дт.*) wink (at), give* (*smb.*) a wink (at).

подмигну́ть *сов. см.* подми́гивать.

подмина́ть, подмя́ть (*вн.*) crush (*smb., smth.*); press down (on).

подмока́ть, подмо́кнуть get* slightly wet.

подмо́кнуть *сов. см.* подмока́ть.

подмора́ж|ивать, подморо́зить 1. (*вн.*) freeze* (*smth.*), touch (*smth.*) with frost; подморо́зить я́блоки freeze* the ápples; доро́гу подморо́зило the road was filmed/cóated with ice; 2. *безл.*: ~ивает it is fréezing; но́чью си́льно подморо́зило there was a hard frost dúring the night.

подморо́зить *сов. см.* подмора́живать.

подмоско́вный near Móscow *после сущ.*, in the vicínity of Móscow *после сущ.*

подмо́стки *мн.* **1.** (*настил*) scáffold *sg*, scáffolding *sg*; **2.** (*сцена*) stage *sg*.

подмо́ченн|ый *разг.* damp, slíghtly wet; *перен.* dámaged; ~ая репута́ция damaged reputátion.

подмочи́ть *сов. см.* подма́чивать.

подмыв|а́ть, подмы́ть (*вн.*) **1.** give* (*smb., smth.*) a wash; **2.** (*размывать*) undermíne (*smth.*); **3.** *тк. несов. безл. разг.* (*о непреодолимом желании что-л. делать*): меня́ ~а́ло сказа́ть ему́ I had a great mind to tell him. ~а́ться, подмы́ться have* a wash, wash onesélf.

подмы́ть *сов. см.* подмыва́ть 1, 2. ~ся *сов. см.* подмыва́ться.

подмы́шка *ж.* (*в косв. падежах пишется раздельно*) ármpit; под мы́шкой únder *one's* arm.

подмы́шник *м.* dréss-presérver, dréss-shield.

подмя́ть *сов. см.* подмина́ть.

поднебе́с|ный of the sky *после сущ.*, celéstial; в ~ой вышине́ high in the héavens.

поднебе́сье *с.* skies *pl*, héavens *pl*; в ~ on high.

поднево́льный **1.** (*зависимый*) depéndent, bound; я челове́к ~ I am not my own máster; **2.** (*принудительный*) forced; ~ труд forced lábour.

поднести́ *сов. см.* подноси́ть.

поднима́ть, подня́ть (*вн.*) **1.** lift (*smth.*), raise (*smth.*); ~ тя́жесть lift a weight; подня́ть бага́ж на ли́фте take* the lúggage up in the lift; подня́ть ру́ку raise *one's* hand; подня́ть го́лову lift up *one's* head; ~ флаг hoist a flag; **2.** (*подбирать с земли, с пола*) pick up (*smth.*); ~ плато́к pick up a hándkerchief; **3.** (*заставлять встать*) get* (*smb.*) up; (*побуждать отправиться*) get* (*smb.*) to go; ~ кого́-л. в ата́ку take* *smb.* óver the top, lead* *smb.* in a charge; **4.** (*воодушевлять на что-л.*) rouse (*smb.*), stímulate (*smb.*), inspíre (*smb.*); ~ кого́-л. на по́двиг inspíre *smb.* to heróic áction; **5.** (*увеличивать, повышать*) raise (*smth.*); *перен.* enhánce (*smth.*); ~ квалифика́цию рабо́чих train wórkers to a hígher level; ~ цены на това́ры raise the price of goods; ~ настрое́ние кому́-л. put* *smb.* in the right mood; ~ дух кому́-л. raise *smb.'s* spírits; **6.** *в сочетании с некоторыми существительными:* подня́ть восста́ние start an úprising; raise the stándard of revólt; ~ трево́гу raise the alárm; ~ хо́хот raise a laugh; **7.** (*вспахивать*) plough up (*smth.*); ~ целину́ break* new/fresh ground, cúltivate vírgin land; ◇ подня́ть глаза́ lift *one's* eyes; ~ пе́тли mend ládders; ~ ру́ку на кого́-л. lift *one's* hand agáinst *smb.*; подня́ть кого́-л. на́ смех make* a láughing-stock of *smb.* ~ся, подня́ться **1.** rise*; баро́метр подня́лся the barómeter has rísen; **2.** (*всходить*) go* up; (*на гору*) climb, ascénd; ~ся по ле́стнице go* upstáirs; ~ся на второ́й эта́ж go* up to the first floor; ~ся на самолёте go* up in an áeroplane; ~ся ввысь (*о птицах*) soar; **3.** (*вставать с постели*) get* up, rise*; **4.** (*возникать, начинаться*) aríse*; подняла́сь вьюга a snówstorm arose; подня́лся шум there was a lot of noise; **5.** *тк. несов.* (*о дороге и т. п.*) climb, rise*; **6.** *тк. несов.* (*выделяться своей высотой*) tówer.

поднови́ть *сов. см.* подновля́ть.

подновля́ть, поднови́ть (*вн.*) rénovate (*smth.*), repáir (*smth.*), fréshen up (*smth.*).

подногóтн|ая *ж. разг.* cárefully guárded sécrets *pl*, inside informátion; знать всю ~ую кого́-л. know* évery líttle thing abóut *smb.*

подно́жи|е *с.* **1.** foot*; у ~я горы́ at the foot of the móuntain; **2.** (*пьедестал*) pédestal.

подно́жк|а *ж.* **1.** (*экипажа, трамвая*) step, fóotboard; (*автомобиля*) rúnning-board; **2.** *разг.* (*удар ногой*) trip; подста́вить ~у кому́-л. trip *smb.* up.

подно́жный: ~ корм fórage crop, grázing; пусти́ть скот на ~ корм graze cáttle.

подно́с *м.* tray; (*металлический тж.*) sálver; ча́йный ~ téa-tray.

подноси́ть, поднести́ **1.** (*вн.*) lift (*smb., smth.*), raise (*smb., smth.*) (*приносить*) cárry (*smth.*), bring* (*smth.*); поднести́ ло́жку ко рту a spoon to *one's* mouth; поднести́ ве́щи к по́езду cárry the lúggage to the train; **2.** (*вн. дт.; дарить*) presént (*smb.* with); **3.** (*вн., рд.; угощать*) give* (*smth.*), bring* (*smth.*).

подноше́ние *с.* (*подарок*) presént.

подня́тие *с.* ráising.

подня́ть *сов. см.* поднима́ть. ~ся *сов. см.* поднима́ться 1, 2, 3, 4.

подо *см.* под.

подоб|а́ть *несов. обыкн. безл.* (*дт.*) becóme* (*smb.*), befít (*smb.*); так поступа́ть вам не ~ает it does not becóme you to act like that. ~а́ющий próper, súitable; becóming *attr.*

подо́би|е *с.* **1.** similárity; resémblance, líkeness; от него́ не оста́лось и ~я пре́жнего челове́ка he is a mere shádow of his fórmer self; **2.** *мат.* similárity.

подо́бн|о **1.** *нареч.* like; **2.** *в знач. предлога* (*дт.*) just as, like. ~ый **1.** (*дт.; сходный*) símilar (to), like; поступа́ть ~ым же о́бразом act in a símilar mánner; **2.** (*такой*) such; of this/that kind *such сущ.*, like this/that *после сущ.*; ~ого ро́да фа́кты such facts; он ничего́ ~ого не говори́л he said nóthing of the sort, he said no such thing; я ничего́ ~ого не ви́дел I have néver seen ánything like that; **3.** *мат.* similar; ~ые треуго́льники símilar tríangles; ◇ ничего́ ~ого nóthing of the kind; и тому́ ~ое (*сокр. и т. п.*) and so on, and so forth, et cétera (*сокр.* etc.).

подобостра́ст|ие *с.* servílity, fáwning; относи́ться с ~ием к кому́-л. fawn upón *smb.*, kowtów to *smb.* ~ный sérvile, fáwning.

подобра́ть(ся) *сов. см.* подбира́ть(ся).

подобре́ть *сов. см.* добре́ть.

подобру́-поздоро́ву: уходи́те ~! go while the góing is good!

подогна́ть *сов. см.* подгоня́ть.

подогну́ть(ся) *сов. см.* подгиба́ть(ся).

подогре́в *м. тех.* wárming up; (*специальным устройством*) prehéating. ~а́ние *с.* héating, wárming up. ~а́тель *м.* prehéater.

подогрева́ть, подогре́ть (*вн.*) warm up (*smth.*); *перен.* stir up (*smb., smth.*), rouse (*smb., smth.*).

подогре́ть *сов. см.* подогрева́ть.

пододвига́ть, пододви́нуть (*вн.*) move up (*smth.*), push (*smth.*) néarer; ~ таре́лку кому́-л. push a plate towards *smb.* ~ся, пододви́нуться come* néarer/clóser, move up.

пододви́нуть(ся) *сов. см.* пододвига́ть(ся).

пододея́льник *м.* blánket cóver/slip, quilt cóver/slip.

подожд|а́ть *сов.* **1.** (*вн., рд.*) wait (for); он немно́го ~а́л he wáited for a líttle while; ~и́те! wait a móment!; **2.** (+ *инф., с тв.*) *разг.* (*повременить с чем-л.*) postpóne (+ -ing, *smth.*).

подозва́ть *сов. см.* подзыва́ть.

подозрев|а́ть *несов.* (*вн., о пр.*) suspéct (*smb., smth.*); ~ кого́-л. в преступле́нии suspéct *smb.* of a crime; он ничего́ не ~ает he suspécts nóthing.

подозре́н|ие *с.* suspícion; по ~ию on suspícion; вызыва́ть ~ aróuse suspícion; навлека́ть на себя́ ~ incúr *smb.'s* suspícion; относи́ться к кому́-л. с ~ем be* súspicious of *smb.*; ◇ быть под ~ем be* únder suspícion, be* suspécted.

подозри́тельн|о **1.** *нареч.* suspíciously; **2.** *в знач. сказ. безл.* it is suspícious. ~ость *ж.* suspíciousness, suspícion. ~ый **1.** (*внушающий подозрение*) suspícious; ~ая ли́чность suspícious/shády cháracter; **2.** (*недоверчивый*) suspícious, distrústful, mistrústful; он сде́лался ~ым he becáme suspícious.

подо́йник *м.* mílk-pail.

подойти́ *сов. см.* подходи́ть.

подоко́нник *м.* window-sill.

подо́л *м.* skirts, hem of a skirt.

подо́лгу (for) a long time; ~ гости́ть у *кого-л.* pay* *smb.* long visits; ~ отсу́тствовать stay away for long intervals; я ~ проси́живал на берегу́ мо́ря I used to sit on the seashore for hours.

подо́нки *мн.* dregs; *перен. тж.* scum *sg*, riff-raff *sg*; ~ о́бщества the dregs of society.

подопе́чн|ый *прил.* 1. under the care of a guardian *после сущ.*; ~ая террито́рия trust territory; 2. *в знач. сущ. м.* ward.

подоплёка *ж.* hidden motive, underlying reason.

подо́пытн|ый experimental; ~ое по́ле experimental plot; ~ые живо́тные experimental animals.

подорва́ть *сов. см.* подрыва́ть II. ~ся *сов. см.* подрыва́ться.

подорожа́ть *сов.* rise in price, become more expensive.

подоро́жник *м.* plantain.

подоси́новик *м.* (*гриб*) orange-cap boletus.

подосла́ть *сов. см.* подсыла́ть.

подоспе́ть *сов. разг.* arrive/come* in time, be* in time.

подостла́ть *сов. см.* подстила́ть.

подоткну́ть *сов. см.* подтыка́ть.

подотря́д *м. зоол.* suborder.

подотчётн|ость *ж.* accountability. ~ый 1. (*выдаваемый с условием последующего отчёта*) to be accounted for *после сущ.*; ~ые де́ньги money to be accounted for; 2. (*дт.; обязанный отчитываться*) accountable (to).

подо́хнуть *сов.* die; (*о человеке разг.*) croak.

подохо́дный: ~ нало́г income-tax.

подо́шва *ж.* 1. (*обуви, ноги*) sole; 2. (*горы*) foot*; (*фундамента, рельса*) base.

подпада́ть, подпа́сть (под *вн.*) fall* (under); ~ под чьё-л. влия́ние fall* under *smb.'s* influence.

подпа́ивать, подпои́ть (*вн.*) *разг.* make* (*smb.*) drunk/tipsy, ply (*smb.*) with drink.

подпа́ливать, подпали́ть (*вн.*) *разг.* 1. (*поджигать*) set* fire (to); 2. (*слегка обжигать*) scorch (*smth.*).

подпали́ть *сов. см.* подпа́ливать.

подпа́сть *сов. см.* подпада́ть.

подпева́ла *м. и ж. разг.* yes-man*, henchman*.

подпева́ть *несов.* (*дт.*) join in (with), accompany (*smb.*), pick up the tune; *перен. разг.* echo (*smb.*).

подпере́ть *сов. см.* подпира́ть.

подпи́|ливать, подпили́ть (*вн.*) 1. (*распиливать снизу не до конца*) make* a cut in/at the base (of); подпили́ть де́рево make* a cut at the base of a tree; 2. (*срезая пилой, укорачивать*) shorten (*smth.*); ~ но́жки стола́ shorten the legs of a table.

подпили́ть *сов. см.* подпи́ливать.

подпира́ть, подпере́ть (*вн.*) prop up (*smth.*).

подписа́ть(ся) *сов. см.* подпи́сывать(ся).

подпи́с|ка *ж.* 1. subscription; ~ на газе́ту subscription to a newspaper; получа́ть журна́лы по ~ке have* magazines sent to one (on subscription); 2. (*письменное обязательство*) written undertaking. ~ной subscription *attr.*; ~ное изда́ние subscribers' edition; <> ~ной лист subscription list.

подпи́счик *м.* subscriber; ~и газе́т subscribers to newspapers.

подпи́сывать, подписа́ть (*вн.*) 1. (*ставить подпись*) sign (*smth.*); ~ докуме́нт sign a document; ~ догово́р sign a treaty; 2. (*приписывать что-л.*) add (*smth.*), write* (*smth.*); подписа́ть ещё не́сколько строк add a few more lines; 3. (*включать в число подписчиков*) subscribe (*smb.*); подписа́ть кого́-л. на газе́ту take* *smb.'s* subscription to a newspaper. ~ся, подписа́ться 1. (*ставить свою подпись*) sign (*smth.*); 2. (*на вн.*) subscribe (to); подписа́ться на газе́ту subscribe to a

newspaper; <> я гото́в обе́ими рука́ми подписа́ться под э́тим I fully endorse that.

по́дпись *ж.* 1. (*действие*) signing; докуме́нт на ~ document to be signed; 2. (*фамилия*) signature; ста́вить свою́ ~ write*/affix one's signature; за ~ю кого́-л. signed by *smb.*, bearing *smb.'s* signature, over *smb.'s* signature; 3. (*надпись*) inscription; (*в кино*) subtitle.

подплыва́ть, подплы́ть (к *дт.*) swim* up (to); (*о судах*) sail up (to), steam up (to); approach (*smth.*), near (*smth.*).

подплы́ть *сов. см.* подплыва́ть.

подпо́лзать *сов. см.* подпа́лывать.

подполза́ть, подползти́ 1. (к *дт.*) creep/crawl up (to); 2. (под *вн.*) crawl under (*smth.*).

подползти́ *сов. см.* подполза́ть.

подполко́вник *м.* lieutenant-colonel.

подпо́ль|е *с.* 1. (*подвал*) cellar; 2. (*конспиративное положение*) the underground; уходи́ть в ~ go* underground. ~ный underground; ~ная типогра́фия secret printing-press. ~щик *м.*, ~щица *ж.* underground (political) worker.

подпо́р|а *ж.*, ~ка *ж.* support, prop.

подпо́чв|а *ж.* subsoil, substratum. ~енный subsoil *attr.*, subterranean; ~енная вода́ ground water.

подпоя́сать(ся) *сов. см.* подпоя́сывать(ся).

подпоя́сывать, подпоя́сать (*вн.*) belt (*smth.*), fasten (*smb.'s*) belt. ~ся, подпоя́саться put* on one's belt; (*тв.*) tie (*smth.*) round one's waist.

подпра́вить *сов. см.* подправля́ть.

подправля́ть, подпра́вить (*вн.*) 1. touch up (*smth.*), put* (*smth.*) right, adjust (*smth.*); (*приводить в порядок*) put* (*smth.*) to rights; 2. *разг.* (*восстанавливать здоровье*) put* (*smb.*) right, make* (*smb.*) well.

подпру́га *ж.* saddle-girth.

подпры́гивать *несов.* jump up and down; (*о лодке на волнах*) bob; (*о мяче и т. п.*) bounce.

подпры́гнуть *сов.* give* a jump.

подпуска́ть, подпусти́ть (*вн.*) let* (*smb., smth.*) come near.

подпусти́ть *сов. см.* подпуска́ть.

подраба́тывать, подрабо́тать *разг.* 1. (*вн.; проводить дополнительную работу*) work (*smth.*) up, elaborate (*smth.*); 2. (*вн., рд.; зарабатывать дополнительно*) earn (*smth.*) on the side, earn a little extra.

подрабо́тать *сов. см.* подраба́тывать.

подра́внивать, подровня́ть (*вн.*) trim (*smth.*).

подража́|ние *с.* imitation; (*манерам, голосу и т. п.*) mimicry. ~тель *м.* imitator; (*имитатор*) mimic, mimicker.

подража́тель|ный imitative; ~ная жи́вопись imitative painting. ~ство *с.* imitation, tendency to imitate.

подража́ть *несов.* (*дт.*) imitate (*smb., smth.*).

подразделе́ние *с.* 1. subdivision; 2. *воен.* subunit, smaller unit.

подраздели́ть *сов. см.* подразделя́ть.

подразделя́ть, подраздели́ть (*вн.*) subdivide (*smth.*). ~ся *несов.* (на *вн.*) subdivide (into).

подразумева́ть *несов.* (*вн.*) imply (*smth.*), mean* (*smth.*). ~ся *несов.* (под *тв.*) be* implied (by), be* meant (by); э́то само́ собо́й подразумева́лось that was understood.

подраст|а́ть, подрасти́ grow* up; (*о человеке тж.*) get* a little older. ~а́ющий: ~а́ющее поколе́ние the rising generation.

подрасти́ *сов. см.* подраста́ть.

подра́ться *сов. см.* дра́ться 1.

подре́зать *сов. см.* подреза́ть.

подреза́ть, подре́зать (*вн.*) cut* (*smth.*), clip (*smth.*), trim (*smth.*); (*о деревьях тж.*) prune (*smth.*); <> подре́зать кры́лья кому́-л. clip *smb.'s* wings.

подрисова́ть *сов. см.* подрисо́вывать.

подрисо́вывать, подрисова́ть (*вн.*) 1. (*добавлять к*

рисунку) add (*smth.*); 2. (*подправлять*) touch up (*smth.*).

подробн|ость ж. détail. ~ый détailed, circumstántial; дать ~ый отчёт о чём-л. give* a détailed accóunt of *smth.*, repórt on *smth.* in détail.

подровнять *сов. см.* подравнивать.

подросток *м.* adoléscent; téenager *разг.*

подрубать I, подрубить (*вн.*) 1. (*дерево и т. п.*) undercút* (*smth.*), notch (*smth.*) at the base; 2. (*укорачивать*) shórten (*smth.*), chop the end off (*smth.*).

подрубать II, подрубить (*вн.*; *подшивать*) hem (*smth.*).

подрубить I, II *сов. см.* подрубать I, II.

подруга *ж.* (girl-)friend; (*по школе*) schóolmate; (*детских игр*) pláymate; ◇ ~ жизни compánion in life, hélpmate, devóted wife*.

подружиться *сов.* (с *тв.*) make* friends (with), strike* up a friendship (with), form a friendship (with).

подруливать, подрулить 1. steer; 2. *ав.* táxi.

подрулить *сов. см.* подруливать.

подрумянивать, подрумянить (*вн.*) 1. rédden (*smth.*); 2. (*румянами*) rouge (*smth.*); 3. (*делать поджаристым*) make* (*smth.*) (a gólden) brown. ~ся, подрумяниться 1. be* flushed, be* red; 2. (*румянами*) rouge onesélf; 3. (*о пирогах и т. п.*) get* brown.

подрумянить(ся) *сов. см.* подрумянивать(ся).

подручный *прил.* 1. that comes to hand *после сущ.*; hándy; 2. *в знач. сущ. м.* assistant, appréntice.

подрыв *м.* blówing up, blásting; *перен.* undermíning; ~ górной порóды rock blásting.

подрывать I, подрыть (*вн.*) dig* (*smth.*), dig* the earth from benéath (*smth.*); (*делать глубже*) déepen (*smth.*).

подрывать II, подорвать (*вн.*) (*взрывать*) blow* up (*smth.*), dýnamite (*smth.*); (*породу*) blast (*smth.*); *перен.* undermíne (*smth.*); ~ мост blow* up a bridge; подорвать своё здорóвье undermíne *one's* health; подорвать авторитéт *кого-л.* undermíne *smb.'s* authórity/prestíge. ~ся, подорваться be* blown up; *перен.* be* undermíned.

подрывн|ой blásting; *перен.* undermíning, subvérsive; ~ая деятельность subvérsive activity.

подрыть *сов. см.* подрывать I.

подряд I *м.* cóntract.

подряд II *нареч.* rúnning; in succéssion; in a row; четыре дня, ряза ~ four days, times rúnning; прозвучáло ~ два выстрела two shots rang out in (quick) succéssion; три урóка ~ three léssons in a row.

подрядчик *м.* contráctor.

подсаживать *сов. см.* подсаживать.

подсаживать, подсадить 1. (*вн.*; *помогать сесть*) help (*smb.*), give* (*smb.*) a hand up; ~ кого-л. в вагóн help *smb.* into a cárriage; ~ кого-л. на лóшадь help *smb.* into the sáddle, help *smb.* on to a horse; (*в. к дт.*; *сажать к кому-л.*) plant (*smb.* on); 3. (*вн.*) *разг.* (*брать на телегу и т. п.*) give* (*smth.*) a lift; 4. (*вн.*, *рд.*; *растение*) plant some more (*smth.*); подсадить (*ещё*) капусты plant some more cábbages.

подсаживаться, подсесть (к *дт.*) take* a seat (beside, by) sit* down (beside, by).

подсаливать, подсолить (*вн.*) put* some more salt (in, into).

подсвечник *м.* cándlestick.

подсемейство *с.* биол. súbfamily.

подсесть *сов. см.* подсаживаться.

подсинить *сов. см.* синить.

подскáбливать, подскоблить (*вн.*) scrape off (*smth.*); (*написанное*) scratch (*smth.*) out.

подсказáть *сов. см.* подсказывать.

подсказывать, подсказáть (*вн.*) 1. (*незаметно шептать кому-л.*) prompt (*smth.*); не ~! no prompting!; 2. (*наводить на мысль*) suggést (*smth.*).

подскакáть *сов. см.* подскáкивать I.

подскáкивать I, подскакáть gállop up, come* gálloping up.

подскáкивать II, подскочить 1. (к *дт.*; *быстро подбегать*) run* up (to); 2. (*подпрыгивать*) jump up and down; *сов. тж.* give* a jump; *перен.* soar, leap*; подскочить от рáдости jump for joy; температýра подскочила the témperature went up.

подскочить *сов. см.* подскáкивать II.

подсластить *сов. см.* подслáщивать.

подслáщивать, подсластить (*вн.*) swéeten (*smth.*), súgar (*smth.*).

подслеповáтый wéak-síghted.

подслýшивать *сов. см.* подслýшивать.

подслýшивать, подслýшать (*вн.*) listen in (to); (*случайно*) overhéar* (*smth.*); *несов. тж.* éavesdrop (on); ~ чужóй разговóр listen in to óther péople's conversátion.

подсмáтривать, подсмотрéть (*вн.*) watch (*smb.*, *smth.*); (*за тв.*) spy (on, upón).

подсмéиваться *несов.* (над *тв.*) laugh (at), make* fun (of).

подсмотрéть *сов.* 1. *см.* подсмáтривать; 2. (*вн.*; *случайно увидеть*) spot (*smb.*, *smth.*), nótice (*smb.*, *smth.*).

подснéжник *м.* snówdrop.

подсóбн|ый subsídiary; личное ~ое хозяйство pérsonal subsídiary plot/hólding; ~ рабóчий assistant.

подсóвывать, подсýнуть 1. (*вн.* под *вн.*) put* (*smth.* únder), tuck (*smth.* únder); 2. (*вн. дт.*) *разг.* (*незаметно подкладывать*) slip (*smth. smth.*); он подсýнул мне бумáгу на пóдпись he súddenly prodúced a páper for me to sign; 3. (*вн. дт.*) *разг.* (*давать что-л. негодное*) palm off (*smth.* on).

подсознáтельный subcónscious.

подсолить *сов. см.* подсáливать.

подсóлнечн|ик *м.* súnflower. ~ый súnflower *attr.*; ~ое мáсло súnflower oil.

подсóлнух *м. разг.* 1. *см.* подсóлнечник; 2. *мн.* (*семечки подсолнечника*) súnflower seeds.

подсóхнуть *сов. см.* подсыхáть.

подспóрье *с. разг.* suppórt, help.

подспýдный látent, hídden.

подстáв|ить *сов. см.* подставлять. ~ка *ж.* stand; (*подпорка*) suppórt, prop.

подстав|лять, подставить 1. (*вн.* под *вн.*) put* (*smth.* únder), place (*smth.* únder); 2. (*вн.*; *придвигать*) move up (*smth.*); put* (*smth.*) near; ~ стул кому-л. move up a chair for *smb.*; 3. (*вн.*; *делать доступным*) óffer (*smth.*); ~ щёку óffer *one's* cheek; 4. (*вн.*; *открывать*) expóse (*smth.*); ~ свой фланг протвнику expóse *one's* flank to the énemy; 5. (*вн.*; *заменять чем-л.*) súbstitute (*smth.*); ◇ подстáвить нóжку кому-л. trip *smb.* up. ~нóй false; ~ный свидéтель false witness; ~нóе лицó ágent, stooge; dúmmy *разг.*

подстакáнник *м.* gláss-hólder.

подстанóвка *ж.* substitútion.

подстáнция *ж.* 1. substátion; 2. (*телефонная*) lócal télephone exchánge.

подстёгивать, подстегнýть (*вн.*) whip up (*smth.*); *перен.* spur (*smb.*) on.

подстегнýть *сов. см.* подстёгивать.

подстелить *сов. разг. см.* подстилáть.

подстерегáть, подстерéчь (*вн.*) lie* in wait (for), be* on the lóokout (for), watch (for), wayláy (*smb.*).

подстерéчь *сов. см.* подстерегáть.

подстилáть, подостлáть, подстелить (*вн.*) spread* (*smth.*).

подстилка *ж.* floor cóvering; (*для скота*) litter.

подстрáивать, подстрóить (*вн.*) 1. build* (*smth.*); 2. (*вн.* под *вн.*) *муз.* tune (*smth.*) to the pitch (of); 3. (*вн.*; *втайне делать что-л.*) rig (*smth.*), arránge (*smth.*); подстрóить пáкость кому-л. play a dirty trick on *smb.*; это всё было подстроено it was a put-up job, the whole thing was rigged.

подстрека́тель *м.* instigator; the man* behind the scenes *разг.* ~ство *с.* instigation, incitement.

подстрека́ть, подстрекну́ть (*вн.*) 1. incite (*smb.*), instigate (*smb.*); ~ *кого-л. к преступле́нию* incite *smb.* to crime; 2. (*возбуждать*) excite (*smth.*); ~ *чьё-л. любопы́тство* excite *smb.'s* curiosity.

подстрекну́ть *сов. см.* подстрека́ть.

подстре́ливать, подстрели́ть (*вн.*) wing (*smth.*), wound (*smth.*).

подстрели́ть *сов. см.* подстре́ливать.

подстрига́ть, подстри́чь (*что-л.*) trim (*smth.*); (*кого-л.*) cut*/trim *smb.'s* hair. ~ся, подстри́чься cut* *one's* hair; (*в парикмахерской*) have* *one's* hair cut; (*не коротко*) have* a trim.

подстри́чь(ся) *сов. см.* подстрига́ть(ся).

подстро́ить *сов. см.* подстра́ивать.

подстро́чн|ый: ~ое примеча́ние footnote; ~ перево́д word-for-word translation.

по́дступ *м.* approach; ~ы к го́роду the approaches to a town; ◇ к нему́ и ~а нет he is so difficult to approach.

подступ|а́ть, подступи́ть approach; слёзы подступи́ли к го́рлу tears came/rose to *one's* eyes. ~а́ться, подступи́ться *разг.* get* near, approach.

подступи́ть(ся) *сов. см.* подступа́ть(ся).

подсуди́мый *м.* the accused, the defendant.

подсу́дн|ый *юр.* within the jurisdiction *после сущ.*; де́ло ~о городско́му суду́ the case comes within the jurisdiction of the city court.

подсу́нуть *сов. см.* подсо́вывать.

подсу́шивать, подсуши́ть (*вн.*) dry (*smth.*) a little. ~ся, подсуши́ться dry a little, get* drier.

подсуши́ть(ся) *сов. см.* подсу́шивать(ся).

подсчёт *м.* 1. (*действие*) counting; ~ голосо́в poll, counting of the votes; 2. *мн.* (*итог расчётов*) calculations; предвари́тельные ~ы preliminary calculations/estimates.

подсчита́ть *сов. см.* подсчи́тывать.

подсчи́тывать, подсчита́ть (*вн.*) count (*smth.*) up, calculate (*smth.*), reckon up (*smth.*); ~ голоса́ count the votes; ~ расхо́ды reckon up the expenses; (*заранее*) calculate/estimate expenses.

подсыла́ть, подосла́ть (*вн.*) send* (*smb.*) for a (secret) purpose.

подосла́ть *сов. см.* подсыла́ть.

подсыпа́ть, подсы́пать 1. (*вн.*, *рд.*) (*прибавлять*) add (*smth.*); (*тайком*) slip (*smth.*) in secretly; 2. (*вн.*; *делать выше*) bank up (*smth.*).

подсыха́ть, подсо́хнуть dry off a little.

подта́лкивать, подтолкну́ть (*вн.*) push (*smb.*, *smth.*), shove (*smb.*, *smth.*); (*локтем*) nudge (*smb.*); *перен.* prompt (*smb.*).

подта́скивать, подтащи́ть (*вн.*) drag (*smth.*), pull (*smth.*).

подтащи́ть *сов. см.* подта́скивать.

подтасо́вка *ж.* fiddling; *перен. тж.* garbling, juggling; ~ фа́ктов juggling with the facts.

подтасо́вывать, подтасова́ть (*вн.*) fiddle (*smth.*); *перен. тж.* garble (*smth.*), juggle (with).

подта́чивать, подточи́ть (*вн.*) 1. (*делать острее*) sharpen (*smth.*); 2. (*разъедать*) eat* (*smth.*) away; (*размывать*) erode (*smth.*); undermine (*smth.*) (*тж. перен.*); боле́знь подточи́ла его́ си́лы the illness undermined his strength.

подтащи́ть *сов. см.* подта́скивать.

подтверди́ть(ся) *сов. см.* подтвержда́ть(ся).

подтвержд|а́ть, подтверди́ть (*вн.*) confirm (*smth.*), corroborate (*smth.*), prove the truth (of), vouch (for); фа́кты подтверди́ли э́ту тео́рию the facts corroborated the theory; ~ приказа́ние confirm an order; ~ получе́ние письма́ acknowledge (receipt of) a letter. ~а́ться, под-

тверди́ться be* confirmed, prove correct; его́ предсказа́ние подтверди́лось his prediction proved correct. ~е́ние *с.* confirmation, corroboration; ~е́ние получе́ния acknowledgement.

подтека́ть, подте́чь (под *вн.*) flow (under), run* (under).

подте́кст *м.* underlying idea, implication.

подтере́ть *сов. см.* подтира́ть.

подте́чь *сов. см.* подтека́ть.

подтира́ть, подтере́ть (*вн.*) wipe (*smth.*) up, mop (*smth.*) up.

подтолкну́ть *сов. см.* подта́лкивать.

подточи́ть *сов. см.* подта́чивать.

подтру́нивать, подтруни́ть (над *тв.*) chaff (*smb.*), banter (*smb.*).

подтруни́ть *сов. см.* подтру́нивать.

подтыка́ть, подоткну́ть (*вн.*) tuck up (*smth.*).

подтя́гивать, подтяну́ть (*вн.*) 1. (*затягивать потуже*) tighten (*smth.*); ~ по́яс tighten *one's* belt; 2. (*подтаскивать*) pull (*smth.*), draw* (*smth.*); 3. (*войска*) bring* up (*smth.*); 4. *разг.* (*заставлять лучше работать и т. п.*) ginger up (*smb.*), pep up (*smb.*); ~ отстаю́щих ginger up the laggards/stragglers; 5. (*подневать*) join in. ~ся, подтяну́ться 1. (*на руках*) pull/haul oneself up; 2. (*о войсках*) come* up, be* brought up; (*о колонне*) close its ranks; резе́рвы подтяну́лись reserves were brought up; 3. *разг.* (*в работе и т. п.*) brace up; (*об отстаю́щих*) catch* up with the rest.

подтя́жки *мн.* (*ед.* подтя́жка *ж.*) braces; suspenders *амер.*

подтя́нут|ость *ж.* bearing; *перен.* smartness, efficiency. ~ый braced; *перен.* smart, efficient.

подтяну́ть(ся) *сов. см.* подтя́гивать(ся).

поду́м|ать *сов.* 1. *см.* ду́мать 1, 4; 2. (*некоторое время*) think* a moment; ~ав, он реши́л идти́ after a moment's thought he decided to go.

поду́мывать *несов. разг.* 1. (о *пр.*) think* (of); 2. (+ инф.; *намереваться*) think* (of, about + -ing).

подурне́ть *сов. см.* дурне́ть.

поду́|ть *сов.* 1. *см.* дуть; 2. (*начать дуть*) begin* to blow; ~л холо́дный ве́тер a cold wind sprang up.

поду́чивать, подучи́ть (*вн.*) *разг.* 1. teach* (*smb.*); (*заучивать*) learn* (*smth.*); 2. (*подговаривать*) egg (*smb.*) on, put* (*smb.*) up to it. ~ся, подучи́ться *разг.* learn*; ему́ необходи́мо ещё подучи́ться he needs to improve his knowledge/skill.

подучи́ть(ся) *сов. см.* поду́чивать(ся).

поду́шк|а *ж.* 1. pillow; (*диванная*) cushion; 2. *тех.* cushion; су́дно на возду́шной ~е hovercraft.

подхали́м *м.* sycophant, toady; bootlicker, lickspittle *разг.* ~ничать *несов.* (перед *тв.*) *разг.* cringe (to, before), fawn (upon), kowtow (to). ~ство *с.* bootlicking, toadying.

подхвати́ть *сов. см.* подхва́тывать.

подхва́тывать, подхвати́ть (*вн.*) 1. (*поднимать*) pick up (*smb.*, *smth.*), hold* up (*smth.*); ~ мешо́к pick up a sack; 2. (*не давать упасть*) catch* (*smb.*, *smth.*); 3. (*брать резким движением*) seize (*smth.*); snatch up (*smth.*); grab (*smb.*, *smth.*) *разг.*; 4. *разг.* (*получать болезнь*) catch* (*smth.*); 5. (*поддерживать, продолжать*) take* up (*smth.*), pick up (*smth.*); ~ инициати́ву follow up *smb.'s* initiative; ~ мысль take* up an idea; 6. (*в пении*) take* up (*smth.*); подхвати́ть пе́сню take* up the song, join in.

подхлестну́ть *сов. см.* подхлёстывать.

подхлёстывать, подхлестну́ть (*вн.*) whip up (*smth.*); *перен. разг.* spur (*smb.*) on.

подхо́д *м.* approach; удо́бный ~ к реке́ convenient way down to the river; у неё нет никако́го ~а к ученика́м she doesn't know how to approach her pupils.

подходи́ть, подойти́ 1. (к *дт.*; *приближаться*) come* up (to), approach (*smb.*, *smth.*); он подошёл к дёвушке he went up to the girl; по́езд подхо́дит к ста́нции the train is appróaching a státion; **2.** (*наступа́ть — о собы́тии, вре́мени и т. п.*) draw* near, near; вре́мя подошло́ к полу́дню it was néaring mídday; рабо́та подхо́дит к концу́ the work is néaring complétion; **3.** (*к дт.; принима́ться за что-л., приступа́ть к чему́-л.*) procéed (to), appróach (*smth.*); подойти́ к изуче́нию дробе́й procéed to the stúdy of décimals; **4.** (*относи́ться как-либо*) appróach; подойти́ объекти́вно к оце́нке рабо́ты take* an objéctive áttitude/appróach in júdging the work; **5.** (*быть го́дным*) suit; (*по разме́ру*) fit; э́та рабо́та ему́ не подхо́дит it isn't the right work for him; ◇ ~ к концу́ be* néarly óver, be* néaring its end, cóme* to an end.

подходя́щ|ий súitable, próper; ~ моме́нт the right móment; он са́мое ~ее лицо́ для э́той до́лжности he is the most súitable man for the job.

подча́с sómetimes, at times.

подчёркивать, подчеркну́ть (*вн.*) **1.** underlíne (*smth.*), underscóre (*smth.*); **2.** (*особо выделя́ть*) émphasize (*smth.*), stress (*smth.*), lay* émphasis (on).

подчеркну́ть *сов. см.* подчёркивать.

подчине́н|ие *с.* subordinátion (*тж. грам.*); (*повинове́ние*) obédience, submíssion; быть в ~ии у кого́-л. be* *smb.'s* subórdinate.

подчине́нн|ость *ж.* subordinátion. ~ый *прил.* **1.** subórdinate (*тж. грам.*); (*подвла́стный*) súbject; **2.** *в знач. сущ. м.* subórdinate.

подчини́ть(ся) *сов. см.* подчиня́ть(ся).

подчиня́ть, подчини́ть **1.** (*вн.; покоря́ть*) súbjugate (*smb.*), subdúe (*smb.*), bring* (*smb.*) into subjéction; **2.** (*вн. дт.; ста́вить в зави́симость*) subórdinate (*smb., smth.* to), make* (*smth.*) obédient (to); ~ кого́-л. своему́ влия́нию gain an ínfluence óver *smb.*; **3.** (*вн. дт.; ста́вить под чьё-л. руково́дство*) place (*smb., smth.* únder); подчинённые кому́-л. войска́ the troops únder *smb.'s* commánd; **4.** (*дт.*) *грам.* subórdinate (to). ~ся, подчини́ться (*дт.*) submít (to), yield (to), obéy (*smb., smth.*); ~ся зако́ну obéy the law; ~ся рассу́дку yield to réason; ~ся си́ле submít/yield to force; ~ся чужо́му влия́нию submít to anóther's ínfluence; ~ся чу́вству obéy a féeling.

подчи́стить *сов. см.* подчища́ть.

подчища́ть, подчи́стить (*вн.*) **1.** clean up (*smth.*); **2.** (*соска́бливать напи́санное*) eráse (*smth.*), rub off (*smth.*).

подшéфный affíliated, adópted; spónsored by.

подшива́ть, подши́ть (*вн.*) **1.** (*пришива́ть с изна́нки, сни́зу*) sew* (*smth.*) in/on; (*обувь*) sole (*smth.*); ~ подкла́дку к пальто́ sew*/put* a líning ínto a coat, line a coat; **2.** (*подо́л и т. п.*) hem (*smth.*); **3.** (*бума́ги*) file (*smth.*); ~ докуме́нт к де́лу add a dócument to the file.

подши́вка *ж.* **1.** (*де́йствие*) bórdering, édging; (*обуви*) sóling; (*бума́г*) fíling; **2.** (*компле́кт газе́т и т. п.*) file.

подши́ть *сов. см.* подшива́ть.

подшути́ть *сов. см.* подшу́чивать.

подшу́чивать, подшути́ть (*над тв.*) make* fun of (*smb.*), play a práctical joke (on).

подъе́зд *м.* **1.** (*вход в зда́ние*) éntrance, porch; **2.** (*путь к чему́-л.*) appróaches *pl.*

подъездн|о́й appróach *attr.*; ~а́я алле́я dríveway.

подъезжа́ть, подъе́хать (к дт.) drive* up (to); (*верхо́м*) ride* up (to); *перен. разг.* have* a go (at).

подъём *м.* **1.** (*де́йствие*) lífting, ráising, hóisting; (*в го́ру*) ascént, climb; (*воды́*) rísing, rise; **2.** (*рост, разви́тие*) úpswing, úpsurge, rise; ~ промы́шленности expánsion/úpswing of índustry; ~ нау́ки vígorous devélopment of science; на ~е on the úpgrade; **3.** (*воодушевле́ние*) animátion, enthúsiasm; чу́вство ~а féeling of ́elevátion; **4.** (*го́ры*) ascént, slope; **5.** (*ноги́, о́буви*)

ínstep; ◇ тяжёл на ~ a slów-stárter, hard to budge; лёгок на ~ always réady, quick off the mark.

подъёмн|ик *м.* **1.** lift, élevator drag; (*в гора́х*) ski--lift; **2.** (*кран*) hoist, crane. ~ый lífting *attr.*; ~ая маши́на lift, élevator; ~ый кран crane; ~ая си́ла cárrying/ lífting capácity; ~ый мост dráwbridge; ◇ ~ые де́ньги reséttlement allówance *sg.*

подъе́хать *сов. см.* подъезжа́ть.

подыма́ть *несов. см.* поднима́ть.

поды́скать *сов. см.* поды́скивать.

поды́скивать, подыска́ть (*вн.*) seek* out (*smth.*); *сов. тж.* find* (*smth.*); *несов. тж.* try to find* (*smth.*), be* on the look out (for).

подыто́живать, подыто́жить (*вн.*) **1.** (*вычисля́ть о́бщую су́мму*) add up (*smth.*), tótal up (*smth.*); **2.** (*обобща́ть*) sum up (*smth.*); ~ свои́ впечатле́ния sum up *one's* impréssions.

подыто́жить *сов. см.* подыто́живать.

подыша́ть *сов.* have* a breath of air; (*на вн.*) breathe (on).

поеди́нок *м.* dúel.

поёживаться *несов.* hunch *one's* shóulders, hunch up.

по́езд *м.* train; е́здить ~ом go* by train.

пое́здить *сов.* trável wídely.

пое́здк|а *ж.* trip, jóurney; (*гастро́льная*) tour; (*рейс*) trip; соверша́ть ~у go* for a trip/jóurney; make* a trip/jóurney; соверша́ть гастро́льную ~у по Фра́нции tour the France.

пое́сть *сов.* **1.** eat*; (*вн., рд.*) have* (*smth.*) to eat, have* (*smth.*); ~ су́пу have* some soup; пло́тно ~ have* a good meal; **2.** (*вн.*) *разг.* (*съесть всё*) eat* all the (*smth.*), scoff (*smth.*).

пое́х|ать *сов.* **1.** go*; (*о сре́дствах передвиже́ния*) begin* to move; ~ по́ездом, трамва́ем и т. п. go* by train, tram *etc.*; ~ (со) сле́дующим по́ездом take* the next train; ~ напра́во turn off to the right; ну, ~али! let's start!; **2.** (*покати́ться*) start móving; кни́ги ~али со стола́ the books slid off the táble.

пожа́дничать *сов. см.* жа́дничать.

пожале́ть *сов. см.* жале́ть.

пожа́ловать *сов. см.* жа́ловать 1, 3.

пожа́ловаться *сов. см.* жа́ловаться.

пожа́луй (*вероя́тно*) perháps, véry líkely; (*должно́ быть*) I daresáy; ~, ты прав I daresáy; I think so.

пожа́луйста **1.** please; да́йте мне ещё хле́ба, ~! may I have some more bread, please?; входи́те, ~ come in, please; сади́тесь, ~ won't you sit down?; **2.** (*при выраже́нии согла́сия*) cértainly; by all means; мо́жно войти́? — Пожа́луйста! may I come in? — Please, do!; мо́жно я возьму́ ва́шу кни́гу? — Пожа́луйста! may I take your book? — Cértainly!, By all means!; **3.** (*в отве́т на выра́женную благода́рность*) not at all!; don't méntion it!, you're wélcome!

пожа́р *м.* fire; conflagrátion (*тж. перен.*); в до́ме ~ the house is on fire; ~ войны́ the fires of war; ◇ как на ~ in a flýing húrry; не на ~ the place ísn't on fire. ~ище *с.* site of a fire, destrúction left by fire; fire-ravaged remáins *pl.* ~ник *м.* fireman*. ~ный *прил.* **1.** fire *attr.*; ~ная трево́га fire-alarm; ~ная маши́на fire-engine; ~ная кома́нда fire-brigade; ~ная часть fire-station; ~ная ле́стница fire-escape; ~ный кран fire-hydrant; **2.** *в знач. сущ. м.* fireman*; ◇ на вся́кий ~ный слу́чай just in case (of need); сде́лать что-л. в ~ном поря́дке do* smth. in great haste.

пожа́тие *с.* hándshake, hándclasp.

пожа́ть I *сов. см.* пожима́ть.

пожа́ть II *сов. см.* пожина́ть.

пожева́ть *сов.* chew.

пожела́ни|е *с.* wish; наилу́чшие ~я best wishes, all good wíshes.

пожела́ть *сов. см.* жела́ть.

пожелте́лый yéllow, yéllowed.

пожелтѐть *сов. см.* желтѐть 1.

поженѝться *сов. разг.* get* márried.

поже́ртвование *с.* donátion, contribútion.

поже́ртвовать *сов. см.* же́ртвовать.

пожив|а́ть *несов.:* как вы ~а́ете? how are you gétting on?

поживѝться *сов. (тв.) разг.* prófit (by), reap a prófit.

пожѝзненн|ый life *attr.;* for life *после сущ.;* ~ая пѐнсия life pénsion.

пожило́й élderly.

пожима́ть, пожа́ть *(вн.)* shake* *(smth.),* press *(smth.);* онѝ пожа́ли друг дру́гу ру́ки they shook hands; ◇ ~ плеча́ми shrug *one's* shóulders.

пожина́ть, пожа́ть *(вн.)* reap *(smth.) (тж. перен.);* ~ плоды́ свои́х трудо́в reap the fruits of *one's* lábour; ◇ ~ ла́вры reap/win* the láurels; что посѐешь, то и пожнѐшь *посл.* we reap as we sow, we reap what we have sown.

пожира́ть *несов. (вн.)* devóur *(smb., smth.) (тж. перен.);* ◇ ~ кого́-л. глаза́ми devóur *smb.* with *one's* eyes.

пожѝтк|и *мн. разг.* things, belóngings; со всѐми ~ами bag and bággage.

пожѝть *сов.* 1: live; ~ год на ю́ге spend* a year in the south; поживѐм — уви́дим *погов.* we shall see what we shall see; 2. *разг. (наслади́ться жи́знью)* enjóy life; ~ в своѐ удово́льствие see* life, have* a good time.

по́з|а *ж.* pose, pósture; áttitude *(тж. перен.);* приня́ть ~у assúme a pose.

позаба́вить *сов. (вн.)* amúse *(smb.),* entertáin *(smth.).* ~ся *сов. (тв.)* amúse onesélf (with).

позабо́титься *сов. см.* забо́титься.

позабы́ть *сов. (вн.,* о *пр.)* forgét* (all abóut) *(smb., smth.).*

позави́довать *сов. см.* зави́довать.

поза́втракать *сов. см.* за́втракать.

позавчера́ *разг.* the day befóre yésterday.

позади́ 1. *нареч.* behínd, at the back; далеко́ ~ far behínd; 2. *нареч. (в про́шлом)* behínd, óver; 3. *предлог (рд.)* behínd; сидѐть ~ всех sit* behínd éveryone; ◇ оста́вить кого́-л. ~ leave* *smb.* behínd.

позаи́мствовать *сов. (вн.)* bórrow *(smth.).*

позанима́ться *сов. разг.* work, do* some work.

позапро́шлый befóre last *после сущ.;* ~ год the year befóre last.

позва́ть *сов. см.* звать 1, 2.

позволѐни|е *с.* permíssion, leave; проси́ть ~я уйти́ ask permíssion to go; с ва́шего ~я with your permíssion/leave; ◇ с ~я сказа́ть an apólogy for; э́та, ~я сказа́ть, пьѐса this apólogy for a play, this play — if such it may be called.

позволи́тельный permíssible.

позво́лить *сов. см.* позволя́ть.

позволя́ть, позво́лить 1. *(дт. вн., дт. + инф.)* allów *(smb. smth., smb. + to inf)*, permít *(smb. smth., smb. + to inf);* 2. *(дт. + инф.; дава́ть возмо́жность)* make* it póssible (for *smb. + to inf),* énable *(smb. + to inf);* но́вая тѐхника позво́лит досро́чно вы́полнить план the new machínery will make it póssible to fulfíl the plan ahéad of schédule; ѐсли врѐмя позво́лит if there is time, if time allóws; ◇ позво́лить себѐ что́-л. 1) vénture *smth.*, take* the líberty (of + -ing); 2) *(быть в состоя́нии сде́лать что́-л.)* allów onesélf *smth.;* он мно́гое себѐ позволя́ет he takes a good mány líberties.

позвони́ть *сов. см.* звони́ть.

позвон|о́к *м.* vértebra *(pl* -ae). ~о́чник *м.* spine, báckbone. ~о́чный vértebral, spinal; ~о́чный столб vertebral/spinal cólumn; ~о́чные живо́тные vértebrates.

по́здн|ий late; ~ прихо́д late arrival; ~ие цветы́ late flówers; ~ урожа́й late hárvest; ~ей о́сенью in late

а́utumn; до ~ей но́чи late into the night; са́мое ~ее в суббо́ту Sáturday at the látest.

по́здно 1. *нареч.* late; ~ но́чью late at night; ~ ложи́ться go* to bed late, sit*/stay up late; ~ верну́ться домо́й come* home late; 2. *в знач. сказ. безл.* it is too late.

поздоро́ваться *сов. см.* здоро́ваться.

поздоровѐть *сов. см.* здоровѐть.

поздоро́в|иться *сов. разг.:* ему́ не ~ится he will get into tróuble, he will be for it.

поздрави́тельн|ый congrátulatory; ~ая телегра́мма grééting telegram.

поздра́в|ить *сов. см.* поздравля́ть. ~лѐние *с.* congratulátion; принести́ ~лѐния кому́-л. óffer *one's* congratulátions to *smb.*

поздравля́ть, поздра́вить *(вн. с тв.)* congrátulate *(smb. on, upón);* ~ кого́-л. с днѐм рожде́ния wish *smb.* mány háppy retúrns (of the day); ~ кого́-л. с Но́вым го́дом wish *smb.* a háppy New Year.

позеленѐть *сов. см.* зеленѐть 2.

поземѐльный land *attr.;* ~ нало́г lánd-tax.

позѐр *м.* pláy-actor, húmbug, poséur.

по́зже *(сравнит. ст. нареч.* по́здно) láter.

по-зи́мнему as in winter; одѐт ~ dressed in winter clothes.

пози́ровать *несов.* 1. pose; ~ для портрѐта sit* for *one's* pórtrait; 2. *(рисова́ться)* put* on airs, try for effect, strike* áttitudes.

пози́тив *м. фото* pósitive.

позити́вный pósitive.

позитро́н *м. физ.* pósitron.

позицио́нн|ый posítional, posítion *attr.;* ~ая война́ posítional/trench wárfare.

пози́ция *ж.* posítion; *(отноше́ние тж.)* áttitude.

познава́ем|ость *ж.* cognoscibílity; ~ ми́ра the possibílity of knówing the world. ~ый knówable, cognóscible, cógnizable.

познава́тельн|ый cógnitive; ~ая спосо́бность cognítion; ~ое значе́ние иску́сства the infórmative válue of art, the power of art to infórm.

познава́ть, позна́ть *(вн.)* 1. *(приобрета́ть зна́ния)* percéive *(smth.); филос.* cógnize *(smth.); (хорошо́ узна́вать)* get* to know *(smb., smth.),* get* acquáinted (with); ~ зако́ны приро́ды percéive the laws of náture; 2. *(испы́тывать, пережива́ть)* know* *(smth.),* expérience *(smth.);* ~ го́речь отступле́ния know* the bítterness of deféat; ~ ра́дость свобо́ды expérience the joy of fréedom. ~ся *несов.* be* known; друзья́ познаю́тся в бедѐ *посл.* a friend in need is a friend indéed.

познако́мить(ся) *сов. см.* знако́мить(ся).

позна́ни|е *с.* 1. knówledge; *филос.* cognítion; тео́рия ~я théory of knówledge; 2. *мн. (совоку́пность зна́ний)* knówledge *sg.*

позна́ть *сов. см.* познава́ть.

позоло́т|а *ж.* gilt, gílding. ~и́ть *сов. см.* золоти́ть.

позоло́ченный gílded, gilt.

позо́р *м.* shame, disgráce, ínfamy. ~ить, опозо́рить *(вн.)* disgráce *(smb., smth.),* dishónour *(smb., smth.); (срами́ть)* put* *(smb.)* to shame. ~иться, опозо́риться disgráce onesélf. ~ный disgráceful, shámeful; ◇ пригвозди́ть кого́-л. к ~ному столбу́ píllory *smb.*, hold* *smb.* up to públic scorn.

позы́в *м. (к дт.)* desíre (for), inclinátion (for); ~ к рво́те féeling of náusea.

позывн|о́й signal *attr.;* ~ы́е *мн.* cáll-sign *sg.*

поигра́ть *сов.* play a little; have* a game.

поимённо by name. ~ый: ~ый спи́сок list of names, nóminal list/roll.

поименова́ть *сов. (вн.)* name *(smb., smth.).*

пои́мка *ж.* cátching; cápture; ~ на мѐсте преступле́ния cátching in the act.

поинтересова́ться *сов.* (*тв.*) show* an ínterest (in), be* ínterested (in).

по́иск *м. воен.* recónnaissance raid; *мор. тж.* sweep.

поиска́ть *сов.* (*вн.*) have* a look (for).

по́иски *мн.* 1. search *sg*, quest *sg*; hunt *sg разг.*; ~ но́вых форм the quest for new forms; отпра́виться на ~ кого́-л. set* out in search of *smb.*; 2. *геол.* prospécting *sg.*

пои́стине indéed, in truth, trúly; ~ гига́нтские разме́ры корабля́ the trúly gigántic size of the ship.

пои́ть *несов.* (*вн.*) give* (*smb.*) a drink; (*скот*) wáter (*smth.*); ~ кого́-л. ча́ем give* (*smb.*) sóme tea; ~ кого́-л. вино́м give* *smb.* wine to drink.

пойло *с.* swill, mash; (*для свине́й*) hóg-wash; pígswill.

пойма́ть *сов. см.* лови́ть.

пойти́ *сов.* 1. *см.* идти́ 6, 7, 8, 13, 20—25; 2. (*нача́ть идти́*) set* off, go* off; ~ пешко́м set* off on foot; 3. (*нача́ть дви́гаться*) begín* to move; start; по́езд пошёл the train stárted; 4. (*нача́ть те́чь*) begín to come/flow; 5. (*об оса́дках*) begín* to fall; пошёл снег it began to snow.

пока́ 1. *нареч.* (*в да́нный моме́нт*) for the présent; (*на не́которое вре́мя*) for the time béing; (*тем вре́менем*) méanwhile; (*до сих пор*) as yet; э́того ~ доста́точно that is enóugh for the time béing; никаки́х новосте́й ~ нет no news as yet; 2. *союз* (*в то вре́мя как*) while; 3. *союз* (*до того́ вре́мени как*) till, untíl; он не придёт, ~ вы его́ не пригласи́те he will not come till you invíte him, he will not come till he is invíted; ◇ ~ что so far; ~ что он не даёт отве́та so far he gives no ánswer; ~! *разг.* býe-for-nów!, býe-býe!, see you (soon)!, chéerio!

пока́з *м.* shówing, demonstrátion; displáy; ~ но́вого кинофи́льма shówing of a new film.

показа́ни|е *с.* 1. téstimony, évidence; (*пи́сьменное под прися́гой*) affidávit, deposítion; дава́ть ~я téstify, bear* téstimony, give* évidence; 2. (*измери́тельных прибо́ров*) réading.

показа́тель *м.* 1. proof, índicator; *обы́кн. мн.* (*нагля́дное выраже́ние в ци́фрах*) índex (*pl* índices); ~ культу́рного у́ровня índicator of the cúltural lével; 2. *мат.* expónent, índex. **~ный** 1. (*характе́рный*) signíficant; 2. (*организо́ванный для всео́бщего ознакомле́ния*) demonstrátion *attr.*; 3. (*образцо́вый*) módel *attr.*

показ|а́ть *сов. см.* пока́зывать. **~а́ться** *сов. см.* пока́зываться *и* каза́ться. **~но́й** ostentátious, put on; for show *по́сле сущ.*

показу́ха *ж. разг. неодобр.* window-dréssing.

пока́зыв|ать, **показа́ть** 1. (*вн.*) show* (*smth.*); (*демонстри́ровать*) démonstrate (*smth.*), perfórm (*smth.*); ~ кому́-л. доро́гу show* *smb.* the way; ~ фо́кус perfórm/démonstrate a trick; ~ пье́су show*/perfórm a play; 2. (*на вн.; ука́зывать*) point (to), índicate (*smth.*); ~ глаза́ми на что́-л. índicate *smth.* with one's eyes, índicate *smth.* with a look; ~ руко́й на окно́ point to the window; 3. (*вн.; разъясня́ть*) expláin (*smth.*); 4. (*вн.; проявля́ть каки́е-л. ка́чества*) displáy (*smth.*), show* (*smth.*); (*реко́рд, вре́мя и т. п.*) achíeve (*smth.*); ~ хра́брость displáy/show* cóurage; ~ лу́чший результа́т в бе́ге achíeve the best resúlt in the rúnning events; ~ реко́рдную ско́рость beat*/break*/top the speed récord; 5. (*вн.; об измери́тельных прибо́рах*) show* (*smth.*), read* (*smth.*), índicate (*smth.*); 6. (*на вн.; дава́ть показа́ния*) téstify (agáinst), give* évidence (agáinst); 7. (*дт.*) *разг.* (*проу́чивать*) show* (*smb.*), teach* (*smb.*) a lésson; я вам покажу́! I'll teach you!; ◇ показа́ть себя́ show* onesélf; но́са не ~ not show* one's face; показа́ть приме́р show* an exámple; показа́ть язы́к put* out one's tongue. **~аться**, **показа́ться** 1. (*станови́ться ви́дным, проявля́ться*) appéar, come* in sight; наконе́ц показа́лся бе́рег the shore came in sight at last; 2. (*явля́ться, приходи́ть куда́-л.*) show* onesélf, appéar; он нигде́ не

~ается he néver goes ánywhere; он бои́тся показа́ться вам на глаза́ he is afráid to appéar in front of you; ~ться врачу́ see* a dóctor.

пока́лыв|ать *несов. разг.* 1. prick; 2. *безл.*: у меня́ ~ает в боку́ I have the stitch.

покапри́зничать be* tróublesome, give* a líttle tróuble.

покара́ть *сов. см.* кара́ть.

поката́ть *сов.* (*вн.*) 1. roll (*smth.*) for a while; 2. (*повози́ть*) take* (*smth.*) for a short ride/drive. **~ся** *сов.* take* a ride, go* for a short ride/drive.

покати́ть *сов.* 1. (*вн.*) roll (*smth.*); 2. *разг.* (*бы́стро пое́хать*) speed* awáy/off. **~ся** *сов.* 1. roll (*по накло́нной пло́скости*) roll (down); ма́чик покати́лся под стол the ball rolled únder the táble; ~ся с горы́ roll downhill; 2. (*дви́нуться, пое́хать*) drive* off; drive*; 3. (*о слеза́х, по́те*) roll down; ◇ ~ся со́ смеху rock with láughter.

пока́т|ость *ж.* slope, íncline. **~ый** slóping; ~ый лоб retréating fórehead; ~ые пле́чи slóping shóulders.

покача́ть *сов.* 1. (*вн.; не́которое вре́мя*) rock (*smb., smth.*) for a while; ~ ребёнка dándle a child*; 2. (*тв.; качну́ть не́сколько раз*) shake* (*smth.*); ~ голово́й shake* one's head; **~ся** *сов.* rock; (*на каче́лях и т. n.*) swing*.

пока́чивать *несов.* 1. (*вн., тв.*) rock slíghtly; 2. *безл.* it's ráther rough. **~ся** *несов.* rock; (*пошатыва́ться*) stágger, tótter, be* unstéady on one's legs; ~ся на волна́х rock on the waves; ~ся в кре́сле rock onesélf (in one's chair; идти́ пока́чиваясь walk unstéadily, roll/stump alóng.

покачн|у́ть *сов.* (*вн.*) give* (*smth.*) a push; (*накрени́ть*) tip (*smth.*), tip (*smth.*) up. **~у́ться** *сов.* sway, lurch; *перен.* take* a turn for the worse; дела́ ~у́лись things are lóoking bad/black.

пока́шливать *несов.* have* a slight cough.

пока́йн|ие *с.* 1. (*и́споведь*) conféssion; (*наказа́ние*) pénance; 2. (*раска́яние*) repéntance; ◇ отпусти́ть ду́шу на ~ let* *smb.* alóne, leave* *smb.* in peace. **~ный** repéntant, pénitent.

пока́яться *сов. см.* ка́яться 1, 2.

поквит|а́ться *сов. разг.* be* quits; (*с тв.*) be*/get* éven (with); я ещё с тобо́й ~а́юсь! I'll be/get éven with you yet!, I'll pay you out one day!

покида́ть, **поки́нуть** (*вн.*) (*уходи́ть от кого́-л.*) desért (*smb.*); abándon (*smb.*), forsáke* (*smb.*); (*уходи́ть отку́да-л.*) leave* (*smth.*), quit (*smth.*); его́ все поки́нули he was abándoned by éveryone; поки́нуть го́род leave* (the) town; поки́нуть сце́ну leave*/quit the stage; поки́нуть дру́га forsáke* a friend; си́лы поки́нули меня́ my strength failed me.

поки́нуть *сов. см.* покида́ть.

покладая́: рабо́тать не ~ рук work without réspite, press on with one's work.

покла́дистый oblíging, éasy-going, complíant.

покла́жа *ж. разг.* (*груз*) load; (*бага́ж*) lúggage.

поклёп *м. разг.* slánder, cálumny; возводи́ть ~ на кого́-л. slánder *smb.*, smear *smb.*

покло́н *м.* 1. bow; 2. (*приве́т*) regárds *pl*, best wishes *pl*; передáть ~ кому́-л. send* *smb.* one's regárds; передáйте ~ ва́шему бра́ту remémber me to your bróther; ◇ идти́ на ~ к кому́-л. go* cap in hand to *smb.* **~е́ние** *с.* 1. wórship; 2. (*преклоне́ние*) admirátion, adorátion.

поклони́ться *сов. см.* кла́няться.

покло́нн|ик *м.*, **~ица** *ж.* admírer.

поклоня́ться *несов.* (*дт.*) wórship (*smb., smth.*), adóre (*smb., smth.*).

покля́сться *сов. см.* кля́сться.

поко́иться *несов.* 1. (*на пр.; опира́ться*) rest (on, upón), be* based (on), repóse (upón, on); 2. (*споко́йно лежа́ть*) repóse, lie*.

поко́|й *м.* 1. (*тишина*) quíetness, stíllness; 2. (*неподвижность*) immobílity; 3. (*спокойствие*) peace, tranquíllity; больно́му необходи́м по́лный ~ the pátient needs compléte rest; 4. *уст.* (*комната*) apártment; ◇ не дава́ть ~я кому́-л. give* smb. no peace; оставля́ть кого́-л. в ~e leave* smb. in peace; смути́ть чей-л. ~ distúrb smb.'s peace of mind; уйти́ на ~ retíre; ве́чный ~ rest etérnal; приёмный ~ recéption ward.

поко́йн|ик *м.* dead pérson; (*при упоминании об умершем*) the decéased. **~ица** *ж.* dead wóman*.

поко́йницкая *ж.* mórtuary.

поко́йн|ый *прил.* 1. (*спокойный*) quíet, calm; 2. (*умерший*) the late; 3. *в знач. сущ. м. см.* поко́йник; ◇ ~ой но́чи good night; бу́дьте ~ы you may be sure.

поколеба́ть *сов. см.* колеба́ть. **~ся** *сов. см.* колеба́ться 2, 4.

поколе́ни|e *с.* generátion; молодо́е ~ the yóunger/new/next generátion; на́ше ~ the présent generátion; ◇ из ~я в ~ from generátion to generátion.

поколоти́ть *сов. разг.* 1. (*вн.; побить*) beat* (smb.), give* (smb.) a béating/thráshing; 2. (*по дт.; постучать*) hámmer (on, at).

поко́нчить *сов.* (с *тв.*) 1. (*довести до конца*) fínish with (smth.); ~ с рабо́той be through with one's work; 2. (*прекратить*) put* an end (to), do* awáy (with); ◇ ~ с собо́й commít suícide.

покоре́ние *с.* cónquest; *перен. тж.* táming; ~ ко́смоса the cónquest of óuter space.

покори́тель *м.* cónqueror; ◇ ~ серде́ц lády-killer. **~ница** *ж.*: **~ница серде́ц** chármer (of men).

покори́ть(ся) *сов. см.* покоря́ть(ся).

покорми́ть *сов.* (*вн.*) feed* (smb., smth.).

поко́рн|о submíssively, húmbly; ~ благодарю́ thank you kíndly. **~ость** *ж.* submíssiveness; (*послушание*) submíssion, obédience. **~ый** submíssive, obédient, húmble; ◇ ваш ~ый слуга́ your obédient sérvant; слуга́ ~ый! I beg to díffer!

покоро́бить(ся) *сов. см.* коро́бить(ся).

покоря́ть, покори́ть (*вн.*) 1. (*силой подчинять*) cónquer (smb., smth.), subdúe (smb., smth.); *перен. тж.* tame (smth.), hárness (smth.); 2. (*пленять*) win* smb.'s heart, vánquish (smb.); ◇ ~ сердца́ win* all hearts. **~ся, покори́ться** (*дт.*) submít (to), surrénder (to); (*обстоятельствам тж.*) resígn onesélf (to); ~ся судьбе́ resígn onesélf to fate.

поко́с *м.* 1. (*косьба*) mówing, hay hárvest, háymaking; второ́й ~ sécond mówing; 2. (*время косьбы*) háymaking time; 3. (*луг*) háyfield, grássland.

покоси́ться *сов. см.* коси́ться 1. и 2. (*искривиться*) be* léaning óver/sídeways; дом покоси́лся the house is léaning óver.

покра́жа *ж. разг.* theft.

покра́сить *сов. см.* кра́сить 1.

покрасне́ть *сов. см.* красне́ть 1, 2.

покри́кивать *несов.* (*на вн.*) call out, útter cries; (*на вн.; бранить*) tell* (smth.) off, réprimand (smth.).

покро́в *м.* cóver; *перен. тж.* cloak, shroud; сне́жный ~ blánket of snow; ◇ под ~ом темноты́, но́чи únder cóver of dárkness, night.

покрови́тель *м.* pátron, protéctor, spónsor. **~ница** *ж.* pátroness, protéctress.

покрови́тельственн|ый 1. pátronizing; ~ тон pátronizing tone; 2. *эк.*: **~ая систе́ма** protéctionism; ~ тари́ф protéctive táriff; ◇ ~ая окра́ска *биол.* protéctive cólouring.

покрови́тельство *с.* pátronage, protéction; взять кого́-л. под своё ~ take* smb. únder one's protéction/wing. **~вать** *несов.* (*дт.*) pátronize (smb., smth.), protéct (smb., smth.).

покро́й *м.* style, cut, fáshion; ◇ все на оди́н ~ all of the same páttern/style.

покроши́ть *сов.* (*вн., рд.*) crúmble a little (smth.).

покружи́ть *сов.* 1. roam abóut/aróund; 2. (*вн.*) spin* (smth.) round. **~ся** *сов.* turn round and round; (*о птицах и т. п.*) fly* aróund, círcle, wheel.

покрути́ть *сов.* (*вн., тв.*) twist (smth.). **~ся** *сов.* go* round.

покрыва́ло *с.* cloth; (*вуаль*) veil; (*для постели*) cóverlet, cóunterpane.

покрыва́ть, покры́ть (*вн.*) 1. (*закрывать чем-л., накрывать*) cóver (smth.); (*крышей*) roof (smth.); ~ желе́зом cóver with íron; ~ дом черепи́цей roof a house with tiles; 2. (*краской и т. п.*) coat (smth.); paint (smth.); ~ что-л. ла́ком várnish smth., cóver smth. with várnish; 3. (*усеивать поверхность чем-л., окутывать*) cóver (smth.); ве́тер покры́л пруд ме́лкой ря́бью a breeze ríppled the súrface of the pond; ~ мгло́ю shroud in dárkness; кра́сные пя́тна покры́ли её лицо́ her face broke out in red spots; 4. (*заглушать*) drown (smth.); 5. (*возмещать*) pay* off (smth.), dischárge (smth.); ~ расхо́ды meet*/cóver the expénses; ~ убы́тки cóver one's lósses, make* up for one's lósses; 6. (*скрывать, укрывать*) hush up (smth.); protéct (smth.); ~ свои́х сообщников protéct one's assóciates; 7. (*расстояние*) cóver (smth.); лы́жники покры́ли диста́нцию за 15 мину́т the skiers cóvered the distance in fiftéen mínutes; ◇ ~ сла́вой cóver with glóry. **~ся, покры́ться** (*тв.*) becóme*/be* cóvered (with); не́бо покры́лось ту́чами the sky becáme clóudy, héavy clouds gáthered in the sky; его́ лицо́ покры́лось пя́тнами his face became blótchy.

покры́тие *с.* 1. (*действие*) cóvering; (*краской*) cóating; (*дорог*) súrfacing; (*долгов*) páyment, dischárge; ~ кры́ши róofing; 2. (*материал*) súrface; доро́жное ~ road súrface.

покры́ть *сов. см.* покрыва́ть *и* крыть. **~ся** *сов. см.* покрыва́ться.

покры́шка *ж.* 1. *разг.* (*крышка*) lid; 2 (*шины*) týre(-cover); (*мяча*) cóver (smth.).

покупа́тель *м.*, **~ница** *ж.* búyer, púrchaser; (*в магазине тж.*) cústomer. **~ный** púrchasing; **~ная способность** населе́ния the púrchasing pówer of the populátion; ~ная си́ла рубля́ the púrchasing pówer of the róuble. **~ский** búyer's, púrchaser's.

покупа́ть, купи́ть (*вн.*) 1. (*приобретать*) buy* (smth.), púrchase (smth.); 2. (*подкупать*) buy* (smb.), bribe (smb.).

поку́пк|а *ж.* 1. (*действие*) búying, púrchasing; 2. (*приобретённая вещь*) púrchase; вы́годная ~ a bárgain; де́лать ~и go* shópping, do* the shópping, make* some púrchases.

покупн|о́й 1. bought, púrchased; 2. (*покупательный*) púrchasing; ~ая спосо́бность púrchasing pówer.

покури́ть *сов.* have* a smoke; дава́йте поку́рим! let's have a smoke!

покус|а́ть *сов.* (*вн.*) bite* (smb., smth.); (*ужалить*) sting* (smb., smth.); его́ ~а́ли пчёлы he got bádly stung by bees.

покуси́ться *сов. см.* покуша́ться.

покусыв|ать *несов.* (*вн.*) *разг.* bite* (smth.); моро́з ~ает щёки the frost makes one's cheeks burn, the frost nips one's cheeks.

поку́шать *сов.* eat*.

покуш|а́ться, покуси́ться (**на** *вн.*) attémpt (smth.); (*посягать*) encróach (upón), try to take (smth.); ~ на чью-л. жизнь make* an attémpt on smb.'s life. **~е́ние** *с.* attémpt; (*посягательство*) encróachment; ~е́ние на чью-л. жизнь attémpt on smb.'s life; ~е́ние на свобо́ду attémpt to restríct líberty.

пол I *м.* (*настил*) floor; настила́ть ~ lay* a floor; натира́ть ~ pólish the floor.

пол II *м. биол.* sex; ребёнок мужско́го (же́нского) ~a male (fémale) child*; ◇ прекра́сный ~ *шутл.* fair sex; си́льный ~ *шутл.* the strónger/stérner sex.

пол- *в сложн.* half-.

пол|á *ж.* flap; ◇ из-под ~ы́ on the sly; продавáть из-под ~ы́ sell* únder the cóunter.

полагáть *несов.* think*, belíeve; ~áют, что он в Москвé he is suppósed to be in Móscow; нáдо ~, что он придёт it may be presúmed that he will come, he will presúmably come.

полагáться I *несов.* **1.:** так ~áется that's the way things are done; it is the cústomary/úsual thing; здесь курйть не ~áется one is not supposed to smoke here; так поступáть не ~áется you shóuldn't do that; **2.** (*дт.*; *причитаться*) be* due (to); за рабóту емý ~áется 200 рублéй he is to recéive two húndred róubles for the work he has done; скóлько мне ~áется? how much is due to me?

полаг|áться II, положйться (на *вн.*) relý (upón), depénd (upón); я ~áюсь на вас I depénd/relý upón you; ~ на чьё-л. мнéние defér to *smb.'s* opínion; на негó нельзя́ положйться you can't depénd/relý on him, he is not to be relíed on.

полáд|ить *сов.* (с *тв.*) *разг.* come* to an understánding (with); онй не ~или мéжду собóй they dídn't get on.

полáкомиться *сов. см.* лáкомиться.

полбеды́ *в знач. сказ.* a small loss; э́то ещё ~ it is not so véry sérious.

полвéка *м.* half a céntury.

полгóда *м.* half a year; six months *pl.*

полдéла *с. разг.* half the work; э́то ещё ~! that's not all!; that's ónly half the báttle!

пóлдень *м.* noon, mídday, nóonday; рóвно в ~ at the stroke of noon; ◇ зá ~ áfter/past mídday; in the afternóon.

полднéвный mídday *attr.*

пóлдни|к *м.* (afternóon) tea. ~чать *несов. разг.* have* one's afternóon tea.

полдорóг|и *ж.* half-wáy; ◇ остановйться на ~е stop half-wáy.

полдю́жины *ж.* half a dózen.

пóл|е *с.* **1.** field (*тж. перен.*); ~ под пáром fállow field; спортйвное ~ pláying field(s); ~ дéятельности sphere of actívity, field of áction; магнйтное ~ magnétic field; **2.** (*фон*) ground; свéтлые цветá на тёмном ~ light cólours on a dark ground; **3.** *обыкн. мн.* (*у книги и т. п.*) márgin *sg*; замéтки на ~áх márginal notes; **4.** *мн.* (*шляпы*) brim *sg*; ◇ ~ зрéния field of vísion; ~ сражéния báttle-field, field (of báttle); одйн в ~ не вóин *посл.* ≈ one man no man.

полевóд *м.* field-crop grówer, cúltivator. ~ство *с.* field-crop grówing/cultivátion. ~ческий field-crop *attr.*

полев|óй field *attr.*; ~ы́е цветы́ wild/field flówers; ~ы́е рабóты field work *sg*; ~ стан field camp; ~ гóспиталь field hóspital; ~áя пóчта field póst-office; ~áя артиллéрия field artíllery; ◇ шпат fél(d)spar; ~áя сýмка field bag.

полегóньку *разг.* little by líttle; by éasy stáges.

полегчáть *сов. см.* легчáть.

полежáть *сов.* (*о человеке*) lie* down (for a while); (*о вещах*) remáin, stay.

полезащйт|ый ~ое лесонасаждéние field-protéctive afforestátion; ~ая леснáя полосá afforestátion belt, wind-break.

полéзн|ый 1. úseful; (*для здоровья*) good*; ~ая пйща nóurishing/whólesome food; сочетáть ~ое с прия́тным combíne búsiness with pléasure; **2.** *mex.* úseful, efféctive; ~ая нагрýзка pay load; ~ая плóщадь úseful space; ◇ чем могý быть полéзен? what can I do for you?

полéзть *сов.* **1.** (*начать лезть*) begín* to climb; ~ в вóду get* ínto the wáter; **2.** (*в вн.*; *в стол и т. п.*) put* one's hand (ínto); ~ в кармáн put* *one's* hand ínto *one's* pócket; ~ в шкаф rúmmage in a cúpboard.

полемизйровать *несов.* (с *тв.*) árgue (with), pólemize (with).

полéмика *ж.* polémics *pl*, dispúte, cóntroversy.

полемйческий polémic(al).

поленйться *сов.* (+ *инф.*) be* too lázy (+ to *inf*).

полéно *с.* log.

полéсье *с.* márshy scrub.

полёт *м.* flight; ~ на дáльнее расстоя́ние long-dístance flight; ~ в кóсмос space flight; ~ на Лунý flight to the Moon, Moon flight; самолёт прóбыл в пять часóв the áircraft was in the air for five hours; фигýрные ~ы aerobátics, stunt flýing *sg*; ◇ ~ фантáзии flight of imaginátion; вид с птйчьего ~а bird's-eye view.

полетáть *сов.* fly* (for a while).

полет|éть *сов.* **1.** fly* up, take* wing; (*о самолёте*) take* off, becóme* áirborne; (*на самолёте*) fly*, make* a flight; **2.** *разг.* (*упасть*) túmble, fall*; всё ~éло со столá éverything went flýing off the táble; **3.** (*стремительно двинуться*) dash off; go* dáshing/rúshing/spéeding; **4.** (*о письмах, донесениях и т. п.*) flash, fly*, be* flashed; **5.** (*быстро распространяться*) flash round; **6.** (*о времени*) дни ~éли the days flashed by.

по-лéтнему as in súmmer.

полечйть *сов.* (*вн.*) treat (*smb.*), give* (*smb.*) some tréatment. ~ся *сов.* take* a cure, have* some tréatment.

полéчь *сов.* **1.** *разг.* (*лечь*) lie* down; **2.** (*быть убитым*) be* killed; **3.** (*о растениях*) lie* flat, be* fláttened, be* béaten down.

пóлзать *несов.* creep*, crawl; (*перед тв.*) *перен.* cringe (to), fawn (upón); kowtów (to).

ползкóм on *one's* hands and knees, on all fours, cráwling.

ползтй *несов.* **1.** crawl; (*о насекомых и т. п. тж.*) creep*; **2.** (*медленно передвигаться, распространяться*) creep*, spread*; чёрные тýчи ползлй по нéбу black clouds spread acróss the sky; **3.** (*скользить*) slide*; **4.** (*медленно литься, течь*) tríckle, ooze; **5.** (*о времени*) creep* by; **6.** *разг.* (*расползаться — о ткани*) go* to pieces.

ползýч|ий cráwling, créeping; ~ие растéния créepers.

полúв *м.* wátering, sprínkling.

полив|áть, полúть **1.** (*вн.*) (*улицы, растения*) wáter (*smth.*); (*на руки*) pour (*smth.*) on; **2.:** дождь ~áет it is póuring; ◇ ~ грязью когó-л. fling*/throw* mud at *smb.* ~áться, полúться wáter óver onesélf.

поливинилхлорúд *м.* polyvinýlchlóride, PVC.

поливитамúны *мн.* polyvítamin táblets.

полúвка *ж.* wátering.

поливнóй 1. (*применяющий искусственное орошение*) irrigátion *attr.*; **2.** (*нуждающийся в поливке*) requíring irrigátion *после сущ.*

полúвочный wátering *attr.*

полигáмия *ж.* polýgamy.

полиглóт *м.* pólyglot.

полигóн *м. воен.* shóoting-range; (*для испытания оружия*) experiméntal range, próving ground.

полиграфйческ|ий prínting *attr.*; ~ая промы́шленность prínting índustry; ~ комбинáт (múltiple) prínting plant.

полиграфúя *ж.* prínting índustry.

поликлúника *ж.* (out-pátient's) polyclínic.

полимéры *мн.* pólymers.

полиня́лый fáded, discóloured.

полиня́ть *сов. см.* линя́ть.

полиомиелúт *м. мед.* poliomyelítis.

полúп *м.* **1.** *зоол.* pólyp; **2.** *мед.* pólypus (*pl* -ses, -pi).

полировáл|ьный pólishing; ~ая машúна pólishing-machine; ~ая пáста pólish.

полирóванный pólished.

полировáть, отполировáть (*вн.*) pólish (*smth.*); (*металл*) búrnish (*smth.*), buff (*smth.*).

полиро́в|ка *ж.* 1. (*действие*) pólishing; (*металла*) búrnishing; 2. (*глянец*) pólish, gloss, búrnish. **~очный** pólishing. **~щик** *м.* pólisher.

по́лис *м.* (insúrance) pólicy.

полисеми́я *ж. лингв.* pólysemy.

политбюро́ *с. нескл.* Political Buréau.

полите́хникум *м.* polytéchnic school.

политехни́ческ|ий polytéchnical; **~ое** обуче́ние polytéchnical tráining; **~ое** образова́ние polytéchnical educátion.

политзаключённый *м.* political prísoner.

поли́тик *м.* politícian.

поли́тик|а *ж.* pólitics; (*линия поведения*) pólicy; интересова́ться **~ой** be* ínterested in pólitics.

политика́н *м. презр.* corrúpt politícian; wírepuller; (*интриган*) intríguer. **~ство** *с. презр.* wírepulling, political manóeuvring; pláying pólitics.

полити́ческ|ий political; **~** де́ятель politícian, political léader/figure; **~ие** права́ political rights; **~ая** борьба́ political strúggle; **~ая** акти́вность масс mass political activity; **~** строй political sýstem; **~ая** ка́рта ми́ра political map of the world.

полити́чный pólitic, sagácious, shrewd.

политрабо́тник *м. ист.* párty man.

политру́к *м. ист.* political instrúctor.

политу́ра *ж.* French pólish.

поли́ть *сов.* 1. *см.* полива́ть; 2. (*начать лить*) begín* to pour; поли́л дождь it began to pour with rain. **~ся** 1. *см.* полива́ться; 2. (*начать литься*) start/come* póuring; (*из крана*) start rúnning.

политэконо́мия *ж.* political ecónomy.

полице́йский *прил.* 1. police *attr.*; 2. *в знач. сущ. м.* políceman*.

поли́ция *ж.* police.

поли́чн|ое *с.*: пойма́ть кого́-л. с **~ым** take*/catch* *smb.* red-hánded.

полишине́л|ь *м.* Punch, Punchinéllo; ◇ секре́т **~я** ópen sécret.

полиэтиле́н *м. хим.* polyéthylene. **~овый** polyéthylene *attr.*, pólythene *attr.*; **~овые** изде́лия polyéthylene árticles.

полк *м.* 1. régiment; 2. *разг.* (*множество*) múltitude; régiments *pl.*

по́лка I *ж.* 1. shelf*; кни́жная **~** bóokshelf*; 2. (*в железнодорожном вагоне*) berth; ни́жняя **~** lówer berth.

по́лка II *ж.* (*огорода*) wéeding.

полко́вник *м.* cólonel.

полково́дец *м.* géneral mílitary léader.

полков|о́й regiméntal; **~о́е** зна́мя regiméntal bánner.

полне́ть, пополне́ть grow* stout, get* fat; put* on weight.

полни́ть *несов.* (*вн.*) make* (*smb.*) look fat.

по́лно *в знач. сказ.* 1.' (+ *инф.*) (*довольно*) that's enóugh!, that will do!; **~** вам рабо́тать you have done enóugh work; 2. (*как возражение*) what an idéa!, don't (be so silly)!, you shóuldn't!

полно́ *разг.* (*много*) full; в ко́мнате бы́ло **~** наро́ду the room was full of people, the room was packed (to overflówing).

полнове́сн|ый full-wéight *attr.*; (*крупный*) mássive; *перен.* full-blóoded, substántial; **~ое** зерно́ héavy-eared grain; **~ые** до́воды wéighty árguments.

полновла́стный sóvereign; **~** хозя́ин ábsolute máster.

полново́дн|ый full-flówing; **~ая** река́ full-flówing ríver.

полново́дье *с.* high wáter.

полнокро́в|ие *с. мед.* pléthora. **~ный** full-blóoded (*тж. перен.*); (*здоровый, цветущий*) robúst.

полнолу́ние *с.* full moon.

полнометра́жный full-léngth *attr.*; **~** фильм full-léngth film.

полномо́чи|е *с.* authórity; plénary pówers *pl*; *юр.* próxy; предоста́вить кому́-л. **~я** fúrnish *smb.* with full pówers; передава́ть свои́ **~я** délegate *one's* pówers; превыше́ние **~й** excéeding *one's* commíssion.

полномо́чный plenipoténtiary; **~** представи́тель plenipoténtiary.

полнопра́в|ие *с.* equálity; full rights *pl.* **~ный** enjóying full rights *после сущ.*; **~ный** член семьи́ an équal mémber of the fámily.

по́лностью fúlly, complétely; ◇ целико́м и **~** complétely, root and branch, from top to bóttom; уничто́жить целико́м и **~** destróy root and branch.

полнот|а́ *ж.* 1. (*тучность*) stóutness, córpulence; (*чрезмерная*) obésity; 2. (*полная мера*) fúllness, compléteness; **~** вла́сти fúllness of pówer; ◇ от **~ы́** се́рдца, души́ out of the fúllness of *one's* heart.

полноце́нн|ый 1. full-válue; **~ая** валю́та strong cúrrency; 2. (*обладающий необходимыми качествами*) full-blóoded, sound; **~ое** произведе́ние work of real válue, full-blóoded work.

полно́чный mídnight *attr.*

по́лночь *ж.* mídnight; в **~** at mídnight; ◇ за́ áfter/past mídnight.

по́лн|ый 1. (*наполненный*) full; (*набитый тж.*) packed; у́лицы **~ы** наро́ду the streets are crówded, the streets are full of people; я́щик по́лон книг (кни́гами) the box is full of books; 2. (*исчерпывающий, доведённый до конца*) compléte; **~ое** собра́ние сочине́ний compléte works *pl*; **~ая** побе́да compléte víctory; **~** отчёт compléte accóunt; 3. (*тучный*) stout, plump; **~** со затме́ние tótal eclípse; в **~ом** цвету́ in full bloom/blóssom; в **~ом** поря́дке in good/pérfect órder; **~ая** луна́ full moon; **~ое** неве́жество útter ígnorance; **~ая** тишина́ ábsolute stíllness.

по́лным-полно́ crammed full (of).

по́ло *с. нескл. спорт.* pólo.

пол-оборо́та *м. нескл.* hálf-turn.

полови́к *м.* mat.

полови́н|а *ж.* half*; **~** до́ма half (of) a house; в **~е** ма́я in the míddle of May; **~** седьмо́го half past six; в **~е** седьмо́го at half past six. **~ка** *ж.* half*. **~ный** half; плати́ть в **~ном** разме́ре pay* half (of) the sum. **~чатый** ambívalent, ambíguous, cómpromise *attr.*; приня́ть **~чатое** реше́ние take* a cómpromise decísion.

полови́ца *ж.* flóor-board.

поло́вник *м.* ládle.

полово́дь|е *с.* fréshet, flood; весе́ннее **~** the spring fréshet(s); пери́од **~я** flóod-time.

полов|о́й I (*для пола*) floor *attr.*; **~а́я** тря́пка flóor-cloth; **~а́я** щётка broom.

полов|о́й II *биол.* sex *attr.*; (*связанный с отношениями полов*) séxual; **~ы́е** кле́тки sex cells; **~ое** чу́вство séxual féeling; ◇ **~а́я** зре́лость púberty.

по́лог *м.* cánopy, cúrtain (*тж. перен.*).

поло́г|ий slóping; **~** бе́рег slóping bank/shore. **~ость** *ж.* slope, declívity.

положе́ни|е *с.* 1. (*местонахождение*) position; определи́ть **~** су́дна detérmine a ship's position, locáte a ship; 2. (*поза*) position, pósture; в сидя́чем **~и** in a sítting position/pósture; 3. (*состояние*) state; (*условия жизни*) condítion; situátion; быть на нелега́льном **~и** be* in híding, be* óperating illégally; **~** веще́й state of things/affáirs; каково́ **~** веще́й? what is the state of affáirs?, how do things stand?; **~** рабо́чих the condítion of the wórkers; он нахо́дится в тяжёлом **~и** his position is sérious, he is in a véry sérious position; быть в стеснён-ном **~и** be* hard up, be* in straits; крити́ческое **~** crítical situátion; 4. (*обстановка общественной жизни*) situátion; междунаро́дное **~** internátional situátion; 5. (*место в обществе*) státus, position; служе́бное **~** official státus, státus at work; **~** в о́бществе place/role in society; 6. (*режим*) state; чрезвыча́йное **~** state of emérgency; 7. (*свод правил*) regulátions *pl*, rules *pl*; ~ о подохо́дном нало́ге íncome tax regulátions *pl*; ~ о вы́борах eléction regulátions *pl*; 8. (*тезис*) prínciple; основны́е ~я main prínciples.

поло́женный (*установленный*) gíven, appóinted, fixed; когда́ ~ срок прошёл áfter the appóinted time; в ~ час at the appóinted/estáblished hour.

поло́жим let us say, let us assúme; ~, что вы пра́вы let's assúme you are right.

положи́тельн|о 1. (*утвердительно*) pósitively; отве́тить ~ ánswer in the affírmative; 2. (*совершенно*) ábsolutely; он ~ ничего́ не понима́ет he understánds ábsolutely nóthing. ~ый 1. (*утвердительный*) pósitive, affírmative; ~ый отве́т affírmative ánswer; ~ый о́тзыв fávourable respónse; 2. (*полезный, заслуживающий одобрения*) pósitive; ~ый результа́т pósitive resúlt; ~ый геро́й pósitive cháracter; 3. *мат.*, *физ.* pósitive; ~ая величина́ pósitive quántity; ~ое электри́чество pósitive electrícity; ◇ ~ая сте́пень сравне́ния *грам.* pósitive degrée.

положи́ть *сов. см.* класть 1. ~ся *сов. см.* полага́ться II.

по́лоз *м.* rúnner.

полома́ть *сов.* (*вн.*) break* (*smth.*). ~ся *сов.* 1. break*; (*о машинах и т. п.*) break* down; 2. *разг.* (*кривляться, ломаться некоторое время*) hedge (for a while), play hárd-to-gét.

поло́мка *ж.* bréakage.

поло́мойка *ж. разг.* chárwoman*.

полоса́ *ж.* 1. (*ткани, металла и т. п.*) strip; 2. (*широкая черта, линия*) stripe; 3. (*какого-л. пространства, земли*) strip, stretch; ~ лу́нного све́та ríbbon of móonlight, móonway; 4. (*пояс, зона*) zone, belt; черноземная ~ black earth belt; лесна́я ~ fórest belt; 5. (*промежуток времени*) périod; са́мая счастли́вая ~ мое́й жи́зни the háppiest périod of my life; ~ нена́стной пого́ды spell of wet wéather; 6. *полигр.* page. ~тый striped.

полоск|а́ *ж.*: в ~у striped.

полоска́|ние *с.* 1. (*белья, рта*) rínsing; (*горла*) gárgling; 2. (*раствор*) gárgle, móuth-wash. ~тельница *ж.* slóp-basin.

полоска́ть *несов.* (*вн.*) rinse (*smth.*); (*горло*) gárgle (*smth.*); ~ рот rinse (out) *one's* mouth. ~ся *несов.* 1. (*плескаться в воде*) splash abóut, flap abóut; 2. (*колебаться от ветра*) flap.

по́лость *ж. анат.* cávity; брюшна́я ~ abdóminal cávity.

полоте́нечн|ый: ~ая ткань tówelling.

полоте́нце *с.* tówel.

полотёр *м.* flóor-polisher.

полотни́щ|е *с.* width, cloth, breadth; па́рус в четы́ре ~а sail of four cloths.

полотн|о́ *с.* 1. (*ткань*) línen; 2. (*картина художника*) cánvas; 3. (*дорожная насыпь*) róad-bed; железнодоро́жное ~ pérmanent way; 4. (*конвейера и т. п.*) belt, ríbbon; ◇ бле́дный как ~ pale as death. ~я́ный línen; ~яная простыня́ línen sheet.

поло́ть *несов.* (*вн.*) weed (*smth.*).

полоу́м|ие *с. разг.* imbecílity. ~ный *разг.* méntally defícient, morónic, half-wítted.

полпути́ *м.*: на ~ halfwáy; он встре́тил меня́ на ~ к ва́шему до́му he met me halfwáy to your house; верну́ться с ~ turn back halfwáy, turn back when the jóurney is half óver.

полсло́ва *с.*: ни ~ от него́ не услы́шишь you can néver get a word out of him; вы мне нужны́ на ~ I would like a word with you.

полти́нник *м. разг.* fifty cópecks; (*монета*) fifty-cópeck piece.

полтора́ one and a half; ~ го́да a year and a half; в ~

ра́за бо́льше half as much agáin; в ~ ра́за да́льше half as far agáin; ◇ ни два ни ~ néither here nor there.

полтора́ста one húndred and fifty.

полу- *в сложн.* half-, sémi-.

полуботи́нки *мн.* (*ед.* полуботи́нок *м.*) (wálking) shoes; low shoes *амер.*

полуго́д|ие *с.* hálf-yéar, half a year; six months *pl*; уче́бное ~ cóllege hálf-yéar; seméster *амер.* ~и́чный six months'; for a périod of six months *после сущ.*

полугодов|а́лый six months old, hálf-yéar old. ~о́й hálf-yéarly; (*рассчитанный на полгода*) síx-month *attr.*; ~о́й отчёт hálf-yéarly repórt.

полуголо́дн|ый half-stárved; ~ое существова́ние half-stárved existence.

полугра́мотный sémi-líterate, ígnorant.

полу́да *ж.* tínning.

полу́денн|ый mídday *attr.*; ~ час the hour of noon; ~ зной the mídday heat; ◇ ~ая ли́ния *астр.* merídian line.

полуди́кий sémi-bárbarous, hálf-sávage.

полуживо́й hálf-déad; ~ от го́лода hálf-déad with húnger; ~ от стра́ха more dead than alíve with fright.

полузабы́тый half-forgótten.

полузабы́ть|ё *с.* sémi-cónsciousness; он лежа́л в ~и́ he was lýing in a state of sémi-cónsciousness.

полузащи́т|а *ж. спорт.* hálf-backs *pl*. ~ник *м. спорт.* hálf-back.

полукро́в|ка *ж. с.-х.* hálf-breed. ~ный *с.-х.* hálf-bred; ~ная ло́шадь hálf-bred horse.

полукру́г *м.* sémicircle; (*луны*) créscent. ~лый semicírcular.

полулежа́ть *несов.* reclíne.

полуме́ра *ж.* half-méasure.

полумёртвый half-dead.

полуме́сяц *м.* hálf-móon; (*серп*) créscent.

полуме́сячный fórtnight's; ~ окла́д two weeks' sálary.

полумра́к *м.* gloom, sémi-dárkness.

полуно́чный mídnight *attr.*

полуобнажённый half-náked.

полуоборо́т *м.* hálf-turn.

полуоде́тый half-dréssed.

полуокру́жность *ж.* sémi-circúmference.

полуосвещённый half-líghted, póorly líghted.

полуо́стров *м.* península. ~но́й penínsular.

полуоткры́тый hálf-ópen, slíghtly ópen, ajár.

полуофициа́льный sémi-official.

полупальто́ *с нескл.* short coat.

полуподва́л *м.* sémi-básement.

полупроводни́к *м. физ.* semicondúctor.

полупроводнико́вый semicondúctor *attr.*

полупрозра́чный sémi-transpárent.

полупусты́ня *ж.* sémi-désert.

полуразде́тый half-undréssed.

полуразру́шенный half-rúined, dilápidated.

полусве́т *м.* dim light, half light.

полусло́в|о *с. см.* полслова; ◇ прерва́ть кого́-л. на ~е not let *smb.* finish; останови́ться на ~е break* off abrúptly, not finish what *one* was sáying; поня́ть кого́-л. с ~а be* quick to understánd *smb.*, grasp *smb.'s* méaning at once, take* the hint.

полусме́рт|ь *ж.*: испуга́ться до ~и be* fríghtened to death; изби́ть кого́-л. до ~и beat* *smb.* within an inch of his, her life.

полу|со́н *м.* dró́wsiness, sléepiness, sómnolence; в ~сне́ half asléep. ~со́нный dró́wsy, sléepy, sómnolent.

полуста́нок *м.* halt, wáyside státion.

полутёмный póorly líghted, dim.

полуте́нь *ж.* light shádow; penúmbra.

полуто́н *м.* 1. *муз.* sémitone; 2. (*о цвете, краске*) hálf-tone, hálf-tint.

полу́торка *ж. разг.* óne-and-a-hálf-ton ló́rry, truck *амер.*

полутьма́ ж. sémi-dárkness, gloom.

полуфабрика́т м. sémi-fínished próduct; мн. (проду́кты) prepáred foods, convénience foods.

полуфин|а́л м. спорт. semifinal. **~а́льный** спорт. semifínal attr.

получасов|о́й half-hóur attr., half an hour's; **~а́я** бесе́да half an hour's conversátion.

получа́тель м., **~ница** ж. recípient; (адреса́т) addressée.

получа́ть, получи́ть (вн.) recéive (smth.); get* (smth.); (добива́ться тж.) obtáin (smth.); получи́ть письмо́ recéive a létter; ~ газе́ту take* a páper; ~ зарпла́ту recéive one's wáges; ~ до́ступ к чему́-л. get* admíssion to smth.; получи́ть сре́днее, вы́сшее образова́ние recéive/have* a sécondary, hígher educátion; получи́ть профессу́ру be* appóinted to a proféssorship; ~ повыше́ние get* promótion; получи́ть на́сморк catch*/get* a cold; получи́ть вы́говор be* réprimanded; получи́ть чьё-л. согла́сие obtáin/get* smb.'s consént; получи́ть призна́ние recéive recognítion. **~ся, получи́ться** come* out; что получи́лось? what was the resúlt of it?, what came of it?; результа́ты получи́лись соверше́нно неожи́данные the resúlts were quite unexpécted; мо́жет быть, из него́ полу́чится хоро́ший музыка́нт he may make a fine musícian, he may turn out a fine musícian.

получи́ть(ся) сов. см. получа́ть(ся).

полуша́ри|е с. hémisphere; **~я** головно́го мо́зга the cérebral hémispheres; се́верное, ю́жное ~ nórthern, sóuthern hémisphere.

полушерстяно́й half-wóolen, wóol-míxture attr.

полушу́бок м. short shéepskin coat, shéepskin jácket.

полцены́ ж. half-príce; за ~ at half-price, dirt-chéap.

полчаса́ м. half an hour; ка́ждые ~ évery half hour; часы́ быот ка́ждые ~ the clock strikes the half-hóurs; че́рез ~ in half an hour; прийти́ за ~ до нача́ла come* half an hour before the beginning; сде́лать что-л. за ~ do* smth. in half an hour.

полчи́ще с. horde; перен. тж. swarm.

по́л|ый 1. (пусто́й внутри́) hóllow; 2. (разли́вшийся весно́й) flood attr.; была́ **~ая** вода́ the ríver was in full flood.

полы́нь ж. бот. wórmwood.

полынья́ ж. polýnia, patch of ópen wáter in ice.

по́льз|а ж. prófit, use; (хоро́ший результа́т) bénefit, good; для о́бщей **~ы** for the públic bénefit/wealth/good; э́то принесёт большу́ю **~у** that will be of great use; кака́я вам от э́того ~? what good will that do you?; ◇ в **~у** кого́-л., чего́-л. in fávour of smb., smth.; реша́ть вопро́с в чью-л. **~у** decíde a quéstion in smb.'s fávour; он говори́л в ва́шу **~у** he spoke in your fávour; э́то говори́т не в ва́шу **~у** it is not to your crédit; идти́ на **~у** кому́-л. do* smb. good; лече́ние пошло́ ему́ на **~у** the cure did him good.

по́льзовани|е с. use; отда́ть что-л. во вре́менное ~ кому́-л. allów smb. témporary use of smth.; предме́ты ли́чного **~я** árticles of pérsonal use.

по́льзоваться несов. (тв.) 1. use (smth.), make* use (of); 2. (испо́льзовать) take* advántage (of), prófit (by), aváil onesélf (of); ~ слу́чаем aváil onesélf of the opportúnity; 3. (облада́ть) enjóy (smth.); пье́са по́льзуется успе́хом the play is a succéss.

по́лька I ж. (же́нщина) Pólish wóman*, Pole.

по́лька II ж. (та́нец) pólka.

по́льский Pólish; ~ язы́к Pólish, the Pólish lánguage.

польсти́ть сов. см. льстить. **~ся** сов. (на вн.) be* témpted (by).

польщённый fláttered.

полюби́ть сов. 1. (вн.) becóme* fond (of), take* a líking (to); (влюби́ться) fall* in love (with); 2. (вн., + инф.; пристрасти́ться) grow*/becóme* fond (of + -ing), take* a líking (to), becóme* attáched (to), take* a fáncy (to), take* (to + -ing); ~ му́зыку becóme* fond of músic; ~ Москву́ becóme* attáched to Móscow.

полюбова́ться сов. 1. см. любова́ться; 2. разг. ирон.: полюбу́йтесь на себя́! just look at yoursélf!

полюбо́вн|ый ámicable; **~ое** соглаше́ние ámicable séttlement.

полюбопы́тствовать сов. inquíre; be* ínterested enóugh.

по́люс м. pole; Се́верный ~ North Pole; Ю́жный ~ South Pole; положи́тельный, отрица́тельный ~ эл. pósitive, négative pole.

поля́к м. Pole.

поля́на ж. fórest méadow, glade.

поляриза́ция ж. физ. polarizátion.

поля́рник м. pólar explórer.

поля́рность ж. polárity.

поля́рн|ый pólar; árctic; перен. diamétrically oppósed; **~ая** ста́нция pólar státion; **~ая** экспеди́ция pólar expedítion; ◇ ~ день, **~ая** ночь pólar day, night; Поля́рный круг pólar círcle; Поля́рная звезда́ the póle-star, the North Star.

пома́да ж. pomáde; губна́я ~ lípstick.

пома́зать сов. см. ма́зать 1. **~ся** сов. см. ма́заться 1, 3.

пома́лкивать несов. разг. keep* quíet, hold* one's tongue, keep mum.

помани́ть сов. см. мани́ть 1.

пома́рка ж. corréction.

помаха́ть сов. (тв.) wave (smth.); ~ шля́пой wave one's hat; ~ на проща́нье wave goodbýe.

пома́хивать несов. (тв.) swing* (smth.); ~ тро́сточкой swing* one's stick; ~ хвосто́м (о соба́ке) wag its tail; (о ло́шади) swing*/swish its tail.

поме́длить сов. wait (a little); ~ немно́го wait awhíle; ~ с отве́том pause befóre ánswering, deláy one's ánswer.

поменя́ть сов. (вн.) разг. change (smth.). **~ся** сов. (тв.) exchánge (smth.).

помере́щиться сов. см. мере́щиться.

помёрзнуть сов. разг. 1. (о расте́ниях) be* killed by frost, be fróst-bítten; 2. (провести́ не́которое вре́мя на моро́зе) be* out in the cold.

поме́рить сов. (вн.) try on (smth.).

поме́риться сов. см. ме́риться.

поме́ркнуть сов. см. ме́ркнуть.

помертве́лый déathly pale.

помертве́ть сов. мертве́ть 2.

помести́ть сов. см. помеща́ть. **~ся** сов. см. помеща́ться 1, 2.

поме́стье с. estáte.

по́месь ж. cróssbreed, hýbrid; перен. разг. míxture.

поме́сячный mónthly; ~ дохо́д mónthly retúrns pl.

помёт м. 1. dróppings pl; 2. (припло́д) brood; (о поро́сятах) fárrow.

помёт|а ж. note. **~ить** сов. см. помеча́ть.

поме́х|а ж. 1. híndrance, impédiment, óbstacle; быть **~ой** be* in the way; 2. мн. interférence sg.

помеча́ть, поме́тить (вн.) mark (smth.); (о да́те) date (smth.); ~ га́лочкой mark with a tick.

помеча́ть сов. dream* for a while, indúlge in dreams.

поме́шанный прил. 1. mad, crázy, insáne; (на пр.) перен. mad (on), crázy (about); он поме́шан на спо́рте he's mad on sport; 2. в знач. сущ. м. mádman*.

помеша́тельство с. insánity; mádness; перен. тж. cráziness.

помеша́ть I сов. см. меша́ть I.

помеша́ть II сов. 1. см. меша́ть II 1; 2. (вн.; не́которое вре́мя, слегка́) stir (smth.) (a little, for a while).

помеша́ться сов. go* mad; (на пр.) перен. разг. be* mad (abóut, on), be* crázy (abóut, óver).

помещ|а́ть, помести́ть (вн.) 1. (поста́вить, положи́ть куда́-л.) put* (smth.), place (smth.); ~ кни́ги на пóлку put* the books on a shelf*; **2.** (*предоставлять помещение*) put* (*smb.*), accómmodate (*smb.*); помести́ть тури́стов в гости́ницу accómmodate/put* tóurists in a hotél; **3.** (*вкладывать*) invést (*smth.*), depósit (*smth.*); ~ капитáл invést cápital; ~ свои́ дéньги в сбербáнк depósit one's móney with the sávings-bank; **4.** (*публиковать где-л.*) put* (*smth.*), públish (*smth.*); помести́ть статью́ в газéте put* an árticle in a néwspaper; помести́ть объявлéние в газéте place/put* an advértisement in a néwspaper. ~áться, помести́ться **1.** (*вмещаться*) get* in; (*о вещах*) go* in, fit in; здесь все не помести́тся there is not enóugh room here for éverybody; **2.** (*поселяться*) instáll onesélf, take* up one's lódging; **3.** *тк. несов.* (*находиться*) be* situated. ~éние *с.* **1.** (*капитала*) invéstment, invésting; (*объявление и т. п.*) pútting, plácing; **2.** (*здание*) building, house; prémises *pl*; жило́е ~éние dwélling-house; living quárters *pl*.

помéщи|к *м.* lándowner, lándlord. ~ца *ж.* the místress of the estáte. ~чий lándowner's; ~чий дом mánor(-house); ~чья сóбственность на зéмлю lánded estátes *pl*.

помидóр *м.* tomáto (*pl -oes*).

поми́лов|ание *с.* párdon; forgíveness. ~ать *сов.* párdon (*smb.*), show* mércy (to, on).

поми́мо (*рд.*) **1.** (*кроме*) apárt (from), besídes; ~ други́х соображéний apárt from óther réasons, óther réasons apárt; **2.** (*без ведома*) withóut smb.'s knówledge; э́то бы́ло сдéлано ~ меня́ it was done withóut my knówledge, I had nóthing tó do with it.

поми́н *м.:* и в ~е нет there is no trace of it; и ~у нет о ком-л., о чём-л. one néver méntions/speaks of smb., smth.; not a méntion of smb., smth.

поми́н|áть, помяну́ть (*вн.*) **1.** (*вспоминать*) recáll (*smb., smth.*), méntion (*smb., smth.*); **2.** (*устраивать поминки*) commémorate (*smb.*); ◇ ~áй, как звáли he has vánished ínto thin air, it's the last you'll see of him.

поми́нки *мн.* commémorative feast *sg*.

помину́тн|о **1.** évery mínute; **2.** (*часто, беспрестанно*) contínually, cónstantly. ~ый **1.** (*исчисляемый по минутам*) pér-mínute; per mínute *после сущ.*; **2.** (*частый*) cónstant, contínual.

помири́ть *сов. см.* мири́ть. ~ся *сов. см.* мири́ться 1.

по́мнить *несов.* (*вн., о пр.*) remémber (*smb., smth.*), bear*/keep* in mind (*smb., smth.*); ◇ не ~ себя́ be* besíde onesélf; ~ себя́ от рáдости be* besíde onesélf with joy; be* transpórted with joy. ~ся *несов.* **1.:** мне пóмнится э́тот день I remémber that day; **2.:** пóмнится *в знач. вводн. сл.* I remémber.

помнóгу *разг.* much, a good deal; in plénty, in large quántities/númbers.

помножáть, помно́жить (*вн. на вн.*) múltiply (*smth. by smth.*); ~ четы́ре на пять múltiply four by five.

помно́жить *сов. см.* помножáть *и* мно́жить 1.

помогáть, помóчь **1.** (*дт.*) help (*smb.*), assíst (*smb.*), aid (*smb.*); ~ кому́-л. деньгáми assíst smb. with móney, give* smb. fináncial aid; ~ кому́-л. в бедé assíst smb. in misfórtune; ~ кому́-л. сóветом assíst smb. with one's advíce, give* smb. the bénefit of one's advíce; помóчь кому́-л. перейти́ у́лицу help smb. acróss the street; ~ кому́-л. в рабóте help smb. in his, her work; э́то дéлу не помóжет that won't do ány good, that won't help mátters; **2.** (*оказывать нужное действие*) be* efféctive; лекáрство ему́ не помоглó the médicine did him no good.

по-мóему **1.** (*по моему мнению*) to my mind, in my opínion, as I see it; **2.** (*по моему желанию*) (in) my way.

помóи *мн.* slops; gárbage *sg*.

помóй|ка *ж. разг.* rúbbish heap; césspit. ~ный: ~ное ведрó slóp-pail, gárbage can, dústbin; ~ная я́ма césspit, rúbbish pit.

помóл *м.* **1.** (*действие*) grínding, mílling; **2.** (*качество размола*) grade; мукá крýпного, грýбого ~а cóarse-ground flour.

помоли́ться *сов. см.* моли́ться 1.

помолодéть *сов. см.* молодéть.

помолчáть *сов.* keep* quíet; be* sílent (for a while).

помóрщить *сов.* (*вн.*) wrínkle (*smth.*) slíghtly. ~ся *сов.* make* a (wry) face.

помóст *м.* dáis, plátform; stage; (*настил*) plánking.

помóч|и *мн.* **1.** hárness *sg*; **2.** (*подтяжки*) bráces; suspénders *амер.*; ◇ води́ть когó-л. на ~áх keep* smb. in léading-strings.

помочи́ть *сов.* (*вн.*) wet (*smth.*), soak (*smth.*).

помóчь *сов. см.* помогáть.

помóщн|ик *м.*, ~ица *ж.* assístant, hélper.

пóмощ|ь *ж.* help, assístance, aid; взывáть о ~и сгу for help; медици́нская ~ médical aid; юриди́ческая ~ légal assístance; ◇ с ~ью, при ~и чегó-л. with (the aid of).

пóмпа I *ж.* (*торжественность*) pomp, state.

пóмпа II *ж.* (*насос*) pump.

помпóн *м.* rómpon.

помрачнéть *сов. см.* мрачнéть.

помути́ться *сов. см.* мути́ться 2.

помутнéние *с.* clóuding, dímming; (*жидкости*) clóudiness, múddiness.

помутнéть *сов. см.* мутнéть.

помýчить *сов.* (*вн.*) tease (*smb.*), tormént (*smth.*), make* (*smb.*) súffer. ~ся *сов.* súffer; (*над тв.*) have* tróuble (with).

помчáть *сов.* **1.** (*вн.*) cárry (*smth.*) off; **2.** *разг. см.* помчáться. ~ся *сов.* run*, rush; ~ся стрелóй dart off.

пóмысел *м.* thought; (*намерение*) design, inténtion.

помы́слить *сов. см.* помышля́ть.

помы́ть(ся) *сов. см.* мы́ть(ся).

помышля́ть, помы́слить (*о пр.*) think* (abóut).

помяну́ть *сов. см.* поминáть.

помя́тый crúmpled, creased; *перен.* flábby, púffy.

помя́ть *сов.* (*вн.*) **1.** (*измять*) crúmple (*smth.*), crush (*smth.*); (*траву*) trámple (*smth.*); ~ плáтье crúmple a dress; **2.** (*повредить*) dámage (*smth.*), knock (*smth.*), dent (*smth.*). ~ся *сов.* **1.** (*измяться*) be* crúmpled, be* crushed; *перен.* be* flábby, be* púffy; **2.** *разг.* (*поколебаться*) shift one's feet hésitantly; díther; *перен. тж.* hésitate.

понаблюдáть *сов.* keep* watch (for a while); (*вн., за тв.*) keep* an eye (on).

понадéяться *сов.* (*на вн.*) relý (on), count (on).

понáдоб|иться *сов.* be* nécessary, be* néeded; ему́ не ~ся э́та кни́га he will not need this book; дéнег мне бóльше не ~ся I shall not need ány more móney; éсли ~ся if nécessary; вáше присýтствие не ~ся your présence will not be requíred; на э́то ~ся мнóго врéмени it will take a long time to do it.

понапрáсну *разг.* **1.** (*бесполезно*) in vain; **2.** (*зря*) for nóthing.

понаслы́шке *разг.* by héarsay.

по-настоя́щему próperly, réally, in the right way.

по-нáшему **1.** (*по нашему мнению*) in our opínion, as we see it; **2.** (*по нашему желанию*) (in) our way.

поневóле *разг.* willy-nílly, whéther one likes it or not, agáinst one's will.

понедéльник *м.* Mónday.

понедéльн|о per week. ~ый wéekly.

понемнóгу **1.** (*небольшими количествами*) a líttle; **2.** (*постепенно*) líttle by líttle, grádually; **3.** *разг.* (*сносно*) abóut the same, not so bad.

понести́ *сов. см.* нести́ I 1, 2, 3, 5, 6. ~сь *сов. см.* нести́сь I.

пóни *м. нескл.* rópу.

пониж|áть, пони́зить (*вн.*) **1.** lówer (*smth.*), redúce (*smth.*); ~ давлéние redúce/léssen préssure; ~ напряжéние lówer the vóltage; 2. *разг.* (*по службе*) degráde (*smb.*); demóte (*smb.*), redúce (*smb.*) in rank; ◇ понизить гóлос lówer one's voice. ~áться, понизиться 1. (*стать более низким*) becóme* lówer, come* lówer, descénd a líttle; 2. (*уменьшаться*) be* redúced; (*о ценах тж.*) fall*, drop; 3. (*звучать ниже, тише*) go* down, drop, sink*. ~éние *с.* (*падение*) drop, fall; (*по службе*) demótion, redúction in rank; ~éние цен redúction/cut in príces; fall in príces; ~éние уровня воды́ fall/súbsidence of the wáter-level.

пони́женн|ый belów-áverage, low; *перен.* depréssed, despóndent; ~ая температу́ра low témperature; ~ые трéбования belów-áverage requírements; у негó ~ое настроéние he is in low spírits.

пони́зить(ся) *сов. см.* понижáть(ся).

пóнизу low; (*внизу*) belów, benéath; (*снизу*) undernéath.

поникáть, пони́кнуть (*прям. и перен.*) droop, wilt; пони́кнуть головóй hang* one's head.

пони́кнуть *сов. см.* поникáть.

пониманиe *с.* 1. (*способность осмыслять что-л.*) understánding, comprehénsion; (*осознание*) realizátion 2. (*представление*) concéption; упрощённое ~ *чего-л.* over-símplified concéption of *smth.*; 3. (*толкование*) interpretátion.

поним|áть, поня́ть (*вн.*) 1. understánd (*smb., smth.*), comprehénd (*smb., smth.*); (*сознавать*) réalize (*smth.*); я не совсéм пóнял, что он сказáл I didn't quite catch what he said; ~áю! I see!; 2. *тк. несов.* (*вн., в пр.*; *быть знатоком чего-л.*) understánd* (*smth.*); be* a good judge (of); ~ му́зыку understánd* músic; ◇ дать кому́-л. поня́ть, что... give* *smb.* to understánd that...; не пóнял! I'm not with you.

по-нóвому in a new way; from a new ángle; начáть жить ~ begín* a new life, start life afrésh.

понóс *м.* diarrhóea.

поноси́ть I *сов.* (*вн.*) 1. (*носить некоторое время*) cárry (*smb., smth.*) (for a while); 2. (*одежду*) wear* (*smth.*) (for a while); э́то пальтó я ещё поношу́ I can go on wéaring this coat a bit lónger.

поноси́ть II *несов.* (*вн.*; *бранить*) curse (*smb., smth.*), abúse (*smb., smth.*), slánder (*smb.*), defáme (*smb., smth.*).

понóшенный worn, shábby, thréadbare; the worse for wear *predic.*; *перен.* díssipated.

понрáвиться *сов. см.* нрáвиться.

понтóн *м.* pontóon; (*мост*) pontóon-bridge. ~ный pontóon *attr.*; ~ный мост pontóon-bridge.

понужд|áть, пону́дить (*вн.*) force (*smb.*), compél (*smb.*); impél (*smb.*). ~éние *с.* compúlsion.

понукáть *несов.* (*вн.*) urge (*smth.*) on; *перен.* húrry (*smb.*), nag (*smb.*); ~ лóшадь urge a horse fórward.

пону́р|ить *сов.* (*вн.*) droop (*smth.*), bend* (*smth.*); ~ гóлову hang* one's head. ~иться *сов.* hang* one's head, look dejécted; (*склониться*) droop. ~ый dówncast, depréssed, dejécted, dísmal; ~ый вид dówncast appéarance.

пóнчик *м.* dóughnut.

пону́не *книжн.* up to nów.

поню́|хать *сов. см.* ню́хать. ~шка *ж.* a pinch of snuff; ◇ пропáсть ни за ~шку табаку́ símply throw* one's life awáy.

поня́т|ие 1. *филос.* cóncept; ~ прибáвочной стóимости the cóncept of súrplus válue; 2. (*представление, осведомлённость*) concéption, nótion, idéa; ~ добрá и зла idéa of good and évil; имéть я́сное ~ о чём-л. have* a clear idéa/concéption of *smth.*; 3. *обыкн. мн.* (*совокупность взглядов на что-л.*) outlook *sg*, comprehénsion *sg.* ~йный concéptual. ~ливый intélligent, bright, quíck-witted.

поня́тн|о 1. *нареч.* cléarly, pláinly, intélligibly; 2. *в* знач. вводн. сл. разг. of course, náturally; I see *разг.* ~ый 1. (*ясный, вразумительный*) clear, intélligible, comprehénsible; 2. (*имеющий основание*) understándable, jústifiable; ◇ ~ое дéло, ~ая вещь náturally; поня́тно? are you with me?

поня́ть *сов. см.* понимáть 1.

пообéдать *сов. см.* обéдать.

пообещáть *сов.* (*вн., + инф.*) prómise (*smth.*, + to *inf.*)

пóодаль at a dístance, fúrther off.

поодинóчке one at a time, one by one.

по-осéннему as in áutumn.

поочерёдн|о in turn, by turns. ~ый in turns *после сущ.*

поощр|éние *с.* encóuragement; (*награда*) awárd, rewárd. ~и́тельный encóuragement *attr.*; stímulatory; (*выражающий поощрение*) encóuraging.

поощри́ть *сов. см.* поощря́ть.

поощря́ть, поощри́ть (*вн.*) encóurage (*smb., smth.*).

поп *м. разг.* priest.

попадáние *с.* hit; ~ в цель hítting the tárget, áccurate shóoting; прямóе ~ diréct hit.

попадáть *сов.* fall* one áfter the óther.

попад|áть, попáсть 1. (*в вн.; тж. в вн.; достигать чего-л.*) hit* (*smb., smth.; smb., smth.* with), strike* (*smb., smth.; smb., smth.* with); кáмень попáл в окнó a stone struck/hit the window; попáсть кáмнем в окнó hit* the window with a stone; попáсть ногóй в стрéмя get* one's foot* ínto the stírrup; пу́ля попáла ему́ в плечó a búllet struck him in the shóulder; 2. (*в вн.; проникать, пробираться куда-л.*) get* (ínto); попáсть в дом get* ínto the house; 3. (*достигать какого-л. места*) get* (to), reach; как тудá попáсть? how does one get there?; как попáсть на стáнцию? what's the best way (to get) to the station?; мы попáли домóй тóлько вéчером we dídn't get home till évening; 4. (*в, на, под вн.; оказываться в каких-л. обстоятельствах, условиях*) get* (ínto), come* to be (in); попáсть под суд be* brought to tríal; попáсть в плен be* táken prísoner; попáсть под машину be* run óver by a car; попáсть в бедý be* in tróuble; 5. (*в, на вн.; на работу, учёбу и т. п.*) get* (ínto); be* admítted (to); попáсть в институ́т be* admítted to the institute; 6. *безл.* (*дт.*) *разг.*: емý попадёт за э́то he'll get it; ◇ дéлать что-л. как попáло do* a thing ányhow. ~ся, попáсться 1. get*; (*быть пойманным*) get* caught; 2. *разг.* (*повстречаться*) come* acróss; (*о людях*) run* ínto; мне никогдá не попадáлась такáя кни́га I have néver come acróss a book of that sort; ◇ попáсться на глазá кому́-л. meet* *smb.'s* eye.

попáрно in pairs, two and two, by two.

поп-áрт *м.* pop art, pópular art.

попáсть(ся) *сов. см.* попадáть(ся).

попеня́ть *сов. см.* пеня́ть.

попéрек acróss.

поперемéнно altérnately, by turns, in turns.

поперéч|ина *ж.* cróss-beam, cróss-piece. ~ник *м.* diámeter. ~ный tránsverse, cross-; ~ное сечéние tránsverse séction, cróss-séction; ~ная ли́ния tránsverse line; ~ная бáлка tránsverse beam.

поперхну́ться *сов.* choke, have* a fit of splúttering; ~ чáем choke in one's tea.

попéрчить *сов. см.* пéрчить.

попечéни|е *с.* charge, care; быть на чьём-л. ~и be* in *smb.'s* charge.

попечи́тель *м.*, ~ница *ж.* guárdian, trustée. ~ство *с.* guárdianship, trustéeship.

попирáть *несов.* (*вн.*) víolate (*smth.*), trámple (on); ~ чьи-л. правá víolate *smb.'s* rights.

попи́ть *сов. разг.* have* a drink.

поплáвать *сов.* have*/take* a swim.

поплавóк *м.* float.

поплáкать *сов.* have* a cry, shed* a few tears.

поплати́ться *сов. см.* плати́ться.

поплести́сь *сов.* trudge alóng; drag *oneself* alóng.

поплы́ть *сов.* begín* to swim; (*о лодке*) begín* to move.

попляса́ть *сов.* dance; ◇ ты у меня́ попля́шешь I'll make you hop.

попо́йка *ж. разг.* drínking-bout, spree.

попола́м in two, in half; разре́зать *что-л.* ~ cut* *smth.* in two/half; дели́ть с *кем-л.* расхо́ды ~ share expénses with *smb.*; go* halves/fifty-fifty with *smb.*; они́ деля́т при́были ~ they go halves in the prófits; ◇ с гре- хо́м ~ áfter a fáshion, só-so.

поползнове́ние *с.* inclinátion, hánkering; féeble éffort.

пополне́ние *с.* 1. (*действие*) replénishment; ~ библио- те́ки но́выми кни́гами addition of new books to a library; 2. (*о войсках*) reinfórcements *pl*, fresh fórces *pl*; (*о кадрах*) additional staff; fresh blood *идиом.*

попо́лнеть *сов. см.* полне́ть.

попо́лнить(ся) *сов. см.* пополня́ть(ся).

пополня́ть, попо́лнить (*вн.*) replénish (*smth.*); (*людьми*) reinfórce (*smth.*); ~ свои́ зна́ния add to one's knówledge; ~ соста́в служа́щих engáge additional staff; ~ библиоте́ку но́выми кни́гами add new books to a library; enrich a library. ~ся, попо́лниться (*запасами*) be* replénished; (*людьми*) be* reinfórced; (*знаниями*) be* enriched; (*о суммах*) be* ádded.

пополу́дни in the afternóon, p.m. (post merídiem); в три часа́ ~ at 3 p.m.

пополу́ночи áfter midnight, a.m. (ánte merídiem); в три часа́ ~ at 3 a.m.

попо́мн|ить *сов.* (*вн.*) *разг.* remémber (*smth.*); я те- бе́ э́то ~ю! I'll be éven with you yet!, I'll pay you out for that!; ~и(те) моё сло́во! mark my words!

попо́на *ж.* hórse-cloth.

поправи́м|ый that can be put right *после сущ.*; améndable, remédiable; ~ая оши́бка améndable érror.

поправ|ить(ся) *сов. см.* поправля́ть(ся). ~ка *ж.* 1. (*исправление*) corréction; (*дополнение*) améndment; вноси́ть ~ки (*в текст*) make* corréctions; (*в законо- проект и т. п.*) make* améndments; ~ка к законопро- е́кту amendment to a bill; 2. (*здоровья*) recóvery; де́ло у него́ идёт на ~ку he is on the mend, he is recovering.

поправля́ть, попра́вить (*вн.*) 1. (*чинить*) mend (*smth.*), put* (*smth.*) right; 2. (*исправлять*) corréct (*smb., smth.*); ~ ученика́ corréct a púpil; ~ текст corréct a text; 3. (*приводить в порядок*) adjúst (*smth.*), put*/set* (*smth.*) straight; ~ пла́тье adjúst one's dress; ~ га́лстук set* one's tie straight; ~ во́лосы put* one's hair straight; 4. (*улучшать, восстанавливать*) impróve (*smth.*), put* (*smth.*) right; ~ здоро́вье impróve one's health; дела́ попра́вить уже́ нельзя́ it's too late to rémedy mátters. ~ся, попра́виться 1. (*исправлять свою ошибку в сказанном*) corréct oneself; 2. (*улучшаться*) impróve; дела́ поправля́ются things are impróving, things are lóoking up; 3. (*выздоравливать*) recóver, get* well; 4. *разг.* (*полнеть*) put* on weight, gain in weight; вы о́чень попра́вились you have put on a lot of weight.

попрактикова́ться *сов.* práctise a little, have* some práctice.

по-пре́жнему as befóre; (*как всегда*) as úsual.

попрёк *м. разг.* repróach; ве́чные ~и etérnal nágging.

попрека́ть, попрекну́ть (*вн.*) *разг.* repróach (*smb.*), nag (*smb.*).

попрекну́ть *сов. см.* попрека́ть.

по́прище *с.* field, walk of life.

попро́б|овать *сов.* 1. *см.* про́бовать; 2. *разг.*: ~уйте! just you try!

попроси́ть *сов. см.* проси́ть 1, 2, 3. ~ся *сов. см.* проси́ться.

по́просту *разг.* simply; straight out; ~ говоря́ fránkly spéaking.

попрошай|ка *м. и ж. разг.* cádger, béggar. ~ничать *несов. разг.* cadge, beg.

попроща́ться *сов. см.* проща́ться.

попры́г|ать *сов.* jump, jump abóut; (*на одной ноге*) hop, hop abóut. ~ун *м.*, ~у́нья *ж. разг.* fidget, réstless spirit.

попря́тать *сов.* (*вн.*) *разг.* hide* (*smth.*). ~ся *сов. разг.* hide* oneself; ~ся от дождя́ take* cóver from the rain.

попуга́й *м.* párrot.

попуга́ть *сов.* (*вн.*) fríghten (*smb.*) a little, scare (*smb.*).

попу́дрить *сов.* (*вн.*) pówder (*smth.*). ~ся *сов.* pówder one's face.

популяриз|а́тор *м.* pópularizer. ~а́ция *ж.* popularizátion. ~и́ровать, ~ова́ть *несов. и сов.* (*вн.*) pópularize (*smth.*).

популя́рн|ость *ж.* populárity; по́льзоваться широ́- кой ~остью enjóy wide populárity, be* widely pópular; он снискал себе́ ~ среди́ студе́нтов he made himself pópular with the stúdents. ~ый pópular; ~ая пе́сня pópular song; ~ые ле́кции pópular léctures; ~ое изложе́- ние pópular presentátion.

попурри́ *с. нескл.* pot-póurri.

попусти́тельство *с.* connívance. ~вать *несов.* (*дт.*) connive (at), wink (at), shut*/close one's eyes (to).

по́пусту *разг.* in vain, to no púrpose; вре́мя ~ тра́- тить waste one's time.

попу́тн|о while one is abóut it, in pássing; on one's way. ~ый 1. (*в одном и том же направлении*) in the same diréction *после сущ.*; ~ый ве́тер fair wind; ~ая ма- ши́на pássing car; 2. (*встречающийся на пути*) on the way *после сущ.*; 3. (*производимый одновременно с чем-л.*) simultáneous; ~ый вопро́с incidéntal quéstion.

попу́тч|ик *м.*, ~ица *ж.* féllow-tráveller.

попыта́ть *сов.* (*вн.*) *разг.* try (*smth.*); ◇ ~ сча́стья try one's luck.

попыта́ться *сов. см.* пыта́ться.

попы́тк|а *ж.* attémpt; (*усилие*) endéavour; тще́тные ~и vain endéavours; ◇ ~ не пы́тка *погов.* ≈ nóthing vénture, nóthing win/have/gain; there is no harm in trýing.

попя́т|иться *сов. см.* пя́титься. ~ный: идти́ на ~ный go* back on one's word, back out.

по́ра *ж.* pore.

пор|а́ *ж.* 1. time, périod, séason; ночна́я ~ night- -time; осе́нняя ~ áutumn; сенокосна́я ~ háymaking time, háy-time; дождли́вая ~ ráiny séason; 2. *в знач. сказ.* it is time; давно́ ~ it is high time; ~ обе́дать it is time for dinner; ◇ до ~ы до вре́мени up to a cértain time; for just so long; с каки́х пор? since when?; с да́вних пор from the éarliest times; в ту по́ру at that time; в э́ту по́ру at this/that time; на пе́рвых ~а́х at first; с той ~ы from that time on; since then, éver since; до тех пор until; до каки́х пор? how long?; с э́тих пор from now on, from then on; до сих пор 1) (*о времени*) up to now; 2) (*до этого места*) up to here; в са́мую по́ру in the nick of time, just at the right time.

порабо́та|ть *сов.* do* some work; сла́вно ~ли well done!

поработи́тель *м.* ensláver; oppréssor; (*завоеватель*) cónqueror.

поработи́ть *сов. см.* порабоща́ть.

порабощ|а́ть, поработи́ть (*вн.*) ensláve (*smth.*), súbjugate (*smth.*). ~е́ние *с.* enslávement, subjugátion.

поравня́ться *сов.* (*с тв.*) come* up (to), draw* lével (with).

пора́довать(ся) *сов. см.* ра́довать(ся).

пораж|а́ть, порази́ть (*вн.*) 1. (*наносить удар*) strike* a blow (at); (*пулей и т. п.*) hit* (*smb., smth.*);

(*кинжалом, ножом и т. п.*) stab (*smb., smth.*); (*разбивать*) deféat (*smb., smth.*); 2. (*о болезни*) afféct (*smth.*); нéкоторые гáзы ~áют лёгкие cértain gáses afféct the lungs; 3. (*удивлять*) strike* (*smb.*), astónish (*smb.*). ~áться, поразѝться be* struck/astónished.

пораже́н|ец *м.* deféatist. ~ие *с.* 1. (*разгром*) deféat, rout; нанести́ ~ие deféat, inflíct a deféat; 2. (*болезненное повреждение*) afféction, dámage; ◇ ~ие в правáх disfránchisement. ~чество *с.* deféatism.

порази́тельн|о strík̇ingly (*тж.*); онá ~ красѝва she is strík̇ingly béautiful. ~ый wónderful, astónishing, amázing, strík̇ing; ~ая пáмять wónderful mémory; ~ое схóдство strík̇ing/wónderful líkeness.

порази́ть(ся) *сов. см.* поражáть(ся).

поразмы́слить *сов.* (*о пр.*) *разг.* think* (*smth.*) óver, turn (*smth.*) óver in one's mind.

по-рáзному in different ways.

пораста́ть, порасти́ (*вн.*) becóme*/be* overgrówn (with), be* dótted with clumps (of); порасти́ травóй becóme* overgrówn with grass, acquíre a cóvering of grass.

порасти́ *сов. см.* пораста́ть.

пореде́ть *сов. см.* реде́ть.

поре́з *м.* cut.

поре́зать 1. (*вн.*; *поранить*) cut* (*smth.*); ~ рýку ножóм cut* one's hand with a knife*; 2. (*вн.*) *разг.* (*зарезать всех, многих*) kill (*smb., smth.*); 3. (*вн., рд.*; *нарезать в каком-л. количестве*) cut* some (*smth.*); ~ колбасы́ cut* some sáusage. ~ся *сов.* cut* onesélf.

поре́й *м.* leek.

порекомендова́ть *сов.* (*вн.*) recomménd (*smb., smth.*).

порист|ость *ж.* porósity, pórousness. ~ый pórous.

порица́|ние *с.* cénsure; выноси́ть ~ кому-л. pass cénsure on *smb.* ~ть *несов.* (*вн.*) cénsure (*smb., smth.*), blame (*smb., smth.*).

по́рка I *ж.* (*платья и т. п.*) unpíck̇ing.

по́рка II *ж. разг.* (*наказание*) flógging.

по́ровну équally, in équal shares/parts; дели́ть расхóды ~ share expénses équally.

поро́г *м.* 1. thréshold, dóorstep; перешагну́ть чéрез ~ cross the thréshold; 2. (*речной*) rápids *pl*; днепрóвские ~и the Dníeper rápids; 3. (*наименьшая величина чего-л.*) thréshold, limit; ~ сознáния thréshold of cónsciousness; ~ излучéния radiátion cút-off; ◇ на ~ не пускáть *кого-л.* not allów *smb.* ínto one's house.

поро́да *ж.* 1. (*домашних животных*) breed, stock; *разг.* (*породистость*) blood, bréeding; 2. (*растений*) type, sort; (*категория людей*) type, kind; э́та ~ людéй this sort of péople. 4. *уст.* (*происхождение*) breed, stock; 5. *геол.* rock.

породи́ст|ость *ж.* bréeding, blood, race. ~ый thóroughbred; pédigree *attr.*; ~ая лóшадь blóod-horse.

породи́ть *сов. см.* порожда́ть.

породни́ть *сов. см.* родни́ть 1. ~ся *сов. см.* родни́ться 1.

порожд|а́ть, породи́ть (*вн.*) génerate (*smth.*); give* rise to (*smth.*); (*о чувствах и т. п. тж.*) cause (*smth.*), evóke (*smth.*), give* rise (to). ~éние *с.* óutcome, resúlt.

поро́жн|ий *разг.* émpty; ~ий рейс émpty run; ◇ перелива́ть из пустóго в ~ее ≈ waste words, waste time in úseless debáte. ~я́к *м. ж.-д.* émpties *pl.* ~яко́м *разг.* émpty, not lóaded.

поро́знь séparately; apárt; жить ~ live séparately; входи́ть ~ énter one by one.

порозове́ть *сов. см.* розове́ть 1.

поро́й now and then; at tímes.

поро́к *м.* 1. (*недостаток*) deféct, fault; více; бéдность не ~ póverty is no crime/disgráce; 2. (*физический недостаток*) defórmity; deféct; ◇ ~ сéрдца válvular diséase of the heart.

пороло́н *м.* (fléxible polyuretháne) foam; pórolon. ~овый foam *attr.*; pórolon *attr.*

поросёнок *м.* súck̇ing-pig; píglet; жáреный ~ roast pig.

пороси́ться, опороси́ться fárrow.

по́росль *ж.* 1. shoots *pl*; young growth (*тж. перен.*); 2. (*заросль*) thícket.

порося́|тина *ж.* pork; ~чий pig's.

поро́ть I, распоро́ть (*вн.*) (*платье и т. п.*) unpíck (*smth.*); (*разрывать*) rip (*smth.*).

поро́ть II, вы́пороть (*вн.*) *разг.* (*бить*) flog (*smb.*), whip (*smb.*), give* (*smb.*) a thráshing/flógging.

поро́ть III *несов.*: ~ вздор, чушь talk nónsense/rot, talk through one's hat.

по́рох *м.* (gún)powder; охóтничий ~ spórting powder; ◇ держáть ~ сухи́м keep* one's powder dry; не хватáет ~у *кому-л.* smb. lacks the énergy; ~ трáтить дáром waste one's powder and shot.

порохов|о́й (gún)powder *attr.*; ◇ ~áя бóчка powder-bárrel.

пороч|ить, опоро́чить (*вн.*) 1. (*позорить*) discrédit (*smb., smth.*); bring* discrédit/disrepúte (upón), disgráce (*smb.*); ~ чьё-л. и́мя blast smb.'s reputátion; 2. (*признавать плохим*) dispárage (*smth.*), run* (*smth.*) down; pull (*smth.*) to píeces *разг.* ~ный 1. vícious, depráved; ~ный человéк immóral pérson; ~ное поведéние vícious cónduct; 2. (*неправильный*) fáulty, unsóund; ◇ ~ный круг vícious círcle.

поро́ша *ж.* fresh/loose snow; néwly-fállen snow.

порошкообра́зный pówdery, powder-like.

порошо́к *м.* pówder.

поро́ю *см.* поро́й.

порт *м.* port; морскóй ~ séaport; речнóй ~ ríver port; торгóвый ~ commércial/tráḋing port; входи́ть в ~ come* ínto port.

порта́л *м. архит.* pórtal.

портати́вн|ый pórtable; ~ая пи́шущая маши́нка pórtable týpewriter.

портве́йн *м.* port.

по́ртик *м.* pórtico (*pl* -oes, -os).

по́ртить, испо́ртить (*вн.*) 1. (*приводить в негодность*) spoil* (*smth.*), ruin (*smth.*); ~ мотóр ruin an éngine; ~ чью-л. рабóту spoil* smb.'s work; ~ здорóвье ruin/impáir one's health; ~ зрéние spoil* one's eyes; испóртить себé желýдок ruin/upsét one's digéstion; испóртить жизнь кому-л. ruin smb.'s life; 2. (*делать неприятным*) spoil* (*smth.*); ~ настроéние кому-л. spoil*/upsét smb.'s mood; 3. (*оказывать дурное влияние*) corrúpt (*smth.*), have* a bad effect (on); (*баловать*) spoil* (*smth.*); ~ детéй spoil*/indúlge one's children. ~ся, испо́ртиться 1. (*становиться негодным*) spoil*, get* spoiled; get* out of órder; (*о пище*) go* off, go*/turn bad; мои́ часы́ испóртились my watch is out of órder; ры́ба легкó пóртится fish éasily goes bad; 2. (*становиться неприятным*) declíne, detériorate; (*о погоде*) break* up; у негó испóртился харáктер his témper/disposítion has changed for the worse; у меня́ испóртилось настроéние I'm upsét/depréssed; 3. (*приобретать дурные наклонности*) degénerate, be* ruined; devélop a flaw.

портни́ха *ж.* dréssmaker.

портно́вский táilor's.

портно́й *м.* táilor; дáмский ~ ládies' táilor.

портня́жный táilor's.

порто́в|ый port *attr.*; ~ые сбóры port chárges; ~ гóрод séaport; ~ые рабóчие dóckers.

по́рто-фра́нко *с. нескл. торг.* free port.

портре́т *м.* 1. pórtrait; ~ во весь рост fúll-length

pórtrait; писáть чей-л. ~ paint smb.'s pórtrait; 2. разг. (подобие кого-л.) líkeness, ímage; он ~ своегó отцá he is the líving ímage of his fáther; 3. (описание персонажа в романе и т. п.) pícture. ~ист м. pórtrait-painter. ~ный pórtrait attr.; ~ная жúвопись pórtrait-painting, pórtraiture.

портсигáр м. cigarétte-case.

португáл|ец м. Portuguése. ~ка ж. Portuguése wóman*.

португáльский Portuguése; ~ язы́к Portuguése, the Portuguése lánguage.

портупéя ж. sword-belt; (плечевая) shóulder-belt.

портфéл|ь м. 1. (сумка) brief-case, bag; 2. (министерский) portfólio (pl -os), ministérial post; распределéние ~ей appóintment of mínisters; 3. перен.: редакцибнный ~ matérial in the éditor's hands.

портьéра ж. cúrtain, drápery; hángings pl; (над дверью тж.) portière, dóor-curtain.

портя́нка ж. fóot-cloth.

порубúть сов. (вн.) 1. (вырубить всё, многое) fell (smth.); 2. (изрубить) chip (smth.); (зарубить) cut* down (smb., smth.).

поругáние с. óutrage, ínsult; (осквернение) profanátion, desecrátion.

порýганный óutraged; (осквернённый) profáned, désecrated.

поругáть сов. (вн.) scold (smb.), tell* (smb.) off, give* (smb.) a télling-off. ~ся сов. 1. (с тв.) quárrel (with), have* a quárrel/row/squábble (with); 2. (ругаться некоторое время) make* a row/fuss.

порýк|а ж. guarantée, pledge; ◇ взять кого-л. на ~и go* bail for smb., bail smb. out; отпустúть кого-л. на ~и let* smb. out on bail, admít smb. to bail.

по-рýсски in Rússian; (в русском стиле) in the Rússian way; Rússian style; говорúть ~ speak* Rússian.

поруч|áть, поручúть 1. (дт. вн., дт. + инф.) charge (smb. with, smb. + to inf), commíssion (smb. with, smb. + to inf); емý бы́ло порученó э́то сдéлать he was charged with the task, he was charged/commíssioned to do it; 2. (дт. вн.; вверять) entrúst (smb. with); ей бы́ло порученó воспитáние ребёнка she was entrústed with the care of the child*. ~éние с. míssion, commíssion, assígnment; (мелкое) érrand; выполня́ть ~éние be* on a míssion; по ~éнию кого-л. on instrúctions from smb., on the instrúctions of smb.

поручúтель м. guárantor, spónsor. ~ство с. guarantée; (залог) bail.

поручúть сов. см. поручáть.

поручúться сов. см. ручáться.

порýчни мн. (ед. пóручень м.) hánd-rails.

порхáть, порхнýть flútter, flit; fly* abóut.

порхнýть сов. см. порхáть.

порцибнный à la carte.

пóрци|я ж. pórtion; (кушанья тж.) hélping; двe ~и салáта sálad for two; три ~и морóженого three íces.

пóрча ж. spóiling; (повреждение) dámage; (ухудшение) deteriorátion.

пóршень м. píston.

поршнев|óй píston attr.; ~óе кольцó píston ring.

поры́в м. 1. (ветра) gust, blast; 2. (внезапное проявление чувства, настроения) ímpulse, gust, burst, óutburst; поддáться минýтному ~у give* way to a mómentary ímpulse; ~ гнéва gust/burst of ánger.

порывáть, порвáть (вн.) break* off (smth.); порвáть дипломатúческие отношéния break* off diplomátic relátions; порвáть связи с кем-л. break* off relátions with smb., break* with smb.

порывáться несов. (+ инф.) try (+ to inf), endéavour (+ to inf).

поры́вист|ость ж. 1. (ветра) gústiness; 2. (человека) impetuósity, impétuousness. ~ый 1. (неровный) gústy; ~ый вéтер gústy wind; 2. (резкий) jérky, abrúpt;

~ые движéния jérky móvements; 3. (пылкий) impétuous; ~ая натýра impétuous náture/cháracter.

порыжéлый rústy-brówn, réddish.

порыжéть сов. см. рыжéть 1.

поры́ться сов. разг. rúmmage; ~ в кармáнах rúmmage in one's póckets; ◇ ~ в пáмяти search one's mémory.

поря́дковый órdinal; ~ нóмер órdinal númber, índex númber.

поря́дком разг. 1. (очень) prétty, considerably, ráther, a good deal; 2. (как следует) próperly, thóroughly.

поря́д|ок м. 1. órder; приводúть свои делá в ~ put*/set* one's affáirs in órder; 2. (система общественного устройства) órder, regíme; стáрый ~ old órder of things, old regíme; установúть нóвый ~ set* up a new órder; 3. (обычай, обыкновение) cústom; по заведённому ~у accórding to the estáblished cústom; 4. (последовательность) órder; алфавúтный ~ alphabétical órder; в ~е óчереди on the queue sýstem; по ~у in succéssion, one áfter anóther; 5. (способ, метод) órder, mánner; (правила) rules pl; в организóванном ~е in an órganized way; в ~е обсуждéния for púrposes of discússion; в ~е предложéния as a suggéstion; ~ голосовáния vóting procédure; ~ утверждéния проéктов procédure to be fóllowed befóre a próject is sánctioned; судéбным ~ком by órder of the court; 6. (построение, строй) órder; боевóй ~ órder of báttle; ◇ в ~ке in órder; всё в ~ке éverything is in órder, éverything is all right; éverything is O.K. амер.; не в ~ке out of órder; здесь чтó-то не в ~ке there is sómething wrong here; у негó гóрло не в ~ке there is sómething wrong with his throat; для ~ка for form's sake; ~ дня agénda; в обы́чном ~ке in the nórmal way; в ~ке вещéй in the náture of things; ~ком вы́ше, на ~ вы́ше a cut abóve, in a dífferent world.

поря́дочн|о 1. (честно, благородно) décently, hónestly; вести себя́ ~ beháve décently; 2. разг. (довольно много) a fair bit; идтú ещё ~ it's a prétty long way yet; there is still a fair bit to go; ждать пришлóсь ~ we had to wait a fáirly long time. ~ость ж. décency, hónesty. ~ый 1. (честный) décent, hónest; ~ый человéк décent pérson; 2. (значительный) considerable; ~ый морóз hard frost; на расстоя́ние quite a dístance; ~ый кусóк quite a large piece; ~ый дохóд fáirly good íncome, substántial íncome.

посадúть сов. см. садúть и сажáть.

посáдка ж. 1. (растений) plánting; 2. обыкн. мн. (посаженные растения) beds, plántings; 3. (самолёта) lánding; слепáя ~ blind lánding; 4. (в поезд, самолёт) bóarding; (на пароход) embarkátion; ещё не началáсь the pássengers are not yet allówed to board the train; 5. (манера держаться в седле) seat, pósture.

посáдочн|ый 1. с.-х. plánting attr.; ~ картóфель plánting potáto (pl -oes); 2. (служащий для посадки на поезд и т. п.) bóarding attr.; ~ талóн (к билéту) bóarding card; ~ трап gángway; 3. ав. lánding attr.; ~ая площáдка lánding ground/place; ~ знак lánding mark.

посвáтаться сов. см. свáтаться.

посвежéть сов. см. свежéть.

посветúть сов. 1. см. светúть 2; 2. (светить некоторое время) shine* (for a while), give* a líttle light.

посветлéть сов. см. светлéть 1.

посвúстывать несов. whístle (sóftly).

по-свóему in one's own way.

посвящ|áть, посвятúть 1. (вн. ~оes), inítiate (smb. into), let* (smb. into); посвятúть дрýга в свою тáйну confíde one's sécret to a friend; 2. (вн. дт.; труд, время) devóte (smth. to), dédicate (smth. to), give* up (smth. to); ~ себя́ наýке devóte onesélf to science; заседáние бы́ло ~енó пáмяти Гóголя the méeting was held in mémory/commemorátion of Gógol; 3. (вн. дт.; литературное произведение и т. п.) dédicate (smth. to). ~ение с. 1. (в тайны и т. п.) initiátion (ínto); 2. (литературного произведения) dedicátion.

посéв м. 1. (действие) sówing; 2. (то, что посеяно) crop; озимые ~ы winter crops; яровые ~ы spring crops. ~нóй sówing; ~ная кампáния sówing campáign; ~ная плóщадь área únder crops/cultivátion, crop área.

поседéть сов. см. седéть.

поселéн|ец м. 1. séttler; 2. (сосланный) éxile, deportée. ~ие с. 1. séttlement; 2. (высылка) deportátion.

поселúть(ся) сов. см. поселять(ся).

поселкóвый víllage attr.

посёлок м. séttlement; дáчный ~ subúrban estáte, súmmer-cóttage commúnity.

поселять, поселúть (вн.) (на новые земли) séttle (smb.); (в новые дома) instáll (smb.). ~ся, поселúться (на новых землях) séttle (в новой квартире) move in.

посеребрúть сов. см. серебрúть.

посередúне 1. нареч. in the míddle; 2. предлог (рд.) in the míddle (of).

посерéть сов. см. серéть 1.

посетúтель м., ~ница ж. vísitor, cáller; чáстый ~ fréquent vísitor.

посетúть сов. см. посещáть.

посéтовать сов. см. сéтовать.

посещáемость ж. atténdance; хорóшая ~ good* atténdance.

посещ|áть, посетúть (вн.) vísit (smb., smth.) (тж. перен.); call on (smb.); (лекции и т. п.) atténd; чáсто ~ когó-л. be* a fréquent vísitor to smb.'s house. ~éние с. vísit; (официальное) call; (лекции и т.п.) atténdance (at).

посéять сов. см. сéять.

посидéть сов. sit* (for a while).

посúльн|ый within one's pówers после сущ.; эта задáча ему вполнé ~a the task is well within his pówers; оказáть ~ую пóмощь do* what one can.

посинéть сов. см. синéть 1.

поскакáть сов. 1. (начать передвигаться скачками) hop awáy; 2. (о лошади) gállop awáy; 3. (скакать некоторое время) gállop (for a while), have* a gállop.

поскользнý|ться сов. slip; он ~лся he slipped, his foot slipped.

поскóльку since, inasmúch as, so far as, as far as.

послаблéни|е с. relaxátion, indúlgence; никакúх ~й no léniency.

послáн|ец м. méssenger, énvoy. ~ие с. méssage. ~ник м. дип. énvoy; (посольства, миссии) the mínister.

послáть сов. см. посылáть.

пóсле 1. нареч. áfterwards, láter; 2. предлог (рд.) áfter; (с тех пор как) since; он придёт ~ рабóты he will come áfter work; мы не вúдели егó ~ егó болéзни we háven't seen him since he was ill; ~ всех last; он вýступил ~ всех he spoke last.

послевоéнный postwár.

послéди|ть сов. (за тв.) watch (smb., smth.) (for a while); ~ глазáми за кем-л. fóllow smb. with one's eyes.

послéдн|ий прил. 1. last; ~ день óтпуска last day of a hóliday; в ~ раз for the last time; в ~ие пять лет он óчень постарéл he has aged considerably óver the last/past five years; в сáмый ~ момéнт at the last móment; 2. (самый новый) the látest; одéт по ~ей мóде (véry) fáshionably dressed; стрóить по ~ему слóву тéхники build* on (extrémely) módern lines; ~ие нóвости the látest news; 3. (только что упомянутый) the látter; 4. (окончательный, решающий) fínal; это моё ~ее слóво that is all I have to say; 5. (плохой, худший) worst; (бранный) vílest; ~ человéк the lówest of the low; ругáть когó-л. ~ими словáми call smb. the vílest names (one can think of); 6. в знач. сущ. one's all; ◇ до ~его to the útmost; за ~ее врéмя látely.

послéдователь м. fóllower, adhérent. ~ность ж. 1. (непрерывность) succéssion, séquence; 2. (логичность) consístency. ~ный 1. (непрерывно следующий один за другим) succéssive, consécutive; 2. (логичный) consístent; ~ный вывод consístent conclúsion.

послéдовать сов. см. слéдовать 1, 2, 3.

послéдстви|е с. cónsequence, resúlt; ~ болéзни the resúlt of an íllness; ◇ остáвить жáлобу без ~й ignóre a compláint.

послéдующи|й fóllowing, súbsequent; ~е события súbsequent evénts.

послезáвтра the day áfter tomórrow.

послелóг м. лингв. póstposition.

послеобéденный áfter-dinner attr.

послеслóвие с. épilogue.

послóвиц|а ж. próverb; войтú в ~у becóme* a próverb, becóme* provérbial.

послужúть сов. 1. см. служúть 5, 6, 7; 2. (служить некоторое время) serve (for a time).

послужнóй: ~ спúсок sérvice récord.

послушáние с. obédience.

послýш|ать сов. 1. см. слýшать 1, 2, 5, 6, 7; 2. (вн.) (некоторое время) listen (to) (for a while); ~ лéкцию atténd a lécture; ~ певцá listen to a sínger; ~ больнóго sound a pátient. ~аться сов. см. слýшаться 1, 2. ~ный obédient, dócile.

послýшаться сов. см. слýшаться.

посмáтривать несов.: ~ по сторонáм glance/look round from time to time; ~ на часý glance/look at one's watch from time to time.

посмéиваться несов. chúckle; (над тв.) twit (smb.), chaff (smb.), make* géntle fun (of); pull smb.'s leg идиом.

посмéнн|о in shifts; рабóтать ~ work in shifts. ~ый shift attr.

посмéртный pósthumous.

посмéть сов. см. сметь.

посмéшище с. láughing-stock; быть всеóбщим ~м be* a láughing-stock, be* a fígure of fun; выставлять когó-л. на ~ make* a láughing-stock of smb., guy smb.

посмеяться сов. 1. (некоторое время) give* a (short) laugh; have* a laugh; 2. (над тв.) laugh (at).

посмотрéть сов. см. смотрéть 1—10. ~ся сов. см. смотрéться 1.

посóбие с. 1. (денежная помощь) allówance, grant, bénefit; ~ по врéменной нетрудоспосóбности témporary disabílity allówance; ~ по инвалúдности disability pénsion; 2. (учебник) téxtbook, mánual; 3. (предмет, необходимый при обучении) aid.

посóбни|к м. неодобр. accómplice. ~чество с. assísting; (в преступлении) complícity.

посовéтовать(ся) сов. см. совéтовать(ся).

посóл м. ambássador; Чрезвычáйный и Полномóчный ~ Ambássador Extraórdinary and Plenipoténtiary.

посолúть сов. см. солúть.

посóль|ский (относящийся к послу) ambassadórial; (относящийся к посольству) émbassy attr. ~ство с. émbassy.

пóсох м. staff*; (пастушеский) crook.

посóхнуть сов. dry up; (о цветах, листьях тж.) wíther.

поспáть сов. sleep*, have* a sleep/nap; ~ пóсле обéда have* an áfter-dinner nap.

поспевáть I, поспéть 1. (созревать) rípen; яблоки поспéли the ápples are ripe; 2. разг. (быть готовым для еды) be* réady.

поспевáть II, поспéть разг. (успевать) be* in time (for); не поспéть к пóезду miss the train; ~ за кем-л. keep* pace with smb., keep* up with smb.

поспéть I, II сов. см. поспевáть I, II.

поспешúть сов. см. спешúть 1.

поспе́шн|ость ж. haste. ~ый há́sty, precípitate; ~ое реше́ние há́sty decísion; ~ый отъе́зд abrúpt depárture.

поспо́рить сов. 1. см. спо́рить; 2. (спорить некоторое время) á́rgue for a while; 3. (с тв.; вступить в соревнование) compéte (with); он мо́жет ~ с лу́чшими игрока́ми he can hold his own with the best plá́yers.

посрами́ть сов. см. посрамля́ть.

посрамля́ть, посрами́ть (вн.) shame (smb.), cóver (smb.) with shame.

посреди́ 1. нареч. in the míddle; 2. предлог (рд.) in the míddle (of); ~ реки́ in the míddle of the rí́ver, in midstré́am.

посреди́не см. посереди́не.

посре́дник м. 1. (торговый) á́gent, míddleman*; 2. (в споре) intermé́diary, gó́-between; (в переговорах) mé́diator.

посре́дни|чать несов. разг. mé́diate. ~чество с. mediá́tion; (содействие примирению тж.) intercéssion.

посре́дственн|о нареч. 1. indífferently; 2. в знач. сущ. с. нескл. (отметка) fair. ~ость ж. mediócrity. ~ый mé́diocre, undistí́nguished; ~ые зна́ния mé́diocre/ indífferent knó́wledge sg.

посре́дство|м с.: при ~е кого́-л., че́рез ~ кого́-л. through smb., thanks to smb.; при ~е чего́-л., че́рез ~ чего́-л. by means of smth.

посре́дством by means of, with the aid of.

поссо́рить(ся) сов. см. ссо́рить(ся).

пост I м. post; наблюда́тельный ~ observá́tion post; прове́рка ~о́в inspé́ction of the guard; ◇ на ~у́ at one's post; умере́ть на (своём) ~у́ die at one's post.

пост II м. церк. fast(ing).

поста́вить I сов. см. ста́вить.

поста́вить II сов. см. поставля́ть.

поста́вк|а ж. delí́very, supplý́; госуда́рственные ~и delí́veries to the state.

поставля́ть, поста́вить (вн.) delí́ver (smth.), supplý́ (smth.). ~щи́к м. delí́verer, supplí́er; (продуктов тж.) purvé́yor.

постаме́нт м. pé́destal, base.

постанови́ть сов. см. постановля́ть.

постано́вка ж. 1. (театральная) prodú́ction, stá́ging; 2. (проблемы и т. п.) pó́siting, propó́unding; ~ вопро́са the way a próblem is stá́ted/put/posed; 3. (дела и т. п.) organizá́tion; 4.: ~ го́лоса voice trá́ining.

постановле́ние с. 1. (решение) resolú́tion, decísion; ~ о́бщего собра́ния decísion of a gé́neral mé́eting; 2. (распоряжение) decré́e.

постановля́ть, постанови́ть (вн.) 1. (решать) decíde (smth.), resó́lve (smth.); 2. (издавать постановление) decré́e (smth.), ená́ct (smth.).

постано́вщик м. театр. prodú́cer, diré́ctor, stá́ge-má́nager.

постара́ться сов. см. стара́ться.

поста́реть сов. см. старе́ть 1.

по-ста́рому in the old way; as of old, as befó́re.

постели́ть сов. см. постила́ть.

посте́ль ж. 1. (кровать) bed; 2. (спальные принадлежности) bed-clothes, bé́dding. ~ный bed attr.; ~ное бельё bé́d-linen; sheets and pí́llow-cases pl; ~ный режи́м confí́nement to bed.

постепе́нн|о grá́dually, lí́ttle by lí́ttle, bit by bit. ~ость ж. grá́dualness; ~ый grá́dual.

постесня́ться сов. см. стесня́ться 2.

постига́ть, пости́гнуть, пости́чь (вн.) 1. (понимать) comprehé́nd (smth.), understá́nd* (smth.), grasp (smth.); пости́чь та́йны приро́ды learn* ná́ture's sécrets; 2. (случаться с кем-л.) overtá́ke* (smb.), befá́ll* (smb.); его́ пости́гло несча́стье he has had a misfó́rtune.

пости́гнуть сов. см. постига́ть.

постиж|е́ние с. comprehé́nsion, understá́nding. ~и́мый comprehé́nsible, understá́ndable.

постила́ть, постла́ть, разг. постели́ть (вн.) spread*

(smth.); постла́ть ска́терть на стол put* a cloth on the tá́ble; ~ посте́ль make* a bed.

постира́ть сов. (вн.) wash (smth.), do* some wá́shing.

пости́ться несов. fast.

пости́чь сов. см. постига́ть.

постла́ть сов. см. постила́ть и стлать 1.

по́стн|ый 1. without meat or milk после сущ.; ~ суп mé́atless soup; ~ое ма́сло vé́getable oil; 2. разг. (нежирный) lean; ~ое мя́со lean meat; 3. разг. (хмурый, скучный) gló́omy, dí́smal; ~ое лицо́ dí́smal face; 4. разг. (ханжеский) sanctimó́nious, smug; ~ вид sanctimó́nious air.

постово́й прил. 1. on pó́int-duty после сущ.; ~ милиционе́р milí́tiaman* on point dú́ty; 2. в знач. сущ. м. pó́intsman*; (о солдате) sé́ntry.

посто́льку inasmú́ch as, in so far as; ~ поско́льку so far as.

посторони́ться сов. см. сторони́ться 1.

посторо́нн|ий прил. 1. (чужой) strange; ~ челове́к strá́nger, outsí́der; 2. (не собственный) ó́utside attr.; of ó́thers после сущ.; без ~ей по́мощи withó́ut á́ny ó́utside help; 3. (не имеющий прямого отношения к чему-л.) incidé́ntal; ~ие разгово́ры incidé́ntal discú́ssion sg; 4. в знач. сущ. м. strá́nger; при ~их in front of strá́ngers; ~им вход воспрещён unaú́thorized pé́rsons not admí́tted.

постоя́нн|о á́lways, cónstantly, contínually. ~ый 1. cónstant, sté́ady, contínuous; ~ые ве́тры cónstant winds; ~ое наблюде́ние cónstant observá́tion; 2. (всегдашний) ré́gular, habí́tual; ~ые покупа́тели ré́gular cú́stomers; ~ый посети́тель habí́tual ví́sitor; 3. (не временный) pé́rmanent, invá́riable; ~ый а́дрес pé́rmanent á́ddress; ~ое местожи́тельство pé́rmanent ré́sidence; 4. (верный) sté́ady; быть ~ым в свои́х взгля́дах hold* fast to one's opínions; ◇ ~ая а́рмия stá́nding/ré́gular á́rmy; ~ая величина́ мат. cónstant; ~ый капита́л эк. cónstant/fixed cá́pital; ~ый ток diré́ct cú́rrent.

постоя́нство с. cónstancy, sté́adfastness; (неизменность) regulá́rity.

постоя́ть сов. 1. (стоять некоторое время) stand* (for a while); (побыть где-л.) stay; 2. (за вн.; защитить) stand* up (for); ~ за себя́ stand* up for onesé́lf, hold* one's own; 3.: посто́й(те)! just a mí́nute!, wait a bit!

пострада́вший м. ví́ctim.

пострада́ть сов. см. страда́ть 3, 4, 5.

постри́чь сов. (что-л.) cut* (smth.); (кого́-л.) cut* smb.'s hair, give* smb. a há́ircut. ~ся сов. have* one's hair cut.

построе́ние с. 1. constrú́ction; ~ треуго́льника drá́wing/constrú́ction of a trí́angle; ~ фра́зы constrú́ction of a sé́ntence; ~ рома́на constrú́ction of a nó́vel; 2. воен. formá́tion.

постро́ить сов. см. стро́ить. ~ся сов. см. стро́иться 1, 2, 5.

постро́йка ж. 1. (действие) bú́ilding, eré́cting, constrú́ction; 2. (место, где строят) bú́ilding site; 3. (здание) bú́ilding, strú́cture.

постскри́птум м. pó́stscript (сокр. P. S.).

посту́кивать несов. knock, tap, rap.

поступа́тельн|ый ó́nward, fó́rward, progré́ssive; ~ое разви́тие progré́ssive devé́lopment; ~ое движе́ние физ. translá́tional mó́tion.

поступа́ть, поступи́ть 1 (действовать) act, do*; он не знал, как поступи́ть he dí́dn't know how to act; 2. (с тв.; по отношению к кому-л., чему-л.) treat (smb., smth.) bá́dly; 3. (в вн.; в учебное заведе́ние, на службу) é́nter (smth.); (в армию) enlí́st (in); ~ на рабо́ту take* a job; она́ поступи́ла секретарём she is emplóyed as a sé́cretary; 4. (доходить по назначению) come*, be* recéived; поступи́ло заявле́ние an applicá́tion has been recéived/filed; к нам поступи́ла жа́лоба а compláint has been lodged with us; дело поступило в суд the case has come befóre the court; в продажу поступила новая партия товаров there is some fresh stock on sale.

поступа́ться, поступи́ться (*тв.*) give* up (*smth.*), forgó* (*smth.*); ~ свои́м пра́вом waive *one's* right; ~ свои́ми интере́сами go* agáinst *one's* ínterests.

поступи́ть *сов.* (*дт.*) поступа́ть.

поступи́ться *сов. см.* поступа́ться.

посту́пок *м.* áction, act, deed; сме́лый ~ brave deed, act of brávery.

по́ступь *ж.* walk, step; march (*тж. перен.*); пла́вная ~ gráceful walk; ~ вре́мени the march of time.

постуча́ть *сов.* tap, knock (at), (*громко*) bang, pound. ~ся *сов.* knock.

постфа́ктум post fáctum, áfter the evént.

постыди́ться *сов.* (*рд.*, + *инф.*) be* ashámed (in front of, + to *inf*); ~ чужи́х люде́й be* ashámed in front of strángers.

посты́дный shámeful, disgráceful.

посты́лый *разг.* háteful.

посу́да *ж.* 1. *собир.* (plates and) díshes *pl*; столо́вая ~ tábleware; ча́йная ~ téa-things; ку́хонная ~ kítchen uténsils *pl*; ме́дная ~ cópper-ware; 2. *разг.* (*сосуд*) contáiner; bóttle.

посу́дина *ж. разг.* véssel, old tub.

посуди́ть *сов.*: посуди́ сам judge for yoursélf.

посу́дн|ый: ~ шкаф chína-closet, cúpboard; ~ое полоте́нце dísh-cloth, tea/dish tówel; ~ый магази́н chína-shop.

посчастли́в|иться *сов. безл.* (*дт.*): мне (нам *и т. д.*) ~илось (+ *инф.*) I was (we were, *etc.*) lúcky/fórtunate enóugh (+ to *inf*); I (we, *etc.*) had the good luck/fórtune (+ to *inf*).

посчит|а́ть *сов.* (*вн.*) count (*smb., smth.*); ~а́й! work it out! ~а́ться *сов.* (с *тв.*) 1. (*свести́ счёты с кем-л.*) get* éven (with); 2. (*приня́ть во внима́ние*) take* accóunt (of).

посыла́ть, посла́ть (*вн.*) send* (*smb., smth.*), dispátch (*smth.*); ~ кого́-л. за врачо́м send* smb. for the dóctor; ~ кого́-л. в командиро́вку send* smb. on a mission/búsiness trip; ~ что-л. по по́чте send* smth. by post; ~ де́ньги по по́чте, по телегра́фу remít móney.

посы́лка *ж.* 1. (*де́йствие*) sénding, dispátching; 2. (*почто́вая*) párcel; 3. *филос.* prémise; ◇ быть на ~х run* érrands.

посы́льн|ый *прил.* 1. dispátch *attr.*; ~ое су́дно dispátch-boat, dispátch-vessel; 2. *в знач. сущ. м.* méssenger.

посыпа́ть *сов. см.* посыпа́ть.

посыпа́ть, посы́пать (*вн.*) 1. sprínkle (*smth.*): ~ хлеб со́лью sprínkle the bread with salt, sprínkle salt on the bread; ~ пиро́жное са́харом dust a cake with súgar; 2. (*усе́ивать, покрыва́ть*) strew* (*smth.*); ~ пол опи́лками strew* the floor with sáwdust.

посы́п|аться *сов.* begín* to fall, fall*; *перен. разг.* rain; ли́стья ~ались leaves begán to fall; на него́ ~ались уда́ры blows rained upón him; на меня́ ~ались вопро́сы I was shówered with quéstions.

посяга́тельство *с.* (*на вн.*) encróachment (on, upón), infríngement (on, upón); ~ на чьи-л. права́ encróachment upón *smb.'s* rights.

посяг|а́ть, посягну́ть (*на вн.*) encróach (on, upón), infrínge (on, upón); ~ на чьи-л. права́ encróach/infrínge upón *smb.'s* rights. ~ну́ть *сов. см.* посяга́ть.

пот *м.* sweat, perspirátion; ◇ ~ом и кро́вью by/with *one's* (own) sweat and blood.

потайно́й sécret, hídden; ~ ход sécret pássage.

потака́ть *несов.* (*дт.*) *разг.* indúlge (*smb., smth.*); pánder (to), give* way (to); ~ чьим-л. капри́зам indúlge *smb.'s* whims.

потанцева́ть *сов.* have* a dance, dance.

потасо́вка *ж. разг.* (*дра́ка*) brawl, fight.

пота́ш *м.* pótash.

по-тво́ему 1. (*по тво́ему мне́нию*) in your opínion, to your mind; как ~? what do you think?, what is your opínion? 2. (*по тво́ему жела́нию*) as you like, as you wish; (*по тво́ему сове́ту*) as you advíse; я сде́лал ~ I did as you told me; пусть бу́дет ~! be it your (own) way!

потво́рство *с.* indúlgence. ~вать *несов.* (*дт.*) indúlge (*smth.*), pánder (to).

потёмк|и *мн.* dárkness *sg*; ◇ быть в ~ах be* in the dark; чужа́я душа́ — ~ *посл.* the heart of anóther is a dark fórest, the húman heart is a mýstery.

потемне́ть *сов. см.* темне́ть 1, 2.

потенциа́л *м.* poténtial; экономи́ческий ~ económic poténtial; ра́зность ~ов poténtial dífference.

потенциа́льный poténtial *attr.*

потепле́ние *с.* rise in témperature; наступи́ло ~ it grew wármer; насту́пит ~ it will be wármer, the cold snap will be óver.

потепле́ть *сов. см.* тепле́ть.

потере́ться *сов. см.* тере́ться 1, 3.

потерпе́вший *прил.* 1. *юр.* that has súffered loss, ínjury, *etc. после сущ.*; 2. *в знач. сущ.*: ~ от пожа́ра víctim of a fire; ~ от наводне́ния flood víctim.

потерпе́ть *сов.* 1. (*терпели́во выноси́ть что-л.*) éxercise pátience, be* pátient; 2. (*вн.; испыта́ть, перенести́ что-л.*) súffer (*smth.*); ~ убы́тки súffer lósses; ~ круше́ние meet* with disáster.

потёртый shábby, thréadbare.

поте́р|я *ж.* loss; ~ вре́мени loss/waste of time; ~и уби́тыми fátal cásualties; ~ созна́ния swoon, fáinting fit, loss of cónsciousness; ~ па́мяти loss of mémory, amnésia. ~янный 1. (*расстро́енный*) dismáyed, upsét; 2. (*смущённый*) confúsed, embárrassed; 3. *разг.* (*опусти́вшийся*) degráded, disréputable.

потеря́ть(ся) *сов. см.* теря́ть(ся).

потесни́ть *сов. см.* тесни́ть.

поте́ть, вспоте́ть, запоте́ть 1. *сов.* вспоте́ть sweat, perspíre, break* out in a sweat; 2. *сов.* запоте́ть (*об о́кнах и т. п.*) be* damp, sweat, ooze móisture; 3. *тк. несов.* (*над тв.*) *разг.* (*труди́ться над чем-л.*) wréstle (with), sweat (at), lábour (at); ~ над зада́чей wréstle with a próblem.

поте́ха *ж.* fun, amúsement; (*смешно́е происше́ствие*) fúnny thing.

потеша́ть *несов.* (*вн.*) amúse (*smb.*), divért (*smb.*). ~ся *несов.* 1. amúse onesélf; 2. (*над тв.; насмеха́ться*) make* fun (of), mock (at) (*smb.*).

поте́ш|ить(ся) *сов. см.* те́шить(ся). ~ный *разг.* fúnny, cómical.

потира́ть *несов.* (*вн.*) rub (*smth.*); ~ ру́ки rub *one's* hands.

потихо́ньку *разг.* 1. (*ме́дленно*) slówly; 2. (*неслы́шно*) quíetly; 3. (*та́йно*) sécretly, on the sly.

по́тн|ый swéaty, perspíring; ~ые ру́ки swéaty/clámmy hands.

пото́к *м.* 1. flood, tórrent; (*све́та и т. п.*) flow, stream (*тж. перен.*); весе́нние ~и spring tórrents; ~ во́здуха air flow; ~ слов flow of words; ~ слёз flood of tears; ~ руга́тельств tórrent/shówer/stream of abúse; людско́й ~ stream of péople; магни́тный ~ magnétic flux; 2. (*непреры́вное произво́дство*) flów-production; 3. (*гру́ппа уча́щихся*) group.

потолкова́ть *сов. разг.* talk, have* a talk.

потол|о́к *м.* céiling (*тж. перен.*); ко́мната с высо́ким ~о́м room with a high céiling, high-céilinged room; достига́ть ~ка́ *ав.* reach its céiling; ◇ взять что-л. с ~ка́ cook/dream* smth. up.

потолсте́ть *сов. см.* толсте́ть.

пото́м (*по́сле*) áfterwards; (*по́зже*) láter on; (*зате́м*) then.

пото́м|ок *м.* 1. descéndant, óffspring; 2. *мн.* (*лю́ди* *будущих поколений*) descéndants; postérity *sg.* ~ственный heréditary. ~ство *с.* 1. (*молодое поколение*) prógeny; оставить многочисленное ~ство leave* mány descéndants; 2. *собир.* (*потомки*) postérity.

потому́ 1. *нареч.* thérefore, that is why; 2. *союз:* ~ что becáuse; for *поэт.*

потону́ть *сов. см.* тону́ть.

пото́п *м.* flood, déluge.

потопи́ть *сов. см.* топи́ть III.

потопта́ть *сов.* (*вн.*) trámple down (*smth.*), tread* down (*smth.*).

поторапливать *несов.* (*вн.*) *разг.* húrry (*smb.*) up, urge (*smb.*) on. ~ся *несов. разг.* make* haste, get* a shift on.

потропи́ть(ся) *сов. см.* торопи́ть(ся).

поточн|ый: ~ое произво́дство mass/line prodúction.

потра́ва *ж.* dámage to crops.

потрави́ть *сов.* (*вн.*) 1. (*посевы*) spoil* (*smth.*), dámage (*smth.*); (*о скоте*) trámple down (*smth.*); 2. (*истребить*) póison (*smth.*), kill off (*smth.*).

потра́тить(ся) *сов. см.* тра́тить(ся).

потреби́тель *м.* consúmer. ~ный: ~ная сто́имость *эк.* use válue.

потреби́тельск|ий consúmer *attr.*, consúmer's; ~ое о́бщество co-óperative socíety; ~ие това́ры consúmer goods.

потреби́ть *сов. см.* потребля́ть.

потребле́ни|е *с.* consúmption; това́ры широ́кого ~я consúmer goods.

потре́бност|ь *ж.* need, want, requírement; у него́ небольши́е ~и he is a man of few wants; ~ в сырье́ need for raw matérial; культу́рные ~и cúltural needs/requírements/expectátions.

потре́бовать *сов. см.* тре́бовать 1, 3, 4. ~ся *сов. см.* тре́боваться.

потрево́жить *сов. см.* трево́жить 2.

потрёпанн|ый shábby, thréadbare; *перен.* (*о войсках*) báttered; (*о человеке*) séedy; ~ое пальто́ shábby coat; ~ая кни́га táttered book; име́ть ~ вид look worn out, look séedy.

потрепа́ть *сов. см.* трепа́ть 1, 2, 3. ~ся *сов. см.* трепа́ться 2.

потре́скаться *сов. см.* тре́скаться.

потре́скивать *несов.* cráckle.

потро́гать *сов.* (*вн.*) touch (*smb., smth.*) once or twice, feel* (*smth.*).

потро|ха́ *мн.* éntrails; (*гусиные*) gíblets; суп с гуси́ными ~ха́ми gíblet soup; ◇ со все́ми ~ха́ми bag and bággage. ~ши́ть (*вн.*) разг. дисembówel (*smth.*); (*птицу*) draw* (*smth.*); (*рыбу*) gut (*smth.*), clean (*smth.*).

потру|ди́ться *сов.* 1. (*поработать*) do* some work, work; 2. (+ *инф.*; *счесть нужным*) take* the tróuble (+ to *inf*); он да́же не ~ился сообщи́ть мне he didn't éven take the tróuble to infórm me; ~и́тесь закры́ть дверь! would you mind clósing the door!

потряс|а́ть, потрясти́ 1. (*вн., тв.*) shake* (*smth.*); (*оружием и т. п.*) brándish (*smth.*), flóurish (*smth.*); 2. (*вн.; заставлять дрожать*) shake* (*smth.*), make* (*smth.*) quíver/vibráte/trémble; уда́р гро́ма потря́с во́здух a clap of thúnder made the air quíver; потря́с зда́ние an explósion shook the building; 3. (*вн.; производить большое впечатление*) shake* (*smth.*), have* a deep efféct (on), stágger (*smb.*); get* únder *smb.'s* skin *идиом.*; он был потрясён тем, что услы́шал he was stággered by what he heard; ~ зри́телей impréss an áudience. ~а́ющий stággering; ~а́ющие но́вости stággering news; ~а́ющее зре́лище astónishing spéctacle. ~е́ние *с.* 1. shock; не́рвное ~е́ние nérvous shock; 2. (*коренная ломка*) uphéaval.

потрясти́ *сов. см.* потряса́ть.

потря́хивать *несов.* (*вн., тв.*) shake* (*smth.*).

поту́ги *мн.* 1. (*родовые*) trávail *sg*; pangs of chíldbirth; lábour *sg*; 2. (*бесплодные попытки*) vain attémpts.

поту́пить *сов.:* ~ взор cast* down one's eyes, look down; ~ го́лову hang* one's head. ~ся *сов.* lówer one's eyes/head.

потускне́лый dimmed; (*о металлах тж.*) tárnished.

потускне́ть *сов. см.* тускне́ть.

потуха́ние *с.* extínction.

потуха́ть, поту́хнуть (*о свете, огне*) go* out; die out; (*об огне тж.*) burn* out.

поту́хнуть *сов. см.* потуха́ть *и* ту́хнуть I.

поту́хш|ий extínct; *перен.* lácklustre; ~ вулка́н extínct volcáno; ~ие глаза́ dim/lácklustre eyes.

потучне́ть *сов. см.* тучне́ть.

потуши́ть *сов. см.* туши́ть I.

потяга́ться *сов.* (с *тв.*) *разг.* tússle (with), conténd (with).

потя́гиваться, потяну́ться stretch onesélf.

потян|у́ть *сов.* 1. (*вн.*) pull (*smb., smth.*); ~ кого́-л. за рука́в pluck (at) *smb.'s* sleeve; 2. *безл.*: его́ ~у́ло домо́й he felt an urge/lónging to go home. ~у́ться *сов.* 1. *см.* потя́гиваться; 2.: он ~у́лся че́рез стол he leaned óver the táble; все за ним ~у́лись éverybody fóllowed him; ~у́лись до́лгие зи́мние вечера́ the long winter évenings have set in.

поу́жинать *сов. см.* у́жинать.

поумне́ть *сов. см.* умне́ть.

поутру́ *разг.* in the (éarly) mórning.

поуч|а́ть *несов.* (*вн.*) lécture (*smb.*). ~е́ние *с.* 1. (*действие*) edificátion; 2. (*наставление*) lécture, hómily, sérmon.

поучи́тельный instrúctive; (*назидательный*) édifying; ~ приме́р instrúctive exámple; ~ сове́т instrúctive advice; ~ тон édifying tone.

поха́б|ный *разг.* fílthy, dírty, obscéne. ~щина *ж. разг.* filth; obscénities *pl.*

похвал|а́ *ж.* praise; рассы́паться в ~а́х кому́-л. sing* *smb.'s* práises.

похвали́ть(ся) *сов. см.* хвали́ть(ся).

похвальба́ *ж. разг.* brágging, bóasting.

похва́льн|ый 1. (*содержащий в себе похвалу*) appróving; of praise *после сущ.*; ~ая гра́мота certíficate of appróval; 2. (*заслуживающий похвалы*) láudable, práiseworthy, comméndable; ~ое усе́рдие comméndable zeal.

похва́стать(ся) *сов. см.* хва́стать(ся).

похити́тель *м.* (*вещей*) stéaler; (*людей*) kídnapper; (*самолётов и т.п.*) híjacker.

похи́тить *сов. см.* похища́ть.

похищ|а́ть, похи́тить (*вн.*) (*вещи*) steal* (*smth.*); (*людей*) kídnap (*smb.*); (*самолёт и т. п.*) híjack (*smth.*). ~е́ние *с.* (*вещей*) stéaling; (*людей*) kídnapping; (*самолётов и т. п.*) híjacking.

похлёбка *ж.* (thick) soup.

похло́пать *сов. см.* хло́пать.

похлопота́ть *сов. см.* хлопота́ть 2, 3.

похло́пывать *несов.* (*вн.*) pat (*smb.*); ~ кого́-л. по плечу́ pat *smb.* on the back.

похме́лье *с.* háng-over; ◇ в чужо́м пиру́ ~ táking the rap for sómebody else, shóuldering óther péople's sins.

похо́д *м.* 1. (*передвижение*) march; вы́ступить в ~ march out, take* the field; 2. (*массовая организованная прогулка*) excúrsion, tour, óuting; (*пешком тж.*) wálking tour, hike; отпра́виться в двухдне́вный ~ go* off on a twó-day excúrsion; 3. (*военная кампания*) campáign; 4. (*кампания*) drive; ~ за эконо́мию ecónomy drive.

похода́тайствовать *сов. см.* хода́тайствовать.

походи́ть I *сов.* (*некоторое время*) walk (for a while); ~ по го́роду go* for a walk round town.

походи́ть II *несов.* (на *вн.*; *быть похожим*) resémble (*smb.*), look/be* like (*smb.*).

похо́дка *ж.* walk; у неё лёгкая ~ she is light-fóoted.

похо́дн|ый **1.** march *attr.*, márching; ~ поря́док march órder/formátion; дви́гаться ~ым поря́дком march; **2.** (*предназначенный для похода*) field *attr.*; camp *attr.*; ~ая крова́ть camp-béd; **3.** (*передвижной*) field *attr.*, móbile; ~ая ку́хня field kítchen; ~ го́спиталь field-hóspital.

похо́дя *разг.* (*торопливо*) in haste, on the move; (*заодно*) in pássing; (*между прочим*) for no partícular réason, óff-hándedly.

похожде́ние *с.* advénture.

похо́ж|ий resémbling, like, símilar; alíke *predic.*; быть ~им друг на дру́га resémble one anóther, be* símilar/alíke; вы все друг на дру́га ~и you are all alíke; он похо́ж на своего́ отца́ he takes áfter his fáther; на кого́ он похо́ж? who is he like?; он на себя́ не похо́ж ≈ you'd néver récognize him; ◇ э́то совсе́м на вас не ~е that's not at all like you; э́то на него́ ~е it's just like him; э́то ни на что не ~е it's unthínkable; I never heard of such a thing; ~е на то, что... it looks as if...; ~ на то, что пойдёт дождь it looks like rain; на кого́ вы ~и! just look at yoursélf!; они́ ~и как две ка́пли воды́ they are as like as two peas.

похолода́ние *с.* fall in témperature; наступи́ло ~ it has grown cólder, a cold snap/spell has set in.

похолода́|ть *сов. безл.:* ~ло it grew cólder.

похолоде́ть *сов. см.* холоде́ть.

похорони́ть *сов. см.* хорони́ть.

похоро́нн|ый fúneral; *перен. разг.* funéreal, dísmal; ~ая проце́ссия fúneral procéssion; ~ое бюро́ úndertaker's óffice; ~ марш fúneral march; ~ое выраже́ние лица́ a funéreal face.

по́хороны *мн.* fúneral *sg*, búrial *sg*.

похороше́ть *сов. см.* хороше́ть.

похохота́ть *сов.* laugh, have* a laugh.

похуде́ть *сов. см.* худе́ть.

поцелова́ть(ся) *сов. см.* целова́ть(ся).

поцелу́й *м.* kiss.

почасов|о́й hóur-to-hour; by the hour *после сущ.*; ~ гра́фик рабо́ты hóur-to-hour tíme-table of work; ~а́я опла́та páyment by the hour.

поча́ток *м. бот.* ear; ~ кукуру́зы córn-cob.

по́чв|а *ж.* **1.** soil; обрабо́тка ~ы soil cultivátion; плодоро́дие ~ы soil fertílity; **2.** *горн.* béd-rock; **3.** (*основание, основа*) ground, foundátion; чу́вствовать под собо́й твёрдую ~у be* on sure/firm ground; выбива́ть ~у из-под ног cut* the ground from únder *smb.'s* feet; подгото́вить ~у prepáre the ground, pave the way; э́ти утвержде́ния не име́ют под собо́й никако́й ~ы these assértions are gróundless; теря́ть под собо́й ~у be*/get* out of *one's* depth; ◇ на ~е *чего-л.* due to *smth.*, ówing to *smth.*

по́чвенн|ый soil *attr.*; ~ слой soil láyer; ~ая ка́рта soil map.

почвове́д *м.* soil scíentist. ~ение *с.* soil science.

почём *разг.* (*по какой цене*) how much?, how much is it?; ◇ ~ знать who knows?; ~ я зна́ю? how do I know?

почему́ **1.** *вопр.* why?; **2.** *относ.* that's why.

почему́|-либо, ~-нибудь for some réason (or óther); éсли он ~ не прие́дет if, for some réason, he dóesn't come.

почему́-то for some réason; он ~ э́того не хо́чет for some réason he dóesn't want it.

по́черк *м.* hánd(writing); *перен.* mánner; ме́лкий ~ small hand; писа́ть ме́лким ~ом write* (a) small (hand); у него́ о́чень хоро́ший ~ he writes a véry good hand; неразбо́рчивый ~ illégible hand/hándwriting.

почерне́ть *сов. см.* черне́ть 1.

почерпну́ть *сов.* (*вн.*) *разг.* scoop up (*smth.*); *перен.*

draw* (*smth.*), take* (*smth.*), deríve (*smth.*); ~ материа́л из первоисто́чников draw* on original sóurces.

почерстве́ть *сов. см.* черстве́ть 2.

почеса́ть *сов. см.* чеса́ть 1. ~ся *сов. см.* чеса́ться 1.

по́чест|ь *ж.* hónour; воздава́ть ~и кому́-л. pay*/do* hónour to *smb.*

почёсывать *несов.* (*вн.*) *разг.* scratch (*smth.*). ~ся *несов. разг.* scratch onesélf.

почёт *м.* hónour, respéct, estéem; по́льзоваться ~ом be* held in high estéem; учёные у нас в большо́м ~е scientists are held in great respéct/hónour in our cóuntry; ~ный **1.** (*пользующийся почётом*) hónoured; ~ный гость guest of hónour, hónoured guest; **2.** (*избираемый в знак почёта*) hónorary; ~ное зва́ние hónorary títle; **3.** (*делающий честь кому-л.*) hónourable; ~ная обя́занность hónourable dúty; **4.** (*не нарушающий достоинства*) hónourable.

по́чечн|ый kidney *attr.*; nephrític; ~ ка́мень kidney-stone; ~ое са́ло suet.

почи́н *м.* **1.** (*инициатива*) inítiative; по со́бственному ~у on *one's* own inítiative; **2.** *разг.* (*начало*) start, begínning; для ~а to start with.

почини́ть *сов. см.* чини́ть I 1.

почи́нка *ж.* repáiring, ménding; repáir-job.

почи́стить *сов.* (*вн.*) clean (*smth.*); (*щёткой*) brush (*smth.*); ~ сапоги́ pólish *one's* boots; ~ зу́бы clean/brush *one's* teeth. ~ся *сов.* have* a wash and brúsh-up, clean onesélf up.

почита́тель *м.*, ~ница *ж.* admírer.

почита́ть I *сов.* (*читать некоторое время*) read* (for a while).

почита́ть II *несов.* (*вн.*; *уважать*) hónour (*smb.*, *smth.*), respéct (*smb.*, *smth.*), estéem (*smb.*, *smth.*).

почи́тывать *несов.* (*вн.*) *разг.* read* (*smth.*) (now and then); ~ кни́жки browse óver *one's* books.

по́чка I *ж.* **1.** *бот.* bud, shoot; **2.** *биол.* gémma (*pl* -ae).

по́чка II *ж.* **1.** *анат.* kidney; **2.** *мн. кул.* kidneys.

по́чт|а *ж.* **1.** post; (*почтовое отделение*) póst-office; ~ рабо́тала пло́хо póstal sérvices were bad/errátic; пойти́ на ~у go* to the póst-office; **2.** (*почтовая служба*) post, mail; отпра́вить письмо́ по ~е send* a létter by post/mail, post/mail a létter; вече́рняя ~ évening post; **3.** (*корреспонденция*) post, mail.

почтальо́н *м.* póstman*.

почта́мт *м.* póst-office; гла́вный ~ Main Póst-Office.

почте́н|ие *с.* respéct; относи́ться с ~ием к кому́-л. treat *smb.* with respéct, have* respéct for *smb.*, respéct *smb.* ~ный **1.** wórthy; (*о возрасте*) vénerable; ~ная нару́жность wórthy appéarance; ~ный стари́к vénerable old man*; **2.** *разг.* (*значительный*) consíderable, respéctable.

почти́ álmost, néarly; э́то ~ то́ же са́мое it's álmost the same thing; мы ~ до́ма we're néarly home; ~ всегда́ álmost álways; ~ никогда́ hárdly éver; ~ ничего́ scárcely ánything, next to nóthing; ~ никого́ hárdly ányone, next to nóbody; рабо́та ~ зако́нчена the work is álmost compléted; э́то ~ невозмо́жно it is álmost impóssible.

почти́тельн|ость *ж.* respéct, déference. ~ый **1.** respéctful, deferéntial; ~ый сын dútiful son; **2.** *разг.* (*значительный*) consíderable; на ~ом расстоя́нии at a respéctful dístance.

почти́ть *сов.* (*вн.*) **1.** (*оказывать почёт*) pay*/do* hómage (to); ~ чью-л. па́мять встава́нием rise* in mémory of *smb.*; **2.** (*оказать честь*) hónour (*smth.*); ~ кого́-л. свои́м прису́тствием hónour *smb.* with/by *one's* présence.

почто́в|ый póstal; post *attr.*; ~ я́щик létter-box; ~ая бума́га nóte-paper, létter-páper; ~ая откры́тка póstcard; ~ая ма́рка (póstage) stamp; ~ое отделе́ние (branch) póst-office; ~ по́езд mail train; ~ парохо́д máil-boat; ~ые расхо́ды póstage *sg*.

почу́вствовать *сов. см.* чу́вствовать.

почу́диться *сов. см.* чу́диться.

пошатну́ть *сов. (вн.; прям. и перен.)* shake* *(smth.)*; ~ чьи-л. убежде́ния shake* *smb.'s* convictions. ~ся *сов. (наклониться)* lurch, give* a lurch; *(о людях тж.)* stagger; *перен.* be* shaken; его́ здоро́вье пошатну́лось his health is shaken.

поша́тыв|ать *несов. безл.*: его́ ~ает he is unsteady on his legs. ~аться *несов.* stagger, reel to and fro; идти́ по у́лице ~аясь go* reeling down the street.

пошеве́ливать *несов. (вн., тв.)* stir *(smth.)*. ~ся *несов.*: пошеве́ливайтесь! get a move on!

пошеве́ли́ть *сов. (вн., тв.)* stir *(smth.)*; ~ ли́стья stir the leaves; ~ кры́льями stir *one's* wings. ~ся *сов.* stir; не сметь ~ся not dare to stir.

пошевельну́ть *сов. (вн., тв.)* stir *(smth.)*; он и па́льцем не пошевельнёт, что́бы ей помо́чь he wouldn't stir/lift a finger to help her. ~ся *сов.* stir.

поши́б *м. разг.* manner; они́ о́ба одного́ ~а they are both of the same breed/stamp.

пошлин|а *ж.* duty; облага́ть что-л. ~ой impose a duty on *smth.*

по́шл|ость *ж.* 1. shallowness; *(узость)* small-mindedness; *(банальность)* triteness, banality; 2. *(замечание, выражение)* trite/commonplace remark; *(пошлый поступок)* low act; *(непристойность)* vulgarity. ~ый 1. *(низкий)* shallow, petty; ~ый челове́к shallow person; 2. *(банальный)* trite, commonplace, banal; *(грубый, непристойный)* vulgar, low.

пошля́к *м. разг.* shallow person.

поштопать *сов. (вн.)* darn *(smth.)*.

пошту́чн|ый by the piece *после сущ.*; ~ая опла́та payment by the piece; ~ая прода́жа loose sale.

пошуме́ть *сов.* make* a bit of noise.

пошути́ть *сов. см.* шути́ть.

поща́д|а *ж.* mercy; проси́ть ~ы cry/beg/ask for mercy; без ~ы without mercy.

пощади́ть *сов. см.* щади́ть.

пощекота́ть *сов. см.* щекота́ть.

пощёчин|а *ж.* slap in the face *(тж. перен.)*; box on the ear; получи́ть ~у receive a slap in the face.

пощу́пать *сов. см.* щу́пать.

поэ́зия *ж.* poetry.

поэ́ма *ж.* poem.

поэ́т *м.* poet. ~е́сса *ж.* poetess. ~ика *ж.* poetics *pl.*

поэти́ческ|ий poetic(al); ~ая во́льность poetic licence; ~ дар poetic talent; ~ое произведе́ние poetical work.

поэти́чный poetical.

поэ́тому therefore, that is why, consequently.

появи́ться *сов. см.* появля́ться.

появле́ние *с.* appearance; *(книги тж.)* publication.

появля́ться, появи́ться appear; *(о людях тж.)* put* in an appearance, show* up; *(на поверхности)* emerge; в темноте́ появи́лась фигу́ра a figure loomed up in the darkness; появи́лась наде́жда there was a hope.

по́яс *м.* 1. belt, girdle; *(юбки, брюк)* waist-band; 2. *(талия)* waist; по ~ up to the waist; по ~ в воде́ waist-deep in water; 3 *геогр.* belt, zone; аркти́ческий ~ frigid zone; ◇ спаса́тельный ~ life-belt; кла́няться в ~ кому́-л. make* a deep/low bow to *smb.*

поясн|е́ние *с.* explanation. ~и́тельный explanatory.

поясни́ть *сов. см.* поясня́ть.

пояснии́ц|а *ж.* loins *pl*; small of the back; боль в ~е pains in the small of the back.

поясн|о́й: ~ реме́нь waist-belt; *(портупея)* sword-belt; ~ портре́т half-length portrait; ~а́я ва́нна hip-bath; ~о́е вре́мя zone time.

поясни́ть, поясни́ть *(вн.)* explain *(smth.)*.

праба́бушка *ж.* great-grandmother.

пра́вд|а *ж.* 1. *(истина)* truth; говори́ть всю ~у speak* the whole truth; го́лая ~ naked/unvarnished truth; 2. *(правдивость)* truthfulness, truth; 3. *разг. (правота)*

rightness; ~ на ва́шей стороне́ you are right; 4. *(справедливость)* justice; 5. *в знач. сказ.* be* true; ~ ли, что он отказа́лся пое́хать? is it true that he refused to go?; 6. *в знач. вводн. сл.* true, admittedly; он, ~, не знал э́того admittedly he didn't know that; 7. *в знач. союза (хотя)* though; ◇ по ~е говоря́, по ~е сказа́ть to tell the truth, the truth is; все́ми ~ами и непра́вдами by hook or by crook; не ~ ли? isn't it?; смотре́ть ~е в глаза́ face (up) to the truth. ~и́вость *ж.* truthfulness, veracity. ~и́вый 1. *(содержащий в себе правду)* true, truthful; ~и́вый расска́з true story.

правдоподо́бный plausible, probable.

пра́ведн|ик *м.* righteous person. ~ый righteous; *(справедливый)* just.

пра́вил|о *с.* 1. rule; граммати́ческое ~ rule of grammar; 2. *обыкн. мн. (положения, служащие руководством)* regulations; ~а вну́треннего распоря́дка rules and regulations; ~а игры́ the rules of the game; соблюда́ть ~а игры́ observe the rules of the game; play according to the rules; ~а у́личного движе́ния traffic regulations, rules of the road; 3. *(образ мыслей, норма поведения)* principle, maxim; взять себе́ за ~ make* it a rule; он взял себе́ за ~ ходи́ть в библиоте́ку ка́ждый день he made it a rule to go to the library every day; ◇ как *(общее)* ~ as a *(general)* rule; по всем ~ам properly.

пра́вильн|о *нареч. (без ошибок)* correctly; *(верно)* rightly; говори́ть ~ speak* correctly; поступа́ть ~ act rightly; 2. *в знач. сказ. разг.* it is correct; *(как восклицание)* quite right!, that's right! ~ый 1. *(соответствующий правилам)* correct; *(закономерный)* regular; ~ое произноше́ние correct pronunciation; ~ый глаго́л regular verb; 2. *(верный, точный)* right, correct; сде́лать ~ый вы́вод из чего́-л. draw* the right conclusion from *smth.*; ~ый отве́т correct/right answer; 3. *(настоящий)* proper, real; 4. *(равномерный)* regular; ~ое бие́ние се́рдца regular pulse; 5. *(симметричный)* well-proportioned, symmetrical; ~ые черты́ лица́ regular features; 6. *мат.* regular.

прави́тель *м.* ruler.

прави́тельственн|ый government *attr.*, governmental; ~ые учрежде́ния government offices; ~ая делега́ция government delegation; ~ая награ́да government award; ~ое сообще́ние government statement.

прави́тельство *с.* government; administration *амер.*

пра́вить I *несов. (тв.)* 1. *(руководить)* rule *(smb., smth.)*; govern *(smb., smth.)*; 2. *(лошадьми, автомаши́ной)* drive* *(smth.)*; *(судном, яхтой)* steer *(smth.)*.

пра́вить II *несов. (вн.)* 1. *(исправлять ошибки)* correct *(smth.)*; ~ корректу́ру read* proofs; 2. *(выпрямля́ть)* straighten *(smth.)*; *(точить, острить)* sharpen *(smth.)*, set* *(smth.)*; ~ бри́тву sharpen/strop a razor.

пра́вка *ж.* 1. *(исправление ошибок)* correcting; ~ корректу́ры proof-correcting, proof-reading; 2. *(бритвы)* stropping, sharpening, setting.

правле́ни|е *с.* 1. *(управление государством)* government; о́браз ~я form of government; 2. *(выборный орган)* (management) board; быть чле́ном ~я be* on the board.

пра́вну|к *м.* great-grandson. ~чка *ж.* great-granddaughter.

пра́в|о I *с.* 1. right; име́ть ~ have* a right, be* entitled; име́ть ~ го́лоса have* the vote; ~ на труд the right to work; ~ да́вности *юр.* (positive) prescription, prescriptive right; 2. *тк. ед. (наука)* law; уголо́вное ~ criminal law; обы́чное ~ customary/common law; изуча́ть ~ study law; read* for the bar; 3. *мн. разг. (свиде́тельство)* licence; ◇ по ~у by right; на ~а́х кого́-л. (in the exercise of) one's rights as *smb.*; на ра́вных ~а́х enjoying/exercising equal rights.

пра́во II *вводн. сл.* really, truly, indeed; я, ~, не зна́ю, что мне де́лать I really don't know what to do.

правобере́жный right-bank *attr.*

правове́рный órthodox.

правов|о́й légal; ~ые отноше́ния relátions góverned by law.

правоме́рный legítimate; ~ вы́вод legítimate conclúsion.

правомо́чный *юр.* cómpetent, áuthorized.

правонаруш|е́ние *с. юр.* offénce, infríngement of the law. ~и́тель *м.* offénder, delínquent.

правописа́ние *с.* spélling, orthógraphy.

правосла́в|ие *с.* the Órthodox/Greek Church, Órthodoxy. ~ный *прил.* 1. Órthodox; 2. *в знач. сущ. м.* a mémber of the Órthodox Church.

правосу́дие *с.* jústice; отправля́ть ~ admínister jústice.

правот|а́ *ж.* ríghtness, sóundness, corréctness; доказа́ть чью-л. ~у́ prove that *smb.* is right.

правофланго́вый *прил.* 1. ríght-flank, ríght-wing; 2. *в знач. сущ. м.* ríght-flank man*; (*передовик*) pácesetter, pácemaker.

пра́в|ый I *прил.* 1. right, ríght-hand; ~ая рука́ right hand; ~ая нога́ right foot*; ~ бе́рег реки́ the ríght (-hand) bank of a ríver; ~ я́щик стола́ the ríght-hand drawer; на ~ой стороне́ on the ríght(-hand) side; 2. *полит.* Ríght-wing; ~ые ли́деры социа́л-демокра́тии the Right sócial-democrátic léaders; 3. *в знач. сущ. м.* Ríght-winger, Ríghtist.

пра́в|ый II 1. (*правильный*) right; вы ~ы you are right; 2. (*справедливый*) just; стоя́ть за ~ое де́ло uphóld* a just cause.

пра́вящ|ий rúling; ~ие кла́ссы the rúling clásses; ~ая па́ртия the párty in pówer.

пра́дед *м.*, праде́душка *м.* gréat-grándfather.

пра́зднеств|о *с.* celebrátion, festívity; (*пир.*) feast; наро́дные ~а nátional celebrátions.

пра́здник *м.* 1. hóliday, féstival; национа́льный ~ nátional hóliday/féstival; пое́хать домо́й на ~и go* home for the hólidays; 2. (*веселье*) celebrátion, entertáinment, festívity; семе́йный ~ fámily celebrátion; ◇ бу́дет и на на́шей у́лице ~ we shall have our day, our day will come.

пра́здничн|о ~ый 1. féstively. féstival *attr.*; (*устраиваемый в честь праздника тж.*) in celebrátion of the féstival *после сущ.*; ~ый салю́т salúte in celebrátion of the féstival; ~ый конце́рт gála cóncert; 2. (*нарядный*) féstive; (*о людях*) célebrating; ~ое пла́тье féstive dress/attíre; 3. (*торжественно-радостный*) féstive; hóliday *attr.*, gála *attr.*; ~ое настрое́ние hóliday/féstive mood.

пра́зднов|ание *с.* celebrátion. ~ать, отпра́здновать (*вн.*) célebrate (*smth.*); ~ать день рожде́ния célebrate *one's* bírthday.

пра́здность *ж.* ídleness.

праздношата́ющийся *м. разг.* lóafer, ídler.

пра́здн|ый ídle; *перен. тж.* fútile, póintless; ~ разгово́р ídle talk; ~ое любопы́тство ídle curiósity.

пра́ктик *м.* practícian, práctical man*.

пра́ктик|а *ж.* 1. práctice; изучи́ть что-л. на ~e learn* *smth.* by práctice; применя́ть что-л. на ~e put* *smth.* into práctice; 2. (*приёмы и навыки*) práctical expérience; у него́ больша́я ~ по строи́тельству желе́зных доро́г he has had long práctical expérience of/in building ráilways; 3. (*студенческая, учебная*) práctical work; проходи́ть ~у do práctical work, take* *one's* prácticals; 4. *уст.* (*врачебная, юридическая*) práctice; врач с большо́й ~ой a dóctor with a large práctice. ~а́нт *м.* tráinee, práctical stúdent.

практикова́ть *несов.* (*вн.*) práctise (*smth.*). ~ся, напрактикова́ться 1. (*в пр.; упражняться*) práctise (*smth.*); ~ся в мета́нии ядра́ práctise pútting the shot; 2. *тк. несов.* (*применяться на практике*) be* práctised/used/applied; (*делаться*) be* done.

пра́ктикум *м.* práctical work; práctical stúdies *pl.*

практици́зм *м.* practicálity, prácticalness.

практи́ческ|ий práctical; ~ая де́ятельность práctical actívity; ~ое примене́ние зна́ний práctical applicátion of (*one's*) knówledge; ~ о́пыт práctical expérience; не име́ть ~ой це́нности be* of no práctical válue.

практи́чн|ость *ж.* practicálity; ~ тка́ни the práctical advántages of a fábric; ~ый práctical; ~ый челове́к práctical pérson; ~ый цвет práctical cólour.

пра́порщик *м.* 1. práporschik (*intermediate rank approximating to warrant officer*); 2. *ист.* énsign.

прах *м.* 1. dust; 2. (*останки*) remáins *pl;* (*после сожжения*) áshes *pl;* ◇ мир ~у его́! may he rest in peace!; отрясти́ ~ от свои́х ног shake* the dust from *one's* feet; пойти́ ~ом go* to rack and ruin.

пра́ч|ечная *ж.* láundry. ~ка *ж.* láundress.

пра́щур *м.* áncestor, fórefather.

праязы́к *м. лингв.* párent lánguage.

преа́мбула *ж.* preámble.

пребыва́ни|е *с.* stay; sójourn *книжн.;* ~ у вла́сти ténure of óffice; ме́сто постоя́нного ~я pérmanent résidence/dómicile; ме́сто ~я прави́тельства the seat of góvernment.

пребыва́ть *несов.* be*; ~ в неве́дении относи́тельно чего-л. be*/remáin in ígnorance of *smth.*, be* in the dark abóut *smth.*

превали́ровать *несов.* (над *тв.*) prepónderate (óver), take* préference (óver).

превзойти́ *сов. см.* превосходи́ть.

превозмога́ть, превозмо́чь (*вн.*) overcóme* (*smth.*).

превозноси́ть *сов. см.* превозноси́ть.

превознести́ *сов. см.* превозноси́ть.

превозноси́ть, превознести́ (*вн.*) praise (*smb., smth.*) to the skies, extól (*smb., smth.*), laud (*smb., smth.*).

превосходи́тельство *с.* éxcellency.

превосходи́ть, превзойти́ 1. (*вн. тв., вн. в пр.; обнаруживать превосходство*) excél (*smb.* in, at), surpáss (*smb.* in), transcénd (*smb.* in); ~ кого-л. тало́нтом surpáss/transcénd *smb.* in tálent; ~ кого-л. чи́сленностью outnúmber *smb.*, be* supérior in númbers to *smb.*; 2. (*вн.; превышать*) surpáss (*smth.*), excéed (*smth.*); превзойти́ все ожида́ния surpáss/excéed all expectátions; превзойти́ самого́ себя́ surpáss onesélf.

превосхо́дн|о éxcellently; (*как восклицание*) spléndid! ~ый éxcellent, fine, spléndid; first-ráte *разг.;* ~ая пого́да spléndid wéather; ◇ ~ая сте́пень *грам.* supérlative degrée.

превосхо́дство *с.* superiórity.

преврати́ть(ся) *сов. см.* превраща́ть(ся).

преврати́ть *во* wróngly; ~ истолко́вывать что-л. misintérpret *smth.*, put* a false constrúction on *smth.;* ~ понима́ть что-л. misunderstánd* *smth.* ~ость *ж.* 1. (*ложность*) wróngness, fálsity; 2. *мн.* (*изменчивость*) vicíssitudes; ~ости судьбы́ the vicíssitudes of life, the ups and downs of life. ~ый 1. (*ложный*) wrong, false; ~ое толкова́ние misinterpretátion; ~ое мне́ние false opínion; 2. (*изменчивый*) chángeable, fíckle, incónstant.

превраща́ть, преврати́ть (*вн. в вн.*) change (*smb., smth.* into), turn (*smb., smth.* into), convért (*smth.* into); (*в порошок, в пыль*) redúce (*smth.* to); (*химически*) resólve (*smth.* into); ~ что-л. в шу́тку laugh *smth.* off, make* a joke of *smth.* ~ться (*в вн.*) change (to, into), turn (to, into), be* convérted (to, into); (*в порошок, в пыль*) be* redúced (to); ◇ преврати́ться в слух be* all ears. ~е́ние *с.* 1. (*действие*) túrning, convérsion; *биол.* transmutátion; 2. (*неожиданное изменение*) metamórphosis (*pl* -ses), change.

превы́сить *сов. см.* превыша́ть.

превыша́ть, превы́сить (*вн.*) excéed (*smth.*); превы́сить реко́рд beat* the récord; ~ власть, полномо́чия excéed *one's* pówers, go* beyónd *one's* pówers; ~ свой креди́т overdráw *one's* accóunt.

превы́ше: ~ всего́ the híghest considerátion.

превыше́ние *с.* 1. (*действие*) excéeding, overstépping; 2. (*излишек*) excéss; (*кредита*) óverdraft.

прегра́да *ж.* óbstacle, bárrier; *перен. тж.* impédiment, bar.

прегради́ть *сов. см.* прегражда́ть.

прегражда́ть, прегради́ть (*вн.*) bar (*smth.*), block (*smth.*); ~ путь bar the way; ~ до́ступ воде́ stop the wáter cóming in.

пред *см.* перед.

предава́ть, преда́ть (*вн.*) 1. (*изменять*) betráy (*smb., smth.*); (*выдавать тж.*) surrénder (*smb.*); 2. (*подвергать чему-л.*) subjéct (*smb.*), commít (*smb.*), hand óver (*smth.*); ~ кого́-л. суду́ commít *smb.* for tríal; ◇ ~ кого́-л. земле́ commít/consign a bódy to the grave/earht; ~ огню́ commít to the flames; ~ го́род огню́ и мечу́ waste a cíty with fíre and sword. ~ся, преда́ться (*дт.*) give* onesélf up (to), abándon onesélf (to); ~ся мечта́м give* onesélf up to réverie; ~ся печа́ли give* way to grief; ~ся поро́кам indúlge in vice; ~ся пья́нству take* to drink.

преда́ние I *с.* (*действие*) committing; ~ суду́ committal for tríal.

преда́ние II *с.* (*рассказ*) legend; (*поверье*) tradítion.

преданн|ость *ж.* devótion, dedicátion. ~ый devóted; он ему́ пре́дан всей душо́й he is whólly devóted to him; и́скренне ~ый вам (*в конце письма*) yours trúly/sincérely.

преда́тель *м.* betráyer, tráitor. ~ница *ж.* tráitress. ~ский tréacherous (*тж. перен.*); (*коварный*) tráitorous, perfídious; ~ский уда́р tréacherous blow; ~ство *с.* betráyal, tréachery; (*измена родине*) tréason.

преда́ть(ся) *сов. см.* предава́ть(ся).

предвари́тельн|о as a prelíminary, first; (*заранее*) beforehand. ~ный 1. prelíminary; (*неоконченный тж.*) téntative; ~ые перегово́ры prelíminary negotiátions, prelíminaries; 2. (*заблаговременный*) advánce *attr.*; in advánce *после сущ.*; ~ая прода́жа биле́тов advánce bóoking; ~ое сле́дствие prelíminary investigátion; ~ое заключе́ние detÉntion únder remánd.

предве́стник *м.* precúrsor, fórerunner, hárbinger, hérald; ~ бу́ри fórerunner of a storm; ~ весны́ hárbinger of spring.

предвещ|а́ть *несов.* (*вн.*) foretéll* (*smth.*), présage (*smth.*), porténd (*smth.*); (*быть признаком чего-л.*) betóken (*smth.*); тёмные ту́чи ~а́ли грозу́ the dark clouds présaged/thréatened a storm; э́то ничего́ хоро́шего не ~а́ет it bodes no good; всё ~а́ло успе́х éverything betókened succéss.

предвзя́т|ость *ж.* 1. preconcéived náture; 2. (*предубеждение*) preposséssion, préjudice. ~ый preconcéived; ~ое мне́ние preconcéived opínion.

предви́дение *с.* prevísion.

предви́деть *несов.* (*вн.*) foresée* (*smth.*); ~ собы́тия foresée* evénts. ~ся *несов.* be* expécted.

предвкуси́ть *сов. см.* предвкуша́ть.

предвкуш|а́ть, предвкуси́ть (*вн.*) look fórward (to), antícipate (*smth.*); ~ удово́льствие antícipate the pléasure. ~е́ние *с.* (pléasurable) anticipátion; в ~е́нии чего́-л. in pléasurable anticipátion of *smth.*

предводи́тель *м.* chief, léader. ~ство *с.* commánd, léadership.

предвое́нный pre-wár.

предвосхи́тить *сов. см.* предвосхища́ть.

предвосхища́ть, предвосхи́тить (*вн.*) antícipate (*smth.*); ~ собы́тия antícipate evénts.

предвы́борн|ый eléction *attr.*, eléctoral; ~ая кампа́ния eléction campáign.

предго́рье *с.* fóothills *pl.*

преде́л *м.* 1. (*граница*) límit; в ~ах го́рода within the cíty límits; в ~ах страны́ within the cóuntry; вы́ехать за ~ы страны́ leave* the cóuntry; 2. *мн.* (*промежуток*

времени): в ~ах трёх ме́сяцев within three months; 3. *мн.* (*границы, рамки дозволенного*) bounds *pl*; в ~ах возмо́жного within the bounds of possibílity; в ~ах учти́вости within the bounds of políteness; 4. (*последняя степень чего-л.*) límit; ~ высоты́ máximum height; ~ про́чности (últimate) strength; ~ ско́рости speed límit; всему́ есть ~ there is a límit to éverything; 5. (*высшая ступень чего-л.*) height, ácme, súmmit; ~ соверше́нства ácme of perféction; ~ жела́ний súmmit of one's desíres; 6. *мат.* límit.

преде́льн|ый máximum *attr.*, límit *attr.*, límiting; ~ во́зраст máximum age, age límit; ~ая ско́рость máximum/top speed; ~ срок tíme-límit; ~ые уси́лия útmost éfforts; ~ая нагру́зка máximum load.

предзнаменова́ние *с.* ómen, présage, pórtent; до́брое ~ good ómen; дурно́е ~ ill ómen.

предика́т *м.* prédicate. ~и́вный predícative; ~и́вное прилага́тельное predícative ádjective.

предисло́вие *с.* préface, fóreword, introdúction.

предлага́ть, предложи́ть 1. (*дт., вн.; предоставлять*) óffer (*smb. smth.*); предложи́ть кому́-л. свои́ услу́ги óffer *smb.* one's sérvices; предложи́ть кому́-л. ча́ю óffer *smb.* tea; 2. (*вн.; на рассмотрение, на выбор*) propóse (*smth.*), suggést (*smth.*); ~ план де́йствий propóse a course of áction; ~ кандидату́ру propóse a cándidate; put* up/fórward a cándidate; 3. (*дт. + инф.; приглашать кого-л. заняться чем-л.*) invíte (*smb.* + to *inf.*), suggést (that *smb.* should + *inf.*); он предложи́л ей танцева́ть he invited her to dance; 4. (*дт. вн.; задавать*) put* (*smth.* to), set* (*smb. smth.*); предложи́ть кому́-л. вопро́с put* a quéstion to *smb.*; предложи́ть кому́-л. тру́дную зада́чу set* *smb.* a difficult próblem; 5. (*дт. + инф.; предписывать*) órder (*smb.* + to *inf.*).

предло́г I *м.* (*повод*) prétext, excúse, plea; под ~ом чего́-л. únder/on the prétext of *smth.*, on the plea of *smth.*; иска́ть ~ look for an excúse; найти́ ~ find* a prétext.

предло́г II *м. грам.* preposítion.

предложе́ни|е I *с.* 1. (*действие*) óffer, suggéstion; 2. (*для обсуждения, рассмотрения*) propósal, suggéstion; (*на собрании*) mótion; ми́рные ~я peace propósals; внести́ ~ propóse/move a mótion; вы́сказаться за да́нное ~ speak* for the mótion, suppórt the mótion; 3. (*о браке*) propósal; сде́лать ~ кому́-л. propóse to *smb.*; 4. *эк.* supplý; спрос превыша́ет ~ demánd excéeds supplý.

предложе́ние II *с. грам.* séntence; (*часть сложного предложения*) clause.

предложи́ть *сов. см.* предлага́ть.

предло́жный *грам.* preposítional; ~ паде́ж lócative/preposítional case.

предма́йск|ий before May Day *после сущ.*; in hónour of May Day *после сущ.*

предме́стье *с.* súburb.

предме́т *м.* 1. óbject, thing; 2. (*вещь*) árticle; ~ы ро́скоши árticles of lúxury; ~ы пе́рвой необходи́мости the nécessaries of life; ~ы дома́шнего обихо́да hóusehold árticles; 3. (*тема*) súbject, tópic; ~ы нау́чного иссле́дования súbjects of reséarch; ~ ле́кции súbject/theme of a lécture; 4. (*цикл знаний*) súbject; каки́е ~ы он преподаёт? what súbjects does he teach?; 5.: быть ~ом насме́шек be* an óbject of rídicule; ◇ на ~ чего́-л. in órder to/for. ~ный súbject *attr.*; ~ный указа́тель índex (*pl* -exes, -ices); ~ный катало́г súbject cátalogue.

предназнача́ть, предназна́чить (*вн. для рд.*) inténd (*smb., smth.* for), mean* (*smb., smth.* for); (*суммы*) allót (*smth.* to), assign (*smth.* to), éarmark (*smth.* for).

предназна́чить *сов. см.* предназнача́ть.

преднаме́ренн|о inténtionally, delíberately. ~ость *ж.* premeditátion, fórethought. ~ый preméditated; inténtional; afórethought *после сущ.*

предо *см.* перед.

предобе́денный befóre dínner *после сущ.*

пре́док *м.* áncestor.

предоперацио́нный preóperative.

предопредели́ть *сов. см.* предопределя́ть.

предопределя́ть, предопредели́ть (*вн.*) predetérmine (*smth.*).

предоста́вить *сов. см.* предоставля́ть.

предоставл|я́ть, предоста́вить 1. (*вн. дт.; дава́ть*) give* (*smb. smth.*), let* (*smb.*) have (*smth.*); (*права и т. п.*) grant (*smb. smth.*); ~ что-л. в чьё-л. распоряже́ние put*/place *smth.* at *smb.'s* dispósal; ~ кому́-л. о́тпуск grant *smb.* leave; 2. (*дт. + инф.; дава́ть возмо́жность сде́лать*) leave* it (to *smb.* + to *inf*), allów (*smb.* + to *inf*); предоста́вьте реша́ть э́то мне leave* it to me to decíde; я ~я́ю вам суди́ть, прав я и́ли нет I leave it to you to decíde whéther I am right; ~ что-л. на чьё-л. усмотре́ние leave* *smth.* to *smb.'s* discrétion; ◇ ~ самому́ себе́ leave* *smb.* to his, her own devíces; предоста́вить сло́во кому́-л. give* *smb.* the floor, allów *smb.* to speak.

предостере|га́ть, предостере́чь (*вн. от рд.*) warn (*smb.* agáinst), cáution (*smb.* agáinst); ~ кого́-л. от опа́сности warn *smb.* of a dánger. ~га́ющий wárning, cáutionary, admónitory; ~га́ющий тон wárning tone. ~же́ние *с.* wárning, cáution.

предостере́чь *сов. см.* предостерега́ть.

предосторо́жност|ь *ж.* 1. cáution; ме́ры ~и precáutionary méasures; приня́ть все ме́ры ~и take* due precáutions, take* évery precáution; 2. (*ме́ра*) precáution; несмотря́ на все на́ши ~и in spite of all our precáutions.

предосуди́тельный reprehénsible, blámeworthy.

предотврати́ть *сов. см.* предотвраща́ть.

предотвраща́|ть, предотврати́ть (*вн.*) avért (*smth.*), prevént (*smth.*), ward off (*smth.*); ~ опа́сность avért a dánger. ~е́ние *с.* prevéntion; ~е́ние войны́ prevéntion of war.

предохран|е́ние *с.* protéction, preservátion. ~и́тель *м.* sáfety devíce; руже́йный ~и́тель sáfety, catch; электри́ческий ~и́тель sáfety fuse.

предохрани́тельн|ый protéctive; sáfety *attr.*; *мед.* prophyláctic, prevéntive; ~ая окра́ска живо́тных protéctive cólouring of ánimals; ~ кла́пан sáfety-valve; ~ые ме́ры prevéntive méasures.

предохрани́ть *сов. см.* предохраня́ть.

предохраня́ть, предохрани́ть (*вн.*) protéct (*smb., smth.*), presérve (*smb., smth.*).

предписа́ние *с.* órder.

предписа́ть *сов. см.* предпи́сывать.

предпи́сывать, предписа́ть (*вн.*) órder (*smth.*).

предплѐчье *с. анат.* fórearm.

предполага́ть, предположи́ть 1. (*вн.*) suppóse (*smth.*), presúme (*smth.*); (*допуска́ть тж.*) assúme (*smth.*); предположи́м, что э́то так let's assúme that this is the case; 2. *тк. несов.* (+ *инф.; име́ть наме́рение*) inténd (+ to *inf*), cóntemplate (+ -ing), expéct (+ to *inf*); 3. *тк. несов.* (*вн.; име́ть свои́м усло́вием*) (pre)suppóse (*smth.*). ~ся *несов.* be* expécted, be* suppósed; (*намеча́ться*) be* cóntemplated.

предполож|е́ние *с.* 1. (*дога́дка*) supposítion, conjécture; стро́ить ~е́ния make* supposítions; 2. (*наме́рение*) suggéstion, plan. ~и́тельный hypothétical.

предположи́ть *сов. см.* предполага́ть 1.

предпосле́дний last but one; penúltimate *книжн.*; ~ но́мер газе́ты the last but one íssue of the newspaper.

предпосы́лк|а *ж.* 1. (*усло́вие*) preréquisite, precondítion; ~ успе́ха preréquisite of succéss; 2. (*исхо́дный пункт како́го-л. рассужде́ния*) prémise; теорети́ческие ~и theorétical prémises.

предпоче́сть *сов. см.* предпочита́ть.

предпоч|ита́ть, предпоче́сть 1. (*вн. дт.; призна́вать преиму́щество*) prefér (*smth.* to); 2. (+ *инф.; вы-*

би́рать) prefér (+ to *inf*), choose* (+ to *inf*); я предпочёл бы оста́ться до́ма I would ráther stay at home. ~те́ние *с.* préference. ~ти́тельный préferable.

предпра́здничный befóre the hóliday *после сущ.*

предприи́мчив|ость *ж.* énterprise, inítiative. ~ый énterprising.

предпринима́тель *м.* 1. ówner/head of a firm, ówner of a fáctory; (*работода́тель*) emplóyer; 2. (*делец*) búsinessman*, búsiness óperator. ~ский ówner's; emplóyer's; (*свойственный предпринима́телю*) búsinessman's.

предпринима́ть, предприня́ть (*вн.*) undertáke* (*smth.*).

предприня́ть *сов. см.* предпринима́ть.

предприя́тие *с.* 1. (*предпри́нятое де́ло*) undertáking; (*риско́ванное*) vénture; 2. (*промы́шленное*) énterprise; (*заво́д тж.*) fáctory, works; ма́лое ~ small énterprise; совме́стное ~ joint vénture.

предрасполага́ть, предрасположи́ть (*вн.*) 1. (*настра́ивать кого́-л.*) dispóse (*smb.*); 2. *тк. несов.* (*спосо́бствовать чему́-л.*) predispóse (*smb.*).

предрасположе́ние *с.*, предрасполо́женность *ж.* predisposítion.

предрасполо́женный predispósed; ~ к ревмати́зму predispósed to rhéumatism.

предрасположи́ть *сов. см.* предрасполага́ть 1.

предрассве́тный of appróaching dawn *после сущ.*, that precédes the dawn *после сущ.*

предрассу́док *м.* préjudice.

предреша́ть, предреши́ть (*вн.*) 1. decíde (*smth.*) in advánce, decíde (*smth.*) befórehand; 2. (*зара́нее определя́ть*) prédetermine (*smth.*), detérmine (*smth.*) befórehand.

предреши́ть *сов. см.* предреша́ть.

председа́тель *м.* 1. cháirman*; ~ собра́ния cháirman* of a méeting; 2. (П.) (*в соста́ве назва́ния главы́ госуда́рства, прави́тельства*) Cháirman*. ~ский cháirman's; заня́ть ~ское ме́сто take* the chair. ~ство *с.* cháirmanship; под ~ством кого́-л. únder the cháirmanship of *smb.*

председа́тельствовать *несов.* 1. (*в пр.; быть председа́телем колхо́за и т. п.*) be* cháirman* (of); 2. (*на собра́нии*) presíde, be* in the chair, take* the chair.

председа́тельствующий *м.* cháirman*.

предсе́рдие *с. анат.* áuricle.

предсказа́|ние *с.* 1. (*де́йствие*) predícting, foretélling; ~ пого́ды wéather fórecasting; 2. (*то, что предска́зано*) predíction, próphecy. ~тель *м.* foretéller, prognósticator.

предска́зывать, предсказа́ть (*вн.*) foretéll* (*smth.*), próphesy (*smth.*); predíct (*smth.*), fórecast* (*smth.*); ~ бу́дущее predíct the fúture; ~ собы́тия predíct/próphesy evénts; ~ пого́ду fórecast* the wéather; ~ со́лнечное затме́ние predíct an eclípse.

предсме́ртн|ый death *attr.*; ~ая аго́ния death ágony.

представа́ть, предста́ть (*перед тв.*) appéar (befóre).

представи́тель *м.*, ~ница *ж.* representátive; (*фи́рмы тж.*) ágent; (*вырази́тель чьих-л. интере́сов*) spókesman*; торго́вый ~ trade representátive; ~ министе́рства иностра́нных дел representátive of the Mínistry for Fóreign Affáirs; (*в А́нглии*) Fóreign Óffice spókesman*; ~ный 1. representátive; ~ные учрежде́ния representátive institútions; 2. (*соли́дный*) impósing, impréssive, dígnified; ~ная вне́шность impósing appéarance.

представи́тельство *с.* 1. representátion; (*фи́рмы*) óffice, ágency; 2. (*учрежде́ние*): торго́вое ~ Trade Delegátion.

предста́вить *сов. см.* представля́ть 1—4, 8—11. ~ся *сов. см.* представля́ться.

представле́ни|е *с.* 1. (*предъявле́ние*) presentátion, prodúction; 2. (*театра́льное*) perfórmance; дневно́е ~

matinée; 3. (*понимание, знание*) idéa, nótion; иметь смутное ~ о чём-л. have* a vague idéa of smth.; не иметь никакого ~я о чём-л. have* not the fáintest idéa of smth.; составить себе правильное ~ о чём-л. form a true nótion of smth.

предста́вленный represénted *после сущ.*

представл|я́ть, предста́вить 1. (*вн.; подавать куда--л.*) presént (smth.), hand in (smth.); предста́вить отчёт presént a repórt; 2. (*вн.; предъявлять*) prodúce (smth.); предста́вить спра́вку prodúce/show* a certíficate; предста́вить удостовере́ние ли́чности prodúce identificátion pápers; 3. (*вн. дт.; знакомить*) introdúce (smb. to), presént (smb. to); 4. (*вн. к; признав достойным чего-л., ходатайствовать о чём-л.*) recomménd (smb., smth. for); ~ кого́-л. к награ́де recomménd smb. for a decorátion; 5. *тк. несов.* (*вн.; быть, являться кем-л., чем-л.*) be* (smb., smth.); что он собо́й ~ет? what kind of pérson is he?; 6. *тк. несов.* (*вн.; быть представителем*) represént (smb., smth.); 7. *тк. несов.* (*вн.; выражать, защищать чьи-л. интересы*) represént (smth.); 8. (*вн.; на сцене*) act (smth.), show* (smth.); 9. (*вн.; изображать, копировать*) imitate (smb., smth.); 10. (*вн.; мысленно воспроизводить*) imágine (smth.), fáncy (smth.); 11. (*вн.; доставлять, причинять*) presént (smth.), óffer (smth.); ~ большие затрудне́ния presént great difficulties. ~я́ться, предста́виться 1. (*знакомиться*) introdúce oneself; 2. (*являться, возникать*) presént itself, occúr; слу́чай ско́ро предста́вился an opportúnity soon presénted itself; ему́ предста́вились у́жасы войны́ he imágined the hórrors of war; 3. (*тв.*) *разг.* (*притворяться*) preténd (+ to *inf*); ~я́ться больны́м preténd to be ill, feign síckness.

предста́ть *сов. см.* представа́ть.

предсто|я́ть *несов.* (*дт.*) lie* ahéad (of); нам ~и́т интере́сная рабо́та we are góing to have some ínteresting work; ~и́т ещё мно́гое сде́лать there is a lot of work to do, a lot of work lies ahéad of us. ~я́щий forthcoming, impénding.

предубежде́ние *с.* préjudice, bías; относи́ться к кому́-л. с ~м be* préjudiced agáinst smb.

предубеждённый préjudiced, bías(s)ed.

предугада́ть *сов. см.* предуга́дывать.

предуга́дывать, предугада́ть (*вн.*) foresée* (smth.).

предуда́рный *лингв.* pretónic; ~ слог, гла́сный prétone.

предупреди́тельн|ость *ж.* atténtiveness, considerátion, obligingness. ~ый 1. (*предохраняющий*) prevéntive; ~ые ме́ры prevéntive méasures; 2. (*о человеке*) atténtive, considerate, obliging; он всегда́ так предупреди́телен he is álways so considerate.

предупреди́ть *сов. см.* предупрежда́ть.

предупрежд|а́ть, предупреди́ть (*вн.*) 1. (*заранее извещать*) nótify (smb.); give* (smb.) nótice (of); (*предостерегать*) warn (smb.); ~ за две неде́ли give* two weeks' nótice; ~ кого́-л. об опа́сности warn smb. of a dánger, give* wárning of dánger to smb.; 2. (*предотвращать*) prevént (smth.); предупреди́ть несча́стные слу́чаи prevént áccidents; 3. (*опережать*) anticipate (smth.); ~ собы́тия anticipate evénts; ~ чьи-л. жела́ния anticipate smb.'s wíshes. ~е́ние *с.* 1. (*действие*) notificátion, wárning; prevéntion; anticipátion; ~е́ние об опа́сности dánger wárning; 2. (*предупреждающее замечание*) nótice, wárning; сде́лать кому́-л. ~е́ние об увольне́нии give* smb. nótice (of dismíssal).

предусма́тривать, предусмотре́ть (*вн.*) 1. (*заранее учитывать возможность чего-л.*) foresée* (smth.); 2. *тк. несов.* (*обусловливать*) provide (for), envísage (smth.), stípulate (smth.).

предусмотре́ть *сов. см.* предусма́тривать I.

предусмотри́тельн|ость *ж.* fóresight, fórethought.

~ый foresééing, fár-seeing; (*осторожный*) prúdent; быть ~ым be* fár-seeing, look ahéad.

предчу́вств|ие *с.* preséntiment, premonítion; (*тяжёлое*) fóreboding, misgíving; ~ опа́сности preséntiment of dánger. ~овать *несов.* (*вн.*) have* a preséntiment/ fóreboding (of, abóut); он ~овал беду́ he had misgívings, he felt sómething térrible would háppen; я ~ую, что мы бу́дем друзья́ми I have a féeling we are góing to be friends.

предше́ственн|ик *м.*, ~ица *ж.* 1. fórerunner, precúrsor; 2. (*по должности*) prédecessor.

предше́ств|овать *несов.* (*дт.*) precéde (smth.). ~ующий precéding.

предъяви́тел|ь *м.* béarer; чек на ~я cheque páyable to béarer; ~ и́ска pláintiff.

предъяв|и́ть *сов. см.* предъявля́ть. ~ле́ние *с.* (*документов, билетов и т. п.*) presentátion, prodúction; по ~ле́нии on presentátion; плати́ть по ~ле́нии pay* on demánd; ~ле́ние и́ска brínging a suit; ~ле́ние тре́бований máking of demánds.

предъявля́ть, предъяви́ть (*вн.*) 1. (*показывать*) presént (smth.), prodúce (smth.); ~ па́спорт presént/ prodúce/show* one's pássport; 2. (*заявлять о чём-л.*) bring* (smth.); ~ кому́-л. обвине́ние bring* an accusátion agáinst smb.; ~ тре́бование к кому́-л. make* a demánd on smb.

предыду́щий precéding, prévious; ~ ора́тор the prévious spéaker.

преем|ник *м.* succéssor. ~ственность *ж.* succéssion, continúity; ~ственность в иску́сстве continúity in art; ~ственность в рабо́те continúity of work. ~ственный succéssive; based on succéssion *после сущ.*

пре́жде 1. *нареч.* (*раньше*) before, fórmerly; (*сначала*) first; 2. *предлог* (*рд.*) before; ◇ ~ всего́ first of all, to begín with; ~ чем before.

преждевре́менн|о prematúrely, before the próper time. ~ый prematúre, untimely, éarly; ~ая смерть untímely/premature death; ~ые ро́ды premature birth *sg.*

пре́жн|ий fórmer; в ~ее вре́мя in fórmer times.

президе́нт *м.* président. ~ский presidéntial; ~ские вы́боры presidéntial eléctions.

прези́диум *м.* presidium; Прези́диум Акаде́мии нау́к Presídium of the Acádemy of Sciences; избра́ть ~ для веде́ния собра́ния eléct a presídium to condúct a méeting.

презира́ть *несов.* (*вн.*) 1. (*относиться с презрением*) despíse (smb., smth.), scorn (smb., smth.), hold* (smb., smth.) in contémpt; он презира́ет тру́сов he despíses cówards; 2. (*пренебрегать*) disregárd (smb., smth.), disdáin (smb., smth.); ~ опа́сность disregárd dánger.

презре́н|ие *с.* 1. (*чувство пренебрежения, неуважения*) contémpt, scorn; относи́ться с ~ием к кому́-л. hold* smb. in contémpt; 2. (*к дт.; пренебрежительное отношение*) disregárd (for, of), disdáin (for). ~ный contémptible, déspicable; ◇ ~ный мета́лл *шутл.* filthy lúcre.

презри́тельн|ость *ж.* contémpt, disdáin. ~ый contémptuous, scórnful, disdáinful.

преиму́щественн|о máinly, chíefly. ~ый 1. prímary, príncipal; 2. *юр.* preferéntial; príority *attr.*; ~ое пра́во préference.

преиму́ществ|о *с.* 1. (*превосходство*) advántage; зна́ние языко́в — его́ большо́е ~ knowledge of languages is a great advántage/ásset to him; 2. (*привилегия*) préference; ◇ по ~у chíefly, máinly, for the most part.

преиспо́лненный (*рд.*) full (of); ~ реши́мости fírmly resólved.

прейскура́нт *м.* price-list, cátalogue; ~ы ро́зничных цен rétail cátalogues.

преклоне́ние *с.* (*перед тв.*) wórship (of), réverence (for), admirátion (for).

преклонн|ый advánced; ~ вóзраст old age; человéк ~ого вóзраста pérson of advánced years.

преклонЯ́ться *несов.* (перед *тв.*) wórship (*smb., smth.*), revére (*smb., smth.*), admíre (*smb., smth.*).

прекослóвить *несов.* (*дт.*) contradíct (*smb.*); talk back (at) *разг.*

прекрáсн|о 1. *нареч.* béautifully; я всё э́то ~ знáю I know all that pérfectly well, I am well awáre of that; 2. *в знач. сказ.* it is wónderful/spléndid; 3. *в знач. частицы* éxcellent, spléndid. ~ый *прил.* 1. (*красивый*) béautiful, fine, lóvely; 2. (*отличный*) éxcellent, first-ráte; быть в ~ом настроéнии be* in wónderful spírits; 3. *в знач. сущ.* с. the béautiful; ◇ в одни́н ~ый день one fine day.

прекра|ти́ть(ся) *сов. см.* прекращáть(ся). ~щáть, прекрати́ть (*вн.*) stop (*smth.*), end (*smth.*), cease (*smth.*); ~щáть рабóту cease work; прекрати́ть свЯ́зи с кем-л. break* off relátions with *smb.*, cease one's connéctions with *smb.*; ~щáть платежи́ stop/suspénd páyments; прекрати́ть переговóры break* off negotiátions; ~щáть прéния halt a debáte; прекрати́ть дéло в судé stop a case; прекрати́ть испытáния Я́дерного орýжия stop/cease tésting núclear wéapons; ~щáть войнý end/stop the war; ~щáть огóнь *воен.* cease fire. ~щáться, прекрати́ться stop, cease, end. ~щéние *с.* cessátion, stópping, énding; ~щéние воéнных дéйствий cessátion of hostílities.

прелéстный chárming, delíghtful.

прéлесть *ж.* 1. charm, fascinátion; 2. *мн.* (*приятные явления*) delíghts; 3. *в знач. сказ.*: э́то прóсто ~! it's símply lóvely!; какáя ~! it's exquísite!, how sweet!

прелом|и́ть(ся) *сов. см.* преломлЯ́ть(ся). ~лéние *с.* *физ.* refráction, bénding; *перен.* interpretátion; ~лéние лучéй refráction (of rays).

преломлЯ́ть, преломи́ть (*вн.*) *физ.* refráct (*smth.*); *перен.* intérpret (*smth.*). ~ся, преломи́ться *физ.* be* refrácted; *перен.* be* intérpreted.

прéлый rótten; (*пропитанный гнилой сыростью*) músty.

прельсти́ть(ся) *сов. см.* прельщáть(ся).

прельщáть, прельсти́ть (*вн.*) 1. (*очаровывать*) fáscinate (*smb.*), cáptivate (*smb.*); 2. (*соблазнять*) attráct (*smb.*), tempt (*smb.*), entíce (*smb.*), lure (*smb.*); ~ когó-л. обещáниями tempt *smb.* with prómises. ~ся, прельсти́ться be* enticed, be* allúred, be* témpted.

прелЮ́дия *ж.* prélude.

премиáльн|ый bónus *attr.*; ~ая систéма оплáты трудá bónus sýstem; ~ые дéньги bónus (móney) *sg.*

премировáние *с.* 1. (*выдача премии кому-л.*) gíving bónuses; 2. (*за выдающиеся качества*) awárding prízes.

премировáть *несов. и сов.* (*вн.*) 1. (*выдавать премию кому-л.*) give* (*smb.*) a bónus; 2. (*отмечать что-л. премией*) award (*smth.*) a prize.

прéми|я *ж.* 1. prize; получи́ть пéрвую ~ю get* the first prize; 2. (*за перевыполнение плана*) bónus; 3. *фин.* (*страховая*) prémium; 4. *эк.* (*экспортная*) bóunty.

премýдр|ость *ж.* 1. *уст.* wísdom; 2. *разг. ирон.* mýsteries *pl*; невеликá ~ that's not véry dífficult. ~ый 1. *уст.* wise; 2. (*трудный*) abstrúse, invólved.

премьéр *м.* 1. *см.* премьéр-мини́стр; 2. *театр.* léading man*/áctor.

премьéра *ж.* first perfórmance, first night, première.

премьéр-мини́стр *м.* prime mínister, prémier.

премьéрша *ж.* *театр. разг.* léading lády.

пренебре|гáть, пренебрéчь (*тв.*) 1. (*относиться с презрением*) ignóre (*smb., smth.*), scorn (*smb., smth.*), look down (on); 2. (*оставлять без внимания*) ignóre (*smth.*), negléct (*smth.*); ~ совéтом negléct advíce; ~ опáсностью ignóre dánger. ~жéние *с.* 1. (*презрительно-высокомерное отношение*) contémpt, disrespéct; вы́сказать своё ~жéние к кому-л. show* one's disrespéct for *smb.*; с ~жéнием упоминáть о ком-л. speak* slíghtingly of *smb.*; 2. (*отсутствие должного внима-*

ния) contémpt; отнести́сь с ~жéнием к чему-л. treat *smth.* with contémpt.

пренебрежи́тельн|о scórnfully, slíghtingly, disdáinfully; ~ отзывáться о чём-л. refér slíghtingly to *smth.* ~ый scórnful, disdáinful; ~ый тон disdáinful/dispáraging tone; ~ый óтзыв scórnful cómment.

пренебрéчь *сов. см.* пренебрегáть.

прéния *мн.* discússion *sg*, debáte *sg*; откры́ть ~ по доклáду ópen the debáte on the repórt; вы́ступить в ~х speak* in a debáte, take* part in a debáte.

преобладáние *с.* prévalence, predóminance; (*перевес*) prepónderance.

преоблад|áть *несов.* (над *тв.*, среди́ *рд.*) predóminate (óver), preváil (óver); (*иметь перевес*) prepónderate. ~áющий predóminant, preváiling.

преображ|áть, преобрази́ть (*вн.*) change (*smth., smth.*), transfórm (*smb., smth.*), transfígure (*smb., smth.*). ~áться, преобрази́ться change, be* transfórmed/transfígured. ~éние *с.* transformátion, transfigurátion.

преобрази́ть(ся) *сов. см.* преображáть(ся).

преобразовá|ние *с.* 1. (*действие*) transformátion, reorganizátion; ~ приро́ды the remáking of náture; ~ постоя́нного тóка в переме́нный convérsion of diréct cúrrent into álternating cúrrent; 2. (*коренное изменение*) transformátion, rádical refórm, fundaméntal change; революЮ́ционные ~ния revolútionary refórms/chánges. ~тель *м.* 1. transfórmer, remáker; (*реформатор*) refórmer; 2. *эл.*, *физ.* convérter.

преобразовáть(ся) *сов. см.* преобразóвывать(ся).

преобразóвывать, преобразовáть (*вн.*) 1. transfórm (*smth.*), change (*smth.*); (*реорганизовывать*) reórganize (*smth.*); ~ приро́ду remáke* náture; 2. *тех.* convért (*smth.*); *мат.* transpóse (*smth.*); преобразовáть переме́нный ток в постоя́нный convért álternating cúrrent into diréct cúrrent; преобразовáть алгебраи́ческое выраже́ние transpóse an algebráical expréssion. ~ся, преобразовáться 1. be* transfórmed, be* changed; (*реорганизовываться*) be* reórganized; 2. *тех.* be* convérted; *мат.* be* transpósed.

преодол|евáть, преодолéть (*вн.*) overcóme* (*smth.*), surmóunt (*smth.*); (*превозмогать*) máster (*smth.*), get* the bétter (of), cónquer (*smth.*), fight* down (*smth.*); ~евáть расстоя́ние overcóme* dístance; преодолéть трýдности overcóme* dífficulties; преодолéть чьё-л. сопротивлéние overcóme* *smb.'s* resístance. ~éние *с.* overcóming, surmóunting; для ~éния трýдностей to overcóme* dífficulties.

преодолéть *сов. см.* преодолевáть.

преодоли́м|ый surmóuntable; легкó ~ое препЯ́тствие éasily surmóuntable óbstacle.

препарáт *м.* preparátion; витами́нные ~ы vítamin preparátions.

препинáни|е *с.*: знáки ~я punctuátion marks; стáвить знáки ~я púnctuate.

препирáтельство *с.* altercátion, dispúte, wrángle, squábble.

препирáться *несов.* (с *тв.*) áltercate (with), wrángle (with), squábble (with); ~ из-за мелочéй squábble óver trífles.

преподавáние *с.* téaching.

преподавáтель *м.*, ~ница *ж.* téacher. ~ский téacher's; ~ский коллекти́в téaching bódy.

преподавáть *несов.* teach*; ~ хи́мию teach* chémistry; ~ в институ́те teach*/lécture at an ínstitute.

преподнести́ *сов. см.* преподноси́ть.

преподноси́ть, преподнести́ 1. (*вн. дт.*) presént (*smth.* to, *smb.* with); ~ кому-л. словáрь presént a díctionary to *smth.*, presént *smb.* with a díctionary; 2. (*вн. дт.*) *разг.* (*делать или сообщать что-л. неожиданное*) give* (*smb. smth.*); преподнести́ кому-л. сюрпри́з give* *smb.* a surpríse; преподнести́ кому-л. неприЯ́тную но́вость break* the news to smb.; **3.** (вн.; представля́ть, изобража́ть в како́м-л. ви́де) presént (smth.), put* (smth.) acróss; преподнести́ материа́л жи́во и увлека́тельно put* one's matérial acróss in a lívely, ínteresting form.

преподноше́ние с. **1.** (де́йствие) presentátion; **2.** (пода́рок) présent, gíft.

препроводи́тельн|ый: ~ое письмо́ létter of advíce, cóvering létter.

препроводи́ть сов. см. препровожда́ть.

препровожд|а́ть, препроводи́ть (вн.) escórt (smb.), send* (smb.) únder éscort; (докуме́нты и т. п.) fórward (smth.). ~е́ние с. **1.** escórting; (докуме́нтов и т. п.) fórwarding; **2.:** ~е́ние вре́мени pástime, divérsion; для ~е́ния вре́мени to pass (awáy) the time.

препя́тств|ие с. **1.** óbstacle, bárrier; перен. тж. híndrance, impédiment; преодоле́ть все ~ия surmóunt/overcóme* all óbstacles; **2.** спорт. óbstacle; (барье́р) húrdle; (для скачек) jump; бег с ~иями húrdle-race; the húrdles pl. ~овать несов. (вн.) prevént (smb., smth.) (ста́вить препя́тствия) hínder (smb., smth.), block (smth.), creáte óbstacles (to).

прерва́ть(ся) сов. см. прерыва́ть(ся).

пререка́ния мн. (ед. пререка́ние с.) altercátion sg, wrángle sg, árgument; вступи́ть в ~ с кем-л. start an árgument with smb.

пререка́ться несов. (с тв.) áltercate (with), wrángle (with).

пре́рии мн. (ед. пре́рия ж.) práiries.

прерыва́тель м. тех. interrúpter, cóntact-breaker.

прерыва́ть, прерва́ть (вн.) interrúpt (smb., smth.); (связь, знако́мство) break* off (smth.); (тишину́, молча́ние) break* (smth.); ~ перегово́ры break* off negotiátions; прерва́ть путеше́ствие break* one's jóurney; ~ молча́ние break* the sílence; прерва́ть разгово́р interrúpt the conversátion; (переста́ть разгова́ривать) stop tálking. ~ся, прерва́ться be* interrúpted; (о го́лосе) break*, break* off.

прерыва́ющийся chóking, fáltering; ~ го́лос fáltering voice.

преры́вист|ый intermíttent, interrúpted, fáltering; ~ые зву́ки intermíttent sounds.

пресека́ть, пресе́чь (вн.) stop (smth.), curb (smth.), put* a stop (to); пресе́чь зло curb évil; пресе́чь злоупотребле́ния put* a stop to abúses. ~ся, пресе́чься stop.

пресе́чь(ся) сов. см. пресека́ть(ся).

пресле́довани|е с. **1.** (пого́ня) pursúit, chásing; **2.** (гоне́ние) persecútion; ма́ния ~я persecútion mánia.

пресле́довать несов. (вн.) **1.** (гна́ться) pursúe (smb., smth.), chase (smb., smth.); **2.** (подверга́ть гоне́ниям) pérsecute (smb.), hound (smb.); **3.** (му́чить) haunt (smb.), obséss (smb.); его́ пресле́дует мысль he is háunted by the thought; **4.** (стреми́ться к чему́-л.) pursúe (smth.); ~ цель pursúe an aim/óbject; ~ свои́ интере́сы pursúe one's own ínterests; **5.** юр. (предава́ть суду́) prósecute (smb.); ~ кого́-л. суде́бным поря́дком take* légal áction agáinst smb., prósecute smb.

пресловутый ирон. notórious.

пресмыка́ться несов. (перед тв.) презр. cringe (to, befóre), fawn (on, upón), gróvel (to, befóre).

пресмыка́ющееся с. зоол. réptile.

пресново́дн|ый fréshwater; ~е ры́бы fréshwater fish.

пре́сный (о воде́) fresh; (о хле́бе) unléavened; (о пи́ще) insípid, tásteless, flávourless; перен. insípid, vápid, bland.

пресс м. press; штампо́вочный ~ stámping/púnching press.

пресс|а ж. **1.** the press; по о́тзывам ~ы júdging from press cómment, accórding to what the néwspapers say; **2.** собир. (журнали́сты) the press, préssmen; места́ для ~ы préss-box sg, préss-gallery sg.

пресс-атташе́ м. нескл. préss-attaché.

пресс-бюро́ с. нескл. press óffice/céntre.

пресс-конфере́нция ж. préss-cónference.

прессо́ванн|ый pressed; ~ое се́но pressed hay.

прессова́ть, спрессова́ть (вн.) press (smth.).

пресс-папье́ с. нескл. blótter.

пресс-слу́жба ж. press sérvice.

пресс-це́нтр м. press céntre.

престаре́л|ый áged; ~е лю́ди the áged.

прести́ж м. prestíge; подня́ть ~ raise prestíge; роня́ть ~ lose* prestíge. ~ный prestíge attr.; of prestíge по́сле сущ.

престо́л м. **1.** throne; взойти́ на ~ ascénd the throne; све́ргнуть кого́-л. с ~а depóse smb., dethróne smb.; **2.** (в це́ркви) áltar, commúnion-table; ◇ па́пский ~ the Hóly See.

преступле́ние с. crime (тж. перен.); юр. félony; соверши́ть ~ commit a crime/félony.

престу́пн|ик м., ~ица ж. críminal; вое́нный ~ war críminal. ~ость ж. **1.** criminálity, críminal náture; ~ость за́мысла the críminal náture of the plan; **2.** (наличие, коли́чество преступле́ний) crime; борьба́ с ~остью prevéntion of crime. ~ый críminal; ~ая небре́жность críminal negléct; ~ый мир the únderworld.

пресы́тить(ся) сов. см. пресыща́ть(ся).

пресыщ|а́ть, пресы́тить (вн. тв.) sate (smb. with), sátiate (smb. with); перен. súrfeit (smb. with), cloy (smb. with). ~а́ться, пресы́титься (тв.) be* sáted/sátiated (with); перен. be* súrfeited (with); be* fed up (with) разг. ~е́ние с. satíety, súrfeit; есть до ~е́ния eat* to replétion.

пресы́щенный sátiated; перен. súrfeited, blóated.

претвори́ть(ся) сов. см. претворя́ть(ся).

претворя́ть, претвори́ть (вн. в вн.) convért (smth. ínto); ~ свои́ пла́ны в жизнь put* one's plans ínto práctice/life. ~ся, претвори́ться **1.** (в вн.; перевоплоща́ться) be* transfórmed; **2.** (осуществля́ться на де́ле) be* réalized, matérialize; его́ мечты́ претвори́лись в жизнь his dreams came true.

претенде́нт м. cláimant (to); ~ы на зва́ние чемпио́на the chállengers for a chámpion títle.

претендова́ть несов. (на вн.) **1.** (домога́ться чего́-л.) seek* (smth.), lay* claim (to), claim (smth.); ~ на получе́ние учёной сте́пени claim/seek* a degrée; ~ на дру́жбу с кем-л. seek* smb.'s fríendship; **2.** (приписывая себе́ какое-л. ка́чество, добива́ться призна́ния э́того ка́чества) aspíre (to), have* preténsions (to); ~ на остроу́мие aspíre to wit; ~ на учёность have* preténsions to léarning.

прете́нзи|я ж. **1.** (тре́бование) claim; (жалоба) compláint; зако́нная ~ légal claim; предъявля́ть ~ю expréss dissatisfáction; заявля́ть ~ю make* a claim, put* in a claim; **2.** (стремле́ние произвести́ впечатле́ние) preténsion; челове́к без ~й unassúming pérson; челове́к с ~ями preténtious pérson; ◇ быть в ~и на кого́-л. have* a gríevance agáinst smb.; have* a bone to pick with smb. идиом.

претерпева́ть, претерпе́ть (вн.) **1.** (пережива́ть, испы́тывать) súffer (smth.); ~ лише́ния súffer hárdships; **2.** (подверга́ться чему́-л.) undergó* (smth.); ~ измене́ния undergó* chánges.

претерпе́ть сов. см. претерпева́ть.

прети́ть несов. (дт.) disgúst (smth.), be* repúgnant (to), make* (smb.) sick.

преткнове́ни|е с.: ка́мень ~я stúmbling-block.

преть, сопре́ть **1.** сов. сопре́ть (гнить) rot; **2.** сов. упре́ть разг. (вари́ться) stew.

преувеличе́ние с. exaggerátion, overstátement.

преувели́ченный exággerated.

преувели́чивать, преувели́чить (вн.) exággerate (smth.), mágnify (smth.), overstáte (smth.); (переоце́нивать) overéstimate (smth.), overráte (smth.); ~ чьи-л. досто́инства overéstimate/overráte smb.'s mérits.

преувели́чить сов. см. преувели́чивать.

преуменьш|а́ть, преуме́ньши́ть (вн.) mínimize (smth.); (недооценивать) underéstimate (smth.), underráte (smth.). **~е́ние** с. minimizátion; underestimátion.

преуме́ньшить сов. см. преуменьша́ть.

преуспева́ть, преуспе́ть 1. (в пр.; добиваться успеха в чём-л.) succéed (in), be* succéssful (in); 2. тк. несов. (процветать) prósper.

преуспе́ть сов. см. преуспева́ть 1.

пре́фикс м. грам. préfix. **~ация** ж. грам. prefixion.

преходя́щий tránsitory, tránsient, ephémeral, mómentary.

прецеде́нт м. précedent.

при 1. (около, возле) at, near, by; ~ доро́ге by the road; ~ ста́нции near the státion; 2. (в непосредственной связи с чем-л.) attáched to; гара́ж ~ до́ме gárage attáched to the house; я́сли ~ заво́де núrsery at the fáctory; 3. (в присутствии кого-л.) in the présence of, befóre, in front of; он сказа́л э́то ~ мне he said it in my présence; 4. (во время, в эпоху) dúring; in the time of; (о правительстве, политической системе и т.п.) únder; ~ жи́зни Пу́шкина dúring the life of Púshkin; ~ феодали́зме únder féudalism; 5. (с собой) with; у него́ все де́ньги ~ себе́ he has all the móney with him; 6. (при обозначении обстоятельства образа действия) by, on, when; чита́ть ~ дневно́м све́те read* by dáylight; ~ вхо́де в помеще́ние when/on éntering the prémises; 7. (при наличии чего-л.; при ком-л.) with; for; ~ всём мо́ём уваже́нии к вам with all due respéct to you; ~ всех его́ зна́ниях for all his léarning; ~ по́мощи друзе́й with the help of one's friends; де́ти нахо́дятся ~ ма́тери the children are with their móther.

приба́в|ить(ся) сов. см. прибавля́ть(ся). **~ка** ж. íncrease, augmentátion; ~ка зарпла́ты íncrease/rise in wáges. **~ле́ние** с. addítion; (увеличение) íncrease; ~ле́ние в ве́се íncrease in weight; ~ле́ние семе́йства addítion to one's fámily.

прибавля́ть, приба́вить 1. (вн., рд.) add (smth.); приба́вить са́хару в чай put* some more súgar in one's tea; 2. (вн., рд.; увеличивать) incréase (smth.); ~ зарпла́ту кому́-л. raise smb.'s sálary; приба́вить ша́гу quícken one's pace, húrry up; 3. разг.: ~ в ве́се gain weight, put* on weight. **~ся**, приба́виться 1. (появляться в добавление к чему-л.) be* ádded; приба́вились но́вые неприя́тности fúrther tróubles were at hand; 2. обыкн. безл. incréase; (о воде) rise*; день приба́вился the days are gétting lónger; рабо́ты приба́вилось there is more work to be done; 3. разг.: ~ся в ве́се gain weight, put* on weight.

приба́вочн|ый эк. súrplus attr.; ~ая сто́имость súrplus válue; ~ проду́кт súrplus próduct; ~ труд súrplus lábour.

прибалти́йский Báltic.

прибега́ть I, прибежа́ть come* rúnning, run*; прибежа́ть пе́рвым get* there first.

прибега́ть II, прибе́гнуть (к дт.) resórt (to), have* recóurse (to); прибе́гнуть к реши́тельным ме́рам resórt to strong tough méasures; прибе́гнуть к сове́там друзе́й seek* the advíce of one's friends.

прибе́гнуть сов. см. прибега́ть II.

прибежа́ть сов. см. прибега́ть I.

прибе́жище с. réfuge; находи́ть ~ в чём-л. take* refuge in smth.

приберега́ть, прибере́чь (вн.) put* (smth.) by; прибере́чь де́ньги на поку́пку чего́-л. put* some móney by for (búying) smth., save up for smth.

прибере́чь сов. см. приберега́ть.

прибива́ть, приби́ть (вн.) 1. (гвоздями) nail (smth.), fásten (smth.) with nails; 2. (придавливать книзу) flátten (smth.); (о пыли) lay* (smth.); град приби́л посе́вы к земле́ the hail fláttened the crops; 3. (си-

лой ветра, воды и т. п.) cárry (smth.); (к берегу) wash (smb., smth.) ashóre; бо́чку приби́ло к бе́регу the bárrel was washed ashóre.

прибира́ть, прибра́ть (вн.) разг. 1. (приводить в порядок) tídy (smth.), put*/set* things in órder; прибра́ть ко́мнату tídy a room, put* a room in órder; 2. (прятать) put* (smth.) awáy; ◇ прибра́ть кого́-л. к рука́м estáblish one's ínfluence óver smb., take* smb. in hand; прибра́ть к рука́м что́-л. get* a grip/hold of smth. **~ся**, прибра́ться разг. put* things in órder.

прибра́ть сов. см. прибира́ть.

приближ|а́ть, прибли́зить (вн., вн. к дт.) bring* (smb., smth.) clóser/néarer (to); (перен. тж.) put* (smth.) into clóser cóntact (with), give* (smth.) clóser ties (with). **~а́ться**, прибли́зиться 1. (к дт.; подходить ближе) appróach (smb., smth.), come*/draw* néar(er) (to); мы ~а́емся к Москве́ we are appróaching/néaring Móscow, we are gétting near Móscow; мы ~а́емся к свое́й це́ли we are néaring our goal; 2. (по времени) appróach, draw* near/on; ночь ~а́ется night is dráwing near/on; 3. (к дт.; приобретать сходство с чем-л.) appróximate (to), be* cómparable (to); э́то ~а́ется к и́стине it appróximates to the truth, it is sómewhere near the truth; ~а́ться к лу́чшим образца́м be* cómparable to the finest exámples. **~е́ние** с. 1. appróach; ~е́ние весны́ the appróach of spring; 2. мат. approximátion.

приближённость ж. мат. appróximate náture.

приближённ|ый I мат. appróximate; ~ое вычисле́ние appróximate calculátion.

приближённый II прил. 1. (о людях) close; 2. в знач. сущ. м. fávourite.

приблизи́тельн|о appróximately, róughly; (о времени, количестве) abóut. **~ый** appróximate.

прибли́зить(ся) сов. см. приближа́ть(ся).

прибо́й м. surf; bréakers pl.

прибо́р м. 1. ínstrument, apparátus, devíce, appliance; оптíческие ~ы óptical ínstruments; измери́тельный ~ méasuring ínstrument; 2. (комплект, набор предметов) set.

приборострое́ние с. ínstrument-máking.

прибра́ть(ся) сов. см. прибира́ть(ся).

прибре́жный shore attr.; near the shore после сущ.; (у моря тж.) cóastal; (у реки) ríverside attr.

прибыва́ть, прибы́ть 1. arríve, come*; по́езд прибы́л во́время the train got in on time; 2. (быть доставленным) arríve, be* delívered; прибыла́ корреспонде́нция some mail has arríved; 3. (увеличиваться) incréase; (о воде) rise*.

при́быль ж. 1. (доход) prófit, gain; приноси́ть ~ yield/show* a prófit; 2. (увеличение) íncrease, íncrement; ~ населе́ния the íncrease of populátion. **~ный** prófitable, lúcrative, páying; ~ное предприя́тие prófitable énterprise.

прибы́ти|е с. arríval; по ~и on arríval.

прибы́ть сов. см. прибыва́ть.

прива́л м. 1. (остановка) stópping, stop, halt; сде́лать ~ make* a halt, bívouac; 2. (место отдыха) stópping-place, bívouac.

прива́ливать, привали́ть 1. (вн. к дт.; прислонять) lean* (smth. agáinst); 2. мор. (причаливать) moor; 3.: како́е сча́стье ему́ привали́ло! what a stroke of luck for him!

привали́ть сов. см. прива́ливать.

привезти́ сов. см. привози́ть.

привере́д|ливый разг. fastídious, fínical, fússy. **~ник** м., **~ница** ж. разг. fastídious pérson.

привере́дничать несов. разг. be* fastídious, be* hard to please.

привер́жен|ец м. adhérent, suppórter, fóllower; ~ старины́ traditionalist. **~ность** ж. devótion; (склонность, расположение) prediléction (for), enthúsiasm (for), bent (for). **~ный** devóted, lóyal; (склонный, расположенный) inclíned (to).

привернýть *сов. см.* привёртывать.

привёртывать, привернýть *(вн.)* 1. *(завинчивать)* screw *(smth.)*; ~ гáйку screw (up) a nut; 2. *(вертя, уменьшать)* turn *(smth.)* down; привернýть газ turn down the gas.

привéсить *сов. см.* привéшивать.

привестú *сов. см.* приводúть.

привéт *м.* gréetings *pl*, regárds *pl*; передáйте ~ вáшему брáту remémber me to your bróther, my kind regárds to your bróther; с сердéчным ~ом yours sincérely.

привéтлив|ость *ж.* affabílity, gráciousness, friendliness. ~ый áffable, grácious, fríendly; ~ый хозяин áffable host.

привéтственн|ый wélcoming; ~ая речь speech of wélcome, sálutary addréss.

привéтстви|е *с.* 1. gréeting; *(военных)* salúte; обмéняться ~ями exchánge gréetings, greet one anóther; 2. *(устное или письменное обращение)* méssage of gréeting; gréetings *pl*; послáть ~ юбилярý send* gréetings to *smb.* on his, her annivérsary.

привéтствовать *несов.* *(вн.)* 1. greet *(smb.)*, wélcome *(smb.)*; hail *(smb.)*; *(шумными возгласами)* cheer *(smb.)*; 2. *воен.* salúte *(smb.)*; 3. *(одобрять)* wélcome *(smth.)*, appláud *(smth.)*; ~ чью-л. инициатúву wélcome *smb.'s* initiative.

привéшивать, привéсить *(вн.)* suspénd *(smth.)*, hang* *(smth.)* on.

прививáть, привúть 1. *(вн.)* с.-х. graft *(smth.)*; 2. *(вн.; акклиматизировать растения)* acclímatize *(smth.)*; 3. *(дт. вн.)* мед. inóculate *(smb.* agáinst*)*; привúть кому-л. óспу váccinate *smb.*; 4. *(вн. дт.; заставлять усвоить)* instíll *(smth.* in*)*; inculcate *(smth.* in, upón*)*; implánt *(smth.* in*)*; привúть кому-л. культýрные навыки introdúce *smb.* to art and cúlture. ~ся, привúться 1. с.-х. take*; 2. *(акклиматизироваться)* becóme* acclímatized; 3. *(о вакцине)* take* (efféct); óспа привилáсь the vaccinátion has táken efféct; 4. *(входить в привычку)* take* root, becóme* estáblished; *(о моде)* catch* on; эти словá привилúсь в рýсском языкé these words have táken root in the Rússian lánguage.

привúвка *ж.* 1. с.-х. gráfting; ~ плодóвых дерéвьев gráfting of frúit-trees; 2. *мед.* inoculátion; *(оспы)* vaccinátion.

привидéние *с.* ghost, spéctre, apparítion; spook *разг.*

привилегирóванный prívileged, fávoured.

привилéгия *ж.* prívilege.

привинтúть *сов. см.* привúнчивать.

привúнчивать, привинтúть *(вн.)* screw *(smth.)* on.

привúть(ся) *сов. см.* прививáть(ся).

прúвкус *м.* *(прям. и перен.)* suggéstion (of), touch (of).

привлекáтельный attráctive; *(о человеке тж.)* engáging.

привлекáть, привлéчь 1. *(вн.)* attráct *(smb., smth.)*, draw* *(smb., smth.)*; ~ чьё-л. внимáние attráct/draw* *smb.'s* atténtion; 2. *(вн.; к участию в чём-л.)* enlíst *(smb.)*, draw* *(smb.)*; ~ кого-л. на свою стóрону win* *smb.* óver to *one's* side; 3.: ~ кого-л. к судý bring*/to/put* on trial *(smb.)*, take* *(smb.)* to court, take* *(légal)* áction agáinst *smb.*; ~ кого-л. к отвéтственности call *smb.* to account.

привлéчь *сов. см.* привлекáть.

прúвод I *м. юр.* arrést, táking into cústody.

прúвод II *м. тех.* drive.

приводúть, привестú 1. *(вн.; доставлять)* bring* *(smb., smth.)*, take* *(smb., smth.)*; привестú детéй домóй bring*/take* the chíldren home; привестú сýдно в гáвань bring* a ship into hárbour; 2. *(вн.; указывать дорогу куда-л.)* lead* *(smb., smth.)*, bring* *(smb., smth.)*; следы привелú охóтников к норé the tracks led the húnters to a búrrow; 3. *(вн.; служить поводом для прихода куда-л.)* bring* *(smb.)*; гóре привелó её сюдá it was misfórtune that brought her here; 4. *(вн. к дт.; к выводу, решению и т. п.)* lead* *(smb.* to*)*; привестú к прáвильному заключéнию lead* to a corréct conclúsion; нóвые фáкты привелú к вáжному открытию new facts led to an impórtant discóvery; 5.: ~ кого-л. в отчáяние drive* *smb.* to despáir; ~ кого-л. в хорóшее настроéние put* *smb.* in a good* mood; 6.: ~ что-л. в готóвность make* *smth.* réady; ~ что-л. в дéйствие set* *smth.* góing, put* *smth.* into operátion; ~ что-л. в исполнéние cárry out *smth.*, put* *smth.* into efféct; 7. *(вн. к дт.; быть причиной чего-л.)* lead* *(smb.* to*)*, resúlt (in), bring* abóut *(smth.)*; привестú кого-л. к гúбели lead* *smb.* to destrúction; resúlt in *smb.'s* death; привестú к пýтанице cause confúsion; 8. *(вн.; ссылаться на что-л.)* cite *(smth.)*, quote *(smth.)*, addúce *(smth.)*; ~ доказáтельства addúce proof; ~ цитáту quote a pássage; ~ примéр give* an exámple; ~ что-л. в примéр quote *smth.* as an exámple/illustrátion; ~ кого-л. в примéр hold* *smb.* up as an exámple; ◇ привестú кого-л. в себя 1) *(из состояния обморока)* revive *smb.*, bring* *smb.* round; 2) *(из задумчивости)* bring* *smb.* back to reálity, rouse *smb.*; привестú к одномý, к óбщему знаменáтелю redúce to a cómmon denóminator; это не приведёт ни к чемý хорóшему it will lead to no good, it will have no good resúlt.

приводнéние *с.* lánding on wáter; *(космического корабля)* splásh-down.

приводнúться *сов.* land/alíght on wáter; *(о космическом корабле)* splash down.

приводнóй *тех.* dríving *attr.*; ~ ремéнь dríving-belt; ~ шкив dríver.

привóз *м.* 1. brínging (in); 2. *(то, что привезено)* delívery.

привозúть, привезтú *(вн.)* bring* *(smb., smth.)* (in).

привозн|óй impórted; ~ые товáры impórted goods.

привóй *м. с.-х.* graft, scion.

привóль|е *с.* 1. *(свободное пространство)* ópen space, vast expánse; степнýе ~я the vast expánses of the steppes; 2. *(свобода)* fréedom, spáciousness. ~ный 1. *(о местности, пространстве)* ópen, spácious, fár-flúng; 2. *(свободный)* free; ~ное житьё cárefree life.

привратн|úк *м.*, ~ица *ж.* gáte-keeper, dóor-keeper.

привставáть, привстáть half rise* (to greet *smb.*), make* as if to rise.

привстáть *сов. см.* привставáть.

привходящи|й atténdant; ~е обстоятельства atténdant círcumstances.

привыкáть, привыкнуть *(к дт., + инф.)* get* used to *(smb., smth., + -ing)*, get*/grow* accústomed (to *smb., smth.,* to + -ing); он привык рáно вставáть he is used/accústomed to rísing éarly; ~ к дисциплúне accústom onesélf to díscipline; дéти скóро к нам привыкли the chíldren soon got used to us; я не привык к этому I'm not used to it.

привыкнуть *сов. см.* привыкáть.

привыч|ка *ж.* hábit; *(умение)* knack; сúла ~ки force of hábit; дéлать что-л. по ~ке do* *smth.* from mere hábit, do* *smth.* from sheer force of hábit; приобрестú ~ку grow*/get* into the hábit of dóing *smth.*; fall* into the way of dóing *smth.* ~ный 1. *(вошедший в привычку)* habítual; *(обычный)* úsual, cústomary; для меня это дéло ~ное I'm used to it; 2. *(привыкший)* accústomed (to), used (to); *(умелый)* práctised, trained.

привязанн|ость *ж.* attáchment, afféction; *(тяготение, склонность)* inclinátion, bent. ~ый *(преданный)* attáched; быть ~ым к кому-л. be* déeply attáched to *smb.*

привязчивый *разг.* 1. *(любящий)* afféctionate, lóyal; 2. *(надоедливый)* tróublesome, tíresome.

привязывать, привязáть *(вн.)* 1. fásten *(smb.,*

smth.), bind* (*smb.*, *smth.*); tie (*smb.*, *smth.*) (*тж. перен.*); ~ лóшадь téther a horse; ~ собáку chain/tie up a dog; ~ лóдку к столбý fásten a boat to a post; 2. (*внушать кому-л. чувство симпатии*) attách (*smb.*); привязáть к себé кого-л. win* *smb.*'s afféctions, gain *smb.*'s goodwill. ~ся, привязáться (к *дт.*) 1. (*чувствовать привязанность к кому-л.*) becóme* attáched (to), becóme* fond (of); за лéто он óчень привязáлся к товáрищам by the time the súmmer was óver he had becóme véry much attáched to his friends; 2. *разг.* (*приставать к кому-л.*) péster (*smb.*), bóther (*smb.*), make* a núisance of one*self* (to); 3. *разг.* (*придираться к чему-л.*) pick on (*smth.*); 4. *разг.* (*следовать*) start fóllowing (*smb.*), tack itsélf on (to), tag alóng (with); ко мне привязáлась какáя-то собáка a stray dog tacked itsélf on to me.

при́вяз|ь ж. (*для собаки*) leash, lead; (*для пасущегося животного*) téther; держáть собáку на ~и keep* a dog on the lead (*на поводке*); keep* a dog chained up (*у дома*).

пригвождáть, пригвоздить (*вн. к дт.*) pin (*smth.* to); *перен.* rívet (*smb.* to); пригвоздить кого-л. к мéсту rívet *smb.* to the spot.

пригвоздить *сов. см.* пригвождáть.

пригибáть, пригнýть (*вн.*) bend* (*smth.*). ~ся, пригнýться bend* down.

приглядéть *сов. см.* приглáживать.

приглáживать, приглáдить (*вн.*) smooth (*smth.*); ~ вóлосы smooth one*'s* hair.

приглас|и́тельный: ~ билéт invitátion card. ~и́ть *сов. см.* приглашáть.

приглаш|áть, пригласи́ть (*вн.*) 1. (*просить прийти*) invíte (*smb.*); пригласи́ть кого-л. на вéчер invíte *smb.* to a párty; пригласи́ть врачá call in a dóctor, send* for a dóctor; 2. (*просить выполнить какую-л. работу*) requést *smb.*'s sérvices, bring* in (*smb.*), híre (*smb.*); пригласи́ть консультáнта ask for proféssional advíce; пригласи́ть учи́теля requést the sérvices of a téacher, híre a téacher. ~éние *с.* invitátion; яви́ться по ~éнию come* by invitátion.

приглуш|áть, приглуши́ть (*вн.*) 1. (*слегка заглушать*) múffle (*smth.*); 2. *разг.* (*огонь*) damp (*smth.*) down; 3. *разг.* (*ослаблять, облегчать*) alláy (*smth.*), déaden (*smth.*); 4. *разг.* (*подавлять*) cramp (*smth.*). ~и́ть *сов. см.* приглушáть.

приглядéть(ся) *сов. см.* приглядывать(ся).

приглядывать, приглядéть *разг.* 1. (за *тв.*) look (áfter), watch (óver); ~ за детьми́ keep* an eye on the children; 2. (*вн.*; *подыскивать*) spot (*smth.*), pick out (*smth.*). ~ся, приглядéться *разг.* (к *дт.*) 1. (*внимательно всматриваться*) stare (at), look hard/close (at); (*изучать*) obsérve (*smb.*, *smth.*); 2. (*привыкать*) get* used to (*smth.*); (*становиться привычным*) pall (on).

приглян|ýться *сов.* (*дт.*) *разг.* take* a líking/fáncy (to); онá мне ~ýлась I took a fáncy to her.

пригнáть *сов. см.* пригонять.

пригнýть(ся) *сов. см.* пригибáть(ся).

пригов|áривать, приговори́ть 1. (*вн. к дт.*; *выносить приговор*) séntence (*smb.* to), condémn (*smb.* to); ~ кого-л. к тюрéмному заключéнию séntence *smb.* to imprísonment; ~ кого-л. к смéртной кáзни séntence/condémn *smb.* to death; 2. *тк. несов.* (*вн.*) *разг.* (*говорить*) keep* on sáying (*smth.*), múrmur (*smth.*).

приговóр *м.* vérdict, júdgement, séntence; приводи́ть ~ в исполнéние éxecute júdgement, cárry out the séntence. ·

приговори́ть *сов. см.* приговáривать 1.

пригоди́ться *сов.* be* of use, be* úseful, come* in úseful/hándy.

пригóдн|ость ж. fitness, suitabílity, úsefulness; (*о вещах тж.*) utílity, usabílity. ~ый fit, súitable, úseful; (*о вещах тж.*) úsable.

пригоня́ть, пригнáть 1. (*вн.*) (*приводить, подгоняя*) drive* (*smb.*, *smth.*) in, herd (*smb.*, *smth.*) in; 2. (*вн. к дт.*; *прилаживать*) adjúst (*smth.* to), fit (*smth.* on).

пригор|áть, пригорéть be* (slíghtly) burnt; молокó пригорéло the milk is burnt. ~éлый (slíghtly) burnt.

пригорéть *сов. см.* пригорáть.

при́город *м.* súburb. ~ный subúrban; (*о транспорте тж.*) lócal; ~ная желéзная дорóга subúrban line; ~ный пóезд lócal train; ~ное движéние lócal tráffic.

пригóрок *м.* híllock.

приго́ршн|я ж. hándful; ~ями by the hándful, in hándfuls; пóлными ~ями lávishly, abúndantly; набрáть в ~ю воды́ take* some wáter in one*'s* cupped hands.

пригорю́ниться *сов. разг.* grow* sad.

приготáвливать, приготóвить (*вн.*) 1. prepáre (*smb.*, *smth.*), make* (*smb.*, *smth.*) réady; get* (*smb.*, *smth.*) réady; приготóвить кого-л. к экзáменам prepáre/coach *smb.* for examinátions; ~ постéль make* a bed; 2. (*работая, осваивать что-л.*) learn* (*smth.*); ~ роль learn* a part; ~ урóки do* one*'s* hómework; 3. (*стряпать*) make* (*smth.*), cook (*smth.*); приготóвить обéд make* dínner. ~ся приготóвиться get* réady, prepáre; приготóвиться к отъéзду get* réady to leave; приготóвиться к прыжкý get* réady to jump/spring.

приготови́тельный prepáratory, prelíminary.

приготóвить(ся) *сов. см.* приготáвливать(ся).

приготов|лéние *с.* preparátion. ~ля́ть(ся) *несов. см.* приготáвливать(ся).

пригревáть, пригрéть (*вн.*) warm (*smb.*, *smth.*); *перен. разг.* (*приютить*) shélter (*smb.*); (*обласкать*) be* kind (to); ◇ пригрéть змею́ на груди́ nóurish a víper in one*'s* bósom.

пригрéть *сов. см.* пригревáть.

пригрози́ть *сов.* (*дт.*) thréaten (*smb.*); ~ кому́-л. судóм thréaten *smb.* with court procéedings; ~ кому́-л. пáльцем wag/shake* one*'s* finger at *smb.*

придавáть, придáть 1. (*вн.*; *прибавлять*) add (*smb.*, *smth.*); *воен.* attách (*smb.*, *smth.*); 2. (*рд.*; *увеличивать, усиливать*) lend* (*smth.*); ~ бóдрости и си́лы lend* vígour and énergy; 3. (*вн.*; *качество, форму и т. п.*) give* (*smth.*), impárt (*smth.*), lend* (*smth.*); ~ вкус чему́-л. give* rélish to *smth.*; ~ лицý стрóгое выражéние give* the face a sevére expréssion, make* the face look sevére; 4. (*вн.*; *вкладывать тот или иной смысл*) attách (*smth.*); ~ чему́-л. серьёзное значéние attách great impórtance to *smth.*

придави́ть *сов.* (*вн.*) weight (*smth.*) down, hold* (*smb.*, *smth.*) down, press (*smth.*) agáinst; (*прищемить*) squeeze (*smth.*).

придáное *с.* 1. (*имущество*) dówry; (*одежда, бельё*) trousseau; 2. (*комплект белья для новорождённого*) layétte, set of báby clothes.

придáток *м.* 1. appéndage; 2. *анат.* appéndix.

придáточн|ый *анат.*, *бот.* appendícular; ◇ ~ое предложéние *грам.* subórdinate clause.

придáть *сов. см.* придавáть.

придáч|а ж. 1. (*действие*) gíving, ádding; *воен.* attáching, attáchment; 2. (*то, что прибавлено, придано*) *перен.* into the bárgain; в ~у in addítion; дать что-л. в ~у give* *smth.* éxtra.

придвигáть, придви́нуть (*вн.*) bring* up (*smth.*), draw* up (*smth.*); придви́нуть стул draw* up a chair. ~ся, придви́нуться come* near, appróach.

придви́нуть(ся) *сов. см.* придвигáть(ся).

придéлать *сов. см.* придéлывать.

придéлывать, придéлать (*вн. к дт.*) fix (*smth.* to); придéлать рýчку к корзи́нке fix a hándle to a básket.

придéрживать, придержáть (*вн.*) 1. hold* (*smth.*);

(*замедлять, задерживать*) check (*smth.*); ~ лóшадь hold*/rein in a horse; 2. *разг.* (*не расходовать*) hold* (*smth.*) back, resérve (*smth.*); (*не пускать в оборот*) withhóld* (*smth.*); ~ товáр withhóld* goods.

придéрживаться *несов.* 1. (*за вн.*; *держаться за что-л.*) hold* on (to); 2. (*рд.*; *держаться ближе к чему-л.*) keep* (to); ~ прáвой (лéвой) стороны keep* to the right (left); 3. (*рд.*; *следовать чему-л.*) adhére (to), stick* (to), abíde* (by); ~ мнéния be* of the opínion, adhére/stick* to the opínion; ~ одногó с *кем-л.* мнéния be* of the same opínion as *smb.*; ~ полítики мíра adhére to a pólicy of peace; ~ тéкста stick* to the text.

придíра *м. и ж. разг.* fáultfinder; cáptious féllow.

придирáться, придрáться (к *дт.*) find* fault (with), pick (on).

придíр|ка *ж.* quíbble, cávil. ~чивый cáptious, cárping, fáultfinding; ~чивый крítик cávilling/fastídious crític; ~чивая крítика cárping críticism.

придрáться *сов. см.* придирáться.

придýмать *сов. см.* придýмывать.

придýмывать, придýмать 1. (*вн.,* + *инф.*; *изобретать, догадываться сделать что-л.*) invént (*smth.*); have* the idéa (of + -ing); (*догадываться*) guess (*smth.*); Это лýчшее, что я мог придýмать it's the best thing I can think of; Это ты неплóхо придýмал! that's not a bad idéa of yours!; 2. (*вн.; сочинять*) make* up (*smth.*), invént (*smth.*); придýмать отговóрку find*/invént an excúse.

придурь *ж. разг.:* с ~ю (a bit) dótty; off one's head.

придушíть *сов.* (*вн.*) *разг.* stránge (*smb., smth.*), thróttle (*smb., smth.*), choke (*smb., smth.*).

придыхá|ние *с. лингв.* aspirátion. ~тельный *лингв.:* ~тельный соглáсный áspirate.

приедáться, приéсться (*дт.*) *разг.* (*прям. и перен.*) pall (on); мне Это приéлось I'm fed up with it, I'm tíred of it.

приéзд *м.* arríval, cóming.

приезж|áть, приéхать arríve, come*. ~áющий *м.* new arríval, néwcomer, vísitor.

приезж|ий *прил.* 1.: ~ая трýппа tóuring cómpany; 2. *в знач. сущ. м.* néwcomer, vísitor.

приём *м.* 1. (*в учебное заведение, профсоюз и т. п.*) admíssion (to), enrólment (in); 2. (*гостей, посетителей, больных и т. п.*) recéption; 3. (*товаров*) accéptance; 4. (*гостеприимство*) wélcome, recéption; оказывать *кому-л.* рáдушный ~ give* *smb.* a héarty wélcome/recéption; 5. (*телеграмм, радиосообщений и т. п.*) recéiving, recéption; 6. (*доза*) dose; у меня остáлось аспирíна на одíн ~ I have ónly one dose of áspirin left; 7. (*способ*) méthod, way, technique; рáзные ~ы лечéния dífferent méthods of tréatment; лóвкий ~ cléver trick; 8. (*отдельное действие*) go, sítting, stage; он прочёл пьéсу в одíн ~ he read the play at one sítting/go; сдéлать что-л. в нéсколько ~ов do* smth. in stáges.

приéмлем|ый accéptable; ~ое предложéние accéptable óffer/propositíon.

приёмник *м.* (*принимающее устройство*) recéiver; (*радиоприёмник тж.*) rádio; ~ излучéния radiátion sénsor/detéctor.

приём|ный *прил.* 1. recéption *attr.*; ~ день recéption day; ~ые часы recéption hours; (*врача*) consúlting hours; ~ые экзáмены éntrance examinátions; ~ая комíссия examíng bódy, the examíners; 2. *тех., радио* recéiving *attr.*; ~ая радиостáнция recéiving státion; 3. *в знач. сущ. ж.* wáiting-room; (*кабинет врача*) consúlting-room, súrgery; ◇ ~ сын adópted son; ~ая дочь adópted dáughter; ~ отéц fóster-father; ~ая мать fóster-mother.

приём|очный recéiving *attr.* ~щик *м.,* ~щица *ж.* recéiving clerk.

приёмыш *м. разг.* adópted child*.

приéсться *сов. см.* приедáться.

приéхать *сов. см.* приезжáть.

прижáть(ся) *сов. см.* прижимáть(ся).

прижéчь *сов. см.* прижигáть.

приживáться, прижíться 1. séttle down, make* onesélf at home; 2. (*о растениях*) take*/strike roots 3. (*привыкнуть*) becóme*/get* acclímatized.

прижигáние *с.* cauterizátion, cáuterizing, cáutery.

прижигáть, прижéчь (*вн.*) cáuterize (*smth.*), sear (*smth.*); прижéчь рáну йóдом disinféct a wound with íodine.

прижимáть, прижáть 1. (*вн. к дт.*) press (*smb., smth.* to), squeeze (*smb., smth.* to), clasp (*smb., smth.* to); ~ когó-л. к грудú hug/press *smb.* to one's heart, hold* *smb.* tight; 2. (*вн.*) *разг.* (*притеснять*) restríct (*smb.*), put* the screw on (*smb.*), clamp down (on); ◇ ~ когó-л. к стéнке drive* *smb.* ínto a córner. ~ся, прижáться (к *дт.*) cúddle up (to), snúggle up (to), cling* close (to); ~ся к стенé stand* close to a wall, flátten one's back agáinst a wall.

прижúмистый *разг.* clóse-fisted, stíngy.

прижíться *сов. см.* приживáться.

приз *м.* prize; взять пéрвый ~ take*/win* the first prize; переходящий ~ challenge prize.

призадýматься *сов.* be*/becóme* thóughtful, be* lost in thought.

призвáни|е *с.* 1. (*склонность*) vocátion, cálling, bent, inclinátion; имéть ~ к жívописи have* an áptitude/taste/turn for páinting; слéдовать своемý ~ю fóllow one's bent; чýвствовать ~ к наýке feel* a cálling for science; он учíтель по ~ю he is cut out to be a téacher, his vocátion is téaching; 2. (*предназначение*) míssion, task.

призвáть *сов. см.* призывáть.

приземíст|ый 1. thicksét, squat, stócky; ~ пáрень stócky féllow; 2. (*низкий*) lów-built, squat; ~ые дóмики lów-built hóuses.

приземлéние *с.* tóuch-down, lánding.

приземлíться *сов. см.* приземляться.

приземляться, приземлíться touch down, land, alíght.

призёр *м.* príze-winner; ~ Олимпíйских игр Olýmpic príze-winner.

прúзма *ж.* prism. ~тúческий prismátic.

признавáть, признáть (*вн.*) 1. recógnize (*smb., smth.*); признáть нейтралитéт госудáрства recógnize a cóuntry's neutrálity; 2. (*соглашаться с чем-л.*) acknówledge (*smth.*), admít (*smth.*), own (*smth.*); ~ чью--л. правотý admít *smb.* is right; ~ свою ошíбку acknówledge one's mistáke; признáть себя побеждённым acknówledge one's deféat; 3. (*приходить к какому-л. заключению*) decláre (*smb., smth.*); ~ чью-л. рабóту отлíчной decláre/consider *smb.'s* work éxcellent; признáть себя винóвным plead guílty; ~ся, признáться (*дт. в пр.*) conféss (*smth.*), admít (*smth.* to); подсудúмые признáлись the accúsed pléaded guílty; признáться *кому-л.* в любвú decláre one's love to *smb.*; признáться во всём own up, make* a clean breast of it; ◇ признáться (*сказать*)... I conféss..., I must say...

прúзнак *м.* sign, indicátion; не подавáть ~ов жúзни show* no sign of life; ~и отравлéния sýmptoms of póisoning; ~и недовóльства signs of discontént; по всем ~ам éverything goes to show.

признáни|е *с.* 1. (*действие*) conféssion, avówal; ~ в любвú declarátion of love; 2. (*выражение своего положительного отношения*) acknówledgement, admíssion; ~ чьей-л. правоты acknówledgement that *smb.* is right; 3. (*слова признающегося в чём-л.*) conféssion; выслушать чьё-л. ~ listen to *smb.'s* conféssion; 4. (*общественное уважение*) recognítion, acknówledgement; он пóльзуется всеóбщим ~ем his reputátion is génerally recógnized, he has a univérsal reputátion; заслужúть всеóбщее ~ mérit univérsal acknówledgement.

при́знанный recógnized, acknówledged; ~ тала́нт recógnized tálent.

призна́тельн|ость ж. grátitude, grátefulness, thánkfulness. ~ый gráteful, thánkful.

призна́ть(ся) сов. см. признава́ть(ся).

призов|о́й prize attr.; ~ы́е места́ спорт. príze-winning pláces.

при́зра|к м. phántom, spéctre; (привидение тж.) ghost, apparítion; гоня́ться за ~ками catch* at shádows. ~чный 1. phantásmal, ghóstly; ~чное виде́ние ghóstly vísion; 2. (мнимый) unréal, illúsory; 3. (неясный, зыбкий) illúsive, shádowy.

призы́в м. 1. (действие) call; ~ на действи́тельную вое́нную слу́жбу cáll-up (for áctive mílitary sérvice); 2. (просьба, мольба) appéal, call; ~ на по́мощь call for help; 3. (лозунг) appéal, slógan; 4. собир. (лица, одновременно призванные на военную службу) cáll-up, draft.

призыв|а́ть, призва́ть 1. (вн.; звать) call (smb.); ~ на по́мощь call/appéal for help; 2. (вн.; на военную службу) call (smb.) up, conscrípt (smb.); 3. (вн. к дт., вн. + инф.; привлекать к важному делу) call (upón smb. + to inf); 4. (вн. к дт.) call (smb. to), appéal (to smb. for); призва́ть кого́-л. к поря́дку call smb. to órder; призва́ть к споко́йствию appéal for calm. ~а́ться несов. разг. be* called up. ~ни́к м. pérson who has been called up; dráftée амер. ~но́й cáll-up attr.; ~но́й во́зраст cáll-up age; ~но́й пункт cáll-up/enlístment óffice; ~на́я коми́ссия cáll-up commíssion.

призы́вный: ~ крик call.

при́иск м. mine; золоты́е ~и góld-fields.

прииска́ть сов. см. прии́скивать.

прии́скивать, прииска́ть (вн.) разг. find* (smth.); несов. тж. look (for).

прийти́ сов. см. приходи́ть.

прийти́сь сов. см. приходи́ться 1—5.

прика́з м. órder; (бумага с распоряжением) printed órder; по ~у кого́-л. by órder of smb.; ~ по войска́м órder of the day; ~ о наступле́нии órder to attáck; ~ есть ~! órders are órders!

прика́з|а́ние с. instrúction, órder. ~а́ть сов. см. прика́зывать.

прика́з|ывать, приказа́ть (дт. + инф.) órder (smb. + to inf), commánd (smb. + to inf); приказа́ть кому́-л. сде́лать что́-л. órder smb. to do smth.; ему́ бы́ло прика́зано яви́ться на сле́дующий день he was órdered to repórt next day; как прика́жете вас понима́ть? how am I expécted to take your remárk?; что прика́жете? what can I do for you?; ◇ приказа́ть до́лго жить die, depárt (from) this life.

прика́лывать, приколо́ть (вн.) pin (smth.), fásten (smth.) with a pin; приколо́ть цвето́к к пла́тью pin a flówer to one's dress.

прика́рмливать несов. (вн.) feed* (smb., smth.) up; ~ грудно́го ребёнка молоко́м súpplement a báby's diet with milk.

прикаса́ться, прикосну́ться (к дт.) touch (smb., smth.); па́льцы его́ слегка́ прикосну́лись к стру́нам his fingers ran líghtly óver the strings.

прикати́ть сов. 1. (вн.; катя, приблизить) roll (smth.); 2. разг. (приехать) drive* in; ~ся сов. roll.

прики́дывать, прики́нуть разг. 1. (вн., рд.; прибавлять) add (smth.); 2. (вн.; определять вес) feel* (smth.); weigh (smth.) róughly, try the weight (of); ~ что́-л. на руке́ heft smth.; 3. (вн.; делать приблизительный подсчёт) réckon (smth.) up; ~ что́-л. в уме́ réckon up smth. in one's head.

прики́дываться, прики́нуться (тв.) разг. preténd (to be smth.), sham (smth.); ~ больны́м sham ill, preténd to be ill; ~ простачко́м play the símpleton.

прики́нуть сов. см. прики́дывать.

прики́нуться сов. см. прики́дываться.

прикла́д м. (оружия) butt, búttstock.

прикладн|о́й applíed; ~ые нау́ки applíed sciences; ~ое иску́сство applíed art(s) (pl).

прикла́дывать, приложи́ть (вн. к дт.) put* (smth. to); applý (smth. to); приложи́ть ру́ку ко лбу put* one's hand to one's fórehead; приложи́ть к у́ху тру́бку put* the recéiver to one's ear. ~ся, приложи́ться 1. (тв. к дт.; приближаться вплотную к чему-л.) applý (smth. to); приложи́ться гла́зом к замо́чной сква́жине applý one's eye to the kéyhole; 2. (к дт.; почтительно целовать) kiss (smb., smth.); 3. (нацеливаться) take* aim.

прикле́ивать, прикле́ить (вн.) stick* (smth.), glue (smth.), paste (smth.). ~ся, прикле́иться stick*, get* stuck, bond.

прикле́ить(ся) сов. см. прикле́ивать(ся).

приклепа́ть сов. см. приклёпывать.

приклёпывать, приклепа́ть (вн.) rivet (smth.).

приклони́ть сов. см. приклоня́ть.

приклоня́ть, приклони́ть: не́где го́лову приклони́ть have* nówhere to lay one's head.

приключён|ие с. advénture; (происшествие) íncident. ~ческий advénture attr.; ~ческий рома́н nóvel of advénture, advénture nóvel.

прикова́ть сов. см. прико́вывать.

прико́вывать, прикова́ть (вн.) 1. chain (smb., smth.); перен. tie (smb., smth.); страх прикова́л его́ к ме́сту fear róoted him to the spot, he was róoted to the spot by fear; быть прико́ванным к посте́ли be* tied to one's bed, be* bédridden; 2. (привлекать) attráct (smth.), rivet (smth.); ~ к себе́ всео́бщее внима́ние attráct éverybody's atténtion.

прико́л м. post; ◇ на ~е (о судах) tied up, at (their) móorings; стоя́ть на ~е 1) be* laid up; 2) (бездействовать) stand* ídle.

прикола́чивать, приколоти́ть (вн.) nail (smth.) up/down, fásten (smth.) with nails.

приколоти́ть сов. см. прикола́чивать.

приколо́ть сов. см. прика́лывать.

прикомандирова́ть сов. (вн. к дт.) attách (smb. to).

прико́рм м. 1. (действие) féeding up; 2. (то, чем прикармливают) éxtra feed. ~ка ж. см. прико́рм.

прикорну́ть сов. разг. snúggle (up); (вздремнуть) take* a nap.

прикоснове́ние с. touch; лёгкое ~ light touch.

прикосну́ться сов. см. прикаса́ться.

прикраси́ть сов. см. прикра́шивать.

прикра́сы мн. (ед. прикра́са ж.) разг. embéllishment sg, embróidery sg; рассказа́ть что́-л. без прикра́с tell* smth. without ány embróidery.

прикра́шивать, прикра́сить (вн.) embéllish (smth.); embróider (smth.).

прикреп|и́ть(ся) сов. см. прикрепля́ть(ся). ~ле́ние с. 1. attáchment; (булавкой, кнопкой) fástening; 2. (регистрация) registrátion.

прикрепля́ть, прикрепи́ть (вн. к дт.) 1. (прикалывать) fásten (smth. to), nail (smth. to); ~ что́-л. була́вками kiss (smth.), fásten (smth. with pins; 2. (передавать в чьё-л. ведение) attách (smb. to); 3. (принимать на учёт) régister (smb. at). ~ся, прикрепи́ться 1. fásten; 2. (регистрироваться) régister; прикрепи́ться к поликли́нике régister at a polyclínic.

прикри́кивать, прикри́кнуть (на вн.) shout (at).

прикри́кнуть сов. см. прикри́кивать.

прикрути́ть сов. см. прикру́чивать.

прикру́чивать, прикрути́ть 1. (вн. к дт.) tie (smth. to), bind* (smth. to); fásten (smth. to); 2. (вн.) разг. (газ, фитиль в лампе и т. п.) turn (smth.) down.

прикрыва́ть, прикры́ть (вн.) 1. (закрывать) cóver (smth.); 2. (скрывать) cóver up (smth.), disguíse (smth.), concéal (smth.); 3. (заслонять) screen (smb., smth.), shield (smb., smth.); 4. (защищать войсками) cóver (smth.); ~ отступле́ние cóver a retréat; 5. (неплотно закрывать) draw* (smth.) to, close (smth.) lightly, half close (smth.); 6. разг. (прекращать) close (smth.) down, wind* up (smth.). ~ся, прикрыться 1. (тв.) cóver onesélf (with); 2. (скрывать, маскировать) concéal one's inténtions; 3. (заслоняться) shield onesélf; 4. (неплотно закрываться) close lightly; 5. разг. (ликвидироваться) close down.

прикрыт|ие с. 1. (действие) concéalment, shíelding, protéction; для ~ия чего-л. to concéal/protéct smth.; 2. (защита, охрана) cóver, protéction; (войска) cóvering force; под ~ием чего-л. protécted by smth.; 3. (сооружения, предметы, укрывающие от чего-л.) shélter.

прикрыть(ся) сов. см. прикрывáть(ся).

прикупáть, прикупить (вн., рд.) buy* (some more) (smth.), get* (some more) (smth.); прикупить ещё метр ткáни buy* anóther métre of cloth.

прикупить сов. см. прикупáть.

прикýривать, прикурить light* a cigarétte; ~ у кого-л. take* a light from smb.; разрешите прикурить! can you give me a light, please!

прикурить сов. см. прикýривать.

прикусить сов. см. прикусывать.

прикусывать, прикусить (вн.) bite* (smth.); прикусить язык bite* one's tongue; перен. keep* one's mouth shut.

прилáв|ок м. cóunter; рабóтник ~ка shop assistant, cóunter-hand.

прилагáтельн|ый: имя ~ое грам. ádjective.

прилагáть, приложить (вн.) 1. (присоединять к чему-л.) appénd (smth.), attách (smth.); (к письму тж.) enclóse (smth.); 2. (применять) exért (smth.); ~ усилия make* évery éffort, do* all one can, exért all one's pówers; он не приложил никакóго старáния he took no pains at all.

прилáдить сов. см. прилáживать.

прилáживать, прилáдить (вн. к дт.) fix (smth. to), fit (smth. to).

приласкáть сов. (вн.) pet (smb., smth.), caréss (smb., smth.), fóndle (smb., smth.); (проявить нежность) show* kindness (to), be* nice (to). ~ся сов. (к дт.) make* up (to), coax afféction (from).

прилег|áть (к дт.) 1. (примыкать) adjóin (smth.); сад ~áет к рекé the gárden adjóins the ríver, the gárden bórders on the ríver; 2. (об одежде) fit snúgly (on), cling* (to).

прилежáние с. díligence, índustry.

прилежáщ|ий мат. adjácent; ~ие углы adjácent ángles.

прилéжный díligent, indústrious, assíduous.

прилеп|ить(ся) сов. см. прилепля́ть(ся). ~ля́ть, прилепить (вн. к дт.) stick* (smth. to, on); (клеем тж.) paste (smth. to, on), glue (smth. to, on). ~ля́ться (к дт.) stick* (to).

прилёт м. arríval, cóming.

прилетáть, прилетéть 1. arríve, come*; 2. разг. (примчаться) rush in/up, fly* in.

прилетéть сов. см. прилетáть.

прилéчь сов. 1. lie* down (for a while); (привалиться) lean* (on); 2. (пригнуться — о траве и т. п.) droop; (осесть — о пыли) séttle.

прилив м. 1. (морской) rísing tide, flood tide; ~ и отлив rise and fall of the tide, ebb and flow of the tide; 2. (поступление, приток) ínflux; 3. (приток крови) rush; afflux научн.; 4. (нарастание, усиление чего-л.) surge, úpsurge; ~ рáдости surge of joy.

прилипáть, прилипнуть (к дт.) stick* (to), adhére (to); перен. разг. glue/press onesélf (to); (приставать) péster (smth.).

прилип|нуть сов. см. прилипáть. ~чивый 1. sticking, adhésive; перен. разг. (заразительный) inféctious, cátching; 2. разг. (надоедливый) bóring, tíresome; ~чивый человéк pest, bore.

прилистник м. бот. stipule.

прилич|ие с. décency, propríety, decórum; для ~ия for décency's/form's sake, for the sake of décency; соблюдáть ~ия obsérve the propríeties. ~но décently; он ~но вы́глядит he looks fáirly well. ~ный 1. (пристойный) décent; décorous, séemly; (порядочный) respéctable; 2. разг. (хороший) décent, pássable; good enóugh predic.; (изрядный) fair; ~ная зарплáта fair wáges; ~ная сýмма tidy sum.

прилож|éние с. 1. (к журналу, газете) súpplement; (к книге, докладу и т. п.) appéndix (pl -ices); 2. грам. apposítion. ~ить сов. см. приклáдывать и прилагáть. ~иться сов. см. приклáдываться.

прилунéние с. lánding on the moon, moon/lúnar lánding.

прилун|иться сов. см. прилуня́ться. ~я́ться, прилуниться land on the moon.

прильнýть сов. см. льнуть 1.

примáнивать, приманить (вн.) entíce (smb., smth.), lure (smb., smth.), attráct (smb., smth.).

приманить сов. см. примáнивать.

примáнка ж. bait; перен. allúrement, lure, attráction.

примелькáться сов. разг. becóme* famíliar.

примен|éние с. 1. applicátion; (употребление) use, emplóyment; ~ нóвых мéтодов произвóдства emplóyment of new méthods of prodúction; достóйный лýчшего ~éния wórthy of bétter applicátion; 2. (к условиям, местности) adaptátion. ~имость ж. applicabílity; ~имость тéхники úsefulness of the machínery. ~имый ápplicable; вполнé ~имый спóсоб quite féasible méthod. ~ительно with/in réference to. ~ить(ся) сов. см. применя́ть(ся).

применя́ть, применить (вн.) applý (smth.); (использовать) use (smth.). ~ся, применя́ться (к дт.) adápt onesélf (to), confórm (to).

примéр м. exámple; (частный случай) ínstance; (образец) módel; ~ мýжества exámple of cóurage; великодýшия exámple of generósity; слéдовать чьемý-л. ~у fóllow smb.'s exámple; по ~у кого-л. fóllowing the exámple of smb.; для ~а as an exámple (to óthers); ◇ к ~у for exámple, for ínstance; не в ~ 1) (в отличие) unlíke; 2) (гораздо): не в ~ умнée much cléverer (than).

примерзáть, примёрзнуть (к дт.) freeze* on (to).

примёрзнуть сов. см. примерзáть.

примéр|ка ж. trýing on, fitting; сдéлать ~ку have* a fitting.

примéрн|о 1. (отлично) exemplá“rily; 2. (приблизительно) appróximately, abóut. ~ый 1. (образцовый) módel attr.; exémplary; ~ое поведéние exémplary cónduct; 2. (приблизительный) appróximate; ~ый подсчёт расхóдов appróximate éstimate of expénditure.

примеря́ть, примéрить (вн.) try (smth.) on.

примéсь ж. admíxture; перен. тж. touch, tinge.

примéт|а ж. 1. sign, tóken; осóбые ~ы distínctive marks; 2. (предзнаменование) ómen, sign; дурнáя (хорóшая) ~ bad (good) ómen; ◇ имéть кого-л. на ~е have* smb. in view.

приметáть сов. см. примётывать.

примéт|ить сов. см. примечáть. ~ный 1. (заметный) percéptible; 2. (выделяющийся среди других) conspícuous; ~ный человéк conspícuous pérson.

примётывать, приметáть (вн.) tack (smth.), baste (smth.).

примечáни|е с. note, annotátion; (сноска) fóotnote; составля́ть ~я к тéксту ánnotate a text; снабдить текст ~ями províde a text with notes, ánnotate a text.

примечáтельный outstánding, nóteworthy.

примечáть, примéтить (вн.) разг. nótice (smb., smth.), obsérve (smb., smth.), note (smb., smth.); (запоминать) make* a méntal note (of).

примешáть сов. см. примéшивать.

примéшивать, примешáть (вн., рд. к дт.) mix (smth. ínto), add (smth. to).

приминⷵа́ть, примⷵя́ть (*вн.*) flátten (*smth.*), tread* (*smth.*) down. ~ся, примⷵя́ться be* trámpled down.

примирён|ец *м.* conciliator. ~ие *с.* conciliátion, reconciliátion, réconcilement. ~ческий concíliatory. ~чество *с.* spírit of conciliátion.

примири́тель *м.* conciliator, réconciler, péace-maker. ~ный reconcíliatory, conciliating.

примирⷵи́ть *сов. см.* примирⷵя́ть. ~и́ться *сов. см.* примирⷵя́ться *и* мири́ться 2. ~я́ть, примири́ть (*вн. с тв.* 1. (*мирить*) réconcile (*smb.* with); примири́ть сосе́дей réconcile the néighbours, make* it up betwéen the néighbours; 2. (*заставлять терпимо относиться*) réconcile (*smb., smth.* to); ~я́ть две то́чки зре́ния réconcile two points of view. ~я́ться, примири́ться (с *тв.*) 1. *разг.* (*мириться*) make* it up (with), be* réconciled (with); 2. (*свыкаться с чем-л.*) becóme* réconciled (to), réconcile onesélf (to); примири́ться с судьбо́й réconcile onesélf to one's fate/lot, make* the best of it.

примити́вный primitive.

примкну́ть *сов. см.* примыка́ть 2.

примо́лкнуть *сов. разг.* becóme*/fall* sílent.

примо́рский séaside *attr.*, cóastal; máritime *научн.*; ~ го́род séaside town.

примо́рье *с.* coast; líttoral *книжн.*

примости́ться *сов. разг.* find* a place (on), perch onesélf (on).

примо́чк|а *ж.* lótion; де́лать ~у apply lótion, bathe the affécted part.

при́мула *ж. бот.* prímula, prímrose.

при́мус *м.* prímus(-stove).

примча́ться *сов.* come* rúnning, come* téaring alóng, rush in.

примык|а́ть, примкну́ть (к *дт.*) 1. *тк. несов.* (*находиться рядом*) adjóin (*smth.*), bórder (on, upón), be* adjácent (to); дом ~а́ет к шко́ле the house adjóins the school; 2. (*присоединяться*) join (*smb., smth.*); *перен. тж.* becóme* assóciated (with), go* alóng (with).

примⷵя́ть(ся) *сов. см.* приминⷵа́ть(ся).

принадлеж|а́ть *несов.* 1. (*дт.; быть чьей-л. собственностью*) belóng (to); 2. (*дт.; являться чьим-л. творением*) be* the work (of); э́та карти́на ~и́т ки́сти Ре́пина this picture is by Répin, this picture is the work of Répin; им ~и́т честь э́того откры́тия the crédit for this discóvery belóngs to them; 3. (*дт.; быть свойственным кому-л., чему-л.*) belóng (to), be* a féature (of); хи́мии ~и́т большо́е бу́дущее the chémical índustry has a great fúture; 4. (к *дт.; входить в состав чего-л.*) belóng (to); be* númbered (amóng); он ~и́т к числу́ лу́чших писа́телей на́шей эпо́хи he is one of the best writers of our time.

принадле́жност|ь *ж.* 1. (*предмет*) árticle, accéssory; ~и туале́та tóilet árticles/accéssories; посте́льные ~и bédding *sg*; рыболо́вные ~и fishing táckle *sg*; 2. (*неотъемлемое свойство*) élement, esséntial quálity; 3. (*к организации и т. п.*). mémbership (of), belónging (to).

принаряди́ть *сов.* (*вн.*) *разг.* dress (*smb.*) up, get* (*smb.*) up, deck (*smb.*) out. ~ся *сов. разг.* dress/get* onesélf up.

принести́ *сов. см.* приноси́ть.

принижⷵа́ть, прини́зить (*вн.*) 1. (*унижать*) lówer (*smb.*), húmble (*smb.*), humíliate (*smth.*); 2. (*роль, значение*) belíttle (*smth.*), dispárage (*smth.*).

прини́женн|ость *ж.* humílity, húmbleness. ~ый 1. (*выражающий смирение*) humíliated; 2. (*унизительный*) humíliating.

прини́зить *сов. см.* принижⷵа́ть.

приⷵня́ть, примⷵя́ть 1. *брать, получать*) accépt (*smth.*), take* (*smth.*); ~ пода́рки accépt gifts; 2. (*вн.; брать под своё командование, вступать в управление предприятием и т. п.*) take* óver (*smth.*);

(*пост, должность*) assúme (*smth.*); приⷵня́ть ро́ту take* óver a cómpany; приня́ть заво́д take* óver a fáctory, take* charge of a fáctory; 3. (*вн.; включать в состав чего-л.*) admít (*smth.*), accépt (*smth.*); (*на работу*) engáge (*smb.*), take* (*smb.*) on; его́ при́няли в университе́т he was admítted to the univérsity; приня́ть на рабо́ту пять челове́к engáge five pérsons; 4. (*вн.; посети́телей, гостей и т. п.*) recéive (*smb., smth.*); ~ делега́цию recéive a delegátion; приня́ть посла́ recéive an ambássador; ~ госте́й recéive guests; хорошо́ приня́ть кого́-л. give* *smb.* a good recéption; приня́ть больно́го recéive a pátient; 5. (*вн.; проявлять какое-л. отношение к чему-л.*) recéive (*smth.*) take* (*smth.*), treat (*smth.*); они́ с восто́ргом при́няли э́ту весть they recéived the news enthusiástically; ~ (что-л. благоскло́нно и т. п.) recéive (*smth.*); приня́ть (предложе́ние) accépt an óffer/propósal; ~ чьи-л. усло́вия agrée to *smb.'s* conditions, accépt *smb.'s* terms; 7. (*вн.; утверждать голосованием*) pass (*smth.*), cárry (*smth.*), adópt (*smth.*); приня́ть резолю́цию pass/cárry a resolútion; 8. (*вн.; по радио, телеграфу, телефону*) take* (down) (*smth.*); приня́ть телефоногра́мму take* (down) (telephone) méssage; 9. (*вн.) в сочетании с сущ.* take* (*smth.*); ~ уча́стие в чём-л. take* part in *smth.*; 10. (*вн.; учение, религию*) adópt (*smth.*), embráce (*smth.*); 11. (*вн.; вид, форму*) assúme (*smth.*); при́нял (пра́здничный вид) the town was decked out for the hóliday, the town looked véry féstive; их отноше́ния при́няли чи́сто официа́льный хара́ктер their relátions assúmed a púrely fórmal cháracter; 12. (*вн., рд.; какое-л. лекарство*) take* (*smth.*); ~ миксту́ру take* one's médicine; 13. (*вн.; подвергаться какой-л. процедуре*) take* (*smth.*); ~ ва́нну have* a bath; 14. (*вн. за вн.; счесть по ошибке за другого, другое*) (mis)take* (*smb., smth.* for); при́няли за кого́-то друго́го he was (mis)táken for sómebody else; ◇ ~ во внима́ние чьё-л. мне́ние take* *smb.'s* opinion into considerátion; ~ что-л. бли́зко к се́рдцу take* *smth.* to heart; ~ что-л. всерьёз take* *smth.* sériously; ~ на себя́ мно́го обя́занностей undertáke* mány dúties, load onesélf with responsibílities; ~ ребёнка (*при родах*) assíst at the birth (of a child). ~ся, приня́ться 1. (за *вн.; приступать к чему-л.*) begín* (*smth.*); set* abóut (*smth.*); приня́ться за рабо́ту set* to work; 2. (за *вн.*) *разг.* (*воздействовать*) take* (*smb.*) in hand, get* to work on (*smb.*); 3. (*давать ростки*) take* root; (*о вакцине*) take*.

приноравⷵливать, приноро́вить (*вн.* к *дт.*) *разг.* 1. adjúst (*smth.* to), adápt (*smth.* to); 2. (*приурочивать*) arránge (*smth.*) to, fit in (with). ~ся, приноро́виться (к *дт.*) *разг.* adápt onesélf (to), accómmodate onesélf (to); acquíre/get* the knack (of).

приноро́вить(ся) *сов. см.* приноравⷵливать(ся).

приноси́ть, принести́ (*вн.*) 1. bring* (*smb., smth.*); (*в руках, на руках тж.*) cárry (*smb., smth.*); fetch (*smth.*); принести́ ве́щи домо́й bring* the lúggage home; принести́ отве́т bring* a replý; 2. (*родить — о животных*) prodúce (*smth.*), have* (*smth.*); ко́шка принесла́ трёх котя́т the cat had three kíttens; 3. (*давать урожай*) bear* (*smth.*), yield (*smth.*); 4. (*давать в результате*) yield (*smth.*), bring* (*smth.*); ~ дохо́д yield a prófit; ~ по́льзу кому́-л. bénefit *smb.*; ~ вред кому́-л. bring* /do* *smb.* harm; 5.: принести́ что-л. в дар présent *smth.* as a gift; принести́ благода́рность кому́-л. thank *smb.*, expréss one's thanks/grátitude to *smb.*; принести́ кля́тву swear an oath, make* a vow; ◇ ~ сча́стье кому́-л. bring* *smb.* luck; ~ несча́стье кому́-л. bring* *smb.* ill luck.

принуди́тельный compúlsory, forced; ~ труд forced lábour.

прину́дить *сов. см.* принужда́ть.

принужд|а́ть, прину́дить (*вн.*) compél (*smb.*), force (*smb.*). ~е́ние *с.* compúlsion, coércion; де́лать что-л. по

~ению do* *smth.* únder compúlsion; дéлать *что-л.* без ~ения do* *smth.* of *one's* own free will.

принуждённ|ость *ж.* constráint. ~ый constráined; (*о манерах*) stiff; ~ая улыбка forced smile.

принц *м.* prínce. ~éсса *ж.* princéss.

прúнцип *м.* prínciple; основнúе ~ы геомéтрии first prínciples of geómetry; ◇ из ~а on prínciple.

принципиáльн|о (*из принципа*) on prínciple; (*в принципе*) in prínciple. ~ость *ж.* adhérence to prínciple. ~ый **1.** (*вытекающий из принципов*) of prínciple *после сущ.*, concérning prínciple *после сущ.*; ~ый вопрóс a mátter of prínciple; ~ые соображéния considerátions of prínciple; **2.** (*руководствующийся принципами*) príncipled; ~ый человéк príncipled pérson; man*, wóman* of prínciple.

принятие *с.* accéptance, adóption.

прúнятый accépted; ~ порядок the accépted sýstem, the úsual way of dóing things.

принять(ся) *сов. см.* принимáть(ся).

приободрúть(ся) *сов. см.* приободрять(ся).

приободрять, приободрúть (*вн.*) encóurage (*smb.*), héarten (*smb.*). ~ся, приободрúться take* cóurage, take* heart, cheer up.

приобрести́ *сов. см.* приобретáть.

приобрет|áть, приобрести́ (*вн.*) acquíre (*smth.*); (*покупать тж.*) buy* (*smth.*); ~ знáния acquíre/attáin knówledge; ~ óпыт acquíre/gain expérience. ~éние *с.* acquírement; acquisítion; (*покупка тж.*) púrchase.

приобщ|áть, приобщúть (*вн. к дт.*) **1.** (*знакомить с чем-л.*) make* (*smb.*) famíliar (with), acquáint (*smb.* with); **2.** (*присоединять*) annéx (*smth.* to), appénd (*smth.* to), attách (*smth.* to). ~áться, приобщúться (к дт.) be* drawn (ínto), becóme* famíliar (with), get* to know (*smth.*). ~éние *с.* (к дт.) famíliarizing (with); dráwing (ínto).

приобщúть(ся) *сов. см.* приобщáть(ся).

приодéть (*вн.*) *разг.* dress (*smb.*) up, get* (*smb.*) up. ~ся *сов. разг.* dress/get* onesélf up.

приостанáвливать, приостановúть (*вн.*) hold* up (*smth.*), check (*smth.*); (*откладывать*) suspénd (*smth.*); шторм приостановúл движéние эскáдры the squádron was held up by a storm. ~ся, приостановúться stop (for a while), pause.

приостановúть(ся) *сов. см.* приостанáвливать(ся).

приотворúть(ся) *сов. см.* приотворять(ся).

приотворять, приотворúть (*вн.*) ópen (*smth.*) slíghtly; ~ дверь set* the door ajár. ~ся, приотворúться hálf-ópen, ópen slíghtly.

приоткрывáть, приоткрыть (*вн.*) ópen (*smth.*) a líttle (way); приоткрыть окнó ópen the wíndow a líttle (way). ~ся, приоткрыться ópen a líttle (way).

приоткрыть(ся) *сов. см.* приоткрывáть(ся).

припадáть, припáсть **1.** (к дт.; *прижиматься*) press close (to), cling* close (to); **2.** (на *вн.*; *опускаться*) drop (on); ~ на колéно drop on one knee; **3.** *тк. несов. разг.* (*прихрамывать*) limp, be* lame.

припáдок *м.* fit, attáck; (*очень сильный*) pároxysm; ~ гнéва fit of ánger, óutburst of pássion; сердéчный ~ heart attáck; нéрвный ~ nérvous attáck.

припаивáть, припаять (*вн. к дт.*) sólder (*smth.* to). ~ся, припаяться join/fuse togéther.

припáйка *ж.* **1.** (*действие*) sóldering; **2.** (*припаянная часть*) sóldered joint.

припасáть, припасти́ (*вн.*) *разг.* lay up (*smth.*) in store.

припасти́ *сов. см.* припасáть.

припáсть *сов. см.* припадáть 1, 2.

припáсы *мн.* **1.** stores; supplíes; (*съестные*) provísions; **2.** *воен.* ammunítion *sg.*

припаять(ся) *сов. см.* припáивать(ся).

припéв *м.* refráin.

припевáючи *разг.:* жить ~ live in clóver.

припёк *м.* the heat of the sun; на ~e right in the sun, in the heat of the sun.

припёка *ж.:* сбóку ~ out of place; redúndant.

припекáть, припéчь (*о солнце*) be* béating down.

приперéть *сов. см.* припирáть.

припéчь *сов. см.* припекáть.

припирáть, приперéть (*вн.*) *разг.* **1.** (*прижимать*) press (*smb.*, *smth.*); squéeze (*smb.*, *smth.*); **2.** (*закрывать*) block (*smth.*); ◇ приперéть когó-л. к стенé drive* *smb.* ínto a córner.

приписáть(ся) *сов. см.* припúсывать(ся).

припúска *ж.* **1.** addítion; (к письму) póstscript; **2.** (*регистрация*) registrátion; **3.** *обыкн. мн.* (*ложные показатели выполнения плана*) úpward distórtion (of resúlts achíeved).

припúсывать, приписáть **1.** (*вн.*; к заранее написанному*) add (*smth.*); **2.** (*вн.*; *причислять к чему-л.*) régister (*smb.*); **3.** (*вн. дт.*; *считать следствием чего-л.*) attríbute (*smth.* to); **4.** (*вн. дт.*; *считать принадлежащим кому-л.*) ascríbe (*smth.* to), impúte (*smth.* to).

приплáта *ж.* éxtra páyment.

приплати́ть *сов. см.* приплáчивать.

приплáчивать, приплати́ть (*вн.*) pay* (*smth.*) éxtra.

приплести́сь *сов. разг.* stágger (there), drag onesélf.

приплóд *м.* lítter, óffspring.

приплывáть, приплыть come* swímming; (*о корабле*) sail up, come* in; ~ к бéрегу reach the shore.

приплыть *сов. см.* приплывáть.

приплюснутый flat.

приплясывать *несов.* jig up and down; dance, hop.

приподнимáть, приподнять (*вн.*) raise (*smb.*, *smth.*) a líttle, lift (*smth.*) a líttle. ~ся, приподнимáться raise onesélf, hálf-rise*; (*в кресле, постели*) sit* up; приподниматься на цыпочках stand* on típtoe.

приподнят|ость *ж.* elátion, (state of) excítement. ~ый eláted, excíted; (*о стиле речи*) élevated; ~ое настроéние elátion; быть в ~ом настроéнии be* eláted, be* in high spírits.

приподнять(ся) *сов. см.* приподнимáть(ся).

приподымáть(ся) *несов. разг. см.* приподнимáть(ся).

припóй *м. тех.* sólder.

приползáть, приползти́ crawl (there).

приползти́ *сов. см.* приползáть.

припоминáть, припóмнить (*вн.*) remémber (*smb.*, *smth.*), recáll (*smth.*).

припóмнить *сов.* **1.** *см.* припоминáть; .**2.** (*вн. дт.*) *разг.* remínd (*smb.* of).

приправ|а *ж.* séasoning, flávouring, rélish. ~ить *сов. см.* приправлять.

приправлять, припрáвить (*вн.*; *пищу*) séason (*smth.*), flávour (*smth.*).

припрятать *сов.* (*вн.*) *разг.* hide* (*smth.*); (*убрать на хранение*) put* (*smth.*) áway; store (*smth.*) up.

припýгивать, припугнуть (*вн.*) *разг.* scare (*smb.*), intímidate (*smb.*).

припугнуть *сов. см.* припýгивать.

припýдривать, припýдрить (*вн.*) put* a líttle pówder (on). ~ся, припýдриться put* on a líttle pówder.

припýдрить(ся) *сов. см.* припýдривать(ся).

прúпуск *м. тех.* allówance.

припускáть, припусти́ть *разг.* **1.** (*вн.*; *заставлять бежать быстрее*) give* free rein to (*smb.*); (*побежать быстрее*) mend *one's* pace; **3.** (*вн.*; *в шитье*) let* (*smth.*) out; припусти́ть *что-л.* на швы let* smth. out at the seams. ~ся, припусти́ться put* on speed, speed* up, .mend *one's* pace.

припусти́ть(ся) *сов. см.* припускáть(ся).

припухáть, припýхнуть swell*.

припýх|лость *ж.* swélling. ~лый swóllen. ~нуть *сов. см.* припухáть.

прираба́тывать, **прирабо́тать** (*вн.*, *рд.*) make*/earn (*smth.*) éxtra.

прирабо́тать *сов. см.* прираба́тывать.

при́работок *м.* éxtra éarnings *pl.*

прира́внивать I, **приравня́ть** (*вн.* к *дт.*; *уподоблять*) equáte (*smb.*, *smth.* with), put*/place (*smb.*, *smth.*) on the same fóoting/lével (as).

прира́внивать II, **прировня́ть** (*вн.*; *выравнивать*) lével (*smth.*).

приравня́ть *сов. см.* прира́внивать I.

прираста́ть, **прирасти́** I. (к *дт.*; *срастаться*) grow* (on to); *перен.* becóme* déeply attáched (to); 2. (*увеличиваться*) incréase; (*о капитале тж.*) accrúe.

прирасти́ *сов. см.* прираста́ть.

прираще́ние *с.* 1. (*увеличение*) íncrease; 2. *мат.* íncrement.

приревнова́ть *сов.* get* jéalous.

прире́зать *сов. см.* прире́зать.

прире́зать, **прире́зать** (*вн.*) 1. (*перерезать горло*) kill (*smb.*, *smth.*), cut* the throat (of); 2. (*землю*) allót (*smth.*) addítionally.

прировня́ть *сов. см.* прира́внивать II.

приро́д|а *ж.* 1. náture; *закон* ~ы law of náture; 2. (*совокупность естественных условий*) phýsico--geográphical féatures, phýsical báckground, nátural life; *северная* ~ the nátural life of the North; nórthern scénery; 3. (*места вне города*) lándscape, scénery, cóuntry(side); 4. (*сущность*) náture; (*характер тж.*) cháracter, disposítion; *человеческая* ~ húman náture; *он весёлый по* ~е he is náturally chéerful; *он добрый по* ~е he is of a kíndly disposítion; ◇ *от* ~ы from birth; *слепой от* ~ы blind from birth, born blind; *в* ~е вещей in the náture of things; *игра* ~ы freak of náture. ~ный 1. (*естественный*) nátural; ~ные богатства nátural resóurces; 2. (*врождённый*) nátive, nátural, innáte; ~ный талáнт nátural/innáte gift; ~ный ум móther wit.

прирождённый 1. (*врождённый*) innáte, inbórn; 2. (*имеющий все данные для какой-л. деятельности*) born; ~ орáтор a born órator.

прирост *м.* íncrement, íncrease; ~ населéния íncrement of populátion; ~ дохóдов от произвóдства íncrement of íncome from índustry.

прируч|а́ть, **приручи́ть** (*вн.*) tame (*smb.*, *smth.*); domésticate (*smth.*). ~éние *с.* táming. ~и́ть *сов. см.* приручáть.

приса́живаться, **присе́сть** take* a seat, sit* down.

присва́ивать, **присво́ить** 1. (*вн.*; *завладевать*) apprópriate (*smth.*), take* posséssion (of); 2. (*вн.*; *выдавать за своё*) árrogate (*smth.*) to onesélf, lay* (false) claim (to), usúrp (*smth.*); 3. (*вн. дт.*; *предоставлять*) confér (*smth.* on); ~ кому-л. стéпень дóктора confér a dóctor's degrée on *smb.*

при́свист *м.* 1. (*свист*) whístle; 2. (*свистящий призвук*) síbilance; *говорить с* ~ом síbilate.

присви́стнуть *сов.* give* a whístle.

присви́стывать *несов.* 1. whístle; 2. (*говорить с присвистом*) síbilate.

присвоéние *с.* 1. appropriátion; 2. (*звания и т. п.*) awárding, conférment.

присво́ить *сов. см.* присва́ивать.

приседа́ние *с.* bénding down, squátting; (*упражнение*) knée-bend.

приседа́ть, **присе́сть** (*на корточки*) squat; (*от страха*) cówer.

присе́ст *м.*: в одúн ~, за одúн ~ at a sítting, at a stretch, at one go.

присе́сть *сов. см.* приседáть и приса́живаться.

при́сказка *ж.* introdúction to a tale.

приск|а́ть, **присќать** *сов.* 1. (*приблизиться скачками*) hop, come* hópping up; ~ на однóй ногé hop (on one leg); *воробéй* ~áл a spárrow came hópping up; 2. (*приблизиться вскачь — о лошади, всаднике*) gállop up, come*

gálloping up; 3. *разг.* (*быстро прибыть*) come* téaring óver.

прискорб|ие *с. уст.* sórrow, grief, woe; ◇ с глубóким ~ием with profóund/deep regrét. ~ный sad, sórrowful, móurnful; ~ный случай sad/mélancholy occásion.

прискуч|ить *сов.* (*дт.*) *разг.* bore (*smb.*), wéary (*smb.*); ему́ всё это о́чень ~ило he's sick and tíred of it, he is bóred with it.

присла́ть *сов. см.* присыла́ть.

прислони́ть(ся) *сов. см.* прислоня́ть(ся).

прислоня́ть, **прислони́ть** (*вн.* к *дт.*) place (*smth.* agáinst), lean* (*smth.* agáinst), rest (*smth.* agáinst). ~ся, прислони́ться (к *дт.*) lean* (agáinst), rest (agáinst).

прислу́га *ж.* 1. sérvant, maid; *приходящая* ~ chárwoman*; 2. *собир. уст.* (*слуги*) sérvants *pl*, doméstics *pl*; 3. *собир. воен.* crew.

прислуж|ивать *несов.* (*дт.*) *уст.* serve (*smb.*), wait on (*smb.*), atténd (*smb.*). ~иваться *несов. уст.* (к *дт.*) try to get into *smb.*'s good gráces, be* subsérvient (to). ~ник *м. разг.* láckey. ~ничество *с. презр.* subsérvience.

прислу́шаться *сов. см.* прислу́шиваться.

прислу́шиваться, **прислу́шаться** (к *дт.*) 1. (*вслушиваться*) lísten atténtively (to); 2. (*принимать к сведению*) heed (*smth.*), lísten (to), pay* atténtion (to), lend* an ear (to); прислу́шаться к мнéнию специалúстов lísten to éxpert opínion.

присма́тривать, **присмотре́ть** 1. (за *тв.*) keep* an eye (on); (*проявлять заботу*) look (áfter), watch (óver); ~ за детьмú keep* an eye on the chíldren; look áfter the chíldren; 2. (*вн.*; *подыскивать*) look (for), look out (for), *сов. тж.* find* (*smth.*). ~ся, присмотрéться (к *дт.*) 1. (*пристально всматриваться*) look atténtively (at); watch (*smb.*, *smth.*) clósely; ~ся к человéку see* what a man* is made of; 2. (*осваиваться, привыкать*) get*/grow* accústomed (to), get* used (to).

присмире́ть *сов.* sóber down; (*притихнуть*) quíeten down, subside, becóme subdúed, grow quíet.

присмо́тр *м.* care, atténdance; (*надзор*) supervísion, survéillance; ~ за детьмú care of the chíldren; *быть под* чьим-л. ~ом be* únder *smb.*'s surveíllance; оста́вить кого-л. без ~а leave* *smb.* withóut atténdance.

присмотре́ть *сов.* 1. *см.* присма́тривать 1; 2. (*подыскать*) find* (*smth.*), spot (*smth.*). ~ся *сов. см.* присма́триваться.

присни́ться *сов. см.* сни́ться.

присоедин|е́ние *с.* 1. ádding; 2. (*включение в состав*) jóining; 3. *эл.* connécting up, connéction. ~и́ть(ся) *сов. см.* присоединя́ть(ся).

присоединя́ть, **присоедини́ть** (*вн.*) 1. (*прибавлять* к *чему-л.*) add (*smth.*); 2. (*включать в состав кого-л., чего-л.*) join (*smth.*), make* (*smth.*) a part (of); 3. *эл.* connéct (*smth.*), link up (*smth.*). ~ся, присоедини́ться (к *дт.*) 1. join up (with); 2. (*поддерживать мнение и т. п.*) suppórt (*smb.*, *smth.*), back (*smb.*) up; ~ся к мнéнию кого-л. suppórt *smb.*'s opínion.

присо́хнуть *сов. см.* присыха́ть.

приспе́шник *м.* accómplice.

приспоса́бливать, **приспосо́бить** (*вн.* к *дт.*) fit up (*smth.* for), adjúst (*smth.* for), adápt (*smth.* for). ~ся, приспосо́биться 1. adápt onesélf, adjúst onesélf; приспосóбиться к обстоя́тельствам adápt onesélf to círcumstances; 2. *презр.* (*о политическом деятеле*) trim.

приспосо́бить(ся) *сов. см.* приспоса́бливать(ся).

приспосо́бленец *м. презр.* tíme-server, trímmer.

приспособле́ние *с.* 1. (*действие*) adaptátion, adjústment; (к *климату*) acclimatizátion; 2. (*прибор, механизм*) device, appliance.

приспосо́бленность *ж.* fítness, suitabílity.

приспособле́нче|ский *презр.* tíme-serving *attr.*;

~ская поли́тика tíme-serving pólicy. ~ство *с. презр.* tíme--serving.

приспособля́емость *ж.* adaptability.

приспособля́ть(ся) *несов. см.* приспосáблять(ся).

приспуска́ть, приспусти́ть *(вн.)* lówer *(smth.)* a little; приспусти́ть флаг put* a flag at half mast.

приспусти́ть *сов. см.* приспускáть.

пристава́ние *с. (надоедáние)* péstering, bádgering.

пристава́ть, приста́ть (к *дт.*) 1. *(прилипáть)* stick* (to), adhére (to); 2. *разг. (надоедáть)* péster *(smb.),* bádger *(smb.),* wórry *(smb.);* 3. *разг. (присоединя́ться к кому-л.)* join *(smb.),* take*/join up (with); 4. *(причáливать)* come* in (to), put* in (to); ~ к бéрегу put* in to the shore.

пристáвить *сов. см.* пристáвлять.

пристáвка *ж.* 1. *тех.* exténsion, adápter; 2. *грам.* préfix.

пристав|ля́ть, пристáвить *(вн.* к *дт.)* 1. *(встáвить вплотну́ю)* put* *(smth.* agáinst); *(прислоня́ть)* lean* *(smth.* agáinst); ~ лéстницу к стенé lean*/prop a ládder agáinst the wall; 2. *(настáвлять)* add on *(smth.* to); 3. *разг. (назначáть для ухóда)* leave* in charge (of). ~нóй attáched; ~ная лéстница ládder.

пристáвочн|ый with a préfix *после сущ.*; ~ые глагóлы verbs with préfixes.

пристáльн|о fíxedly, inténtly; stéadily; ~ смотрéть на что-л. look hard/inténtly at smth. ~ый fixed, intént, stéady; ~ый взгляд stéady/intént gaze; ~ое внимáние close atténtion.

пристáнище *с.* shélter, home, réfuge, háven.

при́стань *ж.* pier, quay; *(грузовáя)* wharf*; *перен.* háven; ти́хая ~ safe réfuge.

приста́ть *сов. см.* пристава́ть.

пристёгивать, пристегну́ть *(вн.)* fásten *(smth.);* *(на пу́говицу)* bútton *(smth.)* (up). ~ся, пристегну́ться be* fástened; fásten; *(на пу́говицу)* be* búttoned up; bútton up.

пристегну́ть(ся) *сов. см.* пристёгиваться.

пристежнóй: ~ воротни́к detáchable cóllar.

пристóйн|о décently, próperly, décorously. ~ый décent, próper, décorous, séemly.

пристрáивать, пристрóить *(вн.)* 1. *(к здáнию)* add *(smth.);* 2. *(помещáть куда-л.)* set* *(smth.),* fix *(smth.);* 3. *разг. (на рабóту и т. п.)* find* a place; fix *(smb.)* up as. ~ся, пристрóиться *разг. (помещáться, располагáться где-л.)* perch, find* a perch, find* a place for *oneself.*

пристрáстие *с.* 1. *(си́льная склóнность, влечéние)* bent, pássion; líking for; ~ к му́зыке bent/pássion for músic; 2. *(необъекти́вное отношéние)* partiálity, bías; ◇ допрóс с ~м interrogátion under tórture.

пристрасти́ться *сов.* (к *дт.)* becóme* pássionately fond (of), concéive a líking (for); make* keen on.

пристрáстн|о unfáirly, with partiálity; суди́ть о чём--л. ~ take* a bías(s)ed view of smth. ~ость *ж.* bías, partiálity. ~ый pártial; unfáir, bías(s)ed; ~ое отношéние bías(s)ed áttitude.

пристрáчивать, пристрочи́ть *(вн.)* stitch *(smth.)* on (with a séwing-machíne).

пристрéливать I, пристрели́ть *(вн.; убивáть)* shoot* *(smb., smth.),* kill *(smb., smth.).*

пристрéливать II, пристреля́ть *(вн.; устанáвливать прáвильный прицéл)* find* the range (of). ~ся, пристреля́ться find* the range.

пристрели́ть *сов. см.* пристрéливать I.

пристрéлка *ж.* ránging fire.

пристрéлочный trial *attr.;* ~ вы́стрел tríal shot.

пристреля́ть *сов. см.* пристрéливать II. ~ся *сов. см.* пристрéливаться.

пристрóить(ся) *сов. см.* пристрáивать(ся).

пристрóйка *ж.* ánnex, wing, exténtion, óut-house.

пристрочи́ть *сов. см.* пристрáчивать.

пристру́нивать, приструни́ть *(вн.) разг.* put* smb. in órder, clamp down (on), take in hand.

приструни́ть *сов. см.* пристру́нивать.

присту́кивать, присту́кнуть *(тв.)* tap *(smth.);* *(каблукáми)* click *(smth.).*

присту́кнуть *сов. см.* присту́кивать.

при́ступ *м.* 1. *(припáдок)* fit, attáck; ~ кáшля fit of cóughing; ~ лихорáдки attáck of féver; 2. *(атáка, штурм)* assáult, stórming.

приступáть, приступи́ть (к *дт.)* *(начинáть)* begin* *(smth.),* start *(smth.);* set* abóut *(smth.);* *(переходи́ть к чему-л.)* procéed (to); приступи́ть к исполнéнию свои́х обя́занностей énter upón one's dúties, take* up one's dúties; приступи́ть к дéлу make* a start, get* down to work/búsiness. ~ся, приступи́ться *разг.* come* near; ◇ к нему́ не присту́пишься he's inaccéssible.

приступи́ть(ся) *сов. см.* приступáть(ся).

пристыди́ть *сов. (вн.)* shame *(smb.),* put* *(smb.)* to shame.

присуди́ть *сов. см.* присуждáть.

присуждáть, присуди́ть 1. *(вн.* к *дт., вн. дт.)* séntence *(smb.* to), condémn *(smb.* to); присуди́ть когó--л. к штрáфу séntence smb. to pay a fine; 2. *(вн. дт.; прéмию и т. п.)* award *(smb. smth.).*

прису́тстви|е *с.* présence; в ~и когó-л. in *smb.'s* présence; в ~и други́х in the présence of óthers; ◇ ~ ду́ха présence of mind; сохраня́ть (теря́ть) ~ ду́ха retáin (lose*) *one's* présence of mind; он потеря́л ~ ду́ха his présence of mind failed him.

прису́тствов|ать *несов.* be* présent, atténd; на приёме ~ало 50 человéк fifty péople atténded the recéption.

прису́щ|ий *(дт.)* inhérent (in), intrínsic (in); с ~м ему́ юмором with the húmour so charactéristic of him.

присылáть, присла́ть *(вн.)* send* *(smb., smth.).*

присы́пать *сов. см.* присыпáть.

присыпáть, присы́пать *(вн. тв.)* sprínkle *(smth.* with), pówder *(smth.* with), dust *(smth.* with).

присы́пка *ж. (порошóк)* pówder.

присыхáть, присóхнуть (к *дт.)* stick* (to), dry (on).

прися́г|а *ж.* oath; приводи́ть когó-л. к ~е put* smb. on (his) oath, swear* *(smb.)* in; принимáть ~у take* the oath; давáть ~у make* a vow; под ~ой on/únder oath.

присягáть, присягну́ть swear*, take*/make* an oath.

присягну́ть *сов. см.* присягáть.

притаи́ться *сов.* hide* *(oneself),* lie* hídden.

прита́птывать, притоптáть *(вн.)* trámple *(smth.);* *(каблукáми)* tap with one's heels; ~ травý trámple down the grass.

притáскивать, притащи́ть *(вн.)* 1. bring* *(smth.)* in, fetch *(smth.);* *(с трудóм)* drag *(smth.)* in, haul *(smth.)* in; 2. *разг. (приводи́ть с собóй)* bring* *(smb.)* alóng; *(наси́льно)* drag *(smb.)* in. ~ся, притащи́ться *разг.* come* alóng, tótter in/up; drag *oneself* alóng.

притащи́ть(ся) *сов. см.* притáскивать(ся).

притвори́ться *сов. см.* притворя́ться.

притвори́ться I, II *сов. см.* притворя́ться I, II.

притвóрн|о: ~ согласи́ться preténd to agrée; ~ улыбáться feign, affécted, preténded; ~ое равноду́шие feigned indífference.

притвóр|ство *с.* sham, preténce. ~щик *м.,* ~щица *ж.* hýpocrite.

притворя́ть, притвори́ть *(вн.)* close *(smth.),* shut* *(smth.).*

притворя́ться I, притвори́ться *(закрывáться)* close, shut*.

притворя́ться II, притвори́ться *(прики́дываться)* feign, símulate, sham, preténd; ~ больны́м feign íllness; ~ мёртвым preténd to be dead.

притерпéться *сов.* (к *дт.) разг.* get* accústomed (to), get* used (to).

притёрт|ый ground, clóse-fitting; ~ая пробка ground stópper.

притесн|éние с. oppréssion (*тж. мн.*), restríction. ~итель м. oppréssor.

притесни́ть *сов. см.* притесня́ть.

притесня́ть, притесни́ть (*вн.*) oppréss (*smb.*), deal* hárdly (with); crack down (on) *разг.*

притиха́ть, прити́хнуть 1. (*умолкать*) grow* quíet, die down; 2. (*становиться тише*) die down, abáte, slácken.

прити́хнуть *сов. см.* притиха́ть.

приткну́ться *сов. разг.* find* a place; (*на ночь*) put* up.

прито́к м. 1. (*прибытие, поступление*) ínflux; ~ това́ров ínflux of goods; ~ воздуха (in)flow of air; ~ средств íncrease of funds; 2. (*усиление чего-л., подъём*) surge, revíval; ~ сил surge of strength, fresh vígour; 3. (*реки*) tríbutary.

притоло́ка ж. líntel.

прито́м besídes, moreóver.

прито́н м. den; haunt; dive; háng-out *амер.*

притопну́ть *сов. см.* прито́пывать 1.

притопта́ть *сов. см.* притáптывать.

прито́пывать, притопну́ть 1. stamp; ~ ного́й stamp *one's* foot*; 2. *тк. несов.* (*стучать ногами в такт чему-л.*) tap *one's* foot*.

при́торн|ость ж. overswéetness, síckly swéetness; *перен.* sáccharine; óiliness. ~ый oversweét, síckly sweet, clóying; *перен.* súgary, óily; ~ая улыбка súgary smile.

притра́гиваться, притро́нуться (к *дт.*) touch (*smth.*).

притро́нуться *сов. см.* притра́гиваться.

притупи́ть(ся) *сов. см.* притупля́ть(ся).

притупля́ть, притупи́ть (*вн.*) blunt (*smth.*), take* the edge off (*smth.*); *перен.* dull (*smth.*), blunt (*smth.*). ~ся, притупи́ться lose* its edge/point; (*о лезвиях*) get* dull/blunt; *перен.* becóme* blúnted/dull, becóme less keen.

при́тча ж. párable; говори́ть ~ми speak* in párables; что за ~? what a strange thing!; ◇ ~ во язы́цах the talk of the town.

притяга́тельный attráctive, magnétic.

притя́гивать, притяну́ть 1. (*вн.*) draw* (*smb.*, *smth.*), pull (*smb.*, *smth.*); (*о магните*) attráct (*smth.*); ~ кого́-л. к себе́ hug/squéeze *smb.*; 2. (*вн. к дт.*) *разг.* (*обязывать*) call (*smb.* to), súmmon (*smb.* to); ◇ э́тот довод притя́нут за́ волосы the árgument is far-fétched.

притяжа́тельн|ый *грам.* posséssive; ~ое местоиме́ние posséssive prónoun.

притяже́ние с. attráction; земно́е ~ terréstrial grávity; лу́нное ~ lúnar grávity.

притяза́ние с. claim; (*необоснованное*) preténsion.

притяну́ть *сов. см.* притя́гивать.

приукра́сить(ся) *сов. см.* приукра́шивать(ся).

приукра́шивать, приукра́сить (*вн.*) *разг.* 1. décorate (*smth.*), bríghten up (*smth.*); приукра́сить ко́мнату bríghten up a room; 2. (*представлять в более красивом виде*) embróider (*smth.*), embéllish (*smth.*). ~ся, приукра́ситься *разг.* impróve *one's* looks; (*становиться ярче*) take* on a bríghter hue.

приуменьша́ть, приуме́ньшить (*вн.*) léssen (*smth.*), redúce (*smth.*) a little.

приуме́ньшить *сов. см.* приуменьша́ть.

приумножа́ть, приумно́жить (*вн.*) (fúrther) incréase (*smth.*), (fúrther) augmént (*smth.*). ~ся, приумно́житься (fúrther) incréase.

приумно́жить(ся) *сов. см.* приумножа́ть(ся).

приуны́ть *сов. разг.* look dówncast/glum, feel* dejécted/upsét, be*/becóme* dispírited.

приуро́чивать, приуро́чить (*вн. к дт.*) time (*smth.*) to coincíde (with), arránge (*smth.* for); приуро́чить от-

пуск к нача́лу о́сени arránge *one's* hóliday for the begínning of áutumn.

приуро́чить *сов. см.* приуро́чивать.

приуса́дебный: ~ уча́сток земли́ plot of land attáched to the house; órchard.

приуча́ть, приучи́ть (*вн. к дт.*; *вн. + инф.*) accústom (*smb.* to), inúre (*smb.* to); (*тренировать*) train (*smb.*, *smth.* + to *inf*); ~ себя́ к хо́лоду inúre onesélf to cold; ~ кого́-л. регуля́рно занима́ться get* *smb.* ínto the hábit of stúdying/práctising régularly. ~ся, приучи́ться (+ *инф.*) get* used (to + -ing), get*/grow* accústomed (to + -ing).

приучи́ть(ся) *сов. см.* приуча́ть(ся).

прифранти́ться *сов. разг.* dress/get* onesélf up.

прифронтов|о́й fórward-area *attr.*; ~ая полоса́ fórward área.

прихва́рывать, прихворну́ть *разг.* feel* unwéll, feel* out of sorts, feel* póorly.

прихвастну́ть *сов. разг.* boast a little, brag a little.

прихвати́ть *сов. см.* прихва́тывать.

прихва́тывать, прихвати́ть *разг.* 1. (*вн.*; *зажимать*) grip (*smth.*); 2. (*вн.*; *привязывать*) tie (*smth.*) up, fásten (*smth.*); 3. (*вн., рд.*; *брать с собой*) take* (*smb.*, *smth.* with); 4. (*вн.*; *слегка подмораживать*) touch (*smth.*); нип (*smth.*).

прихворну́ть *сов. см.* прихва́рывать.

при́хвостень м. *презр.* tóady, líckspittle.

прихлеба́тель м. *разг.* spónger, párasite. ~ский *разг.* spónging *attr.* ~ство с. *разг.* spónging.

прихлёбывать *несов.* (*вн.*) *разг.* sip (*smth.*); ~ чай sip *one's* tea.

прихло́пнуть *сов. см.* прихло́пывать 1, 2, 3.

прихло́пывать, прихло́пнуть 1. (по *дт.*; *ударять ладонью по чему-л.*) slap (*smth.*); 2. (*вн.*; *закрывать со стуком*) slam (*smth.*); 3. (*вн.*) *разг.* (*прищемлять*) nip (*smth.*), catch* (*smth.*), squéeze (*smth.*); 4. *тк. несов.* (*сопровождать что-л. хлопками*) clap.

прихо́д м. 1. (*действие*) cóming, arríval; ~ к вла́сти cóming to pówer; 2. (*доход, поступление*) recéipts *pl*, retúrns *pl*; ~ и расхо́д íncome and expénditure; 3. *церк.* párish.

приходи́ть, прийти́ 1. come*, arríve; прийти́ домо́й come* home; по́езд пришёл с небольши́м опозда́нием the train came in ráther late; он пришёл прости́ться с ни́ми he came to say good-bye to them; посы́лка должна́ прийти́ че́рез неде́лю the párcel should arríve in a week's time; 2. (*наступать*) come*, arríve; пришла́ весна́ spring has come; 3. (*возникать, появляться*) appéar; постепе́нно к нему́ пришла́ уве́ренность he grádually acquíred cónfidence; 4. (к *дт.*; *добиваться*) come* (to), arríve (at); ~ к заключе́нию, вы́воду arríve at the conclúsion, come* to the conclúsion; 5. *в сочета́нии с существи́тельными*: ~ в отча́яние fall*/sink* ínto despáir; ~ в восхище́ние be* delíghted; ~ в я́рость get*/fly* ínto a rage; ~ в негодова́ние be*/feel* indígnant (at); ◇ прийти́ на ум come* to mind; прийти́ кому́-л. в го́лову énter smb.'s head; прийти́ в себя́ come* to *one's* sénses; (*опомниться*) recóver *one's* wits; прийти́ в чу́вство come* to onesélf; прийти́ на по́мощь come* to the réscue, come* to smb.'s aid/help; ~ к концу́ come* to an end. ~сь, прийти́сь 1. (*соответствовать чему-л.*) fit; боти́нки пришли́сь по ноге́ the shoes fitted well; 2. (*совпадать с чем-л.*) fall*; Но́вый год пришёлся на четве́рг New Year fell on a Thúrsday; 3. *безл.* (*быть необходимым*) мне пришло́сь э́то сде́лать I had to do it; 4. *безл.* (*дт.*; *случаться*) one has occásion to; ему́ тяжело́ пришло́сь he had a hard time; мне приходи́лось с ни́ми встреча́ться I have had occásion to meet them; I have met them on occásions; 5. (*причита́ться*): на ка́ждого пришло́сь по десяти́ рубле́й each one had to pay ten róubles; 6. *тк. несов.* (*дт.*; *быть в родственных отношениях*) be* reláted (to); он мне прихо́дится дя́дей he is my úncle; они́ мне прихо́дятся бли́зкими ро́дственниками they are near rélatives of mine; ◇ прийти́сь кому́-л. по вку́су suit *smb.'s* taste; прийти́сь кста́ти prove úseful, turn up just at the right mо́ment; где придётся where *one* can; как придётся how *one* can; что придётся what *one* can.

прихо́дн|ый: ~ая кни́га recéipt book, lédger.

прихо́довать, заприхо́довать (*вн.*) crédit (*smth.*).

прихо́до-расхо́дн|ый: ~ая кни́га accóunt-book, lédger.

прихо́дск|ий párish *attr.*; ~ая це́рковь párish church.

приходя́щ|ий non-résident; ~ая домрабо́тница a dáily (wóman*), home help.

прихо́жая ж. ánte-room, ántechamber, hall.

прихора́шиваться *несов. разг.* smárten *oneself* up, preen *oneself*; doll *oneself* up.

прихотли́в|ость ж. 1. capríciousness; fastídiousness; 2. (*причудливость*) whimsicálity. ~ый 1. (*капризный*) caprícious; fínical, fastídious; ~ый ребёнок fínical child*; 2. (*причудливый*) fánciful, odd, bizárre, whímsical.

при́хоть ж. capríce, fáncy, whim.

прихра́мыв|ать *несов.* hóbble, limp; идти́ ~ая hóbble alóng.

прице́л *м.* 1. (*ружья*) báck-sight; (*орудия*) sight; опти́ческий ~ telescópic sight; 2. (*прицеливание*) aim; взять кого́-л., что́-л. на ~ take* aim at *smb.*, *smth.*; get* *smb.*, *smth.* in one's sights (*тж. перен.*).

прице́ливаться, прице́литься (в *вн.*) take* aim (at), aim (at).

прице́литься *сов. см.* прице́ливаться.

прице́льн|ый áiming *attr.*; ~ое приспособле́ние áiming device.

прице́ниваться, прицени́ться (к *дт.*) *разг.* ask/inquíre the price (of).

прицени́ться *сов. см.* прице́ниваться.

прице́п *м.* tráiler; тяга́ч с ~ом tráctor (únit) and tráiler.

прицепи́ть(ся) *сов. см.* прицепля́ть(ся).

прицепля́ть, прицепи́ть 1. (*вн. к дт.*; *сцеплять*) hook (*smth.* on to); ж.-д. cóuple (*smth.* to); прицепи́ть ваго́н к по́езду cóuple a cárriage to a train; 2. (*вн.*) *разг.* (*прикалывать*) pin on (*smth.*), fásten on (*smth.*); прицепи́ть бант pin on a ríbbon. ~ся, прицепи́ться (к *дт.*) 1. (*к чему́-л. движущемуся*) hang* on (to); attách *oneself* on (*тж. перен.*); 2. (*приставать к чему́-л., повисать*) catch* (on), cling* (to); *перен. разг.* (*о болезни*) inféct (*smb.*); (*надоедать*) péster (*smb.*); 3. *разг.* (*придираться*) pick on (*smth.*), pounce on (*smth.*); прицепи́ться к сло́ву pick on a chance remárk; не́ к чему прицепи́ться there is nóthing to find fault with.

прицепно́й tráil-type *attr.*; ~ ваго́н tráiler.

прича́л *м.* 1. (*действие*) móoring, fástening; 2. (*место*) móorage, berth; 3. (*канат*) móoring rope, móoring line.

прича́ливать, прича́лить 1. (*вн.*) moor (*smth.*); (*большие корабли*) berth (*smth.*); 2. (*к дт.*; *приставать*) tie up (at, to).

прича́лить *сов. см.* прича́ливать.

прича́льн|ый móoring *attr.*; ~ кана́т móoring rope; ~ые кана́ты móorings *pl.*

прича́стие *с. грам.* párticiple; ~ настоя́щего вре́мени présent párticiple; ~ проше́дшего вре́мени past párticiple.

прича́стность ж. participátion (in), invólvement (in); ~ к преступле́нию participátion in a crime.

прича́стный I (к *дт.*) particípating (in), invólved (in); concérned (with); ~ к преступле́нию invólved/ímplicated in a crime.

прича́стный II *грам.* participíal; ~ оборо́т participíal constrúction.

причём 1. *нареч.* why; ~ тут э́то? what's that got to

do with it?; 2. *союз* moreóver, and what's more; передаётся *тж.* через present participle; он не согласи́лся со мной, ~ тут же сказа́л, что передаёт де́ло в суд he did not agrée with me, sáying that he would refér the mátter to the court.

причёсанный with tídy hair *после сущ.*

причеса́ть(ся) *сов. см.* причёсывать(ся).

причёска ж. 1. (*действие*) háirdressing; 2. hair style; háir-do *разг.*; ему́ нра́вится её ~ he likes the way she does her hair.

причёсывать, причеса́ть (*вн.*) do* (*smth.*); ~ го́лову do* one's hair; причеса́ть кого́-л. do* *smb.'s* hair. ~ся, причеса́ться do* one's hair; (*у парикмахера*) have* one's hair done, have* a háir-do.

причи́н|а ж. 1. cause; ~ и сле́дствие cause and efféct; ~ пожа́ра cause of a fire; 2. (*основание*) réason; без вся́кой ~ы for no réason whatéver; не без ~ы not without réason; нет ~ы отка́зываться there is no réason to refúse; неуважи́тельная ~ poor/lame excúse; по неуважи́тельной ~e without válid excúse; ◇ по той (*просто́й*) ~e, что... for the símple réason that...

причини́ть *сов. см.* причиня́ть.

причиня́ть, причини́ть (*вн.*) cause (*smth.*); ~ убы́тки cause lósses; ~ вред чему́-л. do* dámage to *smth.*, do* ínjury to *smth.*; ~ вред кому́-л. cause *smb.* dámage, inflíct ínjury on *smb.*, do* harm to *smb.*; причини́ть кому́-л. неприя́тность make* tróuble for *smb.*

причи́слить *сов. см.* причисля́ть.

причисля́ть, причи́слить ~ к *дт.* 1. (*прибавля́ть*) add (*smth.* to); 2. (*назнача́ть*) attách (*smb.* to); 3. (*относи́ть к числу́ кого́-л.*) rank (*smb.* amóng, in), númber (*smb.* amóng); ~ кого́-л. к вели́ким писа́телям rank *smb.* amóng the great writers. ~ся *несов.* (к *дт.*) belóng (to).

причита́ние *с.* lamentátion.

причита́ть *несов.* 1. compláin, moan; 2. (*исполнять обрядовые песни-плачи*) lamént, wail, keen.

причита́|ться *несов.* be* due; с вас ~ется пять рубле́й you are to pay five róubles.

причмо́кивать, причмо́кнуть smack one's lips.

причмо́кнуть *сов. см.* причмо́кивать.

причу́д|а ж. whim, fad, caprice, vágary; ~ливый 1. (*затейливый*) quaint, whímsical, fánciful; 2. *разг.* (*капризный*) caprícious, whímsical.

пришвартова́ть(ся) *сов. см.* пришварто́вывать(ся).

пришварто́вывать, пришвартова́ть (*вн.*) *мор., ав.* make* (*smth.*) fast, moor (*smth.*). ~ся, пришвартова́ться *мор., ав.* moor; (*о больши́х корабля́х*) berth.

пришле́ц *м.* néwcomer, stránger.

пришепётывать *несов. разг.* lisp.

пришёптывать *несов.* whisper.

пришиблённый dejécted; (*униженный*) dówntrodden, humíliated.

пришива́ть, приши́ть (*вн. к дт.*) 1. sew* (*smth.* on, to); 2. (*приколачивать*) nail (*smth.* to), fix/fásten (*smth.*) with nails (to).

пришивно́й sewn on; ~ воротни́к attáched cóllar.

приши́ть *сов. см.* пришива́ть.

пришко́льный school *attr.*; ~ уча́сток school grounds *pl.*

при́шлый strange.

пришпи́ливать, пришпи́лить (*вн.*) pin (*smth.*), fásten (*smth.*).

пришпи́лить *сов. см.* пришпи́ливать.

пришпо́ривать, пришпо́рить (*вн.*) spur (*smth.*), put* spurs (to); *перен. разг.* spur (*smb.*) on, urge (*smb.*) on.

пришпо́рить *сов. см.* пришпо́ривать.

прищёлкивать, прищёлкнуть: ~ па́льцами snap one's fingers; ~ языко́м click one's tongue.

прищёлкнуть *сов. см.* прищёлкивать.

прищеми́ть *сов.* (*вн.*) pinch (*smth.*), nip (*smth.*); ~

себе па́лец две́рью pinch/catch*/squeeze *one's* finger in the door.

прищу́ривать, прищу́рить: ~ глаза́ *см.* прищу́риваться. ~ся, прищу́риться screw up *one's* eyes, na'rrow *one's* eyes.

прищу́рить(ся) *сов. см.* прищу́ривать(ся).

прию́т *м.* she'lter, asy'lum, re'fuge; найти́ ~ find* she'lter.

приюти́ть *сов.* (*вн.*) give* she'lter (to), she'lter (*smb.*). ~ся *сов.* find* she'lter, take* she'lter; (*поместиться*) find* a place, squeeze in; (*расположиться*) ne'stle.

прия́тель *м.* 1. friend; 2. *разг.* (*обращение*) chum, old chap. ~ница *ж.* (girl-)friend. ~ский friendly; быть в ~ских отноше́ниях с кем-л. be* on friendly terms with *smb.*

прия́тн|о 1. *нареч.* ple'asantly, agre'eably; 2. *в знач. сказ. безл.* it is ple'asant; ему́ бы́ло ~, что... he was glad that... ~ый ple'asant, agre'eable; ~ый за́пах nice smell; ~ое воспомина́ние ple'asing/gra'tifying me'mory; ~ые но́вости good* news; ~ое лицо́ nice face; ~ое зре́лище ple'asing sight.

про *разг.* 1. (*относительно, о*) abo'ut, of; говори́ть ~ друзе́й talk abo'ut friends; 2. (*для*) for; ◇ ~ себя́ to *one*self; он сказа́л э́то ~ себя́ he said it to himself.

проанализи́ровать *сов.* (*вн.*) a'nalyse (*smth.*).

про́б|а *ж.* 1. (*испытание*) tri'al; test; ~ голосо́в voice tri'al; ~ сил tri'al of strength; 2. (*образец чего-л., взятый для анализа*) sa'mple; взять ~y take* a sa'mple; 3. (*относительное содержание благородного металла*) ca'rat; 4. (*клеймо*) ha'llmark; ◇ на ~y on tri'al; ~ пера́ literary de'but; вы́сшей ~ы of the first wa'ter; ни́зкой ~ы of the lo'west/worst type; ме́тод проб и оши́бок me'thod of tri'al and e'rror.

пробе́г *м.* 1. run; ~ при поса́дке *ав.* la'nding run; 2. *спорт.* race; лы́жный ~ ski-race; 3. (*расстояние, пройденное автомашиной и т. п.*) mi'leage; *ж.-д. тж.* run.

пробега́ть *сов.* 1. run* abo'ut; 2. (*вн.*) *разг.* (*пропустить что-л. из-за беготни*) miss (*smth.*) with all *one's* ru'nning abo'ut.

пробега́ть, пробежа́ть 1. run*; пробежа́ть ми́мо до́ма run* past the house; 2. (*вн.; бегом преодолевать какое-л. расстояние*) run* (*smth.*), co'ver (*smth.*); (*о лошади*) trot (*smth.*); 3. (*быстро проезжать, проплывать, проноситься*) pass; (*появившись, быстро исчезать*) go*, pass; дрожь пробежа́ла у него́ по спине́ a cold shi'ver went down his back; 4. (*о времени*) fly* past; 5. (*вн.*) *разг.* (*бегло прочитывать*) run* through (*smth.*), go* o'ver (*smth.*), scan (*smth.*); пробежа́ть газе́ты glance/skim through ne'wspapers.

пробежа́ть *сов. см.* пробега́ть.

пробежа́ться *сов.* 1. have* a run, go* for a run; ~ по са́ду have* a run in the ga'rden; 2. *разг.* (*быстро провести пальцами по чему-л.*) run* (*one's* fingers) o'ver.

пробе́жка *ж.* run; (*самолёта*) (take-off) run.

пробе́л *м.* 1. (*пропуск*) blank, e'mpty space; 2. (*упущение*) gap, flaw; воспо́лнить ~ы своего́ образова́ния fill up the gaps in *one's* educa'tion.

пробива́ть, проби́ть (*вн.*) 1. (*делать отверстие*) pierce (*smth.*), make* a hole/o'pening (in); проби́ть сте́ну make* a hole in a wall; ~ отве́рстие make* a hole; пу́ля проби́ла дверь a bu'llet pierced the door; 2. *разг.* (*прокладывать*) make* (*smth.*), o'pen up (*smth.*), clear (*smth.*); ~ проби́ть себе́ доро́гу make* *one's* way in the world. ~ся, проби́ться 1. (*прокладывать себе путь*) force *one's* way, break* through; проби́ться сквозь толпу́ force/e'lbow/push/sho'ulder *one's* way through the crowd; полк проби́лся к реке́ the regiment broke through to the ri'ver; 2. (*о растительности*) shoot* forth/out; ◇ проби́ться в лю́ди fight* *one's* way to the top.

пробивн|о́й 1. pe'netrating; ~а́я си́ла pe'netrating

---

po'wer; 2. *разг.* (*настойчивый*) go'-getting, thru'sting; ~ па́рень go'-getter.

пробира́ть, пробра́ть (*вн.*) *разг.* 1. (*ругать*) rate (*smb.*), scold (*smb.*), give* (*smb.*) a good ta'lking-to; 2. (*о холоде*) freeze* (*smb.*), chill (*smb.*); моро́з пробра́л меня́ до косте́й I was chilled to the bone; 3. (*о страхе*) overco'me* (*smb.*); ◇ его́ ниче́м не пробере́шь no'thing makes the sli'ghtest impre'ssion on him.

пробира́ться, пробра́ться 1. (*с трудом проходить*) make* *one's* way; (*сквозь толпу́*) stru'ggle through a crowd; 2. (*проходить тайком*) steal*/sneak in; пробра́ться в ко́мнату edge (*one's* way) i'nto a room.

проби́рка *ж.* te'st-tube, te'st-glass.

проби́ть *сов.* бить 9 и пробива́ть. ~ся *сов.* 1. *см.* пробива́ться; 2. *разг.* (*потратить много усилий*) stru'ggle.

про́бк|а *ж.* 1. *тк. ед.* (*материал*) cork; 2. (*для бутылок*) cork; (*стеклянная*) sto'pper; *тех.* plug; 3. *эл.* fuse, ci'rcuit-breaker, cu't-out; ~ перегоре́ла the fuse has blown; поста́вить но́вую ~у put* in a new fuse, change the fuse; 4. (*затор*) jam; ◇ он глуп как ~ ≈ he's as stu'pid as an owl; he's an u'tter blo'ckhead. ~овый cork *attr.*; ◇ ~овый дуб co'rk-oak.

пробле́м|а *ж.* pro'blem; разреши́ть ~у solve a pro'blem.

проблема́тика *ж.* pro'blems *pl.*

проблема́тич|еский, ~ный proble'matical.

про́блеск *м.* (*прям. и перен.*) gleam, gli'mmer; ~и наде́жды gleam/gli'mmer of hope; ~и созна́ния lu'cid i'ntervals.

проблужда́ть *сов.* wa'nder, roam, rove.

про́бный tri'al *attr.*, test *attr.*; ~ полёт test flight; ~ пробе́г test run; (*автомобиля тж.*) road test; ~ уро́к trial le'sson; ◇ ~ ка́мень to'uchstone; ~ шар fe'eler.

про́бовать, попро́бовать 1. (*вн.; испытывать*) try (*smb., smth.*), test (*smb., smth.*); 2. (*на вкус*) taste (*smth.*), sa'mple (*smth.*); попро́бовать всего́ понемно́жку sa'mple a li'ttle of e'verything; 3. (+ *инф.*) пыта́ться сде́лать что-л.) try (+ to *inf*), atte'mpt (+ to *inf*).

прободе́ние *с. мед.* perfora'tion.

пробо́ин|а *ж.* hole, rent; (*в стене тж.*) breach, gap; получи́ть ~у be* holed.

пробол|е́ть I *сов.* be* ill; он ~е́л три неде́ли he was ill for three weeks.

проболе́ть II *сов.* (*о какой-л. части тела*) give* tro'uble; ра́неная рука́ проболи́т недо́лго the i'njured hand will not give tro'uble for long.

проболта́ть *сов. разг.* (*провести какое-л. время в болтовне*) cha'tter (for a while). ~ся *сов. разг.* (*проговориться*) blab, let* out a se'cret, blurt it out.

пробо́р *м.* pa'rting; прямо́й ~ mi'ddle pa'rting; косо́й ~ side pa'rting.

пробормота́ть *сов. см.* бормота́ть.

пробра́ть *сов. см.* пробира́ть.

пробра́ться *сов. см.* пробира́ться.

пробуди́ть(ся) *сов. см.* пробужда́ть(ся).

пробужд|а́ть, пробуди́ть (*вн.*) (a)ro'use (*smb., smth.*), awa'ken (*smb., smth.*); (*чувства тж.*) awa'ke (*smb.*); ~ кого́-л. к акти́вной де́ятельности rouse *smb.* to a'ction. ~а́ться, пробуди́ться (*о людях*) wake* up, awa'ke*; (*о природе*) awa'ken, revi've; *перен.* (*о чувствах, интересе и т. п.*) be* awa'kened, be* roused, be* stirred up. ~е́ние *с.* awa'kening; ~е́ние приро́ды the awa'kening of Na'ture.

пробура́вить *сов. см.* пробура́вливать.

пробура́вливать, пробура́вить (*вн.*) bore (*smth.*), drill (*smth.*), pe'rforate (*smth.*).

пробури́ть *сов. см.* бури́ть.

пробурча́ть *сов. см.* бурча́ть 1.

пробы́ть *сов.* stay, rema'in; ско́лько вре́мени вы здесь пробу́дете? how long will you be here?

прова́л *м.* 1. (*действие*) collapse, fa'lling in; 2. (*уг-*

лубление почвы) depréssion; **3.** (*неудача*) fáilure, crash, fiásco; flop *разг.*; **4.** (*памяти*) blank, bláck-out; **5.** (*раскрытие подпольной организации*) expósure, discóvery.

прова́ливать, провали́ть (*вн.*) **1.** (*дело, предприятие и т. п.*) bring* abóut the fáilure (of), wreck (*smth.*); ruin (*smth.*); **2.** (*отвергать*) turn (*smb., smth.*) down; провали́ть кандида́та turn down a cándidate; провали́ть предложе́ние turn down a propósal; **3.** (*на экзамене*) fail (*smb.*); **4.** (*раскрывать подпольную организацию*) expóse (*smb., smth.*), give* awáy (*smb., smth.*). **~ся, провали́ться 1.** (*падать*) fall*, fall* down, túmble down; провали́ться в я́му fall* down a hole; **2.** (*обрушиваться*) collápse; (*о поле, потолке и т. п. тж.*) fall* in, cave in; кры́ша провали́лась the roof has fállen in; **3.** *разг.* (*терпеть неудачу*) fail, miscárry, fall* through; **4.** (*быть обнаруженным — о подпольной организации*) be* expósed; **5.** *разг.* (*на экзамене*) fail, flunk it, not make* the grade; **6.** *разг.* (*исчезать*) disappéar, vánish; ◇ как сквозь зе́млю провали́лся vánished ínto thin air.

провали́ть(ся) *сов. см.* **прова́ливать(ся)**.

прованса́ль *м.* (*соус*) mayonnáise; капу́ста ~ cábbage píckled with grapes and bérries.

прова́нск|ий: ~ое ма́сло ólive oil.

прова́ривать, провари́ть (*вн.*) boil (*smth.*) thóroughly. **~ся, провари́ться** boil, be* bóiling.

провари́ть(ся) *сов. см.* **прова́ривать(ся)**.

прове́дать *сов. см.* **прове́дывать**.

проведе́ние *с.* **1.** (*дорог*) constrúction, búilding; (*прокладка труб, кабеля*) láying; (*электричества, канализации в помещении*) installátion; **2.** (*осуществление*) cárrying out, realizátion; ~ в жизнь чего́-л. pútting *smth.* ínto efféct; **3.** (*законопроекта*) cárrying, adóption.

прове́дывать, прове́дать *разг.* **1.** (*вн.; навещать*) call on (*smb.*), go* and see* (*smb.*); **2.** (*вн., о пр.; узнавать*) learn* (*smth.*), find* (*smth.*) out.

провезти́ *сов. см.* **провози́ть**.

прове́ивать, прове́ять (*вн.*) wínnow (*smth.*).

провентили́ровать *сов. см.* **вентили́ровать**.

прове́р|енный reliable; of próven reliability после *сущ.* **~ить(ся)** *сов. см.* **проверя́ть(ся)**. **~ка** *ж.* **1.** (*контроль*) chécking, inspéction, examinátion; chéck-up *разг.*; ~ка отчётности chécking of récords/accóunts; ~ка докумéнтов examinátion/inspéction of pápers; ~ка исполнéния chécking the execútion of órders; **2.** (*испытание*) tésting, examinátion; ~ка знáний учащихся examinátion of púpils; ~ка мотóра tésting of an éngine; вы́держать ~ку врéмени stand* the test of time.

проверну́ть *сов. см.* **проверты́вать**.

проверты́вать, проверну́ть (*вн.*) **1.** *разг.* (*пробуравливать*) bore through (*smth.*); **2.** (*перемалывать*) grind* (*smth.*); проверну́ть мя́со grind* meat.

проверя́ть, прове́рить (*вн.*) **1.** check (*smth.*), vérify (*smth.*); ~ счетá check/áudit the accóunts; ~ решéние задáчи vérify the solútion; ~ билéты, про́пуск check/exámine the tíckets, pass; **2.** (*обследовать*) exámine (*smth.*), inspéct (*smth.*); check up (on) *разг.*; ~ рабóту exámine the work; **3.** (*испытывать*) test (*smth.*), check (*smth.*); ~ часы́ check *one's* watch; ~ тормозá check the brakes. **~ся, прове́риться** *разг.* **1.** (*проходить проверку*) be* exámined; прове́риться у врачá be* exámined by a dóctor, go* and see* a dóctor; **2.** (*в каком-л. списке*) check *one's* name; прове́риться в спи́ске избирáтелей check *one's* name in the vóting régister.

провести́ *сов. см.* **проводи́ть I** 1—8, 10.

прове́тривать, прове́трить (*вн.*) (*помещение*) véntilate (*smth.*), air (*smth.*); (*вещи*) air (*smth.*). **~ся, прове́триться 1.** (*о помещении, вещах*) be* áired; **2.** (*о людях*) have* a breath of fresh air; *перен.* have* a change of scene.

прове́трить(ся) *сов. см.* **прове́тривать(ся)**.

прове́ять *сов. см.* **прове́ивать**.

прови́дение *с.* prevísion, fóresight.

прови́зия *ж.* fóod-stuffs *pl*, provísions *pl*.

прови́зор *м.* phármacist, chémist.

провин|и́ться *сов.* (*в пр.*) be* guílty (of), be* at fault (in); в чём ты ~и́лся перед ним? what has he got agáinst you?; ~ перед кем-л. owe *smb.* an apólogy.

провинци|а́л *м.*, ~а́лка *ж.* províncial. ~а́льный províncial.

прови́нция *ж.* **1.** (*область*) próvince; **2.** (*местность вдалеке от крупных центров*) the próvinces *pl*.

провиса́ть, прови́снуть sag, be* wéighed down.

провисе́ть *сов.* hang* for a time, stay up.

прови́снуть *сов. см.* **провиса́ть**.

про́вод *м.* wíre; телегрáфные ~а́ télegraph wíres.

проводи́мость *ж. физ.* conductívity.

проводи́ть I, провести́ 1. (*вн.; направляя, помогáть пройти*) take* (*smth.*), lead* (*smb.*), escórt (*smb.*); conduct (*smth.*); провести́ ребёнка чéрез у́лицу take* a child* acróss the street; провести́ лóдку чéрез поро́ги steer a boat through rápids; **2.** (*тв. по дт.; делать скользя́щее движéние*) pass (*smth.* óver); провести́ ладо́нью по лбу pass *one's* hand óver *one's* fórehead; **3.** (*вн.; обознача́ть*) draw* (*smth.*); провести́ черту́ draw* a line; провести́ грани́цу draw* a bóundary; **4.** (*вн.; прокла́дывать, сооружáть*) build* (*smth.*); install (*smth.*); ~ желéзную доро́гу build* a ráilway; ~ водопрово́д, электри́чество lay* on wáter, electrícity; **5.** (*вн.; мысль, идéю*) devélop (*smth.*), propóund (*smth.*); **6.** (*вн.; добива́ться утверждéния*) cárry through (*smth.*), get* (*smth.*) accépted; провести́ предложéние get* a propósal accépted; **7.** (*вн.; осуществля́ть*) cárry out (*smth.*), conduct (*smth.*); ~ незави́симую внéшнюю полúтику pursúe independent fóreign pólicy; ~ собрáние hold* a méeting; ~ кампáнию conduct a campáign; ~ о́пыт cárry out an expériment; ~ испытáние conduct a test; ~ репетúцию hold*/have* a rehéarsal; ~ убо́рку урожáя bring* in a hárvest; **8.** (*вн.; врéмя*) spend* (*smth.*), pass (*smth.*); провести́ лéто на ю́ге spend* a súmmer in the south; вéсело провести́ прáздники have* a good time on hólidays; **9.** *тк. несов.* (*вн.; быть прово́дником электри́ческого тока и т. п.*) conduct (*smth.*); метáллы проводят электри́чество métals conduct electrícity; **10.** (*вн.*) *разг.* (*обманывать*) fool (*smb.*), cheat (*smb.*); его́ не проведёшь you can't fool him; ◇ провести́ что́-л. в жизнь put* *smth.* ínto práctice.

проводи́ть II *сов. см.* **провожáть**.

прово́дка *ж.* **1.** (*судов*) stéering; (*желéзной доро́ги, канáла*) constrúction, búilding; (*водопрово́да, электри́чества*) installátion, láying-on; **2.** (*сеть проводо́в*) wíres *pl*, wíring.

проводни́к I *м.* (*электри́ческого тока, теплоты́ и т. п.*) conductor; *перен.* béarer; водá — прекрáсный ~ звýка wáter is an éxcellent conductor of sound.

проводни́к II *м.* **1.** (*провожáтый*) guide; **2.** (*в поéзде*) atté(n)dant; stéward *амер.*

про́воды *мн.* farewéll *sg*, léave-taking *sg*, sénd-off *sg*.

провожáтый *м.* éscort, guide.

провожáть, проводи́ть (*вн.*) **1.** (*сопровождáть*) accómpany (*smb.*), go* (*with*); (*уезжáющего*) see* (*smb.*) off; ~ кого́-л. домо́й see*/accómpany/take* *smb.* home; ~ кого́-л. до дверéй see* *smb.* out; ~ кого́-л. на вокзáл see* *smb.* to the státion; **2.** (*отправля́ть кудá-л.*) send* (*smb.*) off; проводи́ть сы́на в áрмию send* *one's* son off to the ármy; **3.** (*выражáть своё отношéние к уходя́щему*) see* (*smb.*) off; проводи́ть кого́-л. аплодисмéнтами clap *smb.* as he, she leaves; ◇ проводи́ть кого́-л. глазáми fóllow *smb.* with *one's* eyes, watch *smb.* go.

прово́з *м.* tránsport, cárriage; платúть за ~ pay* the cárriage.

провозгласи́ть *сов. см.* провозглаша́ть.

провозглаш|а́ть, провозгласи́ть (*вн.*) procláim (*smth.*); (*тост*) propóse (*smth.*); ~ респу́блику procláim a repúblic; ~ *кого-л.* победи́телем procláim *smb.* the wínner; ~éние *с.* proclamátion; ~éние незави́симости declarátion of indepéndence; ~éние то́ста propósing of a toast.

провози́ть, провезти́ (*вн.*) cárry (*smb., smth.*), get* (*smb., smth.*) through; (*контрабанду и т. п.*) smúggle (*smth.*).

провоз|и́ться *сов. разг.* 1. (*с тв.*) be* búsy (with); весь день ~ с больны́м spend* all day lóoking áfter a sick pérson; 2. (*провести время в возне, шалостях*) fool aróund; де́ти ~и́лись весь ве́чер the children fooled aróund all the évening.

провока́тор *м.* agént provocatéur; stóol-pigeon *разг.*

провокацио́нный provocátive.

провока́ция *ж.* provocátion.

про́волока *ж.* wire.

проволо́ч|ка *ж. разг.* deláy, procrastinátion, hóld-up; без вся́ких ~ек withóut ány deláys/hóld-ups.

про́волочн|ый wíre *attr.*; ~ое загражде́ние bárbed-wire entánglements *pl.*

прово́рн|о 1. (*быстро*) quíckly; 2. (*ловко*) déxterously, adróitly. ~ый 1. (*быстрый*) quick, brisk; ~ый шаг brisk walk; 2. (*ловкий*) adróit, ágile, déxterous, slick; ~ый па́рень ágile féllow.

проворова́ться *сов. разг.* be* caught embézzling/stéaling; be* caught with *one's* hand in the till *идиом.*

прово́рство *с.* 1. (*быстрота*) quíckness, prómptness; 2. (*ловкость*) adróitness, agility.

проворча́ть *сов.* grúmble, mútter; (*о собаке*) growl.

провоци́ровать *несов. и сов.* (*сов. тж.* спровоци́ровать) (*вн.*) provóke (*smb., smth.*).

провя́лить *сов. см.* вя́лить.

прогада́ть *сов. см.* прога́дывать.

прога́дывать, прогада́ть *разг.* miscálculate, slip up; back the wrong horse *идиом.*; я прогада́л I'm the lóser.

прога́лина *ж. разг.* 1. cléaring, glade; 2. (*промежуток*) gap.

проги́б *м.* 1. (*действие*) ságging; 2. (*прогнувшееся место*) defléction, sag.

прогиба́ться, прогну́ться sag, be* weighed down, cave in.

прогла́дить *сов.* 1 *см.* прогла́живать; 2. (*гладить в течение какого-л. времени*) iron, be* íroning.

прогла́живать, прогла́дить (*вн.*) íron (*smth.*).

прогла́тывать, проглоти́ть (*вн.; прям. и перен.*) swállow (*smth.*); проглоти́ть оскорбле́ние swállow/stómach an affrónt/ínsult.

проглоти́ть *сов. см.* прогла́тывать.

прогляде́ть *сов.* 1. *см.* прогля́дывать 1; 2. (*вн.*) *разг.* (*не заметить*) miss (*smb., smth.*); (*пропустить*) overlóok (*smth.*); ~ оши́бку not nótice a mistáke; ~ в пье́се са́мое гла́вное miss the whole point of the play.

прогля́дывать, прогляде́ть, прогляну́ть 1. *сов.* прогляде́ть (*вн.*) *разг.* (*просматривать*) glance (through), skim (through); ~ кни́гу glance/skim through a book; 2. *сов.* прогляну́ть (*показываться*) break*/peep through; со́лнце прогляну́ло сквозь облака́ the sun broke through the clouds.

прогляну́ть *сов. см.* прогля́дывать 2.

прогна́ть *сов. см.* прогоня́ть.

прогнива́ть, прогни́ть rot to píeces, be* rótten to the core.

прогни́ть *сов. см.* прогнива́ть.

прогно́з *м.* fórecast, predíction; *мед.* prognósis; ~ пого́ды wéather-forecast.

прогнози́ров|ание *с.* fórecasting. ~ать *несов. и сов.* (*вн.*) fórecast (*smth.*).

прогну́ться *сов. см.* прогиба́ться.

проговáриваться, проговори́ться let* it out, blurt it out; let* the cat out of the bag *идиом.*

проговор|и́ть *сов.* 1. (*вн.; сказать*) say* (*smth.*); 2. (*долго разговаривать*) talk; мы ~и́ли це́лый ве́чер we talked all the évening. ~и́ться *сов. см.* проговáриваться.

проголода́ться *сов.* be*/get* húngry.

проголосова́ть *сов. см.* голосова́ть.

прогоня́ть, прогна́ть (*вн.*) 1. (*стадо*) drive* (*smth.*); 2. (*заставлять уйти*) turn (*smb.*) out of doors, drive* (*smb.*) out/away; *перен.* bánish (*smth.*), dispél (*smth.*); ве́тер прогна́л ту́чи the wind dispélled the clouds; прогна́ть ску́ку dispél bóredom; 3. *разг.* (*увольнять*) sack (*smb.*), dismíss (*smb.*).

прогорáть, прогоре́ть 1. (*обращаться в угли*) burn* away/out, burn* to áshes; дрова́ в пе́чке прогоре́ли the wood in the stove has burned out; 2. (*портиться от огня*) get* (all) burnt; 3. *разг.* (*разоряться*) fail, go* bánkrupt.

прогоре́ть *сов. см.* прогорáть.

прого́рклый rank, ráncid.

прого́ркнуть *сов. см.* го́ркнуть.

програ́мм|а *ж.* 1. prógramme, prógram *амер.*; (*курса тж.*) sýllabus; (*в театре*) théatre prógramme; ~ по матема́тике mathemátics sýllabus; ~ радиопереда́ч на сего́дня today's bróadcasting prógramme; ~ расчёта реа́ктора reáctor code; принима́ть ~у adópt a prógramme; составля́ть ~y draw* up a prógramme; 2. *вчт.*: ~ для вычисли́тельной маши́ны compúter prógramme; паке́т програ́мм sóftware páckage.

программи́ров|ание *с.* prógramming. ~ать, запрограмми́ровать (*вн.*) prógramme (*smth.*), prógram (*smth.*) *амер.*

программи́ст *м.* prógrammer.

програ́ммн|ый 1. (*о политической программе*) programmátic, prógramme *attr.*; ~ докуме́нт programmátic dócument; 2. (*об учебной программе*) sýllabus *attr.*; 3.: ~ое управле́ние prógrammed/compúter contról; ~ое обеспе́чение sóftware; ~ая совмести́мость sóftware compatibility; ~ое обуче́ние prógrammed léarning.

прогрева́ть, прогре́ть (*вн.*) warm (*smth.*), heat (*smth.*). ~ся, прогре́ться get*/becóme* warm, warm up.

прогреме́ть *сов. см.* греме́ть.

прогре́сс *м.* prógress; ~ нау́ки the prógress of science; ~ в те́хнике prógress in enginéering, téchnical prógress; ~и́вный progréssive; ~и́вные убежде́ния, взгля́ды progréssive views.

прогресси́ровать *несов.* progréss, advánce, make* héadway; (*о болезни*) devélop.

прогре́ссия *ж. мат.* progréssion; арифмети́ческая ~ arithmétical progréssion; геометри́ческая ~ geométrical progréssion.

прогре́ть(ся) *сов. см.* прогрева́ть(ся).

прогрыза́ть, прогры́зть (*вн.*) gnaw through (*smth.*).

прогры́зть *сов. см.* прогрыза́ть.

прогуде́ть *сов. см.* гуде́ть.

прогу́л *м.* ábsence from work; ◇ вы́нужденный ~ enfórced ídleness.

прогу́л|ивать, прогуля́ть 1. (*проводить какое-л. время гуляя*) walk; прогуля́ть всё у́тро be* out wálking all the mórning; 2. (*не выходить на работу*) stay awáy from work; 3. (*вн.*) (*пропускать что-л.*) miss (*smth.*); ~ уро́ки play trúant; прогуля́ть у́жин miss súpper, come* in too late for súpper. ~иваться, прогуля́ться walk, stroll, take* a walk. ~ка *ж.* óuting; (*пешком тж.*) walk, stroll; (*верхом, на велосипеде*) ride; (*в автомобиле*) drive; (*в лодке*) row; (*под парусами*) sail.

прогу́лочн|ый excúrsion *attr.*; ~ ка́тер excúrsion launch; ~ая па́луба prómenade deck.

прогу́льщик *м.*, ~ица *ж.* shírker; (*об учащихся*) trúant, slácker.

прогуля́ть(ся) *сов. см.* прогу́ливать(ся).

продава́ть, прода́ть *(вн.)* 1. sell* *(smth.)*; прода́ть что-л. дёшево (до́рого) sell* *smth.* cheap (dear); ~ что-л. кому́-л. sell* *smb. smth.*, sell* *smth.* to *smb.*; ~ что-л. в креди́т sell* *smth.* on crédit; ~ что-л. за нали́чный расчёт sell* *smth.* for cash; ~ что-л. о́птом (в ро́зницу) sell* *smth.* whólesale (rétail); 2. *(предавать)* betráy *(smb.)* for móney; sell* *(smb.)* down the river идио́м. ~ся, прода́ться 1. *тк. несов.* be* on/for sale; дом продаётся the house is for sale; 2. *(дт.; совершать предательство)* sell* onesélf (to).

прода́в|е́ц *м.* séller; *(в магазине)* sálesman*, shópman*. ~щи́ца *ж.* séller; *(в магазине)* sáleswoman*, shóp-girl; ~щи́ца цвето́в flówer-girl.

прода́ж|а *ж.* sale; поступи́ть в ~у come* on the márket; быть в ~е be* on/for sale. ~ный 1. sale *attr.*, sélling *attr.*; ~ная цена́ sale price; 2. *(предназначенный для продажи)* for sale *после сущ.*; 3. *(подкупный)* mércenary, vénal; ~ная печа́ть vénal press.

прода́лбливать, продолби́ть *(вн.)* pierce *(smth.)*, pérforate *(smth.)*, make* a hole (in).

прода́ть *сов. см.* продава́ть. ~ся *сов. см.* продава́ться 2.

продви́г|а́ть, продви́нуть *(вн.)* 1. *(двигать)* move *(smth.)* fórward; 2. *(выдвигать, повышать)* promóte *(smb.)*, advánce *(smb.)*; 3. *разг. (содействовать скорейшему выполнению чего-л.)* help *(smth.)* fórward, give* *(smth.)* a push; ~ де́ло help má́tters fórward. ~а́ться, продви́нуться 1. advánce, move fórward; ~а́ться вперёд make* héadway/prógress, get* on; 2. *(по службе)* rise* in one's proféssion; 3. *разг. (приближаться к завершению)* progréss; рабо́та ~а́ется the work is progréssing.

продвиже́ние *с.* 1. advá́ncement; prógress; 2. *(по службе)* promótion, preférment.

продви́нуть(ся) *сов. см.* продвига́ть(ся).

продева́ть, проде́ть *(вн.)* thread *(smth.)*; ~ ни́тку в иго́лку thread a néedle.

продеклами́ровать *сов. см.* деклами́ровать 1.

проде́л|ать *сов. см.* проде́лывать. ~ка *ж.* trick; *(шаловливая)* prank; *(мошенническая)* swindle, tríckery.

проде́лывать, проде́лать *(вн.)* 1. *(пробивать)* make* *(smth.)*; проде́лать небольшо́е отве́рстие в стене́ make* a small ópening/hole in the wall; 2. *(выполнять, делать)* do* *(smth.)*, perfórm *(smth.)*, cárry out *(smth.)*; 3. *(совершать какую-л. проделку)* do* *(smth.)*, play *(smth.)*. .

продемонстри́ровать *сов. (вн.)* displáy *(smth.)*, show* *(smth.)*.

продержа́ть *сов. (вн.)* keep* *(smb., smth.)*; *(на руках)* hold* *(smb., smth.)*; ~ окно́ откры́тым весь день keep* the window ópen all day. ~ся *сов.* stay; *(не сдаваться)* hold* out; по́сле взры́ва кора́бль продержа́лся на плаву́ то́лько час áfter the explósion the ship stayed afló́at for ónly an hour.

проде́ть *сов. см.* продева́ть.

продешеви́ть *сов. (вн.)* sell* *(smth.)* cheap, make* a bad bárgain.

продикто́вать *сов. см.* диктова́ть.

продира́ть, продра́ть *(вн.) разг.* tear* *(smth.)*, wear* *(smth.)* out; ◇ продра́ть глаза́ *разг.* wake* up, get* one's eyes ópen. ~ся, продра́ться *разг.* 1. be* torn, be* worn out; 2. *(пробираться)* force/shóulder one's way.

продл|ева́ть, продли́ть *(вн.)* prolóng *(smth.)*, exténd *(smth.)*; ~ жизнь prolóng life; продли́ть о́тпуск exténd one's leave. ~е́ние *с.* prolongátion, exténsion, renéwal. ~и́ть *сов. см.* продлева́ть. ~и́ться *сов. см.* дли́ться.

продлённ|ый: ~ день exténded day; гру́ппа ~ого дня exténded-day group/class.

продово́льств|енный food *attr.*; ~ магази́н food shop, gró́cery. ~ие *с.* provisions *pl*, fó́od-stuffs *pl*.

продолби́ть *сов. см.* прода́лбливать.

продолгова́тый óblong.

продолжа́тель *м.* contí́nuer, succéssor.

продолж|а́ть, продо́лжить 1. *(вн., + инф.)* contí́nue *(smth., + to inf, + -ing)*, cárry on *(with, + -ing)*, go* on *(with, + -ing)*; продо́лжить cárry on with one's work; ~ заня́тия cárry on one's stú́dies, go* on with one's stú́dies; ~ путеше́ствие contí́nue/pursúe one's jó́urney; ~ рабо́тать contí́nue working, go* on with one's work; ~ разгово́р contí́nue a conversá́tion; он ~а́л хохота́ть he went on láughing; 2. *(вн.; продлевать, увеличивать)* exténd *(smth.)*, cárry on (with), go* on (with); продо́лжить курс лече́ния go* on with the tréatment. ~а́ться, продо́лжиться last, contí́nue, go* on; перегово́ры всё ещё ~а́ются the negotiá́tions are still gó́ing on. ~е́ние *с.* continuá́tion; *(книги тж.)* séquel; ~е́ние сле́дует to be contí́nued; ◇ в ~е́ние *(рд.)* dúring *(smth.)*; в ~е́ние всего́ дня all day long; в ~е́ние всей неде́ли (dúring) the whole week.

продолжи́тельн|ость *ж.* durá́tion, contí́nuance; ~ дня length of the day; ~ путеше́ствия durá́tion of a jó́urney; ~ челове́ческой жи́зни length of hú́man life. ~ый long; ~ая зима́ long/protrá́cted winter; на ~ое вре́мя for a considerable length of time.

продо́лжить(ся) *сов. см.* продолжа́ть(ся).

продо́льн|ый longitúdinal, léngthwise; ~ая пила́ ríp-saw; ~ разре́з *(на чертеже)* longitúdinal séction.

продра́ть(ся) *сов. см.* продира́ть(ся).

продро́гнуть *сов.* be* chilled to the bone.

продув|а́ть, проду́ть *(вн.)* 1. *(дуя, прочищать)* clean *(smth.)* with compréssed air; *тех.* scá́venge *(smth.)*; 2. *тк. несов. разг. (обдувать со всех сторон)* make* a draught (through); ве́тер ~а́л пала́тку the wind played fréely through the tent; 3. *безл.*: его́ проду́ло he has caught a chill.

проду́вка *ж. тех.* blówing, scá́venging.

продувно́й *разг. (хитрый)* sly, sharp.

проду́вочный *тех.* scá́venging.

проду́кт *м.* 1. pró́duct; ~ы се́льского хозя́йства agricú́ltural prodúce *sg*; 2. *обыкн. мн. (съестные)* provisions, food pró́ducts, fó́od-stuffs.

продукти́вн|ость *ж.* productí́vity; ~ труда́ productí́vity of lá́bour; ~ се́льского хозя́йства productí́vity of ágriculture. ~ый 1. *(производительный)* productí́ve, efficient; 2. *(о сельскохозяйственных животных)* prodú́cing; 3. *лингв.* prodú́ctive; ~ый су́ффикс prodú́ctive sú́ffix.

проду́ктовый: ~ магази́н food shop, gró́cery.

продуктообме́н *м.* exchá́nge of pró́ducts.

проду́кци|я *ж.* prodú́ction, óutput, yield; годова́я ~ фа́брики á́nnual prodú́ction/óutput of a fá́ctory; гото́вая ~ finished pró́ducts *pl*; себесто́имость ~и cost of prodú́ction.

проду́м|анный considered; ~ отве́т considered á́nswer. ~ать *сов. см.* проду́мывать.

проду́мывать, проду́мать *(вн.)* think* out *(smth.)*, think* *(smth.)* óver; проду́мывать вопро́с think* the má́tter óver; проду́мать план think* out a plan.

проду́ть *сов. см.* продува́ть 1, 3.

продыря́вить *сов. (вн.) разг.* make* a hole (in). ~ся *сов. разг.* 1. *(стать дырявым — о лодке и т. п.)* get* holed; 2. *(износиться)* wear* í́nto holes.

продю́сер *м.* prodú́cer.

проеда́ть, прое́сть *(вн.)* 1. *(грызя, поедая, проделать дыру)* eat* *(smth.)*; *(о кислотах и т. п. тж.)* corró́de *(smth.)*, eat* awá́y *(smth.)*; 2. *разг. (тратить на еду)* spend* *(smth.)* on food; мы прое́ли все свои́ де́ньги we spent all our móney on food.

прое́зд *м.* 1. *(действие)* drive, jó́urney; пла́та за ~ fare; плати́ть за ~ pay* one's fare; 2. *(место, где можно проехать)* pá́ssage, thó́roughfare; нет ~а по thó́roughfare, no through road.

прое́зд|ить *сов.* 1. *см.* проезжа́ть 4; 2. *(провести какое-л. время в езде)* trá́vel; он ~ил всю неде́лю he trávelled for a whole week, he spent a whole week trávelling.

проездно́й: ~ биле́т tícket.

прое́здом on *one's* way (to), pássing through.

проезжа́ть, прое́хать, прое́здить 1. *сов.* прое́хать go*, pass; (*на машине, автобусе*) drive*; (*на лошади*) ride*; прое́хать у́лицу drive* the length of a street; прое́хать посёлком go* through a víllage; по́езд прое́хал че́рез тунне́ль the train passed through a túnnel; 2. *сов.* прое́хать (*вн.; покрывать какое-л. расстояние*) do* (*smth.*), cóver (*smth.*); две́сти киломе́тров он прое́хал за дво́е су́ток he did two húndred kílometres in two days; 3. *сов.* прое́хать (*вн.; пропускать нужную остановку*) pass (*smth.*), miss (*smth.*); прое́хать ста́нцию miss *one's* státion; 4. *сов.* прое́здить (*вн.*) *разг.* (*тратить на поездку*) spend* (*smth.*) on the jóurney; прое́здить сто рубле́й spend* a húndred róubles on the jóurney.

прое́зж|ий *прил.* 1. (*годный для езды*) fit for tráffic *после сущ.*; ~ая доро́га road fit for tráffic; ~ая часть у́лицы cárriage-way; 2. *в знач. сущ. м.* tráveller.

прое́кт *м.* 1. (*план какого-л. сооружения*) design, plan; разраба́тывать ~ draw* up a plan, map out a próject; 2. (*предварительный текст какого-л. документа*) draft; ~ соглаше́ния draft agréement; ~ зако́на Bill; ~ резолю́ции draft resolútion; 3. (*замысел*) scheme, próject.

проекти́рование *с.* desígning, plánning.

проекти́ровать I, спроекти́ровать 1. (*вн.; составлять проект*) design (*smth.*), plan (*smth.*); 2. *тк. несов.* (*вн., + инф.; предполагать*) plan (*smth., + to inf*), cóntemplate (*smth., + -ing*).

проекти́ровать II *несов.* (*вн.; чертить проекцию; передавать на экран проекцию*) próject (*smth.*).

проекти́ров|ка *ж. см.* проекти́рование. ~щик *м.* designer.

прое́ктн|ый design *attr.*; (*предусмотренный проектом*) projécted; ~ые организа́ции design organizátions; ~ая мо́щность projécted capácity.

проекто́р *м.* projéctor.

проекцио́нный projéction *attr.*; ~ аппара́т projéctor; ~ фона́рь (*детский*) mágic lántern.

прое́кция *ж.* projéction.

проём *м.* ópening, áperture.

прое́сть *сов. см.* проеда́ть.

прое́хать *сов. см.* проезжа́ть 1, 2, 3. ~ся *сов. разг.* have* a ride, go* for a ride.

прожа́ривать, прожа́рить (*вн.*) roast (*smth.*) well; (*на сковороде*) fry (*smth.*) well. ~ся, прожа́риться roast well; мя́со прожа́рилось the meat is well róasted, the meat has róasted through.

прожа́рить(ся) *сов. см.* прожа́ривать(ся).

прожд|а́ть *сов.* (*вн., рд.*) wait (for); он ~а́л его́ це́лый час he wáited a whole hour for him.

прожева́ть *сов. см.* прожёвывать.

прожёвывать, прожева́ть (*вн.*) chew/másticate (*smth.*) thóroughly.

прожектёр *м. ирон.* concóctor of idéas/schemes, cástle-builder. ~ство *с. ирон.* háre-brained schemes/plans *pl*; búilding cástles in the air *идиом.*

прожёктор *м.* séarchlight.

проже́чь *сов. см.* прожига́ть.

прожива́ть, прожи́ть 1. *тк. несов.* (*жить где-л.*) live, resíde; 2. (*вн.; тратить на существование*) spend* (*smth.*).

прожига́ть, проже́чь (*вн.*) burn* (*smth.*); *перен.* sear (*smb., smth.*); ~ дыру́ в чём-л. burn* a hole in *smth*.

прожи́лка *ж.* vein; (*в камне, металле тж.*) streak.

прожи́т|ие *с.*: на ~ to live on. ~очный: ~очный ми́нимум living-wage, subsístence wage.

прожи́ть *сов.* 1. *см.* прожива́ть 2; 2. (*просуществовать какое-л. время*) live; ~ 90 лет live nínety years; 3.

(*провести некоторое время где-л.*) spend* (*smth.*); ~ всё ле́то на да́че spend* all the súmmer in the cóuntry.

прожо́рлив|ость *ж.* vorácity, voráciousness. ~ый vorácious.

прожужжа́ть *сов.* buzz, hum, drone; ◇ ~ у́ши кому́--л. tell* *smb.* óver and óver agáin, din *smth.* into *smb.'s* ears.

про́з|а *ж.* (*прям. и перен.*) prose; писа́ть ~ой write* prose; стихотворе́ние в ~е prose póem; póem in prose; ~ жи́зни the prose of life.

проза́ик *м.* próse-writer.

прозаи́ч|еский 1. prose *attr.*; ~ перево́д prose translátion; 2. (*скучный*) prosáic, dull, unínteresting; 3. (*практический*) práctical, prosáic. ~ный prosáic, cómmonplace.

прозва́ние *с. см.* про́звище.

прозва́ть *сов. см.* прозыва́ть.

прозвен|е́ть *сов.* make* a tínkle; ring* (shrílly); (*послышаться*) sound; ~е́л звоно́к a bell rang shrílly; гне́вная но́тка ~е́ла в его́ го́лосе there was a trace of ánger in his voice.

про́звище *с.* níckname; дать ~ кому́-л. níckname *smb.*; получи́ть ~ be* nícknamed.

прозвони́ть *сов.* ring* (out).

прозвуча́ть *сов. см.* звуча́ть.

прозева́ть *сов. см.* прозёвывать *и* зева́ть 3.

прозёвывать, прозева́ть (*вн.*) miss (*smth.*); прозева́ть удо́бный моме́нт miss an opportúnity, let* slip an opportunity.

прозимова́ть *сов. см.* зимова́ть.

прозорли́в|ость *ж.* clárity of vísion, far-síghtedness. ~ый shrewd, far-síghted.

прозра́чн|ость *ж.* transpárence, transpárency (*тж. перен.*); limpídity; (*о стиле*) lucídity. ~ый transparent (*тж. перен.*); (*о воздухе, воде тж.*) límpid, pellúcid; (*о стиле*) lúcid; ~ое стекло́ clear glass; ~ое пла́тье flímsy dress; ~ намёк transpárent hint/allúsion.

прозре́ва́ть, прозре́ть regáin *one's* sight; *перен.* cléarly understánd*, see* things cléarly.

прозре́ть *сов. см.* прозрева́ть.

прозыва́ть, прозва́ть (*вн.*) níckname (*smb., smth.*), dub (*smb., smth.*).

прозяба́ние *с.* vegetátion, végetable life.

прозяба́ть *несов.* végetate, lead* an áimless/unevéntful life.

прозя́бнуть *сов. разг.* get* chilled (to the bone).

проигра́ть *сов.* 1. *см.* прои́грывать; 2. (*провести какое-л. время, играя во что-л.*) play; ~ в футбо́л це́лый день play fóotball all day. ~ся *сов.* прои́грываться.

прои́грыватель *м.* récord-player.

прои́грывать, проигра́ть 1. (*вн.; терпеть поражение в чём-л.*) lose* (*smth.*); проигра́ть па́ртию в ша́хматы lose* a game of chess; проигра́ть пари́ lose* a bet/wáger; кома́нда проигра́ла со счётом 2 : 0 the team lost two nil; проигра́ть суде́бный проце́сс lose* a court case; 2. (*вн.; лишиться чего-л. в игре*) lose* (*smth.*); gámble awáy (*smth.*); проигра́ть пе́шку lose* a pawn; 3. (*терпеть ущерб от чего-л.*) súffer, be* spoiled (by); ~ в чём-л. мне́нии sink* in *smb.'s* (good) opínion; пье́са проигра́ла от плохо́й поста́новки the play was spoiled by poor prodúction; 4. (*вн.*) *разг.* (*исполнять*) play (*smth.*). ~ся, проигра́ться *разг.* lose* all *one's* móney.

прои́грыш *м.* loss; *спорт.* deféat; остава́ться в ~е be* the lóser; у него́ ~ в сто рубле́й he has lost a húndred róubles.

произведе́ни|е *с.* 1. work; ~ иску́сства work of art; гениа́льное ~ brílliant work, work of génius; литерату́рное ~ líterary work; и́збранные ~я selécted works; 2. *мат.* próduct.

произвести́ *сов. см.* производи́ть.

производи́тель *м.* 1. *эк.* prodúcer; 2. *с.-х.* síre; жеребе́ц-~ stúd-horse; ◇ ~ рабо́т superinténdent.

производи́тель|ость *ж.* productívity, prodúctive capácity; (*машины тж.*) thróughput; ~ труда́ lábour productívity, productívity/efficiency of lábour. ~ый prodúctive; ~ый труд prodúctive work; ~ые си́лы *эк.* prodúctive fórces.

производи́ть, произвести́ (*вн.*) 1. (*делать, совершать*) make* (*smth.*), cárry out (*smth.*); ~ ремо́нт cárry out repáirs; ~ вычисле́ние make* a calculátion; ~ о́пыт cárry out an expériment; ~ киносъёмку film; ~ сле́дствие condúct an investigátion; 2. (*изготовлять, вырабатывать*) prodúce (*smth.*); ~ това́ры ма́ссового потребле́ния prodúce/make* consúmer goods; ~ пшени́цу prodúce wheat; 3. (*вызывать, делать*) prodúce (*smth.*), make* (*smth.*); ~ впечатле́ние на кого́-л. make*/prodúce an impréssion on smb.; 4. (*родить*) bring* forth (*smth.*), bear* (*smth.*); 5. (*вн. в вн.; присваивать звание*) make* (*smb. smth.*); произвести́ кого́-л. в офице́ры make* smb. an ófficer; ◇ произвести́ на свет bring* into the world. ~ся *несов.* 1. (*изготовляться*) be* prodúced, be* in prodúction; 2. (*происходить*) take* place, procéed.

производн|ый *прил.* 1. derívative; ~ое сло́во derívative; ~ая величина́ derived quántity; 2. *в знач. сущ. ж. мат.* derívative.

производственн|ик *м.*, ~ица *ж.* prodúction wórker.

производственн|ый prodúction *attr.*; ~ план prodúction prógramme; ~ проце́сс prócess of prodúction; ◇ ~ые отноше́ния *эк.* prodúction relátions.

произво́дств|о *с.* 1. (*процесс*) prodúction; (*изготовление тж.*) manufácture; сре́дства ~а means of prodúction; ~ ста́ли steel manufácture; ~ бума́ги páper prodúction; 2. (*отрасль промышленности*) índustry; сталелите́йное ~ steel índustry; 3. (*фабрика, завод*) fáctory; рабо́тать на ~e work at a fáctory/plant.

произво́л *м.* 1. déspotism, týranny; 2. (*необоснованность*) árbitrariness; ◇ оставля́ть кого́-л. на ~ судьбы́ leave* smb. to the mércy of fate.

произво́льн|о 1. (*по своему усмотрению*) at will, at one's own chóosing; 2. (*необоснованно, без доказательств*) árbitrarily. ~ый 1. (*свободный*) (*самовольный*) árbitrary; ~ые отступле́ния от тре́бований зако́на árbitrary depártures from what is required by law; 3. (*лишённый доказательств*) árbitrary, unfóunded; ~ое толкова́ние чего́-л. árbitrary interpretátion of smth.; ~ый вы́вод árbitrary conclúsion.

произнести́ *сов. см.* произноси́ть.

произно|си́ть, произнести́ (*вн.*) 1. (*артикулировать*) pronóunce (*smth.*); (*отчётливо*) artículate (*smth.*); пра́вильно ~ что-л. pronóunce smth. corréctly; 2. (*говорить*) say* (*smth.*), útter (*smth.*); ~ речь make*/delíver a speech; не произнести́ ни одного́ сло́ва not say/útter a world; 3. (*оглашать*) pronóunce. ~ше́ние *с.* pronunciátion; (*артикуляция*) articulátion; пра́вильное ~ше́ние corréct pronunciátion.

произойти́ *сов. см.* происходи́ть 1, 2.

проиллюстри́ровать *сов.* (*вн.; прям. и перен.*) illustrate (*smth.*).

проинструкти́ровать *сов.* (*вн.*) give* (*smb.*) instrúctions.

проинтервьюи́ровать *сов.* (*вн.*) interview (*smth.*).

проинформи́ровать *сов.* (*вн.*) infórm (*smb.*).

про́иски *мн.* intrígues; wírepulling *sg;* únderhand práctices; schéming *sg.*

происходи́ть, произойти́ 1. (*случаться*) take* place, háppen, occúr; произошли́ больши́е измене́ния great chánges have táken place; что там происхо́дит? what is góing on there?; де́йствие происхо́дит в Волгогра́де the scene is set in Vólgograd; 2. (*от рд.; возникать как следствие чего-л.*) occúr (through), resúlt (from), be* due (to); 3. *тк. несов.* (*от, из рд.; быть какого-л. про-*

исхожде́ния) come* (of), spring* (from); ~ из крестья́н come* of péasant stock.

происхожде́ни|е 1. (*возникновение*) órigin; ~ ви́дов órigin of spécies; сло́во гре́ческого ~я word of Greek órigin; 2. (*принадлежность по рождению*) birth, órigin, extráction; (*о вещах*) próvenance; ру́сский, англича́нин по ~ю Rússian, English by birth.

происше́ств|ие *с.* event, íncident; без ~ий unevéntfully, withóut íncident.

пройдо́ха *м. и ж. разг.* old fox, cráfty/wíly/ártful pérson.

про́йма *ж.* árm-hole.

пройти́ *сов. см.* проходи́ть I. ~сь *сов. см.* проха́живаться.

прок *м. разг.* use; из э́того ~у не бу́дет it's no use, it won't do ány good.

прока́за I *ж.* (*шалость*) prank, trick, mónkey-trick.

прока́за II *ж.* (*болезнь*) léprosy.

прока́з|ить, напрока́зить *разг. см.* прока́зничать. ~ник *м.*, ~ница *ж.* ráscal; míschievous/róguish pérson; (*о ребёнке тж.*) náughty child*, young ráscal.

прока́зничать, напрока́зничать play pranks, get* up to míschief.

прока́ливать, прокали́ть (*вн.*) cálcine (*smth.*), anneál (*smth.*). ~ся, прокали́ться be* cálcined/anneáled.

прока́лывать, проколо́ть (*вн.*) 1. prick (*smth.*), pierce (*smth.*) through; (*продырявливать*) pérforate (*smth.*); ~ нары́в lance/drain an ábscess; 2. (*колющим оружием*) pierce (*smb., smth.*); проколо́ть кого́-л. штыко́м run* smb. through with a báyonet.

прока́т I *м.* (*передача имущества во временно́е пользование*) hire; внести́ пла́ту за ~ роя́ля pay* for the hire of a piáno.

прока́т II *м. тех.* 1. (*действие*) rólling; 2. (*изделие*) rolled goods, rolled métal. ~а́ть *сов. см.* прока́тывать.

прокати́ть *сов.* 1. (*вн.; в автомобиле и т. п.*) take* (*smb.*) for a dríve; 2. (*вн.; шар, мяч и т. п.*) roll (*smth.*) (along, about); 3. *разг.* (*промчаться мимо*) ride* by, flash by. ~ся *сов.* 1. (*проехаться*) go* for a ride/drive; take* a ride/drive; ~ся на парохо́де go* for a short trip by boat; 2. (*о шаре, мяче и т. п.*) roll (along, about); 3. (*о звуках*) roll, rúmble, mútter.

прока́т|ка *ж. тех.* rólling. ~ный *тех.* 1. (*относящийся к изготовлению проката*) rólling; ~ный стан rólling mill; ~ный цех rólling shop/depártment; 2. (*изготовленный путём проката*) rolled; ~ная сталь rolled steel.

прока́тчик *м.* rólling-mill óperator, róller.

прока́тывать, прокати́ть (*вн.*) *тех.* roll (*smth.*); (*в листы*) láminate (*smth.*).

прока́шляться *сов.* clear one's throat.

прокипе́ть *сов.* be* thóroughly boiled.

прокипяти́ть *сов.* (*вн.*) boil (*smth.*); (*стерилизовать*) stérilize (*smth.*); ~ молоко́ boil milk.

прокиса́ть, проки́снуть turn sour.

проки́снуть *сов. см.* прокиса́ть.

прокла́дка *ж.* 1. (*действие*) láying; ~ труб láying of pipes; ~ ка́беля cáble-laying; 2. (*слой*) pácking; gásket; wásher; рези́новая ~ rúbber wásher.

прокла́дывать, проложи́ть (*вн.*) 1. (*дорогу и т. п.*) build* (*smth.*), lay* (*smth.*); ~ тро́пу че́рез лес ópen/cut* a path through a fórest, blaze a trail through a fórest; 2. (*вкладывать что-л. между чем-л.*) pack (*smth.* with, in); проложи́ть стекля́нную посу́ду соло́мой pack glássware in straw; ~ себе́ доро́гу make* one's way (in life); проложи́ть доро́гу, путь чему́-л. pave the way for smth.

проклама́ция *ж.* léaflet.

прокле́ивать, прокле́ить (*вн.*) smear/coat (*smth.*) with glue/paste.

проклéить *сов. см.* проклéивать.

проклинáть, проклясть (*вн.*) curse (*smb.*, *smth.*).

проклясть *сов. см.* проклинáть.

проклят|ие *с.* 1. curse; 2. *в знач. межд.:* ~! damn!, damnátion! ~ый damned, accúrsed.

прокóл *м.* púncture, small hole.

проколóть *сов. см.* прокáлывать.

прокомментúровать *сов.* (*вн.*) cómment (on).

прокомпостúровать *сов. см.* компостúровать.

проконспектúровать *сов. см.* конспектúровать.

проконсультúровать(ся) *сов. см.* консультúровать(ся).

проконтролúровать *сов. см.* контролúровать.

прокопáть *сов.* (*вн.*) dig* (*smth.*).

прокормúть *сов.* (*вн.*) feed* (*smb.*, *smth.*), keep* (*smb.*, *smth.*). ~ся *сов. разг.* live (on), subsíst (on).

прокорректúровать *сов. см.* корректúровать.

прокрáдываться, прокрáсться steal* ín(to), creep* ín(to); прокрáсться в кóмнату steal* into a room.

прокрáсться *сов. см.* прокрáдываться.

прокричáть *сов.* 1. shout; *перен.* trúmpet; 2. (*кричать какое-л. время*) shout (for a time); ◇ ~ ýши кому́-л. о чём-л. din *smth.* into *smb.'s* ears, tell* *smb.* abóut *smth.* óver and óver agáin.

прокуратýра *ж.* públic prósecutor's óffice/depártment.

прокурóр *м.* públic prósecutor; Генерáльный ~ Prósecutor-Géneral. ~ский públic prósecutor's.

прокусúть *сов. см.* прокýсывать.

прокýсывать, прокусúть (*вн.*) bite* through (*smth.*).

проламывать, проломúть (*вн.*) break* (*smth.*); (*продырявливать*) make* a hole (in), hole (*smth.*); проломúть дверь make* a hole in a door. ~ся, проломúться break*.

пролегáть *несов.* pass, lie*/run* acróss.

пролеж|áть *сов.* lie*; ~ в постéли три мéсяца stay in bed for three months; письмó ~áло на пóчте бóльше мéсяца the létter lay at the póst-office for óver a month.

пролежень *м.* bédsore.

пролезáть, пролéзть (в *вн.*) get* through (*smth.*), squeeze through (*smth.*); *перен.* insínuate onesélf (ínto), worm onesélf (ínto); пролéзть в полуоткры́тую дверь get* through the half-ópen door.

пролéзть *сов. см.* пролезáть.

пролёт I *м.* (*самолёта, птиц*) flight.

пролёт II *м.* 1. (*открытое пространство*) gap; 2. (*лестницы*) well, wéll-hole; 3. (*моста*) span; мост с одни́м ~ом síngle-span bridge; 4. *архит.* bay, ópening; 5. *разг.* (*перегон*) dístance betwéen two státions, stage.

пролетариáт *м.* proletáriat.

пролетáрий *м.* proletárian.

пролетáрский proletárian.

пролетáть, пролетéть 1. (*летя, миновать что-л.*) fly* past/óver/by; самолёт пролетéл над гóродом a jet flew óver the town; пролетéть чéрез пусты́ню fly* acróss a désert; 2. (*вн.; летя, продвинуться на какое-л. расстояние*) fly* (*smth.*); самолёт пролетéл ты́сячу киломéтров the plane flew/cóvered a thóusand kílometres; 3. *разг.* (*быстро проезжать*) dash (alóng, through); пóезд пролетéл ми́мо стáнции the train dashed through the státion; 4. (*о времени*) fly* (by, alóng); дни пролетéли the days flew by; он не замéтил, как пролетéл вéчер the évening was óver befóre he nóticed it.

пролетéть *сов. см.* пролетáть.

пролúв *м.* strait; straits *pl*; sound.

проливáть, пролúть (*вн.*) spill* (*smth.*); (*кровь, слёзы*) shed* (*smth.*); ~ свою́ кровь за *кого-л., что-л.* shed *one's* blood for *smb., smth.* ~ся, пролúться spill*; водá пролилáсь на скáтерть the wáter spilt óver the táble-cloth.

пролúть(ся) *сов. см.* проливáть(ся).

пролог *м.* prólogue.

проложúть *сов. см.* прокла́дывать.

пролóм *м.* break, gap, breach.

проломúть(ся) *сов. см.* проламывать(ся).

промáзать *сов.* 1. (*вн.; маслом*) oil (*smth.*), lúbricate (*smth.*), grease (*smth.*); 2. (*вн.; замазкой*) pútty (*smth.*); 3. *разг.* (*промахнуться*) miss.

промáлывать, промолóть (*вн.*) grind* (*smth.*).

промáсленн|ый oiled, greased; (*запачканный маслом*) gréasy; ~ая бумáга oiled páper.

прóмах *м.* 1. (*при стрельбе, ударе*) miss; стрелять без ~а néver miss; 2. (*ошибка*) blúnder, slip; сдéлать ~ make* a blúnder; ◇ дать ~ come* to grief *идиом.*; он мáлый не ~ he's got his wits abóut him, he has plénty of gúmption.

промахнýться *сов.* 1. (*не попасть в цель*) miss (*one's* aim); (*при стрельбе тж.*) shoot* wide of the mark; 2. *разг.* (*ошибиться*) make* a blúnder, slip up, trip up.

промáчивать, промочúть (*вн.*) wet (*smth.*), drench (*smth.*); промочúть нóги get* *one's* feet wet.

промедлéни|е *с.* deláy, procrastinátion; без вся́ких ~й withóut a móment's deláy; ~ смéрти подóбно deláy may mean death.

промéдлить *сов.* línger, procrástinate; (*не сделать вовремя*) be* late.

промежýт|ок *м.* 1. (*пространство*) interval, distance, gap, space; 2. (*время*) interval; ~ в дéсять лет interval of ten years. ~очный intermédiate; ~очная стáдия intermédiate stage.

промельк|нýть *сов.* 1. (*прям. и перен.*) flash; у меня́ ~нýла мысль the though flashed through my mind; 2. (*о времени*) fly* by; лéто ~нýло the súmmer flew by; 3. (*обнаружиться*): в егó словáх ~нýла насмéшка there was a glímmer/tinge of sárcasm in his words.

промéн|ять *сов.* (*вн. на кого-л.*) 1. (*обменять*) exchánge (*smth.* for), bárter (*smth.* for); 2. (*предпочесть*) change (*smb.* for); ни на когó тебя́ не ~я́ю I want nóbody but you; I wóuldn't change you for ányone in the world; ◇ ~ кукýшку на я́стреба *погов.* change bad for worse.

промерзáть, промёрзнуть 1. (*покрываться льдом*) freeze*, be* frózen up; земля́ глубокó промёрзла the earth was frózen deep belów the súrface; 2. *разг.* (*зябнуть*) be* chilled; он промёрз до костéй he got chilled to the bone.

промёрз|лый frózen. ~нуть *сов. см.* промерзáть.

промóзглый damp, dank; (*о погоде тж.*) raw.

промокáтельн|ый: ~ая бумáга blótting páper.

промок|áть I, промóкнуть 1. get* wet/soaked/drenched; промóкнуть до костéй get* wet to the skin/bónes, get* wet through, be* drenched to the skin; пальтó промóкло насквóзь the coat is sóaking wet, the coat is wet through; у негó промóкли нóги he got his feet wet; 2. *тк. несов.* (*пропускать воду*) let* wáter through/in; э́то пальтó ~áет this coat is not wáterproof.

промокáть II, промокнýть (*вн.*) blot (*smth.*).

промóкнуть *сов. см.* промокáть I, 1.

промокнýть *сов. см.* промокáть II.

промóлвить *сов.* (*вн.*) say* (*smth.*), útter (*smth.*).

промолóть *сов. см.* промáлывать.

промолч|áть *сов.* 1. (*не ответить, ничего не сказать*) give* no ánswer, hold* *one's* peace; 2. (*молчать в течение какого-л. времени*) be* sílent; он весь вéчер ~áл he didn't say a word all the évening.

промочúть *сов. см.* промáчивать.

промтовáрный: ~ магази́н clóthing and géneral shop.

промтовáры *мн.* manufáctured (consúmer) goods.

промчáться *сов.* 1. (*быстро проехать, проскакать и т. п.*) rush past, fly* past; ~ стрелóй dart/shoot* past; 2. (*о времени*) fly* by, rush by.

промывáние *с.* wáshing; (*раны*) báthing.

промыва́ть, промы́ть (вн.) wash (smth.); (глаза, рану) bathe (smth.); (золото и т. п.) pan (smth.).

про́мыс|ел м. 1. (занятие) trade, craft; охо́тничий ~ húnting; 2. обыкн. мн. (предприятие добывающего типа) mine sg, field sg; золоты́е ~лы góld-fields; нефтяны́е ~лы óil-fields; соляны́е ~лы sált-works, sált-mines. ~ло́вый: ~ло́вая коопера́ция prodúcers' co-óperative society; ~ло́вый зверь fúr-bearing ánimals pl; ~ло́вая ры́ба indústrial fish; ~ло́вый флот fishing fleet.

промы́ть сов. см. промыва́ть.

промы́шленник м. manufácturer, indústrialist.

промы́шленн|ость ж. índustry. ~ый indústrial; ~ое предприя́тие indústrial estáblishment; ~ый центр indústrial céntre; ~ый райо́н indústrial área; ~ый потенциа́л страны́ the cóuntry's indústrial poténtial.

промышля́ть несов. (тв., вн.) make* a líving (out of), engáge in (smth.); ~ охо́той make* a líving out of húnting.

промя́млить сов. см. мя́млить 1.

пронести́ сов. см. проноси́ть I. ~сь сов. см. проноси́ться I.

пронза́ть, пронзи́ть (вн.) pierce (smb., smth.), run* (smb., smth.) through; ~ кого́-л. мечо́м run* smb. through with one's sword; ◇ пронзи́ть кого́-л. взгля́дом give* smb. a píercing glance.

пронзи́тельный 1. (о звуке) shrill, piercing; 2. (о взгляде) pénetrating, keen.

пронзи́ть сов. см. пронза́ть.

прониза́ть сов. см. прони́зывать.

прони́зыв|ать, пронизáть (вн.) pierce (smb., smth.), pénetrate (smb., smth.). ~ающий pénetrating; ~ающий хо́лод pénetrating cold.

проника́ть, прони́кнуть (в вн.) 1. pénetrate (smth.); (пробираться) get* (ínto) (в); луч све́та пронúк в ко́мнату a ray of light pénetrated the room; прони́кнуть в дом get* ínto a house; 2. (распространя́ться) spread* (амо́ng). ~ся, прони́кнуться (тв.) be* imbúed (with), be* filled (with); прони́кнуться реши́мостью be* filled with determinátion.

проникнове́н|ие с. 1. (действие) penetrátion; (распространение) spread; 2. см. проникнове́нность. ~ность ж. emótion, móving sincérity. ~ный pénetrating, móving.

прони́кнутый imbúed (with).

прони́кнуть(ся) сов. см. проника́ть(ся).

пронима́ть, проня́ть (вн.) разг. (производить большое впечатление) move (smb.), make* an impréssion (on), get* únder smb.'s skin; (о страхе) strike* (smb.); ◇ его́ ниче́м не проймёшь you can't get at him.

проница́ем|ость ж. permeability. ~ый pérmeable, pérvious.

проница́тельн|ость ж. ínsight, acúmen, shréwdness. ~ый acúte, shrewd; (о глазах тж.) sharp; ~ый взор pénetrating eye; ~ый ум acúte brain.

проноси́ть I, пронести́ 1. (вн.) cárry (smb., smth.); 2. обыкн. безл. pass; ту́чу пронесло́ the cloud has blown óver.

проноси́ть II сов. (вн.; носить в течение какого-л. времени) cárry (smb., smth.); (одежду) wear* (smth.); це́лый день ~ ребёнка на рука́х cárry a child* about all day; ~ костю́м не́сколько сезо́нов wear* a suit séveral séasons, make* a suit last séveral séasons.

проноси́ться I, пронести́сь 1. (очень быстро проезжать, пролетать) rush past/by, dash past/by, fly* past/by; перен. (о мыслях и т. п.) flash; маши́на пронесла́сь ми́мо до́ма a car dashed past the house; 2. (о времени) fly* by; 3. (быстро распространяться) spread* like wildfire; пронёсся слух there is a rúmour abróad, rúmours are flýing abóut.

проноси́ться II сов. 1. (прийти в ветхость от носки) wear* out; 2. (пробыть в носке в течение какого-

-л. времени) last; костю́м проноси́лся три го́да the suit lásted three years.

пронумерова́ть сов. см. нумерова́ть.

проны́р|а м. и ж. разг. púshing/púshful pérson, púsher. ~ливый púshing, cráfty, sly.

проню́хать сов. (вн., о пр.) разг. nose out (smth.), get* wind (of).

проня́ть сов. см. пронима́ть.

проо́браз м. prótotype.

пропага́нд|а ж. téaching, propagátion, promótion; propagánda; техни́ческая ~ téchnical informátion; антирелигио́зная ~ anti-relígious téaching. ~и́ровать несов. (вн.) própagate (smth.), propagándize (smth.), spread* (smth.). ~и́ст м., ~и́стка ж. propagándist. ~и́стский propagánda attr.; ~и́стская рабо́та propagánda work.

пропада́ть, пропа́сть 1. (теряться) disappéar, vánish, be* míssing; пропа́ла кни́га со стола́ the book has disappéared from the desk; 2. (переставать появляться где-л.) disappéar, be* míssing; он ушёл и пропа́л на неде́лю after he left he was míssing for a week; куда́ он пропа́л? where has he disappéared to?; 3. (исчезать) disappéar; пропа́сть из ви́ду disappéar from view; голоса́ пропа́ли вдали́ the vóices died awáy in the distance; 4. (погибать) die, be* killed; come* to a bad end; я пропа́л! it's all up with me!, I've had it!; 5. (проходить бесполезно, безрезультатно) be* wásted, come* to nóthing; на́ши уси́лия не пропаду́т our éfforts won't be wásted; все его́ уси́лия пропа́ли да́ром all his éfforts went for nóthing; весь день пропа́л the whole day has been wásted; ◇ пиши́ пропа́ло give up all hope.

пропа́жа ж. 1. (действие) loss; 2. (предмет) missing thing.

пропа́лывать, прополо́ть (вн.) weed (smth.).

пропа́ст|ь ж. 1. (обрыв) précipice; (бездна) gulf, abýss; перен. gulf, yáwning gap; на краю́ ~и on the brink of a précipice; перен. on the verge of disáster; 2. (рд.) разг. (множество) a lot (of), lots (of), a great deal (of); у меня́ ~ дел I have lots/heaps of things to do; ~ наро́ду ány amóunt of péople, lots of péople.

пропа́сть сов. см. пропада́ть.

пропа́хнуть сов. 1. (тв.) begin* to reek (of), pick up the smell (of); 2. разг. (испортиться) begin* to smell (bad).

пропа́шка ж. с.-х. plóughing.

пропашн|о́й с.-х.: ~о́й тра́ктор rów-crop tráctor; ~ы́е культу́ры tilled crops.

пропащ|ий разг. 1. lost; 2. (неудавшийся) hópeless; ~ее де́ло hópeless job; 3. (дурной, неисправимый) hópeless, incúrable; past redémption после сущ.; ~ челове́к lost soul.

пропека́ть, пропе́чь (вн.) bake (smth.) to a turn. ~ся, пропе́чься be* baked to a turn, be* baked through.

пропе́ллер м. propéller.

пропе́ть сов. 1. см. петь 1, 3, 4; 2. (петь в течение какого-л. времени) sing* (for a while).

пропе́чь(ся) сов. см. пропека́ть(ся).

пропива́ть, пропи́ть (вн.) drink* (smth.) awáy, spend*/squánder (smth.) on drink.

пропи́ск(ся) сов. см. пропи́сывать(ся).

пропи́ск|а ж. (résidence) registrátion; получи́ть (постоя́нную) ~у acquíre the right of (pérmanent) résidence; перен. becóme (pérmanently) estáblished.

пропис|но́й 1. (о буквах) cápital; 2. (общеизвестный): ~ы́е и́стины cópy-book máxims, trúisms.

пропи́сывать, прописа́ть 1. (вн.; регистрировать) régister (smb., smth.); ~ па́спорт régister one's pássport; прописа́ть но́вого жильца́ régister a new ténant; 2. (вн., + инф.; назначать лекарство, лечение) prescríbe (smth.), recomménd (+ -ing). ~ся, прописа́ться get* régistered.

про́пись ж. hándwriting sámple.

про́писью wrítten out (in words); написа́ть су́мму ~ write* out the amóunt in words.

пропита́ние *с.* food, sústenance; зараба́тывать себе́ на ~ earn one's líving, earn enóugh to buy food.

пропита́ть(ся) *сов. см.* пропи́тывать(ся).

пропи́тывать, пропита́ть *(вн. тв.)* sáturate *(smth.* with), ímpregnate *(smth.* with), pérmeate *(smth.* with); во́здух пропи́тан за́пахом мо́ря the air has the tang of the sea in it. **~ся,** пропита́ться *(тв.)* be* sáturated (with), be* ímpregnated (with), be* pérmeated (with).

пропи́ть *сов. см.* пропива́ть.

пропи́хивать, пропихну́ть *(вн.) разг.* push *(smth.)* through.

пропихну́ть *сов. см.* пропи́хивать.

пропища́ть *сов. см.* пища́ть.

пропла́вать *сов.* swim*; *(о судне)* sail; ~ це́лый час swim* for a whole hour; ~ всю жизнь матро́сом be* a sáilor all one's life.

пропла́кать *сов.* weep* (for a time); ◇ ~ (все) глаза́ sob one's eyes out.

проплыва́ть, проплы́ть 1. swim*; *(о судне)* sail; *(о предметах)* drift; проплы́ть до середи́ны реки́ swim* ínto mídstream; ло́дка проплыла́ ещё немно́го и останови́лась the boat drífted a little fúrther and stopped; 2. *(вн.; преодолевать какое-л. расстояние)* swim* *(smth.),* do* *(smth.),* cóver *(smth.); (о судне)* sail *(smth.);* проплы́ть ты́сячу ме́тров swim* a thóusand métres; они́ проплы́ли на парохо́де 500 киломе́тров they did five húndred kílometres by boat; 3. *(вн.; миновать что-л.)* swim* past *(smth.); (о судне)* sail past *(smth.),* pass *(smth.);* мы проплы́ли ма́як we sailed past a líghthouse; 4. *(проходить)* float, flit; пе́ред его́ глаза́ми проплы́ли карти́ны далёкого де́тства chíldhood mémories flóated through his mind.

проплы́ть *сов. см.* проплыва́ть.

пропове́д|ник *м.* 1. préacher; 2. *(учения, теории)* expónent. **~овать** *несов. (вн.)* 1. preach *(smth.);* 2. *(учение, теорию)* própagate *(smth.).*

про́поведь *ж.* 1. sérmon *(тж. перен.);* 2. *(распространение какого-л. учения, теории)* préaching, propagátion, spréading.

прополá́скивать, прополоска́ть *(вн.)* rinse *(smth.);* прополоска́ть рот rinse (out) one's mouth; прополоска́ть бельё rinse the línen.

пропол|зáть, проползти́ creep*, crawl. **~ти́** *сов. см.* пропол́зать.

пропо́лка *ж.* wéeding.

прополоскáть *сов. см.* прополáскивать.

прополóть *сов. см.* пропáлывать.

пропорционáльн|ый 1. propórtional; пря́мо **~ые** величи́ны dírectly propórtional quántities; обра́тно **~ые** величи́ны ínversely propórtional quántities; сре́днее **~ое** *мат.* the mean propórtional; вес пря́мо пропорционáлен объёму the weight is dírectly propórtional to the vólume; 2. *(соразмерный чему-л.)* well-propórtional; **~ая** фигу́ра well-propórtioned figure.

пропóрция *ж.* propórtion, rátio; арифмети́ческая ~ arithmétical propórtion; геометри́ческая ~ geométrical propórtion.

пропотéть *сов.* 1. *(сильно вспотеть)* perspíre/sweat fréely; ~ от лекáрства be* put in a sweat by the médicine; 2. *разг. (пропитаться потом)* be* soaked in sweat.

прóпуск *м.* 1. *(документ)* pass, pérmit; 2. *(пароль)* pássword; 3. *(в тексте)* omíssion; *(незаполненное место)* gap; 4. *(занятий и т. п.)* non-atténdance, ábsence; он посеща́ет заня́тия без **~ов** he néver mísses a lésson.

пропуск|áть, пропусти́ть 1. *(вн.; давать проникнуть)* let* in *(smth.),* admít *(smth.);* што́ра не **~ает** све́та the blind keeps the light out; ~ во́ду let* in wáter; 2. *(вн.; обслуживать, обрабатывать)* hándle *(smb.),* cáter (for), serve *(smb.);* столóвая **~ает** за день ты́сячу

челове́к the cafetéria cáters for a thóusand péople a day; 3. *(вн. через вн.)* put* *(smth.* through); пропусти́ть ток че́рез реостáт put* cúrrent through the rhéostat; 4. *(вн.; давать пройти, проехать)* let* *(smb.)* pass, let* *(smb.)* go; *(давать дорогу)* make* way (for); *(впускать куда--л.)* admít *(smb.),* let* *(smb.)* in; пропусти́ть дете́й впере́д let* the chíldren go first; пропусти́ть же́нщину с ребёнком make* way for a wóman* with a child*; пропусти́ть кого́-л. на вы́ставку admít smb. to an exhibítion; 5. *(вн.) разг. (разрешать к напечатанию, к постановке)* pass *(smth.);* 6. *(вн.) спорт.* miss *(smth.),* let* *(smth.)* through; пропусти́ть мяч в воро́та let* the ball ínto the goal; 7. *(вн.; упускать)* let* *(smth.)* pass, miss *(smth.);* пропусти́ть удо́бный слу́чай miss a good chance; пропусти́ть срок let* the time-límit expíre; 8. *(вн.; при переписывании, исполнении)* omít *(smth.),* leave* *(smth.)* out; *(при чтении)* skip *(smth.);* он пропусти́л две стро́чки he left out two lines; 9. *(вн.; не являться)* miss *(smth.);* ма́льчик пропусти́л два уро́ка the boy has missed two léssons.

пропускн|óй: **~ая** спосо́бность capácity; *(о станке и т. п.)* thróugh-put; **~ая** спосо́бность желе́зных доро́г cárrying capácity of the ráilways.

пропусти́ть *сов. см.* пропускáть.

прорáб *м.* superinténdent.

прорабáтывать, проработáть *(вн.) разг.* 1. *(подробно изучать)* exámine *(smth.);* ~ вопрóс look ínto a quéstion; 2. *(подвергать суровой критике)* put* *(smb.)* through the mill.

проработáть *сов.* 1. *см.* прорабáтывать; 2. *(работать в течение какого-л. времени)* work; он проработáл там два го́да he worked there for two years.

прорастáть, прорасти́ sprout.

прорасти́ *сов. см.* прорастáть.

прорвáть *сов. см.* прорывáть I. **~ся** *сов. см.* прорывáться.

прорéзать *сов. см.* прорезáть.

прорезáть, прорéзать *(вн.)* cut* through *(smth.);* *(пропиливать)* cut* a hole (in), make* a slot (in).

прорéзаться *сов. см.* прорезáться.

прорез|áться, прорéзаться *(о зубах)* cut*; у ребён-ка **~áются** зу́бы the child* is téething, the child* is cútting its teeth.

прорези́ненн|ый rúbberized; **~ая** ткань rúbberized fábric.

прóрезь *ж.* slit; slot; *(в оружии)* notch, áperture.

проре́ктор *м.* proréctor.

прорепети́ровать *сов. см.* репети́ровать.

прорецензи́ровать *сов. см.* рецензи́ровать.

проржáветь *сов.* get* rústy.

прорóк *м.* próphet.

пророни́ть *сов. (вн.)* útter *(smth.);* не ~ ни сло́ва not útter/say* a word; ◇ не ~ (ни) слези́нки not shed a (síngle) tear.

проро́че|ский prophétic. **~ство** *с.* próphecy. **~ствовать** *несов.* próphesy.

проро́чить, напроро́чить *(вн.)* próphesy *(smth.),* predíct *(smth.).*

прорубáть, проруби́ть *(вн.)* cut* through *(smth.),* hew* through *(smth.);* ~ сте́ну cut* through a wall; ~ про́секу в лесу́ cut*/hew* a pássage/ride through a wood.

проруби́ть *сов. см.* прорубáть.

прóрубь *ж.* ópening/hole in the ice, íce-hole.

прорыв *м.* 1. *(действие):* ~ плоти́ны búrsting/bréaching of a dam; ~ фро́нта bréak-through; 2. *(прорванный участок)* breach; задéлать ~ в плоти́не repáir a breach in a dam; ~ в ли́нии оборо́ны проти́вника breach in the énemy's defénces; 3. *(невыполнение плана и т. п.)* lag, bad patch; вы́вести цех из **~а** get* the depártment óver a bad patch; ~ в рабóте lag.

прорывáть I, прорвáть *(вн.)* 1. tear* *(smth.);* прорвать чулок tear* one's stócking; 2. (разрушать преграду) break* through (smth.); прорвать плотину breach/burst* a dam.

прорывать II, прорыть (вн.) dig* (smth.); прорыть канаву dig* a trench; прорыть тоннель drive* a túnnel (through).

прорываться, прорваться 1. (рваться) tear*, break*; прорвался кулёк, и конфеты рассыпались the bag broke and all the sweets feel out; 2. (лопаться) break*, burst*; нарыв прорвался the ábscess has burst; 3.: плотина прорвалась the dam has burst; 4. (прокладывать себе путь) break* through; прорваться из окружения break* out of encírclement.

прорыть сов. см. прорывать II.

прорычать сов. см. рычать.

просачиваться, просочиться (в вн.) pércolate (into), seep through (into); ínfiltrate (smth.) (тж. перен.).

просверливать, просверлить (вн.) bore (smth.), drill (smth.), pérforate (smth.); просверлить отверстие drill a hole; просверлить дверь drill (a hole) through/in a door.

просверлить сов. см. просверливать.

просвет м. 1. (светлая полоса на тёмном фоне) break, ópening, rift; перен. gleam/glímmer of hope; 2. (промежуток между близко расположенными предметами) gap; 3. архит. bay, áperture.

просветитель м. enlíghtener, lúminary. ~ный educátional. ~ство с. 1. educátional actívities pl. 2. ист. enlíghtenment.

просветить I сов. см. просвещать.

просветить II сов. см. просвечивать 1.

просветиться сов. см. просвещаться.

просветление с. 1. enlíghtenment, clárity; 2. (ясность сознания) lúcid ínterval.

просветлеть сов. 1. (о погоде) clear (up), becóme* bright(er); 2. (о сознании) becóme* lúcid/clear.

просвечивание с. radióscopy; ~ лёгких X-ráy examinátion of the lungs.

просвечивать, просветить 1. (вн.) X-ráy (smb., smth.); 2. тк. несов. (быть прозрачным) be* translúcent, show* the light (through it); 3. тк. несов. (виднеться сквозь что-л.) be* seen.

просвещ|ать, просветить (вн.) enlíghten (smb.), infórm (smb.). ~аться, просветиться be* enlíghtened, be* infórmed. ~ение с. enlíghtenment; (образование) educátion; ◇ эпоха Просвещения Age of Enlíghtenment.

просвещённ|ость ж. cúlture. ~ый enlíghtened, well-infórmed, cúltivated.

просвистеть сов. whístle.

проседь ж.: волосы с ~ю gréying hair, hair tinged/streaked with grey.

просеивать, просеять (вн.; муку, песок) sift (smth.), screen (smth.); (зерно) wínnow (smth.).

просека ж. ride, path.

просёло|к м. cárt-road, cárt-track. ~чный: ~чная дорога см. просёлок.

просеять сов. см. просеивать.

просигнализировать сов. sígnal.

просигналить сов. см. сигналить.

просидеть сов. см. просиживать.

просиживать, просидеть 1. (в течение какого-л. времени) sit*; ~ часами sit* for hours; просидеть дома stay at home; просидеть весь вечер за книгами spend* the whole évening óver one's books; просидеть с больным до позднего вечера sit* up (late) with a sick pérson; 2. (вн.) разг. (протирать, продавливать) wear* out the seat (of).

просить, попросить 1. (вн., рд., о пр., + инф.; обращаться с просьбой) ask (for); ~ помощи ask for help; ~ разрешения ask permíssion; 2. (за вн.; хлопотать, вступаться) intercéde (for); 3. (вн., приглашать, звать) invíte (smb.); ~ гостей к столу invíte one's guests

to táble; директор вас просит к себе the diréctor wants to see you; 4. тк. несов. разг. (нищенствовать) beg. ~ся, попроситься 1. ask (for); дети просятся на улицу the children want to go out; 2. (просить о зачислении куда-л.) ask to be táken on; ~ся на работу ask to be gíven work.

проси|ять, сов. shine*; перен. beam, bríghten, smile bróadly; ~ от счастья be* rádiant with háppiness; лицо его ~яло от радости his face bríghtened with joy; он ~ял от удовольствия he beamed with pléasure.

проскакать сов. gállop; ~ мимо gállop by; ~ по улице gállop down the street.

проскакивать, проскочить 1. (быстро пробегать) dart past; rush by; 2. (проникать, пробираться) slip through, get* through.

проскланять сов. см. склонять II.

проскользнуть сов. slip, steal*; перен. flash; ~ по коридору steal*/slip down the pássage.

проскочить сов. см. проскакивать.

проскрипеть сов. см. скрипеть.

прослав|ить(ся) сов. см. прославлять(ся). ~ленный fámous, célebrated; ~ленный герой célebrated héro.

прославлять, прославить (вн.) glórify (smb., smth.), crown (smb., smth.) with glóry, win* fame (for). ~ся, прославиться (тв.) becóme* fámous (for, through); win* fame/renówn (by).

проследить сов. 1. (вн.; выследить) get* on smb.'s track; 2. (вн.; исследовать, изучить) trace (smth.); 3. (за тв.; проверить) check up (on), keep* track (of).

прослезиться сов. shed* a few tears.

прослойка ж. 1. láyer; 2. геол. seam; 3. (часть общества) séction, strátum (pl stráta), láyer.

прослужить сов. 1. (в течение какого-л. времени) work; (в армии) serve; 2. (об одежде, вещах и т. п.) last; пальто прослужит ещё одну зиму the óvercoat will last anóther winter.

прослушать сов. см. прослушивать.

прослушивать, прослушать (вн.) 1. (воспринимать слухом) lísten (to); прослушать концерт по радио lísten to the (whole) cóncert óver the rádio; ~ магнитофонные записи lísten to tápe-recórdings; 2. мед. examíne (smb., smth.); 3. разг. (не слышать) not catch (smth.), miss (smth.); я прослушал то, что вы сказали I dídn't catch what you said.

прослыть сов. см. слыть.

прослышать сов. (о пр.) разг. hear* (of).

просмаливать, просмолить (вн.) tar (smth.) thóroughly; просмолить верёвку tar a rope.

просматривать, просмотреть (вн.) 1. (бегло прочитывать) look óver (smth.), look through (smth.), scan (smth.); ~ газеты look through the néwspapers; бегло просмотреть книгу glance/skim through a book; 2. (ознакамливаться) run* through (smth.), go* through (smth.), examíne (smth.), see* (smth.); ~ новый фильм see* a new film; 3. (пропускать, не замечать) overlóok (smth.); ~ ошибку overlóok an érror; ◇ все глаза просмотреть watch and wait. ~ся несов. (быть видимым) be* vísible.

просмолить сов. см. просмаливать.

просмотр м. 1. víewing; (рукописей и т. п.) examinátion; предварительный ~ фильма film préview; 2. (пропущенная ошибка) óversight, érror.

просмотреть сов. см. просматривать.

проснуться сов. см. просыпаться I.

просо с. míllet.

просовывать, просунуть (вн. в вн.) thrust* (smth. through, out), push (smth. into, through); ~ голову в окно thrust* one's head through/out of the window.

просодия ж. лит. prósody.

просохнуть сов. см. просыхать.

просочиться сов. см. просачиваться.

просп|ать сов. 1. см. просыпать I; 2. (спать в течение какого-л. времени) sleep* (for a time); он ~а́л три часа́ he slept (for) three hours. ~а́ться сов. разг. sleep* it off.

проспе́кт I м. (улица) ávenue; Не́вский ~ the Névsky Prospékt.

проспе́кт II м. (план) prospéctus; bóoklet, fólder.

проспо́рить сов. 1. (вн.; проиграть) lose* (smth.), lose* a bet/wáger; 2. (в течение некоторого времени) árgue.

проспряга́ть сов. см. спряга́ть.

просро́ченн|ый overdúe, expíred; ~ биле́т expíred tícket, tícket no lónger válid; ~ па́спорт expíred pássport, out-of-dáte pássport; ~ые платежи́ overdúe páyments.

просро́ч|ивать, просро́чить (вн.) deláy (smth.); просро́чить платежи́ be* behínd with one's páyments. ~ить сов. см. просро́чивать. ~ка ж. (отпуска) overstáying; (документа) expirátion; (платежа) deláy.

проста́вить сов. см. проставля́ть.

проставля́ть, проста́вить (вн.) put* (smth.) down, write* (smth.); проста́вить да́ту на докуме́нте date a dócument; проста́вить в журна́ле оце́нки put* down the marks in the régister.

проста́ивать, простоя́ть 1. (проводить какое-л. время стоя) stand*, keep*/be* stánding; он простоя́л неподви́жно ещё пять мину́т he stood mótionless for anóther five mínutes; 2. (быть на стоянке, в лагере и т. п.) stay, stop; по́езд простоя́л у светофо́ра це́лый час the train was held up by the signals for a whole hour; 3. (бездействовать) be* ídle, lie* ídle; (о заводе, фабрике и т. п.) be* at a stándstill, stand* ídle; 4. (оставаться без изменения) stay, remáin; хоро́шая пого́да до́лго не простои́т the good wéather will not last long; 5. (сохраняться) stand*; дом простои́т ещё лет сто the house will stand anóther céntury.

проста́к м. símpleton, nóddy.

простега́ть сов. см. простёгивать.

простёгивать, простега́ть (вн.) quilt (smth.).

просте́йшие мн. зоол. protozóa.

просте́нок м. pier, space betwéen the windows.

простир|а́ться несов. exténd (тж. перен.); stretch; леса́ ~а́ются на ты́сячи киломе́тров the fórests stretch for thóusands of kilómetres.

прости́тельный párdonable, excúsable.

проститу́|тка ж. próstitute, stréetwalker. ~ция ж. prostitútion.

прост|и́ть сов. 1. см. проща́ть; 2.: ~и́те (меня́)! (как вежливое предупреждение) excúse me!, I beg your párdon!

прости́ться сов. см. проща́ться.

про́сто нареч. 1. (легко) símply; éasily; э́то де́лается о́чень ~ it is véry éasily done; 2. в знач. усил. частицы разг. sheer, pure; э́то ~ безу́мие it's sheer mádness; 3. в знач. ограничительной частицы разг. símply; он ~ глуп he is símply stúpid; ◇ ~-на́просто símply; ~ так 1) (обыкновенно) quite órdinarily; 2) (бесцельно) for no spécial réason.

простова́тый разг. simple-mínded; (бесхитростный) guíleless.

простоду́ш|ие с. open-héartedness, simple-héartedness. ~ный open-héarted, simple-héarted, unsophísticated.

прост|о́й I 1. (несложный) símple, éasy; ~а́я зада́ча símple próblem; 2. (однородный, несоставной): ~ое предложе́ние грам. símple séntence; ~о́е число́ мат. prime númber; 3. (безыскусственный) unaffécted, símple; ~ое пла́тье símple dress; 4. (обыкновенный) cómmon, símple, plain, órdinary; ~ые лю́ди órdinary péople; (простодушные, нецеремонные) plain/hómely/unpreténtious péople; ~а́я пи́ща plain food; ~ сме́ртный órdinary mórtal; 5. (недалёкий, наивный) símple; ◇ ~ым гла́зом with the náked eye; ~ое письмо́ létter sent by órdinary mail.

просто́й II м. (станков и т. п.) stóppage, stánding ídle; (рабочих) ídle time; (судна, вагона) demúrrage.

простоква́ша ж. sour clótted milk, yóghourt.

простона́ть сов. 1. см. стона́ть 1; 2. (издать стон) give*/útter a groan; 3. (стонать в течение какого-л. времени) groan; ра́неный простона́л всю ночь the wóunded man* groaned all night.

просто́р м. 1. expánse, spáciousness; 2. (свобода, раздолье) fréedom, scope.

просторе́ч|ие с. cómmon speech. ~ный cómmon, low-collóquial.

просто́рный róomy, wide, spácious.

простосерде́ч|ие с. open-héartedness, simple-héartedness. ~ный open-héarted, simple-héarted, ingénuous, ártless.

простота́ ж. simplícity; (безыскусственность) unafféctedness; ~ нра́вов simplícity of cústom, símple way of life.

простофи́ля м. и ж. разг. símpleton, goof.

простоя́ть сов. см. проста́ивать.

простра́нный 1. (обширный) exténsive, vast; 2. (подробный) léngthy, long; (многословный) prólix, diffúse, verbóse.

простра́нственный spátial.

простра́нств|о с. 1. space; бесконе́чное ~ ínfinite space; 2. (большой участок поверхности) térritory, área; 3. (промежуток между чем-л.) space; свобо́дное ~ ме́жду окно́м и две́рью the space betwéen the window and the door; ◇ боя́знь ~а agoraphóbia.

простре́л м. lumbágo.

простре́ливать, прострели́ть (вн.) 1. shoot* through (smth.); прострели́ть себе́ ру́ку put* a búllet through one's hand; 2. тк. несов. (поражать огнём какой-л. участок) cóver (smth.). ~ся несов. be* in the line of fire, be* expósed to fire.

прострели́ть сов. см. простре́ливать 1.

построчи́ть сов. (вн.) stitch (smth.), báck-stitch (smth.).

просту́д|а ж. cold, chill. ~и́ть(ся) сов. см. простужа́ть(ся).

простужа́ть, простуди́ть (вн.) let* (smb.) catch cold; не простуди́те его́ take care he dóesn't catch cold, don't let him get a cold; простуди́ть дете́й let* the children catch cold; простуди́ть го́рло give* onesélf a sore throat. ~ся, простуди́ться catch* cold, get* a cold.

проступа́ть, проступи́ть break* out, ooze out; (становиться видимым) show* through; на его́ лбу проступи́ла испа́рина small beads of perspirátion broke out on his fórehead; под си́льным зага́ром на его́ щека́х проступи́л румя́нец the flush in his cheeks showed through his deep súnburn.

проступи́ть сов. см. проступа́ть.

просту́пок м. misdéed, offénse; юр. misdeméanour.

простыва́ть, просты́ть разг. 1. (остывать) get* cold; 2. (простужаться) catch* a chill; ◇ а его́ (и) след просты́л he has vánished withóut a trace.

простыня́ ж. sheet; махро́вая ~ báth-towel.

просты́ть сов. см. простыва́ть.

просу́нуть сов. см. просо́вывать.

просу́шивать, просуши́ть (вн.) dry (smth.); ~ оде́жду one's clothes. ~ся, просуши́ться get* (quite) dry.

просуши́ть(ся) сов. см. просу́шивать(ся).

просу́шка ж. разг. drýing; (дров) séasoning.

просущество́вать сов. subsíst; (продлиться) last, endúre, contínue.

просчёт м. miscalculátion, misréckoning; (промах тж.) blúnder.

просчита́ть(ся) сов. см. просчи́тывать(ся).

просчи́тывать, просчита́ть (вн.) 1. (производить подсчёт) count (smth.); 2. (делать ошибки при счёте) make* a mistáke (in cóunting), miscóunt (smth.), miscálculate (smth.). ~ся, просчита́ться 1. (делать *ошибки при счёте*) make* a mistáke (in cóunting), miscálculate; он просчитáлся на дéсять рублéй he is ten róubles out (in his réckoning); 2. (*ошибáться в предположéниях*) miscálculate, be* out in one's réckoning.

просы́п м. разг.: спать без ~y sleep* sóundly, sleep* like a top/log.

просыпáть сов. см. просыпáть II.

просыпáть I, проспáть 1. (*просыпáться позже, чем нужно*) oversléep*; он проспáл и опоздáл на пóезд he overslépt and missed his train; 2. (*вн.*) разг. (*пропускáть*) miss (*smth.*); проспáть стáнцию go* past one's státion while one is asléep.

просыпáть II, просы́пать (*вн.*) spill* (*smth.*).

просыпáться сов. см. просыпáться II.

просыпáться I, проснýться wake* up; awáke* (*тж. перен.*).

просыпáться II, просы́паться spill*, get* spilt.

просыхáть, просóхнуть dry, get* dry; дорóги просóхли the roads have dried.

просьб|а ж. requést; (*мольбá*) entréaty; по чьей-л. ~е at smb.'s requést; у меня к вам ~ I should like to ask you a fávour; ~ не курить! please, do not smoke!, you are requésted not to smoke; ~ не шумéть! silence!

протáлина ж. thawed patch.

протáлкивать, протолкнýть (*вн.*) push (*smb., smth.*) through/into; *перен. разг.* speed* up (*smth.*), éxpedite (*smth.*); протолкнýть дéло give* things a push. **~ся**, протолкнýться разг. force/élbow one's way through.

протанцевáть сов. 1. (*вн.; исполнить танец*) dance (*smth.*); 2. (*танцевáть в течение какого-л. времени*) dance; ~ до утрá dance all night.

протáпливать, протопи́ть (*вн.*) 1. heat (*smth.*) próperly, make* (*smth.*) réally hot; 2. тк. несов. (*топи́ть иногдá или понемнóгу*) heat (*smth.*) up a líttle, take* the chill (of).

протáптывать, протоптáть (*вн.*) tread* (*smth.*); протоптáть дорóжку tread* a path.

протаскáть сов. разг. cárry (*smth.*).

протáскивать, протащи́ть (*вн.*) 1. (*тащить*) drag (*smth.*), cárry (*smth.*); 2. (*проносить через что-л.*) manóeuvre (*smth.*), júggle (*smth.*); 3. разг. (*подвергáть критике*) pillory (*smb.*).

протащи́ть сов. см. протáскивать.

протéз м. prosthétic appliance; (*конечностей*) artifical limb.

протези́ст м. prósthetist; (*зубнóй*) déntal mechánic.

протек|áть, протéчь 1. (*о рекáх*) flow, run*; 2. (*просáчиваться*) come* through; водá ~áет в трюм wáter is cóming through into the hold; 3. (*пропускáть вóду*) leak, spring* a leak; кры́ша ~áет the roof leaks; 4. (*о времени, событиях*) pass, elápse, slip awáy; 5. (*о процéссе и т. п.*) go* on, procéed; болéзнь ~áет без осложнéний the illness is táking a nórmal course.

протекторáт м. protéctorate.

протéкция ж. pátronage, ínfluence.

протерéть(ся) сов. см. протирáть(ся).

протéст м. prótest; вы́ступить с ~ом make* a prótest; заяви́ть реши́тельный ~ make* a strong prótest.

протестáнт м., **~ка** ж. Prótestant. **~ский** Prótestant. **~ство** с. Prótestantism.

протестовáть несов. (против рд.) protést (agáinst); come out.

протéчь сов. см. протекáть.

против предлог (рд.) 1. (*напротив*) ópposite, fácing; сидéть друг ~ друга sit* ópposite/fácing one anóther; 2. (*навстречу движéнию чего-л.*) agáinst; плыть ~ течéния swim* against the cúrrent; ~ вéтра against the wind, with a héadwind; 3. (*вопреки*) cóntrary to, against; сидéть ~ всех ожидáний cóntrary to expectátion; поступáть ~ прáвил act cóntrary to the rules; дéлать что-л. ~ своегó желáния do* smth. against one's will; поступи́ть ~ сóвести go* agáinst one's cónscience; 4.

(*враждéбно по отношéнию к кому-л., чему-л.*) agáinst; дéйствовать ~ неприя́теля óperate against the énemy; он настрóен ~ меня́ he has sómething against me; 5. (*для борьбы́ с кем-л., чем-л.*) agáinst; лекáрство ~ гри́ппа rémedy for influénza; срéдство ~ мóли móth-killer; 6. (*по отношéнию к чему-л.*) to; дéсять шáнсов ~ одногó, что вы вы́играете пáртию ten to one you'll win the game; 7. (*по сравнéнию*) (as) compáred with, as against; рост продýкции ~ прóшлого гóда growth of óutput as against the prévious year; 8. в знач. сказ. (*не в пóльзу кого-л., чего-л.*) against; и совсéм я не ~ I'm not against it by ány means; 9. в знач. сущ. с. con; знать все за и ~ know* all the pros and cons; ◇ ничегó не имéть ~ чего-л. have* nóthing against smth.; я ничегó не имéю ~ э́того I have nóthing against it, I have no objéction, I don't mind.

противень м. óven/róasting pan, gríddle.

противи́тельный: ~ союз грам. advérsative conjúnction.

проти́виться, воспроти́виться (*дт.*) be* oppósed (to), objéct (to); (*сопротивля́ться*) resíst (*smb., smth.*).

проти́вник м. 1. oppónent; (*враг*) énemy; (*в спóре, состязáнии*) ádversary, oppónent, antágonist; 2. тк. ед. собир. (*неприя́тельское вóйско*) énemy.

проти́вно 1. нареч. disgústing; (*неприя́тно*) unpléasant; 2. в знач. сказ. безл. it is disgústing; мне ~ говори́ть об э́том I can't bear to speak abóut it; ~ смотрéть it is disgústing to watch.

проти́вн|ый I прил. 1. (*противоположный*) cóntrary; ~ вéтер ádverse/cóntrary wind; 2. (*враждéбный*) ópposite, ádverse; ~ая сторонá (*в судé*) the oppósing/ádverse párty, the óther side; 3. в знач. сущ. с. the cóntrary; доказáтельством от ~ого by the rule of cóntraries; ◇ в ~ом слýчае ótherwise.

проти́в|ный II (*отврати́тельный, гáдкий*) disgústing, lóathsome, offénsive; ~ зáпах offénsive/lóathsome smell; он ей ~ен she can't bear (the sight of) him, she finds him repéllent.

противоáтомн|ый anti-núclear; ~ая защи́та anti-núclear defénce.

противовéс м. тех. cóunterweight, cóunterpoise; *перен.* cóunterbalance; ◇ в ~ чему-л. to counterbálance smth.

противовоздýшн|ый anti-áircraft; ~ая оборóна anti-áircraft defénce.

противогáз м. gás-mask, respirátor.

противодéйств|ие с. counteráction; оказáть ~ чему-л. take* áction against smth. **~овать** несов. (*дт.*) counteráct (*smth.*); act against (*smb.*).

противоестéственный unnátural.

противозакóнный illégal, unláwful.

противопожáрный fire-prevéntion attr.

противопокáзанный мед. contra-índicated.

противополóжност|ь ж. 1. cóntrast, opposítion; ~ мнéний cóntrast of ópinion(s); ~ интерéсов oppósing ínterests; 2. (*что-л. несхóдное, кто-л. несхóдный с другим по кáчествам, свóйствам*) ópposite, cóntrast; пóлная ~ quite the ópposite; он пóлная ~ своемý брáту he is the exáct ópposite of his bróther; ~и схóдятся extrémes meet; 3. филос. ópposite; единство ~éй the únity of ópposites; ◇ в ~ кому-л., чему-л. cóntrary to smb., smth., unlíke smb., smth.

противополóжн|ый 1. (*располóженный напротив*) ópposite; в ~ом направлéнии in the ópposite diréction; он шёл по ~ой сторонé úлицы he was pássing on the ópposite pávement; 2. (*несхóдный*) ópposite, oppósing, cóntrary; ~ые взгля́ды ópposite views.

противопостáвить сов. см. противопоставля́ть.

противопоставля́ть, противопостáвить (*вн. дт.*) 1. (*срáвнивать*) contrást (*smb., smth.* with); 2. (*направ-*

лять *против*) set* (*smb., smth.* agáinst), cóunterpose (*smb., smth.* to), oppóse (*smb., smth.* to).

противоракётн|ый anti-míssile; ~ая оборóна anti-míssile defénce.

противоречи́в|ость ж. contradíctoriness; ~ показáний contradíctoriness of the évidence, conflícting évidence. **~ый** contradíctory, conflícting; ~ые показáния conflícting évidence *sg*; ~ые заявлéния contradíctory státements.

противорéч|ие с. contradíction; дух ~ия spírit of contradíction, contradíctious spírit; ~ интерéсов clash of ínterests.

противорéч|ить *несов.* (*дт.*) 1. (*возражáть кому́-л.*) contradíct (*smb.*), gainsáy* (*smb.*); 2. (*не соотвéтствовать чему́-л.*) contradíct (*smth.*), be* at váriance (with), run* cóunter (to); э́ти заявлéния ~ат друг дру́гу these státements contradíct each óther; вáши свéдения ~ат фáктам your informátion is at váriance with the facts.

противостоя́ние с. *астр.* oppositíon.

противосто|я́ть *несов.* (*дт.*) 1. (*выдéрживать*) withstánd* (*smth.*), hold* out agáinst (*smth.*); (*сопротивля́ться*) resíst (*smth.*); ~ вéтру withstánd* the wind, stand* up to the wind; ~ атáке withstánd* an attáck; hold* out agáinst an attáck; 2. (*находи́ться в противорéчии с чем-л.*) be* oppósed (to), stand* in oppositíon (to); э́тому мнéнию ~я́ло другóе anóther opínion stood in oppositíon to this one.

противотáнков|ый anti-tánk; ~ое ружьё anti-tánk run.

противохими́ческ|ий anti-gás; ~ая защи́та anti-gás protéction.

противоя́дие с. ántidote (to, for).

протирáть, протерéть (*вн.*) 1. (*продыря́вить трéнием*) wear* (*smth.*) out/through/awáy; 2. (*вытирáть*) rub (*smth.*) dry, wipe (*smth.*) clean; протерéть окнó тря́пкой wipe a window with a cloth; 3. (*растирáя, пропускáть сквозь решетó и т. п.*) rub (*smth.*) through, grate (*smth.*). **~ся,** протерéться wear* out/through.

проти́скивать, проти́снуть (*вн.*) squeeze (*smth.*) in, poke (*smth.*) in. **~ся,** проти́снуться squeeze *one's* way (through).

проти́снуть(ся) *сов. см.* проти́скивать(ся).

проткну́ть *сов. см.* протыкáть.

протóк м. 1. (*реки́*) chánnel; 2. *анат.* duct.

протокóл м. 1. mínutes *pl*; (*заседáния судá*) récord; (*заседáния парлáмента*) the jóurnals *pl*; ~ допрóса récord of examinátion; 2. (*докумéнт, удостоверя́ющий какóй-л. факт*) certíficate; 3. (*акт о нарушéнии обще́ственного поря́дка*) (official) repórt; составля́ть ~ draw* up a repórt; 4. *дип.* prótocol.

протоколи́ровать *несов. и сов.* (*вн.*) keep* the mínutes (of), mínute (*smth.*).

протокóльный 1.: ~ отдéл *дип.* prótocol depártment; 2. (*о стиле*) légal.

протолкну́ть(ся) *сов. см.* протáлкивать(ся).

протóн м. *физ.* próton.

протопи́ть *сов. см.* протáпливать 1.

протоплáзма ж. *биол.* prótoplasm.

протоптáть *сов. см.* протáптывать.

проторённ|ый béaten, dríven-óver; (*протоптáнный*) well-tródden; ◇ идти́ по ~ой дорóжке keep* to the béaten track.

прототи́п м. prótotype.

протóчн|ый 1. flówing, rúnning; ~ая водá flówing wáter; 2. (*не со стоя́чей водóй*) well-dráined, spríng-fed; ~ пруд well-dráined pond.

протрезви́ться *сов. см.* протрезвля́ться.

протрезвля́ться, протрезви́ться becóme* sóber.

протруби́ть *сов. см.* труби́ть.

протухáть, проту́хнуть go* bad.

проту́хнуть *сов. см.* протухáть и ту́хнуть II.

проту́хший foul, rótten; bad; (*о мя́се тж.*) táinted.

протыкáть, проткну́ть (*вн.*) pierce (through) (*smb., smth.*); (*шпáгой*) run* (*smb., smth.*) through.

протя́гивать, протяну́ть (*вн.*) 1. (*натя́гивать*) stretch (*smth.*); верёвку протяну́ли чéрез двор they stretched a rope acróss the yard; ~ телефóнную ли́нию eréct a télephone line; 2. (*вытя́гивать*) stretch out (*smth.*); протяну́ть ру́ку за чéм-л. stretch/hold* out *one's* hand for *smth.*; reach for *smth.*; ~ ру́ку кому́-л. hold* out *one's* hand to *smb.*; ~ кому́-л. ру́ку пóмощи óffer *smb.* a hélping hand; 3. (*предлагáть*) óffer (*smth.*), hold* out (*smth.*); он протяну́л ей кошелёк he held out a purse to her; 4. (*заставля́ть дли́тельно звучáть*) sustáin (*smth.*), draw* out (*smth.*); (*говори́ть медленно*) drawl; протяну́ть нóту hold*/sustáin a note; 5. *разг.* (*затя́гивать, задéрживать*) prolóng (*smth.*), drag out (*smth.*); протяну́ть дéло drag out an affáir; 6. *разг.* (*существовáть*) last; он дóлго не протя́нет he won't last long; ◇ протяну́ть нóги kick the búcket. **~ся,** протяну́ться 1. (*в прострáнстве*) exténd, stretch; дорóга протяну́лась на ты́сячи киломéтров the road stretched for thóusands of kílometres; 2. (*о рукáх*) stretch out, reach out; (*о ногáх*) stretch out; 3. *разг.* (*продолжáться*) last, go* on.

протяжéни|е с. extént; (*в длину́ тж.*) length; на ~и всегó пути́ óver the whole length of the road, all alóng the road; на всём ~и throughóut (its) extént; ◇ на ~и чегó-л. for *smth.*; на ~и мнóгих лет, вексóв for (the space of) mány years, cénturies.

протяжённость ж. 1. *см.* протяжéние; 2. *филос.* exténsion.

протя́жны|й slow, língering; (*о крике*) long, long dráwn-out; (*о гóлосе*) dráwling; ~ напéв língering mélody; говори́ть ~м гóлосом talk in a dráwling/síngsong voice.

протяну́ть(ся) *сов. см.* протя́гивать(ся).

проучи́ть *сов.* (*вн.*) 1. *разг.* (*наказáть*) teach* (*smb.*) a good lésson; 2. (*учить в течéние какóго-л. времени*) (*что-л.*) stúdy (*smth.*); (*когó-л.*) teach* (*smb.*); ~ урóки весь вéчер spend* the whole évening óver/at *one's* hómework; всю жизнь ~ детéй spend* *one's* whole life téaching children. **~ся** *сов.* stúdy; ~ся в шкóле нéсколько лет atténd school for séveral years.

профáн м. ignorámus; быть ~ом в чём-л. not know the first thing abóut *smth.*

профан|áция ж. profanátion, desecrátion. **~и́ровать** *несов. и сов.* (*вн.*) profáne (*smth.*), désecrate (*smth.*).

профбилéт м. tráde-union card.

профбюрó с. *нескл.* tráde-union buréau.

профгрупóрг м. (*вы́борный руководи́тель профсою́зной гру́ппы*) tráde-union group órganizer.

профгру́ппа ж. tráde-union group.

профессионáл м. proféssional.

профессионáльн|ый proféssional; ~ые болéзни occupátional/indústrial diséases; ~ игрóк proféssional (pláyer); ~ое образовáние vocátional tráining; ◇ ~ сою́з trade únion.

профéсси|я ж. proféssion; (*людéй физи́ческого трудá тж.*) trade; врач по ~и dóctor by proféssion.

профéссор м. proféssor. **~ский** professórial; **~ское** звáние the títle of proféssor. **~ство** с. proféssorship.

профессу́р|а ж. 1. (*дóлжность*) proféssorship; получи́ть ~у be* appóinted to a proféssorship; 2. *собир.* the proféssors *pl*, the proféssorate.

профилáктика ж. 1. *мед.* prophyláxis, prevéntive tréatment; 2. *тех.* máintenance chéck-up.

профилакти́ческий prophyláctic, prevéntive.

профилактóрий м. preventórium.

прóфиль м. 1. (*лицá*) prófile, síde-face; в ~ in prófile; 2. *тех.* prófile; (*фóрма*) shape; 3. (*совоку́пность типи́ческих черт*) type, cháracter; ~ вýза type of cóllege.

профильтровáть *сов.* (*вн.*) filter (*smth.*).

профко́м *м.* lócal tráde-union commíttee.

профо́рг *м.* (вы́борный руководи́тель профсою́зной гру́ппы) tráde-union group órganizer.

профорганиза́ция *ж.* lócal tráde-union organizátion.

профориента́ция *ж.* (ориента́ция в вы́боре профе́ссии) caréer-guidance.

профо́рм|а *ж. разг.* formálity; для ~ы as a mátter of form, for form's sake, for the sake of appéarances.

профрабо́тник *м.* tráde-union wórker.

профсою́з *м.* trade únion. ~ный tráde-union *attr.*; ~ное собра́ние tráde-union méeting; ~ный биле́т tráde--union card.

профтехучи́лище *с.* (профессиона́льно-техни́ческое учи́лище) vocátional téchnical school.

прожива́ться, пройти́сь walk, stroll; pace up; ~ по у́лице walk up and down the street; ~ по ко́мнате pace up and down the room; ◇ пройти́сь на чей-л. счёт, пройти́сь по чьему́-л. а́дресу have* a dig at *smb.*

прохла́да *ж.* cool, cóolness, fréshness; вече́рняя ~ the cool of évening; у́тренняя ~ the éarly mórning cool, the cóolness of the éarly mórning air.

прохлади́тельны|й refréshing, cóoling; ~е напи́тки non-alcohólic drinks, soft drinks.

прохлади́ться *сов. см.* прохлажда́ться 1.

прохла́дн|о 1. *нареч.* cóolly; *перен. разг.* unenthusiástically, unrespónsively; **2.** *в знач. сказ. безл.* (о пого́де) it is cool, it is chílly; сего́дня ~ it's cool todáy; **3.** *в знач. сказ. безл.* (дт.; об ощуще́нии прохла́ды): ему́ бы́ло ~ he felt chílly. ~ый cool, fresh; *перен. разг.* cool, unrespónsive; ~ый ве́тер cool wind, fresh breeze; ~ое отноше́ние к това́рищу cool áttitude to a friend.

прохла́дц|а *ж.:* с ~ей 1) (без усе́рдия) withóut cáring; 2) (равноду́шно) indífferently, cóolly; де́лать что-л. с ~ей take* one's time óver *smth.*, do* *smth.* withóut máking much éffort.

прохлажда́ться, прохлади́ться *разг.* **1.** (освежа́ться) take* the air; **2.** *тк. несов.* (безде́льничать) take* things éasy, idle one's time awáy; **3.** *тк. несов.* (ме́дленно де́лать что-л.) loaf (abóut), take* one's time, dáwdle.

прохо́д *м.* pássage; (в аудито́рии) aisle, gángway; (го́рный) pass; оставля́ть ~ leave* a pássage-way; ◇ ~а нет от кого́-л. *smb.* gives one no peace; ~а не дава́ть кому́-л. give* *smb.* no peace; ни ~а, ни прое́зда not a chance of gétting through.

прохо́димец *м. разг.* rogue, ráscal.

прохо́дим|ость *ж.* **1.** (доро́г) practicabílity; **2.** *мед.* permeabílity; **3.** (тра́нспорта) cross-cóuntry abílity; автомоби́ль повы́шенной ~ости cross-cóuntry véhicle. ~ый pássable, prácticable.

проходи́ть I, пройти́ 1. pass; ~ ми́мо pass by; ~ че́рез pass through; он прошёл незаме́тно he passed by unobsérved; пройти́ по́ мосту́ cross a bridge; посети́тели прошли́ в кабине́т the vísitors went/passed ínto the stúdy; доро́га прохо́дит о́коло дере́вни the road pásses close to the víllage; **2.** (вн.; како́е-л. расстоя́ние) cóver (*smth.*), do* (*smth.*); (о тра́нспорте тж.) trável (*smth.*); мы прошли́ два́дцать киломе́тров не остана́вливаясь we did twénty kílometres withóut stópping; за час по́езд прошёл то́лько 50 киломе́тров the train trávelled ónly fífty kílometres in an hour; **3.** (вн.; минова́ть, оставля́ть позади́ себя́) pass (*smth.*), pass through (*smth.*); (по оши́бке) miss (*smth.*); заговори́вшись, пройти́ поворо́т доро́ги miss one's túrning while tálking; **4.** (распространя́ться — о слуха́х и т. п.) go* round, get* aróund; по дере́вне прошёл слух, что... a rúmour went round the víllage that...; **5.** (продвига́ться че́рез что-л.) go* through; шкаф не пройдёт в дверь the wárdrobe won't go through the door; **6.** (проса́чиваться) go* through, seep through; **7.** (вн., че́рез вн.; подверга́ться чему́-л.) go* through, endúre (*smth.*), expérience (*smth.*); ~ че́рез тяжёлые испыта́ния go*

through an ordéal; **8.** (о вре́мени) pass, slip awáy, elápse; мно́го лет прошло́ с тех пор years have elápsed since then; дни прохо́дят незаме́тно the days slip by; как вре́мя бы́стро прохо́дит! how time does fly!; **9.** (зака́нчиваться с каки́м-л. результа́том) go* off; докла́д прошёл уда́чно the lécture was a succéss, the lécture went off well; конце́рт прошёл хорошо́ the cóncert was a succéss; **10.** (вн.; заверша́ть како́й-л. курс) take* (*smth.*), do* (*smth.*); ~ пра́ктику do* one's práctical tráining; пройти́ курс лече́ния undergó*/take* a course of tréatment; **11.** (прекраща́ться) stop; (о бо́ли) pass off, go* off; дождь прошёл it has stopped ráining; головна́я боль у него́ прошла́ his héadache has passed off; **12.** (быть утверждённым) pass, be* adópted, be* appróved; резолю́ция прошла́ the resolútion has been passed/adópted; прое́кт прошёл the design has been accépted; **13.** *разг.* (быть при́нятым, и́збранным) be* accépted; его́ кандидату́ра прошла́ his cándidature has been accépted/appróved; **14.** (вн.) *разг.* (изуча́ть) go* (*smth.*), stúdy (*smth.*); ~ теорети́ческую грамма́тику stúdy theorétical grámmar; ◇ э́то не пройдёт that won't do/work.

проход|и́ть II *сов.* (провести́ како́е-л. вре́мя в ходьбе́) walk, tramp; он пять часо́в ~и́л по́ лесу he tramped abóut in the fórest for five hours.

прохо́дка *ж. горн.* (вертика́льная) sínking; (горизонта́льная) drífting, dríving.

проходна́я *ж.* gátekeeper's óffice.

проходн|о́й communicáting; ~ые ко́мнаты communicáting rooms; ◇ ~а́я бу́дка éntrance-gate; ~ двор communicáting yard.

прохо́дчик *м.* cútter, drífter.

прохожде́ние *с.* pássing, pássage.

прохо́жий *прил.* **1.** pássing; **2.** *в знач. сущ. м.* pásser-by.

прохрипе́ть *сов. см.* хрипе́ть.

процвета́ть *с.* flóurishing/thríving state; (благосостоя́ние тж.) prospérity.

процвета́ть *несов.* flóurish, thríve*; (экономи́чески тж.) prósper.

процеди́ть *сов. см.* проце́живать.

процеду́р|а *ж.* **1.** procédure; ~ голосова́ния vóting procédure; ~ подписа́ния догово́ра procédure for signing a tréaty; **2.** *мед.* (проце́сс лече́ния) tréatment; ходи́ть на ~ы take* tréatments, go* for tréatment.

проце́живать, процеди́ть (вн.) **1.** filter (*smth.*), strain (*smth.*); **2.:** процеди́ть что-л. сквозь зу́бы mútter/say* betwéen one's teeth.

проце́нт *м.* **1.** (со́тая до́ля) per cent; три ~а three per cent; вы́полнить план на сто ~ов fulfil the plan one húndred per cent; **2.** (до́ля це́лого без указа́ния числа́) percéntage; то́лько небольшо́й ~ студе́нтов отсу́тствовал ónly a small percéntage of the stúdents was absent; **3.** *мат.* interest; просты́е (сло́жные) ~ы símple (cómpound) interest *sg*; **4.** (дохо́д с капита́ла) interest; учётный ~ díscount rate; сберега́тельный банк пла́тит три ~а го́довых the sávings-bank pay three per cent interest per ánnum. ~ный **1.** (вы́раженный в проце́нтах) percéntage *attr.*; **2.** (принося́щий проце́нты) interest-bearing; ~ные бума́ги interest-bearing secúrities; ~ные начисле́ния interest chárges.

проце́сс *м.* **1.** (ход разви́тия чего́-л.) prócess; в ~е разви́тия in the prócess of devélopment; хими́ческий ~ chémical prócess; в ~е игры́ in the course of the game; **2.** *мед.:* ~ в лёгких tuberculósis of the lungs; **3.** *юр.* légal procéedings *pl*; (суде́бное де́ло) case; гражда́нский ~ láwsuit, suit; уголо́вный ~ (críminal) tríal; нача́ть суде́бный ~ про́тив кого́-л. bring*/énter an áction agáinst *smb.*, institute procéedings agáinst *smb.*, sue *smb.*

проце́ссия *ж.* procéssion.

процити́ровать *сов. см.* цити́ровать.

прочеса́ть *сов. см.* прочёсывать.

прочéсть *сов. см.* читáть.

прочёсывать, прочесáть (*вн.*) 1. comb (*smth.*) out; (*шерсть*) tease (*smth.*); 2. *разг.* (*тщательно осматривать местность*) comb (*smth.*); прочесáть лес comb a wood.

проч|ий *прил.* 1. óther; 2. *в знач. сущ. с.:* и ~ee et cétera, etc., and the rest, and so on; и всё ~ee and éverything else; помúмо всегó ~его on top of all this, apárt from éverything else; 3. *в знач. сущ. мн.:* все ~ие all the óthers; ◇ мéжду ~им by the by, by the way.

прочúстить *сов. см.* прочищáть.

прочитáть *сов. см.* читáть.

прочищáть, прочúстить (*вн.*) 1. clear (*smth.*), clear (*smth.*) out, clean (*smth.*) out; (*кишечник тж.*) purge (*smth.*); ~ трýбку clean out one's pipe; 2. (*делать более редким — лес, заросли и т. п.*) thin out (*smth.*).

прóчн|о sólidly, fírmly, secúrely; ~ устрóиться estáblish one*self* fírmly/secúrely; стрóить ~ build* próperly/sólidly. ~ость ж. strength, cohésion; (*здания тж.*) stability; (*одежды, обуви и т. п.*) durability; (*знаний*) sóundness, reliability; (*дружбы*) strength, stability. ~ый (*крепкий*) strong, dúrable; (*устойчивый*) stáble; *перен.* endúring, lásting; ~ый фундáмент sólid/dúrable foundátion; ~ая мéбель substántial fúrniture; ~ая обувь dúrable/strong shoes *pl*; ~ая матéрия dúrable cloth; ~ый мир lásting peace; ~ый союз stáble alliance; ~ая семья united fámily; ~ые знáния sound knówledge.

прочýвствовать *сов.* (*вн.*) 1. (*воспринять чувствами что-л.*) feel* (*smth.*); 2. (*пережить, испытать*) live (*smth.*), live through (*smth.*).

прочь awáy, off; ~ с дорóги! get out of the way!; рýки ~! hands off!; ◇ не ~ (+ *инф.*) wóuldn't mind (+ -ing), have* no objéction to (+ -ing), be* not avérse to (+ -ing); я не ~ I don't mind; он не ~ пойтú he wóuldn't mind góing; он не ~ вúпить чáшку кóфе he wouldn't mind a cup of cóffee.

прошéдш|ий *прил.* 1. last; ~ей зимóй last winter; 2. *в знач. сущ. с.* the past; ◇ ~ee врéмя *грам.* the past tense.

прошептáть *сов. см.* шептáть.

прошéстви|е *с.:* по ~и (*рд.*) áfter the lapse (of); (*о сроке*) on expíry (of); по ~и стóльких лет áfter the lapse of so mány years; по ~и срóка on expíry of the term, when the term expíres.

прошивáть, прошúть (*вн.*) sew* (*smth.*) on; (*делать швы*) stitch (*smth.*).

прошúть *сов. см.* прошивáть. ·

прошлогóдний last year's; of the year befóre *после сущ.*

прóшл|ое *с.* the past; далёкое ~ the remóte past; недáвнее ~ the récent past; отойтú в ~ pass awáy. ~ый (*прошедший*) past; (*предыдущий*) last; в ~ые временá in bygone days; на ~ой недéле last week; в ~ом годý last year; дéло ~ое a thing of the past.

прошмыгнýть *сов.* (*в вн.*) *разг.* steal* (into), slip (into).

проштудúровать *сов. см.* штудúровать.

прощáй(те) goodbýe!; farewéll!

прощáльный пáрting; farewéll *attr.*; ~ визúт párting visit; ~ поцелýй párting kiss; ~ обéд farewéll dínner.

прощáние *с.* párting, farewéll, léave-taking; ◇ на ~ in párting; помахáть на ~ wave goodbýe.

прощáть, простúть 1. (*вн.*) forgíve* (*smb., smth.*), párdon (*smb., smth.*); 2. (*вн. дт.*): освобождáть от обязáтельства) reléase (*smb.* from), remít (*smth.* of); простúть долг комý-л. remít *smb.'s* debt.

прощáться, простúться, попрощáться (с *тв.*) say* goodbýe (to); take* one's leave (of), bid* farewéll (to); bid* (*smb.*) farewéll; он попрощáлся и ушёл he said goodbýe and went awáy.

прощéни|е *с.* forgíveness, párdon; просúть ~я у когó-л. ask/beg *smb.'s* párdon; (*за что-л. серьёзное*)

ask/beg *smb.'s* forgíveness; ◇ прошý ~я I beg your párdon.

прощýпать *сов. см.* прощýпывать.

прощýпывать, прощýпать (*вн.*) feel* (*smth.*), touch (*smth.*); *несов. тж.* grope for (*smth.*); *перен.* sound (*smb.*); ~ путь feel* the way. ~ся *несов.* can* be felt, be* nóticeable to the touch.

проэкзаменовáть(ся) *сов. см.* экзаменовáть(ся).

проявúтель *м. фото* devéloper.

прояв|úть(ся) *сов. см.* проявлять(ся). ~лéние *с.* 1. manifestátion, displáy; ~лéние хрáбрости displáy of cóurage; 2. *фото* devélopment.

проявлять, проявúть (*вн.*) 1. show* (*smth.*), displáy (*smth.*); проявúть большúе знáния evínce great léarning; проявúть большýю актúвность displáy great actívity; проявúть забóту о ком-л. show* concérn for *smb.*; проявúть большýю хрáбрость exhíbit/displáy great cóurage; ~ нетерпéние show* impátience; ~ нерешúтельность hésitate; 2. *фото* devélop (*smth.*); ~ плёнку devélop a film; ~ снúмок devélop a phóto; ◇ проявúть себя show* one's worth; он проявúл себя талáнтливым руководúтелем he showed himsélf to be a first-ráte léader. ~ся, проявúться 1. show* itsélf, manifést itsélf; 2. *фото* be* devéloped, devélop.

прояснúться *сов. см.* проясняться.

проясня|ться, проясниться 1. (*становиться ясным, хорошо видимым*) show* up cléarly/distínctly, becóme* distínct; 2. (*о погоде*) clear (up); 3. (*становиться понятным*) clárify, becóme* clear; положéние проясни́лось the situation has clárified; 4. (*о лице*) light* up, brighten; 5. (*о сознании*) clear, becóme* lúcid/clear; постепéнно мои мысли прояснúлись grádually my mind cleared.

пруд *м.* pond. ~úть *несов.* (*вн.*) pond (*smth.*) back, pond (*smth.*) up; ◇ хоть пруд ~ú чего-л. loads of *smth.*; дéнег у негó — хоть пруд ~ú he's rólling in móney, he has pots/tons of móney.

пружúн|а *ж.* (*прям. и перен.*) spring; часовáя ~ wátch-spring; глáвная ~ máinspring; ◇ нажáть на все ~ы pull évery string, leave* no stone untúrned; быть как на ~ах have* springs in one's heels. ~истый spríngly, resílient; (*о движениях тела*) súpple, lithe.

пружúн|ить *несов.* 1. be* resílient; 2. (*вн.; напрягáть*) flex (*smth.*); ~ мышцы flex one's múscles. ~иться *несов.* be* spríngly, yield spríngily. ~ный spring *attr.*; ~ный матрáс spring máttress.

прусáк *м.* (*таракан*) cóckroach.

прут *м.* 1. twig, switch, rod; 2. (*металлический стержень*) rod.

прыг|ать *несов.* 1. jump, leap*; (*о детях*) skip; (*на одной ноге*) hop; ~ с парашютом make* párachute jumps; 2. (*о мяче*) bounce, rebóund; 3. *разг.* (*вздрагивать*) twitch, jump; сéрдце егó ~ало от рáдости his heart leaped for joy, his heart bóunded with joy.

прыгнуть *сов.* take* a leap/jump.

прыгýн *м.* 1. (*спортсмен*) júmper; 2. (*о ребёнке*) júmping jack, grásshopper.

прыжóк *м.* jump, leap; (*с упором*) vault; ~ в высотý high jump; ~ в длинý long jump; ~ с разбéга rúnning jump; ~ в вóду dive; ~ с трамплúна (*на лыжах*) ski-jump.

прýткий *разг.* lívely, ágile, nímble.

прыть *ж. разг.* 1. (*быстрота*) speed, rápid pace; 2. (*проворство*) énergy, go, vim; ◇ бежáть во всю ~ go* for all *one* is worth; откýда ~ взялáсь! where did the énergy come from?

прыщ *м.* pímple; pústule *мед.* ~áвый *разг.* pímpled.

прядéние *с.* spínning.

прядúльн|ый spínning *attr.*; ~ая машúна spínning-machine, spínning-frame; ~ая фáбрика spínning-mill, spínning-factory.

прядúльщ|ик *м.*, ~ица *ж.* spínner.

прядь ж. lock; (*женских волос тж.*) tress.

пряжа ж. yarn; кручёная ~ twist (yarn); шерстяная ~ woollen yarn.

пряжка ж. buckle; (*застёжка*) clasp; ~ для пояса belt-buckle.

прялка ж. (*ручная*) distaff; (*с колесом*) spinning--wheel.

прям|ая ж. straight line; проводить ~ую draw* a straight line; по ~ой in a bee-line, as the crow flies; лететь по ~ой на юг make* a bee-line for the south; конечная ~ *ав.* final leg.

прям|о *нареч.* 1. straight; держаться ~ hold* oneself straight; идти ~ go* straight; 2. (*непосредственно*) straight; идти ~ к цели go*/fly* straight to the mark/target; приступить ~ к делу come* straight to the point; спать на полу sleep* on the bare floor; 3. (*откровенно*) plainly, bluntly, frankly; говорить ~ talk straight; 4. *в знач. усил. частицы разг.* (*совершенно — при сущ.*) real; (*при прил.*) really; это ~ наказание! it's a downright ordeal/nuisance!; это ~ удивительно it's really amazing; я ~ не знаю, что делать I really don't know what to do; 5. *в знач. усил. частицы разг.* (*как раз*) right, directly; ~ напротив directly/right/just opposite; ~ в лоб right in the forehead; ударить *кого-л.* ~ в лицо hit* *smb.* full in the face; попадать ~ в цель hit* the mark, strike* home. ~ой 1. straight; ~ая линия straight line; ~ые волосы straight hair *sg*; 2. (*обеспечивающий непосредственную связь*) through, direct; ~ое сообщение through traffic; ~ой поезд through train; говорить по ~ому проводу speak* by direct line; 3. (*непосредственный*) direct; ~ые выборы direct elections; ~ые указания direct instructions; 4. (*откровенный, правдивый*) straightforward; ~ой человек straightforward person; ~ой ответ straightforward answer; 5. (*явный, открытый*) open, obvious; ~ой вызов open challenge; ~ой обман obvious trickery; 6. (*безусловный, действительный*) sheer; ~ая необходимость sheer necessity; ~ой смысл поступить так there is every reason to act like that; ◇ ~ой ворот upright collar; ~ая дорога, ~ой путь к *чему-л.* direct road to *smth.*, highroad to *smth.*; ~ая речь *грам.* direct speech; ~ой угол *мат.* right angle; ~ая кишка *анат.* rectum; в ~ом смысле слова in the ordinary sense of the word; ~ая линия родства direct line of descent; ~ое попадание direct hit.

прямолинейн|ость ж. 1. straightness of line; 2. (*прямота*) straightforwardness; 3. (*отсутствие гибкости*) rigidity. ~ый 1. (*расположенный по прямой линии*) rectilineal, rectilinear; 2. (*открытый, прямой*) straightforward; ~ый человек straightforward person; 3. (*односторонний, негибкий*) rigid, inflexible.

прямота ж. straightforwardness, direct manner, plain dealing.

прямоугольн|ик м. rectangle. ~ый rectangular; ~ый треугольник right-angled triangle.

пряник м. gingerbread; медовый ~ honeycake.

прян|ость ж. spice. ~ый spicy.

прясть, спрясть (*вн.*) spin* (*smth.*); ~ пряжу spin* yarn; ~ на прялке spin* on a spinning-wheel.

прят|ать, спрятать (*вн.*) 1. hide* (*smth.*), conceal (*smth.*); ~ ключи hide* the keys; ~ улыбку conceal a smile; 2. (*класть для сохранности*) put* away (*smth.*); ~ шубу на лето put* away a fur-coat for the summer. ~аться, спрятаться hide*; (*укрываться от чего-л.*) keep* under cover. ~ки *мн.* hide-and-seek *sg*; играть в ~ки play hide-and-seek; *перен.* play a shifty game.

псалом *м.* psalm.

псарня ж. kennel.

псевдо- *в сложн.* pseudo-.

псевдонаучный pseudo-scientific.

псевдоним pseudonym, assumed name; (*литературный*) pen-name, nom de plume.

психиатр *м.* psychiatrist.

психиатрическ|ий psychiatric; ~ая больница mental hospital, lunatic asylum.

психиатрия ж. psychiatry.

психика ж. mentality, psychology, mind.

психическ|и mentally; ~ больной mental patient/case. ~ий mental, psychological; ~ое расстройство mental derangement; ◇ ~ая атака psychological attack.

психоз *м.* psychosis.

психолог *м.* psychologist.

психологический psychological; ~ роман psychological novel.

психология ж. psychology.

психопат *м.* psychopath, a mental case; nut-case *разг.*

пташка ж. (small) bird; ранняя ~ early bird.

птенец *м.* fledgeling, nestling.

птица ж. bird; *собир.* birds *pl*, fowl(s).

птицевод *м.* poultry farmer. ~ство *с.* poultry farming. ~ческий poultry *attr.*; ~ческая ферма poultry farm.

птицелов *м.* fowler.

птицефабрика ж. integrated poultry farm.

пти|чий bird *attr.*; ~чье гнездо bird's nest; ~ корм birdseed; ◇ ~ двор poultry yard/run; жить на ~чьих правах live* a precarious existence.

птичк|а ж. 1. small bird; 2. *разг.* (*пометка*) tick; пометить *что-л.* ~ой tick off *smth.*

птичн|ик м. 1. (*помещение*) poultry house; 2. (*работник*) poultry-keeper. ~ица ж. poultry-maid.

ПТУ *с. нескл. см.* профтехучилище.

публика ж. *собир.* 1. public; (*в театре и т. п. тж.*) audience; широкая ~ the general public, the public at large; 2. *разг.* (*люди, народ*) people.

публикация ж. 1. (*действие*) publication; 2. (*то, что опубликовано*) published work; 3. (*объявление*) advertisement.

публиковать, опубликовать (*вн.*) publish (*smth.*).

публицист *м.* publicist, journalist. ~ика ж. journalism, publicistic writing. ~ический journalistic, publicistic.

публичн|о in public; (*открыто*) openly, publicly. ~ый public; ~ая речь public speech.

пугало *с.* (*в огороде и т. п.*) scarecrow; *перен.* bogy, bugbear.

пуган|ый frightened; ◇ ~ая ворона и куста боится *посл.* a burnt child dreads the fire, once bit twice shy.

пугать, испугать (*вн.*) frighten (*smth.*), alarm (*smth.*); *сов. тж.* startle (*smth.*), give* (*smth.*) a fright; (*угрожать*) threaten (*smth.*). ~ся, испугаться (*рд.*) be*/feel* frightened (of), take* fright (at); *сов. тж.* get* a fright; не пугайтесь! don't be frightened!; испугаться до смерти be* scared to death; лошади испугались the horses took fright; испугаться *чьего-л.* вида be* shocked by *smb.'s* appearance.

пугливый timorous, timid; (*выражающий испуг*) apprehensive; (*о лошади*) nervous.

пугови|ца ж. button; застегнуться на все ~цы button up one's coat. ~чный button *attr.*; ~чное производство button manufacture.

пудель *м.* poodle.

пудинг *м.* pudding.

пудра ж. powder; ◇ сахарная ~ confectioner's/powdered sugar.

пудреница ж. powder-case.

пудрить, напудрить (*вн.*) powder (*smth.*); ~ лицо powder one's face. ~ся, напудриться powder oneself, put* powder on one's face.

пузырёк *м.* 1. (*в жидкости*) bubble, bead; 2. (*бутылочка*) phial.

пузырь *м.* 1. bubble; 2. (*волдырь*) blister; 3. *анат.* bladder.

пук *м.* bundle; (*цветов*) bunch.

пулемёт *м.* machíne-gun; ручнóй ~ light machíne-gun. ~ный machíne-gun *attr.*; ~ная рóта machine-gun cómpany. ~чик *м.* machíne-gunner.

пульверизáтор *м.* spray, spráyer, púlverizer; ~ для духóв scént-spray.

пульс *м.* pulse; пощýпать ~ feel* *smb.'s* pulse; частотá ~áция *ж.* pulsátion, pulse. ~и́ровать *несов.* pulsáte, pulse, beat*; (*сильно*) throb.

пульт *м.* 1. (*подставка для нот*) músic-stand; 2. *тех.* contról desk/pánel; cónsole; ~ управлéния шлюзами slúice-gate contról room; ~ электростáнции pówer-station contról room; диспéтчерский ~ contról desk.

пýля *ж.* búllet.

пункт *м.* 1. (*место в пространстве*) point, spot; сáмый востóчный ~ нáшей страны́ the éasternmost point of our cóuntry; стратеги́ческий ~ stratégic point; 2. (*место, помещение, приспособленное для какой-л. работы и т. п.*) post, óffice, státion; 3. (*раздел документа, статьи*) páragraph, ítem, point; послéдний ~ пя́той статьи́ договóра the last páragraph of árticle 5 of the tréaty; основны́е ~ы доклáда the main points in the repórt; 4. (*отдельный момент в развитии чего-л.*) point; 5. *полигр.* point; ◇ по ~ам point by point, in détail.

пунктир *м.* dótted line; начерти́ть *что-л.* ~ом dot *smth.* ~ный dótted; ~ная ли́ния dótted line.

пунктуáльн|ость *ж.* punctuálity. ~ый púnctual.

пунктуáция *ж. грам.* punctuátion, póinting.

пýнкция *ж. мед.* púncture.

пунсóн *ж. полигр.* punch; (engráver's) point.

пунцóвый crímson.

пунш *м.* punch.

пуп|овина *ж. анат.* umbílical cord. ~óк *м.* nável.

пургá *ж.* blízzard, snów-storm.

пури́зм *м.* púrism.

пýрпур *м.* púrple.

пурпýр|ный, ~овый púrple.

пуск *м.* stárting; (*машины тж.*) sétting in mótion; (*домны*) firing; (*ракеты*) láunch(ing).

пускáй *см.* пусть.

пускáть, пусти́ть (*вн.*) 1. (*отпускать*) let* (*smb., smth.*) go; (*давать свободу тж.*) set* (*smb., smth.*) free; (*разрешать*) let* (*smb.*); пусти́ть пти́цу на вóлю set* a bird free; пусти́ть ребёнка гуля́ть let* a child* go out for a walk; 2. (*впускать, пропускать*) let* (*smb.*) in; ~ когó-л. ночевáть let* *smb.* stay the night; ~ жильцóв take* in lódgers; 3.(*приводить в действие*) start (*smth.*); (*машину тж.*) set* (*smth.*) góing, put*/set* (*smth.*) in mótion; ~ мотóр start an éngine; ~ ракéту fire a rócket; (*космическую*) launch a rócket; 4. (*пар, газ и т. п.*) turn on (*smth.*); ~ фонтáны turn on the fóuntains; ~ вóду в вáнну turn on the bath; ~ вóду в канáл let* wáter into a canál; 5. (*заставлять двигаться*) start (*smth.*) off, send* (*smth.*) off; ~ лóшадь галóпом start (off) *one's* horse at a gállop; 6. (*бросать*) throw* (*smth.*); (*несильно*) toss (*smth.*); ~ кáмни в когó-л. throw* stones at *smb.*; 7. (*обращать для какой-л. надобности*) put* (*smth.*); ~ *что-л.* в продáжу put* *smth.* on sale, reléase *smth.* for sale; 8. *разг.* (*распространять*) spread* (*smth.*); ~ слух set* a rúmour abóut/aflóat; 9. (*давать ростки*) put* out (*smth.*); ~ ростки́ put* out shoots; ◇ ~ кровь комý-л. bleed* *smb.*; ~ *что-л.* в обращéние put* *smth.* into circulátion; ~ *что-л.* ко дну send* *smth.* to the bóttom; ~ в ход все срéдства leave* no stone untúrned, neglect no means. ~ся, пусти́ться 1. (*отправляться*) start, set* out; пусти́ться в путь start/set* out on *one's* jóurney; пусти́ться бежáть take* to *one's* heels; пусти́ться вдогóнку за кем-л. set* off/out in pursúit of *smb.*; 2. (*в вн.; начинать что-л.*) start (*smth.*), embárk on (*smth.*); пусти́ться во все подрóбности go*/énter into all the détails; ~ся в пляс dance, fling* onesélf into a dance; ~ся в рискóванное предприя́тие

go* in for a rísky undertáking; ~ся в объяснéния énter into explanátions; 3. (*на вн.; отваживаться*) resórt (to), risk (*smth.*).

пуск|óй stárting *attr.*; (*для запуска ракет*) láunching *attr.*; ~ механи́зм stárting méchanism/device, stárter; ~óе ракéтное устрóйство rócket-launching device, láuncher; ~áя площáдка láunching pad.

пустельгá *ж.* windhover, késtrel.

пустéть, опустéть becóme* émpty; (*становиться безлюдным*) becóme* desérted.

пусти́ть(ся) *сов. см.* пускáть(ся).

пýсто *в знач. сказ. безл.* 1. it is émpty; (*безлюдно*) it is desérted; в кóмнате бы́ло ~ the room was émpty; the room looked émpty; 2. (*о чувстве*): на душé у негó бы́ло ~ he felt used up, he felt void of all féeling; ◇ то рýсто, то ~ either too much or too little.

пуст|овáть *несов.* be*/stand* émpty; помещéние ~ýет the building is stánding émpty.

пустоголóвый *разг.* empty-héaded, shállow.

пустозвóн *м. разг.* windbag. ~ство *с.* verbósity, vérbiage, wórdiness, mere talk.

пуст|óй *прил.* 1. (*ничем не заполненный*) émpty; (*полый*) hóllow; (*незанятый*) vácant; (*безлюдный*) desérted; (*свободный от занятий*) free; ~ая корóбка émpty box; ~ дом desérted house; ~ урóк free lésson; ~ие щи cábbage soup without any meat; 2. (*несерьёзный, ограниченный*) shállow, émpty; ~ человéк shállow pérson; 3. (*бессодержательный*) émpty, hóllow; (*неосновательный*) unfóunded; ~ие словá mere/émpty words; ~ие обещáния hóllow prómises; ~ая отговóрка mere excúse; ~ие развлечéния fútile amúsements; 4. (*ничтожный*) trívial, slight; 5. *в знач. сущ. с.* nóthing, a mere nóthing; (*вздор*) rúbbish; ◇ ~ое мéсто nonéntity; с ~ыми рукáми empty-hánded.

пустослóв|ие *с.* émpty chátter, twáddle. ~ить *несов. разг.* chátter.

пустотá *ж.* émptiness (*тж. перен.*); (*незаполненное пространство*) hóllowness; *физ.* vácuum.

пустоцвéт *м.* stérile flówer; *перен.* fáilure.

пýстошь *ж.* waste ground.

пусты́нный 1. (*необитаемый*) désert; 2. (*безлюдный*) desérted, lónely.

пусты́ня *ж.* désert; wílderness *поэт.*

пусты́рь *м.* waste ground.

пусть 1. *частица передаётся посредством гл.* let (+ *инф.*) ~ развлекáются let them amúse themsélves; ~ бýдет так! véry well!; just as you like!, have it your own way!; ~ он идёт let him go; скажи́те ей, ~ помбет посýду tell her she had bétter wash the dishes; 2. *частица* (*ладно, так и быть*) all right; ну ~, я соглáсен all right, I agrée; 3. *союз* (*допустим, хотя*) suppóse, éven though; ~ он оши́бся, но оши́бку мóжно испрáвить well, what if he is mistáken — can't the mistáke be réctified?, he may be mistáken, but the mistáke isn't irrévocable, is it?; 4. *союз* (*хотя бы, даже*) éven.

пустя́к *м.* 1. trífle, bagatélle; занимáться ~áми waste time on trífles; ссóриться из-за ~ов quárrel óver nóthing, quárrel óver a mere trífle; обижáться из-за ~á take* offénce at a mere trífle; 2. *обыкн. мн.* (*вздор*) nónsense *sg*; онá говори́ла ~и, неумéстно смея́лась her talk was nonsénsical, her láughter irrélevant; 3. *обыкн. мн. в знач. сказ.* (*неважно*) néver mind!; ~и, всё уля́дится néver mind, éverything will be all right; ~и для негó э́то пáра ~ов it's mere child's play for him.

пуст|яковый, ~я́чный *разг.* trífling; ~я́ковое дéло trifling mátter.

пýтан|ик *м. разг.* múddler, múddle-head. ~ица *ж.* 1. (*неразбериха*) múddle, confúsion; у негó большáя ~ица в головé his mind is one big múddle; 2. (*запутанность в расположении чего-л.*) maze.

пýтан|ый 1. (*запутанный*) meándering, wínding, zígzag; ~ след зáйца the meándering tracks of a hare;

~ые во́лосы dishévelled/rúffled hair *sg*; 2. (*сбивчивый, нелогичный*) confúsed, stúmbling, incohérent; он вы́слушал мою́ ~ую речь he let me tell my incohérent stóry.

пу́т|ать *несов.* 1. (*вн.; приводить в беспорядок*) tángle (*smth.*); (*бумаги*) múddle (*smth.*) up, mix (*smth.*) up; ~ ни́тки tángle threads; ~ во́лосы rúffle hair; (*вн.; сбивать с толку*) confúse (*smb.*); 3. (*говорить сбивчиво*) get* mixed up, mix things up; не ~ай, говори́ пря́мо! don't beat abóut the bush, out with it!; 4. (*вн.; смешивать с кем-л., чем-л.*) take* (*smb., smth.*) for; ~ имена́ confúse names, múddle up names; я ~аю вас с ва́шим бра́том I take you for your bróther, I confúse you with your bróther; 5. (*вн. в вн.*) *разг.* (*вовлекать кого-л. в неприятное дело*) mix (*smb.*) up (in), ímplicate (*smb.* in), invólve (*smb.* in); 6. (*вн.; надевать путы на ноги лошади*) hóbble (*smth.*). ~аться *несов. разг.* 1. (*приходить в беспорядок*) get* tángled; 2. (*сбиваться, ошибаться*) get* confúsed, get* múddled, lose* the thread of one's thoughts; 3. (*вмешиваться*) interfére, méddle; не ~айтесь не в своё де́ло don't interfére in what does not concérn you, don't méddle in óther péople's affáirs.

путёвка *ж.* 1. pass; ~ в санато́рий pass to a sanatórium; туристи́ческая ~ place in a tóurist group; 2. (*водителя транспорта*) itínerary, schédule.

путеводи́тель *м.* guíde(-book); ~ по музе́ю muséum guide.

путево́дн|ый guíding; ◇ ~ая звезда́ guíding star, lódestar.

путев|о́й 1. ráilway *attr.*, line *attr.*; ~ обхо́дчик tráckwalker; 2. (*относящийся к путешествию*) trável *attr.*, trávelling, itínerary; ~ы́е запи́ски trável notes.

путе́ец *м.* 1. (*инженер*) ráilway enginéer; 2. (*работник службы пути*) ráilwayman*.

путём I *нареч.* próper(ly); cohérently.

путём II *предлог* (*рд.*; *посредством*) by means of, by.

путеше́ственн|ик *м.*, ~ица *ж.* tráveller.

путеше́ствие *с.* jóurney; (*по морю*) vóyage; (*экскурсия, поездка*) trip.

путеше́ствовать *несов.* trável; (*по морю тж.*) vóyage; ~ по стране́ trável abóut/round the cóuntry; ~ вокру́г све́та go*/trável round the world.

пути́на *ж.* fishing séason.

пу́тн|ик *м.*, ~ица *ж.* tráveller, wáyfarer.

пу́тн|ый *прил. разг.* 1. sénsible, wórthwhíle, judícious; 2. *в знач. сущ. с.*: ничего́ ~ого из него́ не вы́йдет he will néver make good, he will néver amóunt to much.

путч *м.* putsch, coup.

пу́ты *мн.* clog *sg*, hóbble *sg*; *перен.* bonds, chains, fétters.

пут|ь *м.* 1. (*дорога*) way, route; во́дный ~ wáter-way; морско́й ~ sea route; вели́кие торго́вые ~и́ the great trade routes; возду́шные ~и́ áir-routes; 2. (*железнодорожная колея*) ráilway track/line, pérmanent way; 3. (*путешествие*) jóurney, way; счастли́вого ~и́! pléasant/good jóurney!; на обра́тном ~и́ on the way back; 4. (*направление, маршрут*) way, course; их ~и́ разошли́сь each took his own course, their ways párted/séparated; 5. (*направление деятельности*) road, path; он на пра́вильном ~и́ he is on the right road; 6. (*способ*) way; means *pl*; ми́рным ~ём by péaceful means, péacefully; 7. *мн. анат.* tract *sg*, duct *sg*; ◇ после́дний ~ last jóurney; ~и́ сообще́ния means of communicátion; ~ сле́дования route; на ~и́ к чему́-л., по ~и́ чего́-л. on the road/way to *smth.*; быть на ~и́ к чему́-л. be* on the road/way to *smth.*; по ~и́ on the way; нам с ва́ми не по ~и́ our ways are not yours; идти́ свои́м ~ём go* one's own way, take* one's own course; напра́вить кого́-л. на ~ и́стины put* *smb.* on the right road.

пух *м.* 1. down; (*на лице тж.*) fuzz; (*на материи*) fluff, nap; 2. *бот.* down, pubéscence; ◇ ни ~а ни пера́! ≈ good luck!; разби́ть в ~ и прах rout complétely.

пу́хлый plump, chúbby.

пу́хнуть *несов.* swell*.

пухо́вка *ж.* pówder-puff.

пухо́вый down *attr.*; made of down *после сущ.*

пучегла́зый *разг.* góggle-eyed.

пучи́на *ж.* 1. (*морская бездна*) the deep; 2. (*в болоте*) the depths *pl*.

пучо́к *м.* 1. little búndle; (*цветов*) pósy, bunch, nósegay; 2. (*лучей*) péncil of (light-)rays, light-pencil; 3. (*причёска*) bun, knot; 4. *физ.* beam; ~ нейтро́нов néutron beam.

пу́шечн|ый gun *attr.*, cánnon *attr.*; ~ая стрельба́ gún-fire; ◇ ~ое мя́со cánnon-fodder.

пуши́нка *ж.* bit of fluff; ~ сне́га féather of snow, féathery snów-flake.

пуши́ст|ый fluffy, dówny; ~ые во́лосы fluffy hair *sg*; ~ котёнок flúffy (líttle) kítten.

пу́шка *ж.* cánnon, gun.

пушн|и́на *ж. собир.* furs *pl*, pelts *pl*. ~о́й fur *attr.*; ~о́й зверь fúr-bearing ánimal, fúr-bearer; ~о́й про́мысел fúr-trade.

пушо́к *м.* fluff, down; (*на плодах*) bloom.

пу́ща *ж.* dense fórest; (*заповедник*) fórest presérve.

пущ|ий: для ~ей ва́жности to enhánce the efféct; to look impórtant.

пчел|а́ *ж.* bee; рабо́чая ~ wórker bee. ~и́ный bee's; bee *attr.*; ~и́ный рой swarm of bees; ~и́ный мёд pure hóney.

пчелово́д *м.* bée-keeper, ápiarist, apicúlturist. ~ство *с.* bée-keeping, ápiculture. ~ческий bée-keeping *attr.*

пче́льник *м.* ápiary.

пшени́|ца *ж.* wheat. ~чный whéaten; ~чная мука́ whéaten flour; ~чный хлеб whéaten bread.

пшённ|ый míllet *attr.*; ~ая ка́ша míllet púdding.

пшено́ *с.* míllet.

пы́жик *м.* 1. (*животное*) young réindeer; 2. (*мех*) young réindeer skin, déerskin.

пыл *м.* férvour, árdour, méttle; охлади́ть чей-л. ~ cool *smb.'s* árdour; ~ в ~у́ сраже́ния, спо́ра *и т. п.* in the heat of the báttle, of debáte, *etc.*; с пы́лу, с жа́ру píping hot.

пыл|а́ть *несов.* 1. flame, blaze; дом ~а́ет the house is on fire, the house is abláze; 2. (*светиться*) be* aglów/abláze (with light); 3. (*о лице*) glow; 4.: ~ гне́вом blaze with ánger; ~ негодова́нием burn* with indignátion; ~ стра́стью be* consúmed with pássion.

пылесо́с *м.* vácuum cléaner.

пыли́нка *ж.* speck/párticle of dust.

пыли́ть, напыли́ть raise the dust. ~ся *несов.* get* dústy, colléct the dust.

пы́лк|ий árdent, férvent, férvid, impétuous; ~ое воображе́ние férvid imaginátion; ~ая любо́вь árdent love; ~ая речь fíery/véhement speech. ~ость *ж.* árdour, férvour, fire, pássion, impetuósity.

пыль *ж.* dust; (*водяная*) spray; выбива́ть ~ из чего́-л. beat* the dust out of *smth.*; ◇ пуска́ть в глаза́ throw* dust in *smb.'s* eyes.

пы́льник I *м. бот.* ánther.

пы́льник II *м. разг.* (*плащ*) light ráincoat; dúster *амер.*

пы́льн|ый dústy; ~ ковёр dústy cárpet, cárpet thick with dust; ~ая доро́га dústy road; ~ городо́к dústy town.

пыльца́ *ж. бот.* póllen.

пыре́й *м. бот.* cóuch-grass.

пыта́ть *несов.* (*вн.*) tórture (*smb.*), tormént (*smb.*). ~ся, попыта́ться try, endéavour, attémpt.

пы́тк|а *ж.* tórture, tórment; *перен. тж.* ánguish; подверга́ть кого́-л. ~е put* *smb.* to tórture; ору́дие ~и instrument of tórture.

пытли́вый cúrious, keen, séarching; ~ ум

keen/séarching mind; ~ взгляд cúrious/séarching look, keen/séarching eyes *pl.*

пыхт|е́ть *несов. разг.* 1. (*тяжело дышать*) pant; puff and blow; (*над тв.*) *перен.* sweat óver (*smth.*); ~ над зада́чей sweat óver a próblem; 2. (*о машинах*) puff; парово́з ~е́л, ме́дленно поднима́ясь в го́ру the éngine puffed slówly up the hill.

пы́шет: он ~ здоро́вьем he's búrsting with health, he's the pícture of health; печь ~ жа́ром the stove is thrówing out a treméndous heat.

пы́шка *ж.* 1. (*булка*) dóughnut, bun; 2. *разг.* (*о женщине*) dúmpling.

пы́шн|ость *ж.* spléndour, súmptuousness; (*великолепие*) magníficence. **~ый** 1. flúffy, fléecy, féathery; (*о волосах*) thick, spléndid; (*о хлебе и т. п.*) light; (*полный*) plump; 2. (*роскошный*) spléndid, magníficent, respléndent; (*о растительности тж.*) luxúriant; 3. (*высокопарный*) high-flown, infláted, vápid.

пьедеста́л *м.* pédestal.

пье́ксы *мн.* (*ед.* пье́кса *ж.*) skí-boots.

пье́са *ж.* 1. *театр.* play; 2. *муз.* piece.

пьяне́ть, опьяне́ть be*/get* drunk/típsy/fúddled; (*от рд.*) *перен.* be* intóxicated (with).

пьян|и́ть, опьяни́ть (*вн.*) make* (*smb.*) drunk/típsy/fúddled; *перен.* intóxicate (*smb.*); его́ ~я́т успе́хи he is intóxicated/drunk with success.

пья́ница *м. и ж.* drúnkard, tóper, típpler.

пья́нка *ж. разг.* binge, dríŋk-up.

пья́нство *с.* drúnkenness, álcoholism. **~вать** *несов.* drink* (héavily).

пья́ный *прил.* 1. drunk, típsy; 2. *в знач. сущ. м.* drunk.

пэр *м.* peer.

пюпи́тр *м.* músic-stand; (*для книг*) bóokrest.

пюре́ *с. нескл.* puráe, mash; карто́фельное ~ mashed potátoes.

пяд|ь *ж.*: ни ~и not an inch; семи́ ~е́й во лбу ≈ wise as Sólomon.

па́льцы *мн.* (*для вышивания*) támbour-frame *sg*; (*для кружев*) láce-frame *sg.*

пят|а́ *ж.* 1. *уст.* heel; 2. (*опорная часть чего-л.*) abútment; ◇ до пят down to *one's* ánkles; ходи́ть за кем-л. по ~а́м tread* on *smb.'s* heels; гна́ться за кем-л. по ~а́м fóllow hard/close/fast on *smb.'s* heels, be* at/upón the heels of *smb.*; быть под ~о́й у кого́-л. be* únder the heel of *smb.*; с головы́ до пят from top to toe.

пята́|к *м. разг.* five-copeck piece. **~чо́к** *м. разг.* 1. *см.* пята́к; 2. (*тупой конец морды у свиньи*) snout; 3. (*небольшая площадка*) ring, patch.

пятёрк|а *ж.* 1. (*цифра*) a five; 2. (*школьная отметка*) five, "excellent"; учени́к получи́л ~у the púpil got an "éxcellent"; 3. *разг.* (*денежный знак*) five-rouble note.

пя́теро five; нас ~ there are five of us.

пятёрочн|ик *м.*, **~ица** *ж. разг.* éxcellent púpil.

пятибо́рье *с. спорт.* pentáthlon.

пятидесятиле́т|ие *с.* 1. (*период*) fifty years *pl*; 2. (*годовщина*) fíftieth anniérsary. **~ний** 1. (*о сроке*) fifty-year *attr.*; of fifty years *после сущ.*; врач с ~ним ста́жем dóctor of fifty years' stánding; 2. (*о возрасте*) fifty-year-óld; of fifty *после сущ.*; ~ний мужчи́на man* of fifty.

пятидеся́т|ый fíftieth; ~ые го́ды the fifties.

пятиконе́чн|ый pentágonal, five-póinted; ~ая звезда́ five-pointed star.

пятикра́тн|ый quíntuple; (*увеличенный в пять раз*) fívefold; в ~ом разме́ре five times the amóunt, fívefold, five times óver.

пятиле́т|ие *с.* 1. (*период*) five-year périod; 2. (*годовщина*) fifth anniérsary. **~ка** *ж.* 1. (*пятилетие*) five-year périod; 2. (*пятилетний план*) five-year plan. **~ний** 1. (*о сроке*) five-year *attr.*; of five years *после*

сущ.; **~ний** план five-year plan; 2. (*о возрасте*) five--year-óld; of five *после сущ.*; **~ний** ребёнок five-year-óld child*.

пятиме́сячный 1. (*о сроке*) five months'; five-month *attr.*; 2. (*о возрасте*) five-month-óld; of five months *после сущ.*; ~ ребёнок five-month-óld child*.

пятисо́тый five-húndredth.

пятисто́пный *лит.* pentámeter *attr.*; ~ ямб iámbic pentámeter.

пя́титься, попя́титься back awáy, move/step/draw* back, retréat; (*о лошади*) back* to *one's* heels.

пятиуго́льн|ик *м.* péntagon. **~ый** pentágonal.

пятичасово́й 1. five-hour *attr.*; of five hours *после сущ.*; 2. *разг.* (*назначенный на пять часов*) five-o'clock *attr.*; ~ по́езд five-o'clock train.

пя́тк|а *ж.* heel; ◇ у него́ душа́ в ~и ушла́ his heart sank, his heart leapt into his mouth; лиза́ть ~и кому́-л. lick *smb.'s* boots; пока́зывать ~и show* a clean pair of heels, take* to *one's* heels.

пятнадцатиле́тний 1. (*о сроке*) fiftéen-year *attr.*; of fiftéen years *после сущ.*; 2. (*о возрасте*) fiftéen-year--óld; of fiftéen *после сущ.*

пятна́дцатый fiftéenth.

пятна́дцать fiftéen.

пятна́ть, запятна́ть (*вн.*) stain (*smth.*), spot (*smth.*); *перен.* súlly (*smb., smth.*), soil (*smth.*), tárnish (*smth.*); ~ чью́-л. репута́цию cast* a slur on *smb.'s* reputátion; запятна́ть свою́ репута́цию soil *one's* reputátion; запятна́ть свою́ честь, своё и́мя bring* dishónour upón *one's* name.

пятни́ст|ый spótted, spéckled, móttled; **~ая** ко́шка tábby/bríndled cat.

пятни́ц|а *ж.* Fríday; в ~у on Fríday; по ~ам on Fríday, évery Fríday; ◇ у него́ семь пя́тниц на неде́ле he is incéssantly chánging his mind, he dóesn't know his own mind.

пятно́ *с.* spot, stain; (*чернильное*) blot, blur, blotch; *перен.* blot, slur, stígma (*pl* -mas, -mata); со́лнечные пя́тна sún-spots; выводи́ть пя́тна remóve stains; ◇ и на со́лнце есть пя́тна *посл.* ≈ there is nóthing pérfect in the world.

пятновыводи́тель *м.* spót-remóver.

пято́к *м. разг.* five.

пя́тый fifth.

пять five.

пятьдеся́т fifty.

пятьсо́т five húndred.

пятью five times.

Р

раб *м.*, **~а́** *ж.* slave.

рабко́р *м.* wórker correspóndent, néwspaper contríbutor.

рабовладе́лец *м.* sláve-owner.

рабовладе́льческий sláve-holder *attr.*; ~ строй sláve--holding sýstem.

раболе́п|ие *с.* servílity. **~ный** sérvile. **~ство** *с.* servílity.

раболе́пствовать *несов.* (*перед тв.*) cringe (to), trúckle (to), fawn (upón), kowtów (to).

рабо́т|а *ж.* 1. work, lábour; (*механизма*) wórking, fúnctioning; физи́ческая ~ phýsical work/lábour; ~ дви́гателя fúnctioning of an éngine; ~ мы́сли what is góing on in *smb.'s* mind; 2. (*занятие, труд на каком-л. предприятии*) work, job; поступи́ть на ~y start work, take* a job; снять кого́-л. с ~ы dismíss *smb.*, dischárge *smb.*; уйти́ с ~ы по со́бственному жела́нию quit the job at one's own will; вы́йти на ~у come* to work; без ~ы out of work, unemplóyed; **3.** *мн. (деятельность по обработке чего-л.)* work *sg*, operátions, *(принудительные)* lábour *sg*; строи́тельные ~ы búilding (work), búilding operátions; **4.** *(то, что подлежит обработке)* work, job; разда́ть всем ~у give* out work to éverybody, give* éverybody a job; **5.** *(продукт труда)* work; печа́тные ~ы públished works; вы́ставка рабо́т худо́жника exhibítion of an ártist's work; **6.** *(качество, способ исполнения)* cráftsmanship, quálity; чья э́то ~? who was this made/done by?; вещь превосхо́дной ~ы piece of supérb cráftsmanship; ◇ взять кого́-л. в ~у take* smb. in hand.

рабо́т|ать *несов.* **1.** *(трудиться, состоять где-л. на службе)* work; ~ в по́ле work in the fields; ~ на заво́де work at a fáctory; **2.** *(тв.; выполнять обязанности кого-л.)* be* *(smth.)*, work (as); ~ меха́ником be* a mechánic; **3.** *(над тв.)* work (at, on); ~ над диссерта́цией work on one's thésis; **4.** *(с тв.; воспитывать)* teach* *(smb.)*, train *(smth.)*; ~ с детьми́ teach* chíldren; ~ с ка́драми train personnél; **5.** *(на вн.)* work (for), work for the bénefit (of); *перен.* be* on smb.'s side, be* wórking in smb.'s fávour; **6.**: *(тв.; действовать чем-л.)* use *(smth.)*, work (with); ~ мо́лотом use a hámmer; ~ локтя́ми use one's élbows; **7.** *(о механизмах, агрегатах)* óperate, work; run*, go*; мото́р рабо́тает безотка́зно the éngine works pérfectly; телефо́н не ~ает the télephone is out of órder; **8.** *(на пр.; действовать с помощью тех или иных материалов и т. п.)* work (on), óperate (on), use *(smth.)*, run* (on); заво́д ~ает на ме́стном сырье́ the fáctory úses lócal raw matérials; мото́р ~ает на ди́зельном то́пливе the éngine runs on díesel fuel; **9.** *(действовать — об органах тела)* fúnction, óperate; его́ желу́док не ~ает his stómach is out of órder, his stómach is not fúnctioning próperly; **10.** *(быть в действии, быть открытым)* óperate, be* ópen; заво́д ~ает в три сме́ны the fáctory works/óperates on a thrée-shift sýstem; библиоте́ка ~ает с двух до восьми́ (часо́в) the líbrary is ópen from two till eight; телегра́ф ~ает кру́глые су́тки the télegraph óffice is ópen day and night; ◇ ~ над собо́й strive* to impróve, cúltivate one's abílities. ~ **аться** *несов. безл.*: по утра́м хорошо́ ~ается it's éasier to work in the mórnings; мне сего́дня не ~ается somehow I can't (get on with my) work todáy.

рабо́тн|ик *м.* **1.** wórker; ~ тра́нспорта tránsport wórker; ~ики у́мственного труда́ bráin-workers; ~ посо́льства émbassy employée; émbassy official; **2.** *уст. (батрак)* fárm-lábourer, fárm-hand; hired man* *амер.* ~**ица** *ж.* wórker; wórking wóman*; ◇ дома́шняя ~ица hóusemaid, (doméstic) sérvant; help *разг.*

работода́тель *м.* emplóyer.
работорго́в|ец *м.* sláve-trader. ~**ля** *ж.* sláve-trade.
работоспосо́бн|ость *ж.* capácity for work. ~**ый 1.** *(трудоспособный)* áble-bódied; **2.** *(усидчивый)* indústrious.
рабо́тяга *м. и ж. разг.* slógger, hard wórker; *(перен. тж.)* wórkhorse.
рабо́тящий *разг.* hárd-working, indústrious.
рабо́че-крестья́нский Wórkers' and Péasants'.
рабо́ч|ий I *м.* wórker; wórkman*; ~**ие** и слу́жащие indústrial, óffice and proféssional wórkers.
рабо́ч|ий II *прил.* **1.** wórking *attr.*; wórkers'; ~**ий** класс wórking class; ~**ая** молодёжь wórking/wórking-class youth; young wórkers *pl*; ~**ее** движе́ние wórking-class móvement; ~ посёлок wórkers' séttlement; *(современный, благоустроенный)* fáctory hóusing estáte; **2.** *(производящий полезную работу)* work *attr.*, wórking *attr.*; ~ скот dráught-animals *pl*; ~**ая** ло́шадь dráy-horse; ~**ие** пчёлы wórker-bees; **3.** *(предназначенный для работы)* wórking *attr.*; ~ день wórking day, wórkday; ~**ее** вре́мя wórking time; wórking hours *pl*; ~ костю́м wórking clothes *pl*; ~**ее** ме́сто place for work;

4. *(служащий руководством для проведения работы)* wórking *attr.*; ~ чертёж wórking dráwing; **5.** *тех.* wórking *attr.*; ~ие ча́сти маши́ны wórking parts of a machine; ◇ ~ие ру́ки hands, óperatives; ~**ая** си́ла *эк.* mánpower, lábour pówer; в ~ем поря́дке in the course of the work, on the job.

ра́бск|ий 1. *(тяжёлый, непосильный)* slave *attr.*; ~ труд slave lábour; **2.** *(свойственный рабу)* sérvile, slávish; ~**ая** поко́рность sérvile submíssion; ~**ое** подража́ние slávish imitátion.

ра́бство *с.* slávery; *(состояние раба тж.)* sérvitude, bóndage.

рабы́ня *ж.* slave, bóndwoman*.
равви́н *м.* rábbi.
ра́венств|о *с.* equálity; ~ очко́в tie; знак ~а a sign of equálity.

равне́ние *с.* dréssing, alígnment; ~ нале́во, напра́во! left, right dress!

равни́на *ж.* plain.
равни́нный flat.
равно́ 1. *нареч.* équally; **2.** *в знач. сказ. (дт.)* équal *(smth.)*; три плюс два ~ пяти́ three and two équal/make five; **3.** *в знач. союза*: а ~ и, ~ как (и) no less than; э́то каса́ется меня́, а ~ и вас this concérns you no less than me; ◇ всё ~ all the same; *(во всяком случае)* ányhow; мне всё ~ it's all the same to me; it's all one to me; it makes no dífference to me; I don't care; я всё ~ приду́ I'll come in ány case.

равнобе́дренный *мат.* isósceles; ~ треуго́льник isósceles tríangle.

равнове́си|е *с.* bálance *(тж. перен.)*; equilíbrium; *(душевное)* poise, compósure; сохраня́ть ~ keep* one's bálance, be* in equilíbrium; теря́ть ~ lose* one's bálance; полити́ческое ~ bálance of pówer; вы́вести кого́-л. из состоя́ния ~я throw* smb. off his, her bálance, destróy smb.'s poise/compósure.

равноде́йствующ|ий: ~**ая** си́ла *физ.* resúltant force.

равноде́нств|енный equinóctial; ~**ие** *с.* équinox; весе́ннее ~ие vérnal équinox; осе́ннее ~ие autúmnal équinox; то́чка ~ия equinóctial point.

равноду́ш|ие *с.* indífference; ~но indífferently; *(безучастно)* with indífference. ~**ный** indífferent; остава́ться ~ным к чему́-л. remáin unmóved by smth., be* indífferent to smth.

равнопра́в|ащий, ~**ный** equívalent, equipóllent.

равноме́рн|ый éven; *(ритмичный)* stéady, rhýthmical; ~ое посту́кивание stéady tápping; ~ шаг méasured tread; ~ое движе́ние, ускоре́ние úniform mótion, accelerátion.

равнопра́в|ие *с.* équal rights *pl*, equálity. ~**ный** équal; *(о людях тж.)* of équal stánding *после сущ.*; háving équal rights *после сущ.*; ~**ный** догово́р équal tréaty; быть ~ным с кем-л. enjóy équal rights with smb.

равноси́льн|ый 1. *(равной силы)* of équal strength *после сущ.*; **2.** *(равнозначный)* equívalent; э́то ~о изме́не it amóunts to tréachery.

равносторо́нний *мат.* equiláteral; ~ треуго́льник equiláteral tríangle.

равноуго́льный *мат.* equiángular.

равноце́нн|ый of équal válue *после сущ.*; ~**ые** ве́щи árticles of équal válue; ~**ые** рабо́тники équally úseful mémbers of the staff.

ра́вн|ый équal; *(одинаковый тж.)* the same; с ~**ой** ско́ростью at the same speed; не име́ть себе́ ~ых по чему́-л. be* unrívalled in smth.; на ~ых усло́виях on équal terms; при про́чих ~ых усло́виях óther things béing équal; относи́ться к кому́-л. как к ~ому treat smb. as an équal; ◇ ~ым о́бразом, в ~ой ме́ре équally, just as much, to the same extént; в ~ой ме́ре винова́т just as much to blame.

равня́ть, сравня́ть 1. *(вн.; делать равным)* make* *(smb., smth.)* équal; сравня́ть счёт *спорт.* équalize; **2.**

(вн. с тв.; *считать одинаковым по качествам, достоинствам и т. п.*) equáte (*smb., smth.* with).

равня́ться *несов.* 1. (с тв.) *разг.* (*считать себя равным кому-л.*) compáre (with), compéte (with); никто́ не мо́жет ~ с ним nóbody can compéte with him, he has no ríval;, 2. (по дт.; *в строю*) dress (on); 3. (по дт., на вн.; *стараться следовать чьему-л. примеру*) émulate (*smb.*); 4. (дт.; *быть равным*) be* équal (to); (*быть равносильным*) amóunt (to); три́жды три равня́ется девяти́ three threes are nine, three times three is nine.

рагу́ *с. нескл.* ragóut, stew.

рад *в знач. сказ.* (что, дт., + инф.) glad (that, + to *inf*); (я) ~ вас ви́деть, я вам ~ (I am) glad to see you; я ~ его́ прие́зду I am glad he has come; он ~ слу́чаю he is glad of the opportúnity; ◇ я и сам не ~ I regrét it mysélf, I'm not háppy abóut it mysélf; ~ стара́ться! it's a pléasure!; он и ~ стара́ться nóthing pléases him bétter, he enjóys dóing it; ~-ра́дёхонек, ~-ра́дёшенек enchánted, delíghted.

рада́р *м.* rádar. ~ный rádar *attr.*; ~ная ста́нция rádar státion; ~ная устано́вка rádar installátion.

ра́ди for the sake (of); ~ меня́, вас, него́ for my, your, his sake; ~ кого́? who for?; ~ кого́ стара́ться? is it worth while?; ~ чего́?, чего́ ~? what for?; шу́тки ~ (just) for fun; ◇ ~ бо́га, бо́га ~, ~ всего́ свято́го for God's/góodness' sake.

радиа́льный rádial.

радиа́тор *м.* rádiator.

радиа́ция *ж.* radiátion; а́томная, со́лнечная ~ núclear, sólar radiátion.

ра́дий *м. хим.* rádium.

радика́л I *м.* rádical.

радика́л II *м. мат., хим.* rádical.

радика́льный rádical; (*решительный тж.*) drástic; ~ые измене́ния rádical chánges; ~ые ме́ры drástic méasures.

ра́дио *с. нескл.* rádio, wíreless; передава́ть по ~ bróadcast; слу́шать ~ lísten to the rádio; включи́ть ~ switch on the rádio.

радиоакти́вность *ж.* radioactívity. ~ый radioáctive; ~ые вещества́ radioáctive matérials; ~ые изото́пы radioáctive ísotopes, radioísotops; ~ые оса́дки radioáctive fáll-out *sg*; ~ые отхо́ды radioáctive waste *sg*; ~ое заражé́ние radioáctive contaminátion.

радиовеща́ние *с.* bróadcasting. ~гра́мма *ж.* wíreless méssage, rádiogram. ~журна́л *м.* régular (rádio) féature. ~зо́нд *м.* rádiosonde. ~коммента́тор *м.* rádio cómmentator.

радио́ла *ж.* rádio-grámophone, rádiogram.

радиола́мпа *ж.* rádio valve.

радио́лог *м.* radiólogist.

радиоло́гия *ж.* radiólogy; медици́нская ~ núclear médicine; физи́ческая ~ radiológical phýsics.

радиолока́тор *м.* radiolocátor. ~цио́нный rádar *attr.*, radiolocátion *attr.*; ~цио́нные прибо́ры rádar devíces. ~ция *ж.* radiolocátion, rádar.

радиолюби́тель *м.* ámateur rádio óperator; rádio ham *разг.* ~ма́як *м.* rádio béacon. ~метри́ст *м.* rádar óperator. ~наведéние *с.* rádio guídance/contról. ~обору́дование *с.* wíreless/rádio equipment. ~о́черк *м.* féature prógramme. ~пеленга́тор *м.* rádio diréction-finder. ~переда́тчик *м.* transmítting set, transmítter. ~переда́ча *ж.* rádio transmíssion, bróadcast. ~поме́хи *мн.* rádio interférence *sg*. ~постано́вка *ж.* bróadcast/rádio play. ~приёмник *м.* rádio(-set), rádio receíver. ~репорта́ж *м.* (wíreless/rádio) cómmentary. ~связь *ж.* wíreless/rádio communicátion/cóntact. ~сёть *ж.* rádio net/nétwork. ~слу́шатель *м.* (rádio) lístener. ~спекта́кль *м.* rádio play. ~ста́нция *ж.* wíreless/rádio státion. ~сту́дия *с.* bróadcasting stúdio. ~телегра́ф *м.* radio-télegraph. ~телеско́п *м.* radio-télescope. ~телефо́н *м.* radio-télephone,

rádiophone. ~те́хник *м.* rádioman. ~те́хника *ж.* rádio engínéering. ~у́зел *м.* lócal bróadcasting céntre.

радиофика́ция *ж.* rádio installátion. ~ци́ровать *несов. и сов.* (вн.) instáll rádio (in).

радиоце́нтр *м.* rádio bróadcasting and communicátion céntre.

радиоэлектро́ника *ж.* rádio electrónics.

ради́ровать *несов. и сов.* rádio; send* a rádio méssage.

ради́ст *м.*, ~ка *ж.* rádio óperator.

ра́диус *м.* rádius (*pl* -dii); ~ де́йствия range/rádius of áction.

ра́довать, обра́довать, пора́довать (вн.) gládden (*smb.*); make* (*smb.*) háppy; ~ се́рдце кому́-л. gládden *smb.'s* heart; меня́ ~ют его́ успе́хи I rejóice at his succéss; меня́ э́то ниско́лько не ~ует that gives me no pléasure. ~оваться, обра́доваться, пора́доваться be* pleased/glad/delíghted; (дт.) rejóice (at, óver); ~ова́ться побе́де rejóice óver víctory; душа́ ~уется it is símply a pléasure.

ра́достный jóyful; glad; он шёл ~ и весёлый he strode alóng mérry and rejóicing; ~ое изве́стие jóyful/glad news; с ~ым лицо́м with joy in *one's* eyes, lóoking delíghted.

ра́дость *ж.* joy; вне себя́ от ~и besíde *one*sélf with joy; ~ жи́зни óptimism, joy of life; пры́гать от ~и jump/leap* for joy; кака́я ~! how lóvely!, how wónderful!; еди́нственная ~ в жи́зни the ónly joy (left) in *one's* life; ◇ с ~ью with pléasure; на ~ях in *one's* joy.

ра́дуга *ж.* ráinbow.

раду́жный iridéscent; *перен.* rádiant, bright; ~ые перспекти́вы glówing próspects; быть в са́мом ~ом настрое́нии be* in a héavenly/beatífic mood; ви́деть, представля́ть что-л. в ~ом све́те have* a rádiant/glówing picture of *smth.*; ◇ ~ая оболо́чка (глаза́) íris.

раду́шие *с.* cordiálity; проявля́ть ~ displáy/show a córdial regárd. ~ный córdial; ~ный приём córdial recéption.

раз I *м.* 1. time; оди́н ~ once; два ~а twice; три ~а three times; ещё ~ once more, agáin; повтори́те ещё ~! say it agáin, please!; ка́ждый ~, как évery time; whenéver; 2. *нескл.* (*при счёте*) one; ◇ (в) друго́й ~ some óther time; до друго́го ~а for anóther time; ино́й ~ sómetimes; не ~ more than once, repéatedly; ни ~у не... néver; ~-друго́й once or twice; ~ за ~ом agáin and agáin; ~ и навсегда́ once and for all; как ~ just, exáctly; в са́мый ~ 1) (*вовремя*) (it's) just (the) right (time); 2) (*впору*) it's just right; ~ на ~ не прихо́дится it's not álways the same; you néver know what may turn up; ~ от ~у лу́чше (ху́же) bétter and bétter (worse and worse) évery time; вот те(бе) ~! you don't say so!, well!, néver!

раз II *нареч.* one day; once; ка́к-то ~ one day.

раз III *союз разг.* since; ~ вы так говори́те... since you say so...; ~ (э́то) так... this being so..., this being the case...

разба́вить *сов. см.* разбавля́ть.

разбавля́ть, разба́вить (вн. тв.) dilúte (*smth.* with).

разба́заривать, разба́зарить (вн.) waste (*smth.*), squánder (*smth.*) (*тж. перен.*).

разба́зарить *сов. см.* разба́заривать.

разболе́ться I, разболе́ться *разг.* (*о человеке*) be*/get* próperly ill.

разба́ливаться II, разболе́ться *разг.* (*об органах, частях тела*) ache; у меня́ разболе́лась голова́ I have a héadache.

разба́лтывать I, разболта́ть (вн.) *разг.* 1. (*встряхивать*) shake* (*smth.*); (*размешивать*) stir (*smth.*); 2. (*расшатывать*) work (*smth.*) loose; разболта́ть га́йку work a nut loose.

разба́лтывать II, разболта́ть (вн.) *разг.* (*разглашать*) let* (*smth.*) out, give* (*smth.*) awáy.

разба́лтываться, разболта́ться *разг.* get* loose; *перен. (о человеке)* get* slack.

разбе́г *м.* run; ~ при взлёте táke-off run; де́лать ~ make*/take* one's run; ◇ с ~у перепры́гнуть че́рез что-л. take* a rúnning jump óver *smth.*; с ~у бро́ситься в во́ду take* a rúnning jump ínto the wáter.

разбе́гаться *сов. разг.* start rúnning abóut.

разбе́|а́ться, разбежа́ться 1. *(в разные стороны)* scátter, dispérse; де́ти разбежа́лись в ра́зные сто́роны the chíldren scáttered in várious diréctions; 2. *(набирать скорость для прыжка)* make*/take* one's run; ◇ глаза́ ~а́ются one dóesn't know what to look at first, it makes you dízzy.

разбежа́ться *сов. см.* разбега́ться.

разбереди́ть *сов. см.* береди́ть.

разбива́ть, разби́ть *(вн.)* 1. *(раскалывать)* break* *(smth.)*, shátter *(smth.) (тж. перен.)*; разби́ть окно́, таре́лку break* a wíndow, a plate; разби́ть чью-л. жизнь ruin *smb.'s* life; разби́ть чьи-л. наде́жды shátter *smb.'s* hopes; разби́ть се́рдце кому́-л. break* *smb.'s* heart; 2. *(повреждать, ушибать)* knock *(smth.)*, hurt* *(smth.)*; *(сильно)* frácture *(smth.)*; разби́ть себе́ коле́но hurt* one's knee; разби́ть го́лову frácture one's skull; 3. *(наносить поражение)* beat* *(smb., smth.)*, deféat *(smb., smth.); перен.* shátter *(smb., smth.)*; на́голову разби́ть врага́ rout the énemy; 4. *(делить на части)* break* up *(smth. into)*; divíde *(smth. into)*; *(распределять)* allót *(smth.)*; 5. *(распланировав, сажать)* lay* out *(smth.)*; разби́ть сад, парк lay* out a gárden, park; 6.: разби́ть ла́герь make* a camp; разби́ть пала́тку pitch a tent; 7. *(лишать движения)*: его́ разби́л парали́ч he was struck down by parálysis. ~ся, разби́ться 1. *(раскалываться)* break*; *(о самолёте)* crash; *(о корабле)* be* wrecked; *перен.* be* wrécked/sháttered; стака́н разби́лся the glass broke; ~ся о бе́рег break* against the shore; 2. *(ушибаться)* hurt* onesélf *(severely/badly)*, be* bádly hurt; он упа́л с ло́шади и разби́лся he fell off his horse and was bádly hurt; 3. *(на вн.; делиться)* break* up *(into)*; ~ся на гру́ппы break* up ínto groups.

разбинтова́ть(ся) *сов. см.* разбинто́вывать(ся).

разбинто́вывать, разбинтова́ть *(вн.)* unbándage *(smb., smth.)*. ~ся, разбинтова́ться 1. *(снимать с себя бинт)* unbándage onesélf, take* off one's bándage(s); 2. *(о бинте)* come* unbándaged.

разбира́тельство *с.* examinátion, investigátion; суде́бное ~ héaring.

разбир|а́ть, разобра́ть *(вн.)* 1. *(брать всё по частям, по одному)* sort out *(smth.)* amóng themsélves; *(раскупать)* buy* up *(smth.)*; весь това́р разобра́ли в како́й-нибудь час all the goods went in an hour or so; 2. *(сортировать)* sort out; разобра́ть сва́ленные кни́ги sort out the heap of books; 3. *(на части)* disassémble *(smth.)*, take* *(smth.)* apárt; dismántle *(smth.)*; *(разрушать)* pull *(smth.)* down; ~ часы́ take* a watch to píeces; ~ кры́шу dismántle a roof; ~ мото́р, винто́вку strip an éngine, rífle; 4. *(рассматривать)* discúss *(smth.)*, go* óver/ínto *(smth.)*; ~ де́ло *(в суде)* try a case; 5. *грам. (по частям речи)* parse *(smth.)*; *(по членам предложения)* ánalyse *(smth.)*; 6. *(различать)* make* *(smth.)* out; *(написанное, сказанное тж.)* understánd* *(smth.)*; в темноте́ ничего́ нельзя́ бы́ло разобра́ть one could make out nóthing in the dárkness; ~ по склада́м spell* out; ~ но́ты read* músic; хорошо́ ~ по́черки be* good* at réading hándwriting; ничего́ не могу́ разобра́ть в э́том I can make nóthing of it, I can't make head or tail of it; 7. *разг. (о чувствах, страстях и т. п.)* overcóme*; меня́ ~ет смех I can't help láughing; 8. *тк. несов. разг.*: не ~я indiscríminately, without stópping to choose. ~а́ться, разобра́ться 1. *тк. несов. (разниматься на части)* disassémble, come* apárt; 2. *разг. (раскладывать вещи)* unpáck; 3. *(в пр.; анализировать что-л.)* go*/look ínto *(smth.)*, exámine *(smth.)*.

(различать, понимать) understánd* *(smth.)*; хорошо́ ~а́ться в чём-л. have* a good* understánding of *smth.*

разбитно́й *разг.* smart, wide awáke; он па́рень ~ he's a smart chap.

разби́т|ый 1. *(расколотый на куски)* bróken; ~ая ча́шка bróken cup; 2. *(повреждённый, испорченный)* báttered; ~ роя́ль báttered/cracked piáno; ~ го́лос cracked voice; ~ое лицо́ báttered face; 3. *(побеждённый)* róuted, sháttered; 4. *(погибший)* ruined, sháttered; ~ая жизнь ruined life; 5. *(усталый, ослабевший)* worn/whacked out *predic.*, out of sorts *predic.*

разби́ть *сов. см.* разбива́ть *и* бить 6. ~ся *сов. см.* разбива́ться.

разбогате́ть *сов. см.* богате́ть.

разбо́й *м.* róbbery, ráiding; ~ на большо́й доро́ге *(прям. и перен.)* híghway róbbery. ~ник *м.* 1. róbber; *перен.* thug, cútthroat; ~ник с большо́й доро́ги híghwayman; 2. *разг. (сорванец)* scamp, ráscal. ~ничать *несов.* 1. *(грабить)* rob, loot, plúnder; 2. *(бесчинствовать)* commít (all kinds of) óutrages. ~ничий róbber's; *(свойственный разбойнику)* gángster-like, múrderous; ~ничий прито́н den of thieves; ~ничье нападе́ние múrderous attáck.

разболе́ться I, II *сов. см.* разба́ливаться I, II.

разболта́ть I, II *сов. см.* разба́лтывать I, II.

разболта́ться I *сов. см.* разба́лтываться I.

разболта́ться II *сов. см. (увлечься болтовнёй)* start cháttering/tálking ninetéen to the dózen.

разбомби́ть *сов. (вн.)* bomb *(smth.)* to bits, destróy *(smth.)* from the air; *(город и т. п.)* blitz *(smth.)*.

разбо́р *м.* 1. *(рассмотрение)* investigátion, examinátion; *(статьи и т. п.)* revíew, análysis; ~ де́ла investigátion of a case; 2. *грам. (по частям речи)* pársing; *(по членам предложения)* análysis; 3. *разг.*: без ~а indiscríminately, without distínction; с ~ом with discriminátion. ~ка *ж.* 1. *(на части)* disassémbling; *(оружия тж.)* strípping; 2. *(сортировка)* sórting. ~ный séctional; ~ная ме́бель séctional fúrniture; ~ный дом séctional/prefábricated house.

разбо́рчив|ость *ж.* 1. discriminátion; 2. *(привередливость)* fastídiousness; 3. *(почерка и т. п.)* legibility. ~ый 1. discríminating; 2. *(привередливый)* fastídious; ~ый покупа́тель fastídious cústomer; 3. *(чёткий)* légible.

разбрани́ть *сов. (вн.) разг.* give* *(smb.)* a sound scólding.

разбра́сывать, разброса́ть *(вн.)* 1. scátter *(smth.)*; *(удобрение и т. п.)* spread* *(smth.)*; 2. *разг.*: ~ ве́щи leave* one's things all óver the place. ~ся *несов.* go* in for too mány things at once; squánder one's énergies.

разбреда́ться, разбрести́сь wánder off *(somewhere)*; *перен. (о мыслях)* wánder, stray.

разбрести́сь *сов. см.* разбреда́ться.

разбро́д *м.* confúsion.

разбро́санный 1. *(по дт.)* scáttered *(about, all over)*; 2. *(расположенный в беспорядке, без плана)* scáttered; dótted here and there *после сущ.*; 3. *разг. (беспорядочный)* vague, scáttered, confúsed.

разброса́ть *сов. см.* разбра́сывать.

разбры́згать *сов. см.* разбры́згивать.

разбры́згивать, разбры́згать *(вн.)* splash abóut, sprinkle *(smth.)* abóut.

разбуди́ть *сов. см.* буди́ть.

разбуха́ние *с.* swélling.

разбуха́ть, разбу́хнуть swell*; *перен. разг.* becóme* infláted.

разбу́хнуть *сов. см.* разбуха́ть *и* бу́хнуть II.

разбушева́ться *сов.* 1. rage; *(о ветре тж.)* blow* like fúry; *(о море тж.)* get* rough, run* high; 2. *разг. (о человеке)* start láshing out.

разва́л *м.* 1. disintegrátion, decáy, collápse; *(разруха)* wrécking; ~ рабо́ты wrécking/rúining of the work; 2. *разг. (беспорядок)* mess, túrmoil.

разва́ливать, развали́ть (*вн.*) 1. (*рассыпать что-л. сложенное*) pull (*smth.*) apárt, scátter (*smth.*); (*постройку*) pull (*smth.*) down; 2. (*приводить в упадок*) wreck (*smth.*), ruin (*smth.*); развали́ть де́ло let* éverything go to rack and ruin. ~ся, развали́ться 1. (*разрушаться*) fall* apárt, fall* to píeces; (*о постройке*) collápse, fall* down; 2. (*приходить в упадок*) go* to píeces, be* ruined; хозя́йство развали́лось the ecónomy went to píeces; 3. *разг.* (*сидеть*) sprawl, lounge.

разва́лина *ж.* 1. *обыкн. мн.* ruin; 2. *разг.* (*о человеке*) wreck, ruin.

развали́ть(ся) *сов. см.* разва́ливать(ся).

разва́ривать, развари́ть (*вн.*) boil (*smth.*) soft. ~ся, развари́ться be* próperly cooked; (*чрезмерно*) be* overcóoked/overdóne.

развари́ть(ся) *сов. см.* разва́ривать(ся).

ра́зве 1. *частица* (*правда?*) réally?; ~ он прие́хал? oh, has he come?; ~ вы не зна́ете? didn't you know?; ~ мо́жно? how can you?; (*да*) ~ я могу́..? how can I póssibly..?; ~ его́ заста́вишь..? as if one could make him (+ *inf*); 2. *частица* (*может быть*) perháps; ~ почита́ть что-нибудь I might perháps read sómething; 3. *союз* (*если не*) unléss; ~ (*что, только*) заболе́ю unléss I fall ill.

развев|а́ть *несов.* (*вн.*) blow* (*smth.*) abóut; ве́тер ~а́л знамёна the bánners were stréaming in the wind. ~а́ться *несов.* flútter, fly*; с ~а́ющимися знамёнами with flýing cólours.

разве́дать *сов. см.* разве́дывать.

разведе́ние *с.* (*животных*) bréeding, réaring; (*растений*) grówing, cultivátion; ~ ове́ц shéep-breeding; ~ садо́в gárden-making.

разведённый *прил.* 1. divórced; 2. *в знач. сущ. м.* divórced pérson, divorcée.

разве́дк|а *ж.* 1. *геол.* explóring, prospécting; ~ буре́нием próbing; вести́ ~у explóre; 2. *воен.* recónnaissance; произвести́ ~у make* a recónnaissance; он посла́л двух бойцо́в в ~у he sent out two men on recónnaissance; 3. (*войсковая группа*) recónnaissance únit; patról; 4. (*организация, учреждение*) intélligence/sécret sérvice.

разве́дочн|ый 1. explóring *attr.*, prospécting *attr.*; ~ые рабо́ты prospécting work *sg*; 2. *воен.* recónnaissance *attr.*

развед|чик *м.* 1. *воен.* scout; 2. (*агент разведки*) sécret sérvice man*/ágent; 3. (*специалист по разведке недр*) explórer, prospéctor; 4. (*самолёт*) recónnaissance áircraft/plane. ~чица *ж.* 1. *воен.* (*wóman**) scout; 2. (*агент разведки*) sécret sérvice wóman*/ágent.

разве́дывательн|ый intélligence *attr.*, recónnaissance *attr.*; ~ отде́л, intélligence séction; ~ые да́нные, ~ые све́дения intélligence (dáta); ~ полёт recónnaissance flight.

разве́дывать, разве́дать 1. (*вн. о пр., про вн.*) *разг.* (*разузнавать*) (try to) find* (*smth.*) out; 2. (*вн.*) *воен.* reconnóitre (*smth.*); 3. (*вн.*) *геол.* explóre (*smth.*), prospéct (*smth.*).

развезти́ *сов. см.* развози́ть.

развенчанный dethróned; debúnked *разг.*; ~ геро́й cást-off héro; ~ куми́р bróken ídol.

развенча́ть *сов. см.* развенчивать.

развенчивать, развенча́ть (*вн.*) dethróne (*smb.*); defláte (*smth.*); debúnk (*smb., smth.*) *разг.*

развёрнут|ый 1. unfólded; 2. (*подробный*) détailed; 3. (*широкий*) full-scále, áll-out, comprehénsive; 4. *воен.* deplóyed.

разверну́ть *сов. см.* развёртывать *и* развора́чивать 3. ~ся *сов. см.* развёртываться.

развёрстка *ж.* appórtionment, allótment; (*налога*) asséssment.

развёртка I *ж. мат.* evólvent; ~ криво́й evolútion of curve.

развёртка II *ж.* (*инструмент*) réamer.

развёртывание *с.* 1. (*развитие*) devélopment; 2. *воен.* deplóyment.

развёртывать, разверну́ть (*вн.*) 1. (*скатанное*) unróll (*smth.*); (*сложенное*) unfóld (*smth.*); разверну́ть ковёр unróll a cárpet; 2. (*завёрнутое*) unwráp (*smth.*); разверну́ть поку́пку unwráp a púrchase; 3. *воен.* deplóy (*smth.*); 4. (*проявлять в полной мере*) displáy (*smth.*); 5. (*осуществлять в широких размерах*) devélop (*smth.*); разверну́ть строи́тельство launch a búilding drive, build* on a large scale; 6. (*повёртывать*) turn (*smth.*) round; разверну́ть маши́ну turn a car round. ~ся, разверну́ться 1. (*о скатанном*) come* unrólled; (*о сложенном*) come* unfólded; ковёр разверну́лся the cárpet came unrólled; 2. (*о завёрнутом*) come* undóne; свёрток разверну́лся the roll came undóne; 3. *воен.* deplóy; 4. (*проявлять свои силы, способности и т. п.*) show* what *one* can do, launch out; 5. (*принимать широкий размах*) devélop; 6. (*делать поворот*) turn round; самолёт разверну́лся над ле́сом the áircraft made a turn óver the wood.

развесели́ть *сов.* (*вн.*) cheer (*smb.*) up. ~ся *сов.* cheer up.

развесёлый *разг.* gay, róllicking, jólly.

развесист|ый spréading; ◇ ~ая клю́ква fántasy, fáble.

разве́сить I, II *сов. см.* разве́шивать I, II.

развесно́й sold by weight *после сущ.*

разве́сти(сь) *сов. см.* разводи́ть(ся).

разветви́ться *сов. см.* разветвля́ться.

разветвле́ние *с.* 1. bránching; bifurcátion *научн.*; 2. (*место*) fork; ~ доро́ги road fork; 3. (*ответвление, отрасль*) ramificátion, branch.

разветвлённый rámifide.

разветвля́ться, разветви́ться 1. branch out; 2. (*о дороге и т. п.*) form séveral bránches, fork.

разве́шать *сов. см.* разве́шивать II.

разве́шивать I, разве́сить (*вн.; на весах*) weigh out (*smth.*); разве́сить муку́ weigh out flour.

разве́шивать II, разве́сить, разве́шать (*вн.*) hang* (*smth.*); ~ бельё hang* out clothes, hang* out the wáshing; разве́сить карти́ны put* up páintings; ◇ разве́сить у́ши ≈ lísten open-móuthed, take* it all in.

разве́ять *сов.* (*вн.*) scátter (*smth.*); *перен.* dispél (*smth.*); ~ миф о чём-л. destróy the myth of *smth.* ~ся *сов.* be* scáttered, drift awáy; *перен.* be* dispélled.

развива́ть, разви́ть (*вн.*) 1. devélop (*smth.*); ~ го́лос devélop *one's* voice; ~ мускулату́ру devélop *one's* múscles; ~ па́мять devélop *one's* mémory; ~ интере́с к му́зыке devélop an ínterest in músic; ~ машинострое́ние expánd machine-building; разви́ть бу́рную де́ятельность get* búsy, make* things hum; ~ ско́рость pick up speed; ~ успе́х fóllow up *one's* succéss; *воен.* explóit a succéss; 2. (*раскручивать*) unwínd* (*smth.*); разви́ть верёвку unrável a rope. ~ся, разви́ться 1. devélop; ребёнок о́чень разви́лся the child* has devéloped a great deal; при спу́ске разви́лась больша́я ско́рость speed was high góing downhíll; 2. (*раскручиваться*) come* unwóund; (*о волосах*) come* out of curl.

разви́лина *ж.* fork.

разви́лка *ж.:* ~ доро́г road fork.

развинти́ть(ся) *сов. см.* разви́нчивать(ся).

разви́нченн|ый 1. unscréwed; 2. *разг.* (*неспокойный*) unrestráined; ~ ребёнок réstive child*; 3. *разг.* (*нетвёрдый, вертля́вый*) slóuching; идти́ ~ой похо́дкой slouch alóng.

разви́нчивать, развинти́ть (*вн.*) unscréw (*smth.*). ~ся, развинти́ться be*/come* unscréwed; work loose; *перен.* разг. lose* *one's* grip; у меня́ не́рвы развинти́лись my nerves are in a shócking condítion; он совсе́м развинти́лся he has grown térribly slack, he has lost his grip entírely.

разви́тие *с.* 1. devélopment; ~ собы́тий devélopment of evénts; ~ наро́дного хозя́йства devélopment of the (nátional) ecónomy; ~ о́бщества sócial devélopment,

devélopment of society; 2. (*степень зрелости*) matúrity; óбщее ~ géneral (intelléctual) matúrity; полити́ческое ~ political lével.

развито́й 1. (*физически*) devéloped, matúre; 2. (*достигший высокого уровня*) well/híghly devéloped; 3. (*умственно*) cúltivated, matúre.

разви́ть(ся) *сов. см.* развива́ть(ся).

развлека́тельный trívial, supérficial; púrely for entertáinment *после сущ.*

развлека́ть, **развле́чь** (*вн.*) 1. (*отвлекать*) distráct (*smb.*); 2. (*забавлять*) amúse (*smb.*), entertáin (*smb.*). ~ся, развлека́ться 1. (*отвлекаться от чего-л.*) seek* relaxátion, amúse onesélf; 2. (*веселиться*) enjóy onesélf.

развлече́ние *с.* 1. (*занятие*) amúsement, distráction; 2. (*зрелище и т. п.*) entertáinment.

развле́чь(ся) *сов. см.* развлека́ть(ся).

разво́д *м.* 1. (*расторжение брака*) divórce; дать ~ grant a divórce; agrée to a divórce; получи́ть ~ get* a divórce; 2. (*разведение*): на ~ for bréeding púrposes; *воен.*: ~ карау́лов, часовы́х móunting of the guard, séntries.

разводи́ть, **развести́** (*вн.*) 1. (*куда-л.*) take* (*smb.*); развести́ дете́й по дома́м take* the children to their homes; 2. *воен.* mount (*smb.*, *smth.*), post (*smb.*, *smth.*); развести́ часовы́х post séntries; 3. (*отделять одно от другого*, *раздвигать*) part (*smth.*); (*мост*) raise (*smth.*) ópen; 4. (*расторгать брак*) grant (*smb.*) a divórce; 5. (*растворять*) dissólve (*smth.*); (*разбавлять*) dilúte (*smth.*); 6. (*животных*) breed* (*smth.*), rear (*smth.*), raise (*smth.*); (*растения*) grow* (*smth.*), cúltivate (*smth.*); (*сад и т. п.*) lay* out (*smth.*); 7. (*разжигать*) make* (*smth.*); ◇ ~ рука́ми throw up *one's* hands, make* a hélpless gésture. ~ся, развести́сь get* divórced; (*с тв.*) divórce (*smb.*).

разводно́й: ~ мост ópening bridge, dráwbridge; ~ ра́ечный ключ adjústable spánner.

разво́ды *мн.* (*узоры*) páttern *sg*; (*потёки*) streaks.

развози́ть, **развезти́** 1. (*вн.*) drive* (*smth.*), take* (*smth.*); (*товары*) delíver (*smth.*); развезти́ дете́й по дома́м drive*/take* the children to their homes; 2. *безл. разг.* (*делать труднопроходимым*): доро́гу развезло́ от дождя́ rain had made the road impássable.

разволнова́ть *сов.* (*вн.*) *разг.* upsét* (*smb.*). ~ся *сов. разг.* get* worked up.

развора́чивать, **разворо́тить**, **разверну́ть** (*вн.*) *разг.* 1. *сов.* разворо́тить heave*/pull apárt, (*постройку*) shátter (*smth.*); разворо́тить гру́ду камне́й scátter a heap of stones; 2. *сов.* разворо́тить (*приводить в беспорядок*) turn (*smth.*) upside-dówn; 3. *сов.* разверну́ть *см.* развёртывать.

разворова́ть *сов. см.* разворо́вывать.

разворо́вывать, **разворова́ть** (*вн.*) *разг.* steal* (*smth.*), make* off (with).

разворо́т *м.* 1. *разг.* (*развитие*) devélopment; 2. (*поворот*) (U-)turn; 3. (*внутренняя сторона листа*, *обложки и т. п.*) the insíde.

разворо́тить *сов. см.* развора́чивать 1, 2.

разворoши́ть *сов. см.* вороши́ть.

разворча́ться *сов. разг.* get* into a grúmbling mood.

развра́т *м.* 1. (*распущенность*) léchery, debáuchery; 2. (*испорченность нравов*) deprávity; 3. *разг.* (*избалованность*) vice.

разврати́ть(ся) *сов. см.* развраща́ть(ся).

разврат|**ник** *м.* lécher, rake. ~ница *ж.* lewd wóman*. ~ничать *несов.* lead* a depráved/díssolute life, debáuch onesélf. ~ный dissolute, licéntious.

развращ|**а́ть**, **разврати́ть** (*вн.*) corrúpt (*smth.*). ~а́ться, разврати́ться 1. (*становиться развратным*) give* onesélf up to debáuchery; 2. (*морально разлагаться*) becóme* corrúpted, go* to the bad. ~ённый depráved, corrúpt.

развьюч|**ивать**, **развьючить** (*вн.*) unlóad (*smth.*). ~ить *сов. см.* развьючивать.

развяза́ть(ся) *сов. см.* развязывать(ся).

развя́зк|**а** *ж.* 1. óutcome; (*конец*) end; *лит.* denóuement; наступа́ет ~ the end is in sight; идти́ к ~е reach the climax; де́ло идёт к ~е things are cóming to a head; неожи́данная ~ unexpécted óutcome; 2. (*транспортная*) flýover (road júnction).

развя́зн|**о** *too* fréely; вести́ себя́ ~ be* over-frée. ~ость *ж.* undúe familiárity, offhándedness. ~ый offhánd, over-frée, brash; ~ые мане́ры offhánd mánners; ~ый тон brash tone.

развя́зывать, **развяза́ть** (*вн.*) undó* (*smth.*), untíe (*smth.*); *перен.* líberate (*smth.*); ~ у́зел untíe a knot; ◇ развяза́ть ру́ки кому́-л. give* *smb.* fréedom, leave* *smb.* free; развяза́ть язы́к 1) (*дт.*) make* (*smb.*) talk; 2) (*разговориться*) give* rein to *one's* tongue; развяза́ть войну́ unléash a war. ~ся, развяза́ться 1. (*о завязанном*) come* undóne; 2. (*с тв.*) *разг.* (*освобождаться от кого-л.*, *чего-л.*) get* rid (of); (*с чем-л. тж.*) get* (*smth.*) off *one's* hands.

разгада́ть *сов. см.* разга́дывать.

разга́дка *ж.* solútion.

разга́дывать, **разгада́ть** (*вн.*) 1. (*отгадывать*) solve (*smth.*), guess (*smth.*); разгада́ть зага́дку solve a ríddle; 2. (*понимать кого-л.*, *что-л.*) púzzle (*smb.*, *smth.*) out, get* to the bóttom (of); разгада́ть чьи-л. наме́рения percéive *smb.'s* inténtions.

разга́р *м.* peak, height, climax; рабо́та в (по́лном) ~е work is in full swing; ле́то в са́мом ~е súmmer is at its height.

разгерметиза́ция *ж.* depressurizátion, depréssurizing.

разгерметизи́ровать *сов.* (*вн.*) depréssurize (*smth.*). ~ся *сов.* becóme* depréssurized.

разгиб|**а́ть**, **разогну́ть** (*вн.*) stráighten (*smth.*); рабо́тать, не ~а́я спины́ néver look up from *one's* work. ~а́ться, разогну́ться stráighten up, stand* up straight.

разглаго́льствовать (о *пр.*) *разг.* hold* forth (on).

разгла́живать, **разгла́дить** (*вн.*) 1. smooth (*smth.*) out; 2. (*утюгом*) iron (*smth.*), press (*smth.*). ~ся, разгла́диться: морщи́ны разгла́дились the wrínkles disappéared.

разгласи́ть *сов. см.* разглаша́ть.

разглаш|**а́ть**, **разгласи́ть** (*вн.*) divúlge (*smth.*), make* (*smth.*) known. ~е́ние *с.* divúlgence, spréading.

разгляде́ть *сов.* (*вн.*) make* out (*smth.*); *перен.* percéive (*smth.*).

разгля́дывать *несов.* (*вн.*) exámine (*smb.*, *smth.*).

разгне́ванный enráged; fúrious; ~ челове́к enráged/wráthful pérson; ~ взгляд fúrious glance.

разгне́вать *сов.* (*вн.*) infúriate (*smb.*). ~ся *сов.* fly* into a pássion/rage.

разгова́рив|**ать** *несов.* 1. speak*, talk; (*с тв.*) speak* (to), talk (to); я не с ва́ми ~аю! I'm not spéaking to you!; с кем (э́то) вы ~али? who's that you were tálking to?; ~ с сами́м собо́й talk to onesélf; он сли́шком мно́го ~ает he talks too much; ~ о му́зыке talk abóut músic; 2. (*с тв.*) *разг.* (*поддерживать общение с кем-л.*) be* on spéaking terms (with); мы с ним не ~аем we are not on spéaking terms.

разгово́р *м.* 1. talk, conversátion; име́ть кру́пный ~ с кем-л. have* words with *smb.*; перемени́ть те́му ~а change the súbject; и никаки́х ~ов! and there's an end of it!; 2. *обыкн. мн. разг.* (*молва*, *пересуды*) góssip, títtle-tattle; ◇ без ли́шних ~ов withóut wásting words, withóut more adó.

разгово́р|**иться** *сов. разг.* 1. (*с тв.*) get* into talk (with); 2. (*увлечься разговором*) becóme* tálkative; он наконе́ц ~и́лся at last he found his tongue.

разгово́рник *м.* conversátion book, phráse-book.

разгово́рн|**ый** collóquial; ~ые слова́ colloquialisms.

разгово́рчивый tálkative, commúnicative.

разгóн *м.* 1. dispérsal; (*парла́мента и т. п.*) dissolútion; 2. (*разбег*) run, moméntum; с ~а full tilt.

разгоня́ть, разогна́ть 1. (*вн.; заставлять разойти́сь в разные стороны*) dispérse (*smb., smth.*), break* up (*smb., smth.*); ~ демонстра́цию break* up a demonstrátion; 2. (*вн.; ликвидировать*) break* up (*smth.*), dissólve (*smth.*); 3. (*вн.; рассеивать*) dispérse (*smth.*), drive* away (*smth.*); *перен. тж.* dispél (*smth.*); ве́тер разогна́л ту́чи the wind blew away the clouds; разогна́ть тоску́ drive* away one's depréssion; 4. (*ускорять ход*) get* up speed, speed* alóng; (*вн.*) speed* up (*smth.*); 5. (*вн.*) *разг.* (*увольнять*) sack (*smb.*), get* rid (of). ~ся, разогна́ться get* up speed, gain moméntum; (*о бегуне*) get* ínto one's stride.

разгора́живать, разгороди́ть (*вн.*) partítion (*smth.*). ~ся, разгороди́ться (с *тв.*) partition/divíde onesélf off (from).

разгора́ться, разгоре́ться 1. flare up, get* well alíght; дрова́ разгоре́лись the wood begán to burn well; 2. (*становиться красным от возбуждения*) begin* to glow; её щёки разгоре́лись her cheeks begán to glow, her cheeks flushed; 3. (*увлекаться*) becóme* enthusiástic/éager; 4. (*становиться сильным, напряжённым*) becóme* inténse/héated; спор разгоре́лся the discússion becáme héated; стра́сти разгоре́лись féeling ran high; ◇ у него́ глаза́ разгоре́лись his eyes shone, an éager look came ínto his eyes.

разгоре́ться *сов. см.* разгора́ться.

разгороди́ть(ся) *сов. см.* разгора́живать(ся).

разгоряче́нный (óver)héated; (*о лице*) flushed.

разгоряче́ть *сов. см.* горячи́ть. ~ся *сов.* 1. get* (too) hot, becóme* (óver)héated; 2. *см.* горячи́ться.

разгра́б|ить (*вн.*) rob (*smth.*), plúnder (*smth.*); ~ склад rob a wárehouse. ~ле́ние *с.* plúnder.

разграниче́ние *с.* demarcátion, delimitátion.

разграни́чивать, разграни́чить (*вн.*) delímit (*smth.*); *перен. тж.* differéntiate (between), draw* a line/distínction (between); ~ поня́тия differéntiate between the concéptions; ~ обя́занности decíde who is to be respónsible for what.

разграни́чить *сов. см.* разграни́чивать.

разграфи́ть *сов. см.* разграфля́ть.

разграфля́ть, разграфи́ть (*вн.*) rule (*smth.*).

разгреба́ть, разгрести́ (*вн.*) rake (*smth.*) away/asíde, scátter (*smth.*).

разгрести́ *сов. см.* разгреба́ть.

разгро́м *м.* 1. crúshing deféat, rout; ~ врага́ rout of the énemy; 2. (*разорение, опустошение*) devastátion, wrécking; ~ го́рода devastátion of a cíty; 3. *разг.* (*беспорядок*) hávoc, mess; в ко́мнате был по́лный ~ the room was in a state of útter hávoc.

разгроми́ть *сов. см.* громи́ть.

разгружа́ть, разгрузи́ть (*вн.*) unlóad (*smth.*), dischárge (*smth.*); *перен. разг.* relíeve (*smb.*). ~ся, разгрузи́ться be* unlóaded; *перен. разг.* dispose of some of one's work.

разгрузи́ть(ся) *сов. см.* разгружа́ть(ся).

разгру́зка *ж.* unlóading, dischárging.

разгрыза́ть, разгры́зть (*вн.*) crunch (*smth.*), bite (*smth.*) in two; (*орех*) crack (*smth.*).

разгры́зть *сов. см.* разгрыза́ть.

разгу́л *м.* 1. (*уха́рство*) éscapades *pl*; (*пьянство*) órgy, caróusing, débauch; binge *разг.*; 2. (*безудержное проявление чего-л.*) órgy, ónslaught; ~ реа́кции órgy of reáction.

разгу́лив|ать *несов. разг.* walk abóut; stroll abóut. ~аться, разгуля́ться *разг.* 1. (*давать себе волю*) get* góing; (*о ветре и т. п.*) break* loose; разгуля́лась непого́да the storm broke loose; 2. (*становиться ясным, солнечным*) clear up; пого́да, день ~а́ется it's beginning to clear up; 3. (*переставать хотеть спать*) not feel

like sléeping ány more; ребёнок разгуля́лся the child* is over-excíted.

разгу́льный *разг.* wild; ~ о́браз жи́зни wild/fast life.

разгуля́ться *сов. разг.* 1. *см.* разгу́ливаться; 2. (*увлечься развлечениями*) let* onesélf go; (*кутить*) live it up, have* a real binge.

раздава́ть, разда́ть (*вн. дт.*) distríbute (*smth.* amóng), hand out (*smth.* amóng); pass/hand (*smth.*) round.

раздава́ться I, разда́ться (*звучать*) be* heard; (*о выстрелах, криках тж.*) ring* out; разда́лся стук в дверь there was a knock at the door; разда́лся крик a cry was heard.

раздава́ться II, разда́ться 1. (*расступаться*) make* way; 2. *разг.*: он разда́лся в плеча́х he has bróadened out acróss the shóulders; она́ разда́лась в та́лии her wáistline has expánded.

раздави́ть *сов.* (*вн.*) crush (*smb., smth.*).

разда́ривать, раздари́ть (*вн.*) give* (*smth.*) away.

раздари́ть *сов. см.* разда́ривать.

разда́точный distríbuting; distribútion *attr.*; ~ пункт distribútion céntre.

разда́ть *сов. см.* раздава́ть.

разда́ться I, II *сов. см.* раздава́ться I, II.

разда́ча *ж.* distribútion.

раздва́ивать, раздво́ить (*вн.*) divíde (*smth.*) ínto two, split* (*smth.*) in two. ~ся, раздво́иться fork; bifurcate *научн.*; *перен.* split* apárt, súffer a split.

раздви́г|ать, раздви́нуть (*вн.*) 1. (*занавески, ветки и т. п.*) draw* (*smth.*), part (*smth.*); 2. (*отодвигать в стороны*) move (*smth.*) aside, move (*smth.*) back; раздви́нуть сту́лья move the chairs back; 3. (*заставлять расступиться*) clear a way through (*smth.*); ~ толпу́ push one's way through the crowd. ~а́ться, раздви́нуться 1. part; 2. *тк. несов.* (*быть раздвижным*) expánd; стол ~а́ется the táble expánds.

раздвижно́й: ~ за́навес draw cúrtain; ~ стол expánding táble.

раздви́нуть *сов. см.* раздвига́ть. ~ся *сов. см.* раздвига́ться 1.

раздво́ить(ся) *сов. см.* раздва́ивать(ся).

раздева́лка *ж. разг.* clóak-room, dréssing-room *амер.*

раздева́ть, разде́ть (*вн.*) 1. undréss (*smb.*); 2. *разг.* (*грабить*) strip (*smb.*) of his clothes. ~ся, разде́ться undréss; разде́ньтесь до по́яса strip (down) to the waist.

разде́л *м.* 1. (*действие*) divísion; 2. (*часть*) part, séction.

разде́лать(ся) *сов. см.* разде́лывать(ся).

разделе́ние *с.* divísion; ~ труда́ divísion of lábour.

раздели́тельн|ый dividing, séparative; ~ая черта́ dividing line; ◇ ~ сою́з *грам.* disjúnctive conjúnction.

раздели́ть *сов. см.* разделя́ть. ~ся *сов. см.* разделя́ться 1, 2.

разде́лывать, разде́лать 1. (*вн.; обрабатывать каким-л. образом*) prepáre (*smth.*), dress (*smth.*); ~ ту́шу dress a cárcass; 2.: разде́лать что-л. под дуб, под кра́сное де́рево *и т. п.* give* smth. an oak, mahógany, *etc.* finish; ~ разде́лать кого-л. под оре́х make* smb. smart. ~ся, разде́латься (с *тв.*) *разг.* 1. (*кончать с кем-л. какие-л. дела, освобождаться от чего-л.*) have* done (with); разде́латься с долга́ми séttle one's debts; 2. (*расправляться*) get* éven (with), fix (*smb.*); я с ним разде́лаюсь! I'll fix him!

разде́льн|о 1. séparately; 2. (*отчётливо*) distínctly. ~ый 1. séparate; 2. (*отчётливый*) distínct; 3. (*о правописании*) séparate.

раздел|я́ть, раздели́ть (*вн.*) 1. (*делить*) divíde (*smth.*); раздели́ть что-л. попола́м, на ча́сти divíde smth. in two, ínto parts; раздели́ть 12 на 3 divíde twelve by three; 2. (*разобщать*) séparate (*smb., smth.*); толпа́ раздели́ла нас the crowd came betwéen us, the crowd cut us off from each óther; нас ~ет про́пасть there is a gulf (fixed) betwéen us; **3.** (*участь, мнение и т. п.*) share (*smth.*); ~ чью-л. ра́дость share *smb.'s* joy. **~я́ться,** раздели́ться **1.** break* up, split* up; отря́д раздели́лся попола́м the detáchment split up ínto two groups; **2.** (*расходиться в чём-л.*) be* divíded; голоса́ раздели́лись the votes were divíded; мне́ния раздели́лись opínions differed; **3.** *тк. несов.* (*распределяться по группам и т. п.*) fall* ínto (*smth.*).

разде́тый undréssed; (*без пальто*) without a coat *после сущ.*

разде́ть(ся) *сов. см.* раздева́ть(ся).

раздир|а́ть, разодра́ть (*вн.*) **1.** *разг.* (*рвать на части*) tear* (*smth.*) up; tear* a hole (in); **2.** *тк. несов.* (*вызывать внутренние противоречия*) tear* (*smth.*) apárt, split* (*smth.*) from top to bóttom; **3.** *тк. несов.* (*причинять страдания*) tear* (*smb., smth.*), rend* (*smb., smth.*); го́ре ~а́ло его́ се́рдце his heart was torn with grief/sórrow, grief was cláwing at his heart.

раздобре́ть *сов. разг.* (*располнеть*) grow* stout/córpulent.

раздобы́ть *сов.* (*вн.*) *разг.* get* (*smth.*), get* hold (of).

раздо́лье *с.* **1.** (*простор*) spáciousness; ópen spáces *pl,* expánse; како́е ~! how spácious!; **2.** *разг.* (*полная свобода*) scope, fréedom. **~ный** *разг.* **1.** spácious, far-flúng; ~ная степь the wide and rólling steppe; **2.** (*свободный*) great, cárefree; ~ная жизнь cárefree life.

раздо́р *м.* díscord, dissénsion; bíckering *разг.;* се́ять ~ sow* (the seeds of) dissénsion; прекрати́ть ~ы stop the bíckering; ◇ я́блоко ~а the ápple of díscord.

раздоса́довать *сов.* (*вн.*) vex (*smb.*), annóy (*smb.*). **~ся** *сов. разг.* get* annóyed, lose* one's témper.

раздраж|а́ть, раздражи́ть (*вн.*) írritate (*smb., smth.*). **~а́ться,** раздражи́ться be* írritated, lose* one's témper. **~а́ющий** írritating. **~е́ние** *с.* irritátion; кра́йнее ~е́ние exasperátion. **~ённый** exásperated, írritated, spúnky *амер.*

раздражи́тель *м.* írritant.

раздражи́тель|ость *ж.* irritabílity. **~ый** írritable.

раздражи́ть(ся) *сов. см.* раздража́ть(ся).

раздразни́ть *сов.* (*вн.*) tease (*smb., smth.*), provóke (*smb., smth.*); ~ соба́ку tease a dog; ~ аппети́т tíckle/whet the áppetite; ~ любопы́тство provóke *smb.'s* curiósity.

раздроби́ть(ся) *сов. см.* раздробля́ть(ся) *и* дроби́ть(ся).

раздро́бленн|ость *ж.* disúnity, disrúption, disuníted state, séparateness. **~ый 1.** crushed, bróken; (*о кости*) splíntered; **2.** (*расчленённый*) disuníted, párcelled up.

раздробля́ть, раздроби́ть **1.** break* (*smth.*), crush (*smth.*); (*кость*) splínter (*smth.*); ему́ раздроби́ло ру́ку his hand was crushed; **2.** (*расчленять*) disuníte (*smth.*), párcel (*smth.*) up; **~ся,** раздроби́ться **1.** (*разбиваться*) fly* to píeces, crúmble; ка́мень раздроби́лся the rock flew to píeces; **2.** (*делиться на части, группы*) split* up, be* split up.

раздува́ть, разду́ть (*вн.*) **1.** (*огонь*) fan (*smth.*) (*тж. перен.*); **2.** *безл.:* у него́ разду́ло щёку he has a swóllen cheek/face; **3.** *разг.* (*чрезмерно увеличивать*) infláte (*smth.*); **4.** *разг.* (*преувеличивать*) enlárge upón (*smth.*), exággerate (*smth.*). **~ся,** разду́ться swell*; (*о парусе*) bíllow; карма́ны разду́лись the póckets begán to bulge.

разду́м|ать *сов.* (+ *инф.*) change one's mind (abóut + -ing); think* bétter of it; я ~ал идти́ I (have) decíded not to go; I have changed my mind abóut góing.

разду́мыв|ать *несов.* think*, pónder; (*колебаться*) hésitate; не ~ая without a móment's hesitátion.

разду́мь|е *с.* meditátion, thought; по́сле до́лгого ~я áfter prolónged meditátion; погрузи́ться в ~ be* lost in thought; в глубо́ком ~ deep/plúnged in thought.

разду́т|ый *разг.* **1.** (*вздутый*) swóllen; **2.** (*ветром*)

bíllowing; **3.** (*непомерно увеличенный*) infláted; ~ые шта́ты overstáffing.

разду́ть(ся) *сов. см.* раздува́ть(ся).

разева́ть, рази́нуть (*вн.*) *разг.* ópen (*smth.*) wide; ◇ рази́нуть рот от удивле́ния be* open-móuthed with astónishment; что ты рот рази́нул? what are you stánding there gáping for?

разжа́лобить *сов.* (*вн.*) move (*smb.*) to píty. **~ся** *сов. разг.* give* in to píty, be* soft.

разжа́ть(ся) *сов. см.* разжима́ть(ся).

разжева́ть *сов. см.* разжёвывать.

разжёвывать, разжева́ть **1.** (*вн.*) chew (*smth.*), másticate (*smth.*); **2.** (*вн. дт.*) *разг.* (*растолковывать*) spóonfeed* (*smth.* to), particularize (*smth.* to).

разже́чь *сов. см.* разжига́ть.

разжига́ть, разже́чь (*вн.*) light* (*smth.*), kíndle (*smth.*); *перен.* infláme (*smth.*); разже́чь костёр get* the cámp-fire góing; ~ не́нависть stir up hátred, fomént hátred.

разжиж|а́ть *несов.* (*вн.*) dilúte (*smth.*), wáter (*smth.*) down. **~е́ние** *с.* dilútion.

разжима́ть, разжа́ть (*вн.*) ópen (*smth.*); (*губы, зубы*) part (*smth.*); ~ кула́к unclénch one's fist; не ~ губ not ópen one's mouth; разжа́ть пружи́ну reléase a spring. **~ся,** разжа́ться (*о губах*) part, ópen; (*о пружине*) expánd; (*о руке, кулаке*) reláx, unclénch.

разжире́ть *сов. см.* жире́ть.

раззадо́ривать, раззадо́рить (*вн.*) *разг.* rouse (*smb.*), egg (*smb.*) on.

раззадо́рить *сов. см.* раззадо́ривать.

раззвони́ть *сов.* (*о пр.*) *разг.* trúmpet (*smth.*); procláim (*smth.*) from the hóuse-tops.

рази́нуть *сов. см.* разева́ть.

рази́ня *м. и ж. разг.* dáy-dreamer, goof.

рази́тельн|ый stríking; ~ приме́р stríking exámple; ~ые переме́ны stríking chánges.

рази́ть I, срази́ть (*вн.; ударять*) strike* (*smb., smth.*); *перен.* crush (*smth.*).

рази́|ть II *несов.* (*тв.*) *разг.* (*пахнуть*) reek (of); от него́ ~т во́дкой he reeks of vódka.

разлага́ть, разложи́ть **1.** (*вн. на вн.*) *хим.* decompóse (*smth.* ínto); *мат.* expánd (*smth.* ínto); *физ.* (*силу*) resólve (*smth.* ínto); **2.** (*вн.; морально*) demóralize (*smb.*), corrúpt (*smb.*). **~ся,** разложи́ться **1.** *хим.* decompóse; *мат.* expánd; *физ.* (*о силе*) be* resólved; (*гнить*) decáy; (*о трупе*) decompóse; **3.** (*морально*) degénerate.

разлага́ющ|е: де́йствовать ~ be* demóralizing, have* a demóralizing efféct. **~ий** demóralizing.

разла́д *м.* díscord; (*отсутствие согласованности*) lack of co-órdinátion; вноси́ть ~ sow* dissénsion.

разла́диться *сов. см.* разла́живаться.

разла́живаться, разла́диться be* not góing well; go* wrong; отноше́ния разла́дились reláations are not what they were.

разла́мывать, разломи́ть, разлома́ть (*вн.*) **1.** *сов.* разломи́ть break* (*smth.*); **2.** *сов.* разлома́ть pull (*smth.*) down. **~ся,** разломи́ться, разлома́ться **1.** *сов.* разломи́ться break*; **2.** *сов.* разлома́ться fall* to píeces; **3.** *тк. несов. разг.* (*сильно болеть — о голове*) be* splítting.

разлени́ться *сов. разг.* becóme* lázy, get* slack.

разлета́ться, разлете́ться **1.** (*улетать в разные стороны*) fly* awáy; (*рассеиваться*) dispérse; бума́ги разлете́лись по всей ко́мнате the pápers flew all over the room; **2.** (*расходиться, разъезжаться*) go* off; *перен. разг.* (*быстро распространяться*) flash round; **3.** *разг.* (*разбившись, рассыпаться на части*) fly* to píeces; *перен.* (*исчезать*) dissólve; разлете́ться вдре́безги break* ínto smitheréens.

разлете́ться *сов. см.* разлета́ться.

разле́чься *сов. разг.* stretch onesélf out; sprawl.

разли́в м. (*половодье*) flood; (*вина*) bóttling.

разлива́тельн|ый: ~ая ло́жка ládle, sóup-ladle.

разлива́ть, разли́ть (*вн.*) 1. (*проливать*) spill* (*smth.*); 2. (*наливать*) pour (*smth.*) out; (*по бутыл-кам*) bóttle (*smth.*); ◇ их водо́й не разольёшь they are bósom friends, they are véry thick with one anóther. ~ся, разли́ться 1. (*проливаться*) spill*; молоко́ разлило́сь the milk has run óver; 2. (*выходить из берегов*) overflów its banks; 3. (*распространяться*) spread*, flood; сла́бый румя́нец разли́лся по его́ щека́м a faint flush spread óver his cheeks; 4. *тк. несов.* (*петь звон-ко*) pour out *one's* song; (*говорить много*) decláim; (*плакать*) sob.

разлив|о́й: ~о́е пи́во draught beer; ~о́е молоко́ unbóttled milk.

разлинова́ть *сов.* (*вн.*) rule (*smth.*).

разли́ть *сов. см.* разлива́ть. ~ся *сов. см.* разлива́ть-ся 1, 2, 3.

различа́ть, различи́ть (*вн.*) 1. (*распознавать*) make* (*smb., smth.*) out, discérn (*smb., smth.*); 2. (*ви-деть разницу*) distínguish (betwéen); tell* (*smb., smth.*) apárt. ~ся *несов.* (*тв.*) díffer (in), be* distínguished (by).

различи́|е с. distínction; не де́лать ~я ме́жду кем--л., чем-л. not discríminate betwéen *smb., smth.*, not make* distínctions betwéen *smb., smth.*; ◇ зна́ки ~я bádges of rank; без ~я irréspective of, regárdless of.

различи́ть *сов. см.* различа́ть.

разли́чный 1. (*несходный*) díffering, dífferent; 2. (*разнообразный*) várious, divérse.

разложе́ние с. 1. (*действие*) decomposítion; (*трупа тж.*) putrefáction; 2. *мат.* expánsion; *физ.* (*сил*) resolútion; 3. (*моральное*) corrúption, demoralizátion.

разложи́ть(ся) *сов. см.* разлага́ть(ся) *и* раскла́ды-вать(ся).

разло́м м. 1. (*действие*) bréaking; 2. (*место разло-ма*) break, frácture.

разлома́ть *сов. см.* разла́мывать 2. ~ся *сов. см.* разла́мываться 2.

разлом|и́ть *сов. см.* разла́мывать 1; ~и́ться *сов. см.* разла́мываться 1.

разлу́к|а ж. (*с тв.*) 1. separátion (from); жить в ~е live apárt; 2. (*расставание*) párting.

разлуча́ть, разлучи́ть (*вн. с тв.*) séparate (*smb.* from). ~ся, разлучи́ться (*с тв.*) part (with).

разлучи́ть(ся) *сов. см.* разлуча́ть(ся).

разлюб|и́ть *сов.* stop lóving (*smb.*); get* tíred (of); он меня́ ~и́л he no lónger cares for me.

размагни́|тить(ся) *сов. см.* размагни́чивать(ся). ~чивать, размагни́тить (*вн.*) demágnetize (*smth.*); (*суд-но*) degáuss (*smth.*); *перен. разг.* cool *smb.'s* enthúsiasm. ~чиваться, размагни́титься get*/becóme* demágnetized; *перен. разг.* cool off, have* a féeling of lét-down.

разма́зать(ся) *сов. см.* разма́зывать(ся).

размазня́ *разг.* 1. ж. (*жидкая каша*) thin gruel, pap; 2. *м. и ж.* (*о человеке*) dítherer, slóppy créature, sap.

разма́зывать, разма́зать (*вн.*) 1. smear (*smth.*); 2. *разг.* (*растягивать*) spread* (*smth.*) out, drag (*smth.*) out. ~ся, разма́заться (*по дт.*) be* spread/smeared (óver).

размалева́ть *сов.* (*вн.*) *разг.* daub (*smth.*).

разма́лывать, размоло́ть (*вн.*) grind* (*smth.*). ~ся, размоло́ться be* ground.

разма́тывать, размота́ть (*вн.*) unwínd* (*smth.*). ~ся, размота́ться come* unwóund.

разма́х м. 1. (*колебание*) swing; 2.: ~ кры́льев wíng--spread, wíng-span; 3. (*охват, масштаб*) scope, range, extént; челове́к широ́кого ~а man* of imaginátion, man* on a large scale; ◇ уда́рить кого́-л. со всего́ ~y strike* *smb.* with all *one's* strength/might; уда́риться со всего́ ~y обо что-л. cánnon ínto *smth.*, hit* *smth.* at full speed.

разма́хивать *несов.* (*тв.*) swing* (*smth.*), brándish (*smth.*); ~ рука́ми wave *one's* hands abóut, gestículate.

размахну́ться *сов.* swing* back *one's* arm.

разма́чивать, размочи́ть (*вн.*) soak (*smth.*), sóften (*smth.*) by sóaking/stéeping; размочи́ть сухари́ в моло-ке́ soak rusks in milk.

разма́шистый *разг.* swínging; ~ шаг pówerful/swínging stride; ~ жест swéeping gésture; ~ по́-черк bold hánd(writing).

размежева́ние с. demarcátion; delimitátion (*тж. пе-рен.*).

размежева́ть(ся) *сов. см.* размежёвывать(ся).

размежёвывать, размежева́ть (*вн.*) démarcate (*smth.*); delímit (*smth.*) (*тж. перен.*); ~ зе́млю démarcate land; размежева́ть фу́нкции define the fúnctions. ~ся, размежева́ться (*прям. и перен.*) séparate, dissóciate onesélf.

размельча́ть, размельчи́ть (*вн.*) crush (*smth.*) ínto píeces; размельчи́ть что-л. в порошо́к crush/pound *smth.* ínto pówder, púlverize (*smth.*).

размельчи́ть *сов. см.* размельча́ть.

разме́нивать, разменя́ть (*вн.*) change (*smth.*). ~ся, разменя́ться *разг.* exchánge; *перен.* frítter awáy *one's* strength/resóurces.

разме́нн|ый: ~ая моне́та small change.

разменя́ть(ся) *сов. см.* разме́нивать(ся).

разме́р м. 1. (*величина чего-л. в одном или не-скольких измерениях*) size; diménsions *pl*; дом огро́м-ных ~ов house of enórmous size; ~ уча́стка size/diménsions of a plot; 2. (*величина денежной сум-мы*) amóunt; ~ зарпла́ты, проце́нта rate of wáges, ínterest; ~ пе́нсии scale of pénsion; ~ капиталовложе́ний amóunt of cápital invésted; 3. (*мерка, номер какого-л. изделия*) size; ~ о́буви, костю́ма size of fóotwear/suit; 4. (*степень*) extént, scale; в небыва́лых ~ах on a large scale; ~ бе́дствия extént of a disáster; 5. *лит.* métre; 6. *муз.* méasure, time.

разме́ренн|ый méasured; régular; stéady; ~ ритм régular rhýthm; ~ шаг méasured tread; ~ые движе́ния well-régulated móvements.

размести́ *сов. см.* размета́ть I.

размести́ть *сов. см.* размеща́ть(ся).

размета́ть I, размести́ (*вн.*) (*очищать от чего-л.*) sweep* (*smth.*); (*убирать что-л.*) sweep* (*smth.*) awáy; размести́ снег sweep* the snow awáy.

размета́ть II *сов.* 1. (*вн.*) (*разбросать*) scátter (*smth.*); 2. (*широко раскинуть руки, ноги*) exténd (*smth.*), spread* out (*smth.*).

размет|ить *сов. см.* размеча́ть. ~ка ж. márking. ~чик м. márker.

размеча́ть, разме́тить (*вн.*) mark (*smth.*), mark (*smth.*) out.

размечта́ться *сов.* (*о пр.*) *разг.* be* lost in dreams (abóut), give* onesélf up to dreams (of).

размеша́ть *сов. см.* разме́шивать II.

разме́шивать I, размеси́ть (*вн.*) knead (*smth.*).

разме́шивать II, размеша́ть (*вн.*) stir (*smth.*), mix (*smth.*); размеша́ть са́хар в ча́е stir *one's* tea.

размещ|а́ть, размести́ть (*вн.*) 1. put* (*smth.*), place (*smth.*); (*кого-л. по комнатам*) assign rooms (to); (*войска*) quárter (*smb., smth.*); 2. (*распределять меж-ду многими*) place (*smth.*), assign (*smth.*); размести́ть зака́зы place órders. ~а́ться, размести́ться take* *one's* place; (*в каком-л. помещении*) be* quártered/accóm-modated. ~е́ние с. 1. plácing; (*по комнатам*) allocá-tion; 2. (*порядок, система расположения чего-л.*) arrángement.

размина́ть, размя́ть (*вн.*) 1. knead (*smth.*); (*карто-фель*) mash (*smth.*); 2. *разг.*: размя́ть но́ги stretch *one's* legs. ~ся, размя́ться 1. (*делаться мягким*) becóme* soft, sóften up; 2. *разг.* (*о человеке*) límber up.

размини́рование *с.* demíning.

размини́ровать *несов. и сов.* (*вн.*) demíne (*smth.*), clear (*smth.*) of mines.

размы́нка *ж. разг.* límbering up; wórk-out *амер.*

размину́ться *сов. разг.* 1. (*разойтись в пути*) miss one anóther; 2. (*с тв.; пройти мимо*) pass (*smb., smth.*).

размнож|а́ть, размно́жить (*вн.; документ и т. п.*) make* cópies (of); ~а́ться, размно́житься 1. múltiply; 2. *тк. несов.* биол. reprodúce; (*о животных*) breed*; (*о растениях*) própagate; (*о рыбах*) spawn. ~е́ние *с.* 1. (*документов и т. п.*) máking cópies of; (*на ксероксе*) xéroxing; 2. биол. reprodúction.

размно́жить *сов. см.* размножа́ть. ~ся *сов. см.* размножа́ться 1.

размозжи́ть *сов.* (*вн.*) smash (*smth.*); ~ кому-л. го́лову smash *smb.'s* skull; ~ себе́ го́лову break* *one's* head.

размока́ть, размо́кнуть be* soaked through, becóme* sódden.

размо́кнуть *сов. см.* размока́ть.

размо́кший sódden, sóggy.

размо́л *м.* mílling.

размо́лвка *ж.* misunderstánding, tiff; ме́жду ни́ми, у них произошла́ ~ they have had a tiff.

размоло́ть(ся) *сов. см.* разма́лывать(ся).

размор|и́ть *сов.* (*вн.*) *разг.* make* (*smb.*) feel dazed/bemúsed; меня́ ~и́ло от жары́ I feel quite dazed by the heat.

размота́ть(ся) *сов. см.* разма́тывать(ся).

размо́тка *ж.* unwínding, unréeling.

размочи́ть *сов. см.* разма́чивать.

размы́в *м.* erósion.

размыва́ть, размы́ть 1. (*вн.*) eróde (*smth.*), wash (*smth.*) awáy; река́ размы́ла берега́ the ríver has washed awáy its banks; 2. *безл.:* доро́гу размы́ло the road is swamped/flóoded.

размыка́ть, разомкну́ть (*вн.*) (*шлюзы и т. п.*) ópen (*smth.*); эл. break* (*smth.*); воен. exténd (*smth.*), ópen (*smth.*). ~ся, разомкну́ться come* apárt; ópen.

размы́ть *сов. см.* размыва́ть.

размышле́ни|е *с.* refléction, meditátion; по зре́лом ~и on matúre considerátion; погрузи́ться в ~я be* lost/deep in thought, be* plunged in meditátion; э́то наво́дит на ~я that makes *one* think.

размышля́ть *несов.* (*о пр.*) refléct (on), méditate (on), pónder (óver, on), think* (óver) óver.

размягч|а́ть, размягчи́ть (*вн.; прям. и перен.*) sóften (*smb., smth.*). ~а́ться, размягчи́ться, becóme* soft; sóften (*тж. перен.*). ~е́ние *с.* sóftening; ~е́ние мо́зга sóftening of the brain. ~и́ть(ся) *сов. см.* размягча́ть(ся).

размяка́ть, размя́кнуть grow* soft; *перен. разг.* (*о человеке*) be* sóftened, melt.

размя́кнуть *сов. см.* размяка́ть.

размя́ть(ся) *сов. см.* размина́ть(ся).

разнаря́дка *ж.* órder, wárrant.

разна́шивать, разноси́ть (*вн.*) break* (*smth.*) in, wear* (*smth.*) in; но́вые боти́нки на́до разноси́ть new boots need bréaking in. ~ся, разноси́ться: боти́нки разноси́лись the boots are quite cómfortable now.

разнести́ *сов. см.* разноси́ть I. ~сь *сов. см.* разноси́ться I.

разнима́ть, разня́ть (*вн.*) 1. (*разъединять*) part (*smth.*); 2. (*дерущихся*) séparate (*smb.*); 3. *тех.* dismántle (*smth.*), take* (*smth.*) apárt.

ра́зниться *несов.* differ; ~ во вку́сах differ in *one's* tastes.

ра́зниц|а *ж.* dífference; ~ лет dífference in age; вся ~ в том, что... the ónly dífference is that...; с той ~ей, что... the dífference béing that...; ◇ больша́я ~ it makes a great dífference; кака́я ~? what dífference does it make?, what's the dífference?; без ~ы makes no dífference.

разнобо́й *м. разг.* lack of co-ordinátion; inconsístency.

разнови́дность *ж.* varíety.

разногла́сие *с.* 1. dissénsion, dífference, disagréement; 2. (*противоречие*) discrépancy; ~ в показа́ниях conflícting évidence.

разноголо́с|ица *ж. разг.* 1. (*нестройное пение*) discórdance; 2. (*разногласие*) dífference; discrépancy; ~ый discórdant.

разнокали́берн|ый 1. of dífferent cálibre(s) *после сущ.*; 2. *разг.* (*неоднородный, разных размеров и т. п.*) heterogéneous, mixed.

разнома́стный dífferent-cóloured, unmátched; (*о картах*) of dífferent suits *после сущ.*

разнообра́зи|е *с.* varíety, divérsity; ~ форм varíety of forms; вноси́ть ~ в жизнь break* the monótony of *one's* life; ◇ для ~я for a change.

разнообра́з|ить *несов.* (*вн.*) váry (*smth.*), divérsify (*smth.*). ~ный divérse; váried; ~ные расте́ния mány sorts of plants.

разнорабо́чий *м.* géneral wórker; ódd-job man*.

разноречи́в|ый conflícting, contradíctory; ~ые слу́хи conflícting rúmours.

разноро́дный heterogéneous.

разно́с *м.* 1. (*доставка*) delívery; 2. *разг.* (*выговор*) dréssing-down, sláting.

разноси́ть I, разнести́ (*вн.*) 1. (*доставлять*) delíver (*smth.*); разнести́ пи́сьма адреса́там delíver létters; 2. (*обнося, раздавать что-л.*) distríbute (*smth.*), hand round (*smth.*); 3. (*записывать в разные места*) énter (*smth.*); ~ счета́ по кни́гам make* up the books; 4. *разг.* (*рассеивать*) scátter (*smth.*), dispérse (*smth.*); ве́тер разнёс обры́вки бума́ги the wind scáttered the strips of páper; 5. *разг.* (*разглашать*) spread* (*smth.*); ~ но́вости, слу́хи spread* news, rúmours; 6. *разг.* (*разрывать, разбивать*) shátter (*smth.*), wreck (*smth.*); бу́ря разнесла́ ло́дку в ще́пки the storm knocked the boat to píeces; 7. *разг.* (*разрушать*) destróy (*smth.*); 8. *разг.* (*ругать*) slate (*smb., smth.*), tear* (*smth.*) to pieces.

разноси́ть II *сов. см.* разна́шивать.

разноси́ться I, разнести́сь 1. (*распространяться*) spread*; 2. (*о звуке*) resóund.

разноси́ться II *сов. см.* разна́шиваться.

разносн|ый 1. ~ая кни́га recéipt-book; 2. *разг.* (*резко критикующий*) anníhilating, sláshing; ~ая статья́ в газе́те anníhilating néwspaper árticle.

разносторо́нн|ий 1. mány-síded; (*о человеке тж.*) vérsatile; ~ее образова́ние áll-round educátion; *мат.:* ~ треуго́льник scaléne tríangle; ~ость *ж.* mány-sídedness; versatílity; ~ость зна́ний váried/univérsal knówledge, wíde-ranging erudítion.

ра́зност|ь *ж. мат.* dífference; ◇ ра́зные ~и all sorts of things.

разно́счик *м.* pédlar, háwker; ~ газе́т néws-vendor, néws-boy.

разноцве́тный of dífferent cólours *после сущ.*; (*пёстрый*) párticoloured, pátterned.

разношёрстн|ый mótley; *перен. разг.* mixed; ~ая толпа́ mixed crowd, íll-matched bunch.

разноязы́чный pólyglot.

разну́зданный unbrídled; *перен. разг.* wild, rówdy, ungóvernable.

разнузда́ть(ся) *сов. см.* разну́здывать(ся).

разну́здывать, разнузда́ть (*вн.*) unbrídle (*smth.*); *перен. разг.* unléash (*smb., smth.*). ~ся, разнузда́ться slip the brídle; *перен. разг.* run* ríot/wild.

ра́зн|ый *прил.* 1. (*разнообразный*) várious, váried, divérse; of all sorts *после сущ.*; мы с ним ~ые лю́ди we are símply dífferent péople; ~ые мне́ния conflícting opínions; в ~ое вре́мя at dífferent times (of the day, year); ~ого рóда слýхи all sorts of rúmours; ~ой величины́ of different sízes; мы говори́ли о совершéнно ~ых вещáх we were not éven tálking abóut the same thing; 2. *в знач. сущ. с.* várious things *pl.*

разня́ть *сов. см.* разнимáть.

разоби́деть *сов. (вн.) разг.* bítterly offénd (*smb.*). ~ся *сов. разг.* take* great offénce, be* véry much put out.

разоблач|áть, разоблачи́ть (*вн.*) expóse (*smb.*, *smth.*), unmásk (*smb.*). ~áться, разоблачи́ться be* expósed, come* to light. ~éние *с.* expósure. ~и́тель *м.* denúnciator. ~и́ть(ся) *сов. см.* разоблачáть(ся).

разобрáть *сов. см.* разбирáть 1-7. ~ся *сов. см.* разбирáться 2, 3.

разобщ|áть, разобщи́ть (*вн.*) 1. break* up (*smb.*, *smth.*); *перен.* estránge (*smb.*); 2. (*прерывать общение*) dissóciate (*smb.*). ~áться, разобщи́ться becóme* dissóciated, get* out of touch. ~éние *с.* 1. bréaking up; *перен.* estrángement; 2. (*отсутствие связи, общения*) dissociátion. ~ённость *ж.* isolátion, estrángement. ~ённый ísolated, estránged.

рáзовый síngle; ~ биле́т síngle ticket, óne-way ticket; ~ прóпуск pass válid for one atténdance ónly.

разогнáть(ся) *сов. см.* разгоня́ть(ся).

разогнýть(ся) *сов. см.* разгибáть(ся).

разогревáть, разогре́ть (*вн.*) heat (*smth.*) up; *разг.* (*вызывать ощущение тепла*) warm (*smb.*, *smth.*) up. ~ся, разогрéться becóme*/get* hot; *разг.* (*согреваться*) get* warm.

разогре́ть(ся) *сов. см.* разогревáть(ся).

разоде́тый *разг.* dressed up, dolled up.

разоде́ть *сов. (вн.) разг.* dress/doll (*smb.*) up. ~ся *сов. разг.* be* dressed/dolled/figged up.

разодрáть *сов. см.* раздирáть.

разодрáться *сов. разг.* (*сильно подраться*) have* a próper scrap/fight.

разозли́ть *сов. (вн.)* make* (*smb.*) fúrious. ~ся *сов.* (на *вн.*) get* fúrious (with); get* mad (with) *разг.*

разойти́сь *сов. см.* расходи́ться.

рáзом *разг.* 1. (*одновременно*) at once, togéther, at the same time; 2. (*в один приём*) all at once, in one go; 3. (*мгновенно*) in a flash.

разомкнýть(ся) *сов. см.* размыкáть(ся).

разонрáвиться *сов. (дт.) разг.* lose* all *one's* attráction (for), cease to be attráctive (to).

разóрванный 1. (*рваный*) torn; with a hole in it *после сущ.*; 2. (*отрывочный*) disjóinted, disconnécted.

разорвáть *сов. см.* разрывáть I. ~ся *сов. см.* разрывáться.

разор|éние *с.* ruin; (*разрушение*) devastátion, rávaging, píllaging. ~ённый ruined; ~ённый войнóй wár-rávaged, dévastated. ~и́тельный rúinous.

разори́ть(ся) *сов. см.* разоря́ть(ся).

разоруж|áть, разоружи́ть (*вн.*) disárm (*smb.*, *smth.*) (*тж. перен.*); ~áться, разоружи́ться disárm. ~éние *с.* disármament; всеóбщее и пóлное ~éние géneral and compléte disármament. ~и́ть(ся) *сов. см.* разоружáть(ся).

разоря́ть, разори́ть (*вн.*) 1. (*разрушать*) dévastate (*smth.*), rávage (*smth.*), píllage (*smth.*); 2. (*лишать имущества*) ruin (*smb.*). ~ся, разори́ться ruin onesélf.

разослáть *сов. см.* рассылáть.

разостлáть(ся) *сов. см.* расстилáть(ся).

разохóтиться *сов.* (на *вн.*; + *инф.*) *разг.* take* a víolent fáncy (to; for + -ing).

разочарова́ние *с.* (*в пр.*) disillúsionment (with), disenchántment (with); ~ в жи́зни disillúsion with life.

разочарóванный disillúsioned, disappóinted; ~ человéк disillúsioned/disappóinted pérson; ~ тон tone of disappóintment.

разочаровáть(ся) *сов. см.* разочарóвывать(ся).

разочарóвывать, разочаровáть (*вн. в пр.*) disappóint (*smb.* in); (*лишать иллюзий*) disillúsion (*smb.* with, abóut), destróy *smb.'s* illúsions (abóut). ~ся, разочаровáться (*в пр.*) be* disappóinted (in), be* disillúsioned (with).

разрабáтывать, разрабóтать (*вн.*) 1. (*делать пригодным для чего-л.*) prepáre (*smth.*); (*почву тж.*) cúltivate (*smth.*); *перен.* devélop (*smth.*), cúltivate (*smth.*); 2. (*подготавливать*) work (*smth.*) out, eláborate (*smth.*); 3. (*усовершенствовать*) work up (*smth.*); train (*smth.*); разрабóтать гóлос train the voice to perféction; 4. *горн.* (*выбирать без остáтка*) exháust (*smth.*); рудни́к пóлностью разрабóтан the mine is exháusted; 5. *тк. несов. горн.* (*эксплуати́ровать*) mine (*smth.*), work (*smth.*).

разрабóтать *сов. см.* разрабáтывать 1, 2, 3, 4.

разрабóтк|а *ж.* 1. (*вопроса и т. п.*) wórking out, elaborátion; 2. (*полезных ископаемых*) míning, extráction; ~ апати́тов míning of ápatites; 3. (*способ добычи*) míning; откры́тая ~ ópen-cast míning; 4. *обыкн. мн.* (*место добычи*) fields, wórkings; торфяны́е ~и peat wórkings.

разрáвнивать, разровня́ть (*вн.*) lével (*smth.*).

разражáться, разрази́ться 1. break*; (*о беде и т.п.*) descénd upón; (*тв.*) break* loose (in), reléase (*smth.*); 2. (*тв.*; *бурно выражать чувства*) burst* (into), burst* out (+ -ing); разрази́ться смéхом burst* out láughing; разрази́ться слезáми burst* into tears; разрази́ться брáнью delíver (onesélf of) a stream of cúrses.

разрази́ться *сов. см.* разражáться.

разрастáться, разрасти́сь grow*, spread*; *перен. тж.* expánd.

разрасти́сь *сов. см.* разрастáться.

разревéться *сов. разг.* howl, start hówling.

разреди́ть *сов. см.* разрежáть.

разрежáть, разреди́ть (*вн.*) 1. (*растения*) thin (*smth.*); 2. (*воздух*) rárefy (*smth.*).

разрежённ|ость *ж.*: ~ вóздуха rárefied átmosphere. ~ый 1. (*менее частый*) thinned out; ~ые посéвы thinned out crops; 2. (*менее насыщенный*) rárefied; ~ый газ, вóздух rárefied gas, air.

разрéз *м.* 1. (*надрез*) cut; (*вдоль*) slit; 2. (*на чертеже*) séction; ◇ ~ глаз set/shape of the eyes; в э́том ~е táken from this áspect/ángle.

разрезáть *сов. см.* разрезáть и рéзать 1.

разрез|áть, разрéзать (*вн.*) 1. cut* (*smth.*); (*вдоль*) slit* (*smth.*); 2. (*вскрывать часть тела*) make* an incísion (in). ~нóй: ~нóй нож páper-knife*.

разреш|áть, разреши́ть 1. (*вн. дт., дт. + инф.*; *позволять*) allów (*smb. smth.*, *smb.* + to inf), permít (*smb. smth.*, *smb.* + to inf), let* (*smb. smth.*, *smb.* + inf); врач разреши́л емý встать с постéли the dóctor allówed him to get up; отéц не ~áет емý чáсто ходи́ть в кинó his fáther does not let him go to the cínema óften; 2. (*вн.*; *допускать*) pass (*smth.*); ~ кни́гу к печáти pass a book for the press; 3. (*вн.*; *находить правильный ответ*) solve (*smth.*); разреши́ть проблéму solve a próblem; 4. (*вн.*; *устранять, разъяснять*) séttle (*smth.*); разреши́ть спор séttle an árgument; разреши́ть сомнéния séttle doubts; 5.: разреши́(те) мне (+ *инф.*) may I (+ inf)?; разреши́те считáть заседáние откры́тым I now decláre the méeting ópen; разреши́те пройти́! excúse me!, may I pass?; разреши́те закури́ть? do you mind if I smoke? ~áться, разреши́ться 1. (*быть решённым*) be* solved, be* séttled; вопрóс разреши́лся óчень легкó the mátter was séttled/solved quite éasily; все егó сомнéния разреши́лись all his doubts disappéared; 2. (*завершáться чем-л.*) be* séttled; дéло наконéц разреши́лось finally the mátter was séttled; 3. *тк. несов. безл.* (*быть позволенным*) be* allówed; здесь кури́ть ~áется smóking is allówed here. ~éние *с.* 1. (*позволение*) permíssion; 2. (документ) pérmit; ~éние на въезд в страну́ pérmit to énter the cóuntry; 3. (вопроса, спора, сомнения) séttlement, séttling.

разреши́ть сов. см. разреша́ть. **~ся** сов. см. разреша́ться 1, 2.

разрисова́ть сов. см. разрисо́вывать.

разрисо́вывать, разрисова́ть (вн.) draw* all óver (smth.); разрисова́ть все сте́ны цвета́ми draw* flówers all óver the walls.

разровня́ть сов. см. разра́внивать.

разро́зненн|ый 1. (неполный) odd; incompléte; **~ые тома́** odd vólumes; **~ компле́кт** incompléte colléction, odd set; 2. (разъединённый) ísolated.

разро́знить сов. (вн.) spoil* (smth.), break* (smth.).

разруб|а́ть, разруби́ть (вн.) (вдоль) split* (smth.); (на части) chop (smth.) up, cut* (smth.) up; **~ что-л. попола́м** cut*/split* smth. in two/halves. **~и́ть** сов. см. разруба́ть.

разруга́ть сов. (вн.) разг. scold (smb.); (дать неодобрительный отзыв) attáck (smb., smth.), slate (smb., smth.). **~ся** сов. (с тв.) разг. quárrel (with), have* a row (with).

разрумя́н|ить сов. (вн.) rédden (smb., smth.). **~иться** сов. (от рд.) (от стыда) blush (with); flush (with); (от быстрого движения) be* flushed (from); **она́ ~илась от моро́за** her face was glówing from the frost.

разру́ха ж. disorganizátion, disrúption.

разруш|а́ть, разру́шить (вн.) 1. destróy (smth.), demólish (smth.); wreck (smth.) (тж. перен.); **разру́шить что-л. до основа́ния** raze smth. to the ground; **разруша́ть госуда́рственный аппара́т** wreck the machínery of State; 2. (портить) ruin (smth.); **~ здоро́вье** ruin one's health; 3. (губить, расстраивать) wreck (smth.); **разру́шить все его́ пла́ны** wreck all his plans; **разру́шить наде́жды** shátter hopes. **~а́ться, разру́шиться** 1. (превращаться в развалины) collápse, be* demólished; 2. (приходить в полный упадок) collápse; 3. (не осуществляться) be* ruined, be* wrecked. **~е́ние** с. destrúction, demolítion, collápse; перен. ruin.

разру́шен|ный wrecked; **~ное зда́ние** wrecked building; **зда́ние бы́ло ~о** the building was destróyed.

разруши́тельный destrúctive.

разру́шить(ся) сов. см. разруша́ть(ся).

разры́в м. 1. (связей и т. п.) rúpture, bréaking off; **~ дипломати́ческих отноше́ний** rúpture of diplomátic relátions; **между ни́ми произошёл ~** they have bróken off their relátions; 2. (действие) bréaking, frácture; (снаряда, котла и т. п.) burst, búrsting; **испыта́ние материа́лов на ~** ténsile test; **~ се́рдца** heart fáilure; 3. (промежуток) gap; 4. (отсутствие связи) gap; **~ между тео́рией и пра́ктикой** gap betwéen théory and práctice.

разрыва́ть I, разорва́ть 1. (вн.) tear* (smth.) up; (твёрдое тело) break* (smth.); перен. тж. shátter (smth.); **разорва́ть письмо́** tear* up a létter; **разорва́ть что-л. на куски́** tear*/rip smth. to píeces; 2. (вн.; прорывать что-л.) tear* (smth.), rip (smth.); slit* (smth.); **перча́тка была́ разо́рвана** the glove was torn/slit; 3. (вн.; растерзать) tear* (smb., smth.) to píeces, maul (smth.); 4. (вн.; взрывом разносить на части) blow* (smth.) to píeces, shátter (smth.); **котёл разорва́ло** the bóiler blew up; 5. (вн.; прекращать действие чего-л.) break* off (smth.); **разорва́ть дипломати́ческие отноше́ния** break* off diplomátic relátions; 6. (с тв.; порывать) séver relátions (with), break* (with); **разорва́ть с про́шлым** break* with the past.

разрыва́ть II, разры́ть (вн.) 1. dig* (smth.) up; (кучу) scátter (smth.); (могилу) ópen (smth.); 2. разг. (в поисках чего-л.) turn (smth.) upside-dówn, ransáck (smth.).

разрыв|а́ться, разорва́ться 1. be* torn; **у меня́ разо́рвалось пальто́** my coat is torn; 2. (взрываться) burst*;

снаря́д разорва́лся the shell burst; 3. (прекращаться, нарушаться) be* sévered, cease (to exíst); **◇ у меня́ се́рдце ~а́ется...** it breaks my heart...

разрывн|о́й explósive; **~а́я пу́ля** explósive búllet.

разрыда́ться сов. burst* into sobs.

разры́ть сов. см. разрыва́ть II.

разрыхли́ть сов. см. разрыхля́ть.

разрыхля́ть, разрыхли́ть (вн.) lóosen (smth.).

разря́д I м. 1. (группа, категория) type, sort; **он принадлежа́л к ~у люде́й о́чень до́брых** he was a véry kind sort of pérson; 2. (степень квалификации) grade; **то́карь тре́тьего ~а** third-grade túrner; **спортсме́н пе́рвого ~а** first-grade áthlete.

разря́д II м. эл. dischárge.

разряди́ть I, II сов. см. разряжа́ть I, II.

разряди́ться I, II сов. см. разряжа́ться I, II.

разря́дка ж. 1. (действие) dischárge; 2. (ослабление напряжения) relief of ténsion (in); **~ междунаро́дной напряжённости** relaxátion of internátional ténsion; détente; 3. полигр. spácing.

разря́дник I м. эл. dischárger, arréster.

разря́дник II м. разг. (спортсмен, имеющий разряд) pérson with a sports ráting.

разряжа́ть I, разряди́ть (вн.) разг. (наряжать) dress (smb.) up, deck (smb.) out.

разряжа́ть II, разряди́ть (вн.) 1. (оружие) unlóad (smth.); (стрелять) dischárge (smth.); 2. физ. dischárge (smth.); **~ аккумуля́тор** use up a báttery; 3. (уменьшать напряжённость) relíeve (smth.), reláx (smth.), calm (smth.); **take* the heat out of** (smth.); разряди́ть напряжённость междунаро́дной обстано́вки relíeve internátional ténsion.

разряжа́ться I, разряди́ться разг. (наряжаться) dress up.

разряжа́ться II, разряди́ться 1. физ. run* down, be* used up; **аккумуля́тор разряди́лся** the báttery has no cúrrent in it; 2. (ослабевать) reláx, be* relíeved/redúced, abáte; **разряди́лось не́рвное напряже́ние** the nérvous ténsion was relíeved.

разубеди́ть(ся) сов. см. разубежда́ть(ся).

разубежда́ть, разубеди́ть (вн. в пр.) dissuáde (smb. from + -ing). **~ся, разубеди́ться** (в пр.) change one's mind (abóut).

разува́ть, разу́ть (вн.) take* off smb.'s shoes, boots. **~ся, разу́ться** take* off one's shoes, boots.

разуве́рить(ся) сов. см. разуверя́ть(ся).

разуверя́ть, разуве́рить (вн. в пр.) disillúsion (smb. of). **~ся, разуве́риться** (в пр.) lose* one's faith (in).

разузнава́ть, разузна́ть (вн.) find* (smth.) out; несов. тж. make* inquíries (abóut).

разузна́ть сов. см. разузнава́ть.

разукра́сить сов. (вн.) разг. décorate (smth.).

разукрупни́ть сов. см. разукрупня́ть.

разукрупня́ть, разукрупни́ть (вн.) разг. break* (smth.) up into smáller únits.

ра́зум м. réason; (ум) mind, íntellect; **челове́ческий ~** the (húman) mind; **◇ у меня́ ум за ~ захо́дит** I am at my wit's end (what to do).

разуме́ть несов. (вн.) mean* (smth.). **~ся** несов. 1. be* understóod/meant; 2.: **разуме́ется** в знач. вводн. сл. of course, cértainly; **он, разуме́ется, придёт** he is sure to come.

разу́мн|ый réasonable; (о поступке) wise; (рациональный) rátional; **~ое существо́** rátional béing; **~ челове́к** wise/réasonable pérson; **~ые до́воды** réasonable árguments; **~ее всего́ бы́ло бы...** the wísest course would be...

разу́т|ый shóeless, bárefoot; **ходи́ть ~ым** go* abóut without shoes, go* abóut bárefoot.

разу́ть(ся) сов. см. разува́ть(ся).

разу́чивать, разучи́ть (вн.) learn* (smth.); **разучи́ть скрипи́чный этю́д** learn* a víolin stúdy. **~ся, разучи́ться**

(+ *инф.*) forgét* (how + to *inf*); разучи́ться танцева́ть forgét* how to dance.

разучи́ть(ся) *сов. см.* разу́чивать(ся).

разъеда́ть, разъе́сть (*вн.*) eat* (*smth.*) awáy; corróde (*smth.*) (*тж. перен.*).

разъедин|е́ние *с.* 1. separátion; 2. эл. disconnéction. ~и́ть(ся) *сов. см.* разъединя́ть(ся).

разъединя́ть, разъедини́ть (*вн.*) 1. séparate (*smb., smth.*), part (*smth.*); 2. эл. disconnéct (*smth.*), break* (*smth.*); нас разъедини́ли (*по телефону*) we were cut off. ~ся, разъедини́ться come* apárt; эл. becóme* disconnécted.

разъе́зд *м.* 1. (*отъезд*) depárture; ~ делега́тов depárture of délegates; 2. *мн.* (*поездка*) trável; он всегда́ в ~ах he's álways on the move; 3. *ж.-д.* pássing-track; dóuble-track séction; (*остановочный пункт*) small júnction; 4. *воен.* móunted patról.

разъезж|а́ть *несов.* trável abóut; (*на машине*) drive* abóut; ~ по стране́ trável abóut the cóuntry; ~ по дела́м слу́жбы trável on búsiness. ~а́ться, разъе́хаться 1. (*уезжать*) leave*, go* awáy; ~а́ться по дома́м leave* for *one's* respéctive homes; ~а́ться на кани́кулы go* awáy for the hólidays; 2. (*с тв.; разлучаться*) séparate (from), part (from); 3. *разг.* (*скользя, расходиться*) slide* apárt; но́ги ~а́ются *one's* feet slide apárt; 4. (*рваться от ветхости*) wear* thin.

разъе́сть *сов. см.* разъеда́ть.

разъе́хаться *сов.* 1. *см.* разъезжа́ться; 2. (*с тв.; проехать мимо*) pass (*smb., smth.*); 3. (*разминуться*) miss each óther.

разъяр|ённый infúriated, frénzied; túrbulent, ráging. ~и́ть(ся) *сов. см.* разъяря́ть(ся).

разъяря́ть, разъяри́ть (*вн.*) stir (*smb.*) to fúry/frénzy. ~ся, разъяри́ться becóme* fúrious/enráged, fly* into a rage.

разъясн|е́ние *с.* explanátion, clarificátion; (*истолкование*) interpretátion. ~и́тельный explánatory.

разъясни́ть(ся) *сов. см.* разъясня́ть(ся).

разъясня́ть, разъясни́ть (*вн. дт.*) expláin (*smth.* to), make* (*smth.*) clear (to). ~ся, разъясни́ться becóme* clear.

разыгра́ть(ся) *сов. см.* разы́грывать(ся).

разы́грывать, разыгра́ть (*вн.*) 1. (*исполнять*) perfórm (*smth.*), play (*smth.*); разыгра́ть спекта́кль perfórm a play; *перен.* put* on an act; 2. *спорт.* (*выполнять какую-л. комбинацию*) play (*smth.*); хорошо́ разыгра́ть мяч play the ball well; 3. (*приводить игру к концу*) bring* (*smth.*) to a conclúsion; round off (*smth.*); остроу́мно разыгра́ть па́ртию в ша́хматы bring* a game of chess to a másterly conclúsion; 4. (*в лотерею*) ráffle (*smth.*); (*по жребию*) draw* lots (for); 5. (*изображать собой кого-л., что-л.*) play the...; feign (*smth.*); разыгра́ть проста́чка play the símpleton; 6. *разг.* (*одурачивать*) pull *smb.'s* leg; ◇ разыгра́ть дурака́ make* a fool of onesélf. ~ся, разыгра́ться 1. (*о детях*) romp; (*о животных*) frisk, gámbol; 2. *разг.* (*начинать играть непринуждённо*) warm up, get* into *one's* stride; 3. (*проявляться с силой*) be* ráging; разыгра́лись собы́тия things begán to háppen; стра́сти разыгра́лись féelings ran high; бу́ря разыгра́лась the storm was ráging.

разыска́ть(ся) *сов. см.* разы́скивать(ся).

разы́скивать, разыска́ть (*вн.*) look (for); search (for); *сов. тж.* find* (*smb., smth.*). ~ся, разыска́ться turn up, be* found; ~ся мили́цией be* wánted by milítia/police.

рай *м.* héaven, páradise; здесь ~! this is héaven!; мы живём как в раю́ this place is a páradise; ◇ земно́й ~ an éarthly páradise.

райисполко́м *м.* (*исполни́тельный комите́т райо́нного Сове́та наро́дных депута́тов*) Exécutive (Committee) of the Dístrict Sóviet (of Péople's Députies).

райо́н *м.* 1. (*местность*) área, région; промы́шлен-

ный ~ indústrial área; земледе́льческий ~ agricúltural área; ю́жные ~ы страны́ sóuthern áreas/régions of the cóuntry; 2. (*часть населённого пункта*) dístrict; рабо́чий ~ wórking-class dístrict; 3. (*рд.; место действия*) área (of); ~ вое́нных де́йствий operátions área; ~ затопле́ния flóoded área; 4. (*административно-территориальная единица в России*) dístrict; 5. (*рд.; место, прилегающее к чему-л.*) région, locálity.

райони́ров|ание *с.* division into dístricts. ~ать *несов. и сов.* (*вн.*) divide (*smth.*) into dístricts.

райо́нный dístrict *attr.*

ра́йск|ий héavenly; у них ~ая жизнь they have a héavenly life, theirs is a blíssful exístence; ~ая пти́ца bird-of-páradise.

райсове́т *м.* (*райо́нный Сове́т наро́дных депута́тов*) Dístrict Sóviet (of Péople's Députies).

рак I *м. зоол.* cráyfish, cráwfish; ◇ кра́сный как ~ red as a lóbster; покрасне́ть как ~ go* red as a lóbster; я ему́ покажу́ где ~и зиму́ют I'll teach him!, I'll have his guts (for gárters).

рак II *м.* 1. (*злокачественная опухоль*) cáncer; 2. (*болезнь растений*) cánker.

раке́та I *ж.* 1. (*фейерверк*) rócket; (*для освещения местности*) flare; 2. (*летательный аппарат*) rócket; косми́ческая ~ space rócket; трёхступе́нчатая ~ thrée-stage rócket; 3. *воен.* (*боевой снаряд*) rócket, ballístic míssile; крыла́тая ~ cruíse míssile; 4. (*судно*) (pássenger-cárrying) hýdrofoil.

раке́та II *ж. см.* раке́тка.

раке́тка *ж. спорт.* rácket; (*для настольного тенниса*) bat.

раке́тница *ж.* flare/signal pístol.

раке́тно-косми́ческий spáce-rócket *attr.*

раке́тно-я́дерный núclear-rócket *attr.*

раке́тн|ый I rócket *attr.*; (*с ракетным двигателем*) jet(-propélled), rócket-propélled; ~ая те́хника rócketry; ~ая ба́за rócket base; ~ дви́гатель jet éngine; ~ые войска́ rócket troops/fórces.

раке́тн|ый II *спорт.* rácket *attr.*; ~ая се́тка strings of a rácket.

ракетодро́м *м.* láunching site; (*для космических ракет*) spácedrome.

ракетоноси́тель *м.* rócket cárrier.

ракетоно́сный míssile-cárrying, rócket-ármed; míssile *attr.*

ракетострое́ние *с.* rócket búilding.

раке́тчик *м.* míssileman.

раки́та *ж. бот.* bríttle wíllow.

раки́тник *м. бот.* broom.

ра́ковина *ж.* 1. shell; ~ ули́тки snail shell; 2. ушна́я ~ extérnal ear; ~ под кра́ном sink; умыва́льная ~ wásh-bowl.

ра́ковый I cráyfish *attr.*

ра́ковый II 1. *мед.* cáncerous; cáncer *attr.*; 2. *бот.* cánkerous.

ра́курс *м.* foreshórtening; в ~е foreshórtened.

раку́шка *ж.* cóckle-shell.

ра́лли *с.* rálly.

ра́м|а *ж.* frame; дверна́я ~ dóor-frame, dóor-casing; вну́тренняя ~ окна́ ínner sash; вста́вить карти́ну в ~у frame a pícture.

ра́мк|а *ж.* 1. frame; *перен.* sétting; в ~е framed; 2. *мн.* (*пределы*) límits; frámework *sg*; в ~ах Организа́ции Объединённых На́ций within the frámework of the United Nátions; 3. *радио* (*антенна*) frame áerial.

ра́мочн|ый frame *attr.*; ◇ ~ая анте́нна *радио* frame áerial.

ра́мпа *ж. театр.* fóotlights *pl.*

ра́н|а *ж.* wound; перевяза́ть ~у dress a wound; душе́вная ~ wound (to *one's* féelings), emótional shock.

ранг *м.* rank; дипломати́ческие ~и diplomátic ranks; капита́н I-го ~а cáptain.

рангоут *м. мор.* masts and spars *pl.*

ранее *см.* **раньше** 2, 4.

ранение *с.* 1. (*действие*) wóunding; 2. (*рана*) wound; получить тяжёлое ~ be* sevérely wóunded.

раненый *прил.* 1. wóunded, ínjured; 2. *в знач. сущ. м.* wóunded man*; *мн.* the wóunded; cásualties.

ранец *м.* (*солдатский*) háversack, knápsack; (*школьный*) sátchel.

ранить *несов. и сов.* (*вн.*) wound (*smb.*); *перен. тж.* hurt* (*smb.*); ~ *кого-л.* в ногу wound *smb.* in the leg.

ранн|ий early; ~яя óсень éarly áutumn; ~им утром in the éarly mórning, éarly in the mórning; ~ей весной in (the) éarly spring, éarly in spring; ~яя пшеница éarly-ripening wheat; ◇ из молодых, да ~! he's beginning éarly!

рано 1. *нареч.* éarly; ~ утром éarly (in the mórning); 2. *в знач. сказ. безл.* it is éarly; ещё слишком ~ it is too éarly; обéдать ещё ~ it is too éarly for dínner yet; ◇ ~ или поздно sóoner or láter.

рант *м.* welt; сапоги на ~у wélted boots.

рантов|ой wélted; ~ая обувь wélted fóot-wear.

рантье *м. нескл.* réntier, stóckholder, fúnd-holder.

рань *ж. разг.:* в такую ~ at such an ungódly hour.

раньше 1. (*сравнит. ст. от нареч.* **рано**) éarlier; как можно ~ (*о часе*) as éarly as póssible; (*о дате*) as soon as póssible; 2. (*до какого-л. момента, срока*) before, until; не вернусь ~ вечера I shall not be back before évening; 3. (*прежде другого*) before; он пришёл ~ всех he was the first to arríve, he arríved before ánybody else; 4. (*в прежнее время*) fórmerly, before; ~ здесь стояли деревянные дома there used to be wóoden hóuses here before; ◇ ~ времени too soon/éarly; волноваться ~ времени wórry befórehand.

рапира *ж.* foil.

рапорт *м.* repórt; отдавáть ~ repórt; принимáть ~ recéive a repórt.

рапортовáть *несов. и сов.* (*дт. о пр.*) repórt (*smth.* to).

рапсóдия *ж.* rhápsody.

рáса *ж.* race.

рас|изм *м.* rácialism. ~ист *м.* rácist, rácialist. ~истский rácialist *attr.*

раскабалить(ся) *сов. см.* **раскабалять(ся)**.

раскабаля|ть, **раскабалить** (*вн.*) emáncipate (*smb.*). ~ся, раскабалиться emáncipate onesélf.

раскáиваться, **раскáяться** (*в пр.*) repént (*smth.*); (*испытывать сожаление*) regrét (*smth.*); раскáяться в своих поступках repént one's misdéeds.

раскалённ|ый scórching, búrning hot; (*от солнца тж.*) tórrid; ~ая печь overhéated/hot stove; ~ые угли red-hot coals.

раскалить(ся) *сов. см.* **раскалять(ся)**.

раскáлывать, **расколоть** (*вн.*) split* (*smth.*); (*тж. перен.*); cleave* (*smth.*); (*орехи*) crack (*smth.*). ~ся, расколоться split* (*тж. перен.*); (*об орехе*) crack.

раскаля|ть, **раскалить** (*вн.*) (*огнём*) heat (*smth.*); (*о солнце тж.*) make* (*smth.*) scórching hot. ~ся, раскаляться be* scórching hot.

раскапризничаться *сов.* becóme* véry náughty, play up; act up *амер.*

раскáпывать, **раскопáть** (*вн.*) 1. enlárge (*smth.*) (by dígging); (*копая, обнаружить*) dig* (*smth.*) up, unéarth (*smth.*); 2. (*производить раскопки*) éxcavate (*smth.*); 3. *разг.* (*разыскивать, находить*) unéarth (*smth.*), dig* up (*smth.*); где вы раскопáли эту рукопись? where did you unéarth that mánuscript?

раскáт *м.* 1. peal; (*отражённый*) reverberátion; 2. *мн.* (*гул*) roar *sg*, rúmble *sg*; peals.

раскатáть *сов. см.* **раскáтывать** 1.

раскáтистый resóunding; ~ смех rúmbling laugh; ~ удáр грóма revérberating peal/clap of thúnder.

раскатиться *сов.* 1. (*покатиться в разные сторо-*

ны) roll abóut; 2. (*набрать скорость*) gáther speed; 3. (*прозвучать*) boom.

раскáтывать, **раскатáть** 1. (*вн.*) roll (*smth.*); 2. *тк. несов. разг.* (*разъезжать*) drive* all óver.

раскачáть *сов. см.* **раскáчивать** 1, 2, 4. ~ся, *сов. см.* **раскáчиваться** 1, 3.

раскáчив|ать, **раскачáть** 1. (*вн.; заставлять качаться*) rock (*smth.*); swing* (*smth., smth.*); раскачáть качéли get* a swing góing well; 2. (*вн.; расшатывать*) lóosen, shake* loose; 3. *тк. несов.* (*тв.; производить колебательные движения*) swing* (*smth.*); 4. (*вн.*) *разг.* (*пробуждать к действию*) stir (*smth.*) to áction; его трудно раскачáть he is hard to rouse. ~аться, раскачáться 1. swing*; rock; качéли раскачáлись the swing begán to move; 2. *тк. несов. разг.* (*переваливаться с боку на бок*) be* swáying/swinging/rócking; ходить ~аясь roll alóng, have* a rólling gait; 3. *разг.* (*выходить из состояния апатии*) get* stárted; он óчень мéдленно ~ается he can't get stárted, he's a slow stárter.

раскáшляться *сов.* have* a fit of cóughing.

раскáяние *с.* repéntance.

раскáяться *сов. см.* **раскáиваться**.

расквартировáть *сов.* (*вн.*) quárter (*smb., smth.*), bíllet (*smb., smth.*).

расквитáться *сов.* (*с тв.*) *разг.* séttle accóunts (with); *перен. тж.* get* éven (with), be* quits (with).

раскидáть *сов. см.* **раскидывать** 1.

раскидистый spréading.

раскидывать, **раскидáть**, **раскинуть** (*вн.*) 1. *сов.* раскидáть scátter (*smth.*); 2. *сов.* раскинуть spread* (*smth.*); (*палатку, лагерь*) pitch (*smth.*); ◇ раскинуть умóм think* it óver. ~ся, раскинуться *разг.* sprawl; раскинуться на диване sprawl on a sófa.

раскинуть *сов. см.* **раскидывать** 2. ~ся *сов.* 1. *см.* **раскидываться**; 2. be* spread (óver); гóрод раскинулся широкó the town is spread óver a wide área.

раскладнóй fólding, collápsible.

раскладушка *ж. разг.* cámp-bed.

расклáдывать, **разложить** (*вн.*) 1. lay* (*smth.*) out; 2. (*расстилать*) spread* (*smth.*); 3.: ~ костёр make* a fire; 4. (*распределять*) appórtion (*smth.*), sort (*smth.*) out, distríbute (*smth.*). ~ся, разложиться (*распаковывать вещи*) unpáck.

расклáниваться, **раскланяться** bow.

раскланяться *сов. см.* **расклáниваться**.

расклéивать, **расклéить** (*вн.*) paste (*smth.*); (*афиши и т. п.*) stick up (*smth.*), post (up) (*smth.*); ~ листóвки stick* up pámphlets. ~ся, расклéиться 1. (*о склеенном*) come* unstúck; 2. (*о здоровье*) go* to píeces; я чтó-то совсéм расклéился I've gone all to píeces.

расклéить(ся) *сов. см.* **расклéивать(ся)**.

раскóванн|о uninhibitedly; чувствовать себя ~ feel* uninhibited/reláxed. ~ость *ж.* uninhibitedness. ~ый uninhibited.

расковáть *сов.* (*вн.*) 1. (*лошадь*) unshóe (*smth.*); 2. (*освободить от цепей*) unsháckle (*smth., smth.*).

раскóл *м.* 1. split, disúnity; 2. *рел.* schism.

расколóть(ся) *сов. см.* **раскáлывать(ся)**.

раскóльни|к *м.* 1. (*тот, кто вносит разлад*) splítter, díssident; 2. *рел.* dissénter. ~ческий 1. (*вносящий разлад*) splítting, bréakaway; 2. *рел.* dissénters'.

раскопáть *сов. см.* **раскáпывать**.

раскóпки *мн.* excavátions.

раскормить *сов.* (*вн.*) feed* up (*smb., smth.*).

раскóсый slánting.

раскошёл|иваться, **раскошéлиться** *разг.* lóosen one's púrse-strings; fork out. ~иться *сов. см.* **раскошéливаться**.

раскрáдывать, **раскрáсть** (*вн.*) steal* (*smth.*), plúnder (*smth.*).

раскрáивать, **раскрóить** (*вн.*) cut* (*smth.*) out; ~ матéрию на костюм cut* out a suit.

раскра́с|ить *сов. см.* раскра́шивать. ~ка *ж.* 1. (*действие*) páinting, cólouring; 2. (*расцветка*) cólours *pl*, colorátion.

раскрасне́вшийся flushed.

раскрасне́ться *сов.* flush, be* flushed, glow.

раскра́сть *сов. см.* раскра́дывать.

раскра́шенный cóloured; (*bríghtly*) páinted.

раскра́шивать, раскра́сить (*вн.*) paint (*smth.*), cólour (*smth.*); ~ что́-л. под де́рево grain (*smth.*); ~ что́-л. под мра́мор márble (*smth.*).

раскрепости́ть(ся) *сов. см.* раскрепоща́ть(ся).

раскрепощ|а́ть, раскрепости́ть (*вн.*) emáncipate (*smb.*). ~а́ться, раскрепости́ться be* emáncipated. ~е́ние *с.* emancipátion.

раскритикова́ть *сов.* (*вн.*) séverely críticize (*smb.*, *smth.*); ~ статью́ slate an árticle, invéigh agáinst an árticle.

раскрича́ться *сов. разг.* 1. (*начать сильно кричать*) start shóuting; 2. (*на вн.; наброситься с бранью*) bawl (at), béllow (at).

раскро́ить *сов. см.* раскра́ивать.

раскроши́ть *сов.* (*вн.*) crúmble (*smth.*), púlverize (*smth.*). ~ся *сов.* crúmble.

раскрути́ть(ся) *сов. см.* раскру́чивать(ся).

раскру́чивать, раскрути́ть (*вн.*) untwíst (*smth.*). ~ся, раскрути́ться come* untwísted.

раскрыва́ть, раскры́ть (*вн.*) 1. (*открывать*) ópen (*smth.*); раскры́ть шкаф ópen a cúpboard; раскры́ть воро́та ópen a gate; раскры́ть паке́т ópen a párcel; ~ зо́нтик ópen an umbrélla, put* up an umbrélla; раскры́ть кни́гу ópen a book; 2. (*обнажать*) expóse (*smth.*); (*часть тела тж.*) bare (*smth.*); 3. (*объяснять скрытый смысл чего-л.*) revéal (*smth.*); раскры́ть та́йну unrável a mýstery; раскры́ть смысл вопро́са revéal the éssence of the mátter; 4. (*обнаруживать*) discóver (*smth.*), uncóver (*smth.*), detéct (*smth.*); ◇ раскры́ть чью́-л. игру́ see* through *smb.'s* game. ~ся, раскры́ться 1. (*открываться*) ópen; (*случайно*) come* ópen; 2. (*обнажаться*) expóse onesélf, uncóver onesélf; 3. (*представать взору*) be* revéaled; spread* out (befóre); 4. (*обнаруживать свою сущность*) revéal onesélf; tell* one's stóry; 5. (*обнаруживаться*) come* out, come* to light.

раскры́тие *с.* 1. ópening; 2. (*тайны*) revelátion, unfólding; 3. (*преступления и т. п.*) expósure; detéction.

раскры́ть(ся) *сов. см.* раскрыва́ть(ся).

раскупа́ть, раскупи́ть (*вн.*) buy* up (*smth.*); това́р неме́дленно раскупи́ли the goods were sold out in no time. ~ся *несов.* sell* stéadily; go* like hot cakes *разг.*

раскупи́ть *сов. см.* раскупа́ть.

раску́поривать, раску́порить (*вн.*) ópen (*smth.*); (*бутылки тж.*) uncórk (*smth.*).

раску́порить *сов. см.* раску́поривать.

раску́рив|ать, раскури́ть 1. (*вн.; разжигать папиросу и т. п.*) get* (*smth.*) próperly líghted; раскури́ть трубку get* one's pipe góing; 2. *тк. несов. разг.* (*проводить время в курении*) pass the time smóking; де́ло ждёт, а он стои́т и ~ает he stands there smóking when there's work to be done! ~аться, раскури́ться light próperly, get* góing.

раскури́ть *сов. см.* раску́ривать 1. ~ся *сов. см.* раску́риваться.

раскуси́ть *сов.* 1. *см.* раску́сывать; 2. (*вн.*) *разг.* (*распознать*) get* smb.'s méasure, size (*smb.*) up, see* through (*smb.*).

раску́сывать, раскуси́ть (*вн.*) bite* (*smth.*), bite* through (*smth.*).

раску́тать(ся) *сов. см.* раску́тывать(ся).

раску́тывать, раску́тать (*вн.*) unwráp (*smb.*, *smth.*). ~ся, раску́таться unwráp onesélf.

ра́сов|ый rácial; race *attr.*; ~ при́знак rácial characterístic; ~ые предрассу́дки race préjudices.

распа́д *м.* disintegrátion, decáy; ~ ядра́ núclear disintegrátion.

распада́ться, распа́сться 1. fall* apárt; disíntegrate; (*об атомах и т. п. тж.*) decáy; 2. (*утрачивать целостность*) break* up, fall* apárt, disíntegrate; *перен.* break* down.

распа́ивать, распая́ть (*вн.*) unsólder (*smth.*). ~ся, распая́ться come* unsóldered, melt apárt.

распакова́ть(ся) *сов. см.* распако́вывать(ся).

распако́вывать, распакова́ть (*вн.*) unpáck (*smth.*). ~ся, распакова́ться unpáck.

распали́ть(ся) *сов. см.* распаля́ть(ся).

распаля́ть, распали́ть (*вн.*) *разг.* make* (*smth.*) burn, fan (*smth.*) ínto a blaze; (*раскалять*) make* (*smth.*) búrning hot, overhéat (*smth.*); *перен.* fire (*smb.*, *smth.*), infláme (*smb.*, *smth.*), incíte (*smb.*). ~ся, распали́ться *разг.* be*/get* overhéated, becóme* búrning hot; *перен.* be* fired/roused; blaze (with).

распа́рывать, распоро́ть (*вн.*) rip (*smth.*) ópen; ~ пла́тье unpíck a dress. ~ся, распоро́ться come* undóne; пла́тье распоро́лось the dress is góing/splítting at the seams.

распа́сться *сов. см.* распада́ться.

распаха́ть *сов. см.* распа́хивать I.

распа́хивать I, распаха́ть (*вн.*) plough (*smth.*) up; распаха́ть целину́ plough up vírgin land.

распа́хивать II, распахну́ть (*вн.*) fling*/throw* (*smth.*) ópen; широко́ распахну́ть дверь fling* the door wide ópen; распахну́ть пальто́ throw* ópen one's coat. ~ся, распахну́ться fly* ópen.

распахну́ть *сов. см.* распа́хивать II. ~ся *сов. см.* распа́хиваться.

распа́шка *ж.* plóughing up.

распашо́нка *ж. разг.* báby's vest.

распая́ть(ся) *сов. см.* распа́ивать(ся).

распева́ть *несов. разг.* sing*, pass the time sínging.

распека́ть, распе́чь (*вн.*) *разг.* scold (*smb.*), tell* (*smb.*) off, give* (*smb.*) a wígging.

распелена́ть *сов.* (*вн.*) unswáddle (*smb.*). ~ся *сов.* come*/get* unwrápped.

распе́ться *сов. разг.* 1. (*увлечься пением*) sing* awáy; 2. (*о птицах*) burst* ínto song; 3. (*начать петь свободно, без затруднений*) warm up, get* ínto good voice.

распеча́тать(ся) *сов. см.* распеча́тывать(ся).

распеча́тывать, распеча́тать (*вн.*) (*запечатанное*) unséal (*smth.*), break* the seals (of); (*заклеенное*) ópen (*smth.*); распеча́тать письмо́ unséal a létter. ~ся, распеча́таться come* unstúck/unséaled.

распе́чь *сов. см.* распека́ть.

распива́ть, распи́ть (*вн.*) *разг.* 1. drink* (*smth.*) (*together*); распи́ть буты́лку вина́ émpty a bóttle of wine; 2. *тк. несов.* (*пить долго, медленно*) línger óver (*smth.*).

распи́ливать, распили́ть (*вн.*) saw* (*smth.*) up.

распили́ть *сов. см.* распи́ливать.

расписа́ни|е *с.* tíme-table, schédule; соста́вить ~ work out a tíme-table; по ~ю accórding to schédule; по́езд идёт по ~ю the train is rúnning to time; шта́тное ~ list of staff.

расписа́ть *сов. см.* распи́сывать. ~ся *сов.* 1. *см.* распи́сываться; 2. *разг.* (*писать с увлечением*) get*/be* absórbed in wríting.

распи́ск|а *ж.* 1. (*действие*): ~ стен décorating the walls; 2. (*документ*) recéipt (for); сдать что́-л. под ~у кому́-л. make* smb. sign for smth.; дать кому́-л. ~у give* smb. a recéipt.

расписно́й *разг.* décorated, páinted.

распи́сывать, расписа́ть (*вн.*) 1. (*выписывать, переписывать*) cópy out (*smth.*); 2. (*распределять*) assign (smth.); (записывать последовательность чего-л.) schédule (smth.); ~ что-л. по книгам énter smth. in the books/lédgers; 3. (красками) décorate (smth.), paint (smth.); 4. разг. (излагать что-л., приукрашивая) give a glówing description of smth. ~ся, расписáться 1. (давать подпись) sign (one's name); перен. acknówledge; displáy; ~ся в получéнии чего-л. recéipt smth., sign for smth.; ~ся в своём невéжестве displáy one's ígnorance; 2. (с тв.) разг. (регистрировать свой брак) régister one's márriage; он расписáлся с нéю they have régistered their márriage.

распить сов. см. распивáть 1.

распихáть сов. см. распихивать.

распихивать, распихáть (вн.) разг. 1. (расталкивать) push one's way (through); 2. (рассовывать) shove (smth.).

расплáв|ить(ся) сов. см. расплавлять(ся). ~ленный mólten.

расплавлять, расплáвить (вн.) melt (smth.). ~ся, расплáвиться melt.

расплáкаться сов. burst* ínto tears, burst* out crýing.

распланировать сов. (вн.) plan (smth.); (сад и m.n.) lay* out (smth.).

распланировáть сов. см. планировáть.

распластáться сов. throw* onesélf flat.

расплáт|а ж. 1. páyment; 2. (кара, возмездие) retribútion, púnishment; настáл час ~ы the day of réckoning has come.

расплатиться сов. см. расплáчиваться.

расплáчиваться, расплатиться 1. (с тв.) pay* (smb.); séttle accóunts (with) (тж. перен.); 2. (за вн.; нести наказание) pay* (for).

расплескáть(ся) сов. см. расплёскивать(ся).

расплёскивать, расплескáть (вн.) spill* (smth.). ~ся, расплескáться spill*; spill* óver.

расплести(сь) сов. см. расплетáть(ся).

расплетáть, расплести (вн.) unpláit (smth.); ~ кóсу unpláit one's hair. ~ся, расплестись come* unpláited.

расплод|ить сов. (вн.; прям. и перен.) breed* (smth.). ~иться сов. (прям. и перен.) breed*; много мышéй и т. п. the place is overrún with mice etc.

расплывáться, расплыться 1. (растекаться) flow, run*; 2. (утрачивать отчётливые очертания) becóme* blurred, blur; 3. разг. (полнеть) becóme* fat; 4.: ~ в улыбку smile bróadly; егó лицó расплылóсь в улыбке a broad smile spread óver his face.

расплывчатый blurred, indistinct; перен. vague.

расплывшийся разг. flábby.

расплыться сов. см. расплывáться.

расплющивать, расплющить (вн.) flátten (smth.). ~ся, расплющиться flátten.

расплющить(ся) сов. см. расплющивать(ся).

распознавáть, распознáть (вн.) récognize (smb., smth.); (различать) discérn (smb., smth.); ~ болéзнь díagnose a diséase; ~ чьи-л. намéрения discóver smb.'s inténtions.

распознáть сов. см. распознавáть.

располагáть I, расположить 1. (вн.; размещать) dispóse (smth.), arránge (smth.); дом располóжен на ропé the house is situated on a hill; ~ что-л. в алфавитном порядке arránge smth. in alphabétical órder; 2. (вн. к дт.; вызывать симпатию) make* (smb., smth.) well dispósed (towárds); ~ к себé make* a good impréssion, win* fávour.

располагáть II несов. 1. (тв.; иметь в распоряжении) dispóse (of); have* (smb., smth.) (at one's dispósal); ~ врéменем have* time at one's dispósal; мóжете ~ мнóю (как хотите) I am (complétely) at your dispósal; 2. (вн. к дт.; способствовать чему-л.) make* (smb.) inclíned (to), be* condúcive (to).

располаг|áться, расположиться séttle down; (о войсках) be* státioned; (усаживаться, ложиться) make*

onesélf cómfortable; ~ лáгерем encámp, pitch camp; ~ писáть séttle down to write; ~ на óтдых sit* down for a rest; ~áйтесь как дóма make yoursélf at home.

располагáющ|ий líkeable, attráctive; ~ая внéшность líkeable appéarance.

расползáться, расползтись 1. (в разные стороны) crawl off (in different diréctions); 2. разг. (рваться от ветхости) fall* to píeces; (о материи тж.) be* thréadbare.

расползтись сов. см. расползáться.

расположéни|е с. 1. (размещение) arrángement; 2. (нахождение, пребывание) situation; воен. positíon(s); 3. (порядок размещения чего-л.) arrángement, láy-out; стрáнное ~ кóмнат strange láy-out of the rooms; 4. (симпатия) sýmpathies pl, regárd; заслужить, снискáть чью-л. ~ win* smb.'s regárd/sýmpathies; gain smb.'s fávour; пóльзоваться чьим-л. ~ем be* in fávour with smb.; 5. (к дт.; склонность) líking (for), taste (for); inclinátion (tóward); (восприимчивость) téndency (to); ~ к чтéнию líking for réading; ~ к болéзни, полнотé téndency to fall ill, to get fat; 6. разг. (настроение) mood; не имéть ~я (+ инф.) be* in no mood (+ to inf.); ◇ ~ дýха frame of mind, mood; быть в хорóшем ~и дýха be* in good spirits.

располóж|енный 1. (находящийся) situated; воен. locáted, státioned, pósted; 2. (к дт.; питающий симпатию) dispósed (to, towárds); он к вам óчень ~ен he is extrémely well dispósed towárds you; 3. (к дт.; + инф.; склонный к чему-л.) inclíned (to, + to inf.); я совершéнно не ~ен занимáться этими делáми I have no inclinátion at all to deal with these mátters.

расположить сов. см. располагáть I. ~ся сов. см. располагáться.

распорóть сов. см. распáрывать и порóть 1. ~ся сов. см. распáрываться.

распорядитель м. superinténdent; (на празднике) máster of cérémonies. ~ный práctical, búsinesslike; (об учреждении) administrative.

распорядиться сов. см. распоряжáться 1, 3.

распоряд|ок м. routíne, procédure; ~ дня dáily routíne; прáвила внýтреннего ~ка regulátions.

распоряжáться, распорядиться 1. (отдавать распоряжение) give* instrúctions; сов. тж. see* (that); распорядиться сдéлать, принести, убрáть что-л. have* smth. done, brought, táken awáy; распорядиться об уплáте дéнег see* that the móney is paid; 2. тк. несов. (тв.; управлять, ведать) be* in charge (of); mánage (smth.), run* (smth.); ~ как у себя дóма beháve as if the place belónged to one; 3. (тв.; находить применение чему-л.) dispóse (of), do* (with); распорядитесь моими деньгáми, как найдёте нýжным dispóse of my móney as you think fit.

распоряжéни|е с. (приказание) instrúction; (постановление, приказ) órder; по чьему-л. ~ю by órder of smb.; до осóбого ~я pénding spécial instrúctions; ◇ в ~ когó-л., чегó-л. at smb.'s, smth's dispósal; получить что-л. в своё ~ have* smth. placed at one's dispósal; предостáвить что-л. в чьё-л. ~ place smth. at smb.'s dispósal; имéть в своём ~и have* at one's dispósal.

распоя́с|аться сов. take* off one's belt; перен. разг. let* onesélf go; он окончáтельно ~ался he has got complétely out of hand, he has passed all bounds.

распрáва ж. harsh/sávage tréatment; reprísals pl; кровáвая ~ mássacre; ◇ у меня с ним ~ коротká I'll make short work of him.

распрáвить сов. см. расправлять. ~ся I, II сов. см. расправляться I, II.

расправлять, расправить (вн.) 1. (разглаживать) smooth out (smth.); 2. (распрямлять) stráighten (smth.); ~ плéчи square one's shóulders.

расправля́ться I, распрáвиться (разглаживаться) smooth out.

расправля́ться II, распра́виться (с *тв.*) deal* (with), make* short work (of).

распределе́ние *с.* distribútion; (*размещение*) allocátion, assígnment; ~ обя́занностей, рабо́ты distribútion/allocátion of dúties, work; ~ своего́ вре́мени plánning *one's* tíme-table; ~ роле́й в пье́се cásting; ~ хими́ческих элеме́нтов в земно́й коре́ distribútion of chémical élements in the earth's crust; ~ специали́стов assígnment of spécialists.

распредели́тельн|ый distríbutive; distríbuting; ~ая доска́ switch-board; ~ пункт distríbuting céntre; ~ вал cám-shaft.

распредели́ть *сов. см.* распределя́ть.

распределя́ть, распредели́ть (*вн.*) 1. (*делить между кем-л.*) distríbute (*smth.*); (*размещать*) állocate (*smb., smth.*), assígn (*smb.*); распредели́ть рабо́ту ме́жду чле́нами брига́ды divíde up work amóng the team; ~ обя́занности állocate dúties; ~ ро́ли в пье́се cast* a play; распредели́ть рабо́чих по уча́сткам assígn wórkers to the várious séctions; 2. (*систематизировать*) sýstematize (*smth.*).

распродава́ть, распрода́ть (*вн.*) sell* (*smth.*); (*оставшееся*) sell* off (*smth.*).

распрода́жа *ж.* sale; sélling off.

распрода́ть *сов. см.* распродава́ть.

распростере́ться *сов. см.* распростира́ться.

распростёрт|ый 1. (*раскрытый*) outspréad; с ~ыми объя́тиями with ópen arms; 2. (*лежащий*) próstrate.

распростира́ться, распростере́ться 1. (*падать, раскинув руки*) prostráte *onesélf*; 2. (*занимать большое пространство*) spread*, stretch, exténd.

распрости́ться *сов.* (с *тв.*) *разг.* take* leave (of); say* goodbýe (to); *перен.* bid* farewéll (to).

распростране́ние *с.* 1. (*действие*) spréading, disseminátion; 2. (*распространённость*) prévalence; име́ть большо́е ~ be* wídespread; (*о методах и т. п.*) be* wídely práctised; ◇ ~ я́дерного ору́жия proliferátion of núclear wéapons.

распространённ|ый wídespread; (*о животных, растениях*) wídely distríbuted; ~ое мне́ние wídespread opínion; ◇ ~ое предложе́ние *грам.* exténded séntence.

распространи́ть(ся) *сов. см.* распространя́ть(ся).

распространя́ть, распространи́ть (*вн.*) 1. (*делать широко известным*) spread* (*smth.*); ~ слу́хи spread* rúmours; 2. (*раздавать, продавать*) distríbute (*smth.*); ~ кни́ги distríbute books; 3. (*расширять круг действия чего-л.*) exténd (*smth.*); ~ де́йствие зако́на на *что-л.* enlárge the scope of a law to cóver *smth.* ~ся, распространи́ться 1. (*до рд.*; *достигать определённых пределов*) exténd (to); 2. (*расширять круг своего действия*) spread*; (*на вн.*; *о законе и т. п.*) cóver (*smb., smth.*), applý (to); 3. (*становиться известным*) spread*; get* abóut *разг.*; 4. *разг.* (*пространно рассказывать*) expátiate, hold* forth.

распроща́ться *сов. см.* распрости́ться.

ра́спря *ж.* díscord, strife.

распряга́ть, распря́чь (*вн.*) unhárness (*smth.*).

распрями́ть(ся) *сов. см.* распрямля́ть(ся).

распрямля́ть, распрями́ть (*вн.*) stráighten (*smth.*); ~ про́волоку stráighten a piece of wíre; ~ пле́чи square *one's* shóulders. ~ся, распрями́ться stráighten up, stand* up straight.

распря́чь *сов. см.* распряга́ть.

распуска́ть, распусти́ть (*вн.*) 1. (*отпускать*) dismíss (*smb., smth.*); (*об организациях, войсках*) disbánd (*smth.*), dissólve (*smth.*); ~ шко́льников на кани́кулы dismíss schóolchildren for the hólidays; ~ собра́ние close a méeting; ~ коми́ссию disbánd a commíssion; ~ парла́мент dissólve párliament; 2. (*развязывать, ослаблять*) lóosen (*smth.*); 3. (*развёртывать, расправлять*) spread* (*smth.*), unfúrl (*smth.*); ~ паруса́ spread* its sails; ~ во́лосы let* *one's* hair down, undó* *one's* hair;

~ кры́лья, хвост spread* its wings, tail; 4. (*вязаную вещь*) undó* (*smth.*); 5. *разг.* (*ослаблять требовательность*) let* (*smb.*) get out of hand; распусти́ть ребёнка spoil* a child; 6. *разг.* (*распространять*) set* (*smth.*) aflóat; ~ слух set* a rúmour aflóat; 7. *разг.* (*растворять*) dissólve (*smth.*); ◇ распусти́ть ню́ни whine, start whíning. ~ся, распусти́ться 1. (*о растениях*) come* out; (*о цветах, листьях тж.*) ópen, unfóld; сире́нь распусти́лась the lilac is out, the lilac has come out; 2. *разг.* (*о волосах*) come* down; 3. *разг.* (*о вязаных вещах*) come* undóne; unrável; 4. *разг.* (*терять выдержку*) lose* *one's* grip; get* slack, go* to seed; 5. *разг.* (*в отношении дисциплины*) get* out of hand; его́ ученики́ распусти́лись his púpils have got quite out of hand.

распусти́ть(ся) *сов. см.* распуска́ть(ся).

распу́тать(ся) *сов. см.* распу́тывать(ся).

распу́тица *ж.* (time of) impássable/flóoded roads, flood séason.

распу́тывать, распу́тать (*вн.*; *прям. и перен.*) unrável (*smth.*); disentángle (*smth.*); распу́тать у́зел get* a knot undóne; распу́тать де́ло unrável the affáir, get* to the bóttom of things. ~ся, распу́таться 1. come* undóne; *перен.* be* cleared up; де́ло в конце́ концо́в распу́талось the mátter was evéntually cleared up; 2. (с *тв.*) *разг.* (*освобождаться от кого-л., чего-л.*) get* rid (of), shake* off (*smth.*).

распу́тье *с.* cróss-roads *pl*; ◇ на ~ at the cróss-roads; at the párting of the ways.

распуха́ть, распу́хнуть swell*; *перен.* bulge.

распу́хнуть *сов. см.* распуха́ть.

распу́щенн|ость *ж.* 1. (*недисциплинированность*) lack of díscipline, láxity; sláckness; 2. (*безнравственность*) dissóluteness; declíne, decádence. ~ый 1. ~ые во́лосы untídy hair; с ~ыми волоса́ми with *one's* hair down; 2. (*недисциплинированный*) undísciplined, wild; ~ые де́ти undísciplined chíldren; 3. (*безнравственный*) dissolute.

распыле́ние *с.* 1. (*превращение в пыль*) pulverizátion; 2. (*жидкости*) spráying, átomizing; 3. (*рассредоточивание*) dispérsing, dispérsal; (*своих сил, средств*) fríttering awáy.

распыли́тель *м.* átomizer, spray.

распыли́ть(ся) *сов. см.* распыля́ть(ся).

распыля́ть, распыли́ть (*вн.*) 1. (*превращать в пыль*) pówder (*smth.*), púlverize (*smth.*); 2. (*жидкость*) spray (*smth.*), átomize (*smth.*); 3. (*рассредоточивать*) dispérse (*smb., smth.*), scátter (*smth., smth.*). ~ся, распыли́ться 1. (*превращаться в пыль*) turn to dust/pówder; 2. (*рассредоточиваться*) be* dispérsed; (*о силах, средствах*) be* fríttered awáy.

расса́д|а *ж.* séedlings *pl*; ~ цветно́й капу́сты cáuliflower séedlings; сажа́ть ~у plant séedlings.

расса́дить *сов. см.* расса́живать.

расса́дник *м.* 1. *с.-х.* (*питомник*) séed-bed, núrsery; 2. (*рд.*; *средоточие чего-л.*) céntre (of); (*в отрицательном смысле тж.*) hótbed (of); ~ зара́зы hótbed of inféction.

расса́живать, рассади́ть (*вн.*) 1. (*по местам*) seat (*smb.*); рассади́ть госте́й seat *one's* guests; 2. (*сажать порознь*) séparate (*smth.*); рассади́ть шалуно́в séparate the misbehá́vers; 3. (*растения*) plant out (*smth.*); рассади́ть клубни́ку plant out stráwberries. ~ся, рассе́сться take* *one's* seats.

расса́сываться, рассоса́ться resólve; be* resólved; *перен. разг.* dispérse.

рассвести́ *сов. см.* рассвета́ть.

рассве́т *м.* dáybreak; dawn (*тж. перен.*); на ~е at dawn.

рассвет|а́ть, рассвести́: ~а́ет day is bréaking; рассвело́ it grew light; day came.

рассвирепе́ть *сов. см.* свирепе́ть.

рассе́длать *сов.* (*вн.*) unsáddle (*smth.*).

рассе́ивать, **рассе́ять** (*вн.*) 1. dispérse (*smth.*), scátter (*smth.*); рассе́ять свет diffúse/diffráct light; 2. (*разгонять в разные стороны*) break* up (*smb.*, *smth.*); *перен.* (*устранять что-л. неприятное*) dispél (*smth.*), clear up (*smth.*); рассе́ять толпу́ break* up a crowd; рассе́ять подозре́ния, сомне́ния clear up suspícions, doubts; 3. (*отвлекать от неприятных мыслей и т. п.*) divért (*smb.*), take* (*smb.*) out of himsélf; рассе́ять чьё-л. го́ре take* *smb.'s* mind off his, her tróubles/sórrows. **~ся**, **рассе́яться** 1. dispérse; (*о свете*) becóme* diffúse; 2. (*расходиться в разные стороны*) scátter; (*о тумане, дыме*) clear, lift; (*о тучах тж.*) be* blown awáy; *перен.* (*о неприятном чувстве и т. п.*) disappéar, be* dispélled; тоска́ рассе́ялась the sádness disappéared; рассе́яться как дым vánish like smoke; 3. (*отвлекаться от чего-л. неприятного*) find* distráction; вам на́до рассе́яться you need distráction/divérsion.

рассека́ть, **рассе́чь** (*вн.*) 1. cleave* (*smth.*), split* (*smth.*); 2. (*наносить рану*) cut* (*smth.*); 3. (*разделять, пересекать*) cut* (*smth.*) in two, split* (*smth.*).

рассе́лина *ж.* cleft, fissure; ~ в скале́ fissure in a cliff.

рассели́ть(ся) *сов. см.* рассе́ля́ть(ся).

рассе́лять, **рассели́ть** (*вн.*) 1. (*размещать, поселив где-л.*) séttle (*smth.*); 2. (*поселять порознь*) séparate (*smb.*). **~ся**, **рассели́ться** 1. (*размещаться*) take* up *one's* séttle; 2. (*поселяться порознь*) séparate.

рассерд|и́ть *сов.* (*вн.*) make* (*smb.*) ángry, annóy (*smth.*). **~и́ться** *сов.* (*на вн.*) be* ángry (with); за что вы на него́ ~и́лись? what makes you so ángry with him?

рассе́сться *сов. см.* расса́живаться.

рассе́чь *сов. см.* рассека́ть.

рассе́яние *с.* dispérsion.

рассе́янн|о ábsent-míndedly, ábsently. **~ость** *ж.* 1. (*невнимательность*) ábsent-míndedness, ábsence of mind; 2. (*разбросанность*) dispérsedness, scátteredness. **~ый** 1. (*разбросанный, несосредоточенный*) scáttered, dispérsed; **~ый** свет diffúsed light; 2. (*невнимательный*) ábsent-mínded; (*выражающий рассеянность*) abstrácted, inatténtive.

рассе́ять(ся) *сов. см.* рассе́ивать(ся).

расска́з *м.* 1. stóry, tale; (*описание*) accóunt, descríption; ~ очеви́дца first-hand accóunt; чей-л. ~ interrúpt *smb.'s* stóry; 2. (*литературный жанр*) short stóry.

рассказа́ть *сов. см.* расска́зывать.

расска́зч|ик *м.*, **~ица** *ж.* nárrátor, tálker; (*артист*) stóry-teller.

расска́зывать, **рассказа́ть** (*вн.*) tell* (*smth.*); reláte (*smth.*), nárrate (*smth.*); ~ кому́-л. о случи́вшемся tell* *smb.* what happened; ~ да́льше go* on with *one's* stóry; рассказа́ть занима́тельную исто́рию reláte/descríbe an interesting íncident.

расслаби́ть *сов. см.* расслабля́ть.

расслабле́нн|ость *ж.* wéakness; (*ненапряжённость*) relaxátion. **~ый** weak, féeble, limp; (*ненапряжённый*) reláxed.

расслабля́ть, **рассла́бить** (*вн.*) wéaken (*smb.*, *smth.*); (*снимать напряжение*) reláx (*smth.*); ~ мы́шцы reláx (the múscles).

рассла́ивать, **расслои́ть** (*вн.*) strátify (*smth.*) (*тж. перен.*); séparate (*smth.*); (*тесто*) arránge (*smth.*) in láyers. **~ся**, **расслои́ться** be* strátified (*тж. перен.*); (*о тесте*) becóme fláky; *тех.* láminate.

рассле́дование *с.* investigátion, inquiry (into); назна́чить ~ set* up an investigátion, appóint an inquiry; произвести́ ~ make*/cárry out an investigátion.

рассле́довать *несов. и сов.* (*вн.*) invéstigate (*smth.*), inquíre (into), look (into), examíne (*smth.*); ~ де́ло invéstigate a case.

расслое́ние *с.* stratificátion (*тж. перен.*); laminátion; (*теста*) láyering.

расслои́ть(ся) *сов. см.* рассла́ивать(ся).

расслы́ш|ать *сов.* (*вн.*) hear* (*smth.*), catch* (*smth.*); я не ~ал, что он сказа́л I dídn't quite catch what he said; прости́те, я не ~ал sórry — I dídn't quite hear.

рассма́тривать, **рассмотре́ть** 1. *тк. несов.* (*вн. как; считать*) regárd (*smth.* as), consíder (*smth.* to be); 2. *тк. несов.* (*вн.; разглядывать*) look (at); внима́тельно, при́стально ~ что-л. scrútinize *smth.*; ~ иллюстра́ции look at the píctures/illustrátions; ~ что-л. в микроско́п look at *smth.* through a mícroscope, examíne *smth.* únder a mícroscope; 3. (*вн.; обсуждать*) consíder (*smth.*), examíne (*smth.*); ~ де́ло (*в суде*) try* a case.

рассмеши́ть *сов.* (*вн.*) make* (*smb.*) laugh.

рассмея́ться *сов.* laugh, burst* out láughing.

рассмотре́ни|е *с.* examinátion; (*оценка тж.*) considerátion; ~ де́ла considerátion of a case; (*в суде*) trial; вторичное ~ чего́-л. reconsiderátion; представля́ть что-л. на ~ submit *smth.* for considerátion; при ближа́йшем ~и on clóser examinátion.

рассмотре́ть *сов.* 1. *см.* рассма́тривать 3; 2. (*вн.; различить*) discérn (*smth.*), make* (*smth.*) out.

рассова́ть *сов. см.* рассо́вывать.

рассо́вывать, **рассова́ть** (*вн. в вн.*) *разг.* shove (*smth.* into); ~ что-л. по карма́нам shove *smth.* into *one's* várious póckets.

рассо́л *м.* brine, píckle; огуре́чный ~ juice of sálted cúcumbers.

рассо́льник *м.* rassólnik (*meat or fish soup with salted cucumbers*).

рассо́рить *сов.* (*вн.*) *разг.* make* míschief (betwéen), set* (*smb.*) at lóggerheads. **~ся** *сов. разг.* quárrel, fall* out.

рассортирова́ть *сов.* (*вн.*) sort (*smth.*) out, clássify (*smth.*).

рассоса́ться *сов. см.* расса́сываться.

рассо́хнуться *сов. см.* рассыха́ться.

расспра́шивать, **расспроси́ть** (*вн.*) quéstion (*smb.*).

расспроси́ть *сов. см.* расспра́шивать.

расспро́сы *мн.* cross-quéstioning *sg*, quéstions.

рассредото́ч|ение *с. воен.* dispérsal. **~ивать**, **рассредото́чить** (*вн.*) *воен.* dispérse (*smb.*, *smth.*). **~иваться**, **рассредото́читься** *воен.* dispérse, break* up (ínto small únits).

рассредото́чить(ся) *сов. см.* рассредото́чивать(ся).

рассро́ч|ивать, **рассро́чить**: ~ платёж кому́-л. (*за купленное*) allów *smb.* to pay by instálments; рассро́чить платёж до́лга кому́-л. allów *smb.* to pay back a debt grádually. **~ить** *сов. см.* рассро́чивать. **~ка** *ж.*: **~ка** платежа́ consént to páyment in instálments; плати́ть в ~ку, ~кой pay* in/by instálments; покупа́ть что-л. в ~ку buy* *smth.* on the instálment sýstem; продава́ть что-л. в ~ку sell* *smth.* on the instálment sýstem.

расстава́ни|е *с.* párting; при ~и at párting.

расстава́ться, **расста́ться** (*с тв.*) 1. part (with); расста́ться с кем-л. навсегда́ part with *smb.* foréver; 2. (*покидать какое-л. место*) leave* (*smth.*), quit (*smth.*); расста́ться с родны́м го́родом quit *smth.'s* home town; 3. (*отказываться от чего-л.*) give* up (*smth.*), relínquish (*smth.*); ~ с мы́слью give* up the idéa; ~ с привы́чкой relínquish a hábit; он не расстаётся с кни́гой he is néver withóut a book in his hands.

расста́вить *сов. см.* расставля́ть.

расставля́ть, **расста́вить** (*вн.*) 1. (*ставить*) place (*smth.*, *smth.*), arránge (*smth.*); расста́вить кни́ги в шкафу́ place/arránge books in a bóokcase; ~ се́ти set* nets; 2. (*распределять для исполнения работы*) distríbute (*smb.*, *smth.*); állocate (*smb.*, *smth.*); ~ си́лы distríbute *one's* fórces; ~ часовы́х post séntries; ~ люде́й állocate (dúties to) personnél; 3. (*раздвигать*) exténd (smth.); ~ нóги set* one's feet apárt; ~ рýки exténd one's arms horizóntally; 4. разг. (платье и т. п.) let* (smth.) out.

расстанóвк|а ж. 1. arrángement; 2. (распределение для исполнения работы) distribútion, allocátion; ~ сил distribútion/líne-up of fórces; ~ кáдров distribútion/plácing of personnél/cadres; 3. (пауза) páuses pl; говорúть с ~ой make* próper páuses, speak* in méasured tones.

расстáться сов. см. расставáться.

расстёгивать, расстегнýть (вн.) undó* (smth.), unfásten (smth.); (застёгнутое на пýговицы тж.) unbútton (smth.). ~ся, расстегнýться 1. (о чём-л.) come* undóne/unfástened/unbúttoned; 2. (о ком-либо) unbútton one's coat etc.

расстегнýть(ся) сов. см. расстёгивать(ся).

расстилáть, разостлáть (вн.) spread* (smth.), ~ся, разостлáться spread* out.

расстоя́ни|е с. dístance; перен. gap; на большóм ~и at a great dístance; на небольшóм ~и a short way off; на ~и 10 киломéтров ten kílometres awáy/dístant; ◇ держáть кого-л. на почтúтельном ~и keep* smb. at arm's length, keep* smb. at a dístance.

расстрáивать, расстрóить (вн.) 1. (нарушать порядок чего-л.) disórganize (smth.), throw* (smth.) ínto confúsion, break* up (smth.); 2. (причинять ущерб) ruin (smth.); wreck (smth.); 3. (мешать осуществлению чего-л.) upsét* (smth.), spoil* (smth.); расстрóить чьи-л. плáны upsét* smb.'s plans; 4. (приводить в болезненное состояние) upsét* (smth.); расстрóить здорóвье undermíne one's health; 5. (музыкальный инструмент) put*/make* (smth.) òut of tune; ~ пиани́но make* a piáno out of tune; 6. (огорчать) upsét* (smth.). ~ся, расстрóиться 1. (терять правильность построения) break* up, lose* formátion, be* thrown ínto confúsion; 2. (приходить в упадок) go* to píeces; break* down, fail; хозя́йство расстрóилось the ecónomy went to píeces; 3. (нарушаться, прерываться) collápse, break* down; (не осуществляться) miscárry; игрá расстрóилась the game was spoiled; поéздка расстрóилась the trip went wrong, the trip miscárried/failed; 4. (приходить в болезненное состояние) fail, collápse; егó здорóвье расстрóилось his health failed; 5. (о музыкальном инструменте) get* out of tune; скрúпка расстрóилась the violín is out of tune; 6. (огорчаться) be* upsét, be* put out, be* discóuraged.

расстрéл м. 1. (действие) shóoting down; 2. (казнь) shóoting; приговорúть кого-л. к ~у séntence smb. to be shot.

расстрéливать, расстрелять (вн.) 1. (казнить) shoot* (smb.); 2. (подвергать сильному обстрелу) rake (smb., smth.) with fire; (молну) shoot* down (smb., smth.), fire (on); ~ кого-л. из пулемёта gun down smb.

расстреля́ть сов. см. расстрéливать.

расстрóенн|ый 1. (беспорядочный) disórganized, disórdered; ~ые ряды́ bróken ranks; 2. (приведённый в упадок) ruined; ~ое хозя́йство ruined ecónomy; 3. (приведённый в болезненное состояние) disórdered; ~ое здорóвье disórdered health; ~ые нéрвы disórdered nerves; 4. (о музыкальном инструменте) òut-of-túne; рояль расстрóен the piáno is out of tune, the piáno needs túning; 5. (огорчённый) upsét; tróubled, distréssed; он óчень расстрóен he's térribly upsét.

расстрóить(ся) сов. см. расстрáивать(ся).

расстрóйство с. disórder; upsétting; ~ желýдка stómach disórder, indigéstion.

расступ|áться, расступúться make* way (for). ~úться сов. см. расступáться.

расстыковáть(ся) сов. см. расстыкóвывать(ся).

расстыкóвка ж. undócking.

расстыкóвывать, расстыковáть (вн.) undóck (smth.). ~ся, расстыковáться undóck.

рассудúтельн|ость ж. réasonableness. ~ый rátional, sóber.

рассуд|úть сов. 1. (вн.; разрешить спор) judge (smb., smth.); ~úте нас be the judge betwéen us; 2. (решить) decíde.

рассýд|ок м. understánding, réason; (здравый смысл) cómmon sense; в пóлном ~ке in full posséssion of one's fáculties; гóлос ~ка the voice of réason; ~ку вопрекú cóntrary to cómmon sense.

рассýдочный rátional.

рассужд|áть несов. 1. (мыслить) réason; 2. (приводить доводы) discúss; 3. (о пр.) разг. (возражать) árgue (about); не ~áя without a word; не ~! don't árgue! ~éние с. 1. réasoning; прáвильное ~éние correct réasoning; 2. обыкн. мн. разг. (высказывание) discússion sg; пустúться в ~éния start discússing mátters, start a léngthy discússion; 3. (возражение) árgument; без ~éний! no árguing!

рассчúтанный (умышленный) delíberate; (размеренный) cálculated, planned.

рассчитáть сов. см. рассчúтывать 1, 4. ~ся сов. см. рассчúтываться 1, 2, 3, 5.

рассчúтыв|ать, рассчитáть, расчéсть 1. (вн.; вычислять) cálculate (smth.); (определять, задумывать что-л.) plan (smth.); have* (smth.) taped разг.; (правильно соразмерять) time (smth.), gauge (smth.); не рассчитáть своúх сил overráte one's strength; 2. тк. несов. (на вн., + инф.; надеяться) depénd (upón), relý (on, upón), count (on); (полагаться на кого-л., что-л.) look fórward (to); мóжете ~ на меня́ you may depénd upón me; я ~ал на егó пóмощь I counted on his help; 3. тк. несов. (предполагать) inténd, mean*; 4. (вн.; увольнять) dischárge (smth.), pay* off (smth.). ~аться, рассчитáться, расчéсться 1. (в ресторане и т. п.) pay* the bill; (с тв.) séttle up (with); 2. (с тв.) разг. (сводить счёты, мстить) be*/get* éven (with); 3. разг. (увольняться) leave*, give* up the job; 4. тк. несов. (за вн.; нести ответственность) pay* (for); ~áться за своú прострýпки pay* for one's áctions; 5. сов. рассчитáться (в строю) númber; по порáдку номерóв рассчитáйсь! númber!

рассылáть, разослáть (вн.) send* (smb., smth.), send* out (smb., smth.).

рассы́лка ж. distribútion.

рассы́льный м. méssenger.

рассы́пать сов. см. рассыпáть.

рассыпáть, рассы́пать (вн.) 1. (просыпать) spill* (smth.); (разбрасывать) strew* (smth.); рассы́пать cáхар spill* the súgar; 2. (распределять, насыпая) pour (smth.) out; рассы́пать мукý по мешкáм pour the flour out ínto sacks.

рассыпáться сов. см. рассыпáться.

рассыпáться, рассы́паться 1. (о сыпучем, мелких предметах) spill*, scátter; бýсы рассы́пались по всемý пóлу the beads scáttered all óver the floor; 2. (разваливаться) go* to píeces, crúmble; рассыпáться в пыль crúmble to dust; 3. (рассредоточиться) scátter; 4. разг.: ~ в похвалáх кому-л. shówer práises on smb.; ~ в любéзностях be* effúsively políte; ~ в извинéниях be* profúse in one's apólogies.

рассыпнóй loose.

рассы́пчатый crúmbly, fríable; (о тесте) short.

рассыхáться, рассóхнуться dry up, shrink*.

расталкивать, растолкáть (вн.) разг. 1. push (smb.) apárt, push (smb.) awáy; ~ толпý push one's way through a crowd; 2. (спящего) shake* (smb.).

растáпливать I, растопúть (вн.; печь и т. п.) light* (smth.).

растáпливать II, растопúть (вн.; плавить) melt (smth.).

растáпливаться I, растопúться (о печи) light*.

растáпливаться II, растопúться (плавиться) melt.

растаска́ть *сов. разг. см.* раста́скивать 1.

раста́скивать, растащи́ть, растаска́ть (*вн.*) 1. pull (*smth.*) apárt, break* (*smth.*) up; (*разворовывать*) steal* (*smth.*); 2. *сов.* растащи́ть *разг.* (*разнимать кого-л.*) drag (*smb.*) apárt.

раста́чивать, расточи́ть (*вн.*) bore (*smth.*) out; ~ отве́рстие bore the hole wíder, déeper.

растащи́ть *сов. см.* раста́скивать.

раста́ять *сов.* thaw; melt (*тж. перен.*).

раство́р *м.* 1. solútion; во́дный ~ áqueous solútion; 2.: строи́тельный ~ mórtar. ~е́ние *с.* dissólving.

раствор|и́мый *хим.* sóluble. ~и́тель *м. хим.* sólvent.

раствори́ть I, II *сов. см.* растворя́ть I, II.

раствори́ться I, II *сов. см.* растворя́ться I, II.

растворя́ть I, раствори́ть (*вн.; открывать*) ópen (*smth.*).

растворя́ть II, раствори́ть (*вн.*) dissólve (*smth.*); (*разбавлять*) dilúte (*smth.*), wéaken (*smth.*); раствори́ть и́звесть в воде́ dissólve lime in wáter.

растворя́ться I, раствори́ться (*открываться*) ópen.

растворя́ться II, раствори́ться dissólve; *перен.* (*исчезать*) melt (awáy), dissólve.

растека́ться, расте́чься spread* (óver); *перен.* drift awáy.

расте́ние *с.* plant.

растениево́дство *с.* plánt-growing, plánt-raising.

растере́ть(ся) *сов. см.* растира́ть(ся).

растёрзанн|ый *разг.* báttered, dishévelled; *перен.* tormént ed; в ~ом ви́де in a dishévelled state.

растерза́ть *сов.* (*вн.*) 1. tear* (*smb., smth.*) to pieces, maul (*smb., smth.*); 2. *разг.* (*растрепать*) dishével (*smb.*); 3. (*нравственно измучить*) tear* (*smth.*), tormént (*smb., smth.*).

расте́рянн|о in bewílderment. ~ость *ж.* bewílderment, perpléxity. ~ый bewíldered, perpléxed; с ~ым ви́дом lóoking bewíldered/perpléxed.

растеря́ть *сов.* (*вн.*) lose* (*smth.*). ~ся *сов.* 1. (*потеряться*) be* lost; 2. (*от волнения и т. п.*) be* bewíldered; ~ся от неожи́данности be* táken abáck; he ~ся keep* *one's* head.

расти́ *несов.* grow*; (*становиться старше*) grow* up; (*увеличиваться*) incréase; (*совершенствоваться*) grow*, devélop.

растира́ть, растере́ть (*вн.*) 1. (*превращать в порошок*) grind* (*smth.*) fine; 2. (*тереть, размазывать*) rub (*smth.*), spread* (*smth.*); 3. (*массажировать*) rub (*smb.*) down, masságe (*smb., smth.*). ~ся, растере́ться 1. (*измельчаться*) be* ground to pówder; 2. (*обтираться*) rub onesélf (down).

расти́тельн|ость *ж.* 1. (*растения*) vegétation; ~ Кавка́за the vegetátion of the Cáucasus; 2. (*волосы*) hair; лишённый ~ости háirless. ~ый plant *attr.*, végetable; ~ый мир végetable kíngdom, plant life; ~ая пи́ща végetable food; ~ое ма́сло végetable oil.

расти́ть *несов.* (*вн.*) raise (*smb., smth.*); grow* (*smth.*); ~ дете́й raise chíldren, bring* up chíldren; ~ ка́дры train persónnel.

растолка́ть *сов. см.* раста́лкивать.

растолкова́ть *сов. см.* растолко́вывать.

растолко́вывать, растолкова́ть (*вн. дт.*) expláin (*smth. to*).

растоло́чь *сов. см.* толо́чь.

растолсте́ть *сов.* grow* stout, put* on flesh.

растопи́ть I, II *сов. см.* раста́пливать I, II.

растопи́ться I, II *сов. см.* раста́пливаться I, II.

расто́пка *ж.* 1. (*действие*) lighting, kíndling; 2. *собир. разг.* (*лучина и т. п.*) kíndling.

растопта́ть *сов.* (*вн.*) crush (*smth.*) underfóot, trámple (*smth.*).

растопы́р|ивать, растопы́рить (*вн.*) *разг.* spread*

(*smth.*); растопы́рить па́льцы spread* *one's* fíngers. ~ить *сов. см.* растопы́ривать.

расторга́ть, расто́ргнуть (*вн.*) cáncel (*smth.*), dissólve (*smth.*), annúl (*smth.*); ~ брак dissólve a márriage; ~ догово́р cáncel a tréaty.

расто́ргнуть *сов. см.* расторга́ть.

расторже́ние *с.* dissolútion, annúlment, cancellátion.

растороп|ность *ж.* efficiency, prómptitude. ~ный efficient, prompt.

расточа́ть, расточи́ть (*вн.*) 1. (*растрачивать*) waste (*smth.*), squánder (*smth.*); 2. (*щедро дарить*) lávish (*smth.*); be* lávish (of); ~ похвалы́ кому́-л. lávish práises on *smb.*

расточи́тель *м.*, ~ница *ж.* squánderer, spéndthrift. ~ность *ж.* extrávagance, wástefulness. ~ный extrávagant, wásteful. ~ство *с. см.* расточи́тельность.

расточи́ть I *сов. см.* расточа́ть.

расточи́ть II *сов. см.* раста́чивать.

растрави́ть *сов. см.* растравля́ть.

растравля́ть, растрави́ть (*вн.*) írritate (*smth.*); *перен. разг.* revíve (*smth.*); растравля́ть ра́ну distúrb/írritate the wound; *перен.* rub salt in a wound; растрави́ть чьё-л. го́ре revíve *smb.'s* grief.

растра́т|а *ж.* squándering, waste; (*кража*) embézzlement. ~ить *сов. см.* растра́чивать. ~чик *м.* embézzler.

растра́чивать, растра́тить (*вн.*) 1. wáste (*smth.*), squánder (*smth.*) (*тж. перен.*); растра́тить все де́ньги squánder all *one's* móney; растра́тить си́лы waste *one's* strength/énergy; 2. (*чужие деньги*) embézzle (*smth.*).

растрезво́нить *сов. см.* трезво́нить 2.

растрёпанный 1. dishévelled; 2. (*о книгах и т. п.*) táttered, dóg-eared.

растрепа́ть *сов.* (*вн.*) *разг.* 1. (*приводить в беспоря́док*) rúffle (*smth.*), disarránge (*smth.*); ~ кому́-л. во́лосы rúmple *smb.'s* hair; 2. (*приводить в негодность*) make* a mess (of); ~ся *сов.* 1. (*о волосах*) be* dishévelled; 2. (*о книге и т. п.*) be* táttered, be* fálling to pieces.

растреска́ться *сов.* crack, be* cracked; (*о коже тж.*) be*/get* chapped.

растро́ганный touched, moved; ~ до слёз moved to tears.

растро́гать *сов.* (*вн.*) touch (*smb.*), move (*smb.*); ~ кого́-л. до слёз move *smb.* to tears. ~ся *сов.* be* moved/touched.

растряс|ти́ *сов.* 1. (*вн.; раскидать*) strew* (*smth.*); 2. *безл.: его́* ~ло́ he is bádly sháken, he has had a bad sháking.

растя́гивать, растяну́ть (*вн.*) 1. (*вытягивать*) stretch (*smth.*), растяну́ть перча́тки stretch a pair of gloves; 2. (*лишать упругости*) wear* (*smth.*) out, strain (*smth.*); растяну́ть рези́ну wear* out the elástic; 3. (*повреждать*) strain (*smth.*); растяну́ть свя́зки pull the lígaments; 4. (*размещать на большом пространстве*) exténd (*smth.*); (*цепочкой*) string* (*smth.*) out; 5. (*затягивать, задерживать*) protráct (*smth.*), prolóng (*smth.*); spin* (*smth.*) out *разг.*; растяну́ть сро́ки се́ва deláy the sówing, hold* up the sówing; 6. (*медленно произносить*) drawl (*smth.*); ~ слова́ drawl. ~ся, растяну́ться 1. (*удлиняться*) stretch; 2. (*терять упру́гость*) be* worn out; 3. (*о связках и т. п.*) be* strained/pulled; (*о кисти, щиколотке тж.*) be* sprained; 4. (*располагаться на большом пространстве*) exténd; (*цепочкой*) be* strung out; 5. *разг.* (*ложиться вытянувшись*) stretch out (full length); 6. (*затягиваться*) drag on; рабо́та растяну́лась на неде́лю the work dragged on for a whole week.

растяже́ние *с.* strain; ~ свя́зок strained lígaments.

растяжи́мый strétchable, ténsile; elástic (*тж. перен.*).

растя́нутый **1.** élongated, exténded; (*об одежде*) stretched; **2.** (*излишне длинный и скучный*) long-winded, prólix, tédious; ~ расска́з long-winded stóry, tédious tale.

растяну́ть *сов. см.* растя́гивать. ~ся *сов.* **1.** *см.* растя́гиваться; **2.** *разг.* (*упасть*) fall* (full length).

растя́па *м. и ж. разг.* múddler, blúnderer.

расфасова́ть *сов. см.* расфасо́вывать.

расфасо́вка *ж.* pácking, páckaging; ~ това́ров páckaging of goods.

расфасо́вывать, расфасова́ть (*вн.*) páckage (*smth.*); ~ муку́ páckage flour.

расформирова́ть *сов. см.* расформиро́вывать.

расформиро́вывать, расформирова́ть (*вн.*) disbánd (*smth.*), break* (*smth.*) up.

расфранчённый dressed/dólled up.

расха́живать *несов.* stroll/sáunter up and down; ~ по ко́мнате stroll up and down the room.

расхва́ливать, расхвали́ть (*вн.*) praise (*smb., smth.*); расхвали́ть до небе́с кого́-л. laud smb. to the skies.

расхвали́ть *сов. см.* расхва́ливать.

расхва́рываться, расхвора́ться *разг.* be* thóroughly ill.

расхва́статься *сов. разг.* boast, brag.

расхвата́ть, расхвати́ть *сов. см.* расхва́тывать.

расхва́тывать, расхвата́ть, расхвати́ть (*вн.*) *разг.* snatch up (*smth.*); (*раскупать тж.*) buy* (*smth.*) up.

расхвора́ться *сов. см.* расхва́рываться.

расхити́тель *м.* plúnderer.

расхи́тить *сов. см.* расхища́ть.

расхищ|а́ть, расхи́тить (*вн.*) plúnder (*smth.*), misapprópriate (*smth.*). ~е́ние *с.* plúndering, misappropriátion.

расхля́банн|ость *ж. разг.* **1.** unstéadiness; **2.** (*недисциплини́рованность*) láxity. ~ый *разг.* **1.** sháky, wéak-jóinted; ~ая похо́дка slóuching walk; **2.** (*недисциплини́рованный*) lax.

расхо́д *м.* **1.** (*затрата, издержки*) expénse; *мн. тж.* expénditure *sg*, óutlay *sg*; госуда́рственные ~ы State expénditure; доро́жные ~ы trávelling expénses; прихо́д и ~ íncome and expénditure; **2.** (*потребление*) consúmption; ~ ма́сла oil consúmption; **3.** (*графа в бухгалтерской книге*) expénditure; ◇ вводи́ть кого́-л. в ~ put* smb. to expénse; спи́сывать что́-л. в ~ write* smth. off (as a loss).

расходи́ться, разойти́сь **1.** (*уходить в разные стороны*) dispérse; (*о толпе, собрании и т. п. тж.*) break* up; ~ по дома́м go* home; го́сти разошли́сь в 12 часо́в the párty broke up at twelve; **2.** (*рассеиваться, исчезать*) dispérse; ту́чи разошли́сь the clouds dispérsed; **3.** (*с тв.; не встречаться в пути*) miss (*smb.*); **4.** (*встретившись, давать пройти*) pass (each óther); **5.** (*прекращать общение, знакомство*) part; (*с тв.*) break* (with), séparate (from); (*разводиться*) divórce (*smb.*); разойти́сь со ста́рым дру́гом break* with an old friend; **6.** (*с тв. в пр.; не соглашаться*) disagrée (with smb. in, óver), differ (with, from smb. óver, in); ~ с ке́м-л. во мне́ниях disagrée with smb.; ~ с ке́м-л. в оце́нке чего́-л. differ from smb. in one's estimátion of smth.; **7.** (*разветвляться*) divérge; (*о дорогах тж.*) fork; *перен.* (*не совпадать*) differ; за дере́вней доро́га разошла́сь the road forked óutside the víllage; мне́ния разошли́сь opínions differed; **8.** (*разъединяться*): по́лы пальто́ расходя́тся the coat dóesn't meet in front; полови́цы разошли́сь the flóor-boards have shrunk; **9.** (*распродаваться, раскупаться*) sell*; be* sold; **10.** (*тратиться*) go*; де́ньги разошли́сь на ра́зные мело́чи the móney went on all kinds of líttle things.

расходн|ый expénse *attr.*; ~ая кни́га accóunt-book.

расходова́ние *с.* **1.** expénditure; **2.** (*потребление*) consúmption.

расхо́д|овать, израсхо́довать (*вн.*) **1.** (*тратить*)

spend* (*smth.*), expénd (*smth.*); **2.** *разг.* (*потреблять*) consúme (*smth.*), use (*smth.*); мото́р ~ует мно́го горю́чего the éngine úses a lot of fuel.

расхожде́ние *с.* divérgence; (*несоответствие*) discrépancy; ~ во мне́ниях difference/divérgence of opínion.

расхола́живать, расхолоди́ть (*вн.*) disenchánt (*smb.*), damp smb.'s enthúsiasm.

расхолоди́ть *сов. см.* расхола́живать.

расхоте́|ть *сов.* (*рд. + инф.*) *разг.* no lónger want (*smth., + to inf*) lose* all desíre (for, + to inf); он ~л спать he lost all desíre to sleep. ~ться *сов. безл. разг.*: мне ~лось спать, есть *и т. п.* I'm not sléepy, húngry, *etc.* ány more.

расхохота́ться *сов.* burst* out láughing; гро́мко ~ roar with láughter, burst* ínto peals of láughter.

расхрабри́ться *сов. разг.* grow* bold.

расцара́п|ать *сов.* scratch (*smth.*); он ~ал себе́ всё лицо́ he got his face all scratched.

расцвести́ *сов. см.* расцвета́ть.

расцве́т *м.* (*цветение*) blóoming, blóssoming; *перен.* blóssoming forth, gólden age; ~ литерату́ры, культу́ры blóssoming forth of líterature, cúlture; бу́рный ~ vígorous/exúberant growth; в ~е сил in one's prime/héyday; в ~е тво́рческих сил at the peak of one's creátive ability.

расцвет|а́ть, расцвести́ bloom, blóssom; *перен.* (*хорошеть*) blóssom out; (*веселеть*) bríghten up; becóme* rádiant; (*достигать высокой степени развития*) flóurish, blóssom forth; ро́зы ~а́ют the róses are just cóming out; ро́зы расцвели́ the róses are in full bloom.

расцвети́ть *сов.* (*вн.*) *разг.* make* (*smth.*) bright.

расцве́тка *ж. разг.* cólour scheme; пёстрая ~ bright cólour scheme.

расцелова́ть *сов.* (*вн.*) kiss (*smb., smth.*). ~ся *сов.* kiss each óther.

расцени|ва́ть, расцени́ть (*вн.*) **1.** (*определять стоимость*) éstimate (*smth.*), válue (*smth.*); (*определять цену*) price (*smth.*); расцени́ть това́р price goods; **2.** (*относиться к чему-л. каким-л. образом*) appráise (*smth.*), regárd (*smth.*); ~ что́-л. как кру́пную оши́бку regárd smth. as a grave érror; как вы ~ете его́ поведе́ние? what do you make of his behávíour?

расцени́ть *сов. см.* расце́нивать.

расце́нка *ж.* **1.** (*действие*) valuátion; **2.** (*цена*) príces *pl*; (*оплата*) rate.

расцепи́ть(ся) *сов. см.* расцепля́ть(ся).

расцепля́ть, расцепи́ть (*вн.*) unhóok (*smth.*); (*вагоны*) uncóuple (*smth.*). ~ся, расцепи́ться get*/come* unhóoked; (*о вагонах*) get* uncóupled.

расчеса́ть(ся) *сов. см.* расчёсываться.

расчёска *ж. разг.* comb.

расчеста́ть *сов. см.* расчита́ть 1, 4. ~ся *сов. разг. см.* рассчи́тываться 1, 2, 3.

расчёсывать, расчеса́ть (*вн.*) **1.** (*волосы*) comb (*smth.*); (*лён, шерсть*) card (*smth.*); **2.** (*ногтями*) scratch (*smth.*) (till it is sore). ~ся, расчеса́ться comb one's hair.

расчёт *м.* **1.** (*вычисление*) calculátion, computátion; ~ вре́мени tíming; ~ про́чности calculátion of the strength; приблизи́тельный ~ estimátion, éstimate; то́чный ~ áccurate calculátions *pl*; (*о цене*) exáct éstimate; производи́ть ~ы make* calculátions, compúte; **2.** (*уплата денег*) páyment, accóunt; в оконча́тельный ~ in séttlement; произвести́ ~ séttle up; **3.** (*увольнение*): взять ~ resígn; дать ~ кому́-л. pay* off smb.; получи́ть ~ be* dischárged; **4.** (*наказание, расплата*): с ним у меня́ бу́дет коро́ткий ~ he'll get short shrift from me; **5.** (*намерение, предположение*) expectátion; ~ оказа́лся пра́вильным it worked out as expécted; э́то не входи́ло в мои́ ~ы I had not allówed for that; в его́ ~ы не входи́ло... he did not réckon with...; обману́ться в свои́х ~ах miscálculate; 6. *разг.* (*польза, выгода*) advántage; мне нет никакóго ~a ждать I have nóthing to gain by wáiting; 7. *воен.* (*люди*) crew, detáchment; squad, (mánning) détail *амер.*; ◇ из ~a cóunting, réckoning; из ~a по десятú рублéй на человéка at the rate of ten róubles per head; из ~a срéднего зарабóтка on a básis of the áverage éarnings; быть в ~е с кем-л. have* séttled accóunts with smb.; be* quits with smb.; тепéрь мы с вáми в ~е now we're quits; принимáть что-л. в ~ take* smth. into considerátion/accóunt.

расчётлив|ость *ж.* (*бережливость*) thríftiness; (*осмотрительность*) prúdence. ~ый (*бережливый*) thrífty; (*осторожный*) prúdent, cálculating.

расчётн|ый 1.: ~ая вéдомость páy-sheet; ~ая кнúжка páy-book; ~ балáнс bálance of páyments; 2. *тех.* ráted; ~ая мóщность ráted capácity.

расчи́стить(ся) *сов. см.* расчищáть(ся).

расчи́стка *ж.* cléaring.

расчихáться *сов. разг.* sneeze víolently, have* a snéezing fit.

расчищáть, расчи́стить (*вн.*) clear (smth.). ~ся, расчи́ститься clear.

расчлени́ть *сов. см.* расчленя́ть.

расчленя́ть, расчлени́ть (*вн.*) divíde (smth.); (*разбивать на составные элементы*) break* (smth.) down.

расчýвствоваться *сов. разг.* give* way to one's féelings, becóme* effúsive.

расшали́ться *сов.* get* véry pláyful.

расша́ркаться *сов. см.* расша́ркиваться.

расша́ркиваться, расша́ркаться (*перед тв.*) bow (to); *перен.* bow and scrape (to), fawn (upón).

расша́танный (*о·предмете*) ríckety, sháky; *перен.* wéakened, flágging, críppled; (*о здоровье, нервах*) debílitated.

расшата́ть(ся) *сов. см.* расша́тывать(ся).

расша́тывать, расшата́ть (*вн.*) lóosen (smth.), shake* (smth.) loose; *перен.* crípple (smth.), wéaken (smth.), undermíne (smth.); расшата́ть стул make* a chair sháky; расшата́ть здорóвье crípple one's health. ~ся, расша́тываться get* loose; (*о мебели*) be* ríckety/sháky; *перен.* be* wéakened, be* underminéd.

расшевéливать, расшевели́ть (*вн.*) *разг.* stir (smth.) up, rouse (smb.).

расшевели́ть *сов. см.* расшевéливать.

расшибáть, расшиби́ть (*вн.*) *разг.* hurt* (smth.), bruise (smth.). ~ся, расшиби́ться *разг.* hurt*/bruise onesélf; ◇ расшиби́ться в лепёшку lay* onesélf out.

расши́ть(ся) *сов. см.* расшивáть(ся).

расшивáть, расши́ть (*вн.*) 1. *разг.* (*распарывать*) unpíck (smth.); 2. (*вышивать чем-л.*) embróider (in, with).

расшире́ние *с.* 1. wídening, bróadening; (*увеличение в числе, объёме*) íncrease, expánsion; ~ ýлицы wídening of a street; ~ экономи́ческих свя́зей expánsion of trade; ~ (*объёма*) произвóдства expánsion of prodúction; ~ кругозóра bróadening of one's óutlook; ~ сéрдца dilátion/dilatátion of the heart; 2. (*расширенная часть чего-л.*) exténsion in width, enlárged séction.

расши́ренн|ый exténded, enlárged; ~ые зрачки́ diláted púpils; ~ое толковáние exténded interpretátion; ~ое воспроизвóдство exténded reprodúction.

расши́рить(ся) *сов. см.* расширя́ть(ся).

расширя́ть, расши́рить (*вн.*) 1. wíden (smth.), bróaden (smth.); ~ дорóгу, ýлицу wíden a road, a street; ~ отвéрстие enlárge an ópening; 2. (*увеличивать в числе, объёме*) íncrease (smth.), enlárge (smth.), expánd (smth.); ~ ассортимéнт хлéбных издéлий íncrease the variety of breads; 3. (*делать более обширным*) bróaden (smth.), expánd (smth.), exténd (smth.); ~ кругозóр bróaden one's óutlook; ~ сфéру влия́ния exténd the sphere of ínfluence. ~ся, расши́риться 1. wíden; егó глазá расши́рились his eyes wídened; 2. (*увеличиваться*)

be* enlárged/expánded; 3. (*становиться более обши́рным*) bróaden, incréase, becóme* wíder; егó кругозóр расши́рился his óutlook has bróadened.

расши́тый embróidered.

расши́ть *сов. см.* расшивáть.

расшифровáть *сов. см.* расшифрóвывать.

расшифрóвывать, расшифровáть (*вн.*) decípher (smth.), decóde (smth.); *перен.* intérpret (smth.).

расшнуровáть *сов. см.* расшнурóвывать.

расшнурóвывать, расшнуровáть (*вн.*) unláce (smth.).

расшумéться *сов. разг.* be*/get* nóisy, make* an úproar.

расщéдри|ться *сов. разг.* show* one's generósity; он ~лся и... in a fit of generósity, he...

расщéлина *ж.* 1. (*ущелье в горах*) crévice, físsure; 2. (*трещина*) crack.

расщеп|и́ть(ся) *сов. см.* расщепля́ть(ся). ~лéние *с.* disintegrátion, splítting; ~лéние áтома átom físsion/splítting, splítting of the átom.

расщепля́ть, расщепи́ть (*вн.*) 1. split* (smth.); (*раздроблять в щепы*) splínter (smth.); 2. *хим.* decompóse (smth.), break* (smth.) down; 3. *физ.* split* (smth.); расщепи́ть áтом split* the átom. ~ся, расщепи́ться 1. split*; splínter; 2. *хим.* decompóse, break* down; 3. *физ.* split*.

ратификациóнн|ый: ~ые грáмоты *дип.* ínstruments of ratificátion.

ратифи|кáция *ж.* ratificátion. ~ци́ровать *несов. и сов.* (*вн.*) rátify (smth.).

рáтовать *несов.* (*за вн., против рд.*) fight* (for, against); (*за вн.*) ádvocate (smth.).

рáтуша *ж.* town hall.

рáунд *м. спорт.* round.

рафинáд *м.* lump súgar. ~ный: ~ный завóд súgar-refinery.

рафини́ровать *несов. и сов.* (*вн.*) refíne (smth.).

рахи́т *м.* ríckets; rachítis *научн.*

рахити́ч|еский, ~ный ríckety.

рациóн *м.* rátion; (*для скота*) dáily díet.

рационализáтор *м.* prodúction-rátionalizer.

рационализáторск|ий ~ое предложéние rationalizátion propósal/suggéstion.

рационализáция *ж.* rationalizátion.

рационáльн|ый rátional; ~ое испóльзование оборýдования rátional use of equípment; ~ые чи́сла *мат.* rátional quántities.

рáция *ж.* rádio transmítter-recéiver, transcéiver; rádio *разг.*

рванýть *сов.* 1. (*вн.*) jerk (smth.); 2. *разг.* (*резко тронуться с места*) start with a jerk. ~ся *сов. разг.* start with a jerk, give* a súdden plunge; (*броситься*) rush, dash.

рвáн|ый 1. (*разорванный на части*) bróken, slashed; 2. (*порванный, с дырами*) torn; ~ые сапоги́ worn boots; 3. (*с неровными краями*) jagged; ~ая рáна lácerated wound.

рвать I *несов.* (*вн.*) 1. (*выдёргивать*) pull (smth.); (*стаскивать*) pull (smth.) off; (*цветы и т. п.*) pick (smth.); ~ что-л. из чьих-л. рук snatch/grab smth. from smb.; 2. (*на части*) tear* (smth.), rend* (smth.); ~ письмó tear* up a létter; 3. (*порывать связи и т. п.*) break* off (smth.); ~ отношéния с кем-л. break* off relátions with smb.; ◇ ~ зýбы common-л. pull smb.'s teeth; ~ на себé вóлосы tear* one's hair; ~ и метáть storm and rage.

рвать II *несов. безл. разг.*: егó рвёт he is vómiting, he is púking *амер. сленг.*

рвáться *несов.* 1. (*разрываться*) tear*; (*о нитке*) break*; ~ от прикоснóвения tear* at a touch; 2. (*нарушаться — о связях и т. п.*) be* bróken; 3. (*взрываться*) burst*; 4. (*вырываться*) strúggle to get free/loose; 5. (*стремиться*) be* lónging (for); ~ в бой be* éager/thírsting for báttle.

рвач *м. разг.* grábber.

рва́чество *с. разг.* grábbing, the grásping hábit.

рве́ние *с.* zeal.

рвот|а *ж.* vómiting; púke *амер. сленг.* ~ный emétic.

рдеть *несов.* glow.

ре *с. нескл. муз.* re, ray, D.

реабилита́ция *ж.* rehabilitátion.

реабилити́ровать *несов. и сов.* (*вн.*) rehabílitate (*smb.*). ~ся *несов. и сов.* be* rehabílitated.

реаги́ровать *несов.* 1. (на *вн.*) reáct (to); (*проявля́ть своё отношение к чему-л. тж.*) respónd (to); 2. *хим.* reáct (to).

реакти́в *м. хим.* reágent.

реакти́вн|ый 1. *хим.* reáctive; 2. *физиол.* respónsive; 3. *физ.* jet *attr.*; ~ое движение jet propúlsion; ~ дви́гатель jet éngine; ~ самолёт jet(-propélled) áircraft.

реа́ктор *м.* 1. *эл.* reáctor, chóking coil; 2. *хим.* reáction véssel; 3. *физ.* reáctor; а́томный ~ atómic/núclear reáctor.

реакционе́р *м.* reáctionary.

реакцио́нный reáctionary.

реа́кция I *ж.* reáction; bácklash *разг.*; (*отклик*) respónse.

реа́кция II *ж. полит.* reáction; *собир.* (*о людях*) the reáctionaries *pl.*

реализа́ция *ж.* realizátion; (*продажа тж.*) sélling, sale; ~ проду́кции sale/realizátion of próducts.

реали́зм *м.* réalism; крити́ческий ~ *иск.* crítical réalism.

реализова́ть *несов. и сов.* (*вн.*) réalize (*smth.*); (*продавать тж.*) sell* (*smth.*); ~ це́нные бума́ги convért secúrities; ~ иму́щество sell* one's próperty.

реали́ст *м.* réalist. ~и́ческий 1. realístic; 2. (*основанный на принципах реализма*) réalist.

реа́льн|ость *ж.* reálity; объекти́вная ~ вне́шнего ми́ра the objéctive reálity of the extérnal world. ~ый 1. (*действительный*) cóncrete; (*подлинный*) real, génuine, áctual; 2. (*основанный на учёте реальных условий*) realístic; (*осуществимый*) prácticable; ◇ ~ая зарпла́та real wáges *pl.*

реанима́ция *ж. мед.* reanimátion.

ребёнок *м.* child*; грудно́й ~ súckling; báby *разг.*

ребро́ *с.* 1. rib; 2. (*край, кромка*) edge; ◇ поста́вить вопро́с ~м put* the quéstion squárely.

ре́бус *м.* rébus; *перен.* ríddle.

ребя́т|а *мн.* 1. children; 2. *разг.* (*молодые люди, парни*) boys, lads. ~ишки *мн. разг.* kiddies.

ребя́че|ский child's, childish; (*незрелый, детский тж.*) púerile; ~ская вы́ходка childish trick. ~ство *с.* childishness, puerílity.

ребя́читься *несов. разг.* be* childish, act like a child.*

рёв *м.* 1. roar; (*звериный тж.*) béllow; ~ мото́ров roar of éngines; ~ бу́ри roar of the storm; 2. *разг.* (*плач*) howl; подня́ть ~ raise a howl.

рева́нш *м.* revénge; матч-~ *шахм.* retúrn match; взять ~ have* one's revénge.

реванши́ст *м.* revénge-séeker. ~ский revánchist, revénge-séeking.

реве́нь *м. бот.* rhúbarb.

рев|е́ть *несов.* 1. roar; (*о зверях тж.*) béllow; всю ночь ~е́ла бу́ря the storm roared all night; 2. *разг.* (*громко плакать*) howl.

ревизиони́зм *м.* revísionism.

ревизио́нн|ый inspéction *attr.*, áuditing; ~ая коми́ссия áuditing commission.

реви́зия *ж.* 1. (*обследование*) inspéction; (*бухгалтерская*) áuditing; 2. (*пересмотр теории*) revísion, revísing.

ревизова́ть *несов. и сов.* (*вн.*) 1. (*обследовать*)

inspéct (*smth.*); (*бухгалтерские книги*) áudit (*smth.*); 2. (*пересматривать теорию*) revíse (*smth.*).

ревизо́р *м.* inspéctor.

ревмат|и́зм *м.* rhéumatism, rheumátics. ~и́ческий rheumátic.

ревма́: ~ реве́ть *разг.* howl dísmally.

ревни́вый jéalous.

ревнова́ть *несов.* be* jéalous; он ревну́ет жену́ к своему́ дру́гу he is jéalous of his friend.

ре́вностный zéalous.

ре́вность *ж.* jéalousy.

револьве́р *м.* revólver.

революционе́р *м.* revolútionary, revolútionist.

революционизи́ровать *несов. и сов.* (*вн.*) revolútionize (*smb., smth.*).

революцио́нн|о: ~ настро́енный revolútionary-mínded, revolútionary; ~ый revolútionary.

револю́ция *ж.* revolútion; пролета́рская ~ proletárian revolútion.

рега́лия *ж. обыкн. мн. разг.* regália; быть при всех ~х be* in one's full regália.

ре́гби *с. нескл. спорт.* rúgby (fóotball).

регби́ст *м.* rúgby pláyer.

регенерати́вный regénerative.

регенера́ция *ж.* regenerátion; (*резины*) recláiming.

ре́гент *м.* régent. ~ство *с.* régency.

региона́льн|ый régional; ~ое соглаше́ние régional agréement; ~ пакт régional pact.

регистра́т|ор *м.* régistering clerk. ~у́ра *ж.* régistry óffice.

регистра́ция *ж.* registrátion.

регистри́ровать *несов.* (*вн.*) 1. régister (*smb., smth.*); 2. (*брак, рождение и т. п.*) régister (*smth.*); 3. (*отмечать какое-л. явление*) recórd (*smth.*). ~ся *несов.* 1. régister; 2. (*о браке*) régister one's márriage.

регла́мент *м.* tíme-limit; устана́вливать ~ fix a tíme-limit; соблюда́ть ~ obsérve the tíme-limit.

регламента́ция *ж.* regulátion.

регламенти́ровать *несов. и сов.* (*вн.*) régulate (*smth.*).

регре́сс *м.* régress, retrogréssion. ~и́ровать *несов.* retrogréss.

регули́рование *с.* regulátion, adjústment; ~ движе́ния тра́ffic-contròl, hándling of tráffic.

регули́ровать *несов.* (*вн.*) régulate (*smth.*); (*механизм тж.*) adjúst (*smth.*); (*уличное движение*) contról (*smth.*).

регулиро́вщик *м.* adjúster; (*уличного движения*) tráffic-contròller.

регуля́рн|ость *ж.* regulárity. ~ый régular; ~ая а́рмия régular/stándard ármy; ~ые войска́ régular troops.

регуля́тор *м.* régulator, góvernor.

редакти́ров|ать *несов. и сов.* (*сов. тж.* отредакти́ровать) (*вн.*) 1. (*проверять и исправлять текст*) édit (*smth.*); ~ ру́копись édit a mánuscript; 2. *тк. несов.* (*руководить изданием*) édit (*smth.*); газе́ту ~ал изве́стный журнали́ст the páper was édited by a fámous jóurnalist; 3. (*формулировать*) word (*smth.*).

реда́ктор *м.* éditor; гла́вный ~ éditor-in-chief; отве́тственный ~ mánaging éditor. ~ский éditorial.

редакцио́нн|ый editórial; ~ая колле́гия editórial board; ~ая обрабо́тка éditing; ~ая статья́ editórial.

реда́кци|я *ж.* 1. (*редактирование*) éditing; 2. (*руководство изданием*) éditorship; под ~ей кого́-л. édited by *smb.*, únder the éditorship of *smb.*; 3. (*формулировка*) wórding; но́вая ~ резолю́ции new wórding of the resolútion; 4. (*вариант произведения*) vérsion, edítion; но́вая ~ рома́на a new vérsion of a nóvel; 5. (*коллектив работников*) the éditors *pl*; гла́вная ~ chief editórial board; письмо́ в ~ю létter to the éditor; 6. (*помещение*) editórial óffice(s).

реде́ть, пореде́ть thin; (*о лесе, волосах*) get

thinner; (*о тучах и т. п.*) dispérse, drift awáy; (*уменьшаться*) be* depléted, thin out.

реди́с *м.* gárden rádish. **~ка** *ж.* 1. *см.* реди́с; 2. (*отдельный корешок*) rádish.

ре́дк|ий 1. (*нечастый, негустой*) thin, sparse; (*неплотный — о ткани*) gáuzy; lóosely-woven; ~ лес sparse wóodland/fórest; ~ие во́лосы sparse/thínning hair *sg*; ~ие зу́бы widely-spaced teeth; 2. (*происходящий через большие промежутки времени*) rare, infréquent; ~ гость rare guest; ~ие вы́стрелы occásional shots; 3. (*исключительный*) excéptional, rare, unúsual; ~ие спосо́бности excéptional abílities.

ре́дко séldom, rárely; ~ ви́деться séldom meet*, not óften meet*.

ре́дкостный rare, excéptional.

ре́дкость *ж.* 1. (*редкое явление*) rárity; 2. (*редкая вещь*) rárity, curiósity; ◇ на ~ excéptionally, uncómmonly; не ~ it is not unúsual/uncómmon.

редуци́рованный *лингв.* redúced.

рее́стр *м.* schédule.

ре́дьк|а *ж.* (black) rádish; ◇ э́то мне надое́ло ху́же го́рькой ~и I'm sick and tíred of it.

режи́м *м.* 1. (*государственный строй*) regíme; 2. (*распорядок жизни, труда и т. п.*) routíne, régimen; ~ дня dáily tíme-table; ~ пита́ния díet; больни́чный ~ hóspital régimen; 3. (*условия*) regíme, régimen; conditions *pl*; ◇ ~ эконо́мии regíme of ecónomy, ecónomy drive.

режиссёр *м.* diréctor; (*в англ. театре тж.*) prodúcer; помо́щник ~а stáge-manager, assístant prodúcer; (*в кино*) députy diréctor.

режиссу́ра *ж.* 1. (*руководство постановкой спектакля, фильма*) diréction; 2. *собир.* (*руководители*) diréctors *pl*.

ре́жущ|ий cútting; ~ие инструме́нты cútting tools; ~ая боль acúte pain.

ре́зать, разреза́ть, заре́зать, вы́резать, сре́зать 1. *сов.* разреза́ть (*вн.*) cut* (*smth.*); (*ломтями тж.*) slice (*smth.*); ~ пиро́г cut*/slice a pie; ~ мя́со carve meat; ~ мета́лл cut* métal; 2. *тк. несов.* (*об острых предметах*) cut*; нож не ре́жет the knife* won't cut; 3. *сов.* заре́зать (*вн.; убивать*) kill (*smb., smth.*); (*скот*) sláughter (*smth.*); 4. *сов.* вы́резать (*по дт., на пр.*) carve (on), engráve (on); ~ по де́реву cut on/in wood; 5. *тк. несов.* (*причинять боль*) cut*; верёвка ре́жет ру́ку the rope cuts one's hand; 6. *сов.* сре́зать (*вн.*) *спорт.* slice (*smth.*); ~ мяч slice a ball; ◇ ~ глаз offénd the eye; у́хо ре́жет it offénds the ear. ~ся *несов.:* у ребёнка ре́жутся зу́бы the báby is cútting its teeth.

резви́ться *несов.* gámbol, frisk abóut.

ре́зв|ость *ж.* 1. pláyfulness; 2. (*скорость*) speed; показа́ть хоро́шую ~ (*о лошади*) show* a good time. **~ый** 1. pláyful, frísky; 2. (*быстрый в беге*) fast.

резеда́ *ж.* *бот.* mignonétte.

резёрв *м.* resérve.

резерви́ровать *несов. и сов.* (*вн.*) resérve (*smth.*).

резёрвн|ый resérve *attr.*; ~ фонд resérve fund; ~ые войска́ resérves *pl*.

резервуа́р *м.* réservoir; (*бак*) tank.

резе́ц *м.* 1. (*инструмент*) chísel; (*режущая часть*) cútter; 2. (*зуб*) incísor.

резиде́н|т *м.* 1. résident; 2. (*иностранец*) fóreign résident; 3. (*тайный представитель разведки в иностранном государстве*) fixed-post spy. **~ция** *ж.* résidence.

рези́н|а *ж.* rúbber. **~ка** *ж.* 1. (*для стирания*) eráser, rúbber; 2. (*тесёмка*) elástic. **~овый** rúbber *attr.*; *перен.* elástic; ~овая о́бувь rúbber fóotwear.

ре́зка *ж.* cútting.

ре́зк|ий 1. sharp; ~ ве́тер sharp/bíting wind; 2. (*неприятно действующий на органы чувств*): ~ го́лос harsh voice; ~ свет harsh/bright light; ~ за́пах púngent

smell; 3. (*отчётливый*) cléan-cut, sharp; ~ие черты́ лица́ cléan-cut féatures; 4. (*внезапный*) súdden, unexpécted; ~ое похолода́ние súdden/sharp drop in témperature; 5. (*порывистый — о движениях*) quick, energétic; 6. (*грубый, дерзкий*) blunt, abrúpt, sharp; ~ отве́т blunt ánswer; ~ие возраже́ния sharp objéctions.

ре́зк|о shárply, hárshly; (*грубо*) blúntly. **~ость** *ж.* 1. definítion, clárity, shárpness; ~ость кра́сок inténsity of cólour(s); 2. (*грубость*) blúntness, abrúptness; 3. (*грубое слово*) harsh words *pl*; наговори́ть ~остей кому́-л. be* véry sharp/blunt with *smb.*

резно́й carved; (*сквозной*) frétted.

резня́ *ж.* sláughter, cárnage, mássacre.

резолю́ция *ж.* resolútion.

резона́нс *м.* résonance; *перен.* efféct.

резона́тор *м.* *физ., тех.* sóunding-board.

резо́нный *разг.* réasonable.

результа́т *м.* resúlt, óutcome; ◇ в ~е as a resúlt. **~и́вный** efféctive.

ре́зус-фа́ктор *м.* *мед.* Rhésus fáctor.

резчи́к *м.* cárver.

резь *ж.* sharp pain/irritátion; (*в желудке*) cólic; gríping pains *pl*.

резьба́ *ж.* 1. (*вырезывание*) cárving; ~ по де́реву wood-carving; 2. (*рисунок, узор*) cárving; 3. (*нарезка*) thread.

резюм|е́ *с.* *нескл.* súmmary, résumé; **~и́ровать** *несов. и сов.* (*вн.*) sum (*smth.*) up, súmmarize (*smth.*).

рей *м.* *мор.* yard.

рейд I *м.* *мор.* róad(stead).

рейд II *м.* 1. *воен.* raid; 2. (*обследование*) spót-check, swoop.

ре́йка *ж.* 1. lath; 2. (*брусок с делениями*) rod; землеме́рная ~ survéying rod; водоме́рная ~ depth gauge.

рейс *м.* trip, run; flight; *мор. тж.* vóyage; пе́рвый ~ (*нового судна*) máiden trip/vóyage; обра́тный ~ retúrn jóurney/vóyage.

ре́йсовый régular-route; ~ авто́бус lócal/long-distance bus.

рейсфе́дер *м.* rúling-pen, cóntour-pen.

рейсши́на *ж.* T-square.

ре́йтинг *м.* ráting.

рейту́зы *мн.* 1. tights; 2. (*для верховой езды*) clóse-fitting ríding-breeches.

рейхста́г *м.* Réichstag.

рек|а́ *ж.* ríver; вверх (вниз) по ~е́ up (down) the ríver.

ре́квием *м.* réquiem.

реквизи́ровать *несов. и сов.* (*вн.*) requisítion (*smth.*); (*для военных целей тж.*) commandéer (*smth.*).

реквизи́т *м.* *театр.* próperties *pl*; props *pl разг.*

реквизи́тор *м.* próperty-man.

реквизи́ция *ж.* requisítioning; (*в военное время тж.*) commandéering.

рекла́ма *ж.* advértisement; (*мероприятие тж.*) publícity; светова́я ~ eléctric sign; театра́льная ~ théatre bill.

реклами́ровать *несов. и сов.* (*вн.*) ádvertise (*smth.*); (*чрезмерно расхваливать тж.*) boost (*smb., smth.*), play up (*smth.*).

рекла́мный ádvertising; publícity *attr.*

рекогносци́р|овать *несов. и сов.* (*вн.*) *воен.* reconnóitre (*smth.*). **~о́вка** *ж.* *воен.* recónnaissance.

рекоменда́|тельный: ~тельное письмо́ létter of recommendátion; credéntials *pl*. **~ция** *ж.* recommendátion.

рекоменд|ова́ть *несов. и сов.* (*вн. тж.* прекомендова́ть) recomménd (*smb., smth.*). **~ова́ться** *несов.:* ~у́ется... it is advísable...; не ~у́ется it is not recomménded.

реконструи́ровать *несов. и сов.* (*вн.*) reconstrúct (*smth.*); (*воссоздавать что-л. по сохранившимся опи-*

саниям и т. п. тж.) restóre (*smth.*). ~ся *несов. и сов.* be* reconstrúcted.

реконстру́кция *ж.* reconstrúction; (*воссоздание по сохранившимся описаниям тж.*) restorátion.

реко́рд *м.* récord; поста́вить ~ make* a récord, set* up a récord.

рекорди́ст *м., ~ка ж.* 1. chámpion; (*животное тж.*) prize-winner; 2. (*тот, кто увлекается рекордами*) pót-hunter.

реко́рдный récord *attr.*; в ~ срок in récord time.

рекордсме́н *м., ~ка ж.* récord-holder, chámpion.

ре́ктор *м.* réctor; ~ университе́та réctor, head of a univérsity.

ректора́т *м.* univérsity administrátion; (*помещение*) réctor's óffice.

реле́ *с. нескл. эл.* rélay.

религио́зный relígious.

рели́гия *ж.* relígion.

рели́квия *ж.* rélic.

релье́ф *м.* relief. ~но vívidly; cléarly; ~но выделя́ться stand* out in relief. ~ный raised, embóssed; *перен.* vívid, stríking.

рельс *м.* rail; сходи́ть с ~ов be* deráiled; ◇ поста́вить *что-л.* на ~ы get* smth. stárted. ~овый rail *attr.*; ~овый путь track.

рема́рка *ж.* note; *meamp.* stáge-direction.

ремённый léather *attr.*; ~ привод bélt-drive.

реме́нь *м.* 1. strap; (*пояс*) belt; 2. *mex.* belt.

реме́сленник *м.* 1. cráftsman*; 2. (*тот, кто работает по шаблону*) drudge, dábbler; (*о писателе*) háck-writer.

реме́сленн|ый 1. craft *attr.*; ~ое произво́дство craft índustry; 2. (*примитивный, неискусный*) bótched-up; 3. (*шаблонный*) sóulless, uncreátive, stándardized; (*о литературной работе тж.*) hack *attr.*

ремесло́ *с.* craft; (*профессия*) trade; сапо́жное ~ shóemaking; пло́тничное ~ cárpentry.

ремо́нт *м.* repáirs *pl*; (*побелка, окраска дома, квартиры*) décorating; decorátions *pl*; находи́ться в ~е be* únder repáir. ~и́ровать, отремонти́ровать (*вн.*) repáir (*smth.*); (*белить, красить дом, квартиру*) décorate (*smth.*). ~ный repáir *attr.*; ~ная мастерска́я repáir shop.

ренега́т *м.* rénegade, túrncoat. ~ство *с.* deféction, apóstasy.

ре́нта *ж. эк.* rent; земе́льная ~ gróund-rent.

рента́бель|ость *ж.* prófitableness. ~ый páying; ~ое хозя́йство góing concérn.

рентге́н *м.* 1. (*просвечивание*) X-ray photógraphy; 2. *физ.* Röntgen.

рентге́нов: ~ы лучи́ X-rays.

рентге́новский X-ray; ~ кабине́т X-ray room; ~ сни́мок rádiograph, X-ray phótograph.

рентгено́лог *м.* radiólogist.

рентгеноскопи́я *ж.* radióscopy, X-ray examinátion.

реоргани́з|а́ция *ж.* reorganizátion. ~ова́ть *несов. и сов.* (*вн.*) reórganize (*smth.*). ~ова́ться *несов. и сов.* reórganize.

реоста́т *м.* rhéostat.

ре́па *ж.* túrnip.

репара́ции *мн.* (*ед. репара́ция ж.*) reparátions.

репарацио́нн|ый reparátion *attr.*; ~ые платежи́ reparátion páyments.

репатри|а́нт *м.* repátriate. ~а́ция *ж.* repatriátion.

репатрии́ровать *несов. и сов.* (*вн.*) repátriate (*smb.*). ~ся *несов. и сов.* be* repátriated.

репе́й *м.*, ~ник *м.* agrímony, búrdock.

репертуа́р *м.* répertoire.

репети́|ровать, прорепети́ровать (*вн.*) 1. (*выступление*) rehéarse (*smth.*); 2. (*ученика*) coach (*smb.*). ~ция *ж.* rehéarsal; генера́льная ~ция dress rehéarsal.

ре́плика *ж.* 1. remárk, replý; (*возражение*) retórt; 2. *meamp.* cue.

репорта́ж *м.* repórting; (*сообщение*) repórt; (*во время игры*) cómmentary.

репортёр *м.* repórter.

репресс|и́вный représsive. ~и́ровать *несов. и сов.* (*вн.*) take* représsive áction (agáinst).

репре́ссия *ж.* représsion.

репроду́ктор *м.* lóudspéaker.

репроду́кция *ж.* reprodúction.

репти́лия *ж. зоол.* réptile.

репута́ция *ж.* reputátion; незапя́тнанная ~ spótless reputátion.

ре́пчатый: ~ лук ónion.

ресни́цы *мн.* (*ед. ресни́ца ж.*) éyelashes.

респира́тор *м.* réspirator, gás-mask.

респу́блика *ж.* repúblic; наро́дная демократи́ческая ~ Péople's Democrátic Repúblic; буржуа́зная ~ bóurgeois repúblic.

республика́н|ец *м.* repúblican. ~ский repúblican.

рессо́р|а *ж.* spring. ~ный sprung, spring-suppórted.

реставра́тор *м.* restórer; ~ ста́рых карти́н restórer of old pictures.

реставра́ция *ж.* restorátion.

реставри́ровать *несов. и сов.* (*вн.*) restóre (*smth.*).

рестора́н *м.* réstaurant. ~ный réstaurant *attr.*

ресу́рсы *мн.* resóurces.

рети́вый zéalous, árdent; (*резвый*) spríghtly.

рето́рта *ж.* retórt.

ретрансли́ровать *несов. и сов.* (*вн.*) *радио* retransmít (*smth.*).

ретрансля́ция *ж. радио* retransmíssion.

ретроспекти́ва *ж.* 1. retrospéctive review; 2. *кино* retrospéctive show.

ретушёр *м.* retóucher.

ретуши́ровать *несов. и сов.* (*вн.*) retóuch (*smth.*).

ре́тушь *ж.* retóuching.

рефера́т *м.* 1. súmmary, synópsis (*pl* -ses); 2. (*доклад*) páper, éssay.

рефере́ндум *м.* referéndum.

рефере́нт *м.* advíser, éxpert.

рефле́кс *м.* réflex; коле́нные ~ы knée-jerks; pátellar réflexes *научн.*; усло́вный ~ conditioned réflex.

рефле́ктор *м.* 1. (*отражатель лучей*) refléctor; 2. (*обогревательный прибор*) bówl-fire, eléctric fire with a refléctor.

рефо́рма *ж.* refórm.

реформа́тор *м.* refórmer.

реформа́ция *ж. ист.* the Reformátion.

реформи́зм *м.* refórmism.

реформи́ровать *несов. и сов.* (*вн.*) refórm (*smth.*).

реформи́ст *м.* refórmist.

рефрижера́тор *м.* 1. refrígerator; 2. (*часть холоди́льной машины*) eváporator. ~ный refrígerator *attr.*; ~ное су́дно refrígerator (ship).

рецензе́нт *м.* (*книг*) revíewer; (*рукописей*) réader. ~и́ровать, прорецензи́ровать (*вн.*) (*книги*) revíew (*smth.*); (*рукописи*) read* (*smth.*).

реце́нзия *ж.* review; (*на рукопись*) opínion.

реце́пт *м.* prescríption; (*способ приготовления чего-л.*) récipe; *перен. тж.* fórmula (*pl* -ae); гото́вый ~ réady-máde fórmula; cút-and-dríed instrúctions *pl.*

рециди́в *м.* 1. sét-back, recúrrence; 2. *мед.* relápse; 3. *юр.* recidivátion, sécond offence; bácksliding *разг.*

рецидиви́ст *м.* recidivist, old offénder, repéater.

рече|во́й speech *attr.*; ~ые на́выки speech hábits.

рече́ние *с.* expréssion.

речи́стый *разг.* vóluble; (*говорливый*) tálkative.

речитати́в *м. муз.* recitative; ◇ говори́ть, чита́ть ~ом chant.

ре́чка *ж.* small ríver, stream.

речни́к *м.* ríver-tránsport wórker.

речн|о́й ríver *attr.*; (*о живущих в реках тж.*) flúvial

научн.; ~бе су́дно ríver-boat; ~бе сообще́ние ríver navigátion; ~ые расте́ния flúvial plants.

реч|ь ж. 1. (*способность говорить*) speech; о́рганы ~и órgans of speech; разви́тие ~и speech tráining; 2. (*язык*) speech; у́стная ~ óral speech; ру́сская ~ Rússian speech, spóken Rússian; 3. (*произношение*) speech, way of spéaking; о́кающая ~ mánner of stréssing the o's in *one's* speech; 4. *разг.* (*беседа, разговор*) talk; ~ идёт о том, чтобы... it is a quéstion/mátter of...; слу́чай, о кото́ром идёт ~ the case in quéstion; о чём ~? what are you tálking abóut?; об э́том и ~и не́ было it was not éven méntioned; об э́том ~ that's not what we are tálking abóut; об э́том не мо́жет быть и ~и that is out of the quéstion; завести́ ~ о чём-л. begin* to speak of *smth.*; пусты́е ~и émpty talk *sg*; 5. (*выступление*) speech; обличи́тельная ~ denunciátion; вы́ступить с ~ью, произнести́ ~ make*/delíver a speech; обрати́ться с ~ью к кому-л. address *smb.*

реш|а́ть, **реши́ть** 1. (+ *инф.*; *приходить к какому-л. выводу*) decíde (+ to *inf*), make* up *one's* mind (+ to *inf*), resólve (+ to *inf*); он реши́л оста́ться до́ма he decíded to stay at home; вы са́ми должны́ ~ it is for you to decíde; 2. (*вн.,* + *инф.*; *принимать решение*) decíde (*smth.,* + to *inf*); реши́ть де́ло в чью-л. по́льзу decíde (the mátter) in *smb.'s* fávour; они́ реши́ли перевы́полнить план they decíded to overfulfíl the plan; 3. (*вн.*; *определять искомое*) solve (*smth.*); work out (*smth.*); ~ зада́чи, приме́ры solve próblems, exámples; ~ кроссво́рд do* a cróssword púzzle; 4. (*вн.*; *выполнять*) solve (*smth.*); *несов. тж.* táckle (*smth.*), work on (*smth.*); реши́ть пробле́му solve a próblem; ◇ реши́ть чью-л. судьбу́, у́часть decíde *smb.'s* fate/fúture; реши́ть судьбу́, у́часть чего-л. decíde the fate of *smth.*; ~а́ться, реши́ться 1. (*на вн.,* + *инф.;* *принимать решение*) decíde (on, + to *inf*), make* up *one's* mind (+ to *inf*); реши́ться на отча́янный посту́пок decíde on a désperate course of áction; реши́ться на тако́й шаг make* up *one's* mind to (take) such a step; не реши́ться на кра́йние ме́ры hésitate to take extréme méasures; не могу́ реши́ться на э́то I can't bring mysélf to do it; не ~а́юсь сказа́ть кому-л. I can't bring mysélf to tell *smb.*; ~а́йтесь! make up your mind!; 2. (*определяться*) be* decíded; за́втра реши́тся его́ де́ло his case will be decíded tomórrow; 3. *тк. несов.* come* out, be* solved; зада́ча легко́ ~а́ется the próblem is éasily solved; зада́ча не ~а́ется the próblem won't come out.

реша́ющ|ий decísive; ~ая си́ла decísive force; ~ моме́нт decísive/crúcial móment; ◇ с ~им го́лосом with the right to vote (*at a congress, conference, etc.*).

реше́ние с. 1. decísion; (*постановление тж.*) resolútion; (*суда*) vérdict, júdg(e)ment; принима́ть ~ come* to a decísion, arríve at a decísion, make*/reach a decísion; выноси́ть ~ pronóunce júdg(e)ment, pronóunce its vérdict; 2. (*ответ к задаче и т. п.*) solútion (of), ánswer (to).

реше́тк|а ж. (*в стене*) grille; (*ограда тж.*) ráilings *pl*; (*деревянная*) láttice, tréllis; (*на окне*) bars *pl*; ◇ посади́ть, упря́тать кого-л. за ~у put* *smb.* behínd bars.

реше́т|о с. sieve; ◇ чудеса́ в ~é a fantástic tale.

решётчатый, **решётчаты|й** láttice *attr*.

реши́мость ж. determinátion, resolútion, resólve.

реши́тельн|о 1. (*смело*) resólutely; (*категорически*) categórically/flátly; ~ отрица́ть что-л. categórically dený *smth.*; быть ~ про́тив чего-л. be* útterly oppósed to *smth.*; 2. (*совершенно*) ábsolutely; ~ ничего́ не де́лать, не знать и т. д. do*, know* ábsolutely nothing. **~ость** ж. 1. (*смелость в принятии решений*) determinátion, resolútion; 2. (*категоричность*) decísiveness, finálity. **~ый** 1. (*смелый, энергичный*) resólute, decíded, detérmined; ~ый челове́к resólute/detérmined pérson; ~ые ме́ры resólute méasures; 2. (*решающий, категори-*

ческий) decísive; (*окончательный*) fínal, últimate; ~ый отве́т fínal replý; ~ый тон résolute tone; с са́мым ~ым ви́дом with an expréssion of the útmost determinátion; с ~ым наме́рением уе́хать with *one's* mind fírmly made up to leave; ~ый бой decísive báttle/áction.

реши́ть *сов. см.* реша́ть. **~ся** *сов. см.* реша́ться 1, 2.

реэвакуа́ция ж. retúrn from evacuátion.

реэ́кспорт м. re-éxport.

ре́я ж. *см.* рей.

ре́ять *несов.* 1. (*плавно двигаться*) glide alóng, drift alóng; 2. (*парить*) hóver; 3. (*развеваться*) stream, fly*.

ржа́в|еть, заржа́веть rust, be* rústy. **~чина** ж. rust; цве́та ~чины rúst-coloured. **~ый** rústy.

ржан|о́й rye *attr.*; ~ ко́лос ear of rye; ~а́я мука́ rye flour; ~ хлеб rye bread.

ржать *несов.* neigh, whínny.

рибонуклеи́нов|ый: ~ая кислота́ (РНК) ribonúcleic ácid, RNA.

ри́га ж. thréshing barn/floor.

ри́за ж. 1. chásuble; (*царское одеяние*) robes *pl*; véstments *pl*; 2. (*накладка на иконе*) ríza, métal móunting.

рикоше́т м. rícochet. ~ом: пу́ля попа́ла в него́ ~ом the bùllet hit him on the rebóund.

ри́мск|ий Róman; ◇ ~ нос Róman nose; ~ое пра́во *юр.* Róman law; ~ая це́рковь Róman Church; ~ие ци́фры Róman númerals.

ринг м. *спорт.* ring.

ри́нуться *сов.* dash, hurl onesélf, charge; ~ в ата́ку hurl onesélf ínto the attáck.

рис м. rice.

риск м. 1. risk, házard; с ~ом для жи́зни at the risk of *one's* life; идти́ на ~ risk it, take* a chance; подве́ргать ~у кого-л. endánger *smb.*, jéopardize *smb.*; гру́ппа ~а risk group; 2. (*действие наудачу*) táking risks/chánces; ◇ ~ — благоро́дное де́ло ≈ nóthing vénture, nóthing have; на свой страх и ~ at *one's* own risk.

рискн|у́ть *сов.* 1. *см.* рискова́ть; 2. (+ *инф.*, на *вн.*; *отважиться*) vénture (+ to *inf*, *smth.*); он ~ул спроси́ть её об э́том he véntured to ask her abóut it.

риско́ванный rísky; ~ шаг rísky step.

рискова́ть, рискну́ть 1. (*подвергаться риску*) take* a risk/chance; лу́чше не ~ bétter not risk it; не хоте́ть ~ be* unwílling to take risks; 2. (*тв.*) risk (*smb., smth.*); jéopardize (*smb., smth.*); ~ жи́знью, голово́й risk *one's* life, neck; ~ здоро́вьем, репута́цией jéopardize *one's* health, reputátion.

рисова́|льщик м. gráphic ártist. ~ние с. dráwing; учи́ться ~нию learn* how to draw.

рисова́ть, нарисова́ть (*вн.*) draw* (*smth.*); (*красками*) paint (*smth.*); *перен.* portráy (*smth.*), depíct (*smth.*); ~ карандашо́м, перо́м draw* in péncil, in ink; ~ с нату́ры draw*/paint from life; ~ портре́т draw*/paint a pórtrait. **~ся** *несов.* 1. (*виднеться*) be* óutlined/silhoué́tted; 2. (*дт.; представляться*) présent itsélf (to); 3. (*тв.; стараться показать себя с выгодной стороны*) show* off (*smth.*).

рисо́вка ж. shówing-off.

ри́сов|ый rice *attr.*; ~ое по́ле rice field; ~ая ка́ша (thin) rice púdding.

рису́н|ок м. dráwing; (*очертание*) óutline; (*узор*) design, páttern; ~ карандашо́м péncil-drawing; ~ перо́м pén-and-ink dráwing; по ~кам кого-л. áfter the designs of *smb.*

ритм м. rhýthm.

ри́тмика ж. 1. (*система и характер ритма*) rhýthms *pl*, rhýthmical páttern; 2. (*учение о ритме*) rhýthmics, théory of rhýthm; 3. (*система физических упражнений*) eurhýthmics.

ритми́ч|еский rhýthmical. **~ность** ж. rhýthm. **~ный** rhýthmical.

рито́р|ика ж. rhétoric. **~и́ческий** rhetórical; ◇ **~и́ческий вопро́с** rhetórical quéstion.

ритуа́л м. rítual.

риф I м. (*подводная скала*) reef.

риф II м. *мор.* reef; **брать ~ы** take* in reefs.

рифлёный (*о железе*) córrugated.

ри́фма ж. rhyme; **мужска́я, же́нская ~** másculine, féminine rhyme.

рифмова́ть *несов.* (*вн.*) rhyme (*smth.*). **~ся** *несов.* rhyme.

рифмоплёт м. *разг.* rhýmer, rhýmester.

ро́ба ж. óveralls *pl.*

робе́ть *несов.* be* tímid; (*перед тв.*) quail (before); **не робе́й(те)!** don't be shy!; don't be scared!

ро́бк|ий tímid; (*застенчивый*) shy; **~ челове́к** shy/tímid pérson; ◇ **он не ~ого деся́тка** he has plénty of pluck, he's not éasily scared.

ро́бост|ь ж. timídity; (*застенчивость*) shýness; **от ~и он не мог говори́ть** he was too shy to speak.

ро́бот м. róbot.

ров м. ditch, dyke; (*крепостной*) moat.

рове́сн|ик м., **~ица** ж. contémporary; **они́ ~ики** they are the same age; **он мне ~** he's my age.

ро́вн|о *нареч.* 1. (*равномерно*) évenly, régularly; (*одинаково*) équally; **би́ться ~** (*о сердце*) beat* évenly; **~ дыша́ть** breathe régularly/stéadily; 2. (*гладко*) smóothly; 3. *в знач. частицы* (*точно*) exáctly, precísely; **~ в два, три** *и т. д.* **часа́** at two, three, *etc.* sharp; **~ де́сять рубле́й** exáctly ten róubles; 4. *в знач. частицы разг.* (*совершенно*): **он ~ ничего́ не понима́ет** he dóesn't understánd a thing; **это ~ ничего́ не зна́чит** that means nóthing whatéver. **~ый** 1. (*гладкий*) éven, lével, smooth; **~ая доро́га** lével/smooth road; 2. (*прямой*) straight; **~ая ли́ния** straight line; 3. (*одинаковый*) équal, éven; (*равномерный*) régular; **~ый зага́р** éven tan; **~ый кли́мат** équable clímate; **~ый го́лос** lével tones *pl*; **~ым ша́гом** with méasured tread; 4. (*уравновешенный*) équable, éven; **~ый хара́ктер** éven disposítion, équable témper; ◇ **~ый счёт** round fígures *pl*; **для ~ого счёта** to make a round sum; **~ым счётом ничего́!** nóthing whatéver!; **не ро́вен, не ровён час** you néver know.

ровня́ м. *и* ж. *разг.* équal; **он ей не ~** he's not good enóugh for her.

ровня́ть, сровня́ть (*вн.*) make* (*smth.*) éven, lével (*smth.*) off; **~ что-л. катко́м** roll *smth.* smooth.

рог м. 1. horn; (*олений*) ántler; 2. (*музыкальный инструмент*) horn; ◇ **брать быка́ за ~а́** take* the bull by the horns.

рога́тк|а ж. 1. (*на дороге*) bárrier; *воен.* knífe-rest; *перен.* (*препятствие*) óbstacle; 2. (*метательная*) cátapult; **стреля́ть из ~и** shoot* *one's* cátapult.

рога́тый horned; **кру́пный ~ скот** cáttle; **ме́лкий ~ скот** goats and sheep.

рогови́ца ж. *анат.* córnea.

рогов|о́й horn *attr.*; **~ые очки́** hórn-rimmed spéctacles.

рого́жа ж. mátting.

род м. 1. (*семейный*) fámily, kin; 2. (*происхождение, рождение*) birth, órigin, stock; (*поколение*) generátion; **ста́рого ~а** of a old stock; **из ~а в ~** from one generátion to anóther; 3. (*сорт, вид*) sort, kind; 4. *биол.* génus; 5. *грам.* génder; **мужско́й, же́нский, сре́дний ~** másculine, féminine, néuter (génder); **существи́тельное мужско́го ~а** a másculine noun; ◇ **~ челове́ческий** mankínd, humánity, the húman race; **ему́ 30 лет от ~у** he is thírty years of age; **двадцати́ лет от ~у** at the age of twénty; **ему́ на ~у́ напи́сано** he was déstined (to); **без ~у, без пле́мени** withóut kith or kin; **~ войск** arm of the sérvice; **вся́кого ~а** all sorts/kind (of); **что-нибудь в**

э́том ~е sómething of the sort/kind; **в своём ~е** in *one's* way; **своего́ ~а**, в не́котором ~е a sort/kind (of).

роди́льн|ица ж. wóman* who has just had a báby. **~ый: ~ый дом** matérnity hóspital.

роди́м|ый *прил. см.* родно́й 1; ◇ **~ое пятно́** birth-mark.

ро́дин|а ж. 1. nátive land, mótherland, móther cóuntry, hómeland; (*место рождения*) birth-place; **любо́вь к ~е** love of cóuntry; 2. (*место происхождения растения, животного*) land, home.

роди́нка ж. birth-mark, mole.

роди́тели *мн.* párents.

роди́тельный: ~ паде́ж *грам.* génitive case.

роди́тельск|ий párents', paréntal; **~ комите́т** párents' commítee; **~ое собра́ние** párents' méeting; **~ дом** *one's* párents' home/house.

род|и́ть *несов. и сов.* 1. (*вн.*) give* birth (to); *перен. тж.* give* rise (to); **~ сы́на, дочь** bear* a son, a dáughter; **она́ то́лько что ~и́ла** she has just gíven birth; **она́ ещё не ~и́ла** the báby hásn't been born yet; 2. *разг.* (*давать урожай*) yield; **~ в чём мать ~и́ла** stárk-náked. **~и́ться** *несов. и сов.* 1. be* born; *перен.* (*возникать*) aríse*, spring* up; **~и́ться слепы́м** be* born blind; **у него́ ~и́лся сын** his wife has just had a báby-boy; **у меня́ ~и́лась мысль** (+ *инф.*) I had the idéa (of + -*ing*); **~и́лось подозре́ние** a suspícion aróuse; 2. (*произрастать*) grow*.

родни́к м. spring. **~о́вый** spring *attr.*

род|ни́ть, **породни́ть** (*вн.*) 1. *сов.* породни́ть uníte (*smb.*); 2. *сов.* сродни́ть draw* (*smb.*) togéther, creáte a bond/affínity (betwéen); 3. *тк. несов.* (*сближать*) make* (*smb.*) alíke. **~ся, породни́ться** (*с тв.*) 1. mix (with), intermíngle (with), becóme* related (to); 2. *тк. несов.* (*сближаться*) becóme* akín (with), grow*/draw* togéther.

родн|о́й *прил.* 1. (*по крови*) *one's* own; (*не приёмный, не двоюродный*) *one's* real; (*являющийся родственником*) of *one's* own fámily/blood *после сущ.*; **~а́я сестра́** *one's* own síster; **~ челове́к** pérson of *one's* own fámily; 2. (*о месте*) nátive; **~ дом** *one's* nátive/own home; **~ го́род** *one's* home town; 3. (*дорогой, близкий сердцу*) dear, dárling; 4. *в знач. сущ. мн.* *one's* rélatives/relátions; (*домашние*) *one's* péople; ◇ **~ язы́к** nátive lánguage, móther-tongue.

родня́ ж. 1. *собир.* (*родственники*) rélatives *pl*, relátions *pl*; 2. *разг.* (*родственник*) rélative, relátion; **он мне ~** we are reláted.

родов|о́й I 1. fámily *attr.*; **~ строй** tríbal sýstem; **~а́я месть** vendétta, blóodfeud; 2. *биол.* genéric; 3. *грам.* génder *attr.*; **~ые оконча́ния** génder infléctions.

родов|о́й II birth *attr.*; **~ые му́ки** birth-pains.

ро́дом by birth; **он ~ из Москвы́, с Кавка́за** he comes from Móscow, from the Cáucasus.

родонача́льник м. progénitor, stock; *перен.* fóunder, fáther.

родосло́вная ж. pédigree.

родстве́нни|к м., **~ца** ж. rélative, relátion; **ближа́йшие ~ки** close rélatives.

родстве́нн|ый 1. fámily *attr.*; of the fámily *после сущ.*; **~ые свя́зи** fámily ties; 2. (*тёплый, сердечный*) córdial; 3. (*сходный*) kíndred, akín *predic.*; **~ые нау́ки** reláted/állied sciences; **~ые языки́** reláted lánguages.

родств|о́ *с.* 1. relátionship; **быть в ~е́ с кем-л.** be* reláted to *smb.*; 2. *собир. разг.* (*родственники*) fámily; rélatives *pl*; 3. (*сходство*) affínity.

род|ы́ *мн.* (child)birth *sg*, háving a child *sg*; confínement *sg*; **у неё бы́ли тяжёлые ~** she had a dífficult confínement; **она́ о́чень похоро́шела по́сле ~ов** she looks wónderful since she had her child.

ро́ж|а I ж. *разг.* face; **ну и ~!** what a mug! ◇ **ко́рчить ~и кому́-л.** pull/make* fáces at *smb.*

рожа II ж. (болезнь) erysípelas, Rose, St. Ánthony's fire.

рожáть несов. разг. have* a báby, give* birth.

рождáемость ж. birth-rate.

рожд|áть несов. (вн.) give* birth (to); bear* (smb.); перен. give* rise (to). **~áться** несов. be* born; перен. aríse*; spring* up. **~éние** с. birth; с сáмого моегó **~éния** éver since I was born; от **~éния** from birth; день **~éния** birthday; мéсто **~éния** bírthplace; дáта **~éния** dáte of birth; ◇ по **~éнию** by birth.

рождéственский Chrístmas attr., Xmas attr.

Рождествó с. Chrístmas, Xmas.

рожéница ж. (женщина в период родов) wóman* in childbirth; (родившая) néwly-máde móther.

рожóк м. 1. (музыкальный инструмент) horn; англúйский **~** ténor óboe, cor angláis; 2. (детский) féeding-bottle; 3. (для обуви) shóe-horn.

рожь ж. rye.

рóз|а ж. rose; ◇ **~** ветрóв метеор. wind-rose. **~ан** м. разг. rose. **~áрий** м. róse-garden, rosárium.

рóзга ж. rod, birch.

розéтка ж. 1. (украшение) rosétte; 2. (блюдце для варенья) small jam dish; 3. эл.: штéпсельная **~** plug (receptácle).

розмарúн м. бот. rósemary.

рóзни|ца ж. rétail goods; ◇ продавáть в **~цу** sell* rétail. **~чный** rétail attr.; **~чная** торгóвля rétail trade; **~чные** цéны rétail príces.

рознь ж. 1. (вражда) díscord; 2. в знач. сказ. (дт.): человéк человéку **~** all men are not alíke.

розовéть, **порозовéть** 1. (становиться розовым) turn pink; (покрываться румянцем) blush pink, blush; 2. тк. несов. (виднеться) show* pink.

розовощёкий pínk-cheeked, rósy-cheeked.

рóзов|ый 1. (о растении) rose attr.; **~** куст róse--bush; **~ое** мáсло áttar of róses; 2. (розового цвета) pink; перен. rósy; **~ая** лéнточка pink ríbbon; **~ые** щёки rósy/pink cheeks; **~** свет rósy light; **~ые** мечты́ róse--coloured dreams; ◇ вúдеть всё в **~ом** свéте, смотрéть на всё сквозь **~ые** очкú see* éverything through róse--coloured spéctacles.

рóзыгрыш м. 1. (лотереи) dráwing; draw; 2. (состязание) tóurnament, mátch(es) (for); **~** Кýбка Россúи по футбóлу the Rússian Fóotball Cup competítion.

рóзыск м. 1. search, quest; 2. юр. investigátion, search; ◇ уголóвный **~** críminal investigátion depártment.

роúться несов. swarm; перен. crowd; мы́сли роя́тся в головé thoughts crowd ínto one's mind.

рой м. swarm; перен. host; **~** воспоминáний host of recolléctions.

рок м. fate.

роков|óй fátal; **~ая** ошúбка fátal mistáke.

рóкот м. múrmuring; (раскатистый шум) rúmble, roar; **~** волн roar of the waves.

рокотáть несов. múrmur; (раскатисто) roar, crash; (о голосе) rúmble, boom.

рóлик м. 1. róller; (у мебели) cástor; 2. (для электропроводки) block. **~овый** róller attr.; **~овый** подшúпник róller béaring; **~овые** конькú róller skates; **~овая** доскá skáteboard.

рол|ь ж. 1. (драматический образ) role, part; в **~и** Гáмлета вы́ступил... the part of Hámlet was táken/ácted by...; игрáть **~** отцá play the (part of the) fáther; 2. (текст) part; lines pl; забы́ть свою́ **~** forget* one's lines/words; 3. (рд.; работа в качестве кого-л.) job, role; вам придётся взять на себя́ **~** перевóдчика you will have to take on the job of intérpreter; 4. (мера влияния, значения) role; **~** лúчности в истóрии the role of the indivídual in hístory; **~** вы́ступила в **~и** act as, play the part of; игрáть **~** 1) (иметь значение) play a part; be* of impórtance, count; 2) (рд.; быть кем-л., чем-л.) be*; э́то обстоя́тельство не игрáет большóй **~и**

this círcumstance hásn't much signíficance; войтú в **~** get* ínto the way of things, begín* to cope.

ром м. rum.

ромáн м. 1. (произведение) nóvel; (героического жанра) románce; 2. разг. (любовные отношения) (lóve-)affair; ◇ он герóй не моегó **~а** he's by no means my idéal.

романúст I м. (писатель) nóvelist.

романúст II м. (филолог) spécialist in Románce philólogy. **~ика** ж. Románce philólogy.

ромáнс м. song; (название инструментальной пьесы) románce.

ромáнск|ий Románce, Románic; **~ие** языкú Románce lánguages.

романтúзм м. románticism.

романтик м. romántic.

романтика ж. románticism; (чего-л. тж.) the romántic side (of).

романт|úческий, **~úчный** romántic.

ромáшка ж. бот. óx-eye dáisy; (аптечная) cámomile.

ромб м. rhomb; в вúде **~а** díamond-sháped, rhómbic.

ромштéкс м. кул. rump steak.

роня́ть, **уронúть** (вн.) 1. (нечаянно выпускать из рук) drop (smth.); let* (smth.) fall; (сталкивать) knock (smth.) off; **~** вéщи из рук drop things; кнúги со столá knock books off a táble; 2. тк. несов. (терять) shed* (smth.), lose* (smth.); **~** лúстья shed* its leaves; **~** пéрья moult, shed* its féathers; 3. (бессильно опускать вниз) drop (smth.), let* (smth.); **~** гóлову на грудь let one's head fall on one's chest; 4. (небрежно произносить) let* fall (smth.); **~** замечáние let* fall a remárk; 5. (унижать, умалять) lówer (smb., smth.); **~** своё достóинство lówer one's dígnity; **~** себя́ в чьих-л. глазáх lówer onesélf in smb.'s eyes/estimátion; ◇ **~** слёзы shed* tears.

рóпот м. múrmur, múrmur of discontént; **~** ручья́ múrmur of a stream.

роптáть несов. (на вн.) múrmur (against), grúmble (at).

рос|á ж. dew. **~úнка** ж. déw-drop; ◇ у меня́ мáковой **~úнки** во рту не́ бы́ло ≈ I háven't had a bite all day. **~úстый** déwy, dew-sprinkled.

роскóшный 1. (отличающийся роскошью) magníficent, luxúrious; 2. разг. (очень хороший) spléndid; 3. разг. (пышно растущий) luxúriant, lush.

рóскошь ж. 1. (внешнее великолепие) magnífícence, spléndour; 2. (излишество в жизненных удобствах) lúxury; 3. (изобилие — о растительности) luxúriance, lúshness.

рóслый tall, well-grówn; **~** пáрень strápping/búrly féllow.

рóспись ж. 1. (действие) páinting; **~** потолкá céiling páinting; 2. (стенная живопись) múrals pl, fréscoes pl.

рóспуск м. (учеников) dismíssal; (армии, организации и т. п.) disbándment; (парламента) dissolútion.

россúйский Rússian.

рóссказни мн. разг. tales.

рóссыпь ж. (золота, алмазов и т. п.) depósit.

рост м. 1. growth; (увеличение) íncrease, rise; (площади) exténsion; (совершенствование) devélopment; **~** населéния growth of populátion; **~** материáльного благосостоя́ния íncrease in matérial well-béing; твóрческий **~** артúста ártist's devélopment; 2. (вышина) height; (человека тж.) státure; быть **~ом с кого-л.** be* smb.'s height; высóкого **~а** tall; срéднего **~а** of middle height; мáленького **~а** short; в **~** человéка as high as a man; ◇ шить, покупáть на **~** allów for growth when máking, búying; по **~у** accórding to height; отдавáть дéньги в **~** lend* móney on ínterest; во весь **~** 1) (выпрямившись) stánding up straight; 2) (на фотографии) full length; встать во весь **~** stand* up, draw* onesélf up to one's full height.

ро́стбиф м. кул. roast beef.

ростовщи́|к м. úsurer, móney-lender. ~ческий usúrious. ~чество с. úsury.

рост|о́к м. sprout; shoot (тж. перен.); пуска́ть ~ки́ sprout.

ро́счерк м. flóurish; ◇ одни́м ~ом пера́ with a stroke of the pen.

рот м. mouth; во рту́ бы́ло су́хо one's mouth felt dry; ~ до уше́й an enórmous mouth; с откры́тым ртом open-móuthed; с рази́нутым ртом, рази́нув ~ agápe, open-móuthed; зева́ть во весь ~ yawn cávernously; ◇ не брать в ~ чего-л. néver touch smth.; в ~ не возьмёшь it's uneátable; еда́ в ~ нейдёт the food sticks in my throat; не сметь рта откры́ть not dare to ópen one's mouth; разжева́ть и в ~ положи́ть spell* smth. out for smb.; хлопо́т по́лон ~ be* up to one's neck in wórry.

ро́та ж. cómpany.

рота́тор м. (rótary sténcil) dúplicator.

ро́тный прил. 1. cómpany attr.; 2. в знач. сущ. м. cómpany commánder.

ротозе́й м. разг. 1. (зевака) býstander; ónlooker; 2. (разиня) dáy-dreamer. ~ничать несов. разг. stand* and gape. ~ство с. разг. dáy-dreaming.

ро́тор м. тех. rótor.

ро́ща ж. grove, copse.

роя́л|ь м. grand piáno; игра́ть на ~е play the piáno; сесть за ~ sit* down at the piáno; у ~я at the piáno.

РСФСР (Росси́йская Сове́тская Федерати́вная Социалисти́ческая Респу́блика) RSFSR (Rússian Sóviet Féderative Sócialist Repúblic).

рту́тный mércury attr.; (содержащий ртуть тж.) mercúric; ~ термо́метр mércury thermómeter.

ртуть ж. mércury, quícksilver; ◇ гремучая ~ fúlminate of mércury.

руба́нок м. plane.

руба́ха ж. shirt.

руба́шка ж. 1. (мужская) shirt; (женская) slip, chemíse; ночна́я ~ (мужская) níght-shirt; (женская) níght-dress, níght-gown; ни́жняя ~ únderwear, pántislip; 2. тех. jácket.

рубе́ж м. 1. (граница) bórder, bóundary; 2. воен. line; ◇ за ~о́м abróad; выезжа́ть за ~ go* abróad.

рубе́ц м. 1. (шрам) scar; (от удара хлыстом и т. п.) weal; 2. (шов) hem; 3. (отдел желудка жвачных животных) paunch; (кушанье) (plain) tripe.

руби́льник м. эл. ~ (knífe-)switch, cút-out.

руби́н м. rúby. ~овый 1. (сделанный из рубина) rúby attr.; 2. (цвета рубина) rúby(-coloured).

руби́ть несов. (вн.) 1. (разрубать) chop (smth.); (измельчать) mince (smth.), chop (smth.) fine; ~ дрова́ chop wood; ~ капу́сту chop cábbage; 2. (деревья) fell (smth.); ~ строево́й лес fell tímber; 3. (поражать холодным оружием) cut* (smb.) down, sábre (smb.); 4. горн. cut* (smth.), hew* (smth.); ~ у́голь cut* coal; 5. разг. (говорить, действовать резко) give* it to smb. straight from the shóulder, not mince mátters. ~ся несов. fight* (with cold steel).

ру́бище с. rags pl, tátters pl.

ру́бка I ж. 1. (на мелкие куски) chópping (up), míncing; 2. (деревьев) félling.

ру́бка II ж. мор. déck-house; рулева́я ~ whéel-house; боева́я ~ cónning-tower.

рублёвый óne-rouble attr.

рубле́н|ый chopped, minced; ~ бифште́кс hámburger.

рубл|ь м. róuble; сто ~е́й one húndred róubles.

ру́брика ж. 1. (заглавие) héading; 2. (раздел) subdivísion, cólumn.

ру́гань ж. abúse, swéaring, náme-calling.

руга́тель|ный abúsive. ~ство с. curse, oath.

руга́ть, вы́ругать (вн.) swear* (at), curse (smb.), scold (smb.); (порицать) run* (smb., smth.) down. ~ся

несов. 1. swear*; 2. (с тв.; переругиваться) hurl abúse at each óther, call each óther names.

руда́ ж. ore.

рудиме́нтарный rudiméntary; ~ о́рган rudiméntary/ vestígial órgan.

рудни́к м. mine, pit. ~о́вый mine attr., pit attr.

рудни́чный míning; ~ газ fire-damp.

руди|ы́ míning; (содержащий руду) ore attr.; ~ые месторожде́ния depósits of ore.

рудоно́сный óre-bearing.

руже́йный gun attr., rifle attr.; ~ вы́стрел rífle-shot.

ружь|ё с. gun; дробово́е ~ shót-gun; двуство́льное ~ dóuble-bárrelled gun; ◇ под ~ём únder arms.

руи́на ж. 1. мн. ruins; 2. разг. (немощный человек) wreck.

рук|а́ ж. 1. (кисть) hand; (от кисти до плеча) arm; в ~е́ in one's hand; за́ руку by the hand; взя́ться за́ руки join hands; ~а́ми не тро́гать! (please) do not touch!; брать кого-л. на́ руки take* smb. in one's arms; держа́ть кого-л. на ~а́х hold* smb. in one's arms; кре́пко держа́ть кого-л. за́ ~у hold tight to the arm; по пра́вую (ле́вую) ру́ку от чего-л. to the right (the left) of smth.; 2. (почерк) hand, hándwriting; э́то не его́ ~ that's not his hand; ◇ быть в чьих-л. ~а́х be* at smb.'s mércy; э́то мне на́ руку that suits me down to the ground; у него́ на ~а́х больша́я семья́ he has a large fámily on his hands; все кни́ги на ~а́х the books are all out; по ~а́м! done!, it's a bárgain!; брать кого-л. под руку take* smb.'s arm; вести́ кого-л. под руку walk árm-in-árm with smb.; не говори́те под руку! don't put me off my stroke!; ~ попа́сться кому-л. под руку come* in smb.'s way; что попадётся под руку ánything one can lay hands upon; под ~о́й, под ~а́ми at/to hand, hándy, withín éasy reach; с ~и́ кому-л. convénient for smb.; ~ об руку hand in hand; ру́ки вверх! hands up!; ру́ки прочь от кого-л., чего-л.! hands off smb., smth.!; ~ не дро́гнет у кого-л. (+ инф.) smb. wóuldn't hésitate (+ to inf), smb. wóuldn't think twice (abóut + -ing); ру́ки опусти́лись у кого-л. smb. (has) lost all ínterest; ~ не поднима́ется у кого-л. (+ инф.) smb. cánnot bring himsélf (+ to inf); ~о́й пода́ть a stone's throw (from); подáть ру́ку по́мощи кому-л. exténd a hélping hand to smb.; быть у кого-л. пра́вой ~о́й be* smb.'s right hand; быть без кого-л., чего-л. как без рук feel* hélpless withóut smb., smth.; брать кого-л. в ру́ки take* smb. in hand; брать что-л. в свои́ ру́ки take* smth. into one's own hands; брать себя́ в ру́ки pull onesélf togéther, contról onesélf; держа́ть себя́ в ~а́х keep* onesélf in hand; игра́ть в четы́ре ~и́ play dúets; выдать что-л. на́ руки кому-л. give* smth. to smb. to take awáy; получи́ть что-л. на́ руки recéive smth. in pérson; в со́бственные руки (надпись) for pérsonal delívery ónly; дать по ~а́м кому-л. гар smb. óver the knúckles; отпуска́ть что-л. в одни́ ру́ки serve smth. per cústomer; в на́ших ~а́х in our hands; передава́ть что-л. из рук в ру́ки, с рук на́ руки pass smth. from hand to hand; из рук вон пло́хо thóroughly bad; на ско́рую ру́ку in a húrry; от ~и́ by hand; писа́ть что-л. от ~и́ write* smth. in long hand; ходи́ть по ~а́м be* passed from hand to hand; с рук сбыть кого-л., что-л. get* rid of smth.; э́то его́ рук де́ло that's his hándiwork; ему́ и кни́ги в ру́ки that's his strong point; ма́стер на все ру́ки Jack of all trádes.

рука́в м. 1. (одежды) sleeve; 2. (реки) arm, branch; 3. (шланг) hose; ◇ спустя́ ~а́ in a slípshod mánner.

рукави́цы мн. (ед. рукави́ца ж.) míttens.

руководи́тель м. léader, head; ~ отде́ла depártment/séction head; худо́жественный ~ árt-adviser; нау́чный ~ supervísor; кла́ссный ~ form máster; (о женщине) form místress; ~ орке́стра artístic diréctor.

руководи́ть несов. (тв.) 1. lead* (smb., smth.), guide (smb., smth.); ~ заня́тиями, рабо́той condúct/súpervise stúdies, work; ~ радиокружко́м run* an ámateur rádio group; 2. (управлять) be* in charge (of), be* at the head (of), head (smth.); ~ отде́лом head a depártment.

руково́дств|о с. 1. (де́йствие) guidance, léadership; supervision; операти́вное ~ efficient mánagement; 2. (то, чем сле́дует руково́дствоваться) guide; приня́ть что-л. к ~y take* smth. as a guiding prínciple; 3. (книга) hándbook, mánual; 4. собир. (руководи́тели) léaders pl, léadership.

руково́дствоваться несов. (тв.) be* guided (by); ~ чьи́ми-л. указа́ниями act in accórdance with smb.'s instrúctions.

руководя́щ|ий 1. léading; ~ рабо́тник exécutive; pérson in charge; 2.: ~ие указа́ния géneral instrúctions.

рукоде́|лие с. néedlework, fáncy-work. ~льница ж. néedlewoman*.

рукомо́йник м. hánging wásh-hand can.

рукопа́шный прил. 1. hánd-to-hánd; ~ бой hánd-to-hánd fight(ing); 2. в знач. сущ. ж. hánd-to-hánd fight.

рукопи́сн|ый mánuscript; ~ые те́ксты hánd-written texts, mánuscripts.

ру́копись ж. mánuscript; (напеча́танная на маши́нке тж.) týpescript; полигр. (оригина́л для набо́ра) cópy.

рукоплеск|а́ния мн. clápping sg, appláuse sg. ~а́ть несов. (дт.) clap (smb., smth.), appláud (smb., smth.).

рукопожа́ти|е с. hándshake, hánd-clasp; обменя́ться ~ями shake* hands.

рукоя́|тка ж., ~ть ж. hándle; (рыча́г тж.) léver; ~ кинжа́ла hilt; ~ револьве́ра butt of a revólver; ~ затво́ра óperating léver; по са́мую ~тку to the hilt.

рулев|о́й прил. 1. rúdder attr., stéering attr.; ~о́е устро́йство stéering gear; 2. в знач. сущ. м. hélmsman*, man* at the wheel.

руле́т м. 1. (о́корок) boned ham/gámmon; 2. (кушанье) roll; мясно́й ~ méat-roll; 3. (конди́терский) swiss-roll.

руле́тка ж. (измери́тельная) tápe-measure.

рули́ть несов. ав. táxi.

руло́н м. roll.

рул|ь м. (су́дна) rúdder; helm (тж. перен.); (автомаши́ны) (stéering-)wheel; (велосипе́да) hándle-bars pl; ~ поворо́та ав. rúdder; ~ высоты́ ав. élevator; ~ тра́ктора tráctor stéering-wheel; пра́вить ~ём steer; стоя́ть, сиде́ть за ~ём be* at the wheel; стать за ~ take* the helm; ◇ без ~я́ и без ветри́л rúdderless; without aim or diréction.

румб м. мор. (cómpass) point.

румы́н м., ~ка ж. Rumánian. ~ский Rumánian; ~ский язы́к Rumánian, the Rumánian lánguage.

румя́на мн. rouge sg.

румя́н|ец м. (high) cólour; (от стыда́, волне́ния) flush; зали́ться ~цем be* suffúsed with cólour.

румя́н|ить, зарумя́нить, нарумя́нить (вн.) 1. сов. зарумя́нить (покрыва́ть румя́нцем) rédden (smth.), flush (smth.); 2. сов. нарумя́нить (кра́сить щёки) rouge (smth.); 3. сов. зарумя́нить (окра́шивать в а́лый цвет) rédden (smth.); ~иться, зарумя́ниться, нарумя́ниться 1. сов. зарумя́ниться (покрыва́ться румя́нцем) flush, turn red; 2. сов. нарумя́ниться (кра́ситься) use rouge; 3. сов. зарумя́ниться (окра́шиваться в а́лый цвет) turn red, be* suffúsed with red; 4. сов. зарумя́ниться (поджа́риваться) get* brown.

румя́ный rósy, pink; (о челове́ке) pínk-cheeked, rúddy-faced, rúbicund.

руно́ с. fleece; ◇ золото́е ~ gólden fleece.

ру́ны мн. (ед. ру́на ж.) runes.

ру́пор м. lóudhailer; mégaphone; перен. móuthpiece, spókesman*.

руса́лка ж. wáter-nymph, mérmaid.

руси́зм м. a bórrowing from Rússian.

руси́ст м. spécialist in Rússian philólogy.

ру́сло с. (river-)bed; chánnel; перен. course, groove; жизнь вхо́дит в своё ~ life is resúming its nátural course.

ру́сский I м. Rússian.

ру́сск|ий II прил. Rússian; ~ язы́к Rússian, the Rússian lánguage; ~ая литерату́ра Rússian literature; ~ая исто́рия Rússian history; ◇ ~ое ма́сло clárified bútter; ~ая печь Rússian stove; говори́ть, сказа́ть ~им языко́м speak*, say* pláinly.

ру́сый light brown; (о челове́ке тж.) with líght-brown hair по́сле сущ.

рути́н|а ж. routíne; stagnátion; hídebound ways pl. ~ный stale.

ру́хлядь ж. собир. разг. lúmber, junk; (оде́жда) old clothes pl.

ру́хну|ть сов. collápse (тж. перен.); (о кры́ше, потолке́ тж.) fall* in; он ~л на зе́млю как подко́шенный he collápsed in a heap on the ground; на́ши наде́жды ~ли our hopes were dashed to the ground.

руча́тельств|о с. guarantée, gúaranty; с ~ом за испра́вность guaranteed in wórking órder; с ~ом на два го́да with a twó-year guarantée.

руч|а́ться, поручи́ться (за кого́-л.) ánswer (for); (за что-л.) guarantée (smth.); ~а́юсь, что сде́лаю э́то I'll do it; ~а́юсь, что вам э́того не сде́лать I defý you to do it; до́ктор не ~а́лся за исхо́д опера́ции the dóctor would give no guarantée as to the resúlt of the operátion.

ручеёк м. bróoklet, stréamlet.

руч|е́й м. brook, rill; лить слёзы в три ~ья́ shed* floods of tears.

ру́чка ж. 1. (рукоя́тка) hándle; (кру́глая) knob; ~ две́ри dóor-handle; (кру́глая) dóor-knob; 3. (ме́бели) arm; 4. (для пера́) pén-holder; (с перо́м) pen.

ручн|о́й 1. (для рук) hand attr.; ~ бага́ж hand lúggage; ~ы́е часы́ wrist-watch sg; 2. (производи́мый рука́ми) mánual; ~ труд mánual lábour; э́то ~а́я рабо́та it's done by hand; 3. (обслу́живаемый вручну́ю) hand attr.; hánd-óperated; ~ то́рмоз hánd-brake; ~а́я пила́ hánd-saw; 4. (приручённый) tame; ◇ ~а́я прода́жа 1) (в апте́ке) sale without prescrіption; 2) (торго́вля с рук) sale without wéighing, sale of páckaged goods.

ру́ш|иться несов. collápse; be* fálling down; перен. be* sháttered; дом ~ится the house is fálling down; его́ наде́жды ~ились his hopes were sháttered.

ры́ба ж. fish; ◇ ни ~ ни мя́со insípid; чу́вствовать себя́ как ~ в воде́ feel* quite at home.

рыба́к м. fisherman*.

рыба́лк|а ж. разг. fishing (trip); пое́хать на ~у go* fishing.

рыба́|цкий, ~чий fishing attr.; fisherman's; ~чья ло́дка fishing-boat. ~чить несов. fish. ~чка ж. 1. fisherwoman*; 2. (жена́ рыбака́) fisherman's wife*.

рыбёшка ж. разг. small fry, little fish.

ры́б|ий прил. перен. cold-blóoded; ~ жир cód-liver oil; ~ клей fish-glue; ~ьи глаза́ códlike glance. ~ный fish attr.; ~ная кость fish bone; ~ный про́мысел fishery; ~ная промы́шленность fish industry; ~ный садо́к fish-pond; ~ные консе́рвы tinned/canned fish.

рыбово́д|ство с. fish-breeding; fish-farming. ~ческий fish-breeding attr.; fish-farming attr.; ~ческое хозя́йство fish-farm.

рыболо́в м. fisherman*; (с удочкой) ángler.

рыболове́цкий fishing attr.

рыболо́в|ный fishing attr.; ~ сезо́н fishing séason; ~ные се́ти fishing nets; ~ флот fishing fleet. ~ство с. fishing.

рыбообраба́тывающий fish-processing; ~ комбина́т fish-processing plant/fáctory.

рыво́к м. 1. jerk, tug; перен. spurt; 2. (в тяжёлой атле́тике) snatch.

рыга́ть, рыгну́ть belch.

рыгну́ть сов. см. рыга́ть.

рыда́ни|е *с.* sob; *мн.* sobs; sóbbing *sg*; разрази́ться ~ями burst* out sóbbing.

рыда́ть *несов.* sob.

рыжеборо́дый red-béarded.

рыжеволо́сый red-háired, sándy(-háired).

рыже́ть, порыже́ть 1. turn réddish-brown, get* rústy; 2. *тк. несов.* (*виднеться*) show* réddish-brown.

ры́жий *прил.* 1. red-háired; (*о волосах*) red; (*о лошади*) chéstnut; (*выцветший*) réddish-brown, rúst-coloured; 2. *в знач. сущ. м. разг.* (*клоун*) clown.

ры́жик *м.* (*гриб*) sáffron milk cap.

рык *м.* roar; льви́ный ~ the roar of a líon.

ры́ло *с.* 1. snout; 2. *груб.* (*лицо*) mug; (*единица счёта*) head.

ры́н|ок *м.* márket; (*место тж.*) márket-place; вну́тренний ~ doméstic márket; ~ки сбы́та márkets. ~очный márket *attr.*; ~очная торго́вля márket trade; ~очная цена́ márket price.

рыса́к *м.* trótter.

рыси́ст|ый: ~ая ло́шадь trótter; ~ые испыта́ния trótting ráces.

рыска́ть *несов.* 1. (*по дт.*) hunt abóut (*smth.*), scóur (*smth.*); (*бродить*) roam (*smth.*), rove (through); ~ ле́су scóur the fórest; ~ по бе́регу roam the shore; 2. *мор.* swerve.

рысцо́й *разг.* at a jóg-trot.

рысь|ю I *ж.* (*аллюр*) trot; ме́лкая (кру́пная) ~ light (long) trot; ◇ на ~я́х at a trot.

рысь II *ж.* (*животное*) lynx.

ры́сью at a trot; идти́ ~ trot.

ры́твина *ж.* hóllow.

рыть *несов.* (*вн.*) 1. dig* (*smth.*); (*рылом*) root (in); 2. *разг.* (*разбрасывать, перемешивать что-л.*) rúmmage (*smth.*); ◇ ~ я́му кому́-л. make* tróuble for smb. ~ся *несов.* dig*; root; (*в вещах*) rúmmage.

рыхле́ть *несов.* 1. becóme* fríable; 2. *разг.* (*о человеке*) run* to seed, get* flábby.

рыхли́ть *несов.* loosen (*smth.*), hoe (*smth.*).

ры́хлый 1. crúmbly, fríable; (*о грунте тж.*) loose; ~ снег soft snow; 2. *разг.* (*о человеке*) flábby.

ры́цар|ский kníghtly; *перен.* chívalrous; ~ о́рден *ист.* órder of knighthood; ~ посту́пок chívalrous áction; ◇ ~ рома́н románce. ~ство *с.* knighthood; *перен.* chívalry; времена́ ~ства the age of chívalry.

ры́царь *м. ист.* knight (*тж. перен.*); стра́нствующий ~ knight érrant.

рыча́г *м.* léver (*тж. перен.*); ~ управле́ния contról-lever.

рыча́ние *с.* grówling, snárling.

рыча́ть, прорыча́ть growl, snarl.

рья́ный zéalous.

рэ́кет *м.* rácket; занима́ться ~ом óperate/run* a rácket.

рэкети́р *м.* racketéer.

рюкза́к *м.* rúcksack, knápsack.

рю́мка *ж.* glass.

ряби́на I *ж.* 1. (*плод*) rówan, áshberry; 2. (*дерево*) rówan-tree, móuntain ash.

ряби́на II *ж.* (*щербина*) pit; (*от оспы*) póck-mark.

ряб|и́ть *несов.* 1. (*вн.*) rípple (*smth.*); ветеро́к ~и́т во́ду a breeze rípples the wáter; 2. *безл.*: у меня́ ~и́т в глаза́х I am dázzled.

рябо́й 1. pítted; (*от оспы*) póck-marked; 2. (*с пятнами другого цвета*) dáppled.

ря́бчик *м.* házel-grouse.

рябь *ж.* (*на воде*) rípple.

ряд *м.* 1. row; ~ кре́сел row of chairs; ~ за ~ом row upón row; 2. (*шеренга*) file; 3. (*места в театре, кино и т. п.*) row; 4. (*совокупность явлений*): дли́нный ~ дней days that dragged on one áfter the óther; 5. (*некоторое количество чего-л.*) séries, númber; в ~е стран in a númber of cóuntries; це́лый ~ причи́н a séries of

cáuses; в це́лом ~е слу́чаев in a númber of cáses; ~ поколе́ний mány generátions; 6. *мн.* (*состав, среда*) rank *sg*; служи́ть в ~а́х Сове́тской А́рмии serve in the Sóviet Army; 7. (*ларьки, прилавки для торговли*) stalls *pl*, row of stalls; моло́чный ~ milk stalls; ры́бный ~ fish stalls; ◇ из ~а вон выходя́щий outstánding; out of the géneral run; из ~а вон выходя́щий слу́чай a quite excéptional case.

рядов|о́й *прил.* 1. órdinary; ~о́е явле́ние cómmon/éveryday occúrrence; 2. *воен.* ránk-and-file; 3. *с.-х.* row *attr.*; in rows *после сущ.*; 4. *в знач. сущ. м. воен.* prívate (sóldier); man*.

ря́дом 1. (*возле, около*) besíde; сесть ~ с кем-л. sit* down next to smb.; он сиде́л ~ he was sítting close by; они́ сиде́ли ~ they sat side by side; 2. (*по соседству*) next door, next; дом ~ с теа́тром the house next door to the théatre; он живёт ~ he lives next door; 3. (*очень близко*) near, close by.

ря́женка *ж.* ryázhenka (*baked fermented milk*).

ря́са *ж.* cássock, frock.

ря́ска *ж. бот.* dúckweed.

С

с, со 1. from; off; встать со сту́ла rise* from *one's* chair; сверну́ть с доро́ги turn off the road; ве́тер с мо́ря wind from/off the sea; прие́хать с Украи́ны arríve from the Ukráine; 2. (*при временных оборотах*) at, with; from; с утра́ до но́чи from mórning till night; вы́ехать с рассве́том start out at dawn; с ка́ждым ча́сом (with) évery hour; 3. (*при причинных оборотах*) from, with, through, out of, in; с испу́га out of fright; с непривы́чки through lack of práctice; с позволе́ния роди́телей with *one's* párents' permíssion; уста́ть с доро́ги be* tíred from the jóurney; 4. (*при обозначении лица, предмета, с которого получают, требуют*) from; on; (*при обозначении единиц*) per; получи́ть де́ньги с покупа́теля take* móney from a cústomer; взима́ть по́шлину с това́ра charge dúty on goods; 50 це́нтнеров с гекта́ра fifty céntners per héctare; 5. (*при обозначении манеры, способа действия*) with, by; корми́ть с ло́жки feed* with a spoon; взять с бо́ю take* by storm; лете́ть со ско́ростью зву́ка fly* at the speed of sound; 6. (*при выражении совместности*) and; with; повида́ть отца́ с ма́терью see* *one's* fáther and móther; дождь со сне́гом rain mixed with snow; нас с детьми́ семь челове́к there are séven of us with the children; 7. (*при обозначении дополнительного количества*) and; два с полови́ной two and a half; 8. (*при обозначении содержимого*) of; буты́лка с молоко́м bóttle of milk; 9. (*при обозначении обоюдного действия, взаимоотношения*) with; спо́рить с дру́гом árgue with a friend; познако́мить кого́-л. с де́вушкой introdúce smb. to a girl; 10. (*при выражении цели действия*): яви́ться с докла́дом come* in to repórt; обрати́ться с про́сьбой make* a request; 11. (*выражает приблизительную меру*) (for) abóut; отдохну́ть с полчаса́ rest (for) abóut half an hour; 12. (*при сравнениях*) the size of; as much as; ма́льчик ро́стом с отца́ a boy as tall as his fáther; о́пухоль величино́й с гре́цкий оре́х a túmor the size of a wálnut.

са́бля *ж.* sábre.

сабота́ж *м.* sábotage. ~ник *м.* sabotéur.

саботи́ровать *несов. и сов.* 1. (*вн.*) sábotage (*smth.*); 2. *тк. несов.* (*заниматься саботажем*) adópt sábotage táctics, commít sábotage.

са́ван *м.* shroud; сне́жный ~ blánket of snow.

са́га *ж.* sága.

сагити́ровать *сов. см.* агити́ровать 2.

сад *м.* gárden; ◇ ботани́ческий ~ botánical gárdens *pl*; зоологи́ческий ~ zoológical gárdens *pl*, zoo; зи́мний ~ wínter gárden, consérvatory.

сади́ть, посади́ть (*вн.*) *разг.* plant (*smth.*).

сади́ться, сесть 1. sit* down, seat *one*sélf; ~ на стул sit* down on a chair; ~ за стол sit* down at táble; сади́тесь! won't you sit down?, take a seat!; ся́дьте! sit down!; сесть верхо́м 1) (*на лошадь*) mount a horse, get* on a horse; 2) (*на стул и т. п.*) sit* astríde a chair *etc.*; сесть в ва́нну get* ínto the bath; сесть в посте́ли sit* up in bed; **2.** (*занимать место для поездки*): ~ в по́езд, трамва́й, авто́бус get* on a train, tram, bus; ~ в маши́ну get* ínto a car; ~ на парохо́д, самолёт board a ship, plane; **3.** (*за, на вн.,* + *инф.; приступать к какому-л. делу*) séttle down (to, + to *inf*), take* (*smth.*); ~ за рабо́ту séttle down to work; ~ за руль take* the wheel; ~ на вёсла take* the oars; **4.** *разг.* (*быть лишённым свободы*) be*/get* put awáy, be* imprísoned; сесть в тюрьму́ get* put in príson, be* gáoled; сесть на гауптва́хту be* confíned to the guárdroom; **5.** (*следовать какому-л. режиму*) start (*smth.*), take* up (*smth.*); сесть на дие́ту start díeting; **6.** (*о птице, насекомом*) alight, perch; (*о самолёте, парашютисте*) land; **7.** (*о светилах*) set*; **8.** (*оседать*) séttle; **9.** (*суживаться, укорачиваться*) shrink*; мате́рия се́ла the matérial has shrunk; ◇ сесть на́ голову кому́-л. jump on *smb.*; сесть на мель run* agróund; *перен. тж.* come* unstúck; сесть на я́йца begin* to sit.

са́днить *несов.* sting*.

садо́вник *м.* gárdener.

садово́д *м.* gárdener, horticúlturist. **~ство** *с.* gárdening, hórticulture.

садо́вый 1. gárden *attr.*; (*о растении тж.*) cúltivated; **2.** (*садоводческий*) horticúltural.

садо́к *м.* **1.** (*живорыбный*) físhpond, tank; **2.** (*для животных*) pen; hátchery; **3.** *охот.* trap.

са́ж|а *ж.* soot; в ~e sóoty, smútty.

сажа́ть, посади́ть 1. (*вн.; просить занять место*) seat (*smb.*); ~ госте́й за стол seat *one's* guests at táble; **2.** (*вн.; помогать сесть*) put* (*smb.*); ~ кого́-л. на по́езд put* *smb.* on the train; *воен.* entráin *smb.*; ~ кого́-л. на су́да (*вн.; вести на посадку*) land (*smth.*); ~ самолёт land a plane; **4.** (*вн. за, на вн., вн.* + *инф.; заставлять что-л. делать*) put* (*smb.* to); make* (*smb.* + *inf*); ~ кого́-л. за рабо́ту put* *smb.* to work; ~ кого́-л. на вёсла make* *smb.* row; **5.** (*вн.; помещать куда-л., лишая свободы*) lock (*smb.*) up; ~ кого́-л. под аре́ст put* *smb.* únder arrést; ~ соба́ку на цепь chain up a dog; ~ пти́цу в кле́тку cage a bird; **6.** (*вн.; растения*) plant (*smth.*); ~ карто́фель plant potátoes; ◇ ~ ку́рицу на я́йца set* a hen on eggs.

са́женец *м. с.-х.* séedling; sápling.

са́жень *ж.* sázhen (*7 feet*); морска́я ~ fáthom.

саза́н *м.* (*рыба*) wild carp, sazán.

са́йка *ж.* (*булка*) roll.

саквоя́ж *м.* trávelling-bag.

саксофо́н *м.* sáxophone.

сала́зк|и *мн.* **1.** (*hánd*)sleigh *sg*, tobóggan *sg*; ката́ться на ~ax tobóggan, go* tobógganing; **2.** *тех.* slide rails; cárrier *sg*.

сала́ка *ж.* (*рыба*) sprat.

сала́т *м.* **1.** (*растение*) léttuce; **2.** (*кушанье*) sálad; ~ из све́жей капу́сты cóleslaw. **~ник** *м.*, **~ница** *ж.* sálad-bowl. **~ный, ~овый** (*о цвете*) líght-green.

са́ло *с.* fat; (*топлёное свиное*) lard; (*нутряное говяжье и бараньё*) suet.

сало́н *м.* **1.** (*в гостинице, отеле*) lounge; (*на парохо́де и т. п.*) salóon; **2.** (*литературный*) sálon; **3.** (*зал для демонстрации и продажи одежды, обуви*) sále-room, shów-room; **4.**: худо́жественный ~ art gállery; ◇ ~-ваго́н lounge car.

салфе́тка *ж.* (*táble*)-nápkin; (*скатерть*) small táblecloth; бума́жная ~ páper nápkin.

са́льдо *с. нескл. бухг.* bálance.

са́льн|ый 1. (*из сала*) tállow; ~ая свеча́ tállow cándle; **2.** (*жирный*) gréasy; **3.** (*непристойный*) dírty, obscéne; ◇ ~ые же́лезы *анат.* sebáceous glands.

салю́т *м.* salúte; произвести́ ~ fire a salúte.

салютова́ть *несов. и сов.* (*дт.*) salúte (*smb.*); ~ кому́-л. фла́гом dip the flag to *smb.*

сам, сама́, само́, са́ми *переводится в зависимости от лица, числа и рода* myself, *pl* oursélves; yoursélf, *pl* yoursélves; himsélf, hersélf, itsélf, *pl* themsélves (*обыкн. ставится в конце предложения*); вы э́то ~и зна́ете you know that yoursélf; вы ~и зна́ете, что... you know véry well that...; я э́то сде́лаю I will do it mysélf; он ~ во всём винова́т it is all his own fault; опери́ровал ~ профе́ссор the operátion was perfórmed by the proféssor himsélf; он ~ учи́тель, а она́ врач he is a téacher, and she is a dóctor; ◇ ~ по себе́ 1) (*самостоятельно*) indepéndently, by onesélf; 2) (*как таковой*) in himsélf, in itsélf; 3) *в знач. сказ.* one thing... anóther; э́то говори́т ~ó за себя́ it speaks for itsélf; ~о собóй разуме́ется it goes without sáying, it stands to réason; э́то уж ~ó собóй but, of course!; that goes without sáying!

сама́ *см.* сам.

са́мбо *с. нескл.* unármed self-defénce.

саме́ц *м.* male; (*об олене, зайце, кролике*) buck; (*о слоне, ките*) bull; (*о птице*) cock, mále-bird.

са́ми *см.* сам.

са́мка *ж.* fémale; (*об олене, зайце, кролике*) doe; (*о слоне, ките, тюлене*) cow; (*о птице*) hen(-bird).

само́ *см.* сам.

само- *в сложн.* self-, auto-.

самоана́лиз *м.* introspéction, self-examinátion.

самобичева́ние *с.* self-condemnátion, self-repróach, self-tórture.

самобы́тн|ость *ж.* originálity. **~ый** oríginal, distínctive; ~ая культу́ра distínctive cúlture, cúlture that is distínctly oríginal.

самова́р *м.* samovár; поста́вить ~ heat the samovár.

самовла́ст|ие *с.* autócracy. **~ный** despótic, autocrátic.

самовлюблённый concéited, self-sátisfied.

самовнуше́ние *с.* auto-suggéstion.

самово́льн|о without permíssion. **~ый 1.** (*своенравный*) self-willed, wílful; (*о поведении, поступках*) árbitrary; high-hánded; **2.** (*без разрешения*) unáuthorized; without permíssion *после сущ.*; ~ая отлу́чка ábsence withóut leave.

самовоспламене́ние *с.* **1.** (*самовозгорание*) spontáneous combústion; **2.** (*в двигателях и т. п.*) self-ígnition, spontáneous ígnition.

самовосхвале́ние *с.* self-glorificátion, self-práise.

самого́н *м.*, **~ка** *ж.* illícit spírits *pl*, hóme-brew.

самодви́жущийся automótive.

самоде́льный home-máde.

самодержа́в|ие *с.* autócracy. **~ный** autocrátic.

самоде́ржец *м.* áutocrat.

самоде́ятельн|ость *ж.* **1.** inítiative; **2.** (*художественное, театральное и т. п. творчество*) ámateur work/activity; худо́жественная ~ ámateur artístic work; ве́чер ~ости ámateur concert; кружо́к худо́жественной ~ости ámateur group; выступле́ние ~ости ámateur perfórmance. **~ый 1.** ámateur *attr.*; ~ое иску́сство ámateur art; ~ый спекта́кль ámateur perfórmance (of a play); **2.** *эк.* indepéndently emplóyed.

самодисципли́на *ж* self-díscipline.

самодовле́ющий self-suffícing.

самодово́ль|ный self-sátisfied, complácent, smug; ~ вид self-sátisfied air; ~ная улы́бка complácent smile. **~ство** *с.* complácency, smúgness, self-satisfáction.

самоду́р *м.* pétty týrant. **~ство** *с.* pétty týranny.

самозащи́та ж. self-defénce.

самозва́н|ец м. impóstor, preténder. **~ство** с. impósture. **~ый** self-stýled.

самокри́т|ика ж. self-críticism. **~и́ческий, ~и́чный** self-crítical.

самолёт м. áircraft, áeroplane; plane разг. **~ный** áircraft attr.

самолёто-вы́лет м. flight.

самолётостро́ение с. áircraft constrúction.

самолюби́вый proud; (обидчивый) tóuchy.

самолю́бие с. pride, self-estéem; ло́жное ~ false pride; заде́ть чье́-л. ~ wound smb.'s pride/vánity.

самомне́ние с. (self-)concéit; челове́к с больши́м ~м concéited pérson; pérson with a high opínion of himsélf.

самонаводя́щийся воен. self-gúided; ~ снаря́д self-gúided míssile.

самонаде́янн|о concéitedly, presúmptuously, pérkily. **~ость** ж. concéit, presúmption. **~ый** concéited, presúmptuous, self-assértive, búmptious.

самооблада́ние с. self-commánd, self-contról, self-posséssion.

самообма́н м. self-decéption.

самообольще́ние с. delúsion; (ложная уверенность) over-cónfidence.

самооборо́на ж. self-defénce.

самообразова́ние с. self-educátion.

самообслу́живани|е с. hélping onesélf; (в магазинах и т. п.) self-sérvice; столо́вая ~я self-sérvice réstaurant, help-yoursélf réstaurant; магази́н ~я self-sérvice shop, súpermarket; (гастроном) food súpermarket.

самоограниче́ние с. self-restráint.

самоопредел|е́ние с. self-determinátion. **~и́ться** сов. см. самоопределя́ться.

самоопределя́ться, самоопредели́ться 1. (в обществе) find* a place for onesélf in life; 2. (получать самостоятельность) gain indepéndence.

самопроки́дывающийся tip attr., típping.

самоопыле́ние с. бот. self-fertilizátion.

самоотве́рженн|о dédicatedly, disínterestedly; sélflessly. **~ость** ж. dedicátion; sélflessness. **~ый** dédicated; sélfless; ~ый труд dédicated/sélfless work; ~ый по́двиг sélfless achíevement.

самоотво́д м. withdráwal of one's cándidature.

самопи́ска ж. разг. fóuntain-pen.

самопи́шущий régistering, (self-)recórding.

самопоже́ртвование с. self-sácrifice.

самопозна́ние с. self-knówledge.

самопроизво́льный spontáneous.

самореклáма ж. self-advértisement.

саморо́док м. núgget; перен. oríginal génius, nátive tálent.

самосва́л м. (автомашина) tip/típper lorry; dúmp-truck амер.

самосозна́ние с. self-awáreness.

самосохране́ние с. self-preservátion.

самостоя́тельн|ость ж. indepéndence. **~ый** indepéndent; (совершаемый своими силами тж.) oríginal; **~ый** челове́к indepéndent pérson; **~ая** рабо́та oríginal work.

самосу́д м. lýnching, mob múrder.

самотёк м. drift, laissez-fáire; пусти́ть де́ло на ~ let* mátters drift, let* mátters take care of themsélves. **~ом** of its own accórd, left to itsélf.

самоуби́й|ство с. súicide; поко́нчить жизнь ~ством commit súicide. **~ца** м. и ж. súicide.

самоуваже́ние с. self-estéem.

самоуве́ренн|о over-cónfidently; with great self-cónfidence. **~ость** ж. (self-)assúrance, over-cónfidence; cocksúre разг.; **~ый** челове́к over-cónfident pérson; **~ый** тон self-assúred tone.

самоуниже́ние с. self-humiliátion.

самоуправл|е́ние с. self-góvernment. **~я́ющийся** self-góverning.

самоупра́вство с. high-hándedness, árbitrariness.

самоусоверше́нствование с. self-perféction, perfécting the self.

самоуспоко́енность ж. smúgness, complácency.

самоустрани́ться сов. см. самоустраня́ться.

самоустраня́ться, самоустрани́ться (от рд.) abándon (smth.), shirk (smth.).

самоучи́тель м. téxtbook for self-instrúction, téach-yoursélf book.

самоучк|а м. и ж. разг. self-éducated/self-táught pérson; слéсарь-~ práctical mechánic. **~ой** разг.: научи́ться чему-л. ~ой learn* smth. by onesélf.

самохва́льство с. разг. self-advértising, bóasting.

самохо́дный self-propélled.

самоцве́т м. (драгоценный камень) précious stone; (поделочный камень) ornaméntal stone.

самоце́ль ж. end in itsélf.

самочу́вствие с. géneral condítion; как ва́ше ~? how do you feel in géneral?

самши́т м. bóxwood. **~овый** bóxwood attr.

cáм|ый 1. the véry (тж. тот ~); тот же ~ the same; ~ факт the véry fact; на ~ом верху́ at the véry top, right at the top; в ~ом низу́ at the véry bóttom, right at the bóttom; на ~ом берегу́ реки́ (о здании, деревьях и т. п.) right on the ríver; (о человеке, животном) right on the bank of the ríver; на ~ом углу́ (о здании, деревьях и т. п.) right on the córner; (о человеке, животном) just at the córner; к ~ому берегу́ close to the bank, shore etc.; в ~ом нача́ле at the véry beginning; с ~ого нача́ла from the véry beginning, first; в ~ой середи́не, в ~ую середи́ну right in the middle; в ~ом деле! réally!, indéed!; на ~ом деле in reálity, réally; в ~ раз (вовремя) in the nick of time; это вам в ~ раз (впору) it fits you perféctly!; 2. (служит для образования превосходной степени) the most; ~ высо́кий the híghest; ~ тру́дный the most dífficult; ~ лу́чший the véry best; ~ое гла́вное... the great thing is...; это ~ое гла́вное that's the most impórtant of all, that's the main thing.

санато́р|ий м. sanatórium, health céntre. **~ный** sanatórium attr.

сандáлии мн. (ед. сандáлия ж.) sándals.

сáни мн. sledge sg, sleigh sg; sled sg амер.

санитáр м. male nurse; воен. médical órderly.

санитáрия ж. sanitátion.

санитáрка ж. júnior nurse; воен. (girl) médical órderly.

санитáрн|ый 1. sánitary; ~ое состоя́ние го́рода sánitary condítions in a town; ~ врач héalth-officer; 2. (относящийся к медицинской службе в армии) médical; ~ая маши́на ámbulance; ~ самолёт ámbulance-plane; ~ по́езд hóspital train; ~ батальо́н médical battálion; ~ инстру́ктор médical instrúctor; ~ая су́мка first-áid bag; ~ая часть médical únit.

сáнки мн. разг. 1. см. сáни; 2. см. салáзки 1.

санкциони́ровать несов. и сов. (вн.) sánction (smth.).

сáнкция ж. sánction.

сáнный sleigh attr.; ~ путь sléigh-road.

сано́вник м. dígnitary.

санскри́т м. Sánscrit. **~ский** Sánscrit.

сантéхника ж. sánitary equípment (and techníques).

сантигрáмм м. céntigramme.

сантимéтр м. 1. céntimetre; 2. (лента для измерения) tápe(-measure).

санýзел м. tóilet facílities pl, báthroom and lávatory.

сап м. вет. glánders pl.

сáп|а ж.: ти́хой ~ой on the sly, on the quiet.

сапёр м. engíneer, sápper. **~ный** 1. engíneer attr., sápper attr.; ~ный батальо́н engíneer battálion; 2. (относящийся к военно-инженерным работам) enginéering; ~ные лопа́тки dígging tools; ~ные рабо́ты engi-néering works.

сапо́г|и *мн.* (*ед.* сапо́г *м.*) boots, tóp-boots; ◇ быть под ~о́м у кого́-л. be* únder *smb.'s* heel.

сапо́жн|ик *м.* 1. shóemaker; 2. *разг.* (*о неумелом человеке*) búngler. ~ый shoe *attr.*; ~ая щётка shoe brush; ~ый крем shoe polish.

сапфи́р *м.* sápphire.

сара́й *м.* 1. shed; 2. *разг.* (*о большой неую́тной ко́мнате*) barn.

саранча́ *ж.* lócust.

сарафа́н *м.* 1. (*национальная женская одежда*) sarafán; 2. (*летнее платье*) sún-frock, sún-dress.

сарде́лька *ж.* sáusage.

сарди́н(к)а *ж.* sardíne.)

са́ржа *ж. текст.* serge.

сарка́|зм *м.* sárcasm. ~сти́ческий sarcástic.

сарко́ма *ж. мед.* sarcóma.

саркофа́г *м.* sarcóphagus.

сата́н|а *ж.* Sátan. ~и́нский satánic.

сателли́т *м.* sátellite.

сати́н *м.* satéen. ~овый satéen *attr.*

сати́р|а *ж.* sátire. ~ик *м.* sátirist. ~и́ческий satírical; ~и́ческие купле́ты satírical cóuplets.

Сату́рн *м. астр.* Sáturn.

сафья́н *м.* morócco. ~ный, ~овый morócco *attr.*

са́хар *м.* súgar.

сахари́н *м.* sáccharin.

са́харистый sáccharine.

са́харница *ж.* súgar-bowl.

са́харный súgar *attr.*; (*сладкий*) súgary; (*приторный тж.*) sáccharine; ~ заво́д súgar-refinery.

сахароваре́ние *с.* súgar refining.

сахаро́за *ж. хим.* súcrose, sáccharose.

сачо́к *м.* (*для ло́вли насекомых*) bútterfly-net; (*для ло́вли ры́бы*) lánding-net.

сба́вить *сов. см.* сбавля́ть.

сбавля́ть, сба́вить (*вн.*) 1. (*отнима́ть часть от общего количества*) take* off (*smth.*); сба́вить 10 рубле́й take* off ten róubles; 2. (*уменьшать величину или количество чего-л.*) redúce (*smth.*); ~ в ве́се lose* weight; ~ це́ну redúce the price; сба́вить шаг slow down, slow *one's* pace.

сбаланси́ровать *сов.* regáin *one's* bálance.

сбе́гать *сов. разг.* (*куда-л.*) run* (to); (*за тв.*) run* and get*/fetch (*smb., smth.*)

сбега́ть, сбежа́ть 1. (*спуска́ться бего́м*) run* down; 2. (*стека́ть — о жидкости*) run* down, flow down; (*исчезать — об улыбке и т. п.*) vánish, drain; 3. (*совершать побег*) run* awáy; *разг.* (*избавля́ться от чего́-л. неприя́тного*) dodge; сбежа́ть из тюрьмы́ break* gaol, break* out of príson; сбежа́ть с уро́ков dodge léssons; 4. *тк. несов.* (*о доро́ге, тропи́нке и т. п.*) run* down. ~ся, сбежа́ться 1. come* rúnning (up); 2. *тк. несов.* (*сходи́ться в одно́м пу́нкте*) join, link up.

сбежа́ть *сов. см.* сбега́ть 1, 2, 3. **~ся** *сов. см.* сбега́ться 1.

сбербанк *м.* (*сберега́тельный банк*) sávings bank.

сберега́тельн|ый ~ый банк, ~ая ка́сса sávings bank; ~ая кни́жка sávings book.

сбере|га́ть, сбере́чь (*вн.*) 1. (*сохраня́ть в це́лости*) look áfter (*smth.*), save (*smth.*); ~ си́лы consérve *one's* strength/énergies; 2. (*уберега́ть от ущерба, по́рчи*) protéct (*smth.*); 3. (*огражда́ть от опа́сности*) save (*smb., smth.*); 4. (*копить*) save (*smth.*) up. ~же́ние *с.* 1. sáving; 2. *обыкн. мн.* (*накопленная су́мма де́нег*) sávings.

сбере́чь *сов. см.* сберега́ть.

сбер|ка́сса *ж.* sávings bank. **~кни́жка** *ж.* sávings book; положи́ть де́ньги на ~кни́жку put* móney into the sávings bank.

сбива́ть, сбить (*вн.*) 1. (*ударом*) knock (*smb.,*

smth.) off/down; ~ самолёт bring* down a plane; ~ кого́-л. с ног knock *smb.* down; 2. (*путать*) confúse (*smth.*); ~ кого́-л. со сле́да put* *smb.* off the scent; 3. (*масло*) churn (*smth.*); (*сливки*) whip (*smth.*); (*яйца*) beat* (*smth.*) up; 4. (*сколачивать*) knock (*smth.*) togéther; 5. (*стаптывать*): ~ каблуки́ run*/wear* *one's* heels down. ~ся, сби́ться 1. (*сдвигаться с места*) be* awrý; be*/get* pushed asíde; 2. (*отклоня́ться от чего́-л.*) lose* (*one's* way); сби́ться со сле́да lose* the trail; сби́ться со счёта lose* count; 3. (*ошиба́ться, пу́тать*) get* confúsed; (*в слова́х*) flóunder; 4. (*собира́ться вме́сте*) húddle (up/togéther); ◇ сби́ться с пути́ go* astráy; сби́ться с ног be* run off *one's* feet.

сби́вчивый múddled, incohérent; ~ отве́т múddled reply.

сби́т|ый 1. (*повреждённый ударом*) dámaged, báttered; 2. *разг.* (*сто́птанный*) dówn-at-héel; ~ые сапоги́ dówn-at-héel boots; 3. (*вспе́ненный*) whipped; ~ые сли́вки whipped cream *sg*; ◇ кре́пко сбит well-knít.

сбить(ся) *сов. см.* сбива́ть(ся).

сближ|а́ть, сбли́зить 1. (*вн.*) bring* (*smb., smth.*) clóser (to each óther); 2. (*вн. с тв.; находи́ть схо́дство, подо́бие*) líken (*smb., smth.* to). ~а́ться, сбли́зиться 1. draw* clóser to one anóther; (*подходи́ть*) appróach; 2. (*с тв.; станови́ться друзья́ми*) becóme* friends (with), becóme íntimate (with). ~е́ние *с.* 1. (*ли́чное*) grówing íntimacy; 2. *полит.* dráwing clóser; rapprochement; 3. *воен.* (*приближе́ние*) appróach; 4. (*схо́дство*) resémblance, growing similárity.

сбли́зить(ся) *сов. см.* сближа́ть(ся).

сбо́ку (*где-л.*) at/on one side; (*откуда-л.*) from the side; ~ от кого́-л. a little to the side of *smb.*

сболтну́ть *сов.* (*вн.*) *разг.* blurt (*smth.*) out.

сбор *м.* 1. (*собирание*) colléction; ~ нало́гов colléction of táxes; ~ све́дений colléction of informátion; 2. (*урожа́я*) hárvest, gáthering, pícking; ~ я́блок, табака́ á́pple, tobácco hárvest/picking; ~ хло́пка, ча́я cótton, tea pícking; ~ виногра́да grápe-gathering; 3. (*общее количество чего-л. собранного*) yield; валово́й ~ зерна́ gross grain yield; 4. (*взимаемые или собранные деньги*) dúty; dues *pl*; тамо́женный ~ cústoms dúties *pl*; 5. (*выручка от прода́жи биле́тов*) bóx-office tákings *pl*; (*на стадио́не и т. п.*) gátemoney; по́лный ~ (*в теа́тре и т. п.*) full house; де́лать ~ы (*о пье́се*) be* dóing well; де́лать по́лные ~ы play to full hóuses; 6. (*людей*) assémbly; ~ на демонстра́цию assémbly for those táking part in the demonstrátion; ме́сто ~а assémbly point; вре́мя ~а time of assémbly; 7. (*собрание*) gáthering, méeting; 8. *мн.* (*приготовле́ния*) preparátions; 9. *воен.* (*periódical*) tráining; ◇ все в ~е éveryone's here, all are assémbled.

сбо́рище *с. разг.* 1. crowd, assémblage; 2. (*схо́дка*) gáthering.

сбо́рка I *ж.* (*монта́ж*) assémbly; ~ станка́ assémbly of a lathe; ~ домо́в assémbly of búildings.

сбо́рка II *ж.* (*мелкая скла́дка на одежде*) pleat; *мн.* gáthers.

сбо́рная *ж.* combíned team/side; ю́ношеская ~ Москвы́ combíned Móscow youth team; all-Móscow youth team; ~ Украи́ны the Ukraine team.

сбо́рник *м.* colléction; (*стихо́в*) anthólogy; ~ зада́ч book of (mathemátical) próblems.

сбо́рн|ый 1. (*явля́ющийся ме́стом сбо́ра*) assémbly *attr.*, rállying; ~ пункт assémbly point; 2. (*состоя́щий из лиц, со́бранных из ра́зных мест*) combíned; ~ая кома́нда combíned team/side; ~ отря́д combíned detáchment; 3. (*состоя́щий из разноро́дных часте́й, элеме́нтов*) miscelláneous; scratch *разг.*; ~ая програ́мма miscelláneous prógramme; 4. (*собира́емый из часте́й*) pre-fábricated; ~ дом pre-fábricated/assémbly-line house; ~ые железобето́нные констру́кции pre-fábricated reinfórced cóncrete élements.

сборочн|ый assémbly *attr.*; ~ые рабóты assémbly work *sg*; ~ конвéйер assémbly line; ~ цех assémbly shop/room.

сбóрщик *м.* 1. colléctor; ~ хлóпка cótton pícker; 2. *mex.* fítter, assémbly wórker.

сбрáсывать, **сбрóсить** (*вн.*) 1. (*бросáть вниз*) throw* (*smth.*) down; ~ что-л. с грузовикá на зéмлю throw* *smth.* out of a lórry on to the ground; ~ бóмбы drop bombs; ~ снег с крыши clear a roof of snow; сбрóсить с себя нóшу throw*/fling* down *one's* búrden; сбрóсить седокá (*о лóшади*) throw* its ríder; ~ протúвника в рéку *воен.* hurl the énemy into the ríver; 2. (*свергáть*) overthrów* (*smb., smth.*); сбрóсить úго cast*/throw* off the yoke; 3. *разг.* (*снимáть с себя*) shed* (*smth.*), throw* off (*smth.*); сбрóсить пальтó throw* off *one's* coat; сбрóсить с себя кóжу (*о змее*) shed* its skin; ◇ сбрóсить со счетóв disregárd; ~ся, сбрóситься throw* onesélf down; (*с рд.*) throw* onesélf (off).

сбривáть, **сбрить** (*вн.*) shave* off (*smth.*).

сбрить *сов. см.* сбривáть.

сброд *м. собир. разг.* ríff-raff, rábble.

сбрóсить(ся) *сов. см.* сбрáсывать(ся).

сброшюровáть *сов. см.* брошюровáть.

сбрýя *ж.* hárness.

сбывáть, **сбыть** (*вн.*) 1. (*продавáть*) sell* (*smth.*); 2. *разг.* (*отдéлываться от когó-л., чегó-л.*) get* rid (of).

сбывáться, **сбыться** come* true; надéжды сбылись *one's* hopes came true.

сбыт *м.* sale; рынок ~а márket; находúть ~ find* a márket, be* in demánd.

сбыть *сов. см.* сбывáть.

сбыться *сов. см.* сбывáться.

свáдебный wédding *attr.*

свáдьб|а *ж.* wédding; сыгрáть ~у célebrate a wédding.

свáйн|ый pile *attr.*; ~ые опóры мостá bridge piles; ~ мóлот píle-driver; ~ые пострóйки píle-buildings.

свáливать, **свалúть** (*вн.*) 1. knock (*smb., smth.*) down; вéтер свалúл дéрево the wind knocked down a tree; свалúть с ног knock *smb.* off his, her feet; пýля свалúла егó he was struck down by a búllet; 2. (*сбрáсывать что-л. тяжёлое*) dump (*smth.*), throw* (*smth.*) down; *перен.* cast* aside (*smth.*); свалúть нóшу с плеч throw* down *one's* búrden; свалúть дровá с грузовикá throw* firewood out of a lórry; свалúть с себя хлóпоты cast* aside *one's* wórries; 3. (*вн. на вн.*) *разг.* (*перекладывать на когó-л.*) shift (*smth.* on to), push (*smth.* on to); он свалúл все делá на меня he pushed all the work on to me; онú свалúли винý на негó they threw/shifted the blame on to him; 4. (*беспорядочно склáдывать в однó мéсто*) dump (*smth.*), chuck (*smth.*) down; ~ что-л. в кýчу dump *smth.* in a heap, pile up *smth.*; ◇ свалúть лес fell tímber; свалúть с больнóй головы на здорóвую blame sómebody else for *one's* own tróubles; ~ся, свалúться 1. (*пáдать*) fall*; (*валúться, обрушиваться*) collápse, tópple; свалúться с крыши fall* off a roof; дéрево мягко свалúлось в сугрóб the tree tóppled géntly into a snówdrift; 2. *разг.* (*заболéвать*) fall* ill.

свалúть *сов. см.* свáливать *и* валúть I. ~ся *сов. см.* свáливаться.

свáлка *ж.* 1. (*мýсора*) dúst-heap; 2. *разг.* (*дрáка*) scúffle, tússle.

свалять *сов. см.* валять 3.

сваляться *сов.* be*/becóme* mátted.

свáривать, **сварúть** (*вн.*) *mex.* weld (*smth.*). ~ся, свáриваться *mex.* weld, be* wélded.

сварúть(ся) *сов. см.* варúть(ся) *и* свáривать(ся).

свáрка *ж. mex.* wélding.

сварлúвый cantánkerous, quárrelsome; (*о жéнщине*) shréwish.

сварн|óй *mex.* wélded; ~áя констрýкция wélded strúcture.

свáр|очный wélding *attr.* ~щик *м.* wélder.

свáтаться, **посвáтаться** (к *дт.*, за *вн.*) propóse (to), ask (*smb.*) to márry one.

свáя *ж.* pile.

свéдени|е *с.* 1. (*извéстие, сообщéние о чём-л.*) piece/item of informátion; *мн.* informátion *sg*; 2. *мн.* (*знáния*) knówledge *sg*; элементáрные ~я по фúзике elementáry knówledge of phýsics; 3.: принимáть что-л. к ~ю make* a note of *smth.*; до нáшего ~я дошлó... it has come to our nótice...; доводúть до чегó-л. ~я bring* to *smb.'s* nótice, nótify *smb.*; довожý до вáшего ~я, что... I have to infórm you that...; ◇ к вáшему ~ю *в знач. вводн. сл.* for your informátion.

свéдущий well-infórmed; (*в какóй-л. óбласти*) well-vérsed (in), expérienced (in).

свежевáть, **освежевáть** (*вн.*) flay (*smth.*), skin (*smth.*).

свежезамóроженный quick-frozen.

свéжест|ь *ж.* fréshness; (*прохлáда*) cool, cóolness; ◇ не пéрвой ~и 1) not véry fresh; 2) (*об одéжде*) not véry clean.

свеж|éть, **посвежéть** 1. get* chílly; на ýлице ~éет it is gétting chílly; вéтер ~éет the wind is fréshening; 2. (*о человéке*) look frésher/bétter, feel* bétter/fítter.

свéж|ий 1. fresh; ~ее мясо fresh meat; ~ хлеб new/fresh bread; ~ие нóвости fresh news; the látest news; со ~ими сúлами with renéwed vígour; 2. (*прохлáдный*) cool; (*холóдный*) chílly, cold; ◇ ~б в пáмяти fresh in *smb.'s* mémory; на ~ую гóлову сдéлать что-л. do* *smth.* when *one's* brain is fresh.

свежó 1. *нареч.* fresh(ly); cóolly; 2. *в знач. сказ. безл.* it is cool; it is chílly; здесь ~ it is chílly (in) here.

свезтú I *сов. см.* свозúть I.

свезтú II *сов.* (*вн.*; *отвезтú и привезтú обрáтно*) take (*smth.*) (and bring* him, her back).

свёкла *ж.* 1. (*растéние*) beet(s); 2. *собир.* (*съедóбные кóрни*) béetroot; ◇ кормовáя ~ mángel-wúrzel; сáхарная ~ súgar-beet.

свеклóви|ца *ж.* beet, súgar-beet. ~чный beet *attr.* (*относящийся к разведéнию свеклóвицы*) béet-growing; ~чный сáхар beet súgar.

свекловóд|ство *с.* (súgar-)beet grówing. ~ческий béet-growing *attr.*

свеклокопáтель *м.* beet hárvester.

свеклоубóрочный béet-harvesting *attr.*; ~ комбáйн beet cómbine.

свекóльн|ик *м.* 1. (*ботвá*) béet-leaves *pl*; 2. (*суп*) béetroot soup (*made from beetroot and beet-leaves*). ~ый béetroot *attr.*

свёкор *м.* fáther-in-law (*pl* fáthers-) (*husband's father*).

свекрóвь *ж.* móther-in-law (*pl* móthers-) (*husband's mother*).

свергáть, **свéргнуть** (*вн.*) overthrów* (*smb., smth.*); ◇ свéргнуть úго чегó-л. throw*/cast* off the yoke of *smth.*

свéргнуть *сов. см.* свергáть.

свержéние *с.* óverthrow.

свéр|ить *сов. см.* сверять. ~ка *ж.* chécking; (*тéкста тж.*) collátion.

сверк|áть, **сверкнýть** spárkle, flash; ослепúтельно ~ glare; егó глазá ~áют от рáдости his eyes spárkle with joy; он гнéвно сверкнýл глазáми his eyes flashed ángrily; мóлния ~нýла there was a flash of líghtning.

сверкнýть *сов. см.* сверкáть.

сверлúль|ный drílling; ~ станóк drílling machine. ~щик *м.* dríller.

сверл|úть *несов.* (*вн.*) 1. drill (*smth.*), bore (*smth.*); ~ зуб *разг.* drill a tooth*; 2. (*пристáльно вглядывати-*

ся): он ~и́л меня́ глаза́ми his eyes seemed to go right through me.

сверло́ с. *тех.* drill.

сверло́вщик м. driller.

сверля́щий 1. (*о боли и т.п.*) gnáwing; 2. (*о звуке*) shrill, píercing.

сверну́ть(ся) *сов. см.* свёртывать(ся).

сверста́ть *сов. см.* верста́ть.

сверстн|**ик** м., **~ица** ж.: он мой ~ he's just my age; мы, они́ ~ики, ~ицы we, they are just the same age.

свёрток м. búndle, pácket.

свёртывание с. 1. (*скатывание*) rólling up; 2. (*ограничение производства и т. п.*) curtáilment, discontínuing; (*временное прекращение*) témporary clósure; 3. (*молока*) túrning, cúrdling; (*крови*) coagulátion, cúrdling.

свёртывать, **сверну́ть** 1. (*вн.; скатывать трубкой*) roll (smth.) up; (*о листьях, лепестках*) close (smth.), fold (smth.); сверну́ть ковёр roll up a cárpet; сверну́ть папиро́су roll a cigarétte; 2. (*вн.; сокращать, ограничивать*) curtáil (smth.), discontínue (smth.); (*временно прекращать*) témporarily close (smth.); сверну́ть произво́дство cut* down prodúction; 3. (*повёртывать куда-л.*) turn; сверну́ть с доро́ги turn off the road; сверну́ть нале́во turn left; ◇ программы голову́; сверну́ть кому́-л. ◇ wring* smb.'s neck. ~ся, сверну́ться 1. curl up, roll up; (*о змее*) coil up; ~ся клубко́м roll onesélf into a ball; curl up in a ball; 2. (*о молоке*) turn, cúrdle; (*о крови*) coágulate, cúrdle; 3. (*сокращаться*) be* redúced/ curtáiled/discontínued; (*временно прекращать свою деятельность*) témporarily close down.

сверх 1. (*поверх чего-л.*) óver; 2. (*помимо, кроме чего-л.*) in addítion to; ~ програ́ммы in addítion to the prógramme; 3. (*выше, более чего-л.*) beyónd; рабо́тать ~ сил work beyónd one's strength; ~ пла́на óver and abóve the plan; 4. (*вопреки чему-л.*) cóntrary to; ~ ожида́ний beyónd all expectátion.

сверх- *в сложн.* súper-, últra-.

сверхзвуков|**о́й** *физ.* supersónic; полёты на ~ых ско́ростях flights at supersónic speeds.

сверхмо́щный superpówerful.

сверхни́зк|**ий** véry/éxtra low; ~ие температу́ры véry low témperatures.

сверхпла́нов|**ый** in excess of plan *после сущ*, óver and abóve the plan *после сущ*; ~ые накопле́ния accumulátions in excéss of plan.

сверхпри́быль ж. *эк.* superprófits *pl*, excess prófits *pl*.

сверхсекре́тный tóp-secret.

сверхскоростно́й superfást.

сверхсро́чн|**ый** 1.: ~ая вое́нная слу́жба re-enlístment; оста́ться на ~ую (вое́нную) слу́жбу stay on as a re-enlísted man*; 2. *разг.* (*крайне спешный*) éxtra úrgent.

све́рху 1. from abóve; (*считая сверху*) from the top; 2. (*наверху*) on top; ◇ смотре́ть на кого́-л. ~ вниз look down on smb.; ~ до́низу 1) from top to bóttom; 2) (*от верховья до устья реки*) throughóut its length.

сверхуро́чн|**о** óvertime; рабо́тать ~ work óvertime. ~ый прил. 1. óvertime attr.; 2. *в знач. сущ. мн.* óvertime (pay) *sg*.

сверхшта́тный supernúmerary.

сверхъесте́ственный supernátural.

сверчо́к м. cricket.

сверя́ть, **све́рить** (*вн.*) check (smth.); (*текст тж.*) collàte (smth.).

све́сить *сов.*: ~ но́ги let* one's feet dángle; он сиде́л све́сив но́ги he sat there, his feet dángling.

све́ситься *сов.* 1. (*повиснуть*) dángle; 2. (*наклониться*) overháng*; (*о человеке*) lean* óver.

свести́ I *сов. см.* своди́ть I.

свести́ II *сов. разг. см.* своди́ть II.

свести́сь *сов. см.* своди́ться.

свет I м. light; при ~е луны́, свечи́ by the light of the moon, cándle; ско́рость ~а velócity of light; встать спино́й к ~у stand* with one's back to the light; ◇ чуть ~, ни ~ ни заря́ at dáybreak; пролива́ть ~ на что́-л. throw*/shed* light on smth.; в ~е чего́-л. in the light of smth.; ви́деть всё в друго́м ~е take* one's own pecúliar view of things; предста́вить что́-л. в вы́годном ~е put* smth. in a fávourable light, displáy smth. to advántage; невзви́деть ~а от чего́-л. be* half blínded by smth.

свет II м. 1. (*мир*) the world; по всему́ ~у all the world óver, all óver the world; 2. (*общество*) socíety, world; э́то всему́ ~у изве́стно éveryone knows that; ◇ появля́ться на ~ be* born; вы́йти в ~ come* out, appéar; всё на ~е the whole wide world; ни за что на ~е not for the world; на том ~е in the next world; сжить кого́-л. со ~а, со ~у drive* smb. to his, her grave; руга́ть кого́-л. на чём ~ сто́ит curse smb. like hell, swear blue múrder at smb.; нет на ~е кого́-л. smb. is gone.

свет|**а́ть** *несов. безл.* ~а́ет day is bréaking; ~а́ло day was bréaking, dáybreak came.

свети́ло с. 1. lúminary; небе́сное ~ celéstial/héavenly bódy; 2. (*знаменитый человек*) lúminary, a great/léading light; ~ медици́ны a léading light in médicine.

свети́льник м. líghting applíance.

свет|**и́ть**, посвети́ть 1. *тк. несов.* shine*; 2 (*дт.*) hold* a light (for); ~ кому́-л. фонарём hold* a lántern for smb. ~и́ться *несов.* 1. shine* (*быть освещённым*) be* líghted; 2. (*выделяться белизной*) show*, show* through; 3. (*тв.; выражать — о лице, глазах*) shine* (with), glow (with); её лицо́ ~и́лось ра́достью her face shone with joy.

свет|**ле́ть**, посветле́ть 1. bríghten up; (*о небе*) get* lighter; (*после дождя*) clear up; его́ взгляд ~е́ет his face clears; 2. *тк. несов.* (*виднеться*) show*.

светло́ 1. *нареч.* bríghtly; 2. *в знач. сказ. безл.* it is light; мне ~ his light enóugh for me.

светло- *в сложн.* light-; светло-голубо́й light-blúe.

светловоло́сый fáir(-háired).

све́тл|**ый** 1. bright, light; ~ день bright day; ~ая ко́мната light/bright room; 2. (*не тёмного цвета*) light-coloured; (*о волосах*) fair; ~ое пла́тье light-coloured dress; 3. (*чистый, прозрачный*) clear; 4. (*радостный*) glad, háppy, rádiant; ~ое чу́вство buóyant féeling, féeling of gládness; ~ое бу́дущее bright fúture; 5. (*умиротворённый, просветлённый*) content, seréne, untróubled; 6. (*прекрасный, благородный*) bright, fine; 7. (*ясный*) lúcid, clear; ~ ум lúcid mind; ~ая голова́ clear head; ◇ ~ый *полигр.* light(-face) type.

светля́к м. *зоол.* fíre-fly, glów-worm.

светов|**о́й** light *attr.*; ~а́я волна́ light wave.

светозащи́тн|**ый**: ~ые очки́ protéctive glásses/ góggles.

светоко́пия ж. print; си́няя ~ blúe-print.

светолече́ние с. photothérapy, light thérapy.

светолюби́вый *бот.* líght-demanding.

светомаскиро́вка ж. bláck-out.

светонепроница́емый líght-proof.

светоте́нь ж. *жив.* chiaroscúro.

светоте́хника ж. líghting enginéering.

светофи́льтр м. *физ.* ray fílter, light fílter.

светофо́р м. tráffic lights *pl*; ж.-д. cólour-light sígnal.

све́точ м. *книжн.* lúminary, léading light.

светочувстви́тельн|**ый** líght-sensitive; ~ая бума́га photográphic páper.

све́тск|**ий** 1. fáshionable; ~ое о́бщество (high) socíety; ~ челове́к man* of fáshion; ~ие мане́ры corréct mánners; ~ разгово́р políte conversátion; 2. (*не церковный*) secúlar, lay.

светя́щийся lúminous.

свеч|а́ ж. 1. cándle; 2. (единица измерения силы света) cándle(-power); ла́мпочка в пятьдеся́т ~е́й fífty cándle(-power) bulb; 3. тех. plug; запа́льная ~ spárk(ing) plug; 4. (взлёт мяча) lób-shot, skýer.

свече́ние с. luminéscence, phosphoréscence; fluoréscence.

све́чка ж. см. свеча́ 1, 3, 5.

све́шать сов. см. ве́шать II.

свива́ть, свить (вн.) 1. (соединять, скручивая) twist (smth.), plait (smth.); 2. (изготовлять, скручивая) make* (smth.); свить гнездо́ build* a nest; 3. (свёртывать трубкой) roll (smth.), roll (smth.) up. ~ся, сви́ться coil; roll up.

свида́н|ие с. 1. méeting, ínterview; (влюблённых) réndezvous; date амер. разг.; назнача́ть кому́-л. ~ fix/make* an appóintment with smb.; 2. (в тюрьме и т. п.) vísit; ◇ до ~ия! goodbýe!; до ско́рого ~ия! see you soon!

свиде́те|ль м., ~льница ж. wítness; ~ защи́ты, обвине́ния wítness for the defénce, prosecútion; брать, призыва́ть кого́-л. в ~и call smb. to wítness; быть ~лем чего́-л. wítness smth.; be* the wítness of smth.

свиде́тельск|ий: ~ие показа́ния téstimony sg.

свиде́тельство с. 1. (показание) téstimony; 2. (доказательство) évidence; 3. (документ) certíficate; ~ о рожде́нии, сме́рти, бра́ке birth, death, márriage certíficate.

свиде́тельствовать несов. 1. (о пр.) (подтверждать) téstify (to); bear* téstimony (to); (рассказывать) show* (smth.); 2. (давать свидетельские показания) give* évidence, téstify; (официально подтверждать) affírm; 3. (вн.; удостоверять подлинность чего-л.) wítness (smth.).

свина́рка ж. píg-tender.

свина́рник м. pígsty; pígpen амер.

свине́ц м. lead.

сви́нина ж. pork.

сви́нка I ж. small pig; ◇ морска́я ~ guínea-pig.

сви́нка II ж. (болезнь) mumps.

свиново́д м. píg-breeder. ~ство с. píg-breeding. ~ческий píg-breeding attr.; ~ческая фе́рма píg-breeding farm.

свин|о́й pig attr.; (из свинины) pork attr.; ~а́я ко́жа pígskin; ~о́е ры́ло snout; ~ хлев pígsty; ~а́я отбивна́я (котлета) pórk-chop.

свинома́тка ж. с.-х. bróod-sow.

свинофе́рма ж. píggery.

свин|ский разг. 1. (грязный, невежественный) squálid; 2. (низкий, подлый) foul, disgústing, swínish. ~ство с. разг. 1. (грязь, беспорядок) squálor, filth; 2. (низкий поступок) foul/swínish/dírty trick; како́е ~ство! how mean!

свинцо́в|ый 1. lead attr.; перен. léaden; ~ сли́ток bar of lead; ~ взгляд léaden/bróoding stare; 2. (о цвете) léaden; ~ые ту́чи léaden clouds.

свинь|я́ ж. 1. pig; hog амер.; (самка) sow; 2. разг. (о человеке) pig, swíne; ◇ подложи́ть ~ю́ кому́-л. play a dírty/mean trick on smb.

свире́ль ж. reed (-pipe).

свирепе́ть, рассвирепе́ть grow* sávage/fúrious; сов. тж. fly* ínto a rage.

свире́пость ж. ferócity, fíerceness; (бури и т. п.) fúry.

свире́пствовать несов. 1. wreak one's fúry, spread* térror; 2. (о стихийном бедствии и т. п.) rage, play hávoc; (о болезнях и т. п. тж.) be* rife, be* rámpant.

свире́пый 1. (кровожадный) ferócious; 2. (злобный, жестокий) sávage; 3. (выражающий злобу) ferócious; 4. (очень сильный в своём проявлении) fierce.

свиса́ть несов. hang* down; (о полях шляпы, ветвях и т. п.) droop.

свист м. whistle, whístling; ◇ худо́жественный ~ cóncert whístling.

свиста́ть, свисте́ть несов. whistle; (о птицах тж.) pipe; (о пуле) whistle, whine.

сви́стнуть сов. give* a whistle.

свисто́к м. whístle.

сви́та ж. suite, rétinue.

сви́тер м. swéater, púllover.

сви́ток м. roll, scroll.

свить сов. см. вить и свива́ть. ~ся сов. см. свива́ться.

свихну́ться сов. разг. 1. (помешаться) be*/go* nuts; 2. (сбиться с правильного пути) go* wrong, go* astráy.

свия́зь ж. зоол. widgeon.

свобо́д|а ж. freedom, líberty; ~ сло́ва, печа́ти, собра́ний, сою́зов fréedom of speech, the press, assémbly, associátion; предоставля́ть кому́-л. ~у вы́бора, де́йствий give* smb. a free hand; выпусти́ть кого́-л. на ~у reléase smb., set* smb. free; на ~е at líberty, at large; (на досуге) at one's ease, at one's léisure.

свобо́дно 1. нареч. (легко) éasily; ~ говори́ть по-францу́зски speak* French flúently; держа́ться ~ beháve náturally; 2. нареч. (просторно — об одежде): сиде́ть ~ fit lóosely, be* loose; 3. в знач. сказ. безл.; в ваго́не бы́ло ~ there was plénty of room in the cárriage.

свобо́д|ный 1. free; (непринуждённый) nátural, éasy; ~ наро́д free péople; ~ная жизнь life of fréedom; ~ челове́к free man*; ~ное дыха́ние éasy bréathing; 2. (незанятый) free; (о месте и т. п. тж.) vácant, disengáged; (о деньгах, времени) spare; to spare после сущ.; э́то ме́сто ~но? is this seat free?, is this seat engáged?; тут мно́го ~ных мест there are plénty of seats here; телефо́н ~ен no one is úsing the télephone; ~ные де́ньги spare cash sg; ~ное от заня́тий вре́мя spare time; у меня́ не быва́ет ни одно́й ~ной мину́ты I néver have a free móment; 3. (не представляющий препятствия) clear; 4. (незаполненный) uncrówded; ~ трамва́й uncrówded tram; 5. (об одежде) loose, éasy-fítting; 6.: кни́га не ~на от недоста́тков the book is not withóut faults.

свободолюби́вый fréedom-loving.

свод м. 1. (совокупность текстов и т. п.) táble, súmmary; ~ зако́нов státute-book; 2. архит. vault; (моста) arch; (печи) crown.

своди́ть I, свести́ (вн.) 1. (вести вниз) take* (smb.) down; (поддерживая) help (smb.) down; 2. (соединять) bring* (smth.) togéther; ~ что-л. в табли́цу tábulate smth.; 3. (доводить до чего-л.) redúce (smth.); ~ что-л. к ми́нимуму redúce smth. to a mínimum, bring* smth. down to a mínimum; ~ разгово́р на что-л., к чему́-л. turn the conversátion to smth.; ~ всё к шу́тке treat éverything as a joke; 4. (удалять) remóve (smth.); (пятно тж.) take* (smth.) out; 5. (судорогой): у него́ свело́ но́гу he has cramp in his leg; 6. разг. (рисунок) trace (smth.); ◇ ~ счёты с кем-л. séttle scores with smb., square accóunts with smb.; ~ концы́ с конца́ми make* both ends meet; не ~ глаз с кого-л., чего-л. not take one's eyes off smb., smth.; ~ кого-л. с ума́ drive* smb. mad.

своди́ть II сов. (вн.; отвести и привести обратно) take* (smb.) (and bring*) him, her back.

своди́ться, свести́сь (к дт.) come* (to); boil down (to) разг.; ~ к нулю́ come* to naught; ~ к одному́ и тому́ же come* to the same thing.

сво́дка ж. súmmary, repórt, súrvey; ~ пого́ды wéather súmmary, wéather-repórt.

сво́дн|ый 1. (объединяющий какие-л. данные) consólidated; ~ отчёт consólidated repórt, súmmary; 2. (составленный из нескольких самостоятельных единиц) combíned; ~ орке́стр combíned órchestra; 3. (о родстве) step-; ~ брат stépbrother; ~ая сестра́ stépsister.

сводчатый váulted.

своё см. свой.

своеволие с. self-will.

своевольный self-willed, héadstrong.

своевременн|о in good time. ~ый tímely, ópportune.

своенрав|ие с. wílfulness, wáywardness. ~ный self-willed, wílful, wáyward.

своеобраз|ие с. peculiárity, distínguishing féature; (*оригинальность*) originálity. ~ный 1. pecúliar, síngular; (*оригинальный*) original; ~ная прелесть spécial/uníque charm, charm of *one's* own; 2. (*своего рода, как бы*) a kind of.

свозить I, **свезти** (*вн.*) 1. (*в одно место*) bring* (*smth.*) togéther; 2. (*вниз*) bring* (*smb., smth.*) down (from); 3. (*увозить*) take* (*smth.*) awáy; свезти хлеб с поля cart the grain.

свозить II *сов. см.* свезти II.

свой см. свой.

сво|й, **своя**, **своё**, **свои** *притяж. мест.* 1. *переводится в зависимости от лица, числа и рода* my, pl our; your; his, her, its, pl their; *неопр.* one's; (*собственный*) one's own; он признал ~ю ошибку he admitted his mistáke; у меня есть ~ экземпляр I have a cópy of my own; 2. *в знач. сущ. с.* one's own; стоять на ~ём stick* to *one's* guns идиом.; настоять на ~ём insíst on háving *one's* own way; получить ~ё get* *one's* due; (*по заслугам*) get* *one's* desérts; 3. *в знач. сущ. мн.* (*родные*) one's péople; (*друзья*) friends; ◇ в ~ём роде in his, her, its way; сам не ~ not *onesélf*; сам не ~ от *чего-л.* crázy with *smth.*; брать ~ё have* its efféct, take* its toll; годы берут ~ё the years are táking their toll; сказáть ~ё слово make* *one's* mark; идти ~ей дорогой go* *one's* own way; рассказáть ~ими словами tell* in *one's* own words; умерéть ~ей смертью die a nátural death.

свойственн|ый characterístic; со ~ой ему искренностью он... with characterístic sincérity he...; это ему ~о that's his way; человéку ~о ошибáться to err is húman; не ~ кому-л. uncharacterístic of *smb.*, unúsual for *smb.*; это ему не ~о it's not like him; зависть ему не ~а it's not in his náture to énvy ányone.

свойство с. characterístic; (*достоинство тж.*) quálity; *физ., хим.* próperty.

свойство с. márriage relátionship; affínity.

свора ж. 1. *собир.* (*охотничьи собаки одного хозяина*) team; 2. *собир.* (*стая собак, волков и т. п.*) pack (*тж. перен.*).

сворачивать, **своротить** (*вн.*) *разг.* 1. (*сдвигать*) move (*smth.*), heave* (*smth.*); 2. см. свёртывать 1, 2.

своротить *сов. см.* сворáчивать.

своя см. свой.

своя|к м. bróther-in-law (*pl* bróthers-) (*husband of wife's sister*). ~ченица ж. sister-in-law (*pl* sísters-) (*wife's sister*).

свыкáться, **свыкнуться** (с *тв.*) get* accústomed/used (to), hábituate *onesélf* (to); свыкнуться с мыслью, что... get* used to the idea that...

свыкнуться *сов. см.* свыкáться.

свысокá háughtily; смотрéть на *кого-л.*, относиться к *кому-л.* ~ look down on *smb.*

свыше 1. *нареч.* from abóve; 2. *предлог* (*рд.*) óver; (*сверх*) in excéss of; ~ ста человéк more than a húndred péople; это ~ мойх сил it is beyónd my pówers, it is more than I can do.

связанн|ый 1. (*соединённый*) connécted, reláted; 2. *хим.* combíned, fixed; 3. *физ.* látent.

связáть *сов. см.* связывать и вязáть 1, 2. ~ся *сов. см.* связываться.

связист м. communicátions enginéer; *воен.* sígnaller.

связка ж. 1. búndle; ~ ключéй bunch of keys; ~ книг búndle of books; 2. *анат.* c(h)ord, cópula; 3. *грам.* cópula.

связни́к м. *разг. см.* связнóй 3.

связн|ой *прил.* 1. liáison *attr.*; dispátch *attr.*; 2. *в знач. сущ. м.* méssenger; 3. *в знач. сущ. м.* (*в развéдке*) go-betwéen, cóurier ágent.

связн|ость ж. cohérence. ~ый cohérent; ~ая речь cohérent speech.

связующ|ий connécting; ~ее вещество bónding ágent, adhésive; ~ее звенó connécting link.

связывать, **связáть** 1. (*вн.; скреплять концы чего-л.*) tie (*smth.*) togéther, knot (*smth.*); ~ узлóм knot the ends togéther; 2. (*вн.; скреплять предметы*) tie (*smth.*) up, bind* (*smth.*); ~ что-л. в узел make* a búndle of *smth.*; ~ свои вéщи make* a búndle of *one's* things; ~ что-л. в один пакéт make* one párcel of *smth.*; 3. (*вн.; спутывать*) bind* (*smb., smth.*); *перен. тж.* tie (*smb.*) down, restríct (*smb., smth.*); связáть престýпника bind* the críminal; связáть когó-л. обещáнием take* a prómise from *smb.*; 4. (*вн.; устанáвливать сообщéние*) link up (*smth.*), connéct (*smth.*); 5. (*вн. с тв.; устанáвливать связь с кем-л., чем-л.*) put* (*smb.*) in touch (with); 6. (*вн.; сближáть когó-л.*) bind* (*smb.*) togéther; судьбá их связáла fate had bound them togéther; 7. (*вн.; объединять, соединять*) uníte (*smth.*); 8. (*вн. с тв.; сочетáть*) combíne (*smth.* with); 9. (*вн.; устанáвливать зависимость*) connéct (*smth.*), link (*smth.*); ◇ связáть свою судьбý с кем-л. throw* in *one's* lot with *smb.*; ~ когó-л. по рукáм и ногáм tie *smb.'s* hands; связáть себé рýки tie *one's* hands, tie *onesélf.* ~ся, связáться (с *тв.*) 1. tie themsélves togéther; 2. (*устанáвливать общéние*) get* in touch/cóntact (with); (*по телефóну, по рáдио*) get* through (to); радистка связáлась с бáзой и передалá радиогрáмму the wíreless óperator called up base and sent a méssage; связáться с рабóчими крýпного завóда get* in touch with wórkers at a big fáctory; 3. *разг.* (*сближáться*) take* up (with); лýчше с ним не ~ся bétter have nóthing whatéver to do with him; 4. *разг.* (*брáться за что-л. трýдное*) get* invólved (in, with).

связ|ь ж. 1. (*взаимная зависимость*) connéction, cóntact; ~ тeóрии и прáктики the connéction betwéen théory and práctice; 2. (*общéние*) relátion, cóntact; (*узы*) ties *pl*; ~ с мáссами cóntact with the másses; дрýжеская ~ friendly relátions *pl*; деловые ~и búsiness relátions; торгóвые ~и мéжду стрáнами trade relátions betwéen cóuntries; потерять ~ с кем-л. lose* touch/cóntact with *smb.*; держáть ~ с кем-л. keep* in touch with *smb.*; 3. *мн.* (*знакóмые*) connéctions; 4. (*любóвная*) liáison; 5. (*срéдства сообщéния*) communicátion; *воен.* íntercommunicátion; sígnals *pl*; министéрство ~и Mínistry of Communicátions; отделéние ~и póst-and--télegraph óffice; 6. *mex.* tie; cóupling; ◇ в ~и с чем-л. in connéction with *smth.*; (*вслéдствие*) ówing to *smth.*; в ~и с этим, в этой ~и in this connéction; выходить на ~ make* cóntact.

святилище с. (*рд.*) shrine (of).

свято réverently; ~ соблюдáть что-л. scrúpulously obsérve *smth.*; ~ хранить пáмять о ком-л. hold* the mémory of *smb.* sácred.

свят|ой *прил.* 1. hóly; (*перед именем*) Saint; (*священный*) sácred; для негó нет ничегó ~óго nóthing is sácred to him; 2. *в знач. сущ. м.* saint.

святость ж. sánctity.

святотáтство с. sácrilege.

свя́точный Chrístmas *attr.*; ~ рассказ Chrístmas stóry.

святóша м. и ж. prig, hýpocrite.

святыня ж. sácred thing; (*место*) sácred place; *перен. тж.* sácred posséssion.

священн|ик м. priest; (*протестáнтский*) clérgyman*. ~ый sácred; *рел.* hóly; ~ая войнá hóly war; ~ый долг sácred dúty.

сгиб м. bend; ~ лóктя crook of *one's* arm; ~ колéна knee(-joint); ~ газéты crease/fold of a néwspaper.

сгибáть, **согнýть** (*вн.*) bend* (*smth.*); (*склáдывать*) fold (smth.); перен. bow (smb.); ~ пáльцы bend* one's fingers; гóды согнýли егó the years have bowed his shóulders; несчáстья (не) согнýли егó his misfórtunes have (not) brought him low. ~ся, согнýться bend*; ~ся под тя́жестью чего-л. bend*/sag benéath the weight of smth., be* weighed down by smth.

сглáдить(ся) сов. см. сглáживать(ся).

сглáживать, сглáдить (вн.) 1. (делать гладким) smooth (smth.) out; 2. (уничтожать, разглаживая) smooth awáy (smth.); ~ морщи́ны smooth awáy wrínkles; 3. (смягчать, ослаблять) smooth óver (smth.); ~ проти́воречия smooth óver contradíctions. ~ся, сглáдиться 1. (становиться гладким) smooth out; 2. (становиться незаметным, исчезать) wear* off.

сгнить сов. см. гнить.

сгноить сов. см. гноить.

сговáриваться, сговори́ться (с тв.) 1. (условливаться) arránge (with); сговори́ться с кем-л. о встрéче arránge a méeting with smb., arránge to meet smb.; 2. (достигать взаимного понимания) come* to an understánding (with), reach an understánding (with).

сгóвор м. (договорённость) understánding; (тайный) conspíracy; быть в ~е с кем-л. be* in league/collúsion with smb.

сговори́ться сов. см. сговáриваться.

сговóрчивый complíant, plíable.

сгонять, согнáть (вн.) 1. (с места) drive* (smb., smth.) out/awáy; согнáть мýху brush awáy a fly; 2. (удалять) remóve (smth.); согнáть веснýшки remove fréckles; 3. (в одно место) drive* (smth.) together, round up (smth.); согнáть стáдо на опýшку round up a herd on the edge of the wood.

сгорáние с. combústion.

сгорáть, сгорéть 1. burn*; перен. wear* onesélf out; дом сгорéл the house was burnt down; самолёт сгорéл the plane burned up; дровá сгорéли the wood burned out/awáy; 2. (высыхать — о растительности) wíther, shrível; 3. (преть, гнить) rot, be* ruined/spoiled; 4. (от рд.) испытывать сильные чувства) burn* (with); ~ со стыдá burn* with shame.

сгорб|ить(ся) сов. см. гóрбить(ся). ~ленный hunched, cróoked.

сгорéть сов. см. сгорáть и горéть I.

сгорячá in the heat of the móment.

сгребáть, сгрести́ (вн.) (лопатой) shóvel (smth.); (граблями) rake (smth.); (руками) gáther (smth.) up.

сгрести́ сов. см. сгребáть.

сгружáть, сгрузи́ть (вн.) unlóad (smth.).

сгрузи́ть сов. см. сгружáть.

сгруппировáть(ся) сов. см. группировáть(ся).

сгуби́ть сов. см. губи́ть.

сгусти́ть(ся) сов. см. сгущáть(ся).

сгýсток м. 1. clot; перен. concentrátion; 2. физ. clúster, bunch.

сгущ|áть, сгусти́ть (вн.) condénse (smth.); ◇ ~ крáски pile it on, exággerate; ~ атмосфéру creáte a strained átmosphere. ~áться, сгусти́ться 1. thícken; 2. (о сумерках, темноте) déepen; ◇ атмосфéра ~áется the plot thíckens.

сгущённ|ый: ~ое молокó condénsed milk.

сдавáть, сдать 1. (вн.; передавать) hand (smth.) óver; (о продуктах труда) hand (smth.) in, delíver (smth.); ~ делá кому-л. turn óver one's dúties to smb.; сдать станóк в отли́чном состоя́нии hand óver the lathe in excellent condition; ~ что-л. в эксплуатáцию make* smth. aváilable; сдать хлеб госудáрству delíver grain to the State; 2. (вн.; отдавать, помещать куда-л.) hand (smth.) in; (возвращать тж.) retúrn (smth.); сдать пальтó на вéшалку put* one's coat in the clóakroom;

сдать кни́гу в библиотéку retúrn a book to the líbrary; сдать орýжие hand in one's wéapons; он сдал ей три рубля́ he gave her three róubles change; 3. (вн.; внаём) let* (smth.); (в аренду) lease (smth.); 4. (вн.; проходить испытания в знаниях, умении что-л. делать) take* (smth.); ~ экзáмены take*/sit* one's examinátions; сдать экзáмены pass one's examinátions; сдать матемáтику pass in mathemátics; ~ нóрмы по плáванию take* a swímming test; 5. (вн.; отдавать неприятелю) surrénder (smth.); ~ гóрод surrénder a town; 6. разг. (слабеть) wéaken, begín* to fail; он си́льно сдал пóсле болéзни he has been véry weak since his íllness; он си́льно сдал за послéднее врéмя he has aged considerably of late; глазá начáли ~ one's sight is fáiling, one's sight is begínning to fail; 7. разг. (портиться) crack up; мотóр сдаёт the éngine is begínning to crack up.

сдавáться, сдáться 1. surrénder, give* onesélf up; 2. (отступать перед трудностями) give* up, give* in; ~ перед невзгóдами give* in when hard pressed; 3. (уступать) give* in, give* way; (на вн.) give* in (to), yield (to).

сдави́ть сов. см. сдáвливать.

сдáвленный (о голосе, крике) chóking.

сдáвливать, сдави́ть (вн.) squeeze (smb., smth.); constríct (smth.).

сдáточный delívery attr.; ~ пункт delívery point.

сдать сов. см. сдавáть.

сдáться сов. см. сдавáться.

сдáч|а ж. 1. (передача) hánding óver; delívery; 2. (внаём) létting, léasing; 3. (капитуляция) surrénder; 4. (деньги) change; получи́ть ~у get* one's change; давáть ~и give* change; перен. give* as good as one gets, ánswer in kind.

сдвиг м. 1. (перемещение) displácement, shift; 2. (улучшение) advánce, pósitive move/devélopment.

сдвигáть, сдви́нуть (вн.) 1. (с места) move (smth.), shift (smth.); сдви́нуть шля́пу на затылок push back one's hat; егó с мéста не сдви́нешь перен. he won't budge; 2. (сближать) bring*/push (smth.) togéther; ~ брóви knit* one's brows. ~ся, сдви́нуться 1. move, budge; не сдви́нуться с мéста make* no héadway; 2. (приближаться друг к другу) come*/draw* togéther, contráct.

сдви́нуть(ся) сов. см. сдвигáть(ся).

сдéлать(ся) сов. см. дéлать(ся).

сдéлк|а ж. deal; bárgain разг.; заключи́ть ~у do*/negótiate a deal; ◇ ~ с сóвестью cómpromise with one's cónscience.

сдéльно: рабóтать ~ do* piece-work.

сдéльно-прогресси́вный progréssive píece-rate(s).

сдéль|ный: ~ная оплáта трудá páyment by the job/piece; ~ная рабóта píece-work. ~щик м. разг. píece-worker. ~щина ж. píece-work.

сдёргивать, сдёрнуть (вн.) jerk (smth.) off, pull (smth.) off.

сдéржанн|о in a resérved mánner; (холодно) cóldly. ~ость ж. restráint, self-contról. ~ый 1. resérved; (владéющий собой) self-contrólled; 2. (подавляемый) restráined; ~ое волнéние restráined emótion/excítement.

сдержáть(ся) сов. см. сдéрживать(ся).

сдéрживать, сдержáть (вн.) 1. (противостоять чему-л.) withstánd* (smth.), stand* up (to); сдержáть напóр проти́вника withstánd* the énemy's préssure; 2. (останавливать) restráin (smb., smth.), hold* (smb., smth.) in check, contról (smb., smth.); перен. тж. curb (smth.); ~ лóшадь contról a horse, hold* in a horse; сдержáть себя́ restráin/contról onesélf; сдержáть слóво, обещáние keep* one's word, prómise. ~ся, сдержáться restráin/contról/check onesélf.

сдёрнуть сов. см. сдёргивать.

сдирáть, содрáть (вн.) 1. (снимать верхний слой чего-л.) tear* (smth.) off, rip (smth.) off; содрáть шкýру с медвéдя flay a bear; содрáть корý с дéрева bark/strip a tree; **2.** *разг.* (*царапать кожу*) graze (*smth.*); **3.** *разг.* (*срывать*) snatch (*smth.*) off.

сдо́б|а *ж.* **1.** (*в тесте*) shórtening; **2.** *собир.* (*булки*) fáncy bread; buns *pl.* ~**ный:** ~ная бу́лка bun; ~ное те́сто short pástry.

сдружи́ться *сов.* (с *тв.*) make*/becóme* friends (with.)

сдува́ть, сдуть (*вн.*) blow* (*smth.*) off.

сду́ру *разг.:* он ~ согласи́лся *и т. д.* he was stúpid/daft enóugh to agrée *etc.*

сдуть *сов. см.* сдува́ть.

сё: то и сё this and that; ни то ни сё néither one thing nor the óther; ни с того́ ни с сего́ for no appárent réason.

сеа́нс *м.* **1.** show(ing); (*в кино тж.*) perfórmance; (*у художника*) sítting; ~ одновреме́нной игры́ в ша́хматы display of múlti-board chéss-play; **2.** (*лечения и т. п.*) tréatment, séssion.

себе́ *разг.* just; он ~ идёт вперёд he just walks on; ◇ ничего́ ~! not bad!; та́к ~! só-so!

себе́ *см.* себя́.

себесто́имост|ь *ж. эк.* (prime) cost; по ~и at cost (price); сниже́ние ~и проду́кции cútting/redúction of prodúction costs.

себя́ (*дт., пр.* себе́, *тв.* собо́й, собо́ю) onesélf; заста́вить уважа́ть, люби́ть ~ make* onesélf respécted, loved; он о́чень дово́лен собо́й he is véry pleased with himsélf; ◇ он о́чень хоро́ш собо́й he is véry góod-lóoking; сам собо́й (*самостоятельно*) of itsélf; про ~ **1)** (*еле слышно*) to onesélf; **2)** (*мысленно*) inwardly; не в себе́ out of one's mind; от ~ (*лично*) pérsonally; он у ~ (*дома*) he is in, he is at home; (*в комнате*) he is in his room; принима́ть кого́-л. у ~ (*дома*) recéive *smb.* in one's home; (*в комнате*) recéive *smb.* in one's room; к себе́ (*домой*) home; (*в комнату*) to one's room; пригласи́ть кого́-л. к себе́ invíte *smb.* to come and see one; по себе́ (*по силам*) to suit onesélf; мне не по себе́ **1)** (*нездоровится*) I am out of sorts; **2)** (*неудобно, неловко*) I feel áwkward; от э́того мне ста́ло не по себе́ it made me feel áwkward/unéasy.

себялю́бие *с.* sélfishness, self-lóve, égoism.

сев *м.* sówing; вре́мя ~а séed-time, sówing séason.

се́вер *м.* the north; на ~ (to the) north; к ~у от (to the) north of; на ~е in the north, up north. ~**ный** nórthern*; в ~ном направле́нии in a nórtherly diréction, nórthwards; ~**ный** ве́тер north wind.

североатланти́ческий Nórth-Atlántic.

се́веро-восто́|к *м.* north-éast. ~**чный** north-éastern; в ~чном направле́нии in a north-éasterly diréction; ~**чный** ве́тер north-éast wind, northéaster.

се́веро-за́пад *м.* north-wést. ~**ный** north-wéstern; в ~ном направле́нии in a north-wésterly diréction; ~**ный** ве́тер north-wést wind, northwéster.

северя́нин *м.* nórtherner.

севооборо́т *м. с.-х.* rotátion of crops, crop rotátion.

севрю́га *ж.* sevrúga, stéllate stúrgeon.

сегме́нт *м.* ségment.

сего́дня *нареч.* **1.** todáy; ~ у́тром this mórning; ~ ве́чером this évening; (*после наступления темноты*) tonight; **2.** в знач. сущ. с. нескл. todáy; the présent day; на ~ for todáy; (*в настоящее время*) up to the présent; ◇ не ~-за́втра ány day now.

сего́дняшн|ий *прил.* todáy's; présent-day *attr.;* ◇ жить ~им днём **1)** (*не отрываться от настоящего*) live in the présent; **2)** (*не думая о будущем*) live for the day.

седа́лищный *анат.* sciátic.

седе́ть, поседе́ть go*/turn grey.

седе́ющий gréying; (*с проседью*) grízzled.

седина́ *ж.* **1.** grey hair; **2.** *тк. ед.* (*проседь в мехе*) grey flecks *pl;* **3.** *тк. ед.* (*серовато-белый налёт на чём-л.*) film of grey.

седла́ть, оседла́ть (*вн.*) sáddle (*smth.*).

седло́ *с.* sáddle.

седлови́на *ж.* sáddle.

седоборо́дый grey-béarded.

сед|о́й (*о волосах*) grey, white; (*о человеке*) grey-háired, white-háired; с ~ы́ми виска́ми grey about the témples; ◇ ~а́я старина́ hóary antíquity.

седо́к *м.* **1.** (*всадник, верховой*) ríder; **2.** (*в экипаже*) fare, pássenger.

седьм|о́й the séventh; ◇ быть на ~о́м не́бе be* in the séventh héaven.

сезо́н *м.* séason; (*время созревания чего-л.*) time; быть оде́тым не по ~у be* unsúitably dressed for the time of year. ~**ник** *м.* séasonal wórker. ~**ный 1.** séasonal; ~ные рабо́ты séasonal work *sg;* ~ный рабо́чий séasonal wórker; **2.** (*годный на весь сезон*) séason *attr.;* ~ный биле́т séason-ticket.

сей this; до сего́ вре́мени till this móment; до ~ поры́ up to now; по ~ день, по сию́ по́ру to this day; по сю сто́рону on the near side; ◇ сию́ мину́ту diréctly, just a sécond.

сейм *м.* Seym.

се́йнер *м.* séiner. ~**ный** séiner *attr.*

сейсми́ка *ж.* seismícity.

сейсми́ческий séismic.

сейсмо́граф *м.* séismograph.

сейсмогра́фия *ж.* seismógraphy.

сейсмоло́гия *ж.* seismólogy.

сейф *м.* safe.

сейча́с 1. (*теперь*) now, at présent, at the présent móment; ~ я за́нят I'm busy now; **2.** (*только что, недавно*) just now, a móment agó; он ~ здесь был he was here a móment agó; **3.** (*скоро*) in a móment, just; ~ приду́ I'm just cóming; **4.** (*немедленно*) diréctly, at once.

се́канс *м. мат.* sécant.

секре́т *м.* **1.** sécret; по ~у in cónfidence; под больши́м ~ом únder the seal of sécrecy, in strict cónfidence; не де́лать ~а из чего́-л. make* no sécret of *smth.;* держа́ть в ~е keep* a sécret; **2.** (*потайное устройство в механизме*) sécret device.

секретариа́т *м.* secrétariat(e).

секрета́рский secretárial.

секрета́рь *м.* sécretary; ~ собра́ния sécretary to the méeting; госуда́рственный ~ Sécretary of State.

секрете́р *м.* secretáire.

секре́тничать *несов. разг.* **1.** (*держать в секрете*) keep* things sécret; make* a sécret of éverything; **2.** (*шептаться*) whísper.

секре́тн|ый sécret; (*о сведениях, изданиях тж.*) clássified; ~ докуме́нт sécret/clássified dócument; ~**ая** рабо́та sécret work.

секре́ция *ж. физиол.* secrétion.

секс *м.* sex.

сексоло́гия *ж.* sexólogy.

секста́нт *м. тех.* séxtant.

сексте́т *м. муз.* sextét.

сексуа́льн|ый 1. (*половой*) séxual; ~ые отноше́ния séxual relátions; **2.** (*чувственный*) séxy *разг.;* ~ая де́вушка séxy girl; ~ая привлека́тельность sex appéal.

се́кта *ж.* sect.

секта́нт *м.,* ~**ка** *ж.* (*прям. и перен.*) sectárian, dissénter. ~**ский** (*прям. и перен.*) sectárian. ~**ство** *с.* (*прям. и перен.*) sectárianism.

се́ктор *м.* **1.** séctor; **2.** (*отдел учреждения*) (spécialized) depártment.

секу́нд|а *ж.* sécond; ◇ в одну́ ~у in one/a sécond; ~ в ~у **1)** (*точно в срок*) right on time; **2)** (*одновременно*) at the same instant; одну́ ~у just a sécond/móment.

секунда́нт *м.* sécond.

секу́ндн|ый sécond *attr.;* ~**ая** стре́лка sécond hand.

секундоме́р *м.* stóp-watch, séconds cóunter.

секу́щая *ж. мат.* sécant.

секцио́нн|ый séctional; ~ые заседа́ния séction méetings; ~ инкуба́тор séctional íncubator; ~ая постро́йка séctional constrúction.

се́кци|я ж. séction; (съезда, конференции) commíttee; ~ ло́дочного спо́рта bóating séction; ~и жило́го до́ма séctions of a block of flats; рабо́та совеща́ния по ~ям the committee work of a cónference, a cónference's work in committee.

селёдка ж. разг. см. сельдь.

селёдочн|ица ж. long dish. ~ый hérring attr.

селезёнка ж. анат. spleen.

се́лезень м. drake.

селекци|оне́р м. seléctionist; plánt-breeder; (животных) stóck-breeder. ~о́нный seléction attr.; plánt-breeding attr.; ~о́нные семена́ selécted seeds.

селе́кция ж. с.-х. seléction, bréeding.

селе́ние с. séttlement; (село, деревня) víllage.

селеноло́гия ж. selenólogy.

се́ли мн. (ед. сель м.) mud flows.

сели́тра ж. хим. sáltpetre.

сели́ться несов. séttle.

сел|о́ с. víllage; на ~é in the cóuntryside; ◇ ни к ~у́ ни к го́роду quite irrélevantly.

сельдере́й м. бот. célery.

сельд|ь ж. hérring; ◇ как ~и в бо́чке ≈ (packed) like sardínes.

селько́р м. rúral correspóndent.

се́льск|ий rúral; ~ая ме́стность the cóuntry(síde), cóuntry/rúral locálity; ~ая молодёжь young péople of the cóuntryside; ~ young cóuntryfolk; ~ учи́тель víllage téacher; ~ое хозя́йство ágriculture, fárming.

сельскохозя́йственн|ый agricúltural; farm attr.; ~ое сырьё raw matérials prodúced by ágriculture; ~ые това́ры farm/agrícultural próduce sg; ~ инвента́рь farm equípment.

сельсове́т м. (се́льский Сове́т наро́дных депута́тов) Víllage Sóviet (of Péople's Députies).

сема́нтика ж. лингв. 1. (значение, смысл слова) méaning; 2. (наука) semántics.

семафо́р м. sémaphore; (железнодорожный тж.) sígnal.

сёмга ж. sálmon.

семе́йн|ый fámily attr., home attr.; ~ челове́к fámily man*, wóman*; ~ое положе́ние fámily státus; ~ая жизнь hómelife; ~ круг fámily círcle; ~ые дела́ fámily/prívate affáirs.

семе́йственн|ость ж. (порочный метод подбора кадров) népotism. ~ый 1. fámily attr., domésticated; 2. (характеризующийся семейственностью) népotic.

семе́йство с. fámily.

семени́ть несов. разг. take* short steps, mince (one's steps), trip alóng.

семенно́й seed attr.; ~ фонд seed stock.

семеново́д м. séedsman*.

семеново́д|ство с. seed fárming/gtówing. ~ческий séed-growing.

семёрка ж. 1. (цифра) a séven; 2. карт. the séven (of).

се́меро séven; нас ~ there are séven of us.

семе́стр м. term; seméster амер.

сёмечко с. 1. seed; 2. мн. (семена подсолнечника) súnflower seeds.

семидесятиле́т|ие с. 1. (период) séventy years pl; 2. (годовщина) séventieth annivérsary. ~ний 1. (о сроке) séventy-year attr.; of séventy years после сущ.; 2. (о возрасте) séventy-year-óld; of séventy после сущ.

семидеся́т|ый séventieth; ~ые го́ды the séventies.

семидне́вный séven-day attr., a week's.

семикра́тный sévenfold.

семиле́тний 1. (о сроке) séven-year attr.; of séven years после сущ.; Семиле́тняя война́ the Séven Years'

War; 2. (о возрасте) séven-year-óld; of séven после сущ.

семиме́сячный 1. (о сроке) séven months'; séven-month attr.; 2. (о возрасте) séven-month-óld; of séven months после сущ.

семина́р м. séminar.

семина́рия ж. séminary.

семисо́тый séven-húndredth.

семистру́нный séven-stringed, héptachord.

семи́т м. Sémite. ~и́ческий, ~ский Semític; ~ские языки́ Semític lánguages.

семиуго́льник м. héptagon.

семичасово́й 1. séven-hour attr.; of séven hours после сущ.; ~ рабо́чий день séven-hour wórking day; 2. разг. (назначенный на семь часов) séven-o'clock attr.; ~ по́езд séven-o'clock train.

семнадцатиле́тний 1. (о сроке) seventéen-year attr.; of seventéen years после сущ.; 2. (о возрасте) seventéen-year-óld; of seventéen после сущ.

семна́дцатый seventéenth.

семна́дцать seventéen.

семь séven; ◇ ~ раз отме́рь, оди́н отре́жь посл. ≈ look befóre you leap.

се́мьдесят séventy.

семьсо́т séven húndred.

семь|я́ ж. fámily; больша́я ~ large fámily; ◇ в ~é не без уро́да ≈ there's a black sheep in évery flock.

семьяни́н м. fámily man*; хоро́ший ~ devóted húsband and fáther.

се́мя с. 1. seed (тж. перен.); семена́ для посе́ва sówing seeds; семена́ раздо́ра the seeds of díscord; 2. физиол. sémen, sperm.

сена́ж м. háylage.

сена́т м. sénate. ~ор м. sénator.

се́ни мн. (storm) porch sg, lóbby sg.

сенно́й hay attr.

се́но с. hay; коси́ть ~ mow* hay.

сено|ва́л м. háyloft. ~копни́тель м. háy-stacker.

сеноко́с м. 1. háymaking; быть на ~е be* máking hay; 2. (время косьбы) háymaking time, mówing time; 3. (луг, место косьбы) háyfield.

сено|коси́лка ж. mówing machíne. ~суши́лка ж. háy-drier.

сенсацио́нн|ый sensátional; ~ые но́вости sensátional news.

сенса́ци|я ж. sensátion; вы́звать ~ю make* a sensátion.

сенте́нция ж. máxim, senténtious útterance.

сентиментали́зм м. sentiméntalism.

сентимента́льн|ость ж. sentimentálity. ~ый sentiméntal.

сентя́бр|ь м. Septémber; в ~é э́того го́да this/in Septémber; в ~é про́шлого го́да last Septémber; last year in Septémber; в ~é бу́дущего го́да next Septémber.

сентя́брьский Septémber attr.

сень ж. книж. cánopy; ◇ под ~ю чего-л. 1) shéltered by smth., in the shade of smth.; 2) (под защитой) únder the protéction of smth.

сепара́тный séparate.

сепара́тор м. с.-х., тех. séparator.

се́пия ж. 1. (моллюск) cúttlefish; 2. (краска) sépia.

сеп|сис м. мед. septicáemia, sépsis. ~ти́ческий мед. séptic.

се́ра ж. 1. хим. súlphur; 2. (ушная) éar-wax, cerúmen.

серб м., ~ка ж. Sérbian. ~ский Sérbian.

сербскохорва́тский Sérbo-Cróatian; ~ язы́к Sérbo-Cróatian, the Sérbo-Cróatian lánguage.

серва́нт м. sídeboard.

серви́з м. set, sérvice; ча́йный ~ tea set/sérvice; столо́вый ~ dínner set/sérvice.

сервир|ова́ть несов. и сов. (вн.) lay* (smth.); (по-

давать) serve (*smth.*). ~**бка** ж. 1. (*действие*) láying; sérving; 2. (*убранство стола*) arrángement.

серде́чник I *м. разг.* 1. (*больной*) héart-case, héart-sufferer; 2. (*врач*) heart spécialist.

серде́чник II *м. mex.* core.

серде́чно-сосу́дистый cárdio-váscular.

серде́чн|ый 1. (*относящийся к сердцу*) heart *attr.*, cárdiac; ~**ая мы́шца** heart múscle; ~**ое сре́дство** cárdiac; 2. (*добрый, отзывчивый*) warm-héarted, óut-going; 3. (*исполненный доброжелательства*) héarty, córdial; ~ **прие́м** córdial recéption; ~**ая встре́ча** héarty wélcome; 4. (*искренний*) sincére, héartfelt; 5. (*любовный*) of the heart *сущ.*, love *attr.*; ~**ые дела́** love affáirs; ~**ая дра́ма** emótional crísis.

серди́т|ый 1. ángry; (*о характере*) bad-témpered; ~ **го́лос** ángry vóice; ~**ое лицо́** ángry face; **быть ~ым на кого́-л., что́-л.** be* ángry cross with *smb.*, abóut *smth.*; 2. *разг.* (*о приправе и т. п.*) hot, strong.

серди́ть *несов.* (*вн.*) ánger (*smb.*), make* (*smb.*) ángry. ~**ся** *несов.* (*на кого́-л.*) be* ángry/cross (with *smb.*); (*на что́-л.*) be* ángry/cross (abóut *smth.*).

сердобо́льный *разг.* ténder-héarted.

се́рдц|е *с.* heart; **больно́е ~** weak heart; **прижа́ть ру́ки к ~у** press/put* *one's* hands to *one's* heart; **схвати́ться за ~** clutch at *one's* heart; **черство́е ~** héartless náture; ◇ ~ **ра́дуется** it gláddens *one's* heart, it's a joy; **от всего́ ~а** with all *one's* heart; **всем ~ем** with all *one's* heart, from the bóttom of *one's* heart; ~ **боли́т** I'm sick at heart; ~ **оборвало́сь у кого́-л.** *smb.'s* heart missed a beat; **он мне (пришёлся) по́ ~у** I took a líking to him; **он мне не по́ ~у** he is not the sort of man I care for; **в ~а́х, с ~ем** in a fit of ánger/irritátion; **от чи́стого ~а** sincérely; **положа́ ру́ку на́ ~** quite fránkly; **брать кого́-л. за́ ~** touch/move *smb.* déeply.

сердцебие́ние *с.* palpitátion (of the heart).

сердцеви́на ж. 1. (*ствола или корня растения*) pith, márrow, héartwood; 2. (*ореха*) kérnel, (*яблока, груши и т. п.*) core; 3. (*середина чего́-л.*) míddle, céntre; *перен.* heart; 4. (*сущность чего́-л.*) core, heart, kérnel.

серебри́стый 1. sílvery; ~ **то́поль** sílver póplar; 2. (*мелодично-звонкий*) sílvery.

серебри́ть, посеребри́ть (*вн.*) sílver (*smth.*). ~**ся** *несов.* 1. (*становиться серебристым*) be* sílvered; 2. (*выделяться своим блеском*) gleam sílver.

серебро́ *с.* 1. sílver; *собир.* (*серебряные вещи тж.*) sílverware; 2. *собир.* (*разменная монета*) sílver.

сере́бряный sílver *attr.*; *перен.* sílvery; ~ **слито́к** bar of sílver; ~**ая жи́ла** sílver vein; ~**ые изде́лия** sílver-work; ~**ые ло́жки** sílver spoons; ~ **и́ней** sílver frost; ~ **звон** sílvery peals *pl*; ◇ ~**ая сва́дьба** sílver wédding.

середи́на ж. 1. (*о месте*) míddle, céntre; 2. (*о времени*) míddle; ~ **ле́та** míddle of súmmer; 3. (*промежуточная позиция в чём-л.*) míddle way/course; **ха́лфway house** *идиом.*; (*умеренность*) moderátion.

середня́к *м.* míddle péasant.

серёжка ж. 1. éar-ring; 2. (*соцветие*) cátkin; **améntum** *научн.*

серена́да ж. serenáde.

сере́ть, посере́ть 1. (*становиться серым*) turn grey; 2. *тк. несов.* (*виднеться*) loom grey.

сержа́нт *м.* sérgeant.

сери́йн|ый sérial; ~**ое произво́дство** sérial/mass prodúction.

се́рия ж. séries; (*фильма*) part.

се́рна ж. *зоол.* chámois.

серни́ст|ый 1. súlphur *attr.*; ~**ые удобре́ния** súlphur fértilizers; 2. *хим.* súlphur *attr.*, súlphurous; ~**ая кислота́** súlphurous ácid.

се́рн|ый 1. súlphur *attr.*; ~ **колчеда́н** súlphur pýrite; 2. *хим.* súlphúric; ~**ая кислота́** sulphúric ácid.

сероводоро́д *м. хим.* hýdrogen súlfide.

сероглазый gréy-eyed.

сероуглеро́д *м. хим.* bisúlphide of cárbon.

серп *м.* síckle; ~ **и мо́лот** hámmer and síckle; ◇ ~ **луны́** créscent.

серпанти́н *м.* 1. (*бумажная лента*) stréamer; 2. (*извилистая дорога*) winding road; háirpin bends *pl.*

се́р|ый grey; *перен.* (*бесцветный*) dull, drab, cólourless; (*необразованный*) ígnorant; ~**ые глаза́** grey eyes; ~ **в я́блоках** dápple-grey; ~ **день** grey/dréary/dull day; ~**ая жизнь** dréary/dull life; ~**ая литерату́ра** cólourless writing.

серьга́ ж. 1. éar-ring; 2. *mex.* sháckle, lug, link.

серьёзн|о *нареч.* 1. sériously; (*важно*) grávely; **поду́мать о чём-л.** give* sérious thought to *smth.*; ~ **заболе́ть** fall* sériously ill; **я говорю́** ~ (*не шучу́*) I mean it, I'm in éarnest; **сказа́ть** ~ say* grávely; 2. *в знач. вводн. сл.* (*в самом деле*) réally; ~? réally?; **вы э́то** ~? are you sérious?, do you mean it? ~**ость** ж. sériousness; (*важность, опасность*) grávity. ~**ый** sérious; (*важный, опасный*) grave; ~**ый челове́к** sérious pérson; ~**ое отноше́ние к рабо́те** sérious áttitude to *one's* work; ~**ое де́ло** mátter of great impórtance; ~**ые недоста́тки** sérious/májor defécts; **э́то** ~**ый разгово́р!** now you are tálking!; ~**ая боле́знь** sérious íllness; ~**ый вид, тон** sérious air, tone.

се́ссия ж. 1. séssion; 2.: **экзаменацио́нная ~** examinátions *pl.*

сестра́ ж. 1. síster; 2. (*в лечебных учреждениях*) (trained) nurse; **ста́ршая ~** (núrsing) síster.

сестра́-хозя́йка ж. mátron.

сесть *сов. см.* сади́ться.

се́тка ж. 1. net; (*металлическая*) screen; (*мелкая*) wíre-gauze; (*на кровати*) wíre máttress; (*в вагоне*) rack; ~ **для воло́с** háir-net; 2. *разг.* (*сумка*) string-bag; 3. (*тарифная и т. п.*) scale.

се́товать, посе́товать (*на вн.*) compláin (of), lamént (*smth.*).

се́ттер *м.* (*собака*) sétter.

сетча́тка ж. *анат.* rétina.

сеть ж. 1. net; 2. (*дорог, линий связи, учрежде́ний и т. п.*) nétwork, sýstem; **железнодоро́жная ~** ráilway sýstem; **электри́ческая ~** eléctrical sýstem.

сече́ние *с.* séction, cross séction, prófile; (*проволоки*) gauge.

се́чка ж. 1. (*нож*) chópper; 2. (*нарубленная соло́ма*) chopped straw.

сечь, вы́сечь (*вн.*) 1. (*розгами, плетью и т. п.*) birch (*smb.*), flog (*smb.*), give* *smb.* a flógging/thráshing; 2. *тк. несов.* (*рубить*) cut* (*smth.*); 3. *разг.* (*понимать*) dig* (*smth.*), catch* on (to). ~**ся** *несов.* 1. (*о волоса́х*) split*; 2. (*о тка́ни*) fray.

се́ялка ж. séeding-machine, séeder, drill; **рядова́я ~** séed-drill.

се́янец *м. с.-х.* séedling.

се́ять, посе́ять (*вн.*) sow* (*smth.*) (*тж. перен.*); ~ **рожь, ове́с** sow* rye, oats; ~ **раздо́ры** sow* díscord; ◇ **что посе́ешь, то и пожнёшь** *погов.* we reap as we have sown.

сжа́литься *сов.* relént; (*над тв.*) take* píty (on).

сжа́тие *с.* compréssion.

сжа́т|ый 1. (*уплотнённый давлением*) compréssed; ~ **во́здух** compréssed air; 2.: ~**ые кулаки́** clenched fists; 3. (*краткий*) brief; (*об изложении и т. п.*) concíse, pithy; **в ~ые сро́ки** in the shórtest póssible time.

сжать I *сов. см.* жать II.

сжать II *сов. см.* сжима́ть. ~**ся** *сов. см.* сжима́ться.

сжечь *сов. см.* сжига́ть.

сжива́ть, сжить (*вн.*) oust (*smb.*). ~**ся, сжи́ться** (*с тв.*) *разг.* get* used (to); **сжи́ться с мы́слью** get* used to the idéa.

сжига́ние *с.* búrning; *mex.* incinerátion; (*кремация*) cremátion.

сжига́ть, сжечь (*вн.*) 1. burn* (*smth.*); (*в крематории*) cremáte (*smb.*); сжечь письмо́ burn* a létter; сжечь дом burn* the house down; сжечь спи́ну на со́лнце burn* *one's* back in the sun; сжечь пироги́ burn* the pies; 2. (*сушить — о солнце*) scorch (*smth.*); ◇ сжечь свои́ корабли́ burn* *one's* boats.

сжим|а́ть, сжать (*вн.*) 1. (*давлением уменьшать объём*) compréss (*smth.*); squeeze (*smth.*); *перен.* cut* down (*smth.*), redúce (*smth.*); ~ пружи́ну compréss a spring; сжать сро́ки в объёме) tíghten the schédule; 2. (*сдавливать, стискивать*) press (*smb., smth.*), squeeze (*smb., smth.*); (*стеснять*) trap (*smth.*); сжать чью-л. ру́ку press/squeeze *smb.'s* hand; ~ кого́-л. в объя́тиях hug *smb.*; ~ кольцо́ окруже́ния *воен.* tíghten the ring (of troops), close in; 3. (*горло, грудь*) make* (*smth.*) contráct/tíghten; 4. (*плотно соединять*) compréss (*smth.*); ~ кулаки́ clench *one's* fists. ~а́ться, сжа́ться 1. (*уменьшаться в объёме*) be* compréssed; (*сокращаться, сдвинувшись*) contráct; 2. (*ёжиться*) shrink*; húddle up; сжа́ться от испу́га shrink* with fear; 3. (*плотно соединяться*) compréss; его́ рука́ сжа́лась в кула́к he clenched his fist invóluntarily; 4. (*о горле, груди*) tíghten; *перен.* be* wrung; се́рдце ~а́ется от жа́лости *one's* heart is wrung with píty.

сжи́ть(ся) *сов. см.* сжива́ть(ся).

сза́ди 1. *нареч.* (*позади*) behínd, at the back; (*с задней стороны*) from behínd; вид ~ rear view; 2. *предлог* (*рд.*) behínd.

сзыва́ть, созва́ть (*вн.*) call (*smb.*), súmmon (*smb.*); (*гостей*) invíte (*smth.*), ask (*smb.*).

си *с. нескл. муз.* si, te, B.

сиби́рск|ий Sibérian; ◇ ~ая я́зва ánthrax; ~ая ко́шка Pérsian cat.

сиби́р|я́к *м.*, ~я́чка *ж.* Sibérian.

си́вый grey.

сиг *м.* lake white-fish.

сига́ра *ж.* cigár.

сигаре́та *ж.* cigarétte.

сигна́л *м.* 1. (*условный знак*) signal (*тж. перен.*); ~ бе́дствия distréss signal; ~ возду́шной трево́ги áir-raid alért/wárning; ~ сбо́ра signal to assémble; ~ы то́чного вре́мени time signals; доро́жные ~ы tráffic signals; светово́й ~ light signal; дать ~ signal; (*звуковой*) sound *one's* horn; 2. (*сообщение*) notificátion, wárning; прислу́шиваться к ~ам с мест pay* atténtion to notifications from the próvinces.

сигнализ|а́ция *ж.* 1. signalling; ~ флажка́ми flag signalling; железнодоро́жная ~ ráilway signalling; 2. (*приспособление*) alárm sýstem; 3. (*система сигналов*) signal sýstem. ~и́ровать *несов. и сов.* (*сов. тж.* просигнализи́ровать) signal; *перен.* send* a méssage, warn.

сигна́лить, просигна́лить signal; nótify, warn.

сигна́л|ьный signal *attr.*; ~ вы́стрел signal shot; ~ные раке́ты flares, Véry lights, signal róckets; ◇ ~ экземпля́р *полигр.* advánce cópy. ~щик *м.* signaller; signaler *амер.*; búgler. ⋅

сиде́лка *ж.* (sick-)nurse.

сиде́нье *с.* seat.

сиде́ть *несов.* 1. sit*, be* séated; (*о птицах*) perch, roost; ~ на сту́ле sit* on a chair; ~ в седле́ sit* in the sáddle, sit* a horse; 2. (*за, над тж., на пр.; делать что-л.*) sit* (óver, at); ~ над уро́ками sit* at *one's* léssons; ~ на вёслах take* the oars, row; 3. (*находиться*) be*; ~ без де́ла have* nóthing to do; ~ до́ма stay at home; ~ под аре́стом be* únder arrést; ~ на дие́те be* on a díet; ~ без де́нег have* no móney, be* short of móney; ~ по ноча́м sit* up (at night); 4. (*об одежде*) fit, sit*; хорошо́ ~ sit* well; ~ мешко́м hang* bádly; 5. (*о судне*) глубоко́ (неглубоко́) ~ draw* much (líttle) wáter; ◇ ~ сложа́ ру́ки idle *one's* time awáy; ~ на я́йцах sit* (on eggs).

сид|е́ться *несов. безл.*: ему́ не ~ится на ме́сте 1)

(*на стуле и т. п.*) he can't keep still; 2) (*в каком-л. месте*) he can't stay in one place; ему́ не ~ится до́ма he can't stay at home.

сидр *м.* cíder.

сидя́ч|ий sítting; (*о работе, жизни*) sédentary; ~ие места́ seats.

сие *см.* сей.

си́зый blúe-grey, dóve-coloured; ~ го́лубь rock pígeon/dove; ~ нос blue nose; ~ тума́н blúe-grey mist.

сил|а *ж.* 1. (*физическая энергия*) strength; облада́ть огро́мной ~ой be* enórmously strong; напря́чь все ~ы strain évery múscle; изо всех сил with all *one's* might; 2. (*физическое воздействие, насилие*) force; ~ой ору́жия by force of arms; поли́тика с пози́ции ~ы position-of-strength pólicy; 3. (*духовная*) pówer, strength, énergy; ~ во́ли strength of will, will-power; 4. (*энергия, мощность*) pówer, capácity; ~ тя́жести grávity; подъёмная ~ кра́на lifting capácity of a crane; 5. (*правомочность*) force; име́ть зако́нную ~у be* válid; не име́ть зако́нной ~ы be* null and void; вступа́ть в ~у come* into force; теря́ть ~у becóme* inválid; 6. (*могущество, авторитет*) pówer; (*способность влиять тж.*) force; ~ убежде́ния force of convíction; ~ приме́ра the pówer of exámple; 7. *разг.* (*сущность, смысл*) the point; the crux of the mátter; 8. (*интенсивность, напряжённость*) force, pówer, inténsity; ~ зву́ка vólume of sound; ~ све́та inténsity of light; ~ взры́ва force of an explósion; ~ тала́нта pówer of tálent; 9. (*источник какой-л. деятельности, могущества*) force; 10. обыкн. мн. (*материальное начало*) fórces; ~ы приро́ды nátural fórces; людски́е ~ы mánpower *sg*; 11. обыкн. мн. (*часть общества*) fórces; прогресси́вные ~ы progréssive fórces; реакцио́нные ~ы reáctionary fórces; 12. мн. (*войска*) fórces; сухопу́тные ~ы land fórces; ~ы обо́их проти́вников, обе́их сторо́н the oppósing fórces; ◇ в ~у чего́-л. ówing to smth., by vírtue of smth.; от ~ы at the outside; в ме́ру сил, по ме́ре сил as much as *one* is áble; э́то мне под ~у, э́то в мои́х ~ах that I can do; всё, что в мои́х ~ах éverything in my pówer; э́то мне не под ~у it is beyónd my pówers; быть в ~ах сде́лать что-л. be* áble to do smth.; я не в ~ах расста́ться с ним I can't bear to part with him; есть че́рез ~у force *oneself* to eat; все́ми ~ами with all *one's* strength; про́бовать ~ы в чём-л. try *one's* hand at smth.; вы́ше чьих-л. сил too much for smth.; beyónd smth.; что есть ~ы, что бы́ло сил for all *one* is worth.

сила́ч *м.* strong man*; быть ~о́м be* véry strong, have* gigántic strength.

сплика́ты *мн.* sílicates.

силико́новый sílicone *attr.*

си́литься *несов.* (+ *инф.*) *разг.* try (+ to *inf*), strive* (+ to *inf*).

силлаби́ческий *лит.* syllábic.

силлоги́зм *м.* sýllogism.

сило́в|о́й 1. pówer *attr.*; 2. *спорт.* invólving strength после *сущ.*; ~ые упражне́ния wéight-lifting éxercises; ~ приём bódy-check.

си́лой by force.

сил|о́к *м.* snare; ста́вить ~ки́ set* snares.

си́лос *м.* (*корм*) sílage. ~ный sílage *attr.*; ~ные корма́ sílage *sg*; ~ная я́ма sílage pit, pit sílo.

силосова́ть *несов. и сов.* (*вн.*) *с.-х.* sílo (*smth.*), sílage (*smth.*).

силуэ́т *м.* silhouétte.

си́льно 1. pówerfully; ~ боле́ть (*причинять боль*) hurt* bádly, be* véry páinful; (*быть больным*) be* véry ill; ~ уда́рить кого́-л. hit* smb. hard; ~ уда́рить кулако́м по́ столу́ thump the táble; 2. (*очень*) véry; ~ испуга́ться, проголода́ться и т. д. be* véry fríghtened, húngry *etc.*; ~ люби́ть love déarly, love véry much.

сильноде́йствующий pótent, pówerful.

си́льн|ый 1. strong; (*мощный*) pówerful; ~ челове́к

strong man*; ~ая рука́ strong arm; ~ уда́р pówerful blow; ~ ток pówerful cúrrent; ~ая а́рмия strong a´rmy; 2. (убеди́тельный) pówerful; ~ые до́воды со́gent árguments; ~ая пье́са pówerful play; 3. (мора́льно усто́йчивый) strong; ~ая нату́ра strong cháracter; челове́к ~ой во́ли stróng-willed pérson; 4. (значи́тельный, большо́й): ~ ве́тер high wind; ~ дождь héavy rain; ~ моро́з sevére frost; ~ая боль víolent pain; 5. (о чу́вствах, жела́ниях) víolent, inténse; ~ое увлече́ние чем-л. víolent enthúsiasm for smth.; 6. (хорошо́ знающий, уме́ющий) strong, good*; ~ учени́к good* púpil; ~ плове́ц strong swímmer; он силён в исто́рии his fórte is hístory; ◇ ~ые слова́, выраже́ния strong words, expréssions; ~ая сторона́ кого́-л. one's strong point.

си́мвол м. sýmbol.

символ|изи́ровать несов. и сов. (вн.) sýmbolize (smth.). ~и́зм м. sýmbolism. ~и́ческий symbólic.

симме́три|чный symmétrical. ~ия ж. sýmmetry.

симпатизи́р|овать несов. (дт.) like (smb.); я ему́ не ~ую I have not much líking for him.

симпати́чный nice, líkable.

симпа́ти|я ж. 1. (чу́вство) líking, afféction; чу́вствовать ~ю к кому́-л. have* a líking for smb., take* a líking (to); относи́ться с ~ей к кому́-л. like smb.; 2. разг. (предме́т симпа́тии, любви́) one's swéetheart.

симпо́зиум м. sympósium (pl -ums, -sia).

симпто́м м. sýmptom. ~ати́чный symptomátic.

симул|и́ровать несов. и сов. (вн.) símulate (smth.); sham (smth.) разг.; ~ боле́знь malínger; ~ глухоту́ sham déafness, preténd to be deaf. ~я́нт м. malíngerer. ~я́ция ж. simulátion.

симфони́ческ|ий symphónic; ~ие этю́ды symphónic stúdies; ~ конце́рт sýmphony cóncert; ◇ ~ орке́стр sýmphony orchéstra.

симфо́ния ж. (прям. и перен.) sýmphony; ~ ля мажо́р sýmphony in A májor.

синаго́га ж. sýnagogue.

синдика́т м. sýndicate.

синдро́м м. sýndrome.

синева́ ж. 1. (си́ний цвет) (dárk-)blue; 2. (си́нее простра́нство) blue/ázure expánse; ◇ ~ под глаза́ми blue shádows únder one's eyes.

синегла́зый blúe-eyed; with déep-blue eyes после сущ.

синера́ма ж. Cineráma.

сине́ть, посине́ть 1. (станови́ться си́ним) becóme*/turn blue; 2. тк. несов. (видне́ться) show* blue.

си́н|ий (dárk-)blue; ~яя кра́ска dárk-blue paint; ~ костю́м návy-blue suit; ~ие глаза́ déep-blue eyes; ◇ ~ чуло́к blúe-stocking.

сини́льн|ый: ~ая кислота́ хим. hydrocyánic ácid.

сини́ть, подсини́ть: ~ бельё blue the línen.

сини́ца ж. tit, títmouse*; tómtit разг.

сино́д м. sýnod.

сино́ним м. лингв. sýnonym. ~и́ческий, ~и́чный лингв. synónymous.

сино́птик м. wéather fórecaster.

сино́ним м. лингв. sýnonym. ~и́ческий, ~и́чный лингв. synónymous.

сино́птик м. wéather fórecaster.

сино́птика ж. synóptic meteoró́logy, wéather fórecasting.

синопти́ческ|ий wéather attr., meteorológical; ~ие усло́вия meteorológical condítions; ◇ ~ая ка́рта wéather map.

си́нтакс|ис м. sýntax. ~и́ческий syntáctic.

си́нтез м. sýnthesis (pl -ses).

синтези́ровать несов. и сов. (вн.) sýnthesize (smth.).

синтези́ровать несов. и сов. (вн.) sýnthesize (smth.).

синте́тика ж. собир. synthétics pl, synthétic goods pl.

синтети́ческ|ий synthétic; ~ ме́тод иссле́дования synthétic méthod of inquíry; ~ каучу́к synthétic rúbber; ~ое волокно́ synthétic fíbre; ~ие языки́ synthétic lánguages.

си́нус м. 1. мат. sine; 2. анат. sínus.

синхрониза́ция м. тех. synchronizátion.

синхронизи́ровать несов. и сов. (вн.) тех. sýnchronize (smth.), bring* (smth.) ínto step.

синхро́н|ный sýnchronous; ~ое пла́вание sýnchronized swímming; ~ перево́д simultáneous translátion/ínterpreting.

синхрофазотро́н м. próton sýnchrotron.

си́нька ж. 1. (кра́ска) (wáshing) blue; 2. (светоко́пия) blue print.

синя́к м. brúise; ~ под гла́зом black eye; ◇ ~и под глаза́ми blue shádows únder one's eyes.

сиони́зм м. Zíonism. ~и́ст м. Zíonist.

сипе́ть несов. wheeze.

си́плый húsky.

сире́на ж. síren.

сире́нев|ый lílac; ~ куст lílac bush; пла́тье ~ого цве́та lílac(-coloured) dress.

сире́нь ж. lílac.

сир|и́ец м., ~и́йка ж. Sýrian. ~и́йский Sýrian.

Си́риус м. астр. Sírius, Dog Star.

сиро́п м. sýrup.

сирота́ м. и ж. órphan.

сиротли́вый lónely; перен. forlórn.

сиро́т|ский órphan's; ~ дом órphanage. ~ство с. órphanhood.

систе́м|а ж. sýstem; (техни́ческое устро́йство тж.) design; ~ воспита́ния sýstem of educátion; привести́ в ~у свои́ наблюде́ния sýstematize/clássify one's observátions; ~ языка́ grammátical sýstem of a lánguage; корнева́я ~ расте́ния root sýstem; ~ о́рганов наро́дного образова́ния públic educátion sýstem; рабо́тать в ~е Акаде́мии нау́к work in one of the institútions of the Acádemy of Sciences; избира́тельная ~ eléctoral sýstem; десяти́чная ~ счисле́ния décimal sýstem; экономи́ческая, полити́ческая ~ económic, polítical sýstem.

система́т|изи́ровать несов. и сов. (вн.) sýstematize (smth.). ~и́ческий systemátic.

си́тец м. prínted cótton; (вощёный) chintz; cálico амер.

си́то с. sieve.

ситуа́ция ж. situátion.

си́тцев|ый prínted cótton attr.; ~ое пла́тье prínted cótton dress.

сифили́с м. sýphilis.

сифо́н м. síphon.

сиюмину́тный mómentary; (неме́дленный) ínstant.

сия́ см. сей.

сия́ни|е с. rádiance; (орео́л) hálo; перен. (вели́чие) brílliance; (счастли́вое выраже́ние глаз, лица́) bríghtness; в ~и сла́вы in a blaze of glóry; ◇ се́верное ~ nórthern lights pl, Auróra Boreális.

сия́ть несов. 1. shine*; (сверка́ть тж.) gleam; со́лнце сия́ет the sun is shíning; 2. (о челове́ке) beam, be* rádiant; (о глаза́х) shine*; ~ от ра́дости beam with joy, be* rádiant with joy; его́ глаза́ сия́ют his eyes are shíning.

сказ м. лит. tale; ◇ вот тебе́ и весь ~ разг. that's the long and the short of it.

сказа́ние с. stóry, légend.

сказа́ть сов. см. говори́ть 2; ◇ тру́дно ~ it is hard to say; что он хо́чет э́тим ~? what does he mean by that?; скажи́те пожа́луйста! fáncy!; не́чего ~! indéed!, there's no denýing the fact; неве́роятно, скажи́те cértainly, that's a fact; ска́зано — сде́лано no sóoner said than done; не скажу́, что́бы... I wóuldn't say...; так ~ so to speak.

сказа́ться сов. см. ска́зываться.

сказ́итель *м.*, **~ница** *ж.* stóry-teller.

сказк|а *ж.* fáiry tale/stóry; наро́дные **~и** fólk-tales; расска́зывать **~и** tell* fáiry tales/stóries; как в **~е** (it's) like a fáiry tale.

сказочн|ик *м.* téller of fáiry tales, stóryteller. **~ый** 1. fáiry-tale *attr.*; **~ый** сюже́т fáiry-tale theme; 2. (*невероятный*) incrédible, fábulous; **~ое** бога́тство fábulous wealth; . **~ая** красота́ wóndrous béauty; **~ая** страна́ fáiryland, enchánted land.

сказу́емое *с. грам.* prédicate.

сказываться, **сказа́ться** 1. (на *пр.*; *отражаться*) tell* (on); 2. (*тв.*) *разг.* (*представляться*) make* onesélf out to be (*smb.*, *smth.*); сказа́ться больны́м plead illness.

скака́лка *ж.* skípping-rope.

скак|а́ть *несов.* 1. (*прыгать*) skip, jump; (*на одной ноге*) hop; (*отскакивать*) bounce; **~** че́рез верёвочку skip óver a rope; 2. (*верхом*) gállop; **~а́л** во весь дух .the hórseman* gálloped for all he was worth; 3. *разг.* (*резко изменяться*) be* (véry) unstéady, keep* chópping and chánging; баро́метр ска́чет the glass is véry unstéady.

скаков|о́й race *attr.*; **~а́я** ло́шадь rácehorse; **~** ипподро́м rácecourse.

скаку́н *м.* (*конь*) rácer.

скал|а́ *ж.* rock; (*отвесная, обыкн. прибрежная*) cliff. **~и́стый** rócky.

ска́лить *несов.*: **~** зу́бы 1) bare *one's* teeth; 2) *разг.* (*смеяться*) laugh, grin.

ска́лка *ж.* (*для теста*) rólling-pin.

ска́лывать, **сколо́ть** (*вн.*) 1. (*сбивать*) chip (*smth.*) off, break* (*smth.*) off; сколо́ть лёд с тротуа́ра chip ice off the pávement; 2. (*скреплять булавкой и т. п.*) pin (*smth.*) togéther.

скаме́йка *ж. см.* скамья́.

скамь|я́ *ж.* bench; ◇ со шко́льной **~и** from *one's* schóol-days, (éver) since *one* was at school; **~** подсуди́мых the dock; попа́сть на **~ю** подсуди́мых find* onesélf in the dock.

сканда́л *м.* 1. scándal; 2. (*ссора, сцена*) row; устро́ить **~** make* a row, kick up a row.

скандали́ст *м.* tróublemaker.

скандалить, **наскандали́ть** kick up a row.

скандальн|ый 1. scándalous, disgráceful; **~ое** происше́ствие disgráceful occúrrence; 2. *разг.* (*любящий скандалить*) quárrelsome; **~** челове́к rówdy/quárrelsome pérson.

скандина́в *м.*, **~ка** *ж.* Scandinávian. **~ский** Scandinávian; **~ские** языки́ Scandinávian lánguages.

скандировать *несов.* (*вн.*) 1. scan (*smth.*); 2. (*громко и отчётливо произносить слова*) chant (*smth.*).

ска́пливать, **скопи́ть** (*вн.*) save (*smth.*), accúmulate (*smth.*). **~ся**, **скопи́ться** accúmulate; pile up; (*о людях*) gáther, crowd round.

скарлати́на *ж.* scárlet féver.

ска́рмливать, **скорми́ть** (*вн.*) use up (*smth.*) (on féeding).

скат I *м.* 1. (*пологий спуск*) slope; (*крыши*) pitch; 2. (*приспособление для скатывания чего-л.*) ramp, slide.

скат II *м.* (*колесо автомобиля*) wheel.

скат III *м.* (*рыба*) skate.

ската́ть *сов. см.* ска́тывать I.

ска́терть *ж.* táblecloth; ◇ **~ю** доро́га! good ríddance!

скати́ть *сов. см.* ска́тывать II. **~ся** *сов. см.* ска́тываться.

ска́тывать I, **ската́ть** (*вн.*) roll (*smth.*) (up).

ска́тывать II, **скати́ть** (*вн.*) (*спускать вниз*) roll (*smth.*) down. **~ся**, **скати́ться** roll down; (*на санках*) slíde* down; (*на велосипеде, машине*) run* down; *перен.* grávitate (towárds).

скафа́ндр *м.* díving suit; (*космонавта*) fúll-pressure suit, spáce suit.

ска́чк|а *ж.* 1. (*быстрый бег лошади*) (hórse-)race; 2. *мн.* (*состязания верховых лошадей*) the ráces; **~и** с препя́тствиями stéeplechase *sg.*

скачкообра́зн|ость *ж.* spasmódic náture. **~ый** unéven, spasmódic devélopment.

скачо́к *м.* 1. (*прыжок*) jump, leap, bound; 2. (*резкое изменение чего-л.*) súdden leap/change; 3. *филос.* leap.

ска́шивать I, **скоси́ть** (*вн.*) 1. (*траву*) mow* (*smth.*); *перен.* cut* down (*smb.*, *smth.*); 2. (*губить, убивать многих*) wipe* out (*smb.*).

ска́шивать II, **скоси́ть** (*вн.*) 1. (*делать косым*) knock (*smth.*) sídeways, twist (*smth.*); 2. (*повёртывать вбок*) turn (*smth.*); **~** глаза́ squint.

скважина *ж.* 1. (*щель*) chink, slit; 2. (*буровая*) drill/bore hole, bóring well; нефтяна́я **~** oil well; 3. *физ., геол.* pore.

сквер *м.* (públic) gárden.

сквернослóвие *с.* foul lánguage.

сквернослóвить *несов.* swear*, use foul lánguage.

скверн|ый bad*; násty, unpléasant; (*гадкий*) foul; **~** за́пах bad* smell; **~ая** исто́рия unpléasant affáir; **~ая** пого́да foul wéather.

скво́з|ить *несов.* 1. *безл.*: здесь **~и́т** there's a draught here, it is dráughty here; 2. (*просвечивать*) come*, peep; 3. (*виднеться*) show*; *перен.* (*обнаруживаться*) can* be felt/detécted; в его́ слова́х **~и́ло** недово́льство a note of displéasure could be detécted in his voice.

сквозн|ой through; **~ое** отве́рстие hole; **~а́я** ра́на pérforating/púnctured wound; **~** ве́тер draught; **~** по́езд through train; **~** гра́фик comprehénsive tímetable.

сквозня́к *м.* draught; сиде́ть на **~е** sit* in a draught.

сквозь through.

скворе́ц *м.* stárling.

скворе́чник *м.* stárling-box.

скеле́т *м.* skéleton; *перен.* frámework.

скепт|ик *м.* scéptic. **~ици́зм** *м.* scépticism. **~и́ческий** scéptical.

ске́рцо *с. нескл. муз.* schérzo.

ски́дк|а *ж.* 1. (*уменьшение суммы*) díscount, rébate; продава́ть что-л. со **~ой** sell* *smth.* at a díscount; (*продажа товаров со* **~ой** на 20 проце́нтов allów a twénty per cent rébate on púrchases; 2. (*на вн.*; *снижение требований*) allówances *pl*; де́лать **~у** на что-л. make* allówances for *smth.*

ски́дывать, **ски́нуть** (*вн.*) 1. throw* (*smth.*) down; *перен. разг.* (*свергать*) overthrów* (*smb.*, *smth.*); 2. *разг.* (*снимать*) throw* off (*smth.*); (*лишаться чего-л.*) shed* (*smth.*) (*тж. перен.*); 3. *разг.* (*уменьшать*) cut* down (*smth.*); 4. *разг.* (*сбавлять в цене*) knock (*smth.*) off.

ски́нуть *сов. см.* ски́дывать.

ски́петр *м.* scéptre.

скипида́р *м.* túrpentine.

скирд *м.*, **~а́** *ж.* rick, stack.

скирдова́ть, **заскирдова́ть** (*вн.*) stack (*smth.*).

скиса́ть, **ски́снуть** turn sóur; *перен. разг.* lose* heart, mope, get* down in the mouth.

ски́снуть *сов. см.* скиса́ть.

скита́|лец *м.* wánderer, róamer. **~ние** *с.* wándering, róaming.

скита́ться *несов.* wánder (abóut), roam.

скиф *м.*, **~ский** Scýthian.

склад I *м.* 1. (*запас чего-л.*) store, stock; **~** ору́жия store of wéapons; 2. (*помещение*) wárehouse, stórehouse; депо́т **~** (*тж. воен.*); лесно́й **~** tímber-yard.

склад II *м.* (*свойство*) kind; **~** жи́зни way of life; **~** ума́ mentálity; лю́ди осо́бого **~а** péople of a spécial mould; péople of a cértain stamp.

скла́дк|а ж. 1. fold; (*бантовая*) pleat; (*заглаженная*) crease; в ~y pléated; ю́бка в ~y pléated skirt; 2. (*морщина*) wrinkle; 3. *геол.* fléxure, fold.

скла́дно smóothly; (*удачно тж.*) nícely.

складно́й fólding; (*о мебели тж.*) collápsible; ~ нож clásp-knife*; ~ стул fólding chair.

скла́дный 1. *разг.* (*стройный*) well-búilt, well-knít; 2. (*о рассказе, тексте*) well-róunded, smooth, neat.

скла́дчин|а ж. clúbbing (togéther); устро́ить ~y club one's resóurces (togéther); купи́ть что-л. в ~y club togéther for smth., share the cost of smth.

скла́дывать, сложи́ть (*вн.*) 1. (*класть что-л. в одно место*) pile (smth.) up; (*в чемодан и т. п.*) put* (smth.); (*вещи для отъезда*) pack (smth.); сложи́ть се́но one's things in a rúcksack; сложи́ть чемода́н pack a case; 2. *мат.* add (smth.) (up); сложи́ть два с пятью́ add two and five; 3. (*собирать из частей*) assémble (smth.), put* (smth.) togéther; 4. (*возводить путём кладки*) build* (smth.); сложи́ть печь build* a stove; 5. (*сгибать*) fold (smth.); fold up (smth.); ~ что-л. вдво́е, попола́м fold smth. in two, half; сложи́ть газе́ту fold up a néwspaper; сложи́ть стул fold up a chair; сложи́ть ру́ки на груди́ fold one's arms on one's chest; 6. (*сочинять*) compóse (smth.), make* (smth.); сложи́ть пе́сню compóse a song; ◇ сложи́ть го́лову lay* down one's life; сложи́ть ору́жие lay* down arms; сиде́ть сложа́ ру́ки sit* twíddling one's thumbs. ~ся, сложи́ться 1. form; y него́ ещё не сложи́лся хара́ктер his cháracter hásn't formed yet; гу́бы его́ сложи́лись в улы́бку his lips formed a smile; 2. (*принимать тот или иной оборот*) shape, turn out, devélop; обстоя́тельства сложи́лись неблагоприя́тно círcumstances took an unfávourable turn; 3. *разг.* (*устраивать складчину*) club togéther.

скле́ивать, скле́ить (*вн.*) stick* (smth.) togéther, glue (smth.) togéther; *перен.* patch up (smth.). ~ся, скле́иться stick*, stick* togéther; *перен. разг.* work out, go*.

скле́ить(ся) *сов. см.* скле́ивать(ся).

склеп м. (búrial) vault.

склепа́ть *сов. см.* склёпывать.

склёпка ж. 1. (*действие*) ríveting; 2. (*место*) rívet.

склёпывать, склепа́ть (*вн.*) rívet (smth.).

склеро́з м. *мед.* sclerósis; ~ сосу́дов hárdening of the árteries.

скло́ка ж. squábble, squábbling; pétty intrígues pl.

склон м. slope; ~ горы́ móuntainside; hillside; ◇ на ~e лет in one's declíning years, in the évening of life.

склоне́ние с. *грам.* declénsion.

склони́ть *сов. см.* склоня́ть 1, 2. ~ся *сов. см.* склоня́ться 1, 2, 3.

склонн|ость ж. 1. (*одарённость*) bent, áptitude, inclinátion; ~ к му́зыке bent for músic; ~ к жи́вописи áptitude for páinting, turn for páinting; 2. (*предрасположенность к чему-л.*) téndency; y него́ ~ к полноте́ he is inclíned to put on weight; 3. (*симпатия*) fóndness. ~ый (к *дт.*) inclíned (to).

склоня́ть I, склони́ть 1. (*вн.; наклонять*) bend* (smth.); ~ знамёна lówer the stándards/bánners; 2. (*вн.* к *дт.*, на *вн.*, + *инф.; уговаривать*) persuáde (smb. + to *inf*); urge (smb. + to *inf*); ~ кого́-л. на свою́ сто́рону win* smb. óver.

склоня́ть II, просклоня́ть (*вн.*) *грам.* declíne (smth.).

склоня́|ться I, склони́ться 1. (*наклоняться*) bend* óver; (*перед тв.*) *перен.* bow (befóre, to); 2. (к *дт.*) принима́ть, признава́ть что-л.) be* inclíned (to), tend (towárds); я ~́юсь к ва́шему мне́нию, мы́сли I am inclíned to the opínion (that); 3. (*о солнце*) go* down.

склоня́ться II *несов. грам.* be* declíned.

скля́нка ж. phíal.

скоба́ ж. 1. stáple, cramp; 2. (*проволочная*) brace; 3. (*на каблуке*) tip.

ско́бк|а ж. brácket; откры́ть ~и ópen the bráckets; закры́ть ~и close the bráckets; в ~ax in bráckets; *перен.* in parénthesis; поста́вить, заключи́ть сло́во в ~и put* a word betwéen bráckets, brácket a word; вы́нести за ~и о́бщий мно́житель take* the cómmon múltiplier out of the bráckets; ◇ в ~ax заме́тим be it said parenthétically.

скобли́ть *несов.* (*вн.*) scrape (smth.); (*чистить тж.*) scour (smth.).

скобян|о́й: ~ые това́ры hárdware sg.

ско́ванность ж. restráint, inhibítion pl; háng-up *разг.*

скова́ть *сов. см.* ско́вывать.

сковорода́ ж., сковоро́дка ж. frýing-pan; skíllet *амер.*

ско́вывать, скова́ть (*вн.*) 1. (*соединять ковкой*) forge (smth.) togéther; 2. (*надевать кандалы, оковы*) sháckle (smb., smth.), fétter (smb., smth.); *перен. тж.* páralyse (smth.); страх скова́л его́ движе́ния he was páralysed with fear; 3. *воен.* páralyse (smb.), hold* down (smb.); ~ проти́вника páralyse the énemy; 4. (*покрывать льдом*) bind* (smth.); лёд, моро́з скова́л ре́ку the ríver is íce-bound.

скола́чивать, сколоти́ть (*вн.*) knock (smth.) up; *перен. разг.* (*создавать*) get* (smth.) togéther.

сколоти́ть *сов. см.* скола́чивать.

сколо́ть *сов. см.* ска́лывать.

скольже́ние с. slíding.

скользи́ть, скользну́ть 1. slide*; (*не иметь устойчивости*) slide* abóut; 2. (*плавно двигаться*) glide; 3. (*о взгляде и т. п.*) rove.

скольз|кий 1. slíppery; *перен. тж.* dángerous; вступи́ть на ~ путь be* on slíppery ground; 2. (*двусмысленный*) délicate, dúbious; dícey *разг.* ~ко в знач. сказ. безл. it is slíppery.

скользну́ть *сов.* 1. *см.* скользи́ть; 2. (*быстро, незаметно пройти*) slip. 3. (*по дт.; слегка задеть — о пуле и т. п.*) graze (smth.).

ско́лько 1. *мест. и нареч.* (*какое количество?*) (*с сущ. в ед. ч.*) how much?; (*с сущ. во мн. ч.*) how mány?; ~ э́то сто́ит? how much is it?, what does it cost?; ~ сто́ит каранда́ш и т. д.? what does the péncil, etc. cost?; ~ вре́мени? what's the time?; 2. *мест. и нареч.* (*какое большое количество!*) how mány!; ~ раз я вам говори́л! how mány times have I told you!; 3. *нареч.* (*в какой мере, насколько*) as far as; ~ я зна́ю as far as I know; ◇ ~ ни... no mátter how much...; не сто́лько... ~... not so much... as...; сто́лько... ~ и... as much... as...; ~ уго́дно as much, as mány as you like; ány amóunt (of).

ско́лько-нибудь 1. *мест. и нареч.* (*некоторое количество*) some, just a few, just a líttle; не бу́дет ли у вас ~ ме́лочи? have you ány small change?; can you let me have a few cóppers?; 2. *нареч.* (*в той или иной мере*) to some extént, in ány way, a líttle.

скомбини́ровать *сов. см.* комбини́ровать.

ско́мкать *сов. см.* ко́мкать.

скомпонова́ть *сов. см.* компонова́ть.

скомпромети́ровать *сов. см.* компромети́ровать.

сконструи́ровать *сов. см.* конструи́ровать.

сконфу́|женный embárrassed. ~зить(ся) *сов. см.* конфу́зить(ся).

сконцентри́ровать(ся) *сов. см.* концентри́ровать(ся).

сконча́ться *сов.* die.

скопи́ровать *сов. см.* копи́ровать.

скоп|и́ть *сов. см.* ска́пливать(ся). ~ле́ние с. 1. (*действие*) accumulátion; 2. (*большое количество кого-л., чего-л.*) jam, congéstion; ~ле́ние наро́да crowd.

скорбе́ть *несов.* (*о пр.*) mourn (óver, for).

ско́рбный móurnful, sólemn.

скорбь ж. grief, sórrow.

скоре́е 1. (*сравнит. ст. прил.* ско́рый *и нареч.*

ско́ро more quíckly; quícker; ~! húrry up!, be quick!; как мо́жно ~ as quíckly as póssible, as fast as you can; **2.** (*верне́е, точне́е*) ráther; **3.** (*охо́тнее*) would ráther; ~ умрём, чем сдади́мся we would ráther/sóoner die than surrénder; **4.** (*бо́льше*) (in fact,) ráther; он ~ высо́кого ро́ста he is, in fact, ráther tall; он ~ похо́ж на отца́ he is more like his fáther; ◇ ~ всего́ most líkely.

скорлуп|а́ *ж.* shell; оре́ховая ~ nútshell; ◇ уйти́ в свою́ ~у́ retíre ínto *one's* shell.

скорми́ть *сов. см.* ска́рмливать.

скорня́к *м.* fúrrier, fúr-dresser.

ско́ро 1. *нареч.* (*бы́стро*) fast, quickly; **2.** *нареч.* (*вско́ре*) soon; я ~ приду́ I won't be long; не ~ not véry soon, not for a long time; он не ~ вернётся he won't be back for a long time; **3.** *в знач. сказ.* it will soon be; ночь it will soon be night; ~ весна́ soon it will be spring, spring will soon be here.

скорова́рка *ж.* préssure cóoker.

скорогово́рк|а *ж.* **1.** rápid speech; **2.** (*тру́дное сочета́ние слов*) tóngue-twister. ~ой: говори́ть ~ой gábble.

ско́ропись *ж.* cúrsive.

скоропо́ртящийся périshable.

скоропости́жн|о súddenly; сконча́ться ~ die súddenly. ~ый súdden; ~ая смерть súdden death.

скороспе́л|ый 1. éarly matúring/rípe, éarly; ~ые я́блоки éarly ápples; **2.** *разг.* (*поспе́шный*) hásty, prémature; ~ое реше́ние hásty decísion.

скоростн|о́й high-speed, fast; ~о́й бег на конька́х spéed skáting; ~о́й спуск (на лы́жах) downhíll/álpine skíing; ~а́я пла́вка high-speed mélting.

ско́рость *ж.* speed, rate; *mex., физ.* velócity; больша́я (небольша́я) ~ high (low) speed; со ~ю... at the rate (of)...; развива́ть ~, е́хать с большо́й ~ю go*/drive* fast; ~ хо́да speed.

скоросшива́тель *м.* fólder.

скорота́ть *сов. см.* корота́ть.

скорохо́д *м.* fast rúnner; (*о конькобе́жце*) spéed-skater; (*о лы́жнике*) rácing skíer.

скорпио́н *м.* **1.** *зоол.* scórpion; **2.** (*знак зодиа́ка*) Scórpio.

ско́рчить *сов. см.* ко́рчить 1. ~ся *сов. см.* ко́рчиться.

ско́р|ый 1. (*бы́стрый*) fast; ~ым ша́гом at a brisk walk; ~ по́езд fast train; **2.** (*бли́зкий по вре́мени*) forthcóming, impénding; в ~ом вре́мени soon, befóre long, shórtly; до ~ого свида́ния! see you soon!; ◇ ~ая по́мощь 1) (*организа́ция*) first-aid; 2) (*автомоби́ль*) ámbulance; на ~ую ру́ку in a rush; пое́сть на ~ую ру́ку snatch a bite; snatch a meal.

скос *м.* slope.

скоси́ть I, II *сов. см.* коси́ть I, II *и* ска́шивать I, II.

скот *м. собир.* lívestock, cáttle; племенно́й ~ bréeding stock, pédigree cáttle. ~и́на *ж. собир. разг.* ánimals *pl*; (*об отде́льном живо́тном*) ánimal; **2.** *бран.* beast, brute.

скóтн|ик *м.* cáttle-man*. ~ица *ж.* cáttle-woman*. ~ый: ~ый двор stóckyard; (*во́зле до́ма*) fármyard.

скотобо́йня *ж.* sláughter-house.

скотово́д *м.* cáttle-breeder, stóck-breeder. ~ство *с.* stóck-breeding, cáttle-breeding, stóck-raising, cáttle-raising. ~ческий stóck-breeding *attr.*, cáttle-breeding *attr.*

скот|ский cáttle *attr.*; *перен.* brútish, béstial. ~ство *с.* **1.** brútishness, bestiálity; **2.** *разг.* (*гру́бость, бескульту́рье*) barbárity, squálor; (*по́длость*) bóorishness, lóutishness.

скра́дывать *несов.* (*вн.*) concéal (*smth.*).

скра́сить *сов. см.* скра́шивать.

скра́шивать, скра́сить (*вн.*) sóften (*smth.*), bríghten (*smth.*).

скребо́к *м.* scráper.

скре́жет *м.* grínding; ~ зубо́вный gnáshing of teeth. ~а́ть *несов.* grind*; ~а́ть зуба́ми gnash *one's* teeth.

скрепи́ть *сов. см.* скрепля́ть.

скре́пка *ж.* clip (for páper), fástener.

скрепля́ть, скрепи́ть (*вн.*) **1.** fásten (*smth.*) (togéther); (*ско́бой*) cramp (*smth.*); (*болта́ми*) bolt (*smth.*); *перен.* consólidate (*smth.*); ~ у́зы дру́жбы tíghten the bonds of fríendship; **2.** (*удостове́рить*) seal (*smth.*); ~ что-л. по́дписью sign *smth.*; ◇ скрепя́ се́рдце with the útmost relúctance.

скрести́ *несов.* (*вн.*) **1.** scratch (*smth.*); **2.** (*чи́стить*) scóur (*smth.*), scrape (*smth.*); **3.** *разг.* (*беспоко́ить*) wórry (*smth.*), nag (at), gnaw (at); у него́ на се́рдце скребёт he is wórried at heart. ~сь *несов.* scratch.

скрести́(сь) *сов. см.* скре́щивать(ся).

скреще́ние *с.* cróssing; (*у́лиц тж.*) interséction.

скре́щивание *с. биол.* cróssing, cróss-breeding.

скре́щивать, скрести́ть (*вн.*) cross (*smth.*) (*тж. биол.*); скрести́ть ру́ки на груди́ fold *one's* arms; скрести́ть штыки́ cross báyonets; ◇ скрести́ть шпа́ги swords. ~ся, скрести́ться 1. (*пересека́ться*) cross; *перен. тж.* come* ínto cónflict; 2. *биол.* interbréed*.

скриви́ть(ся) *сов. см.* криви́ть(ся).

скрип *м.* creak, créaking, squeak, squéaking; (*пера*) scratch; (*сне́га, песка́ под нога́ми*) crunch.

скрипа́ч *м.* víolinist; (*у́личный*) fíddler.

скрипе́ть, проскрипе́ть, скри́пнуть 1. creak, squeak; (*о пере, сне́ге под нога́ми*) crunch; ~ зуба́ми grind*/grit *one's* teeth; **2.** (*издава́ть скрипу́чие зву́ки*) útter harsh cries; (*говори́ть ре́зким го́лосом*) rasp.

скрипи́чн|ый víolin *attr.*; ~ые стру́ны víolin strings; ~ конце́рт víolin concérto; ~ ключ *муз.* tréble/G clef.

скри́пк|а *ж.* víolin; fíddle *разг.*; игра́ть на ~е play the víolin; игра́ть пе́рвую ~у play first víolin; *перен.* play a léading part; игра́ть втору́ю ~у play sécond fíddle.

скри́пнуть *сов. см.* скрипе́ть.

скрипу́ч|ий *разг.* créaking; (*о го́лосе*) gráting, squéaky; (*о сапога́х*) squéaky; (*о пере*) scrátchy; (*о сне́ге, песке́*) crisp; ◇ ~ее де́рево два ве́ка стои́т ≈ a créaking door/gate hangs lóngest.

скро́ить *сов. см.* кро́ить.

скро́мн|ик *м.*, ~ица *ж. разг.* módest pérson.

скромнич|ать *несов.* be* overmódest; не ~ай(-те) don't be so módest!

скро́мн|о módestly; жить (о́чень) ~ live in a small way, live módestly; ~ одева́ться dress quíetly. ~ость *ж.* módesty. ~ый **1.** módest, unassúming; (*сде́ржанный в обраще́нии, поведе́нии тж.*) restráined; **2.** (*просто́й*) unpreténtious, símple; (*о еде́*) frúgal; ~ый наря́д símple attíre/clothes; ~ый о́браз жи́зни frúgal life; **3.** (*уме́ренный*) móderate, módest; ~ая цена́ móderate price; у него́ ~ый за́работок he is not éarning much.

скрупулёзный scrúpulous.

скрути́ть *сов. см.* скру́чивать.

скру́чивать, скрути́ть (*вн.*) **1.** (*свива́ть, свёртывать*) twist (*smth.*); (*папиро́су*) roll (*smth.*); **2.** (*свя́зывать*) bind* (*smb., smth.*) tíghtly; скрути́ть кому́-л. ру́ки fásten/bind* *smb.'s* hands tíghtly; **3.** *разг.* get* (*smb.*) down; боле́знь его́ скрути́ла his íllness is gétting him down.

скрыва́ть, скрыть (*вн.*) **1.** hide* (*smth.*), concéal (*smth.*); следы́ преступле́ния cóver up all tráces of the crime; ~ свои́ недоста́тки hide* *one's* faults; ~ свои́ чу́вства disguíse *one's* féelings; ~ свою́ ра́дость hide* *one's* joy; **2.** (*ута́ивать*) keep* (*smth.*) back; ~ своё и́мя refúse to revéal *one's* name; ~ свои́ наме́рения concéal *one's* inténtions; не ~ чего́-л. make* no bones abóut *smth.*, fránkly admit *smth.*; не скро́ю от вас... I will not concéal/keep from you...; не скрыть, что... not disguíse the fact that...; нельзя́ скрыть there is no disguísing; **3.** *тк. несов.* (*заключа́ть в себе́*) concéal (*smth.*). ~ся *несов.* **1.** (*пря́таться*) hide*, be* in híding; (*избега́ть* *встречи*) keep* out of sight; **2.** *разг.* (*держать что-л. в тайне*) conceal the fact; **3.** (*о чём-л. внешне незаметном*) be* concealed; **4.** (*корениться в чём-л.*) lie*.

скры́тнич|ать *несов. разг.* be* secretive; не ~áйте! out with it, don't be so secretive!

скры́тн|ость *ж.* **1.** secretiveness; **2.** *разг.* (*тайна*) secrecy, concealment. **~ый 1.** secretive; **2.** (*тайный*) secret.

скры́т|ый hidden, concealed; *физ.* latent; **~ая** угро́за hidden/veiled threat; **~ые** возмо́жности latent/hidden possibilities.

скрыть *сов. см.* скрыва́ть 1, 2. **~ся** *сов.* **1.** hide*, conceal oneself; (*сбежать*) escape; (*уйти незаметно*) slip away; **2.** (*исчезнуть*) vanish, disappear; со́лнце скры́лось за ту́чами clouds hid the sun; от него́ ничто́ не мо́жет **~ся** nothing escapes his notice.

скрю́чить(ся) *сов. см.* крю́чить(ся).

скря́га *м. и ж.* miser, skinflint.

скря́жничать *несов. разг.* be* a miser/skinflint; pinch and screw.

скуде́ть *несов. см.* оскудева́ть.

ску́д|ный meagre, scanty; (*бедный чем-л.*) poor (in); **~ное** освеще́ние dim/wretched light; **~ные** запа́сы чего́-л. scanty stock of *smth.*; **~ные** све́дения scant(y) information *sg.* **~ость** *ж.* meagreness, scantiness; (*бедность*) poverty.

ску́к|а *ж.* boredom; (*однообразие*) tedium; от **~и** from sheer boredom; кака́я ~! what a bore!; нагоня́ть **~у** на *кого-л.* bore *smb.*

скула́ *ж.* cheekbone; выдаю́щиеся ску́лы high/prominent cheekbones.

скула́ст|ый high-cheekboned; ~ челове́к person with high cheekbones; **~ое** лицо́ broad face.

скули́ть *несов.* whine, whimper.

скульпт|ор *м.* sculptor. **~у́ра** *ж.* sculpture; (*произведение скульптуры тж.*) statue, figure, piece of sculpture. **~у́рный** sculptural; **~у́рная** мастерска́я sculptor's studio; **~у́рное** изображе́ние statue.

ску́мбрия *ж.* (*рыба*) mackerel.

скунс *м.* (*животное и мех*) skunk.

скупа́ть, скупи́ть (*вн.*) buy* (*smth.*) up; ~ о́птом buy* up wholesale.

скупи́ть *сов. см.* скупа́ть.

скуп|и́ться *несов.* (*на вн., + инф.*) stint (*smth.*); ~ на де́ньги grudge the money; не ~ на похвалы́ not stint *one's* praises; не **~и́сь**, не **~и́тесь**! don't be mean/stingy!

ску́пка *ж.* buying up.

скуп|о́й *прил.* **1.** mean, miserly, stingy, close-fisted; **2.** (*скудный*) ungenerous; **~áя** по́чва niggardly/ungenerous soil; ~ свет dim light; **3.** (*на вн., в пр.; сдержанный*) restrained (in), sparing (of); ~ на слова́ reticent, taciturn; chary of *one's* words; ~ на похвалы́ restrained in *one's* praise, not given to praising; **4.** *в знач. сущ. м.* miser; skinflint.

ску́пость *ж.* **1.** meanness, miserliness, stinginess; **2.** (*необилие*) scantiness; ~ кра́сок sparing use of colour.

ску́пщик *м.* buyer-up.

скуч|а́ть *несов.* **1.** be* bored; **2.** (*о, по пр., по дт.*) miss (*smb., smth.*); он о́чень **~а́ет** обо мне he misses me very much; ~ по до́му be* homesick, miss *one's* home-life; **~áющий** weary, bored; **~áющий** вид weary air.

скученн|о close together; жить ~ live in crowded conditions. **~ость** *ж.* congestion; (*населения тж.*) **~ый** dense, congested, crowded.

ску́чиваться, ску́читься *разг.* huddle together; ~ вокру́г cluster round.

ску́читься *сов. см.* ску́чиваться.

ску́чн|о 1. *нареч.:* ~ говори́ть be* a dull speaker; ~ говори́ть, расска́зывать о чём-л. bore *smb.* to death talking about *smth.*; **2.** *в знач. сказ. безл.* it is boring; ~ сиде́ть без де́ла it is dull/boring doing nothing; как э́то ~! what a bore!; **3.** *в знач. сказ. безл. (дт.):* мне ~ I am

bored. **~ый 1.** (*вызывающий скуку*) dull, boring, tedious; (*о занятии тж.*) tiresome; **~ый** разгово́р dull conversation; **~ый** челове́к bore; **2.** (*выражающий, испытывающий скуку*) bored; (*грустный*) sad; **~ое** лицо́ bored expression.

ску́шать *сов.* (*вн., рд.*) eat* (*smth.*) up; (*об обеде и т. п.*) have* (*smth.*).

слаба́к *м. разг.* weakling, softy.

слаб|е́ть *несов.* weaken; grow*/get* weak(er); (*о ветре, буре*) subside, abate; мои́ си́лы **~е́ют** I am getting weaker and weaker. **~е́ющий** failing, enfeebled; (*о ветре, буре*) slackening; abating; **~е́ющие** ру́ки enfeebled hands; **~е́ющее** зре́ние failing sight.

слаби́тельное *с.* laxative, purgative.

слаб|и́ть *несов. безл.:* его́ **~и́т** he has diarrhoea.

сла́бо 1. weakly, feebly; (*о завязанном*) loosely; **2.** (*плохо*) poorly; ~ знать что-л. be* weak in *smth.*

слабово́лие *с.* weakness of will, weak will.

слабово́льный weak-willed.

слабоси́льный 1. (*недостаточно сильный физически*) weak, feeble; **2.** (*небольшой мощности*) underpowered; low-power *attr.*

сла́бость *ж.* **1.** weakness; (*физическая тж.*) feebleness; ~ зре́ния weak eyesight; ~ во́ли weakness/lack of will; чу́вствовать (каку́ю-то) ~ feel* (rather) weak/poorly; чу́вствовать ~ в нога́х be* weak on *one's* legs, feel* rather tottery; прояви́ть ~ show* a lack of determination; **2.** (*к дт.*) *разг.* (*склонность, расположение*) weakness (for); пита́ть ~ к кому́-л. have* a soft spot in *one's* heart for *smb.*

слабоу́м|ие *с.* feeblemindedness; ста́рческое ~ dotage, senile dementia. **~ный** feebleminded, weak-minded.

слабохара́ктерн|ость *ж.* lack of character. **~ый** weak-willed.

сла́б|ый 1. weak; feeble; (*болезненный*) delicate; **~ое** се́рдце weak heart; ~ ребёнок delicate child*; **~ые** ру́ки feeble hands; **~ая** во́ля weak will; **~ая** а́рмия weak army; **2.** (*имеющий небольшую мощность — о моторах и т. п.*) low-power *attr.*; **3.** (*некрепкий, ненасыщенный*) weak; **~ое** лека́рство weak/mild medicine; ~ чай weak tea; **4.** (*небольшой по силе, неотчётливый*) faint; ~ свет dim light; ~ ве́тер light/gentle breeze; ~ое тече́ние gentle current; ~ след faint mark/track; **~ая** улы́бка faint smile; **~ая** попы́тка feeble attempt; **5.** (*недостаточный, плохой*) weak, poor; **~ая** па́мять bad*/poor memory; ~ учени́к weak pupil*; **6.** (*малоубедительный, несовершенный*) feeble; **~ое** доказа́тельство feeble argument; **7.** (*нетугой*) slack, loose; ◇ **~ое** ме́сто, **~ая** сторона́ weak point; **~ая** стру́нка weak spot.

сла́в|а *ж.* **1.** glory; distinctions *pl*; трудова́я ~ reputation for work; **2.** (*известность*) fame, reputation, name; **3.** *разг.* (*репутация*) reputation; по́льзоваться дурно́й **~ой** have* a bad reputation, be* in bad repute; **4.** *разг.* (*слухи, толки, молва*) rumour; ходи́ла ~, что... it was rumoured that...; ◇ во **~у** *кого-л., чего-л.* for the glory of *smb., smth.*; одна́ ~, что... *разг.* it's all talk that...; ~ бо́гу! thank God/heavens/goodness!; на **~у** splendidly, excellently.

слави́ст *м.* Slavist, Slavonic scholar. **~ика** *ж.* slavonic studies *pl.*

сла́вить *несов.* (*вн.*) glorify (*smth.*), do* honour (to), heap distinctions (on). **~ся** *несов.* (*тв.*) be*-famous/famed (for); have* a reputation/name (for); **сла́вься!** glory (to)!

сла́вн|о splendidly, very well; ~ отдохну́ть have* a splendid rest; провести́ вре́мя, о́тпуск have* a lovely time, holiday. **~ый 1.** glorious; **2.** *разг.* (*хороший*) very nice; fine; **~ая** де́вушка very nice girl; **~ый** па́рень fine chap.

славяни́зм *м.* **1.** (*заимствование неславянского языка из какого-л. славянского языка*) Slavism, borrowing from a Slavonic language; **2.** (*заимствование* *в русском языке из церковнославянского языка)* word derived from Church Slavónic.

слав│яни́н *м.*, **~я́нка** *ж.* Slav.

славя́нск│ий Slavónic, Slávic; **~ие языки́** Slavónic lánguages.

слага́емое *с.* 1. *мат.* ítem; 2. *(составная часть)* compónent, constítuent.

слага́ть, сложи́ть *(вн.)* 1. *(сочинять)* compóse *(smth.)*, make* *smth.*); 2. *(освобождать от чего-л.):* ~ с себя́ обя́занности resígn; ~ с себя́ вся́кую отве́тственность decline all responsibility. **~ся** *несов. (из рд.)* consíst (of), be* made up (of).

слад *м. разг.:* с ним никако́го **~у** нет he is quite unmánageable.

сла́дить *сов. разг.* 1. *(вн.)* arránge *(smth.)*; 2. *(с тв.; справиться)* mánage *(smb, smth.)*, hándle *(smb, smth.)*; cope (with); мне с ним не ~ I can't mánage him; I can't cope with him; мне с э́тим не ~ it is too much for me.

сла́дк│ий *прил.* 1. sweet; *перен. (льстивый, угодливый)* hóneyed, súgary; **~ие я́блоки** sweet ápples; 2. *разг. (о жизни, судьбе)* éasy, soft; 3. *(приятный)* sweet; ~ сон sound/sweet sleep; ~ звук sweet sound; 4. *в знач. сущ. с.* sweets *pl,* sweet things *pl; разг. (десерт)* sweet course, dessért; переста́ть есть **~ое** stop éating sweet things.

сла́дко 1. *нареч.* swéetly; 2. *в знач. сказ. безл.* it is sweet/good; во рту ~ it tastes sweet.

сладкое́жка *м. и ж. разг.:* он ~ he has a sweet tooth.

сла́достный sweet.

сладостра́ст│ие *с.* sensuálity. **~ный** sénsual; *(томный)* volúptuous.

сла́дость *ж.* 1. swéetness; 2. *мн.* sweets, swéetmeats; cándies *амер.;* 3. *(наслаждение)* delíghts *pl.*

сла́женный co-órdinated; *(о пении)* harmónious.

сла́зить *сов. (вниз)* go* down (into); *(вверх)* climb up to; ~ в по́греб go* down ínto the céllar; ~ на черда́к climb up to the áttic.

сла́лом *м. спорт.* slálom.

слан│ец *м.* shale, schist; горю́чие **~цы** oil/bitúminous shale *sg.* **~цевый** shale *attr.*

сла́сти *мн. см.* сла́дость 2.

слать *несов. (вн.)* send* *(smb, smth.)*.

слаща́в│ый súgary, sáccharine; **~ая улы́бка** fúlsome smile.

сле́ва *(откуда-л.)* from the left; *(где-л.)* on/to the left (of); ~ напра́во from left to right; ~ от него́ to his left, on his left side; ~ от доро́ги on the left (of the road).

слегка́ slíghtly, géntly.

след *м.* 1. *(отпечаток)* ímprint; *(человека)* trace, fóotprint; *(колёс, саней, животных)* trace, track; 2. *(остаток чего-л.)* trace; *(характерный отпечаток)* sign; *(результат чего-л.)* mark; **~ы** слёз tráces of tears; никако́го ~а не оста́лось no trace remáins; ни ~á not a véstige; 3. *(раны, ожога и т. п.)* mark, weal, scar; ◇ идти́ по чьим-л. **~ам** 1) fóllow in the tracks of *smb.;* 2) *(следовать учению и т. п.)* fóllow in *smb.'s* fóotsteps, fóllow in the wake of *smb.;* напа́сть на чей-л. ~ get* on the track of *smb.;* его́ и ~ просты́л he has vánished ínto thin air; пройти́ без ~á vánish complétely.

следи́ть I *несов.* (за тв.) 1. watch *(smb, smth.)*, fóllow *(smb, smth.)*; ~ глаза́ми за кем-л. watch *smb.,* fóllow *smb.* with *one's* eyes; при́стально ~ за кем-л. keep* a sharp eye on *smb.;* ~ за полётом птиц watch the birds flýing; 2. *(наблюдать за ходом чего-л.)* fóllow *(smth.)*, keep* up (with); ~ за разви́тием собы́тий obsérve the course of evénts; ~ за успе́хами нау́ки keep* abréast of science; ~ за разгово́рами fóllow the conversátion; 3. *(присматривать, заботиться)* see* (to); ~ за детьми́ see* to the children; ~ за рабо́той superinténd the work; ~ за поря́дком maintáin órder; ~ за

са́дом look áfter the gárden; 4. *(наблюдать с целью разоблачения)* keep* *(smb.)* únder observátion, survéil *(smb.)*, spy (on); *(на улице)* shádow *(smb.)*; ◇ ~ за собо́й look áfter *onesélf* próperly; *(заботиться о своём внешнем виде)* dress with care.

следи́ть II, наследи́ть *разг.* *(оставить следы)* leave* dírty fóotmarks; *(тв.)* make* a mess (with).

следова́ни│е *с.:* по́езд да́льнего **~я** long-dístance train.

сле́дователь *м.* examining mágistrate, preliminary invéstigator.

сле́довательно cónsequently, hence.

след│овать, после́довать 1. *(за тв.; идти, ехать следом)* fóllow *(smb.)*; *перен.* fóllow in *smb.'s* fóotsteps; ~ по пята́м за кем-л. dog *smb.'s* steps, fóllow *smb.* abóut; 2. *(за тв.; наступать после чего-л.)* come* (áfter), fóllow *(smth.)*; собы́тия **~овали** одно́ за други́м evénts fóllowed in quick succéssion; 3. *(дт.; руководствоваться чем-л.)* fóllow *(smb., smth.)*; ~ приме́ру кого́-л. fóllow *smb.'s* exámple; ~ сове́там врача́ fóllow the dóctor's advíce; ~ мо́де keep* up with the fáshion; 4. *тк. несов. (двигаться)* procéed; ~ по назначе́нию procéed to *one's* destinátion; по́езд **~ует** до Москвы́ the train goes as far as Móscow; 5. *тк. несов. (из рд.; вытекать)* fóllow; из э́того **~ует,** что... it fóllows that...; из одного́ предположе́ния **~ует** друго́е one assúmption leads to anóther; 6. *тк. несов. (дт.; причитаться)* be* due (to); ско́лько с меня́ **(~ует)?** how much have I to pay?; *(в магазине)* what will/does this come to?; ему́ заплати́ли, что **~ова**ло he got what was due to him; 7. *тк. несов. безл. (нужно)* it should be; ~ет по́мнить it should be borne in mind; вам **~овало бы**... you ought (to)...; *(в прошлом)* you ought to have...; **~овало** ожида́ть, что...; it was to be expécted that...; как и **~овало** ожида́ть... as was to be expécted...; э́того **~овало** ожида́ть that was to be expécted; не ~ет ду́мать... it should not be conclúded...; кому́ ~ет to the próper pérson; обраща́ться куда́ ~ет applý to the próper quárter; ◇ как ~ет próperly; отдохну́ть как ~ет have* a real rest.

сле́дом immédiately áfter.

следопы́т *м.* 1. *(охотник)* trácker; 2. *(отыскивающий следы былых исторических событий)* tráil-seeker, páthfinder.

сле́дственн│ый invéstigatory; ~ материа́л évidence; **~ые** о́рганы invéstigating authórities; **~ая** коми́ссия committee of inquíry.

сле́дствие I *с. (результат)* cónsequence, resúlt; **~м** э́того бы́ло то, что... the cónsequence/resúlt was that...

сле́дствие II *с. (расследование)* inquíry; ◇ он нахо́дится под **~м** his case is únder investigátion.

сле́дуем│ый due; ~ая мне су́мма the sum due to me.

сле́дующ│ий the fóllowing; *(из многих)* the next; **~им** о́бразом as fóllows; *(в)* ~ раз next time; на ~ день the next day; **~!** *(при вызове)* next (please)!

слежа́ться *сов.* becóme* fírmly packed, séttle.

слежка *ж.* shádowing.

слез│а́ *ж.* tear; *перен.* drop; в **~а́х** in tears; зали́ться **~а́ми** burst* ínto tears; залива́ться **~а́ми** be* drowned in tears; пла́кать го́рькими **~а́ми** weep* bítter tears; доводи́ть кого́-л. до слёз redúce *smb.* to tears; говори́ть сквозь слёзы speak*/say* with tears in *one's* voice; сме́яться до слёз laugh till *one* cries; laugh till the tears come; до слёз бо́льно, оби́дно, что... it's héartrending that...; мне бы́ло оби́дно до слёз I could have cried; **~а́ми** го́рю не помо́жешь it's no use crýing (óver spilt milk); сме́яться сквозь слёзы laugh and cry at the same time, smile through *one's* tears.

слеза́ть, слезть 1. *(спускаться)* come* down, get* down, climb down; *(со стула и т. п.)* get* off; слезть с де́рева climb down a tree; ~ с ло́шади dismóunt; 2. *разг. (с поезда и т. п.)* get* off; 3. *разг. (о краске, коже и т. п.)* come* off, peel.

слези́нка ж. téar-drop.

слез|и́ться несов. wáter; его́ глаза́ ~я́тся от ве́тра the wind is máking his eyes wáter. ~ли́вый téarful; перен. sentiméntal.

слёзн|ый 1. анат. láchrymal; 2. разг. téarful; ~ая жа́лоба, мольба́ húmble compláint, práyer.

слезотече́ние с. epíphora; вызыва́ть ~ make* one's eyes wáter.

слезоточи́вый 1. (слезящийся) wátery, rhéumy; 2. (вызывающий слёзы): ~ газ téar-gas.

слезть сов. см. слезать.

слезя́щийся wátery.

слепе́нь м. зоол. hórse-fly.

слепе́ц м. blind man*.

слепи́ть I несов. (вн.) (мешать видеть) blind (smb.); (о свете) dázzle (smth.).

слепи́ть II сов. см. лепить 2.

сле́пнуть, ослепнуть lose* one's sight, go*/becóme* blind.

сле́по blíndly; ~ повинова́ться кому-л. obéy smb. blíndly; ~ сле́довать чему-л. fóllow smth. blíndly.

слеп|о́й прил. 1. blind; ~ на оди́н глаз blind in one eye; ~ от рождения blind from birth; ~о́е повинове́ние blind/implícit obédience; ~а́я любо́вь blind love; ~ слу́чай the mérest chance; ~ ме́тод печа́тания на маши́нке tóuch-type sýstem; ~ полёт blind flying; 2. в знач. сущ. м. blind man*; ж. blind wóman*; мн. собир. the blind; ◇ ~ая кишка́ анат. blind gut, cáecum.

слепо́к м. cast; перен. réplica; ~ с ключа́ impréssion of a key.

слепорождённый blind from birth после сущ., born blind после сущ.

слепота́ ж. blíndness.

слеса́рн|ый fítter's; ~ая мастерска́я tool shop.

слесарь м. fítter; ~-инструмента́льщик tóol-maker; ~-санте́хник plúmber.

слёт м. 1. (птиц) flight; 2. (собрание) rálly.

слет|а́ть I сов. 1. (на самолёте) fly*; 2. разг. (сбегать) run*; ми́гом ~а́ю I'll be back in no time.

слет|а́ть II, слете́ть 1. fly* down; 2. (падать) fall* off; бума́ги слете́ли со стола́ the pápers were blown off the táble; 3. (улетать) fly* awáy. ~а́ться, слете́ться come* flying, fly* togéther; flock in (тж. перен.).

слете́ть сов. см. слетать II. ~ся сов. см. слетаться.

слечь сов. take* to one's bed, be* laid up.

сли́ва ж. 1. (плод) plum; 2. (дерево) plúm-tree.

слива́ть, слить (вн.) 1. (смешивать) mix (smth.); 2. (отливать) pour (smth.) off; 3. (соединять посредством литья) fuse (smth.); 4. (соединять в одно целое) amálgamate (smth.), merge (smth.); (неразрывно связывать) merge (smth.), blend (smth.). ~ся, сли́ться 1. (соединяться в один поток) flow togéther; (о реках) join; 2. (о красках, звуках) blend, merge; ~ся с фо́ном melt ínto the báckground; ~ся воеди́но becóme* one.

сли́вки мн. cream sg; снять ~ с молока́ skim the milk, take* the cream off the milk; ◇ снима́ть ~ take* the cream.

сли́вовый plum attr.

сли́вочн|ик м. créam-jug. ~ый cream attr.; ~ое ма́сло bútter; ~ое моро́женое ice-cream.

слиза́ть сов. см. сли́зывать.

сли́зистый 1. slímy; 2. анат. múcous.

слизну́ть сов. см. сли́зывать.

слизня́к м. зоол. slug.

сли́зывать, слиза́ть, слизну́ть (вн.) lick (smth.) off.

слизь ж. slime, múcus.

слип|а́ться, сли́пнуться 1. stick* togéther; 2.: глаза́ ~а́ются от сна one can hárdly keep one's eyes ópen.

сли́пнуться сов. см. слипа́ться.

сли́тн|о as one word; togéther. ~ый 1. sólid; ~ый гул confúsed hum, stéady din; 2. (о написании слов) as one word после сущ., sólid predic.

сли́ток м. íngot.

слить(ся) сов. см. сливать(ся).

слич|а́ть, сличи́ть (вн.) compáre (smth.), colláte (smth.). ~е́ние с. compárison, collátion.

сличи́ть сов. см. сличать.

сли́шком too; ~ мно́го too much; не ~ умён no génius; ~ (сильно) люби́ть кого-л. be* too fond of smb.; ~ си́льно нажа́ть press too hard; э́то уж ~! that réally is too much!; I call that the límit! разг.

слия́ние с. 1. (рек) cónfluence, júnction; 2. (объединение) amalgamátion, mérging.

словак м. Slóvak, Slovákian.

словарн|ый léxical; díctionary attr.; ~ состав языка́ vocábulary, word stock; ~ запа́с vocábulary; ~ая рабо́та díctionary work.

словарь м. 1. díctionary; (специальных слов) glóssary; 2. тк. ед. (запас слов) vocábulary.

слова́|цкий Slóvak, Slovákian; ~ язык Slóvak, the Slóvak lánguage. ~чка ж. Slóvak, Slovákian.

словен|ец м., ~ка ж. Slovéne, Slovénian. ~ский Slovénian; ~ский язык Slovénian, the Slovénian lánguage.

слове́сный vérbal, óral.

слóвник м. wórd-list.

слóвно 1. союз (как) like; 2. частица (как будто) as if, as though.

слóв|о с. 1. word; во́время ска́занное ~ a word in séason; понима́ть без слов understánd* without a word háving been spóken; ни ~а! not a word!; моё ~ твёрдо when I say a thing, I mean it; ве́рить кому-л. на́ слово take* smb.'s word for it; take* it on trust; рома́нс на ~а́ Пу́шкина song to words from Púshkin; на два ~а! may I have a word with you?; мне на́до сказа́ть вам два ~а! a word in your ear!; 2. (речь, язык) lánguage; 3.: проси́ть ~а ask to speak, ask for the floor; ~ име́ет товарищ Ивано́в Cómrade Ivanóv will now speak, Cómrade Ivanóv has the floor; ~ за ва́ми, тепе́рь за ва́ми ~ it is for you to decíde; после́днее ~ за защи́той the defence has the last word; после́днее ~ оста́лось за ним he had the last word; 4. (повествование) tale, stóry; «Сло́во о полку́ Игореве» "The Song of Ígor's Campáign"; ◇ ~ в ~ word for word; ~ за́ слово one thing led to anóther; на ~а́х (устно) by word of mouth; то́лько на ~а́х in word ónly; не на ~а́х, а на де́ле ≈ not mérely in words but with deeds; нет слов, чтобы вы́разить... words fail to expréss...; я не нахожу́ слов, чтобы... I have no words to...; слов нет (правда, конечно) there's no denýing, of course; нóвое ~ в чём-л. fresh depárture in smth., mílestone in smth.; advance in smth.; к ~у (сказáть) by the by; к ~у пришло́сь but that's by the way; завод обо́рудован по после́днему ~у те́хники the plant has all the látest equípment.

слóвом in a word, in short.

словообразов|а́ние с. wórd-formation. ~а́тельный wórd-formative.

словоохо́тливый tálkative, loquácious, gárrulous.

словосочета́ние с. combinátion of words; усто́йчивое ~ set expréssion; свобо́дное ~ free combinátion of words.

слог I м. (часть слова) sýllable.

слог II м. уст. (стиль) style.

слогово́й syllábic.

слоён|ый fláky; púff-pastry attr.; ~ пиро́г púff-pastry pie; ~ое те́сто puff paste.

сложе́ни|е с. 1. (действие) formátion; 2. мат. addition; 3. (тела) build; челове́к кре́пкого ~я stúrdy pérson.

сложи́ть I сов. см. скла́дывать и класть 2.

сложи́ть II сов. см. слагать.

сложи́ться сов. см. скла́дываться.

сло́жно íntricately, in a complicated mánner.

сложноподчинённ|**ый** *лингв.*: ~ое предложение cómplex séntence.

сложносочинённ|**ый** *лингв.*: ~ое предложение cómpound/co-órdinated séntence.

сложн|**ость** *ж.* íntricacy, compléxity; (*трудность*) dífficulty. **~ый 1.** (*состоящий из нескольких частей*) cómpound, cómposite; ~ые вещества cómpounds; ~ое слово cómpound word; ~ое предложение cómplex séntence; ~ое число cómpound númber; ~ые проценты cómpound ínterest *sg*; **2.** (*многообразный*) cómplex; ~ая наука cómplex scíence; ~ый характер cómplex cháracter; **3.** (*трудный*) dífficult, invólved, cómplicated (*запутанный*) íntricate; ~ый вопрос cómplicated quéstion/mátter; ~ая обстановка cómplicated situátion; **4.** (*замысловатый*) íntricate; ~ый орнамент íntricate ornamentátion.

слойст|**ый** fláky; ~ые облака láyer cloud *sg*, strátus *sg*.

сло|**й** *м.* **1.** láyer; (*краски*) coat; **2.** *геол.* strátum (*pl* -ta), láyer (*тж. перен.*); различные ~и общества the várious stráta of society.

слойка *ж. разг.* púff(-pastry).

слом *м.* (*машин и т. п.*) bréaking, dismántling; (*домов*) púlling down, demolítion; предназначено на ~ (*о машинах и т. п.*) to be used for scrap; (*о домах*) to be pulled down.

сломать *сов. см.* ломать 1, 3, 4, 5. **~ся** *сов. см.* ломаться 1, 3, 4, 5.

сломить *сов.* (*вн.*) break* (*smth.*); ~ сопротивление кого-л. break* down *smb.'s* resistance.

слон *м.* **1.** élephant; **2.** *шахм.* bíshop; ◇ ~á не приметить miss the óbvious; ~ёнок *м.* élephant-calf*; báby-elephant *разг.* ~иха *ж.*ców-elephant; shé-elephant *разг.*

слонóв|**ый** élephant's; (*похожий на слона*) elephántine; ◇ ~ая кость ívory; ~ая болезнь *мед.* elephantíasis.

слоняться *несов. разг.* (*тж.* ~ без дела) loaf abóut, lóiter.

слуга *м.* sérvant (*тж. перен.*); (*лакей тж.*) mánservant, man*.

служанка *ж* sérvant-girl, hóusemaid.

служащий *прил.* **1.** óffice *attr.*; **2.** *в знач. сущ. м.* employée, óffice wórker, white-collar wórker.

служб|**а** *ж.* **1.** (*действие*) sérvice; ~ в армии sérvice in the ármy; срок ~ы аккумулятора, станка *и т. п.*) sérvice life of a báttery, lathe, *etc.*; **2.** (*работа, должность*) work, job; поступить на ~у begín* wórking, take* a job; **3.** (*исполнение воинских обязанностей*) mílitary sérvice; **4.** (*специальная область работы*) sérvice, depártment; ~ связи sígnal sérvice; communicátion sérvice; ~ движения ж.-д. tráffic depártment; **5.** (*богослужение*) (divíne) sérvice; отстоять ~у atténd sérvice; ◇ не в ~у, а в дружбу as a pérsonal fávour.

служебн|**ый 1.** official, óffice *attr.*; ~ые обязанности official dúties; ~ые помещения óffice prémises; ~ое время, ~ые часы óffice hours; ~ое положение official position, position at work; **2.** (*вспомогательный*) auxíliary; ~ое слово *лингв.* línk-word.

служение *с.* sérvice.

служитель *м.* atténdant; ~ искусства vótary of art; ~ культа mínister of relígion.

служить, послужить **1.** *тк. несов.* (*работать по найму*) work; **2.** *тк. несов.* (*быть военным*) serve; **3.** *тк. несов.* (*дт.; выполнять чью-л. волю*) serve (*smb., smth.*), work (for); ~ и нашим и вашим run* with the hare and hunt with the hounds; **4.** *тк. несов.* (*дт.; работать на благо кого-л., чего-л.*) serve (*smb., smth.*); ~ Родине serve *one's* cóuntry; devóte/dédicate onesélf to *one's* cóuntry; **5.** (*дт.; выполнять своё назначение*) be* úseful (to); **6.** (*тв., для рд.; использоваться*) be* used (as, for), serve (as, for); **7.** (*тв.; быть, являться*) be*; ~ примером be* an exámple; ~ предлогом serve as a

prétext; **8.** *тк. несов.* (*совершать богослужение*) officiate; **9.** *тк. несов.* (*о собаках*) beg.

слукавить *сов. см.* лукавить.

слух *м.* **1.** (*музыкальный*) héaring; (*для музыки*) ear (for músic); острый ~ keen héaring; у него хороший ~ he has a good ear (for músic); у него плохой ~ he has no ear (for músic); играть по ~у play by ear; **2.** (*весть, известие*) news; **3.** *мн.* (*толки, молва*) rúmour *sg*; по ~ам accórding to rúmour, rúmour has it (that); ходят ~и it is rúmoured (that); носятся ~и (что) rúmours are aflóat (that); ◇ ~ом земля полнится *погов.* news flies quíckly; он весь обратился в ~ he becáme all ears.

слухов|**ой 1.** áuditory, acóustic; ~ нерв *анат.* áuditory/acóustic nerve; ~ые восприятия áural impréssions; **2.** (*служащий для слушания*): ~ аппарат héaring aid; ◇ ~ое окно dórmer window.

случа|**й** *м.* **1.** (*происшествие*) occúrrence, evént, íncident; несчастный ~ áccident; **2.** (*явление, факт, обстоятельство*) case; смертельный ~ fátal case; fatálity; небывалый ~ remárkable case; в некоторых ~ях in some cáses; **3.** (*возможность*) opportúnity, chance, occásion; пользоваться всяким удобным ~ем néver miss an opportúnity; иметь ~ get* a chance; **4.** (*случайность*) chance; ◇ в ~е чего-л. in case of *smth.*, in the evént of *smth.*; в ~е войны in the evént of war; if there is a war; в ~е смерти кого-л. in the evént of *smb.'s* death; в ~е необходимости in case of need/necéssity; в ~е крайней необходимости in an emérgency; в ~е чего should ánything háppen; в этом ~е in that case; ни в коем ~е in no case, on no accóunt, by no means, únder no círcumstances; по ~ю чего-л. on the occásion of *smth.*; при ~е when opportúnity óffers, should an opportúnity aríse; купить что-л. по ~ю get* *smth.* by chance.

случайн|**о** *нареч.* **1.** by chance, by áccident, accidéntally; ~ быть где-л. háppen to be sómewhere; ~ встретиться с кем-л. háppen to meet *smb.*; ~ найти что-л., наткнуться на что-л. chance upón *smth.*; **2.** *в знач. вводн. сл. разг.* by ány chance; вы, ~, не знаете? do you by ány chance know?; если..., вы его увидите... if you (should) háppen to see him...; ◇ не ~ (что) it is no mere chance (that); это не ~! ≈ there is sómething behínd it! **~ость** *ж.* **1.** chance/accidéntal náture, fortúity; ~ость встречи accidéntal náture of an encóunter; (*непредвиденное обстоятельство*) chance, coíncidence; по счастливой ~ости lúckily, by good fórtune, by a háppy/lúcky chance; по несчастной ~ости as ill luck would have it; чистая ~ость the mérest chance, a pure chance/áccident; **3.** *филос.* chance; áccident, mátter of chance, chance occúrrence. **~ый 1.** (*возникший непредвиденно*) chance *attr.*, accidéntal; ~ая встреча chance/accidéntal méeting; ~ое знакомство chance acquáintance; ~ый попутчик chance compánion; ~ое совпадение coíncidence; ~ая ошибка a mere slip; **2.** (*появляющийся от случая к случаю*) occásional, sporádic, cásual; ~ый заработок sporádic éarnings *pl*; ~ый посетитель cásual vísitor; **3.** (*незакономерный*) fortúitous, accidéntal; ~ое явление chance phenómenon, áccident.

случать, случить (*вн.*) mate (*smth.*), pair (*smth.*), cóuple (*smth.*).

случ|**аться**, случиться **1.** háppen; occúr; ничего не случилось nóthing has háppened; что (с вами) случилось? what's the mátter (with you)?; с ним случилось несчастье he has had a misfórtune; **2.:** ~áется áccidents will háppen; ~áется, что он... he sómetimes...; случилось так, что... it so háppened that...; ~áлось ли вам (+ *инф.*)? did you éver háppen (+ to *inf*)?

случивш|**ееся** *с.* occúrrence; сообщить кому-л. о ~емся tell* *smb.* what has háppened.

случить *сов. см.* случать.

случиться *сов. см.* случаться.

случка *ж.* máting, páiring, cóupling.

слушатель *м.*, ~ница *ж.* **1.** (*слушающий*) lístener, héarer; *мн. собир.* áudience *sg*; 2. (*учащийся*) stúdent; ~ воéнной акадéмии stúdent at a mílitary acádemy.

слýш|ать, послýшать (*вн.*) 1. lísten (to); ~ мýзыку lísten to músic; ~ лéкцию lísten to a lécture; я ~аю! (*по телефóну*) húllo!; вы ~аете? (*по телефóну*) are you there?; 2. (*о врачé*) exámine smb.'s chest; áuscultate (*smb.*) *научн.*; 3. *тк. несов.* (*разбирáть судéбное дéло*) hear* (*smth.*), try (*smth.*); (*публи́чно заслýшивать чьé--л. сообщéние*) hear* (*smth.*); ~ дéло о крáже со взлóмом try a case of búrglary; ~ отчёт hear* a repórt; 4. *тк. несов.* (*присýтствовать на лéкциях*) atténd (*smth.*), go* (to); ~ курс вы́сшей математики atténd/take* a course in higher mathemátics; 5. (*слéдовать чьим-л. совéтам, прóсьбам*) pay* atténtion (to), lísten (to), lísten to smb.'s advíce, take* nótice (of); он никогó не ~ает he won't lísten to ánybody's advíce, he takes no nótice of ányone; 6. *разг.* (*повиновáться*) obéy (*smb.*); (*об управля́емых механи́змах тж.*) respónd (to); ~ руля́ (*о сýдне*) ánswer the helm; 7. *повел.*: ~ай(те)! I say!; look here!; 8. *тк. несов.*: ~аю! (*отвéт подчинённого*) véry good! ~аться, послýшаться (*рд.*) 1. (*повиновáться*) obéy (*smb.*); (*быть послýшным*) be* obédient (to); не ~аться disobéy; (*быть непослýшным*) be* disobédient; 2.: ~аться совéтов когó-л. take* smb.'s advíce; 3. *тк. несов.* (*о судéбном дéле*) be* tried; дéло бýдет ~аться зáвтра the case comes up for héaring tomórrow, the case comes on tomórrow.

слыть, прослы́ть (*тв.*, *за вн.*) have* the reputátion of béing (*smth.*), be* considered (*smth.*), be* repúted to be (*smth.*); он слывёт хорóшим рабóтником he is repúted/said to be a good wórker.

слыхáть *несов.* (*о пр.*) *разг.* hear* (abóut, of).

слы́ш|ать, услы́шать 1. (*вн.*; *воспринимáть слýхом*) hear* (*smth.*); ~ стук hear* a knock; ~ крик hear* a shout; ~ похвалы́ hear* praise; 2. *тк. несов.* (*обладáть слýхом*) hear*; плóхо ~ be* hard of héaring; не ~у вас I can't hear you; 3. (*вн.*, *о пр.*, *про вн.*; *имéть какие-л. свéдения*) hear* (of, abóut); 4. *тк. несов.* (*вн.*) *разг.* (*ощущáть*) feel* (*smth.*); ~ зáпах feel*/nótice a smell, catch* a whiff; (*прия́тный*) smell* the frágrance; ◇ он об э́том и ~ не хóчет he won't hear of it. ~аться, послы́шаться 1. be* heard; ~ится смех láughter can be heard; мне послы́шался чéй-то гóлос I thought I heard a voice; послы́шался тóпот ног the stámping of feet was heard; 2. *разг.* (*чýвствоваться*) be* felt; в егó словáх ~ится рáдость one can sense the joy in his words, there is joy in his voice.

слы́шим|ость *ж.* 1. audibílity; 2. (*по телефóну, рáдио*) recéption; ~ плохáя! (*по телефóну*) the line is bad! ~ый áudible.

слы́шно *в знач. сказ. безл.* 1. (*мóжно слы́шать*) one can hear; ~, как шелестя́т ли́стья one can hear the leaves rústling; ~ бы́ло, как маши́на въéхала во двор the car could be heard cóming ínto the yard; емý ~ he can hear; мне ничегó не ~ I can't hear a thing; 2. (*о пр.*, *про вн.*; *имéются извéстия*): о нём давнó ничегó не ~ nóthing has been heard of him for áges, there has been no news of him for a long time.

слы́ш|ный 1. áudible; едвá ~ное пéние bárely áudible sínging, the faint sound of sínging; 2. *в знач. сказ.*: ~ен гóлос, шум *и т. п.* a voice, a noise, *etc.* can be heard.

слюдá *ж.* míca.

слюнá *ж.* salíva, spíttal; spit *разг.*

слю́нки *мн.*: у негó ~ текýт his mouth is wátering; от э́того ~ текýт it makes one's mouth wáter.

слюня́вый slóbbery, dríbbling, slávering.

сля́коть *ж.* slush, míre; на дворé ~ it's véry slúshy outside.

смáз|ать(ся) *сов. см.* смáзывать(ся). ~ка *ж.* 1. sméaring; (*жи́ром*) gréasing; (*мáслом*) óiling, lubricátion; 2. (*вещество́*) grease, lúbricant, lúbricator.

смазли́вый *разг.* prétty, cute.

смáзочн|ый lúbricating; ~ое веществó, ~ материáл lúbricant.

смáзчик *м.* gréaser, lúbricator.

смáзывать, смáзать 1. (*вн. тв.*) smear (*smth.* with); (*жи́ром*) grease (*smth.* with); (*мáслом*) oil (*smth.* with), lúbricate (*smth.* with); ~ что-л. йóдом paint smth. with iodine; 2. (*вн.*) стирáть, размáзывать) wipe (*smth.*) off; смáзать крáску рукавóм wipe the paint off on one's sleeve, smear the paint with one's sleeve; 3. (*вн.*) *разг.* (*смягчáть, лишáть остроты́, определённости*) slur (óver); (*пóртить*) make* a mess (of); ~ недостáтки gloss óver the defécts. ~ся, смáзаться 1. (*стирáться*) be* sméared, get* rubbed/wiped off; крáска смáзалась the paint got rubbed off; 2. *разг.* (*лишáться чёткости, остроты́*) be* blurred, be* glossed óver, be* slurred (óver).

смаковáть *несов.* (*вн.*) *разг.* sávour (*smth.*), smack one's lips (óver); *перен.* rélish (*smth.*), revel (in).

смáлец *м.* lard.

смáнивать, смани́ть (*вн.*) 1. lure (*smb.*, *smth.*), entíce (*smb.*, *smth.*); 2. (*перемáнивать*) lure (*smb.*) awáy.

смани́ть *сов. см.* смáнивать.

смастери́ть *сов. см.* мастери́ть.

смáтывать, смотáть (*вн.*) reel (*smth.*) in.

смáхивать I, смахнýть (*вн.*) off, flick (*smth.*) off; (*отгоня́ть*) brush (*smth.*) awáy, flick (*smth.*) awáy; смахнýть пыль flick off the dust.

смáхивать II *несов.* (*на вн.*) *разг.* (*быть похóжим*) be*/look ráther like (*smb.*, *smth.*).

смахнýть *сов. см.* смáхивать I.

смáчивать, смочи́ть (*вн.*) móisten (*smth.*).

смежáть, смежи́ть: ~ глазá shut* one's eyes, close one's eyes.

смежи́ть *сов. см.* смежáть.

смéжн|ость *ж.* contigúity, ~ый adjóining, adjácent, contíguous; ~ые кóмнаты adjóining rooms; ~ые наýки overlápping scíences; ~ые предприя́тия clósely connécted énterprises; ~ые óтрасли промы́шленности állied/reláted índustries; ◇ ~ые углы́ *мат.* adjácent ángles.

смекáлистый *разг.* bright.

смекáлка *ж.* *разг.* áptitude; (*сообрази́тельность*) quick wits *pl*; gúmption.

смекáть, смекнýть *разг.* see* (the point), catch* on, twig.

смекнýть *сов. см.* смекáть.

смелéть, осмелéть grow* bold, take* heart, be* embóldened.

смéл|о bóldly; (*без колебáний, сомнéний*) sáfely; ~ могý сказáть I can sáfely say, I can say with cónfidence; ~ скáзано! that's a bold státement!; э́то сли́шком ~ скáзано that is góing a little too far. ~ость *ж.* bóldness, audácity, cóurage; ◇ брать на себя́ ~ость сдéлать что--л. vénture to do smth., take* the líberty of dóing smth.; ~ость гóрода берёт *погов.* ≈ cóurage wins. ~ый bold, dáring, courágeous; ~ый наéздник dáring hórseman*/ríder; ~ый взгляд bold glance; ~ое утверждéние dáring/bold státement; быть ~ым в решéниях be* bold in táking decísions.

смельчáк *м.* dáredevil, plúcky féllow.

смéн|а *ж.* 1. change; (*замéна*) replácement; ~ дня и нóчи alternátion of night and day; ~ впечатлéний ever-chánging impréssions *pl*; ~ караýла *воен.* relíef/chánging of the guard; 2. (*промежýток врéмени*) shift, spell, turn; *воен.* dúty, watch; 3. (*грýппа людéй, рабóчих*) shift; (*отдыхáющих*) néwcomers *pl*; 4. (*подрастáющее поколéние*) replácement, young generátion; (*свéжие силы*) fresh blood; 5. (*комплéкт одéжды*) change, spare set; ~ белья́ change of únderwear; ◇ приходи́ть на ~у комý-л. take* over from smb., succéed smb.

смени́ть(ся) *сов. см.* сменя́ть(ся).

сме́нн|ый 1. (*связанный с работой по сменам*) shift *attr.*; ~ ма́стер shift fóreman*; ~ое зада́ние stint, work for one shift; ~ая брига́да new shift; 2. (*периодически сменяемый*) chángeable, remóvable; ~ое колесо́ remóvable wheel.

сме́нщ|ик *м.*, ~ица *ж.* relíef, replácement.

сменя́емость *ж.* replaceabílity.

сменя́ть, смени́ть (*вн.*) 1. (*заменять*) change (*smth.*); смени́ть бельё change *one's* únderclothes; (*постельное*) change the béd-linen; 2. (*снимать с какого--л. поста*) change (*smb., smth.*), replace (*smb., smth.*); смени́ть руково́дство на строи́тельстве put* new men in charge of a búilding próject; 3. (*начинать действовать вместо кого-л.*) relíeve (*smb.*), take* óver (from); смени́ть часовы́х relíeve the guard(s); смени́ть кого́-л. на дежу́рстве take* óver *smb.'s* watch; 4. (*появляться на месте чего-л. исчезнувшего*) replace (*smth.*), superséde (*smth.*); ве́чер смени́л жа́ркий день the scórching day gave way to évening. ~ся, смени́ться 1. (*сменять друг друга на какой-л. должности*) be* changed/replaced; 2. (*освобождаться от несения каких-л. обязанностей*) be* relíeved; смени́ться с дежу́рства come* off dúty; я смени́лся то́лько к ве́черу I wásn't relíeved till évening; 3. (*тв.*) (*заменяться чем-л.*) be* replaced (by); страх смени́лся наде́ждой fear turned to hope; день бы́стро смени́лся но́чью the day fled ínto night.

смерза́ться, смёрзнуться freeze* togéther.

смёрзнуться *сов. см.* смерза́ться.

сме́рить *сов.* 1. *см.* ме́рить 1; 2: ~ что́-л. взгля́дом judge *smth.* by eye; ~ кого́-л. взгля́дом eye *smb.* from head to foot.

смерк|а́ться, смёркнуться grow* dusk; ~а́ется it is grówing dusk.

смёркнуться *сов. см.* смерка́ться.

смерте́льно mórtally; ~ ра́неный mórtally/fátally wóunded; ~ скуча́ть be* bored to death; ~ уста́ть be* dead tíred.

смерте́льн|ый 1. fátal; (*об оружии, яде*) déadly; (*грозящий гибелью*) mórtal; ~ая ра́на mórtal wound; ~ уда́р fátal/mórtal blow; находи́ться в ~ой опа́сности be* in dánger of *one's* life; 2. (*сопутствующий смерти*) death *attr.*, déathly; of death *после сущ.*; ~ая бле́дность déathly pállor; 3. (*очень сильный*) mórtal; ~ая оби́да mórtal offénce/ínsult; ~ая ску́ка útter bóredom; ◇ ~ враг mórtal énemy; ~ая вражда́ mórtal énmity.

сме́рт|ость *ж.* mortálity; (*количество случаев смерти тж.*) déath-rate. ~ый *прил.* 1. death *attr.*; of death *после сущ.*; ~ый час mórtal hour; ~ое ло́же déathbed; ~ый слу́чай fátal case; 2. (*подверженный смерти*) mórtal; все лю́ди ~ы all men are mórtal; 3. (*приводящий к смерти*) death *attr.*; (*приводящий к гибели*) mórtal; ~ый пригово́р séntence of death, déath--sentence; ~ая казнь cápital púnishment; ~ый бой mórtal cómbat; 4. (*крайний, предельный*) mórtal; ~ая ску́ка killing bóredom; 5. *в знач. сущ. м.* mórtal; просты́е ~ые mere mórtals.

смертоно́сный léthal; (*гибельный*) déadly.

смерт|ь *ж.* death; идти́ на ве́рную ~ go* to *one's* death; умере́ть голо́дной ~ю die of starvátion; до са́мой ~и till *one's* dýing day; я э́того до са́мой ~и не забу́ду I'll remémber it till my dýing day; ◇ поги́бнуть ~ю геро́я die like a héro; пасть ~ю хра́брых die váliantly; до́ смерти to death; надоеда́ть кому́-л. до́ смерти péster *smb.* to death; мне до́ смерти хо́чется спать, есть, пить I'm dýing for a sleep, some food, a drink; смотре́ть, гляде́ть ~и в глаза́ face death; быть при са́мой ~и be* near to death; be* at death's door *идиом.*; как ~ бле́дный pale as death; как ~ побледне́ть go* white as a sheet, go* déathly pale.

смерч *м.* whírlwind; (*на суше тж.*) tornádo; (*небольшой*) dust dévil; (*водяной*) wáter-spout.

смеси́ть *сов. см.* меси́ть.

смести́ *сов. см.* смета́ть I.

смести́ть(ся) *сов. см.* смеща́ть(ся).

смесь *ж.* míxture; шокола́дная ~ (*конфеты*) assórted chócolates; ◇ горю́чая ~ míxture (of fuel and air).

сме́та *ж.* éstimate; ~ расхо́дов éstimate of expénditure.

смета́на *ж.* sóured cream.

смет|а́ть I, смести́ (*вн.*) (*рукой, щёткой и т. п.*) brush (*smth.*) off; (*метлой*) sweep* (*smth.*) up; (*о ветре*) blow* (*smth.*) off; *перен.* sweep* (*smth.*) aside; ~а́я всё на своём пути́ cárrying éverything befóre it.

смета́ть II *сов. см.* смётывать *и* мета́ть II.

смётка *ж. разг.* áptitude, gúmption, quick-wíttedness.

сметли́в|ость *ж.* resóurcefulness, shréwdness. ~ый resóurceful, shrewd, keen-wítted, ingénious.

сме́тн|ый ~ые ассигнова́ния búdget allówances; ~ые предположе́ния éstimated expénse *sg.*

смётывать, смета́ть (*вн.*) baste (*smth.*), tack (*smth.*) togéther.

сметь, посме́ть (+ *инф.*) dare* (+ *inf*); сме́ю сказа́ть I vénture to say; не ~! don't you dare!; как вы сме́ете! how dare you!

смех *м.* láughter; (*один звук*) laugh; он не мог удержа́ться от ~а he cóuldn't help láughing; взрыв ~а burst of láughter; ◇ ~а ра́ди, для ~а just for fun; мне, ему́ не до ~а it is no láughing mátter for me, him; I am, he is in no láughing mood; ~у бы́ло it was (véry) fúnny; it was a scream *разг.*; и ~ и грех you cóuldn't help láughing, though it wásn't so fúnny; ~ да и то́лько it's pérfectly ridículous; как на ~ as if to mock us (them, me).

смехотво́рный ridículous, láughable, absúrd.

сме́шанн|ый mixed; (*о породе тж.*) crossed, móngrel; ~ репертуа́р mixed répertoire; ◇ ~ лес mixed fórest; ~ое число́ *мат.* mixed númber.

смеш|а́ть *сов. см.* сме́шивать. ~а́ться *сов.* 1. *см.* сме́шиваться; 2. *разг.* (*смутиться*) be* embárrassed/confúsed. ~е́ние *с.* 1. (*действие*) míxing; 2. (*путаница*) confúsion; 3. (*смесь*) blend.

сме́шивать, смеша́ть 1. mix (*smth.*); (*сорта, краски и т. п.*) blend (*smth.*); 2. (*нарушать порядок расположения чего-л.*) scátter (*smth.*); ~ ка́рты shúffle the cards; 3. (*путать, не различать*) mix (*smb., smth.*) up, confúse (*smb., smth.*), múddle (*smth.*). ~ся, смеша́ться 1. (*о чём-л. разнородном*) mix, blend; спирт смеша́лся с водо́й the álcohol mixed with the wáter; 2. (*располагаться беспорядочно, вперемешку*) míngle; (*путаться*) get* mixed up; (*скрываться, исчезать*) míngle, disappéar; смеша́ться с толпо́й disappéar/melt ínto the crowd; 3. (*утрачивать стройность, ясность*) becóme* confúsed; его́ мы́сли смеша́лись his thoughts were in confúsion, his mind was in a whirl; 4. (*утрачивать боевой порядок*) break* ranks, be* thrown ínto disórder.

смеши́ть *несов.* (*вн.*) make* (*smb.*) laugh; (*забавлять*) amúse (*smb.*).

смешли́в|ость *ж.* desíre/réadiness to laugh, risibílity. ~ый rísible, láughing; éasily amúsed *после сущ.*

смешно́ 1. *нареч.* fúnnily, fúnny; (*нелепо*) adsúrdly, cómically; ~ вы́глядеть look fúnny; ~ говори́ть speak* fúnnily/amúsingly; ~ одева́ться dress absúrdly; ~ звуча́ть sound fúnny; 2. *в знач. сказ. безл.* it is absúrd/ridículous; ~ ду́мать, что... it would be absúrd to suppóse...; ~ сказа́ть strange to say; ~ смотре́ть на него́ he looks ridículous; мне ~ I am simply amúsed; мне (совсе́м) не ~ I don't find it all fúnny.

смеш|но́й 1. (*забавный*) fúnny; ~на́я исто́рия amúsing stóry; 2. (*нелепый*) ridículous; он мне ~о́н he makes me laugh; выставля́ть кого́-л. в ~о́м ви́де make* *smb.* look ridículous; ста́вить кого́-л. в ~о́е положе́ние

place *smb.* in an absúrd posítion; ◇ до ~нóго ridícu-
lously, absúrdly.

смешóк *м.* 1. chúckle; 2. *мн. разг.* (*насмешки,
шутки*) jokes, jeers.

смещ|áть, сместúть (*вн.*) 1. displáce (*smth.*); *перен.*
confúse (*smth.*); 2. (*увольнять*) dischárge (*smth.*). ~áть-
ся, сместúться be* displáced; *перен.* change. ~éние *с.* 1.
displácement; 2. (*понятий*) confúsion; 3. (*с должности*)
dischárge; 4. *радио* bías; 5. *геол.* heave, dislocátion.

смея́ться *несов.* 1. laugh; ~ шýтке laugh at a joke; ~
исподтишка́ в кула́к laugh in *one's* sleeve; глаза́ её вéсело смея́лись her eyes were bright with láughter; 2.
(*над тв.; издеваться*) laugh (at); make* fun (of); над
кем смеётесь? who are you láughing at?; 3. *разг.* (*говорить несерьёзно, шутить*) joke; ◇ хорошо́ смеётся
тот, кто смеётся после́дним he laughs lóngest/best who
laughs last.

смире́н|ие *с.* humílity, méekness; (*покорность*)
resignátion. ~ный húmble, meek; (*покорный*) resígned.

смири́тельн|ый: ~ая руба́шка stráit-jacket; наде́ть
~ую руба́шку на кого́-л. put* *smb.* into a stráit-jacket.

смири́ть(ся) *сов. см.* смиря́ть(ся).

смирн|о 1. quíetly; сиде́ть ~ sit* still; 2. (*военная
команда*): ~! (*после команды «вольно»*) atténtion!;
'shun! (*после команды «равняйсь!»*) eyes front!; 3. (*на-
вытяжку*): стоя́ть ~ stand* at atténtion. ~ый quíet;
(*кроткий*) mild, submíssive, meek.

смир|я́ть, смири́ть (*вн.*) subdúe (*smth.*); ~ го́рдость
húmble/cónquer *one's* pride; ~ гнев subdúe *one's* ánger.
~я́ться, смири́ться ,1. (*покоряться обстоятельствам*)
submít; 2. (*с тв.; примиряться с чем-л.*) resign onesélf
(to), acquiésce (in); смири́ться с мы́слью о сме́рти
resign onesélf to the thought of death.

смодели́ровать *сов.* (*вн.*) make* a módel (of), módel
(*smth.*).

смоква *ж.* fig.

смóкинг *м.* dínner-jacket; tuxédo *амер., tux разг.*

смокóвница *ж.* fig tree.

смол|á *ж.* 1. résin; сосно́вая ~ pine résin; 2. (*полу-
чаемая синтетически*) tar, pitch; каменноу́гольная ~
cóal-tar; синтети́ческие смо́лы synthétic résins. ~ёный
tarred. ~и́стый résinous; ~и́стое де́рево resíniferous tree;
~и́стый за́пах résinous smell. ~и́ть *несов.* (*вн.*) tar
(*smth.*).

смолк|áть, смóлкнуть 1. (*о звуках*) die awáy; пе́сня
смóлкла the song died awáy; не ~áя incéssantly,
uninterrúptedly; 2. (*переставать говорить, петь и т.
п.*) relápse into sílence; be* hushed; пти́цы смóлкли the
birds stopped sínging.

смóлкнуть *сов. см.* смолка́ть.

смóлоду *разг.* 1. (*с юных лет*) from *one's* youth; 2.
(*в молодости*) in *one's* youth.

смолоти́ть *сов. см.* молоти́ть.

смолóть *сов. см.* молóть.

смолча́ть *сов. разг.* hold* *one's* tongue, not ánswer,
make* no replý.

смоль *ж.*: чёрный как ~ jet-black.

смоля́н|óй 1. résin *attr.*; (*смолистый*) résinous; 2.
(*относящийся к производству смолы, получаемый из
смолы*) tar *attr.*; ~ые масла́ tar oils; 3. (*о волосах*) jet-
-black.

смонти́ровать *сов. см.* монти́ровать.

сморка́ться, вы́сморкаться blow* *one's* nose.

сморóдин|а *ж.* 1. *собир.* cúrrants *pl*; бе́лая, кра́с-
ная, чёрная ~ white, red, black cúrrants; 2. (*об отдельной ягоде*) cúrrant; 3. (*кустарник*) cúrrant (bush); куст
~ы cúrrant bush.

сморчóк *м.* (*гриб*) morél.

смóрщенный wrínkled; (*о яблоке и т. п.*) shrívelled;
(*об одежде*) crúmpled.

смóрщить *сов. см.* мóрщить 2, 3. ~ся *сов. см.* мóр-
щиться 2, 3.

смотáть *сов. см.* сма́тывать.

смотр *м.* revíew; ~ де́тской худо́жественной самодé-
ятельности children's ámateur tálent revíew.

смотре́ть, посмотре́ть 1. (*на, в вн.*) look (at, ínto)
(*тж. перен.*); (*пристально*) gaze (at, ínto); ~ в окно́
(*изнутри*) look out of the wíndow; (*снаружи*) look
through the wíndow; ~ на часы́ look at *one's* watch; ~
вдаль gaze/stare ínto the dístance; ~ кому́-л. (*прямо*) в
глаза́ look *smb.* (straight) in the eye, face *smb.*; ~ под
но́ги look where *one* is góing; ~ вперёд look ahéad; ~ в
бу́дущее face the fúture, look ahéad; 2. (*в вн.; пользоваться оптическими приборами*) look (through), use
(*smth.*); ~ в телеско́п look through a télescope; 3. (*на
вн.; относиться каким-л. образом*) regárd (*smth.*),
look (at); как вы смо́трите на э́то? what is your
opínion?, what do you think of it?; 4. (*на вн.; обраща́ть
внима́ние*) take* nótice (of); что на него́ ~! néver mind
him!; 5. (*на вн.; принимать за кого-л., что-л.*) regárd
(*smb., smth.*), treat (*smb., smth.*); ~ на кого́-л. как на...
regárd *smb.* as...; смотри́те на меня́ тепе́рь как на ва́-
шего отца́ treat me as your fáther; 6. (*за тв.; заботиться*) look áfter (smb.), take* care (of); ~ за поря́дком
keep* órder; ~ за рабо́тами superinténd the work; ~ за
до́мом look áfter the house; ~ за детьми́ look áfter the
children; 7. (*вн.; осматривать с целью ознакомления*)
look óver (*smth.*), have* a look (at); ~ но́вую кварти́ру
look óver a new flat; 8. (*вн.; знакомиться с содержани-
ем чего-л.*) look (at, through); ~ ру́копись look through
a mánuscript; ~ кни́гу look at a book; 9. (*вн.; быть зри-
телем*) see* (*smth.*); ~ но́вый фильм see* a new film;
10. (*вн.; больных*) exámine (*smb., smth.*); 11. *тк. несов.* (*на, в вн.; быть обращённым*) look out (on), look
on (to), overlóok (*smth.*); 12. *тк. несов.*: ~ во́лком
scowl; 13. *тк. несов.*: смотри́(те)! look!; (*берегитесь*)
look out!; (*будьте осторожны*) take care!; смотри́(те)
не забу́дь(те), не упади́(те) *и т. д.* mind you don't
forget, fall, *etc.*; ◇ на́до бы́ло ра́ньше ~ you should
have thought abóut that before; ~ в о́ба keep* *one's* eyes
ópen; ~ не́ на что it (he, she, *etc.*) is not worth lóoking
at; ~ с наде́ждой на кого́-л., что-л. place *one's* hopes in
smb., smth.; ~ опа́сности в глаза́ look dánger in the
face; смотря́ как it depénds; смотря́ где, когда́ it
depénds where, when; смотря́ по чему́-л. accórding to
smth.; смотря́ по обстоя́тельствам that depénds on the
círcumstances; куда́ он смо́трит? what's he thínking of?
~ся, посмотре́ться 1. (*в вн.*) look at onesélf (in),
exámine onesélf (in); ~ся в зе́ркало look at onesélf in the
glass; 2. *тк. несов. безл.* be* accéptable to the eye;
фильм хорошо́ смо́трится the film is vísually efféctive; 3.
тк. несов. разг. (*производить впечатление*) prodúce
an efféct, look efféctive.

смотри́тель *м.* wátchman*, kéeper; ~ маяка́ líghthouse kéeper.

смотров|óй 1. (*служащий для наблюдения*) obser-
vátion *attr.*; ~óe окно́ péep-hole; 2. (*относящийся к
смотру*) inspéction *attr.*, revíew *attr.*

смочи́ть *сов. см.* сма́чивать.

смочь *сов. см.* мочь.

смошéнничать *сов. см.* мошéнничать.

смрад *м.* stench, stink.

смра́дный stínking.

смуглоли́цый dúsky (-faced).

смугл|ый brown, dark, dúsky; (*о человеке*) dárk-
-skinned; ~ цвет лица́ dark compléxion; ~ые ру́ки brown
arms.

сму́та *ж.* 1. tróuble, strife; 2. *разг.* (*раздоры*)
díscord; 3. (*тревога*) anxíety, confúsion.

смути́ть(ся) *сов. см.* смуща́ть(ся).

сму́тн|о *нареч.* váguely; ~ представля́ть себе́
что-л. have* a vague/házy idéa of smth.; 2. *в знач.
сказ. безл.:* ~ у меня́ на душе́ I feel tróubled/depréssed.
~ый 1. (*мятежный*) tróubled; ~ая пора́ tróubled

days/times *pl*; **2.** (*тревожный, беспокойный*) ánxious, distúrbing; **3.** (*неясный, неопределённый*) vague, házy, dim; ~ое представлéние vague/dim/házy idéa.

смутья́н *м. разг.* tróublemaker.

смущ|а́ть, смути́ть (*вн.*) **1.** (*вызывать волнение, тревогу*) upsét* (*smb.*); distúrb (*smb.*); ~ чей-л. душéвный покóй distúrb *smb.'s* peace of mind; **2.** (*приводить в замешательство*) embárrass (*smb.*), confúse (*smb.*), disconcért (*smb.*); (*вызывать сомнения*) wórry (*smb.*); смути́ть кого-л. похвалóй embárrass *smb.* with praise; э́то извéстие смути́ло всех éveryone was disconcérted at the news. ~а́ться, смути́ться be* embárrassed, be* confúsed; нискóлько, ничýть не ~а́ясь not a bit embárrassed, quíte/all unabáshed. ~е́ние *с.* embárrassment, confúsion; в ~е́нии in embárrassment; от ~е́ния in *one's* confúsion; приводи́ть кого-л. в ~е́ние embárrass *smb.*; (*волновать*) upsét* *smb.*; приходи́ть в ~е́ние be* embárrassed/confúsed.

смущённый embárrassed, uncómfortable.

смыва́ть, смыть (*вн.*) **1.** wash (*smth.*) awáy/off, wash out (*smth.*); *перен.* remóve (*smth.*), expúnge (*smth.*); ~ пятнó wash out/off a stain; смыть с себя́ позóр cleanse *onesélf* of the shame/disgráce; **2.** (*сносить водой*) wash (*smb., smth.*) off/awáy; егó смы́ло волнóй (*с судна*) he was washed óverboard; (*с берега*) he was washed ínto the wáter by a wave. ~ся, смы́ться come* off, wash out; *перен.* be* remóved.

смык|а́ть, сомкнýть (*вн.*) close (*smth.*); *воен., спорт.* close up (*smth.*); ~ вéки close *one's* eyes; ◇ не сомкнýть глаз not sleep a wink, not have a wink of sleep; сомкнýть ряды́ close *one's* ranks. ~а́ться, сомкнýться **1.** (*соприкасаться, соединяться*) join, link up, make* cóntact; (*становиться вплотную друг к другу*) close up, gáther round; *перен.* rálly, uníte; **2.** (*закрываться*) close; у меня́ глаза́ ~а́ются от устáлости I can hárdly keep my eyes ópen.

смысл *м.* **1.** sense; (*значение тж.*) méaning; в перенóсном ~е in a fígurative sense; в извéстном ~е in a sense; улови́ть ~ grasp the sense; **2.** (*основание, цель*) point; ~ жи́зни méaning of life; есть ~ съéздить тудá it might be worthwhíle to go there; нет ~а, не имéет ~а проси́ть об э́том there's no point in ásking for that; нам нет никакóго ~а éхать тудá there's no point in our góing there; ◇ в пóлном ~е слóва in the true/full sense of the word; в ~е чего-л. as regárds *smth.*

смы́сл|ить *несов. разг.* **1.** understánd*; дитя́ ещё ничегó не ~ит the child* dóesn't yet understánd; **2.** (в *пр.*; *разбираться*) understánd* (*smth.*), be* versed (in); ~ в тéхнике be* téchnically mínded.

смыслов|óй semántic; ~ы́е оттéнки shades of méaning.

смыть(ся) *сов. см.* смыва́ть(ся).

смы́чка *ж.* **1.** *тех.* joint, cóupling; **2.** (*союз*) cóntact, alliance, féllowship.

смычкóв|ый bow *attr.*; ~ые музыка́льные инструмéнты bow ínstruments; (*в оркестре*) the strings.

смычóк *м.* bow.

смышлёный *разг.* bright.

смягч|а́ть, смягчи́ть (*вн.*) **1.** (*лишать твёрдости*) make* (*smth.*) soft, sóften (*smth.*); **2.** (*делать менее суровым, строгим*) móllify (*smb.*), sóften (*smb., smth.*); **3.** (*ослаблять, умерять*) móderate (*smth.*); (*делать менее грубым, резким*) tone (*smth.*) down; ~ чей-л. гнев móllify *smb.*; ~ удáр déaden/cúshion the blow; *перен.* sóften/témper the blow; смягчи́ть приговóр mítigate the séntence; **4.** *лингв.* pálatalize (*smth.*). ~а́ться, смягчи́ться **1.** (*делаться эластичным*) becóme* soft; **2.** (*делаться менее суровым, строгим*) relént, sóften; **3.** (*ослабевать, уменьшаться*) dimínish, abáte; **4.** (*о погоде, климате*) grow* mílder; **5.** *лингв.* be* pálatalized. ~а́ющие sóftening; ~а́ющий веществá emóllients,

sóftening ágents; ~а́ющее винý обстоя́тельство exténuating/mítigating círcumstance.

смягчéние *с.* **1.** sóftening; **2.** (*гнева и т. п.*) mollificátion; **3.** (*ослабление*) moderátion; ~ пригóвора mitigátion of the séntence; ~ междунарóдной напряжённости relaxátion of internátional ténsion; **4.** *лингв.* palatalizátion.

смягчи́ть(ся) *сов. см.* смягча́ть(ся).

смятéние *с.* **1.** confúsion, perturbátion; ~ чувств perturbátion; приходи́ть в ~ be* pertúrbed; приводи́ть когó-л. в ~ pertúrb *smb.*; **2.** (*паника*) pánic, disarráy.

смять *сов.* (*вн.*) **1.** (*мять*) (up), crush (*smth.*), crease (*smth.*); ~ плáтье rúmple/crúmple a dress; ~ письмó screw up a létter; **2.** (*растения*) crush (*smth.*), flátten (*smth.*); ~ травý trámple/tread* down the grass; ~ овёс flátten the oats; **3.** (*сломить чьё-л. сопротивление*) crush (*smb., smth.*), smash (*smb., smth.*). ~ся *сов.* **1.** be* crúmpled; **2.** (*превратиться в комок*) be* smashed/crushed.

снабди́ть *сов. см.* снабжа́ть.

снабжа́ть, снабди́ть (*вн. тв.*) supplý (*smb., smth.* with), fúrnish (*smb., smth.* with), províde (*smb., smth.* with); ~ когó-л. деньга́ми províde *smb.* with móney; ~ когó-л. всем необходи́мым fúrnish *smb.* with what he, she needs; supplý *smb.'s* needs; ~ áрмию продовóльствием supplý an ármy with provísions, fúrnish an ármy with supplíes; ~ фáбрику электри́чеством supplý a fáctory with cúrrent; delíver power to a fáctory; ~ кни́гу примечáниями ánnotate a book; снабди́ть станóк автомати́ческим управлéнием áutomate a lathe.

снабжéнец *м.* supplý ágent.

снабжéние *с.* supplý, provísion; ~ продовóльствием fóod-supply.

снáдобье *с.* rémedy; stuff *разг.*

снáйпер *м.* sníper, shárp-shooter.

снарýжи 1. on the óutside; **2.** (*по внешнему виду*) óutwardly; **3.** (*извне*) from the óutside; (*вне пределов чего-л.*) óutside.

снаря́д *м.* **1.** *воен.* prójectile; (*артиллерийский тж.*) shell; разры́вы ~ов shéll-bursts; **2.** (*техническое устройство, машина*) machíne, apparátus; буровóй ~ drílling machíne; **3.** *спорт.* apparátus; упражнéния на ~ax apparátus work *sg.*

снаряди́ть(ся) *сов. см.* снаряжа́ть(ся).

снаряж|áть, снаряди́ть (*вн.*) **1.** fit out (*smb., smth.*), equíp (*smb., smth.*); снаряди́ть экспеди́цию на Сéвер fit out an expedítion for the North; снаряди́ть сýдно fit out a ship; **2.** *разг.* (*посылать*) send* (*smb.*), pack (*smb.*) off. ~áться, снаряди́ться *разг.* fit *onesélf* out. ~éние *с.* **1.** (*действие*) equípping; **2.** *собир.* (*совокупность необходимых приспособлений*) equípment, óutfit; лы́жное ~éние skíing óutfit.

снасть *ж.* **1.** *собир.* gear, táckle; рыболóвная ~ físhing-tackle; **2.** *мор. горе*; *мн. собир. тж.* rígging *sg.*

снача́ла 1. (*сперва*) first; (*первое время*) at first; ~ нáдо... (you must) first...; **2.** (*снова*) all óver agáin.

снег *м.* snow; мóкрый ~ sleet; ~ идёт it is snówing, it snows; занесённый ~ом snówbound; покры́тый ~ом snów-covered; одéтый ~ом snów-clad; ◇ (свали́ться) как ~ нá голову (come*) like a bolt from the blue.

снеги́рь *м.* búllfinch.

снеговик *м.* snówman.

снеговóй snow *attr.*; (*о горах*) snów-capped; ~ покрóв láyer of snow; ~áя ли́ния snówline.

снегозадержáние *с.* snow reténtion.

снегоочисти́тель *м.* (*машина*) snówplough, snówplow *амер.*

снегопáд *м.* snówfall.

снегýрочка *ж.* the Snów-Maiden.

снежи́нка *ж.* snówflake.

снéжн|ый 1. snow *attr.*; (*обильный снегом*) snówy; (*покрытый снегом*) snów-covered, snów-laden, snówy;

~ая зима́ snówy wínter; ~ая поля́на snów-covered/snówy field; 2. (похожий на снег) snówy; ~ая белизна́ snówy white; ◇ ~ая ба́ба см. снегови́к; ~ый челове́к уéti.

снеж|о́к м. 1. light snow; идёт ~ it is snówing a líttle; 2. (снежный ком) snówball; 3. мн. (игра) snówballs; игра́ть в ~ки́ snówball, throw* snówballs.

снести́ I сов. (вн.) 1. см. сноси́ть I; 2. (отнести́ куда́-л.) take* (smth.), cárry (smth.); 3. (в одно́ ме́сто) bring* (smth.).

снести́ II сов. см. нести́ II.

снести́сь I сов. см. сноси́ться I.

снести́сь II сов. см. нести́сь II.

снето́к м. (рыба) smelt.

сниж|а́ть, сни́зить (вн.) 1. redúce (smth.), bring* (smth.) down, lówer (smth.); (о ценах тж.) cut* (smth.); ~ давле́ние redúce préssure; ~ ско́рость redúce speed; ~ себесто́имость проду́кции redúce prodúction costs; ~ тре́бования к чему́-л. be* less exácting with regárd to smth.; ~ тре́бования к кому́-л. demánd less of smb.; 2. (самолёт) bring* (smth.) lówer. ~а́ться, сни́зиться 1. (уменьшаться) drop, fall* (о ценах) fall*, come* down; температу́ра сни́зилась the témperature has fállen; 2. (спускаться) come* down, descénd; (о самолёте тж.) redúce áltitude. ~е́ние с. 1. lówering; (температуры) fall; (уменьшение) redúction; ~е́ние цен redúction/cut in prices; ~е́ние зарпла́ты wáge-cut; ~е́ние себесто́имости проду́кции lówering (of) prodúction costs; ~е́ние те́мпов slówdown, slówing down; 2. (самолёта) descént; вести́ самолёт на ~е́ние bring* in a plane to land.

сни́женн|ый redúced; ~ые це́ны redúced prices.

сни́зить(ся) сов. см. снижа́ть(ся).

снизойти́ сов. см. снисходи́ть.

сни́зу 1. (с нижней стороны) from belów; (считая снизу) from the bóttom; (внизу) underneáth; ~ вверх úpwards; 2. (со стороны народных масс) from belów; ◇ ~ до́верху from top to bóttom; смотре́ть на кого́-л. ~ вверх look up to smb.

снима́ть, снять (вн.) 1. take* off (smth.), remóve (smth.); ~ кни́гу с по́лки take* a book off the shelf*; ~ карти́ну со стены́ take* down a pícture; ~ телефо́нную тру́бку lift the recéiver; ~ ска́терть со стола́ take* off the táblecloth; снять ча́йник с плиты́ take* the kéttle off the stove; ~ дверь с пе́тель remóve a door from its hínges; букси́рный парохо́д снял их с ме́ли they were táken off the sándbank by a tug; снять строи́тельные леса́ take* down the scáffolding; 2. (одежду, покров и т. п.) take* (smth.) off; снять пальто́ take* off one's coat; снять ту́фли take* off one's shoes; снять очки́ take* off one's glásses; 3. (избавлять от чего́-л.): снять блока́ду, оса́ду raise a blockáde, siege; снять вы́говор с кого́-л. cáncel smb.'s réprimand; снять обвине́ние с кого́-л. exónerate smb.; 4. (освобождать себя от чего́-л.) discárd (smth.), free onesélf (of); снять с себя́ отве́тственность free onesélf of responsibílity; 5. (стирая, срезая, удаляя что-л.) remóve (smth.), rub off (smth.); снять грим remóve one's máke-up; ~ шку́ру с медве́дя skin a bear; 6. (собирать, убирать) gáther (smth.), pick (smth.); ~ урожа́й gáther in the hárvest; ~ я́блоки pick ápples; 7. воен. (отводить, отзывать) remóve (smb.), recáll (smb.); (убив, связав, удаляя откуда́-л.) get* rid of (smb.); (выстрелом) pick (smb.) off; ~ часово́го (своего) remóve a séntry; (вражеского) cárry off a séntry; 8. (освобождать от какого-л. дела) dismíss (smb.); ~ кого́-л. с рабо́ты relíeve smb. of his dúties/óffice; dismíss smb.; 9. (отменять) withdráw* (smth.); снять своё предложе́ние withdráw* one's propósal; (в законодательном органе) withdráw* one's mótion; ~ пье́су с репертуа́ра take* off a play; 10. (точно воспроизводить) cópy (smth.); ~ ко́пию с докуме́нта make* a cópy of a dócument; ~ план кре́пости make* a plan of a fórtress; 11. (фотографировать) phótograph

(smb., smth.), take* smb.'s phótograph; ~ фильм shoot* a film; 12. (брать внаём) take* (smth.), rent (smth.); ~ да́чу rent a place in the cóuntry; ◇ снять го́лову с кого́-л. 1) (строго наказать) give* smb. hell, have* smb.'s head; 2) (ставить в неловкое положение) put* smb. in a térrible spot; снять показа́ния take* smb.'s évidence; снять допро́с make* an interrogátion; ~ показа́ние счёт-чика take* a réading of the méter; как руко́й сня́ло it vánished as if by mágic. ~ся, сня́ться 1. (отделяться) come* off; дверь сняла́сь с пе́тель the door came off its hínges; 2. (об одежде) come* off; перча́тка легко́ сня-ла́сь the glove came off éasily; капюшо́н легко́ снима́ет-ся the hood is éasy to take off; 3. (о судне): ~ся с я́коря weigh ánchor; 4. (покидать какое-л. место): ~ся с би-ва́ка break* camp; 5. (принимать участие в киносъём-ке) act in a film, appéar befóre the cámera; 6. (фото-графироваться) be* phótographed, have* one's phótograph táken; ◇ ~ся с учёта take* one's name off the régister.

сни́мок м. phóto(graph); люби́тельский ~ snápshot.

сниска́ть сов. (вн.) win* (smth.), gain (smth.); ~ уваже́ние win*/gain respéct.

снисходи́тельн|о 1. (нестрого) indúlgently, léniently; with forbéarance после сущ.; 2. (свысока) condescéndingly; ~ разгова́ривать с кем-л. talk down to smb. ~ость ж. 1. (отсутствие строгости) léniency, indúlgence; 2. (покровительственное высокомерие) condescénsion. ~ый 1. (нестрогий) lénient, indúlgent; бу́дьте ~ы к нему́ don't be too hard on him, let him down líghtly; 2. (относящийся свысока) condescénding, pátronizing.

снисходи́ть, снизойти́ (к дт.) show* condescénsion (to), condescénd (to), stoop (to); ~ к чьей-л. про́сьбе grácious ly concéde smb.'s request; ~ до разгово́ров с кем-л. deign to speak to smb.

снисхожде́ние с. 1. (к дт.) léniency (towárds); име́ть ~ к нео́пытности кого́-л. show* indúlgence for smb.'s inexpérience; 2. (высокомерное отношение) condescénsion.

сни́ться, присни́ться dream*, have* a dream; мне сня́тся стра́нные сны I have strange dreams; мне сни-лось, что... I dreamed...; вы мне сни́лись I dreamed abóut you, I had a dream abóut you.

сно́ва agáin; once agáin, once more; anéw поэт.; ~ встре́титься meet* agáin; ~ посети́ть кого́-л., что-л. revísit smb., smth.; ~ отпра́виться в путь resúme one's jóurney.

снова́ть несов. (двигаться) scúrry.

сновиде́ние с. dream.

сногсшиба́тельный разг. stúnning; (поразитель-ный) stággering, astóunding, fábulous.

сноп м. sheaf*; перен. shaft, beam; ~ искр shówer of sparks; ~ луче́й shaft of light; ◇ как ~ повали́ться, упа́сть go* down like a ninepin.

сноповяза́лка ж. bínder.

сноро́вка ж. knack, skill.

снос I м. 1. (ветром, течением) drift; ~ ве́тром мор. léeway; 2. (разрушение) demólition; дом предназ-на́чен к ~у the house is to be pulled down.

снос II м. (износ): э́тому ~у нет разг. it will last for éver.

сноси́ть I, снести́ (вн.) 1. (вниз) bring* (smb., smth.) down; 2. (относить) cárry (smth.); кора́бль сно́сит ве́тром, тече́нием на юг the ship is béing cárried south by the wind, cúrrent; 3. (срывая, сбивать) cárry/sweep* awáy (smb., smth.); (ветром) blow* (smb., smth.) off; бу́рей снесло́ кры́шу the roof was blown off by the storm; ме́льницу снесло́ водо́й the mill was swept awáy by the flood; 4. (срезая, срубать) cut* (smth.) off, séver (smth.); снести́ кому́-л. го́лову cut* off smb.'s head; 5. (разрушать) demólish (smth.), pull (smth.) down; 6. (терпеть) bear* (smth.); ◇ ему не ~ головы́ he'll come to grief.

сноси́ть II сов. (вн.) разг. (износи́ть) wear* (smth.) out.

сноси́ться, снести́сь (с тв.) commúnicate (with); ~ пи́сьменно commúnicate by létter; ~ ме́жду собо́й, друг с дру́гом keep* in touch (with one anóther); ~ с кем-л. по телефо́ну speak* to smb. óver the télephone.

сно́ска ж. fóotnote.

сно́сн|о tólerably; fáirly well; (как ответ) só-so, fair to míddling; ~ пообе́дать have* a fáirly décent dínner; ~ провести́ вре́мя have* a fáirly good time. ~ый (терпи́мый) tólerable; (неплохо́й) fáirly good.

снотво́рн|ый прил. 1. soporífic; ~ое сре́дство soporífic, sléeping draught; 2. в знач. сущ. с. soporífic, sléeping pill.

сноха́ ж. dáughter-in-law (pl dáughters-).

сноше́ния мн. déalings, relátions.

сня́тие с. remóval; ~ взыска́ния remíssion of pénalty; ~ блока́ды ráising of the blockáde.

снят|о́й: ~о́е молоко́ skim milk.

сня́ть(ся) сов. см. снима́ть(ся).

со см. с.

соа́втор м. colláborator, co-áuthor; мн. тж. joint áuthors. ~ство с. collaborátion, co-áuthorship.

соба́к|а ж. dog; (го́нчая) hound; дворо́вая, цепна́я ~ wátch-dog; ◇ ~ на се́не dog in the mánger; уста́ть как ~ be* dog-tíred; он на э́том ~у съел he knows the súbject ínside out, he knows all there is to know abóut that; вот где ~ зары́та that's where the tróuble lies; ~е соба́чья смерть погов. the dog shall die a dog's death; с ~ами не сы́щешь кого́-л. you can't find smb. ánywhere.

собаково́д м. dóg-breeder. ~ство с. dóg-breeding.

соба́|чий 1. cánine; dog attr.; ~ лай bárking (of a dog); ~чья пре́данность cánine devótion; ~чья конура́ dog kénnel; ~ оше́йник dóg-collar; 2. разг. (тяжёлый) dog's, rótten; ~чья жизнь dog's life; ◇ ~ хо́лод périshing/béastly cold.

соба́чка ж. 1. líttle dog; 2. mex. pawl, catch; 3. (ору́жия) trígger.

собезья́нничать сов. см. обезья́нничать I.

собесе́дник м. interlócutor; the pérson smb. is tálking to; мн. the spéakers; он интере́сный ~ he's ínteresting to talk to, he's éxellent cómpany; он ску́чный ~ he is a bore, he has no conversátion.

собесе́дование с. ínterview.

собира́тель м. colléctor; ~ ма́рок stámp-collector. ~ный грам. colléctive; ~ные имена́ существи́тельные colléctive nouns.

собир|а́ть, собра́ть (вн.) 1. (сосредото́чивать в одно́м ме́сте) gáther (smth., smb.), colléct (smb., smth.); (живо́тных) round up (smth.); (созыва́ть) assémble (smb., smth.); собра́ть уча́стников экску́рсии assémble a párty of síghtseers, get* togéther the péople for the excúrsion; 2. (скла́дывать в одно́ ме́сто) put* (smth.) togéther, pack (smth.); (о чём-л. упа́вшем) pick (smth.) up; ~ кни́ги в портфе́ль pack the books ínto one's bríefcase; ~ с по́лу бума́ги pick some pápers up off the floor; 3. разг. (упако́вывать) pack (smth.); собра́ть чемода́н pack a súitcase; 4. разг. (приготовля́ть, снаряжа́ть кого́-л.) prepáre (smb.); ~ кого́-л. в доро́гу get* smb. réady for a jóurney; 5. разг.: собра́ть на стол lay* the táble; 6. (соединя́ть) gáther (smth.) up; ~ во́лосы в ко́су braid/plait one's hair; 7. (де́лать сбо́рки) pleat (smth.), take* (smth.) in; собра́ть пла́тье в та́лии take* a skirt in at the waist; 8. (соединя́ть и скрепля́ть отде́льные ча́сти чего́-л.) assémble (smth.); ~ стано́к assémble a lathe; ~ дом из кру́пных бло́ков assémble a búilding out of large precást strúctural élements; 9. (коллекциони́ровать) colléct (smth.); (копи́ть де́ньги) save (smth.) up; собра́ть библиоте́ку colléct a líbrary; собра́ть колле́кцию ма́рок make* a colléction of stamps;

10. (вн.; получа́ть в како́м-л. коли́честве) colléct (smth.); ~ чле́нские взно́сы colléct dues; ~ све́дения colléct/gáther informátion; 11. (вн; подбира́ть, срыва́ть) pick (smth.), gáther (smth.); (снима́ть с поле́й и т. п.) hárvest (smth.); ~ я́годы pick bérries; собра́ть корзи́ну грибо́в pick/gáther a básketful of múshrooms; ~ хво́рост gáther twigs/sticks; ~ лека́рственные расте́ния gáther medícinal herbs; ~ урожа́й take*/get* in the hárvest; 12. (напряга́ть си́лы, спосо́бности) cóncentrate (smth.), múster (smth.); собра́ть после́дние си́лы rálly one's flágging strength; собра́ть всё своё му́жество screw up one's cóurage. ~а́ться, собра́ться 1. (сходи́ться и т. п.) gáther, get* togéther; мы собра́ли́сь здесь, что́бы... we are assémbled here to...; we are gáthered togéther here to...; мы ~а́емся ка́ждую сре́ду we meet évery Wédnesday; не все ещё собрали́сь they háven't all come yet; подождём, пока́ все соберу́тся let us wait till éveryone is here; 2. (гото́виться) get* réady; ~а́ться в доро́гу get* réady for a jóurney; 3. (надвига́ться) be* cóming/appróaching; ~а́ется гроза́ thúnder is appróaching, a storm is gáthering; 4. (+ инф; намерева́ться) inténd (+ to inf, + -ing), be* góing (+ to inf); be* abóut (+ to inf); я ~а́юсь (е́хать) в Москву́ I am thínking of góing to Móscow; он не ~а́ется здесь остава́ться he does not cóntemplate/inténd stáying here; я и не ~а́лся е́хать туда́ I had no inténtion of góing there; я как раз ~а́лся позвони́ть вам I was just abóut to télephone you; 5: ~а́ться с мы́слями colléct one's thoughts; ~а́ться с си́лами súmmon (up) one's strength; ◇ собра́ться с ду́хом pluck/screw up one's cóurage.

соблаговоли́ть сов. (+ инф.) ирон. deign (+ to inf).

собла́зн м. temptátion; вводи́ть кого́-л. в ~ lead* smb. into temptátion.

соблазни́тель м. témpter; (обольсти́тель) sedúcer. ~ный 1. (зама́нчивый) témpting; 2. (возбужда́ющий чу́вственность) sedúctive.

соблазни́ть(ся) сов. см. соблазня́ть(ся).

соблазня́ть, соблазни́ть 1. (вн. тв.; прельща́ть) tempt (smb. with); ~ кого́-л. лёгким за́работком tempt smb. with éasy wáges; 2. (вн. на вн., вн. + инф.; склоня́ть к чему́-л.) tempt (smb. into, smb. + -ing). ~ся, соблазни́ться 1. (тв., на вн.; прельща́ться чем-л.) be* témpted (by); 2. (+ инф.; не устоя́ть пе́ред чем-л.) be* témpted (ínto + -ing).

соблюд|а́ть, соблюсти́ (вн.) obsérve (smth.), keep* (smth., to), adhére (to); ~ зако́н obsérve the law; ~ о́чередь wait one's turn; ~ поря́док act in an órderly fáshion; ~ пра́вила keep (to) the rules; ~ эконо́мию práctise ecónomy. ~е́ние с. obsérvance (of), adhérence (to).

соблюсти́ сов. см. блюсти́ и соблюда́ть.

собо́й см. себя́.

соболе́знование с. condólence; выража́ть ~ кому́-л. óffer smb. one's condólences.

соболе́зновать несов. (дт.) condóle (with), sýmpathize (with).

собо́лий sáble attr.; ~ мех sáble.

соболи́ный sáble attr.; ~ запове́дник sáble resérve.

со́боль м. (живо́тное и мех) sáble.

собо́р м. 1. (храм) cathédral; 2. церк. (собра́ние) cóuncil.

собо́ю см. себя́.

собра́ние с. 1. méeting, gáthering; assémbly (тж. госуда́рственный о́рган); провести́ ~ condúct a méeting; 2. (колле́кция) colléction; 3. (произведе́ний): по́лное ~ сочине́ний Пу́шкина the compléte works of Púshkin.

собра́т м. féllow; ~ по профе́ссии cólleague; ~ по ору́жию bróther-in-arms; ~ по перу́ bróther-wríter.

собра́ть(ся) сов. см. собира́ть(ся).

со́бственн|ик м. ówner, propríetor; земе́льный ~ lándowner, lánded propríetor; ме́лкий земе́льный ~ small hólder; он тако́й ~! разг. he's véry acquísitive! ~ица ж. propríetress, ówner.

со́бственническ|ий 1. о́wner's; of о́wnership *после сущ.*; ~ие права́ rights of о́wnership; 2. (*свойственный собственнику*) acquísitive; ~ инсти́нкт propríetary ínstinct.

со́бственно 1. *вводн. сл.* áctually; ~ говоря́ stríctly spéaking; в чём, ~, де́ло? what is áctually the mátter?; 2. *в знач. частицы* próper, in the full sense.

со́бственнору́чн|о with *one's* own hand(s); ~ постро́ить дом build* a house with *one's* own hands. ~ый made/done with *one's* own hand(s) *после сущ.*; (*о написанном*) áutograph *attr.*; ~ая по́дпись áutograph.

со́бственн|ость ж. 1. (*имущество*) próperty; госуда́рственная ~ State próperty; próperty of the State; ча́стная ~ prívate próperty; 2. (*на зем.; принадлежность кому-л.*) о́wnership of land; пра́во ~ости на *что-л.* próperty rights to *smth.*, right of о́wnership of *smth.* ~ый own; свой ~ый *one's* own; ~ый дом *one's* own house, a prívate house; спра́виться ~ыми си́лами mánage on *one's* own (resóurces); по ~ому жела́нию as one wíshes; в ~ом смы́сле in the true sense; ◇ ~ый корреспонде́нт our own correspóndent; и́мя ~ое *грам.* próper name.

собы́ти|е *с.* evént; междунаро́дные ~я world evénts; следи́ть за ~ями fóllow the course of evénts, keep* up with evénts; э́то це́лое ~ it's quite an evént.

сова́ *ж.* owl.

сова́ть, су́нуть (*вн.*) *разг.* 1. (*вкладывать внутрь*) push (*smth.*), put* (*smth.*); ~ ру́ки в карма́ны push/put* *one's* hands in *one's* póckets; 2. (*класть что-л. небрежно, торопливо*) push (*smth.*), shove (*smth.*); ~ кни́ги на по́лку shove books on a shelf*; 3. (*подавать кому-л. небрежно, торопливо*) thrust* (*smth.*); ~ ру́ку óffer *one's* hand cásually; thrust* out *one's* hand; ~ что-л. кому́-л. в ру́ки thrust* *smth.* ínto *smb.'s* hands. ~ся, су́нуться *разг.* 1. plunge; 2. (*принима́ться*) try; 3. (*в вн.; вмешиваться*) intrúde (in), poke *one's* nose (ínto); ~ся не в своё де́ло poke *one's* nose ínto óther péople's business; не су́йся, куда́ не про́сят! don't go where you are not wánted; 4. (*к дт. с тв.; приставать*) bóther (*smb.* with).

соверша́ть, соверши́ть (*вн.*) 1. accómplish (*smth.*); (*преступление*) commít (*smth.*), pérpetrate (*smth.*); соверши́ть (боево́й) по́двиг perfórm a feat (of arms); ~ оши́бку make* a mistáke, commít an érror; (*грубую*) commít/pérpetrate a blúnder; ~ поса́дку (*о самолёте*) make* a lánding; ~ чудеса́ work wónders; 2. (*оформлять*) conclúde (*smth.*), make* (*smth.*); ~ сде́лку make*/strike* a bárgain. ~ся, соверши́ться take* place, occúr, háppen.

соверше́нно quite, pérfectly; ~ ве́рно! quite right!; ~ го́лый stark náked; ~ неожи́данно quite unexpéctedly.

совершенноле́т|ие *с.* cóming of age, majórity; до его́ ~ия till he comes of age; till his cóming of age; till he attáins his majórity. ~ний of age *после сущ.*

соверше́нн|ый I 1. (*превосходный*) pérfect; 2. (*полный*) ábsolute, útter; ~ая пра́вда ábsolute truth; ~ идио́т útter fool, pérfect ídiot.

соверше́нный II: ~ вид *грам.* perféctive áspect.

соверше́нств|о *с.* perféction; дости́гнуть ~а attáin perféction; в ~е pérfectly.

соверше́нствование *с.* impróvement.

соверше́нствовать, усоверше́нствовать (*вн.*) impróve (*smth.*); ~ свои́ зна́ния impróve *one's* knówledge; ~ но́вую маши́ну make* impróvements to a new car, perféct a new módel. ~ся, усоверше́нствоваться impróve onesélf; усоверше́нствоваться в англи́йском языке́ impróve *one's* Énglish.

соверши́ть(ся) *сов. см.* соверша́ть(ся).

сове́стно: ~ сказа́ть I am ashámed to say; ему́ ~ призна́ться he is ashámed to admít; мне ~ за него́ I am ashámed of him; как вам не ~! you ought to be ashámed of yoursélf; мне ~ ста́ло I felt ashámed/sórry.

со́вест|ь *ж.* cónscience; чи́стая ~ good/clear cónscience; ~ му́чает *кого́-л. smb.* has pangs of cónscience; у него́ нечи́стая ~ he has a bad/guílty cónscience; потеря́ть ~ abándon cónscience; ◇ для успоко́ения ~и to make quite sure; по (чи́стой) ~и fránkly; по ~и говоря́ to tell the truth; на ~ 1) (*добросовестно*) consciéntiously, well; 2) (*на веру*) on trust; не за страх, а за ~ not as an obligátion but for love of *one's* work/job; со споко́йной ~ью with an éasy/clear cónscience; поступа́ть про́тив свое́й ~и go* against *one's* cónscience; на́до, пора́ и ~ знать there's a límit; ~ заговори́ла у *кого́-л. smb.'s* cónscience begán to prick him; ~и хвати́ло у *кого́-л.* (+ *инф.*) *smb.* had the cheek/gall/nerve (+ to *inf*).

Сове́т *м.* (*орган государственной власти в СССР*) Sóviet; Сове́т наро́дных депута́тов Sóviet of Péople's Députies.

сове́т I *м.* 1. (*административный или обществен-ный орган*) cóuncil; Сове́т Мини́стров Cóuncil of Mínisters; 2. (*совещание*) cóuncil; семе́йный ~ fámily cóuncil; держа́ть ~ hold* a méeting.

сове́т II *м.* (*наставление*) advíce; cóunsel; по ~у кого́-л. on *smb.'s* advíce; сле́довать ~у кого́-л. fóllow *smb.'s* advíce.

сове́тник *м.* 1. advíser; 2. (*должность, чин*) cóunsellor; ~ посо́льства, ми́ссии Cóunsellor of the Émbassy, Legátion; вое́нный ~ mílitary advíser.

сове́т|овать, посове́товать 1. (*вн. дт., дт. + инф.*) advíse (*smb. smth., smb.* + to *inf*); 2. с *отриц.* (*дт. + инф.*) *разг.* (*предостерегать от чего-л.*) advíse (*smb.* not + to *inf*), warn (*smb.* against + -ing); он нам не ~ал ходи́ть туда́ he warned us against góing there. ~аться, посове́товаться 1. (с *тв.*) consúlt (*smb.*), ask the advíce (of); ~аться с юри́стом consúlt a solícitor, take* légal advíce; 2. (*совещаться*) discúss, go* ínto cóuncil.

сове́тский Sóviet; Сове́тский Сою́з the Sóviet Únion.

сове́тчик *м.* advíser.

совеща́ние *с.* cónference.

совеща́тельный delíberative, consúltative; ~ го́лос deliberative voice; ~ о́рган consúltative bódy.

совеща́ться *несов.* (о *пр.*) delíberate (on, óver); (с *тв.*) confér (with), hold* a cónference (with).

сови́ный owl's; (*как у совы́*) ówlish.

совлада́ть *сов.* (с *тв.*) *разг.* contról (*smb., smth.*); get* the bétter (of); ~ с собо́й contról onesélf; он не смог ~ с собо́й he was unáble to contról himsélf.

совлада́|лец *м.*, ~лица *ж.* joint о́wner. ~ние *с.* joint о́wnership.

совмести́м|ость *ж.* compatíbility. ~ый compátible, consístent.

совмести́тельств|о *с.* plúralism; рабо́тать по ~у plúralize; рабо́тать секретарём по ~у combíne the job of sécretary with óther work.

совмести́ть(ся) *сов. см.* совмеща́ть(ся).

совме́стн|о jóintly, in cómmon, togéther with; ~ владе́ть *чем-л.* have* joint о́wnership of *smth.*; де́йствовать ~ co-óperate, act in combinátion; ~ с *кем-л.* togéther with *smb.* ~ый joint, combíned; ~ое обуче́ние co-educátion; ~ое предприя́тие joint vénture; ~ая рабо́та collaborátion, work togéther; ~ое заседа́ние joint séssion; ~ое владе́ние *чем-л.* joint о́wnership of *smth.*; ~ая жизнь life togéther; ~ые де́йствия joint áction *sg*; *воен.* combíned operátions; ~ые уси́лия combíned/joint éfforts.

совмещ|а́ть, совмести́ть (*вн.*) 1. combíne (*smth.*); ~ в себе́ combíne; ~ рабо́ту с учёбой combíne work and stúdy; 2. *мат.* superpóse (*smth.*). ~а́ться, совмести́ться 1. (*сочетаться с чем-л.*) combíne, be* combíned; 2. (*совпадать по времени*) coincíde; 3. *мат.* (*совпадать*) be* superpósed, match. ~е́ние *с.* 1. combinátion; ~е́ние не́скольких должносте́й hólding séveral jobs; ~е́ние не́скольких профе́ссий combíning of séveral proféssions; 2. *мат.* superposítion, mátching.

сово́к *м.* scoop; (*для сора*) dústpan.

совоку́пн|ость ж. totálity, ággregate, tótal combinátion; в ~ости in the ággregate; ~ фа́ктов tótal combinátion of facts, the facts táken as a whole; ~ доказа́тельств the totálity of évidence. ~ый joint, combíned.

совпад|а́ть, совпа́сть (с тв.) 1. coincíde (with); 2. (*оказываться общим*) concúr (with); (*о данных и т. п. тж.*) tálly (with); 3. (*соединяться*) uníte (with). ~е́ние с. 1. (*одновременность*) coíncidence; 2. (*общность*) concúrrence; ~е́ние интере́сов concúrrence of ínterests; 3. (*сочетание*) combinátion; ~е́ние обстоя́тельств combinátion of evénts.

совпа́сть сов. см. совпада́ть.

соврати́ть сов. см. совраща́ть.

совра́ть сов. см. врать.

совраща́ть, соврати́ть (*вн.*) pervért (*smb.*), sedúce (*smb.*); ◇ ~ кого́-л. с пути́ и́стинного lead* *smb.* astráy.

совреме́нн|ик м. contémporary. ~ость ж. 1. modérnity, contemporanéity; 2. (*эпоха*) our/módern times pl, módern life. ~ый 1. (*дт.*; *того же времени*) contémporary (with); 2. (*теперешний*) módern; of todáy *после сущ.*; ~ая эпо́ха our/módern times pl; ~ая молодёжь the young péople of todáy; 3. (*отвечающий требованиям своего времени*) módern, contémporary, úp-to-dáte; ~ое обору́дование úp-to-dáte equípment.

совсе́м quite, (*полностью*) totálly, entírely; (*навсегда*) for good; ~ ма́ло a véry little; ~ но́вый brand-néw; ~ молодёжь quite young; ~ друго́й quite a different; ~ друго́е sómething quite different; ~ не... not at all...; он ~ не го́рдый he is not at all proud; он ~ не врач he is not a dóctor at all; я его́ ~ не зна́ю I don't know him at all; я э́того ~ не ожида́л I did not expéct that in the least, that was the last thing I expécted; у меня́ ~ нет вре́мени I háven't a móment to spare; э́то ~ не то that's not it; вы ~ не то говори́те (, что на́до) that is not what you ought to say; ~ не тако́й, как... quite unlíke...; он ~ не тако́й глу́пый he is by no means so stúpid.

совхо́з м. state farm, sovkhóz. ~ный státe-farm *attr.*, sovkhóz *attr.*

согбе́нный bowed.

согла́си|е 1. (*разрешение*) consént, assént; получи́ть ~ кого́-л. obtáin *smb.'s* consént; с о́бщего ~я by cómmon consént; кивну́ть (голово́й) в знак ~я nod assént; 2. (*единомыслие*) agréement; 3. (*единодушие*) hármony, accórd; жить в по́лном ~и live in pérfect hármony.

согласи́ться сов. см. соглаша́ться.

согла́сно 1. *нареч.* in hármony; петь ~ sing* harmóniously; 2. *предлог* (*дт.*) accórding to; ~ предписа́нию accórding to the instrúction; ◇ ~ с чем-л. in accórdance with smth.

согла́сный I *прил. лингв.* 1. cónsonant; 2. *в знач. сущ. м.* cónsonant.

согла́с|ный II 1.: быть ~ным на что-л. agrée to smth.; вы ~ны идти́? are you willing to go?; быть ~ным с кем-л., чем-л. agrée with smb., smth., be* in agréement with smb., smth.; я (вполне́) с ва́ми ~ен I (fúlly) agrée with you; я ~ен с его́ мне́нием I am quite in agréement with his opínion; все с э́тим ~ны éveryone agrées on this point; все ~ны? does éverybody agrée?; ~ен! agréed!; ~ен, но... gránted, but...; 2. (*гармоничный*) harmónious.

согласова́ние с. 1. co-ordinátion; ~ де́йствий co-ordinátion; 2. *грам.* agréement, cóncord; ~ времён séquence of ténses.

согласо́ванн|о in co-ordinátion. ~ость ж. co-ordinátion. ~ый co-órdinated, concérted; ~ые де́йствия concérted áction sg; ~ая рабо́та téamwork.

согласова́ть сов. (*вн. с тв.*) 1. co-órdinate (*smth.* with); ~ расписа́ние движе́ния поездо́в с прибы́тием парохо́дов co-órdinate the train tímetable with the arríval of ships; 2. (*выработать единое мнение*) get*

agréement (on *smth.* with), fix (*smth.* with); ~ план де́йствий get* agréement on a plan of áction; 3. *грам.* make* (*smth.*) agrée (with). ~ся *несов. и сов.* (с тв.) 1. (*сообразоваться*) be* in confórmity (with); 2. *тк. несов. грам.* agrée (with).

соглаша́тель м. class collaborátor; *перен.* conciliator, cómpromiser. ~ский of class collaborátion *после сущ.*; ~ская поли́тика pólicy of class collaborátion. ~ство с. class collaborátion; *перен.* cómpromise.

соглаш|а́ться, согласи́ться 1. (на *вн.*, + *инф.*; *давать согласие*) agrée (to, + to *inf*), consént (to, + to *inf*), assént (to, + to *inf*); ~ на опера́цию agrée to an operátion; он до́лго не ~а́лся it was a long time before he would agrée, he held out for a long time; ~а́йтесь скоре́е! make up your mind!; он согласи́лся пое́хать с на́ми he agréed/consénted to go with us; согласи́тесь, что... you will admít that...; 2. (с тв.; *признавать правильным*) agrée (with); согласи́ться с мне́нием това́рища agrée with *one's* friends' opínion.

соглаше́ни|е с. agréement; по ~ю с кем-л. by agréement with smb.; по взаи́мному ~ю by mútual agréement/consént; прийти́ к ~ю come* to an agréement/understánding; arríve at an agréement/understánding; ~е о товарообме́не bárter agréement.

согна́ть сов. см. сгоня́ть.

со́гнутый crooked, bent; (*сгорбленный*) stooped.

согну́ть(ся) сов. см. сгиба́ть(ся).

согрева́ть, согре́ть (*вн.*) warm (*smb.*, *smth.*), heat (*smth.*); *перен.* (*утешать*) cómfort (*smb.*); (*оживлять*) inspíre (*smth.*); ~ ру́ки make* *one's* hands warm; ~ во́ду heat the wáter. ~ся, согре́ться get* warm; ко́мната ещё не согре́лась the room hásn't got warm yet.

согрева́ющий: ~ компре́сс hot cómpress.

согре́ть(ся) сов. см. согрева́ть(ся).

согреши́ть сов. см. греши́ть 1.

со́да ж. sóda; питьева́я ~ báking sóda; ~ для сти́рки washing sóda; каусти́ческая ~ cáustic sóda.

содействи|е с. assístance; при ~и кого́-л. with *smb.'s* assístance.

соде́йствовать *несов. и сов.* (кому́-л.) assíst (*smb.*); (чему́-л.) fúrther (*smth.*), contríbute (to), promóte (*smth.*).

содержа́ни|е с. 1. (*действие*) máintenance, úpkeep; ~ а́рмии máintenance of an ármy; расхо́ды по ~ю máintenance costs, expénses of úpkeep; 2. (*зарплата*) pay, sálary; 3. (*ассигнование*) allówance; 4. (*тема*) theme, súbject; ~ кни́ги súbject of a book; ~ о́перы theme of an ópera; ~ разгово́ра what the conversátion is/was abóut; кра́ткое ~ súmmary; 5. (*оглавление*) cóntents pl; 6. (*смысл, сущность чего-л.*) súbstance, cóntent, éssence; еди́нство фо́рмы и ~я únity of form and cóntent; 7. *разг.* (*содержимое*) cóntents pl; (*то, из чего состоит что-л.*) súbstance, stuff; esséntial ingrédients pl; 8. (*наличие какого-л. вещества*) cóntent; ~ вла́ги в атмосфе́ре móisture cóntent of the átmosphere.

содержа́тельн|ость ж. ríchness of cóntent, píthiness. ~ый profóund, sérious, píthy; ~ый челове́к interesting man*, wóman*; ~ая кни́га píthy/substántial book.

содержа́ть *несов.* (*вн.*) 1. (*обеспечивать*) maintáin (*smb.*), suppórt (*smb.*), keep* (*smb.*); ~ семью́ suppórt a fámily; он до́лжен ~ свои́х роди́телей he has his parents to keep, he has to maintáin his párents; 2. (*держать*) keep* (*smb.*, *smth.*); ~ что-л. в испра́вности keep* smth. in (wórking) órder; ~ кого́-л. под стра́жей hold*/keep* smb. únder arrést; 3. (*заключать в себе*) contáin (*smth.*); о́вощи содержа́т витами́ны végetables contáin vítamins. ~ся *несов.* 1. be* kept; 2. (*входить в состав чего-л.*): в э́той го́рной поро́де соде́ржится мно́го желе́за there is a high percéntage of iron in this rock; в э́той кни́ге соде́ржатся ну́жные све́дения this book contáins the informátion we need.

содержи́мое *с.* cóntents *pl.*

со́довый sóda *attr.*; ~ая вода́ sóda (-water).

содокла́д *м.* suppórting páper, sécond repórt. ~чик *м.* sécond spéaker.

содо́м *м. разг.* úproar, row.

содра́ть *сов. см.* сдира́ть.

содрог|**а́ние** *с.* shúdder; приводи́ть *кого-л.* в ~ make* *smb.* shúdder. ~а́ться, содрогну́ться shúdder; земля́ ~а́лась от взры́вов the earth rocked with the explósions; ~а́ться от у́жаса shúdder with hórror. ~ну́ться *сов. см.* содрога́ться.

содру́жество *с.* 1. cóncord, hármony; (*сотрудничество*) co-operátion; ~ на́ций co-operátion betwéen nátions; Брита́нское ~ на́ций Brítish Cómmonwealth (of Nátions); 2. (*общество, объединение*) associátion; ~ худо́жников ártists' associátion.

со́ев|**ый** sóya *attr.*; sóybean *attr.*; ~ые бобы́ sóya beans, sóybeans; ~ая мука́ sóya flour; ~ые конфе́ты sóya sweets; ~ое ма́сло sóybean oil; ~ый со́ус soy sauce.

соедине́ни|**е** *с.* 1. (*действие*) jóining, connécting; ~ проводо́в connécting of lines/wíres; 2. (*место*) júnction, connéction; (*стык, шов*) join; 3. (*крупная войсковая единица*) formátion; та́нковые ~я tank formátions; 4. *хим.* combinátion, cómpound. .

соединённый united, joint, combíned; ~ые си́лы combíned fórces.

соедини́тельн|**ый** 1. connécting, cóupling; ~ая пла́нка connécting plate; ~ая му́фта *тех.* connéctor, sleeve; 2. *лингв.* connécting; ~ гла́сный connécting vówel; 3. *грам.* connéctive; ~ сою́з cópulative conjúnction; ◇ ~ая ткань *биол.* connéctive tíssue.

соедини́ть(ся) *сов. см.* соединя́ть(ся).

соедин|**я́ть**, соедини́ть (*вн.*) 1. (*скреплять*) join/connéct (*smth.*); (*together*) cóuple (*smth.*), link (*smth.*); *перен.* bind* (*smb., smth.*); ~ провода́ connéct wíres/lines; 2. (*устанавливать сообщение*) connéct (*smth.*), link up (*smth.*); (*при телефонных переговорах*) put* (*smth.*) through; ~ два го́рода автостра́дой link up two towns with a mótorway/híghway; 3. (*объединять*) connéct (*smb., smth.*); соедини́ть си́лы join fórces; 4. (*сочетать*) combíne (*smth., smth.*), link (*smth.*); ~ тео́рию с пра́ктикой combíne théory with práctice. ~я́ться, соедини́ться 1. (*скрепляться*) join, connéct; (*о металлах*) fuse; *перен.* be* jóined/bound; провода́ соедини́лись the wíres/lines joined; 2. (*при помощи средств связи*) get* through, make* cóntact; соедини́ться с *кем-л.* по телефо́ну get* *smb.* on the télephone; 3. (*объединяться*) uníte, combíne; (*о войсках*) link up, join up; 4. (*сочетаться*) combíne, uníte. 5. *хим.* combíne, uníte.

сожале́ни|**е** *с.* 1. (*о пр.; чувство печали, огорчения*) regrét (for); с ~ем regrétfully; 2. (*к дт.; жалость, сострадание*) píty (for); из ~я к кому́-л. out of píty for *smb.*; досто́йный ~я (*внушающий жалость*) (gréatly) to be píted; (*прискорбный*) to be deplóred; ◇ к ~ю unfórtunately.

сожале́ть *несов.* (о *пр.*) 1. (*испытывать сожаление*) regrét (*smth.*), be* sórry (abóut); ~ о случи́вшемся regrét the íncident; 2. (*испытывать жалость*) píty (*smb.*), be* sórry (for).

сожра́ть *сов. см.* жрать.

созва́ниваться, созвони́ться *разг.* call (one anóther) up, get* in touch by phone.

созва́ть *сов. см.* созыва́ть *и* сзыва́ть.

созве́здие *с.* constellátion; *перен.* gálaxy.

созвони́ться *сов. см.* созва́ниваться.

созву́ч|**ие** *с.* cónsonance. ~ный cónsonant; in hármony *после сущ.*; ~ный эпо́хе in tune with the times.

создава́ть, созда́ть (*вн.*) creáte (*smb., smth.*), make* (*smb., smth.*); (*вызывать появление чего-л.*) cause (*smth.*); ~ симфо́нию compóse/write* a sýmphony; ~ спекта́кль prodúce a play; ~ коми́ссию set up a committee; ~ усло́вия для рабо́ты creáte condítions for work; ~ впечатле́ние creáte/prodúce an impréssion. ~ся, создава́ться be* creáted; (*возникать*) aríse*; создаётся впечатле́ние, что... there seems to be an impréssion that...; у меня́ создало́сь впечатле́ние... I am únder the impréssion...

созда́ние *с.* 1. (*действие*) creátion, máking; 2. (*произведение*) (piece of) work, creátion; ~ ге́ния the work of a génius; 3. (*существо*) creáture.

созда́тель *м.* creátor; (*учения, теории*) fóunder, originátor.

созда́ть(ся) *сов. см.* создава́ть(ся).

созерца́|**ние** *с.* contemplátion. ~тельный cóntemplative.

созерца́ть *несов.* (*вн.*) cóntemplate (*smb., smth.*).

созида́|**ние** *с.* creátion; па́фос ~ния creátive inspirátion. ~тель *м.* creátor. ~тельный creátive, constrúctive; ~тельный труд creátive work.

созида́ть *несов.* (*вн.*) creáte (*smth.*).

сознава́ть, созна́ть (*вн.*) 1. réalize (*smth.*), be* awáre/cónscious (of), be* alíve (to); ~ свой долг be* awáre of one's dúty; ~ свою́ оши́бку réalize one's mistáke; ~ опа́сность be* alíve to the dánger; 2. *тк. несов.* (*воспринимать окружающее*) be* cónscious; больно́й ничего́ не созна́ёт the pátient is uncónscious. ~ся, созна́ться conféss; (в *пр.*) acknówledge (*smth.*), admit (*smth.*); вино́вный созна́лся the cúlprit has conféssed; на́до созна́ться, нельзя́ не созна́ться it must be conféssed.

созна́ни|**е** *с.* 1. cónsciousness; (*мыслительная деятельность*) awáreness, mind, mentálity; кла́ссовое ~ class-cónsciousness; потеря́ть ~ lose* cónsciousness; приводи́ть *кого-л.* в ~ restóre *smb.* to cónsciousness; bring* *smb.* to, bring* *smb.* round *разг.*; приходи́ть в ~ regáin cónsciousness; come* to *разг.*; без ~я faint; он без ~я he is uncónscious; больно́й в ~и the pátient is cónscious; 2. (*ясное понимание чего-л.*) awáreness, realizátion; в ~и своего́ превосхо́дства cónscious of one's superiórity; ~ опа́сности realizátion of dánger; ~ до́лга awáreness of dúty; ◇ до поте́ри ~я till one is blue in the face; жить в чём-л. ~и live in *smb.'s* mind.

созна́тельн|**о** 1. cónsciously; (*добросовестно*) consciéntiously; он ~ пошёл на риск he took the risk cónsciously; 2. (*обдуманно*) deliberately. ~ость *ж.* 1. cónsciousness, awáreness; 2. (*понимание*) (fúllness of) understánding, wísdom. ~ый 1. cónscious; (*осмысленный*) matúre; ~ый во́зраст the age of matúrity; ~ые го́ды of жи́зни matúre years; 2. (*правильно понимающий окружающее*): ~ое отноше́ние к чему́-л. réasoned áttitude to *smth.*; 3. (*обдуманный*) deliberate; ~ый посту́пок deliberate áction.

созна́ть *сов. см.* сознава́ть 1. ~ся *сов. см.* сознава́ться.

созрева́ние *с.* rípening, matúring.

созрева́ть, созре́ть rípen; matúre (*тж. перен.*).

созре́ть *сов. см.* созрева́ть.

созы́в *м.* cálling, convocátion.

созыва́ть, созва́ть (*вн.*) 1. (*приглашать*) call (*smth.*) togéther, súmmon (*smb.*); (*гостей*) invíte (*smb.*); созва́ть друзе́й invíte one's friends; 2. (*съезд и т. п.*) call (*smth.*), convéne (*smth.*), hold* (*smth.*); созва́ть конфере́нцию call/convéne a cónference; созва́ть конси́лиум hold* a consultátion.

соизво́лить *сов.* (+ *инф.*) *ирон.* deign (+ to *inf*), be* pleased (+ to *inf*).

соизмери́м|**ый** comménsurable; *перен. тж.* cómparable; ~ые величи́ны comménsurable quántities; ~ые поня́тия cómparable concéptions.

соиска́ние *с.*: предста́вить диссерта́цию на ~ учё́ной сте́пени до́ктора нау́к presént/submít one's thésis for a dóctor's degrée.

со́йка *ж. зоол.* jay.

сойти́ *сов. см.* сходи́ть I.

сойти́сь *сов. см.* сходи́ться.

сок *м.* juice; (*деревьев*) sap; берёзовый ~ birch sap; ◇ выжима́ть все ~и из *кого-л.* sweat *smb.*, work *smb.* to death; в са́мом ~у́ in the prime of life, in *one's* prime.

соковыжима́лка *ж.* squéezer, júicer.

со́кол *м.* 1. fálcon; 2. *мн.* (*о лётчиках*) éagles, hawks; 3. (*о красивом, смелом человеке*) líon, pródigy; ◇ гол как со́кол ≈ poor as a church mouse, poor as a rat, poor as Job.

соколи́ный 1. fálcon's; 2. (*гордый, смелый*) éagle *attr.*

сократи́ть(ся) *сов. см.* сокраща́ть(ся).

сокращ|а́ть, сократи́ть (*вн.*) 1. (*укорачивать*) shórten (*smth.*), cut* down (*smth.*); (*слово*) abbréviate (*smth.*); (*текст*) abrídge (*smth.*); сократи́ть путь shórten the journey; сократи́ть сро́ки строи́тельства cut* down building time; 2. (*уменьшать*) redúce (*smth.*), curtáil (*smth.*); ~ расхо́ды cut*/keep* down expénditure; redúce/curtáil expénditure/expénses; retrénch; ~ штат(ы) redúce staff; 3. *разг.* (*увольнять*) make* (*smb.*) redúndant, dischárge (*smb.*); 4. *мат.* cáncel (*smth.*) out, elíminate (*smth.*). ~а́ться, сократи́ться 1. (*делаться короче*) shórten, grow* short(er), be* shórtened; путь сократи́тся на две́сти киломе́тров the journey will be shórtened by two húndred kílometres; 2. (*уменьшаться*) be* redúced, dimínish; расхо́ды ~а́ются expénses are béing redúced; 3. *физиол.* (*сжиматься*) contráct; 4. *мат.* cáncel out.

сокраще́ни|е *с.* 1. (*укорочение*) shórtening; (*в тексте*) abrídgement; для ~я вре́мени to save time; для ~я пути́ to redúce the journey; 2. (*уменьшение*) redúction, curtáilment; ~ на де́сять проце́нтов redúction of ten per cent; всеобщее ~ вооруже́ний géneral redúction of ármaments; ~ штáтов staff redúction; cútting down (of) the estáblishment; по ~ю штáтов ówing to redúction of staff; 3. (*сокращённое обозначение*) abbreviátion; 4. (*пропуск в тексте*) abrídgement; изда́ние с ~ями abrídged edítion; 5. *разг.* (*увольнение*) redúndancy, dischárge; 6. *физиол.* contráction; ~ се́рдца sýstole; 7. *мат.* cancellátion.

сокращённ|ый in abbréviated form. ~ый 1. shórtened, redúced, curtáiled; ~ый рабо́чий день shórtened wórking day; ~ое изда́ние abrídged edítion; ~ое изложе́ние dígest, shórtened vérsion; 2. (*обозначенный начальными буквами*) abbréviated; ~ое сло́во abbréviated word.

сокрове́нн|ый ínnermost, sécret; (*дорогой*) chérished; ~ая мечта́ chérished dream.

сокро́вищ|е *с.* tréasure; (*богатства земных недр, лесов и т. п.*) ríches *pl*; ~а мирово́й культу́ры tréasures/ríches of world cúlture; ◇ ни за какие ~а not for the world. ~ница *ж.* tréasury; ~ница зна́ний tréasury of knówledge.

сокруша́ть, сокруши́ть (*вн.*) 1. (*разбивать*) smash (*smth.*), shátter (*smth.*); *перен. тж.* destróy (*smb., smth.*); 2. (*печалить*) distréss (*smb.*). ~ся *несов.* (*о пр.*) grieve (for, óver); be* distréssed (about).

сокрушённ|о móurnfully. ~ый sad, gríeving.

сокруши́тельный crúshing, sháttering; críppling; уда́р crúshing blow.

сокруши́ть *сов. см.* сокруша́ть.

сокры́тие *с.* concéalment.

соку́рсн|ик *м.*, ~ица *ж.* féllow stúdent; он был мои́м ~иком he was in my year at cóllege.

солга́ть *сов. см.* лгать.

солда́т *м.* sóldier (*тж. перен.*); prívate (sóldier); *мн. тж.* the men.

солда́тик *м.* (*игрушечный*) tin sóldier, toy sóldier.

соле́ние *с.* (*действие*) sálting, píckling.

солён|ый 1. salt; (*о воздухе, ветре*) sálty, bríny, bráckish; ~ое о́зеро salt lake; 2. (*обладающий вкусом соли*) sálty; salt; ~ые слёзы sálty tears; 3. (*засоленный*) sálted, píckled; ~ые грибы́ múshrooms in brine; ~ая ка-

пу́ста píckled cábbage, sáuerkraut; ~ые огурцы́ píckled cúcumbers; ~ое мя́со salt/corned beef.

соле́нье *с. обыкн. мн.* píckles.

солидаризи́роваться *несов. и сов.* (с *тв.*) join (with), make* cómmon cause (with).

солида́рн|ость *ж.* solidárity; из ~ости as a demonstrátion of solidárity; чу́вство ~ости sense of solidárity, féllow-feeling. ~ый 1. united; быть ~ым с кем-л. agrée with *smb.*, be* in agréement with *smb.*; 2. *юр.*: ~ая отве́тственность joint liability.

соли́дн|ый 1. (*прочный, крепкий*) sólid, substántial; ~ое зда́ние substántial building; 2. (*основательный, глубокий*) thórough, exténsive, consíderable; ~ые зна́ния thórough/wide knówledge *sg*; ~ журна́л sérious magazíne; 3. (*серьёзный, значительный*) estáblished, sérious, récognized; ~ учёный sérious/estáblished scíentist; ~ое учрежде́ние récognized institútion; 4. (*важный, представительный*) impréssive, impósing, wéighty; ~ челове́к impréssive pérson; ~ тон lófty tone; 5. (*крупный, полный*) mássive, big; 6. (*не очень молодой*): ~ во́зраст fair age; 7. *разг.* (*значительный по величине*) fáirsized, consíderable; ~ая су́мма sízeable amóunt, consíderable sum of móney.

соли́ст *м.*, ~ка *ж.* sóloist.

соли́ть, посоли́ть (*вн.*) salt (*smth.*); (*консервировать тж.*) pickle (*smth.*); ~ суп salt *one's* soup; ~ огурцы́ salt/pickle cúcumbers.

со́лнечн|ый 1. sun *attr.*; sólar *научн.*; ~ спектр *астр.* sólar spéctrum; ~ое затме́ние eclipse of the sun; sólar eclípse; ~ луч súnbeam; ~ свет súnlight, súnshine; ~ая коро́на *астр.* sólar coróna, the sun's coróna; 2. (*освещённый, согретый солнцем*) súnny; ~ая пого́да súnny wéather; ~ день súnny day; ~ая сторона́ the súnny side; ◇ ~ая систе́ма sólar sýstem; ~ое сплете́ние *анат.* sólar pléxus; ~ые су́тки sólar day; ~ уда́р súnstroke; ~ые часы́ súndial *sg*.

со́лнц|е *с.* sun; на ~ in the sun; гре́ться на ~ bask in the sun, sun *onesélf*; ~ по ~у by the sun; до ~а befóre súnrise; ме́сто под ~ем a place in the sun.

солнцепёк *м.* heat of the sun; на ~е right in the sun, in the heat of the sun.

солнцестоя́ние *с. астр.* sólstice; ле́тнее (зи́мнее) ~ súmmer (winter) sólstice.

со́ло *с. нескл.* 1. sólo; ~ для скри́пки violín sólo; 2. *в знач. нареч.* sólo; peть ~ sing* sólo.

солове́|й *м.* nightingale; ~ья ба́снями не ко́рмят *посл.* ≈ fine words bútter no pársnips, it is no use préaching to a húngry man.

солови́ный nightingale's.

соло́м|а *ж.* straw; (*для крыш*) thatch. ~енный 1. straw *attr.*; ~енная шля́па straw hat; ~енная кры́ша thatched roof; 2. (*о цвете*) stráw-coloured; ◇ ~енная вдова́ grass widow.

соло́минк|а *ж.* straw; ◇ хвата́ться за ~у clutch at a straw; утопа́ющий и за ~у хвата́ется *посл.* a dró wning man cátches/clútches at a straw.

солони́на *ж.* corned beef; *мор.* (salt) junk.

соло́нка *ж.* sáltcellar, sáltshaker *амер.*

со́лоно: ему́ ~ пришло́сь he had a (prétty) hard time, he has been through the mill.

солончако́вый *м.* sáline land.

солончако́в|ый sáline; ~ая по́чва sáline soil.

соль I *ж.* salt (*тж. перен.*); столо́вая ~ táble salt; ка́менная ~ rock salt; в э́том вся ~!, that's the whole point!, that's the béauty of it; ◇ а́ттическая ~ Áttic salt/wit; ~ земли́ the salt of the earth.

соль II *с. нескл. муз.* soh, sol, G.

со́льн|ый sólo *attr.*; ~ но́мер a sólo; ~ая па́ртия sólo part.

сольфе́джио *с. нескл. муз.* solféggio.

соля́нка *ж.* solyánka (*meat or fish soup with salted cucumbers and olives*).

соля́н|о́й salt *attr.*; ~ые пласты́ sáline depósits; ~ раство́р salt solútion; ~ые разрабо́тки salt wórkings.

соля́н|ый: ~ая кислота́ *хим.* hydrochlóric ácid.

соля́рий *м.* solárium (*pl* -ia).

сом *м.* (*рыба*) shéatfish, silúrus.

со́мкнут|ый: ~ строй *воен.* close órder; ~ыми ряда́ми in sérried ranks.

сомкну́ть(ся) *сов. см.* смыка́ть(ся).

сомнев|а́ться *несов.* 1. (*в пр.*) doubt (*smb., smth.*), have* doubts (abóut), quéstion (*smth.*); ~а́юсь I have my doubts; ~а́юсь, что... I don't believe (that)...; не ~ в чём-л. have* no doubts as to *smth.*, not quéstion *smth.*; мо́жете не ~! don't wórry!; 2. (*испы́тывать затрудне́ния, колеба́ния*) be* in doubt.

сомне́ни|е *с.* 1. (*неуве́ренность в и́стинности чего́-л.*) doubt; нет ~я, что он придёт he is sure to come; в э́том не мо́жет быть никако́го ~я there can be no doubt abóut that; 2. (*затрудне́ние, недоуме́ние*) doubtful point, próblem; разреши́ть все ~я solve all próblems; ◇ без ~я no doubt, undóubtedly; вне вся́кого ~я beyónd all mánner of doubt.

сомни́тельн|о 1. *нареч.* dóubtfully, dúbiously; 2. *в знач. сказ. безл.* it is dóubtful. ~ый 1. (*недостове́рный*) quéstionable, dúbious; ~ая тео́рия quéstionable théory; 2. (*двусмы́сленный*) dóubtful, ambíguous; ~ый комплиме́нт ambíguous cómpliment; 3. (*подозри́тельный*) dúbious, shády; ~ые дела́ dúbious transáctions; ~ая ли́чность shády cháracter.

сомно́житель *м. мат.* fáctor.

сон *м.* 1. (*состоя́ние*) sleep; slúmber *поэт.*; во сне in one's sleep; меня́ кло́нит ко сну I am sléepy; он со сна ничего́ не по́нял he was too sléepy to understánd ánything; погрузи́ться в глубо́кий ~ fall* into a deep/sound sleep; 2. (*сновиде́ние*) dream; ви́деть ~ have* a dream; ви́деть во сне что́-л. dream* abóut/of *smth.*; как во сне as in a dream; ◇ сквозь ~ half-asléep, in a doze; спать сном пра́ведника sleep* the sleep of the just; сна ни в одно́м глазу́ нет cóuldn't feel less like sleep; засну́ть ве́чным сном go* to etérnal rest.

сонасле́дник *м. юр.* cohéir; *мн.* joint heirs.

сона́та *ж. муз.* sonáta.

соне́т *м. лит.* sónnet.

сонли́в|ость *ж.* sléepiness, dró́wsiness; sómnolence *книжн.* ~ый sléepy; (*со́нный тж.*) dró́wsy.

сонм *м.* múltitude.

со́нн|ый 1. sléepy, dró́wsy; *перен.* slúggish, sómnolent, lístless; в ~ом состоя́нии in a sléepy state, half asléep; ~ вид dró́wsy appéarance; 2. (*спя́щий*) sléeping; разбуди́ть ~ых дете́й wake* up the sléeping children; ◇ ~ая боле́знь *мед.* sléeping-sickness; ~ая арте́рия *анат.* caró́tid (ártery); как ~ая му́ха ≈ like a tíred bútterfly.

со́ня 1. *м. и ж. разг.* sléepyhead; 2. *ж.* (*живо́тное*) dórmouse.

сообража́|ть *несов.* (*вн.*) 1. (*понима́ть*) understánd* (*smth.*); (*быть све́дущим в чём-л.*) know* (*smth.*); (*бы́стро, мгнове́нно*) be* quick (about); в уpтаke; пло́хо ~ not be véry bright; я что́-то пло́хо ~ю I don't quite grasp the point; 2. (*стара́ться поня́ть что́-л.*) try to think out (*smth.*); (*рассужда́ть*) think*.

соображе́ни|е *с.* 1. (*спосо́бность сообража́ть*) wit, sense; 2. (*мне́ние, сужде́ние*) opínion, view; вы́сказать свои́ ~я state one's opínions; 3. *обы́кн. мн.* (*мы́сленные пла́ны, расчёты*) considerátion, réason; такти́ческие ~я táctical considerátions; из э́тих ~й for these réasons; по тем и́ли ины́м ~ям for one réason or anóther.

сообрази́тельн|ость *ж.* quick thínking; quick wits *pl*, ingenúity; у него́ не хвата́ет ~ости сде́лать э́то he hasn't got the wit/sense to do it. ~ый quick-wítted, bright.

сообраз|и́ть *сов.* réalize; (*приду́мать*) think* out (*smth.*); да́йте мне ~! let me think!; он бы́стро ~и́л, что... he réalized ínstantly that...

сообра́зн|о: ~ с (*тв.*) in confórmity (with), in accórdance (with). ~ый (с *тв.*) in kéeping (with); ◇ ни с чем не ~ абсу́рд; э́то ни с чем не ~о! it just dóesn't make sense!

сообраз|ова́ть *несов. и сов.* (*вн. с тв.*) co-órdinate (*smth.* with). ~ова́ться *несов. и сов.* (с *тв.*) confórm (to); (*счита́ться*) take* (*smth.*) ínto accóunt; де́йствовать, ~у́ясь с обстоя́тельствами, усло́виями act in accórdance with círcumstances, condítions.

сообща́ jóintly, togéther; ~ с кем-л. togéther with *smb.*, conjóintly with *smb.*; де́йствовать ~ act in únison; рабо́тать ~ work togéther, work as a group/team; мы ~ реши́ли we have come to the joint conclúsion.

сообщ|а́ть, сообщи́ть 1. (*вн. дт., дт. о пр.; уведомля́ть*) infórm (*smb.* abóut), let* (*smb.*) know (*smth.*), commúnicate (*smth.* to), repórt (*smth.* to); (*по ра́дио*) annóunce (*smth.*); сообщи́ть свой а́дрес знако́мым let* one's friends know one's address; ~ изве́стие give the news; (*неприя́тное*) break* the news; ~ све́дения give*/send* informátion; газе́ты ~а́ют, что... the pápers say...; как ~а́ют газе́ты accórding to the pápers; нам ~а́ют из ... accórding to informátion recéived (from)...; 2. (*вн. дт.; придава́ть*) impárt (*smth.* to); ~ магни́тное сво́йство mágnetize. ~а́ться *несов.* 1.: как уже́ ~а́лось as préviously repórted; 2. (*с тв.; быть соединённым*) commúnicate (with), be* in communicátion (with); ~а́ться ме́жду собо́й commúnicate; 3. (*подде́рживать сноше́ние*) commúnicate.

сообще́ни|е *с.* 1. communicátion; (*изве́стие тж.*) annóuncement, repórt; (*официа́льное*) по ~ю, согла́сно ~ю as repórted; 2. (*связь*) communicátion; железнодоро́жное ~ rail communicátion; прямо́е железнодоро́жное ~ diréct rail communicátion.

сообще́ств|о *с.* associátion; ◇ в ~е с кем-л. in conjúnction with *smb.*

сообщи́ть *сов. см.* сообща́ть.

соо́бщни|к *м.*, ~ца *ж.* accómplice, conféderate. ~чество *с.* complícity.

сооруди́ть *сов. см.* сооружа́ть.

сооруж|а́ть, сооруди́ть (*вн.*) 1. eréct (*smth.*); 2. *разг.* (*мастери́ть*) fix up (*smth.*). ~е́ние *с.* 1. (*де́йствие*) eréction, constrúction; 2. (*строе́ние*) édifice, strúcture.

соотве́тственн|о 1. *нареч.* correspóndingly, accórdingly; 2. *предло́г* (*дт.*) in confórmity (with). ~ый 1. (*дт.; соотве́тствующий*) próper (to), correspónding (to); 2. (*подходя́щий*) próper, súitable.

соотве́тстви|е *с.* confórmity, correspóndence, hármony, accórd; ~ ме́жду частя́ми hármony of the várious parts; ◇ в ~и с чем-л. in confórmity with *smth.*; в ~и с э́тим accórdingly; приводи́ть что-л. в ~ с чем-л. bring* *smth.* into line with *smth.*

соотве́тств|овать *несов.* (*дт.*) correspónd (to, with), confórm (to, with), be* in accórdance/hármony/kéeping (with); (*тре́бованиям, це́ли*) meet* (*smth.*), ánswer (*smth.*); ~ действи́тельности be* true; э́то не ~ует действи́тельности it is not in accórdance with the facts; ~ описа́нию ánswer the descríption; ~ тре́бованиям meet* the requírements; ~ эпо́хе be* in keeping with the périod.

соотве́тствующ|ий correspónding; (*приго́дный*) súitable; (*надлежа́щий*) apprópriate, próper; ~им о́бразом accórdingly; принима́ть ~ие ме́ры take* due/próper méasures, take* apṕrópriate áction.

сооте́чественн|ик *м.* compátriot, cóuntryman*. ~ица *ж.* compátriot, cóuntrywoman*.

соотноше́ние *с.* correlátion, alígnment.

сопе́рн|ик *м.*, ~ица *ж.* rival; не име́ть ~иков be* unrivalled, have* no rival.

сопе́рнич|ать *несов.* (с *тв.*) 1. (*стреми́ться превзойти́ кого́-л.*) compéte (with), conténd (with), vie (with); ~ с *кем-л.* в искусстве шахматной игры́ compéte with *smb.* in the art of chess; 2. (*быть равным по достоинству*) compéte (with), rival (*smth.*). ~ество *с.* rívalry.

сопе́ть *несов.* breathe hard (through *one's* nose), snúffle.

со́пка *ж.* (cóne-shaped) hill; (*вулкан*) volcáno.

со́пли *мн. груб.* snot *sg.*

сопло́ *с. тех.* nózzle.

соподчине́ние *с. грам.* co-ordinátion.

сопоста́вить *сов. см.* сопоставля́ть.

сопоставле́ние *с.* compárison, correlátion, collátion.

сопоставля́ть, сопоста́вить (*вн.*) compáre (*smth.*), córrelate (*smth.*), colláte (*smth.*); ~ показа́ния свиде́телей compáre the évidence.

сопра́но *с. нескл.* sopráno.

сопре́ть *сов. см.* преть 1.

соприкаса́|ться, соприкосну́ться (с *тв.*) 1. (*дотрагиваться*) touch (*smth.*), come* ínto cóntact (with); 2. *тк. несов.* (*иметь смежные границы*) be* contíguous (to), bórder (on); *перен.* be* on the verge (of); земе́льные уча́стки ~аются the plots bórder on each óther; 3. *тк. несов.* (*иметь отношение к чему-л.*) concérn (*smth.*), have* a béaring (on); на́ши интере́сы ни в чём не ~а́ются we have no ínterests in cómmon; 4. (*общаться*) come* ínto cóntact (with), have* to do with, be* invólved (with).

соприкоснове́ни|е *с.* 1. contigúity; 2. (*взаимная связь*) cóntact; входи́ть в ~ с кем-л., чем-л. make* cóntact with *smb., smth.*; 3. *воен.* cóntact; вступа́ть в ~ с проти́вником estáblish cóntact with the énemy; ◇ то́чки ~я points of cóntact; у нас нет никаки́х то́чек ~я there is no cómmon ground betwéen us, there is no cóntact betwéen us.

соприкосну́ться *сов. см.* соприкаса́ться 1, 4.

сопроводи́тельн|ый 1. (*о документе и т. п.*) accómpanying; ~ое письмо́ cóvering létter; 2. (*сопровождающий кого-л., что-л.*) escórting.

сопроводи́ть *сов. см.* сопровожда́ть.

сопровожд|а́ть, сопроводи́ть (*вн.*) accómpany (*smb., smth.*); (*для охраны*) escórt (*smb.*). ~а́ться *несов.* (*тв.*) 1. be* accómpanied (by); 2. (*быть снабжён-ным чем-л.*) be* províded (with), be* fúrnished (with). ~а́ющий *прил.* 1. accómpanying; 2. *в знач. сущ. м.* éscort. ~е́ние *с.* 1.: в ~е́нии кого-л. accómpanied by *smb.*; (*для охраны*) escórted by *smb.*; 2. *муз.* accómpaniment; в ~е́нии скри́пки, роя́ля to the accómpaniment of a violín, piáno, with violín, piáno accómpaniment.

сопрома́т *м. разг.* (*сопротивле́ние материа́лов*) stúdy of strength of matérials.

сопротивле́ни|е *с.* 1. resístance, opposítion; ~ проти́вника énemy resístance; встреча́ть ~ со стороны́ кого-л. encóunter opposítion from *smb.*; ока́зывать ~ óffer resístance; 2. *физ.* resístance; ~ во́здуха air resístance; ~ материа́лов 1) *тех.* strength of matérials; 2) (*наука*) stúdy of strength of matérials; ◇ идти́ по ли́нии наиме́ньшего ~я take* the line of least resístance.

сопротивля́ться *несов.* (*дт.*) resíst (*smb., smth.*); ~ на́тиску врага́ stand* up to the énemy's ónslaught; ~ боле́зни resíst diséase; не ~ óffer/make* no resístance.

сопряж|ённый 1. (с *тв.*; *связанный*) atténded (by); э́то ~ено́ с больши́ми затрудне́ниями that will entáil great dífficulties; 2. *мат., хим.* cónjugate; *тех.* cóupled, connécted.

сопу́тств|овать *несов.* (*дт.*; *прям. и перен.*) accómpany (*smb., smth.*), atténd (*smb., smth.*); ему́ ~овала уда́ча succéss atténded his éfforts. ~ующий атте́ндант; ~ующие обстоя́тельства atténdant círcumstances.

сор *м.* rúbbish, lítter; вы́мести ~ из ко́мнаты sweep*

a room clean; ◇ выноси́ть ~ из избы́ ≈ wash *one's* dírty línen in públic.

соразме́р|ить *сов. см.* соразмеря́ть. ~но (*дт.*) in propórtion (to). ~ность *ж.* proportionálity. ~ный proportionate.

соразмеря́ть, соразме́рить (*вн.* с *тв.*) régulate (*smth.*) in propórtion (to), adjúst (*smth.* to).

сора́тник *м.* bróther-in-árms; (*товарищ по какой-л. деятельности тж.*) assóciate.

сорване́ц *м. разг.* mádcap; (*о девочке тж.*) romp, tómboy, hóyden.

сорва́ть *сов. см.* срыва́ть I.

сорва́ться *сов. см.* срыва́ться.

сорвиголова́ *м. и ж. разг.* dáre-devil.

соревнова́ни|е *с.* 1. competítion, cóntest; 2. *мн.* (*спортивная встреча*) tóurnament *sg*, ~я по пла́ванию swímming tóurnament.

соревнова́ться *несов.* (с *тв.*) compéte (with), conténd (with), vie (with).

сориенти́ровать *сов.* (*вн.*) órientate (*smth.*), contról the áttitude (of); *перен.* give* *smb.* gúidance. ~ся *сов.* (*прям. и перен.*) get*/find* *one's* béarings.

сори́нка *ж.* speck of dust.

сор|и́ть *несов.* (*тв.*) 1. make* a mess (with); не ~и́(те) на́ пол don't lítter the floor; 2. *разг.* (*тратить безрассудно*) squánder (*smth.*); ~ деньга́ми throw* *one's* móney about.

со́рн|ый: ~ая ку́ча heap of swéepings; ~ая трава́ weed. ~я́к *м.* weed.

со́рок *forty.*

соро́ка *ж.* (*птица*) mágpie.

сорокале́т|ие *с.* 1. (*период*) forty years *pl*; 2. (*годовщина*) fórtieth anníversary. ~ний 1. (*о сроке*) forty-year *attr.*; of forty years *после сущ.*; 2. (*о возрасте*) forty-year-óld; of forty *после сущ.*

сороков|о́й fórtieth; ~ы́е го́ды the fórties.

сороконо́жка *ж. разг.* céntipede.

соро́чк|а *ж.* (*мужская*) shirt; (*женская*) slip, chemíse; ночна́я ~ (*мужская*) níght-shirt; (*женская*) níght-gown; ◇ роди́ться в ~е ≈ be* born with a sílver spoon in *one's* mouth.

сорт *м.* 1. (*категория товара*) grade, quálity; (*разновидность*) kind; мука́ пе́рвого ~а high-grade flour; сукно́ вы́сшего ~а tóp-quality cloth; конфе́ты двух ~óв sweets of two kinds; 2. (*разновидность растения*) varíety; скороспе́лые ~á я́блок éarly-ripening varíety of ápple; 3. *разг.* (*вид, род*) kind, sort; ◇ пе́рвый ~ first-ráte.

сорти́ровать *несов.* (*вн.*) sort (*smth.*), grade (*smth.*), clássify (*smth.*); (*тж. перен.*); ~ зерно́ sort grain.

сортиро́в|ка *ж.* (*действие*) sórting, gráding, classifying. ~очный sórting; ~очный цех sórting shop; ~очная ста́нция *ж.-д.* márshalling yard. ~щик *м.*, ~щица *ж.* sórter.

сортов|о́й high-quálity *attr.*, spécial-quálity *attr.*; ~о́е стекло́ spécial-quality glass; ~а́я мука́ high-quality flour; ~ые семена́ selécted seeds; ~о́е зерно́ high-quality grain; ◇ ~о́е желе́зо séction/prófile/strúctural iron.

сос|а́ть *несов.* 1. (*вн.*) suck (*smth.*); 2. *безл.:* у меня́ ~ёт под ло́жечкой I have a sínking sensátion in the pit of my stomach; 3. (*вн.*; *причинять душевную боль*) gnaw (*smb.*), nag (*smb.*); тоска́ ~ёт меня́ grief is gnáwing at my héart.

, сосе́д *м.*, ~ка *ж.* néighbour; ~ сле́ва, спра́ва *one's* néighbour on the left, right. ~ний néighbouring; the next; ~ний дом the néxt-door house; он живёт в ~нем до́ме he lives next door; ~няя ко́мната the next room; ~няя фе́рма néighbouring farm. ~ский the néighbours'; ~ская дочь the girl next door; ~ский огоро́д the néighbours' allótment. ~ство *с.* néighbourhood; прия́тное ~ство pléasant néighbour(s); по ~ству in the néighbourhood.

соси́ска *ж.* (*chippoláta*) sáusage; fránkfurter *амер.*

со́ска *ж.* cómforter; báby's dúmmy; (*надеваемая на бутылочку*) nípple.

соска́кивать, соскочи́ть (с *рд.*) 1. (*прыгать*) jump off (*smth.*), jump down (from); соскочи́ть с ло́шади jump off *one's* horse; ~ со сту́ла leap* up from *one's* chair; 2. (*падать*) come* off (*smth.*).

соска́льзывать, соскользну́ть slide* (down); (*быстро сходить с чего-л.*) slip off.

соскользну́ть *сов. см.* соска́льзывать.

соскочи́ть *сов. см.* соска́кивать.

соску́читься *сов.* 1. (+ *инф.*; *почувствовать скуку*) get* bored (with); grow* wéary (of + -ing); 2. (о *пр.*, о *дт.*; *затосковать*) miss (*smb., smth.*); ~ по родны́м miss *one's* fámily, feel* hómesick; ~ по рабо́те miss *one's* work.

сослага́тельн|ый: ~ое наклоне́ние *грам.* subjúnctive mood.

сосла́ть *сов. см.* ссыла́ть.

сосла́ться *сов. см.* ссыла́ться.

ссо́слепу in *one's* blíndness.

сосло́в|ие *с. ист.* estáte; órder; тре́тье ~ third estáte; купе́ческое ~ the mérchants *pl.* ~ный group *attr.*; ~ные предрассу́дки group préjudices.

сослужи́в|ец *м.*, ~ица *ж.* cólleague.

сослужи́ть *сов.:* ~ слу́жбу 1) (*оказать услугу*) do* a sérvice/fávour; 2) (*принести пользу*) play a úseful role.

сосн|а́ *ж.* pine(-tree). ~о́вый pine *attr.*; (*из сосны*) pínewood *attr.*; ~о́вый бор pine fórest; ~о́вый стол deal táble.

сосня́к *м.* 1. (*лес*). pine wood, stand of pines; 2. *собир.* (*брёвна*) pine logs *pl.*

сосо́к *м.* nípple.

сосредото́чен|ие *с.* concentrátion. ~но with concentrátion, inténtly; ~но слу́шать lísten inténtly. ~ность *ж.* concentrátion. ~ный 1. (*напряжённый*) cóncentrated, inténse, intént; ~ное внима́ние cóncentrated atténtion; 2. (*погружённый в мысли*) atténtive, absórbed; ~ный взгляд absórbed expréssion; ◇ ~ный ого́нь *воен.* cóncentrated fire.

сосредото́чивать, сосредото́чить (*вн.*) cóncentrate (*smth.*); (*о внимании, взгляде тж.*) fócus (*smth.*); сосредото́чить внима́ние на чём-л. fócus/cóncentrate atténtion on *smth.* ~ся, сосредото́читься 1. (*о войсках, огне*) be* cóncentrated; 2. (на *пр.*) cóncentrate (on).

сосредото́чить(ся) *сов. см.* сосредото́чивать(ся).

соста́в *м.* 1. (*совокупность элементов*) compositión; ~ по́чвы soil compositión; определи́ть ~ микстуры ánalyse a míxture; входи́ть в ~ чего-л. be*/form part of *smth.*; 2. (*соединение, смесь*) míxture, cómpound; 3. (*совокупность людей*) cómplement; входи́ть в ~ делега́ции be* a mémber of the delegátion; вводи́ть кого-л. в ~ коми́ссии make* *smth.* a mémber of a commíssion; inclúde *smb.* in a commíssion; гру́ппа, в ~ кото́рой входя́т... a group inclúding...; быть в по́лном ~е have* a full cómplement; ~ исполни́телей *театр.* cast; 4. (*лица, составляющие какую-л. категорию*) staff; руководя́щий ~ managérial staff/personnél; офице́рский ~ ófficer personnél, commíssioned staff; рядово́й и сержа́нтский ~ non-commíssioned ófficers and óther ranks *pl*; enlísted men/personnél *амер.*; профе́ссорско-препода́вательский ~ téaching staff; 5. *ж.-д.* (*поезд*) train; пода́ть ~ на ста́нцию shunt a train ínto a státion; ◇ подвижно́й ~ rólling-stock; в ~е (consísting) of; коми́ссия в ~е трёх челове́к a commíssion (consísting) of three péople; ~ преступле́ния *юр.* córpus delícti; the facts of the crime.

соста́витель *м.* compíler.

соста́вить(ся) *сов. см.* составля́ть(ся).

составле́ние *с.* 1. (*из частей*) formátion; ~ по́езда márshalling of a train; 2. (*сочинение*) máking,

compositión; (*словаря, учебника*) compíling; (*плана, проекта*) wórking out.

составля́ть, соста́вить (*вн.*) 1. (*ставить вместе*) put* (*smth.*) togéther; соста́вить сту́лья в у́гол put* the chairs togéther in the córner; 2. (*образовывать что-л.*) make* (*smth.*); form (*smth.*); ~ уравне́ние make* an equátion; ~ предложе́ние *грам.* form/constrúct a séntence; ~ по́езд márshal a train; 3. (*создавать*) make* (*smth.*), compóse (*smth.*); (*словарь, учебник*) compíle (*smth.*); ~ план make* a plan, draw* up a plan; ~ письмо́ compóse a létter; ~ протоко́л draw* up a státement; ~ спи́сок make* a list; 4. (*группу, коллектив*) form (*smth.*); ~ тру́ппу form a cómpany; вы должны́ соста́вить мне компа́нию you must keep me cómpany; 5. (*собирать, приобретать постепенно*) build* up (*smth.*), collect (*smth.*); ~ библиоте́ку build* up a líbrary; 6. (*создавать путём наблюдений*) form (*smth.*); ~ мне́ние form an opínion; ~ себе́ представле́ние form a concéption, get* an idéa; 7. (*давать в итоге*) tótal (*smth.*), make* (*smth.*), come* to (*smth.*); ~ в сре́днем áverage; э́то соста́вит значи́тельную су́мму it will come to a consíderable sum; 8. (*являться*) be*; э́то не соста́вит труда́ that will be no tróuble. ~ся, соста́виться 1. (*образовываться, организовываться*) be* formed; 2. (*скапливаться постепенно*) accúmulate; 3. (*получаться в итоге, в сумме*) amóunt to.

составн|о́й 1. (*сложный*) cómposite, cómpound; (*о мачтах и т. п.*) séctional; 2. (*входящий в состав чего-л.*) constítuent, compónent; ~ая часть, ~ элеме́нт compónent/constítuent (part); (*смеси*) ingrédient; ~ые элеме́нты воды́ constítuent élements of wáter.

соста́рить(ся) *сов. см.* ста́рить(ся).

состоя́ни|е *с.* 1. condítion, state; ~ войны́ state of war; ~ здоро́вья state of health; в хоро́шем ~и in good* condítion; (*о больном*) dóing well; в плохо́м ~и in a bad* state; прийти́ в него́дное ~ be* in bad* repáir, be* out of repáir; 2. *физ.* state; газообра́зное ~ gáseous state; 3. (*богатство*) fórtune; ◇ быть в ~и сде́лать что-л. be* cápable of dóing *smth.*

состоя́тельн|ость *ж.* 1. (*обеспеченность*) prospérity; (*платёжеспособность*) sólvency; 2. (*обоснованность*) solídity, strength, reliabílity. ~ый 1. (*обеспеченный*) well-to-do; (*платёжеспособный*) sólvent; 2. (*обоснованный*) well-fóunded, relíable.

состо|я́ть *несов.* 1. (*из рд.*; *иметь в своём составе*) consíst (of); кварти́ра ~и́т из трёх ко́мнат the flat consísts of three rooms; семья́ ~и́т из четырёх челове́к there are four péople in the fámily; 2. (*в пр.*; *заключаться*) consíst (in); be*; ра́зница ~и́т в том, что... the difference is that...; 3. (*быть в составе*) be*; ~ в профсою́зе belóng to a trade únion; ~ при ком-л. be* attáched to *smb.*; ~ на действи́тельной слу́жбе be*/serve on the áctive list. ~я́ться *сов.* take* place, be* held; (*о сделке*) come* off; не ~я́ться not come off, not take place.

сострада́|ние *с.* compássion; испы́тывать ~ к кому́-л. have* compássion for *smth.*; из ~ния к кому-л. out of compássion for *smth.*; вызыва́ть ~ aróuse compássion. ~тельный compássionate.

состри́ть *сов. см.* остри́ть II.

состря́пать *сов. см.* стря́пать.

состыкова́ть *сов.* (*вн.*) join (*smth.*); (*о космических корабля́х*) dock (*smth.*). ~ся *сов.* join; (*о космических корабля́х*) dock, be* docked.

состяза́ние *с.* cóntest, competítion; (*спортивное тж.*) match; ~ в остроу́мии cóntest of wit; ~ в бе́ге race; ~ в пла́вании swímming cóntest/race; ~ на пе́рвенство страны́ по футбо́лу match for the nátional fóotball chámpionship.

состяза́ться *несов.* compéte; ~ в бе́ге race; ~ в остроу́мии try to outjést/outshíne one anóther.

сосу́д *м.* véssel.

сосу́дистый váscular.

сосу́лька ж. ícicle.

сосунóк м. súckling.

сосуществов|áние с. coexístence; ми́рное ~ péaceful coexístence. ~áть несов. coexíst.

сосчита́ть сов. см. счита́ть I 1, 2. ~ся сов. см. счита́ться 1.

сотворéни|е с. creátion; от ~я ми́ра since the world begán, since the beginning of time.

сотвори́ть сов. см. твори́ть.

сотка́ть сов. см. тка́ть.

сóтня ж. 1. a húndred; 2. мн. разг. (множество) húndreds; 3. ист. (казачья) squádron (of Cóssacks).

сотова́рищ м. cólleague.

сотови́дный hóneycomb attr., céllular.

сóтов|ый 1. hóneycomb attr., ~ мёд cómb-honey; 2. (сотовидный) hóneycomb attr., céllular.

сотру́дн|ик м., ~ица ж. 1. (тот, кто работает совместно с кем-л.) colláborator, hélper; 2. (служащий) employée, mémber of the staff; ◇ нау́чный ~ scientífic/reséarch wórker.

сотру́днич|ать несов. 1. (с тв.) co-óperate (with), colláborate (with); 2. (быть сотрудником) work; ~ в газéте work on a páper. ~ество с. 1. co-operátion, collaborátion; экономи́ческое, культу́рное ~ество económic, cúltural co-operátion; 2. (работа где-л.) work; (в газете) contríbuting; contríbutions pl.

сотряс|а́ть несов. (вн.) shake* (smth.). ~а́ться несов. shake*. ~éние с. sháking, vibrátion; (от одного удара) shock; ~éние мóзга concússion of the brain.

сóты мн. hóneycomb sg.

сóт|ый húndredth; ~ киломéтр the húndredth kílometre; ~ая дóля чего-л. a húndredth part of smth.; однá ~ая one húndredth.

сóус м. sauce; (мясная подливка) grávy; ◇ под други́м ~ом with a different dréssing, in a different wrápper. ~ник м. sáuce-boat.

соуча́ст|ие с. participátion; (в преступлении) complícity. ~ник м., ~ница ж. colláborator, co-wórker; (преступления) accómplice.

софá ж. sófa.

сохá ж. wóoden plough.

сóхнуть несов. 1. dry, get* dry; 2. (пересыхать) dry up; becóme* parched; 3. (испаряться) dry up, eváporate; 4. (погибать — о растениях) wither, shrível; 5. разг. (худеть, чахнуть) pine, waste awáy; (по пр.) pine (for).

сохранéние с. conservátion; preservátion; ~ энéргии conservátion of énergy; ~ ми́ра preservátion of peace; взять что-л. на ~ take* smth. for safekéeping; дать что-л. на ~ кому-л. give* smb. smth. for safekéeping.

сохрани́вшийся survíving, extánt; хорошó ~ (о человеке) well-presérved.

сохрани́ть сов. см. сохраня́ть 1, 2, 3, 4. ~ся сов. см. сохраня́ться 1, 2, 3.

сохра́нн|ость ж. sáfety, safekéeping, preservátion; в пóлной ~ости pérfectly safe. ~ый safe.

сохраня́ть, сохрани́ть (вн.) 1. (не давать чему-л. пропасть) presérve (smth.); несов. тж. look áfter (smth.); 2. (не нарушать) maintáin (smth.), keep* up (smth.); ~ поря́док maintáin órder; ~ мир presérve/maintáin peace; ~ хорóшие отношéния maintáin good relátions; 3. (не лишаться чего-л.) presérve (smth.), keep* (smth.), retáin (smth.) (тж. перен.); сохрани́ть своё здорóвье presérve one's health, keep* fit; ~ спокóйствие presérve one's calm; за собóй прáво resérve the right; ~ си́лу (о законе и т. п.) remáin in force; сохрани́ть лу́чшие воспоминáния о ком-л., чём-л. have* the pléasantest mémories of smth., smth.; ~ пáмять о ком-л. presérve/retáin a mémory of smth., чтo-л. на пáмять о ком-л. keep* smth. in mémory of smth., keep* smth. as a sóuvenir of smth.; 4. (беречь от порчи,

уничтожéния, опасности) protéct (smb., smth.); сохрани́ть одéжду от мóли protéct clothes from the moth; 5. тк. несов. разг. (помещать для хранения) keep* (smth.); ~ продýкты в холоди́льнике keep* food in the refrigerator. ~ся, сохрани́ться 1. remáin, be* presérved; стари́нное здáние хорошó сохрани́лось the áncient búilding was well presérved, the áncient búilding had lásted well; 2. (не портиться — о продуктах) keep*; 3. разг. (о человеке) wear* well; он хорошó сохрани́лся he is/looks young for his age; 4. тк. несов. (храниться где-л.) be* kept.

соцвéтие с. бот. flóscule, racéme.

социáл-демокрáт м. Sócial Démocrat. ~и́ческий sócial-democrátic. ~ия ж. Sócial Demócracy.

социализ|áция ж. socializátion.

социал|и́зм м. sócialism. ~и́ст м. sócialist.

социалисти́ческ|ий sócialist; ~ая систéма, ~ строй sócialist sýstem.

социáльно-бытов|óй: ~ые услóвия condítions of dáily life.

социáльно-экономи́ческий socioecónomic, sócial and económic.

социáльн|ый sócial; ~ые наýки sócial scíences; ~ое положéние sócial position/státus/stánding; ~ое происхождéние sócial órigin; ◇ ~ое обеспéчение sócial secúrity.

социó|лог м. sociólogist. ~лóгия ж. sociólogy.

соцстрáх м. sócial insúrance.

сочéльник м. (рождественский) Christmas Eve; в ~ on Christmas Eve.

сочетáни|е с. combinátion; ~ крáсок cólour combinátion; ~ слов word combinátion, phrase; ~ теóрии и прáктики combíning/wédding of théory and práctice; в ~и с чем-л. cóupled with smth., in combinátion with smth.

сочет|áть несов. и сов. (вн.) combíne (smth.); ~ в себé be* a combinátion of; ~ теóрию с прáктикой combíne/wed théory and práctice. ~áться несов. и сов. 1. combíne; в нём ~áются энéргия и ум he combínes énergy with brains; 2. тк. несов. (гармонировать) match, blend.

сочинéние с. 1. (действие) compósing, composítion; 2. (литературное произведение) work; 3. (школьное) composítion, éssay; 4. грам. co-ordinátion.

сочини́тельный грам. co-órdinating; ~ сою́з co--órdinating conjúnction.

сочини́ть сов. см. сочиня́ть.

сочиня́ть, сочини́ть (вн.) 1. write* (smth.); (музыку) compóse (smth.); ~ стихи́ write* póetry; 2. (выдумывать) invént (smth.), make* up (smth.); (о детях) tell* stóries/fibs; разг. (лгать) make* it up.

сочи́ться несов. ooze (out), trickle; ~ крóвью bleed*, ooze blood.

сóчн|ость ж. júiciness, súcculence. ~ый 1. júicy, súcculent; 2. (о рте, губах) full, blóoming; 3. (о красках) rich; (о растительности) lush; 4. (о стиле, языке) full-blóoded, rich.

сочу́вственн|о sympathétically, with sýmpathy; отнести́сь ~ к кому-л. be* kind to smth.; отнести́сь ~ к гóрю когo-л. sýmpathize with smb. in his, her grief. ~ый sympathétic; ~ый взгляд sympathétic glance; ~ый óтклик sympathétic respónse.

сочу́встви|е с. sýmpathy; ~ чужóму гóрю sýmpathy for anóther's grief; из ~я out of sýmpathy (for); не встречáть, не находи́ть ~я meet* with no sýmpathy.

сочу́вствовать несов. (дт.) sympathíze (with), feel* (for); ~ чему-л. гóрю feel* for smb.'s grief, sýmpathize with smb. in his, her grief; ~ чьим-л. взглядам be* in sýmpathy with smb.'s idéas; не ~ кому-л., чему-л. have* no sýmpathy for smth., smth.

сочу́вствующий прил. 1. sympathétic; 2. в знач. сущ. м. sýmpathizer.

сощу́рить *сов.*: ~ глаза́ screw up *one's* eyes. ~ся *сов.* screw up *one's* eyes.

сою́з *м.* 1. (*единение*) únion, alliance; 2. (*объедине-ние для совместных действий*) alliance; заключи́ть ~ énter into an alliance; 3. (*государственное объединение*) únion; Сою́з Сове́тских Социалисти́ческих Респу́блик the Únion of Sóviet Sócialist Repúblics; 4. (*обществен-ная организация*) únion; ~ писа́телей writers' únion; 5. *грам.* conjúnction.

сою́з|ик *м.*, ~ица *ж.* álly. ~ический allíed; ~иче-ские обяза́тельства *one's* undertákings/pledges as an álly.

сою́зно-республика́нский Únion-Repúblic *attr.*

сою́зн|ый 1. allíed; ~ые держа́вы allíed pówers; 2. (*относящийся к СССР*) Únion *attr.*; of the Únion *после сущ.*; ~ая респу́блика Únion Repúblic.

со́я *ж.* sóybean, sóya bean.

спад *м.* abátement; ~ произво́дства fálling-off of prodúction.

спада́ть, спасть 1. (*с рд.*; *падать*) fall* (from); 2. (*уменьшаться*) abáte; (*о воде тж.*) sink*; жара́ спа́ла the heat abáted; о́пухоль спа́ла the swélling went down; 3. *тк. несов.* (*свисать*) hang* down.

спазм *м.*, спа́зма *ж. мед.* spasm.

спазмати́ческий spasmódic.

спа́ивать I, спая́ть (*вн.*) sólder (*smth.*); *перен.* uníte (*smth.*), weld (*smth.*) togéther.

спа́ивать II, спои́ть (*вн.*) *разг.* 1. (*поить допьяна*) make* (*smb.*) drunk; 2. (*приучать к пьянству*) make* a drínker/drúnkard (of).

спа́йка *ж.* 1. (*действие*) sóldering; 2. (*место соеди-нения*) sóldered joint, seam; 3. *мед.* cómmissure, adhésion.

спали́ть *сов. см.* пали́ть I 3.

спа́льник *м. разг.* (*спальный мешок*) sléeping-bag.

спа́льн|ый sléeping; ~ ваго́н sléeping-car, sléeper; ~ое ме́сто sléeping-berth.

спа́льня *ж.* bédroom.

спанье́ *с. разг.* sléep(ing).

спа́ренный cóupled, paired, twin, dúplex.

спа́ржа *ж.* aspáragus.

спа́ривать, спа́рить (*вн.*) cóuple (*smth.*), pair (*smth.*).

спа́рить *сов. см.* спа́ривать.

спартакиа́да *ж.* sports féstival.

спарта́н|ец *м.*, ~ка *ж.*, ~ский Spártan.

спа́рывать, спа́роть (*вн.*) cut* off (*smth.*), unpíck (*smth.*).

спаса́ние *с.* réscuing, life-saving, réscue-work.

спаса́тель *м.* réscuer. ~ный life(-saving); réscue *attr.*, escápe *attr.*; ~ круг life-buoy; ~ная шлю́пка life-boat; (*на корабле*) séa-boat.

спас|а́ть, спасти́ (*вн.*) save (*smb.*, *smth.*), réscue (*smb.*, *smth.*); ~ жизнь кому́-л. save *smb.'s* life; ~ уто-па́ющего réscue a dró́wning pérson; réscue/save *smb.* from dró́wning; ~и́те! help!; ~ люде́й (*во время бедст-вия*) save péople's lives; ~ иму́щество réscue/sálvage próperty; ◇ ~ положе́ние save the situátion. ~а́ться, спасти́сь escápe; ~а́ться бе́гством flee* to sáfety, take* réfuge in flight; спасти́сь от пресле́дования succéed in escáping, get* awáy; ~а́ться, выбросившись с парашю́-том párachute to sáfety; он едва́ спа́сся he had a nárrow escápe; ~а́йся, кто мо́жет! fly for your lives!

спасе́ни|е *с.* 1. (*действие*) réscuing, sáving; 2. (*воз-можность спастись*) escápe, sáfety; иска́ть ~я в бе́гст-ве seek* sáfety in flight; быть обя́занным свои́м ~ем ко-му́-л., чему́-л. owe *one's* sáfety to *smb.*, *smth.*; ~я нет there is no escápe; 3. (*то, что спасает*) salvátion; в э́том на́ше еди́нственное ~ that is our sole salvátion; ◇ ложь во ~ white/sáving lie.

спасённый *прил.* 1. réscued; (*об имуществе тж.*)

sálvaged; 2. *в знач. сущ. м.* the réscued man*; *мн.* the réscued, the survívors.

спаси́бо thank you, thanks; большо́е (вам) ~! thank you véry much!; большо́е ~ (за) mány thanks (for); и на том ~ let us be thánkful for small mércies; and thank góodness for that; ◇ де́лать что́-л. за ~ do* *smth.* for nóthing.

спаси́тель *м.* réscuer, delíverer, sáviour. ~ный sálutary; ~ое сре́дство sure rémedy, wónder-working rémedy.

спасова́ть *сов. см.* пасова́ть I.

спасти́(сь) *сов. см.* спаса́ть(ся).

спасть *сов. см.* спада́ть 1, 2.

спать *несов.* sleep* (*тж. перен.*); slúmber *поэт.*; идти́, ложи́ться ~ go* to bed; укла́дывать кого́-л. ~ put* *smb.* to bed; он спит как уби́тый he sleeps like a log; спи́те споко́йно! sleep well! ~ся *несов. безл. разг.*: мне не спи́тся I can't get to sleep; на во́здухе хорошо́ спи́тся one sleeps well in the ópen air; хорошо́ спи́тся под у́тро the best sleep comes just befóre mórning.

спа́янн|ость *ж.* únity, cohésion, team spírit. ~ый uníted.

спая́ть *сов. см.* спа́ивать I.

спева́ться, спе́ться 1. get* used to sínging togéther; 2. *разг.* (*достигать согласия в чём-л.*) fit in with each óther; спе́ться с кем-л. fit in well with *smb.*; они́ отли́ч-но спели́сь they get on perféctly.

спе́вка *ж.* choir práctice.

спек|а́ться, спе́чься *тех.* coágulate; (*об угле*) cake.

спекта́кль *м.* perfórmance, show; *перен.* sight, displáy.

спектр *м.* spéctrum (*pl* -ra). ~а́льный *физ.* spéctral; ~а́льный ана́лиз spéctrum análysis.

спекули́ровать *несов.* (*тв.*, на *пр.*) 1. spéculate (in, on); 2. (*использовать в своих целях*) take* advántage (of), explóit (*smth.*); cash in (on) *разг.*

спекуля́нт *м.*, ~ка *ж.* spéculator, profitéer; (*на чёр-ном рынке*) black marketéer.

спекуляти́вн|ый black-márket *attr.*; ~ая цена́ black--márket price.

спекуля́ция *ж.* speculátion, black márketing, profitéering; (на *пр.*) *перен.* exploíting (*smth.*); cáshing-in (on) *разг.*

спелена́ть *сов. см.* пелена́ть.

спелео́лог *м.* speleólogist; (*спортсмен*) pot-holer; spelúnker *амер.*

спелеол|оги́ческий speleológical. ~о́гия *ж.* speleólogy.

спе́л|ость *ж.* rípeness. ~ый ripe.

спе́рва́ *разг.* at first.

спе́реди *разг.* (*с передней стороны*) from the front; (*впереди*) in front; вид ~ front view.

спе́рма *ж. физиол.* sperm. ~тозо́ид *м. физиол.* spermatozóon.

спёртый *разг.* bad*, foul; здесь о́чень ~ во́здух it's véry stúffy/close in here.

спеси́вый árrogant, háughty.

спесь *ж.* árrogance, háughtiness; сбить ~ с кого́-л. take* *smb.* down a peg.

спеть I *сов. см.* петь 1, 3.

спеть II *несов.* (*созревать*) rípen.

спе́ться *сов. см.* спева́ться.

спех *м. разг.*: мне не к ~у I'm in no húrry; э́то не к ~у there's no húrry.

специализ|а́ция *ж.* specializátion. ~и́ровать *несов. и сов.* (*вн.*) 1. (*обучать какой-л. специальности*) give* (*smb.*) spécialized tráining; 2. (*предназначать для ра-боты в какой-л. специальной области*) cóncentrate (*smth.*). ~и́роваться *несов. и сов.* (по *дт.*, в, на *пр.*) spécialize (in).

специали́ст *м.*, ~ка *ж.* éxpert, spécialist.

специа́льн|о 1. proféssionally; занима́ться чем-л. ~

make* a spécial stúdy of *smth.*, go* in for *smth.* proféssionally; 2. *разг.* (*намеренно*) spécially; ~ для вас for your spécial bénefit; я пришёл ~ для того, чтобы увидеть вас I came spécially to see you. ~ость ж. (spécialized) field; (*профессия тж.*) proféssion line; рабо́тать не по ~ости not be dóing the job *one* was trained for. ~ый spécial; (*требующий профессиональных зна́ний тж.*) spécialized; ~ый вы́пуск газе́ты spécial/éxtra edítion; по ~ому зака́зу to órder; ~ые те́рмины spécial/téchnical terms; ~ые уче́бные заведе́ния spécial/spécialized schools; э́тот вопро́с сли́шком специа́лен this quéstion is too spécialized.

специ́фика ж. specífic féatures *pl*, specífic cháracter.

специфика́ция ж. specificátion.

специфи́ческ|ий specífic, characterístic; ~ие осо́бенности иску́сства characterístic féatures of art.

спе́ция ж. spice.

спецо́вка ж. *разг. см.* спецоде́жда.

спецоде́жда ж. wórking clothes *pl*, óveralls *pl*, bóiler-suit.

спечь *сов.* (*вн.*) *разг.* bake (*smth.*).

спе́чься *сов. см.* спека́ться.

спе́шивать, спе́шить (*вн.*) dismóunt (*smb.*, *smth.*). ~ся, спе́шиться dismóunt.

спе́шить *сов. см.* спе́шивать.

спеш|и́ть, поспеши́ть 1. húrry, hásten; ~ вперёд húrry/push on; ~ на по́мощь *кому́-л.* hásten to the help of *smb.*; ~ на по́езд húrry to the státion; (*боя́ться опозда́ть*) be* afráid of míssing *one's* train; ве́чно ~ be* álways in a húrry; не ~и́те! don't be in a húrry!; он поспеши́л домо́й he húrried home; (*торопли́во*) вниз he ran quíckly downstáirs; 2. *тк. несов.* (*о часа́х*) be* fast; ~ на де́сять мину́т be* ten mínutes fast; ◇ поспеши́шь — люде́й насмеши́шь *посл.* ≈ haste makes waste; more haste less speed; не ~а́ unhúrriedly, delíberately.

спеши́ться *сов. см.* спе́шиваться.

спе́шк|а ж. *разг.* húrry, rush; в ~е in *one's* haste; в ~е о нём забы́ли in the húrry he was overlóoked.

спе́шн|о in a húrry, úrgently, withóut deláy; ~ вы́ехать leave* in a great húrry. ~ый 1. (*сро́чный*) préssing, úrgent; (*о вре́мени тж.*) búsy; ~ая рабо́та rush job, úrgent work; ~ое де́ло préssing/úrgent búsiness; ~ый зака́з úrgent órder; 2. (*торопли́вый*) húrried, rápid.

спива́ться, спи́ться becóme* a habítual drúnkard, take* to the bóttle.

спидо́метр *м.* speedómeter.

спики́ровать *сов. ав.* dive, go* ínto a dive; ~ на цель dive on the tárget.

спи́ливать, спили́ть (*вн.*) 1. saw* (*smth.*) off; спили́ть верху́шку де́рева saw* off the top of a tree; 2. (*напи́льником*) file down (*smth.*).

спили́ть *сов. см.* спи́ливать.

спин|а́ ж. back; согну́ть спи́ну bend* *one's* back; на ~е́ on *one's* back; стоя́ть, сиде́ть ~о́й к све́ту stand*, sit* with *one's* back to the light; уда́р кому́-л. в спи́ну stab *smb.* in the back; ◇ за ~о́й у кого́-л. behind *smb.'s* back; испыта́ть что́-л. на со́бственной ~е́ have* been through *smth.* onesélf; рабо́тать не разгиба́я ~ы́ work all the hours that are made; поверну́ться ~о́й к кому́-л., чему́-л. turn *one's* back ón *smb.*, *smth.*

спи́нк|а ж. back; с прямо́й ~ой (*о ме́бели*) stráight-backed.

спи́ннинг *м.* 1. (*спо́соб уже́ния ры́бы*) spínning; 2. (*снасть*) spínning táckle.

спиннинги́ст *м.* spínner.

спинно́й spínal, dórsal; ~ плавни́к dórsal fin; ~ мозг spínal cord; ~ хребе́т spine, spínal cólumn.

спинномозгово́й of the spínal cord *после сущ.*

спира́ль ж. spíral; (*пружи́на*) spíral spring. ~ный spíral; ~ная ли́ния spíral; ~ная пружи́на spíral/coil spring.

спирт *м.* álcohol, spírit; денатури́рованный ~

méthylated spírit. ~но́е *в знач. сущ. с. разг.* spírits *pl*, hard líquor. ~но́й *прил.* alcohólic; ~ны́е напи́тки alcohólic drinks.

спирто́вка ж. spírit-lamp.

спиртово́й alcohólic, spírituous; (*пригото́вленный со спи́ртом*) spírit *attr.*, álcohol *attr.*

списа́ть(ся) *сов. см.* спи́сывать(ся).

спи́сок *м.* 1. (*пе́речень*) list; ~ избира́телей régister of vóters; ~ ли́чного соста́ва *воен.* múster-roll; ~ абоне́нтов (*телефо́нной се́ти*) télephone diréctory/book; ~ уби́тых и ра́неных cásualty list; зна́читься в спи́сках be* on the books/list; соста́вить ~ draw* up a list, make* out a list; 2. (*докуме́нт*) récord; 3. (*рукопи́сная ко́пия*) cópy.

спи́сывать, списа́ть 1. (*вн.*; *перепи́сывать*) cópy (*smth.*); спи́сывать расписа́ние ле́кций cópy out the lécture tímetable; 2. (*вн.*; *что-л. у кого́-л.*) cópy (*smth.*); crib (*smth.*) *разг.*; списа́ть сочине́ние у това́рища crib a friend's éssay; 3. (*с рд.*; *воспо́льзоваться как прототи́пом*) use (*smb.*, *smth.*) as a módel; 4. (*вн.*; *запи́сывать как изрождо́дованное*) write* (*smth.*) off; списа́ть задо́лженность write* off a debt; списа́ть устаре́лое обору́дование write* off óbsolete equípment; 5. (*вн.*) *мор.* dischárge (*smb.*). ~ся, списа́ться 1. (*с та.*) write* (to), get* in touch (with) by létter; 2. *мор.* be* dischárged.

спи́ться *сов. см.* спива́ться.

спи́хивать, спихну́ть (*вн.*) *разг.* push (*smth.*), shove (*smth.*); *перен.* get* rid (of), kick (*smb.*) out.

спихну́ть *сов. см.* спи́хивать.

спи́ца ж. 1. (*вяза́льная*) knítting-needle; 2. (*колеса́*) spoke; ◇ он после́дняя, пя́тая ~ в колесни́це he dóesn't count; he is the fifth wheel of the coach.

спи́чечн|ый match *attr.*: ~ая коро́бка mátch-box.

спи́чк|а ж. match; заже́чь ~у light* a match; ◇ худо́й как ~ as thin as a mátch-stick.

сплав I *м.* (*мета́ллов*) álloy; ~ ме́ди с зо́лотом álloy of cópper and gold.

сплав II *м.* (*ле́са*) flóating; (*в плота́х*) ráfting; ~ ле́са по реке́ the flóating/ráfting of tímber.

спла́вить, II *сов. см.* сплавля́ть I, II.

сплавля́ть I, спла́вить (*вн.*; *мета́ллы*) fuse (*smth.*), álloy (*smth.*) (*тж. перен.*); спла́вить желе́зо с хро́мом álloy iron and chrómium.

сплавля́ть II, спла́вить (*вн.*) (*лес*) float (*smth.*); (*в плота́х*) raft (*smth.*); *перен. разг.* get* rid (of).

сплавн|о́й I, II flóated, ráfted; ~ лес flóated/ráfting timber; 2. (*приго́дный для спла́ва*) flóatable; ~а́я река́ flóatable ríver.

спла́вщик *м.* (*ле́са*) ráfter.

сплани́ровать I, II *сов. см.* плани́ровать I, II.

спла́чивать, сплоти́ть (*вн.*) 1. (*скрепля́ть*) join (*smth.*), bind* (*smth.*); (*сбива́ть в плоты́*) raft (*smth.*); 2. (*смыка́ть*) close up (*smth.*); 3. (*объедина́ть*) uníte (*smb.*, *smth.*), rálly (*smb.*, *smth.*), ~ся, сплоти́ться (*объедина́ться*) rálly, uníte.

сплести́(сь) *сов. см.* сплета́ть(ся).

сплета́ть, сплести́ (*вн.*) 1. weave* (*smth.*); сплести́ вено́к make* a wreath; 2. (*соединя́ть*) splice (*smth.*); (*ру́ки*) lock (*smth.*); (*во́лосы*) plait (*smth.*); *перен.* interwéave* (*smth.*), interlóck (*smth.*). ~ся, сплести́сь be* interwóven, be* interláced (*тж. перен.*); (*о ветвя́х тж.*) be* tángled; (*о рука́х, пальца́х*) be* locked, lock.

сплете́ние с. 1. júnction; *анат.* pléxus; ~ арте́рий knot of árteries; 2. (*ветве́й, корне́й*) tángle; *перен.* blénding; míxture; ~ обстоя́тельств míxture/combinátion of círcumstances.

сплетн|ик *м.*, ~ица ж. góssip, táleteller; зло́стный ~ invéterate góssip, scándalmonger. ~ичать, насплётничать góssip, talk scándal.

сплётн|я ж. piece of góssip; *мн.* góssip *sg*, títtle-tattle *sg*; злы́е ~и scándal *sg*, báckbiting *sg*.

сплеча straight from the shóulder; *перен.* cárelessly, in an offhánd mánner.

сплоти́ть(ся) *сов. см.* спла́чивать(ся).

сплохов|а́ть *сов. разг.* make* a blúnder; slip up; ~а́л на э́тот раз! slipped up that time!

сплоче́ние *с.* uníting, rállying (round), stíffening.

сплочённ|ость *ж.* cohésion, solidárity. ~ый 1. (*сомкнутый*) close-pácked interlócking; ~ыми ряда́ми shóulder to shóulder; 2. (*дружный*) united; ~ый коллекти́в united colléctive.

сплошн|о́й 1. sólid; (*распространяющийся на всё*) áll-round, óverall; (*непрерывный*) contínuous, unbróken; ~а́я стена́ sólid wall; ~а́я ма́сса sólid mass; ~ лёд sólid ice; ~ лес unbróken fórest; ~а́я электрифика́ция húndred per cent electrificátion; 2. *разг.* (*не содержащий ничего другого*) sheer, pure; ~ бред sheer delírium; ~ вздор sheer nónsense; ~ые неприя́тности nóthing but tróuble, incéssant tróuble.

сплошь complétely, entírely; (*без перерыва*) unintérruptedly; ~ усе́янный *чем-л.* thíckly strewn with *smth.*; ◇ ~ да ря́дом on évery hand, at évery step.

сплутова́ть *сов. см.* плутова́ть.

сплы|ть *сов. разг.*: бы́ло да ~ло there was — once upón a time; it's no more.

сплю́щенный fláttened; (*о пальцах, носе*) flat; ~ болт fláttened bolt; ~ че́реп nárrow skull.

сплю́щивать, сплю́щить (*вн.*) flátten (*smth.*). ~ся, **сплю́щиться** becóme* flat.

сплю́щить(ся) *сов. см.* сплю́щивать(ся).

спляса́ть *сов. см.* пляса́ть.

сподви́жник *м.* féllow campáigner.

спозара́нку *разг.* (*рано утром*) éarly in the mórning; (*очень рано*) so éarly.

спо́йть *сов. см.* спа́ивать II.

споко́йно 1. *нареч.* cálmly, quíetly, péacefully; (*о душевном состоянии тж.*) serénely, tránquilly, ~! stéady!; ~ спать sleep* péacefully; спи́те ~! sleep well!; 2. *в знач. сказ. безл.* (*об обстановке*) it is quíet/péaceful; 3. *в знач. сказ. безл.*: на душе́ ~ *one's* mind is at rest.

споко́йн|ый 1. (*тихий, небурный*) calm, tránquil; ~ое мо́ре calm sea; 2. (*не испытывающий волнения*) at ease *predic.*, éasy in *one's* mind *predic.*; быть ~ым feel* at ease; бу́дьте ~ы! don't wórry!; за него́ я споко́ен I have no fears for him, I'm quite éasy in my mind abóut him; 3. (*выражающий спокойствие*) calm, quíet; ~ тон calm voice; ~ые движе́ния calm móvements; 4. (*отличающийся спокойствием*) péaceful, quíet; ~ая бесе́да péaceful conversátion, quíet chat; 5. (*уравновешенный, сдержанный*) plácid, quíet; ~ ребёнок plácid/seréne child*; ~ая ло́шадь plácid/quíet horse; 6. (*ничем не тревожимый*) péaceful, tránquil; ~ая жизнь péaceful life; ~ сон tránquil/péaceful sleep; 7. (*приятный для глаза*) réstful, sóothing; ~ цвет réstful/sóothing cólour; 8. *разг.* (*удобный*) cómfortable; ~ая о́бувь cómfortable shoes; ◇ ~ой но́чи! good night!

споко́йстви|е *с.* 1. (*покой и тишина*) quíet, repóse, calm, stíllness; тишина́ и ~ quíet + calm and tranquíllity; 2. (*порядок*) peace, públic órder; наруша́ть ~ break*/distúrb the peace; наруше́ние обще́ственного ~я breach of the peace; 3. (*отсутствие волнений, тревог*) serénity, tranquíllity; ~ ду́ха, душе́вное ~ peace of mind.

споко́н: ~ ве́ку, ~ веко́в *разг.* from time immemórial.

спола́скивать, сполосну́ть (*вн.*) rinse (*smth.*), rinse out (*smth.*).

сполза́ть, сползти́ 1. come* down; 2. *разг.* (*с трудом спускаться*) scrámble down/out; 3. (*медленно стекать*) roll down, tríckle down; 4. (*постепенно сдвигаться, смещаться*) slip down; ша́пка у него́ сползла́ на заты́лок his hat slipped back off his fórehead.

сползти́ *сов. см.* сполза́ть.

сполна́ in full.

сполосну́ть *сов. см.* спола́скивать.

спо́нсор *м.* spónsor.

спор *м.* árgument, dispúte; (*обсуждение*) discússion; ◇ ~у нет undóubtedly, of course, it is self-évident.

спо́ра *ж.* *биол.* spore.

споради́ческий sporádic.

спор|ить, поспо́рить 1. (*с тв. о пр.*) árgue (with *smb.* abóut), dispúte (with *smb.* óver, abóut); have* an árgument (with *smb.* abóut); они́ до́лго ~или they had a long árgument; о вку́сах не ~ят there's no accóunting for taste, tastes díffer, éveryone to his taste; 2. (*с тв.*: *заключать пари*) bet* (*smb.*), have* 'a bet (with); 3. (*сопротивляться*) conténd; (*состязаться тж.*) compéte.

спор|и́ться *несов. разг.* (*удаваться*) come* off, turn out well; рабо́та ~ся the work is góing fine; у него́ всё ~ся éverything he puts his hand to turns out well.

спо́рный dispútable, debátable, controvérsial; ~ вопро́с controvérsial quéstion; ~ пункт dispútable/moot point.

споро́ть *сов. см.* спа́рывать.

спорт *м.* sport (*тж. перен.*); sports *pl*; зи́мний ~ winter sports; занима́ться ~ом go* in for sport.

спорти́вн|ый 1. sports *attr.*; ~ые и́гры games; ~ая площа́дка sports ground; ~ костю́м sports kit; ~ инвента́рь sports equípment; ~ое состяза́ние spórting cóntest, match; 2. (*похожий на спортсмена*) athlétic(-looking), óutdoor; име́ть ~ вид look athlétic, have* an óutdoor look; ◇ из ~ого интере́са for the fun of the thing, to test *one's* prówess.

спортсме́н *м.* spórtsman*, áthlete. ~ка *ж.* spórtswoman*, áthlete.

спорхну́ть *сов.* flútter, flútter down; *перен.* dart, spring*.

спо́рщ|ик *м.*, ~ица *ж.* *разг.* árguer, dispútant; он ужа́сный ~ he loves árguing.

спо́рый *разг.* quick; prófitable.

спо́соб *м.* way, méthod, mode; ~ выраже́ния mode of expréssion; ~ употребле́ния way to use; (*надпись*) diréctions for use; ~ произво́дства mode/méthod of prodúction; таки́м ~ом in this way; други́м ~ом in a different way, dífferently; каки́м бы то ни́ бы́ло ~ом one way or anóther.

спосо́б|ность *ж.* 1. ability, pówer; ~ дви́гаться ability/pówer to move; 2. *обыкн. мн.* (*природные дарования*) ability *sg*, áptitude *sg*; ~ности к языка́м lánguage ability *sg*, a tálent for lánguages *sg*; ~ к матема́тике áptitude/gift for mathemátics; челове́к с больши́ми ~ностями extrémely áble pérson, man* of great ability/abílities. ~ный (*к дт.*, *на вн.*) cápable (of); ~ный к труду́ able-bódied; ~ный на же́ртвы cápable of sácrifice; он ~ен рабо́тать день и ночь he is cápable of wórking day and night; он ~ен на всё he is cápable of ánything; 2. (*одарённый*) cléver, áble; ~ный студе́нт gífted stúdent; о́чень ~ная де́вочка véry cléver/bright little girl.

спосо́бствовать *несов.* (*дт.*) contríbute (to), condúce (to), be* condúcive (to), promóte (*smth.*); ~ распростране́нию зна́ний promóte léarning; ~ разви́тию aid/facílitate devélopment; ~ сча́стью *кого-л.* contríbute to *smb.'s* háppiness; be* condúcive to *smb.'s* háppiness; ~ кому́-л. в чём-л. further *smb.'s* aspirátions; о́чень ~ чему́-л. be* gréatly condúcive to *smth.*, do* much to promóte *smth.*

споткну́ться *сов. см.* спотыка́ться 1, 2, 3.

спотык|а́ться, споткну́ться 1. (*о вн.*) stúmble (óver), trip (óver); 2. *разг.* (*встречать препятствие, затруднение*) hésitate, stop short; 3. *разг.* (*допускать ошибку*) go* wrong, trip up; 4. *тк. несов.* (*идти с трудом*) lurch alóng, stágger alóng; идти́ ~а́ясь stúmble alóng.

спохвати́ться *сов. см.* спохва́тываться.

спохва́тываться, спохвати́ться *разг.* réalize,

remémber; спохвати́вшись on sécond thoughts; он во́время спохвати́лся he réalized befóre it was too late.

спра́ва (откуда-л.) from the right; (где-л.) on/to the right (of); ~ от него́ to his right, on his right side; ~ от доро́ги on the right (of the road).

справедли́в|о jústly; (беспристрастно тж.) fáirly, impártially; поступа́ть ~ be* just/fair, do* the right thing; суди́ть ~ be* fair in one's júdgements. ~ость ж. 1. jústice; (беспристрастие тж.) fáirness, impartiálity; чу́вство ~ости sense of jústice; ~ости ра́ди for fáirness' sake; 2. (правильность) corréctness; ◇ на́до отда́ть ему́ ~ость to give him his due, to do him jústice. ~ый 1. just; (беспристрастный тж.) fair, impártial; он стро́гий, но ~ый челове́к he is a stern but just man*; ~ый судья́ fair/impártial judge; ~ый суд fair tríal; ~ое тре́бование just demand; 2. (имеющий законное основание) jústifiable, wárranted, just; ~ый гнев jústifiable ánger; 3. (соответствующий истине) corréct, jústified, right; ~ое замеча́ние jústified remárk; ~ое сужде́ние corréct réasoning/árgument.

спра́вить сов. см. справля́ть.

спра́виться сов. см. справля́ться.

спра́вк|а ж. 1. (действие) réference; 2. (сведения) informátion; обраща́ться за ~ами applý for informátion; 3. (документ) réference, certíficate; ~ с ме́ста рабо́ты réference from (one's place of) work.

справля́ть, спра́вить (вн.) разг. célebrate (smth.), keep* (smth.); ~ день рожде́ния célebrate one's birthday; ~ новосе́лье hold* a hóuse-warming párty.

справл|я́ться, спра́виться 1. (с тв.; выполнять, осуществлять) mánage (with), cope (with); ~ с рабо́той cope with one's work; он хорошо́ ~я́ется со свои́м де́лом he is dóing well; бы́стро, легко́ ~ с чем-л. make* short work of smth.; я сам спра́влюсь I can do it aló́ne/mysélf; он с э́тим не спра́вится he'll néver be áble to mánage it; 2. (с тв.; быть в состоянии побороть) contról (smth.); (заставлять слушаться) mánage (smb., smth.); с ним тру́дно спра́виться he is hard to mánage; 3. (о пр.; осведомляться) inquíre (áfter); ~ о здоро́вье inquíre áfter smb.'s health; ~ в словаре́ consúlt a díctionary; ~ у кого́-л. о чём-л. find* out smth. from smb.; ◇ спра́виться с собо́й contról onesélf, take* a grip on onesélf.

справочн|ик м. réference book; железнодоро́жный ~ ráilway-guide; телефо́нный ~ télephone diréctory. ~ый réference attr.; ~ое бюро́ informátion búreau; ~ая литерату́ра réference books pl.

спра́шив|ать, спроси́ть 1. (вн.) ask (smb., smth.); (о пр.; осведомляться) inquíre (about, áfter), ask (about, áfter); спроси́ть фами́лию ask smb.'s name; спроси́ть о по́езде ask about a train; вас не ~ают! who asked you?; 2. (вн.; вызывать учащегося) quéstion (smb., smth.); ~ уро́к ask quéstions on the work (that was) set; стро́го ~ be* véry exácting; 3. (вн.; рд.; просить) ask (for); ~ у кого́-л. разреше́ния, сове́та ask smb.'s permíssion, advíce; 4. (вн.; желать видеть) ask (for); меня́ никто́ не ~ал? were there ány calls for me?; 5. (вн.) разг. (требовать какую-л. плату) charge (smth.), ask (smth.); ~ с кого́-л. де́сять рубле́й за что-л. chárge smb. ten róubles for smth.; 6. (с рд.; требовать ответственности) make* (smb.) ánswer; с вас за э́то спро́сят you will have to ánswer for that. ~аться, спроси́ться разг. 1. (у рд.; просить разрешения) ask smb.'s permíssion/leave; уйти́, ни у кого́ не спроси́сь leave* without ásking ányone's permíssion; 2. тк. несов.: ~ается в знач. вводн. сл. one would like to know; 3. безл. (с рд.; будет потребован ответ): за э́то с тебя́ спро́сится you will have to ánswer for that.

спрессова́ть сов. см. прессова́ть.

спринт м. спорт. sprint, dash.

спри́нтер м. спорт. sprínter.

спринц|ева́ть несов. (вн.) sýringe (smth.). ~о́вка ж. sýringe.

спрова́дить сов. (вн.) разг. get* rid (of), pack (smb.) off.

спровоци́ровать сов. (вн.) provóke (smb., smth.).

спроекти́ровать сов. см. проекти́ровать I 1.

спрос м. 1. (требование) demánd; ~ и предложе́ние supplý and demánd; в большо́м ~e in great demánd; на э́ти това́ры большо́й ~ there is a great demánd for these goods; 2. разг. (ответственность): с вас ~у бо́льше all the more is expécted of you; ◇ без ~а, без ~у withóut ásking (leave).

спроси́ть сов. см. спра́шивать. ~ся сов. см. спра́шиваться 1, 3.

спросо́нок разг. not fúlly awáke; ~ он не разобра́л, в чём де́ло he was too héavy with sleep to make out (what was góing on).

спрут м. зоол. óctopus.

спры́гивать, спры́гнуть (с рд.) jump off (smth.), jump down (from); спры́гнуть со ступе́ньки jump down the steps; спры́гнуть в кана́ву jump ínto a ditch.

спры́гнуть сов. см. спры́гивать.

спры́скивать, спры́снуть (вн.) разг. sprínkle (smth.).

спры́снуть сов. см. спры́скивать.

спряга́ть, проспряга́ть грам. cónjugate. ~ся несов. грам. be* cónjugated.

спряже́ние с. грам. conjugátion.

спрясть сов. см. прясть.

спря́тать(ся) сов. см. пря́тать(ся).

спу́гивать, спугну́ть (вн.) разг. 1. fríghten (smb., smth.) awáy; спугну́ть оле́ня fríghten the deer* awáy; 2. (испугав, помешать чему-л.) put* (smb.) on his, her guard.

спугну́ть сов. см. спу́гивать.

спуд м.: держа́ть что-л. под ~ом keep* smth. hídden awáy; извле́чь, вы́нуть что-л. из-под ~а unéarth smth., réscue smth. from obscúrity; положи́ть что-л. под ~ bury smth.

спуск м. 1. (движение вниз) descént; (опускание) lówering; ~ с горы́ descént of the móuntain, the way down; ~ корабля́ на́ воду láunching; 2. (воды) dráining; 3. (наклонная плоскость) slope; ◇ не дава́ть ~у, ~у кому́-л. permít smb. no líberties; be* tough with smb., crack down on smb.

спуска́ть, спусти́ть (вн.) 1. (перемещать вниз) lówer (smb., smth.), put* (smth.) down, let* (smth.) down; ~ рабо́чих в ша́хту lówer wórkers down the shaft; ~ флаг lówer the flag; ~ схо́дни put* down the gángway; ~ за́навес pull/let* down the cúrtain/blind; спусти́ть кого́-л. с ле́стницы kick smb. downstáirs; 2. (на воду — о корабле) launch (smth.); (о шлюпке) lówer (smth.); 3. (пересылать нижестоящим организациям) send* (smth.) out; спусти́ть директи́ву send* out a diréctive; 4. (выпускать, освобождая от чего-л.) reléase (smth.); ~ соба́ку с поводка́ unléash a dog; ~ соба́к с це́пи let the dogs lose; 5. (жидкость, газ) let* (smth.) out; ~ во́ду drain the wáter off; (из ванны) let* out the wáter, take* out the plug; 6. (освобождать от жидкости, газа) empty (smth.); ~ пруд drain a pond; ~ балло́н let* down a týre; 7.: ши́на спусти́ла the týre has gone down, the týre is flat; 8. разг. (терять в весе) redúce one's weight; спусти́ть пять килогра́ммов lose* five kílograms; 9. разг. (прощать) párdon (smb.); ◇ спусти́ть куро́к pull the trígger; спусти́ть пе́тлю (в вязании) drop a stitch; спустя́ рукава́ in a slipshod mánner, ányhow. ~ся, спусти́ться 1. come* down, go* down, descénd; (в нижний этаж) come*/go* downstáirs; ~ся по ле́стнице, ступе́нькам come*/go* down the stairs, steps; descénd the stairs, steps; ~ся в по́греб go* down to the céllar; ~ся с горы́ come* down a hill; ~ся с де́рева climb down a tree; ~ся по верёвке let* onesélf down by a rope; ~ся вниз по реке́ go* downstream; чуло́к спусти́лся one's stócking was cóming down; 2. (на вн.; о пти́цах, насеко́мых) séttle (on), alíght (on); (о самолёте) land (on); перен. (о тума́не и т. п.) descénd, spread* óver; ночь спусти́лась на зе́млю night descénded upón the earth; 3. тк. несов. (быть располо́женным накло́нно) slope down (towárds); бе́рег обры́вом спуска́лся к мо́рю the shore sloped/ran down to the sea; 4. тк. несов. (висе́ть) hang*, hang* down; ◇ спусти́ться с облако́в come* down to earth.

спускно́й drain attr.

спуско́в|о́й: ~ крючо́к trígger; ~ механи́зм trígger méchanism; ~áя пружи́на séar-spring.

спусти́ть сов. см. спуска́ть. ~ся сов. см. спуска́ться 1, 2.

спустя́ áfter, láter; немно́го ~ not long áfter; ~ не́сколько дней a few days láter.

спу́танн|ый tángled, disarránged; перен. múddled; (о ре́чи) incohérent; ~ые во́лосы untídy hair sg; ~ые ни́тки tángled threads.

спу́тать сов. 1. (вн.; привести́ в беспоря́док) (en)tángle (smth.); перен. múddle (smth.), confúse (smth.); ~ ни́тки tángle threads; ~ во́лосы кому́-л. disarránge smb.'s hair; 2. (вн.) разг. (сбить с то́лку) confúse (smb.); 3. (вн. с тв.) take* (smth., smb. for); 4. (вн.; ло́шадь) hóbble (smth.); ◇ ~ чьи-л. ка́рты, расчёты, пла́ны upset* smb.'s calculátions, plans. ~ся сов. 1. become* entángled; перен. become* confúsed/múddled, be* in a múddle; 2. разг. (сби́ться) be* mixed up, be* in a múddle; 3. разг. (оши́биться) make* a mistáke, get* into a múddle.

спу́тни|к м. 1. compánion; (по путеше́ствию тж.) fellow-tráveller; 2. (рд.; то, что сопу́тствует чему́-л.) compánion (of); 3. (небе́сное те́ло) sátellite; 4. (иску́сственный) spútnik, artificial Earth sátellite. ~ца ж. см. спу́тник 1.

спья́на, спья́ну разг. while drunk.

спя́чка ж. 1. (у живо́тных): зи́мняя ~ hibernátion; 2. (у люде́й) léthargy, sléepiness.

спя́щ|ий прил. 1. sléeping; притворя́ться ~им feign sleep, preténd to be asléep; 2. в знач. сущ. м. sléeper, sléeping man*.

сраба́тывать, сработа́ть разг. work, span into áction.

сраба́тываться, сработа́ться (достига́ть согласо́ванности в рабо́те) fall* into step, work in hármony; они́ не срабо́тались they are not wórking as a team, they háven't got into step.

сраба́танность ж. (согласо́ванность в рабо́те) good téamwork, co-ordinátion.

сраба́танный (изно́шенный) worn, wórn-out; ~ мото́р wórn-out éngine.

срабо́тать сов. см. сраба́тывать.

сработа́ться I, II сов. см. сраба́тываться I, II.

сравне́ни|е с. 1. compárison; 2. (фигу́ра ре́чи) símile; ~я грам. degrées of compárison; в ~и, по ~ю с кем-л., чем-л. in compárison with smb., smth.; значи́тельное увеличе́ние по ~ю с про́шлым го́дом considerable íncrease compáred with last year; не идёт ни в како́е ~ с кем-л., чем-л. it cánnot be compáred with smb., smth., there can be no compárison between smb., smth.; вне вся́кого ~я beyónd/out of all compárison.

сра́внивать I, сравни́ть (вн. с тв.; сопоставля́ть) compáre (smb., smth. with).

сра́внивать II, сравни́ть (вн. с тв.; де́лать равны́м) make* (smb., smth.) équal; сравни́ть расхо́д с дохо́дом bálance íncome and expénditure.

сра́внивать III, сровня́ть (вн.; де́лать ро́вным) lével (smth.) off; make* (smth.) flush/lével; ◇ сровня́ть что́-л. с землёй raze smth. to the ground.

сра́вниваться, сровня́ться (с тв.) 1. merge (with); 2. разг. (ока́зываться ря́дом) draw* lével (with).

сравни́тельн|о comparatively; ~ с кем-л., чем-л. compáred with smb., smth. ~ый compárative; ~ый ме́тод иссле́дования compárative méthod of inquiry; ◇ ~ая сте́пень грам. compárative degrée.

сравни́ть сов. см. сра́внивать I. ~ся сов. (с тв.) be* compáred (with); не мо́жет ~ся с кем-л., чем-л. bears no compárison with smb., smth.

сравня́ть сов. см. сра́внивать II и равня́ть. ~ся сов. (с тв.) be* the équal (of).

сраж|а́ть, срази́ть (вн.) 1. (убива́ть) strike* (smb., smth.) down; перен. overcóme* (smb.); пу́ля срази́ла бойца́ the sóldier was struck down by a búllet; боле́знь его́ срази́ла he was laid low by íllness; 2. (поража́ть) astóund (smb.); ~а́ться, срази́ться fight*; (в вн.) разг. (игра́ть) have* a báttle (at); ~а́ться с врага́ми fight* the énemy; срази́ться в ша́хматы have* a báttle at chess. ~е́ние с. báttle; ~е́ние на, под... the báttle of...; дать ~е́ние give* báttle; проигра́ть ~е́ние lose* a báttle.

срази́ть сов. см. сража́ть и рази́ть I. ~ся сов. см. сража́ться.

сра́зу 1. (немедленно) at once, immédiately, ínstantly; у него́ ~ измени́лось настрое́ние his mood changed at once; 2. (ря́дом) just; наш ла́герь ~ за ре́чкой our camp is just acróss the river; 3. (в оди́н приём) all at once; мо́жете заплати́ть не всё ~ you néedn't pay it all at once; 4. (одновре́менно) simultáneously; все ~ all togéther; говори́те не все ~! don't all speak at once; one at a time, please!

срам м. разг. shame.

срами́ть, осрами́ть (вн.) разг. 1. (позо́рить) disgráce (smb.); 2. тк. несов. (стыди́ть) tell* (smb.) off, rate (smb.) sóundly. ~ся, осрами́ться разг. disgráce onesélf.

сраста́ться, срасти́сь 1. grow* togéther; (о ко́сти) knit*, mend; 2. (с тв.; неразры́вно соединя́ться) becóme* a part (of).

срасти́сь сов. см. сраста́ться.

срасти́ть сов. см. сра́щивать.

сра́щивание с. 1. jóining; (деревя́нных часте́й) jóinting; (тро́сов, проводо́в) splicing; (косте́й) knitting; 2. (слия́ние) fúsing, amalgamátion.

сред|а́ I ж. 1. (окруже́ние) envíronment; surróundings pl; географи́ческая ~ geográphical envíronment; рабо́чая ~ wórking-class envíronment/surróundings; литерату́рная, худо́жественная ~ líterary, artístic envíronment; в на́шей ~е́ in our circle(s)/set; в ~е́ учёных amóng scíentists, in the scientific world; охра́на окружа́ющей ~ы́ protéction of the envíronment; 2. физ., хим. médium.

среда́ II ж. (день неде́ли) Wédnesday; по ~м on Wédnesdays.

среди́ 1. (в окруже́нии) amóng; amíd, amídst кни́жн.; ~ нас, вас amóng us, you; in our, your midst; 2. (в середи́не) in the middle (of); стоя́ть ~ ко́мнаты stand* in the middle of the room; встать ~ но́чи get* up in the middle of the night.

средиземномо́рски|й Mediterránean; ~е стра́ны the Mediterránean cóuntries.

сре́дне разг. fair to míddling, só-so; (скро́мно) móderately.

среднеазиа́тский Céntral Asiátic.

средневеко́вый mediéval; of the Middle Áges по́сле сущ.

средневеко́вье с. the Middle Áges pl.

среднегодов|о́й áverage ánnual; ~áя температу́ра áverage ánnual témperature; ~ сбор зерна́ áverage ánnual grain yield/hárvest.

сре́дн|ее с.: не́что ~ something in betwéen; в ~ем on an áverage; составля́ть в ~ем áverage, come* to; вы́ше (ни́же) ~его abóve (belów) the áverage.

среднеме́сячный áverage mónthly; ~ за́работок áverage mónthly wage.

среднесу́точный áverage dáily.

сре́дн|ий 1. (*по месту, времени*) míddle; ~ee окно́ míddle window; 2. (*о размере, весе и т. п.*) míddle, médium, áverage; ~ей величины́, ~его разме́ра médium-size(d) *attr.*; боксёр ~его ве́са míddle-weight bóxer; ~ рост médium/áverage height; челове́к ~его ро́ста a man* of áverage/médium height; 3. *мат.* mean; (*в статистике*) áverage; ~яя ско́рость áverage speed; ~яя температу́ра áverage/mean témperature; ~яя но́рма вы́работки áverage óutput quóta; 4. *разг.* (*посредственный*) órdinary, áverage; ~ие спосо́бности áverage abílities; ~ие актёры órdinary áctors; ◇ Сре́дний Восто́к the Míddle East; ~ие века́ the Míddle Áges; ~ па́лец míddle fínger; ~ee у́хо *анат.* the míddle ear; ~ee образова́ние sécondary educátion; ~яя шко́ла sécondary school; high school *амер.*; челове́к ~их лет míddle-aged pérson.

средото́чие *с.* céntre, hub.

сре́дств|о *с.* 1. means *pl*; ~a передвиже́ния convéyance *sg*; means of convéyance; раке́тно-я́дерные ~a сре́дней да́льности médium-range núclear wéapons/míssiles; все́ми ~ами by évery means; для него́ все ~a хороши́ he'll stop at nóthing; 2. (*лекарство*) rémedy; перевя́зочные ~a dréssings; dréssing matérial *sg*; 3. *мн.* (*деньги, материальные ценности*) means; ~a существова́ния means of subsístence/lívelihood; отпуска́ть больши́е де́нежные ~a assígn large sums (of móney); по ~ам (well) withín *one's* means; не по ~ам beyónd *one's* means.

средь *см.* среди́.

срез *м.* 1. cut; 2. (*для микроанализа*) microscópic séction.

сре́зать *сов. см.* среза́ть *и* ре́зать 6.

среза́ть, сре́зать (*вн.*) 1. cut* (*smth.*); (*отрезать*) cut* (*smth.*) off/awáy; (*ветви тж.*) lop (*smth.*); 2. *разг.* (*на экзамене*) fail (*smb.*); 3. (*резко обрывать чью-л. речь*) shut* (*smb.*) up; ◇ сре́зать мяч *спорт.* slice a ball; сре́зать у́гол take* a short cut.

сре́заться *сов. разг.* (*на экзамене*) fail, flunk.

срисова́ть *сов. см.* срисо́вывать.

срисо́вывать, срисова́ть (*вн.*) сóру (*smth.*).

сровня́ть *сов. см.* сра́внивать III *и* ровня́ть. ~ся *сов. см.* сра́вниваться.

сродни́ (*дт.*) *разг.* reláted (to); *перен.* akín (to); он мне ~ we are reláted; he is a relátion of mine.

сродни́ть *сов. см.* родни́ть 2. ~ся *сов.* (с *тв.*) becóme véry close (to), take* (to); (*свыкнуться*) get* fond (of).

сродство́ *с.* affínity.

срок *м.* 1. (*промежуток времени*) périod; term; (*тюремного заключения тж.*) stretch *разг.*; ~ опла́ты пять дней to be paid withín five days; в кратча́йший ~ within the shórtest póssible time, in a véry short (space of) time; по истече́нии ~a when the term expíres; даю́ вам ~y три часа́ you have three hours; 2. (*предельный момент*) déadline, date, time; ~ исполне́ния déadline, time allówed; ~ платежа́ date fixed for páyment; в ~ in/on time; до ~a befóre (its) time, éarly; к ~y to time; яви́ться к ~y arríve on time; пришёл ~ the móment has arríved; поста́вить рабо́ту в ~ do* the work in time; все ~и прошли́ time ran out long agó; ◇ на ~ for a cértain périod; дай(те) ~! give me time!; (*как угроза*) just you wait!

сро́чн|о *нареч.* úrgently; ~ вы́ехать leave* in a húrry; ему́ понадо́бился э́тот уче́бник he needs this téxtbook úrgently, he is in úrgent need of this téxtbook; на́до ~ иска́ть сре́дства *и т. п.* a means, *etc.* must be found withóut deláy; э́то на́до ~ сде́лать it must be done withóut deláy, ~ый 1. (*спешный*) préssing, úrgent; ~ое де́ло úrgent búsiness; ~ый зака́з préssing órder; ~ая телегра́мма expréss télegram; ~ая доста́вка prompt delívery; в ~ом поря́дке withóut deláy; приня́ть ~ые ме́ры take* úrgent méasures; 2. (*производимый в опреде-*

ле́нный срок) fixed-term *attr.*; fixed-date *attr.*; ~ый платёж fixed-date páyment; ~ый вклад depósit accóunt.

сруб *м.* 1. (*действие*) félling; 2. (*деревянное сооружение*) frame of logs; (*шахты*) crib; (*бревенчатая постройка*) log house/cábin.

сруба́ть, сруби́ть (*вн.*) (*деревья*) fell (*smth.*); cut* (*smth.*) down; (*ветки, сучья*) chop (*smth.*) off; (*голову тж.*) cut* (*smth.*) off.

сруби́ть *сов. см.* сруба́ть.

срыв *м.* upsétting; wrécking; (*неудача*) bréakdown, fáilure; ~ пла́на, рабо́ты upsétting/wrécking of the plan, work; ~ перегово́ров bréakdown of negotiátions.

срыва́ть I, сорва́ть 1. (*вн.; что-л. растущее*) pick (*smth.*); сорва́ть цвето́к pick a flówer; сорва́ть ве́тку сире́ни break* off a sprig of lílac; сорва́ть я́блоко pick an ápple; 2. (*вн.; сдёргивать*) tear* off; break* (*smth.*) off; сорва́ть замо́к tear* off a lock; сорва́ть с себя́, с кого́-л. ша́пку snatch *one's*, *smb.'s* hat off; 3. (*вн.; повреждать*) strip (*smth.*); сорва́ть резьбу́ strip a thread; 4. (*вн.; мешать осуществлению чего-л.*) upsét* (*smth.*), wreck (*smth.*); (*что-л. плохое*) frustráte (*smth.*), foil (*smth.*); сорва́ть рабо́ту upsét* the work; сорва́ть уро́к upsét* a lésson; ~ перегово́ры wreck the negotiátions; сорва́ть за́говор foil/frustráte a plot, rénder a plot abórtive; 5. (*вн. на пр.*) *разг.* (*вымещать*) vent (*smth.* on); сорва́ть зло на ком-л. blow* off at *smb.*; ◇ сорва́ть го́лос strain/lose* *one's* voice; сорва́ть заве́су с чего́-л. rip the tráppings/cóvers off *smth.*, take* the lid off *smth.*

срыва́ть II, срыть (*вн.; разрывая, уничтожать*) lével (*smth.*).

срыва́ться, сорва́ться 1. (*о чём-л. прикреплённом или висящем*) come* off; дверь сорвала́сь с пе́тель the door has come off its hínges; 2. (*обрушиваться*) break* off, dislódge itsélf; 3. (*падать, потеряв опору*) lose* *one's* grip/fóothold, slip off; 4. (*разрываться привязь, путы*) break* loose; соба́ка сорвала́сь с це́пи the dog broke loose from its chain; 5. (*поспешно покидать своё место*) spring* up from; сорва́ться с ме́ста start up; 6.: сорва́ться с языка́ escápe *one's* lips; 7. *разг.* (*не удаваться*) miscárry, break* down, fail; сорвало́сь! it's all up!; ◇ его́ го́лос сорва́лся his voice broke; как с це́пи сорва́лся ≈ like a bull at a gate.

срыть *сов. см.* срыва́ть II.

сса́дина *ж.* scratch, graze, abrásion.

ссади́ть I *сов. см.* сса́живать.

ссади́ть II *сов.* (*вн.; поцарапать*) scratch (*smth.*); ~ себе́ ру́ку scratch *one's* hand.

сса́живать, ссади́ть (*вн.*) 1. (*помогать сойти вниз*) lift (*smb.*) down, help (*smb.*) down; 2. (*высаживать с поезда и т. п.*) put* (*smb.*) off.

ссо́р|а *ж.* quárrel; (*мелочная*) tiff, squábble; быть в ~e с кем-л. have* quárreled with *smb.*; ме́жду ни́ми произошла́ ~ из-за чего́-то they quárrelled óver *smth.*

ссо́рить, поссо́рить (*вн.*) set* (*smb.*) at lóggerheads, put* (*smb.*) agáinst each óther, cause a quárrel betwéen (*smb.*). ~ся, поссо́риться (с *тв.*) quárrel (with); (*из-за мелочей*) squábble (with).

ссо́хнуться *сов. см.* ссыха́ться.

СССР (*Сою́з Сове́тских Социалисти́ческих Респу́блик*) USSR (Únion of Sóviet Sócialist Repúblics).

ссу́д|а *ж.* loan. ~и́ть *сов. см.* ссужа́ть.

ссужа́ть, ссуди́ть (*вн. тв., вн. дт.*) lend* (*smb. smth.*), loan (*smb. smth.*).

ссыла́ть, сосла́ть (*вн.*) éxile (*smb.*), depórt (*smb.*).

ссыла́ться, сосла́ться (*на вн.*) quote (*smb., smth.*) as an authórity, cite (*smth.*); (*оправдываться*) plead (*smth.*); ~ на боле́знь, головну́ю боль, уста́лость plead íllness, héadache, fatígue.

ссы́лк|а I *ж.* (*изгнание*) éxile, transportátion; в ~e in éxile.

ссы́лка II *ж.* (*указание источника*) réference (to).

ссы́льный *прил.* 1. éxiled; 2. *в знач. сущ. м.* éxile, deportée.

ссыпа́ть *сов. см.* ссыпа́ть.

ссып|а́ть, ссы́пать (*вн.*) pour (*smth.*); ~ зерно́ в мешки́ pour/put* corn ínto sacks, sack corn.

ссыха́ться, ссо́хнуться shrink*.

стабилиз|а́тор *м. тех.* stábilizer; вертика́льный ~ *ав. fin.* ~а́ция *ж.* stabilizátion; ~а́ция валю́ты stabilizátion of cúrrency. ~и́ровать *несов. и сов.* (*вн.*) stábilize (*smth.*). ~и́роваться *несов. и сов.* be* stábilized, becóme* stáble. ~ова́ть(ся) *несов. и сов. см.* стабилизи́ровать(ся).

стаби́льн|ость *ж.* stability. ~ый stáble.

ста́вень *м. см.* ста́вни.

ста́вить, поста́вить (*вн.*) 1. (*заставлять кого-л. принять стоячее положение*) stand* (*smth.*), make* (*smb.*) stand up; поста́вить ребёнка на стул stand* the child* on a chair; 2. (*назначать для выполнения чего-л.*) put* (*smth.*); *разг.* (*назначать на должность*) appóint (*smth.*); ~ кого́-л. на пост put* smb. on dúty; ~ кого́-л. к станку́ put*/set* smb. to work at a lathe; 3. (*располагать, размещать*) put* (*smth.*), státion (*smth.*); ~ кого́-л. в ряд make* smb. stand in a row; 4. (*приводить кого́-л. в какое-л. состояние*) put* (*smth.*); ~ кого́-л. в неловкое, безвы́ходное положе́ние put* smb. in an áwkward, a hópeless position; 5. (*помещать, устанавливать что-л.*) put* (*smth.*), place (*smth.*), set* (*smth.*); (*вертикально тж.*) stand* (*smth.*); ~ что-л. в шкаф put* smth. in a cúpboard; ~ ча́йник put* the kéttle on; ~ цветы́ в во́ду put* the flówers in wáter; ~ столб plant/fix a post; ~ па́мятник кому́-л. put* up a mónument to smb., eréct a mónument to smb.; 6. (*делать ставку — в азартных играх*) stake (*smth.*), bet* (*smth.*); ~ на ло́шадь back a horse; ~ на ло́шадь де́сять рубле́й put* ten róubles on a horse; 7. (*приводить в нужное положение*) set* (*smth.*); ~ часы́ set* a clock/watch; ~ го́лос кому́-л. place smb.'s voice; 8. (*устанавливать*) instáll (*smth.*), fix (*smth.*); ~ телефо́н, ва́нну *и т. п.* instáll a télephone, bath *etc.*; ~ ми́ны lay* mines; 9. (*о лечебном средстве и т. п.*) apply (*smth.*); ~ ба́нки кому́-л. cup smb.; ~ пия́вки apply léeches; 10. (*прикреплять*) put* (*smth.*) on; ~ подмётку put* a sole on; ~ подкла́дку put*/fit a líning in; 11. (*изображать на письме*) put* (*smth.*); (*об отметках*) give* (*smth.*); ~ то́чку put* a full stop; 12. *разг.* (*строить*) put* (*smth.*) up, build* (*smth.*); 13. (*налаживать, организовывать*) órganize (*smth.*); (*осуществлять*) make* (*smth.*); ~ о́пыты make* expériments; 14. (*осуществлять постановку на сцене*) stage (*smth.*); put* (*smth.*) on the stage, diréct (*smth.*); ~ пье́су diréct a play; 15. (*выдвигать, предлагать*) propóse (*smth.*), move (*smth.*); ~ вопро́с на голосова́ние put* the quéstion to the vote; 16.: ~ что-л. кому́-л. в вину́ place/put* the blame for smth. on smb.; ~ кому́-л. зада́чу set* smb. a task; ~ кого́-л. в приме́р hold* smb. up as an exámple; ~ усло́вия lay* down condítions; поста́вить себе́ цель set* onesélf the aim; ◇ ~ реко́рд set* a récord; ~ на вид кому́-л. officially críticize/admónish smb.; ~ всё на ка́рту stake one's all; ни в грош не ~, ни во что не ~ (*что-л.*) attách not the slíghtest impórtance to smth.; (*кого́-л.*) have* no regárd for smb.; ~ что-л. вы́ше всего́ rate smth. abóve éverything; ~ кого́-л. на ноги set* smb. on his, her feet; ~ вопро́с state/pósit/propóund a quéstion.

ста́вк|а I *ж.* 1. (*оклад*) rate; ~ зарпла́ты rate of wáges; по вы́сшей ~e at the híghest rate; 2. (*в азартных играх*) stake; 3. (*ставка, расчёт, ориентация*) relíance (on); де́лать ~у на кого́-л., что-л. relý/count on smb., smth.

ста́вка II *ж. воен.* héadquárters; ~ главнокома́ндующего Géneral Héadquárters, G.H.Q.

ста́вк|а III *ж.*: о́чная ~ confrontátion; устро́ить кому́-л. о́чную ~у с... confrónt smb. with...

ста́вленник *м.* créature, protégé.

ста́вни *мн.* (*ед.* ста́вень *м.*, ста́вня *ж.*) shútters.

ставри́да *ж.* (*рыба*) horse máckerel.

стадио́н *м.* stádium (*pl* -dia).

ста́дия *ж.* stage.

ста́дный gregárious; ~ инсти́нкт herd/gregárious ínstinct.

ста́до *с.* herd; (*овец, коз*) flock; ~ коро́в herd of cows.

стаж *м.* (length of) sérvice; трудово́й ~ length of sérvice; ~ нау́чной рабо́ты time spent on scientífic work; пятиле́тний ~ five years sérvice.

стажёр *м.* práctical stúdent, fieldworker; (*в университете*) spécial stúdent.

стажирова́ться *несов.* be* on tríal; (*для приобретения опыта*) do* fieldwork, be* on a spécial course.

стажиро́вка *ж.* 1. (*проверочный период*) périod of tríal; 2. (*приобретение опыта*) práctical stúdy, fieldwork.

ста́йер *м.* lóng-distance man*; (*в беге*) lóng-distance rúnner. ~ский lóng-distance *attr.*; ~ская диста́нция lóng-distance evént.

стака́н *м.* glass, túmbler; ~ воды́ glass of wáter.

сталева́р *м.* stéelworker.

сталелите́йный: ~ заво́д steel fóundry, stéelworks; ~ цех steel fóundry.

сталепрока́тный stéel-rolling *attr.*

ста́лкивать, столкну́ть 1. (*вн.*) push (*smb., smth.*) (off); столкну́ть кого́-л., что-л. в во́ду push smb., smth. ínto the wáter; столкну́ть кого́-л. с ме́ста push smb. awáy; 2. (*вн.*; *заставлять удариться*) knock (*smb., smth.*) togéther; *перен.* cause a clash (betwéen); столкну́ть билья́рдные шары́ make* one bílliard ball hit anóther; столкну́ть кого́-л. лба́ми knock smb.'s heads togéther; *перен.* set* smb. at lóggerheads; 3. (*с тв.*; *заставлять встретиться*) bring* (*smb.*) ínto cóntact (with); *перен.* bring* (*smb.*) up agáinst (*smth.*) ~ся, столкну́ться (*с тв.*) 1. (*ударяться друг о друга*) collíde (with); run*/cánnon ínto each óther; *перен.* (*вступать в конфликт*) clash (with); льди́ны столкну́лись the floes collíded; их интере́сы столкну́лись their ínterests clashed; 2. (*встречаться*) come* acróss one anóther, run* ínto each óther, run* ínto (*smb.*); *перен.* be* confrónted/faced (with), run* ínto (*smth.*); мы столкну́лись в двери́х we ran ínto each óther in the dóorway; столкну́ться с действи́тельностью be* faced with reálity, be* confrónted with the facts of life.

сталь *ж.* steel; высокока́чественная ~ high-grade steel; ~но́й steel *attr.*; (*о цвете*) stéel-grey; *перен.* of steel *после сущ.*; ~ные констру́кции steel constrúction *sg*; ~но́й челове́к man* of steel; ~на́я во́ля will of íron, íron will; ~ные не́рвы nerves of steel.

стаме́ска *ж.* chísel.

стан I *м. книжн.* (*туловище человека*) figure.

стан II *м.* 1. (*место стоянки полевых бригад*) camp; 2. (*воюющая сторона*) camp (*тж. перен.*).

стан III *м. тех.* mill.

станда́рт *м.* 1. stándard; (*типовая форма организации чего-л.*) stándard méthod; 2. (*шаблон, трафарет*) cliché, stéreotype; stock tricks *pl*.

стандартиз|а́ция *ж.* standardizátion. ~и́ровать *несов. и сов.* (*вн.*) stándardize.

стандартн|ый 1. stándard *attr.*; (*о предметах широкого потребления*) máss-produced, stándardized; ~ые строи́тельные дета́ли únified strúctural élements; ~ дом stándard/stándardized house; ~ая ме́бель máss-produced fúrniture; 2. *разг.* (*шаблонный*) trite, cómmonplace.

стани́ца *ж.* stanítsa (*large Cossack village*).

станко́в|ый 1. lathe *attr.*; machine-tool *attr.*; 2. *воен.*: ~ пулемёт (médium/héavy) machine-gun; ~ое ору́жие héavy wéapons *pl*; 3. *иск.*: ~ая жи́вопись éasel-painting.

станкостро|éние *с.* machine-tool construction. **~йтельный** machine-tool *attr.*

становйться I, стать 1. (*располагаться стоя*) stand*; стать у стены stand* by the wall; стать в ряд form a row; стать на своё место go* back to one's place; *перен.* fall* into place; стать в очередь за *чем-л.* form a queue (for), queue up (for); стать на стул get* up on a chair; 2. (*приступать к какой-л. работе*) take* up one's position; стать за прилавок go* behind the counter; стать на пост take* up one's post; 3. (*размещаться*): стать лагерем pitch camp; 4. (*вставать*) stand*; ~ на колéни kneel* down; ~ на цыпочки poise oneself on típtoe; ~ на руки do* a hand-stand; ◇ стать во главé *чего-л.* becóme léader of *smth.*, take* óver the léadership of *smth.*; стать в позу strike* an áttitude; стать на лёд go* on the ice; стать на лыжи start skíing; стать на учёт régister; стать на якорь drop ánchor; стать у власти take* pówer.

становйться II, стать (*делаться*) becóme*; (*кем-л., чем-л., каким-л. тж.*) get*, grow*; ~ учителем *и т. п.* becóme* a téacher, *etc.*; ~ подозрйтельным *и т. п.* becóme*/get*/grow* suspícious *etc.*; всем стало скучно éveryone was bored; опять стало тихо sílence reigned/fell once more; нам стало жалко его we were/felt sórry for him; ему стало холодно (*теперь*) he is cold; (*в прошлом*) he felt cold; становится темно, холодно, жарко it is becóming/gétting/grówing dark, cold, hot.

становлéни|е *с.* formátion; ~ характера móulding/formátion of cháracter; в процéссе ~я in the máking.

становóй: ~ хребéт *перен.* báckbone.

станóк *м.* 1. (*для работы*) bench; (*механический*) machine(-tool); печáтный ~ prínting-press; столярный ~ jóiner's bench; 2. (*опора*) móunt(ing).

стáнсы *мн.* stánzas.

станцибнный státion *attr.*

стáнция *ж.* státion; опытная ~ *с.-х.* experiméntal státion; ◇ электрйческая ~ pówer station, pówer plant.

стáпел|ь *м.* building-berth; stocks *pl*; на ~e on the stocks; сходить со ~я, ~ей come* off the stocks.

стáптывать, стоптáть (*вн.*) wear* out (*smth.*); ~ каблукй wear* the heels down.

старáни|е *с.* éffort, endéavour; приложйть все ~я do* one's best, exért one's best éfforts.

старáтель *м.* góld-digger.

старáтельн|о cárefully, páinstakingly. **~ость** *ж.* applicátion; (*прилежание*) díligence. **~ый** páinstaking; (*прилежный*) díligent.

старáться, постарáться 1. (*делать что-л. с усердием*) try, do* one's best; ~ изо всех сил do* one's véry best, try with all one's might; (+ *инф.*; *прилагать усилия*) try (+ to *inf*), endéavour (+ to *inf*), do* one's best (+ to *inf*); ~ выиграть врéмя play for time.

старéйшина *м. ист.* élder.

старéть, постарéть, устарéть 1. *сов.* постарéть age; grow*/get* old; 2. *сов.* устарéть be*/becóme* óbsolete.

стáрец *м.* old man*; élder.

старéющий áging, ágeing.

старйк *м.* old man*.

старикáн *м.* old boy/chap/féllow.

старикóвск|ий old man's; **~ая** похóдка óld-mánnish walk.

старин|á 1. *ж.* (*о времени*) old times *pl*; в ~ý in times past, in ólden days; in the old days; 2. *ж.* (*старинные вещи, обычаи*) rélic of the past; 3. *м. разг.* (*в обращении*) old man*/féllow/chap; ◇ тряхнýть ~óй bring* back one's young days.

старйнк|а *ж.:* по ~е in the old way, as in the old times.

старйнн|ый old; (*древний*) áncient; **~ые** вéщи antiques; **~ая** мéбель antíque/périod fúrniture; **~ая** одéжда périod/histórical cóstume.

стáрить, состáрить (*вн.*) age (*smb.*); (*делать старообразным*) make* (*smb.*) look old. **~ся, состáриться** get*/grow*/becóme* old.

старичóк *м.* (*little*) old man*.

старожйл *м.* old résident.

старомóдный old-fáshioned.

старообрáзный óld-looking.

стáроста *м.* léader; ~ клáсса form cáptain; ~ кýрса course léader.

стáрост|ь *ж.* 1. old age; к ~и, под ~ when one is gétting old; в ~и in one's old age; 2. (*ветхость, изношенность*) age; ◇ ~ не рáдость *посл.* it's not much pléasure to be old.

старт *м.* 1. start; (*ракеты тж.*) blást-off; (*самолёта*) táke-off; брать ~ start; *перен.* (*начинать что-л. удачно*) make* a (good) start; дать ~ give* the signal to start; 2. (*место*) stárting line, start; выходйть на ~ go* to the stárting line.

стáртер *м. спорт., тех.* stárter.

стартовáть *несов. и сов.* start; (*о ракете тж.*) blast off; (*о самолёте*) take* off; *перен.* (*начинаться*) ópen, start.

стáртов|ый 1. *спорт.* stárting *attr.*; ~ сигнáл stárting signal; ~ пистолéт stárting/stárter's pistol; **~ые** дорóжки stárting lanes; 2. *ав.* láunching *attr.*; **~ая** площáдка для зáпуска ракéт rócket láunching pad.

стару|ха *ж.* old wóman*. **~шечий** old wóman's. **~шка** *ж.* (*little*) old wóman*, old soul.

стáрческий sénile.

стáрш|ий *прил.* 1. (*по возрасту*) ólder; (*из всех*) óldest; (*о детях*) élder; (*из всех*) éldest; ~ брат élder bróther; ~ сын the éldest son; 2. (*по положению*) sénior; **~ая** медицйнская сестрá sénior nurse; ~ офицéр sénior ófficer; ~ лейтенáнт first lieuténant; 3. (*близкий к концу обучения*) sénior; **~ие** клáссы sénior/úpper forms; ~ курс sénior year; 4. *в знач. сущ. м.* (*начальник*) chief, man* in charge; кто здесь ~? who is in charge here?; 5. *в знач. сущ. мн.* (*взрослые*) adúlts, one's élders.

старшинá *м.* 1. *воен.* sérgeant májor; first sérgeant *амер.*; 2. *мор.* pétty ófficer.

старшинств|ó *с.* seniórity; по ~ý by seniórity.

стáр|ый *прил.* 1. old; по ~ой пáмяти for the sake of old times; 2. *в знач. сущ. с.* (the) old; борьбá ~ого с нóвым the strúggle betwéen the old and the new; принáться за ~ое fall* back into one's old ways; ◇ кто ~ое помянет, томý глаз вон ≈ let bygones be bygones; человéк ~ого закáла a man* of the old school; Стáрый Свет the Old World; ~ стиль Old Style.

старьё *с. собир. разг.* old stuff/junk; (*старое платье*) old clothes *pl.*

старьёвщик *м.* rág-and-bóne man*.

стáскивать, стащйть (*вн.*) pull (*smth.*) (off); (*силой тж.*) drag (*smth.*) (off); ~ перчáтку pull/draw* off a glove; ~ *кого-л.* с кровáти pull/drag *smb.* out of bed.

стáтика *ж.* státics.

статйст *м. театр.* súper, wálker-on.

статйст|ик *м.* statistícian. **~ика** *ж.* statístics; **~ика** внéшней торгóвли fóreign trade statístics.

статистйческ|ий statístic(al); **~ие** дáнные statistics, statístical data; ~ отчёт statístical repórt.

статйческий státic.

стáтн|ый well-propórtioned, shápely; **~ая** фигýра shápely figure.

стáтус *м.* státus; правовóй ~ légal státus; ~ незавйсимого госудáрства státus of indepéndent státe.

стáтус-квó *м. нескл.* státus quo.

статуэтка *ж.* statuétte, figurine.

стáтуя *ж.* státue.

стать I *сов.* 1. *см.* становйться I; 2. (*остановиться*) stop; лóшадь стáла the horse stopped; часы стáли the watch/clock has stopped; река стала the river is frozen óver, the river is íce-bound.

стать II *сов.* 1. *см.* станови́ться II; 2. (+ *инф.; начать*) begin* (+ to *inf.*, + -ing); (*приобрести привычку*) have* táken (to + -ing); он стал чита́ть письмо́ he begán réading the létter; он стал чита́ть в посте́ли he has táken to réading in bed; 3. (+ *инф.; для образова́ния бу́дущего вре́мени*): не ста́ну чита́ть I won't read; что ты ста́нешь де́лать? what will you do?; 4. (с *тв.; случи́ться*): что с ним ста́ло? what has háppened to him?; 5. *безл.* (*рд.*): его́ не ста́ло he is no more; ⟡ ста́ло быть (*итак*) so, thus; (*сле́довательно*) cónsequently, it fóllows that.

стат | **ь** III *ж.* (*телосложе́ние*) physique, build; ⟡ под ~ 1) (*подобен чему́-л.*) like smth.; 2) (*в соотве́тствии с кем-л., чем-л.*) be* fitting to smb., smth.; с како́й ~и? what on earth for?, why should I, he, etc.?; с како́й ~и мне, ему́ *и т. д.* идти́ туда́? why (on earth) should I, he, etc. go there?

ста́ться *сов. разг.* háppen; что с ним сталось? what has becóme of him?; ⟡ мо́жет ~, что я задержу́сь I may be deláyed; всё мо́жет ~ ánything may háppen.

статья́ *ж.* 1. (*газе́тная и т. п.*) árticle; 2. (*пункт*) páragraph, ítem, clause; (*зако́на, уста́ва*) clause; ~ догово́ра árticle/clause of a tréaty; 3. (*разде́л бюдже́та*) ítem; ~ бюдже́та ítem in the búdget; статьи́ расхо́да ítems of expénditure; прихо́дная ~ crédit ítem; ~ дохо́да source of íncome; ⟡ по всем ~м on all counts; это осо́бая ~ that belóngs in quite anóther cátegory/héading.

стациона́р *м.* 1. pérmanent estáblishment; 2. (*лече́бное учрежде́ние*) hóspital, ín-patient depártment. ~ный 1. pérmanent; 2. (*в больни́це*) ín-patient *attr.*; ~ный больно́й ín-patient; 3. *тех.* státionary, fixed, státic.

стача́ть *сов. см.* тача́ть.

стачечный strike *attr.*

ста́чка *ж.* strike.

стащи́ | **ть** *сов.* 1. *см.* ста́скивать; 2. (*вн.*) *разг.* (*укра́сть*) pílfer (*smth.*), filch (*smth.*), steal* (*smth.*); *шутл.* bag (*smth.*); кто ~л мой каранда́ш? who's bagged my péncil?

ста́я *ж.* (*птиц*) flock; (*живо́тных*) pack; (*рыб*) shoal, school; *перен.* flock.

ста́ять *сов.* melt.

ствол *м.* 1. (*де́рева*) trunk; (*то́нкий тж.*) stem; 2. (*стрелко́вого ору́дия*) bárrel; (*миномёта*) tube.

ство́рка *ж.* leaf*; (*буфе́та и т. п.*) door.

створча́т | **ый** fólding; ~ые две́ри fólding doors.

стеари́н *м.* stéarin. ~овый stéarin *attr.*; ~овые све́чи stéarin cándles.

сте́бель *м.* (*травы́*) stalk; (*цвето́к*) stem.

стёган | **ый** quílted, wádded; ~ая ку́ртка wádded jácket; ~ое одея́ло quilt.

стега́ть I, **стегну́ть** (*вн.; хлеста́ть*) lash (*smb., smth.*).

стега́ть II *несов.* (*вн.; проши́вать*) quilt (*smth.*).

стегну́ть *сов. см.* стега́ть I.

стеж | **о́к** *м.* stitch; де́лать ~ки́ take* stítches.

стека́ть, стечь 1. pour down; (*ка́плями*) tríckle down; ~ с кры́ши pour down from the roof; по скло́ну pour/flow down a slope/híllside; дать воде́ стечь let* the wáter drain off; 2. *тк. несов.* (*о реке́, ручье́*) flow down, run* down. ~ся, сте́чься join; *перен.* come* togéther, gáther; мно́го наро́ду стекло́сь на пло́щадь a large crowd gáthered in the square.

стекло́ *с.* glass; *собир.* (*изде́лия*) glássware; ветрово́е ~ (*в автомаши́не*) wíndscreen, wíndshield; ⟡ увеличи́тельное ~ mágnifying glass.

стекловолокно́ *с.* glass fíbre, fíbre glass.

стеклоду́в *м.* gláss-blower.

стеклопла́стики *мн.* (*ед.* стеклопла́стик *м.*) gláss-fibre plástics.

стёклышко *с.* bit/frágment of glass; ⟡ как ~ чи́стый spick and span, bright as a new pin.

стекля́нн | **ый** 1. glass *attr.*; ~ая ва́за glass vase; ~ шкаф cábinet with glass doors; 2. (*похо́жий на стекло́*) crýstalline; (*о зву́ках*) clear, crýstal-clear; 3. (*о глаза́х, взгля́де*) glássy.

стеко́ль | **ный** glass *attr.*; ~ заво́д gláss-works; ~ная промы́шленность glass índustry/manufácture. ~щик *м.* glázier.

стели́ть(ся) *несов. разг. см.* стла́ть(ся).

стелла́ж *м.* 1. shelves *pl*, stand; 2. (*приспособле́ние для хране́ния чего́-л. в стоя́чем положе́нии*) rack.

сте́лька *ж.* ínsole, sock.

сте́льная: ~ коро́ва cow in/with calf.

сте́лющийся próstrate, tráiling; ~ кедр próstrate cédar.

стемне́ть *сов. см.* темне́ть 1, 2.

стен | **а́** *ж.* wall; за ~о́й the óther side of the wall; в ~а́х within the walls; ме́жду ни́ми вы́росла ~ they becáme estránged; встать ~о́й rise* like one man; как за ка́менной ~о́й safe as hóuses; положи́ться на кого́-л. как на ка́менную сте́ну know* smb. to be útterly trústworthy, have* ábsolute trust in smb.

стенгазе́та *ж.* (*стенна́я газе́та*) wall néwspaper.

стенд *м.* 1. stand; 2. (*устано́вка для испыта́ния маши́н*) test bench; испыта́ть что́-л. на ~е bench-test smth.

сте́нк | **а** *ж.* 1. wall; 2. (*бокова́я сторона́*) side; ~и я́щика sides of a box/drawer; ~и кровено́сных сосу́дов walls of the blood véssels; ⟡ гимнасти́ческая ~ the wáll-bars *pl*.

стенн | **о́й** wall *attr.*, múral; ~ шкаф búilt-in cúpboard/clóset; wall cúpboard; ~а́я жи́вопись múral páinting; múrals *pl*; ~ы́е часы́ wall clock *sg.*

стеногра́мма *ж.* verbátim récord/repórt; ~ докла́да verbátim récord of a speech.

стенографи́ровать *несов.* (*вн.*) take* (*smth.*) down in shórthand.

стеногра́ф | **и́ст** *м.*, ~и́стка *ж.* stenógrapher. ~и́ческий shórthand *attr.*, stenográphic; ~и́ческий отчёт shórthand/verbátim repórt.

стеногра́фия *ж.* stenógraphy, shórthand.

сте́нопись *ж.* múral páinting.

степе́нный staid, sédate, grave.

сте́пен | **ь** *ж.* 1. (*сравни́тельная величина́*) degrée; ~ сжа́тия *газа* compréssion; 2. *тк. ед.* (*ме́ра, преде́л, отноше́ние*) degrée, extént; до изве́стной ~и, до не́которой ~и to a cértain extént; в той и́ли ино́й ~и one way or anóther; в значи́тельной ~и to a considerable extént; до како́й ~и? to what extént?; 3. (*учёное зва́ние*) degrée; ~ до́ктора Dóctor's degrée; ~ кандида́та нау́к Máster's degrée; присужда́ть учёную ~ кому́-л. confér a degrée on smb.; 4. (*разря́д, катего́рия*) class; 5. *мат.* pówer; возводи́ть что́-л. в тре́тью *и т. д.* ~ raise smth. to the third, etc. pówer; ⟡ ро́дственная relátion; в вы́сшей ~и 1) (*о́чень*) extrémely, most; 2) (*совсе́м*) útterly; ни в мале́йшей ~и not in the least.

степно́й steppe *attr.*

степь *ж.* steppe.

стервя́тник *м. зоол.* vúlture.

стереокино́ *с. нескл.* (*стереоскопи́ческое кино́*) thrée-diménsional cínema, 3-D (cínema).

стереомагнитофо́н *м.* stéreo tape recórder.

стереоме́трия *ж.* stereómetry, sólid geómetry.

стереосисте́ма *ж. разг.* stéreo hí-fi.

стереоско́п *м.* stéreoscope.

стереоскопи́ческ | **ий** stereoscópic; ~ое изображе́ние stereoscópic ímage.

стереоти́п *м. полигр.* stéreotype. ~ный *полигр.* stéreotype *attr.*, stéreotyped; *перен. тж.* stock *attr.*; ~ное издáние stéreotype edítion; ~ная фрáза stock/stéreotyped/háckneyed phrase.

стереофи́льм м. (стереоскопи́ческий фильм) 3-D film.

стереофони́ческий stereophónic; ~ звук stereo (phónic) sound.

стерéть сов. см. стирáть I. **~ся** сов. см. стирáться I.

стерéчь несов. (вн.) 1. (охранять) guard (smb., smth.); watch (óver); 2. (подкарáуливать) watch (for).

стерж|ень м. 1. rod, shaft; (опóрный) pívot, spíndle; 2. (растения) core, heart; 3. (главная часть чего-л.) córe, pívot. **~невóй** pívotal; **~невóй** вопрóс pívotal quéstion, key íssue.

стерилизáция ж. sterilizátion.

стерилизовáть несов. и сов. (вн.) sterilize (smth.).

стери́льный 1. (обеззараженный) stérilized; 2. (бесплодный) stérile.

стéрлинг м. stérling. **~овый** stérling attr.

стéрлядь ж. (рыба) stérlet.

стерня́ ж. с.-х. stúbble (field).

стерпéть сов. (вн.) bear* (smth.), endúre (smth.); не ~ lose* pátience; ~ оби́ду sit* down únder an ínsult; он не стерпéл оби́ды he rebélled at the ínsult.

стёртый effáced, oblíterated.

стеснéни|е с. 1. restráint; 2. (затруднённость дыхания) constríction; 3. (неловкость) constráint; говори́ть без **~я** speak* quite fréely; пожáлуйста, без **~й!** make yoursélf quite at home!, don't stand on céremony!

стеснённ|ый 1. (о дыхании) constrícted; (о движениях) cramped; 2. (тяжёлый) dífficult; в **~ых** обстоятельствах in stráitened/redúced círcumstances.

стесни́тельн|ость ж. shýness, áwkwardness. **~ый** 1. (застенчивый) shy, áwkward; 2. (затруднительный) dífficult, restrícted.

стесни́ть сов. см. стеснять.

стесня́ть, стесни́ть (вн.) 1. (лишать простора) confíne (smth.); перен. restríct (smth.); 2. (заставлять потесни́ться) cramp (smb.); вы нас нискóлько не стесни́те you won't inconvénience us in the least, you won't be a bit in the way; я вас не стесню́? won't I be in the way?; 3. (лишать свободы действий) hámper (smb.), hínder (smb.), impéde (smb.); (ограничивать кого-л. в чём-л.) restríct (smb.); ~ кого-л. в срéдствах stint smb. for móney; 4. (лишать непринуждённости) embárrass (smb.); 5. разг. (сдавливать) squeeze (smb.); 6. (горло, грудь) constríct (smth.); перен. oppréss (smb.).

стесн|я́ться, постесня́ться 1. тк. несов. feel* shy (in front of); не **~я́йтесь!** don't be shy/nérvous!; 2. (когó-л.) be* shy (of); (чего-л.; стыдиться) be* ashámed (of); (+ инф.) be* too shy (+ to inf); он вас **~я́ется** you make him shy; он **~я́ется** пу́блики an áudience makes him nérvous, he súffers from stáge-fright; он никогó не **~я́ется** he's as bold as brass, nóbody can make him nérvous; не **~я́йтесь** говори́ть прáвду don't be afráid to tell the truth; не ~ в выражéниях not be óver-níce in one's expréssions, not mince one's words.

стетоскóп м. stéthoscope.

стечéни|е с. cónfluence; ~ нарóда cóncourse; при большóм **~и** нарóда before a vast cóncourse/assémbly; ◇ ~ обстоятельств coíncidence; the círcumstances pl; счастли́вое ~ обстоятельств fórtunate coíncidence; неожи́данное ~ обстоятельств unforeséen coíncidence.

стечь сов. см. стекáть 1. **~ся** сов. см. стекáться.

стилиз|áция ж. stylizátion. **~óванный** stýlized, conventionálized; (манерный) affécted.

стили́стика ж. stylístics, (stúdy of) style.

стилисти́ческ|ий stylístic; **~ая** оши́бка érror of style.

стил|ь I м. style; **~и** в жи́вописи styles in páinting; в рýсском, итальянском и т. д. ~ in the Rússian, Itálian, etc., style; ~ фельетóна satírical style; работáть над **~ем** impróve one's style; ~ руковóдства style of

leadership/mánagement; э́то не в моём ~е that's not my way of dóing things.

стил|ь II м. (способ летосчисления) style; по нóвому (стáрому) **~ю** New (Old) Style.

сти́льный 1. stýlish; 2. разг. (утрированно мóдный) óversmárt; téddy-boy attr.

стиля́га ж. разг. (в 1950-х годах) téddy boy.

сти́мул м. stímulus (pl -li); incéntive.

стимули́ровать несов. и сов. (вн.) stímulate (smth.).

стипендиáт м. gránt-holder, schólarship hólder.

стипéнди|я ж. grant, allówance; получáть **~ю** get* a grant; получи́ть **~ю** за мéсяц recéive one's mónthly allówance.

стирáльн|ый wáshing; **~ая** маши́на wáshing machine; ~ порошóк soap pówder.

стирáть I, стерéть (вн.) 1. (вытирать) wipe off (smth.); (пыль) dust (smth.); (написанное) rub (smth.) out; eráse (smth.); перен. oblíterate (smth.); 2. (повреждáть кóжу) abráde (smth.), rub (smth.) sore; стерéть нóгу rub/make* one's foot sore; ◇ ~ когó-л. с лицá земли́ wipe smb. out, oblíterate smb.; ~ когó-л. в порошóк make* míncemeat of smb.

стирáть II, вы́стирать (вн.) (бельё) wash (smth.), láunder (smth.).

стирáться I, стерéться 1. be* rubbed off; (о напи́санном) be* rubbed out, be* oblíterated/effáced; перен. disappéar; 2. (изнашиваться) wear* smooth, wear* down; (становиться тонким) wear* thin.

стирáться II несов. wash; хорошó ~ wash well.

сти́рк|а ж. wáshing; день **~и** wáshing-day; отдавáть бельё в **~у** give* out one's láundry; брать бельё в **~у** take* in wáshing.

сти́скивать, сти́снуть (вн.) 1. squeeze (smb., smth.); сти́снуть когó-л. в объятиях hold* smb. close, hug smb.; ~ что-л. зубáми bite* smth.; 2. (стеснять гóрло, грудь) constrict (smth.), seize (smth.), grip (smth.) (тж. перен.); 3. (плóтно соединять) clench (smth.); сти́снуть зу́бы grit/set* one's teeth; сти́снув зу́бы grítting one's teeth.

сти́снуть сов. см. сти́скивать.

стих м. 1. verse; в **~áх** in verse; 2. мн. (стихотворéния) póetry sg, verse sg; писáть **~и** write* póetry; **~и** Пу́шкина Púshkin's verse.

стихáть, сти́хнуть 1. (о звуках, шуме) die awáy; кри́ки, шаги́ сти́хли the shouts, fóotsteps died awáy; 2. (замолкáть, умолкáть) becóme quíet; (прекращáть стрельбу́) stop fíring; всё сти́хло a hush fell, all was quíet; 3. (становиться слабее) subsíde, abáte; вéтер стих the wind dropped.

стихи́йн|о spontáneously. **~ость** ж. spontanéity. **~ый** 1. eleméntal, nátural; **~ое** бéдствие nátural disáster; **~ая** си́ла eleméntal/primórdial force; 2. (неорганизóванный) spontáneous; **~ое** движéние spontáneous móvement.

стихи́|я ж. 1. élement; 2. (инстинкт) blind impulse, urge; 3. (не поддающееся регули́рованию явлéние) cháos, ánarchy; ~ конкурéнции the cháos of márket competítion; 4. (привычная среда) élement; в своéй **~и** in one's élement.

сти́хнуть сов. см. стихáть.

стихосложéние с. versificátion; prósody.

стихотворéние с. póem; ~ в прóзе póem in prose.

стихотвóрн|ый poétical; ~ размéр métre; в **~ой** фóрме in verse.

стлать, постлáть, настлáть (вн.) 1. сов. постлáть spread* (smth.); постлáть скáтерть на стол spread* a táblecloth; постлáть постéль make* up a bed; 2. сов. настлáть lay* (smth.); ~ паркéт lay* párquet flóoring; ~ся несов. 1. spread*, spread* out; 2. (о животных, птицах) skim alóng, go* skímming.

сто 1. a húndred; one húndred; считáть дó ста count up to a húndred; ~ рублéй a húndred róubles; ~ двáдцать a húndred and twénty; 2. разг.: ~ раз вам говори́л how mány times have I told you; ~ раз вам говори́ть, повторя́ть? how mány times do you have to be told?

стог м. stack, rick; ~ се́на háystack, háyrick; ~ соло́мы stráwrick.

сто́ик м. stóic.

сто́имост|ь ж. 1. cost; ~ произво́дства cost of prodúction; ~ то́нны зерна́ cost of grain per ton, cost of a ton of grain; о́бщей ~ью в ты́сячу рубле́й to a tótal válue of one thóusand róubles; 2. эк. válue; зако́н ~и law of válue.

сто́|ить несов. 1. (о цене, затрате) cost*; ~ кому́-л. больши́х де́нег cost* smb. a lot of móney; дёшево ~ be* cheap; до́рого ~ be* expénsive, be* dear; ничего́ не ~ be* wórthless; кни́га ~ит два рубля́ the book costs two róubles; 2. (рд.; обладать какой-л. ценностью, значимостью) be* worth (smth.); он ~ит семеры́х ≈ he's worth a dózen óthers; оди́н друго́го ~ит there's nóthing to choose betwéen them; 3. (рд.; быть достойным) be* wórthy (of); (заслуживать) desérve (smth.); 4. (рд.; требовать усилий) take* (smth.); никако́го труда́ не ~ило (+ инф.) it was no tróuble (+ to inf), it was the work of a móment (+ to inf); 5. безл. (+ инф.; имеет смысл) it is (well) worth (+ -ing); э́ту кни́гу ~ит проче́сть this book is (well) worth réading; туда́ ~ит съе́здить the place is well worth a vísit; не ~ит беспоко́ить его́ it's not worth bóthering him; ~ит ли? is it worth it?; 6. безл. (+ инф.; достаточно) one has ónly (+ to inf); ~ит то́лько захоте́ть ... if you réally wánted to, you ...; ◇ э́то де́нег ~ит 1) (оправдывает затраченное) it is worth the móney; 2) (даром не дадут) it costs móney; ничего́ не ~ит (+ инф.) it's a símple mátter (+ to inf).

сто́ческий stóical.

сто́йбище с. nómad encámpment, nómad camp.

сто́йка I ж. 1. (подпорка) úpright, stánchion, strut; 2. (прилавок в столовой, буфете и т. п.) cóunter, bar.

сто́йк|а II ж. воен., спорт. position at atténtion; 2. спорт. (на руках) hándstand; (на голове) héadstand; 3. охот. (о собаке) set; де́лать ~у point.

сто́йк|ий 1. stáble; (твёрдый) firm; (об отравляющих веществах) persístent; ~ая кра́ска fast cólour; 2. (непоколебимый) stéadfast, staunch; ~ хара́ктер strong cháracter; ~ая оборо́на stúbborn defénce. ~о stéadfastly, fírmly; (переносить невзгоды) be* stéadfast in advérsity; ~ обороня́ться put* up a stúbborn defénce. ~ость ж. 1. stabílity; 2. (непоколебимость) tenácity, endúrance, stáying pówer.

сто́йло с. stall.

сто́ймя úpright.

сток м. 1. (действие) flow; 2. (канава, жёлоб) gútter; (труба) wáste-pipe.

стол м. 1. táble; за обе́денным ~ом aróund the dínner-table; 2. (приём пищи) meal; за ~ом (за едой) at táble, at/dúring meals; сади́ться за ~ take* one's seat/place at the táble; встава́ть из-за ~а rise* from the táble; пригласи́ть кого́-л. к ~у invíte smb. to táble; 3. (пища, еда) board; (диета) diet; дома́шний ~ home cóoking; моло́чный, вегетариа́нский ~ milk, vegetárian diet; 4. (отдел в учреждении) depártment, desk; ~ зака́зов órder desk/cóunter.

столб м. post, pole; (каменный) píllar; (воды, ртути) cólumn; ~ ды́ма, пы́ли cólumn/píllar of smoke, dust; пыль стои́т ~ом the air is full of dust; ◇ стоя́ть ~ом, стоя́ть как ~ stand* stóck-still.

столб|е́ц м. cólumn; газе́тные ~цы́ néwspaper cólumns.

столбня́к м. 1. мед. tétanus, lóck-jaw; 2. разг. (состояние оцепенения) trance; в како́м-то ~е́ in a kind of trance.

столбов|о́й: ~а́я доро́га híghroad.

столе́т|ие с. 1. (период) céntury; 2. (годовщина) centénary, centénnial, húndredth annivérsary; ~ со дня рожде́ния Толсто́го the Tólstoy centénary. ~ний

húndred-year-óld, centenárian; ~ние дубы́ céntury--old/centenárian oaks; ~ний стари́к óld man* of a húndred, centenárian; ~ний юбиле́й centénary. ~ник м. бот. agáve, céntury plant.

столи́|ца ж. cápital. ~чный cápital attr.; metropólitan; ~чный го́род cápital (city); ~чный жи́тель inhábitant of the cápital; metropólitan.

столкнове́ние с. 1. collísion; ~ поездо́в train collísion/crash; 2. (противоречие, конфликт) cónflict, clash; ~ интере́сов clash of ínterests; 3. (стычка, бой) clash; вооружённое ~ armed cónflict/clash.

столкну́ть(ся) сов. см. ста́лкивать(ся).

столкова́ться сов. разг. come* to an understánding.

столова́ться несов. (у рд.) board (with).

столо́вая ж. díning-room; (в учреждении, на предприятии и т. п. тж.) cafetéria; canteen; студе́нческая ~ stúdents' díning-room.

столо́в|ый I 1. táble attr.; ~ая ло́жка táble-spoon; ~ое серебро́ sílver plate; ~ прибо́р dínner service/set; ~ое бельё táble-linen; 2. геогр. táble attr.; ~ая гора́ tábleland, mésa.

столо́вый II díning-room attr.; ~ гарниту́р ме́бели díning-room suite.

столп м. архит. píllar (тж. перен.); ~ы́ о́бщества the Estáblishment, píllars of socíety.

столпи́ться сов. crowd.

столпотворе́ние с. túrmoil; bábel; там настоя́щее ~ the place is in a túrmoil.

столь so; ~ ва́жный, мо́щный, незначи́тельный и т. д. so impórtant, pówerful, insigníficant etc.; ~ опа́сное предприя́тие so périlous an undertáking; э́то не ~ ва́жно that's not so impórtant.

сто́лько 1. (с сущ. в ед. ч.) so much; (с сущ. во мн. ч.) so mány; ~ раз, ско́лько ну́жно as óften as requíred; не ~, ско́лько про́шлый раз not so much/mány as last time; ещё ~ (же) the same númber/quántity as befóre; оста́лось ещё ~ же сде́лать there is still as much agáin to do; мне оста́лось ещё ~ же пройти́ I still have as far agáin to go; 2.: он не ~ силён, ско́лько ло́вок he is not so much strong as ágile; он не ~ бо́лен, ско́лько уста́л he is more tíred than ill.

сто́лько-то so much, so mány.

столя́р м. jóiner; cárpenter разг. ~ничать несов. go* in for máking fúrniture. ~ный jóiner's; cárpenter's разг.; ~ное де́ло jóinery, fúrniture-making; ~ный инструме́нт jóiner's tools pl; ◇ ~ный клей jóiner's glue.

стомато́лог м. stomatólogist; déntist.

стоматоло́гия ж. stomatólogy; déntistry.

стометро́вка ж. спорт. (húndred-metre) sprint.

стон м. moan, groan.

стона́ть, простона́ть 1. moan, groan; 2. тк. несов. (страдать под игом кого-л., чего-л.) groan únder the yoke.

стоп stop.

стоп|а́ I ж. (ноги) foot*; ◇ направля́ть свои́ ~ы́ wend one's way; идти́ по ~а́м кого́-л. fóllow in smb.'s fóotsteps.

стопа́ II ж. лит. foot*.

стопа́ III ж. 1. (ряд, кучка) pile; 2. (мера бумаги) ream.

сто́пка I ж. (кучка) pile; ~ тетра́дей pile of éxercise books.

сто́пка II ж. (стаканчик для водки) small (straight) glass, thímble glass.

сто́пор м. stop, detáiner; мор. stópper.

стопроце́нтн|ый húndred-per-cént attr.; ~ая я́вка full atténdance.

сто́птанн|ый wórn-out; ~ые каблуки́ bróken-down heels.

стопта́ть сов. см. ста́птывать.

сторгова́ться сов. agrée upón the price; come* to an

agréement; ~ на ста рубля́х agrée upón one húndred róubles, séttle for one húndred róubles.

сто́рицею: возда́ть *кому-л.* ~ гера́у* *smb.* a húndredfold.

сто́рож *м.* wátchman*; э́та соба́ка — хоро́ший ~ it is a good wátchdog.

сторожев|о́й watch *attr.;* ~ая соба́ка wátchdog; ~ая бу́дка wátchman's shélter; *воен.* séntry-box; ~ая вы́шка wátch-tower; ~ ка́тер patról-launch; ~ое охране́ние *воен.* óutposts *pl;* ~ пост séntry-post.

сторожи́ть *несов.* 1. be* on watch; 2. *(вн.)* guard *(smb., smth.),* keep* watch (óver).

сторо́жка *ж.* lodge; лесна́я ~ fórest wárden's hut.

сторон|а́ *ж.* 1. side; *(направление)* way; сто́роны горизо́нта cárdinal points; сверну́ть в сто́рону ле́са turn in the diréction of the fórest; разойти́сь в ра́зные сто́роны go* off in different diréctions; со всех сторо́н on all sides, on évery hand; в ту сто́рону in that diréction; в каку́ю сто́рону он пошёл? which way did he go?; вам в каку́ю сто́рону? which way are you góing?; в на́шу сто́рону our way; смотре́ть в другу́ю сто́рону look the óther way; смотре́ть в сто́рону *кого-л., чего-л.* look in the diréction of *smb., smth.;* look towárds *smb., smth.;* из ~ы́ в сто́рону from side to side; по ту сто́рону *чего-л.* on the óther side of *smth.,* beyónd *smth.;* на той ~е́ on the óther side; по ~а́м, по о́бе ~ы́ on éither side; по о́бе ~ы́ доро́ги on/alóng both sides of the road; смотре́ть по ~а́м look about one; со ~ы́ *чего-л.* from the diréction of *smth.;* дом не защищён со ~ы́ мо́ря the house is unprotécted on the side néarest/fácing the sea; в ~е́ от доро́ги at a cértain dístance from the road; лес оста́нется в ~е́ you will see the woods in the dístance; сверну́ть в сто́рону turn asíde; с ра́зных сторо́н from all/different diréctions; *(из разных источников)* from várious sóurces; с вну́тренней, нару́жной ~ы́ on the ínside, outsíde; посмотре́ть на *что-л.* со ~ы́ regárd *smth.* in a detáched spírit; 2. *(страна)* land; родна́я ~ nátive land, *one's* own cóuntry; на чужо́й ~е́ on fóreign soil, in fóreign parts; 3. *(вопроса, дела)* áspect; рассма́тривать вопро́с со всех сторо́н consíder a quéstion in all its áspects; си́льные и сла́бые сто́роны докла́да the strong and weak sides/áspects of a repórt; с како́й бы ~ы́ ни посмотре́ть whatéver way you look at it; 4. *(в переговорах, споре, на суде)* side, párty; быть на ~е́ *кого-л.* be* on the side of *smb.;* приня́ть сто́рону *кого-л.,* стать на сто́рону *кого-л.* take* *smb.'s* side, side with *smb.;* ◇ остава́ться в ~е́ hold* onesélf alóof, keep* alóof; держа́ться в ~е́ stand* asíde; на ~е́ élsewhére; прода́ть *что-л.* на́ ~у sell* *smth.* on the side; с чьей-л. ~ы́ on *smb.'s* part; о́чень ми́ло с ва́шей ~ы́ it is véry kind of you; с одно́й ~ы́..., с друго́й ~ы́... on the one hand... on the óther hand...

сторони́ться, посторони́ться 1. stand*/step asíde; посторони́сь! make way there!; 2. *тк. несов.* *(рд.; чужда́ться)* shun *(smb., smth.),* keep* awáy (from); ~ друзе́й shun/avóid *one's* friends.

сторо́нник *м.* suppórter, adhérent; *(чего-л.)* ádvocate, chámpion, uphólder; ~и ми́ра ádvocates/chámpions of peace; его́ немногочи́сленные ~и his small fóllowing.

стороно́й to one side; *перен.* in a róundabout way; идти́ ~ turn asíde; пройти́ ~ pass at a dístance.

сторублёвый húndred-rouble *attr.*

стоскова́ться *сов.* (по *дт., пр.) разг.* pine (for); be* lónging to see *(smb., smth.).*

сто́чн|ый: ~ые во́ды séwage *sg;* ~ая труба́ dráin-pipe; ~ая кана́ва ditch.

стошни́|ть *сов. безл.:* его́ ~и́ло he was sick, he vómited.

стоя́нка *ж.* 1. *(остановка)* stop; десятимину́тная ~ tén-minute stop; 2. *(место временного пребывания)* camp, encámpment; ~ зимо́вщиков winter camp; 3. *(стоя́ние автотранспорта)* párking; *(место, где стоят*

сто|я́ть *несов.* 1. stand*; *(находиться)* be*; приказа́ть *кому-л.* ~ на ме́сте tell* *smb.* to stand still; стул ~и́т на ме́сте the chair is in its úsual place; ~ на нога́х, рука́х, голове́ stand* on *one's* feet, hands, head; ~ на посту́, на часа́х be* on séntry dúty; ~ и смотре́ть, кури́ть, разгова́ривать *и т. д.* stand* lóoking, smóking, tálking, *etc.;* ~ на я́коре lie* at ánchor; по́езд ~и́т у пе́рвой платфо́рмы the train is at plátform one; таре́лки, стака́ны, ча́шки *и т. п.* ~ят на столе́, в шкафу́ the plates, glásses, cups, *etc.* are on the táble, in the cúpboard; ~ на чьём-л. пути́ stand* in *smb.'s* way; 2. *(бездействовать)* be* at a stándstill; часы́ ~ят the clock/watch has stopped; рабо́та ~ит work is at a stándstill; заво́д, маши́на ~и́т the fáctory, the machine is not wórking, the fáctory, the machine is ídle; 3. *(быть неподвижным, не двигаться)* stop; по́езд ~ит де́сять мину́т the train stops (for) ten mínutes; 4. *(быть расположенным)* be* sítuated, stand*, lie*; го́род ~ит на горе́ the town stands on a hill; дом ~и́т с XVIII ве́ка the house has been stánding since the XVIII céntury; 5. *(пе́ред тв.; о задаче и т. п.)* confrónt *(smb.);* пе́ред на́ми ~и́т зада́ча we are faced/confrónted with the próblem/task, we have befóre us the próblem/task; 6. *(быть)* be*; ~ят си́льные моро́зы there are cónstant sevére frosts, the sevére frosts contínue; ~ит хоро́шая пого́да the wéather is good; ~ял тяжёлый за́пах, стра́шный шум *и т. п.* there was an áwful smell, a fríghtful noise, *etc.;* 7. *(быть отмеченным, значиться)* be*; ~ в спи́ске be* on the list; внизу́ ~ит по́дпись there is a sígnature at the end; на пове́стке ~ят два вопро́са there are two quéstions on the agénda; 8. *(за вн.; защищать)* stand* up (for); ~ за пра́вду stand* up for the truth; ◇ ~ во главе́ head, be* at the head (of); ~ у вла́сти be* in pówer, have* the pówer; ~ на своём insíst; stand* *one's* ground; ~ на стра́же ми́ра defénd the cause of peace; ~ над чьей-л. душо́й stand* óver *smth.,* breathe down *smb.'s* neck; ~ за спино́й у *кого-л.* ~ за кем-л. 1) *(быть, иметься)* have* *smth.* behínd one; 2) *(тайно покрови́тельствовать)* be* behínd *smb.*

стоя́ч|ий 1. stánding; ~ воротни́к stánd-up cóllar; 2. *(о воде)* stágnant; ~ие пруды́ stágnant ponds.

сто́ящ|ий *разг.* worthwhíle; ~ая вещь, ~ее де́ло something worth while, a good thing.

страда́ *ж.* hárvest-time.

страда́л|ец *м.,* ~ица *ж.* súfferer.

страда́льческ|ий of súffering *после сущ.;* ~ая жизнь life of súffering/woe; ~ вид look of súffering.

страда́ни|е *с.* súffering *(тж. мн.);* причиня́ть ~я cause/inflíct súffering.

страда́тельный *грам.:* ~ зало́г pássive voice; ~ оборо́т pássive constrúction.

страда́ть, пострада́ть 1. *тк. несов.* *(тв.; какой-л. болезнью)* súffer (from), be* tróubled (by); ~ головны́ми боля́ми súffer from héadaches; ~ самомне́нием súffer from vánity; 2. *тк. несов.* *(от рд.; мучиться)* súffer (from); ~ от зубно́й бо́ли súffer from a tóothache; ~ от любви́ súffer the tórments of love; 3. *(за вн., из-за рд.; претерпевать муки из-за кого-л., чего-л.)* súffer (for); ~ за пра́вду súffer for the truth; 4. *(от рд.; испытывать лишения)* súffer (through), expérience tróuble/difficulties/hárdship (becáuse of); 5. *(от, из-за рд.; терпеть ущерб)* be* dámaged (by), be* impáired (by); 6. *тк. несов. разг. (быть плохим)* be* weak; у него́ страда́ет орфогра́фия he is weak in spélling.

страж *м.* guard.

стра́ж|а *ж.* watch, guard; ◇ быть, стоя́ть на ~е *чего-л.* watch óver *smth.,* stand* guard óver *smth.;* быть, находи́ться под ~ей be* únder guard, be* in cústody; брать *кого-л.* под ~у take* *smb.* into cústody.

стран|а́ ж. cóuntry, land; Страна́ Сове́тов the Land of the Sóviets; по всей ~е́ throughóut the cóuntry; положе́ние в ~е́ the intérnal situátion; в чужо́й ~е́ in fóreign parts; ◇ стра́ны све́та the cárdinal points (of the cómpass).

страни́ц|а ж. 1. page; ~ пе́рвая, втора́я, деся́тая и т. д. page one, two, ten, *etc.*; на пе́рвой ~е on the first page; откры́ть кни́гу на деся́той ~е ópen the book at page ten; 2. (*чего-л., в чём-л.*) leaf*, chápter; лу́чшая ~ чьей-л. жи́зни the finest chápter of *smb.'s* life; ◇ на ~ах на́шей газе́ты in our cólumns; вписа́ть но́вую ~у во что-л. add a fresh page *to smth.*

стра́нн|ик м., ~ица ж. 1. wánderer; 2. *уст.* pílgrim.

стра́нн|о 1. *нареч.* strángely; он ~ ведёт себя́ he is ácting strángely; 2. *в знач. сказ. безл.* it is strange/cúrious/odd; мне ~, что... it strikes me as cúrious that...; ~, что никто́ не зна́ет об э́том it's strange/odd that no one should know abóut it; мне ~ э́то that strikes me as strange; как э́то ни ~ strange though it may seem. ~ость ж. strángeness; (*странная черта́*) óddity; (*странное явле́ние*) strange thing; ~ость взгля́дов strange opínions; челове́к со ~остями ráther eccéntric pérson; queer fish *разг.*; что за ~ость! how queer/fúnny/strange! ~ый 1. strange, odd; queer, fúnny *разг.*; ~ый вы челове́к you're a strange pérson; (*о мужчи́не тж.*) you're a queer chap; мне ка́жется ~ым, что... it strikes me as cúrious that...; са́мое ~ое в э́том то, что... the strángest part of it is that..; ◇ ~ое де́ло! queer!, fúnny!, strange!; ~ое де́ло, я э́того не заме́тил strange to say, I dídn't nótice it.

странове́дение *с.* régional geógraphy; área stúdies *pl.*

стра́нств|ие *с.*, ~ование *с.* wándering. ~овать *несов.* wánder.

стра́нствующ|ий wándering; ~ие музыка́нты strólling musícians.

стра́стно pássionately, with pássion; (*пылко*) árdently, enthusiástically; ~ люби́ть *что-л.* be* inténsely/pássionately fond of *smth.*

страстн|о́й *церк.*: ~а́я неде́ля Hóly Week.

страстн|ость ж. pássion, árdour; ~ нату́ры, хара́ктера pássionate/árdent témperament. ~ый 1. (*пылкий*) impássioned, árdent; ~ая речь impássioned speech; ~ый ора́тор impássioned spéaker; 2. (*увлечённый чем-л.*) enthusiástic; ~ый люби́тель му́зыки a músic enthúsiast; 3. (*способный к си́льной любви́*) pássionate, árdent.

страст|ь I ж. pássion; разжига́ть ~и fire the pássions; ~ к теа́тру pássion for the théatre; цветы́ — моя́ ~ I adóre flówers; мгнове́нная ~ fléeting pássion.

страст|ь II ж. *обыкн. мн. разг.* (*ужас*) hórrors; каки́е ~и! how térrible/hórrible/ghástly!

страте́г *м.* strátegist.

стратеги́ческий stratégic(al).

страте́гия ж. (grand) strátegy (*тж. перен.*); (*наука тж.*) stratégics.

стратона́вт *м.* strátosphere pílot/flíer.

стратоста́т *м.* stratosphéric ballóon. ~сфе́ра ж. strátosphere.

стра́ус *м. зоол.* óstrich.

страх *м.* fear; (*перед бу́дущим тж.*) dread; (*ужас*) térror; ~ сме́рти fear of death; смерте́льный ~ mórtal fear; ~ перед неизве́стностью fear/dread of the unknówn; быть в ~е be* térrified; из ~а перед кем-л., чем-л. for fear of *smb., smth.*; от ~а with fear; от ~а у него́ отня́лся язы́к he was spéechless with térror; натерпе́ться ~у be* térrified, have* a térrible fright; испы́тывать ~ перед кем-л. be* térrified of *smb.*, dread *smb.*; ◇ под ~ом сме́рти únder pain of death; под ~ом суро́вых наказа́ний únder pain of sevére pénalties; у ~а глаза́ велики́ *погов.* fear sees dánger éverywhere; на свой ~ (и риск) at *one's* own risk, on *one's* own responsibílity.

страхова́|ние *с.* insúrance; ~ жи́зни life insúrance; ~ иму́щества insúrance of próperty; ~ от несча́стных слу-

ча́ев áccident insúrance, госуда́рственное ~ State insúrance; социа́льное ~ sócial insúrance. ~тель *м.* insúred (pérson), pólicy-holder.

страх|ова́ть, застрахова́ть 1. (*вн. от рд.*) insúre (*smb., smth.* against) (*тж. перен.*); 2. тк. несов. (*вн.; предохраня́ть*) provide sáfety méasures (for), ensúre the sáfety (of); ~ гимна́ста ensúre the sáfety of a gýmnast. ~ова́ться, застрахова́ться 1. insúre *one's* life; 2. (*быть кра́йне осторо́жным*) keep* on the safe side. ~о́вка ж. insúrance; (*страхова́я пре́мия тж.*) compensátion, indémnity. ~ово́й insúrance *attr.*; ~ово́й по́лис insúrance pólicy; ~ово́й фонд insúrance fund. ~о́вщик *м. разг.* insúrer.

страши́лище *с. разг.* fright.

страш|и́ть *несов.* (*вн.*) fríghten (*smb.*), appál (*smb.*); меня́ ~и́т мысль об э́том I am appálled at the thought of it, I trémble to think of it. ~и́ться *несов.* (*рд.*) fear (*smb., smth.*), dread (*smb., smth.*).

стра́шн|о 1. *нареч.* térribly, áwfully; ~ боя́ться *чего-л.* be* térribly afráid of *smth.*; ~ испуга́ться get* a térrible fright; ~ обра́доваться be* áwfully glad; мне ~ хо́чется (+ *инф.*) I'm símply lónging (+ to *inf*); 2. *в знач. сказ. безл.* (*дт.*): мне ~! I'm afráid!, I'm fríghtened; I'm símply térrified; ~ поду́мать, что... it is an áwful thought that..., it is áwful to think that...; мне ~ поду́мать, что... I can't bear to think...; здесь ~ остава́ться it is dángerous to remáin here. ~ый *прил.* 1. térrible; (*ужа́сный тж.*) fríghtful, dréadful; ~ый расска́з blóod-curdling tale; (*де́тский*) fríghtening stóry; ~ый путь térrible jóurney; 2. *разг.* (*о́чень си́льный*) térrible; ~ый хо́лод térrible cold; ~ая ску́ка dréadful bóredom; ~ый на́сморк fríghtful cold; ~ая боль agónizing/térrible pain; 3. *в знач. сущ. с.*: са́мое ~ое what one dreads most; ◇ сде́лать ~ые глаза́ give* a wárning look.

стрекоза́ ж. drágon-fly.

стрекота́ние *с.* (*насеко́мых*) chírping; (*соро́ки*) chátter (*тж. перен.*); (*мото́ра*) chúgging.

стрекота́ть *несов.* (*о насеко́мых*) chirp, chírrup; (*о соро́ке*) chátter (*тж. перен.*); (*о мото́ре*) chug.

стрел|а́ ж. 1. árrow; *перен. тж.* shaft; пусти́ть ~у́ в кого́-л. shoot* an árrow at *smb.*; 2. (*ве́сов и т. п.*) arm; 3. (*подъёмного кра́на*) jib, crane arm, boom; (*приспособле́ние для подъёма тя́жестей*) dérrick.

стре́лк|а ж. 1. (*часо́в*) hand; (*ко́мпаса*) néedle; (*прибо́ра*) póinter; магни́тная ~ magnétic/dípping néedle; 2. ж.-д. points *pl*; switch; переводи́ть ~у switch óver the points; 3. (*на чертеже́, указа́тельная*) árrow; 4. (*чулка́*) clock.

стрелко́в|ый shóoting; *воен.* rífle *attr.*; (*пехо́тный*) ínfantry *attr.*; ~ая ро́та ínfantry cómpany.

стрело́к *м.* 1. márksman*; хоро́ший, отли́чный ~ good/crack shot; 2. *воен.* ínfantryman*; *ав.* gúnner.

стре́лочник *м.* póintsman*; switchman* *амер.*

стрельб|а́ ж. 1. shóoting, fíring; откры́ть ~у́ ópen fire; ~ прямо́й наво́дкой fire, fire óver ópen sights; ~ непрямо́й наво́дкой indírect fire; 2. *мн. воен.* (*уче́бные вы́стрелы*) shóoting práctice *sg.*

стре́льбище *с.* shóoting-range.

стрельну́ть *сов. см.* стреля́ть 1, 3.

стрел|я́ть, стрельну́ть 1. shoot* (at), fire (at); ~ в цель shoot* at a tárget; do* tárget práctice; ~ из винто́вки, пу́шки *и т. п.* fire a rífle, gun, *etc.*; стой, ~ бу́ду! halt, or I fire!; 2. *тк. несов.* (*вн.; убива́ть на охо́те*) shoot* (*smth.*); ~ у́ток shoot* duck; 3. *безл. разг.* (*о бо́ли*): у меня́ ~́ет в у́хе I have shóoting pains in my ear; ◇ ~ из пу́шки по воробья́м ≈ break* a bútterfly on the wheel; ~ глаза́ми make* eyes. ~я́ться *несов. разг.* 1. (*стреля́ть в себя́*) shoot* onesélf; 2. *уст.* (*на дуэ́ли*) fight* a dúel.

стремгла́в héadlong.

стреми́тельн|о rápidly, véhemently, impétuously; ~ развива́ющаяся жизнь impétuous life. ~ость ж.

(líghtning) speed, impetuósity; (*речи, характера*) véhemence. ~ый 1. (*очень быстрый*) rápid, fást-moving, impétuous; ~ый нáтиск víolent ónslaught; ~ый порýв irrepréssible ímpulse; 2. (*энергичный*) impétuous, dynámic, energétic; ~ый человéк energétic pérson, dynámic personálity; 3. (*выражающий устремлённость к чему-л.*) thrílling, stírring.

стрем|и́ться *несов.* 1. (*стараться попасть куда-л.*) long to go, have* an urge to go, feel* drawn; ~ на юг long to go south; ~ на сцéну feel* drawn to the stage; 2. (*к дт., + инф.*) try to attáin (smth.), strive* (for, áfter); (*к славе, свободе и т. п.*) aspíre (to); ~ к цéли try to attáin one's óbject; ~ к свобóде strive* for fréedom. ~лéние *с.* 1. (*к дт.*) aspirátion (for), desíre (for); в своём ~лéнии к... in his strívings áfter...; ~лéние к счáстью desíre for háppiness; 2. *мн.* (*помыслы, желания*) aspirátions.

стремни́на *ж.* (*реки*) máinstream, fast wáter.

стрéмя *с.* stírrup; вдеть нóгу в ~ put* one's foot in the stírrup.

стремя́нка *ж.* (stép-)ládder.

стренóжить *сов. см.* тренóжить.

стресс *м.* stress.

стрéссовый stress *attr.*

стриж *м.* swift.

стри́жен|ый cut, cropped; (*о деревьях*) clípped; (*об овцах*) sheared, shorn; ~ые вóлосы short hair; ~ая головá cropped head.

стри́жк|а *ж.* 1. (*действие*) cútting; (*овец*) shéaring; (*собак, деревьев*) clípping; маши́нка для ~и clíppers *pl*; shears *pl*; 2. (*способ подстригания волос*) háircut; мóдная ~ fáshionable háircut.

стриптиз *м.* stríptease, strip show.

стричь *несов.* (*вн.*) cut* (smth.); (*собак, деревья*) clip (smth.); (*овец*) shear* (smth.); ~ когó-л. cut* smb.'s hair. ~ся *несов.* have* a háircut, have* one's hair cut.

строгáть *несов.* (*вн.*) plane (smth.); (*изготовлять*) make* (smth.).

строг|ий 1. (*требовательный*) strict; (*суровый тж.*) sevére, stern, rígorous; ~ учи́тель stern/sevére téacher; ~ кри́тик sevére crític; ~ая кри́тика sevére críticism; ~ тон sevére tone/voice; ~ вы́говор sevére réprimand; ~ие мéры rígorous/stern méasures; ~ закóн strict/stríngent law; ~ая дисципли́на strict díscipline; 2. (*выполняемый точно*) strict; ~ая диéта strict díet; ~ая эконóмия strict/rígid ecónomy; ~ поря́док, надзóр strict órder, supervísion; ~ая послéдовательность ábsolute consístency, strict séquence; в ~ом соотвéтствии с чем-л. in strict accórdance with smth.; в ~ом смы́сле слóва in the strict sense of the term; 3. (*морально чистый*) strict, austére, unbénding; ~ие взгля́ды (*на жизнь*) strict views; ~ие нрáвы strict mórals; ~ое поведéние austérity of one's cónduct; 4. (*правильный*) austére, clean, clean-cút; ~ие ли́нии clean/cool lines; ~ие чертá лицá austére féatures; ~ профи́ль clean-cút prófile; 5. (*без украшений*) sevére, restráined, unadórned; ~ костю́м quiet suit; ~ая причёска sevére háirstyle.

строг|о 1. (*сурово*) sevérely, stérnly; ~ наказáть когó-л. púnish smb. sevérely; ~ поговори́ть с кем-л. speak* sevérely to smb.; ~ обращáться с кем-л. treat smb. rígorously; 2. (*точно*) stríctly; ~ вы́держанный стиль consístency of style; 3. (*классически правильно*) sevérely, austérely; ~ одевáться dress sevérely; ◇ ~ воспрещáется stríctly forbídden; ~ говоря́ stríctly spéaking; ~-нáстрого stríctly. ~ость *ж.* 1. stríctness, sevérity; держáть когó-л. в ~ости keep* smb. well in hand; keep* a strict hand óver smb.; поступáть с кем-л. по всей ~ости закóна apply* all the rígours of the law to smb.; 2. *мн. разг.* (*строгие меры*) rígorous/sevére méasures.

строевóй I: ~ лес (stánding) tímber; ~ материáл búilding matérial.

строев|óй II *воен.* 1. drill *attr.*; ~áя подготóвка drill;

~óе учéние fórmal drill; ~ устáв drill regulátions/mánual; 2. (*предназначенный для ведения боевых действий*) cómbatant, frónt-line *attr.*; ~ офицéр cómbatant ófficer; ~áя слýжба frónt-line sérvice.

строéние *с.* 1. (*здание, постройка*) búilding; 2. (*структура*) strúcture.

строи́тель *м.* búilder (*тж. перен.*). ~ный búilding *attr.*, constrúction *attr.*; ~ные материáлы búilding matérials; ~ная площáдка búilding site; ~ная тéхника constrúction enginéering. ~ство *с.* 1. (*процесс*) búilding (*тж. перен.*); constrúction; ~ство жилы́х домóв búilding/eréction of (dwélling) hóuses, hóusing; 2. (*объект*) próject, devélopment.

стрóить, пострóить 1. (*вн.*) build* (smth.) (*тж. перен.*); (*машины и т. п.*) make* (smth.); ~ мост build* a bridge; ~ турби́ны make* túrbines; 2. *мат.* constrúct (smth.); ~ треугóльник constrúct a tríangle; ~ ýгол plot an ángle; 3. (*вн.; создавать, составлять что-л.*) constrúct (smth.), build* up (smth.), make* up (smth.); (*организовать*) órganize (smth.); ~ предложéние, фрáзу constrúct a séntence; ~ лéкцию plan a lécture; 4. (*вн.; намечать мысленно*) devíse (smth.), make* (smth.); ~ плáны build*/make* plans; 5. (*вн. на пр.; основывать на чём-л.*) base (smth. on); ~ свои́ расчёты на чём-л. base one's calculátions on smth., bank on smth.; 6. (*вн.; ставить в строй*) form (smth.), form up (smb., smth.), draw* up (smb., smth.); ~ взвод в две шерéнги form up a platóon in dóuble file; ◇ ~ воздýшные зáмки build* cástles in the air; ~ рóжи make* fáces; ~ из себя́ когó-л. make* onesélf out smb. ~ся, пострóиться 1. (*строить себе что-л.*) build* onesélf a house; 2. (*воздвигаться*) be* únder constrúction, be* góing up; *перен.* (*созидаться*) be* béing built, be* in the máking; 3. *тк. несов.* (*намечаться в уме*) be* made; стрóились предположéния guésses were made (as to), there was much speculátion (as to); 4. *тк. несов.* (*на пр.; основываться*) be* built (on), be* fóunded (on), rest (on); 5. (*становиться в строй*) form, take* up formátion, draw* up.

стро|й *м.* 1. (*ряд, шеренга*) formátion; встать в ~ form up; 2. (*система построения чего-л.*) strúcture, páttern; граммати́ческий ~ языкá grammátical strúcture of a lánguage; ~ мышлéния páttern of thínking; 3. (*система общественного устройства*) sýstem, órder; 4. *муз.* pitch; ◇ вводи́ть что-л. в ~ put* smth. into sérvice, put* smth. into operátion; start óperating smth.; выводи́ть что-л. из ~я put* smth. out of áction; вступáть в ~ (о предприятии*) be* put into operátion; вы́йти из ~я break* down, be* put out of áction.

стрóйка *ж.* 1. (*действие*) búilding, constrúction; 2. (*объект строительства*) (búilding) próject.

строй|ность *ж.* 1. (*фигуры*) grácefulness, slénderness; (*рядов*) órderliness, sýmmetry; 2. (*мысли, изложения*) sýmmetry, grace; 3. (*гармоничность*) hármony, melódiousness; ~ пéния the pérfect hármony of the sínging. ~ный 1. gráceful, shápely, well-propórtioned; (*тонкий*) slénder; ~ая фигýра shápely fígure; ~ая дéвушка slénder girl; ~ый тóполь gráceful póplar; 2. (*правильно расположенный*) symmétrical, régular; ~ые ряды́ régular cólumns; 3. (*чёткий, последовательный*) well-bálanced, órderly; ~ая теóрия well-bálanced théory; 4. (*о звучании*) harmónious; ~ое пéние harmónious sínging.

строкá *ж.* line; нóвая ~ (new) páragraph.

стрóнций *м. хим.* stróntium.

строп *м.* 1. (*аэростата, парашюта*) (stroud) line; 2. (*петля для захвата груза*) sling.

стропи́ло *с.* ráfter.

стропти́вый refráctory, wílful, óbstinate.

строфá *ж. лит.* stánza.

строчи́ть, настрочи́ть 1. *тк. несов.* (*вн.; шить*) stitch (smth.); 2. *разг.* (*писать*) scríbble; 3. *тк. несов. разг.* (*стрелять*) blaze awáy.

стро́чка I ж. см. строка́.

стро́чка II ж. 1. (действие) stítching; 2. (шов) seam.

строчн|о́й: ~а́я бу́ква small létter; полигр. lówer case létter.

стро́ящийся únder constrúction после сущ.

стру́жка ж. 1. sháving; 2. собир. shávings pl.

струи́ться несов. stream (тж. перен.); run* down.

стру́йка ж. см. струя́ 1.

структу́р|а ж. strúcture; организацио́нная ~ scheme of organizátion. ~ный strúctural.

струна́ ж. string; ударя́ть по стру́нам run* one's fingers óver the strings, pluck the strings.

стру́нк|а ж.: чувстви́тельная ~ ténder spot; задева́ть сла́бую ~у кого́-л. touch smb. on a ténder spot; вы́тянуться в ~у stand* (stíffly) eréct; ходи́ть по ~e toe the line.

стру́нный stringed; string attr.; ~ инструме́нт stringed ínstrument; мн. тж. the strings; ~ кварте́т string quartét; ~ орке́стр string órchestra.

струп м. scab.

стру́сить сов. см. тру́сить.

стручко́в|ый legúminous; ~ пе́рец cápsicum; ~ая фасо́ль French beans pl.

стручо́к м. pod.

стру|я́ ж. 1. (текущая) stream; (бьющая) jet, spurt; ~ све́жего во́здуха cúrrent of fresh air; ~ па́ра steam jet; ~ от винта́ ав. (propéller) slípstream; бить ~ёй spurt; 2. (направление, черта) cúrrent; све́жая ~ fresh cúrrent; вноси́ть све́жую ~ю во что́-л. injéct new life into smth.; попа́сть в ~ю swim with the cúrrent.

стря́п|ать, состря́пать (вн.) разг. cook (smth.); перен. concóct (smth.), fábricate (smth.). ~ня́ ж. разг. cóoking; перен. concóction.

стряс|ти́сь сов. (с тв.) разг. háppen (to); с ним ~ла́сь беда́ he is in tróuble; (в прошлом) he got ínto tróuble, tróuble overtóok him; что тут ~ло́сь? what's up?, what's the mátter?

стря́хивать, стряхну́ть (вн.) shake* (smth.) off (тж. перен.); ~ пе́пел с папиро́сы flick the ash off one's cigaré́tte.

стряхну́ть сов. см. стря́хивать.

студе́нт м., ~ка ж. stúdent; (в университе́те тж.) undergráduate; ~-ме́дик médical stúdent; ~-юри́ст láw-stúdent.

студе́нче|ский stúdent's; ~ские го́ды one's cóllege days; ~ское общежи́тие stúdents' hóstel. ~ство с. 1. собир. the stúdents pl, the undergráduates pl; the stúdent bódy; 2. (пребывание в вузе) one's stúdent years pl, one's time at the univérsity; в го́ды моего́ ~ства in my cóllege days.

студёный разг. ícy, chill; ~ го́рный ручей ́ ícy móuntain stream.

сту́день м. áspic jélly; (из рыбы тж.) fish jélly; (из теля́чьих но́жек) calves' foot jélly.

студи́ть, остуди́ть (вн.) разг. cool (smth.), chill (smth.); let* (smth.) get cold; вы́студить ко́мнату make* the room cold.

сту́дия ж. 1. (мастерская) stúdio; 2. (школа) school; бале́тная ~ bállet school; худо́жественная ~ art school; 3. (творческий коллектив) school.

стужа ж. разг. ícy cold.

стук м. knócking; (один удар) knock; (лёгкий) tap; ~ в дверь knóck(ing) at the door; войти́ без ~а come* in withóut knócking; ~ колёс clátter of wheels; ~ копы́т beat of hoofs; ~ пи́шущих маши́нок tápping of týpewriters; ~ посу́ды, ноже́й rátle of plates, cútlery; ~ се́рдца thróbbing/béating of the heart.

сту́кать, сту́кнуть 1. knock; (тихо) tap; сту́кнуть по́ столу bang on the táble; кто́-то ти́хо сту́кнул sómebody tapped on the wíndow; 2. (вн.; ударять) hit* (smb., smth.), strike* (smb., smth.). ~ся, сту́кнуться (о,

обо вн.) knock (against), bang (against); сту́кнуться голово́й обо что́-л. bang/bump one's head agáinst smth.

сту́кн|уть(ся) сов. см. сту́кать(ся).

стул м. 1. chair; 2. мед. stool; ◇ сиде́ть ме́жду двух ~ьев fall* betwéen two stools.

стульча́к м. lávatory seat.

сту́п|а ж. mórtar; ◇ толо́чь во́ду в ~е mill the air.

сту́п|а́ть, ступи́ть 1. tread*, step; 2. тк. несов. (де́лать шаги, идти́) tread*, walk; 3. тк. несов. повел.: ~а́й(те)! go!; ~а́й(те) прочь! take yourself off!; off with you!; ~а́й(те) за ним! fóllow him!; ◇ ша́гу ступи́ть нельзя́ без кого́-л., чего́-л. you dáren't take a step withóut smb., smth.

ступе́нчатый stepped; (о раке́тах) stage attr., múlti-stage attr.

ступе́нь ж. 1. (ле́стницы) step; 2. (э́тап в разви́тии чего́-л.) stage; 3. (степень, уровень) degrée, grade, lével; вы́сшая ~ the híghest lével; подня́ть что́-л. на бо́лее высо́кую ~ raise smth. to a hígher lével; ~ degrée; ◇ ~ раке́ты stage (of a rócket); 4. муз. degrée.

ступе́нька ж. step; (приставно́й ле́стницы тж.) rung; поднима́ться (спуска́ться) по ~м go* up (go* down) the steps.

ступи́ть сов. 1. см. ступа́ть 1; 2. (на вн.; войти́ куда́-л.) énter (smth.), set* foot (on).

ступи́ца ж. hub, boss; ~ колеса́ hub of a wheel, wheel boss.

сту́пка ж. см. сту́па.

ступня́ ж. foot*.

стуч|а́ть несов. tap, knock; (гро́мко) bang, pound; (о копы́тах, колёсах) clátter; (о зуба́х) chátter; (о се́рдце) throb, thud; ~ в дверь knock at the door; ~ кулака́ми в дверь hang/pound on the door with one's fists; ~ молотко́м hámmer; ~ на маши́нке pound away at the týpewriter, bang the týpewriter; он ~и́т зуба́ми от хо́лода his teeth are chátering with cold; дождь ~и́т в окно́ the rain is béating agáinst the wíndow; у меня́ ~и́т в виска́х I have a thróbbing in my témples. ~ться несов. knock; ~ться в дверь knock at the door; (обраща́ться с про́сьбой тж.) make* the rounds (of).

стушева́ться сов. разг. 1. (сгла́диться) melt awáy; (отступи́ть на за́дний план) keep* onesélf in the báckground; 2. (смути́ться, оробе́ть) lose* one's nerve.

стыд м. shame; ~ и позо́р! it's a disgráce!; ~ и позо́р ему́! shame on him!; ~ и срам! for shame!; к вели́кому моему́ ~у́ I must conféss to my shame..., to my shame be it said...; не име́ть ни ~а́ ни со́вести be* dead to shame; потеря́ть вся́кий ~ lose* all sense of shame.

стыд|и́ть несов. (вн.) try to bring (smb.) to a sense of shame, put* (smb.) to shame; ~ кого́-л. за что́-л. repróach smb. for smth., scold smb. for smth. ~и́ться (рд., + инф.) be* ashámed (of, + to inf.); (стесня́ться тж.) be* shy (of); ~и́(те)сь! shame!, you ought to be ashámed of yoursélf!

стыдли́в|ость ж. báshfulness, módesty. ~ый báshful, módest.

сты́дно в знач. сказ. безл.: ~ так поступа́ть, говори́ть you ought to be ashámed of beháving, tálking like that; мне ~ (за себя́) I am ashámed of mysélf; мне ~ за вас I am ashámed of you; мне ~ перед людьми́ I am ashámed to face the world, I am ashámed to look péople in the face; как вам не ~! you ought to be ashámed of yoursélf!, áren't you ashámed (of yoursélf)?; ему́ ничу́ть не ~ he is not a bit ashámed.

стык м. 1. joint; (ли́ния соприкоснове́ния) júnction, bóundary (betwéen); 2. тех. butt, seam.

стыкова́ться несов. join; (о косми́ческих корабля́х) dock, réndezvous.

стыко́вка ж. jóining, línk-up; (о косми́ческих корабля́х) dócking, réndezvous.

сты́нуть, стыть несов. 1. be* gétting cold, cool; пе-

рен. be* cóoling down; 2. (*замерзать*) freeze*, be* frózen.

стычка *ж.* 1. (*бой*) skírmish, brush; 2. (*ссора*) tiff.

стюард *м.* stéward.

стюардёсса *ж.* stéwardess; (*на самолёте тж.*) air hóstess.

стяг *м.* bánner.

стягивать, стянуть (*вн.*) 1. (*затягивать, завязывать*) fásten (*smth.*), make* (*smth.*) fast; ~ тáлию ремнём fasten one's belt tíghtly; ~ мешóк верёвкой tie up a sack; 2. (*соединять концы, края чего-л.*) join (*smth.*), gáther (*smth.*), draw* (*smth.*) togéther; стянуть концы обóрванного прóвода join the bróken ends of wíre; 3. (*собирать в одно место*) cóncentrate (*smb., smth.*), assémble (*smb., smth.*); 4. (*таща, снимать*) pull off (*smth.*), draw* off (*smth.*); pull down (*smth.*); (*сдвигать с места*) move (*smth.*); стянуть скáтерть со столá pull the cloth off the táble; стянуть сапоги pull off one's boots. ~ся, стянуться 1. (*туго затягиваться*) draw* tight; (*поясом и т. п.*) tíghten one's belt; 2. (*смыкаться концами*) join, mend; (*собираться, морщиться*) gáther, crimp, wrínkle; 3. (*собираться в одно место*) cóncentrate.

стяжáтель *м.* móney-grubber, grábber. ~ство *с.* móney-grubbing.

стяжáть *несов. и сов.* (*вн.*) acquíre (*smth.*); (*славу, любовь и т. п.*) win* (*smth.*); ~ извéстность win*/gain renówn.

стянуть *сов.* 1. *см.* **стягивать**; 2. (*вн.*) *разг.* (*украсть*) take* (*smth.*), pinch (*smth.*). ~ся *сов. см.* **стягиваться**.

суббóт|а *ж.* Sáturday. ~ник *м.* subbótnik (*voluntary, unpaid work performed collectively*).

сублимáция *ж.* sublimátion.

субординáция *ж.* (*system of*) seniórity.

субсидировать *несов. и сов.* (*вн.*) súbsidize (*smb., smth.*); ~ стройтельство súbsidize building.

субсидия *ж.* súbsidy.

субтитр *м. кино* súbtitle.

субтрóп|ики *мн.* súbtropical zone *sg.* ~ический súbtropical.

субъéкт *м.* 1. súbject; 2. *разг.* (*о человеке*) indivídual, type.

субъект|ивизм *м.* subjéctivism. ~ивный subjéctive.

сувенир *м.* sóuvenir, kéepsake.

суверенитéт *м.* sóvereignty.

суверéнн|ый sóvereign; ~ое госудáрство sóvereign state.

суворов|ец *м.* púpil at a Suvórov Military Cóllege. ~ский: ~ское училище Suvórov Military Cóllege.

суглинист|ый lóamy; ~ая пóчва lóamy/loam soil.

суглинок *м.* loam.

сугрóб *м.* snówdrift.

сугубо espécially, particularly; exclúsively.

сугубый particular, spécial.

суд *м.* 1. (*государственный орган*) (láw-)court, court of law, court of jústice; ~ низшей инстáнции mínor court; здáние ~á cóurt-house; зал ~á cóurt(-room); 2. (*разбирательство дел*) tríal; на ~é in court, at/dúring the tríal; попáсть под ~ be* brought to tríal; идти под ~ be* prósecuted, be* tried; быть под ~óм be* únder tríal; 3. (*общественный орган*) court; ~ чéсти court of hónour; 4. (*суждение*) júdgement; (*заключение, оценка*) vérdict; ~ нарóда pópular vérdict; ~ потóмства the vérdict of postérity.

судáк *м.* (*рыба*) píke-perch, zánder.

судáн|ец *м.* ~ка *ж.* Sudanése. ~ский Sudanése.

судéбн|ый 1. court *attr.*; (*подлежащий ведению суда тж.*) légal, judícial; ~ые óрганы judicial bódies; ~ое заседáние court séssion; ~ое дéло case; ~ процéсс tríal; ~ое слéдствие judicial inquiry/investigátion; ~ пригово́р court vérdict; ~ая прáктика judicial práctice; ~ые издéр-

жки (láw-)costs; 2. (*связанный с ведением следствия и суда*) forénsic; ~ая медицина médical jurisprúdence, forénsic médicine; ~ая химия forénsic chémistry.

судéйск|ий 1. júdge's; ~ая коллéгия judiciary board; 2. *спорт.* referée's, úmpire's.

судимост|ь *ж.* prévious convíction, criminal récord; имéть две ~и have* two prévious convíctions; снять ~ с когó-л. strike* all prévious convíctions off *smb.'s* récord, ignóre *smb.'s* prévious convíctions.

суд|ить *несов.* 1. (*вн.*) try (*smb.*), judge (*smb.*); 2. (*о пр.; составлять себе мнение*) judge (*smb., smth.*); ~ по внéшнему виду judge by appéarances; éсли ~ по егó словáм... to judge from what he says...; я не могу ~ об этом I'm no judge of that; наскóлько я могу ~ as far as I can judge; не вам ~ меня it is not for you to pass júdgement on me; 3. *спорт.* referée (*smth.*), úmpire (*smth.*); ~ футбóльный матч referée (at) a fóotball match; ◇ судя по чему-л. júdging by *smth.*; судя по всему́ éverything seems to índicate that; судя по его́ словáм accórding to him. ~иться *несов.* 1. go* to law; (*с тв.*) have* légal procéedings (with), lítigate (with); 2. (*иметь судимость*) have* a críminal récord, have* been convícted in court.

сýдно I *с.* véssel; (*морское тж.*) ship; (*малое тж.*) craft (*тж. pl*); (*речное тж.*) boat.

сýдно II *с.* (*для больного*) bédpan.

судовéрфь *ж.* shípyard.

судовладéлец *м.* shíp-owner.

судовождéние *с.* navigátion.

судовóй ship's.

судóк *м.* 1. (*столовый прибор*) crúet(-stand); 2. (*для соусов*) sáuce-boat, dish; 3. *мн.* (*для переноски кушанья*) lúnch-pail *sg.*

судомóйка *ж.* wásher-up, kítchen-help.

судопроизвóдство *с. юр.* légal procédure; légal procéedings *pl.*

судорéмонтн|ый shíp-repair *attr.*; ~ые мастерскúе shíp-repair shops.

сýдоро|га *ж.* convúlsion, cramp; егó лицó стáло сводúть от ~ги his face was seized by a convúlsion. ~жный convúlsive (*тж. перен.*); (*беспокойный, лихорадочный*) héctic.

судострo|éние *с.* shípbuilding. ~итель *м.* shípbuilder. ~ительный shípbuilding *attr.*; ~ительная верфь shípyard; ~ительная промышленность shípbuilding industry.

судоустрóйство *с. юр.* judicial system.

судохóд|ность *ж.* navigability. ~ный návigable; ~ный канáл ship-canal; ~ная рекá návigable ríver. ~ство *с.* navigátion.

судьб|á *ж.* 1. fate; благодарúть ~ý thank fate; thank one's lúcky stars *разг.*; 2. (*участь, доля*) lot, life*; связáть свою́ ~ý с кем-л. throw* in one's lot with *smb.*; устрóить свою́ ~ý arránge one's life; 3. *обыкн. мн.* (*будущность*) fúture *sg*; судьбы человéчества future of humánity/man; ~ видно, не ~! it was not to be!; не ~ нам встрéтиться we are not déstined to meet; какúми ~ми? what brings you here?; вóлею судéб it is one's fate.

судья *м.* 1. judge; нарóдный ~ judge of the Péople's Court; я не ~ в этом дéле I am no judge (of such mátters); вы мне не ~ who are you to judge me?; он вам не ~ it is not him to judge you; 2. *спорт.* referée, úmpire.

суевéр|ие *с.* superstítion. ~ный superstítious.

суетá *ж.* fuss; (*беготня тж.*) bústle; поднялáсь ~ there was a great fuss/bústle.

суетúться *несов.* fuss abóut, bústle.

суетлúв|ость *ж.* réstlessness, fússiness; bústle. ~ый 1. (*беспокойный*) réstless, fússy; 2. (*торопливый*) bústling, flúrried.

сужáть(ся) *несов. см.* **сýживать(ся)**.

сужде́ние *с.* 1. (*мнение*) opínion; (*решение*) júdgement; 2. *лог.* státement, propositíon.

суже́ние *с.* 1. (*действие*) nárrowing, contráction; ~ пищево́да contráction of the gúllet; 2. (*узкое место*) nárrow spot.

су́живать, су́зить (*вн.*) contráct (*smth.*), make* (*smth.*) nárrow; nárrow (*smth.*); *перен. тж.* restríct (*smth.*); су́зить глаза́ nárrow one's eyes. ~ся, су́зиться nárrow; get*/becóme*/grow* nárrow(er); *перен.* be* nárrowed down, be* restrícted; ~ся к концу́ táper.

су́зить(ся) *сов. см.* су́живать(ся).

сук *м.* 1. branch, bough; 2. (*в бревне, доске*) knot.

су́ка *ж.* bitch.

сукно́ *с.* smooth wóollen cloth; ◇ положи́ть что-л. под ~ shelve (*smth.*), pígeon-hole (*smth.*).

сукова́тый knótty, gnarled.

суко́н|ка *ж.* (piece of) cloth. ~ный wóollen cloth *attr.*; ~ное пальто́ wóollen óvercoat; ~ная фа́брика clóth-mill; ◇ ~ный язы́к dull/clúmsy style.

сулема́ *ж. хим.* (corrósive) súblimate.

сул|и́ть *несов.* (*вн. дт.*) prómise (*smb. smth.*), hold* out (*smth.* to); э́то не ~и́т ничего́ хоро́шего it is not (a) véry hópeful (sign); ~ золоты́е го́ры hold* out allúring próspects, prómise the moon.

султа́н I *м.* (*титул*) súltan.

султа́н II *м.* (*украшение*) plume.

сульфа́т *м. хим.* súlphate.

сум|а́ *ж.*; ходи́ть с ~о́й beg one's bread.

сумасбро́д *м.* mádcap, crázy/scátter-bráined féllow. ~ка *ж.* scátter-bráined créature, crázy wóman*.

сумасбро́д|ничать *несов.* beháve wíldly, go* in for mádcap advéntures. ~ный crázy, mad; (*о плане и т. п. тж.*) mádcap *attr.*, wild. ~ство *с.* mádcap/wild beháviour.

сумасше́дший *прил.* 1. mad, crázy; ~ дом lúnatic asýlum; 2. *в знач. сущ. м.* mádman*; *ж.* mádwoman*; как ~ like a mádman*.

сумасше́стви|е *с.* mádness, insánity, lúnacy; ◇ до ~я to distráction; доводи́ть кого́-л. до ~я drive* smb. mad.

сумато́ха *ж.* bústle, húrly-burly, confúsion.

сумбу́р *м.* múddle, túrmoil, confúsion. ~ный confúsed, múddled; ~ные мы́сли múddled thoughts; ~ный челове́к múddle-headed pérson.

су́меречн|ый 1. dim, dark; *перен.* (*мрачный*) glóomy; ~ свет, ~ое вре́мя, ~ая пора́ the twílight, dusk; 2. *зоол.* crepúscular; ~ые живо́тные Crepusculária.

су́мерки *мн.* the twílight *sg*; предрассве́тные ~ the hálf-light of dawn.

суме́|ть *сов.* (+ *инф.*) be* áble (+ to *inf*), mánage (+ to *inf*); он ~ет э́то сде́лать he can do it, he'll mánage it; не ~ fail (+ to *inf*); be* unáble (+ to *inf*); не ~ю вам сказа́ть I'm afráid I can't tell you.

су́мка *ж.* 1. bag; (*для покупок*) shópping-bag; ~ почтальо́на póstman's bag; 2. *анат.*: серде́чная ~ pericárdium; 3. *зоол.* pouch.

су́мм|а *ж.* 1. sum, tótal; ~ трёх чи́сел the sum of the three fígures; в ~е as a whole; составля́ть в ~е что-л. tótal (*smth.*), come* to *smth.*; ~ впечатле́ний the tótal/net impréssion; 2. (*количество денег*) sum, amóunt. ~а́рный 1. tótal; ~а́рное число́ оборо́тов tótal númber of revolútions; 2. (*обобщённый*) géneral, óverall; ~а́рные све́дения géneral informátion *sg*.

сумми́ровать *несов. и сов.* (*вн.*) 1. (*вычислять сумму*) add up (*smth.*); 2. (*обобщать*) sum up (*smth.*), súmmarize (*smth.*).

су́мочка *ж.* (*дамская*) hánd-bag.

су́мрак *м.* dusk, gloom.

су́мрачный glóomy, sómbre; *перен. тж.* dréary.

сумя́тица *ж. разг.* confúsion, túrmoil.

сунду́к *м.* chest; (*дорожный*) trunk.

су́нуть(ся) *сов. см.* сова́ть(ся).

суп *м.* soup.

суперобло́жка *ж.* jácket, book cóver.

суперфосфа́т *м. хим.* superphósphate.

супесо́к *м.* sándy loam.

супесча́н|ый sándy-loam *attr.*; ~ая по́чва sándy loam.

супина́тор *м.* arch suppórt.

супов|о́й soup *attr.*; ~а́я ми́ска (sóup-)turéen.

супру́г *м.* húsband. ~а *ж.* wife*. ~и *мн.* márried cóuple *sg*, húsband and wife.

супру́же|ский matrimónial, cónjugal. ~ство *с.* mátrimony, márried life.

сургу́ч *м.* séaling-wax. ~ный: ~ная печа́ть (wáx-) seal.

сурди́нк|а *ж.* (*у рояля*) dámper; (*у скрипки*) mute; ◇ под ~у on the sly.

суре́пка *ж. бот.* winter-cress.

суро́вость *ж.* sevérity, austérity.

суро́в|ый I 1. sevére, austére; *перен.* sómbre, grim; ~ челове́к harsh/austére pérson; ~ взгляд sevére look; 2. (*крайне строгий*) rígorous, harsh; ~ пригово́р harsh/sevére séntence; 3. (*тяжёлый*) grim; ~ая борьба́ grim strúggle; 4. (*трудный для жизни*) harsh, rígorous, cruel, tough; ~ое мо́ре cruel sea; ~ая зима́ sevére/hard winter; ~ кли́мат rígorous clímate.

суро́в|ый II (*грубый, небелёный*) unbléached, brown; ~ое полотно́ brown Hólland.

суро́к *м. зоол.* mármot; спать как ~ ≈ sleep* like a top.

суррога́т *м.* súbstitute (for). ~ный érsatz; ~ный ко́фе érsatz cóffee.

сурьма́ *ж. хим.* ántimony.

су́слик *м. зоол.* gópher, ground squírrel.

суста́в *м.* jóint. ~но́й: ~но́й ревмати́зм rheumátic féver.

су́тки *мн.* day *sg*, twenty-fóur hours; на тре́тьи ~ on the third day.

суто́лока *ж.* commótion, húrly-burly.

су́точный 1. dáily; díurnal *научн.*; 2. *в знач. сущ. мн.* dáily allówance *sg*.

суту́лить *несов.* (*вн.*) give* (*smth.*) a stoop. ~ся *несов.* have* a stoop, stoop, be* róund-shouldered.

суту́лый róund-shouldered.

сут|ь *ж.* éssence, súbstance; gist; ~ де́ла the gist of the mátter; дойти́ до ~и come* to the point; добра́ться до ~и де́ла get* at the root of things, get* down to bédrock; ◇ по ~и де́ла in reálity, as a mátter of fact.

суфлёр *м.* prómpter. ~ский: ~ская бу́дка prómpter's box, prómpt-box.

суфли́ровать *несов.* prompt.

су́ффикс *м. грам.* súffix.

суха́рь *м.* 1. piece of dried bread; (*сладкий*) rusk; 2. *разг.* (*о человеке*) dry (old) stick.

су́хо 1. *нареч.* drýly, stíffly; ~ поклони́ться кому́-л. bow stíffly to smb.; ~ разгова́ривать с кем-л. convérse drýly with smb.; 2. *в знач. сказ. безл.* it is dry; бы́ло ~ и ве́трено it was dry and wíndy.

сухове́й *м.* dry wind.

сухожи́лие *с.* téndon.

сух|о́й 1. dry; ~и́е дрова́ dry wood *sg*; ~ое се́но dry hay; ~ хлеб stale bread; 2. (*пересохший*) dry, dríed-up; (*о почве*) árid; ~ое ру́сло dríed-up wátercourse; ~и́е гу́бы parched lips; 3. (*лишённый влажности*) dry; ~ая ко́мната dry room; ~ ве́тер dry wind; ~ во́здух dry air; ~ кли́мат dry clímate; ~ое ле́то dry súmmer; 4. (*сушёный*) dried; ~и́е фру́кты dried fruits; 5. *мед.* dry; ~ ка́шель dry cough; ~ плеври́т dry pléurisy; 6. (*о коже, волосах*) dry; 7. (*о растениях*) dry, withered; ~и́е ли́стья dead leaves; ~ая ве́тка withered branch; 8. (*сухощавый*) lean, skínny; 9. (*неласковый, холодный*) alóof, stiff; ~ челове́к ungrácious pérson; ~ приём cold recéption; ~ тон alóof tone; 10. (*неинтересный*) dry, dull, dréary; ~ расскáз dull stóry; ◇ ~бе винó dry wine; ~ закóн prohibítion; ~ паёк dry rátions pl; ~им путём by land; на нём ~ нитки не остáлось he hádn't a dry stitch on.

сухопáрый разг. spare, lean.

сухопýтн|ый land attr., ground attr.; ~ая гранúца land fróntier; ~ые войскá land/ground fórces; ~ трáнспорт land tránsport.

сухостóй м. собир. dead (stánding) wood.

сухость ж. drýness; (засушливость тж.) arídity.

сухощáвый spare, lean.

сучúть несов. 1. (вн.; нитку) spin* (smth.), twist (smth.); 2. (тв.; двигать, перебирать) jerk (smth.), work (smth.); ~ нóжками (о ребёнке) kick.

сучковáтый 1. (о дереве) gnarled; 2. (о палке) knótty.

суч|óк м. 1. twig; 2. (в древесине) knot; ◇ без ~кá без задóринки without a hitch.

сýш|а ж. (dry) land; на ~е и на мóре on land and sea.

сýше (сравнит. ст. прил. сухóй и нареч. сýхо) dríer.

сушёный dried.

сушúлка ж. 1. (аппарат) drýer; 2. (помещение) drýing-room.

сушúльный drýing attr.

сушúть, высушить (вн.) 1. dry (smth.); ~ бельё dry the wáshing; ~ мáлину dry ráspberries; 2. (делать чрезмерно сухим) dry up (smth.), parch (smth.); 3. (мучить) gnaw (smb.); 4. (делать чёрствым, неотзывчивым) hárden (smb., smth.). ~ся, высушиться 1. dry; 2. (сушить на себе мокрую одежду) get* one's wet clothes dry (without táking them off).

сýшка ж. 1. (действие) drýing; 2. (баранка) dry bréad-ring; 3. (для посуды) dráining board.

сушь ж. разг. 1. (засуха) drought; 2. (сухое место) dry spot; 3. (что-л. неинтересное) dry/bóring stuff.

существенн|ый esséntial, intrínsic, matérial, vítal; (крупный) substántial; ~ые изменéния matérial chánges; ~ое значéние vítal impórtance; имéть ~ое значéние be* of vítal impórtance; Это не имéет ~ого значéния it is not so véry impórtant; нет ~ой рáзницы there is no esséntial/intrínsic dífference.

существúтельн|ый: úмя ~ое грам. noun, substántive.

существ|ó I с. (сущность) éssence, súbstance; gist разг.; ~ дéла the point; ~ вопрóса the éssence/gist of the próblem; ◇ по ~ý (говоря) as a mátter of fact; говорúть по ~ý stick* to the facts; отвечáть по ~ý give* a straight ánswer.

существó II с. (живое) béing, créature; любúмое ~ one's best-lóved, one's belóved; чувствовать всем свойм ~м fell* it in one's bones.

существовáни|е с. exístence; (жизнь тж.) life; фóрмы ~я матéрии forms of the exístence of mátter; борьбá за ~ the báttle for survíval.

существ|овáть несов. exíst; (жить тж.) live; ~уют люди, котóрые... there are péople who...; ~ует мнéние, что... some péople think...; не ~ be* non-exístent; для негó не ~ует никакúх препятствий óbstacles do not exíst for him.

существýющ|ий прил. 1. exísting, exístent; in existence после сущ.; лýчший из ~их the best in exístence; 2. в знач. сущ. с.: всё ~ее éverything that/which exists.

сýш|ий: ~ая прáвда the (véry) truth; ~ие пустякú the mérest trífles; ~ее наказáние a régular pest; ~ вздор útter/dównright nónsense.

сýщност|ь ж. éssence; ~ произведéния the éssence of a work; по сáмой своéй ~и by its véry náture; ◇ в ~и (говоря) as a mátter of fact; он в ~и не злой человéк he is not réally unkind.

сфабрикóванный trúmped-up, fáked-up.

сфабриковáть сов. см. фабриковáть.

сфальцевáть сов. см. фальцевáть.

сфальшúвить сов. см. фальшúвить.

сфéр|а ж. sphere; (область тж.) field, realm, domáin, line; ~ дéятельности sphere/field of actívity/áction; Это не егó ~ дéятельности that is not his próvince/line; в своéй ~е on famíliar ground, in one's élement; вне своéй ~ы out of one's sphere/élement; ◇ ~ влияния sphere of influence.

сферúческий 1. sphérical, glóbular, báll-shaped; 2. мат. sphérical.

сфинкс м. sphinx.

сформировáть(ся) сов. см. формировáть(ся).

сформовáть сов. см. формовáть.

сформулúровать сов. (вн.) fórmulate (smth.).

сфотографúровать(ся) сов. см. фотографúровать(ся).

схватúть сов. см. схвáтывать. ~ся сов. см. схвáтываться и хватáться 1.

схвáтк|а ж. 1. (бой) engágement; рукопáшная ~ hánd-to-hánd strúggle/fíghting; 2. (спор, ссора) tússle, fight; 3. мн. (боли) spasms; родовые ~и lábour (pains); 4. (приспособление для крепления) brace.

схвáтывать, схватúть (вн.) 1. (взять, поймать) seize (smth.), grasp (smth.), grip (smth.); схватúть когó-л. зá руку seize smb.'s hand; (силой задерживать) seize (smb.); 3. разг. (болезнь) catch* (smth.); 4. разг. (подмечать и запечатлевать) catch* (smth.), reprodúce (smth.); 5. разг. (быстро понимать) grasp (smth.); ~ смысл grasp the méaning. ~ся, схватúться 1. (за вн.) catch* hold (of); 2. (вступать в борьбу) grápple; (вступать в драку) come* to blows.

схéма ж. 1. (чертёж) díagram; (план) scheme, láy-out; ~ радиоприёмника recéiver círcuit; ~ организáции organizátion chart; 2. (описание чего-л. в общих чертах) plan, óutline; ~ пьéсы óutline of a play; 3. (трафаретная формула) stéreotyped páttern, set of símbols, the bare bones pl; мыслить ~ми think* in stéreotyped ímages.

схематúческий 1. (представленный в виде схемы) schemátic, diagrammátic; óutline attr.; 2. (представленный в упрощённо-обобщённом виде) prímitive, oversímplified.

схематúчн|ость ж. schemátic cháracter. ~ый см. схематúческий 2.

схитрúть сов. см. хитрúть.

схлынуть сов. 1. recéde/withdráw* with a rush, flow back, fall* back; перен. rush, stream; 2. (ослабеть, исчезнуть — о чувстве) pass off, disappéar.

сходúть I, сойтú 1. (с рд.; спускаться) go* down (smth.), come* down (smth.), descénd (smth.); (слезать) get* off (smth.); сходúть с лéстницы go* down the stairs; сойтú с лóшади get* off a horse; 2. (с рд.; о пассажирах) get* off; ~ с пóезда get* off a train; ~ с трамвáя get* off a tram; ~ на бéрег go* ashóre; 3. (с рд.; отходить, уходить) leave* (smth.); (сдвигаться с мéста тж.) go* off (smth.); ~ с дорóги leave* the road, go* off the road; ~ с путú get* out of the way; ~ с рéльсов run* off the rails, leave* the rails, be* deráiled; 4. (с рд.; о краске, грязи, коже и т. п.) come* off (smth.); (о кожице, шелухе) peel off (smth.); (о снеге) vánish (from), melt (off); загáр сошёл с егó лицá his face lost its tan; 5. разг. (заканчиваться успешно) go* off well, turn out all right; сойдёт! it will do!; 6. (за вн.) pass (for); он сойдёт за молодóго he'll pass for a young man*; ◇ сойтú на нет 1) (исчезнуть) fade awáy; 2) (потерять значение) come* to nought/nóthing; ~ с умá go* mad; ~ с умá по ком-л. be* mádly in love with smb.; емý всё схóдит с рук he can get awáy with ánything.

сходúть II сов. (пойти) go*; (за кем-л.) go* and fetch; (за чем-л.) go* and get*.

сходúться, сойтúсь 1. (встречаться, соединяться)

meet*; (*о направлениях*) convérge; они сошлись на полдороге they met half way; пояс не сходится the belt won't fásten; 2. (*собираться*) gáther, come* togéther; сошлись знакомые и друзья it was a gáthering of *one's* friends and acquáintances; 3. (*встречаться для состязания, боя*) meet*; (*об армиях тж.*) close, engáge each óther; 4. (*с тв.; сближаться*) becóme* friends (with); (*вступать в связь*) take* up (with); start líving (with), live togéther; 5. (*в пр., тв.; быть единодушным, сходным*) agrée (in), be* at one (in), have* the same (*smth.*); ~ во взглядах agrée in *one's* views; все сходятся на том, что... éveryone agrées that...; не ~ харáктерами be* unsúited to each óther, not get on; 6. (*совпадать*) tálly; 7. *разг.* (*приходить к соглашению*) agrée; не ~ в цене disagrée abóut the price.

схо́дка *ж. уст.* méeting.

схо́дни *мн.* (*ед.* сходня *ж.*) ramp *sg*; *мор.* gáng-plank *sg*, gángway *sg*.

схо́д|ный 1. (*похожий*) símilar; ~ная черта́ (one) féature in cómmon; 2. *разг.* (*подходящий*) réasonable, accéptable; купи́ть *что-л.* по ~ной цене́ buy* smth. at a réasonable price. **~ство** *с.* similárity, líkeness, resémblance.

схола́ст|ика *ж.* 1. *филос.* scholásticism; 2. (*буквоедство*) pédantry. **~и́ческий** 1. *филос.* scholástic; 2. (*формальный*) pedántic, drýasdust.

схорони́ть *сов. см.* хорони́ть.

сце́н|а *ж.* 1. (*театральные подмостки, театр*) stage; вращáющаяся ~ revólving stage; 2. (*отдельная часть действия*) scene; действие первое, ~ вторáя act one, scene two; 3. (*эпизод*) scene; 4. *разг.* (*ссора*) scene; ~ ре́вности scene of jéalousy; устро́ить ~у *кому-л.* stage a row with *smb.*; ◇ игрáть на ~е act in the théatre; яви́ться, появи́ться на ~е appéar on the scene; сойти со ~ы pass from the scene.

сцена́рий *м.* scenário (*pl* -os), script; scenárist.

сцена́рист *м.* scenário/script wríter.

сцени́ческ|ий 1. (*относящийся к сцене*) scénic; stage *attr.*; ~ие эффекты scénic effects; 2. (*относящийся к представлению в театре*) theátrical; stage *attr.*; *перен. тж.* histriónic; ~ое иску́сство dramátic art.

сцени́чн|ый áctor's; súitable for the stage *после сущ.*; ~ая внешность stage appéarance, áctor's présence; эта пьеса очень ~а this play stáges véry well, this play is véry good théatre.

сцепи́ть(ся) *сов. см.* сцепля́ть(ся).

сцепле́ние *с.* 1. (*действие*) cóupling; 2. (*механизм*) clutch; включáть (выключáть) ~ engáge (disengáge) the clutch; 3. (*состояние*) cohésion, adhésion; ~ молéкул cohésion of mólecules.

сцепля́ть, сцепи́ть (*вн.*) cóuple (*smth.*). **~ся**, сцепи́ться 1. (*соединяться*) be* cóupled up; (*о шестернях*) engáge, mesh; 2. (*случайно зацепляться*) get* caught up togéther; 3. (*о пальцах, руках*) lock, interlóck; (*о зубах*) be* clénched; 4. *разг.* (*вступать в драку, спор, перебранку*) pitch into each óther, have* a sét-to.

сце́пщик *м.* cóupler; brákeman*.

счастли́в|ец *м.* lúcky man*. **~ица** *ж.* lúcky wóman*, girl.

счастли́в|о háppily; ~ отдéлаться get* off líghtly. **~чик** *м. разг. см.* счастли́вец. **~ый** háppy; (*удачливый*) fórtunate, lúcky; ~ый взгляд háppy glance/look; ~ое дéтство háppy childhood; ~ая мысль háppy thought; ~ый билет lúcky/wínning tícket; ~ый случай lúcky chance.

сча́сть|е *с.* 1. háppiness; семéйное ~ fámily háppiness; 2. (*удача*) (good) luck, good fórtune; ◇ к ~ю, по ~ю fórtunately, lúckily; на ~ for luck; не видáть ~я fórtunately/lúckily for me; имéть ~ (+ инф.) have* the good fórtune (+ to *inf*); вáше ~ (*вам повезло*) you were lúcky; какóе ~, что... how fórtunate/lúcky that...

счесть *сов. см.* счита́ть I 6.

счёт *м.* 1. (*действие*) calculátion, réckoning; ~ в умé

méntal aríthmetic; 2. (*результат подсчётов*) resúlt, tótal; *спорт.* score; матч закончился со ~ом 3:1 the match énded with the score at 3:1; 3. (*документ*) bill; ~ за газ и электричество gas and electrícity bill; 4. *бухг.* accóunt; 5. *обыкн. мн.* (*взаимные денежные расчёты*) the accóunt *sg*; 6. *обыкн. мн.* (*взаимные претензии, обиды*) accóunts, scores; личные ~ы prívate grúdges; своди́ть стáрые ~ы pay* off old scores; ◇ без ~у lávishly, fréely; в конéчном ~е when all is said and done; в ~ *чего-л.* to the accóunt of *smth.*; в ~ бу́дущего года towárds next year's prodúction; на чей-л., за чей-л. ~ at *smb.'s* expénse; на чей-л. ~ (*в чей-л. адрес*) at *smb.'s* expénse, aimed at *smb.*; он принимáет это на свой ~ he thinks it reférs to him; за ~ *чего-л.* at the expénse of *smth.*; за ~ сниже́ния себестоимости by lówering prodúction costs; за ~ мобилизáции вну́тренних ресу́рсов by móbilizing intérnal resóurces; за ~ повыше́ния производи́тельности труда́ by incréasing lábour productívity; на этот ~ можно быть споко́йным there is no need for anxiety on that score; это не в ~ that doesn't count; не знать ~а деньгáм be* rólling in móney; знать ~ деньгáм know* the válue of móney; покончить ~ы с кем-л., чем-л. séttle accóunts with *smb.*, *smth.*; предъяви́ть ~ *кому-л., чему-л.* make* a claim on *smb.*, *smth.*; быть у *кого-л.* на хорóшем (плохóм) счету́ be* in good (bad) repúte with *smb.*, be* in *smb.'s* good (bad, black) books; сбрáсывать со счетов not take into considerátion, ignóre; ~а, ~у нет *кому-л., чему-л.* there is no end of/to *smb.*, *smth.*

счёт|ный accóunt *attr.*, accóunting; ~ая лине́йка slide rule.

счетово́д *м.* lédger clerk. **~ство** *с.* bóok-keeping.

счётчик *м.* 1. (*человек*) cóunter; 2. (*аппарат*) méter; cóunter; электри́ческий ~ eléctric méter; ~ Гéйгера Géiger cóunter/tube.

счёт|ы *мн.* ábacus *sg*, cóunting-frame *sg*; считáть на ~ах use an ábacus.

счисле́ни|е *с.* 1. *мат.* numerátion; десяти́чная систéма ~я décimal numerátion; 2. *мор., ав.* réckoning, calculátion; ~ пути́ *мор.* dead réckoning.

счи́стить(ся) *сов. см.* счищáть(ся).

счит|áть I, сосчитáть, счесть 1. *сов.* сосчитáть (*вести счёт*) count; ~ до десяти́ count (up) to ten; ~ на пáльцах count on *one's* fíngers; 2. *сов.* сосчитáть (*вн.*) *определять количество, сумму чего-л.*) count (*smth.*); add up (*smth.*), compúte (*smth.*); (*производить бухгалтерские подсчёты*) do* the accóunts; ~ деньги count móney; ~ пульс count *smb.'s* pulse; 3. *тк. несов.* (*пользоваться какими-л. единицами измерения*) réckon, cálculate; ~ в килогрáммах réckon in kílograms; 4. *тк. несов.* (*принимать за начало отсчёта*) count; пя́тое окнó, ~я от угла́ the fifth window, cóunting from the córner; 5. *тк. несов.* (*вн.; принимать в расчёт при исчислении*) count (*smb., smth.*) ~я в том числé inclúding; не ~я not cóunting; 6. *сов.* счесть (*вн. тж.; полагать*) consíder (*smb. smth.*), regárd (*smb., smth.* as); ~ вопрóс исчéрпанным consíder the quéstion closed; ~ себя́ впрáве... consíder onesélf entítled to...; ~ себя́ прáвым believe onesélf to be in the right; ~ себя́ оби́женным feel* injured; он ~ет вас свои́м дрýгом he regárds you as his friend; ~ свои́м дóлгом consíder it *one's* dúty; ~ необходи́мым, ну́жным (+ *инф.*) consíder it esséntial, nécessary (+ to *inf*); ◇ не ~ дéнег have* plénty of móney, be* rólling in móney; ~ дни, часы́, мину́ты count the days, hours, mínutes.

счита́ть II *сов. см.* счи́тывать.

счит|áться, сосчитáться 1. (*с тв.*) *разг.* (*производить денежные расчёты*) séttle (with), count it up; 2. *тк. несов.* (*с тв.; принимать во внимание*) take* (*smb., smth.*) into considerátion, consíder (*smb., smth.*); с егó мнéнием óчень ~ются his opínion cárries much weight; мы óчень ~емся с егó мнéнием his opínion cárries great weight with us; с ним óчень ~áются he is a great authórity for them; с э́тим нáдо ~ that must be táken ínto considerátion; не ~ с ке́м-л. ignore *smb.*, not consíder *smb.*; не ~ ни с кем have* no considerátion for ányone; ни с чем не ~ stick* at nóthing; с ним э́тим мóжно не ~ he, that can be ignóred; 3. *тк. несов.* (*слыть*) be* considered; он ~áлся хорóшим стрелкóм he was considered a good* shot; ~áется, что... it is considered that...

счи́тывать, счита́ть (*вн.*) collate (*smth.*), check (*smth.*).

счища́ть, чи́стить (*вн.*) clear (*smth.*) awáy, clean (*smth.*) off; (*щёткой, рукой*) brush off (*smth.*); ~ лёд с тротуáров clear the pávement of ice. ~ся, счи́ститься come* off.

сшиба́ть, сшиби́ть (*вн.*) *разг.* knock (*smb.*, *smth.*) down; ~ кого́-л. с ног knock *smb.* down, knock *smb.* off his, her feet.

сшиби́ть *сов. см.* сшиба́ть.

сшива́ть, сшить (*вн.*) 1. stitch (*smth.*), sew* (*smth.*) togéther; 2. *мед.* súture (*smth.*); 3. (*доски, листы металла и т. п.*) join (*smth.*), put* (*smth.*) togéther; ~ лóдку из досóк make* a boat out of planks.

сши́тый sewn; хорошó ~ well-máde suit.

сшить *сов. см.* сшива́ть и шить I.

съеда́ть, съесть (*вн.*) eat* (*smth.*); (*всё без остатка*) eat* up (*smth.*); *перен. тж.* góbble up (*smb.*, *smth.*), swállow up (*smb.*, *smth.*).

съеде́ние *с.*: отдавáть когó-л., чтó-л. на ~ комý-л. deliver *smb.*, *smth.* ínto the hands of *smb.*, leave* *smb.*, *smth.* at the mércy of *smb.*

съедóбн|ый édible; вполнé ~ (quite) éatable; ~ые грибы́ édible fúngi; múshrooms.

съёжиться *сов.* 1. (*сжаться, сморщиться*) shrível; 2. (*скорчиться*) húddle up; 3. (*стать скрюченным, сморщенным*) shrink*, becóme* shrúnken.

съезд *м.* 1. (*прибытие*) arríval; начался́ ~ гостéй the guests begán to arríve; 2. (*собрание*) cóngress; съезд Совéтов Cóngress of Sóviets; ~ профсою́зов tráde-union cóngress; 3. (*спуск*) dríveway, place where one can get off the road; (*у автострады*) láy-by.

съéздить *сов.* go*, make* a trip; ~ зá город make* a trip out of town; мне нáдо ~ в Москвý по дéлу I have to go to Moscow on búsiness.

съéздовский *разг.* cóngress *attr.*

съезжа́ть, съéхать 1. descénd; go* down, come* down; (*скользя*) slide* down; ~ с дорóги get* off the road; ~ с горы́ go* downhíll; 2.: ~ с квартíры move; 3. *разг.* (*сползать*) slide*, slip; ~ нáбок slip sídeways, slip to one side. ~ся, съéхаться 1. (*встречаться*) meet*; 2. (*собираться*) gáther, assémble, come* togéther; гóсти съезжáются the guests are arríving.

съём|ка *ж.* 1. (*планов*) súrvey; глазомéрная ~ field skétching; производíть ~ку чегó-л. súrvey *smth.*, make* a súrvey of *smth.*; 2. (*фотографирование*) photógraphy; 3. (*фильма*) shóoting.

съёмный detáchable, remóvable; ~ замóк pádlock.

съёмочн|ый 1. кино́: ~ процéсс shóoting, fílming; ~ аппарáт (móvie) cámera; ~ая площáдка set; 2. *геод.* súrvey *attr.*; ~ые рабóты на мéстности field survéying.

съёмщик *м.* ténant.

съестн|óй *прил.* 1.: ~ые припáсы provísions, fóod-stuffs; 2. *в знач. сущ. с.* édibles *pl.*

съесть *сов. см.* есть I 1, 4 и съеда́ть; <> собáку ~ на чём-л. be* a past máster at *smth.*, know* *smth.* inside out.

съéхать(ся) *сов. см.* съезжáть(ся).

съéхидничать *сов. см.* ехи́дничать.

съязви́ть *сов. см.* язви́ть.

сы́воротка *ж.* 1. (*молочная*) whey; 2. *биол./мед.* sérum.

сыгра́ть *сов. см.* игра́ть 2, 3, 4; <> ~ шýтку с кем-

-л. play a trick on *smb.* ~ся *сов. муз.* be* pérfectly co-órdinated, make* a good ensémble; *спорт.* achíeve good téamwork.

сы́знова *разг.* all óver agáin; начинáть ~ begín* all óver agáin, start afrésh, make* a fresh start.

сын *м.* son; ~ своегó нарóда his cóuntry's son; ~ своегó врéмени child* of the époch/age. ~и́шка *м.* little boy. ~óвний fílial; ~óвняя привя́занность fílial afféction. ~óк *м. разг.* sónny.

сы́пать *несов.* (*вн.*) pour (*smth.*); (*посыпать*) strew* (*smth.*); (*вн., тв.*) *перен.* pour out (*smth.*); ~ словáми pour out words; ~ острóтами rain wítticisms; <> ~ деньгáми squánder móney. ~ся *несов.* 1. pour; (*просыпаться*) run* out; (*о штукатурке и т. п.*) crúmble; 2. (*идти — о дожде, снеге*) sprinkle down, fall*; 3. (*обрушиваться, поступать во множестве*) rain down; (*звучать отовсюду*) pour out, be* heard on all sides.

сыпнóй: ~ тиф *мед.* týphus, spótted féver.

сыпýч|ий loose, frée-flowing; ~ грунт loose/fríable soil; ~ песóк quicksand; ~ие телá dry súbstances; мéры ~их тел dry (capácity) méasures.

сыпь *ж.* rash, erúption; показáлась ~ a rash broke out.

сыр *м.* cheese; <> как ~ в мáсле катáться live in clóver.

сыр-бóр: вот отчегó ~ загорéлся! so that's what all the fuss is abóut!

сырéть, отсырéть grow*/becóme* damp.

сырéц *м.*: хлóпок-~ raw cótton; шёлк-~ raw silk; кирпи́ч-~ brick clay.

сы́рник *м. кул.* curd frítter.

сы́ро *в знач. сказ. безл.* it is damp.

сыровáр *м.* chéese-maker. ~éние *с.* chéese-making. ~енный chéese-making *attr.* ~ня *ж.* chéese-dairy.

сыроéжка *ж.* (*гриб*) rússula.

сыр|óй 1. (*влажный*) damp; ~óе бельё damp línen; ~ые дровá damp fírewood *sg*; 2. (*имеющий значительную влажность*) damp, moist, húmid; ~óе помещéние damp room; ~ вóздух damp air; ~ вéтер moist wind; ~áя погóда damp wéather; ~óе лéто wet súmmer; 3. (*не подвергшийся варке, кипячению*) raw, uncóoked; ~óе мя́со raw meat; ~ые óвощи raw végetables; пить ~ю́ю вóду drink* unbóiled wáter; 4. (*недоваришийся, недопечённый*) half-dóne, sóggy; ~ хлеб sóggy bread; 5. (*необработанный*) *перен.* in an unfínished state *после сущ*, shóddy.

сырóк *м.* 1. cream cheese; prócessed cheese; 2. (*творожный*) swéetened cóttage cheese.

сы́рость *ж.* dámpness; (*воздуха, климата тж.*) humídity.

сырьё *с.* raw matérial(s).

сыска́ть *сов.* (*вн.*) *разг.* find* (*smth.*).

сы́тн|о: ~ корми́ть когó-л. feed* *smb.* well; ~ накорми́ть когó-л. give* *smb.* a good meal; ~ поéсть have* a substántial meal. ~ый (*питательный*) nutrítious, nóurishing; (*об обеде и т. п.*) sátisfying.

сы́т|ость *ж.* satíety, satiátion. ~ый 1. sátisfied, sáted; я сыт I've had enóugh, I'm full up; 2. *разг.* (*упитанный*) well-nóurished, well-féd; ~ая физионóмия well-nóurished cóuntenance; 3. *разг.* (*богатый*) rich, well-héeled; (*о жизни*) cómfortable; 4. (*богатый едой*) abúndant, fat; 5. *разг.* (*сытый*) fílling; <> я сыт по гóрло I'm fed up (with).

сы́щик *м.* detéctive.

сэконóмить *сов. см.* эконóмить 1, 3.

сюдá here; (*как указание*) this way; иди́те ~ come here; (*как указание*) come this way.

сюжéт *м.* 1. plot, stóry; 2. *разг.* (*тема*) tópic, súbject. ~ный 1. plot *attr.*; 2. (*имеющий сюжет*) intríguing; with a strong plot *после сущ*, that tells a stóry *после сущ*.

сюи́та *ж. муз.* suite.

сюрпри́з *м.* surprise; ах, како́й ~! what a surprise!

сюрту́к *м.* fróck-coat.

сюсю́канье *с. разг.* lisping; *(с детьми́)* báby talk.

сюсю́кать *несов. разг.* lisp; *(с детьми́)* use báby talk.

сяк: и так и ~ this way and that; то так, то ~ sómetimes one way, sómetimes anóther.

Т

та *см.* тот.

таба́к *м.* tobácco; нюхательный ~ snuff.

табаке́рка *ж.* snúff-box.

табаково́д *м.* tobácco-grower. ~ство *с.* tobácco-growing.

таба́нить *несов. (вёслами)* back wáter.

таба́чный 1. tobácco *attr.*; 2. *(о цве́те)* snúff-coloured.

та́бель *м.* 1. *(спи́сок)* táble; 2. *(доска́ для контро́ля)* tíme-board. ~ный: ~ная доска́ tíme-board. ~щик *м.*, ~щица *ж.* tíme-keeper.

табле́тка *ж.* táblet, pill; ~ от головно́й бо́ли héadache táblet.

табли́|ца *ж.* táble. ~чный tábular.

табло́ *с. нескл.* índicator pánel; световое ~ illúminated índicator pánel; информацио́нное ~ informátion board.

та́бор *м.* 1. *(цыга́нский)* band; 2. *разг. (ла́герь)* camp.

табу́н *м. (лошаде́й, оле́ней и т. п.)* herd; *(уток, гусей)* flock *(тж. перен.)*. ~щик *м.* hérdsman*.

табуре́т *м.*, ~ка *ж.* stool.

тавро́ *с.* 1. *(клеймо́)* brand; 2. *(орудие для клейме́ния)* bránding-iron.

тавтоло́гия *ж.* tautólogy.

тага́н *м.* trívet.

таджи́к *м.* Tadjík. ~ский Tadjík; ~ский язы́к Tadjík, the Tadjík language.

таджи́чка *ж.* Tadjík wóman*.

таёжный taigá *attr.*; of the taigá *после сущ.*, in the taigá *после сущ.*

таз I *м. (посу́да)* básin; *(умыва́льный)* wásh-basin; *(для варе́нья)* pan.

таз II *м. анат.* pélvis.

таи́нственн|ость *ж.* mystériousness, mýstery. ~ый 1. mystérious; ~ый посети́тель mystérious vísitor; 2. *(секре́тный)* sécret; 3. *(скрыва́ющий что́-л.)* mystérious, sécretive; с ~ым ви́дом with a mystérious air.

таи́ть *несов. (вн.)* 1. conceál *(smth.)*; *(храни́ть в себе́)* hárbour *(smth.)*; 2. *(заключа́ть в себе́)* hold* *(smth.)*; *(обычно что́-л. плохо́е)* be* fraught (with); ~ в себе́ огро́мные возмо́жности have* enórmous látent possibilities; ◇ не́чего греха́ ~ there's no conceáling the fact (that). ~ся *несов.* 1. *(скрыва́ть что́-л. от други́х)* dissémble, hide* things; не таи́сь fránkly; 2. *(пря́таться, скрыва́ться)* hide*; lie* hídden, lie* conceáled; lurk; ~ся во тьме lurk in the dárkness; 3. *(быть скры́тым, невиди́мым)* be* hídden, be* conceáled; 4. *(быть, име́ться где́-л.)* be*, be* hídden, be* látent.

тайга́ *ж.* taigá.

тайко́м sécretly, surreptítiously; on the quíet *разг.*; уйти́ ~ steal* awáy; ~ от кого́-л. without télling *smb.*

тайм *м. спорт.* half; périod.

та́йн|а *ж.* 1. *(секре́т)* sécret; *(секре́тность)* sécrecy; раскры́ть чужу́ю ~y betráy a sécret; ~ от кого́-л. without télling *smb.*; храни́ть что́-л. в ~e keep* *smth.* sécret; доверя́ть кому́-л. свои́ ~ы take* *smb.* into

one's cónfidence; посвяти́ть кого́-л. в ~y let* *smb.* into a sécret; быть посвящённым в ~y be* in the sécret; ~ успе́ха sécret of success; ~ ремесла́ sécret/trick of the trade; ~ перепи́ски sécrecy/prívacy of correspóndence; служе́бная ~ proféssional sécrecy; 2. *(что́-л. неразга́данное, нея́сное)* mýstery; ~ы приро́ды the mýsteries/sécrets of náture; ~ы ко́смоса the mýsteries of óuter space; ◇ не ~, что... it is no sécret that...; покры́то ~ой wrapped in mýstery.

тайни́к *м.* híding-place; sécret recéss; *перен. тж.* hídden région; в ~áх души́, се́рдца in one's heart of hearts, in the sécrecy of one's heart.

та́йно sécretly, in sécret; ~ от кого́-л. without smb.'s knówledge; unknówn to *smb. разг.*

та́йн|ый 1. sécret; *(скры́тый тж.)* clandéstine; ~ое о́бщество sécret society; ~ враг sécret énemy; ~ая мысль sécret thought; ~ое жела́ние sécret desíre; ~ая поли́ция sécret políce; ~ая аге́нту́ра sécret ágents *pl*; 2. *(сму́тный, таи́нственный)* mystérious, strange; ◇ ~ое голосова́ние bállot, sécret vóting.

тайфу́н *м.* typhóon.

так 1. *нареч. (таки́м о́бразом)* like this/that, in such a way; thus; *(в сравни́тельных предложе́ниях)* so; де́ло обстои́т ~ the facts are as fóllows; ~ прошёл день and thus the day passed; мы сде́лаем ~ this is what we'll do; э́то не ~ де́лается that's not the way to do it; вы э́то не ~ де́лаете you're dóing it wrong; он не ~ де́лал э́то he did it dífferently; де́лать что́-л. не ~ (как на́до) not do *smth.* próperly, do* *smth.* wrong; ~, что́бы не опозда́ть so as not to be late; случи́лось ~, что... it so háppened that...; 2. *нареч. (без после́дствий, да́ром)* like that; э́то тебе́ ~ не пройдёт you won't get awáy with it like that; 3. *нареч. (без осо́бых наме́рений)* just; сказа́л про́сто ~ he just said it; 4. *нареч. (до тако́й сте́пени, насто́лько)* so; он ~ мно́го ходи́л, что уста́л he walked so much that it made him tíred; ~ давно́ such a long time agó, so long agó; ~ ти́хо so quíet; ~ ско́ро so soon; 5. *нареч. (в тако́м слу́чае, тогда́)* then; вы не хоти́те, ~ я пойду́ if you don't want to go, then I will; 6. *частица (ничего́, ничего́ осо́бенного)* nóthing (much); *(при оце́нке чьих́-л. ка́честв)* just; э́та кни́га ~, ничего́ осо́бенного it's just a ráther médiocre book; 7. *частица (сле́довательно, зна́чит)* so, then; *(в нача́ле репли́ки, возобновля́ющей пре́рванный разгово́р)* well, now, so; ~ вы его́ зна́ете? so you know him?; ~ о чём я говори́л? now, what was I sáying?; ~ вы придёте? well, are you cóming?; 8. *союз (всле́дствие э́того, потому́)* so; сего́дня хо́лодно, ~ ты оде́нься потепле́й it's cold today, so dress up wármly; 9. *союз (но, одна́ко)* but; говори́ла я, ~ ты слу́шать не хоте́л I told you, but you wóuldn't listen; э́то ~ усил. *частица* ~это; вот э́то ло́шадь ~ ло́шадь! that's a horse, that is!; 11. *частица (ука́зывает на приблизи́тельное коли́чество)* abóut; лет ~ де́сять тому́ наза́д abóut ten years agó; 12. *частица (наприме́р, к приме́ру)* for instance; ~, наприме́р (thus,) for exámple; ◇ ~ и есть! just as I thought!; ~ и быть! véry well, then!; так себе́ só-so; чу́вствовать себя́ та́к себе́ not feel véry well; ~ и не́ver; он ~ и не пришёл and he néver came; ~ ли (э́то)? indéed?; не ~ ли? didn't (wasn't, *etc.*) he, *etc.*?; ~-то all right, then; ~-то (оно́) ~, но... that's true of course, but...; мы и ~ (уж) опа́здыва́ем we're late as it is; ~ и высо́бо ~! and high time!; как бы не ~! no fear!; ~... как as... as; ~ как as, becáuse, since; ~ что so that; ~ и зна́йте now understánd me; get this straight *разг.*; как на рабо́те, ~ и до́ма both at work and at home, at home as well as at work.

такела́ж *м.* 1. *мор.* rígging; 2. *(для подъёма тяже́стей)* lifting gear. ~ник *м.* rígger; *(строя́щий леса́)* scáffolder.

та́кже too, álso; *(в приве́тствиях)* the same; вас ~ the same to you, I wish you the same; ~... не not... either; а ~ (и) and álso; as well, too *(в конце́ фра́зы)*.

тако́в such; like that; ~ы фа́кты such are the facts; все они́ ~ы they are all alíke; он не ~, как вы ду́маете he is not what you think him; ◇ и был ~ and that was the last we heard of him, and he was gone.

таково́й such; (вышеозначенный) the same; ◇ как ~ as such.

так|о́й мест. 1. (с сущ.) such a, that kind (of); like this после сущ., of that kind после сущ.; (с прил.) such a; so... a; нам ну́жен ~ рабо́тник that's the kind of wórker we need; нам ну́жен тако́й челове́к, кото́рый... we need a pérson who...; 2. (с мест. кто, что, какой) just, exáctly; (с мест. кто-то, что-то) of that kind; кто они́ ~и́е just who are they?, who are they exáctly?; 3. в знач. сущ. с. such a thing; и всё ~о́е and all that sort of thing; ◇ ~-то súch-and-súch a pérson, só-and-só; ~и́м образом 1) in this way; 2) в знач. вводн. сл. thus, so; в ~о́м слу́чае in that case; до ~ степени to such an extént; что ~о́е что-л., кто-л.? what (áctually) is smth., smb.?; что ж ~о́го? what of it?; ещё и не ~о́е быва́ет it's nóthing to what háppens sometimes.

та́кс|а I ж. (расценка) (fixed) rate; пла́та по ~е fíxed-rate páyment.

та́кса II ж. (собака) dáchshund.

такси́ с. нескл. táxi(-cab); грузово́е ~ híre van. ~ст м. táxi dríver.

таксо́метр м. táximeter.

таксофо́н м. públic télephone.

такт I м. 1. муз. bar; попада́ть не в ~ miss the bar, come* in on the wrong bar; 2. разг. (ритм движения) rhythm, the beat; сби́ться с ~а get* out of time, lose* the beat; 3. тех. cýcle; ◇ в ~ in time; не в ~ out of time; держа́ть ~ keep* time; выбива́ть ~ stamp/drum in time (with the músic).

такт II м. (о поведении) tact; челове́к с больши́м ~ом a véry táctful pérson; отсу́тствие ~а táctlessness; держа́ть себя́ с ~ом behave táctfully, be* táctful.

та́к-таки разг. áfter all.

та́ктик м. tactícian.

та́ктика ж. táctics.

такти́ческ|ий táctical; ~ая зада́ча táctical próblem; ~ие разногла́сия disagréement on táctics.

такти́чн|о táctfully, with tact. ~ость ж. tact; ~ость поведе́ния táctful behaviour. ~ый táctful; быть ~ым be* táctful, have* tact; ~ый посту́пок táctful áction.

тала́нт м. 1. tálent, gift; у него́ большо́й ~ he is extrémely tálented; у него́ большо́й математи́ческий ~ he has a real tálent for mathemátics; 2. (человек) brílliant/gífted pérson.

тала́нтлив|ость ж. tálent, brílliance. ~ый 1. tálented, gifted; ~ый арти́ст gifted ártist; 2. (о произведении) tálented.

талисма́н м. tálisman, charm.

та́ли|я ж. waist; ◇ без ~и (о платье) straight; в ~ю (о платье) fitted, wáisted.

тало́н м. 1. cóupon; поса́дочный ~ bóarding card; 2. (в корешке чековой книжки) cóunterfoil.

та́лый 1. (оттаявший) mélting, tháwing; ~ снег mélting snow; (грязный) slush; 2. (о воде) thaw attr.

тальк м. (минерал) talc; (порошок) tálcum pówder.

там нареч. 1. (о месте) there; я бу́ду ~ за́втра I shall be there tomórrow; ~ есть телефо́н there's a télephone there; ~ жа́рко it's hot there; ~ же at the same place; (в ссылке на произведение и т. п.) íbid; ~, где where; 2. (потом, затем) then; ~ ви́дно бу́дет, что де́лать then we'll know what to do; 3. в знач. частицы разг. (выражает пренебрежение) обычно не перево́дится: вся́кие ~ глу́пости all that kind of rot; како́е ~!, куда́ ~! not likely!; ◇ ~ и тут here and there; то тут, то ~ now here, now there.

тамада́ м. tóast-master.

та́мбур м. 1. (пристройка у входных дверей) lóbby; 2. (вагона) (end of the) córridor.

тамо́женн|ик м. cústoms official/ófficer. ~ый cústom(s) attr.; ~ый тари́ф cústoms táriff; ~ая по́шлина cústoms-duty; ~ый осмо́тр cústoms examinátion; проходи́ть ~ый досмо́тр get through cústoms; ~ая поли́тика táriff pólicy; ~ая деклара́ция cústoms declarátion.

тамо́жня ж. cústom-house.

та́мошн|ий разг. lócal; ~ие жи́тели the péople there.

тампо́н м. támpon; wad, pad; ушно́й ~ éar-plug.

та́нгенс м. мат. tángent.

та́ндем м. tándem; они́ рабо́тают в ~е they work in tándem.

та́н|ец м. 1. dance; учи́тель ~цев dáncing máster; уро́к ~цев dáncing lésson; 2. мн. dáncing sg; пойти́ на ~цы go* dáncing, go* to a dance.

танк м. tank.

та́нкер м. tánker.

танке́тка ж. 1. (подошва) wedge sole; 2. мн. (обувь) wédge-soled shoes.

танки́ст м. tánkman*, tank sóldier; (офицер) tánk-officer.

та́нков|ый tank attr., ármoured; ~ое подразделе́ние tank únit.

танкострое́ние с. tank búilding/constrúction.

танцева́льн|ый dance attr.; ~ое иску́сство the art of dáncing; ~ая му́зыка dánce-music; ~ зал dance hall; ~ ве́чер dance, dáncing-párty.

танцева́ть несов. dance; хорошо́ ~ dance well; ~ вальс dance a waltz.

танцо́вщ|ик м., ~ица ж. dáncer.

танцо́р м. dáncer.

та́почки мн. (ед. та́почка ж.) разг. slíppers; (спортивные) gym shoes.

та́ра ж. (ящик) contáiner; (мягкая) pácking.

тарабарщина ж. разг. gíbberish.

тарака́н м. cóckroach; (чёрный тж.) bláck-beetle.

тара́н м. (орудие, предмет) ram; 2. воен. (удар по самолёту и т. п.) rámming attáck; идти́ на ~ ram; 3. воен. (атака) bréak-through (operátion). ~ить несов. (вн.) ram (smth.).

тара́нтул м. зоол. tarántula.

тара́нь ж. roach.

тара́торить несов. разг. chátter, ráttle on, jábber awáy.

тарахте́ть несов. разг. 1. ráttle; 2. (вн.; болтать) ráttle (smth.) off.

тара́щ|ить, вы́таращить разг.: ~ глаза́ stare with búlging eyes; испу́ганно ~a глаза́ eyes wide with fright; ~ глаза́ на кого́-л. stare at smb.

таре́лк|а ж. 1. (посуда) plate; 2. (рд.; содержимое) plate (of); по́лная ~ чего́-л. a pláteful of smth.; 3. мн. муз. cýmbals; 4. тех. disk; ◇ быть не в свое́й ~е be* not quite onesélf; be* off form; fee* ill at ease, feel* out of place; лета́ющая ~ flýing sáucer.

тари́ф м. rate, táriff.

тари́фн|ый táriff attr.; ~ая се́тка distribútion/scale of wage rates; ~ые ста́вки básic wage rates.

таск|а́ть несов. (вн.) 1. см. тащи́ть 1, 2, 3, 4; ~ во́ду fetch wáter; ~ мешки́ heave* sacks; 2. разг. (воровать) steal* (smth.); 3. разг. (носить долгое время) wear* (smth.); он уже́ три го́да ~ает э́тот костю́м he has been wéaring that suit for three years; 4. разг. (носить с собой) cárry (smth.) abóut (with one); ~ письмо́ в карма́не cárry a létter abóut in one's pócket; 5. разг.: ~ кого́-л. за́ волосы, за́ уши pull smb.'s hair, ears; pull smb. by the hair, ears; ◇ он е́ле но́ги ~ает he can hárdly drag himsélf alóng. ~а́ться несов. разг. 1. (ходи́ть, е́здить куда́-л.) traipse, tramp; ~а́ться по го́роду traipse/tramp abóut town; ~а́ться по знако́мым make* the wéary round of one's acquáintances; 2. (странствовать) roam, wánder; 3. (с тв.; носить с собой) keep* (smth.) with one, cárry (smth.) abóut.

тасова́ть несов. (вн.; карты) shúffle (smth.).

ТАСС *м.* (Телегра́фное аге́нтство Сове́тского Сою́за) *ист.* TASS (Télegraph Ágency of the Sóviet Únion).

татáр|ин *м.*, **~ка** *ж.* Tátar. **~ский** Tátar; **~ский язы́к** Tátar, the Tátar lánguage.

татуи́ров|анный tattóoed. **~ать** *несов. и сов.* (*вн.*) tattóo (*smth.*)

татуиро́вка *ж.* 1. (*де́йствие*) tattóoing; 2. (*узо́ры*) tattóo.

тахта́ *ж.* óttoman.

тача́нка *ж.*: пулемётная ~ machine-gun cart.

тача́ть, стача́ть (*вн.*) stitch (*smth.*)

та́чка *ж.* wheel-barrow.

тащи́ть *несов.* (*вн.*) 1. (*воло́чить*) pull (*smth.*), drag (*smth.*); ~ ло́дку в во́ду drag a boat ínto the wáter; ~ что-л. за собо́й drag *smth.* alóng; 2. *разг.* (*нести́ что-л. тяжёлое*) haul (*smth.*) abóut, lug (*smth.*) abóut; с трудо́м ~ чемода́н lug a súitcase abóut; 3. (*тяну́ть за собо́й*) haul (*smth.*), tow (*smth.*); букси́р та́щит ба́ржу the tug is tówing the barge; ~ кого́-л. за́ руку pull *smb.* alóng by the arm; 4. (*извлека́ть, выта́скивать*) pull (*smth.*); ~ ведро́ из коло́дца pull a búcket out of a well, pull up the búcket; ~ зуб pull out a tooth*; 5. *разг.* (*красть*) steal* (*smth.*), lift (*smth.*). **~ся** *несов.* 1. (*воло́читься*) trail alóng; 2. *разг.* (*идти́, е́хать ме́дленно*) procéed slówly; (*о челове́ке тж.*) trudge, tótter; (*о живо́тных*) plod, lábour; 3. *разг.* (*идти́, е́хать куда́-л. без охо́ты*) traipse, make* a jóurney, trek.

та́яние *с.* mélting, tháwing; ~ снего́в mélting of the snow.

та́ять *несов.* 1. melt; (*о сне́ге, льде́ тж.*) thaw; 2. *безл.*: та́ет it is tháwing; 3. (*уменьша́ться, исчеза́ть*) melt awáy; (*о си́лах*) dwíndle; 4. (*ча́хнуть*) waste awáy; 5. (*от рд.*; *умиля́ться*) melt (with); ◇ (так и) та́ет во рту it melts in your mouth.

тварь *ж. уст., разг.* créature (*тж. бран.*).

тверде́ть *несов.* hárden, becóme* hard, set*.

тверди́ть *несов.* (*вн., о пр.*) keep* sáying (*smth.*); (*дт.*) keep* télling (*smb.*); ~ одно́ и то́ же say* the same thing óver and óver agáin.

твёрдо firm(ly); ~ держа́ться stand* firm/fast; (за)по́мнить что-л. néver forgét* *smth.*; ~ заучи́ть что-л. learn *smth.* thóroughly; ~ реши́ть сде́лать что-л. be* firmly detérmined/resólved to do *smth.*; ~ стоя́ть на нога́х be* quite stéady on one's feet; ~ стоя́ть на своём be* firm; stick* to one's guns *разг.*

твердока́менный unyíelding.

твердоло́б|ый dull; thick *разг.*; **~ые консерва́торы** díehard consérvatives.

твёрдость *ж.* 1. hárdness; 2. (*реши́тельность*) firmness; 3. (*сто́йкость*) stéadfastness; ~ ду́ха (móral) fórtitude.

твёрд|ый 1. (*нежи́дкий*) sólid; **~ое те́ло** sólid; 2. (*немя́гкий*) hard; ~ грунт hard ground; **~ое я́блоко** hard ápple; ~ как ка́мень hard as a rock, íron-hard; 3. (*сто́йкий, непоколеби́мый*) stéadfast; (*непрекло́нный*) firm, well-bálanced, stéady; ~ ду́хом челове́к stéadfast pérson; он оста́лся твёрд he remáined firm/unsháken; **~ая во́ля** strong will; ~ хара́ктер firm/bálanced cháracter; **~ая похо́дка** résolute/púrposeful walk; 4. (*усто́йчивый, про́чный*) firm, strong; (*про́чно установи́вшийся*) stáble, estáblished; (*устано́вленный*) fixed; пе́рен. firm; **~ая опо́ра** firm suppórt; **~ая власть** stáble góvernment; ~ поря́док estáblished órder; **~ые це́ны** stáble príces; ~ гра́фик firm tíme-table; **~ое наме́рение, реше́ние** firm inténtion, decísion; ~ое убежде́ние firm convíction; 5. (*я́сный, отчётливый*) sound; (*све́дущий*) strong; в здра́вом уме́ и ~ой па́мяти of sound mind, sound in mind; **~ые зна́ния** sólid léarning/knówledge *sg*; он не о́чень твёрд в матема́тике *и т. п.* he's not véry strong in mathemátics, *etc.*; ◇ знак hard sign; **~ые согла́сные зву́ки** *лингв.* hard cónsonants; стоя́ть ~ой но-

гой have* a firm fóoting; име́ть ~ую по́чву под нога́ми be* on firm ground.

тверды́ня *ж.* strónghold.

твид *м.* tweed. **~овый** tweed *attr.*; **~овый костю́м** tweed suit; я люблю́ ве́щи из ~а I like tweeds.

твоё *притяж. мест. с. см.* твой.

тво́|й *притяж. мест.* 1. (*пе́ред сущ.*) your; (*без сущ.*) yours; ~ дом your house; **~ё пальто́** your óvercoat; **~я́ кни́га** your book; э́то ме́сто моё, а э́то ~ё this is my place, and that is yours; 2. *в знач. сущ. с. разг.* (what is) yours; **~его́ мне не на́до** I want nóthing that is yours; 3. *в знач. сущ. мн.* (*родны́е*) your folk, your péople; приве́т всем ~им my regárds to your péople; ◇ (не) ~ё де́ло it's (none of) your búsiness.

творе́ние *с.* creátion; (*произведе́ние тж.*) másterpiece.

творе́ц *м.* creátor.

твори́тельный: ~ паде́ж *грам.* instruméntal (case).

твор|и́ть *несов.* (*вн.*) 1. (*создава́ть*) create (*smth.*); 2. (*де́лать, соверша́ть*) do* (*smth.*), perfórm (*smth.*); ~ беззако́ния víolate jústice; ~ чудеса́ work wónders. **~и́ться** *несов.* be* góing on; что здесь ~и́тся? what is góing on here?; с ним ста́ло ~и́ться что́-то нела́дное a distúrbing change came óver him, sómething queer is háppening to him.

творо́г *м.* curds *pl*, cóttage cheese.

творо́жник *м. кул.* curd fritter.

тво́рчески creátively; ~ испо́льзовать что-л. make* creátive use of smth.

тво́рческ|ий creátive, constrúctive; **~ие иска́ния** creátive search *sg*, quest for inspirátion *sg*, artístic explorátions; ~ путь худо́жника devélopment of an ártist; ~ ве́чер, отчёт (*музыка́нта*) recítal; (*писа́теля*) réading; **~ая мысль** creátive thought; **~ая де́ятельность** creátive actívities *pl*; **~ая коллекти́в** (creátive) group/team; **~ая командиро́вка** trip to gáther matérial for creátive work; ~ о́тпуск tíme-off (from official dúties) to work in one's own artístic, scientífic field; **~ая си́ла** creátive pówer; ~ успе́х artístic succéss; **~ие го́ды писа́теля** a wríter's prodúctive períod.

тво́рчество *с.* 1. (*де́ятельность*) creátion, creátive work; нау́чное ~ scientífic work; 2. (*со́зданное*) work.

твоя́ *притяж. мест. ж. см.* твой.

те *мест. мн.* those; **те же** the same.

теа́тр *м.* 1. (*род иску́сства*) the théatre; исто́рия ру́сского ~а the history of the Rússian théatre; драмати́ческий ~ the dráma; ~ миниатю́р revúe théatre; эстра́дный ~ músic-hall; ~ ку́кол the púppet théatre, púppetry; 2. (*учрежде́ние*) the théatre, the stage; the théater *амер.*; рабо́тать в ~е work in the théatre; (*об актёре тж.*) be* on the stage; 3. (*зда́ние*) théatre, pláy-house; théater *амер.* 4. (*ме́сто, где происхо́дит что-л.*) théatre; ~ вое́нных де́йствий théatre of operátions.

театра́л *м. ж.* lóver of the théatre, théatregoer; pláygoer; théatergoer *амер.*

театра́льн|ый 1. théatre *attr.*; **~ое иску́сство** the art of the théatre; **~ая кри́тика** dramátic/théatre críticism; **~ые костю́мы** théatre cóstumes; **~ая афи́ша** pláybill; **~ая ка́сса** bóx-office; tícket-office *амер.*; ~ биле́т théatre tícket; 2. (*хара́ктерный для теа́тра*) stage *attr.*; of the stage/théatre *по́сле сущ.*; **~ые усло́вности** stage convéntions, convéntions of the théatre; 3. (*наи́гранный*) histriónic, theátrical; ~ жест theátrical gésture.

теа́тр-сту́дия *м.* experiméntal théatre; fringe théatre *разг.*

тебе́ (*дт., пр. от ли́чн. мест.* ты) you, to you; ~ ну́жно быть там в пять часо́в you've got to be there at five; к ~ пришли́ това́рищи some friends have come to see you.

тебя́ (*рд., вн. от ли́чн. мест.* ты) you.

теза́урус *м.* thesáurus.

те́зис *м.* 1. *лог., филос.* thésis (*pl* théses); 2. (*основ-*

ные положения) main proposítions/points; ~ы докла́да heads of an addréss/speech/repórt.

тёзка *м. и ж.* námesake.

текст *м.* 1. text; (*отрывок тж.*) pássage; 2. (*к му́зыке*) words *pl*; (*оперы*) librétto.

тексти́ль *м. собир.* téxtiles *pl.* ~ный téxtile; ~ная фа́брика téxtile mill; ~ные изде́лия téxtiles. ~щик *м.*, ~щица *ж.* téxtile-worker.

текстуа́льный téxtual.

теку́ч|есть *ж.* 1. *физ.* fluídity; (*металла*) yield; 2. (*непостоянство*) fluctuátion(s); ~ ка́дров fluctuátion in the supplý of trained personnél. ~ий 1. *физ.* flúid; 2. (*проточный — о воде*) flówing, rúnning; 3. (*непостоянный*) flúctuating, unstáble. ~ка *ж. разг.* búsiness routine, chores *pl.*

теку́щ|ий 1. flówing, rúnning; 2. (*настоящий*) cúrrent; (*современный*) présent-day; в ~ем году́ in the cúrrent year; ~ моме́нт the présent situátion; ~ие собы́тия cúrrent events/affáirs; ~ие зада́чи présent-day próblems; 3. (*повседневный*) éveryday; routine *attr.*; ~ие дела́ routine/éveryday mátters; ◇ ~ ремо́нт routine/rúnning repáirs *pl*; ~ счёт cúrrent accóunt.

телеателье́ *с. нескл.* télevision repáir shop.

телеба́шня *ж.* télevision tówer.

телеви́дение *с* télevision, TV.

телевизио́нн|ый télevision *attr.*; ~ая анте́нна TV áerial; ~ая переда́ча télecast.

телеви́зор *м.* télevision set; télly *разг.*, téle *амер.* ~ный télevision *attr.*; ~ный сто́лик télevision táble.

теле́га *ж.* cart, wággon.

телегра́мм|а *ж.* télegram, wíre; (*каблограмма*) cáble; ~-мо́лния expréss-télegram; ~ с опла́ченным отве́том replý-paid télegram; дать ~у send* a télegram/wíre.

телегра́ф *м.* 1. (*система*) télegraph; 2. (*учрежде́ние*) télegraph-office; 3. (*аппарат*) télegraph.

телеграфи́р|овать *несов. и сов.* (*вн., о пр.*) télegraph (*smth.*), wíre (*smth.*); (*по подводному кабелю*) cáble (*smth.*); он не ~овал домо́й he dídn't send any wíre to his home; ~ день вы́езда wíre *one's* day of depárture.

 • телеграфи́ст *м.*, ~ка *ж* télegraph-operator.

телегра́фия *ж.* telégraphy.

телегра́фн|ый telegráphic; télegraph *attr.*; ~ аппара́т telegráphic devíce; ~ая ле́нта (télegraph) tape; ~ое сообще́ние telegráphic méssage, cáble; ~ столб télegraph-pole, télegraph-post; ~ая связь communicátion by télegraph, cáble línk-up; ◇ ~ое аге́нтство news/télegraph ágency.

теле́жка *ж.* 1. light cart; (*ручная*) hánd-cart; 2. *тех.* trólley; (*вагонная*) bógie.

телезри́тель *м.* téleviewer; *мн.* TV áudiences.

те́лекс *м.* télex; посла́ть ~ в Пари́ж télex to Páris; у нас свой ~ we have our own télex facílities.

телеметри́ческ|ий telemétric; ~ие назе́мные ста́нции telémetry ground státions.

 • телемеха́н|ика *ж.* 1. (*управление производственными процессами на расстоянии*) télecontról; 2. (*отрасль науки*) telemechánics. ~и́ческий télecontról *attr.*

телёнок *м.* calf*; (*бычок*) búll-calf*.

телеобъекти́в *м.* telescópic lens.

телепа́т|ия *ж.* telépathy. ~и́ческий telepáthic.

телепереда́ча *ж.* télecast.

телеприёмник *м.* télevision recéiver.

телеско́п *м.* télescope. ~и́ческий telescópic.

теле́сн|ый 1. córporal, bódily; ~ое наказа́ние córporal púnishment; ~ые поврежде́ния bódily ínjuries; ~ого цве́та flésh-coloured; 2. (*материальный*) corpóreal.

телета́йп *м.* téletype, téleprinter. ~ный téletype *attr.*; ~ная ле́нта téletape.

телеуправл|е́ние *с.* remóte contról. ~я́емый remóte-
-contról *attr.*; (*о движущихся объектах*) guíded; ~я́емый снаря́д guíded míssile.

телефо́н *м.* télephone; phone *разг.*; провести́ ~ instáll the télephone; по ~у on/óver the (téle)phone; говори́ть по ~у с кем-л. speak* to *smb.* óver the télephone; вызыва́ть кого́-л. к ~у call *smb.* to the (téle)phone; звони́ть кому́-л. по ~у ring* *smb.* up; подойти́ к ~у ánswer the (téle)phone.

телефо́н-автома́т *м.* 1. (*связь*) públic télephone. 2. (*на улице*) (téle)phone booth/box; call box; (*в помещении*) pay phone; pay státion *амер.*

телефон|и́ровать *несов. и сов.* (*дт., о пр.*) télephone (*smb.*, abóut); ~и́ст *м.* 1. télephone-operator; 2. (*военный связист*) sígnaller. ~и́стка *ж.* télephone-operator.

телефони́я *ж.* teléphony.

телефо́нн|ый télephone *attr.*; telephónic; ~ аппара́т télephone (set); ~ая ста́нция télephone-exchánge; ~ая тру́бка recéiver; ~ая бу́дка (téle)phone/call box; pay státion *амер.*; ~ разгово́р télephone conversátion; ~ое сообще́ние telephónic communicátion; ◇ ~ая кни́га télephone book/diréctory.

телефоногра́мма *ж.* (téle)phoned télegram.

телеце́нтр *м.* (*телевизионный центр*) télevision céntre, TV státion.

телеэкра́н *м.* télevision screen.

тели́ться, отели́ться calve.

тёлка *ж.* héifer.

те́л|о *с.* bódy; геометри́ческие ~á geométrical sólids; температу́ра ~a bódy témperature; быть в ~e be* sleek and well-nóurished; дрожа́ть всем ~ом trémble all óver, trémble in évery limb; ◇ посторо́ннее ~ fóreign bódy; пре́данный душо́й и ~ом devóted bódy and soul; держа́ть кого́-л. в чёрном ~e treat *smb.* rough.

телогре́йка *ж. разг.* wádded jácket.

телодвиже́ние *с.* móvement of the bódy; (*жест*) gésture.

телосложе́ние *с.* build, physíque.

телохрани́тель *м.* bódyguard.

тельня́шка *ж. разг.* sáilor's vest.

те́льце *с.* 1. small bódy; 2. *обыкн. мн.* córpuscle *sg.*

теля́тина *ж.* veal.

теля́тник *м.* (*хлев для телят*) cálf-house, cálf-pen.

теля́тница *ж.* cálf-tender.

теля́|чий 1. calf *attr.*, calve's; ~чьи но́жки calve's foot *sg*; 2. (*из телятины*) veal *attr.*; ~чья отбивна́я veal cútlet; ◇ в ~чьем восто́рге in chíldish glee.

тем I *мест.*: ~ са́мым théreby; с ~, что́бы... in órder to..., for the púrpose (of + -ing).

тем II 1. *нареч.* so much the; ~ лу́чше (ху́же) so much the bétter (the worse); 2. *в составе сложного союза* the; чем скоре́е, ~ лу́чше the sóoner, the bétter; ◇ ~ бо́лее, что... the more so, that...; especially/particularly as...; ~ не ме́нее nevertheléss, nonethéless.

те́м|а *ж.* 1. súbject, theme; (*разговора*) tópic; ~ докла́да súbject of a repórt; на ~ы дня on tópical súbjects; э́то его́ излюбленная ~ it is a fávourite tópic of his; 2. *муз.* theme; ~ с вариа́циями theme with variátions.

тема́тика *ж.* súbjects *pl*, themes *pl.*

темати́ческий 1. súbject *attr.*; concérning a partícular súbject *после сущ.*; ~ план (súbject) prógramme; 2. *муз.* themátic; of theme *после сущ.*

тембр *м.* tímbre, quálity.

теменн|о́й parіétal; ~а́я кость parіétal bone.

те́мень *ж. разг.*: кака́я здесь ~! how dark it is here!

темн|е́ть, потемне́ть, стемне́ть 1. grow* dárk(er); (*о красках, небе*) dárken; 2. *безл.*: ~е́ет it's gr о́wing dark, the day is clósing in, the light is fáiling; 3. *тк. несов.* (*виднеться*) loom dark; вдали́ что́-то ~е́ет there's a dark shape in the distance; ◇ у меня́ ~е́ет в глаза́х éverything is góing dark befóre my eyes.

темни́ть *несов.* 1. (*вн.*) dárken (*smth.*); 2. (*обманывать*) dodge, hide* sómething.

темни́ца *ж.* dúngeon.

темно́ *в знач. сказ. безл.* it is dark.

темно- *в сложн.* dark-.

темноволо́сый dark(-háired).

темногла́зый dark-éyed.

тёмно-зелёный dark-gréen.

темноко́жий dark-skínned.

тёмно-кра́сный dark-réd.

темноли́цый dúsky, dúsky-compléxioned.

тёмно-си́ний dark-blúe, deep-blúe; (*о материи*) navy-blúe.

темнот|а́ *ж.* 1. dárkness, dark; в ~é in the dark; до (наступле́ния) ~ы́ before dark; 2. *разг.* (*невежество*) ígnorance, báckwardness.

тёмн|ый 1. dark; (*о цвете тж.*) deep; ~ая ночь dark night; ~ая ко́мната dark room; ~ые во́лосы dark hair; 2. (*мрачный*) glóomy; 3. (*подозрительный*) shády; ~ая ли́чность shády/dúbious cháracter; ~ое де́ло shády búsiness; 4. (*неясный*) obscúre, vague; ~ое ме́сто (*в тексте*) obscúre pássage; 5. (*невежественный*) ígnorant, beníghted; ◇ ~ое пятно́ stain.

темны́м-темно́ it is pítch-dark.

темп *м.* pace, rate; témpo (*тж. муз.*); ~ а́рии témpo of an ária; ~ бе́га speed; ~ы разви́тия промы́шленности rate of indústrial devélopment; ускоря́ть ~ы quícken the pace; замедля́ть ~ы slácken the pace, slow down.

темпера́мент *м.* 1. témperament; 2. (*внутренний подъём*) zest, inténsity, verve; ◇ с ~ом with treméndous dash. ~ный fórceful, spírited; ~ное исполне́ние spírited/impássioned performance; ~ный актёр fórceful áctor.

температу́р|а *ж.* témperature; ~ во́здуха air témperature; ~ кипе́ния воды́ bóiling point; изме́рить больно́му ~у take* a pátient's témperature. ~ить *несов. разг.* run* a témperature. ~ный témperature *attr.*

те́мя *с. анат.* sínciput; (*макушка*) crown/top of the head.

тенденцио́зн|ость *ж.* tendéntiousness. ~ый tendéntious; (*предвзятый*) bías(s)ed.

тенде́нц|ия *ж.* 1. (*к дт.; склонность*) téndency (to, towárds); име́ть ~ию have* a téndency, tend; 2. (*основная идея*) méssage, theme; 3. (*предвзятая мысль*) bías.

те́ндер *м. ж.-д.* ténder.

тене́в|о́й 1. shády; ~ая сторона́ у́лицы shády side of a street; 2. *иск.* dark; ◇ ~а́я сторона́ чего́-л. dark side of smth.

тенелюби́в|ый sháde-requíring; ~ые расте́ния sháde-requíring plants.

тени́стый shády; ~ сад shády gárden.

те́ннис *м.* ténnis; ◇ насто́льный ~ táble ténnis; píng-pong *разг.* ~и́ст *м.*, ~и́стка *ж.* ténnis-player. ~ный ténnis *attr.*; ~ный мяч ténnis-ball; ~ный корт ténnis-court.

те́нор *м.* 1. ténor; петь ~ом sing* ténor; 2. (*певец*) ténor.

тент *м.* áwning.

тен|ь *ж.* 1. *тк. ед.* (*неосвещённое пространство*) shade; в ~и́ in the shade; в саду́ бы́ло мно́го ~и the gárden was well sháded; 2. *иск.* shade; свет и ~ light and shade; 3. (*отбрасываемая*) shádow (*тж. перен.*); ~и со́сен shádows of píne-trees; ~ неудово́льствия shádow of displéasure; 4. (*слабый след, ничтожная доля чего-л.*) shádow; ~ улы́бки the shádow of a smile; ни ~и пра́вды not a párticle/véstige of truth; ни те́ни сомне́ния not a shádow of doubt; 5. (*силуэт*) figure, shape; 6. (*призрак*) ghost; ◇ ночны́е ~и noctúrnal shádows; броса́ть ~ на кого́-л., что́-л. put* smb., smth. in a bad light; держа́ться, быть в ~и remáin in the background; ходи́ть, сле́довать за кем-л. как ~ fóllow smb. abóut like his, her shádow; от него́ оста́лась одна́ ~ he is the mere shádow of his fórmer self, he is worn to a shádow; ~и под глаза́ми у кого́-л. shádows únder smb.'s eyes.

теоло́гия *ж.* theólogy.

теоре́ма *ж.* théorem.

теоре́тик *м.* théorist.

теорети́ческ|ий theorétical; ~ие иссле́дования theorétical reséarch *sg*; ~ ум theorétical/spéculative mind; ~ая фи́зика theorétical phýsics; ~ие расчёты theorétical calculátions.

тео́ри|я *ж.* théory; в ~и in théory, theorétically.

тепе́реш|ний *разг.* présent; в ~ее вре́мя nówadays.

тепе́рь now; (*в настоящее время*) at présent; (*в наше время*) nówadays; ~, когда́... now that...

тепле́ть, потепле́ть grow* wárm(er).

те́пли|ться *несов.* glímmer (*тж. перен.*), gleam; в нём ещё ~тся наде́жда he still chérishes a faint hope.

тепли́|ца *ж.* hóthouse. ~чный hóthouse *attr.*; ~чная температу́ра hóthouse témperature; ~чные огурцы́ hóthouse cúcumbers; ◇ ~чное расте́ние hóthouse plant, ténder créature.

тепл|о́ I *с.* 1. warmth; *перен. тж.* cordiálity, afféction; держа́ть но́ги в ~é keep* one's feet warm; сиде́ть в ~é be* in the warm; серде́чное ~ sincére afféction; 2. *физ.* heat; 15 гра́дусов ~á fiftéen degrées abóve zéro.

тепло́ II 1. *нареч.* wármly; (*сердечно тж.*) córdially; ~ оде́ваться dress wármly; ~ встре́тить кого́-л. greet smb. wármly/córdially; ~ отзыва́ться о ком-л. be* enthusiástic abóut smb., give* a glówing accóunt of smb.; 2. *в знач. сказ. безл.* it is warm; сего́дня ~ it is warm todáy; в ко́мнате ~ the room is warm; 3. *в знач. сказ. безл.* (*дт.*): мне ~ I am warm.

теплово́з *м.* díesel locomótive.

теплов|о́й *физ.* heat *attr.*; *тех.* thérmal; ~а́я эне́ргия heat/thérmal énergy; ~ дви́гатель heat éngine; ◇ ~а́я сеть (dístrict) céntral héating sýstem; ~ уда́р héat-stroke.

теплоёмкость *ж. физ.* heat/thérmal capácity.

теплоизол|яцио́нный héat-insulation *attr.*, héat-insulating. ~я́ция heat insulátion.

теплопрово́дн|ость *ж. физ.* thérmal condúctivity. ~ый *физ.* héat-condúcting.

теплосто́йк|ий héatproof, héat-resístant; ~ие материа́лы héat-resistant materials.

теплот|а́ *ж.* 1. warmth (*тж. перен.*); серде́чная ~ cordiálity; с ~о́й (*говорить, вспоминать*) with warm féelings; 2. *физ.* heat; скры́тая ~ látent heat; едини́ца измере́ния ~ы́ thérmal únit.

теплотво́р|ный calorífic, héat-prodúcing; ~ая спосо́бность heat válue, héating pówer.

теплоте́хника *ж.* thermotéchnics.

теплотра́сса *ж.* héating main.

теплофика́ция *ж.* céntral héating (of districts, towns).

теплохо́д *м.* mótor-vessel; (*морской тж.*) mótor-ship.

теплоцентра́ль *ж.* héating plant.

теплоэлектроста́нция *ж.* thérmal/heat pówer station.

теплу́шка *ж. разг.* 1. (stóve-)héated goods van; 2. (*тёплое помещение на стадионах и т. п.*) (héated) shélter.

тёпл|ый warm; (*сердечный тж.*) córdial; ~ дождь warm rain; ~ая пого́да warm wéather; ~ая зима́ mild wínter; ~ приём warm/córdial recéption; ~ые слова́ córdial words; чуть ~ lúkewarm; ◇ ~ая компа́ния close círcle; э́то ~ая компа́ния they're as thick as thieves, they are a bunch of rogues.

теплы́нь *ж. разг.* mild wéather; кака́я ~! how warm it is!

терапе́вт *м.* therapéutist, spécialist in intérnal diséases. ~и́ческий therapéutic, therapéutical.

терапи́я *ж.* 1. (*лечение*) thérapy; 2. (*раздел медицины*) therapéutics.

тереби́ть *несов.* (*вн.*) 1. (*дёргать*) keep*

púlling/túgging (at); *перен.* péster (*smb.*); 2. *с-х.:* ~ лён pull flax.

тере́ть *несов.* (*вн.*) 1. rub (*smb.*, *smth.*); 2. (*размельча́ть*) grind* (*smth.*); 3. (*причиня́ть боль — об одежде, обуви*) chafe (*smth.*). ~ся, потере́ться 1. (*тере́ть себя́*) rub oneself; 2. *тж. несов.* (*о пр.; при движе́нии*) rub (*smth.*), chafe (*smth.*); 3. (*о пр.; прикаса́ться головой, спиной*) rub up (against); ~ся об но́ги (*о собаке, кошке*) rub up against *smb.'s* knees; 4. *тж. несов. разг.* (*находи́ться среди́ кого-л.*) hang* abóut.

терза́ние *с.* tórment, ágony.

терза́ть *несов.* (*вн.*) 1. (*рвать*) tear* (*smth.*), maul (*smth.*); 2. (*му́чить*) tormént (*smth.*), tórture (*smth.*), rack (*smth.*). ~ся *несов.* be* in tórment; (*тв.*) be* racked (with).

тёрк|а *ж.* gráter; тере́ть что-л. на ~е grate *smth.*

те́рмин *м.* term.

терминологи́ческий terminológical.

терминоло́гия *ж.* terminólogy.

терми́т I *м.* *зоол.* térmite.

терми́т II *м.* *хим.* thérmite.

терми́тн|ый thérmite *attr.*; ~ая сва́рка thérmite wélding; ~ая бо́мба thérmite bomb.

терми́ческ|ий *физ.*, *тех.* thérmal; ~ая обрабо́тка мета́лла thérmal tréatment of métal, héat-treatment of métal.

термодина́мика *ж.* thermodynámics.

термока́мера *ж.* heat chámber.

термо́метр *м.* thermómeter; медици́нский ~ clínical thermómeter; поста́вить кому́-л. ~ take* *smb.'s* témperature.

терморегуля́тор *м.* témperature-control devíce, thermoregulátor.

те́рмос *м.* thérmos flask/bóttle, flask *амер.*

термоя́дерн|ый thermonúclear; ~ая реа́кция thermonúclear reáction; ~ая эне́ргия thermonúclear énergy; ~ое ору́жие thermonúclear wéapons *pl*; ~ая бо́мба thermonúclear bomb; ~ая война́ thermonúclear war.

тёрн *м.* 1. *собир.* (*я́годы*) sloes *pl*; 2. (*куст*) bláckthorn.

терни́стый thórny; ~ путь thórny path.

тернóв|ник *м.* bláckthorn. ~ый bláckthorn *attr.*; ~ый куст bláckthorn bush; ~ое варе́нье sloe jam.

терпели́в|о pátiently, with pátience. ~ый pátient (*выражающий терпение тж.*) resígned, long-súffering.

терпе́ни|е *с.* pátience; вооружи́ться ~ем arm oneself with pátience; вы́йти из ~я, потеря́ть ~ lose* pátience, get* out of pátience; ~ и труд всё перетру́т pátience and hard work can do ánything.

терпе́ть *несов.* (*вн.*) 1. (*безро́потно переноси́ть*) súffer (*smth.*); бы́ло бо́льно, но пришло́сь ~ it was páinful but *one* had to put up with it; ~ лише́ния súffer privátions/hárdships; приходи́тся ~ it must be borne; 2. (*мири́ться с кем-л., чем-л.*) bear* (*smb.*, *smth.*), tólerate (*smb.*, *smth.*); ~ не могу́ э́того I can't stand/bear/tólerate it, I hate it; ~ не могу́, когда́ мне противоре́чат I hate béing contradícted; он не те́рпит возраже́ния he won't be contradícted; как его́ то́лько те́рпят здесь? how do they put up with him?; 3. (*испы́тывать*) súffer (*smth.*), endúre (*smth.*). (*подверга́ться*) undergó* (*smth.*); ~ пораже́ние súffer deféat, be* deféated; ~ круше́ние meet* disáster; (*о корабле́*) be* wrecked; ~ убы́тки sustáin/súffer lósses, undergó* lósses; ◇ вре́мя те́рпит there is still time; вре́мя не те́рпит time présses; де́ло не те́рпит отлага́тельства there must be no deláy, the mátter is úrgent.

терпи́м|о: относи́ться ~ к кому́-л., чему́-л. be* tólerant of *smb.*, *smth.*; э́то ещё ~ that's still béarable. ~ость *ж.* tólerance; ~ость к чужи́м мне́ниям tólerance towards óther péople's views. ~ый 1. (*допусти́мый*) tólerable, béarable; 2. (*снисходи́тельный*) tólerant.

тёрпк|ий astríngent; (*о за́пахе*) púngent (*тж. перен.*) ~ость *ж.* astríngency; púngency.

терра́с|а *ж.* 1. térrace; располо́женный ~ами térraced; 2. (*часть дома*) verándah; porch *амер.*

террикóн *м.* pit heap.

территориа́льн|ый territórial; ◇ ~ые во́ды territórial wáters.

террито́рия *ж.* térritory.

терро́р *м.* térrorism.

террор|изи́ровать *несов. и сов.* (*вн.*) térrorize (*smb.*). ~и́ст *м.* térrorist. ~исти́ческий terrorístic; ~исти́ческий акт act of térrorism.

тёрт|ый 1. ground, gráted; ~ые кра́ски ground paints; ~ая ре́дька gráted rádish; 2. *разг.* (*быва́лый*) hárd-bitten.

те́рция *ж.* third; больша́я, ма́лая ~ *муз.* májor, mínor third.

тер|я́ть, потеря́ть (*вн.*, *в пр.*) lose* (*smb.*, *smth.*); (*ли́стья, рога́ и т. п.*) shed* (*smth.*); ~ зре́ние, слух lose* sight, héaring; ~ си́лы becóme* weak; ~ вре́мя на что-л. waste time on *smth.*; не ~я́ вре́мени withóut loss of time; не ~я́ вре́мени принима́ться за де́ло, рабо́ту lose* no time in sétting to work; ~ му́жество lose* heart; ~ наде́жду lose* hope; ~ си́лу becóme* inválid, lose* its force; ~ в ве́се lose* weight; ~ в чьих-л. глаза́х lówer oneself in *smb.'s* eyes; ~ в чём-л. мне́нии sink* in *smb.'s* estimátion; ничего́ не ~ (от) lose* nóthing (by); его́ стихи́ ~я́ют в перево́де his póetry lóses a lot in translátion; ◇ ~ го́лову lose* *one's* head/wits; не ~ головы́ keep* *one's* head; ~ по́чву под нога́ми feel* the ground slípping awáy form únder *one's* feet; ~ кого́-л. из ви́ду lose* sight of *smb.*; не́чего ~ кому́-л. *smb.* has nóthing to lose. ~я́ться, потеря́ться 1. (*пропада́ть*) get* lost; 2. (*де́латься незаме́тным*) disappéar; merge; 3. (*о зву́ках, за́пахах*) fade; 4. (*перестава́ть просле́живаться*) be* lost; 5. (*станови́ться слабе́е*) flag, fail, give* out; 6. (*теря́ть прису́тствие ду́ха*) get* flústered; ◇ ~я́ться в дога́дках be* lost in conjécture.

тёс *м.* *собир.* boards *pl.*

теса́к *м.* 1. (*меч*) bróadsword; 2. (*топо́р*) hátchet.

теса́ть *несов.* (*вн.*) 1. cut* (*smth.*), hew* (*smth.*); ~ до́ски cut* planks; 2. (*изготовля́ть*) rough-héw (*smth.*), shape (*smth.*); ◇ ему́ хоть кол на голове́ теши́ there's no gétting it ínto his head, he is so píg-headed.

тесёмка *ж.* tape; (*плетёная*) braid.

тесни́на *ж.* gorge, défile.

тесни́ть, потесни́ть (*вн.*) 1. (*лиша́ть просто́ра*) restríct (*smb.*, *smth.*), be* in the way (of); 2. (*заставля́ть отходи́ть*) drive* (*smb.*) back; *перен.* squeeze out (*smb.*, *smth.*); ~ проти́вника drive* the énemy back. ~ся *несов.* 1. (*толпи́ться*) throng, crowd; 2. (*жить, рабо́тать в тесноте́*) be* crówded togéther, be* overcrówded, endúre a lack of space; *перен.* (*переполня́ть — о чу́вствах и т. п.*) seethe; 3. (*толка́ть*) jóstle.

те́сно 1. *нареч.* clósely, íntimately; ~ прижима́ться к чему́-л. press close against *smth.*; ~ свя́занный с кем-л. clósely/íntimately connécted with *smb.*; ~ сиде́ть not have enóugh room; 2. *в знач. сказ. безл.* it is cramped; здесь о́чень ~ it's véry cramped here; в ваго́не бы́ло ~ the cárriage was packed/crówded; 3. *в знач. сказ. безл.* (*дт.*): ему́ ~ (*ма́ло ме́ста*) he hásn't enóugh room; (*ма́ло свобо́ды*) he feels restrícted, there is no scope for him.

тесно́т|а *ж.* lack of space; (*чего-л.*) smállness, inádequacy; кака́я ~! how crówded it is here!; жить в ~е́ live in crówded condítions, be* cooped up; в ~е́, да не в оби́де *погов.* the more, the mérrier.

те́сн|ый 1. small, póky; *перен.* (*ограни́ченный*) nárrow, tight; ~ая кварти́ра póky flat; ~ круг друзе́й nárrow circle of friends; 2. (*располо́женный бли́зко друг*

к *другу*) tight-packed, crówded, compáct; ~ыми рядáми in close órder, in sérried ranks; 3. (*близкий*) close, íntimate; ~ое соприкоснове́ние close cóntact; ~ое сотру́д- ничество close co-operátion; ~ контáкт close cóntact; ~ая связь close connéction; 4. (*об одежде*) tight, small.

тесо́в|ый board *attr.*; ~ые воро́та board gates.

тест *м.* test. ~и́ровать *несов.* test.

тест|о́ *с.* paste; (*для хлеба*) dough; ◇ из одного́ ~а the same breed; из друго́го ~а quite a different breed/stamp.

тесть *м.* fáther-in-law (*pl* fáthers-) (*wife's father*).

тесьма́ *ж.* braid.

те́терев *м.* blа́ck-cock, héath-cock.

тетёрка *ж.* grey hen.

тетива́ *ж.* 1. (*лука*) bów-string; 2. (*лестницы*) string(er), string-piece.

тётка *ж.* 1. aunt; 2. *разг.* (*женщина*) wóman*.

тетра́дка *ж. см.* тетра́дь.

тетра́дь *ж.* nótebook; éxercise-book (*тж.* шко́льная); ~ в лине́йку líned éxercise-book; ~ для рисова́ния dráwing-book, ské́tch-book.

тётя *ж.* aunt; (*в обращении тж.*) а́unty.

тёфтели *мн. кул.* meat balls.

техми́нимум *м.* requíred mínimum of téchnical knо́wledge; сдава́ть ~ quа́lify in the requíred mínimum of téchnical knо́wledge.

те́хник *м.* téchnícian; ◇ зубно́й ~ déntal mechа́nic.

те́хник|а *ж.* 1. (*область человеческой деятельно- сти*) engineе́ring; technо́logy, indústrial arts; передова́я ~ advа́nced technо́logy; 2. *собир.* (*оборудование*) equípment, machínery, plant; бере́чь ~у look а́fter machínery; боева́я ~ fighting equípment; materiе́l; 3. (*приёмы исполнения*) techníque(s); ~ шахматной игры chess technique; музыка́льная ~ músical technique; ~ рабо́ты operа́tional techniques *pl*; ◇ ~ безопа́сности sáfety devíces, а́ccident prevénition.

те́хникум *м.* téchnical secondary school; строи́тель- ный ~ búilding-trade sécondary school.

техни́ческ|ий 1. téchnical; ~ие усовершенствования téchnical impróvements; ~ая документа́ция téchnical documentа́tion; ~ие на́выки téchnical skills; 2. (*исполь- зуемый в промышленности*) indústrial; ~ие культу́ры indústrial crops; 3. (*связанный с обслуживанием произ- водства*) téchnical; ~ реда́ктор téchnical е́ditor; (*в газе- те*) make-up е́ditor; 4. (*не ответственный*) subо́rdinate, júnior.

техно́лог *м.* technо́logist. ~и́ческий technológical; ~и́ческие тре́бования technológical requírements; ~и́че- ский проце́сс technológical prócess.

техноло́гия *ж.* technо́logy.

техобслу́живани|е *с.* máintenance; ста́нция ~я sérvice stа́tion.

техре́д *м.* téchnical éditor.

тече́ни|е *с.* 1. (*действие*) flow; (*времени, собы- тий*) course; 2. (*струя, поток*) cúrrent, stream; бы́ст- рое ~ swift cúrrent; тёплое (холо́дное) ~ warm (cold) cúrrent; по ~ю with the stream; вверх по ~ю upstréam; вниз по ~ю downstréam; про́тив ~я agа́inst the cúrrent; боро́ться с ~ем fight* the cúrrent; 3. (*направление*) trend, téndency; ~я в иску́сстве trends in art; ◇ в ~ (*рд.*) in the course (of); dúring (*smth.*); в ~ неде́ли, ме́- сяца, го́да in the course of a week, month, year, withín a week, month, year; в ~ до́лгого вре́мени for a long time; в ~ не́которого вре́мени for a while; в ~ всего́, всей... throughóut the...; в ~ всего́ го́да all the year; с ~ем вре́- мени in due course.

те́чка *ж.* heat.

течь I *несов.* 1. (*литься*) flow, run*; с кры́ши течёт the roof is drípping; из её глаз текли́ слёзы her eyes were stréaming with tears; 2. (*пропускать воду*) leak, be* léaky, be* léaking; ло́дка течёт the boat is léaking; 3. (*проходить, совершаться*) pass, pass on; вре́мя те-

чёт бы́стро time pásses quíckly; 4. (*двигаться сплош- ным потоком*) flow.

течь II *ж.* leak; дать ~ (*о судне*) spring* a leak; за- де́лать ~ plug a leak.

те́ш|ить, поте́шить (*вн.*) 1. *разг.* (*забавлять, раз- влекать*) amúse (*smb.*), entertа́in (*smb.*); (*доставлять удовольствие*) flа́tter (*smb.*); ~ взор please the eye; 2. (*утешать*) consо́le (*smb.*), soothe (*smb.*); ~ себя́ на- де́ждами consо́le onesе́lf with hopes. ~иться, поте́шиться (*тв.*) 1. *разг.* (*развлекаться*) amúse onesе́lf (with, at), enjо́y (*smth.*); чем бы дитя́ ни ~лось, лишь бы не пла́- кало *посл.* а́nything to keep him, her quíet; 2. (*уте- шаться*) consо́le onesе́lf (with).

тёща *ж.* mо́ther-in-law (*pl* mо́thers-) (*wife's mother*).

ти́гель *м.* crúcible.

тигр *м.* tíger. ~ёнок *м.* tíger cub. ~и́ца *ж.* tígress. ~о́вый tíger *attr.*

тик I *м.* (*болезнь*) tic.

тик II *м.* (*ткань*) tícking.

тик III *м.* (*дерево*) teak.

ти́канье *с.* tick, tícking.

ти́кать *несов.* tick.

тимофе́евка *ж. бот.* tímothy, herd's grass.

ти́н|а *ж.* slime, ooze. ~истый slímy, о́ozy.

тип *м.* 1. type; ~ корабля́ class of ship; самолёт но́- вого ~а a new type of а́ircraft; 2. *разг.* (*человек*) fé́llow; подозри́тельный ~ suspícious chа́racter.

типа́ж *м.* 1. *тех.* range (of mо́dels), types; 2. *иск.* type(s); 3. *кино* (right) type.

типи́ч|еский týpical. ~ность *ж.* týpicalness; *иск. тж.* represé́ntative/týpical nа́ture. ~ный týpical; *иск. тж.* represé́ntative; ~ный ю́жный го́род týpical só́uthern town; ~ный слу́чай týpical case; э́то ~но для него́ it's just like him.

типов|о́й 1. (*являющийся образцом*) sа́mple *attr.*, mо́del *attr.*; stа́ndard; ~ догово́р mó́del có́ntract; 2. (*стандартный*) stа́ndard, stа́ndardized; ~ое строи́тель- ство stа́ndardized building.

типогра́ф|ия *ж.* prínting-house, prínting-office; the prínter's *разг.* ~ский typográphical, prínter's; ~ская оши́бка prínter's é́rror; ~ская кра́ска prínter's ink.

типу́н *м.* the pip; ◇ тебе́ на язы́к ≈ curse the ton- gue that says it.

тир *м.* shó́oting-gallery.

тира́да *ж.* tirа́de.

тира́ж I *м.* (*займа*) draw; вы́йти в ~ (*об облигации*) be* drawn; *перен.* be* on the shelf*, be* a back nú́mber.

тира́ж II *м.* prínting, nú́mber of có́pies prínted, print run; кла́ссики издаю́тся больши́ми ~а́ми the clа́ssics are pú́blished in large edítions; ~ газе́ты 4 000 000 the né́wspaper is prínted in four míllíon có́pies; весь ~ газе́ты распро́дан the whole íssue of the pа́per is sold out; весь ~ кни́ги распро́дан the whole edítion/prínting of the book is sold out.

тира́н *м.* tу́rant. ~ить *несов.* (*вн.*) *разг.* bú́lly (*smb.*).

тирани́я *ж.* tу́ranny.

тире́ *с. нескл.* dash.

тис *м.* yew(-tree).

ти́скать, ти́снуть (*вн.*) 1. *тк. несов. разг.* (*жать, сжимать*) squeeze (*smb., smth.*); 2. *полигр.* pull (*smth.*).

тиск|и́ *мн.* vice *sg*; *перен.* grip *sg*; зажа́ть в ~ grip in a vice; в ~а́х *чего-л.* in the grip of *smth.*

ти́снуть *сов. см.* ти́скать.

тита́н *м.* 1. títan; ~ы нау́чной мы́сли the títans of science; 2. *хим.* titа́nium; 3. (*кипятильник*) urn. ~и́че- ский titа́nic.

титр *м. кино* súbtitle; (*перед началом фильма*) crédit títle, crédit.

ти́тул *м.* títle.

титуло́ванный títled.

ти́тульный *полигр.* títle *attr.*; ~ лист títle page.

тиф *м. мед.* týphus.

тих|ий 1. (*о звуках*) soft; (*о голосе*) low; ~ стон, шёпот low groan, whísper; ~ смех soft láughter; 2. (*погруженный в тишину*) still, quíet; ~ая ночь still night; 3. (*без шума, суеты*) quíet, tránquil; (*мирный*) péaceful, calm; ~ая улица quíet/secľúded street; у ~ой пристани in a quíet háven; ~ая жизнь péaceful/quíet life; unevéntful life; 4. (*смирный, кроткий*) plácid, géntle; ~ ребёнок quíet child*; ~ нрав plácid disposítion; ~ая грусть géntle grief; 5. (*спокойный*) calm, still, péaceful; ~ая погода calm wéather; ~ая вода still wáter; ~ая река péaceful stream; 6. (*медленный*) slow; ~ ход slow speed; ~им ходом at low speed; ~ шаг slow steps *pl.*

тихо 1. *нареч.* (*негромко*) sóftly; 2. *нареч.* (*без шума*) sílently, nóiselessly; (*без движения, спокойно*) still; ~! quíet!; ~ сидеть *и т. п.* sit*, *etc.* still; жить ~ live péacefully; 3. *нареч.* (*медленно*) slówly; дела идут ~ things are móving slówly; (*в торговле и т. п.*) búsiness is slack; 4. *в знач. сказ.* it is quíet; здесь ~ it's quíet here; в доме ~ it's quíet in the house; 5. *в знач. сказ. безл.* (*о погоде*) it is (véry) still; сегодня ~ there's no wind todáy; на море ~ the sea is calm.

тихоня *м. и ж. разг.* tímid/retíring créature; (*о девочке*) demúre líttle thing.

тихоокеанский Pacific.

тихоходный slow; low-speed *attr.*

тише 1. *сравнит. ст. прил.* тихий *и нареч.* тихо; 2. *в знач. повел. накл.* (*не шумите*) sh!, hush!, quíet there!; (*осторожно*) (be) cáreful!

тишин|а́ ж. sílence, stíllness; (*спокойствие*) calm, peace; ночная ~ the sílence of the night; в ~é in the sílence; нарушать ~ý break* the sílence; просят соблюдáть ~ý sílence, please!

тиш|ь ж. 1. *см.* тишина; 2. (*безветренная погода*) calm; ◇ в ~и́ 1) (*в тихое время*) when it is quíet, dúring a lull; 2) (*в тихом месте*) in a quíet/shéltered spot; ~ да гладь peace and hármony, swéetness and light.

ткань *ж.* 1. (*материя*) fábric, matérial; шёлковая ~ silk; 2. *биол.* tíssue.

ткать, соткать (*вн.*) weave* (*smth.*).

ткацк|ий wéaver's; wéaving *attr.*; ~ая фáбрика wéaving mill; ~ станок (*wéaving*) loom.

ткач *м.,* ~íха *ж.* wéaver.

ткнуть *сов. см.* тыкать.

тление *с.* 1. (*гниение*) decáy; decomposítion; 2. (*слабое горение*) smóuldering.

тленн|ость *ж.* ephemeráliy; ~ый ephémeral.

тлетворный pernícious, báleful.

тлеть *несов.* 1. (*гнить*) decáy, rot, móulder; 2. (*гореть без пламени*) smóulder (*тж. перен.*). ~ся *несов. разг.* smóulder.

тля *ж. зоол.* plánt-louse*; áphis (*pl* áphides) *научн.*

тмин *м.* 1. (*растение*) cáraway; 2. *собир.* (*семена*) cáraway-seeds *pl.*

то I *мест. см.* тот.

то II *союз* 1. (*тогда*) then; *обычно не переводится*; éсли вы не идёте, то я пойду if you don't go, I will; éсли вы не пойдёте, то я тоже не пойду if you don't go I won't éither; 2.: то..., то... now..., now...; то вправо, то влево now right, now left, altérnately right and left; то один, то другой first one, then anóther; не то..., не то... éither...; ~ и дёт, то снег, не то град it might be snówing or háiling, it's sómething betwéen snow and hail; то ли..., то ли éither... or.

-то: в том-то и дéло that's just the point; этого-то я и добивался that is just what I wánted; я-то согласен, но он нет I agrée. He's the one who doesn't; обещáть-то он обещáл, но сдéлает ли он? he said he would, but will he?; тут-то он и... at this, he...

тобой, тобою (*тв. от личн. мест.* ты) you; мы с ~ you and I.

товáр *м.* 1. *эк.* commódity; 2. (*предмет торговли*)

goods *pl*, wares *pl*; ~ы широкого потреблéния consúmer goods; ~ длительного пóльзования consúmer dúrables; ◇ показáть ~ лицóм show* éverything at its best.

товáрищ *м.* 1. friend, cómrade; ~ по рабóте féllow-worker, mate; ~ по оружию compánion-in-árms; ~ по плáванию shípmate; 2. (*в обращении*) Cómrade; ◇ ~ по несчáстью féllow-sufferer.

товáрищеск|ий friendly, cómradely; ~ая взаимопóмощь friendly mútual assístance; ~ матч friendly match.

товáрищество *с.* 1. (*отношения*) cómradeship, compánionship; 2. (*объединение*) associátion; (*фирма*) cómpany.

товáрно-дéнежн|ый: ~ые отношéния commódity-money relátions.

товáрн|ый 1. goods *attr.*; freight *attr. амер.*; ~ые запáсы stock (of goods) *sg*; ~ гóлод goods' shórtage; ~ знак trade mark; ~ склад wárehouse; ~ая стáнция goods státion; freight yard *амер.*; ~ вагóн goods wágon, goods truck; freight car *амер.*; ~ поезд goods train; freight train *амер.*; 2. *эк.* márketable; márket *attr.*; ~ хлеб, ~ое зернó márketable/mérchantable grain; ~ая продýкция commódity óutput; ◇ ~ое производство commódity prodúction.

товаровéд *м.* éxpert on mérchandise. ~ение *с.* the stúdy of mérchandise.

товарообмéн *м.* exchánge of commódities.

товарооборóт *м.* commódity circulátion, trade.

тогдá 1. (*в то время, не теперь*) then; ~ же then, at the time; ~, когдá when; 2. (*в таком случае*) then; *часто не переводится*; устáл? Тогдá отдохни́ are you tíred? Have a rest, then; ◇ ~ как 1) (*наоборот*) whereás; 2) (*хотя*) althóugh.

тогдáшн|ий *разг.* at that time *после сущ.*, of those days *после сущ.*; (*о должностных лицах*) the then; ~яя обстанóвка the situation at that time, the situation then obtáining; ~ие обычаи the cústoms of those days; ~ министр the then mínister.

то́ есть 1. that is to say; (*как поправка, уточнение*) I (you, *etc.*) mean; ~ вы ошиблись you mean, you made a mistáke; 2. (*выражает удивление*) what do you mean?; ~, как — не знáешь? what do you mean, you don't know?

тождéственн|ость *ж.* idéntity. ~ый idéntical (with).

тождество *с.* idéntity.

тóже too, álso; я ~ пойду I'm góing, too; я ~ мнóго испытáл I too have súffered gréatly; я ~! so am I!, so do I!; (*при отрицании*) nor/néither am, do I!; он ~ идёт so is, does, *etc.* he; (*при отрицании*) nor/néither is, does, *etc.* he!; ~ не not... éither; он ~ не глуп he's no fool éither; он ~ не знáет he dóesn't know éither.

ток I *м. физ., эл.* cúrrent; ~ вóздуха áir-current; ~ высóкого (низкого) напряжéния high-tension (lów-tension) cúrrent; ~ высóкой (низкой) частотý high-frequency (lów-frequency) cúrrent.

ток II *м.* (*для молотьбы*) thréshing-floor, bárnyard.

ток III *м. охот.* cóurting place.

токáрн|ый túrning; ~ая мастерскáя túrner's shop; ~ станóк lathe.

тóкарь *м.* túrner; ~ по дéреву wóod-turner; ~ по метáллу métal-turner.

токовáть *несов.* útter the máting call.

токсины *мн.* tóxins.

тол *м.* tólite, T.N.T.

толк *м.* 1. (*смысл*) sense, point; от негó ~у не добьёшься you can't get ány sense out of him; 2. (*польза*) use, point; из этой поéздки не выйдет никакóго ~у there's no point in this jóurney, nóthing will come out of this jóurney; 3. *обыкн. мн.* (*пересуды, разговоры*) talk *sg*; rúmours; (*сплетни*) góssip *sg*; вызвать мнóго ~ов cause a great deal of talk; идýт ~и о том, что... it is rúmoured that...; ◇ без тóлку (*напрасно*) úselessly; и всё без тóлку and all for nóthing; с ~ом efficiently; (*со* *смыслом*) intélligently; сбить *кого-л.* с ~у confúse *smb.*; знать, понимáть ~ в *чём-л.* be* a good judge of *smth.*; be* a connoisséur of *smth.*; сбиться с ~у get* confúsed; не возьму в ~ I can't see, I can't make out.

толк|áть, толкнýть 1. (*вн.*) push (*smb., smth.*), shove (*smb., smth.*); *сов. тж.* give* (*smb., smth.*) a push/shove; толкнýть *кого-л.* локтем nudge *smb.*; **2.** (*вн. на вн., к дт.; побуждать*) ínstigate (*smb.* to), incíte (*smb.* to); кто вас толкнýл на это? who put you up to it?; что вас толкнýло на это? what made you do that?; **3.** (*вн.*) *спорт.* (*кидать*) put* (*smth.*); ~ ядрó put* the shot. **~áться** *несов.* **1.** push; (*толкать друг друга*) push one anóther, jóstle; **2.** *разг.* (*быть, находиться где-л.*) be* аróund, be* knócking about; (*без особого дела*) hang* about. **~нýть(те)** *сов. см.* толкáть.

толкáч *м.* **1.** (*поезда, судна*) púsher; **2.** (*пробивной человек*) fíxer, gó-getter.

толковáние *с.* **1.** interpretátion; (*текста тж.*) réading; дать непрáвильное ~ *чего-л.* misintérpret *smth.*; **2.** (*объяснительный текст*) explanátion; (*на полях*) gloss.

толковáть *несов.* **1.** (*вн.; истолковать*) give* an interpretátion (of); непрáвильно, лóжно ~ *что-л.* intérpret *smth.* wróngly, misintérpret *smth.*; (*поступки, слова тж.*) put* a wrong constrúction on *smth.*; **2.** (*вн. дт.; объяснять*) expláin (*smth.* to); **3.** (*разговаривать*) talk, convérse; что тут мнóго ~! what's the good of tálking!

толкóвый 1. (*о человеке*) cléver, cápable; **2.** (*понятный*) clear; ~ примéр clear exámple; **3.**: ~ словáрь explánatory díctionary.

тóлком *разг.* **1.** (*ясно*) cléarly; я вас ~ не поймý I can't make out what you're trýing to say; говорíте ~ speak so that you can be understóod; **2.** (*серьёзно*) stráight; я ~ вам говорю́ I'm télling you stráight; take it from me!; **3.** (*как следует*) próperly, thóroughly.

толкотня́ *ж. разг.* crush.

толокнó *с.* óatmeal.

толóчь, растолóчь (*вн.*) pound (*smth.*); ◇ ~ вóду в стýпе ≈ beat* the air, mill the wind, cárry wáter in a sieve.

толпá *ж.* crowd.

толпи́ться *несов.* (на, в *пр.*) throng (*smth.*), pack (*smth.*); (в *пр.*; вокрýг *рд.*) crowd (in, aróund); ~ в зáле pack the hall; ~ в дверя́х crowd in the dóorway; ~ у вхóда crowd in front of the éntrance; ~ на плóщади, ýлицах и *т. п.* throng the square, streets, *etc.*

толпóй in a bódy (*в конце фразы*); ~ вы́йти на ýлицу flock ínto the street.

толстéть, потолстéть get* fat/stout, put* on weight.

толсти́ть *несов.* (*вн.*) *разг.* make* (*smb.*) look fat.

толстокóж|ий (*прям. и перен.*) thick-skínned; **~ee** живóтное páchyderm; ~ человéк thick-skínned órange.

тóлст|ый 1. thick; (*о материале тж.*) héavy; **2.** (*о человеке*) fat, stout; ◇ ~ журнáл mónthly, líterary and polítical magazíne; **~ая кишкá** *анат.* large intéstine.

толстя́к *м. разг.* fat/pórtly féllow.

толчёный póunded.

толчея́ *ж. разг.* crowd, crush; (*суета*) húrry-scúrry.

толчóк *м.* **1.** push, jab; (*при езде*) jolt, bump; (*при землетрясении*) shock, trémor; **2.** (*побуждение*) stímulus, incítement, jolt; **3.** (*резкое отталкивающее движение*) púsh-off spring; **4.** *спорт.* clean and jerk.

тóлщ|а *ж.* thíckness, thick láyer; *перен.* the bulk.

тóлще (*сравнит. ст. прил.* тóлстый) thícker; (*о человеке*) fátter, stóuter.

толщинá *ж.* **1.** thíckness; **2.** (*человека*) córpulence.

толь *м.* tár-paper; крóвельный ~ tarred/róofing felt.

тóлько 1. *частица* ónly; я вúдел егó ~ на дня́х I saw him ónly a few days agó; ~ на этот раз just for once; (*сейчáс*) ещё ~ пять часóв it's ónly five o'clóck (now); ~ за 1950 год... in 1950 alóne; ~ в этом слýчае in this case

ónly; ~ потомý, что... just/mérely becáuse...; он вспóмнил об этом ~ тогдá, когдá пришёл в шкóлу he dídn't remémber it until he got to school; **2.** *усил. частица:* когó ~ там нé было! símply éveryone was there!; каки́х ~ звери́й я там не ви́дел! I saw such a lot of ánimals there!; чегó ~ он не испытáл! what that man* has been through!; ~ бы if ónly; ~ бы он пришёл! if ónly he would come!; ~ бы не опоздáть! we símply mústn't be late!; ~ не опáздывай(те) whatéver you do, don't be late!; ~ попрóбуй(те) (это сдéлать)! (*с угрозой*) just you try (to do it)!; откýда ~ это берётся? where can it póssibly come from?; **3.** *союз* (*однако, но*) but; я соглáсен пойти́, ~ не сейчáс I agrée to go, but not now; рáзве ~ (что)... unléss...; **4.** *союз* (*едва*) no sóoner than, as soon as; **5.** *нареч.* just; ◇ смеётся, да и ~ all he does is to laugh; ~~ ónly just; ~ что just (now); я егó ~ что ви́дел I saw him just now; он ~ что пришёл he has just come; как ~ as soon as, the móment; как ~ он придёт as soon as he comes, the móment he comes; ~ егó и ви́дели he was gone in a flash.

том I *м.* vólume; пéрвый ~ vólume one.

том II *пр. от мест.* тот.

томáт *м.* tomáto. **~ный** tomáto *attr.*; ~ный сóус tomáto-sauce; ~ный сок tomáto-juice.

томи́тельн|о: ~ дóлго with ágonizing slówness; там бы́ло ~ скýчно it was térribly bóring there. **~ый** wéarisome; (*мучительный*) ágonizing; **~ая жáжда** ágonies of thirst; **~ая жарá** oppréssive heat; **~ое ожидáние 1)** wéarisome wait; **2)** (*неизвестность*) ágonizing suspénse; **~ая скýка** ágonies of bóredom; **~ая тоскá** inténse lónging.

том|и́ть *несов.* (*вн.*) **1.** tórture (*smb.*), exháust (*smb.*); (*тяготить*) oppréss (*smb.*); егó ~и́т жáжда, жарá *и т. п.* he is tórtured by thirst, heat, *etc.*; не ~и́(те) меня́! don't keep me in suspénse!; **2.** *кул.* stew (*smth.*). **~и́ться** *несов.* **1.** lánguish, pine; ~и́ться от жáжды be* parched with thirst, súffer ágonies of thirst; ~и́ться жáждой *чего-л.* thirst for *smth.*; ~и́ться в заключéнии, в тюрьмé lánguish in príson; ~и́ться в ожидáнии be* in an ágony of suspénse; **2.** *кул.* stew.

тóмн|ость *ж.* lánguor. **~ый** lánguorous, lánguid; ~ый взор lánguid look.

тон *м.* **1.** (*о звуках, цвете*) tone; ни́зкий ~ low tone; высóкие **~á** high tones; свéтлые **~á** light tones/shades; **2.** (*о речи*) tone of voice; tones *pl*; влáстный ~ commánding tones; лáсковый ~ afféctionate tone of voice; говори́ть спокóйным **~ом** speak* cálmly; **3.** (*манера, стиль повествования*) tone, style, mánner; полеми́ческий ~ polémical style; **4.** (*характер, стиль поведения*) style; это считáется хорóшим (плохи́м) **~ом** it's consídered good (bad) form/style; ◇ **~ом** вы́ше, ни́же *муз.* a tone hígher, lówer; *перен.* ráising, lówering *one's* voice; задáть ~ *муз.* set* the pitch, give* the note; **2)** (*показать пример*) lead*/set* the fáshion; **3)** (*дать направление*) give* a lead; повы́сить ~ raise *one's* voice; сбáвить ~ quíeten down; (*говорить менее заносчиво*) pipe down, sing* small; в ~ **1)** (*одинакового цвета*) to match; **2)** (*с той же интонацией*) in tune; не в ~ out of tune (with).

тонáльность *ж. муз.* key; переходи́ть в другýю ~ módulate (ínto anóther key), change key.

тóненький 1. slim, slénder; **2.** (*о голосе*) squéaky; (*о голосе ребёнка, птенца*) píping.

тонизи́ровать *несов. и сов.* (*вн.*) tone up (*smb., smth.*).

тóник *м.* tónic (wáter); джин с **~ом** gin and tónic.

тони́ческий tónic.

тóнк|ий 1. thin (*тж. худой*); (*о материале*) fine; **~ие ни́тки** thin/fine thread *sg*; **~ая бумáга** thin páper; **~ая кни́га** slim vólume; **~ое бельё** fine únderwear; **2.** (*о фигуре, частях тела*) slénder, slim; (*о чертах лица*) refíned, fine; **~ая тáлия** slim waist; **~ая шéя** slénder neck;

~ие па́льцы slénder fíngers; ~ про́филь délicate prófile; 3. (узкий) fine, thin; ~ая ли́ния thin line; 4. (высокий — о звуках) thin, high-pitched; ~ го́лос thin/high-pitched voice; ~ свист high-pitched whistle; 5. (состоя́щий из мельчайших части́ц) fine; ~ая пыль fine dust; 6. (сложный) ingénious, íntricate, éxquisite; (требующий умелого подхода) délicate, trícky; (детальный) exáct; ~ механи́зм ingénious device; ~ая рабо́та fine/éxquisite work; ~ое зна́ние чего-л. exáct knówledge of smth.; 7. (малозаметный) súbtle, fine; ~ оттéнок súbtle shade, nuánce; ~ое различие súbtle/fine distínction; 8. (о вкусе, запахе) délicate; (о пище) dáinty; ~ие ви́на délicate wines; ~ие духи́ súbtle pérfumes; ~ие блю́да dáinty díshes; 9. (изящно-остроумный) súbtle, délicate; ~ намёк géntle hint; ~ ю́мор súbtle húmour; 10. (чувствительный, восприимчивый) keen, acúte; ~ слух keen ear/héaring; ~ое зрéние keen sight; ~ ум percéptive/súbtle mind; ~ худóжественный вкус refíned/discríminating artístic taste; 11. (о человеке) percéptive, kéen-witted; ~ критик percéptive crític; ~ диплома́т astúte/kéen-witted díplomat; ~ наблюда́тель súbtle obsérver; 12. (верный, точный) exáct, súbtle, precíse; ~ая критика súbtle críticism; ~ие наблюдéния precíse observátions; 13. разг. (хитрый) sly, cráfty; ◇ где ~о, там и рвётся погов. the thread breaks where it is wéakest; ~ая кишка́ анат. small intéstine.

то́нко 1. finely; ~ нарéзанный thínly sliced; ~ очи́нненный well-shárpened, sharp-póinted; 2. (утончённо): ~ подмеча́ть что-л. have* a keen eye for smth.; ~ разбира́ться в чём-л. have* a fine understánding of smth.

тонкоко́жий thin-skínned.

тонконо́гий slim-légged.

тонкору́нный fine-fléeced.

то́нкост|ь ж. 1. fineness; (фигуры) slénderness; перен. súbtlety; 2. мн. (подробности) níceties, fine points; refínements; все э́ти ~и all these níceties/súbtleties; знать что-л. до ~ей know* all the ins and outs of smth.

тонкошёрстный 1. (об овцах) fine-fléeced; 2. (сделанный из тонкой шерсти) fine-wool attr.

то́нна ж. ton.

тонна́ж м. tónnage; (судна) shípping.

тонне́ль м. см. тунне́ль.

то́нус м. tone.

тон|у́ть, потону́ть, утону́ть 1. sink*, go* down; (о живом существе тж.) drown; здесь то́нет мно́го народа people are drowned here; я два ра́за в жи́зни ~у́л I was álmost drowned twice in my life; 2. (в пр.; вязнуть, утопать) be* plunged (in); перен. be* lost (in); ~ в снегу́ sink* ínto the snow; дома́ то́нут в зéлени the hóuses are búried in gréenery.

тонфи́льм м. sóund-track.

то́ньше сравнит. ст. прил. то́нкий и нареч. то́нко.

то́ня ж. 1. (место ловли рыбы) físhing-ground; 2. (невод с уловом) haul.

топа́з м. tópaz.

то́пать, то́пнуть 1. (тв.) stamp (smth.); ~ нога́ми stamp one's feet; 2. (при ходьбе, танцах и т. п.) tramp.

топи́ть I несов. (вн.) 1. (печи и т. п.) keep* (smth.) góing; 2. (отапливать помещение) heat (smth.).

топи́ть II несов. (вн.) 1. (плавить) melt (smth.); (сало и т. п.) melt down (smth.), redúce (smth.); 2.: ~ молоко́ heat milk in the óven, bake milk.

топи́ть III, потопи́ть, утопи́ть (вн.) 1. (суда) sink* (smth.); 2. (людей, животных) drown (smb., smth.); перен. (губить) ruin (smb.).

топи́ться I несов. (о печах) burn*.

топи́ться II несов. (плавиться) melt.

топи́ться III, утопи́ться drown onesélf.

то́пка ж. 1. (действие) héating; 2. (часть котла) fúrnace, fíre-box.

то́пкий bóggy.

топлён|ый 1. (перетопленный) clárified; mélted;

~ое ма́сло clárified bútter; 2. (кипячёный) baked; ~ое молоко́ baked milk.

то́пливн|ый fuel attr.; ~ые ресу́рсы страны́ the country's fuel resóurces; ~ кри́зис fuel crísis.

то́пливо с. fuel.

то́пнуть сов. см. то́пать.

топо́граф м. topógrapher. ~и́ческий topográphical; ~и́ческая съёмка topográphical súrvey (work).

топогра́фия ж. topógraphy.

то́поль м. бот. póplar.

топо́р м. axe. ~ик м. hátchet.

топори́ще с. áxe-helve.

топо́рн|ый 1. axe attr.; 2. (грубый, неуклюжий) clúmsy, rough, crude; (о человеке) uncóuth; ~ая рабо́та clúmsy work.

топо́рщиться несов. brístle; (о материи) púcker.

то́пот м. tramp; ко́нский ~ thúd(ding)/clátter of hoofs; hóofbeats pl; ~ ног tramp of feet.

топота́ть несов. разг. 1. tramp, make* a clátter, thud alóng; 2. (топать) stamp vígorously.

топта́ть несов. (вн.) trámple (smth.); ~ траву́ trámple down the grass; ~ нога́ми что-л. trámple smth. únder foot; ~ огонь stamp out a fire; ◇ ~ в грязь кого-л. trámple smb.'s reputátion únder foot; ~ся несов. 1. shift one's feet; (о лошади) stamp; 2. разг. (быть, находи́ться где-л.) hang* abóut, línger; ◇ ~ся на мéсте mark time, make* no prógress.

топь ж. bog, morass.

то́рба ж. nósebag.

торг м. 1. bárgaining, hággling; 2. мн. (аукцион) (públic) sale sg; продава́ть что-л. с ~о́в sell* smth. by áuction.

торга́ш м. разг. húckster (тж. перен.).

торг|ова́ть несов. 1. (тв.) deal* (in); (с тв.) trade (with); (тв.) перен. péddle (smth.); ~ промы́шленными това́рами deal* in indústrial goods; ~ свое́й со́вестью, че́стью sell* one's hónour; 2. (заниматься торговлей) buy* and sell*, trade; (отпускать товары покупателям) serve; ~ вразно́с péddle; 3. (быть открытым для торговли) be* ópen; магази́н ~у́ет до семи́ часо́в the shop is ópen till séven; магази́н сего́дня не ~у́ет the shop is closed todáy. ~ова́ться несов. 1. (с тв.) bárgain (with), hággle óver the price (with); 2. разг. (спорить) árgue.

торго́в|ец м. trádesman*, mérchant; (чем-л.) déaler (in). ~ка ж. (рыночная) márket-woman*.

торго́вля ж. trade; (крупная) cómmerce; госуда́рственная (ро́зничная) ~ State (rétail) trade; ча́стная ~ prívate trade.

торго́во-промы́шленный commércial and indústrial.

торго́в|ый commércial; trade attr.; ~ая сеть commércial nétwork; ~ центр tráding céntre; ~ договор commércial tréaty; ~ое соглашéние trade agréement; ~ая сдéлка deal; ~ капита́л trading cápital; ~ая монопо́лия trade monópoly; ~ая поли́тика trade pólicy; ~ая ма́рка trádemark; ~ое пра́во commércial law; ~ое судно mérchant véssel/ship; ~ флот mércantile maríne, mérchant návy; ~ое дом tr(ding/commércial firm.

торгпрéд м. (торговый представитель) trade representátive. ~ство с. (торговое представительство) Trade Delegátion.

торéц м. 1. (грань) bútt-end; 2. (брусок) (wóoden) páving block.

торжéственн|ость ж. solémnity. ~ый 1. (праздничный) féstive; (пышный) ceremónial, grand; ~ый день gála-day; ~ое заседа́ние grand méeting; ~ая часть official part; the céremonies pl; 2. (величественный, важный) sólemn; (приподнятый) uplífted; ~ый слу́чай sólemn occásion; ~ая кля́тва sólemn oath.

торжеств|ó с. 1. (полная победа) tríumph; 2. (праздество) féstival; мн. celebrátions; семéйное ~ fámily celebrátion; ~á по слу́чаю чего-л. the celebrátions on the occásion of *smth.*; 3. (*радость*) tríumph, exultátion; с ~ом сказáть *что-л.* annóunce *smth.* tríumphantly/exúltantly.

торжеств|овáть *несов.* 1. (*над тв.*; *брать верх*) tríumph (óver); 2. (*вн.*; *радоваться, ликовать*) rejóice (óver, at); ~ побéду rejóice óver a víctory. ~**ующий** tríumphant; (*ликующий*) exúltant; с ~ующим вúдом with an air of tríumph.

тормáшк|и: полетéть вверх ~ами fall* head óver heels.

торможéние *с.* 1. bráking; 2. *физиол.* inhibítion; ~ рефлéксов inhibítion of refléxes.

тóрмоз *м.* 1. (*мн.* тормозá) brake; автоматúческий ~ automátic brake; 2. (*мн.* тóрмозы) (*торможение*) bráking; 3. (*мн.* тóрмозы) (*препятствие, помеха*) híndrance; ~ в рабóте híndrance to work; ◇ на ~áх with the brakes on; спустúть *что-л.* на ~áх let* *smth.* drop quíetly, drop *smth.*

тормозúть *несов.* 1. (*вн.*) brake (*smth.*); apply the brakes (to); 2. (*останавливаться — о машинах*) brake, pull up; 3. (*вн.*; *задерживать движение*) slow down (*smth.*); *перен. тж.* retárd (*smth.*), hold* up (*smth.*), act as a brake (on); ~ рабóту hínder/hámper/impéde work.

тормознóй brake *attr.*, bráking *attr.*; ~ башмáк bráke-shoe.

тормошúть *несов.* (*вн.*) *разг.* tug (at), shake* (*smb.*); *перен.* wórry (*smb.*), péster (*smb.*).

тóрн|ый *разг.* béaten, smooth; ~ая дорóга béaten track.

тороп|úть, поторопúть (*вн.*) húrry (*smb.*), hásten (*smb., smth.*); (*с тв.*) press (for); ~ когó-л. с отвéтом press *smb.* for a replý; ~ когó-л. с отъéздом hásten *smb.'s* depárture; меня тороп**я**т с отъéздом I am béing urged to leave immédiately; не ~úте меня! don't húrry me! ~**úться**, поторопúться be* in a húrry; ~úться на рабóту be* in a húrry to get to *one's* work; ~úться на поезд húrry to catch the train; я óчень ~люсь I'm in a great húrry; ~úтесь! make haste!, húrry up!, get a move on! не ~úться be* in no húrry; не ~ú(те)сь! don't (be in a) húrry, take your time!; он не (óчень) торóпится отвечáть he is in no húrry to replý; ◇ не ~ясь delíberately, without haste.

тороплúв|о húrriedly, hástily. ~**ость** *ж.* haste. ~**ый** húrried; (*совершённый быстро тж.*) hásty.

торóс *м.* íce-hummock. ~**истый** húmmocky; ~**истый** лёд pack ice.

торпéда *ж.* torpédo.

торпедúровать *несов. и сов.* (*вн.*) torpédo (*smth.*) (*тж. перен.*).

торпéдный torpédo *attr.*

тóрс *м.* 1. (*туловище*) trunk; 2. (*статуи*) tórso.

торт *м.* cake.

торф *м.* peat.

торфоразрабóтки *мн.* péatery *sg.*

торфян|úк *м.* (*залежь торфа*) péatbog. ~**óй** peat *attr.*; ~**ое** болóто péatbog; ~**óй** брикéт péat-block.

торч|áть *несов.* 1. stick* up; (*выдаваться*) protrúde, jut out; (*топорщиться, высовываться откуда-л.*) stick* out; ~ в рáзные стóроны stick* out in all diréctions; 2. *разг.* (*находиться где-л.*) hang* abóut, stick* aróund; он вéчно ~úт у меня перед глазáми he álways seems to be there; ~ где-л. цéлый день hang* about sómewhere all day.

торчкóм *разг.* on end, eréct.

торшéр *м.* stándard lamp.

тоск|á *ж.* 1. ánguish, distréss; на сéрдце ~ one feels mélancholy; наводúть ~ý на когó-л. make* *smb.* depréssed; ~ по рóдине hómesickness, nostálgia; с ~óй wístfully; 2. (*скука*) bóredom, tédium; (*уныние*) mísery; какáя ~! how dréary!; там такáя ~! it's sheer mísery there!

тосклúв|о 1. *нареч.* (*уныло*) dréarily; 2. *в знач. сказ. безл.*: ~ бúло в пустúх кóмнатах the émpty rooms were depréssing; 3. *в знач. сказ.* (*дт.*): емý бúло óчень ~ he felt útterly depréssed, he felt véry dréary. ~**ый** 1. (*грустный*) mélancholy; (*унылый тж.*) dréary; ~**ый** взгляд mélancholy glance; ~**ые** глазá sad/wístful eyes; ~**ое** настроéние mood of depréssion; 2. (*наводящий тоску*) depréssing.

тосковáть *несов.* 1. (*грустить*) be* sad/mélancholy; 2. (*по дт.*) *разг.* long (for), pine (for); ~ по дóму be* hómesick.

тост *м.* toast; предлагáть, провозглашáть ~ за когó-л. propóse *smb.'s* health; провозглашáть ~ за что-л. raise *one's* glass to *smth.*

тóстер *м.* tóaster.

тот, та, то, те 1. that; *мн.* those; that one (*без сущ.*); и ~ и другóй both; тем úли другúм спóсобом one way or anóther; не ~, так другóй one or the óther, áпу; ни ~ ни другóй néither; ~, котóрый the one; ~..., котóрый the... who, which; ~ же the same; ~ сáмый the one; он тепéрь не ~ he's quite chánged; 2. (*другой*) the óther; that one; 3. (*какой нужен*) the right; не ~ the wrong; я сел не на ~ пóезд I took the wrong train; ◇ ~ úли другóй éither; на том свéте in the next world; то да сё one thing and anóther; то, что what; я узнáл то, что хотéл I learned what I wánted to know; то, что я узнáл, обрáдовало меня what I learned made me véry glad; (да) и то and that; and... at that; тóлько одúн костюм, да и то стáрый ónly one suit, and that an old one, ónly one suit and an old one at that; не то, не то what; это не то, что мне нáдо that is not what I wánted; не то чтó(бы) (it is) not that; не то чтóбы я хотéл it's not that I want to; он не то что бóлен, а прóсто устáл he's not exáctly ill, he's just tíred; (а) не то or else; всё это тó, да не тó it's not quite what is wánted.

тотáльный tótal.

тó-то 1. (*в том-то и дело*) that's just it; 2. (*вот видите*) ahá!, there you are!, what did I tell you!; 3. (*так вот почему*) so that's why; 4. (*вот уж подлинно*) indéed (*в конце фразы*).

тóтчас at once.

точён|ый *перен.* chíselled; ~**ые** нóги shápely legs; ~**ое** лицó chíselled féatures *pl.*

точúло *с.* (*камень*) whétstone; (*станок*) gríndstone.

точúльщик *м.* knife-grinder.

точúть, наточúть (*вн.*) 1. (*делать острым*) shárpen (*smth.*); (*на круге тж.*) grind* (*smth.*); 2. *тк. несов.* (*изготовлять*) shape (*smth.*) on a lathe, turn (*smth.*) out on a lathe; 3. *тк. несов.* (*разъедать*) eat* awáy (*smth.*); (*металл*) corróde (*smth.*); водá тóчит кáмень contínual drípping wears awáy a stone; 4. *тк. несов.* (*мучить*) gnaw (*smb.*); (*бранить*) nag (*smb.*).

тóчк|а I *ж.* 1. point; (*пятнышко, значок*) dot; пунктúр из тóчек dótted line; наивúсшая ~ гóрного хребтá highest point of a móuntain chain; радиотрансляциóнная ~ rádio reláy státion; торгóвая ~ trade óutlet; ~ кипéния bóiling-point; ~ плавлéния mélting-point; 2. (*знак препинания*) full stop, périod; ~ с запятóй semicólon; 3. *в знач. сказ. разг.* (*конец, довольно*) that'll do!; ◇ сдвúнуть что-л. с мёртвой ~и set* *smth.* in mótion; ~и соприкосновéния points of cóntact; стáвить ~у, ~и над «и» dot the "i's" and cross the "t's"; дойтú до ~и be at the end of *one's* téther; ~ в ~у exáctly, precísely; попáсть в ~у hit* the nail on the head; смотрéть в однý ~у stare fíxedly in front of one.

тóчка II *ж.* 1. (*точение*) shárpening; (*на круге тж.*) grínding; 2. (*на токарном станке*) túrning.

тóчно I *нареч.* exáctly, precísely; (*правильно*) áccurately; (*по времени*) púnctually; ~ определúть что-л. defíne *smth.* precísely; ~ перевестú что-л. make* a fáithful/áccurate translátion of *smth.*, transláte *smth.* áccurately; прибывáть ~ по расписáнию arríve exáctly on time; прийти ~ в назначенное время come*/arrive punctually; ~ так же, как just as, exactly as.

точно II *союз* (*как*) like; (*будто, словно*) as if, as though; ~ глаза ~ угли eyes like coals; ~ он не понимает as if he didn't understand.

точн|ость *ж.* precision, exactness; (*правильность*) accuracy; (*пунктуальность*) punctuality; с ~остью до... to an approximation of...; с ~остью до одного градуса to the nearest degree; с ~остью часового механизма with clockwork precision; ◇ в ~ости exactly; (*буквально*) to the letter; в ~ости исполнить carry out to the letter. **~ый** 1. precise, exact; (*правильный*) accurate; ~ое время exact time; ~ые весы accurate scales; ~ые приборы precision instruments; ~ая копия exact copy; ~ый перевод accurate translation; ~ый расчёт времени accurate timing; ~ый адрес exact address; ~ые инструкции precise instructions; чтобы быть ~ым... to be precise...; 2. (*о человеке*) punctual; ◇ ~ые науки exact sciences.

точь-в-точь exactly.

тошн|ить *несов. безл.*: меня, его *и т. д.* ~ит I feel, he feels, *etc.* sick; меня ~ит от одной мысли (об этом) the very thought (of it) makes me sick.

тошно *в знач. сказ. безл. разг.*: мне, ему *и т. д.* ~ I feel, he feels, *etc.* sick (at heart).

тошнот|а *ж.* nausea; вызывать ~у у кого-л. make* smb. sick; это мне надоело до ~ы I'm sick to death of it.

тошнотворный sickening, nauseating (*тж. перен.*).

тощать, отощать *разг.* waste away, become* gaunt/emaciated.

тощ|ий 1. emaciated, scraggy; (*о человеке тж.*) hollow-cheeked, gaunt; 2. (*скудный*) poor, feeble; meagre; ~ая почва poor soil; ~ая растительность scanty vegetation; ◇ на ~ желудок on an empty stomach.

трава *ж.* grass; ◇ как ~ ≈ tasteless as paper.

травинка *ж.* blade of grass.

трав|ить I *несов.* (*вн.*) 1. (*умерщвлять*) poison (smb., smth.); ~ мышей destroy mice; 2. (*изъязвлять кислотой и т. п.*) make* (smth.) sore; poison (smb., smth.); *перен. разг.* (*мучить*) torment (smth., smb.); 3. *mex.* etch (smth.); 4. (*производить потраву*) damage (smth.); ~ посевы damage young crops; 5. (*на охоте*) hunt (smth.); *перен.* hound (smb.), victimize (smb.), persecute (smb.).

трав|ить II *несов.* (*вн.*) *мор.* ease out (smth.), slacken out (smth.), slack away (smth.).

травиться *несов. разг.* poison oneself, take* poison.

травление *с. mex.* etching.

травля *ж.* hunting; *перен.* hounding, victimization, persecution.

травма *ж. мед.* trauma, injury; психическая ~ (emotional) shock. **~тический** traumatic.

травматология *ж.* traumatology.

травмировать *несов. и сов.* (*вн.*) injure (smb.), damage (smth.).

травопол|е *с.* grassland agriculture/farming. **~ный:** ~ный севооборот grass rotation.

траво|сеяние *с.* grass cultivation; ~стой *м.* stand/ crop of grass.

травоядный *зоол.* herbivorous.

травян|истый grassy; grass *attr.*; *перен. разг.* wishy-washy, watery. **~ой** grassy; grass *attr.*; ~ой покров herbage; ~ые растения grasses; ~ого цвета grass-green *attr.*

трагед|ия *ж.* tragedy; ◇ делать ~ию из чего-л. make* a tragedy of *smth.*

трагизм *м.* 1. (*трагический элемент в произведении*) the spirit of tragedy; 2. (*ужас, безысходность*) the tragedy (of); (*трагическое выражение*) tragedy.

трагик *м.* tragedian.

трагикомедия *ж.* tragicomedy.

трагическ|и tragically; окончиться ~ end in tragedy; относиться ~ к чему-л. see* smth. in a tragic light; не

относитесь к этому так ~! don't be so tragic about it! ~ий tragic; ~ая актриса tragic actress; ~ая гибель tragic death; (*корабля и т. п.*) tragic loss/destruction; ~ое зрелище tragic sight; принять ~ий оборот take* a tragic turn.

трагичн|ость *ж.* tragedy. **~ый** *см.* трагический.

традиционный traditional.

традици|я *ж.* tradition; по ~и to keep* up the tradition; войти в ~ю become* a tradition.

траектория *ж.* trajectory, path.

тракт *м.* highway; ◇ желудочно-кишечный ~ alimentary canal.

трактат *м.* 1. (*научное сочинение*) treatise; 2. (*договор*) treaty.

тракт|овать *несов.* 1. (*о пр.*; *излагать*) treat (of), deal* (with); discuss (smth.); 2. (*вн.*; *истолковывать*) interpret (smth.). **~оваться** *несов.* be* treated; о чём ~уется в этой книге? what is this book about?

трактовка *ж.* interpretation, reading.

трактор *м.* tractor; колёсный ~ wheeled tractor.

тракторист *м.*, **~ка** *ж.* tractor-driver.

тракторн|ый tractor *attr.*; ~ завод tractor works; ~ая колонна column of tractors.

трал *м.* 1. (*рыболовный*) trawl; 2. (*минный*) sweep; 3. (*для исследования дна*) trawl.

тралить *несов.* (*вн.*) 1. trawl (smth.); 2. *воен.*, *мор.* sweep* (smth.); 3. (*исследовать дно*) trawl (smth.).

тральщик *м.* 1. (*рыболовное судно*) trawler; 2. (*рыболов*) trawlerman*; 3. *воен.*, *мор.* mine-sweeper.

трамб|овать *несов.* (*вн.*) ram (smth.). **~овка** *ж.* 1. (*действие*) ramming; 2. (*машина*) rammer, beetle; (*инструмент*) ram.

трамва|й *м.* 1. (*городская электрическая дорога*) tramway, tram service; 2. (*вагон*) tram, tram-car; *амер.* street-car; ехать на ~е get* on the tram; садиться в ~ get* on the tram; ◇ речной ~ river-launch.

трамвайн|ый tram *attr.*; ~ая остановка tram-stop; ~ парк tram-depot.

трамплин *м. спорт.* spring-board; (*лыжный*) ski-jump; *перен.* jumping-off place.

транжир|а *м. и ж. разг.* spendthrift, wastrel. **~ить** *несов.* (*вн.*) *разг.* squander (smth.).

транзистор *м.* 1. (*полупроводник*) transistor; 2. (*приёмник*) transistor radio. **~ный** transistor *attr.*

транзит *м.* transit. **~ный** transit *attr.*; ~ная виза transit visa; ~ные перевозки goods in transit; ~ный билет transit ticket.

транквилизатор *м.* tranquillizer.

транс *м.* trance.

трансатлантический transatlantic.

трансконтинентальный transcontinental.

транскрибировать *несов. и сов.* (*вн.*) *лингв.* transcribe (smth.).

транскрипция *ж. лингв.* transcription.

транслировать *несов. и сов.* (*вн.*) transmit (smth.); broadcast (smth.); ~ концерт broadcast a concert.

транслитерация *ж. лингв.* transliteration.

трансляционн|ый transmitting; ~ая сеть transmitting/broadcasting system.

трансляция *ж.* 1. transmitting, broadcasting; ~ футбольного матча broadcasting of a football match; 2. *разг.* (*то, что передаётся*) broadcast, transmission.

трансмиссия *ж.* transmission.

транспарант *м.* 1. streamer, placard; 2. (*разлинованная бумага*) lined guide-sheet.

транспорт *м.* 1. (*отрасль народного хозяйства*) transport; железнодорожный ~ rail transport; городской ~ urban transport; 2. (*перевозка*) transport, transportation; 3. (*партия грузов*) consignment; 4. *воен.* transport, train; 5. (*судно*) supply ship; (*с войсками*) troop transport, troopship.

транспортёр *м.* 1. *mex.* conveyer; 2. *воен.* carrier.

транспортир *м.* protráctor.

транспортировать *несов. и сов.* (*вн.*) transpórt (*smb., smth.*); convéy (*smb., smth.*).

транспортировка *ж.* transportátion.

транспортник *м.* tránsport wórker.

транспортн|ый tránsport *attr.*; ~ые срéдства means of transportátion; ~ая авиáция air tránsport sérvice; tránsport áircraft *собир. pl.*

трансформáтор *м.* 1. *эл.* transfórmer; 2. (*актёр*) quick-change ártist. ~ный transfórmer *attr.*

трансформáция *ж.* transformátion, convérsion.

трансформировать *несов. и сов.* (*вн.*) transfórm (*smth.*), convért (*smth.*).

траншéя *ж.* trench.

трап *м. мор.* ládder.

трáпеза *ж.* meal.

трапéция *ж.* 1. (*фигура*) trapézium; 2. (*гимнастический снаряд*) trapéze.

трáсса *ж.* 1. (*направление*) route; ~ нефтепровóда route of a pípeline; 2. (*дорога, путь*) road; автомобильная ~ mótor road.

трассирующ|ий *воен.* trácer *attr.*; ~ая пуля trácer (-bullet).

трáта *ж.* 1. (*действие*) spénding; ~ дéнег spénding (of móney); ~ врéмени spénding of time; 2. *обыкн. мн.* (*расход*) expénditure(s); spénding *sg*, expénse *sg*; напрáсная ~ waste, unnécessary expénditure.

трáтить, истрáтить, потрáтить (*вн.*) spend* (*smth.*); (*о времени, энергии тж.*) expénd (*smth.*); ~ напрáсно waste; не ~ слов waste no words. ~ся, истрáтиться, потрáтиться 1. (*расходовать свои деньги*) spend* móney; 2. (*расходоваться*) be* spent, be* used.

трáулер *м.* tráwler.

трáур *м.* móurning; в глубóком ~е in deep móurning; носить ~ по ком-л. be* in móurning for *smb.* ~ный móurning *attr.*; (*похоронный*) fúneral; (*скорбный*) móurnful; ~ный марш fúneral/dead march; ~ная повязка crape band; ~ная рáмка black bórder.

трафарéт *м.* sténcil; *перен.* routíne, set/stéreotyped páttern; (*литературный*) cliché; расписывать по ~у sténcil. ~ный sténcilled; *перен.* convéntional, stéreotyped; háckneyed; ~ная улыбка artificial/convéntional smile; ~ные фрáзы set phráses.

трах bang!

трахéя *ж. анат.* trachéa.

трáхну|ть *сов. разг.* knock, bang; ~ когó-л. по головé knock *smb.* on the head; ~ кулакóм пó столу bang *one's* fist on the táble; чтó-то ~ло there was a bang; ~ из ружья loose* off with a gun.

трахóма *ж. мед.* trachóma.

трéбовани|е *с.* 1. demánd; по пéрвому ~ю as soon as demánded; по ~ю судá by órder of the court; по ~ю публики by públic demánd; по настоятельному ~ю когó-л. at the úrgent requést of *smb.*; останóвка по ~ю (tram, bus) requést stop; 2. (*норма*) requírements, stándards; технологические ~я technológical stándards; отвечáть ~ям чего-л. meet* the requírements of *smth.*; предъявлять высóкие ~я к кому-л. place exácting demánds upón *smb.*; 3. *обыкн. мн.* (*обязательные правила*) stándards, demánds; ~я вéжливости stándards of cóurtesy; 4. *обыкн. мн.* (*потребности, запросы*) requírements, demánds; культýрные ~я óбщества cúltural requírements/needs of society; 5. (*документ*) requisítion, órder.

трéбовательн|ость *ж.* insístence (on a high stándard); ~ к себé self-díscipline; ~ый exácting, demánding; он слишком трéбователен he is too exácting/demánding.

трéб|овать, потрéбовать 1. (*вн., рд. от рд.,* + *инф.,* + *чтобы*) demánd (*smth.* from, of); (*по праву*) claim (*smth.* from); (*ожидать*) require (*smth.* of); ~ прóпуск demánd *smb.'s* pass; ~ повышéния зарплáты demánd

wage íncreases; ~ объяснéния у когó-л. demánd an explanátion from *smb.*; он ~овал сократить объём рабóт he demánded that the amóunt of work should be redúced; он ~овал, чтóбы племянник остáлся в Москвé he demánded that his néphew should stay in Móscow, he insísted on his néphew's stáying in Móscow; вы слишком мнóго ~уете от ребёнка you ask too much of the child*; 2. *тк. несов.* (*рд.,* + *инф.,* + *чтобы; обязывать к чему-л.*) demánd (*smth.*), require (*smth.*); справедливость ~ет сказáть, что... it must be said in jústice that...; этикéт ~овал, чтóбы... étiquette requíred that...; 3. (*рд.; нуждаться*) need (*smth.*), require (*smth.*); эти растéния ~уют мнóго воды these plants require/need plénty of wáter; эта рабóта трéбует большóго искусства this work demánds/requíres great skill; 4. (*вн.; вызывать*) ask (for), call (*вн.*) in; вас ~ует дирéктор the diréctor wants to see you. ~оваться, потрéбоваться be* requíred/néeded; ~уется большóе мужество, чтóбы... much cóurage is requíred to...; ~уется машинистка typíst wánted/needed (*smth.*); на это ~уется мнóго врéмени this takes a lot of time.

требухá *ж.* óffal.

тревóг|а *ж.* 1. (*беспокойство*) alárm, anxíety; быть в ~е be* in a state of anxíety; 2. (*сигнал опасности*) alárm, alért; поднять ~у raise the alárm; боевáя ~ báttle alért; *мор.* géneral quárters; воздýшная ~ áir-raid wárning/alért.

тревóжить, встревóжить, потревóжить (*вн.*) 1. *сов.* встревóжить (*вызывать беспокойство*) alárm (*smb.*), wórry (*smb.*), make* (*smb.*) úneasy; 2. *сов.* потревóжить (*нарушать покой*) distúrb (*smb., smth.*). ~ся, встревóжиться be* úneasy/wórried abóut; becóme*/get* ánxious/nérvous.

тревóжн|ый 1. (*неспокойный*) úneasy, ánxious, distúrbed, tróubled; ~ые мысли tróubled/ánxious thoughts; ~ая ночь ánxious night; ~ момéнт ánxious móment; ~ сон tróubled sleep; ~ взгляд úneasy look; 2. (*тревожащий*) alárming, disquíeting, distúrbing; ~ые слýхи alárming rúmours; ~ые вéсти distúrbing news; 3. (*исполненный опасности*) crítical, ánxious; 4. (*предупреждающий*) alárm *attr.*; ~ые гудки wárning hoots/blasts.

треволнéние *с.* tróuble, bóther.

трéзвенник *м. разг.* teetótaller, tótal abstáiner.

трезвéть, отрезвéть becóme* sóber, sóber down.

трéзво sóberly; ~ относиться к чему-л. take* a sóber/cómmon-sense view of *smth.*

трезвóн *м.* peal (of bells).

трезвóнить, растрезвóнить 1. *тк. несов.* (*о колоколах*) peal; 2. (*вн.*) *разг.* (*разглашать*) trúmpet (*smth.*), proclaím (*smth.*); 3. (*о пр.; распускать слухи*) góssip (abóut).

трéзв|ость *ж.* 1. sobríety, sóber state; 2. (*воздержание*) ábstinence; 3. (*взглядов и т. п.*) bálance, clárity, sóberness; ~ умá cóol-héadedness; 1. (*не пьяный*) sóber; быть в ~ом состоянии be* sóber; 2. *разг.* (*непьющий*) ábstinent; 3. (*здравый, рассудительный*) sóber, sóber-mínded, sane; ~ое отношéние к чему-л. mátter-of-fáct áttitude to *smth.*; человéк ~ого умá sóber-mínded indivídual; ~ый взгляд на вéщи sóber/sénsible view of things.

трек *м. спорт.* track; (*для бега тж.*) cínder-track.

трел|ь *ж.* trill; ~и соловья trílling/júgging of the níghtingale.

трéнер *м.* tráiner; (*спортивной команды тж.*) coach.

трéние *с.* 1. fríction; 2. *мн.* (*разногласия*) fríction *sg.*

тренировáть, натренировáть (*вн.*) train (*smb., smth.*); (*спортсменов, спортивную команду тж.*) coach (*smb., smth.*); ~ пáмять train *one's* mémory. ~ся, натренировáться (*в пр.*) train onesélf (in), práctise (*smth.*), go ínto tráining.

тениро́вк|а ж. tráining; провести́ ~у hold* a práctice; проходи́ть ~у be* in tráining.

трениро́вочный tráining *attr.*; ~ матч práctice-match; ~ костю́м tráck-suit.

трено́га ж. trípod.

трено́жить, стрено́жить *(вн.)* hóbble *(smth.)*.

трено́жник м. см. трено́га.

тре́нькать *несов. разг.* strum.

трёп м. *разг.* talk, twáddle.

трепан|а́ция ж. *мед.* trepanátion; ~ че́репа trepanátion of the skull. **~и́ровать** *несов. и сов. (вн.) мед.* trepán *(smth.)*.

трепа́ть, потрепа́ть *(вн.)* 1. pull *(smth.)* abóut, túmble *(smth.)*, rúmple *(smth.)*; *(волосы тж.)* tóusle *(smth.)*; *(о ветре)* make* *(smth.)* flútter; 2. *(по дт.; похлопывать)* pat *(smb., smth.)*; ~ кого́-л. по плечу́, щеке́ pat *smb.'s* shóulder, cheek; pat *smb.* on the shóulder, cheek; 3. *разг. (одежду, обувь)* wear* out *(smth.)*; *(книгу)* knock *(smth.)* abóut; 4. *тк. несов. (волокно)* scutch *(smth.)*, swíngle *(smth.)*; ◇ ~ кому́-л. не́рвы jar on *smb.'s* nerves, fray *smb.'s* nerves; ~ языко́м jábber. **~ся, потрепа́ться** 1. *тк. несов. (развеваться)* flútter, wave; 2. *разг. (изнашиваться)* wear* out; be* the worse for wear; be*/become táttered.

тре́пет м. 1. *(мелкая дрожь)* quívering, trémbling; *(подёргивание)* twítching; *(о биении сердца)* palpitátion; 2. *(волнение от какого-л. сильного чувства)* excítement; *перен. (проявление чего-л.)* throb, thróbbing, pulsátion; с ~ом éagerly; приводи́ть кого́-л. в ~ throw* *smb.* into a state of anxíety; приводи́ть кого́-л. в ра́достный ~ put* *smb.* into a flútter of joy; 3. *(страх)* trepidátion; приходи́ть в ~ be* seized with trepidátion.

трепета́ть *несов.* 1. *(дрожать)* flútter, quíver; *(биться, содрогаться)* twitch, be* convúlsed; *(о сердце)* pálpitate; *(мерцать)* flícker; 2. *(быть охваченным волнением)* trémble, quíver; *перен. (пробиваться, проявляться)* throb, pulsáte; ~ от сча́стья quíver with joy; 3. *(перед тв., при пр.; за вн.; испытывать страх)* trémble (before, for); ~ за кого́-л. trémble for *smb.*; ~ при мы́сли о чём-л. trémble at the thought of *smth.*

тре́петн|ый 1. quívering; 2. *(тревожный)* ánxious; *(взволнованный)* víbrant; ~ое ожида́ние bréathless expectátion; 3. *(робкий, боязливый)* féarful.

трёпк|а ж. 1. *(волокна)* scútching; 2. *разг. (порка)* thráshing, tróuncing; зада́ть ~у кому́-л. give* *smb.* a thráshing/tróuncing; ◇ ~ не́рвов strain on the nerves.

треск м. 1. *(шум от резких ударов)* crash; ~ огня́ cráckling of the flames; ~ сучьев cráckling of twigs; 2. *разг. (шумиха)* flóurish, fuss, ballyhóo; без шу́ма и ~а withóut any fuss; ◇ с ~ом ignomíniously; пье́са провали́лась с ~ом the play was a compléte flop.

треска́ ж. cód(-fish).

тре́скаться, потре́скаться crack; *(о коже тж.)* chap.

трескотня́ ж. *разг.* cráckle, cráckling; *перен. (болтовня)* chátter, cáckle; ~ пулемётов ráttle of machíne-gun fire.

треску́ч|ий *разг.* 1. cráckling; *(о звуках тж.)* staccáto; *(о голосе)* gráting, harsh; 2. *(высокопарный)* high-flown, pómpous, preténtious; ~ая фра́за high-sóunding phrase; ◇ ~ моро́з rínging/hard frost.

тре́сн|уть *сов.* 1. *(дать трещину)* crack; *(лопнуть)* burst*; 2. *(издать звук)*: что́-то ~уло there was a crácking sound.

трест м. trust.

трете́йский: ~ суд court of arbitrátion; ~ судья́ árbiter.

тре́т|ий the third; ◇ ~его дня the day before yésterday; ~ звоно́к third/final bell; в ~ем лице́ in the third pérson; из ~их рук at third-hand; стра́ны ~ьего ми́ра* Third-World cóuntries.

трети́ровать *несов. (вн.)* treat *(smb.)* slíghtingly, snub *(smb.)*.

трети́чный *геол., мед.* tértiary.

трет|ь ж. a third, one third; две ~и two-thirds.

тре́тье с. *(блюдо)* third course, the sweet; на ~ for the sweet/dessért; for áfters *разг.*

третьекла́сс|ник м. third-form boy. **~ица** ж. third-form girl.

тре́тье|со́ртный third-ráte. **~сте́пенный** trívial; *(низкосортный)* third-ráte.

треуго́льн|ик м. tríangle. **~ый** triángular.

трефо́вый *карт.* of clubs *после сущ.*

тре́фы *мн. карт.* clubs.

трёхгоди́чный three-year *attr.*

трёхгодова́лый three-year-óld; of three *после сущ.*

трёхгра́нный 1. tríple-edged; 2. *мат.* trihédral.

трёхдне́вный three-day *attr.*; в ~ срок (with)in three days.

трёхколёсный three-wheeled; ~ велосипе́д trícycle.

трёхко́мнатный three-room *attr.*; ~ая кварти́ра three-room flat.

трёхле́тний 1. *(о сроке)* three-year *attr.*; of three years *после сущ.*; 2. *(о возрасте)* three-year-óld; of three *после сущ.*; ~ ребёнок three-year-óld child*, child* of three.

трёхме́рный three-diménsional.

трёхме́стный three-séater *attr.*

трёхме́сячный 1. *(о сроке)* three months'; three-month *attr.*; 2. *(о возрасте)* three-months-óld; of three months *после сущ.*; ~ ребёнок three-months-óld báby, báby of three months.

трёхнеде́льный 1. *(о сроке)* three-week *attr.*; ~ о́тпуск three weeks' hóliday; 2. *(о возрасте)* three-weeks-óld; of three weeks *после сущ.*; ~ ребёнок báby of three weeks.

трёхпроце́нтный three-per-cént *attr.*

трёхра́зов|ый: ~ое пита́ние three meals a day.

трёхсло́жн|ый trisyllábic; ~ое сло́во trisýllable.

трёхсо́тый three-húndredth.

трёхсторо́нн|ий 1. three-sided, triláteral; 2. *дип.* tripártite; three-party *attr.*; ~ догово́р three-power tréaty; ~ее соглаше́ние tripártite agréement.

трёхступе́нчат|ый three-stage *attr.*

трёхцве́тный three-colour *attr.*; *(о флаге)* trícolour.

трёхчасово́й 1. three-hour *attr.*; of three hours *после сущ.*; 2. *(назначенный на три часа)* three-o'clock *attr.*

трёхэта́жный three-storey *attr.*; ~ дом three-storey house.

трещ|а́ть *несов.* 1. cráckle; *(о будильнике)* buzz; *(о льде)* crack; *(о барабане)* ráttle; roll; *(о кузнечиках)* chirp; 2. *разг. (болтать)* chátter, jábber; 3. *разг.*: у меня́ голова́ ~и́т I have a splítting héadache.

тре́щин|а ж. crack; *(в земле, скале и т. п. тж.)* físsure, rift; *перен. (неблагополучие в чём-л.)* deféct, something wrong; *(разлад, расхождения)* rift; дать ~у be* cracked; их дру́жба дала́ ~у their fríendship begán to show signs of strain.

трещо́тка ж. 1. ráttle; 2. *разг. (болтун)* chátterbox; 3. *мех.* rátchet; ручна́я ~ rátchet drill.

три three.

трибу́н м. tríbune.

трибу́н|а ж. 1. *(для оратора)* róstrum *(pl* -ra, -rums)*, tríbune, (spéaker's) plátform; *перен.* fórum; подня́ться на ~у mount the róstrum/plátform; 2. *(для зрителей)* stand; ~ы стадио́на the stands.

трибуна́л м. tribúnal; вое́нный ~ mílitary tribúnal.

тригонометри́ческ|ий trigonométric(al); trigonómetry *attr.*; ~ие фу́нкции trigonométrical fúnctions; ~ие табли́цы trigonométrical tábles.

тригономе́трия ж. trigonómetry.

тридевять: за ~ земе́ль far, far awáy, in far distant lands.

тридцатилёт|ие с. 1. (*период*) thírty years *pl*; 2. (*годовщина*) thírtieth annivérsary. **~ний** 1. (*о сроке*) thírty-year *attr.*; of thírty years *после сущ.*; 2. (*о возрасте*) thírty-year-óld; of thírty *после сущ.*

тридцат|ый thírtieth; **~ые** гóды the thírties.

тридцат|ь thírty; в **~й** киломéтрах withín thírty kilometres.

трйер м. с.-х. grain cléaner, gráder.

трйжды three times; thrice *поэт.*; ~ два, три и т. д. three twos, threes, *etc.*

трикó с. нескл. 1. (*шерстяная ткань*) trícot; 2. (*одежда*) tights *pl*; 3. (*женские панталоны*) kníckers *pl.*

трикотáж м. 1. (*ткань*) knítted fábric; (*шерстяной*) jérsey; 2. собир. (*изделия*) knítted goods *pl*, knítwear. **~ный** (machíne-)knítted; (*из шерсти*) jérsey *attr.*; **~ная** фáбрика knítted goods fáctory; **~ная** кóфточка knítted júmper.

трилйстник м. 1. tréfoil; *бот. тж.* red clóver; ~ ползýчий white clóver; 2. (*на эмблемах*) tréfoil.

трйллер м. thríller.

триллиóн м. bíllion; tríllion *амер.*

трилóгия ж. trílogy.

тринадцатилéтний 1. (*о сроке*) thírteen-year *attr.*; of thírteen years *после сущ.*; 2. (*о возрасте*) thírteen-year-óld; of thírteen *после сущ.*

тринáдцатый thírteenth.

тринáдцать thírteen.

трйо с. нескл. trío.

трйста three húndred.

тритóн м. зоол. newt.

триýмф м. tríumph.

триумфáльн|ый triúmphal; (*победный тж.*) triúmphant; **~ая** áрка arch of tríumph; **~ое** шéствие triúmphal procéssion.

трóгательн|о tóuchingly, móvingly. **~ый** tóuching, móving; **~ая** пóвесть móving stóry; **~ая** забóтливость tóuching considerátion.

трóг|ать, трóнуть (*вн.*) 1. touch (*smb., smth.*); рукáми не ~! do not touch!; не ~ когó-л. leave* smb. alóne; 2. (*вызывать сочувствие*) afféct (*smb.*); (*умилять*) touch (*smb.*), move (*smth.*); ~ когó-л. до слёз move smb. to tears; это менá не ~ает it leaves me cold; 3. (*начинать движение*) см. трóгаться; трóгай! you can start!; get góing! разг. **~аться**, трóнуться start, begín* to move; **~аться** в путь set* out; пóезд трóнулся the train stárted; он не трóнулся с мéста he dídn't budge.

трóе three; нас ~ there are three of us.

троебóрье с. спорт. tríple evént, tríple combinátion.

троекрáтн|о three times. **~ый** tríple.

трóйк|а ж. 1. (*цифра, игральная карта*) a three; (*отметка*) "fair", three (out of five); получйть ~у по истóрии get* a "fair" for/in hístory; 2. (*лошадей*) tróika; (*об экипаже тж.*) cárriage and three; 3. (*костюм*) thrée-piece suit.

трóйн|ой tríple; штраф в **~óм** размéре tríple fine; **~óе** прáвило мат. rule of three; **~óй** прыжóк спорт. tríple jump.

трóйня ж. tríplets *pl.*

трóйственный tríple.

троллéйбус м. trólleybus. **~ный** trólleybus *attr.*

тромб м. мед. thrómbus, blood clot.

тромбóн м. trombóne.

трон м. throne; вступйть на ~ ascénd/mount the throne.

трóн|уть сов. 1. см. трóгать; 2. (*вн.; о морозе и т. п.*) touch (*smth.*), afféct (*smth.*); морóзом **~уло** цветы́ the flówers have been touched/nipped by the frost. **~уться** сов. 1. см. трóгаться; 2. разг. (*помешаться*) be* touched; он немнóго **~улся** he is slíghtly touched; 3. разг. (*испортиться*) turn, go* off.

тропá ж. path; (*глухая*) trail.

трóпик м. 1. trópic; ~ Рáка trópic of Cáncer; ~ Козе-

рóга trópic of Cápricorn; 2. мн. (*жаркий пояс*) the trópics.

тропйнка ж. path.

тропйческ|ий trópical; **~ая** лихорáдка júngle féver; ~ пóяс tórrid zone; **~ая** жарá trópical heat.

тропосфéра ж. tróposphere.

трос м. мор., тех. rope.

тростнйк м. reed; (*камыш*) búlrush; ◇ сáхарный ~ súgar-cane.

трóсточка ж., **трость** ж. (wálking-)stick.

тротуáр м. pávement; sídewalk *амер.*

трофéй м. 1. чаще мн. (*военная добыча*) spoils of war; bóoty *sg*; 2. (*вещественная память о какой-л. победе*) tróphy. **~ный** cáptured.

трою́родн|ый: ~ брат, **~ая** сестрá sécond cóusin.

трóйк|ий tríple, thréefold; **~им** óбразом in three ways.

труб|á ж. 1. pipe; (*дымовая*) chímney; (*фабричная тж.*) stack; (*паровоза, парохода*) fúnnel, stack; трубы́ паровóго отоплéния stéam-heating pipes; ~ телескóпа télescope tube; 2. муз. trúmpet; 3. анат. tube; ◇ вы́лететь в **~у́** go* bust, go* smash; crúmble.

трубáч м. trúmpeter.

труб|йть, протрубйть 1. blow*, trúmpet; ~ в трубý blow*/sound the trúmpet; 2. (*звучать*) sound; трубы́ **~я́т** the trúmpets are sóunding; 3. (*вн.; подавать сигнал*) sound (*smth.*); ~ тревóгу sound the alárm; 4. (*о пр.; разглашать*) trúmpet (*smth.*), procláim (*smth.*) (from the hóuse-tops), blare out (*smth.*).

трубк|а ж. 1. tube; (*зажигательная*) fuse; резйновая ~ rúbber tube; рентгéновская ~ X-ray tube; электрóнно-лучевáя ~ (*телевизора*) eléctron-ray tube; cáthode-ray tube; 2. (*телефонная*) recéiver; 3. (*курительная*) pipe; 4. (*свёрток*) roll; свернýть чтó-л. в **~у** roll *smth.* up.

трýбный trúmpet *attr.*; of a trúmpet *после сущ.*

трубопровóд м. pípeline, cónduit.

трубопрокáтный túbe-rolling, pípe-rolling; ~ стан túbe(-rolling) mill.

трубочйст м. chímney-sweep.

трýбочный pipe *attr.*; ~ табáк pipe tobácco.

трýбчатый túbular.

труд м. 1. work, lábour; (*тяжёлый, однообразный*) toil; мн. (*занятия, хлопоты*) affáirs; охрáна **~á** protéction of lábour; 2. (*усилие*) éffort; с **~óм** with dífficulty, with an éffort; не стóило никакóго **~á** сдéлать это it was no tróuble to do it; все **~ы́** остáлись тщéтными all my éfforts were in vain; 3. (*произведение*) work; мн. (*название научных сборников*) transáctions; ◇ давáть себé ~ (+ инф.) take* the tróuble (+ to *inf*); без **~á** without dífficulty, éffortlessly; взять на себá ~ (+ инф.) take* the tróuble (+ to *inf*).

трудйться несов. 1. work; (*тяжело*) toil, lábour; (*над тв.*) be* wórking (on); 2. разг. (*затруднять себя*) bóther, take* the tróuble; он напрáсно трудйтся he is wásting his time; не трудйтесь don't tróuble; (*не пытайтесь*) don't try.

трýдно 1. нареч. with dífficulty; ~ повéрить it is dífficult/hard to belíeve; ~ понáть it is hard to understánd; эту кнйгу ~ купйть this book is véry difficult to get; емý ~ прихóдится he has a hard time; 2. в знач. сказ. безл. it is dífficult/hard; 3. в знач. сказ. безл. (*дт.*) it is hard (for); мне ~ (+ инф.) I have dífficulty (in + -ing), I find it difficult (+ to *inf*).

труднопроизносймый (that is) hard to pronóunce *после сущ.*; unpronóunceable.

труднопроходймый álmost impássable, dífficult (to pass).

трýдн|ость ж. dífficulty; snag, pítfall разг. **~ый** 1. dífficult, hard; (*тяжёлый, изнурительный*) árduous; **~ая** рабóта hard/uphíll work; tough job разг.; **~ая** задáча dífficult task; **~ая** жизнь hard life; **~ое** врéмя dífficult times *pl*; ~ые времена́ hard times; в ~ую мину́ту in time of need, in a tight có́rner, in tróuble; 2. (*с трудо́м под-дающийся воспита́нию*) difficult; ~ый ребёнок dífficult child*; име́ть ~ый хара́ктер be* difficult to get on with; 3. (*мучи́тельный*) páinful; (*о боле́зни*) dángerous.

трудов|о́й 1. lábour *attr.*, wó́rking, work *attr.*; ~ы́е на́выки (work) skills; ~о́е воспита́ние wó́rking educátion, educátion based on work; ~а́я дисципли́на lábour díscipline; ~ стаж length of sérvice; ~о́е законода́тельство lábour legislátion; ~ по́двиг feat of lábour; ~ подъём (lábour) enthúsiasm; 2. (*приобретённый трудо́м*) earned; ~ы́е дохо́ды earned íncome *sg*, íncome from work; 3. (*живу́щий свои́м трудо́м*) wó́rking; ◇ ~а́я кни́жка wó́rk-record card; индивидуа́льная ~а́я де́ятельность indivídual lábour actívity, indivídual énterprise, self--emplóyment.

трудо|де́нь *м.* wó́rk-day (*unit of work in collective farming*); он вы́работал со́рок пять ~дней в э́том ме́ся-це he has fó́rty-five wó́rk-days to his crédit for this month.

трудоёмк|ий lábour-inténsive, labó́rious.

трудо|люби́вый indústrious, díligent. ~лю́бие *с.* índustry, díligence.

трудоспосо́бн|ость *ж.* 1. (*физи́ческая способность к труду́*) abílity to work; поте́ря ~ости disabílity, incapácity, disáblement; 2. (*способность мно́го рабо́-тать*) capácity for work; ~ый áble-bodied; всё ~ое насе-ле́ние the whole áble-bodied populátion.

трудоустро́йство *с.* provísion of emplóyment.

трудя́щ|ийся *прил.* 1. wó́rking; ~иеся ма́ссы the wó́rking péople/másses; 2. *в знач. сущ. мн.* the wó́rking péople.

тру́женик *м.* wó́rker; tó́iler *поэт.*

труни́ть *несов.* (над *тв.*) chaff (*smb.*), pull *smb.'s* leg, kid (*smb.*).

труп *м.* corpse, bó́dy; (*живо́тного*) cárcass. ~ный: ~ный за́пах smell of putrefáction, pú́trid smell; ~ный яд ptó́maine pó́ison.

тру́ппа *ж.* có́mpany, troupe.

трус *м.* có́ward.

тру́сики *мн. см.* трусы́.

тру́сить, стру́сить be* afráid; have*/get* the jítters *разг.*; (перед *тв.*) be* scared (of), shake* in one's shoes (befó́re); не трусь! don't be scared!

труси́ть *несов. разг.* jog alóng, trot; ~ ме́лкой рыс-цо́й go* at a jó́gtrot.

труси́ха *ж. разг.* funk, có́ward.

трусли́в|ый có́wardly; ~ое чу́вство có́wardly fé́eling; ~ взгляд tímorous/ábject glance.

тру́сость *ж.* có́wardice.

трусы́ *мн.* shorts; (*для купа́ния*) swímming trunks; (*ни́жнее бельё*) pants.

трут *м.* tínder.

тру́тень *м.* drone.

труха́ *ж.* dust; (*измельчи́вшееся се́но, соло́ма*) bits of hay; straw; *перен. разг.* rúbbish.

трухля́вый mó́uldering, ró́tten.

трущо́б|а *ж.* 1. (*лесна́я и т. п.*) thícket; 2. (*захолу́-стье*) hole; 3. (*бе́дная, гря́зная окра́ина*) slum; (*жили́-ще*) hó́vel; городски́е ~ы úrban slums.

трюк *м.* trick; stunt; *перен. тж.* ruse, dodge; акро-бати́ческий ~ acrobátic feat. ~а́чество *с. разг.* 1. stúnting; 2. (*в иску́сстве*) gímmickry.

трюм *м.* hold.

трю́фель *м.* 1. (*гриб*) trúffle; 2. *мн.* (*шокола́дные конфе́ты*) trúffle chócolates.

тряпи́чн|ица *ж.* wó́man who is mad on clothes. ~ый rag *attr.*

тря́пка *ж.* 1. rag; полова́я ~ flóor-cloth; пы́льная ~ dú́ster; 2. *мн. разг. ирон.* (*же́нские наря́ды*) clothes; 3. *разг. ирон.* (*о челове́ке*) wet rag, só́fty, jélly-fish.

тряпьё *с. собир.* 1. (*тря́пки, ве́тошь*) rags *pl*; 2. *разг.* (*рва́ная оде́жда*) rags.

тряси́на *ж.* bog, quágmire (*тж. перен.*).

тряск|а *ж.* shá́king, jó́lting. ~ий (*о пово́зке*) jó́lty; (*о доро́ге*) bú́mpy.

трясогу́зка *ж. зоол.* wágtail.

тряс|ти́ *несов.* (*вн., тв.*) 1. shake* (*smth.*); ~ де́ре-во shake* a tree; ~ кому́-л. ру́ку shake* *smb.'s* hand; ~ ковры́ shake* rugs; ~ голово́й shake* one's head; 2. (*при езде́*) jolt (*smb., smth.*), give* (*smb.*) a shá́king; 3. *безл.* (*вызыва́ть дрожь*): его́ ~ёт от хо́лода he is shá́king with cold. ~ти́сь *несов.* 1. (*дрожа́ть*) shake*, trémble; ста́вни ~ли́сь и стуча́ли the shútters shook and rá́ttled; у него́ ~у́тся ру́ки his hands shake; ~ти́сь от стра́ха shake*/trémble with fear; ~ти́сь от хо́лода shíver with cold; 2. (перед *тв.*; *боя́ться*) trémble (befó́re), live in fear (of), dread (*smth.*); 3. (за *вн.*; *опаса́ться*) wó́rry (abó́ut), be* wó́rried (abóut); 4. (над *тв.*; *оберега́ть*) dote (upó́n); (*бере́чь что-л.*) watch (*smth.*); ~ти́сь над ка́ждой копе́йкой watch évery pénny; 5. (*при езде́*) be* jó́lted, have* a shá́king.

тряхн|у́ть *сов. разг.* give* a jolt; нас ~у́ло we felt a sú́dden jolt.

тсс! hush!, sh!; hist! *поэт.*

туале́т *м.* 1. (*пла́тье*) dress; 2. (*стол*) dré́ssing--table; 3. (*убо́рная*) lávatory, tó́ilet. ~ный tó́ilet *attr.*; ~ный сто́лик dré́ssing-table; ~ное мы́ло tó́ilet soap.

туберкулёз *м.* tuberculó́sis; ~ лёгких púlmonary tuberculó́sis. ~ный tubércular, tubérculous; ~ный про-це́сс tubérculous pró́cess; ~ный диспансе́р ТВ prophyláctic céntre.

туви́н|ец *м.*, ~ка *ж.* Tuvínian. ~ский Túva, Tuvínian; ~ский язы́к Tuvínian, the Tuvínian lánguage.

ту́г|о 1. *нареч.* tight, tíghtly; ~ натяну́ть *что-л.* stretch/pull *smth.* taut; ~ затяну́ть по́яс pull one's belt tight; ~ наби́ть мешо́к fill a bag to overfló́wing; ~ наби́-тый tíghtly packed; ~ затя́нутый tíghtly drawn; ~ натя́-нутый кана́т taut rope/cá́ble; 2. *нареч.* (*с трудо́м*): ~ подвига́ться вперёд make* slow pró́gress; 3. *в знач. сказ. безл.*: ему́ ~ прихо́дится he is in a tight có́rner, у него́ ~ с деньга́ми he is hard-préssed for mó́ney, he is hard up (for mó́ney). ~о́й 1. tight; (*ту́го натя́нутый*) taut; ~о́й по́яс tight belt; 2. (*с трудо́м поддаю́щийся како́му-л. возде́йствию*) stiff; ~а́я пружи́на pó́werful/stiff spring; 3. (*о мысли́тельных способно-стях*) slow; ◇ ~о́й на́ ухо hard of hé́aring.

тугопла́вкий refrá́ctory.

тугоу́хий rá́ther deaf, hard of hé́aring.

туда́ there; (*по тому́ направле́нию*) in that diréction; мы идём не ~ we're gó́ing in the wrong diréction; ◇ ~ и обра́тно there and back; ~ и сюда́ éverywhere; и ~ и сюда́ 1) to and fro; 2) (*и так и сяк*) first one way, then anó́ther; то ~, то сюда́ back and forth, to and fro; ни ~ ни сюда́ né́ither back nor fó́rward, stuck fast; ~ ему́ и доро́га! ≈ serve(s) him right!

тужи́ть *несов.* (о, по *пр.*) *разг.* grieve (óver).

тужу́рка *ж.* (dó́uble-bré́asted) jácket.

туз *м.* ace; *перен. разг.* bígwig, big noise, celébrity.

тузе́м|ец *м.*, ~ка *ж.* nátive. ~ный nátive.

тук-ту́к *разг.* rá́t-tát(-tát).

ту́ловище *с.* trunk.

тулу́п *м.* shé́epskin coat.

тулья́ *ж.* crown (*of a hat*).

тума́н *м.* mist; (*густо́й*) fog; сего́дня ~ it is místy/fó́ggy todáy; ◇ как в ~е 1) (*нея́сно, сму́тно*) há́zily; 2) (*нея́сно воспринима́емая окружа́ющее*) in a fog; напусти́ть ~ obscú́re the íssue. ~ить *несов.* 1. (*за-темня́ть собо́й — о пы́ли и т. п.*) smudge (*smth.*), obscú́re (*smth.*); 2. (*завола́кивать глаза́*) dim (*smth.*); *перен.* (*мути́ть созна́ние*) fúddle (*smth.*), befó́g (*smth.*). ~иться *несов.* 1. (*застила́ться тума́ном*) be* dimmed, be* obscú́red; 2. (*видне́ться как в тума́не*) loom; 3. (*о глазах*) be* dimmed; *перен.* (*о мыслях, сознании*) be* confúsed/fúddled/clóuded; 4. (*делаться печальным*) cloud.

тума́нн|о 1. *нареч.* (*неясно*) házily, váguely; 2. *в знач. сказ. безл.*: сего́дня ~ it is místy/fóggy todáy. ~ость *ж.* 1. *астр.* nébula; 2. (*неясность*) obscúrity. ~ый 1. místy, fóggy; *перен.* (*расплывчатый*) házy, vague; 2. (*неопределённый, неясный*) vague, házy; он имеет весьма ~ое представле́ние об э́том he has a véry vague concéption of it, his idéas on it are extrémely nébulous; 3. (*о глазах, взгляде*) místy; (*о голове*) fúddled, dazed.

тумб|а *ж.* 1. (*у тротуара*) post; 2. (*подставка*) pédestal. ~очка *ж.* (*ночной столик*) bédside táble.

ту́ндра *ж.* túndra.

тунея́д|ец *м.* párasite, drone. ~ство *с.* párasitism, living on óther people.

тунне́ль *м.* túnnel; пешехо́дный ~ súbway.

тупе́ть *несов.* 1. *см.* тупи́ться; 2. (*глупеть*) becóme* dull/slúggish.

тупи́к *м.* 1. (*улица*) blind álley, cúl-de-sác; 2. *ж.-д.* dead end; 3. (*безвыходное положение*) déadlock, impásse; зайти́ в ~ be* at a déadlock; ◇ ста́вить *кого-л.* в ~ put* *smb.* in a spot; стать в ~ перед *чем-л.* be* put in a spot by *smb.*

тупи́ть *несов.* (*вн.*) blunt (*smth.*). ~ся *несов.* becóme* blunt, lose* its edge.

тупи́ца *м. и ж. разг.* dunce.

ту́по *dúlly*; ~ смотре́ть look vácantly.

туп|о́й 1. blunt; ~а́я пила́ blunt saw; 2. (*широкий*) broad, blunt; 3. (*умственно ограниченный*) dull, dim-witted, obtúse, stólid; ~ челове́к obtúse pérson; ~ое высокоме́рие impénetrable árrogance; 4. (*невырази́тельный*) dull, obtúse; ~ взгляд dull/vácant glance; ~ая улы́бка uncompréhending smile; 5. (*о чувствах, переживаниях и т. п.*) apathétic, lethárgic, slúggish; ~ страх nágging fear; ~ое упря́мство lethárgic óbstinacy; 6. (*безропотный*) submíssive; ~ое повинове́ние dull obédience; 7. (*нерезкий, ноющий*) dull; ~ая боль dull ache; ◇ ~ у́гол *мат.* obtúse ángle.

тупоконе́чный blunt.

тупоно́с|ый blúnt-nosed; ~ые боти́нки squáre-toed shoes.

ту́пость *ж.* (*глупость, бессмысленность*) dúllness, obtúseness.

тупоуго́льный obtúse(-ángled).

тупоу́м|ие *с.* stupídity, obtúseness. ~ный stúpid, obtúse.

тур I *м.* 1. (*один круг танца*) turn (round the room); 2. (*состязания*) round; 3. (*отдельный этап чего-л.*) round, stage.

тур II *м.* 1. (*вымерший бык*) áurochs; 2. (*горный козёл*) íbex (*pl тж.* íbices).

тура́ *ж. разг. см.* ладья́.

турба́за *ж.* tóurist hóstel.

турби́н|а *ж.* túrbine. ~ный túrbine *attr.*

турбовинтово́й *ав.* túrbo-próp *attr.*; ~ самолёт túrbo-prop áircraft; ~ дви́гатель túrbo-prop éngine.

турбогенера́тор *м.* turbogénerator.

турбореакти́вный *ав.* túrbo-jét *attr.*; ~ самолёт túrbo-jet áircraft; ~ дви́гатель túrbo-jet éngine.

туре́цкий Túrkish; ~ язы́к Túrkish, the Túrkish lánguage; ◇ ~ бараба́н bass/big drum.

тури́зм *м.* tóurism, tóuring; (*вид спорта*) wálking, híking; го́рный ~ móuntain wálking.

тури́ст *м.* tóurist; (*участник пеших походов*) híker, wálker. ~и́ческий híking, wálking; ~и́ческий похо́д híking expedition, wálking tour. ~ка *ж.* tóurist; (*участница пеших походов*) híker, wálker. ~ский tóurist *attr.*; ~ский ла́герь tóurist camp.

туркме́н *м.*, ~ка *ж.* Turkmén. ~ский Turkmén; ~ский язы́к Turkmén, the Turkmén lánguage.

тýрман *м.* túmbler(-pigeon).

турне́ *с. нескл.* tour.

турне́пс *м.* túrnip.

турни́к *м.* horizóntal bar.

турнике́т *м.* túrnstile.

турни́р *м.* tóurnament; ~ по хокке́ю с ша́йбой íce-hockey tóurnament. ~ный tóurnament *attr.*; ~ная табли́ца tóurnament list.

ту́рок *м.* Turk.

турча́нка *ж.* Túrkish wóman*.

ту́скл|о 1. *нареч.* dímly; ~ свети́ть give* a poor light; 2. *в знач. сказ. безл.* it is dark/múrky. ~ый 1. (*непрозрачный*) díngy, bléary; grímy; (*потерявший блеск*) dull, tárnished; (*поблёкший*) fáded; ~ое стекло́ grímy window; ~ое серебро́ tárnished sílver; ~ые кра́ски fáded cólours; 2. (*о свете*) dim; ~ый фона́рь dim lamp; ~ый день pállid day; 3. (*невырази́тельный*) dull, vácant; (*о глазах тж.*) lústreless, glássy; ~ый взгляд dull glance; 4. (*бессодержательный*) dréary; ~ая жизнь dréary life.

тускн|е́ть, потускне́ть 1. dim, grow* dim; (*о металле*) tárnish; *перен.* wane, lose* its lústre; 2. (*перед тв.*, *меркнуть*) pale (besíde); всё э́то ~е́ет перед... all this pales besíde...

тут 1. (*о месте*) here; 2. (*о времени*) then; ◇ ~ же then and there; он ~ как ~! there he is!; и всё ~! and that's that!; не ~-то было! but that's not how it turned out!, but no such luck!

ту́тов|ый múlberry *attr.*; ~ое де́рево múlberry tree; ~ая я́года múlberry; ~ шелкопря́д sílkworm.

туф *м.* túfa.

ту́фли *мн.* (*ед.* ту́фля *ж.*) shoes; дома́шние ~ (bédroom) slíppers.

тухл|ый pútrid, bad*, rótten; (*о масле*) ráncid; (*о мясе*) táinted; ~ое яйцо́ rótten/bad* egg.

ту́хнуть I, потухнуть (*гаснуть*) go* out.

ту́хнуть II, протухнуть (*портиться*) go* bad, spoil*.

ту́ч|а *ж.* cloud (*тж. перен.*); ~ пы́ли cloud of dust; ~ комаро́в swarm of mosquítoes; ◇ мра́чный как ~ like a thúndercloud; ~ей like a thúndercloud; сгусти́лись ~и над *кем-л., чем-л. smb., smth.* was únder a thréatening cloud.

тучне́ть, потучне́ть get* fat/stout, put* on flesh.

ту́чн|ость *ж.* 1. (*полнота*) córpulence, obésity; 2. (*земли*) ríchness, fertílity; 3. (*сочность*) luxúriance. ~ый 1. (*полный*) plump; (*о человеке тж.*) córpulent, stout; 2. (*о земле*) rich, fértile, fat; 3. (*сочный, густой*) lush; ~ые луга́ lush méadows.

туш *м. муз.* flóurish.

ту́ша *ж.* cárcass; коро́вья ~ cow's cárcass.

тушева́ть *несов.* (*вн.*) shade (*smth.*); *перен.* tone (*smth.*) down.

тушёвка *ж.* sháding.

тушён|ый stewed; ~ое мя́со stewed/bráised meat.

туши́ть I, потуши́ть (*вн.*; *гасить*) put* out (*smth.*), extínguish (*smth.*); ~ ого́нь put* out a fire; ~ свечу́ blow* out a cándle; ~ ла́мпу extínguish a lamp; ~ свет turn out the light, switch off the light.

туши́ть II *несов.* (*вн.*) *кул.* stew (*smth.*), braise (*smth.*); ~ бара́нину stew mútton. ~ся *несов.* stew.

тушь *ж.* Índian ink.

ту́я *ж. бот.* thúya, thúja.

тща́тельн|ость *ж.* thóroughness, care. ~ый thórough.

тщеду́ш|ость *ж.* féebleness, púniness. ~ный* púny, wéakly.

тщесла́в|ие *с.* concéit, vánity. ~ный concéited, vain.

тщётн|о váinly, in vain; ~ ждать wait in vain. ~ость *ж.* futílity, úselessness. ~ый vain, fútile, unaváiling; ~ые наде́жды vain hopes.

ты (*рд., вн.* тебя́, *дт., пр.* тебе́, *тв.* тобо́й, тобо́ю) you; thou *уст., поэт.*; ◇ быть с *кем-л.* на ты be* on close terms with *smb.*

ты́кать, ткнуть (*тв. в вн.*) thrust* (*smth.* into), poke (*smth.* into), stick* (*smth.* into); ~ па́льцем во *что-л.* thrust*/point a finger in the diréction of *smth.*

ты́ква *ж.* púmpkin.

ты́квенны|й púmpkin *attr.*; gourd *attr.*; семéйство ~х gourd fámily.

тыл *м.* 1. rear; глубóкий ~ the home front; зайти́ в ~ take* in the rear; 2. *обыкн. мн.* (*совокупность вспомогáтельных войсковых частéй*) rear únits.

тылово́й rear *attr.*, logístic; ~ гóспиталь hóspital in the rear.

ты́льн|ый rear *attr.*; ~ая сторонá руки́ the back of the hand.

тын *м.* pálings *pl.*

ты́ся|ча 1. a thóusand; пять, дéсять *и т. д.* ~ч five, ten, *etc.* thóusand; ~ рублéй thóusand róubles; 2. *обыкн. мн.* (*множество*) thóusands.

тысячелéт|ие *с.* 1. (*срок*) a thóusand years *pl*; 2. (*годовщина*) thóusandth annivérsary. ~ний thóusand-year *of a thóusand years после сущ.*

ты́сячн|ый 1. the thóusandth; 2. (*о части*) thóusandth; 3. (*насчитывающий тысячи*): ~ая толпá a crowd thóusands strong, a crowd séveral thóusand strong, thóusands of péople.

тычи́нка *ж. бот.* stámen.

тьма I *ж.* dárkness (*тж. перен.*), the dark; какáя здесь ~! how dark it is here!

тьма II *ж. разг.* (*множество*) másses *pl*; (*сколько угодно*) heaps (of); ~ нарóду hordes of péople.

тьфу pah!, ugh!; ~, прóпасть! damn!

тюбетéйка *ж.* tyubetéika (*skull-cap worn in Central Asia*)

тю́бик *м.* tube.

тюк *м.* bale; (*узел*) búndle.

тю́лев|ый tulle *attr.*; ~ые занавéски lace cúrtains.

тюлéний seal *attr.*; ~ прóмысел seal húnting.

тюлéнь *м.* 1. seal; 2. *разг.* (*увалень*) lump, oaf.

тюль *м.* tulle.

тюльпáн *м.* túlip.

тюрбáн *м.* túrban.

тюрéм|ный príson *attr.*; ~ное заключéние imprísonment; ~ надзирáтель wárder, jáilor, gáoler. ~щик *м.* wárder; *перен.* oppréssor.

тюрк|и *и мн.*Túrki. ~ский Túrkic; ~ские языки́ Túrkic lánguages.

тюрьмá *ж.* príson, gaol.

тюфя́к *м.* máttress.

тя́вкать, тя́вкнуть уар.

тя́вкнуть *сов. см.* тя́вкать.

тя́г|а ж. 1. (*тянущая сила*) draught, tráction; ~ винтá *ав.* propéller thrust; на кóнной ~е hórse-drawn; на трáкторной ~е tráctor-drawn; электри́ческая ~ eléctric tráction; 2. (*в печи и т. п.*) draught; 3. (*к дт.; стремлéние*) lónging (for); (*тяготéние*) thirst (for), cráving (for); ~ к знáниям thirst/cráving for knówledge.

тягáться *несов.* (*с тв.*) *разг.* take* on (*smb.*), compéte (with), méasure *one's* strength (with), tússle (with).

тягáч *м.* tráctor, mechánical horse.

тя́гло *с.* живóе ~ draught ánimals *pl.*

тя́гостн|ый 1. (*трудный*) hard, árduous; ~ труд báck-breaking work; 2. (*мучительный*) páinful, distréssing; ~ое молчáние páinful sílence.

тя́гость *ж.* búrden; быть в ~ *кому-л.* be* a búrden on *smb.*; мне э́то в ~ I find it a great núisance.

тяготéни|е с. 1. *физ.* grávity, gravitátion; земнóе ~ grávity; закóн всеми́рного ~я the law of gravitátion; 2. (*связь*) gravitátion; 3. (*к дт.; влечéние*) léaning (towárds); ~ к мýзыке bent for músic; ~ к знáниям thirst for knówledge.

тяготéть *несов.* 1. (*к дт.*) grávitate (towárds); 2. (*к дт.; быть связанным*) grávitate (towárds), be*

depéndent (on); 3. (*к дт.; испытывать влечéние*) be* drawn (to); 4. (*над тв.; угнетáть, подавлять*) tówer (óver).

тягот|и́ть *несов.* (*вн.; обременять*) be* írksome (to); егó ~и́т сознáние своéй вины, бесси́лия *и т. п.* he is oppréssed by a sense of guilt, inádequacy, *etc.* ~и́ться *несов.* (*тв.*) be* oppréssed (by); ~и́ться одинóчеством be* oppréssed by *one's* lóneliness.

тягу́ч|есть *ж.* (*жидкостей*) viscósity; (*металлов*) ductílity. ~ий 1. (*способный растягиваться*) elástic; 2. (*густой, вязкий*) clínging; (*о жидкости*) víscous; (*о металле*) dúctile; 3. (*томительный*) lóng-drawn-óut; 4. (*о голосе и т. п.*) slow; ~ая речь dráwling speech, slow way of spéaking.

тя́жба *ж. уст.* litigátion.

тяжелéть *несов.* grow* héavy; (*о частях тéла, голове тж.*) begín* to feel héavy.

тяжелó 1. *нареч.* héavily; ~ нагружённый héavily lóaded; 2. *нареч.* (*серьёзно*) sériously; sevérely; ~ бóлен sériously ill; ~ рáнен sevérely wóunded; ~ поплати́ться за *что-л.* pay* déarly/héavily for *smth.*; 3. *в знач. сказ. безл.* (*дт.; трудно*): больнóму ~ the pátient is háving a hard time; мне ~ поднимáться по лéстнице it is hard for me to go upstáirs; 4. *в знач. сказ. безл.* (*дт.; о мрáчном настроéнии*): мне ~ I am sad; у меня ~ на душé I am sad/héavy at heart.

тяжелоатлéт *м.* wéight-lifter.

тяжелове́с *м. спорт.* héavy-weight. ~ный 1. héavy; 2. (*о человéке*) pónderous; 3. (*о здáниях*) mássive.

тяжелово́з *м.* dráught-horse.

тяжёл|ый 1. héavy; ~ чемодáн héavy súitcase; ~ые портьéры héavy cúrtains; ~ые тýчи héavy clouds; ~ые шаги́ héavy fóotsteps; pónderous tread *sg*; ~ стиль héavy style; 2. (*трудный*) hard; dífficult (*тж. о ребёнке*); ~ая рабóта hard work; ~ая дорóга dífficult road; 3. (*затруднённый*) láboured; ~ое дыхáние láboured bréathing; 4. (*затрудни́тельный*) dífficult; (*полный лишéний, забóт*) stréssful, hard; (*мучительный*) páinful; ~ые услóвия dífficult condítions; ~ая жизнь hard life; ~ое врéмя time of tróuble/stress; stréssful days *pl*; ~ая обязанность páinful dúty; ~ая смерть páinful death; 5. (*сильный, глубóкий*) gríevous; (*серьёзный, опáсный*) grave; (*суровый, жестóкий*) sevére; ~ удáр gríevous/sérious blow; ~ вздох deep sigh; ~ое наказáние sevére/héavy púnishment; он в ~ом состоя́нии his condítion is grave; 6. (*тягостный, гнетýщий*) páinful, distréssing; (*о мыслях и т. п. тж.*) sad; (*о взгля́де*) súllen; ~ое зрéлище distréssing sight; ~ое настроéние depréssed state of mind; 7. (*неужи́вчивый*) dífficult; ~ человéк dífficult pérson; 8. (*удушливый*) héavy, close; ~ зáпах héavy smell/frágrance; ~ вóздух close/fétid air; 9. ~ые тáнки héavy tanks; ~ое машиностроéние héavy enginéering; ~ая промы́шленность héavy índustry; ~ая водá héavy wáter; ◇ ~ вес *спорт.* héavy weight; ~ая головá у *кого-л.* has a dull héadache; ~ день hard day; ~ая рукá héavy hand; быть ~ым на подъём be* hard to move.

тя́жест|ь *ж.* 1. *физ.* grávity; си́ла ~и grávity; центр ~и céntre of grávity (*тж. перен.*); 2. (*большой вес*) weight; 3. (*тяжёлый предмéт*) héavy load; 4. (*серьёзность*) grávity; ~ забóт weight of cares, héavy load of cares; ~ обвинéния, преступлéния grávity of the charge, offénce; ~ ули́к weight of évidence; 5. (*что-л. обремени́тельное*) búrden, encúmbrance.

тя́жк|ий héavy; ~ая дóля hard lot; ~ая болéзнь sérious/dángerous íllness; ~ое преступлéние grave/sérious offénce/crime.

тян|ýть *несов.* 1. (*вн.; перемещáть с си́лой*) pull (*smth.*); (*проклáдывать*) lay* (*smth.*); ~ канáт pull a rope; ~ прóвод lay* a wire; ~ *что-л.* в рáзные стóроны tug/pull *smth.* in ópposite diréctions; 2. (*вн.; рýку, шéю*) stretch (*smth.*); ~ рýку к звонкý reach out for the bell; 3. (*вн.; вытя́гивать*) stretch (*smth.*); (*изготовля́ть* *путём вытягивания*) draw* (*smth.*); ~ прóволоку draw* wire; **4.** (*вн.; вести за собой силой*) pull (*smb., smth.*); tow (*smth.*), haul (*smth.*); ~ на буксѝре tow; ~ когó-л. зá руку pull/tug at *smb.'s* hand; **5.** (*вн.*) *разг.* (*заставлять делать что-л.*) make* (*smb.*) go; *перен.* (*склонять к чему-л.*) lead* (*smb.*); ~ когó-л. в кинó make* *smb.* go to the cínema; никтó егó сѝлой не ~ýл nóbody made him go; **6.** (*вн.; влечь*) draw* (*smb.*); меня тя́нет на вóздух I'm lónging for a breath of air; егó тя́нет к мóрю he feels drawn to the sea, the sea calls him; **7.** (*вн.; доставать, вынимать*) pull (*smth.*) out, take* (*smth.*) out; ~ жрéбий draw* lots; **8.** (*вн.; всасывать — жидкость*) suck (*smth.*); **9.** (*обладать тягой*) draw*; трубá хорошó тя́нет the chímney draws well; **10.** (*слабо дуть*): с мóря тя́нет свéжестью cool air drifts in from the sea; от окнá тя́нет хóлодом there is a cold draught from the window; **11.** (*медлить*) deláy; (*вн.; медленно делать что-л.*) take* a long time óver (*smth.*); ~ с отвéтом deláy *one's* replý; **12.** (*вн.; медленно говорить*) drawl (*smth.*); (*протяжно петь*) intóne (*smth.*), drag out (*smth.*); ~ речь speak up!; ~ и мя́млить hem and haw; **13.** (*вн.; экономно расходовать что-л.*) spin* (*smth.*) out; **14.** (*продолжать что-л.*) go* on (with), prolóng (*smth.*); ◇ ~ врéмя take*/bide* *one's* time; hang* fire *идиом.*; ~ когó-л. за душу péster the life out of *smb.*; ~ когó-л. за язы́к pump *smb.*, make* *smb.* talk; ктó вас ~ýл за язы́к? what on earth posséssed you to say that?

тяну́ться *несов.* **1.** (*растягиваться*) stretch; **2.** (*простираться*) exténd, stretch out; на горизóнте тя́нутся гóры móuntains line the horízon; **3.** (*двигаться*) move slówly; (*о тучах, дыме тж.*) drift; **4.** (*за тв.*, *к дт.*; *руками, корпусом*) reach (for); ~ рукáми к комý-л. stretch out *one's* hands towards *smb.*; **5.** (*к дт.*; *стремиться*) strive* (for); (*стараться сравняться*) try to keep up (with); цветóк тя́нется к сóлнцу the flówer turns towards the sun; **6.** (*длиться*) drag on, be* góing on; (*о времени*) pass; creep* (by).

тяну́чка *ж.* tóffee.

тя́пка *ж.* **1.** (*сечка*) chópper; **2.** (*мотыга*) máttock.

тяп-ля́п *разг.* ányhow, in a slipshod way.

У

у 1. (*около, возле*) at; (*рядом*) by, besíde; у окнá by the window; у двéри at/by the door; постáвить часовóго у двéрей post a séntry at the door; у двéри стои́т шкаф there is a cúpboard by/besíde the door; сидéть у окнá sit* at the window; не сидѝте у окнá don't sit by the window; у постéли больнóго at/by the pátient's bédside; у поднóжия горы́ at the foot of the móuntain; у сáмой рекѝ right on the ríver; **2.** (*при обозначении орудия чьей-л. деятельности*) at; у руля́ at the wheel; **3.** (*при обозначении обладателя, владельца чего-л.*): меня́, у них I, they have; у негó, у нeё he, she has; у меня́ мнóго книг I have a lot of books; нóги у негó бы́ли мóкрые his feet were wet; у меня́ нет врéмени I have no time; **4.** (*при обозначении принадлежности*) of; у э́того стýла слóмана нóжка the leg of the chair is bróken; у э́того стýла слóмана нóжка that chair has a bróken leg; **5.** (*при обозначении лица или объекта, у которых что-л. происходит или имеется*) with; at; in; жить, остановѝться у рóдных live, stay with rélatives; у когó он живёт? who is he stáying with?; роя́ль стои́т у негó в кóмнате the piáno is in his room; встрéтиться у когó-л. meet* at *smb.'s* house/place; у когó нам встрéтиться? where are we to meet?; у нас в странé in our/this

cóuntry; у нас на завóде at our fáctory; у нас так не при́нято it is not the cústom in our cóuntry; **6.** (*при указании на источник приобретения чего-л.*) from; взять кни́гу у товáрища get* the book from a friend.

убáвить(ся) *сов. см.* убавля́ть(ся).

убавля́ть, убáвить 1. (*вн., рд.*) redúce (*smth.*); (*укорачивать*) make* it shórter; (*суживать*) take* it in; ~ скóрость redúce speed, slow down; убáвить шáгу shórten *one's* stride; ~ себé гóды make* onesélf yóunger than one; нельзя́ ни убáвить, ни прибáвить ни слóва it's pérfect just as it is; ~ в тáлии take* it in at the waist; **2.** *разг.*: ~ в вéсе redúce *one's* weight; онá убáвила в вéсе she redúced; **~ся,** убáвиться be* redúced; (*становиться меньше*) dwíndle, wane; (*о днях*) get* shórter; (*о луне*) (be* on the) wane; ~ся наполовѝну be* hálved; воды́ (в рекé) убáвилось the ríver is low, the wáter-level has dropped.

убаю́кать *сов. см.* убаю́кивать *и* баю́кать.

убаю́кивать, убаю́кать (*вн., прям. и перен.*) lull (*smb., smth.*).

убегáть, убежáть 1. run* awáy; **2.** (*совершать побег*) escápe, make* a gétaway; (*из тюрьмы́*) break* out of gaol; **3.** (*о кипящей жидкости*) boil óver; **4.** *тк. несов.* (*быстро удаляться*) flee*; (*проноситься*) stream awáy; **5.** *тк. несов.* (*простираться вдаль*) stretch, run*.

убедѝтельн|о 1. convíncingly, persuásively; ~ говорѝть speak* convíncingly, be* véry persuásive; **2.** (*настоятельно*) éarnestly, sériously; ~ прошý this is a véry sérious requést. **~ость** *ж.* persuásiveness. **~ый 1.** (*доказательный*) convíncing; ~ые фáкты convíncing facts; ~ый тон persuásive tone; егó словá óчень ~ы his words cárry convíction; **2.** (*настоятельный*) éarnest; ~ая прóсьба éarnest requést.

убедѝть(ся) *сов. см.* убеждáть(ся).

убежáть *сов. см.* убегáть 1, 2, 3.

убежд|áть, убедѝть 1. (*вн. в пр.; уверять в чём-л.*) convínce (*smb.* of); убедѝть когó-л., что... convínce *smb.* that...; убедѝть когó-л. в необходи́мости поéздки convínce *smb.* that the jóurney is nécessary; (*вн. + инф.; уговаривать*) persuáde (*smb.* + to *inf*); *несов. тж.* try to persuáde (*smb.* + to *inf*), urge (*smb.* + to *inf*); я убедѝл егó поéхать со мной I persuáded him to go with me. **~áться,** убедѝться (*в пр.*) be* convínced (of); (*удостоверяться*) sátisfy onesélf (that, as to), make* sure (that); убедѝться в несостоя́тельности подозрéний sátisfy *one's* suspícions are unfóunded; тепéрь вы сáми убедѝлись now you have seen for yoursélf. **~éние** *с.* **1.** (*действие*) persuásion; никакѝе ~éния не помоглѝ persuásion was unaváiling; дéйствовать ~éнием, а не сѝлой use persuásion ráther than force; поддавáться ~éнию be* ópen to persuásion; **2.** (*твёрдое мнение*) convíction; э́то моё глубóкое ~éние it is my firm convíction; **3.** *мн.* (*мировоззрение*) convíctions, beliefs; политѝческие ~éния political convíctions; меня́ть свои́ ~éния álter *one's* convíctions.

убеждён|о with convíction. **~ость** *ж.* convíction, súreness. **~ый** convínced (of); (*стойкий*) firm, staunch; ~ый протѝвник detérmined oppónent; он убеждён в своéй правотé he is quite sure he is right.

убéжищ|е *с.* **1.** réfuge; shélter; háven *поэт.*; политѝческое ~ political asýlum; прáво ~а a right of asýlum/sánctuary; искáть ~а take* sánctuary, seek* asýlum; **2.** *воен.* dúg-out, shélter.

уберéчь *сов.* (*вн. от рд.*) presérve (*smth.* from), guard (*smth.* agáinst), keep* (*smb., smth.*) safe (from); ~ от чегó-л. неприя́тного protéct (*smb.* from). **~ся** *сов.* (*от рд.*) keep* onesélf safe (from), avóid (*smth.*); ~ся от волнéний avóid excítement/anxíety.

убивáть, убить (*вн.*) **1.** kill (*smb., smth.*); (*злодейски*) múrder (*smb.*); (*при помощи наёмных убѝйц*) assássinate (*smb.*); **2.** (*уничтожать*) destróy (*smth.*), kill (*smth.*); убить надежду destroy a hope; **3.** (*приводить в отчаяние*) knock (*smb.*) flat, annihilate (*smb., smth.*); вы меня убили своим отказом your refusal is a great blow to me; **4.** (*тратить без пользы*) waste (*smth.*), throw* away (*smth.*); ◇ убить время kill time; хоть убей, не пойму! I'll be hanged/damned if I know what it's about! ~ся *несов.* (о *пр.*; из-за *рд.*) *разг.* lament (over), upset* oneself (over).

убийственн|ый 1. (*губительный*) murderous, devastating, deadly; **2.** (*непереносимый*) dreadful; ~ые последствия dreadful/disastrous consequences; ~ климат pernicious climate; **3.** *разг.* (*поразительный*) killing, devastating; ~ая жара killing heat; ~ая тоска agonizing/consuming grief.

убий|ство *с.* murder, killing; (*политическое тж.*) assassination; непредумышленное ~ manslaughter. ~ца *м. и ж.* murder, killer, assassin; (*женщина*) murderess.

убирать, убрать (*вн.*) **1.** take* away (*smth.*), clear away (*smth.*); ~ со стола clear away; **2.** (*изымать, устранять*) remove (*smth.*); **3.** (*собирать урожай*) gather (in) (*smth.*); ~ зерновые harvest the grain crops, bring* in the grain; **4.:** ~ паруса take* in sail; ~ вёсла ship oars; **5.** (*прятать, укладывать*) put* away (*smth.*); ~ бумаги в ящик put* away the papers in the drawer; **6.** (*приводить в порядок*): ~ комнату do*/tidy a room; ~ постель do*/make* a bed; **7.** (*вн. тв.*; *украшать*) adorn (*smth.* with), decorate (*smth.* with). ~ся, убраться *разг.* **1.** (*удаляться*) clear out; make* oneself scarce; убирайся!, убирайтесь! get out!, clear out!; **2.** (*приводить в порядок*) tidy up.

убит|ый прил. 1. dead; (*злодейски*) murdered; **2.** (*подавленный*) broken-hearted; ~ горем heart-broken; **3.** *в знач. сущ. м.* the dead man*; *мн.* the killed; (*при аварии*) fatal casualties; потерять 1000 человек ~ыми lose* a thousand killed; ◇ спать как ~ sleep* like a log/top; be* fast/sound asleep.

убить *сов. см.* убивать.

ублажать, ублажить (*вн.*) *разг.* please (*smb.*), gratify (*smb.*).

ублажить *сов. см.* ублажать.

убогий прил. 1. (*имеющий увечье*) crippled; **2.** (*жалкий, нищенский*) poor, wretched; (*о жилище тж.*) squalid, shabby; **3.** (*малосодержательный*) mediocre, flat, colourless, shoddy; **4.** *в знач. сущ. м.* (*калека*) cripple.

убожество *с.* **1.** (*уродство*) deformity, disablement; **2.** (*бедность, нищета*) poverty, wretchedness; (*жилища тж.*) squalor, shabbiness; **3.** (*ничтожность*) mediocrity, limitation; ~ мысли poverty of mind.

убой *м.* slaughter; вести на ~ lead* to the slaughter; ◇ кормить кого-л. на ~ stuff *smb.* with food, feed* *smb.* like a prize turkey.

убор *м.* attire; ◇ головной ~ hat, head-dress, head gear.

убористый close; ~ шрифт close print; написанный ~ым почерком closely written.

уборка *ж.* **1.** (*урожая*) harvesting; **2.** (*помещения*) cleaning; ~ комнаты doing the room, clearing up.

уборная *ж.* **1.** *театр.* dressing-room; **2.** lavatory, water-closet (*сокр.* W. C.), toilet.

уборочн|ый harvesting; ~ая кампания harvest drive; ~ая машина harvester.

уборщ|ик *м.* cleaner, sweeper. ~ица *ж.* cleaner, charwoman*.

убранство *с.* **1.** decoration(s); **2.** (*одежда*) attire (*тж. перен.*).

убрать(ся) *сов. см.* убирать(ся).

убывать, убыть (*уменьшаться*) be* diminishing; (*о воде в реке*) subside, sink*; (*о луне*) wane.

убыль *ж.* decrease, diminution; (*о воде*) subsidence, abatement; ◇ идти на ~ subside.

убыт|ок *м.* loss; продать что-л. с ~ком sell* *smth.* at a loss; чистый ~ dead loss.

убыточн|ый unprofitable; ~ое дело unprofitable business.

убыть *сов. см.* убывать.

уважаемый respected; (*в обращении*) dear; *ирон.* my dear man, my dear woman.

уваж|ать *несов.* (*вн.*) respect (*smb., smth.*), esteem (*smb., smth.*); honour (*smb.*); глубоко ~ кого-л. have* the greatest respect for *smb.*; ~ старших respect one's elders. ~ение *с.* respect; пользоваться всеобщим ~ением win* the respect of all; питать глубокое ~ение к кому-л. hold* *smb.* in the greatest/deepest respect; относиться к кому-л. без ~ения have* no respect for *smb.*; достойный ~ения worthy of respect; с ~ением (*в письмах*) yours truly.

уважительн|ый valid; good; ~ая причина valid excuse/reason; без ~ых причин without valid excuse.

уважить *сов.* (*вн.*) *разг.* **1.** (*исполнить, выполнить*) comply (with); ~ просьбу кого-л. comply with *smb.'s* request; **2.** (*проявить внимание к кому-л.*) be* nice (to).

увалень *м.* *разг.* lump.

увариваться, увариться 1. *разг.* (*доходить до полной готовности*) cook properly; **2.** (*уменьшаться в объёме*) cook down.

увариться *сов. см.* увариваться.

уведомить *сов. см.* уведомлять.

уведомл|ение *с.* notice, notification; получить ~ о денежном переводе be* notified of the receipt of a money order in one's name. ~ять, уведомить (*вн.*) notify (*smb.*), inform (*smb.*).

увезти *сов. см.* увозить.

увековечивать, увековечить (*вн.*) immortalize (*smb., smth.*), perpetuate (*smth.*); ~ чью-л. память perpetuate *smb.'s* name.

увековечить *сов. см.* увековечивать.

увеличение *с.* **1.** increase, rise; ~ заработной платы increase/rise in wages; ~ темпов производства step-up/increase in the rate of production; ~ государственных доходов increase in revenues; **2.** (*при помощи оптического прибора*) magnification; *фото* enlargement.

увеличивать, увеличить (*вн.*) **1.** increase (*smth.*), augment (*smth.*); (*расширять*) extend (*smth.*); ~ выпуск продукции increase/boost output; поголовье стада increase the head of cattle, increase the herd; **2.** (*оптическим прибором*) magnify (*smth.*); *фото* enlarge (*smth.*). ~ся, увеличиться increase, grow*, augment; (*расширяться*) extend.

увеличитель *м.* *фото.* enlarger.

увеличительн|ый magnifying; ~ое стекло magnifying glass.

увеличить(ся) *сов. см.* увеличивать(ся).

увенчать *сов. см.* венчать 2, 3, 4. ~ся *сов.* (*тв.*) be* crowned (with); ~ся успехом be* crowned with success.

уверение *с.* (*в пр.*) assurance (of), protestation (of).

уверенн|о with confidence, confidently; ~ смотреть вперёд look ahead with confidence; говорить, отвечать ~ speak*, reply with confidence. ~ость *ж.* confidence, assurance, certitude; ~ость в своей правоте certitude of being in the right; ~ость в себе, в своих силах self-confidence; ~ость в завтрашнем дне confidence in the future, sense of security; ~ость в успехе assurance of success; быть в полной ~ости be* fully confident (that); можно с ~остью сказать, что... it is safe to say that... ~ый confident; (*твёрдый тж.*) sure; ~ые движения confident movements; ~ая рука sure hand; ~ый шаг resolute step; ~ый ответ firm answer; ~ый в себе sure of oneself.

уверить *сов. см.* уверять.

увернуться *сов. см.* увёртываться.

уве́ровать *сов.* (в *вн.*) belíeve (in).

увёрт|ка *ж.* evásion, dodge. ~**ливый** ágile; *перен.* slíppery, cráfty; (*уклончивый*) evásive.

увёртываться, уверну́ться (от *рд.*) dodge (*smth.*); eváde (*smth.*); (*из рук*) escápe from *smb.'s* grasp; (*избегать*) give* (*smb.*) the slip; *перен.* eváde the íssue; уверну́ться от уда́ра dodge a blow.

увертю́ра *ж.* óverture.

уверя́ть, уве́рить (*вн.* в *пр.*) assúre (*smb.* of); он хо́чет нас уве́рить... he would have us belíeve...; ~ кого́-л. в свое́й правоте́ assúre *smb.* that *one* is right.

увеселе́ни|е *с.* 1. (*действие*) amúsement; 2. *обыкн. мн.* (*развлечение, зрелище*) amúsement(s); ма́ссовые ~я públic entertáinment(s).

увесели́тельн|ый pléasure *attr.*; ~ая пое́здка pléasure trip.

увеселя́ть *несов.* (*вн.*) entertáin (*smb.*), amúse (*smb.*).

уве́систый 1. (*тяжёлый*) mássive, wéighty; 2. *разг.* (*сильный*) héfty.

увести́ *сов. см.* уводи́ть.

уве́чить *несов.* (*вн.*) maim (*smb.*), crípple (*smb.*), mútilate (*smb.*); *перен.* spoil* (*smth.*). ~ся *несов.* maim *oneself*, crípple oneself.

уве́чье *с.* ínjury.

уве́шать *сов.* (*вн. тв.*) hang* (*smth.* with); ~ сте́ны карти́нами hang* pictures all óver the walls.

увещ|а́ние *с.* exhortátion; (*назидание*) admonítion. ~**а́ть,** ~**ева́ть** *несов.* (*вн.*) exhórt (*smb.*).

увида́ть *сов.* (*вн.*) *разг.* see* (*smb., smth.*). ~ся *сов. разг.* see* each óther.

уви́деть *сов. см.* ви́деть. ~ся *сов. см.* ви́деться.

уви́ливать, увильну́ть (от *рд.*) *разг.* dodge (*smb., smth.*), eváde (*smb., smth.*).

увильну́ть *сов. см.* уви́ливать.

увлажни́ть *сов. см.* увлажня́ть.

увлажня́ть, увлажни́ть (*вн.*) móisten (*smth.*)

увлека́тельн|ый fáscinating, absórbing; ~ое зре́лище enthrálling sight.

увлек|а́ть, увле́чь (*вн.*) 1. (*уводить, уносить с собой*) cárry (*smb., smth.*) awáy; ~ за собо́й lead*; 2. (*каким-л. делом и т. п.*) cárry (*smb.*) awáy, absórb (*smb.*); (*захватывать*) enthrál (*smb.*); рабо́та увлекла́ его́ he was cárried awáy by his work; 3. (*заставлять влюбиться*) fáscinate (*smb.*), infátuate (*smb.*). ~**а́ться, увле́чься** (*тв.*) 1. be* cárried awáy (by), be* enthúsiastic (about); ~а́ться жи́вописью have*/acquíre a pássion for páinting; ~а́ться футбо́лом be*/get* keen on sóccer; вы сли́шком увлекли́сь you are exággerating; 2. (*влюбляться*) fall* (for), take* a fáncy (to); он легко́ ~а́ется he is éasily infátuated. ~**а́ющийся** 1.: ~а́ющийся челове́к enthúsiast; 2. (*влюбчивый*) impréssionable, ámorous.

увлече́н|ие *с.* 1. (*воодушевление, пыл*) exhilarátion, rápture; 2. (*повышенный интерес к чему-л.*) enthúsiasm, pássion; ~ рабо́той pássion for work; рабо́тать с ~ием work enthúsiastically; ~ спо́ртом love of sport; 3. (*тв.*: *влюблённость в кого-л.*) infatuátion (for).

увлечённый enthúsiastic.

увле́чь(ся) *сов. см.* увлека́ть(ся).

уводи́ть, увести́ (*вн.*) 1. (*прочь*) take* (*smb.*) awáy, lead* (*smb.*) awáy; (*куда-л.*) take* (*smb.* to); *перен. тж.* divért (*smth.*); ~ войска́ withdráw* *one's* troops; ~ кого́-л. домо́й take* *smb.* home; 2. (*похищать*) steal* (*smb., smth.*); walk off (with) *разг.*

увози́ть, увезти́ (*вн.*) 1. take* (*smb., smth.*) awáy; увезти́ дете́й к мо́рю take* the chíldren awáy to the séaside; увезти́ свои́ кни́ги take* *one's* books awáy; 2. (*похищать*) cárry off (*smb., smth.*); (*человека тж.*) kídnap (*smb.*).

уво́лить *сов.* 1. *см.* увольня́ть; 2. (*вн.* от *рд.*; *избав-*

лять от чего́-л. неприя́тного) spare (*smb., smth.*); уво́льте меня́ от э́того! spare me that, please! ~ся *сов. см.* увольня́ться.

увольне́ние *с.* dischárge, dismíssal; ~ в запа́с *воен.* tránsfer to the resérve.

увольни́тельная *ж. воен.* leave wárrant.

увольня́ть, уво́лить (*вн.*) dischárge (*smb.*), dismíss (*smb.*); sack (*smb.*), give* (*smb.*) the sack *разг.*; fire (*smb.*) *амер.*; уво́лить кого́-л. по сокраще́нию шта́тов dischárge *smb.* becáuse of staff redúction, decláre *smb.* redúndant; ~ в запа́с *воен.* tránsfer to the resérve. ~ся, уво́литься get* *one's* dischárge, be* dischárged; ~ся в отста́вку retíre.

увы́ alás!

увяда́ть, увя́нуть 1. (*о растениях*) wíther, fade, wilt; 2. (*утрачивать свежесть, молодость*) lose* its bloom, lose* *one's* fréshness/youth; 3. (*терять бодрость*) droop, sag; (*утрачивать яркость*) fade.

увя́дший fáded (*тж. перен.*); (*высохший*) wíthered.

увяза́ть I *несов. см.* увя́зывать.

увяза́ть II, увя́знуть (в *пр.*) get* stuck (in); *перен.* get* in a rut (with, óver), flóunder (in).

увяза́ться *сов. см.* увя́зываться.

увя́знуть *сов. см.* увяза́ть II.

увя́зывать, увяза́ть (*вн.*) 1. (*верёвками*) tie up (*smth.*); 2. (*согласовывать*) tie in (*smth.*), co-órdinate (*smth.*). ~ся, увяза́ться 1. (с *тв.*: *согласовываться*) tie in (with), be* co-órdinated (with); 2. (*за тв.*) *разг.* (*неотступно следовать*) fóllow (*smb.*) abóut, tag alóng (with); за ним увяза́лась соба́ка a dog tagged alóng with him.

увя́нуть *сов. см.* увяда́ть.

угада́ть *сов. см.* уга́дывать.

уга́дывать, угада́ть (*вн.*) 1. guess (*smth.*); вы угада́ли! quite right!; (*в прошедшем*) you were right; 2. *разг.* (*узнавать*) tell* (*smth.*).

уга́р *м.* 1. (*угарный газ*) (cárbon monóxide) fumes *pl*; 2. (*болезненное состояние*) cárbon monóxide póisoning, chárcoal póisoning; у него́ ~ he is súffering from chárcoal póisoning; 3. (*состояние безудержности*) intoxicátion. ~**ный** 1. chóking; (*содержащий угар*) pollúted; 2. (*безудержный*) frénzied; ◇ ~ный газ cárbon monóxide.

угас|а́ние *с.* fáding, fáding awáy. ~**а́ть,** угасну́ть go* out; becóme* extínct; *перен.* fade, die awáy.

уга́снуть *сов. см.* угаса́ть.

углево́д *м. биол.,* *хим.* cárbohýdrate.

углеводоро́д *м. хим.* hýdrocárbon.

углекислота́ *ж. хим.* cárbon dióxide.

углеки́сл|ый *хим.* carbónic-ácid *attr.*; ~ газ cárbon dióxide; ~ые со́ли cárbonates.

углеко́п *м. уст.* cóal-miner.

углеро́д *м. хим.* cárbon.

углеро́дист|ый cárbon *attr.,* carbónic; rich in cárbon *после сущ.*; ~ая сталь carbónic steel.

углова́тый ángular; *перен.* áwkward.

углово́й 1. (*имеющий форму угла*) ángle *attr.*; 2. (*находящийся на углу, в углу*) córner *attr.*; 3. *мат., физ.* ángular; ~ уда́р *спорт.* córner (kick).

угломе́р *м.* goniómeter, ángle gauge.

углуби́ть(ся) *сов. см.* углубля́ть(ся).

углубле́ние *с.* 1. (*действие*) déepening; *перен. тж.* intensificátion; 2. (*впадина*) depréssion, hóllow, dip; (*небольшое*) recéss; 3. *мор.* (*осадка судна*) draught.

углублён|ый 1. súnken; 2. (*основательный, серьёзный*) fundaméntal, profóund; in-dépth *attr.*; ~ое изуче́ние литерату́ры profóund stúdy of líterature; 3. (в *вн.*: *занятый чем-л.*) absórbed (in), engróssed (in).

углубля́ть, углуби́ть (*вн.*) make* (*smth.*) déeper; déepen (*smth.*) (*тж. перен.*); *перен.* (*усиливать*) inténsify (*smth.*); ~ противоре́чия inténsify contradíctions; углуби́ть свои́ зна́ния déepen/exténd one's knówledge. ~ся, углубиться 1. (становиться более глубоким) becóme*/get* déeper, déepen; перен. be* inténsified; 2. (погружаться) go* down, sink*; 3. (в вн.; проникать в глубь чего-л.) get* déeper (into); перен. becóme* absórbed (in).

угляд|е́ть сов. (за тв.) разг. take* próper care (of); не ~ за кем-л. not take próper care of smb.; за всем не ~ишь you cán't keep track of éverything.

угнáть сов. см. угонять. ~ся сов. (за тв.) keep* up (with).

угнетáтель м. oppréssor.

угнет|áть несов. (вн.) oppréss (smb.); (удручать тж.) depréss (smb.); егó ~áли мрáчные мысли black thoughts oppréssed him. ~áющий oppréssive; (удручающий) depréssing; ~áющее впечатлéние depréssing efféct. ~éние с. 1. oppréssion; 2. (подавленное состояние) depréssion. ~ённый 1. oppréssed; ~ённый нарóд oppréssed péople; 2. (удручённый) depréssed; ~ённое настроéние depréssed state of mind.

уговáривать, уговорить (вн. + инф.) persuáde (smb. + to inf), prevaíl (upón + to inf); несов. тж. urge (smb. + to inf), try to persuáde (smb. + to inf); он уговорил меня пойти в теáтр he persuáded me to go to the théatre. ~ся, уговориться (с тв. + инф.) разг. arránge (with, + to inf), come* to an agréement/understánding (with, + to inf).

уговóр м. 1. (взаимное соглашение) agréement, understánding; 2. (убеждение кого-л. в чём-л.) persuásion; пóсле дóлгих ~ов он согласился áfter much persuásion he agréed. ◇ ~ дорóже дéнег погов. ≅ a prómise is a prómise.

уговорить(ся) сов. см. уговáривать(ся).

угóд|а ж.: в ~у кому-л., чему-л. to sátisfy smb., smth.; for the bénefit of smb.

угодить сов. 1. см. угождáть; 2. (в вн.) разг. (попасть) stúmble (into), step (into); (удариться обо что-л.) bump (into); (попасть в какие-л. условия) find* onesélf (in), land (in); ~ под колёса get* run óver; ~ в лужу step ínto a púddle; 2. (тв. в вн.; дт. в вн.) разг. (бросая, стреляя, попасть) hit* (smth. with; smth. in, on), get* (smth. in, on); ~ кому-л. прямо в глаз hit* smb. slap in the eye; ~ кáмнем в стеклó hit* a window with a stone.

угóдливый obséquious.

угóдно 1. в знач. сказ. (дт.): как вам (бýдет) ~ just as you like; что вам ~? what can I do for you?; 2. частица: когó ~ ányone, ánybody (you like); где, кудá ~ wheréver you like; когдá ~ whenéver you like; скóлько ~ plénty (of), ány amóunt (of); всё что ~ ánything you like; пойти на что ~, чтóбы... go* all lengths to...; ◇ éсли ~ perháps; не ~ ли... won't you..., perháps you will...

угóдный (дт.) pléasing (to), in accórdance with the wishes (of).

угóдь|е с. обыкн. мн. land, área; леснýе ~я fórests.

угождáть, угодить (дт., на вн.) please (smb.); на негó не угóдишь there's no pléasing him; на всех не угóдишь you can't sátisfy éverybody; ◇ угодить на чей-л. вкус cáter for smb.'s taste, sátisfy smb.

ýгол м. 1. córner; удáриться об ~ столá knock onesélf on the córner of the táble; завернýть зá ~ turn the córner; за углóм round the córner; на углý on the córner; 2. (часть дома, комнаты) córner, nook; все разбрелись по свойм углáм they all dispérsed to their chósen córners; 3. (приют, пристанище): имéть свой ~ have* a home of one's own; не имéть углá have* no home of one's own; 4. мат. ángle; под прямым углóм at right ángles (to); perpendícular (to); внéшний ~ треугóльника extérnal ángle of a tríangle; ◇ из-за углá (убить, напасть) underhándedly; убийство из-за углá surreptítious killing; под этим углóм зрéния from this point of view; сгладить óстрые углы́ smooth things óver; ходить из углá в ~ pace abóut, stride* abóut.

уголóвник м. (преступник) críminal.

уголóв|ный críminal; ~ное преступлéние félony, críminal offénce; ~ кóдекс críminal code. ~щина ж. разг. 1. (преступление) críminal affáir, láw-breaking, shády actívity; 2. собир. (преступники) críminals pl, the únderworld.

уголóк м. córner; ◇ крáсный ~ informátion room.

ýголь м. coal; дрéвесный ~ chárcoal; сидéть как на ýглях, ýгольях be* on ténterhooks.

ýгольник м. 1. (для черчения) set squáre; 2. тех. ángle-bar; élbow.

ýголь|ный coal attr.; ~ бассéйн cóal-field; ~ая промышленность cóal(-míning) índustry; ◇ ~ая кислотá carbónic ácid.

угонять, угнáть (вн.) 1. drive* (smth.) (awáy); 2. разг. (похищать скот) steal* (smth.).

угоразди|ть сов. разг.: как вас ~ло пойти тудá? what posséssed you to go there?; и чёрт егó ~л! what the dévil made him do it!

угорáть, угорéть be* affécted by (the) fumes; (до смерти) die from cárbon monóxide póisoning.

угорéлый разг.: как ~ like a mádman*; бежáть как ~ run* like blázes/hell.

угорéть сов. см. угорáть.

ýгорь I м. (рыба) eel.

ýгорь II м. (на коже) bláckhead.

угостить сов. см. угощáть.

угощ|áть, угостить (вн. тв.) entertáin (smb. to), treat (smb. to), regále (smb. with.); ~ когó-л. обéдом entertáin smb. to dínner; я ~áю this is on me, I'm stánding treat. ~éние с. 1. (действие) hospitálity, regáling; 2. (то, чем угощают) fare; refréshments pl.

угрож|áть несов. (дт. тв.) thréaten (smb. with.); ему ~áет опáсность he is in dánger; ему ничтó не ~áет he is in no dánger; ~ войнóй thréaten war, cárry the threat of war. ~áющий thréatening, ménacing; ~áющее положéние périlous situátion.

угрóз|а ж. threat; (опасность тж.) ménace; постáвить что-л. под ~у endánger smth., creáte a threat to smth.

угрызéн|ие с.: ~ия сóвести remórse sg, compúnction sg, pricks of cónscience.

угрю́мый glóomy, sómbre; (о человеке тж.) morose.

удáв м. зоол. bóa-constríctor, python.

уда|вáться, удáться 1. be* a succéss, turn out well; не ~ fail, be* abórtive, turn out bádly; операция удалáсь the operátion was a succéss; 2. безл. (дт. + инф.): ему всё ~ётся éverything he does turns out well, éverything he puts his hand to turns out well; мне удалóсь достáть эту книгу I succéeded in gétting the book; мне не удалóсь поéхать тудá I was unáble to go there, I cóuldn't go.

удавить сов. (вн.) strángle (smb., smth.), thróttle (smb., smth.). ~ся сов. разг. hang onesélf.

удалéни|е с. 1. withdráwal; по мéре ~я от... the fúrther one gets from...; 2. (устранение) remóval; 3. (зуба) extráction.

удалённый remóte, dístant.

удалить(ся) сов. см. удалять(ся).

удал|óй dáring, bold; конь ~ méttlesome horse/steed; трóйка ~áя dáshing tróika; пéсня ~áя stírring song.

ýдаль ж. dash, audácity, dáring.

удалять, удалить (вн.) 1. (отдалять) take* (smth.) awáy, remóve (smth.); 2. (устранять) remóve (smth.); (вырывать) take* out (smth.), extráct (smth.); ~ пятнó remóve a stain; ~ зуб extráct a tooth*; 3. (заставлять уйти) send* (smb.) awáy/out, have* (smb.) remóved; он был удалён с пóля he was sent off. ~ся, удалиться 1. (отдаляться) move awáy (from); бéрег постепéнно удалялся the shore recéded; ~ся от тéмы wánder from the súbject; **2.** (уходить) retíre.

удáр м. **1.** blow (тж. перен); (рубящий) chop; (колющий) stab, thrust; (столкновение) ímpact; (звук от толчка, сотрясения) crash, thud; ~ ногóй kick; наносúть ~ кому-л. deal*/strike* smb. a blow; ~ в спúну stab in the back; ~ судьбы́ stroke of fate; однúм ~ом with one stroke; ~ грóма clap of thúnder; ~ кóлокола stroke of a bell; **2.** воен. attáck, thrust; **3.** мед. stroke; ◇ быть в ~е be* in form, be* at one's best; быть под ~ом be* in dánger; стáвить когó-л., чтó-л. под ~ endánger smb., smth.; однúм ~ом двух зáйцев убúть ≈ kill two birds with one stone.

ударéние с. stress; дéлать ~ на чём-л. stress smth.; перен. тж. lay* stress on smth., émphasize smth.

удáрить(ся) сов. см. ударя́ть(ся).

удáрник м. (музыкант) drúmmer; (в симфонúческом оркéстре) ты́mpanist.

ударн|ый I 1. (дéйствующий удáром) percússion attr.; ~ые музыкáльные инструмéнты percússion ínstruments; ~ое бурéние percússion bóring; **2.** (наносящий решающий удáр) shock attr.; ~ батальóн shock battálion; **3.** лингв.: ~ глáсный stressed vówel.

удáрн|ый II 1. (вáжный, срóчный) úrgent, préssing; ~ое задáние top-priórity task; ~ые тéмпы high témpo sg; **2.** (передовóй) shock attr., top-nótch.

удáрять, удáрить **1.** (вн. и вн., по дт.) hit* (smb., smth.); strike* (smb., smth.); (тж. перен.); удáрить когó-л. по лицý strike*/hit* smb. in the face; удáрить пó столу bang on the táble; **2.** (вн.; причинять страдáния) be* a blow (to); **3.** (в вн.; удáром производúть звук) strike* (smth.), beat* (smth.); удáрить в кóлокол ring* a bell; **4.** (вн.; подавáть сигнáл) sound (smth.); удáрить в набáт sound the alárm; **5.** (раздавáться) sound; (грóмко) crash; удáрил гром thúnder crashed, there was a great clap of thúnder; **6.** (внезáпно атаковáть) pounce, strike*; ◇ удáрить по кармáну make* a hole in one's pócket; удáрить в гóлову (опьянúть) go* to one's head; удáрить по рукáм shake* hands on it. ~ся, удáриться **1.** (о, в вн.) strike* (smth.), hit* (smth.); bump ínto (smth.); (ушибáться) knock onesélf; удáриться головóй обо чтó-л. knock/hit* one's head agáinst smth.; мяч удáрился о стéну the ball hit the wall; **2.** (в вн.) разг. (с увлечéнием предавáться чему-л.) plunge (into); ~ся из однóй крáйности в другýю go* from one extréme to the óther.

удáться сов. см. удавáться.

удáча ж. luck, piece of luck; (достижéние) succéss, achíevement; твóрческая ~ artístic achíevement/tríumph.

удáчн|о succéssfully, well. ~ый **1.** (успéшный) succéssful; (подходящий) apt; **2.** (хорóший) good*; ~ый вы́бор háppy choice.

удвáивать, удвóить (вн.) dóuble (smth.), incréase (smth.) a húndred per cent; ~ усúлия redóuble one's éfforts; ~ цéну dóuble the price, raise the price a húndred per cent. ~ся, удвóиться dóuble, incréase twofold.

удвóенн|ый 1. (вдвóе бóльший) dóuble; **2.** (усúленный, увелúченный) redóubled; с ~ой энéргией with redóubled zeal.

удвóить(ся) сов. см. удвáивать(ся).

удéл м. (учáсть) lot, fate.

удéлить сов. см. уделя́ть.

удéльн|ый физ. specífic; ~ вес specífic grávity; перен. share; ~ая теплоёмкость specífic heat.

уделя́ть, уделúть (вн.) (выделя́ть) allót (smth.); (врéмя и т. п.) spare (smth.); ~ комý-л. внимáние give*/grant atténtion to smb.

ýдерж м.: без ~у разг. unrestráinedly; не знать (ни в чём) ~у know* no restráint, álways go* the whole hog.

удержáние с. **1.** hólding; **2.** (дéнег) dedúction; ~ из зарплáты dedúction from one's sálary/wáges.

удержáть(ся) сов. см. удéрживать(ся).

удéрживать, удержáть (вн.) **1.** (от падéния) hold* (smb., smth.); hold* up (smb., smth.); **2.** (сдéрживать) keep* back (smb., smth.), hold* back (smb., smth.); ~ лóшадь hold*/rein in one's horse; **3.** (не отпускáть) keep* (smb.); **4.** (не давáть сдéлать чтó-л.) restráin (smb.); **5.** (не давáть прояви́ться) hold* back (smth.), restráin, représs (smth.); ~ крик stífle a cry; **6.** (сохраня́ть) keep* (smth.); (не сдавáть протúвнику) hold* (smth.); он удержáл за собóй пéрвое мéсто he kept the first place; ~ позúции hold* one's ground, stand* firm; ~ в пáмяти retáin in one's mémory; **7.** (не выплáчивать) dedúct (smth.), keep* back (smth.), withhóld* (smth.). ~ся, удержáться **1.** (устоя́ть) hold* out, hold* one's ground; удержáться на ногáх keep* one's fóoting, keep* one's feet; **2.** (от рд.) keep* (from), refráin (from); удержáться от слёз keep* back one's tears, restráin one's tears; он не мог удержáться от слёз he couldn't refráin from tears.

удесятери́ть(ся) сов. см. удесятеря́ть(ся).

удесятеря́ть, удесятери́ть (вн.) incréase (smth.) ténfold. ~ся, удесятери́ться incréase ténfold.

удешевúть сов. см. удешевля́ть.

удешевля́ть, удешевúть (вн.) make* (smth.) chéaper; (понижáть в ценé) lówer/redúce the price (of).

удивúтельн|о 1. нареч. remárkably, extraórdinarily; (óчень) extrémely; **2.** в знач. сказ. безл. it is astónishing/fúnny/strange; ~! extraórdinary!; ~, что... it's surprising that...; I'm astónished/surprísed that...; не ~, что... no wónder. ~ый **1.** (стрáнный) surprísing, remárkable; **2.** (необыкновéнный) wónderful, márvellous, remárkable; **3.** (чрезвычáйный) extraórdinary.

удивúть(ся) сов. см. удивля́ть(ся).

удивлéние с. astónishment, surpríse; к моемý велúкому ~ю much to my astónishment/surpríse; к óбщему ~ю to éveryone's astónishment; ◇ на ~ spléndidly; (дт.) to smb.'s delight.

удивля́|ть, удивúть (вн.) astónish (smb.), amáze (smb.); surpríse (smb.); меня́ это нискóлько не ~ет I'm not a bit surprísed; это не должнó никогó ~ this will come as a surpríse to nóbody; этим вы никогó не удивúте that won't make much impréssion. ~ться, удивúться (дт.) be* surprísed (at), be* astónished (at), be* amázed (at).

удилá мн. bit sg.

удúлище с. (fishing-)rod.

удирáть, удрáть разг. run* awáy.

удúть несов. (вн.) fish (for).

удлинéние с. **1.** léngthening; **2.** (продлéние) exténsion.

удлинённый long.

удлинúть(ся) сов. см. удлиня́ть(ся).

удлиня́ть, удлинúть (вн.) **1.** (увелúчивать в длинý) make* (smth.) lónger, léngthen (smth.); **2.** (продлевáть) exténd (smth.). ~ся, удлинúться **1.** (увелúчиваться в длинý) léngthen, get*/grow* lónger; **2.** (станови́ться бóлее длúтельным) léngthen; дни удлинúлись the days léngthened.

удмýрт м., ~ка ж. Údmurt. ~ский Údmurt; ~ский язы́к Údmurt, the Údmurt lánguage.

удóбн|о 1. нареч. cómfortably; **2.** в знач. сказ. безл. it is cómfortable; вам ~ здесь? are you cómfortable here?; **3.** в знач. сказ. безл. (подхóдит) it is convénient; ~ ли вам прийтú? is it convénient for you to come?; это вам ~? does that suit you?, will it be convénient for you?; **4.** в знач. сказ. безл. (умéстно, прилúчно) is it póssible?; ~ ли спросúть егó об этом? can he be asked abóut that? ~ый **1.** cómfortable; (для пóльзования) hándy; (пригóдный) súitable; ~ое крéсло cómfortable chair; ~ая пóза cómfortable posítion; устрáивайтесь ~ее make yoursélf quite cómfortable; **2.** (подходящий) convénient; ~ый момéнт ópportune móment; ~ый слýчай (good) opportúnity; назнáчить ~ое для всех врéмя fix a time that suits éverybody.

удобовари́мый digéstible.

удобочитáемый réadable; éasy to read *predic.*

удобрéние *с.* 1. (*дéйствие*) fértilizing, dréssing (with fértilizers); (*навóзом*) manúring; 2. (*вещество*) fértilizer; (*навóз*) manúre.

удóбрить *сов. см.* удобрять.

удобрять, удóбрить (*вн.*) fértilize (*smth.*); (*навóзом*) manúre (*smth.*).

удóбство *о с.* convénience; квартúра со всéми ~ами flat with all módern convéniences.

удовлетворéние *с.* satisfáction, gratificátion; ~ желáний gratificátion of *one's* desíres.

удовлетворённ|ость *ж.* conténtment. ~ый 1. (*довóльный*) conténted; 2. (*осуществлённый*) sátisfied.

удовлетворúтельн|о 1. *нареч.* satisfáctorily; 2. *в знач. сущ. с нескл.* a satisfáctory (mark). ~ый satisfáctory.

удовлетворúть(ся) *сов. см.* удовлетворя́ть(ся).

удовлетворять, удовлетворúть 1. (*вн.; исполня́ть, осуществля́ть*) sátisfy (*smth.*); meet* (*smth.*); ~ потрéбности населéния sátisfy/meet* the públic's needs/requírements; удовлетворúть чью-л. прóсьбу complý with *smb.'s* requést; 2. (*вн.; дéлать довóльным*) contént (*smb.*), sátisfy (*smb.*); успéх не удовлетворúл её she was not contént with her succéss; 3. (*дт.; соотвéтствовать*) meet* (*smth.*), ánswer (*smth.*), sátisfy (*smth.*); ~ чьим-л. трéбованиям ánswer *smb.'s* demánds, come* up to *smb.'s* stándards/requírements; 4. (*вн. тв.; снабжáть*) keep* (*smb., smth.*) supplíed (with). ~ся, удовлетворúться (*тв.*) be* sátisfied (with), be* contént(ed) (with).

удовóльстви|е *с.* 1. pléasure; (*рáдость*) delíght; с ~ем with pléasure; к óбщему ~ю to éverybody's delíght; доставля́ть ~ кому-л. give* *smb.* pléasure; 2. (*развлечéние*) amúsement.

удóд *м.* (*птúца*) hóopoe.

удó|й *м.* 1. (*колúчество*) mílk-yield; сýточный ~ dáily mílk-yield; 2. (*доéние*) mílking; молокó ýтреннего ~я mórning milk.

удóйность *ж.* mílk-yielding capácity.

удорожáние *с.* íncrease in cost.

удорож|áть, удорожúть (*вн.*) incréase the cost (of). ~úть *сов. см.* удорожáть.

удостáивать, удостóить 1. (*вн. рд.; звáния, стéпени и т. п.*) confér (*smth.* on), awárd (*smb. smth.*); удостóить когó-л. звáния Герóя Совéтского Сою́за confér on *smb.* the títle of Héro of the Sóviet Únion; 2. (*вн. тв.*) *часто ирон.* (*окáзывать внимáние*) fávour (*smb.* with), hónour (*smb.* with); не ~ когó-л. отвéтом vouchsáfe *smb.* no ánswer. ~ся, удостóиться 1. (*рд.; звáния, нагрáды*) be* awárded (*smth.*); 2. (*рд.,* + *инф.*) *часто ирон.* be* fávoured (with), have* the good fórtune (+ to *inf*).

удостовéрение *с.* 1. (*дéйствие*) attestátion, certificátion; 2. (*докумéнт*) card, certíficate; ~ лúчности idéntity card; ~ журналúста press card.

удостовéрить(ся) *сов. см.* удостоверя́ть(ся).

удостоверя́ть, удостовéрить (*вн.*) cértify (*smth.*); ~ пóдпись witness a sígnature; ~ лúчность когó-л. idéntify *smb.* ~ся, удостовéриться sátisfy *onesélf*, make* sure, ascertáin.

удостóить(ся) *сов. см.* удостáивать(ся).

удосýжиться *сов.* (+ *инф.*) *разг.* have*/find* time (for + -ing), get* aróund (to + -ing).

удочер|úть *сов. см.* удочеря́ть. ~я́ть, удочерúть (*вн.*) adópt (*smth.*) (as *one's* dáughter).

ýдочк|а *ж.* (fishing-)rod and line; ◇ поймáть когó-л. на ~у catch* *smb.* néatly; попáсться на ~у swállow the bait.

удрáть *сов. см.* удирáть.

удружúть *сов.* (*дт.*) *разг.* 1. (*оказáть услýгу*) do* (*smb.*) a (good) turn; 2. *ирон.* (*причинúть вред*) do* (*smb.*) a bad turn.

удруч|áть, удручúть (*вн.*) depréss (*smb.*); demóralize (*smb.*). ~áющий depréssing. ~ённый depréssed, dejécted, dispírited, low-spírited; ~ённое состоя́ние state of depréssion/dejéction, depréssed state; ~ённый вид dejécted air/look. ~úть *сов. см.* удручáть.

удушúть *сов.* (*вн.*) stífle (*smth., smth.*) (*тж. перен.*); súffocate (*smth.*); (*верёвкой, рукáми*) strángle (*smth.*), thróttle (*smth.*), choke (*smth.*).

удушлúв|ый 1. súffocating, stífling (*тж. перен.*); ~ая жарá stífling/swéltering heat; 2. (*сопровождáющийся удýшьем*) chóking; 3. *хим.* asphýxiating.

удýшье *с.* suffocátion.

уединéние *с.* 1. (*пребывáние в одинóчестве*) sólitude, seclúsion; 2. (*уединённость*) seclúsion, isolátion.

уедин|ённый seclúded, ísolated. ~úться *сов. см.* уединя́ться.

уединя́ться, уединúться seek* sólitude; ísolate *onesélf*; ~ от óбщества retíre from socíety.

уезжáть, уéхать go* awáy, leave*; (*из рд.; откудá-л.*) leave* (*smth.*); (*в, на вн.; кудá-л.*) leave* (for), go* (to); он уéхал he's awáy; онá уéхала из Москвы́ she has left Móscow; он уéхал в дерéвню he's gone to the cóuntry.

уéхать *сов. см.* уезжáть.

уж I *м.* *зоол.* gráss-snake.

уж II 1. *нареч. см.* ужé 1, 2, 3; 2. *усил. частúца* réally; *чáсто не перевóдится*; уж я не знáю I réally don't know; уж éсли if; уж éсли так if that is the case; ну, это уж... but that's...; не так уж плóхо it's not so bad áfter all.

ужáлить *сов. см.* жáлить.

ýжас *м.* 1. (*сúльный страх*) térror, hórror; приходúть в ~ от чегó-л. be* hórrified/appálled by *smth.*; приводúть когó-л. в ~ hórrify *smb.*; к моемý ~у to my hórror; объя́тый ~ом térror-stricken, térror-struck; содрогáться от ~а shúdder with hórror; 2. (*обыкн. рд.; трагúчность*) hórror (of); мы сознавáли весь ~ нáшего положéния we réalized the full hórror of the situátion we were in; 3. *обыкн. мн.* (*стрáшное явлéние*) hórror; ~ы войны́ hórrors of war; 4. (*изумлéние, негодовáние*) hórror; 5. *в знач. нареч. разг.* térribly; ~ как хóлодно! it's hórribly cold!; ◇ какóй ~! what a hórrible thing!; how áwful!, hórrors!

ужас|áть, ужаснýть (*вн.*) hórrify (*smb.*), appál (*smb.*). ~áться, ужаснýться be* hórrified/appálled. ~áющий appálling; (*плохóй тж.*) áwful, ghástly *разг.*

ужáсно 1. *нареч.* áwfully, térribly; 2. *в знач. сказ. разг.* it is térrible.

ужаснýть(ся) *сов. см.* ужасáть(ся).

ужáсн|ый térrible; áwful *разг.*; ~ое гóре, несчáстье térrible grief, misfórtune; ~ слýчай case; térrible íncident; ~ лгун, трус áwful líar, cóward; ~о! áwful!

ýже *сравнит. ст. прил.* ýзкий *и нареч.* ýзко.

ужé 1. *нареч.* (*укáзывает на окончáние дéйствия*) *не перевóдится*; я ~ пообéдал I've had (my) dínner; вы ~ обéдали? have you had dínner?; когдá мы пришлú, он ~ уéхал he had gone when we arríved; 2. *нареч.* (*при словáх, обозначáющих отрéзок врéмени*) quite, véry; он ~ минýты три говорúл he had been spéaking for quite three mínutes; он ~ давнó живёт в Москвé he has been lívíng in Móscow a véry long time; 3. *нареч.* (*укáзывает на бóлее рáнний срок наступлéния чегó-л. ожидáемого*) alréady, by, éven; ~ в концé февраля́ by the end of Fébruary; ~ в 1960 годý alréady in 1960; ~ тепéрь éven now; alréady; 4. *усил. частúца не перевóдится*; ~ порá éхать, начинáть и т. д. (it's) time to go, begín, *etc.*; он ~ давнó кóнчил рабóту he finished the job long agó; ~ не раз agáin and agáin, more than once.

уживáться, ужи́ться (с тв.) get* on (with).

ужи́вчивый accómmodating, éasy-going; éasy to deal with после сущ.

ужи́мки мн. (ед. ужи́мка ж.) grimáces.

у́жин м. súpper. ~ать, поýжинать have* súpper.

ужи́ться сов. см. уживáться.

узаконéние с. legalizátion.

узакóнить сов. (вн.) légalize (smth.); (признавáть прáвильным) acknówledge (smth.).

узбéк м. Uzbék. ~ский Uzbék; ~ский язы́к Uzbék, the Uzbék lánguage.

узбéчка ж. Uzbék wóman*.

узд|á ж. brídle; ◇ держáть когó-л. в ~é keep* smb. únder one's thumb.

уздéчка ж. brídle.

уздцы́: под ~ by the brídle.

ýзел I м. 1. (на верёвке и т. п.) knot; перен. тж. tángle; завя́зывать ~ tie a knot; развя́зывать ~ untíe a knot; ~ противорéчий tángle of contradíctions; 2. (мéсто скрещéния чегó-л.) júnction, céntre; 3. (совокýпность сооружéний) cómplex, céntre; радиотрансляциóнный ~ bróadcasting céntre; 4. анат. knot, protúberance; нéрвный ~ gánglion; 5. тех. assémbly, únit, pack; сбóрка узлóв комбáйна assémbly of combíne-harvester únits; силовóй ~ pówer pack/únit; 6. (свёрток) búndle; ◇ морскóй ~ séaman's knot.

ýзел II м. мор. (мéра скóрости) knot.

ýзк|ий 1. (неширóкий) nárrow; ~ая колея́ nárrow gauge; 2. (тéсный) tight; 3. (ограни́ченный) nárrow, límited, close; ~ круг знакóмых close círcle of acquáintances; ~ая специáльность híghly spécialized proféssion; в ~ом смы́сле слóва in the nárrow sense; 4. (недалёкий) nárrow-minded, límited; ◇ ~ое мéсто в чём-л. wéakest point in smth.; (в произвóдстве) bóttle-neck.

ýзко nárrowly; tíghtly.

узковéдомственный nárrow departméntal; ~ подхóд nárrow departméntal appróach.

узкоколéй|ка ж. разг. nárrow-gauge ráilway. ~ный nárrow-gauge attr.

узкокоры́стный púrely sélfish.

узколóбый low-brówed; перен. разг. nárrow-minded.

узкоплёночный míniature-film attr.; ~ фотоаппарáт míniature-film cámera.

узкоспециáльный stríctly/híghly spécialized.

узлов|óй 1. (явля́ющийся цéнтром): ~áя стáнция (ráilway-)júnction; 2. (основнóй) key attr., nódal; ~ пункт key/fócal point.

узнавáть, узнáть 1. (вн., о пр.; получáть свéдения) hear* (smth.); (из газéт, писем) learn* (smth.); я тóлько что узнáл об э́том I have just heard abóut it; 2. (о пр.; освéдомляться) find* out (smth.), inquíre (about); 3. (вн.; обнарýживать, раскрывáть) find* out (smth.), discóver (smth.); 4. (вн.; получáть и́стинное представлéние о ком-л., чём-л.) get* to know (smb., smth.); 5. (вн.; испы́тывать, пережи́вать) expérience (smth.); 6. (вн.; признавáть) récognize (smb., smth.); он узнáл меня́ по похóдке he récognized me by my walk; егó нельзя́ бы́ло узнáть one would néver have récognized/known him; 7. (определя́ть) réalize (smth.).

узнáть сов. см. узнавáть.

ýзник м. prísoner.

узóр м. páttern, desígn; мн. trácery sg, páttern sg. ~чатый pátterned.

ýзость ж. 1. nárrowness; 2. (ограни́ченность) nárrow-míndedness, péttiness.

узурп|áтор м. кни́жн. usúrper. ~и́ровать несов. и сов. (вн.) usúrp (smth.).

ýзы мн. bonds, ties.

уйгýр м. ~ка ж. Uígur. ~ский Uígur, Uigúrian, Uigúric; ~ский язы́к Uígur, the Uígur lánguage.

уйма ж. разг. lots (of) pl, heaps (of) pl.

уйти́ сов. см. уходи́ть 1 — 8.

укáз м. 1. decrée, édict, ukáse; 2. в знач. сказ. (дт.): э́то мне не ~ that cárries no weight with me; ты мне не ~ you can't órder me abóut.

указáние с. 1. (свéдение о чём-л.) indicátion; 2. (замечáние, разъясня́ющее что-л.) instrúctions pl.

укáзанный spécified, índicated.

указáтель м. 1. (в кни́ге) índex (pl -kes, índices); 2. (спрáвочник): библиографи́ческий ~ bibliográphical list; железнодорóжный ~ ráilway guide; 3. (дорóжный) róad-sign; 4. тех. índicator; (стрéлка) póinter.

указáтельн|ый índicatory; ~ая стрéлка póinter, árrow; ~ое местоимéние грам. demónstrative prónoun; ◇ ~ пáлец índex-finger, fórefinger.

укáзка ж. 1. (пáлочка) póinter; 2. разг. (указáние) órders pl; дéйствовать по чьей-л. ~е cárry out smb.'s órders.

укáзывать, указáть 1. (вн., на вн.; покáзывать) show* (smb., smth.), índicate (smb., smth.), point out (smb., smth.) (тж. перен.); ~ пáльцем на когó-л. point at smb.; перен. point the finger at smb.; указáть комý-л. дорóгу show* smb. the way; ~ на сéвер point (to the) north; ~ на недостáтки point out the defécts; 2. (на когó-л.; ссылáться) point (to smb.), cite (smb.), refér (to smb.); 3. (давáть указáния) give* instrúctions, expláin; как укáзано according to instrúctions, as dirécted.

укатáть сов. см. укáтывать.

укати́ть сов. 1. (вн.) roll (smth.) awáy, push (smth.) awáy; 2. разг. (уéхать) go* off, drive* off. ~ся сов. roll awáy.

укáтывать, укатáть (вн.) roll (smth.).

укачáть сов. см. укáчивать.

укáчив|ать, укачáть (вн.) 1. (ребёнка) rock (smb.); 2. обыкн. безл. егó укачáло he was sick; меня́ ~ает I get sick, I súffer from car (sea, air) síckness.

уклáд м. 1. (жи́зни) strúcture, organizátion; sét-up разг.; 2. эк. mode of prodúction.

уклáдка ж. 1. (фундáмента, рéльсов) láying; (сéна, брёвен) stácking; (вóлос) arránging, sétting; 2. (причёска) set.

уклáдывать, уложи́ть (вн.) 1. lay* (smb.) on, make* (smb.) lie down; (в постéль) put* (smb.) to bed; врач уложи́л егó в постéль the dóctor órdered him to bed; 2. (класть в определённом поря́дке) lay* (smth.); (дровá, брёвна) stack (smth.); 3. (дéлать причёску) arránge (smth.); (о парикмáхере) style (smth.); 4. (вéщи в дорóгу) pack (smth.); уложи́ть вéщи в чемодáн pack one's things in a case; уложи́ть чемодáн pack a case.

уклáдыв|аться I, уложи́ться 1. (в дорóгу) pack; 2. (умещáться) go* in; (о напи́санном) go* into; 3. (успевáть) get*/be* through; уложи́ться в полчасá get* through in half an hour; вы уло́житесь в полчасá? will half an hour be long enóugh?; ◇ э́то не ~áется в головé one can hárdly take it in, it just dóesn't make sense, it's beyónd belíef.

уклáдываться II, улéчься lie* down; улéчься в постéль get* ínto bed; улéчься spat' go* to bed.

уклóн м. 1. íncline, slope, grádient; под ~ dównhill; 2. полит. deviátion; 3. (напрáвленность) bías, émphasis; с техни́ческим ~ом with a téchnical bías/émphasis.

уклон|éние с. deviátion; (от обя́занностей) evásion; (от тéмы) digréssion. ~и́ться сов. см. уклоня́ться.

уклóнчивый evásive; ~ отвéт evásive ánswer.

уклон|я́ться, уклони́ться (от рд.) 1. (отстраня́ться) dodge (smth.), sídestep (smth.); ~ от удáра dodge a blow; 2. (избегáть) eváde (smb., smth.), shirk (smth.); он ~я́ется от встрéчи со мной he avóids me; ~ от отвéтственности, обя́занностей eváde/shirk one's responsibílities, obligátions; ~ от отвéта eváde a quéstion;

3. (*отклоняться от прежнего пути*) déviate (from), veer (off); крéйсер уклони́лся от зáданного кýрса the crúiser was off course; 4. (*отвлекаться*) digréss (from); ~ от тéмы wánder from the point/súbject.

уклю́чина *ж.* rówlock.

укóл *м.* 1. prick; *перен. тж.* pínprick; 2. (*впрыскивание*) injéction; jab *разг.*; сдéлать ~ комý-л. give* smb. an injéction.

уколóть *сов.* (*вн.*) 1. prick (*smb., smth.*); 2. (*обидеть*) sting* (*smb.*); have* a dig (at). ~ся *сов.* prick onesélf.

укомплектовáть *сов.* (*вн.*) 1. (*составить комплект*) compléte (*smth.*), make* up (*smth.*); 2. (*заполнить до комплекта*) bring* (*smth.*) up to full strength.

укóр *м.* repróach; смотрéть с ~ом look repróachfully, have* a look of repróach in *one's* eyes; ◇ ~ы сóвести twínges of cónscience; sting of remórse *sg*; стáвить что-л. в ~ комý-л. hold* *smth.* against *smb.*

укорáчивать, укоротúть (*вн.*) shórten (*smth.*), redúce (*smth.*).

укорени́вшийся (deep-)róoted, deep-séated, ingráined.

укорени́ться *сов. см.* укореня́ться.

укореня́ться, укорени́ться take* root.

укори́зн|**а** *ж.* repróach. **~енный** repróachful.

укори́ть *сов. см.* укоря́ть.

укороти́ть *сов. см.* укорáчивать.

укорóченный shórtened, redúced; ~ рабóчий день redúced wórking day.

укоря́ть, укори́ть (*вн. в пр.*) repróach (*smb.* with).

укóс *м. с.-х.* háy-harvest, hay crop.

украдкой fúrtively, stéalthily; ~ брóсить взгляд на когó-л. steal* a fúrtive glance at *smb.*; смотрéть на когó-либо ~ look at *smb.* stéalthily, steal* a look at *smb.*

украи́н|**ец** *м.*, **~ка** *ж.* Ukráinian. **~ский** Ukráinian; ~ский язы́к Ukráinian, the Ukráinian lánguage.

украсить(ся) *сов. см.* украшáть(ся).

украсть *сов. см.* красть I.

украшáтельство *с.* óverembéllishment, óverdecorátion; (*вычурность*) affectátion.

украш|**áть, украсить** (*вн.*) adórn (*smb., smth.*), décorate (*smth.*); (*речь, слог*) embéllish (*smth.*); *перен.* enrích (*smth.*). **~áться, украситься** be* décorated; (*о речи, слоге*) be* embéllished; *перен.* be* enríched. **~éние** *с.* 1. (*действие*) decorátion, embéllishment; 2. (*предмет*) órnament; *перен.* adórnment.

укреп|**и́ть(ся)** *сов. см.* укрепля́ть(ся). **~лéние** *с.* 1. (*действие*) strengthening, reinfórcement; (*власти, положения и т. п.*) consolidátion; 2. *воен.* (*сооружение*) fortificátion; ли́ния ~лéний line of fortificátions/defénces. **~лённый** *воен.* fórtified; ~лённая ли́ния fórtified defénce line.

укрепля́ть, укрепи́ть (*вн.*) 1. (*делать более прочным*) strengthen (*smth.*) (*тж. перен.*); shore (*smth.*) up; (*делать устойчивым*) fix (*smth.*); 2. (*делать более выносливым*) fórtify (*smth.*); ~ здорóвье fórtify/impróve *one's* health; 3. (*поддерживать морально*) brace (*smb.*) up; 4. (*делать более мощным, сильным*) consolídate (*smth.*), fórtify (*smth.*). **~ся, укрепи́ться** 1. (*делаться более прочным*) be*/becóme* strónger; (*принимать устойчивое положение*) be* fixed; 2. (*становиться более сильным физически и духовно*) be* strengthened; укрепи́ться в свои́х убеждéниях be* confirmed in *one's* belief; укрепи́ться в свои́х намéрениях be* still more detérmined to cárry out *one's* inténtions; 3. (*прочно устанавливаться*) be* estáblished; 4. (*становиться более мощным, влиятельным*) estáblish itsélf; 5. *воен.* consólidate *one's* positions, entrénch onesélf.

укрóмн|**ый** hídden, seclúded; **~ое** местéчко seclúded spot.

укрóп *м. бот.* dill.

укроти́тель *м.*, **~ница** *ж.* (*ánimal*) támer.

укроти́ть *сов. см.* укрощáть.

укрощ|**áть, укроти́ть** (*вн.*) 1. (*животное, строптивого человека*) tame (*smb., smth.*); 2. (*сдерживать*) curb (*smth.*), subdúe (*smth.*); укроти́ть гнев curb *one's* ánger. **~éние** *с.* 1. (*животного*) táming; 2. (*гнева и т. п.*) cúrbing.

укрупнéние *с.* integrátion, amalgamátion, mérging; ~ предприя́тий integrátion of fáctories/énterprises.

укрупнённый íntegrated.

укрупни́ть *сов. см.* укрупня́ть.

укрупня́ть, укрупни́ть (*вн.*) íntegrate (*smth.*), amálgamate (*smth.*).

укрывáтель *м.*, **~ница** *ж.* concéaler; (*краденого*) recéiver. **~ство** *с.* concéalment; (*краденого*) recéiving.

укрывáть, укры́ть (*вн.*) 1. (*укутывать*) cóver (*smb., smth.*); 2. (*прятать, предохранять*) concéal (*smth., smth.*); shélter (*smth.*). **~ся, укры́ться** 1. (*укутываться*) cóver onesélf up; 2. (*прятаться*) take* shélter; be* protécted; *воен.* take* cóver; 3. (*оставаться незамеченным*) escápe; ничтó не укры́лось от егó взгля́да nóthing escáped his eye.

укры́ти|**е** *с.* 1. cóver; (*защита*) protéction; shélter; 2. (*сооружение*) shélter; в ~и únder cóver.

укры́тый shéltered, cóvered.

укры́ть(ся) *сов. см.* укрывáть(ся).

ýксус *м.* vínegar. **~ный** acétic; **~ная кислотá** acétic ácid; **~ная эссéнция** vínegar éssence.

укýс *м.* bite; (*пчелы*) sting; ~ комарá mosquíto-bite; ~ змеи́ snáke-bite; ~ собáки dog's bite.

укуси́|**ть** *сов.* (*вн.*) bite* (*smb., smth.*); (*о пчеле*) sting* (*smb., smth.*); ◇ какáя тебя́ мýха ~ла? what's bítten you?

укýтать(ся) *сов. см.* укýтывать(ся).

укýтывать, укýтать (*вн. в вн.*) wrap (*smb.*) up (in). **~ся, укýтаться** wrap onesélf up.

улáвливать, улови́ть (*вн.*) catch* (*smth.*); улови́ть нóтку чегó-л. catch* a note of *smth.*; улови́ть удóбный момéнт strike* the right móment; улови́ть смысл catch* the méaning.

улáдить(ся) *сов. см.* улáживать(ся).

улáживать, улáдить (*вн.*) séttle (*smth.*); (*отношения, ссору*) patch (*smth.*); ~ дéло séttle an affáir. **~ся, улáдиться** get* séttled; дéло улáдилось the affáir is séttled.

улáмывать, уломáть (*вн.*) *разг.* talk (*smb.*) round; *несов. тж.* try to persuáde (*smb.*); егó пришлóсь дóлго ~, прéжде чем он согласи́лся it took a lot of persuásion to get him to agrée.

ýлей *м.* (bée)hive.

улетéть, улетéть fly* awáy; птúцы улетéли на юг the birds have flown awáy to the south.

улетéть *сов. см.* улетáть.

улетýчиваться, улетýчиться 1. (*о жидкости*) eváporate; (*о запахе*) go*; 2. *разг.* (*исчезать*) vánish.

улетýчиться *сов. см.* улетýчиваться.

улéчься *сов.* 1. *см.* укладываться II; 2. (*о пыли*) séttle; 3. (*стихнуть*) subsíde, abáte, die down.

улизнýть *сов. разг.* slip awáy.

ули́к|**а** *ж.* évidence; прямы́е **~и** diréct évidence *sg*.

ули́тка *ж. зоол.* snail.

ýлиц|**а** *ж.* street; на **~е** in the street; (*вне помещения*) outside, out of doors, outdóors; вы́йти на ~у go* out/outside; войти́ с ~ы come* in (from outdóors); по ~е alóng the street; жить на ~е Кúрова в дóме 12 live at 12, Kírov Street; ◇ вы́гнать когó-л. на ~у turn *smb.* out; очути́ться на ~е be* thrown out on the street.

уличáть, уличи́ть (*вн.*) catch* (*smb.*) out; (*вн. в пр.*) prove (*smb.*) guílty (of); ~ когó-л. во лжи prove *smb.* a líar, catch* *smb.* in a lie; ~ когó-л. в крáже prove *smb.* a thief, expóse *smb.* as a thief.

уличи́ть *сов. см.* уличáть.

у́личн|ый street *attr.*; ~ое движе́ние tráffic; ~ шум the noise of the street.

уло́в *м.* catch.

улови́мый: едва́ ~ álmost impercéptible, scárcely percéptible.

улови́ть *сов. см.* ула́вливать.

уло́вк|а *ж.* trick, súbterfuge, device; dodge *разг.*; ~и не помогли́ tricks were of no avail.

уложи́ть *сов. см.* укла́дывать. ~ся *сов. см.* укла́дываться I.

уломать *сов. см.* ула́мывать.

улучать, улучить (вн.) find* (*smth.*); улучи́ть моме́нт choose* / catch* the móment.

улучи́ть *сов. см.* улучать.

улучш|а́ть, улучшить (вн.) impróve (*smth.*). ~а́ться, улу́чшиться impróve. ~е́ние *с.* impróvement.

улучш|енный impróved. ~ить(ся) *сов. см.* улучша́ть(ся).

улыб|а́ться, улыбну́ться 1. smile; (*дт.*) smile (at); 2. (*дт.*; *благоприятствовать*) smile (upón), favour (*smb.*); жизнь ему́ ~ается life is kind to him; сча́стье ему́ улыбну́лось fórtune smiled upón him; 3. *тк. несов.* (*дт.*) *разг.* (*нравиться*) appéal (to); мне э́то (совсе́м) не ~ается it dóesn't appéal to me a bit; мне совсе́м не ~ается идти́ туда́ I am not at all keen on góing there.

улы́бка *ж.* smile.

улыбну́ться *сов. см.* улыба́ться 1, 2.

ультимати́вный categórical, ultimátum-like, táke-it-or-léave it *attr.*

ультима́тум *м.* ultimátum; предъяви́ть ~ кому́-л. presént *smb.* with an ultimátum.

у́льтра *м. нескл.* (*о политическом деятеле и т. п.*) últra.

у́льтра- *в сложн.* últra-.

ультразву́к *м.* últrasound.

ультразвуково́й ultrasónic.

ультрапра́вый *прил.* 1. far right; of the far right *после сущ.*; 2. *в знач. сущ. мн.* últras, far ríghtists.

ультрасовреме́нный ultra-módern.

ультрафиоле́товый ultravíolet.

ум *м.* mind, íntellect; (*сообразительность*) intélligence; brains *pl*, sense *разг.*; он челове́к большо́го ума́ he has a spléndid mind/íntellect; ◇ быть без ума́ от кого́-л., чего́-л. be* crázy/mad abóut *smb., smth.*; (*быть влюблённым*) be* wíldly in love with *smb.*; бра́ться за ум come* to *one's* sénses; в уме́ méntally; счита́ть в уме́ réckon in *one's* head; реша́ть зада́чи в уме́ do* sums in *one's* head, do* méntal aríthmetic; оди́н в уме́ cárry one; в своём уме́ in *one's* right mind; быть не в своём уме́ be* out of *one's* mind/sénses; в своём ли ты уме́? are you in your right mind/sénses?; у меня́ в уме́ не́ было... it néver éntered my head...; из ума́ вон! I quite forgót!; у меня́ э́то из ума́ нейдёт I can't forget it!; у него́ на уме́ ничего́, кроме... he thinks of nóthing but...; он себе́ на уме́ he is véry shrewd/cánny; he knows how mány beans make five; ско́лько голо́в — сто́лько умо́в so mány men so mány minds; there are as mány different opínions as there are péople in this world; ум хорошо́, а два лу́чше two heads are bétter than one; учи́ть кого́-л. уму́-ра́зуму teach* *smb.* in the way he, she should go; не ва́шего ума́ де́ло! that's beyónd you!; довести́ до ума́ get* *smth.* ínto shape.

умали́ть *сов. см.* умаля́ть.

умалишённый *прил.* 1. mad, lúnatic; 2. *в знач. сущ. м.* mádman*, lúnatic.

умáлчив|ать, умолча́ть (о *пр.*) ignóre (*smth.*), pass (*smth.*) óver in sílence; (*скрывать*) concéal (*smth.*); ◇ об э́том исто́рия ~ает history is sílent on this point.

умаля́ть, умали́ть (вн.) belíttle (*smth.*); ~ чьи-л. заслу́ги belíttle *smb.'s* sérvices.

уме́лец *м.* máster of *one's* trade, skilled cráftsman*.

уме́л|о skilfully, ábly. ~ый áble, skílful, efficient;

(*квалифицированный*) skilled, éxpert; ~ые ру́ки skílful hands; ~ые де́йствия efficient méasures.

уме́ние *с.* abílity, skill.

уменьша́емое *с. мат.* mínuend.

уменьш|а́ть, уме́ньшить (вн.) dimínish (*smth.*), decréase (*smth.*); ~ расхо́ды cut* / lówer costs; (*личные*) redúce *one's* expénses; ~ ско́рость redúce speed, slow down. ~а́ться, уме́ньшиться dimínish, decréase; (*о ветре и т. п.*) drop, abáte; (*об опухоли*) go* down; опа́сность ~а́ется the dánger grows less; боль ~а́ется the pain dimínishes/decréases. ~е́ние *с.* redúction, decréase; (*размера*) diminútion; (*ветра и т. п.*) abátement.

уменьши́тельн|ый 1. diminishing; ~ое стекло́ diminishing glass; 2. *лингв.* dimínutive; ~ое и́мя существи́тельное dimínutive; ~ су́ффикс dimínutive súffix; 3.: ~ое и́мя pet name.

уме́ньшить(ся) *сов. см.* уменьша́ть(ся).

уме́ренн|о móderately; (*бережливо*) spáringly. ~ость *ж.* moderátion. ~ый 1. móderate; ~ая ско́рость móderate speed; 2. *геогр.* témperate; ~ый кли́мат témperate climate; ~ый по́яс témperate zone.

умере́ть *сов. см.* умира́ть.

уме́рить *сов. см.* умеря́ть.

умертви́ть *сов. см.* умерщвля́ть.

уме́рший *м.* the decéased, the dead man*.

умерщвля́ть, умертви́ть (вн.) kill (*smb., smth.*); (*злодейски*) múrder (*smb.*), do* awáy (with); *перен.* choke (*smth.*).

умеря́ть, уме́рить (вн.) móderate (*smth.*); ~ тре́бования móderate *one's* demánds.

умести́ть(ся) *сов. см.* умеща́ть(ся).

уме́стн|о opportúnely; apprópriately; 2. *в знач. сказ. безл.* (+ *инф.*) it may not be out of place (+ to *inf*). ~ый ópportune; apprópriate, pértinent; to the point *predic.*; ~ый вопро́с pértinent quéstion; э́то вполне́ ~ое замеча́ние this remárk is véry much to the point.

уме́|ть *несов.* (+ *инф.*) be* áble (+ to *inf*); *в личн. формах* can; know* how (+ to *inf*); не ~ (+ *инф.*) be* unáble (+ to *inf*); *в личн. формах* cánnot; not know how (+ to *inf*); он ~ет чита́ть стихи́ he reads póetry véry well; она́ ~ет де́лать пече́нье, вари́ть ко́фе *и т. д.* she knows how to make pástry, cóffee, *etc.*; отли́чно ~ де́лать что-л. be* a past máster at dóing *smth.*

умеща́ть, умести́ть (вн.) get* (*smth.*) in/on. ~ся, умести́ться go* in.

умил|е́ние *с.* ténderness, (*sentiméntal*) affection; прийти́ в ~ be* véry touched. ~ённый déeply touched; (*выражающий умиление*) afféctionate. ~и́ть(ся) *сов. см.* умиля́ть(ся).

уми́льный 1. sweet; (*трогательный*) tóuching; 2. (*угодливый*) ingrátiating.

умиля́ть, умили́ть (вн.) touch (*smb.*), move (*smb.*). ~ся, умили́ться be* touched/moved.

умира́ние *с.* dýing; (*смерть*) death; ме́дленное ~ slow death.

умир|а́ть, умере́ть 1. die; *сов. тж.* be* dead; *перен.* die, disappéar; он ~а́ет he is dýing; он у́мер he is dead, he is no more; умере́ть сме́ртью геро́я die a héro's death; умере́ть есте́ственной сме́ртью die a nátural death; 2.: ~ со́ смеху die of/with láughing; ~ от ску́ки be* bored to death; ◇ ~аю есть хочу́! I'm dýing for sómething to eat! ~а́ющий *м.* the dýing man*.

умиротвор|е́ние *с.* reconciliátion. ~и́ть(ся) *сов. см.* умиротворя́ть(ся). ~и́ть, умиротвори́ть (вн.) pácify (*smb.*), appéase (*smb.*). ~и́ться, умиротвори́ться be* réconciled.

умне́ть, поумне́ть grow* wíser, becóme* more intélligent.

у́мник *м. разг.* 1. smart féllow/chap; 2. *ирон.* bright spark; 3. (*о мальчике*) good boy.

у́мниц|а *разг.* 1. *м. и ж.* cléver man*, wóman*; 2. *ж.* (*о девочке*) good girl; будь ~ей! be a good girl!

у́мничать *несов. разг.* try to be cléver.

умнож|а́ть, умно́жить 1. (*вн. на вн.*) *мат.* múltiply (*smth.* by); 2. (*вн.; увеличивать*) incréase (*smth.*), augmént (*smth.*). ~а́ться, умно́житься (*увеличиваться*) incréase. ~е́ние *с.* 1. *мат.* multiplicátion; табли́ца ~е́ния multiplicátion-table; 2. (*увеличение*) incréase.

умно́жить *сов. см.* умножа́ть *и* мно́жить. ~ся *сов. см.* умножа́ться.

у́мн|ый intélligent; (*способный*) cléver; (*толковый*) sénsible, wise; *разг.* (*послушный — о детях*) good*; ◇ ~ая голова́ man* of sense, cléver pérson.

умозаключе́ние *с.* dedúction; conclúsion; ínference.

умозри́тельный *книжн.* spéculative, ábstract.

умоли́ть *сов.* (*вн.*) preváil (upón), persuáde (*smb.*).

у́молк *м.*: без ~у incéssantly.

умолка́ть, умо́лкнуть becóme* sílent; (*о шуме, звуке и т. п.*) stop; *перен.* cease; не умо́лкнет их сла́ва their glóry will néver cease.

умо́лкнуть *сов. см.* умолка́ть.

умолча́ть *сов. см.* ума́лчивать.

умоля́ть *несов.* (*вн.*) beg (*smb.*), implóre (*smb.*), entréat (*smth.*); ~ кого́-л. о проще́нии implóre *smb.'s* forgíveness.

умопомеша́тельств|о *с.* insánity; находи́ться в состоя́нии ~а be* méntally deránged.

умори́тельный *разг.* hilárious, killingly fúnny.

умори́ть *сов.* (*вн.*) *разг.* 1. kill (*smth.*); ~ кого́-л. го́лодом starve *smb.*; 2. (*утомить*) tíre (*smb.*) out; 3.: ~ кого́-л. со́ смеху make* *smb.* néarly die of láughing.

у́мственн|ый méntal; ~ые спосо́бности méntal abílities; intélligence *sg*; ~ труд bráinwork.

умудрённый made wise; ~ о́пытом made wise by expérience.

умудри́ться *сов. см.* умудря́ться.

умудря́ться, умудри́ться (+ *инф.*) *разг.* contríve (+ to *inf*), mánage (+ to *inf*) (*тж. ирон.*).

умча́ть *сов.* (*вн.*) cárry (*smb., smth.*) rápidly awáy. ~ся *сов.* 1. dash awáy/off; (*о лошади, всаднике*) gállop off; (*об автомобиле, велосипедисте, поезде*) set* off at full speed; 2. (*быстро пройти — о времени*) fly* past.

умыва́льник *м.* (*раковина*) wáshbasin, wásh-bowl; (*без крана*) wásh-stand.

умыва́ть, умы́ть (*вн.*) wash (*smb., smth.*); ◇ ~ ру́ки wash *one's* hands of it. ~ся, умы́ться wash (*one's* hands and face), have* a wash.

у́мыс|ел *м.* inténtion, desígn; с ~лом inténtionally; без вся́кого ~ла quite uninténtionally.

умы́ть(ся) *сов. см.* умыва́ть(ся).

умы́шленн|о inténtionally, delíberately, desígnedly. ~ый inténtional, delíberate; ~ое уби́йство preméditated múrder.

унасле́довать *сов.* (*вн.*) (*прям. и перен.*) inhérit (*smth.*).

унести́(сь) *сов. см.* уноси́ть(ся).

универма́г *м.* depártment store.

универса́л *м.* 1. (*работник*) all-róunder; 2. (*тип машины*) estáte-car; *station* wágon *амер.*

универса́льн|ый (*всеобъемлющий*) univérsal; all-róund *attr.*; ~ые зна́ния encyclopáedic knówledge *sg*; 2. (*пригодный для многих целей*) múltipurpose, convértible; ~ое сре́дство univérsal rémedy.

универса́м *м.* supermárket.

универсиа́да *ж.* stúdent games *pl.*

университе́т *м.* univérsity. ~ский univérsity *attr.*

униж|а́ть, уни́зить (*вн.*) humíliate (*smth.*); (*умалять*) belíttle (*smth.*), lówer (*smth.*). ~а́ться, уни́зиться abáse onesélf; ~а́ться до лжи, про́сьбы stoop to lie, to beg. ~е́ние *с.* humiliátion, abásement; дойти́ до тако́го ~е́ния (что...) sink* so low (as to...).

уни́женн|о abjéctly. ~ый 1. (*о человеке*) humíliated;

---

2. (*выражающий унижение*) ábject; ~ая про́сьба ábject entréaty.

унизи́тельный humíliating.

уни́зить(ся) *сов. см.* унижа́ть(ся).

уника́льный excéptional, rare; (*единственный в своём роде*) uníque.

унима́ть, уня́ть (*вн.*) 1. (*успокаивать*) soothe (*smb.*), quíeten (*smb.*); 2. (*прекращать*) stop (*smth.*); (*сдерживать*) restráin (*smth.*), curb (*smth.*). ~ся, уня́ться 1. (*успокаиваться*) grow*/be* quíet; (*о буре, боли*) abáte, die down; 2. (*прекращаться*) stop; 3. (*о чувствах*) cease, be* relíeved; pass/go* off *разг.*

унисо́н *м.* únison; ◇ в ~ in únison; петь в ~ sing* in únison.

унита́з *м.* lávatory pan.

унифика́ция *ж.* unificátion.

унифици́ровать *несов. и сов.* (*вн.*) únify (*smth.*), bring* (*smth.*) into line.

уничтож|а́ть, уничто́жить (*вн.*) 1. destróy (*smb., smth.*) (*тж. перен.*); (*полностью*) anníhilate (*smb., smth.*), wipe out (*smb., smth.*); (*истреблять*) extérminate (*smb., smth.*); ~ следы́ oblíterate the tráces; ~ зло erádicate an évil; 2. (*упразднять*) abólish (*smth.*); 3. *разг.* (*съедать, выпивать*) dispóse (of); 4. (*унижать*) crush (*smb.*). ~а́ющий 1. (*губительный*) destrúctive; 2. (*беспощадный*) scáthing, sláshing, annihilating; ~а́ющая кри́тика scáthing críticism; 3. (*выражающий презрение*) scórnful, withering; ~а́ющий взгляд withering look. ~е́ние *с.* 1. destrúction; (*истребление*) extermination; по́лное ~е́ние útter destrúction; annihilátion; 2. (*упразднение*) abolítion, remóval.

уничто́жить *сов. см.* уничтожа́ть.

уноси́ть, унести́ (*вн.*) 1. take* (*smb., smth.*) awáy; ~ что́-л. с собо́й take* *smth.* with *one*; 2. *разг.* (*похищать*) cárry (*smth.*) off; 3. (*увлекать течением и т. п.*) bear* (*smb., smth.*) awáy, cárry (*smb., smth.*) awáy; (*ветром*) blow* (*smth.*) awáy; ◇ е́ле но́ги унести́ escápe by the skin of *one's* teeth. ~ся, унести́сь 1. (*быстро удаляться*) speed* awáy; (*быстро убегать*) race off; 2. (*о мечтах и т. п.*) be* cárried awáy; мои́ мы́сли унесли́сь в про́шлое my thoughts went back to the past; 3. (*о времени*) fly* past/by.

унты́ *мн.* (*ед.* унт *м.*) fur boots.

уныв|а́ть *несов.* lose* heart, feel*/be* glum; не ~а́й! cheer up!, don't give up!

уны́л|о *нареч.* móurnfully, dólefully; 2. *в знач. сказ. безл.* it is dréary. ~ый 1. (*грустный, мрачный*) mélancholy, dóleful; (*о выражении лица тж.*) wóebegone; 2. (*наводящий уныние*) depréssing, dréary, dísmal; ~ый ландша́фт depréssing lándscape.

уны́ние *с.* despóndency, dejéction, gloom, dówncast mood; впада́ть в ~ becóme* despóndent, give* way to despáir.

уня́ть(ся) *сов. см.* унима́ть(ся).

упа́д *м.*: до ~у till *one* is réady to drop.

упа́док *м.* declíne; (*разложение, оскудение тж.*) decáy; ~ ду́ха depréssion; ~ сил wéakness, debílity; приходи́ть в ~ fall* into decáy.

упа́дочни|ческий décadent; ~чество *с.* décadence.

упа́дочн|ый depréssed; (*об искусстве, культуре и т. п.*) décadent; ~ое настрое́ние despóndency; low spirits *pl.*

упакова́ть *сов. см.* упако́вывать *и* пакова́ть.

упако́вк|а *ж.* 1. (*действие*) pácking; 2. (*материал*) páckaging, cóver; в изя́щной ~е nícely páckaged.

упако́вочный pácking *attr.*

упако́вывать, упакова́ть (*вн.*) pack (*smth.*), pack (*smth.*) up.

упа́сть *сов. см.* па́дать 1, 6, 10.

упере́ть *сов. см.* упира́ть 1. ~ся *сов. см.* упира́ться.

упива́ться, упи́ться 1. *разг.* (*допьяна*) get* drunk; 2. (*тв.; наслаждаться*) rével (in), be* intóxicated (by).

упира́ть, упере́ть 1. (вн. в вн.) set* (smth. on, against); 2. тк. несов. (на вн.; подчёркивать) émphasize (smth.), stress (smth.), lay* stress (on). ~ся, упере́ться 1. (тв. в вн.) lean* (smth. against); ~ся нога́ми во что-л. plant one's feet against smth.; ~ся нога́ми в зе́млю dig* one's heels in, plant one's feet firmly; 2. разг. (сопротивляться) refuse to budge; (упрямиться) stúbbornly refúse; 3. (в вн.) разг. (подходить вплотную к чему-л.) stop (at), come* (to); (зависеть) rest on, turn on.

упи́танн|ость ж. state of nóurishment. ~ый well-nóurished.

упи́ться сов. см. упива́ться.

упла́та ж. páyment.

уплати́ть сов. см. упла́чивать.

упла́чивать, уплати́ть (вн.) pay* (smth.); уплати́ть по счёту pay* the bill.

уплотн|е́ние с. 1. consolidátion, compréssion; (рядов) tíghtening up; 2. (заполнение времени) filling up; ~ рабо́чего дня filling up of the wórking day; 3. мед. infiltrátion. ~и́ть(ся) сов. см. уплотня́ть(ся).

уплотня́ть, уплотни́ть (вн.) 1. (делать более плотным) compréss (smth.), pack (smth.) down, consólidate (smth.); (ряды) tíghten up (smth.); 2. (заполнять целиком) fill up (smth.); уплотни́ть рабо́чий день fill up the wórking day. ~ся, уплотни́ться 1. (становиться плотнее, твёрже) set* firm; be* packed firmly, becóme* compáct; 2. (о рабочем времени) be* filled up.

уплыва́ть, уплы́ть 1. swim* awáy/off; (о судне) sail awáy; (о моторной лодке) move awáy; (о предметах) float/drift awáy; 2. (медленно, плавно удаляться) glide awáy, float awáy.

уплы́ть сов. см. уплыва́ть.

упова́ть несов. (на вн., + инф.) уст. hope (+ to inf), count (on); (полагаться на кого-л.) place one's trust (in).

уподо́бить(ся) сов. см. уподобля́ть(ся).

уподобля́ть, уподо́бить (вн. дт.) líken (smb., smth. to). ~ся, уподо́биться (дт.) be*/look like (smb., smth.), resémble (smb., smth.).

упое́ни|е с. écstasies pl, ráptures pl; в ~и успе́ха flushed with succéss.

упои́тельный rávishing, entráncing.

уполза́ть, уползти́ crawl awáy.

уползти́ сов. см. уполза́ть.

уполномо́ч|енный м. represéntative. ~ивать, уполномо́чить (вн. на вн., вн. + инф.) áuthorize (smb. + to inf), empówer (smb. + to inf).

уполномо́чить сов. см. уполномо́чивать.

упомина́ние с. méntion; (замечание тж.) remárk, réference.

упомина́ть, упомяну́ть (вн. о пр.) méntion (smb., smth.).

упо́мн|ить сов. (вн.) разг. remémber (smth.); всего́ не ~ишь! you can't remémber éverything!

упомяну́ть сов. см. упомина́ть.

упо́р м. suppórt; (предмет тж.) rest; ◇ де́лать ~ на кого-л., что-л., на ком-л., чём-л. lay* stress on smb., smth.; сказа́ть что-л. в ~ say* smth. to smb.'s face; смотре́ть на кого-л. в ~ gaze fíxedly at smb.; стреля́ть в ~ fire at close/point-blánk range, fire point-blánk.

упо́р|ный (настойчивый) persístent, detérmined, stúbborn; (упрямый) óbstinate; ~ные по́иски persístent search sg; ~ный труд hard work; ~ное молча́ние stúbborn sílence; ~ный взгляд stéady glance; ~ное сопротивле́ние detérmined/stout/stúbborn resístance. ~ство с. (настойчивость) persístence, stúbbornness; (упрямство) óbstinacy.

упо́рствовать несов. be* stúbborn; (в пр.) persíst (in).

упорхну́ть сов. flit awáy.

упоря́дочение с. regulátion, stréamlining.

упоря́дочить сов. (вн.) régulate (smth.), put* (smth.) straight, stréamline (smth.). ~ся сов. acquíre sýstem.

употреби́тельн|ый cómmon, fréquently used; ~ые слова́ words in cómmon/éveryday use.

употреб|и́ть сов. см. употребля́ть. ~ле́ние с. use; в большо́м ~ле́нии wídely used; входи́ть в ~ле́ние come* into use; лёгкий в ~ле́нии úser-friendly.

употребля́ть, употреби́ть (вн.) use (smth.); (применять тж.) apply (smth.); ~ все уси́лия exért évery éffort; ◇ ~ во зло чьё-л. дове́рие abúse smb.'s cónfidence.

упра́виться сов. см. управля́ться.

управле́ние с. 1. (действие) operátion, contról; (руководство) mánagement, administrátion, diréction; (государством) góvernment; ~ на расстоя́нии remóte contról; 2. (оркестром, хором) condúcting; под ~м кого-л. condúcted by smb.; 3. (административный орган) board, administrátion; (здание тж.) héad-office; ~ желе́зной доро́ги ráilway administrátion; 4. (совокупность приборов) contróls pl; рулево́е ~ stéering-gear; 5. грам. góvernment; ◇ теря́ть ~ lose* contról.

управле́нческ|ий administrative; ~ие расхо́ды administrative expénses; ~ аппара́т administrative personnél.

управля́емый guíded; ~ снаря́д guíded míssile.

управля́ть несов. (тв.) 1. (регулировать движение, работу чего-л.) óperate (smth.); ~ автомоби́лем drive* a car; ~ корабле́м steer a ship; ~ комба́йном óperate a cómbine; 2. (руководить) diréct (smb., smth.), mánage (smb., smth.); admínister (smth.), run* (smth.); (государством) góvern (smth.), rule (smth.); 3. (направлять чьи-л. поступки) guide (smb.); 4. (оркестром, хором) condúct (smth.); 5. грам. góvern (smth.). ~ся, упра́виться (с тв.) разг. соре (with).

управля́ющий м. mánager; ~ дела́ми búsiness-manager.

упражне́ние с. 1. (действие) éxercising; 2. (задание) éxercise.

упражн|я́ть несов. (вн.) train (smth.), éxercise (smth.). ~я́ться несов. práctise; ~я́ться в францу́зском языке́ práctise one's French; ~я́ться на рояле práctise the piáno.

упраздн|е́ние с. abolítion; (учреждения) clósing. ~и́ть сов. см. упраздня́ть.

упраздня́ть, упраздни́ть (вн.) abólish (smth.), do* awáy (with); (учреждение) close (smth.).

упра́шивать, упроси́ть (вн.) beg (smb.), entréat (smb.); сов. тж. persuáde (smb.).

упрёк м. repróach; мн. тж. recriminátions; с ~ом repróachfully; осыпа́ть кого-л. ~ами heap repróaches on smb., hurl repróaches at smb.; ◇ бро́сить ~ кому-л. repróach smb.; ста́вить что-л. в ~ кому-л. hold* smth. against smb.

упрека́ть, упрекну́ть (вн. в пр.) repróach (smb. with); ~ кого-л. в небре́жности repróach smb. with negléct.

упрекну́ть сов. см. упрека́ть.

упере́ть сов. см. преть 2.

упроси́ть сов. см. упра́шивать.

упрости́ть(ся) сов. см. упроща́ть(ся).

упроче́ние с. consolidátion, stréngthening, secúring; reinfórcing.

упро́чить сов. (вн.) consólidate (smth.), make* (smth.) strónger; reinfórce (smth.); ~ своё положе́ние consólidate one's position.

упрощ|а́ть, упрости́ть (вн.) símplify (smth.); (делать примитивным, обеднять) oversímplify (smth.). ~а́ться, упрости́ться becóme* símpler. ~е́ние с. simplificátion; (обеднение) oversimplificátion.

упру́г|ий elástic, resílient; перен. spríngy; ~ шаг

spríngy stride/walk; ~ое те́ло resílient bódy. ~ость *ж.* elastícity, resílience; преде́л ~ости *физ.* elástic límit.

упря́жка *ж.* 1. team; 2. *см.* у́пряжь.

упряжн|о́й: ~а́я ло́шадь cárriage-horse; (*ломова́я*) cárt-horse.

у́пряжь *ж.* hárness.

упря́мец *м. разг.* stúbborn/óbstinate féllow.

упря́миться *несов.* be* stúbborn; не упря́мься! don't be (so) stúbborn!

упря́м|ство *с.* óbstinacy, stúbbornness. ~ый 1. óbstinate, stúbborn; 2. (*насто́йчивый*) persístent.

упря́тать *сов. разг.* (*тща́тельно спря́тать*) hide* (*smb.*), put* (*smb.*) awáy; *перен.* put* (*smb.*) awáy; ~ кого́-л. в тюрьму́ send* *smb.* to príson.

упуска́ть, упусти́ть (*вн.*) 1. (*дава́ть убежа́ть*) let* (*smb., smth.*) go; (*не удержа́в, выпуска́ть, теря́ть*) lose* hold (of); (*не замеча́ть*) miss (*smth.*), pass óver (*smth.*); упусти́ть коне́ц верёвки let* go the rope; 2. (*не воспо́льзоваться чем-л. во́время*) miss (*smth.*); упусти́ть вре́мя let* the móment pass; miss the boat *идиом.*; упусти́ть возмо́жность, слу́чай miss the opportúnity; не ~ слу́чая let* pass no occásion; ◇ упусти́ть что́-л. из виду lose* sight of *smth.*, overlóok *smth.*

упусти́ть *сов. см.* упуска́ть.

упуще́ние *с.* óversight; (*про́пуск тж.*) omíssion; (*оши́бка тж.*) slip.

ура́ hurráh!, hurráy!

уравне́ние *с.* 1. (*де́йствие*) equalizátion, bálancing; 2. *мат.* equátion.

ура́внивать I, уравня́ть (*вн.; де́лать ра́вным*) make* (*smb.*) équal; lével up (*smth.*), équalize (*smth.*); ~ кого́-л. в права́х give* équal rights to *smb.*

ура́внивать II, уровня́ть (*вн.; де́лать ро́вным*) smooth (*smth.*), lével (*smth.*).

уравнове́сить *сов. см.* уравнове́шивать.

уравнове́ш|енность *ж.* bálance, poise, éven témper. ~ый (*о челове́ке*) well-bálanced.

уравнове́шивать, уравнове́сить (*вн.*) bálance (*smth.*); *перен.* óffset* (*smth.*), cóunterbalance (*smth.*).

уравня́ть *сов. см.* ура́внивать I.

урага́н *м.* (*прям. и перен.*) húrricane. ~ный húrricane *attr.;* ~ный ого́нь wíthering / cóncentrated fíre.

уразуме́ть *сов.* (*вн.*) understánd* (*smth.*), comprehénd (*smth.*).

ура́н *м.* uránium. ~овый uránium *attr.;* ~овая руда́ uránium ore.

урва́ть *сов.* (*вн.*) *разг.* snatch (*smth.*) (*тж. перен.*).

урду́ *м. нескл.* Urdú.

урегули́ровать *сов.* (*вн.*) régulate (*smth.*).

уре́зать *сов. см.* уреза́ть.

уреза́ть, уре́зать (*вн.*) 1. (*укора́чивать*) shórten (*smth.*); 2. (*сокраща́ть, убавля́ть*) redúce (*smth.*); ~ права́ кого́-л. curtáil *smb.'s* rights; ~ расхо́ды cut* down expénses.

урезо́нивать, урезо́нить (*вн.*) make* (*smb.*) see réason, bring* (*smb.*) to réason.

урезо́нить *сов. см.* урезо́нивать.

у́рна *ж.* 1. urn; 2. (*для избира́тельных бюллете́ней*) bállot box; 3. (*для му́сора*) rúbbish bin.

у́ров|ень *м.* lével; (*сте́пень величины́, зна́чимости тж.*) stándard; над ~нем мо́ря abóve séa-level; ~ зарпла́ты stándard of wáges; довое́нный ~ prewár lével; ◇ быть на ~не be* up to stándard; совеща́ние на вы́сшем ~не súmmit cónference, tóp-level cónference, súmmit; на ~не посло́в, мини́стров at ambássador, mínister lével; на высо́ком худо́жественном ~не at a high lével of artístic éxcellence; на ~не лу́чших мировы́х станда́ртов on a lével with the híghest world stándards, confórming to the híghest world stándards; подня́ть что́-л. на до́лжный ~ bring* *smth.* up to stándard.

уровня́ть *сов. см.* ура́внивать II.

уро́д *м.* 1. freak, defórmed/disfígured pérson; 2. (*бе-*

зобра́зный челове́к) úgly créature; он ~! he's hídeous!; 3. (*нра́вственный*) pérvert, mónster.

уроди́|ться *сов.* 1. yield, rípen; хлеб хорошо́ (пло́хо) ~лся the grain crop was good (poor); 2. *разг.* (*появи́ться на свет*) be* born; (*в вн.; роди́ться похо́жим на кого́-л.*) take* áfter (*smb.*); в кого́ он ~лся? where does he get it from?

уро́длив|ый 1. (*с физи́ческим недоста́тком*) defórmed; 2. (*безобра́зный*) úgly, fréakish; ~ наря́д fréakish attíre; 3. (*искажённый, извращённый*) distórted, twísted; ~ое воспита́ние críppling educátion; принима́ть ~ые фо́рмы assúme abnórmal forms.

уро́довать, изуро́довать (*вн.*) 1. disfígure (*smb., smth.*); 2. (*кале́чить*) crípple (*smb.*), mútilate (*smb.*); 3. (*по́ртить*) spoil* (*smb., smth.*); 4. (*нра́вственно*) demóralize (*smb.*), corrúpt (*smth.*).

уро́дство *с.* 1. (*физи́ческий недоста́ток*) defórmity; 2. (*безобра́зие*) úgliness; 3. (*искаже́ние, извраще́ние*) abnormálity.

урожа́й *м.* hárvest; (*коли́чество со́бранного тж.*) crop, yield; ~ овса́ oat crop/yield; ~ я́блок ápple crop; небыва́лый ~ búmper crop; вы́растить хоро́ший ~ grow* a good* crop.

урожа́йн|ость *ж.* yield capácity, productívity. ~ый high-yíelding; ~ый год good year; ~ый сорт high-yíelding spécies.

урожён|ец *м.,* ~ка *ж.* nátive (of).

уро́к *м.* 1. (*прям. и перен.*) lésson; ~ литерату́ры líterature lésson; извле́чь ~ из чего́-л. learn* a lésson from *smth.;* 2. (*зада́ние*) task, éxercise; гото́вить ~и do* one's léssons/hómework; ◇ брать ~и чего́-л. take* léssons in *smth.;* дава́ть ~и give* (prívate) léssons; дать ~ кому́-л. teach* *smb.* a lésson; ~и исто́рии the léssons of hístory.

уро́н *м.* lósses *pl.*

урони́ть *сов. см.* роня́ть 1, 3, 4, 5.

уро́чн|ый appóinted, fixed, detérmined; ~ая рабо́та set task; ~ час the appóinted hour.

урча́ть *несов.* rúmble.

уры́вками *разг.* in snátches; at odd móments.

урю́к *м. собир.* dried ápricot.

ус *м. см.* усы́.

уса́дить *сов. см.* уса́живать.

уса́дьба *ж.* 1. fármstead; 2. (*поме́щичья*) cóuntry-seat; 3. (*колхо́за, совхо́за*) the (céntral) búildings *pl;* 4. (*земля́, за́нятая строе́ниями*) grounds *pl,* estáte; 5. *разг.* (*приуса́дебный уча́сток*) allótment.

уса́живать, усади́ть (*вн.*) 1. (*предлага́ть сесть*) seat (*smb.*); 2. (*вн. за вн.; заставля́ть заня́ться чем-л.*) set* (*smb.* to); ~ кого́-л. за рабо́ту set* *smb.* to work; ~ кого́-л. за шитьё и *т. п.* set* *smb.* to work séwing, *etc.;* 3. *вн.; цвета́ми и т. п.*) plant (*smth.* with).

уса́живаться, усе́сться 1. seat onesélf, take* one's seat; усе́сться на дива́н sit* down on the sófa; 2. (*за вн., + инф.; принима́ться за что-л.*) sit* down (to); усе́сться за рабо́ту sit*/get* down to work; усе́сться за кни́гу séttle down with a book.

уса́тый moustáched; (*о живо́тном*) bewhískered; ~ кот cat with a fine set of whískers.

усва́ивать, усво́ить (*вн.*) 1. (*де́лать привы́чным для себя́*) acquíre (*smth.*); adópt (*smth.*); усво́ить дурну́ю привы́чку acquíre a bad hábit, get* into a bad hábit; 2. (*воспринима́ть*) máster (*smth.*); learn* (*smth.*), assímilate (*smth.*); усво́ить уро́к know* one's lésson; пло́хо ~ что-л. have* a poor grasp of *smth.;* 3. (*о пи́ще и т. п.*) digést (*smth.*), assímilate (*smth.*).

усвое́ние *с.* assimilátion; (*понима́ние тж.*) understánding; (*обы́чаев и т. п.*) acquíring.

усво́ить *сов. см.* усва́ивать.

усе́ивать, усе́ять (*вн. тв.*) strew* (*smth.* with), dot (*smth.* with), stud (*smth.* with); (*разбра́сывать*) lítter (*smth.* with); луга́ усе́яны цвета́ми the méadows are dótted with flówers; нéбо усéяно звёздами the sky is strewn/stúdded with stars.

усéрд|ие с. zeal; (прилежание) díligence, assidúity; с ~ием zéalously. **~ный** zéalous; (прилежный) díligent, assíduous.

усéрдствовать несов. work hard, show* great zeal.

усéсться сов. см. усáживаться.

усечённый 1. мат. trúncated; ~ кóнус trúncated cone; 2. (о рифме) impérfect; ~ дáктиль impérfect dáctyl.

усéять сов. см. усéивать.

усидéть сов. 1. keep* one's seat; трýдно ~ на мéсте it is hard to sit still; 2. (остаться, пробыть где-л.) stay.

усúдчив|ость ж. díligence, persevérance. **~ый** díligent, persevéring.

ýсики мн. (ед. ýсик м.) 1. little moustáche sg; 2. (у насекомых) féelers, anténnae; 3. (у растений) rúnners, téndrils.

усилéние с. 1. intensificátion; stréngthening; 2. радио, эл. amplificátion.

усúленн|ый 1. (увеличенный) cóncentrated; ~ая дóза чего-л. large/dóuble dose of smth.; ~ая рабóта cóncentrated work; ~ое питáние abúndant díet; 2. (неотступный) persistent; ~ые прóсьбы persístent requests.

усúливать, усúлить (вн.) stréngthen (smth.); (повысить интенсивность) inténsify (smth.); усúлить внимáние redóuble one's atténtion; усúлить страдáния, жáжду inténsify/ággravate one's súfferings, thirst; усúлить звук incréase the vólume; ~ся, усúлиться incréase, inténsify; (о звуке) grow* lóuder, swell*; (о ветре, буре) incréase in víolence, mount; дождь усúлился it begán to rain éven hárder.

усúлие с. éffort; сдéлать над собóй ~ make* an éffort; ~ вóли éffort of will.

усилúтель м. эл. bóoster; радио ámplifier; фото intensífier. **~ный** bóoster attr., bóosting; радио ámplifying; фото intensífying.

усúлить(ся) сов. см. усúливать(ся).

ускакáть сов. 1. hop/scámper awáy; 2. (на лошади) gállop awáy.

ускользáть, ускользнýть slip out, slip awáy; перен. slip through one's fingers; ускользнýть из кóмнаты slip out of the room; ~ из рук slip out of one's hands; slip through one's fingers; ускользнýть от кого-л. give* smb. the slip; ускользнýть от внимáния кого-л. escápe smb.'s nótice/atténtion.

ускользнýть сов. см. ускользáть.

ускорéние с. accelerátion, spéed-up; ~ социáльно--экономúческого развúтия accelerátion/spéed-up of sócioeconómic devélopment.

ускóренный rápid; ~ курс inténsive course.

ускорúтель м. accélerator; ракéтный ~ rócket bóoster.

ускóрить(ся) сов. см. ускорять(ся).

ускорять, ускóрить (вн.) 1. (делать более скорым, быстрым) speed* up (smth.); accélerate (smth.); ускóрить шаг quícken/mend one's pace; 2. (приближать наступление чего-л.) hásten (smth.), precípitate (smth.); ускóрить собýтия precípitate the course of evénts; ускóрить отъéзд hásten one's depárture; ~ся, ускóриться 1. (становиться более быстрым) speed* up, be* accélerated, pick up speed; 2. (приближаться во времени) be* hástened, be* precípitated.

услáть сов. (вн.) send* (smth.) awáy.

услéд|úть сов. (за тв.) keep* an eye on (smb., smth.); keep* track (on); за всем не ~úшь you can't keep track of éverything; онá не ~úла за ребёнком she didn't keep an eye on the child*.

услóви|е с. condítion; мн. (договора и т. п.) terms; при ~и, что... on condítion that..., províded...; при такúх ~ях in/únder such círcumstances; жить в хорóших ~ях have* good líving condítions; жить в плохúх ~ях have*

bad líving condítions, be* bádly off for accommodátion; создавáть кому-л. все ~я для чего-л. give* smb. éverything nécessary for smth.; при существýющих ~ях únder exísting condítions.

услóв|иться сов. см. услóвливаться. **~ленный** appóinted; (сигнал и т. п.) prearránged, agréed; ~ленный час appóinted hour/time.

услóвливаться, услóвиться (с тв. о пр., с тв. + инф.) arránge (with smb. abóut, with smb. + to inf); agrée upón (smth.); мы услóвились встрéтиться в дéсять часóв we arránged to meet at ten; ~ о врéмени fix time.

услóвн|о condítionally, provísionally; symbólically; ~ приговорúть кого-л. séntence smb. condítionally. **~ость** ж. convéntion. **~ый** 1. (понятный только условившимся) sécret, agréed; ~ый знак sécret sign; ~ый стук agréed knock; ~ое мéсто agréed/sécret spot; 2. (ограниченный условием) condítional, provísional; ~ое соглáсие provísional agréement; ~ый приговóр suspénded séntence; 3. (не существующий в действительности) convéntional, symbólic; ~ая лúния convéntional line; 4. иск. symbólic; ~ая декорáция symbólic scénery; 5. грам. condítional; ~ое предложéние condítional séntence.

усложнúть(ся) сов. см. усложнять(ся).

усложнять, усложнúть (вн.) cómplicate (smth.). ~ся, усложнúться becóme* cómplicated.

услýг|а ж. 1. sérvice; плохáя ~ dissérvice, bad turn; окажúте мне ~у! do me a fávour!; к ~ам кого-л. at smb.'s dispósal; ~ за ~у one good turn desérves anóther; 2. мн. sérvices; небольшúе ~и odd jobs; ◇ я к вáшим ~ам I'm at your sérvice.

услужúть сов. (дт.) do* (smb.) a good turn, help (smb.).

услýжливый oblíging, accómmodating, hélpful.

услýшать сов. см. слýшать 1, 3.

усмáтрив|ать, усмотрéть (вн. в пр.) see* (smth. in); (обнаруживать) nótice (smth. in); я не ~аю в этом ничегó осóбенного I see nóthing in that.

усмехáться, усмехнýться give* a short laugh, smile slíghtly/irónically.

усмехнýться сов. см. усмехáться.

усмéшк|а ж. slight/irónic/wry smile; (презрительная) sneer, smirk; посмотрéть на кого-л. с ~ой regárd smb. quízzically.

усмир|éние с. (мятежа и т. п.) suppréssion. **~úть(ся)** сов. см. усмирять(ся).

усмирять, усмирúть (вн.) 1. (делать смирным) restráin (smb., smth.); (ребёнка) make* (smb.) be quíet; 2. (мятеж и т. п.) quell (smth.), suppréss (smth.), put* (smth.) down. ~ся, усмирúться quíet down, quíeten down.

усмотрéни|е с.: по ~ю кого-л. at smb.'s discrétion; дéйствовать по своемý ~ю use one's discrétion, act as one thinks best.

усмотрéть сов. см. усмáтривать.

уснýть сов. 1. fall* asléep; 2. (о рыбе) die.

усовершéнствов|ание с. impróvement; кýрсы ~ания refrésher course sg. **~анный** impróved.

усовершéнствовать(ся) сов. см. совершéнствовать(ся).

усомнúться сов. (в пр.) doubt (smth.), feel* / have* some doubts (abóut).

усóхнуть сов. см. усыхáть.

успевáемость ж. prógress.

успев|áть, успéть 1. (+ инф.) have* time (+ to inf); успéть всё сдéлать find* time for éverything; я не ~áю дéлать это I néver have/get time to do it; успéете! you have plénty of time!; 2. (к дт., на вн.) разг. (прибывать к сроку) be* in time (for); успéть на пóезд be* in time to catch the train; не успéть на пóезд miss the train; 3. тк. несов. (в пр., по дт.; хорошо учиться) get* on (in), make* prógress (in); ~ по математике get* on well in mathemátics, make* good prógress in mathemátics, do* véry well in mathemátics; не ~ по физике make* poor prógress in phýsics. ~ающий good; ~ающие ученикú good púpils.

успеётся *сов. безл. разг.* there's plénty of time.

успéть *сов. см.* успевáть 1, 2.

успéх *м.* succéss; (*достижение*) achíevement; *мн.* (*хорошие результаты*) prógress *sg*; имéть ~ be* succéssful, meet* with succéss; (*у публики*) be* a succéss; (*о пьесе тж.*) be* a hit; пóльзоваться ~ом у кого-л. be* pópular with *smb.*; желáю (вам) ~а! good luck (to you)!; как ваши ~и? how are you gétting on?; ◇ с ~ом обходúться без чего-л. get* on véry well without *smth.*; с тем же ~ом я мог бы сидéть дóма *ирон.* I might just as well have stáyed at home.

успéшн|о succéssfuly, well; ~ учúться make* good prógress in one's stúdies; дéйствовать ~ óperate efféctively. ~ый succéssful.

успокáив|ать, успокóить (*вн.*) 1. soothe (*smb.*), calm (*smb.*) down; (*ободрять*) reassúre (*smb.*); могу́ вас успокóить I can set your mind at rest; 2. (*смягчать — боль, горе*) assuáge (*smth.*), relíeve (*smth.*); (*заглушать, устранять*) alláy (*smth.*); это óчень ~ает it is véry sóothing; ~ подозрéние alláy suspícion. ~аться, успокóиться 1. (*подавлять волнение, тревогу*) regáin/recóver one's compósure, calm onesélf, calm down; успокóйтесь! calm yoursélf!; (*не беспокойтесь*) don't wórry!; 2. (*становиться спокойным*) séttle down; дéти успокóились и уснýли the chíldren séttled down and went to sleep; 3. *разг.* (*удовлетворяться достигнутым*) be* sátisfied, leave* it at that; ~аться на достúгнутом rest on one's láurels; я не успокóюсь, покá не сдéлаю этого I shall not rest till I have done it; 4. (*о боли*) go* off, reláx, be* relíeved; (*о ветре, море*) calm down, abáte.

успокоéни|е *с.* reassúrance, relíef; для ~я (нéрвов) for the sake of one's peace of mind.

успокóенность *ж.* complácency.

успокойтельн|ый sóothing, reassúring; ~ое извéстие reassúring news; ~ тон reassúring tone; ~ое срéдство sédative, tránquillizer.

успокóить(ся) *сов. см.* успокáивать(ся).

устá *мн. уст.* lips; mouth *sg*; ◇ из уст в ~ from mouth to mouth; у всех на ~x on éverybody's lips.

устáв *м.* regulátions *pl*; *воен. тж.* mánual; Устáв ООН Chárter of the Uníted Nátions.

устав|áть, устáть get* tíred; устáть с дорóги be* tíred áfter one's jóurney; ◇ не ~áя дéлать что-л. do* *smth.* tírelessly.

устáвить *сов.* 1. *см.* уставлять; 2. *разг.*: ~ глазá на кого-л. stare at *smb.* ~ся *сов.* 1. *см.* уставляться; 2. (*на вн.; устремить взгляд*) stare (at).

уставлять, устáвить 1. (*вн.; размещать*) place (*smth.*); устáвить все кнúги в шкаф put* all the books in the bóokcase; 2. (*вн. тв.; занимать всю поверхность*) cram (*smth.* with), fill (*smth.* with); устáвить пóлку кнúгами cram a shelf with books. ~ся, устáвиться (*размещаться*) have* room; все кнúги устáвились в шкафý there was enóugh room for all the books in the bóokcase.

устáл|ость *ж.* fatígue, tíredness, wéariness. ~ый tíred, wéary.

устáл|ь *ж.*: без ~и indefátigably, tírelessly; не знать ~и be* indefátigable/tíreless.

устанáвливать, установúть (*вн.*) 1. (*ставить, помещать*) instáll (*smth.*); (*налаживать*) set* (*smth.*); ~ турбúну instáll a túrbine; 2. (*осуществлять*) órganize (*smth.*), arránge (*smth.*); установúть наблюдéние set* up a watch; 3. (*вводить в действие*) estáblish (*smth.*), fix (*smth.*); (*правила тж.*) lay* down (*smth.*); установúть цéны fix príces; установúть расписáние make* up a tímetable; 4. (*добиваться осуществления чего-л.*)

estáblish (*smth.*), achíeve (*smth.*); установúть тишинý achíeve sílence; 5. (*определять, доказывать*) estáblish (*smth.*); (*выяснять тж.*) ascertáin (*smth.*); установúть фáкты estáblish/ascertáin the facts; установúть úстину estáblish the truth. ~ся, установúться 1. (*укрепляться, входить в силу*) becóme* estáblished, take* root; 2. (*о погоде*) becóme* séttled, set* in; 3. (*формироваться, складываться*) take* shape.

установúть(ся) *сов. см.* устанáвливать(ся).

устанóвка *ж.* 1. (*действие*) installátion; sétting; arránging; estáblishing; 2. (*устройство, механизм*) installátion; 3. (*направленность*) orientátion, précept, máxim; 4. (*директива, указание*) diréctive; instrúctions *pl.*

установлéние *с.* estáblishment; (*определение*) determinátion.

установленный estáblished.

устаревáть, устарéть be*/becóme* óbsolete.

устарéлый óbsolete.

устарéть *сов. см.* устаревáть *и* старéть 2.

устáть *сов. см.* уставáть.

устилáть, устлáть (*вн. тв.*) cóver (*smth.* with); (*коврами, цветами*) cárpet (*smth.* with), strew* (*smth.* with).

устлáть *сов. см.* устилáть.

ýстн|о órally. ~ый óral, vérbal; ~ый экзáмен óral examinátion; ~ые указáния vérbal instrúctions; ~ая речь spóken lánguage; ~ый счёт cóunting in one's head.

устó|й *с.* 1. (*опора моста*) pile, pier; 2. (*опора, подпорка*) foundátion; 3. *мн.* (*основы*) foundátions; нрáвственные ~и móral prínciples.

устóйчив|ость *ж.* stabílity. ~ый 1. (*способный твёрдо стоять*) stéady; сдéлать стол ~ым make* a táble stéady; 2. (*постоянный*) stáble, stéady; (*неизменный*) estáblished; ~ое равновéсие stáble equilíbrium; ~ая валюта stáble cúrrency; ~ые цéны stéady príces; ~ая погóда séttled/stéady wéather; ~ые урожáи stáble hárvests; 3. (*стойкий*) stáble, stéady; ~ые взгляды stáble/séttled opínions.

устоять *сов.* keep* one's feet; *перен.* hold* out; (*против рд.*) resíst (*smb., smth.*); withstánd* (*smb., smth.*), hold* out (agáinst); не ~ перед чем-л. succúmb to *smth.*, not be áble to resíst *smth.* ~ся *сов.* séttle.

устрáив|ать, устрóить (*вн.*) 1. build* (*smth.*), make* (*smth.*); 2. (*организовывать*) arránge (*smth.*), hold* (*smth.*); have* (*smth.*) *разг.*; устрóить вы́ставку hold* an exhibítion; устрóить обéд give* a dínner; я всё устрóю I'll see to éverything; 3. (*налаживать*) arránge (*smth.*), séttle (*smth.*); устрóить свой делá arránge one's affáirs; 4. *разг.* (*учинять*) make* (*smth.*); устрóить сцéну make* a scene; 5. (*помещать, определять*) fix (*smb.*) up; устрóить кого-л. на рабóту get* *smb.* a job; 6. *разг.* (*содействовать кому-л. в чём-л.*) get* (*smth.*); я вам устрóю встрéчу с ним I'll arránge for you to meet him; устрóить кому-л. билéт в теáтр get* *smb.* a théatre tícket; 7. *разг.* (*быть удобным, подходящим*) suit (*smb.*), be* convénient (for); меня это ~ает that suits me. ~аться, устрóиться 1. (*налаживаться*) come* right; всё устрóится it will all come right; всё устрóилось, как мы хотéли éverything turned out the way we wánted it; 2. (*обосновываться*) set* onesélf up, estáblish onesélf, be* fixed up; как вы устрóились на нóвом мéсте? how do you like your new place?; он хорошó устрóился he's dóing well; 3. (*располагаться, размещаться*) make* onesélf cómfortable, fit in, find* a place, find* room; 4. (*поступать на работу*) get* work.

устранéние *с.* remóval; (*уничтожение*) eliminátion.

устранúть(ся) *сов. см.* устранять(ся).

устранять, устранúть (*вн.*) remóve (*smth.*), elíminate (*smth.*), get* rid of (*smth.*); устранúть недостáтки elíminate/erádicate defécts. ~ся, устранúться (от рд.) hold* alóof (from), withdráw* (from), retíre (from).

устрашáть, устрашúть (*вн.*) intímidate (*smb.*), fríghten (*smb.*). ~ся, устрашúться (*рд.*) be* fríghtened (of).

устрашúть(ся) *сов. см.* устрашáть(ся).

устрем|úть(ся) *сов. см.* устремлять(ся). ~лéние *с.* aspirátion.

устремлять, устремúть (*вн.*) diréct (*smth.*) (*тж. перен.*); fix (*smth.*); ~ взгляд на кого-л., что-л. fix one's eye/gaze on *smb.*, *smth.*; ~ внимáние на что-л. cóncentrate one's atténtion on *smth.* ~ся, устремúться 1. (*ринуться*) rush, dash; (*сверху*) swoop down (on); 2. (*к дт.; на вн.; имéть направлéние*) point (at); (*о взгляде*) be* dirécted (towards), be* fíxed (upón); *перен. тж.* be* cóncentrated (on), aspíre (to).

ýстрица *ж.* óyster.

устрóитель *м.* órganizer.

устрóить(ся) *сов. см.* устрáивать(ся).

устрóйств|о *с.* 1. (*дéйствие*) arránging; для ~а свойх дел to see to one's affáirs; 2. (*строй*) sýstem, sét-up; 3. (*конструкция*) constrúction, design; (*планировка*) arrángement, láy-out; 4. (*механизм, сооружéние*) device, appliance, apparátus.

устýп *м.* ledge, projéction.

уступáть, уступúть 1. (*вн. дт.; отдавáть*) let* (*smb.*) have (*smth.*); (*отдавáть при отступлéнии*) cede (*smth.* to), yield (*smth.* to); ~ дорóгу кому-л. let* *smb.* pass, make* way for *smb.*; ~ мéсто кому-л. give* up one's place to *smb.*; он уступúл свой билéт другу he let his friend have his tícket; ~ территóрию cede térritory; 2. (*дт. в пр.; поддавáться*) yield (to *smb.* óver), give* in (to *smb.* óver), give* way (to *smb.* óver); ~ сúле, давлéнию yield to force, préssure; он никомý ни в чём не устýпит he néver makes concéssions to ányone; 3. (*быть не в состоянии сравняться*): не ~ кому-л. be* just as good as *smb.*, be* in no way inférior to *smb.*; ~ кому-л. в сúле, умé и т. п. not be as strong, cléver, *etc.* as *smb.*; не ~ кому-л. в сúле, умé и т. п. be* just as strong, cléver, *etc.* as *smb.*; be* a match for *smb.*

уступúтельный *грам.* concéssive; ~ союз concéssive conjúnction.

уступúть *сов. см.* уступáть.

устýпк|а *ж.* 1. (*дéйствие*) yíelding; (*территóрии*) céssion; 2. (*компромúсс*) concéssion; идтú на ~и make* concéssions; взаúмные ~и mútual concéssions; give-and-táke *sg*; 3. (*в ценé*) redúction in price.

устýпчив|ость *ж.* compliance, plíancy. ~ый yíelding, plíant, compliant; он ~ый человéк he's véry compliant, he is álways réady to yield.

устыдúть (*вн.*) shame (*smb.*). ~ся *сов.* (*рд.*) be* ashámed (of).

ýстье *с.* mouth; (*отвéрстие тж.*) órifice, ópening.

усугуб|úть(ся) *сов. см.* усугублять(ся).

усугублять, усугубúть (*вн.*) inténsify (*smth.*), redóuble (*smth.*). ~ся, усугубúться incréase, inténsify.

усы́ *мн.* (*ед.* ус *м.*) 1. moustáche; 2. (*животного*) whiskers.

усынов|úть *сов. см.* усыновлять. ~лéние *с.* adóption. ~лять, усыновúть (*вн.*) adópt (*smb.*).

усы́пать *сов. см.* усыпáть.

усыпáть, усы́пать (*вн. тв.; прям. и перен.*) strew* (*smth.* with), cóver (*smth.* with).

усы́пить *сов. см.* усыплять.

усыплять, усыпúть (*вн.*) 1. lull (*smb.*) to sleep; *перен.* lull (*smb.*); ~ подозрéния alláy/lull suspícions; 2. (*наркóзом*) put* (*smb.*) to sleep.

усыхáть, усóхнуть shrível up (*тж. перен.*); (*о лúстве тж.*) wither.

утаúть, утаúть (*вн.*) 1. (*скрывáть*) concéal (*smth.*); (*умáлчивать*) keep* back (*smth.*); ~ фáкты keep* back the facts; 2. (*прятать*) hide* (*smth.*); 3. (*присвáивать*) steal* (*smth.*).

утаúть *сов. см.* утáивать.

утáйк|а *ж. разг.*: без ~и withóut kéeping ánything back.

утáптывать, утоптáть (*вн.*) stamp (*smth.*) down, flátten (*smth.*).

утащúть (*вн.*) 1. take* (*smth.*) awáy, cárry (*smth.*) off; (*волочá*) drag (*smth.*) awáy; 2. *разг.* (*украсть*) walk off (with), pinch (*smth.*).

ýтварь *ж. собир.* uténsils *pl.*

утвердúтельн|о in the affírmative; ~ кивнýть головóй nod assént. ~ый affírmative.

утвердúть *сов. см.* утверждáть 2, 3, 4. ~ся *сов. см.* утверждáться.

утвержд|áть, утвердúть 1. *тк. несов.* (*вн.; настойчиво говорúть*) assért (*smth.*), affírm (*smth.*), maintáin (*smth.*); (*в спóре тж.*) conténd (*smth.*); (*необоснованно*) allége (*smth.*); категорúчески ~ flátly assért, maintáin pósitively; 2. (*вн.; устанáвливать, укреплять*) fírmly estáblish (*smth.*); утвердúть своё госпóдство secúre one's pówer/predóminance; 3. (*вн. в пр.; убеждáть*) stréngthen (*smb.* in), confírm (*smb.* in); 4. (*вн.; принимáть окончáтельное решéние*) confírm (*smth.*), pass (*smth.*), okáy (*smth.*) *разг.*; (*санкционúровать*) confírm (*smth.*); утвердúть проéкт pass a design; утвердúть повéстку дня pass an agénda; утвердúть рекóрд régister a récord; утвердúть когó-л. в дóлжности дирéктора confírm *smb.'s* appóintment as diréctor. ~áться, утвердúться 1. (*укрепляться*) be* fírmly estáblished; 2. (*в пр.; убеждáться*) be* convínced (in); утвердúться в намéрении книжн. be* confírmed in one's inténtion.

утверждéние *с.* 1. (*дéйствие*) confirmátion; ~ когó-либо в дóлжности confirmátion of *smb.'s* appóintment; ~ плáна confirmátion of a plan; 2. (*мысль, положéние*) affirmátion, assértion; (*голослóвное*) allegátion.

утекáть, утéчь (*о жúдкости*) escápe; ◇ мнóго воды́ утеклó с тех пор much wáter has flówed únder the bridges since then.

утёнок *м.* dúckling.

утепл|éние *с.* máking (*smth.*) cóldproof, winterizátion. ~úть *сов. см.* утеплять.

утеплять, утеплúть (*вн.*) make* (*smth.*) cóldproof, winterize (*smth.*).

утерéть(ся) *сов. см.* утирáть(ся).

утерпé|ть *сов.* stop onesélf, hold* out; я едвá ~л, чтóбы не рассмеяться I could hárdly restráin mysélf from láughing; трýдно ~! how could one resíst?

утéря *ж.* loss.

утерять *сов.* (*вн.*) lose* (*smth.*). ~ся *сов.* get* lost.

утёс *м.* rock; (*прибрéжный*) cliff.

утéчка *ж.* leak, léakage; ~ информáции informátion leak.

утéчь *сов. см.* утекáть.

утеш|áть, утéшить (*вн.*) cómfort (*smb.*), consóle (*smb.*). ~áться, утéшиться consóle onesélf; утéшиться мы́слью о том, что... deríve consolátion from the thought that... ~éние *с.* cómfort, consolátion; sólace *поэт.*; слáбое ~éние! that's not much consolátion! ~úтельный consóling, cómforting.

утéшить(ся) *сов. см.* утешáть(ся).

утилизúровать *несов. и сов.* (*вн.*) útilize (*smth.*), find* a use (for).

утилитáрный utilitárian.

утúль *м.*, утильсырьё *с. собир.* scrap, sálvage.

утú|н|ый duck's; ~ые лáпы duck's feet.

утирáть, утерéть (*вн.*) wipe (*smth.*); ~ слёзы wipe awáy one's tears; ◇ утерéть нос кому-л. score off *smb.* ~ся, утерéться wipe one's face.

утихáть, утúхнуть 1. die down, subsíde (*тж. перен.*); (*о звуке*) die awáy; (*о бóли*) abáte, grow* less; 2. (*успокáиваться — о человéке*) becóme* quíet.

утúхнуть *сов. см.* утихáть.

утихомúрить *сов.* (*вн.*) *разг.* pácify (*smb.*, *smth.*);

calm (smb., smth.) down. ~ся сов. разг. calm down; (ослабеть — о действии чего-л.) die down, slácken off.

у́тк|а ж. 1. duck; 2. (ложный слух) cánard; газе́тная ~ néwspaper hoax; пусти́ть ~у start a cánard, put* out a false repórt.

уткну́ть сов. (вн.) разг. búry (smth.); ~ нос в кни́гу búry one's nose in a book. ~ся сов. разг. plunge; búry (тж. перен.); ~ся головóй в подýшку búry one's head in one's píllow; ~ся в кни́гу búry onesélf in a book.

у́тлый frail.

утолще́ние с. thíckening, bulge.

утоли́ть сов. см. утоля́ть.

утоля́ть, утоли́ть (вн.) (жажду) quench (smth.), slake (smth.); (голод) assuáge (smth.); перен. alláy (smth.), allévіate (smth.).

утоми́тельн|ый exháusting, tíring; ~ая рабóта exháusting work.

утом|и́ть(ся) сов. см. утомля́ть(ся). ~ле́ние с. fatigue, wéariness. ~лённый tíred, wéary.

утомл|я́ть, утоми́ть (вн.) tíre (smb.); (сильно) exháust (smb.). ~я́ться, утоми́ться tíre (onesélf); get* tíred; он бы́стро ~я́ется he tíres éasily.

утону́ть сов. см. тонýть и утопáть 1.

утончённый refíned; ~ вкус sophístіcated taste.

утопа́ть, утону́ть (в пр.) 1. (погружаться) sink* (into); перен. be* búried (in); ~ в снегý sink* waist deep into the snow, be* up to one's neck in snow; перен. be* búried in snow; ~ в зéлени, цветáх be* búried in fóliage, flówers; 2. тк. несов. (пользоваться чем-л. в излишестве) wállow (in), roll (in); ~ в богáтстве be* rólling in wealth; ~ в рóскоши be* wállowing in lúxury. ◇ ~ в крови́ wállow in blood.

утопа́ющий м. drówning man*.

утоп|и́зм м. Utópianism, Útopism. ~и́ст м. Utópian.

утопи́ть сов. см. топи́ть III. ~ся сов. см. топи́ться III.

утопи́ческий Utópian.

уто́пия ж. Utópia.

уто́пленн|ик м. drówned man*. ~ица ж. drówned wóman*.

утопта́ть сов. см. утáптывать.

уточн|е́ние с. clóser definítion; (выяснение) verificátion; вноси́ть ~е́ния в формулирóвку make* the wórding/definítion more precíse. ~и́ть сов. см. уточня́ть.

уточни́ть, уточни́ть (вн.) make* (smth.) more áccurate/precíse; (выяснять) find* out (smth.) exáctly, vérify (smth.).

утра́ивать, утро́ить (вн.) tréble (smth.). ~ся, утро́иться tréble, incréase thréefold.

утрамбова́ть сов. (вн.) pound (smth.) flat; (ногами) stamp (smth.) down, tread* (smth.) smooth.

утра́т|а ж. loss. ~ить сов. см. утра́чивать.

утра́чивать, утра́тить (вн.) lose* (smth.).

у́тренн|ий mórning attr.; ~яя заря́ dawn; ~ие замо́розки mórning frosts; ~яя заря́дка mórning éxercises pl.

у́тренник м. 1. (спектакль) matinée; 2. (мороз) mórning frost.

утри́рованный exággerated.

утри́ровать несов. и сов. (вн.) exággerate (smth.); (роль) overáct (smth.).

у́тр|о с. mórning; пять часóв ~á five in the mórning, 5 a. m.; по ~áм in the mórning; (каждое утро) évery mórning; на (следующее) ~ the next mórning; ◇ дóброе ~!, с дóбрым ~ом! good mórning!; с ~á since mórning, (очень рано) first thing in the mórning; он рабóтал с ~á he had been wórking since mórning; нáдо пойти́ на ры́нок с ~á you must go to the márket first thing in the mórning.

утро́б|а ж. bélly; ~ мáтери womb. ~ный úterine.

утро́ить(ся) сов. см. утра́ивать(ся).

у́тром in the mórning; сего́дня ~ this mórning; вчерá, зáвтра ~ yésterday, tomórrow mórning.

утружда́ть несов. (вн.) tróuble (smb.).

утю́|г м. íron. ~жить (вн.) íron (smth.); (костюм и т. п. тж.) press (smth.).

уф phew!

ух oh!; (при обозначении звука) thump!; (о взрывах) crump!, boom!

ухá ж. fish-soup.

ухáб м. pót-hole. ~истый pítted, búmpy.

ухáживать несов. (за тв.) 1. (заботиться) look (áfter); (за больным тж.) nurse (smb.); 2. (за женщиной) court (smb.); woo (smb.) поэт.

ухвати́ть сов. (вн.) seize (smth.); перен. grasp (smth.). ~ся сов. (за вн.) 1. (взяться за что-л.) grasp (smth.), seize (smth.), clutch (smth.), get* hold (of); ~ся за пери́ла grasp the rail; 2. разг. (быстро приняться за что-л.) set* abóut (smth.), get* down (to); 3. разг. (воспользоваться) jump at (smb., smth.); ~ся за мысль jump at the idéa.

ухва́тка ж. разг. 1. (ловкость) knack; 2. (повадка) mánner.

ухитри́ться сов. см. ухитря́ться.

ухитря́ться, ухитри́ться (+ инф.) разг. mánage (+ to inf), contríve (+ to inf).

ухищр|е́ние с. trick, devíce. ~я́ться несов. contríve, scheme; wángle разг.; (хитрить) bluff; ~я́ться всéми спóсобами try évery trick.

ухмыльну́ться сов. см. ухмыля́ться.

ухмыля́ться, ухмыльну́ться разг. smirk, grin.

у́х|о с. ear; ◇ говори́ть нá ухо кому́-л. whísper in smb.'s ear; заткну́ть ýши stop one's ears; в ушáх звени́т there is a rínging in one's ears; слы́шать что-л. свои́ми ушáми hear* smth. with one's own ears; во все ýши слýшать lísten all ears; он и ~ом не ведёт he dóesn't turn a hair; в однó ~ вошлó, в другóе вы́шло it went in at one ear and out at the óther; пó уши влюби́ться fall* head óver heels in love, fall* mádly in love.

ухóд I м. depárture, léaving; (с должности) resignátion; перед (сáмым) ~ом (just) befóre léaving; ~ из семьи́ léaving one's fámily; ~ со сцéны léaving the stage.

ухóд II м. (заботы) care; ~ за посéвами care of crops; ~ за рáнеными care of the wóunded.

уходи́ть, уйти́ 1. (отправляться куда-л.) go* (awáy), depárt; (из, от, с рд.) leave* (smth.); уйти́ домóй leave* for home, go* home; уйти́ на рабóту leave* for work, go* off to work; пóезд ужé ушёл the train has left; ~ в мóре put* out to sea; уйти́ на вёслах row awáy; 2. (от рд.; скрываться, спасаться) escápe (from), get* awáy (from); 3. (от когó-л.; покидать) leave* (smb.); (от чегó-л.) перен. rid* onesélf (of); 4. (переставать заниматься чем-л.) leave*; уйти́ с рабóты leave* one's job; уйти́ в óтпуск go* on leave; уйти́ на пéнсию retíre; ~ со сцéны leave* the stage; 5. (проходить — о времени) pass; врéмя ещё не ушлó it's not too late; 6. (на вн.; расходоваться) go* (on), be* spent (on); на это ухóдит мнóго врéмени that takes a lot of time; все си́лы ухóдят на это one's whole énergy goes on that; 7.: часы́ ушли́ вперёд the watch/clock is fast; за недéлю часы́ ушли́ на пять минýт the watch/clock has gained five minutes in the last week; 8. (в вн.; увлекаться чем-л.) give* onesélf up (to), devóte onesélf (to); уйти́ в наýку devóte onesélf to scíence; с головóй уйти́ во что-л. be* engróssed in smth.; 9. тк. несов. (простираться) stretch, exténd; дорóга ухóдит вдаль the road disappéars into the dístance; ◇ с этим далекó не уйдёшь that won't get you véry far; уйти́ ни с чем get* no satisfáction, leave* empty-hánded; уйти́ в себя́ withdráw* ínto onesélf; уйти́ вперёд forge ahéad; пóчва ушлá из-под ног когó-либо the ground disappéared únder smb.'s feet.

уху́дш|ать, уху́дшить (вн.) make* (smth.) worse; wórsen (smth.); (состояние тж.) ággravate (smth.); ~ дéло make* mátters worse; ~ состоя́ние здорóвья have* a bad efféct on smb.'s health. ~áться, ухудшиться be* (gétting) worse; (о положении, состоянии тж.) be* ággravated; (о качестве) detériorate. ~éние с. change for the worse; (положения, состояния) aggravátion; (качества) deterioration; ~éние отношéний a fálling-off in smb.'s relátions.

ухýдшить(ся) сов. см. ухудшáть(ся).

уцел|éть сов. not be ínjured; (о предметах тж.) be* undámaged; (остаться в живых) survíve; ~ при пожáре survíve a fire, come* through a fire undámaged; пять человéк ~éло five pérsons escáped with their lives; никтó не ~éл there were no survívors; ~ тóлько чýдом have* a miráculous escápe.

уценённ|ый cút-price attr.; redúced in price после сущ.; ~ые товáры goods at redúced príces.

уцепи́ться сов. (за вн.) 1. (зацепиться) catch* hold (of); (схватиться) hold* on (to); cling* (to); 2. разг. (воспользоваться) make* use (of), turn (smth.) to accóunt.

учáствовать несов. (в пр.) take* part (in); párticipate (in).

учáсти|е с. 1. participátion; 2. (сочувствие) sýmpathy (for); отнести́сь с ~ем к кому-л., приня́ть дрýжеское ~ в ком-л. be* kind to smb., befriend smb., take* an ínterest in smb.

участи́ться сов. см. учащáться.

участкóв|ый прил. 1. divísional; ~ая избирáтельная комиссия divísional eléction committee; 2. в знач. сущ. м. разг. (милиционер) dístrict milítia ófficer.

учáстлив|о with sýmpathy. ~ый sympathétic, kind.

учáстник м. partícipant; (член) mémber; ~ состязáния compétitor.

учáст|ок м. 1. (часть земельной площади) plot; строи́тельный ~ búilding plot; ~ обрабóтанной земли́ plot of cúltivated land; 2. (часть поверхности чего-л.) área; поражённые ~ки ткáни affécted áreas (of tíssue); 3. (часть фронта) séctor; 4. (сфера деятельности) field, depártment; отвéтственный ~ работы respónsible field; 5. (административно-территориальное или производственное подразделение) séctor, divísion; précinct амер.

ýчасть ж. fate, lot.

учащáться, участи́ться becóme* more fréquent, incréase in fréquency; (о пульсе) becóme* more rápid, beat* fáster.

учащённ|ый: ~ пульс high pulse rate, rápid pulse; ~ темп héightened rate; ~ое дыхáние rápid bréathing.

учáщийся м. stúdent; (школьник) púpil.

учёб|а ж. stúdies pl; (специальная) tráining; послáть когó-л. на ~у send* smb. to stúdy; (для получения специальности) send* smb. for spécial tráining.

учéбник м. téxtbook; ~ истóрии téxtbook on history, history-book.

учéбн|ый educátional; (школьный тж.) school attr.; воен. tráining attr.; ~ год schóol-year; (в вузе) académic year; ~ое врéмя schóol-hours pl; (в вузе) stúdy-hours pl; ~ое заведéние school, educátional estáblishment; ~ые посóбия téaching aids; educátional equípment sg; ~ план currículum; ~ая стрельбá shóoting práctice.

учéни|е с. 1. (теория) théory, dóctrine, téaching; 2. обыкн. мн. воен. éxercise sg; tráining sg; 3. stúdies pl; (ремеслу) apprénticeship.

учен|и́к м., ~и́ца ж. 1. púpil; 2. (обучающийся какой-л. профессии у кого-л.) appréntice; ~ тóкаря túrner's appréntice; 3. (последователь) discíple, fóllower. ~и́ческий instrúction attr., school attr.; перен. (незрелый) immatúre, begínner's. ~и́чество с. 1. time as a púpil; гóды ~и́чества school years; 2. (обучение ремеслу) apprénticeship.

учён|ость ж. erudítion, léarning. ~ый прил. 1. léarned, érudite; 2. (научный) scientífic; ~ый совéт académic board; ~ая стéпень degrée; 3. (выученный че-

му-л.) trained; (о животных) perfórming; перен. разг. wíser (from expérience); 4. в знач. сущ. м. léarned man*, scíentist, man* of scíence; schólar (гл. образом в области гуманитарных наук).

учёт м. 1. (действие) accóunting, calculátion; (принятие во внимание) considerátion, appreciátion; ~ товáров stóck-taking; магази́н закры́т на ~ the shop is closed for stóck-taking; 2. (регистрация) registrátion; брать когó-л. на ~ régister smb.; снимáть когó-л. с ~а strike* smb. off the régister; ◇ ~ векселéй díscounting. ~ный 1. récord attr.; ~ная кáрточка récord card; 2. фин. díscount attr.

учётч|ик м., ~ица ж. récord-keeper.

учи́лище с. (spécialized) school.

учини́ть сов. см. учиня́ть.

учиня́ть, учини́ть (вн.) разг. make* (smth.); учини́ть распрáву над кем-л. inflict reprísals on smb.; учини́ть сканда́л creáte a row.

учи́тель м., ~ница ж. téacher; шкóльный ~ schóolmaster; шкóльная ~ница schóolmistress; ~ геогрáфии geógraphy téacher; ~ англи́йского языкá Énglish téacher; ~ская ж. téachers' cómmon room. ~ский téachers'. ~ство с. 1. (профессия) téaching; 2. собир. (учителя) téachers pl.

учи́тельствовать несов. be* a téacher, teach*.

учи́тывать, учéсть (вн.) 1. (производить учёт) take* stock (of), count up (smth.); 2. (принимать во внимание) take* (smth.) into considerátion/accóunt, bear* (smth.) in mind, appréciate (smth.); учéсть óпыт предшéственников take* into accóunt the expérience of one's prédecessors; ◇ учéсть вéксель díscount a bill.

учи́ть несов. 1. (когó-л. дт., когó-л. + инф.) teach* (smb., smth.); ~ когó-л. грáмоте teach* smb. to read and write; чемý вас там ýчат? what do they teach you there?; 2. (с союзом что; развивать теорию) teach*; 3. (что-л.; запоминать, усваивать) learn* (smth.); (роль тж.) stúdy (smth.); ~ урóки do* one's léssons; ~ стихотворéние learn* a póem. ~ся несов. 1. (дт.; приобретать знания) learn* (smth.), stúdy (smth.); ~ся мýзыке stúdy músic; ~ся англи́йскому языкý learn* Énglish; 2. (быть учащимся): ~ся в шкóле go* to school; ~ся в университéте stúdy/be* at a univérsity, be* in/at cóllege; ~ся на шофёра train to be a dríver.

учреди́тельн|ый constítuent; ~ое собрáние Constítuent Assémbly.

учреди́ть сов. см. учреждáть.

учрежд|áть, учреди́ть (вн.) 1. found (smth.), set* up (smth.); 2. (вводить) ínstitute (smth.), introdúce (smth.). ~éние с. 1. (действие) fóunding; 2. (организация) institútion, organizátion; госудáрственное ~éние state institútion.

учýять сов. (вн.) разг. scent (smth.); перен. тж. sense (smth.).

ушáт м. tub.

уши́б м. bruise.

ушибáть, ушиби́ть (вн.) hurt* (smth.). ~ся, уши-би́ться hurt* onesélf.

ушиби́ть(ся) сов. см. ушибáть(ся).

ушивáть, уши́ть (вн.) take* in (smth.).

уши́ть сов. см. ушивáть.

ушкó с. 1. (ýхо; 2. (иголки) eye; 3. (сапога) tab.

ушн|óй ear attr.; ~áя сéра éar-wax.

ущéлье с. ravíne, gorge, cányon.

ущеми́ть сов. см. ущемля́ть.

ущемля́ть, ущеми́ть (вн.) 1. (зажимать) pinch (smth.), squeeze (smth.); ущеми́ть пáлец двéрью pinch one's finger in the door; 2. (ограничивать) restríct (smth., smth.), inerfére (with); (оскорблять) wound (smth.), hurt* (smth.); ~ чьё-л. самолю́бие wound smb.'s pride.

уще́рб *м.* dámage; détriment; без ~а для де́ла withóut détriment to *one's* work; ◇ в ~ кому́-л., чему́-л. to the détriment of *smb.*, *smth.*; луна́ на ~е the moon is on the wane. ~ный 1. (*о луне*) wáning; 2. (*о характере и т. п.*) deficient, unbálanced.

ущипну́ть *сов.* (*вн.*) pinch (*smb.*, *smth.*).

ую́т *м.* cómfort. ~ный cósy; (*с удобствами*) cómfortable.

уязви́м|ость *ж.* vulnerabílity. ~ый vúlnerable; ~ое ме́сто vúlnerable/weak spot.

уязви́ть *сов. см.* уязвля́ть.

уязвля́ть, уязви́ть (*вн.*) wound (*smb.*, *smth.*), sting* (*smb.*, *smth.*); э́то замеча́ние уязви́ло его́ he was stung by this remárk.

уясни́ть *сов. см.* уясня́ть.

уясня́ть, уясни́ть (*вн.*) get* (*smth.*) clear, understánd (*smth.*); ~ себе́ положе́ние size up the situátion.

Ф

фа *с. нескл. муз.* fa, F.

фа́брика *ж.* fáctory, mill, plant; бума́жная ~ páper-mill.

фабрика́нт *м.* manufácturer, fáctory-owner.

фабрика́т *м.* manufáctured árticle/próduct.

фабрика́ция *ж.* fabricátion.

фаброкова́ть, сфаброкова́ть (*вн.*) *разг. ирон.* churn (*smth.*) out by the thóusand; manufácture (*smth.*) (*тк. перен.*).

фабри́чн|ый fáctory *attr.*; (*промышленный*) indústrial; ~ гудо́к fáctory hóoter; ~ая ма́рка trádemark; ~ райо́н indústrial dístrict; ~ городо́к fáctory estáte.

фа́була *ж.* plot.

фаво́р *м.*: быть в ~е у кого́-л. be* in *smb.'s* good gráces; быть не в ~е у кого́-л. be* out of fávour with *smb.*, be* in *smb.'s* bad books.

фавори́т *м.*, ~ка *ж.* fávourite.

фаго́т *м. муз.* bassóon.

фа́за *ж.* phase.

фаза́н *м.* phéasant. ~ий phéasant's.

фазотро́н *м. физ.* sýnchro-cýclotron, phásotron.

фа́кел *м.* 1. torch; 2. (*конусообразное пламя*) jet, tongue.

фа́кельщик *м.* (*участник процессии*) tórch-bearer.

факси́мил|е *с. нескл.* 1. facsímile, réplica; 2. (*клише, печатка*) signature stamp; 3. *в знач. неизм. прил. и нареч.* in facsímile; и́здано ~ reprodúced in facsímile. ~ьный facsímile *attr.*; ~ьное изда́ние facsímile edítion.

факт *м.* 1. fact; достове́рный ~ estáblished fact; ~ы — упря́мая вещь there is no gétting awáy from the facts; соверши́вшийся ~ accómplished fact; 2. *в знач. сказ. разг.*: ~! that's fact!; ◇ поста́вить кого́-л. перед соверши́вшимся ~ом presént *smb.* with a fait accomplí.

факти́ческ|и áctually. ~ий áctual; ~ие да́нные the facts; ~ая сторона́ де́ла the fáctual áspect of the case; ~ое положе́ние де́ла the áctual state of affáirs; ~ое призна́ние de fácto recognítion.

фа́ктор *м.* fáctor.

факто́рия *ж.* tráding státion.

факту́ра *ж.* 1. *иск.* téxture; 2. (*характер обработки*) fínish; 3. *торг.* ínvoice.

факультати́вный óptional; eléctive *амер.*

факульте́т *м.* fáculty, depártment; school *амер.*; я учу́сь на юриди́ческом ~е I am in the law depártment, I am réading law. ~ский fáculty *attr.*; ~ское собра́ние fáculty méeting.

фала́нга *ж.* 1. phálanx (*pl* -xes, -nges); *перен.* ranks *pl*; 2. *анат.* phálanx, phálange.

фа́лда *ж.* tail.

фальсифик|а́тор *м.* fálsifier; ~а́торы исто́рии fálsifiers of hístory. ~а́ция *ж.* 1. (*действие*) fórging; (*продуктов*) adulterátion; ~а́ция докуме́нтов fórging of dócuments; 2. (*искажение*) falsificátion, distórtion; ~а́ция истори́ческих фа́ктов distórtion of the histórical facts; 3. (*подделанная вещь*) fake.

фальсифици́ровать *несов. и сов.* (*вн.*) fálsify (*smth.*), twist (*smth.*), distórt (*smth.*), gárble (*smth.*).

фальц *м.* 1. (*выемка*) rábbet; 2. (*паз*) groove, slot; 3. (*место сгиба листа*) fold.

фальцева́ть, сфальцева́ть (*вн.*) 1. *тех.* rábbet (*smth.*); 2. (*сгибать бумажный лист*) fold (*smth.*).

фальце́т *м. муз.* falsétto. ~ом in falsétto, in a falsétto voice.

фальши́вить, сфальши́вить 1. (*притворяться*) be* insincére, be* hypocrítical, preténd; 2. (*фальшиво играть, петь*) sing*, play out of tune; (*на рояле*) play wrong notes.

фальши́вка *ж. разг.* fórgery.

фальши́в|ый 1. (*поддельный*) false, forged; ~ая моне́та false/dud coin; ~ые докуме́нты forged pápers; 2. (*сделанный наподобие подлинного*) imitátion *attr.*; ~ карма́н imitátion pócket; 3. (*неискренний, неестественный*) false, insincére; ~ челове́к insincére pérson; ~ая улы́бка false smile; 4. (*искажающий мелодию*) false; ~ая но́та false/wrong note.

фальшь *ж.* 1. (*неискренность*) preténce, insincérity; (*надуманность*) fálsity; 2. (*в пении и игре на музыкальном инструменте*) sínging, pláying out of tune.

фами́лия *ж.* 1. súrname, name; как ва́ша ~? what is your súrname?; 2. (*род*) fámily.

фами́льн|ый fámily *attr.*; ~ые портре́ты fámily pórtraits; ~ое схо́дство fámily líkeness.

фамилья́рничать *несов.* (*с тв.*) *разг.* be* too famíliar (with).

фамилья́рн|о withóut céremony, unceremóniously. ~ость *ж.* familiárity, unceremóniousness; не допуска́ть ~остей allów no familiárity, stand* on *one's* dígnity; позволя́ть себе́ ~ости be* undúly famíliar. ~ый unceremónious, (too) famíliar.

фанати́зм *м.* fanáticism.

фана́т|ик *м.* fanátic. ~и́ческий, ~и́чный fanátical.

фане́р|а *ж.* 1. venéer, venéering; лист ~ы leaf*/sheet of venéer; 2. (*многослойная*) plýwood. ~ный venéer *attr.*; (*сделанный из фанеры*) plýwood *attr.*; ~ный я́щик plýwood box.

фантазёр *м.*, ~ка *ж.* románcer, dréamer; fántasist.

фантази́ровать *несов.* románce; (*выдумывать тж.*) make* things up.

фанта́з|ия *ж.* 1. (*воображение*) imaginátion, fáncy; 2. (*мечта*) dreams *pl*; 3. *разг.* (*причуда*) cáprice, whim, fántasy; жить в ми́ре ~ий live in a fántasy world; придёт же в го́лову така́я ~! extraórdinary idéas sómetimes pass through *one's* mind; 4. *муз.* fantásia.

фанта́ст *м.* (*о писателе*) science fiction wríter.

фанта́стик|а *ж.* 1. make-believe, fántasy, flight of fáncy; на гра́ни ~и álmost unréal/unbelíevable, bórdering on fántasy; 2. *собир. разг.* (*литературные произведения*) fántasies *pl*, fántasy fiction; нау́чная ~ science fiction.

фантасти́ч|еский 1. (*основанный на фантастике*) fantástic; ~ рома́н fantástic nóvel, románce; 2. (*причудливый, нелепый, странный*) fánciful; fantástic(al), absúrd; ~ вид fánciful appéarance; 3. (*исключительный*) éxcellent; fantástic; он ~ певе́ц he's a fantástic sínger; 4. (*огромный*) fantástic; ~ уще́рб fantástic dámage; 5. (*невероятный, несбыточный*) fantástic, wild, impróbable; ~ прое́кт fantástic/wild próject. ~ность *ж.* incredibílity; absúrdity; improbabílity; imáginary/máke-believe quálity.

фанфа́ра *ж.* 1. *(музыкальный инструмент)* trúmpet; 2. *(сигнал)* trúmpet-call; 3. *муз.* fánfare (of trúmpets), flóurish of trúmpets.

фа́ра *ж.* héadlight, héadlamp.

фарва́тер *м.* (návigating) chánnel, fáirway; ◇ плыть, идти́, находи́ться в ~е кого́-л., чего́-л. fóllow *smb.'s, smth.'s* lead, go* alóng with *smb., smth.*

Фаренге́йт *м.:* термо́метр ~a Fáhrenheit thermómeter.

фарисе́й Phárisee. ~ский Pharisáical; ~ские фра́зы hypocrítical phráses. ~ство *с.* hypócrisy.

фармако́лог *м.* pharmacólogist.

фармаколо́гия *ж.* pharmacólogy.

фармакопе́я *ж.* pharmacopóeia.

фармаце́вт *м.* pharmacéutist, phármacist.

фармацевти́ческий pharmacéutical.

фарс *м.* farce (*тж. перен.*).

фа́ртук *м.* ápron.

фарфо́р *м.* 1. chína, pórcelain; 2. *собир. (изделия)* chína(ware). ~овый chína *attr.*, pórcelain *attr.*; ~овая посу́да chína(ware).

фарцева́ть *несов. разг.* spéculate (in cúrrency, fóreign clothes *etc.*).

фарцо́вщик *м. разг.* spiv, black-marketéer.

фарш *м.* stúffing; *(мясной)* fórce-meat; *(колбасный)* sáusage-meat.

фарширо́ванный stuffed.

фарширова́ть *несов. (вн.)* stuff (*smth.*).

фаса́д *м.* façáde, front.

фасо́ванный páckaged.

фасова́ть *несов. (вн.)* páckage (*smth.*).

фасо́вочн|ый páckaging; ~ая фа́брика páckaging fáctory.

фасо́ль *ж.* 1. *(растение)* háricot bean; зелёная ~ rúnner bean; 2. *собир. (семена)* beans *pl.*

фасо́н *м.* style; *(платья тж.)* cut. ~ный shaped.

фатали́зм *м.* fátalism.

фата́льный 1. fátal; 2. *(обречённый)* resígned; ~ вид air of resignátion.

фа́уна *ж.* fáuna.

фаш|и́зм *м.* fáscism. ~и́ст *м.* fáscist. ~и́стский fáscist.

файнс *м. собир. (изделия)* faiénce, glazed póttery.

февра́л|ь *м.* Fébruary; в ~é э́того го́да this/in Fébruary; в ~é про́шлого го́да last Fébruary; last year in Fébruary; в ~é бу́дущего го́да next Fébruary.

февра́льский Fébruary *attr.*; ◇ Февра́льская револю́ция the Fébruary Revolútion.

федера́льный féderal.

федерати́вный féderative.

федера́ция *ж.* federátion.

фееpи́ч|еский, ~ный enchánting, mágical.

фее́рия *ж.* fáiry-tale play, pántomime; *перен.* enchánting spéctacle/sight.

фейерве́рк *м.* fireworks *pl.*

фельдма́ршал *м.* Field Márshal.

фельдшер *м.* dóctor's assístant, médical atténdant.

фельдъе́герск|ий state méssenger's; ~ая связь cóurier sérvice.

фельдъе́герь *м.* state méssenger.

фельето́н *м.* satírical árticle, néwspaper sátire. ~и́ст *м.* néwspaper sátirist. ~ный of a néwspaper sátire *после сущ; перен. разг.* knóckabout *attr.*

фен *м.* háir-dryer, háir-drier.

феноме́н *м.* phenómenon.

феномена́льный phenómenal, excéptional.

феода́л *м. ист.* féudal lord. ~и́зм *м.* féudalism.

феода́льный féudal.

ферзь *м. шахм.* queen.

фе́рма I *ж.* 1. farm; 2. *(часть хозяйства)* depártment; моло́чная ~ dáiry depártment.

фе́рма II *ж. (конструкция)* truss, (cómpound) gírder.

ферме́нт *м. биол., хим.* énzyme, férment.

фе́рмер *м.* fármer. ~ство *с.* 1. *(занятие)* fárming; 2. *собир. (фермеры)* the fármers.

ферроспла́в *м.* férro-alloy.

фестива́ль *м.* féstival. ~ный féstival *attr.*

фесто́н *м.* 1. *архит.* festóon; 2. *(зубчатая кайма)* scállop.

фетр *м.* felt. ~овый felt *attr.*

фехтова́ль|ный féncing. ~щик *м.* féncer.

фехтов|а́ние *с.* féncing. ~а́ть *несов.* fence.

фе́я *ж.* fáiry.

фиа́лка *ж. бот.* víolet.

фиа́ско *с. нескл.* fiásco; потерпе́ть ~ be* a fáilure.

фибр|а *ж.* fíbre; ◇ все́ми ~ами души́ in all the fibres of *one's* béing. ~овый fíbre *attr.*; ~овый чемода́н fíbre súitcase.

фибро́ма *ж. мед.* fibroid.

фигу́ра *ж.* 1. fígure; 2. *(в танце)* step; *(в полёте)* evolútion; *(на коньках)* fígure; 3. *шахм.* piece; *разг.* chéss-man*; 4. *карт.* cóurt-card.

фигура́льный fígurative.

фигури́ровать *несов.* appéar, fígure.

фигури́ст *м.*, ~ка *ж.* fígure skáter.

фигу́рн|ый 1. shaped; 2. *(об инструменте)* form *attr.*; 3. *(с узором, тиснением)* fígured, ornaméntal; 4. *(исполняемый с фигурами)* fáncy; ~ое ката́ние на конька́х fígure skáting.

фи́зик *м.* phýsicist.

фи́зика *ж.* phýsics; я́дерная ~ núclear phýsics.

физиогно́мика *ж.* physiognómics, physiógnomy.

физио́|лог *м.* physiólogist. ~логи́ческий physiológical; ◇ ~логи́ческий раство́р physiológical solútion. ~ло́гия *ж.* physiólogy.

физионо́мия *ж.* face; *перен. тж.* shape.

физиотерапе́вт *м.* physiothérapist; phýsio *разг.*

физиотерапи́я *ж.* physiothérapy.

физи́ческ|ий 1. phýsical; ~ие сво́йства по́чвы phýsical próperties of the soil; ~ труд phýsical work; ~ая си́ла phýsical strength; ~ая сла́бость phýsical wéakness; 2. *(предназначенный для занятий физикой)* phýsics *attr.*; ~ кабине́т phýsics room/labóratory; ◇ ~ая геогра́фия phýsical geógraphy; ~ая хи́мия phýsical chémistry; ~ая культу́ра phýsical cúlture.

физкульту́р|а *ж.* phýsical cúlture. ~ник *м.*, ~ница *ж.* áthlete, spórtsman*. ~ный phýsical cúlture *attr.*; ~ный пара́д phýsical cúlture paráde; ~ный костю́м track suit.

фикса́ж *м. фото разг.* hýpo.

фикси́ровать *несов. и сов. (сов. тж. зафикси́ровать) (вн.)* 1. fix (*smth.*); ~ фотоплёнку fix a film; 2. *(сосредоточивать)* ~ внима́ние cóncentrate/fix atténtion; 3. *(отмечать, регистрировать)* recórd (*smth.*); ~ собы́тия recórd evénts. ~ся *несов. и сов.* cóncentrate; *(закрепляться)* remáin fixed, lodge.

фикти́вный fictítious; *(поддельный)* forged.

фи́кус *м. бот.* rúbber plant.

фи́кция *ж.* fiction; *(вымышленное положение тж.)* illúsion.

филантро́п *м.* philánthropist. ~и́ческий philánthrópic. ~ия *ж.* philánthropy; занима́ться ~ией philánthropize.

филармо́ни|я *ж.* Philharmónic Society; орке́стр ~и philharmónic órchestra.

филатели́ст *м.* philátelist, stámp-collector. ~и́ческий philátely *attr.*; ~и́ческое о́бщество philátely society.

филе́ *с. нескл.* 1. sírloin; 2. *(кусок мяса, рыбы, очищенной от костей)* fillet.

филёнка *ж.* pánel.

филиа́л *м.* branch, subsídiary; ~ институ́та branch

of an ínstitute; ~ Ма́лого теа́тра sécond stage of the Ма́ly Théatre.

фи́лин *м.* (*птица*) éagle-owl.

фило|лог *м.* philólogist. ~логи́ческий philológical. ~ло́гия *ж.* philólogy.

филосо́ф *м.* philósopher.

филосо́ф|ия *ж.* philósophy; ~ матема́тики philósophy of mathemátics. ~ский philósophic(al); ~ский тракта́т philosóphical tréatise; ~ская по́весть philosóphical tale; ~ские размышле́ния philosóphical meditátions. ◇ ~ский ка́мень philósopher's stone. ~ствовать *несов.* philósophize.

фильм *м.* film, (mótion) pícture; монта́ж ~а éditing of a film.

фильтр *м.* filter. ~а́ция *ж.* fíltering, filtrátion; (*проса́чивание*) séepage. ~ова́ть *несов.* (*вн.*) filter (smth.); *перен. разг.* screen (smb.).

фимиа́м *м.* íncense; *перен.* adulátion; ◇ кури́ть ~ кому-л. laud smb. to the skies, sing* the práises of smb.

фина́|л *м.* 1. énding; end; (*симфонии, оперы*) finále; 2. *спорт.* final; вы́йти в ~ reach the final; игра́ть в ~ле play in the final. ~ли́ст *м.* fínalist. ~льный final; ~льный матч the final; ~льный свисто́к final whístle, no side; ~льный акко́рд final/conclúding chord.

финанс|и́ровать *несов. и сов.* (*вн.*) finánce (smb., smth.); ~ строи́тельство finánce búilding. ~и́ст *м.* fináncier.

фина́нсов|ый fináncial; ~ год fináncial year, fiscal year *амер.*; ~ые затрудне́ния fináncial dífficulties; ~ кри́зис fináncial crísis.

фина́нсы *мн.* finánces.

фи́ник *м.* date. ~овый: ~овая па́льма dáte-palm.

фи́ниш *м.* finish; у ~a at the fínish; пе́рвым прийти́ к ~у fínish first, come* in first. ~и́ровать *несов. и сов.* finish. ~ный: ~ный столб wínning-post; ~ная ле́нта (fínishing) tape; ~ная черта́ fínishing line.

фи́нка I *ж.* Finn, Fínnish wóman*.

фи́нка II *ж. разг.* (*нож*) Fínnish knife*, shéath-knife*.

финн *м.* Finn.

фи́нский Fínnish; ~ язы́к Fínnish, the Fínnish lánguage; ◇ ~ нож Fínnish knife*, shéath-knife*.

фиоле́тов|ый víolet; ~ цвет víolet; ~ые черни́ла víolet ink *sg.*

фио́рд *м.* fiord.

фи́рм|а *ж.* firm. ~енный the firm's own; ~енное блю́до spéciality of the house.

фиста́шк|а *ж.* 1. (*плод*) pistáchio(-nut); 2. (*дерево*) pistáchio-tree. ~овый 1. pistáchio *attr.*; 2. (*о цвете*) pistáchio (green).

фити́ль *м.* wick; (*шнур*) fuse.

флаг *м.* flag; подня́ть, спусти́ть ~ raise, lówer the flag; кора́бль под сове́тским ~ом ship flýing the Sóviet flag; ◇ под ~ом чего-л. únder the flag of smth.; вы́кинуть ~ unfúrl a flag; оста́ться за ~ом get* left behínd (in the race).

флагма́н *м.* 1. (*командующий*) flag-cáptain; 2. (*корабль*) flágship; (*самолёт*) léading áircraft; 3. (*ведущий*) léader. ~ский flag *attr.*; ◇ ~ский кора́бль flágship.

флагшто́к *м.* flágstaff.

флажо́к *м.* small flag; (*páper*) flag; ста́ртовый ~ stárting flag.

флако́н *м.* bóttle; ~ духо́в bóttle of scent.

флама́нд|ец *м.*, ~ка *ж.* Fléming. ~ский Flémish; ~ская шко́ла (*живописи*) Flémish school; ~ский язы́к Flémish, the Flémish lánguage.

фланг *м.* flank; (*бок, сторона тж.*) side. ~овый *прил.* 1. flank *attr.*; 2. *в знач. сущ. м.* the man* on the flank, flánker.

флане́левый flánnet; (*из бумажной фланели*) flannelétte.

флане́ль *ж.* flánnet; (*бумажная*) flannelétte.

фла́нец *м.* flange.

флегм|а *ж.* phlegm. ~а́тик *м.* phlegmátic pérson; apathétic pérson.

флегмат|и́ческий, ~и́чный phlegmátic; apathétic.

флейт|а *ж.* flute. ~и́ст *м.* fláutist, flútist.

флéксия *ж. лингв.* infléxion.

флекти́вный *лингв.* inflécted, infléxional; ~ язы́к inflécted lánguage.

фли́гель *м.* wing; (*стоящий отдельно*) ánnex.

флирт *м.* flirtátion. ~ова́ть *несов.* flirt.

флокс *м. бот.* phlox.

флома́стер *м.* félt(-tip) pen; (*тонкий*) fíneliner.

фло́ра *ж.* flóra.

флот *м.* fleet; (*часть вооружённых сил*) návy; вое́нно-морско́й ~ Návy; Балти́йский ~ Báltic Fleet; служи́ть во, на ~е serve in the Návy; ◇ возду́шный ~ air fleet.

флоти́лия *ж.* fleet; китобо́йная ~ wháling fleet.

флотово́дец *м.* sea cáptain.

фло́тский nával.

флю́гер *м.* wéather-vane; wéathercock; (*о человеке тж.*) trímmer, tíme-server.

флюорогра́фия *ж.* fluorógraphy, phótofluoróscopy.

флюс I *м.* (*опухоль*) gúmboil, swóllen cheek.

флюс II *м. тех.* flux, fúsing ágent.

фля́га *ж.* flask, wáter-bottle.

фойé *с. нескл.* fóyer; ◇ артисти́ческое ~ artists' room.

фок-ма́чта *ж. мор.* fóremast.

фокстерье́р *м.* fóx-térrier.

фокстро́т *м.* fóxtrot, quíck-step.

фо́кус I *м. физ., мед.* fócus; не в ~е out of fócus.

фо́кус II *м.* 1. (*трюк*) trick; 2. (*секрет в устройстве чего-л.*) sécret device; 3. *разг.* (*увёртка*) double-déaling, tríckery; 4. *обыкн. мн. разг.* (*капризы*) fads *pl*; без ~ов! none of your fads!

фо́кусни|к *м.* 1. (*артист*) cónjurer; 2. *разг.* (*ловкач*) tríckster; 3. *разг.* (*капризный человек*) fáddy pérson. ~чать *несов. разг.* be* fáddy, have* fads.

фолиа́нт *м.* large vólume.

фо́льга *ж.* foil.

фолькло́р *м.* fólklore.

фолькло́рист *м.* fólklorist. ~ика *ж.* fólklore stúdies *pl.*

фон *м.* báckground; (*задний план тж.*) báckcloth, báckdrop; на ~е вече́рнего не́ба agáinst (the báckcloth of) the évening sky.

фона́рный lamp *attr.*; ~ столб lámp-post.

фона́рь *м.* 1. lántern; (*сигнальный*) sígnalling lamp; карма́нный электри́ческий ~ fláshlight, eléctric torch; у́личный ~ stréet-lamp; 2. *архит.* bay wíndow; (*просвет в крыше*) lántern (light).

фонд *м.* 1. fund; ~ зарабо́тной пла́ты wáge(s)-fund; валю́тный ~ cúrrency resérve/fund; 2. (*запас*) stock, resérve; жили́щный ~ available hóusing, resérve of accommodátion; 3. *мн.* (*ценные бумаги*) stocks; ~овый 1. resérve *attr.*, fúnded; 2. (*относящийся к совершению сделок*) stóck-exchange *attr.*; ~овая би́ржа stock exchánge.

фоне́ма *ж. лингв.* phóneme.

фоне́т|ика *ж.* phonétics. ~и́ческий phonétic; ~и́ческая транскри́пция phonétic transcríption.

фоно́граф *м.* phónograph.

фоноло́г|ия *ж. лингв.* phonólogy. ~и́ческий phonológical.

фоноте́ка *ж.* récord líbrary.

фонта́н *м.* fóuntain; (*нефти*) gúsher. ~и́ровать *несов.* gush, spout.

фо́р|а *ж.*: дать ~у give* smb. a start.

форе́ль *ж.* trout.

фо́рзац *м. полигр.* flýleaf*.

форм|а ж. 1. form; (*очертания*) shape; ~ и содержа́ние form and cóntent; в ~е ша́ра báll-shaped; 2. (*одежда*) úniform; ~ оде́жды *воен.* dress; оде́тый не по ~е not próperly dressed; 3. *тех.* (*для отли́вки*) mould, cast; ◇ в ~е in good form; не в ~е off form.

формал|и́зм м. fórmalism. **~и́ст** м. fórmalist. **~и́стский, ~исти́ческий** formalístic; ~ое отноше́ние к де́лу formalístic áttitude; ~ое иску́сство formalístic art.

форма́льн|о fórmally; ~ он прав convéntionally spéaking, he is right; подходи́ть к де́лу ~ adópt a bureaucrátic áttitude to the case. **~ость** ж. formálity; (*усло́вие тж.*) technicálity; пуста́я ~ость mere formálity; пренебрега́ть ~остями brush aside technicálities. **~ый** fórmal; ~ое отноше́ние official/convéntional áttitude; ~ый ме́тод fórmal méthod.

форма́т м. fórmat; большо́го ~а lárge-size; ма́лого ~а smáll-size.

форма́ция ж. 1. formátion; (*структура*) strúcture; 2. *геол.* formátion, strátum; ◇ обще́ственно-экономи́ческая ~ sócio-económic formátion.

фо́рменный 1. (*об одежде*) úniform *attr.*; 2. *разг.* (*самый настоящий*) régular, dównright.

формирова́ние с. 1. (*действие*) fórming, formátion; ~ поездо́в máking up of trains; ~ прави́тельства formátion of a góvernment; ~ хара́ктера formátion of cháracter; 2. (*во́инское соединение*) únit.

формирова́ть, сформирова́ть (*вн.*) form (*smth.*); *воен. тж.* raise (*smth.*); ~ прави́тельство form a góvernment; ~ полк form a régiment; ~ железнодоро́жный соста́в make* up a train; ~ хара́ктер form/mould the cháracter. **~ся, сформирова́ться** 1. (*приобретать какую-л. форму*) form; (*физически развиваться тж.*) grow* up; *перен.* take* shape; 2. (*организо́вываться*) be* formed; (*о войсках тж.*) form into únits.

формова́ть, сформова́ть (*вн.*) *тех.* 1. shape (*smth.*), mould (*smth.*); ~ гли́ну módel clay; 2. (*изготовля́ть форму для отли́вки*) make* a mould.

фо́рмула ж. fórmula (*pl* -ae, -as).

формули́ровать *несов. и сов.* (*сов. тж.* сформули́ровать) (*вн.*) fórmulate (*smth.*).

формулиро́вка ж. formulátion, wórding.

формуля́р м. (*библиотечный*) tícket, card.

форпо́ст м. óutpost (*тж. перен.*).

форси́рованн|ый inténsive; рабо́тать ~ыми те́мпами work at high préssure/speed; ◇ ~ марш *воен.* forced march.

форси́ровать *несов. и сов.* (*вн.*) 1. (*ускорять*) speed* up (*smth.*); ~ строи́тельство speed* up building; 2. *воен.* force (*smth.*); ~ ре́ку force a ríver, force a cróssing.

фортепья́нный piáno *attr.*

фортепья́но с. *нескл.* piáno; игра́ть на ~ play the piáno.

фортифика́ция ж. *воен.* fortificátion.

форточк|а ж. ventilátion pane; откры́ть ~у ópen the window.

фо́рум м. fórum.

фосфа́т м. *хим.* phósphate.

фо́сфор м. *хим.* phósphorus. **~ный** 1. *хим.* phosphóric, phósphorous; ~ный за́пах smell of phósphorus; 2. (*подобный фосфору*) phosphoréscent.

фо́то с. *нескл. разг.* (*снимок*) phóto.

фо́то|аппара́т м. cámera. **~ателье́** с. *нескл.* photógrapher's (stúdio). **~бума́га** ж. photográphic páper. **~вы́ставка** ж. photográphic exhibítion, exhibítion of phótographs.

фотогени́чный photogénic.

фото́граф м. photógrapher.

фотографи́ровать, сфотографи́ровать (*вн.*) phótograph (*smb., smth.*), take* a phótograph (of). **~ся, сфотографи́роваться** *разг.* have* one's pícture táken, have* a snáp(shot) táken of onesélf. **~и́че-**

ский photográphic; с ~и́ческой то́чностью with photográphic precísion.

фотографи|я ж. 1. (*искусство*) photógraphy; занима́ться ~ей go* in for photógraphy; цветна́я ~я cólour photógraphy; 2. (*снимок*) phótograph; 3. (*ателье*) photógrapher's (stúdio).

фото|докуме́нт м. documéntary phótograph. **~ка́рточка** ж. phótograph; phóto *разг.* **~ко́нкурс** м. photográphic competítion. **~ко́пия** ж. phótocopy. **~корреспонде́нт** м. (néwspaper) photógrapher. **~лаборато́рия** ж. photográphic láboratory. **~люби́тель** м. ámateur photógrapher. **~монта́ж** м. photomóntage. **~офсе́т** м. photo-offsét. **~пласти́нка** ж. photográphic plate. **~плёнка** ж. film. **~репортёр** м. photógrapher. **~ро́бот** м. phótofit. **~ружьё** с. cámera gun. **~си́нтез** м. photosýnthesis. **~сни́мок** м. phóto(graph). **~сту́дия** ж. photográphic stúdio. **~телегра́мма** ж. pícture télegram, wírephoto. **~телегра́ф** м. phototélegraph. **~фи́ниш** м. phóto-finish. **~хи́мия** ж. photochémistry. **~хро́ника** ж. pictórial revíew. **~элеме́нт** м. photocéll, photoeléctric cell.

фра́з|а ж. phrase; *грам.* séntence; пусты́е ~ы émpty/mere words.

фразеологи́ческий phraseológical.

фразеоло́гия ж. phraseólogy.

фразёрство с. vérbiage, phráse-spinning, phráse-mongering.

фрак м. dréss-coat, táilcoat, tails *разг.*; во ~е in évening-dress.

фракцио́нный fáctional; (*раскольнический тж.*) splítting.

фра́кция I ж. 1. (*организованная группа в парламенте и т. п.*) group; 2. (*обособившаяся часть политической партии*) fáction.

фра́кция II ж. *хим.* fráction.

фрамýга ж. (*окна*) úpper window-pane; (*над две́рью*) tránsom.

франк м. franc.

франт м. dándy, fop.

францýженка ж. Frénchwoman*; она́ ~ she is French.

францýз м. Frénchman*; он ~ he is French. **~ский** French; **~ский язы́к** (the) French, the French lánguage.

фрахт м. *мор., торг.* freight.

фрега́т м. frígate.

фреза́ ж. *тех.* mílling cútter.

фре́зерный *тех.* mílling; ~ стано́к mílling machíne.

фрезер|ова́ть *несов. и сов.* (*вн.*) *тех.* cut* (*smth.*), mill (*smth.*). **~о́вщик** м. mílling-machine óperator.

френч м. túnic.

фре́ска ж. *иск.* frésco (*pl* -os, -oes).

фрикаде́лька ж. fríkkadel; ры́бная ~ fish fríkkadel.

фронт м. front; еди́ный ~ united/cómmon front; на ~е at the front; ~ рабо́т field of operátions; ◇ на два ~а on two fronts.

фронта́льн|ый fróntal; **~ая ата́ка** fróntal/diréct attáck.

фронтов|и́к м. frónt-line sóldier. **~о́й** front *attr.*, frónt-line *attr.*; **~а́я полоса́** front line; **~а́я доро́га** frónt-line road.

фронто́н м. *архит.* pédiment.

фрукт м. обы́кн. мн. fruit. **~о́вый** fruit *attr.*; **~о́вый нож** fruit knife*; **~о́вый сезо́н** fruit séason; **~о́вый сад** órchard.

фтор м. *хим.* flúorine.

фу 1. (*для выражения досады*) oh!; 2. (*для выражения отвращения*) ugh!; 3. (*для выражения устало́сти, облегче́ния*) phew!

фýга ж. *муз.* fugue.

фугáс м. *воен.* lánd-mine. **~ка** ж. *разг.* 1. *см.* фугáс; 2. (*бомба*) (high-explosive) bomb. **~ный** high-explosive *attr.*; **~ный снаря́д** high-explosive prójectile/shell.

фундáмент м. foundátion; *перен. тж.* básis.

фундаментáльн|ый 1. (*прочный, крепкий*) sólid, próper; *перен.* (*глубокий, солúдный*) thórough, sound; ~ая пострóйка próper/sólid búilding; ~ые знáния thórough knówledge *sg*; ~ труд great/májor work; 2. (*основнóй, глáвный*) main; key *attr.*; ~ая библиотéка main líbrary; 3. *разг.* (*обúльный*) prodígious.

функционáльный fúnctional.

функционúровать *несов.* fúnction.

фýнкци|я *ж.* fúnction; выступáть в ~и когó-л., чегó-л. perfórm the fúnction of *smb.*, *smth.*

фунт I *м.* (*мéра вéса*) pound.

фунт II *м.* (*дéнежная едúница*) pound; ~ стéрлингов pound stérling.

фурáж *м.* fórage, fódder.

фурáжка *ж.* (peaked) cap.

фурáжн|ый fórage *attr.*, fódder *attr.*; ~ые фóнды fórage resérves; ~ое зернó fódder grain.

фургóн *м.* 1. (*повóзка*) (cóvered) wág(g)on; 2. (*грузовáя машúна*) van; мéбельный ~ fúrniture-van.

фýрия *ж.* fúry.

фурóр *м.* furóre; произвестú ~ creáte a furóre.

фурýнкул *м.* boil, fúruncle.

фурункулёз *м. мед.* furunculósis.

фут *м.* foot*.

футбóл *м.* (associátion) fóotball; sóccer *разг.* ~úст *м.* fóotballer.

футбóлка *ж.* fóotball-jérsey.

футбóльн|ый fóotball *attr.*; ~ое пóле fóotball field; ~ мяч fóotball; ~ые состязáния fóotball mátches; ~ая комáнда fóotball team.

футля́р *м.* case; ~ для очкóв spéctacle-case; ◇ человéк в ~е man* who keeps himsélf in cótton wool.

футурúзм *м.* fúturism.

фуфáйка *ж.* 1. (*вязаная*) swéater, jérsey; 2. (*стёганая кýртка*) pádded jácket.

фы́ркать, фы́ркнуть 1. snort; 2. *разг.* (*смеяться*) give* (little) snorts of láughter; 3. (*с шýмом выпускáть дым, пар и т. п.*) belch, hiss; 4. *тк. несов.* (*на вн.*) *разг.* (*брюзжáть*) sniff (at), snort (at).

фы́ркнуть *сов. см.* фы́ркать 1, 2, 3; 2. *разг.* (*выразить недовóльство*) snort.

фюзеля́ж *м. ав.* fúselage, hull.

X

хáки *прил. неизм. и с. нескл.* kháki.

халáт *м.* 1. (*востóчный*) robe; 2. (*домáшний*) dréssing-gown; (*купáльный*) báthrobe; (*рабóчий, дéтский*) óverall; (*врачá, худóжника*) smock; (*хирургúческий*) súrgeon's coat.

халáтн|ость *ж.* négligence, láxity. ~ый négligent, slípshod; ~ое отношéние к дéлу don't-cáre áttitude to *one's* work.

халвá *ж.* halvá.

халтýр|а *ж. разг.* 1. (*небрéжная рабóта*) slápdash/cáreless work; 2. (*побóчная рабóта для зарабóтка*) odd jobs *pl*, cátchpenny job; (*побóчный лёгкий зарабóток*) éasy móney, móney made on the side; 3. (*продýкт небрéжной рабóты*) trash; (*о литератýрной рабóте*) pót-boiler; *собир.* háck-work. ~ить *несов. разг.* 1. (*плóхо рабóтать*) do* cáreless work; 2. (*имéть побóчный лёгкий зарабóток*) do* cátchpenny jobs; (*в литератýре*) prodúce pót-boilers, do* háck-work. ~ный *разг.* cátchpenny; (*небрéжный тж.*) slápdash, slípshod. ~щик *м. разг.* bótcher; (*в литератýре тж.*) hack.

хам *м. разг.* boor, lout.

хамелеóн *м.* chaméleon; (*о человéке тж.*) túrncoat.

хáм|ский *разг.* bóorish, lóutish. ~ство *с. разг.* bóorishness, lóutishness.

хан *м. ист.* khan.

хандр|á *ж.* (fit of) depréssion; dejéction, gloom. ~úть *несов.* mope, have* a fit of depréssion.

ханжá *м. и ж. разг.* hýpocrite.

хáнже|ский hypocrítical, sanctimónious. ~ствó *с.* hýpocrisy, sanctimóniousness.

хáос *м.* cháos.

хаóс *м.* (*беспорядок*) cháos, útter confúsion.

хаотúч|еский chaótic. ~ность *ж.* confúsion. ~ный chaótic.

хáпать, хáпнуть (*вн.*) *разг.* 1. grab (*smth.*), snatch (*smth.*); 2. (*воровáть*) filch (*smth.*).

хáпнуть *сов. см.* хáпать.

харáктер *м.* 1. náture, disposítion, cháracter; мя́гкий ~ géntle disposítion/náture/cháracter; тяжёлый ~ dífficult/disagréeable náture/disposítion; дурнóй, плохóй ~ bad* témper; сúльные ~ы strong nátures; не в егó ~е not like him; уж такóй у негó ~! that's the sort of pérson he is!; 2. (*твёрдая, сúльная вóля*) cháracter, will; человéк с ~ом strong-willed pérson; 3. (*свóйства предмéтов, явлéний и т. п.*) náture, cháracter; ~ мéстности náture/cháracter of the locálity; 4. *лит., иск.* cháracter.

характеризовáть *несов. и сов.* (*сов. тж.* охарактеризовáть) (*вн.*) 1. (*давáть характерúстику*) descríbe (*smb.*, *smth.*); delíneate (*smth.*); 2. (*быть характéрным*) cháracterize (*smth.*), be* cháracteristic (of). ~ся *несов.* (*тв.*) be* cháracterized (by).

характерúстик|а *ж.* 1. descríption, delineátion; для ~и когó-л., чегó-л. to descríbe *smb.*, *smth.*; 2. (*официáльный докумéнт*) réference, testimónial; с мéста рабóты réference from *one's* place of work; 3. *мат.* cháracteristic.

характéрн|о *в знач. сказ. безл.:* ~, что... it is signíficant that... ~ый 1. (*с рéзко выраженными осóбенностями*) distínctive, stríking; ~ое лицó distínctive face; 2. (*свóйственный комý-л., чемý-л.*) characterístic, týpical; ~ые черты́ týpical féatures; э́то для негó ~о! it's just like him!; 3. *иск.* cháracter *attr.*; ~ый актёр cháracter áctor.

хáркать, хáркнуть *разг.* hawk, clear *one's* throat.

хáркнуть *сов. см.* хáркать.

хáта *ж.* cóttage; ◇ моя́ ~ с крáю that is nóthing to do with me, it's no búsiness of mine.

хáять *несов.* (*вн.*) *разг.* run* (*smth.*) down.

хвал|á *ж.* praise; ~ и честь емý за то, что... he desérves all póssible praise for.

хвалéбн|ый láudatory; ~ая рецéнзия enthusiástic revíew; ~ая песнь hymn/páean of praise.

хвалёный *ирон.* váunted, bóasted, célebrated.

хвалúть, похвалúть (*вн.*) praise (*smb.*, *smth.*); он рéдко когó хвáлит he séldom práises ányone, he is spáring of praise. ~ся, похвалúться (*тв.*) boast (of); не могý похвалúться больши́ми знáниями в хúмии I can't claim ány great knówledge of chémistry.

хвáстать, похвáстать *разг. см.* хвáстаться. ~ся, похвáстаться (*тв.*) boast (of), brag (of).

хвастлú|вость *ж.* bóastfulness, vainglóriousness. ~вый bóastful, vainglórious, brágging.

хвастовствó *с.* bóasting, brágging.

хвастýн *м.*, ~ья *ж.* bóaster; shów-off *разг.*

хват|áть, хватúть 1. (*вн.*; *брать, захвáтывать*) seize (*smb.*, *smth.*); snatch (*smb.*, *smth.*), grab (*smb.*, *smth.*); (*зубáми*) snap (*smb.*, *smth.*); ~ когó-л. зá руку seize/grab *smb.* by the hand; 2. *тк. несов.* (*вн.*) *разг.* (*ловúть, задéрживать*) stop (*smb.*), seize (*smb.*); 3. *тк. несов.* (*вн.*) *разг.* (*без разбóра приобретáть*) grab (*smth.*); ~ что попáло grab the first thing that comes to hand, grab what *one* can; 4. *безл.* (*рд.*; *быть достáточным*) be* enóugh, be* suffícient; suffíce; ~ комý-л. на мéсяц, недéлю* и т. д. last *smb.* a month, a week, *etc*.; не ~ be* lácking, not be enóugh; ему́, ей не ~áет сил, ума́ (+ *инф*.) he, she hásn't the strength, wit (+ to *inf*); не ~áет вре́мени there is not enóugh time; мне не хвати́ло вре́мени сде́лать э́то I had no time to do it; не ~áет рабо́чих рук there are not enóugh wórkers; у меня́ не ~áет ду́ха пойти́ туда́ I can't bring myself to go there; вас о́чень не ~а́ло you were gréatly missed; 5. *безл. разг*.: на э́то меня́ хва́тит I can stand that; ◇ ~ во́здух gasp for air, take* a great breath of air; э́того ещё не ~а́ло! as if that wásn't enóugh!, that's the límit! ~а́ться, схвати́ться (за *вн*.) 1. *разг*. (*брать, хва-тать руко́й*) snatch (at), catch* (at); 2. *тк. несов*. (*принима́ться*) seize (upón); он ~а́ется за любо́е де́ло he has a go at éverything; ◇ ~а́ться за́ голову cluth *one's* head.

хват | **и́ть** *сов*. 1. хвата́ть 1, 4, 5; 2. (*рд*.) *разг*. (*пе-ренести́, испыта́ть*) go* through (*smth*.), have* to put up with (*smth*.); они́ ~и́ли нема́ло го́ря they have had a lot to put up with; 3. (*вн. тв*.) *разг*. (*уда́рить*) hit* (*smb*. with); ◇ ~ че́рез край go* too far; ~ ли́шнего have* had a drop too much; с него́ ~ит he has had enóugh.

хвати́ться *сов*. (*рд*.) *разг*. (súddenly) miss (*smb*., *smth*.).

хва́тка *ж*. grasp, grip; (*спо́соб, мане́ра де́йствия*) techníque; (*уме́нье*) efficiency; ◇ мёртвая ~ 1) (*у соба́к*) íron grip; 2) (*упо́рство*) búlldog determinátion.

хво́йн | **ый** coníferous; (*добыва́емый из хво́и*) pine *attr*.; ~ое де́рево cónifer; ~ за́пах résinous smell; ~ая ва́нна píne-scented bath.

хвора́ть *несов. разг*. be* ill/póorly.

хво́рост *м. собир*. 1. (*сухи́е ве́тви*) brúshwood; то-пи́ть ~ом use brúshwood as fuel; 2. (*пече́нье*) straw(s).

хворости́на *ж*. switch, branch.

хвост *м*. 1. tail; (*павли́на*) train; (*лиси́цы*) brush; маха́ть ~о́м wag its tail; (*о ло́шади, коро́ве*) swish its tail; 2. (*самолёта и т. п*.) tail; 3. (*проце́ссии, по́езда и т. п*.) táil-end; ~ эшело́на back of a train; ~ коло́нны táil-end of a cólumn; 4. *разг*. (*о́чередь*) queue; line *амер*.; 5. *разг*. (*невыполненная часть како́й-л. рабо́ты*) arréars *pl*. odds and ends; ◇ быть, плести́сь в ~é lag behind, trail at the back.

хвостово́й 1. tail *attr*.; *анат*. cáudal; 2. (*находя́щий-ся в конце́ чего́-л*.) rear *attr*., híndmost.

хвоя́ *ж*. 1. píne-needles *pl*; 2. *собир*. (*ве́тки*) píne--branches *pl*.

хек *м*. (*ры́ба*) hake.

хе́рес *м*. shérry.

хиба́рка *ж*. shánty, hóvel; shack *амер*.

хи́жина *ж*. hut, cábin.

хи́лый *разг*. áiling, púny, síckly.

химиза́ция *ж*. chemicalizátion.

хи́мик *м*. 1. chémist; 2. (*рабо́тник хими́ческой про-мышленности*) chémical (índustry) wórker.

химика́лии, химика́ты *мн*. chémicals.

химиотерапи́я *ж*. chemothérapy.

хими́ческ | **ий** chémical; (*предназна́ченный для за-ня́тий хи́мией тж*.) chémistry *attr*.; ~ие элеме́нты chémical élements; ~ая реа́кция chémical reáction; ~ая лаборато́рия chémical/chémistry láboratory; ~ие удобре́-ния chémical fértilizers; ◇ ~ каранда́ш indélible péncil; ~ие черни́ла víolet ink *sg*.

хи́мия *ж*. chémistry; бытова́я ~ household chémical goods *pl*.

химчи́стка *ж*. dry cléaning; (*приёмный пункт*) dry cléaner's.

хи́на *ж. см*. хини́н.

хи́нди *м. нескл*. Híndi.

хини́н *м*. quiníne.

хинн | **ый** quiníne *attr*.; cinchóna *attr*.; ~ое де́рево cinchóna.

хи́ппи *мн*. híppies.

хире́ть, захире́ть *разг*. lose* *one's* health, droop; lánguish (*тж. перен*.); grow* síckly (*тж. о расте́нии*).

хиру́рг *м*. súrgeon. ~и́ческий súrgical; ~и́ческий больно́й súrgical case; ~и́ческая сестра́ súrgeon's assistant; ~и́ческая опера́ция súrgical operátion. ~и́я *ж*. súrgery.

хитре́ц *м*. cúnning pérson; он ~ he's véry cúnning, he's a cráfty féllow, he's a sly one.

хитрец | **а́** *ж. разг*. cúnning, shréwdness; с ~о́й with a knówledge of the world.

хитри́ть, схитри́ть 1. bluff; (с *тв*.) try to outwít (*smb*.); fool (*smb*.); он схитри́л he pulled a fast one; 2. *разг*. (*проявля́ть ло́вкость в чём-л*.) manóeuvre, contríve, be* ingénious.

хитросплете́ние *с*. 1. (*сло́жное постро́ение*) compléxity; 2. (*уло́вка*) machinátion.

хи́тр | **ость** *ж*. 1. cúnning, slýness; 2. *разг*. (*изобре-та́тельность*) ingenúity; 3. (*уло́вка*) trick, ruse; 4. *разг*. (*скры́тый смысл чего́-л*.) catch. ~ый 1. cúnning, sly, cráfty; ~ая улы́бка cúnning smile; 2. *разг*. (*изобре-та́тельный*) ingénious; 3. *разг*. (*замыслова́тый, сло́ж-ный*) íntricate, invólved, súbtle.

хихи́кать, хихи́кнуть gíggle; (*еха́дно, зло́бно*) snígger.

хихи́кнуть *сов. см*. хихи́кать.

хище́ние *с*. misappropriátion; (*де́нежное тж*.) embézzlement.

хи́щник *м*. (*о зве́ре*) beast of prey; (*о пти́це*) bird of prey; *перен*. prédator, shark; plúnderer, despóiler.

хи́щническ | **ий** 1. prédatory; ~ие инсти́нкты prédatory ínstincts; 2. (*эксплуата́торский*) rapácious; 3. (*безхозя́йственный*) deprédatory; ~ая вы́рубка лесо́в depredátion/despoliátion of fórests; ~ лов ры́бы róbbing the sea of fish, rúthless óverfishing.

хи́щничество *с*. 1. préying on óthers; 2. (*эксплуата́-ция*) rapácity; 3. (*бесхозя́йственность*) deprédation, despoliátion.

хи́щн | **ый** prédatory; (*о челове́ке тж*.) rapácious; ~ые зве́ри prédatory ánimals, beasts of prey; ~ые пти́цы birds of prey; ~ взгляд rapácious gaze.

хладнокро́в | **ие** *с*. equanímity, compósure; сохраня́ть ~ keep* *one's* head. ~ный cool, compósed; (*соверша́е-мый споко́йно*) cold-blóoded.

хлам *м. собир*. lúmber, junk, rúbbish.

хлеб *м*. 1. bread; (*карава́й*) loaf*; ~ с ма́слом bread and bútter; зараба́тывать себе́ на ~ earn *one's* líving, make* a líving; кусо́к ~а crust; 2. (*на корню́*) corn; 3. (*зерно́*) grain; ◇ насу́щный ~ dáily bread; ~-соль hospitálity; встреча́ть кого́-л. ~ом-со́лью give* *smb*. a hóspitable wélcome; ~ у кого́-л. take* the bread out of *smb's* mouth; с ~а на квас перебива́ться live from hand to mouth.

хлеба́ть *несов*. (*вн*.) sup (*smth*.).

хлебну́ть *сов*. (*рд*.) *разг*. have* a drop (of); *перен*. have* a taste (of); ~ го́ря have* known much sórrow.

хле́бница *ж*. bréad-bin.

хле́бн | **ый** 1. bread *attr*.; (*о зерне́*) grain *attr*.; ~ые запа́сы stocks of grain; ~ая торго́вля corn trade; 2. (*оби́льный хле́бом*) rich in grain; по́сле сущ. abúndant; ~ год abúndant/good year for grain; 3. *разг*. (*дохо́дный*) páying, prófitable.

хлебозаво́д *м*. (mechánical) bákery.

хлебозагото́вки *мн*. (*ед*. хлебозагото́вка *ж*.) (State) grain púrchases.

хлебопа́шество *с*. gráin-growing, grain fárming.

хлебопа́шец *м*. (grain) fármer.

хлебопёк *м*. báker.

хлебопе́ | **ка́рный** báking, bréad-making; (*вы́печен-ный из муки́*) bread *attr*. ~че́ние *с*. máking/báking of bread.

хлебопоста́вки *мн*. (*ед*. хлебопоста́вка *ж*.) (State) grain delíveries.

хлебоприёмный: ~ пункт grain recéption céntre.

хлеборо́б *м.* fármer.

хлеборо́дный fértile; ~ край rich gráin-prodúcing área; ~ год good year for corn.

хлебосо́л *м.*, **~ка** *ж.* good host.

хлебосо́ль|ный hóspitable. **~ство** *с.* hospitálity.

хлебоубо́рочн|ый hárvesting; **~ые** маши́ны hárvesting machínes; ~ комба́йн cómbine hárvester.

хлев *м.* cáttle-shed; *разг.* (*о комнате*) pígsty.

хлест|а́ть *несов.* 1. (*вн., по дт.; бить, ударять*) lash (*smb., smth.*), whip (*smb., smth.*); дождь ~а́л в окно́ the rain beat against the window-pane; ве́тер хле́щет в лицо́ the wind láshes *one's* face; 2. (*литься*) gush (from); ~а́л дождь the rain came down in tórrents.

хлёстк|ий 1. stínging, bíting; *перен.* scáthing; **~ая** статья́ scáthing árticle; 2. (*звучный*) rínging, sharp.

хлестну́ть *сов.* (*вн., по дт.*) lash (*smb., smth.*), lash out (at).

хло́пать, **хло́пнуть**, **похло́пать** 1. clap; ~ в ладо́ши clap (*one's* hands); ~ кры́льями flap its wings lóudly; ~ дверьми́ slam/bang the doors; 2. (*вн., по дт.; ударять*) slap (*smb.*); bang (*smth.*); ~ кого́-л. по спине́ slap *smb.* on the back; ◇ ~ глаза́ми look blank; blink. **~ся**, хло́пнуться *разг.* flop down.

хлопково́д *м.* cótton-grower. **~ство** *с.* cótton-growing. **~ческий** cótton-growing *attr.*; **~ческий** райо́н cótton-growing área.

хло́пков|ый cótton *attr.*; **~ые** поля́ cótton fields; **~ое** ма́сло cótton-seed oil.

хлопкоочисти́тельный gínning; ~ заво́д gínning house.

хлопкопряди́льн|ый cótton-spinning *attr.*; **~ое** произво́дство cótton-spinning índustry; **~ая** маши́на spínning-machine.

хлопкосе́ющий cótton-growing.

хлопкоубо́рочн|ый cótton-picking *attr.*; **~ая** маши́на mechánical cótton-picker.

хло́пнуть(ся) *сов. см.* хло́пать(ся).

хло́пок *м.* cótton.

хлопо́к *м.* 1. crack; (*лёгкий*) pop; 2. *мн.* (*аплодисменты*) appláuse *sg*, clápping *sg.*

хлопота́ть, **похлопота́ть** 1. *тк. несов.* (*усердно занима́ться чем-л.*) bústle/hústle abóut; 2. (*о пр., с сою́зом чтобы; добива́ться чего-л.*) make* arrángements (for); see* to it that; 3. (*за вн.; проси́ть за кого́-л.*) put* in a word (for); give* (*smb.*) a lég-up *разг.*

хлопотли́вый 1. (*о человеке*) fússy; 2. (*затрудни́тельный*) tróublesome, trícky.

хлопоты *мн.* tróuble *sg*, (*заботы о ком-л.*) éfforts; без хлопо́т withóut any fuss.

хлопу́шка *ж.* 1. (*для уничтожения мух*) flý-swot; 2. (*игру́шка*) crácker.

хлопча́тник *м. бот.* cótton plant.

хлопчатобума́жн|ый cótton *attr.*; **~ая** фа́брика cótton mill.

хло́пья *мн.* 1. (*снега*) flakes; (*шерсти*) flocks; 2. (*из зёрен*) flakes; кукуру́зные ~ córnflakes.

хлор *м. хим.* chlórine.

хлорвини́ловый vínyl chlóride.

хлоре́лла *ж.* chlorélla.

хлори́ров|ать *сов. и несов.* (*вн.*) chlórinate (*smth.*); **~анная** вода́ chlórinated wáter.

хло́ристый *хим.* chlóride; ~ ка́льций cálcium chloride.

хлорн|ый: **~ая** и́звесть chlóride of lime, chlórinated lime.

хлорофи́лл *м.* chlórophyll.

хлорофо́рм *м.* chlóroform.

хлы́н|уть *сов.* 1. (*политься с силой*) pour; gush forth; pour down; *перен.* rush; **~ул** дождь rain poured down; 2. (*устреми́ться — о лю́дях*) stream, rush, come* póuring in.

хлыст *м.* húnting-crop, switch; (*плётка*) whip.

хло́пать *несов. разг.* squelch, cloop; ◇ ~ но́сом sniff.

хля́стик *м.* belt (*at back of coat*).

хмеле́ть *несов. разг.* get* típsy.

хмель *м.* 1. (*растение*) hop; 2. (*опьянение*) héadiness, intoxicátion. **~но́й** 1. (*опьяняющий*) héady, intóxicating; 2. (*пьяный*) intóxicated, típsy; **~ны́е** ре́чи drúnken/típsy speech *sg.*

хму́р|ить, **нахму́рить:** ~ бро́ви knit* *one's* brows, frown. **~иться**, нахму́риться 1. (*о человеке*) knit* *one's* brows, frown; 2. (*о небе, погоде*) be* óvercast, be* lówering. **~ый** 1. glóomy, sómbre, súllen; 2. (*о погоде, небе*) glóomy, óvercast.

хна *ж.* hénna.

хны́к|анье *с. разг.* whímpering, whíning; *перен. тж.* compláining. **~ать** *несов. разг.* whímper, whine; *перен. тж.* compláin.

хо́бби *с. нескл.* hóbby.

хо́бот *м. зоол.* trunk.

хобото́к *м.* (*у насекомых*) probóscis, féeler.

ход *м.* 1. (*движение*) mótion; (*скорость*) speed, pace; ускóрить ~ incréase speed, go* fáster; по́езд замéдлил ~ the train slowed down; вскочи́ть (спры́гнуть) на ~у́ jump on (jump off) a tram, train, *etc.* while it is móving; по́лный ~ full speed; дать по́лный ~ go* at full speed; остало́сь де́сять киломéтров ~у there are ten more kílometres to go; туда́ три часа́ ~у it will take three hours to get there; весéнний ~ ры́бы run/rúnning of fish in spring; рабо́та идёт по́лным ~ом work is góing full swing; свои́м ~ом únder its own pówer; 2. (*развитие, течéние чего-л.*) course; ~ собы́тий course of evénts; ~ мы́слей train of thought; 3. (*в игре*) move; (*в картах*) turn, lead; ~ пе́шкой pawn move; 4. (*приём, манёвр*) move; дипломати́ческий ~ diplomátic manóeuvre; 5. *тех.* trável, stroke; (*рабочая часть машины*) móvement; ~ по́ршня píston trável/stroke; ~ руля́ wheel trável; рабо́чий ~ дви́гателя wórking stroke of an éngine; 6. (*вход*) éntrance, éntry; ~ со двора́ éntrance through yard; чёрный ~ back way; ◇ на ~у́ 1) (*попутно, мимохо́дом*) on the move, in pássing; 2) (*в движении*) on the go; 3) (*в порядке*) in operátion; с ~у 1) (*не остана́вливаясь*) withóut a pause; 2) (*без подготовки*) straight off; дать ~ де́лу get* things góing, set* mátters móving; *юр.* take* procéedings; не дать ~у кому́-л. not give *smb.* a chance; быть в большо́м ~у́ be* in great demánd, be* in wide use, be* extrémely pópular; пусти́ть что-л. в ~ set* *smth.* góing.

хода́тай *м.* intercéssor. **~ство** *с.* (*о чём-л.*) applicátion (for); (*за кого́-л.*) intercéssion (for *smb.*, on *smb.'s* behálf).

хода́тайствовать, **похода́тайствовать** (*о чём-л.*) apply (for); (*за кого́-л.*) intercéde (for *smb.*, on *smb.'s* behálf).

хо́дики *мн. разг.* wáll-clock *sg.*, wéight-driven clock *sg.*

ходи́ть *нсов.* 1. go*; (*ступать*) walk; ребёнок на́чал ~ с девяти́ мéсяцев the báby begán to walk at nine months; ~ из угла́ в у́гол walk to and fro; ~ в но́гу march in step; ~ гуля́ть go* for a walk; ~ по магази́нам go* shópping; ~ на охо́ту go* húnting; ~ в шко́лу, на рабо́ту go* to school, to work; ~ на лы́жах ski; 2. (*в пр.; носи́ть*) wear* (*smth.*); ~ в чёрном wear* black; он всегда́ хо́дит без шля́пы he néver wears a hat; 3. (*в, на вн.; посеща́ть*) go* (to), atténd (*smth.*); (*к дт.*) vísit (*smb.*), go* to see (*smb.*); ~ в теа́тр go* to the théatre; ~ в го́сти go* vísiting; 4. (*о поездах, парохо́дах и т. п.*) run*; 5. (*о часа́х*) go*; часы́ хорошо́ хо́дят the watch keeps good time; 6. (*делать ход в игре́*) move; (*в картах*) play, lead*; ~ королём *шахм.* move the king; 7. (*за тв.; уха́живать*) look (áfter); ~ за больны́м look áfter a sick pérson.

хо́дкий *разг.* 1. (*часто употребляемый*) cúrrent; 2. (*имеющий большой спрос*) pópular; ~ това́р sáleable commódity; 3. (*быстроходный*) fast.

ходово́й 1. (*связанный с движением*) operátional; ~ые ка́чества автомаши́ны perfórmance of a car; 2. *тех.* (*рабочий*) trávelling *attr.*; ~о́е колесо́ trávelling wheel; ~ винт lead/guide screw; 3. *разг.* (*имеющий наибольший спрос*) pópular; ~ разме́р о́буви pópular size of shoe; 4. *разг.* (*широко распространённый*) cúrrent, pópular.

ходо́к *м.* 1. (*пешеход*) wálker; хоро́ший (плохо́й) ~ good* (bad*) wálker; 2. (*выборный представитель*) délegate.

ходу́|ли *мн.* (*ед.* ходу́ля *ж.*) stilts. ~льный stílted.

ходу́н *м.* *разг.:* ~о́м ходи́ть 1) (*сотрясаться*) shake*; (*о здании и т. п. тж.*) rock; 2) (*о наличии суеты, беспорядка*) be* in a flúrry/whirl; 3) (*о человеке*) be* all of a dither.

ходьб|а́ *ж.* wálking; в пяти́ мину́тах ~ы́ five mínutes' walk.

ходя́ч|ий 1. wálking; ~ больно́й wálking pátient; 2. (*распространённый*) cúrrent; ~ее выраже́ние cúrrent expréssion; ~ее мне́ние preváiling/géneral opínion.

хожде́ние *с.* wálking; (*посещение*) atténding; ◇ име́ть ~ be* in circulátion.

хозрасчёт *м.* operátion on a self-suppórting básis. ~ный self-suppórting (*not supported by funds from the state budget*); ~ное предприя́тие self-suppórting énterprise.

хозя́ин *м.* 1. (*собственник, владелец*) ówner, propríetor; (*сдающий в аренду*) lándlord; (*частный наниматель*) emplóyer; boss *разг.*; 2. (*человек, ведущий хозяйство*) mánager; он плохо́й ~ he's a bad* mánager; хоро́ший ~ good* mánager; 3. (*глава дома, семьи*) head of the house; (*по отношению к гостю*) host; хозя́ева по́ля *спорт.* the home pláyers/team; 4. (*тот, кто имеет власть над кем-л., чем-л.*) máster; ~ положе́ния máster of the situátion; 5. *биол.* host; ◇ быть самому́ себе́ ~ом be* one's own máster.

хозя́йка *ж.* 1. (*собственница, владелица*) propríetress, ówner; (*сдающая в аренду*) lándlady; (*частная нанимательница*) emplóyer, místress; 2. (*ведущая хозяйство*) mánager; хоро́шая ~ good* mánager; 3. (*глава дома, семьи*) místress of the house; (*по отношению к гостю*) hóstess; дома́шняя ~ hóusewife*.

хозя́йничать *несов.* 1. (*вести хозяйство*) keep* house; 2. (*распоряжаться по-своему*) do* as one likes, boss the show; 3. (*руководить заводом, цехом и т. п.*) mánage.

хозя́йск|ий 1. máster's; emplóyer's; 2. (*заботливый*) propríetary, práctical; ~ глаз the eye of the máster; ~им гла́зом with a thrífty eye; 3. (*властный*) másterful; сказа́ть что́-л. ~им то́ном say* *smth.* in a tone of authórity; ◇ де́ло ~ое do as you please, it is for you to decíde.

хозя́йственник *м.* búsiness mánager.

хозя́йственн|ость *ж.* good mánagement, managérial efficiency, thrift. ~ый 1. (*относящийся к экономике*) económic; ~ая жизнь страны́ the económic life of the cóuntry; 2. (*ведающий хозяйством учреждения и т. п.*) managérial; 3. (*служащий для ведения хозяйства*) hóusehold *attr.*; ~ый инвента́рь hóusehold ímplements *pl* /hárdware; ~ые това́ры hóusehold goods; ~ый магази́н ironmónger's, hóusehold shop; ~ое мы́ло láundry/hóusehold soap; 4. (*расчётливый*) práctical, thrífty.

хозя́йство *с.* 1. *эк.* (*способ производства*) económy; просто́е това́рное ~ símple commódity económy; 2. (*производство, экономика*) económy; 3. (*отрасль производства*) branch of prodúction; (*производственная единица*) prodúction únit; лесно́е ~ fórestry; 4. (*оборудование, инвентарь*) equípment, próperty; ~ це́ха

equípment of a shop; ~ фе́рмы próperty of a farm; 5. (*сельскохозяйственная производственная единица*) farm; 6. (*круг обязанностей по дому*) hóusehold dúties *pl*, hóusekeeping; 7. (*предметы, продукты, необходимые в быту*) hóusehold, hóusekeeping equípment.

хозя́йствовани|е *с.* mánaging; ме́тоды ~я méthods of mánagement.

хозя́йствовать *несов.* mánage.

хоккеи́ст *м.* hóckey-player; (*на льду*) íce-hockey pláyer.

хокке́й *м.* *спорт.* (*с шайбой*) ice hóckey; (*на траве*) hóckey; ~ с мячо́м Rússian hóckey, bándy. ~ный *attr.*; íce-hockey *attr.*; ~ная кома́нда íce-hockey team.

хо́леный well-gróomed; (*о руках*) well-képt.

холе́ра *ж.* *мед.* chólera.

холестери́н *м.* cholésterol. ~овый cholésteric.

хо́лить *несов.* (*вн.*) tend (*smb., smth.*).

хо́лка *ж.* wíthers *pl*; (*грива*) mane, crest.

холл *м.* hall.

холм *м.* hill; (*низкий*) mound. ~ик *м.* híllock, knoll. ~истый hílly, rólling, úndulating.

хо́лод *м.* 1. *тк. ед.* cold; *перен.* (*приёма, манер и т. п.*) cóldness; де́сять гра́дусов ~а ten degrées belów zéro; на ~е in the cold; ~ пробежа́л по его́ спине́ a cold shúdder passed down his spine; 2. *мн.* cold weather *sg.*

холода́ть *несов.* *безл.* grow* cold; начина́ет ~ it is beginning to grow cold, the cold weather is cóming.

холоде́ть, **похолоде́ть** 1. be*/get* cold; grow* cold; 2. (*от страха и т. п.*) freeze*; ~ от у́жаса freeze* with hórror.

холоди́льн|ик *м.* refrígerator; fridge *разг.*; ícebox *амер.*; (*склад*) cold store; ваго́н-~ refrígerator car; 2. (*в паровой машине*) condénser. ~ый refrígerating, cóoling; ~ое обору́дование refrígerating machínery; ~ая устано́вка refrígerating plant.

холоди́ть *несов.* 1. (*вн.*; *охлаждать*) make* (*smb., smth.*) cold, chill (*smb., smth.*); 2. (*вн.*; *приводить в состояние оцепенения*) chill (*smth.*), freeze* (*smth.*); ~ кровь make* the blood run cold.

хо́лодно 1. *нареч.* cóldly; 2. *в знач. сказ. безл.* it is cold; сего́дня о́чень ~ it is véry cold todáy; 3. *в знач. сказ.* (*дт.*): ему́ ~ he feels cold.

холоднокро́вный *зоол.* cold-blóoded.

хо́лодность *ж.* cóldness.

холо́дн|ый 1. cold (*тж. перен.*); ~ая вода́ cold wáter; ~ая о́сень cold áutumn; ~ая заку́ска cold snack; ~ кли́мат cold clímate; ~ое се́рдце cold heart; 2. (*об одежде*) thin; ~ое пальто́ thin óvercoat; 3. (*не имеющий отопления*) unhéated; ~ая да́ча unhéated dácha; 4. (*хладнокровный*) cool; (*суровый, недоброжелательный*) cold, frígid; оказа́ть кому́-л. ~ прие́м recéive *smb.* cóldly; ◇ ~ое ору́жие cold steel.

холодо́к *м.* *разг.* 1. cóolness, chill (*тж. перен.*); 2. (*прохладное место, нежаркое время дня*) the cool; 3. (*озноб*) shíver.

холости́ть *несов.* (*вн.*) castráte (*smth.*), geld (*smth.*).

холост|о́й 1. (*неженатый*) unmárried, single; (*свойственный неженатому*) báchelor *attr.*; ~ая жизнь báchelor('s) life; 2. *тех.* idle; ~ ход ídling; 3. *воен.* blank; ~ патро́н blank cártridge; ~ вы́стрел blank shot.

холостя́к *м.* báchelor.

холостя́цк|ий *разг.* báchelor's; ~ая кварти́ра báchelor flat.

холст *м.* 1. línen; (*небелёный*) hólland; 2. (*для живописи, тж. картина*) cánvas.

холщо́вый unbléached línen *attr.*

хому́т *м.* horse cóllar; *перен. разг.* drúdgery.

хор *м.* chórus; (*певческий коллектив тж.*) choir.

хора́л *м.* *муз.* chorále.

хорва́т *м.*, ~ка *ж.* Croátian.

хо́рда *ж.* *мат.* chord.

хорей *м. лит.* tróchee.

хорёк *м. зоол.* pólecat.

хореóграф *м.* choreógrapher.

хореографи́ческий choreográphic.

хореогра́фия *ж.* choreógraphy.

хори́ст *м.* mémber of a chórus, chórister. ~ка *ж.* chórister, chórus girl, chórine *амер.*

хормéйстер *м.* chórus léader.

хоровóд *м.* round dance.

хоров|óй chóral; ~óе пéние chóral sínging; ~áя пéсня chóral piece; ~ кружóк sínging círcle.

хорони́ть, схорони́ть, похорони́ть (*вн.*) búry (*smb., smth.*) (*тж. перен.*); intér (*smb.*).

хорохóриться *несов. разг.* blúster; be* cock-a-hóop.

хорóшенький 1. prétty; (*о предметах*) nice; 2. *разг.* (*хороший*) good*; 3. *разг. upон.* nice.

хорошéнько *разг.* próperly; я и сам ~ не зна́ю I mysélf don't quite know.

хорош|éть, похорошéть grow* more béautiful, impróve (in appéarance); (*о девушке тж.*) get* préttier; онá ~éет с ка́ждым днём she gets préttier évery day.

хорóш|ий *прил.* 1. good*; (*о погоде тж.*) fine; ~ая жизнь agréeable life; ~ее сукнó good* cloth; ~ая пéсня good* song; ~ совéт sound advíce; ~ конéц háppy énding; ~ее лéто good*/fine súmmer; он ~ специали́ст he knows his job; 2. (*о человеке*) good*; 3. (*близкий, инти́мный*) close; ~ знакóмый close acquáintance; 4. *тк. кратк. ф.* (*красивый*) lóvely, béautiful, good-lóoking; онá ~á собóй she is (véry) béautiful; 5. *обыкн. кратк. ф.:* хорóш друг! a nice friend!; хорóш бы ты был, éсли... where would you have been if...; 6. *разг.* (*достаточно большо́й*) good*; ~ие процéнты good* ínterest *sg*; у негó ~ рост he is a good* height; 7. *разг.* (*любимый*) dear, dárling; мой ~, моя́ ~ая dárling; 8. *в знач. сущ. с.:* всегó ~его! goodbýe!; не ждать ничегó ~его от *кого-л.* not expéct ánything much from *smb.*; ничегó ~его тут нет! there's nóthing good abóut it!; что ~его? what's your news?; ◇ ~ее дéло 1) a good thing; 2) *upoн.* I like that!

хорошó 1. *нареч.* well*; ~ ви́деть, слы́шать see*, hear* well; ~ понима́ть understánd* pérfectly; ~ па́хнуть smell* nice/good; ~ закуси́ть have* a good meal; всем ~ извéстно it is cómmon knówledge, éveryone knows; вы ~ сдéлаете, éсли придёте you would do well to come; и ~ сдéлал! and a good thing he did!; 2. *в знач. сказ. безл.* it's nice, it's a good thing; вот ~!, как ~! how nice!; óчень ~! spléndid!; вам бу́дет ~ там you'll like it there, you'll be quite háppy/cómfortable there; ~ на у́лице it's lóvely outdóors; ~ бы вам повида́ться с ним it would be a good thing for you to see him; (как) ~, что вы пришли́ it's a good thing you came; э́то ~! that's good!, that's a good thing!; всё ~, что ~ кончáется all's well that ends well; вам ~ говори́ть! it's all véry well for you to talk!; 3. *в знач. части́цы* (*да, ла́дно*) all right, véry well; ~, ~! all right; 4. *в знач. сущ. с. нескл.* (*отмéтка*) a good (mark).

хóры *мн.* gállery *sg*.

хотéть, захотéть 1. (*рд., + инф.*) want (*smth., + to inf*); óчень ~ be* lónging (for, + to *inf*); ~ ча́ю want tea; ~ пить be* thírsty; ~ есть be* húngry; не ~ (*отказываться*) refúse, be* unwílling; ~ спать be* sléepy, be* réady for bed; мне хóчется спать I am sléepy; ~ ви́деть *кого-л.* want to see *smb.*; ~ учи́ться want to stúdy; хочу́ в дерéвню, на концéрт I want to go to the cóuntry, to a cóncert; хочу́ домóй I want to go home; он придёт, éсли захóчет he'll come if he wants to; захочу́, приду́ I'll come, if I feel like it; что от меня́ хоти́те? what do you want me to do?; что вы хоти́те э́тим сказа́ть? what do you mean (to say) by that?; он никогó слу́шать не хóчет! he won't listen to ányone; он об э́том и слы́шать не хóчет he won't hear of it; хотéл бы я ви́деть, при-

су́тствовать *и т. д.* I should like to see, be présent, *etc.*; хотéл бы я знать I wónder; 2. (*+ инф.; имéть намерéние*) be* abóut (+ to *inf*), mean* (+ to *inf*); ◇ как хоти́те just as you like; éсли хоти́те if you like; что, куда́, когда́ хоти́те whatéver, wheréver, whenéver you like; хоти́те — иди́те, хоти́те — оставáйтесь go or stay, as you like; хóчешь не хóчешь willy-nílly, whéther you like it or not. ~ся, захотéться *безл.* (*рд., + инф.*) want (*smth., + to inf*), feel* like (*smth., + -ing*), feel* inclíned (+ to *inf*); мне не хóчется I don't feel like it; емý не хóчется идти́ he dóesn't want to go; he dóesn't feel inclíned to go; he dóesn't feel like góing; мне, емý хотéлось бы... I should, he would like to...; мне захотéлось пить, есть I felt thírsty, húngry; мне хóчется домóй I want to go home; мне хотéлось бы быть дóма в шесть часóв I should like to be home at six; спаси́бо, мне бóльше ничегó не хóчется no more for me, thank you; не (совсéм) так, как хотéлось бы not (quite) as one could have wished; чегó же тебé хóчется? what do you want, then?

хоть 1. *союз см.* хотя́; 2. *союз* (*éсли хоти́те*) if you like (*в концé фра́зы*); ~ сейча́с! now, if you like; ~ на мéсяц for a month, if you like; приходи́те ~ сегóдня, ~ зáвтра you can come todáy or tomórrow, whichéver suits you; 3. *части́ца* (*то́лько*) just; (*по кра́йней мéре*) at least; подожди́те ~ мину́ту! won't you wait just a mínute?; да́йте ~ пальтó снять! you might let me take my coat off first!; скажи́те ~ слóво! do say sómething!, won't you say a word to me?; да́йте мне ~ мáленький словáрь quite a small díctionary will do for me; I ónly ask for a small díctionary; 4. *части́ца* (*напримéр*); взять ~ э́тот слу́чай here's an exámple of what I mean; take this, for exámple; ~ э́тот мáльчик this boy, now; 5. *части́ца* (*да́же*) éven; жди ~ цéлый день — не дождёшься nóthing will come of it, éven if you wait all day; you can wait all day and nóthing will come of it; ◇ ~ повéситься one might as well hang onesélf; ~ начина́й всё сначáла it makes one want to start all óver agáin; туда́ ~ не ходи́ть! it's not worth góing there!; ~ бы поскорéе конéц! if ónly the end would come!; ~ бы ча́ю где напи́ться! if ónly one could get a cup of tea sómewhere!; ~ бы былá причи́на кака́я it's not as if there were ány real cause; ~ бы что! no efféct!, like wáter off a duck's back.

хотя́ althóugh, though; (*однáко тж.*) but; ~ пóздно, но он... late as it was, he...; он ~ стар, но совершéнно здорóв he may be old, but he is pérfectly héalthy; ~ и груб, но остроу́мный rude, if wítty; ◇ ~ бы 1) (*да́же éсли*) éven if; ~ бы ты и захотéл éхать, тебé не позвóлят they wóuldn't let you go éven if you wánted to; 2) (*да́же, напримéр*) for exámple; ~ бы на нéсколько мину́т if ónly for a few mínutes; ~ бы и так!; (*ну и что ж!*) well, what of it!, suppósing I am, do *etc.*; what if it is?

хохóл *м.* (*у птиц*) crest; (*у людéй*) tópknot, tuft.

хохолóк *м. разг. см.* хохóл.

хóхот *м.* (loud) láughter.

хохотáть *несов.* roar with láughter; ~ до слёз laugh 'till *one* cries, laugh till the tears run down *one's* face, laugh till the tears come; ~ до упáду laugh till *one's* sides ache.

храбрéц *м.* brave man*, man* of cóurage.

храбри́ться *несов. разг.* put* a bold face on it; (*подбадривать себя́*) screw up *one's* cóurage.

храбр|ость *ж.* cóurage, brávery; для ~ости to keep *one's* spírits up; набра́ться ~ости súmmon/pluck up *one's* cóurage. ~ый *прил.* 1. brave, courágeous; 2. *в знач. сущ. м.* brave man*; *мн.* the brave; ◇ не из ~ого деся́тка no héro.

храм *м.* témple; *перен. тж.* shrine.

хранéние *с.* cústody, kéeping; (*товáров*) stórage; отда́ть *что-л.* на ~ store *smth.*; (*о багаже*) leave* *smth.* in the clóakroom; пла́та за ~ stórage charge; (*багажá*) clóakroom charge.

храни́лище с. repósitory; (для жидкостей) réservoir.

храни́тель м. 1. guárdian, custódian; 2. (музея, библиотеки) curátor.

храни́ть несов. (вн.) 1. (беречь, содержать в целости) keep* (smb., smth.), presérve (smth.) (тж. перен.); (от опасности) guard (smb., smth.), presérve (smth.); ~ что-л. в холо́дном ме́сте keep* smth. in a cold place; ~ что-л. в чистоте́ presérve smth. unblémished; ~ та́йну keep* a sécret; ~ что-л. в та́йне keep* smth. sécret; ~ глубо́кое молча́ние maintáin a profóund sílence; ~ что-л. в па́мяти remémber smth., keep*/presérve the mémory of smth.; 2. (соблюдать) keep* up (smth.); ~ тради́ции keep* up traditions.

храп м. snore; (лошади) snort.

храпе́ть несов. snore; (о лошади) snort.

хребе́т м. 1. (позвоночник животного) spine, báckbone; 2. (горный) range; (возвышенности) ridge.

хрен м. hórse-radish.

хрестома́тия ж. réader.

хризанте́ма ж. бот. chrysánthemum.

хрип м. wheeze; мед. crepitátion; предсме́ртный ~ déath-rattle.

хрипе́ть, прохрипе́ть 1. wheeze; 2. разг. (хрипло говорить) be* hoarse, croak.

хри́п|лый hoarse, húsky. ~нуть несов. grow*/becóme* hoarse, lose* one's voice. ~ота́ ж. hóarseness, húskiness; спо́рить до ~оты́ árgue onesélf hoarse.

христиани́н м. Chrístian.

христиа́н|ский Chrístian. ~ство с. Christiánity.

хром м. 1. (металл) chrómium; 2. (кожа) bóxcalf; 3. (краска) chrome.

хром|а́ть несов. limp; перен. разг. be* weak, be* one's weak point; ~ на пра́вую, ле́вую но́гу be* lame in the right, left leg; у него́ ~а́ет правописа́ние разг. his spélling is weak.

хроми́ров|ание с. тех. chrómium-plating. ~анный chrómium-pláted; chrómium attr.; часы́ в ~анном ко́рпусе chrómium-pláted watch. ~а́ть несов. и сов. (вн.) тех. 1. chrómium-plate (smth.); plate (smth.) with chrómium, chrome (smth.); 2. (кожу) chróme-tan (smth.).

хро́мов|ый 1. хим. chrome attr., chrómic; 2. (о коже) bóxcalf attr.; ~ые сапоги́ bóxcalf boots.

хром|о́й прил. 1. lame; ~а́я ного́й lame leg; 2. в знач. сущ. м. crípple.

хромоно́гий lame.

хромосо́ма ж. биол. chrómosome.

хромота́ ж. lámeness.

хро́ник м. chrónic ínvalid.

хро́ника ж. 1. ист. chrónicle; 2. (газетная) news ítems pl; (кино) néwsreel, news film.

хроника́льный fáctual; ~ фильм néwsreel, news film.

хроникёр м. néws-snippets man*.

хрони́ческий chrónic.

хронологи́ческий chronológical.

хроноло́гия ж. chronólogy.

хроно́метр м. chronómeter. ~а́ж м. time stúdy.

хру́пк|ий 1. (ломкий) frágile, bríttle; 2. (слабый, болезненный) frail. ~ость ж. 1. (ломкость) frágility; 2. (болезненность) infírmity; ~ость здоро́вья délicate/frail health, délicate constitútion.

хруст м. crúnching (sound), crunch.

хруста́лик м. анат. crýstalline lens.

хруста́ль м. 1. (стекло) crýstal (glass), cút-glass; 2. (изделие) cút-glass (ware); 3. (горный) rock crýstal. ~ный 1. crýstal; перен. crýstalline, crýstal-clear; 2. (о посуде) cút-glass attr.

хрусте́ть, хру́стнуть crunch.

хру́стнуть сов. см. хрусте́ть.

хрустя́щ|ий: ~ие хле́бцы críspbread sg.

хрю́кать, хрю́кнуть grunt.

хрю́кнуть сов. см. хрю́кать.

хрящ м. анат. cártilage; grístle.

худе́ть, похуде́ть get* thin.

худ|о I с. уст. harm; нет ~а без добра́ посл. ≈ évery cloud has a sílver líning; it's an ill wind that blows nóbody ány good.

ху́до II 1. нареч. bádly, ill*; ~ отзыва́ться о ком-л. speak* ill* of smb.; 2. в знач. сказ. безл.: ему́ пришло́сь ~ he had a bad* time of it; ему́ ~ he's véry bad, he is in a bad* state; больно́му ста́ло ху́же the pátient is worse.

худоба́ ж. léanness, gáuntness.

худо́жественн|ый artístic; ~ о́браз ímage, cháracter; ~ое произведе́ние work of art; ~ая литерату́ра belles-léttres; fíction and póetry; ~ фильм féature film.

худо́жн|ик м. ~ица ж. ártist; (живописец тж.) páinter.

худо́й I (худощавый) thin, lean.

худ|о́й II 1. (плохой) bad*; 2. разг. (дырявый, ветхий) hóley; ~ые сапоги́ worn boots; сапоги́ ~ые the boots are in holes; ~ое ведро́ pail with holes in it; ◇ на ~ коне́ц if the worst comes to the worst; at a pinch; in the last resórt; ~ мир лу́чше до́брой ссо́ры посл. a bad peace is bétter than a good quárrel; ≈ there néver was a good war or a bad peace.

худоща́вый lean, spare.

ху́дш|ий 1. (превосх. ст. прил. худо́й II 1 и плохо́й) the worst; в ~ем слу́чае at the worst; 2. в знач. сущ. с. the worst; пригото́виться к ~ему be* prepáred for the worst.

ху́же (сравнит. ст. прил. худо́й II 1 и плохо́й, нареч. ху́до и пло́хо) worse; (не так хорошо, как кто-л.) not so well as (smb.); он игра́ет ~ сестры́ he dóesn't play so well as his síster; тем ~ so much the worse; (от этого) ~ не бу́дет it can't do ány harm; ~ всего́ то, что... the worst of it is that...

хула́ ж. abúse, detráction.

хулига́н м. hóoligan, rówdy, rough; hóodlum амер.; (о ребёнке) líttle hóoligan, náughty child*. ~ить несов. act like a hóoligan, make* a públic núisance of onesélf. ~ство с. hóoliganism.

хули́тель м. detráctor, abúser, decríer.

хули́ть несов. (вн.) abúse (smb., smth.), decrý (smb., smth.); run* down (smb., smth.) разг.

ху́нта ж. júnta.

хурма́ ж. (плод и дерево) dáte-plum, persímmon.

ху́тор м. fármstead; (казачий) hámlet, small víllage.

Ц

ца́пля ж. зоол. héron.

цара́п|ать, цара́пнуть (вн.) scratch (smth.). ~аться несов. scratch; (царапать друг друга) scratch each óther. ~ина ж. scratch; abrásion научн. ~нуть сов. см. цара́пать.

цари́зм м. tsárism.

цари́|ть несов. reign; перен. тж. preváil; в лесу́ ~т тишина́ sílence reigns in the fórest.

цари́ца ж. queen (тж. перен.); (русская) tsarína.

ца́рский 1. tsar's; ~ ука́з decrée of the tsar; 2. (относящийся к монархии) tsárist; ~ режи́м tsárist góvernment; 3. (роскошный) régal, róyal.

ца́рственный kíngly, régal.

ца́рство с. 1. kíngdom, realm (тж. перен.); расти́тельное, живо́тное ~ végetable, ánimal kíngdom; 2. (царствование) reign.

ца́рствов|ание с. reign. ~ать несов. reign.

ца́рствующий réigning.

царь *м.* king (*тж. перен.*); (*русский*) tsar.

цвести *несов.* 1. bloom, flówer, blóssom, be* in bloom/blóssom; 2. (*процветать*) flóurish; 3. (*быть здоровым, красивым*) be* in blóoming health; 4. (*о стоячей воде*) be* cóvered with dúckweed.

цвет I *м.* (*окраска*) cólour; ~ лица compléxion; красного, синего *и т. д.* ~a red, blue, *etc.*; красить что-л. в жёлтый, зелёный *и т. д.* ~ paint *smth.* yéllow, green, *etc.*

цвет II *м.* 1. обыкн. мн. blóssom *sg*; собир. flówers; живые ~ы flówers; ~ яблони, вишни ápple, chérry blóssom; 2. (*рд.*; *лучшая часть*) the flówer (of); 3. (*период цветения*) bloom, blóssom; в (*полном*) ~у in (full) bloom; ◇ во ~е лет in the prime of life.

цветение *с.* flówering, blóssoming; floréscence *научн.*

цветистый 1. (*покрытый цветами*) flówer-covered; 2. (*пёстрый*) flóral, gáily-pátterned; 3. (*о стиле*) flórid, flówery.

цветник *м.* flówerbed, small flówer gárden; *перен.* gárden.

цветн|ой 1. cóloured; cólour *attr.*; (*о стекле тж.*) stained; ~áя фотография cólour photógraphy; ~ фильм cólour-film; ~óe телевидение cólour télevision; 2. (*о людях*) cóloured; ◇ ~ые металлы non-férrous métals; ~áя капуста cáuliflower.

цветовод *м.* flórist. ~ство *с.* floricúlture.

цветовой cólour *attr.*

цветок *м.* flówer; (*на дереве*) blóssom.

цветомузыка *ж.* cólour músic.

цветоч|ек *м.* (little) flówer; ◇ это ~ки, а ягодки впереди *погов.* there is worse to come.

цветочница *ж.* flówer girl, flówer seller.

цветочн|ый flówer *attr.*; ~ые семена flówer seeds; ~ горшок flówerpot; ~ магазин flórist's (shop); ~ая выставка flówer-show; ~ одеколон flówer-scented Eau-de--Cológne.

цветущ|ий 1. in (full) bloom *после сущ.*; ~ сад gárden in full bloom; 2. (*полный сил*) lústy; (*о девушке*) blóoming; ~ юноша lústy youth; у него ~ вид he looks márvellous/blóoming, he looks a picture of health; 3. (*процветающий*) flóurishing; ~ая страна prósperous cóuntry.

цедить *несов.* (*вн.*) 1. strain (*smth.*); (*фильтровать*) filter (*smth.*); (*наливать медленно*) pour (*smth.*) drop by drop; (*пить медленно*) sip (*smth.*); 3. *разг.*: ~ сквозь зубы, ~ словá grind* out the words.

цедра *ж.* peel; (*высушенная*) dried peel; лимонная ~ (dried) lémon-peel.

цезура *ж. лит.* caesúra.

цейтнот *м.* tíme-trouble; попасть в ~ get* into tíme--trouble.

целебн|ый medícinal; (*о климате и т. п.*) héalthy; ~ое средство rémedy.

целев|ой spécial-purpose *attr.*, góal-óriented; ~áя устанóвка cléar-cut goal, définite orientátion.

целенаправленный góal-directed, góal-óriented, púrposive.

целесообразн|ость *ж.* 1. expédiency; 2. *филос.* púrposefulness. ~ый 1. expédient, réasonable; ~ое использование средств sénsible use of resóurces; 2. *филос.* púrposeful.

целеустремлённ|ость *ж.* púrposefulness, síngleness of púrpose, cónsistency of aim. ~ый púrposeful.

целиком 1. (*в целом виде*) whole, as a whole; проглотить что-л. ~ swállow *smth.* whole; 2. (*совершенно*) entírely; ~ отдаваться чему-л. devóte onesélf entírely to *smth.*

целин|á *ж.* vírgin land/soil; (*нетронутая поверхность чего-л.*) unbróken/untródden expánse; освоение ~ы cultivátion of vírgin land; распахáть ~у plough up vírgin soil; поднятая ~ upturned soil; ~ой, по ~é across cóuntry.

целинн|ый vírgin; ~ые земли vírgin land(s).

целительн|ость *ж.* héaling próperties *pl*, bénefit to health. ~ый héaling, cúrative.

целить, ~ся *несов.* (в *вн.*) aim (at), take* aim (at).

целлофан *м.* céllophane. ~овый céllophane *attr.*

целлулоид *м.* célluloid.

целлюлоза *ж.* céllulose.

целлюлозно-бумажн|ый pulp and páper *attr.*; ~ая промышленность pulp and paper índustry.

целовáть, поцеловáть kiss (*smb., smth.*); ~ кого-л. в губы, в щёку kiss *smb.'s* lips, cheek, kiss *smb.* on the lips, cheek. ~ся, поцеловáться kiss (each óther).

целое *с.* the whole; ~ и ~ое ~ a síngle whole.

целомудр|енный chaste. ~ие *с.* chástity, vírtue.

целостный íntegrated, whole.

целост|ь *ж.* 1. (*неповреждённость*) sáfety; в ~и intáct; сохранить что-л. в ~и keep* smth. safe/intáct; 2. (*внутреннее единство*) íntegrity, whóleness, únity; ◇ в ~и и сохранности safe and sound, pérfectly safe.

цел|ый 1. (*полный*) whole; ~ день all day, the whole day; ~ыми днями, часáми *и т. д.* for days (and days), hours (and hours), *etc.*; ~ час a whole hour; ~ых два, три *и т. д.* часá, дня, гóда two, three, *etc.* whole hours, days, years; ~ых три чáшки three whole cups; по ~ым дням, неделям *и т. д.* for days, weeks, *etc.* on end; ~ ряд a séries; 2. (*неповреждённый*) safe, unhármed; (*о вещах тж.*) intáct; остáться ~ым be* unhármed; уходи, покудá цел go befóre you get hurt; у вас ещё ~á эта чáшка? is that cup of yours still intáct?; ◇ цел и невредим safe and sound.

цель *ж.* 1. (*для стрельбы*) tárget; попáсть в ~ hit* the mark; не попáсть в ~ be* wide of the mark, miss *one's* aim; 2. (*то, к чему стремятся*) aim, púrpose, óbject, goal, end; благородная ~ nóble púrpose; отвечáть цéли ánswer the púrpose; достичь своей цéли achieve/attáin *one's* óbject; иметь ~ю aim (at); с какой ~ю? what for?; с ~ю (+ *инф.*) with the púrpose (of + -ing); с единственной ~ю with the sole púrpose/óbject (of); с этой ~ю with that end in view.

цельнометаллический áll-métal.

цельн|ый 1. (*состоящий из одного куска*) one--piece *attr.*, sólid; 2. (*нетронутый — о снеге*) untródden, vírgin; 3. (*обладающий внутренним единством*) sound, bálanced; ~ человек bálanced pérson; ~ая натура bálanced/sound náture; 4. (*законченный*) compléte; 5. (*неразбавленный*) undilúted; ~ое молоко unskímmed milk.

Цéльси|й Célsius, céntigrade; 10° по ~ю 10° céntigrade, 10°C.

цемент *м.* cemént.

цементировать *несов. и сов.* (*вн.*) cemént (*smth.*); (*сталь*) cáse-harden (*smth.*).

цементн|ый cemént *attr.*; ~ завод cemént fáctory; ~ая плитá cemént slab.

цен|á *ж.* 1. price; (*стоимость*) cost; *перен.* worth, válue; покупнáя ~ púrchase price; повышение цен rise in príces; снижéние цен redúction/cut in príces; ~ на товáры price of goods; ~óй в... cósting *smth.*; 2.: ~óй чего-л. at the cost of *smth.*; ~óй жизни at the cost of *one's* life; ~óй любóй ~óй at ány price, at all costs; ~é нет 1) (*чему-л.*) it is príceless/inváluable; 2) (*кому-л.*) he, she is worth his, her weight in gold; в ~é in price.

ценз *м.* qualificátion; возрастнóй ~ age qualificátion.

цензор *м.* cénsor.

цензура *ж.* cénsorship.

ценитель *м.* judge, connoisséur; ~ живописи connoisséur of páinting.

ценить *несов.* (*вн.*) 1. (*назначать цену*) válue (*smth.*); *перен.* (*давать оценку*) appráise (*smb., smth.*); 2. (*признавать значение кого-л., чего-л.*) appréciate (*smb., smth.*); (*дорожить*) prize (*smb., smth.*). ~ся *несов.* be* válued.

це́нник *м.* price-list.

це́нност|ь *ж.* value; (*ценный предмет*) valuable; представля́ть большу́ю ~ be* of great value; не представля́ть никако́й ~и be* utterly worthless; культу́рные ~и cultural values. ~ный value *attr.*; ~ный ана́лиз value analysis; ~ная ориента́ция value orientation.

це́нн|ый 1. (*о почтовых отправлениях*) registered; ~ая бандеро́ль registered packet; 2. (*дорогой*) expensive; ~ые пода́рки expensive presents; 3. (*имеющий важное значение*) valuable; ~ое предложе́ние valuable suggestion/proposal; ~ое указа́ние valuable instruction.

цент *м.* (*монета*) cent.

це́нтнер *м.* double/metric centner (*100 kilograms*).

центр *м.* centre; в ~е (*города*) in town; идти́ в ~ (*города*) go* into town; быть в ~е внима́ния be* the centre of attention, be* in the limelight.

централиза́ция *ж.* centralization.

централи́зм *м.* centralism.

централизо́ванн|ый centralized; ~ое плани́рование centralized planning.

централизова́ть *несов. и сов.* (*вн.*) centralize (*smth.*).

центра́льн|ый central; Центра́льная А́зия Central Asia; ~ райо́н central district/area; центра́льный комите́т Central Committee; ~ая телефо́нная ста́нция telephone-exchange, central *амер.*; ~ая печа́ть leading newspapers; ~ напада́ющий *спорт.* centre-forward; ~ое отопле́ние central heating; ◇ ~ая не́рвная систе́ма central nervous system.

центрифу́га *ж.* centrifuge.

центробе́жн|ый centrifugal; ~ая си́ла centrifugal force.

центростреми́тельн|ый centripetal; ~ая си́ла centripetal force.

цеп *м. с.-х.* flail.

цепене́ть, оцепене́ть (от *рд.*) go* numb (with); (*от сильного чувства тж.*) stiffen (with); ~ от у́жаса stiffen with horror, go* numb with horror.

це́пк|ий 1. (*о пальцах, когтях*) strong, tenacious; prehensile *зоол.*; 2. (*вязкий*) clinging, cohesive; 3. (*быстро схватывающий*) keen; (*о памяти*) retentive; 4. *разг.* (*упорно добивающийся чего-л.*) dogged, stubborn, tenacious. ~ость *ж.* (*пальцев, когтей*) prehensity; *перен.* tenacity.

цепля́ться *несов.* (за *вн.*) cling* (to) (*тж. перен.*); (*зацепляться*) catch* (on).

цепн|о́й chain *attr.*; ~а́я переда́ча chain drive; ◇ ~а́я ли́ния *мат.* catenary; ~а́я реа́кция chain reaction.

цепо́чка *ж.* chain.

цепо́чкой in line.

цеп|ь *ж.* 1. chain; соба́ка на ~и chained dog; 2. *мн.* (*оковы*) fetters, shackles (*тж. перен.*); 3. (*ряд, вереница*) chain; ~ озёр chain/series of lakes; го́рная ~ mountain range/chain; 4. *воен.* line; стрелко́вая ~ line of infantry; 5. (*рд.*; *непрерывное следование*) sequence, series; ~ собы́тий sequence of events; 6. *физ.* chain; *эл.* circuit.

це́пью in line.

церемо́ниться *несов.* be* polite, stand* on ceremony; не́чего с ним ~ there's no need to stand on ceremony with him.

церемо́н|ия *ж.* ceremony; *мн.* formalities; без ~ий informally; прошу́ без ~ий! make yourself at home!, don't stand on ceremony!

церемо́нный (*утончённо вежливый*) punctilious; (*отвечающий требованиям этикета*) formal; (*чопорный*) ceremonious, stiff.

церковнославя́нский Church Slavonic; ~ язы́к Church Slavonic language.

церко́вный ecclesiastical; (*принадлежащий церкви*) church *attr.*

це́рковь *ж.* church.

цех *м.* (*завода*) shop; (*мастерской*) division, department.

цехово́й shop *attr.*; ~ комите́т shop (trade-union) committee.

циа́н *м. хим.* cyanogen. ~истый cyanic; ~истый ка́лий potassium cyanide, cyanide of potassium.

цивилиз|а́ция *ж.* civilization. ~о́ванный civilized. ~ова́ть *несов. и сов.* (*вн.*) civilize (*smth.*).

цига́рка *ж. разг.* fag.

циге́йка *ж.* beaver lamb.

цика́да *ж. зоол.* cicada.

цикл *м.* cycle; произво́дственный ~ production cycle; ~ ле́кций course of lectures; ~ конце́ртов series of concerts.

цикламе́н *м. бот.* cyclamen, sowbread.

циклева́ть *несов.* (*вн.*) scrape (*smth.*), shave (*smth.*).

цикли́ч|еский cyclic. ~ный cyclic; ~ное разви́тие development in cycles; ~ная организа́ция произво́дства cyclic organization of production.

цикло́ида *ж. мат.* cycloid.

цикло́н *м. метеор.* cyclone.

циклотро́н *м.* cyclotron.

цико́р|ий *м.* chicory; ко́фе с ~ем coffee with chicory.

цили́ндр *м.* 1. *мат., тех.* cylinder; 2. (*шляпа*) top hat, silk hat.

цилиндри́ческ|ий cylindrical; ~ая фо́рма cylindrical shape.

цимба́лы *мн.* dulcimer *sg.*

цинга́ *ж. мед.* scurvy.

цини́зм *м.* cynicism.

ци́ник *м.* cynic.

цини́ч|еский, ~ный 1. cynical; (*наглый*) callous; 2. (*непристойный*) indecent, obscene.

цинк *м.* zinc.

ци́нков|ый zinc *attr.*; ~ купоро́с zinc vitriol; ~ое ведро́ zinc pail.

цино́вка *ж.* rush mat; straw mat(ting).

цирк *м.* circus. ~а́ч *м. разг.* circus performer. ~ово́й circus *attr.*

циркули́ровать *несов.* circulate.

ци́ркуль *м.* (pair of) compasses; дели́тельный ~ dividers *pl.*

циркуля́р *м.* circular. ~ный circular; ~ное письмо́ circular letter.

циркуля́ция *ж.* circulation; ~ нагре́того во́здуха circulation of warm air.

цисте́рна *ж.* 1. tank; (*автомашина*) tanker; (*вагон*) tank wagon; 2. (*водохранилище*) reservoir.

цитаде́ль *ж.* citadel; *перен. тж.* stronghold.

цита́та *ж.* quotation.

цитва́рн|ый: ~ое се́мя worm-seed, santonica.

цити́ровать, процити́ровать (*вн.*) quote (*smth.*).

ци́тра *ж.* cittern, cithern.

ци́трус *м.* citrus. ~овый *прил.* 1. citrus *attr.*; 2. *в знач. сущ. мн. бот.* citrus plants.

цифербла́т *м.* dial; (*часовой тж.*) face.

ци́фра *ж.* figure; (*сумма тж.*) amount.

цифров|о́й: в ~ом выраже́нии expressed in figures; ~ые да́нные figures.

цицеро́ *с. нескл. полигр.* pica.

ЦК (центра́льный комите́т) Central Committee.

цо́канье *с.*: ~ копы́т clatter of hoofs.

цо́кать, цо́кнуть 1. click, clatter; 2. (*о птицах*) jug.

цо́кнуть *сов. см.* цо́кать.

цо́коль *м.* 1. *архит.* plinth, socle; 2. (*лампочки и т. п.*) base. ~ный: ~ный эта́ж ground floor.

цо́кот *м.* (*копыт*) clatter, beat; (*колёс*) rattle.

цу́гом tandem, one behind the other.

цука́т *м.* candied peel/fruit.

цыга́н *м.*, ~ка *ж.* Gípsy. ~ский Gípsy; ~ский язы́к Gípsy, Rómany, the Gípsy lánguage.

цы́пки *мн.* (*ед.* цы́пка *ж.*) rash *sg.*

цыплёнок *м.* chicken.

цы́почк|и *мн.*: на ~ax on típtoe; ходи́ть на ~ax (go* on) típtoe.

цыц sh!; hush!

Ч

чаба́н *м.* shepherd.

чабре́ц *м. бот.* thyme.

ча́вкать *несов.* 1. (*причмокивать*) champ, munch nóisily; 2. (*при ходьбе*) squelch.

чад *м.* fumes *pl*, fug; *перен.* héadiness; быть как в ~у́ be* in a daze.

чади́ть, начади́ть smoke; make* a smoke.

ча́д|о *с.* child*; ~а и домоча́дцы the whole fámily.

чадра́ *ж.* yáshmak.

чаёвничать *несов. разг.* drink*/have* tea, línger óver one's tea.

чаево́д *м.* téa-grower. ~ство *с.* téa-growing. ~ческий téa-growing *attr.*

чаевы́е *мн. разг.* tip *sg*; (*для нескольких*) tips.

чаепи́тие *с. разг.* téa-drinking; (*во время перерыва на работе*) tea break, téa-time.

чаеубо́рочн|ый téa-picking *attr.*; ~ая маши́на téa-picking machine, mechánical téa-picker.

чаи́нка *ж.* téa-leaf*.

чай *м.* 1. tea; завари́ть ~ make* tea; 2. (*чаепитие*) tea; за ча́ем óver tea; за ча́шкой ча́я óver a cup of tea; приглаша́ть, звать *кого-л.* на ~, на ча́шку ча́я invíte *smb.* to tea párty, ask *smb.* in for a cup of tea; ◇ дава́ть *кому-л.* на ~ tip *smb.*

ча́йка *ж.* séagull.

ча́йная *ж.* téaroom, téashop.

ча́йн|ик *м.* (*для кипячения*) kéttle; (*для заварки*) téapot. ~ица *ж.* téa-caddy.

ча́йн|ый tea *attr.*; ~ куст téa-plant; ~ые планта́ции tea plantátions; ~ серви́з téa set/sérvice; ~ая ло́жка téaspoon; ~ое полоте́нце tea tówel, dish tówel *амер.*; ~ый паке́тик tea bag; ~ое си́течко tea stráiner. ◇ ~ая ро́за téa-rose.

чайхана́ *ж.* chaikhaná (*tea-drinking establishment in Central Asia*).

чалма́ *ж.* túrban.

ча́лый (*о лошади*) roan.

чан *м.* vat.

ча́рдаш *м.* (*танец*) czárdas.

ча́рка *ж.* cup, góblet.

чарова́ть *несов.* (*вн.*) charm (*smb.*), bewítch (*smb.*), cast* a spell (óver), enchánt (*smb.*).

чароде́й *м.* wízard, magícian, enchánter. ~ка *ж.* enchántress.

чару́ющ|ий bewítching, enchánting, chárming, delightful; производи́ть ~ее впечатле́ние make* a delightful impréssion; ~ го́лос enchánting voice.

ча́ры *мн.* spell(s); mágic *sg*; (*обаяние*) charms; ~ любви́ charms of love.

час *м.* 1. (*60 минут*) hour; в ~ (in) an hour; за ~ до an hour befóre; в тече́ние ча́са for an hour; на ~ for an hour; на два ~а́ for two hours; с ~ (for) abóut an hour; че́рез ~ in an hour; (*с промежутками в один час*) évery hour; це́лыми ~а́ми for hours, by the hour; 2. (*время по часам*): тепе́рь ~, два ~а́, пять ~о́в it is one, two, five (o'clóck); в ~, два ~а́, пять ~о́в at one, two, five (o'clóck); кото́рый ~? what is the time?; what time is it?;

в кото́ром ~у́? what time?, when?, at what time?; до кото́рого ~а? till when?; (*тепе́рь*) пе́рвый, второ́й, тре́тий *и т. д.* ~ it is past twelve, one, two, *etc.*; 3. (*время, пора*) time, hour; (*время, отводимое на урок*) périod; ~ о́тдыха rést-hour; обе́денный ~ lunch-time, lunch hour; служе́бные ~ы́ óffice-hours; ~ заня́тий wórking hours; ~ы́ досу́га léisure-time *sg*, léisure-hours; дневны́е ~ы́ the day(-time) *sg*; ночны́е ~ы́ the night(-hours); ~ распла́ты the hour of réckoning; 4.: стоя́ть на ~а́x be* on séntry dúty; ◇ ~ от ~у with évery hour; ~ от ~у не ле́гче! things are góing from bad to worse; не в до́брый ~ in an évil hour; с ~у на ~ 1) ány móment; 2) (*с каждым часом*) hóurly; по ~а́м dead on time.

часа́ми for hours.

часо́вня *ж.* chápel, shrine.

часо́в|ой I *прил.* 1. (*длящийся час*) hour's; ~ая бесе́да an hour's talk; 2. *разг.* (*назначенный на час*) the óne-o'clóck; ~ по́езд the óne-o'clóck train; ◇ ~ по́яс time zone.

часо́в|ой II *прил.* 1. (*относящийся к часам*) clock *attr.*, watch *attr.*; ~ механи́зм clóckwork; ~ые стре́лки hands of a clock/watch; по ~ стре́лке clóckwise; про́тив ~ стре́лки cóunter-clóckwise; 2. (*связанный с производством часов*) clock *attr.*, watch *attr.*; ~ заво́д clock fáctory; ~ая мастерска́я wátch-repair shop; ◇ ~ ма́стер, ~ых дел ма́стер wátch-maker.

часо́в|ой III *м.* séntry, séntinel; поста́вить ~ы́х post séntries.

часовщи́к *м.* wátch-maker.

часо́к *м.* hour; на ~ for an hour or so.

часте́нько *разг.* fáirly óften.

части́ца I *ж.* párticle; *перен. тж.* grain.

части́ца II *ж. грам.* párticle.

части́чн|о pártly. ~ый pártial.

ча́стник *м. разг.* prívate tráder; (*ремесленник*) prívate cráftsman*.

частновладе́льческий prívate, prívately owned.

ча́стн|ое *с.* 1. *мат.* quótient; 2.: от ~ого к о́бщему from the partícular to the géneral.

частнопракти́ку́ющий práctising prívately, in prívate práctice *после сущ.*

частнособ́ственническ|ий based on prívate ównership *после сущ.*; (*свойственный частному владельцу*) prívate-owner *attr.*; ~ая психоло́гия prívate-owner psychólogy.

ча́стност|ь *ж.* détail; ◇ в ~и specífically, amóng their númber; я, в ~и I, pérsonally.

ча́стн|ый 1. (*отдельный*) indivídual; (*нехарактерный, исключительный*) spécial, excéptional; ~ вы́вод pártial conclúsion; ~ слу́чай spécial case; 2. (*личный*) prívate; ~ое лицо́ prívate pérson/indivídual; ~ая со́бственность prívate próperty; ~ым о́бразом prívately; э́то его́ ~ое де́ло that's his own búsiness/affáir.

ча́сто 1. óften, fréquently; ~ дыша́ть breathe rápidly; ~ быва́ть в теа́тре óften go* to the théatre; 2. (*густо, плотно*) thíckly, dénsely, clósely.

частоко́л *м.* fence, palisáde.

частота́ *ж.* fréquency; ~ пу́льса pulse rate.

частотный fréquent.

часту́шка *ж.* chastúshka (*ditty on topical, humorous or lyrical theme*).

ча́ст|ый 1. (*быстро сменяющийся*) rápid; ~ пульс quick/fréquent pulse; 2. (*повторяющийся*) fréquent; ~ые уда́ры repéated knócking *sg*, rain of blows *sg*; ~ посети́тель fréquent vísitor; 3. (*густой, плотный*) thick, dense; ~ые зу́бы clóse-set teeth; ~ гре́бень small-tooth comb, fine comb.

част|ь *ж.* 1. (*доля целого*) part; *разг.* (*пай, доля*) share; одна́ пя́тая ~ one fifth; ме́ньшая ~ the smáller part; по ~я́м in parts; плати́ть по ~я́м pay* in instálments; 2. (*составной элемент*) part, compónent; сбо́рка ~е́й assémbly (of parts); ~и те́ла parts of the bódy; 3. (*раздел какого-л. произведения*) part; (*симфонии и т. п.*) móvement; 4. (*войсковая единица*) únit; авиациóнный ~ air únit; ◇ ~и рéчи *грам.* parts of speech; ~и свéта parts of the world; не по моéй ~и not in my line; по э́той ~и in this respéct; бóльшей ~ью, по бóльшей ~и 1) (*главным образом*) for the gréater part; 2) (*обычно*) úsually; разрывáться на ~и try to do ten different jobs at once; рвать *кого-л.* на ~и péster *smb.*

чáстью pártly, in part (of).

часы́ *мн.* clock *sg*; (*карманные, ручные*) watch *sg*; заводи́ть ~ set* a watch/clock; ◇ биологи́ческие ~ biológical rhýthm.

чáхлый 1. (*о растительности*) wílted, síckly; 2. (*о человеке*) púny, síckly.

чáхнуть, зачáхнуть 1. (*о растениях*) wilt, droop; 2. (*о человеке*) pine awáy, grow* weak.

чахóтка *ж. уст.* consúmption.

чахóточный *уст.* consúmptive.

чáш|а *ж.* cup, bowl; ◇ перепóлнить ~у терпéния exháust all pátience; ~ егó терпéния перепóлнилась he reached the límit of his endúrance, he reached the end of his téther. ~ечка *ж.* 1. (*small*) cup; 2. *бот.* cályx; ◇ колéнная ~ечка knée-cap.

чáшка *ж.* 1. cup; (*чайная*) téacup; 2. (*предмет округлой формы*): ~ весóв pan.

чáщ|а *ж.* thícket; в ~е лéса in the heart of the fórest.

чáще more óften; ~ всегó úsually, more óften than not.

чáяни|е *с.* expectátion, hope; (*мечта*) dream; ◇ пáче ~я to *one's* surpríse, cóntrary to *one's* expectátions.

чáять *несов. уст.* expéct, hope; ◇ души́ не ~ в ком-л. wórship *smb.*, dote upón *smb.*

чвáн|иться *несов.* show* off, swank, put* on airs. ~ный supercílious, preténtious. ~ство *с.* supercíliousness, concéit; preténsions *pl.*

чегó *рд. см.* что I.

чей, чья, чьё, чьи whose; ~ э́то нож? whose knife* is this?; ◇ ~ бы то ни́ был whoéver it belóngs to, no mátter whose it is; чья взялá? whose side won?

чек *м.* 1. (*банковский*) cheque; check *амер.*; ~ на 900 рублéй cheque for nine húndred róubles; 2. (*от продавца*) bill; (*талон из кассы*) recéipt, tícket; вы́писать ~ на товáр write* smb. a bill for his, her púrchases; вы́бить ~ в кáссе get* a recéipt/tícket at the cásh-desk.

чекá *ж. тех.* cótter pin; (*оси*) línchpin.

чекáн *м.* stamp.

чекáнить *несов.* (*вн.*) 1. (*изготовлять монеты и т. п.*) coin (*smth.*); (*вн. на пр.*; *наносить рисунки*) engráve (*smth.* on), stamp (*smth.* on), chase (*smth.* on); 2. rap out; ~ кáждое слóво pronóunce évery word cléarly; ~ шаг march smártly; 3. *тех.* (*швы, заклёпки*) caulk (*smth.*).

чекáнка *ж.* engráving, chásing.

чекáнный 1. (*служащий для чеканки*) engráving, chásing; 2. (*изготовленный чеканкой*) engráved, chased; 3. (*чёткий*) clear; firm; ~ шаг firm/méasured tread; ~ слог cléar-cut/crisp style.

чéков|ый: ~ая кни́жка bank/chéquebook, chéckbook *амер.*

чёлка *ж.* fórelock; (*подстриженная*) fringe.

чёлн *м.* (*дуг-out*) canóe, boat; *поэт.* bark.

челнóк *м.* 1. *см.* чёлн; 2. *тех.* shúttle.

человéк *м.* man*, húman béing; (*лицо*) pérson; (*мужчина тж.*) man*; (*женщина тж.*) wóman*; молодóй ~ young man*; он хорóший ~ he is a nice man*/pérson; онá хорóший ~ she is a nice wóman/pérson; рýсский ~ a pérson of Rússian blood; ýмный ~ wise man*, wóman*; пять ~ five pérsons/péople; ~ пять abóut five pérsons/péople; шесть ~ детéй six chíldren; нас бы́ло семь ~ there were séven of us; по десяти́ рублéй на, с ~а ten róubles a head; ни оди́н ~, ни одногó ~а no one, nóbody, not a síngle

pérson; для непривы́чного ~а to one not accústomed; ◇ правá ~а húman rights.

человеколюби́вый benévolent.

человеколю́бие *с.* benévolence, good will.

человеконенави́стн|ик *м.* misánthropist, mísanthrope, mán-hater. ~ический misanthrópic, mán-háting. ~ичество *с.* misánthropy.

человекообрáзн|ый ánthropoid; ~ые обезья́ны ánthropoid apes.

человé|еский 1. húman; 2. (*гуманный*) humáne, consíderate; ~еское обращéние humáne/consíderate tréatment; ◇ ~ фáктор húman fáctor/élement. ~ество *с.* humánity, mankínd. ~ность *ж.* humánity. ~ный humáne.

чéлюсть *ж.* jaw.

чем I *мест. тв. от* что I.

чем II *союз* 1. (*при сравнит. ст.*) than; лýчше, бли́же, вы́ше, ~ bétter, néarer, táller than; 2. ~..., тем... the... the...; ~ скорéе, тем лýчше the sóoner the bétter; 3. (*вместо того, чтобы*) instéad of; ~ сидéть без дéла, ты бы пошёл гуля́ть why don't you go out for a walk instéad of hánging abóut dóing nóthing?

чём *пр. от* что I.

чемодáн *м.* súitcase. ~чик *м.* small súitcase.

чемпиóн *м.* chámpion; ~ ми́ра по тéннису world ténnis chámpion.

чемпионáт *м.* chámpionship; ~ Еврóпы по футбóлу Européan fóotball chámpionship.

чемý *дт. от* что I.

чепéц *м.* cap.

чепухá *ж. разг.* 1. (*вздор*) nónsense; 2. (*пустяк*) a mere trífle/nóthing, nóthing to speak of; trífles *pl*; (*хлам*) rúbbish.

чéпчик *м.* cap.

черви́в|ый mággoty, wórm-eaten; ~ое я́блоко mággoty ápple.

червóн|ый I: ~ое зóлото high-carat gold.

червóнный II *карт.* of hearts *после сущ.*; ~ валéт knave of hearts.

червотóчина *ж.* wórm-hole; *перен.* flaw.

чéрви *мн. карт.* hearts.

червь *м.*, червя́к *м.* worm.

червячóк *м.* small worm.

чердáк *м.* áttic; (*комната тж.*) gárret.

черёд *м. разг.* turn; настáл егó ~ his time/turn has come; тепéрь ваш ~ it is your turn now; ◇ идти́ свои́м черёдом take* its course.

чередовáние *с.* alternátion, rotátion, ínterchange.

чередовáть *несов.* (*вн. с тв.*) álternate (*smth.* with). ~ся *несов.* álternate, ínterchange; ~ся мéжду собóй álternate with each óther.

чéрез 1. acróss, óver; (*сквозь*) through; by way of, via; перейти́ ~ мост go* óver/acróss the bridge, cross the bridge; ~ окнó through the window; ~ лес, гóрод *и т. д.* through the fórest, the town, *etc.*; éхать на юг ~ Москвý trável south vía Móscow; 2. (*при помощи, при посредстве*) through; (*применяя что-л.*) with; оповести́ть о чём-л. ~ газéту make* *smth.* known through the press; писáть слóво ~ дефи́с write* the word with a hýphen; 3. (*минуя какой-л. промежуток пространства или времени*) évery óther; (*перед числом*) évery; ~ день évery óther day; ~ два, три дня évery two, three days; ~ две ступéньки two steps at a time; писáть ~ стрóчку write* on évery óther line; (*на пишущей машинке*) use dóuble-spácing; 4. (*по истечении какого-л. срока*) in; láter (*с гл. в прошедшем времени*); ~ год in a year; он приéхал ~ год he arríved a year láter; ~ ты́сячу лет in a thóusand years, a thóusand years hence; ~ нéкоторое врéмя (some time) láter.

черёмуха *ж.* 1. (*ягода*) bird-chérry; 2. (*дерево*) bird-cherry tree.

черенóк *м.* 1. (*рукоятка*) haft; 2. *сад.* graft.

чéреп *м.* skull.

черепа́х|а *ж.* 1. tórtoise; (*морская*) túrtle; 2. *собир.* (*роговые пластинки панциря*) tórtoise-shell. ~овый 1. (*из черепахи*) túrtle *attr.*; ~овый суп túrtle soup; 2. (*из панциря черепахи*) tórtoise-shell *attr.*

черепа́|ший tórtoise *attr.*; *перен.* snail's; ~шьим ша́гом at a snail's pace.

черепи́|ца *ж.* 1. *собир.* tiles *pl*; кры́тый ~цей tiled; 2. (*отдельная плитка*) tile. ~чный tile *attr.*; (*сделанный из черепицы*) tiled; ~чная кры́ша tiled roof.

че́реп|о́й cránial; ~а́я коро́бка *анат.* cránium (*pl* -nia), skull.

че́реп|о́к *м.* crock; разлете́ться в ~ки́ fly* to bits/píeces.

чересчу́р (much) too; ~ добросо́вестный much too consciéntious, consciéntious to a fault; э́то уж ~! that's (a líttle) too much!

чере́шня *ж.* chérry; (*дерево тж.*) chérry-tree.

черке́с *м.* Circássian. ~ский Circássian; ~ский язы́к Circássian, the Circássian lánguage.

черке́шенка *ж.* Circássian.

черкну́ть *сов.* (*вн.*) *разг.* 1. scratch (*smth.*); 2. (*быстро написать*) scríbble (*smth.*); ~ не́сколько слов, слове́чко *кому-л.* drop *smb.* a line.

черне́ть, почерне́ть 1. (*становиться чёрным*) get* black; blácken; 2. *тк. несов.* (*виднеться*) show* black.

черни́ка *ж.* 1. *собир.* bílberries *pl*, whórtleberries *pl*; 2. (*об отдельной ягоде и растении*) bílberry, whórtleberry.

черни́ла *мн.* ink *sg*; писа́ть ~ми write* in ink.

черни́льн|ица *ж.* ínkpot; (*на подставке*) ínkstand. ~ый ink *attr.*; ~ое пятно́ ínk-spot, ínk-stain; ~ый прибо́р ínkstand.

черни́ть, очерни́ть (*вн.*) blácken (*smb., smth.*), slánder (*smb., smth.*), smear (*smb., smth.*).

чёрно-бе́л|ый black-and-white *attr.*; ~ое изображе́ние bláck-and-white pícture.

черно|боро́дый bláck-bearded; with a black beard *после сущ.* ~бро́вый bláck-browed.

чернобу́рка *ж.* *разг.* sílver fox.

черно-бу́р|ый bláck-brown; ~ая лиси́ца sílver fox.

черновиќ *м.* rough draft/cópy.

черново́й rough; draft *attr.*

черно|воло́сый bláck-haired. ~гла́зый bláck-eyed, dárk-eyed.

черного́р|ец *м.*, ~ка *ж.* Montenégrin.

чернозём *м.* black soil, chérnozem. ~ный bláck-soil *attr.*, chérnozem *attr.*

черноко́жий *прил.* 1. bláck-skinned; 2. *в знач. сущ. м.* Black.

чернолесье *с.* decíduous fórest.

черномо́рский Black Sea *attr.*

чернорабо́чий *м.* unskilled lábourer.

черносли́в *м. собир.* prunes *pl*.

чернота́ *ж.* bláckness.

чернота́л *м.* bay/láurel wíllow.

чёрн|ый *прил.* 1. black; *перен.* dark; ~ая кра́ска black paint; ~ая неблагода́рность, за́висть black ingrátitude, énvy; 2. (*неглавный, подсобный*) back *attr.*; ~ ход báckdóor, back éntrance; ~ая ле́стница backstáirs; 3. (*неквалифицированный*) rough; ~ая рабо́та rough/unskilled work; spade work *идиом.*; 4. *в знач. сущ. с.* black (*без артикля*); оде́тый в ~ое, в ~ом dressed in black; вам идёт ~ое black suits you; 5. *в знач. сущ. мн. шахм.* Black *sg*; ◇ ~ хлеб black/rye bread; ~ ко́фе black cóffee; ~ая икра́ black cáviar; ~ая сморо́дина blackcúrrant; ~ая ма́гия black art/mágic; ~ый ры́нок black márket; ~ые мета́ллы férrous métals; ~ым по бе́лому in black and white; быть в ~ом спи́ске be on the blácklist.

черпа́к *м.* (*ковшик*) scoop; (*экскаватора и т. п.*) búcket.

чёрпать *несов.* (*вн.*) scoop (*smth.*); (*ведром из коло́дца, пруда и т. п.*) draw* (*smth.*); *перен.* deríve (*smth.*); ~ си́лы, зна́ния deríve strength, knówledge.

черстве́ть, зачерстве́ть, очерстве́ть, почерстве́ть 1. *сов.* зачерстве́ть, почерстве́ть get* stale; 2. *сов.* очерстве́ть, почерстве́ть (*о человеке*) grow* cállous, hárden.

чёрствый 1. (*о хлебе*) stale; 2. (*бездушный*) cállous, hard; ~ челове́к cállous/hard pérson; ~ приём harsh recéption.

чёрт *м.* dévil; ~! oh, damn/hell!; к ~у! to hell with it! иди́те к ~у! go to hell!; go to the dévil!; како́го ~а what the dévil/blázes/hell!; чем ~ не шу́тит! you néver know!, you néver can tell!; сам ~ не разберёт there's no máking head or tail of it; ~ зна́ет тако́е! outrágeous!; ни черта́ не понима́ю! I don't understánd a thing!; что за ~! what the dévil!; не так стра́шен ~, как его́ малю́ют *посл.* the dévil is not so térrible as he is páinted; (*не так плох*) the dévil is not so black as he is páinted.

черт|а́ *ж.* 1. (*линия*) line; 2. (*граница, предел*) bóundary; (*города*) límits *pl*; 3. *обыкн. мн.* ~ы́ лица́ féatures, traits; 4. (*свойство, особенность*) féature, trait, characterístic; ~а́ хара́ктера отличи́тельная ~ distínctive féature; семе́йная, фами́льная ~ fámily trait; ◇ в о́бщих ~а́х in óutline, without góing into détails; за ~о́й бе́дности belów the póverty line.

чертёж *м.* dráwing.

чертёжн|ик *м.*, ~ица *ж.* dráughtsman*. ~ый dráwing *attr.*; ~ая доска́ dráwing-board; ~ая бума́га dráwing páper.

черти́ть, начерти́ть (*вн.*) draw* (*smth.*); ~ план draw* a plan.

черто́вск|и *разг.* dévilishly, héllishly; ~ далеко́ it's a hell of a long way; я ~ го́лоден I'm dévilishly húngry. ~ий *разг.* dévilish, héllish.

чертополо́х *м. бот.* thístle(s).

чёрточка *ж.* 1. line; 2. (*дефис*) hýphen; 3. (*характера*) féature, trait.

чертыха́ться *несов. разг.* swear*.

черче́ние *с.* dráwing; техни́ческое ~ mechánical dráwing.

чеса́ть, почеса́ть (*вн.*) 1. (*скрести*) scratch (*smth.*); 2. *тк. несов.* (*причёсывать*) comb (*smth.*); 3. *тк. несов.* (*лён, хлопок*) card (*smth.*); ◇ ~ язы́к (-о́м) chátter. ~ся, почеса́ться 1. scratch onesélf; 2. *тк. несов.* (*зудеть*) itch; 3. *тк. несов. разг.* (*причёсываться*) do* one's hair; ◇ у него́ ру́ки чешутся (+ *инф.*) he's ítching (+ to *inf.*).

чесно́к *м. бот.* gárlic.

чесо́тка *ж.* the itch; (*у животных*) the mange.

че́ствование *с.* (*рд.*) celebrátion (in hónour of).

че́ствовать *несов.* (*вн.*) fête (*smb.*); célebrate in *smb.'s* hónour.

че́стн|о hónestly; ~ отвеча́ть на вопро́с ánswer a question hónestly; он ~ призна́л, что... he fránkly admítted that...; поступи́ть ~ do* the hónest thing; поступа́ть ~ по отноше́нию к кому-л. act fáirly by *smb.* ~ость *ж.* hónesty; (*правдивость тж.*) íntegrity. ~ый hónest; ~ые лю́ди fair-mínded péople; ~ые глаза́ hónest eyes; ~ые наме́рения hónest inténtions; ~ый за́работок hónest wage; ~ое и́мя good name; ◇ ~ое сло́во! hónestly!, upón my word!, hónest (it is) *разг.*; дава́ть ~ое сло́во give* one's word.

честолюби́вый ambítious.

честолю́бие *с.* ambítion.

чест|ь *ж.* hónour; де́ло ~и mátter of hónour; ◇ в ~ кого-л., чего-л. in hónour of *smb., smth.*; с ~ью вы́полнить что-л. hónourably fulfíl *smth.*; вы́йти с ~ью из чего-л. emérge with flýing cólours; счита́ю за ~ I consíder it an hónour; э́то де́лает вам ~ it does you crédit; пора́ и ~ знать it's time to stop; (*о гостях*) it's time to be góing; отдава́ть ~ кому-л. salúte *smb.*

чета́ *ж.* cóuple, pair; супру́жеская ~ márried couple;

◇ не ~ *кому-л.* not smb.'s kind (at all), not in smb.'s style.

четве́рг *м.* Thúrsday; ◇ по́сле до́ждичка в ~ one fine day.

четвере́ньк|и *мн. разг.*: на ~ах on all fours; стать на ~ get* on to all fours.

четвёрка *ж.* 1. *(цифра)* a four; 2. *(отметка)* four out of five, a "good"; 3. *(лодка)* fóur(-oar boat); 4. *(лошадей)* fóur-in-hánd; 5. *(игральная карта)* the four (of).

че́тверо four; нас ~ there are four of us.

четвероно́гий *прил.* 1. fóur-footed; 2. *в знач. сущ. с.* quádruped.

четверости́шие *с.* quátrain.

четвёртый the fourth.

че́тверт|ь *ж.* 1. quárter; ~ ве́ка quárter of a century; ~ сто́имости quárter of the cost; ~ я́блока quárter of an ápple; ~ часа́ quárter of an hour; ~ пе́рвого a quárter past twelve; без ~и час a quárter to one; 2. *(часть учебного года)* term; 3. *муз. (нота)* crótchet, quárter-note.

четвертьфина́л *м. спорт.* the quárter-finals *pl.*

чётки *мн.* rósary *sg.*

чётк|ий 1. *(отчётливый)* clear, distínct; *(разборчивый)* légible; ~ое изображе́ние clear ímage; ~ по́черк clear/légible hándwriting; 2. *(о звуках)* distínct; 3. *(точный)* precíse; ~ая формулиро́вка precíse wórding; 4. *(хорошо организованный)* púnctual, efficient; ~ое исполне́ние распоряже́ний prompt fulfílment of instrúctions. ~ость *ж.* 1. *(отчётливость)* clárity; *(разборчивость)* legibílity; 2. *(звуков)* distínctness; ~ость произноше́ния clear articulátion; 3. *(точность)* precísion; *(точность исполнения)* efficiency, prómptness.

чётн|ый éven; ~ые чи́сла éven númbers.

четы́ре four; ◇ на все ~ сто́роны wherever one likes.

четы́режды four times; ~ пять — два́дцать four times five is twénty; four fives are/make twenty.

четы́реста four húndred.

четырёхгоди́чный fóur-year *attr.*

четырёхгодова́лый fóur-year óld; of four *после сущ.*

четырёхгра́нн|ик *м.* tetrahédron. ~ый tetrahédral.

четырёхдне́вный fóur-day *attr.*

четырёхкра́тн|ый fóurfold; в ~ом разме́ре four times the amóunt.

четырёхлет|ие *с.* 1. *(период)* four years *pl,* fóur-year périod; 2. *(годовщина)* fourth anníversary. ~ний 1. *(о сроке)* fóur-year *attr.*; of four years *после сущ.*; 2. *(о возрасте)* fóur-year-óld; of four *после сущ.*

четырёхме́стн|ый fóur-seater *attr.*; ~ая каю́та fóur-berth cábin/státe-room; ~ое купе́ compártment for four.

четырёхме́сячный 1. *(о сроке)* four month's; fóur-month *attr.*; 2. *(о возрасте)* fóur-month-óld; of four months *после сущ.*

четырёхмото́рный fóur-éngined.

четырёхсо́тый four húndredth.

четырёхсто́пный *лит.*: ~ ямб iámbic tetrámeter.

четырёхсторо́нний quadriláteral.

четырёхуго́льн|ик *м.* quádrangle. ~ый quadrángular.

четырёхэта́жный fóur-storey *attr.*

четы́рнадцатиле́тний 1. *(о сроке)* fóurteen-year *attr.*; of fourtéen years *после сущ.*; 2. *(о возрасте)* fourtéen-year-óld; of fourtéen *после сущ.*

четы́рнадцатый fourtéenth.

четы́рнадцать fourtéen.

чех *м.* Czech.

чехарда́ *ж.* léap-frog; *перен. разг.* chópping and chánging; министе́рская ~ cábinet reshúffling.

чехо́л *м.* cóver; *(футляр)* case; *(для мебели)* slíp-cóver, dúst-cover.

чехослова́цкий Czécho-Slovák(ian).

чечеви́|ца *ж.* léntil. ~чный léntil *attr.*

чече́н|ец *м.,* ~ка *ж.* Chéchen. ~ский Chéchen; ~ский язы́к Chéchen, the Chéchen lánguage.

че́ш|ка *ж.* Czech wóman*. ~ский Czech; ~ский язы́к Czech, the Czech lánguage.

чешуя́ *ж.* scales *pl.*

чи́бис *м. (птица)* péwit, lápwing.

чиж *м. (птица)* sískin.

чи́жик *м.* 1. *см.* чиж; 2. *(детская игра)* típ-cat.

чили́ец *м.* Chílean.

чили́йский Chílean.

чин *м.* rank.

чина́ра *ж.* plane tree.

чини́ть I, очини́ть, почини́ть *(вн.)* 1. *сов.* почини́ть *(исправлять)* repáir *(smth.)*, mend *(smth.)*; 2. *сов.* очини́ть *(делать острым)* shárpen *(smth.)*; ~ каранда́ш shárpen a pencil.

чини́ть II *несов. (устраивать)*; ~ *кому-л.* препя́тствия put* óbstacles in smb.'s way; ~ суд и распра́ву adminíster jústice.

чи́нн|о decorously, ceremóniously, in a dígnified mánner. ~ый dígnified, décorous, ceremónious.

чино́вни|к *м.* 1. *(government)* official; 2. *(бюрократ)* búreaucrat. ~ческий 1. official('s); 2. *(бюрократический)* bureaucrátic.

чи́псы *мн.* potáto crisps.

чи́рей *м. разг.* boil.

чири́к|ать *несов.* chirp, twítter. ~нуть *сов.* give* a chirp.

чи́рк|ать, чи́ркнуть; ~ спи́чкой strike* a match. ~нуть *сов. см.* чи́ркать.

чиро́к *м. (птица)* teal.

чи́сленн|ость *ж.* size; *(о войсках)* strength; ~ населе́ния size of the populátion; ~остью в сто челове́к númbering a húndred pérsons, one húndred strong. ~ый numérical; име́ть ~ое превосхо́дство *(над)* be* supérior in númbers (to), have* numérical superiórity (óver).

числи́тель *м.* númerator. ~ное *с. грам.* númeral; коли́чественное ~ое cárdinal númber; поря́дковое ~ое órdinal númber. ~ный: и́мя числи́тельное *грам.* númeral.

чи́слит|ься *несов.* 1. *(иметься)* be*; *(за тв.; считаться за кем-л.)* be* to smb.'s accóunt; кни́га ~ся за мной the book is in my name; 2. *(значиться, состоять)* be* régistered (as); ~ больны́м be* on the sick list/leave; ~ в спи́ске be* on the list, be* lísted; 3. *(считаться)* be* consídered.

числ|о́ *с.* 1. númber; *(тж. грам.)*; це́лое ~ whole númber; ~ мест *(в аудитории, театре и т. п.)* séating capácity; в ~е́ прису́тствующих amóng those présent; в ~е́ про́чих amóng óthers; в том ~е́ inclúding; он не из ~а́ тех, кото́рые... he is not one (+ to inf) 2. *(дата)* date; пе́рвое, второ́е и т. д. *(месяца)* the first, sécond, *etc.* (day of the month); в пе́рвых, после́дних чи́слах октября́ и т. д. éarly, late in Octóber, *etc.*; како́е сего́дня ~? what is the day of the month?; ◇ без ~а́ in cóuntless númbers.

числово́й numérical.

чи́стильщик *м.* cléaner; ~ сапо́г bóotblack, shóeblack.

чи́стить *несов. (вн.)* 1. clean *(smth.)*; *(щёткой)* brush *(smth.)*; *(посуду, металл)* scóur *(smth.)*, scrub *(smth.)*; *(лошадь)* cúrry *(smth.)*; ~ башмаки́ shine*/pólish one's shoes; ~ (себе́) зу́бы clean/do* one's teeth; 2. *(фрукты, овощи)* peel *(smth.)*; *(орехи)* shell *(smth.)*; *(рыбу)* scale *(smth.)*. ~ся *несов.* 1. clean onesélf up; 2.: хорошо́ ~ся clean well.

чи́стк|а *ж.* 1. cléaning; *(щёткой)* brúshing; *(посуды, металла)* scóuring, scrúbbing; ~ о́буви boot pólishing; отдава́ть что-л. в ~у send* smth. to the cléaner's; 2. *(фруктов, овощей)* péeling; *(орехов)* shélling.

чи́сто 1. *нареч. (опрятно, аккуратно)* néatly; ~ вы́мытый well-wáshed; ~ у́бранная ко́мната neat/clean room; ~ сделанный néatly done; 2. *нареч.* (*подлинно*) trúly, púrely; ~ по-матери́нски just like a móther; ~ матери́нское отноше́ние a trúly matérnal áttitude; 3. *в знач. сказ. безл.* it is clean.

чистово́й fair, clean; ~ экземпля́р fair cópy.

чистокро́вный thóroughbred, púrebred.

чистопло́тный clean; *перен.* pure.

чистописа́ние *с.* calligraphy.

чистосерде́чный frank, sincére, open-héarted.

чистота́ *ж.* cléanliness; *перен.* púrity; ~ кра́сок, ли́ний púrity of cólour, line.

чист|ый 1. clean; 2. (*неразбавленный, без приме́си*) pure; ~ спирт raw spírits *pl*, pure álcohol; 3. (*пустой, свободный*) clear; (*о пространстве*) ópen; (*неиспользованный*) new, fresh; ~ое по́ле ópen fields *pl*; ~ая страни́ца clean/fresh page; 4. (*нравственно безупре́чный*) pure, high-mínded, hónest; 5. *разг.* (*совершенный, подлинный*) sheer; ~ая пра́вда the símple truth; ~ое муче́ние sheer tórture; 6. (*о доходе и т. п.*) net, clear; ~ая при́быль clear/net prófit; ~ вес net weight; ◇ принима́ть *что-л.* за ~ую моне́ту take* *smth.* at its face válue, accépt *smth.* in all good faith.

чита́ль|ный ~ зал réading-room. **~ня** *ж.* réading-room.

чита́тель *м.* réader. **~ский** réader's; **~ская конфере́нция** réader's cónference.

чита́ть, прочесть, прочита́ть (*вн.*) read* (*smth.*); ~ про себя́ read* to onesélf; ~ вслух read* alóud; ~ ле́кцию give* a lécture; ~ ле́кции lécture; ~ исто́рию США lécture on the history of the USA; ~ докла́д read* a páper; ~ стихи́ recíte póetry; ◇ ~ наставле́ния *кому-л.* lécture *smb.*; ~ в чьих-л. сердца́х read* *smb.'s* heart(s); ~ ме́жду строк read* between the lines.

чита́ться *несов.* read*; легко́ ~ be*/make* éasy réading, read* éasily.

чи́тка *ж.* réading.

чиха́нье *с.* snéezing.

чиха́ть, чихну́ть sneeze.

чихну́ть *сов. см.* чиха́ть.

чи́ще *сравнит. ст. прил.* чи́стый *и нареч.* чи́сто.

член *м.* 1. (*часть тела*) limb; 2. (*часть какого-л. целого*) part; гла́вные ~ы предложе́ния main parts of a séntence; ~ пропо́рции term of a propórtion; 3. (*организа́ции и т. п.*) mémber; (*учёного общества тж.*) féllow; ~ профсою́за tráde-union mémber; ~ па́ртии Párty mémber; действи́тельный ~ mémber; почётный ~ hónorary mémber; ~ы семьи́ mémbers of the fámily; 4. *грам.* (*артикль*) árticle.

член-корреспонде́нт *м.* correspónding mémber.

членоразде́льн|о cléarly, distinctly. **~ый** artículate, distinct; ~ая речь artículate speech.

чле́нский mémbership *attr.*; ~ биле́т mémbership card; ~ взнос dues *pl*.

чмо́к|ать, чмо́кнуть 1. make* a súcking sound; (*губами от удовольствия*) smack one's lips; (*понукая лоша́дь*) chuck; 2. (*издавать хлю́пающие звуки*) squelch; грязь ~ала под нога́ми the mud squelched underfóot; 3. (*вн.*) *разг.* (*звучно целовать*) kiss (*smb.*); ~ кого́-л. в щёку give* *smb.* a smácking kiss on the cheek. **~нуть** *сов. см.* чмо́кать.

чо́каться, чо́кнуться clink glásses.

чо́кнуться *сов. см.* чо́каться.

чо́порный prim, punctílious; (*напыщенный*) stiff, convéntional.

чрева́тый prégnant, fraught; ~ тяжёлыми после́дствиями fraught with grave cónsequences; ~ опа́сностью fraught with dánger.

чревовеща́ние *с.* ventríloquism.

чрезвыча́йн|о extrémely, excéptionally. **~ый** 1. extraórdinary, excéptional; ~ое происше́ствие emérgency; 2. (*экстренный*) emérgency *attr.*; ~ые ме́ры emérgency méasures;

~ое положе́ние state of emérgency; ~ые полномо́чия emérgency pówers.

чрезме́рн|о too, excéssively. **~ый** excéssive, inórdinate.

чте́ние *с.* 1. (*действие*) réading; 2. (*читаемый текст*) réading-matter.

чтец *м.* réader; (*артист тж.*) recíter.

чтить *сов.* (*вн.*) hold* (*smb., smth.*) in estéem, revére (*smb., smth.*); свя́то ~ па́мять *кого-л.* hold* the mémory of *smb.* sácred.

что I *мест.* (*рд.* чего́, *дт.* чему́, *вн.* что, *тв.* чем, *пр.* о чём) 1. what; ~ вы сказа́ли, купи́ли? what did you say, buy?; ~ с ва́ми? what's the mátter with you?; а э́то ~ тако́е? and what is this?; чем вы нас пора́дуете? what's your good news?; чем объясни́ть э́то? what's the explanátion of it?; чем могу́ служи́ть?, чем я могу́ быть вам поле́зен? what can I do for you?; в чём его́ обвиня́ют-ли? what is he accúsed of?; за ~? what for?, why?; за ~ вы его́ оби́дели? why did you hurt his féelings?; на ~ вы наде́етесь? what are you cóunting on?; ~ то́лку, по́льзы в э́том? what's the good/use of that?; 2. *в знач. нареч.* (*почему*) why?, what... for?; ~ он так кричи́т? why is he shóuting, what is he shóuting for?; 3. (*сколько*) what?; ~ сто́ит э́та кни́га? what does that book cost?; 4. *разг.* (*что-нибудь*) sómething, ánything; е́сли ~ случи́тся if ánything should háppen; 5. *относ.* what; (*который*) that; (*и это*) which; он зна́ет, ~ ему́ ну́жно he knows what he wants; я зна́ю, ~ вы име́ете в виду́ I know what you mean; я не зна́ю, ~ взять и ~ оста́вить I don't know what to take and what to leave; э́то всё, ~ я могу́ сказа́ть that is all (that) I can say; всё (то), ~ everything (that); всё то, ~ ну́жно everything *one* needs; дом, ~ сто́ит на берегу́ the house that stands on the bank; он не отве́тил, ~ меня́ удиви́ло he did not ánswer, which surprísed me; ◇ ~ уго́дно, ~ попа́ло, ~ придётся ánything; ~ бы́ло сил with all *one's* might; бежа́ть ~ есть ду́ху run* as fast as *one* can; ни за ~ néver; not for the world; ни за ~ не догада́етесь you'll néver guess; ни за ~ не пойду́ туда́ I wóuldn't go there for the world; ~ вы! 1) (*неужели?*) you don't say so!; 2) (*отнюдь нет!*) not a bit of it!, oh, come!; ~ за ме́ня... as far as I am concérned...; ну и ~ ж(е)! all right!, why not?; ~ говори́ть! of course!; oh, yes!; ~ э́то за де́рево? what is (the name of) that tree?; ~ э́то за кни́ги? what books are those?; ~ (там) за шум? what is that noise?; ~ ли perháps; пойти́ в кино́, ~ ли? what shall I do? go to the cínema?; взять такси́, ~ ли? suppóse I take a táxi?; ~ ни стро́чка, то оши́бка there is not a síngle line without a mistáke; ~ ни день, пого́да меня́ется the wéather is néver the same two days rúnning; ~ бы ни случи́лось whatéver háppens; ни при чём nóthing to do with it; ни за ~ ни про ~ (all) for nóthing; здесь не на ~ сесть there is nóthing to sit on here; на ~ (уж), уж на ~ though; уж на ~ до́брый, а рассерди́лся though he is, he lost his témper; с чего́ бы ему́...? why should he...?; с чего́ вы взя́ли, ~ я бо́лен? what put it into your head that I was ill?

что II *союз* 1. that (*часто опускается*); он сказа́л, ~ придёт he said he would come; я слы́шал, ~ он хоро́ший специали́ст I understánd (that) he is an éxpert; я наде́юсь, ~ вы не отка́жете I trust/hope you will not refúse; чемода́н тако́й тяжёлый, ~ я не могу́ подня́ть его́ the case is so héavy I can't lift it; то, ~ он спосо́бный, никто́ не отрица́ет no one deníes his ability; меня́ не удивля́ет, ~ он простуди́лся I am not surprísed that he caught cold; 2. (*ли... ли*) whéther... or; ~ ты пойдёшь, ~ я — всё равно́ it makes no dífference whéther you go or I do.

чтоб *см.* чтобы.

чтобы 1. *союз* (*цели*) so as to, in órder to; so that; он наде́л очки́, ~ лу́чше ви́деть he put on his spéctacles so as to see bétter; встать ра́но, ~ попа́сть на по́езд get* up éarly (in órder) to catch the train; ~ не разбудить его so as not to wake him; я подвинусь, ~ вам бы́ло лу́чше ви́дно I'll move so that you can see bétter; **2.** *союз (изъяснительный)* that (*smb.*) should; *передаётся тж. оборотом с инфинитивом*; я предлага́ю, ~ докла́д сде́лал он I suggest that he should give the lécture; я хоте́л бы, ~ докла́д сде́лал он I should like him to give the lécture; скажи́те ему́, ~ он ушёл tell him to go awáy; он наста́ивает на том, ~ пойти́ he insists on góing; не мо́жет быть, ~ он э́то сказа́л he cóuldn't have said that!; **3.** *частица*: ~ э́того бо́льше не́ было! it must néver háppen agáin!; ◇ без того́ ~ withóut (+ -ing); для того́ ~, с тем ~, так ~ so that; вме́сто того́ ~ instéad of (+ -ing).

что́-либо, что́-нибудь something; (*в вопросе и при отрицании*) ánything; два часа́ с чем-нибудь óver two hours; нет ли чего́-нибудь почита́ть? have you ánything for me to read?

что́-то I *мест.* sómething.

что́-то II *нареч. разг.* **1.** (*в некоторой степени*) ráther, a bit; quite; мне ~ нездоро́вится I don't feel quite well sómehow; вы ~ невеселы́ you seem (a bit) depréssed; **2.** (*почему-то*) sómehow, for some réason; мне ~ не ве́рится sómehow I can't believe; ~ не по́мню I don't seem to remémber, I'm afráid I don't remémber; **3.** (*приблизительно*) abóut, sómething like.

чу hark!, listen!

чуб *м.* fórelock.

чува́ш *м.*, **~ка** *ж.* Chuvásh. **~ский** Chuvásh; ~ский язы́к Chuvásh, the Chuvásh lánguage.

чу́вственн|ость *ж.* sensuálity. **~ый** sénsual; sense *attr.*; **~ое восприя́тие** 'sense percéption.

чувстви́тель|ость *ж.* **1.** (*восприимчивость*) sensitívity; **2.** (*впечатлительность*) sénsitiveness, sensibílity; **3.** (*сентиментальность*) sentimentálity. **~ый 1.** (*восприимчивый*) sénsitive; **~ая ко́жа** sénsitive skin; **~ый прибо́р** sénsitive apparátus; **~ое ме́сто** ténder spot; **2.** (*впечатлительный*) sénsitive; **3.** (*сентиментальный*) sentiméntal; **4.** *разг.* (*ощутимый*) appréciable; **~ый уда́р** sevére/bódy blow; **~ая утра́та** déeply-felt loss.

чу́вство *с.* **1.** sense; (*ощущение*) sensátion; (*переживание, отношение*) féeling; (*эмоция*) emótion; пять чувств the five sénses; о́рганы чувств sense órgans; ~ бо́ли, хо́лода, го́лода sensátion of pain, cold, húnger; ~ го́рдости féeling of pride; ~ оби́ды sense of ínjury; ~ до́лга, отве́тственности, че́сти, ю́мора, ме́ры sense of dúty, responsibílity, hónour, húmour, propórtion; ~ но́вого sense of the new; ~ со́бственного досто́инства (féeling of) self-respéct; зло́бе ~ reséntment; **2.** (*сознание*) cónsciousness; приходи́ть в ~ recóver cónsciousness; приводи́ть кого́-л. в ~ bring* *smb.* round; быть без чувств be* uncónscious; па́дать без чувств fall* uncónscious to the ground; faint; лиша́ться чувств lose* cónsciousness; **3.** (*любовь*) féeling, love.

чу́вств|овать, почу́вствовать (*вн.*) **1.** feel* (*smth.*); (*воспринимать чутьём тж.*) sense (*smth.*); ~ го́лод, уста́лость, ра́дость *и т. д.* feel* húnger, exháustion, joy *etc.*; он ~овал, как к нему́ возвраща́ются си́лы he felt his strength retúrning; ~ отве́тственность за *что-л.* feel* responsibílity for *smth.*; ~ прису́тствие *кого-л.* sense *smb.'s* présence; **2.** (*осознавать*) feel* (*smth.*), be* aware (of); ◇ ~ себя́ feel*; ~ себя́ больны́м feel* ill; как вы себя́ ~уете? how do you feel?; дава́ть кому́-л. ~ *что-л.* make* *smb.* feel *smth.*; дава́ть себя́ ~ make* itsélf felt. **~оваться** *несов.* be* nóticeable, one can feel; в его́ слова́х ~уется уве́ренность one can feel the cónfidence in his words; ~уется влия́ние среды́ the influence of *smb.'s* surroundings is nóticeable.

чугу́н *м.* **1.** cast íron; **2.** (*сосуд*) cást-iron kéttle/pot. **~ный** cást-iron *attr.*, íron *attr.*

чугунолите́йн|ый iron *attr.*; **~ое произво́дство** iron prodúction; ~ цех íron fóundry.

чуда́к *м.* eccéntric, crank, strange pérson; како́й вы ~! how cránky you are!

чуда́чество *с.* eccentrícity; strángeness; *мн.* fúnny ways.

чуда́чка *ж. см.* чуда́к.

чуде́сный 1. (*сверхъестественный*) miráculous; **2.** (*замечательный*) wónderful, márvellous, spléndid; ~ наро́д spléndid/wónderful péople.

чу́д|иться, почу́диться *обыкн. безл.*: мне ~ится (*зрелище, звук*) I seem to see, hear; (*представляется*) I imágine mysélf; мне почу́дилось it seemed to me; мне почу́дилось, что кто́-то идёт I thought I heard sómebody cóming.

чудн|о́ *разг.* **1.** *нареч.* strángely; **2.** *в знач. сказ. безл.* it is fúnny/strange; ~! fúnny!; queer! **~о́й** *разг.* queer, strange; (*смешной*) fúnny.

чу́дный wónderfull, márvellous, spléndid.

чу́д|о *с.* míracle; (*что-л. небывалое тж.*) wónder; (*о человеке*) pródigy, páragon; ~еса́ геро́изма, те́хники míracles of héroism, téchnical achíevement; он спа́сся каки́м-то ~ом he had a miráculous escápe; твори́ть ~еса́ work wónders; она́ ~ как хороша́! she's divínely béautiful!

чудо́вищ|е *с.* mónster (*тж. о человеке*); monstrósity. **~ный** mónstrous; (*огромный, гигантский*) huge, enórmous; **~ное преступле́ние** abóminable crime/offénce; **~ный аппети́т** treméndous áppetite.

чудоде́йственный miráculous.

чужби́н|а *ж.* strange/álien land; fóreign parts *pl*; на ~е in a strange land; in fóreign parts.

чужда́ться *несов.* (*рд.*) shun (*smb., smth.*), avóid (*smb., smth.*).

чужд|ый 1. (*дт., для рд.*: *противоположный по духу, сущности*) álien (to), fóreign (to); **~ая идеоло́гия** álien ideólogy; он ~ нам челове́к he is not one of us; он мне соверше́нно чужд we have nóthing whatéver in cómmon; честолю́бие ему́ ~о ambítion is álien/fóreign to his náture; **2.** (*рд.; лишённый чего-л.*) devóid (of), free (from); челове́к, ~ честолю́бия a man* devóid of ambítion.

чужезе́мец *м.* fóreigner.

чуж|о́й *прил.* **1.** (*принадлежащий другому*) óther péople's; anóther's; belónging to sómeone else *после сущ.*; ~áя со́бственность óther péople's próperty; э́то ~áя кни́га this book is not mine, this book dóesn't belóng to me; под ~и́м и́менем únder an assúmed name; на ~ счёт at sómeone élse's expénse; ще́дрость за ~ счёт vicárious generósity; **2.** (*чуждый, посторонний*) strange, unfamíliar; ~ие лю́ди strángers; он нам ~ he is not one of us; ~ мужчи́на, ~áя же́нщина stránger, strange man*, wóman*; **3.** (*не являющийся родиной*) strange, fóreign, álien; (*иностранный*) fóreign; ~ язы́к fóreign lánguage; ~ие обы́чаи strange/álien cústoms; **4.** *в знач. сущ. с.* óther péople's próperty; **5.** *в знач. сущ. м.* stránger; ◇ знать *что-л.* с ~и́х слов learn* *smth.* from héarsay; повторя́ть, расска́зывать с ~и́х слов repéat what *one* has heard, repéat what *one* has been told; ~и́ми рука́ми де́лать *что-л.* get* *smth.* done for *one*.

чуко́тский 1. Chukótka *attr.*; **2.** Chúkchi; ~ язы́к Chúkchi lánguage.

чу́кча *м. и ж.* Chúkchi.

чула́н *м.* stóreroom, bóxroom; clóset.

чулки́ *мн.* (*ед.* чуло́к *м.*) stóckings.

чуло́чн|ый **~ые изде́лия** hósiery *sg*; ~ая фа́брика stócking fáctory.

чум *м.* ráw-hide tent.

чума́ *ж.* plague; (*у собак*) distémper.

чума́зый *разг.* grímy.

чумно́й 1. plague *attr.*; **2.** (*заражённый чумой*) plágue-infécted.

чура́ться *несов.* (*ед.*) shun (*smb.*), fight* shy (of).

чурба́н *м.* **1.** block; **2.** *бран.* blóckhead.

чу́рка ж. small block, billet.

чу́ткий 1. (*восприимчивый*) keen, sénsitive; **2.** (*чувствительный, быстро реагирующий*) sénsitive; **3.** (*отзывчивый*) sympathétic, respónsive; ~ това́рищ sympathétic friend; ~ подхо́д sympathétic appróach; ◇ ~ сон light sleep/slúmber.

чу́тк|о (*внимательно*) kéenly; ~ относи́ться к кому́-л. treat smb. with sýmpathy/understánding. **~ость** ж. **1.** (*восприимчивость*) sensitívity; (*слуха и т. п. тж.*) kéenness; **2.** (*отзывчивость*) sýmpathy, understánding; проявля́ть ~ость show* considerátion.

чу́точк|а ж. разг.: ни ~и (не) not a bit, not in the least. **~у** a little, a tíny bit; подожди́(те) ~у! wait just a móment!

чуть 1. нареч. (*едва*) scárcely, hárdly; (*еле*) bárely; (*немного*) a little; ~ ви́дно bárely vísible; ~ живо́й half-déad; ~ заме́тный bárely percéptible; ~ заме́тная улы́бка the ghost of a smile; **2.** союз scárcely, hárdly; ◇ ~ бы́ло не... álmost; ~ (ли) не ве́ры néarly; ~ не весь álmost the whole; ~ что 1) (*если что-л. случится*) on the slíghtest prétext; 2) (*почти*) néarly.

чутьё с. (*у животных*) scent, nose; перен. intuítion, ínstinct, flair.

чуть-чу́ть just a little.

чу́чело с. **1.** (*животного*) stuffed ánimal; (*птицы*) stuffed bird; **2.** (*пугало*) scárecrow (*тж. перен.*).

чушь ж. разг. nónsense, rúbbish.

чу́|ять несов. (вн). **1.** (*о животных*) scent (smth.); **2.** разг. (*чувствовать, ощущать*) feel* (smth.); **3.** разг. (*чувствовать интуитивно*) sense (smth.); (*догадываться*) guess (smth.), suspéct (smth.); ~ло моё се́рдце! my heart told me!; ~ет моё се́рдце, что... I have a preséntiment that...; ◇ ног под собо́й не ~ 1) (*от радости, волнения*) be* wálking on air; 2) (*от усталости*) be* whacked out.

чьё, чьи, чья см. чей.

Ш

ша́баш м. **1.** рел. Sábbath; **2.** witches' sábbath; перен. тж. órgy.

шаблóн м. témplet; (*трафарет*) sténcil; páttern (*тж. перен.*); по ~у on convéntional lines, accórding to páttern. **~ность** ж. перен. tríteness, banálity. **~ный** stándard; перен. тж. convéntional, trite.

шаг м. **1.** step; (*крупный*) stride; (*как мера длины*) pace; мн. (*звук шагов*) (fóot)steps; больши́ми ~а́ми with long strides; идти́ больши́ми ~а́ми stride*/swing* alóng; **2.** (*действие, поступок*) step; необду́манный ~ thóughtless step; де́лать, предпринима́ть ~ take* step; **3.** mex. (*винта, нарезки*) pitch; ◇ пе́рвые ~и first steps; éarly stage sg; сде́лать ~ take* a step; ~ за ~ом step by step; на ка́ждом ~у́ at évery step; два ~а́ (*очень близко*) it is ónly a step; в двух ~а́х от чего́-л. a few steps awáy from smth.; не отходи́ть ни на ~ от кого́-л. néver move from smb.'s side; ни ~у! stay where you are!; ни ~у да́льше! not another step!; ~у не сде́лать для кого́-л., чего́-л. ≈ not lift a finger to help smb., smth.; ~ом марш! quick march!

шаг|а́ть несов. **1.** (*делать шаги*) step; **2.** (*ходить размеренным шагом*) stride*, pace; **3.** (*развиваться*) make* prógress; бы́стро ~ по пути́ прогре́сса make* rápid strides alóng the road of prógress; **4.** (*через вн.; переступать*) step (acróss, óver). **~ающий** mex. self-propélled. **~ну́ть** сов. step, take* a step; ~ну́ть че́рез поро́г step across the thréshold; ◇ далеко́ ~ну́ть go* far.

ша́гом at a walk; (*о лошади*) at a wálking pace; идти́ ~ procéed at a walk.

шагоме́р м. pedómeter.

ша́йба ж. **1.** mex. wásher; (*прокладка*) spácer; **2.** спорт. puck.

ша́йка I ж. (*группа*) gang.

ша́йка II ж. (*для воды*) small tub.

шака́л м. зоол. jáckal.

шала́нда ж. **1.** scow; **2.** shalánda (*flat-bottomed Black Sea fishing-boat*).

шала́ш м. tent/shélter of bránches.

шал|и́ть несов. **1.** fool abóut; (*о детях тж.*) be* náughty; **2.** разг. (*неправильно действовать*) give* tróuble, be* tróublesome; ◇ нет, ~и́шь! no, you don't!

шаловли́вый míschievous, pránkish, pláyful.

шалопа́й м. разг. góod-for-nóthing, ne'er-do-well.

ша́лость ж. prank.

шалу́н м. scamp; (*о ребёнке тж.*) imp.

шалу́нья ж. см. шалу́н.

шалфе́й м. бот. sage.

ша́лый разг. mad, crázy.

шаль ж. shawl.

шальн|о́й 1. mad; **2.:** ~а́я пу́ля stray búllet.

шама́н м. sháman, médicine-man*.

ша́мкать несов. разг. múmble.

шампа́нское с. champágne.

шампиньо́н м. field múshroom.

шампу́нь м. shampóo.

шанс м. chance; больши́е ~ы на успе́х every próspect of succéss; ма́ло ~ов на успе́х not much hope of succéss; не име́ть никаки́х ~ов not have the slíghtest chance.

шанта́ж м. bláckmail.

шантаж|и́ровать несов. (вн.) bláckmail (smb.). **~и́ст** м. bláckmailer.

ша́пка ж. **1.** hat; ~ воло́с mop/shock of hair; ~-уша́нка hat with éar-flaps; мехова́я ~ fur hat; **2.** (*заголовок в газете*) héadline; **3.** (*верх чего-л.*) crown, top; ◇ ~-невиди́мка cap of invisibility; ~ми закида́ем it'll be a wálk-óver; на во́ре ~ гори́т guílty cónscience gives itsélf awáy.

ша́почка ж. cap; ◇ Кра́сная ~ Little Red Ríding Hood.

ша́почн|ый hat attr.; ◇ ~ое знако́мство bówing acquáintance; прийти́ к ~ому разбо́ру arríve when the show/párty is óver.

шар м. **1.** ball; билья́рдный ~ bílliard-ball; **2.** мат. sphere, globe; ◇ земно́й ~ the globe; хоть ~о́м покати́ bare as a bone, not a thing (in the house).

шара́да ж. charáde.

шара́хаться, шара́хнуться разг. **1.** start, recóil; (*о лошади тж.*) shy; ~ в сто́рону plunge to the side; ~ из стороны́ в сто́рону plunge from side to side; **2.** тж. несов. (*от рд.; сторониться, избегать*) shun (smb.), keep* awáy (from).

шара́хнуться сов. см. шара́хаться 1.

шарж м. caricatúre. **~и́ровать** несов. caricatúre, exággerate; (*об актёре*) overáct.

шар-зо́нд м. sóunding ballóon.

ша́рик м. ball; глóбуле научн.; ◇ кровяны́е ~и blood córpuscles. **~овый:** ~овая ру́чка báll-point (pen), bíro.

шарикоподши́пник м. ball-béaring. **~овый** báll-béaring attr.

ша́рить несов. fúmble, rúmmage; ~ в карма́не feel*/fúmble in one's pócket.

ша́рк|ать, ша́ркнуть: ~ нога́ми shúffle (one's feet). **~нуть** сов. см. ша́ркать.

шарлата́н м. chárlatan, impóstor; (*о докторе тж.*) quack. **~ство** с. impósture, hócus-pócus; (*в медицине тж.*) quáckery.

шарма́н|ка ж. bárrel-organ, hánd-organ. **~щик** м. órgan-grinder.

шарни́р *м. тех.* hinge.

шарова́ры *мн.* wide tróusers; (*спортивные*) tráck-suit tróusers.

шарови́дный glóbe-shaped.

шаров|о́й sphérical, glóbular, báll-shaped; ~а́я мо́лния ball lightning.

шарообра́зный glóbe-shaped.

шарф *м.* scarf*, múffler.

шасси́ *с. нескл. тех.* 1. cárriage, únderframe; ~ автомоби́ля chássis; 2. (*самолёта*) úndercarriage.

шата́ние *с.* 1. (*качание*) swáying, swínging; 2. *разг.* (*бесцельная ходьба*) róaming; 3. (*непостоянство, колебание*) vacillátion, wávering; shílly-shallying *разг.*

шат|а́ть *несов.* 1. (*вн.*) sway (*smth.*), rock (*smth.*); 2. *безл.*: его́ ~а́ет he is réeling/stággering. ~а́ться *несов.* 1. (*качаться из стороны в сторону*) sway, swing*, rock; 2. (*покачиваться при ходьбе*) stágger; ~а́сь встать (*на́ ноги*) stágger to one's feet; 3. (*о мебели и т. п.*) be* sháky; (*о зубе*) be* loose, be* cóming out; *перен.* be* sháken, be* rócking on its foundátions; 4. *разг.* (*бродить без дела*) roam; где ты ~а́ешься? where do you spend your time?

шате́н *м.* brówn-háired man*. ~ка *ж.* wóman* with brown/áuburn hair.

шатёр *м.* tent.

шатк|ий unstáble; (*неустойчивый*) rískety: (*о походке*) unstéady; *перен.* (*необоснованный*) sháky; (*непостоянный*) wávering, upstáble; ~ая ле́стница rískety stairs; ~ до́вод sháky árgument; ~ое положе́ние precárious position.

шату́н *м. тех.* connécting-rod.

шафра́н *м. бот.* sáffron.

шах I *м.* (*титул*) Shan.

шах II *м. шахм.* check.

шахмати́ст *м.* chéss-player.

ша́хматн|ый chess *attr.*; ~ая доска́ chéssboard; ~ые фигу́ры chéssmen; ~ turnip chess tóurnament; в ~ом поря́дке arránged chéssboard fáshion, stággered.

ша́хматы *мн.* 1. (*игра*) chess *sg*; 2. (*фигуры*) chéssmen; (*полный комплект*) set of chéssmen.

ша́хта *ж.* 1. (*предприятие*) mine, pit; у́гольная ~ cóal-mine; 2. (*колодец, ствол*) shaft.

шахтёр *м.* míner. ~ский míner's, míners'.

ша́шечн|ый draught *attr.*; ~ая доска́ dráught-board.

ша́шк|а I *ж.* 1. dráughtsman*; 2. *мн.* (*игра*) draughts; игра́ть в ~и play draughts.

ша́шка II *ж.* (*оружие*) sword.

шашлы́к *м.* shashlík, mútton grilled on a spit.

шва́бра *ж. мор.*

швартов *м. мор.* móoring-line; отда́ть ~ы cast* off.

швед *м.*, ~ка *ж.* Swede. ~ский Swédish; ~ский язы́к Swédish, the Swédish lánguage.

швей|ик *м.* clóthing-industry wórker. ~ый séwing *attr.*; ~ая маши́на séwing-machine; ~ая фа́брика clóthing fáctory; ~ые изде́лия clóthing *sg.*

швейца́р *м.* dóor-keeper, hall pórter.

швейца́р|ец *м.*, ~ка *ж.* Swiss. ~ский Swiss; ~ский сыр gruyère.

швея́ *ж.* séamstress. ~-мотори́стка *ж.* eléctric séwing-machine operator.

швырну́ть *сов. см.* швыря́ть.

швыр|я́ть, швырну́ть 1. (*вн., тв.*; *бросать*) fling* (*smth.*); 2. *обыкн. безл.*: ло́дку ~я́ло на волна́х the boat was tóssing/rócking on the waves; ◇ ~ деньга́ми squánder one's móney, throw* one's móney awáy. ~я́ться *несов.* (*тв.*) *разг.* 1. (*бросаться*) fling* (*smth.*) (at one anóther); 2. (*не дорожить*) throw* (*smth.*) awáy.

шевел|и́ть, шевельну́ть 1. (*вн.*; *приводить в лёгкое движение*) move (*smth.*), stir (*smth.*) (*тж. перен.*); 2. (*тв.*; *слегка двигать*) stir (*smth.*); 3. *тк. несов.* (*шуршать*) rústle; 4. *тк. несов.*: ~ се́но turn/ted hay; ◇ он па́льцем не шевельнёт he wóuldn't lift a finger; шевели́

вёслами! get a move on! ~ться, шевельну́ться 1. stir (*тж. перен.*); move; не ~сь without stírring/móving; mótionless; ли́стья шевеля́тся от ве́тра the leaves stir in the breeze; 2. *тк. несов.*: ~сь! look lívely!

шевельну́ть *сов. см.* шевели́ть 1, 2. ~ся *сов. см.* шевели́ться 1.

шевелю́ра *ж.* head of hair; пы́шная ~ fine head of hair.

шевро́ *с. нескл.* kid. ~вый kid *attr.*

шеде́вр *м.* másterpiece.

шезло́нг *м.* déck-chair.

ше́йка *ж.* neck.

ше́йный neck *attr.*; ~ позвоно́к júgular vértebra.

ше́лест *м.* rústle.

шелесте́ть *несов.* rústle.

шёлк *м.* silk; *перен.* vélvet; (*о человеке*) géntleness itsélf; ~-сыре́ц raw silk; иску́сственный ~ artificial/ráyon silk; на шелку́ sílk-lined; ◇ в долгу́ как в шелку́ up to one's neck in debt.

шелкови́нка *ж.* silk thread.

шелкови́стый sílky.

шелкови́чный: ~ червь sílkworm.

шелково́д *м.* sílkworm bréeder, sílk-grower. ~ство *с.* sílkworm bréeding, silk cúlture, sériculture. ~ческий sériculture *attr.*

шёлковый 1. silk *attr.*; 2. (*напоминающий шёлк*) sílky; sílken *поэт.*; 3. *разг.* (*кроткий, послушный*) swéet-tempered.

шелкопря́д *м.* 1. sílkworm, sílkworm moth; bómbyx *зоол.*; 2. (*вредитель деревьев*): сосно́вый ~ pine moth; непа́рный ~ Gýpsy moth.

шёлкотка́цк|ий silk-weaving; ~ая фа́брика sílk-weaving fáctory.

шелохн|у́ться *сов.* stir; стоя́ть не ~у́вшись stand* mótionless, stand* véry still.

шелуха́ *ж.* husk; *перен.* rúbbish; карто́фельная ~ potáto péelings *pl.*

шелуши́ть *несов.* (*вн.*) 1. husk (*smth.*), peel (*smth.*); 2. (*заставлять шелушиться*) make* (*smth.*) peel. ~ся *несов.* peel.

шельмова́ть, ошельмова́ть (*вн.*) *разг.* throw* mud (at), bláckguard (*smb.*).

шепеля́в|ить *несов.* lisp. ~ый lísping.

шепну́ть *сов. см.* шепта́ть.

шёпот *м.* whisper.

шёпотом in a whisper; говори́ть ~ speak* in a whisper; (*о нескольких людях*) speak*/talk in whispers; сказа́ть что-л. ~ whisper *smth.*

шепта́ть, шепну́ть, прошепта́ть (*вн.*) whisper (*smth.*); ~ на́ ухо кому́-л. whisper in *smb.'s* ear. ~ся *несов.* whisper.

шере́нг|а *ж.* 1. rank; в две ~и in two ranks; 2. (*длинный ряд предметов*) line, row; ◇ стоя́ть в одно́й ~е с кем-л. 1) take* part with *smb.*; 2) (*иметь одинаковое достоинство*) rank with *smb.*

шерохова́т|ость *ж.* róughness; *перен.* unévenness, blémish. ~ый rough; *перен.* (*о стиле*) unpólished, inádequate.

шерсти́нка *ж.* wóollen thread; (*волосок*) hair.

шерстопряди́льн|ый wóol-spinning; ~ая фа́брика wóol-spinning fáctory.

шерсть *ж.* 1. (*овцы*) wool; (*собаки*) hair; (*кошки*) fur; 2. (*пряжа*) wool; 3. (*ткань*) cloth, wóollen matérial/stuff; wórsted.

шерстян|о́й wóollen; ~ые тка́ни wóollens, wóollen goods; ~о́е пла́тье wóollen dress.

шерша́в|ый rough; ~ые ру́ки rough hands; ~ая ткань cóarse-téxtured/twéedy cloth.

ше́ршень *м. зоол.* hórnet.

шест *м.* pole; прыжо́к с ~о́м póle-jump.

ше́ствие *с.* procéssion; *перен.* march, prógress.

ше́ствовать *несов.* march (sólemnly).

шестерёнка *ж.* см. шестерня́.

шестёрка *ж.* 1. (*цифра*) a six; 2. *ав.* flight of six (planes); 3. (*упряжка*) team of six hórses; 4. (*лодка*) six-oar boat; 5. (*игра́льная ка́рта*) the six (of).

шестерня́ *ж. тех.* gear, cóg-wheel; (*ме́ньшее колесо́ из па́ры*) pínion; (*велосипе́да*) cháin-wheel.

ше́стеро six; нас ~ there are six of us.

шестигра́нник *м.* héxahédron.

шестидесятилет|ие *с.* 1. (*пери́од*) síxty years *pl*; 2. (*годовщи́на*) síxtieth anníversary. ~ний 1. (*о сро́ке*) síxty-year *attr.*; of síxty years *по́сле сущ.*; 2. (*о во́зрасте*) síxty-year-óld; of síxty *по́сле сущ.*

шестидеся́т|ый síxtieth; ~ые го́ды the síxties.

шестикра́тн|ый síxfold; в ~ом разме́ре síxfold.

шестиле́тний 1. (*о сро́ке*) síx-year *attr.*; of six years *по́сле сущ.*; 2. (*о во́зрасте*) síx-year-óld; of six *по́сле сущ.*

шестимеся́чный 1. (*о сро́ке*) six months'; síx-month *attr.*; 2. (*о во́зрасте*) síx-month-óld; of six months *по́сле сущ.*

шестинеде́льный 1. (*о сро́ке*) síx-week *attr.*; 2. (*о во́зрасте*) síx-week-óld; of six weeks *по́сле сущ.*

шестисо́тый síx-húndredth.

шестиуго́льн|ик *м.* héxagon. ~ый hexágonal.

шестнадцатиле́тний 1. (*о сро́ке*) síxtéen-year *attr.*; of síxtéen years *по́сле сущ.*; 2. (*о во́зрасте*) síxtéen-year-óld; of síxtéen *по́сле сущ.*

шестна́дцатый síxtéenth.

шестна́дцать síxtéen.

шесто́й sixth.

шесть six.

шестьдеся́т síxty.

шестьсо́т six húndred.

шеф *м.* 1. *разг.* chief; 2.: ~по́вар chef, héad-cook; 3. (*предприя́тие, взя́вшее ше́фство*) spónsor, pátron.

шеф|ский vóluntary-assístance *attr.* ~ство *с.* spónsorship, pátronage; взять ~ство над кем-л. give* vóluntary assístance to *smb.* ~ствовать *несов.* (над *тв.*) be* pátron (of), give* vóluntary assístance (to), spónsor (*smb., smth.*).

шея *ж.* neck; ◇ бро́ситься на ше́ю кому́-л. throw*/fling* one's arms round *smb.'s* neck; fall* on *smb.'s* neck; дать кому́-л. по ше́е give* *smb.* a thráshing; гнать кого́-л. в ше́ю, в три ше́и kick *smb.* out; получи́ть по ше́е get* it in the neck; слома́ть себе́ ше́ю break* one's neck; сиде́ть у кого́-л. на ше́е live at *smb.'s* expénse, live on *smb.*

ши́ворот *м.*: взять кого́-л. за ~ take* *smb.* by the scruff of the neck; ~-навы́ворот the wrong way round.

шизофрени́я *ж. мед.* schizophrénia.

шик *м.* smártness; (*ло́вкий приём*) spécial touch/way; с ~ом in style; како́й ~! how smart!

шика́рный smart; (*превосхо́дный*) spléndid.

ши́кать, ши́кнуть *разг.* 1. (на *вн.*) hush (*smb.*) down, sílence (*smb.*); 2. (на *вн.*; на птиц, живо́тных) shoo (*smth.*); 3. (*дт.*; выража́ть неодобре́ние) hiss (*smb.*).

ши́кнуть *сов.* см. ши́кать.

ши́л|о *с.* awl; ◇ ~а в мешке́ не утаи́шь ≈ múrder will out.

шимпанзе́ *с. нескл. зоол.* chimpanzée.

ши́на *ж.* 1. (*на колесе́*) týre; 2. *мед.* splint.

шине́ль *ж.* gréatcoat, óvercoat.

шинкова́ть *несов.* (*вн.*) slice (*smth.*), shred* (*smth.*); ~ капу́сту shred* cábbage.

шиньо́н *м.* chignón, háirpiece.

шип *м.* 1. (*колю́чка*) thorn; 2. (*на подко́вах, обу́ви и т. п.*) stud; 3. *тех.* ténon.

шипе́ние *с.* híssing.

шипе́ть *несов.* hiss; (*о жа́рящемся*) sízzle; (*о напи́тке*) fizz.

шипо́вник *м.* dóg-rose, wild rose; (*я́годы*) hips *pl.*

шипу́ч|ий (*о напи́тках*) fízzy, spárkling. ~ка *ж. разг.* fizz.

шипя́щий híssing; (*о жа́рящемся*) sízzling; ◇ ~ звук, ~ согла́сный *лингв.* síbilant.

ши́ре (*сравнит. ст. прил.* широ́кий *и наре́ч.* широ́ко) wíder, bróader.

ширин|а́ *ж.* width; ~о́й в два ме́тра two métres wide; име́ть два ме́тра в ~у́ be* two métres wide.

ши́рит|ься *несов.* spread* (out); *перен. тж.* incréase its scope.

ши́рма *ж.* screen; *перен.* cloak, cóver.

широ́к|ий 1. wide, broad; *перен. тж.* exténsive; ~ие пле́чи broad shóulders; ~ просто́р wide expánse; ~ая колея́ broad gauge; ~ая улы́бка broad smile; ~ие поля́ spácious/wide fields; (*шля́пы*) broad brim *sg*; ~ие пла́ны exténsive plans; ~ кругозо́р wide óutlook; в ~ом масшта́бе on a lávish/broad scale; в ~ом смы́сле сло́ва in the broad sense of the word; 2. (*просто́рный — об оде́жде*) loose; too wide; ~ пиджа́к loose jácket; пальто́ ~о́ в плеча́х the coat is too wide on/in the shóulders; 3. (*разма́шистый*) vígorous; *перен.* (*ниче́м не стеснённый*) lávish, génerous; ~ шаг vígorous/swínging stride; ~ая нату́ра expánsive/génerous náture; ~ое гостеприи́мство lávish/líberal hospitálity; 4. (*ма́ссовый, охва́тывающий мно́гое*) broad, exténsive, géneral; ~ое обобще́ние swéeping státement/generalizátion; ~ие ма́ссы the broad másses; ~ие круги́ (населе́ния) wide séctions of the populátion; ~ая пу́блика the géneral públic, the públic at large; ~ое распростране́ние wide circulátion; (*ме́тода*) exténsive applicátion; получи́ть ~ое распростране́ние be* in wide use; (*о кни́ге*) be* wídely read; (*о ме́тоде*) be* wídely applíed; ◇ ~ экра́н wide screen; ~им фро́нтом on a broad front; сде́лать ~ жест make* a grand gésture.

широко́ wídely, bróadly; ~ откры́тый, раскры́тый wide ópen; ~ распространённый wídespread; ~ изве́стный wídely known; ~ раскры́ть глаза́ ópen one's eyes wide; жить ~ live on a lávish scale; ~ толкова́ть, понима́ть что́-л. intérpret *smth.* lóosely; ~ образо́ванный челове́к pérson of wide léarning; ~ смотре́ть на ве́щи take* a broad view of things.

широковеща́тельн|ый 1. *ра́дио* bróadcasting *attr.*; 2. *иро́н.* (*обеща́ющий мно́гое*) hígh-sounding; ~ая деклара́ция hígh-sounding declarátion.

ширококоле́йный *ж.-д.* bróad-gauge.

широколи́цый bróad-faced.

широкопле́чий bróad-shóuldered.

широкопо́лый 1. full-skirted; 2. (*о шля́пе*) bróad-brimmed.

широкофо́рматный wide-frame *attr.*; ~ фильм wide-frame film.

широкоэкра́нный wide-screen *attr.*; ~ кинотеа́тр wide-screen cínema; ~ фильм wide-screen film.

широта́ *ж.* 1. breadth, width, wídeness; ~ взгля́дов bróadmindedness; ~ кругозо́ра wide range of ínterests; ~ охва́та (wide) scope, span, sweep; 2. *геогр.* látitude.

ширь *ж.* expánse; ◇ разверну́ться во всю ~ devélop to its full extént.

ши́тый 1. (*сши́тый*) sewn; 2. (*вы́шитый*) embróidered; ~ зо́лотом embróidered in gold.

шить, сшить 1. (*вн.*) sew* (*smth.*); (*оде́жду*) make* (*smth.*); ~ себе́ костю́м 1) (*в ателье́*) have* a suit made; 2) (*само́й*) make* onesélf a suit, ~ сапоги́ make* boots; ~ на маши́нке (*что́-л.*) do* it on the (séwing-) machine; (*рабо́тать*) use a séwing-machine; 2. *тк. несов.* (*тв.*; *вышива́ть*) embróider (in).

шитьё *с.* 1. séwing; (*рукоде́лие тж.*) néedlework; 2. (*вы́шивка*) embróidery.

ши́фер *м.* 1. slate; 2. (*кро́вельный материа́л*) asbéstos cemént. ~ный 1. slate *attr.*; 2. asbéstos-cemént *attr.*

шифр *м.* 1. (*тайно́пись*) code, cípher; (*напи́сан-*

ный) ~ом (written) in code/cípher; 2. (библиотечный) préss-mark.

шифрóванный code attr., cípher attr., códed.

шифровáть несов. (вн.) cípher (smth.).

шифрóвка ж. 1. (действие) cípher-work; 2. разг. (текст) code.

шишка ж. 1. (хвойных деревьев) cone; елóвая ~ fír--cone; 2. (округлая выпуклость) bump, lump; 3. разг. (важная особа) big noise/pot; VIP; ирон. bígwig.

шкалá ж. 1. (система чисел) scale; 2. (циферблат в различных приборах) dial, índicator pánel.

шкатýлка ж. box, cásket.

шкаф м. cúpboard, clóset.

шквал м. squall; (орудийный) bárrage. ~истый gústy.

шквáрки мн. crácklings.

шквóрень м. pin; (автомобиля) king pin.

шкив м. púlley; (блока) sheave.

шкúпер м. 1. bárge-skípper; 2. (на морских судах) bóatswain, bó'sun.

шкóл|а ж. school; (здание тж.) school búilding; schóolhouse; воскрéсная ~ Súnday school; срéдняя ~ sécondary school; начáльная ~ elémentary/prímary school; ходúть в ~у atténd school, go* to school; пройтú хорóшую ~у have* been well trained; перен. have* learned in the school of expérience; пройтú сурóвую ~у have* learned by bítter/hard expérience; рýсская ~ жúвописи Rússian school of páinting; ◇ вýсшая ~ hígher school, hígher educátional institútion; univérsity, cóllege.

шкóльн|ик м. schóolboy; мн. schóolchildren. ~ица ж. schóolgirl; мн. schóolchildren.

шкóльн|ый school attr.; ~ товáрищ schóolmate, schóolfellow; ~ые принадлéжности school appliances; дéти ~ого вóзраста chíldren of school age.

шкýр|а ж. 1. skin; (скота, лошадей тж.) hide; (с мехом тж.) pelt; медвéжья ~ béar-skin; 2. разг. (кожура) peel; ◇ спасáть свою ~у save one's skin; я не хотéл бы быть в егó ~е I wóuldn't be in his shoes for ánything; дрожáть за свою ~у think* of one's own skin; спускáть ~у с когó-л. skin smb. alíve; на своéй ~е узнáть, почýвствовать что-л. know* smth. from expérience.

шкýрн|ик м. разг. self-séeker, caréerist. ~ый разг. sélfish, sórdid; ~ые интерéсы sélfish ínterests.

шлагбáум м. bárrier.

шлак м. 1. (расплавленная масса) slag, dross; 2. (окалина) clínker; 3. мн. мед. résidue(s).

шлакобетóн м. slag cóncrete.

шланг м. hose.

шлем м. hélmet.

шлемофóн м. éarphone hélmet.

шлёпанцы мн. (ед. шлёпанец м.) разг. bédroom slíppers.

шлёп|ать, шлёпнуть 1. (вн., по дт.) slap (smth.), smack (smth.); 2. (тв.; хлопать) flap (smth.), make* a flápping sound (with); 3. тк. несов. разг.: ~ по водé, грязи splash through the wáter, mud. ~аться, шлёпнуться разг. flop/plop down. ~нуть сов. см. шлёпать 1, 2. ~нуться сов. см. шлёпаться.

шлепóк м. slap, smack.

шлея ж. bréech-band, bréeching.

шлифовáль|ный grínding; (полирующий) pólishing. ~щик м. grínder; (алмазов) pólisher.

шлифовáть несов. (вн.) grind* (smth.); (шкуркой) sándpaper (smth.); (полировать) pólish (smth.) (тж. перен.).

шлюз м. lock, sluice; проходúть чéрез ~ы go* through the locks.

шлюзовáть несов. и сов. (вн.) 1. (реку) build* locks (on); 2. (суда) pass (smth.) through a lock.

шлюпка ж. (ship's) boat.

шляп|а ж. 1. hat; в ~е with one's hat on; быть в ~е have* one's hat on; без ~ы withóut a hat; hátless, báre-

-héaded; надéть ~у put* on one's hat; снять ~у take* off one's hat; 2. (о человеке) dúffer, bóoby.

шляпка ж. 1. (дамская) hat; 2. (гвоздя) (náil-)head; 3. (гриба) cap.

шмель м. búmble-bee.

шмыгать, шмыгнýть разг. dart, run* abóut; ~ нóсом sniff.

шмыгнýть сов. разг. 1. см. шмыгать; 2. (быстро проскользнуть, проскочить) dart, slip.

шнúцель м. кул. schnítzel (fillet of pork or veal).

шнур м. cord; (провод тж.) flex.

шнуровáть несов. (вн.) lace up (smth.).

шнурóвка ж. lácing.

шнурóк м. lace; ~ для ботúнок shóelace, bóot-lace.

шнырять несов. разг. dart abóut; (высматривать) snoop aróund, prowl, be* on the prowl; ◇ ~ глазáми peer this way and that.

шов м. 1. seam; без шва séamless; 2. (хирургический) stitch; 3. тех. seam, joint, júnction; ◇ наложúть ~ put* in stítches; снять швы take* out the stítches; стоять рýки по швам stand* at atténtion; трещáть по всем швам go*/fall* to pieces.

шовин|úзм м. cháuvinism, jíngoism. ~úст м. cháuvinist. ~úстический chauvinístic.

шок м. мед. shock.

шокúровать несов. (вн.) shock (smb.).

шоколáд м. chócolate. ~ка ж. разг. bar of chócolate. ~ный 1. chócolate attr.; ~ные конфéты chócolates; 2. (о цвете) dark-brówn, chócolate-brown.

шомпол м. (для чистки) cléaning rod; (для забивки) rámrod.

шóрник м. sáddler, hárness-maker.

шóрох м. rústle.

шóрты мн. shorts.

шóры мн. blínkers; ◇ взять когó-л. в ~ put* blínkers on smb.

шоссé с. нескл. (high-)road, híghway.

шоссéйн|ый road attr.; ~ая дорóга macádamized road.

шотлáндец м. Scot, Scótsman*.

шотлáндка I ж. Scótswoman*.

шотлáндка II ж. (ткань) tártan.

шотлáндский Scóttish; Scotch разг.

шóу нескл. с. show. ~-бúзнес м. show búsiness; shówbiz разг.

шофёр м. dríver; (служебной легковой машины тж.) cháuffeur; ~ таксú táxi dríver. ~ский dríver's.

шпáга ж. (small) sword.

шпагáт м. 1. twine, string; 2. спорт. the splits pl.

шпаклевáть несов. (вн.) pútty (smth.).

шпаклёвка ж. pútty, filler.

шпáла ж. ж.-д. sléeper, tie.

шпалéр|а ж. (ед. шпалéра ж.) 1. (для вьющихся растений) tréllis; (для деревьев) espálier; 2. (ряды деревьев) lines of trees; 3.: стоять ~ами be* lined up.

шпангóут м. мор., ав. frame.

шпаргáлка ж. разг. crib.

шпат м. мин. spar.

шпенёк м. prong.

шпик I м. (сало) fat back.

шпик II м. разг. (шпион) police spy, snóoper.

шпиль м. 1. stéeple, spíre; 2. мор. cápstan.

шпúльк|а ж. (для волос) háirpin; перен. dig; подпустúть ~у комý-л. have* a sly dig at smb.

шпинáт м. spínach.

шпингалéт м. wíndow bolt.

шпиóн м. spy.

шпионáж м. espionáge.

шпиóн|ить несов. spy. ~ский spy attr.; ~ский зáговор espionáge plot.

шпиц м. (собака) Pomeránian.

шпóр|а ж. spur; дать лóшади ~ы spur one's horse.

шприц *м.* sýringe.

шпро́ты *мн.* (*консервы*) sprats in oil.

шпу́лька *ж.* spool, bóbbin.

шрам *м.* scar.

шрапне́ль *м. воен.* shrápnel (shell).

шрифт *м.* type, print; кру́пный ~ large print/type; ме́лкий ~ small print/type.

штаб *м.* 1. héadquárters *pl*, H. Q.; (*личный состав*) staff; ~ а́рмии ármy héadquárters; нача́льник ~a chief of staff; 2. (*руководящий орган чего-л.*) héadquárters, command.

шта́бель *м.* stack, pile.

штаб-кварти́ра *ж.* héadquárters *pl.*

штабно́й staff *attr.*

штамп *м.* 1. (*печать*) stamp; поста́вить ~ stamp it; 2. *тех.* punch; 3. (*шаблон*) cliché; (*литературный тж.*) stóck-phrase.

штампо́ванн|ый 1. préss-work *attr.*; ~ая дета́ль pressed compónent; 2. (*избитый, шаблонный*) trite, stéreotyped.

штампова́ть *несов.* (*вн.*) 1. (*ставить штамп*) stamp (*smth.*); 2. *тех.* punch (*smth.*), stamp (*smth.*); (*большие детали*) press (*smth.*); 3. *разг.* (*делать что-л. по готовым образцам*) prodúce (*smth.*) mechánically, churn (*smth.*) out.

шта́нга *ж.* 1. *тех.* bar; 2. (*в тяжёлой атлетике*) bárbell; 3. *спорт. разг.* (*боковая стойка ворот*) góal-post.

штанги́ст *м.* wéight-lifter.

штани́на *ж. разг.* tróuser leg.

штаны́ *мн. разг.* tróusers.

шта́пель *м.* 1. stáple; 2. (*волокно*) stáple fibre; 3. *разг.* (*ткань*) stáple-fibre fábric. ~ное волокно́ stáple fibre; ~ные тка́ни stáple-fibre fábrics.

штат I *м.* (*административно-территориальная единица*) state.

штат II *м.* 1. (*личный состав*) staff, estáblishment; состоя́ть в ~ be* on the staff; 2. *мн.* (*штатное расписание*) list of staff.

штати́в *м.* suppórt; (*треножник*) trípod.

шта́тн|ый pérmanent; on the staff *после сущ.*; он ~ сотру́дник he is on the staff; ~ая до́лжность pérmanent appóintment.

шта́тский *прил.* 1. civílian; 2. *в знач. сущ. м.* civílian.

штемпелева́ть *несов.* (*вн.*) (*rúbber-*)stamp (*smth.*); (*письмо, бандероль и т. п.*) póstmark (*smth.*).

ште́мпель *м.* stamp; почто́вый ~ póstmark.

ште́псель *м.* (*eléctric*) plug. ~ный plug *attr.*; ~ная ви́лка twó-pin plug.

штиль *м.* calm.

штифт *м. тех.* pin.

што́льня *ж. горн.* ádit.

што́пан|ый darned; ~ые чулки́ darned stóckings.

што́пать *несов.* (*вн.*) darn (*smth.*), mend (*smth.*); ~ чулки́ darn stóckings.

што́пка *ж.* 1. (*действие*) dárning; 2. *разг.* (*нитки*) dárning-thread; (*шерстяные нитки*) dárning-wool; 3. *разг.* (*заштопанное место*) darn.

што́пор *м.* 1. córkscrew; 2. *ав.* spin; táil-spin; входи́ть в ~ go* into a spin. ~ом in a spin.

што́ра *ж.* blind.

шторм *м.* gale, storm.

штормо́вка *ж.* ánorak, wéatherproof jácket.

штормово́й gale *attr.*, storm *attr.*; (*бывающий при шторме*) stórmy.

штраф *м.* fine, pénalty; брать ~ с *кого-л.* fine *smb.*; наложи́ть ~ impóse a fine.

штрафно́й pénalty *attr.*; ~ уда́р *спорт.* pénalty kick; ~ батальо́н pénal battálion.

штрафова́ть, оштрафова́ть (*вн.*) fine (*smb.*).

штрейкбре́хер *м.* stríke-breaker; scab, bláckleg *разг.* ~ство *с.* stríke-breaking.

штрек *м. горн.* drift.

штрих *м.* stroke; (*на карте*) hachúre; *перен.* (*черта*) touch, détail, féature.

штрихова́ть, заштрихова́ть (*вн.*) shade (*smth.*); (*карту*) hatch (*smth.*).

штрихо́вка *ж.* sháding.

штуди́ровать, проштуди́ровать (*вн.*) stúdy (*smth.*) thóroughly, learn* (*smth.*).

штук|а *ж.* 1. (*в счёте*) *не переводится*; де́сять штук ten; штук де́сять abóut ten; де́сять штук яи́ц ten eggs; по рублю́ за ~у one róuble each; 2. *разг.* (*выходка, проделка и т. п.*) trick; в то́м-то и ~ that's just it!; вот так ~! look at that now!; тут-тут!; э́то всё его́ ~и it's all his dóing; 3. *разг.* (*предмет, дело*) thing; что э́то за ~ там лежи́т? what's that (thing) óver there?; что э́то за ~? what's that?

штукату́р *м.* plásterer.

штукату́р|ить, оштукату́рить (*вн.*) pláster (*smth.*). ~ка *ж.* 1. (*действие*) plástering; 2. (*материал*) pláster; ◇ суха́я ~ка pláster board. ~ный pláster *attr.*; ~ные рабо́ты plástering *sg.*

штукова́ть *несов.* (*вн.*) mend invísibly.

штурва́л *м.* stéering-wheel; *ав.* contról cólumn.

штурва́льный *прил.* 1. wheel *attr.*, stéering; 2. *в знач. сущ. м.* hélmsman*, whéelsman*.

штурм *м.* (*рд.*) assáult (on); взять ~ом take* by storm/assáult.

шту́рман *м.* návigator, návigating ófficer; (*на речном теплоходе*) mate.

штурмова́ть *несов.* (*вн.*) 1. storm (*smth.*); 2. *разг.* (*беспорядочно осаждать*) rush (*smth.*); 3. (*упорно овладевать*) cónquer (*smth.*).

штурмови́к *м.* assáult-plane.

штурмово́й assáult *attr.*

штучн|ый: ~ая прода́жа sale óver the cóunter; ~ това́р goods sold séparately, goods sold by the piece; ~ая опла́та páyment by the piece.

штык *м.* báyonet; ◇ идти́ в ~и́ make* a báyonet charge; встреча́ть *кого-л., что-л.* в ~и́ give* *smb., smth.* a hóstile recéption. ~ово́й báyonet *attr.*; ~ова́я ата́ка báyonet charge.

шу́ба *ж.* fúr-coat; (*на меху*) fúr-lined coat.

шуга́ *ж.* sludge ice.

шу́лер *м.* cárd-sharper; *разг.* (*мошенник*) swíndler.

шум *м.* 1. noise; (*чего-л. тж.*) sound (of); без ~a nóiselessly; подня́ть ~ make* a noise; ~ ле́са múrmur of the fórest; ~ ве́тра sound of the wind; 2. *разг.* (*оживлённое обсуждение*) stir; подня́ть ~ вокру́г *чего-л.* make* a fuss abóut *smth.*; наде́лать мно́го ~a cause a stir/sensátion; 3. *разг.* (*громкая ссора*) row, báwling; 4. *мед.*: ~ в се́рдце cárdiac múrmur; ◇ ~ в уша́х búzzing in the ears; мно́го ~a из ничего́ much adó about nóthing.

шум|е́ть *несов.* 1. make* a noise; (*о деревьях*) múrmur, rústle; (*о море*) roar; múrmur; 2. *разг.* (*излишне много говорить о чём-л.*) make* a song/fuss, talk a lot; 3. *разг.* (*вызывать толки*) cause a stir; 4. *разг.* (*браниться*) kick up a row; ◇ у меня́ ~и́т в голове́, в уша́х there is a búzzing in my ears, I have nóises in my ears.

шуми́х|а *ж. разг.* fuss, ballyhóo; поднима́ть, создава́ть ~у вокру́г *чего-л.* make* a rácket abóut *smth.*, raise a húe-and-cry óver *smth.*

шумли́вый 1. nóisy; 2. (*оживлённый*) bústling; 3. *разг.* (*напыщенный*) hígh-sounding.

шу́мн|о 1. *нареч.* nóisily; ~ обсужда́ть *что-л.* discúss *smth.* nóisily; 2. *в знач. сказ. безл.* it is nóisy; на у́лице уже́ ~ и лю́дно the street is nóisy and crówded alréady. ~ый 1. nóisy; (*восторженный*) upróarious; ~ая компа́ния nóisy group; 2. (*оживлённый*) bústling; ~ая у́лица bústling street; 3. (*производящий сенсацию*) impréssive, sensátional; ~ый успе́х sensátional/treméndous succéss.

шумо́вка *ж.* skímmer.
шумово́й sound *attr.*
шумо́к *м. разг.:* под ~ on the quíet.
шу́рин *м.* bróther-in-law (*pl* bróthers-) (*wife's brother*).
шуру́п *м.* screw.
шурф *м. горн.* prospécting pit, bore pit.
шурш|а́ть *несов.* rústle; ли́стья ~а́т под нога́ми the leaves rústle underfóot; ~ бума́гой rústle páper.
шу́стрый *разг.* bright, smart, cléver.
шут *м.* 1. jéster, fool; *перен.* buffóon; 2. *разг.:* на кой ~? why the dévil?
шути́ть, пошути́ть 1. (*весело говорить, поступать*) joke, jest, have* fun; 2. (*над тв.; насмехаться*) play a joke (on), pull (*smb.'s*) leg; 3. (*говорить, поступать не всерьёз*) joke; вы шу́тите! you're jóking!; я не шучу́ I'm sérious, I'm not jóking/fóoling; 4. (*тв.; относиться несерьёзно, пренебрегать*) trifle (with); ◇ ~ с огнём play with fire.
шу́тк|а *ж.* joke; ◇ в ~у, ~и ра́ди for fun; не на ~у рассерди́ться be* dównright ángry; в сто́рону jóking apárt; кро́ме шу́ток sériously, now!; с ним ~и пло́хи he's an ill man to quárrel with.
шутли́вый 1. jócular, facétious; 2. (*имеющий характер шутки*) húmorous, witty; 3. (*совершаемый ради шутки*) facétious, flíppant.
шутни́к *м.* wag.
шутов|ско́й jéster's; ~ска́я вы́ходка a piece of buffóonery. ~ство́ *с.* clówning, buffóonery.
шу́точн|ый cómic, facétious; ~ая пе́сня cómic song; ◇ де́ло не ~ое no trífling matter, no trífle.
шутя́ 1. (*ради шутки*) jókingly; facétiously; 2. (*легко*) éasily; ~ не ~ in all sériousness.
шушу́каться *несов. разг.* whísper; ~ по угла́м whisper in the báckground.
шхе́ры *мн.* skérries.
шху́на *ж.* schóoner.
пш hush!

Щ

щавёлев|ый sórrel *attr.*; ~ые щи sórrel soup; ◇ ~ая кислота́ *хим.* oxálic ácid.
щаве́ль *м.* sórrel.
щад|и́ть, пощади́ть (*вн.*) spare (*smb., smth.*); let* (*smb.*) off *разг.*; не ~ (*своих*) сил (*чтобы*)... spare no éffort/pains to...; ~ чью-л. самолюбие spare *smb.'s* vánity; щадя́щий чью-л. жизнь spare *smb.'s* life; не ~я жи́зни cáreless of *one's* life.
ще́бень *м.* 1. bróken/crushed stone, róad-metal; 2. *геол.* detrítus.
щ́ебет *м.* twitter, twittering.
щебета́ние *с.* twittering, twitter.
щебета́ть *несов.* twitter.
щегол *м.* (*птица*) góldfinch.
щеголева́тый módish; (*о человеке тж.*) dándified, dápper.
щёголь *м.* dandy, fop.
щегольну́ть *сов. см.* щеголя́ть 2, 3.
щего́ль|ско́й 1. (*очень нарядный*) élegant, smart; swish *разг.*; ~ костю́м élegant suit; 2. (*молодцеватый*) stýlish, dáshing, jáunty. ~ство́ *с.* 1. (*пристрастие к изысканным вещам*) fóppishness; 2. (*хвастовство*) shówing off, (love of) displáy.
щеголя́ть, щегольну́ть 1. *тк. несов.* (*нарядно одеваться*) dress smártly, dress up; 2. (*в пр.*) *разг.* (*ходить щегольски одетым*) make* a splash, cut* a dash;

~ в но́вом костю́ме sport a new suit; 3. (*тв.*) *разг.* (*хвастаться*) show* off (*smth.*), flaunt (*smth.*); ~ свои́ми зна́ниями paráde *one's* knówledge.
щедр|о génerously, lávishly; ~ вознагражда́ть кого́-л. reward *smb.* hándsomely; ~ одари́ть кого́-л. be* lávish in *one's* gifts to *smb.* ~ость *ж.* generósity, liberálity; (*обилие*) lávishness. ~ый génerous, open-hánded; ~ый челове́к open-hánded pérson; ~ые дары́ rich/spléndid gifts; ~ый на обеща́ния génerous with *one's* prómises; ~ый на похвалы́ lávish in/of práises; ◇ ~ой руко́й with a bóuntiful hand.
щек|а́ *ж.* cheek; ◇ за о́бе ~и уплета́ть что-л. stuff onesélf with *smth.*
щеко́лда *ж.* latch.
щекота́ть, пощекота́ть 1. (*вн.*) tickle (*smb., smth.*) (*тж. перен.*); ~ чьё-л. самолюбие tickle *smb.'s* vánity; 2. *безл.:* у меня́ щеко́чет в го́рле there is a tíckling in my throat.
щеко́тк|а *ж.* tíckling; боя́ться ~и be* tícklish.
щекотли́вый tícklish, délicate; ~ вопро́с tícklish próblem, délicate íssue.
ще́лка *ж.* chink.
щёлк|ать, щёлкнуть 1. (*вн.; давать кому-л. щелчки*) flick (*smb.*), flip (*smb.*); ~ кого́-л. по́ носу flick/flip *smb.* on the nose; 2. (*производить отрывистый звук*) click, snap; ~ па́льцами snap *one's* fingers; ~ языко́м click *one's* tongue; ~али вы́стрелы there was a ráttle of firing/shots; ~ (*о животном*) snap its teeth; он ~ает зуба́ми от хо́лода his teeth are cháttering with cold; ~ ключо́м turn the key with a click; 3. (*вн.; орехи, семечки*) crack (*smth.*); 4. (*о птицах*) trill.
щёлкнуть *сов. см.* щёлкать.
щёлок *м.* álkaline solútion.
щелочно́й álkaline; ~ раство́р álkaline solútion.
щёлочь *ж. хим.* álkali.
щелчо́к *м.* click; (*пальцами*) snap; (*выстрела*) crack; *перен. разг.* ínsult, slight, blow; ~ по́ носу flick/flip on the nose.
щель *ж.* 1. chink, crack, físsure; (*расщелина*) crévice; 2. *анат.* glóttis; 3. *тех.* áperture; 4. *воен.* slit trench.
щем|и́ть *несов.* 1. (*вн.; сжимать*) constríct (*smth.*); 2. *безл.* (*болеть, ныть*) ache, feel* constrícted; ◇ ~ ду́шу, се́рдце, грудь oppréss/wring* the heart. ~я́щий oppréssive.
щени́ться, ощени́ться whelp; (*о собаках*) pup, have* púppies.
щено́к *м.* púppy (*тж. перен.*); (*у диких зверей*) cub.
щепа́ *ж.* chips *pl*, shávings *pl*; (*кровельная*) shíngles *pl*.
щепети́льн|ость *ж.* 1. punctíliousness, scrúpulousness; 2. (*деликатность*) tríckiness, délicacy. ~ый 1. punctílious, scrúpulous; ~ый челове́к scrúpulous/punctílious pérson; 2. (*деликатный*) trícky, délicate; ~ое положе́ние délicate situátion.
ще́пк|а *ж.* chip, splínter; худо́й как ~ as thin as a lath/rake; ◇ лес ру́бят — ~и летя́т you can't make an ómelet without bréaking eggs.
щепо́тка *ж.*, щепо́ть *ж.* pinch; ~ табаку́ pinch of tobácco; ~ со́ли pinch of salt.
щерба́тый chipped, pitted; ~ рот mouth with séveral teeth míssing.
щерби́на *ж.* 1. pit, scratch; 2. (*рябинка на лице*) scar, róck-mark; 3. (*отверстие вместо зуба*) gap.
щети́н|а *ж.* brístles *pl*; *перен.* spíky/brístly súrface. ~истый brístly. ~иться, ощети́ниться brístle up.
щётка *ж.* 1. brush; (*головная*) (háir)brush; 2. (*над копытом у лошади*) fétlock; 3. *эл.* brush.
щи *мн.* cábbage-soup *sg.*
щи́колотк|а *ж.* ánkle; по ~у ánkle-deep.
щипа́ть, щипну́ть (*вн.*) 1. pinch (*smb., smth.*); 2.

(*вызывать ощущение боли, жжения*) burn* (*smth.*), make* (*smth.*) smart/sting; (*о морозе*) nip (*smth.*); 3. (*дёргать, теребить*) pluck (*smth.*); ~ ус, ухо tug/pull at one's moustáche, ear; 4. *тк. несов.* (*траву, листья*) níbble (*smth.*); 5. *тк. несов.* (*птицу*) pluck (*smth.*). ~ся *несов.* 1. pinch; 2. (*щипать друг друга*) pinch one anóther.

щипну́ть *сов. см.* щипа́ть 1, 2, 3.

щипóк *м.* pinch, nip.

щипцы́ *мн.* píncers; tongs; (*для завивки*) wávers, cúrling tongs/irons; (*для сахара*) (súgar-)tongs.

щи́пчики *мн.* twéezers.

щит *м.* 1. *ист.* shield; 2. (*для предохранения, ограждения*) shield, screen; (*для построек, настила*) sheet; фанéрный ~ sheet of plýwood; 3. *зоол.* shell; 4. (*доска, стенд*) board; (*для рекламы*) bíllboard, hóarding; сигнáльный ~ *ж.-д.* tárget; 5. *тех.* pánel; ~ управлéния contról pánel; распределéтельный ~ switchboard; ◇ поднять *кого-л.* на ~ laud *smb.* to the skies; вернýться на ~é retúrn home deféated; вернýться со ~óм return home victórious.

щитовидн|ый: ~ая железá *анат.* thýroid gland.

щу́ка *ж.* (*рыба*) pike.

щуп *м.* probe.

щу́пальца *мн.* (*ед.* щу́пальце *с.*) téntacles; (*усики*) féelers, anténnae.

щу́пать, пощу́пать (*вн.*) feel* (*smth.*); ~ пульс feel* *smb.'s* pulse; ~ карма́н pat *one's* pócket.

щу́плый *разг.* púny.

щу́рить *несов.*: ~ глазá nárrow *one's* eyes, screw up *one's* eyes. ~ся *несов.* 1. (*о человеке*) screw up *one's* eyes; ~ся от сóлнца screw up *one's* eyes in the súnlight, squint in the súnlight; 2. (*о глазах*) nárrow.

Э

э eh!

эбони́т *м.* ébonit. ~овый ébonite *attr.*

эвакуациóнный evacuátion *attr.*; ~ пункт evacuátion céntre.

эвакуа́ци|я *ж.* evacuátion; проводи́ть мáссовую ~ю населéния carry out mass evacuátion of the populátion.

эваку́ровать *несов. и сов.* (*вн.*) evácuate (*smb., smth.*). ~ся *несов. и сов.* evácuate.

эвкали́пт *м.* eucalýptus. ~овый eucalýptus *attr.*

ЭВМ (*электрóнная вычисли́тельная маши́на*) (electrónic) compúter.

эволюциóнн|ый evolútionary; ~ое учéние dóctrine of evolútion.

эволю́ция *ж.* evolution.

эвфеми́зм *м.* éuphemism.

эгé ohó!

эги́д|а *ж.* áegis; под ~ой *чего-л.*, *кого-л.* únder the áegis of *smth.*, *smb.*

эгои́зм *м.* égo(t)ism; sélfishness.

эгои́ст *м.* égo(t)ist.

эгоисти́ч|еский, ~ный sélfish, ego(t)ístical, self-céntred.

эгои́стка *ж.* sélfish wóman*, girl.

эй! hi!

экватор *м.* equátor; *мор. тж.* the Line; к сéверу от ~а north of the equátor; ◇ небéсный ~ *астр.* celéstial equátor. ~иáльный equatórial; ~иáльный круг equatórial circle; ~иáльные стрáны equatórial cóuntries.

эквивалéнт *м.* equívalent. ~ный (*дт.*) equívalent (to).

эквилибри́ст *м.* equílibrist, rópe-walker. ~ика *ж.*

bálancing tricks *pl*, rópe-walking; *перен. ирон.* bálancing act.

экзальтáция *ж.* exaltátion.

экзáмен *м.* examinátion; exám *разг.*; *перен.* test; ~ на аттестáт зрéлости final school examinátion; school finals *pl разг.*; ~ по математике examinátion in mathemátics; государственные ~ы finals; graduátion examinátions.

экзаменáтор *м.* exáminer.

экзаменациóнный examinátion *attr.*; ~ билéт examinátion páper.

экзаменовáть, проэкзаменовáть (*вн. по дт.*) exámine (*smb. in*). ~ся, проэкзаменовáться (*по дт.*) be* exámined (in); take* an examinátion (in).

экзéма *ж.* éczema.

экземпля́р *м.* 1. (*книги, документа и т. п.*) cópy; в двух ~ах in dúplicate; в трёх ~ах in tríplicate; в четырёх ~ах in quadrúplicate; 2. (*отдельный представитель*) spécimen, represéntative; 3. (*о человеке*) spécimen.

экзóт|ика *ж.* exótica, exótic óbjects, lócal cólour. ~и́ческий, ~и́чный exótic.

эки́вок *м.* 1. ambigúity, dóuble-edged remárk; 2. (*тонкость, замысловатость*) súbtlety, íntricacy.

эк|шáп *разг.* what a; ~ шалун! what an imp!; ~а нéвидаль! nóthing márvellous abóut that!

экипáж I *м.* (*коляска*) cárriage.

экипáж II *м.* (*личный состав*) crew; ~ корабля́ ship's cómplement; ~ тáнка tánk-crew.

экипир|овáть *несов. и сов.* (*вн.*) equíp (*smb., smth.*), fit (*smb., smth.*) out. ~овáться *несов. и сов.* fit onesélf out. ~óвка *ж.* 1. (*действие*) fitting out; 2. (*снаряжение*) equípment.

эклéкт|ик *м.* ecléctic. ~и́ческий, ~и́чный ecléctical.

эклипт|ика *ж.* *астр.* eclíptic. ~и́ческий *астр.* eclíptic.

экóлог *м.* ecólogist.

экологи́ческий ecológical.

экология *ж.* ecólogy.

экономика *ж.* 1. (*совокупность производственных отношений*) ecónomy; 2. (*структура хозяйственной жизни*) ecónomics; ~ трáнспорта ecónomics of tránsport; 3. (*научная дисциплина*) ecónomics.

экономи́ст *м.* ecónomist.

экономить, сэкономить 1. (*вн.; разумно расходовать*) be* ecónomical (with), ecónomize (*smth.*); ~ врéмя и труд save time and lábour; 2. *тк. несов.* (*максимально сокращать расходы*) ecónomize; 3. (*на, в пр.; получать выгоду*) ecónomize (on); ~ на материáлах ecónomize/save on matérials.

экономи́ческ|ий ecónomic; ~ие закóны ecónomic laws; ~ райóн ecónomic área; ~ая геогрáфия ecónomic geógraphy; ~ журнáл magazíne on ecónomics; ~ кри́зис ecónomic crísis; ~ое стимули́рование provísion of ecónomic/fináncial incéntives.

экономи́чн|ый ecónomical; ~ое строи́тельство ecónomical building.

экономи|я *ж.* ecónomy; (*выгода*) sáving (in, of); режи́м ~и ecónomy drive; ◇ полити́ческая ~ polítical ecónomy.

экономный ecónomical; (*о человеке*) thrífty.

экрáн *м.* 1. (*для защиты*) screen, shield; теплозащи́тный ~ heat shield; 2. (*для изображения*) screen; *перен.* the screen.

экраниз|áция *ж.* fílming; ~ óперы fílming of an ópera. ~и́ровать *несов. и сов.* (*вн.*) film (*smth.*), make* a film vérsion (of).

экскавáтор *м.* éxcavator; шагáющий ~ self-propélled/drágline éxcavator. ~ный éxcavator *attr.*; ~ный ковш éxcavator búcket. ~щик *м.* éxcavator man*.

экскурс *м.* digréssion, excúrsus.

экскурсáнт *м.*, ~ка *ж.* excúrsionist.

экскурсио́нн|ый excúrsion *attr.*; **~ое бюро́** excúrsion(s) óffice.

экску́рсия *ж.* 1. excúrsion; **~ в музе́й** excúrsion to a muséum; 2. (*группа туристов*) excúrsion párty, tóurist group.

экскурсово́д *м.* guide.

экспанси́вн|ость *ж.* expánsiveness, effúsiveness. **~ый** expánsive, effúsive.

экспа́нсия *ж.* expánsion.

экспеди́ция *ж.* 1. (*поездка с заданием*) expedítion; 2. (*группа лиц*) expedítion, párty; **спаса́тельная ~** réscue párty; 3. (*отправка чего-л.*) dispátch; 4. (*отдел доставки*) dispátch óffice; dispátches *pl.*

экспериме́нт *м.* expériment.

эксперимента́льн|ый experiméntal; **~ые да́нные** experiméntal dáta; **~ые живо́тные** experiméntal ánimals; **~ая медици́на** experiméntal médicine.

эксперимент|а́тор *м.* experímenter. **~и́рование** *с.* experimentátion; **~и́ровать** *несов.* expériment.

экспе́рт *м.* éxpert; (*на суде*) éxpect wítness; **заключе́ние ~ов** éxperts' repórt, éxpert opínion.

эксперти́з|а *ж.* 1. examinátion/appráisal by éxperts; **производи́ть ~у** cárry out an examinátion; 2. (*комиссия*) (commission of) éxperts.

экспе́ртн|ый éxpert *attr.*; **~ая коми́ссия** commíssion of éxperts.

эксплуата́тор *м.* explóiter. **~ский** explóiting, parasítical.

эксплуатацио́нный óperating; máintenance *attr.*

эксплуата́|ция *ж.* 1. exploitátion; 2. (*природных богатств*) exploitátion; (*железных дорог, машин и т. п.*) operátion; (*домов, квартир*) máintenance; **сдава́ть что-л. в ~ю** put* ínto operátion.

эксплуати́рование *с.* explóiting, exploitátion.

эксплуати́ровать *несов.* (*вн.*) 1. explóit (*smb.*); 2. (*использовать природные богатства*) explóit (*smth.*), use (*smth.*); (*машины и т. п.*) óperate (*smth.*), run* (*smth.*).

экспози́ция *ж.* 1. *лит., муз.* exposítion; 2. (*показ*) displáy, láy-out; 3. *фото* expósure.

экспон|а́т *м.* exhíbit. **~и́ровать** *несов. и сов.* (*вн.*) 1. exhíbit (*smth.*); 2. *фото* expóse (*smth.*).

э́кспорт *м.* éxport.

экспортёр *м.* expórter.

экспорти́ровать *несов. и сов.* (*вн.*) expórt (*smth.*).

э́кспортный éxport *attr.*

экспре́сс *м.* expréss; **~-по́чта** úrgent mail; expréss delívery.

экспресси́вный expréssive.

экспре́сси|я *ж.* expréssion, expréssiveness; **чита́ть с ~ей** read* with expréssion.

экспро́мт *м.* imprómptu, improvisátion. **~ом** imprómptu, on the spur of the móment; **произнести́ речь ~ом** make* an imprómptu speech, speak* extémpore, extémporize.

экспропри|а́тор *м.* exprópriator. **~а́ция** *ж.* expropriátion. **~и́ровать** *несов. и сов.* (*вн.*) exprópriate (*smth.*).

экста́з *м.* écstasy; **впада́ть, приходи́ть в ~** go* ínto écstasies.

экстенси́вный exténsive.

экстерн *м.* extérnal stúdent; **держа́ть экза́мены ~ом** sit* one's examinátions as an extérnal stúdent.

экстерриториа́льн|ость *ж. юр.* exterritoriálity. **~ый** *юр.* exterritórial.

экстраваѓа́нтный eccéntric, bizárre, prepósterous.

экстра́кт *м.* éxtract.

экстраордина́рный extraórdinary.

экстреми́ст *м.* extrémist. **~ский** extrémist *attr.*

э́кстренн|о úrgently. **~ый** 1. (*спешный*) úrgent; **~ый отъе́зд** úrgent depárture; **~ая телегра́мма** úrgent télegram; 2. (*чрезвычайный, непредвиденный*) spécial;

~ый вы́пуск газе́ты spécial edítion of a néwspaper; **~ый слу́чай** emérgency; **в ~ых слу́чаях** in an emérgency, in case of emérgency.

эксце́нтрик I *м.* (*артист*) clown, cómic (áctor).

эксце́нтрик II *м. тех.* eccéntric, cam.

эксцентри́ч|еский eccéntric; *театр.* cómic; **~ный** eccéntric.

эксце́сс *м.* excéss; (*нарушение порядка тж.*) óutrage.

эласти́чн|ость *ж.* elastícity, resílience; *перен.* flexibílity. **~ый** elástic, resílient, súpple; spríngy; *перен.* fléxible; **~ая пружи́на** resílient spring; **~ые движе́ния** súpple móvements; **~ые носки́** stretch socks.

элева́тор *м.* élevator.

элега́нтн|ость *ж.* élegance. **~ый** élegant.

эле́гия *ж.* élegy; *перен. тж.* mélancholy.

электриз|а́ция *ж.* 1. *физ.* electrificátion; 2. *мед.* eléctrical tréatment. **~ова́ть** *несов. и сов.* (*вн.*) 1. *физ.* eléctrify (*smth.*) (*тж. перен.*); 2. *мед.* treat (*smb., smth.*) with electrícity, give* (*smb., smth.*) eléctrical tréatment. **~ова́ться** *несов. и сов. физ.* be* eléctrified.

эле́ктрик *м. разг.* electrícian; **инжене́р-~** eléctrical engíneer.

электри́к *прил. неизм.*: **цвет ~** eléctric blue.

электрифи|ка́ция *ж.* electrificátion; **~ всей страны́** electrificátion of the whole cóuntry. **~ци́ровать** *несов. и сов.* (*вн.*) eléctrify (*smth.*).

электри́ческ|ий eléctric; **~ заря́д** eléctric charge; **~ ток** eléctric cúrrent, electrícity; **~ая батаре́я** eléctric báttery; **~ая цепь** eléctric(al) círcuit; **~ мото́р** eléctric mótor.

электри́чество *с.* 1. electrícity; 2. (*освещение*) eléctric light.

электри́чка *ж. разг.* (*железная дорога*) eléctric ráilway; (*поезд*) (eléctric) train.

электро- *в сложн.* eléctric, eléctro-.

электроакусти́ческий eléctro-acóustic.

электробри́тва *ж.* eléctric rázor/sháver.

электрово́з *м.* eléctric locomótive.

электрогита́ра *ж.* eléctric guitár.

электро́д *м.* eléctrode.

электродви́гатель *м.* eléctric mótor.

электродви́жущ|ий electromótive; **~ая си́ла** electromótive force.

электродо́йлка *ж.* eléctric mílker.

электродо́йка *ж.* eléctric mílking.

электроизмери́тельн|ый electrométric; **~ые прибо́ры** eléctric méters.

электрокардиогра́мма *ж.* eléctrocárdiogram.

электрола́мповый eléctric-bulb *attr.*

электролече́бный eléctrical-treatment *attr.*, eléctro-thérapy *attr.*

электролече́ние *с.* eléctrical tréatment, eléctro-thérapy.

электро́лиз *м. хим.* electrólysis.

электромагни́т *м.* eléctromágnet. **~ный** eléctromagnétic.

электромеха́ника *ж.* electromechánics.

электромехани́ческий electromechánical.

электромонтёр *м.* electrícian.

электромото́р *м.* eléctric mótor.

электромузыка́льный: **~ инструме́нт** eléctric músical ínstrument.

электро́н *м. физ.* eléctron.

электронагрева́тельн|ый: **~ые прибо́ры** eléctric héaters.

электро́ника *ж.* electrónics.

электро́нно-вычисли́тельный electrónic compúter *attr.*

электро́нн|ый eléctron *attr.*, electrónic; **~ая ла́мпа** eléctron tube; **~ая му́зыка** electrónic músic; **~ая па́мять** electrónic mémory, mémory tube; **~ мозг** electrónic brain;

~ые счётно-реша́ющие и управля́ющие устро́йства compúters and cóntrol sýstems.

электрооборӳдование *с.* eléctrical equípment.

электропереда́ч|а *ж.* eléctrical transmíssion; ма́чта ~и eléctric pýlon.

электропе́чь *ж.* eléctric fúrnace.

электропое́зд *м.* eléctric train.

электрополотёр *м.* eléctric flóor-pólisher.

электроприбо́р *м.* eléctrical applíance.

электропрово́дка *ж.* (eléctric) wíring.

электропрово́дность *ж.* eléctrical condúctívity.

электросва́р|ка *ж.* eléctric wélding. ~щик *м.* eléctric wélder.

электросе́ть *ж.* eléctrical transmíssion nétwork, grid; (*в доме*) wíring.

электроста́нция *ж.* eléctric pówerstátion.

электротабло́ *с. нескл.* annúnciator pánel.

электроте́хн|ик *м.* electrícian. ~ика *ж.* eléctrical engineéring. ~и́ческий eléctrical, electrotéchnical; ~и́ческая промы́шленность eléctrical índustry.

электрохи́мия *ж.* eléctrochémistry.

электрошо́к *м.* eléctroshock (thérapy).

электроэне́ргия *ж.* eléctric pówer.

элеме́нт *м.* 1. élement; 2. *собир. или мн.* (*представители какой-л. общественной среды*) élements; прогресси́вные ~ы о́бщества the progréssive élements of society; 3. *эл.* cell.

элемента́рн|ый 1. eleméntary; ~ая матема́тика eleméntary mathemátics; он не мог поня́ть ~ых веще́й the símplest things were a mýstery to him; ~ые пра́вила ве́жливости eleméntary rules of políteness; 2. (*поверхностный*) superfícial; ~ взгляд на ве́щи shállow óutlook; 3. *хим.* élement *attr.*; 4. *физ.* eleméntary; ~ые части́цы eleméntary párticles.

элики́р *м.* elíxir; зубно́й ~ móuth-wash; грудно́й ~ cough mixture.

эли́та *ж. собир.* 1. (*лучшие растения, животные и т. п.*) best spécimens; 2. (*лучшие представители общества*) élite.

э́ллинг *м.* 1. *мор.* slípway; 2. *ав.* hángar; 3. *спорт.* bóathouse.

э́ллипс *м.* 1. *мат.* ellípse; 2. *лингв.* ellípsis (*pl* -ses).

эллипти́ческий ellíptic(al).

эльф *м. миф.* elf*.

эма́лев|ый enámel *attr.*; ~ые кра́ски enámels.

эмалиро́ванн|ый enámel(led); ~ая посу́да enámel-ware.

эмалирова́ть *несов.* (*вн.*) enámel (*smth.*).

эма́ль *ж.* enámel.

эмансип|а́ция *ж.* emancipátion. ~и́рованный emáncipated.

эмба́рго *с. нескл. юр.* embárgo; наложи́ть ~ на что-л. place an embárgo on *smth.*

эмбле́ма *ж.* émblem.

эмбриоло́гия *ж.* embryólogy.

эмбрио́н *м. биол.* émbryo (*pl* -os).

эмбриона́льн|ый *биол.* embryónic; в ~ом состоя́нии in émbryo.

эмигра́нт *м.*, ~ка *ж.* émigrant; (*политический тж.*) émigré.

эмигра́ц|ия *ж.* 1. emigrátion; (*вынужденная*) éxile; находи́ться в ~ии live in éxile; 2. *собир.* (*эмигранты*) émigrants; (*политические тж.*) émigrés.

эмигри́ровать *несов. и сов.* émigrate.

эмисса́р *м.* émissary.

эми́ссия I *ж. фин.* íssue.

эми́ссия II *ж. физ.* emíssion.

эмоциона́льный emótional.

эмо́ция *ж.* emótion.

эмпири́зм *м. филос.* empíricism.

эмпириокритици́зм *м. филос.* empírio-críticism.

эмпири́ческий empírical.

эму́льсия *ж.* emúlsion.

эмфа́за *ж. лит., лингв.* émphasis.

эмфати́ческий *лит., лингв.* emphátic.

эндокри́нн|ый: ~ые же́лезы éndocrine glands.

эндокриноло́гия *ж.* endocrinólogy.

э́ндшпиль *м. шахм.* énd-game.

энерге́т|ик *м.* pówer enginéer. ~ика *ж.* energétics, pówer engineéring. ~и́ческий pówer *attr.*

энерги́чный energétic, vígorous.

эне́рги|я *ж.* énergy; (*способность производить работу тж.*) pówer; затра́та ~и expénditure of énergy; взя́ться за что-л. с ~ей devóte/diréct all *one's* énergy to *smth.*; put* *one's* back ínto *smth.*

энергосисте́мы *мн.* (*ед.* энергосисте́ма *ж.*) pówer grids.

энн|ый N x; ~ое число́ a cértain númber, x; ~ го́род the town of N; ~ая су́мма a cértain sum.

энтомоло́гия *ж.* entomólogy.

энтузи|а́зм *м.* enthúsiasm. ~а́ст *м.*, ~а́стка *ж.* enthúsiast.

энциклопеди́ст *м.* 1. *ист.* Encyclopáedist; 2. (*всесторонне образованный человек*) pérson of encyclopáedic knówledge.

энциклопеди́ческ|ий encyclopáedic; ~ие позна́ния univérsal/encyclopáedic knówledge *sg*; ~ слова́рь encyclopáedic díctionary.

энциклопе́дия *ж.* encyclopáedia; ◇ ходя́чая ~ wálking encyclopáedia, mine of information.

эпиго́н *м.* (mere) ímitator.

эпигра́мма *ж.* épigram.

эпи́граф *м.* épigraph.

эпидемиоло́гия *ж.* epidemiólogy.

эпидеми́ческий epidémic.

эпиде́мия *ж.* epidémic.

эпизо́д *м.* épisode; (*случай тж.*) íncident.

эпизоди́ческий episódical.

эпиле́п|сия *ж. мед.* épilepsy. ~тик *м.* epiléptic.

эпило́г *м.* épilogue.

эпистоля́рный epístolary.

эпита́фия *ж.* épitaph.

эпи́тет *м.* épithet.

эпице́нтр *м.* épicentre.

эпи́ческ|ий épic; ~ая поэ́ма épic.

эпокси́дн|ый epóxy *attr.*, époxide; ~ая смола́ epóxy résin.

эполе́ты *мн.* (*ед.* эполе́т *м.*) épaulet(te)s.

эпопе́я *ж.* épic.

э́пос *м.* 1. (*повествовательный род литературы*) nárrative líterature; 2. (*совокупность народных героических песен, легенд*) épos.

эпо́х|а *ж.* 1. (*большой промежуток времени*) age; ~ Возрожде́ния the Áge of the Renáissance; 2. (*период существования чего-л.*) périod; 3. (*момент, связанный с переломом в развитии чего-л.*) époch; соста́вить, сде́лать ~у constitute an époch, be*/represént a lándmark.

эпоха́льн|ый epóchal, époch-making; ~ое собы́тие époch-making evént.

э́ра *ж.* éra; в пе́рвом ве́ке до на́шей э́ры in the first céntury B. C.; в пе́рвом ве́ке на́шей э́ры in the first céntury A. D.

эритроци́ты *мн.* (*ед.* эритроци́т *м.*) erýthrocites.

эро́зия *ж.* erósion; ~ по́чвы soil erósion.

эро́тика *ж.* sensuálity.

эроти́ч|еский, ~ный erótic.

эруди́рованный well-réad, well-infórmed, érudite.

эруди́ция *ж.* erudítion, léarning.

эска́др|а *ж. мор.* squádron. ~енный *мор.* squádron *attr.*

эскадри́лья *ж. ав.* squádron.

эскадро́н *м. воен.* troop of cávalry.

эскала́тор *м.* éscalator, móving stáirway.

эскалáция *ж.* escalátion.

эскúз *м.* sketch; (*скульптуры*) módel; (*литературного, музыкального произведения*) draft, prelíminary vérsion. ~ный rough, prelíminary; ~ный проéкт rough draft.

эскимó *с. нескл.* chóc-ice.

эскимóс *м.* Éskimo. ~ка *ж.* Éskimo wóman*. ~ский Éskimo *attr.*

эскóрт *м.* éscort. ~ировать *несов.* (*вн.*) escórt (*smb., smth.*).

эсмúнец *м.* destróyer.

эсперáнто *с. нескл.* Esperánto.

эссéнция *ж.* éssence.

эстакáда *ж.* tréstle; (*для причала судов тж.*) pier.

эстáмп *м.* print.

эстафéт|а *ж. спорт.* rélay-race; принять ~у у кого-л. take* up the torch from *smb.* ~ный rélay *attr.*; ~ная пáлочка báton.

эстéт|ика *ж.* 1. aesthétics; 2. (*красота чего-л.*) aesthétic/artístic béauty. ~ический aesthétic. ~ичный aesthétically béautiful.

эстóн|ец *м.*, ~ка *ж.* Estónian. ~ский Estónian; ~ский язык Estónian, the Estónian lánguage.

эстрáд|а *ж.* 1. (*помост*) plátform; 2. (*вид искусства*) variety. ~ный variety *attr.*

эта *см.* э́тот.

этáж *м.* 1. stórey; (*с порядковым числительным*) floor; нúжний, пéрвый ~ ground floor; вторóй, трéтий и т. д. ~ first, sécond, *etc.* floor; дом в 20 ~éй twenty-storey building; 2. (*ряд предметов, расположенных горизонтально*) tier, láyer.

этажéрка *ж.* bóokstand.

-этáжный *в сложн.* -stóried, -stórey(ed); семиэтáжный séven-storey, séven-storied.

этак *разг.* in this way, like this; и так и ~ éither way; ни так ни ~ néither way.

этакий *разг.* such a; (*такой*) what a.

эталóн *м.* stándard; *перен.* módel; ~ мéтра stándard métre.

этáп *м.* stage; на совремéнном ~е at the présent stage.

эти *мест. мн.* these, those.

этика *ж.* éthics.

этикéт *м.* etiquétte.

этикéтка *ж.* lábel.

этил *м. хим.* éthyl.

этилéн *м. хим.* ethyléne.

этимологúческий etymológical; ~ словáрь etymológical díctionary.

этимолóгия *ж.* etymólogy.

этúческий, этúчный éthical.

этнúческий éthnic.

этнографúческ|ий ethnográphic(al); ~ая кáрта ethnográphical map.

этногрáфия *ж.* ethnógraphy.

Это I *частица* 1. *передаётся оборотом* it's... who; ~ он написáл такóе хорóшее сочинéние? was he the one who wrote such a good éssay?; ~ вас я застáл с папирóсой? was it you (whom) I saw smóking a cigarétte?; ~ он вас имéет в виду he means you; 2. *усил.:* что ~ вы? what's come óver you?; как ~ всё случúлось? how did it all háppen?; что ~ он не идёт? I wónder what's kéeping him; как ~ мóжно! how can you?

Это II *мест. см.* э́тот.

Это|т, эта, это, эти *мест.* 1. this; *мн.* these; ~ или тот дом? this house or that one óver there?; в ~м годý this year; это сáмое глáвное that's the great thing; на ~м сáмом мéсте on this véry spot; я возьму себé вот э́ту картúну I'll take this picture; 2. *в знач. сущ.* this one; 3. (*указывает на предмет, лицо и т. п., названные в предшествующем повествовании*) the, this, that; 4. *в знач. сущ.* (*последний из названных*) the látter; 5. *в*

знач. *сущ. с. нескл.* that, this; it; Э́то не он that ísn't him, it's not him; Э́то егó сестрá this/that is his síster; (*в ответе*) it's his síster; Э́то хорошó that's a good thing; Э́то было так неожúданно it was all so súdden; ◇ при ~м incidéntally, besídes, in addítion.

этюд *м.* 1. (*рисунок*) sketch; 2. *лит.* éssay; 3. *муз.* stúdy, étude; 4. (*упражнение*) éxercises *pl.*

этюдник *м.* páinter's case.

эфемéрный ephémeral.

эфéс *м.* swórd-hilt.

эфиóп *м.*, ~ка *ж.* Ethíopian.

эфúр *м.* 1. éther; в ~е on the air; передавáть что-л. в ~ bróadcast *smth.*; 2. *хим.* éther. ~ный ethéreal (*тж. перен.*); ~ное мáсло esséntial/vólatile oil.

эффéкт *м.* 1. efféct; производúть ~ prodúce an efféct; 2. *мн.* effécts *pl*; шумовúе ~ы sound effécts; 3. (*результат*) efféct.

эффектúвн|ость *ж.* efféctiveness; *эк.* efficiency; ~ капиталовложéний efficiency of invéstments. ~ый efféctive, efféctual; *эк.* efficient; ~ая мóщность efféctive pówer; ~ые мéры efféctual méasures.

эффéктный efféctive, stríking; (*рассчитанный на эффект*) shówy.

эх oh!; эх, ты! what a féllow (wóman, *etc.*)!; (*укоризненно*) you're a fine one, you are!

э́хо *с.* écho.

эхолóт *м.* écho (depth) sóunder.

эшафóт *м.* scáffold.

эшелóн *м.* 1. échelon; *ав.* lével; 2. (*поезд*) train; (*автоколонна*) cólumn, cónvoy.

Ю

юбилéй *м.* annivérsary; (*празднование*) celebrátion; пятидесятилéтний ~ júbilee, fíftieth annivérsary; столéтний ~ centénary. ~ный: ~ная дáта annivérsary; ~ное издáние annivérsary/bírthday edítion; júbilee edítion; ~ная сéссия annivérsary séssion.

юбилЯр *м.* héro of the day.

юбк|а *ж.* skirt; ◇ держáться за чью-л. ~у *шутл.* be* tied to smb.'s ápron-strings.

ювелúр *м.* jéweller. ~ный jéwelry *attr.*; jéweller's; *перен.* éxquisite; ~ные издéлия jéwelry; ~ный магазúн jéweller's (shop); ~ная рабóта éxquisite wórkmanship.

юг *м.* the south; на юг (to the) south; к ~у от... (to the) south of...; на ~е in the south, down south.

юго-востóк *м.* south-éast.

юго-востóчн|ый south-éast; ~ое направлéние south-éast diréction; ~ вéтер south-éast wind, southéaster.

юго-зáпад *м.* south-wést.

юго-зáпадн|ый south-wést; ~ое направлéние south-wést diréction; ~ вéтер south-wést wind, southwéster.

югослáв *м.* Júgoslav. ~ский Júgoslav.

южáн|ин *м.*, ~ка *ж.* sóutherner.

южнее fárther south.

южн|ый south, sóuthern*; ~ бéрег south coast; ~ вéтер south wind; ~ клúмат sóuthern clímate; ~ое сóлнце the sóuthern sun; ~ темперáмент sóuthern fire; ◇ ~ пóлюс магнúта *физ.* south-seeking pole of a mágnet.

юзом *разг.* in(to) a skid.

юлá *ж.* 1. (*волчок*) top; 2. *разг.* (*о вертлявом человеке*) fidget.

юлúть *несов. разг.* 1. (*вертеться*) dance abóut, jig aróund; 2. (*перед тв.; лебезить*) dance atténdance (on); 3. (*ловчить, хитрить*) wríggle.

юмор *м.* húmour. ~úст *м.* húmourist. ~истúческий

húmorous; ~исти́ческие расска́зы húmorous stóries; ~исти́ческая но́та в го́лосе a húmorous note in smb.'s voice.

ю́нга *м.* ship's boy.

юне́ц *м.* youth.

юнио́р *м.* júnior, áge-group compétitor; соревнова́ния среди́ ~ов áge-group competítions/évents, júnior evénts.

ю́нкер *м. ист.* ófficer cadét.

юнна́т *м.* young náturalist.

ю́ность|ь *ж.* 1. youth; в дни ~и in one's youth, in the days of one's youth; 2. *собир.* young péople, youth.

ю́нош|а *м.* youth. ~еский yóuthful. ~ество *с.* 1. *собир.* young péople, youth; 2. (*юность*) youth.

ю́н|ый young; (*свойственный юности*) yóuthful; ~ во́зраст youth; с ~ых лет (éver) since one was a child*; теа́тр ~ого зри́теля young péople's théatre.

Юпи́тер *м.* Júpiter.

юпи́тер *м. разг.* (*осветительный прибор*) Júpiter lamp, flóodlight.

юр *м.*: на ~у́ in a próminent situátion/place.

юриди́ческ|ий légal; (*связанный с правовыми нормами тж.*) jurídical; ~ институ́т law school/institute; ~ факульте́т depártment of law, láw-faculty; до́ктор ~их нау́к Dóctor of Laws; ◇ ~ая консульта́ция légal advíce buréau; ~ое лицо́ jurídical pérson.

юрисди́кция *ж.* jurisdíction.

юрисконсульт *м.* légal advíser.

юриспруде́нция *ж.* jurisprúdence, law.

юри́ст *м.* láwyer.

ю́рк|ий nímble, adróit, ágile; *перен. разг.* sharp, énterprising; ~ая мышь nímble mouse*; ~ как бе́лка nímble as a squírrel.

юркну́ть *сов.* dart; (*о мыши тж.*) whisk.

юро́д|ивый *прил.* 1. mad, feeblemínded; 2. *в знач. сущ. м.* God's/holy fool. ~ство *с.* 1. feeblemíndedness, mádness; 2. (*поступок*) aberrátion, ídiocy. ~ствовать *несов.* 1. (*быть юродивым*) be*; 2. (*совершать нелепые поступки*) act like a mádman*.

ю́рский *геол.* Jurássic.

ю́рта *ж.* yúrta (*nomad tent*).

юсти́ция *ж.* jústice.

ют *м. мор.* quárter-deck.

юти́ться *несов.* 1. (*помещаться на небольшой площади — о доме, селении*) perch, néstle; 2. (*тесниться — о людях*) húddle; 3. (*иметь пристанище*) make* one's quárters, live cooped up; ~ у знако́мых take* shélter in a friend's house.

Я

я *личн. мест.* 1. (*рд., вн.* меня́, *дт.* мне, *тв.* мной, мно́ю, *пр.* обо мне́) I; э́то я! it's me!; э́то я сде́лал I did it/that; э́то я ему́ сказа́л it was I who told him; 2. *в знач. сущ. с. нескл.* the self, the égo; ◇ не я бу́ду, е́сли не добью́сь своего́! I'll get my way — you see if I don't!; я тебя́, его́ *и т. д.*! I'll give it to you, him, *etc.*!

я́бед|а *м. и ж. разг. см.* я́бедник. ~ник *м.* sneak; (*у детей тж.*) télltale. ~ничать *несов.* (*на вн.*) infórm (on); (*о детях*) tell* tales (abóut), sneak (abóut).

я́блок|о *с.* ápple; ◇ ада́мово ~ Ádam's ápple; глазно́е ~ éyeball; ~ раздо́ра ápple of discord, bone of conténtion; ~у не́где упа́сть there is hárdly room to move; ~ от я́блони недалеко́ па́дает *посл.* like móther, like dáughter; в ~ах dáppled.

я́блонев|ый ápple attr.; ~ая ве́тка ápple bough; ~ сад ápple órchard.

я́блоня *ж.* ápple-tree.

я́блочко *с.* yáblochko (*sailor's dance*).

я́блочн|ый ápple attr.; ~ое варе́нье ápple jam; ~ пиро́г ápple-pie, ápple-tart.

яви́ть *сов. см.* явля́ть. ~ся *сов. см.* явля́ться 1, 2, 3.

я́вка *ж.* 1. présence, atténdance; ~ в суд présence in court; ~ обяза́тельна atténdance compúlsory; 2. (*место*) sécret addréss, safe house; (*конспиративная встреча*) sécret méeting.

явле́ние *с.* 1. phenómenon (*pl* -na); thing *разг.*; (*событие*) occúrrence; ~ приро́ды nátural phenómenon; отра́дное ~ encóuraging sýmptom/phenómenon; ре́дкое ~ unúsual occúrrence/phenómenon; стра́нное ~ strange thing; 2. (*появление*) appéarance; 3. *театр.* scene; ~ пе́рвое, второ́е *и т. д.* scene one, two, *etc.*; 4. *филос.* phenómenon (*pl* -na).

явля́ть, **яви́ть** (*вн.; показывать*) show* (*smth.*); ~ собо́й приме́р му́жества be* an exámple of cóurage. ~ся, **яви́ться** 1. (*приходить, прибывать*) come*, turn up; (*по официальному вызову*) appéar, repórt; заче́м вы сюда́ яви́лись? why did you come here?; ~ в суд appéar in court; 2. (*появляться*) appéar; (*рождаться*) come* into the world; у меня́ яви́лась мысль it occúrred to me; у меня́ яви́лось жела́ние I felt a desíre; 3. (*оказываться*) be*; просту́да яви́лась причи́ной его́ боле́зни the cause of his íllness was a chill, his íllness was caused by a chill; 4. *тк. несов.* (*быть, представлять собой*) be*.

я́вн|о óbviously. ~ый 1. (*открытый, не тайный*) ópen, óvert; ~ая вражда́ ópen énmity; 2. (*очевидный для всех*) óbvious, pátent; ~ая ложь óbvious lie.

я́вочн|ый sécret attr.; ~ая кварти́ра sécret addréss; ◇ ~ым поря́дком without prévious permíssion.

я́вственный clear, distínct.

я́вств|овать *несов.* be* óbvious; из всех показа́ний ~ует... the évidence shows cléarly..., it is óbvious from the évidence given; как ~ует из его́ слов as his words cléarly prove.

явь *ж.* reálity.

я́гель *м. бот.* réindeer moss.

ягнёнок *м.* lamb; кро́ткий как ~ meek as a lamb.

ягни́ться *несов.* lamb, yean.

я́год|а *ж.* bérry; *собир.* small fruit; собира́ть ~ы go* bérrying; ◇ одного́ по́ля ~ birds of a féather.

я́годица *ж.* búttock.

я́годн|ик *м.* 1. (*место*) patch of bérries; (*культивированный*) smáll-fruit plantátion; 2. (*ягодный куст*) bérry, fruit bush; 3. *разг.* (*о человеке*) bérry-gatherer. ~ый bérry attr.; ~ый сок bérry-juice.

ягуа́р *м.* jáguar.

яд *м.* 1. póison (*тж. перен.*); (*змеиный тж.*) vénom; ~ сомне́ния the póison of doubt; 2. (*злость, ехидство*) vénom; ~ его́ слов the vénom of his words.

я́дерн|ый núclear; ~ая реа́кция núclear reáction; ~ая эне́ргия núclear énergy; ~ое ору́жие núclear wéapons pl; ~ое горю́чее núclear fuel; ◇ ~ реа́ктор núclear reáctor; ~ая фи́зика núclear phýsics; ~ая держа́ва núclear pówer.

ядови́т|ый 1. póisonous, vénomous; ~ гриб tóadstool, póisonous fúngus; ~ое расте́ние póison(ous) plant; ~ая змея́ vénomous/póisonous snake; ~ газ póison/tóxic gas; 2. (*злобный*) vénomous; ~ язы́к vénomous tongue.

ядрёный *разг.* 1. (*о плодах*) fine, júicy; 2. (*здоровый, крепкий*) lústy, robúst; 3. (*свежий, бодрящий*) invigorating, bóisterous.

я́дрица *ж.* búckwheat.

ядро́ *с.* 1. (*плода*) kérnel; ~ оре́ха kérnel of a nut; 2. (*внутренняя часть чего-л.*) core, heart; (*клетки и т. п.*) núcleus; ~ древеси́ны heart of tímber, héart-wood; ~ а́тома atómic núcleus; 3. (*наиболее важная часть чего-л.*) gist, súbstance; 4. (*пушечное*) róund-shot, cánnon-ball; 5. *спорт.* shot.

я́зва *ж.* 1. úlcer; *перен.* (*бич*) pest; 2. *разг.* (*ехидный человек*) víper; ◇ ~ желу́дка gástric úlcer.

язви́тельн|ый cáustic, bíting; ~ое замеча́ние bíting

remárk; ~ отвéт stínging retórt; ~ человéк cáustic/sarcástic pérson; ~ая крúтика bíting críticism.

язвúть, съязвúть sneer, say* snéeringly; ~ на чей-л. счёт take* the rise out of *smb.*

язык *м.* 1. tongue; показáть ~ кому-л. 1) (*врачу*) show* *smb.* one's tongue; 2. (*дразня*) put* out one's tongue at *smb.*; злой ~ wícked/bítter tongue; 2. (*кушанье*) tongue; 3. (*речь*) lánguage; роднóй ~ móther-tongue; one's own lánguage; разговóрный ~ collóquial speech; нóвые ~и módern lánguages; дрéвние ~и áncient lánguages; 4. (*стиль*) style, lánguage; кнúга напúсана хорóшим ~óм the book is well wrítten; 5. (*пленный*) information prísoner; ◇ ~ к гортáни прилúп у кого-л. *smb.'s* tongue stuck/cleaved to the roof of his, her mouth; ~ хорошó подвéшен у кого-л. *smb.* has a réady tongue; ~ чéшется у кого-л. *smb.* is ítching to speak; держáть ~ за зубáми keep* a still tongue in *one's* head; придержáть ~ hold* *one's* tongue; сорвалóсь (слóво) с ~á one néver meant to say it.

языковéд *м.* línguist. **~ение** *с.* linguístics. **~ческий** linguístic, linguístics *attr.*

языковóй linguístic.

языкóвый tongue *attr.*

языкознáние *с.* linguístics.

языческий págan, héathen. **~ество** *с.* páganism. **~ник** *м.* págan, héathen.

язычóк *м.* 1. *анат.* úvula (*pl* -ae); 2.: ~ ботúнка bóot-tongue; ~ плáмени tongue of flame.

яичко *с. анат.* tésticle.

яичники *мн.* (*ед.* яúчник *м.*) *анат.* óvaries.

яúчница *ж.* (*глазунья*) fried eggs *pl*; (*болтунья*) scrámbled eggs *pl.*

яúчный egg *attr.*; ~ порошóк égg-powder; ~ая скорлупá égg-shell.

яйцевúдный égg-shaped.

яйцеклéтка *ж.* égg-cell.

яйцó *с.* 1. *биол.* óvum (*pl* óva); ◇ носúться с кем-л., чем-л. как кýрица с ~óм fuss óver *smb., smth.* like an old hen; выеденного ~á не стóит not worth a rap; яйца кýрицу не ýчат *посл.* don't teach your grándmother to suck eggs.

якобы osténsibly; он ~ пóнял he seemed to understánd, he said he understóod; одúн из них ~ инженéр one of them is supposed to be an enginéer; он пришёл ~ для тогó, чтóбы рабóтать he came here osténsibly to work.

якорный ánchor *attr.*; ~ая цепь ánchor chain; ~ая стоянка ánchorage.

якорь *м.* 1. *мор.* ánchor; стоять на ~е lie* at ánchor; 2. *эл.* ármature, rótor; ◇ ~ спасéния *one's* sheet ánchor.

якýт *м.*, **~ка** *ж.* Yakút. **~ский** Yakút; ~ский язык Yakút, the Yakút lánguage.

якшáться *несов.* (с *тв.*) *разг.* hóbnob (with).

ялик *м.* skiff.

яловая: ~ корóва dry cow.

яма *ж.* pit; hole (*тж. перен.*); (*низина*) hóllow; угóльная ~ cóal-bunker; ◇ вóлчья ~ tráp-hole.

ямб *м. лит.* iámbus. **~úческий** iámbic.

ямочка *ж.* dímple; ~ой dímpled*.

ямщúк *м.* cóachman*.

январский Jánuary *attr.*; ~ хóлод the cold of Jánuary.

январь *м.* Jánuary; в ~é этого гóда this/in Jánuary; в ~é прóшлого гóда last Jánuary, last year in Jánuary; в ~é бýдущего гóда next Jánuary.

янки *мн. нескл.* Yánkee.

янтáрный 1. ámber *attr.*; 2. (*о цвете*) ámber(-coloured).

янтáрь *м.* ámber.

япóнец *м.*, **~ка** *ж.* Japanése. **~ский** Japanése; ~ский язык Japanése, the Japanése lánguage.

яркий 1. (*о свете*) bright, pówerful; ~ая лáмпа pówerful/bright lamp; 2. (*о цвете*) bright, vívid; ~ие лéнты bright ríbbons; 3. (*выдающийся*) stríking, brílliant; ~ талáнт brílliant tálents *pl*; 4. (*убедительный*) vívid, impréssive; ~ примéр stríking/vívid exámple.

ярко brílliantly, bríghtly; ~ выраженный pronóunced; ~ раскрáшенный híghly cóloured; ~ свидéтельствовать о чём-л. afford stríking évidence of *smth.* **~ость** *ж.* brílliance, bríghtness; vívidness.

ярлык *м.* (*прям. и перен.*) lábel.

ярмарка *ж.* fair.

ярмó *с.* yoke; (*бремя*) búrden.

яровизáция *ж. с.-х.* vernalizátion. **~úровать** *несов. и сов.* (*вн.*) *с.-х.* vérnalize (*smth.*).

яровóй *прил.* 1. spring *attr.*; ~ сев spring sówing; ~ая пшенúца spring wheat; ~óе пóле spring-sown field; 2. *в знач. сущ. мн.* spring crops.

яростный 1. fúrious, fierce; 2. (*о стихиях*) víolent; ~ые вóлны reléntless waves; 3. (*чрезмерный, крайний в своём проявлении*) frénzied, frántic.

ярость *ж.* rage, fúry; (*бешенство*) frénzy; вне себя от ~и besíde *onesélf* with rage.

ярус *м.* 1. stórey; (*в театре*) circle; вторóй ~ úpper circle; 2. (*один из горизонтальных рядов чего-л.*) tier, láyer.

ярый 1. (*яростный*) víolent, fúrious; 2. (*крайний в своём проявлении*) fierce; 3. (*страстно преданный чему-л.*) zéalous, rábid.

ясельный dáy-nursery *attr.*; ~ ребёнок dáy-nursery child*; дéти ~ого вóзраста children of dáy-nursery age.

ясень *м.* ash(-tree).

ясли *мн.* 1. mánger *sg*; 2. (*учреждение*) (day) núrsery *sg*, crèche *sg.*

ясно 1. *нареч.* cléarly, distínctly; ~ вúдеть, сознавáть see*/réalize cléarly; ~ выраженный cléarly expréssed; корóтко и ~! that's that!; ~ представлять себé что-л. see* *smth.* with the útmost clárity; 2. *в знач. сказ. безл.* (*о безоблачной погоде*) the sky is clear; сегóдня ~ и теплó todáy it is bright and warm; 3. *в знач. сказ. безл.* (*понятно*) it is clear; былó ~, что... it was clear that...; ~! I see!; ~? is that clear?

ясновúдение *с.* 1. clairvóyance; sécond sight; 2. (*тонкая проницательность*) ínsight. **~ящий** clairvóyant, intúitive.

ясность *ж.* cléarness, clárity; (*мысли, выражения, слога*) lucídity; вносúть ~ во что-л. clear up *smth.*, sort out *smth.*; вносúть ~ в обстанóвку clear up the situátion.

~ый 1. (*яркий*) bright; 2. (*безоблачный, светлый*) clear; (*о погоде*) fine; ~ая ночь clear night; ~ый день fine day; 3. (*спокойный, чистый*) seréne; ~ый взгляд clear/seréne glance; 4. (*отчётливый*) clear, distínct; 5. (*понятный*) lúcid, clear; 6. (*логичный, очевидный*) clear; (*способный логично мыслить*) lúcid; ◇ ~ее ~ого it is as clear as dáylight.

яства *мн.* feast *sg*, víands.

ястреб *м.* hawk.

ястребúный 1. hawk's; hawk *attr.*; 2. (*как у ястреба*) háwklike; ~ взгляд píercing glance.

яхонт *м. уст.* 1. (*рубин*) rúby; 2. (*сапфир*) sápphire.

яхта *ж.* yacht.

яхт-клуб *м.* yácht-club.

ячéйка *ж.* cell.

ячмéнный 1. bárley *attr.*; ~ое зернó grain of bárley, bárley-corn; ~ая крупá bárley; ~ая кáша bárley-milk.

ячмéнь I *м.* (*злак*) bárley.

ячмéнь II *м.* (*на глазу*) sty.

ячневый fíne-barley *attr.*

яшма *ж.* jásper.

ящерица *ж.* lízard.

ящик *м.* 1. box; (*упаковочный*) pácking-case; 2. (*выдвижной*) drawer; ◇ чёрный ~ black box.

ящур *м. мед.* fóot-and-móuth diséase.

NTC'S FOREIGN LANGUAGE DICTIONARIES
The Best, By Definition

Spanish/English
Cervantes-Walls Spanish & English
Diccionario Básico Norteamericano
NTC's Beginner's Spanish & English
NTC's Dictionary of Common Mistakes in Spanish
NTC's Dictionary of Spanish False Cognates
The Dictionary of Chicano Spanish
NTC's Easy Spanish Bilingual Dictionary
Vox Compact Spanish & English
Vox Everyday Spanish & English
Vox Modern Spanish & English (Thumb-indexed & Plain-edged)
Vox Super-Mini Spanish & English
Vox Traveler's Spanish & English

Spanish/Spanish
Diccionario Practico de la Lengua Enspañola del Nuevo Mundo
Vox Diccionario Escolar de la Lengua Española

French/English
NTC's New College French & English
NTC's Beginner's French & English
NTC's Dictionary of Canadian French
NTC's Dictionary of Faux Amis
NTC's Dictionary of French Faux Pas
NTC's Easy French Bilingual Dictionary
NTC's French & English Business

German/English
NTC's Easy German Bilingual Dictionary
Klett's Modern German & English

Klett's Super-Mini German & English
NTC's Beginner's German & English
NTC's Dictionary of German False Cognates
Schöffler-Weiss German & English

Italian/English
NTC's Beginner's Italian & English
NTC's Easy Italian Bilingual Dictionary
Zanichelli New College Italian & English
Zanichelli Super-Mini Italian & English

Other Foreign Languages
NTC's Bulgarian & English
NTC's Compact Korean & English
NTC's Compact Russian & English
NTC's New College Greek & English
NTC's New Japanese-English Character
NTC's Romanian & English
NTC's Vietnamese & English
The Wiedza Powszechna Compact Polish & English
Easy Chinese Phrasebook & Dictionary
Languages of the World on CD-ROM

For Juveniles
French Picture Dictionary
German Picture Dictionary
Spanish Picture Dictionary
Let's Learn French Picture Dictionary
Let's Learn German Picture Dictionary
Let's Learn Hebrew Picture Dictionary
Let's Learn Italian Picture Dictionary
Let's Learn Portuguese Picture Dictionary
Let's Learn Spanish Picture Dictionary

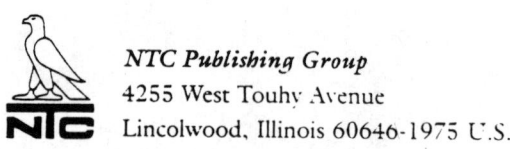
NTC Publishing Group
4255 West Touhy Avenue
Lincolwood, Illinois 60646-1975 U.S.A.